Complete your drug reference library with these 5 essential volumes!

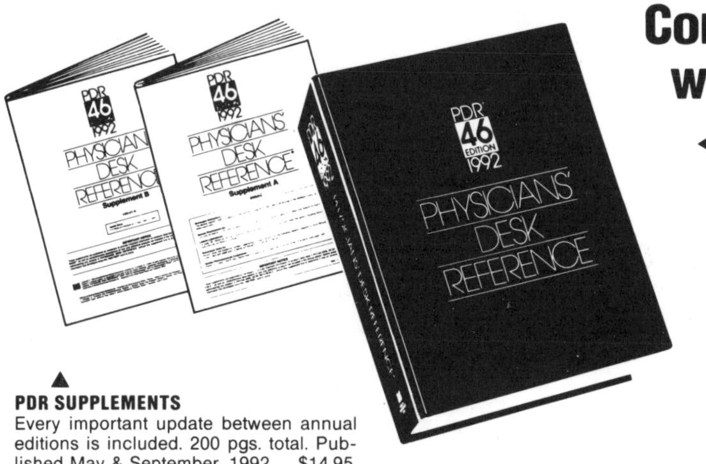

▲ **PDR SUPPLEMENTS**
Every important update between annual editions is included. 200 pgs. total. Published May & September, 1992. $14.95. Payment must accompany order.

◀ **1992 PHYSICIANS' DESK REFERENCE®** Scores of new drugs have been added making previous volumes obsolete. Features include four complete indices • full-color, actual-size photographs • fast, accurate look-ups of all FDA-required information • use-in-pregnancy ratings • and much more. 2,500 pgs. Published December, 1991. $54.95.

1992 PDR FOR NONPRESCRIPTION DRUGS® ▶
Vital information on OTC drug products: ingredients, indications, drug interactions, dosage, administration, and more. Four complete indices, full-color photo section. 400 pgs. Published March, 1992. $35.95.

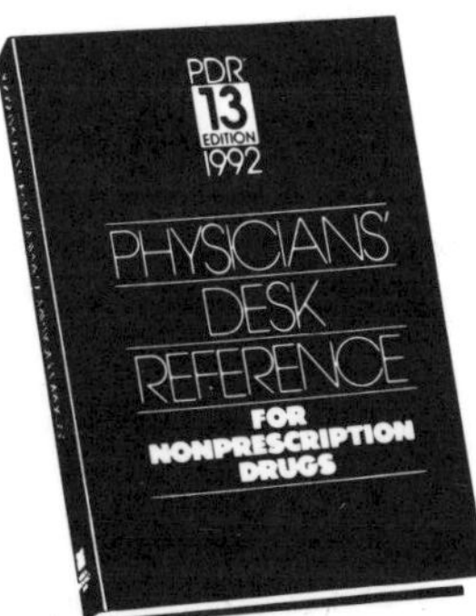

◀ **1992 PDR FOR OPHTHALMOLOGY®**
Complete directory of drug and product information relating to Optometry and Ophthalmology: specialized instrumentation, equipment, lenses, product photographs, color grids for rapid product and drug identification, color-blind test. 260 pgs. Published October, 1991. $39.95.

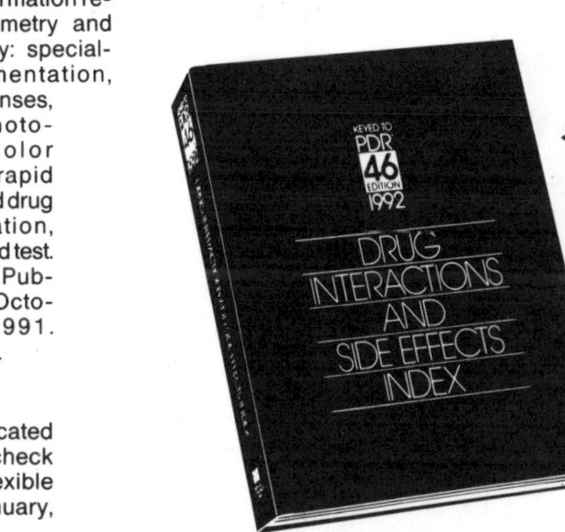

◀ **1992 PDR DRUG INTERACTIONS & SIDE EFFECTS INDEX®**
The perfect companion volume to make your PDR a more powerful reference tool than ever before! Includes food interactions. 1260 pgs. Published January, 1992 $36.95.

◀ **1992 PDR INDICATIONS INDEX™**
Gives full range of drugs specifically indicated for precise clinical situations. Double-check prescriptions, identify alternatives. Flexible binding 4" x 7". 360 pgs. Published January, 1992. $20.95.

See other side for electronic products.

DETACH ALONG DOTTED LINE AND MAIL.

USE THIS CARD TO ORDER PDR PRINT AND ELECTRONIC PRODUCTS

PDR Library

Send ______ copies of **1992 Physicians' Desk Reference®** .... 092031 $54.95 each
Send ______ copies of 1992 PDR for Ophthalmology® .... 092023 $39.95 each
Send ______ copies of 1992 PDR Supplements A 092080
(may not be billed) and B .... 092098 $14.95 set
Send ______ copies of 1992 PDR Drug Interactions and Side Effects Index® .... 092049 $36.95 each
Send ______ copies of 1992 PDR Indications Index™ .... 092056 $20.95 each
Send ______ copies of 1992 PDR for Nonprescription Drugs® .. 092064 $35.95 each

☐ SAVE TIME AND MONEY EVERY YEAR AS A SUBSCRIBER. Check here to enter a standing order for future editions of the publications ordered. Next year we'll confirm your order, and you are guaranteed to receive the lowest price available.

Electronic PDR

☐ Pocket PDR .... $299.00 each

PDR® on CD-ROM. Satisfaction guaranteed.
☐ Complete PDR Library plus The Merck Manual, #1M1 .... $895.00 each
☐ The complete PDR Library, #1P1 .... $595.00 each
Check Format: ☐ 5¼" diskettes ☐ 3½" diskettes
Equipment required: IBM PC/XT/AT-compatible or PS/2 computer, DOS 3.1 or later, MS-DOS CD-ROM Extensions, 640K main memory, CD-ROM drive.

☐ PDR Drug Interactions and Side Effects Diskettes™. Satisfaction guaranteed. .... $219.00 each
Check Format: ☐ 5¼" diskettes ☐ 3½" diskettes
Equipment required: IBM PC/XT/AT-compatible or PS/2 computer, DOS 3.1 or later, 640K main memory, hard disk.

For fastest service call toll free
1-800-232-7379,
or **FAX YOUR ORDER:**
201-573-4956
(Do not mail a confirmation order in addition to this fax.)

CHECK METHOD OF PAYMENT:
☐ Payment enclosed (shipping and handling are free).
☐ Check ☐ VISA ☐ MasterCard

Account # ______ Exp. Date Mo. ______ Yr. ______

Signature ______

☐ Bill me later. Add $3.95 shipping and handling per unit.

Residents of NJ, IL, IA, CA, VA, and KY please add sales tax. Orders shipped in USA only.

Purchase of reference materials for professional use may be tax deductible.

Name ______

Address ______

City ______ St. ______ Zip ______

Occupation ______

Put the power of PDR®
in the palm of your hand with . . .

POCKET PDR™

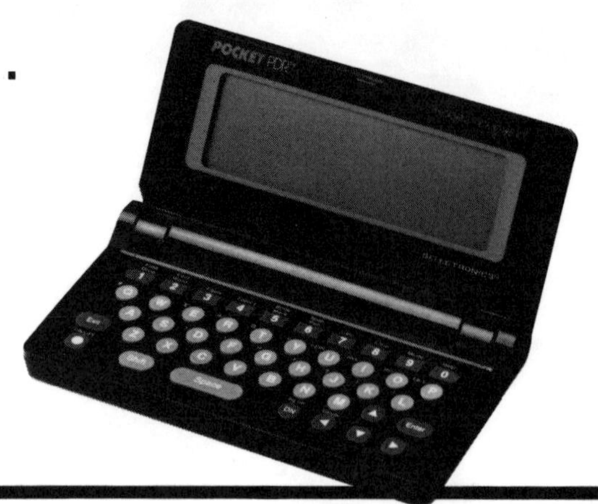

Instant access to indications, contraindications, warnings, adverse reactions, dosage and how-supplied information on every Rx Drug in PDR. This convenient, easy-to-use pocket-sized electronic data bank folds down to 6" long x 3" wide, less than 1" thick — and weighs just 10 ounces. Use it for fast, on-the-spot look ups — for accurate, up-to-date information. As simple to use as a pocket calculator, the POCKET PDR gives you the information you need, when and where you need it!

Also available with The Merck Manual!

Now with built-in Indications Index!

Put the power of PDR on your personal computer!

◀ PDR® on CD-ROM
Fast, fail-safe access to the complete text of all 5 PDR volumes in one integrated program! Complete prescribing information on nearly 3,000 pharmaceuticals. Put the power of today's technology —and the vital information of a complete drug reference library — to work for you as never before!

PDR® Drug Interactions and Side Effects Diskettes™ ▶
Search 5,000 brand and generic listings found in the PDR Library. Check 2,500 side effects as quickly as you can name the reaction. Find approved alternatives for more than 2,000 indications whenever you pinpoint a problem prescription.

Use the order form on the reverse side.

NO POSTAGE NECESSARY IF MAILED IN THE UNITED STATES

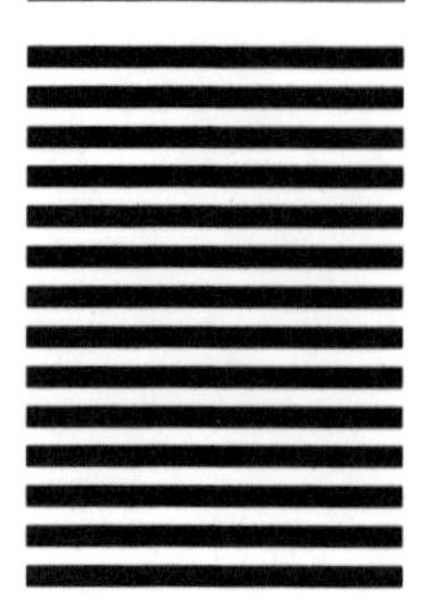

BUSINESS REPLY MAIL

FIRST CLASS MAIL PERMIT NO. 28 MONTVALE NJ

POSTAGE WILL BE PAID BY ADDRESSEE

Physicians' Desk Reference
Medical Economics Data
P.O. Box 430
MONTVALE NJ 07645-9880

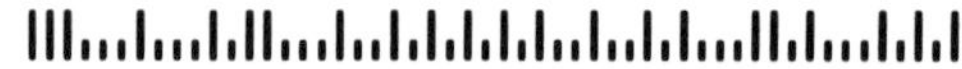

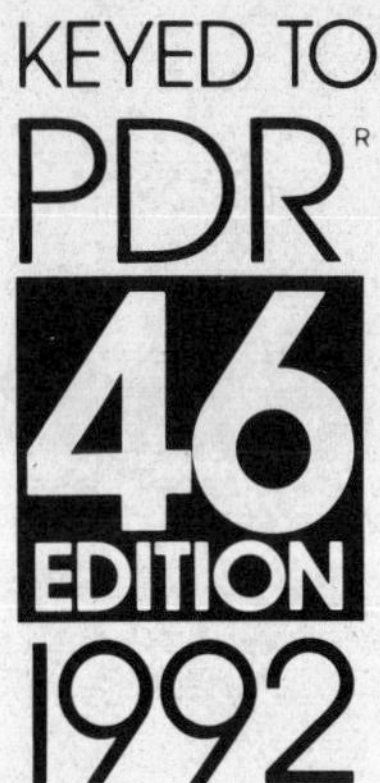

DRUG INTERACTIONS AND SIDE EFFECTS INDEX®

INTERACTIONS 1
FOOD INTERACTIONS CROSS-REFERENCE . 1057
SIDE EFFECTS 1061

EDITOR • MUKESH MEHTA, R.Ph.

ISBN 1-56363-004-4

MEDICAL ECONOMICS DATA

Foreword

Welcome to the 1992 edition of PDR Drug Interactions and Side Effects Index®. We are confident that this publication will prove to be a valuable resource for you in determining potential drug interactions and side effects. In order to help you utilize this cross-reference index to its fullest potential, we offer the following suggestions:

1. To identify potential interactions with a given drug, turn to the white (Interactions) section of the book, in which drugs are listed alphabetically by brand name. Look up the heading for the brand in question. Under it, you'll find first a summary of all the therapeutic drug classes with which the drug may interact, then a list of each compound—and each brand name of the compound—included in those classes. The likely result of co-administration is listed for each compound, as well as each brand's page number in the appropriate PDR® volume. Following the list of interactive compounds is a similar list of any potentially interactive foods.

2. To check for interactions with a particular dietary item turn to the blue (Food Interactions Cross-reference) section. Here foods are listed in alphabetical order. Under each food heading is a list of all brand name drugs citing a possible interaction, together with a brief description of the results and, for further reference, the brand's PDR page number.

3. For information on side effects, turn to the pink (Side Effects) section, in which more than 2,500 distinct reactions are listed alphabetically. Find the heading that best describes the side effect, and underneath it you'll find an alphabetical list of every brand name drug with which it has been associated. To help identify the most likely offenders, incidence data are included whenever found in the official labeling. For further review, each product's PDR page number is also included.

NOTE: All entries in the Index are derived directly from the FDA-sanctioned prescribing information published by PDR. The only products listed in the Index are those described in PDR and its companion volumes; and the only facts presented are those found in approved product labeling.

Although all three PDR volumes have been carefully sifted for pertinent facts during compilation of the Index, please remember that the publisher does not guarantee that the listings are totally complete or accurate. Use this Index only as a convenient cross-reference. Consult the underlying PDR text, as well as the medical literature, for definitive information. Citations refer to the 1992 editions of PDR and PDR For Ophthalmology® and the 1991 edition of PDR For Nonprescription Drugs®, published in March. The PDR Index of Drug Interations and Side Effects is updated once a year, concurrently with publication of the annual edition of PDR.

To assist you in identifying the full range of the prescribing alternatives for any given diagnosis, PDR publishes another cross-reference text, the PDR Indications Index™. In this convenient, pocket-sized book, the entries are arranged alphabetically by diagnosis or indication. Indicated products are cited by brand and generic name, and keyed with the appropriate PDR page number.

MEDICAL ECONOMICS DATA

SECTION 1

Interactions Index

Listed on this and the following pages is a catalogue of interactions found during a review of each product description in PDR®, PDR For Nonprescription Drugs®, and PDR For Ophthalmology®. The list is arranged alphabetically by brand or, when applicable, generic name. Only fully described products are included.

Whenever appropriate, each brand-name heading is followed by a summary of the major pharmaceutical categories, such as "antihypertensives" or "tranquilizers," with which the product is reported to interact. Beneath this summmary is an alphabetical list of the compounds in the cited categories. The potential effect of concurrent administration with the drug in question is reported in parentheses immediately after each compound's name. This is followed by an alphabetical list of brands of the compound described in PDR and its companion volumes. Page numbers refer to the product information found in the 1992 editions of PDR and PDR For Ophthalmology and the 1991 edition of PDR For Nonprescription Drugs. Symbols denoting the subsidiary PDR volumes appear in the bottom margin.

Following the list of interaction compounds is a similar list of interactive foods. Potential effects are summarized in parentheses after each item. Interactions with alcohol are reported as drug interactions, rather than food interactions.

The Index notes only interactions cited in official prescribing information as published by PDR. Cross-sensitivity reactions and effects on laboratory results are not included.

A AND D OINTMENT
(Petrolatum, Lanolin) .... ▣ 692
No interactions described in labeling.

AKWA TEARS OINTMENT
(Mineral Oil, Petrolatum, White) ...... ⊙ 208
No interactions described in labeling.

AKWA TEARS SOLUTION
(Polyvinyl Alcohol) .... ⊙ 208
No interactions described in labeling.

AMO VITRAX SOLUTION
(Sodium Hyaluronate) .... ⊙ 236
No interactions described in labeling.

AMVISC PLUS
(Sodium Hyaluronate) .... ⊙ 323
No interactions described in labeling.

A.P.L.
(Chorionic Gonadotropin) 2431
No interactions described in labeling.

A-200 LICE CONTROL SPRAY AND KIT
(Pyrethroids) 2189
No interactions described in labeling.

A-200 PEDICULICIDE SHAMPOO & GEL
(Pyrethrins) 2189
No interactions described in labeling.

A.R.M. ALLERGY RELIEF MEDICINE CAPLETS
(Chlorpheniramine Maleate, Phenylpropanolamine Hydrochloride) .... ▣ 615
May interact with phenylpropanolamine containing anorectics and certain other agents. Compounds in these categories include:

Alcohol (Do not use concomitantly).

Phenylpropanolamine Containing Anorectics (Effect not specified).

A/T/S TOPICAL GEL AND TOPICAL SOLUTION
(Erythromycin) 1089
May interact with:

Concomitant Topical Acne Therapy (Potential for cumulative irritant effect).

AVC CREAM
(Sulfanilamide) 1322
No interactions described in labeling.

AVC SUPPOSITORIES
(Sulfanilamide) 1322
No interactions described in labeling.

ABBOKINASE
(Urokinase) 503
May interact with anticoagulants and certain other agents. Compounds in these categories include:

Aspirin (Altered platelet function).
Products include:
- Alka-Seltzer Effervescent Antacid and Pain Reliever 1568
- Alka-Seltzer Extra Strength Effervescent Antacid and Pain Reliever 1570
- Alka-Seltzer (Flavored) Effervescent Antacid and Pain Reliever 1569
- Alka-Seltzer Plus Cold Medicine .... ▣ 623
- Alka-Seltzer Plus Night-Time Cold Medicine .... ▣ 623
- Alka Seltzer Plus Sinus Allergy Medicine .... ▣ 624
- Anacin Coated Analgesic Caplets 2417
- Anacin Coated Analgesic Tablets 2417
- Anacin Maximum Strength Analgesic Coated Tablets 2417
- Maximum Strength Arthritis Pain Formula By the Makers of Anacin Analgesic Tablets and Caplets 2418
- Arthritis Pain Formula by the Makers of Anacin Analgesic Tablets and Caplets .... ▣ 747
- Arthritis Strength BC Powder .... ▣ 516
- Ascriptin A/D Caplets 1850
- Regular Strength Ascriptin Tablets 1850
- Azdōne Tablets 844
- BC Powder .... ▣ 517
- BC Cold Powder .... ▣ 517
- Children's Bayer Chewable Aspirin .... ▣ 564
- Genuine Bayer Aspirin Tablets & Caplets .... ▣ 564
- Maximum Bayer Aspirin Tablets & Caplets .... ▣ 566
- Bayer Plus Aspirin Tablets .... ▣ 567
- Therapy Bayer Aspirin Caplets .... ▣ 568
- 8 Hour Bayer Timed-Release Aspirin .... ▣ 566
- Arthritis Strength Bufferin Analgesic Caplets 744
- Extra Strength Bufferin Analgesic Tablets 745
- Bufferin Analgesic Tablets and Caplets 743
- Cama Arthritis Pain Reliever .... ▣ 685
- Damason-P 1356
- Easprin 1719
- Ecotrin Enteric Coated Aspirin Maximum Strength Tablets and Caplets 2189
- Ecotrin Enteric Coated Aspirin Regular Strength Tablets and Caplets 2189
- Empirin Aspirin .... ▣ 541
- Empirin with Codeine Phosphate Nos. 2, 3 & 4 764
- Equagesic Tablets 2451
- Excedrin Extra-Strength Analgesic Tablets & Caplets 749
- 4-Way Cold Tablets 750
- Fiorinal Capsules 2007
- Fiorinal with Codeine Capsules 2008
- Fiorinal Tablets 2007
- Lortab ASA Tablets 2414
- Momentum Muscular Backache Formula .... ▣ 751
- Norgesic 1314
- Norwich Extra-Strength Aspirin .... ▣ 546
- Norwich Regular Strength Aspirin ▣ 547
- P-A-C Analgesic Tablets .... ▣ 669
- Percodan 951
- Robaxisal Tablets 1872
- Sine-Off Sinus Medicine Tablets-Aspirin Formula .... ▣ 722
- Soma Compound w/Codeine Tablets 2390
- Soma Compound Tablets 2389
- St. Joseph Adult Chewable Aspirin (81 mg.) .... ▣ 703
- Synalgos-DC Capsules 2525
- Talwin Compound 2072
- Ursinus Inlay-Tabs .... ▣ 691

Vanquish Analgesic Caplets [ND] 574
Zorprin Tablets 698

Dicumarol (Increased risk of hemorrhage). Products include:
Dicumarol Tablets 516

Heparin Calcium (Increased risk of hemorrhage). Products include:
Calciparine Injection 925

Heparin Sodium (Increased risk of hemorrhage). Products include:
Heparin Lock Flush Solution 2456
Heparin Sodium Vials 1264
Heparin Sodium Injection 2457
Heparin Sodium Injection, USP, Sterile Solution 2342

Indomethacin (Altered platelet function). Products include:
Indocin 1487

Indomethacin Sodium Trihydrate (Altered platelet function). Products include:
Indocin I.V. 1490

Phenylbutazone (Altered platelet function). Products include:
Butazolidin Capsules & Tablets 1027

Warfarin Sodium (Increased risk of hemorrhage). Products include:
Coumadin Injection & Tablets 944
Panwarfin Tablets 547

ABBOKINASE OPEN-CATH

(Urokinase) 505
No interactions described in labeling.

ACCUTANE CAPSULES

(Isotretinoin) 1878
May interact with:

Vitamin A (Additive Vitamin A toxicity). Products include:
Aquasol A Vitamin A Capsules, USP 615
Aquasol A Parenteral, USP 615
Bugs Bunny Children's Chewable Vitamins (Sugar Free) [ND] 625
Bugs Bunny With Extra C Children's Chewable Vitamins (Sugar Free) [ND] 626
Bugs Bunny/Flintstones [ND] 625
Flintstones Children's Chewable Vitamins With Extra C [ND] 626
Flintstones Children's Chewable Vitamins Plus Iron [ND] 625
Lazer Creme 1770
Myadec [ND] 640
Natalins Rx 1391
Natalins Tablets 1391
Ocuvite Vitamin and Mineral Supplement ⊙ 312
One-A-Day Essential Vitamins [ND] 627
One-A-Day Maximum Formula Vitamins and Minerals [ND] 627
One-A-Day Plus Extra C Vitamins [ND] 627
Stressgard Stress Formula Vitamins [ND] 628
Tri-Vi-Flor 1.0 mg Vitamins with Fluoride Chewable Tablets 1400
Tri-Vi-Flor Drops 1400
Tri-Vi-Sol Vitamin Drops [ND] 614
Tri-Vi-Sol Vitamin Drops with Iron [ND] 614
Vicon Forte Capsules 2416
Vicon Plus [ND] 682
Vi-Daylin ADC Vitamins Drops 1980
Vi-Daylin ADC Vitamins + Iron Drops 1980
Vi-Daylin/F ADC Vitamins Drops With Fluoride 1981
Vi-Daylin/F ADC Vitamins + Iron Drops With Fluoride 1981
Vi-Zac [ND] 682
Within Women's Formula Multivitamin with Calcium, Extra Iron and Zinc [ND] 628
Zymacap Capsules [ND] 670

Food Interactions

Dairy products (Increases oral absorption of isotretinoin).

Food, unspecified (Increases oral absorption of isotretinoin).

ACETAMINOPHEN UNISERTS SUPPOSITORIES

(Acetaminophen) 2374
No interactions described in labeling.

ACHROMYCIN V CAPSULES

(Tetracycline Hydrochloride) 1193
May interact with oral anticoagulants, penicillins, antacids, oral contraceptives, and certain other agents. Compounds in these categories include:

Aluminum Carbonate Gel (Impaired absorption of tetracycline). Products include:
Basaljel 2438

Aluminum Hydroxide (Impaired absorption of tetracycline). Products include:
Cama Arthritis Pain Reliever [ND] 685
Gaviscon Extra Strength Relief Formula Liquid Antacid [ND] 594
Gaviscon Extra Strength Relief Formula Antacid Tablets [ND] 594
Gaviscon Liquid Antacid [ND] 594
Gelusil Liquid & Tablets [ND] 639
Extra Strength Maalox Plus Suspension 1850
Maalox TC Suspension 1851
Maalox Plus Tablets [ND] 655
Extra Strength Maalox Plus Tablets 1850
Nephrox Suspension [ND] 563
WinGel Liquid & Tablets [ND] 761

Aluminum Hydroxide Gel (Impaired absorption of tetracycline). Products include:
ALternaGEL Liquid 1154
Aludrox Oral Suspension 2428
Amphojel Suspension 2429
Amphojel Suspension without Flavor 2429
Mylanta Liquid 1155
Mylanta Double Strength Liquid 1155

Aluminum Hydroxide Gel, Dried (Impaired absorption of tetracycline). Products include:
Alu-Tab/Alu-Cap 1309
Amphojel Tablets 2429
Ascriptin A/D Caplets 1850
Regular Strength Ascriptin Tablets 1850
Gaviscon Antacid Tablets [ND] 593
Gaviscon-2 Antacid Tablets [ND] 594
Mylanta Tablets 1155
Mylanta Double Strength Tablets 1155

Amoxicillin (Interference with bactericidal action of penicillin). Products include:
Amoxil 2193
Augmentin Tablets, Powder for Oral Suspension, and Chewable Tablets 2198

Ampicillin Sodium (Interference with bactericidal action of penicillin). Products include:
Unasyn 1965

Azlocillin Sodium (Interference with bactericidal action of penicillin).
No products indexed under this heading.

Bacampicillin Hydrochloride (Interference with bactericidal action of penicillin). Products include:
Spectrobid Tablets & Powder for Oral Suspension 1961

Carbenicillin Disodium (Interference with bactericidal action of penicillin).

Carbenicillin Indanyl Sodium (Interference with bactericidal action of penicillin). Products include:
Geocillin Tablets 1951

Dicumarol (Depressed plasma prothombin activity; downward adjustment of anticoagulant dosage may be necessary). Products include:
Dicumarol Tablets 516

Dihydroxyaluminum Sodium Carbonate (Impaired absorption of tetracycline). Products include:
Rolaids [ND] 743

Ethinyl Estradiol (Reduced efficacy and increased incidence of breakthrough bleeding). Products include:
Brevicon 2304
Demulen 2161
Estinyl Tablets 2085
Jenest-28 Tablets 1636
Levlen/Tri-Levlen 665
Lo/Ovral Tablets 2471
Lo/Ovral-28 Tablets 2476
Loestrin 1728
Modicon 1667
Nordette-21 Tablets 2481
Nordette-28 Tablets 2483
Norethin 2133
Norinyl 2304
Norlestrin 1746
Ortho-Cyclen Tablets 1658
Ortho-Novum 1667
Ovcon 1391
Ovral Tablets 2490
Ovral-28 Tablets 2491
Levlen/Tri-Levlen 665
Tri-Norinyl 2304
Triphasil-21 Tablets 2527
Triphasil-28 Tablets 2532

Ethynodiol Diacetate (Reduced efficacy and increased incidence of breakthrough bleeding). Products include:
Demulen 2161

Levonorgestrel (Reduced efficacy and increased incidence of breakthrough bleeding). Products include:
Levlen/Tri-Levlen 665
Nordette-21 Tablets 2481
Nordette-28 Tablets 2483
Norplant System 2484
Levlen/Tri-Levlen 665
Triphasil-21 Tablets 2527
Triphasil-28 Tablets 2532

Magaldrate (Impaired absorption of tetracycline). Products include:
Riopan Antacid Chew Tablets [ND] 754
Riopan Antacid Chew Tablets in Rollpacks [ND] 754
Riopan Antacid Suspension 2421
Riopan Antacid Swallow Tablets 2421
Riopan Plus Chew Tablets 2422
Riopan Plus Chew Tablets in Rollpack 2422
Riopan Plus 2 Chew Tablets, Mint Flavor, Cherry Flavor 2422
Riopan Plus Suspension 2422
Riopan Plus 2 Suspension, Mint Flavor, Cherry Flavor 2422

Magnesium Hydroxide (Impaired absorption of tetracycline). Products include:
Aludrox Oral Suspension 2428
Ascriptin A/D Caplets 1850
Regular Strength Ascriptin Tablets 1850
Di-Gel Antacid/Anti-Gas [ND] 697
Gelusil Liquid & Tablets [ND] 639
Haley's M-O, Regular & Flavored [ND] 569
Extra Strength Maalox Plus Suspension 1850
Maalox TC Suspension 1851
Maalox Plus Tablets [ND] 655
Extra Strength Maalox Plus Tablets 1850
Mylanta Liquid 1155
Mylanta Tablets 1155
Mylanta Double Strength Liquid 1155
Mylanta Double Strength Tablets 1155
Concentrated Phillips' Milk of Magnesia [ND] 573
Phillips' Milk of Magnesia Liquid [ND] 572
Phillips' Milk of Magnesia Tablets [ND] 573
WinGel Liquid & Tablets [ND] 761

Magnesium Oxide (Impaired absorption of tetracycline). Products include:
Bayer Plus Aspirin Tablets [ND] 567
Beelith Tablets 659
Bufferin Analgesic Tablets and Caplets [ND] 524
Cama Arthritis Pain Reliever [ND] 685
Mag-Ox 400 673
Uro-Mag 673

Mestranol (Reduced efficacy and increased incidence of breakthrough bleeding). Products include:
Enovid 2161
Norethin 2133
Norinyl 2304
Ortho-Novum 1667

Mezlocillin Sodium (Interference with bactericidal action of penicillin). Products include:
Mezlin 1597
Mezlin Pharmacy Bulk Package 1599

Nafcillin Sodium (Interference with bactericidal action of penicillin). Products include:
Unipen 2533

Norethindrone (Reduced efficacy and increased incidence of breakthrough bleeding). Products include:
Brevicon 2304
Jenest-28 Tablets 1636
Micronor Tablets 1667
Modicon 1667
Norethin 2133
Norinyl 2304
Norlutin 1755
Nor-Q D Tablets 2304
Ortho-Novum 1667
Ovcon 1391
Tri-Norinyl 2304

Norethynodrel (Reduced efficacy and increased incidence of breakthrough bleeding). Products include:
Enovid 2161

Norgestimate (Reduced efficacy and increased incidence of breakthrough bleeding). Products include:
Ortho-Cyclen Tablets 1658

Norgestrel (Reduced efficacy and increased incidence of breakthrough bleeding). Products include:
Lo/Ovral Tablets 2471
Lo/Ovral-28 Tablets 2476
Ovral Tablets 2490
Ovral-28 Tablets 2491
Ovrette Tablets 2492

Penicillin G Potassium (Interference with bactericidal action of penicillin). Products include:
Pfizerpen for Injection 1957

Penicillin G Procaine (Interference with bactericidal action of penicillin). Products include:
Bicillin C-R Injection 2438
Bicillin C-R 900/300 Injection 2440
Pfizerpen-AS Aqueous Suspension 1959
Wycillin Injection 2537
Wycillin Injection and Probenecid Tablets 2539

Penicillin G Sodium (Interference with bactericidal action of penicillin).
No products indexed under this heading.

Penicillin G, Benzathine (Interference with bactericidal action of penicillin). Products include:
Bicillin C-R Injection 2438
Bicillin C-R 900/300 Injection 2440
Bicillin L-A Injection 2442

Penicillin V Potassium (Interference with bactericidal action of penicillin).
No products indexed under this heading.

Ticarcillin Disodium (Interference with bactericidal action of penicillin). Products include:
Ticar for Injection 2236
Timentin for Injection 2239

Warfarin Sodium (Depressed plasma prothombin activity; downward adjustment of anticoagulant dosage may be necessary). Products include:
Coumadin Injection & Tablets 944
Panwarfin Tablets 547

Food Interactions

Dairy products (Interferes with absorption of oral forms of tetracycline).

Food, unspecified (Interferes with absorption of oral forms of tetracycline).

ACHROMYCIN OPHTHALMIC OINTMENT 1%
(Tetracycline Hydrochloride) ⊙ 307
No interactions described in labeling.

ACHROMYCIN OPHTHALMIC SUSPENSION 1%
(Tetracycline Hydrochloride) ⊙ 308
No interactions described in labeling.

ACID MANTLE CREME
(Aluminum Acetate) ▣ 684
No interactions described in labeling.

ACI-JEL THERAPEUTIC VAGINAL JELLY
(Acetic Acid, Oxyquinoline Sulfate) 1652
No interactions described in labeling.

ACLOVATE CREAM
(Alclometasone Dipropionate) 1053
No interactions described in labeling.

ACLOVATE OINTMENT
(Alclometasone Dipropionate) 1053
No interactions described in labeling.

ACNOMEL CREAM
(Resorcinol, Sulfur) ▣ 615
No interactions described in labeling.

ACTIBINE
(Yohimbine Hydrochloride) 900
May interact with antidepressant drugs and certain other agents. Compounds in these categories include:

Amitriptyline Hydrochloride (Concurrent use is not recommended). Products include:
- Elavil 2269
- Endep Tablets 1927
- Etrafon 2087
- Limbitrol 1933
- Triavil Tablets 1556

Amoxapine (Concurrent use is not recommended). Products include:
- Asendin Tablets 1196

Bupropion Hydrochloride (Concurrent use is not recommended). Products include:
- Wellbutrin Tablets 821

Desipramine Hydrochloride (Concurrent use is not recommended). Products include:
- Norpramin Tablets 1340

Doxepin Hydrochloride (Concurrent use is not recommended). Products include:
- Sinequan 1960

Fluoxetine Hydrochloride (Concurrent use is not recommended). Products include:
- Prozac Pulvules 920

Imipramine Hydrochloride (Concurrent use is not recommended). Products include:
- Tofranil Ampuls 1038
- Tofranil Tablets 1039

Imipramine Pamoate (Concurrent use is not recommended). Products include:
- Tofranil-PM Capsules 1041

Isocarboxazid (Concurrent use is not recommended). Products include:
- Marplan Tablets 1906

Maprotiline Hydrochloride (Concurrent use is not recommended). Products include:
- Ludiomil Tablets 874

Nortriptyline Hydrochloride (Concurrent use is not recommended). Products include:
- Pamelor 2019

Phenelzine Sulfate (Concurrent use is not recommended). Products include:
- Nardil 1742

Protriptyline Hydrochloride (Concurrent use is not recommended). Products include:
- Vivactil Tablets 1567

Tranylcypromine Sulfate (Concurrent use is not recommended). Products include:
- Parnate Tablets 2222

Trazodone Hydrochloride (Concurrent use is not recommended). Products include:
- Desyrel and Desyrel Dividose 1404

Trimipramine Maleate (Concurrent use is not recommended). Products include:
- Surmontil Capsules 2524

ACTIDIL SYRUP
(Triprolidine Hydrochloride) ▣ 538
May interact with:

Alcohol (Concurrent use not recommended).

ACTIDIL TABLETS
(Triprolidine Hydrochloride) ▣ 538
May interact with:

Alcohol (Concurrent use not recommended).

ACTIFED CAPSULES
(Pseudoephedrine Hydrochloride, Triprolidine Hydrochloride) ▣ 539
May interact with monoamine oxidase inhibitors and certain other agents. Compounds in these categories include:

Alcohol (Concurrent use not recommended).

Furazolidone (Concurrent administration is not recommended). Products include:
- Furoxone 1855

Isocarboxazid (Concurrent administration is not recommended). Products include:
- Marplan Tablets 1906

Phenelzine Sulfate (Concurrent administration is not recommended). Products include:
- Nardil 1742

Selegiline Hydrochloride (Concurrent administration is not recommended). Products include:
- Eldepryl 2250

Tranylcypromine Sulfate (Concurrent administration is not recommended). Products include:
- Parnate Tablets 2222

ACTIFED PLUS CAPLETS
(Acetaminophen, Pseudoephedrine Hydrochloride, Triprolidine Hydrochloride) ▣ 539
May interact with monoamine oxidase inhibitors and certain other agents. Compounds in these categories include:

Alcohol (Concurrent use not recommended).

Furazolidone (Concurrent use not recommended). Products include:
- Furoxone 1855

Isocarboxazid (Concurrent use not recommended). Products include:
- Marplan Tablets 1906

Phenelzine Sulfate (Concurrent use not recommended). Products include:
- Nardil 1742

Selegiline Hydrochloride (Concurrent use not recommended). Products include:
- Eldepryl 2250

Tranylcypromine Sulfate (Concurrent use not recommended). Products include:
- Parnate Tablets 2222

ACTIFED PLUS TABLETS
(Acetaminophen, Pseudoephedrine Hydrochloride, Triprolidine Hydrochloride) ▣ 540
May interact with monoamine oxidase inhibitors and certain other agents. Compounds in these categories include:

Alcohol (Concurrent use not recommended).

Furazolidone (Concurrent use not recommended). Products include:
- Furoxone 1855

Isocarboxazid (Concurrent use not recommended). Products include:
- Marplan Tablets 1906

Phenelzine Sulfate (Concurrent use not recommended). Products include:
- Nardil 1742

Selegiline Hydrochloride (Concurrent use not recommended). Products include:
- Eldepryl 2250

Tranylcypromine Sulfate (Concurrent use not recommended). Products include:
- Parnate Tablets 2222

ACTIFED WITH CODEINE COUGH SYRUP
(Codeine Phosphate, Triprolidine Hydrochloride, Pseudoephedrine Hydrochloride) 752
May interact with central nervous system depressants, monoamine oxidase inhibitors, and certain other agents. Compounds in these categories include:

Alcohol (Increased CNS depression).

Alfentanil Hydrochloride (Increased CNS depression). Products include:
- Alfenta Injection 1131

Alprazolam (Increased CNS depression). Products include:
- Xanax Tablets 2367

Aprobarbital (Increased CNS depression). Products include:
- Alurate Elixir 1883

Buprenorphine (Increased CNS depression).
No products indexed under this heading.

Buspirone Hydrochloride (Increased CNS depression). Products include:
- BuSpar 1401

Butabarbital (Increased CNS depression). Products include:
- Pyridium Plus 1764

Butalbital (Increased CNS depression). Products include:
- Esgic-Plus Tablets 1002
- Esgic Tablets & Capsules 1001
- Fioricet Tablets 2006
- Fiorinal Capsules 2007
- Fiorinal with Codeine Capsules 2008
- Fiorinal Tablets 2007
- Phrenilin 838
- Sedapap Tablets 50 mg/650 mg 1360

Chlordiazepoxide (Increased CNS depression). Products include:
- Libritabs Tablets 1930
- Limbitrol 1933
- Menrium Tablets 1934

Chlordiazepoxide Hydrochloride (Increased CNS depression). Products include:
- Librax Capsules 1929
- Librium Capsules 1931
- Librium Injectable 1932

Chlorpromazine (Increased CNS depression). Products include:
- Thorazine 2234

Chlorprothixene (Increased CNS depression). Products include:
- Taractan Tablets 1920

Chlorprothixene Hydrochloride (Increased CNS depression). Products include:
- Taractan 1920

Clorazepate Dipotassium (Increased CNS depression). Products include:
- Tranxene 556

Codeine (Increased CNS depression). Products include:
- Calcidrine Syrup 506

Codeine Polistirex (Increased CNS depression).
No products indexed under this heading.

Dezocine (Increased CNS depression).

Diazepam (Increased CNS depression). Products include:
- Valium Injectable 1937
- Valium Tablets 1939
- Valrelease Capsules 1923

Droperidol (Increased CNS depression). Products include:
- Inapsine Injection 1140
- Innovar Injection 1141

Enflurane (Increased CNS depression). Products include:
- Ethrane 599

Estazolam (Increased CNS depression). Products include:
- ProSom Tablets 554

Ethchlorvynol (Increased CNS depression). Products include:
- Placidyl Capsules 553

Ethinamate (Increased CNS depression).
No products indexed under this heading.

Fentanyl (Increased CNS depression). Products include:
- Duragesic Transdermal System 1133

Fentanyl Citrate (Increased CNS depression). Products include:
- Innovar Injection 1141
- Sublimaze Injection 1146

Fluphenazine Decanoate (Increased CNS depression). Products include:
- Prolixin Decanoate 1795

Fluphenazine Enanthate (Increased CNS depression). Products include:
- Prolixin Enanthate 1796

Fluphenazine Hydrochloride (Increased CNS depression). Products include:
- Prolixin Elixir 1793
- Prolixin Injection 1791
- Prolixin Oral Concentrate 1792
- Prolixin Tablets 1793

Flurazepam Hydrochloride (Increased CNS depression). Products include:
- Dalmane Capsules 1927

Furazolidone (Enhanced effect of MAO inhibitors). Products include:
- Furoxone 1855

Glutethimide (Increased CNS depression).
No products indexed under this heading.
Haloperidol (Increased CNS depression). Products include:
Haldol Injection, Tablets and Concentrate 1373
Haloperidol Decanoate (Increased CNS depression). Products include:
Haldol Decanoate 1375
Hydrocodone Bitartrate (Increased CNS depression). Products include:
Anexsia 5/500 Tablets 2196
Anexsia 7.5/650 Tablets 2197
Azdōne Tablets 844
Codiclear DH Syrup 845
Codimal DH Syrup 846
Damason-P 1356
Hycodan Syrup, Tablets 927
Hycomine Compound Tablets 929
Hycomine Syrup 927
Hycotuss Expectorant Syrup 930
Hydrocet Capsules 835
Lortab ASA Tablets 2414
Lortab 2412
Ru-Tuss with Hydrocodone 694
Triaminic Expectorant DH 1995
Vicodin Tablets 1187
Vicodin ES Tablets 1189
Zydone Capsules 941
Hydrocodone Polistirex (Increased CNS depression). Products include:
Tussionex Extended-Release Suspension 988
Hydroxyzine Hydrochloride (Increased CNS depression). Products include:
Atarax Tablets & Syrup 1941
Marax Tablets & DF Syrup 1954
Vistaril Intramuscular Solution 1970
Isocarboxazid (Enhanced effect of MAO inhibitors). Products include:
Marplan Tablets 1906
Isoflurane (Increased CNS depression). Products include:
Forane 600
Ketamine Hydrochloride (Increased CNS depression). Products include:
Ketalar 1726
Levorphanol Tartrate (Increased CNS depression). Products include:
Levo-Dromoran 1906
Lorazepam (Increased CNS depression). Products include:
Ativan Injection 2432
Ativan Tablets 2434
Loxapine Hydrochloride (Increased CNS depression). Products include:
Loxitane 1213
Loxapine Succinate (Increased CNS depression). Products include:
Loxitane Capsules 1213
Meperidine Hydrochloride (Increased CNS depression). Products include:
Demerol 2047
Mepergan Injection 2479
Mephobarbital (Increased CNS depression). Products include:
Mebaral Tablets 2061
Meprobamate (Increased CNS depression). Products include:
Deprol Tablets 2382
Equagesic Tablets 2451
Miltown Tablets 2386
PMB 200 and PMB 400 2504
Mesoridazine (Increased CNS depression). Products include:
Serentil 686
Methadone Hydrochloride (Increased CNS depression). Products include:
Dolophine Hydrochloride Ampoules & Vials 1260
Dolophine Hydrochloride Tablets 1261
Methadone Hydrochloride Diskets 1284
Methadone Hydrochloride Oral Solution & Tablets 1987
Methohexital Sodium (Increased CNS depression). Products include:
Brevital Sodium Vials 1248
Methoxyflurane (Increased CNS depression).
No products indexed under this heading.
Methyldopa (Diminished antihypertensive effect). Products include:
Aldoclor Tablets 1413
Aldomet Oral 1415
Aldoril Tablets 1418
Methyldopate Hydrochloride (Diminished antihypertensive effect). Products include:
Aldomet Ester HCl Injection 1417
Midazolam Hydrochloride (Increased CNS depression). Products include:
Versed Injection 1924
Molindone Hydrochloride (Increased CNS depression). Products include:
Moban Tablets & Concentrate 932
Morphine Sulfate (Increased CNS depression). Products include:
Astramorph/PF Injection, USP (Preservative-Free) 618
Duramorph 960
Infumorph 200 and Infumorph 500 Sterile Solutions 962
MS Contin Tablets 1814
MSIR 1817
Oramorph SR (Morphine Sulfate Sustained Release Tablets) 1988
Roxanol 1991
Opium Alkaloids (Increased CNS depression). Products include:
B & O No. 15A & No. 16A Supprettes 2395
Pantopon Injectable 1911
Oxazepam (Increased CNS depression). Products include:
Serax Capsules 2522
Serax Tablets 2522
Oxycodone Hydrochloride (Increased CNS depression). Products include:
Percocet Tablets 950
Percodan 951
Roxicodone Tablets, Oral Solution & Intensol (Oxycodone) 1992
Tylox Capsules 1382
Pentobarbital Sodium (Increased CNS depression). Products include:
Nembutal Sodium Capsules 534
Nembutal Sodium Solution 536
Nembutal Sodium Suppositories 538
Perphenazine (Increased CNS depression). Products include:
Etrafon 2087
Triavil Tablets 1556
Trilafon 2123
Phenelzine Sulfate (Enhanced effect of MAO inhibitors). Products include:
Nardil 1742
Phenobarbital (Increased CNS depression). Products include:
Arco-Lase Plus Tablets 607
Bellergal-S Tablets 1998
Bronkolixir ■ 761
Bronkotabs Tablets ■ 762
Donnatal 1858
Donnatal Extentabs 1859
Donnatal Tablets 1858
Donnazyme Tablets 1860
Kinesed Tablets 2272
Phenobarbital Elixir and Tablets 1293
Primatene Tablets-P Formula 2421
Quadrinal Tablets 1183
Tedral SA 1765
Prazepam (Increased CNS depression). Products include:
Centrax 1693
Prochlorperazine (Increased CNS depression). Products include:
Compazine 2201
Promethazine Hydrochloride (Increased CNS depression). Products include:
Mepergan Injection 2479
Phenergan with Codeine 2497
Phenergan with Dextromethorphan 2499
Phenergan Injection 2493
Phenergan Suppositories 2496
Phenergan Syrup 2495
Phenergan Tablets 2496
Phenergan VC 2500
Phenergan VC with Codeine 2501
Propofol (Increased CNS depression). Products include:
Diprivan Injection 2267
Propoxyphene Hydrochloride (Increased CNS depression). Products include:
Darvon 1256
Wygesic Tablets 2540
Propoxyphene Napsylate (Increased CNS depression). Products include:
Darvon-N/Darvocet-N 1254
Quazepam (Increased CNS depression). Products include:
Doral Tablets 2383
Reserpine (Diminished antihypertensive effect). Products include:
Diupres Tablets 1461
Hydromox R Tablets 1209
Hydropres Tablets 1485
Renese-R Tablets 1786
Salutensin/Salutensin-Demi 719
Ser-Ap-Es Tablets 881
Serpasil Tablets 883
Serpasil-Apresoline Tablets 884
Serpasil-Esidrix Tablets 886
Secobarbital Sodium (Increased CNS depression). Products include:
Seconal Sodium Pulvules 1296
Selegiline Hydrochloride (Enhanced effect of MAO inhibitors). Products include:
Eldepryl 2250
Sufentanil Citrate (Increased CNS depression). Products include:
Sufenta Injection 1147
Temazepam (Increased CNS depression). Products include:
Restoril Capsules 2023
Thiamylal Sodium (Increased CNS depression). Products include:
Surital Ampoules, Steri-Vials 1764
Thioridazine Hydrochloride (Increased CNS depression). Products include:
Mellaril 2011
Thiothixene (Increased CNS depression). Products include:
Navane Capsules and Concentrate 1954
Navane Intramuscular 1956
Tranylcypromine Sulfate (Enhanced effect of MAO inhibitors). Products include:
Parnate Tablets 2222
Triazolam (Increased CNS depression). Products include:
Halcion Tablets 2340
Trifluoperazine Hydrochloride (Increased CNS depression). Products include:
Stelazine 2226

ACTIFED SYRUP

(Pseudoephedrine Hydrochloride, Triprolidine Hydrochloride) ■ 540
May interact with monoamine oxidase inhibitors and certain other agents. Compounds in these categories include:

Alcohol (Concurrent use not recommended).
Furazolidone (Concurrent administration is not recommended). Products include:
Furoxone 1855
Isocarboxazid (Concurrent administration is not recommended). Products include:
Marplan Tablets 1906
Phenelzine Sulfate (Concurrent administration is not recommended). Products include:
Nardil 1742
Selegiline Hydrochloride (Concurrent administration is not recommended). Products include:
Eldepryl 2250
Tranylcypromine Sulfate (Concurrent administration is not recommended). Products include:
Parnate Tablets 2222

ACTIFED TABLETS

(Pseudoephedrine Hydrochloride, Triprolidine Hydrochloride) ■ 540
May interact with monoamine oxidase inhibitors and certain other agents. Compounds in these categories include:

Alcohol (Concurrent use not recommended).
Furazolidone (Concurrent administration is not recommended). Products include:
Furoxone 1855
Isocarboxazid (Concurrent administration is not recommended). Products include:
Marplan Tablets 1906
Phenelzine Sulfate (Concurrent administration is not recommended). Products include:
Nardil 1742
Selegiline Hydrochloride (Concurrent administration is not recommended). Products include:
Eldepryl 2250
Tranylcypromine Sulfate (Concurrent administration is not recommended). Products include:
Parnate Tablets 2222

ACTIFED 12-HOUR CAPSULES

(Pseudoephedrine Hydrochloride, Triprolidine Hydrochloride) ■ 539
May interact with monoamine oxidase inhibitors and certain other agents. Compounds in these categories include:

Alcohol (Concurrent use not recommended).
Furazolidone (Concurrent administration is not recommended). Products include:
Furoxone 1855
Isocarboxazid (Concurrent administration is not recommended). Products include:
Marplan Tablets 1906
Phenelzine Sulfate (Concurrent administration is not recommended). Products include:
Nardil 1742
Selegiline Hydrochloride (Concurrent administration is not recommended). Products include:
Eldepryl 2250
Tranylcypromine Sulfate (Concurrent administration is not recommended). Products include:
Parnate Tablets 2222

ACTIGALL CAPSULES

(Ursodiol) 2280
May interact with bile acid sequestering agents, lipid-lowering drugs, estrogens, oral contraceptives, and

certain other agents. Compounds in these categories include:

Aluminum Carbonate Gel (Interferes with the action of Actigall by reducing its absorption). Products include:
- Basaljel 2438

Aluminum Hydroxide (Interferes with the action of Actigall by reducing its absorption). Products include:
- Cama Arthritis Pain Reliever ▣ 685
- Gaviscon Extra Strength Relief Formula Liquid Antacid ▣ 594
- Gaviscon Extra Strength Relief Formula Antacid Tablets ▣ 594
- Gaviscon Liquid Antacid ▣ 594
- Gelusil Liquid & Tablets ▣ 639
- Extra Strength Maalox Plus Suspension 1850
- Maalox TC Suspension 1851
- Maalox Plus Tablets ▣ 655
- Extra Strength Maalox Plus Tablets 1850
- Nephrox Suspension ▣ 563
- WinGel Liquid & Tablets ▣ 761

Aluminum Hydroxide Gel (Interferes with the action of Actigall by reducing its absorption). Products include:
- ALternaGEL Liquid 1154
- Aludrox Oral Suspension 2428
- Amphojel Suspension 2429
- Amphojel Suspension without Flavor 2429
- Mylanta Liquid 1155
- Mylanta Double Strength Liquid 1155

Aluminum Hydroxide Gel, Dried (Interferes with the action of Actigall by reducing its absorption). Products include:
- Alu-Tab/Alu-Cap 1309
- Amphojel Tablets 2429
- Ascriptin A/D Caplets 1850
- Regular Strength Ascriptin Tablets 1850
- Gaviscon Antacid Tablets ▣ 593
- Gaviscon-2 Antacid Tablets ▣ 594
- Mylanta Tablets 1155
- Mylanta Double Strength Tablets 1155

Chlorotrianisene (May counteract the effectiveness of Actigall). Products include:
- TACE 12 and 25 mg 1353

Cholestyramine (Interferes with the action of Actigall by reducing its absorption; may counteract the effectiveness of Actigall). Products include:
- Cholybar 1705
- Questran Light 711
- Questran Powder 710

Clofibrate (May counteract the effectiveness of Actigall). Products include:
- Atromid-S Capsules 2435

Colestipol Hydrochloride (Interferes with the action of Actigall by reducing its absorption; may counteract the effectiveness of Actigall). Products include:
- Colestid Granules 2328

Dienestrol (May counteract the effectiveness of Actigall). Products include:
- Ortho Dienestrol Cream 1664

Diethylstilbestrol (May counteract the effectiveness of Actigall). Products include:
- Diethylstilbestrol Tablets 1258

Estradiol (May counteract the effectiveness of Actigall). Products include:
- Emcyt Capsules 1161
- Estrace 1385
- Estrace Vaginal Cream 1388
- Estraderm Transdermal System 866

Estrogens, Conjugated (May counteract the effectiveness of Actigall). Products include:
- Mediatric Capsules 2476
- PMB 200 and PMB 400 2504
- Premarin Intravenous 2508
- Premarin with Methyltestosterone 2515
- Premarin Tablets 2510
- Premarin Vaginal Cream 2512

Estrogens, Esterified (May counteract the effectiveness of Actigall). Products include:
- Estratest 2245
- Menrium Tablets 1934

Estropipate (May counteract the effectiveness of Actigall). Products include:
- Ogen 540

Ethinyl Estradiol (May counteract the effectiveness of Actigall). Products include:
- Brevicon 2304
- Demulen 2161
- Estinyl Tablets 2085
- Jenest-28 Tablets 1636
- Levlen/Tri-Levlen 665
- Lo/Ovral Tablets 2471
- Lo/Ovral-28 Tablets 2476
- Loestrin 1728
- Modicon 1667
- Nordette-21 Tablets 2481
- Nordette-28 Tablets 2483
- Norethin 2133
- Norinyl 2304
- Norlestrin 1746
- Ortho-Cyclen Tablets 1658
- Ortho-Novum 1667
- Ovcon 1391
- Ovral Tablets 2490
- Ovral-28 Tablets 2491
- Levlen/Tri-Levlen 665
- Tri-Norinyl 2304
- Triphasil-21 Tablets 2527
- Triphasil-28 Tablets 2532

Ethynodiol Diacetate (May counteract the effectiveness of Actigall). Products include:
- Demulen 2161

Gemfibrozil (May counteract the effectiveness of Actigall). Products include:
- Lopid Capsules and Tablets 1736

Levonorgestrel (May counteract the effectiveness of Actigall). Products include:
- Levlen/Tri-Levlen 665
- Nordette-21 Tablets 2481
- Nordette-28 Tablets 2483
- Norplant System 2484
- Levlen/Tri-Levlen 665
- Triphasil-21 Tablets 2527
- Triphasil-28 Tablets 2532

Lovastatin (May counteract the effectiveness of Actigall). Products include:
- Mevacor Tablets 1505

Mestranol (May counteract the effectiveness of Actigall). Products include:
- Enovid 2161
- Norethin 2133
- Norinyl 2304
- Ortho-Novum 1667

Norethindrone (May counteract the effectiveness of Actigall). Products include:
- Brevicon 2304
- Jenest-28 Tablets 1636
- Micronor Tablets 1667
- Modicon 1667
- Norethin 2133
- Norinyl 2304
- Norlutin 1755
- Nor-Q D Tablets 2304
- Ortho-Novum 1667
- Ovcon 1391
- Tri-Norinyl 2304

Norethynodrel (May counteract the effectiveness of Actigall). Products include:
- Enovid 2161

Norgestimate (May counteract the effectiveness of Actigall). Products include:
- Ortho-Cyclen Tablets 1658

Norgestrel (May counteract the effectiveness of Actigall). Products include:
- Lo/Ovral Tablets 2471
- Lo/Ovral-28 Tablets 2476
- Ovral Tablets 2490
- Ovral-28 Tablets 2491
- Ovrette Tablets 2492

Polyestradiol Phosphate (May counteract the effectiveness of Actigall). Products include:
- Estradurin 2452

Probucol (May counteract the effectiveness of Actigall). Products include:
- Lorelco Tablets 1333

Quinestrol (May counteract the effectiveness of Actigall). Products include:
- Estrovis 1721

ACTIMMUNE
(INTERFERON GAMMA-1B) 1046
May interact with:

Bone Marrow Depressants, unspecified (Caution should be exercised when administering with other potentially myelosuppressive agents).

ACTIVASE
(Alteplase, Recombinant) 1047
May interact with oral anticoagulants, platelet inhibitors, and certain other agents. Compounds in these categories include:

Aspirin (Increased risk of bleeding). Products include:
- Alka-Seltzer Effervescent Antacid and Pain Reliever 1568
- Alka-Seltzer Extra Strength Effervescent Antacid and Pain Reliever 1570
- Alka-Seltzer (Flavored) Effervescent Antacid and Pain Reliever 1569
- Alka-Seltzer Plus Cold Medicine ▣ 623
- Alka-Seltzer Plus Night-Time Cold Medicine ▣ 623
- Alka Seltzer Plus Sinus Allergy Medicine ▣ 624
- Anacin Coated Analgesic Caplets 2417
- Anacin Coated Analgesic Tablets 2417
- Anacin Maximum Strength Analgesic Coated Tablets 2417
- Maximum Strength Arthritis Pain Formula By the Makers of Anacin Analgesic Tablets and Caplets 2418
- Arthritis Pain Formula by the Makers of Anacin Analgesic Tablets and Caplets ▣ 747
- Arthritis Strength BC Powder ▣ 516
- Ascriptin A/D Caplets 1850
- Regular Strength Ascriptin Tablets 1850
- Azdōne Tablets 844
- BC Powder ▣ 517
- BC Cold Powder ▣ 517
- Children's Bayer Chewable Aspirin ▣ 564
- Genuine Bayer Aspirin Tablets & Caplets ▣ 564
- Maximum Bayer Aspirin Tablets & Caplets ▣ 566
- Bayer Plus Aspirin Tablets ▣ 567
- Therapy Bayer Aspirin Caplets ▣ 568
- 8 Hour Bayer Timed-Release Aspirin ▣ 566
- Arthritis Strength Bufferin Analgesic Caplets 744
- Extra Strength Bufferin Analgesic Tablets 745
- Bufferin Analgesic Tablets and Caplets 743
- Cama Arthritis Pain Reliever ▣ 685
- Damason-P 1356
- Easprin 1719
- Ecotrin Enteric Coated Aspirin Maximum Strength Tablets and Caplets 2189
- Ecotrin Enteric Coated Aspirin Regular Strength Tablets and Caplets 2189
- Empirin Aspirin ▣ 541
- Empirin with Codeine Phosphate Nos. 2, 3 & 4 764
- Equagesic Tablets 2451
- Excedrin Extra-Strength Analgesic Tablets & Caplets 749
- 4-Way Cold Tablets 750
- Fiorinal Capsules 2007
- Fiorinal with Codeine Capsules 2008
- Fiorinal Tablets 2007
- Lortab ASA Tablets 2414
- Momentum Muscular Backache Formula ▣ 751
- Norgesic 1314
- Norwich Extra-Strength Aspirin ▣ 546
- Norwich Regular Strength Aspirin ▣ 547
- P-A-C Analgesic Tablets ▣ 669
- Percodan 951
- Robaxisal Tablets 1872
- Sine-Off Sinus Medicine Tablets-Aspirin Formula ▣ 722
- Soma Compound w/Codeine Tablets 2390
- Soma Compound Tablets 2389
- St. Joseph Adult Chewable Aspirin (81 mg.) ▣ 703
- Synalgos-DC Capsules 2525
- Talwin Compound 2072
- Ursinus Inlay-Tabs ▣ 691
- Vanquish Analgesic Caplets ▣ 574
- Zorprin Tablets 698

Azlocillin Sodium (Increased risk of bleeding).
- No products indexed under this heading.

Carbenicillin Indanyl Sodium (Increased risk of bleeding). Products include:
- Geocillin Tablets 1951

Choline Magnesium Trisalicylate (Increased risk of bleeding). Products include:
- Trilisate 1822

Diclofenac Sodium (Increased risk of bleeding). Products include:
- Voltaren Ophthalmic Sterile Ophthalmic Solution ◉ 268
- Voltaren Tablets 1042

Dicumarol (Increased risk of bleeding). Products include:
- Dicumarol Tablets 516

Diflunisal (Increased risk of bleeding). Products include:
- Dolobid Tablets 1465

Dipyridamole (Increased risk of bleeding). Products include:
- Persantine Tablets 683

Fenoprofen Calcium (Increased risk of bleeding). Products include:
- Nalfon Pulvules & Tablets 919

Flurbiprofen (Increased risk of bleeding). Products include:
- Ansaid Tablets 2319

Heparin Calcium (Increased risk of bleeding). Products include:
- Calciparine Injection 925

Heparin Sodium (Increased risk of bleeding). Products include:
- Heparin Lock Flush Solution 2456
- Heparin Sodium Vials 1264
- Heparin Sodium Injection 2457
- Heparin Sodium Injection, USP, Sterile Solution 2342

Ibuprofen (Increased risk of bleeding). Products include:
- Advil Cold & Sinus Caplets (formerly CoAdvil) 2416
- Advil Ibuprofen Tablets and Caplets 2416
- Children's Advil Suspension 2426
- CoAdvil ▣ 748
- Dristan Sinus Caplets 2419
- Haltran Tablets ▣ 668
- Ibuprofen ▣ 631
- Medipren ibuprofen Caplets and Tablets 1362
- Midol 200 Cramp Relief Formula ▣ 570
- Motrin Tablets 2351
- Motrin IB Caplets and Tablets ▣ 736
- Nuprin Ibuprofen/Analgesic Tablets & Caplets 752
- PediaProfen Suspension 1363
- Rufen Tablets 691
- Trendar Ibuprofen Tablets ▣ 756

Indomethacin (Increased risk of bleeding). Products include:
- Indocin 1487

Indomethacin Sodium Trihydrate (Increased risk of bleeding). Products include:
- Indocin I.V. 1490

(▣ Described in PDR For Nonprescription Drugs) (◉ Described in PDR For Ophthalmology)

Ketoprofen (Increased risk of bleeding). Products include:
- Orudis Capsules ... 2488

Magnesium Salicylate (Increased risk of bleeding). Products include:
- Doan's - Extra-Strength Analgesic ▣ 549
- Doan's - Regular Strength Analgesic ... ▣ 549
- Mobigesic Analgesic Tablets ... ▣ 507

Meclofenamate Sodium (Increased risk of bleeding). Products include:
- Meclomen Capsules ... 1739

Mefenamic Acid (Increased risk of bleeding). Products include:
- Ponstel ... 1758

Mezlocillin Sodium (Increased risk of bleeding). Products include:
- Mezlin ... 1597
- Mezlin Pharmacy Bulk Package ... 1599

Nafcillin Sodium (Increased risk of bleeding). Products include:
- Unipen ... 2533

Naproxen (Increased risk of bleeding). Products include:
- Naprosyn ... 2297

Naproxen Sodium (Increased risk of bleeding). Products include:
- Anaprox and Anaprox DS Tablets ... 2288

Penicillin G Procaine (Increased risk of bleeding). Products include:
- Bicillin C-R Injection ... 2438
- Bicillin C-R 900/300 Injection ... 2440
- Pfizerpen-AS Aqueous Suspension 1959
- Wycillin Injection ... 2537
- Wycillin Injection and Probenecid Tablets ... 2539

Penicillin G, Benzathine (Increased risk of bleeding). Products include:
- Bicillin C-R Injection ... 2438
- Bicillin C-R 900/300 Injection ... 2440
- Bicillin L-A Injection ... 2442

Phenylbutazone (Increased risk of bleeding). Products include:
- Butazolidin Capsules & Tablets ... 1027

Piroxicam (Increased risk of bleeding). Products include:
- Feldene Capsules ... 1777

Salsalate (Increased risk of bleeding). Products include:
- Disalcid ... 1310
- Mono-Gesic Tablets ... 846
- Salflex ... 839

Sulindac (Increased risk of bleeding). Products include:
- Clinoril Tablets ... 1433

Ticarcillin Disodium (Increased risk of bleeding). Products include:
- Ticar for Injection ... 2236
- Timentin for Injection ... 2239

Tolmetin Sodium (Increased risk of bleeding). Products include:
- Tolectin (200, 400 and 600 mg) .. 1379

Warfarin Sodium (Increased risk of bleeding). Products include:
- Coumadin Injection & Tablets ... 944
- Panwarfin Tablets ... 547

ACUTRIM 16 HOUR STEADY CONTROL APPETITE SUPPRESSANT
(Phenylpropanolamine Hydrochloride) ... ▣ 548
See **Acutrim Late Day Strength Appetite Suppressant**

ACUTRIM LATE DAY STRENGTH APPETITE SUPPRESSANT
(Phenylpropanolamine Hydrochloride) ... ▣ 548
May interact with antihypertensives, antidepressant drugs, and alpha adrenergic stimulants. Compounds in these categories include:

Acebutolol Hydrochloride (Concurrent use not recommended). Products include:
- Sectral Capsules ... 2520

Amitriptyline Hydrochloride (Concurrent use not recommended). Products include:
- Elavil ... 2269
- Endep Tablets ... 1927
- Etrafon ... 2087
- Limbitrol ... 1933
- Triavil Tablets ... 1556

Amoxapine (Concurrent use not recommended). Products include:
- Asendin Tablets ... 1196

Atenolol (Concurrent use not recommended). Products include:
- Tenoretic Tablets ... 1105
- Tenormin Tablets and I.V. Injection 1107

Benazepril Hydrochloride (Concurrent use not recommended). Products include:
- Lotensin Tablets ... 872

Betaxolol Hydrochloride (Concurrent use not recommended). Products include:
- Betoptic Sterile Ophthalmic Solution ... 569
- Betoptic S Sterile Ophthalmic Suspension ... 570
- Kerlone Tablets ... 2172

Bupropion Hydrochloride (Concurrent use not recommended). Products include:
- Wellbutrin Tablets ... 821

Captopril (Concurrent use not recommended). Products include:
- Capoten ... 2255
- Capozide ... 2258

Carteolol Hydrochloride (Concurrent use not recommended). Products include:
- Cartrol Tablets ... 507

Clonidine (Concurrent use not recommended). Products include:
- Catapres-TTS ... 677

Clonidine Hydrochloride (Concurrent use not recommended). Products include:
- Catapres Tablets ... 676
- Combipres Tablets ... 678

Deserpidine (Concurrent use not recommended). Products include:
- Enduronyl ... 518
- Harmonyl Tablets ... 528
- Oreticyl ... 545

Desipramine Hydrochloride (Concurrent use not recommended). Products include:
- Norpramin Tablets ... 1340

Diazoxide (Concurrent use not recommended). Products include:
- Hyperstat I.V. Injection ... 2095
- Proglycem ... 649

Doxazosin Mesylate (Concurrent use not recommended). Products include:
- Cardura Tablets ... 1941

Doxepin Hydrochloride (Concurrent use not recommended). Products include:
- Sinequan ... 1960

Enalapril Maleate (Concurrent use not recommended). Products include:
- Vaseretic Tablets ... 1559
- Vasotec Tablets ... 1564

Enalaprilat (Concurrent use not recommended). Products include:
- Vasotec I.V. ... 1562

Esmolol Hydrochloride (Concurrent use not recommended). Products include:
- Brevibloc Injection ... 942

Felodipine (Concurrent use not recommended). Products include:
- Plendil Extended-Release Tablets ... 1526

Fluoxetine Hydrochloride (Concurrent use not recommended). Products include:
- Prozac Pulvules ... 920

Fosinopril Sodium (Concurrent use not recommended). Products include:
- Monopril Tablets ... 1406

Guanabenz Acetate (Concurrent use not recommended). Products include:
- Wytensin Tablets ... 2542

Guanethidine Monosulfate (Concurrent use not recommended). Products include:
- Esimil Tablets ... 864
- Ismelin Tablets ... 869

Hydralazine Hydrochloride (Concurrent use not recommended). Products include:
- Apresazide Capsules ... 854
- Apresoline Hydrochloride Parenteral (Ampuls) ... 856
- Apresoline Hydrochloride Tablets .. 855
- Apresoline-Esidrix Tablets ... 857
- Ser-Ap-Es Tablets ... 881
- Serpasil-Apresoline Tablets ... 884

Imipramine Hydrochloride (Concurrent use not recommended). Products include:
- Tofranil Ampuls ... 1038
- Tofranil Tablets ... 1039

Imipramine Pamoate (Concurrent use not recommended). Products include:
- Tofranil-PM Capsules ... 1041

Indapamide (Concurrent use not recommended). Products include:
- Lozol Tablets ... 1843

Isocarboxazid (Concurrent use not recommended). Products include:
- Marplan Tablets ... 1906

Isradipine (Concurrent use not recommended). Products include:
- DynaCirc Capsules ... 2004

Labetalol Hydrochloride (Concurrent use not recommended). Products include:
- Normodyne Injection ... 2108
- Normodyne Tablets ... 2110
- Normozide Tablets ... 2112
- Trandate HCT Tablets ... 579
- Trandate Injection ... 577
- Trandate Tablets ... 579

Lisinopril (Concurrent use not recommended). Products include:
- Prinivil Tablets ... 1538
- Prinzide Tablets ... 1540
- Zestoretic ... 2274
- Zestril Tablets ... 2277

Maprotiline Hydrochloride (Concurrent use not recommended). Products include:
- Ludiomil Tablets ... 874

Mecamylamine Hydrochloride (Concurrent use not recommended). Products include:
- Inversine Tablets ... 1492

Methyldopa (Concurrent use not recommended). Products include:
- Aldoclor Tablets ... 1413
- Aldomet Oral ... 1415
- Aldoril Tablets ... 1418

Methyldopate Hydrochloride (Concurrent use not recommended). Products include:
- Aldomet Ester HCl Injection ... 1417

Metoprolol Tartrate (Concurrent use not recommended). Products include:
- Lopressor Ampuls ... 1032
- Lopressor HCT Tablets ... 1034
- Lopressor Tablets ... 1032

Metyrosine (Concurrent use not recommended). Products include:
- Demser Capsules ... 1460

Minoxidil (Concurrent use not recommended). Products include:
- Loniten Tablets ... 2346
- Rogaine Topical Solution ... 2357

Nadolol (Concurrent use not recommended). Products include:
- Corgard Tablets ... 701
- Corzide Tablets ... 702

Nicardipine Hydrochloride (Concurrent use not recommended). Products include:
- Cardene Capsules ... 2290

Nitroglycerin (Concurrent use not recommended). Products include:
- Deponit NTG Transdermal Delivery System ... 2143
- Minitran Transdermal Delivery System ... 1312
- Nitro-Bid Ointment ... 1339
- Nitro-Bid Capsules ... 1338
- Nitrodisc ... 2176
- Nitro-Dur (nitroglycerin) Transdermal Infusion System ... 1164
- Nitrogard Tablets ... 1004
- Nitrolingual Spray ... 1846
- Nitrostat Tablets ... 1743
- Transderm-Nitro Transdermal Therapeutic System ... 2283

Nortriptyline Hydrochloride (Concurrent use not recommended). Products include:
- Pamelor ... 2019

Penbutolol Sulfate (Concurrent use not recommended). Products include:
- Levatol ... 1832

Phenelzine Sulfate (Concurrent use not recommended). Products include:
- Nardil ... 1742

Phenoxybenzamine Hydrochloride (Concurrent use not recommended). Products include:
- Dibenzyline Capsules ... 2207

Phentolamine Mesylate (Concurrent use not recommended). Products include:
- Regitine ... 878

Phenylpropanolamine Containing Anorectics (Concurrent use not recommended).

Pindolol (Concurrent use not recommended). Products include:
- Visken Tablets ... 2036

Prazosin Hydrochloride (Concurrent use not recommended). Products include:
- Minipress Capsules ... 1778
- Minizide Capsules ... 1779

Propranolol Hydrochloride (Concurrent use not recommended). Products include:
- Inderal ... 2459
- Inderal LA Long Acting Capsules 2461
- Inderide Tablets ... 2463
- Inderide LA Long Acting Capsules .. 2465

Protriptyline Hydrochloride (Concurrent use not recommended). Products include:
- Vivactil Tablets ... 1567

Ramipril (Concurrent use not recommended). Products include:
- Altace Capsules ... 1086

Rauwolfia Serpentina (Concurrent use not recommended). Products include:
- Raudixin Tablets ... 1803
- Rauzide Tablets ... 1804

Rescinnamine (Concurrent use not recommended).
- No products indexed under this heading.

Reserpine (Concurrent use not recommended). Products include:
- Diupres Tablets ... 1461
- Hydromox R Tablets ... 1209
- Hydropres Tablets ... 1485
- Renese-R Tablets ... 1786
- Salutensin/Salutensin-Demi ... 719
- Ser-Ap-Es Tablets ... 881

Serpasil Tablets 883
Serpasil-Apresoline Tablets 884
Serpasil-Esidrix Tablets 886

Sodium Nitroprusside (Concurrent use not recommended). Products include:
Nipride I.V. Infusion 1909

Terazosin Hydrochloride (Concurrent use not recommended). Products include:
Hytrin Tablets 529

Timolol Maleate (Concurrent use not recommended). Products include:
Blocadren Tablets 1429
Timolide Tablets 1547
Timoptic in Ocudose 1552
Timoptic Sterile Ophthalmic Solution 1550

Tranylcypromine Sulfate (Concurrent use not recommended). Products include:
Parnate Tablets 2222

Trazodone Hydrochloride (Concurrent use not recommended). Products include:
Desyrel and Desyrel Dividose 1404

Trimethaphan Camsylate (Concurrent use not recommended). Products include:
Arfonad Ampuls 1887

Trimipramine Maleate (Concurrent use not recommended). Products include:
Surmontil Capsules 2524

ACUTRIM II MAXIMUM STRENGTH APPETITE SUPPRESSANT

(Phenylpropanolamine Hydrochloride) .... ▣ 548
See **Acutrim Late Day Strength Appetite Suppressant**

ADAGEN INJECTION

(Pegademase Bovine) 967
May interact with:

Vidarabine Monohydrate (Concomitant use can substantially alter activities of Adagen). Products include:
Vira-A for Injection 1766
Vira-A Ophthalmic Ointment, 3% 1767

ADALAT CAPSULES (10 MG AND 20 MG)

(Nifedipine) 1587
May interact with beta blockers, cardiac glycosides, oral anticoagulants, and certain other agents. Compounds in these categories include:

Acebutolol Hydrochloride (Increased likelihood of congestive heart failure, severe hypotension, or exacerbation of angina). Products include:
Sectral Capsules 2520

Atenolol (Increased likelihood of congestive heart failure, severe hypotension, or exacerbation of angina). Products include:
Tenoretic Tablets 1105
Tenormin Tablets and I.V. Injection 1107

Betaxolol Hydrochloride (Increased likelihood of congestive heart failure, severe hypotension, or exacerbation of angina). Products include:
Betoptic Sterile Ophthalmic Solution 569
Betoptic S Sterile Ophthalmic Suspension 570
Kerlone Tablets 2172

Carteolol Hydrochloride (Increased likelihood of congestive heart failure, severe hypotension, or exacerbation of angina). Products include:
Cartrol Tablets 507

Cimetidine (Increased peak nifedipine plasma levels). Products include:
Tagamet Tablets 2228

Cimetidine Hydrochloride (Increased peak nifedipine plasma levels). Products include:
Tagamet 2228

Deslanoside (Increased digoxin levels).
No products indexed under this heading.

Dicumarol (Increased prothrombin time). Products include:
Dicumarol Tablets 516

Digitoxin (Increased digoxin levels). Products include:
Crystodigin Tablets 1253

Digoxin (Increased digoxin levels). Products include:
Lanoxicaps 772
Lanoxin Elixir Pediatric 775
Lanoxin Injection 778
Lanoxin Injection Pediatric 781
Lanoxin Tablets 783

Esmolol Hydrochloride (Increased likelihood of congestive heart failure, severe hypotension, or exacerbation of angina). Products include:
Brevibloc Injection 942

Labetalol Hydrochloride (Increased likelihood of congestive heart failure, severe hypotension, or exacerbation of angina). Products include:
Normodyne Injection 2108
Normodyne Tablets 2110
Normozide Tablets 2112
Trandate HCT Tablets 579
Trandate Injection 577
Trandate Tablets 579

Metoprolol Tartrate (Increased likelihood of congestive heart failure, severe hypotension, or exacerbation of angina). Products include:
Lopressor Ampuls 1032
Lopressor HCT Tablets 1034
Lopressor Tablets 1032

Nadolol (Increased likelihood of congestive heart failure, severe hypotension, or exacerbation of angina). Products include:
Corgard Tablets 701
Corzide Tablets 702

Penbutolol Sulfate (Increased likelihood of congestive heart failure, severe hypotension, or exacerbation of angina). Products include:
Levatol 1832

Pindolol (Increased likelihood of congestive heart failure, severe hypotension, or exacerbation of angina). Products include:
Visken Tablets 2036

Propranolol Hydrochloride (Increased likelihood of congestive heart failure, severe hypotension, or exacerbation of angina). Products include:
Inderal 2459
Inderal LA Long Acting Capsules 2461
Inderide Tablets 2463
Inderide LA Long Acting Capsules 2465

Ranitidine Hydrochloride (Produces smaller, non-significant increases in peak nifedipine plasma levels and AUC). Products include:
Zantac Injection and Zantac Injection Premixed 1063
Zantac 1065

Timolol Maleate (Increased likelihood of congestive heart failure, severe hypotension, or exacerbation of angina). Products include:
Blocadren Tablets 1429
Timolide Tablets 1547
Timoptic in Ocudose 1552
Timoptic Sterile Ophthalmic Solution 1550

Warfarin Sodium (Increased prothrombin time). Products include:
Coumadin Injection & Tablets 944
Panwarfin Tablets 547

ADENOCARD INJECTION

(Adenosine) 1007
May interact with xanthine bronchodilators and certain other agents. Compounds in these categories include:

Aminophylline (The effects of adenosine are antagonized). Products include:
Amesec .... ▣ 682
Aminophyllin Tablets 2153

Caffeine-containing medications (The effects of adenosine are antagonized).

Carbamazepine (Potential for higher degrees of heart block). Products include:
Tegretol Chewable Tablets 654
Tegretol Suspension 656
Tegretol Tablets 654

Dipyridamole (Potentiates the effects). Products include:
Persantine Tablets 683

Dyphylline (The effects of adenosine are antagonized). Products include:
Dilor 2079
Dilor-G Tablets & Liquid 2079
Lufyllin Elixir 2384
Lufyllin & Lufyllin-400 Tablets 2384
Lufyllin-GG Elixir & Tablets 2385

Theophylline (The effects of adenosine are antagonized). Products include:
Bronkaid Tablets .... ▣ 757
Bronkolixir .... ▣ 761
Bronkotabs Tablets .... ▣ 762
Constant-T Tablets 1029
Marax Tablets & DF Syrup 1954
Primatene Tablets 2421
Quibron Capsules 713
Quibron-T 714
Quibron-T/SR 716
Theolair Liquid 1317
Theo-Organidin Elixir 2391

Theophylline Anhydrous (The effects of adenosine are antagonized). Products include:
Aerolate 994
Primatene Tablets-M Formula .... ▣ 753
Primatene Tablets-Regular Formula 2421
Respbid Tablets 684
Slo-bid Gyrocaps 1847
T-PHYL (Uniphyl) 200 mg Tablets 1820
Tedral SA 1765
Theo-24 2179
Theo-Dur Sprinkle 1168
Theo-Dur Extended-Release Tablets 1166
Theolair Tablets 1317
Theolair-SR Tablets 1319
TheoX Extended-Release Tablets 841
Uniphyl 400 mg Tablets 1823

Theophylline Calcium Salicylate (The effects of adenosine are antagonized). Products include:
Quadrinal Tablets 1183

Theophylline Sodium Glycinate (The effects of adenosine are antagonized). Products include:
Asbron G 1997

ADIPEX-P TABLETS AND CAPSULES

(Phentermine Hydrochloride) 1019
May interact with monoamine oxidase inhibitors, insulin, and certain other agents. Compounds in these categories include:

Alcohol (May result in adverse drug interaction).

Furazolidone (Contraindication; hypertensive crisis may result). Products include:
Furoxone 1855

Guanethidine Monosulfate (Decreased hypotensive effect of guanethidine). Products include:
Esimil Tablets 864
Ismelin Tablets 869

Insulin, Human (Insulin requirement may be altered).
No products indexed under this heading.

Insulin, Human Isophane Suspension (Insulin requirement may be altered). Products include:
Humulin N, 100 Units 1270

Insulin, Human NPH (Insulin requirement may be altered). Products include:
Insulatard NPH Human 1627
Novolin N 1627
Novolin N PenFill Cartridges 1628
Novolin N Prefilled 1628

Insulin, Human Regular (Insulin requirement may be altered). Products include:
Humulin BR, 100 Units 1268
Humulin R, 100 Units 1272
Novolin R 1627
Novolin R PenFill Cartridges 1628
Novolin R Prefilled 1629
Velosulin Human 1628

Insulin, Human, Zinc Suspension (Insulin requirement may be altered). Products include:
Humulin L, 100 Units 1268
Humulin U, 100 Units 1272
Novolin L 1627

Insulin, NPH (Insulin requirement may be altered). Products include:
NPH, 40 & 100 Units 1273
Beef NPH, 100 Units 1274
Pork NPH, 100 Units 1275
Insulatard NPH 1626
NPH Insulin 1626
NPH Purified Pork Isophane Insulin 1626

Insulin, Regular (Insulin requirement may be altered). Products include:
Regular, 40 & 100 Units 1273
Beef Regular, 100 Units 1275
Pork Regular, 100 Units 1275
Pork Regular (Concentrated), 500 Units 1276
Regular Insulin 1625
Regular Purified Pork Insulin 1626
Velosulin 1627

Insulin, Zinc Crystals (Insulin requirement may be altered). Products include:
NPH, 40 & 100 Units 1273

Insulin, Zinc Suspension (Insulin requirement may be altered). Products include:
Lente, 40 & 100 Units 1272
Protamine, Zinc, 40 & 100 Units 1273
Lente Iletin I 1272
Beef Lente, 100 Units 1274
Beef Protamine Zinc, 100 Units 1274
Pork Lente, 100 Units 1275
Pork, Protamine, Zinc, 100 Units 1275
Lente Insulin 1626
Lente Purified Pork Insulin 1626
Semilente Insulin 1625
Ultralente Insulin 1626

Isocarboxazid (Contraindication; hypertensive crisis may result). Products include:
Marplan Tablets 1906

Phenelzine Sulfate (Contraindication; hypertensive crisis may result). Products include:
Nardil 1742

Selegiline Hydrochloride (Contraindication); hypertensive crisis may result). Products include:

Eldepryl ... 2250

Tranylcypromine Sulfate (Contraindication); hypertensive crisis may result). Products include:

Parnate Tablets ... 2222

ADRENALIN CHLORIDE SOLUTION 1:100 & 1:1,000

(Epinephrine) ... 1689

May interact with tricyclic antidepressants, halogenated hydrocarbon anesthetics, cardiac glycosides, and certain other agents. Compounds in these categories include:

Amitriptyline Hydrochloride (Potentiation of epinephrine). Products include:

Elavil ... 2269
Endep Tablets ... 1927
Etrafon ... 2087
Limbitrol ... 1933
Triavil Tablets ... 1556

Amoxapine (Potentiation of epinephrine). Products include:

Asendin Tablets ... 1196

Chlorpheniramine Maleate (Potentiation of epinephrine). Products include:

A.R.M. Allergy Relief Medicine Caplets ... ■ 615
Alka-Seltzer Plus Cold Medicine ... ■ 623
Allerest ... ■ 559
Ana-Kit Anaphylaxis Emergency Treatment Kit ... 1100
BC Cold Powder Multi-Symptom Formula ... ■ 517
Brexin L.A. Capsules ... 2078
Cerose-DM ... 2443
Cheracol Plus Head Cold/Cough Formula ... ■ 667
Chlor-Trimeton Allergy Syrup, Tablets & Long-Acting Repetabs Tablets ... ■ 693
Chlor-Trimeton Decongestant ... ■ 694
Comhist LA Capsules ... 1618
Allergy-Sinus Comtrex Multi-Symptom Allergy Sinus Formula Tablets & Caplets ... 746
Comtrex Multi-Symptom Cold Reliever Tablets/Caplets/Liqui-Gels/Liquid ... 745
Day-Night Comtrex ... 747
Contac Continuous Action Decongestant/Antihistamine Capsules ■ 710
Contac Maximum Strength Continuous Action Decongestant/Antihistamine Caplets ... ■ 709
Contac Severe Cold and Flu Formula Caplets ... ■ 711
Coricidin 'D' Decongestant Tablets ... ■ 695
Coricidin Demilets Tablets for Children ... ■ 696
Coricidin Tablets ... ■ 695
Deconamine ... 663
Demazin Nasal Decongestant/Antihistamine Repetabs Tablets & Syrup ... ■ 697
Dorcol Children's Liquid Cold Formula ... ■ 686
Dristan Decongestant/Antihistamine/Analgesic Coated Caplets ... ■ 749
Dristan Cold Nasal Decongestant/Antihistamine/ Analgesic Coated Tablets ... 2419
Dristan Advanced Formula Decongestant/Antihistamine/Analgesic Tablets ... ■ 749
Extendryl ... 994
4-Way Cold Tablets ... 750
Fedahist Gyrocaps ... 2145
Fedahist Timecaps ... 2145
Hycomine Compound Tablets ... 929
Isoclor Timesule Capsules ... ■ 561
Kronofed-A ... 970
Medi-Flu Caplet, Liquid ... ■ 640
Naldecon Syrup, Tablets, Pediatric Drops and Pediatric Syrup ... 709
Nolamine Tablets ... 838
Novafed A Capsules ... 1342
Novahistine DH ... 1342
Novahistine Elixir ... ■ 596
Ornade Spansule Capsules ... 2221
Orthoxicol Cough Syrup ... ■ 668
PediaCare Allergy Relief Formula Liquid ... 1362
PediaCare Cough-Cold Formula Liquid ... 1362
PediaCare Night Rest Cough-Cold Formula Liquid ... 1362
PediaCare 6-12 Cough-Cold Formula Chewable Tablets ... 1362
Pyrroxate Capsules ... ■ 669
Quelidrine Syrup ... 556
Ru-Tuss II Capsules ... 693
Ru-Tuss Tablets ... 693
Ryna ... ■ 741
Sinarest Tablets & Extra Strength Tablets ... ■ 562
Sine-Off Maximum Strength Allergy/Sinus Formula Caplets ... ■ 721
Sine-Off Sinus Medicine Tablets-Aspirin Formula ... ■ 722
Singlet Tablets ... ■ 598
Sinulin ... 840
Sinutab Maximum Strength ... ■ 641
St. Joseph Nighttime Cold Medicine ... ■ 705
Sudafed Plus Liquid ... ■ 544
Sudafed Plus Tablets ... ■ 545
Teldrin Timed-Release Allergy Capsules, 12 mg ... 2192
TheraFlu Flu and Cold Medicine ... ■ 687
Triaminic Allergy Tablets ... ■ 688
Triaminic Chewables ... ■ 688
Triaminic Cold Tablets ... ■ 688
Triaminic Nite Light ... ■ 689
Triaminic Syrup ... ■ 689
Triaminic-12 Tablets ... ■ 690
Triaminicin Tablets ... ■ 690
Triaminicol Multi-Symptom Cold Tablets ... ■ 691
Triaminicol Multi-Symptom Relief ■ 691
Tylenol Allergy Sinus Medication Caplets and Gelcaps, Maximum Strength ... 1372
Children's Tylenol Cold Liquid Formula and Chewable Tablets ... 1368
Tylenol Cold & Flu Hot Medication, Packets ... 1369
Tylenol Cold Medication Caplets and Tablets ... 1370
Tylenol Cold Medication, Effervescent Tablets ... 1369
Vicks Children's NyQuil ... ■ 664
Vicks Formula 44 Cough Medicine ... ■ 661
Vicks Formula 44M Multi-Symptom Cough Medicine ... ■ 662
Vicks Pediatric Formula 44m Multi-Symptom Cough & Cold Medicine ... ■ 663

Chlorpheniramine Polistirex (Potentiation of epinephrine). Products include:

Tussionex Extended-Release Suspension ... 988

Chlorpheniramine Tannate (Potentiation of epinephrine). Products include:

Rynatan ... 2387
Rynatuss ... 2388

Clomipramine Hydrochloride (Potentiation of epinephrine). Products include:

Anafranil Capsules ... 650

Cyclopropane (Concurrent administration is contraindicated).

Desipramine Hydrochloride (Potentiation of epinephrine). Products include:

Norpramin Tablets ... 1340

Deslanoside (Concurrent use not recommended).

No products indexed under this heading.

Digitoxin (Concurrent use not recommended). Products include:

Crystodigin Tablets ... 1253

Digoxin (Concurrent use not recommended). Products include:

Lanoxicaps ... 772
Lanoxin Elixir Pediatric ... 775
Lanoxin Injection ... 778
Lanoxin Injection Pediatric ... 781
Lanoxin Tablets ... 783

Diphenhydramine Citrate (Potentiation of epinephrine). Products include:

Alka-Seltzer Plus Night-Time Cold Medicine ... ■ 623
Bufferin AF Nite Time Analgesic/Sleeping Aid Caplets ... 744
Excedrin P.M. Analgesic/Sleeping Aid Tablets, Caplets and Liquid ... 749

Diphenhydramine Hydrochloride (Potentiation of epinephrine). Products include:

Benadryl Anti-Itch Cream ... ■ 635
Benadryl Capsules ... 1691
Benadryl Decongestant Elixir ... ■ 635
Benadryl Decongestant ... ■ 635
Benadryl Elixir ... ■ 636
Benadryl Kapseals ... 1691
Benadryl 25 Kapseals ... ■ 636
Benadryl Parenteral ... 1692
Benadryl Plus ... ■ 636
Benadryl Plus Nighttime ... ■ 637
Benadryl Spray, Maximum Strength ... ■ 637
Benadryl Spray, Regular Strength ■ 637
Benadryl Steri-Vials, Ampoules, and Steri-Dose Syringe ... 1692
Benadryl 25 Tablets ... ■ 636
Benylin Cough Syrup ... ■ 637
Benylin Decongestant ... ■ 638
Caladryl Cream, Lotion, Spray ... ■ 638
Miles Nervine Nighttime Sleep-Aid ■ 627
Nytol Tablets ... ■ 517
Sleep-ettes-D Tablets ... ■ 653
Sleep-eze 3 Tablets ... ■ 755
Sleepinal Night-time Sleep Aid Capsules ... ■ 734
Sominex Caplets and Tablets ... ■ 722
Sominex Liquid ... ■ 723
Sominex Pain Relief Formula ... ■ 723
Tylenol Cold Night Time Medication Liquid ... 1371
Tylenol PM, Extra Strength Caplets and Tablets ... 1368
Unisom Dual Relief Nighttime Sleep Aid/Analgesic ... 1774
Ziradryl Lotion ... ■ 643

Doxepin Hydrochloride (Potentiation of epinephrine). Products include:

Sinequan ... 1960

Enflurane (Concurrent administration is contraindicated). Products include:

Ethrane ... 599

Halothane (Concurrent administration is contraindicated). Products include:

Fluothane ... 2453

Imipramine Hydrochloride (Potentiation of epinephrine). Products include:

Tofranil Ampuls ... 1038
Tofranil Tablets ... 1039

Imipramine Pamoate (Potentiation of epinephrine). Products include:

Tofranil-PM Capsules ... 1041

Isoflurane (Concurrent administration is contraindicated). Products include:

Forane ... 600

Maprotiline Hydrochloride (Potentiation of epinephrine). Products include:

Ludiomil Tablets ... 874

Mercurial Diuretics (Heart sensitized to arrythmias angina pain)).

Methoxyflurane (Concurrent administration is contraindicated).

No products indexed under this heading.

Nortriptyline Hydrochloride (Potentiation of epinephrine). Products include:

Pamelor ... 2019

Protriptyline Hydrochloride (Potentiation of epinephrine). Products include:

Vivactil Tablets ... 1567

Thyroxine Sodium (Potentiation of epinephrine).

No products indexed under this heading.

Trimipramine Maleate (Potentiation of epinephrine). Products include:

Surmontil Capsules ... 2524

ADRIAMYCIN PFS

(Doxorubicin Hydrochloride) ... 561

May interact with:

Cyclophosphamide (Serious irreversible myocardial toxicity; exacerbation of cyclophosphamide-induced hemorrhagic cystitis). Products include:

Cytoxan for Injection ... 726
Neosar for Injection ... 566

Cytarabine (Combination therapy results in necrotizing colitis, typhilitis, bloody stools and severe infections). Products include:

Cytosar-U Sterile Powder ... 2329

Mercaptopurine (Enhanced hepatotoxicity of 6-mercaptopurine). Products include:

Purinethol Tablets ... 800

ADRIAMYCIN RDF

(Doxorubicin Hydrochloride) ... 562

May interact with:

Cyclophosphamide (Exacerbation of cyclophosphamide-induced hemorrhagic cystitis). Products include:

Cytoxan for Injection ... 726
Neosar for Injection ... 566

Cytarabine (Combination therapy results in necrotizing colitis, typhilitis, bloody stools and severe infections). Products include:

Cytosar-U Sterile Powder ... 2329

Mercaptopurine (Enhanced hepatotoxicity of 6-mercaptopurine). Products include:

Purinethol Tablets ... 800

ADSORBONAC 2% AND 5%

(Sodium Chloride) ... ⊙ 210

No interactions described in labeling.

ADSORBOTEAR

(Povidone) ... ⊙ 210

No interactions described in labeling.

ADVANCE PREGNANCY TEST

(HCG Monoclonal Antibody) ... ■ 773

No interactions described in labeling.

ADVIL COLD & SINUS CAPLETS (FORMERLY COADVIL)

(Ibuprofen, Pseudoephedrine Hydrochloride) ... 2416

May interact with antihypertensives, antidepressant drugs, and aspirin and acetaminophen containing products. Compounds in these categories include:

Acebutolol Hydrochloride (Effects not specified). Products include:

Sectral Capsules ... 2520

Acetaminophen (Effects not specified). Products include:

Acetaminophen Uniserts Suppositories ... 2374
Actifed Plus Caplets ... ■ 539
Actifed Plus Tablets ... ■ 540
Alka-Seltzer Advanced Formula Antacid & Non-Aspirin Pain Reliever ... ■ 620
Allerest ... ■ 559

Aspirin Free Anacin Maximum Strength Acetaminophen Film Coated Caplets 2417
Aspirin Free Anacin Maximum Strength Acetaminophen Film Coated Tablets 2417
Anacin-3 Regular Strength Acetaminophen Film Coated Tablets ▣ 746
Anexsia 5/500 Tablets 2196
Anexsia 7.5/650 Tablets 2197
Benadryl Plus ▣ 636
Benadryl Plus Nighttime ▣ 637
Bufferin AF Nite Time Analgesic/Sleeping Aid Caplets 744
Allergy-Sinus Comtrex Multi-Symptom Allergy Sinus Formula Tablets & Caplets 746
Cough Formula Comtrex 746
Comtrex Multi-Symptom Cold Reliever Tablets/Caplets/Liqui-Gels/Liquid 745
Day-Night Comtrex 747
Non-Drowsy Comtrex 747
Congespirin For Children Aspirin Free Chewable Cold Tablets 748
Contac Cough & Sore Throat Formula ▣ 712
Contac Jr. Children's Cold Medicine ▣ 712
Contac Nighttime Cold Medicine ▣ 713
Contac Severe Cold and Flu Formula Caplets ▣ 711
Contac Sinus Caplets Maximum Strength Non-Drowsy Formula ▣ 710
Contac Sinus Tablets Maximum Strength Non-Drowsy Formula ▣ 710
Coricidin 'D' Decongestant Tablets ▣ 695
Coricidin Demilets Tablets for Children ▣ 696
Coricidin Tablets ▣ 695
Darvon-N/Darvocet-N 1254
Datril Extra-Strength Analgesic Tablets 748
Dimetapp Plus Caplets ▣ 675
Dorcol Children's Fever & Pain Reducer ▣ 686
Dristan Decongestant/Antihistamine/Analgesic Coated Caplets ▣ 749
Dristan Cold Nasal Decongestant/Antihistamine/Analgesic Coated Tablets 2419
Dristan Advanced Formula Decongestant/Antihistamine/Analgesic Tablets ▣ 749
Maximum Strength Dristan Decongestant/Analgesic Coated Caplets ▣ 750
No Drowsiness Dristan Cold Nasal Decongestant/Analgesic Coated Caplets 2420
Drixoral Plus Extended-Release Tablets ▣ 699
Drixoral Sinus ▣ 700
Esgic-Plus Tablets 1002
Esgic Tablets & Capsules 1001
Aspirin Free Excedrin Analgesic Caplets 748
Excedrin Extra-Strength Analgesic Tablets & Caplets 749
Excedrin P.M. Analgesic/Sleeping Aid Tablets, Caplets and Liquid 749
Sinus Excedrin Analgesic, Decongestant Tablets & Caplets 750
4-Way Cold Tablets 750
Feverall Sprinkle Caps 2374
Feverall Suppositories 2374
Fioricet Tablets 2006
Hycomine Compound Tablets 929
Hydrocet Capsules 835
Isocom Capsules 1629
Liquiprin ▣ 618
Lortab 2412
Lurline PMS Tablets 972
Medi-Flu Caplet, Liquid ▣ 640
Maximum Strength Midol Multi-Symptom Menstrual Formula ▣ 571
Maximum Strength Midol PMS Premenstrual Syndrome Formula ▣ 570
Regular Strength Midol Multi-Symptom Menstrual Formula ▣ 570
Midrin Capsules 836
Ornex Caplets ▣ 618
Children's Panadol Chewable Tablets, Liquid, Infants' Drops ▣ 571
Junior Strength Panadol ▣ 571
Maximum Strength Panadol Tablets and Caplets ▣ 572
Percocet Tablets 950
Percogesic Analgesic Tablets ▣ 660
Phenaphen with Codeine Capsules 1865
Phenaphen-650 with Codeine Tablets 1866
Phrenilin 838
Prēmsyn PMS Capsules & Caplets ▣ 547
Pyrroxate Capsules ▣ 669
Robitussin Night Relief ▣ 677
Sedapap Tablets 50 mg/650 mg 1360
Sinarest ▣ 562
Sine-Aid Maximum Strength Sinus Headache Caplets 1365
Sine-Aid Maximum Strength Sinus Headache Tablets 1365
Sine-Off Maximum Strength Allergy/Sinus Formula Caplets ▣ 721
Sine-Off Maximum Strength No Drowsiness Formula Caplets ▣ 722
Singlet Tablets ▣ 598
Sinulin 840
Sinutab Maximum Strength ▣ 641
Sinutab Maximum Strength Without Drowsiness Tablets & Caplets ▣ 642
Sinutab Regular Strength Without Drowsiness Formula ▣ 641
Sominex Pain Relief Formula ▣ 723
St. Joseph Aspirin-Free Fever Reducer for Children Chewable Tablets, Liquid & Infant Drops ▣ 704
St. Joseph Cold Tablets for Children ▣ 704
St. Joseph Nighttime Cold Medicine ▣ 705
Sudafed Sinus Caplets ▣ 545
Sudafed Sinus Tablets ▣ 545
Talacen 2070
Tempra, Acetaminophen ▣ 613
TheraFlu Flu and Cold Medicine ▣ 687
Triaminicin Tablets ▣ 690
Tylenol acetaminophen Children's Chewable Tablets & Elixir 1366
Tylenol Allergy Sinus Medication Caplets and Gelcaps, Maximum Strength 1372
Tylenol with Codeine 1381
Children's Tylenol Cold Liquid Formula and Chewable Tablets 1368
Tylenol Cold & Flu Hot Medication, Packets 1369
Tylenol Cold & Flu No Drowsiness Hot Medication, Packets 1371
Tylenol Cold Medication Caplets and Tablets 1370
Tylenol Cold Medication, Effervescent Tablets 1369
Tylenol Cold Medication No Drowsiness Formula Caplets 1370
Tylenol Cold Night Time Medication Liquid 1371
Tylenol Cough Medication Liquid, Maximum Strength 1372
Tylenol Cough Medication Liquid with Decongestant, Maximum Strength 1372
Tylenol, Extra Strength, acetaminophen Adult Liquid Pain Reliever 1367
Tylenol, Extra Strength, acetaminophen Gelcaps, Caplets, Tablets 1367
Tylenol, Infants' Drops 1366
Tylenol, Junior Strength, acetaminophen Coated Caplets, Grape and Fruit Chewable Tablets 1366
Tylenol, Maximum Strength, Sinus Medication Gelcaps, Caplets and Tablets 1373
Tylenol, Regular Strength, acetaminophen Tablets and Caplets 1367
Tylenol PM, Extra Strength Caplets and Tablets 1368
Tylox Capsules 1382
Unisom Dual Relief Nighttime Sleep Aid/Analgesic 1774
Vanquish Analgesic Caplets ▣ 574
Vicks Daycare ▣ 660
Vicks Formula 44M Multi-Symptom Cough Medicine ▣ 662
Vicks NyQuil Nighttime Colds Medicine-Original & Cherry Flavor ▣ 664
Vicodin Tablets 1187
Vicodin ES Tablets 1189
Wygesic Tablets 2540
Zydone Capsules 941

Amitriptyline Hydrochloride (Effects not specified). Products include:
Elavil 2269
Endep Tablets 1927
Etrafon 2087
Limbitrol 1933
Triavil Tablets 1556

Amoxapine (Effects not specified). Products include:
Asendin Tablets 1196

Aspirin (Effects not specified). Products include:
Alka-Seltzer Effervescent Antacid and Pain Reliever 1568
Alka-Seltzer Extra Strength Effervescent Antacid and Pain Reliever 1570
Alka-Seltzer (Flavored) Effervescent Antacid and Pain Reliever 1569
Alka-Seltzer Plus Cold Medicine ▣ 623
Alka-Seltzer Plus Night-Time Cold Medicine ▣ 623
Alka Seltzer Plus Sinus Allergy Medicine ▣ 624
Anacin Coated Analgesic Caplets 2417
Anacin Coated Analgesic Tablets 2417
Anacin Maximum Strength Analgesic Coated Tablets 2417
Maximum Strength Arthritis Pain Formula By the Makers of Anacin Analgesic Tablets and Caplets 2418
Arthritis Pain Formula by the Makers of Anacin Analgesic Tablets and Caplets ▣ 747
Arthritis Strength BC Powder ▣ 516
Ascriptin A/D Caplets 1850
Regular Strength Ascriptin Tablets 1850
Azdōne Tablets 844
BC Powder ▣ 517
BC Cold Powder ▣ 517
Children's Bayer Chewable Aspirin ▣ 564
Genuine Bayer Aspirin Tablets & Caplets ▣ 564
Maximum Bayer Aspirin Tablets & Caplets ▣ 566
Bayer Plus Aspirin Tablets ▣ 567
Therapy Bayer Aspirin Caplets ▣ 568
8 Hour Bayer Timed-Release Aspirin ▣ 566
Arthritis Strength Bufferin Analgesic Caplets 744
Extra Strength Bufferin Analgesic Tablets 745
Bufferin Analgesic Tablets and Caplets 743
Cama Arthritis Pain Reliever ▣ 685
Damason-P 1356
Easprin 1719
Ecotrin Enteric Coated Aspirin Maximum Strength Tablets and Caplets 2189
Ecotrin Enteric Coated Aspirin Regular Strength Tablets and Caplets 2189
Empirin Aspirin ▣ 541
Empirin with Codeine Phosphate Nos. 2, 3 & 4 764
Equagesic Tablets 2451
Excedrin Extra-Strength Analgesic Tablets & Caplets 749
4-Way Cold Tablets 750
Fiorinal Capsules 2007
Fiorinal with Codeine Capsules 2008
Fiorinal Tablets 2007
Lortab ASA Tablets 2414
Momentum Muscular Backache Formula ▣ 751
Norgesic 1314
Norwich Extra-Strength Aspirin ▣ 546
Norwich Regular Strength Aspirin ▣ 547
P-A-C Analgesic Tablets ▣ 669
Percodan 951
Robaxisal Tablets 1872
Sine-Off Sinus Medicine Tablets-Aspirin Formula ▣ 722
Soma Compound w/Codeine Tablets 2390
Soma Compound Tablets 2389
St. Joseph Adult Chewable Aspirin (81 mg.) ▣ 703
Synalgos-DC Capsules 2525
Talwin Compound 2072
Ursinus Inlay-Tabs ▣ 691
Vanquish Analgesic Caplets ▣ 574
Zorprin Tablets 698

Atenolol (Effects not specified). Products include:
Tenoretic Tablets 1105
Tenormin Tablets and I.V. Injection 1107

Benazepril Hydrochloride (Effects not specified). Products include:
Lotensin Tablets 872

Betaxolol Hydrochloride (Effects not specified). Products include:
Betoptic Sterile Ophthalmic Solution 569
Betoptic S Sterile Ophthalmic Suspension 570
Kerlone Tablets 2172

Bupropion Hydrochloride (Effects not specified). Products include:
Wellbutrin Tablets 821

Captopril (Effects not specified). Products include:
Capoten 2255
Capozide 2258

Carteolol Hydrochloride (Effects not specified). Products include:
Cartrol Tablets 507

Clonidine (Effects not specified). Products include:
Catapres-TTS 677

Clonidine Hydrochloride (Effects not specified). Products include:
Catapres Tablets 676
Combipres Tablets 678

Deserpidine (Effects not specified). Products include:
Enduronyl 518
Harmonyl Tablets 528
Oreticyl 545

Desipramine Hydrochloride (Effects not specified). Products include:
Norpramin Tablets 1340

Diazoxide (Effects not specified). Products include:
Hyperstat I.V. Injection 2095
Proglycem 649

Doxazosin Mesylate (Effects not specified). Products include:
Cardura Tablets 1941

Doxepin Hydrochloride (Effects not specified). Products include:
Sinequan 1960

Enalapril Maleate (Effects not specified). Products include:
Vaseretic Tablets 1559
Vasotec Tablets 1564

Enalaprilat (Effects not specified). Products include:
Vasotec I.V. 1562

Esmolol Hydrochloride (Effects not specified). Products include:
Brevibloc Injection 942

Felodipine (Effects not specified). Products include:
Plendil Extended-Release Tablets 1526

Fluoxetine Hydrochloride (Effects not specified). Products include:
Prozac Pulvules 920

Fosinopril Sodium (Effects not specified). Products include:
Monopril Tablets 1406

Guanabenz Acetate (Effects not specified). Products include:
Wytensin Tablets 2542

Guanethidine Monosulfate (Effects not specified). Products include:
Esimil Tablets 864
Ismelin Tablets 869

Hydralazine Hydrochloride (Effects not specified). Products include:
Apresazide Capsules 854
Apresoline Hydrochloride Parenteral (Ampuls) 856
Apresoline Hydrochloride Tablets 855
Apresoline-Esidrix Tablets 857
Ser-Ap-Es Tablets 881
Serpasil-Apresoline Tablets 884

Imipramine Hydrochloride (Effects not specified). Products include:
Tofranil Ampuls 1038
Tofranil Tablets 1039

Imipramine Pamoate (Effects not specified). Products include:
Tofranil-PM Capsules ... 1041
Isocarboxazid (Effects not specified). Products include:
Marplan Tablets ... 1906
Isradipine (Effects not specified). Products include:
DynaCirc Capsules ... 2004
Labetalol Hydrochloride (Effects not specified). Products include:
Normodyne Injection ... 2108
Normodyne Tablets ... 2110
Normozide Tablets ... 2112
Trandate HCT Tablets ... 579
Trandate Injection ... 577
Trandate Tablets ... 579
Lisinopril (Effects not specified). Products include:
Prinivil Tablets ... 1538
Prinzide Tablets ... 1540
Zestoretic ... 2274
Zestril Tablets ... 2277
Maprotiline Hydrochloride (Effects not specified). Products include:
Ludiomil Tablets ... 874
Mecamylamine Hydrochloride (Effects not specified). Products include:
Inversine Tablets ... 1492
Methyldopa (Effects not specified). Products include:
Aldoclor Tablets ... 1413
Aldomet Oral ... 1415
Aldoril Tablets ... 1418
Methyldopate Hydrochloride (Effects not specified). Products include:
Aldomet Ester HCl Injection ... 1417
Metoprolol Tartrate (Effects not specified). Products include:
Lopressor Ampuls ... 1032
Lopressor HCT Tablets ... 1034
Lopressor Tablets ... 1032
Metyrosine (Effects not specified). Products include:
Demser Capsules ... 1460
Minoxidil (Effects not specified). Products include:
Loniten Tablets ... 2346
Rogaine Topical Solution ... 2357
Nadolol (Effects not specified). Products include:
Corgard Tablets ... 701
Corzide Tablets ... 702
Nicardipine Hydrochloride (Effects not specified). Products include:
Cardene Capsules ... 2290
Nitroglycerin (Effects not specified). Products include:
Deponit NTG Transdermal Delivery System ... 2143
Minitran Transdermal Delivery System ... 1312
Nitro-Bid Ointment ... 1339
Nitro-Bid Capsules ... 1338
Nitrodisc ... 2176
Nitro-Dur (nitroglycerin) Transdermal Infusion System ... 1164
Nitrogard Tablets ... 1004
Nitrolingual Spray ... 1846
Nitrostat Tablets ... 1743
Transderm-Nitro Transdermal Therapeutic System ... 2283
Nortriptyline Hydrochloride (Effects not specified). Products include:
Pamelor ... 2019
Penbutolol Sulfate (Effects not specified). Products include:
Levatol ... 1832
Phenelzine Sulfate (Effects not specified). Products include:
Nardil ... 1742
Phenoxybenzamine Hydrochloride (Effects not specified). Products include:
Dibenzyline Capsules ... 2207
Phentolamine Mesylate (Effects not specified). Products include:
Regitine ... 878
Pindolol (Effects not specified). Products include:
Visken Tablets ... 2036
Prazosin Hydrochloride (Effects not specified). Products include:
Minipress Capsules ... 1778
Minizide Capsules ... 1779
Propranolol Hydrochloride (Effects not specified). Products include:
Inderal ... 2459
Inderal LA Long Acting Capsules ... 2461
Inderide Tablets ... 2463
Inderide LA Long Acting Capsules ... 2465
Protriptyline Hydrochloride (Effects not specified). Products include:
Vivactil Tablets ... 1567
Ramipril (Effects not specified). Products include:
Altace Capsules ... 1086
Rauwolfia Serpentina (Effects not specified). Products include:
Raudixin Tablets ... 1803
Rauzide Tablets ... 1804
Rescinnamine (Effects not specified).
No products indexed under this heading.
Reserpine (Effects not specified). Products include:
Diupres Tablets ... 1461
Hydromox R Tablets ... 1209
Hydropres Tablets ... 1485
Renese-R Tablets ... 1786
Salutensin/Salutensin-Demi ... 719
Ser-Ap-Es Tablets ... 881
Serpasil Tablets ... 883
Serpasil-Apresoline Tablets ... 884
Serpasil-Esidrix Tablets ... 886
Sodium Nitroprusside (Effects not specified). Products include:
Nipride I.V. Infusion ... 1909
Terazosin Hydrochloride (Effects not specified). Products include:
Hytrin Tablets ... 529
Timolol Maleate (Effects not specified). Products include:
Blocadren Tablets ... 1429
Timolide Tablets ... 1547
Timoptic in Ocudose ... 1552
Timoptic Sterile Ophthalmic Solution ... 1550
Tranylcypromine Sulfate (Effects not specified). Products include:
Parnate Tablets ... 2222
Trazodone Hydrochloride (Effects not specified). Products include:
Desyrel and Desyrel Dividose ... 1404
Trimethaphan Camsylate (Effects not specified). Products include:
Arfonad Ampuls ... 1887
Trimipramine Maleate (Effects not specified). Products include:
Surmontil Capsules ... 2524

ADVIL IBUPROFEN TABLETS AND CAPLETS
(Ibuprofen) ... 2416
No interactions described in labeling.

AEROBID INHALER SYSTEM
(Flunisolide) ... 995
No interactions described in labeling.

AEROLATE JR. T.D. CAPSULES
(Theophylline Anhydrous) ... 994
No interactions described in labeling.

AEROLATE LIQUID
(Theophylline Anhydrous) ... 994
No interactions described in labeling.

AEROLATE SR. T.D. CAPSULES
(Theophylline Anhydrous) ... 994
No interactions described in labeling.

AEROLATE III T.D. CAPSULES
(Theophylline Anhydrous) ... 994
No interactions described in labeling.

AFRIN CHERRY SCENTED NASAL SPRAY 0.05%
(Oxymetazoline Hydrochloride) ... ▣ 692
No interactions described in labeling.

AFRIN CHILDREN'S STRENGTH NOSE DROPS 0.025%
(Oxymetazoline Hydrochloride) ... ▣ 692
No interactions described in labeling.

AFRIN MENTHOL NASAL SPRAY, 0.05%
(Oxymetazoline Hydrochloride) ... ▣ 692
No interactions described in labeling.

AFRIN NASAL SPRAY 0.05% AND NASAL SPRAY PUMP
(Oxymetazoline Hydrochloride) ... ▣ 692
No interactions described in labeling.

AFRIN NOSE DROPS 0.05%
(Oxymetazoline Hydrochloride) ... ▣ 692
No interactions described in labeling.

AFRIN SALINE MIST
(Sodium Chloride) ... ▣ 692
No interactions described in labeling.

AFRIN TABLETS
(Pseudoephedrine Sulfate) ... ▣ 693
May interact with antihypertensives and antidepressant drugs. Compounds in these categories include:
Acebutolol Hydrochloride (Concurrent use not recommended). Products include:
Sectral Capsules ... 2520
Amitriptyline Hydrochloride (Concurrent use not recommended). Products include:
Elavil ... 2269
Endep Tablets ... 1927
Etrafon ... 2087
Limbitrol ... 1933
Triavil Tablets ... 1556
Amoxapine (Concurrent use not recommended). Products include:
Asendin Tablets ... 1196
Atenolol (Concurrent use not recommended). Products include:
Tenoretic Tablets ... 1105
Tenormin Tablets and I.V. Injection 1107
Benazepril Hydrochloride (Concurrent use not recommended). Products include:
Lotensin Tablets ... 872
Betaxolol Hydrochloride (Concurrent use not recommended). Products include:
Betoptic Sterile Ophthalmic Solution ... 569
Betoptic S Sterile Ophthalmic Suspension ... 570
Kerlone Tablets ... 2172
Bupropion Hydrochloride (Concurrent use not recommended). Products include:
Wellbutrin Tablets ... 821
Captopril (Concurrent use not recommended). Products include:
Capoten ... 2255
Capozide ... 2258
Carteolol Hydrochloride (Concurrent use not recommended). Products include:
Cartrol Tablets ... 507
Clonidine (Concurrent use not recommended). Products include:
Catapres-TTS ... 677
Clonidine Hydrochloride (Concurrent use not recommended). Products include:
Catapres Tablets ... 676
Combipres Tablets ... 678
Deserpidine (Concurrent use not recommended). Products include:
Enduronyl ... 518
Harmonyl Tablets ... 528
Oreticyl ... 545
Desipramine Hydrochloride (Concurrent use not recommended). Products include:
Norpramin Tablets ... 1340
Diazoxide (Concurrent use not recommended). Products include:
Hyperstat I.V. Injection ... 2095
Proglycem ... 649
Doxazosin Mesylate (Concurrent use not recommended). Products include:
Cardura Tablets ... 1941
Doxepin Hydrochloride (Concurrent use not recommended). Products include:
Sinequan ... 1960
Enalapril Maleate (Concurrent use not recommended). Products include:
Vaseretic Tablets ... 1559
Vasotec Tablets ... 1564
Enalaprilat (Concurrent use not recommended). Products include:
Vasotec I.V. ... 1562
Esmolol Hydrochloride (Concurrent use not recommended). Products include:
Brevibloc Injection ... 942
Felodipine (Concurrent use not recommended). Products include:
Plendil Extended-Release Tablets ... 1526
Fluoxetine Hydrochloride (Concurrent use not recommended). Products include:
Prozac Pulvules ... 920
Fosinopril Sodium (Concurrent use not recommended). Products include:
Monopril Tablets ... 1406
Guanabenz Acetate (Concurrent use not recommended). Products include:
Wytensin Tablets ... 2542
Guanethidine Monosulfate (Concurrent use not recommended). Products include:
Esimil Tablets ... 864
Ismelin Tablets ... 869
Hydralazine Hydrochloride (Concurrent use not recommended). Products include:
Apresazide Capsules ... 854
Apresoline Hydrochloride Parenteral (Ampuls) ... 856
Apresoline Hydrochloride Tablets ... 855
Apresoline-Esidrix Tablets ... 857
Ser-Ap-Es Tablets ... 881
Serpasil-Apresoline Tablets ... 884
Imipramine Hydrochloride (Concurrent use not recommended). Products include:
Tofranil Ampuls ... 1038
Tofranil Tablets ... 1039

Imipramine Pamoate (Concurrent use not recommended). Products include:
Tofranil-PM Capsules ... 1041

Indapamide (Concurrent use not recommended). Products include:
Lozol Tablets ... 1843

Isocarboxazid (Concurrent use not recommended). Products include:
Marplan Tablets ... 1906

Isradipine (Concurrent use not recommended). Products include:
DynaCirc Capsules ... 2004

Labetalol Hydrochloride (Concurrent use not recommended). Products include:
Normodyne Injection ... 2108
Normodyne Tablets ... 2110
Normozide Tablets ... 2112
Trandate HCT Tablets ... 579
Trandate Injection ... 577
Trandate Tablets ... 579

Lisinopril (Concurrent use not recommended). Products include:
Prinivil Tablets ... 1538
Prinzide Tablets ... 1540
Zestoretic ... 2274
Zestril Tablets ... 2277

Maprotiline Hydrochloride (Concurrent use not recommended). Products include:
Ludiomil Tablets ... 874

Mecamylamine Hydrochloride (Concurrent use not recommended). Products include:
Inversine Tablets ... 1492

Methyldopa (Concurrent use not recommended). Products include:
Aldoclor Tablets ... 1413
Aldomet Oral ... 1415
Aldoril Tablets ... 1418

Methyldopate Hydrochloride (Concurrent use not recommended). Products include:
Aldomet Ester HCl Injection ... 1417

Metoprolol Tartrate (Concurrent use not recommended). Products include:
Lopressor Ampuls ... 1032
Lopressor HCT Tablets ... 1034
Lopressor Tablets ... 1032

Metyrosine (Concurrent use not recommended). Products include:
Demser Capsules ... 1460

Minoxidil (Concurrent use not recommended). Products include:
Loniten Tablets ... 2346
Rogaine Topical Solution ... 2357

Nadolol (Concurrent use not recommended). Products include:
Corgard Tablets ... 701
Corzide Tablets ... 702

Nicardipine Hydrochloride (Concurrent use not recommended). Products include:
Cardene Capsules ... 2290

Nitroglycerin (Concurrent use not recommended). Products include:
Deponit NTG Transdermal Delivery System ... 2143
Minitran Transdermal Delivery System ... 1312
Nitro-Bid Ointment ... 1339
Nitro-Bid Capsules ... 1338
Nitrodisc ... 2176
Nitro-Dur (nitroglycerin) Transdermal Infusion System ... 1164
Nitrogard Tablets ... 1004
Nitrolingual Spray ... 1846
Nitrostat Tablets ... 1743
Transderm-Nitro Transdermal Therapeutic System ... 2283

Nortriptyline Hydrochloride (Concurrent use not recommended). Products include:
Pamelor ... 2019

Penbutolol Sulfate (Concurrent use not recommended). Products include:
Levatol ... 1832

Phenelzine Sulfate (Concurrent use not recommended). Products include:
Nardil ... 1742

Phenoxybenzamine Hydrochloride (Concurrent use not recommended). Products include:
Dibenzyline Capsules ... 2207

Phentolamine Mesylate (Concurrent use not recommended). Products include:
Regitine ... 878

Pindolol (Concurrent use not recommended). Products include:
Visken Tablets ... 2036

Prazosin Hydrochloride (Concurrent use not recommended). Products include:
Minipress Capsules ... 1778
Minizide Capsules ... 1779

Propranolol Hydrochloride (Concurrent use not recommended). Products include:
Inderal ... 2459
Inderal LA Long Acting Capsules ... 2461
Inderide Tablets ... 2463
Inderide LA Long Acting Capsules ... 2465

Protriptyline Hydrochloride (Concurrent use not recommended). Products include:
Vivactil Tablets ... 1567

Ramipril (Concurrent use not recommended). Products include:
Altace Capsules ... 1086

Rauwolfia Serpentina (Concurrent use not recommended). Products include:
Raudixin Tablets ... 1803
Rauzide Tablets ... 1804

Rescinnamine (Concurrent use not recommended).
No products indexed under this heading.

Reserpine (Concurrent use not recommended). Products include:
Diupres Tablets ... 1461
Hydromox R Tablets ... 1209
Hydropres Tablets ... 1485
Renese-R Tablets ... 1786
Salutensin/Salutensin-Demi ... 719
Ser-Ap-Es Tablets ... 881
Serpasil Tablets ... 883
Serpasil-Apresoline Tablets ... 884
Serpasil-Esidrix Tablets ... 886

Sodium Nitroprusside (Concurrent use not recommended). Products include:
Nipride I.V. Infusion ... 1909

Terazosin Hydrochloride (Concurrent use not recommended). Products include:
Hytrin Tablets ... 529

Timolol Maleate (Concurrent use not recommended). Products include:
Blocadren Tablets ... 1429
Timolide Tablets ... 1547
Timoptic in Ocudose ... 1552
Timoptic Sterile Ophthalmic Solution ... 1550

Tranylcypromine Sulfate (Concurrent use not recommended). Products include:
Parnate Tablets ... 2222

Trazodone Hydrochloride (Concurrent use not recommended). Products include:
Desyrel and Desyrel Dividose ... 1404

Trimethaphan Camsylate (Concurrent use not recommended). Products include:
Arfonad Ampuls ... 1887

Trimipramine Maleate (Concurrent use not recommended). Products include:
Surmontil Capsules ... 2524

AGORAL
(Mineral Oil) ... ▣ 634
May interact with stool softener laxatives. Compounds in this category include:

Docusate Calcium (Concomitant administration is not recommended). Products include:
Doxidan Capsules ... ▣ 736
Surfak Capsules ... ▣ 737

Docusate Potassium (Concomitant administration is not recommended). Products include:
Dialose Capsules ... ▣ 577
Dialose Plus Capsules ... ▣ 577
Kasof Capsules ... ▣ 579

Docusate Sodium (Concomitant administration is not recommended). Products include:
Anticon ... ▣ 629
Colace ... 1403
Correctol Laxative Tablets ... ▣ 696
Dialose Tablets ... 1154
Dialose Plus Tablets ... 1154
Extra Gentle Ex-Lax ... ▣ 687
Feen-A-Mint Laxative Pills and Chocolated Mint Tablets ... ▣ 702
Ferro-Sequels ... 1203
Geriplex-FS Kapseals ... ▣ 639
Geriplex-FS Liquid ... ▣ 639
Modane Plus Tablets ... ▣ 504
Peri-Colace ... 1409
Peritinic Tablets ... ▣ 589
Phillips' LaxCaps ... ▣ 572
Senokot-S Tablets ... 1820

AGORAL, MARSHMALLOW FLAVOR
(Mineral Oil, Phenolphthalein) ... ▣ 634
See **Agoral**

AGORAL, RASPBERRY FLAVOR
(Mineral Oil, Phenolphthalein) ... ▣ 634
See **Agoral**

AKARPINE OPHTHALMIC SOLUTION
(Pilocarpine Hydrochloride) ... ⊙ 201
No interactions described in labeling.

AK-CHLOR STERILE OPHTHALMIC OINTMENT & SOLUTION
(Chloramphenicol) ... ⊙ 201
No interactions described in labeling.

AK-CIDE STERILE OPHTHALMIC OINTMENT & SUSPENSION
(Prednisolone Acetate, Sulfacetamide Sodium) ... ⊙ 202
No interactions described in labeling.

AK-CON
(Naphazoline Hydrochloride) ... ⊙ 202
May interact with monoamine oxidase inhibitors. Compounds in this category include:

Furazolidone (Severe hypertensive crisis). Products include:
Furoxone ... 1855

Isocarboxazid (Severe hypertensive crisis). Products include:
Marplan Tablets ... 1906

Phenelzine Sulfate (Severe hypertensive crisis). Products include:
Nardil ... 1742

Selegiline Hydrochloride (Severe hypertensive crisis). Products include:
Eldepryl ... 2250

Tranylcypromine Sulfate (Severe hypertensive crisis). Products include:
Parnate Tablets ... 2222

AK-CON-A
(Naphazoline Hydrochloride, Pheniramine Maleate) ... ⊙ 203
May interact with monoamine oxidase inhibitors. Compounds in this category include:

Furazolidone (Severe hypertensive crisis). Products include:
Furoxone ... 1855

Isocarboxazid (Severe hypertensive crisis). Products include:
Marplan Tablets ... 1906

Phenelzine Sulfate (Severe hypertensive crisis). Products include:
Nardil ... 1742

Selegiline Hydrochloride (Severe hypertensive crisis). Products include:
Eldepryl ... 2250

Tranylcypromine Sulfate (Severe hypertensive crisis). Products include:
Parnate Tablets ... 2222

AK-DEX 0.05% OINTMENT
(Dexamethasone Sodium Phosphate) ... ⊙ 203
No interactions described in labeling.

AK-DEX 0.1% SOLUTION
(Dexamethasone Sodium Phosphate) ... ⊙ 203
No interactions described in labeling.

AK-DILATE SOLUTION 2.5% AND 10%
(Phenylephrine Hydrochloride) ... ⊙ 203
May interact with monoamine oxidase inhibitors and tricyclic antidepressants. Compounds in these categories include:

Amitriptyline Hydrochloride (Potentiation of adrenergic agents). Products include:
Elavil ... 2269
Endep Tablets ... 1927
Etrafon ... 2087
Limbitrol ... 1933
Triavil Tablets ... 1556

Amoxapine (Potentiation of adrenergic agents). Products include:
Asendin Tablets ... 1196

Clomipramine Hydrochloride (Potentiation of andrenergic agents). Products include:
Anafranil Capsules ... 650

Desipramine Hydrochloride (Potentiation of adrenergic agents). Products include:
Norpramin Tablets ... 1340

Doxepin Hydrochloride (Potentiation of adrenergic agents). Products include:
Sinequan ... 1960

Furazolidone (May result in exaggerated adrenergic effects). Products include:
Furoxone ... 1855

Imipramine Hydrochloride (Potentiation of adrenergic agents). Products include:
Tofranil Ampuls ... 1038
Tofranil Tablets ... 1039

Imipramine Pamoate (Potentiation of adrenergic agents). Products include:
Tofranil-PM Capsules ... 1041

Isocarboxazid (May result in exaggerated adrenergic effects). Products include:
Marplan Tablets ... 1906

Maprotiline Hydrochloride (Potentiation of adrenergic agents). Products include:
- Ludiomil Tablets ... 874

Nortriptyline Hydrochloride (Potentiation of adrenergic agents). Products include:
- Pamelor ... 2019

Phenelzine Sulfate (May result in exaggerated adrenergic effects). Products include:
- Nardil ... 1742

Protriptyline Hydrochloride (Potentiation of adrenergic agents). Products include:
- Vivactil Tablets ... 1567

Selegiline Hydrochloride (May result in exaggerated adrenergic effects). Products include:
- Eldepryl ... 2250

Tranylcypromine Sulfate (May result in exaggerated adrenergic effects). Products include:
- Parnate Tablets ... 2222

Trimipramine Maleate (Potentiation of adrenergic agents). Products include:
- Surmontil Capsules ... 2524

AK-FLUOR INJECTION 10% AND 25%
(Fluorescein Sodium) ... ⊙ 204
No interactions described in labeling.

AKINETON INJECTION
(Biperiden) ... 1171
May interact with tricyclic antidepressants, phenothiazines, antihistamines, neuromuscular blocking agents, and certain other agents. Compounds in these categories include:

Amitriptyline Hydrochloride (Central anticholinergic syndrome). Products include:
- Elavil ... 2269
- Endep Tablets ... 1927
- Etrafon ... 2087
- Limbitrol ... 1933
- Triavil Tablets ... 1556

Amoxapine (Central anticholinergic syndrome). Products include:
- Asendin Tablets ... 1196

Astemizole (Central anticholinergic syndrome). Products include:
- Hismanal Tablets ... 1138

Azatadine Maleate (Central anticholinergic syndrome). Products include:
- Optimine Tablets ... 2115
- Trinalin Repetabs Tablets ... 1170

Bromodiphenhydramine Hydrochloride (Central anticholinergic syndrome).
No products indexed under this heading.

Brompheniramine Maleate (Central anticholinergic syndrome). Products include:
- Alka Seltzer Plus Sinus Allergy Medicine ... 624
- Atrohist Sprinkle Capsules ... 558
- Bromfed Capsules (Timed Release) ... 1615
- Bromfed Syrup ... 628
- Bromfed ... 1615
- Dimetane Decongestant ... 673
- Dimetane ... 672
- Dimetane-DC Cough Syrup ... 1857
- Dimetane-DX Cough Syrup ... 1858
- Dimetapp Elixir ... 673
- Dimetapp DM Elixir ... 674
- Dimetapp Extentabs ... 674
- Dimetapp Plus Caplets ... 675
- Dimetapp Tablets ... 675
- Drixoral Antihistamine/Nasal Decongestant Syrup ... 698

Chlorpheniramine Maleate (Central anticholinergic syndrome). Products include:
- A.R.M. Allergy Relief Medicine Caplets ... 615
- Alka-Seltzer Plus Cold Medicine ... 623
- Allerest ... 559
- Ana-Kit Anaphylaxis Emergency Treatment Kit ... 1100
- BC Cold Powder Multi-Symptom Formula ... 517
- Brexin L.A. Capsules ... 2078
- Cerose-DM ... 2443
- Cheracol Plus Head Cold/Cough Formula ... 667
- Chlor-Trimeton Allergy Syrup, Tablets & Long-Acting Repetabs Tablets ... 693
- Chlor-Trimeton Decongestant ... 694
- Comhist LA Capsules ... 1618
- Allergy-Sinus Comtrex Multi-Symptom Allergy Sinus Formula Tablets & Caplets ... 746
- Comtrex Multi-Symptom Cold Reliever Tablets/Caplets/Liqui-Gels/Liquid ... 745
- Day-Night Comtrex ... 747
- Contac Continuous Action Decongestant/Antihistamine Capsules ... 710
- Contac Maximum Strength Continuous Action Decongestant/Antihistamine Caplets ... 709
- Contac Severe Cold and Flu Formula Caplets ... 711
- Coricidin 'D' Decongestant Tablets ... 695
- Coricidin Demilets Tablets for Children ... 696
- Coricidin Tablets ... 695
- Deconamine ... 663
- Demazin Nasal Decongestant/Antihistamine Repetabs Tablets & Syrup ... 697
- Dorcol Children's Liquid Cold Formula ... 686
- Dristan Decongestant/Antihistamine/ Analgesic Coated Caplets ... 749
- Dristan Cold Nasal Decongestant/Antihistamine/ Analgesic Coated Tablets ... 2419
- Dristan Advanced Formula Decongestant/Antihistamine/ Analgesic Tablets ... 749
- Extendryl ... 994
- 4-Way Cold Tablets ... 750
- Fedahist Gyrocaps ... 2145
- Fedahist Timecaps ... 2145
- Hycomine Compound Tablets ... 929
- Isoclor Timesule Capsules ... 561
- Kronofed-A ... 970
- Medi-Flu Caplet, Liquid ... 640
- Naldecon Syrup, Tablets, Pediatric Drops and Pediatric Syrup ... 709
- Nolamine Tablets ... 838
- Novafed A Capsules ... 1342
- Novahistine DH ... 1342
- Novahistine Elixir ... 596
- Ornade Spansule Capsules ... 2221
- Orthoxicol Cough Syrup ... 668
- PediaCare Allergy Relief Formula Liquid ... 1362
- PediaCare Cough-Cold Formula Liquid ... 1362
- PediaCare Night Rest Cough-Cold Formula Liquid ... 1362
- PediaCare 6-12 Cough-Cold Formula Chewable Tablets ... 1362
- Pyrroxate Capsules ... 669
- Quelidrine Syrup ... 556
- Ru-Tuss II Capsules ... 693
- Ru-Tuss Tablets ... 693
- Ryna ... 741
- Sinarest Tablets & Extra Strength Tablets ... 562
- Sine-Off Maximum Strength Allergy/Sinus Formula Caplets ... 721
- Sine-Off Sinus Medicine Tablets-Aspirin Formula ... 722
- Singlet Tablets ... 598
- Sinulin ... 840
- Sinutab Maximum Strength ... 641
- St. Joseph Nighttime Cold Medicine ... 705
- Sudafed Plus Liquid ... 544
- Sudafed Plus Tablets ... 545
- Teldrin Timed-Release Allergy Capsules, 12 mg ... 2192
- TheraFlu Flu and Cold Medicine ... 687
- Triaminic Allergy Tablets ... 688
- Triaminic Chewables ... 688
- Triaminic Cold Tablets ... 688
- Triaminic Nite Light ... 689
- Triaminic Syrup ... 689
- Triaminic-12 Tablets ... 690
- Triaminicin Tablets ... 690
- Triaminicol Multi-Symptom Cold Tablets ... 691
- Triaminicol Multi-Symptom Relief ... 691
- Tylenol Allergy Sinus Medication Caplets and Gelcaps, Maximum Strength ... 1372
- Children's Tylenol Cold Liquid Formula and Chewable Tablets ... 1368
- Tylenol Cold & Flu Hot Medication, Packets ... 1369
- Tylenol Cold Medication Caplets and Tablets ... 1370
- Tylenol Cold Medication, Effervescent Tablets ... 1369
- Vicks Children's NyQuil ... 664
- Vicks Formula 44 Cough Medicine ... 661
- Vicks Formula 44M Multi-Symptom Cough Medicine ... 662
- Vicks Pediatric Formula 44m Multi-Symptom Cough & Cold Medicine ... 663

Chlorpheniramine Polistirex (Central anticholinergic syndrome). Products include:
- Tussionex Extended-Release Suspension ... 988

Chlorpheniramine Tannate (Central anticholinergic syndrome). Products include:
- Rynatan ... 2387
- Rynatuss ... 2388

Chlorpromazine (Central anticholinergic syndrome). Products include:
- Thorazine ... 2234

Chlorprothixene (Central anticholinergic syndrome). Products include:
- Taractan Tablets ... 1920

Chlorprothixene Hydrochloride (Central anticholinergic syndrome). Products include:
- Taractan ... 1920

Clemastine Fumarate (Central anticholinergic syndrome). Products include:
- Tavist Syrup ... 2033
- Tavist Tablets ... 2035
- Tavist-D Tablets ... 2035

Clomipramine Hydrochloride (Central anticholinergic syndrome). Products include:
- Anafranil Capsules ... 650

Clorazepate Dipotassium (Central anticholinergic syndrome). Products include:
- Tranxene ... 556

Clozapine (Central anticholinergic syndrome). Products include:
- Clozaril Tablets ... 2000

Cyproheptadine Hydrochloride (Central anticholinergic syndrome). Products include:
- Periactin ... 1525

Desipramine Hydrochloride (Central anticholinergic syndrome). Products include:
- Norpramin Tablets ... 1340

Dexchlorpheniramine Maleate (Central anticholinergic syndrome). Products include:
- Polaramine ... 2116

Diphenhydramine Citrate (Central anticholinergic syndrome). Products include:
- Alka-Seltzer Plus Night-Time Cold Medicine ... 623
- Bufferin AF Nite Time Analgesic/ Sleeping Aid Caplets ... 744
- Excedrin P.M. Analgesic/Sleeping Aid Tablets, Caplets and Liquid ... 749

Diphenhydramine Hydrochloride (Central anticholinergic syndrome). Products include:
- Benadryl Anti-Itch Cream ... 635
- Benadryl Capsules ... 1691
- Benadryl Decongestant Elixir ... 635
- Benadryl Decongestant ... 635
- Benadryl Elixir ... 636
- Benadryl Kapseals ... 1691
- Benadryl 25 Kapseals ... 636
- Benadryl Parenteral ... 1692
- Benadryl Plus ... 636
- Benadryl Plus Nighttime ... 637
- Benadryl Spray, Maximum Strength ... 637
- Benadryl Spray, Regular Strength ... 637
- Benadryl Steri-Vials, Ampoules, and Steri-Dose Syringe ... 1692
- Benadryl 25 Tablets ... 636
- Benylin Cough Syrup ... 637
- Benylin Decongestant ... 638
- Caladryl Cream, Lotion, Spray ... 638
- Miles Nervine Nighttime Sleep-Aid ... 627
- Nytol Tablets ... 517
- Sleep-ettes-D Tablets ... 653
- Sleep-eze 3 Tablets ... 755
- Sleepinal Night-time Sleep Aid Capsules ... 734
- Sominex Caplets and Tablets ... 722
- Sominex Liquid ... 723
- Sominex Pain Relief Formula ... 723
- Tylenol Cold Night Time Medication Liquid ... 1371
- Tylenol PM, Extra Strength Caplets and Tablets ... 1368
- Unisom Dual Relief Nighttime Sleep Aid/Analgesic ... 1774
- Ziradryl Lotion ... 643

Diphenylpyraline Hydrochloride (Central anticholinergic syndrome).
No products indexed under this heading.

Doxepin Hydrochloride (Central anticholinergic syndrome). Products include:
- Sinequan ... 1960

Fluphenazine Decanoate (Central anticholinergic syndrome). Products include:
- Prolixin Decanoate ... 1795

Fluphenazine Enanthate (Central anticholinergic syndrome). Products include:
- Prolixin Enanthate ... 1796

Fluphenazine Hydrochloride (Central anticholinergic syndrome). Products include:
- Prolixin Elixir ... 1793
- Prolixin Injection ... 1791
- Prolixin Oral Concentrate ... 1792
- Prolixin Tablets ... 1793

Haloperidol (Central anticholinergic syndrome). Products include:
- Haldol Injection, Tablets and Concentrate ... 1373

Haloperidol Decanoate (Central anticholinergic syndrome). Products include:
- Haldol Decanoate ... 1375

Imipramine Hydrochloride (Central anticholinergic syndrome). Products include:
- Tofranil Ampuls ... 1038
- Tofranil Tablets ... 1039

Imipramine Pamoate (Central anticholinergic syndrome). Products include:
- Tofranil-PM Capsules ... 1041

Loxapine Hydrochloride (Central anticholinergic syndrome). Products include:
- Loxitane ... 1213

Loxapine Succinate (Central anticholinergic syndrome). Products include:
- Loxitane Capsules ... 1213

Maprotiline Hydrochloride (Central anticholinergic syndrome). Products include:
- Ludiomil Tablets ... 874

Meperidine Hydrochloride (Central anticholinergic syndrome). Products include:
- Demerol ... 2047
- Mepergan Injection ... 2479

Mesoridazine (Central anticholinergic syndrome). Products include:
- Serentil ... 686

Methdilazine Hydrochloride (Central anticholinergic syndrome). Products include:
- Tacaryl Syrup & Tablets ... 2409

Molindone Hydrochloride (Central anticholinergic syndrome). Products include:
- Moban Tablets & Concentrate ... 932

Nortriptyline Hydrochloride (Central anticholinergic syndrome). Products include:
- Pamelor ... 2019

Perphenazine (Central anticholinergic syndrome). Products include:
- Etrafon ... 2087
- Triavil Tablets ... 1556
- Trilafon ... 2123

Prochlorperazine (Central anticholinergic syndrome). Products include:
- Compazine ... 2201

Promethazine Hydrochloride (Central anticholinergic syndrome). Products include:
- Mepergan Injection ... 2479
- Phenergan with Codeine ... 2497
- Phenergan with Dextromethorphan 2499
- Phenergan Injection ... 2493
- Phenergan Suppositories ... 2496
- Phenergan Syrup ... 2495
- Phenergan Tablets ... 2496
- Phenergan VC ... 2500
- Phenergan VC with Codeine ... 2501

Protriptyline Hydrochloride (Central anticholinergic syndrome). Products include:
- Vivactil Tablets ... 1567

Pyrilamine Maleate (Central anticholinergic syndrome syndrome). Products include:
- Codimal ... 846
- 4-Way Fast Acting Nasal Spray - Original Formula (regular & mentholated) & Metered Spray Pump (regular) ... 751
- Maximum Strength Midol Multi-Symptom Menstrual Formula ... ▣ 571
- Maximum Strength Midol PMS Premenstrual Syndrome Formula ... ▣ 570
- Regular Strength Midol Multi-Symptom Menstrual Formula ... ▣ 570
- Prefrin-A ... ⊚ 255
- Prēmsyn PMS Capsules & Caplets ▣ 547
- Primatene Tablets-M Formula ... 2421
- Robitussin Night Relief ... ▣ 677
- Ru-Tuss with Hydrocodone ... 694
- Triaminic Expectorant DH ... 1995
- Triaminic Oral Infant Drops ... 1996

Pyrilamine Tannate (Central anticholinergic syndrome). Products include:
- Rynatan ... 2387

Quinidine Gluconate (Central anticholinergic syndrome). Products include:
- Quinaglute Dura-Tabs Tablets ... 663

Quinidine Polygalacturonate (Central anticholinergic syndrome). Products include:
- Cardioquin Tablets ... 1812

Quinidine Sulfate (Central anticholinergic syndrome). Products include:
- Quinidex Extentabs ... 1868

Terfenadine (Central anticholinergic syndrome). Products include:
- Seldane Tablets ... 1349
- Seldane-D Extended-Release Tablets ... 1350

Thioridazine Hydrochloride (Central anticholinergic syndrome). Products include:
- Mellaril ... 2011

Thiothixene (Central anticholinergic syndrome). Products include:
- Navane Capsules and Concentrate 1954
- Navane Intramuscular ... 1956

Trifluoperazine Hydrochloride (Central anticholinergic syndrome). Products include:
- Stelazine ... 2226

Trimeprazine Tartrate (Central anticholinergic syndrome). Products include:
- Temaril Tablets, Syrup and Spansule Sustained Release Capsules 1085

Trimipramine Maleate (Central anticholinergic syndrome). Products include:
- Surmontil Capsules ... 2524

Tripelennamine Hydrochloride (Central anticholinergic syndrome). Products include:
- PBZ Tablets & Elixir ... 1037
- PBZ-SR Tablets ... 1037

Triprolidine Hydrochloride (Central anticholinergic syndrome). Products include:
- Actidil ... ▣ 538
- Actifed Capsules ... ▣ 539
- Actifed Plus Caplets ... ▣ 539
- Actifed Plus Tablets ... ▣ 540
- Actifed with Codeine Cough Syrup.. 752
- Actifed Syrup ... ▣ 540
- Actifed Tablets ... ▣ 540
- Actifed 12-Hour Capsules ... ▣ 539

AKINETON TABLETS
(Betaxolol Hydrochloride) ... 1171
See **Akineton Injection**

AK-MYCIN OINTMENT
(Erythromycin) ... ⊚ 204
No interactions described in labeling.

AK-NACL 5% OINTMENT & SOLUTION
(Sodium Chloride) ... ⊚ 204
No interactions described in labeling.

AK-PENTOLATE
(Cyclopentolate Hydrochloride) ... ⊚ 204
No interactions described in labeling.

AK-POLY-BAC OINTMENT
(Bacitracin Zinc, Polymyxin B Sulfate) ... ⊚ 205
No interactions described in labeling.

AK-PRED
(Prednisolone Sodium Phosphate) .. ⊚ 205
No interactions described in labeling.

AK-SPORE H.C. OINTMENT
(Hydrocortisone, Neomycin Sulfate, Polymyxin B Sulfate) ... ⊚ 206
No interactions described in labeling.

AK-SPORE H. C. SUSPENSION
(Hydrocortisone, Neomycin Sulfate, Polymyxin B Sulfate) ... ⊚ 206
No interactions described in labeling.

AK-SPORE OINTMENT
(Bacitracin Zinc, Neomycin Sulfate, Polymyxin B Sulfate) ... ⊚ 205
No interactions described in labeling.

AK-SPORE SOLUTION
(Gramicidin, Neomycin Sulfate, Polymyxin B Sulfate) ... ⊚ 205
No interactions described in labeling.

AK-SULF
(Sulfacetamide Sodium) ... ⊚ 207
May interact with silver preparations. Compounds in this category include:

Silver Nitrate (Sulfacetamide solutions are incompatible with silver preparations).

AK-TAINE
(Proparacaine Hydrochloride) ... ⊚ 207
No interactions described in labeling.

AK-TROL OINTMENT & SUSPENSION
(Dexamethasone, Neomycin Sulfate, Polymyxin B Sulfate) ... ⊚ 207
No interactions described in labeling.

ALBALON SOLUTION WITH LIQUIFILM
(Naphazoline Hydrochloride) ... ⊚ 238
May interact with monoamine oxidase inhibitors, tricyclic antidepressants, and certain other agents. Compounds in these categories include:

Amitriptyline Hydrochloride (May potentiate the pressor effect of naphazoline). Products include:
- Elavil ... 2269
- Endep Tablets ... 1927
- Etrafon ... 2087
- Limbitrol ... 1933
- Triavil Tablets ... 1556

Amoxapine (May potentiate the pressor effect of naphazoline). Products include:
- Asendin Tablets ... 1196

Clomipramine Hydrochloride (May potentiate the pressor effect of naphazoline). Products include:
- Anafranil Capsules ... 650

Desipramine Hydrochloride (May potentiate the pressor effect of naphazoline). Products include:
- Norpramin Tablets ... 1340

Doxepin Hydrochloride (May potentiate the pressor effect of naphazoline). Products include:
- Sinequan ... 1960

Furazolidone (Severe hypertensive crisis). Products include:
- Furoxone ... 1855

Imipramine Hydrochloride (May potentiate the pressor effect of naphazoline). Products include:
- Tofranil Ampuls ... 1038
- Tofranil Tablets ... 1039

Imipramine Pamoate (May potentiate the pressor effect of naphazoline). Products include:
- Tofranil-PM Capsules ... 1041

Isocarboxazid (Severe hypertensive crisis). Products include:
- Marplan Tablets ... 1906

Maprotiline Hydrochloride (May potentiate the pressor effect of naphazoline). Products include:
- Ludiomil Tablets ... 874

Nortriptyline Hydrochloride (May potentiate the pressor effect of naphazoline). Products include:
- Pamelor ... 2019

Phenelzine Sulfate (Severe hypertensive crisis). Products include:
- Nardil ... 1742

Protriptyline Hydrochloride (May potentiate the pressor effect of naphazoline). Products include:
- Vivactil Tablets ... 1567

Selegiline Hydrochloride (Severe hypertensive crisis). Products include:
- Eldepryl ... 2250

Tranylcypromine Sulfate (Severe hypertensive crisis). Products include:
- Parnate Tablets ... 2222

Trimipramine Maleate (May potentiate the pressor effect of naphazoline). Products include:
- Surmontil Capsules ... 2524

ALBALON-A LIQUIFILM
(Antazoline Phosphate, Naphazoline Hydrochloride) ... ⊚ 238
May interact with monoamine oxidase inhibitors. Compounds in this category include:

Furazolidone (Severe hypertensive crisis). Products include:
- Furoxone ... 1855

Isocarboxazid (Severe hypertensive crisis). Products include:
- Marplan Tablets ... 1906

Phenelzine Sulfate (Severe hypertensive crisis). Products include:
- Nardil ... 1742

Selegiline Hydrochloride (Severe hypertensive crisis). Products include:
- Eldepryl ... 2250

Tranylcypromine Sulfate (Severe hypertensive crisis). Products include:
- Parnate Tablets ... 2222

ALBUMINAR-5, ALBUMIN (HUMAN) U.S.P. 5%
(Albumin (Human)) ... 608
No interactions described in labeling.

ALBUMINAR-25, ALBUMIN (HUMAN) U.S.P. 25%
(Albumin (Human)) ... 608
No interactions described in labeling.

ALCAINE
(Proparacaine Hydrochloride) ... ⊚ 210
No interactions described in labeling.

ALDACTAZIDE
(Spironolactone, Hydrochlorothiazide) ... 2150
May interact with potassium-depleting corticosteroids, loop diuretics, glucocorticoids, diuretics, insulin, oral hypoglycemic agents, potassium sparing diuretics, cardiac glycosides, ACE inhibitors, thiazides, antigout agents, general anesthetics, lithium preparations, and certain other agents. Compounds in these categories include:

ACTH (Concomitant administration may result in hypokalemia).

Allopurinol (Dosage adjustment may be necessary). Products include:
- Zyloprim Tablets ... 830

Amiloride Hydrochloride (Concomitant administration has been associated with severe hyperkalemia and may induce dilutional hyponatremia). Products include:
- Midamor Tablets ... 1508
- Moduretic Tablets ... 1510

Benazepril Hydrochloride (Concomitant administration has been associated with severe hyperkalemia). Products include:
- Lotensin Tablets ... 872

Bendroflumethiazide (Concomitant administration has been associated with severe hyperkalemia; concomitant administration may induce dilutional hyponatremia). Products include:
- Corzide Tablets ... 702
- Naturetin Tablets ... 1789
- Rauzide Tablets ... 1804

Betamethasone Acetate (Concomitant administration may result in hypokalemia). Products include:
- Celestone Soluspan Suspension ... 2081

Betamethasone Sodium Phosphate (Concomitant administration may result in hypokalemia). Products include:
- Celestone Soluspan Suspension ... 2081

Bumetanide (Concomitant administration may result in hypokalemia and may induce dilutional hyponatremia). Products include:

Bumex ... 1895

Captopril (Concomitant administration has been associated with severe hyperkalemia). Products include:

Capoten ... 2255
Capozide ... 2258

Chlorothiazide (Concomitant administration has been associated with severe hyperkalemia and may induce dilutional hyponatremia). Products include:

Aldoclor Tablets ... 1413
Diupres Tablets ... 1461
Diuril Oral ... 1464

Chlorothiazide Sodium (Concomitant administration has been associated with severe hyperkalemia and may induce dilutional hyponatremia). Products include:

Diuril Sodium Intravenous ... 1463

Chlorpropamide (Dosage adjustment of hypoglycemics may be necessary). Products include:

Diabinese Tablets ... 1775

Chlorthalidone (Concomitant administration may induce dilutional hyponatremia). Products include:

Combipres Tablets ... 678
Tenoretic Tablets ... 1105
Thalitone Tablets ... 687

Cortisone Acetate (Concomitant administration may result in hypokalemia). Products include:

Cortone Acetate Sterile Suspension ... 1437
Cortone Acetate Tablets ... 1439

Deslanoside (Resultant hypokalemia may exaggerate the effects of digitalis therapy).

No products indexed under this heading.

Dexamethasone (Concomitant administration may result in hypokalemia). Products include:

AK-Trol Ointment & Suspension ... ⊙ 207
Decadron Elixir ... 1445
Decadron Tablets ... 1447
Decaspray Topical Aerosol ... 1459
Dexacidin ... ⊙ 272
Maxidex Sterile Ophthalmic Suspension ... ⊙ 223
Maxitrol Ophthalmic Ointment/Suspension ... ⊙ 223
TobraDex Ophthalmic Suspension and Ointment ... ⊙ 228

Dexamethasone Acetate (Concomitant administration may result in hypokalemia). Products include:

Dalalone D.P. Injectable ... 999
Decadron-LA Sterile Suspension ... 1457

Dexamethasone Sodium Phosphate (Concomitant administration may result in hypokalemia). Products include:

AK-Dex ... ⊙ 203
Decadron Phosphate Respihaler ... 1454
Decadron Phosphate Sterile Ophthalmic Ointment ... 1453
Decadron Phosphate Sterile Ophthalmic Solution ... 1453
Decadron Phosphate Topical Cream ... 1455
Decadron Phosphate Turbinaire ... 1456
Maxidex Sterile Ophthalmic Ointment ... ⊙ 222
NeoDecadron Sterile Ophthalmic Ointment ... 1517
NeoDecadron Sterile Ophthalmic Solution ... 1518
NeoDecadron Topical Cream ... 1518

Digitoxin (Resultant hypokalemia may exaggerate the effects of digitalis therapy). Products include:

Crystodigin Tablets ... 1253

Digoxin (Resultant hypokalemia may exaggerate the effects of digitalis therapy). Products include:

Lanoxicaps ... 772
Lanoxin Elixir Pediatric ... 775
Lanoxin Injection ... 778
Lanoxin Injection Pediatric ... 781
Lanoxin Tablets ... 783

Enalapril Maleate (Concomitant administration has been associated with severe hyperkalemia). Products include:

Vaseretic Tablets ... 1559
Vasotec Tablets ... 1564

Enalaprilat (Concomitant administration has been associated with severe hyperkalemia). Products include:

Vasotec I.V. ... 1562

Enflurane (Exercise caution). Products include:

Ethrane ... 599

Ethacrynic Acid (Concomitant administration may result in hypokalemia and may induce dilutional hyponatremia). Products include:

Edecrin Tablets ... 1468

Fosinopril Sodium (Concomitant administration has been associated with severe hyperkalemia). Products include:

Monopril Tablets ... 1406

Furosemide (Concomitant administration may result in hypokalemia and may induce dilutional hyponatremia). Products include:

Lasix ... 1093

Glipizide (Dosage adjustment of hypoglycemics may be necessary). Products include:

Glucotrol ... 1952

Glyburide (Dosage adjustment of hypoglycemics may be necessary). Products include:

DiaBeta ... 1091
Micronase Tablets ... 2350

Hydrocortisone (Concomitant administration may result in hypokalemia). Products include:

AK-Spore H.C. ... ⊙ 206
Bactine Hydrocortisone Anti-Itch Cream ... ▣ 625
CaldeCORT Anti-Itch Hydrocortisone Spray ... ▣ 560
Carmol HC Cream 1% ... 2296
Cortaid Spray ... ▣ 735
Cortenema ... 2244
Cortisporin Ointment ... 758
Cortisporin Ophthalmic Ointment Sterile ... 758
Cortisporin Ophthalmic Suspension Sterile ... 759
Cortisporin Otic Solution Sterile ... 760
Cortisporin Otic Suspension Sterile ... 760
Cortizone-5 Creme & Ointment ... ▣ 732
Dermolate Anti-Itch Cream ... ▣ 697
Eldecort Cream 1.0% ... 1113
Eldecort Cream 1.0% and 2.5% ... 1113
Fungoid HC Creme ... 1770
Hydrocortone Tablets ... 1482
Hytone ... 909
LazerSporin-C Solution ... 1770
Massengill Medicated Soft Cloth Towelettes ... 2192
Nutracort Cream & Lotion ... 1684
PediOtic Suspension Sterile ... 797
Synacort Creams 1%, 2.5% ... 2296
Vanoxide-HC Acne Lotion ... 911
Vioform-Hydrocortisone Cream and Mild Cream ... 889
Vioform-Hydrocortisone Ointment ... 889
VōSoL HC Otic Solution ... 2392
Vytone Cream 1% ... 911

Hydrocortisone Acetate (Concomitant administration may result in hypokalemia). Products include:

Analpram-HC Rectal Cream 1% and 2.5% ... 970
Anusol-HC Cream ... 1690
Anusol-HC Suppositories ... 1691
Caldecort ... ▣ 560
Carmol HC Cream 1% ... 2296
Chloromycetin Hydrocortisone Ophthalmic ... 1694
Coly-Mycin S Otic w/Neomycin & Hydrocortisone ... 1708
Cortaid ... ▣ 735
Cortef Feminine Itch Cream ... ▣ 735
Corticaine ... ▣ 682
Cortifoam ... 1827
Cortisporin Cream ... 757
Epifoam ... 1828
Gynecort 5 Creme ... ▣ 556
Hydrocortone Acetate Sterile Suspension ... 1479
Lanacort 5 Creme and Ointment ... ▣ 557
Mantadil Cream ... 789
Ophthocort ... ⊙ 301
Orabase HCA Oral Paste ... 890
Pramosone Cream, Lotion & Ointment ... 971
ProctoCream-HC ... 1834
Proctofoam-HC ... 1835

Hydrocortisone Sodium Phosphate (Concomitant administration may result in hypokalemia). Products include:

Hydrocortone Phosphate Injection, Sterile ... 1481

Hydrocortisone Sodium Succinate (Concomitant administration may result in hypokalemia). Products include:

Solu-Cortef Sterile Powder ... 2361

Hydroflumethiazide (Concomitant administration has been associated with severe hyperkalemia and may induce dilutional hyponatremia). Products include:

Diucardin Tablets ... 2450
Saluron ... 718
Salutensin/Salutensin-Demi ... 719

Indapamide (Concomitant administration may induce dilutional hyponatremia). Products include:

Lozol Tablets ... 1843

Indomethacin (Concomitant administration has been associated with severe hyperkalemia). Products include:

Indocin ... 1487

Indomethacin Sodium Trihydrate (Concomitant administration has been associated with severe hyperkalemia). Products include:

Indocin I.V. ... 1490

Insulin, Human (Dosage adjustment of insulin may be necessary).

No products indexed under this heading.

Insulin, Human Isophane Suspension (Dosage adjustment of insulin may be necessary). Products include:

Humulin N, 100 Units ... 1270

Insulin, Human NPH (Dosage adjustment of insulin may be necessary). Products include:

Insulatard NPH Human ... 1627
Novolin N ... 1627
Novolin N PenFill Cartridges ... 1628
Novolin N Prefilled ... 1628

Insulin, Human Regular (Dosage adjustment of insulin may be necessary). Products include:

Humulin BR, 100 Units ... 1268
Humulin R, 100 Units ... 1272
Novolin R ... 1627
Novolin R PenFill Cartridges ... 1628
Novolin R Prefilled ... 1629
Velosulin Human ... 1628

Insulin, Human, Zinc Suspension (Dosage adjustment of insulin may be necessary). Products include:

Humulin L, 100 Units ... 1268
Humulin U, 100 Units ... 1272
Novolin L ... 1627

Insulin, NPH (Dosage adjustment of insulin may be necessary). Products include:

NPH, 40 & 100 Units ... 1273
Beef NPH, 100 Units ... 1274
Pork NPH, 100 Units ... 1275
Insulatard NPH ... 1626
NPH Insulin ... 1626
NPH Purified Pork Isophane Insulin ... 1626

Insulin, Regular (Dosage adjustment of insulin may be necessary). Products include:

Regular, 40 & 100 Units ... 1273
Beef Regular, 100 Units ... 1275
Pork Regular, 100 Units ... 1275
Pork Regular (Concentrated), 500 Units ... 1276
Regular Insulin ... 1625
Regular Purified Pork Insulin ... 1626
Velosulin ... 1627

Insulin, Zinc Crystals (Dosage adjustment of insulin may be necessary). Products include:

NPH, 40 & 100 Units ... 1273

Insulin, Zinc Suspension (Dosage adjustment of insulin may be necessary). Products include:

Lente, 40 & 100 Units ... 1272
Protamine, Zinc, 40 & 100 Units ... 1273
Lente Iletin I ... 1272
Beef Lente, 100 Units ... 1274
Beef Protamine Zinc, 100 Units ... 1274
Pork Lente, 100 Units ... 1275
Pork, Protamine, Zinc, 100 Units ... 1275
Lente Insulin ... 1626
Lente Purified Pork Insulin ... 1626
Semilente Insulin ... 1625
Ultralente Insulin ... 1626

Isoflurane (Exercise caution). Products include:

Forane ... 600

Ketamine Hydrochloride (Exercise caution). Products include:

Ketalar ... 1726

Lisinopril (Concomitant administration has been associated with severe hyperkalemia). Products include:

Prinivil Tablets ... 1538
Prinzide Tablets ... 1540
Zestoretic ... 2274
Zestril Tablets ... 2277

Lithium Carbonate (Potential for lithium toxicity). Products include:

Eskalith ... 2214
Lithane Tablets ... 1596
Lithium Carbonate Capsules & Tablets ... 1984
Lithobid Tablets ... 870

Lithium Citrate (Potential for lithium toxicity). Products include:

Cibalith-S ... 870

Methohexital Sodium (Exercise caution). Products include:

Brevital Sodium Vials ... 1248

Methoxyflurane (Exercise caution).

No products indexed under this heading.

Methyclothiazide (Concomitant administration has been associated with severe hyperkalemia and may induce dilutional hyponatremia). Products include:

Enduron Tablets ... 517
Enduronyl ... 518

Methylprednisolone Acetate (Concomitant administration may result in hypokalemia). Products include:

Depo-Medrol Sterile Aqueous Suspension ... 2334

Methylprednisolone Sodium Succinate (Concomitant administration may result in hypokalemia). Products include:

Solu-Medrol Sterile Powder ... 2363

Metolazone (Concomitant administration may induce dilutional hyponatremia). Products include:

Diulo ... 2129
Mykrox ½ mg Tablets ... 984
Zaroxolyn Tablets ... 989

Norepinephrine Bitartrate (Reduced vascular responsiveness to norepinephrine). Products include:
- Levophed Bitartrate Injection 2054

Polythiazide (Concomitant administration has been associated with severe hyperkalemia and may induce dilutional hyponatremia). Products include:
- Minizide Capsules 1779
- Renese Tablets 1785
- Renese-R Tablets 1786

Potassium Acid Phosphate (Concurrent administration may cause hyperkalemia). Products include:
- K-Phos M.F. Tablets 659
- K-Phos Original Formula 'Sodium Free' Tablets 660
- K-Phos No. 2 Tablets 659

Potassium Bicarbonate (Concurrent administration may cause hyperkalemia). Products include:
- Alka-Seltzer Advanced Formula Antacid & Non-Aspirin Pain Reliever .... ▣ 620
- Alka-Seltzer Effervescent Antacid ▣ 622
- K-Lyte 707
- Klorvess Effervescent Granules........ 2010
- Klorvess Effervescent Tablets 2011

Potassium Chloride (Concurrent administration may cause hyperkalemia). Products include:
- Chlor-3 Condiment 994
- K-Dur Microburst Release System (potassium chloride, USP) E.R. Tablets 1163
- K-Lor Powder Packets 531
- K-Lyte 707
- K-Norm Capsules 982
- K-Tab Filmtab 532
- Kato Potassium Supplement 1114
- Klor-Con 8/Klor-Con 10 Extended-release Tablets 2374
- Klorvess Effervescent Granules........ 2010
- Klorvess Effervescent Tablets 2011
- Klorvess 10% Liquid 2010
- Klotrix 708
- Kolyum Liquid 983
- Micro-K 1863
- Micro-K LS Packets 1864
- NuLYTELY 699
- Oral Rehydration Salts, Citrate 1150
- Rum-K Syrup 995
- Slow-K Tablets 2281
- Ten-K Controlled-Release Tablets........ 2282
- Thermotabs .... ▣ 619

Potassium Citrate (Concurrent administration may cause hyperkalemia). Products include:
- Alka-Seltzer Effervescent Antacid .. 1570
- K-Lyte 707
- Polycitra Syrup 2424
- Polycitra-K 2424
- Polycitra-LC—Sugar-Free 2424
- Ricelyte, Rice-Based Oral Electrolyte Maintenance Solution .... ▣ 613

Potassium Gluconate (Concurrent administration may cause hyperkalemia). Products include:
- Kolyum Liquid 983

Potassium Phosphate, Dibasic (Concurrent administration may cause hyperkalemia). Products include:
- Neutra-Phos 2423

Potassium Phosphate, Monobasic (Concurrent administration may cause hyperkalemia). Products include:
- K-Phos M.F. Tablets 659
- K-Phos Neutral Tablets 660
- Neutra-Phos 2423

Prednisolone Acetate (Concomitant administration may result in hypokalemia). Products include:
- AK-Cide Sterile Ophthalmic Ointment & Suspension .... ⊙ 202
- Blephamide Liquifilm Sterile Ophthalmic Suspension 586
- Blephamide S.O.P. Sterile Ophthalmic Ointment 586
- Cetapred Ointment .... ⊙ 220
- ⅛% Econopred & 1% Econopred Plus .... ⊙ 217
- Isopto Cetapred Suspension .... ⊙ 220
- Metimyd .... ⊙ 306
- Poly-Pred Liquifilm .... ⊙ 250
- Pred Forte .... ⊙ 252
- Pred Mild .... ⊙ 254
- Pred-G Liquifilm Sterile Ophthalmic Suspension .... ⊙ 252
- Pred-G S.O.P. Sterile Ophthalmic Ointment .... ⊙ 253
- Vasocidin Ointment .... ⊙ 275

Prednisolone Sodium Phosphate (Concomitant administration may result in hypokalemia). Products include:
- AK-Pred .... ⊙ 205
- Hydeltrasol Injection, Sterile 1476
- Inflamase .... ⊙ 274
- Pediapred Oral Liquid 987
- Vasocidin Ophthalmic Solution .... ⊙ 276

Prednisolone Tebutate (Concomitant administration may result in hypokalemia). Products include:
- Hydeltra-T.B.A. Sterile Suspension 1478

Prednisone (Concomitant administration may result in hypokalemia). Products include:
- Deltasone Tablets 2332

Probenecid (Dosage adjustment may be necessary). Products include:
- Benemid Tablets 1426
- ColBENEMID Tablets 1436
- Wycillin Injection and Probenecid Tablets 2539

Propofol (Exercise caution). Products include:
- Diprivan Injection 2267

Ramipril (Concomitant administration has been associated with severe hyperkalemia). Products include:
- Altace Capsules 1086

Sulfinpyrazone (Dosage adjustment may be necessary). Products include:
- Anturane 853

Tolazamide (Dosage adjustment of hypoglycemics may be necessary). Products include:
- Tolinase Tablets 2365

Tolbutamide (Dosage adjustment of hypoglycemics may be necessary). Products include:
- Orinase Tablets 2354

Triamcinolone (Concomitant administration may result in hypokalemia).
- No products indexed under this heading.

Triamcinolone Acetonide (Concomitant administration may result in hypokalemia). Products include:
- Aristocort A 1010
- Azmacort Inhaler 1837
- Kenalog Cream, Lotion & Ointment 2401
- Kenalog-10 Injection 2402
- Kenalog-40 Injection 2403
- Kenalog in Orabase 604
- Kenalog Spray 2401
- Mycolog II Cream and Ointment 2407
- Mytrex Cream & Ointment 2080
- Nasacort Nasal Inhaler 1844

Triamcinolone Diacetate (Concomitant administration may result in hypokalemia). Products include:
- Aristocort Suspension 1008

Triamcinolone Hexacetonide (Concomitant administration may result in hypokalemia). Products include:
- Aristospan Suspension 1011

Triamterene (Concomitant administration has been associated with severe hyperkalemia and may induce dilutional hyponatremia). Products include:
- Dyazide Capsules 2208
- Dyrenium Capsules 2210
- Maxzide 1215

Tubocurarine Chloride (Increased responsiveness to tubocurarine).
- No products indexed under this heading.

ALDACTONE (Spironolactone) 2152
May interact with potassium-depleting corticosteroids, diuretics, antihypertensives, potassium sparing diuretics, general anesthetics, ganglionic blocking agents, ACE inhibitors, thiazides, and certain other agents. Compounds in these categories include:

Acebutolol Hydrochloride (Potentiated antihypertensive effects). Products include:
- Sectral Capsules 2520

Amiloride Hydrochloride (Potentiated diuretic effects; may cause or aggravate hyponatremia; do not administer concurrently). Products include:
- Midamor Tablets 1508
- Moduretic Tablets 1510

Atenolol (Potentiated antihypertensive effects). Products include:
- Tenoretic Tablets 1105
- Tenormin Tablets and I.V. Injection 1107

Benazepril Hydrochloride (Severe hyperkalemia; potentiated antihypertensive effects). Products include:
- Lotensin Tablets 872

Bendroflumethiazide (Potentiated diuretic and antihypertensive effects; may cause or aggravate hyponatremia). Products include:
- Corzide Tablets 702
- Naturetin Tablets 1789
- Rauzide Tablets 1804

Betaxolol Hydrochloride (Severe hyperkalemia; potentiated antihypertensive effects). Products include:
- Betoptic Sterile Ophthalmic Solution 569
- Betoptic S Sterile Ophthalmic Suspension 570
- Kerlone Tablets 2172

Bumetanide (Potentiated diuretic effects; may cause or aggravate hyponatremia). Products include:
- Bumex 1895

Captopril (Severe hyperkalemia; potentiated antihypertensive effects). Products include:
- Capoten 2255
- Capozide 2258

Carteolol Hydrochloride (Potentiated antihypertensive effects). Products include:
- Cartrol Tablets 507

Chlorothiazide (Potentiated diuretic and antihypertensive effects; may cause or aggravate hyponatremia). Products include:
- Aldoclor Tablets 1413
- Diupres Tablets 1461
- Diuril Oral 1464

Chlorothiazide Sodium (Potentiated diuretic and antihypertensive effects; may cause or aggravate hyponatremia). Products include:
- Diuril Sodium Intravenous 1463

Chlorthalidone (Potentiated diuretic and antihypertensive effects; may cause or aggravate hyponatremia). Products include:
- Combipres Tablets 678
- Tenoretic Tablets 1105
- Thalitone Tablets 687

Clonidine (Potentiated antihypertensive effects). Products include:
- Catapres-TTS 677

Clonidine Hydrochloride (Potentiated antihypertensive effects). Products include:
- Catapres Tablets 676
- Combipres Tablets 678

Deserpidine (Potentiated antihypertensive effects). Products include:
- Enduronyl 518
- Harmonyl Tablets 528
- Oreticyl 545

Diazoxide (Potentiated antihypertensive effects). Products include:
- Hyperstat I.V. Injection 2095
- Proglycem 649

Digoxin (Digitalis toxicity). Products include:
- Lanoxicaps 772
- Lanoxin Elixir Pediatric 775
- Lanoxin Injection 778
- Lanoxin Injection Pediatric 781
- Lanoxin Tablets 783

Doxazosin Mesylate (Severe hyperkalemia; potentiated antihypertensive effects). Products include:
- Cardura Tablets 1941

Enalapril Maleate (Potentiated antihypertensive effects; severe hyperkalemia). Products include:
- Vaseretic Tablets 1559
- Vasotec Tablets 1564

Enalaprilat (Potentiated antihypertensive effects; severe hyperkalemia). Products include:
- Vasotec I.V. 1562

Enflurane (Exercise caution). Products include:
- Ethrane 599

Esmolol Hydrochloride (Potentiated antihypertensive effects). Products include:
- Brevibloc Injection 942

Ethacrynic Acid (Potentiated diuretic effects; may cause or aggravate hyponatremia). Products include:
- Edecrin Tablets 1468

Felodipine (Severe hyperkalemia; potentiated antihypertensive effects). Products include:
- Plendil Extended-Release Tablets.... 1526

Fosinopril Sodium (Severe hyperkalemia; potentiated antihypertensive effects). Products include:
- Monopril Tablets 1406

Furosemide (Potentiated diuretic and antihypertensive effects; may cause or aggravate hyponatremia). Products include:
- Lasix 1093

Guanabenz Acetate (Potentiated antihypertensive effects). Products include:
- Wytensin Tablets 2542

Guanethidine Monosulfate (Potentiated antihypertensive effects). Products include:
- Esimil Tablets 864
- Ismelin Tablets 869

Hydralazine Hydrochloride (Potentiated antihypertensive effects). Products include:
- Apresazide Capsules 854
- Apresoline Hydrochloride Parenteral (Ampuls) 856
- Apresoline Hydrochloride Tablets .. 855
- Apresoline-Esidrix Tablets 857
- Ser-Ap-Es Tablets 881
- Serpasil-Apresoline Tablets 884

Hydrochlorothiazide (Potentiated diuretic and antihypertensive effects; may cause or aggravate hyponatremia). Products include:
- Aldactazide 2150
- Aldoril Tablets 1418
- Apresazide Capsules 854
- Apresoline-Esidrix Tablets 857
- Capozide 2258
- Dyazide Capsules 2208

(▣ Described in PDR For Nonprescription Drugs)

(⊙ Described in PDR For Ophthalmology)

Esidrix Tablets 863
Esimil Tablets 864
HydroDIURIL Tablets 1484
Hydropres Tablets 1485
Inderide Tablets 2463
Inderide LA Long Acting Capsules .. 2465
Lopressor HCT Tablets 1034
Maxzide 1215
Moduretic Tablets 1510
Normozide Tablets 2112
Oretic Tablets 544
Oreticyl 545
Prinzide Tablets 1540
Ser-Ap-Es Tablets 881
Serpasil-Esidrix Tablets 886
Timolide Tablets 1547
Trandate HCT Tablets 579
Vaseretic Tablets 1559
Zestoretic 2274

Hydroflumethiazide (Potentiated diuretic and antihypertensive effects; may cause or aggravate hyponatremia). Products include:
Diucardin Tablets 2450
Saluron 718
Salutensin/Salutensin-Demi 719

Indapamide (Potentiated diuretic and antihypertensive effects; may cause or aggravate hyponatremia). Products include:
Lozol Tablets 1843

Indomethacin (Severe hyperkalemia). Products include:
Indocin 1487

Indomethacin Sodium Trihydrate (Severe hyperkalemia). Products include:
Indocin I.V. 1490

Isoflurane (Exercise caution). Products include:
Forane 600

Isradipine (Severe hyperkalemia; potentiated antihypertensive effects). Products include:
DynaCirc Capsules 2004

Ketamine Hydrochloride (Exercise caution). Products include:
Ketalar 1726

Labetalol Hydrochloride (Potentiated antihypertensive effects). Products include:
Normodyne Injection 2108
Normodyne Tablets 2110
Normozide Tablets 2112
Trandate HCT Tablets 579
Trandate Injection 577
Trandate Tablets 579

Lisinopril (Potentiated antihypertensive effects; severe hyperkalemia). Products include:
Prinivil Tablets 1538
Prinzide Tablets 1540
Zestoretic 2274
Zestril Tablets 2277

Mecamylamine Hydrochloride (Potentiated antihypertensive effects; reduce mecamylamine dosage by at least 50 percent). Products include:
Inversine Tablets 1492

Methohexital Sodium (Exercise caution). Products include:
Brevital Sodium Vials 1248

Methoxyflurane (Exercise caution).
No products indexed under this heading.

Methyclothiazide (Potentiated diuretic and antihypertensive effects; may cause or aggravate hyponatremia). Products include:
Enduron Tablets 517
Enduronyl 518

Methyldopa (Potentiated antihypertensive effects). Products include:
Aldoclor Tablets 1413
Aldomet Oral 1415
Aldoril Tablets 1418

Methyldopate Hydrochloride (Potentiated antihypertensive effects). Products include:
Aldomet Ester HCl Injection 1417

Metolazone (Potentiated diuretic and antihypertensive effects; may cause or aggravate hyponatremia). Products include:
Diulo 2129
Mykrox ½ mg Tablets 984
Zaroxolyn Tablets 989

Metoprolol Tartrate (Potentiated antihypertensive effects). Products include:
Lopressor Ampuls 1032
Lopressor HCT Tablets 1034
Lopressor Tablets 1032

Metyrosine (Potentiated antihypertensive effects). Products include:
Demser Capsules 1460

Minoxidil (Potentiated antihypertensive effects). Products include:
Loniten Tablets 2346
Rogaine Topical Solution 2357

Nadolol (Potentiated antihypertensive effects). Products include:
Corgard Tablets 701
Corzide Tablets 702

Nicardipine Hydrochloride (Potentiated antihypertensive effects). Products include:
Cardene Capsules 2290

Nitroglycerin (Potentiated antihypertensive effects). Products include:
Deponit NTG Transdermal Delivery System 2143
Minitran Transdermal Delivery System 1312
Nitro-Bid Ointment 1339
Nitro-Bid Capsules 1338
Nitrodisc 2176
Nitro-Dur (nitroglycerin) Transdermal Infusion System 1164
Nitrogard Tablets 1004
Nitrolingual Spray 1846
Nitrostat Tablets 1743
Transderm-Nitro Transdermal Therapeutic System 2283

Norepinephrine Bitartrate (Reduced vascular responsiveness to norepinephrine). Products include:
Levophed Bitartrate Injection 2054

Penbutolol Sulfate (Potentiated antihypertensive effects). Products include:
Levatol 1832

Phenoxybenzamine Hydrochloride (Potentiated antihypertensive effects). Products include:
Dibenzyline Capsules 2207

Phentolamine Mesylate (Potentiated antihypertensive effects). Products include:
Regitine 878

Pindolol (Potentiated antihypertensive effects). Products include:
Visken Tablets 2036

Polythiazide (Potentiated diuretic and antihypertensive effects; may cause or aggravate hyponatremia). Products include:
Minizide Capsules 1779
Renese Tablets 1785
Renese-R Tablets 1786

Potassium Acid Phosphate (May cause hyperkalemia; cardiac irregularities, possibly fatal). Products include:
K-Phos M.F. Tablets 659
K-Phos Original Formula 'Sodium Free' Tablets 660
K-Phos No. 2 Tablets 659

Potassium Bicarbonate (May cause hyperkalemia; cardiac irregularities, possibly fatal). Products include:
Alka-Seltzer Advanced Formula Antacid & Non-Aspirin Pain Reliever .... ▣ 620
Alka-Seltzer Effervescent Antacid ▣ 622
K-Lyte 707
Klorvess Effervescent Granules 2010
Klorvess Effervescent Tablets 2011

Potassium Chloride (May cause hyperkalemia; cardiac irregularities, possibly fatal). Products include:
Chlor-3 Condiment 994
K-Dur Microburst Release System (potassium chloride, USP) E.R. Tablets 1163
K-Lor Powder Packets 531
K-Lyte 707
K-Norm Capsules 982
K-Tab Filmtab 532
Kato Potassium Supplement 1114
Klor-Con 8/Klor-Con 10 Extended-release Tablets 2374
Klorvess Effervescent Granules 2010
Klorvess Effervescent Tablets 2011
Klorvess 10% Liquid 2010
Klotrix 708
Kolyum Liquid 983
Micro-K 1863
Micro-K LS Packets 1864
NuLYTELY 699
Oral Rehydration Salts, Citrate 1150
Rum-K Syrup 995
Slow-K Tablets 2281
Ten-K Controlled-Release Tablets 2282
Thermotabs .... ▣ 619

Potassium Citrate (May cause hyperkalemia; cardiac irregularities, possibly fatal). Products include:
Alka-Seltzer Effervescent Antacid .. 1570
K-Lyte 707
Polycitra Syrup 2424
Polycitra-K 2424
Polycitra-LC—Sugar-Free 2424
Ricelyte, Rice-Based Oral Electrolyte Maintenance Solution .... ▣ 613

Potassium Gluconate (May cause hyperkalemia; cardiac irregularities, possibly fatal). Products include:
Kolyum Liquid 983

Potassium Phosphate, Dibasic (May cause hyperkalemia; cardiac irregularities, possibly fatal). Products include:
Neutra-Phos 2423

Potassium Phosphate, Monobasic (May cause hyperkalemia; cardiac irregularities, possibly fatal). Products include:
K-Phos M.F. Tablets 659
K-Phos Neutral Tablets 660
Neutra-Phos 2423

Prazosin Hydrochloride (Potentiated antihypertensive effects). Products include:
Minipress Capsules 1778
Minizide Capsules 1779

Propofol (Exercise caution). Products include:
Diprivan Injection 2267

Propranolol Hydrochloride (Potentiated antihypertensive effects). Products include:
Inderal 2459
Inderal LA Long Acting Capsules 2461
Inderide Tablets 2463
Inderide LA Long Acting Capsules .. 2465

Ramipril (Severe hyperkalemia; potentiated antihypertensive effects). Products include:
Altace Capsules 1086

Rauwolfia Serpentina (Potentiated antihypertensive effects). Products include:
Raudixin Tablets 1803
Rauzide Tablets 1804

Rescinnamine (Potentiated antihypertensive effects).
No products indexed under this heading.

Reserpine (Potentiated antihypertensive effects). Products include:
Diupres Tablets 1461
Hydromox R Tablets 1209
Hydropres Tablets 1485
Renese-R Tablets 1786
Salutensin/Salutensin-Demi 719
Ser-Ap-Es Tablets 881
Serpasil Tablets 883
Serpasil-Apresoline Tablets 884
Serpasil-Esidrix Tablets 886

Sodium Nitroprusside (Potentiated antihypertensive effects). Products include:
Nipride I.V. Infusion 1909

Terazosin Hydrochloride (Potentiated antihypertensive effects). Products include:
Hytrin Tablets 529

Timolol Maleate (Potentiated antihypertensive effects). Products include:
Blocadren Tablets 1429
Timolide Tablets 1547
Timoptic in Ocudose 1552
Timoptic Sterile Ophthalmic Solution 1550

Triamterene (Potentiated diuretic effects; may cause or aggravate hyponatremia; do not administer concurrently). Products include:
Dyazide Capsules 2208
Dyrenium Capsules 2210
Maxzide 1215

Trimethaphan Camsylate (Potentiated antihypertensive effects; reduce trimethaphan dosage by at least 50 percent). Products include:
Arfonad Ampuls 1887

ALDOCLOR TABLETS
(Methyldopa, Chlorothiazide) 1413
May interact with antihypertensives, general anesthetics, corticosteroids, insulin, lithium preparations, oral hypoglycemic agents, non-steroidal anti-inflammatory agents, barbiturates, narcotic analgesics, and certain other agents. Compounds in these categories include:

Acebutolol Hydrochloride (Potentiation of antihypertensive effect). Products include:
Sectral Capsules 2520

ACTH (Hypokalemia may result).
No products indexed under this heading.

Alcohol (Aggravates orthostatic hypotension).

Alfentanil Hydrochloride (Aggravates orthostatic hypotension). Products include:
Alfenta Injection 1131

Aprobarbital (Aggravates orthostatic hypotension). Products include:
Alurate Elixir 1883

Atenolol (Potentiation of antihypertensive effect). Products include:
Tenoretic Tablets 1105
Tenormin Tablets and I.V. Injection 1107

Benazepril Hydrochloride (Potentiation of antihypertensive effect). Products include:
Lotensin Tablets 872

Bendroflumethiazide (Potentiation of antihypertensive effect). Products include:
Corzide Tablets 702
Naturetin Tablets 1789
Rauzide Tablets 1804

Betamethasone Acetate (Hypokalemia may result). Products include:
Celestone Soluspan Suspension 2081

Betamethasone Sodium Phosphate (Hypokalemia may result). Products include:
Celestone Soluspan Suspension 2081

Betaxolol Hydrochloride (Potentiation of antihypertensive effect). Products include:
Betoptic Sterile Ophthalmic Solution 569
Betoptic S Sterile Ophthalmic Suspension 570

Kerlone Tablets 2172

Buprenorphine (Aggravates orthostatic hypotension).
No products indexed under this heading.

Butabarbital (Aggravates orthostatic hypotension). Products include:
Pyridium Plus 1764

Butalbital (Aggravates orthostatic hypotension). Products include:
Esgic-Plus Tablets 1002
Esgic Tablets & Capsules 1001
Fioricet Tablets 2006
Fiorinal Capsules 2007
Fiorinal with Codeine Capsules 2008
Fiorinal Tablets 2007
Phrenilin 838
Sedapap Tablets 50 mg/650 mg .. 1360

Captopril (Potentiation of antihypertensive effect). Products include:
Capoten 2255
Capozide 2258

Carteolol Hydrochloride (Potentiation of antihypertensive effects). Products include:
Cartrol Tablets 507

Chlorothiazide Sodium (Potentiation of antihypertensive effect). Products include:
Diuril Sodium Intravenous 1463

Chlorpropamide (Dosage adjustment of the antidiabetic drug may be required). Products include:
Diabinese Tablets 1775

Chlorthalidone (Potentiation of antihypertensive effect). Products include:
Combipres Tablets 678
Tenoretic Tablets 1105
Thalitone Tablets 687

Clonidine (Potentiation of antihypertensive effect). Products include:
Catapres-TTS 677

Clonidine Hydrochloride (Potentiation of antihypertensive effect). Products include:
Catapres Tablets 676
Combipres Tablets 678

Codeine (Aggravates orthostatic hypotension). Products include:
Calcidrine Syrup 506

Codeine Phosphate (Aggravates orthostatic hypotension). Products include:
Actifed with Codeine Cough Syrup.. 752
Cheracol Cough Syrup 1853
Codimal PH Syrup 846
Dimetane-DC Cough Syrup 1857
Empirin with Codeine Phosphate Nos. 2, 3 & 4 764
Fiorinal with Codeine Capsules 2008
Isoclor Expectorant 982
Naldecon CX Adult Liquid .... ▣ 521
Novahistine DH 1342
Novahistine Expectorant 1343
Nucofed Capsules 2219
Nucofed Expectorant 2219
Nucofed Pediatric Expectorant 2220
Nucofed Syrup 2219
Phenaphen with Codeine Capsules 1865
Phenaphen-650 with Codeine Tablets 1866
Phenergan with Codeine 2497
Phenergan VC with Codeine 2501
Robitussin A-C Syrup 1875
Robitussin-DAC Syrup 1875
Ryna .... ▣ 741
Soma Compound w/Codeine Tablets 2390
Triaminic Expectorant w/Codeine .. 1996
Tussi-Organidin Liquid 2391
Tylenol with Codeine 1381

Codeine Polistirex (Aggravates orthostatic hypotension).
No products indexed under this heading.

Cortisone Acetate (Hypokalemia may result). Products include:
Cortone Acetate Sterile Suspension 1437
Cortone Acetate Tablets 1439

Deserpidine (Potentiation of antihypertensive effect). Products include:
Enduronyl 518
Harmonyl Tablets 528
Oreticyl 545

Dexamethasone (Hypokalemia may result). Products include:
AK-Trol Ointment & Suspension .... ⊙ 207
Decadron Elixir 1445
Decadron Tablets 1447
Decaspray Topical Aerosol 1459
Dexacidin .... ⊙ 272
Maxidex Sterile Ophthalmic Suspension .... ⊙ 223
Maxitrol Ophthalmic Ointment/Suspension .... ⊙ 223
TobraDex Ophthalmic Suspension and Ointment .... ⊙ 228

Dexamethasone Acetate (Hypokalemia may result). Products include:
Dalalone D.P. Injectable 999
Decadron-LA Sterile Suspension 1457

Dexamethasone Sodium Phosphate (Hypokalemia may result). Products include:
AK-Dex .... ⊙ 203
Decadron Phosphate Respihaler 1454
Decadron Phosphate Sterile Ophthalmic Ointment 1453
Decadron Phosphate Sterile Ophthalmic Solution 1453
Decadron Phosphate Topical Cream 1455
Decadron Phosphate Turbinaire 1456
Maxidex Sterile Ophthalmic Ointment .... ⊙ 222
NeoDecadron Sterile Ophthalmic Ointment 1517
NeoDecadron Sterile Ophthalmic Solution 1518
NeoDecadron Topical Cream 1518

Dezocine (Aggravates orthostatic hypotension).

Diazoxide (Potentiation of antihypertensive effects). Products include:
Hyperstat I.V. Injection 2095
Proglycem 649

Diclofenac Sodium (May result in reduced diuretic effect). Products include:
Voltaren Ophthalmic Sterile Ophthalmic Solution .... ⊙ 268
Voltaren Tablets 1042

Doxazosin Mesylate (Potentiation of antihypertensive effect). Products include:
Cardura Tablets 1941

Enalapril Maleate (Potentiation of antihypertensive effect). Products include:
Vaseretic Tablets 1559
Vasotec Tablets 1564

Enalaprilat (Potentiation of antihypertensive effect). Products include:
Vasotec I.V. 1562

Enflurane (May require reduced dose of anesthetics). Products include:
Ethrane 599

Esmolol Hydrochloride (Potentiation of antihypertensive effect). Products include:
Brevibloc Injection 942

Etodolac (May result in reduced diuretic effect). Products include:
Lodine Capsules 2468

Felodipine (Potentiation of antihypertensive effect). Products include:
Plendil Extended-Release Tablets.... 1526

Fenoprofen Calcium (May result in reduced diuretic effects). Products include:
Nalfon Pulvules & Tablets 919

Fentanyl (Aggravates orthostatic hypotension). Products include:
Duragesic Transdermal System........ 1133

Fentanyl Citrate (Aggravates orthostatic hypotension). Products include:
Innovar Injection 1141
Sublimaze Injection 1146

Flurbiprofen (May result in reduced diuretic effect). Products include:
Ansaid Tablets 2319

Fosinopril Sodium (Potentiation of antihypertensive effect). Products include:
Monopril Tablets 1406

Furosemide (Potentiation of antihypertensive effect). Products include:
Lasix 1093

Glipizide (Dosage adjustment of the antidiabetic drug may be required). Products include:
Glucotrol 1952

Glyburide (Dosage adjustment of the antidiabetic drug may be required). Products include:
DiaBeta 1091
Micronase Tablets 2350

Guanabenz Acetate (Potentiation of antihypertensive effect). Products include:
Wytensin Tablets 2542

Guanethidine Monosulfate (Potentiation of antihypertensive effect). Products include:
Esimil Tablets 864
Ismelin Tablets 869

Hydralazine Hydrochloride (Potentiation of antihypertensive effect). Products include:
Apresazide Capsules 854
Apresoline Hydrochloride Parenteral (Ampuls) 856
Apresoline Hydrochloride Tablets .. 855
Apresoline-Esidrix Tablets 857
Ser-Ap-Es Tablets 881
Serpasil-Apresoline Tablets 884

Hydrochlorothiazide (Potentiation of antihypertensive effect). Products include:
Aldactazide 2150
Aldoril Tablets 1418
Apresazide Capsules 854
Apresoline-Esidrix Tablets 857
Capozide 2258
Dyazide Capsules 2208
Esidrix Tablets 863
Esimil Tablets 864
HydroDIURIL Tablets 1484
Hydropres Tablets 1485
Inderide Tablets 2463
Inderide LA Long Acting Capsules .. 2465
Lopressor HCT Tablets 1034
Maxzide 1215
Moduretic Tablets 1510
Normozide Tablets 2112
Oretic Tablets 544
Oreticyl 545
Prinzide Tablets 1540
Ser-Ap-Es Tablets 881
Serpasil-Esidrix Tablets 886
Timolide Tablets 1547
Trandate HCT Tablets 579
Vaseretic Tablets 1559
Zestoretic 2274

Hydrocodone Bitartrate (Aggravates orthostatic hypotension). Products include:
Anexsia 5/500 Tablets 2196
Anexsia 7.5/650 Tablets 2197
Azdone Tablets 844
Codiclear DH Syrup 845
Codimal DH Syrup 846
Damason-P 1356
Hycodan Syrup, Tablets 927
Hycomine Compound Tablets 929
Hycomine Syrup 927
Hycotuss Expectorant Syrup 930
Hydrocet Capsules 835
Lortab ASA Tablets 2414
Lortab 2412
Ru-Tuss with Hydrocodone 694
Triaminic Expectorant DH 1995
Vicodin Tablets 1187
Vicodin ES Tablets 1189
Zydone Capsules 941

Hydrocodone Polistirex (Aggravates orthostatic hypotension). Products include:
Tussionex Extended-Release Suspension 988

Hydrocortisone (Hypokalemia may result). Products include:
AK-Spore H.C. .... ⊙ 206
Bactine Hydrocortisone Anti-Itch Cream .... ▣ 625
CaldeCORT Anti-Itch Hydrocortisone Spray .... ▣ 560
Carmol HC Cream 1% 2296
Cortaid Spray .... ▣ 735
Cortenema 2244
Cortisporin Ointment 758
Cortisporin Ophthalmic Ointment Sterile 758
Cortisporin Ophthalmic Suspension Sterile 759
Cortisporin Otic Solution Sterile 760
Cortisporin Otic Suspension Sterile 760
Cortizone-5 Creme & Ointment ..... ▣ 732
Dermolate Anti-Itch Cream .... ▣ 697
Eldecort Cream 1.0% 1113
Eldecort Cream 1.0% and 2.5% 1113
Fungoid HC Creme 1770
Hydrocortone Tablets 1482
Hytone 909
LazerSporin-C Solution 1770
Massengill Medicated Soft Cloth Towelettes 2192
Nutracort Cream & Lotion 1684
PediOtic Suspension Sterile 797
Synacort Creams 1%, 2.5% 2296
Vanoxide-HC Acne Lotion 911
Vioform-Hydrocortisone Cream and Mild Cream 889
Vioform-Hydrocortisone Ointment.. 889
VōSoL HC Otic Solution 2392
Vytone Cream 1% 911

Hydrocortisone Acetate (Hypokalemia may result). Products include:
Analpram-HC Rectal Cream 1% and 2.5% 970
Anusol-HC Cream 1690
Anusol-HC Suppositories 1691
Caldecort .... ▣ 560
Carmol HC Cream 1% 2296
Chloromycetin Hydrocortisone Ophthalmic 1694
Coly-Mycin S Otic w/Neomycin & Hydrocortisone 1708
Cortaid .... ▣ 735
Cortef Feminine Itch Cream .... ▣ 735
Corticaine .... ▣ 682
Cortifoam 1827
Cortisporin Cream 757
Epifoam 1828
Gynecort 5 Creme .... ▣ 556
Hydrocortone Acetate Sterile Suspension 1479
Lanacort 5 Creme and Ointment .. ▣ 557
Mantadil Cream 789
Ophthocort .... ⊙ 301
Orabase HCA Oral Paste 890
Pramosone Cream, Lotion & Ointment 971
ProctoCream-HC 1834
Proctofoam-HC 1835

Hydrocortisone Sodium Phosphate (Hypokalemia may result). Products include:
Hydrocortone Phosphate Injection, Sterile 1481

Hydrocortisone Sodium Succinate (Hypokalemia may result). Products include:
Solu-Cortef Sterile Powder 2361

Hydroflumethiazide (Potentiation of antihypertensive effect). Products include:
Diucardin Tablets 2450
Saluron 718
Salutensin/Salutensin-Demi 719

Ibuprofen (May result in reduced diuretic effects). Products include:
Advil Cold & Sinus Caplets (formerly CoAdvil) 2416
Advil Ibuprofen Tablets and Caplets 2416
Children's Advil Suspension 2426
CoAdvil .... ▣ 748
Dristan Sinus Caplets 2419
Haltran Tablets .... ▣ 668
Ibuprofen .... ▣ 631

Medipren ibuprofen Caplets and Tablets 1362
Midol 200 Cramp Relief Formula.. ▣ 570
Motrin Tablets........ 2351
Motrin IB Caplets and Tablets .... ▣ 736
Nuprin Ibuprofen/Analgesic Tablets & Caplets 752
PediaProfen Suspension........ 1363
Rufen Tablets 691
Trendar Ibuprofen Tablets........ ▣ 756

Indapamide (Potentiation of antihypertensive effect). Products include:
Lozol Tablets 1843

Indomethacin (May result in reduced diuretic effects). Products include:
Indocin 1487

Indomethacin Sodium Trihydrate (May result in reduced diuretic effects). Products include:
Indocin I.V. 1490

Insulin, Human (May alter insulin requirements).
No products indexed under this heading.

Insulin, Human Isophane Suspension (May alter insulin requirements). Products include:
Humulin N, 100 Units 1270

Insulin, Human NPH (May alter insulin requirements). Products include:
Insulatard NPH Human........ 1627
Novolin N........ 1627
Novolin N PenFill Cartridges........ 1628
Novolin N Prefilled 1628

Insulin, Human Regular (May alter insulin requirements). Products include:
Humulin BR, 100 Units 1268
Humulin R, 100 Units 1272
Novolin R........ 1627
Novolin R PenFill Cartridges........ 1628
Novolin R Prefilled........ 1629
Velosulin Human 1628

Insulin, Human, Zinc Suspension (May alter insulin requirements). Products include:
Humulin L, 100 Units 1268
Humulin U, 100 Units........ 1272
Novolin L 1627

Insulin, NPH (May alter insulin requirements). Products include:
NPH, 40 & 100 Units........ 1273
Beef NPH, 100 Units........ 1274
Pork NPH, 100 Units........ 1275
Insulatard NPH 1626
NPH Insulin 1626
NPH Purified Pork Isophane Insulin 1626

Insulin, Regular (May alter insulin requirements). Products include:
Regular, 40 & 100 Units........ 1273
Beef Regular, 100 Units........ 1275
Pork Regular, 100 Units 1275
Pork Regular (Concentrated), 500 Units 1276
Regular Insulin 1625
Regular Purified Pork Insulin 1626
Velosulin 1627

Insulin, Zinc Crystals (May alter insulin requirements). Products include:
NPH, 40 & 100 Units........ 1273

Insulin, Zinc Suspension (May alter insulin requirements). Products include:
Lente, 40 & 100 Units 1272
Protamine, Zinc, 40 & 100 Units.... 1273
Lente Iletin I........ 1272
Beef Lente, 100 Units........ 1274
Beef Protamine Zinc, 100 Units...... 1274
Pork Lente, 100 Units........ 1275
Pork, Protamine, Zinc, 100 Units.... 1275
Lente Insulin........ 1626
Lente Purified Pork Insulin 1626
Semilente Insulin 1625
Ultralente Insulin 1626

Isoflurane (May require reduced dose of anesthetics). Products include:
Forane........ 600

Isradipine (Potentiation of antihypertensive effect). Products include:
DynaCirc Capsules 2004

Ketamine Hydrochloride (May require reduced dose of anesthetics). Products include:
Ketalar 1726

Ketoprofen (May result in reduced diuretic effects). Products include:
Orudis Capsules........ 2488

Ketorolac Tromethamine (May result in reduced diuretic effect). Products include:
Toradol IM Injection 2302

Labetalol Hydrochloride (Potentiation of antihypertensive effect). Products include:
Normodyne Injection 2108
Normodyne Tablets 2110
Normozide Tablets 2112
Trandate HCT Tablets 579
Trandate Injection 577
Trandate Tablets 579

Levorphanol Tartrate (Aggravates orthostatic hypotension). Products include:
Levo-Dromoran........ 1906

Lisinopril (Potentiation of antihypertensive effect). Products include:
Prinivil Tablets 1538
Prinzide Tablets........ 1540
Zestoretic 2274
Zestril Tablets 2277

Lithium Carbonate (High risk of lithium toxicity). Products include:
Eskalith 2214
Lithane Tablets........ 1596
Lithium Carbonate Capsules & Tablets 1984
Lithobid Tablets 870

Lithium Citrate (High risk of lithium toxicity). Products include:
Cibalith-S........ 870

Mecamylamine Hydrochloride (Potentiation of antihypertensive effect). Products include:
Inversine Tablets 1492

Meclofenamate Sodium (May result in reduced diuretic effects). Products include:
Meclomen Capsules 1739

Mefenamic Acid (May result in reduced diuretic effects). Products include:
Ponstel 1758

Meperidine Hydrochloride (Aggravates orthostatic hypotension). Products include:
Demerol 2047
Mepergan Injection 2479

Mephobarbital (Aggravates orthostatic hypotension). Products include:
Mebaral Tablets 2061

Methadone Hydrochloride (Aggravates orthostatic hypotension). Products include:
Dolophine Hydrochloride Ampoules & Vials 1260
Dolophine Hydrochloride Tablets 1261
Methadone Hydrochloride Diskets.. 1284
Methadone Hydrochloride Oral Solution & Tablets........ 1987

Methohexital Sodium (May require reduced dose of anesthetics). Products include:
Brevital Sodium Vials........ 1248

Methoxyflurane (May require reduced dose of anesthetics).
No products indexed under this heading.

Methyclothiazide (Potentiation of antihypertensive effect). Products include:
Enduron Tablets........ 517
Enduronyl 518

Methyldopate Hydrochloride (Potentiation of antihypertensive effect). Products include:
Aldomet Ester HCl Injection 1417

Methylprednisolone Acetate (Hypokalemia may result). Products include:
Depo-Medrol Sterile Aqueous Suspension........ 2334

Methylprednisolone Sodium Succinate (Hypokalemia may result). Products include:
Solu-Medrol Sterile Powder........ 2363

Metolazone (Potentiation of antihypertensive effect). Products include:
Diulo 2129
Mykrox ½ mg Tablets 984
Zaroxolyn Tablets 989

Metoprolol Tartrate (Potentiation of antihypertensive effect). Products include:
Lopressor Ampuls 1032
Lopressor HCT Tablets 1034
Lopressor Tablets 1032

Metyrosine (Potentiation of antihypertensive effect). Products include:
Demser Capsules........ 1460

Minoxidil (Potentiation of antihypertensive effect). Products include:
Loniten Tablets........ 2346
Rogaine Topical Solution 2357

Morphine Sulfate (Aggravates orthostatic hypotension). Products include:
Astramorph/PF Injection, USP (Preservative-Free) 618
Duramorph 960
Infumorph 200 and Infumorph 500 Sterile Solutions........ 962
MS Contin Tablets........ 1814
MSIR 1817
Oramorph SR (Morphine Sulfate Sustained Release Tablets)........ 1988
Roxanol 1991

Nadolol (Potentiation of antihypertensive effect). Products include:
Corgard Tablets 701
Corzide Tablets 702

Naproxen (May result in reduced diuretic effects). Products include:
Naprosyn........ 2297

Naproxen Sodium (May result in reduced diuretic effects). Products include:
Anaprox and Anaprox DS Tablets.... 2288

Nicardipine Hydrochloride (Potentiation of antihypertensive effects). Products include:
Cardene Capsules 2290

Nitroglycerin (Potentiation of antihypertensive effect). Products include:
Deponit NTG Transdermal Delivery System 2143
Minitran Transdermal Delivery System 1312
Nitro-Bid Ointment 1339
Nitro-Bid Capsules 1338
Nitrodisc 2176
Nitro-Dur (nitroglycerin) Transdermal Infusion System 1164
Nitrogard Tablets........ 1004
Nitrolingual Spray 1846
Nitrostat Tablets 1743
Transderm-Nitro Transdermal Therapeutic System 2283

Norepinephrine Bitartrate (May decrease arterial responsiveness to norepinephrine). Products include:
Levophed Bitartrate Injection........ 2054

Opium Alkaloids (Aggravates orthostatic hypotension). Products include:
B & O No. 15A & No. 16A Supprettes 2395
Pantopon Injectable 1911

Oxycodone Hydrochloride (Aggravates orthostatic hypotension). Products include:
Percocet Tablets 950
Percodan 951
Roxicodone Tablets, Oral Solution & Intensol (Oxycodone) 1992
Tylox Capsules 1382

Penbutolol Sulfate (Potentiation of antihypertensive effects). Products include:
Levatol 1832

Pentobarbital Sodium (Aggravates orthostatic hypotension). Products include:
Nembutal Sodium Capsules 534
Nembutal Sodium Solution 536
Nembutal Sodium Suppositories...... 538

Phenobarbital (Aggravates orthostatic hypotension). Products include:
Arco-Lase Plus Tablets 607
Bellergal-S Tablets 1998
Bronkolixir .... ▣ 761
Bronkotabs Tablets........ ▣ 762
Donnatal 1858
Donnatal Extentabs........ 1859
Donnatal Tablets 1858
Donnazyme Tablets 1860
Kinesed Tablets 2272
Phenobarbital Elixir and Tablets...... 1293
Primatene Tablets-P Formula........ 2421
Quadrinal Tablets 1183
Tedral SA 1765

Phenoxybenzamine Hydrochloride (Potentiation of antihypertensive effect). Products include:
Dibenzyline Capsules 2207

Phentolamine Mesylate (Potentiation of antihypertensive effect). Products include:
Regitine 878

Phenylbutazone (May result in reduced diuretic effects). Products include:
Butazolidin Capsules & Tablets........ 1027

Pindolol (Potentiation of antihypertensive effect). Products include:
Visken Tablets........ 2036

Piroxicam (May result in reduced diuretic effects). Products include:
Feldene Capsules........ 1777

Polythiazide (Potentiation of antihypertensive effect). Products include:
Minizide Capsules 1779
Renese Tablets 1785
Renese-R Tablets........ 1786

Prazosin Hydrochloride (Potentiation of antihypertensive effect). Products include:
Minipress Capsules........ 1778
Minizide Capsules 1779

Prednisolone Acetate (Hypokalemia may result). Products include:
AK-Cide Sterile Ophthalmic Ointment & Suspension........ ◉ 202
Blephamide Liquifilm Sterile Ophthalmic Suspension........ 586
Blephamide S.O.P. Sterile Ophthalmic Ointment........ 586
Cetapred Ointment .... ◉ 220
⅛% Econopred & 1% Econopred Plus .... ◉ 217
Isopto Cetapred Suspension........ ◉ 220
Metimyd........ ◉ 306
Poly-Pred Liquifilm .... ◉ 250
Pred Forte........ ◉ 252
Pred Mild........ ◉ 254
Pred-G Liquifilm Sterile Ophthalmic Suspension .... ◉ 252
Pred-G S.O.P. Sterile Ophthalmic Ointment .... ◉ 253
Vasocidin Ointment .... ◉ 275

Prednisolone Sodium Phosphate (Hypokalemia may result). Products include:
AK-Pred .... ◉ 205
Hydeltrasol Injection, Sterile........ 1476
Inflamase........ ◉ 274
Pediapred Oral Liquid 987
Vasocidin Ophthalmic Solution .... ◉ 276

Prednisolone Tebutate (Hypokalemia may result). Products include:
Hydeltra-T.B.A. Sterile Suspension 1478

Prednisone (Hypokalemia may result). Products include:
- Deltasone Tablets 2332

Propofol (May require reduced dose of anesthetics). Products include:
- Diprivan Injection 2267

Propoxyphene Hydrochloride (Aggravates orthostatic hypotension). Products include:
- Darvon 1256
- Wygesic Tablets 2540

Propoxyphene Napsylate (Aggravates orthostatic hypotension). Products include:
- Darvon-N/Darvocet-N 1254

Propranolol Hydrochloride (Potentiation of antihypertensive effect). Products include:
- Inderal 2459
- Inderal LA Long Acting Capsules 2461
- Inderide Tablets 2463
- Inderide LA Long Acting Capsules 2465

Ramipril (Potentiation of antihypertensive effect). Products include:
- Altace Capsules 1086

Rauwolfia Serpentina (Potentiation of antihypertensive effect). Products include:
- Raudixin Tablets 1803
- Rauzide Tablets 1804

Rescinnamine (Potentiation of antihypertensive effect).
- No products indexed under this heading.

Reserpine (Potentiation of antihypertensive effect). Products include:
- Diupres Tablets 1461
- Hydromox R Tablets 1209
- Hydropres Tablets 1485
- Renese-R Tablets 1786
- Salutensin/Salutensin-Demi 719
- Ser-Ap-Es Tablets 881
- Serpasil Tablets 883
- Serpasil-Apresoline Tablets 884
- Serpasil-Esidrix Tablets 886

Secobarbital Sodium (Aggravates orthostatic hypotension). Products include:
- Seconal Sodium Pulvules 1296

Sodium Nitroprusside (Potentiation of antihypertensive effect). Products include:
- Nipride I.V. Infusion 1909

Sufentanil Citrate (Aggravates orthostatic hypotension). Products include:
- Sufenta Injection 1147

Sulindac (May result in reduced diuretic effects). Products include:
- Clinoril Tablets 1433

Terazosin Hydrochloride (Potentiation of antihypertensive effect). Products include:
- Hytrin Tablets 529

Thiamylal Sodium (Aggravates orthostatic hypotension). Products include:
- Surital Ampoules, Steri-Vials 1764

Timolol Maleate (Potentiation of antihypertensive effect). Products include:
- Blocadren Tablets 1429
- Timolide Tablets 1547
- Timoptic in Ocudose 1552
- Timoptic Sterile Ophthalmic Solution 1550

Tolazamide (Dosage adjustment of the antidiabetic drug may be required). Products include:
- Tolinase Tablets 2365

Tolbutamide (Dosage adjustment of the antidiabetic drug may be required). Products include:
- Orinase Tablets 2354

Tolmetin Sodium (May result in reduced diuretic effects). Products include:
- Tolectin (200, 400 and 600 mg) 1379

Triamcinolone (Hypokalemia may result).
- No products indexed under this heading.

Triamcinolone Acetonide (Hypokalemia may result). Products include:
- Aristocort A 1010
- Azmacort Inhaler 1837
- Kenalog Cream, Lotion & Ointment 2401
- Kenalog-10 Injection 2402
- Kenalog-40 Injection 2403
- Kenalog in Orabase 604
- Kenalog Spray 2401
- Mycolog II Cream and Ointment 2407
- Mytrex Cream & Ointment 2080
- Nasacort Nasal Inhaler 1844

Triamcinolone Diacetate (Hypokalemia may result). Products include:
- Aristocort Suspension 1008

Triamcinolone Hexacetonide (Hypokalemia may result). Products include:
- Aristospan Suspension 1011

Trimethaphan Camsylate (Potentiation of antihypertensive effect). Products include:
- Arfonad Ampuls 1887

Tubocurarine Chloride (Increased responsiveness to tubocurarine).
- No products indexed under this heading.

ALDOMET ESTER HCL INJECTION
(Methyldopate Hydrochloride) 1417
May interact with general anesthetics, antihypertensives, lithium preparations, and certain other agents. Compounds in these categories include:

Acebutolol Hydrochloride (Potentiation of antihypertensive effect). Products include:
- Sectral Capsules 2520

Atenolol (Potentiation of antihypertensive effect). Products include:
- Tenoretic Tablets 1105
- Tenormin Tablets and I.V. Injection 1107

Benazepril Hydrochloride (Potentiation of antihypertensive effect). Products include:
- Lotensin Tablets 872

Bendroflumethiazide (Potentiation of antihypertensive effect). Products include:
- Corzide Tablets 702
- Naturetin Tablets 1789
- Rauzide Tablets 1804

Betaxolol Hydrochloride (Potentiation of antihypertensive effect). Products include:
- Betoptic Sterile Ophthalmic Solution 569
- Betoptic S Sterile Ophthalmic Suspension 570
- Kerlone Tablets 2172

Captopril (Potentiation of antihypertensive effect). Products include:
- Capoten 2255
- Capozide 2258

Carteolol Hydrochloride (Potentiation of antihypertensive effect). Products include:
- Cartrol Tablets 507

Chlorothiazide (Potentiation of antihypertensive effect). Products include:
- Aldoclor Tablets 1413
- Diupres Tablets 1461
- Diuril Oral 1464

Chlorothiazide Sodium (Potentiation of antihypertensive effect). Products include:
- Diuril Sodium Intravenous 1463

Chlorthalidone (Potentiation of antihypertensive effect). Products include:
- Combipres Tablets 678
- Tenoretic Tablets 1105
- Thalitone Tablets 687

Clonidine (Potentiation of antihypertensive effect). Products include:
- Catapres-TTS 677

Clonidine Hydrochloride (Potentiation of antihypertensive effect). Products include:
- Catapres Tablets 676
- Combipres Tablets 678

Deserpidine (Potentiation of antihypertensive effect). Products include:
- Enduronyl 518
- Harmonyl Tablets 528
- Oreticyl 545

Diazoxide (Potentiation of antihypertensive effect). Products include:
- Hyperstat I.V. Injection 2095
- Proglycem 649

Doxazosin Mesylate (Potentiation of antihypertensive effect). Products include:
- Cardura Tablets 1941

Enalapril Maleate (Potentiation of antihypertensive effect). Products include:
- Vaseretic Tablets 1559
- Vasotec Tablets 1564

Enalaprilat (Potentiation of antihypertensive effects). Products include:
- Vasotec I.V. 1562

Enflurane (May require reduced dose of anesthetics). Products include:
- Ethrane 599

Esmolol Hydrochloride (Potentiation of antihypertensive effect). Products include:
- Brevibloc Injection 942

Felodipine (Potentiation of antihypertensive effect). Products include:
- Plendil Extended-Release Tablets 1526

Fosinopril Sodium (Potentiation of antihypertensive effect). Products include:
- Monopril Tablets 1406

Furosemide (Potentiation of antihypertensive effect). Products include:
- Lasix 1093

Guanabenz Acetate (Potentiation of antihypertensive effect). Products include:
- Wytensin Tablets 2542

Guanethidine Monosulfate (Potentiation of antihypertensive effect). Products include:
- Esimil Tablets 864
- Ismelin Tablets 869

Hydralazine Hydrochloride (Potentiation of antihypertensive effect). Products include:
- Apresazide Capsules 854
- Apresoline Hydrochloride Parenteral (Ampuls) 856
- Apresoline Hydrochloride Tablets 855
- Apresoline-Esidrix Tablets 857
- Ser-Ap-Es Tablets 881
- Serpasil-Apresoline Tablets 884

Hydrochlorothiazide (Potentiation of antihypertensive effect). Products include:
- Aldactazide 2150
- Aldoril Tablets 1418
- Apresazide Capsules 854
- Apresoline-Esidrix Tablets 857
- Capozide 2258
- Dyazide Capsules 2208
- Esidrix Tablets 863
- Esimil Tablets 864
- HydroDIURIL Tablets 1484
- Hydropres Tablets 1485
- Inderide Tablets 2463
- Inderide LA Long Acting Capsules 2465
- Lopressor HCT Tablets 1034
- Maxzide 1215
- Moduretic Tablets 1510
- Normozide Tablets 2112
- Oretic Tablets 544
- Oreticyl 545
- Prinzide Tablets 1540
- Ser-Ap-Es Tablets 881
- Serpasil-Esidrix Tablets 886
- Timolide Tablets 1547
- Trandate HCT Tablets 579
- Vaseretic Tablets 1559
- Zestoretic 2274

Hydroflumethiazide (Potentiation of antihypertensive effect). Products include:
- Diucardin Tablets 2450
- Saluron 718
- Salutensin/Salutensin-Demi 719

Indapamide (Potentiation of antihypertensive effect). Products include:
- Lozol Tablets 1843

Isoflurane (May require reduced dose of anesthetics). Products include:
- Forane 600

Isradipine (Potentiation of antihypertensive effect). Products include:
- DynaCirc Capsules 2004

Ketamine Hydrochloride (May require reduced dose of anesthetics). Products include:
- Ketalar 1726

Labetalol Hydrochloride (Potentiation of antihypertensive effect). Products include:
- Normodyne Injection 2108
- Normodyne Tablets 2110
- Normozide Tablets 2112
- Trandate HCT Tablets 579
- Trandate Injection 577
- Trandate Tablets 579

Lisinopril (Potentiation of antihypertensive effects). Products include:
- Prinivil Tablets 1538
- Prinzide Tablets 1540
- Zestoretic 2274
- Zestril Tablets 2277

Lithium Carbonate (Potential for lithium toxicity). Products include:
- Eskalith 2214
- Lithane Tablets 1596
- Lithium Carbonate Capsules & Tablets 1984
- Lithobid Tablets 870

Lithium Citrate (Potential for lithium toxicity). Products include:
- Cibalith-S 870

Mecamylamine Hydrochloride (Potentiation of antihypertensive effect). Products include:
- Inversine Tablets 1492

Methohexital Sodium (May require reduced dose of anesthetics). Products include:
- Brevital Sodium Vials 1248

Methoxyflurane (May require reduced dose of anesthetics).
- No products indexed under this heading.

Methyclothiazide (Potentiation of antihypertensive effect). Products include:
- Enduron Tablets 517
- Enduronyl 518

Methyldopa (Potentiation of antihypertensive effect). Products include:
- Aldoclor Tablets 1413
- Aldomet Oral 1415
- Aldoril Tablets 1418

Metolazone (Potentiation of antihypertensive effect). Products include:
- Diulo 2129
- Mykrox ½ mg Tablets 984
- Zaroxolyn Tablets 989

Metoprolol Tartrate (Potentiation of antihypertensive effect). Products include:
Lopressor Ampuls ... 1032
Lopressor HCT Tablets ... 1034
Lopressor Tablets ... 1032

Metyrosine (Potentiation of antihypertensive effect). Products include:
Demser Capsules ... 1460

Minoxidil (Potentiation of antihypertensive effect). Products include:
Loniten Tablets ... 2346
Rogaine Topical Solution ... 2357

Nadolol (Potentiation of antihypertensive effect). Products include:
Corgard Tablets ... 701
Corzide Tablets ... 702

Nicardipine Hydrochloride (Potentiation of antihypertensive effect). Products include:
Cardene Capsules ... 2290

Nitroglycerin (Potentiation of antihypertensive effect). Products include:
Deponit NTG Transdermal Delivery System ... 2143
Minitran Transdermal Delivery System ... 1312
Nitro-Bid Ointment ... 1339
Nitro-Bid Capsules ... 1338
Nitrodisc ... 2176
Nitro-Dur (nitroglycerin) Transdermal Infusion System ... 1164
Nitrogard Tablets ... 1004
Nitrolingual Spray ... 1846
Nitrostat Tablets ... 1743
Transderm-Nitro Transdermal Therapeutic System ... 2283

Penbutolol Sulfate (Potentiation of antihypertensive effect). Products include:
Levatol ... 1832

Phenoxybenzamine Hydrochloride (Potentiation of antihypertensive effect). Products include:
Dibenzyline Capsules ... 2207

Phentolamine Mesylate (Potentiation of antihypertensive effect). Products include:
Regitine ... 878

Pindolol (Potentiation of antihypertensive effect). Products include:
Visken Tablets ... 2036

Polythiazide (Potentiation of antihypertensive effect). Products include:
Minizide Capsules ... 1779
Renese Tablets ... 1785
Renese-R Tablets ... 1786

Prazosin Hydrochloride (Potentiation of antihypertensive effect). Products include:
Minipress Capsules ... 1778
Minizide Capsules ... 1779

Propofol (May require reduced dose of anesthetics). Products include:
Diprivan Injection ... 2267

Propranolol Hydrochloride (Potentiation of antihypertensive effect). Products include:
Inderal ... 2459
Inderal LA Long Acting Capsules ... 2461
Inderide Tablets ... 2463
Inderide LA Long Acting Capsules ... 2465

Ramipril (Potentiation of antihypertensive effect). Products include:
Altace Capsules ... 1086

Rauwolfia Serpentina (Potentiation of antihypertensive effect). Products include:
Raudixin Tablets ... 1803
Rauzide Tablets ... 1804

Rescinnamine (Potentiation of antihypertensive effect).
No products indexed under this heading.

Reserpine (Potentiation of antihypertensive effect). Products include:
Diupres Tablets ... 1461
Hydromox R Tablets ... 1209
Hydropres Tablets ... 1485
Renese-R Tablets ... 1786
Salutensin/Salutensin-Demi ... 719
Ser-Ap-Es Tablets ... 881
Serpasil Tablets ... 883
Serpasil-Apresoline Tablets ... 884
Serpasil-Esidrix Tablets ... 886

Sodium Nitroprusside (Potentiation of antihypertensive effect). Products include:
Nipride I.V. Infusion ... 1909

Terazosin Hydrochloride (Potentiation of antihypertensive effect). Products include:
Hytrin Tablets ... 529

Timolol Maleate (Potentiation of antihypertensive effect). Products include:
Blocadren Tablets ... 1429
Timolide Tablets ... 1547
Timoptic in Ocudose ... 1552
Timoptic Sterile Ophthalmic Solution ... 1550

Trimethaphan Camsylate (Potentiation of antihypertensive effect). Products include:
Arfonad Ampuls ... 1887

ALDOMET ORAL SUSPENSION

(Methyldopa) ... 1415
May interact with antihypertensives, general anesthetics, lithium preparations, and certain other agents. Compounds in these categories include:

Acebutolol Hydrochloride (Potentiation of antihypertensive effect). Products include:
Sectral Capsules ... 2520

Atenolol (Potentiation of antihypertensive effect). Products include:
Tenoretic Tablets ... 1105
Tenormin Tablets and I.V. Injection 1107

Benazepril Hydrochloride (Potentiation of antihypertensive effect). Products include:
Lotensin Tablets ... 872

Bendroflumethiazide (Potentiation of antihypertensive effect). Products include:
Corzide Tablets ... 702
Naturetin Tablets ... 1789
Rauzide Tablets ... 1804

Betaxolol Hydrochloride (Potentiation of antihypertensive effect). Products include:
Betoptic Sterile Ophthalmic Solution ... 569
Betoptic S Sterile Ophthalmic Suspension ... 570
Kerlone Tablets ... 2172

Captopril (Potentiation of antihypertensive effect). Products include:
Capoten ... 2255
Capozide ... 2258

Carteolol Hydrochloride (Potentiation of antihypertensive effect). Products include:
Cartrol Tablets ... 507

Chlorothiazide (Potentiation of antihypertensive effect). Products include:
Aldoclor Tablets ... 1413
Diupres Tablets ... 1461
Diuril Oral ... 1464

Chlorothiazide Sodium (Potentiation of antihypertensive effect). Products include:
Diuril Sodium Intravenous ... 1463

Chlorthalidone (Potentiation of antihypertensive effect). Products include:
Combipres Tablets ... 678
Tenoretic Tablets ... 1105
Thalitone Tablets ... 687

Clonidine (Potentiation of antihypertensive effect). Products include:
Catapres-TTS ... 677

Clonidine Hydrochloride (Potentiation of antihypertensive effect). Products include:
Catapres Tablets ... 676
Combipres Tablets ... 678

Deserpidine (Potentiation of antihypertensive effect). Products include:
Enduronyl ... 518
Harmonyl Tablets ... 528
Oreticyl ... 545

Diazoxide (Potentiation of antihypertensive effect). Products include:
Hyperstat I.V. Injection ... 2095
Proglycem ... 649

Doxazosin Mesylate (Potentiation of antihypertensive effect). Products include:
Cardura Tablets ... 1941

Enalapril Maleate (Potentiation of antihypertensive effect). Products include:
Vaseretic Tablets ... 1559
Vasotec Tablets ... 1564

Enalaprilat (Potentiation of antihypertensive effect). Products include:
Vasotec I.V. ... 1562

Enflurane (May require reduced dose of anesthetics). Products include:
Ethrane ... 599

Esmolol Hydrochloride (Potentiation of antihypertensive effect). Products include:
Brevibloc Injection ... 942

Felodipine (Potentiation of antihypertensive effect). Products include:
Plendil Extended-Release Tablets ... 1526

Fosinopril Sodium (Potentiation of antihypertensive effect). Products include:
Monopril Tablets ... 1406

Furosemide (Potentiation of antihypertensive effect). Products include:
Lasix ... 1093

Guanabenz Acetate (Potentiation of antihypertensive effect). Products include:
Wytensin Tablets ... 2542

Guanethidine Monosulfate (Potentiation of antihypertensive effect). Products include:
Esimil Tablets ... 864
Ismelin Tablets ... 869

Hydralazine Hydrochloride (Potentiation of antihypertensive effect). Products include:
Apresazide Capsules ... 854
Apresoline Hydrochloride Parenteral (Ampuls) ... 856
Apresoline Hydrochloride Tablets ... 855
Apresoline-Esidrix Tablets ... 857
Ser-Ap-Es Tablets ... 881
Serpasil-Apresoline Tablets ... 884

Hydrochlorothiazide (Potentiation of antihypertensive effect). Products include:
Aldactazide ... 2150
Aldoril Tablets ... 1418
Apresazide Capsules ... 854
Apresoline-Esidrix Tablets ... 857
Capozide ... 2258
Dyazide Capsules ... 2208
Esidrix Tablets ... 863
Esimil Tablets ... 864
HydroDIURIL Tablets ... 1484
Hydropres Tablets ... 1485
Inderide Tablets ... 2463
Inderide LA Long Acting Capsules ... 2465
Lopressor HCT Tablets ... 1034
Maxzide ... 1215
Moduretic Tablets ... 1510
Normozide Tablets ... 2112
Oretic Tablets ... 544
Oreticyl ... 545
Prinzide Tablets ... 1540
Ser-Ap-Es Tablets ... 881
Serpasil-Esidrix Tablets ... 886
Timolide Tablets ... 1547
Trandate HCT Tablets ... 579
Vaseretic Tablets ... 1559
Zestoretic ... 2274

Hydroflumethiazide (Potentiation of antihypertensive effect). Products include:
Diucardin Tablets ... 2450
Saluron ... 718
Salutensin/Salutensin-Demi ... 719

Indapamide (Potentiation of antihypertensive effect). Products include:
Lozol Tablets ... 1843

Isoflurane (May require reduced dose of anesthetics). Products include:
Forane ... 600

Isradipine (Potentiation of antihypertensive effect). Products include:
DynaCirc Capsules ... 2004

Ketamine Hydrochloride (May require reduced dose of anesthetics). Products include:
Ketalar ... 1726

Labetalol Hydrochloride (Potentiation of antihypertensive effect). Products include:
Normodyne Injection ... 2108
Normodyne Tablets ... 2110
Normozide Tablets ... 2112
Trandate HCT Tablets ... 579
Trandate Injection ... 577
Trandate Tablets ... 579

Lisinopril (Potentiation of antihypertensive effect). Products include:
Prinivil Tablets ... 1538
Prinzide Tablets ... 1540
Zestoretic ... 2274
Zestril Tablets ... 2277

Lithium Carbonate (Potential for lithium toxicity). Products include:
Eskalith ... 2214
Lithane Tablets ... 1596
Lithium Carbonate Capsules & Tablets ... 1984
Lithobid Tablets ... 870

Lithium Citrate (Potential for lithium toxicity). Products include:
Cibalith-S ... 870

Mecamylamine Hydrochloride (Potentiation of antihypertensive effect). Products include:
Inversine Tablets ... 1492

Methohexital Sodium (May require reduced dose of anesthetics). Products include:
Brevital Sodium Vials ... 1248

Methoxyflurane (May require reduced dose of anesthetics).
No products indexed under this heading.

Methyclothiazide (Potentiation of antihypertensive effect). Products include:
Enduron Tablets ... 517
Enduronyl ... 518

Methyldopate Hydrochloride (Potentiation of antihypertensive effect). Products include:
Aldomet Ester HCl Injection ... 1417

Metolazone (Potentiation of antihypertensive effect). Products include:
Diulo ... 2129
Mykrox ½ mg Tablets ... 984
Zaroxolyn Tablets ... 989

Metoprolol Tartrate (Potentiation of antihypertensive effect). Products include:
Lopressor Ampuls ... 1032
Lopressor HCT Tablets ... 1034
Lopressor Tablets ... 1032

Metyrosine (Potentiation of antihypertensive effect). Products include:
Demser Capsules ... 1460

Minoxidil (Potentiation of antihypertensive effect). Products include:
Loniten Tablets ... 2346
Rogaine Topical Solution ... 2357

Nadolol (Potentiation of antihypertensive effect). Products include:
- Corgard Tablets ... 701
- Corzide Tablets ... 702

Nicardipine Hydrochloride (Potentiation of antihypertensive effect). Products include:
- Cardene Capsules ... 2290

Nitroglycerin (Potentiation of anithypertensive effect). Products include:
- Deponit NTG Transdermal Delivery System ... 2143
- Minitran Transdermal Delivery System ... 1312
- Nitro-Bid Ointment ... 1339
- Nitro-Bid Capsules ... 1338
- Nitrodisc ... 2176
- Nitro-Dur (nitroglycerin) Transdermal Infusion System ... 1164
- Nitrogard Tablets ... 1004
- Nitrolingual Spray ... 1846
- Nitrostat Tablets ... 1743
- Transderm-Nitro Transdermal Therapeutic System ... 2283

Penbutolol Sulfate (Potentiation of antihypertensive effect). Products include:
- Levatol ... 1832

Phenoxybenzamine Hydrochloride (Potentiation of antihypertensive effect). Products include:
- Dibenzyline Capsules ... 2207

Phentolamine Mesylate (Potentiation of antihypertensive effect). Products include:
- Regitine ... 878

Pindolol (Potentiation of antihypertensive effect). Products include:
- Visken Tablets ... 2036

Polythiazide (Potentiation of antihypertensive effect). Products include:
- Minizide Capsules ... 1779
- Renese Tablets ... 1785
- Renese-R Tablets ... 1786

Prazosin Hydrochloride (Potentiation of antihypertensive effect). Products include:
- Minipress Capsules ... 1778
- Minizide Capsules ... 1779

Propofol (May require reduced dose of anesthetics). Products include:
- Diprivan Injection ... 2267

Propranolol Hydrochloride (Potentiation of antihypertensive effect). Products include:
- Inderal ... 2459
- Inderal LA Long Acting Capsules ... 2461
- Inderide Tablets ... 2463
- Inderide LA Long Acting Capsules .. 2465

Ramipril (Potentiation of antihypertensive effect). Products include:
- Altace Capsules ... 1086

Rauwolfia Serpentina (Potentiation of antihypertensive effect). Products include:
- Raudixin Tablets ... 1803
- Rauzide Tablets ... 1804

Rescinnamine (Potentiation of antihypertensive effect).
- No products indexed under this heading.

Reserpine (Potentiation of antihypertensive effect). Products include:
- Diupres Tablets ... 1461
- Hydromox R Tablets ... 1209
- Hydropres Tablets ... 1485
- Renese-R Tablets ... 1786
- Salutensin/Salutensin-Demi ... 719
- Ser-Ap-Es Tablets ... 881
- Serpasil Tablets ... 883
- Serpasil-Apresoline Tablets ... 884
- Serpasil-Esidrix Tablets ... 886

Sodium Nitroprusside (Potentiation of antihypertensive effect). Products include:
- Nipride I.V. Infusion ... 1909

Terazosin Hydrochloride (Potentiation of antihypertensive effect). Products include:
- Hytrin Tablets ... 529

Timolol Maleate (Potentiation of antihypertensive effect). Products include:
- Blocadren Tablets ... 1429
- Timolide Tablets ... 1547
- Timoptic in Ocudose ... 1552
- Timoptic Sterile Ophthalmic Solution ... 1550

Trimethaphan Camsylate (Potentiation of antihypertensive effect). Products include:
- Arfonad Ampuls ... 1887

ALDOMET TABLETS
(Methyldopa) ... 1415
- See **Aldomet Oral Suspension**

ALDORIL TABLETS
(Methyldopa, Hydrochlorothiazide) ... 1418
May interact with corticosteroids, antihypertensives, general anesthetics, insulin, non-steroidal anti-inflammatory agents, barbiturates, narcotic analgesics, oral hypoglycemic agents, lithium preparations, cardiac glycosides, and certain other agents. Compounds in these categories include:

Acebutolol Hydrochloride (Potentiation of antihypertensive effect). Products include:
- Sectral Capsules ... 2520

ACTH (Hypokalemia may result).
- No products indexed under this heading.

Alcohol (Aggravates orthostatic hypotension).

Alfentanil Hydrochloride (Aggravates orthostatic hypotension). Products include:
- Alfenta Injection ... 1131

Aprobarbital (Aggravates orthostatic hypotension). Products include:
- Alurate Elixir ... 1883

Atenolol (Potentiation of antihypertensive effect). Products include:
- Tenoretic Tablets ... 1105
- Tenormin Tablets and I.V. Injection 1107

Benazepril Hydrochloride (Potentiation of antihypertensive effect). Products include:
- Lotensin Tablets ... 872

Bendroflumethiazide (Potentiation of antihypertensive effect). Products include:
- Corzide Tablets ... 702
- Naturetin Tablets ... 1789
- Rauzide Tablets ... 1804

Betamethasone Acetate (Hypokalemia may result). Products include:
- Celestone Soluspan Suspension ... 2081

Betamethasone Sodium Phosphate (Hypokalemia may result). Products include:
- Celestone Soluspan Suspension ... 2081

Betaxolol Hydrochloride (Potentiation of antihypertensive effect). Products include:
- Betoptic Sterile Ophthalmic Solution ... 569
- Betoptic S Sterile Ophthalmic Suspension ... 570
- Kerlone Tablets ... 2172

Buprenorphine (Aggravates orthostatic hypotension).
- No products indexed under this heading.

Butabarbital (Aggravates orthostatic hypotension). Products include:
- Pyridium Plus ... 1764

Butalbital (Aggravates orthostatic hypotension). Products include:
- Esgic-Plus Tablets ... 1002
- Esgic Tablets & Capsules ... 1001
- Fioricet Tablets ... 2006
- Fiorinal Capsules ... 2007
- Fiorinal with Codeine Capsules ... 2008
- Fiorinal Tablets ... 2007
- Phrenilin ... 838
- Sedapap Tablets 50 mg/650 mg .. 1360

Captopril (Potentiation of antihypertensive effect). Products include:
- Capoten ... 2255
- Capozide ... 2258

Carteolol Hydrochloride (Potentiation of antihypertensive effect). Products include:
- Cartrol Tablets ... 507

Chlorothiazide (Potentiation of antihypertensive effect). Products include:
- Aldoclor Tablets ... 1413
- Diupres Tablets ... 1461
- Diuril Oral ... 1464

Chlorothiazide Sodium (Potentiation of antihypertensive effect). Products include:
- Diuril Sodium Intravenous ... 1463

Chlorpropamide (Dosage adjustment of the antidiabetic drug may be required). Products include:
- Diabinese Tablets ... 1775

Chlorthalidone (Potentiation of antihypertensive effect). Products include:
- Combipres Tablets ... 678
- Tenoretic Tablets ... 1105
- Thalitone Tablets ... 687

Clonidine (Potentiation of antihypertensive effect). Products include:
- Catapres-TTS ... 677

Clonidine Hydrochloride (Potentiation of antihypertenisve effect). Products include:
- Catapres Tablets ... 676
- Combipres Tablets ... 678

Codeine (Aggravates orthostatic hypotension). Products include:
- Calcidrine Syrup ... 506

Codeine Phosphate (Aggravates orthostatic hypotension). Products include:
- Actifed with Codeine Cough Syrup.. 752
- Cheracol Cough Syrup ... 1853
- Codimal PH Syrup ... 846
- Dimetane-DC Cough Syrup ... 1857
- Empirin with Codeine Phosphate Nos. 2, 3 & 4 ... 764
- Fiorinal with Codeine Capsules ... 2008
- Isoclor Expectorant ... 982
- Naldecon CX Adult Liquid ... ▣ 521
- Novahistine DH ... 1342
- Novahistine Expectorant ... 1343
- Nucofed Capsules ... 2219
- Nucofed Expectorant ... 2219
- Nucofed Pediatric Expectorant ... 2220
- Nucofed Syrup ... 2219
- Phenaphen with Codeine Capsules 1865
- Phenaphen-650 with Codeine Tablets ... 1866
- Phenergan with Codeine ... 2497
- Phenergan VC with Codeine ... 2501
- Robitussin A-C Syrup ... 1875
- Robitussin-DAC Syrup ... 1875
- Ryna ... ▣ 741
- Soma Compound w/Codeine Tablets ... 2390
- Triaminic Expectorant w/Codeine .. 1996
- Tussi-Organidin Liquid ... 2391
- Tylenol with Codeine ... 1381

Codeine Polistirex (Aggravates orthostatic hypotension).
- No products indexed under this heading.

Cortisone Acetate (Hypokalemia may result). Products include:
- Cortone Acetate Sterile Suspension ... 1437
- Cortone Acetate Tablets ... 1439

Deserpidine (Potentiation of antihypertensive effect). Products include:
- Enduronyl ... 518
- Harmonyl Tablets ... 528
- Oreticyl ... 545

Deslanoside (Hypokalemia may exaggerate cardiac toxicity of digitalis).
- No products indexed under this heading.

Dexamethasone (Hypokalemia may result). Products include:
- AK-Trol Ointment & Suspension ... ⊙ 207
- Decadron Elixir ... 1445
- Decadron Tablets ... 1447
- Decaspray Topical Aerosol ... 1459
- Dexacidin ... ⊙ 272
- Maxidex Sterile Ophthalmic Suspension ... ⊙ 223
- Maxitrol Ophthalmic Ointment/Suspension ... ⊙ 223
- TobraDex Ophthalmic Suspension and Ointment ... ⊙ 228

Dexamethasone Acetate (Hypokalemia may result). Products include:
- Dalalone D.P. Injectable ... 999
- Decadron-LA Sterile Suspension ... 1457

Dexamethasone Sodium Phosphate (Hypokalemia may result). Products include:
- AK-Dex ... ⊙ 203
- Decadron Phosphate Respihaler ... 1454
- Decadron Phosphate Sterile Ophthalmic Ointment ... 1453
- Decadron Phosphate Sterile Ophthalmic Solution ... 1453
- Decadron Phosphate Topical Cream ... 1455
- Decadron Phosphate Turbinaire ... 1456
- Maxidex Sterile Ophthalmic Ointment ... ⊙ 222
- NeoDecadron Sterile Ophthalmic Ointment ... 1517
- NeoDecadron Sterile Ophthalmic Solution ... 1518
- NeoDecadron Topical Cream ... 1518

Dezocine (Aggravates orthostatic hypotension).

Diazoxide (Potentiation of antihypertensive effect). Products include:
- Hyperstat I.V. Injection ... 2095
- Proglycem ... 649

Diclofenac Sodium (May result in reduced diuretic effect). Products include:
- Voltaren Ophthalmic Sterile Ophthalmic Solution ... ⊙ 268
- Voltaren Tablets ... 1042

Digitoxin (Hypokalemia may exaggerate cardiac toxicity of digitalis). Products include:
- Crystodigin Tablets ... 1253

Digoxin (Hypokalemia may exaggerate cardiac toxicity of digitalis). Products include:
- Lanoxicaps ... 772
- Lanoxin Elixir Pediatric ... 775
- Lanoxin Injection ... 778
- Lanoxin Injection Pediatric ... 781
- Lanoxin Tablets ... 783

Doxazosin Mesylate (Potentiation of antihypertensive effect). Products include:
- Cardura Tablets ... 1941

Enalapril Maleate (Potentiation of antihypertensive effect). Products include:
- Vaseretic Tablets ... 1559
- Vasotec Tablets ... 1564

Enalaprilat (Potentiation of antihypertensive effect). Products include:
- Vasotec I.V. ... 1562

Enflurane (May require reduced dose of anesthetics). Products include:
- Ethrane ... 599

Esmolol Hydrochloride (Potentiation of antihypertenisive effect). Products include:
Brevibloc Injection 942

Etodolac (May result in reduced diuretic effect). Products include:
Lodine Capsules 2468

Felodipine (Potentiation of antihypertensive effect). Products include:
Plendil Extended-Release Tablets 1526

Fenoprofen Calcium (May result in reduced diuretic effects). Products include:
Nalfon Pulvules & Tablets 919

Fentanyl (Aggravates orthostatic hypotension). Products include:
Duragesic Transdermal System 1133

Fentanyl Citrate (Aggravates orthostatic hypotension). Products include:
Innovar Injection 1141
Sublimaze Injection 1146

Flurbiprofen (May result in reduced diuretic effect). Products include:
Ansaid Tablets 2319

Fosinopril Sodium (Potentiation of antihypertensive effect). Products include:
Monopril Tablets 1406

Furosemide (Potentiation of antihypertensive effect). Products include:
Lasix 1093

Glipizide (Dosage adjustment of the antidiabetic drug may be required). Products include:
Glucotrol 1952

Glyburide (Dosage adjustment of the antidiabetic drug may be required). Products include:
DiaBeta 1091
Micronase Tablets 2350

Guanabenz Acetate (Potentiation of antihypertensive effect). Products include:
Wytensin Tablets 2542

Guanethidine Monosulfate (Potentiation of antihypertensive effect). Products include:
Esimil Tablets 864
Ismelin Tablets 869

Hydralazine Hydrochloride (Potentiation of antihypertensive effect). Products include:
Apresazide Capsules 854
Apresoline Hydrochloride Parenteral (Ampuls) 856
Apresoline Hydrochloride Tablets .. 855
Apresoline-Esidrix Tablets 857
Ser-Ap-Es Tablets 881
Serpasil-Apresoline Tablets 884

Hydrocodone Bitartrate (Aggravates orthostatic hypotension). Products include:
Anexsia 5/500 Tablets 2196
Anexsia 7.5/650 Tablets 2197
Azdone Tablets 844
Codiclear DH Syrup 845
Codimal DH Syrup 846
Damason-P 1356
Hycodan Syrup, Tablets 927
Hycomine Compound Tablets 929
Hycomine Syrup 927
Hycotuss Expectorant Syrup 930
Hydrocet Capsules 835
Lortab ASA Tablets 2414
Lortab 2412
Ru-Tuss with Hydrocodone 694
Triaminic Expectorant DH 1995
Vicodin Tablets 1187
Vicodin ES Tablets 1189
Zydone Capsules 941

Hydrocodone Polistirex (Aggravates orthostatic hypotension). Products include:
Tussionex Extended-Release Suspension 988

Hydrocortisone (Hypokalemia may result). Products include:
AK-Spore H.C. .... ◉ 206
Bactine Hydrocortisone Anti-Itch Cream .... ND 625
CaldeCORT Anti-Itch Hydrocortisone Spray .... ND 560
Carmol HC Cream 1% 2296
Cortaid Spray .... ND 735
Cortenema 2244
Cortisporin Ointment 758
Cortisporin Ophthalmic Ointment Sterile 758
Cortisporin Ophthalmic Suspension Sterile 759
Cortisporin Otic Solution Sterile 760
Cortisporin Otic Suspension Sterile 760
Cortizone-5 Creme & Ointment .... ND 732
Dermolate Anti-Itch Cream .... ND 697
Eldecort Cream 1.0% 1113
Eldecort Cream 1.0% and 2.5% 1113
Fungoid HC Creme 1770
Hydrocortone Tablets 1482
Hytone 909
LazerSporin-C Solution 1770
Massengill Medicated Soft Cloth Towelettes 2192
Nutracort Cream & Lotion 1684
PediOtic Suspension Sterile 797
Synacort Creams 1%, 2.5% 2296
Vanoxide-HC Acne Lotion 911
Vioform-Hydrocortisone Cream and Mild Cream 889
Vioform-Hydrocortisone Ointment .. 889
VōSoL HC Otic Solution 2392
Vytone Cream 1% 911

Hydrocortisone Acetate (Hypokalemia may result). Products include:
Analpram-HC Rectal Cream 1% and 2.5% 970
Anusol-HC Cream 1690
Anusol-HC Suppositories 1691
Caldecort .... ND 560
Carmol HC Cream 1% 2296
Chloromycetin Hydrocortisone Ophthalmic 1694
Coly-Mycin S Otic w/Neomycin & Hydrocortisone 1708
Cortaid .... ND 735
Cortef Feminine Itch Cream .... ND 735
Corticaine .... ND 682
Cortifoam 1827
Cortisporin Cream 757
Epifoam 1828
Gynecort 5 Creme .... ND 556
Hydrocortone Acetate Sterile Suspension 1479
Lanacort 5 Creme and Ointment .. ND 557
Mantadil Cream 789
Ophthocort .... ◉ 301
Orabase HCA Oral Paste 890
Pramosone Cream, Lotion & Ointment 971
ProctoCream-HC 1834
Proctofoam-HC 1835

Hydrocortisone Sodium Phosphate (Hypokalemia may result). Products include:
Hydrocortone Phosphate Injection, Sterile 1481

Hydrocortisone Sodium Succinate (Hypokalemia may result). Products include:
Solu-Cortef Sterile Powder 2361

Hydroflumethiazide (Potentiation of antihypertensive effect). Products include:
Diucardin Tablets 2450
Saluron 718
Salutensin/Salutensin-Demi 719

Ibuprofen (May result in reduced diuretic effects). Products include:
Advil Cold & Sinus Caplets (formerly CoAdvil) 2416
Advil Ibuprofen Tablets and Caplets 2416
Children's Advil Suspension 2426
CoAdvil .... ND 748
Dristan Sinus Caplets 2419
Haltran Tablets .... ND 668
Ibuprofen .... ND 631
Medipren ibuprofen Caplets and Tablets 1362
Midol 200 Cramp Relief Formula .. ND 570
Motrin Tablets 2351
Motrin IB Caplets and Tablets .... ND 736
Nuprin Ibuprofen/Analgesic Tablets & Caplets 752
PediaProfen Suspension 1363
Rufen Tablets 691
Trendar Ibuprofen Tablets .... ND 756

Indapamide (Potentiation of antihypertensive effect). Products include:
Lozol Tablets 1843

Indomethacin (May result in reduced diuretic effects). Products include:
Indocin 1487

Indomethacin Sodium Trihydrate (May result in reduced diuretic effects). Products include:
Indocin I.V. 1490

Insulin, Human (Insulin requirement may be altered).
No products indexed under this heading.

Insulin, Human Isophane Suspension (Insulin requirement may be altered). Products include:
Humulin N, 100 Units 1270

Insulin, Human NPH (Insulin requirement may be altered). Products include:
Insulatard NPH Human 1627
Novolin N 1627
Novolin N PenFill Cartridges 1628
Novolin N Prefilled 1628

Insulin, Human Regular (Insulin requirement may be altered). Products include:
Humulin BR, 100 Units 1268
Humulin R, 100 Units 1272
Novolin R 1627
Novolin R PenFill Cartridges 1628
Novolin R Prefilled 1629
Velosulin Human 1628

Insulin, Human, Zinc Suspension (Insulin requirement may be altered). Products include:
Humulin L, 100 Units 1268
Humulin U, 100 Units 1272
Novolin L 1627

Insulin, NPH (Insulin requirement may be altered). Products include:
NPH, 40 & 100 Units 1273
Beef NPH, 100 Units 1274
Pork NPH, 100 Units 1275
Insulatard NPH 1626
NPH Insulin 1626
NPH Purified Pork Isophane Insulin 1626

Insulin, Regular (Insulin requirement may be altered). Products include:
Regular, 40 & 100 Units 1273
Beef Regular, 100 Units 1275
Pork Regular, 100 Units 1275
Pork Regular (Concentrated), 500 Units 1276
Regular Insulin 1625
Regular Purified Pork Insulin 1626
Velosulin 1627

Insulin, Zinc Crystals (Insulin requirement may be altered). Products include:
NPH, 40 & 100 Units 1273

Insulin, Zinc Suspension (Insulin requirement may be altered). Products include:
Lente, 40 & 100 Units 1272
Protamine, Zinc, 40 & 100 Units 1273
Lente Iletin I 1272
Beef Lente, 100 Units 1274
Beef Protamine Zinc, 100 Units 1274
Pork Lente, 100 Units 1275
Pork, Protamine, Zinc, 100 Units 1275
Lente Insulin 1626
Lente Purified Pork Insulin 1626
Semilente Insulin 1625
Ultralente Insulin 1626

Isoflurane (May require reduced dose of anesthetics). Products include:
Forane 600

Isradipine (Potentiation of antihypertensive effect). Products include:
DynaCirc Capsules 2004

Ketamine Hydrochloride (May require reduced dose of anesthetics). Products include:
Ketalar 1726

Ketoprofen (May result in reduced diuretic effects). Products include:
Orudis Capsules 2488

Ketorolac Tromethamine (May result in reduced diuretic effect). Products include:
Toradol IM Injection 2302

Labetalol Hydrochloride (Potentiation of antihypertensive effect). Products include:
Normodyne Injection 2108
Normodyne Tablets 2110
Normozide Tablets 2112
Trandate HCT Tablets 579
Trandate Injection 577
Trandate Tablets 579

Levorphanol Tartrate (Aggravates orthostatic hypotension). Products include:
Levo-Dromoran 1906

Lisinopril (Potentiation of antihypertensive effect). Products include:
Prinivil Tablets 1538
Prinzide Tablets 1540
Zestoretic 2274
Zestril Tablets 2277

Lithium Carbonate (High risk of lithium toxicity). Products include:
Eskalith 2214
Lithane Tablets 1596
Lithium Carbonate Capsules & Tablets 1984
Lithobid Tablets 870

Lithium Citrate (High risk of lithium toxicity). Products include:
Cibalith-S 870

Mecamylamine Hydrochloride (Potentiation of antihypertensive effect). Products include:
Inversine Tablets 1492

Meclofenamate Sodium (May result in reduced diuretic effects). Products include:
Meclomen Capsules 1739

Mefenamic Acid (May result in reduced diuretic effects). Products include:
Ponstel 1758

Meperidine Hydrochloride (Aggravates orthostatic hypotension). Products include:
Demerol 2047
Mepergan Injection 2479

Mephobarbital (Aggravates orthostatic hypotension). Products include:
Mebaral Tablets 2061

Methadone Hydrochloride (Aggravates orthostatic hypotension). Products include:
Dolophine Hydrochloride Ampoules & Vials 1260
Dolophine Hydrochloride Tablets 1261
Methadone Hydrochloride Diskets .. 1284
Methadone Hydrochloride Oral Solution & Tablets 1987

Methohexital Sodium (May require reduced dose of anesthetics). Products include:
Brevital Sodium Vials 1248

Methoxyflurane (May require reduced dose of anesthetics).
No products indexed under this heading.

Methyclothiazide (Potentiation of antihypertensive effect). Products include:
Enduron Tablets 517
Enduronyl 518

Methyldopate Hydrochloride (Potentiation of antihypertensive effect). Products include:
Aldomet Ester HCl Injection 1417

Methylprednisolone Acetate (Hypokalemia may result). Products include:
- Depo-Medrol Sterile Aqueous Suspension 2334

Methylprednisolone Sodium Succinate (Hypokalemia may result). Products include:
- Solu-Medrol Sterile Powder 2363

Metolazone (Potentiation of antihypertensive effect). Products include:
- Diulo 2129
- Mykrox ½ mg Tablets 984
- Zaroxolyn Tablets 989

Metoprolol Tartrate (Potentiation of antihypertensive effect). Products include:
- Lopressor Ampuls 1032
- Lopressor HCT Tablets 1034
- Lopressor Tablets 1032

Metyrosine (Potentiation of antihypertensive effect). Products include:
- Demser Capsules 1460

Minoxidil (Potentiation of antihypertensive effect). Products include:
- Loniten Tablets 2346
- Rogaine Topical Solution 2357

Morphine Sulfate (Aggravates orthostatic hypotension). Products include:
- Astramorph/PF Injection, USP (Preservative-Free) 618
- Duramorph 960
- Infumorph 200 and Infumorph 500 Sterile Solutions 962
- MS Contin Tablets 1814
- MSIR 1817
- Oramorph SR (Morphine Sulfate Sustained Release Tablets) 1988
- Roxanol 1991

Nadolol (Potentiation of antihypertensive effect). Products include:
- Corgard Tablets 701
- Corzide Tablets 702

Naproxen (May result in reduced diuretic effects). Products include:
- Naprosyn 2297

Naproxen Sodium (May result in reduced diuretic effects). Products include:
- Anaprox and Anaprox DS Tablets 2288

Nicardipine Hydrochloride (Potentiation of antihypertensive effect). Products include:
- Cardene Capsules 2290

Nitroglycerin (Potentiation of antihypertensive effect). Products include:
- Deponit NTG Transdermal Delivery System 2143
- Minitran Transdermal Delivery System 1312
- Nitro-Bid Ointment 1339
- Nitro-Bid Capsules 1338
- Nitrodisc 2176
- Nitro-Dur (nitroglycerin) Transdermal Infusion System 1164
- Nitrogard Tablets 1004
- Nitrolingual Spray 1846
- Nitrostat Tablets 1743
- Transderm-Nitro Transdermal Therapeutic System 2283

Norepinephrine Bitartrate (Decreased arterial responsiveness to norepinephrine). Products include:
- Levophed Bitartrate Injection 2054

Opium Alkaloids (Aggravates orthostatic hypotension). Products include:
- B & O No. 15A & No. 16A Supprettes 2395
- Pantopon Injectable 1911

Oxycodone Hydrochloride (Aggravates orthostatic hypotension). Products include:
- Percocet Tablets 950
- Percodan 951
- Roxicodone Tablets, Oral Solution & Intensol (Oxycodone) 1992
- Tylox Capsules 1382

Penbutolol Sulfate (Potentiation of antihypertensive effect). Products include:
- Levatol 1832

Pentobarbital Sodium (Aggravates orthostatic hypotension). Products include:
- Nembutal Sodium Capsules 534
- Nembutal Sodium Solution 536
- Nembutal Sodium Suppositories 538

Phenobarbital (Aggravates orthostatic hypotension). Products include:
- Arco-Lase Plus Tablets 607
- Bellergal-S Tablets 1998
- Bronkolixir ..... ⊞ 761
- Bronkotabs Tablets ..... ⊞ 762
- Donnatal 1858
- Donnatal Extentabs 1859
- Donnatal Tablets 1858
- Donnazyme Tablets 1860
- Kinesed Tablets 2272
- Phenobarbital Elixir and Tablets 1293
- Primatene Tablets-P Formula 2421
- Quadrinal Tablets 1183
- Tedral SA 1765

Phenoxybenzamine Hydrochloride (Potentiation of antihypertensive effect). Products include:
- Dibenzyline Capsules 2207

Phentolamine Mesylate (Potentiation of antihypertensive effect). Products include:
- Regitine 878

Phenylbutazone (May result in reduced diuretic effects). Products include:
- Butazolidin Capsules & Tablets 1027

Pindolol (Potentiation of antihypertensive effect). Products include:
- Visken Tablets 2036

Piroxicam (May result in reduced diuretic effects). Products include:
- Feldene Capsules 1777

Polythiazide (Potentiation of antihypertensive effect). Products include:
- Minizide Capsules 1779
- Renese Tablets 1785
- Renese-R Tablets 1786

Prazosin Hydrochloride (Potentiation of antihypertensive effect). Products include:
- Minipress Capsules 1778
- Minizide Capsules 1779

Prednisolone Acetate (Hypokalemia may result). Products include:
- AK-Cide Sterile Ophthalmic Ointment & Suspension ..... ◉ 202
- Blephamide Liquifilm Sterile Ophthalmic Suspension 586
- Blephamide S.O.P. Sterile Ophthalmic Ointment 586
- Cetapred Ointment ..... ◉ 220
- ⅛% Econopred & 1% Econopred Plus ..... ◉ 217
- Isopto Cetapred Suspension ..... ◉ 220
- Metimyd ..... ◉ 306
- Poly-Pred Liquifilm ..... ◉ 250
- Pred Forte ..... ◉ 252
- Pred Mild ..... ◉ 254
- Pred-G Liquifilm Sterile Ophthalmic Suspension ..... ◉ 252
- Pred-G S.O.P. Sterile Ophthalmic Ointment ..... ◉ 253
- Vasocidin Ointment ..... ◉ 275

Prednisolone Sodium Phosphate (Hypokalemia may result). Products include:
- AK-Pred ..... ◉ 205
- Hydeltrasol Injection, Sterile 1476
- Inflamase ..... ◉ 274
- Pediapred Oral Liquid 987
- Vasocidin Ophthalmic Solution ..... ◉ 276

Prednisolone Tebutate (Hypokalemia may result). Products include:
- Hydeltra-T.B.A. Sterile Suspension 1478

Prednisone (Hypokalemia may result). Products include:
- Deltasone Tablets 2332

Propofol (May require reduced dose of anesthetics). Products include:
- Diprivan Injection 2267

Propoxyphene Hydrochloride (Aggravates orthostatic hypotension). Products include:
- Darvon 1256
- Wygesic Tablets 2540

Propoxyphene Napsylate (Aggravates orthostatic hypotension). Products include:
- Darvon-N/Darvocet-N 1254

Propranolol Hydrochloride (Potentiation of antihypertensive effect). Products include:
- Inderal 2459
- Inderal LA Long Acting Capsules 2461
- Inderide Tablets 2463
- Inderide LA Long Acting Capsules 2465

Ramipril (Potentiation of antihypertensive effect). Products include:
- Altace Capsules 1086

Rauwolfia Serpentina (Potentiation of antihypertensive effect). Products include:
- Raudixin Tablets 1803
- Rauzide Tablets 1804

Rescinnamine (Potentiation of antihypertensive effect).
- No products indexed under this heading.

Reserpine (Potentiation of antihypertensive effect). Products include:
- Diupres Tablets 1461
- Hydromox R Tablets 1209
- Hydropres Tablets 1485
- Renese-R Tablets 1786
- Salutensin/Salutensin-Demi 719
- Ser-Ap-Es Tablets 881
- Serpasil Tablets 883
- Serpasil-Apresoline Tablets 884
- Serpasil-Esidrix Tablets 886

Secobarbital Sodium (Aggravates orthostatic hypotension). Products include:
- Seconal Sodium Pulvules 1296

Sodium Nitroprusside (Potentiation of antihypertensive effect). Products include:
- Nipride I.V. Infusion 1909

Sufentanil Citrate (Aggravates orthostatic hypotension). Products include:
- Sufenta Injection 1147

Sulindac (May result in reduced diuretic effects). Products include:
- Clinoril Tablets 1433

Terazosin Hydrochloride (Potentiation of antihypertensive effect). Products include:
- Hytrin Tablets 529

Thiamylal Sodium (Aggravates orthostatic hypotension). Products include:
- Surital Ampoules, Steri-Vials 1764

Timolol Maleate (Potentiation of antihypertensive effect). Products include:
- Blocadren Tablets 1429
- Timolide Tablets 1547
- Timoptic in Ocudose 1552
- Timoptic Sterile Ophthalmic Solution 1550

Tolazamide (Dosage adjustment of the antidiabetic drug may be required). Products include:
- Tolinase Tablets 2365

Tolbutamide (Dosage adjustment of the antidiabetic drug may be required). Products include:
- Orinase Tablets 2354

Tolmetin Sodium (May result in reduced diuretic effects). Products include:
- Tolectin (200, 400 and 600 mg) 1379

Triamcinolone (Hypokalemia may result).
- No products indexed under this heading.

Triamcinolone Acetonide (Hypokalemia may result). Products include:
- Aristocort A 1010
- Azmacort Inhaler 1837
- Kenalog Cream, Lotion & Ointment 2401
- Kenalog-10 Injection 2402
- Kenalog-40 Injection 2403
- Kenalog in Orabase 604
- Kenalog Spray 2401
- Mycolog II Cream and Ointment 2407
- Mytrex Cream & Ointment 2080
- Nasacort Nasal Inhaler 1844

Triamcinolone Diacetate (Hypokalemia may result). Products include:
- Aristocort Suspension 1008

Triamcinolone Hexacetonide (Hypokalemia may result). Products include:
- Aristospan Suspension 1011

Trimethaphan Camsylate (Potentiation of antihypertensive effect). Products include:
- Arfonad Ampuls 1887

Tubocurarine Chloride (Increased responsiveness to tubocurarine).
- No products indexed under this heading.

ALFENTA INJECTION

(Alfentanil Hydrochloride) 1131

May interact with central nervous system depressants and certain other agents. Compounds in these categories include:

Alprazolam (Enhances CNS and cardiovascular effects). Products include:
- Xanax Tablets 2367

Aprobarbital (Enhances CNS and cardiovascular effects). Products include:
- Alurate Elixir 1883

Buprenorphine (Enhances CNS and cardiovascular effects).
- No products indexed under this heading.

Buspirone Hydrochloride (Enhances CNS and cardiovascular effects). Products include:
- BuSpar 1401

Butabarbital (Enhances CNS and cardiovascular effects). Products include:
- Pyridium Plus 1764

Butalbital (Enhances CNS and cardiovascular effects). Products include:
- Esgic-Plus Tablets 1002
- Esgic Tablets & Capsules 1001
- Fioricet Tablets 2006
- Fiorinal Capsules 2007
- Fiorinal with Codeine Capsules 2008
- Fiorinal Tablets 2007
- Phrenilin 838
- Sedapap Tablets 50 mg/650 mg 1360

Chlordiazepoxide (Enhances CNS and cardiovascular effects). Products include:
- Libritabs Tablets 1930
- Limbitrol 1933
- Menrium Tablets 1934

Chlordiazepoxide Hydrochloride (Enhances CNS and cardiovascular effects). Products include:
- Librax Capsules 1929
- Librium Capsules 1931
- Librium Injectable 1932

Chlorpromazine (Enhances CNS and cardiovascular effects). Products include:
- Thorazine 2234

Chlorprothixene (Enhances CNS and cardiovascular effects). Products include:
- Taractan Tablets 1920

Chlorprothixene Hydrochloride (Enhances CNS and cardiovascular effects). Products include:
- Taractan 1920

Clorazepate Dipotassium (Enhances CNS and cardiovascular effects). Products include:
- Tranxene 556

Codeine (Enhances CNS and cardiovascular effects). Products include:
- Calcidrine Syrup 506

Codeine Phosphate (Enhances CNS and cardiovascular effects). Products include:
- Actifed with Codeine Cough Syrup .. 752
- Cheracol Cough Syrup 1853
- Codimal PH Syrup 846
- Dimetane-DC Cough Syrup 1857
- Empirin with Codeine Phosphate Nos. 2, 3 & 4 764
- Fiorinal with Codeine Capsules 2008
- Isoclor Expectorant 982
- Naldecon CX Adult Liquid .... ▣ 521
- Novahistine DH 1342
- Novahistine Expectorant 1343
- Nucofed Capsules 2219
- Nucofed Expectorant 2219
- Nucofed Pediatric Expectorant 2220
- Nucofed Syrup 2219
- Phenaphen with Codeine Capsules 1865
- Phenaphen-650 with Codeine Tablets 1866
- Phenergan with Codeine 2497
- Phenergan VC with Codeine 2501
- Robitussin A-C Syrup 1875
- Robitussin-DAC Syrup 1875
- Ryna .... ▣ 741
- Soma Compound w/Codeine Tablets 2390
- Triaminic Expectorant w/Codeine .. 1996
- Tussi-Organidin Liquid 2391
- Tylenol with Codeine 1381

Codeine Polistirex (Enhances CNS and cardiovascular effects).
- No products indexed under this heading.

Dezocine (Enhances CNS and cardiovascular effects).

Diazepam (Enhances CNS and cardiovascular effects; vasodilation, hypotension, delayed recovery). Products include:
- Valium Injectable 1937
- Valium Tablets 1939
- Valrelease Capsules 1923

Droperidol (Enhances CNS and cardiovascular effects). Products include:
- Inapsine Injection 1140
- Innovar Injection 1141

Enflurane (Enhances CNS and cardiovascular effects). Products include:
- Ethrane 599

Erythromycin (Inhibits Alfenta clearance and may increase or prolong respiratory depression). Products include:
- A/T/S Topical Gel and Topical Solution 1089
- AK-Mycin Ointment .... ⊙ 204
- Benzamycin Topical Gel 907
- E-Mycin Tablets 688
- ETS-2% 1685
- ERYC 1720
- Erycette (erythromycin 2%) Topical Solution 1678
- Ery-Tab Tablets 521
- Erythromycin Base Filmtab 525
- Erythromycin Delayed-Release Capsules, USP 526
- Ilotycin Ophthalmic Ointment 915
- PCE Dispertab Tablets 549
- Pediazole 1973
- T-Stat 2.0% Topical Solution and Pads 2409
- Theramycin Z Topical Solution 2% 1410

Erythromycin Estolate (Inhibits Alfenta clearance and may increase or prolong respiratory depression). Products include:
- Ilosone 913

Erythromycin Ethylsuccinate (Inhibits Alfenta clearance and may increase or prolong respiratory depression). Products include:
- E.E.S. 522
- EryPed 519
- Pediazole 1973

Erythromycin Gluceptate (Inhibits Alfenta clearance and may increase or prolong respiratory depression). Products include:
- Ilotycin Gluceptate, IV, Vials 915

Erythromycin Stearate (Inhibits Alfenta clearance and may increase or prolong respiratory depression). Products include:
- Erythrocin Stearate Filmtab 523

Estazolam (Enhances CNS and cardiovascular effects). Products include:
- ProSom Tablets 554

Ethchlorvynol (Enhances CNS and cardiovascular effects). Products include:
- Placidyl Capsules 553

Ethinamate (Enhances CNS and cardiovascular effects).
- No products indexed under this heading.

Fentanyl (Enhances CNS and cardiovascular effects). Products include:
- Duragesic Transdermal System 1133

Fentanyl Citrate (Enhances CNS and cardiovascular effects). Products include:
- Innovar Injection 1141
- Sublimaze Injection 1146

Fluphenazine Decanoate (Enhances CNS and cardiovascular effects). Products include:
- Prolixin Decanoate 1795

Fluphenazine Enanthate (Enhances CNS and cardiovascular effects). Products include:
- Prolixin Enanthate 1796

Fluphenazine Hydrochloride (Enhances CNS and cardiovascular effects). Products include:
- Prolixin Elixir 1793
- Prolixin Injection 1791
- Prolixin Oral Concentrate 1792
- Prolixin Tablets 1793

Flurazepam Hydrochloride (Enhances CNS and cardiovascular effects). Products include:
- Dalmane Capsules 1927

Glutethimide (Enhances CNS and cardiovascular effects).
- No products indexed under this heading.

Haloperidol (Enhances CNS and cardiovascular effects). Products include:
- Haldol Injection, Tablets and Concentrate 1373

Haloperidol Decanoate (Enhances CNS and cardiovascular effects). Products include:
- Haldol Decanoate 1375

Hydrocodone Bitartrate (Enhances CNS and cardiovascular effects). Products include:
- Anexsia 5/500 Tablets 2196
- Anexsia 7.5/650 Tablets 2197
- Azdone Tablets 844
- Codiclear DH Syrup 845
- Codimal DH Syrup 846
- Damason-P 1356
- Hycodan Syrup, Tablets 927
- Hycomine Compound Tablets 929
- Hycomine Syrup 927
- Hycotuss Expectorant Syrup 930
- Hydrocet Capsules 835
- Lortab ASA Tablets 2414
- Lortab 2412
- Ru-Tuss with Hydrocodone 694
- Triaminic Expectorant DH 1995
- Vicodin Tablets 1187
- Vicodin ES Tablets 1189
- Zydone Capsules 941

Hydrocodone Polistirex (Enhances CNS and cardiovascular effects). Products include:
- Tussionex Extended-Release Suspension 988

Hydroxyzine Hydrochloride (Enhances CNS and cardiovascular effects). Products include:
- Atarax Tablets & Syrup 1941
- Marax Tablets & DF Syrup 1954
- Vistaril Intramuscular Solution 1970

Isoflurane (Enhances CNS and cardiovascular effects). Products include:
- Forane 600

Ketamine Hydrochloride (Enhances CNS and cardiovascular effects). Products include:
- Ketalar 1726

Levorphanol Tartrate (Enhances CNS and cardiovascular effects). Products include:
- Levo-Dromoran 1906

Lorazepam (Enhances CNS and cardiovascular effects). Products include:
- Ativan Injection 2432
- Ativan Tablets 2434

Loxapine Hydrochloride (Enhances CNS and cardiovascular effects). Products include:
- Loxitane 1213

Loxapine Succinate (Enhances CNS and cardiovascular effects). Products include:
- Loxitane Capsules 1213

Meperidine Hydrochloride (Enhances CNS and cardiovascular effects). Products include:
- Demerol 2047
- Mepergan Injection 2479

Mephobarbital (Enhances CNS and cardiovascular effects). Products include:
- Mebaral Tablets 2061

Meprobamate (Enhances CNS and cardiovascular effects). Products include:
- Deprol Tablets 2382
- Equagesic Tablets 2451
- Miltown Tablets 2386
- PMB 200 and PMB 400 2504

Mesoridazine (Enhances CNS and cardiovascular effects). Products include:
- Serentil 686

Methadone Hydrochloride (Enhances CNS and cardiovascular effects). Products include:
- Dolophine Hydrochloride Ampoules & Vials 1260
- Dolophine Hydrochloride Tablets ... 1261
- Methadone Hydrochloride Diskets .. 1284
- Methadone Hydrochloride Oral Solution & Tablets 1987

Methohexital Sodium (Enhances CNS and cardiovascular effects). Products include:
- Brevital Sodium Vials 1248

Methoxyflurane (Enhances CNS and cardiovascular effects).
- No products indexed under this heading.

Midazolam Hydrochloride (Enhances CNS and cardiovascular effects). Products include:
- Versed Injection 1924

Molindone Hydrochloride (Enhances CNS and cardiovascular effects). Products include:
- Moban Tablets & Concentrate 932

Morphine Sulfate (Enhances CNS and cardiovascular effects). Products include:
- Astramorph/PF Injection, USP (Preservative-Free) 618
- Duramorph 960
- Infumorph 200 and Infumorph 500 Sterile Solutions 962
- MS Contin Tablets 1814
- MSIR 1817
- Oramorph SR (Morphine Sulfate Sustained Release Tablets) 1988
- Roxanol 1991

Opium Alkaloids (Enhances CNS and cardiovascular effects). Products include:
- B & O No. 15A & No. 16A Supprettes 2395
- Pantopon Injectable 1911

Oxazepam (Enhances CNS and cardiovascular effects). Products include:
- Serax Capsules 2522
- Serax Tablets 2522

Oxycodone Hydrochloride (Enhances CNS and cardiovascular effects). Products include:
- Percocet Tablets 950
- Percodan 951
- Roxicodone Tablets, Oral Solution & Intensol (Oxycodone) 1992
- Tylox Capsules 1382

Pentobarbital Sodium (Enhances CNS and depressant effects). Products include:
- Nembutal Sodium Capsules 534
- Nembutal Sodium Solution 536
- Nembutal Sodium Suppositories 538

Perphenazine (Enhances CNS and cardiovascular effects). Products include:
- Etrafon 2087
- Triavil Tablets 1556
- Trilafon 2123

Phenobarbital (Enhances CNS and cardiovascular effects). Products include:
- Arco-Lase Plus Tablets 607
- Bellergal-S Tablets 1998
- Bronkolixir .... ▣ 761
- Bronkotabs Tablets .... ▣ 762
- Donnatal 1858
- Donnatal Extentabs 1859
- Donnatal Tablets 1858
- Donnazyme Tablets 1860
- Kinesed Tablets 2272
- Phenobarbital Elixir and Tablets 1293
- Primatene Tablets-P Formula 2421
- Quadrinal Tablets 1183
- Tedral SA 1765

Prazepam (Enhances CNS and cardiovascular effects). Products include:
- Centrax 1693

Prochlorperazine (Enhances CNS and cardiovascular effects). Products include:
- Compazine 2201

Promethazine Hydrochloride (Enhances CNS and cardiovascular effects). Products include:
- Mepergan Injection 2479
- Phenergan with Codeine 2497
- Phenergan with Dextromethorphan 2499
- Phenergan Injection 2493
- Phenergan Suppositories 2496
- Phenergan Syrup 2495
- Phenergan Tablets 2496
- Phenergan VC 2500
- Phenergan VC with Codeine 2501

Propofol (Enhances CNS and cardiovascular effects). Products include:
- Diprivan Injection 2267

Propoxyphene Hydrochloride (Enhances CNS and cardiovascular effects). Products include:
- Darvon 1256
- Wygesic Tablets 2540

Propoxyphene Napsylate (Enhances CNS and cardiovascular effects). Products include:
- Darvon-N/Darvocet-N 1254

Quazepam (Enhances CNS and cardiovascular effects). Products include:
Doral Tablets 2383
Secobarbital Sodium (Enhances CNS and cardiovascular effects). Products include:
Seconal Sodium Pulvules 1296
Sufentanil Citrate (Enhances CNS and cardiovascular effects). Products include:
Sufenta Injection 1147
Temazepam (Enhances CNS and cardiovascular effects). Products include:
Restoril Capsules 2023
Thiamylal Sodium (Enhances CNS and cardiovascular effects). Products include:
Surital Ampoules, Steri-Vials 1764
Thioridazine Hydrochloride (Enhances CNS and cardiovascular effects). Products include:
Mellaril 2011
Thiothixene (Enhances CNS and cardiovascular effects). Products include:
Navane Capsules and Concentrate 1954
Navane Intramuscular 1956
Triazolam (Enhances CNS and cardiovascular effects). Products include:
Halcion Tablets 2340
Trifluoperazine Hydrochloride (Enhances CNS and cardiovascular effects). Products include:
Stelazine 2226

ALFERON N INJECTION
(Interferon Alfa-N3 (Human Leukocyte Derived)) 1809
No interactions described in labeling.

ALKA-MINTS CHEWABLE ANTACID
(Calcium Carbonate) .... ▣ 620
No interactions described in labeling.

ALKA-SELTZER ADVANCED FORMULA ANTACID & NON-ASPIRIN PAIN RELIEVER
(Acetaminophen, Calcium Carbonate, Citric Acid, Sodium Bicarbonate, Potassium Bicarbonate) .... ▣ 620
No interactions described in labeling.

ALKA-SELTZER EFFERVESCENT ANTACID
(Sodium Bicarbonate, Citric Acid, Potassium Bicarbonate) 1570
No interactions described in labeling.

ALKA-SELTZER EFFERVESCENT ANTACID AND PAIN RELIEVER
(Aspirin, Sodium Bicarbonate, Citric Acid) 1568
No interactions described in labeling.

ALKA-SELTZER EXTRA STRENGTH EFFERVESCENT ANTACID AND PAIN RELIEVER
(Aspirin, Sodium Bicarbonate, Citric Acid) 1570
No interactions described in labeling.

ALKA-SELTZER (FLAVORED) EFFERVESCENT ANTACID AND PAIN RELIEVER
(Aspirin, Sodium Bicarbonate, Citric Acid) 1569
No interactions described in labeling.

ALKA-SELTZER PLUS COLD MEDICINE
(Phenylpropanolamine Hydrochloride, Chlorpheniramine Maleate, Aspirin) .... ▣ 623
May interact with hypnotics and sedatives, tranquilizers, anticoagulants, antihypertensives, antidepressant drugs, and certain other agents. Compounds in these categories include:

Acebutolol Hydrochloride (Effect not specified). Products include:
Sectral Capsules 2520
Alcohol (May increase drowsiness effect).
Alprazolam (May increase drowsiness effect). Products include:
Xanax Tablets 2367
Amitriptyline Hydrochloride (Effect not specified). Products include:
Elavil 2269
Endep Tablets 1927
Etrafon 2087
Limbitrol 1933
Triavil Tablets 1556
Amoxapine (Effect not specified). Products include:
Asendin Tablets 1196
Atenolol (Effect not specified). Products include:
Tenoretic Tablets 1105
Tenormin Tablets and I.V. Injection 1107
Benazepril Hydrochloride (Effect not specified). Products include:
Lotensin Tablets 872
Bendroflumethiazide (Effect not specified). Products include:
Corzide Tablets 702
Naturetin Tablets 1789
Rauzide Tablets 1804
Betaxolol Hydrochloride (Effect not specified). Products include:
Betoptic Sterile Ophthalmic Solution 569
Betoptic S Sterile Ophthalmic Suspension 570
Kerlone Tablets 2172
Bupropion Hydrochloride (Effect not specified). Products include:
Wellbutrin Tablets 821
Buspirone Hydrochloride (May increase drowsiness effect). Products include:
BuSpar 1401
Captopril (Effect not specified). Products include:
Capoten 2255
Capozide 2258
Carteolol Hydrochloride (Effect not specified). Products include:
Cartrol Tablets 507
Chlordiazepoxide (May increase drowsiness effect). Products include:
Libritabs Tablets 1930
Limbitrol 1933
Menrium Tablets 1934
Chlordiazepoxide Hydrochloride (May increase drowsiness effect). Products include:
Librax Capsules 1929
Librium Capsules 1931
Librium Injectable 1932
Chlorothiazide (Effect not specified). Products include:
Aldoclor Tablets 1413
Diupres Tablets 1461
Diuril Oral 1464
Chlorothiazide Sodium (Effect not specified). Products include:
Diuril Sodium Intravenous 1463
Chlorpromazine (May increase drowsiness effect). Products include:
Thorazine 2234
Chlorprothixene (May increase drowsiness effect). Products include:
Taractan Tablets 1920
Chlorprothixene Hydrochloride (May increase drowsiness effect). Products include:
Taractan 1920
Chlorthalidone (Effect not specified). Products include:
Combipres Tablets 678
Tenoretic Tablets 1105
Thalitone Tablets 687
Clonidine (Effect not specified). Products include:
Catapres-TTS 677
Clonidine Hydrochloride (Effect not specified). Products include:
Catapres Tablets 676
Combipres Tablets 678
Clorazepate Dipotassium (May increase drowsiness effect). Products include:
Tranxene 556
Deserpidine (Effect not specified). Products include:
Enduronyl 518
Harmonyl Tablets 528
Oreticyl 545
Desipramine Hydrochloride (Effect not specified). Products include:
Norpramin Tablets 1340
Diazepam (May increase drowsiness effect). Products include:
Valium Injectable 1937
Valium Tablets 1939
Valrelease Capsules 1923
Diazoxide (Effect not specified). Products include:
Hyperstat I.V. Injection 2095
Proglycem 649
Dicumarol (Effect not specified). Products include:
Dicumarol Tablets 516
Doxazosin Mesylate (Effect not specified). Products include:
Cardura Tablets 1941
Doxepin Hydrochloride (Effect not specified). Products include:
Sinequan 1960
Droperidol (May increase drowsiness effect). Products include:
Inapsine Injection 1140
Innovar Injection 1141
Enalapril Maleate (Effect not specified). Products include:
Vaseretic Tablets 1559
Vasotec Tablets 1564
Enalaprilat (Effect not specified). Products include:
Vasotec I.V. 1562
Esmolol Hydrochloride (Effect not specified). Products include:
Brevibloc Injection 942
Estazolam (May increase drowsiness effect). Products include:
ProSom Tablets 554
Ethchlorvynol (May increase drowsiness effect). Products include:
Placidyl Capsules 553
Ethinamate (May increase drowsiness effect).
No products indexed under this heading.
Felodipine (Effect not specified). Products include:
Plendil Extended-Release Tablets 1526
Fluoxetine Hydrochloride (Effect not specified). Products include:
Prozac Pulvules 920
Fluphenazine Decanoate (May increase drowsiness effect). Products include:
Prolixin Decanoate 1795
Fluphenazine Enanthate (May increase drowsiness effect). Products include:
Prolixin Enanthate 1796
Fluphenazine Hydrochloride (May increase drowsiness effect). Products include:
Prolixin Elixir 1793
Prolixin Injection 1791
Prolixin Oral Concentrate 1792
Prolixin Tablets 1793
Flurazepam Hydrochloride (May increase drowsiness effect). Products include:
Dalmane Capsules 1927
Fosinopril Sodium (Effect not specified). Products include:
Monopril Tablets 1406
Furosemide (Effect not specified). Products include:
Lasix 1093
Glutethimide (May increase drowsiness effect).
No products indexed under this heading.
Guanabenz Acetate (Effect not specified). Products include:
Wytensin Tablets 2542
Guanethidine Monosulfate (Effect not specified). Products include:
Esimil Tablets 864
Ismelin Tablets 869
Haloperidol (May increase drowsiness effect). Products include:
Haldol Injection, Tablets and Concentrate 1373
Haloperidol Decanoate (May increase drowsiness effect). Products include:
Haldol Decanoate 1375
Heparin Calcium (Effect not specified). Products include:
Calciparine Injection 925
Heparin Sodium (Effect not specified). Products include:
Heparin Lock Flush Solution 2456
Heparin Sodium Vials 1264
Heparin Sodium Injection 2457
Heparin Sodium Injection, USP, Sterile Solution 2342
Hydralazine Hydrochloride (Effect not specified). Products include:
Apresazide Capsules 854
Apresoline Hydrochloride Parenteral (Ampuls) 856
Apresoline Hydrochloride Tablets .. 855
Apresoline-Esidrix Tablets 857
Ser-Ap-Es Tablets 881
Serpasil-Apresoline Tablets 884
Hydrochlorothiazide (Effect not specified). Products include:
Aldactazide 2150
Aldoril Tablets 1418
Apresazide Capsules 854
Apresoline-Esidrix Tablets 857
Capozide 2258
Dyazide Capsules 2208
Esidrix Tablets 863
Esimil Tablets 864
HydroDIURIL Tablets 1484
Hydropres Tablets 1485
Inderide Tablets 2463
Inderide LA Long Acting Capsules .. 2465
Lopressor HCT Tablets 1034
Maxzide 1215
Moduretic Tablets 1510
Normozide Tablets 2112
Oretic Tablets 544
Oreticyl 545
Prinzide Tablets 1540
Ser-Ap-Es Tablets 881
Serpasil-Esidrix Tablets 886
Timolide Tablets 1547
Trandate HCT Tablets 579
Vaseretic Tablets 1559
Zestoretic 2274
Hydroflumethiazide (Effect not specified). Products include:
Diucardin Tablets 2450
Saluron 718
Salutensin/Salutensin-Demi 719
Hydroxyzine Hydrochloride (May increase drowsiness effect). Products include:
Atarax Tablets & Syrup 1941
Marax Tablets & DF Syrup 1954

Vistaril Intramuscular Solution.......... 1970

Imipramine Hydrochloride (Effect not specified). Products include:
- Tofranil Ampuls 1038
- Tofranil Tablets 1039

Imipramine Pamoate (Effect not specified). Products include:
- Tofranil-PM Capsules 1041

Indapamide (Effect not specified). Products include:
- Lozol Tablets 1843

Isocarboxazid (Effect not specified). Products include:
- Marplan Tablets 1906

Isradipine (Effect not specified). Products include:
- DynaCirc Capsules 2004

Labetalol Hydrochloride (Effect not specified). Products include:
- Normodyne Injection 2108
- Normodyne Tablets 2110
- Normozide Tablets 2112
- Trandate HCT Tablets 579
- Trandate Injection 577
- Trandate Tablets 579

Lisinopril (Effect not specified). Products include:
- Prinivil Tablets 1538
- Prinzide Tablets 1540
- Zestoretic 2274
- Zestril Tablets 2277

Lorazepam (May increase drowsiness effect). Products include:
- Ativan Injection 2432
- Ativan Tablets 2434

Loxapine Hydrochloride (May increase drowsiness effect). Products include:
- Loxitane 1213

Loxapine Succinate (May increase drowsiness effect). Products include:
- Loxitane Capsules 1213

Maprotiline Hydrochloride (Effect not specified). Products include:
- Ludiomil Tablets 874

Mecamylamine Hydrochloride (Effect not specified). Products include:
- Inversine Tablets 1492

Meprobamate (May increase drowsiness effect). Products include:
- Deprol Tablets 2382
- Equagesic Tablets 2451
- Miltown Tablets 2386
- PMB 200 and PMB 400 2504

Mesoridazine Besylate (May increase drowsiness effect).

Methyclothiazide (Effect not specified). Products include:
- Enduron Tablets 517
- Enduronyl 518

Methyldopa (Effect not specified). Products include:
- Aldoclor Tablets 1413
- Aldomet Oral 1415
- Aldoril Tablets 1418

Methyldopate Hydrochloride (Effect not specified). Products include:
- Aldomet Ester HCl Injection 1417

Metolazone (Effect not specified). Products include:
- Diulo 2129
- Mykrox ½ mg Tablets 984
- Zaroxolyn Tablets 989

Metoprolol Tartrate (Effect not specified). Products include:
- Lopressor Ampuls 1032
- Lopressor HCT Tablets 1034
- Lopressor Tablets 1032

Metyrosine (Effect not specified). Products include:
- Demser Capsules 1460

Midazolam Hydrochloride (May increase drowsiness effect). Products include:
- Versed Injection 1924

Minoxidil (Effect not specified). Products include:
- Loniten Tablets 2346
- Rogaine Topical Solution 2357

Molindone Hydrochloride (May increase drowsiness effect). Products include:
- Moban Tablets & Concentrate 932

Nadolol (Effect not specified). Products include:
- Corgard Tablets 701
- Corzide Tablets 702

Nicardipine Hydrochloride (Effect not specified). Products include:
- Cardene Capsules 2290

Nitroglycerin (Effect not specified). Products include:
- Deponit NTG Transdermal Delivery System 2143
- Minitran Transdermal Delivery System 1312
- Nitro-Bid Ointment 1339
- Nitro-Bid Capsules 1338
- Nitrodisc 2176
- Nitro-Dur (nitroglycerin) Transdermal Infusion System 1164
- Nitrogard Tablets 1004
- Nitrolingual Spray 1846
- Nitrostat Tablets 1743
- Transderm-Nitro Transdermal Therapeutic System 2283

Nortriptyline Hydrochloride (Effect not specified). Products include:
- Pamelor 2019

Oxazepam (May increase drowsiness effect). Products include:
- Serax Capsules 2522
- Serax Tablets 2522

Penbutolol Sulfate (Effect not specified). Products include:
- Levatol 1832

Perphenazine (May increase drowsiness effect). Products include:
- Etrafon 2087
- Triavil Tablets 1556
- Trilafon 2123

Phenelzine Sulfate (Effect not specified). Products include:
- Nardil 1742

Phenoxybenzamine Hydrochloride (Effect not specified). Products include:
- Dibenzyline Capsules 2207

Phentolamine Mesylate (Effect not specified). Products include:
- Regitine 878

Pindolol (Effect not specified). Products include:
- Visken Tablets 2036

Polythiazide (Effect not specified). Products include:
- Minizide Capsules 1779
- Renese Tablets 1785
- Renese-R Tablets 1786

Prazepam (May increase drowsiness effect). Products include:
- Centrax 1693

Prazosin Hydrochloride (Effect not specified). Products include:
- Minipress Capsules 1778
- Minizide Capsules 1779

Prochlorperazine (May increase drowsiness effect). Products include:
- Compazine 2201

Promethazine Hydrochloride (May increase drowsiness effect). Products include:
- Mepergan Injection 2479
- Phenergan with Codeine 2497
- Phenergan with Dextromethorphan 2499
- Phenergan Injection 2493
- Phenergan Suppositories 2496
- Phenergan Syrup 2495
- Phenergan Tablets 2496
- Phenergan VC 2500
- Phenergan VC with Codeine 2501

Propofol (May increase drowsiness effect). Products include:
- Diprivan Injection 2267

Propranolol Hydrochloride (Effect not specified). Products include:
- Inderal 2459
- Inderal LA Long Acting Capsules 2461
- Inderide Tablets 2463
- Inderide LA Long Acting Capsules 2465

Protriptyline Hydrochloride (Effect not specified). Products include:
- Vivactil Tablets 1567

Quazepam (May increase drowsiness effect). Products include:
- Doral Tablets 2383

Ramipril (Effect not specified). Products include:
- Altace Capsules 1086

Rauwolfia Serpentina (Effect not specified). Products include:
- Raudixin Tablets 1803
- Rauzide Tablets 1804

Rescinnamine (Effect not specified).
- No products indexed under this heading.

Reserpine (Effect not specified). Products include:
- Diupres Tablets 1461
- Hydromox R Tablets 1209
- Hydropres Tablets 1485
- Renese-R Tablets 1786
- Salutensin/Salutensin-Demi 719
- Ser-Ap-Es Tablets 881
- Serpasil Tablets 883
- Serpasil-Apresoline Tablets 884
- Serpasil-Esidrix Tablets 886

Secobarbital Sodium (May increase drowsiness effect). Products include:
- Seconal Sodium Pulvules 1296

Sodium Nitroprusside (Effect not specified). Products include:
- Nipride I.V. Infusion 1909

Temazepam (May increase drowsiness effect). Products include:
- Restoril Capsules 2023

Terazosin Hydrochloride (Effect not specified). Products include:
- Hytrin Tablets 529

Thioridazine Hydrochloride (May increase drowsiness effect). Products include:
- Mellaril 2011

Thiothixene (May increase drowsiness effect). Products include:
- Navane Capsules and Concentrate 1954
- Navane Intramuscular 1956

Timolol Maleate (Effect not specified). Products include:
- Blocadren Tablets 1429
- Timolide Tablets 1547
- Timoptic in Ocudose 1552
- Timoptic Sterile Ophthalmic Solution 1550

Tranylcypromine Sulfate (Effect not specified). Products include:
- Parnate Tablets 2222

Trazodone Hydrochloride (Effect not specified). Products include:
- Desyrel and Desyrel Dividose 1404

Triazolam (May increase drowsiness effect). Products include:
- Halcion Tablets 2340

Trifluoperazine Hydrochloride (May increase drowsiness effect). Products include:
- Stelazine 2226

Trimethaphan Camsylate (Effect not specified). Products include:
- Arfonad Ampuls 1887

Trimipramine Maleate (Effect not specified). Products include:
- Surmontil Capsules 2524

Warfarin Sodium (Effect not specified). Products include:
- Coumadin Injection & Tablets 944
- Panwarfin Tablets 547

ALKA-SELTZER PLUS NIGHT-TIME COLD MEDICINE

(Phenylpropanolamine Hydrochloride, Diphenhydramine Hydrochloride, Aspirin) .... ◙ 623

May interact with hypnotics and sedatives, tranquilizers, anticoagulants, and certain other agents. Compounds in these categories include:

Acebutolol Hydrochloride (Effect not specified). Products include:
- Sectral Capsules 2520

Alcohol (Increases the drowsiness effect).

Alprazolam (May increase drowsiness effect). Products include:
- Xanax Tablets 2367

Amitriptyline Hydrochloride (Effect not specified). Products include:
- Elavil 2269
- Endep Tablets 1927
- Etrafon 2087
- Limbitrol 1933
- Triavil Tablets 1556

Amoxapine (Effect not specified). Products include:
- Asendin Tablets 1196

Atenolol (Effect not specified). Products include:
- Tenoretic Tablets 1105
- Tenormin Tablets and I.V. Injection 1107

Bendroflumethiazide (Effect not specified). Products include:
- Corzide Tablets 702
- Naturetin Tablets 1789
- Rauzide Tablets 1804

Bupropion Hydrochloride (Effect not specified). Products include:
- Wellbutrin Tablets 821

Buspirone Hydrochloride (May increase drowsiness effect). Products include:
- BuSpar 1401

Captopril (Effect not specified). Products include:
- Capoten 2255
- Capozide 2258

Carteolol Hydrochloride (Effect not specified). Products include:
- Cartrol Tablets 507

Chlordiazepoxide (May increase drowsiness effect). Products include:
- Libritabs Tablets 1930
- Limbitrol 1933
- Menrium Tablets 1934

Chlordiazepoxide Hydrochloride (May increase drowsiness effect). Products include:
- Librax Capsules 1929
- Librium Capsules 1931
- Librium Injectable 1932

Chlorothiazide (Effect not specified). Products include:
- Aldoclor Tablets 1413
- Diupres Tablets 1461
- Diuril Oral 1464

Chlorothiazide Sodium (Effect not specified). Products include:
- Diuril Sodium Intravenous 1463

Chlorpromazine (May increase drowsiness effect). Products include:
- Thorazine 2234

Chlorprothixene (May increase drowsiness effect). Products include:
- Taractan Tablets 1920

Chlorprothixene Hydrochloride (May increase drowsiness effect). Products include:
- Taractan 1920

Chlorthalidone (Effect not specified). Products include:
- Combipres Tablets 678
- Tenoretic Tablets 1105
- Thalitone Tablets 687

Clonidine (Effect not specified). Products include:
Catapres-TTS 677
Clonidine Hydrochloride (Effect not specified). Products include:
Catapres Tablets 676
Combipres Tablets 678
Clorazepate Dipotassium (May increase drowsiness effect). Products include:
Tranxene 556
Deserpidine (Effect not specified). Products include:
Enduronyl 518
Harmonyl Tablets 528
Oreticyl 545
Desipramine Hydrochloride (Effect not specified). Products include:
Norpramin Tablets 1340
Diazepam (May increase drowsiness effect). Products include:
Valium Injectable 1937
Valium Tablets 1939
Valrelease Capsules 1923
Diazoxide (Effect not specified). Products include:
Hyperstat I.V. Injection 2095
Proglycem 649
Dicumarol (Effect not specified). Products include:
Dicumarol Tablets 516
Doxepin Hydrochloride (Effect not specified). Products include:
Sinequan 1960
Droperidol (May increase drowsiness effect). Products include:
Inapsine Injection 1140
Innovar Injection 1141
Enalapril Maleate (Effect not specified). Products include:
Vaseretic Tablets 1559
Vasotec Tablets 1564
Enalaprilat (Effect not specified). Products include:
Vasotec I.V. 1562
Esmolol Hydrochloride (Effect not specified). Products include:
Brevibloc Injection 942
Estazolam (May increase drowsiness effect). Products include:
ProSom Tablets 554
Ethchlorvynol (May increase drowsiness effect). Products include:
Placidyl Capsules 553
Ethinamate (May increase drowsiness effect).
No products indexed under this heading.
Fluoxetine Hydrochloride (Effect not specified). Products include:
Prozac Pulvules 920
Fluphenazine Decanoate (May increase drowsiness effect). Products include:
Prolixin Decanoate 1795
Fluphenazine Enanthate (May increase drowsiness effect). Products include:
Prolixin Enanthate 1796
Fluphenazine Hydrochloride (May increase drowsiness effect). Products include:
Prolixin Elixir 1793
Prolixin Injection 1791
Prolixin Oral Concentrate 1792
Prolixin Tablets 1793
Flurazepam Hydrochloride (May increase drowsiness effect). Products include:
Dalmane Capsules 1927
Furosemide (Effect not specified). Products include:
Lasix 1093
Glutethimide (May increase drowsiness effect).
No products indexed under this heading.
Guanabenz Acetate (Effect not specified). Products include:
Wytensin Tablets 2542
Guanethidine Monosulfate (Effect not specified). Products include:
Esimil Tablets 864
Ismelin Tablets 869
Haloperidol (May increase drowsiness effect). Products include:
Haldol Injection, Tablets and Concentrate 1373
Haloperidol Decanoate (May increase drowsiness effect). Products include:
Haldol Decanoate 1375
Heparin Calcium (Effect not specified). Products include:
Calciparine Injection 925
Heparin Sodium (Effect not specified). Products include:
Heparin Lock Flush Solution 2456
Heparin Sodium Vials 1264
Heparin Sodium Injection 2457
Heparin Sodium Injection, USP, Sterile Solution 2342
Hydralazine Hydrochloride (Effect not specified). Products include:
Apresazide Capsules 854
Apresoline Hydrochloride Parenteral (Ampuls) 856
Apresoline Hydrochloride Tablets 855
Apresoline-Esidrix Tablets 857
Ser-Ap-Es Tablets 881
Serpasil-Apresoline Tablets 884
Hydrochlorothiazide (Effect not specified). Products include:
Aldactazide 2150
Aldoril Tablets 1418
Apresazide Capsules 854
Apresoline-Esidrix Tablets 857
Capozide 2258
Dyazide Capsules 2208
Esidrix Tablets 863
Esimil Tablets 864
HydroDIURIL Tablets 1484
Hydropres Tablets 1485
Inderide Tablets 2463
Inderide LA Long Acting Capsules 2465
Lopressor HCT Tablets 1034
Maxzide 1215
Moduretic Tablets 1510
Normozide Tablets 2112
Oretic Tablets 544
Oreticyl 545
Prinzide Tablets 1540
Ser-Ap-Es Tablets 881
Serpasil-Esidrix Tablets 886
Timolide Tablets 1547
Trandate HCT Tablets 579
Vaseretic Tablets 1559
Zestoretic 2274
Hydroflumethiazide (Effect not specified). Products include:
Diucardin Tablets 2450
Saluron 718
Salutensin/Salutensin-Demi 719
Hydroxyzine Hydrochloride (May increase drowsiness effect). Products include:
Atarax Tablets & Syrup 1941
Marax Tablets & DF Syrup 1954
Vistaril Intramuscular Solution 1970
Imipramine Hydrochloride (Effect not specified). Products include:
Tofranil Ampuls 1038
Tofranil Tablets 1039
Imipramine Pamoate (Effect not specified). Products include:
Tofranil-PM Capsules 1041
Indapamide (Effect not specified). Products include:
Lozol Tablets 1843
Isocarboxazid (Effect not specified). Products include:
Marplan Tablets 1906
Labetalol Hydrochloride (Effect not specified). Products include:
Normodyne Injection 2108
Normodyne Tablets 2110
Normozide Tablets 2112
Trandate HCT Tablets 579
Trandate Injection 577
Trandate Tablets 579
Lisinopril (Effect not specified). Products include:
Prinivil Tablets 1538
Prinzide Tablets 1540
Zestoretic 2274
Zestril Tablets 2277
Lorazepam (May increase drowsiness effect). Products include:
Ativan Injection 2432
Ativan Tablets 2434
Loxapine Hydrochloride (May increase drowsiness effect). Products include:
Loxitane 1213
Loxapine Succinate (May increase drowsiness effect). Products include:
Loxitane Capsules 1213
Maprotiline Hydrochloride (Effect not specified). Products include:
Ludiomil Tablets 874
Mecamylamine Hydrochloride (Effect not specified). Products include:
Inversine Tablets 1492
Meprobamate (May increase drowsiness effect). Products include:
Deprol Tablets 2382
Equagesic Tablets 2451
Miltown Tablets 2386
PMB 200 and PMB 400 2504
Mesoridazine Besylate (May increase drowsiness effect).
Methyclothiazide (Effect not specified). Products include:
Enduron Tablets 517
Enduronyl 518
Methyldopa (Effect not specified). Products include:
Aldoclor Tablets 1413
Aldomet Oral 1415
Aldoril Tablets 1418
Methyldopate Hydrochloride (Effect not specified). Products include:
Aldomet Ester HCl Injection 1417
Metolazone (Effect not specified). Products include:
Diulo 2129
Mykrox ½ mg Tablets 984
Zaroxolyn Tablets 989
Metoprolol Tartrate (Effect not specified). Products include:
Lopressor Ampuls 1032
Lopressor HCT Tablets 1034
Lopressor Tablets 1032
Metyrosine (Effect not specified). Products include:
Demser Capsules 1460
Midazolam Hydrochloride (May increase drowsiness effect). Products include:
Versed Injection 1924
Minoxidil (Effect not specified). Products include:
Loniten Tablets 2346
Rogaine Topical Solution 2357
Molindone Hydrochloride (May increase drowsiness effect). Products include:
Moban Tablets & Concentrate 932
Nadolol (Effect not specified). Products include:
Corgard Tablets 701
Corzide Tablets 702
Nicardipine Hydrochloride (Effect not specified). Products include:
Cardene Capsules 2290
Nitroglycerin (Effect not specified). Products include:
Deponit NTG Transdermal Delivery System 2143
Minitran Transdermal Delivery System 1312
Nitro-Bid Ointment 1339
Nitro-Bid Capsules 1338
Nitrodisc 2176
Nitro-Dur (nitroglycerin) Transdermal Infusion System 1164
Nitrogard Tablets 1004
Nitrolingual Spray 1846
Nitrostat Tablets 1743
Transderm-Nitro Transdermal Therapeutic System 2283
Nortriptyline Hydrochloride (Effect not specified). Products include:
Pamelor 2019
Oxazepam (May increase drowsiness effect). Products include:
Serax Capsules 2522
Serax Tablets 2522
Penbutolol Sulfate (Effect not specified). Products include:
Levatol 1832
Perphenazine (May increase drowsiness effect). Products include:
Etrafon 2087
Triavil Tablets 1556
Trilafon 2123
Phenelzine Sulfate (Effect not specified). Products include:
Nardil 1742
Phenoxybenzamine Hydrochloride (Effect not specified). Products include:
Dibenzyline Capsules 2207
Phentolamine Mesylate (Effect not specified). Products include:
Regitine 878
Pindolol (Effect not specified). Products include:
Visken Tablets 2036
Polythiazide (Effect not specified). Products include:
Minizide Capsules 1779
Renese Tablets 1785
Renese-R Tablets 1786
Prazepam (May increase drowsiness effect). Products include:
Centrax 1693
Prazosin Hydrochloride (Effect not specified). Products include:
Minipress Capsules 1778
Minizide Capsules 1779
Prochlorperazine (May increase drowsiness effect). Products include:
Compazine 2201
Promethazine Hydrochloride (May increase drowsiness effect). Products include:
Mepergan Injection 2479
Phenergan with Codeine 2497
Phenergan with Dextromethorphan 2499
Phenergan Injection 2493
Phenergan Suppositories 2496
Phenergan Syrup 2495
Phenergan Tablets 2496
Phenergan VC 2500
Phenergan VC with Codeine 2501
Propofol (May increase drowsiness effect). Products include:
Diprivan Injection 2267
Propranolol Hydrochloride (Effect not specified). Products include:
Inderal 2459
Inderal LA Long Acting Capsules 2461
Inderide Tablets 2463
Inderide LA Long Acting Capsules 2465
Protriptyline Hydrochloride (Effect not specified). Products include:
Vivactil Tablets 1567
Quazepam (May increase drowsiness effect). Products include:
Doral Tablets 2383
Rauwolfia Serpentina (Effect not specified). Products include:
Raudixin Tablets 1803
Rauzide Tablets 1804
Rescinnamine (Effect not specified).
No products indexed under this heading.

Reserpine (Effect not specified). Products include:
- Diupres Tablets 1461
- Hydromox R Tablets 1209
- Hydropres Tablets 1485
- Renese-R Tablets 1786
- Salutensin/Salutensin-Demi 719
- Ser-Ap-Es Tablets 881
- Serpasil Tablets 883
- Serpasil-Apresoline Tablets 884
- Serpasil-Esidrix Tablets 886

Secobarbital Sodium (May increase drowsiness effect). Products include:
- Seconal Sodium Pulvules 1296

Sodium Nitroprusside (Effect not specified). Products include:
- Nipride I.V. Infusion 1909

Temazepam (May increase drowsiness effect). Products include:
- Restoril Capsules 2023

Terazosin Hydrochloride (Effect not specified). Products include:
- Hytrin Tablets 529

Thioridazine Hydrochloride (May increase drowsiness effect). Products include:
- Mellaril 2011

Thiothixene (May increase drowsiness effect). Products include:
- Navane Capsules and Concentrate 1954
- Navane Intramuscular 1956

Timolol Maleate (Effect not specified). Products include:
- Blocadren Tablets 1429
- Timolide Tablets 1547
- Timoptic in Ocudose 1552
- Timoptic Sterile Ophthalmic Solution 1550

Tranylcypromine Sulfate (Effect not specified). Products include:
- Parnate Tablets 2222

Trazodone Hydrochloride (Effect not specified). Products include:
- Desyrel and Desyrel Dividose 1404

Triazolam (May increase drowsiness effect). Products include:
- Halcion Tablets 2340

Trifluoperazine Hydrochloride (May increase drowsiness effect). Products include:
- Stelazine 2226

Trimethaphan Camsylate (Effect not specified). Products include:
- Arfonad Ampuls 1887

Trimipramine Maleate (Effect not specified). Products include:
- Surmontil Capsules 2524

Warfarin Sodium (Effect not specified). Products include:
- Coumadin Injection & Tablets 944
- Panwarfin Tablets 547

ALKA SELTZER PLUS SINUS ALLERGY MEDICINE

(Phenylpropanolamine Bitartrate, Aspirin, Brompheniramine Maleate) 624

May interact with hypnotics and sedatives, tranquilizers, oral anticoagulants, antihypertensives, antidepressant drugs, and certain other agents. Compounds in these categories include:

Acebutolol Hydrochloride (Effect not specified). Products include:
- Sectral Capsules 2520

Alcohol (Increases the drowsiness effect).

Alprazolam (Increases the drowsiness effect). Products include:
- Xanax Tablets 2367

Amitriptyline Hydrochloride (Effect not specified). Products include:
- Elavil 2269
- Endep Tablets 1927
- Etrafon 2087
- Limbitrol 1933
- Triavil Tablets 1556

Amoxapine (Effect not specified). Products include:
- Asendin Tablets 1196

Atenolol (Effect not specified). Products include:
- Tenoretic Tablets 1105
- Tenormin Tablets and I.V. Injection 1107

Benazepril Hydrochloride (Effect not specified). Products include:
- Lotensin Tablets 872

Bendroflumethiazide (Effect not specified). Products include:
- Corzide Tablets 702
- Naturetin Tablets 1789
- Rauzide Tablets 1804

Betaxolol Hydrochloride (Effect not specified). Products include:
- Betoptic Sterile Ophthalmic Solution 569
- Betoptic S Sterile Ophthalmic Suspension 570
- Kerlone Tablets 2172

Bupropion Hydrochloride (Effect not specified). Products include:
- Wellbutrin Tablets 821

Buspirone Hydrochloride (Increases the drowsiness effect). Products include:
- BuSpar 1401

Captopril (Effect not specified). Products include:
- Capoten 2255
- Capozide 2258

Carteolol Hydrochloride (Effect not specified). Products include:
- Cartrol Tablets 507

Chlordiazepoxide (Increases the drowsiness effect). Products include:
- Libritabs Tablets 1930
- Limbitrol 1933
- Menrium Tablets 1934

Chlordiazepoxide Hydrochloride (Increases the drowsiness effect). Products include:
- Librax Capsules 1929
- Librium Capsules 1931
- Librium Injectable 1932

Chlorothiazide (Effect not specified). Products include:
- Aldoclor Tablets 1413
- Diupres Tablets 1461
- Diuril Oral 1464

Chlorothiazide Sodium (Effect not specified). Products include:
- Diuril Sodium Intravenous 1463

Chlorpromazine (Increases the drowsiness effect). Products include:
- Thorazine 2234

Chlorprothixene (Increases the drowsiness effect). Products include:
- Taractan Tablets 1920

Chlorprothixene Hydrochloride (Increases the drowsiness effect). Products include:
- Taractan 1920

Chlorthalidone (Effect not specified). Products include:
- Combipres Tablets 678
- Tenoretic Tablets 1105
- Thalitone Tablets 687

Clonidine (Effect not specified). Products include:
- Catapres-TTS 677

Clonidine Hydrochloride (Effect not specified). Products include:
- Catapres Tablets 676
- Combipres Tablets 678

Clorazepate Dipotassium (Increases the drowsiness effect). Products include:
- Tranxene 556

Deserpidine (Effect not specified). Products include:
- Enduronyl 518
- Harmonyl Tablets 528
- Oreticyl 545

Desipramine Hydrochloride (Effect not specified). Products include:
- Norpramin Tablets 1340

Diazepam (Increases the drowsiness effect). Products include:
- Valium Injectable 1937
- Valium Tablets 1939
- Valrelease Capsules 1923

Diazoxide (Effect not specified). Products include:
- Hyperstat I.V. Injection 2095
- Proglycem 649

Dicumarol (Effect not specified). Products include:
- Dicumarol Tablets 516

Doxazosin Mesylate (Effect not specified). Products include:
- Cardura Tablets 1941

Doxepin Hydrochloride (Effect not specified). Products include:
- Sinequan 1960

Droperidol (Increases the drowsiness effect). Products include:
- Inapsine Injection 1140
- Innovar Injection 1141

Enalapril Maleate (Effect not specified). Products include:
- Vaseretic Tablets 1559
- • Vasotec Tablets 1564

Enalaprilat (Effect not specified). Products include:
- Vasotec I.V. 1562

Esmolol Hydrochloride (Effect not specified). Products include:
- Brevibloc Injection 942

Estazolam (Increases the drowsiness effect). Products include:
- ProSom Tablets 554

Ethchlorvynol (Increases the drowsiness effect). Products include:
- Placidyl Capsules 553

Ethinamate (Increases the drowsiness effect).
- No products indexed under this heading.

Felodipine (Effect not specified). Products include:
- Plendil Extended-Release Tablets 1526

Fluoxetine Hydrochloride (Effect not specified). Products include:
- Prozac Pulvules 920

Fluphenazine Decanoate (Increases the drowsiness effect). Products include:
- Prolixin Decanoate 1795

Fluphenazine Enanthate (Increases the drowsiness effect). Products include:
- Prolixin Enanthate 1796

Fluphenazine Hydrochloride (Increases the drowsiness effect). Products include:
- Prolixin Elixir 1793
- Prolixin Injection 1791
- Prolixin Oral Concentrate 1792
- Prolixin Tablets 1793

Flurazepam Hydrochloride (Increases the drowsiness effect). Products include:
- Dalmane Capsules 1927

Fosinopril Sodium (Effect not specified). Products include:
- Monopril Tablets 1406

Furosemide (Effect not specified). Products include:
- Lasix 1093

Glutethimide (Increases the drowsiness effect).
- No products indexed under this heading.

Guanabenz Acetate (Effect not specified). Products include:
- Wytensin Tablets 2542

Guanethidine Monosulfate (Effect not specified). Products include:
- Esimil Tablets 864
- Ismelin Tablets 869

Haloperidol (Increases the drowsiness effect). Products include:
- Haldol Injection, Tablets and Concentrate 1373

Haloperidol Decanoate (Increases the drowsiness effect). Products include:
- Haldol Decanoate 1375

Hydralazine Hydrochloride (Effect not specified). Products include:
- Apresazide Capsules 854
- Apresoline Hydrochloride Parenteral (Ampuls) 856
- Apresoline Hydrochloride Tablets 855
- Apresoline-Esidrix Tablets 857
- Ser-Ap-Es Tablets 881
- Serpasil-Apresoline Tablets 884

Hydrochlorothiazide (Effect not specified). Products include:
- Aldactazide 2150
- Aldoril Tablets 1418
- Apresazide Capsules 854
- Apresoline-Esidrix Tablets 857
- Capozide 2258
- Dyazide Capsules 2208
- Esidrix Tablets 863
- Esimil Tablets 864
- HydroDIURIL Tablets 1484
- Hydropres Tablets 1485
- Inderide Tablets 2463
- Inderide LA Long Acting Capsules 2465
- Lopressor HCT Tablets 1034
- Maxzide 1215
- Moduretic Tablets 1510
- Normozide Tablets 2112
- Oretic Tablets 544
- Oreticyl 545
- Prinzide Tablets 1540
- Ser-Ap-Es Tablets 881
- Serpasil-Esidrix Tablets 886
- Timolide Tablets 1547
- Trandate HCT Tablets 579
- Vaseretic Tablets 1559
- Zestoretic 2274

Hydroflumethiazide (Effect not specified). Products include:
- Diucardin Tablets 2450
- Saluron 718
- Salutensin/Salutensin-Demi 719

Hydroxyzine Hydrochloride (Increases the drowsiness effect). Products include:
- Atarax Tablets & Syrup 1941
- Marax Tablets & DF Syrup 1954
- Vistaril Intramuscular Solution 1970

Imipramine Hydrochloride (Effect not specified). Products include:
- Tofranil Ampuls 1038
- Tofranil Tablets 1039

Imipramine Pamoate (Effect not specified). Products include:
- Tofranil-PM Capsules 1041

Indapamide (Effect not specified). Products include:
- Lozol Tablets 1843

Isocarboxazid (Effect not specified). Products include:
- Marplan Tablets 1906

Isradipine (Effect not specified). Products include:
- DynaCirc Capsules 2004

Labetalol Hydrochloride (Effect not specified). Products include:
- Normodyne Injection 2108
- Normodyne Tablets 2110
- Normozide Tablets 2112
- Trandate HCT Tablets 579
- Trandate Injection 577
- Trandate Tablets 579

Lisinopril (Effect not specified). Products include:
- Prinivil Tablets 1538
- Prinzide Tablets 1540
- Zestoretic 2274
- Zestril Tablets 2277

Lorazepam (Increases the drowsiness effect). Products include:
- Ativan Injection 2432
- Ativan Tablets 2434

Loxapine Hydrochloride (Increases the drowsiness effect). Products include:
- Loxitane 1213

Loxapine Succinate (Increases the drowsiness effect). Products include:
- Loxitane Capsules 1213

Maprotiline Hydrochloride (Effect not specified). Products include:
- Ludiomil Tablets 874

Mecamylamine Hydrochloride (Effect not specified). Products include:
- Inversine Tablets 1492

Meprobamate (Increases the drowsiness effect). Products include:
- Deprol Tablets 2382
- Equagesic Tablets 2451
- Miltown Tablets 2386
- PMB 200 and PMB 400 2504

Mesoridazine Besylate (Increases the drowsiness effect).

Methyclothiazide (Effect not specified). Products include:
- Enduron Tablets 517
- Enduronyl 518

Methyldopa (Effect not specified). Products include:
- Aldoclor Tablets 1413
- Aldomet Oral 1415
- Aldoril Tablets 1418

Methyldopate Hydrochloride (Effect not specified). Products include:
- Aldomet Ester HCl Injection 1417

Metolazone (Effect not specified). Products include:
- Diulo 2129
- Mykrox ½ mg Tablets 984
- Zaroxolyn Tablets 989

Metoprolol Tartrate (Effect not specified). Products include:
- Lopressor Ampuls 1032
- Lopressor HCT Tablets 1034
- Lopressor Tablets 1032

Metyrosine (Effect not specified). Products include:
- Demser Capsules 1460

Midazolam Hydrochloride (Increases the drowsiness effect). Products include:
- Versed Injection 1924

Minoxidil (Effect not specified). Products include:
- Loniten Tablets 2346
- Rogaine Topical Solution 2357

Molindone Hydrochloride (Increases the drowsiness effect). Products include:
- Moban Tablets & Concentrate 932

Nadolol (Effect not specified). Products include:
- Corgard Tablets 701
- Corzide Tablets 702

Nicardipine Hydrochloride (Effect not specified). Products include:
- Cardene Capsules 2290

Nitroglycerin (Effect not specified). Products include:
- Deponit NTG Transdermal Delivery System 2143
- Minitran Transdermal Delivery System 1312
- Nitro-Bid Ointment 1339
- Nitro-Bid Capsules 1338
- Nitrodisc 2176
- Nitro-Dur (nitroglycerin) Transdermal Infusion System 1164
- Nitrogard Tablets 1004
- Nitrolingual Spray 1846
- Nitrostat Tablets 1743
- Transderm-Nitro Transdermal Therapeutic System 2283

Nortriptyline Hydrochloride (Effect not specified). Products include:
- Pamelor 2019

Oxazepam (Increases the drowsiness effect). Products include:
- Serax Capsules 2522
- Serax Tablets 2522

Penbutolol Sulfate (Effect not specified). Products include:
- Levatol 1832

Perphenazine (Increases the drowsiness effect). Products include:
- Etrafon 2087
- Triavil Tablets 1556
- Trilafon 2123

Phenelzine Sulfate (Effect not specified). Products include:
- Nardil 1742

Phenoxybenzamine Hydrochloride (Effect not specified). Products include:
- Dibenzyline Capsules 2207

Phentolamine Mesylate (Effect not specified). Products include:
- Regitine 878

Pindolol (Effect not specified). Products include:
- Visken Tablets 2036

Polythiazide (Effect not specified). Products include:
- Minizide Capsules 1779
- Renese Tablets 1785
- Renese-R Tablets 1786

Prazepam (Increases the drowsiness effect). Products include:
- Centrax 1693

Prazosin Hydrochloride (Effect not specified). Products include:
- Minipress Capsules 1778
- Minizide Capsules 1779

Prochlorperazine (Increases the drowsiness effect). Products include:
- Compazine 2201

Promethazine Hydrochloride (Increases the drowsiness effect). Products include:
- Mepergan Injection 2479
- Phenergan with Codeine 2497
- Phenergan with Dextromethorphan 2499
- Phenergan Injection 2493
- Phenergan Suppositories 2496
- Phenergan Syrup 2495
- Phenergan Tablets 2496
- Phenergan VC 2500
- Phenergan VC with Codeine 2501

Propofol (Increases the drowsiness effect). Products include:
- Diprivan Injection 2267

Propranolol Hydrochloride (Effect not specified). Products include:
- Inderal 2459
- Inderal LA Long Acting Capsules 2461
- Inderide Tablets 2463
- Inderide LA Long Acting Capsules .. 2465

Protriptyline Hydrochloride (Effect not specified). Products include:
- Vivactil Tablets 1567

Quazepam (Increases the drowsiness effect). Products include:
- Doral Tablets 2383

Ramipril (Effect not specified). Products include:
- Altace Capsules 1086

Rauwolfia Serpentina (Effect not specified). Products include:
- Raudixin Tablets 1803
- Rauzide Tablets 1804

Rescinnamine (Effect not specified).
- No products indexed under this heading.

Reserpine (Effect not specified). Products include:
- Diupres Tablets 1461
- Hydromox R Tablets 1209
- Hydropres Tablets 1485
- Renese-R Tablets 1786
- Salutensin/Salutensin-Demi 719
- Ser-Ap-Es Tablets 881
- Serpasil Tablets 883
- Serpasil-Apresoline Tablets 884
- Serpasil-Esidrix Tablets 886

Secobarbital Sodium (Increases the drowsiness effect). Products include:
- Seconal Sodium Pulvules 1296

Sodium Nitroprusside (Effect not specified). Products include:
- Nipride I.V. Infusion 1909

Temazepam (Increases the drowsiness effect). Products include:
- Restoril Capsules 2023

Terazosin Hydrochloride (Effect not specified). Products include:
- Hytrin Tablets 529

Thioridazine Hydrochloride (Increases the drowsiness effect). Products include:
- Mellaril 2011

Thiothixene (Increases the drowsiness effect). Products include:
- Navane Capsules and Concentrate 1954
- Navane Intramuscular 1956

Timolol Maleate (Effect not specified). Products include:
- Blocadren Tablets 1429
- Timolide Tablets 1547
- Timoptic in Ocudose 1552
- Timoptic Sterile Ophthalmic Solution 1550

Tranylcypromine Sulfate (Effect not specified). Products include:
- Parnate Tablets 2222

Trazodone Hydrochloride (Effect not specified). Products include:
- Desyrel and Desyrel Dividose 1404

Triazolam (Increases the drowsiness effect). Products include:
- Halcion Tablets 2340

Trifluoperazine Hydrochloride (Increases the drowsiness effect). Products include:
- Stelazine 2226

Trimethaphan Camsylate (Effect not specified). Products include:
- Arfonad Ampuls 1887

Trimipramine Maleate (Effect not specified). Products include:
- Surmontil Capsules 2524

Warfarin Sodium (Effect not specified). Products include:
- Coumadin Injection & Tablets 944
- Panwarfin Tablets 547

ALKERAN TABLETS
(Melphalan) 754
No interactions described in labeling.

ALLBEE WITH C CAPLETS
(Vitamin B Complex With Vitamin C) .... ▣ 670
No interactions described in labeling.

ALLBEE C-800 PLUS IRON TABLETS
(Ferrous Fumarate, Vitamin B Complex With Vitamin C) .... ▣ 670
May interact with tetracyclines. Compounds in this category include:

Demeclocycline Hydrochloride (Iron products interfere with absorption of oral tetracyclines). Products include:
- Declomycin Capsules, Tablets 1199

Doxycycline Calcium (Iron products interfere with absorption of oral tetracyclines).
- No products indexed under this heading.

Doxycycline Hyclate (Iron products interfere with absorption of oral tetracyclines). Products include:
- Doryx Capsules 1717
- Vibramycin Hyclate Capsules 1787
- Vibramycin Hyclate Intravenous 1968
- Vibra-Tabs Film Coated Tablets 1787

Doxycycline Monohydrate (Iron products interfere with absorption of oral tetracyclines). Products include:
- Monodox Capsules 1630
- Vibramycin Monohydrate for Oral Suspension 1787

Methacycline Hydrochloride (Iron products interfere with absorption of oral tetracyclines).
- No products indexed under this heading.

Minocycline Hydrochloride (Iron products interfere with absorption of oral tetracyclines). Products include:
- Minocin Intravenous 1221
- Minocin Oral Suspension 1224
- Minocin Pellet-Filled Capsules 1222

Oxytetracycline Hydrochloride (Iron products interfere with absorption of oral tetracyclines). Products include:
- Terra-Cortril Ophthalmic Suspension 1963
- Terramycin Capsules 1786
- Terramycin Intramuscular Solution 1964
- Terramycin with Polymyxin B Sulfate Ophthalmic Ointment 1965

Tetracycline Hydrochloride (Iron products interfere with absorption of oral tetracyclines). Products include:
- Achromycin V Capsules 1193
- Achromycin Ophthalmic Ointment 1% .... ⊙ 307
- Achromycin Ophthalmic Suspension 1% .... ⊙ 308
- Topicycline for Topical Solution 1856

ALLBEE C-800 TABLETS
(Vitamin B Complex With Vitamin C) .... ▣ 670
No interactions described in labeling.

ALLEREST CHILDREN'S CHEWABLE TABLETS
(Chlorpheniramine Maleate, Phenylpropanolamine Hydrochloride) .... ▣ 559
See **Allerest Maximum Strength Tablets**

ALLEREST HEADACHE STRENGTH TABLETS
(Acetaminophen, Chlorpheniramine Maleate, Phenylpropanolamine Hydrochloride) .... ▣ 559
See **Allerest Maximum Strength Tablets**

ALLEREST 12 HOUR CAPLETS
(Chlorpheniramine Maleate, Phenylpropanolamine Hydrochloride) .... ▣ 559
See **Allerest Maximum Strength Tablets**

ALLEREST MAXIMUM STRENGTH TABLETS
(Chlorpheniramine Maleate, Phenylpropanolamine Hydrochloride) .... ▣ 559
May interact with monoamine oxidase inhibitors, central nervous system depressants, and certain other agents. Compounds in these categories include:

Alcohol (Concurrent use produces additive effects).

Alfentanil Hydrochloride (Concurrent use produces additive effects). Products include:
- Alfenta Injection 1131

Alprazolam (Concurrent use produces additive effects). Products include:
- Xanax Tablets 2367

Aprobarbital (Concurrent use produces additive effects). Products include:
- Alurate Elixir ... 1883

Buprenorphine (Concurrent use produces additive effects).
- No products indexed under this heading.

Buspirone Hydrochloride (Concurrent use produces additive effects). Products include:
- BuSpar ... 1401

Butabarbital (Concurrent use produces additive effects). Products include:
- Pyridium Plus ... 1764

Butalbital (Concurrent use produces additive effects). Products include:
- Esgic-Plus Tablets ... 1002
- Esgic Tablets & Capsules ... 1001
- Fioricet Tablets ... 2006
- Fiorinal Capsules ... 2007
- Fiorinal with Codeine Capsules ... 2008
- Fiorinal Tablets ... 2007
- Phrenilin ... 838
- Sedapap Tablets 50 mg/650 mg .. 1360

Chlordiazepoxide (Concurrent use produces additive effects). Products include:
- Libritabs Tablets ... 1930
- Limbitrol ... 1933
- Menrium Tablets ... 1934

Chlordiazepoxide Hydrochloride (Concurrent use produces additive effects). Products include:
- Librax Capsules ... 1929
- Librium Capsules ... 1931
- Librium Injectable ... 1932

Chlorpromazine (Concurrent use produces additive effects). Products include:
- Thorazine ... 2234

Chlorprothixene (Concurrent use produces additive effects). Products include:
- Taractan Tablets ... 1920

Chlorprothixene Hydrochloride (Concurrent use produces additive effects). Products include:
- Taractan ... 1920

Clorazepate Dipotassium (Concurrent use produces additive effects). Products include:
- Tranxene ... 556

Codeine (Concurrent use produces additive effects). Products include:
- Calcidrine Syrup ... 506

Codeine Phosphate (Concurrent use produces additive effects). Products include:
- Actifed with Codeine Cough Syrup.. 752
- Cheracol Cough Syrup ... 1853
- Codimal PH Syrup ... 846
- Dimetane-DC Cough Syrup ... 1857
- Empirin with Codeine Phosphate Nos. 2, 3 & 4 ... 764
- Fiorinal with Codeine Capsules ... 2008
- Isoclor Expectorant ... 982
- Naldecon CX Adult Liquid ... ▣ 521
- Novahistine DH ... 1342
- Novahistine Expectorant ... 1343
- Nucofed Capsules ... 2219
- Nucofed Expectorant ... 2219
- Nucofed Pediatric Expectorant ... 2220
- Nucofed Syrup ... 2219
- Phenaphen with Codeine Capsules 1865
- Phenaphen-650 with Codeine Tablets ... 1866
- Phenergan with Codeine ... 2497
- Phenergan VC with Codeine ... 2501
- Robitussin A-C Syrup ... 1875
- Robitussin-DAC Syrup ... 1875
- Ryna ... ▣ 741
- Soma Compound w/Codeine Tablets ... 2390
- Triaminic Expectorant w/Codeine .. 1996
- Tussi-Organidin Liquid ... 2391
- Tylenol with Codeine ... 1381

Codeine Polistirex (Concurrent use produces additive effects).
- No products indexed under this heading.

Dezocine (Concurrent use produces additive effects).

Diazepam (Concurrent use produces additive effects). Products include:
- Valium Injectable ... 1937
- Valium Tablets ... 1939
- Valrelease Capsules ... 1923

Droperidol (Concurrent use produces additive effects). Products include:
- Inapsine Injection ... 1140
- Innovar Injection ... 1141

Enflurane (Concurrent use produces additive effects). Products include:
- Ethrane ... 599

Estazolam (Concurrent use produces additive effects). Products include:
- ProSom Tablets ... 554

Ethchlorvynol (Concurrent use produces additive effects). Products include:
- Placidyl Capsules ... 553

Ethinamate (Concurrent use produces additive effects).
- No products indexed under this heading.

Fentanyl (Concurrent use produces additive effects). Products include:
- Duragesic Transdermal System ... 1133

Fentanyl Citrate (Concurrent use produces additive effects). Products include:
- Innovar Injection ... 1141
- Sublimaze Injection ... 1146

Fluphenazine Decanoate (Concurrent use produces additive effects). Products include:
- Prolixin Decanoate ... 1795

Fluphenazine Enanthate (Concurrent use produces additive effects). Products include:
- Prolixin Enanthate ... 1796

Fluphenazine Hydrochloride (Concurrent use produces additive effects). Products include:
- Prolixin Elixir ... 1793
- Prolixin Injection ... 1791
- Prolixin Oral Concentrate ... 1792
- Prolixin Tablets ... 1793

Flurazepam Hydrochloride (Concurrent use produces additive effects). Products include:
- Dalmane Capsules ... 1927

Furazolidone (Concurrent use is not recommended). Products include:
- Furoxone ... 1855

Glutethimide (Concurrent use produces additive effects).
- No products indexed under this heading.

Haloperidol (Concurrent use produces additive effects). Products include:
- Haldol Injection, Tablets and Concentrate ... 1373

Haloperidol Decanoate (Concurrent use produces additive effects). Products include:
- Haldol Decanoate ... 1375

Hydrocodone Bitartrate (Concurrent use produces additive effects). Products include:
- Anexsia 5/500 Tablets ... 2196
- Anexsia 7.5/650 Tablets ... 2197
- Azdone Tablets ... 844
- Codiclear DH Syrup ... 845
- Codimal DH Syrup ... 846
- Damason-P ... 1356
- Hycodan Syrup, Tablets ... 927
- Hycomine Compound Tablets ... 929
- Hycomine Syrup ... 927
- Hycotuss Expectorant Syrup ... 930
- Hydrocet Capsules ... 835
- Lortab ASA Tablets ... 2414
- Lortab ... 2412
- Ru-Tuss with Hydrocodone ... 694
- Triaminic Expectorant DH ... 1995
- Vicodin Tablets ... 1187
- Vicodin ES Tablets ... 1189
- Zydone Capsules ... 941

Hydrocodone Polistirex (Concurrent use produces additive effects). Products include:
- Tussionex Extended-Release Suspension ... 988

Hydroxyzine Hydrochloride (Concurrent use produces additive effects). Products include:
- Atarax Tablets & Syrup ... 1941
- Marax Tablets & DF Syrup ... 1954
- Vistaril Intramuscular Solution ... 1970

Isocarboxazid (Concurrent use is not recommended). Products include:
- Marplan Tablets ... 1906

Isoflurane (Concurrent use produces additive effects). Products include:
- Forane ... 600

Ketamine Hydrochloride (Concurrent use produces additive effects). Products include:
- Ketalar ... 1726

Levorphanol Tartrate (Concurrent use produces additive effects). Products include:
- Levo-Dromoran ... 1906

Lorazepam (Concurrent use produces additive effects). Products include:
- Ativan Injection ... 2432
- Ativan Tablets ... 2434

Loxapine Hydrochloride (Concurrent use produces additive effects). Products include:
- Loxitane ... 1213

Loxapine Succinate (Concurrent use produces additive effects). Products include:
- Loxitane Capsules ... 1213

Meperidine Hydrochloride (Concurrent use produces additive effects). Products include:
- Demerol ... 2047
- Mepergan Injection ... 2479

Mephobarbital (Concurrent use produces additive effects). Products include:
- Mebaral Tablets ... 2061

Meprobamate (Concurrent use produces additive effects). Products include:
- Deprol Tablets ... 2382
- Equagesic Tablets ... 2451
- Miltown Tablets ... 2386
- PMB 200 and PMB 400 ... 2504

Mesoridazine (Concurrent use produces additive effects). Products include:
- Serentil ... 686

Methadone Hydrochloride (Concurrent use produces additive effects). Products include:
- Dolophine Hydrochloride Ampoules & Vials ... 1260
- Dolophine Hydrochloride Tablets ... 1261
- Methadone Hydrochloride Diskets .. 1284
- Methadone Hydrochloride Oral Solution & Tablets ... 1987

Methohexital Sodium (Concurrent use produces additive effects). Products include:
- Brevital Sodium Vials ... 1248

Methoxyflurane (Concurrent use produces additive effects).
- No products indexed under this heading.

Midazolam Hydrochloride (Concurrent use produces additive effects). Products include:
- Versed Injection ... 1924

Molindone Hydrochloride (Concurrent use produces additive effects). Products include:
- Moban Tablets & Concentrate ... 932

Morphine Sulfate (Concurrent use produces additive effects). Products include:
- Astramorph/PF Injection, USP (Preservative-Free) ... 618
- Duramorph ... 960
- Infumorph 200 and Infumorph 500 Sterile Solutions ... 962
- MS Contin Tablets ... 1814
- MSIR ... 1817
- Oramorph SR (Morphine Sulfate Sustained Release Tablets) ... 1988
- Roxanol ... 1991

Opium Alkaloids (Concurrent use produces additive effects). Products include:
- B & O No. 15A & No. 16A Supprettes ... 2395
- Pantopon Injectable ... 1911

Oxazepam (Concurrent use produces additive effects). Products include:
- Serax Capsules ... 2522
- Serax Tablets ... 2522

Oxycodone Hydrochloride (Concurrent use produces additive effects). Products include:
- Percocet Tablets ... 950
- Percodan ... 951
- Roxicodone Tablets, Oral Solution & Intensol (Oxycodone) ... 1992
- Tylox Capsules ... 1382

Pentobarbital Sodium (Concurrent use produces additive effects). Products include:
- Nembutal Sodium Capsules ... 534
- Nembutal Sodium Solution ... 536
- Nembutal Sodium Suppositories ... 538

Perphenazine (Concurrent use produces additive effects). Products include:
- Etrafon ... 2087
- Triavil Tablets ... 1556
- Trilafon ... 2123

Phenelzine Sulfate (Concurrent use is not recommended). Products include:
- Nardil ... 1742

Phenobarbital (Concurrent use produces additive effects). Products include:
- Arco-Lase Plus Tablets ... 607
- Bellergal-S Tablets ... 1998
- Bronkolixir ... ▣ 761
- Bronkotabs Tablets ... ▣ 762
- Donnatal ... 1858
- Donnatal Extentabs ... 1859
- Donnatal Tablets ... 1858
- Donnazyme Tablets ... 1860
- Kinesed Tablets ... 2272
- Phenobarbital Elixir and Tablets ... 1293
- Primatene Tablets-P Formula ... 2421
- Quadrinal Tablets ... 1183
- Tedral SA ... 1765

Prazepam (Concurrent use produces additive effects). Products include:
- Centrax ... 1693

Prochlorperazine (Concurrent use produces additive effects). Products include:
- Compazine ... 2201

Promethazine Hydrochloride (Concurrent use produces additive effects). Products include:
- Mepergan Injection ... 2479
- Phenergan with Codeine ... 2497
- Phenergan with Dextromethorphan 2499
- Phenergan Injection ... 2493
- Phenergan Suppositories ... 2496
- Phenergan Syrup ... 2495
- Phenergan Tablets ... 2496
- Phenergan VC ... 2500
- Phenergan VC with Codeine ... 2501

Propofol (Concurrent use produces additive effects). Products include:
- Diprivan Injection ... 2267

Propoxyphene Hydrochloride (Concurrent use produces additive effects). Products include:
- Darvon ... 1256
- Wygesic Tablets ... 2540

Propoxyphene Napsylate (Concurrent use produces additive effects). Products include:
- Darvon-N/Darvocet-N ... 1254

Quazepam (Concurrent use produces additive effects). Products include:
- Doral Tablets ... 2383

Secobarbital Sodium (Concurrent use produces additive effects). Products include:
- Seconal Sodium Pulvules ... 1296

Selegiline Hydrochloride (Concurrent use is not recommended). Products include:
- Eldepryl ... 2250

Sufentanil Citrate (Concurrent use produces additive effects). Products include:
- Sufenta Injection ... 1147

Temazepam (Concurrent use produces additive effects). Products include:
- Restoril Capsules ... 2023

Thiamylal Sodium (Concurrent use produces additive effects). Products include:
- Surital Ampoules, Steri-Vials ... 1764

Thioridazine Hydrochloride (Concurrent use produces additive effects). Products include:
- Mellaril ... 2011

Thiothixene (Concurrent use produces additive effects). Products include:
- Navane Capsules and Concentrate 1954
- Navane Intramuscular ... 1956

Tranylcypromine Sulfate (Concurrent use is not recommended). Products include:
- Parnate Tablets ... 2222

Triazolam (Concurrent use produces additive effects). Products include:
- Halcion Tablets ... 2340

Trifluoperazine Hydrochloride (Concurrent use produces additive effects). Products include:
- Stelazine ... 2226

ALLEREST NO DROWSINESS TABLETS
(Acetaminophen, Pseudoephedrine Hydrochloride) ... ◘ 559
See **Allerest Maximum Strength Tablets**

ALLEREST SINUS PAIN FORMULA
(Acetaminophen, Chlorpheniramine Maleate, Phenylpropanolamine Hydrochloride) ... ◘ 559
See **Allerest Maximum Strength Tablets**

ALLERGAN EYEWASH
(Benzalkonium Chloride) ... ⊙ 238
No interactions described in labeling.

ALLERGENIC EXTRACTS, DIAGNOSIS AND/OR IMMUNOTHERAPY
(Allergenic Extracts) ... 650
No interactions described in labeling.

ALLERGY DROPS
(Naphazoline Hydrochloride) ... ⊙ 258
No interactions described in labeling.

ALPHA KERI MOISTURE RICH BODY OIL
(Emollient) ... ◘ 524
No interactions described in labeling.

ALPHA KERI MOISTURE RICH CLEANSING BAR
(Emollient) ... ◘ 524
No interactions described in labeling.

ALPHATREX CREAM, OINTMENT & LOTION
(Betamethasone Dipropionate) ... 2076
No interactions described in labeling.

ALTACE CAPSULES
(Ramipril) ... 1086
May interact with potassium sparing diuretics, diuretics, potassium-depleting corticosteroids, lithium preparations, and certain other agents. Compounds in these categories include:

Amiloride Hydrochloride (May result in excessive reduction of blood pressure after initiation of therapy; increased risk of hyperkalemia). Products include:
- Midamor Tablets ... 1508
- Moduretic Tablets ... 1510

Bendroflumethiazide (May result in excessive reduction of blood pressure after initiation of therapy). Products include:
- Corzide Tablets ... 702
- Naturetin Tablets ... 1789
- Rauzide Tablets ... 1804

Bumetanide (May result in excessive reduction of blood pressure after initiation of therapy). Products include:
- Bumex ... 1895

Chlorothiazide (May result in excessive reduction of blood pressure after initiation of therapy). Products include:
- Aldoclor Tablets ... 1413
- Diupres Tablets ... 1461
- Diuril Oral ... 1464

Chlorothiazide Sodium (May result in excessive reduction of blood pressure after initiation of therapy). Products include:
- Diuril Sodium Intravenous ... 1463

Chlorthalidone (May result in excessive reduction of blood pressure after initiation of therapy). Products include:
- Combipres Tablets ... 678
- Tenoretic Tablets ... 1105
- Thalitone Tablets ... 687

Ethacrynic Acid (May result in excessive reduction of blood pressure after initiation of therapy). Products include:
- Edecrin Tablets ... 1468

Furosemide (May result in excessive reduction of blood pressure after initiation of therapy). Products include:
- Lasix ... 1093

Hydrochlorothiazide (May result in excessive reduction of blood pressure after initiation of therapy). Products include:
- Aldactazide ... 2150
- Aldoril Tablets ... 1418
- Apresazide Capsules ... 854
- Apresoline-Esidrix Tablets ... 857
- Capozide ... 2258
- Dyazide Capsules ... 2208
- Esidrix Tablets ... 863
- Esimil Tablets ... 864
- HydroDIURIL Tablets ... 1484
- Hydropres Tablets ... 1485
- Inderide Tablets ... 2463
- Inderide LA Long Acting Capsules .. 2465
- Lopressor HCT Tablets ... 1034
- Maxzide ... 1215
- Moduretic Tablets ... 1510
- Normozide Tablets ... 2112
- Oretic Tablets ... 544
- Oreticyl ... 545
- Prinzide Tablets ... 1540
- Ser-Ap-Es Tablets ... 881
- Serpasil-Esidrix Tablets ... 886
- Timolide Tablets ... 1547
- Trandate HCT Tablets ... 579
- Vaseretic Tablets ... 1559
- Zestoretic ... 2274

Hydroflumethiazide (May result in excessive reduction of blood pressure after initiation of therapy). Products include:
- Diucardin Tablets ... 2450
- Saluron ... 718
- Salutensin/Salutensin-Demi ... 719

Indapamide (May result in excessive reduction of blood pressure after initiation of therapy). Products include:
- Lozol Tablets ... 1843

Lithium Carbonate (Increased serum lithium levels). Products include:
- Eskalith ... 2214
- Lithane Tablets ... 1596
- Lithium Carbonate Capsules & Tablets ... 1984
- Lithobid Tablets ... 870

Lithium Citrate (Increased serum lithium levels). Products include:
- Cibalith-S ... 870

Methyclothiazide (May result in excessive reduction of blood pressure after initiation of therapy). Products include:
- Enduron Tablets ... 517
- Enduronyl ... 518

Metolazone (May result in excessive reduction of blood pressure after initiation of therapy). Products include:
- Diulo ... 2129
- Mykrox ½ mg Tablets ... 984
- Zaroxolyn Tablets ... 989

Polythiazide (May result in excessive reduction of blood pressure after initiation of therapy). Products include:
- Minizide Capsules ... 1779
- Renese Tablets ... 1785
- Renese-R Tablets ... 1786

Potassium Acid Phosphate (Increased risk of hyperkalemia). Products include:
- K-Phos M.F. Tablets ... 659
- K-Phos Original Formula 'Sodium Free' Tablets ... 660
- K-Phos No. 2 Tablets ... 659

Potassium Bicarbonate (Increased risk of hyperkalemia). Products include:
- Alka-Seltzer Advanced Formula Antacid & Non-Aspirin Pain Reliever ... ◘ 620
- Alka-Seltzer Effervescent Antacid ◘ 622
- K-Lyte ... 707
- Klorvess Effervescent Granules ... 2010
- Klorvess Effervescent Tablets ... 2011

Potassium Chloride (Increased risk of hyperkalemia). Products include:
- Chlor-3 Condiment ... 994
- K-Dur Microburst Release System (potassium chloride, USP) E.R. Tablets ... 1163
- K-Lor Powder Packets ... 531
- K-Lyte ... 707
- K-Norm Capsules ... 982
- K-Tab Filmtab ... 532
- Kato Potassium Supplement ... 1114
- Klor-Con 8/Klor-Con 10 Extended-release Tablets ... 2374
- Klorvess Effervescent Granules ... 2010
- Klorvess Effervescent Tablets ... 2011
- Klorvess 10% Liquid ... 2010
- Klotrix ... 708
- Kolyum Liquid ... 983
- Micro-K ... 1863
- Micro-K LS Packets ... 1864
- NuLYTELY ... 699
- Oral Rehydration Salts, Citrate ... 1150
- Rum-K Syrup ... 995
- Slow-K Tablets ... 2281
- Ten-K Controlled-Release Tablets ... 2282
- Thermotabs ... ◘ 619

Potassium Citrate (Increased risk of hyperkalemia). Products include:
- Alka-Seltzer Effervescent Antacid .. 1570
- K-Lyte ... 707
- Polycitra Syrup ... 2424
- Polycitra-K ... 2424
- Polycitra-LC—Sugar-Free ... 2424
- Ricelyte, Rice-Based Oral Electrolyte Maintenance Solution ... ◘ 613

Potassium Gluconate (Increased risk of hyperkalemia). Products include:
- Kolyum Liquid ... 983

Potassium Phosphate, Dibasic (Increased risk of hyperkalemia). Products include:
- Neutra-Phos ... 2423

Potassium Phosphate, Monobasic (Increased risk of hyperkalemia). Products include:
- K-Phos M.F. Tablets ... 659
- K-Phos Neutral Tablets ... 660
- Neutra-Phos ... 2423

Spironolactone (May result in excessive reduction of blood pressure after initiation of therapy; increased risk of hyperkalemia). Products include:
- Aldactazide ... 2150
- Aldactone ... 2152

Triamterene (May result in excessive reduction of blood pressure after initiation of therapy; increased risk of hyperkalemia). Products include:
- Dyazide Capsules ... 2208
- Dyrenium Capsules ... 2210
- Maxzide ... 1215

Food Interactions

Food, unspecified (The rate of absorption is reduced not the extent of absorption).

ALTERNA LOW PROTEIN MILK SUBSTITUTE
(Dietary Supplement) ... 1971
No interactions described in labeling.

ALTERNAGEL LIQUID
(Aluminum Hydroxide) ... 1154
May interact with tetracyclines. Compounds in this category include:

Demeclocycline Hydrochloride (Should not be taken concurrently). Products include:
- Declomycin Capsules, Tablets ... 1199

Doxycycline Calcium (Should not be taken concurrently).
No products indexed under this heading.

Doxycycline Hyclate (Should not be taken concurrently). Products include:
- Doryx Capsules ... 1717
- Vibramycin Hyclate Capsules ... 1787
- Vibramycin Hyclate Intravenous ... 1968
- Vibra-Tabs Film Coated Tablets ... 1787

Doxycycline Monohydrate (Should not be taken concurrently). Products include:
- Monodox Capsules ... 1630
- Vibramycin Monohydrate for Oral Suspension ... 1787

Methacycline Hydrochloride (Should not be taken concurrently).
No products indexed under this heading.

Minocycline Hydrochloride (Should not be taken concurrently). Products include:
- Minocin Intravenous ... 1221
- Minocin Oral Suspension ... 1224
- Minocin Pellet-Filled Capsules ... 1222

Oxytetracycline (Should not be taken concurrently). Products include:
- Terramycin Intramuscular Solution 1964
- Urobiotic-250 Capsules ... 1968

Oxytetracycline Hydrochloride (Should not be taken concurrently). Products include:
- Terra-Cortril Ophthalmic Suspension 1963
- Terramycin Capsules 1786
- Terramycin Intramuscular Solution 1964
- Terramycin with Polymyxin B Sulfate Ophthalmic Ointment 1965

Tetracycline Hydrochloride (Should not be taken concurrently). Products include:
- Achromycin V Capsules 1193
- Achromycin Ophthalmic Ointment 1% .... ⊙ 307
- Achromycin Ophthalmic Suspension 1% .... ⊙ 308
- Topicycline for Topical Solution 1856

ALTOCAPS-400 CAPSULES
(Vitamin E) .... ⊞ 516
No interactions described in labeling.

ALU-CAP CAPSULES
(Aluminum Hydroxide Gel, Dried) 1309
May interact with tetracyclines. Compounds in this category include:

Demeclocycline Hydrochloride (Impaired absorption of tetracycline). Products include:
- Declomycin Capsules, Tablets 1199

Doxycycline Calcium (Impaired absorption of tetracycline).
- No products indexed under this heading.

Doxycycline Hyclate (Impaired absorption of tetracycline). Products include:
- Doryx Capsules 1717
- Vibramycin Hyclate Capsules 1787
- Vibramycin Hyclate Intravenous 1968
- Vibra-Tabs Film Coated Tablets 1787

Doxycycline Monohydrate (Impaired absorption of tetracycline). Products include:
- Monodox Capsules 1630
- Vibramycin Monohydrate for Oral Suspension 1787

Methacycline Hydrochloride (Impaired absorption of tetracycline).
- No products indexed under this heading.

Minocycline Hydrochloride (Impaired absorption of tetracycline). Products include:
- Minocin Intravenous 1221
- Minocin Oral Suspension 1224
- Minocin Pellet-Filled Capsules 1222

Oxytetracycline (Impaired absorption of tetracycline). Products include:
- Terramycin Intramuscular Solution 1964
- Urobiotic-250 Capsules 1968

Oxytetracycline Hydrochloride (Impaired absorption of tetracycline). Products include:
- Terra-Cortril Ophthalmic Suspension 1963
- Terramycin Capsules 1786
- Terramycin Intramuscular Solution 1964
- Terramycin with Polymyxin B Sulfate Ophthalmic Ointment 1965

Tetracycline Hydrochloride (Impaired absorption of tetracycline). Products include:
- Achromycin V Capsules 1193
- Achromycin Ophthalmic Ointment 1% .... ⊙ 307
- Achromycin Ophthalmic Suspension 1% .... ⊙ 308
- Topicycline for Topical Solution 1856

ALUDROX ORAL SUSPENSION
(Aluminum Hydroxide, Magnesium Hydroxide) 2428
May interact with tetracyclines. Compounds in this category include:

Demeclocycline Hydrochloride (Avoid concurrent administration). Products include:
- Declomycin Capsules, Tablets 1199

Doxycycline Calcium (Avoid concurrent administration).
- No products indexed under this heading.

Doxycycline Hyclate (Avoid concurrent administration). Products include:
- Doryx Capsules 1717
- Vibramycin Hyclate Capsules 1787
- Vibramycin Hyclate Intravenous 1968
- Vibra-Tabs Film Coated Tablets 1787

Doxycycline Monohydrate (Avoid concurrent administration). Products include:
- Monodox Capsules 1630
- Vibramycin Monohydrate for Oral Suspension 1787

Methacycline Hydrochloride (Avoid concurrent administration).
- No products indexed under this heading.

Minocycline Hydrochloride (Avoid concurrent administration). Products include:
- Minocin Intravenous 1221
- Minocin Oral Suspension 1224
- Minocin Pellet-Filled Capsules 1222

Oxytetracycline (Avoid concurrent administration). Products include:
- Terramycin Intramuscular Solution 1964
- Urobiotic-250 Capsules 1968

Oxytetracycline Hydrochloride (Avoid concurrent administration). Products include:
- Terra-Cortril Ophthalmic Suspension 1963
- Terramycin Capsules 1786
- Terramycin Intramuscular Solution 1964
- Terramycin with Polymyxin B Sulfate Ophthalmic Ointment 1965

Tetracycline Hydrochloride (Avoid concurrent administration). Products include:
- Achromycin V Capsules 1193
- Achromycin Ophthalmic Ointment 1% .... ⊙ 307
- Achromycin Ophthalmic Suspension 1% .... ⊙ 308
- Topicycline for Topical Solution 1856

ALUPENT INHALATION AEROSOL
(Metaproterenol Sulfate) 674
See **Alupent Inhalation Solution**

ALUPENT INHALATION SOLUTION
(Metaproterenol Sulfate) 674
May interact with monoamine oxidase inhibitors, tricyclic antidepressants, and sympathomimetic aerosol brochodilators. Compounds in these categories include:

Albuterol (Possible potentiation of adrenergic effects with beta adrenergic aerosol bronchodilators). Products include:
- Proventil Inhalation Aerosol 2117
- Ventolin Inhalation Aerosol and Refill 583

Amitriptyline Hydrochloride (The action of beta adrenergic agonists on the vascular system may be potentiated). Products include:
- Elavil 2269
- Endep Tablets 1927
- Etrafon 2087
- Limbitrol 1933
- Triavil Tablets 1556

Amoxapine (The action of beta adrenergic agonists on the vascular system may be potentiated). Products include:
- Asendin Tablets 1196

Bitolterol Mesylate (Possible potentiation of adrenergic effects with beta adrenergic aerosol bronchodilators). Products include:
- Tornalate 2074

Clomipramine Hydrochloride (The action of beta adrenergic agonists on the vascular system may be potentiated). Products include:
- Anafranil Capsules 650

Desipramine Hydrochloride (The action of beta adrenergic agonists on the vascular system may be potentiated). Products include:
- Norpramin Tablets 1340

Doxepin Hydrochloride (The action of beta adrenergic agonists on the vascular system may be potentiated). Products include:
- Sinequan 1960

Furazolidone (The action of beta adrenergic agonists on the vascular system may be potentiated). Products include:
- Furoxone 1855

Imipramine Hydrochloride (The action of beta adrenergic agonists on the vascular system may be potentiated). Products include:
- Tofranil Ampuls 1038
- Tofranil Tablets 1039

Imipramine Pamoate (The action of beta adrenergic agonists on the vascular system may be potentiated). Products include:
- Tofranil-PM Capsules 1041

Isocarboxazid (The action of beta adrenergic agonists on the vascular system may be potentiated). Products include:
- Marplan Tablets 1906

Isoetharine (Possible potentiation of adrenergic effects with beta adrenergic aerosol bronchodilators). Products include:
- Arm-a-Med Isoetharine Inhalation Solution, USP 616
- Bronkometer Aerosol 2042
- Bronkosol Solution 2042

Isoproterenol Hydrochloride (Possible potentiation of adrenergic effects with beta adrenergic aerosol bronchodilators). Products include:
- Isuprel Hydrochloride Injection 1:5000 2050
- Isuprel Hydrochloride Mistometer .. 2051
- Isuprel Hydrochloride Solution 1:200 & 1:100 2052
- Norisodrine Aerotrol 540

Maprotiline Hydrochloride (The action of beta adrenergic agonists on the vascular system may be potentiated). Products include:
- Ludiomil Tablets 874

Nortriptyline Hydrochloride (The action of beta adrenergic agonists on the vascular system may be potentiated). Products include:
- Pamelor 2019

Phenelzine Sulfate (The action of beta adrenergic agonists on the vascular system may be potentiated). Products include:
- Nardil 1742

Pirbuterol Acetate (Possible potentiation of adrenergic effects with beta adrenergic aerosol bronchodilators). Products include:
- Maxair Inhaler 1311

Protriptyline Hydrochloride (The action of beta adrenergic agonists on the vascular system may be potentiated). Products include:
- Vivactil Tablets 1567

Selegiline Hydrochloride (The action of beta adrenergic agonists on the vascular system may be potentiated). Products include:
- Eldepryl 2250

Terbutaline Sulfate (Possible potentiation of adrenergic effects with beta adrenergic aerosol bronchodilators). Products include:
- Brethaire Inhaler 1024
- Brethine Ampuls 1026
- Brethine Tablets 1026
- Bricanyl Injection 1324
- Bricanyl Tablets 1325

Tranylcypromine Sulfate (The action of beta adrenergic agonists on the vascular system may be potentiated). Products include:
- Parnate Tablets 2222

Trimipramine Maleate (The action of beta adrenergic agonists on the vascular system may be potentiated). Products include:
- Surmontil Capsules 2524

ALUPENT SYRUP
(Metaproterenol Sulfate) 674
See **Alupent Inhalation Solution**

ALUPENT TABLETS
(Metaproterenol Sulfate) 674
See **Alupent Inhalation Solution**

ALURATE ELIXIR
(Aprobarbital) 1883
May interact with central nervous system depressants, monoamine oxidase inhibitors, oral anticoagulants, corticosteroids, and certain other agents. Compounds in these categories include:

Alcohol (Increased CNS depressant effects).

Alfentanil Hydrochloride (Increased CNS depressant effect). Products include:
- Alfenta Injection 1131

Alprazolam (Increased CNS depressant effect). Products include:
- Xanax Tablets 2367

Betamethasone Acetate (Enhanced metabolism of corticosteroids). Products include:
- Celestone Soluspan Suspension 2081

Betamethasone Sodium Phosphate (Enhanced metabolism of corticosteroids). Products include:
- Celestone Soluspan Suspension 2081

Buprenorphine (Increased CNS depressant effect).
- No products indexed under this heading.

Buspirone Hydrochloride (Increased CNS depressant effect). Products include:
- BuSpar 1401

Butabarbital (Increased CNS depressant effect). Products include:
- Pyridium Plus 1764

Butalbital (Increased CNS depressant effect). Products include:
- Esgic-Plus Tablets 1002
- Esgic Tablets & Capsules 1001
- Fioricet Tablets 2006
- Fiorinal Capsules 2007
- Fiorinal with Codeine Capsules 2008
- Fiorinal Tablets 2007
- Phrenilin 838
- Sedapap Tablets 50 mg/650 mg .. 1360

Chlordiazepoxide (Increased CNS depressant effect). Products include:
- Libritabs Tablets 1930
- Limbitrol 1933
- Menrium Tablets 1934

Chlordiazepoxide Hydrochloride (Increased CNS depressant effect). Products include:
Librax Capsules ... 1929
Librium Capsules ... 1931
Librium Injectable ... 1932

Chlorpromazine (Increased CNS depressant effect). Products include:
Thorazine ... 2234

Chlorprothixene (Increased CNS depressant effect). Products include:
Taractan Tablets ... 1920

Chlorprothixene Hydrochloride (Increased CNS depressant effect). Products include:
Taractan ... 1920

Chlorprothixene Lactate (Increased CNS depressant effect). Products include:
Taractan Concentrate ... 1920

Clorazepate Dipotassium (Increased CNS depressant effect). Products include:
Tranxene ... 556

Codeine (Increased CNS depressant effect). Products include:
Calcidrine Syrup ... 506

Codeine Phosphate (Increased CNS depressant effect). Products include:
Actifed with Codeine Cough Syrup.. 752
Cheracol Cough Syrup ... 1853
Codimal PH Syrup ... 846
Dimetane-DC Cough Syrup ... 1857
Empirin with Codeine Phosphate Nos. 2, 3 & 4 ... 764
Fiorinal with Codeine Capsules ... 2008
Isoclor Expectorant ... 982
Naldecon CX Adult Liquid ... ▣ 521
Novahistine DH ... 1342
Novahistine Expectorant ... 1343
Nucofed Capsules ... 2219
Nucofed Expectorant ... 2219
Nucofed Pediatric Expectorant ... 2220
Nucofed Syrup ... 2219
Phenaphen with Codeine Capsules 1865
Phenaphen-650 with Codeine Tablets ... 1866
Phenergan with Codeine ... 2497
Phenergan VC with Codeine ... 2501
Robitussin A-C Syrup ... 1875
Robitussin-DAC Syrup ... 1875
Ryna ... ▣ 741
Soma Compound w/Codeine Tablets ... 2390
Triaminic Expectorant w/Codeine .. 1996
Tussi-Organidin Liquid ... 2391
Tylenol with Codeine ... 1381

Codeine Polistirex (Increased CNS depressant effect).
No products indexed under this heading.

Cortisone Acetate (Enhanced metabolism of corticosteroids). Products include:
Cortone Acetate Sterile Suspension ... 1437
Cortone Acetate Tablets ... 1439

Dexamethasone (Enhanced metabolism of corticosteroids). Products include:
AK-Trol Ointment & Suspension ... ◉ 207
Decadron Elixir ... 1445
Decadron Tablets ... 1447
Decaspray Topical Aerosol ... 1459
Dexacidin ... ◉ 272
Maxidex Sterile Ophthalmic Suspension ... ◉ 223
Maxitrol Ophthalmic Ointment/Suspension ... ◉ 223
TobraDex Ophthalmic Suspension and Ointment ... ◉ 228

Dexamethasone Acetate (Enhanced metabolism of corticosteroids). Products include:
Dalalone D.P. Injectable ... 999
Decadron-LA Sterile Suspension ... 1457

Dexamethasone Sodium Phosphate (Enhanced metabolism of corticosteroids). Products include:
AK-Dex ... ◉ 203
Decadron Phosphate Respihaler ... 1454
Decadron Phosphate Sterile Ophthalmic Ointment ... 1453
Decadron Phosphate Sterile Ophthalmic Solution ... 1453
Decadron Phosphate Topical Cream ... 1455
Decadron Phosphate Turbinaire ... 1456
Maxidex Sterile Ophthalmic Ointment ... ◉ 222
NeoDecadron Sterile Ophthalmic Ointment ... 1517
NeoDecadron Sterile Ophthalmic Solution ... 1518
NeoDecadron Topical Cream ... 1518

Dezocine (Increased CNS depressant effect).

Diazepam (Increased CNS depressant effect). Products include:
Valium Injectable ... 1937
Valium Tablets ... 1939
Valrelease Capsules ... 1923

Dicumarol (Decreased anticoagulant response). Products include:
Dicumarol Tablets ... 516

Droperidol (Increased CNS depressant effect). Products include:
Inapsine Injection ... 1140
Innovar Injection ... 1141

Enflurane (Increased CNS depressant effect). Products include:
Ethrane ... 599

Estazolam (Increased CNS depressant effect). Products include:
ProSom Tablets ... 554

Estradiol (Decreased effect of estradiol). Products include:
Emcyt Capsules ... 1161
Estrace ... 1385
Estrace Vaginal Cream ... 1388
Estraderm Transdermal System ... 866

Estrone (Decreased effect of estrone). Products include:
Ogen ... 540

Ethchlorvynol (Increased CNS depressant effect). Products include:
Placidyl Capsules ... 553

Ethinamate (Increased CNS depressant effect).
No products indexed under this heading.

Fentanyl (Increased CNS depressant effect). Products include:
Duragesic Transdermal System ... 1133

Fentanyl Citrate (Increased CNS depressant effect). Products include:
Innovar Injection ... 1141
Sublimaze Injection ... 1146

Fluphenazine Decanoate (Increased CNS depressant effect). Products include:
Prolixin Decanoate ... 1795

Fluphenazine Enanthate (Increased CNS depressant effect). Products include:
Prolixin Enanthate ... 1796

Fluphenazine Hydrochloride (Increased CNS depressant effect). Products include:
Prolixin Elixir ... 1793
Prolixin Injection ... 1791
Prolixin Oral Concentrate ... 1792
Prolixin Tablets ... 1793

Flurazepam Hydrochloride (Increased CNS depressant effect). Products include:
Dalmane Capsules ... 1927

Furazolidone (Increased effect of Alurate). Products include:
Furoxone ... 1855

Glutethimide (Increased CNS depressant effect).
No products indexed under this heading.

Griseofulvin (Decreased griseofulvin blood level). Products include:
Fulvicin P/G Tablets ... 2090
Fulvicin P/G 165 & 330 Tablets ... 2091
Fulvicin-U/F Tablets ... 2092
Grifulvin V (griseofulvin microsize) Tablets/Suspension ... 1678
Grisactin ... 2454
Grisactin Ultra Tablets ... 2455
Gris-PEG Tablets, 125 mg & 250 mg ... 1083

Haloperidol (Increased CNS depressant effect). Products include:
Haldol Injection, Tablets and Concentrate ... 1373

Haloperidol Decanoate (Increased CNS depressant effect). Products include:
Haldol Decanoate ... 1375

Hydrocodone Bitartrate (Increased CNS depressant effect). Products include:
Anexsia 5/500 Tablets ... 2196
Anexsia 7.5/650 Tablets ... 2197
Azdōne Tablets ... 844
Codiclear DH Syrup ... 845
Codimal DH Syrup ... 846
Damason-P ... 1356
Hycodan Syrup, Tablets ... 927
Hycomine Compound Tablets ... 929
Hycomine Syrup ... 927
Hycotuss Expectorant Syrup ... 930
Hydrocet Capsules ... 835
Lortab ASA Tablets ... 2414
Lortab ... 2412
Ru-Tuss with Hydrocodone ... 694
Triaminic Expectorant DH ... 1995
Vicodin Tablets ... 1187
Vicodin ES Tablets ... 1189
Zydone Capsules ... 941

Hydrocodone Polistirex (Increased CNS depressant effect). Products include:
Tussionex Extended-Release Suspension ... 988

Hydrocortisone (Enhanced metabolism of corticosteroids). Products include:
AK-Spore H.C. ... ◉ 206
Bactine Hydrocortisone Anti-Itch Cream ... ▣ 625
CaldeCORT Anti-Itch Hydrocortisone Spray ... ▣ 560
Carmol HC Cream 1% ... 2296
Cortaid Spray ... ▣ 735
Cortenema ... 2244
Cortisporin Ointment ... 758
Cortisporin Ophthalmic Ointment Sterile ... 758
Cortisporin Ophthalmic Suspension Sterile ... 759
Cortisporin Otic Solution Sterile ... 760
Cortisporin Otic Suspension Sterile 760
Cortizone-5 Creme & Ointment ... ▣ 732
Dermolate Anti-Itch Cream ... ▣ 697
Eldecort Cream 1.0% ... 1113
Eldecort Cream 1.0% and 2.5% ... 1113
Fungoid HC Creme ... 1770
Hydrocortone Tablets ... 1482
Hytone ... 909
LazerSporin-C Solution ... 1770
Massengill Medicated Soft Cloth Towelettes ... 2192
Nutracort Cream & Lotion ... 1684
PediOtic Suspension Sterile ... 797
Synacort Creams 1%, 2.5% ... 2296
Vanoxide-HC Acne Lotion ... 911
Vioform-Hydrocortisone Cream and Mild Cream ... 889
Vioform-Hydrocortisone Ointment .. 889
VōSoL HC Otic Solution ... 2392
Vytone Cream 1% ... 911

Hydrocortisone Acetate (Enhanced metabolism of corticosteroids). Products include:
Analpram-HC Rectal Cream 1% and 2.5% ... 970
Anusol-HC Cream ... 1690
Anusol-HC Suppositories ... 1691
Caldecort ... ▣ 560
Carmol HC Cream 1% ... 2296
Chloromycetin Hydrocortisone Ophthalmic ... 1694
Coly-Mycin S Otic w/Neomycin & Hydrocortisone ... 1708
Cortaid ... ▣ 735
Cortef Feminine Itch Cream ... ▣ 735
Corticaine ... ▣ 682
Cortifoam ... 1827
Cortisporin Cream ... 757
Epifoam ... 1828
Gynecort 5 Creme ... ▣ 556
Hydrocortone Acetate Sterile Suspension ... 1479
Lanacort 5 Creme and Ointment .. ▣ 557
Mantadil Cream ... 789
Ophthocort ... ◉ 301
Orabase HCA Oral Paste ... 890
Pramosone Cream, Lotion & Ointment ... 971
ProctoCream-HC ... 1834
Proctofoam-HC ... 1835

Hydrocortisone Sodium Phosphate (Enhanced metabolism of corticosteroids). Products include:
Hydrocortone Phosphate Injection, Sterile ... 1481

Hydrocortisone Sodium Succinate (Enhanced metabolism of corticosteroids). Products include:
Solu-Cortef Sterile Powder ... 2361

Hydroxyzine Hydrochloride (Increased CNS depressant effect). Products include:
Atarax Tablets & Syrup ... 1941
Marax Tablets & DF Syrup ... 1954
Vistaril Intramuscular Solution ... 1970

Isocarboxazid (Increased effect of Alurate). Products include:
Marplan Tablets ... 1906

Isoflurane (Increased CNS depressant effect). Products include:
Forane ... 600

Ketamine Hydrochloride (Increased CNS depressant effect). Products include:
Ketalar ... 1726

Levorphanol Tartrate (Increased CNS depressant effect). Products include:
Levo-Dromoran ... 1906

Lorazepam (Increased CNS depressant effect). Products include:
Ativan Injection ... 2432
Ativan Tablets ... 2434

Loxapine Hydrochloride (Increased CNS depressant effect). Products include:
Loxitane ... 1213

Loxapine Succinate (Increased CNS depressant effect). Products include:
Loxitane Capsules ... 1213

Meperidine Hydrochloride (Increased CNS depressant effect). Products include:
Demerol ... 2047
Mepergan Injection ... 2479

Mephobarbital (Increased CNS depressant effect). Products include:
Mebaral Tablets ... 2061

Meprobamate (Increased CNS depressant effect). Products include:
Deprol Tablets ... 2382
Equagesic Tablets ... 2451
Miltown Tablets ... 2386
PMB 200 and PMB 400 ... 2504

Mesoridazine (Increased CNS depressant effect). Products include:
Serentil ... 686

Methadone Hydrochloride (Increased CNS depressant effect). Products include:
Dolophine Hydrochloride Ampoules & Vials ... 1260
Dolophine Hydrochloride Tablets ... 1261
Methadone Hydrochloride Diskets .. 1284
Methadone Hydrochloride Oral Solution & Tablets ... 1987

Methohexital Sodium (Increased CNS depressant effect). Products include:
Brevital Sodium Vials ... 1248

Methoxyflurane (Increased CNS depressant effect).
No products indexed under this heading.

Methylprednisolone Acetate (Enhanced metabolism of corticosteroids). Products include:
Depo-Medrol Sterile Aqueous Suspension ... 2334

Methylprednisolone Sodium Succinate (Enhanced metabolism of corticosteroids). Products include:
- Solu-Medrol Sterile Powder 2363

Midazolam Hydrochloride (Increased CNS depressant effect). Products include:
- Versed Injection 1924

Molindone Hydrochloride (Increased CNS depressant effect). Products include:
- Moban Tablets & Concentrate 932

Morphine Sulfate (Increased CNS depressant effect). Products include:
- Astramorph/PF Injection, USP (Preservative-Free) 618
- Duramorph 960
- Infumorph 200 and Infumorph 500 Sterile Solutions 962
- MS Contin Tablets 1814
- MSIR 1817
- Oramorph SR (Morphine Sulfate Sustained Release Tablets) 1988
- Roxanol 1991

Opium Alkaloids (Increased CNS depressant effect). Products include:
- B & O No. 15A & No. 16A Supprettes 2395
- Pantopon Injectable 1911

Oxazepam (Increased CNS depressant effect). Products include:
- Serax Capsules 2522
- Serax Tablets 2522

Oxycodone Hydrochloride (Increased CNS depressant effect). Products include:
- Percocet Tablets 950
- Percodan 951
- Roxicodone Tablets, Oral Solution & Intensol (Oxycodone) 1992
- Tylox Capsules 1382

Pentobarbital Sodium (Increased CNS depressant effect). Products include:
- Nembutal Sodium Capsules 534
- Nembutal Sodium Solution 536
- Nembutal Sodium Suppositories 538

Perphenazine (Increased CNS depressant effect). Products include:
- Etrafon 2087
- Triavil Tablets 1556
- Trilafon 2123

Phenelzine Sulfate (Increased effect of Alurate). Products include:
- Nardil 1742

Phenobarbital (Decreased anticoagulant activity; increased CNS depressant effect). Products include:
- Arco-Lase Plus Tablets 607
- Bellergal-S Tablets 1998
- Bronkolixir .... ▣ 761
- Bronkotabs Tablets .... ▣ 762
- Donnatal 1858
- Donnatal Extentabs 1859
- Donnatal Tablets 1858
- Donnazyme Tablets 1860
- Kinesed Tablets 2272
- Phenobarbital Elixir and Tablets 1293
- Primatene Tablets-P Formula 2421
- Quadrinal Tablets 1183
- Tedral SA 1765

Phenytoin (Decreased barbiturate blood levels). Products include:
- Dilantin Infatabs 1710
- Dilantin-30 Pediatric/Dilantin-125 Suspension 1713

Phenytoin Sodium (Decreased barbiturate blood levels). Products include:
- Dilantin Kapseals 1708
- Dilantin Parenteral 1712
- Dilantin with Phenobarbital Kapseals 1715

Prazepam (Increased CNS depressant effect). Products include:
- Centrax 1693

Prednisolone Acetate (Enhanced metabolism of corticosteroids). Products include:
- AK-Cide Sterile Ophthalmic Ointment & Suspension .... ⊛ 202
- Blephamide Liquifilm Sterile Ophthalmic Suspension 586
- Blephamide S.O.P. Sterile Ophthalmic Ointment 586
- Cetapred Ointment .... ⊛ 220
- ⅛% Econopred & 1% Econopred Plus .... ⊛ 217
- Isopto Cetapred Suspension .... ⊛ 220
- Metimyd .... ⊛ 306
- Poly-Pred Liquifilm .... ⊛ 250
- Pred Forte .... ⊛ 252
- Pred Mild .... ⊛ 254
- Pred-G Liquifilm Sterile Ophthalmic Suspension .... ⊛ 252
- Pred-G S.O.P. Sterile Ophthalmic Ointment .... ⊛ 253
- Vasocidin Ointment .... ⊛ 275

Prednisolone Sodium Phosphate (Enhanced metabolism of corticosteroids). Products include:
- AK-Pred .... ⊛ 205
- Hydeltrasol Injection, Sterile 1476
- Inflamase .... ⊛ 274
- Pediapred Oral Liquid 987
- Vasocidin Ophthalmic Solution .... ⊛ 276

Prednisolone Tebutate (Enhanced metabolism of corticosteroids). Products include:
- Hydeltra-T.B.A. Sterile Suspension 1478

Prednisone (Enhanced metabolism of corticosteroids). Products include:
- Deltasone Tablets 2332

Prochlorperazine (Increased CNS depressant effect). Products include:
- Compazine 2201

Progesterone (Decreased effect of progesterone).
- No products indexed under this heading.

Promethazine Hydrochloride (Increased CNS depressant effect). Products include:
- Mepergan Injection 2479
- Phenergan with Codeine 2497
- Phenergan with Dextromethorphan 2499
- Phenergan Injection 2493
- Phenergan Suppositories 2496
- Phenergan Syrup 2495
- Phenergan Tablets 2496
- Phenergan VC 2500
- Phenergan VC with Codeine 2501

Propofol (Increased CNS depressant effect). Products include:
- Diprivan Injection 2267

Propoxyphene Hydrochloride (Increased CNS depressant effect). Products include:
- Darvon 1256
- Wygesic Tablets 2540

Propoxyphene Napsylate (Increased CNS depressant effect). Products include:
- Darvon-N/Darvocet-N 1254

Quazepam (Increased CNS depressant effect). Products include:
- Doral Tablets 2383

Secobarbital Sodium (Increased CNS depressant effect). Products include:
- Seconal Sodium Pulvules 1296

Selegiline Hydrochloride (Increased effect of Alurate). Products include:
- Eldepryl 2250

Sodium Valproate (Decreased barbiturate metabolism).

Sufentanil Citrate (Increased CNS depressant effect). Products include:
- Sufenta Injection 1147

Temazepam (Increased CNS depressant effect). Products include:
- Restoril Capsules 2023

Thiamylal Sodium (Increased CNS depressant effect). Products include:
- Surital Ampoules, Steri-Vials 1764

Thioridazine Hydrochloride (Increased CNS depressant effect). Products include:
- Mellaril 2011

Thiothixene (Increased CNS depressant effect). Products include:
- Navane Capsules and Concentrate 1954
- Navane Intramuscular 1956

Tranylcypromine Sulfate (Increased effect of Alurate). Products include:
- Parnate Tablets 2222

Triamcinolone (Enhanced metabolism of corticosteroids).
- No products indexed under this heading.

Triamcinolone Acetonide (Enhanced metabolism of corticosteroids). Products include:
- Aristocort A 1010
- Azmacort Inhaler 1837
- Kenalog Cream, Lotion & Ointment 2401
- Kenalog-10 Injection 2402
- Kenalog-40 Injection 2403
- Kenalog in Orabase 604
- Kenalog Spray 2401
- Mycolog II Cream and Ointment 2407
- Mytrex Cream & Ointment 2080
- Nasacort Nasal Inhaler 1844

Triamcinolone Diacetate (Enhanced metabolism of corticosteroids). Products include:
- Aristocort Suspension 1008

Triamcinolone Hexacetonide (Enhanced metabolism of corticosteroids). Products include:
- Aristospan Suspension 1011

Triazolam (Increased CNS depressant effect). Products include:
- Halcion Tablets 2340

Trifluoperazine Hydrochloride (Increased CNS depressant effect). Products include:
- Stelazine 2226

Valproic Acid (Decreased barbiturate metabolism). Products include:
- Depakene Capsules & Syrup 511

Warfarin Sodium (Decreased anticoagulant response). Products include:
- Coumadin Injection & Tablets 944
- Panwarfin Tablets 547

ALU-TAB TABLETS
(Aluminum Hydroxide Gel, Dried) 1309
See **Alu-Cap Capsules**

AMEN
(Medroxyprogesterone Acetate) 833
No interactions described in labeling.

AMERICAINE ANESTHETIC LUBRICANT
(Benzocaine) 972
No interactions described in labeling.

AMERICAINE HEMORRHOIDAL OINTMENT
(Benzocaine) .... ▣ 558
No interactions described in labeling.

AMERICAINE OTIC TOPICAL ANESTHETIC EAR DROPS
(Benzocaine) 973
No interactions described in labeling.

AMERICAINE TOPICAL ANESTHETIC FIRST AID OINTMENT
(Benzocaine) .... ▣ 559
No interactions described in labeling.

AMERICAINE TOPICAL ANESTHETIC SPRAY
(Benzocaine) .... ▣ 559
No interactions described in labeling.

AMESEC
(Aminophylline, Ephedrine Hydrochloride) .... ▣ 682
May interact with monoamine oxidase inhibitors. Compounds in this category include:

Furazolidone (Effect not specified). Products include:
- Furoxone 1855

Isocarboxazid (Effect not specified). Products include:
- Marplan Tablets 1906

Phenelzine Sulfate (Effect not specified). Products include:
- Nardil 1742

Selegiline Hydrochloride (Effect not specified). Products include:
- Eldepryl 2250

Tranylcypromine Sulfate (Effect not specified). Products include:
- Parnate Tablets 2222

AMICAR SYRUP, TABLETS, AND INJECTION
(Aminocaproic Acid) 1194
No interactions described in labeling.

AMIKIN INJECTABLE
(Amikacin Sulfate) 602
May interact with aminoglycosides, cephalosporins, penicillins, and certain other agents. Compounds in these categories include:

Amoxicillin (Significant mutual inactivation). Products include:
- Amoxil 2193
- Augmentin Tablets, Powder for Oral Suspension, and Chewable Tablets 2198

Amphotericin B (Increased risk of toxicity). Products include:
- Fungizone Cream, Lotion and Ointment 2261
- Fungizone Intravenous 2262

Ampicillin Sodium (Significant mutual inactivation). Products include:
- Unasyn 1965

Azlocillin Sodium (Significant mutual inactivation).
- No products indexed under this heading.

Bacampicillin Hydrochloride (Significant mutual inactivation). Products include:
- Spectrobid Tablets & Powder for Oral Suspension 1961

Bacitracin (Increased risk of toxicity). Products include:
- Baciguent Antibiotic Ointment .... ▣ 735
- Bactine First Aid Antibiotic Ointment .... ▣ 625
- Campho-Phenique Triple Antibiotic Ointment Plus Pain Reliever ▣ 758
- Lanabiotic Ointment .... ▣ 556
- Mycitracin .... ▣ 737

Carbenicillin Disodium (Significant mutual inactivation).

Carbenicillin Indanyl Sodium (Significant mutual inactivation). Products include:
- Geocillin Tablets 1951

Cefaclor (Increased nephrotoxicity; elevated creatinine). Products include:
- Ceclor Pulvules & Suspension 1251

Cefadroxil Monohydrate (Increased nephrotoxicity; elevated creatinine). Products include:
- Duricef 1405
- Ultracef Capsules, Tablets & Oral Suspension 722

Cefamandole Nafate (Increased nephrotoxicity; elevated creatinine). Products include:
- Mandol Vials, Faspak & ADD-Vantage 1281

Cefazolin Sodium (Increased nephrotoxicity; elevated creatinine). Products include:
- Ancef Injection 2194
- Kefzol Vials, Faspak & ADD-Vantage 1279

Cefixime (Increased nephrotoxicity; elevated creatinine). Products include:
- Suprax 1235

Cefmetazole Sodium (Increased nephrotoxicity; elevated creatinine). Products include:
- Zefazone Sterile Powder 2372

Cefonicid Sodium (Increased nephrotoxicity; elevated creatinine). Products include:
- Monocid Injection 2217

Cefoperazone Sodium (Increased nephrotoxicity; elevated creatinine). Products include:
- Cefobid Intravenous/Intramuscular 1943
- Cefobid Pharmacy Bulk Package - Not for Direct Infusion 1945

Ceforanide (Increased nephrotoxicity; elevated creatinine).
- No products indexed under this heading.

Cefotaxime Sodium (Increased nephrotoxicity; elevated creatinine). Products include:
- Claforan Sterile Injection 1089

Cefotetan (Increased nephrotoxicity; elevated creatinine). Products include:
- Cefotan 2265

Cefoxitin Sodium (Increased nephrotoxicity; elevated creatinine). Products include:
- Mefoxin 1498
- Mefoxin Premixed Intravenous Solution 1500

Ceftazidime (Increased nephrotoxicity; elevated creatinine). Products include:
- Ceptaz for Injection 1057
- Fortaz 1060
- Tazicef for Injection 2231
- Tazidime Vials, Faspak & ADD-Vantage 1299

Ceftizoxime Sodium (Increased nephrotoxicity; elevated creatinine). Products include:
- Cefizox Injection 1012

Ceftriaxone Sodium (Increased nephrotoxicity; elevated creatinine). Products include:
- Rocephin Injectable Vials, ADD-Vantage 1914

Cefuroxime Axetil (Increased nephrotoxicity; elevated creatinine). Products include:
- Ceftin Tablets 575

Cefuroxime Sodium (Increased nephrotoxicity; elevated creatinine). Products include:
- Kefurox Vials, Faspak & ADD-Vantage 1277
- Zinacef 1066

Cephalexin (Increased nephrotoxicity; elevated creatinine). Products include:
- Keflex Pulvules, Oral Suspension & Pediatric Drops 916

Cephaloridine (Increased risk of toxicity).

Cephalothin Sodium (Increased nephrotoxicity; elevated creatinine).

Cephapirin Sodium (Increased nephrotoxicity; elevated creatinine).
- No products indexed under this heading.

Cephradine (Increased nephrotoxicity; elevated creatinine). Products include:
- Velosef Capsules and for Oral Suspension 606

Cisplatin (Increased risk of toxicity). Products include:
- Platinol 737
- Platinol-AQ Injection 738

Colistin Sulfate (Increased risk of toxicity). Products include:
- Coly-Mycin S For Oral Suspension 1708
- Coly-Mycin S Otic w/Neomycin & Hydrocortisone 1708

Ethacrynic Acid (Ototoxicity; enhanced aminoglycoside toxicity). Products include:
- Edecrin Tablets 1468

Furosemide (Ototoxicity; enhanced aminoglycoside toxicity). Products include:
- Lasix 1093

Gentamicin Sulfate (Increased nephrotoxicity). Products include:
- Garamycin Injectable 2093
- Garamycin Ophthalmic ⊙ 305
- Genoptic Liquifilm Sterile Ophthalmic Solution ⊙ 247
- Genoptic S.O.P. Sterile Ophthalmic Ointment ⊙ 247
- Gentacidin Ointment ⊙ 273
- Gentacidin Solution ⊙ 273
- Gentak Ointment & Solution ⊙ 208
- G-myticin Creme and Ointment 0.1% 1770
- Pred-G Liquifilm Sterile Ophthalmic Suspension ⊙ 252
- Pred-G S.O.P. Sterile Ophthalmic Ointment ⊙ 253

Kanamycin Sulfate (Increased nephrotoxicity). Products include:
- Kantrex Injection 601
- Kantrex Pediatric Injection 601

Mezlocillin Sodium (Significant mutual inactivation). Products include:
- Mezlin 1597
- Mezlin Pharmacy Bulk Package 1599

Nafcillin Sodium (Significant mutual inactivation). Products include:
- Unipen 2533

Paromomycin Sulfate (Increased risk of toxicity). Products include:
- Humatin Capsules 1726

Penicillin G Potassium (Significant mutual inactivation). Products include:
- Pfizerpen for Injection 1957

Penicillin G Procaine (Significant mutual inactivation). Products include:
- Bicillin C-R Injection 2438
- Bicillin C-R 900/300 Injection 2440
- Pfizerpen-AS Aqueous Suspension 1959
- Wycillin Injection 2537
- Wycillin Injection and Probenecid Tablets 2539

Penicillin G Sodium (Significant mutual inactivation).
- No products indexed under this heading.

Penicillin G, Benzathine (Significant mutual inactivation). Products include:
- Bicillin C-R Injection 2438
- Bicillin C-R 900/300 Injection 2440
- Bicillin L-A Injection 2442

Penicillin V Potassium (Significant mutual inactivation).
- No products indexed under this heading.

Polymyxin B Sulfate (Increased risk of toxicity). Products include:
- AK-Poly-Bac Ointment ⊙ 205
- AK-Spore H.C. ⊙ 206
- AK-Spore ⊙ 205
- AK-Trol Ointment & Suspension ⊙ 207
- Aquaphor Antibiotic Formula 662
- Bactine First Aid Antibiotic Ointment ▣ 625
- Campho-Phenique Triple Antibiotic Ointment Plus Pain Reliever ▣ 758
- Cortisporin Cream 757
- Cortisporin Ointment 758
- Cortisporin Ophthalmic Ointment Sterile 758
- Cortisporin Ophthalmic Suspension Sterile 759
- Cortisporin Otic Solution Sterile 760
- Cortisporin Otic Suspension Sterile 760
- Dexacidin ⊙ 272
- Lanabiotic Ointment ▣ 556
- LazerSporin-C Solution 1770
- Maxitrol Ophthalmic Ointment/Suspension ⊙ 223
- Mycitracin ▣ 737
- Neosporin Cream 792
- Neosporin G.U. Irrigant Sterile 793
- Neosporin Ointment 793
- Maximum Strength Neosporin Ointment 793
- Neosporin Ophthalmic Ointment Sterile 793
- Neosporin Ophthalmic Solution Sterile 794
- Ophthocort ⊙ 301
- PediOtic Suspension Sterile 797
- Polymyxin B Sulfate, Aerosporin Brand Sterile Powder 798
- Poly-Pred Liquifilm ⊙ 250
- Polysporin Ointment ▣ 543
- Polysporin Ophthalmic Ointment Sterile 798
- Polysporin Powder ▣ 543
- Polysporin Spray ▣ 543
- Polytrim Ophthalmic Solution Sterile 588
- Terramycin with Polymyxin B Sulfate Ophthalmic Ointment 1965

Streptomycin Sulfate (Increased nephrotoxicity).
- No products indexed under this heading.

Ticarcillin Disodium (Significant mutual inactivation). Products include:
- Ticar for Injection 2236
- Timentin for Injection 2239

Tobramycin Sulfate (Increased nephrotoxicity). Products include:
- Nebcin Vials, Hyporets & ADD-Vantage 1286

Vancomycin Hydrochloride (Increased risk of toxicity). Products include:
- Vancocin HCl, Oral Solution & Pulvules 1304
- Vancocin HCl, Vials & ADD-Vantage 1302

Viomycin (Increased risk of toxicity).

AMINO-CERV
(Urea Preparations) 1613
No interactions described in labeling.

AMINOHIPPURATE SODIUM INJECTION
(Aminohippurate Sodium) 1421
May interact with sulfonamides and certain other agents. Compounds in these categories include:

Bendroflumethiazide (Renal clearance measurements impaired). Products include:
- Corzide Tablets 702
- Naturetin Tablets 1789
- Rauzide Tablets 1804

Chlorothiazide (Renal clearance measurements impaired). Products include:
- Aldoclor Tablets 1413
- Diupres Tablets 1461
- Diuril Oral 1464

Chlorothiazide Sodium (Renal clearance measurements impaired). Products include:
- Diuril Sodium Intravenous 1463

Chlorpropamide (Renal clearance measurements impaired). Products include:
- Diabinese Tablets 1775

Glipizide (Renal clearance measurements impaired). Products include:
- Glucotrol 1952

Glyburide (Renal clearance measurements impaired). Products include:
- DiaBeta 1091
- Micronase Tablets 2350

Hydrochlorothiazide (Renal clearance measurements impaired). Products include:
- Aldactazide 2150
- Aldoril Tablets 1418
- Apresazide Capsules 854
- Apresoline-Esidrix Tablets 857
- Capozide 2258
- Dyazide Capsules 2208
- Esidrix Tablets 863
- Esimil Tablets 864
- HydroDIURIL Tablets 1484
- Hydropres Tablets 1485
- Inderide Tablets 2463
- Inderide LA Long Acting Capsules 2465
- Lopressor HCT Tablets 1034
- Maxzide 1215
- Moduretic Tablets 1510
- Normozide Tablets 2112
- Oretic Tablets 544
- Oreticyl 545
- Prinzide Tablets 1540
- Ser-Ap-Es Tablets 881
- Serpasil-Esidrix Tablets 886
- Timolide Tablets 1547
- Trandate HCT Tablets 579
- Vaseretic Tablets 1559
- Zestoretic 2274

Hydroflumethiazide (Renal clearance measurements impaired). Products include:
- Diucardin Tablets 2450
- Saluron 718
- Salutensin/Salutensin-Demi 719

Methyclothiazide (Renal clearance measurements impaired). Products include:
- Enduron Tablets 517
- Enduronyl 518

Polythiazide (Renal clearance measurements impaired). Products include:
- Minizide Capsules 1779
- Renese Tablets 1785
- Renese-R Tablets 1786

Probenecid (Tubular secretion of PAH depressed). Products include:
- Benemid Tablets 1426
- ColBENEMID Tablets 1436
- Wycillin Injection and Probenecid Tablets 2539

Procaine Hydrochloride (Renal clearance measurements impaired). Products include:
- Novocain Hydrochloride for Spinal Anesthesia 2065

Sulfamethizole (Renal clearance measurements impaired). Products include:
- Thiosulfil Forte Tablets 2526
- Urobiotic-250 Capsules 1968

Sulfamethoxazole (Renal clearance measurements impaired). Products include:
- Azo Gantanol Tablets 1887
- Bactrim DS Tablets 1891
- Bactrim I.V. Infusion 1889
- Bactrim 1891
- Gantanol 1899
- Septra 813
- Septra I.V. Infusion 808
- Septra I.V. Infusion ADD-Vantage Vials 810
- Septra 813

Sulfasalazine (Renal clearance measurements impaired). Products include:
- Azulfidine Tablets, EN-tabs, Oral Suspension 1157

Sulfinpyrazone (Renal clearance measurements impaired). Products include:
- Anturane 853

Sulfisoxazole (Renal clearance measurements impaired). Products include:
- Azo Gantrisin Tablets 1888
- Gantrisin Tablets 1901

Pediazole 1973

Sulfisoxazole Diolamine (Renal clearance measurements impaired). Products include:
- Gantrisin Ophthalmic Ointment/ Solution 1900

Tolazamide (Renal clearance measurements impaired). Products include:
- Tolinase Tablets 2365

Tolbutamide (Renal clearance measurements impaired). Products include:
- Orinase Tablets 2354

AMINOPHYLLIN TABLETS
(Aminophylline) 2153
May interact with oral contraceptives, sympathomimetic bronchodilators, macrolide antibiotics, and certain other agents. Compounds in these categories include:

Albuterol (Potential for toxic synergism). Products include:
- Proventil Inhalation Aerosol 2117
- Ventolin Inhalation Aerosol and Refill 583

Albuterol Sulfate (Potential for toxic synergism). Products include:
- Proventil Repetabs Tablets 2120
- Proventil Solutions for Inhalation 0.5% and 0.083% 2118
- Proventil Syrup 2119
- Proventil Tablets 2120
- Ventolin 583

Allopurinol (Increased serum theophylline levels at high-dose of allopurinol). Products include:
- Zyloprim Tablets 830

Bitolterol Mesylate (Potential for toxic synergism). Products include:
- Tornalate 2074

Carbamazepine (Decreased serum theophylline levels). Products include:
- Tegretol Chewable Tablets 654
- Tegretol Suspension 656
- Tegretol Tablets 654

Cimetidine (Increased serum theophylline levels). Products include:
- Tagamet Tablets 2228

Cimetidine Hydrochloride (Increased serum theophylline levels). Products include:
- Tagamet 2228

Ephedrine Hydrochloride (Potential for toxic synergism). Products include:
- Amesec .... ⊡ 682
- Primatene Tablets-M Formula 2421
- Primatene Tablets-P Formula 2421
- Primatene Tablets-Regular Formula 2421
- Quadrinal Tablets 1183
- Quelidrine Syrup 556
- Tedral SA 1765

Ephedrine Sulfate (Potential for toxic synergism). Products include:
- Bronkaid Tablets .... ⊡ 757
- Bronkolixir .... ⊡ 761
- Bronkotabs Tablets .... ⊡ 762
- Marax Tablets & DF Syrup 1954
- Pazo Hemorrhoid Ointment & Suppositories 752
- Vicks Vatronol Nose Drops .... ⊡ 666

Ephedrine Tannate (Potential for toxic synergism). Products include:
- Rynatuss 2388

Epinephrine (Potential for toxic synergism). Products include:
- Ana-Kit Anaphylaxis Emergency Treatment Kit 1100
- Bronkaid Mist .... ⊡ 757
- EpiPen 843
- Marcaine Hydrochloride 0.5% with Epinephrine 1:200,000 (as bitartrate) 958
- Marcaine Hydrochloride with Epinephrine 1:200,000 2055
- Primatene Mist 2420
- Sus-Phrine Injection 1006
- Xylocaine with Epinephrine Injections 637

Epinephrine Hydrochloride (Potential for toxic synergism). Products include:
- Adrenalin Chloride Solution 1:100 & 1:1,000 1689
- Epifrin .... ⊙ 244
- Glaucon .... ⊙ 218

Erythromycin (Increased theophylline serum levels). Products include:
- A/T/S Topical Gel and Topical Solution 1089
- AK-Mycin Ointment .... ⊙ 204
- Benzamycin Topical Gel 907
- E-Mycin Tablets 688
- ETS-2% 1685
- ERYC 1720
- Erycette (erythromycin 2%) Topical Solution 1678
- Ery-Tab Tablets 521
- Erythromycin Base Filmtab 525
- Erythromycin Delayed-Release Capsules, USP 526
- Ilotycin Ophthalmic Ointment 915
- PCE Dispertab Tablets 549
- Pediazole 1973
- T-Stat 2.0% Topical Solution and Pads 2409
- Theramycin Z Topical Solution 2% 1410

Erythromycin Estolate (Increased theophylline serum levels). Products include:
- Ilosone 913

Erythromycin Ethylsuccinate (Increased theophylline serum levels). Products include:
- E.E.S. 522
- EryPed 519
- Pediazole 1973

Erythromycin Gluceptate (Increased theophylline serum levels). Products include:
- Ilotycin Gluceptate, IV, Vials 915

Erythromycin Stearate (Increased theophylline serum levels). Products include:
- Erythrocin Stearate Filmtab 523

Ethinyl Estradiol (Increased serum theophylline levels). Products include:
- Brevicon 2304
- Demulen 2161
- Estinyl Tablets 2085
- Jenest-28 Tablets 1636
- Levlen/Tri-Levlen 665
- Lo/Ovral Tablets 2471
- Lo/Ovral-28 Tablets 2476
- Loestrin 1728
- Modicon 1667
- Nordette-21 Tablets 2481
- Nordette-28 Tablets 2483
- Norethin 2133
- Norinyl 2304
- Norlestrin 1746
- Ortho-Cyclen Tablets 1658
- Ortho-Novum 1667
- Ovcon 1391
- Ovral Tablets 2490
- Ovral-28 Tablets 2491
- Levlen/Tri-Levlen 665
- Tri-Norinyl 2304
- Triphasil-21 Tablets 2527
- Triphasil-28 Tablets 2532

Ethylnorepinephrine Hydrochloride (Potential for toxic synergism). Products include:
- Bronkephrine Injection 2042

Ethynodiol Diacetate (Increased serum theophylline levels). Products include:
- Demulen 2161

Halothane (Potential for sinus tachycardia or ventricular arrhythmias). Products include:
- Fluothane 2453

Isoetharine (Potential for toxic synergism). Products include:
- Arm-a-Med Isoetharine Inhalation Solution, USP 616
- Bronkometer Aerosol 2042
- Bronkosol Solution 2042

Isoproterenol Hydrochloride (Potential for toxic synergism). Products include:
- Isuprel Hydrochloride Injection 1:5000 2050
- Isuprel Hydrochloride Mistometer .. 2051
- Isuprel Hydrochloride Solution 1:200 & 1:100 2052
- Norisodrine Aerotrol 540

Levonorgestrel (Increased serum theophylline levels). Products include:
- Levlen/Tri-Levlen 665
- Nordette-21 Tablets 2481
- Nordette-28 Tablets 2483
- Norplant System 2484
- Levlen/Tri-Levlen 665
- Triphasil-21 Tablets 2527
- Triphasil-28 Tablets 2532

Lithium Carbonate (Increased renal excretion of lithium). Products include:
- Eskalith 2214
- Lithane Tablets 1596
- Lithium Carbonate Capsules & Tablets 1984
- Lithobid Tablets 870

Mestranol (Increased serum theophylline levels). Products include:
- Enovid 2161
- Norethin 2133
- Norinyl 2304
- Ortho-Novum 1667

Metaproterenol Sulfate (Potential for toxic synergism). Products include:
- Alupent 674
- Arm-a-Med Metaproterenol Sulfate Inhalation Solution, USP 617
- Metaprel Inhalation Aerosol Bronchodilator 2014
- Metaprel Inhalation Solution 2015
- Metaprel 2015
- Metaproterenol Sulfate Inhalation Solution, USP 912

Norethindrone (Increased serum theophylline levels). Products include:
- Brevicon 2304
- Jenest-28 Tablets 1636
- Micronor Tablets 1667
- Modicon 1667
- Norethin 2133
- Norinyl 2304
- Norlutin 1755
- Nor-Q D Tablets 2304
- Ortho-Novum 1667
- Ovcon 1391
- Tri-Norinyl 2304

Norethynodrel (Increased serum theophylline levels). Products include:
- Enovid 2161

Norgestimate (Increased serum theophylline levels). Products include:
- Ortho-Cyclen Tablets 1658

Norgestrel (Increased serum theophylline levels). Products include:
- Lo/Ovral Tablets 2471
- Lo/Ovral-28 Tablets 2476
- Ovral Tablets 2490
- Ovral-28 Tablets 2491
- Ovrette Tablets 2492

Phenobarbital (Decreased serum theophylline levels). Products include:
- Arco-Lase Plus Tablets 607
- Bellergal-S Tablets 1998
- Bronkolixir .... ⊡ 761
- Bronkotabs Tablets .... ⊡ 762
- Donnatal 1858
- Donnatal Extentabs 1859
- Donnatal Tablets 1858
- Donnazyme Tablets 1860
- Kinesed Tablets 2272
- Phenobarbital Elixir and Tablets 1293
- Primatene Tablets-P Formula 2421
- Quadrinal Tablets 1183
- Tedral SA 1765

Phenytoin (Decreased theophylline and phenytoin serum levels). Products include:
- Dilantin Infatabs 1710
- Dilantin-30 Pediatric/Dilantin-125 Suspension 1713

Phenytoin Sodium (Decreased theophylline and phenytoin serum levels). Products include:
- Dilantin Kapseals 1708
- Dilantin Parenteral 1712
- Dilantin with Phenobarbital Kapseals 1715

Pirbuterol Acetate (Potential for toxic synergism). Products include:
- Maxair Inhaler 1311

Propranolol Hydrochloride (Decreased serum theophylline levels). Products include:
- Inderal 2459
- Inderal LA Long Acting Capsules 2461
- Inderide Tablets 2463
- Inderide LA Long Acting Capsules .. 2465

Rifampin (Decreased serum theophylline levels). Products include:
- Rifadin 1345
- Rifamate Capsules 1347
- Rimactane Capsules 879

Terbutaline Sulfate (Potential for toxic synergism). Products include:
- Brethaire Inhaler 1024
- Brethine Ampuls 1026
- Brethine Tablets 1026
- Bricanyl Injection 1324
- Bricanyl Tablets 1325

Troleandomycin (Increased theophylline serum levels). Products include:
- Tao Capsules 1963

AMOXIL CAPSULES, POWDER FOR ORAL SUSPENSION & CHEWABLE TABLETS
(Amoxicillin) 2193
May interact with:

Probenecid (Concurrent administration delays excretion of amoxicillin). Products include:
- Benemid Tablets 1426
- ColBENEMID Tablets 1436
- Wycillin Injection and Probenecid Tablets 2539

AMOXIL PEDIATRIC DROPS, POWDER FOR ORAL SUSPENSION
(Amoxicillin) 2193
See **Amoxil Capsules, Powder for Oral Suspension & Chewable Tablets**

AMPHOJEL SUSPENSION
(Aluminum Hydroxide Gel) 2429
May interact with tetracyclines. Compounds in this category include:

Demeclocycline Hydrochloride (Concurrent administration should be avoided). Products include:
- Declomycin Capsules, Tablets 1199

Doxycycline Calcium (Concurrent administration should be avoided).
No products indexed under this heading.

Doxycycline Hyclate (Concurrent administration should be avoided). Products include:
- Doryx Capsules 1717
- Vibramycin Hyclate Capsules 1787
- Vibramycin Hyclate Intravenous 1968
- Vibra-Tabs Film Coated Tablets 1787

Doxycycline Monohydrate (Concurrent administration should be avoided). Products include:
- Monodox Capsules 1630
- Vibramycin Monohydrate for Oral Suspension 1787

Methacycline Hydrochloride (Concurrent administration should be avoided).
No products indexed under this heading.

Minocycline Hydrochloride (Concurrent administration should be avoided). Products include:
- Minocin Intravenous 1221
- Minocin Oral Suspension 1224
- Minocin Pellet-Filled Capsules 1222

Oxytetracycline (Concurrent administration should be avoided). Products include:
- Terramycin Intramuscular Solution 1964
- Urobiotic-250 Capsules 1968

Oxytetracycline Hydrochloride (Concurrent administration should be avoided). Products include:
- Terra-Cortril Ophthalmic Suspension 1963
- Terramycin Capsules 1786
- Terramycin Intramuscular Solution 1964
- Terramycin with Polymyxin B Sulfate Ophthalmic Ointment 1965

Tetracycline Hydrochloride (Concurrent administration should be avoided). Products include:
- Achromycin V Capsules 1193
- Achromycin Ophthalmic Ointment 1% ..... ⊙ 307
- Achromycin Ophthalmic Suspension 1% ..... ⊙ 308
- Topicycline for Topical Solution 1856

AMPHOJEL SUSPENSION WITHOUT FLAVOR
(Aluminum Hydroxide Gel) 2429
See **Amphojel Suspension**

AMPHOJEL TABLETS
(Aluminum Hydroxide Gel) 2429
See **Amphojel Suspension**

ANACIN COATED ANALGESIC CAPLETS
(Aspirin, Caffeine) 2417
No interactions described in labeling.

ANACIN COATED ANALGESIC TABLETS
(Aspirin, Caffeine) 2417
No interactions described in labeling.

ANACIN MAXIMUM STRENGTH ANALGESIC COATED TABLETS
(Aspirin, Caffeine) 2417
No interactions described in labeling.

ASPIRIN FREE ANACIN MAXIMUM STRENGTH ACETAMINOPHEN FILM COATED CAPLETS
(Acetaminophen) 2417
No interactions described in labeling.

ASPIRIN FREE ANACIN MAXIMUM STRENGTH ACETAMINOPHEN FILM COATED TABLETS
(Acetaminophen) 2417
No interactions described in labeling.

ANADROL-50 TABLETS
(Oxymetholone) 2287
May interact with insulin, oral hypoglycemic agents, anticoagulants, corticosteroids, and certain other agents. Compounds in these categories include:

ACTH (Concomitant administration may add to the edema).

Betamethasone Acetate (Concomitant administration may add to the edema). Products include:
- Celestone Soluspan Suspension 2081

Betamethasone Sodium Phosphate (Concomitant administration may add to the edema). Products include:
- Celestone Soluspan Suspension 2081

Chlorpropamide (Oral hypoglycemic dosage may need adjustment). Products include:
- Diabinese Tablets 1775

Cortisone Acetate (Concomitant administration may add to the edema). Products include:
- Cortone Acetate Sterile Suspension 1437
- Cortone Acetate Tablets 1439

Dexamethasone (Concomitant administration may add to the edema). Products include:
- AK-Trol Ointment & Suspension ..... ⊙ 207
- Decadron Elixir 1445
- Decadron Tablets 1447
- Decaspray Topical Aerosol 1459
- Dexacidin ..... ⊙ 272
- Maxidex Sterile Ophthalmic Suspension ..... ⊙ 223
- Maxitrol Ophthalmic Ointment/Suspension ..... ⊙ 223
- TobraDex Ophthalmic Suspension and Ointment ..... ⊙ 228

Dexamethasone Acetate (Concomitant administration may add to the edema). Products include:
- Dalalone D.P. Injectable 999
- Decadron-LA Sterile Suspension 1457

Dexamethasone Sodium Phosphate (Concomitant administration may add to the edema). Products include:
- AK-Dex ..... ⊙ 203
- Decadron Phosphate Respihaler 1454
- Decadron Phosphate Sterile Ophthalmic Ointment 1453
- Decadron Phosphate Sterile Ophthalmic Solution 1453
- Decadron Phosphate Topical Cream 1455
- Decadron Phosphate Turbinaire 1456
- Maxidex Sterile Ophthalmic Ointment ..... ⊙ 222
- NeoDecadron Sterile Ophthalmic Ointment 1517
- NeoDecadron Sterile Ophthalmic Solution 1518
- NeoDecadron Topical Cream 1518

Dicumarol (Increased sensitivity to anticoagulants; may need to decrease anticoagulant dosage). Products include:
- Dicumarol Tablets 516

Glipizide (Oral hypoglycemic dosage may need adjustment). Products include:
- Glucotrol 1952

Glyburide (Oral hypoglycemic dosage may need adjustment). Products include:
- DiaBeta 1091
- Micronase Tablets 2350

Heparin Calcium (Increased sensitivity to anticoagulants; may need to decrease anticoagulant dosage). Products include:
- Calciparine Injection 925

Heparin Sodium (Increased sensitivity to anticoagulants; may need to decrease anticoagulant dosage). Products include:
- Heparin Lock Flush Solution 2456
- Heparin Sodium Vials 1264
- Heparin Sodium Injection 2457
- Heparin Sodium Injection, USP, Sterile Solution 2342

Hydrocortisone (Concomitant administration may add to the edema). Products include:
- AK-Spore H.C. ..... ⊙ 206
- Bactine Hydrocortisone Anti-Itch Cream ..... ▣ 625
- CaldeCORT Anti-Itch Hydrocortisone Spray ..... ▣ 560
- Carmol HC Cream 1% 2296
- Cortaid Spray ..... ▣ 735
- Cortenema 2244
- Cortisporin Ointment 758
- Cortisporin Ophthalmic Ointment Sterile 758
- Cortisporin Ophthalmic Suspension Sterile 759
- Cortisporin Otic Solution Sterile 760
- Cortisporin Otic Suspension Sterile 760
- Cortizone-5 Creme & Ointment ..... ▣ 732
- Dermolate Anti-Itch Cream ..... ▣ 697
- Eldecort Cream 1.0% 1113
- Eldecort Cream 1.0% and 2.5% 1113
- Fungoid HC Creme 1770
- Hydrocortone Tablets 1482
- Hytone 909
- LazerSporin-C Solution 1770
- Massengill Medicated Soft Cloth Towelettes 2192
- Nutracort Cream & Lotion 1684
- PediOtic Suspension Sterile 797
- Synacort Creams 1%, 2.5% 2296
- Vanoxide-HC Acne Lotion 911
- Vioform-Hydrocortisone Cream and Mild Cream 889
- Vioform-Hydrocortisone Ointment 889
- VōSoL HC Otic Solution 2392
- Vytone Cream 1% 911

Hydrocortisone Acetate (Concomitant administration may add to the edema). Products include:
- Analpram-HC Rectal Cream 1% and 2.5% 970
- Anusol-HC Cream 1690
- Anusol-HC Suppositories 1691
- Caldecort ..... ▣ 560
- Carmol HC Cream 1% 2296
- Chloromycetin Hydrocortisone Ophthalmic 1694
- Coly-Mycin S Otic w/Neomycin & Hydrocortisone 1708
- Cortaid ..... ▣ 735
- Cortef Feminine Itch Cream ..... ▣ 735
- Corticaine ..... ▣ 682
- Cortifoam 1827
- Cortisporin Cream 757
- Epifoam 1828
- Gynecort 5 Creme ..... ▣ 556
- Hydrocortone Acetate Sterile Suspension 1479
- Lanacort 5 Creme and Ointment ..... ▣ 557
- Mantadil Cream 789
- Ophthocort ..... ⊙ 301
- Orabase HCA Oral Paste 890
- Pramosone Cream, Lotion & Ointment 971
- ProctoCream-HC 1834
- Proctofoam-HC 1835

Hydrocortisone Sodium Phosphate (Concomitant administration may add to the edema). Products include:
- Hydrocortone Phosphate Injection, Sterile 1481

Hydrocortisone Sodium Succinate (Concomitant administration may add to the edema). Products include:
- Solu-Cortef Sterile Powder 2361

Insulin, Human (Insulin dosage may need adjustment).
- No products indexed under this heading.

Insulin, Human Isophane Suspension (Insulin dosage may need adjustment). Products include:
- Humulin N, 100 Units 1270

Insulin, Human NPH (Insulin dosage may need adjustment). Products include:
- Insulatard NPH Human 1627
- Novolin N 1627
- Novolin N PenFill Cartridges 1628
- Novolin N Prefilled 1628

Insulin, Human Regular (Insulin dosage may need adjustment). Products include:
- Humulin BR, 100 Units 1268
- Humulin R, 100 Units 1272
- Novolin R 1627
- Novolin R PenFill Cartridges 1628
- Novolin R Prefilled 1629
- Velosulin Human 1628

Insulin, Human, Zinc Suspension (Insulin dosage may need adjustment). Products include:
- Humulin L, 100 Units 1268
- Humulin U, 100 Units 1272
- Novolin L 1627

Insulin, NPH (Insulin dosage may need adjustment). Products include:
- NPH, 40 & 100 Units 1273
- Beef NPH, 100 Units 1274
- Pork NPH, 100 Units 1275
- Insulatard NPH 1626
- NPH Insulin 1626
- NPH Purified Pork Isophane Insulin 1626

Insulin, Regular (Insulin dosage may need adjustment). Products include:
- Regular, 40 & 100 Units 1273
- Beef Regular, 100 Units 1275
- Pork Regular, 100 Units 1275
- Pork Regular (Concentrated), 500 Units 1276
- Regular Insulin 1625
- Regular Purified Pork Insulin 1626
- Velosulin 1627

Insulin, Zinc Crystals (Insulin dosage may need adjustment). Products include:
- NPH, 40 & 100 Units 1273

Insulin, Zinc Suspension (Insulin dosage may need adjustment). Products include:
- Lente, 40 & 100 Units 1272
- Protamine, Zinc, 40 & 100 Units 1273
- Lente Iletin I 1272
- Beef Lente, 100 Units 1274
- Beef Protamine Zinc, 100 Units 1274
- Pork Lente, 100 Units 1275
- Pork, Protamine, Zinc, 100 Units 1275
- Lente Insulin 1626
- Lente Purified Pork Insulin 1626
- Semilente Insulin 1625
- Ultralente Insulin 1626

Methylprednisolone Acetate (Concomitant administration may add to the edema). Products include:
- Depo-Medrol Sterile Aqueous Suspension 2334

Methylprednisolone Sodium Succinate (Concomitant administration may add to the edema). Products include:
- Solu-Medrol Sterile Powder 2363

Prednisolone Acetate (Concomitant administration may add to the edema). Products include:
- AK-Cide Sterile Ophthalmic Ointment & Suspension ..... ⊙ 202
- Blephamide Liquifilm Sterile Ophthalmic Suspension 586
- Blephamide S.O.P. Sterile Ophthalmic Ointment 586
- Cetapred Ointment ..... ⊙ 220
- ⅛% Econopred & 1% Econopred Plus ..... ⊙ 217
- Isopto Cetapred Suspension ..... ⊙ 220
- Metimyd ..... ⊙ 306
- Poly-Pred Liquifilm ..... ⊙ 250
- Pred Forte ..... ⊙ 252
- Pred Mild ..... ⊙ 254
- Pred-G Liquifilm Sterile Ophthalmic Suspension ..... ⊙ 252
- Pred-G S.O.P. Sterile Ophthalmic Ointment ..... ⊙ 253
- Vasocidin Ointment ..... ⊙ 275

Prednisolone Sodium Phosphate (Concomitant administration may add to the edema). Products include:
- AK-Pred ..... ⊙ 205
- Hydeltrasol Injection, Sterile 1476
- Inflamase ..... ⊙ 274
- Pediapred Oral Liquid 987
- Vasocidin Ophthalmic Solution ..... ⊙ 276

Prednisolone Tebutate (Concomitant administration may add to the edema). Products include:
- Hydeltra-T.B.A. Sterile Suspension 1478

Prednisone (Concomitant administration may add to the edema). Products include:
- Deltasone Tablets 2332

Tolazamide (Oral hypoglycemic dosage may need adjustment). Products include:
- Tolinase Tablets 2365

Tolbutamide (Oral hypoglycemic dosage may need adjustment). Products include:
- Orinase Tablets 2354

(▣ Described in PDR For Nonprescription Drugs) (⊙ Described in PDR For Ophthalmology)

Triamcinolone (Concomitant administration may add to the edema).
- No products indexed under this heading.

Triamcinolone Acetonide (Concomitant administration may add to the edema). Products include:
- Aristocort A ... 1010
- Azmacort Inhaler ... 1837
- Kenalog Cream, Lotion & Ointment 2401
- Kenalog-10 Injection ... 2402
- Kenalog-40 Injection ... 2403
- Kenalog in Orabase ... 604
- Kenalog Spray ... 2401
- Mycolog II Cream and Ointment ... 2407
- Mytrex Cream & Ointment ... 2080
- Nasacort Nasal Inhaler ... 1844

Triamcinolone Diacetate (Concomitant administration may add to the edema). Products include:
- Aristocort Suspension ... 1008

Triamcinolone Hexacetonide (Concomitant administration may add to the edema). Products include:
- Aristospan Suspension ... 1011

Warfarin Sodium (Increased sensitivity to anticoagulants; may need to decrease anticoagulant dosage). Products include:
- Coumadin Injection & Tablets ... 944
- Panwarfin Tablets ... 547

ANAFRANIL CAPSULES
(Clomipramine Hydrochloride) ... **650**
May interact with sympathomimetic aerosal brochodilators, anticholinergics, central nervous system depressants, monoamine oxidase inhibitors, and certain other agents. Compounds in these categories include:

Albuterol (Effect not specified; close supervision and careful adjustment of dosage are required). Products include:
- Proventil Inhalation Aerosol ... 2117
- Ventolin Inhalation Aerosol and Refill ... 583

Albuterol Sulfate (Effect not specified; close supervision and careful adjustment of dosage are required). Products include:
- Proventil Repetabs Tablets ... 2120
- Proventil Solutions for Inhalation 0.5% and 0.083% ... 2118
- Proventil Syrup ... 2119
- Proventil Tablets ... 2120
- Ventolin ... 583

Alcohol (Anafranil may exaggerate patients' response to alcohol).

Alfentanil Hydrochloride (Anafranil may exaggerate patients' response to CNS depressants). Products include:
- Alfenta Injection ... 1131

Alprazolam (Anafranil may exaggerate patients' response to CNS depressants). Products include:
- Xanax Tablets ... 2367

Aprobarbital (Anafranil may exaggerate patients' response to CNS depressants). Products include:
- Alurate Elixir ... 1883

Atropine Sulfate (Effect not specified; close supervision and careful adjustment of dosage are required). Products include:
- Arco-Lase Plus Tablets ... 607
- Atropine Sulfate Sterile Ophthalmic Solution and S.O.P. Sterile Ophthalmic Ointment ... ⊙ 239
- Donnagel ... ⊞ 675
- Donnagel-PG ... 1858
- Donnatal ... 1858
- Donnatal Extentabs ... 1859
- Donnatal Tablets ... 1858
- Donnazyme Tablets ... 1860
- Isopto Atropine ... ⊙ 218
- Lomotil ... 2174
- Motofen Tablets ... 836
- Ru-Tuss Tablets ... 693
- Urised Tablets ... 2396

Belladonna Alkaloids (Effect not specified; close supervision and careful adjustment of dosage are required). Products include:
- Bellergal-S Tablets ... 1998
- Hyland's Bed Wetting Tablets ... ⊞ 728
- Hyland's Teething Tablets ... ⊞ 728
- Kinesed Tablets ... 2272

Benztropine Mesylate (Effect not specified; close supervision and careful adjustment of dosage are required). Products include:
- Cogentin ... 1435

Biperiden (Effect not specified; close supervision and careful adjustment of dosage are required). Products include:
- Akineton ... 1171

Buprenorphine (Anafranil may exaggerate patients' response to CNS depressants).
- No products indexed under this heading.

Buspirone Hydrochloride (Anafranil may exaggerate patients' response to CNS depressants). Products include:
- BuSpar ... 1401

Butabarbital (Anafranil may exaggerate patients' response to CNS depressants). Products include:
- Pyridium Plus ... 1764

Butalbital (Anafranil may exaggerate patients' response to CNS depressants). Products include:
- Esgic-Plus Tablets ... 1002
- Esgic Tablets & Capsules ... 1001
- Fioricet Tablets ... 2006
- Fiorinal Capsules ... 2007
- Fiorinal with Codeine Capsules ... 2008
- Fiorinal Tablets ... 2007
- Phrenilin ... 838
- Sedapap Tablets 50 mg/650 mg ... 1360

Chlordiazepoxide (Anafranil may exaggerate patients' response to CNS depressants). Products include:
- Libritabs Tablets ... 1930
- Limbitrol ... 1933
- Menrium Tablets ... 1934

Chlordiazepoxide Hydrochloride (Anafranil may exaggerate patients' response to CNS depressants). Products include:
- Librax Capsules ... 1929
- Librium Capsules ... 1931
- Librium Injectable ... 1932

Chlorpromazine (Anafranil may exaggerate patients' response to CNS depressants). Products include:
- Thorazine ... 2234

Chlorprothixene (Anafranil may exaggerate patients' response to CNS depressants). Products include:
- Taractan Tablets ... 1920

Chlorprothixene Hydrochloride (Anafranil may exaggerate patients' response to CNS depressants). Products include:
- Taractan ... 1920

Cimetidine (May increase plasma concentration of clomipramine). Products include:
- Tagamet Tablets ... 2228

Cimetidine Hydrochloride (May increase plasma concentration of clomipramine). Products include:
- Tagamet ... 2228

Clidinium Bromide (Effect not specified; close supervision and careful adjustment of dosage are required). Products include:
- Librax Capsules ... 1929
- Quarzan Capsules ... 1937

Clonidine (Pharmacological effects of clonidine blocked). Products include:
- Catapres-TTS ... 677

Clonidine Hydrochloride (Pharmacological effects of clonidine blocked). Products include:
- Catapres Tablets ... 676
- Combipres Tablets ... 678

Clorazepate Dipotassium (Anafranil may exaggerate patients' response to CNS depressants). Products include:
- Tranxene ... 556

Codeine (Anafranil may exaggerate patients' response to CNS depressants). Products include:
- Calcidrine Syrup ... 506

Codeine Phosphate (Anafranil may exaggerate patients' response to CNS depressants). Products include:
- Actifed with Codeine Cough Syrup.. 752
- Cheracol Cough Syrup ... 1853
- Codimal PH Syrup ... 846
- Dimetane-DC Cough Syrup ... 1857
- Empirin with Codeine Phosphate Nos. 2, 3 & 4 ... 764
- Fiorinal with Codeine Capsules ... 2008
- Isoclor Expectorant ... 982
- Naldecon CX Adult Liquid ... ⊞ 521
- Novahistine DH ... 1342
- Novahistine Expectorant ... 1343
- Nucofed Capsules ... 2219
- Nucofed Expectorant ... 2219
- Nucofed Pediatric Expectorant ... 2220
- Nucofed Syrup ... 2219
- Phenaphen with Codeine Capsules 1865
- Phenaphen-650 with Codeine Tablets ... 1866
- Phenergan with Codeine ... 2497
- Phenergan VC with Codeine ... 2501
- Robitussin A-C Syrup ... 1875
- Robitussin-DAC Syrup ... 1875
- Ryna ... ⊞ 741
- Soma Compound w/Codeine Tablets ... 2390
- Triaminic Expectorant w/Codeine .. 1996
- Tussi-Organidin Liquid ... 2391
- Tylenol with Codeine ... 1381

Codeine Polistirex (Anafranil may exaggerate patients' response to CNS depressants).
- No products indexed under this heading.

Dezocine (Anafranil may exaggerate patients' response to CNS depressants).

Diazepam (Anafranil may exaggerate patients' response to CNS depressants). Products include:
- Valium Injectable ... 1937
- Valium Tablets ... 1939
- Valrelease Capsules ... 1923

Dicyclomine Hydrochloride (Effect not specified; close supervision and careful adjustment of dosage are required). Products include:
- Bentyl ... 1322

Digoxin (Potential for adverse effects due to displacement of either drug from protein binding site). Products include:
- Lanoxicaps ... 772
- Lanoxin Elixir Pediatric ... 775
- Lanoxin Injection ... 778
- Lanoxin Injection Pediatric ... 781
- Lanoxin Tablets ... 783

Dobutamine Hydrochloride (Effect not specified; close supervision and careful adjustment of dosage are required). Products include:
- Dobutrex Solution Vials ... 1259

Dopamine Hydrochloride (Effect not specified; close supervision and careful adjustment of dosage are required). Products include:
- Intropin Injection ... 930

Droperidol (Anafranil may exaggerate patients' response to CNS depressants). Products include:
- Inapsine Injection ... 1140
- Innovar Injection ... 1141

Enflurane (Anafranil may exaggerate patients' response to CNS depressants). Products include:
- Ethrane ... 599

Ephedrine Hydrochloride (Effect not specified; close supervision and careful adjustment of dosage are required). Products include:
- Amesec ... ⊞ 682
- Primatene Tablets-M Formula ... 2421
- Primatene Tablets-P Formula ... 2421
- Primatene Tablets-Regular Formula ... 2421
- Quadrinal Tablets ... 1183
- Quelidrine Syrup ... 556
- Tedral SA ... 1765

Ephedrine Sulfate (Effect not specified; close supervision and careful adjustment of dosage are required). Products include:
- Bronkaid Tablets ... ⊞ 757
- Bronkolixir ... ⊞ 761
- Bronkotabs Tablets ... ⊞ 762
- Marax Tablets & DF Syrup ... 1954
- Pazo Hemorrhoid Ointment & Suppositories ... 752
- Vicks Vatronol Nose Drops ... ⊞ 666

Ephedrine Tannate (Effect not specified; close supervision and careful adjustment of dosage are required). Products include:
- Rynatuss ... 2388

Epinephrine (Effect not specified; close supervision and careful adjustment of dosage are required). Products include:
- Ana-Kit Anaphylaxis Emergency Treatment Kit ... 1100
- Bronkaid Mist ... ⊞ 757
- EpiPen ... 843
- Marcaine Hydrochloride 0.5% with Epinephrine 1:200,000 (as bitartrate) ... 958
- Marcaine Hydrochloride with Epinephrine 1:200,000 ... 2055
- Primatene Mist ... 2420
- Sus-Phrine Injection ... 1006
- Xylocaine with Epinephrine Injections ... 637

Epinephrine Bitartrate (Effect not specified; close supervision and careful adjustment of dosage are required). Products include:
- AsthmaHaler Mist Epinephrine Bitartrate Bronchodilator ... ⊞ 616
- Bronkaid Mist Suspension ... ⊞ 757
- Primatene Mist Suspension ... 2421

Epinephrine Hydrochloride (Effect not specified; close supervision and careful adjustment of dosage are required). Products include:
- Adrenalin Chloride Solution 1:100 & 1:1,000 ... 1689
- Epifrin ... ⊙ 244
- Glaucon ... ⊙ 218

Estazolam (Anafranil may exaggerate patients' response to CNS depressants). Products include:
- ProSom Tablets ... 554

Ethchlorvynol (Anafranil may exaggerate patients' response to CNS depressants). Products include:
- Placidyl Capsules ... 553

Ethinamate (Anafranil may exaggerate patients' response to CNS depressants).
- No products indexed under this heading.

Fentanyl (Anafranil may exaggerate patients' response to CNS depressants). Products include:
- Duragesic Transdermal System ... 1133

Fentanyl Citrate (Anafranil may exaggerate patients' response to CNS depressants). Products include:
- Innovar Injection ... 1141
- Sublimaze Injection ... 1146

Fluoxetine Hydrochloride (May increase plasma concentration of clomipramine). Products include:
- Prozac Pulvules ... 920

Fluphenazine Decanoate (Anafranil may exaggerate patients' response to CNS depressants). Products include:
- Prolixin Decanoate ... 1795

Fluphenazine Enanthate (Anafranil may exaggerate patients' response to CNS depressants). Products include:
- Prolixin Enanthate ... 1796

Fluphenazine Hydrochloride (Anafranil may exaggerate patients' response to CNS depressants). Products include:
- Prolixin Elixir ... 1793
- Prolixin Injection ... 1791
- Prolixin Oral Concentrate ... 1792
- Prolixin Tablets ... 1793

Flurazepam Hydrochloride (Anafranil may exaggerate patients' response to CNS depressants). Products include:
- Dalmane Capsules ... 1927

Furazolidone (Concurrent therapy is contraindicated, or should not be used within 14 days before or after treatment with MAOI). Products include:
- Furoxone ... 1855

Glutethimide (Anafranil may exaggerate patients' response to CNS depressants).
- No products indexed under this heading.

Glycopyrrolate (Effect not specified; close supervision and careful adjustment of dosage are required). Products include:
- Robinul Forte Tablets ... 1873
- Robinul Injectable ... 1873
- Robinul Tablets ... 1873

Guanethidine Monosulfate (Pharmacological effects of guanethidine blocked). Products include:
- Esimil Tablets ... 864
- Ismelin Tablets ... 869

Haloperidol (Increases plasma concentration of clomipramine). Products include:
- Haldol Injection, Tablets and Concentrate ... 1373

Haloperidol Decanoate (Increases plasma concentration of clomipramine). Products include:
- Haldol Decanoate ... 1375

Hydrocodone Bitartrate (Anafranil may exaggerate patients' response to CNS depressants). Products include:
- Anexsia 5/500 Tablets ... 2196
- Anexsia 7.5/650 Tablets ... 2197
- Azdone Tablets ... 844
- Codiclear DH Syrup ... 845
- Codimal DH Syrup ... 846
- Damason-P ... 1356
- Hycodan Syrup, Tablets ... 927
- Hycomine Compound Tablets ... 929
- Hycomine Syrup ... 927
- Hycotuss Expectorant Syrup ... 930
- Hydrocet Capsules ... 835
- Lortab ASA Tablets ... 2414
- Lortab ... 2412
- Ru-Tuss with Hydrocodone ... 694
- Triaminic Expectorant DH ... 1995
- Vicodin Tablets ... 1187
- Vicodin ES Tablets ... 1189
- Zydone Capsules ... 941

Hydrocodone Polistirex (Anafranil may exaggerate patients' response to CNS depressants). Products include:
- Tussionex Extended-Release Suspension ... 988

Hydroxyzine Hydrochloride (Anafranil may exaggerate patients' response to CNS depressants). Products include:
- Atarax Tablets & Syrup ... 1941
- Marax Tablets & DF Syrup ... 1954
- Vistaril Intramuscular Solution ... 1970

Hyoscyamine (Effect not specified; close supervision and careful adjustment of dosage are required). Products include:
- Cystospaz Tablets ... 2395
- Urised Tablets ... 2396

Hyoscyamine Sulfate (Effect not specified; close supervision and careful adjustment of dosage are required). Products include:
- Arco-Lase Plus Tablets ... 607
- Cystospaz-M Capsules ... 2395
- Donnagel ... ▣ 675
- Donnagel-PG ... 1858
- Donnatal ... 1858
- Donnatal Extentabs ... 1859
- Donnatal Tablets ... 1858
- Donnazyme Tablets ... 1860
- Kutrase Capsules ... 2146
- Levsin/Levsinex ... 2147
- Ru-Tuss Tablets ... 693

Ipratropium Bromide (Effect not specified; close supervision and careful adjustment of dosage are required). Products include:
- Atrovent Inhalation Aerosol ... 675

Isocarboxazid (Concurrent therapy is contraindicated, or should not be used within 14 days before or after treatment with MAOI). Products include:
- Marplan Tablets ... 1906

Isoflurane (Anafranil may exaggerate patients' response to CNS depressants). Products include:
- Forane ... 600

Isoproterenol Hydrochloride (Effect not specified; close supervision and careful adjustment of dosage are required). Products include:
- Isuprel Hydrochloride Injection 1:5000 ... 2050
- Isuprel Hydrochloride Mistometer .. 2051
- Isuprel Hydrochloride Solution 1:200 & 1:100 ... 2052
- Norisodrine Aerotrol ... 540

Ketamine Hydrochloride (Anafranil may exaggerate patients' response to CNS depressants). Products include:
- Ketalar ... 1726

Levorphanol Tartrate (Anafranil may exaggerate patients' response to CNS depressants). Products include:
- Levo-Dromoran ... 1906

Lorazepam (Anafranil may exaggerate patients' response to CNS depressants). Products include:
- Ativan Injection ... 2432
- Ativan Tablets ... 2434

Loxapine Hydrochloride (Anafranil may exaggerate patients' response to CNS depressants). Products include:
- Loxitane ... 1213

Loxapine Succinate (Anafranil may exaggerate patients' response to CNS depressants). Products include:
- Loxitane Capsules ... 1213

Mepenzolate Bromide (Effect not specified; close supervision and careful adjustment of dosage are required). Products include:
- Cantil Tablets ... 1326

Meperidine Hydrochloride (Anafranil may exaggerate patients' response to CNS depressants). Products include:
- Demerol ... 2047
- Mepergan Injection ... 2479

Mephobarbital (Anafranil may exaggerate patients' response to CNS depressants). Products include:
- Mebaral Tablets ... 2061

Meprobamate (Anafranil may exaggerate patients' response to CNS depressants). Products include:
- Deprol Tablets ... 2382
- Equagesic Tablets ... 2451
- Miltown Tablets ... 2386
- PMB 200 and PMB 400 ... 2504

Mesoridazine (Anafranil may exaggerate patients' response to CNS depressants). Products include:
- Serentil ... 686

Metaproterenol Sulfate (Effect not specified; close supervision and careful adjustment of dosage are required). Products include:
- Alupent ... 674
- Arm-a-Med Metaproterenol Sulfate Inhalation Solution, USP ... 617
- Metaprel Inhalation Aerosol Bronchodilator ... 2014
- Metaprel Inhalation Solution ... 2015
- Metaprel ... 2015
- Metaproterenol Sulfate Inhalation Solution, USP ... 912

Metaraminol Bitartrate (Effect not specified; close supervision and careful adjustment of dosage are required). Products include:
- Aramine Injection ... 1424

Methadone Hydrochloride (Anafranil may exaggerate patients' response to CNS depressants). Products include:
- Dolophine Hydrochloride Ampoules & Vials ... 1260
- Dolophine Hydrochloride Tablets 1261
- Methadone Hydrochloride Diskets .. 1284
- Methadone Hydrochloride Oral Solution & Tablets ... 1987

Methohexital Sodium (Anafranil may exaggerate patients' response to CNS depressants). Products include:
- Brevital Sodium Vials ... 1248

Methoxamine Hydrochloride (Effect not specified; close supervision and careful adjustment of dosage are required). Products include:
- Vasoxyl Injection ... 819

Methoxyflurane (Anafranil may exaggerate patients' response to CNS depressants).
- No products indexed under this heading.

Methylphenidate Hydrochloride (May increase plasma concentration of clomipramine). Products include:
- Ritalin ... 880

Midazolam Hydrochloride (Anafranil may exaggerate patients' response to CNS depressants). Products include:
- Versed Injection ... 1924

Molindone Hydrochloride (Anafranil may exaggerate patients' response to CNS depressants). Products include:
- Moban Tablets & Concentrate ... 932

Morphine Sulfate (Anafranil may exaggerate patients' response to CNS depressants). Products include:
- Astramorph/PF Injection, USP (Preservative-Free) ... 618
- Duramorph ... 960
- Infumorph 200 and Infumorph 500 Sterile Solutions ... 962
- MS Contin Tablets ... 1814
- MSIR ... 1817
- Oramorph SR (Morphine Sulfate Sustained Release Tablets) ... 1988
- Roxanol ... 1991

Norepinephrine Bitartrate (Effect not specified; close supervision and careful adjustment of dosage are required). Products include:
- Levophed Bitartrate Injection ... 2054

Opium Alkaloids (Anafranil may exaggerate patients' response to CNS depressants). Products include:
- B & O No. 15A & No. 16A Supprettes ... 2395
- Pantopon Injectable ... 1911

Oxazepam (Anafranil may exaggerate patients' response to CNS depressants). Products include:
- Serax Capsules ... 2522
- Serax Tablets ... 2522

Oxybutynin Chloride (Effect not specified; close supervision and careful adjustment of dosage are required). Products include:
- Ditropan ... 1332

Oxycodone Hydrochloride (Anafranil may exaggerate patients' response to CNS depressants). Products include:
- Percocet Tablets ... 950
- Percodan ... 951
- Roxicodone Tablets, Oral Solution & Intensol (Oxycodone) ... 1992
- Tylox Capsules ... 1382

Pentobarbital Sodium (Anafranil may exaggerate patients' response to CNS depressants). Products include:
- Nembutal Sodium Capsules ... 534
- Nembutal Sodium Solution ... 536
- Nembutal Sodium Suppositories ... 538

Perphenazine (Anafranil may exaggerate patients' response to CNS depressants). Products include:
- Etrafon ... 2087
- Triavil Tablets ... 1556
- Trilafon ... 2123

Phenelzine Sulfate (Concurrent therapy is contraindicated, or should not be used within 14 days before or after treatment with MAOI). Products include:
- Nardil ... 1742

Phenobarbital (Increases plasma concentration of clomipramine). Products include:
- Arco-Lase Plus Tablets ... 607
- Bellergal-S Tablets ... 1998
- Bronkolixir ... ▣ 761
- Bronkotabs Tablets ... ▣ 762
- Donnatal ... 1858
- Donnatal Extentabs ... 1859
- Donnatal Tablets ... 1858
- Donnazyme Tablets ... 1860
- Kinesed Tablets ... 2272
- Phenobarbital Elixir and Tablets ... 1293
- Primatene Tablets-P Formula ... 2421
- Quadrinal Tablets ... 1183
- Tedral SA ... 1765

Phenylephrine Bitartrate (Effect not specified; close supervision and careful adjustment of dosage are required).
- No products indexed under this heading.

Phenylephrine Hydrochloride (Effect not specified; close supervision and careful adjustment of dosage are required). Products include:
- AK-Dilate Solution 2.5% and 10% ... ⊙ 203
- Atrohist Sprinkle Capsules ... 558
- Cerose-DM ... 2443
- Codimal ... 846
- Comhist LA Capsules ... 1618
- Congespirin For Children Aspirin Free Chewable Cold Tablets ... 748
- Cyclomydril ... ⊙ 216
- Deconsal Sprinkle Capsules ... 559
- Dimetane Decongestant ... ▣ 673
- Dristan Decongestant/Antihistamine/ Analgesic Coated Caplets ... ▣ 749
- Dristan Cold Nasal Decongestant/ Antihistamine/ Analgesic Coated Tablets ... 2419
- Dristan Advanced Formula Decongestant/Antihistamine/ Analgesic Tablets ... ▣ 749
- Dristan Nasal Spray, Menthol ... 2419
- Dristan Nasal Spray, Regular and Regular with Metered Pump ... 2419

Entex Capsules 1623
Entex Liquid 1623
Sinus Excedrin Analgesic, Decongestant Tablets & Caplets 750
Extendryl 994
4-Way Fast Acting Nasal Spray - Original Formula (regular & mentholated) & Metered Spray Pump (regular) 751
Hycomine Compound Tablets 929
Murocoll-2 Sterile Ophthalmic Solution ◉ 261
Mydfrin 2.5% ◉ 224
Naldecon Syrup, Tablets, Pediatric Drops and Pediatric Syrup 709
Neo-Synephrine Hydrochloride 1% Carpuject 2063
Neo-Synephrine Hydrochloride 1% Injection 2063
Neo-Synephrine Hydrochloride (Ophthalmic) 2064
Neo-Synephrine ▣ 759
Nōstril Nasal Decongestant ▣ 520
Novahistine Elixir ▣ 596
Phenergan VC 2500
Phenergan VC with Codeine 2501
Prefrin Liquifilm Vasoconstrictor and Lubricant Eye Drops ◉ 254
Prefrin-A ◉ 255
Quelidrine Syrup 556
Relief Vasoconstrictor and Lubricant Eye Drops ◉ 256
Robitussin Night Relief ▣ 677
Ru-Tuss with Hydrocodone 694
Ru-Tuss Tablets 693
Vasosulf ◉ 279
Vicks Sinex ▣ 665
Zincfrin ◉ 230

Phenylephrine Tannate (Effect not specified; close supervision and careful adjustment of dosage are required). Products include:

Rynatan 2387
Rynatuss 2388

Phenylpropanolamine Hydrochloride (Effect not specified; close supervision and careful adjustment of dosage are required). Products include:

A.R.M. Allergy Relief Medicine Caplets ▣ 615
Acutrim ▣ 548
Allerest ▣ 559
BC Cold Powder ▣ 517
Cheracol Plus Head Cold/Cough Formula ▣ 667
Codimal Expectorant 846
Comtrex Multi-Symptom Cold Reliever Tablets/Caplets/Liqui-Gels/Liquid 745
Contac Continuous Action Decongestant/Antihistamine Capsules ▣ 710
Contac Maximum Strength Continuous Action Decongestant/Antihistamine Caplets ▣ 709
Contac Severe Cold and Flu Formula Caplets ▣ 711
Coricidin 'D' Decongestant Tablets ▣ 695
Coricidin Demilets Tablets for Children ▣ 696
Demazin Nasal Decongestant/Antihistamine Repetabs Tablets & Syrup ▣ 697
Dexatrim ▣ 733
Dimetane-DC Cough Syrup 1857
Dimetapp Elixir ▣ 673
Dimetapp DM Elixir ▣ 674
Dimetapp Extentabs ▣ 674
Dimetapp Plus Caplets ▣ 675
Dimetapp Tablets ▣ 675
Entex Capsules 1623
Entex LA Tablets 1623
Entex Liquid 1623
4-Way Cold Tablets 750
Hycomine Syrup 927
Naldecon CX Adult Liquid ▣ 521
Naldecon DX Adult Liquid ▣ 521
Naldecon DX Children's Syrup ▣ 522
Naldecon DX Pediatric Drops ▣ 522
Naldecon EX Children's Syrup ▣ 522
Naldecon EX Pediatric Drops ▣ 523
Naldecon Syrup, Tablets, Pediatric Drops and Pediatric Syrup 709
Nolamine Tablets 838
Nolex LA Tablets 838
Ornade Spansule Capsules 2221
Orthoxicol Cough Syrup ▣ 668
Propagest 839
Pyrroxate Capsules ▣ 669
Robitussin-CF ▣ 676
Ru-Tuss II Capsules 693
Ru-Tuss with Hydrocodone 694
Ru-Tuss Tablets 693
Sine-Off Sinus Medicine Tablets-Aspirin Formula ▣ 722
Sinulin 840
St. Joseph Cold Tablets for Children ▣ 704
Tavist-D Tablets 2035
Triaminic Allergy Tablets ▣ 688
Triaminic Chewables ▣ 688
Triaminic Cold Tablets ▣ 688
Triaminic Expectorant ▣ 688
Triaminic Expectorant w/Codeine 1996
Triaminic Expectorant DH 1995
Triaminic Oral Infant Drops 1996
Triaminic Syrup ▣ 689
Triaminic-12 Tablets ▣ 690
Triaminic-DM Syrup ▣ 689
Triaminicin Tablets ▣ 690
Triaminicol Multi-Symptom Cold Tablets ▣ 691
Triaminicol Multi-Symptom Relief ▣ 691
Tuss-Ornade Liquid 2242
Tuss-Ornade Spansule Capsules 2242
Tylenol Cold Medication, Effervescent Tablets 1369

Pirbuterol Acetate (Effect not specified; close supervision and careful adjustment of dosage are required). Products include:

Maxair Inhaler 1311

Prazepam (Anafranil may exaggerate patients' response to CNS depressants). Products include:

Centrax 1693

Prochlorperazine (Anafranil may exaggerate patients' response to CNS depressants). Products include:

Compazine 2201

Procyclidine Hydrochloride (Effect not specified; close supervision and careful adjustment of dosage are required). Products include:

Kemadrin Tablets 771

Promethazine Hydrochloride (Anafranil may exaggerate patients' response to CNS depressants). Products include:

Mepergan Injection 2479
Phenergan with Codeine 2497
Phenergan with Dextromethorphan 2499
Phenergan Injection 2493
Phenergan Suppositories 2496
Phenergan Syrup 2495
Phenergan Tablets 2496
Phenergan VC 2500
Phenergan VC with Codeine 2501

Propantheline Bromide (Effect not specified; close supervision and careful adjustment of dosage are required). Products include:

Pro-Banthīne Tablets 2141

Propofol (Anafranil may exaggerate patients' response to CNS depressants). Products include:

Diprivan Injection 2267

Propoxyphene Hydrochloride (Anafranil may exaggerate patients' response to CNS depressants). Products include:

Darvon 1256
Wygesic Tablets 2540

Propoxyphene Napsylate (Anafranil may exaggerate patients' response to CNS depressants). Products include:

Darvon-N/Darvocet-N 1254

Pseudoephedrine Hydrochloride (Effect not specified; close supervision and careful adjustment of dosage are required). Products include:

Actifed Capsules ▣ 539
Actifed Plus Caplets ▣ 539
Actifed Plus Tablets ▣ 540
Actifed with Codeine Cough Syrup 752
Actifed Syrup ▣ 540
Actifed Tablets ▣ 540
Actifed 12-Hour Capsules ▣ 539
Advil Cold & Sinus Caplets (formerly CoAdvil) 2416
Allerest ▣ 559
Anatuss LA Tablets 1359
Benadryl Decongestant Elixir ▣ 635
Benadryl Decongestant ▣ 635
Benadryl Plus ▣ 636
Benadryl Plus Nighttime ▣ 637
Benylin Decongestant ▣ 638
Brexin L.A. Capsules 2078
Bromfed Capsules (Timed Release) 1615
Bromfed Syrup ▣ 628
Bromfed 1615
CoAdvil ▣ 748
Allergy-Sinus Comtrex Multi-Symptom Allergy Sinus Formula Tablets & Caplets 746
Cough Formula Comtrex 746
Comtrex Multi-Symptom Cold Reliever Tablets/Caplets/Liqui-Gels/Liquid 745
Day-Night Comtrex 747
Non-Drowsy Comtrex 747
Congess 994
Congestac Caplets ▣ 617
Contac Jr. Children's Cold Medicine ▣ 712
Contac Nighttime Cold Medicine ▣ 713
Contac Sinus Caplets Maximum Strength Non-Drowsy Formula ▣ 710
Contac Sinus Tablets Maximum Strength Non-Drowsy Formula ▣ 710
Deconamine 663
Deconsal II Tablets 559
Dimacol Caplets ▣ 672
Dimetane-DX Cough Syrup 1858
Dorcol Children's Cough Syrup ▣ 685
Dorcol Children's Decongestant Liquid ▣ 685
Dorcol Children's Liquid Cold Formula ▣ 686
Maximum Strength Dristan Decongestant/Analgesic Coated Caplets ▣ 750
No Drowsiness Dristan Cold Nasal Decongestant/Analgesic Coated Caplets 2420
Dristan Sinus Caplets 2419
Sinus Excedrin Analgesic, Decongestant Tablets & Caplets ▣ 533
Fedahist Gyrocaps 2145
Fedahist Timecaps 2145
Guaifed 1615
Guaifed Syrup ▣ 629
Isoclor Expectorant 982
Isoclor Timesule Capsules ▣ 561
Kronofed-A 970
Medi-Flu Caplet, Liquid ▣ 640
Novafed A Capsules 1342
Novafed Capsules 1342
Novahistine DH 1342
Novahistine DMX ▣ 595
Novahistine Expectorant 1343
Nucofed Capsules 2219
Nucofed Expectorant 2219
Nucofed Pediatric Expectorant 2220
Nucofed Syrup 2219
Ornex Caplets ▣ 618
PediaCare Allergy Relief Formula Liquid 1362
PediaCare Cough-Cold Formula Liquid 1362
PediaCare Infants' Oral Decongestant Drops 1362
PediaCare Night Rest Cough-Cold Formula Liquid 1362
PediaCare 6-12 Cough-Cold Formula Chewable Tablets 1362
Robitussin-DAC Syrup 1875
Robitussin-PE ▣ 677
Rondec 1975
Rondec-DM 1976
Rondec-TR Tablet 1975
Ru-Tuss DE Tablets 694
Ryna ▣ 741
Seldane-D Extended-Release Tablets 1350
Sinarest ▣ 562
Sine-Aid Maximum Strength Sinus Headache Caplets 1365
Sine-Aid Maximum Strength Sinus Headache Tablets 1365
Sine-Off Maximum Strength Allergy/Sinus Formula Caplets ▣ 721
Sine-Off Maximum Strength No Drowsiness Formula Caplets ▣ 722
Singlet Tablets ▣ 598
Sinutab Maximum Strength ▣ 641
Sinutab Maximum Strength Without Drowsiness Tablets & Caplets ▣ 642
Sinutab Regular Strength Without Drowsiness Formula ▣ 641
St. Joseph Nighttime Cold Medicine ▣ 705
Sudafed Children's Liquid ▣ 543
Sudafed Cough Syrup ▣ 543
Sudafed Plus Liquid ▣ 544
Sudafed Plus Tablets ▣ 545
Sudafed Sinus Caplets ▣ 545
Sudafed Sinus Tablets ▣ 545
Sudafed Tablets, 30 mg ▣ 544
Sudafed Tablets, Adult Strength, 60 mg ▣ 544
Sudafed 12 Hour Capsules ▣ 545
TheraFlu Flu and Cold Medicine ▣ 687
Triaminic Nite Light ▣ 689
Tylenol Allergy Sinus Medication Caplets and Gelcaps, Maximum Strength 1372
Children's Tylenol Cold Liquid Formula and Chewable Tablets 1368
Tylenol Cold & Flu Hot Medication, Packets 1369
Tylenol Cold & Flu No Drowsiness Hot Medication, Packets 1371
Tylenol Cold Medication Caplets and Tablets 1370
Tylenol Cold Medication No Drowsiness Formula Caplets 1370
Tylenol Cold Night Time Medication Liquid 1371
Tylenol Cough Medication Liquid with Decongestant, Maximum Strength 1372
Tylenol, Maximum Strength, Sinus Medication Gelcaps, Caplets and Tablets 1373
Ursinus Inlay-Tabs ▣ 691
Vicks Children's NyQuil ▣ 664
Vicks Daycare ▣ 660
Vicks Formula 44D Decongestant Cough Medicine ▣ 662
Vicks Formula 44M Multi-Symptom Cough Medicine ▣ 662
Vicks NyQuil Nighttime Colds Medicine-Original & Cherry Flavor ▣ 664
Vicks Pediatric Formula 44 Cough & Congestion Medicine ▣ 663
Vicks Pediatric Formula 44m Multi-Symptom Cough & Cold Medicine ▣ 663

Pseudoephedrine Sulfate (Effect not specified; close supervision and careful adjustment of dosage are required). Products include:

Afrin Tablets ▣ 693
Chlor-Trimeton Decongestant ▣ 694
Disophrol Chronotab Sustained-Action Tablets ▣ 698
Drixoral Antihistamine/Nasal Decongestant Syrup ▣ 698
Drixoral Non-Drowsy Formula ▣ 699
Drixoral Plus Extended-Release Tablets ▣ 699
Drixoral Sinus ▣ 700
Drixoral Sustained-Action Tablets ▣ 698
Sinutab Allergy Formula Sustained Action Tablets ▣ 640
Trinalin Repetabs Tablets 1170

Quazepam (Anafranil may exaggerate patients' response to CNS depressants). Products include:

Doral Tablets 2383

Scopolamine Hydrobromide (Effect not specified; close supervision and careful adjustment of dosage are required). Products include:

Donnagel ▣ 675
Donnagel-PG 1858
Donnatal 1858
Donnatal Extentabs 1859
Donnatal Tablets 1858
Donnazyme Tablets 1860
Isopto Hyoscine ◉ 222
Murocoll-2 Sterile Ophthalmic Solution ◉ 261
Ru-Tuss Tablets 693

Scopolamine Preparations (Effect not specified; close supervision and careful adjustment of dosage are required). Products include:

Transderm Scōp Transdermal Therapeutic System 887

Secobarbital Sodium (Anafranil may exaggerate patients' response to CNS depressants). Products include:
Seconal Sodium Pulvules ... 1296

Selegiline Hydrochloride (Concurrent therapy is contraindicated, or should not be used within 14 days before or after treatment with MAOI). Products include:
Eldepryl ... 2250

Sufentanil Citrate (Anafranil may exaggerate patients' response to CNS depressants). Products include:
Sufenta Injection ... 1147

Temazepam (Anafranil may exaggerate patients' response to CNS depressants). Products include:
Restoril Capsules ... 2023

Terbutaline Sulfate (Effect not specified; close supervision and careful adjustment of dosage are required). Products include:
Brethaire Inhaler ... 1024
Brethine Ampuls ... 1026
Brethine Tablets ... 1026
Bricanyl Injection ... 1324
Bricanyl Tablets ... 1325

Thiamylal Sodium (Anafranil may exaggerate patients' response to CNS depressants). Products include:
Surital Ampoules, Steri-Vials ... 1764

Thioridazine Hydrochloride (Anafranil may exaggerate patients' response to CNS depressants). Products include:
Mellaril ... 2011

Thiothixene (Anafranil may exaggerate patients' response to CNS depressants). Products include:
Navane Capsules and Concentrate 1954
Navane Intramuscular ... 1956

Tranylcypromine Sulfate (Concurrent therapy is contraindicated, or should not be used within 14 days before or after treatment with MAOI). Products include:
Parnate Tablets ... 2222

Triazolam (Anafranil may exaggerate patients' response to CNS depressants). Products include:
Halcion Tablets ... 2340

Tridihexethyl Chloride (Effect not specified; close supervision and careful adjustment of dosage are required).
No products indexed under this heading.

Trifluoperazine Hydrochloride (Anafranil may exaggerate patients' response to CNS depressants). Products include:
Stelazine ... 2226

Trihexyphenidyl Hydrochloride (Effect not specified; close supervision and careful adjustment of dosage are required). Products include:
Artane ... 1195

Warfarin Sodium (Potential for adverse effects due to displacement of either drug from protein binding site). Products include:
Coumadin Injection & Tablets ... 944
Panwarfin Tablets ... 547

ANA-KIT ANAPHYLAXIS EMERGENCY TREATMENT KIT

(Epinephrine Hydrochloride, Chlorpheniramine Maleate) ... 1100
May interact with tricyclic antidepressants, sympathomimetic aerosal brochodilators, and certain other agents. Compounds in these categories include:

Albuterol (Additive effects may be detrimental to the patient). Products include:
Proventil Inhalation Aerosol ... 2117
Ventolin Inhalation Aerosol and Refill ... 583

Albuterol Sulfate (Additive effects may be detrimental to the patient). Products include:
Proventil Repetabs Tablets ... 2120
Proventil Solutions for Inhalation 0.5% and 0.083% ... 2118
Proventil Syrup ... 2119
Proventil Tablets ... 2120
Ventolin ... 583

Amitriptyline Hydrochloride (Potentiation of epinephrine). Products include:
Elavil ... 2269
Endep Tablets ... 1927
Etrafon ... 2087
Limbitrol ... 1933
Triavil Tablets ... 1556

Amoxapine (Potentiation of epinephrine). Products include:
Asendin Tablets ... 1196

Chlorpheniramine Polistirex (Potentiation of epinephrine). Products include:
Tussionex Extended-Release Suspension ... 988

Chlorpheniramine Tannate (Potentiation of epinephrine). Products include:
Rynatan ... 2387
Rynatuss ... 2388

Clomipramine Hydrochloride (Potentiation of epinephrine). Products include:
Anafranil Capsules ... 650

Desipramine Hydrochloride (Potentiation of epinephrine). Products include:
Norpramin Tablets ... 1340

Dexchlorpheniramine Maleate (Potentiation of epinephrine). Products include:
Polaramine ... 2116

Diphenhydramine Citrate (Potentiation of epinephrine). Products include:
Alka-Seltzer Plus Night-Time Cold Medicine ... ◘ 623
Bufferin AF Nite Time Analgesic/Sleeping Aid Caplets ... 744
Excedrin P.M. Analgesic/Sleeping Aid Tablets, Caplets and Liquid ... 749

Diphenhydramine Hydrochloride (Potentiation of epinephrine). Products include:
Benadryl Anti-Itch Cream ... ◘ 635
Benadryl Capsules ... 1691
Benadryl Decongestant Elixir ... ◘ 635
Benadryl Decongestant ... ◘ 635
Benadryl Elixir ... ◘ 636
Benadryl Kapseals ... 1691
Benadryl 25 Kapseals ... ◘ 636
Benadryl Parenteral ... 1692
Benadryl Plus ... ◘ 636
Benadryl Plus Nighttime ... ◘ 637
Benadryl Spray, Maximum Strength ... ◘ 637
Benadryl Spray, Regular Strength ◘ 637
Benadryl Steri-Vials, Ampoules, and Steri-Dose Syringe ... 1692
Benadryl 25 Tablets ... ◘ 636
Benylin Cough Syrup ... ◘ 637
Benylin Decongestant ... ◘ 638
Caladryl Cream, Lotion, Spray ... ◘ 638
Miles Nervine Nighttime Sleep-Aid ◘ 627
Nytol Tablets ... ◘ 517
Sleep-ettes-D Tablets ... ◘ 653
Sleep-eze 3 Tablets ... ◘ 755
Sleepinal Night-time Sleep Aid Capsules ... ◘ 734
Sominex Caplets and Tablets ... ◘ 722
Sominex Liquid ... ◘ 723
Sominex Pain Relief Formula ... ◘ 723
Tylenol Cold Night Time Medication Liquid ... 1371
Tylenol PM, Extra Strength Caplets and Tablets ... 1368
Unisom Dual Relief Nighttime Sleep Aid/Analgesic ... 1774
Ziradryl Lotion ... ◘ 643

Dobutamine Hydrochloride (Additive effects may be detrimental to the patient). Products include:
Dobutrex Solution Vials ... 1259

Dopamine Hydrochloride (Additive effects may be detrimental to the patient). Products include:
Intropin Injection ... 930

Doxepin Hydrochloride (Potentiation of epinephrine). Products include:
Sinequan ... 1960

Ephedrine Hydrochloride (Additive effects may be detrimental to the patient). Products include:
Amesec ... ◘ 682
Primatene Tablets-M Formula ... 2421
Primatene Tablets-P Formula ... 2421
Primatene Tablets-Regular Formula ... 2421
Quadrinal Tablets ... 1183
Quelidrine Syrup ... 556
Tedral SA ... 1765

Ephedrine Sulfate (Additive effects may be detrimental to the patient). Products include:
Bronkaid Tablets ... ◘ 757
Bronkolixir ... ◘ 761
Bronkotabs Tablets ... ◘ 762
Marax Tablets & DF Syrup ... 1954
Pazo Hemorrhoid Ointment & Suppositories ... 752
Vicks Vatronol Nose Drops ... ◘ 666

Ephedrine Tannate (Additive effects may be detrimental to the patient). Products include:
Rynatuss ... 2388

Epinephrine (Additive effects may be detrimental to the patient). Products include:
Ana-Kit Anaphylaxis Emergency Treatment Kit ... 1100
Bronkaid Mist ... ◘ 757
EpiPen ... 843
Marcaine Hydrochloride 0.5% with Epinephrine 1:200,000 (as bitartrate) ... 958
Marcaine Hydrochloride with Epinephrine 1:200,000 ... 2055
Primatene Mist ... 2420
Sus-Phrine Injection ... 1006
Xylocaine with Epinephrine Injections ... 637

Epinephrine Bitartrate (Additive effects may be detrimental to the patient). Products include:
AsthmaHaler Mist Epinephrine Bitartrate Bronchodilator ... ◘ 616
Bronkaid Mist Suspension ... ◘ 757
Primatene Mist Suspension ... 2421

Imipramine Hydrochloride (Potentiation of epinephrine). Products include:
Tofranil Ampuls ... 1038
Tofranil Tablets ... 1039

Imipramine Pamoate (Potentiation of epinephrine). Products include:
Tofranil-PM Capsules ... 1041

Isoproterenol Hydrochloride (Additive effects may be detrimental to the patient). Products include:
Isuprel Hydrochloride Injection 1:5000 ... 2050
Isuprel Hydrochloride Mistometer .. 2051
Isuprel Hydrochloride Solution 1:200 & 1:100 ... 2052
Norisodrine Aerotrol ... 540

Maprotiline Hydrochloride (Potentiation of epinephrine). Products include:
Ludiomil Tablets ... 874

Metaproterenol Sulfate (Additive effects may be detrimental to the patient). Products include:
Alupent ... 674
Arm-a-Med Metaproterenol Sulfate Inhalation Solution, USP ... 617
Metaprel Inhalation Aerosol Bronchodilator ... 2014
Metaprel Inhalation Solution ... 2015
Metaprel ... 2015
Metaproterenol Sulfate Inhalation Solution, USP ... 912

Metaraminol Bitartrate (Additive effects may be detrimental to the patient). Products include:
Aramine Injection ... 1424

Methoxamine Hydrochloride (Additive effects may be detrimental to the patient). Products include:
Vasoxyl Injection ... 819

Norepinephrine Bitartrate (Additive effects may be detrimental to the patient). Products include:
Levophed Bitartrate Injection ... 2054

Nortriptyline Hydrochloride (Potentiation of epinephrine). Products include:
Pamelor ... 2019

Phenylephrine Bitartrate (Additive effects may be detrimental to the patient).
No products indexed under this heading.

Phenylephrine Hydrochloride (Additive effects may be detrimental to the patient). Products include:
AK-Dilate Solution 2.5% and 10% ... ⊚ 203
Atrohist Sprinkle Capsules ... 558
Cerose-DM ... 2443
Codimal ... 846
Comhist LA Capsules ... 1618
Congespirin For Children Aspirin Free Chewable Cold Tablets ... 748
Cyclomydril ... ⊚ 216
Deconsal Sprinkle Capsules ... 559
Dimetane Decongestant ... ◘ 673
Dristan Decongestant/Antihistamine/Analgesic Coated Caplets ... ◘ 749
Dristan Cold Nasal Decongestant/Antihistamine/Analgesic Coated Tablets ... 2419
Dristan Advanced Formula Decongestant/Antihistamine/Analgesic Tablets ... ◘ 749
Dristan Nasal Spray, Menthol ... 2419
Dristan Nasal Spray, Regular and Regular with Metered Pump ... 2419
Entex Capsules ... 1623
Entex Liquid ... 1623
Sinus Excedrin Analgesic, Decongestant Tablets & Caplets ... 750
Extendryl ... 994
4-Way Fast Acting Nasal Spray - Original Formula (regular & mentholated) & Metered Spray Pump (regular) ... 751
Hycomine Compound Tablets ... 929
Murocoll-2 Sterile Ophthalmic Solution ... ⊚ 261
Mydfrin 2.5% ... ⊚ 224
Naldecon Syrup, Tablets, Pediatric Drops and Pediatric Syrup ... 709
Neo-Synephrine Hydrochloride 1% Carpuject ... 2063
Neo-Synephrine Hydrochloride 1% Injection ... 2063
Neo-Synephrine Hydrochloride (Ophthalmic) ... 2064
Neo-Synephrine ... ◘ 759
Nōstril Nasal Decongestant ... ◘ 520
Novahistine Elixir ... ◘ 596
Phenergan VC ... 2500
Phenergan VC with Codeine ... 2501
Prefrin Liquifilm Vasoconstrictor and Lubricant Eye Drops ... ⊚ 254
Prefrin-A ... ⊚ 255
Quelidrine Syrup ... 556
Relief Vasoconstrictor and Lubricant Eye Drops ... ⊚ 256
Robitussin Night Relief ... ◘ 677
Ru-Tuss with Hydrocodone ... 694
Ru-Tuss Tablets ... 693
Vasosulf ... ⊚ 279
Vicks Sinex ... ◘ 665
Zincfrin ... ⊚ 230

Phenylephrine Tannate (Additive effects may be detrimental to the patient). Products include:
Rynatan ... 2387
Rynatuss ... 2388

Phenylpropanolamine Hydrochloride (Additive effects may be detrimental to the patient). Products include:

A.R.M. Allergy Relief Medicine Caplets ▣ 615
Acutrim ▣ 548
Allerest ▣ 559
BC Cold Powder ▣ 517
Cheracol Plus Head Cold/Cough Formula ▣ 667
Codimal Expectorant 846
Comtrex Multi-Symptom Cold Reliever Tablets/Caplets/Liqui-Gels/Liquid 745
Contac Continuous Action Decongestant/Antihistamine Capsules ▣ 710
Contac Maximum Strength Continuous Action Decongestant/Antihistamine Caplets ▣ 709
Contac Severe Cold and Flu Formula Caplets ▣ 711
Coricidin 'D' Decongestant Tablets ▣ 695
Coricidin Demilets Tablets for Children ▣ 696
Demazin Nasal Decongestant/Antihistamine Repetabs Tablets & Syrup ▣ 697
Dexatrim ▣ 733
Dimetane-DC Cough Syrup 1857
Dimetapp Elixir ▣ 673
Dimetapp DM Elixir ▣ 674
Dimetapp Extentabs ▣ 674
Dimetapp Plus Caplets ▣ 675
Dimetapp Tablets ▣ 675
Entex Capsules 1623
Entex LA Tablets 1623
Entex Liquid 1623
4-Way Cold Tablets 750
Hycomine Syrup 927
Naldecon CX Adult Liquid ▣ 521
Naldecon DX Adult Liquid ▣ 521
Naldecon DX Children's Syrup ▣ 522
Naldecon DX Pediatric Drops ▣ 522
Naldecon EX Children's Syrup ▣ 522
Naldecon EX Pediatric Drops ▣ 523
Naldecon Syrup, Tablets, Pediatric Drops and Pediatric Syrup 709
Nolamine Tablets 838
Nolex LA Tablets 838
Ornade Spansule Capsules 2221
Orthoxicol Cough Syrup ▣ 668
Propagest 839
Pyrroxate Capsules ▣ 669
Robitussin-CF ▣ 676
Ru-Tuss II Capsules 693
Ru-Tuss with Hydrocodone 694
Ru-Tuss Tablets 693
Sine-Off Sinus Medicine Tablets-Aspirin Formula ▣ 722
Sinulin 840
St. Joseph Cold Tablets for Children ▣ 704
Tavist-D Tablets 2035
Triaminic Allergy Tablets ▣ 688
Triaminic Chewables ▣ 688
Triaminic Cold Tablets ▣ 688
Triaminic Expectorant ▣ 688
Triaminic Expectorant w/Codeine 1996
Triaminic Expectorant DH 1995
Triaminic Oral Infant Drops 1996
Triaminic Syrup ▣ 689
Triaminic-12 Tablets ▣ 690
Triaminic-DM Syrup ▣ 689
Triaminicin Tablets ▣ 690
Triaminicol Multi-Symptom Cold Tablets ▣ 691
Triaminicol Multi-Symptom Relief ▣ 691
Tuss-Ornade Liquid 2242
Tuss-Ornade Spansule Capsules 2242
Tylenol Cold Medication, Effervescent Tablets 1369

Pirbuterol Acetate (Additive effects may be detrimental to the patient). Products include:

Maxair Inhaler 1311

Protriptyline Hydrochloride (Potentiation of epinephrine). Products include:

Vivactil Tablets 1567

Pseudoephedrine Hydrochloride (Additive effects may be detrimental to the patient). Products include:

Actifed Capsules ▣ 539
Actifed Plus Caplets ▣ 539
Actifed Plus Tablets ▣ 540
Actifed with Codeine Cough Syrup 752
Actifed Syrup ▣ 540
Actifed Tablets ▣ 540
Actifed 12-Hour Capsules ▣ 539
Advil Cold & Sinus Caplets (formerly CoAdvil) 2416
Allerest ▣ 559
Anatuss LA Tablets 1359
Benadryl Decongestant Elixir ▣ 635
Benadryl Decongestant ▣ 635
Benadryl Plus ▣ 636
Benadryl Plus Nighttime ▣ 637
Benylin Decongestant ▣ 638
Brexin L.A. Capsules 2078
Bromfed Capsules (Timed Release) 1615
Bromfed Syrup ▣ 628
Bromfed 1615
CoAdvil ▣ 748
Allergy-Sinus Comtrex Multi-Symptom Allergy Sinus Formula Tablets & Caplets 746
Cough Formula Comtrex 746
Comtrex Multi-Symptom Cold Reliever Tablets/Caplets/Liqui-Gels/Liquid 745
Day-Night Comtrex 747
Non-Drowsy Comtrex 747
Congess 994
Congestac Caplets ▣ 617
Contac Jr. Children's Cold Medicine ▣ 712
Contac Nighttime Cold Medicine ▣ 713
Contac Sinus Caplets Maximum Strength Non-Drowsy Formula ▣ 710
Contac Sinus Tablets Maximum Strength Non-Drowsy Formula ▣ 710
Deconamine 663
Deconsal II Tablets 559
Dimacol Caplets ▣ 672
Dimetane-DX Cough Syrup 1858
Dorcol Children's Cough Syrup ▣ 685
Dorcol Children's Decongestant Liquid ▣ 685
Dorcol Children's Liquid Cold Formula ▣ 686
Maximum Strength Dristan Decongestant/Analgesic Coated Caplets ▣ 750
No Drowsiness Dristan Cold Nasal Decongestant/Analgesic Coated Caplets 2420
Dristan Sinus Caplets 2419
Sinus Excedrin Analgesic, Decongestant Tablets & Caplets ▣ 533
Fedahist Gyrocaps 2145
Fedahist Timecaps 2145
Guaifed 1615
Guaifed Syrup ▣ 629
Isoclor Expectorant 982
Isoclor Timesule Capsules ▣ 561
Kronofed-A 970
Medi-Flu Caplet, Liquid ▣ 640
Novafed A Capsules 1342
Novafed Capsules 1342
Novahistine DH 1342
Novahistine DMX ▣ 595
Novahistine Expectorant 1343
Nucofed Capsules 2219
Nucofed Expectorant 2219
Nucofed Pediatric Expectorant 2220
Nucofed Syrup 2219
Ornex Caplets ▣ 618
PediaCare Allergy Relief Formula Liquid 1362
PediaCare Cough-Cold Formula Liquid 1362
PediaCare Infants' Oral Decongestant Drops 1362
PediaCare Night Rest Cough-Cold Formula Liquid 1362
PediaCare 6-12 Cough-Cold Formula Chewable Tablets 1362
Robitussin-DAC Syrup 1875
Robitussin-PE ▣ 677
Rondec 1975
Rondec-DM 1976
Rondec-TR Tablet 1975
Ru-Tuss DE Tablets 694
Ryna ▣ 741
Seldane-D Extended-Release Tablets 1350
Sinarest ▣ 562
Sine-Aid Maximum Strength Sinus Headache Caplets 1365
Sine-Aid Maximum Strength Sinus Headache Tablets 1365
Sine-Off Maximum Strength Allergy/Sinus Formula Caplets ▣ 721
Sine-Off Maximum Strength No Drowsiness Formula Caplets ▣ 722
Singlet Tablets ▣ 598
Sinutab Maximum Strength ▣ 641
Sinutab Maximum Strength Without Drowsiness Tablets & Caplets ▣ 642
Sinutab Regular Strength Without Drowsiness Formula ▣ 641
St. Joseph Nighttime Cold Medicine ▣ 705
Sudafed Children's Liquid ▣ 543
Sudafed Cough Syrup ▣ 543
Sudafed Plus Liquid ▣ 544
Sudafed Plus Tablets ▣ 545
Sudafed Sinus Caplets ▣ 545
Sudafed Sinus Tablets ▣ 545
Sudafed Tablets, 30 mg ▣ 544
Sudafed Tablets, Adult Strength, 60 mg ▣ 544
Sudafed 12 Hour Capsules ▣ 545
TheraFlu Flu and Cold Medicine ▣ 687
Triaminic Nite Light ▣ 689
Tylenol Allergy Sinus Medication Caplets and Gelcaps, Maximum Strength 1372
Children's Tylenol Cold Liquid Formula and Chewable Tablets 1368
Tylenol Cold & Flu Hot Medication, Packets 1369
Tylenol Cold & Flu No Drowsiness Hot Medication, Packets 1371
Tylenol Cold Medication Caplets and Tablets 1370
Tylenol Cold Medication No Drowsiness Formula Caplets 1370
Tylenol Cold Night Time Medication Liquid 1371
Tylenol Cough Medication Liquid with Decongestant, Maximum Strength 1372
Tylenol, Maximum Strength, Sinus Medication Gelcaps, Caplets and Tablets 1373
Ursinus Inlay-Tabs ▣ 691
Vicks Children's NyQuil ▣ 664
Vicks Daycare ▣ 660
Vicks Formula 44D Decongestant Cough Medicine ▣ 662
Vicks Formula 44M Multi-Symptom Cough Medicine ▣ 662
Vicks NyQuil Nighttime Colds Medicine-Original & Cherry Flavor ▣ 664
Vicks Pediatric Formula 44 Cough & Congestion Medicine ▣ 663
Vicks Pediatric Formula 44m Multi-Symptom Cough & Cold Medicine ▣ 663

Pseudoephedrine Sulfate (Additive effects may be detrimental to the patient). Products include:

Afrin Tablets ▣ 693
Chlor-Trimeton Decongestant ▣ 694
Disophrol Chronotab Sustained-Action Tablets ▣ 698
Drixoral Antihistamine/Nasal Decongestant Syrup ▣ 698
Drixoral Non-Drowsy Formula ▣ 699
Drixoral Plus Extended-Release Tablets ▣ 699
Drixoral Sinus ▣ 700
Drixoral Sustained-Action Tablets ▣ 698
Sinutab Allergy Formula Sustained Action Tablets ▣ 640
Trinalin Repetabs Tablets 1170

Sodium Levothyroxine (Potentiation of epinephrine).

No products indexed under this heading.

Terbutaline Sulfate (Additive effects may be detrimental to the patient). Products include:

Brethaire Inhaler 1024
Brethine Ampuls 1026
Brethine Tablets 1026
Bricanyl Injection 1324
Bricanyl Tablets 1325

Trimeprazine Tartrate (Potentiation of epinephrine). Products include:

Temaril Tablets, Syrup and Spansule Sustained Release Capsules 1085

Trimipramine Maleate (Potentiation of epinephrine). Products include:

Surmontil Capsules 2524

Tripelennamine Hydrochloride (Potentiation of epinephrine). Products include:

PBZ Tablets & Elixir 1037
PBZ-SR Tablets 1037

ANALPRAM-HC RECTAL CREAM 1% AND 2.5%
(Hydrocortisone Acetate, Pramoxine Hydrochloride) 970
No interactions described in labeling.

ANAPROX AND ANAPROX DS TABLETS
(Naproxen Sodium) 2288
May interact with oral anticoagulants, oral hypoglycemic agents, sulfonamides, beta blockers, lithium preparations, hydantoin anticonvulsants, and certain other agents. Compounds in these categories include:

Acebutolol Hydrochloride (Reduced antihypertensive effect). Products include:

Sectral Capsules 2520

Atenolol (Reduced antihypertensive effect). Products include:

Tenoretic Tablets 1105
Tenormin Tablets and I.V. Injection 1107

Betaxolol Hydrochloride (Reduced antihypertensive effect). Products include:

Betoptic Sterile Ophthalmic Solution 569
Betoptic S Sterile Ophthalmic Suspension 570
Kerlone Tablets 2172

Carteolol Hydrochloride (Reduced antihypertensive effect). Products include:

Cartrol Tablets 507

Chlorpropamide (Chlorpropamide toxicity). Products include:

Diabinese Tablets 1775

Dicumarol (Prothrombin time may be affected). Products include:

Dicumarol Tablets 516

Esmolol Hydrochloride (Reduced antihypertensive effect). Products include:

Brevibloc Injection 942

Ethotoin (Hydantoin toxicity). Products include:

Peganone Tablets 551

Furosemide (Natriuretic effect of furosemide inhibited). Products include:

Lasix 1093

Glipizide (Glipizide toxicity). Products include:

Glucotrol 1952

Glyburide (Glyburide toxicity). Products include:

DiaBeta 1091
Micronase Tablets 2350

Labetalol Hydrochloride (Reduced antihypertensive effect). Products include:

Normodyne Injection 2108
Normodyne Tablets 2110
Normozide Tablets 2112
Trandate HCT Tablets 579
Trandate Injection 577
Trandate Tablets 579

Lithium Carbonate (Increased plasma lithium concentration). Products include:

Eskalith 2214
Lithane Tablets 1596
Lithium Carbonate Capsules & Tablets 1984
Lithobid Tablets 870

Lithium Citrate (Increased plasma lithium concentration). Products include:

Cibalith-S 870

Mephenytoin (Hydantoin toxicity). Products include:
- Mesantoin Tablets ... 2013

Methotrexate Sodium (Methotrexate toxicity may be enhanced). Products include:
- Methotrexate Tablets, Parenteral, LPF Parenteral ... 1217
- Rheumatrex Methotrexate Dose Pack ... 1234

Metoprolol Tartrate (Reduced antihypertensive effect). Products include:
- Lopressor Ampuls ... 1032
- Lopressor HCT Tablets ... 1034
- Lopressor Tablets ... 1032

Nadolol (Reduced antihypertensive effect). Products include:
- Corgard Tablets ... 701
- Corzide Tablets ... 702

Penbutolol Sulfate (Reduced antihypertensive effect). Products include:
- Levatol ... 1832

Phenytoin (Hydantoin toxicity). Products include:
- Dilantin Infatabs ... 1710
- Dilantin-30 Pediatric/Dilantin-125 Suspension ... 1713

Phenytoin Sodium (Hydantoin toxicity). Products include:
- Dilantin Kapseals ... 1708
- Dilantin Parenteral ... 1712
- Dilantin with Phenobarbital Kapseals ... 1715

Pindolol (Reduced antihypertensive effect). Products include:
- Visken Tablets ... 2036

Probenecid (Increased Naproxen anion). Products include:
- Benemid Tablets ... 1426
- ColBENEMID Tablets ... 1436
- Wycillin Injection and Probenecid Tablets ... 2539

Propranolol Hydrochloride (Reduced antihypertensive effect). Products include:
- Inderal ... 2459
- Inderal LA Long Acting Capsules ... 2461
- Inderide Tablets ... 2463
- Inderide LA Long Acting Capsules .. 2465

Sulfamethizole (Sulfamethizole toxicity). Products include:
- Thiosulfil Forte Tablets ... 2526
- Urobiotic-250 Capsules ... 1968

Sulfamethoxazole (Sulfamethoxazole toxicity). Products include:
- Azo Gantanol Tablets ... 1887
- Bactrim DS Tablets ... 1891
- Bactrim I.V. Infusion ... 1889
- Bactrim ... 1891
- Gantanol ... 1899
- Septra ... 813
- Septra I.V. Infusion ... 808
- Septra I.V. Infusion ADD-Vantage Vials ... 810
- Septra ... 813

Sulfasalazine (Sulfasalazine toxicity). Products include:
- Azulfidine Tablets, EN-tabs, Oral Suspension ... 1157

Sulfinpyrazone (Sulfinpyrazone toxicity). Products include:
- Anturane ... 853

Sulfisoxazole (Sulfisoxazole toxicity). Products include:
- Azo Gantrisin Tablets ... 1888
- Gantrisin Tablets ... 1901
- Pediazole ... 1973

Sulfisoxazole Diolamine (Sulfisoxazole toxicity). Products include:
- Gantrisin Ophthalmic Ointment/Solution ... 1900

Timolol Maleate (Reduced antihypertensive effect). Products include:
- Blocadren Tablets ... 1429
- Timolide Tablets ... 1547
- Timoptic in Ocudose ... 1552
- Timoptic Sterile Ophthalmic Solution ... 1550

Tolazamide (Tolazamide toxicity). Products include:
- Tolinase Tablets ... 2365

Tolbutamide (Tolbutamide toxicity). Products include:
- Orinase Tablets ... 2354

Warfarin Sodium (Prothrombin time may be affected). Products include:
- Coumadin Injection & Tablets ... 944
- Panwarfin Tablets ... 547

ANATUSS LA TABLETS
(Guaifenesin, Pseudoephedrine Hydrochloride) ... 1359
May interact with veratrum alkaloids, monoamine oxidase inhibitors, beta blockers, catecholamine depleting drugs, and certain other agents. Compounds in these categories include:

Acebutolol Hydrochloride (Potentiates the effects of sympathomimetics). Products include:
- Sectral Capsules ... 2520

Atenolol (Potentiates the effects of sympathomimetics). Products include:
- Tenoretic Tablets ... 1105
- Tenormin Tablets and I.V. Injection 1107

Betaxolol Hydrochloride (Potentiates the effects of sympathomimetics). Products include:
- Betoptic Sterile Ophthalmic Solution ... 569
- Betoptic S Sterile Ophthalmic Suspension ... 570
- Kerlone Tablets ... 2172

Carteolol Hydrochloride (Potentiates the effects of sympathomimetics). Products include:
- Cartrol Tablets ... 507

Cryptenamine Preparations (Reduced antihypertensive effect).

Deserpidine (Reduced antihypertensive effect). Products include:
- Enduronyl ... 518
- Harmonyl Tablets ... 528
- Oreticyl ... 545

Esmolol Hydrochloride (Potentiates the effects of sympathomimetics). Products include:
- Brevibloc Injection ... 942

Furazolidone (Potentiates the effects of sympathomimetics; concurrent use is contraindicated). Products include:
- Furoxone ... 1855

Guanethidine Monosulfate (Reduced antihypertensive effect). Products include:
- Esimil Tablets ... 864
- Ismelin Tablets ... 869

Isocarboxazid (Potentiates the effects of sympathomimetics; concurrent use is contraindicated). Products include:
- Marplan Tablets ... 1906

Labetalol Hydrochloride (Potentiates the effects of sympathomimetics). Products include:
- Normodyne Injection ... 2108
- Normodyne Tablets ... 2110
- Normozide Tablets ... 2112
- Trandate HCT Tablets ... 579
- Trandate Injection ... 577
- Trandate Tablets ... 579

Mecamylamine Hydrochloride (Reduced antihypertensive effect). Products include:
- Inversine Tablets ... 1492

Methyldopa (Reduced antihypertensive effect). Products include:
- Aldoclor Tablets ... 1413
- Aldomet Oral ... 1415
- Aldoril Tablets ... 1418

Methyldopate Hydrochloride (Reduced antihypertensive effect). Products include:
- Aldomet Ester HCl Injection ... 1417

Metoprolol Tartrate (Potentiates the effects of sympathomimetics). Products include:
- Lopressor Ampuls ... 1032
- Lopressor HCT Tablets ... 1034
- Lopressor Tablets ... 1032

Nadolol (Potentiates the effects of sympathomimetics). Products include:
- Corgard Tablets ... 701
- Corzide Tablets ... 702

Penbutolol Sulfate (Potentiates the effects of sympathomimetics). Products include:
- Levatol ... 1832

Phenelzine Sulfate (Potentiates the effects of sympathomimetics; concurrent use is contraindicated). Products include:
- Nardil ... 1742

Pindolol (Potentiates the effects of sympathomimetics). Products include:
- Visken Tablets ... 2036

Propranolol Hydrochloride (Potentiates the effects of sympathomimetics). Products include:
- Inderal ... 2459
- Inderal LA Long Acting Capsules ... 2461
- Inderide Tablets ... 2463
- Inderide LA Long Acting Capsules .. 2465

Rauwolfia Serpentina (Reduced antihypertensive effect). Products include:
- Raudixin Tablets ... 1803
- Rauzide Tablets ... 1804

Rescinnamine (Reduced antihypertensive effect).
- No products indexed under this heading.

Reserpine (Reduced antihypertensive effect). Products include:
- Diupres Tablets ... 1461
- Hydromox R Tablets ... 1209
- Hydropres Tablets ... 1485
- Renese-R Tablets ... 1786
- Salutensin/Salutensin-Demi ... 719
- Ser-Ap-Es Tablets ... 881
- Serpasil Tablets ... 883
- Serpasil-Apresoline Tablets ... 884
- Serpasil-Esidrix Tablets ... 886

Selegiline Hydrochloride (Potentiates the effects of sympathomimetics; concurrent use is contraindicated). Products include:
- Eldepryl ... 2250

Timolol Maleate (Potentiates the effects of sympathomimetics). Products include:
- Blocadren Tablets ... 1429
- Timolide Tablets ... 1547
- Timoptic in Ocudose ... 1552
- Timoptic Sterile Ophthalmic Solution ... 1550

Tranylcypromine Sulfate (Potentiates the effects of sympathomimetics; concurrent use is contraindicated). Products include:
- Parnate Tablets ... 2222

BABY ANBESOL TEETHING GEL ANESTHETIC
(Benzocaine) ... 2418
No interactions described in labeling.

ANBESOL GEL ANTISEPTIC-ANESTHETIC
(Benzocaine) ... 2417
No interactions described in labeling.

ANBESOL GEL ANTISEPTIC-ANESTHETIC - MAXIMUM STRENGTH
(Benzocaine) ... 2417
No interactions described in labeling.

ANBESOL LIQUID ANTISEPTIC-ANESTHETIC
(Benzocaine) ... 2417
No interactions described in labeling.

ANBESOL LIQUID ANTISEPTIC-ANESTHETIC - MAXIMUM STRENGTH
(Benzocaine) ... 2417
No interactions described in labeling.

ANCEF INJECTION
(Cefazolin Sodium) ... 2194
May interact with:

Probenecid (Increased and prolonged cephalosporin blood levels). Products include:
- Benemid Tablets ... 1426
- ColBENEMID Tablets ... 1436
- Wycillin Injection and Probenecid Tablets ... 2539

ANCOBON CAPSULES
(Flucytosine) ... 1886
May interact with:

Amphotericin B (Antifungal synergism). Products include:
- Fungizone Cream, Lotion and Ointment ... 2261
- Fungizone Intravenous ... 2262

Cytosine Arabinoside (Inactivation of Ancobon's antifungal activity). Products include:
- CytoGam ... 891

Drugs That Impair Glomerular Filtration (Biological half-life of Ancobon may be prolonged).

ANDROID-10 TABLETS
(Methyltestosterone) ... 1111
May interact with oral anticoagulants, insulin, and certain other agents. Compounds in these categories include:

Dicumarol (Decreased anticoagulant requirements). Products include:
- Dicumarol Tablets ... 516

Insulin, Human (Concurrent use may decrease blood glucose and insulin requirements).
- No products indexed under this heading.

Insulin, Human Isophane Suspension (Concurrent use may decrease blood glucose and insulin requirements). Products include:
- Humulin N, 100 Units ... 1270

Insulin, Human NPH (Concurrent use may decrease blood glucose and insulin requirements). Products include:
- Insulatard NPH Human ... 1627
- Novolin N ... 1627
- Novolin N PenFill Cartridges ... 1628
- Novolin N Prefilled ... 1628

Insulin, Human Regular (Concurrent use may decrease blood glucose and insulin requirements). Products include:
- Humulin BR, 100 Units ... 1268
- Humulin R, 100 Units ... 1272
- Novolin R ... 1627
- Novolin R PenFill Cartridges ... 1628
- Novolin R Prefilled ... 1629
- Velosulin Human ... 1628

Insulin, Human, Zinc Suspension (Concurrent use may decrease blood glucose and insulin requirements). Products include:
- Humulin L, 100 Units ... 1268
- Humulin U, 100 Units ... 1272
- Novolin L ... 1627

Insulin, NPH (Concurrent use may decrease blood glucose and insulin requirements). Products include:
- NPH, 40 & 100 Units ... 1273
- Beef NPH, 100 Units ... 1274
- Pork NPH, 100 Units ... 1275

- Insulatard NPH ... 1626
- NPH Insulin ... 1626
- NPH Purified Pork Isophane Insulin ... 1626

Insulin, Regular (Concurrent use may decrease blood glucose and insulin requirements). Products include:
- Regular, 40 & 100 Units ... 1273
- Beef Regular, 100 Units ... 1275
- Pork Regular, 100 Units ... 1275
- Pork Regular (Concentrated), 500 Units ... 1276
- Regular Insulin ... 1625
- Regular Purified Pork Insulin ... 1626
- Velosulin ... 1627

Insulin, Zinc Crystals (Concurrent use may decrease blood glucose and insulin requirements). Products include:
- NPH, 40 & 100 Units ... 1273

Insulin, Zinc Suspension (Concurrent use may decrease blood glucose and insulin requirements). Products include:
- Lente, 40 & 100 Units ... 1272
- Protamine, Zinc, 40 & 100 Units ... 1273
- Lente Iletin I ... 1272
- Beef Lente, 100 Units ... 1274
- Beef Protamine Zinc, 100 Units ... 1274
- Pork Lente, 100 Units ... 1275
- Pork, Protamine, Zinc, 100 Units ... 1275
- Lente Insulin ... 1626
- Lente Purified Pork Insulin ... 1626
- Semilente Insulin ... 1625
- Ultralente Insulin ... 1626

Oxyphenbutazone (Elevated serum levels of oxyphenbutazone).

Warfarin Sodium (Decreased anticoagulant requirements). Products include:
- Coumadin Injection & Tablets ... 944
- Panwarfin Tablets ... 547

ANDROID-25 TABLETS
(Methyltestosterone) ... 1111
See **Android-10 Tablets**

ANECTINE FLO-PACK
(Succinylcholine Chloride) ... 755
May interact with beta blockers, preanesthetic medications, monoamine oxidase inhibitors, oral contraceptives, and certain other agents. Compounds in these categories include:

Acebutolol Hydrochloride (Enhances neuromuscular blocking action). Products include:
- Sectral Capsules ... 2520

Anticancer Drugs, unspecified (Prolong respiratory depression).

Aprotinin (Enhances neuromuscular blocking action).

Atenolol (Enhances neuromuscular blocking action). Products include:
- Tenoretic Tablets ... 1105
- Tenormin Tablets and I.V. Injection 1107

Betaxolol Hydrochloride (Enhances neuromuscular blocking action). Products include:
- Betoptic Sterile Ophthalmic Solution ... 569
- Betoptic S Sterile Ophthalmic Suspension ... 570
- Kerlone Tablets ... 2172

Carteolol Hydrochloride (Enhances neuromuscular blocking action). Products include:
- Cartrol Tablets ... 507

Chloroquine Hydrochloride (Enhances neuromuscular blocking action). Products include:
- Aralen Hydrochloride Injection ... 2038

Chloroquine Phosphate (Enhances neuromuscular blocking action). Products include:
- Aralen Phosphate with Primaquine Phosphate Tablets ... 2040
- Aralen Phosphate Tablets ... 2039

Chlorpromazine (Prolongs respiratory depression). Products include:
- Thorazine ... 2234

Diazepam (Synergistic or antagonistic effect). Products include:
- Valium Injectable ... 1937
- Valium Tablets ... 1939
- Valrelease Capsules ... 1923

Diethyl Ether (Enhances neuromuscular blocking action).

Doxorubicin Hydrochloride (Low pseudocholinesterase levels). Products include:
- Adriamycin PFS ... 561
- Adriamycin RDF ... 562
- Doxorubicin Hydrochloride for Injection, USP ... 622
- Doxorubicin Hydrochloride Injection, USP ... 848
- Rubex ... 739

Droperidol (Synergistic or antagonistic effect). Products include:
- Inapsine Injection ... 1140
- Innovar Injection ... 1141

Echothiophate Iodide (Prolongs respiratory depression). Products include:
- Phospholine Iodide ... ◉ 315

Esmolol Hydrochloride (Enhances neuromuscular blocking action). Products include:
- Brevibloc Injection ... 942

Ethinyl Estradiol (Prolongs respiratory depression). Products include:
- Brevicon ... 2304
- Demulen ... 2161
- Estinyl Tablets ... 2085
- Jenest-28 Tablets ... 1636
- Levlen/Tri-Levlen ... 665
- Lo/Ovral Tablets ... 2471
- Lo/Ovral-28 Tablets ... 2476
- Loestrin ... 1728
- Modicon ... 1667
- Nordette-21 Tablets ... 2481
- Nordette-28 Tablets ... 2483
- Norethin ... 2133
- Norinyl ... 2304
- Norlestrin ... 1746
- Ortho-Cyclen Tablets ... 1658
- Ortho-Novum ... 1667
- Ovcon ... 1391
- Ovral Tablets ... 2490
- Ovral-28 Tablets ... 2491
- Levlen/Tri-Levlen ... 665
- Tri-Norinyl ... 2304
- Triphasil-21 Tablets ... 2527
- Triphasil-28 Tablets ... 2532

Ethynodiol Diacetate (Prolongs respiratory depression). Products include:
- Demulen ... 2161

Fentanyl Citrate (Synergistic or antagonistic effect). Products include:
- Innovar Injection ... 1141
- Sublimaze Injection ... 1146

Furazolidone (Prolongs respiratory depression). Products include:
- Furoxone ... 1855

Gentamicin Sulfate (Enhances neuromuscular blocking action). Products include:
- Garamycin Injectable ... 2093
- Garamycin Ophthalmic ... ◉ 305
- Genoptic Liquifilm Sterile Ophthalmic Solution ... ◉ 247
- Genoptic S.O.P. Sterile Ophthalmic Ointment ... ◉ 247
- Gentacidin Ointment ... ◉ 273
- Gentacidin Solution ... ◉ 273
- Gentak Ointment & Solution ... ◉ 208
- G-myticin Creme and Ointment 0.1% ... 1770
- Pred-G Liquifilm Sterile Ophthalmic Suspension ... ◉ 252
- Pred-G S.O.P. Sterile Ophthalmic Ointment ... ◉ 253

Hydroxychloroquine Sulfate (Prolongs respiratory depression). Products include:
- Plaquenil Sulfate Tablets ... 2067

Isocarboxazid (Prolongs respiratory depression). Products include:
- Marplan Tablets ... 1906

Isoflurane (Enhances neuromuscular blocking action). Products include:
- Forane ... 600

Labetalol Hydrochloride (Enhances neuromuscular blocking action). Products include:
- Normodyne Injection ... 2108
- Normodyne Tablets ... 2110
- Normozide Tablets ... 2112
- Trandate HCT Tablets ... 579
- Trandate Injection ... 577
- Trandate Tablets ... 579

Levonorgestrel (Prolongs respiratory depression). Products include:
- Levlen/Tri-Levlen ... 665
- Nordette-21 Tablets ... 2481
- Nordette-28 Tablets ... 2483
- Norplant System ... 2484
- Levlen/Tri-Levlen ... 665
- Triphasil-21 Tablets ... 2527
- Triphasil-28 Tablets ... 2532

Lidocaine Hydrochloride (Enhances neuromuscular blocking action). Products include:
- Anestacon Solution ... 2394
- Bactine Antiseptic/Anesthetic First Aid Spray ... ▣ 624
- Decadron Phosphate with Xylocaine Injection, Sterile ... 1451
- Xylocaine Injections ... 637
- Xylocaine Injections for Ventricular Arrhythmias ... 639
- Xylocaine 2% Jelly ... 643
- 4% Xylocaine-MPF Sterile Solution 641
- Xylocaine 2% Viscous Solution ... 646

Lithium Carbonate (Enhances neuromuscular blocking action). Products include:
- Eskalith ... 2214
- Lithane Tablets ... 1596
- Lithium Carbonate Capsules & Tablets ... 1984
- Lithobid Tablets ... 870

Magnesium Sulfate Injection (Enhances neuromuscular blocking action).

Mestranol (Prolongs respiratory depression). Products include:
- Enovid ... 2161
- Norethin ... 2133
- Norinyl ... 2304
- Ortho-Novum ... 1667

Metoprolol Tartrate (Enhances neuromuscular blocking action). Products include:
- Lopressor Ampuls ... 1032
- Lopressor HCT Tablets ... 1034
- Lopressor Tablets ... 1032

Nadolol (Enhances neuromuscular blocking action). Products include:
- Corgard Tablets ... 701
- Corzide Tablets ... 702

Neostigmine Bromide (Prolongs respiratory depression). Products include:
- Prostigmin Tablets ... 1121

Neostigmine Methylsulfate (Prolongs respiratory depression). Products include:
- Prostigmin Injectable ... 1120

Norethindrone (Prolongs respiratory depression). Products include:
- Brevicon ... 2304
- Jenest-28 Tablets ... 1636
- Micronor Tablets ... 1667
- Modicon ... 1667
- Norethin ... 2133
- Norinyl ... 2304
- Norlutin ... 1755
- Nor-Q D Tablets ... 2304
- Ortho-Novum ... 1667
- Ovcon ... 1391
- Tri-Norinyl ... 2304

Norethynodrel (Prolongs respiratory depression). Products include:
- Enovid ... 2161

Norgestimate (Prolongs respiratory depression). Products include:
- Ortho-Cyclen Tablets ... 1658

Norgestrel (Prolongs respiratory depression). Products include:
- Lo/Ovral Tablets ... 2471
- Lo/Ovral-28 Tablets ... 2476
- Ovral Tablets ... 2490
- Ovral-28 Tablets ... 2491
- Ovrette Tablets ... 2492

Oxytocin (Injection) (Enhances neuromuscular blocking action). Products include:
- Oxytocin Injection ... 2492
- Pitocin Injection, Ampoules, Steri-Dose Syringes ... 1757

Oxytocin (Nasal Spray) (Enhances neuromuscular blocking action).
- No products indexed under this heading.

Pancuronium Bromide Injection (Prolongs respiratory depression).
- No products indexed under this heading.

Penbutolol Sulfate (Enhances neuromuscular blocking action). Products include:
- Levatol ... 1832

Pentobarbital Sodium (Barbituric acid may be precipitated; succinylcholine may be hydrolyzed; synergistic or antagonistic effect). Products include:
- Nembutal Sodium Capsules ... 534
- Nembutal Sodium Solution ... 536
- Nembutal Sodium Suppositories ... 538

Phenelzine Sulfate (Enhances neuromuscular blocking action). Products include:
- Nardil ... 1742

Pindolol (Enhances neuromuscular blocking action). Products include:
- Visken Tablets ... 2036

Procainamide Hydrochloride (Enhances neuromuscular blocking action). Products include:
- Procan SR Tablets ... 1760
- Pronestyl Capsules and Tablets ... 1800
- Pronestyl Injection ... 1798
- Pronestyl-SR Tablets ... 1801

Propanidid (Enhances neuromuscular blocking action).

Propranolol Hydrochloride (Enhances neuromuscular blocking action). Products include:
- Inderal ... 2459
- Inderal LA Long Acting Capsules ... 2461
- Inderide Tablets ... 2463
- Inderide LA Long Acting Capsules .. 2465

Quinidine Gluconate (Enhances neuromuscular blocking action). Products include:
- Quinaglute Dura-Tabs Tablets ... 663

Quinidine Polygalacturonate (Enhances neuromuscular blocking action). Products include:
- Cardioquin Tablets ... 1812

Quinidine Sulfate (Enhances neuromuscular blocking action). Products include:
- Quinidex Extentabs ... 1868

Quinine (Enhances neuromuscular blocking action).

Secobarbital Sodium (Synergistic or antagonistic effect). Products include:
- Seconal Sodium Pulvules ... 1296

Selegiline Hydrochloride (Prolongs respiratory depression). Products include:
- Eldepryl ... 2250

Timolol Maleate (Enhances neuromuscular blocking action). Products include:
- Blocadren Tablets ... 1429
- Timolide Tablets ... 1547
- Timoptic in Ocudose ... 1552

Timoptic Sterile Ophthalmic Solution 1550

Tranylcypromine Sulfate (Prolongs respiratory depression). Products include:

Parnate Tablets 2222

Trimethaphan Camsylate (Enhances neuromuscular blocking action). Products include:

Arfonad Ampuls 1887

ANECTINE INJECTION
(Succinylcholine Chloride) **755**
See **Anectine Flo-Pack**

ANESTACON SOLUTION
(Lidocaine Hydrochloride) **2394**
No interactions described in labeling.

ANEXSIA 5/500 TABLETS
(Hydrocodone Bitartrate, Acetaminophen) **2196**
May interact with central nervous system depressants, monoamine oxidase inhibitors, tricyclic antidepressants, anticholinergics, narcotic analgesics, neuromuscular blocking agents, tranquilizers, and certain other agents. Compounds in these categories include:

Alcohol (Additive CNS depression).

Alfentanil Hydrochloride (Additive CNS depression). Products include:

Alfenta Injection 1131

Alprazolam (Additive CNS depression). Products include:

Xanax Tablets 2367

Amitriptyline Hydrochloride (Effect of either agent may be increased). Products include:

Elavil 2269
Endep Tablets 1927
Etrafon 2087
Limbitrol 1933
Triavil Tablets 1556

Amoxapine (Effect of either agent may be increased). Products include:

Asendin Tablets 1196

Aprobarbital (Additive CNS depression). Products include:

Alurate Elixir 1883

Atropine Sulfate (Possible paralytic ileus). Products include:

Arco-Lase Plus Tablets 607
Atropine Sulfate Sterile Ophthalmic Solution and S.O.P. Sterile Ophthalmic Ointment ..... ⊙ 239
Donnagel ..... ⊞ 675
Donnagel-PG 1858
Donnatal 1858
Donnatal Extentabs 1859
Donnatal Tablets 1858
Donnazyme Tablets 1860
Isopto Atropine ..... ⊙ 218
Lomotil 2174
Motofen Tablets 836
Ru-Tuss Tablets 693
Urised Tablets 2396

Belladonna Alkaloids (Possible paralytic ileus). Products include:

Bellergal-S Tablets 1998
Hyland's Bed Wetting Tablets ..... ⊞ 728
Hyland's Teething Tablets ..... ⊞ 728
Kinesed Tablets 2272

Benztropine Mesylate (Possible paralytic ileus). Products include:

Cogentin 1435

Biperiden (Possible paralytic ileus). Products include:

Akineton 1171

Buprenorphine (Additive CNS depression).

No products indexed under this heading.

Buspirone Hydrochloride (Additive CNS depression). Products include:

BuSpar 1401

Butabarbital (Additive CNS depression). Products include:

Pyridium Plus 1764

Butalbital (Additive CNS depression). Products include:

Esgic-Plus Tablets 1002
Esgic Tablets & Capsules 1001
Fioricet Tablets 2006
Fiorinal Capsules 2007
Fiorinal with Codeine Capsules 2008
Fiorinal Tablets 2007
Phrenilin 838
Sedapap Tablets 50 mg/650 mg 1360

Chlordiazepoxide (Additive CNS depression). Products include:

Libritabs Tablets 1930
Limbitrol 1933
Menrium Tablets 1934

Chlordiazepoxide Hydrochloride (Additive CNS depression). Products include:

Librax Capsules 1929
Librium Capsules 1931
Librium Injectable 1932

Chlorpromazine (Additive CNS depression). Products include:

Thorazine 2234

Chlorprothixene (Additive CNS depression). Products include:

Taractan Tablets 1920

Chlorprothixene Hydrochloride (Additive CNS depression). Products include:

Taractan 1920

Clidinium Bromide (Possible paralytic ileus). Products include:

Librax Capsules 1929
Quarzan Capsules 1937

Clomipramine Hydrochloride (Effect of either agent may be increased). Products include:

Anafranil Capsules 650

Clorazepate Dipotassium (Additive CNS depression). Products include:

Tranxene 556

Clozapine (Additive CNS depression). Products include:

Clozaril Tablets 2000

Codeine (Additive CNS depression). Products include:

Calcidrine Syrup 506

Codeine Phosphate (Additive CNS depression). Products include:

Actifed with Codeine Cough Syrup 752
Cheracol Cough Syrup 1853
Codimal PH Syrup 846
Dimetane-DC Cough Syrup 1857
Empirin with Codeine Phosphate Nos. 2, 3 & 4 764
Fiorinal with Codeine Capsules 2008
Isoclor Expectorant 982
Naldecon CX Adult Liquid ..... ⊞ 521
Novahistine DH 1342
Novahistine Expectorant 1343
Nucofed Capsules 2219
Nucofed Expectorant 2219
Nucofed Pediatric Expectorant 2220
Nucofed Syrup 2219
Phenaphen with Codeine Capsules 1865
Phenaphen-650 with Codeine Tablets 1866
Phenergan with Codeine 2497
Phenergan VC with Codeine 2501
Robitussin A-C Syrup 1875
Robitussin-DAC Syrup 1875
Ryna ..... ⊞ 741
Soma Compound w/Codeine Tablets 2390
Triaminic Expectorant w/Codeine 1996
Tussi-Organidin Liquid 2391
Tylenol with Codeine 1381

Codeine Polistirex (Additive CNS depression).

No products indexed under this heading.

Desipramine Hydrochloride (Effect of either agent may be increased). Products include:

Norpramin Tablets 1340

Dezocine (Additive CNS depression).

Diazepam (Additive CNS depression). Products include:

Valium Injectable 1937
Valium Tablets 1939
Valrelease Capsules 1923

Dicyclomine Hydrochloride (Possible paralytic ileus). Products include:

Bentyl 1322

Doxepin Hydrochloride (Effect of either agent may be increased). Products include:

Sinequan 1960

Droperidol (Additive CNS depression). Products include:

Inapsine Injection 1140
Innovar Injection 1141

Enflurane (Additive CNS depression). Products include:

Ethrane 599

Estazolam (Additive CNS depression). Products include:

ProSom Tablets 554

Ethchlorvynol (Additive CNS depression). Products include:

Placidyl Capsules 553

Ethinamate (Additive CNS depression).

No products indexed under this heading.

Ethopropazine Hydrochloride (Possible paralytic ileus).

Fentanyl (Additive CNS depression). Products include:

Duragesic Transdermal System 1133

Fentanyl Citrate (Additive CNS depression). Products include:

Innovar Injection 1141
Sublimaze Injection 1146

Fluphenazine Decanoate (Additive CNS depression). Products include:

Prolixin Decanoate 1795

Fluphenazine Enanthate (Additive CNS depression). Products include:

Prolixin Enanthate 1796

Fluphenazine Hydrochloride (Additive CNS depression). Products include:

Prolixin Elixir 1793
Prolixin Injection 1791
Prolixin Oral Concentrate 1792
Prolixin Tablets 1793

Flurazepam Hydrochloride (Additive CNS depression). Products include:

Dalmane Capsules 1927

Furazolidone (Effect of either agent may be increased). Products include:

Furoxone 1855

Glutethimide (Additive CNS depression).

No products indexed under this heading.

Glycopyrrolate (Possible paralytic ileus). Products include:

Robinul Forte Tablets 1873
Robinul Injectable 1873
Robinul Tablets 1873

Haloperidol (Additive CNS depression). Products include:

Haldol Injection, Tablets and Concentrate 1373

Haloperidol Decanoate (Additive CNS depression). Products include:

Haldol Decanoate 1375

Hydrocodone Polistirex (Additive CNS depression). Products include:

Tussionex Extended-Release Suspension 988

Hydroxyzine Hydrochloride (Additive CNS depression). Products include:

Atarax Tablets & Syrup 1941
Marax Tablets & DF Syrup 1954
Vistaril Intramuscular Solution 1970

Hyoscyamine (Possible paralytic ileus). Products include:

Cystospaz Tablets 2395
Urised Tablets 2396

Hyoscyamine Sulfate (Possible paralytic ileus). Products include:

Arco-Lase Plus Tablets 607
Cystospaz-M Capsules 2395
Donnagel ..... ⊞ 675
Donnagel-PG 1858
Donnatal 1858
Donnatal Extentabs 1859
Donnatal Tablets 1858
Donnazyme Tablets 1860
Kutrase Capsules 2146
Levsin/Levsinex 2147
Ru-Tuss Tablets 693

Imipramine Hydrochloride (Effect of either agent may be increased). Products include:

Tofranil Ampuls 1038
Tofranil Tablets 1039

Imipramine Pamoate (Effect of either agent may be increased). Products include:

Tofranil-PM Capsules 1041

Ipratropium Bromide (Possible paralytic ileus). Products include:

Atrovent Inhalation Aerosol 675

Isocarboxazid (Effect of either agent may be increased). Products include:

Marplan Tablets 1906

Isoflurane (Additive CNS depression). Products include:

Forane 600

Ketamine Hydrochloride (Additive CNS depression). Products include:

Ketalar 1726

Levorphanol Tartrate (Additive CNS depression). Products include:

Levo-Dromoran 1906

Lorazepam (Additive CNS depression). Products include:

Ativan Injection 2432
Ativan Tablets 2434

Loxapine Hydrochloride (Additive CNS depression). Products include:

Loxitane 1213

Loxapine Succinate (Additive CNS depression). Products include:

Loxitane Capsules 1213

Maprotiline Hydrochloride (Effect of either agent may be increased). Products include:

Ludiomil Tablets 874

Mepenzolate Bromide (Possible paralytic ileus). Products include:

Cantil Tablets 1326

Meperidine Hydrochloride (Additive CNS depression). Products include:

Demerol 2047
Mepergan Injection 2479

Mephobarbital (Additive CNS depression). Products include:

Mebaral Tablets 2061

Meprobamate (Additive CNS depression). Products include:

Deprol Tablets 2382
Equagesic Tablets 2451
Miltown Tablets 2386
PMB 200 and PMB 400 2504

Mesoridazine (Additive CNS depression). Products include:

Serentil 686

Methadone Hydrochloride (Additive CNS depression). Products include:

Dolophine Hydrochloride Ampoules & Vials 1260
Dolophine Hydrochloride Tablets 1261
Methadone Hydrochloride Diskets 1284
Methadone Hydrochloride Oral Solution & Tablets 1987

Methohexital Sodium (Additive CNS depression). Products include:
- Brevital Sodium Vials 1248

Methoxyflurane (Additive CNS depression).
- No products indexed under this heading.

Midazolam Hydrochloride (Additive CNS depression). Products include:
- Versed Injection 1924

Molindone Hydrochloride (Additive CNS depression). Products include:
- Moban Tablets & Concentrate 932

Morphine Sulfate (Additive CNS depression). Products include:
- Astramorph/PF Injection, USP (Preservative-Free) 618
- Duramorph 960
- Infumorph 200 and Infumorph 500 Sterile Solutions 962
- MS Contin Tablets 1814
- MSIR 1817
- Oramorph SR (Morphine Sulfate Sustained Release Tablets) 1988
- Roxanol 1991

Nortriptyline Hydrochloride (Effect of either agent may be increased). Products include:
- Pamelor 2019

Opium Alkaloids (Additive CNS depression). Products include:
- B & O No. 15A & No. 16A Supprettes 2395
- Pantopon Injectable 1911

Oxazepam (Additive CNS depression). Products include:
- Serax Capsules 2522
- Serax Tablets 2522

Oxybutynin Chloride (Possible paralytic ileus). Products include:
- Ditropan 1332

Oxycodone Hydrochloride (Additive CNS depression). Products include:
- Percocet Tablets 950
- Percodan 951
- Roxicodone Tablets, Oral Solution & Intensol (Oxycodone) 1992
- Tylox Capsules 1382

Oxyphenonium Bromide (Possible paralytic ileus).

Pentobarbital Sodium (Additive CNS depression). Products include:
- Nembutal Sodium Capsules 534
- Nembutal Sodium Solution 536
- Nembutal Sodium Suppositories 538

Perphenazine (Additive CNS depression). Products include:
- Etrafon 2087
- Triavil Tablets 1556
- Trilafon 2123

Phenelzine Sulfate (Effect of either agent may be increased). Products include:
- Nardil 1742

Phenobarbital (Additive CNS depression). Products include:
- Arco-Lase Plus Tablets 607
- Bellergal-S Tablets 1998
- Bronkolixir .... ▣ 761
- Bronkotabs Tablets .... ▣ 762
- Donnatal 1858
- Donnatal Extentabs 1859
- Donnatal Tablets 1858
- Donnazyme Tablets 1860
- Kinesed Tablets 2272
- Phenobarbital Elixir and Tablets 1293
- Primatene Tablets-P Formula 2421
- Quadrinal Tablets 1183
- Tedral SA 1765

Prazepam (Additive CNS depression). Products include:
- Centrax 1693

Prochlorperazine (Additive CNS depression). Products include:
- Compazine 2201

Procyclidine Hydrochloride (Possible paralytic ileus). Products include:
- Kemadrin Tablets 771

Promethazine Hydrochloride (Additive CNS depression). Products include:
- Mepergan Injection 2479
- Phenergan with Codeine 2497
- Phenergan with Dextromethorphan 2499
- Phenergan Injection 2493
- Phenergan Suppositories 2496
- Phenergan Syrup 2495
- Phenergan Tablets 2496
- Phenergan VC 2500
- Phenergan VC with Codeine 2501

Propantheline Bromide (Possible paralytic ileus). Products include:
- Pro-Banthīne Tablets 2141

Propofol (Additive CNS depression). Products include:
- Diprivan Injection 2267

Propoxyphene Hydrochloride (Additive CNS depression). Products include:
- Darvon 1256
- Wygesic Tablets 2540

Propoxyphene Napsylate (Additive CNS depression). Products include:
- Darvon-N/Darvocet-N 1254

Protriptyline Hydrochloride (Effect of either agent may be increased). Products include:
- Vivactil Tablets 1567

Quazepam (Additive CNS depression). Products include:
- Doral Tablets 2383

Scopolamine Hydrobromide (Possible paralytic ileus). Products include:
- Donnagel .... ▣ 675
- Donnagel-PG 1858
- Donnatal 1858
- Donnatal Extentabs 1859
- Donnatal Tablets 1858
- Donnazyme Tablets 1860
- Isopto Hyoscine .... ⊙ 222
- Murocoll-2 Sterile Ophthalmic Solution .... ⊙ 261
- Ru-Tuss Tablets 693

Scopolamine Preparations (Possible paralytic ileus). Products include:
- Transderm Scōp Transdermal Therapeutic System 887

Secobarbital Sodium (Additive CNS depression). Products include:
- Seconal Sodium Pulvules 1296

Selegiline Hydrochloride (Effect of either agent may be increased). Products include:
- Eldepryl 2250

Sufentanil Citrate (Additive CNS depression). Products include:
- Sufenta Injection 1147

Temazepam (Additive CNS depression). Products include:
- Restoril Capsules 2023

Thiamylal Sodium (Additive CNS depression). Products include:
- Surital Ampoules, Steri-Vials 1764

Thioridazine Hydrochloride (Additive CNS depression). Products include:
- Mellaril 2011

Thiothixene (Additive CNS depression). Products include:
- Navane Capsules and Concentrate 1954
- Navane Intramuscular 1956

Tranylcypromine Sulfate (Effect of either agent may be increased). Products include:
- Parnate Tablets 2222

Triazolam (Additive CNS depression). Products include:
- Halcion Tablets 2340

Tridihexethyl Chloride (Possible paralytic ileus).
- No products indexed under this heading.

Trifluoperazine Hydrochloride (Additive CNS depression). Products include:
- Stelazine 2226

Trihexyphenidyl Hydrochloride (Possible paralytic ileus). Products include:
- Artane 1195

Trimipramine Maleate (Effect of either agent may be increased). Products include:
- Surmontil Capsules 2524

ANEXSIA 7.5/650 TABLETS

(Hydrocodone Bitartrate, Acetaminophen) 2197

May interact with central nervous system depressants, monoamine oxidase inhibitors, tricyclic antidepressants, anticholinergics, narcotic analgesics, neuromuscular blocking agents, tranquilizers, and certain other agents. Compounds in these categories include:

Alcohol (Additive CNS depression).

Alfentanil Hydrochloride (Additive CNS depression). Products include:
- Alfenta Injection 1131

Alprazolam (Additive CNS depression). Products include:
- Xanax Tablets 2367

Amitriptyline Hydrochloride (Effect of either agent may be increased). Products include:
- Elavil 2269
- Endep Tablets 1927
- Etrafon 2087
- Limbitrol 1933
- Triavil Tablets 1556

Amoxapine (Effect of either agent may be increased). Products include:
- Asendin Tablets 1196

Aprobarbital (Additive CNS depression). Products include:
- Alurate Elixir 1883

Atropine Sulfate (Possible paralytic ileus). Products include:
- Arco-Lase Plus Tablets 607
- Atropine Sulfate Sterile Ophthalmic Solution and S.O.P. Sterile Ophthalmic Ointment .... ⊙ 239
- Donnagel .... ▣ 675
- Donnagel-PG 1858
- Donnatal 1858
- Donnatal Extentabs 1859
- Donnatal Tablets 1858
- Donnazyme Tablets 1860
- Isopto Atropine .... ⊙ 218
- Lomotil 2174
- Motofen Tablets 836
- Ru-Tuss Tablets 693
- Urised Tablets 2396

Belladonna Alkaloids (Possible paralytic ileus). Products include:
- Bellergal-S Tablets 1998
- Hyland's Bed Wetting Tablets .... ▣ 728
- Hyland's Teething Tablets .... ▣ 728
- Kinesed Tablets 2272

Benztropine Mesylate (Possible paralytic ileus). Products include:
- Cogentin 1435

Biperiden (Possible paralytic ileus). Products include:
- Akineton 1171

Buprenorphine (Additive CNS depression).
- No products indexed under this heading.

Buspirone Hydrochloride (Additive CNS depression). Products include:
- BuSpar 1401

Butabarbital (Additive CNS depression). Products include:
- Pyridium Plus 1764

Butalbital (Additive CNS depression). Products include:
- Esgic-Plus Tablets 1002
- Esgic Tablets & Capsules 1001
- Fioricet Tablets 2006
- Fiorinal Capsules 2007
- Fiorinal with Codeine Capsules 2008
- Fiorinal Tablets 2007
- Phrenilin 838
- Sedapap Tablets 50 mg/650 mg .. 1360

Chlordiazepoxide (Additive CNS depression). Products include:
- Libritabs Tablets 1930
- Limbitrol 1933
- Menrium Tablets 1934

Chlordiazepoxide Hydrochloride (Additive CNS depression). Products include:
- Librax Capsules 1929
- Librium Capsules 1931
- Librium Injectable 1932

Chlorpromazine (Additive CNS depression). Products include:
- Thorazine 2234

Chlorprothixene (Additive CNS depression). Products include:
- Taractan Tablets 1920

Chlorprothixene Hydrochloride (Additive CNS depression). Products include:
- Taractan 1920

Clidinium Bromide (Possible paralytic ileus). Products include:
- Librax Capsules 1929
- Quarzan Capsules 1937

Clomipramine Hydrochloride (Effect of either agent may be increased). Products include:
- Anafranil Capsules 650

Clorazepate Dipotassium (Additive CNS depression). Products include:
- Tranxene 556

Clozapine (Additive CNS depression). Products include:
- Clozaril Tablets 2000

Codeine (Additive CNS depression). Products include:
- Calcidrine Syrup 506

Codeine Phosphate (Additive CNS depression). Products include:
- Actifed with Codeine Cough Syrup.. 752
- Cheracol Cough Syrup 1853
- Codimal PH Syrup 846
- Dimetane-DC Cough Syrup 1857
- Empirin with Codeine Phosphate Nos. 2, 3 & 4 764
- Fiorinal with Codeine Capsules 2008
- Isoclor Expectorant 982
- Naldecon CX Adult Liquid .... ▣ 521
- Novahistine DH 1342
- Novahistine Expectorant 1343
- Nucofed Capsules 2219
- Nucofed Expectorant 2219
- Nucofed Pediatric Expectorant 2220
- Nucofed Syrup 2219
- Phenaphen with Codeine Capsules 1865
- Phenaphen-650 with Codeine Tablets 1866
- Phenergan with Codeine 2497
- Phenergan VC with Codeine 2501
- Robitussin A-C Syrup 1875
- Robitussin-DAC Syrup 1875
- Ryna .... ▣ 741
- Soma Compound w/Codeine Tablets 2390
- Triaminic Expectorant w/Codeine .. 1996
- Tussi-Organidin Liquid 2391
- Tylenol with Codeine 1381

Codeine Polistirex (Additive CNS depression).
- No products indexed under this heading.

Desipramine Hydrochloride (Effect of either agent may be increased). Products include:
- Norpramin Tablets 1340

Dezocine (Additive CNS depression).

Diazepam (Additive CNS depression). Products include:
- Valium Injectable ... 1937
- Valium Tablets ... 1939
- Valrelease Capsules ... 1923

Dicyclomine Hydrochloride (Possible paralytic ileus). Products include:
- Bentyl ... 1322

Doxepin Hydrochloride (Effect of either agent may be increased). Products include:
- Sinequan ... 1960

Droperidol (Additive CNS depression). Products include:
- Inapsine Injection ... 1140
- Innovar Injection ... 1141

Enflurane (Additive CNS depression). Products include:
- Ethrane ... 599

Estazolam (Additive CNS depression). Products include:
- ProSom Tablets ... 554

Ethchlorvynol (Additive CNS depression). Products include:
- Placidyl Capsules ... 553

Ethinamate (Additive CNS depression).
- No products indexed under this heading.

Ethopropazine Hydrochloride (Possible paralytic ileus).

Fentanyl (Additive CNS depression). Products include:
- Duragesic Transdermal System ... 1133

Fentanyl Citrate (Additive CNS depression). Products include:
- Innovar Injection ... 1141
- Sublimaze Injection ... 1146

Fluphenazine Decanoate (Additive CNS depression). Products include:
- Prolixin Decanoate ... 1795

Fluphenazine Enanthate (Additive CNS depression). Products include:
- Prolixin Enanthate ... 1796

Fluphenazine Hydrochloride (Additive CNS depression). Products include:
- Prolixin Elixir ... 1793
- Prolixin Injection ... 1791
- Prolixin Oral Concentrate ... 1792
- Prolixin Tablets ... 1793

Flurazepam Hydrochloride (Additive CNS depression). Products include:
- Dalmane Capsules ... 1927

Furazolidone (Effect of either agent may be increased). Products include:
- Furoxone ... 1855

Glutethimide (Additive CNS depression).
- No products indexed under this heading.

Glycopyrrolate (Possible paralytic ileus). Products include:
- Robinul Forte Tablets ... 1873
- Robinul Injectable ... 1873
- Robinul Tablets ... 1873

Haloperidol (Additive CNS depression). Products include:
- Haldol Injection, Tablets and Concentrate ... 1373

Haloperidol Decanoate (Additive CNS depression). Products include:
- Haldol Decanoate ... 1375

Hydrocodone Polistirex (Additive CNS depression). Products include:
- Tussionex Extended-Release Suspension ... 988

Hydroxyzine Hydrochloride (Additive CNS depression). Products include:
- Atarax Tablets & Syrup ... 1941
- Marax Tablets & DF Syrup ... 1954
- Vistaril Intramuscular Solution ... 1970

Hyoscyamine (Possible paralytic ileus). Products include:
- Cystospaz Tablets ... 2395
- Urised Tablets ... 2396

Hyoscyamine Sulfate (Possible paralytic ileus). Products include:
- Arco-Lase Plus Tablets ... 607
- Cystospaz-M Capsules ... 2395
- Donnagel ... ⊞ 675
- Donnagel-PG ... 1858
- Donnatal ... 1858
- Donnatal Extentabs ... 1859
- Donnatal Tablets ... 1858
- Donnazyme Tablets ... 1860
- Kutrase Capsules ... 2146
- Levsin/Levsinex ... 2147
- Ru-Tuss Tablets ... 693

Imipramine Hydrochloride (Effect of either agent may be increased). Products include:
- Tofranil Ampuls ... 1038
- Tofranil Tablets ... 1039

Imipramine Pamoate (Effect of either agent may be increased). Products include:
- Tofranil-PM Capsules ... 1041

Ipratropium Bromide (Possible paralytic ileus). Products include:
- Atrovent Inhalation Aerosol ... 675

Isocarboxazid (Effect of either agent may be increased). Products include:
- Marplan Tablets ... 1906

Isoflurane (Additive CNS depression). Products include:
- Forane ... 600

Ketamine Hydrochloride (Additive CNS depression). Products include:
- Ketalar ... 1726

Levorphanol Tartrate (Additive CNS depression). Products include:
- Levo-Dromoran ... 1906

Lorazepam (Additive CNS depression). Products include:
- Ativan Injection ... 2432
- Ativan Tablets ... 2434

Loxapine Hydrochloride (Additive CNS depression). Products include:
- Loxitane ... 1213

Loxapine Succinate (Additive CNS depression). Products include:
- Loxitane Capsules ... 1213

Maprotiline Hydrochloride (Effect of either agent may be increased). Products include:
- Ludiomil Tablets ... 874

Mepenzolate Bromide (Possible paralytic ileus). Products include:
- Cantil Tablets ... 1326

Meperidine Hydrochloride (Additive CNS depression). Products include:
- Demerol ... 2047
- Mepergan Injection ... 2479

Mephobarbital (Additive CNS depression). Products include:
- Mebaral Tablets ... 2061

Meprobamate (Additive CNS depression). Products include:
- Deprol Tablets ... 2382
- Equagesic Tablets ... 2451
- Miltown Tablets ... 2386
- PMB 200 and PMB 400 ... 2504

Mesoridazine (Additive CNS depression). Products include:
- Serentil ... 686

Methadone Hydrochloride (Additive CNS depression). Products include:
- Dolophine Hydrochloride Ampoules & Vials ... 1260
- Dolophine Hydrochloride Tablets ... 1261
- Methadone Hydrochloride Diskets ... 1284
- Methadone Hydrochloride Oral Solution & Tablets ... 1987

Methohexital Sodium (Additive CNS depression). Products include:
- Brevital Sodium Vials ... 1248

Methoxyflurane (Additive CNS depression).
- No products indexed under this heading.

Midazolam Hydrochloride (Additive CNS depression). Products include:
- Versed Injection ... 1924

Molindone Hydrochloride (Additive CNS depression). Products include:
- Moban Tablets & Concentrate ... 932

Morphine Sulfate (Additive CNS depression). Products include:
- Astramorph/PF Injection, USP (Preservative-Free) ... 618
- Duramorph ... 960
- Infumorph 200 and Infumorph 500 Sterile Solutions ... 962
- MS Contin Tablets ... 1814
- MSIR ... 1817
- Oramorph SR (Morphine Sulfate Sustained Release Tablets) ... 1988
- Roxanol ... 1991

Nortriptyline Hydrochloride (Effect of either agent may be increased). Products include:
- Pamelor ... 2019

Opium Alkaloids (Additive CNS depression). Products include:
- B & O No. 15A & No. 16A Supprettes ... 2395
- Pantopon Injectable ... 1911

Oxazepam (Additive CNS depression). Products include:
- Serax Capsules ... 2522
- Serax Tablets ... 2522

Oxybutynin Chloride (Possible paralytic ileus). Products include:
- Ditropan ... 1332

Oxycodone Hydrochloride (Additive CNS depression). Products include:
- Percocet Tablets ... 950
- Percodan ... 951
- Roxicodone Tablets, Oral Solution & Intensol (Oxycodone) ... 1992
- Tylox Capsules ... 1382

Oxyphenonium Bromide (Possible paralytic ileus).

Pentobarbital Sodium (Additive CNS depression). Products include:
- Nembutal Sodium Capsules ... 534
- Nembutal Sodium Solution ... 536
- Nembutal Sodium Suppositories ... 538

Perphenazine (Additive CNS depression). Products include:
- Etrafon ... 2087
- Triavil Tablets ... 1556
- Trilafon ... 2123

Phenelzine Sulfate (Effect of either agent may be increased). Products include:
- Nardil ... 1742

Phenobarbital (Additive CNS depression). Products include:
- Arco-Lase Plus Tablets ... 607
- Bellergal-S Tablets ... 1998
- Bronkolixir ... ⊞ 761
- Bronkotabs Tablets ... ⊞ 762
- Donnatal ... 1858
- Donnatal Extentabs ... 1859
- Donnatal Tablets ... 1858
- Donnazyme Tablets ... 1860
- Kinesed Tablets ... 2272
- Phenobarbital Elixir and Tablets ... 1293
- Primatene Tablets-P Formula ... 2421
- Quadrinal Tablets ... 1183
- Tedral SA ... 1765

Prazepam (Additive CNS depression). Products include:
- Centrax ... 1693

Prochlorperazine (Additive CNS depression). Products include:
- Compazine ... 2201

Procyclidine Hydrochloride (Possible paralytic ileus). Products include:
- Kemadrin Tablets ... 771

Promethazine Hydrochloride (Additive CNS depression). Products include:
- Mepergan Injection ... 2479
- Phenergan with Codeine ... 2497
- Phenergan with Dextromethorphan 2499
- Phenergan Injection ... 2493
- Phenergan Suppositories ... 2496
- Phenergan Syrup ... 2495
- Phenergan Tablets ... 2496
- Phenergan VC ... 2500
- Phenergan VC with Codeine ... 2501

Propantheline Bromide (Possible paralytic ileus). Products include:
- Pro-Banthīne Tablets ... 2141

Propofol (Additive CNS depression). Products include:
- Diprivan Injection ... 2267

Propoxyphene Hydrochloride (Additive CNS depression). Products include:
- Darvon ... 1256
- Wygesic Tablets ... 2540

Propoxyphene Napsylate (Additive CNS depression). Products include:
- Darvon-N/Darvocet-N ... 1254

Protriptyline Hydrochloride (Effect of either agent may be increased). Products include:
- Vivactil Tablets ... 1567

Quazepam (Additive CNS depression). Products include:
- Doral Tablets ... 2383

Scopolamine Hydrobromide (Possible paralytic ileus). Products include:
- Donnagel ... ⊞ 675
- Donnagel-PG ... 1858
- Donnatal ... 1858
- Donnatal Extentabs ... 1859
- Donnatal Tablets ... 1858
- Donnazyme Tablets ... 1860
- Isopto Hyoscine ... ⊙ 222
- Murocoll-2 Sterile Ophthalmic Solution ... ⊙ 261
- Ru-Tuss Tablets ... 693

Scopolamine Preparations (Possible paralytic ileus). Products include:
- Transderm Scōp Transdermal Therapeutic System ... 887

Secobarbital Sodium (Additive CNS depression). Products include:
- Seconal Sodium Pulvules ... 1296

Selegiline Hydrochloride (Effect of either agent may be increased). Products include:
- Eldepryl ... 2250

Sufentanil Citrate (Additive CNS depression). Products include:
- Sufenta Injection ... 1147

Temazepam (Additive CNS depression). Products include:
- Restoril Capsules ... 2023

Thiamylal Sodium (Additive CNS depression). Products include:
- Surital Ampoules, Steri-Vials ... 1764

Thioridazine Hydrochloride (Additive CNS depression). Products include:
- Mellaril ... 2011

Thiothixene (Additive CNS depression). Products include:
- Navane Capsules and Concentrate 1954
- Navane Intramuscular ... 1956

Tranylcypromine Sulfate (Effect of either agent may be increased). Products include:
- Parnate Tablets ... 2222

Triazolam (Additive CNS depression). Products include:
- Halcion Tablets ... 2340

Tridihexethyl Chloride (Possible paralytic ileus).
- No products indexed under this heading.

Trifluoperazine Hydrochloride (Additive CNS depression). Products include:
- Stelazine ... 2226

Trihexyphenidyl Hydrochloride (Possible paralytic ileus). Products include:
- Artane ... 1195

Trimipramine Maleate (Effect of either agent may be increased). Products include:
- Surmontil Capsules ... 2524

ANSAID TABLETS
(Flurbiprofen) ... 2319

May interact with antacids, oral hypoglycemic agents, diuretics, beta blockers , anticoagulants, and certain other agents. Compounds in these categories include:

Acebutolol Hydrochloride (Potential interference with hypotensive effect). Products include:
- Sectral Capsules ... 2520

Aluminum Carbonate Gel (Possible reduction in rate of absorption in geriatric subjects). Products include:
- Basaljel ... 2438

Aluminum Hydroxide (Possible reduction in rate of absorption in geriatric subjects). Products include:
- Cama Arthritis Pain Reliever ... ◘ 685
- Gaviscon Extra Strength Relief Formula Liquid Antacid ... ◘ 594
- Gaviscon Extra Strength Relief Formula Antacid Tablets ... ◘ 594
- Gaviscon Liquid Antacid ... ◘ 594
- Gelusil Liquid & Tablets ... ◘ 639
- Extra Strength Maalox Plus Suspension ... 1850
- Maalox TC Suspension ... 1851
- Maalox Plus Tablets ... ◘ 655
- Extra Strength Maalox Plus Tablets 1850
- Nephrox Suspension ... ◘ 563
- WinGel Liquid & Tablets ... ◘ 761

Aluminum Hydroxide Gel (Possible reduction in rate of absorption in geriatric subjects). Products include:
- ALternaGEL Liquid ... 1154
- Aludrox Oral Suspension ... 2428
- Amphojel Suspension ... 2429
- Amphojel Suspension without Flavor ... 2429
- Mylanta Liquid ... 1155
- Mylanta Double Strength Liquid ... 1155

Aluminum Hydroxide Gel, Dried (Possible reduction in rate of absorption in geriatric subjects). Products include:
- Alu-Tab/Alu-Cap ... 1309
- Amphojel Tablets ... 2429
- Ascriptin A/D Caplets ... 1850
- Regular Strength Ascriptin Tablets 1850
- Gaviscon Antacid Tablets ... ◘ 593
- Gaviscon-2 Antacid Tablets ... ◘ 594
- Mylanta Tablets ... 1155
- Mylanta Double Strength Tablets ... 1155

Amiloride Hydrochloride (Flurbiprofen may interfere with diuretic effect). Products include:
- Midamor Tablets ... 1508
- Moduretic Tablets ... 1510

Aspirin (Lowers serum flurbiprofen concentrations by 50%). Products include:
- Alka-Seltzer Effervescent Antacid and Pain Reliever ... 1568
- Alka-Seltzer Extra Strength Effervescent Antacid and Pain Reliever ... 1570
- Alka-Seltzer (Flavored) Effervescent Antacid and Pain Reliever ... 1569
- Alka-Seltzer Plus Cold Medicine ... ◘ 623
- Alka-Seltzer Plus Night-Time Cold Medicine ... ◘ 623
- Alka Seltzer Plus Sinus Allergy Medicine ... ◘ 624
- Anacin Coated Analgesic Caplets ... 2417
- Anacin Coated Analgesic Tablets ... 2417
- Anacin Maximum Strength Analgesic Coated Tablets ... 2417
- Maximum Strength Arthritis Pain Formula By the Makers of Anacin Analgesic Tablets and Caplets ... 2418
- Arthritis Pain Formula by the Makers of Anacin Analgesic Tablets and Caplets ... ◘ 747
- Arthritis Strength BC Powder ... ◘ 516
- Ascriptin A/D Caplets ... 1850
- Regular Strength Ascriptin Tablets 1850
- Azdōne Tablets ... 844
- BC Powder ... ◘ 517
- BC Cold Powder ... ◘ 517
- Children's Bayer Chewable Aspirin ... ◘ 564
- Genuine Bayer Aspirin Tablets & Caplets ... ◘ 564
- Maximum Bayer Aspirin Tablets & Caplets ... ◘ 566
- Bayer Plus Aspirin Tablets ... ◘ 567
- Therapy Bayer Aspirin Caplets ... ◘ 568
- 8 Hour Bayer Timed-Release Aspirin ... ◘ 566
- Arthritis Strength Bufferin Analgesic Caplets ... 744
- Extra Strength Bufferin Analgesic Tablets ... 745
- Bufferin Analgesic Tablets and Caplets ... 743
- Cama Arthritis Pain Reliever ... ◘ 685
- Damason-P ... 1356
- Easprin ... 1719
- Ecotrin Enteric Coated Aspirin Maximum Strength Tablets and Caplets ... 2189
- Ecotrin Enteric Coated Aspirin Regular Strength Tablets and Caplets ... 2189
- Empirin Aspirin ... ◘ 541
- Empirin with Codeine Phosphate Nos. 2, 3 & 4 ... 764
- Equagesic Tablets ... 2451
- Excedrin Extra-Strength Analgesic Tablets & Caplets ... 749
- 4-Way Cold Tablets ... 750
- Fiorinal Capsules ... 2007
- Fiorinal with Codeine Capsules ... 2008
- Fiorinal Tablets ... 2007
- Lortab ASA Tablets ... 2414
- Momentum Muscular Backache Formula ... ◘ 751
- Norgesic ... 1314
- Norwich Extra-Strength Aspirin ... ◘ 546
- Norwich Regular Strength Aspirin ◘ 547
- P-A-C Analgesic Tablets ... ◘ 669
- Percodan ... 951
- Robaxisal Tablets ... 1872
- Sine-Off Sinus Medicine Tablets-Aspirin Formula ... ◘ 722
- Soma Compound w/Codeine Tablets ... 2390
- Soma Compound Tablets ... 2389
- St. Joseph Adult Chewable Aspirin (81 mg.) ... ◘ 703
- Synalgos-DC Capsules ... 2525
- Talwin Compound ... 2072
- Ursinus Inlay-Tabs ... ◘ 691
- Vanquish Analgesic Caplets ... ◘ 574
- Zorprin Tablets ... 698

Atenolol (Potential interference with hypotensive effect). Products include:
- Tenoretic Tablets ... 1105
- Tenormin Tablets and I.V. Injection 1107

Bendroflumethiazide (Flurbiprofen may interfere with diuretic effect). Products include:
- Corzide Tablets ... 702
- Naturetin Tablets ... 1789
- Rauzide Tablets ... 1804

Betaxolol Hydrochloride (Potential interference with hypotensive effect). Products include:
- Betoptic Sterile Ophthalmic Solution ... 569
- Betoptic S Sterile Ophthalmic Suspension ... 570
- Kerlone Tablets ... 2172

Bumetanide (Flurbiprofen may interfere with diuretic effect). Products include:
- Bumex ... 1895

Carteolol Hydrochloride (Potential interference with hypotensive effect). Products include:
- Cartrol Tablets ... 507

Chlorothiazide (Flurbiprofen may interfere with diuretic effect). Products include:
- Aldoclor Tablets ... 1413
- Diupres Tablets ... 1461
- Diuril Oral ... 1464

Chlorothiazide Sodium (Flurbiprofen may interfere with diuretic effect). Products include:
- Diuril Sodium Intravenous ... 1463

Chlorpropamide (Slight reduction in blood sugar concentrations). Products include:
- Diabinese Tablets ... 1775

Chlorthalidone (Flurbiprofen may interfere with diuretic effect). Products include:
- Combipres Tablets ... 678
- Tenoretic Tablets ... 1105
- Thalitone Tablets ... 687

Cimetidine (Small increase in the AUC of flurbiprofen). Products include:
- Tagamet Tablets ... 2228

Cimetidine Hydrochloride (Small increase in the AUC of flurbiprofen). Products include:
- Tagamet ... 2228

Dicumarol (Possible serious clinical bleeding). Products include:
- Dicumarol Tablets ... 516

Dihydroxyaluminum Sodium Carbonate (Possible reduction in rate of absorption in geriatric subjects). Products include:
- Rolaids ... ◘ 743

Esmolol Hydrochloride (Potential interference with hypotensive effect). Products include:
- Brevibloc Injection ... 942

Ethacrynic Acid (Flurbiprofen may interfere with diuretic effect). Products include:
- Edecrin Tablets ... 1468

Furosemide (Flurbiprofen may interfere with diuretic effect). Products include:
- Lasix ... 1093

Glipizide (Slight reduction in blood sugar concentrations). Products include:
- Glucotrol ... 1952

Glyburide (Slight reduction in blood sugar concentrations). Products include:
- DiaBeta ... 1091
- Micronase Tablets ... 2350

Heparin Calcium (Possible serious clinical bleeding). Products include:
- Calciparine Injection ... 925

Heparin Sodium (Possible serious clinical bleeding). Products include:
- Heparin Lock Flush Solution ... 2456
- Heparin Sodium Vials ... 1264
- Heparin Sodium Injection ... 2457
- Heparin Sodium Injection, USP, Sterile Solution ... 2342

Hydrochlorothiazide (Flurbiprofen may interfere with diuretic effect). Products include:
- Aldactazide ... 2150
- Aldoril Tablets ... 1418
- Apresazide Capsules ... 854
- Apresoline-Esidrix Tablets ... 857
- Capozide ... 2258
- Dyazide Capsules ... 2208
- Esidrix Tablets ... 863
- Esimil Tablets ... 864
- HydroDIURIL Tablets ... 1484
- Hydropres Tablets ... 1485
- Inderide Tablets ... 2463
- Inderide LA Long Acting Capsules .. 2465
- Lopressor HCT Tablets ... 1034
- Maxzide ... 1215
- Moduretic Tablets ... 1510
- Normozide Tablets ... 2112
- Oretic Tablets ... 544
- Oreticyl ... 545
- Prinzide Tablets ... 1540
- Ser-Ap-Es Tablets ... 881
- Serpasil-Esidrix Tablets ... 886
- Timolide Tablets ... 1547
- Trandate HCT Tablets ... 579
- Vaseretic Tablets ... 1559
- Zestoretic ... 2274

Hydroflumethiazide (Flurbiprofen may interfere with diuretic effect). Products include:
- Diucardin Tablets ... 2450
- Saluron ... 718
- Salutensin/Salutensin-Demi ... 719

Indapamide (Flurbiprofen may interfere with diuretic effect). Products include:
- Lozol Tablets ... 1843

Labetalol Hydrochloride (Potential interference with hypotensive effect). Products include:
- Normodyne Injection ... 2108
- Normodyne Tablets ... 2110
- Normozide Tablets ... 2112
- Trandate HCT Tablets ... 579
- Trandate Injection ... 577
- Trandate Tablets ... 579

Magaldrate (Possible reduction in rate of absorption in geriatric subjects). Products include:
- Riopan Antacid Chew Tablets ... ◘ 754
- Riopan Antacid Chew Tablets in Rollpacks ... ◘ 754
- Riopan Antacid Suspension ... 2421
- Riopan Antacid Swallow Tablets ... 2421
- Riopan Plus Chew Tablets ... 2422
- Riopan Plus Chew Tablets in Rollpack ... 2422
- Riopan Plus 2 Chew Tablets, Mint Flavor, Cherry Flavor ... 2422
- Riopan Plus Suspension ... 2422
- Riopan Plus 2 Suspension, Mint Flavor, Cherry Flavor ... 2422

Magnesium Hydroxide (Possible reduction in rate of absorption in geriatric subjects). Products include:
- Aludrox Oral Suspension ... 2428
- Ascriptin A/D Caplets ... 1850
- Regular Strength Ascriptin Tablets 1850
- Di-Gel Antacid/Anti-Gas ... ◘ 697
- Gelusil Liquid & Tablets ... ◘ 639
- Haley's M-O, Regular & Flavored .. ◘ 569
- Extra Strength Maalox Plus Suspension ... 1850
- Maalox TC Suspension ... 1851
- Maalox Plus Tablets ... ◘ 655
- Extra Strength Maalox Plus Tablets 1850
- Mylanta Liquid ... 1155
- Mylanta Tablets ... 1155
- Mylanta Double Strength Liquid ... 1155
- Mylanta Double Strength Tablets ... 1155
- Concentrated Phillips' Milk of Magnesia ... ◘ 573
- Phillips' Milk of Magnesia Liquid ... ◘ 572
- Phillips' Milk of Magnesia Tablets ◘ 573
- WinGel Liquid & Tablets ... ◘ 761

Magnesium Oxide (Possible reduction in rate of absorption in geriatric subjects). Products include:
- Bayer Plus Aspirin Tablets ... ◘ 567
- Beelith Tablets ... 659
- Bufferin Analgesic Tablets and Caplets ... ◘ 524
- Cama Arthritis Pain Reliever ... ◘ 685
- Mag-Ox 400 ... 673
- Uro-Mag ... 673

Methyclothiazide (Flurbiprofen may interfere with diuretic effect). Products include:
- Enduron Tablets ... 517
- Enduronyl ... 518

Metolazone (Flurbiprofen may interfere with diuretic effect). Products include:
- Diulo ... 2129
- Mykrox ½ mg Tablets ... 984
- Zaroxolyn Tablets ... 989

Metoprolol Tartrate (Potential interference with hypotensive effect). Products include:
- Lopressor Ampuls ... 1032
- Lopressor HCT Tablets ... 1034
- Lopressor Tablets ... 1032

Nadolol (Potential interference with hypotensive effect). Products include:
Corgard Tablets 701
Corzide Tablets 702

Penbutolol Sulfate (Potential interference with hypotensive effect). Products include:
Levatol 1832

Pindolol (Potential interference with hypotensive effect). Products include:
Visken Tablets 2036

Polythiazide (Flurbiprofen may interfere with diuretic effect). Products include:
Minizide Capsules 1779
Renese Tablets 1785
Renese-R Tablets 1786

Propranolol Hydrochloride (Potential interference with hypotensive effect). Products include:
Inderal 2459
Inderal LA Long Acting Capsules 2461
Inderide Tablets 2463
Inderide LA Long Acting Capsules .. 2465

Sodium Bicarbonate (Possible reduction in rate of absorption in geriatric subjects). Products include:
Alka-Seltzer Advanced Formula Antacid & Non-Aspirin Pain Reliever .... ▣ 620
Alka-Seltzer Effervescent Antacid ▣ 622
Alka-Seltzer Effervescent Antacid and Pain Reliever 1568
Alka-Seltzer Extra Strength Effervescent Antacid and Pain Reliever .... ▣ 623
Alka-Seltzer (Flavored) Effervescent Antacid and Pain Reliever .. ▣ 621
Arm & Hammer Pure Baking Soda .... ▣ 548
Ceo-Two Rectal Suppositories 671
Citrocarbonate Antacid .... ▣ 668
Massengill Liquid Concentrate 2191
NuLYTELY 699

Spironolactone (Flurbiprofen may interfere with diuretic effect). Products include:
Aldactazide 2150
Aldactone 2152

Timolol Maleate (Potential interference with hypotensive effect). Products include:
Blocadren Tablets 1429
Timolide Tablets 1547
Timoptic in Ocudose 1552
Timoptic Sterile Ophthalmic Solution 1550

Tolazamide (Slight reduction in blood sugar concentrations). Products include:
Tolinase Tablets 2365

Tolbutamide (Slight reduction in blood sugar concentrations). Products include:
Orinase Tablets 2354

Triamterene (Flurbiprofen may interfere with diuretic effect). Products include:
Dyazide Capsules 2208
Dyrenium Capsules 2210
Maxzide 1215

Warfarin Sodium (Possible serious clinical bleeding). Products include:
Coumadin Injection & Tablets 944
Panwarfin Tablets 547

Food Interactions

Food, unspecified (Alters the rate of absorption but does not affect the extent of drug availability).

ANTABUSE TABLETS
(Disulfiram) 2429
May interact with oral anticoagulants and certain other agents. Compounds in these categories include:

Alcohol (Contraindication).

Dicumarol (Prolonged prothrombin time). Products include:
Dicumarol Tablets 516

Isoniazid (Potential for the appearance of unsteady gait or marked changes in mental status). Products include:
INH Tablets 868
Rifamate Capsules 1347

Metronidazole (Psychotic reactions due to combined toxicity). Products include:
Flagyl I.V. RTU 2131
Flagyl Tablets 2170
MetroGel 903
Protostat Tablets 1674

Metronidazole Hydrochloride (Psychotic reactions due to combined toxicity). Products include:
Flagyl I.V. 2131

Paraldehyde (Contraindicated).

Phenytoin (Phenytoin intoxication). Products include:
Dilantin Infatabs 1710
Dilantin-30 Pediatric/Dilantin-125 Suspension 1713

Phenytoin Sodium (Phenytoin intoxication). Products include:
Dilantin Kapseals 1708
Dilantin Parenteral 1712
Dilantin with Phenobarbital Kapseals 1715

Warfarin Sodium (Prolonged prothrombin time). Products include:
Coumadin Injection & Tablets 944
Panwarfin Tablets 547

ANTHRA-DERM OINTMENT 1%, ½%, ¼%, 1/10%
(Anthralin) 907
No interactions described in labeling.

ANTICON
(Docusate Sodium, Casanthranol) .. ▣ 629
No interactions described in labeling.

ANTILIRIUM INJECTABLE
(Physostigmine Salicylate) 998
May interact with:

Atropine Sulfate (Atropine antagonizes the action of Physostigmine). Products include:
Arco-Lase Plus Tablets 607
Atropine Sulfate Sterile Ophthalmic Solution and S.O.P. Sterile Ophthalmic Ointment .... ⊙ 239
Donnagel .... ▣ 675
Donnagel-PG 1858
Donnatal 1858
Donnatal Extentabs 1859
Donnatal Tablets 1858
Donnazyme Tablets 1860
Isopto Atropine .... ⊙ 218
Lomotil 2174
Motofen Tablets 836
Ru-Tuss Tablets 693
Urised Tablets 2396

Decamethonium (Concurrent adminsitration contraindicated).

Succinylcholine Chloride (Concurrent administration contraindicated). Products include:
Anectine 755

ANTIVENIN (BLACK WIDOW SPIDER)
(Black Widow Spider Antivenin (Equine)) 1422
No interactions described in labeling.

ANTIVENIN (CROTALIDAE) POLYVALENT
(Antivenin (Crotalidae) Polyvalent) 2430
May interact with beta blockers. Compounds in this category include:

Acebutolol Hydrochloride (Potential for increased severity of acute and prolonged anaphylaxis). Products include:
Sectral Capsules 2520

Atenolol (Potential for increased severity of acute and prolonged anaphylaxis). Products include:
Tenoretic Tablets 1105
Tenormin Tablets and I.V. Injection 1107

Betaxolol Hydrochloride (Potential for increased severity of acute and prolonged anaphylaxis). Products include:
Betoptic Sterile Ophthalmic Solution 569
Betoptic S Sterile Ophthalmic Suspension 570
Kerlone Tablets 2172

Carteolol Hydrochloride (Potential for increased severity of acute and prolonged anaphylaxis). Products include:
Cartrol Tablets 507

Esmolol Hydrochloride (Potential for increased severity of acute and prolonged anaphylaxis). Products include:
Brevibloc Injection 942

Labetalol Hydrochloride (Potential for increased severity of acute and prolonged anaphylaxis). Products include:
Normodyne Injection 2108
Normodyne Tablets 2110
Normozide Tablets 2112
Trandate HCT Tablets 579
Trandate Injection 577
Trandate Tablets 579

Metoprolol Tartrate (Potential for increased severity of acute and prolonged anaphylaxis). Products include:
Lopressor Ampuls 1032
Lopressor HCT Tablets 1034
Lopressor Tablets 1032

Nadolol (Potential for increased severity of acute and prolonged anaphylaxis). Products include:
Corgard Tablets 701
Corzide Tablets 702

Penbutolol Sulfate (Potential for increased severity of acute and prolonged anaphylaxis). Products include:
Levatol 1832

Pindolol (Potential for increased severity of acute and prolonged anaphylaxis). Products include:
Visken Tablets 2036

Propranolol Hydrochloride (Potential for increased severity of acute and prolonged anaphylaxis). Products include:
Inderal 2459
Inderal LA Long Acting Capsules 2461
Inderide Tablets 2463
Inderide LA Long Acting Capsules .. 2465

Timolol Maleate (Potential for increased severity of acute and prolonged anaphylaxis). Products include:
Blocadren Tablets 1429
Timolide Tablets 1547
Timoptic in Ocudose 1552
Timoptic Sterile Ophthalmic Solution 1550

ANTIVERT, ANTIVERT/25 TABLETS, ANTIVERT/25 CHEWABLE TABLETS & ANTIVERT/50 TABLETS
(Meclizine Hydrochloride) 1940
May interact with:

Alcohol (Avoid alcohol).

ANTURANE CAPSULES
(Sulfinpyrazone) 853
May interact with oral anticoagulants, salicylates, oral hypoglycemic agents, insulin, and certain other agents. Compounds in these categories include:

Aspirin (Uricosuric action antagonized). Products include:
Alka-Seltzer Effervescent Antacid and Pain Reliever 1568
Alka-Seltzer Extra Strength Effervescent Antacid and Pain Reliever 1570
Alka-Seltzer (Flavored) Effervescent Antacid and Pain Reliever 1569
Alka-Seltzer Plus Cold Medicine .... ▣ 623
Alka-Seltzer Plus Night-Time Cold Medicine .... ▣ 623
Alka Seltzer Plus Sinus Allergy Medicine .... ▣ 624
Anacin Coated Analgesic Caplets 2417
Anacin Coated Analgesic Tablets 2417
Anacin Maximum Strength Analgesic Coated Tablets 2417
Maximum Strength Arthritis Pain Formula By the Makers of Anacin Analgesic Tablets and Caplets 2418
Arthritis Pain Formula by the Makers of Anacin Analgesic Tablets and Caplets .... ▣ 747
Arthritis Strength BC Powder .... ▣ 516
Ascriptin A/D Caplets 1850
Regular Strength Ascriptin Tablets 1850
Azdone Tablets 844
BC Powder .... ▣ 517
BC Cold Powder .... ▣ 517
Children's Bayer Chewable Aspirin .... ▣ 564
Genuine Bayer Aspirin Tablets & Caplets .... ▣ 564
Maximum Bayer Aspirin Tablets & Caplets .... ▣ 566
Bayer Plus Aspirin Tablets .... ▣ 567
Therapy Bayer Aspirin Caplets .... ▣ 568
8 Hour Bayer Timed-Release Aspirin .... ▣ 566
Arthritis Strength Bufferin Analgesic Caplets 744
Extra Strength Bufferin Analgesic Tablets 745
Bufferin Analgesic Tablets and Caplets 743
Cama Arthritis Pain Reliever .... ▣ 685
Damason-P 1356
Easprin 1719
Ecotrin Enteric Coated Aspirin Maximum Strength Tablets and Caplets 2189
Ecotrin Enteric Coated Aspirin Regular Strength Tablets and Caplets 2189
Empirin Aspirin .... ▣ 541
Empirin with Codeine Phosphate Nos. 2, 3 & 4 764
Equagesic Tablets 2451
Excedrin Extra-Strength Analgesic Tablets & Caplets 749
4-Way Cold Tablets 750
Fiorinal Capsules 2007
Fiorinal with Codeine Capsules 2008
Fiorinal Tablets 2007
Lortab ASA Tablets 2414
Momentum Muscular Backache Formula .... ▣ 751
Norgesic 1314
Norwich Extra-Strength Aspirin .... ▣ 546
Norwich Regular Strength Aspirin ▣ 547
P-A-C Analgesic Tablets .... ▣ 669
Percodan 951
Robaxisal Tablets 1872
Sine-Off Sinus Medicine Tablets-Aspirin Formula .... ▣ 722
Soma Compound w/Codeine Tablets 2390
Soma Compound Tablets 2389
St. Joseph Adult Chewable Aspirin (81 mg.) .... ▣ 703
Synalgos-DC Capsules 2525

Talwin Compound 2072
Ursinus Inlay-Tabs ▣ 691
Vanquish Analgesic Caplets ▣ 574
Zorprin Tablets 698

Chlorpropamide (Potentiated). Products include:
Diabinese Tablets 1775

Choline Magnesium Trisalicylate (Uricosuric action antagonized). Products include:
Trilisate 1822

Dicumarol (Action of coumarin-type anticoagulants may be accentuated). Products include:
Dicumarol Tablets 516

Diflunisal (Uricosuric action antagonized). Products include:
Dolobid Tablets 1465

Glipizide (Potentiated). Products include:
Glucotrol 1952

Glyburide (Potentiated). Products include:
DiaBeta 1091
Micronase Tablets 2350

Insulin, Human (Potentiated).
No products indexed under this heading.

Insulin, Human Isophane Suspension (Potentiated). Products include:
Humulin N, 100 Units 1270

Insulin, Human NPH (Potentiated). Products include:
Insulatard NPH Human 1627
Novolin N 1627
Novolin N PenFill Cartridges 1628
Novolin N Prefilled 1628

Insulin, Human Regular (Potentiated). Products include:
Humulin BR, 100 Units 1268
Humulin R, 100 Units 1272
Novolin R 1627
Novolin R PenFill Cartridges 1628
Novolin R Prefilled 1629
Velosulin Human 1628

Insulin, Human, Zinc Suspension (Potentiated). Products include:
Humulin L, 100 Units 1268
Humulin U, 100 Units 1272
Novolin L 1627

Insulin, NPH (Potentiated). Products include:
NPH, 40 & 100 Units 1273
Beef NPH, 100 Units 1274
Pork NPH, 100 Units 1275
Insulatard NPH 1626
NPH Insulin 1626
NPH Purified Pork Isophane Insulin 1626

Insulin, Regular (Potentiated). Products include:
Regular, 40 & 100 Units 1273
Beef Regular, 100 Units 1275
Pork Regular, 100 Units 1275
Pork Regular (Concentrated), 500 Units 1276
Regular Insulin 1625
Regular Purified Pork Insulin 1626
Velosulin 1627

Insulin, Zinc Crystals (Potentiated). Products include:
NPH, 40 & 100 Units 1273

Insulin, Zinc Suspension (Potentiated). Products include:
Lente, 40 & 100 Units 1272
Protamine, Zinc, 40 & 100 Units 1273
Lente Iletin I 1272
Beef Lente, 100 Units 1274
Beef Protamine Zinc, 100 Units 1274
Pork Lente, 100 Units 1275
Pork, Protamine, Zinc, 100 Units 1275
Lente Insulin 1626
Lente Purified Pork Insulin 1626
Semilente Insulin 1625
Ultralente Insulin 1626

Magnesium Salicylate (Uricosuric action antagonized). Products include:
Doan's - Extra-Strength Analgesic ▣ 549
Doan's - Regular Strength Analgesic ▣ 549
Mobigesic Analgesic Tablets ▣ 507

Salsalate (Uricosuric action antagonized). Products include:
Disalcid 1310
Mono-Gesic Tablets 846
Salflex 839

Sulfisoxazole (Potentiated). Products include:
Azo Gantrisin Tablets 1888
Gantrisin Tablets 1901
Pediazole 1973

Tolazamide (Potentiated). Products include:
Tolinase Tablets 2365

Tolbutamide (Potentiated). Products include:
Orinase Tablets 2354

Warfarin Sodium (Action of coumarin-type anticoagulants may be accentuated). Products include:
Coumadin Injection & Tablets 944
Panwarfin Tablets 547

ANTURANE TABLETS
(Sulfinpyrazone) 853
See **Anturane Capsules**

ANUSOL HEMORRHOIDAL SUPPOSITORIES
(Balsam Peru, Bismuth Subgallate) ▣ 634
No interactions described in labeling.

ANUSOL OINTMENT
(Balsam Peru, Pramoxine Hydrochloride, Zinc Oxide) ▣ 634
No interactions described in labeling.

ANUSOL-HC CREAM
(Hydrocortisone Acetate) 1690
No interactions described in labeling.

ANUSOL-HC SUPPOSITORIES
(Hydrocortisone Acetate) 1691
No interactions described in labeling.

APLISOL (TUBERCULIN PPD, DILUTED)
(Tuberculin, Purified Protein Derivative For Mantoux Test) 2550
No interactions described in labeling.

APLITEST (TUBERCULIN PPD, MULTIPLE-PUNCTURE DEVICE)
(Tuberculin, Purified Protein Derivative, Multiple Puncture Device) 2551
May interact with corticosteroids and immunosuppressive agents. Compounds in these categories include:

Azathioprine (Sensitivity may decrease or disappear). Products include:
Imuran 768

Betamethasone Acetate (Sensitivity may decrease or disappear). Products include:
Celestone Soluspan Suspension 2081

Betamethasone Sodium Phosphate (Sensitivity may decrease or disappear). Products include:
Celestone Soluspan Suspension 2081

Cortisone Acetate (Sensitivity may decrease or disappear). Products include:
Cortone Acetate Sterile Suspension 1437
Cortone Acetate Tablets 1439

Cyclosporine (Sensitivity may decrease or disappear). Products include:
Sandimmune 2024

Dexamethasone (Sensitivity may decrease or disappear). Products include:
AK-Trol Ointment & Suspension ◉ 207
Decadron Elixir 1445
Decadron Tablets 1447
Decaspray Topical Aerosol 1459
Dexacidin ◉ 272
Maxidex Sterile Ophthalmic Suspension ◉ 223
Maxitrol Ophthalmic Ointment/Suspension ◉ 223
TobraDex Ophthalmic Suspension and Ointment ◉ 228

Dexamethasone Acetate (Sensitivity may decrease or disappear). Products include:
Dalalone D.P. Injectable 999
Decadron-LA Sterile Suspension 1457

Dexamethasone Sodium Phosphate (Sensitivity may decrease or disappear). Products include:
AK-Dex ◉ 203
Decadron Phosphate Respihaler 1454
Decadron Phosphate Sterile Ophthalmic Ointment 1453
Decadron Phosphate Sterile Ophthalmic Solution 1453
Decadron Phosphate Topical Cream 1455
Decadron Phosphate Turbinaire 1456
Maxidex Sterile Ophthalmic Ointment ◉ 222
NeoDecadron Sterile Ophthalmic Ointment 1517
NeoDecadron Sterile Ophthalmic Solution 1518
NeoDecadron Topical Cream 1518

Hydrocortisone (Sensitivity may decrease or disappear). Products include:
AK-Spore H.C. ◉ 206
Bactine Hydrocortisone Anti-Itch Cream ▣ 625
CaldeCORT Anti-Itch Hydrocortisone Spray ▣ 560
Carmol HC Cream 1% 2296
Cortaid Spray ▣ 735
Cortenema 2244
Cortisporin Ointment 758
Cortisporin Ophthalmic Ointment Sterile 758
Cortisporin Ophthalmic Suspension Sterile 759
Cortisporin Otic Solution Sterile 760
Cortisporin Otic Suspension Sterile 760
Cortizone-5 Creme & Ointment ▣ 732
Dermolate Anti-Itch Cream ▣ 697
Eldecort Cream 1.0% 1113
Eldecort Cream 1.0% and 2.5% 1113
Fungoid HC Creme 1770
Hydrocortone Tablets 1482
Hytone 909
LazerSporin-C Solution 1770
Massengill Medicated Soft Cloth Towelettes 2192
Nutracort Cream & Lotion 1684
PediOtic Suspension Sterile 797
Synacort Creams 1%, 2.5% 2296
Vanoxide-HC Acne Lotion 911
Vioform-Hydrocortisone Cream and Mild Cream 889
Vioform-Hydrocortisone Ointment 889
VōSoL HC Otic Solution 2392
Vytone Cream 1% 911

Hydrocortisone Acetate (Sensitivity may decrease or disappear). Products include:
Analpram-HC Rectal Cream 1% and 2.5% 970
Anusol-HC Cream 1690
Anusol-HC Suppositories 1691
Caldecort ▣ 560
Carmol HC Cream 1% 2296
Chloromycetin Hydrocortisone Ophthalmic 1694
Coly-Mycin S Otic w/Neomycin & Hydrocortisone 1708
Cortaid ▣ 735
Cortef Feminine Itch Cream ▣ 735
Corticaine ▣ 682
Cortifoam 1827
Cortisporin Cream 757
Epifoam 1828
Gynecort 5 Creme ▣ 556
Hydrocortone Acetate Sterile Suspension 1479
Lanacort 5 Creme and Ointment ▣ 557
Mantadil Cream 789
Ophthocort ◉ 301
Orabase HCA Oral Paste 890
Pramosone Cream, Lotion & Ointment 971
ProctoCream-HC 1834
Proctofoam-HC 1835

Hydrocortisone Sodium Phosphate (Sensitivity may decrease or disappear). Products include:
Hydrocortone Phosphate Injection, Sterile 1481

Hydrocortisone Sodium Succinate (Sensitivity may decrease or disappear). Products include:
Solu-Cortef Sterile Powder 2361

Immune Globulin (Human) (Sensitivity may decrease or disappear). Products include:
MICRhoGAM Rh_0(D) Immune Globulin (Human) 1650
RhoGAM Rh_0(D) Immune Globulin (Human) 1651

Immune Globulin Intravenous (Human) (Sensitivity may decrease or disappear). Products include:
Gamimune N Immune Globulin Intravenous (Human) 1572
Gammagard Immune Globulin, Intravenous (Human) 658
Iveegam 1129
Sandoglobulin I.V. 2027

Methylprednisolone Acetate (Sensitivity may decrease or disappear). Products include:
Depo-Medrol Sterile Aqueous Suspension 2334

Methylprednisolone Sodium Succinate (Sensitivity may decrease or disappear). Products include:
Solu-Medrol Sterile Powder 2363

Muromonab-CD3 (Sensitivity may decrease or disappear). Products include:
Orthoclone OKT3 Sterile Solution 1645

Prednisolone Acetate (Sensitivity may decrease or disappear). Products include:
AK-Cide Sterile Ophthalmic Ointment & Suspension ◉ 202
Blephamide Liquifilm Sterile Ophthalmic Suspension 586
Blephamide S.O.P. Sterile Ophthalmic Ointment 586
Cetapred Ointment ◉ 220
⅛% Econopred & 1% Econopred Plus ◉ 217
Isopto Cetapred Suspension ◉ 220
Metimyd ◉ 306
Poly-Pred Liquifilm ◉ 250
Pred Forte ◉ 252
Pred Mild ◉ 254
Pred-G Liquifilm Sterile Ophthalmic Suspension ◉ 252
Pred-G S.O.P. Sterile Ophthalmic Ointment ◉ 253
Vasocidin Ointment ◉ 275

Prednisolone Sodium Phosphate (Sensitivity may decrease or disappear). Products include:
AK-Pred ◉ 205
Hydeltrasol Injection, Sterile 1476
Inflamase ◉ 274
Pediapred Oral Liquid 987
Vasocidin Ophthalmic Solution ◉ 276

Prednisolone Tebutate (Sensitivity may decrease or disappear). Products include:
Hydeltra-T.B.A. Sterile Suspension 1478

Prednisone (Sensitivity may decrease or disappear). Products include:
Deltasone Tablets 2332

Triamcinolone (Sensitivity may decrease or disappear).
No products indexed under this heading.

Triamcinolone Acetonide (Sensitivity may decrease or disappear). Products include:
Aristocort A 1010

(▣ Described in PDR For Nonprescription Drugs) (◉ Described in PDR For Ophthalmology)

Azmacort Inhaler 1837
Kenalog Cream, Lotion & Ointment 2401
Kenalog-10 Injection 2402
Kenalog-40 Injection 2403
Kenalog in Orabase 604
Kenalog Spray 2401
Mycolog II Cream and Ointment 2407
Mytrex Cream & Ointment 2080
Nasacort Nasal Inhaler 1844

Triamcinolone Diacetate (Sensitivity may decrease or disappear). Products include:
Aristocort Suspension 1008

Triamcinolone Hexacetonide (Sensitivity may decrease or disappear). Products include:
Aristospan Suspension 1011

APRESAZIDE CAPSULES (Hydralazine Hydrochloride, Hydrochlorothiazide) **854**
May interact with monoamine oxidase inhibitors, corticosteroids, antihypertensives, insulin, narcotic analgesics, barbiturates, cardiac glycosides, non-steroidal anti-inflammatory agents, and certain other agents. Compounds in these categories include:

Acebutolol Hydrochloride (Additive or potentiated action). Products include:
Sectral Capsules 2520

ACTH (Hypokalemia).
No products indexed under this heading.

Alcohol (May potentiate orthostatic hypotension).

Alfentanil Hydrochloride (May potentiate orthostatic hypotension). Products include:
Alfenta Injection 1131

Aprobarbital (May potentiate orthostatic hypotension). Products include:
Alurate Elixir 1883

Atenolol (Additive or potentiated action). Products include:
Tenoretic Tablets 1105
Tenormin Tablets and I.V. Injection 1107

Benazepril Hydrochloride (Additive or potentiated action). Products include:
Lotensin Tablets 872

Bendroflumethiazide (Additive or potentiated action). Products include:
Corzide Tablets 702
Naturetin Tablets 1789
Rauzide Tablets 1804

Betamethasone Acetate (Concomitant use may result in hypokalemia). Products include:
Celestone Soluspan Suspension 2081

Betamethasone Sodium Phosphate (Concomitant use may result in hypokalemia). Products include:
Celestone Soluspan Suspension 2081

Betaxolol Hydrochloride (Additive or potentiated action). Products include:
Betoptic Sterile Ophthalmic Solution 569
Betoptic S Sterile Ophthalmic Suspension 570
Kerlone Tablets 2172

Buprenorphine (May potentiate orthostatic hypotension).
No products indexed under this heading.

Butabarbital (May potentiate orthostatic hypotension). Products include:
Pyridium Plus 1764

Butalbital (May potentiate orthostatic hypotension). Products include:
Esgic-Plus Tablets 1002
Esgic Tablets & Capsules 1001
Fioricet Tablets 2006
Fiorinal Capsules 2007
Fiorinal with Codeine Capsules 2008
Fiorinal Tablets 2007
Phrenilin 838
Sedapap Tablets 50 mg/650 mg .. 1360

Captopril (Additive or potentiated action). Products include:
Capoten 2255
Capozide 2258

Carteolol Hydrochloride (Additive or potentiated action). Products include:
Cartrol Tablets 507

Chlorothiazide (Additive or potentiated action). Products include:
Aldoclor Tablets 1413
Diupres Tablets 1461
Diuril Oral 1464

Chlorothiazide Sodium (Additive or potentiated action). Products include:
Diuril Sodium Intravenous 1463

Chlorthalidone (Additive or potentiated action). Products include:
Combipres Tablets 678
Tenoretic Tablets 1105
Thalitone Tablets 687

Clonidine (Additive or potentiated action). Products include:
Catapres-TTS 677

Clonidine Hydrochloride (Additive or potentiated action). Products include:
Catapres Tablets 676
Combipres Tablets 678

Codeine (May potentiate orthostatic hypotension). Products include:
Calcidrine Syrup 506

Codeine Phosphate (May potentiate orthostatic hypotension). Products include:
Actifed with Codeine Cough Syrup.. 752
Cheracol Cough Syrup 1853
Codimal PH Syrup 846
Dimetane-DC Cough Syrup 1857
Empirin with Codeine Phosphate Nos. 2, 3 & 4 764
Fiorinal with Codeine Capsules 2008
Isoclor Expectorant 982
Naldecon CX Adult Liquid .... ▣ 521
Novahistine DH 1342
Novahistine Expectorant 1343
Nucofed Capsules 2219
Nucofed Expectorant 2219
Nucofed Pediatric Expectorant 2220
Nucofed Syrup 2219
Phenaphen with Codeine Capsules 1865
Phenaphen-650 with Codeine Tablets 1866
Phenergan with Codeine 2497
Phenergan VC with Codeine 2501
Robitussin A-C Syrup 1875
Robitussin-DAC Syrup 1875
Ryna .... ▣ 741
Soma Compound w/Codeine Tablets 2390
Triaminic Expectorant w/Codeine .. 1996
Tussi-Organidin Liquid 2391
Tylenol with Codeine 1381

Codeine Polistirex (May potentiate orthostatic hypotension).
No products indexed under this heading.

Cortisone Acetate (Concomitant use may result in hypokalemia). Products include:
Cortone Acetate Sterile Suspension 1437
Cortone Acetate Tablets 1439

Deserpidine (Additive or potentiated action). Products include:
Enduronyl 518
Harmonyl Tablets 528
Oreticyl 545

Deslanoside (Hypokalemia can exaggerate cardiotoxicity of digitalis).
No products indexed under this heading.

Dexamethasone (Concomitant use may result in hypokalemia). Products include:
AK-Trol Ointment & Suspension .... ◉ 207
Decadron Elixir 1445
Decadron Tablets 1447
Decaspray Topical Aerosol 1459
Dexacidin .... ◉ 272
Maxidex Sterile Ophthalmic Suspension .... ◉ 223
Maxitrol Ophthalmic Ointment/Suspension .... ◉ 223
TobraDex Ophthalmic Suspension and Ointment .... ◉ 228

Dexamethasone Acetate (Concomitant use may result in hypokalemia). Products include:
Dalalone D.P. Injectable 999
Decadron-LA Sterile Suspension 1457

Dexamethasone Sodium Phosphate (Concomitant use may result in hypokalemia). Products include:
AK-Dex .... ◉ 203
Decadron Phosphate Respihaler 1454
Decadron Phosphate Sterile Ophthalmic Ointment 1453
Decadron Phosphate Sterile Ophthalmic Solution 1453
Decadron Phosphate Topical Cream 1455
Decadron Phosphate Turbinaire 1456
Maxidex Sterile Ophthalmic Ointment .... ◉ 222
NeoDecadron Sterile Ophthalmic Ointment 1517
NeoDecadron Sterile Ophthalmic Solution 1518
NeoDecadron Topical Cream 1518

Dezocine (May potentiate orthostatic hypotension).

Diazoxide (Profound hypotensive episodes; additive or potentiated action). Products include:
Hyperstat I.V. Injection 2095
Proglycem 649

Diclofenac Sodium (Concurrent administration may reduce the diuretic, natriuretic and antihypertensive effects of thiazide diuretics). Products include:
Voltaren Ophthalmic Sterile Ophthalmic Solution .... ◉ 268
Voltaren Tablets 1042

Digitoxin (Hypokalemia can exaggerate cardiotoxicity of digitalis). Products include:
Crystodigin Tablets 1253

Digoxin (Hypokalemia can exaggerate cardiotoxicity of digitalis). Products include:
Lanoxicaps 772
Lanoxin Elixir Pediatric 775
Lanoxin Injection 778
Lanoxin Injection Pediatric 781
Lanoxin Tablets 783

Doxazosin Mesylate (Additive or potentiated action). Products include:
Cardura Tablets 1941

Enalapril Maleate (Additive or potentiated action). Products include:
Vaseretic Tablets 1559
Vasotec Tablets 1564

Enalaprilat (Additive or potentiated action). Products include:
Vasotec I.V. 1562

Epinephrine (Pressor responses may be reduced). Products include:
Ana-Kit Anaphylaxis Emergency Treatment Kit 1100
Bronkaid Mist .... ▣ 757
EpiPen 843
Marcaine Hydrochloride 0.5% with Epinephrine 1:200,000 (as bitartrate) 958
Marcaine Hydrochloride with Epinephrine 1:200,000 2055
Primatene Mist 2420
Sus-Phrine Injection 1006
Xylocaine with Epinephrine Injections 637

Epinephrine Bitartrate (Pressor responses may be reduced). Products include:
AsthmaHaler Mist Epinephrine Bitartrate Bronchodilator .... ▣ 616
Bronkaid Mist Suspension .... ▣ 757
Primatene Mist Suspension 2421

Esmolol Hydrochloride (Additive or potentiated action). Products include:
Brevibloc Injection 942

Etodolac (Concurrent administration may reduce the diuretic, natriuretic and antihypertensive effects of thiazide diuretics). Products include:
Lodine Capsules 2468

Felodipine (Additive or potentiated action). Products include:
Plendil Extended-Release Tablets 1526

Fenoprofen Calcium (Concurrent administration may reduce the diuretic, natriuretic and antihypertensive effects of thiazide diuretics). Products include:
Nalfon Pulvules & Tablets 919

Fentanyl (May potentiate orthostatic hypotension). Products include:
Duragesic Transdermal System 1133

Fentanyl Citrate (May potentiate orthostatic hypotension). Products include:
Innovar Injection 1141
Sublimaze Injection 1146

Flurbiprofen (Concurrent administration may reduce the diuretic, natriuretic and antihypertensive effects of thiazide diuretics). Products include:
Ansaid Tablets 2319

Fosinopril Sodium (Additive or potentiated action). Products include:
Monopril Tablets 1406

Furazolidone (Concurrent use requires caution). Products include:
Furoxone 1855

Furosemide (Additive or potentiated action). Products include:
Lasix 1093

Guanabenz Acetate (Additive or potentiated action). Products include:
Wytensin Tablets 2542

Guanethidine Monosulfate (Additive or potentiated action). Products include:
Esimil Tablets 864
Ismelin Tablets 869

Hydrocodone Bitartrate (May potentiate orthostatic hypotension). Products include:
Anexsia 5/500 Tablets 2196
Anexsia 7.5/650 Tablets 2197
Azdone Tablets 844
Codiclear DH Syrup 845
Codimal DH Syrup 846
Damason-P 1356
Hycodan Syrup, Tablets 927
Hycomine Compound Tablets 929
Hycomine Syrup 927
Hycotuss Expectorant Syrup 930
Hydrocet Capsules 835
Lortab ASA Tablets 2414
Lortab 2412
Ru-Tuss with Hydrocodone 694
Triaminic Expectorant DH 1995
Vicodin Tablets 1187
Vicodin ES Tablets 1189
Zydone Capsules 941

Hydrocodone Polistirex (May potentiate orthostatic hypotension). Products include:
Tussionex Extended-Release Suspension 988

Hydrocortisone (Concomitant use may result in hypokalemia). Products include:
AK-Spore H.C. .... ◉ 206

(▣ Described in PDR For Nonprescription Drugs) (◉ Described in PDR For Ophthalmology)

Bactine Hydrocortisone Anti-Itch Cream ▣ 625
CaldeCORT Anti-Itch Hydrocortisone Spray ▣ 560
Carmol HC Cream 1% 2296
Cortaid Spray ▣ 735
Cortenema 2244
Cortisporin Ointment 758
Cortisporin Ophthalmic Ointment Sterile 758
Cortisporin Ophthalmic Suspension Sterile 759
Cortisporin Otic Solution Sterile 760
Cortisporin Otic Suspension Sterile 760
Cortizone-5 Creme & Ointment ▣ 732
Dermolate Anti-Itch Cream ▣ 697
Eldecort Cream 1.0% 1113
Eldecort Cream 1.0% and 2.5% 1113
Fungoid HC Creme 1770
Hydrocortone Tablets 1482
Hytone 909
LazerSporin-C Solution 1770
Massengill Medicated Soft Cloth Towelettes 2192
Nutracort Cream & Lotion 1684
PediOtic Suspension Sterile 797
Synacort Creams 1%, 2.5% 2296
Vanoxide-HC Acne Lotion 911
Vioform-Hydrocortisone Cream and Mild Cream 889
Vioform-Hydrocortisone Ointment 889
VōSoL HC Otic Solution 2392
Vytone Cream 1% 911

Hydrocortisone Acetate (Concomitant use may result in hypokalemia). Products include:
Analpram-HC Rectal Cream 1% and 2.5% 970
Anusol-HC Cream 1690
Anusol-HC Suppositories 1691
Caldecort ▣ 560
Carmol HC Cream 1% 2296
Chloromycetin Hydrocortisone Ophthalmic 1694
Coly-Mycin S Otic w/Neomycin & Hydrocortisone 1708
Cortaid ▣ 735
Cortef Feminine Itch Cream ▣ 735
Corticaine ▣ 682
Cortifoam 1827
Cortisporin Cream 757
Epifoam 1828
Gynecort 5 Creme ▣ 556
Hydrocortone Acetate Sterile Suspension 1479
Lanacort 5 Creme and Ointment ▣ 557
Mantadil Cream 789
Ophthocort ⊙ 301
Orabase HCA Oral Paste 890
Pramosone Cream, Lotion & Ointment 971
ProctoCream-HC 1834
Proctofoam-HC 1835

Hydrocortisone Sodium Phosphate (Concomitant use may result in hypokalemia). Products include:
Hydrocortone Phosphate Injection, Sterile 1481

Hydrocortisone Sodium Succinate (Concomitant use may result in hypokalemia). Products include:
Solu-Cortef Sterile Powder 2361

Hydroflumethiazide (Additive or potentiated action). Products include:
Diucardin Tablets 2450
Saluron 718
Salutensin/Salutensin-Demi 719

Ibuprofen (Concurrent administration may reduce the diuretic, natriuretic and antihypertensive effects of thiazide diuretics). Products include:
Advil Cold & Sinus Caplets (formerly CoAdvil) 2416
Advil Ibuprofen Tablets and Caplets 2416
Children's Advil Suspension 2426
CoAdvil ▣ 748
Dristan Sinus Caplets 2419
Haltran Tablets ▣ 668
Ibuprofen ▣ 631
Medipren ibuprofen Caplets and Tablets 1362
Midol 200 Cramp Relief Formula ▣ 570
Motrin Tablets 2351
Motrin IB Caplets and Tablets ▣ 736
Nuprin Ibuprofen/Analgesic Tablets & Caplets 752
PediaProfen Suspension 1363
Rufen Tablets 691
Trendar Ibuprofen Tablets ▣ 756

Indapamide (Additive or potentiated action). Products include:
Lozol Tablets 1843

Indomethacin (Concurrent administration may reduce the diuretic, natriuretic and antihypertensive effects of thiazide diuretics). Products include:
Indocin 1487

Indomethacin Sodium Trihydrate (Concurrent administration may reduce the diuretic, natriuretic and antihypertensive effects of thiazide diuretics). Products include:
Indocin I.V. 1490

Insulin, Human (Insulin requirements may be altered).
No products indexed under this heading.

Insulin, Human Isophane Suspension (Insulin requirements may be altered). Products include:
Humulin N, 100 Units 1270

Insulin, Human NPH (Insulin requirements may be altered). Products include:
Insulatard NPH Human 1627
Novolin N 1627
Novolin N PenFill Cartridges 1628
Novolin N Prefilled 1628

Insulin, Human Regular (Insulin requirements may be altered). Products include:
Humulin BR, 100 Units 1268
Humulin R, 100 Units 1272
Novolin R 1627
Novolin R PenFill Cartridges 1628
Novolin R Prefilled 1629
Velosulin Human 1628

Insulin, Human, Zinc Suspension (Insulin requirements may be altered). Products include:
Humulin L, 100 Units 1268
Humulin U, 100 Units 1272
Novolin L 1627

Insulin, NPH (Insulin requirements may be altered). Products include:
NPH, 40 & 100 Units 1273
Beef NPH, 100 Units 1274
Pork NPH, 100 Units 1275
Insulatard NPH 1626
NPH Insulin 1626
NPH Purified Pork Isophane Insulin 1626

Insulin, Regular (Insulin requirements may be altered). Products include:
Regular, 40 & 100 Units 1273
Beef Regular, 100 Units 1275
Pork Regular, 100 Units 1275
Pork Regular (Concentrated), 500 Units 1276
Regular Insulin 1625
Regular Purified Pork Insulin 1626
Velosulin 1627

Insulin, Zinc Crystals (Insulin requirements may be altered). Products include:
NPH, 40 & 100 Units 1273

Insulin, Zinc Suspension (Insulin requirements may be altered). Products include:
Lente, 40 & 100 Units 1272
Protamine, Zinc, 40 & 100 Units 1273
Lente Iletin I 1272
Beef Lente, 100 Units 1274
Beef Protamine Zinc, 100 Units 1274
Pork Lente, 100 Units 1275
Pork, Protamine, Zinc, 100 Units 1275
Lente Insulin 1626
Lente Purified Pork Insulin 1626
Semilente Insulin 1625
Ultralente Insulin 1626

Isocarboxazid (Concurrent use requires caution). Products include:
Marplan Tablets 1906

Isradipine (Additive or potentiated action). Products include:
DynaCirc Capsules 2004

Ketoprofen (Concurrent administration may reduce the diuretic, natriuretic and antihypertensive effects of thiazide diuretics). Products include:
Orudis Capsules 2488

Ketorolac Tromethamine (Concurrent administration may reduce the diuretic, natriuretic and antihypertensive effects of thiazide diuretics). Products include:
Toradol IM Injection 2302

Labetalol Hydrochloride (Additive or potentiated action). Products include:
Normodyne Injection 2108
Normodyne Tablets 2110
Normozide Tablets 2112
Trandate HCT Tablets 579
Trandate Injection 577
Trandate Tablets 579

Levorphanol Tartrate (May potentiate orthostatic hypotension). Products include:
Levo-Dromoran 1906

Lisinopril (Additive or potentiated action). Products include:
Prinivil Tablets 1538
Prinzide Tablets 1540
Zestoretic 2274
Zestril Tablets 2277

Lithium Carbonate (Increased risk of lithium toxicity). Products include:
Eskalith 2214
Lithane Tablets 1596
Lithium Carbonate Capsules & Tablets 1984
Lithobid Tablets 870

Lithium Citrate (Increased risk of lithium toxicity). Products include:
Cibalith-S 870

Mecamylamine Hydrochloride (Additive or potentiated action). Products include:
Inversine Tablets 1492

Meclofenamate Sodium (Concurrent administration may reduce the diuretic, natriuretic and antihypertensive effects of thiazide diuretics). Products include:
Meclomen Capsules 1739

Mefenamic Acid (Concurrent administration may reduce the diuretic, natriuretic and antihypertensive effects of thiazide diuretics). Products include:
Ponstel 1758

Meperidine Hydrochloride (May potentiate orthostatic hypotension). Products include:
Demerol 2047
Mepergan Injection 2479

Mephobarbital (May potentiate orthostatic hypotension). Products include:
Mebaral Tablets 2061

Methadone Hydrochloride (May potentiate orthostatic hypotension). Products include:
Dolophine Hydrochloride Ampoules & Vials 1260
Dolophine Hydrochloride Tablets 1261
Methadone Hydrochloride Diskets 1284
Methadone Hydrochloride Oral Solution & Tablets 1987

Methyclothiazide (Additive or potentiated action). Products include:
Enduron Tablets 517
Enduronyl 518

Methyldopa (Additive or potentiated action; concomitant use may cause hemolytic anemia). Products include:
Aldoclor Tablets 1413
Aldomet Oral 1415
Aldoril Tablets 1418

Methyldopate Hydrochloride (Additive or potentiated action; concomitant use may cause hemolytic anemia). Products include:
Aldomet Ester HCl Injection 1417

Methylprednisolone (Concomitant use may result in hypokalemia). Products include:
Medrol 2348

Methylprednisolone Acetate (Concomitant use may result in hypokalemia). Products include:
Depo-Medrol Sterile Aqueous Suspension 2334

Methylprednisolone Sodium Succinate (Concomitant use may result in hypokalemia). Products include:
Solu-Medrol Sterile Powder 2363

Metolazone (Additive or potentiated action). Products include:
Diulo 2129
Mykrox ½ mg Tablets 984
Zaroxolyn Tablets 989

Metoprolol Tartrate (Additive or potentiated action). Products include:
Lopressor Ampuls 1032
Lopressor HCT Tablets 1034
Lopressor Tablets 1032

Metyrosine (Additive or potentiated action). Products include:
Demser Capsules 1460

Minoxidil (Additive or potentiated action). Products include:
Loniten Tablets 2346
Rogaine Topical Solution 2357

Morphine Sulfate (May potentiate orthostatic hypotension). Products include:
Astramorph/PF Injection, USP (Preservative-Free) 618
Duramorph 960
Infumorph 200 and Infumorph 500 Sterile Solutions 962
MS Contin Tablets 1814
MSIR 1817
Oramorph SR (Morphine Sulfate Sustained Release Tablets) 1988
Roxanol 1991

Nadolol (Additive or potentiated action). Products include:
Corgard Tablets 701
Corzide Tablets 702

Naproxen (Concurrent administration may reduce the diuretic, natriuretic and antihypertensive effects of thiazide diuretics). Products include:
Naprosyn 2297

Naproxen Sodium (Concurrent administration may reduce the diuretic, natriuretic and antihypertensive effects of thiazide diuretics). Products include:
Anaprox and Anaprox DS Tablets 2288

Nicardipine Hydrochloride (Additive or potentiated action). Products include:
Cardene Capsules 2290

Nitroglycerin (Additive or potentiated action). Products include:
Deponit NTG Transdermal Delivery System 2143
Minitran Transdermal Delivery System 1312
Nitro-Bid Ointment 1339
Nitro-Bid Capsules 1338
Nitrodisc 2176
Nitro-Dur (nitroglycerin) Transdermal Infusion System 1164
Nitrogard Tablets 1004
Nitrolingual Spray 1846
Nitrostat Tablets 1743
Transderm-Nitro Transdermal Therapeutic System 2283

Norepinephrine Bitartrate (Decreased arterial response to norepinephrine). Products include:
- Levophed Bitartrate Injection ... 2054

Opium Alkaloids (May potentiate orthostatic hypotension). Products include:
- B & O No. 15A & No. 16A Supprettes ... 2395
- Pantopon Injectable ... 1911

Oxycodone Hydrochloride (May potentiate orthostatic hypotension). Products include:
- Percocet Tablets ... 950
- Percodan ... 951
- Roxicodone Tablets, Oral Solution & Intensol (Oxycodone) ... 1992
- Tylox Capsules ... 1382

Pargyline Hydrochloride (Concurrent administration contraindicated).
- No products indexed under this heading.

Penbutolol Sulfate (Additive or potentiated action). Products include:
- Levatol ... 1832

Pentobarbital Sodium (May potentiate orthostatic hypotension). Products include:
- Nembutal Sodium Capsules ... 534
- Nembutal Sodium Solution ... 536
- Nembutal Sodium Suppositories ... 538

Phenelzine Sulfate (Concurrent use requires caution). Products include:
- Nardil ... 1742

Phenobarbital (May potentiate orthostatic hypotension). Products include:
- Arco-Lase Plus Tablets ... 607
- Bellergal-S Tablets ... 1998
- Bronkolixir ... ▣ 761
- Bronkotabs Tablets ... ▣ 762
- Donnatal ... 1858
- Donnatal Extentabs ... 1859
- Donnatal Tablets ... 1858
- Donnazyme Tablets ... 1860
- Kinesed Tablets ... 2272
- Phenobarbital Elixir and Tablets ... 1293
- Primatene Tablets-P Formula ... 2421
- Quadrinal Tablets ... 1183
- Tedral SA ... 1765

Phenoxybenzamine Hydrochloride (Additive or potentiated action). Products include:
- Dibenzyline Capsules ... 2207

Phentolamine Mesylate (Additive or potentiated action). Products include:
- Regitine ... 878

Phenylbutazone (Concurrent administration may reduce the diuretic, natriuretic and antihypertensive effects of thiazide diuretics). Products include:
- Butazolidin Capsules & Tablets ... 1027

Pindolol (Additive or potentiated action). Products include:
- Visken Tablets ... 2036

Piroxicam (Concurrent administration may reduce the diuretic, natriuretic and antihypertensive effects of thiazide diuretics). Products include:
- Feldene Capsules ... 1777

Polythiazide (Additive or potentiated action). Products include:
- Minizide Capsules ... 1779
- Renese Tablets ... 1785
- Renese-R Tablets ... 1786

Prazosin Hydrochloride (Additive or potentiated action). Products include:
- Minipress Capsules ... 1778
- Minizide Capsules ... 1779

Prednisolone Acetate (Concomitant use may result in hypokalemia). Products include:
- AK-Cide Sterile Ophthalmic Ointment & Suspension ... ⊙ 202
- Blephamide Liquifilm Sterile Ophthalmic Suspension ... 586
- Blephamide S.O.P. Sterile Ophthalmic Ointment ... 586
- Cetapred Ointment ... ⊙ 220
- ⅛ % Econopred & 1 % Econopred Plus ... ⊙ 217
- Isopto Cetapred Suspension ... ⊙ 220
- Metimyd ... ⊙ 306
- Poly-Pred Liquifilm ... ⊙ 250
- Pred Forte ... ⊙ 252
- Pred Mild ... ⊙ 254
- Pred-G Liquifilm Sterile Ophthalmic Suspension ... ⊙ 252
- Pred-G S.O.P. Sterile Ophthalmic Ointment ... ⊙ 253
- Vasocidin Ointment ... ⊙ 275

Prednisolone Sodium Phosphate (Concomitant use may result in hypokalemia). Products include:
- AK-Pred ... ⊙ 205
- Hydeltrasol Injection, Sterile ... 1476
- Inflamase ... ⊙ 274
- Pediapred Oral Liquid ... 987
- Vasocidin Ophthalmic Solution ... ⊙ 276

Prednisolone Tebutate (Concomitant use may result in hypokalemia). Products include:
- Hydeltra-T.B.A. Sterile Suspension 1478

Prednisone (Concomitant use may result in hypokalemia). Products include:
- Deltasone Tablets ... 2332

Propoxyphene Hydrochloride (May potentiate orthostatic hypotension). Products include:
- Darvon ... 1256
- Wygesic Tablets ... 2540

Propoxyphene Napsylate (May potentiate orthostatic hypotension). Products include:
- Darvon-N/Darvocet-N ... 1254

Propranolol Hydrochloride (Additive or potentiated action). Products include:
- Inderal ... 2459
- Inderal LA Long Acting Capsules ... 2461
- Inderide Tablets ... 2463
- Inderide LA Long Acting Capsules .. 2465

Ramipril (Additive or potentiated action). Products include:
- Altace Capsules ... 1086

Rauwolfia Serpentina (Additive or potentiated action). Products include:
- Raudixin Tablets ... 1803
- Rauzide Tablets ... 1804

Rescinnamine (Additive or potentiated action).
- No products indexed under this heading.

Reserpine (Additive or potentiated action). Products include:
- Diupres Tablets ... 1461
- Hydromox R Tablets ... 1209
- Hydropres Tablets ... 1485
- Renese-R Tablets ... 1786
- Salutensin/Salutensin-Demi ... 719
- Ser-Ap-Es Tablets ... 881
- Serpasil Tablets ... 883
- Serpasil-Apresoline Tablets ... 884
- Serpasil-Esidrix Tablets ... 886

Secobarbital Sodium (May potentiate orthostatic hypotension). Products include:
- Seconal Sodium Pulvules ... 1296

Selegiline Hydrochloride (Concurrent use requires caution). Products include:
- Eldepryl ... 2250

Sodium Nitroprusside (Additive or potentiated action). Products include:
- Nipride I.V. Infusion ... 1909

Sufentanil Citrate (May potentiate orthostatic hypotension). Products include:
- Sufenta Injection ... 1147

Sulindac (Concurrent administration may reduce the diuretic, natriuretic and antihypertensive effects of thiazide diuretics). Products include:
- Clinoril Tablets ... 1433

Terazosin Hydrochloride (Additive or potentiated action). Products include:
- Hytrin Tablets ... 529

Thiamylal Sodium (May potentiate orthostatic hypotension). Products include:
- Surital Ampoules, Steri-Vials ... 1764

Timolol Maleate (Additive or potentiated action). Products include:
- Blocadren Tablets ... 1429
- Timolide Tablets ... 1547
- Timoptic in Ocudose ... 1552
- Timoptic Sterile Ophthalmic Solution ... 1550

Tolmetin Sodium (Concurrent administration may reduce the diuretic, natriuretic and antihypertensive effects of thiazide diuretics). Products include:
- Tolectin (200, 400 and 600 mg) .. 1379

Tranylcypromine Sulfate (Concurrent use requires caution). Products include:
- Parnate Tablets ... 2222

Triamcinolone (Concomitant use may result in hypokalemia).
- No products indexed under this heading.

Triamcinolone Acetonide (Concomitant use may result in hypokalemia). Products include:
- Aristocort A ... 1010
- Azmacort Inhaler ... 1837
- Kenalog Cream, Lotion & Ointment 2401
- Kenalog-10 Injection ... 2402
- Kenalog-40 Injection ... 2403
- Kenalog in Orabase ... 604
- Kenalog Spray ... 2401
- Mycolog II Cream and Ointment ... 2407
- Mytrex Cream & Ointment ... 2080
- Nasacort Nasal Inhaler ... 1844

Triamcinolone Diacetate (Concomitant use may result in hypokalemia). Products include:
- Aristocort Suspension ... 1008

Triamcinolone Hexacetonide (Concomitant use may result in hypokalemia). Products include:
- Aristospan Suspension ... 1011

Trimethaphan Camsylate (Additive or potentiated action). Products include:
- Arfonad Ampuls ... 1887

Tubocurarine Chloride (Increased responsiveness to tubocurarine).
- No products indexed under this heading.

Food Interactions

Food, unspecified (Enhances gastrointestinal absorption of hydrochlorothiazide).

APRESOLINE HYDROCHLORIDE PARENTERAL (AMPULS)

(Hydralazine Hydrochloride) ... 856

May interact with monoamine oxidase inhibitors and certain other agents. Compounds in these categories include:

Diazoxide (Excessive fall in blood pressure; profound hypotensive episodes). Products include:
- Hyperstat I.V. Injection ... 2095
- Proglycem ... 649

Furazolidone (Use with caution). Products include:
- Furoxone ... 1855

Isocarboxazid (Use with caution). Products include:
- Marplan Tablets ... 1906

Phenelzine Sulfate (Use with caution). Products include:
- Nardil ... 1742

Selegiline Hydrochloride (Use with caution). Products include:
- Eldepryl ... 2250

Tranylcypromine Sulfate (Use with caution). Products include:
- Parnate Tablets ... 2222

APRESOLINE HYDROCHLORIDE TABLETS

(Hydralazine Hydrochloride) ... 855

May interact with monoamine oxidase inhibitors and certain other agents. Compounds in these categories include:

Diazoxide (Profound hypotensive episodes). Products include:
- Hyperstat I.V. Injection ... 2095
- Proglycem ... 649

Epinephrine (Pressor responses to epinephrine may be reduced). Products include:
- Ana-Kit Anaphylaxis Emergency Treatment Kit ... 1100
- Bronkaid Mist ... ▣ 757
- EpiPen ... 843
- Marcaine Hydrochloride 0.5% with Epinephrine 1:200,000 (as bitartrate) ... 958
- Marcaine Hydrochloride with Epinephrine 1:200,000 ... 2055
- Primatene Mist ... 2420
- Sus-Phrine Injection ... 1006
- Xylocaine with Epinephrine Injections ... 637

Epinephrine Bitartrate (Pressor responses to epinephrine may be reduced). Products include:
- AsthmaHaler Mist Epinephrine Bitartrate Bronchodilator ... ▣ 616
- Bronkaid Mist Suspension ... ▣ 757
- Primatene Mist Suspension ... 2421

Furazolidone (Concurrent administration contraindicated). Products include:
- Furoxone ... 1855

Isocarboxazid (Concurrent administration contraindicated). Products include:
- Marplan Tablets ... 1906

Phenelzine Sulfate (Concurrent administration contraindicated). Products include:
- Nardil ... 1742

Selegiline Hydrochloride (Concurrent administration contraindicated). Products include:
- Eldepryl ... 2250

Tranylcypromine Sulfate (Concurrent administration contraindicated). Products include:
- Parnate Tablets ... 2222

Food Interactions

Food, unspecified (Results in higher plasma levels).

APRESOLINE-ESIDRIX TABLETS

(Hydralazine Hydrochloride, Hydrochlorothiazide) ... 857

May interact with monoamine oxidase inhibitors, corticosteroids, antihypertensives, insulin, narcotic analgesics, non-steroidal anti-inflammatory agents, barbiturates, lithium preparations, and cer-

tain other agents. Compounds in these categories include:

Acebutolol Hydrochloride (Additive or potentiated action). Products include:
Sectral Capsules 2520

ACTH (Hypokalemia).
No products indexed under this heading.

Alcohol (May potentiate orthostatic hypotension).

Alfentanil Hydrochloride (May potentiate orthostatic hypotension). Products include:
Alfenta Injection 1131

Aprobarbital (May potentiate orthostatic hypotension). Products include:
Alurate Elixir 1883

Atenolol (Additive or potentiated action). Products include:
Tenoretic Tablets 1105
Tenormin Tablets and I.V. Injection 1107

Benazepril Hydrochloride (Additive or potentiated action). Products include:
Lotensin Tablets 872

Bendroflumethiazide (Additive or potentiated action). Products include:
Corzide Tablets 702
Naturetin Tablets 1789
Rauzide Tablets 1804

Betamethasone Acetate (Hypokalemia). Products include:
Celestone Soluspan Suspension 2081

Betamethasone Sodium Phosphate (Hypokalemia). Products include:
Celestone Soluspan Suspension 2081

Betaxolol Hydrochloride (Additive or potentiated action). Products include:
Betoptic Sterile Ophthalmic Solution 569
Betoptic S Sterile Ophthalmic Suspension 570
Kerlone Tablets 2172

Buprenorphine (May potentiate orthostatic hypotension).
No products indexed under this heading.

Butabarbital (May potentiate orthostatic hypotension). Products include:
Pyridium Plus 1764

Butalbital (May potentiate orthostatic hypotension). Products include:
Esgic-Plus Tablets 1002
Esgic Tablets & Capsules 1001
Fioricet Tablets 2006
Fiorinal Capsules 2007
Fiorinal with Codeine Capsules 2008
Fiorinal Tablets 2007
Phrenilin 838
Sedapap Tablets 50 mg/650 mg .. 1360

Captopril (Additive or potentiated action). Products include:
Capoten 2255
Capozide 2258

Carteolol Hydrochloride (Additive or potentiated action). Products include:
Cartrol Tablets 507

Chlorothiazide (Additive or potentiated action). Products include:
Aldoclor Tablets 1413
Diupres Tablets 1461
Diuril Oral 1464

Chlorothiazide Sodium (Additive or potentiated action). Products include:
Diuril Sodium Intravenous 1463

Chlorthalidone (Additive or potentiated action). Products include:
Combipres Tablets 678
Tenoretic Tablets 1105
Thalitone Tablets 687

Clonidine (Additive or potentiated action). Products include:
Catapres-TTS 677

Clonidine Hydrochloride (Additive or potentiated action). Products include:
Catapres Tablets 676
Combipres Tablets 678

Codeine (May potentiate orthostatic hypotension). Products include:
Calcidrine Syrup 506

Codeine Phosphate (May potentiate orthostatic hypotension). Products include:
Actifed with Codeine Cough Syrup.. 752
Cheracol Cough Syrup 1853
Codimal PH Syrup 846
Dimetane-DC Cough Syrup 1857
Empirin with Codeine Phosphate Nos. 2, 3 & 4 764
Fiorinal with Codeine Capsules 2008
Isoclor Expectorant 982
Naldecon CX Adult Liquid .... ▣ 521
Novahistine DH 1342
Novahistine Expectorant 1343
Nucofed Capsules 2219
Nucofed Expectorant 2219
Nucofed Pediatric Expectorant 2220
Nucofed Syrup 2219
Phenaphen with Codeine Capsules 1865
Phenaphen-650 with Codeine Tablets 1866
Phenergan with Codeine 2497
Phenergan VC with Codeine 2501
Robitussin A-C Syrup 1875
Robitussin-DAC Syrup 1875
Ryna .... ▣ 741
Soma Compound w/Codeine Tablets 2390
Triaminic Expectorant w/Codeine .. 1996
Tussi-Organidin Liquid 2391
Tylenol with Codeine 1381

Codeine Polistirex (May potentiate orthostatic hypotension).
No products indexed under this heading.

Cortisone Acetate (Hypokalemia). Products include:
Cortone Acetate Sterile Suspension 1437
Cortone Acetate Tablets 1439

Deserpidine (Additive or potentiated action). Products include:
Enduronyl 518
Harmonyl Tablets 528
Oreticyl 545

Deslanoside (Increased ventricular irritability).
No products indexed under this heading.

Dexamethasone Acetate (Hypokalemia). Products include:
Dalalone D.P. Injectable 999
Decadron-LA Sterile Suspension 1457

Dexamethasone Sodium Phosphate (Hypokalemia). Products include:
AK-Dex .... ◉ 203
Decadron Phosphate Respihaler 1454
Decadron Phosphate Sterile Ophthalmic Ointment 1453
Decadron Phosphate Sterile Ophthalmic Solution 1453
Decadron Phosphate Topical Cream 1455
Decadron Phosphate Turbinaire 1456
Maxidex Sterile Ophthalmic Ointment .... ◉ 222
NeoDecadron Sterile Ophthalmic Ointment 1517
NeoDecadron Sterile Ophthalmic Solution 1518
NeoDecadron Topical Cream 1518

Dezocine (May potentiate orthostatic hypotension).

Diazoxide (Profound hypotensive episodes; additive or potentiated action). Products include:
Hyperstat I.V. Injection 2095
Proglycem 649

Diclofenac Sodium (May reduce diuretic, natriuretic, and antihypertensive effects of thiazide diuretics). Products include:
Voltaren Ophthalmic Sterile Ophthalmic Solution .... ◉ 268
Voltaren Tablets 1042

Digitoxin (Increased ventricular irritability). Products include:
Crystodigin Tablets 1253

Digoxin (Increased ventricular irritability). Products include:
Lanoxicaps 772
Lanoxin Elixir Pediatric 775
Lanoxin Injection 778
Lanoxin Injection Pediatric 781
Lanoxin Tablets 783

Doxazosin Mesylate (Additive or potentiated action). Products include:
Cardura Tablets 1941

Enalapril Maleate (Additive or potentiated action). Products include:
Vaseretic Tablets 1559
Vasotec Tablets 1564

Enalaprilat (Additive or potentiated action). Products include:
Vasotec I.V. 1562

Esmolol Hydrochloride (Additive or potentiated action). Products include:
Brevibloc Injection 942

Etodolac (May reduce diuretic, natriuretic, and antihypertensive effects of thiazide diuretics). Products include:
Lodine Capsules 2468

Felodipine (Additive or potentiated action). Products include:
Plendil Extended-Release Tablets 1526

Fenoprofen Calcium (May reduce diuretic, natriuretic, and antihypertensive effects of thiazide diuretics). Products include:
Nalfon Pulvules & Tablets 919

Fentanyl (May potentiate orthostatic hypotension). Products include:
Duragesic Transdermal System 1133

Fentanyl Citrate (May potentiate orthostatic hypotension). Products include:
Innovar Injection 1141
Sublimaze Injection 1146

Flurbiprofen (May reduce diuretic, natriuretic, and antihypertensive effects of thiazide diuretics). Products include:
Ansaid Tablets 2319

Fosinopril Sodium (Additive or potentiated action). Products include:
Monopril Tablets 1406

Furazolidone (Concurrent administration contraindicated). Products include:
Furoxone 1855

Furosemide (Additive or potentiated action). Products include:
Lasix 1093

Guanabenz Acetate (Additive or potentiated action). Products include:
Wytensin Tablets 2542

Guanethidine Monosulfate (Additive or potentiated action). Products include:
Esimil Tablets 864
Ismelin Tablets 869

Hydrocodone Bitartrate (May potentiate orthostatic hypotension). Products include:
Anexsia 5/500 Tablets 2196
Anexsia 7.5/650 Tablets 2197
Azdone Tablets 844
Codiclear DH Syrup 845
Codimal DH Syrup 846
Damason-P 1356
Hycodan Syrup, Tablets 927
Hycomine Compound Tablets 929
Hycomine Syrup 927
Hycotuss Expectorant Syrup 930
Hydrocet Capsules 835
Lortab ASA Tablets 2414
Lortab 2412
Ru-Tuss with Hydrocodone 694
Triaminic Expectorant DH 1995
Vicodin Tablets 1187
Vicodin ES Tablets 1189
Zydone Capsules 941

Hydrocodone Polistirex (May potentiate orthostatic hypotension). Products include:
Tussionex Extended-Release Suspension 988

Hydrocortisone (Hypokalemia). Products include:
AK-Spore H.C. .... ◉ 206
Bactine Hydrocortisone Anti-Itch Cream .... ▣ 625
CaldeCORT Anti-Itch Hydrocortisone Spray .... ▣ 560
Carmol HC Cream 1% 2296
Cortaid Spray .... ▣ 735
Cortenema 2244
Cortisporin Ointment 758
Cortisporin Ophthalmic Ointment Sterile 758
Cortisporin Ophthalmic Suspension Sterile 759
Cortisporin Otic Solution Sterile 760
Cortisporin Otic Suspension Sterile 760
Cortizone-5 Creme & Ointment .... ▣ 732
Dermolate Anti-Itch Cream .... ▣ 697
Eldecort Cream 1.0% 1113
Eldecort Cream 1.0% and 2.5% 1113
Fungoid HC Creme 1770
Hydrocortone Tablets 1482
Hytone 909
LazerSporin-C Solution 1770
Massengill Medicated Soft Cloth Towelettes 2192
Nutracort Cream & Lotion 1684
PediOtic Suspension Sterile 797
Synacort Creams 1%, 2.5% 2296
Vanoxide-HC Acne Lotion 911
Vioform-Hydrocortisone Cream and Mild Cream 889
Vioform-Hydrocortisone Ointment.. 889
VōSoL HC Otic Solution 2392
Vytone Cream 1% 911

Hydrocortisone Acetate (Hypokalemia). Products include:
Analpram-HC Rectal Cream 1% and 2.5% 970
Anusol-HC Cream 1690
Anusol-HC Suppositories 1691
Caldecort .... ▣ 560
Carmol HC Cream 1% 2296
Chloromycetin Hydrocortisone Ophthalmic 1694
Coly-Mycin S Otic w/Neomycin & Hydrocortisone 1708
Cortaid .... ▣ 735
Cortef Feminine Itch Cream .... ▣ 735
Corticaine .... ▣ 682
Cortifoam 1827
Cortisporin Cream 757
Epifoam 1828
Gynecort 5 Creme .... ▣ 556
Hydrocortone Acetate Sterile Suspension 1479
Lanacort 5 Creme and Ointment .. ▣ 557
Mantadil Cream 789
Ophthocort .... ◉ 301
Orabase HCA Oral Paste 890
Pramosone Cream, Lotion & Ointment 971
ProctoCream-HC 1834
Proctofoam-HC 1835

Hydrocortisone Sodium Phosphate (Hypokalemia). Products include:
Hydrocortone Phosphate Injection, Sterile 1481

Hydrocortisone Sodium Succinate (Hypokalemia). Products include:
Solu-Cortef Sterile Powder 2361

Hydroflumethiazide (Additive or potentiated action). Products include:
Diucardin Tablets 2450
Saluron 718

(▣ Described in PDR For Nonprescription Drugs) (◉ Described in PDR For Ophthalmology)

Salutensin/Salutensin-Demi 719

Ibuprofen (May reduce diuretic, natriuretic, and antihypertensive effects of thiazide diuretics). Products include:
- Advil Cold & Sinus Caplets (formerly CoAdvil) 2416
- Advil Ibuprofen Tablets and Caplets 2416
- Children's Advil Suspension 2426
- CoAdvil .... ▣ 748
- Dristan Sinus Caplets 2419
- Haltran Tablets .... ▣ 668
- Ibuprofen .... ▣ 631
- Medipren ibuprofen Caplets and Tablets 1362
- Midol 200 Cramp Relief Formula .. ▣ 570
- Motrin Tablets 2351
- Motrin IB Caplets and Tablets .... ▣ 736
- Nuprin Ibuprofen/Analgesic Tablets & Caplets 752
- PediaProfen Suspension 1363
- Rufen Tablets 691
- Trendar Ibuprofen Tablets .... ▣ 756

Indapamide (Additive or potentiated action). Products include:
- Lozol Tablets 1843

Indomethacin (May reduce diuretic, natriuretic, and antihypertensive effects of thiazide diuretics). Products include:
- Indocin 1487

Indomethacin Sodium Trihydrate (May reduce diuretic, natriuretic, and antihypertensive effects of thiazide diuretics). Products include:
- Indocin I.V. 1490

Insulin, Human (Insulin requirements may be altered).
- No products indexed under this heading.

Insulin, Human Isophane Suspension (Insulin requirements may be altered). Products include:
- Humulin N, 100 Units 1270

Insulin, Human NPH (Insulin requirements may be altered). Products include:
- Insulatard NPH Human 1627
- Novolin N 1627
- Novolin N PenFill Cartridges 1628
- Novolin N Prefilled 1628

Insulin, Human Regular (Insulin requirements may be altered). Products include:
- Humulin BR, 100 Units 1268
- Humulin R, 100 Units 1272
- Novolin R 1627
- Novolin R PenFill Cartridges 1628
- Novolin R Prefilled 1629
- Velosulin Human 1628

Insulin, Human, Zinc Suspension (Insulin requirements may be altered). Products include:
- Humulin L, 100 Units 1268
- Humulin U, 100 Units 1272
- Novolin L 1627

Insulin, NPH (Insulin requirements may be altered). Products include:
- NPH, 40 & 100 Units 1273
- Beef NPH, 100 Units 1274
- Pork NPH, 100 Units 1275
- Insulatard NPH 1626
- NPH Insulin 1626
- NPH Purified Pork Isophane Insulin 1626

Insulin, Regular (Insulin requirements may be altered). Products include:
- Regular, 40 & 100 Units 1273
- Beef Regular, 100 Units 1275
- Pork Regular, 100 Units 1275
- Pork Regular (Concentrated), 500 Units 1276
- Regular Insulin 1625
- Regular Purified Pork Insulin 1626
- Velosulin 1627

Insulin, Zinc Crystals (Insulin requirements may be altered). Products include:
- NPH, 40 & 100 Units 1273

Insulin, Zinc Suspension (Insulin requirements may be altered). Products include:
- Lente, 40 & 100 Units 1272
- Protamine, Zinc, 40 & 100 Units 1273
- Lente Iletin I 1272
- Beef Lente, 100 Units 1274
- Beef Protamine Zinc, 100 Units 1274
- Pork Lente, 100 Units 1275
- Pork, Protamine, Zinc, 100 Units 1275
- Lente Insulin 1626
- Lente Purified Pork Insulin 1626
- Semilente Insulin 1625
- Ultralente Insulin 1626

Isocarboxazid (Concurrent administration contraindicated). Products include:
- Marplan Tablets 1906

Isradipine (Additive or potentiated action). Products include:
- DynaCirc Capsules 2004

Ketoprofen (May reduce diuretic, natriuretic, and antihypertensive effects of thiazide diuretics). Products include:
- Orudis Capsules 2488

Ketorolac Tromethamine (May reduce diuretic, natriuretic, and antihypertensive effects of thiazide diuretics). Products include:
- Toradol IM Injection 2302

Labetalol Hydrochloride (Additive or potentiated action). Products include:
- Normodyne Injection 2108
- Normodyne Tablets 2110
- Normozide Tablets 2112
- Trandate HCT Tablets 579
- Trandate Injection 577
- Trandate Tablets 579

Levorphanol Tartrate (May potentiate orthostatic hypotension). Products include:
- Levo-Dromoran 1906

Lisinopril (Additive or potentiated action). Products include:
- Prinivil Tablets 1538
- Prinzide Tablets 1540
- Zestoretic 2274
- Zestril Tablets 2277

Lithium Carbonate (Increased risk of lithium toxicity). Products include:
- Eskalith 2214
- Lithane Tablets 1596
- Lithium Carbonate Capsules & Tablets 1984
- Lithobid Tablets 870

Lithium Citrate (Increased risk of lithium toxicity). Products include:
- Cibalith-S 870

Mecamylamine Hydrochloride (Additive or potentiated action). Products include:
- Inversine Tablets 1492

Meclofenamate Sodium (May reduce diuretic, natriuretic, and antihypertensive effects of thiazide diuretics). Products include:
- Meclomen Capsules 1739

Mefenamic Acid (May reduce diuretic, natriuretic, and antihypertensive effects of thiazide diuretics). Products include:
- Ponstel 1758

Meperidine Hydrochloride (May potentiate orthostatic hypotension). Products include:
- Demerol 2047
- Mepergan Injection 2479

Mephobarbital (May potentiate orthostatic hypotension). Products include:
- Mebaral Tablets 2061

Methadone Hydrochloride (May potentiate orthostatic hypotension). Products include:
- Dolophine Hydrochloride Ampoules & Vials 1260
- Dolophine Hydrochloride Tablets 1261
- Methadone Hydrochloride Diskets .. 1284
- Methadone Hydrochloride Oral Solution & Tablets 1987

Methyclothiazide (Additive or potentiated action). Products include:
- Enduron Tablets 517
- Enduronyl 518

Methyldopa (Additive or potentiated action; hemolytic anemia). Products include:
- Aldoclor Tablets 1413
- Aldomet Oral 1415
- Aldoril Tablets 1418

Methyldopate Hydrochloride (Additive or potentiated action; hemolytic anemia). Products include:
- Aldomet Ester HCl Injection 1417

Methylprednisolone (Hypokalemia). Products include:
- Medrol 2348

Methylprednisolone Acetate (Hypokalemia). Products include:
- Depo-Medrol Sterile Aqueous Suspension 2334

Methylprednisolone Sodium Succinate (Hypokalemia). Products include:
- Solu-Medrol Sterile Powder 2363

Metolazone (Additive or potentiated action). Products include:
- Diulo 2129
- Mykrox ½ mg Tablets 984
- Zaroxolyn Tablets 989

Metoprolol Tartrate (Additive or potentiated action). Products include:
- Lopressor Ampuls 1032
- Lopressor HCT Tablets 1034
- Lopressor Tablets 1032

Metyrosine (Additive or potentiated action). Products include:
- Demser Capsules 1460

Minoxidil (Additive or potentiated action). Products include:
- Loniten Tablets 2346
- Rogaine Topical Solution 2357

Morphine Sulfate (May potentiate orthostatic hypotension). Products include:
- Astramorph/PF Injection, USP (Preservative-Free) 618
- Duramorph 960
- Infumorph 200 and Infumorph 500 Sterile Solutions 962
- MS Contin Tablets 1814
- MSIR 1817
- Oramorph SR (Morphine Sulfate Sustained Release Tablets) 1988
- Roxanol 1991

Nadolol (Additive or potentiated action). Products include:
- Corgard Tablets 701
- Corzide Tablets 702

Naproxen (May reduce diuretic, natriuretic, and antihypertensive effects of thiazide diuretics). Products include:
- Naprosyn 2297

Naproxen Sodium (May reduce diuretic, natriuretic, and antihypertensive effects of thiazide diuretics). Products include:
- Anaprox and Anaprox DS Tablets 2288

Nicardipine Hydrochloride (Additive or potentiated action). Products include:
- Cardene Capsules 2290

Nitroglycerin (Additive or potentiated action). Products include:
- Deponit NTG Transdermal Delivery System 2143
- Minitran Transdermal Delivery System 1312
- Nitro-Bid Ointment 1339
- Nitro-Bid Capsules 1338
- Nitrodisc 2176
- Nitro-Dur (nitroglycerin) Transdermal Infusion System 1164
- Nitrogard Tablets 1004
- Nitrolingual Spray 1846
- Nitrostat Tablets 1743
- Transderm-Nitro Transdermal Therapeutic System 2283

Norepinephrine Bitartrate (Decreased arterial response to norepinephrine). Products include:
- Levophed Bitartrate Injection 2054

Opium Alkaloids (May potentiate orthostatic hypotension). Products include:
- B & O No. 15A & No. 16A Supprettes 2395
- Pantopon Injectable 1911

Oxycodone Hydrochloride (May potentiate orthostatic hypotension). Products include:
- Percocet Tablets 950
- Percodan 951
- Roxicodone Tablets, Oral Solution & Intensol (Oxycodone) 1992
- Tylox Capsules 1382

Penbutolol Sulfate (Additive or potentiated action). Products include:
- Levatol 1832

Pentobarbital Sodium (May potentiate orthostatic hypotension). Products include:
- Nembutal Sodium Capsules 534
- Nembutal Sodium Solution 536
- Nembutal Sodium Suppositories 538

Phenelzine Sulfate (Concurrent administration contraindicated). Products include:
- Nardil 1742

Phenobarbital (May potentiate orthostatic hypotension). Products include:
- Arco-Lase Plus Tablets 607
- Bellergal-S Tablets 1998
- Bronkolixir .... ▣ 761
- Bronkotabs Tablets .... ▣ 762
- Donnatal 1858
- Donnatal Extentabs 1859
- Donnatal Tablets 1858
- Donnazyme Tablets 1860
- Kinesed Tablets 2272
- Phenobarbital Elixir and Tablets 1293
- Primatene Tablets-P Formula 2421
- Quadrinal Tablets 1183
- Tedral SA 1765

Phenoxybenzamine Hydrochloride (Additive or potentiated action). Products include:
- Dibenzyline Capsules 2207

Phentolamine Mesylate (Additive or potentiated action). Products include:
- Regitine 878

Phenylbutazone (May reduce diuretic, natriuretic, and antihypertensive effects of thiazide diuretics). Products include:
- Butazolidin Capsules & Tablets 1027

Pindolol (Additive or potentiated action). Products include:
- Visken Tablets 2036

Piroxicam (May reduce diuretic, natriuretic, and antihypertensive effects of thiazide diuretics). Products include:
- Feldene Capsules 1777

Polythiazide (Additive or potentiated action). Products include:
- Minizide Capsules 1779
- Renese Tablets 1785
- Renese-R Tablets 1786

Prazosin Hydrochloride (Additive or potentiated action). Products include:
- Minipress Capsules 1778
- Minizide Capsules 1779

Prednisolone Acetate (Hypokalemia). Products include:
- AK-Cide Sterile Ophthalmic Ointment & Suspension .... ⊙ 202
- Blephamide Liquifilm Sterile Ophthalmic Suspension 586
- Blephamide S.O.P. Sterile Ophthalmic Ointment 586
- Cetapred Ointment .... ⊙ 220

(▣ Described in PDR For Nonprescription Drugs)

(⊙ Described in PDR For Ophthalmology)

- ⅛% Econopred & 1% Econopred Plus ◉ 217
- Isopto Cetapred Suspension ◉ 220
- Metimyd ◉ 306
- Poly-Pred Liquifilm ◉ 250
- Pred Forte ◉ 252
- Pred Mild ◉ 254
- Pred-G Liquifilm Sterile Ophthalmic Suspension ◉ 252
- Pred-G S.O.P. Sterile Ophthalmic Ointment ◉ 253
- Vasocidin Ointment ◉ 275

Prednisolone Sodium Phosphate (Hypokalemia). Products include:
- AK-Pred ◉ 205
- Hydeltrasol Injection, Sterile 1476
- Inflamase ◉ 274
- Pediapred Oral Liquid 987
- Vasocidin Ophthalmic Solution ◉ 276

Prednisolone Tebutate (Hypokalemia). Products include:
- Hydeltra-T.B.A. Sterile Suspension 1478

Prednisone (Hypokalemia). Products include:
- Deltasone Tablets 2332

Propoxyphene Hydrochloride (May potentiate orthostatic hypotension). Products include:
- Darvon 1256
- Wygesic Tablets 2540

Propoxyphene Napsylate (May potentiate orthostatic hypotension). Products include:
- Darvon-N/Darvocet-N 1254

Propranolol Hydrochloride (Additive or potentiated action). Products include:
- Inderal 2459
- Inderal LA Long Acting Capsules 2461
- Inderide Tablets 2463
- Inderide LA Long Acting Capsules 2465

Ramipril (Additive or potentiated action). Products include:
- Altace Capsules 1086

Rauwolfia Serpentina (Additive or potentiated action). Products include:
- Raudixin Tablets 1803
- Rauzide Tablets 1804

Rescinnamine (Additive or potentiated action).
- No products indexed under this heading.

Reserpine (Additive or potentiated action). Products include:
- Diupres Tablets 1461
- Hydromox R Tablets 1209
- Hydropres Tablets 1485
- Renese-R Tablets 1786
- Salutensin/Salutensin-Demi 719
- Ser-Ap-Es Tablets 881
- Serpasil Tablets 883
- Serpasil-Apresoline Tablets 884
- Serpasil-Esidrix Tablets 886

Secobarbital Sodium (May potentiate orthostatic hypotension). Products include:
- Seconal Sodium Pulvules 1296

Selegiline Hydrochloride (Concurrent administration contraindicated). Products include:
- Eldepryl 2250

Sodium Nitroprusside (Additive or potentiated action). Products include:
- Nipride I.V. Infusion 1909

Sufentanil Citrate (May potentiate orthostatic hypotension). Products include:
- Sufenta Injection 1147

Sulindac (May reduce diuretic, natriuretic, and antihypertensive effects of thiazide diuretics). Products include:
- Clinoril Tablets 1433

Terazosin Hydrochloride (Additive or potentiated action). Products include:
- Hytrin Tablets 529

Thiamylal Sodium (May potentiate orthostatic hypotension). Products include:
- Surital Ampoules, Steri-Vials 1764

Timolol Maleate (Additive or potentiated action). Products include:
- Blocadren Tablets 1429
- Timolide Tablets 1547
- Timoptic in Ocudose 1552
- Timoptic Sterile Ophthalmic Solution 1550

Tolmetin Sodium (May reduce diuretic, natriuretic, and antihypertensive effects of thiazide diuretics). Products include:
- Tolectin (200, 400 and 600 mg) 1379

Tranylcypromine Sulfate (Concurrent administration contraindicated). Products include:
- Parnate Tablets 2222

Triamcinolone (Hypokalemia).
- No products indexed under this heading.

Triamcinolone Acetonide (Hypokalemia). Products include:
- Aristocort A 1010
- Azmacort Inhaler 1837
- Kenalog Cream, Lotion & Ointment 2401
- Kenalog-10 Injection 2402
- Kenalog-40 Injection 2403
- Kenalog in Orabase 604
- Kenalog Spray 2401
- Mycolog II Cream and Ointment 2407
- Mytrex Cream & Ointment 2080
- Nasacort Nasal Inhaler 1844

Triamcinolone Diacetate (Hypokalemia). Products include:
- Aristocort Suspension 1008

Triamcinolone Hexacetonide (Hypokalemia). Products include:
- Aristospan Suspension 1011

Trimethaphan Camsylate (Additive or potentiated action). Products include:
- Arfonad Ampuls 1887

Tubocurarine Chloride (Increased responsiveness to tubocurarine).
- No products indexed under this heading.

Food Interactions

Food, unspecified (Enhances gastrointestinal absorption of hydrochlorothiazide; results in higher plasma levels of hydralazine).

AQUA CARE CREAM
(Urea) ▣ 616
No interactions described in labeling.

AQUA CARE LOTION
(Urea) ▣ 616
No interactions described in labeling.

AQUA-A CREAM
(Moisturizing formula) ▣ 509
No interactions described in labeling.

AQUADERM COMBINATION TREATMENT/MOISTURIZER-(SPF 15 FORMULA)
(Octyl Methoxycinnamate, Oxybenzone) ▣ 509
No interactions described in labeling.

AQUADERM CREAM
(Moisturizing formula) ▣ 509
No interactions described in labeling.

AQUADERM LOTION
(Moisturizing formula) ▣ 509
No interactions described in labeling.

AQUAMEPHYTON INJECTION
(Phytonadione) 1422
May interact with oral anticoagulants. Compounds in this category include:

Dicumarol (Temporary resistance to anticoagulants). Products include:
- Dicumarol Tablets 516

Warfarin Sodium (Temporary resistance to anticoagulants). Products include:
- Coumadin Injection & Tablets 944
- Panwarfin Tablets 547

AQUANIL LOTION
(Cleanser) 1772
No interactions described in labeling.

AQUAPHOR ANTIBIOTIC FORMULA
(Polymyxin B Sulfate, Bacitracin Zinc) 662
No interactions described in labeling.

AQUAPHOR HEALING OINTMENT, ORIGINAL FORMULA
(Ointment base) 662
No interactions described in labeling.

AQUAPHOR NATURAL HEALING FORMULA
(Petrolatum, Mineral Oil) 662
No interactions described in labeling.

AQUASOL A VITAMIN A CAPSULES, USP
(Vitamin A) 615
May interact with oral contraceptives. Compounds in this category include:

Ethinyl Estradiol (Potential for a significant increase in plasma vitamin A levels). Products include:
- Brevicon 2304
- Demulen 2161
- Estinyl Tablets 2085
- Jenest-28 Tablets 1636
- Levlen/Tri-Levlen 665
- Lo/Ovral Tablets 2471
- Lo/Ovral-28 Tablets 2476
- Loestrin 1728
- Modicon 1667
- Nordette-21 Tablets 2481
- Nordette-28 Tablets 2483
- Norethin 2133
- Norinyl 2304
- Norlestrin 1746
- Ortho-Cyclen Tablets 1658
- Ortho-Novum 1667
- Ovcon 1391
- Ovral Tablets 2490
- Ovral-28 Tablets 2491
- Levlen/Tri-Levlen 665
- Tri-Norinyl 2304
- Triphasil-21 Tablets 2527
- Triphasil-28 Tablets 2532

Ethynodiol Diacetate (Potential for a significant increase in plasma vitamin A levels). Products include:
- Demulen 2161

Levonorgestrel (Potential for a significant increase in plasma vitamin A levels). Products include:
- Levlen/Tri-Levlen 665
- Nordette-21 Tablets 2481
- Nordette-28 Tablets 2483
- Norplant System 2484
- Levlen/Tri-Levlen 665
- Triphasil-21 Tablets 2527
- Triphasil-28 Tablets 2532

Mestranol (Potential for a significant increase in plasma vitamin A levels). Products include:
- Enovid 2161
- Norethin 2133
- Norinyl 2304
- Ortho-Novum 1667

Norethindrone (Potential for a significant increase in plasma vitamin A levels). Products include:
- Brevicon 2304
- Jenest-28 Tablets 1636
- Micronor Tablets 1667
- Modicon 1667
- Norethin 2133
- Norinyl 2304
- Norlutin 1755
- Nor-Q D Tablets 2304
- Ortho-Novum 1667
- Ovcon 1391
- Tri-Norinyl 2304

Norethynodrel (Potential for a significant increase in plasma vitamin A levels). Products include:
- Enovid 2161

Norgestimate (Potential for a significant increase in plasma vitamin A levels). Products include:
- Ortho-Cyclen Tablets 1658

Norgestrel (Potential for a significant increase in plasma vitamin A levels). Products include:
- Lo/Ovral Tablets 2471
- Lo/Ovral-28 Tablets 2476
- Ovral Tablets 2490
- Ovral-28 Tablets 2491
- Ovrette Tablets 2492

AQUASOL A PARENTERAL, USP
(Vitamin A) 615
May interact with oral contraceptives. Compounds in this category include:

Ethinyl Estradiol (Potential for a significant increase in plasma vitamin A levels). Products include:
- Brevicon 2304
- Demulen 2161
- Estinyl Tablets 2085
- Jenest-28 Tablets 1636
- Levlen/Tri-Levlen 665
- Lo/Ovral Tablets 2471
- Lo/Ovral-28 Tablets 2476
- Loestrin 1728
- Modicon 1667
- Nordette-21 Tablets 2481
- Nordette-28 Tablets 2483
- Norethin 2133
- Norinyl 2304
- Norlestrin 1746
- Ortho-Cyclen Tablets 1658
- Ortho-Novum 1667
- Ovcon 1391
- Ovral Tablets 2490
- Ovral-28 Tablets 2491
- Levlen/Tri-Levlen 665
- Tri-Norinyl 2304
- Triphasil-21 Tablets 2527
- Triphasil-28 Tablets 2532

Ethynodiol Diacetate (Potential for a significant increase in plasma vitamin A levels). Products include:
- Demulen 2161

Levonorgestrel (Potential for a significant increase in plasma vitamin A levels). Products include:
- Levlen/Tri-Levlen 665
- Nordette-21 Tablets 2481
- Nordette-28 Tablets 2483
- Norplant System 2484
- Levlen/Tri-Levlen 665
- Triphasil-21 Tablets 2527
- Triphasil-28 Tablets 2532

Mestranol (Potential for a significant increase in plasma vitamin A levels). Products include:
- Enovid 2161
- Norethin 2133
- Norinyl 2304
- Ortho-Novum 1667

Norethindrone (Potential for a significant increase in plasma vitamin A levels). Products include:
- Brevicon 2304
- Jenest-28 Tablets 1636
- Micronor Tablets 1667
- Modicon 1667
- Norethin 2133
- Norinyl 2304

Norlutin ... 1755
Nor-Q D Tablets ... 2304
Ortho-Novum ... 1667
Ovcon ... 1391
Tri-Norinyl ... 2304

Norethynodrel (Potential for a significant increase in plasma vitamin A levels). Products include:
Enovid ... 2161

Norgestimate (Potential for a significant increase in plasma vitamin A levels). Products include:
Ortho-Cyclen Tablets ... 1658

Norgestrel (Potential for a significant increase in plasma vitamin A levels). Products include:
Lo/Ovral Tablets ... 2471
Lo/Ovral-28 Tablets ... 2476
Ovral Tablets ... 2490
Ovral-28 Tablets ... 2491
Ovrette Tablets ... 2492

ARALEN HYDROCHLORIDE INJECTION
(Chloroquine Hydrochloride) ... 2038
May interact with:

Hepatotoxic Drugs, unspecified (Concurrent use requires caution).

ARALEN PHOSPHATE WITH PRIMAQUINE PHOSPHATE TABLETS
(Chloroquine Phosphate, Primaquine Phosphate) ... 2040
May interact with:

Bone Marrow Depressants, unspecified (Concurrent administration is contraindicated).

Quinacrine Hydrochloride (Increased toxicity). Products include:
Atabrine Hydrochloride Tablets ... 2041

ARALEN PHOSPHATE TABLETS
(Chloroquine Hydrochloride) ... 2039
May interact with:

Hepatotoxic Drugs, unspecified (Caution should be exercised when used in conjunction with known hepatotoxic drugs).

ARAMINE INJECTION
(Metaraminol Bitartrate) ... 1424
May interact with cardiac glycosides, monoamine oxidase inhibitors, tricyclic antidepressants, and certain other agents. Compounds in these categories include:

Amitriptyline Hydrochloride (Potentiates pressor effect). Products include:
Elavil ... 2269
Endep Tablets ... 1927
Etrafon ... 2087
Limbitrol ... 1933
Triavil Tablets ... 1556

Amoxapine (Potentiates pressor effect). Products include:
Asendin Tablets ... 1196

Clomipramine Hydrochloride (Potentiates pressor effect). Products include:
Anafranil Capsules ... 650

Desipramine Hydrochloride (Potentiates pressor effect). Products include:
Norpramin Tablets ... 1340

Deslanoside (May cause ectopic arrhythmic reaction).
No products indexed under this heading.

Digitoxin (May cause ectopic arrhythmic reaction). Products include:
Crystodigin Tablets ... 1253

Digoxin (May cause ectopic arrhythmic reaction). Products include:
Lanoxicaps ... 772
Lanoxin Elixir Pediatric ... 775
Lanoxin Injection ... 778
Lanoxin Injection Pediatric ... 781
Lanoxin Tablets ... 783

Doxepin Hydrochloride (Potentiates pressor effect). Products include:
Sinequan ... 1960

Furazolidone (Potentiates pressor effect). Products include:
Furoxone ... 1855

Halothane (Concurrent use should be avoided). Products include:
Fluothane ... 2453

Imipramine Hydrochloride (Potentiates pressor effect). Products include:
Tofranil Ampuls ... 1038
Tofranil Tablets ... 1039

Imipramine Pamoate (Potentiates pressor effect). Products include:
Tofranil-PM Capsules ... 1041

Isocarboxazid (Potentiates pressor effect). Products include:
Marplan Tablets ... 1906

Maprotiline Hydrochloride (Potentiates pressor effect). Products include:
Ludiomil Tablets ... 874

Nortriptyline Hydrochloride (Potentiates pressor effect). Products include:
Pamelor ... 2019

Phenelzine Sulfate (Potentiates pressor effect). Products include:
Nardil ... 1742

Protriptyline Hydrochloride (Potentiates pressor effect). Products include:
Vivactil Tablets ... 1567

Selegiline Hydrochloride (Potentiates pressor effect). Products include:
Eldepryl ... 2250

Tranylcypromine Sulfate (Potentiates pressor effect). Products include:
Parnate Tablets ... 2222

Trimipramine Maleate (Potentiates pressor effect). Products include:
Surmontil Capsules ... 2524

ARCO-LASE PLUS TABLETS
(Enzymes, Digestive) ... 607
No interactions described in labeling.

ARCO-LASE TABLETS
(Enzymes, Digestive) ... 607
No interactions described in labeling.

ARFONAD AMPULS
(Trimethaphan Camsylate) ... 1887
May interact with antihypertensives, diuretics, nondepolarizing neuromuscular blocking agents, and certain other agents. Compounds in these categories include:

Acebutolol Hydrochloride (Additive hypotensive effect). Products include:
Sectral Capsules ... 2520

Amiloride Hydrochloride (Enhances ganglionic blocking effects). Products include:
Midamor Tablets ... 1508
Moduretic Tablets ... 1510

Atenolol (Additive hypotensive effect). Products include:
Tenoretic Tablets ... 1105
Tenormin Tablets and I.V. Injection 1107

Atracurium Besylate (Prolonged effects of neuromuscular blocking agents). Products include:
Tracrium Injection ... 817

Benazepril Hydrochloride (Additive hypotensive effect). Products include:
Lotensin Tablets ... 872

Bendroflumethiazide (Enhances ganglionic blocking effects; additive hypotensive effect). Products include:
Corzide Tablets ... 702
Naturetin Tablets ... 1789
Rauzide Tablets ... 1804

Betaxolol Hydrochloride (Additive hypotensive effect). Products include:
Betoptic Sterile Ophthalmic Solution ... 569
Betoptic S Sterile Ophthalmic Suspension ... 570
Kerlone Tablets ... 2172

Bumetanide (Enhances ganglionic blocking effects). Products include:
Bumex ... 1895

Bupivacaine Hydrochloride (Additive hypotensive effect). Products include:
Marcaine Hydrochloride 0.5% with Epinephrine 1:200,000 (as bitartrate) ... 958
Marcaine Hydrochloride with Epinephrine 1:200,000 ... 2055
Marcaine Hydrochloride Injection ... 2055
Marcaine Spinal ... 2058
Sensorcaine ... 631
Sensorcaine-MPF Spinal ... 634

Captopril (Additive hypotensive effect). Products include:
Capoten ... 2255
Capozide ... 2258

Carteolol Hydrochloride (Additive hypotensive effect). Products include:
Cartrol Tablets ... 507

Chlorothiazide (Enhances ganglionic blocking effects; additive hypotensive effect). Products include:
Aldoclor Tablets ... 1413
Diupres Tablets ... 1461
Diuril Oral ... 1464

Chlorothiazide Sodium (Enhances ganglionic blocking effects; additive hypotensive effect). Products include:
Diuril Sodium Intravenous ... 1463

Chlorthalidone (Additive hypotensive effect; enhances ganglionic blocking effects). Products include:
Combipres Tablets ... 678
Tenoretic Tablets ... 1105
Thalitone Tablets ... 687

Clonidine (Additive hypotensive effect). Products include:
Catapres-TTS ... 677

Clonidine Hydrochloride (Additive hypotensive effect). Products include:
Catapres Tablets ... 676
Combipres Tablets ... 678

Deserpidine (Additive hypotensive effect). Products include:
Enduronyl ... 518
Harmonyl Tablets ... 528
Oreticyl ... 545

Diazoxide (Additive hypotensive effect). Products include:
Hyperstat I.V. Injection ... 2095
Proglycem ... 649

Doxazosin Mesylate (Additive hypotensive effect). Products include:
Cardura Tablets ... 1941

Enalapril Maleate (Additive hypotensive effect). Products include:
Vaseretic Tablets ... 1559
Vasotec Tablets ... 1564

Enalaprilat (Additive hypotensive effect). Products include:
Vasotec I.V. ... 1562

Esmolol Hydrochloride (Additive hypotensive effect). Products include:
Brevibloc Injection ... 942

Ethacrynic Acid (Enhances ganglionic blocking effects). Products include:
Edecrin Tablets ... 1468

Felodipine (Additive hypotensive effect). Products include:
Plendil Extended-Release Tablets ... 1526

Fosinopril Sodium (Additive hypotensive effect). Products include:
Monopril Tablets ... 1406

Furosemide (Enhances ganglionic blocking effects; additive hypotensive effect). Products include:
Lasix ... 1093

Guanabenz Acetate (Additive hypotensive effect). Products include:
Wytensin Tablets ... 2542

Guanethidine Monosulfate (Additive hypotensive effect). Products include:
Esimil Tablets ... 864
Ismelin Tablets ... 869

Hydralazine Hydrochloride (Additive hypotensive effect). Products include:
Apresazide Capsules ... 854
Apresoline Hydrochloride Parenteral (Ampuls) ... 856
Apresoline Hydrochloride Tablets ... 855
Apresoline-Esidrix Tablets ... 857
Ser-Ap-Es Tablets ... 881
Serpasil-Apresoline Tablets ... 884

Hydrochlorothiazide (Enhances ganglionic blocking effects; additive hypotensive effect). Products include:
Aldactazide ... 2150
Aldoril Tablets ... 1418
Apresazide Capsules ... 854
Apresoline-Esidrix Tablets ... 857
Capozide ... 2258
Dyazide Capsules ... 2208
Esidrix Tablets ... 863
Esimil Tablets ... 864
HydroDIURIL Tablets ... 1484
Hydropres Tablets ... 1485
Inderide Tablets ... 2463
Inderide LA Long Acting Capsules ... 2465
Lopressor HCT Tablets ... 1034
Maxzide ... 1215
Moduretic Tablets ... 1510
Normozide Tablets ... 2112
Oretic Tablets ... 544
Oreticyl ... 545
Prinzide Tablets ... 1540
Ser-Ap-Es Tablets ... 881
Serpasil-Esidrix Tablets ... 886
Timolide Tablets ... 1547
Trandate HCT Tablets ... 579
Vaseretic Tablets ... 1559
Zestoretic ... 2274

Hydroflumethiazide (Enhances ganglionic blocking effects; additive hypotensive effect). Products include:
Diucardin Tablets ... 2450
Saluron ... 718
Salutensin/Salutensin-Demi ... 719

Indapamide (Enhances ganglionic blocking effects; additive hypotensive effect). Products include:
Lozol Tablets ... 1843

Isradipine (Additive hypotensive effect). Products include:
DynaCirc Capsules ... 2004

Labetalol Hydrochloride (Additive hypotensive effect). Products include:
Normodyne Injection ... 2108
Normodyne Tablets ... 2110
Normozide Tablets ... 2112
Trandate HCT Tablets ... 579
Trandate Injection ... 577
Trandate Tablets ... 579

Lisinopril (Additive hypotensive effect). Products include:
- Prinivil Tablets ... 1538
- Prinzide Tablets ... 1540
- Zestoretic ... 2274
- Zestril Tablets ... 2277

Mecamylamine Hydrochloride (Additive hypotensive effect). Products include:
- Inversine Tablets ... 1492

Methyclothiazide (Enhances ganglionic blocking effects; additive hypotensive effect). Products include:
- Enduron Tablets ... 517
- Enduronyl ... 518

Methyldopa (Additive hypotensive effect). Products include:
- Aldoclor Tablets ... 1413
- Aldomet Oral ... 1415
- Aldoril Tablets ... 1418

Methyldopate Hydrochloride (Additive hypotensive effect). Products include:
- Aldomet Ester HCl Injection ... 1417

Metocurine Iodide (Prolonged effects of neuromuscular blocking agents). Products include:
- Metubine Iodide Vials ... 1285

Metolazone (Enhances ganglionic blocking effects; additive hypotensive effect). Products include:
- Diulo ... 2129
- Mykrox ½ mg Tablets ... 984
- Zaroxolyn Tablets ... 989

Metoprolol Tartrate (Additive hypotensive effect). Products include:
- Lopressor Ampuls ... 1032
- Lopressor HCT Tablets ... 1034
- Lopressor Tablets ... 1032

Metyrosine (Additive hypotensive effect). Products include:
- Demser Capsules ... 1460

Minoxidil (Additive hypotensive effect). Products include:
- Loniten Tablets ... 2346
- Rogaine Topical Solution ... 2357

Nadolol (Additive hypotensive effect). Products include:
- Corgard Tablets ... 701
- Corzide Tablets ... 702

Nicardipine Hydrochloride (Additive hypotensive effect). Products include:
- Cardene Capsules ... 2290

Nitroglycerin (Additive hypotensive effect). Products include:
- Deponit NTG Transdermal Delivery System ... 2143
- Minitran Transdermal Delivery System ... 1312
- Nitro-Bid Ointment ... 1339
- Nitro-Bid Capsules ... 1338
- Nitrodisc ... 2176
- Nitro-Dur (nitroglycerin) Transdermal Infusion System ... 1164
- Nitrogard Tablets ... 1004
- Nitrolingual Spray ... 1846
- Nitrostat Tablets ... 1743
- Transderm-Nitro Transdermal Therapeutic System ... 2283

Pancuronium Bromide Injection (Prolonged effects of neuromuscular blocking agents).
- No products indexed under this heading.

Penbutolol Sulfate (Additive hypotensive effect). Products include:
- Levatol ... 1832

Phenoxybenzamine Hydrochloride (Additive hypotensive effect). Products include:
- Dibenzyline Capsules ... 2207

Phentolamine Mesylate (Additive hypotensive effect). Products include:
- Regitine ... 878

Pindolol (Additive hypotensive effect). Products include:
- Visken Tablets ... 2036

Polythiazide (Enhances ganglionic blocking effects; additive hypotensive effect). Products include:
- Minizide Capsules ... 1779
- Renese Tablets ... 1785
- Renese-R Tablets ... 1786

Prazosin Hydrochloride (Additive hypotensive effect). Products include:
- Minipress Capsules ... 1778
- Minizide Capsules ... 1779

Procainamide Hydrochloride (Additive hypotensive effect). Products include:
- Procan SR Tablets ... 1760
- Pronestyl Capsules and Tablets ... 1800
- Pronestyl Injection ... 1798
- Pronestyl-SR Tablets ... 1801

Procaine Hydrochloride (Additive hypotensive effect). Products include:
- Novocain Hydrochloride for Spinal Anesthesia ... 2065

Propranolol Hydrochloride (Additive hypotensive effect). Products include:
- Inderal ... 2459
- Inderal LA Long Acting Capsules ... 2461
- Inderide Tablets ... 2463
- Inderide LA Long Acting Capsules ... 2465

Ramipril (Additive hypotensive effect). Products include:
- Altace Capsules ... 1086

Rauwolfia Serpentina (Additive hypotensive effect). Products include:
- Raudixin Tablets ... 1803
- Rauzide Tablets ... 1804

Rescinnamine (Additive hypotensive effect).
- No products indexed under this heading.

Reserpine (Additive hypotensive effect). Products include:
- Diupres Tablets ... 1461
- Hydromox R Tablets ... 1209
- Hydropres Tablets ... 1485
- Renese-R Tablets ... 1786
- Salutensin/Salutensin-Demi ... 719
- Ser-Ap-Es Tablets ... 881
- Serpasil Tablets ... 883
- Serpasil-Apresoline Tablets ... 884
- Serpasil-Esidrix Tablets ... 886

Sodium Nitroprusside (Additive hypotensive effect). Products include:
- Nipride I.V. Infusion ... 1909

Spironolactone (Enhances ganglionic blocking effects). Products include:
- Aldactazide ... 2150
- Aldactone ... 2152

Terazosin Hydrochloride (Additive hypotensive effect). Products include:
- Hytrin Tablets ... 529

Tetracaine Hydrochloride (Additive hypotensive effect). Products include:
- Cetacaine Topical Anesthetic ... 850
- Pontocaine Hydrochloride for Spinal Anesthesia ... 2069

Timolol Maleate (Additive hypotensive effect). Products include:
- Blocadren Tablets ... 1429
- Timolide Tablets ... 1547
- Timoptic in Ocudose ... 1552
- Timoptic Sterile Ophthalmic Solution ... 1550

Triamterene (Enhances ganglionic blocking effects). Products include:
- Dyazide Capsules ... 2208
- Dyrenium Capsules ... 2210
- Maxzide ... 1215

Vecuronium Bromide (Prolonged effects of neuromuscular blocking agents). Products include:
- Norcuron ... 1642

ARISTOCORT SUSPENSION (FORTE PARENTERAL)

(Triamcinolone Diacetate) ... 1008

May interact with:

Immunization (Neurological complications; lack of antibody response).

Smallpox Vaccine (Neurological complications; lack of antibody response).

ARISTOCORT SUSPENSION (INTRALESIONAL)

(Triamcinolone Diacetate) ... 1008

See **Aristocort Suspension (Forte Parenteral)**

ARISTOCORT A TOPICAL CREAM

(Triamcinolone Acetonide) ... 1010

No interactions described in labeling.

ARISTOCORT A TOPICAL OINTMENT

(Triamcinolone Acetonide) ... 1010

No interactions described in labeling.

ARISTOSPAN SUSPENSION (INTRA-ARTICULAR)

(Triamcinolone Hexacetonide) ... 1011

May interact with:

Aspirin (Caution is advised in patient with hypoprothrombinemia). Products include:
- Alka-Seltzer Effervescent Antacid and Pain Reliever ... 1568
- Alka-Seltzer Extra Strength Effervescent Antacid and Pain Reliever ... 1570
- Alka-Seltzer (Flavored) Effervescent Antacid and Pain Reliever ... 1569
- Alka-Seltzer Plus Cold Medicine ... ▣ 623
- Alka-Seltzer Plus Night-Time Cold Medicine ... ▣ 623
- Alka Seltzer Plus Sinus Allergy Medicine ... ▣ 624
- Anacin Coated Analgesic Caplets ... 2417
- Anacin Coated Analgesic Tablets ... 2417
- Anacin Maximum Strength Analgesic Coated Tablets ... 2417
- Maximum Strength Arthritis Pain Formula By the Makers of Anacin Analgesic Tablets and Caplets ... 2418
- Arthritis Pain Formula by the Makers of Anacin Analgesic Tablets and Caplets ... ▣ 747
- Arthritis Strength BC Powder ... ▣ 516
- Ascriptin A/D Caplets ... 1850
- Regular Strength Ascriptin Tablets 1850
- Azdone Tablets ... 844
- BC Powder ... ▣ 517
- BC Cold Powder ... ▣ 517
- Children's Bayer Chewable Aspirin ... ▣ 564
- Genuine Bayer Aspirin Tablets & Caplets ... ▣ 564
- Maximum Bayer Aspirin Tablets & Caplets ... ▣ 566
- Bayer Plus Aspirin Tablets ... ▣ 567
- Therapy Bayer Aspirin Caplets ... ▣ 568
- 8 Hour Bayer Timed-Release Aspirin ... ▣ 566
- Arthritis Strength Bufferin Analgesic Caplets ... 744
- Extra Strength Bufferin Analgesic Tablets ... 745
- Bufferin Analgesic Tablets and Caplets ... 743
- Cama Arthritis Pain Reliever ... ▣ 685
- Damason-P ... 1356
- Easprin ... 1719
- Ecotrin Enteric Coated Aspirin Maximum Strength Tablets and Caplets ... 2189
- Ecotrin Enteric Coated Aspirin Regular Strength Tablets and Caplets ... 2189
- Empirin Aspirin ... ▣ 541
- Empirin with Codeine Phosphate Nos. 2, 3 & 4 ... 764
- Equagesic Tablets ... 2451
- Excedrin Extra-Strength Analgesic Tablets & Caplets ... 749
- 4-Way Cold Tablets ... 750
- Fiorinal Capsules ... 2007
- Fiorinal with Codeine Capsules ... 2008
- Fiorinal Tablets ... 2007
- Lortab ASA Tablets ... 2414
- Momentum Muscular Backache Formula ... ▣ 751
- Norgesic ... 1314
- Norwich Extra-Strength Aspirin ... ▣ 546
- Norwich Regular Strength Aspirin ▣ 547
- P-A-C Analgesic Tablets ... ▣ 669
- Percodan ... 951
- Robaxisal Tablets ... 1872
- Sine-Off Sinus Medicine Tablets-Aspirin Formula ... ▣ 722
- Soma Compound w/Codeine Tablets ... 2390
- Soma Compound Tablets ... 2389
- St. Joseph Adult Chewable Aspirin (81 mg.) ... ▣ 703
- Synalgos-DC Capsules ... 2525
- Talwin Compound ... 2072
- Ursinus Inlay-Tabs ... ▣ 691
- Vanquish Analgesic Caplets ... ▣ 574
- Zorprin Tablets ... 698

Immunization (Neurological complications; lack of antibody response).

Smallpox Vaccine (Neurological complications; lack of antibody response).

ARISTOSPAN SUSPENSION (INTRALESIONAL)

(Triamcinolone Diacetate) ... 1011

See **Aristospan Suspension (Intra-articular)**

ARM & HAMMER PURE BAKING SODA

(Sodium Bicarbonate) ... ▣ 548

No interactions described in labeling.

ARM-A-MED ISOETHARINE INHALATION SOLUTION, USP

(Isoetharine) ... 616

May interact with sympathomimetic aerosol brochodilators. Compounds in this category include:

Albuterol (May cause excessive tachycardia). Products include:
- Proventil Inhalation Aerosol ... 2117
- Ventolin Inhalation Aerosol and Refill ... 583

Albuterol Sulfate (May cause excessive tachycardia). Products include:
- Proventil Repetabs Tablets ... 2120
- Proventil Solutions for Inhalation 0.5% and 0.083% ... 2118
- Proventil Syrup ... 2119
- Proventil Tablets ... 2120
- Ventolin ... 583

Dobutamine Hydrochloride (May cause excessive tachycardia). Products include:
- Dobutrex Solution Vials ... 1259

Dopamine Hydrochloride (May cause excessive tachycardia). Products include:
- Intropin Injection ... 930

Ephedrine Hydrochloride (May cause excessive tachycardia). Products include:
- Amesec ... ▣ 682
- Primatene Tablets-M Formula ... 2421
- Primatene Tablets-P Formula ... 2421
- Primatene Tablets-Regular Formula ... 2421
- Quadrinal Tablets ... 1183
- Quelidrine Syrup ... 556
- Tedral SA ... 1765

Ephedrine Sulfate (May cause excessive tachycardia). Products include:
- Bronkaid Tablets ■ 757
- Bronkolixir ■ 761
- Bronkotabs Tablets ■ 762
- Marax Tablets & DF Syrup 1954
- Pazo Hemorrhoid Ointment & Suppositories 752
- Vicks Vatronol Nose Drops ■ 666

Ephedrine Tannate (May cause excessive tachycardia). Products include:
- Rynatuss 2388

Epinephrine (May cause excessive tachycardia). Products include:
- Ana-Kit Anaphylaxis Emergency Treatment Kit 1100
- Bronkaid Mist ■ 757
- EpiPen 843
- Marcaine Hydrochloride 0.5% with Epinephrine 1:200,000 (as bitartrate) 958
- Marcaine Hydrochloride with Epinephrine 1:200,000 2055
- Primatene Mist 2420
- Sus-Phrine Injection 1006
- Xylocaine with Epinephrine Injections 637

Epinephrine Bitartrate (May cause excessive tachycardia). Products include:
- AsthmaHaler Mist Epinephrine Bitartrate Bronchodilator ■ 616
- Bronkaid Mist Suspension ■ 757
- Primatene Mist Suspension 2421

Epinephrine Hydrochloride (May cause excessive tachycardia). Products include:
- Adrenalin Chloride Solution 1:100 & 1:1,000 1689
- Epifrin ◉ 244
- Glaucon ◉ 218

Isoproterenol Hydrochloride (May cause excessive tachycardia). Products include:
- Isuprel Hydrochloride Injection 1:5000 2050
- Isuprel Hydrochloride Mistometer 2051
- Isuprel Hydrochloride Solution 1:200 & 1:100 2052
- Norisodrine Aerotrol 540

Metaproterenol Sulfate (May cause excessive tachycardia). Products include:
- Alupent 674
- Arm-a-Med Metaproterenol Sulfate Inhalation Solution, USP 617
- Metaprel Inhalation Aerosol Bronchodilator 2014
- Metaprel Inhalation Solution 2015
- Metaprel 2015
- Metaproterenol Sulfate Inhalation Solution, USP 912

Metaraminol Bitartrate (May cause excessive tachycardia). Products include:
- Aramine Injection 1424

Methoxamine Hydrochloride (May cause excessive tachycardia). Products include:
- Vasoxyl Injection 819

Norepinephrine Bitartrate (May cause excessive tachycardia). Products include:
- Levophed Bitartrate Injection 2054

Phenylephrine Bitartrate (May cause excessive tachycardia).
- No products indexed under this heading.

Phenylephrine Hydrochloride (May cause excessive tachycardia). Products include:
- AK-Dilate Solution 2.5% and 10% ◉ 203
- Atrohist Sprinkle Capsules 558
- Cerose-DM 2443
- Codimal 846
- Comhist LA Capsules 1618
- Congespirin For Children Aspirin Free Chewable Cold Tablets 748
- Cyclomydril ◉ 216
- Deconsal Sprinkle Capsules 559
- Dimetane Decongestant ■ 673
- Dristan Decongestant/Antihistamine/Analgesic Coated Caplets ■ 749
- Dristan Cold Nasal Decongestant/Antihistamine/Analgesic Coated Tablets 2419
- Dristan Advanced Formula Decongestant/Antihistamine/Analgesic Tablets ■ 749
- Dristan Nasal Spray, Menthol 2419
- Dristan Nasal Spray, Regular and Regular with Metered Pump 2419
- Entex Capsules 1623
- Entex Liquid 1623
- Sinus Excedrin Analgesic, Decongestant Tablets & Caplets 750
- Extendryl 994
- 4-Way Fast Acting Nasal Spray - Original Formula (regular & mentholated) & Metered Spray Pump (regular) 751
- Hycomine Compound Tablets 929
- Murocoll-2 Sterile Ophthalmic Solution ◉ 261
- Mydfrin 2.5% ◉ 224
- Naldecon Syrup, Tablets, Pediatric Drops and Pediatric Syrup 709
- Neo-Synephrine Hydrochloride 1% Carpuject 2063
- Neo-Synephrine Hydrochloride 1% Injection 2063
- Neo-Synephrine Hydrochloride (Ophthalmic) 2064
- Neo-Synephrine ■ 759
- Nōstril Nasal Decongestant ■ 520
- Novahistine Elixir ■ 596
- Phenergan VC 2500
- Phenergan VC with Codeine 2501
- Prefrin Liquifilm Vasoconstrictor and Lubricant Eye Drops ◉ 254
- Prefrin-A ◉ 255
- Quelidrine Syrup 556
- Relief Vasoconstrictor and Lubricant Eye Drops ◉ 256
- Robitussin Night Relief ■ 677
- Ru-Tuss with Hydrocodone 694
- Ru-Tuss Tablets 693
- Vasosulf ◉ 279
- Vicks Sinex ■ 665
- Zincfrin ◉ 230

Phenylephrine Tannate (May cause excessive tachycardia). Products include:
- Rynatan 2387
- Rynatuss 2388

Phenylpropanolamine Hydrochloride (May cause excessive tachycardia). Products include:
- A.R.M. Allergy Relief Medicine Caplets ■ 615
- Acutrim ■ 548
- Allerest ■ 559
- BC Cold Powder ■ 517
- Cheracol Plus Head Cold/Cough Formula ■ 667
- Codimal Expectorant 846
- Comtrex Multi-Symptom Cold Reliever Tablets/Caplets/Liqui-Gels/Liquid 745
- Contac Continuous Action Decongestant/Antihistamine Capsules ■ 710
- Contac Maximum Strength Continuous Action Decongestant/Antihistamine Caplets ■ 709
- Contac Severe Cold and Flu Formula Caplets ■ 711
- Coricidin 'D' Decongestant Tablets ■ 695
- Coricidin Demilets Tablets for Children ■ 696
- Demazin Nasal Decongestant/Antihistamine Repetabs Tablets & Syrup ■ 697
- Dexatrim ■ 733
- Dimetane-DC Cough Syrup 1857
- Dimetapp Elixir ■ 673
- Dimetapp DM Elixir ■ 674
- Dimetapp Extentabs ■ 674
- Dimetapp Plus Caplets ■ 675
- Dimetapp Tablets ■ 675
- Entex Capsules 1623
- Entex LA Tablets 1623
- Entex Liquid 1623
- 4-Way Cold Tablets 750
- Hycomine Syrup 927
- Naldecon CX Adult Liquid ■ 521
- Naldecon DX Adult Liquid ■ 521
- Naldecon DX Children's Syrup ■ 522
- Naldecon DX Pediatric Drops ■ 522
- Naldecon EX Children's Syrup ■ 522
- Naldecon EX Pediatric Drops ■ 523
- Naldecon Syrup, Tablets, Pediatric Drops and Pediatric Syrup 709
- Nolamine Tablets 838
- Nolex LA Tablets 838
- Ornade Spansule Capsules 2221
- Orthoxicol Cough Syrup ■ 668
- Propagest 839
- Pyrroxate Capsules ■ 669
- Robitussin-CF ■ 676
- Ru-Tuss II Capsules 693
- Ru-Tuss with Hydrocodone 694
- Ru-Tuss Tablets 693
- Sine-Off Sinus Medicine Tablets-Aspirin Formula ■ 722
- Sinulin 840
- St. Joseph Cold Tablets for Children ■ 704
- Tavist-D Tablets 2035
- Triaminic Allergy Tablets ■ 688
- Triaminic Chewables ■ 688
- Triaminic Cold Tablets ■ 688
- Triaminic Expectorant ■ 688
- Triaminic Expectorant w/Codeine 1996
- Triaminic Expectorant DH 1995
- Triaminic Oral Infant Drops 1996
- Triaminic Syrup ■ 689
- Triaminic-12 Tablets ■ 690
- Triaminic-DM Syrup ■ 689
- Triaminicin Tablets ■ 690
- Triaminicol Multi-Symptom Cold Tablets ■ 691
- Triaminicol Multi-Symptom Relief ■ 691
- Tuss-Ornade Liquid 2242
- Tuss-Ornade Spansule Capsules 2242
- Tylenol Cold Medication, Effervescent Tablets 1369

Pirbuterol Acetate (May cause excessive tachycardia). Products include:
- Maxair Inhaler 1311

Pseudoephedrine Hydrochloride (May cause excessive tachycardia). Products include:
- Actifed Capsules ■ 539
- Actifed Plus Caplets ■ 539
- Actifed Plus Tablets ■ 540
- Actifed with Codeine Cough Syrup 752
- Actifed Syrup ■ 540
- Actifed Tablets ■ 540
- Actifed 12-Hour Capsules ■ 539
- Advil Cold & Sinus Caplets (formerly CoAdvil) 2416
- Allerest ■ 559
- Anatuss LA Tablets 1359
- Benadryl Decongestant Elixir ■ 635
- Benadryl Decongestant ■ 635
- Benadryl Plus ■ 636
- Benadryl Plus Nighttime ■ 637
- Benylin Decongestant ■ 638
- Brexin L.A. Capsules 2078
- Bromfed Capsules (Timed Release) 1615
- Bromfed Syrup ■ 628
- Bromfed 1615
- CoAdvil ■ 748
- Allergy-Sinus Comtrex Multi-Symptom Allergy Sinus Formula Tablets & Caplets 746
- Cough Formula Comtrex 746
- Comtrex Multi-Symptom Cold Reliever Tablets/Caplets/Liqui-Gels/Liquid 745
- Day-Night Comtrex 747
- Non-Drowsy Comtrex 747
- Congess 994
- Congestac Caplets ■ 617
- Contac Jr. Children's Cold Medicine ■ 712
- Contac Nighttime Cold Medicine ■ 713
- Contac Sinus Caplets Maximum Strength Non-Drowsy Formula ■ 710
- Contac Sinus Tablets Maximum Strength Non-Drowsy Formula ■ 710
- Deconamine 663
- Deconsal II Tablets 559
- Dimacol Caplets ■ 672
- Dimetane-DX Cough Syrup 1858
- Dorcol Children's Cough Syrup ■ 685
- Dorcol Children's Decongestant Liquid ■ 685
- Dorcol Children's Liquid Cold Formula ■ 686
- Maximum Strength Dristan Decongestant/Analgesic Coated Caplets ■ 750
- No Drowsiness Dristan Cold Nasal Decongestant/Analgesic Coated Caplets 2420
- Dristan Sinus Caplets 2419
- Sinus Excedrin Analgesic, Decongestant Tablets & Caplets ■ 533
- Fedahist Gyrocaps 2145
- Fedahist Timecaps 2145
- Guaifed 1615
- Guaifed Syrup ■ 629
- Isoclor Expectorant 982
- Isoclor Timesule Capsules ■ 561
- Kronofed-A 970
- Medi-Flu Caplet, Liquid ■ 640
- Novafed A Capsules 1342
- Novafed Capsules 1342
- Novahistine DH 1342
- Novahistine DMX ■ 595
- Novahistine Expectorant 1343
- Nucofed Capsules 2219
- Nucofed Expectorant 2219
- Nucofed Pediatric Expectorant 2220
- Nucofed Syrup 2219
- Ornex Caplets ■ 618
- PediaCare Allergy Relief Formula Liquid 1362
- PediaCare Cough-Cold Formula Liquid 1362
- PediaCare Infants' Oral Decongestant Drops 1362
- PediaCare Night Rest Cough-Cold Formula Liquid 1362
- PediaCare 6-12 Cough-Cold Formula Chewable Tablets 1362
- Robitussin-DAC Syrup 1875
- Robitussin-PE ■ 677
- Rondec 1975
- Rondec-DM 1976
- Rondec-TR Tablet 1975
- Ru-Tuss DE Tablets 694
- Ryna ■ 741
- Seldane-D Extended-Release Tablets 1350
- Sinarest ■ 562
- Sine-Aid Maximum Strength Sinus Headache Caplets 1365
- Sine-Aid Maximum Strength Sinus Headache Tablets 1365
- Sine-Off Maximum Strength Allergy/Sinus Formula Caplets ■ 721
- Sine-Off Maximum Strength No Drowsiness Formula Caplets ■ 722
- Singlet Tablets ■ 598
- Sinutab Maximum Strength ■ 641
- Sinutab Maximum Strength Without Drowsiness Tablets & Caplets ■ 642
- Sinutab Regular Strength Without Drowsiness Formula ■ 641
- St. Joseph Nighttime Cold Medicine ■ 705
- Sudafed Children's Liquid ■ 543
- Sudafed Cough Syrup ■ 543
- Sudafed Plus Liquid ■ 544
- Sudafed Plus Tablets ■ 545
- Sudafed Sinus Caplets ■ 545
- Sudafed Sinus Tablets ■ 545
- Sudafed Tablets, 30 mg ■ 544
- Sudafed Tablets, Adult Strength, 60 mg ■ 544
- Sudafed 12 Hour Capsules ■ 545
- TheraFlu Flu and Cold Medicine ■ 687
- Triaminic Nite Light ■ 689
- Tylenol Allergy Sinus Medication Caplets and Gelcaps, Maximum Strength 1372
- Children's Tylenol Cold Liquid Formula and Chewable Tablets 1368
- Tylenol Cold & Flu Hot Medication, Packets 1369
- Tylenol Cold & Flu No Drowsiness Hot Medication, Packets 1371
- Tylenol Cold Medication Caplets and Tablets 1370
- Tylenol Cold Medication No Drowsiness Formula Caplets 1370
- Tylenol Cold Night Time Medication Liquid 1371
- Tylenol Cough Medication Liquid with Decongestant, Maximum Strength 1372
- Tylenol, Maximum Strength, Sinus Medication Gelcaps, Caplets and Tablets 1373
- Ursinus Inlay-Tabs ■ 691
- Vicks Children's NyQuil ■ 664
- Vicks Daycare ■ 660
- Vicks Formula 44D Decongestant Cough Medicine ■ 662
- Vicks Formula 44M Multi-Symptom Cough Medicine ■ 662
- Vicks NyQuil Nighttime Colds Medicine-Original & Cherry Flavor ■ 664

Vicks Pediatric Formula 44 Cough & Congestion Medicine ▣ 663
Vicks Pediatric Formula 44m Multi-Symptom Cough & Cold Medicine ▣ 663

Pseudoephedrine Sulfate (May cause excessive tachycardia). Products include:
Afrin Tablets ▣ 693
Chlor-Trimeton Decongestant ▣ 694
Disophrol Chronotab Sustained-Action Tablets ▣ 698
Drixoral Antihistamine/Nasal Decongestant Syrup ▣ 698
Drixoral Non-Drowsy Formula ▣ 699
Drixoral Plus Extended-Release Tablets ▣ 699
Drixoral Sinus ▣ 700
Drixoral Sustained-Action Tablets ▣ 698
Sinutab Allergy Formula Sustained Action Tablets ▣ 640
Trinalin Repetabs Tablets 1170

Terbutaline Sulfate (May cause excessive tachycardia). Products include:
Brethaire Inhaler 1024
Brethine Ampuls 1026
Brethine Tablets 1026
Bricanyl Injection 1324
Bricanyl Tablets 1325

ARM-A-MED METAPROTERENOL SULFATE INHALATION SOLUTION, USP

(Metaproterenol Sulfate) 617
May interact with sympathomimetic aerosal brochodilators. Compounds in this category include:

Albuterol (Effect not specified). Products include:
Proventil Inhalation Aerosol 2117
Ventolin Inhalation Aerosol and Refill 583

Albuterol Sulfate (Effect not specified). Products include:
Proventil Repetabs Tablets 2120
Proventil Solutions for Inhalation 0.5% and 0.083% 2118
Proventil Syrup 2119
Proventil Tablets 2120
Ventolin 583

Dobutamine Hydrochloride (Effect not specified). Products include:
Dobutrex Solution Vials 1259

Dopamine Hydrochloride (Effect not specified). Products include:
Intropin Injection 930

Ephedrine Hydrochloride (Effect not specified). Products include:
Amesec ▣ 682
Primatene Tablets-M Formula 2421
Primatene Tablets-P Formula 2421
Primatene Tablets-Regular Formula 2421
Quadrinal Tablets 1183
Quelidrine Syrup 556
Tedral SA 1765

Ephedrine Sulfate (Effect not specified). Products include:
Bronkaid Tablets ▣ 757
Bronkolixir ▣ 761
Bronkotabs Tablets ▣ 762
Marax Tablets & DF Syrup 1954
Pazo Hemorrhoid Ointment & Suppositories 752
Vicks Vatronol Nose Drops ▣ 666

Ephedrine Tannate (Effect not specified). Products include:
Rynatuss 2388

Epinephrine (Effect not specified). Products include:
Ana-Kit Anaphylaxis Emergency Treatment Kit 1100
Bronkaid Mist ▣ 757
EpiPen 843
Marcaine Hydrochloride 0.5% with Epinephrine 1:200,000 (as bitartrate) 958
Marcaine Hydrochloride with Epinephrine 1:200,000 2055
Primatene Mist 2420
Sus-Phrine Injection 1006
Xylocaine with Epinephrine Injections 637

Epinephrine Bitartrate (Effect not specified). Products include:
AsthmaHaler Mist Epinephrine Bitartrate Bronchodilator ▣ 616
Bronkaid Mist Suspension ▣ 757
Primatene Mist Suspension 2421

Epinephrine Hydrochloride (Effect not specified). Products include:
Adrenalin Chloride Solution 1:100 & 1:1,000 1689
Epifrin ⊙ 244
Glaucon ⊙ 218

Isoproterenol Hydrochloride (Effect not specified). Products include:
Isuprel Hydrochloride Injection 1:5000 2050
Isuprel Hydrochloride Mistometer 2051
Isuprel Hydrochloride Solution 1:200 & 1:100 2052
Norisodrine Aerotrol 540

Metaraminol Bitartrate (Effect not specified). Products include:
Aramine Injection 1424

Methoxamine Hydrochloride (Effect not specified). Products include:
Vasoxyl Injection 819

Norepinephrine Bitartrate (Effect not specified). Products include:
Levophed Bitartrate Injection 2054

Phenylephrine Bitartrate (Effect not specified).
No products indexed under this heading.

Phenylephrine Hydrochloride (Effect not specified). Products include:
AK-Dilate Solution 2.5% and 10% ⊙ 203
Atrohist Sprinkle Capsules 558
Cerose-DM 2443
Codimal 846
Comhist LA Capsules 1618
Congespirin For Children Aspirin Free Chewable Cold Tablets 748
Cyclomydril ⊙ 216
Deconsal Sprinkle Capsules 559
Dimetane Decongestant ▣ 673
Dristan Decongestant/Antihistamine/Analgesic Coated Caplets ▣ 749
Dristan Cold Nasal Decongestant/Antihistamine/ Analgesic Coated Tablets 2419
Dristan Advanced Formula Decongestant/Antihistamine/ Analgesic Tablets ▣ 749
Dristan Nasal Spray, Menthol 2419
Dristan Nasal Spray, Regular and Regular with Metered Pump 2419
Entex Capsules 1623
Entex Liquid 1623
Sinus Excedrin Analgesic, Decongestant Tablets & Caplets 750
Extendryl 994
4-Way Fast Acting Nasal Spray - Original Formula (regular & mentholated) & Metered Spray Pump (regular) 751
Hycomine Compound Tablets 929
Murocoll-2 Sterile Ophthalmic Solution ⊙ 261
Mydfrin 2.5% ⊙ 224
Naldecon Syrup, Tablets, Pediatric Drops and Pediatric Syrup 709
Neo-Synephrine Hydrochloride 1% Carpuject 2063
Neo-Synephrine Hydrochloride 1% Injection 2063
Neo-Synephrine Hydrochloride (Ophthalmic) 2064
Neo-Synephrine ▣ 759
Nōstril Nasal Decongestant ▣ 520
Novahistine Elixir ▣ 596
Phenergan VC 2500
Phenergan VC with Codeine 2501
Prefrin Liquifilm Vasoconstrictor and Lubricant Eye Drops ⊙ 254
Prefrin-A ⊙ 255
Quelidrine Syrup 556
Relief Vasoconstrictor and Lubricant Eye Drops ⊙ 256
Robitussin Night Relief ▣ 677
Ru-Tuss with Hydrocodone 694
Ru-Tuss Tablets 693
Vasosulf ⊙ 279
Vicks Sinex ▣ 665
Zincfrin ⊙ 230

Phenylephrine Tannate (Effect not specified). Products include:
Rynatan 2387
Rynatuss 2388

Phenylpropanolamine Hydrochloride (Effect not specified). Products include:
A.R.M. Allergy Relief Medicine Caplets ▣ 615
Acutrim ▣ 548
Allerest ▣ 559
BC Cold Powder ▣ 517
Cheracol Plus Head Cold/Cough Formula ▣ 667
Codimal Expectorant 846
Comtrex Multi-Symptom Cold Reliever Tablets/Caplets/Liqui-Gels/Liquid 745
Contac Continuous Action Decongestant/Antihistamine Capsules ▣ 710
Contac Maximum Strength Continuous Action Decongestant/ Antihistamine Caplets ▣ 709
Contac Severe Cold and Flu Formula Caplets ▣ 711
Coricidin 'D' Decongestant Tablets ▣ 695
Coricidin Demilets Tablets for Children ▣ 696
Demazin Nasal Decongestant/ Antihistamine Repetabs Tablets & Syrup ▣ 697
Dexatrim ▣ 733
Dimetane-DC Cough Syrup 1857
Dimetapp Elixir ▣ 673
Dimetapp DM Elixir ▣ 674
Dimetapp Extentabs ▣ 674
Dimetapp Plus Caplets ▣ 675
Dimetapp Tablets ▣ 675
Entex Capsules 1623
Entex LA Tablets 1623
Entex Liquid 1623
4-Way Cold Tablets 750
Hycomine Syrup 927
Naldecon CX Adult Liquid ▣ 521
Naldecon DX Adult Liquid ▣ 521
Naldecon DX Children's Syrup ▣ 522
Naldecon DX Pediatric Drops ▣ 522
Naldecon EX Children's Syrup ▣ 522
Naldecon EX Pediatric Drops ▣ 523
Naldecon Syrup, Tablets, Pediatric Drops and Pediatric Syrup 709
Nolamine Tablets 838
Nolex LA Tablets 838
Ornade Spansule Capsules 2221
Orthoxicol Cough Syrup ▣ 668
Propagest 839
Pyrroxate Capsules ▣ 669
Robitussin-CF ▣ 676
Ru-Tuss II Capsules 693
Ru-Tuss with Hydrocodone 694
Ru-Tuss Tablets 693
Sine-Off Sinus Medicine Tablets-Aspirin Formula ▣ 722
Sinulin 840
St. Joseph Cold Tablets for Children ▣ 704
Tavist-D Tablets 2035
Triaminic Allergy Tablets ▣ 688
Triaminic Chewables ▣ 688
Triaminic Cold Tablets ▣ 688
Triaminic Expectorant ▣ 688
Triaminic Expectorant w/Codeine 1996
Triaminic Expectorant DH 1995
Triaminic Oral Infant Drops 1996
Triaminic Syrup ▣ 689
Triaminic-12 Tablets ▣ 690
Triaminic-DM Syrup ▣ 689
Triaminicin Tablets ▣ 690
Triaminicol Multi-Symptom Cold Tablets ▣ 691
Triaminicol Multi-Symptom Relief ▣ 691
Tuss-Ornade Liquid 2242
Tuss-Ornade Spansule Capsules 2242
Tylenol Cold Medication, Effervescent Tablets 1369

Pirbuterol Acetate (Effect not specified). Products include:
Maxair Inhaler 1311

Pseudoephedrine Hydrochloride (Effect not specified). Products include:
Actifed Capsules ▣ 539
Actifed Plus Caplets ▣ 539
Actifed Plus Tablets ▣ 540
Actifed with Codeine Cough Syrup 752
Actifed Syrup ▣ 540
Actifed Tablets ▣ 540
Actifed 12-Hour Capsules ▣ 539
Advil Cold & Sinus Caplets (formerly CoAdvil) 2416
Allerest ▣ 559
Anatuss LA Tablets 1359
Benadryl Decongestant Elixir ▣ 635
Benadryl Decongestant ▣ 635
Benadryl Plus ▣ 636
Benadryl Plus Nighttime ▣ 637
Benylin Decongestant ▣ 638
Brexin L.A. Capsules 2078
Bromfed Capsules (Timed Release) 1615
Bromfed Syrup ▣ 628
Bromfed 1615
CoAdvil ▣ 748
Allergy-Sinus Comtrex Multi-Symptom Allergy Sinus Formula Tablets & Caplets 746
Cough Formula Comtrex 746
Comtrex Multi-Symptom Cold Reliever Tablets/Caplets/Liqui-Gels/Liquid 745
Day-Night Comtrex 747
Non-Drowsy Comtrex 747
Congess 994
Congestac Caplets ▣ 617
Contac Jr. Children's Cold Medicine ▣ 712
Contac Nighttime Cold Medicine ▣ 713
Contac Sinus Caplets Maximum Strength Non-Drowsy Formula ▣ 710
Contac Sinus Tablets Maximum Strength Non-Drowsy Formula ▣ 710
Deconamine 663
Deconsal II Tablets 559
Dimacol Caplets ▣ 672
Dimetane-DX Cough Syrup 1858
Dorcol Children's Cough Syrup ▣ 685
Dorcol Children's Decongestant Liquid ▣ 685
Dorcol Children's Liquid Cold Formula ▣ 686
Maximum Strength Dristan Decongestant/Analgesic Coated Caplets ▣ 750
No Drowsiness Dristan Cold Nasal Decongestant/Analgesic Coated Caplets 2420
Dristan Sinus Caplets 2419
Sinus Excedrin Analgesic, Decongestant Tablets & Caplets ▣ 533
Fedahist Gyrocaps 2145
Fedahist Timecaps 2145
Guaifed 1615
Guaifed Syrup ▣ 629
Isoclor Expectorant 982
Isoclor Timesule Capsules ▣ 561
Kronofed-A 970
Medi-Flu Caplet, Liquid ▣ 640
Novafed A Capsules 1342
Novafed Capsules 1342
Novahistine DH 1342
Novahistine DMX ▣ 595
Novahistine Expectorant 1343
Nucofed Capsules 2219
Nucofed Expectorant 2219
Nucofed Pediatric Expectorant 2220
Nucofed Syrup 2219
Ornex Caplets ▣ 618
PediaCare Allergy Relief Formula Liquid 1362
PediaCare Cough-Cold Formula Liquid 1362
PediaCare Infants' Oral Decongestant Drops 1362
PediaCare Night Rest Cough-Cold Formula Liquid 1362
PediaCare 6-12 Cough-Cold Formula Chewable Tablets 1362
Robitussin-DAC Syrup 1875
Robitussin-PE ▣ 677
Rondec 1975
Rondec-DM 1976
Rondec-TR Tablet 1975
Ru-Tuss DE Tablets 694
Ryna ▣ 741
Seldane-D Extended-Release Tablets 1350
Sinarest ▣ 562
Sine-Aid Maximum Strength Sinus Headache Caplets 1365
Sine-Aid Maximum Strength Sinus Headache Tablets 1365

Sine-Off Maximum Strength Allergy/Sinus Formula Caplets ...... [ND] 721
Sine-Off Maximum Strength No Drowsiness Formula Caplets........ [ND] 722
Singlet Tablets ...... [ND] 598
Sinutab Maximum Strength...... [ND] 641
Sinutab Maximum Strength Without Drowsiness Tablets & Caplets ...... [ND] 642
Sinutab Regular Strength Without Drowsiness Formula ...... [ND] 641
St. Joseph Nighttime Cold Medicine ...... [ND] 705
Sudafed Children's Liquid ...... [ND] 543
Sudafed Cough Syrup ...... [ND] 543
Sudafed Plus Liquid ...... [ND] 544
Sudafed Plus Tablets ...... [ND] 545
Sudafed Sinus Caplets...... [ND] 545
Sudafed Sinus Tablets...... [ND] 545
Sudafed Tablets, 30 mg...... [ND] 544
Sudafed Tablets, Adult Strength, 60 mg...... [ND] 544
Sudafed 12 Hour Capsules...... [ND] 545
TheraFlu Flu and Cold Medicine .... [ND] 687
Triaminic Nite Light ...... [ND] 689
Tylenol Allergy Sinus Medication Caplets and Gelcaps, Maximum Strength...... 1372
Children's Tylenol Cold Liquid Formula and Chewable Tablets 1368
Tylenol Cold & Flu Hot Medication, Packets 1369
Tylenol Cold & Flu No Drowsiness Hot Medication, Packets...... 1371
Tylenol Cold Medication Caplets and Tablets...... 1370
Tylenol Cold Medication No Drowsiness Formula Caplets 1370
Tylenol Cold Night Time Medication Liquid...... 1371
Tylenol Cough Medication Liquid with Decongestant, Maximum Strength...... 1372
Tylenol, Maximum Strength, Sinus Medication Gelcaps, Caplets and Tablets 1373
Ursinus Inlay-Tabs...... [ND] 691
Vicks Children's NyQuil...... [ND] 664
Vicks Daycare ...... [ND] 660
Vicks Formula 44D Decongestant Cough Medicine ...... [ND] 662
Vicks Formula 44M Multi-Symptom Cough Medicine ...... [ND] 662
Vicks NyQuil Nighttime Colds Medicine-Original & Cherry Flavor ...... [ND] 664
Vicks Pediatric Formula 44 Cough & Congestion Medicine.... [ND] 663
Vicks Pediatric Formula 44m Multi-Symptom Cough & Cold Medicine ...... [ND] 663

Pseudoephedrine Sulfate (Effect not specified). Products include:
Afrin Tablets ...... [ND] 693
Chlor-Trimeton Decongestant ...... [ND] 694
Disophrol Chronotab Sustained-Action Tablets ...... [ND] 698
Drixoral Antihistamine/Nasal Decongestant Syrup ...... [ND] 698
Drixoral Non-Drowsy Formula ...... [ND] 699
Drixoral Plus Extended-Release Tablets ...... [ND] 699
Drixoral Sinus ...... [ND] 700
Drixoral Sustained-Action Tablets [ND] 698
Sinutab Allergy Formula Sustained Action Tablets...... [ND] 640
Trinalin Repetabs Tablets 1170

Terbutaline Sulfate (Effect not specified). Products include:
Brethaire Inhaler 1024
Brethine Ampuls 1026
Brethine Tablets...... 1026
Bricanyl Injection...... 1324
Bricanyl Tablets 1325

ARM-A-VIAL SODIUM CHLORIDE AND STERILE WATER FOR INHALATION
(Sodium Chloride) 618
No interactions described in labeling.

ARTANE ELIXIR
(Trihexyphenidyl Hydrochloride)........1195
May interact with:

Levodopa (The usual dose of each may need to be reduced when used concomitantly). Products include:
Larodopa Tablets...... 1905
Sinemet Tablets 952
Sinemet CR Tablets 953

ARTANE SEQUELS
(Trihexyphenidyl Hydrochloride)........1195
See **Artane Elixir**

ARTANE TABLETS
(Trihexyphenidyl Hydrochloride) 1195
See **Artane Elixir**

MAXIMUM STRENGTH ARTHRITIS PAIN FORMULA BY THE MAKERS OF ANACIN ANALGESIC TABLETS AND CAPLETS
(Aspirin, Aluminum Hydroxide, Magnesium Hydroxide)......2418
No interactions described in labeling.

ARTHRITIS STRENGTH BC POWDER
(Aspirin, Salicylamide, Caffeine)...... [ND] 516
No interactions described in labeling.

ASBRON G ELIXIR
(Theophylline Sodium Glycinate, Guaifenesin) 1997
May interact with sympathomimetic bronchodilators and certain other agents. Compounds in these categories include:

Albuterol (Significant increase in side effects). Products include:
Proventil Inhalation Aerosol 2117
Ventolin Inhalation Aerosol and Refill 583

Albuterol Sulfate (Significant increase in side effects). Products include:
Proventil Repetabs Tablets 2120
Proventil Solutions for Inhalation 0.5% and 0.083%...... 2118
Proventil Syrup...... 2119
Proventil Tablets 2120
Ventolin 583

Bitolterol Mesylate (Significant increase in side effects). Products include:
Tornalate...... 2074

Cimetidine (Increased theophylline blood levels). Products include:
Tagamet Tablets 2228

Clindamycin Hydrochloride (Increased theophylline blood levels). Products include:
Cleocin HCl Capsules...... 2322

Clindamycin Palmitate Hydrochloride (Increased theophylline blood levels). Products include:
Cleocin Pediatric Flavored Granules 2324

Clindamycin Phosphate (Increased theophylline blood levels). Products include:
Cleocin Phosphate Injection 2325
Cleocin T Topical 2327

Ephedrine Hydrochloride (Significant increase in side effects). Products include:
Amesec ...... [ND] 682
Primatene Tablets-M Formula 2421
Primatene Tablets-P Formula...... 2421
Primatene Tablets-Regular Formula 2421
Quadrinal Tablets 1183
Quelidrine Syrup 556
Tedral SA 1765

Ephedrine Sulfate (Significant increase in side effects). Products include:
Bronkaid Tablets ...... [ND] 757
Bronkolixir ...... [ND] 761
Bronkotabs Tablets...... [ND] 762
Marax Tablets & DF Syrup...... 1954
Pazo Hemorrhoid Ointment & Suppositories...... 752
Vicks Vatronol Nose Drops ...... [ND] 666

Ephedrine Tannate (Significant increase in side effects). Products include:
Rynatuss 2388

Epinephrine (Significant increase in side effects). Products include:
Ana-Kit Anaphylaxis Emergency Treatment Kit 1100
Bronkaid Mist ...... [ND] 757
EpiPen 843
Marcaine Hydrochloride 0.5% with Epinephrine 1:200,000 (as bitartrate) 958
Marcaine Hydrochloride with Epinephrine 1:200,000 2055
Primatene Mist...... 2420
Sus-Phrine Injection 1006
Xylocaine with Epinephrine Injections...... 637

Epinephrine Bitartrate (Significant increase in side effects). Products include:
AsthmaHaler Mist Epinephrine Bitartrate Bronchodilator ...... [ND] 616
Bronkaid Mist Suspension ...... [ND] 757
Primatene Mist Suspension...... 2421

Epinephrine Hydrochloride (Significant increase in side effects). Products include:
Adrenalin Chloride Solution 1:100 & 1:1,000 1689
Epifrin...... ◉ 244
Glaucon ...... ◉ 218

Erythromycin (Increased theophylline blood levels). Products include:
A/T/S Topical Gel and Topical Solution 1089
AK-Mycin Ointment...... ◉ 204
Benzamycin Topical Gel 907
E-Mycin Tablets 688
ETS-2% 1685
ERYC...... 1720
Erycette (erythromycin 2%) Topical Solution...... 1678
Ery-Tab Tablets 521
Erythromycin Base Filmtab 525
Erythromycin Delayed-Release Capsules, USP...... 526
Ilotycin Ophthalmic Ointment...... 915
PCE Dispertab Tablets 549
Pediazole...... 1973
T-Stat 2.0% Topical Solution and Pads 2409
Theramycin Z Topical Solution 2% 1410

Erythromycin Estolate (Increased theophylline blood levels). Products include:
Ilosone 913

Erythromycin Ethylsuccinate (Increased theophylline blood levels). Products include:
E.E.S...... 522
EryPed 519
Pediazole...... 1973

Erythromycin Gluceptate (Increased theophylline blood levels). Products include:
Ilotycin Gluceptate, IV, Vials 915

Erythromycin Lactobionate (Increased theophylline blood levels).
No products indexed under this heading.

Erythromycin Stearate (Increased theophylline blood levels). Products include:
Erythrocin Stearate Filmtab 523

Ethylnorepinephrine Hydrochloride (Significant increase in side effects). Products include:
Bronkephrine Injection 2042

Furosemide (Increased diuresis). Products include:
Lasix 1093

Hexamethonium (Decreased hexamethonium-induced chronotropic effect).

Isoetharine (Significant increase in side effects). Products include:
Arm-a-Med Isoetharine Inhalation Solution, USP...... 616
Bronkometer Aerosol...... 2042
Bronkosol Solution 2042

Isoproterenol Hydrochloride (Significant increase in side effects). Products include:
Isuprel Hydrochloride Injection 1:5000 2050
Isuprel Hydrochloride Mistometer .. 2051
Isuprel Hydrochloride Solution 1:200 & 1:100 2052
Norisodrine Aerotrol...... 540

Lincomycin Hydrochloride Monohydrate (Increased theophylline blood levels).
No products indexed under this heading.

Lithium Carbonate (Increased excretion of lithium carbonate). Products include:
Eskalith 2214
Lithane Tablets...... 1596
Lithium Carbonate Capsules & Tablets 1984
Lithobid Tablets 870

Metaproterenol Sulfate (Significant increase in side effects). Products include:
Alupent...... 674
Arm-a-Med Metaproterenol Sulfate Inhalation Solution, USP 617
Metaprel Inhalation Aerosol Bronchodilator 2014
Metaprel Inhalation Solution...... 2015
Metaprel 2015
Metaproterenol Sulfate Inhalation Solution, USP...... 912

Pirbuterol Acetate (Significant increase in side effects). Products include:
Maxair Inhaler 1311

Propranolol Hydrochloride (Antagonsim of propranol effect). Products include:
Inderal 2459
Inderal LA Long Acting Capsules 2461
Inderide Tablets 2463
Inderide LA Long Acting Capsules .. 2465

Reserpine (Reserpine-induced tachycardia). Products include:
Diupres Tablets 1461
Hydromox R Tablets...... 1209
Hydropres Tablets...... 1485
Renese-R Tablets...... 1786
Salutensin/Salutensin-Demi 719
Ser-Ap-Es Tablets 881
Serpasil Tablets 883
Serpasil-Apresoline Tablets...... 884
Serpasil-Esidrix Tablets...... 886

Terbutaline Sulfate (Significant increase in side effects). Products include:
Brethaire Inhaler 1024
Brethine Ampuls 1026
Brethine Tablets...... 1026
Bricanyl Injection...... 1324
Bricanyl Tablets 1325

Troleandomycin (Increased theophylline blood levels). Products include:
Tao Capsules...... 1963

ASBRON G INLAY-TABS
(Theophylline Sodium Glycinate, Guaifenesin) 1997
See **Asbron G Elixir**

ASCRIPTIN A/D CAPLETS
(Aluminum Hydroxide Gel, Dried, Aspirin, Magnesium Hydroxide, Calcium Carbonate)......1850
May interact with oral anticoagulants, tetracyclines, and certain other

([ND] Described in PDR For Nonprescription Drugs) (◉ Described in PDR For Ophthalmology)

agents. Compounds in these categories include:

Antiarthritic Drugs, unspecified (Effect not specified).

Antidiabetic Drugs, unspecified (Effect not specified).

Antigout Drugs, unspecified (Effect not specified).

Demeclocycline Hydrochloride (Do not use concomitantly). Products include:

Declomycin Capsules, Tablets 1199

Dicumarol (Do not use concomitantly). Products include:

Dicumarol Tablets 516

Doxycycline Calcium (Do not use concomitantly).

No products indexed under this heading.

Doxycycline Hyclate (Do not use concomitantly). Products include:

Doryx Capsules 1717
Vibramycin Hyclate Capsules 1787
Vibramycin Hyclate Intravenous 1968
Vibra-Tabs Film Coated Tablets 1787

Doxycycline Monohydrate (Do not use concomitantly). Products include:

Monodox Capsules 1630
Vibramycin Monohydrate for Oral Suspension 1787

Methacycline Hydrochloride (Do not use concomitantly).

No products indexed under this heading.

Minocycline Hydrochloride (Do not use concomitantly). Products include:

Minocin Intravenous 1221
Minocin Oral Suspension 1224
Minocin Pellet-Filled Capsules 1222

Oxytetracycline Hydrochloride (Do not use concomitantly). Products include:

Terra-Cortril Ophthalmic Suspension 1963
Terramycin Capsules 1786
Terramycin Intramuscular Solution 1964
Terramycin with Polymyxin B Sulfate Ophthalmic Ointment 1965

Tetracycline Hydrochloride (Do not use concomitantly). Products include:

Achromycin V Capsules 1193
Achromycin Ophthalmic Ointment 1% .... ⊙ 307
Achromycin Ophthalmic Suspension 1% .... ⊙ 308
Topicycline for Topical Solution 1856

Warfarin Sodium (Do not use concomitantly). Products include:

Coumadin Injection & Tablets 944
Panwarfin Tablets 547

REGULAR STRENGTH ASCRIPTIN TABLETS
(Aluminum Hydroxide Gel, Dried, Aspirin, Magnesium Hydroxide, Calcium Carbonate) 1850
May interact with oral anticoagulants, tetracyclines, and certain other agents. Compounds in these categories include:

Antiarthritic Drugs, unspecified (Effect not specified).

Antidiabetic Drugs, unspecified (Effect not specified).

Antigout Drugs, unspecified (Effect not specified).

Demeclocycline Hydrochloride (Do not use concomitantly). Products include:

Declomycin Capsules, Tablets 1199

Dicumarol (Do not use concomitantly). Products include:

Dicumarol Tablets 516

Doxycycline Calcium (Do not use concomitantly).

No products indexed under this heading.

Doxycycline Hyclate (Do not use concomitantly). Products include:

Doryx Capsules 1717
Vibramycin Hyclate Capsules 1787
Vibramycin Hyclate Intravenous 1968
Vibra-Tabs Film Coated Tablets 1787

Doxycycline Monohydrate (Do not use concomitantly). Products include:

Monodox Capsules 1630
Vibramycin Monohydrate for Oral Suspension 1787

Methacycline Hydrochloride (Do not use concomitantly).

No products indexed under this heading.

Minocycline Hydrochloride (Do not use concomitantly). Products include:

Minocin Intravenous 1221
Minocin Oral Suspension 1224
Minocin Pellet-Filled Capsules 1222

Oxytetracycline Hydrochloride (Do not use concomitantly). Products include:

Terra-Cortril Ophthalmic Suspension 1963
Terramycin Capsules 1786
Terramycin Intramuscular Solution 1964
Terramycin with Polymyxin B Sulfate Ophthalmic Ointment 1965

Tetracycline Hydrochloride (Do not use concomitantly). Products include:

Achromycin V Capsules 1193
Achromycin Ophthalmic Ointment 1% .... ⊙ 307
Achromycin Ophthalmic Suspension 1% .... ⊙ 308
Topicycline for Topical Solution 1856

Warfarin Sodium (Do not use concomitantly). Products include:

Coumadin Injection & Tablets 944
Panwarfin Tablets 547

ASENDIN TABLETS
(Amoxapine) 1196
May interact with monoamine oxidase inhibitors, anticholinergics, barbiturates, central nervous system depressants, and certain other agents. Compounds in these categories include:

Alcohol (Enhanced response to alcohol).

Alfentanil Hydrochloride (Enhanced response to central nervous system depressants). Products include:

Alfenta Injection 1131

Alprazolam (Enhanced response to central nervous system depressants). Products include:

Xanax Tablets 2367

Aprobarbital (Enhanced response to barbiturates and central nervous system depressants). Products include:

Alurate Elixir 1883

Atropine Sulfate (Paralytic ileus). Products include:

Arco-Lase Plus Tablets 607
Atropine Sulfate Sterile Ophthalmic Solution and S.O.P. Sterile Ophthalmic Ointment .... ⊙ 239
Donnagel .... ▣ 675
Donnagel-PG 1858
Donnatal 1858
Donnatal Extentabs 1859
Donnatal Tablets 1858
Donnazyme Tablets 1860
Isopto Atropine .... ⊙ 218
Lomotil 2174
Motofen Tablets 836
Ru-Tuss Tablets 693
Urised Tablets 2396

Belladonna Alkaloids (Paralytic ileus). Products include:

Bellergal-S Tablets 1998
Hyland's Bed Wetting Tablets .... ▣ 728
Hyland's Teething Tablets .... ▣ 728
Kinesed Tablets 2272

Benztropine Mesylate (Paralytic ileus). Products include:

Cogentin 1435

Biperiden (Paralytic ileus). Products include:

Akineton 1171

Buprenorphine (Enhanced response to central nervous system depressants).

No products indexed under this heading.

Buspirone Hydrochloride (Enhanced response to central nervous system depressants). Products include:

BuSpar 1401

Butabarbital (Enhanced response to barbiturates and central nervous system depressants). Products include:

Pyridium Plus 1764

Butalbital (Enhanced response to barbiturates and central nervous system depressants). Products include:

Esgic-Plus Tablets 1002
Esgic Tablets & Capsules 1001
Fioricet Tablets 2006
Fiorinal Capsules 2007
Fiorinal with Codeine Capsules 2008
Fiorinal Tablets 2007
Phrenilin 838
Sedapap Tablets 50 mg/650 mg .. 1360

Chlordiazepoxide (Enhanced response to central nervous system depressants). Products include:

Libritabs Tablets 1930
Limbitrol 1933
Menrium Tablets 1934

Chlordiazepoxide Hydrochloride (Enhanced response to central nervous system depressants). Products include:

Librax Capsules 1929
Librium Capsules 1931
Librium Injectable 1932

Chlorpromazine (Enhanced response to central nervous system depressants). Products include:

Thorazine 2234

Chlorprothixene (Enhanced response to central nervous system depressants). Products include:

Taractan Tablets 1920

Chlorprothixene Hydrochloride (Enhanced response to central nervous system depressants). Products include:

Taractan 1920

Cimetidine (Significant increase in serum levels of several tricyclic antidepressants; not documented with Asendin). Products include:

Tagamet Tablets 2228

Cimetidine Hydrochloride (Significant increase in serum levels of several tricyclic antidepressants; not documented with Asendin). Products include:

Tagamet 2228

Clidinium Bromide (Paralytic ileus; enhanced response to central nervous system depressants). Products include:

Librax Capsules 1929
Quarzan Capsules 1937

Clorazepate Dipotassium (Enhanced response to central nervous system depressants). Products include:

Tranxene 556

Codeine (Enhanced response to central nervous system depressants). Products include:

Calcidrine Syrup 506

Codeine Phosphate (Enhanced response to central nervous system depressants). Products include:

Actifed with Codeine Cough Syrup .. 752
Cheracol Cough Syrup 1853
Codimal PH Syrup 846
Dimetane-DC Cough Syrup 1857
Empirin with Codeine Phosphate Nos. 2, 3 & 4 764
Fiorinal with Codeine Capsules 2008
Isoclor Expectorant 982
Naldecon CX Adult Liquid .... ▣ 521
Novahistine DH 1342
Novahistine Expectorant 1343
Nucofed Capsules 2219
Nucofed Expectorant 2219
Nucofed Pediatric Expectorant 2220
Nucofed Syrup 2219
Phenaphen with Codeine Capsules 1865
Phenaphen-650 with Codeine Tablets 1866
Phenergan with Codeine 2497
Phenergan VC with Codeine 2501
Robitussin A-C Syrup 1875
Robitussin-DAC Syrup 1875
Ryna .... ▣ 741
Soma Compound w/Codeine Tablets 2390
Triaminic Expectorant w/Codeine .. 1996
Tussi-Organidin Liquid 2391
Tylenol with Codeine 1381

Codeine Polistirex (Enhanced response to central nervous system depressants).

No products indexed under this heading.

Dezocine (Enhanced response to central nervous system depressants).

Diazepam (Enhanced response to central nervous system depressants). Products include:

Valium Injectable 1937
Valium Tablets 1939
Valrelease Capsules 1923

Dicyclomine Hydrochloride (Paralytic ileus). Products include:

Bentyl 1322

Droperidol (Enhanced response to central nervous system depressants). Products include:

Inapsine Injection 1140
Innovar Injection 1141

Enflurane (Enhanced response to central nervous system depressants). Products include:

Ethrane 599

Estazolam (Enhanced response to central nervous system depressants). Products include:

ProSom Tablets 554

Ethchlorvynol (Enhanced response to central nervous system depressants). Products include:

Placidyl Capsules 553

Ethinamate (Enhanced response to central nervous system depressants).

No products indexed under this heading.

Ethopropazine Hydrochloride (Paralytic ileus).

Fentanyl (Enhanced response to central nervous system depressants). Products include:

Duragesic Transdermal System 1133

Fentanyl Citrate (Enhanced response to central nervous system depressants). Products include:

Innovar Injection 1141
Sublimaze Injection 1146

Fluphenazine Decanoate (Enhanced response to central nervous system depressants). Products include:

Prolixin Decanoate 1795

(▣ Described in PDR For Nonprescription Drugs)

(⊙ Described in PDR For Ophthalmology)

Fluphenazine Enanthate (Enhanced response to central nervous system depressants). Products include:
- Prolixin Enanthate ... 1796

Fluphenazine Hydrochloride (Enhanced response to central nervous system depressants). Products include:
- Prolixin Elixir ... 1793
- Prolixin Injection ... 1791
- Prolixin Oral Concentrate ... 1792
- Prolixin Tablets ... 1793

Flurazepam Hydrochloride (Enhanced response to central nervous system depressants). Products include:
- Dalmane Capsules ... 1927

Furazolidone (Contraindicated; hyperpyretic crises; severe convulsions; death). Products include:
- Furoxone ... 1855

Glutethimide (Enhanced response to central nervous system depressants).
- No products indexed under this heading.

Glycopyrrolate (Paralytic ileus). Products include:
- Robinul Forte Tablets ... 1873
- Robinul Injectable ... 1873
- Robinul Tablets ... 1873

Haloperidol (Enhanced response to central nervous system depressants). Products include:
- Haldol Injection, Tablets and Concentrate ... 1373

Haloperidol Decanoate (Enhanced response to central nervous system depressants). Products include:
- Haldol Decanoate ... 1375

Hydrocodone Bitartrate (Enhanced response to central nervous system depressants). Products include:
- Anexsia 5/500 Tablets ... 2196
- Anexsia 7.5/650 Tablets ... 2197
- Azdone Tablets ... 844
- Codiclear DH Syrup ... 845
- Codimal DH Syrup ... 846
- Damason-P ... 1356
- Hycodan Syrup, Tablets ... 927
- Hycomine Compound Tablets ... 929
- Hycomine Syrup ... 927
- Hycotuss Expectorant Syrup ... 930
- Hydrocet Capsules ... 835
- Lortab ASA Tablets ... 2414
- Lortab ... 2412
- Ru-Tuss with Hydrocodone ... 694
- Triaminic Expectorant DH ... 1995
- Vicodin Tablets ... 1187
- Vicodin ES Tablets ... 1189
- Zydone Capsules ... 941

Hydrocodone Polistirex (Enhanced response to central nervous system depressants). Products include:
- Tussionex Extended-Release Suspension ... 988

Hydroxyzine Hydrochloride (Enhanced response to central nervous system depressants). Products include:
- Atarax Tablets & Syrup ... 1941
- Marax Tablets & DF Syrup ... 1954
- Vistaril Intramuscular Solution ... 1970

Hyoscyamine (Paralytic ileus). Products include:
- Cystospaz Tablets ... 2395
- Urised Tablets ... 2396

Hyoscyamine Sulfate (Paralytic ileus). Products include:
- Arco-Lase Plus Tablets ... 607
- Cystospaz-M Capsules ... 2395
- Donnagel ... ▣ 675
- Donnagel-PG ... 1858
- Donnatal ... 1858
- Donnatal Extentabs ... 1859
- Donnatal Tablets ... 1858
- Donnazyme Tablets ... 1860
- Kutrase Capsules ... 2146
- Levsin/Levsinex ... 2147
- Ru-Tuss Tablets ... 693

Ipratropium Bromide (Paralytic ileus). Products include:
- Atrovent Inhalation Aerosol ... 675

Isocarboxazid (Contraindicated; hyperpyretic crises; severe convulsions; death). Products include:
- Marplan Tablets ... 1906

Isoflurane (Enhanced response to central nervous system depressants). Products include:
- Forane ... 600

Ketamine Hydrochloride (Enhanced response to central nervous system depressants). Products include:
- Ketalar ... 1726

Levorphanol Tartrate (Enhanced response to central nervous system depressants). Products include:
- Levo-Dromoran ... 1906

Lorazepam (Enhanced response to central nervous system depressants). Products include:
- Ativan Injection ... 2432
- Ativan Tablets ... 2434

Loxapine Hydrochloride (Enhanced response to central nervous system depressants). Products include:
- Loxitane ... 1213

Loxapine Succinate (Enhanced response to central nervous system depressants). Products include:
- Loxitane Capsules ... 1213

Mepenzolate Bromide (Paralytic ileus). Products include:
- Cantil Tablets ... 1326

Meperidine Hydrochloride (Enhanced response to central nervous system depressants). Products include:
- Demerol ... 2047
- Mepergan Injection ... 2479

Mephobarbital (Enhanced response to barbiturates and central nervous system depressants). Products include:
- Mebaral Tablets ... 2061

Meprobamate (Enhanced response to central nervous system depressants). Products include:
- Deprol Tablets ... 2382
- Equagesic Tablets ... 2451
- Miltown Tablets ... 2386
- PMB 200 and PMB 400 ... 2504

Mesoridazine (Enhanced response to central nervous system depressants). Products include:
- Serentil ... 686

Methadone Hydrochloride (Enhanced response to central nervous system depressants). Products include:
- Dolophine Hydrochloride Ampoules & Vials ... 1260
- Dolophine Hydrochloride Tablets ... 1261
- Methadone Hydrochloride Diskets ... 1284
- Methadone Hydrochloride Oral Solution & Tablets ... 1987

Methohexital Sodium (Enhanced response to central nervous system depressants). Products include:
- Brevital Sodium Vials ... 1248

Methoxyflurane (Enhanced response to central nervous system depressants).
- No products indexed under this heading.

Midazolam Hydrochloride (Enhanced response to central nervous system depressants). Products include:
- Versed Injection ... 1924

Molindone Hydrochloride (Enhanced response to central nervous system depressants). Products include:
- Moban Tablets & Concentrate ... 932

Morphine Sulfate (Enhanced response to central nervous system depressants). Products include:
- Astramorph/PF Injection, USP (Preservative-Free) ... 618
- Duramorph ... 960
- Infumorph 200 and Infumorph 500 Sterile Solutions ... 962
- MS Contin Tablets ... 1814
- MSIR ... 1817
- Oramorph SR (Morphine Sulfate Sustained Release Tablets) ... 1988
- Roxanol ... 1991

Opium Alkaloids (Enhanced response to central nervous system depressants). Products include:
- B & O No. 15A & No. 16A Supprettes ... 2395
- Pantopon Injectable ... 1911

Oxazepam (Enhanced response to central nervous system depressants). Products include:
- Serax Capsules ... 2522
- Serax Tablets ... 2522

Oxybutynin Chloride (Paralytic ileus). Products include:
- Ditropan ... 1332

Oxycodone Hydrochloride (Enhanced response to central nervous system depressants). Products include:
- Percocet Tablets ... 950
- Percodan ... 951
- Roxicodone Tablets, Oral Solution & Intensol (Oxycodone) ... 1992
- Tylox Capsules ... 1382

Oxyphenonium Bromide (Paralytic ileus).

Pentobarbital Sodium (Enhanced response to barbiturates and central nervous system depressants). Products include:
- Nembutal Sodium Capsules ... 534
- Nembutal Sodium Solution ... 536
- Nembutal Sodium Suppositories ... 538

Perphenazine (Enhanced response to central nervous system depressants). Products include:
- Etrafon ... 2087
- Triavil Tablets ... 1556
- Trilafon ... 2123

Phenelzine Sulfate (Contraindicated; hyperpyretic crises; severe convulsions; death). Products include:
- Nardil ... 1742

Phenobarbital (Enhanced response to barbiturates and central nervous system depressants). Products include:
- Arco-Lase Plus Tablets ... 607
- Bellergal-S Tablets ... 1998
- Bronkolixir ... ▣ 761
- Bronkotabs Tablets ... ▣ 762
- Donnatal ... 1858
- Donnatal Extentabs ... 1859
- Donnatal Tablets ... 1858
- Donnazyme Tablets ... 1860
- Kinesed Tablets ... 2272
- Phenobarbital Elixir and Tablets ... 1293
- Primatene Tablets-P Formula ... 2421
- Quadrinal Tablets ... 1183
- Tedral SA ... 1765

Prazepam (Enhanced response to central nervous system depressants). Products include:
- Centrax ... 1693

Prochlorperazine (Enhanced response to central nervous system depressants). Products include:
- Compazine ... 2201

Procyclidine Hydrochloride (Paralytic ileus). Products include:
- Kemadrin Tablets ... 771

Promethazine Hydrochloride (Enhanced response to central nervous system depressants). Products include:
- Mepergan Injection ... 2479
- Phenergan with Codeine ... 2497
- Phenergan with Dextromethorphan ... 2499
- Phenergan Injection ... 2493
- Phenergan Suppositories ... 2496
- Phenergan Syrup ... 2495
- Phenergan Tablets ... 2496
- Phenergan VC ... 2500
- Phenergan VC with Codeine ... 2501

Propantheline Bromide (Paralytic ileus). Products include:
- Pro-Banthine Tablets ... 2141

Propofol (Enhanced response to central nervous system depressants). Products include:
- Diprivan Injection ... 2267

Propoxyphene Hydrochloride (Enhanced response to central nervous system depressants). Products include:
- Darvon ... 1256
- Wygesic Tablets ... 2540

Propoxyphene Napsylate (Enhanced response to central nervous system depressants). Products include:
- Darvon-N/Darvocet-N ... 1254

Quazepam (Enhanced response to central nervous system depressants). Products include:
- Doral Tablets ... 2383

Scopolamine Hydrobromide (Paralytic ileus). Products include:
- Donnagel ... ▣ 675
- Donnagel-PG ... 1858
- Donnatal ... 1858
- Donnatal Extentabs ... 1859
- Donnatal Tablets ... 1858
- Donnazyme Tablets ... 1860
- Isopto Hyoscine ... ⊙ 222
- Murocoll-2 Sterile Ophthalmic Solution ... ⊙ 261
- Ru-Tuss Tablets ... 693

Scopolamine Preparations (Paralytic ileus). Products include:
- Transderm Scōp Transdermal Therapeutic System ... 887

Secobarbital Sodium (Enhanced response to barbiturates and central nervous system depressants). Products include:
- Seconal Sodium Pulvules ... 1296

Selegiline Hydrochloride (Contraindicated; hyperpyretic crises; severe convulsions; death). Products include:
- Eldepryl ... 2250

Sufentanil Citrate (Enhanced response to central nervous system depressants). Products include:
- Sufenta Injection ... 1147

Temazepam (Enhanced response to central nervous system depressants). Products include:
- Restoril Capsules ... 2023

Thiamylal Sodium (Enhanced response to barbiturates and central nervous system depressants). Products include:
- Surital Ampoules, Steri-Vials ... 1764

Thioridazine Hydrochloride (Enhanced response to central nervous system depressants). Products include:
- Mellaril ... 2011

Thiothixene (Enhanced response to central nervous system depressants). Products include:
- Navane Capsules and Concentrate ... 1954
- Navane Intramuscular ... 1956

Tranylcypromine Sulfate (Contraindicated; hyperpyretic crises; severe convulsions; death). Products include:
- Parnate Tablets ... 2222

(▣ Described in PDR For Nonprescription Drugs)

(⊙ Described in PDR For Ophthalmology)

Triazolam (Enhanced response to central nervous system depressants). Products include:
- Halcion Tablets ... 2340

Tridihexethyl Chloride (Paralytic ileus).
- No products indexed under this heading.

Trifluoperazine Hydrochloride (Enhanced response to central nervous system depressants). Products include:
- Stelazine ... 2226

Trihexyphenidyl Hydrochloride (Paralytic ileus). Products include:
- Artane ... 1195

ASPERCREME CREME & LOTION ANALGESIC RUB
(Trolamine Salicylate) ... ▣ 732
No interactions described in labeling.

ASTHMAHALER MIST EPINEPHRINE BITARTRATE BRONCHODILATOR
(Epinephrine Bitartrate) ... ▣ 616
May interact with antihypertensives and antidepressant drugs. Compounds in these categories include:

Acebutolol Hydrochloride (Concurrent use not recommended). Products include:
- Sectral Capsules ... 2520

Amitriptyline Hydrochloride (Concurrent use not recommended). Products include:
- Elavil ... 2269
- Endep Tablets ... 1927
- Etrafon ... 2087
- Limbitrol ... 1933
- Triavil Tablets ... 1556

Amoxapine (Concurrent use not recommended). Products include:
- Asendin Tablets ... 1196

Atenolol (Concurrent use not recommended). Products include:
- Tenoretic Tablets ... 1105
- Tenormin Tablets and I.V. Injection 1107

Benazepril Hydrochloride (Concurrent use not recommended). Products include:
- Lotensin Tablets ... 872

Betaxolol Hydrochloride (Concurrent use not recommended). Products include:
- Betoptic Sterile Ophthalmic Solution ... 569
- Betoptic S Sterile Ophthalmic Suspension ... 570
- Kerlone Tablets ... 2172

Bupropion Hydrochloride (Concurrent use not recommended). Products include:
- Wellbutrin Tablets ... 821

Captopril (Concurrent use not recommended). Products include:
- Capoten ... 2255
- Capozide ... 2258

Carteolol Hydrochloride (Concurrent use not recommended). Products include:
- Cartrol Tablets ... 507

Clonidine (Concurrent use not recommended). Products include:
- Catapres-TTS ... 677

Clonidine Hydrochloride (Concurrent use not recommended). Products include:
- Catapres Tablets ... 676
- Combipres Tablets ... 678

Deserpidine (Concurrent use not recommended). Products include:
- Enduronyl ... 518
- Harmonyl Tablets ... 528
- Oreticyl ... 545

Desipramine Hydrochloride (Concurrent use not recommended). Products include:
- Norpramin Tablets ... 1340

Diazoxide (Concurrent use not recommended). Products include:
- Hyperstat I.V. Injection ... 2095
- Proglycem ... 649

Doxazosin Mesylate (Concurrent use not recommended). Products include:
- Cardura Tablets ... 1941

Doxepin Hydrochloride (Concurrent use not recommended). Products include:
- Sinequan ... 1960

Enalapril Maleate (Concurrent use not recommended). Products include:
- Vaseretic Tablets ... 1559
- Vasotec Tablets ... 1564

Enalaprilat (Concurrent use not recommended). Products include:
- Vasotec I.V. ... 1562

Esmolol Hydrochloride (Concurrent use not recommended). Products include:
- Brevibloc Injection ... 942

Felodipine (Concurrent use not recommended). Products include:
- Plendil Extended-Release Tablets ... 1526

Fluoxetine Hydrochloride (Concurrent use not recommended). Products include:
- Prozac Pulvules ... 920

Fosinopril Sodium (Concurrent use not recommended). Products include:
- Monopril Tablets ... 1406

Guanabenz Acetate (Concurrent use not recommended). Products include:
- Wytensin Tablets ... 2542

Guanethidine Monosulfate (Concurrent use not recommended). Products include:
- Esimil Tablets ... 864
- Ismelin Tablets ... 869

Hydralazine Hydrochloride (Concurrent use not recommended). Products include:
- Apresazide Capsules ... 854
- Apresoline Hydrochloride Parenteral (Ampuls) ... 856
- Apresoline Hydrochloride Tablets ... 855
- Apresoline-Esidrix Tablets ... 857
- Ser-Ap-Es Tablets ... 881
- Serpasil-Apresoline Tablets ... 884

Imipramine Hydrochloride (Concurrent use not recommended). Products include:
- Tofranil Ampuls ... 1038
- Tofranil Tablets ... 1039

Imipramine Pamoate (Concurrent use not recommended). Products include:
- Tofranil-PM Capsules ... 1041

Indapamide (Concurrent use not recommended). Products include:
- Lozol Tablets ... 1843

Isocarboxazid (Concurrent use not recommended). Products include:
- Marplan Tablets ... 1906

Isradipine (Concurrent use not recommended). Products include:
- DynaCirc Capsules ... 2004

Labetalol Hydrochloride (Concurrent use not recommended). Products include:
- Normodyne Injection ... 2108
- Normodyne Tablets ... 2110
- Normozide Tablets ... 2112
- Trandate HCT Tablets ... 579
- Trandate Injection ... 577
- Trandate Tablets ... 579

Lisinopril (Concurrent use not recommended). Products include:
- Prinivil Tablets ... 1538
- Prinzide Tablets ... 1540
- Zestoretic ... 2274
- Zestril Tablets ... 2277

Maprotiline Hydrochloride (Concurrent use not recommended). Products include:
- Ludiomil Tablets ... 874

Mecamylamine Hydrochloride (Concurrent use not recommended). Products include:
- Inversine Tablets ... 1492

Methyldopa (Concurrent use not recommended). Products include:
- Aldoclor Tablets ... 1413
- Aldomet Oral ... 1415
- Aldoril Tablets ... 1418

Methyldopate Hydrochloride (Concurrent use not recommended). Products include:
- Aldomet Ester HCl Injection ... 1417

Metoprolol Tartrate (Concurrent use not recommended). Products include:
- Lopressor Ampuls ... 1032
- Lopressor HCT Tablets ... 1034
- Lopressor Tablets ... 1032

Metyrosine (Concurrent use not recommended). Products include:
- Demser Capsules ... 1460

Minoxidil (Concurrent use not recommended). Products include:
- Loniten Tablets ... 2346
- Rogaine Topical Solution ... 2357

Nadolol (Concurrent use not recommended). Products include:
- Corgard Tablets ... 701
- Corzide Tablets ... 702

Nicardipine Hydrochloride (Concurrent use not recommended). Products include:
- Cardene Capsules ... 2290

Nitroglycerin (Concurrent use not recommended). Products include:
- Deponit NTG Transdermal Delivery System ... 2143
- Minitran Transdermal Delivery System ... 1312
- Nitro-Bid Ointment ... 1339
- Nitro-Bid Capsules ... 1338
- Nitrodisc ... 2176
- Nitro-Dur (nitroglycerin) Transdermal Infusion System ... 1164
- Nitrogard Tablets ... 1004
- Nitrolingual Spray ... 1846
- Nitrostat Tablets ... 1743
- Transderm-Nitro Transdermal Therapeutic System ... 2283

Nortriptyline Hydrochloride (Concurrent use not recommended). Products include:
- Pamelor ... 2019

Penbutolol Sulfate (Concurrent use not recommended). Products include:
- Levatol ... 1832

Phenelzine Sulfate (Concurrent use not recommended). Products include:
- Nardil ... 1742

Phenoxybenzamine Hydrochloride (Concurrent use not recommended). Products include:
- Dibenzyline Capsules ... 2207

Phentolamine Mesylate (Concurrent use not recommended). Products include:
- Regitine ... 878

Pindolol (Concurrent use not recommended). Products include:
- Visken Tablets ... 2036

Prazosin Hydrochloride (Concurrent use not recommended). Products include:
- Minipress Capsules ... 1778
- Minizide Capsules ... 1779

Propranolol Hydrochloride (Concurrent use not recommended). Products include:
- Inderal ... 2459
- Inderal LA Long Acting Capsules ... 2461
- Inderide Tablets ... 2463
- Inderide LA Long Acting Capsules ... 2465

Protriptyline Hydrochloride (Concurrent use not recommended). Products include:
- Vivactil Tablets ... 1567

Ramipril (Concurrent use not recommended). Products include:
- Altace Capsules ... 1086

Rauwolfia Serpentina (Concurrent use not recommended). Products include:
- Raudixin Tablets ... 1803
- Rauzide Tablets ... 1804

Rescinnamine (Concurrent use not recommended).
- No products indexed under this heading.

Reserpine (Concurrent use not recommended). Products include:
- Diupres Tablets ... 1461
- Hydromox R Tablets ... 1209
- Hydropres Tablets ... 1485
- Renese-R Tablets ... 1786
- Salutensin/Salutensin-Demi ... 719
- Ser-Ap-Es Tablets ... 881
- Serpasil Tablets ... 883
- Serpasil-Apresoline Tablets ... 884
- Serpasil-Esidrix Tablets ... 886

Sodium Nitroprusside (Concurrent use not recommended). Products include:
- Nipride I.V. Infusion ... 1909

Terazosin Hydrochloride (Concurrent use not recommended). Products include:
- Hytrin Tablets ... 529

Timolol Maleate (Concurrent use not recommended). Products include:
- Blocadren Tablets ... 1429
- Timolide Tablets ... 1547
- Timoptic in Ocudose ... 1552
- Timoptic Sterile Ophthalmic Solution ... 1550

Tranylcypromine Sulfate (Concurrent use not recommended). Products include:
- Parnate Tablets ... 2222

Trazodone Hydrochloride (Concurrent use not recommended). Products include:
- Desyrel and Desyrel Dividose ... 1404

Trimethaphan Camsylate (Concurrent use not recommended). Products include:
- Arfonad Ampuls ... 1887

Trimipramine Maleate (Concurrent use not recommended). Products include:
- Surmontil Capsules ... 2524

ASTHMANEFRIN SOLUTION "A" BRONCHODILATOR
(Racepinephrine Hydrochloride) ... ▣ 616
May interact with antihypertensives and antidepressant drugs. Compounds in these categories include:

Acebutolol Hydrochloride (Concurrent use not recommended). Products include:
- Sectral Capsules ... 2520

Amitriptyline Hydrochloride (Concurrent use not recommended). Products include:
- Elavil ... 2269
- Endep Tablets ... 1927
- Etrafon ... 2087
- Limbitrol ... 1933
- Triavil Tablets ... 1556

Amoxapine (Concurrent use not recommended). Products include:
- Asendin Tablets ... 1196

Atenolol (Concurrent use not recommended). Products include:
- Tenoretic Tablets ... 1105
- Tenormin Tablets and I.V. Injection 1107

Benazepril Hydrochloride (Concurrent use not recommended). Products include:
- Lotensin Tablets ... 872

Betaxolol Hydrochloride (Concurrent use not recommended). Products include:
- Betoptic Sterile Ophthalmic Solution ... 569
- Betoptic S Sterile Ophthalmic Suspension ... 570
- Kerlone Tablets ... 2172

Bupropion Hydrochloride (Concurrent use not recommended). Products include:
- Wellbutrin Tablets ... 821

Captopril (Concurrent use not recommended). Products include:
- Capoten ... 2255
- Capozide ... 2258

Carteolol Hydrochloride (Concurrent use not recommended). Products include:
- Cartrol Tablets ... 507

Clonidine (Concurrent use not recommended). Products include:
- Catapres-TTS ... 677

Clonidine Hydrochloride (Concurrent use not recommended). Products include:
- Catapres Tablets ... 676
- Combipres Tablets ... 678

Deserpidine (Concurrent use not recommended). Products include:
- Enduronyl ... 518
- Harmonyl Tablets ... 528
- Oreticyl ... 545

Desipramine Hydrochloride (Concurrent use not recommended). Products include:
- Norpramin Tablets ... 1340

Diazoxide (Concurrent use not recommended). Products include:
- Hyperstat I.V. Injection ... 2095
- Proglycem ... 649

Doxazosin Mesylate (Concurrent use not recommended). Products include:
- Cardura Tablets ... 1941

Doxepin Hydrochloride (Concurrent use not recommended). Products include:
- Sinequan ... 1960

Enalapril Maleate (Concurrent use not recommended). Products include:
- Vaseretic Tablets ... 1559
- Vasotec Tablets ... 1564

Enalaprilat (Concurrent use not recommended). Products include:
- Vasotec I.V. ... 1562

Esmolol Hydrochloride (Concurrent use not recommended). Products include:
- Brevibloc Injection ... 942

Felodipine (Concurrent use not recommended). Products include:
- Plendil Extended-Release Tablets ... 1526

Fluoxetine Hydrochloride (Concurrent use not recommended). Products include:
- Prozac Pulvules ... 920

Fosinopril Sodium (Concurrent use not recommended). Products include:
- Monopril Tablets ... 1406

Guanabenz Acetate (Concurrent use not recommended). Products include:
- Wytensin Tablets ... 2542

Guanethidine Monosulfate (Concurrent use not recommended). Products include:
- Esimil Tablets ... 864
- Ismelin Tablets ... 869

Hydralazine Hydrochloride (Concurrent use not recommended). Products include:
- Apresazide Capsules ... 854
- Apresoline Hydrochloride Parenteral (Ampuls) ... 856
- Apresoline Hydrochloride Tablets ... 855
- Apresoline-Esidrix Tablets ... 857
- Ser-Ap-Es Tablets ... 881
- Serpasil-Apresoline Tablets ... 884

Imipramine Hydrochloride (Concurrent use not recommended). Products include:
- Tofranil Ampuls ... 1038
- Tofranil Tablets ... 1039

Imipramine Pamoate (Concurrent use not recommended). Products include:
- Tofranil-PM Capsules ... 1041

Indapamide (Concurrent use not recommended). Products include:
- Lozol Tablets ... 1843

Isocarboxazid (Concurrent use not recommended). Products include:
- Marplan Tablets ... 1906

Isradipine (Concurrent use not recommended). Products include:
- DynaCirc Capsules ... 2004

Labetalol Hydrochloride (Concurrent use not recommended). Products include:
- Normodyne Injection ... 2108
- Normodyne Tablets ... 2110
- Normozide Tablets ... 2112
- Trandate HCT Tablets ... 579
- Trandate Injection ... 577
- Trandate Tablets ... 579

Lisinopril (Concurrent use not recommended). Products include:
- Prinivil Tablets ... 1538
- Prinzide Tablets ... 1540
- Zestoretic ... 2274
- Zestril Tablets ... 2277

Maprotiline Hydrochloride (Concurrent use not recommended). Products include:
- Ludiomil Tablets ... 874

Mecamylamine Hydrochloride (Concurrent use not recommended). Products include:
- Inversine Tablets ... 1492

Methyldopa (Concurrent use not recommended). Products include:
- Aldoclor Tablets ... 1413
- Aldomet Oral ... 1415
- Aldoril Tablets ... 1418

Methyldopate Hydrochloride (Concurrent use not recommended). Products include:
- Aldomet Ester HCl Injection ... 1417

Metoprolol Tartrate (Concurrent use not recommended). Products include:
- Lopressor Ampuls ... 1032
- Lopressor HCT Tablets ... 1034
- Lopressor Tablets ... 1032

Metyrosine (Concurrent use not recommended). Products include:
- Demser Capsules ... 1460

Minoxidil (Concurrent use not recommended). Products include:
- Loniten Tablets ... 2346
- Rogaine Topical Solution ... 2357

Nadolol (Concurrent use not recommended). Products include:
- Corgard Tablets ... 701
- Corzide Tablets ... 702

Nicardipine Hydrochloride (Concurrent use not recommended). Products include:
- Cardene Capsules ... 2290

Nitroglycerin (Concurrent use not recommended). Products include:
- Deponit NTG Transdermal Delivery System ... 2143
- Minitran Transdermal Delivery System ... 1312
- Nitro-Bid Ointment ... 1339
- Nitro-Bid Capsules ... 1338
- Nitrodisc ... 2176
- Nitro-Dur (nitroglycerin) Transdermal Infusion System ... 1164
- Nitrogard Tablets ... 1004
- Nitrolingual Spray ... 1846
- Nitrostat Tablets ... 1743
- Transderm-Nitro Transdermal Therapeutic System ... 2283

Nortriptyline Hydrochloride (Concurrent use not recommended). Products include:
- Pamelor ... 2019

Penbutolol Sulfate (Concurrent use not recommended). Products include:
- Levatol ... 1832

Phenelzine Sulfate (Concurrent use not recommended). Products include:
- Nardil ... 1742

Phenoxybenzamine Hydrochloride (Concurrent use not recommended). Products include:
- Dibenzyline Capsules ... 2207

Phentolamine Mesylate (Concurrent use not recommended). Products include:
- Regitine ... 878

Pindolol (Concurrent use not recommended). Products include:
- Visken Tablets ... 2036

Prazosin Hydrochloride (Concurrent use not recommended). Products include:
- Minipress Capsules ... 1778
- Minizide Capsules ... 1779

Propranolol Hydrochloride (Concurrent use not recommended). Products include:
- Inderal ... 2459
- Inderal LA Long Acting Capsules ... 2461
- Inderide Tablets ... 2463
- Inderide LA Long Acting Capsules ... 2465

Protriptyline Hydrochloride (Concurrent use not recommended). Products include:
- Vivactil Tablets ... 1567

Ramipril (Concurrent use not recommended). Products include:
- Altace Capsules ... 1086

Rauwolfia Serpentina (Concurrent use not recommended). Products include:
- Raudixin Tablets ... 1803
- Rauzide Tablets ... 1804

Rescinnamine (Concurrent use not recommended).
- No products indexed under this heading.

Reserpine (Concurrent use not recommended). Products include:
- Diupres Tablets ... 1461
- Hydromox R Tablets ... 1209
- Hydropres Tablets ... 1485
- Renese-R Tablets ... 1786
- Salutensin/Salutensin-Demi ... 719
- Ser-Ap-Es Tablets ... 881
- Serpasil Tablets ... 883
- Serpasil-Apresoline Tablets ... 884
- Serpasil-Esidrix Tablets ... 886

Sodium Nitroprusside (Concurrent use not recommended). Products include:
- Nipride I.V. Infusion ... 1909

Terazosin Hydrochloride (Concurrent use not recommended). Products include:
- Hytrin Tablets ... 529

Timolol Maleate (Concurrent use not recommended). Products include:
- Blocadren Tablets ... 1429
- Timolide Tablets ... 1547
- Timoptic in Ocudose ... 1552
- Timoptic Sterile Ophthalmic Solution ... 1550

Tranylcypromine Sulfate (Concurrent use not recommended). Products include:
- Parnate Tablets ... 2222

Trazodone Hydrochloride (Concurrent use not recommended). Products include:
- Desyrel and Desyrel Dividose ... 1404

Trimethaphan Camsylate (Concurrent use not recommended). Products include:
- Arfonad Ampuls ... 1887

Trimipramine Maleate (Concurrent use not recommended). Products include:
- Surmontil Capsules ... 2524

ASTRAMORPH/PF INJECTION, USP (PRESERVATIVE-FREE) (Morphine Sulfate) ... 618

May interact with central nervous system depressants, psychotropics, antihistamines, neuromuscular blocking agents, and certain other agents. Compounds in these categories include:

Alcohol (Potentiation of depressant effects of morphine).

Alfentanil Hydrochloride (Potentiation of depressant effects of morphine). Products include:
- Alfenta Injection ... 1131

Alprazolam (Potentiation of depressant effects of morphine). Products include:
- Xanax Tablets ... 2367

Amitriptyline Hydrochloride (Potentiation of depressant effects of morphine). Products include:
- Elavil ... 2269
- Endep Tablets ... 1927
- Etrafon ... 2087
- Limbitrol ... 1933
- Triavil Tablets ... 1556

Amoxapine (Potentiation of depressant effects of morphine). Products include:
- Asendin Tablets ... 1196

Aprobarbital (Potentiation of depressant effects of morphine). Products include:
- Alurate Elixir ... 1883

Astemizole (Potentiation of depressant effects of morphine). Products include:
- Hismanal Tablets ... 1138

Azatadine Maleate (Potentiation of depressant effects of morphine). Products include:
- Optimine Tablets ... 2115
- Trinalin Repetabs Tablets ... 1170

Bromodiphenhydramine Hydrochloride (Potentiation of depressant effects of morphine).
- No products indexed under this heading.

Brompheniramine Maleate (Potentiation of depressant effects of morphine). Products include:
- Alka Seltzer Plus Sinus Allergy Medicine ... ▣ 624
- Atrohist Sprinkle Capsules ... 558
- Bromfed Capsules (Timed Release) ... 1615
- Bromfed Syrup ... ▣ 628
- Bromfed ... 1615
- Dimetane Decongestant ... ▣ 673
- Dimetane ... ▣ 672
- Dimetane-DC Cough Syrup ... 1857
- Dimetane-DX Cough Syrup ... 1858
- Dimetapp Elixir ... ▣ 673
- Dimetapp DM Elixir ... ▣ 674
- Dimetapp Extentabs ... ▣ 674
- Dimetapp Plus Caplets ... ▣ 675
- Dimetapp Tablets ... ▣ 675
- Drixoral Antihistamine/Nasal Decongestant Syrup ... ▣ 698

Buprenorphine (Potentiation of depressant effects of morphine).
- No products indexed under this heading.

Buspirone Hydrochloride (Potentiation of depressant effects of morphine). Products include:
- BuSpar ... 1401

Butabarbital (Potentiation of depressant effects of morphine). Products include:
- Pyridium Plus ... 1764

Butalbital (Potentiation of depressant effects of morphine). Products include:
- Esgic-Plus Tablets ... 1002
- Esgic Tablets & Capsules ... 1001
- Fioricet Tablets ... 2006
- Fiorinal Capsules ... 2007
- Fiorinal with Codeine Capsules ... 2008
- Fiorinal Tablets ... 2007
- Phrenilin ... 838
- Sedapap Tablets 50 mg/650 mg .. 1360

Chlordiazepoxide (Potentiation of depressant effects of morphine). Products include:
- Libritabs Tablets ... 1930
- Limbitrol ... 1933
- Menrium Tablets ... 1934

Chlordiazepoxide Hydrochloride (Potentiation of depressant effects of morphine). Products include:
- Librax Capsules ... 1929
- Librium Capsules ... 1931
- Librium Injectable ... 1932

Chlorpheniramine Maleate (Potentiation of depressant effects of morphine). Products include:
- A.R.M. Allergy Relief Medicine Caplets ... ▣ 615
- Alka-Seltzer Plus Cold Medicine ... ▣ 623
- Allerest ... ▣ 559
- Ana-Kit Anaphylaxis Emergency Treatment Kit ... 1100
- BC Cold Powder Multi-Symptom Formula ... ▣ 517
- Brexin L.A. Capsules ... 2078
- Cerose-DM ... 2443
- Cheracol Plus Head Cold/Cough Formula ... ▣ 667
- Chlor-Trimeton Allergy Syrup, Tablets & Long-Acting Repetabs Tablets ... ▣ 693
- Chlor-Trimeton Decongestant ... ▣ 694
- Comhist LA Capsules ... 1618
- Allergy-Sinus Comtrex Multi-Symptom Allergy Sinus Formula Tablets & Caplets ... 746
- Comtrex Multi-Symptom Cold Reliever Tablets/Caplets/Liqui-Gels/Liquid ... 745
- Day-Night Comtrex ... 747
- Contac Continuous Action Decongestant/Antihistamine Capsules ▣ 710
- Contac Maximum Strength Continuous Action Decongestant/Antihistamine Caplets ... ▣ 709
- Contac Severe Cold and Flu Formula Caplets ... ▣ 711
- Coricidin 'D' Decongestant Tablets ... ▣ 695
- Coricidin Demilets Tablets for Children ... ▣ 696
- Coricidin Tablets ... ▣ 695
- Deconamine ... 663
- Demazin Nasal Decongestant/Antihistamine Repetabs Tablets & Syrup ... ▣ 697
- Dorcol Children's Liquid Cold Formula ... ▣ 686
- Dristan Decongestant/Antihistamine/Analgesic Coated Caplets ... ▣ 749
- Dristan Cold Nasal Decongestant/Antihistamine/ Analgesic Coated Tablets ... 2419
- Dristan Advanced Formula Decongestant/Antihistamine/Analgesic Tablets ... ▣ 749
- Extendryl ... 994
- 4-Way Cold Tablets ... 750
- Fedahist Gyrocaps ... 2145
- Fedahist Timecaps ... 2145
- Hycomine Compound Tablets ... 929
- Isoclor Timesule Capsules ... ▣ 561
- Kronofed-A ... 970
- Medi-Flu Caplet, Liquid ... ▣ 640
- Naldecon Syrup, Tablets, Pediatric Drops and Pediatric Syrup ... 709
- Nolamine Tablets ... 838
- Novafed A Capsules ... 1342
- Novahistine DH ... 1342
- Novahistine Elixir ... ▣ 596
- Ornade Spansule Capsules ... 2221
- Orthoxicol Cough Syrup ... ▣ 668
- PediaCare Allergy Relief Formula Liquid ... 1362
- PediaCare Cough-Cold Formula Liquid ... 1362
- PediaCare Night Rest Cough-Cold Formula Liquid ... 1362
- PediaCare 6-12 Cough-Cold Formula Chewable Tablets ... 1362
- Pyrroxate Capsules ... ▣ 669
- Quelidrine Syrup ... 556
- Ru-Tuss II Capsules ... 693
- Ru-Tuss Tablets ... 693
- Ryna ... ▣ 741
- Sinarest Tablets & Extra Strength Tablets ... ▣ 562
- Sine-Off Maximum Strength Allergy/Sinus Formula Caplets ... ▣ 721
- Sine-Off Sinus Medicine Tablets-Aspirin Formula ... ▣ 722
- Singlet Tablets ... ▣ 598
- Sinulin ... 840
- Sinutab Maximum Strength ... ▣ 641
- St. Joseph Nighttime Cold Medicine ... ▣ 705
- Sudafed Plus Liquid ... ▣ 544
- Sudafed Plus Tablets ... ▣ 545
- Teldrin Timed-Release Allergy Capsules, 12 mg ... 2192
- TheraFlu Flu and Cold Medicine ... ▣ 687
- Triaminic Allergy Tablets ... ▣ 688
- Triaminic Chewables ... ▣ 688
- Triaminic Cold Tablets ... ▣ 688
- Triaminic Nite Light ... ▣ 689
- Triaminic Syrup ... ▣ 689
- Triaminic-12 Tablets ... ▣ 690
- Triaminicin Tablets ... ▣ 690
- Triaminicol Multi-Symptom Cold Tablets ... ▣ 691
- Triaminicol Multi-Symptom Relief ▣ 691
- Tylenol Allergy Sinus Medication Caplets and Gelcaps, Maximum Strength ... 1372
- Children's Tylenol Cold Liquid Formula and Chewable Tablets ... 1368
- Tylenol Cold & Flu Hot Medication, Packets ... 1369
- Tylenol Cold Medication Caplets and Tablets ... 1370
- Tylenol Cold Medication, Effervescent Tablets ... 1369
- Vicks Children's NyQuil ... ▣ 664
- Vicks Formula 44 Cough Medicine ... ▣ 661
- Vicks Formula 44M Multi-Symptom Cough Medicine ... ▣ 662
- Vicks Pediatric Formula 44m Multi-Symptom Cough & Cold Medicine ... ▣ 663

Chlorpheniramine Polistirex (Potentiation of depressant effects of morphine). Products include:
- Tussionex Extended-Release Suspension ... 988

Chlorpheniramine Tannate (Potentiation of depressant effects of morphine). Products include:
- Rynatan ... 2387
- Rynatuss ... 2388

Chlorpromazine (Potentiation of depressant effects of morphine; increased risk of respiratory depression). Products include:
- Thorazine ... 2234

Chlorprothixene (Potentiation of depressant effects of morphine; increased risk of respiratory depression). Products include:
- Taractan Tablets ... 1920

Chlorprothixene Hydrochloride (Potentiation of depressant effects of morphine; increased risk of respiratory depression). Products include:
- Taractan ... 1920

Clemastine Fumarate (Potentiation of depressant effects of morphine). Products include:
- Tavist Syrup ... 2033
- Tavist Tablets ... 2035
- Tavist-D Tablets ... 2035

Clorazepate Dipotassium (Potentiation of depressant effects of morphine). Products include:
- Tranxene ... 556

Clozapine (Potentiation of depressant effects of morphine; increased risk of respiratory depression). Products include:
- Clozaril Tablets ... 2000

Codeine (Potentiation of depressant effects of morphine). Products include:
- Calcidrine Syrup ... 506

Codeine Phosphate (Potentiation of depressant effects of morphine). Products include:
- Actifed with Codeine Cough Syrup .. 752
- Cheracol Cough Syrup ... 1853
- Codimal PH Syrup ... 846
- Dimetane-DC Cough Syrup ... 1857
- Empirin with Codeine Phosphate Nos. 2, 3 & 4 ... 764
- Fiorinal with Codeine Capsules ... 2008
- Isoclor Expectorant ... 982
- Naldecon CX Adult Liquid ... ▣ 521
- Novahistine DH ... 1342
- Novahistine Expectorant ... 1343
- Nucofed Capsules ... 2219
- Nucofed Expectorant ... 2219
- Nucofed Pediatric Expectorant ... 2220
- Nucofed Syrup ... 2219
- Phenaphen with Codeine Capsules 1865
- Phenaphen-650 with Codeine Tablets ... 1866
- Phenergan with Codeine ... 2497
- Phenergan VC with Codeine ... 2501
- Robitussin A-C Syrup ... 1875
- Robitussin-DAC Syrup ... 1875
- Ryna ... ▣ 741
- Soma Compound w/Codeine Tablets ... 2390
- Triaminic Expectorant w/Codeine .. 1996
- Tussi-Organidin Liquid ... 2391
- Tylenol with Codeine ... 1381

Codeine Polistirex (Potentiation of depressant effects of morphine).
- No products indexed under this heading.

Cyproheptadine Hydrochloride (Potentiation of depressant effects of morphine). Products include:
- Periactin ... 1525

Desipramine Hydrochloride (Potentiation of depressant effects of morphine). Products include:
- Norpramin Tablets ... 1340

Dexchlorpheniramine Maleate (Potentiation of depressant effects of morphine). Products include:
- Polaramine ... 2116

Dezocine (Potentiation of depressant effects of morphine).

Diazepam (Potentiation of depressant effects of morphine). Products include:
- Valium Injectable ... 1937
- Valium Tablets ... 1939
- Valrelease Capsules ... 1923

Diethylpropion Hydrochloride (Potentiation of depressant effects of morphine). Products include:
- Tenuate ... 1354

Diphenhydramine Citrate (Potentiation of depressant effects of morphine). Products include:
- Alka-Seltzer Plus Night-Time Cold Medicine ... ▣ 623
- Bufferin AF Nite Time Analgesic/Sleeping Aid Caplets ... 744
- Excedrin P.M. Analgesic/Sleeping Aid Tablets, Caplets and Liquid ... 749

Diphenhydramine Hydrochloride (Potentiation of depressant effects of morphine). Products include:
- Benadryl Anti-Itch Cream ... ▣ 635
- Benadryl Capsules ... 1691
- Benadryl Decongestant Elixir ... ▣ 635
- Benadryl Decongestant ... ▣ 635
- Benadryl Elixir ... ▣ 636
- Benadryl Kapseals ... 1691
- Benadryl 25 Kapseals ... ▣ 636
- Benadryl Parenteral ... 1692
- Benadryl Plus ... ▣ 636
- Benadryl Plus Nighttime ... ▣ 637
- Benadryl Spray, Maximum Strength ... ▣ 637
- Benadryl Spray, Regular Strength ▣ 637
- Benadryl Steri-Vials, Ampoules, and Steri-Dose Syringe ... 1692
- Benadryl 25 Tablets ... ▣ 636
- Benylin Cough Syrup ... ▣ 637
- Benylin Decongestant ... ▣ 638
- Caladryl Cream, Lotion, Spray ... ▣ 638
- Miles Nervine Nighttime Sleep-Aid ▣ 627
- Nytol Tablets ... ▣ 517
- Sleep-ettes-D Tablets ... ▣ 653
- Sleep-eze 3 Tablets ... ▣ 755
- Sleepinal Night-time Sleep Aid Capsules ... ▣ 734
- Sominex Caplets and Tablets ... ▣ 722
- Sominex Liquid ... ▣ 723
- Sominex Pain Relief Formula ... ▣ 723
- Tylenol Cold Night Time Medication Liquid ... 1371
- Tylenol PM, Extra Strength Caplets and Tablets ... 1368
- Unisom Dual Relief Nighttime Sleep Aid/Analgesic ... 1774
- Ziradryl Lotion ... ▣ 643

Diphenylpyraline Hydrochloride (Potentiation of depressant effects of morphine).
- No products indexed under this heading.

Doxepin Hydrochloride (Potentiation of depressant effects of morphine). Products include:
- Sinequan ... 1960

Droperidol (Potentiation of depressant effects of morphine). Products include:
- Inapsine Injection ... 1140
- Innovar Injection ... 1141

Enflurane (Potentiation of depressant effects of morphine). Products include:
- Ethrane ... 599

Estazolam (Potentiation of depressant effects of morphine). Products include:
- ProSom Tablets ... 554

Ethchlorvynol (Potentiation of depressant effects of morphine). Products include:
- Placidyl Capsules ... 553

Ethinamate (Potentiation of depressant effects of morphine).
- No products indexed under this heading.

Fentanyl (Potentiation of depressant effects of morphine). Products include:
- Duragesic Transdermal System ... 1133

Fentanyl Citrate (Potentiation of depressant effects of morphine). Products include:
- Innovar Injection ... 1141
- Sublimaze Injection ... 1146

Fluphenazine Decanoate (Potentiation of depressant effects of morphine; increased risk of respiratory depression). Products include:
- Prolixin Decanoate ... 1795

Fluphenazine Enanthate (Potentiation of depressant effects of morphine; increased risk of respiratory depression). Products include:
- Prolixin Enanthate ... 1796

Fluphenazine Hydrochloride (Potentiation of depressant effects of morphine; increased risk of respiratory depression). Products include:
- Prolixin Elixir ... 1793
- Prolixin Injection ... 1791
- Prolixin Oral Concentrate ... 1792
- Prolixin Tablets ... 1793

Flurazepam Hydrochloride (Potentiation of depressant effects of morphine). Products include:
- Dalmane Capsules ... 1927

Glutethimide (Potentiation of depressant effects of morphine).
No products indexed under this heading.

Haloperidol (Potentiation of depressant effects of morphine). Products include:
Haldol Injection, Tablets and Concentrate 1373

Haloperidol Decanoate (Potentiation of depressant effects of morphine; increased risk of respiratory depression). Products include:
Haldol Decanoate 1375

Hydrocodone Bitartrate (Potentiation of depressant effects of morphine). Products include:
Anexsia 5/500 Tablets 2196
Anexsia 7.5/650 Tablets 2197
Azdōne Tablets 844
Codiclear DH Syrup 845
Codimal DH Syrup 846
Damason-P 1356
Hycodan Syrup, Tablets 927
Hycomine Compound Tablets 929
Hycomine Syrup 927
Hycotuss Expectorant Syrup 930
Hydrocet Capsules 835
Lortab ASA Tablets 2414
Lortab 2412
Ru-Tuss with Hydrocodone 694
Triaminic Expectorant DH 1995
Vicodin Tablets 1187
Vicodin ES Tablets 1189
Zydone Capsules 941

Hydrocodone Polistirex (Potentiation of depressant effects of morphine). Products include:
Tussionex Extended-Release Suspension 988

Hydroxyzine Hydrochloride (Potentiation of depressant effects of morphine). Products include:
Atarax Tablets & Syrup 1941
Marax Tablets & DF Syrup 1954
Vistaril Intramuscular Solution 1970

Imipramine Hydrochloride (Potentiation of depressant effects of morphine). Products include:
Tofranil Ampuls 1038
Tofranil Tablets 1039

Imipramine Pamoate (Potentiation of depressant effects of morphine). Products include:
Tofranil-PM Capsules 1041

Isocarboxazid (Potentiation of depressant effects of morphine). Products include:
Marplan Tablets 1906

Isoflurane (Potentiation of depressant effects of morphine). Products include:
Forane 600

Ketamine Hydrochloride (Potentiation of depressant effects of morphine). Products include:
Ketalar 1726

Levorphanol Tartrate (Potentiation of depressant effects of morphine). Products include:
Levo-Dromoran 1906

Lithium Carbonate (Potentiation of depressant effects of morphine; increased risk of respiratory depression). Products include:
Eskalith 2214
Lithane Tablets 1596
Lithium Carbonate Capsules & Tablets 1984
Lithobid Tablets 870

Lithium Citrate (Potentiation of depressant effects of morphine; increased risk of respiratory depression). Products include:
Cibalith-S 870

Lorazepam (Potentiation of depressant effects of morphine). Products include:
Ativan Injection 2432
Ativan Tablets 2434

Loxapine Hydrochloride (Potentiation of depressant effects of morphine; increased risk of respiratory depression). Products include:
Loxitane 1213

Loxapine Succinate (Potentiation of depressant effects of morphine). Products include:
Loxitane Capsules 1213

Maprotiline Hydrochloride (Potentiation of depressant effects of morphine). Products include:
Ludiomil Tablets 874

Meperidine Hydrochloride (Potentiation of depressant effects of morphine). Products include:
Demerol 2047
Mepergan Injection 2479

Mephobarbital (Potentiation of depressant effects of morphine). Products include:
Mebaral Tablets 2061

Meprobamate (Potentiation of depressant effects of morphine). Products include:
Deprol Tablets 2382
Equagesic Tablets 2451
Miltown Tablets 2386
PMB 200 and PMB 400 2504

Mesoridazine (Potentiation of depressant effects of morphine; increased risk of respiratory depression). Products include:
Serentil 686

Methadone Hydrochloride (Potentiation of depressant effects of morphine). Products include:
Dolophine Hydrochloride Ampoules & Vials 1260
Dolophine Hydrochloride Tablets 1261
Methadone Hydrochloride Diskets 1284
Methadone Hydrochloride Oral Solution & Tablets 1987

Methdilazine Hydrochloride (Potentiation of depressant effects of morphine). Products include:
Tacaryl Syrup & Tablets 2409

Methohexital Sodium (Potentiation of depressant effects of morphine). Products include:
Brevital Sodium Vials 1248

Methoxyflurane (Potentiation of depressant effects of morphine).
No products indexed under this heading.

Midazolam Hydrochloride (Potentiation of depressant effects of morphine). Products include:
Versed Injection 1924

Molindone Hydrochloride (Potentiation of depressant effects of morphine; increased risk of respiratory depression with neuroleptics). Products include:
Moban Tablets & Concentrate 932

Nortriptyline Hydrochloride (Potentiation of depressant effects of morphine). Products include:
Pamelor 2019

Opium Alkaloids (Potentiation of depressant effects of morphine). Products include:
B & O No. 15A & No. 16A Supprettes 2395
Pantopon Injectable 1911

Oxazepam (Potentiation of depressant effects of morphine). Products include:
Serax Capsules 2522
Serax Tablets 2522

Oxycodone Hydrochloride (Potentiation of depressant effects of morphine). Products include:
Percocet Tablets 950
Percodan 951
Roxicodone Tablets, Oral Solution & Intensol (Oxycodone) 1992
Tylox Capsules 1382

Pentobarbital Sodium (Potentiation of depressant effects of morphine). Products include:
Nembutal Sodium Capsules 534
Nembutal Sodium Solution 536
Nembutal Sodium Suppositories 538

Perphenazine (Potentiation of depressant effects of morphine). Products include:
Etrafon 2087
Triavil Tablets 1556
Trilafon 2123

Phenelzine Sulfate (Potentiation of depressant effects of morphine). Products include:
Nardil 1742

Phenobarbital (Potentiation of depressant effects of morphine). Products include:
Arco-Lase Plus Tablets 607
Bellergal-S Tablets 1998
Bronkolixir ▣ 761
Bronkotabs Tablets ▣ 762
Donnatal 1858
Donnatal Extentabs 1859
Donnatal Tablets 1858
Donnazyme Tablets 1860
Kinesed Tablets 2272
Phenobarbital Elixir and Tablets 1293
Primatene Tablets-P Formula 2421
Quadrinal Tablets 1183
Tedral SA 1765

Pimozide (Potentiation of depressant effects of morphine; increased risk of respiratory depression). Products include:
Orap Tablets 1020

Prazepam (Potentiation of depressant effects of morphine). Products include:
Centrax 1693

Prochlorperazine (Potentiation of depressant effects of morphine; increased risk of respiratory depression). Products include:
Compazine 2201

Promethazine Hydrochloride (Potentiation of depressant effects of morphine; increased risk of respiratory depression). Products include:
Mepergan Injection 2479
Phenergan with Codeine 2497
Phenergan with Dextromethorphan 2499
Phenergan Injection 2493
Phenergan Suppositories 2496
Phenergan Syrup 2495
Phenergan Tablets 2496
Phenergan VC 2500
Phenergan VC with Codeine 2501

Propofol (Potentiation of depressant effects of morphine). Products include:
Diprivan Injection 2267

Propoxyphene Hydrochloride (Potentiation of depressant effects of morphine). Products include:
Darvon 1256
Wygesic Tablets 2540

Propoxyphene Napsylate (Potentiation of depressant effects of morphine). Products include:
Darvon-N/Darvocet-N 1254

Protriptyline Hydrochloride (Potentiation of depressant effects of morphine). Products include:
Vivactil Tablets 1567

Pyrilamine Maleate (Potentiation of depressant effects of morphine). Products include:
Codimal 846
4-Way Fast Acting Nasal Spray - Original Formula (regular & mentholated) & Metered Spray Pump (regular) 751
Maximum Strength Midol Multi-Symptom Menstrual Formula ▣ 571
Maximum Strength Midol PMS Premenstrual Syndrome Formula ▣ 570
Regular Strength Midol Multi-Symptom Menstrual Formula ▣ 570
Prefrin-A ◉ 255
Prēmsyn PMS Capsules & Caplets ▣ 547
Primatene Tablets-M Formula 2421
Robitussin Night Relief ▣ 677
Ru-Tuss with Hydrocodone 694
Triaminic Expectorant DH 1995
Triaminic Oral Infant Drops 1996

Pyrilamine Tannate (Potentiation of depressant effects of morphine). Products include:
Rynatan 2387

Quazepam (Potentiation of depressant effects of morphine). Products include:
Doral Tablets 2383

Secobarbital Sodium (Potentiation of depressant effects of morphine). Products include:
Seconal Sodium Pulvules 1296

Sufentanil Citrate (Potentiation of depressant effects of morphine). Products include:
Sufenta Injection 1147

Temazepam (Potentiation of depressant effects of morphine). Products include:
Restoril Capsules 2023

Terfenadine (Potentiation of depressant effects of morphine). Products include:
Seldane Tablets 1349
Seldane-D Extended-Release Tablets 1350

Thiamylal Sodium (Potentiation of depressant effects of morphine). Products include:
Surital Ampoules, Steri-Vials 1764

Thioridazine Hydrochloride (Potentiation of depressant effects of morphine; increased risk of respiratory depression). Products include:
Mellaril 2011

Thiothixene (Potentiation of depressant effects of morphine; increased risk of respiratory depression). Products include:
Navane Capsules and Concentrate 1954
Navane Intramuscular 1956

Tranylcypromine Sulfate (Potentiation of depressant effects of morphine). Products include:
Parnate Tablets 2222

Triazolam (Potentiation of depressant effects of morphine). Products include:
Halcion Tablets 2340

Trifluoperazine Hydrochloride (Potentiation of depressant effects of morphine; increased risk of respiratory depression). Products include:
Stelazine 2226

Trimeprazine Tartrate (Potentiation of depressant effects of morphine). Products include:
Temaril Tablets, Syrup and Spansule Sustained Release Capsules 1085

Trimipramine Maleate (Potentiation of depressant effects of morphine). Products include:
Surmontil Capsules 2524

Tripelennamine Hydrochloride (Potentiation of depressant effects of morphine). Products include:
PBZ Tablets & Elixir 1037
PBZ-SR Tablets 1037

Triprolidine Hydrochloride (Potentiation of depressant effects of morphine). Products include:
Actidil ▣ 538
Actifed Capsules ▣ 539
Actifed Plus Caplets ▣ 539
Actifed Plus Tablets ▣ 540
Actifed with Codeine Cough Syrup 752
Actifed Syrup ▣ 540
Actifed Tablets ▣ 540
Actifed 12-Hour Capsules ▣ 539

ATABRINE HYDROCHLORIDE TABLETS
(Quinacrine Hydrochloride) 2041
May interact with:

Primaquine Phosphate (Increased toxicity of primaquine; concurrent use is contraindicated). Products include:
- Aralen Phosphate with Primaquine Phosphate Tablets 2040

ATARAX TABLETS & SYRUP
(Hydroxyzine Hydrochloride) 1941
May interact with narcotic analgesics, barbiturates, central nervous system depressants, and certain other agents. Compounds in these categories include:

Alcohol (Potentiated effect of alcohol).

Alfentanil Hydrochloride (Potentiated action of narcotics). Products include:
- Alfenta Injection 1131

Alprazolam (Potentiated action of CNS depressant). Products include:
- Xanax Tablets 2367

Aprobarbital (Potentiated action of barbiturates). Products include:
- Alurate Elixir 1883

Buprenorphine (Potentiated action of narcotics).
- No products indexed under this heading.

Buspirone Hydrochloride (Potentiated action of CNS depressant). Products include:
- BuSpar 1401

Butabarbital (Potentiated action of barbiturates). Products include:
- Pyridium Plus 1764

Butalbital (Potentiated action of barbiturates). Products include:
- Esgic-Plus Tablets 1002
- Esgic Tablets & Capsules 1001
- Fioricet Tablets 2006
- Fiorinal Capsules 2007
- Fiorinal with Codeine Capsules 2008
- Fiorinal Tablets 2007
- Phrenilin 838
- Sedapap Tablets 50 mg/650 mg .. 1360

Chlordiazepoxide (Potentiated action of CNS depressant). Products include:
- Libritabs Tablets 1930
- Limbitrol 1933
- Menrium Tablets 1934

Chlordiazepoxide Hydrochloride (Potentiated action of CNS depressant). Products include:
- Librax Capsules 1929
- Librium Capsules 1931
- Librium Injectable 1932

Chlorpromazine (Potentiated action of CNS depressant). Products include:
- Thorazine 2234

Chlorprothixene (Potentiated action of narcotics). Products include:
- Taractan Tablets 1920

Chlorprothixene Hydrochloride (Potentiated action of narcotics). Products include:
- Taractan 1920

Clorazepate Dipotassium (Potentiated action of CNS depressant). Products include:
- Tranxene 556

Codeine (Potentiated action of narcotics). Products include:
- Calcidrine Syrup 506

Codeine Phosphate (Potentiated action of narcotics). Products include:
- Actifed with Codeine Cough Syrup .. 752
- Cheracol Cough Syrup 1853
- Codimal PH Syrup 846
- Dimetane-DC Cough Syrup 1857
- Empirin with Codeine Phosphate Nos. 2, 3 & 4 764
- Fiorinal with Codeine Capsules 2008
- Isoclor Expectorant 982
- Naldecon CX Adult Liquid .... ▣ 521
- Novahistine DH 1342
- Novahistine Expectorant 1343
- Nucofed Capsules 2219
- Nucofed Expectorant 2219
- Nucofed Pediatric Expectorant 2220
- Nucofed Syrup 2219
- Phenaphen with Codeine Capsules 1865
- Phenaphen-650 with Codeine Tablets 1866
- Phenergan with Codeine 2497
- Phenergan VC with Codeine 2501
- Robitussin A-C Syrup 1875
- Robitussin-DAC Syrup 1875
- Ryna .... ▣ 741
- Soma Compound w/Codeine Tablets 2390
- Triaminic Expectorant w/Codeine .. 1996
- Tussi-Organidin Liquid 2391
- Tylenol with Codeine 1381

Codeine Polistirex (Potentiated action of narcotics).
- No products indexed under this heading.

Dezocine (Potentiated action of narcotics).

Diazepam (Potentiated action of CNS depressant). Products include:
- Valium Injectable 1937
- Valium Tablets 1939
- Valrelease Capsules 1923

Droperidol (Potentiated action of CNS depressant). Products include:
- Inapsine Injection 1140
- Innovar Injection 1141

Enflurane (Potentiated action of CNS depressant). Products include:
- Ethrane 599

Epinephrine (Atarax, if used in cases of overdosage, counteracts pressor action). Products include:
- Ana-Kit Anaphylaxis Emergency Treatment Kit 1100
- Bronkaid Mist .... ▣ 757
- EpiPen 843
- Marcaine Hydrochloride 0.5% with Epinephrine 1:200,000 (as bitartrate) 958
- Marcaine Hydrochloride with Epinephrine 1:200,000 2055
- Primatene Mist 2420
- Sus-Phrine Injection 1006
- Xylocaine with Epinephrine Injections 637

Estazolam (Potentiated action of narcotics). Products include:
- ProSom Tablets 554

Ethchlorvynol (Potentiated action of narcotics). Products include:
- Placidyl Capsules 553

Ethinamate (Potentiated action of narcotics).
- No products indexed under this heading.

Fentanyl (Potentiated action of narcotics). Products include:
- Duragesic Transdermal System 1133

Fentanyl Citrate (Potentiated action of narcotics). Products include:
- Innovar Injection 1141
- Sublimaze Injection 1146

Fluphenazine Decanoate (Potentiated action of CNS depressant). Products include:
- Prolixin Decanoate 1795

Fluphenazine Enanthate (Potentiated action of CNS depressant). Products include:
- Prolixin Enanthate 1796

Fluphenazine Hydrochloride (Potentiated action of CNS depressant). Products include:
- Prolixin Elixir 1793
- Prolixin Injection 1791
- Prolixin Oral Concentrate 1792
- Prolixin Tablets 1793

Flurazepam Hydrochloride (Potentiated action of narcotics). Products include:
- Dalmane Capsules 1927

Glutethimide (Potentiated action of narcotics).
- No products indexed under this heading.

Haloperidol (Potentiated action of CNS depressant). Products include:
- Haldol Injection, Tablets and Concentrate 1373

Haloperidol Decanoate (Potentiated action of CNS depressant). Products include:
- Haldol Decanoate 1375

Hydrocodone Bitartrate (Potentiated action of narcotics). Products include:
- Anexsia 5/500 Tablets 2196
- Anexsia 7.5/650 Tablets 2197
- Azdōne Tablets 844
- Codiclear DH Syrup 845
- Codimal DH Syrup 846
- Damason-P 1356
- Hycodan Syrup, Tablets 927
- Hycomine Compound Tablets 929
- Hycomine Syrup 927
- Hycotuss Expectorant Syrup 930
- Hydrocet Capsules 835
- Lortab ASA Tablets 2414
- Lortab 2412
- Ru-Tuss with Hydrocodone 694
- Triaminic Expectorant DH 1995
- Vicodin Tablets 1187
- Vicodin ES Tablets 1189
- Zydone Capsules 941

Hydrocodone Polistirex (Potentiated action of narcotics). Products include:
- Tussionex Extended-Release Suspension 988

Isoflurane (Potentiated action of CNS depressant). Products include:
- Forane 600

Ketamine Hydrochloride (Potentiated action of narcotics). Products include:
- Ketalar 1726

Levorphanol Tartrate (Potentiated action of narcotics). Products include:
- Levo-Dromoran 1906

Lorazepam (Potentiated action of narcotics). Products include:
- Ativan Injection 2432
- Ativan Tablets 2434

Loxapine Hydrochloride (Potentiated action of CNS depressant). Products include:
- Loxitane 1213

Loxapine Succinate (Potentiated action of narcotics). Products include:
- Loxitane Capsules 1213

Meperidine Hydrochloride (Potentiated action of narcotics). Products include:
- Demerol 2047
- Mepergan Injection 2479

Mephobarbital (Potentiated action of barbiturates). Products include:
- Mebaral Tablets 2061

Meprobamate (Potentiated action of CNS depressant). Products include:
- Deprol Tablets 2382
- Equagesic Tablets 2451
- Miltown Tablets 2386
- PMB 200 and PMB 400 2504

Mesoridazine (Potentiated action of CNS depressant). Products include:
- Serentil 686

Methadone Hydrochloride (Potentiated action of narcotics). Products include:
- Dolophine Hydrochloride Ampoules & Vials 1260
- Dolophine Hydrochloride Tablets 1261
- Methadone Hydrochloride Diskets .. 1284
- Methadone Hydrochloride Oral Solution & Tablets 1987

Methohexital Sodium (Potentiated action of CNS depressant). Products include:
- Brevital Sodium Vials 1248

Methoxyflurane (Potentiated action of CNS depressant).
- No products indexed under this heading.

Midazolam Hydrochloride (Potentiated action of narcotics). Products include:
- Versed Injection 1924

Molindone Hydrochloride (Potentiated action of CNS depressant). Products include:
- Moban Tablets & Concentrate 932

Morphine Sulfate (Potentiated action of narcotics). Products include:
- Astramorph/PF Injection, USP (Preservative-Free) 618
- Duramorph 960
- Infumorph 200 and Infumorph 500 Sterile Solutions 962
- MS Contin Tablets 1814
- MSIR 1817
- Oramorph SR (Morphine Sulfate Sustained Release Tablets) 1988
- Roxanol 1991

Non-narcotic Analgesics (Potentiated action of non-narcotic analgesics).

Opium Alkaloids (Potentiated action of narcotics). Products include:
- B & O No. 15A & No. 16A Supprettes 2395
- Pantopon Injectable 1911

Oxazepam (Potentiated action of CNS depressant). Products include:
- Serax Capsules 2522
- Serax Tablets 2522

Oxycodone Hydrochloride (Potentiated action of narcotics). Products include:
- Percocet Tablets 950
- Percodan 951
- Roxicodone Tablets, Oral Solution & Intensol (Oxycodone) 1992
- Tylox Capsules 1382

Pentobarbital Sodium (Potentiated action of barbiturates). Products include:
- Nembutal Sodium Capsules 534
- Nembutal Sodium Solution 536
- Nembutal Sodium Suppositories 538

Perphenazine (Potentiated action of CNS depressant). Products include:
- Etrafon 2087
- Triavil Tablets 1556
- Trilafon 2123

Phenobarbital (Potentiated action of barbiturates). Products include:
- Arco-Lase Plus Tablets 607
- Bellergal-S Tablets 1998
- Bronkolixir .... ▣ 761
- Bronkotabs Tablets .... ▣ 762
- Donnatal 1858
- Donnatal Extentabs 1859
- Donnatal Tablets 1858
- Donnazyme Tablets 1860
- Kinesed Tablets 2272
- Phenobarbital Elixir and Tablets 1293
- Primatene Tablets-P Formula 2421
- Quadrinal Tablets 1183
- Tedral SA 1765

Prazepam (Potentiated action of CNS depressant). Products include:
- Centrax 1693

Prochlorperazine (Potentiated action of CNS depressant). Products include:
- Compazine 2201

Promethazine Hydrochloride (Potentiated action of CNS depressant). Products include:
- Mepergan Injection 2479
- Phenergan with Codeine 2497
- Phenergan with Dextromethorphan 2499
- Phenergan Injection 2493
- Phenergan Suppositories 2496
- Phenergan Syrup 2495
- Phenergan Tablets 2496
- Phenergan VC 2500
- Phenergan VC with Codeine 2501

Propofol (Potentiated action of narcotics). Products include:
- Diprivan Injection 2267

Propoxyphene Hydrochloride (Potentiated action of narcotics). Products include:
- Darvon 1256
- Wygesic Tablets 2540

Propoxyphene Napsylate (Potentiated action of narcotics). Products include:
- Darvon-N/Darvocet-N 1254

Quazepam (Potentiated action of narcotics). Products include:
- Doral Tablets 2383

Secobarbital Sodium (Potentiated action of barbiturates). Products include:
- Seconal Sodium Pulvules 1296

Sufentanil Citrate (Potentiated action of narcotics). Products include:
- Sufenta Injection 1147

Temazepam (Potentiated action of narcotics). Products include:
- Restoril Capsules 2023

Thiamylal Sodium (Potentiated action of barbiturates). Products include:
- Surital Ampoules, Steri-Vials 1764

Thioridazine Hydrochloride (Potentiated action of CNS depressant). Products include:
- Mellaril 2011

Thiothixene (Potentiated action of CNS depressant). Products include:
- Navane Capsules and Concentrate 1954
- Navane Intramuscular 1956

Triazolam (Potentiated action of narcotics). Products include:
- Halcion Tablets 2340

Trifluoperazine Hydrochloride (Potentiated action of CNS depressant). Products include:
- Stelazine 2226

ATGAM STERILE SOLUTION

(Lubricant) 2320

May interact with corticosteroids, immunosuppressive agents, and certain other agents. Compounds in these categories include:

Azathioprine (When the dose of corticosteroids is reduced, some previously masked reactions to Atgam may appear). Products include:
- Imuran 768

Betamethasone Acetate (When the dose of corticosteroids is reduced, some previously masked reactions to Atgam may appear). Products include:
- Celestone Soluspan Suspension 2081

Betamethasone Sodium Phosphate (When the dose of corticosteroids is reduced, some previously masked reactions to Atgam may appear). Products include:
- Celestone Soluspan Suspension 2081

Cortisone Acetate (When the dose of corticosteroids is reduced, some previously masked reactions to Atgam may appear). Products include:
- Cortone Acetate Sterile Suspension 1437
- Cortone Acetate Tablets 1439

Cyclosporine (When the dose of corticosteroids is reduced, some previously masked reactions to Atgam may appear). Products include:
- Sandimmune 2024

Dexamethasone (When the dose of corticosteroids is reduced, some previously masked reactions to Atgam may appear). Products include:
- AK-Trol Ointment & Suspension .... ⊙ 207
- Decadron Elixir 1445
- Decadron Tablets 1447
- Decaspray Topical Aerosol 1459
- Dexacidin .... ⊙ 272
- Maxidex Sterile Ophthalmic Suspension .... ⊙ 223
- Maxitrol Ophthalmic Ointment/Suspension .... ⊙ 223
- TobraDex Ophthalmic Suspension and Ointment .... ⊙ 228

Dexamethasone Acetate (When the dose of corticosteroids is reduced, some previously masked reactions to Atgam may appear). Products include:
- Dalalone D.P. Injectable 999
- Decadron-LA Sterile Suspension 1457

Dexamethasone Sodium Phosphate (When the dose of corticosteroids is reduced, some previously masked reactions to Atgam may appear). Products include:
- AK-Dex .... ⊙ 203
- Decadron Phosphate Respihaler 1454
- Decadron Phosphate Sterile Ophthalmic Ointment 1453
- Decadron Phosphate Sterile Ophthalmic Solution 1453
- Decadron Phosphate Topical Cream 1455
- Decadron Phosphate Turbinaire 1456
- Maxidex Sterile Ophthalmic Ointment .... ⊙ 222
- NeoDecadron Sterile Ophthalmic Ointment 1517
- NeoDecadron Sterile Ophthalmic Solution 1518
- NeoDecadron Topical Cream 1518

Dextrose Injection (Physical incompatability).

Hydrocortisone (When the dose of corticosteroids is reduced, some previously masked reactions to Atgam may appear). Products include:
- AK-Spore H.C. .... ⊙ 206
- Bactine Hydrocortisone Anti-Itch Cream .... ▣ 625
- CaldeCORT Anti-Itch Hydrocortisone Spray .... ▣ 560
- Carmol HC Cream 1% 2296
- Cortaid Spray .... ▣ 735
- Cortenema 2244
- Cortisporin Ointment 758
- Cortisporin Ophthalmic Ointment Sterile 758
- Cortisporin Ophthalmic Suspension Sterile 759
- Cortisporin Otic Solution Sterile 760
- Cortisporin Otic Suspension Sterile 760
- Cortizone-5 Creme & Ointment .... ▣ 732
- Dermolate Anti-Itch Cream .... ▣ 697
- Eldecort Cream 1.0% 1113
- Eldecort Cream 1.0% and 2.5% 1113
- Fungoid HC Creme 1770
- Hydrocortone Tablets 1482
- Hytone 909
- LazerSporin-C Solution 1770
- Massengill Medicated Soft Cloth Towelettes 2192
- Nutracort Cream & Lotion 1684
- PediOtic Suspension Sterile 797
- Synacort Creams 1%, 2.5% 2296
- Vanoxide-HC Acne Lotion 911
- Vioform-Hydrocortisone Cream and Mild Cream 889
- Vioform-Hydrocortisone Ointment 889
- VōSoL HC Otic Solution 2392
- Vytone Cream 1% 911

Hydrocortisone Acetate (When the dose of corticosteroids is reduced, some previously masked reactions to Atgam may appear). Products include:
- Analpram-HC Rectal Cream 1% and 2.5% 970
- Anusol-HC Cream 1690
- Anusol-HC Suppositories 1691
- Caldecort .... ▣ 560
- Carmol HC Cream 1% 2296
- Chloromycetin Hydrocortisone Ophthalmic 1694
- Coly-Mycin S Otic w/Neomycin & Hydrocortisone 1708
- Cortaid .... ▣ 735
- Cortef Feminine Itch Cream .... ▣ 735
- Corticaine .... ▣ 682
- Cortifoam 1827
- Cortisporin Cream 757
- Epifoam 1828
- Gynecort 5 Creme .... ▣ 556
- Hydrocortone Acetate Sterile Suspension 1479
- Lanacort 5 Creme and Ointment .... ▣ 557
- Mantadil Cream 789
- Ophthocort .... ⊙ 301
- Orabase HCA Oral Paste 890
- Pramosone Cream, Lotion & Ointment 971
- ProctoCream-HC 1834
- Proctofoam-HC 1835

Hydrocortisone Sodium Phosphate (When the dose of corticosteroids is reduced, some previously masked reactions to Atgam may appear). Products include:
- Hydrocortone Phosphate Injection, Sterile 1481

Hydrocortisone Sodium Succinate (When the dose of corticosteroids is reduced, some previously masked reactions to Atgam may appear). Products include:
- Solu-Cortef Sterile Powder 2361

Immune Globulin (Human) (When the dose of corticosteroids is reduced, some previously masked reactions to Atgam may appear). Products include:
- MICRhoGAM Rh$_0$(D) Immune Globulin (Human) 1650
- RhoGAM Rh$_0$(D) Immune Globulin (Human) 1651

Immune Globulin Intravenous (Human) (When the dose of corticosteroids is reduced, some previously masked reactions to Atgam may appear). Products include:
- Gamimune N Immune Globulin Intravenous (Human) 1572
- Gammagard Immune Globulin, Intravenous (Human) 658
- Iveegam 1129
- Sandoglobulin I.V. 2027

Methylprednisolone Acetate (When the dose of corticosteroids is reduced, some previously masked reactions to Atgam may appear). Products include:
- Depo-Medrol Sterile Aqueous Suspension 2334

Methylprednisolone Sodium Succinate (When the dose of corticosteroids is reduced, some previously masked reactions to Atgam may appear). Products include:
- Solu-Medrol Sterile Powder 2363

Muromonab-CD3 (When the dose of corticosteroids is reduced, some previously masked reactions to Atgam may appear). Products include:
- Orthoclone OKT3 Sterile Solution 1645

Prednisolone Acetate (When the dose of corticosteroids is reduced, some previously masked reactions to Atgam may appear). Products include:
- AK-Cide Sterile Ophthalmic Ointment & Suspension .... ⊙ 202
- Blephamide Liquifilm Sterile Ophthalmic Suspension 586
- Blephamide S.O.P. Sterile Ophthalmic Ointment 586
- Cetapred Ointment .... ⊙ 220
- ⅛% Econopred & 1% Econopred Plus .... ⊙ 217
- Isopto Cetapred Suspension .... ⊙ 220
- Metimyd .... ⊙ 306
- Poly-Pred Liquifilm .... ⊙ 250
- Pred Forte .... ⊙ 252
- Pred Mild .... ⊙ 254
- Pred-G Liquifilm Sterile Ophthalmic Suspension .... ⊙ 252
- Pred-G S.O.P. Sterile Ophthalmic Ointment .... ⊙ 253
- Vasocidin Ointment .... ⊙ 275

Prednisolone Sodium Phosphate (When the dose of corticosteroids is reduced, some previously masked reactions to Atgam may appear). Products include:
- AK-Pred .... ⊙ 205
- Hydeltrasol Injection, Sterile 1476
- Inflamase .... ⊙ 274
- Pediapred Oral Liquid 987
- Vasocidin Ophthalmic Solution .... ⊙ 276

Prednisolone Tebutate (When the dose of corticosteroids is reduced, some previously masked reactions to Atgam may appear). Products include:
- Hydeltra-T.B.A. Sterile Suspension 1478

Prednisone (When the dose of corticosteroids is reduced, some previously masked reactions to Atgam may appear). Products include:
- Deltasone Tablets 2332

Triamcinolone (When the dose of corticosteroids is reduced, some previously masked reactions to Atgam may appear).
- No products indexed under this heading.

Triamcinolone Acetonide (When the dose of corticosteroids is reduced, some previously masked reactions to Atgam may appear). Products include:
- Aristocort A 1010
- Azmacort Inhaler 1837
- Kenalog Cream, Lotion & Ointment 2401
- Kenalog-10 Injection 2402
- Kenalog-40 Injection 2403
- Kenalog in Orabase 604
- Kenalog Spray 2401
- Mycolog II Cream and Ointment 2407
- Mytrex Cream & Ointment 2080
- Nasacort Nasal Inhaler 1844

Triamcinolone Diacetate (When the dose of corticosteroids is reduced, some previously masked reactions to Atgam may appear). Products include:
- Aristocort Suspension 1008

Triamcinolone Hexacetonide (When the dose of corticosteroids is reduced, some previously masked reactions to Atgam may appear). Products include:
- Aristospan Suspension 1011

ATIVAN INJECTION

(Lorazepam) 2432

May interact with phenothiazines, barbiturates, monoamine oxidase inhibitors, narcotic analgesics, central nervous system depressants, and certain other agents. Compounds in these categories include:

Alcohol (Additive CNS depressant effects).

Alfentanil Hydrochloride (Additive CNS depressant effects). Products include:
Alfenta Injection ... 1131

Alprazolam (Additive CNS depressant effects). Products include:
Xanax Tablets ... 2367

Aprobarbital (Additive CNS depressant effects). Products include:
Alurate Elixir ... 1883

Buprenorphine (Additive CNS depressant effects).
No products indexed under this heading.

Buspirone Hydrochloride (Additive CNS depressant effects). Products include:
BuSpar ... 1401

Butabarbital (Additive CNS depressant effects). Products include:
Pyridium Plus ... 1764

Butalbital (Additive CNS depressant effects). Products include:
Esgic-Plus Tablets ... 1002
Esgic Tablets & Capsules ... 1001
Fioricet Tablets ... 2006
Fiorinal Capsules ... 2007
Fiorinal with Codeine Capsules ... 2008
Fiorinal Tablets ... 2007
Phrenilin ... 838
Sedapap Tablets 50 mg/650 mg .. 1360

Chlordiazepoxide (Additive CNS depressant effects). Products include:
Libritabs Tablets ... 1930
Limbitrol ... 1933
Menrium Tablets ... 1934

Chlordiazepoxide Hydrochloride (Additive CNS depressant effects). Products include:
Librax Capsules ... 1929
Librium Capsules ... 1931
Librium Injectable ... 1932

Chlorpromazine (Additive CNS depressant effects). Products include:
Thorazine ... 2234

Chlorprothixene (Additive CNS depressant effects). Products include:
Taractan Tablets ... 1920

Chlorprothixene Hydrochloride (Additive CNS depressant effects). Products include:
Taractan ... 1920

Clorazepate Dipotassium (Additive CNS depressant effects). Products include:
Tranxene ... 556

Codeine (Additive CNS depressant effects). Products include:
Calcidrine Syrup ... 506

Codeine Phosphate (Additive CNS depressant effects). Products include:
Actifed with Codeine Cough Syrup.. 752
Cheracol Cough Syrup ... 1863
Codimal PH Syrup ... 846
Dimetane-DC Cough Syrup ... 1857
Empirin with Codeine Phosphate Nos. 2, 3 & 4 ... 764
Fiorinal with Codeine Capsules ... 2008
Isoclor Expectorant ... 982
Naldecon CX Adult Liquid ... ▣ 521
Novahistine DH ... 1342
Novahistine Expectorant ... 1343
Nucofed Capsules ... 2219
Nucofed Expectorant ... 2219
Nucofed Pediatric Expectorant ... 2220
Nucofed Syrup ... 2219
Phenaphen with Codeine Capsules 1865
Phenaphen-650 with Codeine Tablets ... 1866
Phenergan with Codeine ... 2497
Phenergan VC with Codeine ... 2501
Robitussin A-C Syrup ... 1875
Robitussin-DAC Syrup ... 1875
Ryna ... ▣ 741
Soma Compound w/Codeine Tablets ... 2390
Triaminic Expectorant w/Codeine .. 1996
Tussi-Organidin Liquid ... 2391
Tylenol with Codeine ... 1381

Codeine Polistirex (Additive CNS depressant effects).
No products indexed under this heading.

Dezocine (Additive CNS depressant effects).

Diazepam (Additive CNS depressant effects). Products include:
Valium Injectable ... 1937
Valium Tablets ... 1939
Valrelease Capsules ... 1923

Droperidol (Additive CNS depressant effects). Products include:
Inapsine Injection ... 1140
Innovar Injection ... 1141

Enflurane (Additive CNS depressant effects). Products include:
Ethrane ... 599

Estazolam (Additive CNS depressant effects). Products include:
ProSom Tablets ... 554

Ethchlorvynol (Additive CNS depressant effects). Products include:
Placidyl Capsules ... 553

Ethinamate (Additive CNS depressant effects).
No products indexed under this heading.

Fentanyl (Additive CNS depressant effects). Products include:
Duragesic Transdermal System ... 1133

Fentanyl Citrate (Additive CNS depressant effects). Products include:
Innovar Injection ... 1141
Sublimaze Injection ... 1146

Fluphenazine Decanoate (Additive CNS depressant effects). Products include:
Prolixin Decanoate ... 1795

Fluphenazine Enanthate (Additive CNS depressant effects). Products include:
Prolixin Enanthate ... 1796

Fluphenazine Hydrochloride (Additive CNS depressant effects). Products include:
Prolixin Elixir ... 1793
Prolixin Injection ... 1791
Prolixin Oral Concentrate ... 1792
Prolixin Tablets ... 1793

Flurazepam Hydrochloride (Additive CNS depressant effects). Products include:
Dalmane Capsules ... 1927

Furazolidone (Additive CNS depressant effects). Products include:
Furoxone ... 1855

Glutethimide (Additive CNS depressant effects).
No products indexed under this heading.

Haloperidol (Additive CNS depressant effects). Products include:
Haldol Injection, Tablets and Concentrate ... 1373

Haloperidol Decanoate (Additive CNS depressant effects). Products include:
Haldol Decanoate ... 1375

Hydrocodone Bitartrate (Additive CNS depressant effects). Products include:
Anexsia 5/500 Tablets ... 2196
Anexsia 7.5/650 Tablets ... 2197
Azdone Tablets ... 844
Codiclear DH Syrup ... 845
Codimal DH Syrup ... 846
Damason-P ... 1356
Hycodan Syrup, Tablets ... 927
Hycomine Compound Tablets ... 929
Hycomine Syrup ... 927
Hycotuss Expectorant Syrup ... 930
Hydrocet Capsules ... 835
Lortab ASA Tablets ... 2414
Lortab ... 2412
Ru-Tuss with Hydrocodone ... 694
Triaminic Expectorant DH ... 1995
Vicodin Tablets ... 1187
Vicodin ES Tablets ... 1189
Zydone Capsules ... 941

Hydrocodone Polistirex (Additive CNS depressant effects). Products include:
Tussionex Extended-Release Suspension ... 988

Hydroxyzine Hydrochloride (Additive CNS depressant effects). Products include:
Atarax Tablets & Syrup ... 1941
Marax Tablets & DF Syrup ... 1954
Vistaril Intramuscular Solution ... 1970

Isocarboxazid (Additive CNS depressant effects). Products include:
Marplan Tablets ... 1906

Isoflurane (Additive CNS depressant effects). Products include:
Forane ... 600

Ketamine Hydrochloride (Additive CNS depressant effects). Products include:
Ketalar ... 1726

Levorphanol Tartrate (Additive CNS depressant effects). Products include:
Levo-Dromoran ... 1906

Loxapine Hydrochloride (Additive CNS depressant effects). Products include:
Loxitane ... 1213

Loxapine Succinate (Additive CNS depressant effects). Products include:
Loxitane Capsules ... 1213

Meperidine Hydrochloride (Additive CNS depressant effects). Products include:
Demerol ... 2047
Mepergan Injection ... 2479

Mephobarbital (Additive CNS depressant effects). Products include:
Mebaral Tablets ... 2061

Meprobamate (Additive CNS depressant effects). Products include:
Deprol Tablets ... 2382
Equagesic Tablets ... 2451
Miltown Tablets ... 2386
PMB 200 and PMB 400 ... 2504

Mesoridazine (Additive CNS depressant effects). Products include:
Serentil ... 686

Methadone Hydrochloride (Additive CNS depressant effects). Products include:
Dolophine Hydrochloride Ampoules & Vials ... 1260
Dolophine Hydrochloride Tablets ... 1261
Methadone Hydrochloride Diskets .. 1284
Methadone Hydrochloride Oral Solution & Tablets ... 1987

Methohexital Sodium (Additive CNS depressant effects). Products include:
Brevital Sodium Vials ... 1248

Methoxyflurane (Additive CNS depressant effects).
No products indexed under this heading.

Midazolam Hydrochloride (Additive CNS depressant effects). Products include:
Versed Injection ... 1924

Molindone Hydrochloride (Additive CNS depressant effects). Products include:
Moban Tablets & Concentrate ... 932

Morphine Sulfate (Additive CNS depressant effects). Products include:
Astramorph/PF Injection, USP (Preservative-Free) ... 618
Duramorph ... 960
Infumorph 200 and Infumorph 500 Sterile Solutions ... 962
MS Contin Tablets ... 1814
MSIR ... 1817
Oramorph SR (Morphine Sulfate Sustained Release Tablets) ... 1988
Roxanol ... 1991

Opium Alkaloids (Additive CNS depressant effects). Products include:
B & O No. 15A & No. 16A Supprettes ... 2395
Pantopon Injectable ... 1911

Oxazepam (Additive CNS depressant effects). Products include:
Serax Capsules ... 2522
Serax Tablets ... 2522

Oxycodone Hydrochloride (Additive CNS depressant effects). Products include:
Percocet Tablets ... 950
Percodan ... 951
Roxicodone Tablets, Oral Solution & Intensol (Oxycodone) ... 1992
Tylox Capsules ... 1382

Pentobarbital Sodium (Additive CNS depressant effects). Products include:
Nembutal Sodium Capsules ... 534
Nembutal Sodium Solution ... 536
Nembutal Sodium Suppositories ... 538

Perphenazine (Additive CNS depressant effects). Products include:
Etrafon ... 2087
Triavil Tablets ... 1556
Trilafon ... 2123

Phenelzine Sulfate (Additive CNS depressant effects). Products include:
Nardil ... 1742

Phenobarbital (Additive CNS depressant effects). Products include:
Arco-Lase Plus Tablets ... 607
Bellergal-S Tablets ... 1998
Bronkolixir ... ▣ 761
Bronkotabs Tablets ... ▣ 762
Donnatal ... 1858
Donnatal Extentabs ... 1859
Donnatal Tablets ... 1858
Donnazyme Tablets ... 1860
Kinesed Tablets ... 2272
Phenobarbital Elixir and Tablets ... 1293
Primatene Tablets-P Formula ... 2421
Quadrinal Tablets ... 1183
Tedral SA ... 1765

Prazepam (Additive CNS depressant effects). Products include:
Centrax ... 1693

Prochlorperazine (Additive CNS depressant effects). Products include:
Compazine ... 2201

Promethazine Hydrochloride (Additive CNS depressant effects). Products include:
Mepergan Injection ... 2479
Phenergan with Codeine ... 2497
Phenergan with Dextromethorphan 2499
Phenergan Injection ... 2493
Phenergan Suppositories ... 2496
Phenergan Syrup ... 2495
Phenergan Tablets ... 2496
Phenergan VC ... 2500
Phenergan VC with Codeine ... 2501

Propofol (Additive CNS depressant effects). Products include:
Diprivan Injection ... 2267

Propoxyphene Hydrochloride (Additive CNS depressant effects). Products include:
Darvon ... 1256
Wygesic Tablets ... 2540

Propoxyphene Napsylate (Additive CNS depressant effects). Products include:
Darvon-N/Darvocet-N ... 1254

Quazepam (Additive CNS depressant effects). Products include:
Doral Tablets ... 2383

Scopolamine Hydrobromide (Increased incidence of sedation, hallucinations, and irrational behavior). Products include:
Donnagel ... ▣ 675
Donnagel-PG ... 1858
Donnatal ... 1858

Donnatal Extentabs 1859
Donnatal Tablets 1858
Donnazyme Tablets 1860
Isopto Hyoscine .... ⊙ 222
Murocoll-2 Sterile Ophthalmic Solution .... ⊙ 261
Ru-Tuss Tablets 693

Scopolamine Preparations (Increased incidence of sedation, hallucinations, and irrational behavior). Products include:
Transderm Scōp Transdermal Therapeutic System 887

Secobarbital Sodium (Additive CNS depressant effects). Products include:
Seconal Sodium Pulvules 1296

Selegiline Hydrochloride (Additive CNS depressant effects). Products include:
Eldepryl 2250

Sufentanil Citrate (Additive CNS depressant effects). Products include:
Sufenta Injection 1147

Temazepam (Additive CNS depressant effects). Products include:
Restoril Capsules 2023

Thiamylal Sodium (Additive CNS depressant effects). Products include:
Surital Ampoules, Steri-Vials 1764

Thioridazine Hydrochloride (Additive CNS depressant effects). Products include:
Mellaril 2011

Thiothixene (Additive CNS depressant effects). Products include:
Navane Capsules and Concentrate 1954
Navane Intramuscular 1956

Tranylcypromine Sulfate (Additive CNS depressant effects). Products include:
Parnate Tablets 2222

Triazolam (Additive CNS depressant effects). Products include:
Halcion Tablets 2340

Trifluoperazine Hydrochloride (Additive CNS depressant effects). Products include:
Stelazine 2226

ATIVAN TABLETS

(Lorazepam) 2434
May interact with barbiturates and certain other agents. Compounds in these categories include:

Alcohol (Depressant effect).

Aprobarbital (Depressant effect). Products include:
Alurate Elixir 1883

Butabarbital (Depressant effect). Products include:
Pyridium Plus 1764

Butalbital (Depressant effect). Products include:
Esgic-Plus Tablets 1002
Esgic Tablets & Capsules 1001
Fioricet Tablets 2006
Fiorinal Capsules 2007
Fiorinal with Codeine Capsules 2008
Fiorinal Tablets 2007
Phrenilin 838
Sedapap Tablets 50 mg/650 mg .. 1360

Mephobarbital (Depressant effect). Products include:
Mebaral Tablets 2061

Pentobarbital Sodium (Depressant effect). Products include:
Nembutal Sodium Capsules 534
Nembutal Sodium Solution 536
Nembutal Sodium Suppositories 538

Phenobarbital (Depressant effect). Products include:
Arco-Lase Plus Tablets 607
Bellergal-S Tablets 1998
Bronkolixir .... ▣ 761
Bronkotabs Tablets .... ▣ 762
Donnatal 1858
Donnatal Extentabs 1859
Donnatal Tablets 1858
Donnazyme Tablets 1860
Kinesed Tablets 2272
Phenobarbital Elixir and Tablets 1293
Primatene Tablets-P Formula 2421
Quadrinal Tablets 1183
Tedral SA 1765

Secobarbital Sodium (Depressant effect). Products include:
Seconal Sodium Pulvules 1296

Thiamylal Sodium (Depressant effect). Products include:
Surital Ampoules, Steri-Vials 1764

ATRAC-TAIN, MOISTURIZING CREAM

(Urea Peroxide, Lactic Acid) 2285
No interactions described in labeling.

ATRAC-TAIN, MOISTURIZING LOTION

(Urea Peroxide, Lactic Acid) 2285
No interactions described in labeling.

ATROHIST SPRINKLE CAPSULES

(Brompheniramine Maleate, Phenyltoloxamine Citrate, Phenylephrine Hydrochloride) 558
May interact with monoamine oxidase inhibitors, tricyclic antidepressants, beta blockers, veratrum alkaloids, central nervous system depressants, cardiac glycosides, and certain other agents. Compounds in these categories include:

Acebutolol Hydrochloride (Potentiates pressor effect). Products include:
Sectral Capsules 2520

Alcohol (Additive effect).

Alfentanil Hydrochloride (Additive effect). Products include:
Alfenta Injection 1131

Alprazolam (Additive effect). Products include:
Xanax Tablets 2367

Amitriptyline Hydrochloride (Antagonizes phenylephrine effects; additive CNS depressant effect). Products include:
Elavil 2269
Endep Tablets 1927
Etrafon 2087
Limbitrol 1933
Triavil Tablets 1556

Amoxapine (Antagonizes phenylephrine effects; additive CNS depressant effect). Products include:
Asendin Tablets 1196

Aprobarbital (Additive effect). Products include:
Alurate Elixir 1883

Atenolol (Potentiates pressor effect). Products include:
Tenoretic Tablets 1105
Tenormin Tablets and I.V. Injection 1107

Betaxolol Hydrochloride (Potentiates pressor effect). Products include:
Betoptic Sterile Ophthalmic Solution 569
Betoptic S Sterile Ophthalmic Suspension 570
Kerlone Tablets 2172

Buprenorphine (Additive effect).
No products indexed under this heading.

Buspirone Hydrochloride (Additive effect). Products include:
BuSpar 1401

Butabarbital (Additive effect). Products include:
Pyridium Plus 1764

Butalbital (Additive effect). Products include:
Esgic-Plus Tablets 1002
Esgic Tablets & Capsules 1001
Fioricet Tablets 2006
Fiorinal Capsules 2007
Fiorinal with Codeine Capsules 2008
Fiorinal Tablets 2007
Phrenilin 838
Sedapap Tablets 50 mg/650 mg .. 1360

Carteolol Hydrochloride (Potentiates pressor effect). Products include:
Cartrol Tablets 507

Chlordiazepoxide (Additive effect). Products include:
Libritabs Tablets 1930
Limbitrol 1933
Menrium Tablets 1934

Chlordiazepoxide Hydrochloride (Additive effect). Products include:
Librax Capsules 1929
Librium Capsules 1931
Librium Injectable 1932

Chlorpromazine (Additive effect). Products include:
Thorazine 2234

Chlorprothixene (Additive effect). Products include:
Taractan Tablets 1920

Chlorprothixene Hydrochloride (Additive effect). Products include:
Taractan 1920

Clomipramine Hydrochloride (Antagonizes phenylephrine effects; additive CNS depressant effect). Products include:
Anafranil Capsules 650

Clorazepate Dipotassium (Additive effect). Products include:
Tranxene 556

Codeine (Additive effect). Products include:
Calcidrine Syrup 506

Codeine Phosphate (Additive effect). Products include:
Actifed with Codeine Cough Syrup .. 752
Cheracol Cough Syrup 1853
Codimal PH Syrup 846
Dimetane-DC Cough Syrup 1857
Empirin with Codeine Phosphate Nos. 2, 3 & 4 764
Fiorinal with Codeine Capsules 2008
Isoclor Expectorant 982
Naldecon CX Adult Liquid .... ▣ 521
Novahistine DH 1342
Novahistine Expectorant 1343
Nucofed Capsules 2219
Nucofed Expectorant 2219
Nucofed Pediatric Expectorant 2220
Nucofed Syrup 2219
Phenaphen with Codeine Capsules 1865
Phenaphen-650 with Codeine Tablets 1866
Phenergan with Codeine 2497
Phenergan VC with Codeine 2501
Robitussin A-C Syrup 1875
Robitussin-DAC Syrup 1875
Ryna .... ▣ 741
Soma Compound w/Codeine Tablets 2390
Triaminic Expectorant w/Codeine .. 1996
Tussi-Organidin Liquid 2391
Tylenol with Codeine 1381

Codeine Polistirex (Additive effect).
No products indexed under this heading.

Cryptenamine Preparations (Reduced hypotensive effects).

Desipramine Hydrochloride (Antagonizes phenylephrine effects; additive CNS depressant effect). Products include:
Norpramin Tablets 1340

Deslanoside (May increase possibility of cardiac arrhythmias).
No products indexed under this heading.

Dezocine (Additive effect).

Diazepam (Additive effect). Products include:
Valium Injectable 1937
Valium Tablets 1939
Valrelease Capsules 1923

Digitoxin (May increase possibility of cardiac arrhythmias). Products include:
Crystodigin Tablets 1253

Digoxin (May increase possibility of cardiac arrhythmias). Products include:
Lanoxicaps 772
Lanoxin Elixir Pediatric 775
Lanoxin Injection 778
Lanoxin Injection Pediatric 781
Lanoxin Tablets 783

Doxepin Hydrochloride (Antagonizes phenylephrine effects; additive CNS depressant effect). Products include:
Sinequan 1960

Droperidol (Additive effect). Products include:
Inapsine Injection 1140
Innovar Injection 1141

Enflurane (Additive effect). Products include:
Ethrane 599

Esmolol Hydrochloride (Potentiates pressor effect). Products include:
Brevibloc Injection 942

Estazolam (Additive effect). Products include:
ProSom Tablets 554

Ethchlorvynol (Additive effect). Products include:
Placidyl Capsules 553

Ethinamate (Additive effect).
No products indexed under this heading.

Fentanyl (Additive effect). Products include:
Duragesic Transdermal System 1133

Fentanyl Citrate (Additive effect). Products include:
Innovar Injection 1141
Sublimaze Injection 1146

Fluphenazine Decanoate (Additive effect). Products include:
Prolixin Decanoate 1795

Fluphenazine Enanthate (Additive effect). Products include:
Prolixin Enanthate 1796

Fluphenazine Hydrochloride (Additive effect). Products include:
Prolixin Elixir 1793
Prolixin Injection 1791
Prolixin Oral Concentrate 1792
Prolixin Tablets 1793

Flurazepam Hydrochloride (Additive effect). Products include:
Dalmane Capsules 1927

Furazolidone (Prolongs and intensifies anticholinergic effects; concurrent use is contraindicated). Products include:
Furoxone 1855

Glutethimide (Additive effect).
No products indexed under this heading.

Guanethidine Monosulfate (Reduced hypotensive effects). Products include:
Esimil Tablets 864
Ismelin Tablets 869

Haloperidol (Additive effect). Products include:
Haldol Injection, Tablets and Concentrate 1373

Haloperidol Decanoate (Additive effect). Products include:
Haldol Decanoate 1375

Hydrocodone Bitartrate (Additive effect). Products include:
Anexsia 5/500 Tablets 2196
Anexsia 7.5/650 Tablets 2197
Azdōne Tablets 844
Codiclear DH Syrup 845
Codimal DH Syrup 846
Damason-P 1356
Hycodan Syrup, Tablets 927
Hycomine Compound Tablets 929

Hycomine Syrup ... 927
Hycotuss Expectorant Syrup ... 930
Hydrocet Capsules ... 835
Lortab ASA Tablets ... 2414
Lortab ... 2412
Ru-Tuss with Hydrocodone ... 694
Triaminic Expectorant DH ... 1995
Vicodin Tablets ... 1187
Vicodin ES Tablets ... 1189
Zydone Capsules ... 941

Hydrocodone Polistirex (Additive effect). Products include:
Tussionex Extended-Release Suspension ... 988

Hydroxyzine Hydrochloride (Additive effect). Products include:
Atarax Tablets & Syrup ... 1941
Marax Tablets & DF Syrup ... 1954
Vistaril Intramuscular Solution ... 1970

Imipramine Hydrochloride (Antagonizes phenylephrine effects; additive CNS depressant effect). Products include:
Tofranil Ampuls ... 1038
Tofranil Tablets ... 1039

Imipramine Pamoate (Antagonizes phenylephrine effects; additive CNS depressant effect). Products include:
Tofranil-PM Capsules ... 1041

Isocarboxazid (Prolongs and intensifies anticholinergic effects; concurrent use is contraindicated). Products include:
Marplan Tablets ... 1906

Isoflurane (Additive effect). Products include:
Forane ... 600

Ketamine Hydrochloride (Additive effect). Products include:
Ketalar ... 1726

Labetalol Hydrochloride (Potentiates pressor effect). Products include:
Normodyne Injection ... 2108
Normodyne Tablets ... 2110
Normozide Tablets ... 2112
Trandate HCT Tablets ... 579
Trandate Injection ... 577
Trandate Tablets ... 579

Levorphanol Tartrate (Additive effect). Products include:
Levo-Dromoran ... 1906

Lorazepam (Additive effect). Products include:
Ativan Injection ... 2432
Ativan Tablets ... 2434

Loxapine Hydrochloride (Additive effect). Products include:
Loxitane ... 1213

Loxapine Succinate (Additive effect). Products include:
Loxitane Capsules ... 1213

Maprotiline Hydrochloride (Antagonizes phenylephrine effects; additive CNS depressant effect). Products include:
Ludiomil Tablets ... 874

Mecamylamine Hydrochloride (Reduced hypotensive effects). Products include:
Inversine Tablets ... 1492

Meperidine Hydrochloride (Additive effect). Products include:
Demerol ... 2047
Mepergan Injection ... 2479

Mephobarbital (Additive effect). Products include:
Mebaral Tablets ... 2061

Meprobamate (Additive effect). Products include:
Deprol Tablets ... 2382
Equagesic Tablets ... 2451
Miltown Tablets ... 2386
PMB 200 and PMB 400 ... 2504

Mesoridazine (Additive effect). Products include:
Serentil ... 686

Methadone Hydrochloride (Additive effect). Products include:
Dolophine Hydrochloride Ampoules & Vials ... 1260
Dolophine Hydrochloride Tablets ... 1261
Methadone Hydrochloride Diskets .. 1284
Methadone Hydrochloride Oral Solution & Tablets ... 1987

Methohexital Sodium (Additive effect). Products include:
Brevital Sodium Vials ... 1248

Methoxyflurane (Additive effect).
No products indexed under this heading.

Methyldopa (Reduced hypotensive effects). Products include:
Aldoclor Tablets ... 1413
Aldomet Oral ... 1415
Aldoril Tablets ... 1418

Methyldopate Hydrochloride (Reduced hypotensive effect). Products include:
Aldomet Ester HCl Injection ... 1417

Metoprolol Tartrate (Potentiates pressor effect). Products include:
Lopressor Ampuls ... 1032
Lopressor HCT Tablets ... 1034
Lopressor Tablets ... 1032

Midazolam Hydrochloride (Additive effect). Products include:
Versed Injection ... 1924

Molindone Hydrochloride (Additive effect). Products include:
Moban Tablets & Concentrate ... 932

Morphine Sulfate (Additive effect). Products include:
Astramorph/PF Injection, USP (Preservative-Free) ... 618
Duramorph ... 960
Infumorph 200 and Infumorph 500 Sterile Solutions ... 962
MS Contin Tablets ... 1814
MSIR ... 1817
Oramorph SR (Morphine Sulfate Sustained Release Tablets) ... 1988
Roxanol ... 1991

Nadolol (Potentiates pressor effect). Products include:
Corgard Tablets ... 701
Corzide Tablets ... 702

Nortriptyline Hydrochloride (Antagonizes phenylephrine effects; additive CNS depressant effect). Products include:
Pamelor ... 2019

Opium Alkaloids (Additive effect). Products include:
B & O No. 15A & No. 16A Supprettes ... 2395
Pantopon Injectable ... 1911

Oxazepam (Additive effect). Products include:
Serax Capsules ... 2522
Serax Tablets ... 2522

Oxycodone Hydrochloride (Additive effect). Products include:
Percocet Tablets ... 950
Percodan ... 951
Roxicodone Tablets, Oral Solution & Intensol (Oxycodone) ... 1992
Tylox Capsules ... 1382

Penbutolol Sulfate (Potentiates pressor effect). Products include:
Levatol ... 1832

Pentobarbital Sodium (Additive effect). Products include:
Nembutal Sodium Capsules ... 534
Nembutal Sodium Solution ... 536
Nembutal Sodium Suppositories ... 538

Perphenazine (Additive effect). Products include:
Etrafon ... 2087
Triavil Tablets ... 1556
Trilafon ... 2123

Phenelzine Sulfate (Prolongs and intensifies anticholinergic effects; concurrent use is contraindicated). Products include:
Nardil ... 1742

Phenobarbital (Additive effect). Products include:
Arco-Lase Plus Tablets ... 607
Bellergal-S Tablets ... 1998
Bronkolixir ... 761
Bronkotabs Tablets ... 762
Donnatal ... 1858
Donnatal Extentabs ... 1859
Donnatal Tablets ... 1858
Donnazyme Tablets ... 1860
Kinesed Tablets ... 2272
Phenobarbital Elixir and Tablets ... 1293
Primatene Tablets-P Formula ... 2421
Quadrinal Tablets ... 1183
Tedral SA ... 1765

Pindolol (Potentiates pressor effect). Products include:
Visken Tablets ... 2036

Prazepam (Additive effect). Products include:
Centrax ... 1693

Prochlorperazine (Additive effect). Products include:
Compazine ... 2201

Promethazine Hydrochloride (Additive effect). Products include:
Mepergan Injection ... 2479
Phenergan with Codeine ... 2497
Phenergan with Dextromethorphan 2499
Phenergan Injection ... 2493
Phenergan Suppositories ... 2496
Phenergan Syrup ... 2495
Phenergan Tablets ... 2496
Phenergan VC ... 2500
Phenergan VC with Codeine ... 2501

Propofol (Additive effect). Products include:
Diprivan Injection ... 2267

Propoxyphene Hydrochloride (Additive effect). Products include:
Darvon ... 1256
Wygesic Tablets ... 2540

Propoxyphene Napsylate (Additive effect). Products include:
Darvon-N/Darvocet-N ... 1254

Propranolol Hydrochloride (Potentiates pressor effect). Products include:
Inderal ... 2459
Inderal LA Long Acting Capsules ... 2461
Inderide Tablets ... 2463
Inderide LA Long Acting Capsules .. 2465

Protriptyline Hydrochloride (Antagonizes phenylephrine effects; additive CNS depressant effect). Products include:
Vivactil Tablets ... 1567

Quazepam (Additive effect). Products include:
Doral Tablets ... 2383

Reserpine (Reduced hypotensive effects). Products include:
Diupres Tablets ... 1461
Hydromox R Tablets ... 1209
Hydropres Tablets ... 1485
Renese-R Tablets ... 1786
Salutensin/Salutensin-Demi ... 719
Ser-Ap-Es Tablets ... 881
Serpasil Tablets ... 883
Serpasil-Apresoline Tablets ... 884
Serpasil-Esidrix Tablets ... 886

Secobarbital Sodium (Additive effect). Products include:
Seconal Sodium Pulvules ... 1296

Selegiline Hydrochloride (Prolongs and intensifies anticholinergic effects; concurrent use is contraindicated). Products include:
Eldepryl ... 2250

Sufentanil Citrate (Additive effect). Products include:
Sufenta Injection ... 1147

Temazepam (Additive effect). Products include:
Restoril Capsules ... 2023

Thiamylal Sodium (Additive effect). Products include:
Surital Ampoules, Steri-Vials ... 1764

Thioridazine Hydrochloride (Additive effect). Products include:
Mellaril ... 2011

Thiothixene (Additive effect). Products include:
Navane Capsules and Concentrate 1954
Navane Intramuscular ... 1956

Timolol Maleate (Potentiates pressor effect). Products include:
Blocadren Tablets ... 1429
Timolide Tablets ... 1547
Timoptic in Ocudose ... 1552
Timoptic Sterile Ophthalmic Solution ... 1550

Tranylcypromine Sulfate (Prolongs and intensifies anticholinergic effects; concurrent use is contraindicated). Products include:
Parnate Tablets ... 2222

Triazolam (Additive effect). Products include:
Halcion Tablets ... 2340

Trifluoperazine Hydrochloride (Additive effect). Products include:
Stelazine ... 2226

Trimipramine Maleate (Antagonizes phenylephrine effects; additive CNS depressant effect). Products include:
Surmontil Capsules ... 2524

ATROMID-S CAPSULES
(Clofibrate) ... 2435
May interact with anticoagulants and certain other agents. Compounds in these categories include:

Dicumarol (To prevent bleeding complications, anticoagulant dosage should be reduced generally by one-half). Products include:
Dicumarol Tablets ... 516

Heparin Calcium (To prevent bleeding complications, anticoagulant dosage should be reduced generally by one-half). Products include:
Calciparine Injection ... 925

Heparin Sodium (To prevent bleeding complications, anticoagulant dosage should be reduced generally by one-half). Products include:
Heparin Lock Flush Solution ... 2456
Heparin Sodium Vials ... 1264
Heparin Sodium Injection ... 2457
Heparin Sodium Injection, USP, Sterile Solution ... 2342

Lovastatin (Potential for fulminant rhabdomyolysis, myopathy, and acute renal failure). Products include:
Mevacor Tablets ... 1505

Phenytoin (Atromid-S may displace phenytoin from its binding site). Products include:
Dilantin Infatabs ... 1710
Dilantin-30 Pediatric/Dilantin-125 Suspension ... 1713

Phenytoin Sodium (Atromid-S may displace phenytoin from its binding site). Products include:
Dilantin Kapseals ... 1708
Dilantin Parenteral ... 1712
Dilantin with Phenobarbital Kapseals ... 1715

Tolbutamide (Increased hypoglycemic effect; Atromid-S may displace tolbutamide from its binding site). Products include:
Orinase Tablets ... 2354

Warfarin Sodium (To prevent bleeding complications, anticoagulant dosage should be reduced generally by one-half). Products include:
Coumadin Injection & Tablets ... 944
Panwarfin Tablets ... 547

ATROPINE SULFATE STERILE OPHTHALMIC SOLUTION AND S.O.P. STERILE OPHTHALMIC OINTMENT
(Atropine Sulfate) .... ◉ 239
No interactions described in labeling.

ATROVENT INHALATION AEROSOL
(Ipratropium Bromide) 675
No interactions described in labeling.

ATTENUVAX
(Measles Virus Vaccine Live) 1424
May interact with:

Azathioprine (Contraindication). Products include:
- Imuran 768

Cyclosporine (Contraindication). Products include:
- Sandimmune 2024

Immune Globulin (Human) (Contraindication). Products include:
- MICRhoGAM Rh_0(D) Immune Globulin (Human) 1650
- RhoGAM Rh_0(D) Immune Globulin (Human) 1651

Immune Globulin Intravenous (Human) (Contraindication). Products include:
- Gamimune N Immune Globulin Intravenous (Human)........................ 1572
- Gammagard Immune Globulin, Intravenous (Human)........................ 658
- Iveegam 1129
- Sandoglobulin I.V. 2027

Muromonab-CD3 (Contraindication). Products include:
- Orthoclone OKT3 Sterile Solution .. 1645

AUGMENTIN TABLETS, POWDER FOR ORAL SUSPENSION, AND CHEWABLE TABLETS
(Amoxicillin, Clavulanate Potassium) 2198
May interact with:

Allopurinol (Substantially increased incidence of rashes). Products include:
- Zyloprim Tablets 830

Disulfiram (Co-administration should be avoided). Products include:
- Antabuse Tablets.. 2429

Probenecid (Delays amoxicillin excretion). Products include:
- Benemid Tablets 1426
- ColBENEMID Tablets 1436
- Wycillin Injection and Probenecid Tablets 2539

AURALGAN OTIC SOLUTION
(Antipyrine, Benzocaine, Glycerin) 2437
No interactions described in labeling.

AUREOMYCIN OPHTHALMIC OINTMENT 1.0%
(Chlortetracycline Hydrochloride) .. ◉ 308
No interactions described in labeling.

AURUM - THE GOLD LOTION
(Methyl Salicylate, Menthol, Camphor) .... ⊞ 508
No interactions described in labeling.

AVEENO ANTI-ITCH CONCENTRATED LOTION
(Calamine, Pramoxine Hydrochloride)...................................... ⊞ 683
No interactions described in labeling.

AVEENO ANTI-ITCH CREAM
(Calamine, Pramoxine Hydrochloride)...................................... ⊞ 683
No interactions described in labeling.

AXID PULVULES
(Nizatidine) 1246
May interact with:

Aspirin (Increased serum salicylate levels when nizatidine is given concurrently with very high doses (3,900 mg) of aspirin). Products include:
- Alka-Seltzer Effervescent Antacid and Pain Reliever 1568
- Alka-Seltzer Extra Strength Effervescent Antacid and Pain Reliever 1570
- Alka-Seltzer (Flavored) Effervescent Antacid and Pain Reliever 1569
- Alka-Seltzer Plus Cold Medicine .... ⊞ 623
- Alka-Seltzer Plus Night-Time Cold Medicine .... ⊞ 623
- Alka Seltzer Plus Sinus Allergy Medicine .... ⊞ 624
- Anacin Coated Analgesic Caplets 2417
- Anacin Coated Analgesic Tablets 2417
- Anacin Maximum Strength Analgesic Coated Tablets.......................... 2417
- Maximum Strength Arthritis Pain Formula By the Makers of Anacin Analgesic Tablets and Caplets...... 2418
- Arthritis Pain Formula by the Makers of Anacin Analgesic Tablets and Caplets .... ⊞ 747
- Arthritis Strength BC Powder.......... ⊞ 516
- Ascriptin A/D Caplets 1850
- Regular Strength Ascriptin Tablets 1850
- Azdōne Tablets....................................... 844
- BC Powder .... ⊞ 517
- BC Cold Powder .... ⊞ 517
- Children's Bayer Chewable Aspirin .... ⊞ 564
- Genuine Bayer Aspirin Tablets & Caplets .... ⊞ 564
- Maximum Bayer Aspirin Tablets & Caplets .... ⊞ 566
- Bayer Plus Aspirin Tablets............... ⊞ 567
- Therapy Bayer Aspirin Caplets ...... ⊞ 568
- 8 Hour Bayer Timed-Release Aspirin .... ⊞ 566
- Arthritis Strength Bufferin Analgesic Caplets 744
- Extra Strength Bufferin Analgesic Tablets 745
- Bufferin Analgesic Tablets and Caplets 743
- Cama Arthritis Pain Reliever............ ⊞ 685
- Damason-P 1356
- Easprin 1719
- Ecotrin Enteric Coated Aspirin Maximum Strength Tablets and Caplets 2189
- Ecotrin Enteric Coated Aspirin Regular Strength Tablets and Caplets 2189
- Empirin Aspirin.................................. ⊞ 541
- Empirin with Codeine Phosphate Nos. 2, 3 & 4 764
- Equagesic Tablets 2451
- Excedrin Extra-Strength Analgesic Tablets & Caplets 749
- 4-Way Cold Tablets................................ 750
- Fiorinal Capsules 2007
- Fiorinal with Codeine Capsules 2008
- Fiorinal Tablets 2007
- Lortab ASA Tablets............................. 2414
- Momentum Muscular Backache Formula .... ⊞ 751
- Norgesic... 1314
- Norwich Extra-Strength Aspirin...... ⊞ 546
- Norwich Regular Strength Aspirin ⊞ 547
- P-A-C Analgesic Tablets .... ⊞ 669
- Percodan 951
- Robaxisal Tablets................................. 1872
- Sine-Off Sinus Medicine Tablets-Aspirin Formula .... ⊞ 722
- Soma Compound w/Codeine Tablets 2390
- Soma Compound Tablets.................... 2389
- St. Joseph Adult Chewable Aspirin (81 mg.) .... ⊞ 703
- Synalgos-DC Capsules........................ 2525
- Talwin Compound 2072
- Ursinus Inlay-Tabs............................. ⊞ 691
- Vanquish Analgesic Caplets .... ⊞ 574
- Zorprin Tablets 698

Aspirin, Enteric Coated (Increased serum salicylate levels when nizatidine is given concurrently with very high doses (3,900 mg) of aspirin). Products include:
- Therapy Bayer Aspirin Caplets ...... ⊞ 568
- Ecotrin 2189

AYGESTIN TABLETS
(Norethindrone Acetate).....................2437
No interactions described in labeling.

AYR SALINE NASAL DROPS
(Sodium Chloride)............................. ⊞ 507
No interactions described in labeling.

AYR SALINE NASAL MIST
(Sodium Chloride)............................. ⊞ 507
No interactions described in labeling.

AZACTAM FOR INJECTION
(Aztreonam) 2252
May interact with aminoglycosides and certain other agents. Compounds in these categories include:

Amikacin Sulfate (Renal function should be monitored if used concurrently or if higher dosages of aminoglycosides are used). Products include:
- Amikin Injectable 602

Cefoxitin Sodium (Beta-lactamase inducing antibiotics may antagonize aztreonam). Products include:
- Mefoxin 1498
- Mefoxin Premixed Intravenous Solution 1500

Gentamicin Sulfate (Renal function should be monitored if used concurrently or if higher dosages of aminoglycosides are used). Products include:
- Garamycin Injectable 2093
- Garamycin Ophthalmic .... ◉ 305
- Genoptic Liquifilm Sterile Ophthalmic Solution .... ◉ 247
- Genoptic S.O.P. Sterile Ophthalmic Ointment.................................. ◉ 247
- Gentacidin Ointment .... ◉ 273
- Gentacidin Solution........................... ◉ 273
- Gentak Ointment & Solution........... ◉ 208
- G-mycitin Creme and Ointment 0.1% 1770
- Pred-G Liquifilm Sterile Ophthalmic Suspension .... ◉ 252
- Pred-G S.O.P. Sterile Ophthalmic Ointment... ◉ 253

Kanamycin Sulfate (Renal function should be monitored if used concurrently or if higher dosages of aminoglycosides are used). Products include:
- Kantrex Injection 601
- Kantrex Pediatric Injection.................. 601

Streptomycin Sulfate (Renal function should be monitored if used concurrently or if higher dosages of aminoglycosides are used).
- No products indexed under this heading.

Tobramycin (Renal function should be monitored if used concurrently or if higher dosages of aminoglycosides are used). Products include:
- TobraDex Ophthalmic Suspension and Ointment.................................... ◉ 228
- Tobrex Ophthalmic Ointment and Solution 572

Tobramycin Sulfate (Renal function should be monitored if used concurrently or if higher dosages of aminoglycosides are used). Products include:
- Nebcin Vials, Hyporets & ADD-Vantage 1286

AZDŌNE TABLETS
(Hydrocodone Bitartrate, Aspirin)...... 844
May interact with narcotic analgesics, monoamine oxidase inhibitors, tranquilizers, central nervous system depressants, psychotropics, anticholinergics, tricyclic antidepressants, oral anticoagulants, oral hypoglycemic agents, insulin, non-steroidal anti-inflammatory agents, corticosteroids, and certain other agents. Compounds in these categories include:

Alcohol (Additive CNS depression).

Alfentanil Hydrochloride (Additive CNS depression; the dose of one or both agents should be reduced). Products include:
- Alfenta Injection 1131

Alprazolam (Additive CNS depression; the dose of one or both agents should be reduced). Products include:
- Xanax Tablets 2367

Amitriptyline Hydrochloride (Additive CNS depression; the dose of one or both agents should be reduced; increased effect of either hydrocodone or antidepressant). Products include:
- Elavil 2269
- Endep Tablets 1927
- Etrafon 2087
- Limbitrol 1933
- Triavil Tablets 1556

Amoxapine (Additive CNS depression; the dose of one or both agents should be reduced; increased effect of either hydrocodone or antidepressant). Products include:
- Asendin Tablets 1196

Aprobarbital (Additive CNS depression; the dose of one or both agents should be reduced). Products include:
- Alurate Elixir 1883

Atropine Sulfate (May produce paralytic ileus). Products include:
- Arco-Lase Plus Tablets 607
- Atropine Sulfate Sterile Ophthalmic Solution and S.O.P. Sterile Ophthalmic Ointment.................... ◉ 239
- Donnagel .... ⊞ 675
- Donnagel-PG 1858
- Donnatal 1858
- Donnatal Extentabs............................. 1859
- Donnatal Tablets 1858
- Donnazyme Tablets 1860
- Isopto Atropine.................................. ◉ 218
- Lomotil 2174
- Motofen Tablets..................................... 836
- Ru-Tuss Tablets..................................... 693
- Urised Tablets...................................... 2396

Belladonna Alkaloids (May produce paralytic ileus). Products include:
- Bellergal-S Tablets 1998
- Hyland's Bed Wetting Tablets .... ⊞ 728
- Hyland's Teething Tablets .... ⊞ 728
- Kinesed Tablets 2272

Benztropine Mesylate (May produce paralytic ileus). Products include:
- Cogentin 1435

Betamethasone Acetate (Potential for enhanced effect). Products include:
- Celestone Soluspan Suspension 2081

Betamethasone Sodium Phosphate (Potential for enhanced effect). Products include:
- Celestone Soluspan Suspension 2081

Biperiden (May produce paralytic ileus). Products include:
- Akineton 1171

Buprenorphine (Additive CNS depression; the dose of one or both agents should be reduced).
- No products indexed under this heading.

Buspirone Hydrochloride (Additive CNS depression; the dose of one or both agents should be reduced). Products include:
BuSpar 1401

Butabarbital (Additive CNS depression; the dose of one or both agents should be reduced). Products include:
Pyridium Plus 1764

Butalbital (Additive CNS depression; the dose of one or both agents should be reduced). Products include:
Esgic-Plus Tablets 1002
Esgic Tablets & Capsules 1001
Fioricet Tablets 2006
Fiorinal Capsules 2007
Fiorinal with Codeine Capsules 2008
Fiorinal Tablets 2007
Phrenilin 838
Sedapap Tablets 50 mg/650 mg .. 1360

Chlordiazepoxide (Additive CNS depression; the dose of one or both agents should be reduced). Products include:
Libritabs Tablets 1930
Limbitrol 1933
Menrium Tablets 1934

Chlordiazepoxide Hydrochloride (Additive CNS depression; the dose of one or both agents should be reduced). Products include:
Librax Capsules 1929
Librium Capsules 1931
Librium Injectable 1932

Chlorpromazine (Additive CNS depression; the dose of one or both agents should be reduced). Products include:
Thorazine 2234

Chlorpropamide (Aspirin may enhance the effects of oral hypoglycemic agents). Products include:
Diabinese Tablets 1775

Chlorprothixene (Additive CNS depression; the dose of one or both agents should be reduced). Products include:
Taractan Tablets 1920

Chlorprothixene Hydrochloride (Additive CNS depression; the dose of one or both agents should be reduced). Products include:
Taractan 1920

Clidinium Bromide (May produce paralytic ileus). Products include:
Librax Capsules 1929
Quarzan Capsules 1937

Clomipramine Hydrochloride (Additive CNS depression; the dose of one or both agents should be reduced; increased effect of either hydrocodone or antidepressant). Products include:
Anafranil Capsules 650

Clorazepate Dipotassium (Additive CNS depression; the dose of one or both agents should be reduced). Products include:
Tranxene 556

Codeine (Additive CNS depression; the dose of one or both agents should be reduced). Products include:
Calcidrine Syrup 506

Codeine Phosphate (Additive CNS depression; the dose of one or both agents should be reduced). Products include:
Actifed with Codeine Cough Syrup.. 752
Cheracol Cough Syrup 1853
Codimal PH Syrup 846
Dimetane-DC Cough Syrup 1857
Empirin with Codeine Phosphate Nos. 2, 3 & 4 764
Fiorinal with Codeine Capsules 2008
Isoclor Expectorant 982
Naldecon CX Adult Liquid .... ◙ 521
Novahistine DH 1342
Novahistine Expectorant 1343
Nucofed Capsules 2219
Nucofed Expectorant 2219
Nucofed Pediatric Expectorant 2220
Nucofed Syrup 2219
Phenaphen with Codeine Capsules 1865
Phenaphen-650 with Codeine Tablets 1866
Phenergan with Codeine 2497
Phenergan VC with Codeine 2501
Robitussin A-C Syrup 1875
Robitussin-DAC Syrup 1875
Ryna .... ◙ 741
Soma Compound w/Codeine Tablets 2390
Triaminic Expectorant w/Codeine .. 1996
Tussi-Organidin Liquid 2391
Tylenol with Codeine 1381

Codeine Polistirex (Additive CNS depression; the dose of one or both agents should be reduced).
No products indexed under this heading.

Cortisone Acetate (Potential for enhanced effect). Products include:
Cortone Acetate Sterile Suspension 1437
Cortone Acetate Tablets 1439

Desipramine Hydrochloride (Additive CNS depression; the dose of one or both agents should be reduced; increased effect of either hydrocodone or antidepressant). Products include:
Norpramin Tablets 1340

Dexamethasone (Potential for enhanced effect). Products include:
AK-Trol Ointment & Suspension .... ⊙ 207
Decadron Elixir 1445
Decadron Tablets 1447
Decaspray Topical Aerosol 1459
Dexacidin .... ⊙ 272
Maxidex Sterile Ophthalmic Suspension .... ⊙ 223
Maxitrol Ophthalmic Ointment/Suspension .... ⊙ 223
TobraDex Ophthalmic Suspension and Ointment .... ⊙ 228

Dexamethasone Acetate (Potential for enhanced effect). Products include:
Dalalone D.P. Injectable 999
Decadron-LA Sterile Suspension 1457

Dexamethasone Sodium Phosphate (Potential for enhanced effect). Products include:
AK-Dex .... ⊙ 203
Decadron Phosphate Respihaler 1454
Decadron Phosphate Sterile Ophthalmic Ointment 1453
Decadron Phosphate Sterile Ophthalmic Solution 1453
Decadron Phosphate Topical Cream 1455
Decadron Phosphate Turbinaire 1456
Maxidex Sterile Ophthalmic Ointment .... ⊙ 222
NeoDecadron Sterile Ophthalmic Ointment 1517
NeoDecadron Sterile Ophthalmic Solution 1518
NeoDecadron Topical Cream 1518

Dezocine (Additive CNS depression; the dose of one or both agents should be reduced).

Diazepam (Additive CNS depression; the dose of one or both agents should be reduced). Products include:
Valium Injectable 1937
Valium Tablets 1939
Valrelease Capsules 1923

Diclofenac Sodium (Potential for enhanced effect). Products include:
Voltaren Ophthalmic Sterile Ophthalmic Solution .... ⊙ 268
Voltaren Tablets 1042

Dicumarol (Aspirin may enhance the effects of oral anticoagulant). Products include:
Dicumarol Tablets 516

Dicyclomine Hydrochloride (May produce paralytic ileus). Products include:
Bentyl 1322

Doxepin Hydrochloride (Additive CNS depression; the dose of one or both agents should be reduced; increased effect of either hydrocodone or antidepressant). Products include:
Sinequan 1960

Droperidol (Additive CNS depression; the dose of one or both agents should be reduced). Products include:
Inapsine Injection 1140
Innovar Injection 1141

Enflurane (Additive CNS depression; the dose of one or both agents should be reduced). Products include:
Ethrane 599

Estazolam (Additive CNS depression; the dose of one or both agents should be reduced). Products include:
ProSom Tablets 554

Ethchlorvynol (Additive CNS depression; the dose of one or both agents should be reduced). Products include:
Placidyl Capsules 553

Ethinamate (Additive CNS depression; the dose of one or both agents should be reduced).
No products indexed under this heading.

Etodolac (Potential for enhanced effect). Products include:
Lodine Capsules 2468

Fenoprofen Calcium (Potential for enhanced effect). Products include:
Nalfon Pulvules & Tablets 919

Fentanyl (Additive CNS depression; the dose of one or both agents should be reduced). Products include:
Duragesic Transdermal System 1133

Fentanyl Citrate (Additive CNS depression; the dose of one or both agents should be reduced). Products include:
Innovar Injection 1141
Sublimaze Injection 1146

Fluphenazine Decanoate (Additive CNS depression; the dose of one or both agents should be reduced). Products include:
Prolixin Decanoate 1795

Fluphenazine Enanthate (Additive CNS depression; the dose of one or both agents should be reduced). Products include:
Prolixin Enanthate 1796

Fluphenazine Hydrochloride (Additive CNS depression; the dose of one or both agents should be reduced). Products include:
Prolixin Elixir 1793
Prolixin Injection 1791
Prolixin Oral Concentrate 1792
Prolixin Tablets 1793

Flurazepam Hydrochloride (Additive CNS depression; the dose of one or both agents should be reduced). Products include:
Dalmane Capsules 1927

Flurbiprofen (Potential for enhanced effect). Products include:
Ansaid Tablets 2319

Furazolidone (Increased effect of either hydrocodone or MAO inhibitor). Products include:
Furoxone 1855

Glipizide (Aspirin may enhance the effects of oral hypoglycemic agents). Products include:
Glucotrol 1952

Glutethimide (Additive CNS depression; the dose of one or both agents should be reduced).
No products indexed under this heading.

Glyburide (Aspirin may enhance the effects of oral hypoglycemic agents). Products include:
DiaBeta 1091
Micronase Tablets 2350

Glycopyrrolate (May produce paralytic ileus). Products include:
Robinul Forte Tablets 1873
Robinul Injectable 1873
Robinul Tablets 1873

Haloperidol (Additive CNS depression; the dose of one or both agents should be reduced). Products include:
Haldol Injection, Tablets and Concentrate 1373

Haloperidol Decanoate (Additive CNS depression; the dose of one or both agents should be reduced). Products include:
Haldol Decanoate 1375

Hydrocodone Polistirex (Additive CNS depression; the dose of one or both agents should be reduced). Products include:
Tussionex Extended-Release Suspension 988

Hydrocortisone (Potential for enhanced effect). Products include:
AK-Spore H.C. .... ⊙ 206
Bactine Hydrocortisone Anti-Itch Cream .... ◙ 625
CaldeCORT Anti-Itch Hydrocortisone Spray .... ◙ 560
Carmol HC Cream 1% 2296
Cortaid Spray .... ◙ 735
Cortenema 2244
Cortisporin Ointment 758
Cortisporin Ophthalmic Ointment Sterile 758
Cortisporin Ophthalmic Suspension Sterile 759
Cortisporin Otic Solution Sterile 760
Cortisporin Otic Suspension Sterile 760
Cortizone-5 Creme & Ointment .... ◙ 732
Dermolate Anti-Itch Cream .... ◙ 697
Eldecort Cream 1.0% 1113
Eldecort Cream 1.0% and 2.5% 1113
Fungoid HC Creme 1770
Hydrocortone Tablets 1482
Hytone 909
LazerSporin-C Solution 1770
Massengill Medicated Soft Cloth Towelettes 2192
Nutracort Cream & Lotion 1684
PediOtic Suspension Sterile 797
Synacort Creams 1%, 2.5% 2296
Vanoxide-HC Acne Lotion 911
Vioform-Hydrocortisone Cream and Mild Cream 889
Vioform-Hydrocortisone Ointment .. 889
VōSoL HC Otic Solution 2392
Vytone Cream 1% 911

Hydrocortisone Acetate (Potential for enhanced effect). Products include:
Analpram-HC Rectal Cream 1% and 2.5% 970
Anusol-HC Cream 1690
Anusol-HC Suppositories 1691
Caldecort .... ◙ 560
Carmol HC Cream 1% 2296
Chloromycetin Hydrocortisone Ophthalmic 1694
Coly-Mycin S Otic w/Neomycin & Hydrocortisone 1708
Cortaid .... ◙ 735
Cortef Feminine Itch Cream .... ◙ 735
Corticaine .... ◙ 682
Cortifoam 1827
Cortisporin Cream 757
Epifoam 1828
Gynecort 5 Creme .... ◙ 556
Hydrocortone Acetate Sterile Suspension 1479
Lanacort 5 Creme and Ointment .. ◙ 557

Mantadil Cream 789
Ophthocort .... ⊙ 301
Orabase HCA Oral Paste 890
Pramosone Cream, Lotion & Ointment 971
ProctoCream-HC 1834
Proctofoam-HC 1835

Hydrocortisone Sodium Phosphate (Potential for enhanced effect). Products include:
Hydrocortone Phosphate Injection, Sterile 1481

Hydrocortisone Sodium Succinate (Potential for enhanced effect). Products include:
Solu-Cortef Sterile Powder 2361

Hydroxyzine Hydrochloride (Additive CNS depression; the dose of one or both agents should be reduced). Products include:
Atarax Tablets & Syrup 1941
Marax Tablets & DF Syrup 1954
Vistaril Intramuscular Solution 1970

Hyoscyamine (May produce paralytic ileus). Products include:
Cystospaz Tablets 2395
Urised Tablets 2396

Hyoscyamine Sulfate (May produce paralytic ileus). Products include:
Arco-Lase Plus Tablets 607
Cystospaz-M Capsules 2395
Donnagel .... ▣ 675
Donnagel-PG 1858
Donnatal 1858
Donnatal Extentabs 1859
Donnatal Tablets 1858
Donnazyme Tablets 1860
Kutrase Capsules 2146
Levsin/Levsinex 2147
Ru-Tuss Tablets 693

Ibuprofen (Potential for enhanced effect). Products include:
Advil Cold & Sinus Caplets (formerly CoAdvil) 2416
Advil Ibuprofen Tablets and Caplets 2416
Children's Advil Suspension 2426
CoAdvil .... ▣ 748
Dristan Sinus Caplets 2419
Haltran Tablets .... ▣ 668
Ibuprofen .... ▣ 631
Medipren ibuprofen Caplets and Tablets 1362
Midol 200 Cramp Relief Formula .... ▣ 570
Motrin Tablets 2351
Motrin IB Caplets and Tablets .... ▣ 736
Nuprin Ibuprofen/Analgesic Tablets & Caplets 752
PediaProfen Suspension 1363
Rufen Tablets 691
Trendar Ibuprofen Tablets .... ▣ 756

Imipramine Hydrochloride (Additive CNS depression; the dose of one or both agents should be reduced; increased effect of either hydrocodone or antidepressant). Products include:
Tofranil Ampuls 1038
Tofranil Tablets 1039

Imipramine Pamoate (Additive CNS depression; the dose of one or both agents should be reduced; increased effect of either hydrocodone or antidepressant). Products include:
Tofranil-PM Capsules 1041

Indomethacin (Potential for enhanced effect). Products include:
Indocin 1487

Indomethacin Sodium Trihydrate (Potential for enhanced effect). Products include:
Indocin I.V. 1490

Insulin, Human (Aspirin may enhance the effects of insulin).
No products indexed under this heading.

Insulin, Human Isophane Suspension (Aspirin may enhance the effects of insulin). Products include:
Humulin N, 100 Units 1270

Insulin, Human NPH (Aspirin may enhance the effects of insulin). Products include:
Insulatard NPH Human 1627
Novolin N 1627
Novolin N PenFill Cartridges 1628
Novolin N Prefilled 1628

Insulin, Human Regular (Aspirin may enhance the effects of insulin). Products include:
Humulin BR, 100 Units 1268
Humulin R, 100 Units 1272
Novolin R 1627
Novolin R PenFill Cartridges 1628
Novolin R Prefilled 1629
Velosulin Human 1628

Insulin, Human, Zinc Suspension (Aspirin may enhance the effects of insulin). Products include:
Humulin L, 100 Units 1268
Humulin U, 100 Units 1272
Novolin L 1627

Insulin, NPH (Aspirin may enhance the effects of insulin). Products include:
NPH, 40 & 100 Units 1273
Beef NPH, 100 Units 1274
Pork NPH, 100 Units 1275
Insulatard NPH 1626
NPH Insulin 1626
NPH Purified Pork Isophane Insulin 1626

Insulin, Regular (Aspirin may enhance the effects of insulin). Products include:
Regular, 40 & 100 Units 1273
Beef Regular, 100 Units 1275
Pork Regular, 100 Units 1275
Pork Regular (Concentrated), 500 Units 1276
Regular Insulin 1625
Regular Purified Pork Insulin 1626
Velosulin 1627

Insulin, Zinc Crystals (Aspirin may enhance the effects of insulin). Products include:
NPH, 40 & 100 Units 1273

Insulin, Zinc Suspension (Aspirin may enhance the effects of insulin). Products include:
Lente, 40 & 100 Units 1272
Protamine, Zinc, 40 & 100 Units 1273
Lente Iletin I 1272
Beef Lente, 100 Units 1274
Beef Protamine Zinc, 100 Units 1274
Pork Lente, 100 Units 1275
Pork, Protamine, Zinc, 100 Units 1275
Lente Insulin 1626
Lente Purified Pork Insulin 1626
Semilente Insulin 1625
Ultralente Insulin 1626

Ipratropium Bromide (May produce paralytic ileus). Products include:
Atrovent Inhalation Aerosol 675

Isocarboxazid (Increased effect of either hydrocodone or MAO inhibitor). Products include:
Marplan Tablets 1906

Isoflurane (Additive CNS depression; the dose of one or both agents should be reduced). Products include:
Forane 600

Ketamine Hydrochloride (Additive CNS depression; the dose of one or both agents should be reduced). Products include:
Ketalar 1726

Ketoprofen (Potential for enhanced effect). Products include:
Orudis Capsules 2488

Ketorolac Tromethamine (Potential for enhanced effect). Products include:
Toradol IM Injection 2302

Levorphanol Tartrate (Additive CNS depression; the dose of one or both agents should be reduced). Products include:
Levo-Dromoran 1906

Lithium Carbonate (Additive CNS depression; the dose of one or both agents should be reduced). Products include:
Eskalith 2214
Lithane Tablets 1596
Lithium Carbonate Capsules & Tablets 1984
Lithobid Tablets 870

Lithium Citrate (Additive CNS depression; the dose of one or both agents should be reduced). Products include:
Cibalith-S 870

Lorazepam (Additive CNS depression; the dose of one or both agents should be reduced). Products include:
Ativan Injection 2432
Ativan Tablets 2434

Loxapine Hydrochloride (Additive CNS depression; the dose of one or both agents should be reduced). Products include:
Loxitane 1213

Loxapine Succinate (Additive CNS depression; the dose of one or both agents should be reduced). Products include:
Loxitane Capsules 1213

Maprotiline Hydrochloride (Additive CNS depression; the dose of one or both agents should be reduced; increased effect of either hydrocodone or antidepressant). Products include:
Ludiomil Tablets 874

Meclofenamate Sodium (Potential for enhanced effect). Products include:
Meclomen Capsules 1739

Mefenamic Acid (Potential for enhanced effect). Products include:
Ponstel 1758

Mepenzolate Bromide (May produce paralytic ileus). Products include:
Cantil Tablets 1326

Meperidine Hydrochloride (Additive CNS depression; the dose of one or both agents should be reduced). Products include:
Demerol 2047
Mepergan Injection 2479

Mephobarbital (Additive CNS depression; the dose of one or both agents should be reduced). Products include:
Mebaral Tablets 2061

Meprobamate (Additive CNS depression; the dose of one or both agents should be reduced). Products include:
Deprol Tablets 2382
Equagesic Tablets 2451
Miltown Tablets 2386
PMB 200 and PMB 400 2504

Mercaptopurine (Potential for enhanced effect and bone marrow toxicity). Products include:
Purinethol Tablets 800

Mesoridazine (Additive CNS depression; the dose of one or both agents should be reduced). Products include:
Serentil 686

Mesoridazine Besylate (Additive CNS depression; the dose of one or both agents should be reduced).

Methadone Hydrochloride (Additive CNS depression; the dose of one or both agents should be reduced). Products include:
Dolophine Hydrochloride Ampoules & Vials 1260
Dolophine Hydrochloride Tablets 1261
Methadone Hydrochloride Diskets 1284
Methadone Hydrochloride Oral Solution & Tablets 1987

Methohexital Sodium (Additive CNS depression; the dose of one or both agents should be reduced). Products include:
Brevital Sodium Vials 1248

Methoxyflurane (Additive CNS depression; the dose of one or both agents should be reduced).
No products indexed under this heading.

Methylprednisolone Acetate (Potential for enhanced effect). Products include:
Depo-Medrol Sterile Aqueous Suspension 2334

Methylprednisolone Sodium Succinate (Potential for enhanced effect). Products include:
Solu-Medrol Sterile Powder 2363

Midazolam Hydrochloride (Additive CNS depression; the dose of one or both agents should be reduced). Products include:
Versed Injection 1924

Molindone Hydrochloride (Additive CNS depression; the dose of one or both agents should be reduced). Products include:
Moban Tablets & Concentrate 932

Morphine Sulfate (Additive CNS depression; the dose of one or both agents should be reduced). Products include:
Astramorph/PF Injection, USP (Preservative-Free) 618
Duramorph 960
Infumorph 200 and Infumorph 500 Sterile Solutions 962
MS Contin Tablets 1814
MSIR 1817
Oramorph SR (Morphine Sulfate Sustained Release Tablets) 1988
Roxanol 1991

Naproxen (Potential for enhanced effect). Products include:
Naprosyn 2297

Naproxen Sodium (Potential for enhanced effect). Products include:
Anaprox and Anaprox DS Tablets 2288

Nortriptyline Hydrochloride (Additive CNS depression; the dose of one or both agents should be reduced; increased effect of either hydrocodone or antidepressant). Products include:
Pamelor 2019

Opium Alkaloids (Additive CNS depression; the dose of one or both agents should be reduced). Products include:
B & O No. 15A & No. 16A Supprettes 2395
Pantopon Injectable 1911

Oxazepam (Additive CNS depression; the dose of one or both agents should be reduced). Products include:
Serax Capsules 2522
Serax Tablets 2522

Oxybutynin Chloride (May produce paralytic ileus). Products include:
Ditropan 1332

Oxycodone Hydrochloride (Additive CNS depression; the dose of one or both agents should be reduced). Products include:
Percocet Tablets 950
Percodan 951
Roxicodone Tablets, Oral Solution & Intensol (Oxycodone) 1992
Tylox Capsules 1382

Pentobarbital Sodium (Additive CNS depression; the dose of one or both agents should be reduced). Products include:
Nembutal Sodium Capsules 534
Nembutal Sodium Solution 536

Nembutal Sodium Suppositories 538

Perphenazine (Additive CNS depression; the dose of one or both agents should be reduced). Products include:

Etrafon ... 2087
Triavil Tablets ... 1556
Trilafon ... 2123

Phenelzine Sulfate (Additive CNS depression; the dose of one or both agents should be reduced; increased effect of either hydrocodone or MAO inhibitor). Products include:

Nardil ... 1742

Phenobarbital (Additive CNS depression; the dose of one or both agents should be reduced). Products include:

Arco-Lase Plus Tablets ... 607
Bellergal-S Tablets ... 1998
Bronkolixir ... ▣ 761
Bronkotabs Tablets ... ▣ 762
Donnatal ... 1858
Donnatal Extentabs ... 1859
Donnatal Tablets ... 1858
Donnazyme Tablets ... 1860
Kinesed Tablets ... 2272
Phenobarbital Elixir and Tablets ... 1293
Primatene Tablets-P Formula ... 2421
Quadrinal Tablets ... 1183
Tedral SA ... 1765

Phenylbutazone (Potential for enhanced effect). Products include:

Butazolidin Capsules & Tablets ... 1027

Piroxicam (Potential for enhanced effect). Products include:

Feldene Capsules ... 1777

Prazepam (Additive CNS depression; the dose of one or both agents should be reduced). Products include:

Centrax ... 1693

Prednisolone Acetate (Potential for enhanced effect). Products include:

AK-Cide Sterile Ophthalmic Ointment & Suspension ... ⊙ 202
Blephamide Liquifilm Sterile Ophthalmic Suspension ... 586
Blephamide S.O.P. Sterile Ophthalmic Ointment ... 586
Cetapred Ointment ... ⊙ 220
⅛% Econopred & 1% Econopred Plus ... ⊙ 217
Isopto Cetapred Suspension ... ⊙ 220
Metimyd ... ⊙ 306
Poly-Pred Liquifilm ... ⊙ 250
Pred Forte ... ⊙ 252
Pred Mild ... ⊙ 254
Pred-G Liquifilm Sterile Ophthalmic Suspension ... ⊙ 252
Pred-G S.O.P. Sterile Ophthalmic Ointment ... ⊙ 253
Vasocidin Ointment ... ⊙ 275

Prednisolone Sodium Phosphate (Potential for enhanced effect). Products include:

AK-Pred ... ⊙ 205
Hydeltrasol Injection, Sterile ... 1476
Inflamase ... ⊙ 274
Pediapred Oral Liquid ... 987
Vasocidin Ophthalmic Solution ... ⊙ 276

Prednisolone Tebutate (Potential for enhanced effect). Products include:

Hydeltra-T.B.A. Sterile Suspension 1478

Prednisone (Potential for enhanced effect). Products include:

Deltasone Tablets ... 2332

Probenecid (Aspirin may diminish the effects of uricosuric agent). Products include:

Benemid Tablets ... 1426
ColBENEMID Tablets ... 1436
Wycillin Injection and Probenecid Tablets ... 2539

Prochlorperazine (Additive CNS depression; the dose of one or both agents should be reduced). Products include:

Compazine ... 2201

Procyclidine Hydrochloride (May produce paralytic ileus). Products include:

Kemadrin Tablets ... 771

Promethazine Hydrochloride (Additive CNS depression; the dose of one or both agents should be reduced). Products include:

Mepergan Injection ... 2479
Phenergan with Codeine ... 2497
Phenergan with Dextromethorphan 2499
Phenergan Injection ... 2493
Phenergan Suppositories ... 2496
Phenergan Syrup ... 2495
Phenergan Tablets ... 2496
Phenergan VC ... 2500
Phenergan VC with Codeine ... 2501

Propantheline Bromide (May produce paralytic ileus). Products include:

Pro-Banthīne Tablets ... 2141

Propofol (Additive CNS depression; the dose of one or both agents should be reduced). Products include:

Diprivan Injection ... 2267

Propoxyphene Hydrochloride (Additive CNS depression; the dose of one or both agents should be reduced). Products include:

Darvon ... 1256
Wygesic Tablets ... 2540

Propoxyphene Napsylate (Additive CNS depression; the dose of one or both agents should be reduced). Products include:

Darvon-N/Darvocet-N ... 1254

Protriptyline Hydrochloride (Additive CNS depression; the dose of one or both agents should be reduced; increased effect of either hydrocodone or antidepressant). Products include:

Vivactil Tablets ... 1567

Quazepam (Additive CNS depression; the dose of one or both agents should be reduced). Products include:

Doral Tablets ... 2383

Scopolamine Hydrobromide (May produce paralytic ileus). Products include:

Donnagel ... ▣ 675
Donnagel-PG ... 1858
Donnatal ... 1858
Donnatal Extentabs ... 1859
Donnatal Tablets ... 1858
Donnazyme Tablets ... 1860
Isopto Hyoscine ... ⊙ 222
Murocoll-2 Sterile Ophthalmic Solution ... ⊙ 261
Ru-Tuss Tablets ... 693

Scopolamine Preparations (May produce paralytic ileus). Products include:

Transderm Scōp Transdermal Therapeutic System ... 887

Secobarbital Sodium (Additive CNS depression; the dose of one or both agents should be reduced). Products include:

Seconal Sodium Pulvules ... 1296

Selegiline Hydrochloride (Increased effect of either hydrocodone or MAO inhibitor). Products include:

Eldepryl ... 2250

Sufentanil Citrate (Additive CNS depression; the dose of one or both agents should be reduced). Products include:

Sufenta Injection ... 1147

Sulfinpyrazone (Aspirin may diminish the effects of uricosuric agent). Products include:

Anturane ... 853

Sulindac (Potential for enhanced effect). Products include:

Clinoril Tablets ... 1433

Temazepam (Additive CNS depression; the dose of one or both agents should be reduced). Products include:

Restoril Capsules ... 2023

Thiamylal Sodium (Additive CNS depression; the dose of one or both agents should be reduced). Products include:

Surital Ampoules, Steri-Vials ... 1764

Thioridazine Hydrochloride (Additive CNS depression; the dose of one or both agents should be reduced). Products include:

Mellaril ... 2011

Thiothixene (Additive CNS depression; the dose of one or both agents should be reduced). Products include:

Navane Capsules and Concentrate 1954
Navane Intramuscular ... 1956

Tolazamide (Aspirin may enhance the effects of oral hypoglycemic agents). Products include:

Tolinase Tablets ... 2365

Tolbutamide (Aspirin may enhance the effects of oral hypoglycemic agents). Products include:

Orinase Tablets ... 2354

Tolmetin Sodium (Potential for enhanced effect). Products include:

Tolectin (200, 400 and 600 mg) .. 1379

Tranylcypromine Sulfate (Increased effect of either hydrocodone or MAO inhibitor). Products include:

Parnate Tablets ... 2222

Triamcinolone (Potential for enhanced effect).

No products indexed under this heading.

Triamcinolone Acetonide (Potential for enhanced effect). Products include:

Aristocort A ... 1010
Azmacort Inhaler ... 1837
Kenalog Cream, Lotion & Ointment 2401
Kenalog-10 Injection ... 2402
Kenalog-40 Injection ... 2403
Kenalog in Orabase ... 604
Kenalog Spray ... 2401
Mycolog II Cream and Ointment ... 2407
Mytrex Cream & Ointment ... 2080
Nasacort Nasal Inhaler ... 1844

Triamcinolone Diacetate (Potential for enhanced effect). Products include:

Aristocort Suspension ... 1008

Triamcinolone Hexacetonide (Potential for enhanced effect). Products include:

Aristospan Suspension ... 1011

Triazolam (Additive CNS depression; the dose of one or both agents should be reduced). Products include:

Halcion Tablets ... 2340

Tridihexethyl Chloride (May produce paralytic ileus).

No products indexed under this heading.

Trifluoperazine Hydrochloride (Additive CNS depression; the dose of one or both agents should be reduced). Products include:

Stelazine ... 2226

Trihexyphenidyl Hydrochloride (May produce paralytic ileus). Products include:

Artane ... 1195

Trimipramine Maleate (Additive CNS depression; the dose of one or both agents should be reduced; increased effect of either hydrocodone or antidepressant). Products include:

Surmontil Capsules ... 2524

Warfarin Sodium (Aspirin may enhance the effects of oral anticoagulant). Products include:

Coumadin Injection & Tablets ... 944
Panwarfin Tablets ... 547

Food Interactions

Food, unspecified (Slightly delays the absorption of aspirin).

AZMACORT INHALER

(Triamcinolone Acetonide) ... 1837
No interactions described in labeling.

AZO GANTANOL TABLETS

(Sulfamethoxazole, Phenazopyridine Hydrochloride) ... 1887
No interactions described in labeling.

AZO GANTRISIN TABLETS

(Sulfisoxazole, Phenazopyridine Hydrochloride) ... 1888
May interact with oral anticoagulants, oral hypoglycemic agents, and certain other agents. Compounds in these categories include:

Chlorpropamide (Blood sugar-lowering activity of sulfonylureas potentiated). Products include:

Diabinese Tablets ... 1775

Dicumarol (Sulfisoxazole prolongs the prothrombin time). Products include:

Dicumarol Tablets ... 516

Glipizide (Blood sugar-lowering activity of sulfonylureas potentiated). Products include:

Glucotrol ... 1952

Glyburide (Blood sugar-lowering activity of sulfonylureas potentiated). Products include:

DiaBeta ... 1091
Micronase Tablets ... 2350

Methotrexate Sodium (Displacement from protein binding sites). Products include:

Methotrexate Tablets, Parenteral, LPF Parenteral ... 1217
Rheumatrex Methotrexate Dose Pack ... 1234

Sodium Thiopental (Sulfisoxazole competes with thiopental for plasma protein binding).

No products indexed under this heading.

Tolazamide (Blood sugar-lowering activity of sulfonylureas potentiated). Products include:

Tolinase Tablets ... 2365

Tolbutamide (Blood sugar-lowering activity of sulfonylureas potentiated). Products include:

Orinase Tablets ... 2354

Warfarin Sodium (Sulfisoxazole prolongs the prothrombin time). Products include:

Coumadin Injection & Tablets ... 944
Panwarfin Tablets ... 547

AZULFIDINE TABLETS, EN-TABS, ORAL SUSPENSION

(Sulfasalazine) ... 1157
May interact with:

Digitoxin (Reduced absorption of digoxin). Products include:

Crystodigin Tablets ... 1253

Digoxin (Reduced absorption of digoxin). Products include:

Lanoxicaps ... 772
Lanoxin Elixir Pediatric ... 775
Lanoxin Injection ... 778
Lanoxin Injection Pediatric ... 781
Lanoxin Tablets ... 783

Folic Acid (Reduced absorption of folic acid). Products include:

Allbee C-800 Plus Iron Tablets ... ▣ 670

Biotin Forte 3mg. & Extra Strength Biotin Forte 5mg. 2377
Bugs Bunny Children's Chewable Vitamins (Sugar Free) .... ▣ 625
Bugs Bunny With Extra C Children's Chewable Vitamins (Sugar Free) .... ▣ 626
Bugs Bunny Plus Iron Children's Chewable Vitamins (Sugar Free) ▣ 625
Cefol Filmtab 509
Fero-Folic-500 Filmtab 527
Flintstones Children's Chewable Vitamins .... ▣ 625
Flintstones Children's Chewable Vitamins With Extra C .... ▣ 626
Flintstones Children's Chewable Vitamins Plus Iron .... ▣ 625
Iberet-Folic-500 Filmtab 527
Materna Tablets 1214
May-Vita Elixir 1359
Mega-B 607
Nephro-Vite Rx 1826
Niferex-150 Forte Capsules 847
One-A-Day Essential Vitamins .... ▣ 627
One-A-Day Maximum Formula Vitamins and Minerals .... ▣ 627
One-A-Day Plus Extra C Vitamins .. ▣ 627
Pramet FA 1974
Pramilet FA 1974
Sigtab Tablets .... ▣ 669
Stressgard Stress Formula Vitamins .... ▣ 628
STUART PRENATAL Tablets .... ▣ 731
The Stuart Formula Tablets .... ▣ 581
Stuartnatal 1+1 Tablets 2273
Theragran Stress Formula .... ▣ 727
Trinsicon Capsules 2415
Vicon Forte Capsules 2416
Within Women's Formula Multivitamin with Calcium, Extra Iron and Zinc .... ▣ 628
Zenate Tablets 2250
Zymacap Capsules .... ▣ 670

BAL IN OIL AMPULES
(Dimercaprol) 661
May interact with:

Iron Preparations (Concurrent administration with medicinal iron should be avoided). Products include:
Allbee C-800 Plus Iron Tablets .... ▣ 670
Bugs Bunny Children's Chewable Vitamins + Minerals with Iron and Calcium (Sugar Free) .... ▣ 626
Bugs Bunny Plus Iron Children's Chewable Vitamins (Sugar Free) ▣ 625
FemIron Multi-Vitamins and Iron.... ▣ 617
Ferancee Chewable Tablets 1155
Ferancee-HP Tablets 1155
Fergon .... ▣ 758
Fero-Folic-500 Filmtab 527
Fero-Grad-500 Filmtab 528
Fero-Gradumet Filmtab 528
Ferro-Sequels 1203
Flintstones Children's Chewable Vitamins Plus Iron .... ▣ 625
Flintstones Complete With Calcium, Iron & Minerals Children's Chewable Vitamins .... ▣ 626
Geritol Extend Tablets and Caplets .... ▣ 717
Geritol Liquid - High Potency Iron & Vitamin Tonic .... ▣ 717
Iberet Tablets 531
Iberet-500 Liquid 531
Iberet-Folic-500 Filmtab 527
Iberet-Liquid 531
Incremin w/Iron Syrup .... ▣ 588
Irospan 972
Mol-Iron .... ▣ 703
Niferex 847
Niferex-150 Forte Capsules 847
Niferex Forte Elixir 847
Niferex 847
Niferex-PN Tablets 847
One-A-Day Maximum Formula Vitamins and Minerals .... ▣ 627
Peritinic Tablets .... ▣ 589
Poly-Vi-Flor with Iron 1399
Poly-Vi-Flor with Iron Drops 1399
Poly-Vi-Sol Vitamins with Iron, Chewable Tablets and Circus Shapes Chewable .... ▣ 612
Poly-Vi-Sol Vitamins with Iron, Drops .... ▣ 612
SMA Iron Fortified Infant Formula, Concentrated, Ready-to-Feed and Powder .... ▣ 767
Slow Fe Tablets .... ▣ 552
The Stuart Formula Tablets .... ▣ 581
Stuartinic Tablets 1157
Surbex-750 with Iron .... ▣ 503
Tri-Vi-Flor 0.25 mg Vitamins with Iron and Fluoride Drops 1401
Unicap Plus Iron Vitamin Formula Tablets .... ▣ 738
Vi-Daylin ADC Vitamins + Iron Drops 1980
Vi-Daylin Multivitamin + Iron Drops 1981
Vi-Daylin/F ADC Vitamins + Iron Drops With Fluoride 1981
Vi-Daylin/F Multivitamin + Iron Drops With Fluoride 1981
Vi-Daylin Multivitamin + Iron Chewable Tablets 1982
Vi-Daylin/F Multivitamin + Iron Chewable Tablets With Fluoride .. 1982
Vi-Daylin Multivitamin + Iron Liquid 1983

BC POWDER
(Aspirin, Salicylamide, Caffeine) .... ▣ 517
No interactions described in labeling.

BC COLD POWDER MULTI-SYMPTOM FORMULA
(Aspirin, Phenylpropanolamine Hydrochloride, Chlorpheniramine Maleate) .... ▣ 517
May interact with monoamine oxidase inhibitors and certain other agents. Compounds in these categories include:

Alcohol (Concurrent use not recommended).

Furazolidone (Concurrent use not recommended). Products include:
Furoxone 1855

Isocarboxazid (Concurrent use not recommended). Products include:
Marplan Tablets 1906

Phenelzine Sulfate (Concurrent use not recommended). Products include:
Nardil 1742

Selegiline Hydrochloride (Concurrent use not recommended). Products include:
Eldepryl 2250

Tranylcypromine Sulfate (Concurrent use not recommended). Products include:
Parnate Tablets 2222

BC COLD POWDER NON-DROWSY FORMULA
(Aspirin, Phenylpropanolamine Hydrochloride) .... ▣ 517
See **BC Cold Powder Multi-Symptom Formula**

BCG VACCINE, USP (TICE)
(BCG Vaccine) 1632
May interact with immunosuppressive agents and certain other agents. Compounds in these categories include:

Azathioprine (May interfere with development of immune response). Products include:
Imuran 768

Cyclosporine (May interfere with development of immune response). Products include:
Sandimmune 2024

Immune Globulin (Human) (May interfere with development of immune response). Products include:
MICRhoGAM $Rh_o(D)$ Immune Globulin (Human) 1650
RhoGAM $Rh_o(D)$ Immune Globulin (Human) 1651

Immune Globulin Intravenous (Human) (May interfere with development of immune response). Products include:
Gamimune N Immune Globulin Intravenous (Human) 1572
Gammagard Immune Globulin, Intravenous (Human) 658
Iveegam 1129
Sandoglobulin I.V. 2027

Muromonab-CD3 (May interfere with development of immune response). Products include:
Orthoclone OKT3 Sterile Solution .. 1645

B-D GLUCOSE TABLETS
(Dextrose) .... ▣ 512
No interactions described in labeling.

BIO-COR 12, 24, AND 72 COLLAGEN CORNEAL SHIELD
(Collagen) .... ⊙ 260
No interactions described in labeling.

B & O NO. 15A & NO. 16A SUPPRETTES
(Belladonna Extract, Opium Preparations) 2395
No interactions described in labeling.

BSS (15 ML & 30 ML) STERILE IRRIGATION SOLUTION
(Balanced Salt Solution) .... ⊙ 230
No interactions described in labeling.

BSS (250 ML) STERILE IRRIGATION SOLUTION
(Balanced Salt Solution) .... ⊙ 231
No interactions described in labeling.

BSS (500 ML) STERILE IRRIGATION SOLUTION
(Balanced Salt Solution) .... ⊙ 231
No interactions described in labeling.

BSS PLUS (500 ML) STERILE IRRIGATION SOLUTION
(Balanced Salt Solution) .... ⊙ 231
No interactions described in labeling.

BACIGUENT ANTIBIOTIC OINTMENT
(Bacitracin) .... ▣ 735
No interactions described in labeling.

BACTINE ANTISEPTIC/ANESTHETIC FIRST AID SPRAY
(Benzalkonium Chloride, Lidocaine Hydrochloride) .... ▣ 624
No interactions described in labeling.

BACTINE FIRST AID ANTIBIOTIC OINTMENT
(Bacitracin, Neomycin Sulfate, Polymyxin B Sulfate) .... ▣ 625
No interactions described in labeling.

BACTINE HYDROCORTISONE ANTI-ITCH CREAM
(Hydrocortisone) .... ▣ 625
No interactions described in labeling.

BACTRIM DS TABLETS
(Trimethoprim, Sulfamethoxazole) 1891
May interact with thiazides, oral anticoagulants, and certain other agents. Compounds in these categories include:

Bendroflumethiazide (Increased incidence of thrombocytopenia with purpura in elderly). Products include:
Corzide Tablets 702
Naturetin Tablets 1789
Rauzide Tablets 1804

Chlorothiazide (Increased incidence of thrombocytopenia with purpura in elderly). Products include:
Aldoclor Tablets 1413
Diupres Tablets 1461
Diuril Oral 1464

Chlorothiazide Sodium (Increased incidence of thrombocytopenia with purpura in elderly). Products include:
Diuril Sodium Intravenous 1463

Dicumarol (Prolonged prothrombin time). Products include:
Dicumarol Tablets 516

Hydrochlorothiazide (Increased incidence of thrombocytopenia with purpura in elderly). Products include:
Aldactazide 2150
Aldoril Tablets 1418
Apresazide Capsules 854
Apresoline-Esidrix Tablets 857
Capozide 2258
Dyazide Capsules 2208
Esidrix Tablets 863
Esimil Tablets 864
HydroDIURIL Tablets 1484
Hydropres Tablets 1485
Inderide Tablets 2463
Inderide LA Long Acting Capsules .. 2465
Lopressor HCT Tablets 1034
Maxzide 1215
Moduretic Tablets 1510
Normozide Tablets 2112
Oretic Tablets 544
Oreticyl 545
Prinzide Tablets 1540
Ser-Ap-Es Tablets 881
Serpasil-Esidrix Tablets 886
Timolide Tablets 1547
Trandate HCT Tablets 579
Vaseretic Tablets 1559
Zestoretic 2274

Hydroflumethiazide (Increased incidence of thrombocytopenia with purpura in elderly). Products include:
Diucardin Tablets 2450
Saluron 718
Salutensin/Salutensin-Demi 719

Methotrexate Sodium (Increased free methotrexate concentrations). Products include:
Methotrexate Tablets, Parenteral, LPF Parenteral 1217
Rheumatrex Methotrexate Dose Pack 1234

Methyclothiazide (Increased incidence of thrombocytopenia with purpura in elderly). Products include:
Enduron Tablets 517
Enduronyl 518

Phenytoin (Decreased hepatic metabolism of phenytoin). Products include:
Dilantin Infatabs 1710
Dilantin-30 Pediatric/Dilantin-125 Suspension 1713

Phenytoin Sodium (Decreased hepatic metabolism of phenytoin). Products include:
Dilantin Kapseals 1708
Dilantin Parenteral 1712
Dilantin with Phenobarbital Kapseals 1715

Polythiazide (Increased incidence of thrombocytopenia with purpura in elderly). Products include:
Minizide Capsules 1779
Renese Tablets 1785
Renese-R Tablets 1786

Warfarin Sodium (Prolonged prothrombin time). Products include:
Coumadin Injection & Tablets 944
Panwarfin Tablets 547

BACTRIM I.V. INFUSION
(Trimethoprim, Sulfamethoxazole) 1889
May interact with thiazides, oral anticoagulants, and certain other agents. Compounds in these categories include:

Bendroflumethiazide (Increased incidence of thrombocytopenia with purpura in elderly). Products include:
Corzide Tablets 702
Naturetin Tablets 1789
Rauzide Tablets 1804

Chlorothiazide (Increased incidence of thrombocytopenia with purpura in elderly). Products include:
Aldoclor Tablets 1413
Diupres Tablets 1461
Diuril Oral 1464

Chlorothiazide Sodium (Increased incidence of thrombocytopenia with purpura in elderly). Products include:
Diuril Sodium Intravenous 1463

Dicumarol (Prolonged prothrombin time). Products include:
Dicumarol Tablets 516

Hydrochlorothiazide (Increased incidence of thrombocytopenia with purpura in elderly). Products include:
Aldactazide 2150
Aldoril Tablets 1418
Apresazide Capsules 854
Apresoline-Esidrix Tablets 857
Capozide 2258
Dyazide Capsules 2208
Esidrix Tablets 863
Esimil Tablets 864
HydroDIURIL Tablets 1484
Hydropres Tablets 1485
Inderide Tablets 2463
Inderide LA Long Acting Capsules 2465
Lopressor HCT Tablets 1034
Maxzide 1215
Moduretic Tablets 1510
Normozide Tablets 2112
Oretic Tablets 544
Oreticyl 545
Prinzide Tablets 1540
Ser-Ap-Es Tablets 881
Serpasil-Esidrix Tablets 886
Timolide Tablets 1547
Trandate HCT Tablets 579
Vaseretic Tablets 1559
Zestoretic 2274

Hydroflumethiazide (Increased incidence of thrombocytopenia with purpura in elderly). Products include:
Diucardin Tablets 2450
Saluron 718
Salutensin/Salutensin-Demi 719

Methotrexate Sodium (Increased free methotrexate concentrations). Products include:
Methotrexate Tablets, Parenteral, LPF Parenteral 1217
Rheumatrex Methotrexate Dose Pack 1234

Methyclothiazide (Increased incidence of thrombocytopenia with purpura in elderly). Products include:
Enduron Tablets 517
Enduronyl 518

Phenytoin (Decreased hepatic metabolism of phenytoin). Products include:
Dilantin Infatabs 1710
Dilantin-30 Pediatric/Dilantin-125 Suspension 1713

Phenytoin Sodium (Decreased hepatic metabolism of phenytoin). Products include:
Dilantin Kapseals 1708
Dilantin Parenteral 1712
Dilantin with Phenobarbital Kapseals 1715

Polythiazide (Increased incidence of thrombocytopenia with purpura in elderly). Products include:
Minizide Capsules 1779
Renese Tablets 1785
Renese-R Tablets 1786

Warfarin Sodium (Prolonged prothrombin time). Products include:
Coumadin Injection & Tablets 944
Panwarfin Tablets 547

BACTRIM PEDIATRIC SUSPENSION
(Trimethoprim, Sulfamethoxazole) 1891
See **Bactrim DS Tablets**

BACTRIM SUSPENSION
(Trimethoprim, Sulfamethoxazole) 1891
See **Bactrim DS Tablets**

BACTRIM TABLETS
(Trimethoprim, Sulfamethoxazole) 1891
See **Bactrim DS Tablets**

BACTROBAN OINTMENT
(Mupirocin) 2200
No interactions described in labeling.

BALANCED SALT SOLUTION
(Balanced Salt Solution) ◉ 239
No interactions described in labeling.

BALMEX BABY POWDER
(Zinc Oxide) ▣ 590
No interactions described in labeling.

BALMEX EMOLLIENT LOTION
(Lanolin Oil) ▣ 590
No interactions described in labeling.

BALMEX OINTMENT
(Bismuth Subnitrate, Zinc Oxide) ▣ 590
No interactions described in labeling.

BARON-X TABLETS
(Yohimbine Hydrochloride) 650
May interact with antidepressant drugs. Compounds in this category include:

Amitriptyline Hydrochloride (Effect not specified). Products include:
Elavil 2269
Endep Tablets 1927
Etrafon 2087
Limbitrol 1933
Triavil Tablets 1556

Amoxapine (Effect not specified). Products include:
Asendin Tablets 1196

Bupropion Hydrochloride (Effect not specified). Products include:
Wellbutrin Tablets 821

Desipramine Hydrochloride (Effect not specified). Products include:
Norpramin Tablets 1340

Doxepin Hydrochloride (Effect not specified). Products include:
Sinequan 1960

Fluoxetine Hydrochloride (Effect not specified). Products include:
Prozac Pulvules 920

Imipramine Hydrochloride (Effect not specified). Products include:
Tofranil Ampuls 1038
Tofranil Tablets 1039

Imipramine Pamoate (Effect not specified). Products include:
Tofranil-PM Capsules 1041

Isocarboxazid (Effect not specified). Products include:
Marplan Tablets 1906

Maprotiline Hydrochloride (Effect not specified). Products include:
Ludiomil Tablets 874

Nortriptyline Hydrochloride (Effect not specified). Products include:
Pamelor 2019

Phenelzine Sulfate (Effect not specified). Products include:
Nardil 1742

Protriptyline Hydrochloride (Effect not specified). Products include:
Vivactil Tablets 1567

Tranylcypromine Sulfate (Effect not specified). Products include:
Parnate Tablets 2222

Trazodone Hydrochloride (Effect not specified). Products include:
Desyrel and Desyrel Dividose 1404

Trimipramine Maleate (Effect not specified). Products include:
Surmontil Capsules 2524

BASALJEL CAPSULES
(Aluminum Carbonate Gel) 2438
May interact with tetracyclines. Compounds in this category include:

Demeclocycline Hydrochloride (Concurrent oral administration should be avoided). Products include:
Declomycin Capsules, Tablets 1199

Doxycycline Calcium (Concurrent oral administration should be avoided).
No products indexed under this heading.

Doxycycline Hyclate (Concurrent oral administration should be avoided). Products include:
Doryx Capsules 1717
Vibramycin Hyclate Capsules 1787
Vibramycin Hyclate Intravenous 1968
Vibra-Tabs Film Coated Tablets 1787

Doxycycline Monohydrate (Concurrent oral administration should be avoided). Products include:
Monodox Capsules 1630
Vibramycin Monohydrate for Oral Suspension 1787

Methacycline Hydrochloride (Concurrent oral administration should be avoided).
No products indexed under this heading.

Minocycline Hydrochloride (Concurrent oral administration should be avoided). Products include:
Minocin Intravenous 1221
Minocin Oral Suspension 1224
Minocin Pellet-Filled Capsules 1222

Oxytetracycline (Concurrent oral administration should be avoided). Products include:
Terramycin Intramuscular Solution 1964
Urobiotic-250 Capsules 1968

Oxytetracycline Hydrochloride (Concurrent oral administration should be avoided). Products include:
Terra-Cortril Ophthalmic Suspension 1963
Terramycin Capsules 1786
Terramycin Intramuscular Solution 1964
Terramycin with Polymyxin B Sulfate Ophthalmic Ointment 1965

Tetracycline Hydrochloride (Concurrent oral administration should be avoided). Products include:
Achromycin V Capsules 1193
Achromycin Ophthalmic Ointment 1% ◉ 307
Achromycin Ophthalmic Suspension 1% ◉ 308
Topicycline for Topical Solution 1856

BASALJEL SUSPENSION
(Aluminum Carbonate Gel) 2438
See **Basaljel Capsules**

BASALJEL TABLETS
(Aluminum Carbonate Gel) 2438
See **Basaljel Capsules**

BASIS FACIAL CLEANSER (NORMAL TO DRY SKIN)
(Glycerin) ▣ 512
No interactions described in labeling.

BASIS SOAP-COMBINATION SKIN
(Cleanser) ▣ 513
No interactions described in labeling.

BASIS SOAP-EXTRA DRY SKIN
(Cleanser) ▣ 513
No interactions described in labeling.

BASIS SOAP-NORMAL TO DRY SKIN
(Cleanser) ▣ 513
No interactions described in labeling.

BASIS SOAP-SENSITIVE SKIN
(Cleanser) ▣ 513
No interactions described in labeling.

CHILDREN'S BAYER CHEWABLE ASPIRIN
(Aspirin) ▣ 564
May interact with oral anticoagulants and certain other agents. Compounds in these categories include:

Antiarthritic Drugs, unspecified (Effect not specified).

Antidiabetic Drugs, unspecified (Effect not specified).

Dicumarol (Effect not specified). Products include:
Dicumarol Tablets 516

Warfarin Sodium (Effect not specified). Products include:
Coumadin Injection & Tablets 944
Panwarfin Tablets 547

GENUINE BAYER ASPIRIN TABLETS & CAPLETS
(Aspirin) ▣ 564
May interact with oral anticoagulants, antigout agents, and certain other agents. Compounds in these categories include:

Allopurinol (Effect not specified). Products include:
Zyloprim Tablets 830

Antiarthritic Drugs, unspecified (Effect not specified).

Antidiabetic Drugs, unspecified (Effect not specified).

Dicumarol (Effect not specified). Products include:
Dicumarol Tablets 516

Probenecid (Effect not specified). Products include:
Benemid Tablets 1426
ColBENEMID Tablets 1436
Wycillin Injection and Probenecid Tablets 2539

Sulfinpyrazone (Effect not specified). Products include:
Anturane 853

Warfarin Sodium (Effect not specified). Products include:
Coumadin Injection & Tablets 944
Panwarfin Tablets 547

MAXIMUM BAYER ASPIRIN TABLETS & CAPLETS
(Aspirin) ▣ 566
May interact with oral anticoagu-

lants, antigout agents, and certain other agents. Compounds in these categories include:

Allopurinol (Effect not specified). Products include:
Zyloprim Tablets 830
Antiarthritic Drugs, unspecified (Effect not specified).
Antidiabetic Drugs, unspecified (Effect not specified).
Dicumarol (Effect not specified). Products include:
Dicumarol Tablets 516
Probenecid (Effect not specified). Products include:
Benemid Tablets 1426
ColBENEMID Tablets 1436
Wycillin Injection and Probenecid Tablets 2539
Sulfinpyrazone (Effect not specified). Products include:
Anturane 853
Warfarin Sodium (Effect not specified). Products include:
Coumadin Injection & Tablets 944
Panwarfin Tablets 547

BAYER PLUS ASPIRIN TABLETS
(Aspirin) .... ▣ 567
May interact with oral anticoagulants, antigout agents, and certain other agents. Compounds in these categories include:

Allopurinol (Effect not specified). Products include:
Zyloprim Tablets 830
Antiarthritic Drugs, unspecified (Effect not specified).
Antidiabetic Drugs, unspecified (Effect not specified).
Dicumarol (Effct not specified). Products include:
Dicumarol Tablets 516
Probenecid (Effect not specified). Products include:
Benemid Tablets 1426
ColBENEMID Tablets 1436
Wycillin Injection and Probenecid Tablets 2539
Sulfinpyrazone (Effect not specified). Products include:
Anturane 853
Warfarin Sodium (Effct not specified). Products include:
Coumadin Injection & Tablets 944
Panwarfin Tablets 547

THERAPY BAYER ASPIRIN CAPLETS
(Aspirin, Enteric Coated) .... ▣ 568
May interact with oral anticoagulants, antigout agents, and certain other agents. Compounds in these categories include:

Allopurinol (Effect not specified). Products include:
Zyloprim Tablets 830
Antiarthritic Drugs, unspecified (Effect not specified).
Antidiabetic Drugs, unspecified (Effect not specified).
Dicumarol (Effect not specified). Products include:
Dicumarol Tablets 516
Probenecid (Effect not specified). Products include:
Benemid Tablets 1426
ColBENEMID Tablets 1436
Wycillin Injection and Probenecid Tablets 2539
Sulfinpyrazone (Effect not specified). Products include:
Anturane 853
Warfarin Sodium (Effect not specified). Products include:
Coumadin Injection & Tablets 944
Panwarfin Tablets 547

8 HOUR BAYER TIMED-RELEASE ASPIRIN
(Aspirin) .... ▣ 566
May interact with oral anticoagulants, antigout agents, and certain other agents. Compounds in these categories include:

Allopurinol (Effect not specified). Products include:
Zyloprim Tablets 830
Antiarthritic Drugs, unspecified (Effect not specified).
Antidiabetic Drugs, unspecified (Effect not specified).
Dicumarol (Effect not specified). Products include:
Dicumarol Tablets 516
Probenecid (Effect not specified). Products include:
Benemid Tablets 1426
ColBENEMID Tablets 1436
Wycillin Injection and Probenecid Tablets 2539
Sulfinpyrazone (Effect not specified). Products include:
Anturane 853
Warfarin Sodium (Effect not specified). Products include:
Coumadin Injection & Tablets 944
Panwarfin Tablets 547

BAZA CREAM, OCCLUSIVE SKIN PROTECTANT
(Zinc Oxide, Benzethonium Chloride) 2285
No interactions described in labeling.

BECLOVENT INHALATION AEROSOL AND REFILL
(Beclomethasone Dipropionate) 572
No interactions described in labeling.

BECONASE AQ NASAL SPRAY
(Beclomethasone Dipropionate) 574
No interactions described in labeling.

BECONASE INHALATION AEROSOL & REFILL
(Beclomethasone Dipropionate) 574
No interactions described in labeling.

BEELITH TABLETS
(Magnesium Oxide, Vitamin B_6) 659
May interact with tetracyclines. Compounds in this category include:

Demeclocycline Hydrochloride (Concomitant oral administration with any form of tetracycline is not recommended). Products include:
Declomycin Capsules, Tablets 1199
Doxycycline Calcium (Concomitant oral administration with any form of tetracycline is not recommended).
No products indexed under this heading.
Doxycycline Hyclate (Concomitant oral administration with any form of tetracycline is not recommended). Products include:
Doryx Capsules 1717
Vibramycin Hyclate Capsules 1787
Vibramycin Hyclate Intravenous 1968
Vibra-Tabs Film Coated Tablets 1787
Doxycycline Monohydrate (Concomitant oral administration with any form of tetracycline is not recommended). Products include:
Monodox Capsules 1630
Vibramycin Monohydrate for Oral Suspension 1787
Methacycline Hydrochloride (Concomitant oral administration with any form of tetracycline is not recommended).
No products indexed under this heading.
Minocycline Hydrochloride (Concomitant oral administration with any form of tetracycline is not recommended). Products include:
Minocin Intravenous 1221
Minocin Oral Suspension 1224
Minocin Pellet-Filled Capsules 1222
Oxytetracycline Hydrochloride (Concomitant oral administration with any form of tetracycline is not recommended). Products include:
Terra-Cortril Ophthalmic Suspension 1963
Terramycin Capsules 1786
Terramycin Intramuscular Solution 1964
Terramycin with Polymyxin B Sulfate Ophthalmic Ointment 1965
Tetracycline Hydrochloride (Concomitant oral administration with any form of tetracycline is not recommended). Products include:
Achromycin V Capsules 1193
Achromycin Ophthalmic Ointment 1% .... ⊙ 307
Achromycin Ophthalmic Suspension 1% .... ⊙ 308
Topicycline for Topical Solution 1856

BELLERGAL-S TABLETS
(Phenobarbital, Ergotamine Tartrate, Belladonna Alkaloids) 1998
May interact with oral anticoagulants, tricyclic antidepressants, phenothiazines, narcotic analgesics, beta blockers, estrogens, central nervous system depressants, and certain other agents. Compounds in these categories include:

Acebutolol Hydrochloride (Excessive vasoconstriction). Products include:
Sectral Capsules 2520
Alcohol (Potentiated depressant action).
Alfentanil Hydrochloride (Potentiated depressant action). Products include:
Alfenta Injection 1131
Amitriptyline Hydrochloride (Potentiated depressant action; additive anticholinergic effects). Products include:
Elavil 2269
Endep Tablets 1927
Etrafon 2087
Limbitrol 1933
Triavil Tablets 1556
Amoxapine (Potentiated depressant action; additive anticholinergic effects). Products include:
Asendin Tablets 1196
Atenolol (Excessive vasoconstriction). Products include:
Tenoretic Tablets 1105
Tenormin Tablets and I.V. Injection 1107
Betaxolol Hydrochloride (Excessive vasoconstriction). Products include:
Betoptic Sterile Ophthalmic Solution 569
Betoptic S Sterile Ophthalmic Suspension 570
Kerlone Tablets 2172
Buprenorphine (Potentiated depressant action).
No products indexed under this heading.
Carteolol Hydrochloride (Excessive vasoconstriction). Products include:
Cartrol Tablets 507
Chlorotrianisene (Increased metabolism rate of estrogen). Products include:
TACE 12 and 25 mg 1353
Chlorpromazine (Potentiated depressant action). Products include:
Thorazine 2234
Clomipramine Hydrochloride (Potentiated depressant action; additive anticholinergic effects). Products include:
Anafranil Capsules 650
Codeine (Potentiated depressant action). Products include:
Calcidrine Syrup 506
Codeine Phosphate (Potentiated depressant action). Products include:
Actifed with Codeine Cough Syrup.. 752
Cheracol Cough Syrup 1853
Codimal PH Syrup 846
Dimetane-DC Cough Syrup 1857
Empirin with Codeine Phosphate Nos. 2, 3 & 4 764
Fiorinal with Codeine Capsules 2008
Isoclor Expectorant 982
Naldecon CX Adult Liquid .... ▣ 521
Novahistine DH 1342
Novahistine Expectorant 1343
Nucofed Capsules 2219
Nucofed Expectorant 2219
Nucofed Pediatric Expectorant 2220
Nucofed Syrup 2219
Phenaphen with Codeine Capsules 1865
Phenaphen-650 with Codeine Tablets 1866
Phenergan with Codeine 2497
Phenergan VC with Codeine 2501
Robitussin A-C Syrup 1875
Robitussin-DAC Syrup 1875
Ryna .... ▣ 741
Soma Compound w/Codeine Tablets 2390
Triaminic Expectorant w/Codeine .. 1996
Tussi-Organidin Liquid 2391
Tylenol with Codeine 1381
Codeine Polistirex (Potentiated depressant action).
No products indexed under this heading.
Desipramine Hydrochloride (Potentiated depressant action; additive anticholinergic effects). Products include:
Norpramin Tablets 1340
Dezocine (Potentiated depressant action).
Dicumarol (Decreased anticoagulant activity). Products include:
Dicumarol Tablets 516
Dienestrol (Increased metabolism rate of estrogen). Products include:
Ortho Dienestrol Cream 1664
Diethylstilbestrol (Increased metabolism rate of estrogen). Products include:
Diethylstilbestrol Tablets 1258
Divalproex Sodium (Increases metabolism of barbiturate). Products include:
Depakote 512
Dopamine Hydrochloride (Potential for ischemic vasoconstriction; concomitant administration is contraindicated). Products include:
Intropin Injection 930
Doxepin Hydrochloride (Potentiated depressant action; additive anticholinergic effects). Products include:
Sinequan 1960
Doxycycline Calcium (Increased metabolism rate of doxycycline).
No products indexed under this heading.
Doxycycline Hyclate (Increased metabolism rate of doxycycline). Products include:
Doryx Capsules 1717
Vibramycin Hyclate Capsules 1787
Vibramycin Hyclate Intravenous 1968
Vibra-Tabs Film Coated Tablets 1787

Doxycycline Monohydrate (Increased metabolism rate of doxycycline). Products include:
Monodox Capsules 1630
Vibramycin Monohydrate for Oral Suspension 1787

Esmolol Hydrochloride (Excessive vasoconstriction). Products include:
Brevibloc Injection 942

Estazolam (Potentiated depressant action). Products include:
ProSom Tablets 554

Estradiol (Increased metabolism rate of estrogen). Products include:
Emcyt Capsules 1161
Estrace 1385
Estrace Vaginal Cream 1388
Estraderm Transdermal System 866

Estrogens, Conjugated (Increased metabolism rate of estrogen). Products include:
Mediatric Capsules 2476
PMB 200 and PMB 400 2504
Premarin Intravenous 2508
Premarin with Methyltestosterone 2515
Premarin Tablets 2510
Premarin Vaginal Cream 2512

Estrogens, Esterified (Increased metabolism rate of estrogen). Products include:
Estratest 2245
Menrium Tablets 1934

Estropipate (Increased metabolism rate of estrogen). Products include:
Ogen 540

Ethinyl Estradiol (Increased metabolism rate of estrogen). Products include:
Brevicon 2304
Demulen 2161
Estinyl Tablets 2085
Jenest-28 Tablets 1636
Levlen/Tri-Levlen 665
Lo/Ovral Tablets 2471
Lo/Ovral-28 Tablets 2476
Loestrin 1728
Modicon 1667
Nordette-21 Tablets 2481
Nordette-28 Tablets 2483
Norethin 2133
Norinyl 2304
Norlestrin 1746
Ortho-Cyclen Tablets 1658
Ortho-Novum 1667
Ovcon 1391
Ovral Tablets 2490
Ovral-28 Tablets 2491
Levlen/Tri-Levlen 665
Tri-Norinyl 2304
Triphasil-21 Tablets 2527
Triphasil-28 Tablets 2532

Fentanyl (Potentiated depressant action). Products include:
Duragesic Transdermal System 1133

Fentanyl Citrate (Potentiated depressant action). Products include:
Innovar Injection 1141
Sublimaze Injection 1146

Fluphenazine Decanoate (Potentiated depressant action). Products include:
Prolixin Decanoate 1795

Fluphenazine Enanthate (Potentiated depressant action). Products include:
Prolixin Enanthate 1796

Fluphenazine Hydrochloride (Potentiated depressant action). Products include:
Prolixin Elixir 1793
Prolixin Injection 1791
Prolixin Oral Concentrate 1792
Prolixin Tablets 1793

Griseofulvin (Increased metabolism rate of griseofulvin). Products include:
Fulvicin P/G Tablets 2090
Fulvicin P/G 165 & 330 Tablets 2091
Fulvicin-U/F Tablets 2092
Grifulvin V (griseofulvin microsize) Tablets/Suspension 1678
Grisactin 2454
Grisactin Ultra Tablets 2455
Gris-PEG Tablets, 125 mg & 250 mg 1083

Hydrocodone Bitartrate (Potentiated depressant action). Products include:
Anexsia 5/500 Tablets 2196
Anexsia 7.5/650 Tablets 2197
Azdōne Tablets 844
Codiclear DH Syrup 845
Codimal DH Syrup 846
Damason-P 1356
Hycodan Syrup, Tablets 927
Hycomine Compound Tablets 929
Hycomine Syrup 927
Hycotuss Expectorant Syrup 930
Hydrocet Capsules 835
Lortab ASA Tablets 2414
Lortab 2412
Ru-Tuss with Hydrocodone 694
Triaminic Expectorant DH 1995
Vicodin Tablets 1187
Vicodin ES Tablets 1189
Zydone Capsules 941

Hydrocodone Polistirex (Potentiated depressant action). Products include:
Tussionex Extended-Release Suspension 988

Imipramine Hydrochloride (Potentiated depressant action; additive anticholinergic effects). Products include:
Tofranil Ampuls 1038
Tofranil Tablets 1039

Imipramine Pamoate (Potentiated depressant action; additive anticholinergic effects). Products include:
Tofranil-PM Capsules 1041

Labetalol Hydrochloride (Excessive vasoconstriction). Products include:
Normodyne Injection 2108
Normodyne Tablets 2110
Normozide Tablets 2112
Trandate HCT Tablets 579
Trandate Injection 577
Trandate Tablets 579

Levorphanol Tartrate (Potentiated depressant action). Products include:
Levo-Dromoran 1906

Maprotiline Hydrochloride (Potentiated depressant action; additive anticholinergic effects). Products include:
Ludiomil Tablets 874

Meperidine Hydrochloride (Potentiated depressant action). Products include:
Demerol 2047
Mepergan Injection 2479

Mesoridazine (Potentiated depressant action). Products include:
Serentil 686

Methadone Hydrochloride (Potentiated depressant action). Products include:
Dolophine Hydrochloride Ampoules & Vials 1260
Dolophine Hydrochloride Tablets 1261
Methadone Hydrochloride Diskets 1284
Methadone Hydrochloride Oral Solution & Tablets 1987

Metoprolol Tartrate (Excessive vasoconstriction). Products include:
Lopressor Ampuls 1032
Lopressor HCT Tablets 1034
Lopressor Tablets 1032

Morphine Sulfate (Potentiated depressant action). Products include:
Astramorph/PF Injection, USP (Preservative-Free) 618
Duramorph 960
Infumorph 200 and Infumorph 500 Sterile Solutions 962
MS Contin Tablets 1814
MSIR 1817
Oramorph SR (Morphine Sulfate Sustained Release Tablets) 1988
Roxanol 1991

Nadolol (Excessive vasoconstriction). Products include:
Corgard Tablets 701
Corzide Tablets 702

Nortriptyline Hydrochloride (Potentiated depressant action; additive anticholinergic effects). Products include:
Pamelor 2019

Opium Alkaloids (Potentiated depressant action). Products include:
B & O No. 15A & No. 16A Supprettes 2395
Pantopon Injectable 1911

Oxycodone Hydrochloride (Potentiated depressant action). Products include:
Percocet Tablets 950
Percodan 951
Roxicodone Tablets, Oral Solution & Intensol (Oxycodone) 1992
Tylox Capsules 1382

Penbutolol Sulfate (Excessive vasoconstriction). Products include:
Levatol 1832

Perphenazine (Potentiated depressant action). Products include:
Etrafon 2087
Triavil Tablets 1556
Trilafon 2123

Phenytoin (Accelerated effect of phenytoin). Products include:
Dilantin Infatabs 1710
Dilantin-30 Pediatric/Dilantin-125 Suspension 1713

Phenytoin Sodium (Accelerated effect of phenytoin). Products include:
Dilantin Kapseals 1708
Dilantin Parenteral 1712
Dilantin with Phenobarbital Kapseals 1715

Pindolol (Excessive vasoconstriction). Products include:
Visken Tablets 2036

Polyestradiol Phosphate (Increased metabolism rate of estrogen). Products include:
Estradurin 2452

Prochlorperazine (Potentiated depressant action). Products include:
Compazine 2201

Promethazine Hydrochloride (Potentiated depressant action). Products include:
Mepergan Injection 2479
Phenergan with Codeine 2497
Phenergan with Dextromethorphan 2499
Phenergan Injection 2493
Phenergan Suppositories 2496
Phenergan Syrup 2495
Phenergan Tablets 2496
Phenergan VC 2500
Phenergan VC with Codeine 2501

Propoxyphene Hydrochloride (Potentiated depressant action). Products include:
Darvon 1256
Wygesic Tablets 2540

Propoxyphene Napsylate (Potentiated depressant action). Products include:
Darvon-N/Darvocet-N 1254

Propranolol Hydrochloride (Excessive vasoconstriction). Products include:
Inderal 2459
Inderal LA Long Acting Capsules 2461
Inderide Tablets 2463
Inderide LA Long Acting Capsules 2465

Protriptyline Hydrochloride (Potentiated depressant action; additive anticholinergic effects). Products include:
Vivactil Tablets 1567

Quinestrol (Increased metabolism rate of estrogen). Products include:
Estrovis 1721

Quinidine Gluconate (Increased metabolism rate of quinidine). Products include:
Quinaglute Dura-Tabs Tablets 663

Quinidine Polygalacturonate (Increased metabolism rate of quinidine). Products include:
Cardioquin Tablets 1812

Quinidine Sulfate (Increased metabolism rate of quinidine). Products include:
Quinidex Extentabs 1868

Sufentanil Citrate (Potentiated depressant action). Products include:
Sufenta Injection 1147

Thioridazine Hydrochloride (Potentiated depressant action). Products include:
Mellaril 2011

Timolol Maleate (Excessive vasoconstriction). Products include:
Blocadren Tablets 1429
Timolide Tablets 1547
Timoptic in Ocudose 1552
Timoptic Sterile Ophthalmic Solution 1550

Trifluoperazine Hydrochloride (Potentiated depressant action). Products include:
Stelazine 2226

Trimipramine Maleate (Potentiated depressant action; additive anticholinergic effects). Products include:
Surmontil Capsules 2524

Valproic Acid (Increases metabolism of barbiturate). Products include:
Depakene Capsules & Syrup 511

Warfarin Sodium (Decreased anticoagulant activity). Products include:
Coumadin Injection & Tablets 944
Panwarfin Tablets 547

BENADRYL ANTI-ITCH CREAM
(Diphenhydramine Hydrochloride) .. (NP) 635
May interact with:

Diphenhydramine (Concurrent use is not recommended).

BENADRYL CAPSULES
(Diphenhydramine Hydrochloride) 1691
May interact with central nervous system depressants, monoamine oxidase inhibitors, and certain other agents. Compounds in these categories include:

Alcohol (Additive effects).

Alfentanil Hydrochloride (Additive effects). Products include:
Alfenta Injection 1131

Alprazolam (Additive effects). Products include:
Xanax Tablets 2367

Aprobarbital (Additive effects). Products include:
Alurate Elixir 1883

Buprenorphine (Additive effects).
No products indexed under this heading.

Buspirone Hydrochloride (Additive effects). Products include:
BuSpar 1401

Butabarbital (Additive effects). Products include:
Pyridium Plus 1764

Butalbital (Additive effects). Products include:
Esgic-Plus Tablets 1002
Esgic Tablets & Capsules 1001
Fioricet Tablets 2006

Fiorinal Capsules 2007
Fiorinal with Codeine Capsules 2008
Fiorinal Tablets 2007
Phrenilin 838
Sedapap Tablets 50 mg/650 mg .. 1360

Chlordiazepoxide (Additive effects). Products include:
Libritabs Tablets 1930
Limbitrol 1933
Menrium Tablets 1934

Chlordiazepoxide Hydrochloride (Additive effects). Products include:
Librax Capsules 1929
Librium Capsules 1931
Librium Injectable 1932

Chlorpromazine (Additive effects). Products include:
Thorazine 2234

Chlorprothixene (Additive effects). Products include:
Taractan Tablets 1920

Chlorprothixene Hydrochloride (Additive effects). Products include:
Taractan 1920

Chlorprothixene Lactate (Additive effects). Products include:
Taractan Concentrate 1920

Clorazepate Dipotassium (Additive effects). Products include:
Tranxene 556

Codeine (Additive effects). Products include:
Calcidrine Syrup 506

Codeine Phosphate (Additive effects). Products include:
Actifed with Codeine Cough Syrup.. 752
Cheracol Cough Syrup 1853
Codimal PH Syrup 846
Dimetane-DC Cough Syrup 1857
Empirin with Codeine Phosphate Nos. 2, 3 & 4 764
Fiorinal with Codeine Capsules 2008
Isoclor Expectorant 982
Naldecon CX Adult Liquid .... ◘ 521
Novahistine DH 1342
Novahistine Expectorant 1343
Nucofed Capsules 2219
Nucofed Expectorant 2219
Nucofed Pediatric Expectorant 2220
Nucofed Syrup 2219
Phenaphen with Codeine Capsules 1865
Phenaphen-650 with Codeine Tablets 1866
Phenergan with Codeine 2497
Phenergan VC with Codeine 2501
Robitussin A-C Syrup 1875
Robitussin-DAC Syrup 1875
Ryna .... ◘ 741
Soma Compound w/Codeine Tablets 2390
Triaminic Expectorant w/Codeine .. 1996
Tussi-Organidin Liquid 2391
Tylenol with Codeine 1381

Codeine Polistirex (Additive effects).
No products indexed under this heading.

Dezocine (Additive effects).

Diazepam (Additive effects). Products include:
Valium Injectable 1937
Valium Tablets 1939
Valrelease Capsules 1923

Droperidol (Additive effects). Products include:
Inapsine Injection 1140
Innovar Injection 1141

Enflurane (Additive effects). Products include:
Ethrane 599

Estazolam (Additive effects). Products include:
ProSom Tablets 554

Ethchlorvynol (Additive effects). Products include:
Placidyl Capsules 553

Ethinamate (Additive effects).
No products indexed under this heading.

Fentanyl (Additive effects). Products include:
Duragesic Transdermal System........ 1133

Fentanyl Citrate (Additive effects). Products include:
Innovar Injection 1141
Sublimaze Injection 1146

Fluphenazine Decanoate (Additive effects). Products include:
Prolixin Decanoate 1795

Fluphenazine Enanthate (Additive effects). Products include:
Prolixin Enanthate 1796

Fluphenazine Hydrochloride (Additive effects). Products include:
Prolixin Elixir 1793
Prolixin Injection 1791
Prolixin Oral Concentrate 1792
Prolixin Tablets 1793

Flurazepam Hydrochloride (Additive effects). Products include:
Dalmane Capsules 1927

Furazolidone (Anticholinergic effects of antihistamines prolonged and intensified). Products include:
Furoxone 1855

Glutethimide (Additive effects).
No products indexed under this heading.

Haloperidol (Additive effects). Products include:
Haldol Injection, Tablets and Concentrate 1373

Haloperidol Decanoate (Additive effects). Products include:
Haldol Decanoate 1375

Hydrocodone Bitartrate (Additive effects). Products include:
Anexsia 5/500 Tablets 2196
Anexsia 7.5/650 Tablets 2197
Azdōne Tablets 844
Codiclear DH Syrup 845
Codimal DH Syrup 846
Damason-P 1356
Hycodan Syrup, Tablets 927
Hycomine Compound Tablets 929
Hycomine Syrup 927
Hycotuss Expectorant Syrup 930
Hydrocet Capsules 835
Lortab ASA Tablets 2414
Lortab 2412
Ru-Tuss with Hydrocodone 694
Triaminic Expectorant DH 1995
Vicodin Tablets 1187
Vicodin ES Tablets 1189
Zydone Capsules 941

Hydrocodone Polistirex (Additive effects). Products include:
Tussionex Extended-Release Suspension 988

Hydroxyzine Hydrochloride (Additive effects). Products include:
Atarax Tablets & Syrup 1941
Marax Tablets & DF Syrup 1954
Vistaril Intramuscular Solution 1970

Isocarboxazid (Anticholinergic effects of antihistamines prolonged and intensified). Products include:
Marplan Tablets 1906

Isoflurane (Additive effects). Products include:
Forane 600

Ketamine Hydrochloride (Additive effects). Products include:
Ketalar 1726

Levorphanol Tartrate (Additive effects). Products include:
Levo-Dromoran 1906

Lorazepam (Additive effects). Products include:
Ativan Injection 2432
Ativan Tablets 2434

Loxapine Hydrochloride (Additive effects). Products include:
Loxitane 1213

Loxapine Succinate (Additive effects). Products include:
Loxitane Capsules 1213

Meperidine Hydrochloride (Additive effects). Products include:
Demerol 2047
Mepergan Injection 2479

Mephobarbital (Additive effects). Products include:
Mebaral Tablets 2061

Meprobamate (Additive effects). Products include:
Deprol Tablets 2382
Equagesic Tablets 2451
Miltown Tablets 2386
PMB 200 and PMB 400 2504

Mesoridazine (Additive effects). Products include:
Serentil 686

Methadone Hydrochloride (Additive effects). Products include:
Dolophine Hydrochloride Ampoules & Vials 1260
Dolophine Hydrochloride Tablets 1261
Methadone Hydrochloride Diskets .. 1284
Methadone Hydrochloride Oral Solution & Tablets 1987

Methohexital Sodium (Additive effects). Products include:
Brevital Sodium Vials 1248

Methoxyflurane (Additive effects).
No products indexed under this heading.

Midazolam Hydrochloride (Additive effects). Products include:
Versed Injection 1924

Molindone Hydrochloride (Additive effects). Products include:
Moban Tablets & Concentrate 932

Morphine Sulfate (Additive effects). Products include:
Astramorph/PF Injection, USP (Preservative-Free) 618
Duramorph 960
Infumorph 200 and Infumorph 500 Sterile Solutions 962
MS Contin Tablets 1814
MSIR 1817
Oramorph SR (Morphine Sulfate Sustained Release Tablets) 1988
Roxanol 1991

Opium Alkaloids (Additive effects). Products include:
B & O No. 15A & No. 16A Supprettes 2395
Pantopon Injectable 1911

Oxazepam (Additive effects). Products include:
Serax Capsules 2522
Serax Tablets 2522

Oxycodone Hydrochloride (Additive effects). Products include:
Percocet Tablets 950
Percodan 951
Roxicodone Tablets, Oral Solution & Intensol (Oxycodone) 1992
Tylox Capsules 1382

Pentobarbital Sodium (Additive effects). Products include:
Nembutal Sodium Capsules 534
Nembutal Sodium Solution 536
Nembutal Sodium Suppositories...... 538

Perphenazine (Additive effects). Products include:
Etrafon 2087
Triavil Tablets 1556
Trilafon 2123

Phenelzine Sulfate (Anticholinergic effects of antihistamines prolonged and intensified). Products include:
Nardil 1742

Phenobarbital (Additive effects). Products include:
Arco-Lase Plus Tablets 607
Bellergal-S Tablets 1998
Bronkolixir .... ◘ 761
Bronkotabs Tablets .... ◘ 762
Donnatal 1858
Donnatal Extentabs 1859
Donnatal Tablets 1858
Donnazyme Tablets 1860
Kinesed Tablets 2272
Phenobarbital Elixir and Tablets 1293
Primatene Tablets-P Formula 2421

Quadrinal Tablets 1183
Tedral SA 1765

Prazepam (Additive effects). Products include:
Centrax 1693

Prochlorperazine (Additive effects). Products include:
Compazine 2201

Promethazine Hydrochloride (Additive effects). Products include:
Mepergan Injection 2479
Phenergan with Codeine 2497
Phenergan with Dextromethorphan 2499
Phenergan Injection 2493
Phenergan Suppositories 2496
Phenergan Syrup 2495
Phenergan Tablets 2496
Phenergan VC 2500
Phenergan VC with Codeine 2501

Propofol (Additive effects). Products include:
Diprivan Injection 2267

Propoxyphene Hydrochloride (Additive effects). Products include:
Darvon 1256
Wygesic Tablets 2540

Propoxyphene Napsylate (Additive effects). Products include:
Darvon-N/Darvocet-N 1254

Quazepam (Additive effects). Products include:
Doral Tablets 2383

Secobarbital Sodium (Additive effects). Products include:
Seconal Sodium Pulvules 1296

Selegiline Hydrochloride (Anticholinergic effects of antihistamines prolonged and intensified). Products include:
Eldepryl 2250

Sufentanil Citrate (Additive effects). Products include:
Sufenta Injection 1147

Temazepam (Additive effects). Products include:
Restoril Capsules 2023

Thiamylal Sodium (Additive effects). Products include:
Surital Ampoules, Steri-Vials 1764

Thioridazine Hydrochloride (Additive effects). Products include:
Mellaril 2011

Thiothixene (Additive effects). Products include:
Navane Capsules and Concentrate 1954
Navane Intramuscular 1956

Tranylcypromine Sulfate (Anticholinergic effects of antihistamines prolonged and intensified). Products include:
Parnate Tablets 2222

Triazolam (Additive effects). Products include:
Halcion Tablets 2340

Trifluoperazine Hydrochloride (Additive effects). Products include:
Stelazine 2226

BENADRYL DECONGESTANT ELIXIR
(Diphenhydramine Hydrochloride, Pseudoephedrine Hydrochloride) .... ◘ 635
May interact with antihypertensives, antidepressant drugs, and certain other agents. Compounds in these categories include:

Acebutolol Hydrochloride (Concurrent use not recommended). Products include:
Sectral Capsules 2520

Alcohol (Increases drowsiness effect).

Amitriptyline Hydrochloride (Concurrent use not recommended). Products include:
Elavil 2269
Endep Tablets 1927
Etrafon 2087

Limbitrol 1933
Triavil Tablets 1556

Amoxapine (Concurrent use not recommended). Products include:
Asendin Tablets 1196

Atenolol (Concurrent use not recommended). Products include:
Tenoretic Tablets 1105
Tenormin Tablets and I.V. Injection 1107

Benazepril Hydrochloride (Concurrent use not recommended). Products include:
Lotensin Tablets 872

Betaxolol Hydrochloride (Concurrent use not recommended). Products include:
Betoptic Sterile Ophthalmic Solution 569
Betoptic S Sterile Ophthalmic Suspension 570
Kerlone Tablets 2172

Bupropion Hydrochloride (Concurrent use not recommended). Products include:
Wellbutrin Tablets 821

Captopril (Concurrent use not recommended). Products include:
Capoten 2255
Capozide 2258

Carteolol Hydrochloride (Concurrent use not recommended). Products include:
Cartrol Tablets 507

Clonidine (Concurrent use not recommended). Products include:
Catapres-TTS 677

Clonidine Hydrochloride (Concurrent use not recommended). Products include:
Catapres Tablets 676
Combipres Tablets 678

Deserpidine (Concurrent use not recommended). Products include:
Enduronyl 518
Harmonyl Tablets 528
Oreticyl 545

Desipramine Hydrochloride (Concurrent use not recommended). Products include:
Norpramin Tablets 1340

Diazoxide (Concurrent use not recommended). Products include:
Hyperstat I.V. Injection 2095
Proglycem 649

Doxazosin Mesylate (Concurrent use not recommended). Products include:
Cardura Tablets 1941

Doxepin Hydrochloride (Concurrent use not recommended). Products include:
Sinequan 1960

Enalapril Maleate (Concurrent use not recommended). Products include:
Vaseretic Tablets 1559
Vasotec Tablets 1564

Enalaprilat (Concurrent use not recommended). Products include:
Vasotec I.V. 1562

Esmolol Hydrochloride (Concurrent use not recommended). Products include:
Brevibloc Injection 942

Felodipine (Concurrent use not recommended). Products include:
Plendil Extended-Release Tablets 1526

Fluoxetine Hydrochloride (Concurrent use not recommended). Products include:
Prozac Pulvules 920

Fosinopril Sodium (Concurrent use not recommended). Products include:
Monopril Tablets 1406

Guanabenz Acetate (Concurrent use not recommended). Products include:
Wytensin Tablets 2542

Guanethidine Monosulfate (Concurrent use not recommended). Products include:
Esimil Tablets 864
Ismelin Tablets 869

Hydralazine Hydrochloride (Concurrent use not recommended). Products include:
Apresazide Capsules 854
Apresoline Hydrochloride Parenteral (Ampuls) 856
Apresoline Hydrochloride Tablets .. 855
Apresoline-Esidrix Tablets 857
Ser-Ap-Es Tablets 881
Serpasil-Apresoline Tablets 884

Imipramine Hydrochloride (Concurrent use not recommended). Products include:
Tofranil Ampuls 1038
Tofranil Tablets 1039

Imipramine Pamoate (Concurrent use not recommended). Products include:
Tofranil-PM Capsules 1041

Indapamide (Concurrent use not recommended). Products include:
Lozol Tablets 1843

Isocarboxazid (Concurrent use not recommended). Products include:
Marplan Tablets 1906

Isradipine (Concurrent use not recommended). Products include:
DynaCirc Capsules 2004

Labetalol Hydrochloride (Concurrent use not recommended). Products include:
Normodyne Injection 2108
Normodyne Tablets 2110
Normozide Tablets 2112
Trandate HCT Tablets 579
Trandate Injection 577
Trandate Tablets 579

Lisinopril (Concurrent use not recommended). Products include:
Prinivil Tablets 1538
Prinzide Tablets 1540
Zestoretic 2274
Zestril Tablets 2277

Maprotiline Hydrochloride (Concurrent use not recommended). Products include:
Ludiomil Tablets 874

Mecamylamine Hydrochloride (Concurrent use not recommended). Products include:
Inversine Tablets 1492

Methyldopa (Concurrent use not recommended). Products include:
Aldoclor Tablets 1413
Aldomet Oral 1415
Aldoril Tablets 1418

Methyldopate Hydrochloride (Concurrent use not recommended). Products include:
Aldomet Ester HCl Injection 1417

Metoprolol Tartrate (Concurrent use not recommended). Products include:
Lopressor Ampuls 1032
Lopressor HCT Tablets 1034
Lopressor Tablets 1032

Metyrosine (Concurrent use not recommended). Products include:
Demser Capsules 1460

Minoxidil (Concurrent use not recommended). Products include:
Loniten Tablets 2346
Rogaine Topical Solution 2357

Nadolol (Concurrent use not recommended). Products include:
Corgard Tablets 701
Corzide Tablets 702

Nicardipine Hydrochloride (Concurrent use not recommended). Products include:
Cardene Capsules 2290

Nitroglycerin (Concurrent use not recommended). Products include:
Deponit NTG Transdermal Delivery System 2143
Minitran Transdermal Delivery System 1312
Nitro-Bid Ointment 1339
Nitro-Bid Capsules 1338
Nitrodisc 2176
Nitro-Dur (nitroglycerin) Transdermal Infusion System 1164
Nitrogard Tablets 1004
Nitrolingual Spray 1846
Nitrostat Tablets 1743
Transderm-Nitro Transdermal Therapeutic System 2283

Nortriptyline Hydrochloride (Concurrent use not recommended). Products include:
Pamelor 2019

Penbutolol Sulfate (Concurrent use not recommended). Products include:
Levatol 1832

Phenelzine Sulfate (Concurrent use not recommended). Products include:
Nardil 1742

Phenoxybenzamine Hydrochloride (Concurrent use not recommended). Products include:
Dibenzyline Capsules 2207

Phentolamine Mesylate (Concurrent use not recommended). Products include:
Regitine 878

Pindolol (Concurrent use not recommended). Products include:
Visken Tablets 2036

Prazosin Hydrochloride (Concurrent use not recommended). Products include:
Minipress Capsules 1778
Minizide Capsules 1779

Propranolol Hydrochloride (Concurrent use not recommended). Products include:
Inderal 2459
Inderal LA Long Acting Capsules 2461
Inderide Tablets 2463
Inderide LA Long Acting Capsules .. 2465

Protriptyline Hydrochloride (Concurrent use not recommended). Products include:
Vivactil Tablets 1567

Ramipril (Concurrent use not recommended). Products include:
Altace Capsules 1086

Rauwolfia Serpentina (Concurrent use not recommended). Products include:
Raudixin Tablets 1803
Rauzide Tablets 1804

Rescinnamine (Concurrent use not recommended).
No products indexed under this heading.

Reserpine (Concurrent use not recommended). Products include:
Diupres Tablets 1461
Hydromox R Tablets 1209
Hydropres Tablets 1485
Renese-R Tablets 1786
Salutensin/Salutensin-Demi 719
Ser-Ap-Es Tablets 881
Serpasil Tablets 883
Serpasil-Apresoline Tablets 884
Serpasil-Esidrix Tablets 886

Sodium Nitroprusside (Concurrent use not recommended). Products include:
Nipride I.V. Infusion 1909

Terazosin Hydrochloride (Concurrent use not recommended). Products include:
Hytrin Tablets 529

Timolol Maleate (Concurrent use not recommended). Products include:
Blocadren Tablets 1429
Timolide Tablets 1547
Timoptic in Ocudose 1552
Timoptic Sterile Ophthalmic Solution 1550

Tranylcypromine Sulfate (Concurrent use not recommended). Products include:
Parnate Tablets 2222

Trazodone Hydrochloride (Concurrent use not recommended). Products include:
Desyrel and Desyrel Dividose 1404

Trimethaphan Camsylate (Concurrent use not recommended). Products include:
Arfonad Ampuls 1887

Trimipramine Maleate (Concurrent use not recommended). Products include:
Surmontil Capsules 2524

BENADRYL DECONGESTANT KAPSEALS
(Pseudoephedrine Hydrochloride, Diphenhydramine Hydrochloride).... 635
May interact with antihypertensives, antidepressant drugs, and certain other agents. Compounds in these categories include:

Acebutolol Hydrochloride (Concurrent use not recommended). Products include:
Sectral Capsules 2520

Alcohol (Increases drowsiness effect).

Amitriptyline Hydrochloride (Concurrent use not recommended). Products include:
Elavil 2269
Endep Tablets 1927
Etrafon 2087
Limbitrol 1933
Triavil Tablets 1556

Amoxapine (Concurrent use not recommended). Products include:
Asendin Tablets 1196

Atenolol (Concurrent use not recommended). Products include:
Tenoretic Tablets 1105
Tenormin Tablets and I.V. Injection 1107

Benazepril Hydrochloride (Concurrent use not recommended). Products include:
Lotensin Tablets 872

Betaxolol Hydrochloride (Concurrent use not recommended). Products include:
Betoptic Sterile Ophthalmic Solution 569
Betoptic S Sterile Ophthalmic Suspension 570
Kerlone Tablets 2172

Bupropion Hydrochloride (Concurrent use not recommended). Products include:
Wellbutrin Tablets 821

Captopril (Concurrent use not recommended). Products include:
Capoten 2255
Capozide 2258

Carteolol Hydrochloride (Concurrent use not recommended). Products include:
Cartrol Tablets 507

Clonidine (Concurrent use not recommended). Products include:
Catapres-TTS 677

Clonidine Hydrochloride (Concurrent use not recommended). Products include:
Catapres Tablets 676
Combipres Tablets 678

Deserpidine (Concurrent use not recommended). Products include:
Enduronyl ... 518
Harmonyl Tablets ... 528
Oreticyl ... 545

Desipramine Hydrochloride (Concurrent use not recommended). Products include:
Norpramin Tablets ... 1340

Diazoxide (Concurrent use not recommended). Products include:
Hyperstat I.V. Injection ... 2095
Proglycem ... 649

Doxazosin Mesylate (Concurrent use not recommended). Products include:
Cardura Tablets ... 1941

Doxepin Hydrochloride (Concurrent use not recommended). Products include:
Sinequan ... 1960

Enalapril Maleate (Concurrent use not recommended). Products include:
Vaseretic Tablets ... 1559
Vasotec Tablets ... 1564

Enalaprilat (Concurrent use not recommended). Products include:
Vasotec I.V. ... 1562

Esmolol Hydrochloride (Concurrent use not recommended). Products include:
Brevibloc Injection ... 942

Felodipine (Concurrent use not recommended). Products include:
Plendil Extended-Release Tablets ... 1526

Fluoxetine Hydrochloride (Concurrent use not recommended). Products include:
Prozac Pulvules ... 920

Fosinopril Sodium (Concurrent use not recommended). Products include:
Monopril Tablets ... 1406

Guanabenz Acetate (Concurrent use not recommended). Products include:
Wytensin Tablets ... 2542

Guanethidine Monosulfate (Concurrent use not recommended). Products include:
Esimil Tablets ... 864
Ismelin Tablets ... 869

Hydralazine Hydrochloride (Concurrent use not recommended). Products include:
Apresazide Capsules ... 854
Apresoline Hydrochloride Parenteral (Ampuls) ... 856
Apresoline Hydrochloride Tablets ... 855
Apresoline-Esidrix Tablets ... 857
Ser-Ap-Es Tablets ... 881
Serpasil-Apresoline Tablets ... 884

Imipramine Hydrochloride (Concurrent use not recommended). Products include:
Tofranil Ampuls ... 1038
Tofranil Tablets ... 1039

Imipramine Pamoate (Concurrent use not recommended). Products include:
Tofranil-PM Capsules ... 1041

Indapamide (Concurrent use not recommended). Products include:
Lozol Tablets ... 1843

Isocarboxazid (Concurrent use not recommended). Products include:
Marplan Tablets ... 1906

Isradipine (Concurrent use not recommended). Products include:
DynaCirc Capsules ... 2004

Labetalol Hydrochloride (Concurrent use not recommended). Products include:
Normodyne Injection ... 2108
Normodyne Tablets ... 2110
Normozide Tablets ... 2112
Trandate HCT Tablets ... 579
Trandate Injection ... 577
Trandate Tablets ... 579

Lisinopril (Concurrent use not recommended). Products include:
Prinivil Tablets ... 1538
Prinzide Tablets ... 1540
Zestoretic ... 2274
Zestril Tablets ... 2277

Maprotiline Hydrochloride (Concurrent use not recommended). Products include:
Ludiomil Tablets ... 874

Mecamylamine Hydrochloride (Concurrent use not recommended). Products include:
Inversine Tablets ... 1492

Methyldopa (Concurrent use not recommended). Products include:
Aldoclor Tablets ... 1413
Aldomet Oral ... 1415
Aldoril Tablets ... 1418

Methyldopate Hydrochloride (Concurrent use not recommended). Products include:
Aldomet Ester HCl Injection ... 1417

Metoprolol Tartrate (Concurrent use not recommended). Products include:
Lopressor Ampuls ... 1032
Lopressor HCT Tablets ... 1034
Lopressor Tablets ... 1032

Metyrosine (Concurrent use not recommended). Products include:
Demser Capsules ... 1460

Minoxidil (Concurrent use not recommended). Products include:
Loniten Tablets ... 2346
Rogaine Topical Solution ... 2357

Nadolol (Concurrent use not recommended). Products include:
Corgard Tablets ... 701
Corzide Tablets ... 702

Nicardipine Hydrochloride (Concurrent use not recommended). Products include:
Cardene Capsules ... 2290

Nitroglycerin (Concurrent use not recommended). Products include:
Deponit NTG Transdermal Delivery System ... 2143
Minitran Transdermal Delivery System ... 1312
Nitro-Bid Ointment ... 1339
Nitro-Bid Capsules ... 1338
Nitrodisc ... 2176
Nitro-Dur (nitroglycerin) Transdermal Infusion System ... 1164
Nitrogard Tablets ... 1004
Nitrolingual Spray ... 1846
Nitrostat Tablets ... 1743
Transderm-Nitro Transdermal Therapeutic System ... 2283

Nortriptyline Hydrochloride (Concurrent use not recommended). Products include:
Pamelor ... 2019

Penbutolol Sulfate (Concurrent use not recommended). Products include:
Levatol ... 1832

Phenelzine Sulfate (Concurrent use not recommended). Products include:
Nardil ... 1742

Phenoxybenzamine Hydrochloride (Concurrent use not recommended). Products include:
Dibenzyline Capsules ... 2207

Phentolamine Mesylate (Concurrent use not recommended). Products include:
Regitine ... 878

Pindolol (Concurrent use not recommended). Products include:
Visken Tablets ... 2036

Prazosin Hydrochloride (Concurrent use not recommended). Products include:
Minipress Capsules ... 1778
Minizide Capsules ... 1779

Propranolol Hydrochloride (Concurrent use not recommended). Products include:
Inderal ... 2459
Inderal LA Long Acting Capsules ... 2461
Inderide Tablets ... 2463
Inderide LA Long Acting Capsules ... 2465

Protriptyline Hydrochloride (Concurrent use not recommended). Products include:
Vivactil Tablets ... 1567

Ramipril (Concurrent use not recommended). Products include:
Altace Capsules ... 1086

Rauwolfia Serpentina (Concurrent use not recommended). Products include:
Raudixin Tablets ... 1803
Rauzide Tablets ... 1804

Rescinnamine (Concurrent use not recommended).
No products indexed under this heading.

Reserpine (Concurrent use not recommended). Products include:
Diupres Tablets ... 1461
Hydromox R Tablets ... 1209
Hydropres Tablets ... 1485
Renese-R Tablets ... 1786
Salutensin/Salutensin-Demi ... 719
Ser-Ap-Es Tablets ... 881
Serpasil Tablets ... 883
Serpasil-Apresoline Tablets ... 884
Serpasil-Esidrix Tablets ... 886

Sodium Nitroprusside (Concurrent use not recommended). Products include:
Nipride I.V. Infusion ... 1909

Terazosin Hydrochloride (Concurrent use not recommended). Products include:
Hytrin Tablets ... 529

Timolol Maleate (Concurrent use not recommended). Products include:
Blocadren Tablets ... 1429
Timolide Tablets ... 1547
Timoptic in Ocudose ... 1552
Timoptic Sterile Ophthalmic Solution ... 1550

Tranylcypromine Sulfate (Concurrent use not recommended). Products include:
Parnate Tablets ... 2222

Trazodone Hydrochloride (Concurrent use not recommended). Products include:
Desyrel and Desyrel Dividose ... 1404

Trimethaphan Camsylate (Concurrent use not recommended). Products include:
Arfonad Ampuls ... 1887

Trimipramine Maleate (Concurrent use not recommended). Products include:
Surmontil Capsules ... 2524

BENADRYL DECONGESTANT TABLETS
(Diphenhydramine Hydrochloride, Pseudoephedrine Hydrochloride) ... ◘ 635
See **Benadryl Decongestant Kapseals**

BENADRYL ELIXIR
(Diphenhydramine Hydrochloride) ... ◘ 636
May interact with:

Alcohol (Increases drowsiness effect).

BENADRYL KAPSEALS
(Diphenhydramine Hydrochloride) ... 1691
See **Benadryl Capsules**

BENADRYL 25 KAPSEALS
(Diphenhydramine Hydrochloride) ... ◘ 636
May interact with:

Alcohol (Increases drowsiness effect).

BENADRYL PARENTERAL
(Diphenhydramine Hydrochloride) ... 1692
May interact with central nervous system depressants, monoamine oxidase inhibitors, and certain other agents. Compounds in these categories include:

Alcohol (Additive effects).

Alfentanil Hydrochloride (Additive effects). Products include:
Alfenta Injection ... 1131

Alprazolam (Additive effects). Products include:
Xanax Tablets ... 2367

Aprobarbital (Additive effects). Products include:
Alurate Elixir ... 1883

Buprenorphine (Additive effects).
No products indexed under this heading.

Buspirone Hydrochloride (Additive effects). Products include:
BuSpar ... 1401

Butabarbital (Additive effects). Products include:
Pyridium Plus ... 1764

Butalbital (Additive effects). Products include:
Esgic-Plus Tablets ... 1002
Esgic Tablets & Capsules ... 1001
Fioricet Tablets ... 2006
Fiorinal Capsules ... 2007
Fiorinal with Codeine Capsules ... 2008
Fiorinal Tablets ... 2007
Phrenilin ... 838
Sedapap Tablets 50 mg/650 mg ... 1360

Chlordiazepoxide (Additive effects). Products include:
Libritabs Tablets ... 1930
Limbitrol ... 1933
Menrium Tablets ... 1934

Chlordiazepoxide Hydrochloride (Additive effects). Products include:
Librax Capsules ... 1929
Librium Capsules ... 1931
Librium Injectable ... 1932

Chlorpromazine (Additive effects). Products include:
Thorazine ... 2234

Chlorprothixene (Additive effects). Products include:
Taractan Tablets ... 1920

Chlorprothixene Hydrochloride (Additive effects). Products include:
Taractan ... 1920

Clorazepate Dipotassium (Additive effects). Products include:
Tranxene ... 556

Codeine (Additive effects). Products include:
Calcidrine Syrup ... 506

Codeine Phosphate (Additive effects). Products include:
Actifed with Codeine Cough Syrup ... 752
Cheracol Cough Syrup ... 1853
Codimal PH Syrup ... 846
Dimetane-DC Cough Syrup ... 1857
Empirin with Codeine Phosphate Nos. 2, 3 & 4 ... 764
Fiorinal with Codeine Capsules ... 2008
Isoclor Expectorant ... 982
Naldecon CX Adult Liquid ... ◘ 521
Novahistine DH ... 1342
Novahistine Expectorant ... 1343
Nucofed Capsules ... 2219
Nucofed Expectorant ... 2219
Nucofed Pediatric Expectorant ... 2220
Nucofed Syrup ... 2219
Phenaphen with Codeine Capsules ... 1865
Phenaphen-650 with Codeine Tablets ... 1866
Phenergan with Codeine ... 2497
Phenergan VC with Codeine ... 2501

Robitussin A-C Syrup 1875
Robitussin-DAC Syrup 1875
Ryna .... ▣ 741
Soma Compound w/Codeine Tablets 2390
Triaminic Expectorant w/Codeine .. 1996
Tussi-Organidin Liquid 2391
Tylenol with Codeine 1381

Codeine Polistirex (Additive effects).
No products indexed under this heading.

Dezocine (Additive effects).

Diazepam (Additive effects). Products include:
Valium Injectable 1937
Valium Tablets 1939
Valrelease Capsules 1923

Droperidol (Additive effects). Products include:
Inapsine Injection 1140
Innovar Injection 1141

Enflurane (Additive effects). Products include:
Ethrane 599

Estazolam (Additive effects). Products include:
ProSom Tablets 554

Ethchlorvynol (Additive effects). Products include:
Placidyl Capsules 553

Ethinamate (Additive effects).
No products indexed under this heading.

Fentanyl (Additive effects). Products include:
Duragesic Transdermal System 1133

Fentanyl Citrate (Additive effects). Products include:
Innovar Injection 1141
Sublimaze Injection 1146

Fluphenazine Decanoate (Additive effects). Products include:
Prolixin Decanoate 1795

Fluphenazine Enanthate (Additive effects). Products include:
Prolixin Enanthate 1796

Fluphenazine Hydrochloride (Additive effects). Products include:
Prolixin Elixir 1793
Prolixin Injection 1791
Prolixin Oral Concentrate 1792
Prolixin Tablets 1793

Flurazepam Hydrochloride (Additive effects). Products include:
Dalmane Capsules 1927

Furazolidone (Anticholinergic effects of antihistamines prolonged and intensified). Products include:
Furoxone 1855

Glutethimide (Additive effects).
No products indexed under this heading.

Haloperidol (Additive effects). Products include:
Haldol Injection, Tablets and Concentrate 1373

Haloperidol Decanoate (Additive effects). Products include:
Haldol Decanoate 1375

Hydrocodone Bitartrate (Additive effects). Products include:
Anexsia 5/500 Tablets 2196
Anexsia 7.5/650 Tablets 2197
Azdone Tablets 844
Codiclear DH Syrup 845
Codimal DH Syrup 846
Damason-P 1356
Hycodan Syrup, Tablets 927
Hycomine Compound Tablets 929
Hycomine Syrup 927
Hycotuss Expectorant Syrup 930
Hydrocet Capsules 835
Lortab ASA Tablets 2414
Lortab 2412
Ru-Tuss with Hydrocodone 694
Triaminic Expectorant DH 1995
Vicodin Tablets 1187
Vicodin ES Tablets 1189
Zydone Capsules 941

Hydrocodone Polistirex (Additive effects). Products include:
Tussionex Extended-Release Suspension 988

Hydroxyzine Hydrochloride (Additive effects). Products include:
Atarax Tablets & Syrup 1941
Marax Tablets & DF Syrup 1954
Vistaril Intramuscular Solution 1970

Isocarboxazid (Anticholinergic effects of antihistamines prolonged and intensified). Products include:
Marplan Tablets 1906

Isoflurane (Additive effects). Products include:
Forane 600

Ketamine Hydrochloride (Additive effects). Products include:
Ketalar 1726

Levorphanol Tartrate (Additive effects). Products include:
Levo-Dromoran 1906

Lorazepam (Additive effects). Products include:
Ativan Injection 2432
Ativan Tablets 2434

Loxapine Hydrochloride (Additive effects). Products include:
Loxitane 1213

Loxapine Succinate (Additive effects). Products include:
Loxitane Capsules 1213

Meperidine Hydrochloride (Additive effects). Products include:
Demerol 2047
Mepergan Injection 2479

Mephobarbital (Additive effects). Products include:
Mebaral Tablets 2061

Meprobamate (Additive effects). Products include:
Deprol Tablets 2382
Equagesic Tablets 2451
Miltown Tablets 2386
PMB 200 and PMB 400 2504

Mesoridazine (Additive effects). Products include:
Serentil 686

Methadone Hydrochloride (Additive effects). Products include:
Dolophine Hydrochloride Ampoules & Vials 1260
Dolophine Hydrochloride Tablets 1261
Methadone Hydrochloride Diskets .. 1284
Methadone Hydrochloride Oral Solution & Tablets 1987

Methohexital Sodium (Additive effects). Products include:
Brevital Sodium Vials 1248

Methoxyflurane (Additive effects).
No products indexed under this heading.

Midazolam Hydrochloride (Additive effects). Products include:
Versed Injection 1924

Molindone Hydrochloride (Additive effects). Products include:
Moban Tablets & Concentrate 932

Morphine Sulfate (Additive effects). Products include:
Astramorph/PF Injection, USP (Preservative-Free) 618
Duramorph 960
Infumorph 200 and Infumorph 500 Sterile Solutions 962
MS Contin Tablets 1814
MSIR 1817
Oramorph SR (Morphine Sulfate Sustained Release Tablets) 1988
Roxanol 1991

Opium Alkaloids (Additive effects). Products include:
B & O No. 15A & No. 16A Supprettes 2395
Pantopon Injectable 1911

Oxazepam (Additive effects). Products include:
Serax Capsules 2522
Serax Tablets 2522

Oxycodone Hydrochloride (Additive effects). Products include:
Percocet Tablets 950
Percodan 951
Roxicodone Tablets, Oral Solution & Intensol (Oxycodone) 1992
Tylox Capsules 1382

Pentobarbital Sodium (Additive effects). Products include:
Nembutal Sodium Capsules 534
Nembutal Sodium Solution 536
Nembutal Sodium Suppositories 538

Perphenazine (Additive effects). Products include:
Etrafon 2087
Triavil Tablets 1556
Trilafon 2123

Phenelzine Sulfate (Anticholinergic effects of antihistamines prolonged and intensified). Products include:
Nardil 1742

Phenobarbital (Additive effects). Products include:
Arco-Lase Plus Tablets 607
Bellergal-S Tablets 1998
Bronkolixir .... ▣ 761
Bronkotabs Tablets .... ▣ 762
Donnatal 1858
Donnatal Extentabs 1859
Donnatal Tablets 1858
Donnazyme Tablets 1860
Kinesed Tablets 2272
Phenobarbital Elixir and Tablets 1293
Primatene Tablets-P Formula 2421
Quadrinal Tablets 1183
Tedral SA 1765

Prazepam (Additive effects). Products include:
Centrax 1693

Prochlorperazine (Additive effects). Products include:
Compazine 2201

Promethazine Hydrochloride (Additive effects). Products include:
Mepergan Injection 2479
Phenergan with Codeine 2497
Phenergan with Dextromethorphan 2499
Phenergan Injection 2493
Phenergan Suppositories 2496
Phenergan Syrup 2495
Phenergan Tablets 2496
Phenergan VC 2500
Phenergan VC with Codeine 2501

Propofol (Additive effects). Products include:
Diprivan Injection 2267

Propoxyphene Hydrochloride (Additive effects). Products include:
Darvon 1256
Wygesic Tablets 2540

Propoxyphene Napsylate (Additive effects). Products include:
Darvon-N/Darvocet-N 1254

Quazepam (Additive effects). Products include:
Doral Tablets 2383

Secobarbital Sodium (Additive effects). Products include:
Seconal Sodium Pulvules 1296

Selegiline Hydrochloride (Anticholinergic effects of antihistamines prolonged and intensified). Products include:
Eldepryl 2250

Sufentanil Citrate (Additive effects). Products include:
Sufenta Injection 1147

Temazepam (Additive effects). Products include:
Restoril Capsules 2023

Thiamylal Sodium (Additive effects). Products include:
Surital Ampoules, Steri-Vials 1764

Thioridazine Hydrochloride (Additive effects). Products include:
Mellaril 2011

Thiothixene (Additive effects). Products include:
Navane Capsules and Concentrate 1954
Navane Intramuscular 1956

Tranylcypromine Sulfate (Anticholinergic effects of antihistamines prolonged and intensified). Products include:
Parnate Tablets 2222

Triazolam (Additive effects). Products include:
Halcion Tablets 2340

Trifluoperazine Hydrochloride (Additive effects). Products include:
Stelazine 2226

BENADRYL PLUS
(Acetaminophen, Diphenhydramine Hydrochloride, Pseudoephedrine Hydrochloride) .... ▣ 636
May interact with antihypertensives, antidepressant drugs, and certain other agents. Compounds in these categories include:

Acebutolol Hydrochloride (Concurrent use not recommended). Products include:
Sectral Capsules 2520

Alcohol (Increases drowsiness effect).

Amitriptyline Hydrochloride (Concurrent use not recommended). Products include:
Elavil 2269
Endep Tablets 1927
Etrafon 2087
Limbitrol 1933
Triavil Tablets 1556

Amoxapine (Concurrent use not recommended). Products include:
Asendin Tablets 1196

Atenolol (Concurrent use not recommended). Products include:
Tenoretic Tablets 1105
Tenormin Tablets and I.V. Injection 1107

Benazepril Hydrochloride (Concurrent use not recommended). Products include:
Lotensin Tablets 872

Betaxolol Hydrochloride (Concurrent use not recommended). Products include:
Betoptic Sterile Ophthalmic Solution 569
Betoptic S Sterile Ophthalmic Suspension 570
Kerlone Tablets 2172

Bupropion Hydrochloride (Concurrent use not recommended). Products include:
Wellbutrin Tablets 821

Captopril (Concurrent use not recommended). Products include:
Capoten 2255
Capozide 2258

Carteolol Hydrochloride (Concurrent use not recommended). Products include:
Cartrol Tablets 507

Clonidine (Concurrent use not recommended). Products include:
Catapres-TTS 677

Clonidine Hydrochloride (Concurrent use not recommended). Products include:
Catapres Tablets 676
Combipres Tablets 678

Deserpidine (Concurrent use not recommended). Products include:
Enduronyl 518
Harmonyl Tablets 528
Oreticyl 545

Desipramine Hydrochloride (Concurrent use not recommended). Products include:
Norpramin Tablets 1340

Diazoxide (Concurrent use not recommended). Products include:
Hyperstat I.V. Injection 2095
Proglycem 649

Doxazosin Mesylate (Concurrent use not recommended). Products include:
- Cardura Tablets ... 1941

Doxepin Hydrochloride (Concurrent use not recommended). Products include:
- Sinequan ... 1960

Enalapril Maleate (Concurrent use not recommended). Products include:
- Vaseretic Tablets ... 1559
- Vasotec Tablets ... 1564

Enalaprilat (Concurrent use not recommended). Products include:
- Vasotec I.V. ... 1562

Esmolol Hydrochloride (Concurrent use not recommended). Products include:
- Brevibloc Injection ... 942

Felodipine (Concurrent use not recommended). Products include:
- Plendil Extended-Release Tablets ... 1526

Fluoxetine Hydrochloride (Concurrent use not recommended). Products include:
- Prozac Pulvules ... 920

Fosinopril Sodium (Concurrent use not recommended). Products include:
- Monopril Tablets ... 1406

Guanabenz Acetate (Concurrent use not recommended). Products include:
- Wytensin Tablets ... 2542

Guanethidine Monosulfate (Concurrent use not recommended). Products include:
- Esimil Tablets ... 864
- Ismelin Tablets ... 869

Hydralazine Hydrochloride (Concurrent use not recommended). Products include:
- Apresazide Capsules ... 854
- Apresoline Hydrochloride Parenteral (Ampuls) ... 856
- Apresoline Hydrochloride Tablets ... 855
- Apresoline-Esidrix Tablets ... 857
- Ser-Ap-Es Tablets ... 881
- Serpasil-Apresoline Tablets ... 884

Imipramine Hydrochloride (Concurrent use not recommended). Products include:
- Tofranil Ampuls ... 1038
- Tofranil Tablets ... 1039

Imipramine Pamoate (Concurrent use not recommended). Products include:
- Tofranil-PM Capsules ... 1041

Indapamide (Concurrent use not recommended). Products include:
- Lozol Tablets ... 1843

Isocarboxazid (Concurrent use not recommended). Products include:
- Marplan Tablets ... 1906

Isradipine (Concurrent use not recommended). Products include:
- DynaCirc Capsules ... 2004

Labetalol Hydrochloride (Concurrent use not recommended). Products include:
- Normodyne Injection ... 2108
- Normodyne Tablets ... 2110
- Normozide Tablets ... 2112
- Trandate HCT Tablets ... 579
- Trandate Injection ... 577
- Trandate Tablets ... 579

Lisinopril (Concurrent use not recommended). Products include:
- Prinivil Tablets ... 1538
- Prinzide Tablets ... 1540
- Zestoretic ... 2274
- Zestril Tablets ... 2277

Maprotiline Hydrochloride (Concurrent use not recommended). Products include:
- Ludiomil Tablets ... 874

Mecamylamine Hydrochloride (Concurrent use not recommended). Products include:
- Inversine Tablets ... 1492

Methyldopa (Concurrent use not recommended). Products include:
- Aldoclor Tablets ... 1413
- Aldomet Oral ... 1415
- Aldoril Tablets ... 1418

Methyldopate Hydrochloride (Concurrent use not recommended). Products include:
- Aldomet Ester HCl Injection ... 1417

Metoprolol Tartrate (Concurrent use not recommended). Products include:
- Lopressor Ampuls ... 1032
- Lopressor HCT Tablets ... 1034
- Lopressor Tablets ... 1032

Metyrosine (Concurrent use not recommended). Products include:
- Demser Capsules ... 1460

Minoxidil (Concurrent use not recommended). Products include:
- Loniten Tablets ... 2346
- Rogaine Topical Solution ... 2357

Nadolol (Concurrent use not recommended). Products include:
- Corgard Tablets ... 701
- Corzide Tablets ... 702

Nicardipine Hydrochloride (Concurrent use not recommended). Products include:
- Cardene Capsules ... 2290

Nitroglycerin (Concurrent use not recommended). Products include:
- Deponit NTG Transdermal Delivery System ... 2143
- Minitran Transdermal Delivery System ... 1312
- Nitro-Bid Ointment ... 1339
- Nitro-Bid Capsules ... 1338
- Nitrodisc ... 2176
- Nitro-Dur (nitroglycerin) Transdermal Infusion System ... 1164
- Nitrogard Tablets ... 1004
- Nitrolingual Spray ... 1846
- Nitrostat Tablets ... 1743
- Transderm-Nitro Transdermal Therapeutic System ... 2283

Nortriptyline Hydrochloride (Concurrent use not recommended). Products include:
- Pamelor ... 2019

Penbutolol Sulfate (Concurrent use not recommended). Products include:
- Levatol ... 1832

Phenelzine Sulfate (Concurrent use not recommended). Products include:
- Nardil ... 1742

Phenoxybenzamine Hydrochloride (Concurrent use not recommended). Products include:
- Dibenzyline Capsules ... 2207

Phentolamine Mesylate (Concurrent use not recommended). Products include:
- Regitine ... 878

Pindolol (Concurrent use not recommended). Products include:
- Visken Tablets ... 2036

Prazosin Hydrochloride (Concurrent use not recommended). Products include:
- Minipress Capsules ... 1778
- Minizide Capsules ... 1779

Propranolol Hydrochloride (Concurrent use not recommended). Products include:
- Inderal ... 2459
- Inderal LA Long Acting Capsules ... 2461
- Inderide Tablets ... 2463
- Inderide LA Long Acting Capsules ... 2465

Protriptyline Hydrochloride (Concurrent use not recommended). Products include:
- Vivactil Tablets ... 1567

Ramipril (Concurrent use not recommended). Products include:
- Altace Capsules ... 1086

Rauwolfia Serpentina (Concurrent use not recommended). Products include:
- Raudixin Tablets ... 1803
- Rauzide Tablets ... 1804

Rescinnamine (Concurrent use not recommended).
- No products indexed under this heading.

Reserpine (Concurrent use not recommended). Products include:
- Diupres Tablets ... 1461
- Hydromox R Tablets ... 1209
- Hydropres Tablets ... 1485
- Renese-R Tablets ... 1786
- Salutensin/Salutensin-Demi ... 719
- Ser-Ap-Es Tablets ... 881
- Serpasil Tablets ... 883
- Serpasil-Apresoline Tablets ... 884
- Serpasil-Esidrix Tablets ... 886

Sodium Nitroprusside (Concurrent use not recommended). Products include:
- Nipride I.V. Infusion ... 1909

Terazosin Hydrochloride (Concurrent use not recommended). Products include:
- Hytrin Tablets ... 529

Timolol Maleate (Concurrent use not recommended). Products include:
- Blocadren Tablets ... 1429
- Timolide Tablets ... 1547
- Timoptic in Ocudose ... 1552
- Timoptic Sterile Ophthalmic Solution ... 1550

Tranylcypromine Sulfate (Concurrent use not recommended). Products include:
- Parnate Tablets ... 2222

Trazodone Hydrochloride (Concurrent use not recommended). Products include:
- Desyrel and Desyrel Dividose ... 1404

Trimethaphan Camsylate (Concurrent use not recommended). Products include:
- Arfonad Ampuls ... 1887

Trimipramine Maleate (Concurrent use not recommended). Products include:
- Surmontil Capsules ... 2524

BENADRYL PLUS NIGHTTIME
(Acetaminophen, Diphenhydramine Hydrochloride, Pseudoephedrine Hydrochloride) ... ⊞ 637
May interact with antihypertensives, antidepressant drugs, and certain other agents. Compounds in these categories include:

Acebutolol Hydrochloride (Concurrent use not recommended). Products include:
- Sectral Capsules ... 2520

Alcohol (May increase drowsiness effect).

Amitriptyline Hydrochloride (Concurrent use not recommended). Products include:
- Elavil ... 2269
- Endep Tablets ... 1927
- Etrafon ... 2087
- Limbitrol ... 1933
- Triavil Tablets ... 1556

Amoxapine (Concurrent use not recommended). Products include:
- Asendin Tablets ... 1196

Atenolol (Concurrent use not recommended). Products include:
- Tenoretic Tablets ... 1105
- Tenormin Tablets and I.V. Injection ... 1107

Benazepril Hydrochloride (Concurrent use not recommended). Products include:
- Lotensin Tablets ... 872

Bendroflumethiazide (Concurrent use not recommended). Products include:
- Corzide Tablets ... 702
- Naturetin Tablets ... 1789
- Rauzide Tablets ... 1804

Betaxolol Hydrochloride (Concurrent use not recommended). Products include:
- Betoptic Sterile Ophthalmic Solution ... 569
- Betoptic S Sterile Ophthalmic Suspension ... 570
- Kerlone Tablets ... 2172

Bupropion Hydrochloride (Concurrent use not recommended). Products include:
- Wellbutrin Tablets ... 821

Captopril (Concurrent use not recommended). Products include:
- Capoten ... 2255
- Capozide ... 2258

Carteolol Hydrochloride (Concurrent use not recommended). Products include:
- Cartrol Tablets ... 507

Chlorothiazide (Concurrent use not recommended). Products include:
- Aldoclor Tablets ... 1413
- Diupres Tablets ... 1461
- Diuril Oral ... 1464

Chlorothiazide Sodium (Concurrent use not recommended). Products include:
- Diuril Sodium Intravenous ... 1463

Chlorthalidone (Concurrent use not recommended). Products include:
- Combipres Tablets ... 678
- Tenoretic Tablets ... 1105
- Thalitone Tablets ... 687

Clonidine (Concurrent use not recommended). Products include:
- Catapres-TTS ... 677

Clonidine Hydrochloride (Concurrent use not recommended). Products include:
- Catapres Tablets ... 676
- Combipres Tablets ... 678

Deserpidine (Concurrent use not recommended). Products include:
- Enduronyl ... 518
- Harmonyl Tablets ... 528
- Oreticyl ... 545

Desipramine Hydrochloride (Concurrent use not recommended). Products include:
- Norpramin Tablets ... 1340

Diazoxide (Concurrent use not recommended). Products include:
- Hyperstat I.V. Injection ... 2095
- Proglycem ... 649

Doxazosin Mesylate (Concurrent use not recommended). Products include:
- Cardura Tablets ... 1941

Doxepin Hydrochloride (Concurrent use not recommended). Products include:
- Sinequan ... 1960

Enalapril Maleate (Concurrent use not recommended). Products include:
- Vaseretic Tablets ... 1559
- Vasotec Tablets ... 1564

Enalaprilat (Concurrent use not recommended). Products include:
- Vasotec I.V. ... 1562

Esmolol Hydrochloride (Concurrent use not recommended). Products include:
- Brevibloc Injection ... 942

Felodipine (Concurrent use not recommended). Products include:
Plendil Extended-Release Tablets.... 1526

Fluoxetine Hydrochloride (Concurrent use not recommended). Products include:
Prozac Pulvules 920

Fosinopril Sodium (Concurrent use not recommended). Products include:
Monopril Tablets 1406

Furosemide (Concurrent use not recommended). Products include:
Lasix 1093

Guanabenz Acetate (Concurrent use not recommended). Products include:
Wytensin Tablets 2542

Guanethidine Monosulfate (Concurrent use not recommended). Products include:
Esimil Tablets 864
Ismelin Tablets 869

Hydralazine Hydrochloride (Concurrent use not recommended). Products include:
Apresazide Capsules 854
Apresoline Hydrochloride Parenteral (Ampuls) 856
Apresoline Hydrochloride Tablets .. 855
Apresoline-Esidrix Tablets 857
Ser-Ap-Es Tablets 881
Serpasil-Apresoline Tablets 884

Hydrochlorothiazide (Concurrent use not recommended). Products include:
Aldactazide 2150
Aldoril Tablets 1418
Apresazide Capsules 854
Apresoline-Esidrix Tablets 857
Capozide 2258
Dyazide Capsules 2208
Esidrix Tablets 863
Esimil Tablets 864
HydroDIURIL Tablets 1484
Hydropres Tablets 1485
Inderide Tablets 2463
Inderide LA Long Acting Capsules .. 2465
Lopressor HCT Tablets 1034
Maxzide 1215
Moduretic Tablets 1510
Normozide Tablets 2112
Oretic Tablets 544
Oreticyl 545
Prinzide Tablets 1540
Ser-Ap-Es Tablets 881
Serpasil-Esidrix Tablets 886
Timolide Tablets 1547
Trandate HCT Tablets 579
Vaseretic Tablets 1559
Zestoretic 2274

Hydroflumethiazide (Concurrent use not recommended). Products include:
Diucardin Tablets 2450
Saluron 718
Salutensin/Salutensin-Demi 719

Imipramine Hydrochloride (Concurrent use not recommended). Products include:
Tofranil Ampuls 1038
Tofranil Tablets 1039

Imipramine Pamoate (Concurrent use not recommended). Products include:
Tofranil-PM Capsules 1041

Indapamide (Concurrent use not recommended). Products include:
Lozol Tablets 1843

Isocarboxazid (Concurrent use not recommended). Products include:
Marplan Tablets 1906

Isradipine (Concurrent use not recommended). Products include:
DynaCirc Capsules 2004

Labetalol Hydrochloride (Concurrent use not recommended). Products include:
Normodyne Injection 2108
Normodyne Tablets 2110
Normozide Tablets 2112
Trandate HCT Tablets 579
Trandate Injection 577
Trandate Tablets 579

Lisinopril (Concurrent use not recommended). Products include:
Prinivil Tablets 1538
Prinzide Tablets 1540
Zestoretic 2274
Zestril Tablets 2277

Maprotiline Hydrochloride (Concurrent use not recommended). Products include:
Ludiomil Tablets 874

Mecamylamine Hydrochloride (Concurrent use not recommended). Products include:
Inversine Tablets 1492

Methyclothiazide (Concurrent use not recommended). Products include:
Enduron Tablets 517
Enduronyl 518

Methyldopa (Concurrent use not recommended). Products include:
Aldoclor Tablets 1413
Aldomet Oral 1415
Aldoril Tablets 1418

Methyldopate Hydrochloride (Concurrent use not recommended). Products include:
Aldomet Ester HCl Injection 1417

Metolazone (Concurrent use not recommended). Products include:
Diulo 2129
Mykrox ½ mg Tablets 984
Zaroxolyn Tablets 989

Metoprolol Tartrate (Concurrent use not recommended). Products include:
Lopressor Ampuls 1032
Lopressor HCT Tablets 1034
Lopressor Tablets 1032

Metyrosine (Concurrent use not recommended). Products include:
Demser Capsules 1460

Minoxidil (Concurrent use not recommended). Products include:
Loniten Tablets 2346
Rogaine Topical Solution 2357

Nadolol (Concurrent use not recommended). Products include:
Corgard Tablets 701
Corzide Tablets 702

Nicardipine Hydrochloride (Concurrent use not recommended). Products include:
Cardene Capsules 2290

Nitroglycerin (Concurrent use not recommended). Products include:
Deponit NTG Transdermal Delivery System 2143
Minitran Transdermal Delivery System 1312
Nitro-Bid Ointment 1339
Nitro-Bid Capsules 1338
Nitrodisc 2176
Nitro-Dur (nitroglycerin) Transdermal Infusion System 1164
Nitrogard Tablets 1004
Nitrolingual Spray 1846
Nitrostat Tablets 1743
Transderm-Nitro Transdermal Therapeutic System 2283

Nortriptyline Hydrochloride (Concurrent use not recommended). Products include:
Pamelor 2019

Penbutolol Sulfate (Concurrent use not recommended). Products include:
Levatol 1832

Phenelzine Sulfate (Concurrent use not recommended). Products include:
Nardil 1742

Phenoxybenzamine Hydrochloride (Concurrent use not recommended). Products include:
Dibenzyline Capsules 2207

Phentolamine Mesylate (Concurrent use not recommended). Products include:
Regitine 878

Pindolol (Concurrent use not recommended). Products include:
Visken Tablets 2036

Polythiazide (Concurrent use not recommended). Products include:
Minizide Capsules 1779
Renese Tablets 1785
Renese-R Tablets 1786

Prazosin Hydrochloride (Concurrent use not recommended). Products include:
Minipress Capsules 1778
Minizide Capsules 1779

Propranolol Hydrochloride (Concurrent use not recommended). Products include:
Inderal 2459
Inderal LA Long Acting Capsules 2461
Inderide Tablets 2463
Inderide LA Long Acting Capsules .. 2465

Protriptyline Hydrochloride (Concurrent use not recommended). Products include:
Vivactil Tablets 1567

Ramipril (Concurrent use not recommended). Products include:
Altace Capsules 1086

Rauwolfia Serpentina (Concurrent use not recommended). Products include:
Raudixin Tablets 1803
Rauzide Tablets 1804

Rescinnamine (Concurrent use not recommended).
No products indexed under this heading.

Reserpine (Concurrent use not recommended). Products include:
Diupres Tablets 1461
Hydromox R Tablets 1209
Hydropres Tablets 1485
Renese-R Tablets 1786
Salutensin/Salutensin-Demi 719
Ser-Ap-Es Tablets 881
Serpasil Tablets 883
Serpasil-Apresoline Tablets 884
Serpasil-Esidrix Tablets 886

Sodium Nitroprusside (Concurrent use not recommended). Products include:
Nipride I.V. Infusion 1909

Terazosin Hydrochloride (Concurrent use not recommended). Products include:
Hytrin Tablets 529

Timolol Maleate (Concurrent use not recommended). Products include:
Blocadren Tablets 1429
Timolide Tablets 1547
Timoptic in Ocudose 1552
Timoptic Sterile Ophthalmic Solution 1550

Tranylcypromine Sulfate (Concurrent use not recommended). Products include:
Parnate Tablets 2222

Trazodone Hydrochloride (Concurrent use not recommended). Products include:
Desyrel and Desyrel Dividose 1404

Trimethaphan Camsylate (Concurrent use not recommended). Products include:
Arfonad Ampuls 1887

Trimipramine Maleate (Concurrent use not recommended). Products include:
Surmontil Capsules 2524

BENADRYL SPRAY, MAXIMUM STRENGTH
(Diphenhydramine Hydrochloride) .. ▣ 637
May interact with:

Diphenhydramine (Concurrent use is not recommended).

BENADRYL STERI-VIALS, AMPOULES, AND STERI-DOSE SYRINGE
(Diphenhydramine Hydrochloride) 1692
See **Benadryl Parenteral**

BENADRYL 25 TABLETS
(Diphenhydramine Hydrochloride) .. ▣ 636
See **Benadryl 25 Kapseals**

BENEMID TABLETS
(Probenecid) 1426
May interact with oral hypoglycemic agents, salicylates, penicillins, sulfonamides, and certain other agents. Compounds in these categories include:

Acetaminophen (Increased peak plasma concentrations of acetaminophen). Products include:
Acetaminophen Uniserts Suppositories 2374
Actifed Plus Caplets .... ▣ 539
Actifed Plus Tablets .... ▣ 540
Alka-Seltzer Advanced Formula Antacid & Non-Aspirin Pain Reliever .... ▣ 620
Allerest .... ▣ 559
Aspirin Free Anacin Maximum Strength Acetaminophen Film Coated Caplets 2417
Aspirin Free Anacin Maximum Strength Acetaminophen Film Coated Tablets 2417
Anacin-3 Regular Strength Acetaminophen Film Coated Tablets ▣ 746
Anexsia 5/500 Tablets 2196
Anexsia 7.5/650 Tablets 2197
Benadryl Plus .... ▣ 636
Benadryl Plus Nighttime .... ▣ 637
Bufferin AF Nite Time Analgesic/Sleeping Aid Caplets 744
Allergy-Sinus Comtrex Multi-Symptom Allergy Sinus Formula Tablets & Caplets 746
Cough Formula Comtrex 746
Comtrex Multi-Symptom Cold Reliever Tablets/Caplets/Liqui-Gels/Liquid 745
Day-Night Comtrex 747
Non-Drowsy Comtrex 747
Congespirin For Children Aspirin Free Chewable Cold Tablets 748
Contac Cough & Sore Throat Formula .... ▣ 712
Contac Jr. Children's Cold Medicine .... ▣ 712
Contac Nighttime Cold Medicine .... ▣ 713
Contac Severe Cold and Flu Formula Caplets .... ▣ 711
Contac Sinus Caplets Maximum Strength Non-Drowsy Formula .... ▣ 710
Contac Sinus Tablets Maximum Strength Non-Drowsy Formula .... ▣ 710
Coricidin 'D' Decongestant Tablets .... ▣ 695
Coricidin Demilets Tablets for Children .... ▣ 696
Coricidin Tablets .... ▣ 695
Darvon-N/Darvocet-N 1254
Datril Extra-Strength Analgesic Tablets 748
Dimetapp Plus Caplets .... ▣ 675
Dorcol Children's Fever & Pain Reducer .... ▣ 686
Dristan Decongestant/Antihistamine/Analgesic Coated Caplets .... ▣ 749
Dristan Cold Nasal Decongestant/Antihistamine/ Analgesic Coated Tablets 2419
Dristan Advanced Formula Decongestant/Antihistamine/Analgesic Tablets .... ▣ 749
Maximum Strength Dristan Decongestant/Analgesic Coated Caplets .... ▣ 750

No Drowsiness Dristan Cold Nasal Decongestant/Analgesic Coated Caplets ... 2420
Drixoral Plus Extended-Release Tablets ... ◘ 699
Drixoral Sinus ... ◘ 700
Esgic-Plus Tablets ... 1002
Esgic Tablets & Capsules ... 1001
Aspirin Free Excedrin Analgesic Caplets ... 748
Excedrin Extra-Strength Analgesic Tablets & Caplets ... 749
Excedrin P.M. Analgesic/Sleeping Aid Tablets, Caplets and Liquid ... 749
Sinus Excedrin Analgesic, Decongestant Tablets & Caplets ... 750
4-Way Cold Tablets ... 750
Feverall Sprinkle Caps ... 2374
Feverall Suppositories ... 2374
Fioricet Tablets ... 2006
Hycomine Compound Tablets ... 929
Hydrocet Capsules ... 835
Isocom Capsules ... 1629
Liquiprin ... ◘ 618
Lortab ... 2412
Lurline PMS Tablets ... 972
Medi-Flu Caplet, Liquid ... ◘ 640
Maximum Strength Midol Multi-Symptom Menstrual Formula ... ◘ 571
Maximum Strength Midol PMS Premenstrual Syndrome Formula ... ◘ 570
Regular Strength Midol Multi-Symptom Menstrual Formula ... ◘ 570
Midrin Capsules ... 836
Ornex Caplets ... ◘ 618
Children's Panadol Chewable Tablets, Liquid, Infants' Drops ... ◘ 571
Junior Strength Panadol ... ◘ 571
Maximum Strength Panadol Tablets and Caplets ... ◘ 572
Percocet Tablets ... 950
Percogesic Analgesic Tablets ... ◘ 660
Phenaphen with Codeine Capsules 1865
Phenaphen-650 with Codeine Tablets ... 1866
Phrenilin ... 838
Prēmsyn PMS Capsules & Caplets ◘ 547
Pyrroxate Capsules ... ◘ 669
Robitussin Night Relief ... ◘ 677
Sedapap Tablets 50 mg/650 mg ... 1360
Sinarest ... ◘ 562
Sine-Aid Maximum Strength Sinus Headache Caplets ... 1365
Sine-Aid Maximum Strength Sinus Headache Tablets ... 1365
Sine-Off Maximum Strength Allergy/Sinus Formula Caplets ... ◘ 721
Sine-Off Maximum Strength No Drowsiness Formula Caplets ... ◘ 722
Singlet Tablets ... ◘ 598
Sinulin ... 840
Sinutab Maximum Strength ... ◘ 641
Sinutab Maximum Strength Without Drowsiness Tablets & Caplets ... ◘ 642
Sinutab Regular Strength Without Drowsiness Formula ... ◘ 641
Sominex Pain Relief Formula ... ◘ 723
St. Joseph Aspirin-Free Fever Reducer for Children Chewable Tablets, Liquid & Infant Drops ... ◘ 704
St. Joseph Cold Tablets for Children ... ◘ 704
St. Joseph Nighttime Cold Medicine ... ◘ 705
Sudafed Sinus Caplets ... ◘ 545
Sudafed Sinus Tablets ... ◘ 545
Talacen ... 2070
Tempra, Acetaminophen ... ◘ 613
TheraFlu Flu and Cold Medicine ... ◘ 687
Triaminicin Tablets ... ◘ 690
Tylenol acetaminophen Children's Chewable Tablets & Elixir ... 1366
Tylenol Allergy Sinus Medication Caplets and Gelcaps, Maximum Strength ... 1372
Tylenol with Codeine ... 1381
Children's Tylenol Cold Liquid Formula and Chewable Tablets ... 1368
Tylenol Cold & Flu Hot Medication, Packets ... 1369
Tylenol Cold & Flu No Drowsiness Hot Medication, Packets ... 1371
Tylenol Cold Medication Caplets and Tablets ... 1370
Tylenol Cold Medication, Effervescent Tablets ... 1369
Tylenol Cold Medication No Drowsiness Formula Caplets ... 1370
Tylenol Cold Night Time Medication Liquid ... 1371
Tylenol Cough Medication Liquid, Maximum Strength ... 1372
Tylenol Cough Medication Liquid with Decongestant, Maximum Strength ... 1372
Tylenol, Extra Strength, acetaminophen Adult Liquid Pain Reliever ... 1367
Tylenol, Extra Strength, acetaminophen Gelcaps, Caplets, Tablets ... 1367
Tylenol, Infants' Drops ... 1366
Tylenol, Junior Strength, acetaminophen Coated Caplets, Grape and Fruit Chewable Tablets ... 1366
Tylenol, Maximum Strength, Sinus Medication Gelcaps, Caplets and Tablets ... 1373
Tylenol, Regular Strength, acetaminophen Tablets and Caplets ... 1367
Tylenol PM, Extra Strength Caplets and Tablets ... 1368
Tylox Capsules ... 1382
Unisom Dual Relief Nighttime Sleep Aid/Analgesic ... 1774
Vanquish Analgesic Caplets ... ◘ 574
Vicks Daycare ... ◘ 660
Vicks Formula 44M Multi-Symptom Cough Medicine ... ◘ 662
Vicks NyQuil Nighttime Colds Medicine-Original & Cherry Flavor ... ◘ 664
Vicodin Tablets ... 1187
Vicodin ES Tablets ... 1189
Wygesic Tablets ... 2540
Zydone Capsules ... 941

Aminophylline (Falsely high theophylline readings in an in vitro study). Products include:
Amesec ... ◘ 682
Aminophyllin Tablets ... 2153

Amoxicillin (May result in high plasma levels of amoxicillin). Products include:
Amoxil ... 2193
Augmentin Tablets, Powder for Oral Suspension, and Chewable Tablets ... 2198

Ampicillin Sodium (May result in high plasma levels of ampicillin). Products include:
Unasyn ... 1965

Aspirin (Uricosuric action of probenecid antagonized). Products include:
Alka-Seltzer Effervescent Antacid and Pain Reliever ... 1568
Alka-Seltzer Extra Strength Effervescent Antacid and Pain Reliever ... 1570
Alka-Seltzer (Flavored) Effervescent Antacid and Pain Reliever ... 1569
Alka-Seltzer Plus Cold Medicine ... ◘ 623
Alka-Seltzer Plus Night-Time Cold Medicine ... ◘ 623
Alka Seltzer Plus Sinus Allergy Medicine ... ◘ 624
Anacin Coated Analgesic Caplets ... 2417
Anacin Coated Analgesic Tablets ... 2417
Anacin Maximum Strength Analgesic Coated Tablets ... 2417
Maximum Strength Arthritis Pain Formula By the Makers of Anacin Analgesic Tablets and Caplets ... 2418
Arthritis Pain Formula by the Makers of Anacin Analgesic Tablets and Caplets ... ◘ 747
Arthritis Strength BC Powder ... ◘ 516
Ascriptin A/D Caplets ... 1850
Regular Strength Ascriptin Tablets 1850
Azdone Tablets ... 844
BC Powder ... ◘ 517
BC Cold Powder ... ◘ 517
Children's Bayer Chewable Aspirin ... ◘ 564
Genuine Bayer Aspirin Tablets & Caplets ... ◘ 564
Maximum Bayer Aspirin Tablets & Caplets ... ◘ 566
Bayer Plus Aspirin Tablets ... ◘ 567
Therapy Bayer Aspirin Caplets ... ◘ 568
8 Hour Bayer Timed-Release Aspirin ... ◘ 566
Arthritis Strength Bufferin Analgesic Caplets ... 744
Extra Strength Bufferin Analgesic Tablets ... 745
Bufferin Analgesic Tablets and Caplets ... 743
Cama Arthritis Pain Reliever ... ◘ 685
Damason-P ... 1356
Easprin ... 1719
Ecotrin Enteric Coated Aspirin Maximum Strength Tablets and Caplets ... 2189
Ecotrin Enteric Coated Aspirin Regular Strength Tablets and Caplets ... 2189
Empirin Aspirin ... ◘ 541
Empirin with Codeine Phosphate Nos. 2, 3 & 4 ... 764
Equagesic Tablets ... 2451
Excedrin Extra-Strength Analgesic Tablets & Caplets ... 749
4-Way Cold Tablets ... 750
Fiorinal Capsules ... 2007
Fiorinal with Codeine Capsules ... 2008
Fiorinal Tablets ... 2007
Lortab ASA Tablets ... 2414
Momentum Muscular Backache Formula ... ◘ 751
Norgesic ... 1314
Norwich Extra-Strength Aspirin ... ◘ 546
Norwich Regular Strength Aspirin ◘ 547
P-A-C Analgesic Tablets ... ◘ 669
Percodan ... 951
Robaxisal Tablets ... 1872
Sine-Off Sinus Medicine Tablets-Aspirin Formula ... ◘ 722
Soma Compound w/Codeine Tablets ... 2390
Soma Compound Tablets ... 2389
St. Joseph Adult Chewable Aspirin (81 mg.) ... ◘ 703
Synalgos-DC Capsules ... 2525
Talwin Compound ... 2072
Ursinus Inlay-Tabs ... ◘ 691
Vanquish Analgesic Caplets ... ◘ 574
Zorprin Tablets ... 698

Azlocillin Sodium (May result in high plasma levels of azlocillin).
No products indexed under this heading.

Bacampicillin Hydrochloride (May result in high plasma levels of bacampicillin). Products include:
Spectrobid Tablets & Powder for Oral Suspension ... 1961

Bendroflumethiazide (Significant increase in total sulfonamide plasma levels). Products include:
Corzide Tablets ... 702
Naturetin Tablets ... 1789
Rauzide Tablets ... 1804

Carbenicillin Disodium (May result in high plasma levels of carbenicillin).

Carbenicillin Indanyl Sodium (May result in high plasma levels of carbenicillin). Products include:
Geocillin Tablets ... 1951

Chlorothiazide (Significant increase in total sulfonamide plasma levels). Products include:
Aldoclor Tablets ... 1413
Diupres Tablets ... 1461
Diuril Oral ... 1464

Chlorothiazide Sodium (Significant increase in total sulfonamide plasma levels). Products include:
Diuril Sodium Intravenous ... 1463

Chlorpropamide (Significant increase in total sulfonamide plasma levels; increased risk of hypoglycemia). Products include:
Diabinese Tablets ... 1775

Choline Magnesium Trisalicylate (Uricosuric action of probenecid antagonized). Products include:
Trilisate ... 1822

Diflunisal (Uricosuric action of probenecid antagonized). Products include:
Dolobid Tablets ... 1465

Dyphylline (Falsely high theophylline readings in an in vitro study). Products include:
Dilor ... 2079
Dilor-G Tablets & Liquid ... 2079
Lufyllin Elixir ... 2384
Lufyllin & Lufyllin-400 Tablets ... 2384
Lufyllin-GG Elixir & Tablets ... 2385

Glipizide (Significant increase in total sulfonamide plasma levels; increased risk of hypoglycemia). Products include:
Glucotrol ... 1952

Glyburide (Significant increase in total sulfonamide plasma levels; increased risk of hypoglycemia). Products include:
DiaBeta ... 1091
Micronase Tablets ... 2350

Hydrochlorothiazide (Significant increase in total sulfonamide plasma levels). Products include:
Aldactazide ... 2150
Aldoril Tablets ... 1418
Apresazide Capsules ... 854
Apresoline-Esidrix Tablets ... 857
Capozide ... 2258
Dyazide Capsules ... 2208
Esidrix Tablets ... 863
Esimil Tablets ... 864
HydroDIURIL Tablets ... 1484
Hydropres Tablets ... 1485
Inderide Tablets ... 2463
Inderide LA Long Acting Capsules ... 2465
Lopressor HCT Tablets ... 1034
Maxzide ... 1215
Moduretic Tablets ... 1510
Normozide Tablets ... 2112
Oretic Tablets ... 544
Oreticyl ... 545
Prinzide Tablets ... 1540
Ser-Ap-Es Tablets ... 881
Serpasil-Esidrix Tablets ... 886
Timolide Tablets ... 1547
Trandate HCT Tablets ... 579
Vaseretic Tablets ... 1559
Zestoretic ... 2274

Hydroflumethiazide (Significant increase in total sulfonamide plasma levels). Products include:
Diucardin Tablets ... 2450
Saluron ... 718
Salutensin/Salutensin-Demi ... 719

Indomethacin (Increased plasma levels of indomethacin). Products include:
Indocin ... 1487

Indomethacin Sodium Trihydrate (Increased plasma levels of indomethacin). Products include:
Indocin I.V. ... 1490

Ketamine Hydrochloride (Anesthesia prolonged). Products include:
Ketalar ... 1726

Ketoprofen (Increased peak plasma levels of ketoprofen). Products include:
Orudis Capsules ... 2488

Lorazepam (Increased peak plasma levels of lorazepam). Products include:
Ativan Injection ... 2432
Ativan Tablets ... 2434

Magnesium Salicylate (Uricosuric action of probenecid antagonized). Products include:
Doan's - Extra-Strength Analgesic ◘ 549
Doan's - Regular Strength Analgesic ... ◘ 549
Mobigesic Analgesic Tablets ... ◘ 507

Meclofenamate Sodium (Increased peak plasma concentrations of meclofenamate). Products include:
Meclomen Capsules ... 1739

Methotrexate Sodium (Methotrexate toxicity). Products include:
Methotrexate Tablets, Parenteral, LPF Parenteral ... 1217
Rheumatrex Methotrexate Dose Pack ... 1234

Methyclothiazide (Significant increase in total sulfonamide plasma levels). Products include:
Enduron Tablets ... 517
Enduronyl ... 518

Mezlocillin Sodium (May result in high plasma levels of mezlocillin). Products include:
Mezlin ... 1597
Mezlin Pharmacy Bulk Package ... 1599

Nafcillin Sodium (May result in high plasma levels of nafcillin). Products include:
Unipen ... 2533

Naproxen (Increased peak plasma concentrations of naproxen). Products include:
Naprosyn ... 2297

Naproxen Sodium (Increased peak plasma concentrations of naproxen). Products include:
Anaprox and Anaprox DS Tablets ... 2288

Penicillin G Potassium (May result in high plasma levels of penicillin). Products include:
Pfizerpen for Injection ... 1957

Penicillin G Procaine (May result in high plasma levels of penicillin). Products include:
Bicillin C-R Injection ... 2438
Bicillin C-R 900/300 Injection ... 2440
Pfizerpen-AS Aqueous Suspension 1959
Wycillin Injection ... 2537
Wycillin Injection and Probenecid Tablets ... 2539

Penicillin G, Benzathine (May result in high plasma levels of penicillin). Products include:
Bicillin C-R Injection ... 2438
Bicillin C-R 900/300 Injection ... 2440
Bicillin L-A Injection ... 2442

Penicillin V Potassium (May result in high plasma levels of penicillin).
No products indexed under this heading.

Polythiazide (Significant increase in total sulfonamide plasma levels). Products include:
Minizide Capsules ... 1779
Renese Tablets ... 1785
Renese-R Tablets ... 1786

Pyrazinamide (Uricosuric action of probenecid antagonized).
No products indexed under this heading.

Rifampin (Increased peak plasma concentrations of rifampin). Products include:
Rifadin ... 1345
Rifamate Capsules ... 1347
Rimactane Capsules ... 879

Salsalate (Uricosuric action of probenecid antagonized). Products include:
Disalcid ... 1310
Mono-Gesic Tablets ... 846
Salflex ... 839

Sulfamethizole (Significant increase in total sulfonamide plasma levels). Products include:
Thiosulfil Forte Tablets ... 2526
Urobiotic-250 Capsules ... 1968

Sulfamethoxazole (Significant increase in total sulfonamide plasma levels). Products include:
Azo Gantanol Tablets ... 1887
Bactrim DS Tablets ... 1891
Bactrim I.V. Infusion ... 1889
Bactrim ... 1891
Gantanol ... 1899
Septra ... 813
Septra I.V. Infusion ... 808
Septra I.V. Infusion ADD-Vantage Vials ... 810
Septra ... 813

Sulfasalazine (Significant increase in total sulfonamide plasma levels). Products include:
Azulfidine Tablets, EN-tabs, Oral Suspension ... 1157

Sulfinpyrazone (Significant increase in total sulfonamide plasma levels). Products include:
Anturane ... 853

Sulfisoxazole (Significant increase in total sulfonamide plasma levels). Products include:
Azo Gantrisin Tablets ... 1888
Gantrisin Tablets ... 1901
Pediazole ... 1973

Sulfisoxazole Diolamine (Significant increase in total sulfonamide plasma levels). Products include:
Gantrisin Ophthalmic Ointment/Solution ... 1900

Sulindac (Modest reduction in uricosuric action of probenecid). Products include:
Clinoril Tablets ... 1433

Theophylline (Falsely high theophylline readings in an in vitro study). Products include:
Bronkaid Tablets ... ▣ 757
Bronkolixir ... ▣ 761
Bronkotabs Tablets ... ▣ 762
Constant-T Tablets ... 1029
Marax Tablets & DF Syrup ... 1954
Primatene Tablets ... 2421
Quibron Capsules ... 713
Quibron-T ... 714
Quibron-T/SR ... 716
Theolair Liquid ... 1317
Theo-Organidin Elixir ... 2391

Theophylline Anhydrous (Falsely high theophylline readings in an in vitro study). Products include:
Aerolate ... 994
Primatene Tablets-M Formula ... ▣ 753
Primatene Tablets-Regular Formula ... 2421
Respbid Tablets ... 684
Slo-bid Gyrocaps ... 1847
T-PHYL (Uniphyl) 200 mg Tablets 1820
Tedral SA ... 1765
Theo-24 ... 2179
Theo-Dur Sprinkle ... 1168
Theo-Dur Extended-Release Tablets ... 1166
Theolair Tablets ... 1317
Theolair-SR Tablets ... 1319
TheoX Extended-Release Tablets ... 841
Uniphyl 400 mg Tablets ... 1823

Theophylline Calcium Salicylate (Falsely high theophylline readings in an in vitro study). Products include:
Quadrinal Tablets ... 1183

Theophylline Sodium Glycinate (Falsely high theophylline readings in an in vitro study). Products include:
Asbron G ... 1997

Ticarcillin Disodium (May result in high plasma levels of ticarcillin). Products include:
Ticar for Injection ... 2236
Timentin for Injection ... 2239

Tolazamide (Significant increase in total sulfonamide plasma levels; increased risk of hypoglycemia). Products include:
Tolinase Tablets ... 2365

Tolbutamide (Significant increase in total sulfonamide plasma levels; increased risk of hypoglycemia). Products include:
Orinase Tablets ... 2354

BEN-GAY EXTERNAL ANALGESIC PRODUCTS
(Menthol, Methyl Salicylate) ... ▣ 643
No interactions described in labeling.

BENOQUIN CREAM 20%
(Monobenzone) ... 1112
No interactions described in labeling.

BENTYL 10 MG CAPSULES
(Dicyclomine Hydrochloride) ... 1322
May interact with antacids, agents used to treat achlorhydria and/or to test gastric secretion, nitrates and nitrites, monoamine oxidase inhibitors, phenothiazines, antihistamines, narcotic analgesics, tricyclic antidepressants, benzodiazepines, corticosteroids, sympathomimetic aerosal brochodilators, type 1 antiarrhythmic drugs, antiglaucoma agents, anticholinergics, and certain other agents. Compounds in these categories include:

Acetazolamide (Effects of antiglaucoma agents antagonized). Products include:
Diamox Parenteral ... 1200
Diamox Parenteral ... ⊙ 308
Diamox Sequels (Sustained Release) ... 1201
Diamox Sequels (Sustained Release) ... ⊙ 310
Diamox Tablets ... 1200
Diamox Tablets ... ⊙ 308

Acetylcholine Chloride (Effects of antiglaucoma agents antagonized). Products include:
Miochol with Iocare Steri-Tags, Miochol System Pak and Miochol System Pak Plus ... ⊙ 274

Albuterol (Increases certain actions or side effects). Products include:
Proventil Inhalation Aerosol ... 2117
Ventolin Inhalation Aerosol and Refill ... 583

Albuterol Sulfate (Increases certain actions or side effects). Products include:
Proventil Repetabs Tablets ... 2120
Proventil Solutions for Inhalation 0.5% and 0.083% ... 2118
Proventil Syrup ... 2119
Proventil Tablets ... 2120
Ventolin ... 583

Alfentanil Hydrochloride (Increases certain actions or side effects). Products include:
Alfenta Injection ... 1131

Alprazolam (Increases certain actions or side effects). Products include:
Xanax Tablets ... 2367

Aluminum Carbonate Gel (Interferes with the absorption). Products include:
Basaljel ... 2438

Aluminum Hydroxide (Interferes with the absorption). Products include:
Cama Arthritis Pain Reliever ... ▣ 685
Gaviscon Extra Strength Relief Formula Liquid Antacid ... ▣ 594
Gaviscon Extra Strength Relief Formula Antacid Tablets ... ▣ 594
Gaviscon Liquid Antacid ... ▣ 594
Gelusil Liquid & Tablets ... ▣ 639
Extra Strength Maalox Plus Suspension ... 1850
Maalox TC Suspension ... 1851
Maalox Plus Tablets ... ▣ 655
Extra Strength Maalox Plus Tablets 1850
Nephrox Suspension ... ▣ 563
WinGel Liquid & Tablets ... ▣ 761

Aluminum Hydroxide Gel (Interferes with the absorption). Products include:
ALternaGEL Liquid ... 1154
Aludrox Oral Suspension ... 2428
Amphojel Suspension ... 2429
Amphojel Suspension without Flavor ... 2429
Mylanta Liquid ... 1155
Mylanta Double Strength Liquid ... 1155

Aluminum Hydroxide Gel, Dried (Interferes with the absorption). Products include:
Alu-Tab/Alu-Cap ... 1309
Amphojel Tablets ... 2429
Ascriptin A/D Caplets ... 1850
Regular Strength Ascriptin Tablets 1850
Gaviscon Antacid Tablets ... ▣ 593
Gaviscon-2 Antacid Tablets ... ▣ 594
Mylanta Tablets ... 1155
Mylanta Double Strength Tablets ... 1155

Amantadine Hydrochloride (Increases certain actions or side effects). Products include:
Symmetrel Capsules & Syrup ... 936

Amitriptyline Hydrochloride (Increases certain actions or side effects). Products include:
Elavil ... 2269
Endep Tablets ... 1927
Etrafon ... 2087
Limbitrol ... 1933
Triavil Tablets ... 1556

Amoxapine (Increases certain actions or side effects). Products include:
Asendin Tablets ... 1196

Amyl Nitrite (Increases certain actions and side effects).
No products indexed under this heading.

Astemizole (Increases certain actions or side effects). Products include:
Hismanal Tablets ... 1138

Atropine Sulfate (Increases certain actions or side effects). Products include:
Arco-Lase Plus Tablets ... 607
Atropine Sulfate Sterile Ophthalmic Solution and S.O.P. Sterile Ophthalmic Ointment ... ⊙ 239
Donnagel ... ▣ 675
Donnagel-PG ... 1858
Donnatal ... 1858
Donnatal Extentabs ... 1859
Donnatal Tablets ... 1858
Donnazyme Tablets ... 1860
Isopto Atropine ... ⊙ 218
Lomotil ... 2174
Motofen Tablets ... 836
Ru-Tuss Tablets ... 693
Urised Tablets ... 2396

Azatadine Maleate (Increases certain actions or side effects). Products include:
Optimine Tablets ... 2115
Trinalin Repetabs Tablets ... 1170

Belladonna Alkaloids (Increases certain actions or side effects). Products include:
Bellergal-S Tablets ... 1998
Hyland's Bed Wetting Tablets ... ▣ 728
Hyland's Teething Tablets ... ▣ 728
Kinesed Tablets ... 2272

Benztropine Mesylate (Increases certain actions or side effects). Products include:
Cogentin ... 1435

Betamethasone Acetate (Concurrent use in the presence of increased intraocular pressure may be hazardous). Products include:
Celestone Soluspan Suspension ... 2081

Betamethasone Sodium Phosphate (Concurrent use in the presence of increased intraocular pressure may be hazardous). Products include:
Celestone Soluspan Suspension ... 2081

Betaxolol Hydrochloride (Effects of antiglaucoma agents antagonized). Products include:
Betoptic Sterile Ophthalmic Solution ... 569
Betoptic S Sterile Ophthalmic Suspension ... 570
Kerlone Tablets ... 2172

Biperiden (Increases certain actions or side effects). Products include:
Akineton ... 1171

Bromodiphenhydramine Hydrochloride (Increases certain actions or side effects).
No products indexed under this heading.

Brompheniramine Maleate (Increases certain actions or side effects). Products include:
Alka Seltzer Plus Sinus Allergy Medicine ... ▣ 624
Atrohist Sprinkle Capsules ... 558
Bromfed Capsules (Timed Release) ... 1615
Bromfed Syrup ... ▣ 628

Bromfed ... 1615
Dimetane Decongestant ... ⊞ 673
Dimetane ... ⊞ 672
Dimetane-DC Cough Syrup ... 1857
Dimetane-DX Cough Syrup ... 1858
Dimetapp Elixir ... ⊞ 673
Dimetapp DM Elixir ... ⊞ 674
Dimetapp Extentabs ... ⊞ 674
Dimetapp Plus Caplets ... ⊞ 675
Dimetapp Tablets ... ⊞ 675
Drixoral Antihistamine/Nasal Decongestant Syrup ... ⊞ 698

Buprenorphine (Increases certain actions or side effects).
No products indexed under this heading.

Carbachol (Effects of antiglaucoma agents antagonized). Products include:
Isopto Carbachol ... ⊙ 219
MIOSTAT ... ⊙ 233

Chlordiazepoxide (Increases certain actions or side effects). Products include:
Libritabs Tablets ... 1930
Limbitrol ... 1933
Menrium Tablets ... 1934

Chlordiazepoxide Hydrochloride (Increases certain actions or side effects). Products include:
Librax Capsules ... 1929
Librium Capsules ... 1931
Librium Injectable ... 1932

Chlorpheniramine Maleate (Increases certain actions or side effects). Products include:
A.R.M. Allergy Relief Medicine Caplets ... ⊞ 615
Alka-Seltzer Plus Cold Medicine ... ⊞ 623
Allerest ... ⊞ 559
Ana-Kit Anaphylaxis Emergency Treatment Kit ... 1100
BC Cold Powder Multi-Symptom Formula ... ⊞ 517
Brexin L.A. Capsules ... 2078
Cerose-DM ... 2443
Cheracol Plus Head Cold/Cough Formula ... ⊞ 667
Chlor-Trimeton Allergy Syrup, Tablets & Long-Acting Repetabs Tablets ... ⊞ 693
Chlor-Trimeton Decongestant ... ⊞ 694
Comhist LA Capsules ... 1618
Allergy-Sinus Comtrex Multi-Symptom Allergy Sinus Formula Tablets & Caplets ... 746
Comtrex Multi-Symptom Cold Reliever Tablets/Caplets/Liqui-Gels/Liquid ... 745
Day-Night Comtrex ... 747
Contac Continuous Action Decongestant/Antihistamine Capsules ⊞ 710
Contac Maximum Strength Continuous Action Decongestant/Antihistamine Caplets ... ⊞ 709
Contac Severe Cold and Flu Formula Caplets ... ⊞ 711
Coricidin 'D' Decongestant Tablets ... ⊞ 695
Coricidin Demilets Tablets for Children ... ⊞ 696
Coricidin Tablets ... ⊞ 695
Deconamine ... 663
Demazin Nasal Decongestant/Antihistamine Repetabs Tablets & Syrup ... ⊞ 697
Dorcol Children's Liquid Cold Formula ... ⊞ 686
Dristan Decongestant/Antihistamine/Analgesic Coated Caplets ... ⊞ 749
Dristan Cold Nasal Decongestant/Antihistamine/ Analgesic Coated Tablets ... 2419
Dristan Advanced Formula Decongestant/Antihistamine/Analgesic Tablets ... ⊞ 749
Extendryl ... 994
4-Way Cold Tablets ... 750
Fedahist Gyrocaps ... 2145
Fedahist Timecaps ... 2145
Hycomine Compound Tablets ... 929
Isoclor Timesule Capsules ... ⊞ 561
Kronofed-A ... 970
Medi-Flu Caplet, Liquid ... ⊞ 640
Naldecon Syrup, Tablets, Pediatric Drops and Pediatric Syrup ... 709
Nolamine Tablets ... 838
Novafed A Capsules ... 1342
Novahistine DH ... 1342
Novahistine Elixir ... ⊞ 596
Ornade Spansule Capsules ... 2221
Orthoxicol Cough Syrup ... ⊞ 668
PediaCare Allergy Relief Formula Liquid ... 1362
PediaCare Cough-Cold Formula Liquid ... 1362
PediaCare Night Rest Cough-Cold Formula Liquid ... 1362
PediaCare 6-12 Cough-Cold Formula Chewable Tablets ... 1362
Pyrroxate Capsules ... ⊞ 669
Quelidrine Syrup ... 556
Ru-Tuss II Capsules ... 693
Ru-Tuss Tablets ... 693
Ryna ... ⊞ 741
Sinarest Tablets & Extra Strength Tablets ... ⊞ 562
Sine-Off Maximum Strength Allergy/Sinus Formula Caplets ... ⊞ 721
Sine-Off Sinus Medicine Tablets-Aspirin Formula ... ⊞ 722
Singlet Tablets ... ⊞ 598
Sinulin ... 840
Sinutab Maximum Strength ... ⊞ 641
St. Joseph Nighttime Cold Medicine ... ⊞ 705
Sudafed Plus Liquid ... ⊞ 544
Sudafed Plus Tablets ... ⊞ 545
Teldrin Timed-Release Allergy Capsules, 12 mg ... 2192
TheraFlu Flu and Cold Medicine ... ⊞ 687
Triaminic Allergy Tablets ... ⊞ 688
Triaminic Chewables ... ⊞ 688
Triaminic Cold Tablets ... ⊞ 688
Triaminic Nite Light ... ⊞ 689
Triaminic Syrup ... ⊞ 689
Triaminic-12 Tablets ... ⊞ 690
Triaminicin Tablets ... ⊞ 690
Triaminicol Multi-Symptom Cold Tablets ... ⊞ 691
Triaminicol Multi-Symptom Relief ⊞ 691
Tylenol Allergy Sinus Medication Caplets and Gelcaps, Maximum Strength ... 1372
Children's Tylenol Cold Liquid Formula and Chewable Tablets ... 1368
Tylenol Cold & Flu Hot Medication, Packets ... 1369
Tylenol Cold Medication Caplets and Tablets ... 1370
Tylenol Cold Medication, Effervescent Tablets ... 1369
Vicks Children's NyQuil ... ⊞ 664
Vicks Formula 44 Cough Medicine ... ⊞ 661
Vicks Formula 44M Multi-Symptom Cough Medicine ... ⊞ 662
Vicks Pediatric Formula 44m Multi-Symptom Cough & Cold Medicine ... ⊞ 663

Chlorpheniramine Polistirex (Increases certain actions or side effects). Products include:
Tussionex Extended-Release Suspension ... 988

Chlorpheniramine Tannate (Increases certain actions or side effects). Products include:
Rynatan ... 2387
Rynatuss ... 2388

Chlorpromazine (Increases certain actions or side effects). Products include:
Thorazine ... 2234

Clemastine Fumarate (Increases certain actions or side effects). Products include:
Tavist Syrup ... 2033
Tavist Tablets ... 2035
Tavist-D Tablets ... 2035

Clidinium Bromide (Increases certain actions or side effects). Products include:
Librax Capsules ... 1929
Quarzan Capsules ... 1937

Clomipramine Hydrochloride (Increases certain actions or side effects). Products include:
Anafranil Capsules ... 650

Clorazepate Dipotassium (Increases certain actions or side effects). Products include:
Tranxene ... 556

Codeine (Increases certain actions or side effects). Products include:
Calcidrine Syrup ... 506

Codeine Phosphate (Increases certain actions or side effects). Products include:
Actifed with Codeine Cough Syrup .. 752
Cheracol Cough Syrup ... 1853
Codimal PH Syrup ... 846
Dimetane-DC Cough Syrup ... 1857
Empirin with Codeine Phosphate Nos. 2, 3 & 4 ... 764
Fiorinal with Codeine Capsules ... 2008
Isoclor Expectorant ... 982
Naldecon CX Adult Liquid ... ⊞ 521
Novahistine DH ... 1342
Novahistine Expectorant ... 1343
Nucofed Capsules ... 2219
Nucofed Expectorant ... 2219
Nucofed Pediatric Expectorant ... 2220
Nucofed Syrup ... 2219
Phenaphen with Codeine Capsules 1865
Phenaphen-650 with Codeine Tablets ... 1866
Phenergan with Codeine ... 2497
Phenergan VC with Codeine ... 2501
Robitussin A-C Syrup ... 1875
Robitussin-DAC Syrup ... 1875
Ryna ... ⊞ 741
Soma Compound w/Codeine Tablets ... 2390
Triaminic Expectorant w/Codeine .. 1996
Tussi-Organidin Liquid ... 2391
Tylenol with Codeine ... 1381

Codeine Polistirex (Increases certain actions or side effects).
No products indexed under this heading.

Cortisone Acetate (Concurrent use in the presence of increased intraocular pressure may be hazardous). Products include:
Cortone Acetate Sterile Suspension ... 1437
Cortone Acetate Tablets ... 1439

Cyproheptadine Hydrochloride (Increases certain actions or side effects). Products include:
Periactin ... 1525

Demecarium Bromide (Effects of antiglaucoma agents antagonized). Products include:
Humorsol Sterile Ophthalmic Solution ... 1475

Desipramine Hydrochloride (Increases certain actions or side effects). Products include:
Norpramin Tablets ... 1340

Dexamethasone (Concurrent use in the presence of increased intraocular pressure may be hazardous). Products include:
AK-Trol Ointment & Suspension ... ⊙ 207
Decadron Elixir ... 1445
Decadron Tablets ... 1447
Decaspray Topical Aerosol ... 1459
Dexacidin ... ⊙ 272
Maxidex Sterile Ophthalmic Suspension ... ⊙ 223
Maxitrol Ophthalmic Ointment/Suspension ... ⊙ 223
TobraDex Ophthalmic Suspension and Ointment ... ⊙ 228

Dexamethasone Acetate (Concurrent use in the presence of increased intraocular pressure may be hazardous). Products include:
Dalalone D.P. Injectable ... 999
Decadron-LA Sterile Suspension ... 1457

Dexamethasone Sodium Phosphate (Concurrent use in the presence of increased intraocular pressure may be hazardous). Products include:
AK-Dex ... ⊙ 203
Decadron Phosphate Respihaler ... 1454
Decadron Phosphate Sterile Ophthalmic Ointment ... 1453
Decadron Phosphate Sterile Ophthalmic Solution ... 1453
Decadron Phosphate Topical Cream ... 1455
Decadron Phosphate Turbinaire ... 1456
Maxidex Sterile Ophthalmic Ointment ... ⊙ 222
NeoDecadron Sterile Ophthalmic Ointment ... 1517
NeoDecadron Sterile Ophthalmic Solution ... 1518
NeoDecadron Topical Cream ... 1518

Dexchlorpheniramine Maleate (Increases certain actions or side effects). Products include:
Polaramine ... 2116

Dezocine (Increases certain actions or side effects).

Diazepam (Increases certain actions or side effects). Products include:
Valium Injectable ... 1937
Valium Tablets ... 1939
Valrelease Capsules ... 1923

Dichlorphenamide (Effects of antiglaucoma agents antagonized). Products include:
Daranide Tablets ... 1445

Digoxin (Increased serum digoxin levels). Products include:
Lanoxicaps ... 772
Lanoxin Elixir Pediatric ... 775
Lanoxin Injection ... 778
Lanoxin Injection Pediatric ... 781
Lanoxin Tablets ... 783

Dihydroxyaluminum Sodium Carbonate (Interferes with the absorption). Products include:
Rolaids ... ⊞ 743

Diphenhydramine Citrate (Increases certain actions or side effects). Products include:
Alka-Seltzer Plus Night-Time Cold Medicine ... ⊞ 623
Bufferin AF Nite Time Analgesic/Sleeping Aid Caplets ... 744
Excedrin P.M. Analgesic/Sleeping Aid Tablets, Caplets and Liquid ... 749

Diphenhydramine Hydrochloride (Increases certain actions or side effects). Products include:
Benadryl Anti-Itch Cream ... ⊞ 635
Benadryl Capsules ... 1691
Benadryl Decongestant Elixir ... ⊞ 635
Benadryl Decongestant ... ⊞ 635
Benadryl Elixir ... ⊞ 636
Benadryl Kapseals ... 1691
Benadryl 25 Kapseals ... ⊞ 636
Benadryl Parenteral ... 1692
Benadryl Plus ... ⊞ 636
Benadryl Plus Nighttime ... ⊞ 637
Benadryl Spray, Maximum Strength ... ⊞ 637
Benadryl Spray, Regular Strength ⊞ 637
Benadryl Steri-Vials, Ampoules, and Steri-Dose Syringe ... 1692
Benadryl 25 Tablets ... ⊞ 636
Benylin Cough Syrup ... ⊞ 637
Benylin Decongestant ... ⊞ 638
Caladryl Cream, Lotion, Spray ... ⊞ 638
Miles Nervine Nighttime Sleep-Aid ⊞ 627
Nytol Tablets ... ⊞ 517
Sleep-ettes-D Tablets ... ⊞ 653
Sleep-eze 3 Tablets ... ⊞ 755
Sleepinal Night-time Sleep Aid Capsules ... ⊞ 734
Sominex Caplets and Tablets ... ⊞ 722
Sominex Liquid ... ⊞ 723
Sominex Pain Relief Formula ... ⊞ 723
Tylenol Cold Night Time Medication Liquid ... 1371
Tylenol PM, Extra Strength Caplets and Tablets ... 1368
Unisom Dual Relief Nighttime Sleep Aid/Analgesic ... 1774
Ziradryl Lotion ... ⊞ 643

Dipivefrin Hydrochloride (Effects of antiglaucoma agents antagonized). Products include:
Propine with C Cap Compliance Cap ... ⊙ 255

Disopyramide Phosphate (Increases certain actions or side effects). Products include:
Norpace ... 2177

Dobutamine Hydrochloride (Increases certain actions or side effects). Products include:
Dobutrex Solution Vials ... 1259

Dopamine Hydrochloride (Increases certain actions or side effects). Products include:
- Intropin Injection ... 930

Doxepin Hydrochloride (Increases certain actions or side effects). Products include:
- Sinequan ... 1960

Echothiophate Iodide (Effects of antiglaucoma agents antagonized). Products include:
- Phospholine Iodide ... ⊙ 315

Ephedrine Hydrochloride (Effects of antiglaucoma agents antagonized). Products include:
- Amesec ... ▣ 682
- Primatene Tablets-M Formula ... 2421
- Primatene Tablets-P Formula ... 2421
- Primatene Tablets-Regular Formula ... 2421
- Quadrinal Tablets ... 1183
- Quelidrine Syrup ... 556
- Tedral SA ... 1765

Ephedrine Sulfate (Increases certain actions or side effects). Products include:
- Bronkaid Tablets ... ▣ 757
- Bronkolixir ... ▣ 761
- Bronkotabs Tablets ... ▣ 762
- Marax Tablets & DF Syrup ... 1954
- Pazo Hemorrhoid Ointment & Suppositories ... 752
- Vicks Vatronol Nose Drops ... ▣ 666

Ephedrine Tannate (Increases certain actions or side effects). Products include:
- Rynatuss ... 2388

Epinephrine (Increases certain actions or side effects). Products include:
- Ana-Kit Anaphylaxis Emergency Treatment Kit ... 1100
- Bronkaid Mist ... ▣ 757
- EpiPen ... 843
- Marcaine Hydrochloride 0.5% with Epinephrine 1:200,000 (as bitartrate) ... 958
- Marcaine Hydrochloride with Epinephrine 1:200,000 ... 2055
- Primatene Mist ... 2420
- Sus-Phrine Injection ... 1006
- Xylocaine with Epinephrine Injections ... 637

Epinephrine Bitartrate (Effects of antiglaucoma agents antagonized). Products include:
- AsthmaHaler Mist Epinephrine Bitartrate Bronchodilator ... ▣ 616
- Bronkaid Mist Suspension ... ▣ 757
- Primatene Mist Suspension ... 2421

Epinephrine Hydrochloride (Increases certain actions or side effects; effects of antiglaucoma agents antagonized). Products include:
- Adrenalin Chloride Solution 1:100 & 1:1,000 ... 1689
- Epifrin ... ⊙ 244
- Glaucon ... ⊙ 218

Epinephryl Borate (Effects of antiglaucoma agents antagonized).
- No products indexed under this heading.

Erythrityl Tetranitrate (Increases certain actions and side effects). Products include:
- Cardilate Oral/Sublingual Tablets .. 757

Estazolam (Increases certain actions or side effects). Products include:
- ProSom Tablets ... 554

Fentanyl (Increases certain actions or side effects). Products include:
- Duragesic Transdermal System ... 1133

Fentanyl Citrate (Increases certain actions or side effects). Products include:
- Innovar Injection ... 1141
- Sublimaze Injection ... 1146

Fluphenazine Decanoate (Increases certain actions or side effects). Products include:
- Prolixin Decanoate ... 1795

Fluphenazine Enanthate (Increases certain actions or side effects). Products include:
- Prolixin Enanthate ... 1796

Fluphenazine Hydrochloride (Increases certain actions or side effects). Products include:
- Prolixin Elixir ... 1793
- Prolixin Injection ... 1791
- Prolixin Oral Concentrate ... 1792
- Prolixin Tablets ... 1793

Furazolidone (Increases certain actions or side effects). Products include:
- Furoxone ... 1855

Glutamic Acid Hydrochloride (Antagonizes the inhibiting effects on gastric hydrochloric acid).
- No products indexed under this heading.

Glycopyrrolate (Increases certain actions or side effects). Products include:
- Robinul Forte Tablets ... 1873
- Robinul Injectable ... 1873
- Robinul Tablets ... 1873

Hydrocodone Bitartrate (Increases certain actions or side effects). Products include:
- Anexsia 5/500 Tablets ... 2196
- Anexsia 7.5/650 Tablets ... 2197
- Azdone Tablets ... 844
- Codiclear DH Syrup ... 845
- Codimal DH Syrup ... 846
- Damason-P ... 1356
- Hycodan Syrup, Tablets ... 927
- Hycomine Compound Tablets ... 929
- Hycomine Syrup ... 927
- Hycotuss Expectorant Syrup ... 930
- Hydrocet Capsules ... 835
- Lortab ASA Tablets ... 2414
- Lortab ... 2412
- Ru-Tuss with Hydrocodone ... 694
- Triaminic Expectorant DH ... 1995
- Vicodin Tablets ... 1187
- Vicodin ES Tablets ... 1189
- Zydone Capsules ... 941

Hydrocodone Polistirex (Increases certain actions or side effects). Products include:
- Tussionex Extended-Release Suspension ... 988

Hydrocortisone (Concurrent use in the presence of increased intraocular pressure may be hazardous). Products include:
- AK-Spore H.C. ... ⊙ 206
- Bactine Hydrocortisone Anti-Itch Cream ... ▣ 625
- CaldeCORT Anti-Itch Hydrocortisone Spray ... ▣ 560
- Carmol HC Cream 1% ... 2296
- Cortaid Spray ... ▣ 735
- Cortenema ... 2244
- Cortisporin Ointment ... 758
- Cortisporin Ophthalmic Ointment Sterile ... 758
- Cortisporin Ophthalmic Suspension Sterile ... 759
- Cortisporin Otic Solution Sterile ... 760
- Cortisporin Otic Suspension Sterile ... 760
- Cortizone-5 Creme & Ointment ... ▣ 732
- Dermolate Anti-Itch Cream ... ▣ 697
- Eldecort Cream 1.0% ... 1113
- Eldecort Cream 1.0% and 2.5% ... 1113
- Fungoid HC Creme ... 1770
- Hydrocortone Tablets ... 1482
- Hytone ... 909
- LazerSporin-C Solution ... 1770
- Massengill Medicated Soft Cloth Towelettes ... 2192
- Nutracort Cream & Lotion ... 1684
- PediOtic Suspension Sterile ... 797
- Synacort Creams 1%, 2.5% ... 2296
- Vanoxide-HC Acne Lotion ... 911
- Vioform-Hydrocortisone Cream and Mild Cream ... 889
- Vioform-Hydrocortisone Ointment .. 889
- VōSoL HC Otic Solution ... 2392
- Vytone Cream 1% ... 911

Hydrocortisone Acetate (Concurrent use in the presence of increased intraocular pressure may be hazardous). Products include:
- Analpram-HC Rectal Cream 1% and 2.5% ... 970
- Anusol-HC Cream ... 1690
- Anusol-HC Suppositories ... 1691
- Caldecort ... ▣ 560
- Carmol HC Cream 1% ... 2296
- Chloromycetin Hydrocortisone Ophthalmic ... 1694
- Coly-Mycin S Otic w/Neomycin & Hydrocortisone ... 1708
- Cortaid ... ▣ 735
- Cortef Feminine Itch Cream ... ▣ 735
- Corticaine ... ▣ 682
- Cortifoam ... 1827
- Cortisporin Cream ... 757
- Epifoam ... 1828
- Gynecort 5 Creme ... ▣ 556
- Hydrocortone Acetate Sterile Suspension ... 1479
- Lanacort 5 Creme and Ointment .. ▣ 557
- Mantadil Cream ... 789
- Ophthocort ... ⊙ 301
- Orabase HCA Oral Paste ... 890
- Pramosone Cream, Lotion & Ointment ... 971
- ProctoCream-HC ... 1834
- Proctofoam-HC ... 1835

Hydrocortisone Sodium Phosphate (Concurrent use in the presence of increased intraocular pressure may be hazardous). Products include:
- Hydrocortone Phosphate Injection, Sterile ... 1481

Hydrocortisone Sodium Succinate (Concurrent use in the presence of increased intraocular pressure may be hazardous). Products include:
- Solu-Cortef Sterile Powder ... 2361

Hyoscyamine (Increases certain actions or side effects). Products include:
- Cystospaz Tablets ... 2395
- Urised Tablets ... 2396

Hyoscyamine Sulfate (Increases certain actions or side effects). Products include:
- Arco-Lase Plus Tablets ... 607
- Cystospaz-M Capsules ... 2395
- Donnagel ... ▣ 675
- Donnagel-PG ... 1858
- Donnatal ... 1858
- Donnatal Extentabs ... 1859
- Donnatal Tablets ... 1858
- Donnazyme Tablets ... 1860
- Kutrase Capsules ... 2146
- Levsin/Levsinex ... 2147
- Ru-Tuss Tablets ... 693

Imipramine Hydrochloride (Increases certain actions or side effects). Products include:
- Tofranil Ampuls ... 1038
- Tofranil Tablets ... 1039

Imipramine Pamoate (Increases certain actions or side effects). Products include:
- Tofranil-PM Capsules ... 1041

Ipratropium Bromide (Increases certain actions or side effects). Products include:
- Atrovent Inhalation Aerosol ... 675

Isocarboxazid (Increases certain actions or side effects). Products include:
- Marplan Tablets ... 1906

Isoflurophate (Effects of antiglaucoma agents antagonized). Products include:
- Floropryl Sterile Ophthalmic Ointment ... 1473

Isoproterenol Hydrochloride (Increases certain actions or side effects). Products include:
- Isuprel Hydrochloride Injection 1:5000 ... 2050
- Isuprel Hydrochloride Mistometer .. 2051
- Isuprel Hydrochloride Solution 1:200 & 1:100 ... 2052
- Norisodrine Aerotrol ... 540

Isosorbide Dinitrate (Increases certain actions and side effects). Products include:
- Dilatrate-SR ... 1827
- Isordil ... 2467
- Sorbitrate ... 1103

Levobunolol Hydrochloride (Effects of antiglaucoma agents antagonized). Products include:
- Betagan ... ⊙ 239

Levorphanol Tartrate (Increases certain actions or side effects). Products include:
- Levo-Dromoran ... 1906

Lorazepam (Increases certain actions or side effects). Products include:
- Ativan Injection ... 2432
- Ativan Tablets ... 2434

Magaldrate (Interferes with the absorption). Products include:
- Riopan Antacid Chew Tablets ... ▣ 754
- Riopan Antacid Chew Tablets in Rollpacks ... ▣ 754
- Riopan Antacid Suspension ... 2421
- Riopan Antacid Swallow Tablets ... 2421
- Riopan Plus Chew Tablets ... 2422
- Riopan Plus Chew Tablets in Rollpack ... 2422
- Riopan Plus 2 Chew Tablets, Mint Flavor, Cherry Flavor ... 2422
- Riopan Plus Suspension ... 2422
- Riopan Plus 2 Suspension, Mint Flavor, Cherry Flavor ... 2422

Magnesium Hydroxide (Interferes with the absorption). Products include:
- Aludrox Oral Suspension ... 2428
- Ascriptin A/D Caplets ... 1850
- Regular Strength Ascriptin Tablets 1850
- Di-Gel Antacid/Anti-Gas ... ▣ 697
- Gelusil Liquid & Tablets ... ▣ 639
- Haley's M-O, Regular & Flavored .. ▣ 569
- Extra Strength Maalox Plus Suspension ... 1850
- Maalox TC Suspension ... 1851
- Maalox Plus Tablets ... ▣ 655
- Extra Strength Maalox Plus Tablets 1850
- Mylanta Liquid ... 1155
- Mylanta Tablets ... 1155
- Mylanta Double Strength Liquid ... 1155
- Mylanta Double Strength Tablets ... 1155
- Concentrated Phillips' Milk of Magnesia ... ▣ 573
- Phillips' Milk of Magnesia Liquid ... ▣ 572
- Phillips' Milk of Magnesia Tablets ▣ 573
- WinGel Liquid & Tablets ... ▣ 761

Magnesium Oxide (Interferes with the absorption). Products include:
- Bayer Plus Aspirin Tablets ... ▣ 567
- Beelith Tablets ... 659
- Bufferin Analgesic Tablets and Caplets ... ▣ 524
- Cama Arthritis Pain Reliever ... ▣ 685
- Mag-Ox 400 ... 673
- Uro-Mag ... 673

Maprotiline Hydrochloride (Increases certain actions or side effects). Products include:
- Ludiomil Tablets ... 874

Mepenzolate Bromide (Increases certain actions or side effects). Products include:
- Cantil Tablets ... 1326

Meperidine Hydrochloride (Increases certain actions or side effects). Products include:
- Demerol ... 2047
- Mepergan Injection ... 2479

Mesoridazine (Increases certain actions or side effects). Products include:
- Serentil ... 686

Metaproterenol Sulfate (Increases certain actions or side effects). Products include:
- Alupent ... 674
- Arm-a-Med Metaproterenol Sulfate Inhalation Solution, USP ... 617
- Metaprel Inhalation Aerosol Bronchodilator ... 2014

Metaprel Inhalation Solution 2015
Metaprel 2015
Metaproterenol Sulfate Inhalation Solution, USP 912

Metaraminol Bitartrate (Increases certain actions or side effects). Products include:
Aramine Injection 1424

Methadone Hydrochloride (Increases certain actions or side effects). Products include:
Dolophine Hydrochloride Ampoules & Vials 1260
Dolophine Hydrochloride Tablets 1261
Methadone Hydrochloride Diskets .. 1284
Methadone Hydrochloride Oral Solution & Tablets 1987

Methazolamide (Effects of antiglaucoma agents antagonized). Products include:
Neptazane Tablets .... ◉ 311

Methdilazine Hydrochloride (Increases certain actions or side effects). Products include:
Tacaryl Syrup & Tablets 2409

Methoxamine Hydrochloride (Increases certain actions or side effects). Products include:
Vasoxyl Injection 819

Methylprednisolone Acetate (Concurrent use in the presence of increased intraocular pressure may be hazardous). Products include:
Depo-Medrol Sterile Aqueous Suspension 2334

Methylprednisolone Sodium Succinate (Concurrent use in the presence of increased intraocular pressure may be hazardous). Products include:
Solu-Medrol Sterile Powder 2363

Metoclopramide Hydrochloride (Gastrointestinal motility effects of metoclopramide may be antagonized). Products include:
Reglan 1869

Midazolam Hydrochloride (Increases certain actions or side effects). Products include:
Versed Injection 1924

Moricizine Hydrochloride (Increases certain actions or side effects). Products include:
Ethmozine Tablets 946

Morphine Sulfate (Increases certain actions or side effects). Products include:
Astramorph/PF Injection, USP (Preservative-Free) 618
Duramorph 960
Infumorph 200 and Infumorph 500 Sterile Solutions 962
MS Contin Tablets 1814
MSIR 1817
Oramorph SR (Morphine Sulfate Sustained Release Tablets) 1988
Roxanol 1991

Nitroglycerin (Increases certain actions and side effects). Products include:
Deponit NTG Transdermal Delivery System 2143
Minitran Transdermal Delivery System 1312
Nitro-Bid Ointment 1339
Nitro-Bid Capsules 1338
Nitrodisc 2176
Nitro-Dur (nitroglycerin) Transdermal Infusion System 1164
Nitrogard Tablets 1004
Nitrolingual Spray 1846
Nitrostat Tablets 1743
Transderm-Nitro Transdermal Therapeutic System 2283

Norepinephrine Bitartrate (Increases certain actions or side effects). Products include:
Levophed Bitartrate Injection 2054

Nortriptyline Hydrochloride (Increases certain actions or side effects). Products include:
Pamelor 2019

Opium Alkaloids (Increases certain actions or side effects). Products include:
B & O No. 15A & No. 16A Supprettes 2395
Pantopon Injectable 1911

Oxazepam (Increases certain actions or side effects). Products include:
Serax Capsules 2522
Serax Tablets 2522

Oxybutynin Chloride (Increases certain actions or side effects). Products include:
Ditropan 1332

Oxycodone Hydrochloride (Increases certain actions or side effects). Products include:
Percocet Tablets 950
Percodan 951
Roxicodone Tablets, Oral Solution & Intensol (Oxycodone) 1992
Tylox Capsules 1382

Pentaerythritol Tetranitrate (Increases certain actions and side effects). Products include:
Peritrate 1756

Pentagastrin (Antagonizes the inhibiting effects on gastric hydrochloric acid). Products include:
Peptavlon 2563

Perphenazine (Increases certain actions or side effects). Products include:
Etrafon 2087
Triavil Tablets 1556
Trilafon 2123

Phenelzine Sulfate (Increases certain actions or side effects). Products include:
Nardil 1742

Phenylephrine Bitartrate (Increases certain actions or side effects).
No products indexed under this heading.

Phenylephrine Hydrochloride (Increases certain actions or side effects). Products include:
AK-Dilate Solution 2.5% and 10% .... ◉ 203
Atrohist Sprinkle Capsules 558
Cerose-DM 2443
Codimal 846
Comhist LA Capsules 1618
Congespirin For Children Aspirin Free Chewable Cold Tablets 748
Cyclomydril .... ◉ 216
Deconsal Sprinkle Capsules 559
Dimetane Decongestant .... ▣ 673
Dristan Decongestant/Antihistamine/ Analgesic Coated Caplets .... ▣ 749
Dristan Cold Nasal Decongestant/ Antihistamine/ Analgesic Coated Tablets 2419
Dristan Advanced Formula Decongestant/Antihistamine/ Analgesic Tablets .... ▣ 749
Dristan Nasal Spray, Menthol 2419
Dristan Nasal Spray, Regular and Regular with Metered Pump 2419
Entex Capsules 1623
Entex Liquid 1623
Sinus Excedrin Analgesic, Decongestant Tablets & Caplets 750
Extendryl 994
4-Way Fast Acting Nasal Spray - Original Formula (regular & mentholated) & Metered Spray Pump (regular) 751
Hycomine Compound Tablets 929
Murocoll-2 Sterile Ophthalmic Solution .... ◉ 261
Mydfrin 2.5% .... ◉ 224
Naldecon Syrup, Tablets, Pediatric Drops and Pediatric Syrup 709
Neo-Synephrine Hydrochloride 1% Carpuject 2063
Neo-Synephrine Hydrochloride 1% Injection 2063
Neo-Synephrine Hydrochloride (Ophthalmic) 2064
Neo-Synephrine .... ▣ 759
Nōstril Nasal Decongestant .... ▣ 520
Novahistine Elixir .... ▣ 596
Phenergan VC 2500
Phenergan VC with Codeine 2501
Prefrin Liquifilm Vasoconstrictor and Lubricant Eye Drops .... ◉ 254
Prefrin-A .... ◉ 255
Quelidrine Syrup 556
Relief Vasoconstrictor and Lubricant Eye Drops .... ◉ 256
Robitussin Night Relief .... ▣ 677
Ru-Tuss with Hydrocodone 694
Ru-Tuss Tablets 693
Vasosulf .... ◉ 279
Vicks Sinex .... ▣ 665
Zincfrin .... ◉ 230

Phenylephrine Tannate (Increases certain actions or side effects). Products include:
Rynatan 2387
Rynatuss 2388

Phenylpropanolamine Hydrochloride (Increases certain actions or side effects). Products include:
A.R.M. Allergy Relief Medicine Caplets .... ▣ 615
Acutrim .... ▣ 548
Allerest .... ▣ 559
BC Cold Powder .... ▣ 517
Cheracol Plus Head Cold/Cough Formula .... ▣ 667
Codimal Expectorant 846
Comtrex Multi-Symptom Cold Reliever Tablets/Caplets/Liqui-Gels/Liquid 745
Contac Continuous Action Decongestant/Antihistamine Capsules ▣ 710
Contac Maximum Strength Continuous Action Decongestant/ Antihistamine Caplets .... ▣ 709
Contac Severe Cold and Flu Formula Caplets .... ▣ 711
Coricidin 'D' Decongestant Tablets .... ▣ 695
Coricidin Demilets Tablets for Children .... ▣ 696
Demazin Nasal Decongestant/ Antihistamine Repetabs Tablets & Syrup .... ▣ 697
Dexatrim .... ▣ 733
Dimetane-DC Cough Syrup 1857
Dimetapp Elixir .... ▣ 673
Dimetapp DM Elixir .... ▣ 674
Dimetapp Extentabs .... ▣ 674
Dimetapp Plus Caplets .... ▣ 675
Dimetapp Tablets .... ▣ 675
Entex Capsules 1623
Entex LA Tablets 1623
Entex Liquid 1623
4-Way Cold Tablets 750
Hycomine Syrup 927
Naldecon CX Adult Liquid .... ▣ 521
Naldecon DX Adult Liquid .... ▣ 521
Naldecon DX Children's Syrup .... ▣ 522
Naldecon DX Pediatric Drops .... ▣ 522
Naldecon EX Children's Syrup .... ▣ 522
Naldecon EX Pediatric Drops .... ▣ 523
Naldecon Syrup, Tablets, Pediatric Drops and Pediatric Syrup 709
Nolamine Tablets 838
Nolex LA Tablets 838
Ornade Spansule Capsules 2221
Orthoxicol Cough Syrup .... ▣ 668
Propagest 839
Pyrroxate Capsules .... ▣ 669
Robitussin-CF .... ▣ 676
Ru-Tuss II Capsules 693
Ru-Tuss with Hydrocodone 694
Ru-Tuss Tablets 693
Sine-Off Sinus Medicine Tablets-Aspirin Formula .... ▣ 722
Sinulin 840
St. Joseph Cold Tablets for Children .... ▣ 704
Tavist-D Tablets 2035
Triaminic Allergy Tablets .... ▣ 688
Triaminic Chewables .... ▣ 688
Triaminic Cold Tablets .... ▣ 688
Triaminic Expectorant .... ▣ 688
Triaminic Expectorant w/Codeine .. 1996
Triaminic Expectorant DH 1995
Triaminic Oral Infant Drops 1996
Triaminic Syrup .... ▣ 689
Triaminic-12 Tablets .... ▣ 690
Triaminic-DM Syrup .... ▣ 689
Triaminicin Tablets .... ▣ 690
Triaminicol Multi-Symptom Cold Tablets .... ▣ 691
Triaminicol Multi-Symptom Relief ▣ 691
Tuss-Ornade Liquid 2242
Tuss-Ornade Spansule Capsules 2242
Tylenol Cold Medication, Effervescent Tablets 1369

Pilocarpine (Effects of antiglaucoma agents antagonized). Products include:
Ocusert Pilo-20 and Pilo-40 Ocular Therapeutic Systems .... ◉ 256

Pilocarpine Hydrochloride (Effects of antiglaucoma agents antagonized). Products include:
Akarpine Ophthalmic Solution .... ◉ 201
Isopto Carpine .... ◉ 219
Pilocar .... ◉ 275
Pilopine HS Gel .... ◉ 227
Pilostat Sterile Ophthalmic Solution 0.5%, 1%, 2%, 3%, 4%, 5%, 6% .... ◉ 263

Pirbuterol Acetate (Increases certain actions or side effects). Products include:
Maxair Inhaler 1311

Prazepam (Increases certain actions or side effects). Products include:
Centrax 1693

Prednisolone Acetate (Concurrent use in the presence of increased intraocular pressure may be hazardous). Products include:
AK-Cide Sterile Ophthalmic Ointment & Suspension .... ◉ 202
Blephamide Liquifilm Sterile Ophthalmic Suspension 586
Blephamide S.O.P. Sterile Ophthalmic Ointment 586
Cetapred Ointment .... ◉ 220
⅛% Econopred & 1% Econopred Plus .... ◉ 217
Isopto Cetapred Suspension .... ◉ 220
Metimyd .... ◉ 306
Poly-Pred Liquifilm .... ◉ 250
Pred Forte .... ◉ 252
Pred Mild .... ◉ 254
Pred-G Liquifilm Sterile Ophthalmic Suspension .... ◉ 252
Pred-G S.O.P. Sterile Ophthalmic Ointment .... ◉ 253
Vasocidin Ointment .... ◉ 275

Prednisolone Sodium Phosphate (Concurrent use in the presence of increased intraocular pressure may be hazardous). Products include:
AK-Pred .... ◉ 205
Hydeltrasol Injection, Sterile 1476
Inflamase .... ◉ 274
Pediapred Oral Liquid 987
Vasocidin Ophthalmic Solution .... ◉ 276

Prednisolone Tebutate (Concurrent use in the presence of increased intraocular pressure may be hazardous). Products include:
Hydeltra-T.B.A. Sterile Suspension 1478

Prednisone (Concurrent use in the presence of increased intraocular pressure may be hazardous). Products include:
Deltasone Tablets 2332

Procainamide Hydrochloride (Increases certain actions or side effects). Products include:
Procan SR Tablets 1760
Pronestyl Capsules and Tablets 1800
Pronestyl Injection 1798
Pronestyl-SR Tablets 1801

Prochlorperazine (Increases certain actions or side effects). Products include:
Compazine 2201

Procyclidine Hydrochloride (Increases certain actions or side effects). Products include:
Kemadrin Tablets 771

Promethazine Hydrochloride (Increases certain actions or side effects). Products include:
Mepergan Injection 2479
Phenergan with Codeine 2497
Phenergan with Dextromethorphan 2499
Phenergan Injection 2493
Phenergan Suppositories 2496
Phenergan Syrup 2495
Phenergan Tablets 2496

Phenergan VC 2500
Phenergan VC with Codeine 2501

Propafenone Hydrochloride (Increases certain actions or side effects). Products include:
Rythmol Tablets 1184

Propantheline Bromide (Increases certain actions or side effects). Products include:
Pro-Banthīne Tablets 2141

Propoxyphene Hydrochloride (Increases certain actions or side effects). Products include:
Darvon 1256
Wygesic Tablets 2540

Propoxyphene Napsylate (Increases certain actions or side effects). Products include:
Darvon-N/Darvocet-N 1254

Protriptyline Hydrochloride (Increases certain actions or side effects). Products include:
Vivactil Tablets 1567

Pseudoephedrine Hydrochloride (Increases certain actions or side effects). Products include:
Actifed Capsules .... ▣ 539
Actifed Plus Caplets .... ▣ 539
Actifed Plus Tablets .... ▣ 540
Actifed with Codeine Cough Syrup.. 752
Actifed Syrup .... ▣ 540
Actifed Tablets .... ▣ 540
Actifed 12-Hour Capsules .... ▣ 539
Advil Cold & Sinus Caplets (formerly CoAdvil) 2416
Allerest .... ▣ 559
Anatuss LA Tablets 1359
Benadryl Decongestant Elixir .... ▣ 635
Benadryl Decongestant .... ▣ 635
Benadryl Plus .... ▣ 636
Benadryl Plus Nighttime .... ▣ 637
Benylin Decongestant .... ▣ 638
Brexin L.A. Capsules 2078
Bromfed Capsules (Timed Release) 1615
Bromfed Syrup .... ▣ 628
Bromfed 1615
CoAdvil .... ▣ 748
Allergy-Sinus Comtrex Multi-Symptom Allergy Sinus Formula Tablets & Caplets 746
Cough Formula Comtrex 746
Comtrex Multi-Symptom Cold Reliever Tablets/Caplets/Liqui-Gels/Liquid 745
Day-Night Comtrex 747
Non-Drowsy Comtrex 747
Congess 994
Congestac Caplets .... ▣ 617
Contac Jr. Children's Cold Medicine .... ▣ 712
Contac Nighttime Cold Medicine .... ▣ 713
Contac Sinus Caplets Maximum Strength Non-Drowsy Formula .... ▣ 710
Contac Sinus Tablets Maximum Strength Non-Drowsy Formula .... ▣ 710
Deconamine 663
Deconsal II Tablets 559
Dimacol Caplets .... ▣ 672
Dimetane-DX Cough Syrup 1858
Dorcol Children's Cough Syrup .... ▣ 685
Dorcol Children's Decongestant Liquid .... ▣ 685
Dorcol Children's Liquid Cold Formula .... ▣ 686
Maximum Strength Dristan Decongestant/Analgesic Coated Caplets .... ▣ 750
No Drowsiness Dristan Cold Nasal Decongestant/Analgesic Coated Caplets 2420
Dristan Sinus Caplets 2419
Sinus Excedrin Analgesic, Decongestant Tablets & Caplets .... ▣ 533
Fedahist Gyrocaps 2145
Fedahist Timecaps 2145
Guaifed 1615
Guaifed Syrup .... ▣ 629
Isoclor Expectorant 982
Isoclor Timesule Capsules .... ▣ 561
Kronofed-A 970
Medi-Flu Caplet, Liquid .... ▣ 640
Novafed A Capsules 1342
Novafed Capsules 1342
Novahistine DH 1342
Novahistine DMX .... ▣ 595
Novahistine Expectorant 1343
Nucofed Capsules 2219
Nucofed Expectorant 2219
Nucofed Pediatric Expectorant 2220
Nucofed Syrup 2219
Ornex Caplets .... ▣ 618
PediaCare Allergy Relief Formula Liquid 1362
PediaCare Cough-Cold Formula Liquid 1362
PediaCare Infants' Oral Decongestant Drops 1362
PediaCare Night Rest Cough-Cold Formula Liquid 1362
PediaCare 6-12 Cough-Cold Formula Chewable Tablets 1362
Robitussin-DAC Syrup 1875
Robitussin-PE .... ▣ 677
Rondec 1975
Rondec-DM 1976
Rondec-TR Tablet 1975
Ru-Tuss DE Tablets 694
Ryna .... ▣ 741
Seldane-D Extended-Release Tablets 1350
Sinarest .... ▣ 562
Sine-Aid Maximum Strength Sinus Headache Caplets 1365
Sine-Aid Maximum Strength Sinus Headache Tablets 1365
Sine-Off Maximum Strength Allergy/Sinus Formula Caplets .... ▣ 721
Sine-Off Maximum Strength No Drowsiness Formula Caplets .... ▣ 722
Singlet Tablets .... ▣ 598
Sinutab Maximum Strength .... ▣ 641
Sinutab Maximum Strength Without Drowsiness Tablets & Caplets .... ▣ 642
Sinutab Regular Strength Without Drowsiness Formula .... ▣ 641
St. Joseph Nighttime Cold Medicine .... ▣ 705
Sudafed Children's Liquid .... ▣ 543
Sudafed Cough Syrup .... ▣ 543
Sudafed Plus Liquid .... ▣ 544
Sudafed Plus Tablets .... ▣ 545
Sudafed Sinus Caplets .... ▣ 545
Sudafed Sinus Tablets .... ▣ 545
Sudafed Tablets, 30 mg .... ▣ 544
Sudafed Tablets, Adult Strength, 60 mg .... ▣ 544
Sudafed 12 Hour Capsules .... ▣ 545
TheraFlu Flu and Cold Medicine .... ▣ 687
Triaminic Nite Light .... ▣ 689
Tylenol Allergy Sinus Medication Caplets and Gelcaps, Maximum Strength 1372
Children's Tylenol Cold Liquid Formula and Chewable Tablets 1368
Tylenol Cold & Flu Hot Medication, Packets 1369
Tylenol Cold & Flu No Drowsiness Hot Medication, Packets 1371
Tylenol Cold Medication Caplets and Tablets 1370
Tylenol Cold Medication No Drowsiness Formula Caplets 1370
Tylenol Cold Night Time Medication Liquid 1371
Tylenol Cough Medication Liquid with Decongestant, Maximum Strength 1372
Tylenol, Maximum Strength, Sinus Medication Gelcaps, Caplets and Tablets 1373
Ursinus Inlay-Tabs .... ▣ 691
Vicks Children's NyQuil .... ▣ 664
Vicks Daycare .... ▣ 660
Vicks Formula 44D Decongestant Cough Medicine .... ▣ 662
Vicks Formula 44M Multi-Symptom Cough Medicine .... ▣ 662
Vicks NyQuil Nighttime Colds Medicine-Original & Cherry Flavor .... ▣ 664
Vicks Pediatric Formula 44 Cough & Congestion Medicine .... ▣ 663
Vicks Pediatric Formula 44m Multi-Symptom Cough & Cold Medicine .... ▣ 663

Pseudoephedrine Sulfate (Increases certain actions or side effects). Products include:
Afrin Tablets .... ▣ 693
Chlor-Trimeton Decongestant .... ▣ 694
Disophrol Chronotab Sustained-Action Tablets .... ▣ 698
Drixoral Antihistamine/Nasal Decongestant Syrup .... ▣ 698
Drixoral Non-Drowsy Formula .... ▣ 699
Drixoral Plus Extended-Release Tablets .... ▣ 699
Drixoral Sinus .... ▣ 700
Drixoral Sustained-Action Tablets .... ▣ 698
Sinutab Allergy Formula Sustained Action Tablets .... ▣ 640
Trinalin Repetabs Tablets 1170

Pyrilamine Maleate (Increases certain actions or side effects). Products include:
Codimal 846
4-Way Fast Acting Nasal Spray - Original Formula (regular & mentholated) & Metered Spray Pump (regular) 751
Maximum Strength Midol Multi-Symptom Menstrual Formula .... ▣ 571
Maximum Strength Midol PMS Premenstrual Syndrome Formula .... ▣ 570
Regular Strength Midol Multi-Symptom Menstrual Formula .... ▣ 570
Prefrin-A .... ⊙ 255
Prēmsyn PMS Capsules & Caplets .... ▣ 547
Primatene Tablets-M Formula 2421
Robitussin Night Relief .... ▣ 677
Ru-Tuss with Hydrocodone 694
Triaminic Expectorant DH 1995
Triaminic Oral Infant Drops 1996

Pyrilamine Tannate (Increases certain actions or side effects). Products include:
Rynatan 2387

Quazepam (Increases certain actions or side effects). Products include:
Doral Tablets 2383

Quinidine Gluconate (Increases certain actions or side effects). Products include:
Quinaglute Dura-Tabs Tablets 663

Quinidine Polygalacturonate (Increases certain actions or side effects). Products include:
Cardioquin Tablets 1812

Quinidine Sulfate (Increases certain actions or side effects). Products include:
Quinidex Extentabs 1868

Scopolamine Hydrobromide (Increases certain actions or side effects). Products include:
Donnagel .... ▣ 675
Donnagel-PG 1858
Donnatal 1858
Donnatal Extentabs 1859
Donnatal Tablets 1858
Donnazyme Tablets 1860
Isopto Hyoscine .... ⊙ 222
Murocoll-2 Sterile Ophthalmic Solution .... ⊙ 261
Ru-Tuss Tablets 693

Scopolamine Preparations (Increases certain actions or side effects). Products include:
Transderm Scōp Transdermal Therapeutic System 887

Selegiline Hydrochloride (Increases certain actions or side effects). Products include:
Eldepryl 2250

Sodium Bicarbonate (Interferes with the absorption). Products include:
Alka-Seltzer Advanced Formula Antacid & Non-Aspirin Pain Reliever .... ▣ 620
Alka-Seltzer Effervescent Antacid .... ▣ 622
Alka-Seltzer Effervescent Antacid and Pain Reliever 1568
Alka-Seltzer Extra Strength Effervescent Antacid and Pain Reliever .... ▣ 623
Alka-Seltzer (Flavored) Effervescent Antacid and Pain Reliever .... ▣ 621
Arm & Hammer Pure Baking Soda .... ▣ 548
Ceo-Two Rectal Suppositories 671
Citrocarbonate Antacid .... ▣ 668
Massengill Liquid Concentrate 2191
NuLYTELY 699

Sufentanil Citrate (Increases certain actions or side effects). Products include:
Sufenta Injection 1147

Terbutaline Sulfate (Increases certain actions or side effects). Products include:
Brethaire Inhaler 1024
Brethine Ampuls 1026
Brethine Tablets 1026
Bricanyl Injection 1324
Bricanyl Tablets 1325

Terfenadine (Increases certain actions or side effects). Products include:
Seldane Tablets 1349
Seldane-D Extended-Release Tablets 1350

Thioridazine Hydrochloride (Increases certain actions or side effects). Products include:
Mellaril 2011

Timolol Maleate (Effects of anti-glaucoma agents antagonized). Products include:
Blocadren Tablets 1429
Timolide Tablets 1547
Timoptic in Ocudose 1552
Timoptic Sterile Ophthalmic Solution 1550

Tranylcypromine Sulfate (Increases certain actions or side effects). Products include:
Parnate Tablets 2222

Triamcinolone (Concurrent use in the presence of increased intraocular pressure may be hazardous).
No products indexed under this heading.

Triamcinolone Acetonide (Concurrent use in the presence of increased intraocular pressure may be hazardous). Products include:
Aristocort A 1010
Azmacort Inhaler 1837
Kenalog Cream, Lotion & Ointment 2401
Kenalog-10 Injection 2402
Kenalog-40 Injection 2403
Kenalog in Orabase 604
Kenalog Spray 2401
Mycolog II Cream and Ointment 2407
Mytrex Cream & Ointment 2080
Nasacort Nasal Inhaler 1844

Triamcinolone Diacetate (Concurrent use in the presence of increased intraocular pressure may be hazardous). Products include:
Aristocort Suspension 1008

Triamcinolone Hexacetonide (Concurrent use in the presence of increased intraocular pressure may be hazardous). Products include:
Aristospan Suspension 1011

Tridihexethyl Chloride (Increases certain actions or side effects).
No products indexed under this heading.

Trifluoperazine Hydrochloride (Increases certain actions or side effects). Products include:
Stelazine 2226

Trihexyphenidyl Hydrochloride (Increases certain actions or side effects). Products include:
Artane 1195

Trimeprazine Tartrate (Increases certain actions or side effects). Products include:
Temaril Tablets, Syrup and Spansule Sustained Release Capsules 1085

Trimipramine Maleate (Increases certain actions or side effects). Products include:
Surmontil Capsules 2524

Tripelennamine Hydrochloride (Increases certain actions or side effects). Products include:
PBZ Tablets & Elixir 1037
PBZ-SR Tablets 1037

Triprolidine Hydrochloride (Increases certain actions or side effects). Products include:
Actidil ▣ 538
Actifed Capsules ▣ 539
Actifed Plus Caplets ▣ 539
Actifed Plus Tablets ▣ 540
Actifed with Codeine Cough Syrup.. 752
Actifed Syrup ▣ 540
Actifed Tablets ▣ 540
Actifed 12-Hour Capsules ▣ 539

BENTYL INJECTION
(Dicyclomine Hydrochloride) 1322
See **Bentyl 10 mg Capsules**

BENTYL SYRUP
(Dicyclomine Hydrochloride) 1322
See **Bentyl 10 mg Capsules**

BENTYL 20 MG TABLETS
(Dicyclomine Hydrochloride) 1322
See **Bentyl 10 mg Capsules**

BENYLIN COUGH SYRUP
(Diphenhydramine Hydrochloride) ▣ 637
May interact with:

Alcohol (Do not use concomitantly).

BENYLIN DECONGESTANT
(Diphenhydramine Hydrochloride, Pseudoephedrine Hydrochloride) ▣ 638
May interact with antihypertensives, antidepressant drugs, and certain other agents. Compounds in these categories include:

Acebutolol Hydrochloride (Concurrent use not recommended). Products include:
Sectral Capsules 2520

Alcohol (Do not use concomitantly).

Amitriptyline Hydrochloride (Concurrent use not recommended). Products include:
Elavil 2269
Endep Tablets 1927
Etrafon 2087
Limbitrol 1933
Triavil Tablets 1556

Amoxapine (Concurrent use not recommended). Products include:
Asendin Tablets 1196

Atenolol (Concurrent use not recommended). Products include:
Tenoretic Tablets 1105
Tenormin Tablets and I.V. Injection 1107

Benazepril Hydrochloride (Concurrent use not recommended). Products include:
Lotensin Tablets 872

Betaxolol Hydrochloride (Concurrent use not recommended). Products include:
Betoptic Sterile Ophthalmic Solution 569
Betoptic S Sterile Ophthalmic Suspension 570
Kerlone Tablets 2172

Bupropion Hydrochloride (Concurrent use not recommended). Products include:
Wellbutrin Tablets 821

Captopril (Concurrent use not recommended). Products include:
Capoten 2255
Capozide 2258

Carteolol Hydrochloride (Concurrent use not recommended). Products include:
Cartrol Tablets 507

Clonidine (Concurrent use not recommended). Products include:
Catapres-TTS 677

Clonidine Hydrochloride (Concurrent use not recommended). Products include:
Catapres Tablets 676
Combipres Tablets 678

Deserpidine (Concurrent use not recommended). Products include:
Enduronyl 518
Harmonyl Tablets 528
Oreticyl 545

Desipramine Hydrochloride (Concurrent use not recommended). Products include:
Norpramin Tablets 1340

Diazoxide (Concurrent use not recommended). Products include:
Hyperstat I.V. Injection 2095
Proglycem 649

Doxazosin Mesylate (Concurrent use not recommended). Products include:
Cardura Tablets 1941

Doxepin Hydrochloride (Concurrent use not recommended). Products include:
Sinequan 1960

Enalapril Maleate (Concurrent use not recommended). Products include:
Vaseretic Tablets 1559
Vasotec Tablets 1564

Enalaprilat (Concurrent use not recommended). Products include:
Vasotec I.V. 1562

Esmolol Hydrochloride (Concurrent use not recommended). Products include:
Brevibloc Injection 942

Felodipine (Concurrent use not recommended). Products include:
Plendil Extended-Release Tablets 1526

Fluoxetine Hydrochloride (Concurrent use not recommended). Products include:
Prozac Pulvules 920

Fosinopril Sodium (Concurrent use not recommended). Products include:
Monopril Tablets 1406

Guanabenz Acetate (Concurrent use not recommended). Products include:
Wytensin Tablets 2542

Guanethidine Monosulfate (Concurrent use not recommended). Products include:
Esimil Tablets 864
Ismelin Tablets 869

Hydralazine Hydrochloride (Concurrent use not recommended). Products include:
Apresazide Capsules 854
Apresoline Hydrochloride Parenteral (Ampuls) 856
Apresoline Hydrochloride Tablets .. 855
Apresoline-Esidrix Tablets 857
Ser-Ap-Es Tablets 881
Serpasil-Apresoline Tablets 884

Imipramine Hydrochloride (Concurrent use not recommended). Products include:
Tofranil Ampuls 1038
Tofranil Tablets 1039

Imipramine Pamoate (Concurrent use not recommended). Products include:
Tofranil-PM Capsules 1041

Indapamide (Concurrent use not recommended). Products include:
Lozol Tablets 1843

Isocarboxazid (Concurrent use not recommended). Products include:
Marplan Tablets 1906

Isradipine (Concurrent use not recommended). Products include:
DynaCirc Capsules 2004

Labetalol Hydrochloride (Concurrent use not recommended). Products include:
Normodyne Injection 2108
Normodyne Tablets 2110
Normozide Tablets 2112
Trandate HCT Tablets 579
Trandate Injection 577
Trandate Tablets 579

Lisinopril (Concurrent use not recommended). Products include:
Prinivil Tablets 1538
Prinzide Tablets 1540
Zestoretic 2274
Zestril Tablets 2277

Maprotiline Hydrochloride (Concurrent use not recommended). Products include:
Ludiomil Tablets 874

Mecamylamine Hydrochloride (Concurrent use not recommended). Products include:
Inversine Tablets 1492

Methyldopa (Concurrent use not recommended). Products include:
Aldoclor Tablets 1413
Aldomet Oral 1415
Aldoril Tablets 1418

Methyldopate Hydrochloride (Concurrent use not recommended). Products include:
Aldomet Ester HCl Injection 1417

Metoprolol Tartrate (Concurrent use not recommended). Products include:
Lopressor Ampuls 1032
Lopressor HCT Tablets 1034
Lopressor Tablets 1032

Metyrosine (Concurrent use not recommended). Products include:
Demser Capsules 1460

Minoxidil (Concurrent use not recommended). Products include:
Loniten Tablets 2346
Rogaine Topical Solution 2357

Nadolol (Concurrent use not recommended). Products include:
Corgard Tablets 701
Corzide Tablets 702

Nicardipine Hydrochloride (Concurrent use not recommended). Products include:
Cardene Capsules 2290

Nitroglycerin (Concurrent use not recommended). Products include:
Deponit NTG Transdermal Delivery System 2143
Minitran Transdermal Delivery System 1312
Nitro-Bid Ointment 1339
Nitro-Bid Capsules 1338
Nitrodisc 2176
Nitro-Dur (nitroglycerin) Transdermal Infusion System 1164
Nitrogard Tablets 1004
Nitrolingual Spray 1846
Nitrostat Tablets 1743
Transderm-Nitro Transdermal Therapeutic System 2283

Nortriptyline Hydrochloride (Concurrent use not recommended). Products include:
Pamelor 2019

Penbutolol Sulfate (Concurrent use not recommended). Products include:
Levatol 1832

Phenelzine Sulfate (Concurrent use not recommended). Products include:
Nardil 1742

Phenoxybenzamine Hydrochloride (Concurrent use not recommended). Products include:
Dibenzyline Capsules 2207

Phentolamine Mesylate (Concurrent use not recommended). Products include:
Regitine 878

Pindolol (Concurrent use not recommended). Products include:
Visken Tablets 2036

Prazosin Hydrochloride (Concurrent use not recommended). Products include:
Minipress Capsules 1778
Minizide Capsules 1779

Propranolol Hydrochloride (Concurrent use not recommended). Products include:
Inderal 2459
Inderal LA Long Acting Capsules 2461
Inderide Tablets 2463
Inderide LA Long Acting Capsules .. 2465

Protriptyline Hydrochloride (Concurrent use not recommended). Products include:
Vivactil Tablets 1567

Ramipril (Concurrent use not recommended). Products include:
Altace Capsules 1086

Rauwolfia Serpentina (Concurrent use not recommended). Products include:
Raudixin Tablets 1803
Rauzide Tablets 1804

Rescinnamine (Concurrent use not recommended).
No products indexed under this heading.

Reserpine (Concurrent use not recommended). Products include:
Diupres Tablets 1461
Hydromox R Tablets 1209
Hydropres Tablets 1485
Renese-R Tablets 1786
Salutensin/Salutensin-Demi 719
Ser-Ap-Es Tablets 881
Serpasil Tablets 883
Serpasil-Apresoline Tablets 884
Serpasil-Esidrix Tablets 886

Sodium Nitroprusside (Concurrent use not recommended). Products include:
Nipride I.V. Infusion 1909

Terazosin Hydrochloride (Concurrent use not recommended). Products include:
Hytrin Tablets 529

Timolol Maleate (Concurrent use not recommended). Products include:
Blocadren Tablets 1429
Timolide Tablets 1547
Timoptic in Ocudose 1552
Timoptic Sterile Ophthalmic Solution 1550

Tranylcypromine Sulfate (Concurrent use not recommended). Products include:
Parnate Tablets 2222

Trazodone Hydrochloride (Concurrent use not recommended). Products include:
Desyrel and Desyrel Dividose 1404

Trimethaphan Camsylate (Concurrent use not recommended). Products include:
Arfonad Ampuls 1887

Trimipramine Maleate (Concurrent use not recommended). Products include:
Surmontil Capsules 2524

BENYLIN DM
(Dextromethorphan Hydrobromide) ▣ 638
No interactions described in labeling.

BENYLIN EXPECTORANT
(Dextromethorphan Hydrobromide, Guaifenesin) ▣ 638
No interactions described in labeling.

BENZAC 5 & 10 GEL
(Benzoyl Peroxide) 1682
May interact with:

Octyl Dimethyl PABA (Concurrent use with PABA-containing sunscreens may result in transient discoloration of the skin). Products include:
Herpecin-L Cold Sore Lip Balm 833
PreSun 15 Facial Sunscreen ▣ 537

PreSun 8, 15 and 39 Creamy Sunscreens ▣ 537
PreSun 23 Spray Mist ▣ 537
Solbar Plus 15 Cream 1772

BENZAC AC 2½%, 5%, AND 10% WATER-BASE GEL
(Benzoyl Peroxide) 1681
No interactions described in labeling.

BENZAC AC WASH 2½%, 5%, 10% WATER-BASE CLEANSER
(Benzoyl Peroxide) 1681
No interactions described in labeling.

BENZAC W WASH 5 & 10 WATER-BASE CLEANSER
(Benzoyl Peroxide) 1682
See **Benzac 5 & 10 Gel**

BENZAC W 2½, 5 & 10 WATER-BASE GEL
(Benzoyl Peroxide) 1682
See **Benzac 5 & 10 Gel**

5 BENZAGEL (5% BENZOYL PEROXIDE) & 10 BENZAGEL (10% BENZOYL PEROXIDE), ACNE GELS, MICROGEL FORMULA
(Benzoyl Peroxide) 907
No interactions described in labeling.

BENZAMYCIN TOPICAL GEL
(Erythromycin, Benzoyl Peroxide) 907
May interact with:

Clindamycin Palmitate Hydrochloride (Erythromycin antagonist). Products include:
Cleocin Pediatric Flavored Granules 2324

Clindamycin Phosphate (Erythromycin antagonist). Products include:
Cleocin Phosphate Injection 2325
Cleocin T Topical 2327

BENZASHAVE MEDICATED SHAVE CREAM 5% AND 10%
(Benzoyl Peroxide) 1409
No interactions described in labeling.

BENZEDREX INHALER
(Propylhexedrine) ▣ 617
No interactions described in labeling.

BEROCCA PLUS TABLETS
(Vitamins with Minerals) 1894
May interact with:

Levodopa (Decreased efficacy). Products include:
Larodopa Tablets 1905
Sinemet Tablets 952
Sinemet CR Tablets 953

BEROCCA TABLETS
(Vitamins with Minerals, Therapeutic) 1893
May interact with:

Levodopa (Decreased efficacy). Products include:
Larodopa Tablets 1905
Sinemet Tablets 952
Sinemet CR Tablets 953

BETADINE DISPOSABLE MEDICATED DOUCHE
(Povidone Iodine) 1811
No interactions described in labeling.

BETADINE FIRST AID CREAM
(Povidone Iodine) 1811
No interactions described in labeling.

BETADINE MEDICATED DOUCHE
(Povidone Iodine) 1811
No interactions described in labeling.

BETADINE MEDICATED GEL
(Povidone Iodine) 1811
No interactions described in labeling.

BETADINE MEDICATED VAGINAL SUPPOSITORIES
(Povidone Iodine) 1812
No interactions described in labeling.

BETADINE OINTMENT
(Povidone Iodine) 1812
No interactions described in labeling.

BETADINE PRE-MIXED MEDICATED DISPOSABLE DOUCHE
(Povidone Iodine) 1811
No interactions described in labeling.

BETADINE SKIN CLEANSER
(Povidone Iodine) 1812
No interactions described in labeling.

BETADINE SOLUTION
(Povidone Iodine) 1812
No interactions described in labeling.

BETADINE SURGICAL SCRUB
(Povidone Iodine) 1812
No interactions described in labeling.

BETAGAN LIQUIFILM
(Levobunolol Hydrochloride) ⊙ 239
See **Betagan Liquifilm with C Cap Compliance Cap**

BETAGAN LIQUIFILM WITH C CAP COMPLIANCE CAP
(Levobunolol Hydrochloride) ⊙ 239
May interact with $beta_2$ agonists, catecholamine depleting drugs, oral hypoglycemic agents, insulin, sympathomimetic bronchodilators, and certain other agents. Compounds in these categories include:

Acebutolol Hydrochloride (Additive effects on systemic beta-blockade from concomitant therapy with orally administered beta-blockers). Products include:
Sectral Capsules 2520

Albuterol (Betagan may block bronchodilation produced by $beta_2$adrenergic agonists). Products include:
Proventil Inhalation Aerosol 2117
Ventolin Inhalation Aerosol and Refill 583

Albuterol Sulfate (Betagan may block bronchodilation produced by $beta_2$adrenergic agonists). Products include:
Proventil Repetabs Tablets 2120
Proventil Solutions for Inhalation 0.5% and 0.083% 2118
Proventil Syrup 2119
Proventil Tablets 2120
Ventolin 583

Atenolol (Additive effects on systemic beta-blockade from concomitant therapy with orally administered beta-blockers). Products include:
Tenoretic Tablets 1105
Tenormin Tablets and I.V. Injection 1107

Betaxolol Hydrochloride (Additive effects on systemic beta-blockade from concomitant therapy with orally administered beta-blockers). Products include:
Betoptic Sterile Ophthalmic Solution 569
Betoptic S Sterile Ophthalmic Suspension 570
Kerlone Tablets 2172

Bitolterol Mesylate (Betagan may block bronchodilation produced by $beta_2$adrenergic agonists). Products include:
Tornalate 2074

Chlorpropamide (Beta-blockers may mask the signs and symptoms of acute hypoglycemia). Products include:
Diabinese Tablets 1775

Deserpidine (Possible additive effects and production of hypotension and/or bradycardia). Products include:
Enduronyl 518
Harmonyl Tablets 528
Oreticyl 545

Epinephrine (Mydriasis may result from concomitant ocular therapy). Products include:
Ana-Kit Anaphylaxis Emergency Treatment Kit 1100
Bronkaid Mist ▣ 757
EpiPen 843
Marcaine Hydrochloride 0.5% with Epinephrine 1:200,000 (as bitartrate) 958
Marcaine Hydrochloride with Epinephrine 1:200,000 2055
Primatene Mist 2420
Sus-Phrine Injection 1006
Xylocaine with Epinephrine Injections 637

Epinephrine Bitartrate (Mydriasis may result from concomitant ocular therapy). Products include:
AsthmaHaler Mist Epinephrine Bitartrate Bronchodilator ▣ 616
Bronkaid Mist Suspension ▣ 757
Primatene Mist Suspension 2421

Epinephrine Hydrochloride (Mydriasis may result from concomitant ocular therapy). Products include:
Adrenalin Chloride Solution 1:100 & 1:1,000 1689
Epifrin ⊙ 244
Glaucon ⊙ 218

Esmolol Hydrochloride (Additive effects on systemic beta-blockade from concomitant therapy with orally administered beta-blockers). Products include:
Brevibloc Injection 942

Glipizide (Beta-blockers may mask the signs and symptoms of acute hypoglycemia). Products include:
Glucotrol 1952

Glyburide (Beta-blockers may mask the signs and symptoms of acute hypoglycemia). Products include:
DiaBeta 1091
Micronase Tablets 2350

Insulin, Human (Beta-blockers may mask the signs and symptoms of acute hypoglycemia).
No products indexed under this heading.

Insulin, Human Isophane Suspension (Beta-blockers may mask the signs and symptoms of acute hypoglycemia). Products include:
Humulin N, 100 Units 1270

Insulin, Human NPH (Beta-blockers may mask the signs and symptoms of acute hypoglycemia). Products include:
Insulatard NPH Human 1627
Novolin N 1627
Novolin N PenFill Cartridges 1628
Novolin N Prefilled 1628

Insulin, Human Regular (Beta-blockers may mask the signs and symptoms of acute hypoglycemia). Products include:
Humulin BR, 100 Units 1268
Humulin R, 100 Units 1272
Novolin R 1627
Novolin R PenFill Cartridges 1628
Novolin R Prefilled 1629
Velosulin Human 1628

Insulin, Human, Zinc Suspension (Beta-blockers may mask the signs and symptoms of acute hypoglycemia). Products include:
Humulin L, 100 Units 1268
Humulin U, 100 Units 1272
Novolin L 1627

Insulin, NPH (Beta-blockers may mask the signs and symptoms of acute hypoglycemia). Products include:
NPH, 40 & 100 Units 1273
Beef NPH, 100 Units 1274
Pork NPH, 100 Units 1275
Insulatard NPH 1626
NPH Insulin 1626
NPH Purified Pork Isophane Insulin 1626

Insulin, Regular (Beta-blockers may mask the signs and symptoms of acute hypoglycemia). Products include:
Regular, 40 & 100 Units 1273
Beef Regular, 100 Units 1275
Pork Regular, 100 Units 1275
Pork Regular (Concentrated), 500 Units 1276
Regular Insulin 1625
Regular Purified Pork Insulin 1626
Velosulin 1627

Insulin, Zinc Crystals (Beta-blockers may mask the signs and symptoms of acute hypoglycemia). Products include:
NPH, 40 & 100 Units 1273

Insulin, Zinc Suspension (Beta-blockers may mask the signs and symptoms of acute hypoglycemia). Products include:
Lente, 40 & 100 Units 1272
Protamine, Zinc, 40 & 100 Units 1273
Lente Iletin I 1272
Beef Lente, 100 Units 1274
Beef Protamine Zinc, 100 Units 1274
Pork Lente, 100 Units 1275
Pork, Protamine, Zinc, 100 Units 1275
Lente Insulin 1626
Lente Purified Pork Insulin 1626
Semilente Insulin 1625
Ultralente Insulin 1626

Isoproterenol Hydrochloride (Betagan may block bronchodilation produced by $beta_2$adrenergic agonists). Products include:
Isuprel Hydrochloride Injection 1:5000 2050
Isuprel Hydrochloride Mistometer 2051
Isuprel Hydrochloride Solution 1:200 & 1:100 2052
Norisodrine Aerotrol 540

Labetalol Hydrochloride (Additive effects on systemic beta-blockade from concomitant therapy with orally administered beta-blockers). Products include:
Normodyne Injection 2108
Normodyne Tablets 2110
Normozide Tablets 2112
Trandate HCT Tablets 579
Trandate Injection 577
Trandate Tablets 579

Metaproterenol Sulfate (Betagan may block bronchodilation produced by $beta_2$adrenergic agonists). Products include:
Alupent 674
Arm-a-Med Metaproterenol Sulfate Inhalation Solution, USP 617
Metaprel Inhalation Aerosol Bronchodilator 2014
Metaprel Inhalation Solution 2015
Metaprel 2015

Metaproterenol Sulfate Inhalation Solution, USP ... 912

Metoprolol Tartrate (Additive effects on systemic beta-blockade from concomitant therapy with orally administered beta-blockers). Products include:

- Lopressor Ampuls ... 1032
- Lopressor HCT Tablets ... 1034
- Lopressor Tablets ... 1032

Nadolol (Additive effects on systemic beta-blockade from concomitant therapy with orally administered beta-blockers). Products include:

- Corgard Tablets ... 701
- Corzide Tablets ... 702

Pindolol (Additive effects on systemic beta-blockade from concomitant therapy with orally administered beta-blockers). Products include:

- Visken Tablets ... 2036

Pirbuterol Acetate (Betagan may block bronchodilation produced by $beta_2$adrenergic agonists). Products include:

- Maxair Inhaler ... 1311

Propranolol Hydrochloride (Additive effects on systemic beta-blockade from concomitant therapy with orally administered beta-blockers). Products include:

- Inderal ... 2459
- Inderal LA Long Acting Capsules ... 2461
- Inderide Tablets ... 2463
- Inderide LA Long Acting Capsules .. 2465

Rauwolfia Serpentina (Possible additive effects and production of hypotension and/or bradycardia). Products include:

- Raudixin Tablets ... 1803
- Rauzide Tablets ... 1804

Rescinnamine (Possible additive effects and production of hypotension and/or bradycardia).

No products indexed under this heading.

Reserpine (Possible additive effects and production of hypotension and/or bradycardia). Products include:

- Diupres Tablets ... 1461
- Hydromox R Tablets ... 1209
- Hydropres Tablets ... 1485
- Renese-R Tablets ... 1786
- Salutensin/Salutensin-Demi ... 719
- Ser-Ap-Es Tablets ... 881
- Serpasil Tablets ... 883
- Serpasil-Apresoline Tablets ... 884
- Serpasil-Esidrix Tablets ... 886

Terbutaline Sulfate (Betagan may block bronchodilation produced by $beta_2$adrenergic agonists). Products include:

- Brethaire Inhaler ... 1024
- Brethine Ampuls ... 1026
- Brethine Tablets ... 1026
- Bricanyl Injection ... 1324
- Bricanyl Tablets ... 1325

Timolol Maleate (Additive effects on systemic beta-blockade from concomitant therapy with orally administered beta-blockers). Products include:

- Blocadren Tablets ... 1429
- Timolide Tablets ... 1547
- Timoptic in Ocudose ... 1552
- Timoptic Sterile Ophthalmic Solution ... 1550

Tolazamide (Beta-blockers may mask the signs and symptoms of acute hypoglycemia). Products include:

- Tolinase Tablets ... 2365

Tolbutamide (Beta-blockers may mask the signs and symptoms of acute hypoglycemia). Products include:

- Orinase Tablets ... 2354

BETATREX CREAM, OINTMENT & LOTION

(Betamethasone Valerate) ... 2077

No interactions described in labeling.

BETOPTIC STERILE OPHTHALMIC SOLUTION

(Betaxolol Hydrochloride) ... 569

May interact with $beta_2$ agonists, general anesthetics, catecholamine depleting drugs, adrenergic augmenting psychotropics, and certain other agents. Compounds in these categories include:

Acebutolol Hydrochloride (Potential additive effect). Products include:

- Sectral Capsules ... 2520

Atenolol (Potential additive effect). Products include:

- Tenoretic Tablets ... 1105
- Tenormin Tablets and I.V. Injection 1107

Carteolol Hydrochloride (Potential additive effect). Products include:

- Cartrol Tablets ... 507

Deserpidine (Additive effects). Products include:

- Enduronyl ... 518
- Harmonyl Tablets ... 528
- Oreticyl ... 545

Enflurane (Impairment of heart's ability to respond to beta-adrenergically mediated sympathetic reflex stimuli). Products include:

- Ethrane ... 599

Epinephrine (Mydriasis). Products include:

- Ana-Kit Anaphylaxis Emergency Treatment Kit ... 1100
- Bronkaid Mist ... ▣ 757
- EpiPen ... 843
- Marcaine Hydrochloride 0.5% with Epinephrine 1:200,000 (as bitartrate) ... 958
- Marcaine Hydrochloride with Epinephrine 1:200,000 ... 2055
- Primatene Mist ... 2420
- Sus-Phrine Injection ... 1006
- Xylocaine with Epinephrine Injections ... 637

Epinephrine Bitartrate (Mydriasis). Products include:

- AsthmaHaler Mist Epinephrine Bitartrate Bronchodilator ... ▣ 616
- Bronkaid Mist Suspension ... ▣ 757
- Primatene Mist Suspension ... 2421

Epinephrine, Racemic (Mydriasis).

Esmolol Hydrochloride (Potential additive effect). Products include:

- Brevibloc Injection ... 942

Isocarboxazid (Exercise caution when used concomitantly). Products include:

- Marplan Tablets ... 1906

Isoflurane (Impairment of heart's ability to respond to beta-adrenergically mediated sympathetic reflex stimuli). Products include:

- Forane ... 600

Ketamine Hydrochloride (Impairment of heart's ability to respond to beta-adrenergically mediated sympathetic reflex stimuli). Products include:

- Ketalar ... 1726

Labetalol Hydrochloride (Potential additive effect). Products include:

- Normodyne Injection ... 2108
- Normodyne Tablets ... 2110
- Normozide Tablets ... 2112
- Trandate HCT Tablets ... 579
- Trandate Injection ... 577
- Trandate Tablets ... 579

Methohexital Sodium (Impairment of heart's ability to respond to beta-adrenergically mediated sympathetic reflex stimuli). Products include:

- Brevital Sodium Vials ... 1248

Methoxyflurane (Impairment of heart's ability to respond to beta-adrenergically mediated sympathetic reflex stimuli).

No products indexed under this heading.

Metoprolol Tartrate (Potential additive effect). Products include:

- Lopressor Ampuls ... 1032
- Lopressor HCT Tablets ... 1034
- Lopressor Tablets ... 1032

Nadolol (Potential additive effect). Products include:

- Corgard Tablets ... 701
- Corzide Tablets ... 702

Pargyline Hydrochloride (Exercise caution when used concomitantly).

No products indexed under this heading.

Penbutolol Sulfate (Potential additive effect). Products include:

- Levatol ... 1832

Phenelzine Sulfate (Exercise caution when used concomitantly). Products include:

- Nardil ... 1742

Pindolol (Potential additive effect). Products include:

- Visken Tablets ... 2036

Propofol (Impairment of heart's ability to respond to beta-adrenergically mediated sympathetic reflex stimuli). Products include:

- Diprivan Injection ... 2267

Propranolol Hydrochloride (Potential additive effect). Products include:

- Inderal ... 2459
- Inderal LA Long Acting Capsules ... 2461
- Inderide Tablets ... 2463
- Inderide LA Long Acting Capsules .. 2465

Rauwolfia Serpentina (Additive effects). Products include:

- Raudixin Tablets ... 1803
- Rauzide Tablets ... 1804

Rescinnamine (Additive effects).

No products indexed under this heading.

Reserpine (Additive effects). Products include:

- Diupres Tablets ... 1461
- Hydromox R Tablets ... 1209
- Hydropres Tablets ... 1485
- Renese-R Tablets ... 1786
- Salutensin/Salutensin-Demi ... 719
- Ser-Ap-Es Tablets ... 881
- Serpasil Tablets ... 883
- Serpasil-Apresoline Tablets ... 884
- Serpasil-Esidrix Tablets ... 886

Timolol Maleate (Potential additive effect). Products include:

- Blocadren Tablets ... 1429
- Timolide Tablets ... 1547
- Timoptic in Ocudose ... 1552
- Timoptic Sterile Ophthalmic Solution ... 1550

Tranylcypromine Sulfate (Exercise caution when used concomitantly). Products include:

- Parnate Tablets ... 2222

BETOPTIC S STERILE OPHTHALMIC SUSPENSION

(Betaxolol Hydrochloride) ... 570

May interact with catecholamine depleting drugs, adrenergic augmenting psychotropics, beta blockers, and general anesthetics. Compounds in these categories include:

Acebutolol Hydrochloride (Potential for additive effects). Products include:

- Sectral Capsules ... 2520

Atenolol (Potential for additive effects). Products include:

- Tenoretic Tablets ... 1105
- Tenormin Tablets and I.V. Injection 1107

Carteolol Hydrochloride (Potential for additive effects). Products include:

- Cartrol Tablets ... 507

Deserpidine (Potential for additive effects and production of hypotension and/or bradycardia). Products include:

- Enduronyl ... 518
- Harmonyl Tablets ... 528
- Oreticyl ... 545

Enflurane (Impairment of heart's ability to respond to beta-adrenergically mediated sympathetic reflux stimuli). Products include:

- Ethrane ... 599

Esmolol Hydrochloride (Potential for additive effects). Products include:

- Brevibloc Injection ... 942

Isocarboxazid (Exercise caution when used concomitantly). Products include:

- Marplan Tablets ... 1906

Isoflurane (Impairment of heart's ability to respond to beta-adrenergically mediated sympathetic reflux stimuli). Products include:

- Forane ... 600

Ketamine Hydrochloride (Impairment of heart's ability to respond to beta-adrenergically mediated sympathetic reflux stimuli). Products include:

- Ketalar ... 1726

Labetalol Hydrochloride (Potential for additive effects). Products include:

- Normodyne Injection ... 2108
- Normodyne Tablets ... 2110
- Normozide Tablets ... 2112
- Trandate HCT Tablets ... 579
- Trandate Injection ... 577
- Trandate Tablets ... 579

Methohexital Sodium (Impairment of heart's ability to respond to beta-adrenergically mediated sympathetic reflux stimuli). Products include:

- Brevital Sodium Vials ... 1248

Methoxyflurane (Impairment of heart's ability to respond to beta-adrenergically mediated sympathetic reflux stimuli).

No products indexed under this heading.

Metoprolol Tartrate (Potential for additive effects). Products include:

- Lopressor Ampuls ... 1032
- Lopressor HCT Tablets ... 1034
- Lopressor Tablets ... 1032

Nadolol (Potential for additive effects). Products include:

- Corgard Tablets ... 701
- Corzide Tablets ... 702

Pargyline Hydrochloride (Exercise caution when used concomitantly).

No products indexed under this heading.

Penbutolol Sulfate (Potential for additive effects). Products include:

- Levatol ... 1832

Phenelzine Sulfate (Exercise caution when used concomitantly). Products include:

- Nardil ... 1742

Pindolol (Potential for additive effects). Products include:
Visken Tablets 2036

Propofol (Impairment of heart's ability to respond to beta-adrenergically mediated sympathetic reflux stimuli). Products include:
Diprivan Injection 2267

Propranolol Hydrochloride (Potential for additive effects). Products include:
Inderal 2459
Inderal LA Long Acting Capsules 2461
Inderide Tablets 2463
Inderide LA Long Acting Capsules .. 2465

Rauwolfia Serpentina (Potential for additive effects and production of hypotension and/or bradycardia). Products include:
Raudixin Tablets 1803
Rauzide Tablets 1804

Rescinnamine (Potential for additive effects and production of hypotension and/or bradycardia).
No products indexed under this heading.

Reserpine (Potential for additive effects and production of hypotension and/or bradycardia). Products include:
Diupres Tablets 1461
Hydromox R Tablets 1209
Hydropres Tablets 1485
Renese-R Tablets 1786
Salutensin/Salutensin-Demi 719
Ser-Ap-Es Tablets 881
Serpasil Tablets 883
Serpasil-Apresoline Tablets 884
Serpasil-Esidrix Tablets 886

Timolol Maleate (Potential for additive effects). Products include:
Blocadren Tablets 1429
Timolide Tablets 1547
Timoptic in Ocudose 1552
Timoptic Sterile Ophthalmic Solution 1550

Tranylcypromine Sulfate (Exercise caution when used concomitantly). Products include:
Parnate Tablets 2222

BIAVAX II
(Rubella & Mumps Virus Vaccine Live) 1427
May interact with:

Azathioprine (Contraindication). Products include:
Imuran 768

Cyclosporine (Contraindication). Products include:
Sandimmune 2024

Immune Globulin (Human) (Contraindication). Products include:
MICRhoGAM Rh_0(D) Immune Globulin (Human) 1650
RhoGAM Rh_0(D) Immune Globulin (Human) 1651

Immune Globulin Intravenous (Human) (Contraindication). Products include:
Gamimune N Immune Globulin Intravenous (Human) 1572
Gammagard Immune Globulin, Intravenous (Human) 658
Iveegam 1129
Sandoglobulin I.V. 2027

Muromonab-CD3 (Contraindication). Products include:
Orthoclone OKT3 Sterile Solution .. 1645

BICHLORACETIC ACID KAHLENBERG
(Dichloroacetic Acid) 1071
No interactions described in labeling.

BICILLIN C-R INJECTION
(Penicillin G Procaine, Penicillin G, Benzathine) 2438
May interact with tetracyclines and certain other agents. Compounds in these categories include:

Demeclocycline Hydrochloride (May antagonize the bactericidal effect of penicillin). Products include:
Declomycin Capsules, Tablets 1199

Doxycycline Calcium (May antagonize the bactericidal effect of penicillin).
No products indexed under this heading.

Doxycycline Hyclate (May antagonize the bactericidal effect of penicillin). Products include:
Doryx Capsules 1717
Vibramycin Hyclate Capsules 1787
Vibramycin Hyclate Intravenous 1968
Vibra-Tabs Film Coated Tablets 1787

Doxycycline Monohydrate (May antagonize the bactericidal effect of penicillin). Products include:
Monodox Capsules 1630
Vibramycin Monohydrate for Oral Suspension 1787

Methacycline Hydrochloride (May antagonize the bactericidal effect of penicillin).
No products indexed under this heading.

Minocycline Hydrochloride (May antagonize the bactericidal effect of penicillin). Products include:
Minocin Intravenous 1221
Minocin Oral Suspension 1224
Minocin Pellet-Filled Capsules 1222

Oxytetracycline Hydrochloride (May antagonize the bactericidal effect of penicillin). Products include:
Terra-Cortril Ophthalmic Suspension 1963
Terramycin Capsules 1786
Terramycin Intramuscular Solution 1964
Terramycin with Polymyxin B Sulfate Ophthalmic Ointment 1965

Probenecid (Increases serum penicillin levels). Products include:
Benemid Tablets 1426
ColBENEMID Tablets 1436
Wycillin Injection and Probenecid Tablets 2539

Tetracycline Hydrochloride (May antagonize the bactericidal effect of penicillin). Products include:
Achromycin V Capsules 1193
Achromycin Ophthalmic Ointment 1% .... ◎ 307
Achromycin Ophthalmic Suspension 1% .... ◎ 308
Topicycline for Topical Solution 1856

BICILLIN C-R 900/300 INJECTION
(Penicillin G Procaine, Penicillin G, Benzathine) 2440
May interact with tetracyclines and certain other agents. Compounds in these categories include:

Demeclocycline Hydrochloride (May antagonize the bactericidal effect of penicillin). Products include:
Declomycin Capsules, Tablets 1199

Doxycycline Calcium (May antagonize the bactericidal effect of penicillin).
No products indexed under this heading.

Doxycycline Hyclate (May antagonize the bactericidal effect of penicillin). Products include:
Doryx Capsules 1717
Vibramycin Hyclate Capsules 1787
Vibramycin Hyclate Intravenous 1968
Vibra-Tabs Film Coated Tablets 1787

Doxycycline Monohydrate (May antagonize the bactericidal effect of penicillin). Products include:
Monodox Capsules 1630
Vibramycin Monohydrate for Oral Suspension 1787

Methacycline Hydrochloride (May antagonize the bactericidal effect of penicillin).
No products indexed under this heading.

Minocycline Hydrochloride (May antagonize the bactericidal effect of penicillin). Products include:
Minocin Intravenous 1221
Minocin Oral Suspension 1224
Minocin Pellet-Filled Capsules 1222

Oxytetracycline Hydrochloride (May antagonize the bactericidal effect of penicillin). Products include:
Terra-Cortril Ophthalmic Suspension 1963
Terramycin Capsules 1786
Terramycin Intramuscular Solution 1964
Terramycin with Polymyxin B Sulfate Ophthalmic Ointment 1965

Probenecid (Concurrent administration increases and prolongs serum penicillin levels). Products include:
Benemid Tablets 1426
ColBENEMID Tablets 1436
Wycillin Injection and Probenecid Tablets 2539

Tetracycline Hydrochloride (May antagonize the bactericidal effect of penicillin). Products include:
Achromycin V Capsules 1193
Achromycin Ophthalmic Ointment 1% .... ◎ 307
Achromycin Ophthalmic Suspension 1% .... ◎ 308
Topicycline for Topical Solution 1856

BICILLIN L-A INJECTION
(Penicillin G, Benzathine) 2442
May interact with tetracyclines and certain other agents. Compounds in these categories include:

Demeclocycline Hydrochloride (May antagonize the bactericidal effect of penicillin). Products include:
Declomycin Capsules, Tablets 1199

Doxycycline Calcium (May antagonize the bactericidal effect of penicillin).
No products indexed under this heading.

Doxycycline Hyclate (May antagonize the bactericidal effect of penicillin). Products include:
Doryx Capsules 1717
Vibramycin Hyclate Capsules 1787
Vibramycin Hyclate Intravenous 1968
Vibra-Tabs Film Coated Tablets 1787

Doxycycline Monohydrate (May antagonize the bactericidal effect of penicillin). Products include:
Monodox Capsules 1630
Vibramycin Monohydrate for Oral Suspension 1787

Methacycline Hydrochloride (May antagonize the bactericidal effect of penicillin).
No products indexed under this heading.

Minocycline Hydrochloride (May antagonize the bactericidal effect of penicillin). Products include:
Minocin Intravenous 1221
Minocin Oral Suspension 1224
Minocin Pellet-Filled Capsules 1222

Oxytetracycline Hydrochloride (May antagonize the bactericidal effect of penicillin). Products include:
Terra-Cortril Ophthalmic Suspension 1963
Terramycin Capsules 1786
Terramycin Intramuscular Solution 1964
Terramycin with Polymyxin B Sulfate Ophthalmic Ointment 1965

Probenecid (Increases serum penicillin levels). Products include:
Benemid Tablets 1426
ColBENEMID Tablets 1436
Wycillin Injection and Probenecid Tablets 2539

Tetracycline Hydrochloride (May antagonize the bactericidal effect of penicillin). Products include:
Achromycin V Capsules 1193
Achromycin Ophthalmic Ointment 1% .... ◎ 307
Achromycin Ophthalmic Suspension 1% .... ◎ 308
Topicycline for Topical Solution 1856

BICITRA—SUGAR-FREE
(Sodium Citrate, Citric Acid) 2423
May interact with:

Aluminum Carbonate Gel (Concurrent therapy in patients with renal insufficiency should be avoided). Products include:
Basaljel 2438

Aluminum Hydroxide (Concurrent therapy in patients with renal insufficiency should be avoided). Products include:
Cama Arthritis Pain Reliever .... ▣ 685
Gaviscon Extra Strength Relief Formula Liquid Antacid .... ▣ 594
Gaviscon Extra Strength Relief Formula Antacid Tablets .... ▣ 594
Gaviscon Liquid Antacid .... ▣ 594
Gelusil Liquid & Tablets .... ▣ 639
Extra Strength Maalox Plus Suspension 1850
Maalox TC Suspension 1851
Maalox Plus Tablets .... ▣ 655
Extra Strength Maalox Plus Tablets 1850
Nephrox Suspension .... ▣ 563
WinGel Liquid & Tablets .... ▣ 761

Aluminum Hydroxide Gel (Concurrent therapy in patients with renal insufficiency should be avoided). Products include:
ALternaGEL Liquid 1154
Aludrox Oral Suspension 2428
Amphojel Suspension 2429
Amphojel Suspension without Flavor 2429
Mylanta Liquid 1155
Mylanta Double Strength Liquid 1155

Aluminum Hydroxide Gel, Dried (Concurrent therapy in patients with renal insufficiency should be avoided). Products include:
Alu-Tab/Alu-Cap 1309
Amphojel Tablets 2429
Ascriptin A/D Caplets 1850
Regular Strength Ascriptin Tablets 1850
Gaviscon Antacid Tablets .... ▣ 593
Gaviscon-2 Antacid Tablets .... ▣ 594
Mylanta Tablets 1155
Mylanta Double Strength Tablets 1155

BICNU
(Carmustine (BCNU)) 723
No interactions described in labeling.

BICOZENE CREME
(Benzocaine, Resorcinol) .... ▣ 684
No interactions described in labeling.

BILTRICIDE
(Praziquantel) 1589
No interactions described in labeling.

BIOCAL 500 MG TABLET CALCIUM SUPPLEMENT
(Calcium Carbonate) ▣ 625
No interactions described in labeling.

BIPHETAMINE CAPSULES
(Amphetamine Resins) 973
May interact with monoamine oxidase inhibitors, insulin, and certain other agents. Compounds in these categories include:

Furazolidone (Hypertensive crisis may result; concurrent use is contraindicated). Products include:
- Furoxone 1855

Guanethidine Monosulfate (Decreased hypotensive effect of guanethidine). Products include:
- Esimil Tablets 864
- Ismelin Tablets 869

Insulin, Human (Insulin requirements in diabetic patients may be altered).
- No products indexed under this heading.

Insulin, Human Isophane Suspension (Insulin requirements in diabetic patients may be altered). Products include:
- Humulin N, 100 Units 1270

Insulin, Human NPH (Insulin requirements in diabetic patients may be altered). Products include:
- Insulatard NPH Human 1627
- Novolin N 1627
- Novolin N PenFill Cartridges 1628
- Novolin N Prefilled 1628

Insulin, Human Regular (Insulin requirements in diabetic patients may be altered). Products include:
- Humulin BR, 100 Units 1268
- Humulin R, 100 Units 1272
- Novolin R 1627
- Novolin R PenFill Cartridges 1628
- Novolin R Prefilled 1629
- Velosulin Human 1628

Insulin, Human, Zinc Suspension (Insulin requirements in diabetic patients may be altered). Products include:
- Humulin L, 100 Units 1268
- Humulin U, 100 Units 1272
- Novolin L 1627

Insulin, NPH (Insulin requirements in diabetic patients may be altered). Products include:
- NPH, 40 & 100 Units 1273
- Beef NPH, 100 Units 1274
- Pork NPH, 100 Units 1275
- Insulatard NPH 1626
- NPH Insulin 1626
- NPH Purified Pork Isophane Insulin 1626

Insulin, Regular (Insulin requirements in diabetic patients may be altered). Products include:
- Regular, 40 & 100 Units 1273
- Beef Regular, 100 Units 1275
- Pork Regular, 100 Units 1275
- Pork Regular (Concentrated), 500 Units 1276
- Regular Insulin 1625
- Regular Purified Pork Insulin 1626
- Velosulin 1627

Insulin, Zinc Crystals (Insulin requirements in diabetic patients may be altered). Products include:
- NPH, 40 & 100 Units 1273

Insulin, Zinc Suspension (Insulin requirements in diabetic patients may be altered). Products include:
- Lente, 40 & 100 Units 1272
- Protamine, Zinc, 40 & 100 Units 1273
- Lente Iletin I 1272
- Beef Lente, 100 Units 1274
- Beef Protamine Zinc, 100 Units 1274
- Pork Lente, 100 Units 1275
- Pork, Protamine, Zinc, 100 Units 1275
- Lente Insulin 1626
- Lente Purified Pork Insulin 1626
- Semilente Insulin 1625
- Ultralente Insulin 1626

Isocarboxazid (Hypertensive crisis may result; concurrent use is contraindicated). Products include:
- Marplan Tablets 1906

Phenelzine Sulfate (Hypertensive crisis may result; concurrent use is contraindicated). Products include:
- Nardil 1742

Selegiline Hydrochloride (Hypertensive crisis may result; concurrent use is contraindicated). Products include:
- Eldepryl 2250

Tranylcypromine Sulfate (Hypertensive crisis may result; concurrent use is contraindicated). Products include:
- Parnate Tablets 2222

BLENOXANE
(Bleomycin Sulfate) 724
No interactions described in labeling.

BLEPH-10 LIQUIFILM STERILE OPHTHALMIC SOLUTION
(Sulfacetamide Sodium) 586
May interact with silver preparations. Compounds in this category include:

Silver Nitrate (Incompatible).

BLEPH-10 OPHTHALMIC OINTMENT 10%
(Sulfacetamide Sodium) 586
May interact with silver preparations. Compounds in this category include:

Silver Nitrate (Incompatible).

BLEPHAMIDE LIQUIFILM STERILE OPHTHALMIC SUSPENSION
(Prednisolone Acetate, Sulfacetamide Sodium) 586
No interactions described in labeling.

BLEPHAMIDE S.O.P. STERILE OPHTHALMIC OINTMENT
(Prednisolone Acetate, Sulfacetamide Sodium) 586
No interactions described in labeling.

BLOCADREN TABLETS
(Timolol Maleate) 1429
May interact with cardiac glycosides, insulin, oral hypoglycemic agents, catecholamine depleting drugs, calcium channel blockers, non-steroidal anti-inflammatory agents, and certain other agents. Compounds in these categories include:

Bepridil Hydrochloride (AV conduction disturbances; left ventricular failure). Products include:
- Vascor (200, 300 and 400 mg) Tablets 1383

Chlorpropamide (Beta blockers may mask the signs and symptoms of acute hypoglycemia). Products include:
- Diabinese Tablets 1775

Deserpidine (Additive effects; hypotension and/or bradycardia). Products include:
- Enduronyl 518
- Harmonyl Tablets 528
- Oreticyl 545

Deslanoside (Additive effects in prolonging AV conduction time).
- No products indexed under this heading.

Diclofenac Sodium (Blunting of the antihypertensive effect). Products include:
- Voltaren Ophthalmic Sterile Ophthalmic Solution ⊙ 268
- Voltaren Tablets 1042

Digitoxin (Additive effects in prolonging AV conduction time). Products include:
- Crystodigin Tablets 1253

Digoxin (Additive effects in prolonging AV conduction time). Products include:
- Lanoxicaps 772
- Lanoxin Elixir Pediatric 775
- Lanoxin Injection 778
- Lanoxin Injection Pediatric 781
- Lanoxin Tablets 783

Diltiazem Hydrochloride (AV conduction disturbances; left ventricular failure). Products include:
- Cardizem Tablets-30 mg, 60 mg, 90 mg and 120 mg 1329
- Cardizem SR Capsules-60 mg, 90 mg and 120 mg 1327

Etodolac (Blunting of the antihypertensive effect). Products include:
- Lodine Capsules 2468

Felodipine (AV conduction disturbances; left ventricular failure). Products include:
- Plendil Extended-Release Tablets 1526

Fenoprofen Calcium (Blunting of the antihypertensive effect). Products include:
- Nalfon Pulvules & Tablets 919

Flurbiprofen (Blunting of the antihypertensive effect). Products include:
- Ansaid Tablets 2319

Glipizide (Beta blockers may mask the signs and symptoms of acute hypoglycemia). Products include:
- Glucotrol 1952

Glyburide (Beta blockers may mask the signs and symptoms of acute hypoglycemia). Products include:
- DiaBeta 1091
- Micronase Tablets 2350

Ibuprofen (Blunting of the antihypertensive effect). Products include:
- Advil Cold & Sinus Caplets (formerly CoAdvil) 2416
- Advil Ibuprofen Tablets and Caplets 2416
- Children's Advil Suspension 2426
- CoAdvil ▣ 748
- Dristan Sinus Caplets 2419
- Haltran Tablets ▣ 668
- Ibuprofen ▣ 631
- Medipren ibuprofen Caplets and Tablets 1362
- Midol 200 Cramp Relief Formula ▣ 570
- Motrin Tablets 2351
- Motrin IB Caplets and Tablets ▣ 736
- Nuprin Ibuprofen/Analgesic Tablets & Caplets 752
- PediaProfen Suspension 1363
- Rufen Tablets 691
- Trendar Ibuprofen Tablets ▣ 756

Indomethacin (Blunting of the antihypertensive effect). Products include:
- Indocin 1487

Indomethacin Sodium Trihydrate (Blunting of the antihypertensive effect). Products include:
- Indocin I.V. 1490

Insulin, Human (Beta blockers may mask the signs and symptoms of acute hypoglycemia).
- No products indexed under this heading.

Insulin, Human Isophane Suspension (Beta blockers may mask the signs and symptoms of acute hypoglycemia). Products include:
- Humulin N, 100 Units 1270

Insulin, Human NPH (Beta blockers may mask the signs and symptoms of acute hypoglycemia). Products include:
- Insulatard NPH Human 1627
- Novolin N 1627
- Novolin N PenFill Cartridges 1628
- Novolin N Prefilled 1628

Insulin, Human Regular (Beta blockers may mask the signs and symptoms of acute hypoglycemia). Products include:
- Humulin BR, 100 Units 1268
- Humulin R, 100 Units 1272
- Novolin R 1627
- Novolin R PenFill Cartridges 1628
- Novolin R Prefilled 1629
- Velosulin Human 1628

Insulin, Human, Zinc Suspension (Beta blockers may mask the signs and symptoms of acute hypoglycemia). Products include:
- Humulin L, 100 Units 1268
- Humulin U, 100 Units 1272
- Novolin L 1627

Insulin, NPH (Beta blockers may mask the signs and symptoms of acute hypoglycemia). Products include:
- NPH, 40 & 100 Units 1273
- Beef NPH, 100 Units 1274
- Pork NPH, 100 Units 1275
- Insulatard NPH 1626
- NPH Insulin 1626
- NPH Purified Pork Isophane Insulin 1626

Insulin, Regular (Beta blockers may mask the signs and symptoms of acute hypoglycemia). Products include:
- Regular, 40 & 100 Units 1273
- Beef Regular, 100 Units 1275
- Pork Regular, 100 Units 1275
- Pork Regular (Concentrated), 500 Units 1276
- Regular Insulin 1625
- Regular Purified Pork Insulin 1626
- Velosulin 1627

Insulin, Zinc Crystals (Beta blockers may mask the signs and symptoms of acute hypoglycemia). Products include:
- NPH, 40 & 100 Units 1273

Insulin, Zinc Suspension (Beta blockers may mask the signs and symptoms of acute hypoglycemia). Products include:
- Lente, 40 & 100 Units 1272
- Protamine, Zinc, 40 & 100 Units 1273
- Lente Iletin I 1272
- Beef Lente, 100 Units 1274
- Beef Protamine Zinc, 100 Units 1274
- Pork Lente, 100 Units 1275
- Pork, Protamine, Zinc, 100 Units 1275
- Lente Insulin 1626
- Lente Purified Pork Insulin 1626
- Semilente Insulin 1625
- Ultralente Insulin 1626

Isradipine (AV conduction disturbances; left ventricular failure). Products include:
- DynaCirc Capsules 2004

Ketoprofen (Blunting of the antihypertensive effect). Products include:
- Orudis Capsules 2488

Ketorolac Tromethamine (Blunting of the antihypertensive effect). Products include:
- Toradol IM Injection 2302

Meclofenamate Sodium (Blunting of the antihypertensive effect). Products include:
- Meclomen Capsules 1739

Mefenamic Acid (Blunting of the antihypertensive effect). Products include:
- Ponstel 1758

Naproxen (Blunting of the antihypertensive effect). Products include:
- Naprosyn 2297

Naproxen Sodium (Blunting of the antihypertensive effect). Products include:
- Anaprox and Anaprox DS Tablets 2288

Nicardipine Hydrochloride (AV conduction disturbances; left ventricular failure). Products include:
- Cardene Capsules 2290

Nifedipine (Hypotension). Products include:
- Adalat Capsules (10 mg and 20 mg) ... 1587
- Procardia Capsules ... 1781
- Procardia XL Tablets ... 1783

Nimodipine (AV conduction disturbances; left ventricular failure). Products include:
- Nimotop Capsules ... 1607

Phenylbutazone (Blunting of the antihypertensive effect). Products include:
- Butazolidin Capsules & Tablets ... 1027

Piroxicam (Blunting of the antihypertensive effect). Products include:
- Feldene Capsules ... 1777

Rauwolfia Serpentina (Additive effects; hypotension and/or bradycardia). Products include:
- Raudixin Tablets ... 1803
- Rauzide Tablets ... 1804

Rescinnamine (Additive effects; hypotension and/or bradycardia).
- No products indexed under this heading.

Reserpine (Additive effects; hypotension and/or bradycardia). Products include:
- Diupres Tablets ... 1461
- Hydromox R Tablets ... 1209
- Hydropres Tablets ... 1485
- Renese-R Tablets ... 1786
- Salutensin/Salutensin-Demi ... 719
- Ser-Ap-Es Tablets ... 881
- Serpasil Tablets ... 883
- Serpasil-Apresoline Tablets ... 884
- Serpasil-Esidrix Tablets ... 886

Sulindac (Blunting of the antihypertensive effect). Products include:
- Clinoril Tablets ... 1433

Tolazamide (Beta blockers may mask the signs and symptoms of acute hypoglycemia). Products include:
- Tolinase Tablets ... 2365

Tolbutamide (Beta blockers may mask the signs and symptoms of acute hypoglycemia). Products include:
- Orinase Tablets ... 2354

Tolmetin Sodium (Blunting of the antihypertensive effect). Products include:
- Tolectin (200, 400 and 600 mg) .. 1379

Verapamil Hydrochloride (AV conduction disturbances; left ventricular failure). Products include:
- Calan SR Caplets ... 2157
- Calan Tablets ... 2155
- Isoptin Injectable ... 1177
- Isoptin Oral Tablets ... 1179
- Isoptin SR Sustained Release Tablets ... 1181
- Verelan Capsules ... 1243
- Verelan Capsules ... 2535

BONINE TABLETS

(Meclizine Hydrochloride) ... 1773

May interact with hypnotics and sedatives, tranquilizers, and certain other agents. Compounds in these categories include:

Alcohol (May increase drowsiness effect).

Alprazolam (May increase drowsiness effect). Products include:
- Xanax Tablets ... 2367

Buspirone Hydrochloride (May increase drowsiness effect). Products include:
- BuSpar ... 1401

Chlordiazepoxide (May increase drowsiness effect). Products include:
- Libritabs Tablets ... 1930
- Limbitrol ... 1933
- Menrium Tablets ... 1934

Chlordiazepoxide Hydrochloride (May increase drowsiness effect). Products include:
- Librax Capsules ... 1929
- Librium Capsules ... 1931
- Librium Injectable ... 1932

Chlorpromazine (May increase drowsiness effect). Products include:
- Thorazine ... 2234

Chlorprothixene (May increase drowsiness effect). Products include:
- Taractan Tablets ... 1920

Chlorprothixene Hydrochloride (May increase drowsiness effect). Products include:
- Taractan ... 1920

Clorazepate Dipotassium (May increase drowsiness effect). Products include:
- Tranxene ... 556

Diazepam (May increase drowsiness effect). Products include:
- Valium Injectable ... 1937
- Valium Tablets ... 1939
- Valrelease Capsules ... 1923

Droperidol (May increase drowsiness effect). Products include:
- Inapsine Injection ... 1140
- Innovar Injection ... 1141

Estazolam (May increase drowsiness effect). Products include:
- ProSom Tablets ... 554

Ethchlorvynol (May increase drowsiness effect). Products include:
- Placidyl Capsules ... 553

Ethinamate (May increase drowsiness effect).
- No products indexed under this heading.

Fluphenazine Decanoate (May increase drowsiness effect). Products include:
- Prolixin Decanoate ... 1795

Fluphenazine Enanthate (May increase drowsiness effect). Products include:
- Prolixin Enanthate ... 1796

Fluphenazine Hydrochloride (May increase drowsiness effect). Products include:
- Prolixin Elixir ... 1793
- Prolixin Injection ... 1791
- Prolixin Oral Concentrate ... 1792
- Prolixin Tablets ... 1793

Flurazepam Hydrochloride (May increase drowsiness effect). Products include:
- Dalmane Capsules ... 1927

Glutethimide (May increase drowsiness effect).
- No products indexed under this heading.

Haloperidol (May increase drowsiness effect). Products include:
- Haldol Injection, Tablets and Concentrate ... 1373

Haloperidol Decanoate (May increase drowsiness effect). Products include:
- Haldol Decanoate ... 1375

Hydroxyzine Hydrochloride (May increase drowsiness effect). Products include:
- Atarax Tablets & Syrup ... 1941
- Marax Tablets & DF Syrup ... 1954
- Vistaril Intramuscular Solution ... 1970

Lorazepam (May increase drowsiness effect). Products include:
- Ativan Injection ... 2432
- Ativan Tablets ... 2434

Loxapine Hydrochloride (May increase drowsiness effect). Products include:
- Loxitane ... 1213

Loxapine Succinate (May increase drowsiness effect). Products include:
- Loxitane Capsules ... 1213

Meprobamate (May increase drowsiness effect). Products include:
- Deprol Tablets ... 2382
- Equagesic Tablets ... 2451
- Miltown Tablets ... 2386
- PMB 200 and PMB 400 ... 2504

Mesoridazine (May increas drowsiness effect). Products include:
- Serentil ... 686

Midazolam Hydrochloride (May increase drowsiness effect). Products include:
- Versed Injection ... 1924

Molindone Hydrochloride (May increase drowsiness effect). Products include:
- Moban Tablets & Concentrate ... 932

Oxazepam (May increase drowsiness effect). Products include:
- Serax Capsules ... 2522
- Serax Tablets ... 2522

Perphenazine (May increase drowsiness effect). Products include:
- Etrafon ... 2087
- Triavil Tablets ... 1556
- Trilafon ... 2123

Prazepam (May increase drowsiness effect). Products include:
- Centrax ... 1693

Prochlorperazine (May increase drowsiness effect). Products include:
- Compazine ... 2201

Promethazine Hydrochloride (May increase drowsiness effect). Products include:
- Mepergan Injection ... 2479
- Phenergan with Codeine ... 2497
- Phenergan with Dextromethorphan 2499
- Phenergan Injection ... 2493
- Phenergan Suppositories ... 2496
- Phenergan Syrup ... 2495
- Phenergan Tablets ... 2496
- Phenergan VC ... 2500
- Phenergan VC with Codeine ... 2501

Propofol (May increase drowsiness effect). Products include:
- Diprivan Injection ... 2267

Quazepam (May increase drowsiness effect). Products include:
- Doral Tablets ... 2383

Secobarbital Sodium (May increase drowsiness effect). Products include:
- Seconal Sodium Pulvules ... 1296

Temazepam (May increase drowsiness effect). Products include:
- Restoril Capsules ... 2023

Thioridazine Hydrochloride (May increase drowsiness effect). Products include:
- Mellaril ... 2011

Thiothixene (May increase drowsiness effect). Products include:
- Navane Capsules and Concentrate 1954
- Navane Intramuscular ... 1956

Triazolam (May increase drowsiness effect). Products include:
- Halcion Tablets ... 2340

Trifluoperazine Hydrochloride (May increase drowsiness effect). Products include:
- Stelazine ... 2226

BONTRIL SLOW-RELEASE

(Phendimetrazine Tartrate) ... 834

May interact with monoamine oxidase inhibitors, insulin, and certain other agents. Compounds in these categories include:

Furazolidone (Potential for hypertensive crisis). Products include:
- Furoxone ... 1855

Guanethidine Monosulfate (Hypotensive effect of guanethidine may be decreased). Products include:
- Esimil Tablets ... 864
- Ismelin Tablets ... 869

Insulin, Human (Insulin requirement may be altered).
- No products indexed under this heading.

Insulin, Human Isophane Suspension (Insulin requirement may be altered). Products include:
- Humulin N, 100 Units ... 1270

Insulin, Human NPH (Insulin requirement may be altered). Products include:
- Insulatard NPH Human ... 1627
- Novolin N ... 1627
- Novolin N PenFill Cartridges ... 1628
- Novolin N Prefilled ... 1628

Insulin, Human Regular (Insulin requirement may be altered). Products include:
- Humulin BR, 100 Units ... 1268
- Humulin R, 100 Units ... 1272
- Novolin R ... 1627
- Novolin R PenFill Cartridges ... 1628
- Novolin R Prefilled ... 1629
- Velosulin Human ... 1628

Insulin, Human, Zinc Suspension (Insulin requirement may be altered). Products include:
- Humulin L, 100 Units ... 1268
- Humulin U, 100 Units ... 1272
- Novolin L ... 1627

Insulin, NPH (Insulin requirement may be altered). Products include:
- NPH, 40 & 100 Units ... 1273
- Beef NPH, 100 Units ... 1274
- Pork NPH, 100 Units ... 1275
- Insulatard NPH ... 1626
- NPH Insulin ... 1626
- NPH Purified Pork Isophane Insulin ... 1626

Insulin, Regular (Insulin requirement may be altered). Products include:
- Regular, 40 & 100 Units ... 1273
- Beef Regular, 100 Units ... 1275
- Pork Regular, 100 Units ... 1275
- Pork Regular (Concentrated), 500 Units ... 1276
- Regular Insulin ... 1625
- Regular Purified Pork Insulin ... 1626
- Velosulin ... 1627

Insulin, Zinc Crystals (Insulin requirement may be altered). Products include:
- NPH, 40 & 100 Units ... 1273

Insulin, Zinc Suspension (Insulin requirement may be altered). Products include:
- Lente, 40 & 100 Units ... 1272
- Protamine, Zinc, 40 & 100 Units ... 1273
- Lente Iletin I ... 1272
- Beef Lente, 100 Units ... 1274
- Beef Protamine Zinc, 100 Units ... 1274
- Pork Lente, 100 Units ... 1275
- Pork, Protamine, Zinc, 100 Units ... 1275
- Lente Insulin ... 1626
- Lente Purified Pork Insulin ... 1626
- Semilente Insulin ... 1625
- Ultralente Insulin ... 1626

Isocarboxazid (Potential for hypertensive crisis). Products include:
- Marplan Tablets ... 1906

Phenelzine Sulfate (Potential for hypertensive crisis). Products include:
- Nardil ... 1742

Selegiline Hydrochloride (Potential for hypertensive crisis). Products include:
- Eldepryl ... 2250

Tranylcypromine Sulfate (Potential for hypertensive crisis). Products include:
- Parnate Tablets ... 2222

BOROFAX OINTMENT

(Boric Acid) ... ▣ 541

No interactions described in labeling.

BRETHAIRE INHALER

(Terbutaline Sulfate) ... 1024

May interact with monoamine oxi-

dase inhibitors, tricyclic antidepressants, $beta_2$ agonists, sympathomimetic aerosol brochodilators, and certain other agents. Compounds in these categories include:

Acebutolol Hydrochloride (Beta receptor blocking agents and terbutaline sulfate inhibit each other). Products include:
Sectral Capsules 2520

Albuterol (Concomitant therapy with other sympathomimetic aerosol bronchodilator should be avoided). Products include:
Proventil Inhalation Aerosol 2117
Ventolin Inhalation Aerosol and Refill 583

Amitriptyline Hydrochloride (May potentiate action of terbutaline sulfate on vascular system). Products include:
Elavil 2269
Endep Tablets 1927
Etrafon 2087
Limbitrol 1933
Triavil Tablets 1556

Amoxapine (May potentiate action of terbutaline sulfate on vascular system). Products include:
Asendin Tablets 1196

Atenolol (Beta receptor blocking agents and terbutaline sulfate inhibit each other). Products include:
Tenoretic Tablets 1105
Tenormin Tablets and I.V. Injection 1107

Betaxolol Hydrochloride (Beta receptor blocking agents and terbutaline sulfate inhibit each other). Products include:
Betoptic Sterile Ophthalmic Solution 569
Betoptic S Sterile Ophthalmic Suspension 570
Kerlone Tablets 2172

Bitolterol Mesylate (Concomitant therapy with other sympathomimetic aerosol bronchodilator should be avoided). Products include:
Tornalate 2074

Carteolol Hydrochloride (Beta receptor blocking agents and terbutaline sulfate inhibit each other). Products include:
Cartrol Tablets 507

Clomipramine Hydrochloride (May potentiate action of terbutaline sulfate on vascular system). Products include:
Anafranil Capsules 650

Desipramine Hydrochloride (May potentiate action of terbutaline sulfate on vascular system). Products include:
Norpramin Tablets 1340

Doxepin Hydrochloride (May potentiate action of terbutaline sulfate on vascular system). Products include:
Sinequan 1960

Epinephrine (Concomitant administration is not advised). Products include:
Ana-Kit Anaphylaxis Emergency Treatment Kit 1100
Bronkaid Mist .... ▣ 757
EpiPen 843
Marcaine Hydrochloride 0.5% with Epinephrine 1:200,000 (as bitartrate) 958
Marcaine Hydrochloride with Epinephrine 1:200,000 2055
Primatene Mist 2420
Sus-Phrine Injection 1006
Xylocaine with Epinephrine Injections 637

Epinephrine Bitartrate (Concomitant adminmistration is not advised). Products include:
AsthmaHaler Mist Epinephrine Bitartrate Bronchodilator .... ▣ 616
Bronkaid Mist Suspension .... ▣ 757
Primatene Mist Suspension 2421

Epinephrine Hydrochloride (Concomitant administration is not advised). Products include:
Adrenalin Chloride Solution 1:100 & 1:1,000 1689
Epifrin .... ⊙ 244
Glaucon .... ⊙ 218

Esmolol Hydrochloride (Beta receptors blocking agents and terbutaline sulfate inhibit each other). Products include:
Brevibloc Injection 942

Furazolidone (May potentiate action of terbutaline sulfate on vascular system). Products include:
Furoxone 1855

Imipramine Hydrochloride (May potentiate action of terbutaline sulfate on vascular system). Products include:
Tofranil Ampuls 1038
Tofranil Tablets 1039

Imipramine Pamoate (May potentiate action of terbutaline sulfate on vascular system). Products include:
Tofranil-PM Capsules 1041

Isocarboxazid (May potentiate action of terbutaline sulfate on vascular system). Products include:
Marplan Tablets 1906

Isoetharine (Concomitant therapy with other sympathomimetic aerosol bronchodilator should be avoided). Products include:
Arm-a-Med Isoetharine Inhalation Solution, USP 616
Bronkometer Aerosol 2042
Bronkosol Solution 2042

Isoproterenol Hydrochloride (Concomitant therapy with other sympathomimetic aerosol bronchodilator should be avoided). Products include:
Isuprel Hydrochloride Injection 1:5000 2050
Isuprel Hydrochloride Mistometer .. 2051
Isuprel Hydrochloride Solution 1:200 & 1:100 2052
Norisodrine Aerotrol 540

Isoproterenol Sulfate (Concomitant administration is not advised).
No products indexed under this heading.

Labetalol Hydrochloride (Beta receptor blocking agents and terbutaline sulfate inhibit each other). Products include:
Normodyne Injection 2108
Normodyne Tablets 2110
Normozide Tablets 2112
Trandate HCT Tablets 579
Trandate Injection 577
Trandate Tablets 579

Maprotiline Hydrochloride (May potentiate action of terbutaline sulfate on vascular system). Products include:
Ludiomil Tablets 874

Metaproterenol Sulfate (Concomitant therapy with other sympathomimetic aerosol bronchodilator should be avoided). Products include:
Alupent 674
Arm-a-Med Metaproterenol Sulfate Inhalation Solution, USP 617
Metaprel Inhalation Aerosol Bronchodilator 2014
Metaprel Inhalation Solution 2015
Metaprel 2015
Metaproterenol Sulfate Inhalation Solution, USP 912

Metoprolol Tartrate (Beta receptor blocking agents and terbutaline sulfate inhibit each other). Products include:
Lopressor Ampuls 1032
Lopressor HCT Tablets 1034
Lopressor Tablets 1032

Nadolol (Beta receptor blocking agents and terbutaline sulfate inhibit each other). Products include:
Corgard Tablets 701
Corzide Tablets 702

Nortriptyline Hydrochloride (May potentiate action of terbutaline sulfate on vascular system). Products include:
Pamelor 2019

Penbutolol Sulfate (Beta receptor blocking agents and terbutaline sulfate inhibit each other). Products include:
Levatol 1832

Phenelzine Sulfate (May potentiate action of terbutaline sulfate on vascular system). Products include:
Nardil 1742

Pindolol (Beta receptor blocking agents and terbutaline sulfate inhibit each other). Products include:
Visken Tablets 2036

Pirbuterol Acetate (Concomitant therapy with other sympathomimetic aerosol bronchodilator should be avoided). Products include:
Maxair Inhaler 1311

Propranolol Hydrochloride (Beta receptor blocking agents and terbutaline sulfate inhibit each other). Products include:
Inderal 2459
Inderal LA Long Acting Capsules 2461
Inderide Tablets 2463
Inderide LA Long Acting Capsules .. 2465

Protriptyline Hydrochloride (May potentiate action of terbutaline sulfate on vascular system). Products include:
Vivactil Tablets 1567

Selegiline Hydrochloride (May potentiate action of terbutaline sulfate on vascular system). Products include:
Eldepryl 2250

Timolol Maleate (Beta receptor blocking agents and terbutaline sulfate inhibit each other). Products include:
Blocadren Tablets 1429
Timolide Tablets 1547
Timoptic in Ocudose 1552
Timoptic Sterile Ophthalmic Solution 1550

Tranylcypromine Sulfate (May potentiate action of terbutaline sulfate on vascular system). Products include:
Parnate Tablets 2222

Trimipramine Maleate (May potentiate action of terbutaline sulfate on vascular system). Products include:
Surmontil Capsules 2524

BRETHINE AMPULS
(Terbutaline Sulfate) 1026
May interact with sympathomimetic aerosal brochodilators, monoamine oxidase inhibitors, and tricyclic antidepressants. Compounds in these categories include:

Albuterol (Combined effect on cardiovascular system may be deleterious). Products include:
Proventil Inhalation Aerosol 2117
Ventolin Inhalation Aerosol and Refill 583

Albuterol Sulfate (Combined effect on cardiovascular system may be deleterious). Products include:
Proventil Repetabs Tablets 2120
Proventil Solutions for Inhalation 0.5% and 0.083% 2118
Proventil Syrup 2119
Proventil Tablets 2120
Ventolin 583

Amitriptyline Hydrochloride (The action of β-adrenergic agonists on the vascular system may be potentiated). Products include:
Elavil 2269
Endep Tablets 1927
Etrafon 2087
Limbitrol 1933
Triavil Tablets 1556

Amoxapine (The action of β-adrenergic agonists on the vascular system may be potentiated). Products include:
Asendin Tablets 1196

Clomipramine Hydrochloride (The action of β-adrenergic agonists on the vascular system may be potentiated). Products include:
Anafranil Capsules 650

Desipramine Hydrochloride (The action of β-adrenergic agonists on the vascular system may be potentiated). Products include:
Norpramin Tablets 1340

Dobutamine Hydrochloride (Combined effect on cardiovascular system may be deleterious). Products include:
Dobutrex Solution Vials 1259

Dopamine Hydrochloride (Combined effect on cardiovascular system may be deleterious). Products include:
Intropin Injection 930

Doxepin Hydrochloride (The action of β-adrenergic agonists on the vascular system may be potentiated). Products include:
Sinequan 1960

Ephedrine Hydrochloride (Combined effect on cardiovascular system may be deleterious). Products include:
Amesec .... ▣ 682
Primatene Tablets-M Formula 2421
Primatene Tablets-P Formula 2421
Primatene Tablets-Regular Formula 2421
Quadrinal Tablets 1183
Quelidrine Syrup 556
Tedral SA 1765

Ephedrine Sulfate (Combined effect on cardiovascular system may be deleterious). Products include:
Bronkaid Tablets .... ▣ 757
Bronkolixir .... ▣ 761
Bronkotabs Tablets .... ▣ 762
Marax Tablets & DF Syrup 1954
Pazo Hemorrhoid Ointment & Suppositories 752
Vicks Vatronol Nose Drops .... ▣ 666

Ephedrine Tannate (Combined effect on cardiovascular system may be deleterious). Products include:
Rynatuss 2388

Epinephrine (Combined effect on cardiovascular system may be deleterious). Products include:
Ana-Kit Anaphylaxis Emergency Treatment Kit 1100
Bronkaid Mist .... ▣ 757
EpiPen 843
Marcaine Hydrochloride 0.5% with Epinephrine 1:200,000 (as bitartrate) 958
Marcaine Hydrochloride with Epinephrine 1:200,000 2055
Primatene Mist 2420
Sus-Phrine Injection 1006
Xylocaine with Epinephrine Injections 637

Epinephrine Bitartrate (Combined effect on cardiovascular system may be deleterious). Products include:
AsthmaHaler Mist Epinephrine Bitartrate Bronchodilator .... ▣ 616
Bronkaid Mist Suspension .... ▣ 757
Primatene Mist Suspension 2421

Epinephrine Hydrochloride (Combined effect on cardiovascular system may be deleterious). Products include:

Adrenalin Chloride Solution 1:100 & 1:1,000 1689
Epifrin .... ⊙ 244
Glaucon .... ⊙ 218

Furazolidone (The action of β-adrenergic agonists on the vascular system may be potentiated). Products include:

Furoxone 1855

Imipramine Hydrochloride (The action of β-adrenergic agonists on the vascular system may be potentiated). Products include:

Tofranil Ampuls 1038
Tofranil Tablets 1039

Imipramine Pamoate (The action of β-adrenergic agonists on the vascular system may be potentiated). Products include:

Tofranil-PM Capsules 1041

Isocarboxazid (The action of β-adrenergic agonists on the vascular system may be potentiated). Products include:

Marplan Tablets 1906

Isoproterenol Hydrochloride (Combined effect on cardiovascular system may be deleterious). Products include:

Isuprel Hydrochloride Injection 1:5000 2050
Isuprel Hydrochloride Mistometer .. 2051
Isuprel Hydrochloride Solution 1:200 & 1:100 2052
Norisodrine Aerotrol 540

Maprotiline Hydrochloride (The action of β-adrenergic agonists on the vascular system may be potentiated). Products include:

Ludiomil Tablets 874

Metaproterenol Sulfate (Combined effect on cardiovascular system may be deleterious). Products include:

Alupent 674
Arm-a-Med Metaproterenol Sulfate Inhalation Solution, USP 617
Metaprel Inhalation Aerosol Bronchodilator 2014
Metaprel Inhalation Solution 2015
Metaprel 2015
Metaproterenol Sulfate Inhalation Solution, USP 912

Metaraminol Bitartrate (Combined effect on cardiovascular system may be deleterious). Products include:

Aramine Injection 1424

Norepinephrine Bitartrate (Combined effect on cardiovascular system may be deleterious). Products include:

Levophed Bitartrate Injection 2054

Nortriptyline Hydrochloride (The action of β-adrenergic agonists on the vascular system may be potentiated). Products include:

Pamelor 2019

Phenelzine Sulfate (The action of β-adrenergic agonists on the vascular system may be potentiated). Products include:

Nardil 1742

Phenylephrine Bitartrate (Combined effect on cardiovascular system may be deleterious).

No products indexed under this heading.

Phenylephrine Hydrochloride (Combined effect on cardiovascular system may be deleterious). Products include:

AK-Dilate Solution 2.5% and 10% .... ⊙ 203
Atrohist Sprinkle Capsules 558
Cerose-DM 2443
Codimal 846
Comhist LA Capsules 1618
Congespirin For Children Aspirin Free Chewable Cold Tablets 748
Cyclomydril .... ⊙ 216
Deconsal Sprinkle Capsules 559
Dimetane Decongestant .... ⊡ 673
Dristan Decongestant/Antihistamine/Analgesic Coated Caplets .... ⊡ 749
Dristan Cold Nasal Decongestant/Antihistamine/ Analgesic Coated Tablets 2419
Dristan Advanced Formula Decongestant/Antihistamine/Analgesic Tablets .... ⊡ 749
Dristan Nasal Spray, Menthol 2419
Dristan Nasal Spray, Regular and Regular with Metered Pump 2419
Entex Capsules 1623
Entex Liquid 1623
Sinus Excedrin Analgesic, Decongestant Tablets & Caplets 750
Extendryl 994
4-Way Fast Acting Nasal Spray - Original Formula (regular & mentholated) & Metered Spray Pump (regular) 751
Hycomine Compound Tablets 929
Murocoll-2 Sterile Ophthalmic Solution .... ⊙ 261
Mydfrin 2.5% .... ⊙ 224
Naldecon Syrup, Tablets, Pediatric Drops and Pediatric Syrup 709
Neo-Synephrine Hydrochloride 1% Carpuject 2063
Neo-Synephrine Hydrochloride 1% Injection 2063
Neo-Synephrine Hydrochloride (Ophthalmic) 2064
Neo-Synephrine .... ⊡ 759
Nōstril Nasal Decongestant .... ⊡ 520
Novahistine Elixir .... ⊡ 596
Phenergan VC 2500
Phenergan VC with Codeine 2501
Prefrin Liquifilm Vasoconstrictor and Lubricant Eye Drops .... ⊙ 254
Prefrin-A .... ⊙ 255
Quelidrine Syrup 556
Relief Vasoconstrictor and Lubricant Eye Drops .... ⊙ 256
Robitussin Night Relief .... ⊡ 677
Ru-Tuss with Hydrocodone 694
Ru-Tuss Tablets 693
Vasosulf .... ⊙ 279
Vicks Sinex .... ⊡ 665
Zincfrin .... ⊙ 230

Phenylephrine Tannate (Combined effect on cardiovascular system may be deleterious). Products include:

Rynatan 2387
Rynatuss 2388

Phenylpropanolamine Hydrochloride (Combined effect on cardiovascular system may be deleterious). Products include:

A.R.M. Allergy Relief Medicine Caplets .... ⊡ 615
Acutrim .... ⊡ 548
Allerest .... ⊡ 559
BC Cold Powder .... ⊡ 517
Cheracol Plus Head Cold/Cough Formula .... ⊡ 667
Codimal Expectorant 846
Comtrex Multi-Symptom Cold Reliever Tablets/Caplets/Liqui-Gels/Liquid 745
Contac Continuous Action Decongestant/Antihistamine Capsules ⊡ 710
Contac Maximum Strength Continuous Action Decongestant/Antihistamine Caplets .... ⊡ 709
Contac Severe Cold and Flu Formula Caplets .... ⊡ 711
Coricidin 'D' Decongestant Tablets .... ⊡ 695
Coricidin Demilets Tablets for Children .... ⊡ 696
Demazin Nasal Decongestant/Antihistamine Repetabs Tablets & Syrup .... ⊡ 697
Dexatrim .... ⊡ 733
Dimetane-DC Cough Syrup 1857
Dimetapp Elixir .... ⊡ 673
Dimetapp DM Elixir .... ⊡ 674
Dimetapp Extentabs .... ⊡ 674
Dimetapp Plus Caplets .... ⊡ 675
Dimetapp Tablets .... ⊡ 675
Entex Capsules 1623
Entex LA Tablets 1623
Entex Liquid 1623
4-Way Cold Tablets 750
Hycomine Syrup 927
Naldecon CX Adult Liquid .... ⊡ 521
Naldecon DX Adult Liquid .... ⊡ 521
Naldecon DX Children's Syrup .... ⊡ 522
Naldecon DX Pediatric Drops .... ⊡ 522
Naldecon EX Children's Syrup .... ⊡ 522
Naldecon EX Pediatric Drops .... ⊡ 523
Naldecon Syrup, Tablets, Pediatric Drops and Pediatric Syrup 709
Nolamine Tablets 838
Nolex LA Tablets 838
Ornade Spansule Capsules 2221
Orthoxicol Cough Syrup .... ⊡ 668
Propagest 839
Pyrroxate Capsules .... ⊡ 669
Robitussin-CF .... ⊡ 676
Ru-Tuss II Capsules 693
Ru-Tuss with Hydrocodone 694
Ru-Tuss Tablets 693
Sine-Off Sinus Medicine Tablets-Aspirin Formula .... ⊡ 722
Sinulin 840
St. Joseph Cold Tablets for Children .... ⊡ 704
Tavist-D Tablets 2035
Triaminic Allergy Tablets .... ⊡ 688
Triaminic Chewables .... ⊡ 688
Triaminic Cold Tablets .... ⊡ 688
Triaminic Expectorant .... ⊡ 688
Triaminic Expectorant w/Codeine .. 1996
Triaminic Expectorant DH 1995
Triaminic Oral Infant Drops 1996
Triaminic Syrup .... ⊡ 689
Triaminic-12 Tablets .... ⊡ 690
Triaminic-DM Syrup .... ⊡ 689
Triaminicin Tablets .... ⊡ 690
Triaminicol Multi-Symptom Cold Tablets .... ⊡ 691
Triaminicol Multi-Symptom Relief ⊡ 691
Tuss-Ornade Liquid 2242
Tuss-Ornade Spansule Capsules 2242
Tylenol Cold Medication, Effervescent Tablets 1369

Pirbuterol Acetate (Combined effect on cardiovascular system may be deleterious). Products include:

Maxair Inhaler 1311

Protriptyline Hydrochloride (The action of β-adrenergic agonists on the vascular system may be potentiated). Products include:

Vivactil Tablets 1567

Pseudoephedrine Hydrochloride (Combined effect on cardiovascular system may be deleterious). Products include:

Actifed Capsules .... ⊡ 539
Actifed Plus Caplets .... ⊡ 539
Actifed Plus Tablets .... ⊡ 540
Actifed with Codeine Cough Syrup .. 752
Actifed Syrup .... ⊡ 540
Actifed Tablets .... ⊡ 540
Actifed 12-Hour Capsules .... ⊡ 539
Advil Cold & Sinus Caplets (formerly CoAdvil) 2416
Allerest .... ⊡ 559
Anatuss LA Tablets 1359
Benadryl Decongestant Elixir .... ⊡ 635
Benadryl Decongestant .... ⊡ 635
Benadryl Plus .... ⊡ 636
Benadryl Plus Nighttime .... ⊡ 637
Benylin Decongestant .... ⊡ 638
Brexin L.A. Capsules 2078
Bromfed Capsules (Timed Release) 1615
Bromfed Syrup .... ⊡ 628
Bromfed 1615
CoAdvil .... ⊡ 748
Allergy-Sinus Comtrex Multi-Symptom Allergy Sinus Formula Tablets & Caplets 746
Cough Formula Comtrex 746
Comtrex Multi-Symptom Cold Reliever Tablets/Caplets/Liqui-Gels/Liquid 745
Day-Night Comtrex 747
Non-Drowsy Comtrex 747
Congess 994
Congestac Caplets .... ⊡ 617
Contac Jr. Children's Cold Medicine .... ⊡ 712
Contac Nighttime Cold Medicine .... ⊡ 713
Contac Sinus Caplets Maximum Strength Non-Drowsy Formula .... ⊡ 710
Contac Sinus Tablets Maximum Strength Non-Drowsy Formula .... ⊡ 710
Deconamine 663
Deconsal II Tablets 559
Dimacol Caplets .... ⊡ 672
Dimetane-DX Cough Syrup 1858
Dorcol Children's Cough Syrup .... ⊡ 685
Dorcol Children's Decongestant Liquid .... ⊡ 685
Dorcol Children's Liquid Cold Formula .... ⊡ 686
Maximum Strength Dristan Decongestant/Analgesic Coated Caplets .... ⊡ 750
No Drowsiness Dristan Cold Nasal Decongestant/Analgesic Coated Caplets 2420
Dristan Sinus Caplets 2419
Sinus Excedrin Analgesic, Decongestant Tablets & Caplets .... ⊡ 533
Fedahist Gyrocaps 2145
Fedahist Timecaps 2145
Guaifed 1615
Guaifed Syrup .... ⊡ 629
Isoclor Expectorant 982
Isoclor Timesule Capsules .... ⊡ 561
Kronofed-A 970
Medi-Flu Caplet, Liquid .... ⊡ 640
Novafed A Capsules 1342
Novafed Capsules 1342
Novahistine DH 1342
Novahistine DMX .... ⊡ 595
Novahistine Expectorant 1343
Nucofed Capsules 2219
Nucofed Expectorant 2219
Nucofed Pediatric Expectorant 2220
Nucofed Syrup 2219
Ornex Caplets .... ⊡ 618
PediaCare Allergy Relief Formula Liquid 1362
PediaCare Cough-Cold Formula Liquid 1362
PediaCare Infants' Oral Decongestant Drops 1362
PediaCare Night Rest Cough-Cold Formula Liquid 1362
PediaCare 6-12 Cough-Cold Formula Chewable Tablets 1362
Robitussin-DAC Syrup 1875
Robitussin-PE .... ⊡ 677
Rondec 1975
Rondec-DM 1976
Rondec-TR Tablet 1975
Ru-Tuss DE Tablets 694
Ryna .... ⊡ 741
Seldane-D Extended-Release Tablets 1350
Sinarest .... ⊡ 562
Sine-Aid Maximum Strength Sinus Headache Caplets 1365
Sine-Aid Maximum Strength Sinus Headache Tablets 1365
Sine-Off Maximum Strength Allergy/Sinus Formula Caplets .... ⊡ 721
Sine-Off Maximum Strength No Drowsiness Formula Caplets .... ⊡ 722
Singlet Tablets .... ⊡ 598
Sinutab Maximum Strength .... ⊡ 641
Sinutab Maximum Strength Without Drowsiness Tablets & Caplets .... ⊡ 642
Sinutab Regular Strength Without Drowsiness Formula .... ⊡ 641
St. Joseph Nighttime Cold Medicine .... ⊡ 705
Sudafed Children's Liquid .... ⊡ 543
Sudafed Cough Syrup .... ⊡ 543
Sudafed Plus Liquid .... ⊡ 544
Sudafed Plus Tablets .... ⊡ 545
Sudafed Sinus Caplets .... ⊡ 545
Sudafed Sinus Tablets .... ⊡ 545
Sudafed Tablets, 30 mg .... ⊡ 544
Sudafed Tablets, Adult Strength, 60 mg .... ⊡ 544
Sudafed 12 Hour Capsules .... ⊡ 545
TheraFlu Flu and Cold Medicine .... ⊡ 687
Triaminic Nite Light .... ⊡ 689
Tylenol Allergy Sinus Medication Caplets and Gelcaps, Maximum Strength 1372
Children's Tylenol Cold Liquid Formula and Chewable Tablets 1368
Tylenol Cold & Flu Hot Medication, Packets 1369
Tylenol Cold & Flu No Drowsiness Hot Medication, Packets 1371
Tylenol Cold Medication Caplets and Tablets 1370
Tylenol Cold Medication No Drowsiness Formula Caplets 1370
Tylenol Cold Night Time Medication Liquid 1371

Tylenol Cough Medication Liquid with Decongestant, Maximum Strength 1372
Tylenol, Maximum Strength, Sinus Medication Gelcaps, Caplets and Tablets 1373
Ursinus Inlay-Tabs ▣ 691
Vicks Children's NyQuil ▣ 664
Vicks Daycare ▣ 660
Vicks Formula 44D Decongestant Cough Medicine ▣ 662
Vicks Formula 44M Multi-Symptom Cough Medicine ▣ 662
Vicks NyQuil Nighttime Colds Medicine-Original & Cherry Flavor ▣ 664
Vicks Pediatric Formula 44 Cough & Congestion Medicine ▣ 663
Vicks Pediatric Formula 44m Multi-Symptom Cough & Cold Medicine ▣ 663

Pseudoephedrine Sulfate (Combined effect on cardiovascular system may be deleterious). Products include:
Afrin Tablets ▣ 693
Chlor-Trimeton Decongestant ▣ 694
Disophrol Chronotab Sustained-Action Tablets ▣ 698
Drixoral Antihistamine/Nasal Decongestant Syrup ▣ 698
Drixoral Non-Drowsy Formula ▣ 699
Drixoral Plus Extended-Release Tablets ▣ 699
Drixoral Sinus ▣ 700
Drixoral Sustained-Action Tablets ▣ 698
Sinutab Allergy Formula Sustained Action Tablets ▣ 640
Trinalin Repetabs Tablets 1170

Selegiline Hydrochloride (The action of β-adrenergic agonists on the vascular system may be potentiated). Products include:
Eldepryl 2250

Tranylcypromine Sulfate (The action of β-adrenergic agonists on the vascular system may be potentiated). Products include:
Parnate Tablets 2222

Trimipramine Maleate (The action of β-adrenergic agonists on the vascular system may be potentiated). Products include:
Surmontil Capsules 2524

BRETHINE TABLETS
(Terbutaline Sulfate) 1026
May interact with sympathomimetic aerosal brochodilators. Compounds in this category include:

Albuterol (Concomitant use not recommended; combined effect on the cardiovascular system may be deleterious). Products include:
Proventil Inhalation Aerosol 2117
Ventolin Inhalation Aerosol and Refill 583

Albuterol Sulfate (Concomitant use not recommended; combined effect on the cardiovascular system may be deleterious). Products include:
Proventil Repetabs Tablets 2120
Proventil Solutions for Inhalation 0.5% and 0.083% 2118
Proventil Syrup 2119
Proventil Tablets 2120
Ventolin 583

Dobutamine Hydrochloride (Concomitant use not recommended; combined effect on the cardiovascular system may be deleterious). Products include:
Dobutrex Solution Vials 1259

Dopamine Hydrochloride (Concomitant use not recommended; combined effect on the cardiovascular system may be deleterious). Products include:
Intropin Injection 930

Ephedrine Hydrochloride (Concomitant use not recommended; combined effect on the cardiovascular system may be deleterious). Products include:
Amesec ▣ 682
Primatene Tablets-M Formula 2421
Primatene Tablets-P Formula 2421
Primatene Tablets-Regular Formula 2421
Quadrinal Tablets 1183
Quelidrine Syrup 556
Tedral SA 1765

Ephedrine Sulfate (Concomitant use not recommended; combined effect on the cardiovascular system may be deleterious). Products include:
Bronkaid Tablets ▣ 757
Bronkolixir ▣ 761
Bronkotabs Tablets ▣ 762
Marax Tablets & DF Syrup 1954
Pazo Hemorrhoid Ointment & Suppositories 752
Vicks Vatronol Nose Drops ▣ 666

Ephedrine Tannate (Concomitant use not recommended; combined effect on the cardiovascular system may be deleterious). Products include:
Rynatuss 2388

Epinephrine (Concomitant use not recommended; combined effect on the cardiovascular system may be deleterious). Products include:
Ana-Kit Anaphylaxis Emergency Treatment Kit 1100
Bronkaid Mist ▣ 757
EpiPen 843
Marcaine Hydrochloride 0.5% with Epinephrine 1:200,000 (as bitartrate) 958
Marcaine Hydrochloride with Epinephrine 1:200,000 2055
Primatene Mist 2420
Sus-Phrine Injection 1006
Xylocaine with Epinephrine Injections 637

Epinephrine Bitartrate (Concomitant use not recommended; combined effect on the cardiovascular system may be deleterious). Products include:
AsthmaHaler Mist Epinephrine Bitartrate Bronchodilator ▣ 616
Bronkaid Mist Suspension ▣ 757
Primatene Mist Suspension 2421

Epinephrine Hydrochloride (Concomitant use not recommended; combined effect on the cardiovascular system may be deleterious). Products include:
Adrenalin Chloride Solution 1:100 & 1:1,000 1689
Epifrin ⊙ 244
Glaucon ⊙ 218

Isoproterenol Hydrochloride (Concomitant use not recommended; combined effect on the cardiovascular system may be deleterious). Products include:
Isuprel Hydrochloride Injection 1:5000 2050
Isuprel Hydrochloride Mistometer 2051
Isuprel Hydrochloride Solution 1:200 & 1:100 2052
Norisodrine Aerotrol 540

Metaproterenol Sulfate (Concomitant use not recommended; combined effect on the cardiovascular system may be deleterious). Products include:
Alupent 674
Arm-a-Med Metaproterenol Sulfate Inhalation Solution, USP 617
Metaprel Inhalation Aerosol Bronchodilator 2014
Metaprel Inhalation Solution 2015
Metaprel 2015
Metaproterenol Sulfate Inhalation Solution, USP 912

Metaraminol Bitartrate (Concomitant use not recommended; combined effect on the cardiovascular system may be deleterious). Products include:
Aramine Injection 1424

Methoxamine Hydrochloride (Concomitant use not recommended; combined effect on the cardiovascular system may be deleterious). Products include:
Vasoxyl Injection 819

Norepinephrine Bitartrate (Concomitant use not recommended; combined effect on the cardiovascular system may be deleterious). Products include:
Levophed Bitartrate Injection 2054

Phenylephrine Bitartrate (Concomitant use not recommended; combined effect on the cardiovascular system may be deleterious).
No products indexed under this heading.

Phenylephrine Hydrochloride (Concomitant use not recommended; combined effect on the cardiovascular system may be deleterious). Products include:
AK-Dilate Solution 2.5% and 10% ⊙ 203
Atrohist Sprinkle Capsules 558
Cerose-DM 2443
Codimal 846
Comhist LA Capsules 1618
Congespirin For Children Aspirin Free Chewable Cold Tablets 748
Cyclomydril ⊙ 216
Deconsal Sprinkle Capsules 559
Dimetane Decongestant ▣ 673
Dristan Decongestant/Antihistamine/ Analgesic Coated Caplets ▣ 749
Dristan Cold Nasal Decongestant/ Antihistamine/ Analgesic Coated Tablets 2419
Dristan Advanced Formula Decongestant/Antihistamine/ Analgesic Tablets ▣ 749
Dristan Nasal Spray, Menthol 2419
Dristan Nasal Spray, Regular and Regular with Metered Pump 2419
Entex Capsules 1623
Entex Liquid 1623
Sinus Excedrin Analgesic, Decongestant Tablets & Caplets 750
Extendryl 994
4-Way Fast Acting Nasal Spray - Original Formula (regular & mentholated) & Metered Spray Pump (regular) 751
Hycomine Compound Tablets 929
Murocoll-2 Sterile Ophthalmic Solution ⊙ 261
Mydfrin 2.5% ⊙ 224
Naldecon Syrup, Tablets, Pediatric Drops and Pediatric Syrup 709
Neo-Synephrine Hydrochloride 1% Carpuject 2063
Neo-Synephrine Hydrochloride 1% Injection 2063
Neo-Synephrine Hydrochloride (Ophthalmic) 2064
Neo-Synephrine ▣ 759
Nōstril Nasal Decongestant ▣ 520
Novahistine Elixir ▣ 596
Phenergan VC 2500
Phenergan VC with Codeine 2501
Prefrin Liquifilm Vasoconstrictor and Lubricant Eye Drops ⊙ 254
Prefrin-A ⊙ 255
Quelidrine Syrup 556
Relief Vasoconstrictor and Lubricant Eye Drops ⊙ 256
Robitussin Night Relief ▣ 677
Ru-Tuss with Hydrocodone 694
Ru-Tuss Tablets 693
Vasosulf ⊙ 279
Vicks Sinex ▣ 665
Zincfrin ⊙ 230

Phenylephrine Tannate (Concomitant use not recommended; combined effect on the cardiovascular system may be deleterious). Products include:
Rynatan 2387
Rynatuss 2388

Phenylpropanolamine Hydrochloride (Concomitant use not recommended; combined effect on the cardiovascular system may be deleterious). Products include:
A.R.M. Allergy Relief Medicine Caplets ▣ 615
Acutrim ▣ 548
Allerest ▣ 559
BC Cold Powder ▣ 517
Cheracol Plus Head Cold/Cough Formula ▣ 667
Codimal Expectorant 846
Comtrex Multi-Symptom Cold Reliever Tablets/Caplets/Liqui- Gels/ Liquid 745
Contac Continuous Action Decongestant/Antihistamine Capsules ▣ 710
Contac Maximum Strength Continuous Action Decongestant/ Antihistamine Caplets ▣ 709
Contac Severe Cold and Flu Formula Caplets ▣ 711
Coricidin 'D' Decongestant Tablets ▣ 695
Coricidin Demilets Tablets for Children ▣ 696
Demazin Nasal Decongestant/ Antihistamine Repetabs Tablets & Syrup ▣ 697
Dexatrim ▣ 733
Dimetane-DC Cough Syrup 1857
Dimetapp Elixir ▣ 673
Dimetapp DM Elixir ▣ 674
Dimetapp Extentabs ▣ 674
Dimetapp Plus Caplets ▣ 675
Dimetapp Tablets ▣ 675
Entex Capsules 1623
Entex LA Tablets 1623
Entex Liquid 1623
4-Way Cold Tablets 750
Hycomine Syrup 927
Naldecon CX Adult Liquid ▣ 521
Naldecon DX Adult Liquid ▣ 521
Naldecon DX Children's Syrup ▣ 522
Naldecon DX Pediatric Drops ▣ 522
Naldecon EX Children's Syrup ▣ 522
Naldecon EX Pediatric Drops ▣ 523
Naldecon Syrup, Tablets, Pediatric Drops and Pediatric Syrup 709
Nolamine Tablets 838
Nolex LA Tablets 838
Ornade Spansule Capsules 2221
Orthoxicol Cough Syrup ▣ 668
Propagest 839
Pyrroxate Capsules ▣ 669
Robitussin-CF ▣ 676
Ru-Tuss II Capsules 693
Ru-Tuss with Hydrocodone 694
Ru-Tuss Tablets 693
Sine-Off Sinus Medicine Tablets-Aspirin Formula ▣ 722
Sinulin 840
St. Joseph Cold Tablets for Children ▣ 704
Tavist-D Tablets 2035
Triaminic Allergy Tablets ▣ 688
Triaminic Chewables ▣ 688
Triaminic Cold Tablets ▣ 688
Triaminic Expectorant ▣ 688
Triaminic Expectorant w/Codeine 1996
Triaminic Expectorant DH 1995
Triaminic Oral Infant Drops 1996
Triaminic Syrup ▣ 689
Triaminic-12 Tablets ▣ 690
Triaminic-DM Syrup ▣ 689
Triaminicin Tablets ▣ 690
Triaminicol Multi-Symptom Cold Tablets ▣ 691
Triaminicol Multi-Symptom Relief ▣ 691
Tuss-Ornade Liquid 2242
Tuss-Ornade Spansule Capsules 2242
Tylenol Cold Medication, Effervescent Tablets 1369

Pirbuterol Acetate (Concomitant use not recommended; combined effect on the cardiovascular system may be deleterious). Products include:
Maxair Inhaler 1311

Pseudoephedrine Hydrochloride (Concomitant use not recommended; combined effect on the cardiovascular system may be deleterious). Products include:
Actifed Capsules ▣ 539
Actifed Plus Caplets ▣ 539

Actifed Plus Tablets ▣ 540
Actifed with Codeine Cough Syrup.. 752
Actifed Syrup ▣ 540
Actifed Tablets ▣ 540
Actifed 12-Hour Capsules ▣ 539
Advil Cold & Sinus Caplets (formerly CoAdvil) 2416
Allerest ▣ 559
Anatuss LA Tablets 1359
Benadryl Decongestant Elixir ▣ 635
Benadryl Decongestant ▣ 635
Benadryl Plus ▣ 636
Benadryl Plus Nighttime ▣ 637
Benylin Decongestant ▣ 638
Brexin L.A. Capsules 2078
Bromfed Capsules (Timed Release) 1615
Bromfed Syrup ▣ 628
Bromfed 1615
CoAdvil ▣ 748
Allergy-Sinus Comtrex Multi-Symptom Allergy Sinus Formula Tablets & Caplets 746
Cough Formula Comtrex 746
Comtrex Multi-Symptom Cold Reliever Tablets/Caplets/Liqui-Gels/Liquid 745
Day-Night Comtrex 747
Non-Drowsy Comtrex 747
Congess 994
Congestac Caplets ▣ 617
Contac Jr. Children's Cold Medicine ▣ 712
Contac Nighttime Cold Medicine ▣ 713
Contac Sinus Caplets Maximum Strength Non-Drowsy Formula ▣ 710
Contac Sinus Tablets Maximum Strength Non-Drowsy Formula ▣ 710
Deconamine 663
Deconsal II Tablets 559
Dimacol Caplets ▣ 672
Dimetane-DX Cough Syrup 1858
Dorcol Children's Cough Syrup ▣ 685
Dorcol Children's Decongestant Liquid ▣ 685
Dorcol Children's Liquid Cold Formula ▣ 686
Maximum Strength Dristan Decongestant/Analgesic Coated Caplets ▣ 750
No Drowsiness Dristan Cold Nasal Decongestant/Analgesic Coated Caplets 2420
Dristan Sinus Caplets 2419
Sinus Excedrin Analgesic, Decongestant Tablets & Caplets ▣ 533
Fedahist Gyrocaps 2145
Fedahist Timecaps 2145
Guaifed 1615
Guaifed Syrup ▣ 629
Isoclor Expectorant 982
Isoclor Timesule Capsules ▣ 561
Kronofed-A 970
Medi-Flu Caplet, Liquid ▣ 640
Novafed A Capsules 1342
Novafed Capsules 1342
Novahistine DH 1342
Novahistine DMX ▣ 595
Novahistine Expectorant 1343
Nucofed Capsules 2219
Nucofed Expectorant 2219
Nucofed Pediatric Expectorant 2220
Nucofed Syrup 2219
Ornex Caplets ▣ 618
PediaCare Allergy Relief Formula Liquid 1362
PediaCare Cough-Cold Formula Liquid 1362
PediaCare Infants' Oral Decongestant Drops 1362
PediaCare Night Rest Cough-Cold Formula Liquid 1362
PediaCare 6-12 Cough-Cold Formula Chewable Tablets 1362
Robitussin-DAC Syrup 1875
Robitussin-PE ▣ 677
Rondec 1975
Rondec-DM 1976
Rondec-TR Tablet 1975
Ru-Tuss DE Tablets 694
Ryna ▣ 741
Seldane-D Extended-Release Tablets 1350
Sinarest ▣ 562
Sine-Aid Maximum Strength Sinus Headache Caplets 1365
Sine-Aid Maximum Strength Sinus Headache Tablets 1365
Sine-Off Maximum Strength Allergy/Sinus Formula Caplets ▣ 721
Sine-Off Maximum Strength No Drowsiness Formula Caplets ▣ 722
Singlet Tablets ▣ 598
Sinutab Maximum Strength ▣ 641
Sinutab Maximum Strength Without Drowsiness Tablets & Caplets ▣ 642
Sinutab Regular Strength Without Drowsiness Formula ▣ 641
St. Joseph Nighttime Cold Medicine ▣ 705
Sudafed Children's Liquid ▣ 543
Sudafed Cough Syrup ▣ 543
Sudafed Plus Liquid ▣ 544
Sudafed Plus Tablets ▣ 545
Sudafed Sinus Caplets ▣ 545
Sudafed Sinus Tablets ▣ 545
Sudafed Tablets, 30 mg ▣ 544
Sudafed Tablets, Adult Strength, 60 mg ▣ 544
Sudafed 12 Hour Capsules ▣ 545
TheraFlu Flu and Cold Medicine ▣ 687
Triaminic Nite Light ▣ 689
Tylenol Allergy Sinus Medication Caplets and Gelcaps, Maximum Strength 1372
Children's Tylenol Cold Liquid Formula and Chewable Tablets 1368
Tylenol Cold & Flu Hot Medication, Packets 1369
Tylenol Cold & Flu No Drowsiness Hot Medication, Packets 1371
Tylenol Cold Medication Caplets and Tablets 1370
Tylenol Cold Medication No Drowsiness Formula Caplets 1370
Tylenol Cold Night Time Medication Liquid 1371
Tylenol Cough Medication Liquid with Decongestant, Maximum Strength 1372
Tylenol, Maximum Strength, Sinus Medication Gelcaps, Caplets and Tablets 1373
Ursinus Inlay-Tabs ▣ 691
Vicks Children's NyQuil ▣ 664
Vicks Daycare ▣ 660
Vicks Formula 44D Decongestant Cough Medicine ▣ 662
Vicks Formula 44M Multi-Symptom Cough Medicine ▣ 662
Vicks NyQuil Nighttime Colds Medicine-Original & Cherry Flavor ▣ 664
Vicks Pediatric Formula 44 Cough & Congestion Medicine ▣ 663
Vicks Pediatric Formula 44m Multi-Symptom Cough & Cold Medicine ▣ 663

Pseudoephedrine Sulfate (Concomitant use not recommended; combined effect on the cardiovascular system may be deleterious). Products include:
Afrin Tablets ▣ 693
Chlor-Trimeton Decongestant ▣ 694
Disophrol Chronotab Sustained-Action Tablets ▣ 698
Drixoral Antihistamine/Nasal Decongestant Syrup ▣ 698
Drixoral Non-Drowsy Formula ▣ 699
Drixoral Plus Extended-Release Tablets ▣ 699
Drixoral Sinus ▣ 700
Drixoral Sustained-Action Tablets ▣ 698
Sinutab Allergy Formula Sustained Action Tablets ▣ 640
Trinalin Repetabs Tablets 1170

BRETYLOL INJECTION

(Bretylium Tosylate) 923
May interact with cardiac glycosides and certain other agents. Compounds in these categories include:

Deslanoside (Aggravated digitalis toxicity).

Digitoxin (Aggravated digitalis toxicity). Products include:
Crystodigin Tablets 1253

Digoxin (Aggravated digitalis toxicity). Products include:
Lanoxicaps 772
Lanoxin Elixir Pediatric 775
Lanoxin Injection 778
Lanoxin Injection Pediatric 781
Lanoxin Tablets 783

Dopamine Hydrochloride (Concurrent therapy results in increased pressor effects). Products include:
Intropin Injection 930

Norepinephrine Bitartrate (Concurrent therapy results in increased pressor effects). Products include:
Levophed Bitartrate Injection 2054

BREVIBLOC INJECTION

(Esmolol Hydrochloride) 942
May interact with catecholamine depleting drugs and certain other agents. Compounds in these categories include:

Deserpidine (Additive effect). Products include:
Enduronyl 518
Harmonyl Tablets 528
Oreticyl 545

Digoxin (10 to 20% increase in digoxin blood levels). Products include:
Lanoxicaps 772
Lanoxin Elixir Pediatric 775
Lanoxin Injection 778
Lanoxin Injection Pediatric 781
Lanoxin Tablets 783

Morphine Sulfate (Concomitant intravenous morphine therapy results in 46% increase in steady-state esmolol blood levels). Products include:
Astramorph/PF Injection, USP (Preservative-Free) 618
Duramorph 960
Infumorph 200 and Infumorph 500 Sterile Solutions 962
MS Contin Tablets 1814
MSIR 1817
Oramorph SR (Morphine Sulfate Sustained Release Tablets) 1988
Roxanol 1991

Rauwolfia Serpentina (Additive effect). Products include:
Raudixin Tablets 1803
Rauzide Tablets 1804

Rescinnamine (Additive effect).
No products indexed under this heading.

Reserpine (Additive effect). Products include:
Diupres Tablets 1461
Hydromox R Tablets 1209
Hydropres Tablets 1485
Renese-R Tablets 1786
Salutensin/Salutensin-Demi 719
Ser-Ap-Es Tablets 881
Serpasil Tablets 883
Serpasil-Apresoline Tablets 884
Serpasil-Esidrix Tablets 886

Succinylcholine Chloride (Neuromuscular blockade prolonged from 5 to 8 minutes). Products include:
Anectine 755

Warfarin Sodium (Brevibloc should be titrated with caution in patients being treated concurrently with warfarin). Products include:
Coumadin Injection & Tablets 944
Panwarfin Tablets 547

BREVICON 21-DAY TABLETS

(Norethindrone, Ethinyl Estradiol) 2304
May interact with barbiturates, tetracyclines, and certain other agents. Compounds in these categories include:

Ampicillin Sodium (Possibility of reduced efficacy, increased incidence of breakthrough bleeding, and menstrual irregularities). Products include:
Unasyn 1965

Aprobarbital (Reduced efficacy; increased incidence of breakthrough bleeding; menstrual irregularities). Products include:
Alurate Elixir 1883

Butabarbital (Reduced efficacy; increased incidence of breakthrough bleeding; menstrual irregularities). Products include:
Pyridium Plus 1764

Butalbital (Reduced efficacy; increased incidence of breakthrough bleeding; menstrual irregularities). Products include:
Esgic-Plus Tablets 1002
Esgic Tablets & Capsules 1001
Fioricet Tablets 2006
Fiorinal Capsules 2007
Fiorinal with Codeine Capsules 2008
Fiorinal Tablets 2007
Phrenilin 838
Sedapap Tablets 50 mg/650 mg .. 1360

Demeclocycline Hydrochloride (Possibility of reduced efficacy, increased incidence of breakthrough bleeding, and menstrual irregularities). Products include:
Declomycin Capsules, Tablets 1199

Doxycycline Calcium (Possibility of reduced efficacy, increased incidence of breakthrough bleeding, and menstrual irregularities).
No products indexed under this heading.

Doxycycline Hyclate (Possibility of reduced efficacy, increased incidence of breakthrough bleeding, and menstrual irregularities). Products include:
Doryx Capsules 1717
Vibramycin Hyclate Capsules 1787
Vibramycin Hyclate Intravenous 1968
Vibra-Tabs Film Coated Tablets 1787

Doxycycline Monohydrate (Possibility of reduced efficacy, increased incidence of breakthrough bleeding, and menstrual irregularities). Products include:
Monodox Capsules 1630
Vibramycin Monohydrate for Oral Suspension 1787

Griseofulvin (Possibility of reduced efficacy, increased incidence of breakthrough bleeding, and menstrual irregularities). Products include:
Fulvicin P/G Tablets 2090
Fulvicin P/G 165 & 330 Tablets 2091
Fulvicin-U/F Tablets 2092
Grifulvin V (griseofulvin microsize) Tablets/Suspension 1678
Grisactin 2454
Grisactin Ultra Tablets 2455
Gris-PEG Tablets, 125 mg & 250 mg 1083

Mephobarbital (Reduced efficacy; increased incidence of breakthrough bleeding; menstrual irregularities). Products include:
Mebaral Tablets 2061

Methacycline Hydrochloride (Possibility of reduced efficacy, increased incidence of breakthrough bleeding, and menstrual irregularities).
No products indexed under this heading.

Minocycline Hydrochloride (Possibility of reduced efficacy, increased incidence of breakthrough bleeding, and menstrual irregularities). Products include:
Minocin Intravenous 1221
Minocin Oral Suspension 1224
Minocin Pellet-Filled Capsules 1222

Oxytetracycline Hydrochloride (Possibility of reduced efficacy, increased incidence of breakthrough bleeding, and menstrual irregularities). Products include:
Terra-Cortril Ophthalmic Suspension 1963
Terramycin Capsules 1786
Terramycin Intramuscular Solution 1964
Terramycin with Polymyxin B Sulfate Ophthalmic Ointment 1965

Pentobarbital Sodium (Reduced efficacy; increased incidence of breakthrough bleeding; menstrual irregularities). Products include:
- Nembutal Sodium Capsules 534
- Nembutal Sodium Solution 536
- Nembutal Sodium Suppositories...... 538

Phenobarbital (Reduced efficacy; increased incidence of breakthrough bleeding; menstrual irregularities). Products include:
- Arco-Lase Plus Tablets 607
- Bellergal-S Tablets 1998
- Bronkolixir .... ▣ 761
- Bronkotabs Tablets.......... ▣ 762
- Donnatal 1858
- Donnatal Extentabs.......... 1859
- Donnatal Tablets 1858
- Donnazyme Tablets 1860
- Kinesed Tablets 2272
- Phenobarbital Elixir and Tablets...... 1293
- Primatene Tablets-P Formula.......... 2421
- Quadrinal Tablets 1183
- Tedral SA 1765

Phenylbutazone (Reduced efficacy; increased incidence of breakthrough bleeding; menstrual irregularities). Products include:
- Butazolidin Capsules & Tablets........ 1027

Phenytoin Sodium (Reduced efficacy; increased incidence of breakthrough bleeding; menstrual irregularities). Products include:
- Dilantin Kapseals 1708
- Dilantin Parenteral 1712
- Dilantin with Phenobarbital Kapseals 1715

Rifampin (Reduced efficacy; increased incidence of breakthrough bleeding; menstrual irregularities). Products include:
- Rifadin 1345
- Rifamate Capsules 1347
- Rimactane Capsules.......... 879

Secobarbital Sodium (Reduced efficacy; increased incidence of breakthrough bleeding; menstrual irregularities). Products include:
- Seconal Sodium Pulvules 1296

Tetracycline Hydrochloride (Possibility of reduced efficacy, increased incidence of breakthrough bleeding, and menstrual irregularities). Products include:
- Achromycin V Capsules 1193
- Achromycin Ophthalmic Ointment 1% .... ◉ 307
- Achromycin Ophthalmic Suspension 1% .... ◉ 308
- Topicycline for Topical Solution 1856

Thiamylal Sodium (Reduced efficacy; increased incidence of breakthrough bleeding; menstrual irregularities). Products include:
- Surital Ampoules, Steri-Vials.......... 1764

BREVICON 28-DAY TABLETS
(Norethindrone, Ethinyl Estradiol)......2304
See **Brevicon 21-Day Tablets**

BREVITAL SODIUM VIALS
(Methohexital Sodium) 1248
May interact with central nervous system depressants, oral anticoagulants, corticosteroids, and certain other agents. Compounds in these categories include:

Alcohol (Additive effect).

Alfentanil Hydrochloride (Additive effect). Products include:
- Alfenta Injection 1131

Alprazolam (Additive effect). Products include:
- Xanax Tablets 2367

Aprobarbital (Additive effect). Products include:
- Alurate Elixir 1883

Betamethasone Acetate (Barbiturates may influence the absorption and elimination of concomitantly used corticosteroids). Products include:
- Celestone Soluspan Suspension 2081

Betamethasone Sodium Phosphate (Barbiturates may influence the absorption and elimination of concomitantly used corticosteroids). Products include:
- Celestone Soluspan Suspension 2081

Buprenorphine (Additive effect).
- No products indexed under this heading.

Buspirone Hydrochloride (Additive effect). Products include:
- BuSpar 1401

Butabarbital (Additive effect). Products include:
- Pyridium Plus 1764

Butalbital (Additive effect). Products include:
- Esgic-Plus Tablets 1002
- Esgic Tablets & Capsules.......... 1001
- Fioricet Tablets.......... 2006
- Fiorinal Capsules 2007
- Fiorinal with Codeine Capsules 2008
- Fiorinal Tablets.......... 2007
- Phrenilin 838
- Sedapap Tablets 50 mg/650 mg .. 1360

Chlordiazepoxide (Additive effect). Products include:
- Libritabs Tablets 1930
- Limbitrol 1933
- Menrium Tablets 1934

Chlordiazepoxide Hydrochloride (Additive effect). Products include:
- Librax Capsules 1929
- Librium Capsules.......... 1931
- Librium Injectable 1932

Chlorpromazine (Additive effect). Products include:
- Thorazine 2234

Chlorprothixene (Additive effect). Products include:
- Taractan Tablets 1920

Chlorprothixene Hydrochloride (Additive effect). Products include:
- Taractan 1920

Clorazepate Dipotassium (Additive effect). Products include:
- Tranxene 556

Codeine (Additive effect). Products include:
- Calcidrine Syrup.......... 506

Codeine Phosphate (Additive effect). Products include:
- Actifed with Codeine Cough Syrup.. 752
- Cheracol Cough Syrup.......... 1853
- Codimal PH Syrup.......... 846
- Dimetane-DC Cough Syrup 1857
- Empirin with Codeine Phosphate Nos. 2, 3 & 4.......... 764
- Fiorinal with Codeine Capsules 2008
- Isoclor Expectorant.......... 982
- Naldecon CX Adult Liquid .... ▣ 521
- Novahistine DH.......... 1342
- Novahistine Expectorant.......... 1343
- Nucofed Capsules 2219
- Nucofed Expectorant 2219
- Nucofed Pediatric Expectorant 2220
- Nucofed Syrup 2219
- Phenaphen with Codeine Capsules 1865
- Phenaphen-650 with Codeine Tablets 1866
- Phenergan with Codeine.......... 2497
- Phenergan VC with Codeine 2501
- Robitussin A-C Syrup.......... 1875
- Robitussin-DAC Syrup 1875
- Ryna .... ▣ 741
- Soma Compound w/Codeine Tablets 2390
- Triaminic Expectorant w/Codeine .. 1996
- Tussi-Organidin Liquid 2391
- Tylenol with Codeine 1381

Codeine Polistirex (Additive effect).
- No products indexed under this heading.

Cortisone Acetate (Barbiturates may influence the absorption and elimination of concomitantly used corticosteroids). Products include:
- Cortone Acetate Sterile Suspension 1437
- Cortone Acetate Tablets.......... 1439

Dexamethasone (Barbiturates may influence the absorption and elimination of concomitantly used corticosteroids). Products include:
- AK-Trol Ointment & Suspension .... ◉ 207
- Decadron Elixir 1445
- Decadron Tablets.......... 1447
- Decaspray Topical Aerosol 1459
- Dexacidin.......... ◉ 272
- Maxidex Sterile Ophthalmic Suspension.......... ◉ 223
- Maxitrol Ophthalmic Ointment/Suspension .... ◉ 223
- TobraDex Ophthalmic Suspension and Ointment.......... ◉ 228

Dexamethasone Acetate (Barbiturates may influence the absorption and elimination of concomitantly used corticosteroids). Products include:
- Dalalone D.P. Injectable 999
- Decadron-LA Sterile Suspension...... 1457

Dexamethasone Sodium Phosphate (Barbiturates may influence the absorption and elimination of concomitantly used corticosteroids). Products include:
- AK-Dex .... ◉ 203
- Decadron Phosphate Respihaler...... 1454
- Decadron Phosphate Sterile Ophthalmic Ointment.......... 1453
- Decadron Phosphate Sterile Ophthalmic Solution 1453
- Decadron Phosphate Topical Cream 1455
- Decadron Phosphate Turbinaire 1456
- Maxidex Sterile Ophthalmic Ointment .... ◉ 222
- NeoDecadron Sterile Ophthalmic Ointment 1517
- NeoDecadron Sterile Ophthalmic Solution 1518
- NeoDecadron Topical Cream 1518

Dezocine (Additive effect).

Diazepam (Additive effect). Products include:
- Valium Injectable 1937
- Valium Tablets 1939
- Valrelease Capsules 1923

Dicumarol (Barbiturates may influence the absorption and elimination of concomitantly used anticoagulants). Products include:
- Dicumarol Tablets 516

Droperidol (Additive effect). Products include:
- Inapsine Injection.......... 1140
- Innovar Injection.......... 1141

Enflurane (Additive effect). Products include:
- Ethrane.......... 599

Estazolam (Additive effect). Products include:
- ProSom Tablets 554

Ethchlorvynol (Additive effect). Products include:
- Placidyl Capsules.......... 553

Ethinamate (Additive effect).
- No products indexed under this heading.

Fentanyl (Additive effect). Products include:
- Duragesic Transdermal System........ 1133

Fentanyl Citrate (Additive effect). Products include:
- Innovar Injection.......... 1141
- Sublimaze Injection.......... 1146

Fluphenazine Decanoate (Additive effect). Products include:
- Prolixin Decanoate 1795

Fluphenazine Enanthate (Additive effect). Products include:
- Prolixin Enanthate 1796

Fluphenazine Hydrochloride (Additive effect). Products include:
- Prolixin Elixir 1793
- Prolixin Injection.......... 1791
- Prolixin Oral Concentrate.......... 1792
- Prolixin Tablets.......... 1793

Flurazepam Hydrochloride (Additive effect). Products include:
- Dalmane Capsules.......... 1927

Glutethimide (Additive effect).
- No products indexed under this heading.

Haloperidol (Additive effect). Products include:
- Haldol Injection, Tablets and Concentrate 1373

Haloperidol Decanoate (Additive effect). Products include:
- Haldol Decanoate.......... 1375

Halothane (Barbiturates may influence the absorption and elimination of concomitantly used halothane). Products include:
- Fluothane 2453

Hydrocodone Bitartrate (Additive effect). Products include:
- Anexsia 5/500 Tablets.......... 2196
- Anexsia 7.5/650 Tablets 2197
- Azdone Tablets.......... 844
- Codiclear DH Syrup 845
- Codimal DH Syrup.......... 846
- Damason-P.......... 1356
- Hycodan Syrup, Tablets 927
- Hycomine Compound Tablets 929
- Hycomine Syrup.......... 927
- Hycotuss Expectorant Syrup 930
- Hydrocet Capsules 835
- Lortab ASA Tablets.......... 2414
- Lortab.......... 2412
- Ru-Tuss with Hydrocodone 694
- Triaminic Expectorant DH 1995
- Vicodin Tablets.......... 1187
- Vicodin ES Tablets 1189
- Zydone Capsules 941

Hydrocodone Polistirex (Additive effect). Products include:
- Tussionex Extended-Release Suspension.......... 988

Hydrocortisone (Barbiturates may influence the absorption and elimination of concomitantly used corticosteroids). Products include:
- AK-Spore H.C. .... ◉ 206
- Bactine Hydrocortisone Anti-Itch Cream .... ▣ 625
- CaldeCORT Anti-Itch Hydrocortisone Spray .... ▣ 560
- Carmol HC Cream 1% 2296
- Cortaid Spray .... ▣ 735
- Cortenema 2244
- Cortisporin Ointment.......... 758
- Cortisporin Ophthalmic Ointment Sterile 758
- Cortisporin Ophthalmic Suspension Sterile 759
- Cortisporin Otic Solution Sterile 760
- Cortisporin Otic Suspension Sterile 760
- Cortizone-5 Creme & Ointment...... ▣ 732
- Dermolate Anti-Itch Cream .... ▣ 697
- Eldecort Cream 1.0% 1113
- Eldecort Cream 1.0% and 2.5% 1113
- Fungoid HC Creme 1770
- Hydrocortone Tablets 1482
- Hytone 909
- LazerSporin-C Solution 1770
- Massengill Medicated Soft Cloth Towelettes.......... 2192
- Nutracort Cream & Lotion 1684
- PediOtic Suspension Sterile 797
- Synacort Creams 1%, 2.5% 2296
- Vanoxide-HC Acne Lotion.......... 911
- Vioform-Hydrocortisone Cream and Mild Cream 889
- Vioform-Hydrocortisone Ointment.. 889
- VōSoL HC Otic Solution.......... 2392
- Vytone Cream 1% 911

Hydrocortisone Acetate (Barbiturates may influence the absorption and elimination of concomitantly used corticosteroids). Products include:
- Analpram-HC Rectal Cream 1% and 2.5% 970
- Anusol-HC Cream 1690
- Anusol-HC Suppositories 1691

Caldecort ▣ 560
Carmol HC Cream 1% 2296
Chloromycetin Hydrocortisone Ophthalmic 1694
Coly-Mycin S Otic w/Neomycin & Hydrocortisone 1708
Cortaid ▣ 735
Cortef Feminine Itch Cream ▣ 735
Corticaine ▣ 682
Cortifoam 1827
Cortisporin Cream 757
Epifoam 1828
Gynecort 5 Creme ▣ 556
Hydrocortone Acetate Sterile Suspension 1479
Lanacort 5 Creme and Ointment ▣ 557
Mantadil Cream 789
Ophthocort ◉ 301
Orabase HCA Oral Paste 890
Pramosone Cream, Lotion & Ointment 971
ProctoCream-HC 1834
Proctofoam-HC 1835

Hydrocortisone Sodium Phosphate (Barbiturates may influence the absorption and elimination of concomitantly used corticosteroids). Products include:
Hydrocortone Phosphate Injection, Sterile 1481

Hydrocortisone Sodium Succinate (Barbiturates may influence the absorption and elimination of concomitantly used corticosteroids). Products include:
Solu-Cortef Sterile Powder 2361

Hydroxyzine Hydrochloride (Additive effect). Products include:
Atarax Tablets & Syrup 1941
Marax Tablets & DF Syrup 1954
Vistaril Intramuscular Solution 1970

Isoflurane (Additive effect). Products include:
Forane 600

Ketamine Hydrochloride (Additive effect). Products include:
Ketalar 1726

Levorphanol Tartrate (Additive effect). Products include:
Levo-Dromoran 1906

Lorazepam (Additive effect). Products include:
Ativan Injection 2432
Ativan Tablets 2434

Loxapine Hydrochloride (Additive effect). Products include:
Loxitane 1213

Loxapine Succinate (Additive effect). Products include:
Loxitane Capsules 1213

Meperidine Hydrochloride (Additive effect). Products include:
Demerol 2047
Mepergan Injection 2479

Mephobarbital (Additive effect). Products include:
Mebaral Tablets 2061

Meprobamate (Additive effect). Products include:
Deprol Tablets 2382
Equagesic Tablets 2451
Miltown Tablets 2386
PMB 200 and PMB 400 2504

Mesoridazine (Additive effect). Products include:
Serentil 686

Methadone Hydrochloride (Additive effect). Products include:
Dolophine Hydrochloride Ampoules & Vials 1260
Dolophine Hydrochloride Tablets 1261
Methadone Hydrochloride Diskets 1284
Methadone Hydrochloride Oral Solution & Tablets 1987

Methoxyflurane (Additive effect).
No products indexed under this heading.

Methylprednisolone Acetate (Barbiturates may influence the absorption and elimination of concomitantly used corticosteroids). Products include:
Depo-Medrol Sterile Aqueous Suspension 2334

Methylprednisolone Sodium Succinate (Barbiturates may influence the absorption and elimination of concomitantly used corticosteroids). Products include:
Solu-Medrol Sterile Powder 2363

Midazolam Hydrochloride (Additive effect). Products include:
Versed Injection 1924

Molindone Hydrochloride (Additive effect). Products include:
Moban Tablets & Concentrate 932

Morphine Sulfate (Additive effect). Products include:
Astramorph/PF Injection, USP (Preservative-Free) 618
Duramorph 960
Infumorph 200 and Infumorph 500 Sterile Solutions 962
MS Contin Tablets 1814
MSIR 1817
Oramorph SR (Morphine Sulfate Sustained Release Tablets) 1988
Roxanol 1991

Opium Alkaloids (Additive effect). Products include:
B & O No. 15A & No. 16A Supprettes 2395
Pantopon Injectable 1911

Oxazepam (Additive effect). Products include:
Serax Capsules 2522
Serax Tablets 2522

Oxycodone Hydrochloride (Additive effect). Products include:
Percocet Tablets 950
Percodan 951
Roxicodone Tablets, Oral Solution & Intensol (Oxycodone) 1992
Tylox Capsules 1382

Pentobarbital Sodium (Additive effect). Products include:
Nembutal Sodium Capsules 534
Nembutal Sodium Solution 536
Nembutal Sodium Suppositories 538

Perphenazine (Additive effect). Products include:
Etrafon 2087
Triavil Tablets 1556
Trilafon 2123

Phenobarbital (Additive effect). Products include:
Arco-Lase Plus Tablets 607
Bellergal-S Tablets 1998
Bronkolixir ▣ 761
Bronkotabs Tablets ▣ 762
Donnatal 1858
Donnatal Extentabs 1859
Donnatal Tablets 1858
Donnazyme Tablets 1860
Kinesed Tablets 2272
Phenobarbital Elixir and Tablets 1293
Primatene Tablets-P Formula 2421
Quadrinal Tablets 1183
Tedral SA 1765

Phenytoin (Barbiturates may influence the absorption and elimination of concomitantly used diphenylhydantoin). Products include:
Dilantin Infatabs 1710
Dilantin-30 Pediatric/Dilantin-125 Suspension 1713

Phenytoin Sodium (Barbiturates may influence the absorption and elimination of concomitantly used diphenylhydantoin). Products include:
Dilantin Kapseals 1708
Dilantin Parenteral 1712
Dilantin with Phenobarbital Kapseals 1715

Prazepam (Additive effect). Products include:
Centrax 1693

Prednisolone Acetate (Barbiturates may influence the absorption and elimination of concomitantly used corticosteroids). Products include:
AK-Cide Sterile Ophthalmic Ointment & Suspension ◉ 202
Blephamide Liquifilm Sterile Ophthalmic Suspension 586
Blephamide S.O.P. Sterile Ophthalmic Ointment 586
Cetapred Ointment ◉ 220
⅛% Econopred & 1% Econopred Plus ◉ 217
Isopto Cetapred Suspension ◉ 220
Metimyd ◉ 306
Poly-Pred Liquifilm ◉ 250
Pred Forte ◉ 252
Pred Mild ◉ 254
Pred-G Liquifilm Sterile Ophthalmic Suspension ◉ 252
Pred-G S.O.P. Sterile Ophthalmic Ointment ◉ 253
Vasocidin Ointment ◉ 275

Prednisolone Sodium Phosphate (Barbiturates may influence the absorption and elimination of concomitantly used corticosteroids). Products include:
AK-Pred ◉ 205
Hydeltrasol Injection, Sterile 1476
Inflamase ◉ 274
Pediapred Oral Liquid 987
Vasocidin Ophthalmic Solution ◉ 276

Prednisolone Tebutate (Barbiturates may influence the absorption and elimination of concomitantly used corticosteroids). Products include:
Hydeltra-T.B.A. Sterile Suspension 1478

Prednisone (Barbiturates may influence the absorption and elimination of concomitantly used corticosteroids). Products include:
Deltasone Tablets 2332

Prochlorperazine (Additive effect). Products include:
Compazine 2201

Promethazine Hydrochloride (Additive effect). Products include:
Mepergan Injection 2479
Phenergan with Codeine 2497
Phenergan with Dextromethorphan 2499
Phenergan Injection 2493
Phenergan Suppositories 2496
Phenergan Syrup 2495
Phenergan Tablets 2496
Phenergan VC 2500
Phenergan VC with Codeine 2501

Propofol (Additive effect). Products include:
Diprivan Injection 2267

Propoxyphene Hydrochloride (Additive effect). Products include:
Darvon 1256
Wygesic Tablets 2540

Propoxyphene Napsylate (Additive effect). Products include:
Darvon-N/Darvocet-N 1254

Propylene glycol-containing solutions (Additive effect).

Quazepam (Additive effect). Products include:
Doral Tablets 2383

Secobarbital Sodium (Additive effect). Products include:
Seconal Sodium Pulvules 1296

Sufentanil Citrate (Additive effect). Products include:
Sufenta Injection 1147

Temazepam (Additive effect). Products include:
Restoril Capsules 2023

Thiamylal Sodium (Additive effect). Products include:
Surital Ampoules, Steri-Vials 1764

Thioridazine Hydrochloride (Additive effect). Products include:
Mellaril 2011

Thiothixene (Additive effect). Products include:
Navane Capsules and Concentrate 1954
Navane Intramuscular 1956

Triamcinolone (Barbiturates may influence the absorption and elimination of concomitantly used corticosteroids).
No products indexed under this heading.

Triamcinolone Acetonide (Barbiturates may influence the absorption and elimination of concomitantly used corticosteroids). Products include:
Aristocort A 1010
Azmacort Inhaler 1837
Kenalog Cream, Lotion & Ointment 2401
Kenalog-10 Injection 2402
Kenalog-40 Injection 2403
Kenalog in Orabase 604
Kenalog Spray 2401
Mycolog II Cream and Ointment 2407
Mytrex Cream & Ointment 2080
Nasacort Nasal Inhaler 1844

Triamcinolone Diacetate (Barbiturates may influence the absorption and elimination of concomitantly used corticosteroids). Products include:
Aristocort Suspension 1008

Triamcinolone Hexacetonide (Barbiturates may influence the absorption and elimination of concomitantly used corticosteroids). Products include:
Aristospan Suspension 1011

Triazolam (Additive effect). Products include:
Halcion Tablets 2340

Trifluoperazine Hydrochloride (Additive effect). Products include:
Stelazine 2226

Warfarin Sodium (Barbiturates may influence the absorption and elimination of concomitantly used anticoagulants). Products include:
Coumadin Injection & Tablets 944
Panwarfin Tablets 547

BREVOXYL GEL

(Benzoyl Peroxide) 2264
No interactions described in labeling.

BREXIN L.A. CAPSULES

(Chlorpheniramine Maleate, Pseudoephedrine Hydrochloride) 2078
May interact with monoamine oxidase inhibitors, beta blockers, central nervous system depressants, catecholamine depleting drugs, veratrum alkaloids, and certain other agents. Compounds in these categories include:

Acebutolol Hydrochloride (Increases effects of sympathomimetics). Products include:
Sectral Capsules 2520

Alcohol (Additive effect).

Alfentanil Hydrochloride (Additive effect). Products include:
Alfenta Injection 1131

Alprazolam (Additive effect). Products include:
Xanax Tablets 2367

Aprobarbital (Additive effect). Products include:
Alurate Elixir 1883

Atenolol (Increases effects of sympathomimetics). Products include:
Tenoretic Tablets 1105
Tenormin Tablets and I.V. Injection 1107

Betaxolol Hydrochloride (Increases effects of sympathomimetics). Products include:
Betoptic Sterile Ophthalmic Solution 569
Betoptic S Sterile Ophthalmic Suspension 570

Kerlone Tablets 2172

Buprenorphine (Additive effect).
No products indexed under this heading.

Buspirone Hydrochloride (Additive effect). Products include:
BuSpar 1401

Butabarbital (Additive effect). Products include:
Pyridium Plus 1764

Butalbital (Additive effect). Products include:
Esgic-Plus Tablets 1002
Esgic Tablets & Capsules 1001
Fioricet Tablets 2006
Fiorinal Capsules 2007
Fiorinal with Codeine Capsules 2008
Fiorinal Tablets 2007
Phrenilin 838
Sedapap Tablets 50 mg/650 mg .. 1360

Carteolol Hydrochloride (Increases effects of sympathomimetics). Products include:
Cartrol Tablets 507

Chlordiazepoxide (Additive effect). Products include:
Libritabs Tablets 1930
Limbitrol 1933
Menrium Tablets 1934

Chlordiazepoxide Hydrochloride (Additive effect). Products include:
Librax Capsules 1929
Librium Capsules 1931
Librium Injectable 1932

Chlorpromazine (Additive effect). Products include:
Thorazine 2234

Chlorprothixene (Additive effect). Products include:
Taractan Tablets 1920

Chlorprothixene Hydrochloride (Additive effect). Products include:
Taractan 1920

Clorazepate Dipotassium (Additive effect). Products include:
Tranxene 556

Codeine (Additive effect). Products include:
Calcidrine Syrup 506

Codeine Phosphate (Additive effect). Products include:
Actifed with Codeine Cough Syrup.. 752
Cheracol Cough Syrup 1853
Codimal PH Syrup 846
Dimetane-DC Cough Syrup 1857
Empirin with Codeine Phosphate Nos. 2, 3 & 4 764
Fiorinal with Codeine Capsules 2008
Isoclor Expectorant 982
Naldecon CX Adult Liquid .... ▣ 521
Novahistine DH 1342
Novahistine Expectorant 1343
Nucofed Capsules 2219
Nucofed Expectorant 2219
Nucofed Pediatric Expectorant 2220
Nucofed Syrup 2219
Phenaphen with Codeine Capsules 1865
Phenaphen-650 with Codeine Tablets 1866
Phenergan with Codeine 2497
Phenergan VC with Codeine 2501
Robitussin A-C Syrup 1875
Robitussin-DAC Syrup 1875
Ryna .... ▣ 741
Soma Compound w/Codeine Tablets 2390
Triaminic Expectorant w/Codeine .. 1996
Tussi-Organidin Liquid 2391
Tylenol with Codeine 1381

Codeine Polistirex (Additive effect).
No products indexed under this heading.

Cryptenamine Preparations (Reduced antihypertensive effects).

Deserpidine (Reduced antihypertensive effects). Products include:
Enduronyl 518
Harmonyl Tablets 528
Oreticyl 545

Dezocine (Additive effect).

Diazepam (Additive effect). Products include:
Valium Injectable 1937
Valium Tablets 1939
Valrelease Capsules 1923

Droperidol (Additive effect). Products include:
Inapsine Injection 1140
Innovar Injection 1141

Enflurane (Additive effect). Products include:
Ethrane 599

Esmolol Hydrochloride (Increases effects of sympathomimetics). Products include:
Brevibloc Injection 942

Estazolam (Additive effect). Products include:
ProSom Tablets 554

Ethchlorvynol (Additive effect). Products include:
Placidyl Capsules 553

Ethinamate (Additive effect).
No products indexed under this heading.

Fentanyl (Additive effect). Products include:
Duragesic Transdermal System 1133

Fentanyl Citrate (Additive effect). Products include:
Innovar Injection 1141
Sublimaze Injection 1146

Fluphenazine Decanoate (Additive effect). Products include:
Prolixin Decanoate 1795

Fluphenazine Enanthate (Additive effect). Products include:
Prolixin Enanthate 1796

Fluphenazine Hydrochloride (Additive effect). Products include:
Prolixin Elixir 1793
Prolixin Injection 1791
Prolixin Oral Concentrate 1792
Prolixin Tablets 1793

Flurazepam Hydrochloride (Additive effect). Products include:
Dalmane Capsules 1927

Furazolidone (Concurrent therapy is contraindicated; increases effects of sympathomimetics). Products include:
Furoxone 1855

Glutethimide (Additive effect).
No products indexed under this heading.

Haloperidol (Additive effect). Products include:
Haldol Injection, Tablets and Concentrate 1373

Haloperidol Decanoate (Additive effect). Products include:
Haldol Decanoate 1375

Hydrocodone Bitartrate (Additive effect). Products include:
Anexsia 5/500 Tablets 2196
Anexsia 7.5/650 Tablets 2197
Azdone Tablets 844
Codiclear DH Syrup 845
Codimal DH Syrup 846
Damason-P 1356
Hycodan Syrup, Tablets 927
Hycomine Compound Tablets 929
Hycomine Syrup 927
Hycotuss Expectorant Syrup 930
Hydrocet Capsules 835
Lortab ASA Tablets 2414
Lortab 2412
Ru-Tuss with Hydrocodone 694
Triaminic Expectorant DH 1995
Vicodin Tablets 1187
Vicodin ES Tablets 1189
Zydone Capsules 941

Hydrocodone Polistirex (Additive effect). Products include:
Tussionex Extended-Release Suspension 988

Hydroxyzine Hydrochloride (Additive effect). Products include:
Atarax Tablets & Syrup 1941
Marax Tablets & DF Syrup 1954
Vistaril Intramuscular Solution 1970

Isocarboxazid (Concurrent therapy is contraindicated; increases effects of sympathomimetics). Products include:
Marplan Tablets 1906

Isoflurane (Additive effect). Products include:
Forane 600

Ketamine Hydrochloride (Additive effect). Products include:
Ketalar 1726

Labetalol Hydrochloride (Increases effects of sympathomimetics). Products include:
Normodyne Injection 2108
Normodyne Tablets 2110
Normozide Tablets 2112
Trandate HCT Tablets 579
Trandate Injection 577
Trandate Tablets 579

Levorphanol Tartrate (Additive effect). Products include:
Levo-Dromoran 1906

Lorazepam (Additive effect). Products include:
Ativan Injection 2432
Ativan Tablets 2434

Loxapine Hydrochloride (Additive effect). Products include:
Loxitane 1213

Loxapine Succinate (Additive effect). Products include:
Loxitane Capsules 1213

Mecamylamine Hydrochloride (Reduced antihypertensive effects). Products include:
Inversine Tablets 1492

Meperidine Hydrochloride (Additive effect). Products include:
Demerol 2047
Mepergan Injection 2479

Mephobarbital (Additive effect). Products include:
Mebaral Tablets 2061

Meprobamate (Additive effect). Products include:
Deprol Tablets 2382
Equagesic Tablets 2451
Miltown Tablets 2386
PMB 200 and PMB 400 2504

Mesoridazine (Additive effect). Products include:
Serentil 686

Methadone Hydrochloride (Additive effect). Products include:
Dolophine Hydrochloride Ampoules & Vials 1260
Dolophine Hydrochloride Tablets 1261
Methadone Hydrochloride Diskets .. 1284
Methadone Hydrochloride Oral Solution & Tablets 1987

Methohexital Sodium (Additive effect). Products include:
Brevital Sodium Vials 1248

Methoxyflurane (Additive effect).
No products indexed under this heading.

Methyldopa (Reduced antihypertensive effects). Products include:
Aldoclor Tablets 1413
Aldomet Oral 1415
Aldoril Tablets 1418

Methyldopate Hydrochloride (Reduced antihypertensive effects). Products include:
Aldomet Ester HCl Injection 1417

Metoprolol Tartrate (Increases effects of sympathomimetics). Products include:
Lopressor Ampuls 1032
Lopressor HCT Tablets 1034
Lopressor Tablets 1032

Midazolam Hydrochloride (Additive effect). Products include:
Versed Injection 1924

Molindone Hydrochloride (Additive effect). Products include:
Moban Tablets & Concentrate 932

Morphine Sulfate (Additive effect). Products include:
Astramorph/PF Injection, USP (Preservative-Free) 618
Duramorph 960
Infumorph 200 and Infumorph 500 Sterile Solutions 962
MS Contin Tablets 1814
MSIR 1817
Oramorph SR (Morphine Sulfate Sustained Release Tablets) 1988
Roxanol 1991

Nadolol (Increases effects of sympathomimetics). Products include:
Corgard Tablets 701
Corzide Tablets 702

Opium Alkaloids (Additive effect). Products include:
B & O No. 15A & No. 16A Supprettes 2395
Pantopon Injectable 1911

Oxazepam (Additive effect). Products include:
Serax Capsules 2522
Serax Tablets 2522

Oxycodone Hydrochloride (Additive effect). Products include:
Percocet Tablets 950
Percodan 951
Roxicodone Tablets, Oral Solution & Intensol (Oxycodone) 1992
Tylox Capsules 1382

Penbutolol Sulfate (Increases effects of sympathomimetics). Products include:
Levatol 1832

Pentobarbital Sodium (Additive effect). Products include:
Nembutal Sodium Capsules 534
Nembutal Sodium Solution 536
Nembutal Sodium Suppositories 538

Perphenazine (Additive effect). Products include:
Etrafon 2087
Triavil Tablets 1556
Trilafon 2123

Phenelzine Sulfate (Concurrent therapy is contraindicated; increases effects of sympathomimetics). Products include:
Nardil 1742

Phenobarbital (Additive effect). Products include:
Arco-Lase Plus Tablets 607
Bellergal-S Tablets 1998
Bronkolixir .... ▣ 761
Bronkotabs Tablets .... ▣ 762
Donnatal 1858
Donnatal Extentabs 1859
Donnatal Tablets 1858
Donnazyme Tablets 1860
Kinesed Tablets 2272
Phenobarbital Elixir and Tablets 1293
Primatene Tablets-P Formula 2421
Quadrinal Tablets 1183
Tedral SA 1765

Pindolol (Increases effects of sympathomimetics). Products include:
Visken Tablets 2036

Prazepam (Additive effect). Products include:
Centrax 1693

Prochlorperazine (Additive effect). Products include:
Compazine 2201

Promethazine Hydrochloride (Additive effect). Products include:
Mepergan Injection 2479
Phenergan with Codeine 2497
Phenergan with Dextromethorphan 2499
Phenergan Injection 2493
Phenergan Suppositories 2496
Phenergan Syrup 2495
Phenergan Tablets 2496
Phenergan VC 2500
Phenergan VC with Codeine 2501

Propofol (Additive effect). Products include:
Diprivan Injection 2267

Propoxyphene Hydrochloride (Additive effect). Products include:
Darvon 1256

Wygesic Tablets 2540

Propoxyphene Napsylate (Additive effect). Products include:

Darvon-N/Darvocet-N 1254

Propranolol Hydrochloride (Increases effects of sympathomimetics). Products include:

Inderal 2459
Inderal LA Long Acting Capsules 2461
Inderide Tablets 2463
Inderide LA Long Acting Capsules 2465

Quazepam (Additive effect). Products include:

Doral Tablets 2383

Rauwolfia Serpentina (Reduced antihypertensive effects). Products include:

Raudixin Tablets 1803
Rauzide Tablets 1804

Rescinnamine (Reduced antihypertensive effects).

No products indexed under this heading.

Reserpine (Reduced antihypertensive effects). Products include:

Diupres Tablets 1461
Hydromox R Tablets 1209
Hydropres Tablets 1485
Renese-R Tablets 1786
Salutensin/Salutensin-Demi 719
Ser-Ap-Es Tablets 881
Serpasil Tablets 883
Serpasil-Apresoline Tablets 884
Serpasil-Esidrix Tablets 886

Secobarbital Sodium (Additive effect). Products include:

Seconal Sodium Pulvules 1296

Selegiline Hydrochloride (Concurrent therapy is contraindicated; increases effects of sympathomimetics). Products include:

Eldepryl 2250

Sufentanil Citrate (Additive effect). Products include:

Sufenta Injection 1147

Temazepam (Additive effect). Products include:

Restoril Capsules 2023

Thiamylal Sodium (Additive effect). Products include:

Surital Ampoules, Steri-Vials 1764

Thioridazine Hydrochloride (Additive effect). Products include:

Mellaril 2011

Thiothixene (Additive effect). Products include:

Navane Capsules and Concentrate 1954
Navane Intramuscular 1956

Timolol Maleate (Increases effects of sympathomimetics). Products include:

Blocadren Tablets 1429
Timolide Tablets 1547
Timoptic in Ocudose 1552
Timoptic Sterile Ophthalmic Solution 1550

Tranylcypromine Sulfate (Concurrent therapy is contraindicated; increases effects of sympathomimetics). Products include:

Parnate Tablets 2222

Triazolam (Additive effect). Products include:

Halcion Tablets 2340

Trifluoperazine Hydrochloride (Additive effect). Products include:

Stelazine 2226

BRICANYL INJECTION
(Terbutaline Sulfate) 1324
May interact with sympathomimetic bronchodilators, monoamine oxidase inhibitors, tricyclic antidepressants, and beta blockers. Compounds in these categories include:

Acebutolol Hydrochloride (Blocked pulmonary effects; may produce severe asthma attacks in asthmatic patients). Products include:

Sectral Capsules 2520

Albuterol (Deleterious cardiovascular effects). Products include:

Proventil Inhalation Aerosol 2117
Ventolin Inhalation Aerosol and Refill 583

Albuterol Sulfate (Deleterious cardiovascular effects). Products include:

Proventil Repetabs Tablets 2120
Proventil Solutions for Inhalation 0.5% and 0.083% 2118
Proventil Syrup 2119
Proventil Tablets 2120
Ventolin 583

Amitriptyline Hydrochloride (Potentiates terbutaline's vascular effects). Products include:

Elavil 2269
Endep Tablets 1927
Etrafon 2087
Limbitrol 1933
Triavil Tablets 1556

Amoxapine (Potentiates terbutaline's vascular effects). Products include:

Asendin Tablets 1196

Atenolol (Blocked pulmonary effects; may produce severe asthma attacks in asthmatic patients). Products include:

Tenoretic Tablets 1105
Tenormin Tablets and I.V. Injection 1107

Betaxolol Hydrochloride (Blocked pulmonary effects; may produce severe asthma attacks in asthmatic patients). Products include:

Betoptic Sterile Ophthalmic Solution 569
Betoptic S Sterile Ophthalmic Suspension 570
Kerlone Tablets 2172

Bitolterol Mesylate (Deleterious cardiovascular effects). Products include:

Tornalate 2074

Carteolol Hydrochloride (Blocked pulmonary effects; may produce severe asthma attacks in asthmatic patients). Products include:

Cartrol Tablets 507

Clomipramine Hydrochloride (Potentiates terbutaline's vascular effects). Products include:

Anafranil Capsules 650

Desipramine Hydrochloride (Potentiates terbutaline's vascular effects). Products include:

Norpramin Tablets 1340

Doxepin Hydrochloride (Potentiates terbutaline's vascular effects). Products include:

Sinequan 1960

Ephedrine Hydrochloride (Deleterious cardiovascular effects). Products include:

Amesec .... ▣ 682
Primatene Tablets-M Formula 2421
Primatene Tablets-P Formula 2421
Primatene Tablets-Regular Formula 2421
Quadrinal Tablets 1183
Quelidrine Syrup 556
Tedral SA 1765

Ephedrine Sulfate (Deleterious cardiovascular effects). Products include:

Bronkaid Tablets .... ▣ 757
Bronkolixir .... ▣ 761
Bronkotabs Tablets .... ▣ 762
Marax Tablets & DF Syrup 1954
Pazo Hemorrhoid Ointment & Suppositories 752
Vicks Vatronol Nose Drops .... ▣ 666

Ephedrine Tannate (Deleterious cardiovascular effects). Products include:

Rynatuss 2388

Epinephrine (Deleterious cardiovascular effects). Products include:

Ana-Kit Anaphylaxis Emergency Treatment Kit 1100
Bronkaid Mist .... ▣ 757
EpiPen 843
Marcaine Hydrochloride 0.5% with Epinephrine 1:200,000 (as bitartrate) 958
Marcaine Hydrochloride with Epinephrine 1:200,000 2055
Primatene Mist 2420
Sus-Phrine Injection 1006
Xylocaine with Epinephrine Injections 637

Epinephrine Hydrochloride (Deleterious cardiovascular effects). Products include:

Adrenalin Chloride Solution 1:100 & 1:1,000 1689
Epifrin .... ⊙ 244
Glaucon .... ⊙ 218

Esmolol Hydrochloride (Blocked pulmonary effects; may produce severe asthma attacks in asthmatic patients). Products include:

Brevibloc Injection 942

Ethylnorepinephrine Hydrochloride (Deleterious cardiovascular effects). Products include:

Bronkephrine Injection 2042

Furazolidone (Potentiates terbutaline's vascular effects). Products include:

Furoxone 1855

Imipramine Hydrochloride (Potentiates terbutaline's vascular effects). Products include:

Tofranil Ampuls 1038
Tofranil Tablets 1039

Imipramine Pamoate (Potentiates terbutaline's vascular effects). Products include:

Tofranil-PM Capsules 1041

Isocarboxazid (Potentiates terbutaline's vascular effects). Products include:

Marplan Tablets 1906

Isoetharine (Deleterious cardiovascular effects). Products include:

Arm-a-Med Isoetharine Inhalation Solution, USP 616
Bronkometer Aerosol 2042
Bronkosol Solution 2042

Isoproterenol Hydrochloride (Deleterious cardiovascular effects). Products include:

Isuprel Hydrochloride Injection 1:5000 2050
Isuprel Hydrochloride Mistometer 2051
Isuprel Hydrochloride Solution 1:200 & 1:100 2052
Norisodrine Aerotrol 540

Labetalol Hydrochloride (Blocked pulmonary effects; may produce severe asthma attacks in asthmatic patients). Products include:

Normodyne Injection 2108
Normodyne Tablets 2110
Normozide Tablets 2112
Trandate HCT Tablets 579
Trandate Injection 577
Trandate Tablets 579

Maprotiline Hydrochloride (Potentiates terbutaline's vascular effects). Products include:

Ludiomil Tablets 874

Metaproterenol Sulfate (Deleterious cardiovascular effects). Products include:

Alupent 674
Arm-a-Med Metaproterenol Sulfate Inhalation Solution, USP 617
Metaprel Inhalation Aerosol Bronchodilator 2014
Metaprel Inhalation Solution 2015
Metaprel 2015
Metaproterenol Sulfate Inhalation Solution, USP 912

Metoprolol Tartrate (Blocked pulmonary effects; may produce severe asthma attacks in asthmatic patients). Products include:

Lopressor Ampuls 1032
Lopressor HCT Tablets 1034
Lopressor Tablets 1032

Nadolol (Blocked pulmonary effects; may produce severe asthma attacks in asthmatic patients). Products include:

Corgard Tablets 701
Corzide Tablets 702

Nortriptyline Hydrochloride (Potentiates terbutaline's vascular effects). Products include:

Pamelor 2019

Penbutolol Sulfate (Blocked pulmonary effects; may produce severe asthma attacks in asthmatic patients). Products include:

Levatol 1832

Phenelzine Sulfate (Potentiates terbutaline's vascular effects). Products include:

Nardil 1742

Pindolol (Blocked pulmonary effects; may produce severe asthma attacks in asthmatic patients). Products include:

Visken Tablets 2036

Pirbuterol Acetate (Deleterious cardiovascular effects). Products include:

Maxair Inhaler 1311

Propranolol Hydrochloride (Blocked pulmonary effects; may produce severe asthma attacks in asthmatic patients). Products include:

Inderal 2459
Inderal LA Long Acting Capsules 2461
Inderide Tablets 2463
Inderide LA Long Acting Capsules 2465

Protriptyline Hydrochloride (Potentiates terbutaline's vascular effects). Products include:

Vivactil Tablets 1567

Selegiline Hydrochloride (Potentiates terbutaline's vascular effects). Products include:

Eldepryl 2250

Timolol Maleate (Blocked pulmonary effects; may produce severe asthma attacks in asthmatic patients). Products include:

Blocadren Tablets 1429
Timolide Tablets 1547
Timoptic in Ocudose 1552
Timoptic Sterile Ophthalmic Solution 1550

Tranylcypromine Sulfate (Potentiates terbutaline's vascular effects). Products include:

Parnate Tablets 2222

Trimipramine Maleate (Potentiates terbutaline's vascular effects). Products include:

Surmontil Capsules 2524

BRICANYL TABLETS
(Terbutaline Sulfate) 1325
May interact with sympathomimetic bronchodilators, monoamine oxidase inhibitors, tricyclic antidepressants, and beta blockers. Compounds in these categories include:

Acebutolol Hydrochloride (Blocked pulmonary effects; may produce severe asthma attacks in asthmatic patients). Products include:

Sectral Capsules 2520

Albuterol (Deleterious cardiovascular effects). Products include:
- Proventil Inhalation Aerosol 2117
- Ventolin Inhalation Aerosol and Refill 583

Albuterol Sulfate (Deleterious cardiovascular effects). Products include:
- Proventil Repetabs Tablets 2120
- Proventil Solutions for Inhalation 0.5% and 0.083% 2118
- Proventil Syrup 2119
- Proventil Tablets 2120
- Ventolin 583

Amitriptyline Hydrochloride (Potentiates terbutaline's vascular effects). Products include:
- Elavil 2269
- Endep Tablets 1927
- Etrafon 2087
- Limbitrol 1933
- Triavil Tablets 1556

Amoxapine (Potentiates terbutaline's vascular effects). Products include:
- Asendin Tablets 1196

Atenolol (Blocked pulmonary effects; may produce severe asthma attacks in asthmatic patients). Products include:
- Tenoretic Tablets 1105
- Tenormin Tablets and I.V. Injection 1107

Betaxolol Hydrochloride (Blocked pulmonary effects; may produce severe asthma attacks in asthmatic patients). Products include:
- Betoptic Sterile Ophthalmic Solution 569
- Betoptic S Sterile Ophthalmic Suspension 570
- Kerlone Tablets 2172

Bitolterol Mesylate (Deleterious cardiovascular effects). Products include:
- Tornalate 2074

Carteolol Hydrochloride (Blocked pulmonary effects; may produce severe asthma attacks in asthmatic patients). Products include:
- Cartrol Tablets 507

Clomipramine Hydrochloride (Potentiates terbutaline's vascular effects). Products include:
- Anafranil Capsules 650

Desipramine Hydrochloride (Potentiates terbutaline's vascular effects). Products include:
- Norpramin Tablets 1340

Doxepin Hydrochloride (Potentiates terbutaline's vascular effects). Products include:
- Sinequan 1960

Ephedrine Hydrochloride (Deleterious cardiovascular effects). Products include:
- Amesec .... ▣ 682
- Primatene Tablets-M Formula 2421
- Primatene Tablets-P Formula 2421
- Primatene Tablets-Regular Formula 2421
- Quadrinal Tablets 1183
- Quelidrine Syrup 556
- Tedral SA 1765

Ephedrine Sulfate (Deleterious cardiovascular effects). Products include:
- Bronkaid Tablets .... ▣ 757
- Bronkolixir .... ▣ 761
- Bronkotabs Tablets .... ▣ 762
- Marax Tablets & DF Syrup 1954
- Pazo Hemorrhoid Ointment & Suppositories 752
- Vicks Vatronol Nose Drops .... ▣ 666

Ephedrine Tannate (Deleterious cardiovascular effects). Products include:
- Rynatuss 2388

Epinephrine (Deleterious cardiovascular effects). Products include:
- Ana-Kit Anaphylaxis Emergency Treatment Kit 1100
- Bronkaid Mist .... ▣ 757
- EpiPen 843
- Marcaine Hydrochloride 0.5% with Epinephrine 1:200,000 (as bitartrate) 958
- Marcaine Hydrochloride with Epinephrine 1:200,000 2055
- Primatene Mist 2420
- Sus-Phrine Injection 1006
- Xylocaine with Epinephrine Injections 637

Epinephrine Hydrochloride (Deleterious cardiovascular effects). Products include:
- Adrenalin Chloride Solution 1:100 & 1:1,000 1689
- Epifrin .... ◉ 244
- Glaucon .... ◉ 218

Esmolol Hydrochloride (Blocked pulmonary effects; may produce severe asthma attacks in asthmatic patients). Products include:
- Brevibloc Injection 942

Ethylnorepinephrine Hydrochloride (Deleterious cardiovascular effects). Products include:
- Bronkephrine Injection 2042

Furazolidone (Potentiates terbutaline's vascular effects). Products include:
- Furoxone 1855

Imipramine Hydrochloride (Potentiates terbutaline's vascular effects). Products include:
- Tofranil Ampuls 1038
- Tofranil Tablets 1039

Imipramine Pamoate (Potentiates terbutaline's vascular effects). Products include:
- Tofranil-PM Capsules 1041

Isocarboxazid (Potentiates terbutaline's vascular effects). Products include:
- Marplan Tablets 1906

Isoetharine (Deleterious cardiovascular effects). Products include:
- Arm-a-Med Isoetharine Inhalation Solution, USP 616
- Bronkometer Aerosol 2042
- Bronkosol Solution 2042

Isoproterenol Hydrochloride (Deleterious cardiovascular effects). Products include:
- Isuprel Hydrochloride Injection 1:5000 2050
- Isuprel Hydrochloride Mistometer .. 2051
- Isuprel Hydrochloride Solution 1:200 & 1:100 2052
- Norisodrine Aerotrol 540

Labetalol Hydrochloride (Blocked pulmonary effects; may produce severe asthma attacks in asthmatic patients). Products include:
- Normodyne Injection 2108
- Normodyne Tablets 2110
- Normozide Tablets 2112
- Trandate HCT Tablets 579
- Trandate Injection 577
- Trandate Tablets 579

Maprotiline Hydrochloride (Potentiates terbutaline's vascular effects). Products include:
- Ludiomil Tablets 874

Metaproterenol Sulfate (Deleterious cardiovascular effects). Products include:
- Alupent 674
- Arm-a-Med Metaproterenol Sulfate Inhalation Solution, USP 617
- Metaprel Inhalation Aerosol Bronchodilator 2014
- Metaprel Inhalation Solution 2015
- Metaprel 2015
- Metaproterenol Sulfate Inhalation Solution, USP 912

Metoprolol Tartrate (Blocked pulmonary effects; may produce severe asthma attacks in asthmatic patients). Products include:
- Lopressor Ampuls 1032
- Lopressor HCT Tablets 1034
- Lopressor Tablets 1032

Nadolol (Blocked pulmonary effects; may produce severe asthma attacks in asthmatic patients). Products include:
- Corgard Tablets 701
- Corzide Tablets 702

Nortriptyline Hydrochloride (Potentiates terbutaline's vascular effects). Products include:
- Pamelor 2019

Penbutolol Sulfate (Blocked pulmonary effects; may produce severe asthma attacks in asthmatic patients). Products include:
- Levatol 1832

Phenelzine Sulfate (Potentiates terbutaline's vascular effects). Products include:
- Nardil 1742

Pindolol (Blocked pulmonary effects; may produce severe asthma attacks in asthmatic patients). Products include:
- Visken Tablets 2036

Pirbuterol Acetate (Deleterious cardiovascular effects). Products include:
- Maxair Inhaler 1311

Propranolol Hydrochloride (Blocked pulmonary effects; may produce severe asthma attacks in asthmatic patients). Products include:
- Inderal 2459
- Inderal LA Long Acting Capsules 2461
- Inderide Tablets 2463
- Inderide LA Long Acting Capsules .. 2465

Protriptyline Hydrochloride (Potentiates terbutaline's vascular effects). Products include:
- Vivactil Tablets 1567

Selegiline Hydrochloride (Potentiates terbutaline's vascular effects). Products include:
- Eldepryl 2250

Timolol Maleate (Blocked pulmonary effects; may produce severe asthma attacks in asthmatic patients). Products include:
- Blocadren Tablets 1429
- Timolide Tablets 1547
- Timoptic in Ocudose 1552
- Timoptic Sterile Ophthalmic Solution 1550

Tranylcypromine Sulfate (Potentiates terbutaline's vascular effects). Products include:
- Parnate Tablets 2222

Trimipramine Maleate (Potentiates terbutaline's vascular effects). Products include:
- Surmontil Capsules 2524

BROMASE CAPSULES (Proteolytic Enzymes, Vitamin C) 672
May interact with oral anticoagulants. Compounds in this category include:

Dicumarol (Concomitant use is inadvisable). Products include:
- Dicumarol Tablets 516

Warfarin Sodium (Concomitant use is inadvisable). Products include:
- Coumadin Injection & Tablets 944
- Panwarfin Tablets 547

BROMFED CAPSULES (TIMED RELEASE) (Brompheniramine Maleate, Pseudoephedrine Hydrochloride) 1615
May interact with central nervous system depressants, monoamine oxidase inhibitors, beta blockers, veratrum alkaloids, and certain other agents. Compounds in these categories include:

Acebutolol Hydrochloride (Increased sympathomimetic effect). Products include:
- Sectral Capsules 2520

Alcohol (Additive effects).

Alfentanil Hydrochloride (Additive effects). Products include:
- Alfenta Injection 1131

Alprazolam (Additive effects). Products include:
- Xanax Tablets 2367

Aprobarbital (Additive effects). Products include:
- Alurate Elixir 1883

Atenolol (Increased sympathomimetic effect). Products include:
- Tenoretic Tablets 1105
- Tenormin Tablets and I.V. Injection 1107

Betaxolol Hydrochloride (Increased sympathomimetic effect). Products include:
- Betoptic Sterile Ophthalmic Solution 569
- Betoptic S Sterile Ophthalmic Suspension 570
- Kerlone Tablets 2172

Buprenorphine (Additive effects).
- No products indexed under this heading.

Buspirone Hydrochloride (Additive effects). Products include:
- BuSpar 1401

Butabarbital (Additive effects). Products include:
- Pyridium Plus 1764

Butalbital (Additive effects). Products include:
- Esgic-Plus Tablets 1002
- Esgic Tablets & Capsules 1001
- Fioricet Tablets 2006
- Fiorinal Capsules 2007
- Fiorinal with Codeine Capsules 2008
- Fiorinal Tablets 2007
- Phrenilin 838
- Sedapap Tablets 50 mg/650 mg .. 1360

Carteolol Hydrochloride (Increased sympathomimetic effect). Products include:
- Cartrol Tablets 507

Chlordiazepoxide (Additive effects). Products include:
- Libritabs Tablets 1930
- Limbitrol 1933
- Menrium Tablets 1934

Chlordiazepoxide Hydrochloride (Additive effects). Products include:
- Librax Capsules 1929
- Librium Capsules 1931
- Librium Injectable 1932

Chlorpromazine (Additive effects). Products include:
- Thorazine 2234

Chlorprothixene (Additive effects). Products include:
- Taractan Tablets 1920

Chlorprothixene Hydrochloride (Additive effects). Products include:
- Taractan 1920

Clorazepate Dipotassium (Additive effects). Products include:
- Tranxene 556

Codeine (Additive effects). Products include:
- Calcidrine Syrup 506

Codeine Phosphate (Additive effects). Products include:
- Actifed with Codeine Cough Syrup.. 752
- Cheracol Cough Syrup 1853
- Codimal PH Syrup 846
- Dimetane-DC Cough Syrup 1857
- Empirin with Codeine Phosphate Nos. 2, 3 & 4 764
- Fiorinal with Codeine Capsules 2008

Isoclor Expectorant ... 982
Naldecon CX Adult Liquid ... 521
Novahistine DH ... 1342
Novahistine Expectorant ... 1343
Nucofed Capsules ... 2219
Nucofed Expectorant ... 2219
Nucofed Pediatric Expectorant ... 2220
Nucofed Syrup ... 2219
Phenaphen with Codeine Capsules 1865
Phenaphen-650 with Codeine Tablets ... 1866
Phenergan with Codeine ... 2497
Phenergan VC with Codeine ... 2501
Robitussin A-C Syrup ... 1875
Robitussin-DAC Syrup ... 1875
Ryna ... 741
Soma Compound w/Codeine Tablets ... 2390
Triaminic Expectorant w/Codeine .. 1996
Tussi-Organidin Liquid ... 2391
Tylenol with Codeine ... 1381

Codeine Polistirex (Additive effects).
No products indexed under this heading.

Cryptenamine Preparations (Reduced antihypertensive effects).

Dezocine (Additive effects).

Diazepam (Additive effects). Products include:
Valium Injectable ... 1937
Valium Tablets ... 1939
Valrelease Capsules ... 1923

Droperidol (Additive effects). Products include:
Inapsine Injection ... 1140
Innovar Injection ... 1141

Enflurane (Additive effects). Products include:
Ethrane ... 599

Esmolol Hydrochloride (Increased sympathomimetic effect). Products include:
Brevibloc Injection ... 942

Estazolam (Additive effects). Products include:
ProSom Tablets ... 554

Ethchlorvynol (Additive effects). Products include:
Placidyl Capsules ... 553

Ethinamate (Additive effects).
No products indexed under this heading.

Fentanyl (Additive effects). Products include:
Duragesic Transdermal System ... 1133

Fentanyl Citrate (Additive effects). Products include:
Innovar Injection ... 1141
Sublimaze Injection ... 1146

Fluphenazine Decanoate (Additive effects). Products include:
Prolixin Decanoate ... 1795

Fluphenazine Enanthate (Additive effects). Products include:
Prolixin Enanthate ... 1796

Fluphenazine Hydrochloride (Additive effects). Products include:
Prolixin Elixir ... 1793
Prolixin Injection ... 1791
Prolixin Oral Concentrate ... 1792
Prolixin Tablets ... 1793

Flurazepam Hydrochloride (Additive effects). Products include:
Dalmane Capsules ... 1927

Furazolidone (Increased sympathomimetic effect; concurrent therapy is contraindicated). Products include:
Furoxone ... 1855

Glutethimide (Additive effects).
No products indexed under this heading.

Haloperidol (Additive effects). Products include:
Haldol Injection, Tablets and Concentrate ... 1373

Haloperidol Decanoate (Additive effects). Products include:
Haldol Decanoate ... 1375

Hydrocodone Bitartrate (Additive effects). Products include:
Anexsia 5/500 Tablets ... 2196
Anexsia 7.5/650 Tablets ... 2197
Azdone Tablets ... 844
Codiclear DH Syrup ... 845
Codimal DH Syrup ... 846
Damason-P ... 1356
Hycodan Syrup, Tablets ... 927
Hycomine Compound Tablets ... 929
Hycomine Syrup ... 927
Hycotuss Expectorant Syrup ... 930
Hydrocet Capsules ... 835
Lortab ASA Tablets ... 2414
Lortab ... 2412
Ru-Tuss with Hydrocodone ... 694
Triaminic Expectorant DH ... 1995
Vicodin Tablets ... 1187
Vicodin ES Tablets ... 1189
Zydone Capsules ... 941

Hydrocodone Polistirex (Additive effects). Products include:
Tussionex Extended-Release Suspension ... 988

Hydroxyzine Hydrochloride (Additive effects). Products include:
Atarax Tablets & Syrup ... 1941
Marax Tablets & DF Syrup ... 1954
Vistaril Intramuscular Solution ... 1970

Isocarboxazid (Increased sympathomimetic effect; concurrent therapy is contraindicated). Products include:
Marplan Tablets ... 1906

Isoflurane (Additive effects). Products include:
Forane ... 600

Ketamine Hydrochloride (Additive effects). Products include:
Ketalar ... 1726

Labetalol Hydrochloride (Increased sympathomimetic effect). Products include:
Normodyne Injection ... 2108
Normodyne Tablets ... 2110
Normozide Tablets ... 2112
Trandate HCT Tablets ... 579
Trandate Injection ... 577
Trandate Tablets ... 579

Levorphanol Tartrate (Additive effects). Products include:
Levo-Dromoran ... 1906

Lorazepam (Additive effects). Products include:
Ativan Injection ... 2432
Ativan Tablets ... 2434

Loxapine Hydrochloride (Additive effects). Products include:
Loxitane ... 1213

Loxapine Succinate (Additive effects). Products include:
Loxitane Capsules ... 1213

Mecamylamine Hydrochloride (Reduced antihypertensive effects). Products include:
Inversine Tablets ... 1492

Meperidine Hydrochloride (Additive effects). Products include:
Demerol ... 2047
Mepergan Injection ... 2479

Mephobarbital (Additive effects). Products include:
Mebaral Tablets ... 2061

Meprobamate (Additive effects). Products include:
Deprol Tablets ... 2382
Equagesic Tablets ... 2451
Miltown Tablets ... 2386
PMB 200 and PMB 400 ... 2504

Mesoridazine (Additive effects). Products include:
Serentil ... 686

Methadone Hydrochloride (Additive effects). Products include:
Dolophine Hydrochloride Ampoules & Vials ... 1260
Dolophine Hydrochloride Tablets ... 1261
Methadone Hydrochloride Diskets .. 1284
Methadone Hydrochloride Oral Solution & Tablets ... 1987

Methohexital Sodium (Additive effects). Products include:
Brevital Sodium Vials ... 1248

Methoxyflurane (Additive effects).
No products indexed under this heading.

Methyldopa (Reduced antihypertensive effects). Products include:
Aldoclor Tablets ... 1413
Aldomet Oral ... 1415
Aldoril Tablets ... 1418

Methyldopate Hydrochloride (Reduced antihypertensive effects). Products include:
Aldomet Ester HCl Injection ... 1417

Metoprolol Tartrate (Increased sympathomimetic effect). Products include:
Lopressor Ampuls ... 1032
Lopressor HCT Tablets ... 1034
Lopressor Tablets ... 1032

Midazolam Hydrochloride (Additive effects). Products include:
Versed Injection ... 1924

Molindone Hydrochloride (Additive effects). Products include:
Moban Tablets & Concentrate ... 932

Morphine Sulfate (Additive effects). Products include:
Astramorph/PF Injection, USP (Preservative-Free) ... 618
Duramorph ... 960
Infumorph 200 and Infumorph 500 Sterile Solutions ... 962
MS Contin Tablets ... 1814
MSIR ... 1817
Oramorph SR (Morphine Sulfate Sustained Release Tablets) ... 1988
Roxanol ... 1991

Nadolol (Increased sympathomimetic effect). Products include:
Corgard Tablets ... 701
Corzide Tablets ... 702

Opium Alkaloids (Additive effects). Products include:
B & O No. 15A & No. 16A Supprettes ... 2395
Pantopon Injectable ... 1911

Oxazepam (Additive effects). Products include:
Serax Capsules ... 2522
Serax Tablets ... 2522

Oxycodone Hydrochloride (Additive effects). Products include:
Percocet Tablets ... 950
Percodan ... 951
Roxicodone Tablets, Oral Solution & Intensol (Oxycodone) ... 1992
Tylox Capsules ... 1382

Penbutolol Sulfate (Increased sympathomimetic effect). Products include:
Levatol ... 1832

Pentobarbital Sodium (Additive effects). Products include:
Nembutal Sodium Capsules ... 534
Nembutal Sodium Solution ... 536
Nembutal Sodium Suppositories ... 538

Perphenazine (Additive effects). Products include:
Etrafon ... 2087
Triavil Tablets ... 1556
Trilafon ... 2123

Phenelzine Sulfate (Increased sympathomimetic effect; concurrent therapy is contraindicated). Products include:
Nardil ... 1742

Phenobarbital (Additive effects). Products include:
Arco-Lase Plus Tablets ... 607
Bellergal-S Tablets ... 1998
Bronkolixir ... 761
Bronkotabs Tablets ... 762
Donnatal ... 1858
Donnatal Extentabs ... 1859
Donnatal Tablets ... 1858
Donnazyme Tablets ... 1860
Kinesed Tablets ... 2272
Phenobarbital Elixir and Tablets ... 1293
Primatene Tablets-P Formula ... 2421

Quadrinal Tablets ... 1183
Tedral SA ... 1765

Pindolol (Increased sympathomimetic effect). Products include:
Visken Tablets ... 2036

Prazepam (Additive effects). Products include:
Centrax ... 1693

Prochlorperazine (Additive effects). Products include:
Compazine ... 2201

Promethazine Hydrochloride (Additive effects). Products include:
Mepergan Injection ... 2479
Phenergan with Codeine ... 2497
Phenergan with Dextromethorphan 2499
Phenergan Injection ... 2493
Phenergan Suppositories ... 2496
Phenergan Syrup ... 2495
Phenergan Tablets ... 2496
Phenergan VC ... 2500
Phenergan VC with Codeine ... 2501

Propofol (Additive effects). Products include:
Diprivan Injection ... 2267

Propoxyphene Hydrochloride (Additive effects). Products include:
Darvon ... 1256
Wygesic Tablets ... 2540

Propoxyphene Napsylate (Additive effects). Products include:
Darvon-N/Darvocet-N ... 1254

Propranolol Hydrochloride (Increased sympathomimetic effect). Products include:
Inderal ... 2459
Inderal LA Long Acting Capsules ... 2461
Inderide Tablets ... 2463
Inderide LA Long Acting Capsules .. 2465

Quazepam (Additive effects). Products include:
Doral Tablets ... 2383

Reserpine (Reduced antihypertensive effects). Products include:
Diupres Tablets ... 1461
Hydromox R Tablets ... 1209
Hydropres Tablets ... 1485
Renese-R Tablets ... 1786
Salutensin/Salutensin-Demi ... 719
Ser-Ap-Es Tablets ... 881
Serpasil Tablets ... 883
Serpasil-Apresoline Tablets ... 884
Serpasil-Esidrix Tablets ... 886

Secobarbital Sodium (Additive effects). Products include:
Seconal Sodium Pulvules ... 1296

Selegiline Hydrochloride (Increased sympathomimetic effect; concurrent therapy is contraindicated). Products include:
Eldepryl ... 2250

Sufentanil Citrate (Additive effects). Products include:
Sufenta Injection ... 1147

Temazepam (Additive effects). Products include:
Restoril Capsules ... 2023

Thiamylal Sodium (Additive effects). Products include:
Surital Ampoules, Steri-Vials ... 1764

Thioridazine Hydrochloride (Additive effects). Products include:
Mellaril ... 2011

Thiothixene (Additive effects). Products include:
Navane Capsules and Concentrate 1954
Navane Intramuscular ... 1956

Timolol Maleate (Increased sympathomimetic effect). Products include:
Blocadren Tablets ... 1429
Timolide Tablets ... 1547
Timoptic in Ocudose ... 1552
Timoptic Sterile Ophthalmic Solution ... 1550

Tranylcypromine Sulfate (Increased sympathomimetic effect; concurrent therapy is contraindicated). Products include:
Parnate Tablets ... 2222

Triazolam (Additive effects). Products include:
Halcion Tablets 2340

Trifluoperazine Hydrochloride (Additive effects). Products include:
Stelazine 2226

BROMFED SYRUP
(Brompheniramine Maleate, Pseudoephedrine Hydrochloride) 628
May interact with monoamine oxidase inhibitors. Compounds in this category include:

Alcohol (Effect not specified).

Furazolidone (Effect not specified). Products include:
Furoxone 1855

Isocarboxazid (Effect not specified). Products include:
Marplan Tablets 1906

Pargyline Hydrochloride (Effect not specified).
No products indexed under this heading.

Phenelzine Sulfate (Effect not specified). Products include:
Nardil 1742

Selegiline Hydrochloride (Effect not specified). Products include:
Eldepryl 2250

Tranylcypromine Sulfate (Effect not specified). Products include:
Parnate Tablets 2222

BROMFED TABLETS
(Brompheniramine Maleate, Pseudoephedrine Hydrochloride) 1615
See **Bromfed Capsules (Timed Release)**

BROMFED-PD CAPSULES (TIMED RELEASE)
(Brompheniramine Maleate, Pseudoephedrine Hydrochloride) 1615
See **Bromfed Capsules (Timed Release)**

BRONKAID MIST
(Epinephrine) 757
May interact with antihypertensives and antidepressant drugs. Compounds in these categories include:

Acebutolol Hydrochloride (Concurrent use is not recommended without physician's consultation). Products include:
Sectral Capsules 2520

Amitriptyline Hydrochloride (Concurrent use is not recommended without physician's consultation). Products include:
Elavil 2269
Endep Tablets 1927
Etrafon 2087
Limbitrol 1933
Triavil Tablets 1556

Amoxapine (Concurrent use is not recommended without physician's consultation). Products include:
Asendin Tablets 1196

Atenolol (Concurrent use is not recommended without physician's consultation). Products include:
Tenoretic Tablets 1105
Tenormin Tablets and I.V. Injection 1107

Benazepril Hydrochloride (Concurrent use is not recommended without physician's consultation). Products include:
Lotensin Tablets 872

Bendroflumethiazide (Concurrent use is not recommended without physician's consultation). Products include:
Corzide Tablets 702
Naturetin Tablets 1789
Rauzide Tablets 1804

Betaxolol Hydrochloride (Concurrent use is not recommended without physician's consultation). Products include:
Betoptic Sterile Ophthalmic Solution 569
Betoptic S Sterile Ophthalmic Suspension 570
Kerlone Tablets 2172

Bupropion Hydrochloride (Concurrent use is not recommended without physician's consultation). Products include:
Wellbutrin Tablets 821

Captopril (Concurrent use is not recommended without physician's consultation). Products include:
Capoten 2255
Capozide 2258

Carteolol Hydrochloride (Concurrent use is not recommended without physician's consultation). Products include:
Cartrol Tablets 507

Chlorothiazide (Concurrent use is not recommended without physician's consultation). Products include:
Aldoclor Tablets 1413
Diupres Tablets 1461
Diuril Oral 1464

Chlorothiazide Sodium (Concurrent use is not recommended without physician's consultation). Products include:
Diuril Sodium Intravenous 1463

Chlorthalidone (Concurrent use is not recommended without physician's consultation). Products include:
Combipres Tablets 678
Tenoretic Tablets 1105
Thalitone Tablets 687

Clonidine (Concurrent use is not recommended without physician's consultation). Products include:
Catapres-TTS 677

Clonidine Hydrochloride (Concurrent use is not recommended without physician's consultation). Products include:
Catapres Tablets 676
Combipres Tablets 678

Deserpidine (Concurrent use is not recommended without physician's consultation). Products include:
Enduronyl 518
Harmonyl Tablets 528
Oreticyl 545

Desipramine Hydrochloride (Concurrent use is not recommended without physician's consultation). Products include:
Norpramin Tablets 1340

Diazoxide (Concurrent use is not recommended without physician's consultation). Products include:
Hyperstat I.V. Injection 2095
Proglycem 649

Doxazosin Mesylate (Concurrent use is not recommended without physician's consultation). Products include:
Cardura Tablets 1941

Doxepin Hydrochloride (Concurrent use is not recommended without physician's consultation). Products include:
Sinequan 1960

Enalapril Maleate (Concurrent use is not recommended without physician's consultation). Products include:
Vaseretic Tablets 1559
Vasotec Tablets 1564

Enalaprilat (Concurrent use is not recommended without physician's consultation). Products include:
Vasotec I.V. 1562

Esmolol Hydrochloride (Concurrent use is not recommended without physician's consultation). Products include:
Brevibloc Injection 942

Felodipine (Concurrent use is not recommended without physician's consultation). Products include:
Plendil Extended-Release Tablets 1526

Fluoxetine Hydrochloride (Concurrent use is not recommended without physician's consultation). Products include:
Prozac Pulvules 920

Fosinopril Sodium (Concurrent use is not recommended without physician's consultation). Products include:
Monopril Tablets 1406

Furosemide (Concurrent use is not recommended without physician's consultation). Products include:
Lasix 1093

Guanabenz Acetate (Concurrent use is not recommended without physician's consultation). Products include:
Wytensin Tablets 2542

Guanethidine Monosulfate (Concurrent use is not recommended without physician's consultation). Products include:
Esimil Tablets 864
Ismelin Tablets 869

Hydralazine Hydrochloride (Concurrent use is not recommended without physician's consultation). Products include:
Apresazide Capsules 854
Apresoline Hydrochloride Parenteral (Ampuls) 856
Apresoline Hydrochloride Tablets 855
Apresoline-Esidrix Tablets 857
Ser-Ap-Es Tablets 881
Serpasil-Apresoline Tablets 884

Hydrochlorothiazide (Concurrent use is not recommended without physician's consultation). Products include:
Aldactazide 2150
Aldoril Tablets 1418
Apresazide Capsules 854
Apresoline-Esidrix Tablets 857
Capozide 2258
Dyazide Capsules 2208
Esidrix Tablets 863
Esimil Tablets 864
HydroDIURIL Tablets 1484
Hydropres Tablets 1485
Inderide Tablets 2463
Inderide LA Long Acting Capsules 2465
Lopressor HCT Tablets 1034
Maxzide 1215
Moduretic Tablets 1510
Normozide Tablets 2112
Oretic Tablets 544
Oreticyl 545
Prinzide Tablets 1540
Ser-Ap-Es Tablets 881
Serpasil-Esidrix Tablets 886
Timolide Tablets 1547
Trandate HCT Tablets 579
Vaseretic Tablets 1559
Zestoretic 2274

Hydroflumethiazide (Concurrent use is not recommended without physician's consultation). Products include:
Diucardin Tablets 2450
Saluron 718
Salutensin/Salutensin-Demi 719

Imipramine Hydrochloride (Concurrent use is not recommended without physician's consultation). Products include:
Tofranil Ampuls 1038
Tofranil Tablets 1039

Imipramine Pamoate (Concurrent use is not recommended without physician's consultation). Products include:
Tofranil-PM Capsules 1041

Indapamide (Concurrent use is not recommended without physician's consultation). Products include:
Lozol Tablets 1843

Isocarboxazid (Concurrent use is not recommended without physician's consultation). Products include:
Marplan Tablets 1906

Isradipine (Concurrent use is not recommended without physician's consultation). Products include:
DynaCirc Capsules 2004

Labetalol Hydrochloride (Concurrent use is not recommended without physician's consultation). Products include:
Normodyne Injection 2108
Normodyne Tablets 2110
Normozide Tablets 2112
Trandate HCT Tablets 579
Trandate Injection 577
Trandate Tablets 579

Lisinopril (Concurrent use is not recommended without physician's consultation). Products include:
Prinivil Tablets 1538
Prinzide Tablets 1540
Zestoretic 2274
Zestril Tablets 2277

Maprotiline Hydrochloride (Concurrent use is not recommended without physician's consultation). Products include:
Ludiomil Tablets 874

Mecamylamine Hydrochloride (Concurrent use is not recommended without physician's consultation). Products include:
Inversine Tablets 1492

Methyclothiazide (Concurrent use is not recommended without physician's consultation). Products include:
Enduron Tablets 517
Enduronyl 518

Methyldopa (Concurrent use is not recommended without physician's consultation). Products include:
Aldoclor Tablets 1413
Aldomet Oral 1415
Aldoril Tablets 1418

Methyldopate Hydrochloride (Concurrent use is not recommended without physician's consultation). Products include:
Aldomet Ester HCl Injection 1417

Metolazone (Concurrent use is not recommended without physician's consultation). Products include:
Diulo 2129
Mykrox ½ mg Tablets 984
Zaroxolyn Tablets 989

Metoprolol Tartrate (Concurrent use is not recommended without physician's consultation). Products include:
Lopressor Ampuls 1032
Lopressor HCT Tablets 1034
Lopressor Tablets 1032

Metyrosine (Concurrent use is not recommended without physician's consultation). Products include:
Demser Capsules 1460

Minoxidil (Concurrent use is not recommended without physician's consultation). Products include:
Loniten Tablets 2346
Rogaine Topical Solution 2357

Nadolol (Concurrent use is not recommended without physician's consultation). Products include:
Corgard Tablets 701
Corzide Tablets 702

Nicardipine Hydrochloride (Concurrent use is not recommended without physician's consultation). Products include:
Cardene Capsules ... 2290

Nitroglycerin (Concurrent use is not recommended without physician's consultation). Products include:
Deponit NTG Transdermal Delivery System ... 2143
Minitran Transdermal Delivery System ... 1312
Nitro-Bid Ointment ... 1339
Nitro-Bid Capsules ... 1338
Nitrodisc ... 2176
Nitro-Dur (nitroglycerin) Transdermal Infusion System ... 1164
Nitrogard Tablets ... 1004
Nitrolingual Spray ... 1846
Nitrostat Tablets ... 1743
Transderm-Nitro Transdermal Therapeutic System ... 2283

Nortriptyline Hydrochloride (Concurrent use is not recommended without physician's consultation). Products include:
Pamelor ... 2019

Penbutolol Sulfate (Concurrent use is not recommended without physician's consultation). Products include:
Levatol ... 1832

Phenelzine Sulfate (Concurrent use is not recommended without physician's consultation). Products include:
Nardil ... 1742

Phenoxybenzamine Hydrochloride (Concurrent use is not recommended without physician's consultation). Products include:
Dibenzyline Capsules ... 2207

Phentolamine Mesylate (Concurrent use is not recommended without physician's consultation). Products include:
Regitine ... 878

Pindolol (Concurrent use is not recommended without physician's consultation). Products include:
Visken Tablets ... 2036

Polythiazide (Concurrent use is not recommended without physician's consultation). Products include:
Minizide Capsules ... 1779
Renese Tablets ... 1785
Renese-R Tablets ... 1786

Prazosin Hydrochloride (Concurrent use is not recommended without physician's consultation). Products include:
Minipress Capsules ... 1778
Minizide Capsules ... 1779

Propranolol Hydrochloride (Concurrent use is not recommended without physician's consultation). Products include:
Inderal ... 2459
Inderal LA Long Acting Capsules ... 2461
Inderide Tablets ... 2463
Inderide LA Long Acting Capsules ... 2465

Protriptyline Hydrochloride (Concurrent use is not recommended without physician's consultation). Products include:
Vivactil Tablets ... 1567

Ramipril (Concurrent use is not recommended without physician's consultation). Products include:
Altace Capsules ... 1086

Rauwolfia Serpentina (Concurrent use is not recommended without physician's consultation). Products include:
Raudixin Tablets ... 1803
Rauzide Tablets ... 1804

Rescinnamine (Concurrent use is not recommended without physician's consultation).
No products indexed under this heading.

Reserpine (Concurrent use is not recommended without physician's consultation). Products include:
Diupres Tablets ... 1461
Hydromox R Tablets ... 1209
Hydropres Tablets ... 1485
Renese-R Tablets ... 1786
Salutensin/Salutensin-Demi ... 719
Ser-Ap-Es Tablets ... 881
Serpasil Tablets ... 883
Serpasil-Apresoline Tablets ... 884
Serpasil-Esidrix Tablets ... 886

Sodium Nitroprusside (Concurrent use is not recommended without physician's consultation). Products include:
Nipride I.V. Infusion ... 1909

Terazosin Hydrochloride (Concurrent use is not recommended without physician's consultation). Products include:
Hytrin Tablets ... 529

Timolol Maleate (Concurrent use is not recommended without physician's consultation). Products include:
Blocadren Tablets ... 1429
Timolide Tablets ... 1547
Timoptic in Ocudose ... 1552
Timoptic Sterile Ophthalmic Solution ... 1550

Tranylcypromine Sulfate (Concurrent use is not recommended without physician's consultation). Products include:
Parnate Tablets ... 2222

Trazodone Hydrochloride (Concurrent use is not recommended without physician's consultation). Products include:
Desyrel and Desyrel Dividose ... 1404

Trimethaphan Camsylate (Concurrent use is not recommended without physician's consultation). Products include:
Arfonad Ampuls ... 1887

Trimipramine Maleate (Concurrent use is not recommended without physician's consultation). Products include:
Surmontil Capsules ... 2524

BRONKAID MIST SUSPENSION
(Epinephrine Bitartrate) ... ▣ 757
May interact with antihypertensives and antidepressant drugs. Compounds in these categories include:

Acebutolol Hydrochloride (Concurrent use is not recommended without physician's consultation). Products include:
Sectral Capsules ... 2520

Amitriptyline Hydrochloride (Concurrent use is not recommended without physician's consultation). Products include:
Elavil ... 2269
Endep Tablets ... 1927
Etrafon ... 2087
Limbitrol ... 1933
Triavil Tablets ... 1556

Amoxapine (Concurrent use is not recommended without physician's consultation). Products include:
Asendin Tablets ... 1196

Atenolol (Concurrent use is not recommended without physician's consultation). Products include:
Tenoretic Tablets ... 1105
Tenormin Tablets and I.V. Injection 1107

Benazepril Hydrochloride (Concurrent use is not recommended without physician's consultation). Products include:
Lotensin Tablets ... 872

Bendroflumethiazide (Concurrent use is not recommended without physician's consultation). Products include:
Corzide Tablets ... 702
Naturetin Tablets ... 1789
Rauzide Tablets ... 1804

Betaxolol Hydrochloride (Concurrent use is not recommended without physician's consultation). Products include:
Betoptic Sterile Ophthalmic Solution ... 569
Betoptic S Sterile Ophthalmic Suspension ... 570
Kerlone Tablets ... 2172

Bupropion Hydrochloride (Concurrent use is not recommended without physician's consultation). Products include:
Wellbutrin Tablets ... 821

Captopril (Concurrent use is not recommended without physician's consultation). Products include:
Capoten ... 2255
Capozide ... 2258

Carteolol Hydrochloride (Concurrent use is not recommended without physician's consultation). Products include:
Cartrol Tablets ... 507

Chlorothiazide (Concurrent use is not recommended without physician's consultation). Products include:
Aldoclor Tablets ... 1413
Diupres Tablets ... 1461
Diuril Oral ... 1464

Chlorothiazide Sodium (Concurrent use is not recommended without physician's consultation). Products include:
Diuril Sodium Intravenous ... 1463

Chlorthalidone (Concurrent use is not recommended without physician's consultation). Products include:
Combipres Tablets ... 678
Tenoretic Tablets ... 1105
Thalitone Tablets ... 687

Clonidine (Concurrent use is not recommended without physician's consultation). Products include:
Catapres-TTS ... 677

Clonidine Hydrochloride (Concurrent use is not recommended without physician's consultation). Products include:
Catapres Tablets ... 676
Combipres Tablets ... 678

Deserpidine (Concurrent use is not recommended without physician's consultation). Products include:
Enduronyl ... 518
Harmonyl Tablets ... 528
Oreticyl ... 545

Desipramine Hydrochloride (Concurrent use is not recommended without physician's consultation). Products include:
Norpramin Tablets ... 1340

Diazoxide (Concurrent use is not recommended without physician's consultation). Products include:
Hyperstat I.V. Injection ... 2095
Proglycem ... 649

Doxazosin Mesylate (Concurrent use is not recommended without physician's consultation). Products include:
Cardura Tablets ... 1941

Doxepin Hydrochloride (Concurrent use is not recommended without physician's consultation). Products include:
Sinequan ... 1960

Enalapril Maleate (Concurrent use is not recommended without physician's consultation). Products include:
Vaseretic Tablets ... 1559
Vasotec Tablets ... 1564

Enalaprilat (Concurrent use is not recommended without physician's consultation). Products include:
Vasotec I.V. ... 1562

Esmolol Hydrochloride (Concurrent use is not recommended without physician's consultation). Products include:
Brevibloc Injection ... 942

Felodipine (Concurrent use is not recommended without physician's consultation). Products include:
Plendil Extended-Release Tablets ... 1526

Fluoxetine Hydrochloride (Concurrent use is not recommended without physician's consultation). Products include:
Prozac Pulvules ... 920

Fosinopril Sodium (Concurrent use is not recommended without physician's consultation). Products include:
Monopril Tablets ... 1406

Furosemide (Concurrent use is not recommended without physician's consultation). Products include:
Lasix ... 1093

Guanabenz Acetate (Concurrent use is not recommended without physician's consultation). Products include:
Wytensin Tablets ... 2542

Guanethidine Monosulfate (Concurrent use is not recommended without physician's consultation). Products include:
Esimil Tablets ... 864
Ismelin Tablets ... 869

Hydralazine Hydrochloride (Concurrent use is not recommended without physician's consultation). Products include:
Apresazide Capsules ... 854
Apresoline Hydrochloride Parenteral (Ampuls) ... 856
Apresoline Hydrochloride Tablets ... 855
Apresoline-Esidrix Tablets ... 857
Ser-Ap-Es Tablets ... 881
Serpasil-Apresoline Tablets ... 884

Hydrochlorothiazide (Concurrent use is not recommended without physician's consultation). Products include:
Aldactazide ... 2150
Aldoril Tablets ... 1418
Apresazide Capsules ... 854
Apresoline-Esidrix Tablets ... 857
Capozide ... 2258
Dyazide Capsules ... 2208
Esidrix Tablets ... 863
Esimil Tablets ... 864
HydroDIURIL Tablets ... 1484
Hydropres Tablets ... 1485
Inderide Tablets ... 2463
Inderide LA Long Acting Capsules ... 2465
Lopressor HCT Tablets ... 1034
Maxzide ... 1215
Moduretic Tablets ... 1510
Normozide Tablets ... 2112
Oretic Tablets ... 544
Oreticyl ... 545
Prinzide Tablets ... 1540
Ser-Ap-Es Tablets ... 881
Serpasil-Esidrix Tablets ... 886
Timolide Tablets ... 1547
Trandate HCT Tablets ... 579
Vaseretic Tablets ... 1559
Zestoretic ... 2274

Hydroflumethiazide (Concurrent use is not recommended without physician's consultation). Products include:

Diucardin Tablets 2450
Saluron 718
Salutensin/Salutensin-Demi 719

Imipramine Hydrochloride (Concurrent use is not recommended without physician's consultation). Products include:

Tofranil Ampuls 1038
Tofranil Tablets 1039

Imipramine Pamoate (Concurrent use is not recommended without physician's consultation). Products include:

Tofranil-PM Capsules 1041

Indapamide (Concurrent use is not recommended without physician's consultation). Products include:

Lozol Tablets 1843

Isocarboxazid (Concurrent use is not recommended without physician's consultation). Products include:

Marplan Tablets 1906

Isradipine (Concurrent use is not recommended without physician's consultation). Products include:

DynaCirc Capsules 2004

Labetalol Hydrochloride (Concurrent use is not recommended without physician's consultation). Products include:

Normodyne Injection 2108
Normodyne Tablets 2110
Normozide Tablets 2112
Trandate HCT Tablets 579
Trandate Injection 577
Trandate Tablets 579

Lisinopril (Concurrent use is not recommended without physician's consultation). Products include:

Prinivil Tablets 1538
Prinzide Tablets 1540
Zestoretic 2274
Zestril Tablets 2277

Maprotiline Hydrochloride (Concurrent use is not recommended without physician's consultation). Products include:

Ludiomil Tablets 874

Mecamylamine Hydrochloride (Concurrent use is not recommended without physician's consultation). Products include:

Inversine Tablets 1492

Methyclothiazide (Concurrent use is not recommended without physician's consultation). Products include:

Enduron Tablets 517
Enduronyl 518

Methyldopa (Concurrent use is not recommended without physician's consultation). Products include:

Aldoclor Tablets 1413
Aldomet Oral 1415
Aldoril Tablets 1418

Methyldopate Hydrochloride (Concurrent use is not recommended without physician's consultation). Products include:

Aldomet Ester HCl Injection 1417

Metolazone (Concurrent use is not recommended without physician's consultation). Products include:

Diulo 2129
Mykrox ½ mg Tablets 984
Zaroxolyn Tablets 989

Metoprolol Tartrate (Concurrent use is not recommended without physician's consultation). Products include:

Lopressor Ampuls 1032
Lopressor HCT Tablets 1034
Lopressor Tablets 1032

Metyrosine (Concurrent use is not recommended without physician's consultation). Products include:

Demser Capsules 1460

Minoxidil (Concurrent use is not recommended without physician's consultation). Products include:

Loniten Tablets 2346
Rogaine Topical Solution 2357

Nadolol (Concurrent use is not recommended without physician's consultation). Products include:

Corgard Tablets 701
Corzide Tablets 702

Nicardipine Hydrochloride (Concurrent use is not recommended without physician's consultation). Products include:

Cardene Capsules 2290

Nitroglycerin (Concurrent use is not recommended without physician's consultation). Products include:

Deponit NTG Transdermal Delivery System 2143
Minitran Transdermal Delivery System 1312
Nitro-Bid Ointment 1339
Nitro-Bid Capsules 1338
Nitrodisc 2176
Nitro-Dur (nitroglycerin) Transdermal Infusion System 1164
Nitrogard Tablets 1004
Nitrolingual Spray 1846
Nitrostat Tablets 1743
Transderm-Nitro Transdermal Therapeutic System 2283

Nortriptyline Hydrochloride (Concurrent use is not recommended without physician's consultation). Products include:

Pamelor 2019

Penbutolol Sulfate (Concurrent use is not recommended without physician's consultation). Products include:

Levatol 1832

Phenelzine Sulfate (Concurrent use is not recommended without physician's consultation). Products include:

Nardil 1742

Phenoxybenzamine Hydrochloride (Concurrent use is not recommended without physician's consultation). Products include:

Dibenzyline Capsules 2207

Phentolamine Mesylate (Concurrent use is not recommended without physician's consultation). Products include:

Regitine 878

Pindolol (Concurrent use is not recommended without physician's consultation). Products include:

Visken Tablets 2036

Polythiazide (Concurrent use is not recommended without physician's consultation). Products include:

Minizide Capsules 1779
Renese Tablets 1785
Renese-R Tablets 1786

Prazosin Hydrochloride (Concurrent use is not recommended without physician's consultation). Products include:

Minipress Capsules 1778
Minizide Capsules 1779

Propranolol Hydrochloride (Concurrent use is not recommended without physician's consultation). Products include:

Inderal 2459
Inderal LA Long Acting Capsules 2461
Inderide Tablets 2463
Inderide LA Long Acting Capsules .. 2465

Protriptyline Hydrochloride (Concurrent use is not recommended without physician's consultation). Products include:

Vivactil Tablets 1567

Ramipril (Concurrent use is not recommended without physician's consultation). Products include:

Altace Capsules 1086

Rauwolfia Serpentina (Concurrent use is not recommended without physician's consultation). Products include:

Raudixin Tablets 1803
Rauzide Tablets 1804

Rescinnamine (Concurrent use is not recommended without physician's consultation).

No products indexed under this heading.

Reserpine (Concurrent use is not recommended without physician's consultation). Products include:

Diupres Tablets 1461
Hydromox R Tablets 1209
Hydropres Tablets 1485
Renese-R Tablets 1786
Salutensin/Salutensin-Demi 719
Ser-Ap-Es Tablets 881
Serpasil Tablets 883
Serpasil-Apresoline Tablets 884
Serpasil-Esidrix Tablets 886

Sodium Nitroprusside (Concurrent use is not recommended without physician's consultation). Products include:

Nipride I.V. Infusion 1909

Terazosin Hydrochloride (Concurrent use is not recommended without physician's consultation). Products include:

Hytrin Tablets 529

Timolol Maleate (Concurrent use is not recommended without physician's consultation). Products include:

Blocadren Tablets 1429
Timolide Tablets 1547
Timoptic in Ocudose 1552
Timoptic Sterile Ophthalmic Solution 1550

Tranylcypromine Sulfate (Concurrent use is not recommended without physician's consultation). Products include:

Parnate Tablets 2222

Trazodone Hydrochloride (Concurrent use is not recommended without physician's consultation). Products include:

Desyrel and Desyrel Dividose 1404

Trimethaphan Camsylate (Concurrent use is not recommended without physician's consultation). Products include:

Arfonad Ampuls 1887

Trimipramine Maleate (Concurrent use is not recommended without physician's consultation). Products include:

Surmontil Capsules 2524

BRONKAID TABLETS

(Epinephrine, Guaifenesin, Theophylline) .... ▣ 757

May interact with antihypertensives, tricyclic antidepressants, sympathomimetic bronchodilators, and xanthine bronchodilators. Compounds in these categories include:

Product labeling recommends physician's supervision for concurrent administration of these drugs ().

BRONKEPHRINE INJECTION

(Ethylnorepinephrine Hydrochloride) 2042

May interact with sympathomimetic aerosal bronchodilators. Compounds in this category include:

Albuterol (Excessive tachycardia). Products include:

Proventil Inhalation Aerosol 2117
Ventolin Inhalation Aerosol and Refill 583

Albuterol Sulfate (Excessive tachycardia). Products include:

Proventil Repetabs Tablets 2120
Proventil Solutions for Inhalation 0.5% and 0.083% 2118
Proventil Syrup 2119
Proventil Tablets 2120
Ventolin 583

Dobutamine Hydrochloride (Excessive tachycardia). Products include:

Dobutrex Solution Vials 1259

Dopamine Hydrochloride (Excessive tachycardia). Products include:

Intropin Injection 930

Ephedrine Hydrochloride (Excessive tachycardia). Products include:

Amesec .... ▣ 682
Primatene Tablets-M Formula 2421
Primatene Tablets-P Formula 2421
Primatene Tablets-Regular Formula 2421
Quadrinal Tablets 1183
Quelidrine Syrup 556
Tedral SA 1765

Ephedrine Sulfate (Excessive tachycardia). Products include:

Bronkaid Tablets .... ▣ 757
Bronkolixir .... ▣ 761
Bronkotabs Tablets .... ▣ 762
Marax Tablets & DF Syrup 1954
Pazo Hemorrhoid Ointment & Suppositories 752
Vicks Vatronol Nose Drops .... ▣ 666

Ephedrine Tannate (Excessive tachycardia). Products include:

Rynatuss 2388

Epinephrine (Excessive tachycardia). Products include:

Ana-Kit Anaphylaxis Emergency Treatment Kit 1100
Bronkaid Mist .... ▣ 757
EpiPen 843
Marcaine Hydrochloride 0.5% with Epinephrine 1:200,000 (as bitartrate) 958
Marcaine Hydrochloride with Epinephrine 1:200,000 2055
Primatene Mist 2420
Sus-Phrine Injection 1006
Xylocaine with Epinephrine Injections 637

Epinephrine Bitartrate (Excessive tachycardia). Products include:

AsthmaHaler Mist Epinephrine Bitartrate Bronchodilator .... ▣ 616
Bronkaid Mist Suspension .... ▣ 757
Primatene Mist Suspension 2421

Epinephrine Hydrochloride (Excessive tachycardia). Products include:

Adrenalin Chloride Solution 1:100 & 1:1,000 1689
Epifrin .... ⊙ 244
Glaucon .... ⊙ 218

Isoproterenol Hydrochloride (Excessive tachycardia). Products include:

Isuprel Hydrochloride Injection 1:5000 2050
Isuprel Hydrochloride Mistometer .. 2051
Isuprel Hydrochloride Solution 1:200 & 1:100 2052
Norisodrine Aerotrol 540

Metaproterenol Sulfate (Excessive tachycardia). Products include:

Alupent 674
Arm-a-Med Metaproterenol Sulfate Inhalation Solution, USP 617
Metaprel Inhalation Aerosol Bronchodilator 2014
Metaprel Inhalation Solution 2015
Metaprel 2015

Metaproterenol Sulfate Inhalation Solution, USP 912

Metaraminol Bitartrate (Excessive tachycardia). Products include:
Aramine Injection 1424

Methoxamine Hydrochloride (Excessive tachycardia). Products include:
Vasoxyl Injection 819

Norepinephrine Bitartrate (Excessive tachycardia). Products include:
Levophed Bitartrate Injection 2054

Phenylephrine Bitartrate (Excessive tachycardia).
No products indexed under this heading.

Phenylephrine Hydrochloride (Excessive tachycardia). Products include:
AK-Dilate Solution 2.5% and 10% ⊙ 203
Atrohist Sprinkle Capsules 558
Cerose-DM 2443
Codimal 846
Comhist LA Capsules 1618
Congespirin For Children Aspirin Free Chewable Cold Tablets 748
Cyclomydril ⊙ 216
Deconsal Sprinkle Capsules 559
Dimetane Decongestant ▣ 673
Dristan Decongestant/Antihistamine/Analgesic Coated Caplets ▣ 749
Dristan Cold Nasal Decongestant/Antihistamine/ Analgesic Coated Tablets 2419
Dristan Advanced Formula Decongestant/Antihistamine/Analgesic Tablets ▣ 749
Dristan Nasal Spray, Menthol 2419
Dristan Nasal Spray, Regular and Regular with Metered Pump 2419
Entex Capsules 1623
Entex Liquid 1623
Sinus Excedrin Analgesic, Decongestant Tablets & Caplets 750
Extendryl 994
4-Way Fast Acting Nasal Spray - Original Formula (regular & mentholated) & Metered Spray Pump (regular) 751
Hycomine Compound Tablets 929
Murocoll-2 Sterile Ophthalmic Solution ⊙ 261
Mydfrin 2.5% ⊙ 224
Naldecon Syrup, Tablets, Pediatric Drops and Pediatric Syrup 709
Neo-Synephrine Hydrochloride 1% Carpuject 2063
Neo-Synephrine Hydrochloride 1% Injection 2063
Neo-Synephrine Hydrochloride (Ophthalmic) 2064
Neo-Synephrine ▣ 759
Nöstril Nasal Decongestant ▣ 520
Novahistine Elixir ▣ 596
Phenergan VC 2500
Phenergan VC with Codeine 2501
Prefrin Liquifilm Vasoconstrictor and Lubricant Eye Drops ⊙ 254
Prefrin-A ⊙ 255
Quelidrine Syrup 556
Relief Vasoconstrictor and Lubricant Eye Drops ⊙ 256
Robitussin Night Relief ▣ 677
Ru-Tuss with Hydrocodone 694
Ru-Tuss Tablets 693
Vasosulf ⊙ 279
Vicks Sinex ▣ 665
Zincfrin ⊙ 230

Phenylephrine Tannate (Excessive tachycardia). Products include:
Rynatan 2387
Rynatuss 2388

Phenylpropanolamine Hydrochloride (Excessive tachycardia). Products include:
A.R.M. Allergy Relief Medicine Caplets ▣ 615
Acutrim ▣ 548
Allerest ▣ 559
BC Cold Powder ▣ 517
Cheracol Plus Head Cold/Cough Formula ▣ 667
Codimal Expectorant 846
Comtrex Multi-Symptom Cold Reliever Tablets/Caplets/Liqui-Gels/Liquid 745
Contac Continuous Action Decongestant/Antihistamine Capsules ▣ 710
Contac Maximum Strength Continuous Action Decongestant/Antihistamine Caplets ▣ 709
Contac Severe Cold and Flu Formula Caplets ▣ 711
Coricidin 'D' Decongestant Tablets ▣ 695
Coricidin Demilets Tablets for Children ▣ 696
Demazin Nasal Decongestant/Antihistamine Repetabs Tablets & Syrup ▣ 697
Dexatrim ▣ 733
Dimetane-DC Cough Syrup 1857
Dimetapp Elixir ▣ 673
Dimetapp DM Elixir ▣ 674
Dimetapp Extentabs ▣ 674
Dimetapp Plus Caplets ▣ 675
Dimetapp Tablets ▣ 675
Entex Capsules 1623
Entex LA Tablets 1623
Entex Liquid 1623
4-Way Cold Tablets 750
Hycomine Syrup 927
Naldecon CX Adult Liquid ▣ 521
Naldecon DX Adult Liquid ▣ 521
Naldecon DX Children's Syrup ▣ 522
Naldecon DX Pediatric Drops ▣ 522
Naldecon EX Children's Syrup ▣ 522
Naldecon EX Pediatric Drops ▣ 523
Naldecon Syrup, Tablets, Pediatric Drops and Pediatric Syrup 709
Nolamine Tablets 838
Nolex LA Tablets 838
Ornade Spansule Capsules 2221
Orthoxicol Cough Syrup ▣ 668
Propagest 839
Pyrroxate Capsules ▣ 669
Robitussin-CF ▣ 676
Ru-Tuss II Capsules 693
Ru-Tuss with Hydrocodone 694
Ru-Tuss Tablets 693
Sine-Off Sinus Medicine Tablets-Aspirin Formula ▣ 722
Sinulin 840
St. Joseph Cold Tablets for Children ▣ 704
Tavist-D Tablets 2035
Triaminic Allergy Tablets ▣ 688
Triaminic Chewables ▣ 688
Triaminic Cold Tablets ▣ 688
Triaminic Expectorant ▣ 688
Triaminic Expectorant w/Codeine 1996
Triaminic Expectorant DH 1995
Triaminic Oral Infant Drops 1996
Triaminic Syrup ▣ 689
Triaminic-12 Tablets ▣ 690
Triaminic-DM Syrup ▣ 689
Triaminicin Tablets ▣ 690
Triaminicol Multi-Symptom Cold Tablets ▣ 691
Triaminicol Multi-Symptom Relief ▣ 691
Tuss-Ornade Liquid 2242
Tuss-Ornade Spansule Capsules 2242
Tylenol Cold Medication, Effervescent Tablets 1369

Pirbuterol Acetate (Excessive tachycardia). Products include:
Maxair Inhaler 1311

Pseudoephedrine Hydrochloride (Excessive tachycardia). Products include:
Actifed Capsules ▣ 539
Actifed Plus Caplets ▣ 539
Actifed Plus Tablets ▣ 540
Actifed with Codeine Cough Syrup 752
Actifed Syrup ▣ 540
Actifed Tablets ▣ 540
Actifed 12-Hour Capsules ▣ 539
Advil Cold & Sinus Caplets (formerly CoAdvil) 2416
Allerest ▣ 559
Anatuss LA Tablets 1359
Benadryl Decongestant Elixir ▣ 635
Benadryl Decongestant ▣ 635
Benadryl Plus ▣ 636
Benadryl Plus Nighttime ▣ 637
Benylin Decongestant ▣ 638
Brexin L.A. Capsules 2078
Bromfed Capsules (Timed Release) 1615
Bromfed Syrup ▣ 628
Bromfed 1615
CoAdvil ▣ 748
Allergy-Sinus Comtrex Multi-Symptom Allergy Sinus Formula Tablets & Caplets 746
Cough Formula Comtrex 746
Comtrex Multi-Symptom Cold Reliever Tablets/Caplets/Liqui-Gels/Liquid 745
Day-Night Comtrex 747
Non-Drowsy Comtrex 747
Congess 994
Congestac Caplets ▣ 617
Contac Jr. Children's Cold Medicine ▣ 712
Contac Nighttime Cold Medicine ▣ 713
Contac Sinus Caplets Maximum Strength Non-Drowsy Formula ▣ 710
Contac Sinus Tablets Maximum Strength Non-Drowsy Formula ▣ 710
Deconamine 663
Deconsal II Tablets 559
Dimacol Caplets ▣ 672
Dimetane-DX Cough Syrup 1858
Dorcol Children's Cough Syrup ▣ 685
Dorcol Children's Decongestant Liquid ▣ 685
Dorcol Children's Liquid Cold Formula ▣ 686
Maximum Strength Dristan Decongestant/Analgesic Coated Caplets ▣ 750
No Drowsiness Dristan Cold Nasal Decongestant/Analgesic Coated Caplets 2420
Dristan Sinus Caplets 2419
Sinus Excedrin Analgesic, Decongestant Tablets & Caplets ▣ 533
Fedahist Gyrocaps 2145
Fedahist Timecaps 2145
Guaifed 1615
Guaifed Syrup ▣ 629
Isoclor Expectorant 982
Isoclor Timesule Capsules ▣ 561
Kronofed-A 970
Medi-Flu Caplet, Liquid ▣ 640
Novafed A Capsules 1342
Novafed Capsules 1342
Novahistine DH 1342
Novahistine DMX ▣ 595
Novahistine Expectorant 1343
Nucofed Capsules 2219
Nucofed Expectorant 2219
Nucofed Pediatric Expectorant 2220
Nucofed Syrup 2219
Ornex Caplets ▣ 618
PediaCare Allergy Relief Formula Liquid 1362
PediaCare Cough-Cold Formula Liquid 1362
PediaCare Infants' Oral Decongestant Drops 1362
PediaCare Night Rest Cough-Cold Formula Liquid 1362
PediaCare 6-12 Cough-Cold Formula Chewable Tablets 1362
Robitussin-DAC Syrup 1875
Robitussin-PE ▣ 677
Rondec 1975
Rondec-DM 1976
Rondec-TR Tablet 1975
Ru-Tuss DE Tablets 694
Ryna ▣ 741
Seldane-D Extended-Release Tablets 1350
Sinarest ▣ 562
Sine-Aid Maximum Strength Sinus Headache Caplets 1365
Sine-Aid Maximum Strength Sinus Headache Tablets 1365
Sine-Off Maximum Strength Allergy/Sinus Formula Caplets ▣ 721
Sine-Off Maximum Strength No Drowsiness Formula Caplets ▣ 722
Singlet Tablets ▣ 598
Sinutab Maximum Strength ▣ 641
Sinutab Maximum Strength Without Drowsiness Tablets & Caplets ▣ 642
Sinutab Regular Strength Without Drowsiness Formula ▣ 641
St. Joseph Nighttime Cold Medicine ▣ 705
Sudafed Children's Liquid ▣ 543
Sudafed Cough Syrup ▣ 543
Sudafed Plus Liquid ▣ 544
Sudafed Plus Tablets ▣ 545
Sudafed Sinus Caplets ▣ 545
Sudafed Sinus Tablets ▣ 545
Sudafed Tablets, 30 mg ▣ 544
Sudafed Tablets, Adult Strength, 60 mg ▣ 544
Sudafed 12 Hour Capsules ▣ 545
TheraFlu Flu and Cold Medicine ▣ 687
Triaminic Nite Light ▣ 689
Tylenol Allergy Sinus Medication Caplets and Gelcaps, Maximum Strength 1372
Children's Tylenol Cold Liquid Formula and Chewable Tablets 1368
Tylenol Cold & Flu Hot Medication, Packets 1369
Tylenol Cold & Flu No Drowsiness Hot Medication, Packets 1371
Tylenol Cold Medication Caplets and Tablets 1370
Tylenol Cold Medication No Drowsiness Formula Caplets 1370
Tylenol Cold Night Time Medication Liquid 1371
Tylenol Cough Medication Liquid with Decongestant, Maximum Strength 1372
Tylenol, Maximum Strength, Sinus Medication Gelcaps, Caplets and Tablets 1373
Ursinus Inlay-Tabs ▣ 691
Vicks Children's NyQuil ▣ 664
Vicks Daycare ▣ 660
Vicks Formula 44D Decongestant Cough Medicine ▣ 662
Vicks Formula 44M Multi-Symptom Cough Medicine ▣ 662
Vicks NyQuil Nighttime Colds Medicine-Original & Cherry Flavor ▣ 664
Vicks Pediatric Formula 44 Cough & Congestion Medicine ▣ 663
Vicks Pediatric Formula 44m Multi-Symptom Cough & Cold Medicine ▣ 663

Pseudoephedrine Sulfate (Excessive tachycardia). Products include:
Afrin Tablets ▣ 693
Chlor-Trimeton Decongestant ▣ 694
Disophrol Chronotab Sustained-Action Tablets ▣ 698
Drixoral Antihistamine/Nasal Decongestant Syrup ▣ 698
Drixoral Non-Drowsy Formula ▣ 699
Drixoral Plus Extended-Release Tablets ▣ 699
Drixoral Sinus ▣ 700
Drixoral Sustained-Action Tablets ▣ 698
Sinutab Allergy Formula Sustained Action Tablets ▣ 640
Trinalin Repetabs Tablets 1170

Terbutaline Sulfate (Excessive tachycardia). Products include:
Brethaire Inhaler 1024
Brethine Ampuls 1026
Brethine Tablets 1026
Bricanyl Injection 1324
Bricanyl Tablets 1325

BRONKOLIXIR
(Ephedrine Sulfate, Guaifenesin, Phenobarbital, Theophylline) ▣ 761
No interactions described in labeling.

BRONKOMETER AEROSOL
(Isoetharine) 2042
See **Bronkosol Solution**

BRONKOSOL SOLUTION
(Isoetharine) 2042
May interact with sympathomimetic aerosal brochodilators. Compounds in this category include:

Albuterol (Excessive tachycardia). Products include:
Proventil Inhalation Aerosol 2117
Ventolin Inhalation Aerosol and Refill 583

Albuterol Sulfate (Excessive tachycardia). Products include:
Proventil Repetabs Tablets 2120
Proventil Solutions for Inhalation 0.5% and 0.083% 2118
Proventil Syrup 2119
Proventil Tablets 2120
Ventolin 583

Dobutamine Hydrochloride (Excessive tachycardia). Products include:
Dobutrex Solution Vials 1259

Dopamine Hydrochloride (Excessive tachycardia). Products include:

Intropin Injection ... 930

Ephedrine Hydrochloride (Excessive tachycardia). Products include:

Amesec ... ▣ 682
Primatene Tablets-M Formula ... 2421
Primatene Tablets-P Formula ... 2421
Primatene Tablets-Regular Formula ... 2421
Quadrinal Tablets ... 1183
Quelidrine Syrup ... 556
Tedral SA ... 1765

Ephedrine Sulfate (Excessive tachycardia). Products include:

Bronkaid Tablets ... ▣ 757
Bronkolixir ... ▣ 761
Bronkotabs Tablets ... ▣ 762
Marax Tablets & DF Syrup ... 1954
Pazo Hemorrhoid Ointment & Suppositories ... 752
Vicks Vatronol Nose Drops ... ▣ 666

Ephedrine Tannate (Excessive tachycardia). Products include:

Rynatuss ... 2388

Epinephrine (Excessive tachycardia). Products include:

Ana-Kit Anaphylaxis Emergency Treatment Kit ... 1100
Bronkaid Mist ... ▣ 757
EpiPen ... 843
Marcaine Hydrochloride 0.5% with Epinephrine 1:200,000 (as bitartrate) ... 958
Marcaine Hydrochloride with Epinephrine 1:200,000 ... 2055
Primatene Mist ... 2420
Sus-Phrine Injection ... 1006
Xylocaine with Epinephrine Injections ... 637

Epinephrine Bitartrate (Excessive tachycardia). Products include:

AsthmaHaler Mist Epinephrine Bitartrate Bronchodilator ... ▣ 616
Bronkaid Mist Suspension ... ▣ 757
Primatene Mist Suspension ... 2421

Epinephrine Hydrochloride (Excessive tachycardia). Products include:

Adrenalin Chloride Solution 1:100 & 1:1,000 ... 1689
Epifrin ... ◉ 244
Glaucon ... ◉ 218

Isoproterenol Hydrochloride (Excessive tachycardia). Products include:

Isuprel Hydrochloride Injection 1:5000 ... 2050
Isuprel Hydrochloride Mistometer .. 2051
Isuprel Hydrochloride Solution 1:200 & 1:100 ... 2052
Norisodrine Aerotrol ... 540

Metaproterenol Sulfate (Excessive tachycardia). Products include:

Alupent ... 674
Arm-a-Med Metaproterenol Sulfate Inhalation Solution, USP ... 617
Metaprel Inhalation Aerosol Bronchodilator ... 2014
Metaprel Inhalation Solution ... 2015
Metaprel ... 2015
Metaproterenol Sulfate Inhalation Solution, USP ... 912

Metaraminol Bitartrate (Excessive tachycardia). Products include:

Aramine Injection ... 1424

Methoxamine Hydrochloride (Excessive tachycardia). Products include:

Vasoxyl Injection ... 819

Norepinephrine Bitartrate (Excessive tachycardia). Products include:

Levophed Bitartrate Injection ... 2054

Phenylephrine Bitartrate (Excessive tachycardia).

No products indexed under this heading.

Phenylephrine Hydrochloride (Excessive tachycardia). Products include:

AK-Dilate Solution 2.5% and 10% ... ◉ 203
Atrohist Sprinkle Capsules ... 558
Cerose-DM ... 2443
Codimal ... 846
Comhist LA Capsules ... 1618
Congespirin For Children Aspirin Free Chewable Cold Tablets ... 748
Cyclomydril ... ◉ 216
Deconsal Sprinkle Capsules ... 559
Dimetane Decongestant ... ▣ 673
Dristan Decongestant/Antihistamine/Analgesic Coated Caplets ... ▣ 749
Dristan Cold Nasal Decongestant/Antihistamine/Analgesic Coated Tablets ... 2419
Dristan Advanced Formula Decongestant/Antihistamine/Analgesic Tablets ... ▣ 749
Dristan Nasal Spray, Menthol ... 2419
Dristan Nasal Spray, Regular and Regular with Metered Pump ... 2419
Entex Capsules ... 1623
Entex Liquid ... 1623
Sinus Excedrin Analgesic, Decongestant Tablets & Caplets ... 750
Extendryl ... 994
4-Way Fast Acting Nasal Spray - Original Formula (regular & mentholated) & Metered Spray Pump (regular) ... 751
Hycomine Compound Tablets ... 929
Murocoll-2 Sterile Ophthalmic Solution ... ◉ 261
Mydfrin 2.5% ... ◉ 224
Naldecon Syrup, Tablets, Pediatric Drops and Pediatric Syrup ... 709
Neo-Synephrine Hydrochloride 1% Carpuject ... 2063
Neo-Synephrine Hydrochloride 1% Injection ... 2063
Neo-Synephrine Hydrochloride (Ophthalmic) ... 2064
Neo-Synephrine ... ▣ 759
Nōstril Nasal Decongestant ... ▣ 520
Novahistine Elixir ... ▣ 596
Phenergan VC ... 2500
Phenergan VC with Codeine ... 2501
Prefrin Liquifilm Vasoconstrictor and Lubricant Eye Drops ... ◉ 254
Prefrin-A ... ◉ 255
Quelidrine Syrup ... 556
Relief Vasoconstrictor and Lubricant Eye Drops ... ◉ 256
Robitussin Night Relief ... ▣ 677
Ru-Tuss with Hydrocodone ... 694
Ru-Tuss Tablets ... 693
Vasosulf ... ◉ 279
Vicks Sinex ... ▣ 665
Zincfrin ... ◉ 230

Phenylephrine Tannate (Excessive tachycardia). Products include:

Rynatan ... 2387
Rynatuss ... 2388

Phenylpropanolamine Hydrochloride (Excessive tachycardia). Products include:

A.R.M. Allergy Relief Medicine Caplets ... ▣ 615
Acutrim ... ▣ 548
Allerest ... ▣ 559
BC Cold Powder ... ▣ 517
Cheracol Plus Head Cold/Cough Formula ... ▣ 667
Codimal Expectorant ... 846
Comtrex Multi-Symptom Cold Reliever Tablets/Caplets/Liqui-Gels/Liquid ... 745
Contac Continuous Action Decongestant/Antihistamine Capsules ▣ 710
Contac Maximum Strength Continuous Action Decongestant/Antihistamine Caplets ... ▣ 709
Contac Severe Cold and Flu Formula Caplets ... ▣ 711
Coricidin 'D' Decongestant Tablets ... ▣ 695
Coricidin Demilets Tablets for Children ... ▣ 696
Demazin Nasal Decongestant/Antihistamine Repetabs Tablets & Syrup ... ▣ 697
Dexatrim ... ▣ 733
Dimetane-DC Cough Syrup ... 1857
Dimetapp Elixir ... ▣ 673
Dimetapp DM Elixir ... ▣ 674
Dimetapp Extentabs ... ▣ 674
Dimetapp Plus Caplets ... ▣ 675
Dimetapp Tablets ... ▣ 675
Entex Capsules ... 1623
Entex LA Tablets ... 1623
Entex Liquid ... 1623
4-Way Cold Tablets ... 750
Hycomine Syrup ... 927
Naldecon CX Adult Liquid ... ▣ 521
Naldecon DX Adult Liquid ... ▣ 521
Naldecon DX Children's Syrup ... ▣ 522
Naldecon DX Pediatric Drops ... ▣ 522
Naldecon EX Children's Syrup ... ▣ 522
Naldecon EX Pediatric Drops ... ▣ 523
Naldecon Syrup, Tablets, Pediatric Drops and Pediatric Syrup ... 709
Nolamine Tablets ... 838
Nolex LA Tablets ... 838
Ornade Spansule Capsules ... 2221
Orthoxicol Cough Syrup ... ▣ 668
Propagest ... 839
Pyrroxate Capsules ... ▣ 669
Robitussin-CF ... ▣ 676
Ru-Tuss II Capsules ... 693
Ru-Tuss with Hydrocodone ... 694
Ru-Tuss Tablets ... 693
Sine-Off Sinus Medicine Tablets-Aspirin Formula ... ▣ 722
Sinulin ... 840
St. Joseph Cold Tablets for Children ... ▣ 704
Tavist-D Tablets ... 2035
Triaminic Allergy Tablets ... ▣ 688
Triaminic Chewables ... ▣ 688
Triaminic Cold Tablets ... ▣ 688
Triaminic Expectorant ... ▣ 688
Triaminic Expectorant w/Codeine .. 1996
Triaminic Expectorant DH ... 1995
Triaminic Oral Infant Drops ... 1996
Triaminic Syrup ... ▣ 689
Triaminic-12 Tablets ... ▣ 690
Triaminic-DM Syrup ... ▣ 689
Triaminicin Tablets ... ▣ 690
Triaminicol Multi-Symptom Cold Tablets ... ▣ 691
Triaminicol Multi-Symptom Relief ▣ 691
Tuss-Ornade Liquid ... 2242
Tuss-Ornade Spansule Capsules ... 2242
Tylenol Cold Medication, Effervescent Tablets ... 1369

Pirbuterol Acetate (Excessive tachycardia). Products include:

Maxair Inhaler ... 1311

Pseudoephedrine Hydrochloride (Excessive tachycardia). Products include:

Actifed Capsules ... ▣ 539
Actifed Plus Caplets ... ▣ 539
Actifed Plus Tablets ... ▣ 540
Actifed with Codeine Cough Syrup .. 752
Actifed Syrup ... ▣ 540
Actifed Tablets ... ▣ 540
Actifed 12-Hour Capsules ... ▣ 539
Advil Cold & Sinus Caplets (formerly CoAdvil) ... 2416
Allerest ... ▣ 559
Anatuss LA Tablets ... 1359
Benadryl Decongestant Elixir ... ▣ 635
Benadryl Decongestant ... ▣ 635
Benadryl Plus ... ▣ 636
Benadryl Plus Nighttime ... ▣ 637
Benylin Decongestant ... ▣ 638
Brexin L.A. Capsules ... 2078
Bromfed Capsules (Timed Release) ... 1615
Bromfed Syrup ... ▣ 628
Bromfed ... 1615
CoAdvil ... ▣ 748
Allergy-Sinus Comtrex Multi-Symptom Allergy Sinus Formula Tablets & Caplets ... 746
Cough Formula Comtrex ... 746
Comtrex Multi-Symptom Cold Reliever Tablets/Caplets/Liqui-Gels/Liquid ... 745
Day-Night Comtrex ... 747
Non-Drowsy Comtrex ... 747
Congess ... 994
Congestac Caplets ... ▣ 617
Contac Jr. Children's Cold Medicine ... ▣ 712
Contac Nighttime Cold Medicine ... ▣ 713
Contac Sinus Caplets Maximum Strength Non-Drowsy Formula ... ▣ 710
Contac Sinus Tablets Maximum Strength Non-Drowsy Formula ... ▣ 710
Deconamine ... 663
Deconsal II Tablets ... 559
Dimacol Caplets ... ▣ 672
Dimetane-DX Cough Syrup ... 1858
Dorcol Children's Cough Syrup ... ▣ 685
Dorcol Children's Decongestant Liquid ... ▣ 685
Dorcol Children's Liquid Cold Formula ... ▣ 686
Maximum Strength Dristan Decongestant/Analgesic Coated Caplets ... ▣ 750
No Drowsiness Dristan Cold Nasal Decongestant/Analgesic Coated Caplets ... 2420
Dristan Sinus Caplets ... 2419
Sinus Excedrin Analgesic, Decongestant Tablets & Caplets ... ▣ 533
Fedahist Gyrocaps ... 2145
Fedahist Timecaps ... 2145
Guaifed ... 1615
Guaifed Syrup ... ▣ 629
Isoclor Expectorant ... 982
Isoclor Timesule Capsules ... ▣ 561
Kronofed-A ... 970
Medi-Flu Caplet, Liquid ... ▣ 640
Novafed A Capsules ... 1342
Novafed Capsules ... 1342
Novahistine DH ... 1342
Novahistine DMX ... ▣ 595
Novahistine Expectorant ... 1343
Nucofed Capsules ... 2219
Nucofed Expectorant ... 2219
Nucofed Pediatric Expectorant ... 2220
Nucofed Syrup ... 2219
Ornex Caplets ... ▣ 618
PediaCare Allergy Relief Formula Liquid ... 1362
PediaCare Cough-Cold Formula Liquid ... 1362
PediaCare Infants' Oral Decongestant Drops ... 1362
PediaCare Night Rest Cough-Cold Formula Liquid ... 1362
PediaCare 6-12 Cough-Cold Formula Chewable Tablets ... 1362
Robitussin-DAC Syrup ... 1875
Robitussin-PE ... ▣ 677
Rondec ... 1975
Rondec-DM ... 1976
Rondec-TR Tablet ... 1975
Ru-Tuss DE Tablets ... 694
Ryna ... ▣ 741
Seldane-D Extended-Release Tablets ... 1350
Sinarest ... ▣ 562
Sine-Aid Maximum Strength Sinus Headache Caplets ... 1365
Sine-Aid Maximum Strength Sinus Headache Tablets ... 1365
Sine-Off Maximum Strength Allergy/Sinus Formula Caplets ... ▣ 721
Sine-Off Maximum Strength No Drowsiness Formula Caplets ... ▣ 722
Singlet Tablets ... ▣ 598
Sinutab Maximum Strength ... ▣ 641
Sinutab Maximum Strength Without Drowsiness Tablets & Caplets ... ▣ 642
Sinutab Regular Strength Without Drowsiness Formula ... ▣ 641
St. Joseph Nighttime Cold Medicine ... ▣ 705
Sudafed Children's Liquid ... ▣ 543
Sudafed Cough Syrup ... ▣ 543
Sudafed Plus Liquid ... ▣ 544
Sudafed Plus Tablets ... ▣ 545
Sudafed Sinus Caplets ... ▣ 545
Sudafed Sinus Tablets ... ▣ 545
Sudafed Tablets, 30 mg ... ▣ 544
Sudafed Tablets, Adult Strength, 60 mg ... ▣ 544
Sudafed 12 Hour Capsules ... ▣ 545
TheraFlu Flu and Cold Medicine ... ▣ 687
Triaminic Nite Light ... ▣ 689
Tylenol Allergy Sinus Medication Caplets and Gelcaps, Maximum Strength ... 1372
Children's Tylenol Cold Liquid Formula and Chewable Tablets ... 1368
Tylenol Cold & Flu Hot Medication, Packets ... 1369
Tylenol Cold & Flu No Drowsiness Hot Medication, Packets ... 1371
Tylenol Cold Medication Caplets and Tablets ... 1370
Tylenol Cold Medication No Drowsiness Formula Caplets ... 1370
Tylenol Cold Night Time Medication Liquid ... 1371
Tylenol Cough Medication Liquid with Decongestant, Maximum Strength ... 1372

(▣ Described in PDR For Nonprescription Drugs) (◉ Described in PDR For Ophthalmology)

Tylenol, Maximum Strength, Sinus Medication Gelcaps, Caplets and Tablets 1373
Ursinus Inlay-Tabs .... ■ 691
Vicks Children's NyQuil .... ■ 664
Vicks Daycare .... ■ 660
Vicks Formula 44D Decongestant Cough Medicine .... ■ 662
Vicks Formula 44M Multi-Symptom Cough Medicine .... ■ 662
Vicks NyQuil Nighttime Colds Medicine-Original & Cherry Flavor .... ■ 664
Vicks Pediatric Formula 44 Cough & Congestion Medicine .... ■ 663
Vicks Pediatric Formula 44m Multi-Symptom Cough & Cold Medicine .... ■ 663

Pseudoephedrine Sulfate (Excessive tachycardia). Products include:
Afrin Tablets .... ■ 693
Chlor-Trimeton Decongestant .... ■ 694
Disophrol Chronotab Sustained-Action Tablets .... ■ 698
Drixoral Antihistamine/Nasal Decongestant Syrup .... ■ 698
Drixoral Non-Drowsy Formula .... ■ 699
Drixoral Plus Extended-Release Tablets .... ■ 699
Drixoral Sinus .... ■ 700
Drixoral Sustained-Action Tablets ■ 698
Sinutab Allergy Formula Sustained Action Tablets .... ■ 640
Trinalin Repetabs Tablets 1170

Terbutaline Sulfate (Excessive tachycardia). Products include:
Brethaire Inhaler 1024
Brethine Ampuls 1026
Brethine Tablets 1026
Bricanyl Injection 1324
Bricanyl Tablets 1325

BRONKOTABS TABLETS
(Ephedrine Sulfate, Guaifenesin, Phenobarbital, Theophylline) .... ■ 762
No interactions described in labeling.

BUCLADIN-S SOFTAB CHEWABLE TABLETS
(Buclizine Hydrochloride) 2264
No interactions described in labeling.

ARTHRITIS STRENGTH BUFFERIN ANALGESIC CAPLETS
(Aspirin) 744
May interact with:

Antiarthritic Drugs, unspecified (Effect not specified).
Anticoagulant Drugs, unspecified (Effect not specified).
Antidiabetic Drugs, unspecified (Effect not specified).
Antigout Drugs, unspecified (Effect not specified).

EXTRA STRENGTH BUFFERIN ANALGESIC TABLETS
(Aspirin) 745
May interact with:

Antiarthritic Drugs, unspecified (Effect not specified).
Anticoagulant Drugs, unspecified (Effect not specified).
Antidiabetic Drugs, unspecified (Effect not specified).
Antigout Drugs, unspecified (Effect not specified).

BUFFERIN ANALGESIC TABLETS AND CAPLETS
(Aspirin) 743
May interact with:

Aluminum Carbonate Gel (Concurrent administration of nonabsorbable antacids may alter the rate of absorption of aspirin). Products include:
Basaljel 2438

Aluminum Hydroxide (Concurrent administration of nonabsorbable antacids may alter the rate of absorption of aspirin). Products include:
Cama Arthritis Pain Reliever .... ■ 685
Gaviscon Extra Strength Relief Formula Liquid Antacid .... ■ 594
Gaviscon Extra Strength Relief Formula Antacid Tablets .... ■ 594
Gaviscon Liquid Antacid .... ■ 594
Gelusil Liquid & Tablets .... ■ 639
Extra Strength Maalox Plus Suspension 1850
Maalox TC Suspension 1851
Maalox Plus Tablets .... ■ 655
Extra Strength Maalox Plus Tablets 1850
Nephrox Suspension .... ■ 563
WinGel Liquid & Tablets .... ■ 761

Aluminum Hydroxide Gel (Concurrent administration of nonabsorbable antacids may alter the rate of absorption of aspirin). Products include:
ALternaGEL Liquid 1154
Aludrox Oral Suspension 2428
Amphojel Suspension 2429
Amphojel Suspension without Flavor 2429
Mylanta Liquid 1155
Mylanta Double Strength Liquid 1155

Aluminum Hydroxide Gel, Dried (Concurrent administration of nonabsorbable antacids may alter the rate of absorption of aspirin). Products include:
Alu-Tab/Alu-Cap 1309
Amphojel Tablets 2429
Ascriptin A/D Caplets 1850
Regular Strength Ascriptin Tablets 1850
Gaviscon Antacid Tablets .... ■ 593
Gaviscon-2 Antacid Tablets .... ■ 594
Mylanta Tablets 1155
Mylanta Double Strength Tablets 1155

Antiarthritic Drugs, unspecified (Effect not specified).
Anticoagulant Drugs, unspecified (Effect not specified).
Antidiabetic Drugs, unspecified (Effect not specified).
Antigout Drugs, unspecified (Effect not specified).

Dihydroxyaluminum Sodium Carbonate (Concurrent administration of nonabsorbable antacids may alter the rate of absorption of aspirin). Products include:
Rolaids .... ■ 743

Magaldrate (Concurrent administration of nonabsorbable antacids may alter the rate of absorption of aspirin). Products include:
Riopan Antacid Chew Tablets .... ■ 754
Riopan Antacid Chew Tablets in Rollpacks .... ■ 754
Riopan Antacid Suspension 2421
Riopan Antacid Swallow Tablets 2421
Riopan Plus Chew Tablets 2422
Riopan Plus Chew Tablets in Rollpack 2422
Riopan Plus 2 Chew Tablets, Mint Flavor, Cherry Flavor 2422
Riopan Plus Suspension 2422
Riopan Plus 2 Suspension, Mint Flavor, Cherry Flavor 2422

Magnesium Hydroxide (Concurrent administration of nonabsorbable antacids may alter the rate of absorption of aspirin). Products include:
Aludrox Oral Suspension 2428
Ascriptin A/D Caplets 1850
Regular Strength Ascriptin Tablets 1850
Di-Gel Antacid/Anti-Gas .... ■ 697
Gelusil Liquid & Tablets .... ■ 639
Haley's M-O, Regular & Flavored .. ■ 569
Extra Strength Maalox Plus Suspension 1850
Maalox TC Suspension 1851
Maalox Plus Tablets .... ■ 655
Extra Strength Maalox Plus Tablets 1850
Mylanta Liquid 1155
Mylanta Tablets 1155
Mylanta Double Strength Liquid 1155
Mylanta Double Strength Tablets 1155
Concentrated Phillips' Milk of Magnesia .... ■ 573
Phillips' Milk of Magnesia Liquid .... ■ 572
Phillips' Milk of Magnesia Tablets ■ 573
WinGel Liquid & Tablets .... ■ 761

Magnesium Oxide (Concurrent administration of nonabsorbable antacids may alter the rate of absorption of aspirin). Products include:
Bayer Plus Aspirin Tablets .... ■ 567
Beelith Tablets 659
Bufferin Analgesic Tablets and Caplets .... ■ 524
Cama Arthritis Pain Reliever .... ■ 685
Mag-Ox 400 673
Uro-Mag 673

Sodium Bicarbonate (Concurrent administration with absorbable antacids may increase the clearance of salicylates). Products include:
Alka-Seltzer Advanced Formula Antacid & Non-Aspirin Pain Reliever .... ■ 620
Alka-Seltzer Effervescent Antacid ■ 622
Alka-Seltzer Effervescent Antacid and Pain Reliever 1568
Alka-Seltzer Extra Strength Effervescent Antacid and Pain Reliever .... ■ 623
Alka-Seltzer (Flavored) Effervescent Antacid and Pain Reliever .. ■ 621
Arm & Hammer Pure Baking Soda .... ■ 548
Ceo-Two Rectal Suppositories 671
Citrocarbonate Antacid .... ■ 668
Massengill Liquid Concentrate 2191
NuLYTELY 699

BUFFERIN AF NITE TIME ANALGESIC/SLEEPING AID CAPLETS
(Acetaminophen, Diphenhydramine Citrate) 744
May interact with hypnotics and sedatives and tranquilizers. Compounds in these categories include:

Alprazolam (Effect not specified). Products include:
Xanax Tablets 2367

Buspirone Hydrochloride (Effect not specified). Products include:
BuSpar 1401

Chlordiazepoxide (Effect not specified). Products include:
Libritabs Tablets 1930
Limbitrol 1933
Menrium Tablets 1934

Chlordiazepoxide Hydrochloride (Effect not specified). Products include:
Librax Capsules 1929
Librium Capsules 1931
Librium Injectable 1932

Chlorpromazine (Effect not specified). Products include:
Thorazine 2234

Chlorprothixene (Effect not specified). Products include:
Taractan Tablets 1920

Chlorprothixene Hydrochloride (Effect not specified). Products include:
Taractan 1920

Clorazepate Dipotassium (Effect not specified). Products include:
Tranxene 556

Diazepam (Effect not specified). Products include:
Valium Injectable 1937
Valium Tablets 1939
Valrelease Capsules 1923

Droperidol (Effect not specified). Products include:
Inapsine Injection 1140
Innovar Injection 1141

Estazolam (Effect not specified). Products include:
ProSom Tablets 554

Ethchlorvynol (Effect not specified). Products include:
Placidyl Capsules 553

Ethinamate (Effect not specified).
No products indexed under this heading.

Fluphenazine Decanoate (Effect not specified). Products include:
Prolixin Decanoate 1795

Fluphenazine Enanthate (Effect not specified). Products include:
Prolixin Enanthate 1796

Fluphenazine Hydrochloride (Effect not specified). Products include:
Prolixin Elixir 1793
Prolixin Injection 1791
Prolixin Oral Concentrate 1792
Prolixin Tablets 1793

Flurazepam Hydrochloride (Effect not specified). Products include:
Dalmane Capsules 1927

Glutethimide (Effect not specified).
No products indexed under this heading.

Haloperidol (Effect not specified). Products include:
Haldol Injection, Tablets and Concentrate 1373

Haloperidol Decanoate (Effect not specified). Products include:
Haldol Decanoate 1375

Hydroxyzine Hydrochloride (Effect not specified). Products include:
Atarax Tablets & Syrup 1941
Marax Tablets & DF Syrup 1954
Vistaril Intramuscular Solution 1970

Lorazepam (Effect not specified). Products include:
Ativan Injection 2432
Ativan Tablets 2434

Loxapine Hydrochloride (Effect not specified). Products include:
Loxitane 1213

Loxapine Succinate (Effect not specified). Products include:
Loxitane Capsules 1213

Meprobamate (Effect not specified). Products include:
Deprol Tablets 2382
Equagesic Tablets 2451
Miltown Tablets 2386
PMB 200 and PMB 400 2504

Mesoridazine Besylate (Effect not specified).

Midazolam Hydrochloride (Effect not specified). Products include:
Versed Injection 1924

Molindone Hydrochloride (Effect not specified). Products include:
Moban Tablets & Concentrate 932

Oxazepam (Effect not specified). Products include:
Serax Capsules 2522
Serax Tablets 2522

Perphenazine (Effect not specified). Products include:
Etrafon 2087
Triavil Tablets 1556
Trilafon 2123

Prazepam (Effect not specified). Products include:
Centrax 1693

Prochlorperazine (Effect not specified). Products include:
Compazine 2201

Promethazine Hydrochloride (Effect not specified). Products include:
Mepergan Injection 2479
Phenergan with Codeine 2497
Phenergan with Dextromethorphan 2499
Phenergan Injection 2493
Phenergan Suppositories 2496
Phenergan Syrup 2495
Phenergan Tablets 2496
Phenergan VC 2500
Phenergan VC with Codeine 2501

Propofol (Effect not specified). Products include:
Diprivan Injection 2267

Quazepam (Effect not specified). Products include:
Doral Tablets 2383

Secobarbital Sodium (Effect not specified). Products include:
Seconal Sodium Pulvules 1296

Temazepam (Effect not specified). Products include:
Restoril Capsules 2023

Thioridazine Hydrochloride (Effect not specified). Products include:
Mellaril 2011

Thiothixene (Effect not specified). Products include:
Navane Capsules and Concentrate 1954
Navane Intramuscular 1956

Triazolam (Effect not specified). Products include:
Halcion Tablets 2340

Trifluoperazine Hydrochloride (Effect not specified). Products include:
Stelazine 2226

BUGS BUNNY CHILDREN'S CHEWABLE VITAMINS + MINERALS WITH IRON AND CALCIUM (SUGAR FREE)
(Vitamins with Minerals) .... ▣ 626
No interactions described in labeling.

BUGS BUNNY CHILDREN'S CHEWABLE VITAMINS (SUGAR FREE)
(Multivitamins) .... ▣ 625
No interactions described in labeling.

BUGS BUNNY WITH EXTRA C CHILDREN'S CHEWABLE VITAMINS (SUGAR FREE)
(Multivitamins) .... ▣ 626
No interactions described in labeling.

BUGS BUNNY PLUS IRON CHILDREN'S CHEWABLE VITAMINS (SUGAR FREE)
(Vitamins with Iron) .... ▣ 625
No interactions described in labeling.

BUMEX INJECTION
(Bumetanide) 1895
May interact with aminoglycosides, lithium preparations, antihypertensives, and certain other agents. Compounds in these categories include:

Acebutolol Hydrochloride (Antihypertensive effect potentiated). Products include:
Sectral Capsules 2520

Amikacin Sulfate (Potential for ototoxicity and/or nephrotoxicity). Products include:
Amikin Injectable 602

Atenolol (Antihypertensive effect potentiated). Products include:
Tenoretic Tablets 1105
Tenormin Tablets and I.V. Injection 1107

Benazepril Hydrochloride (Antihypertensive effect potentiated). Products include:
Lotensin Tablets 872

Bendroflumethiazide (Antihypertensive effect potentiated). Products include:
Corzide Tablets 702
Naturetin Tablets 1789
Rauzide Tablets 1804

Betaxolol Hydrochloride (Antihypertensive effect potentiated). Products include:
Betoptic Sterile Ophthalmic Solution 569
Betoptic S Sterile Ophthalmic Suspension 570
Kerlone Tablets 2172

Captopril (Antihypertensive effect potentiated). Products include:
Capoten 2255
Capozide 2258

Carteolol Hydrochloride (Antihypertensive effect potentiated). Products include:
Cartrol Tablets 507

Chlorothiazide (Antihypertensive effect potentiated). Products include:
Aldoclor Tablets 1413
Diupres Tablets 1461
Diuril Oral 1464

Chlorothiazide Sodium (Antihypertensive effect potentiated). Products include:
Diuril Sodium Intravenous 1463

Chlorthalidone (Antihypertensive effect potentiated). Products include:
Combipres Tablets 678
Tenoretic Tablets 1105
Thalitone Tablets 687

Clonidine (Antihypertensive effect potentiated). Products include:
Catapres-TTS 677

Clonidine Hydrochloride (Antihypertensive effect potentiated). Products include:
Catapres Tablets 676
Combipres Tablets 678

Deserpidine (Antihypertensive effect potentiated). Products include:
Enduronyl 518
Harmonyl Tablets 528
Oreticyl 545

Diazoxide (Antihypertensive effect potentiated). Products include:
Hyperstat I.V. Injection 2095
Proglycem 649

Doxazosin Mesylate (Antihypertensive effect potentiated). Products include:
Cardura Tablets 1941

Enalapril Maleate (Antihypertensive effect potentiated). Products include:
Vaseretic Tablets 1559
Vasotec Tablets 1564

Enalaprilat (Antihypertensive effect potentiated). Products include:
Vasotec I.V. 1562

Esmolol Hydrochloride (Antihypertensive effect potentiated). Products include:
Brevibloc Injection 942

Felodipine (Antihypertensive effect potentiated). Products include:
Plendil Extended-Release Tablets 1526

Fosinopril Sodium (Antihypertensive effect potentiated). Products include:
Monopril Tablets 1406

Furosemide (Antihypertensive effect potentiated). Products include:
Lasix 1093

Gentamicin Sulfate (Potential for ototoxicity and/or nephrotoxicity). Products include:
Garamycin Injectable 2093
Garamycin Ophthalmic .... ◉ 305
Genoptic Liquifilm Sterile Ophthalmic Solution .... ◉ 247
Genoptic S.O.P. Sterile Ophthalmic Ointment .... ◉ 247
Gentacidin Ointment .... ◉ 273
Gentacidin Solution .... ◉ 273
Gentak Ointment & Solution .... ◉ 208
G-myticin Creme and Ointment 0.1% 1770
Pred-G Liquifilm Sterile Ophthalmic Suspension .... ◉ 252
Pred-G S.O.P. Sterile Ophthalmic Ointment .... ◉ 253

Guanabenz Acetate (Antihypertensive effect potentiated). Products include:
Wytensin Tablets 2542

Guanethidine Monosulfate (Antihypertensive effect potentiated). Products include:
Esimil Tablets 864
Ismelin Tablets 869

Hydralazine Hydrochloride (Antihypertensive effect potentiated). Products include:
Apresazide Capsules 854
Apresoline Hydrochloride Parenteral (Ampuls) 856
Apresoline Hydrochloride Tablets 855
Apresoline-Esidrix Tablets 857
Ser-Ap-Es Tablets 881
Serpasil-Apresoline Tablets 884

Hydrochlorothiazide (Antihypertensive effect potentiated). Products include:
Aldactazide 2150
Aldoril Tablets 1418
Apresazide Capsules 854
Apresoline-Esidrix Tablets 857
Capozide 2258
Dyazide Capsules 2208
Esidrix Tablets 863
Esimil Tablets 864
HydroDIURIL Tablets 1484
Hydropres Tablets 1485
Inderide Tablets 2463
Inderide LA Long Acting Capsules 2465
Lopressor HCT Tablets 1034
Maxzide 1215
Moduretic Tablets 1510
Normozide Tablets 2112
Oretic Tablets 544
Oreticyl 545
Prinzide Tablets 1540
Ser-Ap-Es Tablets 881
Serpasil-Esidrix Tablets 886
Timolide Tablets 1547
Trandate HCT Tablets 579
Vaseretic Tablets 1559
Zestoretic 2274

Hydroflumethiazide (Antihypertensive effect potentiated). Products include:
Diucardin Tablets 2450
Saluron 718
Salutensin/Salutensin-Demi 719

Indapamide (Antihypertensive effect potentiated). Products include:
Lozol Tablets 1843

Indomethacin (Decreased plasma renin activity). Products include:
Indocin 1487

Indomethacin Sodium Trihydrate (Decreased plasma renin activity). Products include:
Indocin I.V. 1490

Isradipine (Antihypertensive effect potentiated). Products include:
DynaCirc Capsules 2004

Kanamycin Sulfate (Potential for ototoxicity and/or nephrotoxicity). Products include:
Kantrex Injection 601
Kantrex Pediatric Injection 601

Labetalol Hydrochloride (Antihypertensive effect potentiated). Products include:
Normodyne Injection 2108
Normodyne Tablets 2110
Normozide Tablets 2112
Trandate HCT Tablets 579
Trandate Injection 577
Trandate Tablets 579

Lisinopril (Antihypertensive effect potentiated). Products include:
Prinivil Tablets 1538
Prinzide Tablets 1540
Zestoretic 2274
Zestril Tablets 2277

Lithium Carbonate (Lithium toxicity). Products include:
Eskalith 2214
Lithane Tablets 1596
Lithium Carbonate Capsules & Tablets 1984
Lithobid Tablets 870

Lithium Citrate (Lithium toxicity). Products include:
Cibalith-S 870

Mecamylamine Hydrochloride (Antihypertensive effect potentiated). Products include:
Inversine Tablets 1492

Methyclothiazide (Antihypertensive effect potentiated). Products include:
Enduron Tablets 517
Enduronyl 518

Methyldopa (Antihypertensive effect potentiated). Products include:
Aldoclor Tablets 1413
Aldomet Oral 1415
Aldoril Tablets 1418

Methyldopate Hydrochloride (Antihypertensive effect potentiated). Products include:
Aldomet Ester HCl Injection 1417

Metolazone (Antihypertensive effect potentiated). Products include:
Diulo 2129
Mykrox ½ mg Tablets 984
Zaroxolyn Tablets 989

Metoprolol Tartrate (Antihypertensive effect potentiated). Products include:
Lopressor Ampuls 1032
Lopressor HCT Tablets 1034
Lopressor Tablets 1032

Metyrosine (Antihypertensive effect potentiated). Products include:
Demser Capsules 1460

Minoxidil (Antihypertensive effect potentiated). Products include:
Loniten Tablets 2346
Rogaine Topical Solution 2357

Nadolol (Antihypertensive effect potentiated). Products include:
Corgard Tablets 701
Corzide Tablets 702

Nicardipine Hydrochloride (Antihypertensive effect potentiated). Products include:
Cardene Capsules 2290

Nitroglycerin (Antihypertensive effect potentiated). Products include:
Deponit NTG Transdermal Delivery System 2143
Minitran Transdermal Delivery System 1312
Nitro-Bid Ointment 1339
Nitro-Bid Capsules 1338
Nitrodisc 2176
Nitro-Dur (nitroglycerin) Transdermal Infusion System 1164
Nitrogard Tablets 1004
Nitrolingual Spray 1846
Nitrostat Tablets 1743
Transderm-Nitro Transdermal Therapeutic System 2283

(▣ Described in PDR For Nonprescription Drugs)

(◉ Described in PDR For Ophthalmology)

Penbutolol Sulfate (Antihypertensive effect potentiated). Products include:
Levatol 1832

Phenoxybenzamine Hydrochloride (Antihypertensive effect potentiated). Products include:
Dibenzyline Capsules 2207

Phentolamine Mesylate (Antihypertensive effect potentiated). Products include:
Regitine 878

Pindolol (Antihypertensive effect potentiated). Products include:
Visken Tablets 2036

Polythiazide (Antihypertensive effect potentiated). Products include:
Minizide Capsules 1779
Renese Tablets 1785
Renese-R Tablets 1786

Prazosin Hydrochloride (Antihypertensive effect potentiated). Products include:
Minipress Capsules 1778
Minizide Capsules 1779

Probenecid (Decreases natriuresis and hyperreninemia). Products include:
Benemid Tablets 1426
ColBENEMID Tablets 1436
Wycillin Injection and Probenecid Tablets 2539

Propranolol Hydrochloride (Antihypertensive effect potentiated). Products include:
Inderal 2459
Inderal LA Long Acting Capsules 2461
Inderide Tablets 2463
Inderide LA Long Acting Capsules .. 2465

Ramipril (Antihypertensive effect potentiated). Products include:
Altace Capsules 1086

Rauwolfia Serpentina (Antihypertensive effect potentiated). Products include:
Raudixin Tablets 1803
Rauzide Tablets 1804

Rescinnamine (Antihypertensive effect potentiated).
No products indexed under this heading.

Reserpine (Antihypertensive effect potentiated). Products include:
Diupres Tablets 1461
Hydromox R Tablets 1209
Hydropres Tablets 1485
Renese-R Tablets 1786
Salutensin/Salutensin-Demi 719
Ser-Ap-Es Tablets 881
Serpasil Tablets 883
Serpasil-Apresoline Tablets 884
Serpasil-Esidrix Tablets 886

Sodium Nitroprusside (Antihypertensive effect potentiated). Products include:
Nipride I.V. Infusion 1909

Streptomycin Sulfate (Potential for ototoxicity and/or nephrotoxicity).
No products indexed under this heading.

Terazosin Hydrochloride (Antihypertensive effect potentiated). Products include:
Hytrin Tablets 529

Timolol Maleate (Antihypertensive effect potentiated). Products include:
Blocadren Tablets 1429
Timolide Tablets 1547
Timoptic in Ocudose 1552
Timoptic Sterile Ophthalmic Solution 1550

Tobramycin (Potential for ototoxicity and/or nephrotoxicity). Products include:
TobraDex Ophthalmic Suspension and Ointment .... ⊙ 228
Tobrex Ophthalmic Ointment and Solution 572

Tobramycin Sulfate (Potential for ototoxicity and/or nephrotoxicity). Products include:
Nebcin Vials, Hyporets & ADD-Vantage 1286

Trimethaphan Camsylate (Antihypertensive effect potentiated). Products include:
Arfonad Ampuls 1887

BUMEX TABLETS
(Bumetanide) 1895
See **Bumex Injection**

BUSPAR
(Buspirone Hydrochloride) 1401
May interact with monoamine oxidase inhibitors and certain other agents. Compounds in these categories include:

Digitoxin (May result in higher blood levels). Products include:
Crystodigin Tablets 1253

Digoxin (May result in higher blood levels). Products include:
Lanoxicaps 772
Lanoxin Elixir Pediatric 775
Lanoxin Injection 778
Lanoxin Injection Pediatric 781
Lanoxin Tablets 783

Furazolidone (Elevated blood pressure). Products include:
Furoxone 1855

Haloperidol (Increased serum haloperidol concentrations). Products include:
Haldol Injection, Tablets and Concentrate 1373

Haloperidol Decanoate (Increased serum haloperidol concentrations). Products include:
Haldol Decanoate 1375

Isocarboxazid (Elevated blood pressure). Products include:
Marplan Tablets 1906

Phenelzine Sulfate (Elevated blood pressure). Products include:
Nardil 1742

Selegiline Hydrochloride (Elevated blood pressure). Products include:
Eldepryl 2250

Tranylcypromine Sulfate (Elevated blood pressure). Products include:
Parnate Tablets 2222

Trazodone Hydrochloride (Possible SGPT elevation). Products include:
Desyrel and Desyrel Dividose 1404

Warfarin Sodium (Single report of prolonged prothrombin time in a patient on other tightly protein bound drugs). Products include:
Coumadin Injection & Tablets 944
Panwarfin Tablets 547

Food Interactions

Food, unspecified (Food may decrease presystemic clearance of buspirone).

BUTAZOLIDIN CAPSULES & TABLETS
(Phenylbutazone) 1027
May interact with non-steroidal anti-inflammatory agents, oral anticoagulants, oral hypoglycemic agents, sulfonamides, barbiturates, insulin, lithium preparations, and certain other agents. Compounds in these categories include:

Aprobarbital (May decrease the half-life of Butazolidin). Products include:
Alurate Elixir 1883

Butabarbital (May decrease the half-life of Butazolidin). Products include:
Pyridium Plus 1764

Butalbital (May decrease the half-life of Butazolidin). Products include:
Esgic-Plus Tablets 1002
Esgic Tablets & Capsules 1001
Fioricet Tablets 2006
Fiorinal Capsules 2007
Fiorinal with Codeine Capsules 2008
Fiorinal Tablets 2007
Phrenilin 838
Sedapap Tablets 50 mg/650 mg .. 1360

Chlorpheniramine Maleate (May decrease the half-life of Butazolidin). Products include:
A.R.M. Allergy Relief Medicine Caplets .... ▣ 615
Alka-Seltzer Plus Cold Medicine .... ▣ 623
Allerest .... ▣ 559
Ana-Kit Anaphylaxis Emergency Treatment Kit 1100
BC Cold Powder Multi-Symptom Formula .... ▣ 517
Brexin L.A. Capsules 2078
Cerose-DM 2443
Cheracol Plus Head Cold/Cough Formula .... ▣ 667
Chlor-Trimeton Allergy Syrup, Tablets & Long-Acting Repetabs Tablets .... ▣ 693
Chlor-Trimeton Decongestant .... ▣ 694
Comhist LA Capsules 1618
Allergy-Sinus Comtrex Multi-Symptom Allergy Sinus Formula Tablets & Caplets 746
Comtrex Multi-Symptom Cold Reliever Tablets/Caplets/LiquiGels/Liquid 745
Day-Night Comtrex 747
Contac Continuous Action Decongestant/Antihistamine Capsules ▣ 710
Contac Maximum Strength Continuous Action Decongestant/Antihistamine Caplets .... ▣ 709
Contac Severe Cold and Flu Formula Caplets .... ▣ 711
Coricidin 'D' Decongestant Tablets .... ▣ 695
Coricidin Demilets Tablets for Children .... ▣ 696
Coricidin Tablets .... ▣ 695
Deconamine 663
Demazin Nasal Decongestant/Antihistamine Repetabs Tablets & Syrup .... ▣ 697
Dorcol Children's Liquid Cold Formula .... ▣ 686
Dristan Decongestant/Antihistamine/Analgesic Coated Caplets .... ▣ 749
Dristan Cold Nasal Decongestant/Antihistamine/ Analgesic Coated Tablets 2419
Dristan Advanced Formula Decongestant/Antihistamine/Analgesic Tablets .... ▣ 749
Extendryl 994
4-Way Cold Tablets 750
Fedahist Gyrocaps 2145
Fedahist Timecaps 2145
Hycomine Compound Tablets 929
Isoclor Timesule Capsules .... ▣ 561
Kronofed-A 970
Medi-Flu Caplet, Liquid .... ▣ 640
Naldecon Syrup, Tablets, Pediatric Drops and Pediatric Syrup 709
Nolamine Tablets 838
Novafed A Capsules 1342
Novahistine DH 1342
Novahistine Elixir .... ▣ 596
Ornade Spansule Capsules 2221
Orthoxicol Cough Syrup .... ▣ 668
PediaCare Allergy Relief Formula Liquid 1362
PediaCare Cough-Cold Formula Liquid 1362
PediaCare Night Rest Cough-Cold Formula Liquid 1362
PediaCare 6-12 Cough-Cold Formula Chewable Tablets 1362
Pyrroxate Capsules .... ▣ 669
Quelidrine Syrup 556
Ru-Tuss II Capsules 693
Ru-Tuss Tablets 693
Ryna .... ▣ 741
Sinarest Tablets & Extra Strength Tablets .... ▣ 562
Sine-Off Maximum Strength Allergy/Sinus Formula Caplets .... ▣ 721
Sine-Off Sinus Medicine Tablets-Aspirin Formula .... ▣ 722
Singlet Tablets .... ▣ 598
Sinulin 840
Sinutab Maximum Strength .... ▣ 641
St. Joseph Nighttime Cold Medicine .... ▣ 705
Sudafed Plus Liquid .... ▣ 544
Sudafed Plus Tablets .... ▣ 545
Teldrin Timed-Release Allergy Capsules, 12 mg 2192
TheraFlu Flu and Cold Medicine .... ▣ 687
Triaminic Allergy Tablets .... ▣ 688
Triaminic Chewables .... ▣ 688
Triaminic Cold Tablets .... ▣ 688
Triaminic Nite Light .... ▣ 689
Triaminic Syrup .... ▣ 689
Triaminic-12 Tablets .... ▣ 690
Triaminicin Tablets .... ▣ 690
Triaminicol Multi-Symptom Cold Tablets .... ▣ 691
Triaminicol Multi-Symptom Relief ▣ 691
Tylenol Allergy Sinus Medication Caplets and Gelcaps, Maximum Strength 1372
Children's Tylenol Cold Liquid Formula and Chewable Tablets 1368
Tylenol Cold & Flu Hot Medication, Packets 1369
Tylenol Cold Medication Caplets and Tablets 1370
Tylenol Cold Medication, Effervescent Tablets 1369
Vicks Children's NyQuil .... ▣ 664
Vicks Formula 44 Cough Medicine .... ▣ 661
Vicks Formula 44M Multi-Symptom Cough Medicine .... ▣ 662
Vicks Pediatric Formula 44m Multi-Symptom Cough & Cold Medicine .... ▣ 663

Chlorpheniramine Polistirex (May decrease the half-life of Butazolidin). Products include:
Tussionex Extended-Release Suspension 988

Chlorpheniramine Tannate (May decrease the half-life of Butazolidin). Products include:
Rynatan 2387
Rynatuss 2388

Chlorpropamide (Potential for increased effects, duration and toxicity of oral antidiabetics). Products include:
Diabinese Tablets 1775

Cholestyramine (Enteral absorption of Butazolidin is reduced). Products include:
Cholybar 1705
Questran Light 711
Questran Powder 710

Cortisone Acetate (Butazolidin may induce hepatic microsomal metabolism of cortisone). Products include:
Cortone Acetate Sterile Suspension 1437
Cortone Acetate Tablets 1439

Diclofenac Sodium (Potential for increased effects, duration and toxicity of NSAIDs). Products include:
Voltaren Ophthalmic Sterile Ophthalmic Solution .... ⊙ 268
Voltaren Tablets 1042

Dicumarol (Potential for increased effects, duration and toxicity of anticoagulants). Products include:
Dicumarol Tablets 516

Digitoxin (Butazolidin may induce hepatic microsomal metabolism of digitoxin). Products include:
Crystodigin Tablets 1253

Divalproex Sodium (Potential for increased effects, duration and toxicity of sodium valproate). Products include:
Depakote 512

Etodolac (Potential for increased effects, duration and toxicity of NSAIDs). Products include:
Lodine Capsules 2468

Fenoprofen Calcium (Potential for increased effects, duration and toxicity of NSAIDs). Products include:
- Nalfon Pulvules & Tablets 919

Flurbiprofen (Potential for increased effects, duration and toxicity of NSAIDs). Products include:
- Ansaid Tablets 2319

Glipizide (Potential for increased effects, duration and toxicity of oral antidiabetics). Products include:
- Glucotrol 1952

Glyburide (Potential for increased effects, duration and toxicity of oral antidiabetics). Products include:
- DiaBeta 1091
- Micronase Tablets 2350

Ibuprofen (Potential for increased effects, duration and toxicity of NSAIDs). Products include:
- Advil Cold & Sinus Caplets (formerly CoAdvil) 2416
- Advil Ibuprofen Tablets and Caplets 2416
- Children's Advil Suspension 2426
- CoAdvil .... ■ 748
- Dristan Sinus Caplets 2419
- Haltran Tablets .... ■ 668
- Ibuprofen .... ■ 631
- Medipren ibuprofen Caplets and Tablets 1362
- Midol 200 Cramp Relief Formula .... ■ 570
- Motrin Tablets 2351
- Motrin IB Caplets and Tablets .... ■ 736
- Nuprin Ibuprofen/Analgesic Tablets & Caplets 752
- PediaProfen Suspension 1363
- Rufen Tablets 691
- Trendar Ibuprofen Tablets .... ■ 756

Indomethacin (Potential for increased effects, duration and toxicity of NSAIDs). Products include:
- Indocin 1487

Indomethacin Sodium Trihydrate (Potential for increased effects, duration and toxicity of NSAIDs). Products include:
- Indocin I.V. 1490

Insulin, Human (Potentiation of insulin effects).
- No products indexed under this heading.

Insulin, Human Isophane Suspension (Potentiation of insulin effects). Products include:
- Humulin N, 100 Units 1270

Insulin, Human NPH (Potentiation of insulin effects). Products include:
- Insulatard NPH Human 1627
- Novolin N 1627
- Novolin N PenFill Cartridges 1628
- Novolin N Prefilled 1628

Insulin, Human Regular (Potentiation of insulin effects). Products include:
- Humulin BR, 100 Units 1268
- Humulin R, 100 Units 1272
- Novolin R 1627
- Novolin R PenFill Cartridges 1628
- Novolin R Prefilled 1629
- Velosulin Human 1628

Insulin, Human, Zinc Suspension (Potentiation of insulin effects). Products include:
- Humulin L, 100 Units 1268
- Humulin U, 100 Units 1272
- Novolin L 1627

Insulin, NPH (Potentiation of insulin effects). Products include:
- NPH, 40 & 100 Units 1273
- Beef NPH, 100 Units 1274
- Pork NPH, 100 Units 1275
- Insulatard NPH 1626
- NPH Insulin 1626
- NPH Purified Pork Isophane Insulin 1626

Insulin, Regular (Potentiation of insulin effects). Products include:
- Regular, 40 & 100 Units 1273
- Beef Regular, 100 Units 1275
- Pork Regular, 100 Units 1275
- Pork Regular (Concentrated), 500 Units 1276
- Regular Insulin 1625
- Regular Purified Pork Insulin 1626
- Velosulin 1627

Insulin, Zinc Crystals (Potentiation of insulin effects). Products include:
- NPH, 40 & 100 Units 1273

Insulin, Zinc Suspension (Potentiation of insulin effects). Products include:
- Lente, 40 & 100 Units 1272
- Protamine, Zinc, 40 & 100 Units 1273
- Lente Iletin I 1272
- Beef Lente, 100 Units 1274
- Beef Protamine Zinc, 100 Units 1274
- Pork Lente, 100 Units 1275
- Pork, Protamine, Zinc, 100 Units 1275
- Lente Insulin 1626
- Lente Purified Pork Insulin 1626
- Semilente Insulin 1625
- Ultralente Insulin 1626

Ketoprofen (Potential for increased effects, duration and toxicity of NSAIDs). Products include:
- Orudis Capsules 2488

Ketorolac Tromethamine (Potential for increased effects, duration and toxicity of NSAIDs). Products include:
- Toradol IM Injection 2302

Lithium Carbonate (Increased serum concentration of lithium). Products include:
- Eskalith 2214
- Lithane Tablets 1596
- Lithium Carbonate Capsules & Tablets 1984
- Lithobid Tablets 870

Lithium Citrate (Increased serum concentration of lithium). Products include:
- Cibalith-S 870

Meclofenamate Sodium (Potential for increased effects, duration and toxicity of NSAIDs). Products include:
- Meclomen Capsules 1739

Mefenamic Acid (Potential for increased effects, duration and toxicity of NSAIDs). Products include:
- Ponstel 1758

Mephobarbital (May decrease the half-life of Butazolidin). Products include:
- Mebaral Tablets 2061

Methohexital Sodium (Potentiation of methotrexate effects). Products include:
- Brevital Sodium Vials 1248

Methotrexate Sodium (Potentiation of methotrexate effects). Products include:
- Methotrexate Tablets, Parenteral, LPF Parenteral 1217
- Rheumatrex Methotrexate Dose Pack 1234

Methylphenidate Hydrochloride (Half-life of Butazolidin is prolonged). Products include:
- Ritalin 880

Naproxen (Potential for increased effects, duration and toxicity of NSAIDs). Products include:
- Naprosyn 2297

Naproxen Sodium (Potential for increased effects, duration and toxicity of NSAIDs). Products include:
- Anaprox and Anaprox DS Tablets 2288

Pentobarbital Sodium (May increase the half-life of Butazolidin). Products include:
- Nembutal Sodium Capsules 534
- Nembutal Sodium Solution 536
- Nembutal Sodium Suppositories 538

Phenobarbital (May decrease the half-life of Butazolidin). Products include:
- Arco-Lase Plus Tablets 607
- Bellergal-S Tablets 1998
- Bronkolixir .... ■ 761
- Bronkotabs Tablets .... ■ 762
- Donnatal 1858
- Donnatal Extentabs 1859
- Donnatal Tablets 1858
- Donnazyme Tablets 1860
- Kinesed Tablets 2272
- Phenobarbital Elixir and Tablets 1293
- Primatene Tablets-P Formula 2421
- Quadrinal Tablets 1183
- Tedral SA 1765

Phenytoin (Potential for increased effects, duration and toxicity of phenytoin). Products include:
- Dilantin Infatabs 1710
- Dilantin-30 Pediatric/Dilantin-125 Suspension 1713

Phenytoin Sodium (Potential for increased effects, duration and toxicity of phenytoin). Products include:
- Dilantin Kapseals 1708
- Dilantin Parenteral 1712
- Dilantin with Phenobarbital Kapseals 1715

Piroxicam (Potential for increased effects, duration and toxicity of NSAIDs). Products include:
- Feldene Capsules 1777

Prednisone (May decrease the half-life of Butazolidin). Products include:
- Deltasone Tablets 2332

Promethazine Hydrochloride (May decrease the half-life of Butazolidin). Products include:
- Mepergan Injection 2479
- Phenergan with Codeine 2497
- Phenergan with Dextromethorphan 2499
- Phenergan Injection 2493
- Phenergan Suppositories 2496
- Phenergan Syrup 2495
- Phenergan Tablets 2496
- Phenergan VC 2500
- Phenergan VC with Codeine 2501

Rifampin (May decrease the half-life of Butazolidin). Products include:
- Rifadin 1345
- Rifamate Capsules 1347
- Rimactane Capsules 879

Secobarbital Sodium (May decrease the half-life of Butazolidin). Products include:
- Seconal Sodium Pulvules 1296

Sulfamethizole (Potential for increased effects, duration and toxicity of sulfonamides). Products include:
- Thiosulfil Forte Tablets 2526
- Urobiotic-250 Capsules 1968

Sulfamethoxazole (Potential for increased effects, duration and toxicity of sulfonamides). Products include:
- Azo Gantanol Tablets 1887
- Bactrim DS Tablets 1891
- Bactrim I.V. Infusion 1889
- Bactrim 1891
- Gantanol 1899
- Septra 813
- Septra I.V. Infusion 808
- Septra I.V. Infusion ADD-Vantage Vials 810
- Septra 813

Sulfasalazine (Potential for increased effects, duration and toxicity of sulfonamides). Products include:
- Azulfidine Tablets, EN-tabs, Oral Suspension 1157

Sulfinpyrazone (Potential for increased effects, duration and toxicity of sulfonamides). Products include:
- Anturane 853

Sulfisoxazole (Potential for increased effects, duration and toxicity of sulfonamides). Products include:
- Azo Gantrisin Tablets 1888
- Gantrisin Tablets 1901
- Pediazole 1973

Sulfisoxazole Diolamine (Potential for increased effects, duration and toxicity of sulfonamides). Products include:
- Gantrisin Ophthalmic Ointment/Solution 1900

Sulindac (Potential for increased effects, duration and toxicity of NSAIDs). Products include:
- Clinoril Tablets 1433

Thiamylal Sodium (May decrease the half-life of Butazolidin). Products include:
- Surital Ampoules, Steri-Vials 1764

Tolazamide (Potential for increased effects, duration and toxicity of oral antidiabetics). Products include:
- Tolinase Tablets 2365

Tolbutamide (Potential for increased effects, duration and toxicity of oral antidiabetics). Products include:
- Orinase Tablets 2354

Tolmetin Sodium (Potential for increased effects, duration and toxicity of NSAIDs). Products include:
- Tolectin (200, 400 and 600 mg) .. 1379

Valproic Acid (Potential for increased effects, duration and toxicity of sodium valproate). Products include:
- Depakene Capsules & Syrup 511

Warfarin Sodium (Potential for increased effects, duration and toxicity of anticoagulants). Products include:
- Coumadin Injection & Tablets 944
- Panwarfin Tablets 547

BUTESIN PICRATE OINTMENT

(Butamben Picrate) 506
No interactions described in labeling.

BUTISOL SODIUM ELIXIR & TABLETS

(Butabarbital Sodium) 2377
May interact with oral anticoagulants, anticoagulants, corticosteroids, central nervous system depressants, monoamine oxidase inhibitors, estrogens, oral contraceptives, and certain other agents. Compounds in these categories include:

Alcohol (Additive CNS depressant effects).

Alfentanil Hydrochloride (Additive CNS depressant effects). Products include:
- Alfenta Injection 1131

Alprazolam (Additive CNS depressant effects). Products include:
- Xanax Tablets 2367

Aprobarbital (Additive CNS depressant effects). Products include:
- Alurate Elixir 1883

Betamethasone Acetate (Enhanced metabolism of corticosteroids; dosage adjustment may be necessary). Products include:
- Celestone Soluspan Suspension 2081

Betamethasone Sodium Phosphate (Enhanced metabolism of corticosteroids; dosage adjustment may be necessary). Products include:
- Celestone Soluspan Suspension 2081

Buprenorphine (Additive CNS depressant effects).
- No products indexed under this heading.

Buspirone Hydrochloride (Additive CNS depressant effects). Products include:
- BuSpar 1401

Butabarbital (Additive CNS depressant effects). Products include:
- Pyridium Plus ... 1764

Butalbital (Additive CNS depressant effects). Products include:
- Esgic-Plus Tablets ... 1002
- Esgic Tablets & Capsules ... 1001
- Fioricet Tablets ... 2006
- Fiorinal Capsules ... 2007
- Fiorinal with Codeine Capsules ... 2008
- Fiorinal Tablets ... 2007
- Phrenilin ... 838
- Sedapap Tablets 50 mg/650 mg ... 1360

Chlordiazepoxide (Additive CNS depressant effects). Products include:
- Libritabs Tablets ... 1930
- Limbitrol ... 1933
- Menrium Tablets ... 1934

Chlordiazepoxide Hydrochloride (Additive CNS depressant effects). Products include:
- Librax Capsules ... 1929
- Librium Capsules ... 1931
- Librium Injectable ... 1932

Chlorotrianisene (Increased metabolism of estradiol). Products include:
- TACE 12 and 25 mg ... 1353

Chlorpromazine (Additive CNS depressant effects). Products include:
- Thorazine ... 2234

Chlorprothixene (Additive CNS depressant effects). Products include:
- Taractan Tablets ... 1920

Chlorprothixene Hydrochloride (Additive CNS depressant effects). Products include:
- Taractan ... 1920

Clorazepate Dipotassium (Additive CNS depressant effects). Products include:
- Tranxene ... 556

Codeine (Additive CNS depressant effects). Products include:
- Calcidrine Syrup ... 506

Codeine Phosphate (Additive CNS depressant effects). Products include:
- Actifed with Codeine Cough Syrup ... 752
- Cheracol Cough Syrup ... 1853
- Codimal PH Syrup ... 846
- Dimetane-DC Cough Syrup ... 1857
- Empirin with Codeine Phosphate Nos. 2, 3 & 4 ... 764
- Fiorinal with Codeine Capsules ... 2008
- Isoclor Expectorant ... 982
- Naldecon CX Adult Liquid ... ▣ 521
- Novahistine DH ... 1342
- Novahistine Expectorant ... 1343
- Nucofed Capsules ... 2219
- Nucofed Expectorant ... 2219
- Nucofed Pediatric Expectorant ... 2220
- Nucofed Syrup ... 2219
- Phenaphen with Codeine Capsules 1865
- Phenaphen-650 with Codeine Tablets ... 1866
- Phenergan with Codeine ... 2497
- Phenergan VC with Codeine ... 2501
- Robitussin A-C Syrup ... 1875
- Robitussin-DAC Syrup ... 1875
- Ryna ... ▣ 741
- Soma Compound w/Codeine Tablets ... 2390
- Triaminic Expectorant w/Codeine ... 1996
- Tussi-Organidin Liquid ... 2391
- Tylenol with Codeine ... 1381

Codeine Polistirex (Additive CNS depressant effects).
- No products indexed under this heading.

Cortisone Acetate (Enhanced metabolism of corticosteroids; dosage adjustment may be necessary). Products include:
- Cortone Acetate Sterile Suspension ... 1437
- Cortone Acetate Tablets ... 1439

Dexamethasone (Enhanced metabolism of corticosteroids; dosage adjustment may be necessary). Products include:
- AK-Trol Ointment & Suspension ... ◉ 207
- Decadron Elixir ... 1445
- Decadron Tablets ... 1447
- Decaspray Topical Aerosol ... 1459
- Dexacidin ... ◉ 272
- Maxidex Sterile Ophthalmic Suspension ... ◉ 223
- Maxitrol Ophthalmic Ointment/Suspension ... ◉ 223
- TobraDex Ophthalmic Suspension and Ointment ... ◉ 228

Dexamethasone Acetate (Enhanced metabolism of corticosteroids; dosage adjustment may be necessary). Products include:
- Dalalone D.P. Injectable ... 999
- Decadron-LA Sterile Suspension ... 1457

Dexamethasone Sodium Phosphate (Enhanced metabolism of corticosteroids; dosage adjustment may be necessary). Products include:
- AK-Dex ... ◉ 203
- Decadron Phosphate Respihaler ... 1454
- Decadron Phosphate Sterile Ophthalmic Ointment ... 1453
- Decadron Phosphate Sterile Ophthalmic Solution ... 1453
- Decadron Phosphate Topical Cream ... 1455
- Decadron Phosphate Turbinaire ... 1456
- Maxidex Sterile Ophthalmic Ointment ... ◉ 222
- NeoDecadron Sterile Ophthalmic Ointment ... 1517
- NeoDecadron Sterile Ophthalmic Solution ... 1518
- NeoDecadron Topical Cream ... 1518

Dezocine (Additive CNS depressant effects).

Diazepam (Additive CNS depressant effects). Products include:
- Valium Injectable ... 1937
- Valium Tablets ... 1939
- Valrelease Capsules ... 1923

Dicumarol (Decreased anticoagulant response). Products include:
- Dicumarol Tablets ... 516

Dienestrol (Increased metabolism of estradiol). Products include:
- Ortho Dienestrol Cream ... 1664

Diethylstilbestrol (Increased metabolism of estradiol). Products include:
- Diethylstilbestrol Tablets ... 1258

Droperidol (Additive CNS depressant effects). Products include:
- Inapsine Injection ... 1140
- Innovar Injection ... 1141

Enflurane (Additive CNS depressant effects). Products include:
- Ethrane ... 599

Estazolam (Additive CNS depressant effects). Products include:
- ProSom Tablets ... 554

Estradiol (Increased metabolism of estradiol). Products include:
- Emcyt Capsules ... 1161
- Estrace ... 1385
- Estrace Vaginal Cream ... 1388
- Estraderm Transdermal System ... 866

Estrogens, Conjugated (Increased metabolism of estradiol). Products include:
- Mediatric Capsules ... 2476
- PMB 200 and PMB 400 ... 2504
- Premarin Intravenous ... 2508
- Premarin with Methyltestosterone ... 2515
- Premarin Tablets ... 2510
- Premarin Vaginal Cream ... 2512

Estrogens, Esterified (Increased metabolism of estradiol). Products include:
- Estratest ... 2245
- Menrium Tablets ... 1934

Estropipate (Increased metabolism of estradiol). Products include:
- Ogen ... 540

Ethchlorvynol (Additive CNS depressant effects). Products include:
- Placidyl Capsules ... 553

Ethinamate (Additive CNS depressant effects).
- No products indexed under this heading.

Ethinyl Estradiol (Increased metabolism of estradiol). Products include:
- Brevicon ... 2304
- Demulen ... 2161
- Estinyl Tablets ... 2085
- Jenest-28 Tablets ... 1636
- Levlen/Tri-Levlen ... 665
- Lo/Ovral Tablets ... 2471
- Lo/Ovral-28 Tablets ... 2476
- Loestrin ... 1728
- Modicon ... 1667
- Nordette-21 Tablets ... 2481
- Nordette-28 Tablets ... 2483
- Norethin ... 2133
- Norinyl ... 2304
- Norlestrin ... 1746
- Ortho-Cyclen Tablets ... 1658
- Ortho-Novum ... 1667
- Ovcon ... 1391
- Ovral Tablets ... 2490
- Ovral-28 Tablets ... 2491
- Levlen/Tri-Levlen ... 665
- Tri-Norinyl ... 2304
- Triphasil-21 Tablets ... 2527
- Triphasil-28 Tablets ... 2532

Ethynodiol Diacetate (Increased metabolism of estradiol). Products include:
- Demulen ... 2161

Fentanyl (Additive CNS depressant effects). Products include:
- Duragesic Transdermal System ... 1133

Fentanyl Citrate (Additive CNS depressant effects). Products include:
- Innovar Injection ... 1141
- Sublimaze Injection ... 1146

Fluphenazine Decanoate (Additive CNS depressant effects). Products include:
- Prolixin Decanoate ... 1795

Fluphenazine Enanthate (Additive CNS depressant effects). Products include:
- Prolixin Enanthate ... 1796

Fluphenazine Hydrochloride (Additive CNS depressant effects). Products include:
- Prolixin Elixir ... 1793
- Prolixin Injection ... 1791
- Prolixin Oral Concentrate ... 1792
- Prolixin Tablets ... 1793

Flurazepam Hydrochloride (Additive CNS depressant effects). Products include:
- Dalmane Capsules ... 1927

Furazolidone (Prolonged barbiturate effects). Products include:
- Furoxone ... 1855

Glutethimide (Additive CNS depressant effects).
- No products indexed under this heading.

Griseofulvin (Decreased griseofulvin blood levels). Products include:
- Fulvicin P/G Tablets ... 2090
- Fulvicin P/G 165 & 330 Tablets ... 2091
- Fulvicin-U/F Tablets ... 2092
- Grifulvin V (griseofulvin microsize) Tablets/Suspension ... 1678
- Grisactin ... 2454
- Grisactin Ultra Tablets ... 2455
- Gris-PEG Tablets, 125 mg & 250 mg ... 1083

Haloperidol (Additive CNS depressant effects). Products include:
- Haldol Injection, Tablets and Concentrate ... 1373

Haloperidol Decanoate (Additive CNS depressant effects). Products include:
- Haldol Decanoate ... 1375

Heparin Calcium (Decreased anticoagulant response). Products include:
- Calciparine Injection ... 925

Heparin Sodium (Decreased anticoagulant response). Products include:
- Heparin Lock Flush Solution ... 2456
- Heparin Sodium Vials ... 1264
- Heparin Sodium Injection ... 2457
- Heparin Sodium Injection, USP, Sterile Solution ... 2342

Hydrocodone Bitartrate (Additive CNS depressant effects). Products include:
- Anexsia 5/500 Tablets ... 2196
- Anexsia 7.5/650 Tablets ... 2197
- Azdōne Tablets ... 844
- Codiclear DH Syrup ... 845
- Codimal DH Syrup ... 846
- Damason-P ... 1356
- Hycodan Syrup, Tablets ... 927
- Hycomine Compound Tablets ... 929
- Hycomine Syrup ... 927
- Hycotuss Expectorant Syrup ... 930
- Hydrocet Capsules ... 835
- Lortab ASA Tablets ... 2414
- Lortab ... 2412
- Ru-Tuss with Hydrocodone ... 694
- Triaminic Expectorant DH ... 1995
- Vicodin Tablets ... 1187
- Vicodin ES Tablets ... 1189
- Zydone Capsules ... 941

Hydrocodone Polistirex (Additive CNS depressant effects). Products include:
- Tussionex Extended-Release Suspension ... 988

Hydrocortisone (Enhanced metabolism of corticosteroids; dosage adjustment may be necessary). Products include:
- AK-Spore H.C. ... ◉ 206
- Bactine Hydrocortisone Anti-Itch Cream ... ▣ 625
- CaldeCORT Anti-Itch Hydrocortisone Spray ... ▣ 560
- Carmol HC Cream 1% ... 2296
- Cortaid Spray ... ▣ 735
- Cortenema ... 2244
- Cortisporin Ointment ... 758
- Cortisporin Ophthalmic Ointment Sterile ... 758
- Cortisporin Ophthalmic Suspension Sterile ... 759
- Cortisporin Otic Solution Sterile ... 760
- Cortisporin Otic Suspension Sterile 760
- Cortizone-5 Creme & Ointment ... ▣ 732
- Dermolate Anti-Itch Cream ... ▣ 697
- Eldecort Cream 1.0% ... 1113
- Eldecort Cream 1.0% and 2.5% ... 1113
- Fungoid HC Creme ... 1770
- Hydrocortone Tablets ... 1482
- Hytone ... 909
- LazerSporin-C Solution ... 1770
- Massengill Medicated Soft Cloth Towelettes ... 2192
- Nutracort Cream & Lotion ... 1684
- PediOtic Suspension Sterile ... 797
- Synacort Creams 1%, 2.5% ... 2296
- Vanoxide-HC Acne Lotion ... 911
- Vioform-Hydrocortisone Cream and Mild Cream ... 889
- Vioform-Hydrocortisone Ointment ... 889
- VōSoL HC Otic Solution ... 2392
- Vytone Cream 1% ... 911

Hydrocortisone Acetate (Enhanced metabolism of corticosteroids; dosage adjustment may be necessary). Products include:
- Analpram-HC Rectal Cream 1% and 2.5% ... 970
- Anusol-HC Cream ... 1690
- Anusol-HC Suppositories ... 1691
- Caldecort ... ▣ 560
- Carmol HC Cream 1% ... 2296
- Chloromycetin Hydrocortisone Ophthalmic ... 1694
- Coly-Mycin S Otic w/Neomycin & Hydrocortisone ... 1708
- Cortaid ... ▣ 735
- Cortef Feminine Itch Cream ... ▣ 735

Corticaine ▣ 682
Cortifoam 1827
Cortisporin Cream 757
Epifoam 1828
Gynecort 5 Creme ▣ 556
Hydrocortone Acetate Sterile Suspension 1479
Lanacort 5 Creme and Ointment ▣ 557
Mantadil Cream 789
Ophthocort ◉ 301
Orabase HCA Oral Paste 890
Pramosone Cream, Lotion & Ointment 971
ProctoCream-HC 1834
Proctofoam-HC 1835

Hydrocortisone Sodium Phosphate (Enhanced metabolism of corticosteroids; dosage adjustment may be necessary). Products include:
Hydrocortone Phosphate Injection, Sterile 1481

Hydrocortisone Sodium Succinate (Enhanced metabolism of corticosteroids; dosage adjustment may be necessary). Products include:
Solu-Cortef Sterile Powder 2361

Hydroxyzine Hydrochloride (Additive CNS depressant effects). Products include:
Atarax Tablets & Syrup 1941
Marax Tablets & DF Syrup 1954
Vistaril Intramuscular Solution 1970

Isocarboxazid (Prolonged barbiturate effects). Products include:
Marplan Tablets 1906

Isoflurane (Additive CNS depressant effects). Products include:
Forane 600

Ketamine Hydrochloride (Additive CNS depressant effects). Products include:
Ketalar 1726

Levonorgestrel (Increased metabolism of estradiol). Products include:
Levlen/Tri-Levlen 665
Nordette-21 Tablets 2481
Nordette-28 Tablets 2483
Norplant System 2484
Levlen/Tri-Levlen 665
Triphasil-21 Tablets 2527
Triphasil-28 Tablets 2532

Levorphanol Tartrate (Additive CNS depressant effects). Products include:
Levo-Dromoran 1906

Lorazepam (Additive CNS depressant effects). Products include:
Ativan Injection 2432
Ativan Tablets 2434

Loxapine Hydrochloride (Additive CNS depressant effects). Products include:
Loxitane 1213

Loxapine Succinate (Additive CNS depressant effects). Products include:
Loxitane Capsules 1213

Meperidine Hydrochloride (Additive CNS depressant effects). Products include:
Demerol 2047
Mepergan Injection 2479

Mephobarbital (Additive CNS depressant effects). Products include:
Mebaral Tablets 2061

Meprobamate (Additive CNS depressant effects). Products include:
Deprol Tablets 2382
Equagesic Tablets 2451
Miltown Tablets 2386
PMB 200 and PMB 400 2504

Mesoridazine (Additive CNS depressant effects). Products include:
Serentil 686

Mestranol (Increased metabolism of estradiol). Products include:
Enovid 2161
Norethin 2133
Norinyl 2304
Ortho-Novum 1667

Methadone Hydrochloride (Additive CNS depressant effects). Products include:
Dolophine Hydrochloride Ampoules & Vials 1260
Dolophine Hydrochloride Tablets 1261
Methadone Hydrochloride Diskets 1284
Methadone Hydrochloride Oral Solution & Tablets 1987

Methohexital Sodium (Additive CNS depressant effects). Products include:
Brevital Sodium Vials 1248

Methoxyflurane (Additive CNS depressant effects).
No products indexed under this heading.

Methylprednisolone (Enhanced metabolism of corticosteroids; dosage adjustment may be necessary). Products include:
Medrol 2348

Methylprednisolone Acetate (Enhanced metabolism of corticosteroids; dosage adjustment may be necessary). Products include:
Depo-Medrol Sterile Aqueous Suspension 2334

Methylprednisolone Sodium Succinate (Enhanced metabolism of corticosteroids; dosage adjustment may be necessary). Products include:
Solu-Medrol Sterile Powder 2363

Midazolam Hydrochloride (Additive CNS depressant effects). Products include:
Versed Injection 1924

Molindone Hydrochloride (Additive CNS depressant effects). Products include:
Moban Tablets & Concentrate 932

Morphine Sulfate (Additive CNS depressant effects). Products include:
Astramorph/PF Injection, USP (Preservative-Free) 618
Duramorph 960
Infumorph 200 and Infumorph 500 Sterile Solutions 962
MS Contin Tablets 1814
MSIR 1817
Oramorph SR (Morphine Sulfate Sustained Release Tablets) 1988
Roxanol 1991

Norethindrone (Increased metabolism of estradiol). Products include:
Brevicon 2304
Jenest-28 Tablets 1636
Micronor Tablets 1667
Modicon 1667
Norethin 2133
Norinyl 2304
Norlutin 1755
Nor-Q D Tablets 2304
Ortho-Novum 1667
Ovcon 1391
Tri-Norinyl 2304

Norethynodrel (Increased metabolism of estradiol). Products include:
Enovid 2161

Norgestimate (Increased metabolism of estradiol). Products include:
Ortho-Cyclen Tablets 1658

Norgestrel (Increased metabolism of estradiol). Products include:
Lo/Ovral Tablets 2471
Lo/Ovral-28 Tablets 2476
Ovral Tablets 2490
Ovral-28 Tablets 2491
Ovrette Tablets 2492

Opium Alkaloids (Additive CNS depressant effects). Products include:
B & O No. 15A & No. 16A Supprettes 2395
Pantopon Injectable 1911

Oxazepam (Additive CNS depressant effects). Products include:
Serax Capsules 2522
Serax Tablets 2522

Oxycodone Hydrochloride (Additive CNS depressant effects). Products include:
Percocet Tablets 950
Percodan 951
Roxicodone Tablets, Oral Solution & Intensol (Oxycodone) 1992
Tylox Capsules 1382

Pentobarbital Sodium (Additive CNS depressant effects). Products include:
Nembutal Sodium Capsules 534
Nembutal Sodium Solution 536
Nembutal Sodium Suppositories 538

Perphenazine (Additive CNS depressant effects). Products include:
Etrafon 2087
Triavil Tablets 1556
Trilafon 2123

Phenelzine Sulfate (Prolonged barbiturate effects). Products include:
Nardil 1742

Phenobarbital (Additive CNS depressant effects). Products include:
Arco-Lase Plus Tablets 607
Bellergal-S Tablets 1998
Bronkolixir ▣ 761
Bronkotabs Tablets ▣ 762
Donnatal 1858
Donnatal Extentabs 1859
Donnatal Tablets 1858
Donnazyme Tablets 1860
Kinesed Tablets 2272
Phenobarbital Elixir and Tablets 1293
Primatene Tablets-P Formula 2421
Quadrinal Tablets 1183
Tedral SA 1765

Phenprocoumon (Decreased anticoagulant effect).

Phenytoin (Variable effect on phenytoin metabolism). Products include:
Dilantin Infatabs 1710
Dilantin-30 Pediatric/Dilantin-125 Suspension 1713

Phenytoin Sodium (Variable effect on phenytoin metabolism). Products include:
Dilantin Kapseals 1708
Dilantin Parenteral 1712
Dilantin with Phenobarbital Kapseals 1715

Polyestradiol Phosphate (Increased metabolism of estradiol). Products include:
Estradurin 2452

Prazepam (Additive CNS depressant effects). Products include:
Centrax 1693

Prednisolone Acetate (Enhanced metabolism of corticosteroids; dosage adjustment may be necessary). Products include:
AK-Cide Sterile Ophthalmic Ointment & Suspension ◉ 202
Blephamide Liquifilm Sterile Ophthalmic Suspension 586
Blephamide S.O.P. Sterile Ophthalmic Ointment 586
Cetapred Ointment ◉ 220
⅛% Econopred & 1% Econopred Plus ◉ 217
Isopto Cetapred Suspension ◉ 220
Metimyd ◉ 306
Poly-Pred Liquifilm ◉ 250
Pred Forte ◉ 252
Pred Mild ◉ 254
Pred-G Liquifilm Sterile Ophthalmic Suspension ◉ 252
Pred-G S.O.P. Sterile Ophthalmic Ointment ◉ 253
Vasocidin Ointment ◉ 275

Prednisolone Sodium Phosphate (Enhanced metabolism of corticosteroids; dosage adjustment may be necessary). Products include:
AK-Pred ◉ 205
Hydeltrasol Injection, Sterile 1476
Inflamase ◉ 274
Pediapred Oral Liquid 987
Vasocidin Ophthalmic Solution ◉ 276

Prednisolone Tebutate (Enhanced metabolism of corticosteroids; dosage adjustment may be necessary). Products include:
Hydeltra-T.B.A. Sterile Suspension 1478

Prednisone (Enhanced metabolism of corticosteroids; dosage adjustment may be necessary). Products include:
Deltasone Tablets 2332

Prochlorperazine (Additive CNS depressant effects). Products include:
Compazine 2201

Promethazine Hydrochloride (Additive CNS depressant effects). Products include:
Mepergan Injection 2479
Phenergan with Codeine 2497
Phenergan with Dextromethorphan 2499
Phenergan Injection 2493
Phenergan Suppositories 2496
Phenergan Syrup 2495
Phenergan Tablets 2496
Phenergan VC 2500
Phenergan VC with Codeine 2501

Propofol (Additive CNS depressant effects). Products include:
Diprivan Injection 2267

Propoxyphene Hydrochloride (Additive CNS depressant effects). Products include:
Darvon 1256
Wygesic Tablets 2540

Propoxyphene Napsylate (Additive CNS depressant effects). Products include:
Darvon-N/Darvocet-N 1254

Quazepam (Additive CNS depressant effects). Products include:
Doral Tablets 2383

Quinestrol (Increased metabolism of estradiol). Products include:
Estrovis 1721

Secobarbital Sodium (Additive CNS depressant effects). Products include:
Seconal Sodium Pulvules 1296

Selegiline Hydrochloride (Prolonged barbiturate effects). Products include:
Eldepryl 2250

Sufentanil Citrate (Additive CNS depressant effects). Products include:
Sufenta Injection 1147

Temazepam (Additive CNS depressant effects). Products include:
Restoril Capsules 2023

Thiamylal Sodium (Additive CNS depressant effects). Products include:
Surital Ampoules, Steri-Vials 1764

Thioridazine Hydrochloride (Additive CNS depressant effects). Products include:
Mellaril 2011

Thiothixene (Additive CNS depressant effects). Products include:
Navane Capsules and Concentrate 1954
Navane Intramuscular 1956

Tranylcypromine Sulfate (Prolonged barbiturate effects). Products include:
Parnate Tablets 2222

Triamcinolone (Enhanced metabolism of corticosteroids; dosage adjustment may be necessary).
No products indexed under this heading.

Triamcinolone Acetonide (Enhanced metabolism of corticosteroids; dosage adjustment may be necessary). Products include:
Aristocort A 1010
Azmacort Inhaler 1837
Kenalog Cream, Lotion & Ointment 2401
Kenalog-10 Injection 2402

Kenalog-40 Injection ... 2403
Kenalog in Orabase ... 604
Kenalog Spray ... 2401
Mycolog II Cream and Ointment ... 2407
Mytrex Cream & Ointment ... 2080
Nasacort Nasal Inhaler ... 1844

Triamcinolone Diacetate (Enhanced metabolism of corticosteroids; dosage adjustment may be necessary). Products include:
Aristocort Suspension ... 1008

Triamcinolone Hexacetonide (Enhanced metabolism of corticosteroids; dosage adjustment may be necessary). Products include:
Aristospan Suspension ... 1011

Triazolam (Additive CNS depressant effects). Products include:
Halcion Tablets ... 2340

Trifluoperazine Hydrochloride (Additive CNS depressant effects). Products include:
Stelazine ... 2226

Valproic Acid (Decreased barbiturate metabolism). Products include:
Depakene Capsules & Syrup ... 511

Warfarin Sodium (Decreased anticoagulant response). Products include:
Coumadin Injection & Tablets ... 944
Panwarfin Tablets ... 547

CAFERGOT SUPPOSITORIES

(Ergotamine Tartrate, Caffeine) ... 1999
No interactions described in labeling.

CAFERGOT TABLETS

(Ergotamine Tartrate, Caffeine) ... 1999
No interactions described in labeling.

CALADRYL CREAM, LOTION, SPRAY

(Calamine, Diphenhydramine Hydrochloride) ... ▣ 638
No interactions described in labeling.

CALAN SR CAPLETS

(Verapamil Hydrochloride) ... 2157
May interact with beta blockers, lithium preparations, nondepolarizing neuromuscular blocking agents, inhalant anesthetics, alpha adrenergic blockers, cardiac glycosides, diuretics, ACE inhibitors, vasodilators, and certain other agents. Compounds in these categories include:

Acebutolol Hydrochloride (Additive effect on lowering blood pressure; additive negative effects on heart rate, atrioventricular conduction, and/or cardiac contractility). Products include:
Sectral Capsules ... 2520

Amiloride Hydrochloride (Additive effect on lowering blood pressure). Products include:
Midamor Tablets ... 1508
Moduretic Tablets ... 1510

Aminophylline (Verapamil may inhibit the clearance and increase the plasma levels of theophylline). Products include:
Amesec ... ▣ 682
Aminophyllin Tablets ... 2153

Atenolol (Additive effect on lowering blood pressure; additive negative effects on heart rate, atrioventricular conduction, and/or cardiac contractility; variable effect in atenolol clearance). Products include:
Tenoretic Tablets ... 1105
Tenormin Tablets and I.V. Injection 1107

Atracurium Besylate (Activity of neuromuscular blocking agents potentiated). Products include:
Tracrium Injection ... 817

Benazepril Hydrochloride (Additive effect on lowering blood pressure). Products include:
Lotensin Tablets ... 872

Bendroflumethiazide (Additive effect on lowering blood pressure). Products include:
Corzide Tablets ... 702
Naturetin Tablets ... 1789
Rauzide Tablets ... 1804

Betaxolol Hydrochloride (Additive effect on lowering blood pressure; additive negative effects on heart rate, atrioventricular conduction, and/or cardiac contractility). Products include:
Betoptic Sterile Ophthalmic Solution ... 569
Betoptic S Sterile Ophthalmic Suspension ... 570
Kerlone Tablets ... 2172

Bumetanide (Additive effect on lowering blood pressure). Products include:
Bumex ... 1895

Captopril (Additive effect on lowering blood pressure). Products include:
Capoten ... 2255
Capozide ... 2258

Carbamazepine (Increased concentrations of carbamazepine). Products include:
Tegretol Chewable Tablets ... 654
Tegretol Suspension ... 656
Tegretol Tablets ... 654

Carteolol Hydrochloride (Additive effect on lowering blood pressure; additive negative effects on heart rate, atrioventricular conduction, and/or cardiac contractility). Products include:
Cartrol Tablets ... 507

Chlorothiazide (Additive effect on lowering blood pressure). Products include:
Aldoclor Tablets ... 1413
Diupres Tablets ... 1461
Diuril Oral ... 1464

Chlorothiazide Sodium (Additive effect on lowering blood pressure). Products include:
Diuril Sodium Intravenous ... 1463

Chlorthalidone (Additive effect on lowering blood pressure). Products include:
Combipres Tablets ... 678
Tenoretic Tablets ... 1105
Thalitone Tablets ... 687

Cimetidine (Possible reduction in verapamil clearance). Products include:
Tagamet Tablets ... 2228

Cimetidine Hydrochloride (Possible reduction in verapamil clearance). Products include:
Tagamet ... 2228

Clonidine (Additive effect on lowering blood pressure). Products include:
Catapres-TTS ... 677

Clonidine Hydrochloride (Additive effect on lowering blood pressure). Products include:
Catapres Tablets ... 676
Combipres Tablets ... 678

Cyclosporine (Possible increase in serum levels of cyclosporine). Products include:
Sandimmune ... 2024

Deslanoside (Chronic verapamil treatment can increase serum digoxin levels and this can result in digitalis toxicity).
No products indexed under this heading.

Diazoxide (Additive effect on lowering blood pressure). Products include:
Hyperstat I.V. Injection ... 2095
Proglycem ... 649

Digitoxin (Chronic verapamil treatment can increase serum digoxin levels and this can result in digitalis toxicity). Products include:
Crystodigin Tablets ... 1253

Digoxin (Chronic verapamil treatment can increase serum digoxin levels and this can result in digitalis toxicity). Products include:
Lanoxicaps ... 772
Lanoxin Elixir Pediatric ... 775
Lanoxin Injection ... 778
Lanoxin Injection Pediatric ... 781
Lanoxin Tablets ... 783

Disopyramide Phosphate (Do not administer concomitantly). Products include:
Norpace ... 2177

Doxazosin Mesylate (May result in a reduction in blood pressure that is excessive in some patients). Products include:
Cardura Tablets ... 1941

Dyphylline (Verapamil may inhibit the clearance and increase the plasma levels of theophylline). Products include:
Dilor ... 2079
Dilor-G Tablets & Liquid ... 2079
Lufyllin Elixir ... 2384
Lufyllin & Lufyllin-400 Tablets ... 2384
Lufyllin-GG Elixir & Tablets ... 2385

Enalapril Maleate (Additive effect on lowering blood pressure). Products include:
Vaseretic Tablets ... 1559
Vasotec Tablets ... 1564

Enalaprilat (Additive effect on lowering blood pressure). Products include:
Vasotec I.V. ... 1562

Enflurane (Excessive cardiovascular depression). Products include:
Ethrane ... 599

Esmolol Hydrochloride (Additive effect on lowering blood pressure; additive negative effects on heart rate, atrioventricular conduction, and/or cardiac contractility). Products include:
Brevibloc Injection ... 942

Ethacrynic Acid (Additive effect on lowering blood pressure). Products include:
Edecrin Tablets ... 1468

Flecainide Acetate (Possible additive effects on myocardial contractility, AV conduction, and repolarization). Products include:
Tambocor Tablets ... 1315

Fosinopril Sodium (Additive effect on lowering blood pressure). Products include:
Monopril Tablets ... 1406

Furosemide (Additive effect on lowering blood pressure). Products include:
Lasix ... 1093

Guanabenz Acetate (Additive effect on lowering blood pressure). Products include:
Wytensin Tablets ... 2542

Guanadrel Sulfate (Additive effect on lowering blood pressure). Products include:
Hylorel Tablets ... 975

Guanethidine Monosulfate (Additive effect on lowering blood pressure). Products include:
Esimil Tablets ... 864
Ismelin Tablets ... 869

Halothane (Excessive cardiovascular depression). Products include:
Fluothane ... 2453

Hydralazine Hydrochloride (Additive effect on lowering blood pressure). Products include:
Apresazide Capsules ... 854
Apresoline Hydrochloride Parenteral (Ampuls) ... 856
Apresoline Hydrochloride Tablets .. 855
Apresoline-Esidrix Tablets ... 857
Ser-Ap-Es Tablets ... 881
Serpasil-Apresoline Tablets ... 884

Hydrochlorothiazide (Additive effect on lowering blood pressure). Products include:
Aldactazide ... 2150
Aldoril Tablets ... 1418
Apresazide Capsules ... 854
Apresoline-Esidrix Tablets ... 857
Capozide ... 2258
Dyazide Capsules ... 2208
Esidrix Tablets ... 863
Esimil Tablets ... 864
HydroDIURIL Tablets ... 1484
Hydropres Tablets ... 1485
Inderide Tablets ... 2463
Inderide LA Long Acting Capsules .. 2465
Lopressor HCT Tablets ... 1034
Maxzide ... 1215
Moduretic Tablets ... 1510
Normozide Tablets ... 2112
Oretic Tablets ... 544
Oreticyl ... 545
Prinzide Tablets ... 1540
Ser-Ap-Es Tablets ... 881
Serpasil-Esidrix Tablets ... 886
Timolide Tablets ... 1547
Trandate HCT Tablets ... 579
Vaseretic Tablets ... 1559
Zestoretic ... 2274

Hydroflumethiazide (Additive effect on lowering blood pressure). Products include:
Diucardin Tablets ... 2450
Saluron ... 718
Salutensin/Salutensin-Demi ... 719

Indapamide (Additive effect on lowering blood pressure). Products include:
Lozol Tablets ... 1843

Isoflurane (Excessive cardiovascular depression). Products include:
Forane ... 600

Labetalol Hydrochloride (Additive effect on lowering blood pressure; additive negative effects on heart rate, atrioventricular conduction, and/or cardiac contractility). Products include:
Normodyne Injection ... 2108
Normodyne Tablets ... 2110
Normozide Tablets ... 2112
Trandate HCT Tablets ... 579
Trandate Injection ... 577
Trandate Tablets ... 579

Lisinopril (Additive effect on lowering blood pressure). Products include:
Prinivil Tablets ... 1538
Prinzide Tablets ... 1540
Zestoretic ... 2274
Zestril Tablets ... 2277

Lithium Carbonate (Possible lowering of serum lithium levels; possible increased sensitivity to effects of lithium). Products include:
Eskalith ... 2214
Lithane Tablets ... 1596
Lithium Carbonate Capsules & Tablets ... 1984
Lithobid Tablets ... 870

Lithium Citrate (Possible lowering of serum lithium levels; possible increased sensitivity to effects of lithium). Products include:
Cibalith-S ... 870

Mecamylamine Hydrochloride (Additive effect on lowering blood pressure). Products include:
Inversine Tablets ... 1492

(▣ Described in PDR For Nonprescription Drugs) (⊙ Described in PDR For Ophthalmology)

Methoxyflurane (Excessive cardiovascular depression).
No products indexed under this heading.

Methyclothiazide (Additive effect on lowering blood pressure). Products include:
Enduron Tablets ... 517
Enduronyl ... 518

Methyldopa (Additive effect on lowering blood pressure). Products include:
Aldoclor Tablets ... 1413
Aldomet Oral ... 1415
Aldoril Tablets ... 1418

Methyldopate Hydrochloride (Additive effect on lowering blood pressure). Products include:
Aldomet Ester HCl Injection ... 1417

Metocurine Iodide (Activity of neuromuscular blocking agents potentiated). Products include:
Metubine Iodide Vials ... 1285

Metolazone (Additive effect on lowering blood pressure). Products include:
Diulo ... 2129
Mykrox ½ mg Tablets ... 984
Zaroxolyn Tablets ... 989

Metoprolol Tartrate (Additive effect on lowering blood pressure; additive negative effects on heart rate, atrioventricular conduction, and/or cardiac contractility; decrease in metoprolol clearance). Products include:
Lopressor Ampuls ... 1032
Lopressor HCT Tablets ... 1034
Lopressor Tablets ... 1032

Metyrosine (Additive effect on lowering blood pressure). Products include:
Demser Capsules ... 1460

Minoxidil (Additive effect on lowering blood pressure). Products include:
Loniten Tablets ... 2346
Rogaine Topical Solution ... 2357

Nadolol (Additive effect on lowering blood pressure; additive negative effects on heart rate, atrioventricular conduction, and/or cardiac contractility). Products include:
Corgard Tablets ... 701
Corzide Tablets ... 702

Pancuronium Bromide Injection (Activity of neuromuscular blocking agents potentiated).
No products indexed under this heading.

Penbutolol Sulfate (Additive effect on lowering blood pressure; additive negative effects on heart rate, atrioventricular conduction, and/or cardiac contractility). Products include:
Levatol ... 1832

Phenobarbital (Verapamil clearance may be increased). Products include:
Arco-Lase Plus Tablets ... 607
Bellergal-S Tablets ... 1998
Bronkolixir ... ▣ 761
Bronkotabs Tablets ... ▣ 762
Donnatal ... 1858
Donnatal Extentabs ... 1859
Donnatal Tablets ... 1858
Donnazyme Tablets ... 1860
Kinesed Tablets ... 2272
Phenobarbital Elixir and Tablets ... 1293
Primatene Tablets-P Formula ... 2421
Quadrinal Tablets ... 1183
Tedral SA ... 1765

Phenoxybenzamine Hydrochloride (Additive effect on lowering blood pressure). Products include:
Dibenzyline Capsules ... 2207

Phentolamine Mesylate (Additive effect on lowering blood pressure). Products include:
Regitine ... 878

Pindolol (Additive effect on lowering blood pressure; additive negative effects on heart rate, atrioventricular conduction, and/or cardiac contractility). Products include:
Visken Tablets ... 2036

Polythiazide (Additive effect on lowering blood pressure). Products include:
Minizide Capsules ... 1779
Renese Tablets ... 1785
Renese-R Tablets ... 1786

Prazosin Hydrochloride (May result in a reduction in blood pressure that is excessive in some patients). Products include:
Minipress Capsules ... 1778
Minizide Capsules ... 1779

Propranolol Hydrochloride (Additive effect on lowering blood pressure; additive negative effects on heart rate, atrioventricular conduction, and/or cardiac contractility; decrease in propranolol clearance). Products include:
Inderal ... 2459
Inderal LA Long Acting Capsules ... 2461
Inderide Tablets ... 2463
Inderide LA Long Acting Capsules ... 2465

Quinidine Gluconate (Hypotension in patients with hypertrophic cardiomyopathy). Products include:
Quinaglute Dura-Tabs Tablets ... 663

Quinidine Polygalacturonate (Hypotension in patients with hypertrophic cardiomyopathy). Products include:
Cardioquin Tablets ... 1812

Quinidine Sulfate (Hypotension in patients with hypertrophic cardiomyopathy). Products include:
Quinidex Extentabs ... 1868

Ramipril (Additive effect on lowering blood pressure). Products include:
Altace Capsules ... 1086

Rifampin (Reduced oral verapamil bioavailability). Products include:
Rifadin ... 1345
Rifamate Capsules ... 1347
Rimactane Capsules ... 879

Spironolactone (Additive effect on lowering blood pressure). Products include:
Aldactazide ... 2150
Aldactone ... 2152

Succinylcholine Chloride (Potentiation of neuromuscular blockers). Products include:
Anectine ... 755

Terazosin Hydrochloride (May result in a reduction in blood pressure that is excessive in some patients). Products include:
Hytrin Tablets ... 529

Theophylline (Verapamil may inhibit the clearance and increase the plasma levels of theophylline). Products include:
Bronkaid Tablets ... ▣ 757
Bronkolixir ... ▣ 761
Bronkotabs Tablets ... ▣ 762
Constant-T Tablets ... 1029
Marax Tablets & DF Syrup ... 1954
Primatene Tablets ... 2421
Quibron Capsules ... 713
Quibron-T ... 714
Quibron-T/SR ... 716
Theolair Liquid ... 1317
Theo-Organidin Elixir ... 2391

Theophylline Anhydrous (Verapamil may inhibit the clearance and increase the plasma levels of theophylline). Products include:
Aerolate ... 994
Primatene Tablets-M Formula ... ▣ 753
Primatene Tablets-Regular Formula ... 2421
Respbid Tablets ... 684
Slo-bid Gyrocaps ... 1847
T-PHYL (Uniphyl) 200 mg Tablets ... 1820
Tedral SA ... 1765
Theo-24 ... 2179
Theo-Dur Sprinkle ... 1168
Theo-Dur Extended-Release Tablets ... 1166
Theolair Tablets ... 1317
Theolair-SR Tablets ... 1319
TheoX Extended-Release Tablets ... 841
Uniphyl 400 mg Tablets ... 1823

Theophylline Calcium Salicylate (Verapamil may inhibit the clearance and increase the plasma levels of theophylline). Products include:
Quadrinal Tablets ... 1183

Theophylline Sodium Glycinate (Verapamil may inhibit the clearance and increase the plasma levels of theophylline). Products include:
Asbron G ... 1997

Timolol Maleate (Additive effect on lowering blood pressure; additive negative effects on heart rate, atrioventricular conduction, and/or cardiac contractility). Products include:
Blocadren Tablets ... 1429
Timolide Tablets ... 1547
Timoptic in Ocudose ... 1552
Timoptic Sterile Ophthalmic Solution ... 1550

Triamterene (Additive effect on lowering blood pressure). Products include:
Dyazide Capsules ... 2208
Dyrenium Capsules ... 2210
Maxzide ... 1215

Vecuronium Bromide (Activity of neuromuscular blocking agents potentiated). Products include:
Norcuron ... 1642

Food Interactions

Food, unspecified (Produces decreased bioavailability (AUC) but a narrower peak-to-trough ratio).

CALAN TABLETS

(Verapamil Hydrochloride) ... 2155
May interact with beta blockers, cardiac glycosides, lithium preparations, diuretics, ACE inhibitors, vasodilators, nondepolarizing neuromuscular blocking agents, inhalant anesthetics, and certain other agents. Compounds in these categories include:

Acebutolol Hydrochloride (Additive negative effects on heart rate, AV conduction and/or cardiac contractility; additive hypotensive effect). Products include:
Sectral Capsules ... 2520

Amiloride Hydrochloride (Additive effect on lowering blood pressure). Products include:
Midamor Tablets ... 1508
Moduretic Tablets ... 1510

Aminophylline (Verapamil may inhibit the clearance and increase the plasma levels of theophylline). Products include:
Amesec ... ▣ 682
Aminophyllin Tablets ... 2153

Atenolol (Additive negative effects on heart rate, AV conduction and/or cardiac contractility; additive hypotensive effect; variable effect in atenolol clearance). Products include:
Tenoretic Tablets ... 1105
Tenormin Tablets and I.V. Injection ... 1107

Atracurium Besylate (Activity of neuromuscular blocking agents potentiated). Products include:
Tracrium Injection ... 817

Benazepril Hydrochloride (Additive effect on lowering blood pressure). Products include:
Lotensin Tablets ... 872

Bendroflumethiazide (Additive effect on lowering blood pressure). Products include:
Corzide Tablets ... 702
Naturetin Tablets ... 1789
Rauzide Tablets ... 1804

Betaxolol Hydrochloride (Additive negative effects on heart rate, AV conduction and/or cardiac contractility; additive hypotensive effect). Products include:
Betoptic Sterile Ophthalmic Solution ... 569
Betoptic S Sterile Ophthalmic Suspension ... 570
Kerlone Tablets ... 2172

Bumetanide (Additive effect on lowering blood pressure). Products include:
Bumex ... 1895

Captopril (Additive effect on lowering blood pressure). Products include:
Capoten ... 2255
Capozide ... 2258

Carbamazepine (Increased carbamazepine concentrations). Products include:
Tegretol Chewable Tablets ... 654
Tegretol Suspension ... 656
Tegretol Tablets ... 654

Carteolol Hydrochloride (Additive negative effects on heart rate, AV conduction, and/or cardiac contractility; additive hypotensive effect). Products include:
Cartrol Tablets ... 507

Chlorothiazide (Additive effect on lowering blood pressure). Products include:
Aldoclor Tablets ... 1413
Diupres Tablets ... 1461
Diuril Oral ... 1464

Chlorothiazide Sodium (Additive effect on lowering blood pressure). Products include:
Diuril Sodium Intravenous ... 1463

Chlorthalidone (Additive effect on lowering blood pressure). Products include:
Combipres Tablets ... 678
Tenoretic Tablets ... 1105
Thalitone Tablets ... 687

Cimetidine (Possible reduction in verapamil clearance). Products include:
Tagamet Tablets ... 2228

Cimetidine Hydrochloride (Possible reduction in verapamil clearance). Products include:
Tagamet ... 2228

Clonidine (Additive effect on lowering blood pressure). Products include:
Catapres-TTS ... 677

Clonidine Hydrochloride (Additive effect on lowering blood pressure). Products include:
Catapres Tablets ... 676
Combipres Tablets ... 678

Cyclosporine (Possible increase in serum levels of cyclosporine). Products include:
Sandimmune ... 2024

Deslanoside (Chronic verapamil treatment can increase serum digoxin levels and this can result in digitalis toxicity).
No products indexed under this heading.

Diazoxide (Additive effect on lowering blood pressure). Products include:
Hyperstat I.V. Injection ... 2095
Proglycem ... 649

Digitoxin (Chronic verapamil treatment can increase serum digoxin levels and this can result in digitalis toxicity). Products include:
- Crystodigin Tablets ... 1253

Digoxin (Chronic verapamil treatment can increase serum digoxin levels and this can result in digitalis toxicity). Products include:
- Lanoxicaps ... 772
- Lanoxin Elixir Pediatric ... 775
- Lanoxin Injection ... 778
- Lanoxin Injection Pediatric ... 781
- Lanoxin Tablets ... 783

Disopyramide Phosphate (Do not administer concomitantly). Products include:
- Norpace ... 2177

Dyphylline (Verapamil may inhibit the clearance and increase the plasma levels of theophylline). Products include:
- Dilor ... 2079
- Dilor-G Tablets & Liquid ... 2079
- Lufyllin Elixir ... 2384
- Lufyllin & Lufyllin-400 Tablets ... 2384
- Lufyllin-GG Elixir & Tablets ... 2385

Enalapril Maleate (Additive effect on lowering blood pressure). Products include:
- Vaseretic Tablets ... 1559
- Vasotec Tablets ... 1564

Enalaprilat (Additive effect on lowering blood pressure). Products include:
- Vasotec I.V. ... 1562

Enflurane (Excessive cardiovascular depression). Products include:
- Ethrane ... 599

Esmolol Hydrochloride (Additive negative effects on heart rate, AV conduction and/or cardiac contractility; additive hypotensive effect). Products include:
- Brevibloc Injection ... 942

Ethacrynic Acid (Additive effect on lowering blood pressure). Products include:
- Edecrin Tablets ... 1468

Flecainide Acetate (Possible additive negative inotropic effect and prolongation of AV conduction). Products include:
- Tambocor Tablets ... 1315

Fosinopril Sodium (Additive effect on lowering blood pressure). Products include:
- Monopril Tablets ... 1406

Furosemide (Additive effect on lowering blood pressure). Products include:
- Lasix ... 1093

Guanabenz Acetate (Additive effect on lowering blood pressure). Products include:
- Wytensin Tablets ... 2542

Guanadrel Sulfate (Additive effect on lowering blood pressure). Products include:
- Hylorel Tablets ... 975

Guanethidine Monosulfate (Additive effect on lowering blood pressure). Products include:
- Esimil Tablets ... 864
- Ismelin Tablets ... 869

Halothane (Excessive cardiovascular depression). Products include:
- Fluothane ... 2453

Hydralazine Hydrochloride (Additive effect on lowering blood pressure). Products include:
- Apresazide Capsules ... 854
- Apresoline Hydrochloride Parenteral (Ampuls) ... 856
- Apresoline Hydrochloride Tablets ... 855
- Apresoline-Esidrix Tablets ... 857
- Ser-Ap-Es Tablets ... 881
- Serpasil-Apresoline Tablets ... 884

Hydrochlorothiazide (Additive effect on lowering blood pressure). Products include:
- Aldactazide ... 2150
- Aldoril Tablets ... 1418
- Apresazide Capsules ... 854
- Apresoline-Esidrix Tablets ... 857
- Capozide ... 2258
- Dyazide Capsules ... 2208
- Esidrix Tablets ... 863
- Esimil Tablets ... 864
- HydroDIURIL Tablets ... 1484
- Hydropres Tablets ... 1485
- Inderide Tablets ... 2463
- Inderide LA Long Acting Capsules ... 2465
- Lopressor HCT Tablets ... 1034
- Maxzide ... 1215
- Moduretic Tablets ... 1510
- Normozide Tablets ... 2112
- Oretic Tablets ... 544
- Oreticyl ... 545
- Prinzide Tablets ... 1540
- Ser-Ap-Es Tablets ... 881
- Serpasil-Esidrix Tablets ... 886
- Timolide Tablets ... 1547
- Trandate HCT Tablets ... 579
- Vaseretic Tablets ... 1559
- Zestoretic ... 2274

Hydroflumethiazide (Additive effect on lowering blood pressure). Products include:
- Diucardin Tablets ... 2450
- Saluron ... 718
- Salutensin/Salutensin-Demi ... 719

Indapamide (Additive effect on lowering blood pressure). Products include:
- Lozol Tablets ... 1843

Isoflurane (Excessive cardiovascular depression). Products include:
- Forane ... 600

Labetalol Hydrochloride (Additive negative effects on heart rate, AV conduction and/or cardiac contractility; additive hypotensive effect). Products include:
- Normodyne Injection ... 2108
- Normodyne Tablets ... 2110
- Normozide Tablets ... 2112
- Trandate HCT Tablets ... 579
- Trandate Injection ... 577
- Trandate Tablets ... 579

Lisinopril (Additive effect on lowering blood pressure). Products include:
- Prinivil Tablets ... 1538
- Prinzide Tablets ... 1540
- Zestoretic ... 2274
- Zestril Tablets ... 2277

Lithium Carbonate (May result in lowering of serum lithium levels and increased sensitivity to the effects of lithium). Products include:
- Eskalith ... 2214
- Lithane Tablets ... 1596
- Lithium Carbonate Capsules & Tablets ... 1984
- Lithobid Tablets ... 870

Lithium Citrate (May result in lowering of serum lithium levels and increased sensitivity to the effects of lithium). Products include:
- Cibalith-S ... 870

Mecamylamine Hydrochloride (Additive effect on lowering blood pressure). Products include:
- Inversine Tablets ... 1492

Methoxyflurane (Excessive cardiovascular depression).
- No products indexed under this heading.

Methyclothiazide (Additive effect on lowering blood pressure). Products include:
- Enduron Tablets ... 517
- Enduronyl ... 518

Methyldopa (Additive effect on lowering blood pressure). Products include:
- Aldoclor Tablets ... 1413
- Aldomet Oral ... 1415
- Aldoril Tablets ... 1418

Methyldopate Hydrochloride (Additive effect on lowering blood pressure). Products include:
- Aldomet Ester HCl Injection ... 1417

Metocurine Iodide (Activity of neuromuscular blocking agents potentiated). Products include:
- Metubine Iodide Vials ... 1285

Metolazone (Additive effect on lowering blood pressure). Products include:
- Diulo ... 2129
- Mykrox ½ mg Tablets ... 984
- Zaroxolyn Tablets ... 989

Metoprolol Tartrate (Additive negative effects on heart rate, AV conduction and/or cardiac contractility; additive hypotensive effect; decrease in metoprolol clearance). Products include:
- Lopressor Ampuls ... 1032
- Lopressor HCT Tablets ... 1034
- Lopressor Tablets ... 1032

Metyrosine (Additive effect on lowering blood pressure). Products include:
- Demser Capsules ... 1460

Minoxidil (Additive effect on lowering blood pressure). Products include:
- Loniten Tablets ... 2346
- Rogaine Topical Solution ... 2357

Nadolol (Additive negative effects on heart rate, AV conduction and/or cardiac contractility; additive hypotensive effect). Products include:
- Corgard Tablets ... 701
- Corzide Tablets ... 702

Pancuronium Bromide Injection (Activity of neuromuscular blocking agents potentiated).
- No products indexed under this heading.

Pargyline Hydrochloride (Additive effect on lowering blood pressure).
- No products indexed under this heading.

Penbutolol Sulfate (Additive negative effects on heart rate, AV conduction, and/or cardiac contractility; additive hypotensive effect). Products include:
- Levatol ... 1832

Phenobarbital (Verapamil clearance may be increased). Products include:
- Arco-Lase Plus Tablets ... 607
- Bellergal-S Tablets ... 1998
- Bronkolixir ◘ 761
- Bronkotabs Tablets ◘ 762
- Donnatal ... 1858
- Donnatal Extentabs ... 1859
- Donnatal Tablets ... 1858
- Donnazyme Tablets ... 1860
- Kinesed Tablets ... 2272
- Phenobarbital Elixir and Tablets ... 1293
- Primatene Tablets-P Formula ... 2421
- Quadrinal Tablets ... 1183
- Tedral SA ... 1765

Phenoxybenzamine Hydrochloride (Additive effect on lowering blood pressure). Products include:
- Dibenzyline Capsules ... 2207

Phentolamine Mesylate (Additive effect on lowering blood pressure). Products include:
- Regitine ... 878

Pindolol (Additive negative effects on heart rate, AV conduction and/or cardiac contractility; additive hypotensive effect). Products include:
- Visken Tablets ... 2036

Polythiazide (Additive effect on lowering blood pressure). Products include:
- Minizide Capsules ... 1779
- Renese Tablets ... 1785
- Renese-R Tablets ... 1786

Prazosin Hydrochloride (May result in a reduction in blood pressure that is excessive in some patients). Products include:
- Minipress Capsules ... 1778
- Minizide Capsules ... 1779

Propranolol Hydrochloride (Additive negative effects on heart rate, AV conduction and/or cardiac contractility; additive hypotensive effect; decrease in propranolol clearance). Products include:
- Inderal ... 2459
- Inderal LA Long Acting Capsules ... 2461
- Inderide Tablets ... 2463
- Inderide LA Long Acting Capsules ... 2465

Quinidine Gluconate (Hypotension in patients with hypertrophic cardiomyopathy; increased quinidine levels). Products include:
- Quinaglute Dura-Tabs Tablets ... 663

Quinidine Polygalacturonate (Hypotension in patients with hypertrophic cardiomyopathy; increased quinidine levels). Products include:
- Cardioquin Tablets ... 1812

Quinidine Sulfate (Hypotension in patients with hypertrophic cardiomyopathy; increased quinidine levels). Products include:
- Quinidex Extentabs ... 1868

Ramipril (Additive effect on lowering blood pressure). Products include:
- Altace Capsules ... 1086

Rifampin (Bioavailability of oral verapamil may be markedly reduced). Products include:
- Rifadin ... 1345
- Rifamate Capsules ... 1347
- Rimactane Capsules ... 879

Spironolactone (Additive effect on lowering blood pressure). Products include:
- Aldactazide ... 2150
- Aldactone ... 2152

Succinylcholine Chloride (Potentiation of neuromuscular blockers). Products include:
- Anectine ... 755

Terazosin Hydrochloride (May result in a reduction in blood pressure that is excessive in some patients). Products include:
- Hytrin Tablets ... 529

Theophylline (Verapamil may inhibit the clearance and increase the plasma levels of theophylline). Products include:
- Bronkaid Tablets ◘ 757
- Bronkolixir ◘ 761
- Bronkotabs Tablets ◘ 762
- Constant-T Tablets ... 1029
- Marax Tablets & DF Syrup ... 1954
- Primatene Tablets ... 2421
- Quibron Capsules ... 713
- Quibron-T ... 714
- Quibron-T/SR ... 716
- Theolair Liquid ... 1317
- Theo-Organidin Elixir ... 2391

Theophylline Anhydrous (Verapamil may inhibit the clearance and increase the plasma levels of theophylline). Products include:
- Aerolate ... 994
- Primatene Tablets-M Formula ◘ 753
- Primatene Tablets-Regular Formula ... 2421
- Respbid Tablets ... 684
- Slo-bid Gyrocaps ... 1847
- T-PHYL (Uniphyl) 200 mg Tablets ... 1820
- Tedral SA ... 1765
- Theo-24 ... 2179
- Theo-Dur Sprinkle ... 1168
- Theo-Dur Extended-Release Tablets ... 1166
- Theolair Tablets ... 1317
- Theolair-SR Tablets ... 1319
- TheoX Extended-Release Tablets ... 841
- Uniphyl 400 mg Tablets ... 1823

Theophylline Calcium Salicylate (Verapamil may inhibit the clearance and increase the plasma levels of theophylline). Products include:

- Quadrinal Tablets 1183

Theophylline Sodium Glycinate (Verapamil may inhibit the clearance and increase the plasma levels of theophylline). Products include:

- Asbron G 1997

Timolol Maleate (Additive negative effects on heart rate, AV conduction and/or cardiac contractility; additive hypotensive effect). Products include:

- Blocadren Tablets 1429
- Timolide Tablets 1547
- Timoptic in Ocudose 1552
- Timoptic Sterile Ophthalmic Solution 1550

Triamterene (Additive effect on lowering blood pressure). Products include:

- Dyazide Capsules 2208
- Dyrenium Capsules 2210
- Maxzide 1215

Vecuronium Bromide (Activity of neuromuscular blocking agents potentiated). Products include:

- Norcuron 1642

CALCIDRINE SYRUP

(Codeine, Calcium Iodide) **506**

May interact with:

Lithium Carbonate (May enhance hypothyroid and goitrogenic effects of either drug). Products include:

- Eskalith 2214
- Lithane Tablets 1596
- Lithium Carbonate Capsules & Tablets 1984
- Lithobid Tablets 870

CALCIJEX CALCITRIOL INJECTION

(Calcitriol) **506**

May interact with magnesium-containing antacids. Compounds in this category include:

Magaldrate (Potential for hypermagnesemia). Products include:

- Riopan Antacid Chew Tablets ■ 754
- Riopan Antacid Chew Tablets in Rollpacks ■ 754
- Riopan Antacid Suspension 2421
- Riopan Antacid Swallow Tablets 2421
- Riopan Plus Chew Tablets 2422
- Riopan Plus Chew Tablets in Rollpack 2422
- Riopan Plus 2 Chew Tablets, Mint Flavor, Cherry Flavor 2422
- Riopan Plus Suspension 2422
- Riopan Plus 2 Suspension, Mint Flavor, Cherry Flavor 2422

Magnesium Carbonate (Potential for hypermagnesemia). Products include:

- Bayer Plus Aspirin Tablets ■ 567
- Gaviscon Extra Strength Relief Formula Liquid Antacid ■ 594
- Gaviscon Extra Strength Relief Formula Antacid Tablets ■ 594
- Gaviscon Liquid Antacid ■ 594
- Marblen ■ 563
- Osti-Derm Lotion 1771

Magnesium Hydroxide (Potential for hypermagnesemia). Products include:

- Aludrox Oral Suspension 2428
- Ascriptin A/D Caplets 1850
- Regular Strength Ascriptin Tablets 1850
- Di-Gel Antacid/Anti-Gas ■ 697
- Gelusil Liquid & Tablets ■ 639
- Haley's M-O, Regular & Flavored ■ 569
- Extra Strength Maalox Plus Suspension 1850
- Maalox TC Suspension 1851
- Maalox Plus Tablets ■ 655
- Extra Strength Maalox Plus Tablets 1850
- Mylanta Liquid 1155
- Mylanta Tablets 1155
- Mylanta Double Strength Liquid 1155
- Mylanta Double Strength Tablets 1155
- Concentrated Phillips' Milk of Magnesia ■ 573
- Phillips' Milk of Magnesia Liquid ■ 572
- Phillips' Milk of Magnesia Tablets ■ 573
- WinGel Liquid & Tablets ■ 761

Magnesium Trisilicate (Potential for hypermagnesemia). Products include:

- Gaviscon Antacid Tablets ■ 593
- Gaviscon-2 Antacid Tablets ■ 594

CALCIMAR INJECTION, SYNTHETIC

(Calcitonin, Synthetic) **1839**

No interactions described in labeling.

CALCIPARINE INJECTION

(Heparin Calcium) **925**

May interact with oral anticoagulants, non-steroidal anti-inflammatory agents, salicylates, cardiac glycosides, high doses of parenteral penicillins, phenothiazines, tetracyclines, antihistamines, platelet inhibitors, cephalosporins with methylthiotetrazole side chains, macrolide antibiotics, and certain other agents. Compounds in these categories include:

Aspirin (Coadministration may result in an additive or synergistic activity and can result in an increased risk of bleeding). Products include:

- Alka-Seltzer Effervescent Antacid and Pain Reliever 1568
- Alka-Seltzer Extra Strength Effervescent Antacid and Pain Reliever 1570
- Alka-Seltzer (Flavored) Effervescent Antacid and Pain Reliever 1569
- Alka-Seltzer Plus Cold Medicine ■ 623
- Alka-Seltzer Plus Night-Time Cold Medicine ■ 623
- Alka Seltzer Plus Sinus Allergy Medicine ■ 624
- Anacin Coated Analgesic Caplets 2417
- Anacin Coated Analgesic Tablets 2417
- Anacin Maximum Strength Analgesic Coated Tablets 2417
- Maximum Strength Arthritis Pain Formula By the Makers of Anacin Analgesic Tablets and Caplets 2418
- Arthritis Pain Formula by the Makers of Anacin Analgesic Tablets and Caplets ■ 747
- Arthritis Strength BC Powder ■ 516
- Ascriptin A/D Caplets 1850
- Regular Strength Ascriptin Tablets 1850
- Azdōne Tablets 844
- BC Powder ■ 517
- BC Cold Powder ■ 517
- Children's Bayer Chewable Aspirin ■ 564
- Genuine Bayer Aspirin Tablets & Caplets ■ 564
- Maximum Bayer Aspirin Tablets & Caplets ■ 566
- Bayer Plus Aspirin Tablets ■ 567
- Therapy Bayer Aspirin Caplets ■ 568
- 8 Hour Bayer Timed-Release Aspirin ■ 566
- Arthritis Strength Bufferin Analgesic Caplets 744
- Extra Strength Bufferin Analgesic Tablets 745
- Bufferin Analgesic Tablets and Caplets 743
- Cama Arthritis Pain Reliever ■ 685
- Damason-P 1356
- Easprin 1719
- Ecotrin Enteric Coated Aspirin Maximum Strength Tablets and Caplets 2189
- Ecotrin Enteric Coated Aspirin Regular Strength Tablets and Caplets 2189
- Empirin Aspirin ■ 541
- Empirin with Codeine Phosphate Nos. 2, 3 & 4 764
- Equagesic Tablets 2451
- Excedrin Extra-Strength Analgesic Tablets & Caplets 749
- 4-Way Cold Tablets 750
- Fiorinal Capsules 2007
- Fiorinal with Codeine Capsules 2008
- Fiorinal Tablets 2007
- Lortab ASA Tablets 2414
- Momentum Muscular Backache Formula ■ 751
- Norgesic 1314
- Norwich Extra-Strength Aspirin ■ 546
- Norwich Regular Strength Aspirin ■ 547
- P-A-C Analgesic Tablets ■ 669
- Percodan 951
- Robaxisal Tablets 1872
- Sine-Off Sinus Medicine Tablets-Aspirin Formula ■ 722
- Soma Compound w/Codeine Tablets 2390
- Soma Compound Tablets 2389
- St. Joseph Adult Chewable Aspirin (81 mg.) ■ 703
- Synalgos-DC Capsules 2525
- Talwin Compound 2072
- Ursinus Inlay-Tabs ■ 691
- Vanquish Analgesic Caplets ■ 574
- Zorprin Tablets 698

Astemizole (Antagonizes the antithrombotic activity of heparin). Products include:

- Hismanal Tablets 1138

Azatadine Maleate (Antagonizes the antithrombotic activity of heparin). Products include:

- Optimine Tablets 2115
- Trinalin Repetabs Tablets 1170

Azlocillin Sodium (Coadministration may result in an additive or synergistic activity and can result in an increased risk of bleeding).

No products indexed under this heading.

Bromodiphenhydramine Hydrochloride (Antagonizes the antithrombotic activity of heparin).

No products indexed under this heading.

Brompheniramine Maleate (Antagonizes the antithrombotic activity of heparin). Products include:

- Alka Seltzer Plus Sinus Allergy Medicine ■ 624
- Atrohist Sprinkle Capsules 558
- Bromfed Capsules (Timed Release) 1615
- Bromfed Syrup ■ 628
- Bromfed 1615
- Dimetane Decongestant ■ 673
- Dimetane ■ 672
- Dimetane-DC Cough Syrup 1857
- Dimetane-DX Cough Syrup 1858
- Dimetapp Elixir ■ 673
- Dimetapp DM Elixir ■ 674
- Dimetapp Extentabs ■ 674
- Dimetapp Plus Caplets ■ 675
- Dimetapp Tablets ■ 675
- Drixoral Antihistamine/Nasal Decongestant Syrup ■ 698

Carbenicillin Indanyl Sodium (Coadministration may result in an additive or synergistic activity and can result in an increased risk of bleeding). Products include:

- Geocillin Tablets 1951

Cefamandole Nafate (Coadministration may result in an additive or synergistic activity and can result in an increased risk of bleeding). Products include:

- Mandol Vials, Faspak & ADD-Vantage 1281

Cefmetazole Sodium (Coadministration may result in an additive or synergistic activity and can result in an increased risk of bleeding). Products include:

- Zefazone Sterile Powder 2372

Cefoperazone Sodium (Coadministration may result in an additive or synergistic activity and can result in an increased risk of bleeding). Products include:

- Cefobid Intravenous/Intramuscular 1943
- Cefobid Pharmacy Bulk Package - Not for Direct Infusion 1945

Cefotetan (Coadministration may result in an additive or synergistic activity and can result in an increased risk of bleeding). Products include:

- Cefotan 2265

Chlorpheniramine Maleate (Antagonizes the antithrombotic activity of heparin). Products include:

- A.R.M. Allergy Relief Medicine Caplets ■ 615
- Alka-Seltzer Plus Cold Medicine ■ 623
- Allerest ■ 559
- Ana-Kit Anaphylaxis Emergency Treatment Kit 1100
- BC Cold Powder Multi-Symptom Formula ■ 517
- Brexin L.A. Capsules 2078
- Cerose-DM 2443
- Cheracol Plus Head Cold/Cough Formula ■ 667
- Chlor-Trimeton Allergy Syrup, Tablets & Long-Acting Repetabs Tablets ■ 693
- Chlor-Trimeton Decongestant ■ 694
- Comhist LA Capsules 1618
- Allergy-Sinus Comtrex Multi-Symptom Allergy Sinus Formula Tablets & Caplets 746
- Comtrex Multi-Symptom Cold Reliever Tablets/Caplets/Liqui-Gels/Liquid 745
- Day-Night Comtrex 747
- Contac Continuous Action Decongestant/Antihistamine Capsules ■ 710
- Contac Maximum Strength Continuous Action Decongestant/Antihistamine Caplets ■ 709
- Contac Severe Cold and Flu Formula Caplets ■ 711
- Coricidin 'D' Decongestant Tablets ■ 695
- Coricidin Demilets Tablets for Children ■ 696
- Coricidin Tablets ■ 695
- Deconamine 663
- Demazin Nasal Decongestant/Antihistamine Repetabs Tablets & Syrup ■ 697
- Dorcol Children's Liquid Cold Formula ■ 686
- Dristan Decongestant/Antihistamine/Analgesic Coated Caplets ■ 749
- Dristan Cold Nasal Decongestant/Antihistamine/ Analgesic Coated Tablets 2419
- Dristan Advanced Formula Decongestant/Antihistamine/Analgesic Tablets ■ 749
- Extendryl 994
- 4-Way Cold Tablets 750
- Fedahist Gyrocaps 2145
- Fedahist Timecaps 2145
- Hycomine Compound Tablets 929
- Isoclor Timesule Capsules ■ 561
- Kronofed-A 970
- Medi-Flu Caplet, Liquid ■ 640
- Naldecon Syrup, Tablets, Pediatric Drops and Pediatric Syrup 709
- Nolamine Tablets 838
- Novafed A Capsules 1342
- Novahistine DH 1342
- Novahistine Elixir ■ 596
- Ornade Spansule Capsules 2221
- Orthoxicol Cough Syrup ■ 668
- PediaCare Allergy Relief Formula Liquid 1362
- PediaCare Cough-Cold Formula Liquid 1362
- PediaCare Night Rest Cough-Cold Formula Liquid 1362
- PediaCare 6-12 Cough-Cold Formula Chewable Tablets 1362
- Pyrroxate Capsules ■ 669
- Quelidrine Syrup 556
- Ru-Tuss II Capsules 693
- Ru-Tuss Tablets 693
- Ryna ■ 741
- Sinarest Tablets & Extra Strength Tablets ■ 562
- Sine-Off Maximum Strength Allergy/Sinus Formula Caplets ■ 721
- Sine-Off Sinus Medicine Tablets-Aspirin Formula ■ 722
- Singlet Tablets ■ 598
- Sinulin 840
- Sinutab Maximum Strength ■ 641

St. Joseph Nighttime Cold Medicine ⊞ 705
Sudafed Plus Liquid ⊞ 544
Sudafed Plus Tablets ⊞ 545
Teldrin Timed-Release Allergy Capsules, 12 mg. 2192
TheraFlu Flu and Cold Medicine ⊞ 687
Triaminic Allergy Tablets ⊞ 688
Triaminic Chewables ⊞ 688
Triaminic Cold Tablets ⊞ 688
Triaminic Nite Light ⊞ 689
Triaminic Syrup ⊞ 689
Triaminic-12 Tablets ⊞ 690
Triaminicin Tablets ⊞ 690
Triaminicol Multi-Symptom Cold Tablets ⊞ 691
Triaminicol Multi-Symptom Relief ⊞ 691
Tylenol Allergy Sinus Medication Caplets and Gelcaps, Maximum Strength 1372
Children's Tylenol Cold Liquid Formula and Chewable Tablets 1368
Tylenol Cold & Flu Hot Medication, Packets 1369
Tylenol Cold Medication Caplets and Tablets 1370
Tylenol Cold Medication, Effervescent Tablets 1369
Vicks Children's NyQuil ⊞ 664
Vicks Formula 44 Cough Medicine ⊞ 661
Vicks Formula 44M Multi-Symptom Cough Medicine ⊞ 662
Vicks Pediatric Formula 44m Multi-Symptom Cough & Cold Medicine ⊞ 663

Chlorpheniramine Polistirex (Antagonizes the antithrombotic activity of heparin). Products include:
Tussionex Extended-Release Suspension 988

Chlorpheniramine Tannate (Antagonizes the antithrombotic activity of heparin). Products include:
Rynatan 2387
Rynatuss 2388

Chlorpromazine (Antagonizes the antithrombotic activity of heparin). Products include:
Thorazine 2234

Choline Magnesium Trisalicylate (Coadministration may result in an additive or synergistic activity and can result in an increased risk of bleeding). Products include:
Trilisate 1822

Clemastine Fumarate (Antagonizes the antithrombotic activity of heparin). Products include:
Tavist Syrup 2033
Tavist Tablets 2035
Tavist-D Tablets 2035

Cyproheptadine Hydrochloride (Antagonizes the antithrombotic activity of heparin). Products include:
Periactin 1525

Demeclocycline Hydrochloride (Loss of pharmacological activity of either or both drugs). Products include:
Declomycin Capsules, Tablets 1199

Deslanoside (Antagonizes the antithrombotic activity of heparin).
No products indexed under this heading.

Dexchlorpheniramine Maleate (Antagonizes the antithrombotic activity of heparin). Products include:
Polaramine 2116

Dextran 40 (Interferes with platelet aggregation reactions).
No products indexed under this heading.

Dextran 70 (Interferes with platelet aggregation reactions). Products include:
Hyskon Hysteroscopy Fluid 1162
Moisture Drops ◉ 258
Tears Naturale II 572

Diclofenac Sodium (Coadministration may result in an additive or synergistic activity and can result in an increased risk of bleeding). Products include:
Voltaren Ophthalmic Sterile Ophthalmic Solution ◉ 268
Voltaren Tablets 1042

Dicumarol (One-stage prothrombin time prolonged). Products include:
Dicumarol Tablets 516

Diflunisal (Coadministration may result in an additive or synergistic activity and can result in an increased risk of bleeding). Products include:
Dolobid Tablets 1465

Digitoxin (Antagonizes the antithrombotic activity of heparin). Products include:
Crystodigin Tablets 1253

Digoxin (Antagonizes the antithrombotic activity of heparin). Products include:
Lanoxicaps 772
Lanoxin Elixir Pediatric 775
Lanoxin Injection 778
Lanoxin Injection Pediatric 781
Lanoxin Tablets 783

Diphenhydramine Citrate (Antagonizes the antithrombotic activity of heparin). Products include:
Alka-Seltzer Plus Night-Time Cold Medicine ⊞ 623
Bufferin AF Nite Time Analgesic/Sleeping Aid Caplets 744
Excedrin P.M. Analgesic/Sleeping Aid Tablets, Caplets and Liquid 749

Diphenhydramine Hydrochloride (Antagonizes the antithrombotic activity of heparin). Products include:
Benadryl Anti-Itch Cream ⊞ 635
Benadryl Capsules 1691
Benadryl Decongestant Elixir ⊞ 635
Benadryl Decongestant ⊞ 635
Benadryl Elixir ⊞ 636
Benadryl Kapseals 1691
Benadryl 25 Kapseals ⊞ 636
Benadryl Parenteral 1692
Benadryl Plus ⊞ 636
Benadryl Plus Nighttime ⊞ 637
Benadryl Spray, Maximum Strength ⊞ 637
Benadryl Spray, Regular Strength ⊞ 637
Benadryl Steri-Vials, Ampoules, and Steri-Dose Syringe 1692
Benadryl 25 Tablets ⊞ 636
Benylin Cough Syrup ⊞ 637
Benylin Decongestant ⊞ 638
Caladryl Cream, Lotion, Spray ⊞ 638
Miles Nervine Nighttime Sleep-Aid ⊞ 627
Nytol Tablets ⊞ 517
Sleep-ettes-D Tablets ⊞ 653
Sleep-eze 3 Tablets ⊞ 755
Sleepinal Night-time Sleep Aid Capsules ⊞ 734
Sominex Caplets and Tablets ⊞ 722
Sominex Liquid ⊞ 723
Sominex Pain Relief Formula ⊞ 723
Tylenol Cold Night Time Medication Liquid 1371
Tylenol PM, Extra Strength Caplets and Tablets 1368
Unisom Dual Relief Nighttime Sleep Aid/Analgesic 1774
Ziradryl Lotion ⊞ 643

Diphenylpyraline Hydrochloride (Antagonizes the antithrombotic activity of heparin).
No products indexed under this heading.

Dipyridamole (Coadministration may result in an additive or synergistic activity and can result in an increased risk of bleeding). Products include:
Persantine Tablets 683

Doxycycline Calcium (Loss of pharmacological activity of either or both drugs).
No products indexed under this heading.

Doxycycline Hyclate (Loss of pharmacological activity of either or both drugs). Products include:
Doryx Capsules 1717
Vibramycin Hyclate Capsules 1787
Vibramycin Hyclate Intravenous 1968
Vibra-Tabs Film Coated Tablets 1787

Doxycycline Monohydrate (Loss of pharmacological activity of either or both drugs). Products include:
Monodox Capsules 1630
Vibramycin Monohydrate for Oral Suspension 1787

Erythromycin (Loss of pharmacological activity of either or both drugs). Products include:
A/T/S Topical Gel and Topical Solution 1089
AK-Mycin Ointment ◉ 204
Benzamycin Topical Gel 907
E-Mycin Tablets 688
ETS-2% 1685
ERYC 1720
Erycette (erythromycin 2%) Topical Solution 1678
Ery-Tab Tablets 521
Erythromycin Base Filmtab 525
Erythromycin Delayed-Release Capsules, USP 526
Ilotycin Ophthalmic Ointment 915
PCE Dispertab Tablets 549
Pediazole 1973
T-Stat 2.0% Topical Solution and Pads 2409
Theramycin Z Topical Solution 2% 1410

Erythromycin Estolate (Loss of pharmacological activity of either or both drugs). Products include:
Ilosone 913

Erythromycin Ethylsuccinate (Loss of pharmacological activity of either or both drugs). Products include:
E.E.S. 522
EryPed 519
Pediazole 1973

Erythromycin Gluceptate (Loss of pharmacological activity of either or both drugs). Products include:
Ilotycin Gluceptate, IV, Vials 915

Erythromycin Stearate (Loss of pharmacological activity of either or both drugs). Products include:
Erythrocin Stearate Filmtab 523

Etodolac (Coadministration may result in an additive or synergistic activity and can result in an increased risk of bleeding). Products include:
Lodine Capsules 2468

Fenoprofen Calcium (Coadministration may result in an additive or synergistic activity and can result in an increased risk of bleeding). Products include:
Nalfon Pulvules & Tablets 919

Fluphenazine Decanoate (Antagonizes the antithrombotic activity of heparin). Products include:
Prolixin Decanoate 1795

Fluphenazine Enanthate (Antagonizes the antithrombotic activity of heparin). Products include:
Prolixin Enanthate 1796

Fluphenazine Hydrochloride (Antagonizes the antithrombotic activity of heparin). Products include:
Prolixin Elixir 1793
Prolixin Injection 1791
Prolixin Oral Concentrate 1792
Prolixin Tablets 1793

Flurbiprofen (Coadministration may result in an additive or synergistic activity and can result in an increased risk of bleeding). Products include:
Ansaid Tablets 2319

Gentamicin Sulfate (Loss of pharmacological activity of either or both drugs). Products include:
Garamycin Injectable 2093
Garamycin Ophthalmic ◉ 305
Genoptic Liquifilm Sterile Ophthalmic Solution ◉ 247
Genoptic S.O.P. Sterile Ophthalmic Ointment ◉ 247
Gentacidin Ointment ◉ 273
Gentacidin Solution ◉ 273
Gentak Ointment & Solution ◉ 208
G-myticin Creme and Ointment 0.1% 1770
Pred-G Liquifilm Sterile Ophthalmic Suspension ◉ 252
Pred-G S.O.P. Sterile Ophthalmic Ointment ◉ 253

Ibuprofen (Coadministration may result in an additive or synergistic activity and can result in an increased risk of bleeding). Products include:
Advil Cold & Sinus Caplets (formerly CoAdvil) 2416
Advil Ibuprofen Tablets and Caplets 2416
Children's Advil Suspension 2426
CoAdvil ⊞ 748
Dristan Sinus Caplets 2419
Haltran Tablets ⊞ 668
Ibuprofen ⊞ 631
Medipren ibuprofen Caplets and Tablets 1362
Midol 200 Cramp Relief Formula ⊞ 570
Motrin Tablets 2351
Motrin IB Caplets and Tablets ⊞ 736
Nuprin Ibuprofen/Analgesic Tablets & Caplets 752
PediaProfen Suspension 1363
Rufen Tablets 691
Trendar Ibuprofen Tablets ⊞ 756

Indomethacin (Coadministration may result in an additive or synergistic activity and can result in an increased risk of bleeding). Products include:
Indocin 1487

Indomethacin Sodium Trihydrate (Coadministration may result in an additive or synergistic activity and can result in an increased risk of bleeding). Products include:
Indocin I.V. 1490

Ketoprofen (Coadministration may result in an additive or synergistic activity and can result in an increased risk of bleeding). Products include:
Orudis Capsules 2488

Ketorolac Tromethamine (Coadministration may result in an additive or synergistic activity and can result in an increased risk of bleeding). Products include:
Toradol IM Injection 2302

Magnesium Salicylate (Coadministration may result in an additive or synergistic activity and can result in an increased risk of bleeding). Products include:
Doan's - Extra-Strength Analgesic ⊞ 549
Doan's - Regular Strength Analgesic ⊞ 549
Mobigesic Analgesic Tablets ⊞ 507

Meclofenamate Sodium (Coadministration may result in an additive or synergistic activity and can result in an increased risk of bleeding). Products include:
Meclomen Capsules 1739

Mefenamic Acid (Coadministration may result in an additive or synergistic activity and can result in an increased risk of bleeding). Products include:
Ponstel 1758

Mesoridazine (Antagonizes the antithrombotic activity of heparin). Products include:
Serentil 686

Methacycline Hydrochloride (Loss of pharmacological activity of either or both drugs).
No products indexed under this heading.

Methdilazine Hydrochloride (Antagonizes the antithrombotic activity of heparin). Products include:
Tacaryl Syrup & Tablets 2409

Mezlocillin Sodium (Coadministration may result in an additive or synergistic activity and can result in an increased risk of bleeding). Products include:
Mezlin 1597
Mezlin Pharmacy Bulk Package 1599

Minocycline Hydrochloride (Loss of pharmacological activity of either or both drugs). Products include:
Minocin Intravenous 1221
Minocin Oral Suspension 1224
Minocin Pellet-Filled Capsules 1222

Moxalactam Disodium (Coadministration may result in an additive or synergistic activity and can result in an increased risk of bleeding).

Nafcillin Sodium (Coadministration may result in an additive or synergistic activity and can result in an increased risk of bleeding). Products include:
Unipen 2533

Naproxen (Coadministration may result in an additive or synergistic activity and can result in an increased risk of bleeding). Products include:
Naprosyn 2297

Naproxen Sodium (Coadministration may result in an additive or synergistic activity and can result in an increased risk of bleeding). Products include:
Anaprox and Anaprox DS Tablets 2288

Neomycin, oral (Loss of pharmacological activity of either or both drugs).

Nicotine Polacrilex (Antagonizes the antithrombotic activity of heparin). Products include:
Nicorette 1335

Nitroglycerin Intravenous (May require higher doses of heparin; close monitoring of the partial thromboplastin time is required). Products include:
Nitro-Bid IV 1338
Nitrostat IV 1744
Tridil Ampuls & Vials 939

Oxytetracycline Hydrochloride (Loss of pharmacological activity of either or both drugs). Products include:
Terra-Cortril Ophthalmic Suspension 1963
Terramycin Capsules 1786
Terramycin Intramuscular Solution 1964
Terramycin with Polymyxin B Sulfate Ophthalmic Ointment 1965

Penicillin G Procaine (Coadministration may result in an additive or synergistic activity and can result in an increased risk of bleeding). Products include:
Bicillin C-R Injection 2438
Bicillin C-R 900/300 Injection 2440
Pfizerpen-AS Aqueous Suspension 1959
Wycillin Injection 2537
Wycillin Injection and Probenecid Tablets 2539

Penicillin G, Benzathine (Coadministration may result in an additive or synergistic activity and can result in an increased risk of bleeding). Products include:
Bicillin C-R Injection 2438
Bicillin C-R 900/300 Injection 2440
Bicillin L-A Injection 2442

Perphenazine (Antagonizes the antithrombotic activity of heparin). Products include:
Etrafon 2087
Triavil Tablets 1556
Trilafon 2123

Phenylbutazone (Coadministration may result in an additive or synergistic activity and can result in an increased risk of bleeding). Products include:
Butazolidin Capsules & Tablets 1027

Piroxicam (Coadministration may result in an additive or synergistic activity and can result in an increased risk of bleeding). Products include:
Feldene Capsules 1777

Polymyxin B Sulfate (Loss of pharmacological activity of either or both drugs). Products include:
AK-Poly-Bac Ointment ..... ◉ 205
AK-Spore H.C. ..... ◉ 206
AK-Spore ..... ◉ 205
AK-Trol Ointment & Suspension ..... ◉ 207
Aquaphor Antibiotic Formula 662
Bactine First Aid Antibiotic Ointment ..... ▣ 625
Campho-Phenique Triple Antibiotic Ointment Plus Pain Reliever ▣ 758
Cortisporin Cream 757
Cortisporin Ointment 758
Cortisporin Ophthalmic Ointment Sterile 758
Cortisporin Ophthalmic Suspension Sterile 759
Cortisporin Otic Solution Sterile 760
Cortisporin Otic Suspension Sterile 760
Dexacidin ..... ◉ 272
Lanabiotic Ointment ..... ▣ 556
LazerSporin-C Solution 1770
Maxitrol Ophthalmic Ointment/Suspension ..... ◉ 223
Mycitracin ..... ▣ 737
Neosporin Cream 792
Neosporin G.U. Irrigant Sterile 793
Neosporin Ointment 793
Maximum Strength Neosporin Ointment 793
Neosporin Ophthalmic Ointment Sterile 793
Neosporin Ophthalmic Solution Sterile 794
Ophthocort ..... ◉ 301
PediOtic Suspension Sterile 797
Polymyxin B Sulfate, Aerosporin Brand Sterile Powder 798
Poly-Pred Liquifilm ..... ◉ 250
Polysporin Ointment ..... ▣ 543
Polysporin Ophthalmic Ointment Sterile 798
Polysporin Powder ..... ▣ 543
Polysporin Spray ..... ▣ 543
Polytrim Ophthalmic Solution Sterile 588
Terramycin with Polymyxin B Sulfate Ophthalmic Ointment 1965

Prochlorperazine (Antagonizes the antithrombotic activity of heparin). Products include:
Compazine 2201

Promethazine Hydrochloride (Antagonizes the antithrombotic activity of heparin). Products include:
Mepergan Injection 2479
Phenergan with Codeine 2497
Phenergan with Dextromethorphan 2499
Phenergan Injection 2493
Phenergan Suppositories 2496
Phenergan Syrup 2495
Phenergan Tablets 2496
Phenergan VC 2500
Phenergan VC with Codeine 2501

Pyrilamine Maleate (Antagonizes the antithrombotic activity of heparin). Products include:
Codimal 846
4-Way Fast Acting Nasal Spray - Original Formula (regular & mentholated) & Metered Spray Pump (regular) 751
Maximum Strength Midol Multi-Symptom Menstrual Formula ..... ▣ 571
Maximum Strength Midol PMS Premenstrual Syndrome Formula ..... ▣ 570
Regular Strength Midol Multi-Symptom Menstrual Formula ..... ▣ 570
Prefrin-A ..... ◉ 255
Prēmsyn PMS Capsules & Caplets ▣ 547
Primatene Tablets-M Formula 2421
Robitussin Night Relief ..... ▣ 677
Ru-Tuss with Hydrocodone 694
Triaminic Expectorant DH 1995
Triaminic Oral Infant Drops 1996

Pyrilamine Tannate (Antagonizes the antithrombotic activity of heparin). Products include:
Rynatan 2387

Salsalate (Coadministration may result in an additive or synergistic activity and can result in an increased risk of bleeding). Products include:
Disalcid 1310
Mono-Gesic Tablets 846
Salflex 839

Streptomycin Sulfate (Loss of pharmacological activity of either or both drugs).
No products indexed under this heading.

Sulindac (Coadministration may result in an additive or synergistic activity and can result in an increased risk of bleeding). Products include:
Clinoril Tablets 1433

Terfenadine (Antagonizes the antithrombotic activity of heparin). Products include:
Seldane Tablets 1349
Seldane-D Extended-Release Tablets 1350

Tetracycline Hydrochloride (Loss of pharmacological activity of either or both drugs). Products include:
Achromycin V Capsules 1193
Achromycin Ophthalmic Ointment 1% ..... ◉ 307
Achromycin Ophthalmic Suspension 1% ..... ◉ 308
Topicycline for Topical Solution 1856

Thioridazine Hydrochloride (Antagonizes the antithrombotic activity of heparin). Products include:
Mellaril 2011

Ticarcillin Disodium (Coadministration may result in an additive or synergistic activity and can result in an increased risk of bleeding). Products include:
Ticar for Injection 2236
Timentin for Injection 2239

Tolmetin Sodium (Coadministration may result in an additive or synergistic activity and can result in an increased risk of bleeding). Products include:
Tolectin (200, 400 and 600 mg) .. 1379

Trifluoperazine Hydrochloride (Antagonizes the antithrombotic activity of heparin). Products include:
Stelazine 2226

Trimeprazine Tartrate (Antagonizes the antithrombotic activity of heparin). Products include:
Temaril Tablets, Syrup and Spansule Sustained Release Capsules 1085

Tripelennamine Hydrochloride (Antagonizes the antithrombotic activity of heparin). Products include:
PBZ Tablets & Elixir 1037
PBZ-SR Tablets 1037

Triprolidine Hydrochloride (Antagonizes the antithrombotic activity of heparin). Products include:
Actidil ..... ▣ 538
Actifed Capsules ..... ▣ 539
Actifed Plus Caplets ..... ▣ 539
Actifed Plus Tablets ..... ▣ 540
Actifed with Codeine Cough Syrup .. 752
Actifed Syrup ..... ▣ 540
Actifed Tablets ..... ▣ 540
Actifed 12-Hour Capsules ..... ▣ 539

Troleandomycin (Loss of pharmacological activity of either or both drugs). Products include:
Tao Capsules 1963

Vitamin C (Antagonizes the antithrombotic activity of heparin). Products include:
Allbee with C Caplets ..... ▣ 670
Allbee C-800 ..... ▣ 670
Bromase Capsules 672
Bugs Bunny Children's Chewable Vitamins (Sugar Free) ..... ▣ 625
Bugs Bunny With Extra C Children's Chewable Vitamins (Sugar Free) ..... ▣ 626
Bugs Bunny Plus Iron Children's Chewable Vitamins (Sugar Free) ▣ 625
Cefol Filmtab 509
Centrum, Jr. (Children's Chewable) + Extra C ..... ▣ 585
Cod Liver Oil Concentrate Tablets with Vitamin C ..... ▣ 694
Ester-C Tablets ..... ▣ 575
Ferancee Chewable Tablets 1155
Ferancee-HP Tablets 1155
Fero-Folic-500 Filmtab 527
Fero-Grad-500 Filmtab 528
Flintstones Children's Chewable Vitamins ..... ▣ 625
Flintstones Children's Chewable Vitamins With Extra C ..... ▣ 626
Flintstones Children's Chewable Vitamins Plus Iron ..... ▣ 625
Halls Vitamin C Drops ..... ▣ 742
Hyland's Vitamin C for Children ..... ▣ 729
ICAPS Plus ..... ◉ 280
Mediatric Capsules 2476
Mol-Iron w/Vitamin C Tablets ..... ▣ 703
Natalins Rx 1391
Natalins Tablets 1391
N'ICE Sugarless Vitamin C Drops .. ▣ 719
Niferex w/Vitamin C Tablets 847
Ocuvite Vitamin and Mineral Supplement ..... ◉ 312
One-A-Day Essential Vitamins ..... ▣ 627
One-A-Day Maximum Formula Vitamins and Minerals ..... ▣ 627
One-A-Day Plus Extra C Vitamins .. ▣ 627
Probec-T Tablets ..... ▣ 581
Stressgard Stress Formula Vitamins ..... ▣ 628
STUART PRENATAL Tablets ..... ▣ 731
The Stuart Formula Tablets 1157
Stuartinic Tablets 1157
Sunkist Children's Chewable Multivitamins - Plus Extra C ..... ▣ 553
Sunkist Vitamin C ..... ▣ 553
Surbex with C ..... ▣ 502
Trinsicon Capsules 2415
Tri-Vi-Flor 1.0 mg Vitamins with Fluoride Chewable Tablets 1400
Tri-Vi-Flor Drops 1400
Tri-Vi-Sol Vitamin Drops ..... ▣ 614
Tri-Vi-Sol Vitamin Drops with Iron ▣ 614
Vicon Forte Capsules 2416
Vicon Plus ..... ▣ 682
Vicon-C ..... ▣ 682
Vi-Daylin ADC Vitamins Drops 1980
Vi-Daylin ADC Vitamins + Iron Drops 1980
Vi-Daylin/F ADC Vitamins Drops With Fluoride 1981
Vi-Daylin/F ADC Vitamins + Iron Drops With Fluoride 1981
Vi-Zac ..... ▣ 682
Within Women's Formula Multivitamin with Calcium, Extra Iron and Zinc ..... ▣ 628
Z-Bec Tablets ..... ▣ 678

Warfarin Sodium (One-stage prothrombin time prolonged). Products include:
Coumadin Injection & Tablets 944
Panwarfin Tablets 547

CALCIUM DISODIUM VERSENATE INJECTION
(Calcium Disodium Edetate) 1309
No interactions described in labeling.

CALDECORT ANTI-ITCH HYDROCORTISONE CREAM
(Hydrocortisone Acetate) ▣ 560
No interactions described in labeling.

CALDECORT ANTI-ITCH HYDROCORTISONE SPRAY
(Hydrocortisone) ▣ 560
No interactions described in labeling.

CALDECORT LIGHT CREAM
(Hydrocortisone Acetate) ▣ 560
No interactions described in labeling.

CALDEROL CAPSULES
(Calcifediol) 1635
May interact with anticonvulsants, cardiac glycosides, and certain other agents. Compounds in these categories include:

Carbamazepine (Affects Calderol requirements in some patients). Products include:
- Tegretol Chewable Tablets 654
- Tegretol Suspension 656
- Tegretol Tablets 654

Cholestyramine (Impaired intestinal absorption of Calderol). Products include:
- Cholybar 1705
- Questran Light 711
- Questran Powder 710

Deslanoside (Hypercalcemia may precipitate cardiac arrhythmias).
- No products indexed under this heading.

Digitoxin (Hypercalcemia may precipitate cardiac arrhythmias). Products include:
- Crystodigin Tablets 1253

Digoxin (Hypercalcemia may precipitate cardiac arrhythmias). Products include:
- Lanoxicaps 772
- Lanoxin Elixir Pediatric 775
- Lanoxin Injection 778
- Lanoxin Injection Pediatric 781
- Lanoxin Tablets 783

Divalproex Sodium (Affects Calderol requirements in some patients). Products include:
- Depakote 512

Ethosuximide (Affects Calderol requirements in some patients). Products include:
- Zarontin Capsules 1768
- Zarontin Syrup 1769

Ethotoin (Affects Calderol requirements in some patients). Products include:
- Peganone Tablets 551

Mephenytoin (Affects Calderol requirements in some patients). Products include:
- Mesantoin Tablets 2013

Methsuximide (Affects Calderol requirements in some patients). Products include:
- Celontin 1692

Paramethadione (Affects Calderol requirements in some patients). Products include:
- Paradione Capsules 548

Phenacemide (Affects Calderol requirements in some patients). Products include:
- Phenurone Tablets 552

Phenobarbital (Affects Calderol requirements in some patients). Products include:
- Arco-Lase Plus Tablets 607
- Bellergal-S Tablets 1998
- Bronkolixir ▣ 761
- Bronkotabs Tablets ▣ 762
- Donnatal 1858
- Donnatal Extentabs 1859
- Donnatal Tablets 1858
- Donnazyme Tablets 1860
- Kinesed Tablets 2272
- Phenobarbital Elixir and Tablets 1293
- Primatene Tablets-P Formula 2421
- Quadrinal Tablets 1183
- Tedral SA 1765

Phensuximide (Affects Calderol requirements in some patients). Products include:
- Milontin Kapseals 1741

Phenytoin (Affects Calderol requirements in some patients). Products include:
- Dilantin Infatabs 1710
- Dilantin-30 Pediatric/Dilantin-125 Suspension 1713

Phenytoin Sodium (Affects Calderol requirements in some patients). Products include:
- Dilantin Kapseals 1708
- Dilantin Parenteral 1712
- Dilantin with Phenobarbital Kapseals 1715

Primidone (Affects Calderol requirements in some patients). Products include:
- Mysoline 2480

Trimethadione (Affects Calderol requirements in some patients). Products include:
- Tridione 557

Valproic Acid (Affects Calderol requirements in some patients). Products include:
- Depakene Capsules & Syrup 511

Vitamin D (Should be withheld during Calderol treatment). Products include:
- Bugs Bunny Children's Chewable Vitamins (Sugar Free) ▣ 625
- Bugs Bunny With Extra C Children's Chewable Vitamins (Sugar Free) ▣ 626
- Bugs Bunny Plus Iron Children's Chewable Vitamins (Sugar Free) ▣ 625
- Calderol Capsules 1635
- Caltrate 600 + Iron & Vitamin D 1198
- Caltrate 600 + Vitamin D 1197
- Caltrate, Jr. Tablets 1198
- Flintstones Children's Chewable Vitamins ▣ 625
- Flintstones Children's Chewable Vitamins With Extra C ▣ 626
- Flintstones Children's Chewable Vitamins Plus Iron ▣ 625
- Natalins Rx 1391
- Natalins Tablets 1391
- One-A-Day Essential Vitamins ▣ 627
- One-A-Day Maximum Formula Vitamins and Minerals ▣ 627
- One-A-Day Plus Extra C Vitamins ▣ 627
- Os-Cal 250+D Tablets ▣ 597
- Os-Cal 500+D Tablets ▣ 597
- Os-Cal Fortified Tablets ▣ 597
- Os-Cal Plus Tablets ▣ 597
- Posture-D 600 mg 2420
- Stressgard Stress Formula Vitamins ▣ 628
- Tri-Vi-Flor 1.0 mg Vitamins with Fluoride Chewable Tablets 1400
- Tri-Vi-Flor Drops 1400
- Tri-Vi-Sol Vitamin Drops ▣ 614
- Tri-Vi-Sol Vitamin Drops with Iron ▣ 614
- Vi-Daylin ADC Vitamins Drops 1980
- Vi-Daylin ADC Vitamins + Iron Drops 1980
- Vi-Daylin/F ADC Vitamins Drops With Fluoride 1981
- Vi-Daylin/F ADC Vitamins + Iron Drops With Fluoride 1981
- Within Women's Formula Multivitamin with Calcium, Extra Iron and Zinc ▣ 628
- Zymacap Capsules ▣ 670

CALDESENE MEDICATED OINTMENT
(Petrolatum, Zinc Oxide) ▣ 560
No interactions described in labeling.

CALDESENE MEDICATED POWDER
(Calcium Undecylenate) ▣ 560
No interactions described in labeling.

CALPHOSAN
(Calcium Glycerophosphate, Calcium Lactate) 1071
No interactions described in labeling.

CALTRATE 600 TABLETS
(Calcium Carbonate) 1197
No interactions described in labeling.

CALTRATE 600 + IRON & VITAMIN D
(Calcium Carbonate, Ferrous Fumarate, Vitamin D) 1198
No interactions described in labeling.

CALTRATE 600 + VITAMIN D
(Calcium Carbonate, Vitamin D) 1197
No interactions described in labeling.

CALTRATE, JR. TABLETS
(Calcium Carbonate, Vitamin D) 1198
No interactions described in labeling.

CAMA ARTHRITIS PAIN RELIEVER
(Aspirin, Aluminum Hydroxide Gel, Dried, Magnesium Oxide) ▣ 685
May interact with oral hypoglycemic agents, oral anticoagulants, and antigout agents. Compounds in these categories include:

Allopurinol (Do not use concomitantly). Products include:
- Zyloprim Tablets 830

Chlorpropamide (Do not use concomitantly). Products include:
- Diabinese Tablets 1775

Dicumarol (Do not use concomitantly). Products include:
- Dicumarol Tablets 516

Glipizide (Do not use concomitantly). Products include:
- Glucotrol 1952

Glyburide (Do not use concomitantly). Products include:
- DiaBeta 1091
- Micronase Tablets 2350

Probenecid (Do not use concomitantly). Products include:
- Benemid Tablets 1426
- ColBENEMID Tablets 1436
- Wycillin Injection and Probenecid Tablets 2539

Sulfinpyrazone (Do not use concomitantly). Products include:
- Anturane 853

Tolazamide (Do not use concomitantly). Products include:
- Tolinase Tablets 2365

Tolbutamide (Do not use concomitantly). Products include:
- Orinase Tablets 2354

Warfarin Sodium (Do not use concomitantly). Products include:
- Coumadin Injection & Tablets 944
- Panwarfin Tablets 547

CAMPHO-PHENIQUE COLD SORE GEL
(Camphor, Phenol) ▣ 758
No interactions described in labeling.

CAMPHO-PHENIQUE LIQUID
(Phenol, Camphor) ▣ 758
No interactions described in labeling.

CAMPHO-PHENIQUE TRIPLE ANTIBIOTIC OINTMENT PLUS PAIN RELIEVER
(Bacitracin, Neomycin Sulfate, Polymyxin B Sulfate) ▣ 758
No interactions described in labeling.

CANTIL TABLETS
(Mepenzolate Bromide) 1326
May interact with antacids, anticholinergics, agents used to treat achlorhydria and/or to test gastric secretion, antiglaucoma agents, corticosteroids, narcotic analgesics, sympathomimetic aerosal bronchodilators, tricyclic antidepressants, type 1 antiarrhythmic drugs, antihistamines, phenothiazines, benzodiazepines, monoamine oxidase inhibitors, and certain other agents. Compounds in these categories include:

Acetazolamide (Effects of antiglaucoma agents antagonized). Products include:
- Diamox Parenteral 1200
- Diamox Parenteral ◉ 308
- Diamox Sequels (Sustained Release) 1201
- Diamox Sequels (Sustained Release) ◉ 310
- Diamox Tablets 1200
- Diamox Tablets ◉ 308

Acetylcholine Chloride (Effects of antiglaucoma agents antagonized). Products include:
- Miochol with Iocare Steri-Tags, Miochol System Pak and Miochol System Pak Plus ◉ 274

Albuterol (Increases certain actions or side effects). Products include:
- Proventil Inhalation Aerosol 2117
- Ventolin Inhalation Aerosol and Refill 583

Albuterol Sulfate (Increases certain actions or side effects). Products include:
- Proventil Repetabs Tablets 2120
- Proventil Solutions for Inhalation 0.5% and 0.083% 2118
- Proventil Syrup 2119
- Proventil Tablets 2120
- Ventolin 583

Alfentanil Hydrochloride (Increases certain actions or side effects). Products include:
- Alfenta Injection 1131

Alprazolam (Increases certain actions or side effects). Products include:
- Xanax Tablets 2367

Aluminum Carbonate Gel (Interferes with the absorption). Products include:
- Basaljel 2438

Aluminum Hydroxide (Interferes with the absorption). Products include:
- Cama Arthritis Pain Reliever ▣ 685
- Gaviscon Extra Strength Relief Formula Liquid Antacid ▣ 594
- Gaviscon Extra Strength Relief Formula Antacid Tablets ▣ 594
- Gaviscon Liquid Antacid ▣ 594
- Gelusil Liquid & Tablets ▣ 639
- Extra Strength Maalox Plus Suspension 1850
- Maalox TC Suspension 1851
- Maalox Plus Tablets ▣ 655
- Extra Strength Maalox Plus Tablets 1850
- Nephrox Suspension ▣ 563
- WinGel Liquid & Tablets ▣ 761

Aluminum Hydroxide Gel (Interferes with the absorption). Products include:
- ALternaGEL Liquid 1154
- Aludrox Oral Suspension 2428
- Amphojel Suspension 2429
- Amphojel Suspension without Flavor 2429
- Mylanta Liquid 1155
- Mylanta Double Strength Liquid 1155

Aluminum Hydroxide Gel, Dried (Interferes with the absorption). Products include:
- Alu-Tab/Alu-Cap 1309
- Amphojel Tablets 2429
- Ascriptin A/D Caplets 1850
- Regular Strength Ascriptin Tablets 1850

Gaviscon Antacid Tablets.................. 593
Gaviscon-2 Antacid Tablets 594
Mylanta Tablets 1155
Mylanta Double Strength Tablets..... 1155

Amantadine Hydrochloride (Increases certain actions or side effects). Products include:
Symmetrel Capsules & Syrup............ 936

Amitriptyline Hydrochloride (Increases certain actions or side effects). Products include:
Elavil 2269
Endep Tablets 1927
Etrafon 2087
Limbitrol 1933
Triavil Tablets 1556

Amoxapine (Increases certain actions or side effects). Products include:
Asendin Tablets 1196

Amyl Nitrite (Increases certain actions or side effects).
No products indexed under this heading.

Astemizole (Increases certain actions or side effects). Products include:
Hismanal Tablets 1138

Atropine Sulfate (Increases certain actions or side effects). Products include:
Arco-Lase Plus Tablets 607
Atropine Sulfate Sterile Ophthalmic Solution and S.O.P. Sterile Ophthalmic Ointment...................... ⊙ 239
Donnagel 675
Donnagel-PG 1858
Donnatal 1858
Donnatal Extentabs.............................. 1859
Donnatal Tablets 1858
Donnazyme Tablets 1860
Isopto Atropine...................................... ⊙ 218
Lomotil 2174
Motofen Tablets 836
Ru-Tuss Tablets 693
Urised Tablets 2396

Azatadine Maleate (Increases certain actions or side effects). Products include:
Optimine Tablets 2115
Trinalin Repetabs Tablets 1170

Belladonna Alkaloids (Increases certain actions or side effects). Products include:
Bellergal-S Tablets 1998
Hyland's Bed Wetting Tablets 728
Hyland's Teething Tablets 728
Kinesed Tablets 2272

Benztropine Mesylate (Increases certain actions or side effects). Products include:
Cogentin 1435

Betamethasone Acetate (Concurrent use in the presence of increased intraocular pressure may be hazardous). Products include:
Celestone Soluspan Suspension 2081

Betamethasone Sodium Phosphate (Concurrent use in the presence of increased intraocular pressure may be hazardous). Products include:
Celestone Soluspan Suspension 2081

Betaxolol Hydrochloride (Effects of antiglaucoma agents antagonized). Products include:
Betoptic Sterile Ophthalmic Solution.. 569
Betoptic S Sterile Ophthalmic Suspension.. 570
Kerlone Tablets...................................... 2172

Biperiden (Increases certain actions or side effects). Products include:
Akineton 1171

Bromodiphenhydramine Hydrochloride (Increases certain actions or side effects).
No products indexed under this heading.

Brompheniramine Maleate (Increases certain actions or side effects). Products include:
Alka Seltzer Plus Sinus Allergy Medicine 624
Atrohist Sprinkle Capsules 558
Bromfed Capsules (Timed Release) 1615
Bromfed Syrup 628
Bromfed.. 1615
Dimetane Decongestant 673
Dimetane.. 672
Dimetane-DC Cough Syrup 1857
Dimetane-DX Cough Syrup 1858
Dimetapp Elixir 673
Dimetapp DM Elixir.............................. 674
Dimetapp Extentabs............................ 674
Dimetapp Plus Caplets 675
Dimetapp Tablets 675
Drixoral Antihistamine/Nasal Decongestant Syrup........................ 698

Buprenorphine (Increases certain actions or side effects).
No products indexed under this heading.

Carbachol (Effects of antiglaucoma agents antagonized). Products include:
Isopto Carbachol .... ⊙ 219
MIOSTAT.. ⊙ 233

Chlordiazepoxide (Increases certain actions or side effects). Products include:
Libritabs Tablets 1930
Limbitrol 1933
Menrium Tablets 1934

Chlordiazepoxide Hydrochloride (Increases certain actions or side effects). Products include:
Librax Capsules 1929
Librium Capsules.................................. 1931
Librium Injectable 1932

Chlorpheniramine Maleate (Increases certain actions or side effects). Products include:
A.R.M. Allergy Relief Medicine Caplets 615
Alka-Seltzer Plus Cold Medicine 623
Allerest.. 559
Ana-Kit Anaphylaxis Emergency Treatment Kit 1100
BC Cold Powder Multi-Symptom Formula 517
Brexin L.A. Capsules............................ 2078
Cerose-DM 2443
Cheracol Plus Head Cold/Cough Formula 667
Chlor-Trimeton Allergy Syrup, Tablets & Long-Acting Repetabs Tablets 693
Chlor-Trimeton Decongestant 694
Comhist LA Capsules.......................... 1618
Allergy-Sinus Comtrex Multi-Symptom Allergy Sinus Formula Tablets & Caplets 746
Comtrex Multi-Symptom Cold Reliever Tablets/Caplets/Liqui-Gels/Liquid.. 745
Day-Night Comtrex 747
Contac Continuous Action Decongestant/Antihistamine Capsules 710
Contac Maximum Strength Continuous Action Decongestant/Antihistamine Caplets 709
Contac Severe Cold and Flu Formula Caplets 711
Coricidin 'D' Decongestant Tablets.. 695
Coricidin Demilets Tablets for Children 696
Coricidin Tablets 695
Deconamine 663
Demazin Nasal Decongestant/Antihistamine Repetabs Tablets & Syrup 697
Dorcol Children's Liquid Cold Formula 686
Dristan Decongestant/Antihistamine/Analgesic Coated Caplets 749
Dristan Cold Nasal Decongestant/Antihistamine/ Analgesic Coated Tablets 2419
Dristan Advanced Formula Decongestant/Antihistamine/ Analgesic Tablets 749
Extendryl 994
4-Way Cold Tablets.............................. 750
Fedahist Gyrocaps................................ 2145
Fedahist Timecaps 2145
Hycomine Compound Tablets 929
Isoclor Timesule Capsules 561
Kronofed-A 970
Medi-Flu Caplet, Liquid 640
Naldecon Syrup, Tablets, Pediatric Drops and Pediatric Syrup.............. 709
Nolamine Tablets.................................. 838
Novafed A Capsules 1342
Novahistine DH...................................... 1342
Novahistine Elixir 596
Ornade Spansule Capsules 2221
Orthoxicol Cough Syrup 668
PediaCare Allergy Relief Formula Liquid 1362
PediaCare Cough-Cold Formula Liquid 1362
PediaCare Night Rest Cough-Cold Formula Liquid 1362
PediaCare 6-12 Cough-Cold Formula Chewable Tablets 1362
Pyrroxate Capsules.............................. 669
Quelidrine Syrup 556
Ru-Tuss II Capsules 693
Ru-Tuss Tablets 693
Ryna 741
Sinarest Tablets & Extra Strength Tablets 562
Sine-Off Maximum Strength Allergy/Sinus Formula Caplets 721
Sine-Off Sinus Medicine Tablets-Aspirin Formula 722
Singlet Tablets 598
Sinulin.. 840
Sinutab Maximum Strength.............. 641
St. Joseph Nighttime Cold Medicine 705
Sudafed Plus Liquid 544
Sudafed Plus Tablets 545
Teldrin Timed-Release Allergy Capsules, 12 mg.................................. 2192
TheraFlu Flu and Cold Medicine 687
Triaminic Allergy Tablets 688
Triaminic Chewables 688
Triaminic Cold Tablets 688
Triaminic Nite Light 689
Triaminic Syrup 689
Triaminic-12 Tablets 690
Triaminicin Tablets 690
Triaminicol Multi-Symptom Cold Tablets 691
Triaminicol Multi-Symptom Relief .. 691
Tylenol Allergy Sinus Medication Caplets and Gelcaps, Maximum Strength.. 1372
Children's Tylenol Cold Liquid Formula and Chewable Tablets 1368
Tylenol Cold & Flu Hot Medication, Packets 1369
Tylenol Cold Medication Caplets and Tablets.. 1370
Tylenol Cold Medication, Effervescent Tablets 1369
Vicks Children's NyQuil...................... 664
Vicks Formula 44 Cough Medicine 661
Vicks Formula 44M Multi-Symptom Cough Medicine 662
Vicks Pediatric Formula 44m Multi-Symptom Cough & Cold Medicine 663

Chlorpheniramine Polistirex (Increases certain actions or side effects). Products include:
Tussionex Extended-Release Suspension.. 988

Chlorpheniramine Tannate (Increases certain actions or side effects). Products include:
Rynatan 2387
Rynatuss 2388

Chlorpromazine (Increases certain actions or side effects). Products include:
Thorazine 2234

Clemastine Fumarate (Increases certain actions or side effects). Products include:
Tavist Syrup.. 2033
Tavist Tablets 2035
Tavist-D Tablets 2035

Clidinium Bromide (Increases certain actions or side effects). Products include:
Librax Capsules 1929
Quarzan Capsules 1937

Clomipramine Hydrochloride (Increases certain actions or side effects). Products include:
Anafranil Capsules 650

Clorazepate Dipotassium (Increases certain actions or side effects). Products include:
Tranxene 556

Codeine (Increases certain actions or side effects). Products include:
Calcidrine Syrup.................................... 506

Codeine Phosphate (Increases certain actions or side effects). Products include:
Actifed with Codeine Cough Syrup.. 752
Cheracol Cough Syrup.......................... 1853
Codimal PH Syrup.................................. 846
Dimetane-DC Cough Syrup 1857
Empirin with Codeine Phosphate Nos. 2, 3 & 4.. 764
Fiorinal with Codeine Capsules 2008
Isoclor Expectorant.............................. 982
Naldecon CX Adult Liquid 521
Novahistine DH...................................... 1342
Novahistine Expectorant.................... 1343
Nucofed Capsules 2219
Nucofed Expectorant 2219
Nucofed Pediatric Expectorant 2220
Nucofed Syrup 2219
Phenaphen with Codeine Capsules 1865
Phenaphen-650 with Codeine Tablets 1866
Phenergan with Codeine.................... 2497
Phenergan VC with Codeine 2501
Robitussin A-C Syrup.......................... 1875
Robitussin-DAC Syrup........................ 1875
Ryna 741
Soma Compound w/Codeine Tablets 2390
Triaminic Expectorant w/Codeine .. 1996
Tussi-Organidin Liquid 2391
Tylenol with Codeine 1381

Codeine Polistirex (Increases certain actions or side effects).
No products indexed under this heading.

Cortisone Acetate (Concurrent use in the presence of increased intraocular pressure may be hazardous). Products include:
Cortone Acetate Sterile Suspension 1437
Cortone Acetate Tablets.................... 1439

Cyproheptadine Hydrochloride (Increases certain actions or side effects). Products include:
Periactin 1525

Demecarium Bromide (Effects of antiglaucoma agents antagonized). Products include:
Humorsol Sterile Ophthalmic Solution.. 1475

Desipramine Hydrochloride (Increases certain actions or side effects). Products include:
Norpramin Tablets 1340

Dexamethasone (Concurrent use in the presence of increased intraocular pressure may be hazardous). Products include:
AK-Trol Ointment & Suspension .... ⊙ 207
Decadron Elixir 1445
Decadron Tablets.................................. 1447
Decaspray Topical Aerosol 1459
Dexacidin.. ⊙ 272
Maxidex Sterile Ophthalmic Suspension.. ⊙ 223
Maxitrol Ophthalmic Ointment/Suspension .... ⊙ 223
TobraDex Ophthalmic Suspension and Ointment.................................... ⊙ 228

Dexamethasone Acetate (Concurrent use in the presence of increased intraocular pressure may be hazardous). Products include:
Dalalone D.P. Injectable 999
Decadron-LA Sterile Suspension...... 1457

Dexamethasone Sodium Phosphate (Concurrent use in the presence of increased intraocular pressure may be hazardous). Products include:
AK-Dex .... ⊙ 203

- Decadron Phosphate Respihaler 1454
- Decadron Phosphate Sterile Ophthalmic Ointment 1453
- Decadron Phosphate Sterile Ophthalmic Solution 1453
- Decadron Phosphate Topical Cream 1455
- Decadron Phosphate Turbinaire 1456
- Maxidex Sterile Ophthalmic Ointment ⊙ 222
- NeoDecadron Sterile Ophthalmic Ointment 1517
- NeoDecadron Sterile Ophthalmic Solution 1518
- NeoDecadron Topical Cream 1518

Dexchlorpheniramine Maleate (Increases certain actions or side effects). Products include:
- Polaramine 2116

Dezocine (Increases certain actions or side effects).

Diazepam (Increases certain actions or side effects). Products include:
- Valium Injectable 1937
- Valium Tablets 1939
- Valrelease Capsules 1923

Dichlorphenamide (Effects of antiglaucoma agents antagonized). Products include:
- Daranide Tablets 1445

Dicyclomine Hydrochloride (Increases certain actions or side effects). Products include:
- Bentyl 1322

Digoxin (Increased serum digoxin levels). Products include:
- Lanoxicaps 772
- Lanoxin Elixir Pediatric 775
- Lanoxin Injection 778
- Lanoxin Injection Pediatric 781
- Lanoxin Tablets 783

Dihydroxyaluminum Sodium Carbonate (Interferes with the absorption). Products include:
- Rolaids ▣ 743

Diphenhydramine Citrate (Increases certain actions or side effects). Products include:
- Alka-Seltzer Plus Night-Time Cold Medicine ▣ 623
- Bufferin AF Nite Time Analgesic/Sleeping Aid Caplets 744
- Excedrin P.M. Analgesic/Sleeping Aid Tablets, Caplets and Liquid 749

Diphenhydramine Hydrochloride (Increases certain actions or side effects). Products include:
- Benadryl Anti-Itch Cream ▣ 635
- Benadryl Capsules 1691
- Benadryl Decongestant Elixir ▣ 635
- Benadryl Decongestant ▣ 635
- Benadryl Elixir ▣ 636
- Benadryl Kapseals 1691
- Benadryl 25 Kapseals ▣ 636
- Benadryl Parenteral 1692
- Benadryl Plus ▣ 636
- Benadryl Plus Nighttime ▣ 637
- Benadryl Spray, Maximum Strength ▣ 637
- Benadryl Spray, Regular Strength ▣ 637
- Benadryl Steri-Vials, Ampoules, and Steri-Dose Syringe 1692
- Benadryl 25 Tablets ▣ 636
- Benylin Cough Syrup ▣ 637
- Benylin Decongestant ▣ 638
- Caladryl Cream, Lotion, Spray ▣ 638
- Miles Nervine Nighttime Sleep-Aid ▣ 627
- Nytol Tablets ▣ 517
- Sleep-ettes-D Tablets ▣ 653
- Sleep-eze 3 Tablets ▣ 755
- Sleepinal Night-time Sleep Aid Capsules ▣ 734
- Sominex Caplets and Tablets ▣ 722
- Sominex Liquid ▣ 723
- Sominex Pain Relief Formula ▣ 723
- Tylenol Cold Night Time Medication Liquid 1371
- Tylenol PM, Extra Strength Caplets and Tablets 1368
- Unisom Dual Relief Nighttime Sleep Aid/Analgesic 1774
- Ziradryl Lotion ▣ 643

Diphenylpyraline Hydrochloride (Increases certain actions or side effects).
- No products indexed under this heading.

Dipivefrin Hydrochloride (Effects of antiglaucoma agents antagonized). Products include:
- Propine with C Cap Compliance Cap ⊙ 255

Disopyramide Phosphate (Increases certain actions or side effects). Products include:
- Norpace 2177

Dobutamine Hydrochloride (Increases certain actions or side effects). Products include:
- Dobutrex Solution Vials 1259

Dopamine Hydrochloride (Increases certain actions or side effects). Products include:
- Intropin Injection 930

Doxepin Hydrochloride (Increases certain actions or side effects). Products include:
- Sinequan 1960

Echothiophate Iodide (Effects of antiglaucoma agents antagonized). Products include:
- Phospholine Iodide ⊙ 315

Ephedrine Hydrochloride (Increases certain actions or side effects). Products include:
- Amesec ▣ 682
- Primatene Tablets-M Formula 2421
- Primatene Tablets-P Formula 2421
- Primatene Tablets-Regular Formula 2421
- Quadrinal Tablets 1183
- Quelidrine Syrup 556
- Tedral SA 1765

Ephedrine Sulfate (Increases certain actions or side effects). Products include:
- Bronkaid Tablets ▣ 757
- Bronkolixir ▣ 761
- Bronkotabs Tablets ▣ 762
- Marax Tablets & DF Syrup 1954
- Pazo Hemorrhoid Ointment & Suppositories 752
- Vicks Vatronol Nose Drops ▣ 666

Ephedrine Tannate (Increases certain actions or side effects). Products include:
- Rynatuss 2388

Epinephrine (Increases certain actions or side effects). Products include:
- Ana-Kit Anaphylaxis Emergency Treatment Kit 1100
- Bronkaid Mist ▣ 757
- EpiPen 843
- Marcaine Hydrochloride 0.5% with Epinephrine 1:200,000 (as bitartrate) 958
- Marcaine Hydrochloride with Epinephrine 1:200,000 2055
- Primatene Mist 2420
- Sus-Phrine Injection 1006
- Xylocaine with Epinephrine Injections 637

Epinephrine Bitartrate (Increases certain actions or side effects; effects of antiglaucoma agents antagonized). Products include:
- AsthmaHaler Mist Epinephrine Bitartrate Bronchodilator ▣ 616
- Bronkaid Mist Suspension ▣ 757
- Primatene Mist Suspension 2421

Epinephrine Hydrochloride (Increases certain actions or side effects; effects of antiglaucoma agents antagonized). Products include:
- Adrenalin Chloride Solution 1:100 & 1:1,000 1689
- Epifrin ⊙ 244
- Glaucon ⊙ 218

Epinephryl Borate (Effects of antiglaucoma agents antagonized).
- No products indexed under this heading.

Erythrityl Tetranitrate (Increases certain actions or side effects). Products include:
- Cardilate Oral/Sublingual Tablets 757

Estazolam (Increases certain actions or side effects). Products include:
- ProSom Tablets 554

Fentanyl (Increases certain actions or side effects). Products include:
- Duragesic Transdermal System 1133

Fentanyl Citrate (Increases certain actions or side effects). Products include:
- Innovar Injection 1141
- Sublimaze Injection 1146

Fluphenazine Decanoate (Increases certain actions or side effects). Products include:
- Prolixin Decanoate 1795

Fluphenazine Enanthate (Increases certain actions or side effects). Products include:
- Prolixin Enanthate 1796

Fluphenazine Hydrochloride (Increases certain actions or side effects). Products include:
- Prolixin Elixir 1793
- Prolixin Injection 1791
- Prolixin Oral Concentrate 1792
- Prolixin Tablets 1793

Furazolidone (Increases certain actions or side effects). Products include:
- Furoxone 1855

Glutamic Acid Hydrochloride (Antagonizes the inhibiting effects on gastric hydrochloric acid).
- No products indexed under this heading.

Glycopyrrolate (Increases certain actions or side effects). Products include:
- Robinul Forte Tablets 1873
- Robinul Injectable 1873
- Robinul Tablets 1873

Hydrocodone Bitartrate (Increases certain actions or side effects). Products include:
- Anexsia 5/500 Tablets 2196
- Anexsia 7.5/650 Tablets 2197
- Azdone Tablets 844
- Codiclear DH Syrup 845
- Codimal DH Syrup 846
- Damason-P 1356
- Hycodan Syrup, Tablets 927
- Hycomine Compound Tablets 929
- Hycomine Syrup 927
- Hycotuss Expectorant Syrup 930
- Hydrocet Capsules 835
- Lortab ASA Tablets 2414
- Lortab 2412
- Ru-Tuss with Hydrocodone 694
- Triaminic Expectorant DH 1995
- Vicodin Tablets 1187
- Vicodin ES Tablets 1189
- Zydone Capsules 941

Hydrocodone Polistirex (Increases certain actions or side effects). Products include:
- Tussionex Extended-Release Suspension 988

Hydrocortisone (Concurrent use in the presence of increased intraocular pressure may be hazardous). Products include:
- AK-Spore H.C. ⊙ 206
- Bactine Hydrocortisone Anti-Itch Cream ▣ 625
- CaldeCORT Anti-Itch Hydrocortisone Spray ▣ 560
- Carmol HC Cream 1% 2296
- Cortaid Spray ▣ 735
- Cortenema 2244
- Cortisporin Ointment 758
- Cortisporin Ophthalmic Ointment Sterile 758
- Cortisporin Ophthalmic Suspension Sterile 759
- Cortisporin Otic Solution Sterile 760
- Cortisporin Otic Suspension Sterile 760
- Cortizone-5 Creme & Ointment ▣ 732
- Dermolate Anti-Itch Cream ▣ 697
- Eldecort Cream 1.0% 1113
- Eldecort Cream 1.0% and 2.5% 1113
- Fungoid HC Creme 1770
- Hydrocortone Tablets 1482
- Hytone 909
- LazerSporin-C Solution 1770
- Massengill Medicated Soft Cloth Towelettes 2192
- Nutracort Cream & Lotion 1684
- PediOtic Suspension Sterile 797
- Synacort Creams 1%, 2.5% 2296
- Vanoxide-HC Acne Lotion 911
- Vioform-Hydrocortisone Cream and Mild Cream 889
- Vioform-Hydrocortisone Ointment 889
- VōSoL HC Otic Solution 2392
- Vytone Cream 1% 911

Hydrocortisone Acetate (Concurrent use in the presence of increased intraocular pressure may be hazardous). Products include:
- Analpram-HC Rectal Cream 1% and 2.5% 970
- Anusol-HC Cream 1690
- Anusol-HC Suppositories 1691
- Caldecort ▣ 560
- Carmol HC Cream 1% 2296
- Chloromycetin Hydrocortisone Ophthalmic 1694
- Coly-Mycin S Otic w/Neomycin & Hydrocortisone 1708
- Cortaid ▣ 735
- Cortef Feminine Itch Cream ▣ 735
- Corticaine ▣ 682
- Cortifoam 1827
- Cortisporin Cream 757
- Epifoam 1828
- Gynecort 5 Creme ▣ 556
- Hydrocortone Acetate Sterile Suspension 1479
- Lanacort 5 Creme and Ointment ▣ 557
- Mantadil Cream 789
- Ophthocort ⊙ 301
- Orabase HCA Oral Paste 890
- Pramosone Cream, Lotion & Ointment 971
- ProctoCream-HC 1834
- Proctofoam-HC 1835

Hydrocortisone Sodium Phosphate (Concurrent use in the presence of increased intraocular pressure may be hazardous). Products include:
- Hydrocortone Phosphate Injection, Sterile 1481

Hydrocortisone Sodium Succinate (Concurrent use in the presence of increased intraocular pressure may be hazardous). Products include:
- Solu-Cortef Sterile Powder 2361

Hyoscyamine (Increases certain actions or side effects). Products include:
- Cystospaz Tablets 2395
- Urised Tablets 2396

Hyoscyamine Sulfate (Increases certain actions or side effects). Products include:
- Arco-Lase Plus Tablets 607
- Cystospaz-M Capsules 2395
- Donnagel ▣ 675
- Donnagel-PG 1858
- Donnatal 1858
- Donnatal Extentabs 1859
- Donnatal Tablets 1858
- Donnazyme Tablets 1860
- Kutrase Capsules 2146
- Levsin/Levsinex 2147
- Ru-Tuss Tablets 693

Imipramine Hydrochloride (Increases certain actions or side effects). Products include:
- Tofranil Ampuls 1038
- Tofranil Tablets 1039

Imipramine Pamoate (Increases certain actions or side effects). Products include:
- Tofranil-PM Capsules 1041

Ipratropium Bromide (Increases certain actions or side effects). Products include:
- Atrovent Inhalation Aerosol ... 675

Isocarboxazid (Increases certain actions or side effects). Products include:
- Marplan Tablets ... 1906

Isoflurophate (Effects of anti-glaucoma agents antagonized). Products include:
- Floropryl Sterile Ophthalmic Ointment ... 1473

Isoproterenol Hydrochloride (Increases certain actions or side effects). Products include:
- Isuprel Hydrochloride Injection 1:5000 ... 2050
- Isuprel Hydrochloride Mistometer .. 2051
- Isuprel Hydrochloride Solution 1:200 & 1:100 ... 2052
- Norisodrine Aerotrol ... 540

Isosorbide Dinitrate (Increases certain actions or side effects). Products include:
- Dilatrate-SR ... 1827
- Isordil ... 2467
- Sorbitrate ... 1103

Levobunolol Hydrochloride (Effects of antiglaucoma agents antagonized). Products include:
- Betagan ... ⊙ 239

Levorphanol Tartrate (Increases certain actions or side effects). Products include:
- Levo-Dromoran ... 1906

Lorazepam (Increases certain actions or side effects). Products include:
- Ativan Injection ... 2432
- Ativan Tablets ... 2434

Magaldrate (Interferes with the absorption). Products include:
- Riopan Antacid Chew Tablets ... ⊡ 754
- Riopan Antacid Chew Tablets in Rollpacks ... ⊡ 754
- Riopan Antacid Suspension ... 2421
- Riopan Antacid Swallow Tablets ... 2421
- Riopan Plus Chew Tablets ... 2422
- Riopan Plus Chew Tablets in Rollpack ... 2422
- Riopan Plus 2 Chew Tablets, Mint Flavor, Cherry Flavor ... 2422
- Riopan Plus Suspension ... 2422
- Riopan Plus 2 Suspension, Mint Flavor, Cherry Flavor ... 2422

Magnesium Hydroxide (Interferes with the absorption). Products include:
- Aludrox Oral Suspension ... 2428
- Ascriptin A/D Caplets ... 1850
- Regular Strength Ascriptin Tablets 1850
- Di-Gel Antacid/Anti-Gas ... ⊡ 697
- Gelusil Liquid & Tablets ... ⊡ 639
- Haley's M-O, Regular & Flavored .. ⊡ 569
- Extra Strength Maalox Plus Suspension ... 1850
- Maalox TC Suspension ... 1851
- Maalox Plus Tablets ... ⊡ 655
- Extra Strength Maalox Plus Tablets 1850
- Mylanta Liquid ... 1155
- Mylanta Tablets ... 1155
- Mylanta Double Strength Liquid ... 1155
- Mylanta Double Strength Tablets ... 1155
- Concentrated Phillips' Milk of Magnesia ... ⊡ 573
- Phillips' Milk of Magnesia Liquid ... ⊡ 572
- Phillips' Milk of Magnesia Tablets ⊡ 573
- WinGel Liquid & Tablets ... ⊡ 761

Magnesium Oxide (Interferes with the absorption). Products include:
- Bayer Plus Aspirin Tablets ... ⊡ 567
- Beelith Tablets ... 659
- Bufferin Analgesic Tablets and Caplets ... ⊡ 524
- Cama Arthritis Pain Reliever ... ⊡ 685
- Mag-Ox 400 ... 673
- Uro-Mag ... 673

Maprotiline Hydrochloride (Increases certain actions or side effects). Products include:
- Ludiomil Tablets ... 874

Meperidine Hydrochloride (Increases certain actions or side effects). Products include:
- Demerol ... 2047
- Mepergan Injection ... 2479

Mesoridazine Besylate (Increases certain actions or side effects).

Metaproterenol Sulfate (Increases certain actions or side effects). Products include:
- Alupent ... 674
- Arm-a-Med Metaproterenol Sulfate Inhalation Solution, USP ... 617
- Metaprel Inhalation Aerosol Bronchodilator ... 2014
- Metaprel Inhalation Solution ... 2015
- Metaprel ... 2015
- Metaproterenol Sulfate Inhalation Solution, USP ... 912

Metaraminol Bitartrate (Increases certain actions or side effects). Products include:
- Aramine Injection ... 1424

Methadone Hydrochloride (Increases certain actions or side effects). Products include:
- Dolophine Hydrochloride Ampoules & Vials ... 1260
- Dolophine Hydrochloride Tablets ... 1261
- Methadone Hydrochloride Diskets .. 1284
- Methadone Hydrochloride Oral Solution & Tablets ... 1987

Methazolamide (Effects of anti-glaucoma agents antagonized). Products include:
- Neptazane Tablets ... ⊙ 311

Methdilazine Hydrochloride (Increases certain actions or side effects). Products include:
- Tacaryl Syrup & Tablets ... 2409

Methoxamine Hydrochloride (Increases certain actions or side effects). Products include:
- Vasoxyl Injection ... 819

Methylprednisolone Acetate (Concurrent use in the presence of increased intraocular pressure may be hazardous). Products include:
- Depo-Medrol Sterile Aqueous Suspension ... 2334

Methylprednisolone Sodium Succinate (Concurrent use in the presence of increased intraocular pressure may be hazardous). Products include:
- Solu-Medrol Sterile Powder ... 2363

Metoclopramide Hydrochloride (Gastrointestinal motility effects of metoclopramide may be antagonized). Products include:
- Reglan ... 1869

Midazolam Hydrochloride (Increases certain actions or side effects). Products include:
- Versed Injection ... 1924

Moricizine Hydrochloride (Increases certain actions or side effects). Products include:
- Ethmozine Tablets ... 946

Morphine Sulfate (Increases certain actions or side effects). Products include:
- Astramorph/PF Injection, USP (Preservative-Free) ... 618
- Duramorph ... 960
- Infumorph 200 and Infumorph 500 Sterile Solutions ... 962
- MS Contin Tablets ... 1814
- MSIR ... 1817
- Oramorph SR (Morphine Sulfate Sustained Release Tablets) ... 1988
- Roxanol ... 1991

Nitroglycerin (Increases certain actions or side effects). Products include:
- Deponit NTG Transdermal Delivery System ... 2143
- Minitran Transdermal Delivery System ... 1312
- Nitro-Bid Ointment ... 1339
- Nitro-Bid Capsules ... 1338
- Nitrodisc ... 2176
- Nitro-Dur (nitroglycerin) Transdermal Infusion System ... 1164
- Nitrogard Tablets ... 1004
- Nitrolingual Spray ... 1846
- Nitrostat Tablets ... 1743
- Transderm-Nitro Transdermal Therapeutic System ... 2283

Norepinephrine Bitartrate (Increases certain actions or side effects). Products include:
- Levophed Bitartrate Injection ... 2054

Nortriptyline Hydrochloride (Increases certain actions or side effects). Products include:
- Pamelor ... 2019

Opium Alkaloids (Increases certain actions or side effects). Products include:
- B & O No. 15A & No. 16A Supprettes ... 2395
- Pantopon Injectable ... 1911

Oxazepam (Increases certain actions or side effects). Products include:
- Serax Capsules ... 2522
- Serax Tablets ... 2522

Oxybutynin Chloride (Increases certain actions or side effects). Products include:
- Ditropan ... 1332

Oxycodone Hydrochloride (Increases certain actions or side effects). Products include:
- Percocet Tablets ... 950
- Percodan ... 951
- Roxicodone Tablets, Oral Solution & Intensol (Oxycodone) ... 1992
- Tylox Capsules ... 1382

Pentaerythritol Tetranitrate (Increases certain actions or side effects). Products include:
- Peritrate ... 1756

Pentagastrin (Antagonizes the inhibiting effects on gastric hydrochloric acid). Products include:
- Peptavlon ... 2563

Perphenazine (Increases certain actions or side effects). Products include:
- Etrafon ... 2087
- Triavil Tablets ... 1556
- Trilafon ... 2123

Phenelzine Sulfate (Increases certain actions or side effects). Products include:
- Nardil ... 1742

Phenylephrine Bitartrate (Increases certain actions or side effects).
- No products indexed under this heading.

Phenylephrine Hydrochloride (Increases certain actions or side effects). Products include:
- AK-Dilate Solution 2.5% and 10% ... ⊙ 203
- Atrohist Sprinkle Capsules ... 558
- Cerose-DM ... 2443
- Codimal ... 846
- Comhist LA Capsules ... 1618
- Congespirin For Children Aspirin Free Chewable Cold Tablets ... 748
- Cyclomydril ... ⊙ 216
- Deconsal Sprinkle Capsules ... 559
- Dimetane Decongestant ... ⊡ 673
- Dristan Decongestant/Antihistamine/Analgesic Coated Caplets ... ⊡ 749
- Dristan Cold Nasal Decongestant/Antihistamine/ Analgesic Coated Tablets ... 2419
- Dristan Advanced Formula Decongestant/Antihistamine/Analgesic Tablets ... ⊡ 749
- Dristan Nasal Spray, Menthol ... 2419
- Dristan Nasal Spray, Regular and Regular with Metered Pump ... 2419
- Entex Capsules ... 1623
- Entex Liquid ... 1623
- Sinus Excedrin Analgesic, Decongestant Tablets & Caplets ... 750
- Extendryl ... 994
- 4-Way Fast Acting Nasal Spray - Original Formula (regular & mentholated) & Metered Spray Pump (regular) ... 751
- Hycomine Compound Tablets ... 929
- Murocoll-2 Sterile Ophthalmic Solution ... ⊙ 261
- Mydfrin 2.5% ... ⊙ 224
- Naldecon Syrup, Tablets, Pediatric Drops and Pediatric Syrup ... 709
- Neo-Synephrine Hydrochloride 1% Carpuject ... 2063
- Neo-Synephrine Hydrochloride 1% Injection ... 2063
- Neo-Synephrine Hydrochloride (Ophthalmic) ... 2064
- Neo-Synephrine ... ⊡ 759
- Nōstril Nasal Decongestant ... ⊡ 520
- Novahistine Elixir ... ⊡ 596
- Phenergan VC ... 2500
- Phenergan VC with Codeine ... 2501
- Prefrin Liquifilm Vasoconstrictor and Lubricant Eye Drops ... ⊙ 254
- Prefrin-A ... ⊙ 255
- Quelidrine Syrup ... 556
- Relief Vasoconstrictor and Lubricant Eye Drops ... ⊙ 256
- Robitussin Night Relief ... ⊡ 677
- Ru-Tuss with Hydrocodone ... 694
- Ru-Tuss Tablets ... 693
- Vasosulf ... ⊙ 279
- Vicks Sinex ... ⊡ 665
- Zincfrin ... ⊙ 230

Phenylephrine Tannate (Increases certain actions or side effects). Products include:
- Rynatan ... 2387
- Rynatuss ... 2388

Phenylpropanolamine Hydrochloride (Increases certain actions or side effects). Products include:
- A.R.M. Allergy Relief Medicine Caplets ... ⊡ 615
- Acutrim ... ⊡ 548
- Allerest ... ⊡ 559
- BC Cold Powder ... ⊡ 517
- Cheracol Plus Head Cold/Cough Formula ... ⊡ 667
- Codimal Expectorant ... 846
- Comtrex Multi-Symptom Cold Reliever Tablets/Caplets/Liqui-Gels/Liquid ... 745
- Contac Continuous Action Decongestant/Antihistamine Capsules ⊡ 710
- Contac Maximum Strength Continuous Action Decongestant/Antihistamine Caplets ... ⊡ 709
- Contac Severe Cold and Flu Formula Caplets ... ⊡ 711
- Coricidin 'D' Decongestant Tablets ... ⊡ 695
- Coricidin Demilets Tablets for Children ... ⊡ 696
- Demazin Nasal Decongestant/Antihistamine Repetabs Tablets & Syrup ... ⊡ 697
- Dexatrim ... ⊡ 733
- Dimetane-DC Cough Syrup ... 1857
- Dimetapp Elixir ... ⊡ 673
- Dimetapp DM Elixir ... ⊡ 674
- Dimetapp Extentabs ... ⊡ 674
- Dimetapp Plus Caplets ... ⊡ 675
- Dimetapp Tablets ... ⊡ 675
- Entex Capsules ... 1623
- Entex LA Tablets ... 1623
- Entex Liquid ... 1623
- 4-Way Cold Tablets ... 750
- Hycomine Syrup ... 927
- Naldecon CX Adult Liquid ... ⊡ 521
- Naldecon DX Adult Liquid ... ⊡ 521
- Naldecon DX Children's Syrup ... ⊡ 522
- Naldecon DX Pediatric Drops ... ⊡ 522
- Naldecon EX Children's Syrup ... ⊡ 522
- Naldecon EX Pediatric Drops ... ⊡ 523
- Naldecon Syrup, Tablets, Pediatric Drops and Pediatric Syrup ... 709
- Nolamine Tablets ... 838
- Nolex LA Tablets ... 838
- Ornade Spansule Capsules ... 2221
- Orthoxicol Cough Syrup ... ⊡ 668
- Propagest ... 839
- Pyrroxate Capsules ... ⊡ 669
- Robitussin-CF ... ⊡ 676
- Ru-Tuss II Capsules ... 693
- Ru-Tuss with Hydrocodone ... 694
- Ru-Tuss Tablets ... 693
- Sine-Off Sinus Medicine Tablets-Aspirin Formula ... ⊡ 722
- Sinulin ... 840

St. Joseph Cold Tablets for Children ▣ 704
Tavist-D Tablets 2035
Triaminic Allergy Tablets ▣ 688
Triaminic Chewables ▣ 688
Triaminic Cold Tablets ▣ 688
Triaminic Expectorant ▣ 688
Triaminic Expectorant w/Codeine 1996
Triaminic Expectorant DH 1995
Triaminic Oral Infant Drops 1996
Triaminic Syrup ▣ 689
Triaminic-12 Tablets ▣ 690
Triaminic-DM Syrup ▣ 689
Triaminicin Tablets ▣ 690
Triaminicol Multi-Symptom Cold Tablets ▣ 691
Triaminicol Multi-Symptom Relief ▣ 691
Tuss-Ornade Liquid 2242
Tuss-Ornade Spansule Capsules 2242
Tylenol Cold Medication, Effervescent Tablets 1369

Pilocarpine (Effects of antiglaucoma agents antagonized). Products include:
Ocusert Pilo-20 and Pilo-40 Ocular Therapeutic Systems ⊙ 256

Pilocarpine Hydrochloride (Effects of antiglaucoma agents antagonized). Products include:
Akarpine Ophthalmic Solution ⊙ 201
Isopto Carpine ⊙ 219
Pilocar ⊙ 275
Pilopine HS Gel ⊙ 227
Pilostat Sterile Ophthalmic Solution 0.5%, 1%, 2%, 3%, 4%, 5%, 6% ⊙ 263

Pirbuterol Acetate (Increases certain actions or side effects). Products include:
Maxair Inhaler 1311

Prazepam (Increases certain actions or side effects). Products include:
Centrax 1693

Prednisolone Acetate (Concurrent use in the presence of increased intraocular pressure may be hazardous). Products include:
AK-Cide Sterile Ophthalmic Ointment & Suspension ⊙ 202
Blephamide Liquifilm Sterile Ophthalmic Suspension 586
Blephamide S.O.P. Sterile Ophthalmic Ointment 586
Cetapred Ointment ⊙ 220
⅛% Econopred & 1% Econopred Plus ⊙ 217
Isopto Cetapred Suspension ⊙ 220
Metimyd ⊙ 306
Poly-Pred Liquifilm ⊙ 250
Pred Forte ⊙ 252
Pred Mild ⊙ 254
Pred-G Liquifilm Sterile Ophthalmic Suspension ⊙ 252
Pred-G S.O.P. Sterile Ophthalmic Ointment ⊙ 253
Vasocidin Ointment ⊙ 275

Prednisolone Sodium Phosphate (Concurrent use in the presence of increased intraocular pressure may be hazardous). Products include:
AK-Pred ⊙ 205
Hydeltrasol Injection, Sterile 1476
Inflamase ⊙ 274
Pediapred Oral Liquid 987
Vasocidin Ophthalmic Solution ⊙ 276

Prednisolone Tebutate (Concurrent use in the presence of increased intraocular pressure may be hazardous). Products include:
Hydeltra-T.B.A. Sterile Suspension 1478

Prednisone (Concurrent use in the presence of increased intraocular pressure may be hazardous). Products include:
Deltasone Tablets 2332

Procainamide Hydrochloride (Increases certain actions or side effects). Products include:
Procan SR Tablets 1760
Pronestyl Capsules and Tablets 1800
Pronestyl Injection 1798
Pronestyl-SR Tablets 1801

Prochlorperazine (Increases certain actions or side effects). Products include:
Compazine 2201

Procyclidine Hydrochloride (Increases certain actions or side effects). Products include:
Kemadrin Tablets 771

Promethazine Hydrochloride (Increases certain actions or side effects). Products include:
Mepergan Injection 2479
Phenergan with Codeine 2497
Phenergan with Dextromethorphan 2499
Phenergan Injection 2493
Phenergan Suppositories 2496
Phenergan Syrup 2495
Phenergan Tablets 2496
Phenergan VC 2500
Phenergan VC with Codeine 2501

Propafenone Hydrochloride (Increases certain actions or side effects). Products include:
Rythmol Tablets 1184

Propantheline Bromide (Increases certain actions or side effects). Products include:
Pro-Banthīne Tablets 2141

Propoxyphene Hydrochloride (Increases certain actions or side effects). Products include:
Darvon 1256
Wygesic Tablets 2540

Propoxyphene Napsylate (Increases certain actions or side effects). Products include:
Darvon-N/Darvocet-N 1254

Protriptyline Hydrochloride (Increases certain actions or side effects). Products include:
Vivactil Tablets 1567

Pseudoephedrine Hydrochloride (Increases certain actions or side effects). Products include:
Actifed Capsules ▣ 539
Actifed Plus Caplets ▣ 539
Actifed Plus Tablets ▣ 540
Actifed with Codeine Cough Syrup 752
Actifed Syrup ▣ 540
Actifed Tablets ▣ 540
Actifed 12-Hour Capsules ▣ 539
Advil Cold & Sinus Caplets (formerly CoAdvil) 2416
Allerest ▣ 559
Anatuss LA Tablets 1359
Benadryl Decongestant Elixir ▣ 635
Benadryl Decongestant ▣ 635
Benadryl Plus ▣ 636
Benadryl Plus Nighttime ▣ 637
Benylin Decongestant ▣ 638
Brexin L.A. Capsules 2078
Bromfed Capsules (Timed Release) 1615
Bromfed Syrup ▣ 628
Bromfed 1615
CoAdvil ▣ 748
Allergy-Sinus Comtrex Multi-Symptom Allergy Sinus Formula Tablets & Caplets 746
Cough Formula Comtrex 746
Comtrex Multi-Symptom Cold Reliever Tablets/Caplets/Liqui-Gels/Liquid 745
Day-Night Comtrex 747
Non-Drowsy Comtrex 747
Congess 994
Congestac Caplets ▣ 617
Contac Jr. Children's Cold Medicine ▣ 712
Contac Nighttime Cold Medicine ▣ 713
Contac Sinus Caplets Maximum Strength Non-Drowsy Formula ▣ 710
Contac Sinus Tablets Maximum Strength Non-Drowsy Formula ▣ 710
Deconamine 663
Deconsal II Tablets 559
Dimacol Caplets ▣ 672
Dimetane-DX Cough Syrup 1858
Dorcol Children's Cough Syrup ▣ 685
Dorcol Children's Decongestant Liquid ▣ 685
Dorcol Children's Liquid Cold Formula ▣ 686
Maximum Strength Dristan Decongestant/Analgesic Coated Caplets ▣ 750
No Drowsiness Dristan Cold Nasal Decongestant/Analgesic Coated Caplets 2420
Dristan Sinus Caplets 2419
Sinus Excedrin Analgesic, Decongestant Tablets & Caplets ▣ 533
Fedahist Gyrocaps 2145
Fedahist Timecaps 2145
Guaifed 1615
Guaifed Syrup ▣ 629
Isoclor Expectorant 982
Isoclor Timesule Capsules ▣ 561
Kronofed-A 970
Medi-Flu Caplet, Liquid ▣ 640
Novafed A Capsules 1342
Novafed Capsules 1342
Novahistine DH 1342
Novahistine DMX ▣ 595
Novahistine Expectorant 1343
Nucofed Capsules 2219
Nucofed Expectorant 2219
Nucofed Pediatric Expectorant 2220
Nucofed Syrup 2219
Ornex Caplets ▣ 618
PediaCare Allergy Relief Formula Liquid 1362
PediaCare Cough-Cold Formula Liquid 1362
PediaCare Infants' Oral Decongestant Drops 1362
PediaCare Night Rest Cough-Cold Formula Liquid 1362
PediaCare 6-12 Cough-Cold Formula Chewable Tablets 1362
Robitussin-DAC Syrup 1875
Robitussin-PE ▣ 677
Rondec 1975
Rondec-DM 1976
Rondec-TR Tablet 1975
Ru-Tuss DE Tablets 694
Ryna ▣ 741
Seldane-D Extended-Release Tablets 1350
Sinarest ▣ 562
Sine-Aid Maximum Strength Sinus Headache Caplets 1365
Sine-Aid Maximum Strength Sinus Headache Tablets 1365
Sine-Off Maximum Strength Allergy/Sinus Formula Caplets ▣ 721
Sine-Off Maximum Strength No Drowsiness Formula Caplets ▣ 722
Singlet Tablets ▣ 598
Sinutab Maximum Strength ▣ 641
Sinutab Maximum Strength Without Drowsiness Tablets & Caplets ▣ 642
Sinutab Regular Strength Without Drowsiness Formula ▣ 641
St. Joseph Nighttime Cold Medicine ▣ 705
Sudafed Children's Liquid ▣ 543
Sudafed Cough Syrup ▣ 543
Sudafed Plus Liquid ▣ 544
Sudafed Plus Tablets ▣ 545
Sudafed Sinus Caplets ▣ 545
Sudafed Sinus Tablets ▣ 545
Sudafed Tablets, 30 mg ▣ 544
Sudafed Tablets, Adult Strength, 60 mg ▣ 544
Sudafed 12 Hour Capsules ▣ 545
TheraFlu Flu and Cold Medicine ▣ 687
Triaminic Nite Light ▣ 689
Tylenol Allergy Sinus Medication Caplets and Gelcaps, Maximum Strength 1372
Children's Tylenol Cold Liquid Formula and Chewable Tablets 1368
Tylenol Cold & Flu Hot Medication, Packets 1369
Tylenol Cold & Flu No Drowsiness Hot Medication, Packets 1371
Tylenol Cold Medication Caplets and Tablets 1370
Tylenol Cold Medication No Drowsiness Formula Caplets 1370
Tylenol Cold Night Time Medication Liquid 1371
Tylenol Cough Medication Liquid with Decongestant, Maximum Strength 1372
Tylenol, Maximum Strength, Sinus Medication Gelcaps, Caplets and Tablets 1373
Ursinus Inlay-Tabs ▣ 691
Vicks Children's NyQuil ▣ 664
Vicks Daycare ▣ 660
Vicks Formula 44D Decongestant Cough Medicine ▣ 662
Vicks Formula 44M Multi-Symptom Cough Medicine ▣ 662
Vicks NyQuil Nighttime Colds Medicine-Original & Cherry Flavor ▣ 664
Vicks Pediatric Formula 44 Cough & Congestion Medicine ▣ 663
Vicks Pediatric Formula 44m Multi-Symptom Cough & Cold Medicine ▣ 663

Pseudoephedrine Sulfate (Increases certain actions or side effects). Products include:
Afrin Tablets ▣ 693
Chlor-Trimeton Decongestant ▣ 694
Disophrol Chronotab Sustained-Action Tablets ▣ 698
Drixoral Antihistamine/Nasal Decongestant Syrup ▣ 698
Drixoral Non-Drowsy Formula ▣ 699
Drixoral Plus Extended-Release Tablets ▣ 699
Drixoral Sinus ▣ 700
Drixoral Sustained-Action Tablets ▣ 698
Sinutab Allergy Formula Sustained Action Tablets ▣ 640
Trinalin Repetabs Tablets 1170

Pyrilamine Maleate (Increases certain actions or side effects). Products include:
Codimal 846
4-Way Fast Acting Nasal Spray - Original Formula (regular & mentholated) & Metered Spray Pump (regular) 751
Maximum Strength Midol Multi-Symptom Menstrual Formula ▣ 571
Maximum Strength Midol PMS Premenstrual Syndrome Formula ▣ 570
Regular Strength Midol Multi-Symptom Menstrual Formula ▣ 570
Prefrin-A ⊙ 255
Prēmsyn PMS Capsules & Caplets ▣ 547
Primatene Tablets-M Formula 2421
Robitussin Night Relief ▣ 677
Ru-Tuss with Hydrocodone 694
Triaminic Expectorant DH 1995
Triaminic Oral Infant Drops 1996

Pyrilamine Tannate (Increases certain actions or side effects). Products include:
Rynatan 2387

Quazepam (Increases certain actions or side effects). Products include:
Doral Tablets 2383

Quinidine Gluconate (Increases certain actions or side effects). Products include:
Quinaglute Dura-Tabs Tablets 663

Quinidine Polygalacturonate (Increases certain actions or side effects). Products include:
Cardioquin Tablets 1812

Quinidine Sulfate (Increases certain actions or side effects). Products include:
Quinidex Extentabs 1868

Scopolamine Hydrobromide (Increases certain actions or side effects). Products include:
Donnagel ▣ 675
Donnagel-PG 1858
Donnatal 1858
Donnatal Extentabs 1859
Donnatal Tablets 1858
Donnazyme Tablets 1860
Isopto Hyoscine ⊙ 222
Murocoll-2 Sterile Ophthalmic Solution ⊙ 261
Ru-Tuss Tablets 693

Scopolamine Preparations (Increases certain actions or side effects). Products include:
Transderm Scōp Transdermal Therapeutic System 887

Selegiline Hydrochloride (Increases certain actions or side effects). Products include:
Eldepryl 2250

Sodium Bicarbonate (Interferes with the absorption). Products include:

- Alka-Seltzer Advanced Formula Antacid & Non-Aspirin Pain Reliever ▣ 620
- Alka-Seltzer Effervescent Antacid ▣ 622
- Alka-Seltzer Effervescent Antacid and Pain Reliever 1568
- Alka-Seltzer Extra Strength Effervescent Antacid and Pain Reliever ▣ 623
- Alka-Seltzer (Flavored) Effervescent Antacid and Pain Reliever ▣ 621
- Arm & Hammer Pure Baking Soda ▣ 548
- Ceo-Two Rectal Suppositories 671
- Citrocarbonate Antacid ▣ 668
- Massengill Liquid Concentrate 2191
- NuLYTELY 699

Sufentanil Citrate (Increases certain actions or side effects). Products include:

- Sufenta Injection 1147

Terbutaline Sulfate (Increases certain actions or side effects). Products include:

- Brethaire Inhaler 1024
- Brethine Ampuls 1026
- Brethine Tablets 1026
- Bricanyl Injection 1324
- Bricanyl Tablets 1325

Terfenadine (Increases certain actions or side effects). Products include:

- Seldane Tablets 1349
- Seldane-D Extended-Release Tablets 1350

Thioridazine Hydrochloride (Increases certain actions or side effects). Products include:

- Mellaril 2011

Timolol Maleate (Effects of anti-glaucoma agents antagonized). Products include:

- Blocadren Tablets 1429
- Timolide Tablets 1547
- Timoptic in Ocudose 1552
- Timoptic Sterile Ophthalmic Solution 1550

Tranylcypromine Sulfate (Increases certain actions or side effects). Products include:

- Parnate Tablets 2222

Triamcinolone (Concurrent use in the presence of increased intraocular pressure may be hazardous).

- No products indexed under this heading.

Triamcinolone Acetonide (Concurrent use in the presence of increased intraocular pressure may be hazardous). Products include:

- Aristocort A 1010
- Azmacort Inhaler 1837
- Kenalog Cream, Lotion & Ointment 2401
- Kenalog-10 Injection 2402
- Kenalog-40 Injection 2403
- Kenalog in Orabase 604
- Kenalog Spray 2401
- Mycolog II Cream and Ointment 2407
- Mytrex Cream & Ointment 2080
- Nasacort Nasal Inhaler 1844

Triamcinolone Diacetate (Concurrent use in the presence of increased intraocular pressure may be hazardous). Products include:

- Aristocort Suspension 1008

Triamcinolone Hexacetonide (Concurrent use in the presence of increased intraocular pressure may be hazardous). Products include:

- Aristospan Suspension 1011

Tridihexethyl Chloride (Increases certain actions or side effects).

- No products indexed under this heading.

Trifluoperazine Hydrochloride (Increases certain actions or side effects). Products include:

- Stelazine 2226

Trihexyphenidyl Hydrochloride (Increases certain actions or side effects). Products include:

- Artane 1195

Trimeprazine Tartrate (Increases certain actions or side effects). Products include:

- Temaril Tablets, Syrup and Spansule Sustained Release Capsules 1085

Trimipramine Maleate (Increases certain actions or side effects). Products include:

- Surmontil Capsules 2524

Tripelennamine Hydrochloride (Increases certain actions or side effects). Products include:

- PBZ Tablets & Elixir 1037
- PBZ-SR Tablets 1037

Triprolidine Hydrochloride (Increases certain actions or side effects). Products include:

- Actidil ▣ 538
- Actifed Capsules ▣ 539
- Actifed Plus Caplets ▣ 539
- Actifed Plus Tablets ▣ 540
- Actifed with Codeine Cough Syrup 752
- Actifed Syrup ▣ 540
- Actifed Tablets ▣ 540
- Actifed 12-Hour Capsules ▣ 539

CAPASTAT SULFATE VIALS

(Capreomycin Sulfate) 1250

May interact with antituberculosis drugs, aminoglycosides, and certain other agents. Compounds in these categories include:

Amikacin Sulfate (Additive ototoxicity and/or nephrotoxicity). Products include:

- Amikin Injectable 602

Colistin Sulfate (Additive ototoxicity and/or nephrotoxicity). Products include:

- Coly-Mycin S For Oral Suspension 1708
- Coly-Mycin S Otic w/Neomycin & Hydrocortisone 1708

Cycloserine (Potential for febrile reactions and abnormal liver function tests). Products include:

- Seromycin Pulvules 1298

Ethambutol Hydrochloride (Potential for febrile reactions and abnormal liver function tests). Products include:

- Myambutol Tablets 1225

Ether (Neuromuscular block enhanced).

Gentamicin Sulfate (Additive ototoxicity and/or nephrotoxicity). Products include:

- Garamycin Injectable 2093
- Garamycin Ophthalmic ⊙ 305
- Genoptic Liquifilm Sterile Ophthalmic Solution ⊙ 247
- Genoptic S.O.P. Sterile Ophthalmic Ointment ⊙ 247
- Gentacidin Ointment ⊙ 273
- Gentacidin Solution ⊙ 273
- Gentak Ointment & Solution ⊙ 208
- G-myticin Creme and Ointment 0.1% 1770
- Pred-G Liquifilm Sterile Ophthalmic Suspension ⊙ 252
- Pred-G S.O.P. Sterile Ophthalmic Ointment ⊙ 253

Isoniazid (Potential for febrile reactions and abnormal liver function tests). Products include:

- INH Tablets 868
- Rifamate Capsules 1347

Kanamycin Sulfate (Additive ototoxicity and/or nephrotoxicity). Products include:

- Kantrex Injection 601
- Kantrex Pediatric Injection 601

Neomycin, oral (Additive ototoxicity and/or nephrotoxicity).

Paromomycin Sulfate (Additive ototoxicity and/or nephrotoxicity). Products include:

- Humatin Capsules 1726

Polymyxin B Sulfate (Additive ototoxicity and/or nephrotoxicity). Products include:

- AK-Poly-Bac Ointment ⊙ 205
- AK-Spore H.C. ⊙ 206
- AK-Spore ⊙ 205
- AK-Trol Ointment & Suspension ⊙ 207
- Aquaphor Antibiotic Formula 662
- Bactine First Aid Antibiotic Ointment ▣ 625
- Campho-Phenique Triple Antibiotic Ointment Plus Pain Reliever ▣ 758
- Cortisporin Cream 757
- Cortisporin Ointment 758
- Cortisporin Ophthalmic Ointment Sterile 758
- Cortisporin Ophthalmic Suspension Sterile 759
- Cortisporin Otic Solution Sterile 760
- Cortisporin Otic Suspension Sterile 760
- Dexacidin ⊙ 272
- Lanabiotic Ointment ▣ 556
- LazerSporin-C Solution 1770
- Maxitrol Ophthalmic Ointment/Suspension ⊙ 223
- Mycitracin ▣ 737
- Neosporin Cream 792
- Neosporin G.U. Irrigant Sterile 793
- Neosporin Ointment 793
- Maximum Strength Neosporin Ointment 793
- Neosporin Ophthalmic Ointment Sterile 793
- Neosporin Ophthalmic Solution Sterile 794
- Ophthocort ⊙ 301
- PediOtic Suspension Sterile 797
- Polymyxin B Sulfate, Aerosporin Brand Sterile Powder 798
- Poly-Pred Liquifilm ⊙ 250
- Polysporin Ointment ▣ 543
- Polysporin Ophthalmic Ointment Sterile 798
- Polysporin Powder ▣ 543
- Polysporin Spray ▣ 543
- Polytrim Ophthalmic Solution Sterile 588
- Terramycin with Polymyxin B Sulfate Ophthalmic Ointment 1965

Rifampin (Potential for febrile reactions and abnormal liver function tests). Products include:

- Rifadin 1345
- Rifamate Capsules 1347
- Rimactane Capsules 879

Streptomycin Sulfate (Additive ototoxicity and/or nephrotoxicity).

- No products indexed under this heading.

Tobramycin Sulfate (Additive ototoxicity and/or nephrotoxicity). Products include:

- Nebcin Vials, Hyporets & ADD-Vantage 1286

Vancomycin Hydrochloride (Additive ototoxicity and/or nephrotoxicity). Products include:

- Vancocin HCl, Oral Solution & Pulvules 1304
- Vancocin HCl, Vials & ADD-Vantage 1302

Viomycin (Additive ototoxicity and/or nephrotoxicity).

CAPITROL SHAMPOO

(Chloroxine) 2396

No interactions described in labeling.

CAPOTEN

(Captopril) 2255

May interact with diuretics, thiazides, ganglionic blocking agents, para-aminobenzoic acid based local anesthetics, potassium sparing diuretics, potassium-depleting corticosteroids, non-steroidal anti-inflammatory agents, beta blockers, nitrates and nitrites, agents causing renin release, inhibitors of endogenous prostaglandin synthesis, and certain other agents. Compounds in these categories include:

Acebutolol Hydrochloride (Less than additive antihypertensive effect). Products include:

- Sectral Capsules 2520

Amiloride Hydrochloride (Hypotension; increased serum potassium). Products include:

- Midamor Tablets 1508
- Moduretic Tablets 1510

Amyl Nitrite (Discontinue before starting captopril; if resumed administer at lower dosage).

- No products indexed under this heading.

Aspirin (Antihypertensive effects of captopril reduced). Products include:

- Alka-Seltzer Effervescent Antacid and Pain Reliever 1568
- Alka-Seltzer Extra Strength Effervescent Antacid and Pain Reliever 1570
- Alka-Seltzer (Flavored) Effervescent Antacid and Pain Reliever 1569
- Alka-Seltzer Plus Cold Medicine ▣ 623
- Alka-Seltzer Plus Night-Time Cold Medicine ▣ 623
- Alka Seltzer Plus Sinus Allergy Medicine ▣ 624
- Anacin Coated Analgesic Caplets 2417
- Anacin Coated Analgesic Tablets 2417
- Anacin Maximum Strength Analgesic Coated Tablets 2417
- Maximum Strength Arthritis Pain Formula By the Makers of Anacin Analgesic Tablets and Caplets 2418
- Arthritis Pain Formula by the Makers of Anacin Analgesic Tablets and Caplets ▣ 747
- Arthritis Strength BC Powder ▣ 516
- Ascriptin A/D Caplets 1850
- Regular Strength Ascriptin Tablets 1850
- Azdōne Tablets 844
- BC Powder ▣ 517
- BC Cold Powder ▣ 517
- Children's Bayer Chewable Aspirin ▣ 564
- Genuine Bayer Aspirin Tablets & Caplets ▣ 564
- Maximum Bayer Aspirin Tablets & Caplets ▣ 566
- Bayer Plus Aspirin Tablets ▣ 567
- Therapy Bayer Aspirin Caplets ▣ 568
- 8 Hour Bayer Timed-Release Aspirin ▣ 566
- Arthritis Strength Bufferin Analgesic Caplets 744
- Extra Strength Bufferin Analgesic Tablets 745
- Bufferin Analgesic Tablets and Caplets 743
- Cama Arthritis Pain Reliever ▣ 685
- Damason-P 1356
- Easprin 1719
- Ecotrin Enteric Coated Aspirin Maximum Strength Tablets and Caplets 2189
- Ecotrin Enteric Coated Aspirin Regular Strength Tablets and Caplets 2189
- Empirin Aspirin ▣ 541
- Empirin with Codeine Phosphate Nos. 2, 3 & 4 764
- Equagesic Tablets 2451
- Excedrin Extra-Strength Analgesic Tablets & Caplets 749
- 4-Way Cold Tablets 750
- Fiorinal Capsules 2007
- Fiorinal with Codeine Capsules 2008
- Fiorinal Tablets 2007
- Lortab ASA Tablets 2414
- Momentum Muscular Backache Formula ▣ 751
- Norgesic 1314
- Norwich Extra-Strength Aspirin ▣ 546
- Norwich Regular Strength Aspirin ▣ 547
- P-A-C Analgesic Tablets ▣ 669
- Percodan 951
- Robaxisal Tablets 1872
- Sine-Off Sinus Medicine Tablets-Aspirin Formula ▣ 722
- Soma Compound w/Codeine Tablets 2390
- Soma Compound Tablets 2389
- St. Joseph Adult Chewable Aspirin (81 mg.) ▣ 703
- Synalgos-DC Capsules 2525

Talwin Compound 2072
Ursinus Inlay-Tabs .... ▣ 691
Vanquish Analgesic Caplets .... ▣ 574
Zorprin Tablets 698

Atenolol (Less than additive antihypertensive effect). Products include:
Tenoretic Tablets 1105
Tenormin Tablets and I.V. Injection 1107

Bendroflumethiazide (Captopril's effect will be augmented). Products include:
Corzide Tablets 702
Naturetin Tablets 1789
Rauzide Tablets 1804

Betaxolol Hydrochloride (Less than additive antihypertensive effect). Products include:
Betoptic Sterile Ophthalmic Solution 569
Betoptic S Sterile Ophthalmic Suspension 570
Kerlone Tablets 2172

Bumetanide (Hypotension). Products include:
Bumex 1895

Carteolol Hydrochloride (Less than additive antihypertensive effect). Products include:
Cartrol Tablets 507

Chlorothiazide (Captopril's effect will be augmented). Products include:
Aldoclor Tablets 1413
Diupres Tablets 1461
Diuril Oral 1464

Chlorothiazide Sodium (Captopril's effect will be augmented). Products include:
Diuril Sodium Intravenous 1463

Chlorthalidone (Hypotension; increased serum potassium). Products include:
Combipres Tablets 678
Tenoretic Tablets 1105
Thalitone Tablets 687

Deserpidine (Use with caution). Products include:
Enduronyl 518
Harmonyl Tablets 528
Oreticyl 545

Diclofenac Sodium (Antihypertensive effects of captopril reduced). Products include:
Voltaren Ophthalmic Sterile Ophthalmic Solution .... ◉ 268
Voltaren Tablets 1042

Erythrityl Tetranitrate (Discontinue before starting captopril; if resumed administer at lower dosage). Products include:
Cardilate Oral/Sublingual Tablets .. 757

Esmolol Hydrochloride (Less than additive antihypertensive effect). Products include:
Brevibloc Injection 942

Ethacrynic Acid (Hypotension). Products include:
Edecrin Tablets 1468

Etodolac (Antihypertensive effects of captopril reduced). Products include:
Lodine Capsules 2468

Fenoprofen Calcium (Antihypertensive effects of captopril reduced). Products include:
Nalfon Pulvules & Tablets 919

Flurbiprofen (Antihypertensive effects of captopril reduced). Products include:
Ansaid Tablets 2319

Furosemide (Hypotension). Products include:
Lasix 1093

Guanethidine Monosulfate (Use with caution). Products include:
Esimil Tablets 864
Ismelin Tablets 869

Hydrochlorothiazide (Captopril's effect will be augmented). Products include:
Aldactazide 2150
Aldoril Tablets 1418
Apresazide Capsules 854
Apresoline-Esidrix Tablets 857
Capozide 2258
Dyazide Capsules 2208
Esidrix Tablets 863
Esimil Tablets 864
HydroDIURIL Tablets 1484
Hydropres Tablets 1485
Inderide Tablets 2463
Inderide LA Long Acting Capsules .. 2465
Lopressor HCT Tablets 1034
Maxzide 1215
Moduretic Tablets 1510
Normozide Tablets 2112
Oretic Tablets 544
Oreticyl 545
Prinzide Tablets 1540
Ser-Ap-Es Tablets 881
Serpasil-Esidrix Tablets 886
Timolide Tablets 1547
Trandate HCT Tablets 579
Vaseretic Tablets 1559
Zestoretic 2274

Hydroflumethiazide (Captopril's effect will be augmented). Products include:
Diucardin Tablets 2450
Saluron 718
Salutensin/Salutensin-Demi 719

Ibuprofen (Antihypertensive effects of captopril reduced). Products include:
Advil Cold & Sinus Caplets (formerly CoAdvil) 2416
Advil Ibuprofen Tablets and Caplets 2416
Children's Advil Suspension 2426
CoAdvil .... ▣ 748
Dristan Sinus Caplets 2419
Haltran Tablets .... ▣ 668
Ibuprofen .... ▣ 631
Medipren ibuprofen Caplets and Tablets 1362
Midol 200 Cramp Relief Formula .. ▣ 570
Motrin Tablets 2351
Motrin IB Caplets and Tablets .... ▣ 736
Nuprin Ibuprofen/Analgesic Tablets & Caplets 752
PediaProfen Suspension 1363
Rufen Tablets 691
Trendar Ibuprofen Tablets .... ▣ 756

Indapamide (Hypotension). Products include:
Lozol Tablets 1843

Indomethacin (Antihypertensive effects of captopril reduced). Products include:
Indocin 1487

Indomethacin Sodium Trihydrate (Antihypertensive effects of captopril reduced). Products include:
Indocin I.V. 1490

Isosorbide Dinitrate (Discontinue before starting captopril; if resumed administer at lower dosage). Products include:
Dilatrate-SR 1827
Isordil 2467
Sorbitrate 1103

Ketoprofen (Antihypertensive effects of captopril reduced). Products include:
Orudis Capsules 2488

Ketorolac Tromethamine (Antihypertensive effects of captopril reduced). Products include:
Toradol IM Injection 2302

Labetalol Hydrochloride (Less than additive antihypertensive effect). Products include:
Normodyne Injection 2108
Normodyne Tablets 2110
Normozide Tablets 2112
Trandate HCT Tablets 579
Trandate Injection 577
Trandate Tablets 579

Mecamylamine Hydrochloride (Use with caution). Products include:
Inversine Tablets 1492

Meclofenamate Sodium (Antihypertensive effects of captopril reduced). Products include:
Meclomen Capsules 1739

Mefenamic Acid (Antihypertensive effects of captopril reduced). Products include:
Ponstel 1758

Methyclothiazide (Captopril's effect will be augmented). Products include:
Enduron Tablets 517
Enduronyl 518

Metolazone (Hypotension). Products include:
Diulo 2129
Mykrox ½ mg Tablets 984
Zaroxolyn Tablets 989

Metoprolol Tartrate (Less than additive antihypertensive effect). Products include:
Lopressor Ampuls 1032
Lopressor HCT Tablets 1034
Lopressor Tablets 1032

Nadolol (Less than additive antihypertensive effect). Products include:
Corgard Tablets 701
Corzide Tablets 702

Naproxen (Antihypertensive effects of captopril reduced). Products include:
Naprosyn 2297

Naproxen Sodium (Antihypertensive effects of captopril reduced). Products include:
Anaprox and Anaprox DS Tablets 2288

Nitroglycerin (Discontinue before starting captopril; if resumed administer at lower dosage). Products include:
Deponit NTG Transdermal Delivery System 2143
Minitran Transdermal Delivery System 1312
Nitro-Bid Ointment 1339
Nitro-Bid Capsules 1338
Nitrodisc 2176
Nitro-Dur (nitroglycerin) Transdermal Infusion System 1164
Nitrogard Tablets 1004
Nitrolingual Spray 1846
Nitrostat Tablets 1743
Transderm-Nitro Transdermal Therapeutic System 2283

Penbutolol Sulfate (Less than additive antihypertensive effect). Products include:
Levatol 1832

Pentaerythritol Tetranitrate (Discontinue before starting captopril; if resumed administer at lower dosage). Products include:
Peritrate 1756

Phenylbutazone (Antihypertensive effects of captopril reduced). Products include:
Butazolidin Capsules & Tablets 1027

Pindolol (Less than additive antihypertensive effect). Products include:
Visken Tablets 2036

Piroxicam (Antihypertensive effects of captopril reduced). Products include:
Feldene Capsules 1777

Polythiazide (Captopril's effect will be augmented). Products include:
Minizide Capsules 1779
Renese Tablets 1785
Renese-R Tablets 1786

Potassium Acid Phosphate (Potential for significant increase in serum potassium). Products include:
K-Phos M.F. Tablets 659
K-Phos Original Formula 'Sodium Free' Tablets 660
K-Phos No. 2 Tablets 659

Potassium Bicarbonate (Potential for significant increase in serum potassium). Products include:
Alka-Seltzer Advanced Formula Antacid & Non-Aspirin Pain Reliever .... ▣ 620
Alka-Seltzer Effervescent Antacid ▣ 622
K-Lyte 707
Klorvess Effervescent Granules 2010
Klorvess Effervescent Tablets 2011

Potassium Chloride (Potential for significant increase in serum potassium). Products include:
Chlor-3 Condiment 994
K-Dur Microburst Release System (potassium chloride, USP) E.R. Tablets 1163
K-Lor Powder Packets 531
K-Lyte 707
K-Norm Capsules 982
K-Tab Filmtab 532
Kato Potassium Supplement 1114
Klor-Con 8/Klor-Con 10 Extended-release Tablets 2374
Klorvess Effervescent Granules 2010
Klorvess Effervescent Tablets 2011
Klorvess 10% Liquid 2010
Klotrix 708
Kolyum Liquid 983
Micro-K 1863
Micro-K LS Packets 1864
NuLYTELY 699
Oral Rehydration Salts, Citrate 1150
Rum-K Syrup 995
Slow-K Tablets 2281
Ten-K Controlled-Release Tablets 2282
Thermotabs .... ▣ 619

Potassium Citrate (Potential for significant increase in serum potassium). Products include:
Alka-Seltzer Effervescent Antacid .. 1570
K-Lyte 707
Polycitra Syrup 2424
Polycitra-K 2424
Polycitra-LC—Sugar-Free 2424
Ricelyte, Rice-Based Oral Electrolyte Maintenance Solution .... ▣ 613

Potassium Gluconate (Potential for significant increase in serum potassium). Products include:
Kolyum Liquid 983

Potassium Phosphate, Dibasic (Potential for significant increase in serum potassium). Products include:
Neutra-Phos 2423

Potassium Phosphate, Monobasic (Potential for significant increase in serum potassium). Products include:
K-Phos M.F. Tablets 659
K-Phos Neutral Tablets 660
Neutra-Phos 2423

Prazosin Hydrochloride (Use with caution). Products include:
Minipress Capsules 1778
Minizide Capsules 1779

Propranolol Hydrochloride (Less than additive antihypertensive effect). Products include:
Inderal 2459
Inderal LA Long Acting Capsules 2461
Inderide Tablets 2463
Inderide LA Long Acting Capsules .. 2465

Rauwolfia Serpentina (Use with caution). Products include:
Raudixin Tablets 1803
Rauzide Tablets 1804

Rescinnamine (Use with caution).
No products indexed under this heading.

Reserpine (Use with caution). Products include:
Diupres Tablets 1461
Hydromox R Tablets 1209
Hydropres Tablets 1485
Renese-R Tablets 1786
Salutensin/Salutensin-Demi 719
Ser-Ap-Es Tablets 881
Serpasil Tablets 883
Serpasil-Apresoline Tablets 884
Serpasil-Esidrix Tablets 886

Spironolactone (Hypotension; increased serum potassium). Products include:
- Aldactazide 2150
- Aldactone 2152

Sulindac (Antihypertensive effects of captopril reduced). Products include:
- Clinoril Tablets 1433

Terazosin Hydrochloride (Use with caution). Products include:
- Hytrin Tablets 529

Timolol Maleate (Less than additive antihypertensive effect). Products include:
- Blocadren Tablets 1429
- Timolide Tablets 1547
- Timoptic in Ocudose 1552
- Timoptic Sterile Ophthalmic Solution 1550

Tolmetin Sodium (Antihypertensive effects of captopril reduced). Products include:
- Tolectin (200, 400 and 600 mg) .. 1379

Triamterene (Hypotension; increased serum potassium). Products include:
- Dyazide Capsules 2208
- Dyrenium Capsules 2210
- Maxzide 1215

Trimethaphan Camsylate (Use with caution). Products include:
- Arfonad Ampuls 1887

Food Interactions

Food, unspecified (Reduces absorption by about 30 to 40 percent).

CAPOZIDE

(Captopril, Hydrochlorothiazide) **2258**

May interact with diuretics, thiazides, ganglionic blocking agents, para-aminobenzoic acid based local anesthetics, lithium preparations, potassium sparing diuretics, potassium-depleting corticosteroids, oral anticoagulants, calcium preparations, cardiac glycosides, non-steroidal anti-inflammatory agents, barbiturates, agents causing renin release, inhibitors of endogenous prostaglandin synthesis, narcotic analgesics, antihypertensives, corticosteroids, preanesthetic medications, general anesthetics, non-depolarizing neuromuscular blocking agents, oral hypoglycemic agents, insulin, monoamine oxidase inhibitors, and certain other agents. Compounds in these categories include:

Acebutolol Hydrochloride (Additive effect). Products include:
- Sectral Capsules 2520

ACTH (Intensified electrolyte depletion, particularly hypokalemia).
- No products indexed under this heading.

Alcohol (Potentation of orthostatic hypotension).

Alfentanil Hydrochloride (Potentiation of orthostatic hypotension). Products include:
- Alfenta Injection 1131

Amiloride Hydrochloride (Precipitous reduction of blood pressure; elevated serum potassium; additive effect). Products include:
- Midamor Tablets 1508
- Moduretic Tablets 1510

Amphotericin B (Intensified electrolyte depletion, particularly hypokalemia). Products include:
- Fungizone Cream, Lotion and Ointment 2261
- Fungizone Intravenous 2262

Aprobarbital (Potentiation of orthostatic hypotension). Products include:
- Alurate Elixir 1883

Aspirin (May reduce the antihypertensive effect of captopril). Products include:
- Alka-Seltzer Effervescent Antacid and Pain Reliever 1568
- Alka-Seltzer Extra Strength Effervescent Antacid and Pain Reliever 1570
- Alka-Seltzer (Flavored) Effervescent Antacid and Pain Reliever 1569
- Alka-Seltzer Plus Cold Medicine .... ⊞ 623
- Alka-Seltzer Plus Night-Time Cold Medicine .... ⊞ 623
- Alka Seltzer Plus Sinus Allergy Medicine .... ⊞ 624
- Anacin Coated Analgesic Caplets 2417
- Anacin Coated Analgesic Tablets 2417
- Anacin Maximum Strength Analgesic Coated Tablets 2417
- Maximum Strength Arthritis Pain Formula By the Makers of Anacin Analgesic Tablets and Caplets 2418
- Arthritis Pain Formula by the Makers of Anacin Analgesic Tablets and Caplets .... ⊞ 747
- Arthritis Strength BC Powder .... ⊞ 516
- Ascriptin A/D Caplets 1850
- Regular Strength Ascriptin Tablets 1850
- Azdōne Tablets 844
- BC Powder .... ⊞ 517
- BC Cold Powder .... ⊞ 517
- Children's Bayer Chewable Aspirin .... ⊞ 564
- Genuine Bayer Aspirin Tablets & Caplets .... ⊞ 564
- Maximum Bayer Aspirin Tablets & Caplets .... ⊞ 566
- Bayer Plus Aspirin Tablets .... ⊞ 567
- Therapy Bayer Aspirin Caplets .... ⊞ 568
- 8 Hour Bayer Timed-Release Aspirin .... ⊞ 566
- Arthritis Strength Bufferin Analgesic Caplets 744
- Extra Strength Bufferin Analgesic Tablets 745
- Bufferin Analgesic Tablets and Caplets 743
- Cama Arthritis Pain Reliever .... ⊞ 685
- Damason-P 1356
- Easprin 1719
- Ecotrin Enteric Coated Aspirin Maximum Strength Tablets and Caplets 2189
- Ecotrin Enteric Coated Aspirin Regular Strength Tablets and Caplets 2189
- Empirin Aspirin .... ⊞ 541
- Empirin with Codeine Phosphate Nos. 2, 3 & 4 764
- Equagesic Tablets 2451
- Excedrin Extra-Strength Analgesic Tablets & Caplets 749
- 4-Way Cold Tablets 750
- Fiorinal Capsules 2007
- Fiorinal with Codeine Capsules 2008
- Fiorinal Tablets 2007
- Lortab ASA Tablets 2414
- Momentum Muscular Backache Formula .... ⊞ 751
- Norgesic 1314
- Norwich Extra-Strength Aspirin ..... ⊞ 546
- Norwich Regular Strength Aspirin ⊞ 547
- P-A-C Analgesic Tablets .... ⊞ 669
- Percodan 951
- Robaxisal Tablets 1872
- Sine-Off Sinus Medicine Tablets-Aspirin Formula .... ⊞ 722
- Soma Compound w/Codeine Tablets 2390
- Soma Compound Tablets 2389
- St. Joseph Adult Chewable Aspirin (81 mg.) .... ⊞ 703
- Synalgos-DC Capsules 2525
- Talwin Compound 2072
- Ursinus Inlay-Tabs .... ⊞ 691
- Vanquish Analgesic Caplets .... ⊞ 574
- Zorprin Tablets 698

Atenolol (Additive effect). Products include:
- Tenoretic Tablets 1105
- Tenormin Tablets and I.V. Injection 1107

Atracurium Besylate (Increased response to relaxant). Products include:
- Tracrium Injection 817

Benazepril Hydrochloride (Additive effect; precipitous reduction of blood pressure; elevated serum potassium). Products include:
- Lotensin Tablets 872

Bendroflumethiazide (Precipitous reduction of blood pressure; captopril's effect will be augmented). Products include:
- Corzide Tablets 702
- Naturetin Tablets 1789
- Rauzide Tablets 1804

Betamethasone Acetate (Intensified electrolyte depletion, particularly hypokalemia). Products include:
- Celestone Soluspan Suspension 2081

Betamethasone Sodium Phosphate (Intensified electrolyte depletion, particularly hypokalemia). Products include:
- Celestone Soluspan Suspension 2081

Betaxolol Hydrochloride (Additive effect; precipitous reduction of blood pressure; elevated serum potassium). Products include:
- Betoptic Sterile Ophthalmic Solution 569
- Betoptic S Sterile Ophthalmic Suspension 570
- Kerlone Tablets 2172

Bumetanide (Precipitous reduction of blood pressure). Products include:
- Bumex 1895

Buprenorphine (Potentiation of orthostatic hypotension).
- No products indexed under this heading.

Butabarbital (Potentiation of orthostatic hypotension). Products include:
- Pyridium Plus 1764

Butalbital (Potentiation of orthostatic hypotension). Products include:
- Esgic-Plus Tablets 1002
- Esgic Tablets & Capsules 1001
- Fioricet Tablets 2006
- Fiorinal Capsules 2007
- Fiorinal with Codeine Capsules 2008
- Fiorinal Tablets 2007
- Phrenilin 838
- Sedapap Tablets 50 mg/650 mg .. 1360

Calcium Carbonate (Potential for hypercalcemia). Products include:
- Alka-Mints Chewable Antacid .... ⊞ 620
- Alka-Seltzer Advanced Formula Antacid & Non-Aspirin Pain Reliever .... ⊞ 620
- Ascriptin A/D Caplets 1850
- Regular Strength Ascriptin Tablets 1850
- Balmex Baby Powder .... ⊞ 590
- Bayer Plus Aspirin Tablets .... ⊞ 567
- Biocal 500 mg Tablet Calcium Supplement .... ⊞ 625
- Bufferin Analgesic Tablets and Caplets .... ⊞ 524
- Caltrate 600 .... ⊞ 583
- Caltrate 600 + Iron .... ⊞ 583
- Caltrate 600 + Vitamin D .... ⊞ 584
- Caltrate, Jr. .... ⊞ 583
- Centrum, Jr. (Children's Chewable) + Extra Calcium .... ⊞ 585
- Di-Gel Antacid/Anti-Gas .... ⊞ 697
- Gerimed Tablets 972
- Marblen .... ⊞ 563
- Natalins Rx 1391
- Natalins Tablets 1391
- Nephro-Calci Tablets 1826
- Os-Cal 500 Chewable Tablets .... ⊞ 596
- Os-Cal 500 Tablets .... ⊞ 597
- Os-Cal 250+D Tablets .... ⊞ 597
- Os-Cal 500+D Tablets .... ⊞ 597
- Pramet FA 1974
- Pramilet FA 1974
- Rolaids (Calcium Rich/Sodium Free) .... ⊞ 744
- Extra Strength Rolaids .... ⊞ 744
- Thermotabs .... ⊞ 619
- Total Formula-2 (multivitamin/multimineral) 2377
- Tums Liquid Extra .... ⊞ 726
- Zenate Tablets 2250

Calcium Chloride (Potential for hypercalcemia).
- No products indexed under this heading.

Calcium Citrate (Potential for hypercalcemia). Products include:
- Citracal Liquitab 1613
- Total Formula-2 (multivitamin/multimineral) 2377

Calcium Glubionate (Potential for hypercalcemia). Products include:
- Neo-Calglucon Syrup 2018

Carteolol Hydrochloride (Additive effect). Products include:
- Cartrol Tablets 507

Chlorothiazide (Precipitous reduction of blood pressure; captopril's effect will be augmented). Products include:
- Aldoclor Tablets 1413
- Diupres Tablets 1461
- Diuril Oral 1464

Chlorothiazide Sodium (Precipitous reduction of blood pressure; captopril's effect will be augmented). Products include:
- Diuril Sodium Intravenous 1463

Chlorpropamide (Thiazide-induced hyperglycemia may require dosage adjustment of antidiabetic drugs). Products include:
- Diabinese Tablets 1775

Chlorthalidone (Additive effect; precipitous reduction of blood pressure; elevated serum potassium). Products include:
- Combipres Tablets 678
- Tenoretic Tablets 1105
- Thalitone Tablets 687

Cholestyramine (Delays or decreases absorption of hydrochlorothiazide). Products include:
- Cholybar 1705
- Questran Light 711
- Questran Powder 710

Clonidine (Additive effect). Products include:
- Catapres-TTS 677

Clonidine Hydrochloride (Additive effect). Products include:
- Catapres Tablets 676
- Combipres Tablets 678

Codeine (Potentiation of orthostatic hypotension). Products include:
- Calcidrine Syrup 506

Codeine Phosphate (Potentiation of orthostatic hypotension). Products include:
- Actifed with Codeine Cough Syrup .. 752
- Cheracol Cough Syrup 1853
- Codimal PH Syrup 846
- Dimetane-DC Cough Syrup 1857
- Empirin with Codeine Phosphate Nos. 2, 3 & 4 764
- Fiorinal with Codeine Capsules 2008
- Isoclor Expectorant 982
- Naldecon CX Adult Liquid .... ⊞ 521
- Novahistine DH 1342
- Novahistine Expectorant 1343
- Nucofed Capsules 2219
- Nucofed Expectorant 2219
- Nucofed Pediatric Expectorant 2220
- Nucofed Syrup 2219
- Phenaphen with Codeine Capsules 1865
- Phenaphen-650 with Codeine Tablets 1866
- Phenergan with Codeine 2497
- Phenergan VC with Codeine 2501
- Robitussin A-C Syrup 1875
- Robitussin-DAC Syrup 1875
- Ryna .... ⊞ 741
- Soma Compound w/Codeine Tablets 2390
- Triaminic Expectorant w/Codeine .. 1996
- Tussi-Organidin Liquid 2391
- Tylenol with Codeine 1381

Codeine Polistirex (Potentiation of orthostatic hypotension).
- No products indexed under this heading.

Colestipol Hydrochloride (Delays or decreases absorption of hydrochlorothiazide). Products include:
- Colestid Granules ... 2328

Cortisone Acetate (Intensified electrolyte depletion, particularly hypokalemia). Products include:
- Cortone Acetate Sterile Suspension ... 1437
- Cortone Acetate Tablets ... 1439

Deserpidine (Additive effect or potentiation; use with caution). Products include:
- Enduronyl ... 518
- Harmonyl Tablets ... 528
- Oreticyl ... 545

Deslanoside (Enhanced possibility of digitalis toxicity).
- No products indexed under this heading.

Dexamethasone Acetate (Intensified electrolyte depletion, particularly hypokalemia). Products include:
- Dalalone D.P. Injectable ... 999
- Decadron-LA Sterile Suspension ... 1457

Dexamethasone Sodium Phosphate (Intensified electrolyte depletion, particularly hypokalemia). Products include:
- AK-Dex ... ⊙ 203
- Decadron Phosphate Respihaler ... 1454
- Decadron Phosphate Sterile Ophthalmic Ointment ... 1453
- Decadron Phosphate Sterile Ophthalmic Solution ... 1453
- Decadron Phosphate Topical Cream ... 1455
- Decadron Phosphate Turbinaire ... 1456
- Maxidex Sterile Ophthalmic Ointment ... ⊙ 222
- NeoDecadron Sterile Ophthalmic Ointment ... 1517
- NeoDecadron Sterile Ophthalmic Solution ... 1518
- NeoDecadron Topical Cream ... 1518

Dezocine (Potentiation of orthostatic hypotension).

Diazepam (Potentiated). Products include:
- Valium Injectable ... 1937
- Valium Tablets ... 1939
- Valrelease Capsules ... 1923

Diazoxide (Enhanced hyperglycemic, hyperuricemic, and antihypertensive effect). Products include:
- Hyperstat I.V. Injection ... 2095
- Proglycem ... 649

Diclofenac Sodium (Antihypertensive effect of captopril may be reduced; reduces diuretic and natriuretic effects). Products include:
- Voltaren Ophthalmic Sterile Ophthalmic Solution ... ⊙ 268
- Voltaren Tablets ... 1042

Dicumarol (Decreased anticoagulant effect). Products include:
- Dicumarol Tablets ... 516

Digitoxin (Enhanced possibility of digitalis toxicity). Products include:
- Crystodigin Tablets ... 1253

Digoxin (Enhanced possibility of digitalis toxicity). Products include:
- Lanoxicaps ... 772
- Lanoxin Elixir Pediatric ... 775
- Lanoxin Injection ... 778
- Lanoxin Injection Pediatric ... 781
- Lanoxin Tablets ... 783

Dopamine Hydrochloride (Decreased response to pressor amines). Products include:
- Intropin Injection ... 930

Doxazosin Mesylate (Additive effect; precipitous reduction of blood pressure; elevated serum potassium). Products include:
- Cardura Tablets ... 1941

Droperidol (Potentiated). Products include:
- Inapsine Injection ... 1140
- Innovar Injection ... 1141

Enalapril Maleate (Additive effect). Products include:
- Vaseretic Tablets ... 1559
- Vasotec Tablets ... 1564

Enalaprilat (Additive effect). Products include:
- Vasotec I.V. ... 1562

Enflurane (Potentiated). Products include:
- Ethrane ... 599

Epinephrine Hydrochloride (Decreased response to pressor amines). Products include:
- Adrenalin Chloride Solution 1:100 & 1:1,000 ... 1689
- Epifrin ... ⊙ 244
- Glaucon ... ⊙ 218

Erythrityl Tetranitrate (Discontinue before starting captopril; if resumed administer at lower dosage). Products include:
- Cardilate Oral/Sublingual Tablets ... 757

Esmolol Hydrochloride (Additive effect). Products include:
- Brevibloc Injection ... 942

Ethacrynic Acid (Precipitous reduction of blood pressure; additive effect). Products include:
- Edecrin Tablets ... 1468

Etodolac (Antihypertensive effect of captopril may be reduced; reduces diuretic and natriuretic effects). Products include:
- Lodine Capsules ... 2468

Felodipine (Additive effect; precipitous reduction of blood pressure; elevated serum potassium). Products include:
- Plendil Extended-Release Tablets ... 1526

Fenoprofen Calcium (Antihypertensive effect of captopril may be reduced; reduces diuretic and natriuretic effects). Products include:
- Nalfon Pulvules & Tablets ... 919

Fentanyl (Potentiation of orthostatic hypotension). Products include:
- Duragesic Transdermal System ... 1133

Fentanyl Citrate (Potentiated; potentiation of orthostatic hypotension). Products include:
- Innovar Injection ... 1141
- Sublimaze Injection ... 1146

Flurbiprofen (Antihypertensive effect of captopril may be reduced; reduces diuretic and natriuretic effects). Products include:
- Ansaid Tablets ... 2319

Fosinopril Sodium (Additive effect; precipitous reduction of blood pressure; elevated serum potassium). Products include:
- Monopril Tablets ... 1406

Furazolidone (Enhanced hypotensive effect). Products include:
- Furoxone ... 1855

Furosemide (Precipitous reduction of blood pressure; additive effect). Products include:
- Lasix ... 1093

Glipizide (Thiazide-induced hyperglycemia may require dosage adjustment of antidiabetic drugs). Products include:
- Glucotrol ... 1952

Glyburide (Thiazide-induced hyperglycemia may require dosage adjustment of antidiabetic drugs). Products include:
- DiaBeta ... 1091
- Micronase Tablets ... 2350

Guanabenz Acetate (Additive effect). Products include:
- Wytensin Tablets ... 2542

Guanethidine Monosulfate (Additive effect or potentiation; use with caution). Products include:
- Esimil Tablets ... 864
- Ismelin Tablets ... 869

Hydralazine Hydrochloride (Additive effect). Products include:
- Apresazide Capsules ... 854
- Apresoline Hydrochloride Parenteral (Ampuls) ... 856
- Apresoline Hydrochloride Tablets ... 855
- Apresoline-Esidrix Tablets ... 857
- Ser-Ap-Es Tablets ... 881
- Serpasil-Apresoline Tablets ... 884

Hydrocodone Bitartrate (Potentiation of orthostatic hypotension). Products include:
- Anexsia 5/500 Tablets ... 2196
- Anexsia 7.5/650 Tablets ... 2197
- Azdone Tablets ... 844
- Codiclear DH Syrup ... 845
- Codimal DH Syrup ... 846
- Damason-P ... 1356
- Hycodan Syrup, Tablets ... 927
- Hycomine Compound Tablets ... 929
- Hycomine Syrup ... 927
- Hycotuss Expectorant Syrup ... 930
- Hydrocet Capsules ... 835
- Lortab ASA Tablets ... 2414
- Lortab ... 2412
- Ru-Tuss with Hydrocodone ... 694
- Triaminic Expectorant DH ... 1995
- Vicodin Tablets ... 1187
- Vicodin ES Tablets ... 1189
- Zydone Capsules ... 941

Hydrocodone Polistirex (Potentiation of orthostatic hypotension). Products include:
- Tussionex Extended-Release Suspension ... 988

Hydrocortisone (Intensified electrolyte depletion, particularly hypokalemia). Products include:
- AK-Spore H.C. ... ⊙ 206
- Bactine Hydrocortisone Anti-Itch Cream ... ▣ 625
- CaldeCORT Anti-Itch Hydrocortisone Spray ... ▣ 560
- Carmol HC Cream 1% ... 2296
- Cortaid Spray ... ▣ 735
- Cortenema ... 2244
- Cortisporin Ointment ... 758
- Cortisporin Ophthalmic Ointment Sterile ... 758
- Cortisporin Ophthalmic Suspension Sterile ... 759
- Cortisporin Otic Solution Sterile ... 760
- Cortisporin Otic Suspension Sterile ... 760
- Cortizone-5 Creme & Ointment ... ▣ 732
- Dermolate Anti-Itch Cream ... ▣ 697
- Eldecort Cream 1.0% ... 1113
- Eldecort Cream 1.0% and 2.5% ... 1113
- Fungoid HC Creme ... 1770
- Hydrocortone Tablets ... 1482
- Hytone ... 909
- LazerSporin-C Solution ... 1770
- Massengill Medicated Soft Cloth Towelettes ... 2192
- Nutracort Cream & Lotion ... 1684
- PediOtic Suspension Sterile ... 797
- Synacort Creams 1%, 2.5% ... 2296
- Vanoxide-HC Acne Lotion ... 911
- Vioform-Hydrocortisone Cream and Mild Cream ... 889
- Vioform-Hydrocortisone Ointment ... 889
- VōSoL HC Otic Solution ... 2392
- Vytone Cream 1% ... 911

Hydrocortisone Acetate (Intensified electrolyte depletion, particularly hypokalemia). Products include:
- Analpram-HC Rectal Cream 1% and 2.5% ... 970
- Anusol-HC Cream ... 1690
- Anusol-HC Suppositories ... 1691
- Caldecort ... ▣ 560
- Carmol HC Cream 1% ... 2296
- Chloromycetin Hydrocortisone Ophthalmic ... 1694
- Coly-Mycin S Otic w/Neomycin & Hydrocortisone ... 1708
- Cortaid ... ▣ 735
- Cortef Feminine Itch Cream ... ▣ 735
- Corticaine ... ▣ 682
- Cortifoam ... 1827
- Cortisporin Cream ... 757
- Epifoam ... 1828
- Gynecort 5 Creme ... ▣ 556
- Hydrocortone Acetate Sterile Suspension ... 1479
- Lanacort 5 Creme and Ointment ... ▣ 557
- Mantadil Cream ... 789
- Ophthocort ... ⊙ 301
- Orabase HCA Oral Paste ... 890
- Pramosone Cream, Lotion & Ointment ... 971
- ProctoCream-HC ... 1834
- Proctofoam-HC ... 1835

Hydrocortisone Sodium Phosphate (Intensified electrolyte depletion, particularly hypokalemia). Products include:
- Hydrocortone Phosphate Injection, Sterile ... 1481

Hydrocortisone Sodium Succinate (Intensified electrolyte depletion, particularly hypokalemia). Products include:
- Solu-Cortef Sterile Powder ... 2361

Hydroflumethiazide (Precipitous reduction of blood pressure; captopril's effect will be augmented). Products include:
- Diucardin Tablets ... 2450
- Saluron ... 718
- Salutensin/Salutensin-Demi ... 719

Hydroxyzine Hydrochloride (Potentiated). Products include:
- Atarax Tablets & Syrup ... 1941
- Marax Tablets & DF Syrup ... 1954
- Vistaril Intramuscular Solution ... 1970

Ibuprofen (Antihypertensive effect of captopril may be reduced; reduces diuretic and natriuretic effects). Products include:
- Advil Cold & Sinus Caplets (formerly CoAdvil) ... 2416
- Advil Ibuprofen Tablets and Caplets ... 2416
- Children's Advil Suspension ... 2426
- CoAdvil ... ▣ 748
- Dristan Sinus Caplets ... 2419
- Haltran Tablets ... ▣ 668
- Ibuprofen ... ▣ 631
- Medipren ibuprofen Caplets and Tablets ... 1362
- Midol 200 Cramp Relief Formula ... ▣ 570
- Motrin Tablets ... 2351
- Motrin IB Caplets and Tablets ... ▣ 736
- Nuprin Ibuprofen/Analgesic Tablets & Caplets ... 752
- PediaProfen Suspension ... 1363
- Rufen Tablets ... 691
- Trendar Ibuprofen Tablets ... ▣ 756

Indapamide (Precipitous reduction of blood pressure; additive effect). Products include:
- Lozol Tablets ... 1843

Indomethacin (Antihypertensive effect of captopril may be reduced; reduces diuretic and natriuretic effects). Products include:
- Indocin ... 1487

Indomethacin Sodium Trihydrate (Antihypertensive effect of captopril may be reduced; reduces diuretic and natriuretic effects). Products include:
- Indocin I.V. ... 1490

Insulin, Human (Thiazide-induced hyperglycemia may require dosage adjustment of antidiabetic drugs).
- No products indexed under this heading.

Insulin, Human Isophane Suspension (Thiazide-induced hyperglycemia may require dosage adjustment of antidiabetic drugs). Products include:
- Humulin N, 100 Units ... 1270

Insulin, Human NPH (Thiazide-induced hyperglycemia may require dosage adjustment of antidiabetic drugs). Products include:
- Insulatard NPH Human ... 1627
- Novolin N ... 1627
- Novolin N PenFill Cartridges ... 1628
- Novolin N Prefilled ... 1628

Insulin, Human Regular (Thiazide-induced hyperglycemia may require dosage adjustment of antidiabetic drugs). Products include:
- Humulin BR, 100 Units 1268
- Humulin R, 100 Units 1272
- Novolin R 1627
- Novolin R PenFill Cartridges 1628
- Novolin R Prefilled 1629
- Velosulin Human 1628

Insulin, Human, Zinc Suspension (Thiazide-induced hyperglycemia may require dosage adjustment of antidiabetic drugs). Products include:
- Humulin L, 100 Units 1268
- Humulin U, 100 Units 1272
- Novolin L 1627

Insulin, NPH (Thiazide-induced hyperglycemia may require dosage adjustment of antidiabetic drugs). Products include:
- NPH, 40 & 100 Units 1273
- Beef NPH, 100 Units 1274
- Pork NPH, 100 Units 1275
- Insulatard NPH 1626
- NPH Insulin 1626
- NPH Purified Pork Isophane Insulin 1626

Insulin, Regular (Thiazide-induced hyperglycemia may require dosage adjustment of antidiabetic drugs). Products include:
- Regular, 40 & 100 Units 1273
- Beef Regular, 100 Units 1275
- Pork Regular, 100 Units 1275
- Pork Regular (Concentrated), 500 Units 1276
- Regular Insulin 1625
- Regular Purified Pork Insulin 1626
- Velosulin 1627

Insulin, Zinc Crystals (Thiazide-induced hyperglycemia may require dosage adjustment of antidiabetic drugs). Products include:
- NPH, 40 & 100 Units 1273

Insulin, Zinc Suspension (Thiazide-induced hyperglycemia may require dosage adjustment of antidiabetic drugs). Products include:
- Lente, 40 & 100 Units 1272
- Protamine, Zinc, 40 & 100 Units 1273
- Lente Iletin I 1272
- Beef Lente, 100 Units 1274
- Beef Protamine Zinc, 100 Units 1274
- Pork Lente, 100 Units 1275
- Pork, Protamine, Zinc, 100 Units 1275
- Lente Insulin 1626
- Lente Purified Pork Insulin 1626
- Semilente Insulin 1625
- Ultralente Insulin 1626

Isocarboxazid (Enhanced hypotensive effect). Products include:
- Marplan Tablets 1906

Isoflurane (Potentiated). Products include:
- Forane 600

Isosorbide Dinitrate (Discontinue before starting captopril; if resumed administer at lower dosage). Products include:
- Dilatrate-SR 1827
- Isordil 2467
- Sorbitrate 1103

Isradipine (Additive effect; precipitous reduction of blood pressure; elevated serum potassium). Products include:
- DynaCirc Capsules 2004

Ketamine Hydrochloride (Potentiated). Products include:
- Ketalar 1726

Ketoprofen (Antihypertensive effect of captopril may be reduced; reduces diuretic and natriuretic effects). Products include:
- Orudis Capsules 2488

Ketorolac Tromethamine (Antihypertensive effect of captopril may be reduced; reduces diuretic and natriuretic effects). Products include:
- Toradol IM Injection 2302

Labetalol Hydrochloride (Additive effect). Products include:
- Normodyne Injection 2108
- Normodyne Tablets 2110
- Normozide Tablets 2112
- Trandate HCT Tablets 579
- Trandate Injection 577
- Trandate Tablets 579

Levorphanol Tartrate (Potentiation of orthostatic hypotension). Products include:
- Levo-Dromoran 1906

Lisinopril (Additive effect). Products include:
- Prinivil Tablets 1538
- Prinzide Tablets 1540
- Zestoretic 2274
- Zestril Tablets 2277

Lithium Carbonate (Increased serum lithium levels and symptoms of lithium toxicity). Products include:
- Eskalith 2214
- Lithane Tablets 1596
- Lithium Carbonate Capsules & Tablets 1984
- Lithobid Tablets 870

Lithium Citrate (Increased serum lithium levels and symptoms of lithium toxicity). Products include:
- Cibalith-S 870

Lorazepam (Potentiated). Products include:
- Ativan Injection 2432
- Ativan Tablets 2434

Mecamylamine Hydrochloride (Additive effect or potentiation; use with caution). Products include:
- Inversine Tablets 1492

Meclofenamate Sodium (Antihypertensive effect of captopril may be reduced; reduces diuretic and natriuretic effects). Products include:
- Meclomen Capsules 1739

Mefenamic Acid (Antihypertensive effect of captopril may be reduced; reduces diuretic and natriuretic effects). Products include:
- Ponstel 1758

Meperidine Hydrochloride (Potentiated; potentiation of orthostatic hypotension). Products include:
- Demerol 2047
- Mepergan Injection 2479

Mephobarbital (Potentiation of orthostatic hypotension). Products include:
- Mebaral Tablets 2061

Metaraminol Bitartrate (Decreased response to pressor amines). Products include:
- Aramine Injection 1424

Methadone Hydrochloride (Potentiation of orthostatic hypotension). Products include:
- Dolophine Hydrochloride Ampoules & Vials 1260
- Dolophine Hydrochloride Tablets 1261
- Methadone Hydrochloride Diskets 1284
- Methadone Hydrochloride Oral Solution & Tablets 1987

Methenamine (Possible decreased effectiveness due to alkalinization of urine). Products include:
- Urised Tablets 2396

Methohexital Sodium (Potentiated). Products include:
- Brevital Sodium Vials 1248

Methoxamine Hydrochloride (Decreased response to pressor amines). Products include:
- Vasoxyl Injection 819

Methoxyflurane (Potentiated).
- No products indexed under this heading.

Methyclothiazide (Precipitous reduction of blood pressure; captopril's effect will be augmented). Products include:
- Enduron Tablets 517
- Enduronyl 518

Methyldopa (Additive effect). Products include:
- Aldoclor Tablets 1413
- Aldomet Oral 1415
- Aldoril Tablets 1418

Methyldopate Hydrochloride (Additive effect). Products include:
- Aldomet Ester HCl Injection 1417

Methylprednisolone Acetate (Intensified electrolyte depletion, particularly hypokalemia). Products include:
- Depo-Medrol Sterile Aqueous Suspension 2334

Methylprednisolone Sodium Succinate (Intensified electrolyte depletion, particularly hypokalemia). Products include:
- Solu-Medrol Sterile Powder 2363

Metocurine Iodide (Increased response to relaxant). Products include:
- Metubine Iodide Vials 1285

Metolazone (Additive effect). Products include:
- Diulo 2129
- Mykrox ½ mg Tablets 984
- Zaroxolyn Tablets 989

Metoprolol Tartrate (Additive effect). Products include:
- Lopressor Ampuls 1032
- Lopressor HCT Tablets 1034
- Lopressor Tablets 1032

Metyrosine (Additive effect). Products include:
- Demser Capsules 1460

Minoxidil (Additive effect). Products include:
- Loniten Tablets 2346
- Rogaine Topical Solution 2357

Morphine Sulfate (Potentiated; potentiation of orthostatic hypotension). Products include:
- Astramorph/PF Injection, USP (Preservative-Free) 618
- Duramorph 960
- Infumorph 200 and Infumorph 500 Sterile Solutions 962
- MS Contin Tablets 1814
- MSIR 1817
- Oramorph SR (Morphine Sulfate Sustained Release Tablets) 1988
- Roxanol 1991

Nadolol (Additive effect). Products include:
- Corgard Tablets 701
- Corzide Tablets 702

Naproxen (Antihypertensive effect of captopril may be reduced; reduces diuretic and natriuretic effects). Products include:
- Naprosyn 2297

Naproxen Sodium (Antihypertensive effect of captopril may be reduced; reduces diuretic and natriuretic effects). Products include:
- Anaprox and Anaprox DS Tablets 2288

Nicardipine Hydrochloride (Additive effect). Products include:
- Cardene Capsules 2290

Nitroglycerin (Discontinue before starting captopril; if resumed administer at lower dosage). Products include:
- Deponit NTG Transdermal Delivery System 2143
- Minitran Transdermal Delivery System 1312
- Nitro-Bid Ointment 1339
- Nitro-Bid Capsules 1338
- Nitrodisc 2176
- Nitro-Dur (nitroglycerin) Transdermal Infusion System 1164
- Nitrogard Tablets 1004
- Nitrolingual Spray 1846
- Nitrostat Tablets 1743
- Transderm-Nitro Transdermal Therapeutic System 2283

Norepinephrine Bitartrate (Possible decreased response to pressor amines). Products include:
- Levophed Bitartrate Injection 2054

Opium Alkaloids (Potentiation of orthostatic hypotension). Products include:
- B & O No. 15A & No. 16A Supprettes 2395
- Pantopon Injectable 1911

Oxycodone Hydrochloride (Potentiation of orthostatic hypotension). Products include:
- Percocet Tablets 950
- Percodan 951
- Roxicodone Tablets, Oral Solution & Intensol (Oxycodone) 1992
- Tylox Capsules 1382

Pancuronium Bromide Injection (Increased response to relaxant).
- No products indexed under this heading.

Penbutolol Sulfate (Additive effect). Products include:
- Levatol 1832

Pentaerythritol Tetranitrate (Discontinue before starting captopril; if resumed administer at lower dosage). Products include:
- Peritrate 1756

Pentobarbital Sodium (Potentiated; potentiation of orthostatic hypotension). Products include:
- Nembutal Sodium Capsules 534
- Nembutal Sodium Solution 536
- Nembutal Sodium Suppositories 538

Phenelzine Sulfate (Enhanced hypotensive effect). Products include:
- Nardil 1742

Phenobarbital (Potentiation of orthostatic hypotension). Products include:
- Arco-Lase Plus Tablets 607
- Bellergal-S Tablets 1998
- Bronkolixir ..... ▣ 761
- Bronkotabs Tablets ..... ▣ 762
- Donnatal 1858
- Donnatal Extentabs 1859
- Donnatal Tablets 1858
- Donnazyme Tablets 1860
- Kinesed Tablets 2272
- Phenobarbital Elixir and Tablets 1293
- Primatene Tablets-P Formula 2421
- Quadrinal Tablets 1183
- Tedral SA 1765

Phenoxybenzamine Hydrochloride (Additive effect). Products include:
- Dibenzyline Capsules 2207

Phentolamine Mesylate (Additive effect). Products include:
- Regitine 878

Phenylbutazone (Antihypertensive effect of captopril may be reduced; reduces diuretic and natriuretic effects). Products include:
- Butazolidin Capsules & Tablets 1027

Phenylephrine Hydrochloride (Decreased response to pressor amines). Products include:
- AK-Dilate Solution 2.5% and 10% ..... ◉ 203
- Atrohist Sprinkle Capsules 558
- Cerose-DM 2443
- Codimal 846
- Comhist LA Capsules 1618
- Congespirin For Children Aspirin Free Chewable Cold Tablets 748
- Cyclomydril ..... ◉ 216
- Deconsal Sprinkle Capsules 559
- Dimetane Decongestant ..... ▣ 673

Dristan Decongestant/Antihistamine/Analgesic Coated Caplets ◙ 749
Dristan Cold Nasal Decongestant/Antihistamine/ Analgesic Coated Tablets 2419
Dristan Advanced Formula Decongestant/Antihistamine/Analgesic Tablets ◙ 749
Dristan Nasal Spray, Menthol 2419
Dristan Nasal Spray, Regular and Regular with Metered Pump 2419
Entex Capsules 1623
Entex Liquid 1623
Sinus Excedrin Analgesic, Decongestant Tablets & Caplets 750
Extendryl 994
4-Way Fast Acting Nasal Spray - Original Formula (regular & mentholated) & Metered Spray Pump (regular) 751
Hycomine Compound Tablets 929
Murocoll-2 Sterile Ophthalmic Solution ⊙ 261
Mydfrin 2.5% ⊙ 224
Naldecon Syrup, Tablets, Pediatric Drops and Pediatric Syrup 709
Neo-Synephrine Hydrochloride 1% Carpuject 2063
Neo-Synephrine Hydrochloride 1% Injection 2063
Neo-Synephrine Hydrochloride (Ophthalmic) 2064
Neo-Synephrine ◙ 759
Nōstril Nasal Decongestant ◙ 520
Novahistine Elixir ◙ 596
Phenergan VC 2500
Phenergan VC with Codeine 2501
Prefrin Liquifilm Vasoconstrictor and Lubricant Eye Drops ⊙ 254
Prefrin-A ⊙ 255
Quelidrine Syrup 556
Relief Vasoconstrictor and Lubricant Eye Drops ⊙ 256
Robitussin Night Relief ◙ 677
Ru-Tuss with Hydrocodone 694
Ru-Tuss Tablets 693
Vasosulf ⊙ 279
Vicks Sinex ◙ 665
Zincfrin ⊙ 230

Pindolol (Additive effect). Products include:
Visken Tablets 2036

Piroxicam (Antihypertensive effect of captopril may be reduced; reduces diuretic and natriuretic effects). Products include:
Feldene Capsules 1777

Polythiazide (Precipitous reduction of blood pressure; captopril's effect will be augmented). Products include:
Minizide Capsules 1779
Renese Tablets 1785
Renese-R Tablets 1786

Prazosin Hydrochloride (Additive effect or potentiation; use with caution). Products include:
Minipress Capsules 1778
Minizide Capsules 1779

Prednisolone Acetate (Intensified electrolyte depletion, particularly hypokalemia). Products include:
AK-Cide Sterile Ophthalmic Ointment & Suspension ⊙ 202
Blephamide Liquifilm Sterile Ophthalmic Suspension 586
Blephamide S.O.P. Sterile Ophthalmic Ointment 586
Cetapred Ointment ⊙ 220
⅛% Econopred & 1% Econopred Plus ⊙ 217
Isopto Cetapred Suspension ⊙ 220
Metimyd ⊙ 306
Poly-Pred Liquifilm ⊙ 250
Pred Forte ⊙ 252
Pred Mild ⊙ 254
Pred-G Liquifilm Sterile Ophthalmic Suspension ⊙ 252
Pred-G S.O.P. Sterile Ophthalmic Ointment ⊙ 253
Vasocidin Ointment ⊙ 275

Prednisolone Sodium Phosphate (Intensified electrolyte depletion, particularly hypokalemia). Products include:
AK-Pred ⊙ 205
Hydeltrasol Injection, Sterile 1476
Inflamase ⊙ 274
Pediapred Oral Liquid 987
Vasocidin Ophthalmic Solution ⊙ 276

Prednisolone Tebutate (Intensified electrolyte depletion, particularly hypokalemia). Products include:
Hydeltra-T.B.A. Sterile Suspension 1478

Prednisone (Intensified electrolyte depletion, particularly hypokalemia). Products include:
Deltasone Tablets 2332

Probenecid (Increased dosage of these agents may be necessary since hydrochlorothiazide may have hyperuricomic effect). Products include:
Benemid Tablets 1426
ColBENEMID Tablets 1436
Wycillin Injection and Probenecid Tablets 2539

Promethazine Hydrochloride (Potentiated). Products include:
Mepergan Injection 2479
Phenergan with Codeine 2497
Phenergan with Dextromethorphan 2499
Phenergan Injection 2493
Phenergan Suppositories 2496
Phenergan Syrup 2495
Phenergan Tablets 2496
Phenergan VC 2500
Phenergan VC with Codeine 2501

Propofol (Potentiated). Products include:
Diprivan Injection 2267

Propoxyphene Hydrochloride (Potentiation of orthostatic hypotension). Products include:
Darvon 1256
Wygesic Tablets 2540

Propoxyphene Napsylate (Potentiation of orthostatic hypotension). Products include:
Darvon-N/Darvocet-N 1254

Propranolol Hydrochloride (Additive effect). Products include:
Inderal 2459
Inderal LA Long Acting Capsules 2461
Inderide Tablets 2463
Inderide LA Long Acting Capsules 2465

Ramipril (Additive effect; precipitous reduction of blood pressure; elevated serum potassium). Products include:
Altace Capsules 1086

Rauwolfia Serpentina (Additive effect or potentiation; use with caution). Products include:
Raudixin Tablets 1803
Rauzide Tablets 1804

Rescinnamine (Additive effect or potentiation; use with caution).
No products indexed under this heading.

Reserpine (Additive effect or potentiation; use with caution). Products include:
Diupres Tablets 1461
Hydromox R Tablets 1209
Hydropres Tablets 1485
Renese-R Tablets 1786
Salutensin/Salutensin-Demi 719
Ser-Ap-Es Tablets 881
Serpasil Tablets 883
Serpasil-Apresoline Tablets 884
Serpasil-Esidrix Tablets 886

Secobarbital Sodium (Potentiation of orthostatic hypotension). Products include:
Seconal Sodium Pulvules 1296

Selegiline Hydrochloride (Enhanced hypotensive effect). Products include:
Eldepryl 2250

Sodium Nitroprusside (Additive effect). Products include:
Nipride I.V. Infusion 1909

Spironolactone (Precipitous reduction of blood pressure; elevated serum potassium; additive effect). Products include:
Aldactazide 2150
Aldactone 2152

Sufentanil Citrate (Potentiation of orthostatic hypotension). Products include:
Sufenta Injection 1147

Sulfinpyrazone (Increased dosage of these agents may be necessary since hydrochlorothiazide may have hyperuricomic effect). Products include:
Anturane 853

Sulindac (Antihypertensive effect of captopril may be reduced; reduces diuretic and natriuretic effects). Products include:
Clinoril Tablets 1433

Terazosin Hydrochloride (Additive effect or potentiation; use with caution). Products include:
Hytrin Tablets 529

Thiamylal Sodium (Potentiation of orthostatic hypotension). Products include:
Surital Ampoules, Steri-Vials 1764

Timolol Maleate (Additive effect). Products include:
Blocadren Tablets 1429
Timolide Tablets 1547
Timoptic in Ocudose 1552
Timoptic Sterile Ophthalmic Solution 1550

Tolazamide (Thiazide-induced hyperglycemia may require dosage adjustment of antidiabetic drugs). Products include:
Tolinase Tablets 2365

Tolbutamide (Thiazide-induced hyperglycemia may require dosage adjustment of antidiabetic drugs). Products include:
Orinase Tablets 2354

Tolmetin Sodium (Antihypertensive effect of captopril may be reduced; reduces diuretic and natriuretic effects). Products include:
Tolectin (200, 400 and 600 mg) 1379

Tranylcypromine Sulfate (Enhanced hypotensive effect). Products include:
Parnate Tablets 2222

Triamcinolone (Intensified electrolyte depletion, particularly hypokalemia).
No products indexed under this heading.

Triamcinolone Acetonide (Intensified electrolyte depletion, particularly hypokalemia). Products include:
Aristocort A 1010
Azmacort Inhaler 1837
Kenalog Cream, Lotion & Ointment 2401
Kenalog-10 Injection 2402
Kenalog-40 Injection 2403
Kenalog in Orabase 604
Kenalog Spray 2401
Mycolog II Cream and Ointment 2407
Mytrex Cream & Ointment 2080
Nasacort Nasal Inhaler 1844

Triamcinolone Diacetate (Intensified electrolyte depletion, particularly hypokalemia). Products include:
Aristocort Suspension 1008

Triamcinolone Hexacetonide (Intensified electrolyte depletion, particularly hypokalemia). Products include:
Aristospan Suspension 1011

Triamterene (Precipitous reduction of blood pressure; elevated serum potassium; additive effect). Products include:
Dyazide Capsules 2208
Dyrenium Capsules 2210
Maxzide 1215

Trimethaphan Camsylate (Additive effect or potentiation; use with caution). Products include:
Arfonad Ampuls 1887

Vecuronium Bromide (Increased response to relaxant). Products include:
Norcuron 1642

Warfarin Sodium (Decreased anticoagulant effect). Products include:
Coumadin Injection & Tablets 944
Panwarfin Tablets 547

CARAFATE TABLETS
(Sucralfate) 1326
May interact with antacids and certain other agents. Compounds in these categories include:

Aluminum Carbonate Gel (Simultaneous administration within one-half hour before or after sucralfate should be avoided; may increase the total body burden of aluminum). Products include:
Basaljel 2438

Aluminum Hydroxide (Simultaneous administration within one-half hour before or after sucralfate should be avoided; may increase the total body burden of aluminum). Products include:
Cama Arthritis Pain Reliever ◙ 685
Gaviscon Extra Strength Relief Formula Liquid Antacid ◙ 594
Gaviscon Extra Strength Relief Formula Antacid Tablets ◙ 594
Gaviscon Liquid Antacid ◙ 594
Gelusil Liquid & Tablets ◙ 639
Extra Strength Maalox Plus Suspension 1850
Maalox TC Suspension 1851
Maalox Plus Tablets ◙ 655
Extra Strength Maalox Plus Tablets 1850
Nephrox Suspension ◙ 563
WinGel Liquid & Tablets ◙ 761

Aluminum Hydroxide Gel (Simultaneous administration within one-half hour before or after sucralfate should be avoided; may increase the total body burden of aluminum). Products include:
ALternaGEL Liquid 1154
Aludrox Oral Suspension 2428
Amphojel Suspension 2429
Amphojel Suspension without Flavor 2429
Mylanta Liquid 1155
Mylanta Double Strength Liquid 1155

Aluminum Hydroxide Gel, Dried (Simultaneous administration within one-half hour before or after sucralfate should be avoided; may increase the total body burden of aluminum). Products include:
Alu-Tab/Alu-Cap 1309
Amphojel Tablets 2429
Ascriptin A/D Caplets 1850
Regular Strength Ascriptin Tablets 1850
Gaviscon Antacid Tablets ◙ 593
Gaviscon-2 Antacid Tablets ◙ 594
Mylanta Tablets 1155
Mylanta Double Strength Tablets 1155

Aminophylline (Reduction in bioavailability of theophylline). Products include:
Amesec ◙ 682
Aminophyllin Tablets 2153

Cimetidine (Reduction in bioavailability of cimetidine). Products include:
Tagamet Tablets 2228

Cimetidine Hydrochloride (Reduction in bioavailability of cimetidine). Products include:
Tagamet 2228

Ciprofloxacin Hydrochloride (Reduction in bioavailability of ciprofloxacin). Products include:
- Ciloxan Sterile Ophthalmic Solution ◉ 214
- Cipro I.V. 1592
- Cipro Tablets 1589

Digitoxin (Reduction in bioavailability of digitoxin). Products include:
- Crystodigin Tablets 1253

Digoxin (Reduction in bioavailability of digoxin). Products include:
- Lanoxicaps 772
- Lanoxin Elixir Pediatric 775
- Lanoxin Injection 778
- Lanoxin Injection Pediatric 781
- Lanoxin Tablets 783

Dihydroxyaluminum Sodium Carbonate (Simultaneous administration within one-half hour before or after sucralfate should be avoided). Products include:
- Rolaids ⊕ 743

Dyphylline (Reduction in bioavailability of theophylline). Products include:
- Dilor 2079
- Dilor-G Tablets & Liquid 2079
- Lufyllin Elixir 2384
- Lufyllin & Lufyllin-400 Tablets 2384
- Lufyllin-GG Elixir & Tablets 2385

Magaldrate (Simultaneous administration within one-half hour before or after sucralfate should be avoided). Products include:
- Riopan Antacid Chew Tablets ⊕ 754
- Riopan Antacid Chew Tablets in Rollpacks ⊕ 754
- Riopan Antacid Suspension 2421
- Riopan Antacid Swallow Tablets 2421
- Riopan Plus Chew Tablets 2422
- Riopan Plus Chew Tablets in Rollpack 2422
- Riopan Plus 2 Chew Tablets, Mint Flavor, Cherry Flavor 2422
- Riopan Plus Suspension 2422
- Riopan Plus 2 Suspension, Mint Flavor, Cherry Flavor 2422

Magnesium Hydroxide (Simultaneous administration within one-half hour before or after sucralfate should be avoided). Products include:
- Aludrox Oral Suspension 2428
- Ascriptin A/D Caplets 1850
- Regular Strength Ascriptin Tablets 1850
- Di-Gel Antacid/Anti-Gas ⊕ 697
- Gelusil Liquid & Tablets ⊕ 639
- Haley's M-O, Regular & Flavored ⊕ 569
- Extra Strength Maalox Plus Suspension 1850
- Maalox TC Suspension 1851
- Maalox Plus Tablets ⊕ 655
- Extra Strength Maalox Plus Tablets 1850
- Mylanta Liquid 1155
- Mylanta Tablets 1155
- Mylanta Double Strength Liquid 1155
- Mylanta Double Strength Tablets 1155
- Concentrated Phillips' Milk of Magnesia ⊕ 573
- Phillips' Milk of Magnesia Liquid ⊕ 572
- Phillips' Milk of Magnesia Tablets ⊕ 573
- WinGel Liquid & Tablets ⊕ 761

Magnesium Oxide (Simultaneous administration within one-half hour before or after sucralfate should be avoided). Products include:
- Bayer Plus Aspirin Tablets ⊕ 567
- Beelith Tablets 659
- Bufferin Analgesic Tablets and Caplets ⊕ 524
- Cama Arthritis Pain Reliever ⊕ 685
- Mag-Ox 400 673
- Uro-Mag 673

Norfloxacin (Reduction in bioavailability of norfloxacin). Products include:
- Chibroxin Sterile Ophthalmic Solution 1431
- Noroxin Tablets 1519

Oxytetracycline (Reduction in bioavailability of oxytetracycline). Products include:
- Terramycin Intramuscular Solution 1964
- Urobiotic-250 Capsules 1968

Oxytetracycline Hydrochloride (Reduction in bioavailability of oxytetracycline). Products include:
- Terra-Cortril Ophthalmic Suspension 1963
- Terramycin Capsules 1786
- Terramycin Intramuscular Solution 1964
- Terramycin with Polymyxin B Sulfate Ophthalmic Ointment 1965

Phenytoin (Reduction in bioavailability of phenytoin). Products include:
- Dilantin Infatabs 1710
- Dilantin-30 Pediatric/Dilantin-125 Suspension 1713

Phenytoin Sodium (Reduction in bioavailability of phenytoin). Products include:
- Dilantin Kapseals 1708
- Dilantin Parenteral 1712
- Dilantin with Phenobarbital Kapseals 1715

Ranitidine Hydrochloride (Reduction in bioavailability of ranitidine). Products include:
- Zantac Injection and Zantac Injection Premixed 1063
- Zantac 1065

Tetracycline Hydrochloride (Reduction in bioavailability of tetracycline). Products include:
- Achromycin V Capsules 1193
- Achromycin Ophthalmic Ointment 1% ◉ 307
- Achromycin Ophthalmic Suspension 1% ◉ 308
- Topicycline for Topical Solution 1856

Theophylline (Reduction in bioavailability of theophylline). Products include:
- Bronkaid Tablets ⊕ 757
- Bronkolixir ⊕ 761
- Bronkotabs Tablets ⊕ 762
- Constant-T Tablets 1029
- Marax Tablets & DF Syrup 1954
- Primatene Tablets 2421
- Quibron Capsules 713
- Quibron-T 714
- Quibron-T/SR 716
- Theolair Liquid 1317
- Theo-Organidin Elixir 2391

Theophylline Anhydrous (Reduction in bioavailability of theophylline). Products include:
- Aerolate 994
- Primatene Tablets-M Formula ⊕ 753
- Primatene Tablets-Regular Formula 2421
- Respbid Tablets 684
- Slo-bid Gyrocaps 1847
- T-PHYL (Uniphyl) 200 mg Tablets 1820
- Tedral SA 1765
- Theo-24 2179
- Theo-Dur Sprinkle 1168
- Theo-Dur Extended-Release Tablets 1166
- Theolair Tablets 1317
- Theolair-SR Tablets 1319
- TheoX Extended-Release Tablets 841
- Uniphyl 400 mg Tablets 1823

Theophylline Calcium Salicylate (Reduction in bioavailability of theophylline). Products include:
- Quadrinal Tablets 1183

Theophylline Sodium Glycinate (Reduction in bioavailability of theophylline). Products include:
- Asbron G 1997

CARBOCAINE HYDROCHLORIDE 3% INJECTION (KODAK)

(Mepivacaine Hydrochloride Injection) 956

See **Carbocaine Hydrochloride 2% with Neo-Cobefrin**

CARBOCAINE HYDROCHLORIDE INJECTION (SANOFI)

(Mepivacaine Hydrochloride Injection) 2043

No interactions described in labeling.

CARBOCAINE HYDROCHLORIDE 2% WITH NEO-COBEFRIN (KODAK)

(Mepivacaine Hydrochloride Injection, Levonordefrin Injection) 956

May interact with monoamine oxidase inhibitors, tricyclic antidepressants, phenothiazines, inhalant anesthetics, and certain other agents. Compounds in these categories include:

Amitriptyline Hydrochloride (Potential for blood pressure alterations). Products include:
- Elavil 2269
- Endep Tablets 1927
- Etrafon 2087
- Limbitrol 1933
- Triavil Tablets 1556

Amoxapine (Potential for blood pressure alterations). Products include:
- Asendin Tablets 1196

Chlorpromazine (Potential for blood pressure alterations). Products include:
- Thorazine 2234

Clomipramine Hydrochloride (Potential for blood pressure alterations). Products include:
- Anafranil Capsules 650

Desipramine Hydrochloride (Potential for blood pressure alterations). Products include:
- Norpramin Tablets 1340

Doxepin Hydrochloride (Potential for blood pressure alterations). Products include:
- Sinequan 1960

Enflurane (Potential for cardiac arrhythmias). Products include:
- Ethrane 599

Fluphenazine Decanoate (Potential for blood pressure alterations). Products include:
- Prolixin Decanoate 1795

Fluphenazine Enanthate (Potential for blood pressure alterations). Products include:
- Prolixin Enanthate 1796

Fluphenazine Hydrochloride (Potential for blood pressure alterations). Products include:
- Prolixin Elixir 1793
- Prolixin Injection 1791
- Prolixin Oral Concentrate 1792
- Prolixin Tablets 1793

Furazolidone (Potential for blood pressure alterations). Products include:
- Furoxone 1855

Halothane (Potential for cardiac arrhythmias). Products include:
- Fluothane 2453

Imipramine Hydrochloride (Potential for blood pressure alterations). Products include:
- Tofranil Ampuls 1038
- Tofranil Tablets 1039

Imipramine Pamoate (Potential for blood pressure alterations). Products include:
- Tofranil-PM Capsules 1041

Isocarboxazid (Potential for blood pressure alterations). Products include:
- Marplan Tablets 1906

Isoflurane (Potential for cardiac arrhythmias). Products include:
- Forane 600

Maprotiline Hydrochloride (Potential for blood pressure alterations). Products include:
- Ludiomil Tablets 874

Mesoridazine Besylate (Potential for blood pressure alterations).

Methoxyflurane (Potential for cardiac arrhythmias).
- No products indexed under this heading.

Nortriptyline Hydrochloride (Potential for blood pressure alterations). Products include:
- Pamelor 2019

Perphenazine (Potential for blood pressure alterations). Products include:
- Etrafon 2087
- Triavil Tablets 1556
- Trilafon 2123

Phenelzine Sulfate (Potential for blood pressure alterations). Products include:
- Nardil 1742

Prochlorperazine (Potential for blood pressure alterations). Products include:
- Compazine 2201

Promethazine Hydrochloride (Potential for blood pressure alterations). Products include:
- Mepergan Injection 2479
- Phenergan with Codeine 2497
- Phenergan with Dextromethorphan 2499
- Phenergan Injection 2493
- Phenergan Suppositories 2496
- Phenergan Syrup 2495
- Phenergan Tablets 2496
- Phenergan VC 2500
- Phenergan VC with Codeine 2501

Protriptyline Hydrochloride (Potential for blood pressure alterations). Products include:
- Vivactil Tablets 1567

Selegiline Hydrochloride (Potential for blood pressure alterations). Products include:
- Eldepryl 2250

Thioridazine Hydrochloride (Potential for blood pressure alterations). Products include:
- Mellaril 2011

Tranylcypromine Sulfate (Potential for blood pressure alterations). Products include:
- Parnate Tablets 2222

Trifluoperazine Hydrochloride (Potential for blood pressure alterations). Products include:
- Stelazine 2226

Trimipramine Maleate (Potential for blood pressure alterations). Products include:
- Surmontil Capsules 2524

CARDENE CAPSULES

(Nicardipine Hydrochloride) 2290

May interact with cardiac glycosides and certain other agents. Compounds in these categories include:

Cimetidine (Increased Cardene plasma levels). Products include:
- Tagamet Tablets 2228

Cimetidine Hydrochloride (Increased Cardene plasma levels). Products include:
- Tagamet 2228

Cyclosporine (Concomitant administration results in elevated plasma cyclosporine levels). Products include:
- Sandimmune 2024

Deslanoside (Potential for altered plasma deslanoside levels).
- No products indexed under this heading.

Digitoxin (Potential for altered plasma digitoxin levels). Products include:
- Crystodigin Tablets 1253

Digoxin (Potential for altered plasma digoxin levels). Products include:
- Lanoxicaps 772
- Lanoxin Elixir Pediatric 775
- Lanoxin Injection 778
- Lanoxin Injection Pediatric 781
- Lanoxin Tablets 783

Fentanyl Citrate (May require increased volume of circulating fluids if severe hypotension were to occur). Products include:
- Innovar Injection 1141
- Sublimaze Injection 1146

CARDILATE ORAL/SUBLINGUAL TABLETS
(Erythrityl Tetranitrate) 757
May interact with:

Alcohol (Enhances hypotensive effects).

CARDIOQUIN TABLETS
(Quinidine Polygalacturonate) 1812
May interact with oral anticoagulants, thiazides, carbonic anhydrase inhibitors, anticholinergics, antiarrhythmics, cardiac glycosides, cholinergic agents, antacids, and certain other agents. Compounds in these categories include:

Acebutolol Hydrochloride (Additive cardiac depressant effects). Products include:
- Sectral Capsules 2520

Acetazolamide (Prolongs half-life). Products include:
- Diamox Parenteral 1200
- Diamox Parenteral .... ⊙ 308
- Diamox Sequels (Sustained Release) 1201
- Diamox Sequels (Sustained Release) .... ⊙ 310
- Diamox Tablets 1200
- Diamox Tablets .... ⊙ 308

Adenosine (Additive cardiac depressant effects). Products include:
- Adenocard Injection 1007

Aluminum Carbonate Gel (Delays quinidine absorption). Products include:
- Basaljel 2438

Aluminum Hydroxide (Delays quinidine absorption). Products include:
- Cama Arthritis Pain Reliever .... ▣ 685
- Gaviscon Extra Strength Relief Formula Liquid Antacid .... ▣ 594
- Gaviscon Extra Strength Relief Formula Antacid Tablets .... ▣ 594
- Gaviscon Liquid Antacid .... ▣ 594
- Gelusil Liquid & Tablets .... ▣ 639
- Extra Strength Maalox Plus Suspension 1850
- Maalox TC Suspension 1851
- Maalox Plus Tablets .... ▣ 655
- Extra Strength Maalox Plus Tablets 1850
- Nephrox Suspension .... ▣ 563
- WinGel Liquid & Tablets .... ▣ 761

Aluminum Hydroxide Gel (Delays quinidine absorption). Products include:
- ALternaGEL Liquid 1154
- Aludrox Oral Suspension 2428
- Amphojel Suspension 2429
- Amphojel Suspension without Flavor 2429
- Mylanta Liquid 1155
- Mylanta Double Strength Liquid 1155

Aluminum Hydroxide Gel, Dried (Delays quinidine absorption). Products include:
- Alu-Tab/Alu-Cap 1309
- Amphojel Tablets 2429
- Ascriptin A/D Caplets 1850
- Regular Strength Ascriptin Tablets 1850
- Gaviscon Antacid Tablets .... ▣ 593
- Gaviscon-2 Antacid Tablets .... ▣ 594
- Mylanta Tablets 1155
- Mylanta Double Strength Tablets 1155

Amiodarone Hydrochloride (Additive cardiac depressant effects). Products include:
- Cordarone Tablets 2446

Atropine Sulfate (Additive vagolytic effect). Products include:
- Arco-Lase Plus Tablets 607
- Atropine Sulfate Sterile Ophthalmic Solution and S.O.P. Sterile Ophthalmic Ointment .... ⊙ 239
- Donnagel .... ▣ 675
- Donnagel-PG 1858
- Donnatal 1858
- Donnatal Extentabs 1859
- Donnatal Tablets 1858
- Donnazyme Tablets 1860
- Isopto Atropine .... ⊙ 218
- Lomotil 2174
- Motofen Tablets 836
- Ru-Tuss Tablets 693
- Urised Tablets 2396

Belladonna Alkaloids (Additive vagolytic effect). Products include:
- Bellergal-S Tablets 1998
- Hyland's Bed Wetting Tablets .... ▣ 728
- Hyland's Teething Tablets .... ▣ 728
- Kinesed Tablets 2272

Bendroflumethiazide (Prolongs quinidine's half-life). Products include:
- Corzide Tablets 702
- Naturetin Tablets 1789
- Rauzide Tablets 1804

Benztropine Mesylate (Additive vagolytic effect). Products include:
- Cogentin 1435

Biperiden (Additive vagolytic effect). Products include:
- Akineton 1171

Bretylium Tosylate (Additive cardiac depressant effects). Products include:
- Bretylol Injection 923

Chlorothiazide (Prolongs quinidine's half-life). Products include:
- Aldoclor Tablets 1413
- Diupres Tablets 1461
- Diuril Oral 1464

Chlorothiazide Sodium (Prolongs quinidine's half-life). Products include:
- Diuril Sodium Intravenous 1463

Clidinium Bromide (Additive vagolytic effect). Products include:
- Librax Capsules 1929
- Quarzan Capsules 1937

Decamethonium (Potentiation of neuromuscular blocking).

Deslanoside (Increased digoxin levels; digoxin toxicity).
- No products indexed under this heading.

Dichlorphenamide (Prolongs quinidine's half-life). Products include:
- Daranide Tablets 1445

Dicumarol (Combination therapy may reduce prothrombin levels and cause bleeding). Products include:
- Dicumarol Tablets 516

Dicyclomine Hydrochloride (Additive vagolytic effect). Products include:
- Bentyl 1322

Digitoxin (Increased digoxin levels; digoxin toxicity). Products include:
- Crystodigin Tablets 1253

Digoxin (Increased digoxin levels; digoxin toxicity). Products include:
- Lanoxicaps 772
- Lanoxin Elixir Pediatric 775
- Lanoxin Injection 778
- Lanoxin Injection Pediatric 781
- Lanoxin Tablets 783

Dihydroxyaluminum Sodium Carbonate (Delays quinidine absorption). Products include:
- Rolaids .... ▣ 743

Disopyramide Phosphate (Additive cardiac depressant effects). Products include:
- Norpace 2177

Edrophonium Chloride (Antagonized by quinidine). Products include:
- Enlon Injection 598
- Tensilon Injectable 1123

Ethopropazine Hydrochloride (Additive vagolytic effect).

Glycopyrrolate (Additive vagolytic effect). Products include:
- Robinul Forte Tablets 1873
- Robinul Injectable 1873
- Robinul Tablets 1873

Hydrochlorothiazide (Prolongs quinidine's half-life). Products include:
- Aldactazide 2150
- Aldoril Tablets 1418
- Apresazide Capsules 854
- Apresoline-Esidrix Tablets 857
- Capozide 2258
- Dyazide Capsules 2208
- Esidrix Tablets 863
- Esimil Tablets 864
- HydroDIURIL Tablets 1484
- Hydropres Tablets 1485
- Inderide Tablets 2463
- Inderide LA Long Acting Capsules .. 2465
- Lopressor HCT Tablets 1034
- Maxzide 1215
- Moduretic Tablets 1510
- Normozide Tablets 2112
- Oretic Tablets 544
- Oreticyl 545
- Prinzide Tablets 1540
- Ser-Ap-Es Tablets 881
- Serpasil-Esidrix Tablets 886
- Timolide Tablets 1547
- Trandate HCT Tablets 579
- Vaseretic Tablets 1559
- Zestoretic 2274

Hydroflumethiazide (Prolongs quinidine's half-life). Products include:
- Diucardin Tablets 2450
- Saluron 718
- Salutensin/Salutensin-Demi 719

Hyoscyamine (Additive vagolytic effect). Products include:
- Cystospaz Tablets 2395
- Urised Tablets 2396

Hyoscyamine Sulfate (Additive vagolytic effect). Products include:
- Arco-Lase Plus Tablets 607
- Cystospaz-M Capsules 2395
- Donnagel .... ▣ 675
- Donnagel-PG 1858
- Donnatal 1858
- Donnatal Extentabs 1859
- Donnatal Tablets 1858
- Donnazyme Tablets 1860
- Kutrase Capsules 2146
- Levsin/Levsinex 2147
- Ru-Tuss Tablets 693

Ipratropium Bromide (Additive vagolytic effect). Products include:
- Atrovent Inhalation Aerosol 675

Lidocaine Hydrochloride (Additive cardiac depressant effects). Products include:
- Anestacon Solution 2394
- Bactine Antiseptic/Anesthetic First Aid Spray .... ▣ 624
- Decadron Phosphate with Xylocaine Injection, Sterile 1451
- Xylocaine Injections 637
- Xylocaine Injections for Ventricular Arrhythmias 639
- Xylocaine 2% Jelly 643
- 4% Xylocaine-MPF Sterile Solution 641
- Xylocaine 2% Viscous Solution 646

Magaldrate (Delays quinidine absorption). Products include:
- Riopan Antacid Chew Tablets .... ▣ 754
- Riopan Antacid Chew Tablets in Rollpacks .... ▣ 754
- Riopan Antacid Suspension 2421
- Riopan Antacid Swallow Tablets 2421
- Riopan Plus Chew Tablets 2422
- Riopan Plus Chew Tablets in Rollpack 2422
- Riopan Plus 2 Chew Tablets, Mint Flavor, Cherry Flavor 2422
- Riopan Plus Suspension 2422
- Riopan Plus 2 Suspension, Mint Flavor, Cherry Flavor 2422

Magnesium Hydroxide (Delays quinidine absorption). Products include:
- Aludrox Oral Suspension 2428
- Ascriptin A/D Caplets 1850
- Regular Strength Ascriptin Tablets 1850
- Di-Gel Antacid/Anti-Gas .... ▣ 697
- Gelusil Liquid & Tablets .... ▣ 639
- Haley's M-O, Regular & Flavored .. ▣ 569
- Extra Strength Maalox Plus Suspension 1850
- Maalox TC Suspension 1851
- Maalox Plus Tablets .... ▣ 655
- Extra Strength Maalox Plus Tablets 1850
- Mylanta Liquid 1155
- Mylanta Tablets 1155
- Mylanta Double Strength Liquid 1155
- Mylanta Double Strength Tablets 1155
- Concentrated Phillips' Milk of Magnesia .... ▣ 573
- Phillips' Milk of Magnesia Liquid .... ▣ 572
- Phillips' Milk of Magnesia Tablets ▣ 573
- WinGel Liquid & Tablets .... ▣ 761

Magnesium Oxide (Delays quinidine absorption). Products include:
- Bayer Plus Aspirin Tablets .... ▣ 567
- Beelith Tablets 659
- Bufferin Analgesic Tablets and Caplets .... ▣ 524
- Cama Arthritis Pain Reliever .... ▣ 685
- Mag-Ox 400 673
- Uro-Mag 673

Mepenzolate Bromide (Additive vagolytic effect). Products include:
- Cantil Tablets 1326

Methazolamide (Prolongs quinidine's half-life). Products include:
- Neptazane Tablets .... ⊙ 311

Methyclothiazide (Prolongs quinidine's half-life). Products include:
- Enduron Tablets 517
- Enduronyl 518

Mexiletine Hydrochloride (Additive cardiac depressant effects). Products include:
- Mexitil Capsules 680

Moricizine Hydrochloride (Additive cardiac depressant effects). Products include:
- Ethmozine Tablets 946

Neostigmine Bromide (Antagonized by quinidine). Products include:
- Prostigmin Tablets 1121

Neostigmine Methylsulfate (Antagonized by quinidine). Products include:
- Prostigmin Injectable 1120

Oxybutynin Chloride (Additive vagolytic effect). Products include:
- Ditropan 1332

Phenobarbital (Reduces quinidine's plasma half-life by 50%). Products include:
- Arco-Lase Plus Tablets 607
- Bellergal-S Tablets 1998
- Bronkolixir .... ▣ 761
- Bronkotabs Tablets .... ▣ 762
- Donnatal 1858
- Donnatal Extentabs 1859
- Donnatal Tablets 1858
- Donnazyme Tablets 1860
- Kinesed Tablets 2272
- Phenobarbital Elixir and Tablets 1293
- Primatene Tablets-P Formula 2421
- Quadrinal Tablets 1183
- Tedral SA 1765

Phenytoin (Reduces quinidine's plasma half-life by 50%). Products include:
- Dilantin Infatabs 1710
- Dilantin-30 Pediatric/Dilantin-125 Suspension 1713

Phenytoin Sodium (Reduces quinidine's plasma half-life by 50%). Products include:
- Dilantin Kapseals 1708
- Dilantin Parenteral 1712
- Dilantin with Phenobarbital Kapseals 1715

Polythiazide (Prolongs quinidine's half-life). Products include:
- Minizide Capsules 1779
- Renese Tablets 1785
- Renese-R Tablets 1786

Procainamide Hydrochloride (Additive cardiac depressant effects). Products include:
- Procan SR Tablets 1760
- Pronestyl Capsules and Tablets 1800
- Pronestyl Injection 1798
- Pronestyl-SR Tablets 1801

Procyclidine Hydrochloride (Additive vagolytic effect). Products include:
- Kemadrin Tablets 771

Propafenone Hydrochloride (Additive cardiac depressant effects). Products include:
- Rythmol Tablets 1184

Propantheline Bromide (Additive vagolytic effect). Products include:
- Pro-Banthine Tablets 2141

Propranolol Hydrochloride (Additive cardiac depressant effects). Products include:
- Inderal 2459
- Inderal LA Long Acting Capsules 2461
- Inderide Tablets 2463
- Inderide LA Long Acting Capsules 2465

Pyridostigmine Bromide (Antagonized by quinidine). Products include:
- Mestinon Injectable 1115
- Mestinon 1116

Quinidine Gluconate (Additive cardiac depressant effects). Products include:
- Quinaglute Dura-Tabs Tablets 663

Quinidine Sulfate (Additive cardiac depressant effects). Products include:
- Quinidex Extentabs 1868

Scopolamine Hydrobromide (Additive vagolytic effect). Products include:
- Donnagel ..... ▣ 675
- Donnagel-PG 1858
- Donnatal 1858
- Donnatal Extentabs 1859
- Donnatal Tablets 1858
- Donnazyme Tablets 1860
- Isopto Hyoscine ..... ⊙ 222
- Murocoll-2 Sterile Ophthalmic Solution ..... ⊙ 261
- Ru-Tuss Tablets 693

Scopolamine Preparations (Additive vagolytic effect). Products include:
- Transderm Scōp Transdermal Therapeutic System 887

Sodium Bicarbonate (Prolongs quinidine's half-life). Products include:
- Alka-Seltzer Advanced Formula Antacid & Non-Aspirin Pain Reliever ..... ▣ 620
- Alka-Seltzer Effervescent Antacid ▣ 622
- Alka-Seltzer Effervescent Antacid and Pain Reliever 1568
- Alka-Seltzer Extra Strength Effervescent Antacid and Pain Reliever ..... ▣ 623
- Alka-Seltzer (Flavored) Effervescent Antacid and Pain Reliever .. ▣ 621
- Arm & Hammer Pure Baking Soda ..... ▣ 548
- Ceo-Two Rectal Suppositories 671
- Citrocarbonate Antacid ..... ▣ 668
- Massengill Liquid Concentrate 2191
- NuLYTELY 699

Succinylcholine Chloride (Potentiation of neuromuscular blocking effect). Products include:
- Anectine 755

Tocainide Hydrochloride (Additive cardiac depressant effects). Products include:
- Tonocard Tablets 1554

Tridihexethyl Chloride (Additive vagolytic effect).
- No products indexed under this heading.

Trihexyphenidyl Hydrochloride (Additive vagolytic effect). Products include:
- Artane 1195

Tubocurarine Chloride (Potentiation of neuromuscular blocking effect).
- No products indexed under this heading.

Verapamil Hydrochloride (Additive cardiac depressant effects). Products include:
- Calan SR Caplets 2157
- Calan Tablets 2155
- Isoptin Injectable 1177
- Isoptin Oral Tablets 1179
- Isoptin SR Sustained Release Tablets 1181
- Verelan Capsules 1243
- Verelan Capsules 2535

Warfarin Sodium (Combination therapy may reduce prothrombin levels and cause bleeding). Products include:
- Coumadin Injection & Tablets 944
- Panwarfin Tablets 547

CARDIZEM TABLETS-30 MG, 60 MG, 90 MG AND 120 MG

(Diltiazem Hydrochloride) 1329
May interact with beta blockers, general anesthetics, cardiac glycosides, and certain other agents. Compounds in these categories include:

Acebutolol Hydrochloride (Potential for additive effects on cardiac conduction). Products include:
- Sectral Capsules 2520

Atenolol (Potential for additive effects on cardiac conduction). Products include:
- Tenoretic Tablets 1105
- Tenormin Tablets and I.V. Injection 1107

Betaxolol Hydrochloride (Potential for additive effects on cardiac conduction). Products include:
- Betoptic Sterile Ophthalmic Solution 569
- Betoptic S Sterile Ophthalmic Suspension 570
- Kerlone Tablets 2172

Carteolol Hydrochloride (Potential for additive effects on cardiac conduction). Products include:
- Cartrol Tablets 507

Cimetidine (May increase peak plasma levels and AUC when administered concurrently). Products include:
- Tagamet Tablets 2228

Cimetidine Hydrochloride (May increase peak plasma levels and AUC when administered concurrently). Products include:
- Tagamet 2228

Deslanoside (Potential for additive effects on cardiac conduction; variable effect on plasma digoxin concentrations).
- No products indexed under this heading.

Digitoxin (Potential for additive effects on cardiac conduction; variable effect on plasma digoxin concentrations). Products include:
- Crystodigin Tablets 1253

Digoxin (Potential for additive effects on cardiac conduction; variable effect on plasma digoxin concentrations). Products include:
- Lanoxicaps 772
- Lanoxin Elixir Pediatric 775
- Lanoxin Injection 778
- Lanoxin Injection Pediatric 781
- Lanoxin Tablets 783

Enflurane (Cardiovascular side effects of anesthetics potentiated). Products include:
- Ethrane 599

Esmolol Hydrochloride (Potential for additive effects on cardiac conduction). Products include:
- Brevibloc Injection 942

Isoflurane (Cardiovascular side effects of anesthetics potentiated). Products include:
- Forane 600

Ketamine Hydrochloride (Cardiovascular side effects of anesthetics potentiated). Products include:
- Ketalar 1726

Labetalol Hydrochloride (Potential for additive effects on cardiac conduction). Products include:
- Normodyne Injection 2108
- Normodyne Tablets 2110
- Normozide Tablets 2112
- Trandate HCT Tablets 579
- Trandate Injection 577
- Trandate Tablets 579

Methohexital Sodium (Cardiovascular side effects of anesthetics potentiated). Products include:
- Brevital Sodium Vials 1248

Methoxyflurane (Cardiovascular side effects of anesthetics potentiated).
- No products indexed under this heading.

Metoprolol Tartrate (Potential for additive effects on cardiac conduction). Products include:
- Lopressor Ampuls 1032
- Lopressor HCT Tablets 1034
- Lopressor Tablets 1032

Nadolol (Potential for additive effects on cardiac conduction). Products include:
- Corgard Tablets 701
- Corzide Tablets 702

Penbutolol Sulfate (Potential for additive effects on cardiac conduction). Products include:
- Levatol 1832

Pindolol (Potential for additive effects on cardiac conduction). Products include:
- Visken Tablets 2036

Propofol (Cardiovascular side effects of anesthetics potentiated). Products include:
- Diprivan Injection 2267

Propranolol Hydrochloride (Potential for additive effects on cardiac conduction; increased propranolol levels). Products include:
- Inderal 2459
- Inderal LA Long Acting Capsules 2461
- Inderide Tablets 2463
- Inderide LA Long Acting Capsules .. 2465

Ranitidine Hydrochloride (Produces smaller increase in plasma levels). Products include:
- Zantac Injection and Zantac Injection Premixed 1063
- Zantac 1065

Timolol Maleate (Potential for additive effects on cardiac conduction). Products include:
- Blocadren Tablets 1429
- Timolide Tablets 1547
- Timoptic in Ocudose 1552
- Timoptic Sterile Ophthalmic Solution 1550

CARDIZEM SR CAPSULES-60 MG, 90 MG AND 120 MG

(Diltiazem Hydrochloride) 1327
May interact with beta blockers, cardiac glycosides, general anesthetics, drugs which undergo biotransformation by cytochrome p-450 mixed function oxidase, and certain other agents. Compounds in these categories include:

Acebutolol Hydrochloride (Concomitant administration may result in additive effects in prolonging AV conduction). Products include:
- Sectral Capsules 2520

Atenolol (Concomitant administration may result in additive effects in prolonging AV conduction). Products include:
- Tenoretic Tablets 1105
- Tenormin Tablets and I.V. Injection 1107

Betaxolol Hydrochloride (Concomitant administration may result in additive effects in prolonging AV conduction). Products include:
- Betoptic Sterile Ophthalmic Solution 569
- Betoptic S Sterile Ophthalmic Suspension 570
- Kerlone Tablets 2172

Carteolol Hydrochloride (Concomitant administration may result in additive effects in prolonging AV conduction). Products include:
- Cartrol Tablets 507

Cimetidine (Increases peak diltiazem plasma levels (58%) and AUC (53%)). Products include:
- Tagamet Tablets 2228

Cimetidine Hydrochloride (Increases peak diltiazem plasma levels (58%) and AUC (53%)). Products include:
- Tagamet 2228

Deslanoside (Additive effects on cardiac conduction; variable effect on plasma digoxin).
- No products indexed under this heading.

Digitoxin (Additive effects on cardiac conduction; variable effect on plasma digoxin). Products include:
- Crystodigin Tablets 1253

Digoxin (Additive effects on cardiac conduction; variable effect on plasma digoxin). Products include:
- Lanoxicaps 772
- Lanoxin Elixir Pediatric 775
- Lanoxin Injection 778
- Lanoxin Injection Pediatric 781
- Lanoxin Tablets 783

Drugs which undergo biotransformation by cytochrome P-450 mixed function oxidase (Coadministration may result in the competitive inhibition of metabolism).

Enflurane (Depression of cardiac contractility, conductivity, automaticity, and vasodilation may be potentiated). Products include:
- Ethrane 599

Esmolol Hydrochloride (Concomitant administration may result in additive effects in prolonging AV conduction). Products include:
- Brevibloc Injection 942

Isoflurane (Depression of cardiac contractility, conductivity, automaticity, and vasodilation may be potentiated). Products include:
- Forane 600

Ketamine Hydrochloride (Depression of cardiac contractility, conductivity, automaticity, and vasodilation may be potentiated). Products include:
- Ketalar 1726

Labetalol Hydrochloride (Concomitant administration may result in additive effects in prolonging AV conduction). Products include:
- Normodyne Injection 2108
- Normodyne Tablets 2110
- Normozide Tablets 2112
- Trandate HCT Tablets 579
- Trandate Injection 577
- Trandate Tablets 579

Methohexital Sodium (Depression of cardiac contractility, conductivity, automaticity, and vasodilation may be potentiated). Products include:
- Brevital Sodium Vials 1248

Methoxyflurane (Depression of cardiac contractility, conductivity, automaticity, and vasodilation may be potentiated).
- No products indexed under this heading.

Metoprolol Tartrate (Concomitant administration may result in additive effects in prolonging AV conduction). Products include:
- Lopressor Ampuls 1032
- Lopressor HCT Tablets 1034
- Lopressor Tablets 1032

Nadolol (Concomitant administration may result in additive effects in prolonging AV conduction). Products include:
- Corgard Tablets 701
- Corzide Tablets 702

Penbutolol Sulfate (Concomitant administration may result in additive effects in prolonging AV conduction). Products include:
- Levatol 1832

Pindolol (Concomitant administration may result in additive effects in prolonging AV conduction). Products include:
- Visken Tablets 2036

Propofol (Depression of cardiac contractility, conductivity, automaticity, and vasodilation may be potentiated). Products include:
- Diprivan Injection 2267

Propranolol Hydrochloride (Concomitant administration may result in additive effects in prolonging AV conduction; increased bioavailability of propranolol by 50%). Products include:
- Inderal 2459
- Inderal LA Long Acting Capsules 2461
- Inderide Tablets 2463
- Inderide LA Long Acting Capsules 2465

Ranitidine Hydrochloride (Produces smaller, nonsignificant increase in plasma levels). Products include:
- Zantac Injection and Zantac Injection Premixed 1063
- Zantac 1065

Timolol Maleate (Concomitant administration may result in additive effects in prolonging AV conduction). Products include:
- Blocadren Tablets 1429
- Timolide Tablets 1547
- Timoptic in Ocudose 1552
- Timoptic Sterile Ophthalmic Solution 1550

CARDURA TABLETS
(Doxazosin Mesylate) 1941
No interactions described in labeling.

CARMOL 20 CREAM
(Urea) ..... ■ 732
No interactions described in labeling.

CARMOL HC CREAM 1%
(Hydrocortisone Acetate) 2296
No interactions described in labeling.

CARMOL 10 LOTION
(Urea) ..... ■ 732
No interactions described in labeling.

CARNITOR
(L-Carnitine) 2188
No interactions described in labeling.

CARTROL TABLETS
(Carteolol Hydrochloride) 507
May interact with calcium channel blockers, insulin, oral hypoglycemic agents, non-steroidal anti-inflammatory agents, sympathomimetic bronchodilators, catecholamine depleting drugs, and general anesthetics. Compounds in these categories include:

Albuterol (Diminished response to therapy with a beta-receptor agonist). Products include:
- Proventil Inhalation Aerosol 2117
- Ventolin Inhalation Aerosol and Refill 583

Albuterol Sulfate (Diminished response to therapy with a beta-receptor agonist). Products include:
- Proventil Repetabs Tablets 2120
- Proventil Solutions for Inhalation 0.5% and 0.083% 2118
- Proventil Syrup 2119
- Proventil Tablets 2120
- Ventolin 583

Bepridil Hydrochloride (Potential for hypotension, AV conduction disturbances and LVF in some patients). Products include:
- Vascor (200, 300 and 400 mg) Tablets 1383

Bitolterol Mesylate (Diminished response to therapy with a beta-receptor agonist). Products include:
- Tornalate 2074

Chlorpropamide (Concomitant administration may result in hypo- or hyperglycemia). Products include:
- Diabinese Tablets 1775

Deserpidine (Possible additive effect). Products include:
- Enduronyl 518
- Harmonyl Tablets 528
- Oreticyl 545

Diclofenac Sodium (Possible blunting of the antihypertensive effect). Products include:
- Voltaren Ophthalmic Sterile Ophthalmic Solution ..... ◉ 268
- Voltaren Tablets 1042

Diltiazem Hydrochloride (Potential for hypotension, AV conduction disturbances and LVF in some patients). Products include:
- Cardizem Tablets-30 mg, 60 mg, 90 mg and 120 mg 1329
- Cardizem SR Capsules-60 mg, 90 mg and 120 mg 1327

Enflurane (Possible exaggeration of hypotension). Products include:
- Ethrane 599

Ephedrine Hydrochloride (Diminished response to therapy with a beta-receptor agonist). Products include:
- Amesec ..... ■ 682
- Primatene Tablets-M Formula 2421
- Primatene Tablets-P Formula 2421
- Primatene Tablets-Regular Formula 2421
- Quadrinal Tablets 1183
- Quelidrine Syrup 556
- Tedral SA 1765

Ephedrine Sulfate (Diminished response to therapy with a beta-receptor agonist). Products include:
- Bronkaid Tablets ..... ■ 757
- Bronkolixir ..... ■ 761
- Bronkotabs Tablets ..... ■ 762
- Marax Tablets & DF Syrup 1954
- Pazo Hemorrhoid Ointment & Suppositories 752
- Vicks Vatronol Nose Drops ..... ■ 666

Ephedrine Tannate (Diminished response to therapy with a beta-receptor agonist). Products include:
- Rynatuss 2388

Epinephrine (Diminished response to therapy with a beta-receptor agonist). Products include:
- Ana-Kit Anaphylaxis Emergency Treatment Kit 1100
- Bronkaid Mist ..... ■ 757
- EpiPen 843
- Marcaine Hydrochloride 0.5% with Epinephrine 1:200,000 (as bitartrate) 958
- Marcaine Hydrochloride with Epinephrine 1:200,000 2055
- Primatene Mist 2420
- Sus-Phrine Injection 1006
- Xylocaine with Epinephrine Injections 637

Epinephrine Hydrochloride (Diminished response to therapy with a beta-receptor agonist). Products include:
- Adrenalin Chloride Solution 1:100 & 1:1,000 1689
- Epifrin ..... ◉ 244
- Glaucon ..... ◉ 218

Ethylnorepinephrine Hydrochloride (Diminished response to therapy with a beta-receptor agonist). Products include:
- Bronkephrine Injection 2042

Etodolac (Possible blunting of the antihypertensive effect). Products include:
- Lodine Capsules 2468

Felodipine (Potential for hypotension, AV conduction disturbances and LVF in some patients). Products include:
- Plendil Extended-Release Tablets 1526

Fenoprofen Calcium (Possible blunting of the antihypertensive effect). Products include:
- Nalfon Pulvules & Tablets 919

Flurbiprofen (Possible blunting of the antihypertensive effect). Products include:
- Ansaid Tablets 2319

Glipizide (Concomitant administration may result in hypo- or hyperglycemia). Products include:
- Glucotrol 1952

Glyburide (Concomitant administration may result in hypo- or hyperglycemia). Products include:
- DiaBeta 1091
- Micronase Tablets 2350

Ibuprofen (Possible blunting of the antihypertensive effect). Products include:
- Advil Cold & Sinus Caplets (formerly CoAdvil) 2416
- Advil Ibuprofen Tablets and Caplets 2416
- Children's Advil Suspension 2426
- CoAdvil ..... ■ 748
- Dristan Sinus Caplets 2419
- Haltran Tablets ..... ■ 668
- Ibuprofen ..... ■ 631
- Medipren ibuprofen Caplets and Tablets 1362
- Midol 200 Cramp Relief Formula ..... ■ 570
- Motrin Tablets 2351
- Motrin IB Caplets and Tablets ..... ■ 736
- Nuprin Ibuprofen/Analgesic Tablets & Caplets 752
- PediaProfen Suspension 1363
- Rufen Tablets 691
- Trendar Ibuprofen Tablets ..... ■ 756

Indomethacin (Possible blunting of the antihypertensive effect). Products include:
- Indocin 1487

Indomethacin Sodium Trihydrate (Possible blunting of the antihypertensive effect). Products include:
- Indocin I.V. 1490

Insulin, Human (Concomitant administration may result in hypo- or hyperglycemia).
- No products indexed under this heading.

Insulin, Human Isophane Suspension (Concomitant administration may result in hypo- or hyperglycemia). Products include:
- Humulin N, 100 Units 1270

Insulin, Human NPH (Concomitant administration may result in hypo- or hyperglycemia). Products include:
- Insulatard NPH Human 1627
- Novolin N 1627
- Novolin N PenFill Cartridges 1628
- Novolin N Prefilled 1628

Insulin, Human Regular (Concomitant administration may result in hypo- or hyperglycemia). Products include:
- Humulin BR, 100 Units 1268
- Humulin R, 100 Units 1272
- Novolin R 1627
- Novolin R PenFill Cartridges 1628
- Novolin R Prefilled 1629
- Velosulin Human 1628

Insulin, Human, Zinc Suspension (Concomitant administration may result in hypo- or hyperglycemia). Products include:
- Humulin L, 100 Units 1268
- Humulin U, 100 Units 1272
- Novolin L 1627

Insulin, NPH (Concomitant administration may result in hypo- or hyperglycemia). Products include:
- NPH, 40 & 100 Units 1273
- Beef NPH, 100 Units 1274
- Pork NPH, 100 Units 1275
- Insulatard NPH 1626
- NPH Insulin 1626
- NPH Purified Pork Isophane Insulin 1626

Insulin, Regular (Concomitant administration may result in hypo- or hyperglycemia). Products include:
- Regular, 40 & 100 Units 1273
- Beef Regular, 100 Units 1275
- Pork Regular, 100 Units 1275
- Pork Regular (Concentrated), 500 Units 1276
- Regular Insulin 1625
- Regular Purified Pork Insulin 1626
- Velosulin 1627

Insulin, Zinc Crystals (Concomitant administration may result in hypo- or hyperglycemia). Products include:
- NPH, 40 & 100 Units 1273

Insulin, Zinc Suspension (Concomitant administration may result in hypo- or hyperglycemia). Products include:
- Lente, 40 & 100 Units 1272
- Protamine, Zinc, 40 & 100 Units 1273
- Lente Iletin I 1272
- Beef Lente, 100 Units 1274
- Beef Protamine Zinc, 100 Units 1274
- Pork Lente, 100 Units 1275
- Pork, Protamine, Zinc, 100 Units 1275
- Lente Insulin 1626
- Lente Purified Pork Insulin 1626
- Semilente Insulin 1625
- Ultralente Insulin 1626

Isoetharine (Diminished response to therapy with a beta-receptor agonist). Products include:
- Arm-a-Med Isoetharine Inhalation Solution, USP 616
- Bronkometer Aerosol 2042
- Bronkosol Solution 2042

Isoflurane (Possible exaggeration of hypotension). Products include:
- Forane 600

Isoproterenol Hydrochloride (Diminished response to therapy with a beta-receptor agonist). Products include:
- Isuprel Hydrochloride Injection 1:5000 ... 2050
- Isuprel Hydrochloride Mistometer .. 2051
- Isuprel Hydrochloride Solution 1:200 & 1:100 ... 2052
- Norisodrine Aerotrol ... 540

Isradipine (Potential for hypotension, AV conduction disturbances and LVF in some patients). Products include:
- DynaCirc Capsules ... 2004

Ketamine Hydrochloride (Possible exaggeration of hypotension). Products include:
- Ketalar ... 1726

Ketoprofen (Possible blunting of the antihypertensive effect). Products include:
- Orudis Capsules ... 2488

Ketorolac Tromethamine (Possible blunting of the antihypertensive effect). Products include:
- Toradol IM Injection ... 2302

Meclofenamate Sodium (Possible blunting of the antihypertensive effect). Products include:
- Meclomen Capsules ... 1739

Mefenamic Acid (Possible blunting of the antihypertensive effect). Products include:
- Ponstel ... 1758

Metaproterenol Sulfate (Diminished response to therapy with a beta-receptor agonist). Products include:
- Alupent ... 674
- Arm-a-Med Metaproterenol Sulfate Inhalation Solution, USP ... 617
- Metaprel Inhalation Aerosol Bronchodilator ... 2014
- Metaprel Inhalation Solution ... 2015
- Metaprel ... 2015
- Metaproterenol Sulfate Inhalation Solution, USP ... 912

Methohexital Sodium (Possible exaggeration of hypotension). Products include:
- Brevital Sodium Vials ... 1248

Methoxyflurane (Possible exaggeration of hypotension).
- No products indexed under this heading.

Naproxen (Possible blunting of the antihypertensive effect). Products include:
- Naprosyn ... 2297

Naproxen Sodium (Possible blunting of the antihypertensive effect). Products include:
- Anaprox and Anaprox DS Tablets.... 2288

Nicardipine Hydrochloride (Potential for hypotension, AV conduction disturbances and LVF in some patients). Products include:
- Cardene Capsules ... 2290

Nifedipine (Potential for hypotension, AV conduction disturbances and LVF in some patients). Products include:
- Adalat Capsules (10 mg and 20 mg) ... 1587
- Procardia Capsules ... 1781
- Procardia XL Tablets ... 1783

Nimodipine (Potential for hypotension, AV conduction disturbances and LVF in some patients). Products include:
- Nimotop Capsules ... 1607

Phenylbutazone (Possible blunting of the antihypertensive effect). Products include:
- Butazolidin Capsules & Tablets ... 1027

Pirbuterol Acetate (Diminished response to therapy with a beta-receptor agonist). Products include:
- Maxair Inhaler ... 1311

Piroxicam (Possible blunting of the antihypertensive effect). Products include:
- Feldene Capsules ... 1777

Propofol (Possible exaggeration of hypotension). Products include:
- Diprivan Injection ... 2267

Rauwolfia Serpentina (Possible additive effect). Products include:
- Raudixin Tablets ... 1803
- Rauzide Tablets ... 1804

Rescinnamine (Possible additive effect).
- No products indexed under this heading.

Reserpine (Possible additive effect). Products include:
- Diupres Tablets ... 1461
- Hydromox R Tablets ... 1209
- Hydropres Tablets ... 1485
- Renese-R Tablets ... 1786
- Salutensin/Salutensin-Demi ... 719
- Ser-Ap-Es Tablets ... 881
- Serpasil Tablets ... 883
- Serpasil-Apresoline Tablets ... 884
- Serpasil-Esidrix Tablets ... 886

Sulindac (Possible blunting of the antihypertensive effect). Products include:
- Clinoril Tablets ... 1433

Terbutaline Sulfate (Diminished response to therapy with a beta-receptor agonist). Products include:
- Brethaire Inhaler ... 1024
- Brethine Ampuls ... 1026
- Brethine Tablets ... 1026
- Bricanyl Injection ... 1324
- Bricanyl Tablets ... 1325

Tolazamide (Concomitant administration may result in hypo- or hyperglycemia). Products include:
- Tolinase Tablets ... 2365

Tolbutamide (Concomitant administration may result in hypo- or hyperglycemia). Products include:
- Orinase Tablets ... 2354

Tolmetin Sodium (Possible blunting of the antihypertensive effect). Products include:
- Tolectin (200, 400 and 600 mg) .. 1379

Verapamil Hydrochloride (Potential for hypotension, AV conduction disturbances and LVF in some patients). Products include:
- Calan SR Caplets ... 2157
- Calan Tablets ... 2155
- Isoptin Injectable ... 1177
- Isoptin Oral Tablets ... 1179
- Isoptin SR Sustained Release Tablets ... 1181
- Verelan Capsules ... 1243
- Verelan Capsules ... 2535

CASTELLANI PAINT
(Basic Fuchsin) ... 1769
No interactions described in labeling.

CATAPRES TABLETS
(Clonidine Hydrochloride) ... 676
May interact with tricyclic antidepressants, barbiturates, hypnotics and sedatives, cardiac glycosides, beta blockers, and certain other agents. Compounds in these categories include:

Acebutolol Hydrochloride (Rapid rise in blood pressure following sudden cessation of Catapres). Products include:
- Sectral Capsules ... 2520

Alcohol (Enhanced CNS-depressive effects).

Amitriptyline Hydrochloride (Enhanced manifestation of corneal lesions (in rats); reduced effect of clonidine). Products include:
- Elavil ... 2269
- Endep Tablets ... 1927
- Etrafon ... 2087
- Limbitrol ... 1933
- Triavil Tablets ... 1556

Amoxapine (Reduced effect of clonidine). Products include:
- Asendin Tablets ... 1196

Aprobarbital (Enhanced CNS-depressive effects). Products include:
- Alurate Elixir ... 1883

Atenolol (Rapid rise in blood pressure following sudden cessation of Catapres). Products include:
- Tenoretic Tablets ... 1105
- Tenormin Tablets and I.V. Injection 1107

Betaxolol Hydrochloride (Rapid rise in blood pressure following sudden cessation of Catapres). Products include:
- Betoptic Sterile Ophthalmic Solution ... 569
- Betoptic S Sterile Ophthalmic Suspension ... 570
- Kerlone Tablets ... 2172

Butabarbital (Enhanced CNS-depressive effects). Products include:
- Pyridium Plus ... 1764

Butalbital (Enhanced CNS-depressive effects). Products include:
- Esgic-Plus Tablets ... 1002
- Esgic Tablets & Capsules ... 1001
- Fioricet Tablets ... 2006
- Fiorinal Capsules ... 2007
- Fiorinal with Codeine Capsules ... 2008
- Fiorinal Tablets ... 2007
- Phrenilin ... 838
- Sedapap Tablets 50 mg/650 mg .. 1360

Carteolol Hydrochloride (Rapid rise in blood pressure following sudden cessation of Catapres). Products include:
- Cartrol Tablets ... 507

Clomipramine Hydrochloride (Enhanced manifestation of corneal lesions (in rats); reduced effect of clonidine). Products include:
- Anafranil Capsules ... 650

Desipramine Hydrochloride (Reduced effect of clonidine). Products include:
- Norpramin Tablets ... 1340

Deslanoside (Sinus bradycardia and atrioventricular block (rare)).
- No products indexed under this heading.

Digitoxin (Sinus bradycardia and atrioventricular block (rare)). Products include:
- Crystodigin Tablets ... 1253

Digoxin (Sinus bradycardia and atrioventricular block (rare)). Products include:
- Lanoxicaps ... 772
- Lanoxin Elixir Pediatric ... 775
- Lanoxin Injection ... 778
- Lanoxin Injection Pediatric ... 781
- Lanoxin Tablets ... 783

Doxepin Hydrochloride (Reduced effect of clonidine). Products include:
- Sinequan ... 1960

Esmolol Hydrochloride (Rapid rise in blood pressure following sudden cessation of Catapres). Products include:
- Brevibloc Injection ... 942

Estazolam (Enhanced CNS-depressive effects). Products include:
- ProSom Tablets ... 554

Ethchlorvynol (Enhanced CNS-depressive effects). Products include:
- Placidyl Capsules ... 553

Ethinamate (Enhanced CNS-depressive effects).
- No products indexed under this heading.

Flurazepam Hydrochloride (Enhanced CNS-depressive effects). Products include:
- Dalmane Capsules ... 1927

Glutethimide (Enhanced CNS-depressive effects).
- No products indexed under this heading.

Imipramine Hydrochloride (Reduced effect of clonidine). Products include:
- Tofranil Ampuls ... 1038
- Tofranil Tablets ... 1039

Imipramine Pamoate (Reduced effect of clonidine). Products include:
- Tofranil-PM Capsules ... 1041

Labetalol Hydrochloride (Rapid rise in blood pressure following sudden cessation of Catapres). Products include:
- Normodyne Injection ... 2108
- Normodyne Tablets ... 2110
- Normozide Tablets ... 2112
- Trandate HCT Tablets ... 579
- Trandate Injection ... 577
- Trandate Tablets ... 579

Lorazepam (Enhanced CNS-depressive effects). Products include:
- Ativan Injection ... 2432
- Ativan Tablets ... 2434

Maprotiline Hydrochloride (Reduced effect of clonidine). Products include:
- Ludiomil Tablets ... 874

Mephobarbital (Enhanced CNS-depressive effects). Products include:
- Mebaral Tablets ... 2061

Methyltestosterone (Enhanced CNS-depressive effects). Products include:
- Android ... 1111
- Estratest ... 2245
- Mediatric Capsules ... 2476
- Metandren Linguets and Tablets ... 875
- Premarin with Methyltestosterone .. 2515
- Testred Capsules ... 1124

Metoprolol Tartrate (Rapid rise in blood pressure following sudden cessation of Catapres). Products include:
- Lopressor Ampuls ... 1032
- Lopressor HCT Tablets ... 1034
- Lopressor Tablets ... 1032

Midazolam Hydrochloride (Enhanced CNS-depressive effects). Products include:
- Versed Injection ... 1924

Nadolol (Rapid rise in blood pressure following sudden cessation of Catapres). Products include:
- Corgard Tablets ... 701
- Corzide Tablets ... 702

Nortriptyline Hydrochloride (Reduced effect of clonidine). Products include:
- Pamelor ... 2019

Penbutolol Sulfate (Rapid rise in blood pressure following sudden cessation of Catapres). Products include:
- Levatol ... 1832

Pentobarbital Sodium (Effect not specified). Products include:
- Nembutal Sodium Capsules ... 534
- Nembutal Sodium Solution ... 536
- Nembutal Sodium Suppositories ... 538

Phenobarbital (Enhanced CNS-depressive effects). Products include:
- Arco-Lase Plus Tablets ... 607
- Bellergal-S Tablets ... 1998
- Bronkolixir ... ▣ 761
- Bronkotabs Tablets ... ▣ 762
- Donnatal ... 1858
- Donnatal Extentabs ... 1859

Donnatal Tablets ... 1858
Donnazyme Tablets ... 1860
Kinesed Tablets ... 2272
Phenobarbital Elixir and Tablets ... 1293
Primatene Tablets-P Formula ... 2421
Quadrinal Tablets ... 1183
Tedral SA ... 1765

Pindolol (Rapid rise in blood pressure following sudden cessation of Catapres). Products include:
Visken Tablets ... 2036

Propofol (Enhanced CNS-depressive effects). Products include:
Diprivan Injection ... 2267

Propranolol Hydrochloride (Rapid rise in blood pressure following sudden cessation of Catapres). Products include:
Inderal ... 2459
Inderal LA Long Acting Capsules ... 2461
Inderide Tablets ... 2463
Inderide LA Long Acting Capsules ... 2465

Protriptyline Hydrochloride (Reduced effect of clonidine). Products include:
Vivactil Tablets ... 1567

Quazepam (Enhanced CNS-depressive effects). Products include:
Doral Tablets ... 2383

Secobarbital Sodium (Enhanced CNS-depressive effects). Products include:
Seconal Sodium Pulvules ... 1296

Temazepam (Enhanced CNS-depressive effects). Products include:
Restoril Capsules ... 2023

Thiamylal Sodium (Enhanced CNS-depressive effects). Products include:
Surital Ampoules, Steri-Vials ... 1764

Timolol Maleate (Rapid rise in blood pressure following sudden cessation of Catapres). Products include:
Blocadren Tablets ... 1429
Timolide Tablets ... 1547
Timoptic in Ocudose ... 1552
Timoptic Sterile Ophthalmic Solution ... 1550

Triazolam (Enhanced CNS-depressive effects). Products include:
Halcion Tablets ... 2340

Trimipramine Maleate (Reduced effect of clonidine). Products include:
Surmontil Capsules ... 2524

CATAPRES-TTS

(Clonidine) ... 677
May interact with tricyclic antidepressants, barbiturates, hypnotics and sedatives, and certain other agents. Compounds in these categories include:

Alcohol (Enhanced CNS-depressive effects).

Amitriptyline Hydrochloride (Enhanced manifestation of corneal lesions (in rats); reduced effect of clonidine). Products include:
Elavil ... 2269
Endep Tablets ... 1927
Etrafon ... 2087
Limbitrol ... 1933
Triavil Tablets ... 1556

Amoxapine (Reduced effect of clonidine). Products include:
Asendin Tablets ... 1196

Aprobarbital (Enhanced CNS-depressive effects). Products include:
Alurate Elixir ... 1883

Butabarbital (Enhanced CNS-depressive effects). Products include:
Pyridium Plus ... 1764

Butalbital (Enhanced CNS-depressive effects). Products include:
Esgic-Plus Tablets ... 1002
Esgic Tablets & Capsules ... 1001
Fioricet Tablets ... 2006
Fiorinal Capsules ... 2007
Fiorinal with Codeine Capsules ... 2008
Fiorinal Tablets ... 2007
Phrenilin ... 838
Sedapap Tablets 50 mg/650 mg ... 1360

Clomipramine Hydrochloride (Enhanced manifestation of corneal lesions (in rats); reduced effect of clonidine). Products include:
Anafranil Capsules ... 650

Desipramine Hydrochloride (Reduced effect of clonidine). Products include:
Norpramin Tablets ... 1340

Doxepin Hydrochloride (Reduced effect of clonidine). Products include:
Sinequan ... 1960

Estazolam (Enhanced CNS-depressive effects). Products include:
ProSom Tablets ... 554

Ethchlorvynol (Enhanced CNS-depressive effects). Products include:
Placidyl Capsules ... 553

Ethinamate (Enhanced CNS-depressive effects).
No products indexed under this heading.

Flurazepam Hydrochloride (Enhanced CNS-depressive effects). Products include:
Dalmane Capsules ... 1927

Glutethimide (Enhanced CNS-depressive effects).
No products indexed under this heading.

Imipramine Hydrochloride (Reduced effect of clonidine). Products include:
Tofranil Ampuls ... 1038
Tofranil Tablets ... 1039

Imipramine Pamoate (Reduced effect of clonidine). Products include:
Tofranil-PM Capsules ... 1041

Lorazepam (Enhanced CNS-depressive effects). Products include:
Ativan Injection ... 2432
Ativan Tablets ... 2434

Maprotiline Hydrochloride (Reduced effect of clonidine). Products include:
Ludiomil Tablets ... 874

Mephobarbital (Enhanced CNS-depressive effects). Products include:
Mebaral Tablets ... 2061

Midazolam Hydrochloride (Enhanced CNS-depressive effects). Products include:
Versed Injection ... 1924

Nortriptyline Hydrochloride (Reduced effect of clonidine). Products include:
Pamelor ... 2019

Pentobarbital Sodium (Enhanced CNS-depressive effects). Products include:
Nembutal Sodium Capsules ... 534
Nembutal Sodium Solution ... 536
Nembutal Sodium Suppositories ... 538

Phenobarbital (Enhanced CNS-depressive effects). Products include:
Arco-Lase Plus Tablets ... 607
Bellergal-S Tablets ... 1998
Bronkolixir ... ▣ 761
Bronkotabs Tablets ... ▣ 762
Donnatal ... 1858
Donnatal Extentabs ... 1859
Donnatal Tablets ... 1858
Donnazyme Tablets ... 1860
Kinesed Tablets ... 2272
Phenobarbital Elixir and Tablets ... 1293
Primatene Tablets-P Formula ... 2421
Quadrinal Tablets ... 1183
Tedral SA ... 1765

Propofol (Enhanced CNS-depressive effects). Products include:
Diprivan Injection ... 2267

Protriptyline Hydrochloride (Reduced effect of clonidine). Products include:
Vivactil Tablets ... 1567

Quazepam (Enhanced CNS-depressive effects). Products include:
Doral Tablets ... 2383

Secobarbital Sodium (Enhanced CNS-depressive effects). Products include:
Seconal Sodium Pulvules ... 1296

Temazepam (Enhanced CNS-depressive effects). Products include:
Restoril Capsules ... 2023

Thiamylal Sodium (Enhanced CNS-depressive effects). Products include:
Surital Ampoules, Steri-Vials ... 1764

Triazolam (Enhanced CNS-depressive effects). Products include:
Halcion Tablets ... 2340

Trimipramine Maleate (Reduced effect of clonidine). Products include:
Surmontil Capsules ... 2524

CECLOR PULVULES & SUSPENSION

(Cefaclor) ... 1251
May interact with certain other agents. Compounds in this category include:

Warfarin Sodium (Rare reports of increased prothrombin time—with or without clinical bleeding—with concomitant use). Products include:
Coumadin Injection & Tablets ... 944
Panwarfin Tablets ... 547

CEENU

(Lomustine (CCNU)) ... 725
No interactions described in labeling.

CEFIZOX INJECTION

(Ceftizoxime Sodium) ... 1012
May interact with aminoglycosides. Compounds in this category include:

Amikacin Sulfate (Concomitant administration may result in possible nephrotoxicity). Products include:
Amikin Injectable ... 602

Gentamicin Sulfate (Concomitant administration may result in possible nephrotoxicity). Products include:
Garamycin Injectable ... 2093
Garamycin Ophthalmic ... ◉ 305
Genoptic Liquifilm Sterile Ophthalmic Solution ... ◉ 247
Genoptic S.O.P. Sterile Ophthalmic Ointment ... ◉ 247
Gentacidin Ointment ... ◉ 273
Gentacidin Solution ... ◉ 273
Gentak Ointment & Solution ... ◉ 208
G-myticin Creme and Ointment 0.1% ... 1770
Pred-G Liquifilm Sterile Ophthalmic Suspension ... ◉ 252
Pred-G S.O.P. Sterile Ophthalmic Ointment ... ◉ 253

Kanamycin Sulfate (Concomitant administration may result in possible nephrotoxicity). Products include:
Kantrex Injection ... 601
Kantrex Pediatric Injection ... 601

Streptomycin Sulfate (Concomitant administration may result in possible nephrotoxicity).
No products indexed under this heading.

Tobramycin Sulfate (Concomitant administration may result in possible nephrotoxicity). Products include:
Nebcin Vials, Hyporets & ADD-Vantage ... 1286

CEFOBID INTRAVENOUS/INTRAMUSCULAR

(Cefoperazone Sodium) ... 1943
May interact with aminoglycosides and certain other agents. Compounds in these categories include:

Alcohol (When ingested within 72 hours, flushing, sweating, headache, and tachycardia have been reported).

Amikacin Sulfate (Nephrotoxicity). Products include:
Amikin Injectable ... 602

Gentamicin Sulfate (Nephrotoxicity). Products include:
Garamycin Injectable ... 2093
Garamycin Ophthalmic ... ◉ 305
Genoptic Liquifilm Sterile Ophthalmic Solution ... ◉ 247
Genoptic S.O.P. Sterile Ophthalmic Ointment ... ◉ 247
Gentacidin Ointment ... ◉ 273
Gentacidin Solution ... ◉ 273
Gentak Ointment & Solution ... ◉ 208
G-myticin Creme and Ointment 0.1% ... 1770
Pred-G Liquifilm Sterile Ophthalmic Suspension ... ◉ 252
Pred-G S.O.P. Sterile Ophthalmic Ointment ... ◉ 253

Kanamycin Sulfate (Nephrotoxicity). Products include:
Kantrex Injection ... 601
Kantrex Pediatric Injection ... 601

Streptomycin Sulfate (Nephrotoxicity).
No products indexed under this heading.

Tobramycin (Nephrotoxicity). Products include:
TobraDex Ophthalmic Suspension and Ointment ... ◉ 228
Tobrex Ophthalmic Ointment and Solution ... 572

Tobramycin Sulfate (Nephrotoxicity). Products include:
Nebcin Vials, Hyporets & ADD-Vantage ... 1286

CEFOBID PHARMACY BULK PACKAGE - NOT FOR DIRECT INFUSION

(Cefoperazone Sodium) ... 1945
May interact with aminoglycosides and certain other agents. Compounds in these categories include:

Alcohol (A disulfiram-like reaction characterized by flushing, sweating, headache, and tachycardia has been reported when alcohol was ingested within 72 hours after Cefobid administration).

Amikacin Sulfate (Potential for nephrotoxicity). Products include:
Amikin Injectable ... 602

Gentamicin Sulfate (Potential for nephrotoxicity). Products include:
Garamycin Injectable ... 2093
Garamycin Ophthalmic ... ◉ 305
Genoptic Liquifilm Sterile Ophthalmic Solution ... ◉ 247
Genoptic S.O.P. Sterile Ophthalmic Ointment ... ◉ 247
Gentacidin Ointment ... ◉ 273
Gentacidin Solution ... ◉ 273
Gentak Ointment & Solution ... ◉ 208
G-myticin Creme and Ointment 0.1% ... 1770
Pred-G Liquifilm Sterile Ophthalmic Suspension ... ◉ 252
Pred-G S.O.P. Sterile Ophthalmic Ointment ... ◉ 253

Kanamycin Sulfate (Potential for nephrotoxicity). Products include:
Kantrex Injection ... 601
Kantrex Pediatric Injection ... 601

Streptomycin Sulfate (Potential for nephrotoxicity).
No products indexed under this heading.

Tobramycin (Potential for nephrotoxicity). Products include:
- TobraDex Ophthalmic Suspension and Ointment ◉ 228
- Tobrex Ophthalmic Ointment and Solution 572

Tobramycin Sulfate (Potential for nephrotoxicity). Products include:
- Nebcin Vials, Hyporets & ADD-Vantage 1286

CEFOL FILMTAB
(Vitamin B Complex With Vitamin C) 509
No interactions described in labeling.

CEFOTAN
(Cefotetan) 2265
May interact with aminoglycosides. Compounds in this category include:

Amikacin Sulfate (Potentiation of nephrotoxicity). Products include:
- Amikin Injectable 602

Gentamicin Sulfate (Potentiation of nephrotoxicity). Products include:
- Garamycin Injectable 2093
- Garamycin Ophthalmic ◉ 305
- Genoptic Liquifilm Sterile Ophthalmic Solution ◉ 247
- Genoptic S.O.P. Sterile Ophthalmic Ointment ◉ 247
- Gentacidin Ointment ◉ 273
- Gentacidin Solution ◉ 273
- Gentak Ointment & Solution ◉ 208
- G-myticin Creme and Ointment 0.1% 1770
- Pred-G Liquifilm Sterile Ophthalmic Suspension ◉ 252
- Pred-G S.O.P. Sterile Ophthalmic Ointment ◉ 253

Kanamycin Sulfate (Potentiation of nephrotoxicity). Products include:
- Kantrex Injection 601
- Kantrex Pediatric Injection 601

Streptomycin Sulfate (Potentiation of nephrotoxicity).
No products indexed under this heading.

Tobramycin Sulfate (Potentiation of nephrotoxicity). Products include:
- Nebcin Vials, Hyporets & ADD-Vantage 1286

CEFTIN TABLETS
(Cefuroxime Axetil) 575
May interact with:

Diphenoxylate Hydrochloride (May prolong and/or worsen pseudomembranous colitis). Products include:
- Lomotil 2174

Paregoric (May prolong and/or worsen pseudomembranous colitis). Products include:
- Donnagel-PG 1858

Probenecid (Increases serum concentration of cefuroxime). Products include:
- Benemid Tablets 1426
- ColBENEMID Tablets 1436
- Wycillin Injection and Probenecid Tablets 2539

Food Interactions

Food, unspecified (Absorption is greater when taken after food).

CELESTONE SOLUSPAN SUSPENSION
(Betamethasone Sodium Phosphate, Betamethasone Acetate) 2081
May interact with:

Aspirin (Use cautiously). Products include:
- Alka-Seltzer Effervescent Antacid and Pain Reliever 1568
- Alka-Seltzer Extra Strength Effervescent Antacid and Pain Reliever 1570
- Alka-Seltzer (Flavored) Effervescent Antacid and Pain Reliever 1569
- Alka-Seltzer Plus Cold Medicine ▣ 623
- Alka-Seltzer Plus Night-Time Cold Medicine ▣ 623
- Alka Seltzer Plus Sinus Allergy Medicine ▣ 624
- Anacin Coated Analgesic Caplets 2417
- Anacin Coated Analgesic Tablets 2417
- Anacin Maximum Strength Analgesic Coated Tablets 2417
- Maximum Strength Arthritis Pain Formula By the Makers of Anacin Analgesic Tablets and Caplets 2418
- Arthritis Pain Formula by the Makers of Anacin Analgesic Tablets and Caplets ▣ 747
- Arthritis Strength BC Powder ▣ 516
- Ascriptin A/D Caplets 1850
- Regular Strength Ascriptin Tablets 1850
- Azdōne Tablets 844
- BC Powder ▣ 517
- BC Cold Powder ▣ 517
- Children's Bayer Chewable Aspirin ▣ 564
- Genuine Bayer Aspirin Tablets & Caplets ▣ 564
- Maximum Bayer Aspirin Tablets & Caplets ▣ 566
- Bayer Plus Aspirin Tablets ▣ 567
- Therapy Bayer Aspirin Caplets ▣ 568
- 8 Hour Bayer Timed-Release Aspirin ▣ 566
- Arthritis Strength Bufferin Analgesic Caplets 744
- Extra Strength Bufferin Analgesic Tablets 745
- Bufferin Analgesic Tablets and Caplets 743
- Cama Arthritis Pain Reliever ▣ 685
- Damason-P 1356
- Easprin 1719
- Ecotrin Enteric Coated Aspirin Maximum Strength Tablets and Caplets 2189
- Ecotrin Enteric Coated Aspirin Regular Strength Tablets and Caplets 2189
- Empirin Aspirin ▣ 541
- Empirin with Codeine Phosphate Nos. 2, 3 & 4 764
- Equagesic Tablets 2451
- Excedrin Extra-Strength Analgesic Tablets & Caplets 749
- 4-Way Cold Tablets 750
- Fiorinal Capsules 2007
- Fiorinal with Codeine Capsules 2008
- Fiorinal Tablets 2007
- Lortab ASA Tablets 2414
- Momentum Muscular Backache Formula ▣ 751
- Norgesic 1314
- Norwich Extra-Strength Aspirin ▣ 546
- Norwich Regular Strength Aspirin ▣ 547
- P-A-C Analgesic Tablets ▣ 669
- Percodan 951
- Robaxisal Tablets 1872
- Sine-Off Sinus Medicine Tablets-Aspirin Formula ▣ 722
- Soma Compound w/Codeine Tablets 2390
- Soma Compound Tablets 2389
- St. Joseph Adult Chewable Aspirin (81 mg.) ▣ 703
- Synalgos-DC Capsules 2525
- Talwin Compound 2072
- Ursinus Inlay-Tabs ▣ 691
- Vanquish Analgesic Caplets ▣ 574
- Zorprin Tablets 698

Aspirin, Enteric Coated (Use cautiously). Products include:
- Therapy Bayer Aspirin Caplets ▣ 568
- Ecotrin 2189

Immunization (Neurological complications).

CELLUFRESH LUBRICANT OPHTHALMIC SOLUTION
(Carboxymethylcellulose Sodium) .. ◉ 243
No interactions described in labeling.

CELLUVISC LUBRICANT OPHTHALMIC SOLUTION
(Carboxymethylcellulose Sodium) .. ◉ 243
No interactions described in labeling.

CELONTIN (HALF STRENGTH) KAPSEALS
(Methsuximide) 1692
See **Celontin Kapseals**

CELONTIN KAPSEALS
(Methsuximide) 1692
May interact with anticonvulsants. Compounds in this category include:

Carbamazepine (Effect not specified; periodic serum level determination may be necessary). Products include:
- Tegretol Chewable Tablets 654
- Tegretol Suspension 656
- Tegretol Tablets 654

Divalproex Sodium (Effect not specified; periodic serum level determination may be necessary). Products include:
- Depakote 512

Ethosuximide (Effect not specified; periodic serum level determination may be necessary). Products include:
- Zarontin Capsules 1768
- Zarontin Syrup 1769

Ethotoin (Effect not specified; periodic serum level determination may be necessary). Products include:
- Peganone Tablets 551

Mephenytoin (Effect not specified; periodic serum level determination may be necessary). Products include:
- Mesantoin Tablets 2013

Paramethadione (Effect not specified; periodic serum level determination may be necessary). Products include:
- Paradione Capsules 548

Phenacemide (Effect not specified; periodic serum level determination may be necessary). Products include:
- Phenurone Tablets 552

Phenobarbital (Increased plasma concentration of phenobarbital). Products include:
- Arco-Lase Plus Tablets 607
- Bellergal-S Tablets 1998
- Bronkolixir ▣ 761
- Bronkotabs Tablets ▣ 762
- Donnatal 1858
- Donnatal Extentabs 1859
- Donnatal Tablets 1858
- Donnazyme Tablets 1860
- Kinesed Tablets 2272
- Phenobarbital Elixir and Tablets 1293
- Primatene Tablets-P Formula 2421
- Quadrinal Tablets 1183
- Tedral SA 1765

Phensuximide (Effect not specified; periodic serum level determination may be necessary). Products include:
- Milontin Kapseals 1741

Phenytoin (Increased plasma concentration of phenytoin). Products include:
- Dilantin Infatabs 1710
- Dilantin-30 Pediatric/Dilantin-125 Suspension 1713

Phenytoin Sodium (Increased plasma concentration of phenytoin). Products include:
- Dilantin Kapseals 1708
- Dilantin Parenteral 1712
- Dilantin with Phenobarbital Kapseals 1715

Primidone (Effect not specified; periodic serum level determination may be necessary). Products include:
- Mysoline 2480

Trimethadione (Effect not specified; periodic serum level determination may be necessary). Products include:
- Tridione 557

Valproic Acid (Effect not specified; periodic serum level determination may be necessary). Products include:
- Depakene Capsules & Syrup 511

CENTRAX CAPSULES
(Prazepam) 1693
May interact with phenothiazines, monoamine oxidase inhibitors, central nervous system depressants, barbiturates, narcotic analgesics, antidepressant drugs, and certain other agents. Compounds in these categories include:

Alcohol (May potentiate the action of Centrax).

Alfentanil Hydrochloride (May potentiate the action of Centrax). Products include:
- Alfenta Injection 1131

Alprazolam (May potentiate the action of Centrax). Products include:
- Xanax Tablets 2367

Amitriptyline Hydrochloride (May potentiate the action of Centrax). Products include:
- Elavil 2269
- Endep Tablets 1927
- Etrafon 2087
- Limbitrol 1933
- Triavil Tablets 1556

Amoxapine (May potentiate the action of Centrax). Products include:
- Asendin Tablets 1196

Aprobarbital (May potentiate the action of Centrax). Products include:
- Alurate Elixir 1883

Buprenorphine (May potentiate the action of Centrax).
No products indexed under this heading.

Bupropion Hydrochloride (May potentiate the action of Centrax). Products include:
- Wellbutrin Tablets 821

Buspirone Hydrochloride (May potentiate the action of Centrax). Products include:
- BuSpar 1401

Butabarbital (May potentiate the action of Centrax). Products include:
- Pyridium Plus 1764

Butalbital (May potentiate the action of Centrax). Products include:
- Esgic-Plus Tablets 1002
- Esgic Tablets & Capsules 1001
- Fioricet Tablets 2006
- Fiorinal Capsules 2007
- Fiorinal with Codeine Capsules 2008
- Fiorinal Tablets 2007
- Phrenilin 838
- Sedapap Tablets 50 mg/650 mg .. 1360

Chlordiazepoxide (May potentiate the action of Centrax). Products include:
- Libritabs Tablets 1930
- Limbitrol 1933
- Menrium Tablets 1934

Chlordiazepoxide Hydrochloride (May potentiate the action of Centrax). Products include:
- Librax Capsules 1929
- Librium Capsules 1931
- Librium Injectable 1932

Chlorpromazine (May potentiate the action of Centrax). Products include:
- Thorazine 2234

Chlorprothixene (May potentiate the action of Centrax). Products include:
- Taractan Tablets 1920

Chlorprothixene Hydrochloride (May potentiate the action of Centrax). Products include:
- Taractan ... 1920

Clorazepate Dipotassium (May potentiate the action of Centrax). Products include:
- Tranxene ... 556

Codeine (May potentiate the action of Centrax). Products include:
- Calcidrine Syrup ... 506

Codeine Phosphate (May potentiate the action of Centrax). Products include:
- Actifed with Codeine Cough Syrup.. 752
- Cheracol Cough Syrup ... 1853
- Codimal PH Syrup ... 846
- Dimetane-DC Cough Syrup ... 1857
- Empirin with Codeine Phosphate Nos. 2, 3 & 4 ... 764
- Fiorinal with Codeine Capsules ... 2008
- Isoclor Expectorant ... 982
- Naldecon CX Adult Liquid ... ▣ 521
- Novahistine DH ... 1342
- Novahistine Expectorant ... 1343
- Nucofed Capsules ... 2219
- Nucofed Expectorant ... 2219
- Nucofed Pediatric Expectorant ... 2220
- Nucofed Syrup ... 2219
- Phenaphen with Codeine Capsules 1865
- Phenaphen-650 with Codeine Tablets ... 1866
- Phenergan with Codeine ... 2497
- Phenergan VC with Codeine ... 2501
- Robitussin A-C Syrup ... 1875
- Robitussin-DAC Syrup ... 1875
- Ryna ... ▣ 741
- Soma Compound w/Codeine Tablets ... 2390
- Triaminic Expectorant w/Codeine .. 1996
- Tussi-Organidin Liquid ... 2391
- Tylenol with Codeine ... 1381

Codeine Polistirex (May potentiate the action of Centrax).
- No products indexed under this heading.

Desipramine Hydrochloride (May potentiate the action of Centrax). Products include:
- Norpramin Tablets ... 1340

Dezocine (May potentiate the action of Centrax).

Diazepam (May potentiate the action of Centrax). Products include:
- Valium Injectable ... 1937
- Valium Tablets ... 1939
- Valrelease Capsules ... 1923

Doxepin Hydrochloride (May potentiate the action of Centrax). Products include:
- Sinequan ... 1960

Droperidol (May potentiate the action of Centrax). Products include:
- Inapsine Injection ... 1140
- Innovar Injection ... 1141

Enflurane (May potentiate the action of Centrax). Products include:
- Ethrane ... 599

Estazolam (May potentiate the action of Centrax). Products include:
- ProSom Tablets ... 554

Ethchlorvynol (May potentiate the action of Centrax). Products include:
- Placidyl Capsules ... 553

Ethinamate (May potentiate the action of Centrax).
- No products indexed under this heading.

Fentanyl (May potentiate the action of Centrax). Products include:
- Duragesic Transdermal System ... 1133

Fentanyl Citrate (May potentiate the action of Centrax). Products include:
- Innovar Injection ... 1141
- Sublimaze Injection ... 1146

Fluoxetine Hydrochloride (May potentiate the action of Centrax). Products include:
- Prozac Pulvules ... 920

Fluphenazine Decanoate (May potentiate the action of Centrax). Products include:
- Prolixin Decanoate ... 1795

Fluphenazine Enanthate (May potentiate the action of Centrax). Products include:
- Prolixin Enanthate ... 1796

Fluphenazine Hydrochloride (May potentiate the action of Centrax). Products include:
- Prolixin Elixir ... 1793
- Prolixin Injection ... 1791
- Prolixin Oral Concentrate ... 1792
- Prolixin Tablets ... 1793

Flurazepam Hydrochloride (May potentiate the action of Centrax). Products include:
- Dalmane Capsules ... 1927

Furazolidone (May potentiate the action of Centrax). Products include:
- Furoxone ... 1855

Glutethimide (May potentiate the action of Centrax).
- No products indexed under this heading.

Haloperidol (May potentiate the action of Centrax). Products include:
- Haldol Injection, Tablets and Concentrate ... 1373

Haloperidol Decanoate (May potentiate the action of Centrax). Products include:
- Haldol Decanoate ... 1375

Hydrocodone Bitartrate (May potentiate the action of Centrax). Products include:
- Anexsia 5/500 Tablets ... 2196
- Anexsia 7.5/650 Tablets ... 2197
- Azdône Tablets ... 844
- Codiclear DH Syrup ... 845
- Codimal DH Syrup ... 846
- Damason-P ... 1356
- Hycodan Syrup, Tablets ... 927
- Hycomine Compound Tablets ... 929
- Hycomine Syrup ... 927
- Hycotuss Expectorant Syrup ... 930
- Hydrocet Capsules ... 835
- Lortab ASA Tablets ... 2414
- Lortab ... 2412
- Ru-Tuss with Hydrocodone ... 694
- Triaminic Expectorant DH ... 1995
- Vicodin Tablets ... 1187
- Vicodin ES Tablets ... 1189
- Zydone Capsules ... 941

Hydrocodone Polistirex (May potentiate the action of Centrax). Products include:
- Tussionex Extended-Release Suspension ... 988

Hydroxyzine Hydrochloride (May potentiate the action of Centrax). Products include:
- Atarax Tablets & Syrup ... 1941
- Marax Tablets & DF Syrup ... 1954
- Vistaril Intramuscular Solution ... 1970

Imipramine Hydrochloride (May potentiate the action of Centrax). Products include:
- Tofranil Ampuls ... 1038
- Tofranil Tablets ... 1039

Imipramine Pamoate (May potentiate the action of Centrax). Products include:
- Tofranil-PM Capsules ... 1041

Isocarboxazid (May potentiate the action of Centrax). Products include:
- Marplan Tablets ... 1906

Isoflurane (May potentiate the action of Centrax). Products include:
- Forane ... 600

Ketamine Hydrochloride (May potentiate the action of Centrax). Products include:
- Ketalar ... 1726

Levorphanol Tartrate (May potentiate the action of Centrax). Products include:
- Levo-Dromoran ... 1906

Lorazepam (May potentiate the action of Centrax). Products include:
- Ativan Injection ... 2432
- Ativan Tablets ... 2434

Loxapine Hydrochloride (May potentiate the action of Centrax). Products include:
- Loxitane ... 1213

Loxapine Succinate (May potentiate the action of Centrax). Products include:
- Loxitane Capsules ... 1213

Maprotiline Hydrochloride (May potentiate the action of Centrax). Products include:
- Ludiomil Tablets ... 874

Meperidine Hydrochloride (May potentiate the action of Centrax). Products include:
- Demerol ... 2047
- Mepergan Injection ... 2479

Mephobarbital (May potentiate the action of Centrax). Products include:
- Mebaral Tablets ... 2061

Meprobamate (May potentiate the action of Centrax). Products include:
- Deprol Tablets ... 2382
- Equagesic Tablets ... 2451
- Miltown Tablets ... 2386
- PMB 200 and PMB 400 ... 2504

Mesoridazine (May potentiate the action of Centrax). Products include:
- Serentil ... 686

Mesoridazine Besylate (May potentiate the action of Centrax).

Methadone Hydrochloride (May potentiate the action of Centrax). Products include:
- Dolophine Hydrochloride Ampoules & Vials ... 1260
- Dolophine Hydrochloride Tablets ... 1261
- Methadone Hydrochloride Diskets .. 1284
- Methadone Hydrochloride Oral Solution & Tablets ... 1987

Methohexital Sodium (May potentiate the action of Centrax). Products include:
- Brevital Sodium Vials ... 1248

Methoxyflurane (May potentiate the action of Centrax).
- No products indexed under this heading.

Midazolam Hydrochloride (May potentiate the action of Centrax). Products include:
- Versed Injection ... 1924

Molindone Hydrochloride (May potentiate the action of Centrax). Products include:
- Moban Tablets & Concentrate ... 932

Morphine Sulfate (May potentiate the action of Centrax). Products include:
- Astramorph/PF Injection, USP (Preservative-Free) ... 618
- Duramorph ... 960
- Infumorph 200 and Infumorph 500 Sterile Solutions ... 962
- MS Contin Tablets ... 1814
- MSIR ... 1817
- Oramorph SR (Morphine Sulfate Sustained Release Tablets) ... 1988
- Roxanol ... 1991

Nortriptyline Hydrochloride (May potentiate the action of Centrax). Products include:
- Pamelor ... 2019

Opium Alkaloids (May potentiate the action of Centrax). Products include:
- B & O No. 15A & No. 16A Supprettes ... 2395
- Pantopon Injectable ... 1911

Oxazepam (May potentiate the action of Centrax). Products include:
- Serax Capsules ... 2522
- Serax Tablets ... 2522

Oxycodone Hydrochloride (May potentiate the action of Centrax). Products include:
- Percocet Tablets ... 950
- Percodan ... 951
- Roxicodone Tablets, Oral Solution & Intensol (Oxycodone) ... 1992
- Tylox Capsules ... 1382

Pentobarbital Sodium (May potentiate the action of Centrax). Products include:
- Nembutal Sodium Capsules ... 534
- Nembutal Sodium Solution ... 536
- Nembutal Sodium Suppositories ... 538

Perphenazine (May potentiate the action of Centrax). Products include:
- Etrafon ... 2087
- Triavil Tablets ... 1556
- Trilafon ... 2123

Phenelzine Sulfate (May potentiate the action of Centrax). Products include:
- Nardil ... 1742

Phenobarbital (May potentiate the action of Centrax). Products include:
- Arco-Lase Plus Tablets ... 607
- Bellergal-S Tablets ... 1998
- Bronkolixir ... ▣ 761
- Bronkotabs Tablets ... ▣ 762
- Donnatal ... 1858
- Donnatal Extentabs ... 1859
- Donnatal Tablets ... 1858
- Donnazyme Tablets ... 1860
- Kinesed Tablets ... 2272
- Phenobarbital Elixir and Tablets ... 1293
- Primatene Tablets-P Formula ... 2421
- Quadrinal Tablets ... 1183
- Tedral SA ... 1765

Prochlorperazine (May potentiate the action of Centrax). Products include:
- Compazine ... 2201

Promethazine Hydrochloride (May potentiate the action of Centrax). Products include:
- Mepergan Injection ... 2479
- Phenergan with Codeine ... 2497
- Phenergan with Dextromethorphan 2499
- Phenergan Injection ... 2493
- Phenergan Suppositories ... 2496
- Phenergan Syrup ... 2495
- Phenergan Tablets ... 2496
- Phenergan VC ... 2500
- Phenergan VC with Codeine ... 2501

Propofol (May potentiate the action of Centrax). Products include:
- Diprivan Injection ... 2267

Propoxyphene Hydrochloride (May potentiate the action of Centrax). Products include:
- Darvon ... 1256
- Wygesic Tablets ... 2540

Propoxyphene Napsylate (May potentiate the action of Centrax). Products include:
- Darvon-N/Darvocet-N ... 1254

Protriptyline Hydrochloride (May potentiate the action of Centrax). Products include:
- Vivactil Tablets ... 1567

Quazepam (May potentiate the action of Centrax). Products include:
- Doral Tablets ... 2383

Secobarbital Sodium (May potentiate the action of Centrax). Products include:
- Seconal Sodium Pulvules ... 1296

Selegiline Hydrochloride (May potentiate the action of Centrax). Products include:
- Eldepryl ... 2250

Sufentanil Citrate (May potentiate the action of Centrax). Products include:
- Sufenta Injection ... 1147

Temazepam (May potentiate the action of Centrax). Products include:
- Restoril Capsules ... 2023

Thiamylal Sodium (May potentiate the action of Centrax). Products include:
- Surital Ampoules, Steri-Vials ... 1764

Thioridazine Hydrochloride (May potentiate the action of Centrax). Products include:
- Mellaril ... 2011

Thiothixene (May potentiate the action of Centrax). Products include:
- Navane Capsules and Concentrate 1954
- Navane Intramuscular ... 1956

Tranylcypromine Sulfate (May potentiate the action of Centrax). Products include:
- Parnate Tablets ... 2222

Trazodone Hydrochloride (May potentiate the action of Centrax). Products include:
- Desyrel and Desyrel Dividose ... 1404

Triazolam (May potentiate the action of Centrax). Products include:
- Halcion Tablets ... 2340

Trifluoperazine Hydrochloride (May potentiate the action of Centrax). Products include:
- Stelazine ... 2226

Trimipramine Maleate (May potentiate the action of Centrax). Products include:
- Surmontil Capsules ... 2524

CENTRAX TABLETS
(Prazepam) ... 1693
May interact with phenothiazines, monoamine oxidase inhibitors, central nervous system depressants, barbiturates, narcotic analgesics, antidepressant drugs, and certain other agents. Compounds in these categories include:

Alcohol (May potentiate the action of Centrax).

Alfentanil Hydrochloride (May potentiate the action of Centrax). Products include:
- Alfenta Injection ... 1131

Alprazolam (May potentiate the action of Centrax). Products include:
- Xanax Tablets ... 2367

Amitriptyline Hydrochloride (May potentiate the action of Centrax). Products include:
- Elavil ... 2269
- Endep Tablets ... 1927
- Etrafon ... 2087
- Limbitrol ... 1933
- Triavil Tablets ... 1556

Amoxapine (May potentiate the action of Centrax). Products include:
- Asendin Tablets ... 1196

Aprobarbital (May potentiate the action of Centrax). Products include:
- Alurate Elixir ... 1883

Buprenorphine (May potentiate the action of Centrax).
- No products indexed under this heading.

Bupropion Hydrochloride (May potentiate the action of Centrax). Products include:
- Wellbutrin Tablets ... 821

Buspirone Hydrochloride (May potentiate the action of Centrax). Products include:
- BuSpar ... 1401

Butabarbital (May potentiate the action of Centrax). Products include:
- Pyridium Plus ... 1764

Butalbital (May potentiate the action of Centrax). Products include:
- Esgic-Plus Tablets ... 1002
- Esgic Tablets & Capsules ... 1001
- Fioricet Tablets ... 2006
- Fiorinal Capsules ... 2007
- Fiorinal with Codeine Capsules ... 2008
- Fiorinal Tablets ... 2007
- Phrenilin ... 838
- Sedapap Tablets 50 mg/650 mg .. 1360

Chlordiazepoxide (May potentiate the action of Centrax). Products include:
- Libritabs Tablets ... 1930
- Limbitrol ... 1933
- Menrium Tablets ... 1934

Chlordiazepoxide Hydrochloride (May potentiate the action of Centrax). Products include:
- Librax Capsules ... 1929
- Librium Capsules ... 1931
- Librium Injectable ... 1932

Chlorpromazine (May potentiate the action of Centrax). Products include:
- Thorazine ... 2234

Chlorprothixene (May potentiate the action of Centrax). Products include:
- Taractan Tablets ... 1920

Chlorprothixene Hydrochloride (May potentiate the action of Centrax). Products include:
- Taractan ... 1920

Clorazepate Dipotassium (May potentiate the action of Centrax). Products include:
- Tranxene ... 556

Codeine (May potentiate the action of Centrax). Products include:
- Calcidrine Syrup ... 506

Codeine Phosphate (May potentiate the action of Centrax). Products include:
- Actifed with Codeine Cough Syrup.. 752
- Cheracol Cough Syrup ... 1853
- Codimal PH Syrup ... 846
- Dimetane-DC Cough Syrup ... 1857
- Empirin with Codeine Phosphate Nos. 2, 3 & 4 ... 764
- Fiorinal with Codeine Capsules ... 2008
- Isoclor Expectorant ... 982
- Naldecon CX Adult Liquid ... ▣ 521
- Novahistine DH ... 1342
- Novahistine Expectorant ... 1343
- Nucofed Capsules ... 2219
- Nucofed Expectorant ... 2219
- Nucofed Pediatric Expectorant ... 2220
- Nucofed Syrup ... 2219
- Phenaphen with Codeine Capsules 1865
- Phenaphen-650 with Codeine Tablets ... 1866
- Phenergan with Codeine ... 2497
- Phenergan VC with Codeine ... 2501
- Robitussin A-C Syrup ... 1875
- Robitussin-DAC Syrup ... 1875
- Ryna ... ▣ 741
- Soma Compound w/Codeine Tablets ... 2390
- Triaminic Expectorant w/Codeine .. 1996
- Tussi-Organidin Liquid ... 2391
- Tylenol with Codeine ... 1381

Codeine Polistirex (May potentiate the action of Centrax).
- No products indexed under this heading.

Desipramine Hydrochloride (May potentiate the action of Centrax). Products include:
- Norpramin Tablets ... 1340

Dezocine (May potentiate the action of Centrax).

Diazepam (May potentiate the action of Centrax). Products include:
- Valium Injectable ... 1937
- Valium Tablets ... 1939
- Valrelease Capsules ... 1923

Doxepin Hydrochloride (May potentiate the action of Centrax). Products include:
- Sinequan ... 1960

Droperidol (May potentiate the action of Centrax). Products include:
- Inapsine Injection ... 1140
- Innovar Injection ... 1141

Enflurane (May potentiate the action of Centrax). Products include:
- Ethrane ... 599

Estazolam (May potentiate the action of Centrax). Products include:
- ProSom Tablets ... 554

Ethchlorvynol (May potentiate the action of Centrax). Products include:
- Placidyl Capsules ... 553

Ethinamate (May potentiate the action of Centrax).
- No products indexed under this heading.

Fentanyl (May potentiate the action of Centrax). Products include:
- Duragesic Transdermal System ... 1133

Fentanyl Citrate (May potentiate the action of Centrax). Products include:
- Innovar Injection ... 1141
- Sublimaze Injection ... 1146

Fluoxetine Hydrochloride (May potentiate the action of Centrax). Products include:
- Prozac Pulvules ... 920

Fluphenazine Decanoate (May potentiate the action of Centrax). Products include:
- Prolixin Decanoate ... 1795

Fluphenazine Enanthate (May potentiate the action of Centrax). Products include:
- Prolixin Enanthate ... 1796

Fluphenazine Hydrochloride (May potentiate the action of Centrax). Products include:
- Prolixin Elixir ... 1793
- Prolixin Injection ... 1791
- Prolixin Oral Concentrate ... 1792
- Prolixin Tablets ... 1793

Flurazepam Hydrochloride (May potentiate the action of Centrax). Products include:
- Dalmane Capsules ... 1927

Furazolidone (May potentiate the action of Centrax). Products include:
- Furoxone ... 1855

Glutethimide (May potentiate the action of Centrax).
- No products indexed under this heading.

Haloperidol (May potentiate the action of Centrax). Products include:
- Haldol Injection, Tablets and Concentrate ... 1373

Haloperidol Decanoate (May potentiate the action of Centrax). Products include:
- Haldol Decanoate ... 1375

Hydrocodone Bitartrate (May potentiate the action of Centrax). Products include:
- Anexsia 5/500 Tablets ... 2196
- Anexsia 7.5/650 Tablets ... 2197
- Azdone Tablets ... 844
- Codiclear DH Syrup ... 845
- Codimal DH Syrup ... 846
- Damason-P ... 1356
- Hycodan Syrup, Tablets ... 927
- Hycomine Compound Tablets ... 929
- Hycomine Syrup ... 927
- Hycotuss Expectorant Syrup ... 930
- Hydrocet Capsules ... 835
- Lortab ASA Tablets ... 2414
- Lortab ... 2412
- Ru-Tuss with Hydrocodone ... 694
- Triaminic Expectorant DH ... 1995
- Vicodin Tablets ... 1187
- Vicodin ES Tablets ... 1189
- Zydone Capsules ... 941

Hydrocodone Polistirex (May potentiate the action of Centrax). Products include:
- Tussionex Extended-Release Suspension ... 988

Hydroxyzine Hydrochloride (May potentiate the action of Centrax). Products include:
- Atarax Tablets & Syrup ... 1941
- Marax Tablets & DF Syrup ... 1954
- Vistaril Intramuscular Solution ... 1970

Imipramine Hydrochloride (May potentiate the action of Centrax). Products include:
- Tofranil Ampuls ... 1038
- Tofranil Tablets ... 1039

Imipramine Pamoate (May potentiate the action of Centrax). Products include:
- Tofranil-PM Capsules ... 1041

Isocarboxazid (May potentiate the action of Centrax). Products include:
- Marplan Tablets ... 1906

Isoflurane (May potentiate the action of Centrax). Products include:
- Forane ... 600

Ketamine Hydrochloride (May potentiate the action of Centrax). Products include:
- Ketalar ... 1726

Levorphanol Tartrate (May potentiate the action of Centrax). Products include:
- Levo-Dromoran ... 1906

Lorazepam (May potentiate the action of Centrax). Products include:
- Ativan Injection ... 2432
- Ativan Tablets ... 2434

Loxapine Hydrochloride (May potentiate the action of Centrax). Products include:
- Loxitane ... 1213

Loxapine Succinate (May potentiate the action of Centrax). Products include:
- Loxitane Capsules ... 1213

Maprotiline Hydrochloride (May potentiate the action of Centrax). Products include:
- Ludiomil Tablets ... 874

Meperidine Hydrochloride (May potentiate the action of Centrax). Products include:
- Demerol ... 2047
- Mepergan Injection ... 2479

Mephobarbital (May potentiate the action of Centrax). Products include:
- Mebaral Tablets ... 2061

Meprobamate (May potentiate the action of Centrax). Products include:
- Deprol Tablets ... 2382
- Equagesic Tablets ... 2451
- Miltown Tablets ... 2386
- PMB 200 and PMB 400 ... 2504

Mesoridazine (May potentiate the action of Centrax). Products include:
- Serentil ... 686

Mesoridazine Besylate (May potentiate the action of Centrax).

Methadone Hydrochloride (May potentiate the action of Centrax). Products include:
- Dolophine Hydrochloride Ampoules & Vials ... 1260
- Dolophine Hydrochloride Tablets ... 1261
- Methadone Hydrochloride Diskets .. 1284
- Methadone Hydrochloride Oral Solution & Tablets ... 1987

Methohexital Sodium (May potentiate the action of Centrax). Products include:
- Brevital Sodium Vials ... 1248

Methoxyflurane (May potentiate the action of Centrax).
- No products indexed under this heading.

Midazolam Hydrochloride (May potentiate the action of Centrax). Products include:
- Versed Injection ... 1924

Molindone Hydrochloride (May potentiate the action of Centrax). Products include:
- Moban Tablets & Concentrate ... 932

Morphine Sulfate (May potentiate the action of Centrax). Products include:
- Astramorph/PF Injection, USP (Preservative-Free) ... 618
- Duramorph ... 960
- Infumorph 200 and Infumorph 500 Sterile Solutions ... 962
- MS Contin Tablets ... 1814
- MSIR ... 1817
- Oramorph SR (Morphine Sulfate Sustained Release Tablets) ... 1988
- Roxanol ... 1991

Nortriptyline Hydrochloride (May potentiate the action of Centrax). Products include:
- Pamelor ... 2019

Opium Alkaloids (May potentiate the action of Centrax). Products include:
- B & O No. 15A & No. 16A Supprettes ... 2395
- Pantopon Injectable ... 1911

Oxazepam (May potentiate the action of Centrax). Products include:
- Serax Capsules ... 2522
- Serax Tablets ... 2522

Oxycodone Hydrochloride (May potentiate the action of Centrax). Products include:
- Percocet Tablets ... 950
- Percodan ... 951
- Roxicodone Tablets, Oral Solution & Intensol (Oxycodone) ... 1992
- Tylox Capsules ... 1382

Pentobarbital Sodium (May potentiate the action of Centrax). Products include:
- Nembutal Sodium Capsules ... 534
- Nembutal Sodium Solution ... 536
- Nembutal Sodium Suppositories ... 538

Perphenazine (May potentiate the action of Centrax). Products include:
- Etrafon ... 2087
- Triavil Tablets ... 1556
- Trilafon ... 2123

Phenelzine Sulfate (May potentiate the action of Centrax). Products include:
- Nardil ... 1742

Phenobarbital (May potentiate the action of Centrax). Products include:
- Arco-Lase Plus Tablets ... 607
- Bellergal-S Tablets ... 1998
- Bronkolixir ... ▣ 761
- Bronkotabs Tablets ... ▣ 762
- Donnatal ... 1858
- Donnatal Extentabs ... 1859
- Donnatal Tablets ... 1858
- Donnazyme Tablets ... 1860
- Kinesed Tablets ... 2272
- Phenobarbital Elixir and Tablets ... 1293
- Primatene Tablets-P Formula ... 2421
- Quadrinal Tablets ... 1183
- Tedral SA ... 1765

Prochlorperazine (May potentiate the action of Centrax). Products include:
- Compazine ... 2201

Promethazine Hydrochloride (May potentiate the action of Centrax). Products include:
- Mepergan Injection ... 2479
- Phenergan with Codeine ... 2497
- Phenergan with Dextromethorphan ... 2499
- Phenergan Injection ... 2493
- Phenergan Suppositories ... 2496
- Phenergan Syrup ... 2495
- Phenergan Tablets ... 2496
- Phenergan VC ... 2500
- Phenergan VC with Codeine ... 2501

Propofol (May potentiate the action of Centrax). Products include:
- Diprivan Injection ... 2267

Propoxyphene Hydrochloride (May potentiate the action of Centrax). Products include:
- Darvon ... 1256
- Wygesic Tablets ... 2540

Propoxyphene Napsylate (May potentiate the action of Centrax). Products include:
- Darvon-N/Darvocet-N ... 1254

Protriptyline Hydrochloride (May potentiate the action of Centrax). Products include:
- Vivactil Tablets ... 1567

Quazepam (May potentiate the action of Centrax). Products include:
- Doral Tablets ... 2383

Secobarbital Sodium (May potentiate the action of Centrax). Products include:
- Seconal Sodium Pulvules ... 1296

Selegiline Hydrochloride (May potentiate the action of Centrax). Products include:
- Eldepryl ... 2250

Sufentanil Citrate (May potentiate the action of Centrax). Products include:
- Sufenta Injection ... 1147

Temazepam (May potentiate the action of Centrax). Products include:
- Restoril Capsules ... 2023

Thiamylal Sodium (May potentiate the action of Centrax). Products include:
- Surital Ampoules, Steri-Vials ... 1764

Thioridazine Hydrochloride (May potentiate the action of Centrax). Products include:
- Mellaril ... 2011

Thiothixene (May potentiate the action of Centrax). Products include:
- Navane Capsules and Concentrate ... 1954
- Navane Intramuscular ... 1956

Tranylcypromine Sulfate (May potentiate the action of Centrax). Products include:
- Parnate Tablets ... 2222

Trazodone Hydrochloride (May potentiate the action of Centrax). Products include:
- Desyrel and Desyrel Dividose ... 1404

Triazolam (May potentiate the action of Centrax). Products include:
- Halcion Tablets ... 2340

Trifluoperazine Hydrochloride (May potentiate the action of Centrax). Products include:
- Stelazine ... 2226

Trimipramine Maleate (May potentiate the action of Centrax). Products include:
- Surmontil Capsules ... 2524

CENTRUM
(Vitamins with Minerals) ... ▣ 584
No interactions described in labeling.

CENTRUM, JR. (CHILDREN'S CHEWABLE) + EXTRA C
(Multivitamins with Minerals) ... ▣ 585
No interactions described in labeling.

CENTRUM, JR. (CHILDREN'S CHEWABLE) + EXTRA CALCIUM
(Multivitamins with Minerals) ... ▣ 585
No interactions described in labeling.

CENTRUM, JR. (CHILDREN'S CHEWABLE) + IRON
(Multivitamins with Minerals) ... ▣ 586
No interactions described in labeling.

CENTRUM LIQUID
(Multivitamins with Minerals) ... ▣ 584
No interactions described in labeling.

CENTRUM SILVER
(Multivitamins with Minerals) ... ▣ 586
No interactions described in labeling.

CEO-TWO RECTAL SUPPOSITORIES
(Sodium Bicarbonate, Potassium Bitartrate) ... 671
No interactions described in labeling.

CĒPACOL ANESTHETIC LOZENGES (TROCHES)
(Benzocaine, Cetylpyridinium Chloride) ... ▣ 592
No interactions described in labeling.

CĒPACOL / CĒPACOL MINT MOUTHWASH/GARGLE
(Cetylpyridinium Chloride) ... ▣ 591
No interactions described in labeling.

CĒPACOL DRY THROAT LOZENGES, CHERRY FLAVOR
(Menthol) ... ▣ 591
No interactions described in labeling.

CĒPACOL DRY THROAT LOZENGES, HONEY-LEMON FLAVOR
(Menthol) ... ▣ 591
No interactions described in labeling.

CĒPACOL DRY THROAT LOZENGES, MENTHOL-EUCALYPTUS FLAVOR
(Menthol) ... ▣ 591
No interactions described in labeling.

CĒPACOL DRY THROAT LOZENGES, ORIGINAL FLAVOR
(Benzyl Alcohol, Cetylpyridinium Chloride) ... ▣ 592
No interactions described in labeling.

CEPASTAT CHERRY FLAVOR SORE THROAT LOZENGES
(Menthol, Phenol) ... ▣ 592
No interactions described in labeling.

CEPASTAT EXTRA STRENGTH SORE THROAT LOZENGES
(Phenol, Menthol) ... ▣ 592
No interactions described in labeling.

CEPHULAC SYRUP
(Lactulose) ... 1331
May interact with:

Aluminum Hydroxide (Desired lactulose-induced drop in colonic pH inhibited). Products include:
- Cama Arthritis Pain Reliever ... ▣ 685
- Gaviscon Extra Strength Relief Formula Liquid Antacid ... ▣ 594
- Gaviscon Extra Strength Relief Formula Antacid Tablets ... ▣ 594
- Gaviscon Liquid Antacid ... ▣ 594
- Gelusil Liquid & Tablets ... ▣ 639
- Extra Strength Maalox Plus Suspension ... 1850
- Maalox TC Suspension ... 1851
- Maalox Plus Tablets ... ▣ 655
- Extra Strength Maalox Plus Tablets 1850
- Nephrox Suspension ... ▣ 563
- WinGel Liquid & Tablets ... ▣ 761

Aluminum Hydroxide Gel (Desired lactulose-induced drop in colonic pH inhibited). Products include:
- ALternaGEL Liquid ... 1154
- Aludrox Oral Suspension ... 2428
- Amphojel Suspension ... 2429
- Amphojel Suspension without Flavor ... 2429
- Mylanta Liquid ... 1155
- Mylanta Double Strength Liquid ... 1155

Aluminum Hydroxide Gel, Dried (Desired lactulose-induced drop in colonic pH inhibited). Products include:
- Alu-Tab/Alu-Cap ... 1309
- Amphojel Tablets ... 2429
- Ascriptin A/D Caplets ... 1850
- Regular Strength Ascriptin Tablets 1850
- Gaviscon Antacid Tablets ... ▣ 593
- Gaviscon-2 Antacid Tablets ... ▣ 594
- Mylanta Tablets ... 1155
- Mylanta Double Strength Tablets ... 1155

Anti-infectives, oral, unspecified (Interference with desired degradation of lactulose; acidification of colonic contents prevented).

Bisacodyl (Other laxatives should not be used). Products include:
- Dulcolax Suppositories ... ▣ 519
- Dulcolax Tablets ... ▣ 519
- Fleet Bisacodyl Enema ... 991
- Fleet Prep Kits ... 993

Calcium Carbonate (Desired lactulose-induced drop in colonic pH inhibited). Products include:
- Alka-Mints Chewable Antacid ... ▣ 620
- Alka-Seltzer Advanced Formula Antacid & Non-Aspirin Pain Reliever ... ▣ 620
- Ascriptin A/D Caplets ... 1850
- Regular Strength Ascriptin Tablets 1850
- Balmex Baby Powder ... ▣ 590
- Bayer Plus Aspirin Tablets ... ▣ 567
- Biocal 500 mg Tablet Calcium Supplement ... ▣ 625
- Bufferin Analgesic Tablets and Caplets ... ▣ 524
- Caltrate 600 ... ▣ 583
- Caltrate 600 + Iron ... ▣ 583
- Caltrate 600 + Vitamin D ... ▣ 584
- Caltrate, Jr. ... ▣ 583
- Centrum, Jr. (Children's Chewable) + Extra Calcium ... ▣ 585
- Di-Gel Antacid/Anti-Gas ... ▣ 697
- Gerimed Tablets ... 972
- Marblen ... ▣ 563
- Natalins Rx ... 1391
- Natalins Tablets ... 1391
- Nephro-Calci Tablets ... 1826
- Os-Cal 500 Chewable Tablets ... ▣ 596
- Os-Cal 500 Tablets ... ▣ 597
- Os-Cal 250+D Tablets ... ▣ 597
- Os-Cal 500+D Tablets ... ▣ 597
- Pramet FA ... 1974
- Pramilet FA ... 1974
- Rolaids (Calcium Rich/Sodium Free) ... ▣ 744
- Extra Strength Rolaids ... ▣ 744
- Thermotabs ... ▣ 619
- Total Formula-2 (multivitamin/multimineral) ... 2377
- Tums Liquid Extra ... ▣ 726
- Zenate Tablets ... 2250

Casanthranol (Other laxatives should not be used). Products include:
- Anticon ... ▣ 629
- Dialose Plus Capsules ... ▣ 577
- Peri-Colace ... 1409

Cascara Sagrada (Other laxatives should not be used). Products include:
- Nature's Remedy Natural Vegetable Laxative ... ▣ 719
- Peri-Colace ... 1409

Castor Oil (Other laxatives should not be used). Products include:
- Emulsoil ... ▣ 633
- Fleet Flavored Castor Oil Emulsion 993
- Fleet Prep Kits ... 993
- Granulex ... 1086
- Hydrisinol Creme & Lotion ... 1770
- Neoloid Emulsified Castor Oil ... 1226
- Nivea Bath Silk Bath Oil ... ▣ 514
- Purge Concentrate ... ▣ 563

Docusate Potassium (Other laxatives should not be used). Products include:
- Dialose Capsules ... ▣ 577
- Dialose Plus Capsules ... ▣ 577
- Kasof Capsules ... ▣ 579

Docusate Sodium (Other laxatives should not be used). Products include:
- Anticon ... ▣ 629

Colace 1403
Correctol Laxative Tablets .... ▣ 696
Dialose Tablets 1154
Dialose Plus Tablets 1154
Extra Gentle Ex-Lax .... ▣ 687
Feen-A-Mint Laxative Pills and Chocolated Mint Tablets .... ▣ 702
Ferro-Sequels 1203
Geriplex-FS Kapseals .... ▣ 639
Geriplex-FS Liquid .... ▣ 639
Modane Plus Tablets .... ▣ 504
Peri-Colace 1409
Peritinic Tablets .... ▣ 589
Phillips' LaxCaps .... ▣ 572
Senokot-S Tablets 1820

Mineral Oil (Other laxatives should not be used). Products include:
AKWA Tears Ointment .... ⊙ 208
Agoral .... ▣ 634
Aqua Care Cream .... ▣ 616
Aqua Care Lotion .... ▣ 616
Aquaphor Antibiotic Formula 662
Aquaphor Healing Ointment, Original Formula 662
Aquaphor Natural Healing Formula 662
Complex 15 Hand & Body Moisturizing Cream .... ▣ 694
Complex 15 Hand & Body Moisturizing Lotion .... ▣ 695
Complex 15 Moisturizing Face Cream .... ▣ 695
Duolube Eye Ointment .... ⊙ 258
Duratears Naturale .... ⊙ 216
Eucerin Dry Skin Care Lotion 662
Eucerin Moisturizing Creme (Unscented) 662
Eucerin Dry Skin Care Lotion (Fragrace-free) .... ▣ 514
Fleet Mineral Oil Enema 992
Fleet Relief 993
Haley's M-O, Regular & Flavored .. ▣ 569
Keri Lotion - Original Formula .... ▣ 535
Lacri-Lube NP Lubricant Ophthalmic Ointment .... ⊙ 249
Lacri-Lube S.O.P. Sterile Ophthalmic Ointment .... ⊙ 249
Nephrox Suspension .... ▣ 563
Nivea Bath Silk Bath Oil .... ▣ 514
Nivea Bath Silk Bath & Shower Gel (Extra-Dry Skin) .... ▣ 514
Nivea Moisturizing Creme .... ▣ 514
Nivea Moisturizing Lotion (Original Formula) .... ▣ 514
Nivea Moisturizing Oil .... ▣ 515
Nivea Skin Oil .... ▣ 515
Nivea Sun After Sun Lotion .... ▣ 515
Nutraderm Cream & Lotion 1684
pHisoDerm For Baby .... ▣ 761
pHisoDerm Skin Cleanser and Conditioner - Regular and Oily .... ▣ 760
Refresh P.M. Lubricant Ophthalmic Ointment .... ⊙ 256
Replens .... ▣ 556
Tears Renewed Ointment .... ⊙ 209
Theraplex ClearLotion 1410

Neomycin, oral (Interference with desired degradation of lactulose; acidification of colonic contents prevented).

Psyllium Preparations (Other laxatives should not be used). Products include:
Effer-Syllium Natural Fiber Bulking Agent 1154
Fiberall Fiber Wafers-Fruit & Nut 851
Fiberall Fiber Wafers - Oatmeal Raisin 851
Fiberall Powder, Natural Flavor 851
Fiberall Powder, Orange Flavor 851
Metamucil Effervescent Sugar Free, Lemon-Lime Flavor 1806
Metamucil Effervescent Sugar Free, Orange Flavor 1806
Metamucil Powder, Orange Flavor .. 1806
Metamucil Powder, Regular Flavor.. 1806
Metamucil Powder, Strawberry Flavor .... ▣ 649
Metamucil Powder, Sugar Free, Orange Flavor 1806
Metamucil Powder, Sugar Free, Regular Flavor .... ▣ 649
Metamucil 1806
Perdiem Fiber Granules 1852
Perdiem Granules 1852
Serutan Toasted Granules .... ▣ 619
Syllact Powder .... ▣ 741

Senna (Other laxatives should not be used).

Senna Concentrates (Other laxatives should not be used). Products include:
Gentle Nature Natural Vegetable Laxative .... ▣ 687
Perdiem Granules 1852
Senna X-Prep Bowel Evacuant Liquid 1073
Senokot 1819
Senokot-S Tablets 1820

CEPTAZ FOR INJECTION
(Ceftazidime) 1057
May interact with aminoglycosides and certain other agents. Compounds in these categories include:

Amikacin Sulfate (Potential for nephrotoxicity following concomitant administration). Products include:
Amikin Injectable 602

Furosemide (Potential for nephrotoxicity following concomitant administration). Products include:
Lasix 1093

Gentamicin Sulfate (Potential for nephrotoxicity following concomitant administration). Products include:
Garamycin Injectable 2093
Garamycin Ophthalmic .... ⊙ 305
Genoptic Liquifilm Sterile Ophthalmic Solution .... ⊙ 247
Genoptic S.O.P. Sterile Ophthalmic Ointment .... ⊙ 247
Gentacidin Ointment .... ⊙ 273
Gentacidin Solution .... ⊙ 273
Gentak Ointment & Solution .... ⊙ 208
G-myticin Creme and Ointment 0.1% 1770
Pred-G Liquifilm Sterile Ophthalmic Suspension .... ⊙ 252
Pred-G S.O.P. Sterile Ophthalmic Ointment .... ⊙ 253

Kanamycin Sulfate (Potential for nephrotoxicity following concomitant administration). Products include:
Kantrex Injection 601
Kantrex Pediatric Injection 601

Streptomycin Sulfate (Potential for nephrotoxicity following concomitant administration).
No products indexed under this heading.

Tobramycin (Potential for nephrotoxicity following concomitant administration). Products include:
TobraDex Ophthalmic Suspension and Ointment .... ⊙ 228
Tobrex Ophthalmic Ointment and Solution 572

Tobramycin Sulfate (Potential for nephrotoxicity following concomitant administration). Products include:
Nebcin Vials, Hyporets & ADD-Vantage 1286

CEREDASE INJECTION
(Alglucerase) 1052
No interactions described in labeling.

CEROSE-DM
(Dextromethorphan Hydrobromide, Chlorpheniramine Maleate, Phenylephrine Hydrochloride) 2443
May interact with antihypertensives, antidepressant drugs, and certain other agents. Compounds in these categories include:

Acebutolol Hydrochloride (Effect not specified). Products include:
Sectral Capsules 2520

Alcohol (Increases drowsiness effect).

Amitriptyline Hydrochloride (Effect not specified). Products include:
Elavil 2269
Endep Tablets 1927
Etrafon 2087
Limbitrol 1933
Triavil Tablets 1556

Amoxapine (Effect not specified). Products include:
Asendin Tablets 1196

Atenolol (Effect not specified). Products include:
Tenoretic Tablets 1105
Tenormin Tablets and I.V. Injection 1107

Benazepril Hydrochloride (Effect not specified). Products include:
Lotensin Tablets 872

Bendroflumethiazide (Effect not specified). Products include:
Corzide Tablets 702
Naturetin Tablets 1789
Rauzide Tablets 1804

Betaxolol Hydrochloride (Effect not specified). Products include:
Betoptic Sterile Ophthalmic Solution 569
Betoptic S Sterile Ophthalmic Suspension 570
Kerlone Tablets 2172

Bupropion Hydrochloride (Effect not specified). Products include:
Wellbutrin Tablets 821

Captopril (Effect not specified). Products include:
Capoten 2255
Capozide 2258

Carteolol Hydrochloride (Effect not specified). Products include:
Cartrol Tablets 507

Chlorothiazide (Effect not specified). Products include:
Aldoclor Tablets 1413
Diupres Tablets 1461
Diuril Oral 1464

Chlorothiazide Sodium (Effect not specified). Products include:
Diuril Sodium Intravenous 1463

Chlorthalidone (Effect not specified). Products include:
Combipres Tablets 678
Tenoretic Tablets 1105
Thalitone Tablets 687

Clonidine (Effect not specified). Products include:
Catapres-TTS 677

Clonidine Hydrochloride (Effect not specified). Products include:
Catapres Tablets 676
Combipres Tablets 678

Deserpidine (Effect not specified). Products include:
Enduronyl 518
Harmonyl Tablets 528
Oreticyl 545

Desipramine Hydrochloride (Effect not specified). Products include:
Norpramin Tablets 1340

Diazoxide (Effect not specified). Products include:
Hyperstat I.V. Injection 2095
Proglycem 649

Doxazosin Mesylate (Effect not specified). Products include:
Cardura Tablets 1941

Doxepin Hydrochloride (Effect not specified). Products include:
Sinequan 1960

Enalapril Maleate (Effect not specified). Products include:
Vaseretic Tablets 1559
Vasotec Tablets 1564

Enalaprilat (Effect not specified). Products include:
Vasotec I.V. 1562

Esmolol Hydrochloride (Effect not specified). Products include:
Brevibloc Injection 942

Felodipine (Effect not specified). Products include:
Plendil Extended-Release Tablets 1526

Fluoxetine Hydrochloride (Effect not specified). Products include:
Prozac Pulvules 920

Fosinopril Sodium (Effect not specified). Products include:
Monopril Tablets 1406

Furosemide (Effect not specified). Products include:
Lasix 1093

Guanabenz Acetate (Effect not specified). Products include:
Wytensin Tablets 2542

Guanethidine Monosulfate (Effect not specified). Products include:
Esimil Tablets 864
Ismelin Tablets 869

Hydralazine Hydrochloride (Effect not specified). Products include:
Apresazide Capsules 854
Apresoline Hydrochloride Parenteral (Ampuls) 856
Apresoline Hydrochloride Tablets .. 855
Apresoline-Esidrix Tablets 857
Ser-Ap-Es Tablets 881
Serpasil-Apresoline Tablets 884

Hydrochlorothiazide (Effect not specified). Products include:
Aldactazide 2150
Aldoril Tablets 1418
Apresazide Capsules 854
Apresoline-Esidrix Tablets 857
Capozide 2258
Dyazide Capsules 2208
Esidrix Tablets 863
Esimil Tablets 864
HydroDIURIL Tablets 1484
Hydropres Tablets 1485
Inderide Tablets 2463
Inderide LA Long Acting Capsules .. 2465
Lopressor HCT Tablets 1034
Maxzide 1215
Moduretic Tablets 1510
Normozide Tablets 2112
Oretic Tablets 544
Oreticyl 545
Prinzide Tablets 1540
Ser-Ap-Es Tablets 881
Serpasil-Esidrix Tablets 886
Timolide Tablets 1547
Trandate HCT Tablets 579
Vaseretic Tablets 1559
Zestoretic 2274

Hydroflumethiazide (Effect not specified). Products include:
Diucardin Tablets 2450
Saluron 718
Salutensin/Salutensin-Demi 719

Imipramine Hydrochloride (Effect not specified). Products include:
Tofranil Ampuls 1038
Tofranil Tablets 1039

Imipramine Pamoate (Effect not specified). Products include:
Tofranil-PM Capsules 1041

Indapamide (Effect not specified). Products include:
Lozol Tablets 1843

Isocarboxazid (Effect not specified). Products include:
Marplan Tablets 1906

Isradipine (Effect not specified). Products include:
DynaCirc Capsules 2004

Labetalol Hydrochloride (Effect not specified). Products include:
Normodyne Injection 2108
Normodyne Tablets 2110
Normozide Tablets 2112
Trandate HCT Tablets 579
Trandate Injection 577
Trandate Tablets 579

Lisinopril (Effect not specified). Products include:
Prinivil Tablets 1538
Prinzide Tablets 1540
Zestoretic 2274
Zestril Tablets 2277

Maprotiline Hydrochloride (Effect not specified). Products include:
Ludiomil Tablets 874

Mecamylamine Hydrochloride (Effect not specified). Products include:
Inversine Tablets 1492

(▣ Described in PDR For Nonprescription Drugs) (⊙ Described in PDR For Ophthalmology)

Methyclothiazide (Effect not specified). Products include:
Enduron Tablets 517
Enduronyl 518

Methyldopa (Effect not specified). Products include:
Aldoclor Tablets 1413
Aldomet Oral 1415
Aldoril Tablets 1418

Methyldopate Hydrochloride (Effect not specified). Products include:
Aldomet Ester HCl Injection 1417

Metolazone (Effect not specified). Products include:
Diulo 2129
Mykrox ½ mg Tablets 984
Zaroxolyn Tablets 989

Metoprolol Tartrate (Effect not specified). Products include:
Lopressor Ampuls 1032
Lopressor HCT Tablets 1034
Lopressor Tablets 1032

Metyrosine (Effect not specified). Products include:
Demser Capsules 1460

Minoxidil (Effect not specified). Products include:
Loniten Tablets 2346
Rogaine Topical Solution 2357

Nadolol (Effect not specified). Products include:
Corgard Tablets 701
Corzide Tablets 702

Nicardipine Hydrochloride (Effect not specified). Products include:
Cardene Capsules 2290

Nitroglycerin (Effect not specified). Products include:
Deponit NTG Transdermal Delivery System 2143
Minitran Transdermal Delivery System 1312
Nitro-Bid Ointment 1339
Nitro-Bid Capsules 1338
Nitrodisc 2176
Nitro-Dur (nitroglycerin) Transdermal Infusion System 1164
Nitrogard Tablets 1004
Nitrolingual Spray 1846
Nitrostat Tablets 1743
Transderm-Nitro Transdermal Therapeutic System 2283

Nortriptyline Hydrochloride (Effect not specified). Products include:
Pamelor 2019

Penbutolol Sulfate (Effect not specified). Products include:
Levatol 1832

Phenelzine Sulfate (Effect not specified). Products include:
Nardil 1742

Phenoxybenzamine Hydrochloride (Effect not specified). Products include:
Dibenzyline Capsules 2207

Phentolamine Mesylate (Effect not specified). Products include:
Regitine 878

Pindolol (Effect not specified). Products include:
Visken Tablets 2036

Polythiazide (Effect not specified). Products include:
Minizide Capsules 1779
Renese Tablets 1785
Renese-R Tablets 1786

Prazosin Hydrochloride (Effect not specified). Products include:
Minipress Capsules 1778
Minizide Capsules 1779

Propranolol Hydrochloride (Effect not specified). Products include:
Inderal 2459
Inderal LA Long Acting Capsules 2461
Inderide Tablets 2463
Inderide LA Long Acting Capsules 2465

Protriptyline Hydrochloride (Effect not specified). Products include:
Vivactil Tablets 1567

Ramipril (Effect not specified). Products include:
Altace Capsules 1086

Rauwolfia Serpentina (Effect not specified). Products include:
Raudixin Tablets 1803
Rauzide Tablets 1804

Rescinnamine (Effect not specified).
No products indexed under this heading.

Reserpine (Effect not specified). Products include:
Diupres Tablets 1461
Hydromox R Tablets 1209
Hydropres Tablets 1485
Renese-R Tablets 1786
Salutensin/Salutensin-Demi 719
Ser-Ap-Es Tablets 881
Serpasil Tablets 883
Serpasil-Apresoline Tablets 884
Serpasil-Esidrix Tablets 886

Sodium Nitroprusside (Effect not specified). Products include:
Nipride I.V. Infusion 1909

Terazosin Hydrochloride (Effect not specified). Products include:
Hytrin Tablets 529

Timolol Maleate (Effect not specified). Products include:
Blocadren Tablets 1429
Timolide Tablets 1547
Timoptic in Ocudose 1552
Timoptic Sterile Ophthalmic Solution 1550

Tranylcypromine Sulfate (Effect not specified). Products include:
Parnate Tablets 2222

Trazodone Hydrochloride (Effect not specified). Products include:
Desyrel and Desyrel Dividose 1404

Trimethaphan Camsylate (Effect not specified). Products include:
Arfonad Ampuls 1887

Trimipramine Maleate (Effect not specified). Products include:
Surmontil Capsules 2524

CERTAIN DRI ANTIPERSPIRANT
(Aluminum Chloride) ▣ 630
No interactions described in labeling.

CERUBIDINE
(Daunorubicin Hydrochloride) 2443
May interact with:

Bone Marrow Depressants, unspecified (Therapy with Cerubidine should not be started in patients with preexisting drug-induced myelosuppression).

CERUMENEX DROPS
(Triethanolamine Polypeptide Oleate-Condensate) 1813
No interactions described in labeling.

CETACAINE TOPICAL ANESTHETIC
(Benzocaine) 850
No interactions described in labeling.

CETAMIDE OINTMENT
(Sulfacetamide Sodium) ⊙ 220
May interact with silver preparations. Compounds in this category include:

Silver Nitrate (Incompatible).

CETAPHIL SKIN CLEANSER
(Cetyl Alcohol) 1682
No interactions described in labeling.

CETAPRED OINTMENT
(Prednisolone Acetate, Sulfacetamide Sodium) ⊙ 220
No interactions described in labeling.

CETYLCIDE GERMICIDAL CONCENTRATE
(Cetyl Dimethyl Ethyl Ammonium Bromide) 850
No interactions described in labeling.

CETYLCIDE-G CONCENTRATE FOR STERILIZATION AND DISINFECTION
(Glutaraldehyde) 850
No interactions described in labeling.

CHAP STICK LIP BALM
(Petrolatum) ▣ 671
No interactions described in labeling.

CHAP STICK PETROLEUM JELLY PLUS
(Petrolatum) ▣ 671
No interactions described in labeling.

CHAP STICK PETROLEUM JELLY PLUS WITH SUNBLOCK 15
(Petrolatum, Oxybenzone, Padimate O (Octyl Dimethyl Paba)) ▣ 671
No interactions described in labeling.

CHAP STICK SUNBLOCK 15 LIP BALM
(Petrolatum, Padimate O (Octyl Dimethyl Paba), Oxybenzone) ▣ 671
No interactions described in labeling.

CHARCOAID
(Charcoal, Activated) ▣ 653
No interactions described in labeling.

CHARCOAL PLUS TABLETS
(Simethicone) 1190
No interactions described in labeling.

CHARCOCAPS
(Charcoal, Activated) ▣ 653
No interactions described in labeling.

CHEMET (SUCCIMER) CAPSULES
(Succimer) 1361
May interact with:

Calcium Disodium Edetate (Concomitant administration is not recommended). Products include:
Calcium Disodium Versenate Injection 1309

CHERACOL COUGH SYRUP
(Guaifenesin, Codeine Phosphate) 1853
No interactions described in labeling.

CHERACOL D COUGH FORMULA
(Dextromethorphan Hydrobromide, Guaifenesin) ▣ 667
No interactions described in labeling.

CHERACOL NASAL SPRAY PUMP
(Oxymetazoline Hydrochloride) ▣ 667
No interactions described in labeling.

CHERACOL PLUS HEAD COLD/COUGH FORMULA
(Phenylpropanolamine Hydrochloride, Dextromethorphan Hydrobromide, Chlorpheniramine Maleate) ▣ 667
May interact with monoamine oxidase inhibitors. Compounds in this category include:

Furazolidone (Concurrent administration is not recommended). Products include:
Furoxone 1855

Isocarboxazid (Concurrent administration is not recommended). Products include:
Marplan Tablets 1906

Phenelzine Sulfate (Concurrent administration is not recommended). Products include:
Nardil 1742

Selegiline Hydrochloride (Concurrent administration is not recommended). Products include:
Eldepryl 2250

Tranylcypromine Sulfate (Concurrent administration is not recommended). Products include:
Parnate Tablets 2222

CHERACOL SORE THROAT SPRAY
(Phenol) ▣ 667
No interactions described in labeling.

CHIBROXIN STERILE OPHTHALMIC SOLUTION
(Norfloxacin) 1431
May interact with oral anticoagulants and certain other agents. Compounds in these categories include:

Aminophylline (Potential elevation of serum theophylline concentrations). Products include:
Amesec ▣ 682
Aminophyllin Tablets 2153

Caffeine (Interferes with the metabolism of caffeine). Products include:
Anacin Coated Analgesic Caplets 2417
Anacin Coated Analgesic Tablets 2417
Anacin Maximum Strength Analgesic Coated Tablets 2417
Cafergot/Cafergot P-B 1999
Esgic-Plus Tablets 1002
Esgic Tablets & Capsules 1001
Aspirin Free Excedrin Analgesic Caplets 748
Excedrin Extra-Strength Analgesic Tablets & Caplets 749
Fioricet Tablets 2006
Fiorinal Capsules 2007
Fiorinal with Codeine Capsules 2008
Fiorinal Tablets 2007
No Doz Fast Acting Alertness Aid Tablets 751
No Doz Maximum Strength Caplets 751
Norgesic 1314
P-A-C Analgesic Tablets ▣ 669
Synalgos-DC Capsules 2525
Vanquish Analgesic Caplets ▣ 574
Vivarin Stimulant Tablets ▣ 726
Wigraine Tablets & Suppositories 1645

Cyclosporine (Elevated serum levels of cyclosporine). Products include:
Sandimmune 2024

Dicumarol (Enhanced effects of anticoagulant). Products include:
Dicumarol Tablets 516

Dyphylline (Potential elevation of serum theophylline concentrations). Products include:
Dilor 2079
Dilor-G Tablets & Liquid 2079
Lufyllin Elixir 2384
Lufyllin & Lufyllin-400 Tablets 2384
Lufyllin-GG Elixir & Tablets 2385

Theophylline (Potential elevation of serum theophylline concentrations). Products include:
Bronkaid Tablets ▣ 757
Bronkolixir ▣ 761
Bronkotabs Tablets ▣ 762
Constant-T Tablets 1029
Marax Tablets & DF Syrup 1954
Primatene Tablets 2421

- Quibron Capsules 713
- Quibron-T 714
- Quibron-T/SR 716
- Theolair Liquid 1317
- Theo-Organidin Elixir 2391

Theophylline Anhydrous (Potential elevation of serum theophylline concentrations). Products include:

- Aerolate 994
- Primatene Tablets-M Formula .... ▣ 753
- Primatene Tablets-Regular Formula 2421
- Respbid Tablets 684
- Slo-bid Gyrocaps 1847
- T-PHYL (Uniphyl) 200 mg Tablets 1820
- Tedral SA 1765
- Theo-24 2179
- Theo-Dur Sprinkle 1168
- Theo-Dur Extended-Release Tablets 1166
- Theolair Tablets 1317
- Theolair-SR Tablets 1319
- TheoX Extended-Release Tablets 841
- Uniphyl 400 mg Tablets 1823

Theophylline Calcium Salicylate (Potential elevation of serum theophylline concentrations). Products include:

- Quadrinal Tablets 1183

Theophylline Sodium Glycinate (Potential elevation of serum theophylline concentrations). Products include:

- Asbron G 1997

Warfarin Sodium (Enhanced effects of anticoagulant). Products include:

- Coumadin Injection & Tablets 944
- Panwarfin Tablets 547

CHILDREN'S ADVIL SUSPENSION

(Ibuprofen) 2426
May interact with oral anticoagulants, thiazides, lithium preparations, and certain other agents. Compounds in these categories include:

Aspirin (Yields a net decrease in anti-inflammatory activity with lowered blood levels of the non-aspirin drug in animal studies). Products include:

- Alka-Seltzer Effervescent Antacid and Pain Reliever 1568
- Alka-Seltzer Extra Strength Effervescent Antacid and Pain Reliever 1570
- Alka-Seltzer (Flavored) Effervescent Antacid and Pain Reliever 1569
- Alka-Seltzer Plus Cold Medicine .... ▣ 623
- Alka-Seltzer Plus Night-Time Cold Medicine .... ▣ 623
- Alka Seltzer Plus Sinus Allergy Medicine .... ▣ 624
- Anacin Coated Analgesic Caplets 2417
- Anacin Coated Analgesic Tablets 2417
- Anacin Maximum Strength Analgesic Coated Tablets 2417
- Maximum Strength Arthritis Pain Formula By the Makers of Anacin Analgesic Tablets and Caplets 2418
- Arthritis Pain Formula by the Makers of Anacin Analgesic Tablets and Caplets .... ▣ 747
- Arthritis Strength BC Powder .... ▣ 516
- Ascriptin A/D Caplets 1850
- Regular Strength Ascriptin Tablets 1850
- Azdone Tablets 844
- BC Powder .... ▣ 517
- BC Cold Powder .... ▣ 517
- Children's Bayer Chewable Aspirin .... ▣ 564
- Genuine Bayer Aspirin Tablets & Caplets .... ▣ 564
- Maximum Bayer Aspirin Tablets & Caplets .... ▣ 566
- Bayer Plus Aspirin Tablets .... ▣ 567
- Therapy Bayer Aspirin Caplets .... ▣ 568
- 8 Hour Bayer Timed-Release Aspirin .... ▣ 566
- Arthritis Strength Bufferin Analgesic Caplets 744
- Extra Strength Bufferin Analgesic Tablets 745
- Bufferin Analgesic Tablets and Caplets 743
- Cama Arthritis Pain Reliever .... ▣ 685
- Damason-P 1356
- Easprin 1719
- Ecotrin Enteric Coated Aspirin Maximum Strength Tablets and Caplets 2189
- Ecotrin Enteric Coated Aspirin Regular Strength Tablets and Caplets 2189
- Empirin Aspirin .... ▣ 541
- Empirin with Codeine Phosphate Nos. 2, 3 & 4 764
- Equagesic Tablets 2451
- Excedrin Extra-Strength Analgesic Tablets & Caplets 749
- 4-Way Cold Tablets 750
- Fiorinal Capsules 2007
- Fiorinal with Codeine Capsules 2008
- Fiorinal Tablets 2007
- Lortab ASA Tablets 2414
- Momentum Muscular Backache Formula .... ▣ 751
- Norgesic 1314
- Norwich Extra-Strength Aspirin .... ▣ 546
- Norwich Regular Strength Aspirin ▣ 547
- P-A-C Analgesic Tablets .... ▣ 669
- Percodan 951
- Robaxisal Tablets 1872
- Sine-Off Sinus Medicine Tablets-Aspirin Formula .... ▣ 722
- Soma Compound w/Codeine Tablets 2390
- Soma Compound Tablets 2389
- St. Joseph Adult Chewable Aspirin (81 mg.) .... ▣ 703
- Synalgos-DC Capsules 2525
- Talwin Compound 2072
- Ursinus Inlay-Tabs .... ▣ 691
- Vanquish Analgesic Caplets .... ▣ 574
- Zorprin Tablets 698

Aspirin, Enteric Coated (Yields a net decrease in anti-inflammatory activity with lowered blood levels of the non-aspirin drug in animal studies). Products include:

- Therapy Bayer Aspirin Caplets .... ▣ 568
- Ecotrin 2189

Bendroflumethiazide (Reduced natriuretic effect). Products include:

- Corzide Tablets 702
- Naturetin Tablets 1789
- Rauzide Tablets 1804

Chlorothiazide (Reduced natriuretic effect). Products include:

- Aldoclor Tablets 1413
- Diupres Tablets 1461
- Diuril Oral 1464

Chlorothiazide Sodium (Reduced natriuretic effect). Products include:

- Diuril Sodium Intravenous 1463

Dicumarol (Potential for excessive bleeding). Products include:

- Dicumarol Tablets 516

Furosemide (Reduced natriuretic effect). Products include:

- Lasix 1093

Hydrochlorothiazide (Reduced natriuretic effect). Products include:

- Aldactazide 2150
- Aldoril Tablets 1418
- Apresazide Capsules 854
- Apresoline-Esidrix Tablets 857
- Capozide 2258
- Dyazide Capsules 2208
- Esidrix Tablets 863
- Esimil Tablets 864
- HydroDIURIL Tablets 1484
- Hydropres Tablets 1485
- Inderide Tablets 2463
- Inderide LA Long Acting Capsules .. 2465
- Lopressor HCT Tablets 1034
- Maxzide 1215
- Moduretic Tablets 1510
- Normozide Tablets 2112
- Oretic Tablets 544
- Oreticyl 545
- Prinzide Tablets 1540
- Ser-Ap-Es Tablets 881
- Serpasil-Esidrix Tablets 886
- Timolide Tablets 1547
- Trandate HCT Tablets 579
- Vaseretic Tablets 1559
- Zestoretic 2274

Hydroflumethiazide (Reduced natriuretic effect). Products include:

- Diucardin Tablets 2450
- Saluron 718
- Salutensin/Salutensin-Demi 719

Lithium Carbonate (Reduced renal lithium clearance and elevation of plasma lithium levels). Products include:

- Eskalith 2214
- Lithane Tablets 1596
- Lithium Carbonate Capsules & Tablets 1984
- Lithobid Tablets 870

Lithium Citrate (Reduced renal lithium clearance and elevation of plasma lithium levels). Products include:

- Cibalith-S 870

Methotrexate Sodium (Enhanced toxicity of methotrexate). Products include:

- Methotrexate Tablets, Parenteral, LPF Parenteral 1217
- Rheumatrex Methotrexate Dose Pack 1234

Methyclothiazide (Reduced natriuretic effect). Products include:

- Enduron Tablets 517
- Enduronyl 518

Polythiazide (Reduced natriuretic effect). Products include:

- Minizide Capsules 1779
- Renese Tablets 1785
- Renese-R Tablets 1786

Warfarin Sodium (Potential for excessive bleeding). Products include:

- Coumadin Injection & Tablets 944
- Panwarfin Tablets 547

Food Interactions

Food, unspecified (Peak plasma levels are somewhat lower (up to 30%) and the time to reach peak levels is slightly prolonged (up to 30 min.)).

CHLOR-3 CONDIMENT

(Potassium Chloride) 994
No interactions described in labeling.

CHLORESIUM OINTMENT

(Chlorophyllin Copper Complex) 1994
No interactions described in labeling.

CHLORESIUM SOLUTION

(Chlorophyllin Copper Complex) 1994
No interactions described in labeling.

CHLOROMYCETIN CREAM, 1%

(Chloramphenicol) 1694
No interactions described in labeling.

CHLOROMYCETIN HYDROCORTISONE OPHTHALMIC

(Chloramphenicol, Hydrocortisone Acetate) 1694
No interactions described in labeling.

CHLOROMYCETIN KAPSEALS

(Chloramphenicol) 1695
May interact with:

Bone Marrow Depressants, unspecified (Concurrent therapy should be avoided).

CHLOROMYCETIN OPHTHALMIC OINTMENT, 1%

(Chloramphenicol) 1696
No interactions described in labeling.

CHLOROMYCETIN OPHTHALMIC SOLUTION

(Chloramphenicol) 1696
No interactions described in labeling.

CHLOROMYCETIN OTIC

(Chloramphenicol) 1697
No interactions described in labeling.

CHLOROMYCETIN PALMITATE, ORAL SUSPENSION

(Chloramphenicol Palmitate) 1697
May interact with:

Bone Marrow Depressants, unspecified (Concurrent therapy should be avoided).

CHLOROMYCETIN SODIUM SUCCINATE

(Chloramphenicol Sodium Succinate) 1698
May interact with:

Bone Marrow Depressants, unspecified (Concurrent therapy should be avoided).

CHLOROPTIC S.O.P.

(Chloramphenicol) .... ⊙ 243
No interactions described in labeling.

CHLOROPTIC STERILE OPHTHALMIC SOLUTION

(Chloramphenicol) .... ⊙ 243
No interactions described in labeling.

CHLOR-TRIMETON ALLERGY SYRUP, TABLETS & LONG-ACTING REPETABS TABLETS

(Chlorpheniramine Maleate) .... ▣ 693
May interact with:

Alcohol (Do not use concomitantly).

CHLOR-TRIMETON DECONGESTANT TABLETS

(Chlorpheniramine Maleate, Pseudoephedrine Sulfate) .... ▣ 694
May interact with antihypertensives, antidepressant drugs, and certain other agents. Compounds in these categories include:

Acebutolol Hydrochloride (Concomitant administration is not recommended). Products include:

- Sectral Capsules 2520

Alcohol (Do not use concomitantly).

Amitriptyline Hydrochloride (Concomitant administration is not recommended). Products include:

- Elavil 2269
- Endep Tablets 1927
- Etrafon 2087
- Limbitrol 1933
- Triavil Tablets 1556

Amoxapine (Concomitant administration is not recommended). Products include:

- Asendin Tablets 1196

Atenolol (Concomitant administration is not recommended). Products include:

- Tenoretic Tablets 1105
- Tenormin Tablets and I.V. Injection 1107

Benazepril Hydrochloride (Concomitant administration is not recommended). Products include:

- Lotensin Tablets 872

Bendroflumethiazide (Concomitant administration is not recommended). Products include:

- Corzide Tablets 702
- Naturetin Tablets 1789
- Rauzide Tablets 1804

Betaxolol Hydrochloride (Concomitant administration is not recommended). Products include:
Betoptic Sterile Ophthalmic Solution ... 569
Betoptic S Sterile Ophthalmic Suspension ... 570
Kerlone Tablets ... 2172

Bupropion Hydrochloride (Concomitant administration is not recommended). Products include:
Wellbutrin Tablets ... 821

Captopril (Concomitant administration is not recommended). Products include:
Capoten ... 2255
Capozide ... 2258

Carteolol Hydrochloride (Concomitant administration is not recommended). Products include:
Cartrol Tablets ... 507

Chlorothiazide (Concomitant administration is not recommended). Products include:
Aldoclor Tablets ... 1413
Diupres Tablets ... 1461
Diuril Oral ... 1464

Chlorothiazide Sodium (Concomitant administration is not recommended). Products include:
Diuril Sodium Intravenous ... 1463

Chlorthalidone (Concomitant administration is not recommended). Products include:
Combipres Tablets ... 678
Tenoretic Tablets ... 1105
Thalitone Tablets ... 687

Clonidine (Concomitant administration is not recommended). Products include:
Catapres-TTS ... 677

Clonidine Hydrochloride (Concomitant administration is not recommended). Products include:
Catapres Tablets ... 676
Combipres Tablets ... 678

Deserpidine (Concomitant administration is not recommended). Products include:
Enduronyl ... 518
Harmonyl Tablets ... 528
Oreticyl ... 545

Desipramine Hydrochloride (Concomitant administration is not recommended). Products include:
Norpramin Tablets ... 1340

Diazoxide (Concomitant administration is not recommended). Products include:
Hyperstat I.V. Injection ... 2095
Proglycem ... 649

Doxazosin Mesylate (Concomitant administration is not recommended). Products include:
Cardura Tablets ... 1941

Doxepin Hydrochloride (Concomitant administration is not recommended). Products include:
Sinequan ... 1960

Enalapril Maleate (Concomitant administration is not recommended). Products include:
Vaseretic Tablets ... 1559
Vasotec Tablets ... 1564

Enalaprilat (Concomitant administration is not recommended). Products include:
Vasotec I.V. ... 1562

Esmolol Hydrochloride (Concomitant administration is not recommended). Products include:
Brevibloc Injection ... 942

Felodipine (Concomitant administration is not recommended). Products include:
Plendil Extended-Release Tablets ... 1526

Fluoxetine Hydrochloride (Concomitant administration is not recommended). Products include:
Prozac Pulvules ... 920

Fosinopril Sodium (Concomitant administration is not recommended). Products include:
Monopril Tablets ... 1406

Furosemide (Concomitant administration is not recommended). Products include:
Lasix ... 1093

Guanabenz Acetate (Concomitant administration is not recommended). Products include:
Wytensin Tablets ... 2542

Guanethidine Monosulfate (Concomitant administration is not recommended). Products include:
Esimil Tablets ... 864
Ismelin Tablets ... 869

Hydralazine Hydrochloride (Concomitant administration is not recommended). Products include:
Apresazide Capsules ... 854
Apresoline Hydrochloride Parenteral (Ampuls) ... 856
Apresoline Hydrochloride Tablets ... 855
Apresoline-Esidrix Tablets ... 857
Ser-Ap-Es Tablets ... 881
Serpasil-Apresoline Tablets ... 884

Hydrochlorothiazide (Concomitant administration is not recommended). Products include:
Aldactazide ... 2150
Aldoril Tablets ... 1418
Apresazide Capsules ... 854
Apresoline-Esidrix Tablets ... 857
Capozide ... 2258
Dyazide Capsules ... 2208
Esidrix Tablets ... 863
Esimil Tablets ... 864
HydroDIURIL Tablets ... 1484
Hydropres Tablets ... 1485
Inderide Tablets ... 2463
Inderide LA Long Acting Capsules ... 2465
Lopressor HCT Tablets ... 1034
Maxzide ... 1215
Moduretic Tablets ... 1510
Normozide Tablets ... 2112
Oretic Tablets ... 544
Oreticyl ... 545
Prinzide Tablets ... 1540
Ser-Ap-Es Tablets ... 881
Serpasil-Esidrix Tablets ... 886
Timolide Tablets ... 1547
Trandate HCT Tablets ... 579
Vaseretic Tablets ... 1559
Zestoretic ... 2274

Hydroflumethiazide (Concomitant administration is not recommended). Products include:
Diucardin Tablets ... 2450
Saluron ... 718
Salutensin/Salutensin-Demi ... 719

Imipramine Hydrochloride (Concomitant administration is not recommended). Products include:
Tofranil Ampuls ... 1038
Tofranil Tablets ... 1039

Imipramine Pamoate (Concomitant administration is not recommended). Products include:
Tofranil-PM Capsules ... 1041

Indapamide (Concomitant administration is not recommended). Products include:
Lozol Tablets ... 1843

Isocarboxazid (Concomitant administration is not recommended). Products include:
Marplan Tablets ... 1906

Isradipine (Concomitant administration is not recommended). Products include:
DynaCirc Capsules ... 2004

Labetalol Hydrochloride (Concomitant administration is not recommended). Products include:
Normodyne Injection ... 2108
Normodyne Tablets ... 2110
Normozide Tablets ... 2112
Trandate HCT Tablets ... 579
Trandate Injection ... 577
Trandate Tablets ... 579

Lisinopril (Concomitant administration is not recommended). Products include:
Prinivil Tablets ... 1538
Prinzide Tablets ... 1540
Zestoretic ... 2274
Zestril Tablets ... 2277

Maprotiline Hydrochloride (Concomitant administration is not recommended). Products include:
Ludiomil Tablets ... 874

Mecamylamine Hydrochloride (Concomitant administration is not recommended). Products include:
Inversine Tablets ... 1492

Methyclothiazide (Concomitant administration is not recommended). Products include:
Enduron Tablets ... 517
Enduronyl ... 518

Methyldopa (Concomitant administration is not recommended). Products include:
Aldoclor Tablets ... 1413
Aldomet Oral ... 1415
Aldoril Tablets ... 1418

Methyldopate Hydrochloride (Concomitant administration is not recommended). Products include:
Aldomet Ester HCl Injection ... 1417

Metolazone (Concomitant administration is not recommended). Products include:
Diulo ... 2129
Mykrox ½ mg Tablets ... 984
Zaroxolyn Tablets ... 989

Metoprolol Tartrate (Concomitant administration is not recommended). Products include:
Lopressor Ampuls ... 1032
Lopressor HCT Tablets ... 1034
Lopressor Tablets ... 1032

Metyrosine (Concomitant administration is not recommended). Products include:
Demser Capsules ... 1460

Minoxidil (Concomitant administration is not recommended). Products include:
Loniten Tablets ... 2346
Rogaine Topical Solution ... 2357

Nadolol (Concomitant administration is not recommended). Products include:
Corgard Tablets ... 701
Corzide Tablets ... 702

Nicardipine Hydrochloride (Concomitant administration is not recommended). Products include:
Cardene Capsules ... 2290

Nitroglycerin (Concomitant administration is not recommended). Products include:
Deponit NTG Transdermal Delivery System ... 2143
Minitran Transdermal Delivery System ... 1312
Nitro-Bid Ointment ... 1339
Nitro-Bid Capsules ... 1338
Nitrodisc ... 2176
Nitro-Dur (nitroglycerin) Transdermal Infusion System ... 1164
Nitrogard Tablets ... 1004
Nitrolingual Spray ... 1846
Nitrostat Tablets ... 1743
Transderm-Nitro Transdermal Therapeutic System ... 2283

Nortriptyline Hydrochloride (Concomitant administration is not recommended). Products include:
Pamelor ... 2019

Penbutolol Sulfate (Concomitant administration is not recommended). Products include:
Levatol ... 1832

Phenelzine Sulfate (Concomitant administration is not recommended). Products include:
Nardil ... 1742

Phenoxybenzamine Hydrochloride (Concomitant administration is not recommended). Products include:
Dibenzyline Capsules ... 2207

Phentolamine Mesylate (Concomitant administration is not recommended). Products include:
Regitine ... 878

Pindolol (Concomitant administration is not recommended). Products include:
Visken Tablets ... 2036

Polythiazide (Concomitant administration is not recommended). Products include:
Minizide Capsules ... 1779
Renese Tablets ... 1785
Renese-R Tablets ... 1786

Prazosin Hydrochloride (Concomitant administration is not recommended). Products include:
Minipress Capsules ... 1778
Minizide Capsules ... 1779

Propranolol Hydrochloride (Concomitant administration is not recommended). Products include:
Inderal ... 2459
Inderal LA Long Acting Capsules ... 2461
Inderide Tablets ... 2463
Inderide LA Long Acting Capsules ... 2465

Protriptyline Hydrochloride (Concomitant administration is not recommended). Products include:
Vivactil Tablets ... 1567

Ramipril (Concomitant administration is not recommended). Products include:
Altace Capsules ... 1086

Rauwolfia Serpentina (Concomitant administration is not recommended). Products include:
Raudixin Tablets ... 1803
Rauzide Tablets ... 1804

Rescinnamine (Concomitant administration is not recommended).
No products indexed under this heading.

Reserpine (Concomitant administration is not recommended). Products include:
Diupres Tablets ... 1461
Hydromox R Tablets ... 1209
Hydropres Tablets ... 1485
Renese-R Tablets ... 1786
Salutensin/Salutensin-Demi ... 719
Ser-Ap-Es Tablets ... 881
Serpasil Tablets ... 883
Serpasil-Apresoline Tablets ... 884
Serpasil-Esidrix Tablets ... 886

Sodium Nitroprusside (Concomitant administration is not recommended). Products include:
Nipride I.V. Infusion ... 1909

Terazosin Hydrochloride (Concomitant administration is not recommended). Products include:
Hytrin Tablets ... 529

Timolol Maleate (Concomitant administration is not recommended). Products include:
Blocadren Tablets ... 1429
Timolide Tablets ... 1547
Timoptic in Ocudose ... 1552
Timoptic Sterile Ophthalmic Solution ... 1550

Tranylcypromine Sulfate (Concomitant administration is not recommended). Products include:
Parnate Tablets ... 2222

Trazodone Hydrochloride (Concomitant administration is not recommended). Products include:
Desyrel and Desyrel Dividose ... 1404

Trimethaphan Camsylate (Concomitant administration is not recommended). Products include:
- Arfonad Ampuls ... 1887

Trimipramine Maleate (Concomitant administration is not recommended). Products include:
- Surmontil Capsules ... 2524

CHLOR-TRIMETON LONG ACTING DECONGESTANT REPETABS TABLETS
(Chlorpheniramine Maleate, Pseudoephedrine Sulfate) ... ■ 694
See **Chlor-Trimeton Decongestant Tablets**

CHOLEDYL PEDIATRIC ELIXIR
(Oxtriphylline) ... 1702
May interact with macrolide antibiotics, oral contraceptives, sympathomimetic bronchodilators, and certain other agents. Compounds in these categories include:

Albuterol (Potential for toxic synergism). Products include:
- Proventil Inhalation Aerosol ... 2117
- Ventolin Inhalation Aerosol and Refill ... 583

Albuterol Sulfate (Potential for toxic synergism). Products include:
- Proventil Repetabs Tablets ... 2120
- Proventil Solutions for Inhalation 0.5% and 0.083% ... 2118
- Proventil Syrup ... 2119
- Proventil Tablets ... 2120
- Ventolin ... 583

Allopurinol (Increased serum theophylline levels). Products include:
- Zyloprim Tablets ... 830

Bitolterol Mesylate (Potential for toxic synergism). Products include:
- Tornalate ... 2074

Cimetidine (Increased serum theophylline levels). Products include:
- Tagamet Tablets ... 2228

Cimetidine Hydrochloride (Increased serum theophylline levels). Products include:
- Tagamet ... 2228

Ephedrine Hydrochloride (Potential for toxic synergism). Products include:
- Amesec ... ■ 682
- Primatene Tablets-M Formula ... 2421
- Primatene Tablets-P Formula ... 2421
- Primatene Tablets-Regular Formula ... 2421
- Quadrinal Tablets ... 1183
- Quelidrine Syrup ... 556
- Tedral SA ... 1765

Ephedrine Sulfate (Potential for toxic synergism). Products include:
- Bronkaid Tablets ... ■ 757
- Bronkolixir ... ■ 761
- Bronkotabs Tablets ... ■ 762
- Marax Tablets & DF Syrup ... 1954
- Pazo Hemorrhoid Ointment & Suppositories ... 752
- Vicks Vatronol Nose Drops ... ■ 666

Ephedrine Tannate (Potential for toxic synergism). Products include:
- Rynatuss ... 2388

Epinephrine (Potential for toxic synergism). Products include:
- Ana-Kit Anaphylaxis Emergency Treatment Kit ... 1100
- Bronkaid Mist ... ■ 757
- EpiPen ... 843
- Marcaine Hydrochloride 0.5% with Epinephrine 1:200,000 (as bitartrate) ... 958
- Marcaine Hydrochloride with Epinephrine 1:200,000 ... 2055
- Primatene Mist ... 2420
- Sus-Phrine Injection ... 1006
- Xylocaine with Epinephrine Injections ... 637

Epinephrine Hydrochloride (Potential for toxic synergism). Products include:
- Adrenalin Chloride Solution 1:100 & 1:1,000 ... 1689
- Epifrin ... ⊙ 244
- Glaucon ... ⊙ 218

Erythromycin (Increased serum theophylline levels). Products include:
- A/T/S Topical Gel and Topical Solution ... 1089
- AK-Mycin Ointment ... ⊙ 204
- Benzamycin Topical Gel ... 907
- E-Mycin Tablets ... 688
- ETS-2% ... 1685
- ERYC ... 1720
- Erycette (erythromycin 2%) Topical Solution ... 1678
- Ery-Tab Tablets ... 521
- Erythromycin Base Filmtab ... 525
- Erythromycin Delayed-Release Capsules, USP ... 526
- Ilotycin Ophthalmic Ointment ... 915
- PCE Dispertab Tablets ... 549
- Pediazole ... 1973
- T-Stat 2.0% Topical Solution and Pads ... 2409
- Theramycin Z Topical Solution 2% 1410

Erythromycin Estolate (Increased serum theophylline levels). Products include:
- Ilosone ... 913

Erythromycin Ethylsuccinate (Increased serum theophylline levels). Products include:
- E.E.S. ... 522
- EryPed ... 519
- Pediazole ... 1973

Erythromycin Gluceptate (Increased serum theophylline levels). Products include:
- Ilotycin Gluceptate, IV, Vials ... 915

Erythromycin Stearate (Increased serum theophylline levels). Products include:
- Erythrocin Stearate Filmtab ... 523

Ethinyl Estradiol (Increased serum theophylline levels). Products include:
- Brevicon ... 2304
- Demulen ... 2161
- Estinyl Tablets ... 2085
- Jenest-28 Tablets ... 1636
- Levlen/Tri-Levlen ... 665
- Lo/Ovral Tablets ... 2471
- Lo/Ovral-28 Tablets ... 2476
- Loestrin ... 1728
- Modicon ... 1667
- Nordette-21 Tablets ... 2481
- Nordette-28 Tablets ... 2483
- Norethin ... 2133
- Norinyl ... 2304
- Norlestrin ... 1746
- Ortho-Cyclen Tablets ... 1658
- Ortho-Novum ... 1667
- Ovcon ... 1391
- Ovral Tablets ... 2490
- Ovral-28 Tablets ... 2491
- Levlen/Tri-Levlen ... 665
- Tri-Norinyl ... 2304
- Triphasil-21 Tablets ... 2527
- Triphasil-28 Tablets ... 2532

Ethylnorepinephrine Hydrochloride (Potential for toxic synergism). Products include:
- Bronkephrine Injection ... 2042

Ethynodiol Diacetate (Increased serum theophylline levels). Products include:
- Demulen ... 2161

Isoetharine (Potential for toxic synergism). Products include:
- Arm-a-Med Isoetharine Inhalation Solution, USP ... 616
- Bronkometer Aerosol ... 2042
- Bronkosol Solution ... 2042

Isoproterenol Hydrochloride (Potential for toxic synergism). Products include:
- Isuprel Hydrochloride Injection 1:5000 ... 2050
- Isuprel Hydrochloride Mistometer .. 2051
- Isuprel Hydrochloride Solution 1:200 & 1:100 ... 2052
- Norisodrine Aerotrol ... 540

Levonorgestrel (Increased serum theophylline levels). Products include:
- Levlen/Tri-Levlen ... 665
- Nordette-21 Tablets ... 2481
- Nordette-28 Tablets ... 2483
- Norplant System ... 2484
- Levlen/Tri-Levlen ... 665
- Triphasil-21 Tablets ... 2527
- Triphasil-28 Tablets ... 2532

Lithium Carbonate (Increased serum theophylline levels). Products include:
- Eskalith ... 2214
- Lithane Tablets ... 1596
- Lithium Carbonate Capsules & Tablets ... 1984
- Lithobid Tablets ... 870

Mestranol (Increased serum theophylline levels). Products include:
- Enovid ... 2161
- Norethin ... 2133
- Norinyl ... 2304
- Ortho-Novum ... 1667

Metaproterenol Sulfate (Potential for toxic synergism). Products include:
- Alupent ... 674
- Arm-a-Med Metaproterenol Sulfate Inhalation Solution, USP ... 617
- Metaprel Inhalation Aerosol Bronchodilator ... 2014
- Metaprel Inhalation Solution ... 2015
- Metaprel ... 2015
- Metaproterenol Sulfate Inhalation Solution, USP ... 912

Norethindrone (Increased serum theophylline levels). Products include:
- Brevicon ... 2304
- Jenest-28 Tablets ... 1636
- Micronor Tablets ... 1667
- Modicon ... 1667
- Norethin ... 2133
- Norinyl ... 2304
- Norlutin ... 1755
- Nor-Q D Tablets ... 2304
- Ortho-Novum ... 1667
- Ovcon ... 1391
- Tri-Norinyl ... 2304

Norethynodrel (Increased serum theophylline levels). Products include:
- Enovid ... 2161

Norgestimate (Increased serum theophylline levels). Products include:
- Ortho-Cyclen Tablets ... 1658

Norgestrel (Increased serum theophylline levels). Products include:
- Lo/Ovral Tablets ... 2471
- Lo/Ovral-28 Tablets ... 2476
- Ovral Tablets ... 2490
- Ovral-28 Tablets ... 2491
- Ovrette Tablets ... 2492

Phenytoin (Decreased theophylline and phenytoin serum levels). Products include:
- Dilantin Infatabs ... 1710
- Dilantin-30 Pediatric/Dilantin-125 Suspension ... 1713

Phenytoin Sodium (Decreased theophylline and phenytoin serum levels). Products include:
- Dilantin Kapseals ... 1708
- Dilantin Parenteral ... 1712
- Dilantin with Phenobarbital Kapseals ... 1715

Pirbuterol Acetate (Potential for toxic synergism). Products include:
- Maxair Inhaler ... 1311

Rifampin (Decreased serum theophylline levels). Products include:
- Rifadin ... 1345
- Rifamate Capsules ... 1347
- Rimactane Capsules ... 879

Terbutaline Sulfate (Potential for toxic synergism). Products include:
- Brethaire Inhaler ... 1024
- Brethine Ampuls ... 1026
- Brethine Tablets ... 1026
- Bricanyl Injection ... 1324
- Bricanyl Tablets ... 1325

Troleandomycin (Increased serum theophylline levels). Products include:
- Tao Capsules ... 1963

CHOLEDYL TABLETS
(Oxtriphylline) ... 1700
May interact with macrolide antibiotics, oral contraceptives, sympathomimetic bronchodilators, and certain other agents. Compounds in these categories include:

Albuterol (Potential for toxic synergism). Products include:
- Proventil Inhalation Aerosol ... 2117
- Ventolin Inhalation Aerosol and Refill ... 583

Albuterol Sulfate (Potential for toxic synergism). Products include:
- Proventil Repetabs Tablets ... 2120
- Proventil Solutions for Inhalation 0.5% and 0.083% ... 2118
- Proventil Syrup ... 2119
- Proventil Tablets ... 2120
- Ventolin ... 583

Allopurinol (Increased serum theophylline levels at high dose of allopurinol). Products include:
- Zyloprim Tablets ... 830

Bitolterol Mesylate (Potential for toxic synergism). Products include:
- Tornalate ... 2074

Cimetidine (Increased serum theophylline levels). Products include:
- Tagamet Tablets ... 2228

Cimetidine Hydrochloride (Increased serum theophylline levels). Products include:
- Tagamet ... 2228

Ephedrine Hydrochloride (Potential for toxic synergism). Products include:
- Amesec ... ■ 682
- Primatene Tablets-M Formula ... 2421
- Primatene Tablets-P Formula ... 2421
- Primatene Tablets-Regular Formula ... 2421
- Quadrinal Tablets ... 1183
- Quelidrine Syrup ... 556
- Tedral SA ... 1765

Ephedrine Sulfate (Potential for toxic synergism). Products include:
- Bronkaid Tablets ... ■ 757
- Bronkolixir ... ■ 761
- Bronkotabs Tablets ... ■ 762
- Marax Tablets & DF Syrup ... 1954
- Pazo Hemorrhoid Ointment & Suppositories ... 752
- Vicks Vatronol Nose Drops ... ■ 666

Ephedrine Tannate (Potential for toxic synergism). Products include:
- Rynatuss ... 2388

Epinephrine (Potential for toxic synergism). Products include:
- Ana-Kit Anaphylaxis Emergency Treatment Kit ... 1100
- Bronkaid Mist ... ■ 757
- EpiPen ... 843
- Marcaine Hydrochloride 0.5% with Epinephrine 1:200,000 (as bitartrate) ... 958
- Marcaine Hydrochloride with Epinephrine 1:200,000 ... 2055
- Primatene Mist ... 2420
- Sus-Phrine Injection ... 1006
- Xylocaine with Epinephrine Injections ... 637

Epinephrine Hydrochloride (Potential for toxic synergism). Products include:
- Adrenalin Chloride Solution 1:100 & 1:1,000 ... 1689
- Epifrin ... ⊙ 244
- Glaucon ... ⊙ 218

Erythromycin (Increased serum theophylline levels). Products include:
- A/T/S Topical Gel and Topical Solution ... 1089

AK-Mycin Ointment ⊙ 204
Benzamycin Topical Gel 907
E-Mycin Tablets 688
ETS-2% 1685
ERYC 1720
Erycette (erythromycin 2%) Topical Solution 1678
Ery-Tab Tablets 521
Erythromycin Base Filmtab 525
Erythromycin Delayed-Release Capsules, USP 526
Ilotycin Ophthalmic Ointment 915
PCE Dispertab Tablets 549
Pediazole 1973
T-Stat 2.0% Topical Solution and Pads 2409
Theramycin Z Topical Solution 2% 1410

Erythromycin Estolate (Increased serum theophylline levels). Products include:
Ilosone 913

Erythromycin Ethylsuccinate (Increased serum theophylline levels). Products include:
E.E.S. 522
EryPed 519
Pediazole 1973

Erythromycin Gluceptate (Increased serum theophylline levels). Products include:
Ilotycin Gluceptate, IV, Vials 915

Erythromycin Stearate (Increased serum theophylline levels). Products include:
Erythrocin Stearate Filmtab 523

Ethinyl Estradiol (Increased serum theophylline levels). Products include:
Brevicon 2304
Demulen 2161
Estinyl Tablets 2085
Jenest-28 Tablets 1636
Levlen/Tri-Levlen 665
Lo/Ovral Tablets 2471
Lo/Ovral-28 Tablets 2476
Loestrin 1728
Modicon 1667
Nordette-21 Tablets 2481
Nordette-28 Tablets 2483
Norethin 2133
Norinyl 2304
Norlestrin 1746
Ortho-Cyclen Tablets 1658
Ortho-Novum 1667
Ovcon 1391
Ovral Tablets 2490
Ovral-28 Tablets 2491
Levlen/Tri-Levlen 665
Tri-Norinyl 2304
Triphasil-21 Tablets 2527
Triphasil-28 Tablets 2532

Ethylnorepinephrine Hydrochloride (Potential for toxic synergism). Products include:
Bronkephrine Injection 2042

Ethynodiol Diacetate (Increased serum theophylline levels). Products include:
Demulen 2161

Isoetharine (Potential for toxic synergism). Products include:
Arm-a-Med Isoetharine Inhalation Solution, USP 616
Bronkometer Aerosol 2042
Bronkosol Solution 2042

Isoproterenol Hydrochloride (Potential for toxic synergism). Products include:
Isuprel Hydrochloride Injection 1:5000 2050
Isuprel Hydrochloride Mistometer 2051
Isuprel Hydrochloride Solution 1:200 & 1:100 2052
Norisodrine Aerotrol 540

Levonorgestrel (Increased serum theophylline levels). Products include:
Levlen/Tri-Levlen 665
Nordette-21 Tablets 2481
Nordette-28 Tablets 2483
Norplant System 2484
Levlen/Tri-Levlen 665
Triphasil-21 Tablets 2527
Triphasil-28 Tablets 2532

Lithium Carbonate (Increased serum theophylline levels). Products include:
Eskalith 2214
Lithane Tablets 1596
Lithium Carbonate Capsules & Tablets 1984
Lithobid Tablets 870

Mestranol (Increased serum theophylline levels). Products include:
Enovid 2161
Norethin 2133
Norinyl 2304
Ortho-Novum 1667

Metaproterenol Sulfate (Potential for toxic synergism). Products include:
Alupent 674
Arm-a-Med Metaproterenol Sulfate Inhalation Solution, USP 617
Metaprel Inhalation Aerosol Bronchodilator 2014
Metaprel Inhalation Solution 2015
Metaprel 2015
Metaproterenol Sulfate Inhalation Solution, USP 912

Norethindrone (Increased serum theophylline levels). Products include:
Brevicon 2304
Jenest-28 Tablets 1636
Micronor Tablets 1667
Modicon 1667
Norethin 2133
Norinyl 2304
Norlutin 1755
Nor-Q D Tablets 2304
Ortho-Novum 1667
Ovcon 1391
Tri-Norinyl 2304

Norethynodrel (Increased serum theophylline levels). Products include:
Enovid 2161

Norgestimate (Increased serum theophylline levels). Products include:
Ortho-Cyclen Tablets 1658

Norgestrel (Increased serum theophylline levels). Products include:
Lo/Ovral Tablets 2471
Lo/Ovral-28 Tablets 2476
Ovral Tablets 2490
Ovral-28 Tablets 2491
Ovrette Tablets 2492

Phenytoin (Decreased theophylline and plenytoin serum levels). Products include:
Dilantin Infatabs 1710
Dilantin-30 Pediatric/Dilantin-125 Suspension 1713

Phenytoin Sodium (Decreased theophylline and phenytoin serum levels). Products include:
Dilantin Kapseals 1708
Dilantin Parenteral 1712
Dilantin with Phenobarbital Kapseals 1715

Pirbuterol Acetate (Potential for toxic synergism). Products include:
Maxair Inhaler 1311

Rifampin (Decreased serum theophylline levels). Products include:
Rifadin 1345
Rifamate Capsules 1347
Rimactane Capsules 879

Terbutaline Sulfate (Potential for toxic synergism). Products include:
Brethaire Inhaler 1024
Brethine Ampuls 1026
Brethine Tablets 1026
Bricanyl Injection 1324
Bricanyl Tablets 1325

Troleandomycin (Increased serum theophylline levels). Products include:
Tao Capsules 1963

CHOLEDYL SA TABLETS
(Oxtriphylline) 1704
May interact with:

Chlordiazepoxide (Chlordiazepoxide-induced fatty acid mobilization). Products include:
Libritabs Tablets 1930
Limbitrol 1933
Menrium Tablets 1934

Chlordiazepoxide Hydrochloride (Chlordiazepoxide-induced fatty acid mobilization). Products include:
Librax Capsules 1929
Librium Capsules 1931
Librium Injectable 1932

Erythromycin (Increased theophylline plasma levels). Products include:
A/T/S Topical Gel and Topical Solution 1089
AK-Mycin Ointment ⊙ 204
Benzamycin Topical Gel 907
E-Mycin Tablets 688
ETS-2% 1685
ERYC 1720
Erycette (erythromycin 2%) Topical Solution 1678
Ery-Tab Tablets 521
Erythromycin Base Filmtab 525
Erythromycin Delayed-Release Capsules, USP 526
Ilotycin Ophthalmic Ointment 915
PCE Dispertab Tablets 549
Pediazole 1973
T-Stat 2.0% Topical Solution and Pads 2409
Theramycin Z Topical Solution 2% 1410

Erythromycin Estolate (Increased theophylline plasma levels). Products include:
Ilosone 913

Erythromycin Ethylsuccinate (Increased theophylline plasma levels). Products include:
E.E.S. 522
EryPed 519
Pediazole 1973

Erythromycin Gluceptate (Increased theophylline plasma levels). Products include:
Ilotycin Gluceptate, IV, Vials 915

Erythromycin Lactobionate (Increased theophylline plasma levels).
No products indexed under this heading.

Erythromycin Stearate (Increased theophylline plasma levels). Products include:
Erythrocin Stearate Filmtab 523

Furosemide (Increased furosemide diuresis). Products include:
Lasix 1093

Hexamethonium (Decreased hexamethonium-induced chronatropic).

Lincomycin Hydrochloride Monohydrate (Increased theophylline plasma levels).
No products indexed under this heading.

Lithium Carbonate (Increased excretion of lithium carbonate). Products include:
Eskalith 2214
Lithane Tablets 1596
Lithium Carbonate Capsules & Tablets 1984
Lithobid Tablets 870

Propranolol Hydrochloride (Propranolol effect antagonized). Products include:
Inderal 2459
Inderal LA Long Acting Capsules 2461
Inderide Tablets 2463
Inderide LA Long Acting Capsules 2465

Reserpine (Reserpine-induced tachycardia). Products include:
Diupres Tablets 1461
Hydromox R Tablets 1209
Hydropres Tablets 1485
Renese-R Tablets 1786
Salutensin/Salutensin-Demi 719
Ser-Ap-Es Tablets 881
Serpasil Tablets 883
Serpasil-Apresoline Tablets 884
Serpasil-Esidrix Tablets 886

Troleandomycin (Increased theophylline plasma levels). Products include:
Tao Capsules 1963

CHOLERA VACCINE
(Cholera Vaccine) 2445
No interactions described in labeling.

CHOLYBAR
(Cholestyramine) 1705
May interact with thyroid preparations, cardiac glycosides, tetracyclines, and certain other agents. Compounds in these categories include:

Chlorothiazide (Delayed or reduced absorption of concomitant administered oral chlorothiazide). Products include:
Aldoclor Tablets 1413
Diupres Tablets 1461
Diuril Oral 1464

Demeclocycline Hydrochloride (Delayed or reduced absorption of concomitant administered oral tetracycline). Products include:
Declomycin Capsules, Tablets 1199

Deslanoside (Delayed or reduced absorption of concomitant administered oral digitalis).
No products indexed under this heading.

Digitoxin (Delayed or reduced absorption of concomitant administered oral digitalis). Products include:
Crystodigin Tablets 1253

Digoxin (Delayed or reduced absorption of concomitant administered oral digitalis). Products include:
Lanoxicaps 772
Lanoxin Elixir Pediatric 775
Lanoxin Injection 778
Lanoxin Injection Pediatric 781
Lanoxin Tablets 783

Doxycycline Calcium (Delayed or reduced absorption of concomitant administered oral tetracycline).
No products indexed under this heading.

Doxycycline Hyclate (Delayed or reduced absorption of concomitant administered oral tetracycline). Products include:
Doryx Capsules 1717
Vibramycin Hyclate Capsules 1787
Vibramycin Hyclate Intravenous 1968
Vibra-Tabs Film Coated Tablets 1787

Doxycycline Monohydrate (Delayed or reduced absorption of concomitant administered oral tetracycline). Products include:
Monodox Capsules 1630
Vibramycin Monohydrate for Oral Suspension 1787

Levothyroxine Sodium (Delayed or reduced absorption of concomitant administered oral thyroid preparations). Products include:
Levothroid Tablets 1003
Levoxine Tablets 904
Synthroid 695

Liothyronine Sodium (Delayed or reduced absorption of concomitant administered oral thyroid preparations). Products include:
Cytomel Tablets 2203

Liotrix (Delayed or reduced absorption of concomitant administered oral thyroid preparations). Products include:
Euthroid 1724

Methacycline Hydrochloride (Delayed or reduced absorption of concomitant administered oral tetracycline).
- No products indexed under this heading.

Minocycline Hydrochloride (Delayed or reduced absorption of concomitant administered oral tetracycline). Products include:
- Minocin Intravenous ... 1221
- Minocin Oral Suspension ... 1224
- Minocin Pellet-Filled Capsules ... 1222

Oxytetracycline Hydrochloride (Delayed or reduced absorption of concomitant administered oral tetracycline). Products include:
- Terra-Cortril Ophthalmic Suspension ... 1963
- Terramycin Capsules ... 1786
- Terramycin Intramuscular Solution 1964
- Terramycin with Polymyxin B Sulfate Ophthalmic Ointment ... 1965

Penicillin G Potassium (Delayed or reduced absorption of concomitant administered oral penicillin G). Products include:
- Pfizerpen for Injection ... 1957

Phenobarbital (Delayed or reduced absorption of concomitant administered oral phenobarbital). Products include:
- Arco-Lase Plus Tablets ... 607
- Bellergal-S Tablets ... 1998
- Bronkolixir ... ▣ 761
- Bronkotabs Tablets ... ▣ 762
- Donnatal ... 1858
- Donnatal Extentabs ... 1859
- Donnatal Tablets ... 1858
- Donnazyme Tablets ... 1860
- Kinesed Tablets ... 2272
- Phenobarbital Elixir and Tablets ... 1293
- Primatene Tablets-P Formula ... 2421
- Quadrinal Tablets ... 1183
- Tedral SA ... 1765

Phenylbutazone (Delayed or reduced absorption of concomitant administered oral phenylbutazone). Products include:
- Butazolidin Capsules & Tablets ... 1027

Tetracycline Hydrochloride (Delayed or reduced absorption of concomitant administered oral tetracycline). Products include:
- Achromycin V Capsules ... 1193
- Achromycin Ophthalmic Ointment 1% ... ◉ 307
- Achromycin Ophthalmic Suspension 1% ... ◉ 308
- Topicycline for Topical Solution ... 1856

Thyroglobulin (Delayed or reduced absorption of concomitant administered oral thyroid preparations). Products include:
- Proloid Tablets ... 1761

Thyroid (Delayed or reduced absorption of concomitant administered oral thyroid preparations). Products include:
- S-P-T "Liquid" Capsules ... 995

Thyroxine (Delayed or reduced absorption of concomitant administered oral thyroid preparations).
- No products indexed under this heading.

Thyroxine Sodium (Delayed or reduced absorption of concomitant administered oral thyroid preparations).
- No products indexed under this heading.

Vitamin A (Cholestyramine may prevent the oral absorption of fat soluble vitamin A). Products include:
- Aquasol A Vitamin A Capsules, USP ... 615
- Aquasol A Parenteral, USP ... 615
- Bugs Bunny Children's Chewable Vitamins (Sugar Free) ... ▣ 625
- Bugs Bunny With Extra C Children's Chewable Vitamins (Sugar Free) ... ▣ 626
- Bugs Bunny/Flintstones ... ▣ 625
- Flintstones Children's Chewable Vitamins With Extra C ... ▣ 626
- Flintstones Children's Chewable Vitamins Plus Iron ... ▣ 625
- Lazer Creme ... 1770
- Myadec ... ▣ 640
- Natalins Rx ... 1391
- Natalins Tablets ... 1391
- Ocuvite Vitamin and Mineral Supplement ... ◉ 312
- One-A-Day Essential Vitamins ... ▣ 627
- One-A-Day Maximum Formula Vitamins and Minerals ... ▣ 627
- One-A-Day Plus Extra C Vitamins ... ▣ 627
- Stressgard Stress Formula Vitamins ... ▣ 628
- Tri-Vi-Flor 1.0 mg Vitamins with Fluoride Chewable Tablets ... 1400
- Tri-Vi-Flor Drops ... 1400
- Tri-Vi-Sol Vitamin Drops ... ▣ 614
- Tri-Vi-Sol Vitamin Drops with Iron ▣ 614
- Vicon Forte Capsules ... 2416
- Vicon Plus ... ▣ 682
- Vi-Daylin ADC Vitamins Drops ... 1980
- Vi-Daylin ADC Vitamins + Iron Drops ... 1980
- Vi-Daylin/F ADC Vitamins Drops With Fluoride ... 1981
- Vi-Daylin/F ADC Vitamins + Iron Drops With Fluoride ... 1981
- Vi-Zac ... ▣ 682
- Within Women's Formula Multivitamin with Calcium, Extra Iron and Zinc ... ▣ 628
- Zymacap Capsules ... ▣ 670

Vitamin D (Cholestyramine may prevent the oral absorption of fat soluble vitamin D). Products include:
- Bugs Bunny Children's Chewable Vitamins (Sugar Free) ... ▣ 625
- Bugs Bunny With Extra C Children's Chewable Vitamins (Sugar Free) ... ▣ 626
- Bugs Bunny Plus Iron Children's Chewable Vitamins (Sugar Free) ▣ 625
- Calderol Capsules ... 1635
- Caltrate 600 + Iron & Vitamin D ... 1198
- Caltrate 600 + Vitamin D ... 1197
- Caltrate, Jr. Tablets ... 1198
- Flintstones Children's Chewable Vitamins ... ▣ 625
- Flintstones Children's Chewable Vitamins With Extra C ... ▣ 626
- Flintstones Children's Chewable Vitamins Plus Iron ... ▣ 625
- Natalins Rx ... 1391
- Natalins Tablets ... 1391
- One-A-Day Essential Vitamins ... ▣ 627
- One-A-Day Maximum Formula Vitamins and Minerals ... ▣ 627
- One-A-Day Plus Extra C Vitamins ... ▣ 627
- Os-Cal 250+D Tablets ... ▣ 597
- Os-Cal 500+D Tablets ... ▣ 597
- Os-Cal Fortified Tablets ... ▣ 597
- Os-Cal Plus Tablets ... ▣ 597
- Posture-D 600 mg ... 2420
- Stressgard Stress Formula Vitamins ... ▣ 628
- Tri-Vi-Flor 1.0 mg Vitamins with Fluoride Chewable Tablets ... 1400
- Tri-Vi-Flor Drops ... 1400
- Tri-Vi-Sol Vitamin Drops ... ▣ 614
- Tri-Vi-Sol Vitamin Drops with Iron ▣ 614
- Vi-Daylin ADC Vitamins Drops ... 1980
- Vi-Daylin ADC Vitamins + Iron Drops ... 1980
- Vi-Daylin/F ADC Vitamins Drops With Fluoride ... 1981
- Vi-Daylin/F ADC Vitamins + Iron Drops With Fluoride ... 1981
- Within Women's Formula Multivitamin with Calcium, Extra Iron and Zinc ... ▣ 628
- Zymacap Capsules ... ▣ 670

Vitamin K (Cholestyramine may prevent the oral absorption of fat soluble vitamin K). Products include:
- One-A-Day Maximum Formula Vitamins and Minerals ... ▣ 627
- Synkayvite Injection ... 1919
- Synkayvite Tablets ... 1920

Warfarin Sodium (Delayed or reduced absorption of concomitant administered oral warfarin). Products include:
- Coumadin Injection & Tablets ... 944
- Panwarfin Tablets ... 547

CHROMAGEN CAPSULES

(Ferrous Fumarate, Vitamin C, Vitamin B_{12}) ... 2078

No interactions described in labeling.

CHRONULAC SYRUP

(Lactulose) ... 1332

May interact with:

Aluminum Hydroxide (Inhibition of lactulose-induced drop in colonic pH). Products include:
- Cama Arthritis Pain Reliever ... ▣ 685
- Gaviscon Extra Strength Relief Formula Liquid Antacid ... ▣ 594
- Gaviscon Extra Strength Relief Formula Antacid Tablets ... ▣ 594
- Gaviscon Liquid Antacid ... ▣ 594
- Gelusil Liquid & Tablets ... ▣ 639
- Extra Strength Maalox Plus Suspension ... 1850
- Maalox TC Suspension ... 1851
- Maalox Plus Tablets ... ▣ 655
- Extra Strength Maalox Plus Tablets 1850
- Nephrox Suspension ... ▣ 563
- WinGel Liquid & Tablets ... ▣ 761

Aluminum Hydroxide Gel (Inhibition of lactulose-induced drop in colonic pH). Products include:
- ALternaGEL Liquid ... 1154
- Aludrox Oral Suspension ... 2428
- Amphojel Suspension ... 2429
- Amphojel Suspension without Flavor ... 2429
- Mylanta Liquid ... 1155
- Mylanta Double Strength Liquid ... 1155

Aluminum Hydroxide Gel, Dried (Inhibition of lactulose-induced drop in colonic pH). Products include:
- Alu-Tab/Alu-Cap ... 1309
- Amphojel Tablets ... 2429
- Ascriptin A/D Caplets ... 1850
- Regular Strength Ascriptin Tablets 1850
- Gaviscon Antacid Tablets ... ▣ 593
- Gaviscon-2 Antacid Tablets ... ▣ 594
- Mylanta Tablets ... 1155
- Mylanta Double Strength Tablets ... 1155

Calcium Carbonate (Inhibition of lactulose-induced drop in colonic pH). Products include:
- Alka-Mints Chewable Antacid ... ▣ 620
- Alka-Seltzer Advanced Formula Antacid & Non-Aspirin Pain Reliever ... ▣ 620
- Ascriptin A/D Caplets ... 1850
- Regular Strength Ascriptin Tablets 1850
- Balmex Baby Powder ... ▣ 590
- Bayer Plus Aspirin Tablets ... ▣ 567
- Biocal 500 mg Tablet Calcium Supplement ... ▣ 625
- Bufferin Analgesic Tablets and Caplets ... ▣ 524
- Caltrate 600 ... ▣ 583
- Caltrate 600 + Iron ... ▣ 583
- Caltrate 600 + Vitamin D ... ▣ 584
- Caltrate, Jr. ... ▣ 583
- Centrum, Jr. (Children's Chewable) + Extra Calcium ... ▣ 585
- Di-Gel Antacid/Anti-Gas ... ▣ 697
- Gerimed Tablets ... 972
- Marblen ... ▣ 563
- Natalins Rx ... 1391
- Natalins Tablets ... 1391
- Nephro-Calci Tablets ... 1826
- Os-Cal 500 Chewable Tablets ... ▣ 596
- Os-Cal 500 Tablets ... ▣ 597
- Os-Cal 250+D Tablets ... ▣ 597
- Os-Cal 500+D Tablets ... ▣ 597
- Pramet FA ... 1974
- Pramilet FA ... 1974
- Rolaids (Calcium Rich/Sodium Free) ... ▣ 744
- Extra Strength Rolaids ... ▣ 744
- Thermotabs ... ▣ 619
- Total Formula-2 (multivitamin/multimineral) ... 2377
- Tums Liquid Extra ... ▣ 726
- Zenate Tablets ... 2250

CIBACALCIN DOUBLE-CHAMBERED SYRINGES

(Calcitonin, Synthetic) ... 859

No interactions described in labeling.

CIBALITH-S

(Lithium Citrate) ... 870

May interact with thiazides, non-steroidal anti-inflammatory agents, phenothiazines, xanthine bronchodilators, ACE inhibitors, and certain other agents. Compounds in these categories include:

Aminophylline (Decreases therapeutic effect of lithium). Products include:
- Amesec ... ▣ 682
- Aminophyllin Tablets ... 2153

Benazepril Hydrochloride (May substantially increase steady-state plasma lithium levels resulting in lithium toxicity). Products include:
- Lotensin Tablets ... 872

Bendroflumethiazide (Provokes lithium toxicity). Products include:
- Corzide Tablets ... 702
- Naturetin Tablets ... 1789
- Rauzide Tablets ... 1804

Caffeine (Decreases therapeutic effect of lithium). Products include:
- Anacin Coated Analgesic Caplets ... 2417
- Anacin Coated Analgesic Tablets ... 2417
- Anacin Maximum Strength Analgesic Coated Tablets ... 2417
- Cafergot/Cafergot P-B ... 1999
- Esgic-Plus Tablets ... 1002
- Esgic Tablets & Capsules ... 1001
- Aspirin Free Excedrin Analgesic Caplets ... 748
- Excedrin Extra-Strength Analgesic Tablets & Caplets ... 749
- Fioricet Tablets ... 2006
- Fiorinal Capsules ... 2007
- Fiorinal with Codeine Capsules ... 2008
- Fiorinal Tablets ... 2007
- No Doz Fast Acting Alertness Aid Tablets ... 751
- No Doz Maximum Strength Caplets 751
- Norgesic ... 1314
- P-A-C Analgesic Tablets ... ▣ 669
- Synalgos-DC Capsules ... 2525
- Vanquish Analgesic Caplets ... ▣ 574
- Vivarin Stimulant Tablets ... ▣ 726
- Wigraine Tablets & Suppositories ... 1645

Captopril (May substantially increase steady-state plasma lithium levels resulting in lithium toxicity). Products include:
- Capoten ... 2255
- Capozide ... 2258

Carbamazepine (Increased risk of neuromuscular side effect). Products include:
- Tegretol Chewable Tablets ... 654
- Tegretol Suspension ... 656
- Tegretol Tablets ... 654

Chlorothiazide (Provokes lithium toxicity). Products include:
- Aldoclor Tablets ... 1413
- Diupres Tablets ... 1461
- Diuril Oral ... 1464

Chlorothiazide Sodium (Provokes lithium toxicity). Products include:
- Diuril Sodium Intravenous ... 1463

Chlorpromazine (Concurrent use of lithium with phenothiazines decreases serum phenothiazine levels). Products include:
- Thorazine ... 2234

Decamethonium (Potentiated).

Diclofenac Sodium (Increases steady state plasma lithium levels). Products include:
- Voltaren Ophthalmic Sterile Ophthalmic Solution ... ◉ 268
- Voltaren Tablets ... 1042

Dyphylline (Decreases therapeutic effect of lithium). Products include:
- Dilor ... 2079
- Dilor-G Tablets & Liquid ... 2079
- Lufyllin Elixir ... 2384
- Lufyllin & Lufyllin-400 Tablets ... 2384
- Lufyllin-GG Elixir & Tablets ... 2385

Enalapril Maleate (May substantially increase steady-state plasma lithium levels resulting in lithium toxicity). Products include:
- Vaseretic Tablets ... 1559
- Vasotec Tablets ... 1564

Enalaprilat (May substantially increase steady-state plasma lithium levels resulting in lithium toxicity). Products include:
- Vasotec I.V. ... 1562

Etodolac (Increases steady state plasma lithium levels). Products include:
- Lodine Capsules ... 2468

Fenoprofen Calcium (Increases steady state plasma lithium levels). Products include:
- Nalfon Pulvules & Tablets ... 919

Fluphenazine Decanoate (Concurrent use of lithium with phenothiazines decreases serum phenothiazine levels). Products include:
- Prolixin Decanoate ... 1795

Fluphenazine Enanthate (Concurrent use of lithium with phenothiazines decreases serum phenothiazine levels). Products include:
- Prolixin Enanthate ... 1796

Fluphenazine Hydrochloride (Concurrent use of lithium with phenothiazines decreases serum phenothiazine levels). Products include:
- Prolixin Elixir ... 1793
- Prolixin Injection ... 1791
- Prolixin Oral Concentrate ... 1792
- Prolixin Tablets ... 1793

Flurbiprofen (Increases steady state plasma lithium levels). Products include:
- Ansaid Tablets ... 2319

Fosinopril Sodium (May substantially increase steady-state plasma lithium levels resulting in lithium toxicity). Products include:
- Monopril Tablets ... 1406

Haloperidol (Encephalopathic syndrome). Products include:
- Haldol Injection, Tablets and Concentrate ... 1373

Haloperidol Decanoate (Encephalopathic syndrome). Products include:
- Haldol Decanoate ... 1375

Hydrochlorothiazide (Provokes lithium toxicity). Products include:
- Aldactazide ... 2150
- Aldoril Tablets ... 1418
- Apresazide Capsules ... 854
- Apresoline-Esidrix Tablets ... 857
- Capozide ... 2258
- Dyazide Capsules ... 2208
- Esidrix Tablets ... 863
- Esimil Tablets ... 864
- HydroDIURIL Tablets ... 1484
- Hydropres Tablets ... 1485
- Inderide Tablets ... 2463
- Inderide LA Long Acting Capsules .. 2465
- Lopressor HCT Tablets ... 1034
- Maxzide ... 1215
- Moduretic Tablets ... 1510
- Normozide Tablets ... 2112
- Oretic Tablets ... 544
- Oreticyl ... 545
- Prinzide Tablets ... 1540
- Ser-Ap-Es Tablets ... 881
- Serpasil-Esidrix Tablets ... 886
- Timolide Tablets ... 1547
- Trandate HCT Tablets ... 579
- Vaseretic Tablets ... 1559
- Zestoretic ... 2274

Hydroflumethiazide (Provokes lithium toxicity). Products include:
- Diucardin Tablets ... 2450
- Saluron ... 718
- Salutensin/Salutensin-Demi ... 719

Ibuprofen (Increases steady state plasma lithium levels). Products include:
- Advil Cold & Sinus Caplets (formerly CoAdvil) ... 2416
- Advil Ibuprofen Tablets and Caplets ... 2416
- Children's Advil Suspension ... 2426
- CoAdvil ... ▣ 748
- Dristan Sinus Caplets ... 2419
- Haltran Tablets ... ▣ 668
- Ibuprofen ... ▣ 631
- Medipren ibuprofen Caplets and Tablets ... 1362
- Midol 200 Cramp Relief Formula .. ▣ 570
- Motrin Tablets ... 2351
- Motrin IB Caplets and Tablets ... ▣ 736
- Nuprin Ibuprofen/Analgesic Tablets & Caplets ... 752
- PediaProfen Suspension ... 1363
- Rufen Tablets ... 691
- Trendar Ibuprofen Tablets ... ▣ 756

Indomethacin (Increases steady state plasma lithium levels). Products include:
- Indocin ... 1487

Indomethacin Sodium Trihydrate (Increases steady state plasma lithium levels). Products include:
- Indocin I.V. ... 1490

Ketoprofen (Increases steady state plasma lithium levels). Products include:
- Orudis Capsules ... 2488

Ketorolac Tromethamine (Increases steady state plasma lithium levels). Products include:
- Toradol IM Injection ... 2302

Lisinopril (May substantially increase steady-state plasma lithium levels resulting in lithium toxicity). Products include:
- Prinivil Tablets ... 1538
- Prinzide Tablets ... 1540
- Zestoretic ... 2274
- Zestril Tablets ... 2277

Meclofenamate Sodium (Increases steady state plasma lithium levels). Products include:
- Meclomen Capsules ... 1739

Mefenamic Acid (Increases steady state plasma lithium levels). Products include:
- Ponstel ... 1758

Mesoridazine (Concurrent use of lithium with phenothiazines decreases serum phenothiazine levels). Products include:
- Serentil ... 686

Methyclothiazide (Provokes lithium toxicity). Products include:
- Enduron Tablets ... 517
- Enduronyl ... 518

Naproxen (Increases steady state plasma lithium levels). Products include:
- Naprosyn ... 2297

Naproxen Sodium (Increases steady state plasma lithium levels). Products include:
- Anaprox and Anaprox DS Tablets ... 2288

Pancuronium Bromide Injection (Potentiated).
- No products indexed under this heading.

Perphenazine (Concurrent use of lithium with phenothiazines decreases serum phenothiazine levels). Products include:
- Etrafon ... 2087
- Triavil Tablets ... 1556
- Trilafon ... 2123

Phenylbutazone (Increases steady state plasma lithium levels). Products include:
- Butazolidin Capsules & Tablets ... 1027

Piroxicam (Increases steady state plasma lithium levels). Products include:
- Feldene Capsules ... 1777

Polythiazide (Provokes lithium toxicity). Products include:
- Minizide Capsules ... 1779
- Renese Tablets ... 1785
- Renese-R Tablets ... 1786

Potassium Iodide (Provokes lithium toxicity). Products include:
- Hyland's C-Plus Cold Tablets ... ▣ 728
- Pima Syrup ... 994
- Quadrinal Tablets ... 1183

Prochlorperazine (Concurrent use of lithium with phenothiazines decreases serum phenothiazine levels). Products include:
- Compazine ... 2201

Promethazine Hydrochloride (Concurrent use of lithium with phenothiazines decreases serum phenothiazine levels). Products include:
- Mepergan Injection ... 2479
- Phenergan with Codeine ... 2497
- Phenergan with Dextromethorphan 2499
- Phenergan Injection ... 2493
- Phenergan Suppositories ... 2496
- Phenergan Syrup ... 2495
- Phenergan Tablets ... 2496
- Phenergan VC ... 2500
- Phenergan VC with Codeine ... 2501

Ramipril (May substantially increase steady-state plasma lithium levels resulting in lithium toxicity). Products include:
- Altace Capsules ... 1086

Sodium Bicarbonate (Decreases therapeutic effect of lithium). Products include:
- Alka-Seltzer Advanced Formula Antacid & Non-Aspirin Pain Reliever ... ▣ 620
- Alka-Seltzer Effervescent Antacid ▣ 622
- Alka-Seltzer Effervescent Antacid and Pain Reliever ... 1568
- Alka-Seltzer Extra Strength Effervescent Antacid and Pain Reliever ... ▣ 623
- Alka-Seltzer (Flavored) Effervescent Antacid and Pain Reliever .. ▣ 621
- Arm & Hammer Pure Baking Soda ... ▣ 548
- Ceo-Two Rectal Suppositories ... 671
- Citrocarbonate Antacid ... ▣ 668
- Massengill Liquid Concentrate ... 2191
- NuLYTELY ... 699

Succinylcholine Chloride (Potentiated). Products include:
- Anectine ... 755

Sulindac (Increases steady state plasma lithium levels). Products include:
- Clinoril Tablets ... 1433

Theophylline (Decreases therapeutic effect of lithium). Products include:
- Bronkaid Tablets ... ▣ 757
- Bronkolixir ... ▣ 761
- Bronkotabs Tablets ... ▣ 762
- Constant-T Tablets ... 1029
- Marax Tablets & DF Syrup ... 1954
- Primatene Tablets ... 2421
- Quibron Capsules ... 713
- Quibron-T ... 714
- Quibron-T/SR ... 716
- Theolair Liquid ... 1317
- Theo-Organidin Elixir ... 2391

Theophylline Anhydrous (Decreases therapeutic effect of lithium). Products include:
- Aerolate ... 994
- Primatene Tablets-M Formula ... ▣ 753
- Primatene Tablets-Regular Formula ... 2421
- Respbid Tablets ... 684
- Slo-bid Gyrocaps ... 1847
- T-PHYL (Uniphyl) 200 mg Tablets 1820
- Tedral SA ... 1765
- Theo-24 ... 2179
- Theo-Dur Sprinkle ... 1168
- Theo-Dur Extended-Release Tablets ... 1166
- Theolair Tablets ... 1317
- Theolair-SR Tablets ... 1319
- TheoX Extended-Release Tablets ... 841
- Uniphyl 400 mg Tablets ... 1823

Theophylline Calcium Salicylate (Decreases therapeutic effect of lithium). Products include:
- Quadrinal Tablets ... 1183

Theophylline Sodium Glycinate (Decreases therapeutic effect of lithium). Products include:
- Asbron G ... 1997

Thioridazine Hydrochloride (Concurrent use of lithium with phenothiazines decreases serum phenothiazine levels). Products include:
- Mellaril ... 2011

Tolmetin Sodium (Increases steady state plasma lithium levels). Products include:
- Tolectin (200, 400 and 600 mg) .. 1379

Trifluoperazine Hydrochloride (Concurrent use of lithium with phenothiazines decreases serum phenothiazine levels). Products include:
- Stelazine ... 2226

CIGARREST TABLETS

(Lobeline Sulfate) ... ▣ 628

No interactions described in labeling.

CILOXAN STERILE OPHTHALMIC SOLUTION

(Ciprofloxacin Hydrochloride) ... ⊙ 214

May interact with xanthine bronchodilators, oral anticoagulants, and certain other agents. Compounds in these categories include:

Aminophylline (Potential for elevated theophylline levels with systemic administration). Products include:
- Amesec ... ▣ 682
- Aminophyllin Tablets ... 2153

Caffeine-containing medications (Interference with caffeine metabolism).

Cyclosporine (Potential for transient elevation in serum creatinine). Products include:
- Sandimmune ... 2024

Dicumarol (Enhanced anticoagulant effect). Products include:
- Dicumarol Tablets ... 516

Dyphylline (Potential for elevated theophylline levels with systemic administration). Products include:
- Dilor ... 2079
- Dilor-G Tablets & Liquid ... 2079
- Lufyllin Elixir ... 2384
- Lufyllin & Lufyllin-400 Tablets ... 2384
- Lufyllin-GG Elixir & Tablets ... 2385

Theophylline (Potential for elevated theophylline levels with systemic administration). Products include:
- Bronkaid Tablets ... ▣ 757
- Bronkolixir ... ▣ 761
- Bronkotabs Tablets ... ▣ 762
- Constant-T Tablets ... 1029
- Marax Tablets & DF Syrup ... 1954
- Primatene Tablets ... 2421
- Quibron Capsules ... 713
- Quibron-T ... 714
- Quibron-T/SR ... 716
- Theolair Liquid ... 1317
- Theo-Organidin Elixir ... 2391

Theophylline Anhydrous (Potential for elevated theophylline levels with systemic administration). Products include:
- Aerolate ... 994
- Primatene Tablets-M Formula ... ▣ 753
- Primatene Tablets-Regular Formula ... 2421
- Respbid Tablets ... 684
- Slo-bid Gyrocaps ... 1847
- T-PHYL (Uniphyl) 200 mg Tablets 1820
- Tedral SA ... 1765
- Theo-24 ... 2179
- Theo-Dur Sprinkle ... 1168
- Theo-Dur Extended-Release Tablets ... 1166
- Theolair Tablets ... 1317
- Theolair-SR Tablets ... 1319
- TheoX Extended-Release Tablets ... 841
- Uniphyl 400 mg Tablets ... 1823

Theophylline Calcium Salicylate (Potential for elevated theophylline levels with systemic administration). Products include:
- Quadrinal Tablets 1183

Theophylline Sodium Glycinate (Potential for elevated theophylline levels with systemic administration). Products include:
- Asbron G 1997

Warfarin Sodium (Enhanced anticoagulant effect). Products include:
- Coumadin Injection & Tablets 944
- Panwarfin Tablets 547

CIPRO I.V.

(Ciprofloxacin) 1592
May interact with oral anticoagulants and certain other agents. Compounds in these categories include:

Aminophylline (Elevated serum theophylline levels and prolongation of its elimination half-life). Products include:
- Amesec ▣ 682
- Aminophyllin Tablets 2153

Caffeine (Reduced clearance of caffeine and prolongation of its serum half-life). Products include:
- Anacin Coated Analgesic Caplets 2417
- Anacin Coated Analgesic Tablets 2417
- Anacin Maximum Strength Analgesic Coated Tablets 2417
- Cafergot/Cafergot P-B 1999
- Esgic-Plus Tablets 1002
- Esgic Tablets & Capsules 1001
- Aspirin Free Excedrin Analgesic Caplets 748
- Excedrin Extra-Strength Analgesic Tablets & Caplets 749
- Fioricet Tablets 2006
- Fiorinal Capsules 2007
- Fiorinal with Codeine Capsules 2008
- Fiorinal Tablets 2007
- No Doz Fast Acting Alertness Aid Tablets 751
- No Doz Maximum Strength Caplets 751
- Norgesic 1314
- P-A-C Analgesic Tablets ▣ 669
- Synalgos-DC Capsules 2525
- Vanquish Analgesic Caplets ▣ 574
- Vivarin Stimulant Tablets ▣ 726
- Wigraine Tablets & Suppositories 1645

Cyclosporine (Potential for transient elevations in serum creatinine). Products include:
- Sandimmune 2024

Dicumarol (Enhanced effects of anticoagulant). Products include:
- Dicumarol Tablets 516

Dyphylline (Elevated serum theophylline levels and prolongation of its elimination half-life). Products include:
- Dilor 2079
- Dilor-G Tablets & Liquid 2079
- Lufyllin Elixir 2384
- Lufyllin & Lufyllin-400 Tablets 2384
- Lufyllin-GG Elixir & Tablets 2385

Probenecid (Interferes with renal tubular secretion and produces an increase in the level of ciprofloxacin). Products include:
- Benemid Tablets 1426
- ColBENEMID Tablets 1436
- Wycillin Injection and Probenecid Tablets 2539

Theophylline (Elevated serum theophylline levels and prolongation of its elimination half-life). Products include:
- Bronkaid Tablets ▣ 757
- Bronkolixir ▣ 761
- Bronkotabs Tablets ▣ 762
- Constant-T Tablets 1029
- Marax Tablets & DF Syrup 1954
- Primatene Tablets 2421
- Quibron Capsules 713
- Quibron-T 714
- Quibron-T/SR 716
- Theolair Liquid 1317
- Theo-Organidin Elixir 2391

Theophylline Anhydrous (Elevated serum theophylline levels and prolongation of its elimination half-life). Products include:
- Aerolate 994
- Primatene Tablets-M Formula ▣ 753
- Primatene Tablets-Regular Formula 2421
- Respbid Tablets 684
- Slo-bid Gyrocaps 1847
- T-PHYL (Uniphyl) 200 mg Tablets 1820
- Tedral SA 1765
- Theo-24 2179
- Theo-Dur Sprinkle 1168
- Theo-Dur Extended-Release Tablets 1166
- Theolair Tablets 1317
- Theolair-SR Tablets 1319
- TheoX Extended-Release Tablets 841
- Uniphyl 400 mg Tablets 1823

Theophylline Calcium Salicylate (Elevated serum theophylline levels and prolongation of its elimination half-life). Products include:
- Quadrinal Tablets 1183

Theophylline Sodium Glycinate (Elevated serum theophylline levels and prolongation of its elimination half-life). Products include:
- Asbron G 1997

Warfarin Sodium (Enhanced effects of anticoagulant). Products include:
- Coumadin Injection & Tablets 944
- Panwarfin Tablets 547

CIPRO TABLETS

(Ciprofloxacin Hydrochloride) 1589
May interact with xanthine bronchodilators, antacids containing aluminium, calcium and magnesium, oral anticoagulants, and certain other agents. Compounds in these categories include:

Aluminum Carbonate Gel (Interferes with absorption of ciprofloxaxin). Products include:
- Basaljel 2438

Aluminum Hydroxide (Interferes with absorption of ciprofloxacin). Products include:
- Cama Arthritis Pain Reliever ▣ 685
- Gaviscon Extra Strength Relief Formula Liquid Antacid ▣ 594
- Gaviscon Extra Strength Relief Formula Antacid Tablets ▣ 594
- Gaviscon Liquid Antacid ▣ 594
- Gelusil Liquid & Tablets ▣ 639
- Extra Strength Maalox Plus Suspension 1850
- Maalox TC Suspension 1851
- Maalox Plus Tablets ▣ 655
- Extra Strength Maalox Plus Tablets 1850
- Nephrox Suspension ▣ 563
- WinGel Liquid & Tablets ▣ 761

Aluminum Hydroxide Gel (Interferes with absorption of ciprofloxacin). Products include:
- ALternaGEL Liquid 1154
- Aludrox Oral Suspension 2428
- Amphojel Suspension 2429
- Amphojel Suspension without Flavor 2429
- Mylanta Liquid 1155
- Mylanta Double Strength Liquid 1155

Aluminum Hydroxide Gel, Dried (Interferes with absorption of ciprofloxacin). Products include:
- Alu-Tab/Alu-Cap 1309
- Amphojel Tablets 2429
- Ascriptin A/D Caplets 1850
- Regular Strength Ascriptin Tablets 1850
- Gaviscon Antacid Tablets ▣ 593
- Gaviscon-2 Antacid Tablets ▣ 594
- Mylanta Tablets 1155
- Mylanta Double Strength Tablets 1155

Aminophylline (Concurrent administration may lead to elevation of plasma theophylline levels and prolongation of its elimination half-life). Products include:
- Amesec ▣ 682
- Aminophyllin Tablets 2153

Cyclosporine (Transient elevations in serum creatinine). Products include:
- Sandimmune 2024

Dicumarol (Enhanced effects of anticoagulant). Products include:
- Dicumarol Tablets 516

Dihydroxyaluminum Sodium Carbonate (Interferes with absorption of ciprofloxaxin). Products include:
- Rolaids ▣ 743

Dyphylline (Concurrent administration may lead to elevation of plasma theophylline levels and prolongation of its elimination half-life). Products include:
- Dilor 2079
- Dilor-G Tablets & Liquid 2079
- Lufyllin Elixir 2384
- Lufyllin & Lufyllin-400 Tablets 2384
- Lufyllin-GG Elixir & Tablets 2385

Iron Preparations (Interferes with absorption of ciprofloxacin). Products include:
- Allbee C-800 Plus Iron Tablets ▣ 670
- Bugs Bunny Children's Chewable Vitamins + Minerals with Iron and Calcium (Sugar Free) ▣ 626
- Bugs Bunny Plus Iron Children's Chewable Vitamins (Sugar Free) ▣ 625
- FemIron Multi-Vitamins and Iron ▣ 617
- Ferancee Chewable Tablets 1155
- Ferancee-HP Tablets 1155
- Fergon ▣ 758
- Fero-Folic-500 Filmtab 527
- Fero-Grad-500 Filmtab 528
- Fero-Gradumet Filmtab 528
- Ferro-Sequels 1203
- Flintstones Children's Chewable Vitamins Plus Iron ▣ 625
- Flintstones Complete With Calcium, Iron & Minerals Children's Chewable Vitamins ▣ 626
- Geritol Extend Tablets and Caplets ▣ 717
- Geritol Liquid - High Potency Iron & Vitamin Tonic ▣ 717
- Iberet Tablets 531
- Iberet-500 Liquid 531
- Iberet-Folic-500 Filmtab 527
- Iberet-Liquid 531
- Incremin w/Iron Syrup ▣ 588
- Irospan 972
- Mol-Iron ▣ 703
- Niferex 847
- Niferex-150 Forte Capsules 847
- Niferex Forte Elixir 847
- Niferex 847
- Niferex-PN Tablets 847
- One-A-Day Maximum Formula Vitamins and Minerals ▣ 627
- Peritinic Tablets ▣ 589
- Poly-Vi-Flor with Iron 1399
- Poly-Vi-Flor with Iron Drops 1399
- Poly-Vi-Sol Vitamins with Iron, Chewable Tablets and Circus Shapes Chewable ▣ 612
- Poly-Vi-Sol Vitamins with Iron, Drops ▣ 612
- SMA Iron Fortified Infant Formula, Concentrated, Ready-to-Feed and Powder ▣ 767
- Slow Fe Tablets ▣ 552
- The Stuart Formula Tablets ▣ 581
- Stuartinic Tablets 1157
- Surbex-750 with Iron ▣ 503
- Tri-Vi-Flor 0.25 mg Vitamins with Iron and Fluoride Drops 1401
- Unicap Plus Iron Vitamin Formula Tablets ▣ 738
- Vi-Daylin ADC Vitamins + Iron Drops 1980
- Vi-Daylin Multivitamin + Iron Drops 1981
- Vi-Daylin/F ADC Vitamins + Iron Drops With Fluoride 1981
- Vi-Daylin/F Multivitamin + Iron Drops With Fluoride 1981
- Vi-Daylin Multivitamin + Iron Chewable Tablets 1982
- Vi-Daylin/F Multivitamin + Iron Chewable Tablets With Fluoride 1982
- Vi-Daylin Multivitamin + Iron Liquid 1983

Magaldrate (Interferes with absorption of ciprofloxacin). Products include:
- Riopan Antacid Chew Tablets ▣ 754
- Riopan Antacid Chew Tablets in Rollpacks ▣ 754
- Riopan Antacid Suspension 2421
- Riopan Antacid Swallow Tablets 2421
- Riopan Plus Chew Tablets 2422
- Riopan Plus Chew Tablets in Rollpack 2422
- Riopan Plus 2 Chew Tablets, Mint Flavor, Cherry Flavor 2422
- Riopan Plus Suspension 2422
- Riopan Plus 2 Suspension, Mint Flavor, Cherry Flavor 2422

Magnesium Hydroxide (Interferes with absorption of ciprofloxacin). Products include:
- Aludrox Oral Suspension 2428
- Ascriptin A/D Caplets 1850
- Regular Strength Ascriptin Tablets 1850
- Di-Gel Antacid/Anti-Gas ▣ 697
- Gelusil Liquid & Tablets ▣ 639
- Haley's M-O, Regular & Flavored ▣ 569
- Extra Strength Maalox Plus Suspension 1850
- Maalox TC Suspension 1851
- Maalox Plus Tablets ▣ 655
- Extra Strength Maalox Plus Tablets 1850
- Mylanta Liquid 1155
- Mylanta Tablets 1155
- Mylanta Double Strength Liquid 1155
- Mylanta Double Strength Tablets 1155
- Concentrated Phillips' Milk of Magnesia ▣ 573
- Phillips' Milk of Magnesia Liquid ▣ 572
- Phillips' Milk of Magnesia Tablets ▣ 573
- WinGel Liquid & Tablets ▣ 761

Magnesium Oxide (Interferes with absorption of ciprofloxaxin). Products include:
- Bayer Plus Aspirin Tablets ▣ 567
- Beelith Tablets 659
- Bufferin Analgesic Tablets and Caplets ▣ 524
- Cama Arthritis Pain Reliever ▣ 685
- Mag-Ox 400 673
- Uro-Mag 673

Probenecid (Interferes with renal tubular secretion of ciprofloxacin). Products include:
- Benemid Tablets 1426
- ColBENEMID Tablets 1436
- Wycillin Injection and Probenecid Tablets 2539

Sucralfate (Substantially interferes with absorption of ciprofloxacin). Products include:
- Carafate Tablets 1326

Theophylline (Concurrent administration may lead to elevation of plasma theophylline levels and prolongation of its elimination half-life). Products include:
- Bronkaid Tablets ▣ 757
- Bronkolixir ▣ 761
- Bronkotabs Tablets ▣ 762
- Constant-T Tablets 1029
- Marax Tablets & DF Syrup 1954
- Primatene Tablets 2421
- Quibron Capsules 713
- Quibron-T 714
- Quibron-T/SR 716
- Theolair Liquid 1317
- Theo-Organidin Elixir 2391

Theophylline Anhydrous (Concurrent administration may lead to elevation of plasma theophylline levels and prolongation of its elimination half-life). Products include:
- Aerolate 994
- Primatene Tablets-M Formula ▣ 753
- Primatene Tablets-Regular Formula 2421
- Respbid Tablets 684
- Slo-bid Gyrocaps 1847
- T-PHYL (Uniphyl) 200 mg Tablets 1820
- Tedral SA 1765
- Theo-24 2179
- Theo-Dur Sprinkle 1168
- Theo-Dur Extended-Release Tablets 1166
- Theolair Tablets 1317
- Theolair-SR Tablets 1319
- TheoX Extended-Release Tablets 841

Uniphyl 400 mg Tablets 1823

Theophylline Calcium Salicylate (Concurrent administration may lead to elevation of plasma theophylline levels and prolongation of its elimination half-life). Products include:

Quadrinal Tablets 1183

Theophylline Sodium Glycinate (Concurrent administration may lead to elevation of plasma theophylline levels and prolongation of its elimination half-life). Products include:

Asbron G 1997

Warfarin Sodium (Enhanced effects of anticoagulant). Products include:

Coumadin Injection & Tablets 944
Panwarfin Tablets 547

Zinc Sulfate (Interferes with absorption of ciprofloxacin). Products include:

Clear Eyes ACR ..... ⊙ 305
Eldertonic 1359
Surbex-750 with Zinc ..... ▣ 503
Vicon Forte Capsules 2416
Visine A.C. Eye Drops ..... ▣ 646
Visine A.C. Eye Drops ..... ⊙ 303
Zincfrin ..... ⊙ 230

Food Interactions

Food, unspecified (Delays the absorption of the drug resulting in peak concentrations that are closer to 2 hours after dosing).

CITRACAL LIQUITAB

(Calcium Citrate) 1613
May interact with:

Aluminum-containing compounds, unspecified (Concurrent use should be avoided in patients with impaired renal function).

CITROCARBONATE ANTACID

(Sodium Bicarbonate, Sodium Citrate) ..... ▣ 668
No interactions described in labeling.

CITRUCEL ORANGE FLAVOR

(Methylcellulose) ..... ▣ 592
No interactions described in labeling.

CITRUCEL REGULAR FLAVOR

(Methylcellulose) ..... ▣ 593
No interactions described in labeling.

CLAFORAN STERILE INJECTION

(Cefotaxime Sodium) 1089
May interact with aminoglycosides. Compounds in this category include:

Amikacin Sulfate (Increased nephrotoxicity). Products include:

Amikin Injectable 602

Gentamicin Sulfate (Increased nephrotoxicity). Products include:

Garamycin Injectable 2093
Garamycin Ophthalmic ..... ⊙ 305
Genoptic Liquifilm Sterile Ophthalmic Solution ..... ⊙ 247
Genoptic S.O.P. Sterile Ophthalmic Ointment ..... ⊙ 247
Gentacidin Ointment ..... ⊙ 273
Gentacidin Solution ..... ⊙ 273
Gentak Ointment & Solution ..... ⊙ 208
G-myticin Creme and Ointment 0.1% 1770
Pred-G Liquifilm Sterile Ophthalmic Suspension ..... ⊙ 252
Pred-G S.O.P. Sterile Ophthalmic Ointment ..... ⊙ 253

Kanamycin Sulfate (Increased nephrotoxicity). Products include:

Kantrex Injection 601
Kantrex Pediatric Injection 601

Streptomycin Sulfate (Increased nephrotoxicity).

No products indexed under this heading.

Tobramycin (Increased nephrotoxicity). Products include:

TobraDex Ophthalmic Suspension and Ointment ..... ⊙ 228
Tobrex Ophthalmic Ointment and Solution 572

Tobramycin Sulfate (Increased nephrotoxicity). Products include:

Nebcin Vials, Hyporets & ADD-Vantage 1286

CLEAR BY DESIGN MEDICATED ACNE GEL

(Benzoyl Peroxide) ..... ▣ 709
No interactions described in labeling.

CLEAR BY DESIGN MEDICATED CLEANSING PADS

(Salicylic Acid) ..... ▣ 709
May interact with:

Concurrent use with other topical acne products may increase dryness or irritation ().

CLEAR EYES ACR

(Zinc Sulfate, Naphazoline Hydrochloride) ..... ⊙ 305
No interactions described in labeling.

CLEARASIL ADULT CARE MEDICATED BLEMISH CREAM

(Sulfur, Resorcinol) ..... ▣ 657
May interact with:

Concomitant Topical Acne Therapy (Simultaneous administration should be avoided).

CLEARASIL 10% BENZOYL PEROXIDE ACNE MEDICATION VANISHING LOTION

(Benzoyl Peroxide) ..... ▣ 658
May interact with:

Concomitant Topical Acne Therapy (Simultaneous administration should be avoided).

CLEARASIL DOUBLE TEXTURED PADS - REGULAR AND MAXIMUM STRENGTH

(Salicylic Acid, Alcohol) ..... ▣ 658
No interactions described in labeling.

CLEARASIL 10% BENZOYL PEROXIDE MAXIMUM STRENGTH ACNE MEDICATION CREAM, TINTED

(Benzoyl Peroxide) ..... ▣ 658
May interact with:

Concomitant Topical Acne Therapy (Simultaneous administration should be avoided).

CLEARASIL 10% BENZOYL PEROXIDE MAXIMUM STRENGTH ACNE MEDICATION CREAM, VANISHING

(Benzoyl Peroxide) ..... ▣ 658
No interactions described in labeling.

CLEARBLUE EASY

(Chorionic Gonadotropin) ..... ▣ 775
No interactions described in labeling.

CLEOCIN HCL CAPSULES

(Clindamycin Hydrochloride) 2322
May interact with nondepolarizing neuromuscular blocking agents and certain other agents. Compounds in these categories include:

Atracurium Besylate (Enhanced action of atracurium). Products include:

Tracrium Injection 817

Diphenoxylate Hydrochloride (Worsened colitis). Products include:

Lomotil 2174

Metocurine Iodide (Enhanced action of metocurine). Products include:

Metubine Iodide Vials 1285

Pancuronium Bromide Injection (Enhanced action of pancuronium).

No products indexed under this heading.

Paregoric (Worsened colitis). Products include:

Donnagel-PG 1858

Vecuronium Bromide (Enhanced action of vecuronium). Products include:

Norcuron 1642

CLEOCIN PEDIATRIC FLAVORED GRANULES

(Clindamycin Palmitate Hydrochloride) 2324
May interact with nondepolarizing neuromuscular blocking agents and certain other agents. Compounds in these categories include:

Atracurium Besylate (Enhanced action of atracurium). Products include:

Tracrium Injection 817

Diphenoxylate Hydrochloride (Worsened colitis). Products include:

Lomotil 2174

Metocurine Iodide (Enhanced action of metocurine). Products include:

Metubine Iodide Vials 1285

Pancuronium Bromide Injection (Enhanced action of pancuronium).

No products indexed under this heading.

Paregoric (Worsened colitis). Products include:

Donnagel-PG 1858

Vecuronium Bromide (Enhanced action of vecuronium). Products include:

Norcuron 1642

CLEOCIN PHOSPHATE IV SOLUTION

(Clindamycin Phosphate) 2325
See **Cleocin Phosphate Sterile Solution**

CLEOCIN PHOSPHATE STERILE SOLUTION

(Clindamycin Phosphate) 2325
May interact with:

Atracurium Besylate (Enhanced action of neuromuscular blocking agents). Products include:

Tracrium Injection 817

Diphenoxylate Hydrochloride (May prolong and/or worsen colitis). Products include:

Lomotil 2174

Erythromycin (Should not be administered concurrently; in vivo antagonism). Products include:

A/T/S Topical Gel and Topical Solution 1089
AK-Mycin Ointment ..... ⊙ 204
Benzamycin Topical Gel 907
E-Mycin Tablets 688
ETS-2% 1685
ERYC 1720
Erycette (erythromycin 2%) Topical Solution 1678
Ery-Tab Tablets 521
Erythromycin Base Filmtab 525
Erythromycin Delayed-Release Capsules, USP 526
Ilotycin Ophthalmic Ointment 915
PCE Dispertab Tablets 549
Pediazole 1973
T-Stat 2.0% Topical Solution and Pads 2409
Theramycin Z Topical Solution 2% 1410

Erythromycin Estolate (Should not be administered concurrently; in vivo antagonism). Products include:

Ilosone 913

Erythromycin Ethylsuccinate (Should not be administered concurrently; in vivo antagonism). Products include:

E.E.S. 522
EryPed 519
Pediazole 1973

Erythromycin Gluceptate (Should not be administered concurrently; in vivo antagonism). Products include:

Ilotycin Gluceptate, IV, Vials 915

Erythromycin Stearate (Should not be administered concurrently; in vivo antagonism). Products include:

Erythrocin Stearate Filmtab 523

Metocurine Iodide (Enhanced action of neuromuscular blocking agents). Products include:

Metubine Iodide Vials 1285

Pancuronium Bromide Injection (Enhanced action of neuromuscular blocking agents).

No products indexed under this heading.

Paregoric (May prolong and/or worsen colitis). Products include:

Donnagel-PG 1858

Succinylcholine Chloride (Enhanced action of neuromuscular blocking agents). Products include:

Anectine 755

Vecuronium Bromide (Enhanced action of neuromuscular blocking agents). Products include:

Norcuron 1642

CLEOCIN T TOPICAL GEL

(Clindamycin Phosphate) 2327
May interact with:

Diphenoxylate Hydrochloride (Worsened colitis). Products include:

Lomotil 2174

Paregoric (Worsened colitis). Products include:

Donnagel-PG 1858

CLEOCIN T TOPICAL LOTION

(Clindamycin Phosphate) 2327
See **Cleocin T Topical Gel**

CLEOCIN T TOPICAL SOLUTION

(Clindamycin Phosphate) 2327
See **Cleocin T Topical Gel**

CLINORIL TABLETS

(Sulindac) 1433
May interact with oral anticoagulants, oral hypoglycemic agents, and certain other agents. Compounds in these categories include:

Aspirin (Increased gastrointestinal reactions). Products include:

Alka-Seltzer Effervescent Antacid and Pain Reliever 1568
Alka-Seltzer Extra Strength Effervescent Antacid and Pain Reliever 1570

Alka-Seltzer (Flavored) Effervescent Antacid and Pain Reliever 1569
Alka-Seltzer Plus Cold Medicine .... ▣ 623
Alka-Seltzer Plus Night-Time Cold Medicine .... ▣ 623
Alka Seltzer Plus Sinus Allergy Medicine .... ▣ 624
Anacin Coated Analgesic Caplets 2417
Anacin Coated Analgesic Tablets 2417
Anacin Maximum Strength Analgesic Coated Tablets 2417
Maximum Strength Arthritis Pain Formula By the Makers of Anacin Analgesic Tablets and Caplets 2418
Arthritis Pain Formula by the Makers of Anacin Analgesic Tablets and Caplets .... ▣ 747
Arthritis Strength BC Powder .... ▣ 516
Ascriptin A/D Caplets 1850
Regular Strength Ascriptin Tablets 1850
Azdone Tablets 844
BC Powder .... ▣ 517
BC Cold Powder .... ▣ 517
Children's Bayer Chewable Aspirin .... ▣ 564
Genuine Bayer Aspirin Tablets & Caplets .... ▣ 564
Maximum Bayer Aspirin Tablets & Caplets .... ▣ 566
Bayer Plus Aspirin Tablets .... ▣ 567
Therapy Bayer Aspirin Caplets .... ▣ 568
8 Hour Bayer Timed-Release Aspirin .... ▣ 566
Arthritis Strength Bufferin Analgesic Caplets 744
Extra Strength Bufferin Analgesic Tablets 745
Bufferin Analgesic Tablets and Caplets 743
Cama Arthritis Pain Reliever .... ▣ 685
Damason-P 1356
Easprin 1719
Ecotrin Enteric Coated Aspirin Maximum Strength Tablets and Caplets 2189
Ecotrin Enteric Coated Aspirin Regular Strength Tablets and Caplets 2189
Empirin Aspirin .... ▣ 541
Empirin with Codeine Phosphate Nos. 2, 3 & 4 764
Equagesic Tablets 2451
Excedrin Extra-Strength Analgesic Tablets & Caplets 749
4-Way Cold Tablets 750
Fiorinal Capsules 2007
Fiorinal with Codeine Capsules 2008
Fiorinal Tablets 2007
Lortab ASA Tablets 2414
Momentum Muscular Backache Formula .... ▣ 751
Norgesic 1314
Norwich Extra-Strength Aspirin .... ▣ 546
Norwich Regular Strength Aspirin ▣ 547
P-A-C Analgesic Tablets .... ▣ 669
Percodan 951
Robaxisal Tablets 1872
Sine-Off Sinus Medicine Tablets-Aspirin Formula .... ▣ 722
Soma Compound w/Codeine Tablets 2390
Soma Compound Tablets 2389
St. Joseph Adult Chewable Aspirin (81 mg.) .... ▣ 703
Synalgos-DC Capsules 2525
Talwin Compound 2072
Ursinus Inlay-Tabs .... ▣ 691
Vanquish Analgesic Caplets .... ▣ 574
Zorprin Tablets 698

Aspirin, Enteric Coated (Increased gastrointestinal reactions). Products include:
Therapy Bayer Aspirin Caplets .... ▣ 568
Ecotrin 2189

Chlorpropamide (Special attention should be paid to patients taking higher doses than those recommended and to patients with renal or metabolic impairment). Products include:
Diabinese Tablets 1775

Cyclosporine (Increased cyclosporine-induced toxicity). Products include:
Sandimmune 2024

DMSO (Reduced efficacy of sulindac; peripheral neuropathy).

Dicumarol (Special attention should be paid to patients taking higher doses than those recommended and to patients with renal or metabolic impairment). Products include:
Dicumarol Tablets 516

Diflunisal (Decreased plasma levels of sulindac). Products include:
Dolobid Tablets 1465

Furosemide (Clinoril may blunt the renal response to I.V. furosemide). Products include:
Lasix 1093

Glipizide (Special attention should be paid to patients taking higher doses than those recommended and to patients with renal or metabolic impairment). Products include:
Glucotrol 1952

Glyburide (Special attention should be paid to patients taking higher doses than those recommended and to patients with renal or metabolic impairment). Products include:
DiaBeta 1091
Micronase Tablets 2350

Methotrexate Sodium (Decreased tubular secretion of methotrexate and potentiation of its toxicity). Products include:
Methotrexate Tablets, Parenteral, LPF Parenteral 1217
Rheumatrex Methotrexate Dose Pack 1234

Probenecid (Increased plasma levels of sulindac; modest reduction in uricosuric action of probenecid). Products include:
Benemid Tablets 1426
ColBENEMID Tablets 1436
Wycillin Injection and Probenecid Tablets 2539

Tolazamide (Special attention should be paid to patients taking higher doses than those recommended and to patients with renal or metabolic impairment). Products include:
Tolinase Tablets 2365

Tolbutamide (Special attention should be paid to patients taking higher doses than those recommended and to patients with renal or metabolic impairment). Products include:
Orinase Tablets 2354

Warfarin Sodium (Special attention should be paid to patients taking higher doses than those recommended and to patients with renal or metabolic impairment). Products include:
Coumadin Injection & Tablets 944
Panwarfin Tablets 547

Food Interactions

Food, unspecified (The peak plasma concentrations of biologically active sulfide metabolite is delayed slightly in the presence of food).

CLOCREAM SKIN PROTECTANT CREAM
(Vitamins A & D) .... ▣ 668
No interactions described in labeling.

CLORPACTIN WCS-90
(Sodium Oxychlorosene) 1073
No interactions described in labeling.

CLOZARIL TABLETS
(Clozapine) 2000
May interact with antihypertensives, belladona products, benzodiazepines, and certain other agents. Compounds in these categories include:

Acebutolol Hydrochloride (Hypotensive effects potentiated). Products include:
Sectral Capsules 2520

Alcohol (Effect not specified).

Alprazolam (Potential for profound collapse and respiratory depression). Products include:
Xanax Tablets 2367

Atenolol (Hypotensive effects potentiated). Products include:
Tenoretic Tablets 1105
Tenormin Tablets and I.V. Injection 1107

Atropine Sulfate (Anticholinergic effects potentiated). Products include:
Arco-Lase Plus Tablets 607
Atropine Sulfate Sterile Ophthalmic Solution and S.O.P. Sterile Ophthalmic Ointment .... ⊙ 239
Donnagel .... ▣ 675
Donnagel-PG 1858
Donnatal 1858
Donnatal Extentabs 1859
Donnatal Tablets 1858
Donnazyme Tablets 1860
Isopto Atropine .... ⊙ 218
Lomotil 2174
Motofen Tablets 836
Ru-Tuss Tablets 693
Urised Tablets 2396

Belladonna Alkaloids (Anticholinergic effects potentiated). Products include:
Bellergal-S Tablets 1998
Hyland's Bed Wetting Tablets .... ▣ 728
Hyland's Teething Tablets .... ▣ 728
Kinesed Tablets 2272

Benazepril Hydrochloride (Hypotensive effects potentiated). Products include:
Lotensin Tablets 872

Bendroflumethiazide (Hypotensive effects potentiated). Products include:
Corzide Tablets 702
Naturetin Tablets 1789
Rauzide Tablets 1804

Betaxolol Hydrochloride (Hypotensive effects potentiated). Products include:
Betoptic Sterile Ophthalmic Solution 569
Betoptic S Sterile Ophthalmic Suspension 570
Kerlone Tablets 2172

Bone Marrow Depressants, unspecified (Increases the risk and/or severity of bone marrow suppression).

Captopril (Hypotensive effects potentiated). Products include:
Capoten 2255
Capozide 2258

Carbamazepine (Concurrent use is contraindicated; increases the risk and/or severity of bone marrow suppression). Products include:
Tegretol Chewable Tablets 654
Tegretol Suspension 656
Tegretol Tablets 654

Carteolol Hydrochloride (Hypotensive effects potentiated). Products include:
Cartrol Tablets 507

Chlordiazepoxide (Potential for profound collapse and respiratory depression). Products include:
Libritabs Tablets 1930
Limbitrol 1933
Menrium Tablets 1934

Chlordiazepoxide Hydrochloride (Potential for profound collapse and respiratory depression). Products include:
Librax Capsules 1929
Librium Capsules 1931
Librium Injectable 1932

Chlorothiazide (Hypotensive effects potentiated). Products include:
Aldoclor Tablets 1413
Diupres Tablets 1461
Diuril Oral 1464

Chlorothiazide Sodium (Hypotensive effects potentiated). Products include:
Diuril Sodium Intravenous 1463

Chlorthalidone (Hypotensive effects potentiated). Products include:
Combipres Tablets 678
Tenoretic Tablets 1105
Thalitone Tablets 687

Clonidine (Hypotensive effects potentiated). Products include:
Catapres-TTS 677

Clonidine Hydrochloride (Hypotensive effects potentiated). Products include:
Catapres Tablets 676
Combipres Tablets 678

Clorazepate Dipotassium (Potential for profound collapse and respiratory depression). Products include:
Tranxene 556

CNS-Active Drugs, unspecified (Caution is advised).

Deserpidine (Hypotensive effects potentiated). Products include:
Enduronyl 518
Harmonyl Tablets 528
Oreticyl 545

Diazepam (Potential for profound collapse and respiratory depression). Products include:
Valium Injectable 1937
Valium Tablets 1939
Valrelease Capsules 1923

Diazoxide (Hypotensive effects potentiated). Products include:
Hyperstat I.V. Injection 2095
Proglycem 649

Digitoxin (Potential for increased plasma levels and adverse effects). Products include:
Crystodigin Tablets 1253

Digoxin (Increase in plasma concentrations resulting in adverse affects). Products include:
Lanoxicaps 772
Lanoxin Elixir Pediatric 775
Lanoxin Injection 778
Lanoxin Injection Pediatric 781
Lanoxin Tablets 783

Doxazosin Mesylate (Hypotensive effects potentiated). Products include:
Cardura Tablets 1941

Enalapril Maleate (Hypotensive effects potentiated). Products include:
Vaseretic Tablets 1559
Vasotec Tablets 1564

Enalaprilat (Hypotensive effects potentiated). Products include:
Vasotec I.V. 1562

Epinephrine Hydrochloride (Possible reverse epinephrine effect). Products include:
Adrenalin Chloride Solution 1:100 & 1:1,000 1689
Epifrin .... ⊙ 244
Glaucon .... ⊙ 218

Esmolol Hydrochloride (Hypotensive effects potentiated). Products include:
Brevibloc Injection 942

Estazolam (Potential for profound collapse and respiratory depression). Products include:
ProSom Tablets 554

Felodipine (Hypotensive effects potentiated). Products include:
Plendil Extended-Release Tablets 1526

Fosinopril Sodium (Hypotensive effects potentiated). Products include:
- Monopril Tablets ... 1406

Furosemide (Hypotensive effects potentiated). Products include:
- Lasix ... 1093

Guanabenz Acetate (Hypotensive effects potentiated). Products include:
- Wytensin Tablets ... 2542

Guanethidine Monosulfate (Hypotensive effects potentiated). Products include:
- Esimil Tablets ... 864
- Ismelin Tablets ... 869

Hydralazine Hydrochloride (Hypotensive effects potentiated). Products include:
- Apresazide Capsules ... 854
- Apresoline Hydrochloride Parenteral (Ampuls) ... 856
- Apresoline Hydrochloride Tablets ... 855
- Apresoline-Esidrix Tablets ... 857
- Ser-Ap-Es Tablets ... 881
- Serpasil-Apresoline Tablets ... 884

Hydrochlorothiazide (Hypotensive effects potentiated). Products include:
- Aldactazide ... 2150
- Aldoril Tablets ... 1418
- Apresazide Capsules ... 854
- Apresoline-Esidrix Tablets ... 857
- Capozide ... 2258
- Dyazide Capsules ... 2208
- Esidrix Tablets ... 863
- Esimil Tablets ... 864
- HydroDIURIL Tablets ... 1484
- Hydropres Tablets ... 1485
- Inderide Tablets ... 2463
- Inderide LA Long Acting Capsules ... 2465
- Lopressor HCT Tablets ... 1034
- Maxzide ... 1215
- Moduretic Tablets ... 1510
- Normozide Tablets ... 2112
- Oretic Tablets ... 544
- Oreticyl ... 545
- Prinzide Tablets ... 1540
- Ser-Ap-Es Tablets ... 881
- Serpasil-Esidrix Tablets ... 886
- Timolide Tablets ... 1547
- Trandate HCT Tablets ... 579
- Vaseretic Tablets ... 1559
- Zestoretic ... 2274

Hydroflumethiazide (Hypotensive effects potentiated). Products include:
- Diucardin Tablets ... 2450
- Saluron ... 718
- Salutensin/Salutensin-Demi ... 719

Hyoscyamine (Anticholinergic effects potentiated). Products include:
- Cystospaz Tablets ... 2395
- Urised Tablets ... 2396

Hyoscyamine Sulfate (Anticholinergic effects potentiated). Products include:
- Arco-Lase Plus Tablets ... 607
- Cystospaz-M Capsules ... 2395
- Donnagel ... ▣ 675
- Donnagel-PG ... 1858
- Donnatal ... 1858
- Donnatal Extentabs ... 1859
- Donnatal Tablets ... 1858
- Donnazyme Tablets ... 1860
- Kutrase Capsules ... 2146
- Levsin/Levsinex ... 2147
- Ru-Tuss Tablets ... 693

Indapamide (Hypotensive effects potentiated). Products include:
- Lozol Tablets ... 1843

Isradipine (Hypotensive effects potentiated). Products include:
- DynaCirc Capsules ... 2004

Labetalol Hydrochloride (Hypotensive effects potentiated). Products include:
- Normodyne Injection ... 2108
- Normodyne Tablets ... 2110
- Normozide Tablets ... 2112
- Trandate HCT Tablets ... 579
- Trandate Injection ... 577
- Trandate Tablets ... 579

Lisinopril (Hypotensive effects potentiated). Products include:
- Prinivil Tablets ... 1538
- Prinzide Tablets ... 1540
- Zestoretic ... 2274
- Zestril Tablets ... 2277

Lorazepam (Potential for profound collapse and respiratory depression). Products include:
- Ativan Injection ... 2432
- Ativan Tablets ... 2434

Mecamylamine Hydrochloride (Hypotensive effects potentiated). Products include:
- Inversine Tablets ... 1492

Methyclothiazide (Hypotensive effects potentiated). Products include:
- Enduron Tablets ... 517
- Enduronyl ... 518

Methyldopa (Hypotensive effects potentiated). Products include:
- Aldoclor Tablets ... 1413
- Aldomet Oral ... 1415
- Aldoril Tablets ... 1418

Methyldopate Hydrochloride (Hypotensive effects potentiated). Products include:
- Aldomet Ester HCl Injection ... 1417

Metolazone (Hypotensive effects potentiated). Products include:
- Diulo ... 2129
- Mykrox ½ mg Tablets ... 984
- Zaroxolyn Tablets ... 989

Metoprolol Tartrate (Hypotensive effects potentiated). Products include:
- Lopressor Ampuls ... 1032
- Lopressor HCT Tablets ... 1034
- Lopressor Tablets ... 1032

Metyrosine (Hypotensive effects potentiated). Products include:
- Demser Capsules ... 1460

Midazolam Hydrochloride (Potential for profound collapse and respiratory depression). Products include:
- Versed Injection ... 1924

Minoxidil (Hypotensive effects potentiated). Products include:
- Loniten Tablets ... 2346
- Rogaine Topical Solution ... 2357

Nadolol (Hypotensive effects potentiated). Products include:
- Corgard Tablets ... 701
- Corzide Tablets ... 702

Nicardipine Hydrochloride (Hypotensive effects potentiated). Products include:
- Cardene Capsules ... 2290

Nitroglycerin (Hypotensive effects potentiated). Products include:
- Deponit NTG Transdermal Delivery System ... 2143
- Minitran Transdermal Delivery System ... 1312
- Nitro-Bid Ointment ... 1339
- Nitro-Bid Capsules ... 1338
- Nitrodisc ... 2176
- Nitro-Dur (nitroglycerin) Transdermal Infusion System ... 1164
- Nitrogard Tablets ... 1004
- Nitrolingual Spray ... 1846
- Nitrostat Tablets ... 1743
- Transderm-Nitro Transdermal Therapeutic System ... 2283

Norepinephrine Bitartrate (Possible reverse epinephrine effect). Products include:
- Levophed Bitartrate Injection ... 2054

Oxazepam (Potential for profound collapse and respiratory depression). Products include:
- Serax Capsules ... 2522
- Serax Tablets ... 2522

Penbutolol Sulfate (Hypotensive effects potentiated). Products include:
- Levatol ... 1832

Phenoxybenzamine Hydrochloride (Hypotensive effects potentiated). Products include:
- Dibenzyline Capsules ... 2207

Phentolamine Mesylate (Hypotensive effects potentiated). Products include:
- Regitine ... 878

Pindolol (Hypotensive effects potentiated). Products include:
- Visken Tablets ... 2036

Polythiazide (Hypotensive effects potentiated). Products include:
- Minizide Capsules ... 1779
- Renese Tablets ... 1785
- Renese-R Tablets ... 1786

Prazepam (Potential for profound collapse and respiratory depression). Products include:
- Centrax ... 1693

Prazosin Hydrochloride (Hypotensive effects potentiated). Products include:
- Minipress Capsules ... 1778
- Minizide Capsules ... 1779

Propranolol Hydrochloride (Hypotensive effects potentiated). Products include:
- Inderal ... 2459
- Inderal LA Long Acting Capsules ... 2461
- Inderide Tablets ... 2463
- Inderide LA Long Acting Capsules ... 2465

Quazepam (Potential for profound collapse and respiratory depression). Products include:
- Doral Tablets ... 2383

Ramipril (Hypotensive effects potentiated). Products include:
- Altace Capsules ... 1086

Rauwolfia Serpentina (Hypotensive effects potentiated). Products include:
- Raudixin Tablets ... 1803
- Rauzide Tablets ... 1804

Rescinnamine (Hypotensive effects potentiated).
- No products indexed under this heading.

Reserpine (Hypotensive effects potentiated). Products include:
- Diupres Tablets ... 1461
- Hydromox R Tablets ... 1209
- Hydropres Tablets ... 1485
- Renese-R Tablets ... 1786
- Salutensin/Salutensin-Demi ... 719
- Ser-Ap-Es Tablets ... 881
- Serpasil Tablets ... 883
- Serpasil-Apresoline Tablets ... 884
- Serpasil-Esidrix Tablets ... 886

Scopolamine Hydrobromide (Anticholinergic effects potentiated). Products include:
- Donnagel ... ▣ 675
- Donnagel-PG ... 1858
- Donnatal ... 1858
- Donnatal Extentabs ... 1859
- Donnatal Tablets ... 1858
- Donnazyme Tablets ... 1860
- Isopto Hyoscine ... ⊙ 222
- Murocoll-2 Sterile Ophthalmic Solution ... ⊙ 261
- Ru-Tuss Tablets ... 693

Scopolamine Preparations (Anticholinergic effects potentiated). Products include:
- Transderm Scōp Transdermal Therapeutic System ... 887

Sodium Nitroprusside (Hypotensive effects potentiated). Products include:
- Nipride I.V. Infusion ... 1909

Terazosin Hydrochloride (Hypotensive effects potentiated). Products include:
- Hytrin Tablets ... 529

Timolol Maleate (Hypotensive effects potentiated). Products include:
- Blocadren Tablets ... 1429
- Timolide Tablets ... 1547
- Timoptic in Ocudose ... 1552
- Timoptic Sterile Ophthalmic Solution ... 1550

Trimethaphan Camsylate (Hypotensive effects potentiated). Products include:
- Arfonad Ampuls ... 1887

Warfarin Sodium (Potential for increased plasma levels and adverse effects). Products include:
- Coumadin Injection & Tablets ... 944
- Panwarfin Tablets ... 547

COCAINE HYDROCHLORIDE TOPICAL SOLUTION

(Cocaine Hydrochloride) ... 620
No interactions described in labeling.

COD LIVER OIL CONCENTRATE CAPSULES

(Cod Liver Oil, Vitamins A & D) ... ▣ 694
No interactions described in labeling.

COD LIVER OIL CONCENTRATE TABLETS

(Cod Liver Oil, Vitamins A & D) ... ▣ 694
No interactions described in labeling.

COD LIVER OIL CONCENTRATE TABLETS WITH VITAMIN C

(Cod Liver Oil, Vitamins A & D, Vitamin C) ... ▣ 694
No interactions described in labeling.

CODICLEAR DH SYRUP

(Guaifenesin, Hydrocodone Bitartrate) ... 845
May interact with narcotic analgesics, hypnotics and sedatives, tranquilizers, central nervous system depressants, and certain other agents. Compounds in these categories include:

Alcohol (Additive CNS depression).

Alfentanil Hydrochloride (Additive CNS depression). Products include:
- Alfenta Injection ... 1131

Alprazolam (Additive CNS depression). Products include:
- Xanax Tablets ... 2367

Aprobarbital (Additive CNS depression). Products include:
- Alurate Elixir ... 1883

Buprenorphine (Additive CNS depression).
- No products indexed under this heading.

Buspirone Hydrochloride (Additive CNS depression). Products include:
- BuSpar ... 1401

Butabarbital (Additive CNS depression). Products include:
- Pyridium Plus ... 1764

Butalbital (Additive CNS depression). Products include:
- Esgic-Plus Tablets ... 1002
- Esgic Tablets & Capsules ... 1001
- Fioricet Tablets ... 2006
- Fiorinal Capsules ... 2007
- Fiorinal with Codeine Capsules ... 2008
- Fiorinal Tablets ... 2007
- Phrenilin ... 838
- Sedapap Tablets 50 mg/650 mg ... 1360

Chlordiazepoxide (Additive CNS depression). Products include:
- Libritabs Tablets ... 1930
- Limbitrol ... 1933
- Menrium Tablets ... 1934

Chlordiazepoxide Hydrochloride (Additive CNS depression). Products include:
- Librax Capsules ... 1929
- Librium Capsules ... 1931

(▣ Described in PDR For Nonprescription Drugs) (⊙ Described in PDR For Ophthalmology)

Librium Injectable 1932

Chlorpromazine (Additive CNS depression). Products include:
Thorazine 2234

Chlorprothixene (Additive CNS depression). Products include:
Taractan Tablets 1920

Chlorprothixene Hydrochloride (Additive CNS depression). Products include:
Taractan 1920

Chlorprothixene Lactate (Additive CNS depression). Products include:
Taractan Concentrate 1920

Clorazepate Dipotassium (Additive CNS depression). Products include:
Tranxene 556

Codeine (Additive CNS depression). Products include:
Calcidrine Syrup 506

Codeine Phosphate (Additive CNS depression). Products include:
Actifed with Codeine Cough Syrup.. 752
Cheracol Cough Syrup 1853
Codimal PH Syrup 846
Dimetane-DC Cough Syrup 1857
Empirin with Codeine Phosphate Nos. 2, 3 & 4 764
Fiorinal with Codeine Capsules 2008
Isoclor Expectorant 982
Naldecon CX Adult Liquid .... ▣ 521
Novahistine DH 1342
Novahistine Expectorant 1343
Nucofed Capsules 2219
Nucofed Expectorant 2219
Nucofed Pediatric Expectorant 2220
Nucofed Syrup 2219
Phenaphen with Codeine Capsules 1865
Phenaphen-650 with Codeine Tablets 1866
Phenergan with Codeine 2497
Phenergan VC with Codeine 2501
Robitussin A-C Syrup 1875
Robitussin-DAC Syrup 1875
Ryna .... ▣ 741
Soma Compound w/Codeine Tablets 2390
Triaminic Expectorant w/Codeine .. 1996
Tussi-Organidin Liquid 2391
Tylenol with Codeine 1381

Codeine Polistirex (Additive CNS depression).
No products indexed under this heading.

Dezocine (Additive CNS depression).

Diazepam (Additive CNS depression). Products include:
Valium Injectable 1937
Valium Tablets 1939
Valrelease Capsules 1923

Droperidol (Additive CNS depression). Products include:
Inapsine Injection 1140
Innovar Injection 1141

Enflurane (Additive CNS depression). Products include:
Ethrane 599

Estazolam (Additive CNS depression). Products include:
ProSom Tablets 554

Ethchlorvynol (Additive CNS depression). Products include:
Placidyl Capsules 553

Ethinamate (Additive CNS depression).
No products indexed under this heading.

Fentanyl (Additive CNS depression). Products include:
Duragesic Transdermal System 1133

Fentanyl Citrate (Additive CNS depression). Products include:
Innovar Injection 1141
Sublimaze Injection 1146

Fluphenazine Decanoate (Additive CNS depression). Products include:
Prolixin Decanoate 1795

Fluphenazine Enanthate (Additive CNS depression). Products include:
Prolixin Enanthate 1796

Fluphenazine Hydrochloride (Additive CNS depression). Products include:
Prolixin Elixir 1793
Prolixin Injection 1791
Prolixin Oral Concentrate 1792
Prolixin Tablets 1793

Flurazepam Hydrochloride (Additive CNS depression). Products include:
Dalmane Capsules 1927

Glutethimide (Additive CNS depression).
No products indexed under this heading.

Haloperidol (Additive CNS depression). Products include:
Haldol Injection, Tablets and Concentrate 1373

Haloperidol Decanoate (Additive CNS depression). Products include:
Haldol Decanoate 1375

Hydrocodone Polistirex (Additive CNS depression). Products include:
Tussionex Extended-Release Suspension 988

Hydroxyzine Hydrochloride (Additive CNS depression). Products include:
Atarax Tablets & Syrup 1941
Marax Tablets & DF Syrup 1954
Vistaril Intramuscular Solution 1970

Isoflurane (Additive CNS depression). Products include:
Forane 600

Ketamine Hydrochloride (Additive CNS depression). Products include:
Ketalar 1726

Levorphanol Tartrate (Additive CNS depression). Products include:
Levo-Dromoran 1906

Lorazepam (Additive CNS depression). Products include:
Ativan Injection 2432
Ativan Tablets 2434

Loxapine Hydrochloride (Additive CNS depression). Products include:
Loxitane 1213

Loxapine Succinate (Additive CNS depression). Products include:
Loxitane Capsules 1213

Meperidine Hydrochloride (Additive CNS depression). Products include:
Demerol 2047
Mepergan Injection 2479

Mephobarbital (Additive CNS depression). Products include:
Mebaral Tablets 2061

Meprobamate (Additive CNS depression). Products include:
Deprol Tablets 2382
Equagesic Tablets 2451
Miltown Tablets 2386
PMB 200 and PMB 400 2504

Mesoridazine (Additive CNS depression). Products include:
Serentil 686

Methadone Hydrochloride (Additive CNS depression). Products include:
Dolophine Hydrochloride Ampoules & Vials 1260
Dolophine Hydrochloride Tablets 1261
Methadone Hydrochloride Diskets .. 1284
Methadone Hydrochloride Oral Solution & Tablets 1987

Methohexital Sodium (Additive CNS depression). Products include:
Brevital Sodium Vials 1248

Methoxyflurane (Additive CNS depression).
No products indexed under this heading.

Midazolam Hydrochloride (Additive CNS depression). Products include:
Versed Injection 1924

Molindone Hydrochloride (Additive CNS depression). Products include:
Moban Tablets & Concentrate 932

Morphine Sulfate (Additive CNS depression). Products include:
Astramorph/PF Injection, USP (Preservative-Free) 618
Duramorph 960
Infumorph 200 and Infumorph 500 Sterile Solutions 962
MS Contin Tablets 1814
MSIR 1817
Oramorph SR (Morphine Sulfate Sustained Release Tablets) 1988
Roxanol 1991

Opium Alkaloids (Additive CNS depression). Products include:
B & O No. 15A & No. 16A Supprettes 2395
Pantopon Injectable 1911

Oxazepam (Additive CNS depression). Products include:
Serax Capsules 2522
Serax Tablets 2522

Oxycodone Hydrochloride (Additive CNS depression). Products include:
Percocet Tablets 950
Percodan 951
Roxicodone Tablets, Oral Solution & Intensol (Oxycodone) 1992
Tylox Capsules 1382

Pentobarbital Sodium (Additive CNS depression). Products include:
Nembutal Sodium Capsules 534
Nembutal Sodium Solution 536
Nembutal Sodium Suppositories 538

Perphenazine (Additive CNS depression). Products include:
Etrafon 2087
Triavil Tablets 1556
Trilafon 2123

Phenobarbital (Additive CNS depression). Products include:
Arco-Lase Plus Tablets 607
Bellergal-S Tablets 1998
Bronkolixir .... ▣ 761
Bronkotabs Tablets .... ▣ 762
Donnatal 1858
Donnatal Extentabs 1859
Donnatal Tablets 1858
Donnazyme Tablets 1860
Kinesed Tablets 2272
Phenobarbital Elixir and Tablets 1293
Primatene Tablets-P Formula 2421
Quadrinal Tablets 1183
Tedral SA 1765

Prazepam (Additive CNS depression). Products include:
Centrax 1693

Prochlorperazine (Additive CNS depression). Products include:
Compazine 2201

Promethazine Hydrochloride (Additive CNS depression). Products include:
Mepergan Injection 2479
Phenergan with Codeine 2497
Phenergan with Dextromethorphan 2499
Phenergan Injection 2493
Phenergan Suppositories 2496
Phenergan Syrup 2495
Phenergan Tablets 2496
Phenergan VC 2500
Phenergan VC with Codeine 2501

Propofol (Additive CNS depression). Products include:
Diprivan Injection 2267

Propoxyphene Hydrochloride (Additive CNS depression). Products include:
Darvon 1256
Wygesic Tablets 2540

Propoxyphene Napsylate (Additive CNS depression). Products include:
Darvon-N/Darvocet-N 1254

Quazepam (Additive CNS depression). Products include:
Doral Tablets 2383

Secobarbital Sodium (Additive CNS depression). Products include:
Seconal Sodium Pulvules 1296

Sufentanil Citrate (Additive CNS depression). Products include:
Sufenta Injection 1147

Temazepam (Additive CNS depression). Products include:
Restoril Capsules 2023

Thiamylal Sodium (Additive CNS depression). Products include:
Surital Ampoules, Steri-Vials 1764

Thiothixene (Additive CNS depression). Products include:
Navane Capsules and Concentrate 1954
Navane Intramuscular 1956

Triazolam (Additive CNS depression). Products include:
Halcion Tablets 2340

Trifluoperazine Hydrochloride (Additive CNS depression). Products include:
Stelazine 2226

CODIMAL DH SYRUP (Hydrocodone Bitartrate, Phenylephrine Hydrochloride, Pyrilamine Maleate) 846
May interact with monoamine oxidase inhibitors, beta blockers, central nervous system depressants, veratrum alkaloids, and certain other agents. Compounds in these categories include:

Acebutolol Hydrochloride (Increases the effects of sympathomimetics). Products include:
Sectral Capsules 2520

Alcohol (May exhibit additive effects).

Alfentanil Hydrochloride (Concurrent use may exhibit additive effects). Products include:
Alfenta Injection 1131

Alprazolam (Concurrent use may exhibit additive effects). Products include:
Xanax Tablets 2367

Aprobarbital (Concurrent use may exhibit additive effects). Products include:
Alurate Elixir 1883

Atenolol (Increases the effects of sympathomimetics). Products include:
Tenoretic Tablets 1105
Tenormin Tablets and I.V. Injection 1107

Betaxolol Hydrochloride (Increases the effects of sympathomimetics). Products include:
Betoptic Sterile Ophthalmic Solution 569
Betoptic S Sterile Ophthalmic Suspension 570
Kerlone Tablets 2172

Buprenorphine (Concurrent use may exhibit additive effects).
No products indexed under this heading.

Buspirone Hydrochloride (Concurrent use may exhibit additive effects). Products include:
BuSpar 1401

Butabarbital (Concurrent use may exhibit additive effects). Products include:
Pyridium Plus 1764

Butalbital (Concurrent use may exhibit additive effects). Products include:
- Esgic-Plus Tablets ... 1002
- Esgic Tablets & Capsules ... 1001
- Fioricet Tablets ... 2006
- Fiorinal Capsules ... 2007
- Fiorinal with Codeine Capsules ... 2008
- Fiorinal Tablets ... 2007
- Phrenilin ... 838
- Sedapap Tablets 50 mg/650 mg ... 1360

Carteolol Hydrochloride (Increases the effects of sympathomimetics). Products include:
- Cartrol Tablets ... 507

Chlordiazepoxide (Concurrent use may exhibit additive effects). Products include:
- Libritabs Tablets ... 1930
- Limbitrol ... 1933
- Menrium Tablets ... 1934

Chlordiazepoxide Hydrochloride (Concurrent use may exhibit additive effects). Products include:
- Librax Capsules ... 1929
- Librium Capsules ... 1931
- Librium Injectable ... 1932

Chlorpromazine (Concurrent use may exhibit additive effects). Products include:
- Thorazine ... 2234

Chlorprothixene (Concurrent use may exhibit additive effects). Products include:
- Taractan Tablets ... 1920

Chlorprothixene Hydrochloride (Concurrent use may exhibit additive effects). Products include:
- Taractan ... 1920

Clorazepate Dipotassium (Concurrent use may exhibit additive effects). Products include:
- Tranxene ... 556

Codeine (Concurrent use may exhibit additive effects). Products include:
- Calcidrine Syrup ... 506

Codeine Phosphate (Concurrent use may exhibit additive effects). Products include:
- Actifed with Codeine Cough Syrup ... 752
- Cheracol Cough Syrup ... 1853
- Codimal PH Syrup ... 846
- Dimetane-DC Cough Syrup ... 1857
- Empirin with Codeine Phosphate Nos. 2, 3 & 4 ... 764
- Fiorinal with Codeine Capsules ... 2008
- Isoclor Expectorant ... 982
- Naldecon CX Adult Liquid ... ◙ 521
- Novahistine DH ... 1342
- Novahistine Expectorant ... 1343
- Nucofed Capsules ... 2219
- Nucofed Expectorant ... 2219
- Nucofed Pediatric Expectorant ... 2220
- Nucofed Syrup ... 2219
- Phenaphen with Codeine Capsules ... 1865
- Phenaphen-650 with Codeine Tablets ... 1866
- Phenergan with Codeine ... 2497
- Phenergan VC with Codeine ... 2501
- Robitussin A-C Syrup ... 1875
- Robitussin-DAC Syrup ... 1875
- Ryna ... ◙ 741
- Soma Compound w/Codeine Tablets ... 2390
- Triaminic Expectorant w/Codeine ... 1996
- Tussi-Organidin Liquid ... 2391
- Tylenol with Codeine ... 1381

Codeine Polistirex (Concurrent use may exhibit additive effects).
- No products indexed under this heading.

Cryptenamine Preparations (Concurrent use may reduce antihypertensive effects).

Deserpidine (Concurrent use may reduce antihypertensive effects). Products include:
- Enduronyl ... 518
- Harmonyl Tablets ... 528
- Oreticyl ... 545

Dezocine (Concurrent use may exhibit additive effects).

Diazepam (Concurrent use may exhibit additive effects). Products include:
- Valium Injectable ... 1937
- Valium Tablets ... 1939
- Valrelease Capsules ... 1923

Droperidol (Concurrent use may exhibit additive effects). Products include:
- Inapsine Injection ... 1140
- Innovar Injection ... 1141

Enflurane (Concurrent use may exhibit additive effects). Products include:
- Ethrane ... 599

Esmolol Hydrochloride (Increases the effects of sympathomimetics). Products include:
- Brevibloc Injection ... 942

Estazolam (Concurrent use may exhibit additive effects). Products include:
- ProSom Tablets ... 554

Ethchlorvynol (Concurrent use may exhibit additive effects). Products include:
- Placidyl Capsules ... 553

Ethinamate (Concurrent use may exhibit additive effects).
- No products indexed under this heading.

Fentanyl (Concurrent use may exhibit additive effects). Products include:
- Duragesic Transdermal System ... 1133

Fentanyl Citrate (Concurrent use may exhibit additive effects). Products include:
- Innovar Injection ... 1141
- Sublimaze Injection ... 1146

Fluphenazine Decanoate (Concurrent use may exhibit additive effects). Products include:
- Prolixin Decanoate ... 1795

Fluphenazine Enanthate (Concurrent use may exhibit additive effects). Products include:
- Prolixin Enanthate ... 1796

Fluphenazine Hydrochloride (Concurrent use may exhibit additive effects). Products include:
- Prolixin Elixir ... 1793
- Prolixin Injection ... 1791
- Prolixin Oral Concentrate ... 1792
- Prolixin Tablets ... 1793

Flurazepam Hydrochloride (Concurrent use may exhibit additive effects). Products include:
- Dalmane Capsules ... 1927

Furazolidone (Concurrent use requires extreme caution; may increase the effects of sympathomimetics). Products include:
- Furoxone ... 1855

Glutethimide (Concurrent use may exhibit additive effects).
- No products indexed under this heading.

Haloperidol (Concurrent use may exhibit additive effects). Products include:
- Haldol Injection, Tablets and Concentrate ... 1373

Haloperidol Decanoate (Concurrent use may exhibit additive effects). Products include:
- Haldol Decanoate ... 1375

Hydrocodone Polistirex (Concurrent use may exhibit additive effects). Products include:
- Tussionex Extended-Release Suspension ... 988

Hydroxyzine Hydrochloride (Concurrent use may exhibit additive effects). Products include:
- Atarax Tablets & Syrup ... 1941
- Marax Tablets & DF Syrup ... 1954
- Vistaril Intramuscular Solution ... 1970

Isocarboxazid (Concurrent use requires extreme caution; may increase the effects of sympathomimetics). Products include:
- Marplan Tablets ... 1906

Isoflurane (Concurrent use may exhibit additive effects). Products include:
- Forane ... 600

Ketamine Hydrochloride (Concurrent use may exhibit additive effects). Products include:
- Ketalar ... 1726

Labetalol Hydrochloride (Increases the effects of sympathomimetics). Products include:
- Normodyne Injection ... 2108
- Normodyne Tablets ... 2110
- Normozide Tablets ... 2112
- Trandate HCT Tablets ... 579
- Trandate Injection ... 577
- Trandate Tablets ... 579

Levorphanol Tartrate (Concurrent use may exhibit additive effects). Products include:
- Levo-Dromoran ... 1906

Lorazepam (Concurrent use may exhibit additive effects). Products include:
- Ativan Injection ... 2432
- Ativan Tablets ... 2434

Loxapine Hydrochloride (Concurrent use may exhibit additive effects). Products include:
- Loxitane ... 1213

Loxapine Succinate (Concurrent use may exhibit additive effects). Products include:
- Loxitane Capsules ... 1213

Mecamylamine Hydrochloride (Concurrent use may reduce antihypertensive effects). Products include:
- Inversine Tablets ... 1492

Meperidine Hydrochloride (Concurrent use may exhibit additive effects). Products include:
- Demerol ... 2047
- Mepergan Injection ... 2479

Mephobarbital (Concurrent use may exhibit additive effects). Products include:
- Mebaral Tablets ... 2061

Meprobamate (Concurrent use may exhibit additive effects). Products include:
- Deprol Tablets ... 2382
- Equagesic Tablets ... 2451
- Miltown Tablets ... 2386
- PMB 200 and PMB 400 ... 2504

Mesoridazine (Concurrent use may exhibit additive effects). Products include:
- Serentil ... 686

Methadone Hydrochloride (Concurrent use may exhibit additive effects). Products include:
- Dolophine Hydrochloride Ampoules & Vials ... 1260
- Dolophine Hydrochloride Tablets ... 1261
- Methadone Hydrochloride Diskets ... 1284
- Methadone Hydrochloride Oral Solution & Tablets ... 1987

Methohexital Sodium (Concurrent use may exhibit additive effects). Products include:
- Brevital Sodium Vials ... 1248

Methoxyflurane (Concurrent use may exhibit additive effects).
- No products indexed under this heading.

Methyldopa (Concurrent use may reduce antihypertensive effects). Products include:
- Aldoclor Tablets ... 1413
- Aldomet Oral ... 1415
- Aldoril Tablets ... 1418

Methyldopate Hydrochloride (Concurrent use may reduce antihypertensive effects). Products include:
- Aldomet Ester HCl Injection ... 1417

Metoprolol Tartrate (Increases the effects of sympathomimetics). Products include:
- Lopressor Ampuls ... 1032
- Lopressor HCT Tablets ... 1034
- Lopressor Tablets ... 1032

Midazolam Hydrochloride (Concurrent use may exhibit additive effects). Products include:
- Versed Injection ... 1924

Molindone Hydrochloride (Concurrent use may exhibit additive effects). Products include:
- Moban Tablets & Concentrate ... 932

Morphine Sulfate (Concurrent use may exhibit additive effects). Products include:
- Astramorph/PF Injection, USP (Preservative-Free) ... 618
- Duramorph ... 960
- Infumorph 200 and Infumorph 500 Sterile Solutions ... 962
- MS Contin Tablets ... 1814
- MSIR ... 1817
- Oramorph SR (Morphine Sulfate Sustained Release Tablets) ... 1988
- Roxanol ... 1991

Nadolol (Increases the effects of sympathomimetics). Products include:
- Corgard Tablets ... 701
- Corzide Tablets ... 702

Opium Alkaloids (Concurrent use may exhibit additive effects). Products include:
- B & O No. 15A & No. 16A Supprettes ... 2395
- Pantopon Injectable ... 1911

Oxazepam (Concurrent use may exhibit additive effects). Products include:
- Serax Capsules ... 2522
- Serax Tablets ... 2522

Oxycodone Hydrochloride (Concurrent use may exhibit additive effects). Products include:
- Percocet Tablets ... 950
- Percodan ... 951
- Roxicodone Tablets, Oral Solution & Intensol (Oxycodone) ... 1992
- Tylox Capsules ... 1382

Penbutolol Sulfate (Increases the effects of sympathomimetics). Products include:
- Levatol ... 1832

Pentobarbital Sodium (Concurrent use may exhibit additive effects). Products include:
- Nembutal Sodium Capsules ... 534
- Nembutal Sodium Solution ... 536
- Nembutal Sodium Suppositories ... 538

Perphenazine (Concurrent use may exhibit additive effects). Products include:
- Etrafon ... 2087
- Triavil Tablets ... 1556
- Trilafon ... 2123

Phenelzine Sulfate (Concurrent use requires extreme caution; may increase the effects of sympathomimetics). Products include:
- Nardil ... 1742

Phenobarbital (Concurrent use may exhibit additive effects). Products include:
- Arco-Lase Plus Tablets ... 607
- Bellergal-S Tablets ... 1998
- Bronkolixir ... ◙ 761
- Bronkotabs Tablets ... ◙ 762
- Donnatal ... 1858
- Donnatal Extentabs ... 1859
- Donnatal Tablets ... 1858
- Donnazyme Tablets ... 1860
- Kinesed Tablets ... 2272
- Phenobarbital Elixir and Tablets ... 1293
- Primatene Tablets-P Formula ... 2421

Quadrinal Tablets 1183
Tedral SA 1765

Pindolol (Increases the effects of sympathomimetics). Products include:
Visken Tablets 2036

Prazepam (Concurrent use may exhibit additive effects). Products include:
Centrax 1693

Prochlorperazine (Concurrent use may exhibit additive effects). Products include:
Compazine 2201

Promethazine Hydrochloride (Concurrent use may exhibit additive effects). Products include:
Mepergan Injection 2479
Phenergan with Codeine 2497
Phenergan with Dextromethorphan 2499
Phenergan Injection 2493
Phenergan Suppositories 2496
Phenergan Syrup 2495
Phenergan Tablets 2496
Phenergan VC 2500
Phenergan VC with Codeine 2501

Propofol (Concurrent use may exhibit additive effects). Products include:
Diprivan Injection 2267

Propoxyphene Hydrochloride (Concurrent use may exhibit additive effects). Products include:
Darvon 1256
Wygesic Tablets 2540

Propoxyphene Napsylate (Concurrent use may exhibit additive effects). Products include:
Darvon-N/Darvocet-N 1254

Propranolol Hydrochloride (Increases the effects of sympathomimetics). Products include:
Inderal 2459
Inderal LA Long Acting Capsules 2461
Inderide Tablets 2463
Inderide LA Long Acting Capsules .. 2465

Quazepam (Concurrent use may exhibit additive effects). Products include:
Doral Tablets 2383

Rauwolfia Serpentina (Concurrent use may reduce antihypertensive effects). Products include:
Raudixin Tablets 1803
Rauzide Tablets 1804

Rescinnamine (Concurrent use may reduce antihypertensive effects).
No products indexed under this heading.

Reserpine (Concurrent use may reduce antihypertensive effects). Products include:
Diupres Tablets 1461
Hydromox R Tablets 1209
Hydropres Tablets 1485
Renese-R Tablets 1786
Salutensin/Salutensin-Demi 719
Ser-Ap-Es Tablets 881
Serpasil Tablets 883
Serpasil-Apresoline Tablets 884
Serpasil-Esidrix Tablets 886

Secobarbital Sodium (Concurrent use may exhibit additive effects). Products include:
Seconal Sodium Pulvules 1296

Selegiline Hydrochloride (Concurrent use requires extreme caution; may increase the effects of sympathomimetics). Products include:
Eldepryl 2250

Sufentanil Citrate (Concurrent use may exhibit additive effects). Products include:
Sufenta Injection 1147

Temazepam (Concurrent use may exhibit additive effects). Products include:
Restoril Capsules 2023

Thiamylal Sodium (Concurrent use may exhibit additive effects). Products include:
Surital Ampoules, Steri-Vials 1764

Thioridazine Hydrochloride (Concurrent use may exhibit additive effects). Products include:
Mellaril 2011

Thiothixene (Concurrent use may exhibit additive effects). Products include:
Navane Capsules and Concentrate 1954
Navane Intramuscular 1956

Timolol Maleate (Increases the effects of sympathomimetics). Products include:
Blocadren Tablets 1429
Timolide Tablets 1547
Timoptic in Ocudose 1552
Timoptic Sterile Ophthalmic Solution 1550

Tranylcypromine Sulfate (Concurrent use requires extreme caution; may increase the effects of sympathomimetics). Products include:
Parnate Tablets 2222

Triazolam (Concurrent use may exhibit additive effects). Products include:
Halcion Tablets 2340

Trifluoperazine Hydrochloride (Concurrent use may exhibit additive effects). Products include:
Stelazine 2226

CODIMAL DM SYRUP

(Dextromethorphan Hydrobromide, Phenylephrine Hydrochloride, Pyrilamine Maleate) 846
See **Codimal DH Syrup**

CODIMAL EXPECTORANT

(Phenylpropanolamine Hydrochloride, Guaifenesin) 846
See **Codimal DH Syrup**

CODIMAL PH SYRUP

(Codeine Phosphate, Phenylephrine Hydrochloride, Pyrilamine Maleate) .. 846
See **Codimal DH Syrup**

COGENTIN INJECTION

(Benztropine Mesylate) 1435
May interact with phenothiazines, tricyclic antidepressants, belladona products, anticholinergics, butyrophenones, and dopamine antagonists. Compounds in these categories include:

Amitriptyline Hydrochloride (Potential for paralytic ileus, hyperthermia and heat stroke). Products include:
Elavil 2269
Endep Tablets 1927
Etrafon 2087
Limbitrol 1933
Triavil Tablets 1556

Amoxapine (Potential for paralytic ileus, hyperthermia and heat stroke). Products include:
Asendin Tablets 1196

Atropine Sulfate (Potential for paralytic ileus, hyperthermia and heat stroke). Products include:
Arco-Lase Plus Tablets 607
Atropine Sulfate Sterile Ophthalmic Solution and S.O.P. Sterile Ophthalmic Ointment .... ⊙ 239
Donnagel .... ▣ 675
Donnagel-PG 1858
Donnatal 1858
Donnatal Extentabs 1859
Donnatal Tablets 1858
Donnazyme Tablets 1860
Isopto Atropine .... ⊙ 218
Lomotil 2174
Motofen Tablets 836
Ru-Tuss Tablets 693
Urised Tablets 2396

Belladonna Alkaloids (Potential for paralytic ileus, hyperthermia and heat stroke). Products include:
Bellergal-S Tablets 1998
Hyland's Bed Wetting Tablets .... ▣ 728
Hyland's Teething Tablets .... ▣ 728
Kinesed Tablets 2272

Biperiden (Potential for paralytic ileus, hyperthermia and heat stroke). Products include:
Akineton 1171

Chlorpromazine (Potential for paralytic ileus, hyperthermia and heat stroke). Products include:
Thorazine 2234

Clidinium Bromide (Potential for paralytic ileus, hyperthermia and heat stroke). Products include:
Librax Capsules 1929
Quarzan Capsules 1937

Clomipramine Hydrochloride (Potential for paralytic ileus, hyperthermia and heat stroke). Products include:
Anafranil Capsules 650

Clozapine (Potential for paralytic ileus, hyperthermia and heat stroke). Products include:
Clozaril Tablets 2000

Desipramine Hydrochloride (Potential for paralytic ileus, hyperthermia and heat stroke). Products include:
Norpramin Tablets 1340

Dicyclomine Hydrochloride (Potential for paralytic ileus, hyperthermia and heat stroke). Products include:
Bentyl 1322

Doxepin Hydrochloride (Potential for paralytic ileus, hyperthermia and heat stroke). Products include:
Sinequan 1960

Fluphenazine Decanoate (Potential for paralytic ileus, hyperthermia and heat stroke). Products include:
Prolixin Decanoate 1795

Fluphenazine Enanthate (Potential for paralytic ileus, hyperthermia and heat stroke). Products include:
Prolixin Enanthate 1796

Fluphenazine Hydrochloride (Potential for paralytic ileus, hyperthermia and heat stroke). Products include:
Prolixin Elixir 1793
Prolixin Injection 1791
Prolixin Oral Concentrate 1792
Prolixin Tablets 1793

Glycopyrrolate (Potential for paralytic ileus, hyperthermia and heat stroke). Products include:
Robinul Forte Tablets 1873
Robinul Injectable 1873
Robinul Tablets 1873

Haloperidol (Potential for paralytic ileus, hyperthermia and heat stroke). Products include:
Haldol Injection, Tablets and Concentrate 1373

Haloperidol Decanoate (Potential for paralytic ileus, hyperthermia and heat stroke). Products include:
Haldol Decanoate 1375

Hyoscyamine (Potential for paralytic ileus, hyperthermia and heat stroke). Products include:
Cystospaz Tablets 2395
Urised Tablets 2396

Hyoscyamine Sulfate (Potential for paralytic ileus, hyperthermia and heat stroke). Products include:
Arco-Lase Plus Tablets 607
Cystospaz-M Capsules 2395
Donnagel .... ▣ 675
Donnagel-PG 1858
Donnatal 1858
Donnatal Extentabs 1859
Donnatal Tablets 1858
Donnazyme Tablets 1860
Kutrase Capsules 2146
Levsin/Levsinex 2147
Ru-Tuss Tablets 693

Imipramine Hydrochloride (Potential for paralytic ileus, hyperthermia and heat stroke). Products include:
Tofranil Ampuls 1038
Tofranil Tablets 1039

Imipramine Pamoate (Potential for paralytic ileus, hyperthermia and heat stroke). Products include:
Tofranil-PM Capsules 1041

Ipratropium Bromide (Potential for paralytic ileus, hyperthermia and heat stroke). Products include:
Atrovent Inhalation Aerosol 675

Maprotiline Hydrochloride (Potential for paralytic ileus, hyperthermia and heat stroke). Products include:
Ludiomil Tablets 874

Mepenzolate Bromide (Potential for paralytic ileus, hyperthermia and heat stroke). Products include:
Cantil Tablets 1326

Mesoridazine (Potential for paralytic ileus, hyperthermia and heat stroke). Products include:
Serentil 686

Metoclopramide Hydrochloride (Potential for paralytic ileus, hyperthermia and heat stroke). Products include:
Reglan 1869

Nortriptyline Hydrochloride (Potential for paralytic ileus, hyperthermia and heat stroke). Products include:
Pamelor 2019

Oxybutynin Chloride (Potential for paralytic ileus, hyperthermia and heat stroke). Products include:
Ditropan 1332

Perphenazine (Potential for paralytic ileus, hyperthermia and heat stroke). Products include:
Etrafon 2087
Triavil Tablets 1556
Trilafon 2123

Pimozide (Potential for paralytic ileus, hyperthermia and heat stroke). Products include:
Orap Tablets 1020

Prochlorperazine (Potential for paralytic ileus, hyperthermia and heat stroke). Products include:
Compazine 2201

Procyclidine Hydrochloride (Potential for paralytic ileus, hyperthermia and heat stroke). Products include:
Kemadrin Tablets 771

Promethazine Hydrochloride (Potential for paralytic ileus, hyperthermia and heat stroke). Products include:
Mepergan Injection 2479
Phenergan with Codeine 2497
Phenergan with Dextromethorphan 2499
Phenergan Injection 2493
Phenergan Suppositories 2496
Phenergan Syrup 2495
Phenergan Tablets 2496
Phenergan VC 2500
Phenergan VC with Codeine 2501

Propantheline Bromide (Potential for paralytic ileus, hyperthermia and heat stroke). Products include:
Pro-Banthīne Tablets 2141

Protriptyline Hydrochloride (Potential for paralytic ileus, hyperthermia and heat stroke). Products include:
Vivactil Tablets 1567

Scopolamine Hydrobromide (Potential for paralytic ileus, hyperthermia and heat stroke). Products include:
Donnagel ▣ 675
Donnagel-PG 1858
Donnatal 1858
Donnatal Extentabs 1859
Donnatal Tablets 1858
Donnazyme Tablets 1860
Isopto Hyoscine ⊙ 222
Murocoll-2 Sterile Ophthalmic Solution ⊙ 261
Ru-Tuss Tablets 693

Scopolamine Preparations (Potential for paralytic ileus, hyperthermia and heat stroke). Products include:
Transderm Scōp Transdermal Therapeutic System 887

Thioridazine Hydrochloride (Potential for paralytic ileus, hyperthermia and heat stroke). Products include:
Mellaril 2011

Tridihexethyl Chloride (Potential for paralytic ileus, hyperthermia and heat stroke).
No products indexed under this heading.

Trifluoperazine Hydrochloride (Potential for paralytic ileus, hyperthermia and heat stroke). Products include:
Stelazine 2226

Trihexyphenidyl Hydrochloride (Potential for paralytic ileus, hyperthermia and heat stroke). Products include:
Artane 1195

Trimipramine Maleate (Potential for paralytic ileus, hyperthermia and heat stroke). Products include:
Surmontil Capsules 2524

COGENTIN TABLETS
(Benztropine Mesylate) 1435
See **Cogentin Injection**

COLACE
(Docusate Sodium) 1403
No interactions described in labeling.

COLBENEMID TABLETS
(Probenecid, Colchicine) 1436
May interact with penicillins, salicylates, sulfonamides, oral hypoglycemic agents, and certain other agents. Compounds in these categories include:

Acetaminophen (Increased plasma concentrations of acetaminophen). Products include:
Acetaminophen Uniserts Suppositories 2374
Actifed Plus Caplets ▣ 539
Actifed Plus Tablets ▣ 540
Alka-Seltzer Advanced Formula Antacid & Non-Aspirin Pain Reliever ▣ 620
Allerest ▣ 559
Aspirin Free Anacin Maximum Strength Acetaminophen Film Coated Caplets 2417
Aspirin Free Anacin Maximum Strength Acetaminophen Film Coated Tablets 2417
Anacin-3 Regular Strength Acetaminophen Film Coated Tablets ▣ 746
Anexsia 5/500 Tablets 2196
Anexsia 7.5/650 Tablets 2197
Benadryl Plus ▣ 636
Benadryl Plus Nighttime ▣ 637
Bufferin AF Nite Time Analgesic/Sleeping Aid Caplets 744
Allergy-Sinus Comtrex Multi-Symptom Allergy Sinus Formula Tablets & Caplets 746
Cough Formula Comtrex 746
Comtrex Multi-Symptom Cold Reliever Tablets/Caplets/Liqui-Gels/Liquid 745
Day-Night Comtrex 747
Non-Drowsy Comtrex 747
Congespirin For Children Aspirin Free Chewable Cold Tablets 748
Contac Cough & Sore Throat Formula ▣ 712
Contac Jr. Children's Cold Medicine ▣ 712
Contac Nighttime Cold Medicine ▣ 713
Contac Severe Cold and Flu Formula Caplets ▣ 711
Contac Sinus Caplets Maximum Strength Non-Drowsy Formula ▣ 710
Contac Sinus Tablets Maximum Strength Non-Drowsy Formula ▣ 710
Coricidin 'D' Decongestant Tablets ▣ 695
Coricidin Demilets Tablets for Children ▣ 696
Coricidin Tablets ▣ 695
Darvon-N/Darvocet-N 1254
Datril Extra-Strength Analgesic Tablets 748
Dimetapp Plus Caplets ▣ 675
Dorcol Children's Fever & Pain Reducer ▣ 686
Dristan Decongestant/Antihistamine/ Analgesic Coated Caplets ▣ 749
Dristan Cold Nasal Decongestant/ Antihistamine/ Analgesic Coated Tablets 2419
Dristan Advanced Formula Decongestant/Antihistamine/ Analgesic Tablets ▣ 749
Maximum Strength Dristan Decongestant/Analgesic Coated Caplets ▣ 750
No Drowsiness Dristan Cold Nasal Decongestant/Analgesic Coated Caplets 2420
Drixoral Plus Extended-Release Tablets ▣ 699
Drixoral Sinus ▣ 700
Esgic-Plus Tablets 1002
Esgic Tablets & Capsules 1001
Aspirin Free Excedrin Analgesic Caplets 748
Excedrin Extra-Strength Analgesic Tablets & Caplets 749
Excedrin P.M. Analgesic/Sleeping Aid Tablets, Caplets and Liquid 749
Sinus Excedrin Analgesic, Decongestant Tablets & Caplets 750
4-Way Cold Tablets 750
Feverall Sprinkle Caps 2374
Feverall Suppositories 2374
Fioricet Tablets 2006
Hycomine Compound Tablets 929
Hydrocet Capsules 835
Isocom Capsules 1629
Liquiprin ▣ 618
Lortab 2412
Lurline PMS Tablets 972
Medi-Flu Caplet, Liquid ▣ 640
Maximum Strength Midol Multi-Symptom Menstrual Formula ▣ 571
Maximum Strength Midol PMS Premenstrual Syndrome Formula ▣ 570
Regular Strength Midol Multi-Symptom Menstrual Formula ▣ 570
Midrin Capsules 836
Ornex Caplets ▣ 618
Children's Panadol Chewable Tablets, Liquid, Infants' Drops ▣ 571
Junior Strength Panadol ▣ 571
Maximum Strength Panadol Tablets and Caplets ▣ 572
Percocet Tablets 950
Percogesic Analgesic Tablets ▣ 660
Phenaphen with Codeine Capsules 1865
Phenaphen-650 with Codeine Tablets 1866
Phrenilin 838
Prēmsyn PMS Capsules & Caplets ▣ 547
Pyrroxate Capsules ▣ 669
Robitussin Night Relief ▣ 677
Sedapap Tablets 50 mg/650 mg 1360
Sinarest ▣ 562
Sine-Aid Maximum Strength Sinus Headache Caplets 1365
Sine-Aid Maximum Strength Sinus Headache Tablets 1365
Sine-Off Maximum Strength Allergy/Sinus Formula Caplets ▣ 721
Sine-Off Maximum Strength No Drowsiness Formula Caplets ▣ 722
Singlet Tablets ▣ 598
Sinulin 840
Sinutab Maximum Strength ▣ 641
Sinutab Maximum Strength Without Drowsiness Tablets & Caplets ▣ 642
Sinutab Regular Strength Without Drowsiness Formula ▣ 641
Sominex Pain Relief Formula ▣ 723
St. Joseph Aspirin-Free Fever Reducer for Children Chewable Tablets, Liquid & Infant Drops ▣ 704
St. Joseph Cold Tablets for Children ▣ 704
St. Joseph Nighttime Cold Medicine ▣ 705
Sudafed Sinus Caplets ▣ 545
Sudafed Sinus Tablets ▣ 545
Talacen 2070
Tempra, Acetaminophen ▣ 613
TheraFlu Flu and Cold Medicine ▣ 687
Triaminicin Tablets ▣ 690
Tylenol acetaminophen Children's Chewable Tablets & Elixir 1366
Tylenol Allergy Sinus Medication Caplets and Gelcaps, Maximum Strength 1372
Tylenol with Codeine 1381
Children's Tylenol Cold Liquid Formula and Chewable Tablets 1368
Tylenol Cold & Flu Hot Medication, Packets 1369
Tylenol Cold & Flu No Drowsiness Hot Medication, Packets 1371
Tylenol Cold Medication Caplets and Tablets 1370
Tylenol Cold Medication, Effervescent Tablets 1369
Tylenol Cold Medication No Drowsiness Formula Caplets 1370
Tylenol Cold Night Time Medication Liquid 1371
Tylenol Cough Medication Liquid, Maximum Strength 1372
Tylenol Cough Medication Liquid with Decongestant, Maximum Strength 1372
Tylenol, Extra Strength, acetaminophen Adult Liquid Pain Reliever 1367
Tylenol, Extra Strength, acetaminophen Gelcaps, Caplets, Tablets 1367
Tylenol, Infants' Drops 1366
Tylenol, Junior Strength, acetaminophen Coated Caplets, Grape and Fruit Chewable Tablets 1366
Tylenol, Maximum Strength, Sinus Medication Gelcaps, Caplets and Tablets 1373
Tylenol, Regular Strength, acetaminophen Tablets and Caplets 1367
Tylenol PM, Extra Strength Caplets and Tablets 1368
Tylox Capsules 1382
Unisom Dual Relief Nighttime Sleep Aid/Analgesic 1774
Vanquish Analgesic Caplets ▣ 574
Vicks Daycare ▣ 660
Vicks Formula 44M Multi-Symptom Cough Medicine ▣ 662
Vicks NyQuil Nighttime Colds Medicine-Original & Cherry Flavor ▣ 664
Vicodin Tablets 1187
Vicodin ES Tablets 1189
Wygesic Tablets 2540
Zydone Capsules 941

Amoxicillin (Elevated plasma concentration of amoxicillin). Products include:
Amoxil 2193
Augmentin Tablets, Powder for Oral Suspension, and Chewable Tablets 2198

Ampicillin Sodium (Elevated plasma concentration of ampicillin). Products include:
Unasyn 1965

Aspirin (Uricosuric action of probenecid antagonized). Products include:
Alka-Seltzer Effervescent Antacid and Pain Reliever 1568
Alka-Seltzer Extra Strength Effervescent Antacid and Pain Reliever 1570
Alka-Seltzer (Flavored) Effervescent Antacid and Pain Reliever 1569
Alka-Seltzer Plus Cold Medicine ▣ 623
Alka-Seltzer Plus Night-Time Cold Medicine ▣ 623
Alka Seltzer Plus Sinus Allergy Medicine ▣ 624
Anacin Coated Analgesic Caplets 2417
Anacin Coated Analgesic Tablets 2417
Anacin Maximum Strength Analgesic Coated Tablets 2417
Maximum Strength Arthritis Pain Formula By the Makers of Anacin Analgesic Tablets and Caplets 2418
Arthritis Pain Formula by the Makers of Anacin Analgesic Tablets and Caplets ▣ 747
Arthritis Strength BC Powder ▣ 516
Ascriptin A/D Caplets 1850
Regular Strength Ascriptin Tablets 1850
Azdone Tablets 844
BC Powder ▣ 517
BC Cold Powder ▣ 517
Children's Bayer Chewable Aspirin ▣ 564
Genuine Bayer Aspirin Tablets & Caplets ▣ 564
Maximum Bayer Aspirin Tablets & Caplets ▣ 566
Bayer Plus Aspirin Tablets ▣ 567
Therapy Bayer Aspirin Caplets ▣ 568
8 Hour Bayer Timed-Release Aspirin ▣ 566
Arthritis Strength Bufferin Analgesic Caplets 744
Extra Strength Bufferin Analgesic Tablets 745
Bufferin Analgesic Tablets and Caplets 743
Cama Arthritis Pain Reliever ▣ 685
Damason-P 1356
Easprin 1719
Ecotrin Enteric Coated Aspirin Maximum Strength Tablets and Caplets 2189
Ecotrin Enteric Coated Aspirin Regular Strength Tablets and Caplets 2189
Empirin Aspirin ▣ 541
Empirin with Codeine Phosphate Nos. 2, 3 & 4 764
Equagesic Tablets 2451
Excedrin Extra-Strength Analgesic Tablets & Caplets 749
4-Way Cold Tablets 750
Fiorinal Capsules 2007
Fiorinal with Codeine Capsules 2008
Fiorinal Tablets 2007
Lortab ASA Tablets 2414
Momentum Muscular Backache Formula ▣ 751
Norgesic 1314
Norwich Extra-Strength Aspirin ▣ 546
Norwich Regular Strength Aspirin ▣ 547
P-A-C Analgesic Tablets ▣ 669
Percodan 951
Robaxisal Tablets 1872
Sine-Off Sinus Medicine Tablets-Aspirin Formula ▣ 722
Soma Compound w/Codeine Tablets 2390
Soma Compound Tablets 2389
St. Joseph Adult Chewable Aspirin (81 mg.) ▣ 703
Synalgos-DC Capsules 2525
Talwin Compound 2072
Ursinus Inlay-Tabs ▣ 691
Vanquish Analgesic Caplets ▣ 574
Zorprin Tablets 698

Azlocillin Sodium (Elevated plasma concentration of azlocillin).
No products indexed under this heading.

Bacampicillin Hydrochloride (Elevated plasma concentration of bacampicillin). Products include:
Spectrobid Tablets & Powder for Oral Suspension 1961

Carbenicillin Disodium (Elevated plasma concentration of carbenicillin).

Carbenicillin Indanyl Sodium (Elevated plasma concentration of carbenicillin). Products include:
Geocillin Tablets 1951

Chlorpropamide (Prolonged or enhanced action of oral sulfonylureas). Products include:
Diabinese Tablets 1775

Choline Magnesium Trisalicylate (Uricosuric action of probenecid antagonized). Products include:
Trilisate 1822

(▣ Described in PDR For Nonprescription Drugs)

(⊙ Described in PDR For Ophthalmology)

Diflunisal (Uricosuric action of probenecid antagonized). Products include:
- Dolobid Tablets ... 1465

Glipizide (Prolonged or enhanced action of oral sulfonylureas). Products include:
- Glucotrol ... 1952

Glyburide (Prolonged or enhanced action of oral sulfonylureas). Products include:
- DiaBeta ... 1091
- Micronase Tablets ... 2350

Indomethacin (Increased plasma levels of indomethacin). Products include:
- Indocin ... 1487

Indomethacin Sodium Trihydrate (Increased plasma levels of indomethacin). Products include:
- Indocin I.V. ... 1490

Ketamine Hydrochloride (Anesthesia prolonged). Products include:
- Ketalar ... 1726

Ketoprofen (Increased plasma concentrations of ketoprofen). Products include:
- Orudis Capsules ... 2488

Lorazepam (Increased plasma concentrations of lorazepam). Products include:
- Ativan Injection ... 2432
- Ativan Tablets ... 2434

Magnesium Salicylate (Uricosuric action of probenecid antagonized). Products include:
- Doan's - Extra-Strength Analgesic ◘ 549
- Doan's - Regular Strength Analgesic ... ◘ 549
- Mobigesic Analgesic Tablets ... ◘ 507

Meclofenamate Sodium (Increased plasma concentrations of meclofenamate). Products include:
- Meclomen Capsules ... 1739

Methotrexate Sodium (In concurrent administration methotrexate dosage should be reduced). Products include:
- Methotrexate Tablets, Parenteral, LPF Parenteral ... 1217
- Rheumatrex Methotrexate Dose Pack ... 1234

Mezlocillin Sodium (Elevated plasma concentration of mezlocillin). Products include:
- Mezlin ... 1597
- Mezlin Pharmacy Bulk Package ... 1599

Nafcillin Sodium (Elevated plasma concentration of nafcillin). Products include:
- Unipen ... 2533

Naproxen (Increased plasma concentrations of naproxen). Products include:
- Naprosyn ... 2297

Naproxen Sodium (Increased plasma concentrations of naproxen). Products include:
- Anaprox and Anaprox DS Tablets ... 2288

Penicillin G Potassium (Elevated plasma concentration of penicillin). Products include:
- Pfizerpen for Injection ... 1957

Penicillin G Procaine (Elevated plasma concentration of penicillin). Products include:
- Bicillin C-R Injection ... 2438
- Bicillin C-R 900/300 Injection ... 2440
- Pfizerpen-AS Aqueous Suspension 1959
- Wycillin Injection ... 2537
- Wycillin Injection and Probenecid Tablets ... 2539

Penicillin G Sodium (Elevated plasma concentration of penicillin).
- No products indexed under this heading.

Penicillin G, Benzathine (Elevated plasma concentration of penicillin). Products include:
- Bicillin C-R Injection ... 2438
- Bicillin C-R 900/300 Injection ... 2440
- Bicillin L-A Injection ... 2442

Penicillin V Potassium (Elevated plasma concentration of penicillin).
- No products indexed under this heading.

Pyrazinamide (Uricosuric action of probenecid antagonized).
- No products indexed under this heading.

Rifampin (Increased plasma concentrations of rifampin). Products include:
- Rifadin ... 1345
- Rifamate Capsules ... 1347
- Rimactane Capsules ... 879

Salsalate (Uricosuric action of probenecid antagonized). Products include:
- Disalcid ... 1310
- Mono-Gesic Tablets ... 846
- Salflex ... 839

Sulfamethizole (Significant increase in total sulfonamide plasma levels). Products include:
- Thiosulfil Forte Tablets ... 2526
- Urobiotic-250 Capsules ... 1968

Sulfamethoxazole (Significant increase in total sulfonamide plasma levels). Products include:
- Azo Gantanol Tablets ... 1887
- Bactrim DS Tablets ... 1891
- Bactrim I.V. Infusion ... 1889
- Bactrim ... 1891
- Gantanol ... 1899
- Septra ... 813
- Septra I.V. Infusion ... 808
- Septra I.V. Infusion ADD-Vantage Vials ... 810
- Septra ... 813

Sulfasalazine (Significant increase in total sulfonamide plasma levels). Products include:
- Azulfidine Tablets, EN-tabs, Oral Suspension ... 1157

Sulfinpyrazone (Significant increase in total sulfonamide plasma levels). Products include:
- Anturane ... 853

Sulfisoxazole (Significant increase in total sulfonamide plasma levels). Products include:
- Azo Gantrisin Tablets ... 1888
- Gantrisin Tablets ... 1901
- Pediazole ... 1973

Sulfisoxazole Diolamine (Significant increase in total sulfonamide plasma levels). Products include:
- Gantrisin Ophthalmic Ointment/Solution ... 1900

Sulindac (Increased plasma levels of sulindac; modest reduction in uricosuric action of probenecid). Products include:
- Clinoril Tablets ... 1433

Ticarcillin Disodium (Elevated plasma concentration of ticarcillin). Products include:
- Ticar for Injection ... 2236
- Timentin for Injection ... 2239

Tolazamide (Prolonged or enhanced action of oral sulfonylureas). Products include:
- Tolinase Tablets ... 2365

Tolbutamide (Prolonged or enhanced action of oral sulfonylureas). Products include:
- Orinase Tablets ... 2354

COLCHICINE AMPOULES
(Colchicine) ... 1252
May interact with central nervous system depressants, sympathomimetic aerosal brochodilators, and certain other agents. Compounds in these categories include:

Albuterol (Potential for increased response to sympathomimetics). Products include:
- Proventil Inhalation Aerosol ... 2117
- Ventolin Inhalation Aerosol and Refill ... 583

Albuterol Sulfate (Potential for increased response to sympathomimetics). Products include:
- Proventil Repetabs Tablets ... 2120
- Proventil Solutions for Inhalation 0.5% and 0.083% ... 2118
- Proventil Syrup ... 2119
- Proventil Tablets ... 2120
- Ventolin ... 583

Alfentanil Hydrochloride (Increased response to central nervous system depressants). Products include:
- Alfenta Injection ... 1131

Alprazolam (Increased response to central nervous system depressants). Products include:
- Xanax Tablets ... 2367

Aprobarbital (Increased response to central nervous system depressants). Products include:
- Alurate Elixir ... 1883

Buprenorphine (Increased response to central nervous system depressants).
- No products indexed under this heading.

Buspirone Hydrochloride (Increased response to central nervous system depressants). Products include:
- BuSpar ... 1401

Butabarbital (Increased response to central nervous system depressants). Products include:
- Pyridium Plus ... 1764

Butalbital (Increased response to central nervous system depressants). Products include:
- Esgic-Plus Tablets ... 1002
- Esgic Tablets & Capsules ... 1001
- Fioricet Tablets ... 2006
- Fiorinal Capsules ... 2007
- Fiorinal with Codeine Capsules ... 2008
- Fiorinal Tablets ... 2007
- Phrenilin ... 838
- Sedapap Tablets 50 mg/650 mg .. 1360

Chlordiazepoxide (Increased response to central nervous system depressants). Products include:
- Libritabs Tablets ... 1930
- Limbitrol ... 1933
- Menrium Tablets ... 1934

Chlordiazepoxide Hydrochloride (Increased response to central nervous system depressants). Products include:
- Librax Capsules ... 1929
- Librium Capsules ... 1931
- Librium Injectable ... 1932

Chlorpromazine (Increased response to central nervous system depressants). Products include:
- Thorazine ... 2234

Chlorprothixene (Increased response to central nervous system depressants). Products include:
- Taractan Tablets ... 1920

Chlorprothixene Hydrochloride (Increased response to central nervous system depressants). Products include:
- Taractan ... 1920

Clorazepate Dipotassium (Increased response to central nervous system depressants). Products include:
- Tranxene ... 556

Codeine (Increased response to central nervous system depressants). Products include:
- Calcidrine Syrup ... 506

Codeine Phosphate (Increased response to central nervous system depressants). Products include:
- Actifed with Codeine Cough Syrup.. 752
- Cheracol Cough Syrup ... 1853
- Codimal PH Syrup ... 846
- Dimetane-DC Cough Syrup ... 1857
- Empirin with Codeine Phosphate Nos. 2, 3 & 4 ... 764
- Fiorinal with Codeine Capsules ... 2008
- Isoclor Expectorant ... 982
- Naldecon CX Adult Liquid ... ◘ 521
- Novahistine DH ... 1342
- Novahistine Expectorant ... 1343
- Nucofed Capsules ... 2219
- Nucofed Expectorant ... 2219
- Nucofed Pediatric Expectorant ... 2220
- Nucofed Syrup ... 2219
- Phenaphen with Codeine Capsules 1865
- Phenaphen-650 with Codeine Tablets ... 1866
- Phenergan with Codeine ... 2497
- Phenergan VC with Codeine ... 2501
- Robitussin A-C Syrup ... 1875
- Robitussin-DAC Syrup ... 1875
- Ryna ... ◘ 741
- Soma Compound w/Codeine Tablets ... 2390
- Triaminic Expectorant w/Codeine .. 1996
- Tussi-Organidin Liquid ... 2391
- Tylenol with Codeine ... 1381

Codeine Polistirex (Increased response to central nervous system depressants).
- No products indexed under this heading.

Dezocine (Increased response to central nervous system depressants).

Diazepam (Increased response to central nervous system depressants). Products include:
- Valium Injectable ... 1937
- Valium Tablets ... 1939
- Valrelease Capsules ... 1923

Dobutamine Hydrochloride (Potential for increased response to sympathomimetics). Products include:
- Dobutrex Solution Vials ... 1259

Dopamine Hydrochloride (Potential for increased response to sympathomimetics). Products include:
- Intropin Injection ... 930

Droperidol (Increased response to central nervous system depressants). Products include:
- Inapsine Injection ... 1140
- Innovar Injection ... 1141

Enflurane (Increased response to central nervous system depressants). Products include:
- Ethrane ... 599

Ephedrine Hydrochloride (Potential for increased response to sympathomimetics). Products include:
- Amesec ... ◘ 682
- Primatene Tablets-M Formula ... 2421
- Primatene Tablets-P Formula ... 2421
- Primatene Tablets-Regular Formula ... 2421
- Quadrinal Tablets ... 1183
- Quelidrine Syrup ... 556
- Tedral SA ... 1765

Ephedrine Sulfate (Potential for increased response to sympathomimetics). Products include:
- Bronkaid Tablets ... ◘ 757
- Bronkolixir ... ◘ 761
- Bronkotabs Tablets ... ◘ 762
- Marax Tablets & DF Syrup ... 1954
- Pazo Hemorrhoid Ointment & Suppositories ... 752
- Vicks Vatronol Nose Drops ... ◘ 666

(◘ Described in PDR For Nonprescription Drugs) (⊙ Described in PDR For Ophthalmology)

Ephedrine Tannate (Potential for increased response to sympathomimetics). Products include:
- Rynatuss ... 2388

Epinephrine (Potential for increased response to sympathomimetics). Products include:
- Ana-Kit Anaphylaxis Emergency Treatment Kit ... 1100
- Bronkaid Mist ... ◘ 757
- EpiPen ... 843
- Marcaine Hydrochloride 0.5% with Epinephrine 1:200,000 (as bitartrate) ... 958
- Marcaine Hydrochloride with Epinephrine 1:200,000 ... 2055
- Primatene Mist ... 2420
- Sus-Phrine Injection ... 1006
- Xylocaine with Epinephrine Injections ... 637

Epinephrine Bitartrate (Potential for increased response to sympathomimetics). Products include:
- AsthmaHaler Mist Epinephrine Bitartrate Bronchodilator ... ◘ 616
- Bronkaid Mist Suspension ... ◘ 757
- Primatene Mist Suspension ... 2421

Epinephrine Hydrochloride (Potential for increased response to sympathomimetics). Products include:
- Adrenalin Chloride Solution 1:100 & 1:1,000 ... 1689
- Epifrin ... ◉ 244
- Glaucon ... ◉ 218

Estazolam (Increased response to central nervous system depressants). Products include:
- ProSom Tablets ... 554

Ethchlorvynol (Increased response to central nervous system depressants). Products include:
- Placidyl Capsules ... 553

Ethinamate (Increased response to central nervous system depressants).
- No products indexed under this heading.

Fentanyl (Increased response to central nervous system depressants). Products include:
- Duragesic Transdermal System ... 1133

Fentanyl Citrate (Increased response to central nervous system depressants). Products include:
- Innovar Injection ... 1141
- Sublimaze Injection ... 1146

Fluphenazine Decanoate (Increased response to central nervous system depressants). Products include:
- Prolixin Decanoate ... 1795

Fluphenazine Enanthate (Increased response to central nervous system depressants). Products include:
- Prolixin Enanthate ... 1796

Fluphenazine Hydrochloride (Increased response to central nervous system depressants). Products include:
- Prolixin Elixir ... 1793
- Prolixin Injection ... 1791
- Prolixin Oral Concentrate ... 1792
- Prolixin Tablets ... 1793

Flurazepam Hydrochloride (Increased response to central nervous system depressants). Products include:
- Dalmane Capsules ... 1927

Glutethimide (Increased response to central nervous system depressants).
- No products indexed under this heading.

Haloperidol (Increased response to central nervous system depressants). Products include:
- Haldol Injection, Tablets and Concentrate ... 1373

Haloperidol Decanoate (Increased response to central nervous system depressants). Products include:
- Haldol Decanoate ... 1375

Hydrocodone Bitartrate (Increased response to central nervous system depressants). Products include:
- Anexsia 5/500 Tablets ... 2196
- Anexsia 7.5/650 Tablets ... 2197
- Azdone Tablets ... 844
- Codiclear DH Syrup ... 845
- Codimal DH Syrup ... 846
- Damason-P ... 1356
- Hycodan Syrup, Tablets ... 927
- Hycomine Compound Tablets ... 929
- Hycomine Syrup ... 927
- Hycotuss Expectorant Syrup ... 930
- Hydrocet Capsules ... 835
- Lortab ASA Tablets ... 2414
- Lortab ... 2412
- Ru-Tuss with Hydrocodone ... 694
- Triaminic Expectorant DH ... 1995
- Vicodin Tablets ... 1187
- Vicodin ES Tablets ... 1189
- Zydone Capsules ... 941

Hydrocodone Polistirex (Increased response to central nervous system depressants). Products include:
- Tussionex Extended-Release Suspension ... 988

Hydroxyzine Hydrochloride (Increased response to central nervous system depressants). Products include:
- Atarax Tablets & Syrup ... 1941
- Marax Tablets & DF Syrup ... 1954
- Vistaril Intramuscular Solution ... 1970

Isoflurane (Increased response to central nervous system depressants). Products include:
- Forane ... 600

Isoproterenol Hydrochloride (Potential for increased response to sympathomimetics). Products include:
- Isuprel Hydrochloride Injection 1:5000 ... 2050
- Isuprel Hydrochloride Mistometer ... 2051
- Isuprel Hydrochloride Solution 1:200 & 1:100 ... 2052
- Norisodrine Aerotrol ... 540

Ketamine Hydrochloride (Increased response to central nervous system depressants). Products include:
- Ketalar ... 1726

Levorphanol Tartrate (Increased response to central nervous system depressants). Products include:
- Levo-Dromoran ... 1906

Lorazepam (Increased response to central nervous system depressants). Products include:
- Ativan Injection ... 2432
- Ativan Tablets ... 2434

Loxapine Hydrochloride (Increased response to central nervous system depressants). Products include:
- Loxitane ... 1213

Loxapine Succinate (Increased response to central nervous system depressants). Products include:
- Loxitane Capsules ... 1213

Meperidine Hydrochloride (Increased response to central nervous system depressants). Products include:
- Demerol ... 2047
- Mepergan Injection ... 2479

Mephobarbital (Increased response to central nervous system depressants). Products include:
- Mebaral Tablets ... 2061

Meprobamate (Increased response to central nervous system depressants). Products include:
- Deprol Tablets ... 2382
- Equagesic Tablets ... 2451
- Miltown Tablets ... 2386
- PMB 200 and PMB 400 ... 2504

Mesoridazine (Increased response to central nervous system depressants). Products include:
- Serentil ... 686

Metaproterenol Sulfate (Potential for increased response to sympathomimetics). Products include:
- Alupent ... 674
- Arm-a-Med Metaproterenol Sulfate Inhalation Solution, USP ... 617
- Metaprel Inhalation Aerosol Bronchodilator ... 2014
- Metaprel Inhalation Solution ... 2015
- Metaprel ... 2015
- Metaproterenol Sulfate Inhalation Solution, USP ... 912

Metaraminol Bitartrate (Potential for increased response to sympathomimetics). Products include:
- Aramine Injection ... 1424

Methadone Hydrochloride (Increased response to central nervous system depressants). Products include:
- Dolophine Hydrochloride Ampoules & Vials ... 1260
- Dolophine Hydrochloride Tablets ... 1261
- Methadone Hydrochloride Diskets ... 1284
- Methadone Hydrochloride Oral Solution & Tablets ... 1987

Methohexital Sodium (Increased response to central nervous system depressants). Products include:
- Brevital Sodium Vials ... 1248

Methoxamine Hydrochloride (Potential for increased response to sympathomimetics). Products include:
- Vasoxyl Injection ... 819

Methoxyflurane (Increased response to central nervous system depressants).
- No products indexed under this heading.

Midazolam Hydrochloride (Increased response to central nervous system depressants). Products include:
- Versed Injection ... 1924

Molindone Hydrochloride (Increased response to central nervous system depressants). Products include:
- Moban Tablets & Concentrate ... 932

Morphine Sulfate (Increased response to central nervous system depressants). Products include:
- Astramorph/PF Injection, USP (Preservative-Free) ... 618
- Duramorph ... 960
- Infumorph 200 and Infumorph 500 Sterile Solutions ... 962
- MS Contin Tablets ... 1814
- MSIR ... 1817
- Oramorph SR (Morphine Sulfate Sustained Release Tablets) ... 1988
- Roxanol ... 1991

Norepinephrine Bitartrate (Potential for increased response to sympathomimetics). Products include:
- Levophed Bitartrate Injection ... 2054

Opium Alkaloids (Increased response to central nervous system depressants). Products include:
- B & O No. 15A & No. 16A Supprettes ... 2395
- Pantopon Injectable ... 1911

Oxazepam (Increased response to central nervous system depressants). Products include:
- Serax Capsules ... 2522
- Serax Tablets ... 2522

Oxycodone Hydrochloride (Increased response to central nervous system depressants). Products include:
- Percocet Tablets ... 950
- Percodan ... 951
- Roxicodone Tablets, Oral Solution & Intensol (Oxycodone) ... 1992
- Tylox Capsules ... 1382

Pentobarbital Sodium (Increased response to central nervous system depressants). Products include:
- Nembutal Sodium Capsules ... 534
- Nembutal Sodium Solution ... 536
- Nembutal Sodium Suppositories ... 538

Perphenazine (Increased response to central nervous system depressants). Products include:
- Etrafon ... 2087
- Triavil Tablets ... 1556
- Trilafon ... 2123

Phenobarbital (Increased response to central nervous system depressants). Products include:
- Arco-Lase Plus Tablets ... 607
- Bellergal-S Tablets ... 1998
- Bronkolixir ... ◘ 761
- Bronkotabs Tablets ... ◘ 762
- Donnatal ... 1858
- Donnatal Extentabs ... 1859
- Donnatal Tablets ... 1858
- Donnazyme Tablets ... 1860
- Kinesed Tablets ... 2272
- Phenobarbital Elixir and Tablets ... 1293
- Primatene Tablets-P Formula ... 2421
- Quadrinal Tablets ... 1183
- Tedral SA ... 1765

Phenylephrine Bitartrate (Potential for increased response to sympathomimetics).
- No products indexed under this heading.

Phenylephrine Hydrochloride (Potential for increased response to sympathomimetics). Products include:
- AK-Dilate Solution 2.5% and 10% ... ◉ 203
- Atrohist Sprinkle Capsules ... 558
- Cerose-DM ... 2443
- Codimal ... 846
- Comhist LA Capsules ... 1618
- Congespirin For Children Aspirin Free Chewable Cold Tablets ... 748
- Cyclomydril ... ◉ 216
- Deconsal Sprinkle Capsules ... 559
- Dimetane Decongestant ... ◘ 673
- Dristan Decongestant/Antihistamine/Analgesic Coated Caplets ... ◘ 749
- Dristan Cold Nasal Decongestant/Antihistamine/Analgesic Coated Tablets ... 2419
- Dristan Advanced Formula Decongestant/Antihistamine/Analgesic Tablets ... ◘ 749
- Dristan Nasal Spray, Menthol ... 2419
- Dristan Nasal Spray, Regular and Regular with Metered Pump ... 2419
- Entex Capsules ... 1623
- Entex Liquid ... 1623
- Sinus Excedrin Analgesic, Decongestant Tablets & Caplets ... 750
- Extendryl ... 994
- 4-Way Fast Acting Nasal Spray - Original Formula (regular & mentholated) & Metered Spray Pump (regular) ... 751
- Hycomine Compound Tablets ... 929
- Murocoll-2 Sterile Ophthalmic Solution ... ◉ 261
- Mydfrin 2.5% ... ◉ 224
- Naldecon Syrup, Tablets, Pediatric Drops and Pediatric Syrup ... 709
- Neo-Synephrine Hydrochloride 1% Carpuject ... 2063
- Neo-Synephrine Hydrochloride 1% Injection ... 2063
- Neo-Synephrine Hydrochloride (Ophthalmic) ... 2064
- Neo-Synephrine ... ◘ 759
- Nōstril Nasal Decongestant ... ◘ 520
- Novahistine Elixir ... ◘ 596
- Phenergan VC ... 2500
- Phenergan VC with Codeine ... 2501
- Prefrin Liquifilm Vasoconstrictor and Lubricant Eye Drops ... ◉ 254
- Prefrin-A ... ◉ 255
- Quelidrine Syrup ... 556
- Relief Vasoconstrictor and Lubricant Eye Drops ... ◉ 256
- Robitussin Night Relief ... ◘ 677
- Ru-Tuss with Hydrocodone ... 694

(◘ Described in PDR For Nonprescription Drugs)

(◉ Described in PDR For Ophthalmology)

Ru-Tuss Tablets ... 693
Vasosulf ... ◉ 279
Vicks Sinex ... ▣ 665
Zincfrin ... ◉ 230

Phenylephrine Tannate (Potential for increased response to sympathomimetics). Products include:
Rynatan ... 2387
Rynatuss ... 2388

Phenylpropanolamine Hydrochloride (Potential for increased response to sympathomimetics). Products include:
A.R.M. Allergy Relief Medicine Caplets ... ▣ 615
Acutrim ... ▣ 548
Allerest ... ▣ 559
BC Cold Powder ... ▣ 517
Cheracol Plus Head Cold/Cough Formula ... ▣ 667
Codimal Expectorant ... 846
Comtrex Multi-Symptom Cold Reliever Tablets/Caplets/Liqui-Gels/Liquid ... 745
Contac Continuous Action Decongestant/Antihistamine Capsules ▣ 710
Contac Maximum Strength Continuous Action Decongestant/Antihistamine Caplets ... ▣ 709
Contac Severe Cold and Flu Formula Caplets ... ▣ 711
Coricidin 'D' Decongestant Tablets ... ▣ 695
Coricidin Demilets Tablets for Children ... ▣ 696
Demazin Nasal Decongestant/Antihistamine Repetabs Tablets & Syrup ... ▣ 697
Dexatrim ... ▣ 733
Dimetane-DC Cough Syrup ... 1857
Dimetapp Elixir ... ▣ 673
Dimetapp DM Elixir ... ▣ 674
Dimetapp Extentabs ... ▣ 674
Dimetapp Plus Caplets ... ▣ 675
Dimetapp Tablets ... ▣ 675
Entex Capsules ... 1623
Entex LA Tablets ... 1623
Entex Liquid ... 1623
4-Way Cold Tablets ... 750
Hycomine Syrup ... 927
Naldecon CX Adult Liquid ... ▣ 521
Naldecon DX Adult Liquid ... ▣ 521
Naldecon DX Children's Syrup ... ▣ 522
Naldecon DX Pediatric Drops ... ▣ 522
Naldecon EX Children's Syrup ... ▣ 522
Naldecon EX Pediatric Drops ... ▣ 523
Naldecon Syrup, Tablets, Pediatric Drops and Pediatric Syrup ... 709
Nolamine Tablets ... 838
Nolex LA Tablets ... 838
Ornade Spansule Capsules ... 2221
Orthoxicol Cough Syrup ... ▣ 668
Propagest ... 839
Pyrroxate Capsules ... ▣ 669
Robitussin-CF ... ▣ 676
Ru-Tuss II Capsules ... 693
Ru-Tuss with Hydrocodone ... 694
Ru-Tuss Tablets ... 693
Sine-Off Sinus Medicine Tablets-Aspirin Formula ... ▣ 722
Sinulin ... 840
St. Joseph Cold Tablets for Children ... ▣ 704
Tavist-D Tablets ... 2035
Triaminic Allergy Tablets ... ▣ 688
Triaminic Chewables ... ▣ 688
Triaminic Cold Tablets ... ▣ 688
Triaminic Expectorant ... ▣ 688
Triaminic Expectorant w/Codeine .. 1996
Triaminic Expectorant DH ... 1995
Triaminic Oral Infant Drops ... 1996
Triaminic Syrup ... ▣ 689
Triaminic-12 Tablets ... ▣ 690
Triaminic-DM Syrup ... ▣ 689
Triaminicin Tablets ... ▣ 690
Triaminicol Multi-Symptom Cold Tablets ... ▣ 691
Triaminicol Multi-Symptom Relief ▣ 691
Tuss-Ornade Liquid ... 2242
Tuss-Ornade Spansule Capsules ... 2242
Tylenol Cold Medication, Effervescent Tablets ... 1369

Pirbuterol Acetate (Potential for increased response to sympathomimetics). Products include:
Maxair Inhaler ... 1311

Prazepam (Increased response to central nervous system depressants). Products include:
Centrax ... 1693

Prochlorperazine (Increased response to central nervous system depressants). Products include:
Compazine ... 2201

Promethazine Hydrochloride (Increased response to central nervous system depressants). Products include:
Mepergan Injection ... 2479
Phenergan with Codeine ... 2497
Phenergan with Dextromethorphan 2499
Phenergan Injection ... 2493
Phenergan Suppositories ... 2496
Phenergan Syrup ... 2495
Phenergan Tablets ... 2496
Phenergan VC ... 2500
Phenergan VC with Codeine ... 2501

Propofol (Increased response to central nervous system depressants). Products include:
Diprivan Injection ... 2267

Propoxyphene Hydrochloride (Increased response to central nervous system depressants). Products include:
Darvon ... 1256
Wygesic Tablets ... 2540

Propoxyphene Napsylate (Increased response to central nervous system depressants). Products include:
Darvon-N/Darvocet-N ... 1254

Pseudoephedrine Hydrochloride (Potential for increased response to sympathomimetics). Products include:
Actifed Capsules ... ▣ 539
Actifed Plus Caplets ... ▣ 539
Actifed Plus Tablets ... ▣ 540
Actifed with Codeine Cough Syrup.. 752
Actifed Syrup ... ▣ 540
Actifed Tablets ... ▣ 540
Actifed 12-Hour Capsules ... ▣ 539
Advil Cold & Sinus Caplets (formerly CoAdvil) ... 2416
Allerest ... ▣ 559
Anatuss LA Tablets ... 1359
Benadryl Decongestant Elixir ... ▣ 635
Benadryl Decongestant ... ▣ 635
Benadryl Plus ... ▣ 636
Benadryl Plus Nighttime ... ▣ 637
Benylin Decongestant ... ▣ 638
Brexin L.A. Capsules ... 2078
Bromfed Capsules (Timed Release) ... 1615
Bromfed Syrup ... ▣ 628
Bromfed ... 1615
CoAdvil ... ▣ 748
Allergy-Sinus Comtrex Multi-Symptom Allergy Sinus Formula Tablets & Caplets ... 746
Cough Formula Comtrex ... 746
Comtrex Multi-Symptom Cold Reliever Tablets/Caplets/Liqui-Gels/Liquid ... 745
Day-Night Comtrex ... 747
Non-Drowsy Comtrex ... 747
Congess ... 994
Congestac Caplets ... ▣ 617
Contac Jr. Children's Cold Medicine ... ▣ 712
Contac Nighttime Cold Medicine ... ▣ 713
Contac Sinus Caplets Maximum Strength Non-Drowsy Formula ... ▣ 710
Contac Sinus Tablets Maximum Strength Non-Drowsy Formula ... ▣ 710
Deconamine ... 663
Deconsal II Tablets ... 559
Dimacol Caplets ... ▣ 672
Dimetane-DX Cough Syrup ... 1858
Dorcol Children's Cough Syrup ... ▣ 685
Dorcol Children's Decongestant Liquid ... ▣ 685
Dorcol Children's Liquid Cold Formula ... ▣ 686
Maximum Strength Dristan Decongestant/Analgesic Coated Caplets ... ▣ 750
No Drowsiness Dristan Cold Nasal Decongestant/Analgesic Coated Caplets ... 2420
Dristan Sinus Caplets ... 2419
Sinus Excedrin Analgesic, Decongestant Tablets & Caplets ... ▣ 533
Fedahist Gyrocaps ... 2145
Fedahist Timecaps ... 2145
Guaifed ... 1615
Guaifed Syrup ... ▣ 629
Isoclor Expectorant ... 982
Isoclor Timesule Capsules ... ▣ 561
Kronofed-A ... 970
Medi-Flu Caplet, Liquid ... ▣ 640
Novafed A Capsules ... 1342
Novafed Capsules ... 1342
Novahistine DH ... 1342
Novahistine DMX ... ▣ 595
Novahistine Expectorant ... 1343
Nucofed Capsules ... 2219
Nucofed Expectorant ... 2219
Nucofed Pediatric Expectorant ... 2220
Nucofed Syrup ... 2219
Ornex Caplets ... ▣ 618
PediaCare Allergy Relief Formula Liquid ... 1362
PediaCare Cough-Cold Formula Liquid ... 1362
PediaCare Infants' Oral Decongestant Drops ... 1362
PediaCare Night Rest Cough-Cold Formula Liquid ... 1362
PediaCare 6-12 Cough-Cold Formula Chewable Tablets ... 1362
Robitussin-DAC Syrup ... 1875
Robitussin-PE ... ▣ 677
Rondec ... 1975
Rondec-DM ... 1976
Rondec-TR Tablet ... 1975
Ru-Tuss DE Tablets ... 694
Ryna ... ▣ 741
Seldane-D Extended-Release Tablets ... 1350
Sinarest ... ▣ 562
Sine-Aid Maximum Strength Sinus Headache Caplets ... 1365
Sine-Aid Maximum Strength Sinus Headache Tablets ... 1365
Sine-Off Maximum Strength Allergy/Sinus Formula Caplets ... ▣ 721
Sine-Off Maximum Strength No Drowsiness Formula Caplets ... ▣ 722
Singlet Tablets ... ▣ 598
Sinutab Maximum Strength ... ▣ 641
Sinutab Maximum Strength Without Drowsiness Tablets & Caplets ... ▣ 642
Sinutab Regular Strength Without Drowsiness Formula ... ▣ 641
St. Joseph Nighttime Cold Medicine ... ▣ 705
Sudafed Children's Liquid ... ▣ 543
Sudafed Cough Syrup ... ▣ 543
Sudafed Plus Liquid ... ▣ 544
Sudafed Plus Tablets ... ▣ 545
Sudafed Sinus Caplets ... ▣ 545
Sudafed Sinus Tablets ... ▣ 545
Sudafed Tablets, 30 mg ... ▣ 544
Sudafed Tablets, Adult Strength, 60 mg ... ▣ 544
Sudafed 12 Hour Capsules ... ▣ 545
TheraFlu Flu and Cold Medicine ... ▣ 687
Triaminic Nite Light ... ▣ 689
Tylenol Allergy Sinus Medication Caplets and Gelcaps, Maximum Strength ... 1372
Children's Tylenol Cold Liquid Formula and Chewable Tablets ... 1368
Tylenol Cold & Flu Hot Medication, Packets ... 1369
Tylenol Cold & Flu No Drowsiness Hot Medication, Packets ... 1371
Tylenol Cold Medication Caplets and Tablets ... 1370
Tylenol Cold Medication No Drowsiness Formula Caplets ... 1370
Tylenol Cold Night Time Medication Liquid ... 1371
Tylenol Cough Medication Liquid with Decongestant, Maximum Strength ... 1372
Tylenol, Maximum Strength, Sinus Medication Gelcaps, Caplets and Tablets ... 1373
Ursinus Inlay-Tabs ... ▣ 691
Vicks Children's NyQuil ... ▣ 664
Vicks Daycare ... ▣ 660
Vicks Formula 44D Decongestant Cough Medicine ... ▣ 662
Vicks Formula 44M Multi-Symptom Cough Medicine ... ▣ 662
Vicks NyQuil Nighttime Colds Medicine-Original & Cherry Flavor ... ▣ 664
Vicks Pediatric Formula 44 Cough & Congestion Medicine ... ▣ 663
Vicks Pediatric Formula 44m Multi-Symptom Cough & Cold Medicine ... ▣ 663

Pseudoephedrine Sulfate (Potential for increased response to sympathomimetics). Products include:
Afrin Tablets ... ▣ 693
Chlor-Trimeton Decongestant ... ▣ 694
Disophrol Chronotab Sustained-Action Tablets ... ▣ 698
Drixoral Antihistamine/Nasal Decongestant Syrup ... ▣ 698
Drixoral Non-Drowsy Formula ... ▣ 699
Drixoral Plus Extended-Release Tablets ... ▣ 699
Drixoral Sinus ... ▣ 700
Drixoral Sustained-Action Tablets ▣ 698
Sinutab Allergy Formula Sustained Action Tablets ... ▣ 640
Trinalin Repetabs Tablets ... 1170

Quazepam (Increased response to central nervous system depressants). Products include:
Doral Tablets ... 2383

Secobarbital Sodium (Increased response to central nervous system depressants). Products include:
Seconal Sodium Pulvules ... 1296

Sufentanil Citrate (Increased response to central nervous system depressants). Products include:
Sufenta Injection ... 1147

Temazepam (Increased response to central nervous system depressants). Products include:
Restoril Capsules ... 2023

Terbutaline Sulfate (Potential for increased response to sympathomimetics). Products include:
Brethaire Inhaler ... 1024
Brethine Ampuls ... 1026
Brethine Tablets ... 1026
Bricanyl Injection ... 1324
Bricanyl Tablets ... 1325

Thiamylal Sodium (Increased response to central nervous system depressants). Products include:
Surital Ampoules, Steri-Vials ... 1764

Thioridazine Hydrochloride (Increased response to central nervous system depressants). Products include:
Mellaril ... 2011

Thiothixene (Increased response to central nervous system depressants). Products include:
Navane Capsules and Concentrate 1954
Navane Intramuscular ... 1956

Triazolam (Increased response to central nervous system depressants). Products include:
Halcion Tablets ... 2340

Trifluoperazine Hydrochloride (Increased response to central nervous system depressants). Products include:
Stelazine ... 2226

Vitamin B_{12} (Colchicine may induce reversible malabsorption of Vitamin B_{12}). Products include:
Allbee C-800 ... ▣ 670
Bugs Bunny Children's Chewable Vitamins (Sugar Free) ... ▣ 625
Bugs Bunny With Extra C Children's Chewable Vitamins (Sugar Free) ... ▣ 626
Bugs Bunny Plus Iron Children's Chewable Vitamins (Sugar Free) ▣ 625
Centrum Silver ... ▣ 586
Ener-B Vitamin B_{12} Nasal Gel Dietary Supplement ... 1617
Flintstones Children's Chewable Vitamins ... ▣ 625
Flintstones Children's Chewable Vitamins With Extra C ... ▣ 626
Flintstones Children's Chewable Vitamins Plus Iron ... ▣ 625
Mega-B ... 607
One-A-Day Essential Vitamins ... ▣ 627

(▣ Described in PDR For Nonprescription Drugs) (◉ Described in PDR For Ophthalmology)

One-A-Day Maximum Formula Vitamins and Minerals ▣ 627
One-A-Day Plus Extra C Vitamins ▣ 627
Orexin Softab Tablets 1157
Stressgard Stress Formula Vitamins ▣ 628
STUART PRENATAL Tablets ▣ 731
The Stuart Formula Tablets 1157
Stuartinic Tablets ▣ 581
Trinsicon Capsules 2415
Troph-Iron Liquid ▣ 619
Trophite Liquid ▣ 619
Vicon Forte Capsules 2416
Within Women's Formula Multivitamin with Calcium, Extra Iron and Zinc ▣ 628
Z-Bec Tablets ▣ 678

COLESTID GRANULES
(Colestipol Hydrochloride) 2328
May interact with tetracyclines, cardiac glycosides, and certain other agents. Compounds in these categories include:

Chlorothiazide (Decreased absorption of chlorothiazide). Products include:
Aldoclor Tablets 1413
Diupres Tablets 1461
Diuril Oral 1464

Chlorothiazide Sodium (Decreased absorption of chlorothiazide). Products include:
Diuril Sodium Intravenous 1463

Demeclocycline Hydrochloride (Significantly decreased absorption of tetracyclines). Products include:
Declomycin Capsules, Tablets 1199

Deslanoside (Possible binding effect).
No products indexed under this heading.

Digitoxin (Possible binding effect). Products include:
Crystodigin Tablets 1253

Digoxin (Possible binding effect). Products include:
Lanoxicaps 772
Lanoxin Elixir Pediatric 775
Lanoxin Injection 778
Lanoxin Injection Pediatric 781
Lanoxin Tablets 783

Doxycycline Calcium (Significantly decreased absorption of tetracyclines).
No products indexed under this heading.

Doxycycline Hyclate (Significantly decreased absorption of tetracyclines). Products include:
Doryx Capsules 1717
Vibramycin Hyclate Capsules 1787
Vibramycin Hyclate Intravenous 1968
Vibra-Tabs Film Coated Tablets 1787

Doxycycline Monohydrate (Significantly decreased absorption of tetracyclines). Products include:
Monodox Capsules 1630
Vibramycin Monohydrate for Oral Suspension 1787

Methacycline Hydrochloride (Significantly decreased absorption of tetracyclines).
No products indexed under this heading.

Minocycline Hydrochloride (Significantly decreased absorption of tetracyclines). Products include:
Minocin Intravenous 1221
Minocin Oral Suspension 1224
Minocin Pellet-Filled Capsules 1222

Oxytetracycline (Significantly decreased absorption of tetracyclines). Products include:
Terramycin Intramuscular Solution 1964
Urobiotic-250 Capsules 1968

Oxytetracycline Hydrochloride (Significantly decreased absorption of tetracyclines). Products include:
Terra-Cortril Ophthalmic Suspension 1963
Terramycin Capsules 1786
Terramycin Intramuscular Solution 1964
Terramycin with Polymyxin B Sulfate Ophthalmic Ointment 1965

Penicillin G Potassium (Significantly decreased absorption of penicillin). Products include:
Pfizerpen for Injection 1957

Propranolol Hydrochloride (May decrease absorption of propranolol). Products include:
Inderal 2459
Inderal LA Long Acting Capsules 2461
Inderide Tablets 2463
Inderide LA Long Acting Capsules 2465

Tetracycline Hydrochloride (Significantly decreased absorption of tetracyclines). Products include:
Achromycin V Capsules 1193
Achromycin Ophthalmic Ointment 1% ⊙ 307
Achromycin Ophthalmic Suspension 1% ⊙ 308
Topicycline for Topical Solution 1856

Vitamin A (Colestipol may prevent absorption of fat-soluble vitamins). Products include:
Aquasol A Vitamin A Capsules, USP 615
Aquasol A Parenteral, USP 615
Bugs Bunny Children's Chewable Vitamins (Sugar Free) ▣ 625
Bugs Bunny With Extra C Children's Chewable Vitamins (Sugar Free) ▣ 626
Bugs Bunny/Flintstones ▣ 625
Flintstones Children's Chewable Vitamins With Extra C ▣ 626
Flintstones Children's Chewable Vitamins Plus Iron ▣ 625
Lazer Creme 1770
Myadec ▣ 640
Natalins Rx 1391
Natalins Tablets 1391
Ocuvite Vitamin and Mineral Supplement ⊙ 312
One-A-Day Essential Vitamins ▣ 627
One-A-Day Maximum Formula Vitamins and Minerals ▣ 627
One-A-Day Plus Extra C Vitamins ▣ 627
Stressgard Stress Formula Vitamins ▣ 628
Tri-Vi-Flor 1.0 mg Vitamins with Fluoride Chewable Tablets 1400
Tri-Vi-Flor Drops 1400
Tri-Vi-Sol Vitamin Drops ▣ 614
Tri-Vi-Sol Vitamin Drops with Iron ▣ 614
Vicon Forte Capsules 2416
Vicon Plus ▣ 682
Vi-Daylin ADC Vitamins Drops 1980
Vi-Daylin ADC Vitamins + Iron Drops 1980
Vi-Daylin/F ADC Vitamins Drops With Fluoride 1981
Vi-Daylin/F ADC Vitamins + Iron Drops With Fluoride 1981
Vi-Zac ▣ 682
Within Women's Formula Multivitamin with Calcium, Extra Iron and Zinc ▣ 628
Zymacap Capsules ▣ 670

Vitamin D (Colestipol may prevent absorption of fat-soluble vitamins). Products include:
Bugs Bunny Children's Chewable Vitamins (Sugar Free) ▣ 625
Bugs Bunny With Extra C Children's Chewable Vitamins (Sugar Free) ▣ 626
Bugs Bunny Plus Iron Children's Chewable Vitamins (Sugar Free) ▣ 625
Calderol Capsules 1635
Caltrate 600 + Iron & Vitamin D 1198
Caltrate 600 + Vitamin D 1197
Caltrate, Jr. Tablets 1198
Flintstones Children's Chewable Vitamins ▣ 625
Flintstones Children's Chewable Vitamins With Extra C ▣ 626
Flintstones Children's Chewable Vitamins Plus Iron ▣ 625
Natalins Rx 1391
Natalins Tablets 1391
One-A-Day Essential Vitamins ▣ 627
One-A-Day Maximum Formula Vitamins and Minerals ▣ 627
One-A-Day Plus Extra C Vitamins ▣ 627
Os-Cal 250+D Tablets ▣ 597
Os-Cal 500+D Tablets ▣ 597
Os-Cal Fortified Tablets ▣ 597
Os-Cal Plus Tablets ▣ 597
Posture-D 600 mg 2420
Stressgard Stress Formula Vitamins ▣ 628
Tri-Vi-Flor 1.0 mg Vitamins with Fluoride Chewable Tablets 1400
Tri-Vi-Flor Drops 1400
Tri-Vi-Sol Vitamin Drops ▣ 614
Tri-Vi-Sol Vitamin Drops with Iron ▣ 614
Vi-Daylin ADC Vitamins Drops 1980
Vi-Daylin ADC Vitamins + Iron Drops 1980
Vi-Daylin/F ADC Vitamins Drops With Fluoride 1981
Vi-Daylin/F ADC Vitamins + Iron Drops With Fluoride 1981
Within Women's Formula Multivitamin with Calcium, Extra Iron and Zinc ▣ 628
Zymacap Capsules ▣ 670

Vitamin K (Colestipol may prevent absorption of fat-soluble vitamins). Products include:
One-A-Day Maximum Formula Vitamins and Minerals ▣ 627
Synkayvite Injection 1919
Synkayvite Tablets 1920

COLGATE JUNIOR FLUORIDE GEL TOOTHPASTE
(Sodium Fluoride) ▣ 554
No interactions described in labeling.

COLGATE MFP FLUORIDE GEL
(Sodium Fluoride) ▣ 554
No interactions described in labeling.

COLGATE MFP FLUORIDE TOOTHPASTE
(Sodium Monofluorophosphate) ▣ 554
No interactions described in labeling.

COLGATE MOUTHWASH TARTAR CONTROL FORMULA
(Sodium Fluoride) ▣ 554
No interactions described in labeling.

COLGATE TARTAR CONTROL FORMULA
(Sodium Fluoride) ▣ 554
No interactions described in labeling.

COLGATE TARTAR CONTROL GEL
(Sodium Fluoride) ▣ 555
No interactions described in labeling.

COLICON DROPS
(Simethicone) ▣ 653
No interactions described in labeling.

COLLAGENASE SANTYL OINTMENT
(Collagen) 1172
May interact with:

Cortisone Acetate (Chronic concurrent use may result in systemic manifestations of hypersensitivity to collagenase). Products include:
Cortone Acetate Sterile Suspension 1437
Cortone Acetate Tablets 1439

COLLYRIUM FOR FRESH EYES
(Boric Acid, Sodium Borate) 2445
No interactions described in labeling.

COLLYRIUM FRESH
(Tetrahydrozoline Hydrochloride, Glycerin) 2445
No interactions described in labeling.

COLY-MYCIN M PARENTERAL
(Colistimethate Sodium) 1706
May interact with:

Decamethonium (Potentiation of neuromuscular blocking effect of Coly-Mycin M).

Ether (Potentiation of neuromuscular blocking effect of Coly-Mycin M).

Furosemide (Potentiation of neuromuscular blocking effect of Coly-Mycin M). Products include:
Lasix 1093

Gallamine (Potentiation of neuromuscular blocking effect of Coly-Mycin M).

Kanamycin Sulfate (Interference with nerve transmission at the neuromuscular junction). Products include:
Kantrex Injection 601
Kantrex Pediatric Injection 601

Neomycin, oral (Interference with nerve transmission at the neuromuscular junction).

Polymyxin Preparations (Interference with nerve transmission at the neuromuscular junction).

Sodium Citrate (Potentiation of neuromuscular blocking effect of Coly-Mycin M). Products include:
Alka-Seltzer Effervescent Antacid 1570
Alka-Seltzer Extra Strength Effervescent Antacid and Pain Reliever 1570
Alka-Seltzer (Flavored) Effervescent Antacid and Pain Reliever 1569
Bicitra—Sugar-Free 2423
Citrocarbonate Antacid ▣ 668
Polycitra 2424
Ricelyte, Rice-Based Oral Electrolyte Maintenance Solution ▣ 613

Streptomycin Sulfate (Interference with nerve transmission at the neuromuscular junction).
No products indexed under this heading.

Succinylcholine Chloride (Potentiation of neuromuscular blocking effect of Coly-Mycin M). Products include:
Anectine 755

Tubocurarine Chloride (Potentiation of neuromuscular blocking effect of Coly-Mycin M).
No products indexed under this heading.

COLY-MYCIN S FOR ORAL SUSPENSION
(Colistin Sulfate) 1708
No interactions described in labeling.

COLY-MYCIN S OTIC W/NEOMYCIN & HYDROCORTISONE
(Colistin Sulfate, Neomycin Sulfate, Hydrocortisone Acetate) 1708
No interactions described in labeling.

COLYTE
(Electrolyte lavage) 1826
May interact with:

Oral Medications (Those administered within one hour of Colyte usage may be flushed from the gastrointestinal tract and not absorbed).

COMBIPRES TABLETS
(Clonidine Hydrochloride, Chlorthalidone) 678
May interact with tricyclic antidepressants, barbiturates, hypnotics and sedatives, cardiac glycosides, antihypertensives, insulin, oral hypoglycemic agents, lithium preparations, narcotic analgesics, and cer-

tain other agents. Compounds in these categories include:

Acebutolol Hydrochloride (Chlorthalidone may add to or potentiate the action of other antihypertensive drugs). Products include:
Sectral Capsules 2520

Alcohol (Orthostatic hypotension; enhanced CNS-depressive effects).

Alfentanil Hydrochloride (Orthostatic hypotension). Products include:
Alfenta Injection 1131

Amitriptyline Hydrochloride (Enhanced manifestation of corneal lesions (in rats); reduced effect of clonidine). Products include:
Elavil 2269
Endep Tablets 1927
Etrafon 2087
Limbitrol 1933
Triavil Tablets 1556

Amoxapine (Reduced effect of clonidine). Products include:
Asendin Tablets 1196

Aprobarbital (Orthostatic hypotension; enhanced CNS-depressive effects). Products include:
Alurate Elixir 1883

Atenolol (Chlorthalidone may add to or potentiate the action of other antihypertensive drugs). Products include:
Tenoretic Tablets 1105
Tenormin Tablets and I.V. Injection 1107

Benazepril Hydrochloride (Chlorthalidone may add to or potentiate the action of other antihypertensive drugs). Products include:
Lotensin Tablets 872

Bendroflumethiazide (Chlorthalidone may add to or potentiate the action of other antihypertensive drugs). Products include:
Corzide Tablets 702
Naturetin Tablets 1789
Rauzide Tablets 1804

Betaxolol Hydrochloride (Chlorthalidone may add to or potentiate the action of other antihypertensive drugs). Products include:
Betoptic Sterile Ophthalmic Solution 569
Betoptic S Sterile Ophthalmic Suspension 570
Kerlone Tablets 2172

Buprenorphine (Orthostatic hypotension).
No products indexed under this heading.

Butabarbital (Orthostatic hypotension; enhanced CNS-depressive effects). Products include:
Pyridium Plus 1764

Butalbital (Orthostatic hypotension; enhanced CNS-depressive effects). Products include:
Esgic-Plus Tablets 1002
Esgic Tablets & Capsules 1001
Fioricet Tablets 2006
Fiorinal Capsules 2007
Fiorinal with Codeine Capsules 2008
Fiorinal Tablets 2007
Phrenilin 838
Sedapap Tablets 50 mg/650 mg 1360

Captopril (Chlorthalidone may add to or potentiate the action of other antihypertensive drugs). Products include:
Capoten 2255
Capozide 2258

Carteolol Hydrochloride (Chlorthalidone may add to or potentiate the action of other antihypertensive drugs). Products include:
Cartrol Tablets 507

Chlorothiazide (Chlorthalidone may add to or potentiate the action of other antihypertensive drugs). Products include:
Aldoclor Tablets 1413
Diupres Tablets 1461
Diuril Oral 1464

Chlorothiazide Sodium (Chlorthalidone may add to or potentiate the action of other antihypertensive drugs). Products include:
Diuril Sodium Intravenous 1463

Chlorpropamide (Higher dosage of oral hypoglycemic agents may be required). Products include:
Diabinese Tablets 1775

Clomipramine Hydrochloride (Enhanced manifestation of corneal lesions (in rats); reduced effect of clonidine). Products include:
Anafranil Capsules 650

Clonidine (Chlorthalidone may add to or potentiate the action of other antihypertensive drugs). Products include:
Catapres-TTS 677

Codeine (Orthostatic hypotension). Products include:
Calcidrine Syrup 506

Codeine Phosphate (Orthostatic hypotension). Products include:
Actifed with Codeine Cough Syrup 752
Cheracol Cough Syrup 1853
Codimal PH Syrup 846
Dimetane-DC Cough Syrup 1857
Empirin with Codeine Phosphate Nos. 2, 3 & 4 764
Fiorinal with Codeine Capsules 2008
Isoclor Expectorant 982
Naldecon CX Adult Liquid ⊡ 521
Novahistine DH 1342
Novahistine Expectorant 1343
Nucofed Capsules 2219
Nucofed Expectorant 2219
Nucofed Pediatric Expectorant 2220
Nucofed Syrup 2219
Phenaphen with Codeine Capsules 1865
Phenaphen-650 with Codeine Tablets 1866
Phenergan with Codeine 2497
Phenergan VC with Codeine 2501
Robitussin A-C Syrup 1875
Robitussin-DAC Syrup 1875
Ryna ⊡ 741
Soma Compound w/Codeine Tablets 2390
Triaminic Expectorant w/Codeine 1996
Tussi-Organidin Liquid 2391
Tylenol with Codeine 1381

Codeine Polistirex (Orthostatic hypotension).
No products indexed under this heading.

Deserpidine (Chlorthalidone may add to or potentiate the action of other antihypertensive drugs). Products include:
Enduronyl 518
Harmonyl Tablets 528
Oreticyl 545

Desipramine Hydrochloride (Reduced effect of clonidine). Products include:
Norpramin Tablets 1340

Deslanoside (Sinus bradycardia and atrioventricular block (rare)).
No products indexed under this heading.

Dezocine (Orthostatic hypotension).

Diazoxide (Chlorthalidone may add to or potentiate the action of other antihypertensive drugs). Products include:
Hyperstat I.V. Injection 2095
Proglycem 649

Digitoxin (Sinus bradycardia and atrioventricular block (rare)). Products include:
Crystodigin Tablets 1253

Digoxin (Sinus bradycardia and atrioventricular block (rare)). Products include:
Lanoxicaps 772
Lanoxin Elixir Pediatric 775
Lanoxin Injection 778
Lanoxin Injection Pediatric 781
Lanoxin Tablets 783

Doxazosin Mesylate (Chlorthalidone may add to or potentiate the action of other antihypertensive drugs). Products include:
Cardura Tablets 1941

Doxepin Hydrochloride (Reduced effect of clonidine). Products include:
Sinequan 1960

Enalapril Maleate (Chlorthalidone may add to or potentiate the action of other antihypertensive drugs). Products include:
Vaseretic Tablets 1559
Vasotec Tablets 1564

Enalaprilat (Chlorthalidone may add to or potentiate the action of other antihypertensive drugs). Products include:
Vasotec I.V. 1562

Esmolol Hydrochloride (Chlorthalidone may add to or potentiate the action of other antihypertensive drugs). Products include:
Brevibloc Injection 942

Estazolam (Enhanced CNS-depressive effects). Products include:
ProSom Tablets 554

Ethchlorvynol (Enhanced CNS-depressive effects). Products include:
Placidyl Capsules 553

Ethinamate (Enhanced CNS-depressive effects).
No products indexed under this heading.

Felodipine (Chlorthalidone may add to or potentiate the action of other antihypertensive drugs). Products include:
Plendil Extended-Release Tablets 1526

Fentanyl (Orthostatic hypotension). Products include:
Duragesic Transdermal System 1133

Fentanyl Citrate (Orthostatic hypotension). Products include:
Innovar Injection 1141
Sublimaze Injection 1146

Flurazepam Hydrochloride (Enhanced CNS-depressive effects). Products include:
Dalmane Capsules 1927

Fosinopril Sodium (Chlorthalidone may add to or potentiate the action of other antihypertensive drugs). Products include:
Monopril Tablets 1406

Furosemide (Chlorthalidone may add to or potentiate the action of other antihypertensive drugs). Products include:
Lasix 1093

Glipizide (Higher dosage of oral hypoglycemic agents may be required). Products include:
Glucotrol 1952

Glutethimide (Enhanced CNS-depressive effects).
No products indexed under this heading.

Glyburide (Higher dosage of oral hypoglycemic agents may be required). Products include:
DiaBeta 1091
Micronase Tablets 2350

Guanabenz Acetate (Chlorthalidone may add to or potentiate the action of other antihypertensive drugs). Products include:
Wytensin Tablets 2542

Guanethidine Monosulfate (Chlorthalidone may add to or potentiate the action of other antihypertensive drugs). Products include:
Esimil Tablets 864
Ismelin Tablets 869

Hydralazine Hydrochloride (Chlorthalidone may add to or potentiate the action of other antihypertensive drugs). Products include:
Apresazide Capsules 854
Apresoline Hydrochloride Parenteral (Ampuls) 856
Apresoline Hydrochloride Tablets 855
Apresoline-Esidrix Tablets 857
Ser-Ap-Es Tablets 881
Serpasil-Apresoline Tablets 884

Hydrochlorothiazide (Chlorthalidone may add to or potentiate the action of other antihypertensive drugs). Products include:
Aldactazide 2150
Aldoril Tablets 1418
Apresazide Capsules 854
Apresoline-Esidrix Tablets 857
Capozide 2258
Dyazide Capsules 2208
Esidrix Tablets 863
Esimil Tablets 864
HydroDIURIL Tablets 1484
Hydropres Tablets 1485
Inderide Tablets 2463
Inderide LA Long Acting Capsules 2465
Lopressor HCT Tablets 1034
Maxzide 1215
Moduretic Tablets 1510
Normozide Tablets 2112
Oretic Tablets 544
Oreticyl 545
Prinzide Tablets 1540
Ser-Ap-Es Tablets 881
Serpasil-Esidrix Tablets 886
Timolide Tablets 1547
Trandate HCT Tablets 579
Vaseretic Tablets 1559
Zestoretic 2274

Hydrocodone Bitartrate (Orthostatic hypotension). Products include:
Anexsia 5/500 Tablets 2196
Anexsia 7.5/650 Tablets 2197
Azdōne Tablets 844
Codiclear DH Syrup 845
Codimal DH Syrup 846
Damason-P 1356
Hycodan Syrup, Tablets 927
Hycomine Compound Tablets 929
Hycomine Syrup 927
Hycotuss Expectorant Syrup 930
Hydrocet Capsules 835
Lortab ASA Tablets 2414
Lortab 2412
Ru-Tuss with Hydrocodone 694
Triaminic Expectorant DH 1995
Vicodin Tablets 1187
Vicodin ES Tablets 1189
Zydone Capsules 941

Hydrocodone Polistirex (Orthostatic hypotension). Products include:
Tussionex Extended-Release Suspension 988

Hydroflumethiazide (Chlorthalidone may add to or potentiate the action of other antihypertensive drugs). Products include:
Diucardin Tablets 2450
Saluron 718
Salutensin/Salutensin-Demi 719

Imipramine Hydrochloride (Reduced effect of clonidine). Products include:
Tofranil Ampuls 1038
Tofranil Tablets 1039

Imipramine Pamoate (Reduced effect of clonidine). Products include:
Tofranil-PM Capsules 1041

Indapamide (Chlorthalidone may add to or potentiate the action of other antihypertensive drugs). Products include:
Lozol Tablets 1843

Insulin, Human (Insulin requirements in diabetic patients may be increased, decreased or unchanged).
No products indexed under this heading.

Insulin, Human Isophane Suspension (Insulin requirements in diabetic patients may be increased, decreased or unchanged). Products include:
Humulin N, 100 Units 1270

Insulin, Human NPH (Insulin requirements in diabetic patients may be increased, decreased or unchanged). Products include:
Insulatard NPH Human 1627
Novolin N 1627
Novolin N PenFill Cartridges 1628
Novolin N Prefilled 1628

Insulin, Human Regular (Insulin requirements in diabetic patients may be increased, decreased or unchanged). Products include:
Humulin BR, 100 Units 1268
Humulin R, 100 Units 1272
Novolin R 1627
Novolin R PenFill Cartridges 1628
Novolin R Prefilled 1629
Velosulin Human 1628

Insulin, Human, Zinc Suspension (Insulin requirements in diabetic patients may be increased, decreased or unchanged). Products include:
Humulin L, 100 Units 1268
Humulin U, 100 Units 1272
Novolin L 1627

Insulin, NPH (Insulin requirements in diabetic patients may be increased, decreased or unchanged). Products include:
NPH, 40 & 100 Units 1273
Beef NPH, 100 Units 1274
Pork NPH, 100 Units 1275
Insulatard NPH 1626
NPH Insulin 1626
NPH Purified Pork Isophane Insulin 1626

Insulin, Regular (Insulin requirements in diabetic patients may be increased, decreased or unchanged). Products include:
Regular, 40 & 100 Units 1273
Beef Regular, 100 Units 1275
Pork Regular, 100 Units 1275
Pork Regular (Concentrated), 500 Units 1276
Regular Insulin 1625
Regular Purified Pork Insulin 1626
Velosulin 1627

Insulin, Zinc Crystals (Insulin requirements in diabetic patients may be increased, decreased or unchanged). Products include:
NPH, 40 & 100 Units 1273

Insulin, Zinc Suspension (Insulin requirements in diabetic patients may be increased, decreased or unchanged). Products include:
Lente, 40 & 100 Units 1272
Protamine, Zinc, 40 & 100 Units 1273
Lente Iletin I 1272
Beef Lente, 100 Units 1274
Beef Protamine Zinc, 100 Units 1274
Pork Lente, 100 Units 1275
Pork, Protamine, Zinc, 100 Units 1275
Lente Insulin 1626
Lente Purified Pork Insulin 1626
Semilente Insulin 1625
Ultralente Insulin 1626

Isradipine (Chlorthalidone may add to or potentiate the action of other antihypertensive drugs). Products include:
DynaCirc Capsules 2004

Labetalol Hydrochloride (Chlorthalidone may add to or potentiate the action of other antihypertensive drugs). Products include:
Normodyne Injection 2108
Normodyne Tablets 2110
Normozide Tablets 2112
Trandate HCT Tablets 579
Trandate Injection 577
Trandate Tablets 579

Levorphanol Tartrate (Orthostatic hypotension). Products include:
Levo-Dromoran 1906

Lisinopril (Chlorthalidone may add to or potentiate the action of other antihypertensive drugs). Products include:
Prinivil Tablets 1538
Prinzide Tablets 1540
Zestoretic 2274
Zestril Tablets 2277

Lithium Carbonate (Reduced renal lithium clearance and increased risk of lithium toxicity). Products include:
Eskalith 2214
Lithane Tablets 1596
Lithium Carbonate Capsules & Tablets 1984
Lithobid Tablets 870

Lithium Citrate (Reduced renal lithium clearance and increased risk of lithium toxicity). Products include:
Cibalith-S 870

Lorazepam (Enhanced CNS-depressive effects). Products include:
Ativan Injection 2432
Ativan Tablets 2434

Maprotiline Hydrochloride (Reduced effect of clonidine). Products include:
Ludiomil Tablets 874

Mecamylamine Hydrochloride (Chlorthalidone may add to or potentiate the action of other antihypertensive drugs). Products include:
Inversine Tablets 1492

Meperidine Hydrochloride (Orthostatic hypotension). Products include:
Demerol 2047
Mepergan Injection 2479

Mephobarbital (Orthostatic hypotension; enhanced CNS-depressive effects). Products include:
Mebaral Tablets 2061

Methadone Hydrochloride (Orthostatic hypotension). Products include:
Dolophine Hydrochloride Ampoules & Vials 1260
Dolophine Hydrochloride Tablets 1261
Methadone Hydrochloride Diskets 1284
Methadone Hydrochloride Oral Solution & Tablets 1987

Methyclothiazide (Chlorthalidone may add to or potentiate the action of other antihypertensive drugs). Products include:
Enduron Tablets 517
Enduronyl 518

Methyldopa (Chlorthalidone may add to or potentiate the action of other antihypertensive drugs). Products include:
Aldoclor Tablets 1413
Aldomet Oral 1415
Aldoril Tablets 1418

Methyldopate Hydrochloride (Chlorthalidone may add to or potentiate the action of other antihypertensive drugs). Products include:
Aldomet Ester HCl Injection 1417

Metolazone (Chlorthalidone may add to or potentiate the action of other antihypertensive drugs). Products include:
Diulo 2129
Mykrox ½ mg Tablets 984
Zaroxolyn Tablets 989

Metoprolol Tartrate (Chlorthalidone may add to or potentiate the action of other antihypertensive drugs). Products include:
Lopressor Ampuls 1032
Lopressor HCT Tablets 1034
Lopressor Tablets 1032

Metyrosine (Chlorthalidone may add to or potentiate the action of other antihypertensive drugs). Products include:
Demser Capsules 1460

Midazolam Hydrochloride (Enhanced CNS-depressive effects). Products include:
Versed Injection 1924

Minoxidil (Chlorthalidone may add to or potentiate the action of other antihypertensive drugs). Products include:
Loniten Tablets 2346
Rogaine Topical Solution 2357

Morphine Sulfate (Orthostatic hypotension). Products include:
Astramorph/PF Injection, USP (Preservative-Free) 618
Duramorph 960
Infumorph 200 and Infumorph 500 Sterile Solutions 962
MS Contin Tablets 1814
MSIR 1817
Oramorph SR (Morphine Sulfate Sustained Release Tablets) 1988
Roxanol 1991

Nadolol (Chlorthalidone may add to or potentiate the action of other antihypertensive drugs). Products include:
Corgard Tablets 701
Corzide Tablets 702

Nicardipine Hydrochloride (Chlorthalidone may add to or potentiate the action of other antihypertensive drugs). Products include:
Cardene Capsules 2290

Nitroglycerin (Chlorthalidone may add to or potentiate the action of other antihypertensive drugs). Products include:
Deponit NTG Transdermal Delivery System 2143
Minitran Transdermal Delivery System 1312
Nitro-Bid Ointment 1339
Nitro-Bid Capsules 1338
Nitrodisc 2176
Nitro-Dur (nitroglycerin) Transdermal Infusion System 1164
Nitrogard Tablets 1004
Nitrolingual Spray 1846
Nitrostat Tablets 1743
Transderm-Nitro Transdermal Therapeutic System 2283

Norepinephrine Bitartrate (Decreased arterial responsiveness to norepinephrine). Products include:
Levophed Bitartrate Injection 2054

Nortriptyline Hydrochloride (Reduced effect of clonidine). Products include:
Pamelor 2019

Opium Alkaloids (Orthostatic hypotension). Products include:
B & O No. 15A & No. 16A Supprettes 2395
Pantopon Injectable 1911

Oxycodone Hydrochloride (Orthostatic hypotension). Products include:
Percocet Tablets 950
Percodan 951
Roxicodone Tablets, Oral Solution & Intensol (Oxycodone) 1992
Tylox Capsules 1382

Papaverine (Drug-induced hepatitis (one case)).

Penbutolol Sulfate (Chlorthalidone may add to or potentiate the action of other antihypertensive drugs). Products include:
Levatol 1832

Pentobarbital Sodium (Orthostatic hypotension; enhanced CNS-depressive effects). Products include:
Nembutal Sodium Capsules 534
Nembutal Sodium Solution 536
Nembutal Sodium Suppositories 538

Phenobarbital (Orthostatic hypotension; enhanced CNS-depressive effects). Products include:
Arco-Lase Plus Tablets 607
Bellergal-S Tablets 1998
Bronkolixir .... ▣ 761
Bronkotabs Tablets .... ▣ 762
Donnatal 1858
Donnatal Extentabs 1859
Donnatal Tablets 1858
Donnazyme Tablets 1860
Kinesed Tablets 2272
Phenobarbital Elixir and Tablets 1293
Primatene Tablets-P Formula 2421
Quadrinal Tablets 1183
Tedral SA 1765

Phenoxybenzamine Hydrochloride (Chlorthalidone may add to or potentiate the action of other antihypertensive drugs). Products include:
Dibenzyline Capsules 2207

Phentolamine Mesylate (Chlorthalidone may add to or potentiate the action of other antihypertensive drugs). Products include:
Regitine 878

Pindolol (Chlorthalidone may add to or potentiate the action of other antihypertensive drugs). Products include:
Visken Tablets 2036

Polythiazide (Chlorthalidone may add to or potentiate the action of other antihypertensive drugs). Products include:
Minizide Capsules 1779
Renese Tablets 1785
Renese-R Tablets 1786

Prazosin Hydrochloride (Chlorthalidone may add to or potentiate the action of other antihypertensive drugs). Products include:
Minipress Capsules 1778
Minizide Capsules 1779

Propofol (Enhanced CNS-depressive effects). Products include:
Diprivan Injection 2267

Propoxyphene Hydrochloride (Orthostatic hypotension). Products include:
Darvon 1256
Wygesic Tablets 2540

Propoxyphene Napsylate (Orthostatic hypotension). Products include:
Darvon-N/Darvocet-N 1254

Propranolol Hydrochloride (Chlorthalidone may add to or potentiate the action of other antihypertensive drugs). Products include:
Inderal 2459
Inderal LA Long Acting Capsules 2461
Inderide Tablets 2463
Inderide LA Long Acting Capsules 2465

Protriptyline Hydrochloride (Reduced effect of clonidine). Products include:
Vivactil Tablets 1567

Quazepam (Enhanced CNS-depressive effects). Products include:
Doral Tablets 2383

Ramipril (Chlorthalidone may add to or potentiate the action of other antihypertensive drugs). Products include:
Altace Capsules 1086

Rauwolfia Serpentina (Chlorthalidone may add to or potentiate the action of other antihypertensive drugs). Products include:
Raudixin Tablets 1803
Rauzide Tablets 1804

Rescinnamine (Chlorthalidone may add to or potentiate the action of other antihypertensive drugs).
No products indexed under this heading.

Reserpine (Chlorthalidone may add to or potentiate the action of other antihypertensive drugs). Products include:
- Diupres Tablets 1461
- Hydromox R Tablets 1209
- Hydropres Tablets 1485
- Renese-R Tablets 1786
- Salutensin/Salutensin-Demi 719
- Ser-Ap-Es Tablets 881
- Serpasil Tablets 883
- Serpasil-Apresoline Tablets 884
- Serpasil-Esidrix Tablets 886

Secobarbital Sodium (Orthostatic hypotension; enhanced CNS-depressive effects). Products include:
- Seconal Sodium Pulvules 1296

Sodium Nitroprusside (Chlorthalidone may add to or potentiate the action of other antihypertensive drugs). Products include:
- Nipride I.V. Infusion 1909

Sufentanil Citrate (Orthostatic hypotension). Products include:
- Sufenta Injection 1147

Temazepam (Enhanced CNS-depressive effects). Products include:
- Restoril Capsules 2023

Terazosin Hydrochloride (Chlorthalidone may add to or potentiate the action of other antihypertensive drugs). Products include:
- Hytrin Tablets 529

Thiamylal Sodium (Orthostatic hypotension; enhanced CNS-depressive effects). Products include:
- Surital Ampoules, Steri-Vials 1764

Timolol Maleate (Chlorthalidone may add to or potentiate the action of other antihypertensive drugs). Products include:
- Blocadren Tablets 1429
- Timolide Tablets 1547
- Timoptic in Ocudose 1552
- Timoptic Sterile Ophthalmic Solution 1550

Tolazamide (Higher dosage of oral hypoglycemic agents may be required). Products include:
- Tolinase Tablets 2365

Tolbutamide (Higher dosage of oral hypoglycemic agents may be required). Products include:
- Orinase Tablets 2354

Triazolam (Enhanced CNS-depressive effects). Products include:
- Halcion Tablets 2340

Trimethaphan Camsylate (Chlorthalidone may add to or potentiate the action of other antihypertensive drugs). Products include:
- Arfonad Ampuls 1887

Trimipramine Maleate (Reduced effect of clonidine). Products include:
- Surmontil Capsules 2524

Tubocurarine Chloride (Increased responsiveness to tubocurarine).
- No products indexed under this heading.

COMHIST LA CAPSULES (Chlorpheniramine Maleate, Phenyltoloxamine Citrate, Phenylephrine Hydrochloride) 1618
May interact with hypnotics and sedatives, tranquilizers, monoamine oxidase inhibitors, and certain other agents. Compounds in these categories include:

Alcohol (Sedative effects additive to CNS depressant effects).

Alprazolam (Sedative effects additive to CNS depressant effects). Products include:
- Xanax Tablets 2367

Buspirone Hydrochloride (Sedative effects additive to CNS depressant effects). Products include:
- BuSpar 1401

Chlordiazepoxide (Sedative effects additive to CNS depressant effects). Products include:
- Libritabs Tablets 1930
- Limbitrol 1933
- Menrium Tablets 1934

Chlordiazepoxide Hydrochloride (Sedative effects additive to CNS depressant effects). Products include:
- Librax Capsules 1929
- Librium Capsules 1931
- Librium Injectable 1932

Chlorpromazine (Sedative effects additive to CNS depressant effects). Products include:
- Thorazine 2234

Clorazepate Dipotassium (Sedative effects additive to CNS depressant effects). Products include:
- Tranxene 556

Diazepam (Sedative effects additive to CNS depressant effects). Products include:
- Valium Injectable 1937
- Valium Tablets 1939
- Valrelease Capsules 1923

Droperidol (Sedative effects additive to CNS depressant effects). Products include:
- Inapsine Injection 1140
- Innovar Injection 1141

Estazolam (Sedative effects additive to CNS depressant effects). Products include:
- ProSom Tablets 554

Ethchlorvynol (Sedative effects additive to CNS depressant effects). Products include:
- Placidyl Capsules 553

Ethinamate (Sedative effects additive to CNS depressant effects).
- No products indexed under this heading.

Fluphenazine Decanoate (Sedative effects additive to CNS depressant effects). Products include:
- Prolixin Decanoate 1795

Fluphenazine Enanthate (Sedative effects additive to CNS depressant effects). Products include:
- Prolixin Enanthate 1796

Fluphenazine Hydrochloride (Sedative effects additive to CNS depressant effects). Products include:
- Prolixin Elixir 1793
- Prolixin Injection 1791
- Prolixin Oral Concentrate 1792
- Prolixin Tablets 1793

Flurazepam Hydrochloride (Sedative effects additive to CNS depressant effects). Products include:
- Dalmane Capsules 1927

Furazolidone (Should not be used). Products include:
- Furoxone 1855

Glutethimide (Sedative effects additive to CNS depressant effects).
- No products indexed under this heading.

Haloperidol (Sedative effects additive to CNS depressant effects). Products include:
- Haldol Injection, Tablets and Concentrate 1373

Haloperidol Decanoate (Sedative effects additive to CNS depressant effects). Products include:
- Haldol Decanoate 1375

Hydroxyzine Hydrochloride (Sedative effects additive to CNS depressant effects). Products include:
- Atarax Tablets & Syrup 1941
- Marax Tablets & DF Syrup 1954
- Vistaril Intramuscular Solution 1970

Isocarboxazid (Should not be used). Products include:
- Marplan Tablets 1906

Lorazepam (Sedative effects additive to CNS depressant effects). Products include:
- Ativan Injection 2432
- Ativan Tablets 2434

Loxapine Hydrochloride (Sedative effects additive to CNS depressant effects). Products include:
- Loxitane 1213

Loxapine Succinate (Sedative effects additive to CNS depressant effects). Products include:
- Loxitane Capsules 1213

Meprobamate (Sedative effects additive to CNS depressant effects). Products include:
- Deprol Tablets 2382
- Equagesic Tablets 2451
- Miltown Tablets 2386
- PMB 200 and PMB 400 2504

Mesoridazine (Sedative effects additive to CNS depressant effects). Products include:
- Serentil 686

Midazolam Hydrochloride (Sedative effects additive to CNS depressant effects). Products include:
- Versed Injection 1924

Molindone Hydrochloride (Sedative effects additive to CNS depressant effects). Products include:
- Moban Tablets & Concentrate 932

Oxazepam (Sedative effects additive to CNS depressant effects). Products include:
- Serax Capsules 2522
- Serax Tablets 2522

Perphenazine (Sedative effects additive to CNS depressant effects). Products include:
- Etrafon 2087
- Triavil Tablets 1556
- Trilafon 2123

Phenelzine Sulfate (Should not be used). Products include:
- Nardil 1742

Prazepam (Sedative effects additive to CNS depressant effects). Products include:
- Centrax 1693

Prochlorperazine (Sedative effects additive to CNS depressant effects). Products include:
- Compazine 2201

Promethazine Hydrochloride (Sedative effects additive to CNS depressant effects). Products include:
- Mepergan Injection 2479
- Phenergan with Codeine 2497
- Phenergan with Dextromethorphan 2499
- Phenergan Injection 2493
- Phenergan Suppositories 2496
- Phenergan Syrup 2495
- Phenergan Tablets 2496
- Phenergan VC 2500
- Phenergan VC with Codeine 2501

Propofol (Sedative effects additive to CNS depressant effects). Products include:
- Diprivan Injection 2267

Quazepam (Sedative effects additive to CNS depressant effects). Products include:
- Doral Tablets 2383

Secobarbital Sodium (Sedative effects additive to CNS depressant effects). Products include:
- Seconal Sodium Pulvules 1296

Selegiline Hydrochloride (Should not be used). Products include:
- Eldepryl 2250

Temazepam (Sedative effects additive to CNS depressant effects). Products include:
- Restoril Capsules 2023

Thioridazine Hydrochloride (Sedative effects additive to CNS depressant effects). Products include:
- Mellaril 2011

Tranylcypromine Sulfate (Should not be used). Products include:
- Parnate Tablets 2222

Triazolam (Sedative effects additive to CNS depressant effects). Products include:
- Halcion Tablets 2340

Trifluoperazine Hydrochloride (Sedative effects additive to CNS depressant effects). Products include:
- Stelazine 2226

COMPAZINE AMPULS (Prochlorperazine) 2201
May interact with central nervous system depressants, oral anticoagulants, thiazides, anticonvulsants, and certain other agents. Compounds in these categories include:

Alcohol (Intensified or prolonged action).

Alfentanil Hydrochloride (Intensified or prolonged action of CNS depressants). Products include:
- Alfenta Injection 1131

Alprazolam (Intensified or prolonged action of CNS depressant). Products include:
- Xanax Tablets 2367

Aprobarbital (Intensified or prolonged action of CNS depressants). Products include:
- Alurate Elixir 1883

Atropine Nitrate, Methyl (Intensification and prolongation of action of atropine).
- No products indexed under this heading.

Atropine Sulfate (Intensification and prolongation of action of atropine). Products include:
- Arco-Lase Plus Tablets 607
- Atropine Sulfate Sterile Ophthalmic Solution and S.O.P. Sterile Ophthalmic Ointment ..... ⊙ 239
- Donnagel ..... ▣ 675
- Donnagel-PG 1858
- Donnatal 1858
- Donnatal Extentabs 1859
- Donnatal Tablets 1858
- Donnazyme Tablets 1860
- Isopto Atropine ..... ⊙ 218
- Lomotil 2174
- Motofen Tablets 836
- Ru-Tuss Tablets 693
- Urised Tablets 2396

Bendroflumethiazide (Orthostatic hypotension that occurs with phenothiazines may be accentuated). Products include:
- Corzide Tablets 702
- Naturetin Tablets 1789
- Rauzide Tablets 1804

Buprenorphine (Intensified or prolonged action of CNS depressant).
- No products indexed under this heading.

Buspirone Hydrochloride (Intensified or prolonged action of CNS depressant). Products include:
- BuSpar 1401

Butabarbital (Intensified or prolonged action of CNS depressant). Products include:
Pyridium Plus 1764

Butalbital (Intensified or prolonged action of CNS depressant). Products include:
Esgic-Plus Tablets 1002
Esgic Tablets & Capsules 1001
Fioricet Tablets 2006
Fiorinal Capsules 2007
Fiorinal with Codeine Capsules 2008
Fiorinal Tablets 2007
Phrenilin 838
Sedapap Tablets 50 mg/650 mg 1360

Carbamazepine (Phenothiazines may lower convulsive threshold; dosage adjustments of anticonvulsants may be necessary). Products include:
Tegretol Chewable Tablets 654
Tegretol Suspension 656
Tegretol Tablets 654

Chlordiazepoxide (Intensified or prolonged action of CNS depressant). Products include:
Libritabs Tablets 1930
Limbitrol 1933
Menrium Tablets 1934

Chlordiazepoxide Hydrochloride (Intensified or prolonged action of CNS depressant). Products include:
Librax Capsules 1929
Librium Capsules 1931
Librium Injectable 1932

Chlorothiazide (Orthostatic hypotension that occurs with phenothiazines may be accentuated). Products include:
Aldoclor Tablets 1413
Diupres Tablets 1461
Diuril Oral 1464

Chlorothiazide Sodium (Orthostatic hypotension that occurs with phenothiazines may be accentuated). Products include:
Diuril Sodium Intravenous 1463

Chlorpromazine (Intensified or prolonged action of CNS depressant). Products include:
Thorazine 2234

Chlorprothixene (Intensified or prolonged action of CNS depressant). Products include:
Taractan Tablets 1920

Chlorprothixene Hydrochloride (Intensified or prolonged action of CNS depressant). Products include:
Taractan 1920

Clorazepate Dipotassium (Intensified or prolonged action of CNS depressant). Products include:
Tranxene 556

Codeine (Intensified or prolonged action of CNS depressant). Products include:
Calcidrine Syrup 506

Codeine Phosphate (Intensified or prolonged action of CNS depressants). Products include:
Actifed with Codeine Cough Syrup 752
Cheracol Cough Syrup 1853
Codimal PH Syrup 846
Dimetane-DC Cough Syrup 1857
Empirin with Codeine Phosphate Nos. 2, 3 & 4 764
Fiorinal with Codeine Capsules 2008
Isoclor Expectorant 982
Naldecon CX Adult Liquid ▣ 521
Novahistine DH 1342
Novahistine Expectorant 1343
Nucofed Capsules 2219
Nucofed Expectorant 2219
Nucofed Pediatric Expectorant 2220
Nucofed Syrup 2219
Phenaphen with Codeine Capsules 1865
Phenaphen-650 with Codeine Tablets 1866
Phenergan with Codeine 2497
Phenergan VC with Codeine 2501
Robitussin A-C Syrup 1875
Robitussin-DAC Syrup 1875
Ryna ▣ 741
Soma Compound w/Codeine Tablets 2390
Triaminic Expectorant w/Codeine 1996
Tussi-Organidin Liquid 2391
Tylenol with Codeine 1381

Codeine Polistirex (Intensified or prolonged action of CNS depressant).
No products indexed under this heading.

Dezocine (Intensified or prolonged action of CNS depressants).

Diazepam (Intensified or prolonged action of CNS depressant). Products include:
Valium Injectable 1937
Valium Tablets 1939
Valrelease Capsules 1923

Dicumarol (Diminished effect of oral anticoagulants). Products include:
Dicumarol Tablets 516

Divalproex Sodium (Phenothiazines may lower convulsive threshold; dosage adjustments of anticonvulsants may be necessary). Products include:
Depakote 512

Droperidol (Intensified or prolonged action of CNS depressant). Products include:
Inapsine Injection 1140
Innovar Injection 1141

Enflurane (Intensified or prolonged action of CNS depressant). Products include:
Ethrane 599

Epinephrine (Reversed epinephrine effect). Products include:
Ana-Kit Anaphylaxis Emergency Treatment Kit 1100
Bronkaid Mist ▣ 757
EpiPen 843
Marcaine Hydrochloride 0.5% with Epinephrine 1:200,000 (as bitartrate) 958
Marcaine Hydrochloride with Epinephrine 1:200,000 2055
Primatene Mist 2420
Sus-Phrine Injection 1006
Xylocaine with Epinephrine Injections 637

Estazolam (Intensified or prolonged action of CNS depressants). Products include:
ProSom Tablets 554

Ethchlorvynol (Intensified or prolonged action of CNS depressant). Products include:
Placidyl Capsules 553

Ethinamate (Intensified or prolonged action of CNS depressant).
No products indexed under this heading.

Ethosuximide (Phenothiazines may lower convulsive threshold; dosage adjustments of anticonvulsants may be necessary). Products include:
Zarontin Capsules 1768
Zarontin Syrup 1769

Ethotoin (Phenothiazines may lower convulsive threshold; dosage adjustments of anticonvulsants may be necessary). Products include:
Peganone Tablets 551

Fentanyl (Intensified or prolonged action of CNS depressants). Products include:
Duragesic Transdermal System 1133

Fentanyl Citrate (Intensified or prolonged action of CNS depressant). Products include:
Innovar Injection 1141
Sublimaze Injection 1146

Fluphenazine Decanoate (Intensified or prolonged action of CNS depressant). Products include:
Prolixin Decanoate 1795

Fluphenazine Enanthate (Intensified or prolonged action of CNS depressant in). Products include:
Prolixin Enanthate 1796

Fluphenazine Hydrochloride (Intensified or prolonged action of CNS depressant). Products include:
Prolixin Elixir 1793
Prolixin Injection 1791
Prolixin Oral Concentrate 1792
Prolixin Tablets 1793

Flurazepam Hydrochloride (Intensified or prolonged action of CNS depressant). Products include:
Dalmane Capsules 1927

Glutethimide (Intensified or prolonged action of CNS depressant).
No products indexed under this heading.

Guanethidine Monosulfate (Concomitant use of phenothiazines may counteract antihypertensive effects of guanethidine). Products include:
Esimil Tablets 864
Ismelin Tablets 869

Haloperidol (Intensified or prolonged action of CNS depressant). Products include:
Haldol Injection, Tablets and Concentrate 1373

Haloperidol Decanoate (Intensified or prolonged action of CNS depressant). Products include:
Haldol Decanoate 1375

Hydralazine Hydrochloride (Inhibited by amphetamines). Products include:
Apresazide Capsules 854
Apresoline Hydrochloride Parenteral (Ampuls) 856
Apresoline Hydrochloride Tablets 855
Apresoline-Esidrix Tablets 857
Ser-Ap-Es Tablets 881
Serpasil-Apresoline Tablets 884

Hydrochlorothiazide (Orthostatic hypotension that occurs with phenothiazines may be accentuated). Products include:
Aldactazide 2150
Aldoril Tablets 1418
Apresazide Capsules 854
Apresoline-Esidrix Tablets 857
Capozide 2258
Dyazide Capsules 2208
Esidrix Tablets 863
Esimil Tablets 864
HydroDIURIL Tablets 1484
Hydropres Tablets 1485
Inderide Tablets 2463
Inderide LA Long Acting Capsules 2465
Lopressor HCT Tablets 1034
Maxzide 1215
Moduretic Tablets 1510
Normozide Tablets 2112
Oretic Tablets 544
Oreticyl 545
Prinzide Tablets 1540
Ser-Ap-Es Tablets 881
Serpasil-Esidrix Tablets 886
Timolide Tablets 1547
Trandate HCT Tablets 579
Vaseretic Tablets 1559
Zestoretic 2274

Hydrocodone Bitartrate (Intensified or prolonged action of CNS depressant). Products include:
Anexsia 5/500 Tablets 2196
Anexsia 7.5/650 Tablets 2197
Azdone Tablets 844
Codiclear DH Syrup 845
Codimal DH Syrup 846
Damason-P 1356
Hycodan Syrup, Tablets 927
Hycomine Compound Tablets 929
Hycomine Syrup 927
Hycotuss Expectorant Syrup 930
Hydrocet Capsules 835
Lortab ASA Tablets 2414
Lortab 2412
Ru-Tuss with Hydrocodone 694
Triaminic Expectorant DH 1995
Vicodin Tablets 1187
Vicodin ES Tablets 1189
Zydone Capsules 941

Hydrocodone Polistirex (Intensified or prolonged action of CNS depressant). Products include:
Tussionex Extended-Release Suspension 988

Hydroflumethiazide (Orthostatic hypotension that occurs with phenothiazines may be accentuated). Products include:
Diucardin Tablets 2450
Saluron 718
Salutensin/Salutensin-Demi 719

Hydroxyzine Hydrochloride (Intensified or prolonged action of CNS depressant). Products include:
Atarax Tablets & Syrup 1941
Marax Tablets & DF Syrup 1954
Vistaril Intramuscular Solution 1970

Isoflurane (Intensified or prolonged action of CNS depressant). Products include:
Forane 600

Ketamine Hydrochloride (Intensified or prolonged action of CNS depressant). Products include:
Ketalar 1726

Levorphanol Tartrate (Intensified or prolonged action of CNS depressant). Products include:
Levo-Dromoran 1906

Lorazepam (Intensified or prolonged action of CNS depressant). Products include:
Ativan Injection 2432
Ativan Tablets 2434

Loxapine Hydrochloride (Intensified or prolonged action of CNS depressant). Products include:
Loxitane 1213

Loxapine Succinate (Intensified or prolonged action of CNS depressants). Products include:
Loxitane Capsules 1213

Meperidine Hydrochloride (Intensified or prolonged action of CNS depressant). Products include:
Demerol 2047
Mepergan Injection 2479

Mephenytoin (Phenothiazines may lower convulsive threshold; dosage adjustments of anticonvulsants may be necessary). Products include:
Mesantoin Tablets 2013

Mephobarbital (Intensified or prolonged action of CNS depressant). Products include:
Mebaral Tablets 2061

Meprobamate (Intensified or prolonged action of CNS depressant). Products include:
Deprol Tablets 2382
Equagesic Tablets 2451
Miltown Tablets 2386
PMB 200 and PMB 400 2504

Mesoridazine (Intensified or prolonged action of CNS depressant). Products include:
Serentil 686

Methadone Hydrochloride (Intensified or prolonged action of CNS depressant). Products include:
Dolophine Hydrochloride Ampoules & Vials 1260
Dolophine Hydrochloride Tablets 1261
Methadone Hydrochloride Diskets 1284
Methadone Hydrochloride Oral Solution & Tablets 1987

Methohexital Sodium (Intensified or prolonged action of CNS depressant). Products include:
Brevital Sodium Vials 1248

Methoxyflurane (Intensified or prolonged action of CNS depressant).
No products indexed under this heading.

Methsuximide (Phenothiazines may lower convulsive threshold; dosage adjustments of anticonvulsants may be necessary). Products include:
Celontin ... 1692

Methyclothiazide (Orthostatic hypotension that occurs with phenothiazines may be accentuated). Products include:
Enduron Tablets ... 517
Enduronyl ... 518

Metrizamide (Phenothiazines may lower convulsive threshold; avoid concurrent use).

Midazolam Hydrochloride (Intensified or prolonged action of CNS depressant). Products include:
Versed Injection ... 1924

Molindone Hydrochloride (Intensified or prolonged action of CNS depressant). Products include:
Moban Tablets & Concentrate ... 932

Morphine Sulfate (Intensified or prolonged action of CNS depressant). Products include:
Astramorph/PF Injection, USP (Preservative-Free) ... 618
Duramorph ... 960
Infumorph 200 and Infumorph 500 Sterile Solutions ... 962
MS Contin Tablets ... 1814
MSIR ... 1817
Oramorph SR (Morphine Sulfate Sustained Release Tablets) ... 1988
Roxanol ... 1991

Opium Alkaloids (Intensified or prolonged action of CNS depressant). Products include:
B & O No. 15A & No. 16A Supprettes ... 2395
Pantopon Injectable ... 1911

Oxazepam (Intensified or prolonged action of CNS depressant). Products include:
Serax Capsules ... 2522
Serax Tablets ... 2522

Oxycodone Hydrochloride (Intensified or prolonged action of CNS depressant). Products include:
Percocet Tablets ... 950
Percodan ... 951
Roxicodone Tablets, Oral Solution & Intensol (Oxycodone) ... 1992
Tylox Capsules ... 1382

Paramethadione (Phenothiazines may lower convulsive threshold; dosage adjustments of anticonvulsants may be necessary). Products include:
Paradione Capsules ... 548

Pentobarbital Sodium (Intensified or prolonged action of CNS depressant). Products include:
Nembutal Sodium Capsules ... 534
Nembutal Sodium Solution ... 536
Nembutal Sodium Suppositories ... 538

Perphenazine (Intensified or prolonged action of CNS depressant). Products include:
Etrafon ... 2087
Triavil Tablets ... 1556
Trilafon ... 2123

Phenacemide (Phenothiazines may lower convulsive threshold; dosage adjustments of anticonvulsants may be necessary). Products include:
Phenurone Tablets ... 552

Phenobarbital (Phenothiazines may lower convulsive threshold; intensified or prolonged CNS depressant action). Products include:
Arco-Lase Plus Tablets ... 607
Bellergal-S Tablets ... 1998
Bronkolixir ... ▣ 761
Bronkotabs Tablets ... ▣ 762
Donnatal ... 1858
Donnatal Extentabs ... 1859
Donnatal Tablets ... 1858
Donnazyme Tablets ... 1860
Kinesed Tablets ... 2272
Phenobarbital Elixir and Tablets ... 1293
Primatene Tablets-P Formula ... 2421
Quadrinal Tablets ... 1183
Tedral SA ... 1765

Phensuximide (Phenothiazines may lower convulsive threshold; dosage adjustments of anticonvulsants may be necessary). Products include:
Milontin Kapseals ... 1741

Phenytoin (Phenytoin toxicity may be precipitated; phenothiazines may lower convulsive threshold; dosage adjustments of anticonvulsant may be necessary). Products include:
Dilantin Infatabs ... 1710
Dilantin-30 Pediatric/Dilantin-125 Suspension ... 1713

Phenytoin Sodium (Phenytoin toxicity may be precipitated; phenothiazines may lower convulsive threshold; dosage adjustments of anticonvulsant may be necessary). Products include:
Dilantin Kapseals ... 1708
Dilantin Parenteral ... 1712
Dilantin with Phenobarbital Kapseals ... 1715

Polythiazide (Orthostatic hypotension that occurs with phenothiazines may be accentuated). Products include:
Minizide Capsules ... 1779
Renese Tablets ... 1785
Renese-R Tablets ... 1786

Prazepam (Intensified or prolonged action of CNS depressant). Products include:
Centrax ... 1693

Primidone (Phenothiazines may lower convulsive threshold; dosage adjustments of anticonvulsants may be necessary). Products include:
Mysoline ... 2480

Promethazine Hydrochloride (Intensified or prolonged action of CNS depressant). Products include:
Mepergan Injection ... 2479
Phenergan with Codeine ... 2497
Phenergan with Dextromethorphan ... 2499
Phenergan Injection ... 2493
Phenergan Suppositories ... 2496
Phenergan Syrup ... 2495
Phenergan Tablets ... 2496
Phenergan VC ... 2500
Phenergan VC with Codeine ... 2501

Propofol (Intensified or prolonged action of CNS depressants). Products include:
Diprivan Injection ... 2267

Propoxyphene Hydrochloride (Intensified or prolonged action of CNS depressant). Products include:
Darvon ... 1256
Wygesic Tablets ... 2540

Propoxyphene Napsylate (Intensified or prolonged action of CNS depressant). Products include:
Darvon-N/Darvocet-N ... 1254

Propranolol Hydrochloride (Concomitant administration results in increased plasma levels of both drugs). Products include:
Inderal ... 2459
Inderal LA Long Acting Capsules ... 2461
Inderide Tablets ... 2463
Inderide LA Long Acting Capsules ... 2465

Quazepam (Intensified or prolonged action of CNS depressants). Products include:
Doral Tablets ... 2383

Secobarbital Sodium (Intensified or prolonged action of CNS depressants). Products include:
Seconal Sodium Pulvules ... 1296

Sufentanil Citrate (Intensified or prolonged action of CNS depressant). Products include:
Sufenta Injection ... 1147

Temazepam (Intensified or prolonged action of CNS depressant). Products include:
Restoril Capsules ... 2023

Thiamylal Sodium (Intensified or prolonged action of CNS depressant). Products include:
Surital Ampoules, Steri-Vials ... 1764

Thioridazine Hydrochloride (Intensified or prolonged action of CNS depressant). Products include:
Mellaril ... 2011

Thiothixene (Intensified or prolonged action of CNS depressant). Products include:
Navane Capsules and Concentrate ... 1954
Navane Intramuscular ... 1956

Triazolam (Intensified or prolonged action of CNS depressant). Products include:
Halcion Tablets ... 2340

Trifluoperazine Hydrochloride (Intensified or prolonged action of CNS depressant). Products include:
Stelazine ... 2226

Trimethadione (Phenothiazines may lower convulsive threshold; dosage adjustments of anticonvulsants may be necessary). Products include:
Tridione ... 557

Valproic Acid (Phenothiazines may lower convulsive threshold; dosage adjustments of anticonvulsants may be necessary). Products include:
Depakene Capsules & Syrup ... 511

Warfarin Sodium (Diminished effect of oral anticoagulants). Products include:
Coumadin Injection & Tablets ... 944
Panwarfin Tablets ... 547

COMPAZINE INJECTION
(Prochlorperazine) ... 2201
See **Compazine Ampuls**

COMPAZINE MULTIPLE-DOSE VIALS
(Prochlorperazine) ... 2201
See **Compazine Ampuls**

COMPAZINE PREFILLED DISPOSABLE SYRINGES
(Prochlorperazine) ... 2201
See **Compazine Ampuls**

COMPAZINE SPANSULE CAPSULES
(Prochlorperazine) ... 2201
See **Compazine Ampuls**

COMPAZINE SUPPOSITORIES
(Prochlorperazine) ... 2201
See **Compazine Ampuls**

COMPAZINE SYRUP
(Prochlorperazine) ... 2201
See **Compazine Ampuls**

COMPAZINE TABLETS
(Prochlorperazine) ... 2201
See **Compazine Ampuls**

COMPLEX 15 HAND & BODY MOISTURIZING CREAM
(Dimethicone, Lecithin) ... ▣ 694
No interactions described in labeling.

COMPLEX 15 HAND & BODY MOISTURIZING LOTION
(Dimethicone, Lecithin) ... ▣ 695
No interactions described in labeling.

COMPLEX 15 MOISTURIZING FACE CREAM
(Dimethicone, Lecithin) ... ▣ 695
No interactions described in labeling.

COMPOUND W GEL
(Salicylic Acid) ... 2418
No interactions described in labeling.

COMPOUND W SOLUTION
(Salicylic Acid) ... 2418
No interactions described in labeling.

ALLERGY-SINUS COMTREX MULTI-SYMPTOM ALLERGY SINUS FORMULA TABLETS & CAPLETS
(Acetaminophen, Chlorpheniramine Maleate, Pseudoephedrine Hydrochloride) ... 746
May interact with hypnotics and sedatives, tranquilizers, and certain other agents. Compounds in these categories include:

Alcohol (Increases drowsiness effect).

Alprazolam (Increases drowsiness effect). Products include:
Xanax Tablets ... 2367

Antidepressant Medications, unspecified (Effect not specified).

Blood Pressure Medications, unspecified (Effect not specified).
No products indexed under this heading.

Buspirone Hydrochloride (Increases drowsiness effect). Products include:
BuSpar ... 1401

Chlordiazepoxide (Increases drowsiness effect). Products include:
Libritabs Tablets ... 1930
Limbitrol ... 1933
Menrium Tablets ... 1934

Chlordiazepoxide Hydrochloride (Increases drowsiness effect). Products include:
Librax Capsules ... 1929
Librium Capsules ... 1931
Librium Injectable ... 1932

Chlorpromazine (Increases drowsiness effect). Products include:
Thorazine ... 2234

Chlorprothixene (Increases drowsiness effect). Products include:
Taractan Tablets ... 1920

Chlorprothixene Hydrochloride (Increases drowsiness effect). Products include:
Taractan ... 1920

Clorazepate Dipotassium (Increases drowsiness effect). Products include:
Tranxene ... 556

Diazepam (Increases drowsiness effect). Products include:
Valium Injectable ... 1937
Valium Tablets ... 1939
Valrelease Capsules ... 1923

Droperidol (Increases drowsiness effect). Products include:
Inapsine Injection ... 1140
Innovar Injection ... 1141

Estazolam (Increases drowsiness effect). Products include:
ProSom Tablets ... 554

Ethchlorvynol (Increases drowsiness effect). Products include:
Placidyl Capsules ... 553

Ethinamate (Increases drowsiness effect).
No products indexed under this heading.

Fluphenazine Decanoate (Increases drowsiness effect). Products include:
Prolixin Decanoate ... 1795

Fluphenazine Enanthate (Increases drowsiness effect). Products include:
Prolixin Enanthate ... 1796

Fluphenazine Hydrochloride (Increases drowsiness effect). Products include:
Prolixin Elixir ... 1793
Prolixin Injection ... 1791
Prolixin Oral Concentrate ... 1792
Prolixin Tablets ... 1793

Flurazepam Hydrochloride (Increases drowsiness effect). Products include:
Dalmane Capsules ... 1927

Glutethimide (Increases drowsiness effect).
No products indexed under this heading.

Haloperidol (Increases drowsiness effect). Products include:
Haldol Injection, Tablets and Concentrate ... 1373

Haloperidol Decanoate (Increases drowsiness effect). Products include:
Haldol Decanoate ... 1375

Hydroxyzine Hydrochloride (Increases drowsiness effect). Products include:
Atarax Tablets & Syrup ... 1941
Marax Tablets & DF Syrup ... 1954
Vistaril Intramuscular Solution ... 1970

Lorazepam (Increases drowsiness effect). Products include:
Ativan Injection ... 2432
Ativan Tablets ... 2434

Loxapine Hydrochloride (Increases drowsiness effect). Products include:
Loxitane ... 1213

Loxapine Succinate (Increases drowsiness effect). Products include:
Loxitane Capsules ... 1213

Meprobamate (Increases drowsiness effect). Products include:
Deprol Tablets ... 2382
Equagesic Tablets ... 2451
Miltown Tablets ... 2386
PMB 200 and PMB 400 ... 2504

Mesoridazine Besylate (Increases drowsiness effect).

Midazolam Hydrochloride (Increases drowsiness effect). Products include:
Versed Injection ... 1924

Molindone Hydrochloride (Increases drowsiness effect). Products include:
Moban Tablets & Concentrate ... 932

Oxazepam (Increases drowsiness effect). Products include:
Serax Capsules ... 2522
Serax Tablets ... 2522

Perphenazine (Increases drowsiness effect). Products include:
Etrafon ... 2087
Triavil Tablets ... 1556
Trilafon ... 2123

Prazepam (Increases drowsiness effect). Products include:
Centrax ... 1693

Prochlorperazine (Increases drowsiness effect). Products include:
Compazine ... 2201

Promethazine Hydrochloride (Increases drowsiness effect). Products include:
Mepergan Injection ... 2479
Phenergan with Codeine ... 2497
Phenergan with Dextromethorphan ... 2499
Phenergan Injection ... 2493
Phenergan Suppositories ... 2496
Phenergan Syrup ... 2495
Phenergan Tablets ... 2496
Phenergan VC ... 2500
Phenergan VC with Codeine ... 2501

Propofol (Increases drowsiness effect). Products include:
Diprivan Injection ... 2267

Quazepam (Increases drowsiness effect). Products include:
Doral Tablets ... 2383

Secobarbital Sodium (Increases drowsiness effect). Products include:
Seconal Sodium Pulvules ... 1296

Temazepam (Increases drowsiness effect). Products include:
Restoril Capsules ... 2023

Thioridazine Hydrochloride (Increases drowsiness effect). Products include:
Mellaril ... 2011

Thiothixene (Increases drowsiness effect). Products include:
Navane Capsules and Concentrate ... 1954
Navane Intramuscular ... 1956

Triazolam (Increases drowsiness effect). Products include:
Halcion Tablets ... 2340

Trifluoperazine Hydrochloride (Increases drowsiness effect). Products include:
Stelazine ... 2226

COUGH FORMULA COMTREX
(Pseudoephedrine Hydrochloride, Acetaminophen, Guaifenesin, Dextromethorphan Hydrobromide) ... 746
May interact with antihypertensives, antidepressant drugs, hypnotics and sedatives, and certain other agents. Compounds in these categories include:

Acebutolol Hydrochloride (Effect not specified). Products include:
Sectral Capsules ... 2520

Alcohol (Increases the drowsiness effect).

Amitriptyline Hydrochloride (Effect not specified). Products include:
Elavil ... 2269
Endep Tablets ... 1927
Etrafon ... 2087
Limbitrol ... 1933
Triavil Tablets ... 1556

Amoxapine (Effect not specified). Products include:
Asendin Tablets ... 1196

Atenolol (Effect not specified). Products include:
Tenoretic Tablets ... 1105
Tenormin Tablets and I.V. Injection ... 1107

Benazepril Hydrochloride (Effect not specified). Products include:
Lotensin Tablets ... 872

Betaxolol Hydrochloride (Effect not specified). Products include:
Betoptic Sterile Ophthalmic Solution ... 569
Betoptic S Sterile Ophthalmic Suspension ... 570
Kerlone Tablets ... 2172

Bupropion Hydrochloride (Effect not specified). Products include:
Wellbutrin Tablets ... 821

Captopril (Effect not specified). Products include:
Capoten ... 2255
Capozide ... 2258

Carteolol Hydrochloride (Effect not specified). Products include:
Cartrol Tablets ... 507

Clonidine (Effect not specified). Products include:
Catapres-TTS ... 677

Clonidine Hydrochloride (Effect not specified). Products include:
Catapres Tablets ... 676
Combipres Tablets ... 678

Deserpidine (Effect not specified). Products include:
Enduronyl ... 518
Harmonyl Tablets ... 528
Oreticyl ... 545

Desipramine Hydrochloride (Effect not specified). Products include:
Norpramin Tablets ... 1340

Diazoxide (Effect not specified). Products include:
Hyperstat I.V. Injection ... 2095
Proglycem ... 649

Doxazosin Mesylate (Effect not specified). Products include:
Cardura Tablets ... 1941

Doxepin Hydrochloride (Effect not specified). Products include:
Sinequan ... 1960

Enalapril Maleate (Effect not specified). Products include:
Vaseretic Tablets ... 1559
Vasotec Tablets ... 1564

Enalaprilat (Effect not specified). Products include:
Vasotec I.V. ... 1562

Esmolol Hydrochloride (Effect not specified). Products include:
Brevibloc Injection ... 942

Estazolam (Effect not specified). Products include:
ProSom Tablets ... 554

Ethchlorvynol (Effect not specified). Products include:
Placidyl Capsules ... 553

Ethinamate (Effect not specified).
No products indexed under this heading.

Felodipine (Effect not specified). Products include:
Plendil Extended-Release Tablets ... 1526

Fluoxetine Hydrochloride (Effect not specified). Products include:
Prozac Pulvules ... 920

Flurazepam Hydrochloride (Effect not specified). Products include:
Dalmane Capsules ... 1927

Fosinopril Sodium (Effect not specified). Products include:
Monopril Tablets ... 1406

Glutethimide (Effect not specified).
No products indexed under this heading.

Guanabenz Acetate (Effect not specified). Products include:
Wytensin Tablets ... 2542

Guanethidine Monosulfate (Effect not specified). Products include:
Esimil Tablets ... 864
Ismelin Tablets ... 869

Hydralazine Hydrochloride (Effect not specified). Products include:
Apresazide Capsules ... 854
Apresoline Hydrochloride Parenteral (Ampuls) ... 856
Apresoline Hydrochloride Tablets ... 855
Apresoline-Esidrix Tablets ... 857
Ser-Ap-Es Tablets ... 881
Serpasil-Apresoline Tablets ... 884

Imipramine Hydrochloride (Effect not specified). Products include:
Tofranil Ampuls ... 1038
Tofranil Tablets ... 1039

Imipramine Pamoate (Effect not specified). Products include:
Tofranil-PM Capsules ... 1041

Isocarboxazid (Effect not specified). Products include:
Marplan Tablets ... 1906

Isradipine (Effect not specified). Products include:
DynaCirc Capsules ... 2004

Labetalol Hydrochloride (Effect not specified). Products include:
Normodyne Injection ... 2108
Normodyne Tablets ... 2110
Normozide Tablets ... 2112
Trandate HCT Tablets ... 579
Trandate Injection ... 577
Trandate Tablets ... 579

Lisinopril (Effect not specified). Products include:
Prinivil Tablets ... 1538
Prinzide Tablets ... 1540
Zestoretic ... 2274
Zestril Tablets ... 2277

Lorazepam (Effect not specified). Products include:
Ativan Injection ... 2432
Ativan Tablets ... 2434

Maprotiline Hydrochloride (Effect not specified). Products include:
Ludiomil Tablets ... 874

Mecamylamine Hydrochloride (Effect not specified). Products include:
Inversine Tablets ... 1492

Methyldopa (Effect not specified). Products include:
Aldoclor Tablets ... 1413
Aldomet Oral ... 1415
Aldoril Tablets ... 1418

Metoprolol Tartrate (Effect not specified). Products include:
Lopressor Ampuls ... 1032
Lopressor HCT Tablets ... 1034
Lopressor Tablets ... 1032

Metyrosine (Effect not specified). Products include:
Demser Capsules ... 1460

Midazolam Hydrochloride (Effect not specified). Products include:
Versed Injection ... 1924

Minoxidil (Effect not specified). Products include:
Loniten Tablets ... 2346
Rogaine Topical Solution ... 2357

Nadolol (Effect not specified). Products include:
Corgard Tablets ... 701
Corzide Tablets ... 702

Nicardipine Hydrochloride (Effect not specified). Products include:
Cardene Capsules ... 2290

Nitroglycerin (Effect not specified). Products include:
Deponit NTG Transdermal Delivery System ... 2143
Minitran Transdermal Delivery System ... 1312
Nitro-Bid Ointment ... 1339
Nitro-Bid Capsules ... 1338
Nitrodisc ... 2176
Nitro-Dur (nitroglycerin) Transdermal Infusion System ... 1164
Nitrogard Tablets ... 1004
Nitrolingual Spray ... 1846
Nitrostat Tablets ... 1743
Transderm-Nitro Transdermal Therapeutic System ... 2283

Nortriptyline Hydrochloride (Effect not specified). Products include:
Pamelor ... 2019

Penbutolol Sulfate (Effect not specified). Products include:
Levatol ... 1832

Phenelzine Sulfate (Effect not specified). Products include:
Nardil ... 1742

Phenoxybenzamine Hydrochloride (Effect not specified). Products include:
Dibenzyline Capsules ... 2207

Phentolamine Mesylate (Effect not specified). Products include:
Regitine 878
Pindolol (Effect not specified). Products include:
Visken Tablets 2036
Prazosin Hydrochloride (Effect not specified). Products include:
Minipress Capsules 1778
Minizide Capsules 1779
Propofol (Effect not specified). Products include:
Diprivan Injection 2267
Propranolol Hydrochloride (Effect not specified). Products include:
Inderal 2459
Inderal LA Long Acting Capsules 2461
Inderide Tablets 2463
Inderide LA Long Acting Capsules .. 2465
Protriptyline Hydrochloride (Effect not specified). Products include:
Vivactil Tablets 1567
Quazepam (Effect not specified). Products include:
Doral Tablets 2383
Ramipril (Effect not specified). Products include:
Altace Capsules 1086
Rauwolfia Serpentina (Effect not specified). Products include:
Raudixin Tablets 1803
Rauzide Tablets 1804
Rescinnamine (Effect not specified).
No products indexed under this heading.
Reserpine (Effect not specified). Products include:
Diupres Tablets 1461
Hydromox R Tablets 1209
Hydropres Tablets 1485
Renese-R Tablets 1786
Salutensin/Salutensin-Demi 719
Ser-Ap-Es Tablets 881
Serpasil Tablets 883
Serpasil-Apresoline Tablets 884
Serpasil-Esidrix Tablets 886
Secobarbital Sodium (Effect not specified). Products include:
Seconal Sodium Pulvules 1296
Sodium Nitroprusside (Effect not specified). Products include:
Nipride I.V. Infusion 1909
Temazepam (Effect not specified). Products include:
Restoril Capsules 2023
Terazosin Hydrochloride (Effect not specified). Products include:
Hytrin Tablets 529
Timolol Maleate (Effect not specified). Products include:
Blocadren Tablets 1429
Timolide Tablets 1547
Timoptic in Ocudose 1552
Timoptic Sterile Ophthalmic Solution 1550
Tranylcypromine Sulfate (Effect not specified). Products include:
Parnate Tablets 2222
Trazodone Hydrochloride (Effect not specified). Products include:
Desyrel and Desyrel Dividose 1404
Triazolam (Effect not specified). Products include:
Halcion Tablets 2340
Trimethaphan Camsylate (Effect not specified). Products include:
Arfonad Ampuls 1887
Trimipramine Maleate (Effect not specified). Products include:
Surmontil Capsules 2524

COMTREX MULTI-SYMPTOM COLD RELIEVER TABLETS/CAPLETS/LIQUI-GELS/LIQUID
(Pseudoephedrine Hydrochloride, Phenylpropanolamine Hydrochloride, Dextromethorphan Hydrobromide, Acetaminophen, Chlorpheniramine Maleate) 745
May interact with hypnotics and sedatives, tranquilizers, and certain other agents. Compounds in these categories include:

Alcohol (Avoid concomitant use).
Alprazolam (Effect not specified). Products include:
Xanax Tablets 2367
Buspirone Hydrochloride (Effect not specified). Products include:
BuSpar 1401
Chlordiazepoxide (Effect not specified). Products include:
Libritabs Tablets 1930
Limbitrol 1933
Menrium Tablets 1934
Chlordiazepoxide Hydrochloride (Effect not specified). Products include:
Librax Capsules 1929
Librium Capsules 1931
Librium Injectable 1932
Chlorpromazine (Effect not specified). Products include:
Thorazine 2234
Chlorprothixene (Effect not specified). Products include:
Taractan Tablets 1920
Chlorprothixene Hydrochloride (Effect not specified). Products include:
Taractan 1920
Clorazepate Dipotassium (Effect not specified). Products include:
Tranxene 556
Diazepam (Effect not specified). Products include:
Valium Injectable 1937
Valium Tablets 1939
Valrelease Capsules 1923
Droperidol (Effect not specified). Products include:
Inapsine Injection 1140
Innovar Injection 1141
Estazolam (Effect not specified). Products include:
ProSom Tablets 554
Ethchlorvynol (Effect not specified). Products include:
Placidyl Capsules 553
Ethinamate (Effect not specified).
No products indexed under this heading.
Fluphenazine Decanoate (Effect not specified). Products include:
Prolixin Decanoate 1795
Fluphenazine Enanthate (Effect not specified). Products include:
Prolixin Enanthate 1796
Fluphenazine Hydrochloride (Effect not specified). Products include:
Prolixin Elixir 1793
Prolixin Injection 1791
Prolixin Oral Concentrate 1792
Prolixin Tablets 1793
Flurazepam Hydrochloride (Effect not specified). Products include:
Dalmane Capsules 1927
Glutethimide (Effect not specified).
No products indexed under this heading.
Haloperidol (Effect not specified). Products include:
Haldol Injection, Tablets and Concentrate 1373
Haloperidol Decanoate (Effect not specified). Products include:
Haldol Decanoate 1375
Hydroxyzine Hydrochloride (Effect not specified). Products include:
Atarax Tablets & Syrup 1941
Marax Tablets & DF Syrup 1954
Vistaril Intramuscular Solution 1970
Lorazepam (Effect not specified). Products include:
Ativan Injection 2432
Ativan Tablets 2434
Loxapine Hydrochloride (Effect not specified). Products include:
Loxitane 1213
Loxapine Succinate (Effect not specified). Products include:
Loxitane Capsules 1213
Meprobamate (Effect not specified). Products include:
Deprol Tablets 2382
Equagesic Tablets 2451
Miltown Tablets 2386
PMB 200 and PMB 400 2504
Mesoridazine Besylate (Effect not specified).
Midazolam Hydrochloride (Effect not specified). Products include:
Versed Injection 1924
Molindone Hydrochloride (Effect not specified). Products include:
Moban Tablets & Concentrate 932
Oxazepam (Effect not specified). Products include:
Serax Capsules 2522
Serax Tablets 2522
Perphenazine (Effect not specified). Products include:
Etrafon 2087
Triavil Tablets 1556
Trilafon 2123
Prazepam (Effect not specified). Products include:
Centrax 1693
Prochlorperazine (Effect not specified). Products include:
Compazine 2201
Promethazine Hydrochloride (Effect not specified). Products include:
Mepergan Injection 2479
Phenergan with Codeine 2497
Phenergan with Dextromethorphan 2499
Phenergan Injection 2493
Phenergan Suppositories 2496
Phenergan Syrup 2495
Phenergan Tablets 2496
Phenergan VC 2500
Phenergan VC with Codeine 2501
Propofol (Effect not specified). Products include:
Diprivan Injection 2267
Quazepam (Effect not specified). Products include:
Doral Tablets 2383
Secobarbital Sodium (Effect not specified). Products include:
Seconal Sodium Pulvules 1296
Temazepam (Effect not specified). Products include:
Restoril Capsules 2023
Thioridazine Hydrochloride (Effect not specified). Products include:
Mellaril 2011
Thiothixene (Effect not specified). Products include:
Navane Capsules and Concentrate 1954
Navane Intramuscular 1956
Triazolam (Effect not specified). Products include:
Halcion Tablets 2340
Trifluoperazine Hydrochloride (Effect not specified). Products include:
Stelazine 2226

DAY-NIGHT COMTREX
(Acetaminophen, Chlorpheniramine Maleate, Dextromethorphan Hydrobromide, Pseudoephedrine Hydrochloride) 747
May interact with hypnotics and sedatives, tranquilizers, and certain other agents. Compounds in these categories include:

Alcohol (Increases drowsiness).
Alprazolam (Effect not specified). Products include:
Xanax Tablets 2367
Antidepressant Medications, unspecified (Effect not specified).
Blood Pressure Medications, unspecified (Effect not specified).
No products indexed under this heading.
Buspirone Hydrochloride (Effect not specified). Products include:
BuSpar 1401
Chlordiazepoxide (Effect not specified). Products include:
Libritabs Tablets 1930
Limbitrol 1933
Menrium Tablets 1934
Chlordiazepoxide Hydrochloride (Effect not specified). Products include:
Librax Capsules 1929
Librium Capsules 1931
Librium Injectable 1932
Chlorpromazine (Effect not specified). Products include:
Thorazine 2234
Chlorprothixene (Effect not specified). Products include:
Taractan Tablets 1920
Chlorprothixene Hydrochloride (Effect not specified). Products include:
Taractan 1920
Clorazepate Dipotassium (Effect not specified). Products include:
Tranxene 556
Diazepam (Effect not specified). Products include:
Valium Injectable 1937
Valium Tablets 1939
Valrelease Capsules 1923
Droperidol (Effect not specified). Products include:
Inapsine Injection 1140
Innovar Injection 1141
Estazolam (Effect not specified). Products include:
ProSom Tablets 554
Ethchlorvynol (Effect not specified). Products include:
Placidyl Capsules 553
Ethinamate (Effect not specified).
No products indexed under this heading.
Fluphenazine Decanoate (Effect not specified). Products include:
Prolixin Decanoate 1795
Fluphenazine Enanthate (Effect not specified). Products include:
Prolixin Enanthate 1796
Fluphenazine Hydrochloride (Effect not specified). Products include:
Prolixin Elixir 1793
Prolixin Injection 1791
Prolixin Oral Concentrate 1792
Prolixin Tablets 1793
Flurazepam Hydrochloride (Effect not specified). Products include:
Dalmane Capsules 1927
Glutethimide (Effect not specified).
No products indexed under this heading.
Haloperidol (Effect not specified). Products include:
Haldol Injection, Tablets and Concentrate 1373

Haloperidol Decanoate (Effect not specified). Products include:
- Haldol Decanoate 1375

Hydroxyzine Hydrochloride (Effect not specified). Products include:
- Atarax Tablets & Syrup 1941
- Marax Tablets & DF Syrup 1954
- Vistaril Intramuscular Solution 1970

Lorazepam (Effect not specified). Products include:
- Ativan Injection 2432
- Ativan Tablets 2434

Loxapine Hydrochloride (Effect not specified). Products include:
- Loxitane 1213

Loxapine Succinate (Effect not specified). Products include:
- Loxitane Capsules 1213

Meprobamate (Effect not specified). Products include:
- Deprol Tablets 2382
- Equagesic Tablets 2451
- Miltown Tablets 2386
- PMB 200 and PMB 400 2504

Mesoridazine Besylate (Effect not specified).

Midazolam Hydrochloride (Effect not specified). Products include:
- Versed Injection 1924

Molindone Hydrochloride (Effect not specified). Products include:
- Moban Tablets & Concentrate 932

Oxazepam (Effect not specified). Products include:
- Serax Capsules 2522
- Serax Tablets 2522

Perphenazine (Effect not specified). Products include:
- Etrafon 2087
- Triavil Tablets 1556
- Trilafon 2123

Prazepam (Effect not specified). Products include:
- Centrax 1693

Prochlorperazine (Effect not specified). Products include:
- Compazine 2201

Promethazine Hydrochloride (Effect not specified). Products include:
- Mepergan Injection 2479
- Phenergan with Codeine 2497
- Phenergan with Dextromethorphan 2499
- Phenergan Injection 2493
- Phenergan Suppositories 2496
- Phenergan Syrup 2495
- Phenergan Tablets 2496
- Phenergan VC 2500
- Phenergan VC with Codeine 2501

Propofol (Effect not specified). Products include:
- Diprivan Injection 2267

Quazepam (Effect not specified). Products include:
- Doral Tablets 2383

Secobarbital Sodium (Effect not specified). Products include:
- Seconal Sodium Pulvules 1296

Temazepam (Effect not specified). Products include:
- Restoril Capsules 2023

Thioridazine Hydrochloride (Effect not specified). Products include:
- Mellaril 2011

Thiothixene (Effect not specified). Products include:
- Navane Capsules and Concentrate 1954
- Navane Intramuscular 1956

Triazolam (Effect not specified). Products include:
- Halcion Tablets 2340

Trifluoperazine Hydrochloride (Effect not specified). Products include:
- Stelazine 2226

NON-DROWSY COMTREX
(Acetaminophen, Dextromethorphan Hydrobromide, Pseudoephedrine Hydrochloride) 747
May interact with:

Antidepressant Medications, unspecified (Effect not specified).

Blood Pressure Medications, unspecified (Effect not specified).
- No products indexed under this heading.

CONCEPTROL CONTRACEPTIVE GEL • SINGLE USE CONTRACEPTIVES
(Nonoxynol-9) .... ▣ 631
No interactions described in labeling.

CONCEPTROL CONTRACEPTIVE INSERTS
(Nonoxynol-9) .... ▣ 631
No interactions described in labeling.

CONDYLOX
(Podofilox) 1630
No interactions described in labeling.

CONGESPIRIN FOR CHILDREN ASPIRIN FREE CHEWABLE COLD TABLETS
(Acetaminophen, Phenylephrine Hydrochloride) 748
No interactions described in labeling.

CONGESS JR. T.D. CAPSULES
(Guaifenesin, Pseudoephedrine Hydrochloride) 994
May interact with monoamine oxidase inhibitors. Compounds in this category include:

Furazolidone (Concurrent administration is contraindicated). Products include:
- Furoxone 1855

Isocarboxazid (Concurrent administration is contraindicated). Products include:
- Marplan Tablets 1906

Phenelzine Sulfate (Concurrent administration is contraindicated). Products include:
- Nardil 1742

Selegiline Hydrochloride (Concurrent administration is contraindicated). Products include:
- Eldepryl 2250

Tranylcypromine Sulfate (Concurrent administration is contraindicated). Products include:
- Parnate Tablets 2222

CONGESS SR. T.D. CAPSULES
(Guaifenesin, Pseudoephedrine Hydrochloride) 994
May interact with monoamine oxidase inhibitors. Compounds in this category include:

Furazolidone (Concurrent administration is contraindicated). Products include:
- Furoxone 1855

Isocarboxazid (Concurrent administration is contraindicated). Products include:
- Marplan Tablets 1906

Phenelzine Sulfate (Concurrent administration is contraindicated). Products include:
- Nardil 1742

Selegiline Hydrochloride (Concurrent administration is contraindicated). Products include:
- Eldepryl 2250

Tranylcypromine Sulfate (Concurrent administration is contraindicated). Products include:
- Parnate Tablets 2222

CONGESTAC CAPLETS
(Guaifenesin, Pseudoephedrine Hydrochloride) .... ▣ 617
May interact with monoamine oxidase inhibitors. Compounds in this category include:

Furazolidone (Concurrent administration is not recommended). Products include:
- Furoxone 1855

Isocarboxazid (Concurrent administration is not recommended). Products include:
- Marplan Tablets 1906

Phenelzine Sulfate (Concurrent administration is not recommended). Products include:
- Nardil 1742

Selegiline Hydrochloride (Concurrent administration is not recommended). Products include:
- Eldepryl 2250

Tranylcypromine Sulfate (Concurrent administration is not recommended). Products include:
- Parnate Tablets 2222

CONSTANT-T TABLETS
(Theophylline Anhydrous) 1029
May interact with catecholamine depleting drugs and certain other agents. Compounds in these categories include:

Cyclamycin (Increased theophylline blood levels).

Deserpidine (Tachycardia). Products include:
- Enduronyl 518
- Harmonyl Tablets 528
- Oreticyl 545

Erythromycin (Increased theophylline blood levels). Products include:
- A/T/S Topical Gel and Topical Solution 1089
- AK-Mycin Ointment .... ⊙ 204
- Benzamycin Topical Gel 907
- E-Mycin Tablets 688
- ETS-2% 1685
- ERYC 1720
- Erycette (erythromycin 2%) Topical Solution 1678
- Ery-Tab Tablets 521
- Erythromycin Base Filmtab 525
- Erythromycin Delayed-Release Capsules, USP 526
- Ilotycin Ophthalmic Ointment 915
- PCE Dispertab Tablets 549
- Pediazole 1973
- T-Stat 2.0% Topical Solution and Pads 2409
- Theramycin Z Topical Solution 2% 1410

Erythromycin Estolate (Increased theophylline blood levels). Products include:
- Ilosone 913

Erythromycin Ethylsuccinate (Increased theophylline blood levels). Products include:
- E.E.S. 522
- EryPed 519
- Pediazole 1973

Erythromycin Gluceptate (Increased theophylline blood levels). Products include:
- Ilotycin Gluceptate, IV, Vials 915

Erythromycin Lactobionate (Increased theophylline blood levels).
- No products indexed under this heading.

Erythromycin Stearate (Increased theophylline blood levels). Products include:
- Erythrocin Stearate Filmtab 523

Furosemide (Increased diuresis). Products include:
- Lasix 1093

Hexamethonium (Decreased chronotropic effect).

Lincomycin Hydrochloride Monohydrate (Increased theophylline blood levels).
- No products indexed under this heading.

Rauwolfia Serpentina (Tachycardia). Products include:
- Raudixin Tablets 1803
- Rauzide Tablets 1804

Rescinnamine (Tachycardia).
- No products indexed under this heading.

Reserpine (Tachycardia). Products include:
- Diupres Tablets 1461
- Hydromox R Tablets 1209
- Hydropres Tablets 1485
- Renese-R Tablets 1786
- Salutensin/Salutensin-Demi 719
- Ser-Ap-Es Tablets 881
- Serpasil Tablets 883
- Serpasil-Apresoline Tablets 884
- Serpasil-Esidrix Tablets 886

Troleandomycin (Increased theophylline blood levels). Products include:
- Tao Capsules 1963

Food Interactions

Food, unspecified (Food ingestion may influence the absorption characteristics).

CONTAC CONTINUOUS ACTION DECONGESTANT/ANTIHISTAMINE CAPSULES
(Chlorpheniramine Maleate, Phenylpropanolamine Hydrochloride) .... ▣ 710
May interact with monoamine oxidase inhibitors, phenylpropanolamine containing anorectics, and certain other agents. Compounds in these categories include:

Alcohol (Do not use concomitantly).

Furazolidone (Effect not specified). Products include:
- Furoxone 1855

Isocarboxazid (Effect not specified). Products include:
- Marplan Tablets 1906

Phenelzine Sulfate (Effect not specified). Products include:
- Nardil 1742

Phenylpropanolamine Containing Anorectics (Effect not specified).

Selegiline Hydrochloride (Effect not specified). Products include:
- Eldepryl 2250

Tranylcypromine Sulfate (Effect not specified). Products include:
- Parnate Tablets 2222

CONTAC COUGH FORMULA
(Dextromethorphan Hydrobromide, Guaifenesin) .... ▣ 711
No interactions described in labeling.

CONTAC COUGH & SORE THROAT FORMULA
(Acetaminophen, Dextromethorphan Hydrobromide, Guaifenesin) .... ▣ 712
May interact with aspirin and acet-

aminophen containing products. Compounds in this category include:

Aspirin (Effect not specified). Products include:
- Alka-Seltzer Effervescent Antacid and Pain Reliever 1568
- Alka-Seltzer Extra Strength Effervescent Antacid and Pain Reliever 1570
- Alka-Seltzer (Flavored) Effervescent Antacid and Pain Reliever 1569
- Alka-Seltzer Plus Cold Medicine .... ▣ 623
- Alka-Seltzer Plus Night-Time Cold Medicine ..... ▣ 623
- Alka Seltzer Plus Sinus Allergy Medicine ..... ▣ 624
- Anacin Coated Analgesic Caplets 2417
- Anacin Coated Analgesic Tablets 2417
- Anacin Maximum Strength Analgesic Coated Tablets 2417
- Maximum Strength Arthritis Pain Formula By the Makers of Anacin Analgesic Tablets and Caplets 2418
- Arthritis Pain Formula by the Makers of Anacin Analgesic Tablets and Caplets ..... ▣ 747
- Arthritis Strength BC Powder ..... ▣ 516
- Ascriptin A/D Caplets 1850
- Regular Strength Ascriptin Tablets 1850
- Azdōne Tablets 844
- BC Powder ..... ▣ 517
- BC Cold Powder ..... ▣ 517
- Children's Bayer Chewable Aspirin ..... ▣ 564
- Genuine Bayer Aspirin Tablets & Caplets ..... ▣ 564
- Maximum Bayer Aspirin Tablets & Caplets ..... ▣ 566
- Bayer Plus Aspirin Tablets ..... ▣ 567
- Therapy Bayer Aspirin Caplets ..... ▣ 568
- 8 Hour Bayer Timed-Release Aspirin ..... ▣ 566
- Arthritis Strength Bufferin Analgesic Caplets 744
- Extra Strength Bufferin Analgesic Tablets 745
- Bufferin Analgesic Tablets and Caplets 743
- Cama Arthritis Pain Reliever ..... ▣ 685
- Damason-P 1356
- Easprin 1719
- Ecotrin Enteric Coated Aspirin Maximum Strength Tablets and Caplets 2189
- Ecotrin Enteric Coated Aspirin Regular Strength Tablets and Caplets 2189
- Empirin Aspirin ..... ▣ 541
- Empirin with Codeine Phosphate Nos. 2, 3 & 4 764
- Equagesic Tablets 2451
- Excedrin Extra-Strength Analgesic Tablets & Caplets 749
- 4-Way Cold Tablets 750
- Fiorinal Capsules 2007
- Fiorinal with Codeine Capsules 2008
- Fiorinal Tablets 2007
- Lortab ASA Tablets 2414
- Momentum Muscular Backache Formula ..... ▣ 751
- Norgesic 1314
- Norwich Extra-Strength Aspirin ..... ▣ 546
- Norwich Regular Strength Aspirin ▣ 547
- P-A-C Analgesic Tablets ..... ▣ 669
- Percodan 951
- Robaxisal Tablets 1872
- Sine-Off Sinus Medicine Tablets-Aspirin Formula ..... ▣ 722
- Soma Compound w/Codeine Tablets 2390
- Soma Compound Tablets 2389
- St. Joseph Adult Chewable Aspirin (81 mg.) ..... ▣ 703
- Synalgos-DC Capsules 2525
- Talwin Compound 2072
- Ursinus Inlay-Tabs ..... ▣ 691
- Vanquish Analgesic Caplets ..... ▣ 574
- Zorprin Tablets 698

CONTAC JR. CHILDREN'S COLD MEDICINE
(Acetaminophen, Dextromethorphan Hydrobromide, Pseudoephedrine Hydrochloride) .... ▣ 712
No interactions described in labeling.

CONTAC MAXIMUM STRENGTH CONTINUOUS ACTION DECONGESTANT/ANTIHISTAMINE CAPLETS
(Chlorpheniramine Maleate, Phenylpropanolamine Hydrochloride) ..... ▣ 709
May interact with monoamine oxidase inhibitors, phenylpropanolamine containing anorectics, and certain other agents. Compounds in these categories include:

Alcohol (Do not use concomitantly).

Furazolidone (Effect not specified). Products include:
- Furoxone 1855

Isocarboxazid (Effect not specified). Products include:
- Marplan Tablets 1906

Phenelzine Sulfate (Effect not specified). Products include:
- Nardil 1742

Phenylpropanolamine Containing Anorectics (Effect not specified).

Selegiline Hydrochloride (Effect not specified). Products include:
- Eldepryl 2250

Tranylcypromine Sulfate (Effect not specified). Products include:
- Parnate Tablets 2222

CONTAC NIGHTTIME COLD MEDICINE
(Acetaminophen, Dextromethorphan Hydrobromide, Doxylamine Succinate, Pseudoephedrine Hydrochloride) .... ▣ 713
May interact with:

Alcohol (Do not use concomitantly).

Antidepressant Medications, unspecified (Effect not specified).

Antihypertensive agents, unspecified (Effect not specified).

CONTAC SEVERE COLD AND FLU FORMULA CAPLETS
(Acetaminophen, Chlorpheniramine Maleate, Dextromethorphan Hydrobromide, Phenylpropanolamine Hydrochloride) ..... ▣ 711
May interact with monoamine oxidase inhibitors, phenylpropanolamine containing anorectics, and certain other agents. Compounds in these categories include:

Alcohol (Do not use concomitantly).

Furazolidone (Effect not specified). Products include:
- Furoxone 1855

Isocarboxazid (Effect not specified). Products include:
- Marplan Tablets 1906

Phenelzine Sulfate (Effect not specified). Products include:
- Nardil 1742

Phenylpropanolamine Containing Anorectics (Effect not specified).

Selegiline Hydrochloride (Effect not specified). Products include:
- Eldepryl 2250

Tranylcypromine Sulfate (Effect not specified). Products include:
- Parnate Tablets 2222

CONTAC SINUS CAPLETS MAXIMUM STRENGTH NON-DROWSY FORMULA
(Acetaminophen, Pseudoephedrine Hydrochloride) ..... ▣ 710
May interact with antihypertensives and antidepressant drugs. Compounds in these categories include:

Acebutolol Hydrochloride (Concurrent use not recommended). Products include:
- Sectral Capsules 2520

Amitriptyline Hydrochloride (Concurrent use not recommended). Products include:
- Elavil 2269
- Endep Tablets 1927
- Etrafon 2087
- Limbitrol 1933
- Triavil Tablets 1556

Amoxapine (Concurrent use not recommended). Products include:
- Asendin Tablets 1196

Atenolol (Concurrent use not recommended). Products include:
- Tenoretic Tablets 1105
- Tenormin Tablets and I.V. Injection 1107

Benazepril Hydrochloride (Concurrent use not recommended). Products include:
- Lotensin Tablets 872

Bendroflumethiazide (Concurrent use not recommended). Products include:
- Corzide Tablets 702
- Naturetin Tablets 1789
- Rauzide Tablets 1804

Betaxolol Hydrochloride (Concurrent use not recommended). Products include:
- Betoptic Sterile Ophthalmic Solution 569
- Betoptic S Sterile Ophthalmic Suspension 570
- Kerlone Tablets 2172

Bupropion Hydrochloride (Concurrent use not recommended). Products include:
- Wellbutrin Tablets 821

Captopril (Concurrent use not recommended). Products include:
- Capoten 2255
- Capozide 2258

Carteolol Hydrochloride (Concurrent use not recommended). Products include:
- Cartrol Tablets 507

Chlorothiazide (Concurrent use not recommended). Products include:
- Aldoclor Tablets 1413
- Diupres Tablets 1461
- Diuril Oral 1464

Chlorothiazide Sodium (Concurrent use not recommended). Products include:
- Diuril Sodium Intravenous 1463

Chlorthalidone (Concurrent use not recommended). Products include:
- Combipres Tablets 678
- Tenoretic Tablets 1105
- Thalitone Tablets 687

Clonidine (Concurrent use not recommended). Products include:
- Catapres-TTS 677

Clonidine Hydrochloride (Concurrent use not recommended). Products include:
- Catapres Tablets 676
- Combipres Tablets 678

Deserpidine (Concurrent use not recommended). Products include:
- Enduronyl 518
- Harmonyl Tablets 528
- Oreticyl 545

Desipramine Hydrochloride (Concurrent use not recommended). Products include:
- Norpramin Tablets 1340

Diazoxide (Concurrent use not recommended). Products include:
- Hyperstat I.V. Injection 2095
- Proglycem 649

Doxazosin Mesylate (Concurrent use not recommended). Products include:
- Cardura Tablets 1941

Doxepin Hydrochloride (Concurrent use not recommended). Products include:
- Sinequan 1960

Enalapril Maleate (Concurrent use not recommended). Products include:
- Vaseretic Tablets 1559
- Vasotec Tablets 1564

Enalaprilat (Concurrent use not recommended). Products include:
- Vasotec I.V. 1562

Esmolol Hydrochloride (Concurrent use not recommended). Products include:
- Brevibloc Injection 942

Felodipine (Concurrent use not recommended). Products include:
- Plendil Extended-Release Tablets 1526

Fluoxetine Hydrochloride (Concurrent use not recommended). Products include:
- Prozac Pulvules 920

Fosinopril Sodium (Concurrent use not recommended). Products include:
- Monopril Tablets 1406

Furosemide (Concurrent use not recommended). Products include:
- Lasix 1093

Guanabenz Acetate (Concurrent use not recommended). Products include:
- Wytensin Tablets 2542

Guanethidine Monosulfate (Concurrent use not recommended). Products include:
- Esimil Tablets 864
- Ismelin Tablets 869

Hydralazine Hydrochloride (Concurrent use not recommended). Products include:
- Apresazide Capsules 854
- Apresoline Hydrochloride Parenteral (Ampuls) 856
- Apresoline Hydrochloride Tablets .. 855
- Apresoline-Esidrix Tablets 857
- Ser-Ap-Es Tablets 881
- Serpasil-Apresoline Tablets 884

Hydrochlorothiazide (Concurrent use not recommended). Products include:
- Aldactazide 2150
- Aldoril Tablets 1418
- Apresazide Capsules 854
- Apresoline-Esidrix Tablets 857
- Capozide 2258
- Dyazide Capsules 2208
- Esidrix Tablets 863
- Esimil Tablets 864
- HydroDIURIL Tablets 1484
- Hydropres Tablets 1485
- Inderide Tablets 2463
- Inderide LA Long Acting Capsules .. 2465
- Lopressor HCT Tablets 1034
- Maxzide 1215
- Moduretic Tablets 1510
- Normozide Tablets 2112
- Oretic Tablets 544
- Oreticyl 545
- Prinzide Tablets 1540
- Ser-Ap-Es Tablets 881
- Serpasil-Esidrix Tablets 886
- Timolide Tablets 1547
- Trandate HCT Tablets 579
- Vaseretic Tablets 1559
- Zestoretic 2274

Hydroflumethiazide (Concurrent use not recommended). Products include:
- Diucardin Tablets 2450
- Saluron 718
- Salutensin/Salutensin-Demi 719

Imipramine Hydrochloride (Concurrent use not recommended). Products include:
- Tofranil Ampuls 1038
- Tofranil Tablets 1039

Imipramine Pamoate (Concurrent use not recommended). Products include:
- Tofranil-PM Capsules 1041

Indapamide (Concurrent use not recommended). Products include:
- Lozol Tablets 1843

Isocarboxazid (Concurrent use not recommended). Products include:
- Marplan Tablets 1906

Isradipine (Concurrent use not recommended). Products include:
- DynaCirc Capsules 2004

Labetalol Hydrochloride (Concurrent use not recommended). Products include:
- Normodyne Injection 2108
- Normodyne Tablets 2110
- Normozide Tablets 2112
- Trandate HCT Tablets 579
- Trandate Injection 577
- Trandate Tablets 579

Lisinopril (Concurrent use not recommended). Products include:
- Prinivil Tablets 1538
- Prinzide Tablets 1540
- Zestoretic 2274
- Zestril Tablets 2277

Maprotiline Hydrochloride (Concurrent use not recommended). Products include:
- Ludiomil Tablets 874

Mecamylamine Hydrochloride (Concurrent use not recommended). Products include:
- Inversine Tablets 1492

Methyclothiazide (Concurrent use not recommended). Products include:
- Enduron Tablets 517
- Enduronyl 518

Methyldopa (Concurrent use not recommended). Products include:
- Aldoclor Tablets 1413
- Aldomet Oral 1415
- Aldoril Tablets 1418

Methyldopate Hydrochloride (Concurrent use not recommended). Products include:
- Aldomet Ester HCl Injection 1417

Metolazone (Concurrent use not recommended). Products include:
- Diulo 2129
- Mykrox ½ mg Tablets 984
- Zaroxolyn Tablets 989

Metoprolol Tartrate (Concurrent use not recommended). Products include:
- Lopressor Ampuls 1032
- Lopressor HCT Tablets 1034
- Lopressor Tablets 1032

Metyrosine (Concurrent use not recommended). Products include:
- Demser Capsules 1460

Minoxidil (Concurrent use not recommended). Products include:
- Loniten Tablets 2346
- Rogaine Topical Solution 2357

Nadolol (Concurrent use not recommended). Products include:
- Corgard Tablets 701
- Corzide Tablets 702

Nicardipine Hydrochloride (Concurrent use not recommended). Products include:
- Cardene Capsules 2290

Nitroglycerin (Concurrent use not recommended). Products include:
- Deponit NTG Transdermal Delivery System 2143
- Minitran Transdermal Delivery System 1312
- Nitro-Bid Ointment 1339
- Nitro-Bid Capsules 1338
- Nitrodisc 2176
- Nitro-Dur (nitroglycerin) Transdermal Infusion System 1164
- Nitrogard Tablets 1004
- Nitrolingual Spray 1846
- Nitrostat Tablets 1743
- Transderm-Nitro Transdermal Therapeutic System 2283

Nortriptyline Hydrochloride (Concurrent use not recommended). Products include:
- Pamelor 2019

Penbutolol Sulfate (Concurrent use not recommended). Products include:
- Levatol 1832

Phenelzine Sulfate (Concurrent use not recommended). Products include:
- Nardil 1742

Phenoxybenzamine Hydrochloride (Concurrent use not recommended). Products include:
- Dibenzyline Capsules 2207

Phentolamine Mesylate (Concurrent use not recommended). Products include:
- Regitine 878

Pindolol (Concurrent use not recommended). Products include:
- Visken Tablets 2036

Polythiazide (Concurrent use not recommended). Products include:
- Minizide Capsules 1779
- Renese Tablets 1785
- Renese-R Tablets 1786

Prazosin Hydrochloride (Concurrent use not recommended). Products include:
- Minipress Capsules 1778
- Minizide Capsules 1779

Propranolol Hydrochloride (Concurrent use not recommended). Products include:
- Inderal 2459
- Inderal LA Long Acting Capsules 2461
- Inderide Tablets 2463
- Inderide LA Long Acting Capsules 2465

Protriptyline Hydrochloride (Concurrent use not recommended). Products include:
- Vivactil Tablets 1567

Ramipril (Concurrent use not recommended). Products include:
- Altace Capsules 1086

Rauwolfia Serpentina (Concurrent use not recommended). Products include:
- Raudixin Tablets 1803
- Rauzide Tablets 1804

Rescinnamine (Concurrent use not recommended).
- No products indexed under this heading.

Reserpine (Concurrent use not recommended). Products include:
- Diupres Tablets 1461
- Hydromox R Tablets 1209
- Hydropres Tablets 1485
- Renese-R Tablets 1786
- Salutensin/Salutensin-Demi 719
- Ser-Ap-Es Tablets 881
- Serpasil Tablets 883
- Serpasil-Apresoline Tablets 884
- Serpasil-Esidrix Tablets 886

Sodium Nitroprusside (Concurrent use not recommended). Products include:
- Nipride I.V. Infusion 1909

Terazosin Hydrochloride (Concurrent use not recommended). Products include:
- Hytrin Tablets 529

Timolol Maleate (Concurrent use not recommended). Products include:
- Blocadren Tablets 1429
- Timolide Tablets 1547
- Timoptic in Ocudose 1552
- Timoptic Sterile Ophthalmic Solution 1550

Tranylcypromine Sulfate (Concurrent use not recommended). Products include:
- Parnate Tablets 2222

Trazodone Hydrochloride (Concurrent use not recommended). Products include:
- Desyrel and Desyrel Dividose 1404

Trimethaphan Camsylate (Concurrent use not recommended). Products include:
- Arfonad Ampuls 1887

Trimipramine Maleate (Concurrent use not recommended). Products include:
- Surmontil Capsules 2524

CONTAC SINUS TABLETS MAXIMUM STRENGTH NON-DROWSY FORMULA
(Acetaminophen, Pseudoephedrine Hydrochloride) ■ 710
May interact with antihypertensives and antidepressant drugs. Compounds in these categories include:

Acebutolol Hydrochloride (Concurrent use not recommended). Products include:
- Sectral Capsules 2520

Amitriptyline Hydrochloride (Concurrent use not recommended). Products include:
- Elavil 2269
- Endep Tablets 1927
- Etrafon 2087
- Limbitrol 1933
- Triavil Tablets 1556

Amoxapine (Concurrent use not recommended). Products include:
- Asendin Tablets 1196

Atenolol (Concurrent use not recommended). Products include:
- Tenoretic Tablets 1105
- Tenormin Tablets and I.V. Injection 1107

Benazepril Hydrochloride (Concurrent use not recommended). Products include:
- Lotensin Tablets 872

Bendroflumethiazide (Concurrent use not recommended). Products include:
- Corzide Tablets 702
- Naturetin Tablets 1789
- Rauzide Tablets 1804

Betaxolol Hydrochloride (Concurrent use not recommended). Products include:
- Betoptic Sterile Ophthalmic Solution 569
- Betoptic S Sterile Ophthalmic Suspension 570
- Kerlone Tablets 2172

Bupropion Hydrochloride (Concurrent use not recommended). Products include:
- Wellbutrin Tablets 821

Captopril (Concurrent use not recommended). Products include:
- Capoten 2255
- Capozide 2258

Carteolol Hydrochloride (Concurrent use not recommended). Products include:
- Cartrol Tablets 507

Chlorothiazide (Concurrent use not recommended). Products include:
- Aldoclor Tablets 1413
- Diupres Tablets 1461
- Diuril Oral 1464

Chlorothiazide Sodium (Concurrent use not recommended). Products include:
- Diuril Sodium Intravenous 1463

Chlorthalidone (Concurrent use not recommended). Products include:
- Combipres Tablets 678
- Tenoretic Tablets 1105
- Thalitone Tablets 687

Clonidine (Concurrent use not recommended). Products include:
- Catapres-TTS 677

Clonidine Hydrochloride (Concurrent use not recommended). Products include:
- Catapres Tablets 676
- Combipres Tablets 678

Deserpidine (Concurrent use not recommended). Products include:
- Enduronyl 518
- Harmonyl Tablets 528
- Oreticyl 545

Desipramine Hydrochloride (Concurrent use not recommended). Products include:
- Norpramin Tablets 1340

Diazoxide (Concurrent use not recommended). Products include:
- Hyperstat I.V. Injection 2095
- Proglycem 649

Doxazosin Mesylate (Concurrent use not recommended). Products include:
- Cardura Tablets 1941

Doxepin Hydrochloride (Concurrent use not recommended). Products include:
- Sinequan 1960

Enalapril Maleate (Concurrent use not recommended). Products include:
- Vaseretic Tablets 1559
- Vasotec Tablets 1564

Enalaprilat (Concurrent use not recommended). Products include:
- Vasotec I.V. 1562

Esmolol Hydrochloride (Concurrent use not recommended). Products include:
- Brevibloc Injection 942

Felodipine (Concurrent use not recommended). Products include:
- Plendil Extended-Release Tablets 1526

Fluoxetine Hydrochloride (Concurrent use not recommended). Products include:
- Prozac Pulvules 920

Fosinopril Sodium (Concurrent use not recommended). Products include:
- Monopril Tablets 1406

Furosemide (Concurrent use not recommended). Products include:
- Lasix 1093

Guanabenz Acetate (Concurrent use not recommended). Products include:
- Wytensin Tablets 2542

Guanethidine Monosulfate (Concurrent use not recommended). Products include:
- Esimil Tablets 864
- Ismelin Tablets 869

Hydralazine Hydrochloride (Concurrent use not recommended). Products include:
- Apresazide Capsules 854
- Apresoline Hydrochloride Parenteral (Ampuls) 856
- Apresoline Hydrochloride Tablets 855
- Apresoline-Esidrix Tablets 857
- Ser-Ap-Es Tablets 881
- Serpasil-Apresoline Tablets 884

Hydrochlorothiazide (Concurrent use not recommended). Products include:
- Aldactazide 2150

Aldoril Tablets 1418
Apresazide Capsules 854
Apresoline-Esidrix Tablets 857
Capozide 2258
Dyazide Capsules 2208
Esidrix Tablets 863
Esimil Tablets 864
HydroDIURIL Tablets 1484
Hydropres Tablets 1485
Inderide Tablets 2463
Inderide LA Long Acting Capsules 2465
Lopressor HCT Tablets 1034
Maxzide 1215
Moduretic Tablets 1510
Normozide Tablets 2112
Oretic Tablets 544
Oreticyl 545
Prinzide Tablets 1540
Ser-Ap-Es Tablets 881
Serpasil-Esidrix Tablets 886
Timolide Tablets 1547
Trandate HCT Tablets 579
Vaseretic Tablets 1559
Zestoretic 2274

Hydroflumethiazide (Concurrent use not recommended). Products include:
Diucardin Tablets 2450
Saluron 718
Salutensin/Salutensin-Demi 719

Imipramine Hydrochloride (Concurrent use not recommended). Products include:
Tofranil Ampuls 1038
Tofranil Tablets 1039

Imipramine Pamoate (Concurrent use not recommended). Products include:
Tofranil-PM Capsules 1041

Indapamide (Concurrent use not recommended). Products include:
Lozol Tablets 1843

Isocarboxazid (Concurrent use not recommended). Products include:
Marplan Tablets 1906

Isradipine (Concurrent use not recommended). Products include:
DynaCirc Capsules 2004

Labetalol Hydrochloride (Concurrent use not recommended). Products include:
Normodyne Injection 2108
Normodyne Tablets 2110
Normozide Tablets 2112
Trandate HCT Tablets 579
Trandate Injection 577
Trandate Tablets 579

Lisinopril (Concurrent use not recommended). Products include:
Prinivil Tablets 1538
Prinzide Tablets 1540
Zestoretic 2274
Zestril Tablets 2277

Maprotiline Hydrochloride (Concurrent use not recommended). Products include:
Ludiomil Tablets 874

Mecamylamine Hydrochloride (Concurrent use not recommended). Products include:
Inversine Tablets 1492

Methyclothiazide (Concurrent use not recommended). Products include:
Enduron Tablets 517
Enduronyl 518

Methyldopa (Concurrent use not recommended). Products include:
Aldoclor Tablets 1413
Aldomet Oral 1415
Aldoril Tablets 1418

Methyldopate Hydrochloride (Concurrent use not recommended). Products include:
Aldomet Ester HCl Injection 1417

Metolazone (Concurrent use not recommended). Products include:
Diulo 2129
Mykrox ½ mg Tablets 984
Zaroxolyn Tablets 989

Metoprolol Tartrate (Concurrent use not recommended). Products include:
Lopressor Ampuls 1032
Lopressor HCT Tablets 1034
Lopressor Tablets 1032

Metyrosine (Concurrent use not recommended). Products include:
Demser Capsules 1460

Minoxidil (Concurrent use not recommended). Products include:
Loniten Tablets 2346
Rogaine Topical Solution 2357

Nadolol (Concurrent use not recommended). Products include:
Corgard Tablets 701
Corzide Tablets 702

Nicardipine Hydrochloride (Concurrent use not recommended). Products include:
Cardene Capsules 2290

Nitroglycerin (Concurrent use not recommended). Products include:
Deponit NTG Transdermal Delivery System 2143
Minitran Transdermal Delivery System 1312
Nitro-Bid Ointment 1339
Nitro-Bid Capsules 1338
Nitrodisc 2176
Nitro-Dur (nitroglycerin) Transdermal Infusion System 1164
Nitrogard Tablets 1004
Nitrolingual Spray 1846
Nitrostat Tablets 1743
Transderm-Nitro Transdermal Therapeutic System 2283

Nortriptyline Hydrochloride (Concurrent use not recommended). Products include:
Pamelor 2019

Penbutolol Sulfate (Concurrent use not recommended). Products include:
Levatol 1832

Phenelzine Sulfate (Concurrent use not recommended). Products include:
Nardil 1742

Phenoxybenzamine Hydrochloride (Concurrent use not recommended). Products include:
Dibenzyline Capsules 2207

Phentolamine Mesylate (Concurrent use not recommended). Products include:
Regitine 878

Pindolol (Concurrent use not recommended). Products include:
Visken Tablets 2036

Polythiazide (Concurrent use not recommended). Products include:
Minizide Capsules 1779
Renese Tablets 1785
Renese-R Tablets 1786

Prazosin Hydrochloride (Concurrent use not recommended). Products include:
Minipress Capsules 1778
Minizide Capsules 1779

Propranolol Hydrochloride (Concurrent use not recommended). Products include:
Inderal 2459
Inderal LA Long Acting Capsules 2461
Inderide Tablets 2463
Inderide LA Long Acting Capsules 2465

Protriptyline Hydrochloride (Concurrent use not recommended). Products include:
Vivactil Tablets 1567

Ramipril (Concurrent use not recommended). Products include:
Altace Capsules 1086

Rauwolfia Serpentina (Concurrent use not recommended). Products include:
Raudixin Tablets 1803
Rauzide Tablets 1804

Rescinnamine (Concurrent use not recommended).
No products indexed under this heading.

Reserpine (Concurrent use not recommended). Products include:
Diupres Tablets 1461
Hydromox R Tablets 1209
Hydropres Tablets 1485
Renese-R Tablets 1786
Salutensin/Salutensin-Demi 719
Ser-Ap-Es Tablets 881
Serpasil Tablets 883
Serpasil-Apresoline Tablets 884
Serpasil-Esidrix Tablets 886

Sodium Nitroprusside (Concurrent use not recommended). Products include:
Nipride I.V. Infusion 1909

Terazosin Hydrochloride (Concurrent use not recommended). Products include:
Hytrin Tablets 529

Timolol Maleate (Concurrent use not recommended). Products include:
Blocadren Tablets 1429
Timolide Tablets 1547
Timoptic in Ocudose 1552
Timoptic Sterile Ophthalmic Solution 1550

Tranylcypromine Sulfate (Concurrent use not recommended). Products include:
Parnate Tablets 2222

Trazodone Hydrochloride (Concurrent use not recommended). Products include:
Desyrel and Desyrel Dividose 1404

Trimethaphan Camsylate (Concurrent use not recommended). Products include:
Arfonad Ampuls 1887

Trimipramine Maleate (Concurrent use not recommended). Products include:
Surmontil Capsules 2524

CORDARONE TABLETS
(Amiodarone Hydrochloride) 2446
May interact with antiarrhythmics, oral anticoagulants, beta blockers, calcium channel blockers, cardiac glycosides, and certain other agents. Compounds in these categories include:

Acebutolol Hydrochloride (Bradycardia, sinus arrest, and AV block potentiated; potentially serious toxicity). Products include:
Sectral Capsules 2520

Adenosine (Bradycardia, sinus arrest, and AV block potentiated; potentially serious toxicity). Products include:
Adenocard Injection 1007

Atenolol (Bradycardia, sinus arrest, and AV block potentiated). Products include:
Tenoretic Tablets 1105
Tenormin Tablets and I.V. Injection 1107

Bepridil Hydrochloride (Bradycardia, sinus arrest, and AV block potentiated). Products include:
Vascor (200, 300 and 400 mg) Tablets 1383

Betaxolol Hydrochloride (Bradycardia, sinus arrest, and AV block potentiated; potentially serious toxicity). Products include:
Betoptic Sterile Ophthalmic Solution 569
Betoptic S Sterile Ophthalmic Suspension 570
Kerlone Tablets 2172

Bretylium Tosylate (Potentially serious toxicity). Products include:
Bretylol Injection 923

Carteolol Hydrochloride (Bradycardia, sinus arrest, and AV block potentiated; potentially serious toxicity). Products include:
Cartrol Tablets 507

Deslanoside (Increased in serum digitalis glycoside levels resulting in clinical toxicity; discontinue or reduce digitalis dosage by 50%).
No products indexed under this heading.

Dicumarol (Potentiated; serious or fatal bleeding). Products include:
Dicumarol Tablets 516

Digitoxin (Increased in serum digitalis glycoside levels resulting in clinical toxicity; discontinue or reduce digitalis dosage by 50%). Products include:
Crystodigin Tablets 1253

Digoxin (Increased in serum digitalis glycoside levels resulting in clinical toxicity; discontinue or reduce digitalis dosage by 50%). Products include:
Lanoxicaps 772
Lanoxin Elixir Pediatric 775
Lanoxin Injection 778
Lanoxin Injection Pediatric 781
Lanoxin Tablets 783

Diltiazem Hydrochloride (Bradycardia, sinus arrest, and AV block potentiated). Products include:
Cardizem Tablets-30 mg, 60 mg, 90 mg and 120 mg 1329
Cardizem SR Capsules-60 mg, 90 mg and 120 mg 1327

Disopyramide Phosphate (Potentially serious toxicity). Products include:
Norpace 2177

Esmolol Hydrochloride (Bradycardia, sinus arrest, and AV block potentiated). Products include:
Brevibloc Injection 942

Felodipine (Bradycardia, sinus arrest, and AV block potentiated). Products include:
Plendil Extended-Release Tablets 1526

Isradipine (Bradycardia, sinus arrest, and AV block potentiated). Products include:
DynaCirc Capsules 2004

Labetalol Hydrochloride (Bradycardia, sinus arrest, and AV block potentiated). Products include:
Normodyne Injection 2108
Normodyne Tablets 2110
Normozide Tablets 2112
Trandate HCT Tablets 579
Trandate Injection 577
Trandate Tablets 579

Lidocaine Hydrochloride (Potentially serious toxicity). Products include:
Anestacon Solution 2394
Bactine Antiseptic/Anesthetic First Aid Spray ▣ 624
Decadron Phosphate with Xylocaine Injection, Sterile 1451
Xylocaine Injections 637
Xylocaine Injections for Ventricular Arrhythmias 639
Xylocaine 2% Jelly 643
4% Xylocaine-MPF Sterile Solution 641
Xylocaine 2% Viscous Solution 646

Metoprolol Tartrate (Bradycardia, sinus arrest, and AV block potentiated). Products include:
Lopressor Ampuls 1032
Lopressor HCT Tablets 1034
Lopressor Tablets 1032

Mexiletine Hydrochloride (Potentially serious toxicity). Products include:
Mexitil Capsules 680

Moricizine Hydrochloride (Bradycardia, sinus arrest, and AV block potentiated; potentially serious toxicity). Products include:
- Ethmozine Tablets 946

Nadolol (Bradycardia, sinus arrest, and AV block potentiated). Products include:
- Corgard Tablets 701
- Corzide Tablets 702

Nicardipine Hydrochloride (Bradycardia, sinus arrest, and AV block potentiated). Products include:
- Cardene Capsules 2290

Nifedipine (Bradycardia, sinus arrest, and AV block potentiated). Products include:
- Adalat Capsules (10 mg and 20 mg) 1587
- Procardia Capsules 1781
- Procardia XL Tablets 1783

Nimodipine (Bradycardia, sinus arrest, and AV block potentiated). Products include:
- Nimotop Capsules 1607

Penbutolol Sulfate (Bradycardia, sinus arrest, and AV block potentiated; potentially serious toxicity). Products include:
- Levatol 1832

Phenytoin (Increased steady state levels). Products include:
- Dilantin Infatabs 1710
- Dilantin-30 Pediatric/Dilantin-125 Suspension 1713

Phenytoin Sodium (Increased steady state levels). Products include:
- Dilantin Kapseals 1708
- Dilantin Parenteral 1712
- Dilantin with Phenobarbital Kapseals 1715

Pindolol (Bradycardia, sinus arrest, and AV block potentiated). Products include:
- Visken Tablets 2036

Procainamide Hydrochloride (Increased steady state levels; bradycardia, sinus arrest, and AV block potentiated; potentially serious toxicity). Products include:
- Procan SR Tablets 1760
- Pronestyl Capsules and Tablets 1800
- Pronestyl Injection 1798
- Pronestyl-SR Tablets 1801

Propafenone Hydrochloride (Bradycardia, sinus arrest, and AV block potentiated; potentially serious toxicity). Products include:
- Rythmol Tablets 1184

Propranolol Hydrochloride (Bradycardia, sinus arrest, and AV block potentiated; potentially serious toxicity). Products include:
- Inderal 2459
- Inderal LA Long Acting Capsules 2461
- Inderide Tablets 2463
- Inderide LA Long Acting Capsules 2465

Quinidine Gluconate (Potentially serious toxicity; increases serum concentration by 33%). Products include:
- Quinaglute Dura-Tabs Tablets 663

Quinidine Polygalacturonate (Potentially serious toxicity; increases serum concentration by 33%). Products include:
- Cardioquin Tablets 1812

Quinidine Sulfate (Potentially serious toxicity; increases serum concentration by 33%). Products include:
- Quinidex Extentabs 1868

Timolol Maleate (Bradycardia, sinus arrest, and AV block potentiated). Products include:
- Blocadren Tablets 1429
- Timolide Tablets 1547
- Timoptic in Ocudose 1552
- Timoptic Sterile Ophthalmic Solution 1550

Tocainide Hydrochloride (Potentially serious toxicity). Products include:
- Tonocard Tablets 1554

Verapamil Hydrochloride (Bradycardia, sinus arrest, and AV block potentiated; potentially serious toxicity). Products include:
- Calan SR Caplets 2157
- Calan Tablets 2155
- Isoptin Injectable 1177
- Isoptin Oral Tablets 1179
- Isoptin SR Sustained Release Tablets 1181
- Verelan Capsules 1243
- Verelan Capsules 2535

Warfarin Sodium (Potentiated; serious or fatal bleeding; increased prothrombin time by 100%). Products include:
- Coumadin Injection & Tablets 944
- Panwarfin Tablets 547

CORGARD TABLETS

(Nadolol) 701

May interact with general anesthetics, insulin, oral hypoglycemic agents, and catecholamine depleting drugs. Compounds in these categories include:

Chlorpropamide (Altered antidiabetic requirement). Products include:
- Diabinese Tablets 1775

Deserpidine (Additive effect; hypotension; excessive bradycardia). Products include:
- Enduronyl 518
- Harmonyl Tablets 528
- Oreticyl 545

Enflurane (Exaggerated hypotension). Products include:
- Ethrane 599

Glipizide (Altered antidiabetic requirement). Products include:
- Glucotrol 1952

Glyburide (Altered antidiabetic requirement). Products include:
- DiaBeta 1091
- Micronase Tablets 2350

Insulin, Human (Altered insulin requirements).
- No products indexed under this heading.

Insulin, Human Isophane Suspension (Altered insulin requirements). Products include:
- Humulin N, 100 Units 1270

Insulin, Human NPH (Altered insulin requirements). Products include:
- Insulatard NPH Human 1627
- Novolin N 1627
- Novolin N PenFill Cartridges 1628
- Novolin N Prefilled 1628

Insulin, Human Regular (Altered insulin requirements). Products include:
- Humulin BR, 100 Units 1268
- Humulin R, 100 Units 1272
- Novolin R 1627
- Novolin R PenFill Cartridges 1628
- Novolin R Prefilled 1629
- Velosulin Human 1628

Insulin, Human, Zinc Suspension (Altered insulin requirements). Products include:
- Humulin L, 100 Units 1268
- Humulin U, 100 Units 1272
- Novolin L 1627

Insulin, NPH (Altered insulin requirements). Products include:
- NPH, 40 & 100 Units 1273
- Beef NPH, 100 Units 1274
- Pork NPH, 100 Units 1275
- Insulatard NPH 1626
- NPH Insulin 1626
- NPH Purified Pork Isophane Insulin 1626

Insulin, Regular (Altered insulin requirements). Products include:
- Regular, 40 & 100 Units 1273
- Beef Regular, 100 Units 1275
- Pork Regular, 100 Units 1275
- Pork Regular (Concentrated), 500 Units 1276
- Regular Insulin 1625
- Regular Purified Pork Insulin 1626
- Velosulin 1627

Insulin, Zinc Crystals (Altered insulin requirements). Products include:
- NPH, 40 & 100 Units 1273

Insulin, Zinc Suspension (Altered insulin requirements). Products include:
- Lente, 40 & 100 Units 1272
- Protamine, Zinc, 40 & 100 Units 1273
- Lente Iletin I 1272
- Beef Lente, 100 Units 1274
- Beef Protamine Zinc, 100 Units 1274
- Pork Lente, 100 Units 1275
- Pork, Protamine, Zinc, 100 Units 1275
- Lente Insulin 1626
- Lente Purified Pork Insulin 1626
- Semilente Insulin 1625
- Ultralente Insulin 1626

Isoflurane (Exaggerated hypotension). Products include:
- Forane 600

Ketamine Hydrochloride (Exaggerated hypotension). Products include:
- Ketalar 1726

Methohexital Sodium (Exaggerated hypotension). Products include:
- Brevital Sodium Vials 1248

Methoxyflurane (Exaggerated hypotension).
- No products indexed under this heading.

Propofol (Exaggerated hypotension). Products include:
- Diprivan Injection 2267

Rauwolfia Serpentina (Additive effect; hypotension; excessive bradycardia). Products include:
- Raudixin Tablets 1803
- Rauzide Tablets 1804

Rescinnamine (Additive effect; hypotension; excessive bradycardia).
- No products indexed under this heading.

Reserpine (Additive effect; hypotension; excessive bradycardia). Products include:
- Diupres Tablets 1461
- Hydromox R Tablets 1209
- Hydropres Tablets 1485
- Renese-R Tablets 1786
- Salutensin/Salutensin-Demi 719
- Ser-Ap-Es Tablets 881
- Serpasil Tablets 883
- Serpasil-Apresoline Tablets 884
- Serpasil-Esidrix Tablets 886

Tolazamide (Altered antidiabetic requirement). Products include:
- Tolinase Tablets 2365

Tolbutamide (Altered antidiabetic requirement). Products include:
- Orinase Tablets 2354

CORICIDIN 'D' DECONGESTANT TABLETS

(Acetaminophen, Chlorpheniramine Maleate, Phenylpropanolamine Hydrochloride) .... (NP) 695

May interact with phenylpropanolamine containing anorectics, antihypertensives, antidepressant drugs, hypnotics and sedatives, tranquilizers, and certain other agents. Compounds in these categories include:

Acebutolol Hydrochloride (Effect not specified). Products include:
- Sectral Capsules 2520

Alcohol (Do not use concomitantly).

Alprazolam (Effect not specified). Products include:
- Xanax Tablets 2367

Amitriptyline Hydrochloride (Effect not specified). Products include:
- Elavil 2269
- Endep Tablets 1927
- Etrafon 2087
- Limbitrol 1933
- Triavil Tablets 1556

Amoxapine (Effect not specified). Products include:
- Asendin Tablets 1196

Atenolol (Effect not specified). Products include:
- Tenoretic Tablets 1105
- Tenormin Tablets and I.V. Injection 1107

Benazepril Hydrochloride (Effect not specified). Products include:
- Lotensin Tablets 872

Bendroflumethiazide (Effect not specified). Products include:
- Corzide Tablets 702
- Naturetin Tablets 1789
- Rauzide Tablets 1804

Betaxolol Hydrochloride (Effect not specified). Products include:
- Betoptic Sterile Ophthalmic Solution 569
- Betoptic S Sterile Ophthalmic Suspension 570
- Kerlone Tablets 2172

Bupropion Hydrochloride (Effect not specified). Products include:
- Wellbutrin Tablets 821

Buspirone Hydrochloride (Effect not specified). Products include:
- BuSpar 1401

Captopril (Effect not specified). Products include:
- Capoten 2255
- Capozide 2258

Carteolol Hydrochloride (Effect not specified). Products include:
- Cartrol Tablets 507

Chlordiazepoxide (Effect not specified). Products include:
- Libritabs Tablets 1930
- Limbitrol 1933
- Menrium Tablets 1934

Chlordiazepoxide Hydrochloride (Effect not specified). Products include:
- Librax Capsules 1929
- Librium Capsules 1931
- Librium Injectable 1932

Chlorothiazide (Effect not specified). Products include:
- Aldoclor Tablets 1413
- Diupres Tablets 1461
- Diuril Oral 1464

Chlorothiazide Sodium (Effect not specified). Products include:
- Diuril Sodium Intravenous 1463

Chlorpromazine (Effect not specified). Products include:
- Thorazine 2234

Chlorprothixene (Effect not specified). Products include:
- Taractan Tablets 1920

Chlorprothixene Hydrochloride (Effect not specified). Products include:
- Taractan 1920

Chlorthalidone (Effect not specified). Products include:
- Combipres Tablets 678
- Tenoretic Tablets 1105
- Thalitone Tablets 687

Clonidine (Effect not specified). Products include:
- Catapres-TTS 677

Clonidine Hydrochloride (Effect not specified). Products include:
- Catapres Tablets 676
- Combipres Tablets 678

Clorazepate Dipotassium (Effect not specified). Products include:
Tranxene ... 556

Deserpidine (Effect not specified). Products include:
Enduronyl ... 518
Harmonyl Tablets ... 528
Oreticyl ... 545

Desipramine Hydrochloride (Effect not specified). Products include:
Norpramin Tablets ... 1340

Diazepam (Effect not specified). Products include:
Valium Injectable ... 1937
Valium Tablets ... 1939
Valrelease Capsules ... 1923

Diazoxide (Effect not specified). Products include:
Hyperstat I.V. Injection ... 2095
Proglycem ... 649

Doxazosin Mesylate (Effect not specified). Products include:
Cardura Tablets ... 1941

Doxepin Hydrochloride (Effect not specified). Products include:
Sinequan ... 1960

Droperidol (Effect not specified). Products include:
Inapsine Injection ... 1140
Innovar Injection ... 1141

Enalapril Maleate (Effect not specified). Products include:
Vaseretic Tablets ... 1559
Vasotec Tablets ... 1564

Enalaprilat (Effect not specified). Products include:
Vasotec I.V. ... 1562

Esmolol Hydrochloride (Effect not specified). Products include:
Brevibloc Injection ... 942

Estazolam (Effect not specified). Products include:
ProSom Tablets ... 554

Ethchlorvynol (Effect not specified). Products include:
Placidyl Capsules ... 553

Ethinamate (Effect not specified).
No products indexed under this heading.

Felodipine (Effect not specified). Products include:
Plendil Extended-Release Tablets ... 1526

Fluoxetine Hydrochloride (Effect not specified). Products include:
Prozac Pulvules ... 920

Fluphenazine Decanoate (Effect not specified). Products include:
Prolixin Decanoate ... 1795

Fluphenazine Enanthate (Effect not specified). Products include:
Prolixin Enanthate ... 1796

Fluphenazine Hydrochloride (Effect not specified). Products include:
Prolixin Elixir ... 1793
Prolixin Injection ... 1791
Prolixin Oral Concentrate ... 1792
Prolixin Tablets ... 1793

Flurazepam Hydrochloride (Effect not specified). Products include:
Dalmane Capsules ... 1927

Fosinopril Sodium (Effect not specified). Products include:
Monopril Tablets ... 1406

Furosemide (Effect not specified). Products include:
Lasix ... 1093

Glutethimide (Effect not specified).
No products indexed under this heading.

Guanabenz Acetate (Effect not specified). Products include:
Wytensin Tablets ... 2542

Guanethidine Monosulfate (Effect not specified). Products include:
Esimil Tablets ... 864
Ismelin Tablets ... 869

Haloperidol (Effect not specified). Products include:
Haldol Injection, Tablets and Concentrate ... 1373

Haloperidol Decanoate (Effect not specified). Products include:
Haldol Decanoate ... 1375

Hydralazine Hydrochloride (Effect not specified). Products include:
Apresazide Capsules ... 854
Apresoline Hydrochloride Parenteral (Ampuls) ... 856
Apresoline Hydrochloride Tablets ... 855
Apresoline-Esidrix Tablets ... 857
Ser-Ap-Es Tablets ... 881
Serpasil-Apresoline Tablets ... 884

Hydrochlorothiazide (Effect not specified). Products include:
Aldactazide ... 2150
Aldoril Tablets ... 1418
Apresazide Capsules ... 854
Apresoline-Esidrix Tablets ... 857
Capozide ... 2258
Dyazide Capsules ... 2208
Esidrix Tablets ... 863
Esimil Tablets ... 864
HydroDIURIL Tablets ... 1484
Hydropres Tablets ... 1485
Inderide Tablets ... 2463
Inderide LA Long Acting Capsules ... 2465
Lopressor HCT Tablets ... 1034
Maxzide ... 1215
Moduretic Tablets ... 1510
Normozide Tablets ... 2112
Oretic Tablets ... 544
Oreticyl ... 545
Prinzide Tablets ... 1540
Ser-Ap-Es Tablets ... 881
Serpasil-Esidrix Tablets ... 886
Timolide Tablets ... 1547
Trandate HCT Tablets ... 579
Vaseretic Tablets ... 1559
Zestoretic ... 2274

Hydroflumethiazide (Effect not specified). Products include:
Diucardin Tablets ... 2450
Saluron ... 718
Salutensin/Salutensin-Demi ... 719

Hydroxyzine Hydrochloride (Effect not specified). Products include:
Atarax Tablets & Syrup ... 1941
Marax Tablets & DF Syrup ... 1954
Vistaril Intramuscular Solution ... 1970

Imipramine Hydrochloride (Effect not specified). Products include:
Tofranil Ampuls ... 1038
Tofranil Tablets ... 1039

Imipramine Pamoate (Effect not specified). Products include:
Tofranil-PM Capsules ... 1041

Indapamide (Effect not specified). Products include:
Lozol Tablets ... 1843

Isocarboxazid (Effect not specified). Products include:
Marplan Tablets ... 1906

Isradipine (Effect not specified). Products include:
DynaCirc Capsules ... 2004

Labetalol Hydrochloride (Effect not specified). Products include:
Normodyne Injection ... 2108
Normodyne Tablets ... 2110
Normozide Tablets ... 2112
Trandate HCT Tablets ... 579
Trandate Injection ... 577
Trandate Tablets ... 579

Lisinopril (Effect not specified). Products include:
Prinivil Tablets ... 1538
Prinzide Tablets ... 1540
Zestoretic ... 2274
Zestril Tablets ... 2277

Lorazepam (Effect not specified). Products include:
Ativan Injection ... 2432
Ativan Tablets ... 2434

Loxapine Hydrochloride (Effect not specified). Products include:
Loxitane ... 1213

Loxapine Succinate (Effect not specified). Products include:
Loxitane Capsules ... 1213

Maprotiline Hydrochloride (Effect not specified). Products include:
Ludiomil Tablets ... 874

Mecamylamine Hydrochloride (Effect not specified). Products include:
Inversine Tablets ... 1492

Meprobamate (Effect not specified). Products include:
Deprol Tablets ... 2382
Equagesic Tablets ... 2451
Miltown Tablets ... 2386
PMB 200 and PMB 400 ... 2504

Mesoridazine Besylate (Effect not specified).

Methyclothiazide (Effect not specified). Products include:
Enduron Tablets ... 517
Enduronyl ... 518

Methyldopa (Effect not specified). Products include:
Aldoclor Tablets ... 1413
Aldomet Oral ... 1415
Aldoril Tablets ... 1418

Methyldopate Hydrochloride (Effect not specified). Products include:
Aldomet Ester HCl Injection ... 1417

Metolazone (Effect not specified). Products include:
Diulo ... 2129
Mykrox ½ mg Tablets ... 984
Zaroxolyn Tablets ... 989

Metoprolol Tartrate (Effect not specified). Products include:
Lopressor Ampuls ... 1032
Lopressor HCT Tablets ... 1034
Lopressor Tablets ... 1032

Metyrosine (Effect not specified). Products include:
Demser Capsules ... 1460

Midazolam Hydrochloride (Effect not specified). Products include:
Versed Injection ... 1924

Minoxidil (Effect not specified). Products include:
Loniten Tablets ... 2346
Rogaine Topical Solution ... 2357

Molindone Hydrochloride (Effect not specified). Products include:
Moban Tablets & Concentrate ... 932

Nadolol (Effect not specified). Products include:
Corgard Tablets ... 701
Corzide Tablets ... 702

Nicardipine Hydrochloride (Effect not specified). Products include:
Cardene Capsules ... 2290

Nitroglycerin (Effect not specified). Products include:
Deponit NTG Transdermal Delivery System ... 2143
Minitran Transdermal Delivery System ... 1312
Nitro-Bid Ointment ... 1339
Nitro-Bid Capsules ... 1338
Nitrodisc ... 2176
Nitro-Dur (nitroglycerin) Transdermal Infusion System ... 1164
Nitrogard Tablets ... 1004
Nitrolingual Spray ... 1846
Nitrostat Tablets ... 1743
Transderm-Nitro Transdermal Therapeutic System ... 2283

Nortriptyline Hydrochloride (Effect not specified). Products include:
Pamelor ... 2019

Oxazepam (Effect not specified). Products include:
Serax Capsules ... 2522
Serax Tablets ... 2522

Penbutolol Sulfate (Effect not specified). Products include:
Levatol ... 1832

Perphenazine (Effect not specified). Products include:
Etrafon ... 2087
Triavil Tablets ... 1556
Trilafon ... 2123

Phenelzine Sulfate (Effect not specified). Products include:
Nardil ... 1742

Phenoxybenzamine Hydrochloride (Effect not specified). Products include:
Dibenzyline Capsules ... 2207

Phentolamine Mesylate (Effect not specified). Products include:
Regitine ... 878

Phenylpropanolamine Containing Anorectics (Product labeling recommends physician's supervision for concurrent administration of these drugs).

Pindolol (Effect not specified). Products include:
Visken Tablets ... 2036

Polythiazide (Effect not specified). Products include:
Minizide Capsules ... 1779
Renese Tablets ... 1785
Renese-R Tablets ... 1786

Prazepam (Effect not specified). Products include:
Centrax ... 1693

Prazosin Hydrochloride (Effect not specified). Products include:
Minipress Capsules ... 1778
Minizide Capsules ... 1779

Prochlorperazine (Effect not specified). Products include:
Compazine ... 2201

Promethazine Hydrochloride (Effect not specified). Products include:
Mepergan Injection ... 2479
Phenergan with Codeine ... 2497
Phenergan with Dextromethorphan 2499
Phenergan Injection ... 2493
Phenergan Suppositories ... 2496
Phenergan Syrup ... 2495
Phenergan Tablets ... 2496
Phenergan VC ... 2500
Phenergan VC with Codeine ... 2501

Propofol (Effect not specified). Products include:
Diprivan Injection ... 2267

Propranolol Hydrochloride (Effect not specified). Products include:
Inderal ... 2459
Inderal LA Long Acting Capsules ... 2461
Inderide Tablets ... 2463
Inderide LA Long Acting Capsules ... 2465

Protriptyline Hydrochloride (Effect not specified). Products include:
Vivactil Tablets ... 1567

Quazepam (Effect not specified). Products include:
Doral Tablets ... 2383

Ramipril (Effect not specified). Products include:
Altace Capsules ... 1086

Rauwolfia Serpentina (Effect not specified). Products include:
Raudixin Tablets ... 1803
Rauzide Tablets ... 1804

Rescinnamine (Effect not specified).
No products indexed under this heading.

Reserpine (Effect not specified). Products include:
Diupres Tablets ... 1461
Hydromox R Tablets ... 1209
Hydropres Tablets ... 1485
Renese-R Tablets ... 1786
Salutensin/Salutensin-Demi ... 719
Ser-Ap-Es Tablets ... 881

Serpasil Tablets 883
Serpasil-Apresoline Tablets 884
Serpasil-Esidrix Tablets 886

Secobarbital Sodium (Effect not specified). Products include:
Seconal Sodium Pulvules 1296

Sodium Nitroprusside (Effect not specified). Products include:
Nipride I.V. Infusion 1909

Temazepam (Effect not specified). Products include:
Restoril Capsules 2023

Terazosin Hydrochloride (Effect not specified). Products include:
Hytrin Tablets 529

Thioridazine Hydrochloride (Effect not specified). Products include:
Mellaril 2011

Thiothixene (Effect not specified). Products include:
Navane Capsules and Concentrate 1954
Navane Intramuscular 1956

Timolol Maleate (Effect not specified). Products include:
Blocadren Tablets 1429
Timolide Tablets 1547
Timoptic in Ocudose 1552
Timoptic Sterile Ophthalmic Solution 1550

Tranylcypromine Sulfate (Effect not specified). Products include:
Parnate Tablets 2222

Trazodone Hydrochloride (Effect not specified). Products include:
Desyrel and Desyrel Dividose 1404

Triazolam (Effect not specified). Products include:
Halcion Tablets 2340

Trifluoperazine Hydrochloride (Effect not specified). Products include:
Stelazine 2226

Trimethaphan Camsylate (Effect not specified). Products include:
Arfonad Ampuls 1887

Trimipramine Maleate (Effect not specified). Products include:
Surmontil Capsules 2524

CORICIDIN DEMILETS TABLETS FOR CHILDREN
(Acetaminophen, Chlorpheniramine Maleate, Phenylpropanolamine Hydrochloride) .... ▣ 696
May interact with monoamine oxidase inhibitors, phenylpropanolamine containing anorectics, and certain other agents. Compounds in these categories include:

Alcohol (Do not use concomitantly).

Furazolidone (Effect not specified). Products include:
Furoxone 1855

Isocarboxazid (Effect not specified). Products include:
Marplan Tablets 1906

Phenelzine Sulfate (Effect not specified). Products include:
Nardil 1742

Phenylpropanolamine Containing Anorectics (Effect not specified).

Selegiline Hydrochloride (Effect not specified). Products include:
Eldepryl 2250

Tranylcypromine Sulfate (Effect not specified). Products include:
Parnate Tablets 2222

CORICIDIN TABLETS
(Acetaminophen, Chlorpheniramine Maleate) .... ▣ 695
See **Coricidin 'D' Decongestant Tablets**

CORRECTOL LAXATIVE TABLETS
(Docusate Sodium, Phenolphthalein, Yellow) .... ▣ 696
No interactions described in labeling.

CORTAID CREAM WITH ALOE
(Hydrocortisone Acetate) .... ▣ 735
No interactions described in labeling.

CORTAID LOTION
(Hydrocortisone Acetate) .... ▣ 735
No interactions described in labeling.

CORTAID OINTMENT WITH ALOE
(Hydrocortisone Acetate) .... ▣ 735
No interactions described in labeling.

CORTAID SPRAY
(Hydrocortisone) .... ▣ 735
No interactions described in labeling.

CORTEF FEMININE ITCH CREAM
(Hydrocortisone Acetate) .... ▣ 735
No interactions described in labeling.

CORTENEMA
(Hydrocortisone) 2244
May interact with:

Aspirin (Concurrent use requires caution in hypoprothrombinemia). Products include:
Alka-Seltzer Effervescent Antacid and Pain Reliever 1568
Alka-Seltzer Extra Strength Effervescent Antacid and Pain Reliever 1570
Alka-Seltzer (Flavored) Effervescent Antacid and Pain Reliever 1569
Alka-Seltzer Plus Cold Medicine .... ▣ 623
Alka-Seltzer Plus Night-Time Cold Medicine .... ▣ 623
Alka Seltzer Plus Sinus Allergy Medicine .... ▣ 624
Anacin Coated Analgesic Caplets 2417
Anacin Coated Analgesic Tablets 2417
Anacin Maximum Strength Analgesic Coated Tablets 2417
Maximum Strength Arthritis Pain Formula By the Makers of Anacin Analgesic Tablets and Caplets 2418
Arthritis Pain Formula by the Makers of Anacin Analgesic Tablets and Caplets .... ▣ 747
Arthritis Strength BC Powder .... ▣ 516
Ascriptin A/D Caplets 1850
Regular Strength Ascriptin Tablets 1850
Azdone Tablets 844
BC Powder .... ▣ 517
BC Cold Powder .... ▣ 517
Children's Bayer Chewable Aspirin .... ▣ 564
Genuine Bayer Aspirin Tablets & Caplets .... ▣ 564
Maximum Bayer Aspirin Tablets & Caplets .... ▣ 566
Bayer Plus Aspirin Tablets .... ▣ 567
Therapy Bayer Aspirin Caplets .... ▣ 568
8 Hour Bayer Timed-Release Aspirin .... ▣ 566
Arthritis Strength Bufferin Analgesic Caplets 744
Extra Strength Bufferin Analgesic Tablets 745
Bufferin Analgesic Tablets and Caplets 743
Cama Arthritis Pain Reliever .... ▣ 685
Damason-P 1356
Easprin 1719
Ecotrin Enteric Coated Aspirin Maximum Strength Tablets and Caplets 2189
Ecotrin Enteric Coated Aspirin Regular Strength Tablets and Caplets 2189
Empirin Aspirin .... ▣ 541
Empirin with Codeine Phosphate Nos. 2, 3 & 4 764
Equagesic Tablets 2451
Excedrin Extra-Strength Analgesic Tablets & Caplets 749
4-Way Cold Tablets 750
Fiorinal Capsules 2007
Fiorinal with Codeine Capsules 2008
Fiorinal Tablets 2007
Lortab ASA Tablets 2414
Momentum Muscular Backache Formula .... ▣ 751
Norgesic 1314
Norwich Extra-Strength Aspirin .... ▣ 546
Norwich Regular Strength Aspirin ▣ 547
P-A-C Analgesic Tablets .... ▣ 669
Percodan 951
Robaxisal Tablets 1872
Sine-Off Sinus Medicine Tablets-Aspirin Formula .... ▣ 722
Soma Compound w/Codeine Tablets 2390
Soma Compound Tablets 2389
St. Joseph Adult Chewable Aspirin (81 mg.) .... ▣ 703
Synalgos-DC Capsules 2525
Talwin Compound 2072
Ursinus Inlay-Tabs .... ▣ 691
Vanquish Analgesic Caplets .... ▣ 574
Zorprin Tablets 698

Aspirin, Enteric Coated (Concurrent use requires caution in hypoprothrombinemia). Products include:
Therapy Bayer Aspirin Caplets .... ▣ 568
Ecotrin 2189

CORTICAINE
(Hydrocortisone Acetate) .... ▣ 682
No interactions described in labeling.

CORTIFOAM
(Hydrocortisone Acetate) 1827
No interactions described in labeling.

CORTISPORIN CREAM
(Polymyxin B Sulfate, Neomycin Sulfate, Hydrocortisone Acetate) 757
No interactions described in labeling.

CORTISPORIN OINTMENT
(Polymyxin B Sulfate, Bacitracin Zinc, Neomycin Sulfate, Hydrocortisone) 758
No interactions described in labeling.

CORTISPORIN OPHTHALMIC OINTMENT STERILE
(Polymyxin B Sulfate, Bacitracin Zinc, Neomycin Sulfate, Hydrocortisone) 758
No interactions described in labeling.

CORTISPORIN OPHTHALMIC SUSPENSION STERILE
(Hydrocortisone, Polymyxin B Sulfate, Neomycin Sulfate) 759
No interactions described in labeling.

CORTISPORIN OTIC SOLUTION STERILE
(Polymyxin B Sulfate, Neomycin Sulfate, Hydrocortisone) 760
No interactions described in labeling.

CORTISPORIN OTIC SUSPENSION STERILE
(Polymyxin B Sulfate, Neomycin Sulfate, Hydrocortisone) 760
No interactions described in labeling.

CORTIZONE-5 CREME & OINTMENT
(Hydrocortisone) .... ▣ 732
No interactions described in labeling.

CORTONE ACETATE STERILE SUSPENSION
(Cortisone Acetate) 1437
May interact with oral anticoagulants, potassium sparing diuretics, and certain other agents. Compounds in these categories include:

Amiloride Hydrochloride (Hypokalemia). Products include:
Midamor Tablets 1508
Moduretic Tablets 1510

Dicumarol (Reponse to dicumarol inhibited). Products include:
Dicumarol Tablets 516

Ephedrine Hydrochloride (Enhanced metabolic clearance of corticosteroids). Products include:
Amesec .... ▣ 682
Primatene Tablets-M Formula 2421
Primatene Tablets-P Formula 2421
Primatene Tablets-Regular Formula 2421
Quadrinal Tablets 1183
Quelidrine Syrup 556
Tedral SA 1765

Ephedrine Sulfate (Enhanced metabolic clearance of corticosteroids). Products include:
Bronkaid Tablets .... ▣ 757
Bronkolixir .... ▣ 761
Bronkotabs Tablets .... ▣ 762
Marax Tablets & DF Syrup 1954
Pazo Hemorrhoid Ointment & Suppositories 752
Vicks Vatronol Nose Drops .... ▣ 666

Ephedrine Tannate (Enhanced metabolic clearance of corticosteroids). Products include:
Rynatuss 2388

Phenobarbital (Enhanced metabolic clearance of corticosteroids). Products include:
Arco-Lase Plus Tablets 607
Bellergal-S Tablets 1998
Bronkolixir .... ▣ 761
Bronkotabs Tablets .... ▣ 762
Donnatal 1858
Donnatal Extentabs 1859
Donnatal Tablets 1858
Donnazyme Tablets 1860
Kinesed Tablets 2272
Phenobarbital Elixir and Tablets 1293
Primatene Tablets-P Formula 2421
Quadrinal Tablets 1183
Tedral SA 1765

Phenytoin (Enhanced metabolic clearance of corticosteroids). Products include:
Dilantin Infatabs 1710
Dilantin-30 Pediatric/Dilantin-125 Suspension 1713

Phenytoin Sodium (Enhanced metabolic clearance of corticosteroids). Products include:
Dilantin Kapseals 1708
Dilantin Parenteral 1712
Dilantin with Phenobarbital Kapseals 1715

Rifampin (Enhanced metabolic clearance of corticosteroids). Products include:
Rifadin 1345
Rifamate Capsules 1347
Rimactane Capsules 879

Spironolactone (Hypokalemia). Products include:
Aldactazide 2150
Aldactone 2152

Triamterene (Hypokalemia). Products include:
Dyazide Capsules 2208
Dyrenium Capsules 2210
Maxzide 1215

Warfarin Sodium (Reponse to warfarin inhibited). Products include:
Coumadin Injection & Tablets 944
Panwarfin Tablets 547

CORTONE ACETATE TABLETS
(Cortisone Acetate) 1439
May interact with oral anticoagulants, potassium sparing diuretics, and certain other agents. Compounds in these categories include:

Amiloride Hydrochloride (Hypokalemia). Products include:
Midamor Tablets 1508
Moduretic Tablets 1510

Aspirin (Aspirin should be used cautiously in conjunction with corticosteroids in hypoprothrombinemia). Products include:

Alka-Seltzer Effervescent Antacid and Pain Reliever 1568
Alka-Seltzer Extra Strength Effervescent Antacid and Pain Reliever 1570
Alka-Seltzer (Flavored) Effervescent Antacid and Pain Reliever 1569
Alka-Seltzer Plus Cold Medicine ◼ 623
Alka-Seltzer Plus Night-Time Cold Medicine ◼ 623
Alka Seltzer Plus Sinus Allergy Medicine ◼ 624
Anacin Coated Analgesic Caplets 2417
Anacin Coated Analgesic Tablets 2417
Anacin Maximum Strength Analgesic Coated Tablets 2417
Maximum Strength Arthritis Pain Formula By the Makers of Anacin Analgesic Tablets and Caplets 2418
Arthritis Pain Formula by the Makers of Anacin Analgesic Tablets and Caplets ◼ 747
Arthritis Strength BC Powder ◼ 516
Ascriptin A/D Caplets 1850
Regular Strength Ascriptin Tablets 1850
Azdone Tablets 844
BC Powder ◼ 517
BC Cold Powder ◼ 517
Children's Bayer Chewable Aspirin ◼ 564
Genuine Bayer Aspirin Tablets & Caplets ◼ 564
Maximum Bayer Aspirin Tablets & Caplets ◼ 566
Bayer Plus Aspirin Tablets ◼ 567
Therapy Bayer Aspirin Caplets ◼ 568
8 Hour Bayer Timed-Release Aspirin ◼ 566
Arthritis Strength Bufferin Analgesic Caplets 744
Extra Strength Bufferin Analgesic Tablets 745
Bufferin Analgesic Tablets and Caplets 743
Cama Arthritis Pain Reliever ◼ 685
Damason-P 1356
Easprin 1719
Ecotrin Enteric Coated Aspirin Maximum Strength Tablets and Caplets 2189
Ecotrin Enteric Coated Aspirin Regular Strength Tablets and Caplets 2189
Empirin Aspirin ◼ 541
Empirin with Codeine Phosphate Nos. 2, 3 & 4 764
Equagesic Tablets 2451
Excedrin Extra-Strength Analgesic Tablets & Caplets 749
4-Way Cold Tablets 750
Fiorinal Capsules 2007
Fiorinal with Codeine Capsules 2008
Fiorinal Tablets 2007
Lortab ASA Tablets 2414
Momentum Muscular Backache Formula ◼ 751
Norgesic 1314
Norwich Extra-Strength Aspirin ◼ 546
Norwich Regular Strength Aspirin ◼ 547
P-A-C Analgesic Tablets ◼ 669
Percodan 951
Robaxisal Tablets 1872
Sine-Off Sinus Medicine Tablets-Aspirin Formula ◼ 722
Soma Compound w/Codeine Tablets 2390
Soma Compound Tablets 2389
St. Joseph Adult Chewable Aspirin (81 mg.) ◼ 703
Synalgos-DC Capsules 2525
Talwin Compound 2072
Ursinus Inlay-Tabs ◼ 691
Vanquish Analgesic Caplets ◼ 574
Zorprin Tablets 698

Dicumarol (Response to dicumarol inhibited). Products include:

Dicumarol Tablets 516

Ephedrine Hydrochloride (Enhanced metabolic clearance of corticosteroids). Products include:

Amesec ◼ 682
Primatene Tablets-M Formula 2421
Primatene Tablets-P Formula 2421
Primatene Tablets-Regular Formula 2421
Quadrinal Tablets 1183
Quelidrine Syrup 556
Tedral SA 1765

Ephedrine Sulfate (Enhanced metabolic clearance of corticosteroids). Products include:

Bronkaid Tablets ◼ 757
Bronkolixir ◼ 761
Bronkotabs Tablets ◼ 762
Marax Tablets & DF Syrup 1954
Pazo Hemorrhoid Ointment & Suppositories 752
Vicks Vatronol Nose Drops ◼ 666

Ephedrine Tannate (Enhanced metabolic clearance of corticosteroids). Products include:

Rynatuss 2388

Phenobarbital (Enhanced metabolic clearance of corticosteroids). Products include:

Arco-Lase Plus Tablets 607
Bellergal-S Tablets 1998
Bronkolixir ◼ 761
Bronkotabs Tablets ◼ 762
Donnatal 1858
Donnatal Extentabs 1859
Donnatal Tablets 1858
Donnazyme Tablets 1860
Kinesed Tablets 2272
Phenobarbital Elixir and Tablets 1293
Primatene Tablets-P Formula 2421
Quadrinal Tablets 1183
Tedral SA 1765

Phenytoin (Enhanced metabolic clearance of corticosteroids). Products include:

Dilantin Infatabs 1710
Dilantin-30 Pediatric/Dilantin-125 Suspension 1713

Phenytoin Sodium (Enhanced metabolic clearance of corticosteroids). Products include:

Dilantin Kapseals 1708
Dilantin Parenteral 1712
Dilantin with Phenobarbital Kapseals 1715

Rifampin (Enhanced metabolic clearance of corticosteroids). Products include:

Rifadin 1345
Rifamate Capsules 1347
Rimactane Capsules 879

Spironolactone (Hypokalemia). Products include:

Aldactazide 2150
Aldactone 2152

Triamterene (Hypokalemia). Products include:

Dyazide Capsules 2208
Dyrenium Capsules 2210
Maxzide 1215

Warfarin Sodium (Reponse to warfarin inhibited). Products include:

Coumadin Injection & Tablets 944
Panwarfin Tablets 547

CORZIDE TABLETS
(Nadolol, Bendroflumethiazide) 702
May interact with general anesthetics, insulin, oral hypoglycemic agents, catecholamine depleting drugs, barbiturates, narcotic analgesics, antihypertensives, oral anticoagulants, antigout agents, cardiac glycosides, corticosteroids, ganglionic blocking agents, para-aminobenzoic acid based local anesthetics, preanesthetic medications, nondepolarizing neuromuscular blocking agents, monoamine oxidase inhibitors, lithium preparations, non-steroidal anti-inflammatory agents, and certain other agents. Compounds in these categories include:

Acebutolol Hydrochloride (Additive effect). Products include:

Sectral Capsules 2520

ACTH (Intensified electrolyte depletion).

No products indexed under this heading.

Alcohol (Potentiation of orthostatic hypotension).

Alfentanil Hydrochloride (Potentiation of orthostatic hypotension). Products include:

Alfenta Injection 1131

Allopurinol (Bendroflumethiazide may raise the level of blood uric acid). Products include:

Zyloprim Tablets 830

Amphotericin B (May intensify electrolyte imbalance, particularly hypokalemia). Products include:

Fungizone Cream, Lotion and Ointment 2261
Fungizone Intravenous 2262

Aprobarbital (Potentiation of orthostatic hypotension). Products include:

Alurate Elixir 1883

Atenolol (Additive effect or potentiation). Products include:

Tenoretic Tablets 1105
Tenormin Tablets and I.V. Injection 1107

Atracurium Besylate (Increased response to muscle relaxants). Products include:

Tracrium Injection 817

Benazepril Hydrochloride (Additive effect or potentiation). Products include:

Lotensin Tablets 872

Betamethasone Acetate (Intensified electrolyte depletion; hypokalemia). Products include:

Celestone Soluspan Suspension 2081

Betamethasone Sodium Phosphate (Intensified electrolyte depletion; hypokalemia). Products include:

Celestone Soluspan Suspension 2081

Betaxolol Hydrochloride (Additive effect or potentiation). Products include:

Betoptic Sterile Ophthalmic Solution 569
Betoptic S Sterile Ophthalmic Suspension 570
Kerlone Tablets 2172

Buprenorphine (Potentiation of orthostatic hypotension).

No products indexed under this heading.

Butabarbital (Potentiation of orthostatic hypotension). Products include:

Pyridium Plus 1764

Butalbital (Potentiation of orthostatic hypotension). Products include:

Esgic-Plus Tablets 1002
Esgic Tablets & Capsules 1001
Fioricet Tablets 2006
Fiorinal Capsules 2007
Fiorinal with Codeine Capsules 2008
Fiorinal Tablets 2007
Phrenilin 838
Sedapap Tablets 50 mg/650 mg 1360

Captopril (Additive effect or potentiation). Products include:

Capoten 2255
Capozide 2258

Carteolol Hydrochloride (Additive effect or potentiation). Products include:

Cartrol Tablets 507

Chlorothiazide (Additive effect or potentiation). Products include:

Aldoclor Tablets 1413
Diupres Tablets 1461
Diuril Oral 1464

Chlorothiazide Sodium (Additive effect or potentiation). Products include:

Diuril Sodium Intravenous 1463

Chlorpropamide (Altered antidiabetic requirements). Products include:

Diabinese Tablets 1775

Chlorthalidone (Additive effect). Products include:

Combipres Tablets 678
Tenoretic Tablets 1105
Thalitone Tablets 687

Cholestyramine (May delay or decrease absorption of bendroflumethiazide). Products include:

Cholybar 1705
Questran Light 711
Questran Powder 710

Clonidine (Additive effect or potentiation). Products include:

Catapres-TTS 677

Clonidine Hydrochloride (Additive effect or potentiation). Products include:

Catapres Tablets 676
Combipres Tablets 678

Codeine (Potentiation of orthostatic hypotension). Products include:

Calcidrine Syrup 506

Codeine Phosphate (Potentiation of orthostatic hypotension). Products include:

Actifed with Codeine Cough Syrup 752
Cheracol Cough Syrup 1853
Codimal PH Syrup 846
Dimetane-DC Cough Syrup 1857
Empirin with Codeine Phosphate Nos. 2, 3 & 4 764
Fiorinal with Codeine Capsules 2008
Isoclor Expectorant 982
Naldecon CX Adult Liquid ◼ 521
Novahistine DH 1342
Novahistine Expectorant 1343
Nucofed Capsules 2219
Nucofed Expectorant 2219
Nucofed Pediatric Expectorant 2220
Nucofed Syrup 2219
Phenaphen with Codeine Capsules 1865
Phenaphen-650 with Codeine Tablets 1866
Phenergan with Codeine 2497
Phenergan VC with Codeine 2501
Robitussin A-C Syrup 1875
Robitussin-DAC Syrup 1875
Ryna ◼ 741
Soma Compound w/Codeine Tablets 2390
Triaminic Expectorant w/Codeine 1996
Tussi-Organidin Liquid 2391
Tylenol with Codeine 1381

Codeine Polistirex (Potentiation of orthostatic hypotension).

No products indexed under this heading.

Colestipol Hydrochloride (May delay or decrease absorption of bendroflumethiazide). Products include:

Colestid Granules 2328

Cortisone Acetate (Intensified electrolyte depletion). Products include:

Cortone Acetate Sterile Suspension 1437
Cortone Acetate Tablets 1439

Deserpidine (Additive effects; potential for hypotension and/or excessive bradycardia). Products include:

Enduronyl 518
Harmonyl Tablets 528
Oreticyl 545

Deslanoside (Enhanced possibility of digitalis toxicity associated with hypokalemia).

No products indexed under this heading.

Dexamethasone (Intensified electrolyte depletion; hypokalemia). Products include:

AK-Trol Ointment & Suspension ⊙ 207
Decadron Elixir 1445
Decadron Tablets 1447
Decaspray Topical Aerosol 1459
Dexacidin ⊙ 272
Maxidex Sterile Ophthalmic Suspension ⊙ 223
Maxitrol Ophthalmic Ointment/Suspension ⊙ 223
TobraDex Ophthalmic Suspension and Ointment ⊙ 228

Dexamethasone Acetate (Intensified electrolyte depletion; hypokalemia). Products include:
Dalalone D.P. Injectable ... 999
Decadron-LA Sterile Suspension ... 1457

Dexamethasone Sodium Phosphate (Intensified electrolyte depletion; hypokalemia). Products include:
AK-Dex ... ⊙ 203
Decadron Phosphate Respihaler ... 1454
Decadron Phosphate Sterile Ophthalmic Ointment ... 1453
Decadron Phosphate Sterile Ophthalmic Solution ... 1453
Decadron Phosphate Topical Cream ... 1455
Decadron Phosphate Turbinaire ... 1456
Maxidex Sterile Ophthalmic Ointment ... ⊙ 222
NeoDecadron Sterile Ophthalmic Ointment ... 1517
NeoDecadron Sterile Ophthalmic Solution ... 1518
NeoDecadron Topical Cream ... 1518

Dezocine (Potentiation of orthostatic hypotension).

Diazepam (Potentiation of preanesthetic agents). Products include:
Valium Injectable ... 1937
Valium Tablets ... 1939
Valrelease Capsules ... 1923

Diazoxide (Enhanced hyperglycemic, hyperuricemic and antihypertensive effects). Products include:
Hyperstat I.V. Injection ... 2095
Proglycem ... 649

Diclofenac Sodium (Potential for reduced diuretic, natriuretic, and antihypertensive effect). Products include:
Voltaren Ophthalmic Sterile Ophthalmic Solution ... ⊙ 268
Voltaren Tablets ... 1042

Dicumarol (Decreased anticoagulant effects). Products include:
Dicumarol Tablets ... 516

Digitoxin (Enhanced possibility of digitalis toxicity associated with hypokalemia). Products include:
Crystodigin Tablets ... 1253

Digoxin (Enhanced possibility of digitalis toxicity associated with hypokalemia). Products include:
Lanoxicaps ... 772
Lanoxin Elixir Pediatric ... 775
Lanoxin Injection ... 778
Lanoxin Injection Pediatric ... 781
Lanoxin Tablets ... 783

Dopamine Hydrochloride (Decreased response to pressor amine). Products include:
Intropin Injection ... 930

Doxazosin Mesylate (Additive effect or potentiation). Products include:
Cardura Tablets ... 1941

Droperidol (Potentiation of preanesthetic agents). Products include:
Inapsine Injection ... 1140
Innovar Injection ... 1141

Enalapril Maleate (Additive effect or potentiation). Products include:
Vaseretic Tablets ... 1559
Vasotec Tablets ... 1564

Enalaprilat (Additive effect or potentiation). Products include:
Vasotec I.V. ... 1562

Enflurane (Potentiation of anesthetic agents agents). Products include:
Ethrane ... 599

Epinephrine Hydrochloride (Decreased response to pressor amine). Products include:
Adrenalin Chloride Solution 1:100 & 1:1,000 ... 1689
Epifrin ... ⊙ 244
Glaucon ... ⊙ 218

Esmolol Hydrochloride (Additive effect or potentiation). Products include:
Brevibloc Injection ... 942

Etodolac (Potential for reduced diuretic, natriuretic, and antihypertensive effect). Products include:
Lodine Capsules ... 2468

Felodipine (Additive effect or potentiation). Products include:
Plendil Extended-Release Tablets ... 1526

Fenoprofen Calcium (Potential for reduced diuretic, natriuretic, and antihypertensive effect). Products include:
Nalfon Pulvules & Tablets ... 919

Fentanyl (Potentiation of orthostatic hypotension). Products include:
Duragesic Transdermal System ... 1133

Fentanyl Citrate (Potentiation of preanesthetic agents). Products include:
Innovar Injection ... 1141
Sublimaze Injection ... 1146

Flurbiprofen (Potential for reduced diuretic, natriuretic, and antihypertensive effect). Products include:
Ansaid Tablets ... 2319

Fosinopril Sodium (Additive effect or potentiation). Products include:
Monopril Tablets ... 1406

Furazolidone (Enhanced hypotensive effects). Products include:
Furoxone ... 1855

Furosemide (Additive effect or potentiation). Products include:
Lasix ... 1093

Glipizide (Altered antidiabetic requirements). Products include:
Glucotrol ... 1952

Glyburide (Altered antidiabetic requirements). Products include:
DiaBeta ... 1091
Micronase Tablets ... 2350

Guanabenz Acetate (Additive effect or potentiation). Products include:
Wytensin Tablets ... 2542

Guanethidine Monosulfate (Potentiated). Products include:
Esimil Tablets ... 864
Ismelin Tablets ... 869

Hydralazine Hydrochloride (Additive effect). Products include:
Apresazide Capsules ... 854
Apresoline Hydrochloride Parenteral (Ampuls) ... 856
Apresoline Hydrochloride Tablets ... 855
Apresoline-Esidrix Tablets ... 857
Ser-Ap-Es Tablets ... 881
Serpasil-Apresoline Tablets ... 884

Hydrochlorothiazide (Additive effect or potentiation). Products include:
Aldactazide ... 2150
Aldoril Tablets ... 1418
Apresazide Capsules ... 854
Apresoline-Esidrix Tablets ... 857
Capozide ... 2258
Dyazide Capsules ... 2208
Esidrix Tablets ... 863
Esimil Tablets ... 864
HydroDIURIL Tablets ... 1484
Hydropres Tablets ... 1485
Inderide Tablets ... 2463
Inderide LA Long Acting Capsules ... 2465
Lopressor HCT Tablets ... 1034
Maxzide ... 1215
Moduretic Tablets ... 1510
Normozide Tablets ... 2112
Oretic Tablets ... 544
Oreticyl ... 545
Prinzide Tablets ... 1540
Ser-Ap-Es Tablets ... 881
Serpasil-Esidrix Tablets ... 886
Timolide Tablets ... 1547
Trandate HCT Tablets ... 579
Vaseretic Tablets ... 1559
Zestoretic ... 2274

Hydrocodone Bitartrate (Potentiation of orthostatic hypotension). Products include:
Anexsia 5/500 Tablets ... 2196
Anexsia 7.5/650 Tablets ... 2197
Azdōne Tablets ... 844
Codiclear DH Syrup ... 845
Codimal DH Syrup ... 846
Damason-P ... 1356
Hycodan Syrup, Tablets ... 927
Hycomine Compound Tablets ... 929
Hycomine Syrup ... 927
Hycotuss Expectorant Syrup ... 930
Hydrocet Capsules ... 835
Lortab ASA Tablets ... 2414
Lortab ... 2412
Ru-Tuss with Hydrocodone ... 694
Triaminic Expectorant DH ... 1995
Vicodin Tablets ... 1187
Vicodin ES Tablets ... 1189
Zydone Capsules ... 941

Hydrocodone Polistirex (Potentiation of orthostatic hypotension). Products include:
Tussionex Extended-Release Suspension ... 988

Hydrocortisone (Intensified electrolyte depletion; hypokalemia). Products include:
AK-Spore H.C. ... ⊙ 206
Bactine Hydrocortisone Anti-Itch Cream ... ▣ 625
CaldeCORT Anti-Itch Hydrocortisone Spray ... ▣ 560
Carmol HC Cream 1% ... 2296
Cortaid Spray ... ▣ 735
Cortenema ... 2244
Cortisporin Ointment ... 758
Cortisporin Ophthalmic Ointment Sterile ... 758
Cortisporin Ophthalmic Suspension Sterile ... 759
Cortisporin Otic Solution Sterile ... 760
Cortisporin Otic Suspension Sterile ... 760
Cortizone-5 Creme & Ointment ... ▣ 732
Dermolate Anti-Itch Cream ... ▣ 697
Eldecort Cream 1.0% ... 1113
Eldecort Cream 1.0% and 2.5% ... 1113
Fungoid HC Creme ... 1770
Hydrocortone Tablets ... 1482
Hytone ... 909
LazerSporin-C Solution ... 1770
Massengill Medicated Soft Cloth Towelettes ... 2192
Nutracort Cream & Lotion ... 1684
PediOtic Suspension Sterile ... 797
Synacort Creams 1%, 2.5% ... 2296
Vanoxide-HC Acne Lotion ... 911
Vioform-Hydrocortisone Cream and Mild Cream ... 889
Vioform-Hydrocortisone Ointment ... 889
VōSoL HC Otic Solution ... 2392
Vytone Cream 1% ... 911

Hydrocortisone Acetate (Intensified electrolyte depletion; hypokalemia). Products include:
Analpram-HC Rectal Cream 1% and 2.5% ... 970
Anusol-HC Cream ... 1690
Anusol-HC Suppositories ... 1691
Caldecort ... ▣ 560
Carmol HC Cream 1% ... 2296
Chloromycetin Hydrocortisone Ophthalmic ... 1694
Coly-Mycin S Otic w/Neomycin & Hydrocortisone ... 1708
Cortaid ... ▣ 735
Cortef Feminine Itch Cream ... ▣ 735
Corticaine ... ▣ 682
Cortifoam ... 1827
Cortisporin Cream ... 757
Epifoam ... 1828
Gynecort 5 Creme ... ▣ 556
Hydrocortone Acetate Sterile Suspension ... 1479
Lanacort 5 Creme and Ointment ... ▣ 557
Mantadil Cream ... 789
Ophthocort ... ⊙ 301
Orabase HCA Oral Paste ... 890
Pramosone Cream, Lotion & Ointment ... 971
ProctoCream-HC ... 1834
Proctofoam-HC ... 1835

Hydrocortisone Sodium Phosphate (Intensified electrolyte depletion; hypokalemia). Products include:
Hydrocortone Phosphate Injection, Sterile ... 1481

Hydrocortisone Sodium Succinate (Intensified electrolyte depletion; hypokalemia). Products include:
Solu-Cortef Sterile Powder ... 2361

Hydroflumethiazide (Additive effect or potentiation). Products include:
Diucardin Tablets ... 2450
Saluron ... 718
Salutensin/Salutensin-Demi ... 719

Hydroxyzine Hydrochloride (Potentiation of preanesthetic agents). Products include:
Atarax Tablets & Syrup ... 1941
Marax Tablets & DF Syrup ... 1954
Vistaril Intramuscular Solution ... 1970

Ibuprofen (Potential for reduced diuretic, natriuretic, and antihypertensive effect). Products include:
Advil Cold & Sinus Caplets (formerly CoAdvil) ... 2416
Advil Ibuprofen Tablets and Caplets ... 2416
Children's Advil Suspension ... 2426
CoAdvil ... ▣ 748
Dristan Sinus Caplets ... 2419
Haltran Tablets ... ▣ 668
Ibuprofen ... ▣ 631
Medipren ibuprofen Caplets and Tablets ... 1362
Midol 200 Cramp Relief Formula ... ▣ 570
Motrin Tablets ... 2351
Motrin IB Caplets and Tablets ... ▣ 736
Nuprin Ibuprofen/Analgesic Tablets & Caplets ... 752
PediaProfen Suspension ... 1363
Rufen Tablets ... 691
Trendar Ibuprofen Tablets ... ▣ 756

Indapamide (Additive effect or potentiation). Products include:
Lozol Tablets ... 1843

Indomethacin (Potential for reduced diuretic, natriuretic, and antihypertensive effect). Products include:
Indocin ... 1487

Indomethacin Sodium Trihydrate (Potential for reduced diuretic, natriuretic, and antihypertensive effect). Products include:
Indocin I.V. ... 1490

Insulin, Human (Altered insulin requirements).
No products indexed under this heading.

Insulin, Human Isophane Suspension (Altered insulin requirements). Products include:
Humulin N, 100 Units ... 1270

Insulin, Human NPH (Altered insulin requirements). Products include:
Insulatard NPH Human ... 1627
Novolin N ... 1627
Novolin N PenFill Cartridges ... 1628
Novolin N Prefilled ... 1628

Insulin, Human Regular (Altered insulin requirements). Products include:
Humulin BR, 100 Units ... 1268
Humulin R, 100 Units ... 1272
Novolin R ... 1627
Novolin R PenFill Cartridges ... 1628
Novolin R Prefilled ... 1629
Velosulin Human ... 1628

Insulin, Human, Zinc Suspension (Altered insulin requirements). Products include:
Humulin L, 100 Units ... 1268
Humulin U, 100 Units ... 1272
Novolin L ... 1627

Insulin, NPH (Altered insulin requirements). Products include:
NPH, 40 & 100 Units ... 1273
Beef NPH, 100 Units ... 1274
Pork NPH, 100 Units ... 1275
Insulatard NPH ... 1626

(▣ Described in PDR For Nonprescription Drugs) (⊙ Described in PDR For Ophthalmology)

NPH Insulin ... 1626
NPH Purified Pork Isophane Insulin ... 1626

Insulin, Regular (Altered insulin requirements). Products include:
Regular, 40 & 100 Units ... 1273
Beef Regular, 100 Units ... 1275
Pork Regular, 100 Units ... 1275
Pork Regular (Concentrated), 500 Units ... 1276
Regular Insulin ... 1625
Regular Purified Pork Insulin ... 1626
Velosulin ... 1627

Insulin, Zinc Crystals (Altered insulin requirements). Products include:
NPH, 40 & 100 Units ... 1273

Insulin, Zinc Suspension (Altered insulin requirements). Products include:
Lente, 40 & 100 Units ... 1272
Protamine, Zinc, 40 & 100 Units ... 1273
Lente Iletin I ... 1272
Beef Lente, 100 Units ... 1274
Beef Protamine Zinc, 100 Units ... 1274
Pork Lente, 100 Units ... 1275
Pork, Protamine, Zinc, 100 Units ... 1275
Lente Insulin ... 1626
Lente Purified Pork Insulin ... 1626
Semilente Insulin ... 1625
Ultralente Insulin ... 1626

Isocarboxazid (Enhanced hypotensive effects). Products include:
Marplan Tablets ... 1906

Isoflurane (Potentiation of anesthetic agents). Products include:
Forane ... 600

Isradipine (Additive effect or potentiation). Products include:
DynaCirc Capsules ... 2004

Ketamine Hydrochloride (Potentiation of anesthetic agents). Products include:
Ketalar ... 1726

Ketoprofen (Potential for reduced diuretic, natriuretic, and antihypertensive effect). Products include:
Orudis Capsules ... 2488

Ketorolac Tromethamine (Potential for reduced diuretic, natriuretic, and antihypertensive effect). Products include:
Toradol IM Injection ... 2302

Labetalol Hydrochloride (Additive effect or potentiation). Products include:
Normodyne Injection ... 2108
Normodyne Tablets ... 2110
Normozide Tablets ... 2112
Trandate HCT Tablets ... 579
Trandate Injection ... 577
Trandate Tablets ... 579

Levorphanol Tartrate (Potentiation of orthostatic hypotension). Products include:
Levo-Dromoran ... 1906

Lisinopril (Additive effect or potentiation). Products include:
Prinivil Tablets ... 1538
Prinzide Tablets ... 1540
Zestoretic ... 2274
Zestril Tablets ... 2277

Lithium Carbonate (Reduced renal clearance and increased risk of lithium toxicity). Products include:
Eskalith ... 2214
Lithane Tablets ... 1596
Lithium Carbonate Capsules & Tablets ... 1984
Lithobid Tablets ... 870

Lithium Citrate (Reduced renal clearance and increased risk of lithium toxicity). Products include:
Cibalith-S ... 870

Lorazepam (Potentiation of preanesthetic agents). Products include:
Ativan Injection ... 2432
Ativan Tablets ... 2434

Mecamylamine Hydrochloride (Potentiated). Products include:
Inversine Tablets ... 1492

Meclofenamate Sodium (Potential for reduced diuretic, natriuretic, and antihypertensive effect). Products include:
Meclomen Capsules ... 1739

Mefenamic Acid (Potential for reduced diuretic, natriuretic, and antihypertensive effect). Products include:
Ponstel ... 1758

Meperidine Hydrochloride (Potentiation of preanesthetic agents). Products include:
Demerol ... 2047
Mepergan Injection ... 2479

Mephobarbital (Potentiation of orthostatic hypotension). Products include:
Mebaral Tablets ... 2061

Metaraminol Bitartrate (Decreased response to pressor amine). Products include:
Aramine Injection ... 1424

Methadone Hydrochloride (Potentiation of orthostatic hypotension). Products include:
Dolophine Hydrochloride Ampoules & Vials ... 1260
Dolophine Hydrochloride Tablets ... 1261
Methadone Hydrochloride Diskets ... 1284
Methadone Hydrochloride Oral Solution & Tablets ... 1987

Methenamine (Possible decreased effectiveness due to alkalinization of the urine). Products include:
Urised Tablets ... 2396

Methenamine Hippurate (Possible decreased effectiveness due to alkalinization of the urine). Products include:
Hiprex Tablets ... 1333
Urex Tablets ... 1321

Methenamine Mandelate (Possible decreased effectiveness due to alkalinization of the urine). Products include:
Mandelamine ... 1738
Uroqid-Acid ... 661

Methohexital Sodium (Potentiation of anesthetic agents). Products include:
Brevital Sodium Vials ... 1248

Methoxamine Hydrochloride (Decreased response to pressor amine). Products include:
Vasoxyl Injection ... 819

Methoxyflurane (Potentiation of anesthetic agents).
No products indexed under this heading.

Methyclothiazide (Additive effect or potentiation). Products include:
Enduron Tablets ... 517
Enduronyl ... 518

Methyldopa (Additive effect or potentiation). Products include:
Aldoclor Tablets ... 1413
Aldomet Oral ... 1415
Aldoril Tablets ... 1418

Methyldopate Hydrochloride (Additive effect or potentiation). Products include:
Aldomet Ester HCl Injection ... 1417

Methylprednisolone (Intensified electrolyte depletion). Products include:
Medrol ... 2348

Methylprednisolone Acetate (Intensified electrolyte depletion). Products include:
Depo-Medrol Sterile Aqueous Suspension ... 2334

Methylprednisolone Sodium Succinate (Intensified electrolyte depletion). Products include:
Solu-Medrol Sterile Powder ... 2363

Metocurine Iodide (Increased response to muscle relaxants). Products include:
Metubine Iodide Vials ... 1285

Metolazone (Additive effect or potentiation). Products include:
Diulo ... 2129
Mykrox ½ mg Tablets ... 984
Zaroxolyn Tablets ... 989

Metoprolol Tartrate (Additive effect or potentiation). Products include:
Lopressor Ampuls ... 1032
Lopressor HCT Tablets ... 1034
Lopressor Tablets ... 1032

Metyrosine (Additive effect or potentiation). Products include:
Demser Capsules ... 1460

Minoxidil (Additive effect or potentiation). Products include:
Loniten Tablets ... 2346
Rogaine Topical Solution ... 2357

Morphine Sulfate (Potentiation of preanesthetic agents). Products include:
Astramorph/PF Injection, USP (Preservative-Free) ... 618
Duramorph ... 960
Infumorph 200 and Infumorph 500 Sterile Solutions ... 962
MS Contin Tablets ... 1814
MSIR ... 1817
Oramorph SR (Morphine Sulfate Sustained Release Tablets) ... 1988
Roxanol ... 1991

Naproxen (Potential for reduced diuretic, natriuretic, and antihypertensive effect). Products include:
Naprosyn ... 2297

Naproxen Sodium (Potential for reduced diuretic, natriuretic, and antihypertensive effect). Products include:
Anaprox and Anaprox DS Tablets ... 2288

Nicardipine Hydrochloride (Additive effect or potentiation). Products include:
Cardene Capsules ... 2290

Nitroglycerin (Additive effect or potentiation). Products include:
Deponit NTG Transdermal Delivery System ... 2143
Minitran Transdermal Delivery System ... 1312
Nitro-Bid Ointment ... 1339
Nitro-Bid Capsules ... 1338
Nitrodisc ... 2176
Nitro-Dur (nitroglycerin) Transdermal Infusion System ... 1164
Nitrogard Tablets ... 1004
Nitrolingual Spray ... 1846
Nitrostat Tablets ... 1743
Transderm-Nitro Transdermal Therapeutic System ... 2283

Norepinephrine Bitartrate (Decreased pressor response). Products include:
Levophed Bitartrate Injection ... 2054

Opium Alkaloids (Potentiation of orthostatic hypotension). Products include:
B & O No. 15A & No. 16A Supprettes ... 2395
Pantopon Injectable ... 1911

Oxycodone Hydrochloride (Potentiation of orthostatic hypotension). Products include:
Percocet Tablets ... 950
Percodan ... 951
Roxicodone Tablets, Oral Solution & Intensol (Oxycodone) ... 1992
Tylox Capsules ... 1382

Pancuronium Bromide Injection (Increased response to muscle relaxants).
No products indexed under this heading.

Penbutolol Sulfate (Additive effect or potentiation). Products include:
Levatol ... 1832

Pentobarbital Sodium (Potentiation of orthostatic hypotension). Products include:
Nembutal Sodium Capsules ... 534
Nembutal Sodium Solution ... 536
Nembutal Sodium Suppositories ... 538

Phenelzine Sulfate (Enhanced hypotensive effects). Products include:
Nardil ... 1742

Phenobarbital (Potentiation of orthostatic hypotension). Products include:
Arco-Lase Plus Tablets ... 607
Bellergal-S Tablets ... 1998
Bronkolixir ... ▣ 761
Bronkotabs Tablets ... ▣ 762
Donnatal ... 1858
Donnatal Extentabs ... 1859
Donnatal Tablets ... 1858
Donnazyme Tablets ... 1860
Kinesed Tablets ... 2272
Phenobarbital Elixir and Tablets ... 1293
Primatene Tablets-P Formula ... 2421
Quadrinal Tablets ... 1183
Tedral SA ... 1765

Phenoxybenzamine Hydrochloride (Additive effect or potentiation). Products include:
Dibenzyline Capsules ... 2207

Phentolamine Mesylate (Additive effect or potentiation). Products include:
Regitine ... 878

Phenylbutazone (Potential for reduced diuretic, natriuretic, and antihypertensive effect). Products include:
Butazolidin Capsules & Tablets ... 1027

Phenylephrine Hydrochloride (Decreased response to pressor amine). Products include:
AK-Dilate Solution 2.5% and 10% ... ⊙ 203
Atrohist Sprinkle Capsules ... 558
Cerose-DM ... 2443
Codimal ... 846
Comhist LA Capsules ... 1618
Congespirin For Children Aspirin Free Chewable Cold Tablets ... 748
Cyclomydril ... ⊙ 216
Deconsal Sprinkle Capsules ... 559
Dimetane Decongestant ... ▣ 673
Dristan Decongestant/Antihistamine/Analgesic Coated Caplets ... ▣ 749
Dristan Cold Nasal Decongestant/Antihistamine/Analgesic Coated Tablets ... 2419
Dristan Advanced Formula Decongestant/Antihistamine/Analgesic Tablets ... ▣ 749
Dristan Nasal Spray, Menthol ... 2419
Dristan Nasal Spray, Regular and Regular with Metered Pump ... 2419
Entex Capsules ... 1623
Entex Liquid ... 1623
Sinus Excedrin Analgesic, Decongestant Tablets & Caplets ... 750
Extendryl ... 994
4-Way Fast Acting Nasal Spray - Original Formula (regular & mentholated) & Metered Spray Pump (regular) ... 751
Hycomine Compound Tablets ... 929
Murocoll-2 Sterile Ophthalmic Solution ... ⊙ 261
Mydfrin 2.5% ... ⊙ 224
Naldecon Syrup, Tablets, Pediatric Drops and Pediatric Syrup ... 709
Neo-Synephrine Hydrochloride 1% Carpuject ... 2063
Neo-Synephrine Hydrochloride 1% Injection ... 2063
Neo-Synephrine Hydrochloride (Ophthalmic) ... 2064
Neo-Synephrine ... ▣ 759
Nōstril Nasal Decongestant ... ▣ 520
Novahistine Elixir ... ▣ 596
Phenergan VC ... 2500
Phenergan VC with Codeine ... 2501
Prefrin Liquifilm Vasoconstrictor and Lubricant Eye Drops ... ⊙ 254
Prefrin-A ... ⊙ 255
Quelidrine Syrup ... 556

Relief Vasoconstrictor and Lubricant Eye Drops ◉ 256
Robitussin Night Relief ▣ 677
Ru-Tuss with Hydrocodone 694
Ru-Tuss Tablets 693
Vasosulf ◉ 279
Vicks Sinex ▣ 665
Zincfrin ◉ 230

Pindolol (Additive effect or potentiation). Products include:
Visken Tablets 2036

Piroxicam (Potential for reduced diuretic, natriuretic, and antihypertensive effect). Products include:
Feldene Capsules 1777

Polythiazide (Additive effect or potentiation). Products include:
Minizide Capsules 1779
Renese Tablets 1785
Renese-R Tablets 1786

Prazosin Hydrochloride (Potentiated). Products include:
Minipress Capsules 1778
Minizide Capsules 1779

Prednisolone Acetate (Intensified electrolyte depletion; hypokalemia). Products include:
AK-Cide Sterile Ophthalmic Ointment & Suspension ◉ 202
Blephamide Liquifilm Sterile Ophthalmic Suspension 586
Blephamide S.O.P. Sterile Ophthalmic Ointment 586
Cetapred Ointment ◉ 220
⅛% Econopred & 1% Econopred Plus ◉ 217
Isopto Cetapred Suspension ◉ 220
Metimyd ◉ 306
Poly-Pred Liquifilm ◉ 250
Pred Forte ◉ 252
Pred Mild ◉ 254
Pred-G Liquifilm Sterile Ophthalmic Suspension ◉ 252
Pred-G S.O.P. Sterile Ophthalmic Ointment ◉ 253
Vasocidin Ointment ◉ 275

Prednisolone Sodium Phosphate (Intensified electrolyte depletion; hypokalemia). Products include:
AK-Pred ◉ 205
Hydeltrasol Injection, Sterile 1476
Inflamase ◉ 274
Pediapred Oral Liquid 987
Vasocidin Ophthalmic Solution ◉ 276

Prednisolone Tebutate (Intensified electrolyte depletion; hypokalemia). Products include:
Hydeltra-T.B.A. Sterile Suspension 1478

Prednisone (Intensified electrolyte depletion; hypokalemia). Products include:
Deltasone Tablets 2332

Probenecid (Bendroflumethiazide may raise the level of blood uric acid). Products include:
Benemid Tablets 1426
ColBENEMID Tablets 1436
Wycillin Injection and Probenecid Tablets 2539

Promethazine Hydrochloride (Potentiation of preanesthetic agents). Products include:
Mepergan Injection 2479
Phenergan with Codeine 2497
Phenergan with Dextromethorphan 2499
Phenergan Injection 2493
Phenergan Suppositories 2496
Phenergan Syrup 2495
Phenergan Tablets 2496
Phenergan VC 2500
Phenergan VC with Codeine 2501

Propofol (Potentiation of anesthetic agents agents). Products include:
Diprivan Injection 2267

Propoxyphene Hydrochloride (Potentiation of orthostatic hypotension). Products include:
Darvon 1256
Wygesic Tablets 2540

Propoxyphene Napsylate (Potentiation of orthostatic hypotension). Products include:
Darvon-N/Darvocet-N 1254

Propranolol Hydrochloride (Additive effect or potentiation). Products include:
Inderal 2459
Inderal LA Long Acting Capsules 2461
Inderide Tablets 2463
Inderide LA Long Acting Capsules 2465

Ramipril (Additive effect or potentiation). Products include:
Altace Capsules 1086

Rauwolfia Serpentina (Additive effects; potential for hypotension and/or excessive bradycardia). Products include:
Raudixin Tablets 1803
Rauzide Tablets 1804

Rescinnamine (Additive effects; potential for hypotension and/or excessive bradycardia).
No products indexed under this heading.

Reserpine (Additive effects; potential for hypotension and/or excessive bradycardia). Products include:
Diupres Tablets 1461
Hydromox R Tablets 1209
Hydropres Tablets 1485
Renese-R Tablets 1786
Salutensin/Salutensin-Demi 719
Ser-Ap-Es Tablets 881
Serpasil Tablets 883
Serpasil-Apresoline Tablets 884
Serpasil-Esidrix Tablets 886

Secobarbital Sodium (Potentiation of orthostatic hypotension). Products include:
Seconal Sodium Pulvules 1296

Selegiline Hydrochloride (Enhanced hypotensive effects). Products include:
Eldepryl 2250

Sodium Nitroprusside (Additive effect or potentiation). Products include:
Nipride I.V. Infusion 1909

Sufentanil Citrate (Potentiation of orthostatic hypotension). Products include:
Sufenta Injection 1147

Sulfinpyrazone (Bendroflumethiazide may raise the level of blood uric acid). Products include:
Anturane 853

Sulindac (Potential for reduced diuretic, natriuretic, and antihypertensive effect). Products include:
Clinoril Tablets 1433

Terazosin Hydrochloride (Additive effect or potentiation). Products include:
Hytrin Tablets 529

Thiamylal Sodium (Potentiation of orthostatic hypotension). Products include:
Surital Ampoules, Steri-Vials 1764

Timolol Maleate (Additive effect or potentiation). Products include:
Blocadren Tablets 1429
Timolide Tablets 1547
Timoptic in Ocudose 1552
Timoptic Sterile Ophthalmic Solution 1550

Tolazamide (Altered antidiabetic requirements). Products include:
Tolinase Tablets 2365

Tolbutamide (Altered antidiabetic requirements). Products include:
Orinase Tablets 2354

Tolmetin Sodium (Potential for reduced diuretic, natriuretic, and antihypertensive effect). Products include:
Tolectin (200, 400 and 600 mg) 1379

Tranylcypromine Sulfate (Enhanced hypotensive effects). Products include:
Parnate Tablets 2222

Triamcinolone (Intensified electrolyte depletion; hypokalemia).
No products indexed under this heading.

Triamcinolone Acetonide (Intensified electrolyte depletion; hypokalemia). Products include:
Aristocort A 1010
Azmacort Inhaler 1837
Kenalog Cream, Lotion & Ointment 2401
Kenalog-10 Injection 2402
Kenalog-40 Injection 2403
Kenalog in Orabase 604
Kenalog Spray 2401
Mycolog II Cream and Ointment 2407
Mytrex Cream & Ointment 2080
Nasacort Nasal Inhaler 1844

Triamcinolone Diacetate (Intensified electrolyte depletion; hypokalemia). Products include:
Aristocort Suspension 1008

Triamcinolone Hexacetonide (Intensified electrolyte depletion; hypokalemia). Products include:
Aristospan Suspension 1011

Trimethaphan Camsylate (Potentiated). Products include:
Arfonad Ampuls 1887

Vecuronium Bromide (Increased response to muscle relaxants). Products include:
Norcuron 1642

Warfarin Sodium (Decreased anticoagulant effects). Products include:
Coumadin Injection & Tablets 944
Panwarfin Tablets 547

COSMEGEN INJECTION
(Dactinomycin) 1440
No interactions described in labeling.

COTAZYM
(Pancrelipase) 1636
No interactions described in labeling.

COUMADIN INJECTION & TABLETS
(Warfarin Sodium) 944
May interact with antihistamines, diuretics, androgens, monoamine oxidase inhibitors, salicylates, sulfonamides, thyroid preparations, barbiturates, oral contraceptives, inhalant anesthetics, corticosteroids, narcotic analgesics, antacids, fluoroquinolone antibiotics, pyrazolon derivatives, and certain other agents. Compounds in these categories include:

Alcohol (Decreased or increased prothrombin time response).

Alfentanil Hydrochloride (Increased prothrombin time response with prolonged use). Products include:
Alfenta Injection 1131

Allopurinol (Increased prothrombin time response). Products include:
Zyloprim Tablets 830

Aluminum Carbonate Gel (Decreased prothrombin time response). Products include:
Basaljel 2438

Aluminum Hydroxide (Decreased prothrombin response). Products include:
Cama Arthritis Pain Reliever ▣ 685
Gaviscon Extra Strength Relief Formula Liquid Antacid ▣ 594
Gaviscon Extra Strength Relief Formula Antacid Tablets ▣ 594
Gaviscon Liquid Antacid ▣ 594
Gelusil Liquid & Tablets ▣ 639
Extra Strength Maalox Plus Suspension 1850
Maalox TC Suspension 1851
Maalox Plus Tablets ▣ 655
Extra Strength Maalox Plus Tablets 1850
Nephrox Suspension ▣ 563
WinGel Liquid & Tablets ▣ 761

Aluminum Hydroxide Gel (Decreased prothrombin time response). Products include:
ALternaGEL Liquid 1154
Aludrox Oral Suspension 2428
Amphojel Suspension 2429
Amphojel Suspension without Flavor 2429
Mylanta Liquid 1155
Mylanta Double Strength Liquid 1155

Aluminum Hydroxide Gel, Dried (Decreased prothrombin time response). Products include:
Alu-Tab/Alu-Cap 1309
Amphojel Tablets 2429
Ascriptin A/D Caplets 1850
Regular Strength Ascriptin Tablets 1850
Gaviscon Antacid Tablets ▣ 593
Gaviscon-2 Antacid Tablets ▣ 594
Mylanta Tablets 1155
Mylanta Double Strength Tablets 1155

Amiloride Hydrochloride (Decreased or increased prothrombin time response). Products include:
Midamor Tablets 1508
Moduretic Tablets 1510

Aminoglutethimide (Decreased prothrombin time response). Products include:
Cytadren Tablets 861

Aminosalicylic Acid (Increased prothrombin time response).

Amiodarone Hydrochloride (Increased prothrombin time response). Products include:
Cordarone Tablets 2446

Antibiotics, unspecified (Increased prothrombin time response).

Antipyrine (Increased prothrombin time response). Products include:
Auralgan Otic Solution 2437

Aprobarbital (Decreased prothrombin time response). Products include:
Alurate Elixir 1883

Aspirin (Increased prothrombin time response). Products include:
Alka-Seltzer Effervescent Antacid and Pain Reliever 1568
Alka-Seltzer Extra Strength Effervescent Antacid and Pain Reliever 1570
Alka-Seltzer (Flavored) Effervescent Antacid and Pain Reliever 1569
Alka-Seltzer Plus Cold Medicine ▣ 623
Alka-Seltzer Plus Night-Time Cold Medicine ▣ 623
Alka Seltzer Plus Sinus Allergy Medicine ▣ 624
Anacin Coated Analgesic Caplets 2417
Anacin Coated Analgesic Tablets 2417
Anacin Maximum Strength Analgesic Coated Tablets 2417
Maximum Strength Arthritis Pain Formula By the Makers of Anacin Analgesic Tablets and Caplets 2418
Arthritis Pain Formula by the Makers of Anacin Analgesic Tablets and Caplets ▣ 747
Arthritis Strength BC Powder ▣ 516
Ascriptin A/D Caplets 1850
Regular Strength Ascriptin Tablets 1850
Azdône Tablets 844
BC Powder ▣ 517
BC Cold Powder ▣ 517
Children's Bayer Chewable Aspirin ▣ 564
Genuine Bayer Aspirin Tablets & Caplets ▣ 564
Maximum Bayer Aspirin Tablets & Caplets ▣ 566
Bayer Plus Aspirin Tablets ▣ 567
Therapy Bayer Aspirin Caplets ▣ 568
8 Hour Bayer Timed-Release Aspirin ▣ 566
Arthritis Strength Bufferin Analgesic Caplets 744

Extra Strength Bufferin Analgesic Tablets 745
Bufferin Analgesic Tablets and Caplets 743
Cama Arthritis Pain Reliever ND 685
Damason-P 1356
Easprin 1719
Ecotrin Enteric Coated Aspirin Maximum Strength Tablets and Caplets 2189
Ecotrin Enteric Coated Aspirin Regular Strength Tablets and Caplets 2189
Empirin Aspirin ND 541
Empirin with Codeine Phosphate Nos. 2, 3 & 4 764
Equagesic Tablets 2451
Excedrin Extra-Strength Analgesic Tablets & Caplets 749
4-Way Cold Tablets 750
Fiorinal Capsules 2007
Fiorinal with Codeine Capsules 2008
Fiorinal Tablets 2007
Lortab ASA Tablets 2414
Momentum Muscular Backache Formula ND 751
Norgesic 1314
Norwich Extra-Strength Aspirin ND 546
Norwich Regular Strength Aspirin ND 547
P-A-C Analgesic Tablets ND 669
Percodan 951
Robaxisal Tablets 1872
Sine-Off Sinus Medicine Tablets-Aspirin Formula ND 722
Soma Compound w/Codeine Tablets 2390
Soma Compound Tablets 2389
St. Joseph Adult Chewable Aspirin (81 mg.) ND 703
Synalgos-DC Capsules 2525
Talwin Compound 2072
Ursinus Inlay-Tabs ND 691
Vanquish Analgesic Caplets ND 574
Zorprin Tablets 698

Astemizole (Decreased protyhrombin time response). Products include:
Hismanal Tablets 1138

Azatadine Maleate (Decreased prothrombin time response). Products include:
Optimine Tablets 2115
Trinalin Repetabs Tablets 1170

Bendroflumethiazide (Decreased or increased prothrombin time response). Products include:
Corzide Tablets 702
Naturetin Tablets 1789
Rauzide Tablets 1804

Betamethasone Acetate (Decreased prothrombin time response). Products include:
Celestone Soluspan Suspension 2081

Betamethasone Sodium Phosphate (Decreased prothrombin time response). Products include:
Celestone Soluspan Suspension 2081

Bromelains (Increased prothrombin time response). Products include:
Bromase Capsules 672

Bromodiphenhydramine Hydrochloride (Decreased prothrombin time response).
No products indexed under this heading.

Brompheniramine Maleate (Decreased prothrombin time response). Products include:
Alka Seltzer Plus Sinus Allergy Medicine ND 624
Atrohist Sprinkle Capsules 558
Bromfed Capsules (Timed Release) 1615
Bromfed Syrup ND 628
Bromfed 1615
Dimetane Decongestant ND 673
Dimetane ND 672
Dimetane-DC Cough Syrup 1857
Dimetane-DX Cough Syrup 1858
Dimetapp Elixir ND 673
Dimetapp DM Elixir ND 674
Dimetapp Extentabs ND 674
Dimetapp Plus Caplets ND 675
Dimetapp Tablets ND 675
Drixoral Antihistamine/Nasal Decongestant Syrup ND 698

Bumetanide (Decreased or increased prothrombin time response). Products include:
Bumex 1895

Buprenorphine (Increased prothrombin time response with prolonged use).
No products indexed under this heading.

Butabarbital (Decreased prothrombin time response). Products include:
Pyridium Plus 1764

Butalbital (Decreased prothrombin time response). Products include:
Esgic-Plus Tablets 1002
Esgic Tablets & Capsules 1001
Fioricet Tablets 2006
Fiorinal Capsules 2007
Fiorinal with Codeine Capsules 2008
Fiorinal Tablets 2007
Phrenilin 838
Sedapap Tablets 50 mg/650 mg 1360

Carbamazepine (Decreased prothrombin time response). Products include:
Tegretol Chewable Tablets 654
Tegretol Suspension 656
Tegretol Tablets 654

Chenodiol (Increased prothrombin time response).
No products indexed under this heading.

Chloral Hydrate (Decreased or increased prothrombin time response).
No products indexed under this heading.

Chlordiazepoxide (Decreased prothrombin time response). Products include:
Libritabs Tablets 1930
Limbitrol 1933
Menrium Tablets 1934

Chlordiazepoxide Hydrochloride (Decreased prothrombin time response). Products include:
Librax Capsules 1929
Librium Capsules 1931
Librium Injectable 1932

Chlorothiazide (Decreased or increased prothrombin time response). Products include:
Aldoclor Tablets 1413
Diupres Tablets 1461
Diuril Oral 1464

Chlorothiazide Sodium (Decreased or increased prothrombin time response). Products include:
Diuril Sodium Intravenous 1463

Chlorpheniramine Maleate (Decreased prothrombin time response). Products include:
A.R.M. Allergy Relief Medicine Caplets ND 615
Alka-Seltzer Plus Cold Medicine ND 623
Allerest ND 559
Ana-Kit Anaphylaxis Emergency Treatment Kit 1100
BC Cold Powder Multi-Symptom Formula ND 517
Brexin L.A. Capsules 2078
Cerose-DM 2443
Cheracol Plus Head Cold/Cough Formula ND 667
Chlor-Trimeton Allergy Syrup, Tablets & Long-Acting Repetabs Tablets ND 693
Chlor-Trimeton Decongestant ND 694
Comhist LA Capsules 1618
Allergy-Sinus Comtrex Multi-Symptom Allergy Sinus Formula Tablets & Caplets 746
Comtrex Multi-Symptom Cold Reliever Tablets/Caplets/Liqui-Gels/Liquid 745
Day-Night Comtrex 747
Contac Continuous Action Decongestant/Antihistamine Capsules ND 710
Contac Maximum Strength Continuous Action Decongestant/Antihistamine Caplets ND 709
Contac Severe Cold and Flu Formula Caplets ND 711
Coricidin 'D' Decongestant Tablets ND 695
Coricidin Demilets Tablets for Children ND 696
Coricidin Tablets ND 695
Deconamine 663
Demazin Nasal Decongestant/Antihistamine Repetabs Tablets & Syrup ND 697
Dorcol Children's Liquid Cold Formula ND 686
Dristan Decongestant/Antihistamine/ Analgesic Coated Caplets ND 749
Dristan Cold Nasal Decongestant/Antihistamine/ Analgesic Coated Tablets 2419
Dristan Advanced Formula Decongestant/Antihistamine/Analgesic Tablets ND 749
Extendryl 994
4-Way Cold Tablets 750
Fedahist Gyrocaps 2145
Fedahist Timecaps 2145
Hycomine Compound Tablets 929
Isoclor Timesule Capsules ND 561
Kronofed-A 970
Medi-Flu Caplet, Liquid ND 640
Naldecon Syrup, Tablets, Pediatric Drops and Pediatric Syrup 709
Nolamine Tablets 838
Novafed A Capsules 1342
Novahistine DH 1342
Novahistine Elixir ND 596
Ornade Spansule Capsules 2221
Orthoxicol Cough Syrup ND 668
PediaCare Allergy Relief Formula Liquid 1362
PediaCare Cough-Cold Formula Liquid 1362
PediaCare Night Rest Cough-Cold Formula Liquid 1362
PediaCare 6-12 Cough-Cold Formula Chewable Tablets 1362
Pyrroxate Capsules ND 669
Quelidrine Syrup 556
Ru-Tuss II Capsules 693
Ru-Tuss Tablets 693
Ryna ND 741
Sinarest Tablets & Extra Strength Tablets ND 562
Sine-Off Maximum Strength Allergy/Sinus Formula Caplets ND 721
Sine-Off Sinus Medicine Tablets-Aspirin Formula ND 722
Singlet Tablets ND 598
Sinulin 840
Sinutab Maximum Strength ND 641
St. Joseph Nighttime Cold Medicine ND 705
Sudafed Plus Liquid ND 544
Sudafed Plus Tablets ND 545
Teldrin Timed-Release Allergy Capsules, 12 mg. 2192
TheraFlu Flu and Cold Medicine ND 687
Triaminic Allergy Tablets ND 688
Triaminic Chewables ND 688
Triaminic Cold Tablets ND 688
Triaminic Nite Light ND 689
Triaminic Syrup ND 689
Triaminic-12 Tablets ND 690
Triaminicin Tablets ND 690
Triaminicol Multi-Symptom Cold Tablets ND 691
Triaminicol Multi-Symptom Relief ND 691
Tylenol Allergy Sinus Medication Caplets and Gelcaps, Maximum Strength 1372
Children's Tylenol Cold Liquid Formula and Chewable Tablets 1368
Tylenol Cold & Flu Hot Medication, Packets 1369
Tylenol Cold Medication Caplets and Tablets 1370
Tylenol Cold Medication, Effervescent Tablets 1369
Vicks Children's NyQuil ND 664
Vicks Formula 44 Cough Medicine ND 661
Vicks Formula 44M Multi-Symptom Cough Medicine ND 662
Vicks Pediatric Formula 44m Multi-Symptom Cough & Cold Medicine ND 663

Chlorpheniramine Polistirex (Decreased prothrombin time response). Products include:
Tussionex Extended-Release Suspension 988

Chlorpheniramine Tannate (Decreased prothrombin time response). Products include:
Rynatan 2387
Rynatuss 2388

Chlorpropamide (Increased prothrombin time response; accumulation of chlorpropamide). Products include:
Diabinese Tablets 1775

Chlorthalidone (Decreased or increased prothrombin time response). Products include:
Combipres Tablets 678
Tenoretic Tablets 1105
Thalitone Tablets 687

Cholestyramine (Decreased prothrombin time response). Products include:
Cholybar 1705
Questran Light 711
Questran Powder 710

Choline Magnesium Trisalicylate (Increased prothrombin time response). Products include:
Trilisate 1822

Chymotrypsin (Increased prothrombin time response).
No products indexed under this heading.

Cimetidine (Increased prothrombin time response). Products include:
Tagamet Tablets 2228

Cimetidine Hydrochloride (Increased prothrombin time response). Products include:
Tagamet 2228

Ciprofloxacin (Increased prothrombin time response).
No products indexed under this heading.

Ciprofloxacin Hydrochloride (Increased prothrombin time response). Products include:
Ciloxan Sterile Ophthalmic Solution ⊙ 214
Cipro I.V. 1592
Cipro Tablets 1589

Clemastine Fumarate (Decreased prothrombin time response). Products include:
Tavist Syrup 2033
Tavist Tablets 2035
Tavist-D Tablets 2035

Clofibrate (Increased prothrombin time response). Products include:
Atromid-S Capsules 2435

Codeine (Increased prothrombin time response with prolonged use). Products include:
Calcidrine Syrup 506

Codeine Phosphate (Increased prothrombin time response with prolonged use). Products include:
Actifed with Codeine Cough Syrup 752
Cheracol Cough Syrup 1853
Codimal PH Syrup 846
Dimetane-DC Cough Syrup 1857
Empirin with Codeine Phosphate Nos. 2, 3 & 4 764
Fiorinal with Codeine Capsules 2008
Isoclor Expectorant 982
Naldecon CX Adult Liquid ND 521
Novahistine DH 1342
Novahistine Expectorant 1343
Nucofed Capsules 2219
Nucofed Expectorant 2219
Nucofed Pediatric Expectorant 2220
Nucofed Syrup 2219
Phenaphen with Codeine Capsules 1865
Phenaphen-650 with Codeine Tablets 1866
Phenergan with Codeine 2497
Phenergan VC with Codeine 2501
Robitussin A-C Syrup 1875

Robitussin-DAC Syrup ... 1875
Ryna ... ▣ 741
Soma Compound w/Codeine Tablets ... 2390
Triaminic Expectorant w/Codeine ... 1996
Tussi-Organidin Liquid ... 2391
Tylenol with Codeine ... 1381

Codeine Polistirex (Increased prothrombin time response with prolonged use).
No products indexed under this heading.

Cortisone Acetate (Decreased prothrombin time response). Products include:
Cortone Acetate Sterile Suspension ... 1437
Cortone Acetate Tablets ... 1439

Cyproheptadine Hydrochloride (Decreased prothrombin time response). Products include:
Periactin ... 1525

Dexamethasone (Decreased prothrombin time response). Products include:
AK-Trol Ointment & Suspension ... ◉ 207
Decadron Elixir ... 1445
Decadron Tablets ... 1447
Decaspray Topical Aerosol ... 1459
Dexacidin ... ◉ 272
Maxidex Sterile Ophthalmic Suspension ... ◉ 223
Maxitrol Ophthalmic Ointment/Suspension ... ◉ 223
TobraDex Ophthalmic Suspension and Ointment ... ◉ 228

Dexamethasone Acetate (Decreased prothrombin time response). Products include:
Dalalone D.P. Injectable ... 999
Decadron-LA Sterile Suspension ... 1457

Dexamethasone Sodium Phosphate (Decreased prothrombin time response). Products include:
AK-Dex ... ◉ 203
Decadron Phosphate Respihaler ... 1454
Decadron Phosphate Sterile Ophthalmic Ointment ... 1453
Decadron Phosphate Sterile Ophthalmic Solution ... 1453
Decadron Phosphate Topical Cream ... 1455
Decadron Phosphate Turbinaire ... 1456
Maxidex Sterile Ophthalmic Ointment ... ◉ 222
NeoDecadron Sterile Ophthalmic Ointment ... 1517
NeoDecadron Sterile Ophthalmic Solution ... 1518
NeoDecadron Topical Cream ... 1518

Dexchlorpheniramine Maleate (Decreased prothrombin time response). Products include:
Polaramine ... 2116

Dextrans (Low Molecular Weight) (Increased prothrombin time response).
No products indexed under this heading.

Dextrothyroxine Sodium (Increased prothrombin time response).
No products indexed under this heading.

Dezocine (Increased prothrombin time response with prolonged use).

Diazoxide (Increased prothrombin time response). Products include:
Hyperstat I.V. Injection ... 2095
Proglycem ... 649

Diflunisal (Increased prothrombin time response). Products include:
Dolobid Tablets ... 1465

Diphenhydramine Citrate (Decreased prothrombin time response). Products include:
Alka-Seltzer Plus Night-Time Cold Medicine ... ▣ 623
Bufferin AF Nite Time Analgesic/Sleeping Aid Caplets ... 744
Excedrin P.M. Analgesic/Sleeping Aid Tablets, Caplets and Liquid ... 749

Diphenhydramine Hydrochloride (Decreased prothrombin time response). Products include:
Benadryl Anti-Itch Cream ... ▣ 635
Benadryl Capsules ... 1691
Benadryl Decongestant Elixir ... ▣ 635
Benadryl Decongestant ... ▣ 635
Benadryl Elixir ... ▣ 636
Benadryl Kapseals ... 1691
Benadryl 25 Kapseals ... ▣ 636
Benadryl Parenteral ... 1692
Benadryl Plus ... ▣ 636
Benadryl Plus Nighttime ... ▣ 637
Benadryl Spray, Maximum Strength ... ▣ 637
Benadryl Spray, Regular Strength ▣ 637
Benadryl Steri-Vials, Ampoules, and Steri-Dose Syringe ... 1692
Benadryl 25 Tablets ... ▣ 636
Benylin Cough Syrup ... ▣ 637
Benylin Decongestant ... ▣ 638
Caladryl Cream, Lotion, Spray ... ▣ 638
Miles Nervine Nighttime Sleep-Aid ▣ 627
Nytol Tablets ... ▣ 517
Sleep-ettes-D Tablets ... ▣ 653
Sleep-eze 3 Tablets ... ▣ 755
Sleepinal Night-time Sleep Aid Capsules ... ▣ 734
Sominex Caplets and Tablets ... ▣ 722
Sominex Liquid ... ▣ 723
Sominex Pain Relief Formula ... ▣ 723
Tylenol Cold Night Time Medication Liquid ... 1371
Tylenol PM, Extra Strength Caplets and Tablets ... 1368
Unisom Dual Relief Nighttime Sleep Aid/Analgesic ... 1774
Ziradryl Lotion ... ▣ 643

Diphenylpyraline Hydrochloride (Decreased prothrombin time response).
No products indexed under this heading.

Disulfiram (Increased prothrombin time response). Products include:
Antabuse Tablets ... 2429

Enflurane (Increased prothrombin time response). Products include:
Ethrane ... 599

Ethacrynic Acid (Decreased or increased prothrombin time response). Products include:
Edecrin Tablets ... 1468

Ethchlorvynol (Decreased prothrombin time response). Products include:
Placidyl Capsules ... 553

Ethinyl Estradiol (Decreased prothrombin time response). Products include:
Brevicon ... 2304
Demulen ... 2161
Estinyl Tablets ... 2085
Jenest-28 Tablets ... 1636
Levlen/Tri-Levlen ... 665
Lo/Ovral Tablets ... 2471
Lo/Ovral-28 Tablets ... 2476
Loestrin ... 1728
Modicon ... 1667
Nordette-21 Tablets ... 2481
Nordette-28 Tablets ... 2483
Norethin ... 2133
Norinyl ... 2304
Norlestrin ... 1746
Ortho-Cyclen Tablets ... 1658
Ortho-Novum ... 1667
Ovcon ... 1391
Ovral Tablets ... 2490
Ovral-28 Tablets ... 2491
Levlen/Tri-Levlen ... 665
Tri-Norinyl ... 2304
Triphasil-21 Tablets ... 2527
Triphasil-28 Tablets ... 2532

Ethynodiol Diacetate (Decreased prothrombin time response). Products include:
Demulen ... 2161

Fenoprofen Calcium (Increased prothrombin time response). Products include:
Nalfon Pulvules & Tablets ... 919

Fentanyl (Increased prothrombin time response with prolonged use). Products include:
Duragesic Transdermal System ... 1133

Fentanyl Citrate (Increased prothrombin time response with prolonged use). Products include:
Innovar Injection ... 1141
Sublimaze Injection ... 1146

Fluoxymesterone (Increased prothrombin time response). Products include:
Halotestin Tablets ... 2341

Furazolidone (Increased prothrombin time response). Products include:
Furoxone ... 1855

Furosemide (Decreased or increased prothrombin time response). Products include:
Lasix ... 1093

Glipizide (Increased prothrombin time response). Products include:
Glucotrol ... 1952

Glucagon (Increased prothrombin time response). Products include:
Glucagon for Injection Vials and Emergency Kit ... 1263

Glutethimide (Decreased prothrombin time response).
No products indexed under this heading.

Glyburide (Increased prothrombin time response). Products include:
DiaBeta ... 1091
Micronase Tablets ... 2350

Griseofulvin (Decreased prothrombin time response). Products include:
Fulvicin P/G Tablets ... 2090
Fulvicin P/G 165 & 330 Tablets ... 2091
Fulvicin-U/F Tablets ... 2092
Grifulvin V (griseofulvin microsize) Tablets/Suspension ... 1678
Grisactin ... 2454
Grisactin Ultra Tablets ... 2455
Gris-PEG Tablets, 125 mg & 250 mg ... 1083

Haloperidol (Decreased prothrombin time response). Products include:
Haldol Injection, Tablets and Concentrate ... 1373

Haloperidol Decanoate (Decreased prothrombin time response). Products include:
Haldol Decanoate ... 1375

Halothane (Increased prothrombin time response). Products include:
Fluothane ... 2453

Hepatotoxic Drugs, unspecified (Increased prothrombin time response).

Hydrochlorothiazide (Decreased or increased prothrombin time response). Products include:
Aldactazide ... 2150
Aldoril Tablets ... 1418
Apresazide Capsules ... 854
Apresoline-Esidrix Tablets ... 857
Capozide ... 2258
Dyazide Capsules ... 2208
Esidrix Tablets ... 863
Esimil Tablets ... 864
HydroDIURIL Tablets ... 1484
Hydropres Tablets ... 1485
Inderide Tablets ... 2463
Inderide LA Long Acting Capsules ... 2465
Lopressor HCT Tablets ... 1034
Maxzide ... 1215
Moduretic Tablets ... 1510
Normozide Tablets ... 2112
Oretic Tablets ... 544
Oreticyl ... 545
Prinzide Tablets ... 1540
Ser-Ap-Es Tablets ... 881
Serpasil-Esidrix Tablets ... 886
Timolide Tablets ... 1547
Trandate HCT Tablets ... 579
Vaseretic Tablets ... 1559
Zestoretic ... 2274

Hydrocodone Bitartrate (Increased prothrombin time response with prolonged use). Products include:
Anexsia 5/500 Tablets ... 2196
Anexsia 7.5/650 Tablets ... 2197
Azdōne Tablets ... 844
Codiclear DH Syrup ... 845
Codimal DH Syrup ... 846
Damason-P ... 1356
Hycodan Syrup, Tablets ... 927
Hycomine Compound Tablets ... 929
Hycomine Syrup ... 927
Hycotuss Expectorant Syrup ... 930
Hydrocet Capsules ... 835
Lortab ASA Tablets ... 2414
Lortab ... 2412
Ru-Tuss with Hydrocodone ... 694
Triaminic Expectorant DH ... 1995
Vicodin Tablets ... 1187
Vicodin ES Tablets ... 1189
Zydone Capsules ... 941

Hydrocodone Polistirex (Increased prothrombin time response with prolonged use). Products include:
Tussionex Extended-Release Suspension ... 988

Hydrocortisone (Decreased prothrombin time response). Products include:
AK-Spore H.C. ... ◉ 206
Bactine Hydrocortisone Anti-Itch Cream ... ▣ 625
CaldeCORT Anti-Itch Hydrocortisone Spray ... ▣ 560
Carmol HC Cream 1% ... 2296
Cortaid Spray ... ▣ 735
Cortenema ... 2244
Cortisporin Ointment ... 758
Cortisporin Ophthalmic Ointment Sterile ... 758
Cortisporin Ophthalmic Suspension Sterile ... 759
Cortisporin Otic Solution Sterile ... 760
Cortisporin Otic Suspension Sterile ... 760
Cortizone-5 Creme & Ointment ... ▣ 732
Dermolate Anti-Itch Cream ... ▣ 697
Eldecort Cream 1.0% ... 1113
Eldecort Cream 1.0% and 2.5% ... 1113
Fungoid HC Creme ... 1770
Hydrocortone Tablets ... 1482
Hytone ... 909
LazerSporin-C Solution ... 1770
Massengill Medicated Soft Cloth Towelettes ... 2192
Nutracort Cream & Lotion ... 1684
PediOtic Suspension Sterile ... 797
Synacort Creams 1%, 2.5% ... 2296
Vanoxide-HC Acne Lotion ... 911
Vioform-Hydrocortisone Cream and Mild Cream ... 889
Vioform-Hydrocortisone Ointment ... 889
VōSoL HC Otic Solution ... 2392
Vytone Cream 1% ... 911

Hydrocortisone Acetate (Decreased prothrombin time response). Products include:
Analpram-HC Rectal Cream 1% and 2.5% ... 970
Anusol-HC Cream ... 1690
Anusol-HC Suppositories ... 1691
Caldecort ... ▣ 560
Carmol HC Cream 1% ... 2296
Chloromycetin Hydrocortisone Ophthalmic ... 1694
Coly-Mycin S Otic w/Neomycin & Hydrocortisone ... 1708
Cortaid ... ▣ 735
Cortef Feminine Itch Cream ... ▣ 735
Corticaine ... ▣ 682
Cortifoam ... 1827
Cortisporin Cream ... 757
Epifoam ... 1828
Gynecort 5 Creme ... ▣ 556
Hydrocortone Acetate Sterile Suspension ... 1479
Lanacort 5 Creme and Ointment ... ▣ 557
Mantadil Cream ... 789
Ophthocort ... ◉ 301
Orabase HCA Oral Paste ... 890
Pramosone Cream, Lotion & Ointment ... 971
ProctoCream-HC ... 1834
Proctofoam-HC ... 1835

Hydrocortisone Sodium Phosphate (Decreased prothrombin time response). Products include:
Hydrocortone Phosphate Injection, Sterile 1481

Hydrocortisone Sodium Succinate (Decreased prothrombin time response). Products include:
Solu-Cortef Sterile Powder..... 2361

Hydroflumethiazide (Decreased or increased prothrombin time response). Products include:
Diucardin Tablets..... 2450
Saluron..... 718
Salutensin/Salutensin-Demi 719

Ibuprofen (Increased prothrombin time response). Products include:
Advil Cold & Sinus Caplets (formerly CoAdvil) 2416
Advil Ibuprofen Tablets and Caplets 2416
Children's Advil Suspension 2426
CoAdvil..... ▣ 748
Dristan Sinus Caplets..... 2419
Haltran Tablets..... ▣ 668
Ibuprofen..... ▣ 631
Medipren ibuprofen Caplets and Tablets 1362
Midol 200 Cramp Relief Formula.. ▣ 570
Motrin Tablets..... 2351
Motrin IB Caplets and Tablets ..... ▣ 736
Nuprin Ibuprofen/Analgesic Tablets & Caplets 752
PediaProfen Suspension..... 1363
Rufen Tablets 691
Trendar Ibuprofen Tablets..... ▣ 756

Indapamide (Decreased or increased prothrombin time response). Products include:
Lozol Tablets 1843

Indomethacin (Increased prothrombin time response). Products include:
Indocin 1487

Indomethacin Sodium Trihydrate (Increased prothrombin time response). Products include:
Indocin I.V. 1490

Influenza Virus Vaccine (Increased prothrombin time response). Products include:
Flu-Imune Influenza Virus Vaccine .. 1204

Isocarboxazid (Increased prothrombin time response). Products include:
Marplan Tablets 1906

Isoflurane (Increased prothrombin time response). Products include:
Forane..... 600

Levonorgestrel (Decreased prothrombin time response). Products include:
Levlen/Tri-Levlen..... 665
Nordette-21 Tablets..... 2481
Nordette-28 Tablets..... 2483
Norplant System 2484
Levlen/Tri-Levlen..... 665
Triphasil-21 Tablets..... 2527
Triphasil-28 Tablets..... 2532

Levorphanol Tartrate (Increased prothrombin response with proloned use). Products include:
Levo-Dromoran..... 1906

Levothyroxine Sodium (Increased prothrombin time response). Products include:
Levothroid Tablets 1003
Levoxine Tablets 904
Synthroid..... 695

Liothyronine Sodium (Increased prothrombin time response). Products include:
Cytomel Tablets 2203

Liotrix (Increased prothrombin time response). Products include:
Euthroid..... 1724

Lovastatin (Increased prothrombin time response). Products include:
Mevacor Tablets..... 1505

Magaldrate (Decreased prothrombin time response). Products include:
Riopan Antacid Chew Tablets..... ▣ 754
Riopan Antacid Chew Tablets in Rollpacks..... ▣ 754
Riopan Antacid Suspension..... 2421
Riopan Antacid Swallow Tablets 2421
Riopan Plus Chew Tablets 2422
Riopan Plus Chew Tablets in Rollpack..... 2422
Riopan Plus 2 Chew Tablets, Mint Flavor, Cherry Flavor 2422
Riopan Plus Suspension 2422
Riopan Plus 2 Suspension, Mint Flavor, Cherry Flavor 2422

Magnesium Hydroxide (Decreased prothrombin time response). Products include:
Aludrox Oral Suspension 2428
Ascriptin A/D Caplets 1850
Regular Strength Ascriptin Tablets 1850
Di-Gel Antacid/Anti-Gas ..... ▣ 697
Gelusil Liquid & Tablets ..... ▣ 639
Haley's M-O, Regular & Flavored .. ▣ 569
Extra Strength Maalox Plus Suspension..... 1850
Maalox TC Suspension 1851
Maalox Plus Tablets ..... ▣ 655
Extra Strength Maalox Plus Tablets 1850
Mylanta Liquid 1155
Mylanta Tablets 1155
Mylanta Double Strength Liquid 1155
Mylanta Double Strength Tablets 1155
Concentrated Phillips' Milk of Magnesia ..... ▣ 573
Phillips' Milk of Magnesia Liquid.... ▣ 572
Phillips' Milk of Magnesia Tablets ▣ 573
WinGel Liquid & Tablets ..... ▣ 761

Magnesium Oxide (Decreased prothrombin time response). Products include:
Bayer Plus Aspirin Tablets..... ▣ 567
Beelith Tablets 659
Bufferin Analgesic Tablets and Caplets ..... ▣ 524
Cama Arthritis Pain Reliever..... ▣ 685
Mag-Ox 400 673
Uro-Mag..... 673

Magnesium Salicylate (Increased prothrombin time response). Products include:
Doan's - Extra-Strength Analgesic ▣ 549
Doan's - Regular Strength Analgesic..... ▣ 549
Mobigesic Analgesic Tablets..... ▣ 507

Mefenamic Acid (Increased prothrombin time response). Products include:
Ponstel 1758

Meperidine Hydrochloride (Increased prothrombin time response with prolonged use). Products include:
Demerol 2047
Mepergan Injection 2479

Mephobarbital (Decreased prothrombin time response). Products include:
Mebaral Tablets 2061

Meprobamate (Decreased prothrombin time response). Products include:
Deprol Tablets..... 2382
Equagesic Tablets 2451
Miltown Tablets 2386
PMB 200 and PMB 400 2504

Mestranol (Decreased prothrombin time response). Products include:
Enovid..... 2161
Norethin..... 2133
Norinyl 2304
Ortho-Novum..... 1667

Methadone Hydrochloride (Increased prothrombin time response with proloned use). Products include:
Dolophine Hydrochloride Ampoules & Vials 1260
Dolophine Hydrochloride Tablets 1261
Methadone Hydrochloride Diskets .. 1284
Methadone Hydrochloride Oral Solution & Tablets..... 1987

Methdilazine Hydrochloride (Decreased prothrombin time response). Products include:
Tacaryl Syrup & Tablets 2409

Methoxyflurane (Increased prothrombin time response).
No products indexed under this heading.

Methyclothiazide (Decreased or increased prothrombin time response). Products include:
Enduron Tablets..... 517
Enduronyl 518

Methyldopa (Increased prothrombin time response). Products include:
Aldoclor Tablets 1413
Aldomet Oral 1415
Aldoril Tablets..... 1418

Methyldopate Hydrochloride (Increased prothrombin time response). Products include:
Aldomet Ester HCl Injection 1417

Methylphenidate Hydrochloride (Increased prothrombin time response). Products include:
Ritalin 880

Methylprednisolone Acetate (Decreased prothrombin time response). Products include:
Depo-Medrol Sterile Aqueous Suspension..... 2334

Methylprednisolone Sodium Succinate (Decreased prothrombin time response). Products include:
Solu-Medrol Sterile Powder..... 2363

Methyltestosterone (Increased prothrombin time response). Products include:
Android 1111
Estratest 2245
Mediatric Capsules 2476
Metandren Linguets and Tablets..... 875
Premarin with Methyltestosterone .. 2515
Testred Capsules..... 1124

Metolazone (Decreased or increased prothrombin time response). Products include:
Diulo 2129
Mykrox ½ mg Tablets 984
Zaroxolyn Tablets 989

Metronidazole (Increased prothrombin time response). Products include:
Flagyl I.V. RTU..... 2131
Flagyl Tablets 2170
MetroGel 903
Protostat Tablets..... 1674

Metronidazole Hydrochloride (Increased prothrombin time response). Products include:
Flagyl I.V. 2131

Miconazole (Increased prothrombin time response). Products include:
Monistat I.V. 1143

Morphine Sulfate (Increased prothrombin time response with prolonged use). Products include:
Astramorph/PF Injection, USP (Preservative-Free) 618
Duramorph..... 960
Infumorph 200 and Infumorph 500 Sterile Solutions..... 962
MS Contin Tablets..... 1814
MSIR 1817
Oramorph SR (Morphine Sulfate Sustained Release Tablets) 1988
Roxanol 1991

Nafcillin Sodium (Decreased prothrombin time response). Products include:
Unipen 2533

Nalidixic Acid (Increased prothrombin time response). Products include:
NegGram..... 2062

Naproxen (Increased prothrombin time response). Products include:
Naprosyn..... 2297

Naproxen Sodium (Increased prothrombin time response). Products include:
Anaprox and Anaprox DS Tablets.... 2288

Norethindrone (Decreased prothrombin time response). Products include:
Brevicon..... 2304
Jenest-28 Tablets 1636
Micronor Tablets 1667
Modicon..... 1667
Norethin..... 2133
Norinyl 2304
Norlutin 1755
Nor-Q D Tablets 2304
Ortho-Novum..... 1667
Ovcon 1391
Tri-Norinyl..... 2304

Norethynodrel (Decreased prothrombin time response). Products include:
Enovid..... 2161

Norfloxacin (Increased prothrombin time response). Products include:
Chibroxin Sterile Ophthalmic Solution..... 1431
Noroxin Tablets 1519

Norgestimate (Decreased prothrombin time response). Products include:
Ortho-Cyclen Tablets 1658

Norgestrel (Decreased prothrombin time response). Products include:
Lo/Ovral Tablets 2471
Lo/Ovral-28 Tablets..... 2476
Ovral Tablets..... 2490
Ovral-28 Tablets 2491
Ovrette Tablets 2492

Ofloxacin (Increased prothrombin time response). Products include:
Floxin Tablets 1652

Opium Alkaloids (Increased prothrombin time response with prolonged use). Products include:
B & O No. 15A & No. 16A Supprettes 2395
Pantopon Injectable 1911

Oxandrolone (Increased prothrombin time response).
No products indexed under this heading.

Oxycodone Hydrochloride (Increased prothrombin time response with prolonged use). Products include:
Percocet Tablets 950
Percodan..... 951
Roxicodone Tablets, Oral Solution & Intensol (Oxycodone) 1992
Tylox Capsules 1382

Oxymetholone (Increased prothrombin time response). Products include:
Anadrol-50 Tablets..... 2287

Oxyphenbutazone (Increased prothrombin time response).

Paraldehyde (Decreased prothrombin time response).

Pentobarbital Sodium (Decreased prothrombin time response). Products include:
Nembutal Sodium Capsules 534
Nembutal Sodium Solution 536
Nembutal Sodium Suppositories..... 538

Pentoxifylline (Increased prothrombin time response). Products include:
Trental 1099

Phenelzine Sulfate (Increased prothrombin time response). Products include:
Nardil 1742

Phenobarbital (Decreased prothrombin time response; accumulation of phenobarbital). Products include:
Arco-Lase Plus Tablets 607
Bellergal-S Tablets 1998

Bronkolixir ▣ 761
Bronkotabs Tablets ▣ 762
Donnatal 1858
Donnatal Extentabs 1859
Donnatal Tablets 1858
Donnazyme Tablets 1860
Kinesed Tablets 2272
Phenobarbital Elixir and Tablets 1293
Primatene Tablets-P Formula 2421
Quadrinal Tablets 1183
Tedral SA 1765

Phenylbutazone (Increased prothrombin time response). Products include:
Butazolidin Capsules & Tablets 1027

Phenytoin (Accumulation of phenytoin; increased prothrombin time response). Products include:
Dilantin Infatabs 1710
Dilantin-30 Pediatric/Dilantin-125 Suspension 1713

Phenytoin Sodium (Accumulation of phenytoin; increased prothrombin time response). Products include:
Dilantin Kapseals 1708
Dilantin Parenteral 1712
Dilantin with Phenobarbital Kapseals 1715

Polythiazide (Decreased or increased prothrombin time response). Products include:
Minizide Capsules 1779
Renese Tablets 1785
Renese-R Tablets 1786

Prednisolone Acetate (Decreased prothrombin time response). Products include:
AK-Cide Sterile Ophthalmic Ointment & Suspension ⊙ 202
Blephamide Liquifilm Sterile Ophthalmic Suspension 586
Blephamide S.O.P. Sterile Ophthalmic Ointment 586
Cetapred Ointment ⊙ 220
⅛% Econopred & 1% Econopred Plus ⊙ 217
Isopto Cetapred Suspension ⊙ 220
Metimyd ⊙ 306
Poly-Pred Liquifilm ⊙ 250
Pred Forte ⊙ 252
Pred Mild ⊙ 254
Pred-G Liquifilm Sterile Ophthalmic Suspension ⊙ 252
Pred-G S.O.P. Sterile Ophthalmic Ointment ⊙ 253
Vasocidin Ointment ⊙ 275

Prednisolone Sodium Phosphate (Decreased prothrombin time response). Products include:
AK-Pred ⊙ 205
Hydeltrasol Injection, Sterile 1476
Inflamase ⊙ 274
Pediapred Oral Liquid 987
Vasocidin Ophthalmic Solution ⊙ 276

Prednisolone Tebutate (Decreased prothrombin time response). Products include:
Hydeltra-T.B.A. Sterile Suspension 1478

Prednisone (Decreased prothrombin time response). Products include:
Deltasone Tablets 2332

Primidone (Decreased prothrombin time response). Products include:
Mysoline 2480

Promethazine Hydrochloride (Decreased prothrombin time response). Products include:
Mepergan Injection 2479
Phenergan with Codeine 2497
Phenergan with Dextromethorphan 2499
Phenergan Injection 2493
Phenergan Suppositories 2496
Phenergan Syrup 2495
Phenergan Tablets 2496
Phenergan VC 2500
Phenergan VC with Codeine 2501

Propafenone Hydrochloride (Increased prothrombin time response). Products include:
Rythmol Tablets 1184

Propoxyphene Hydrochloride (Increased prothrombin time response with prolonged use). Products include:
Darvon 1256
Wygesic Tablets 2540

Propoxyphene Napsylate (Increased prothrombin time response with prolonged use). Products include:
Darvon-N/Darvocet-N 1254

Pyrazolones (Increased prothrombin time response).

Pyrilamine Maleate (Decreased prothrombin time response). Products include:
Codimal 846
4-Way Fast Acting Nasal Spray - Original Formula (regular & mentholated) & Metered Spray Pump (regular) 751
Maximum Strength Midol Multi-Symptom Menstrual Formula ▣ 571
Maximum Strength Midol PMS Premenstrual Syndrome Formula ▣ 570
Regular Strength Midol Multi-Symptom Menstrual Formula ▣ 570
Prefrin-A ⊙ 255
Prēmsyn PMS Capsules & Caplets ▣ 547
Primatene Tablets-M Formula 2421
Robitussin Night Relief ▣ 677
Ru-Tuss with Hydrocodone 694
Triaminic Expectorant DH 1995
Triaminic Oral Infant Drops 1996

Pyrilamine Tannate (Decreased prothrombin time response). Products include:
Rynatan 2387

Quinidine Gluconate (Increased prothrombin time response). Products include:
Quinaglute Dura-Tabs Tablets 663

Quinidine Polygalacturonate (Increased prothrombin time response). Products include:
Cardioquin Tablets 1812

Quinidine Sulfate (Increased prothrombin time response). Products include:
Quinidex Extentabs 1868

Quinine Sulfate (Increased prothrombin time response). Products include:
Legatrin ▣ 556
Quinamm Tablets 1344
Q-vel Muscle Relaxant Pain Reliever ▣ 552

Ranitidine Hydrochloride (Decreased or increased prothrombin time response). Products include:
Zantac Injection and Zantac Injection Premixed 1063
Zantac 1065

Rifampin (Decreased prothrombin time response). Products include:
Rifadin 1345
Rifamate Capsules 1347
Rimactane Capsules 879

Salsalate (Increased prothrombin time response). Products include:
Disalcid 1310
Mono-Gesic Tablets 846
Salflex 839

Secobarbital Sodium (Decreased prothrombin time response). Products include:
Seconal Sodium Pulvules 1296

Selegiline Hydrochloride (Increased prothrombin time response). Products include:
Eldepryl 2250

Spironolactone (Decreased or increased prothrombin time response). Products include:
Aldactazide 2150
Aldactone 2152

Stanozolol (Increased prothrombin time response). Products include:
Winstrol Tablets 2075

Streptokinase (Concurrent use is not recommended and may be hazardous). Products include:
Kabikinase (Streptokinase) 1162
Streptase for Infusion 635

Sucralfate (Decreased prothrombin time response). Products include:
Carafate Tablets 1326

Sufentanil Citrate (Increased prothrombin time response with prolonged use). Products include:
Sufenta Injection 1147

Sulfamethizole (Increased prothrombin time response). Products include:
Thiosulfil Forte Tablets 2526
Urobiotic-250 Capsules 1968

Sulfamethoxazole (Increased prothrombin time response). Products include:
Azo Gantanol Tablets 1887
Bactrim DS Tablets 1891
Bactrim I.V. Infusion 1889
Bactrim 1891
Gantanol 1899
Septra 813
Septra I.V. Infusion 808
Septra I.V. Infusion ADD-Vantage Vials 810
Septra 813

Sulfasalazine (Increased prothrombin time response). Products include:
Azulfidine Tablets, EN-tabs, Oral Suspension 1157

Sulfinpyrazone (Increased prothrombin time response). Products include:
Anturane 853

Sulfisoxazole (Increased prothrombin time response). Products include:
Azo Gantrisin Tablets 1888
Gantrisin Tablets 1901
Pediazole 1973

Sulfisoxazole Diolamine (Increased prothrombin time response). Products include:
Gantrisin Ophthalmic Ointment/Solution 1900

Sulindac (Increased prothrombin time response). Products include:
Clinoril Tablets 1433

Tamoxifen Citrate (Increased prothrombin time response). Products include:
Nolvadex Tablets 1102

Terfenadine (Decreased prothrombin time response). Products include:
Seldane Tablets 1349
Seldane-D Extended-Release Tablets 1350

Thiamylal Sodium (Decreased prothrombin time response). Products include:
Surital Ampoules, Steri-Vials 1764

Thyroglobulin (Increased prothrombin time response). Products include:
Proloid Tablets 1761

Thyroid (Increased prothrombin time response). Products include:
S-P-T "Liquid" Capsules 995

Thyroxine (Increased prothrombin time response).
No products indexed under this heading.

Thyroxine Sodium (Increased prothrombin time response).
No products indexed under this heading.

Tolazamide (Increased prothrombin time response). Products include:
Tolinase Tablets 2365

Tolbutamide (Increased prothrombin time response; accumulation of tolbutamide). Products include:
Orinase Tablets 2354

Tranylcypromine Sulfate (Increased prothrombin time response). Products include:
Parnate Tablets 2222

Trazodone Hydrochloride (Decreased prothrombin time response). Products include:
Desyrel and Desyrel Dividose 1404

Triamcinolone (Decreased prothrombin time response).
No products indexed under this heading.

Triamcinolone Acetonide (Decreased prothrombin time response). Products include:
Aristocort A 1010
Azmacort Inhaler 1837
Kenalog Cream, Lotion & Ointment 2401
Kenalog-10 Injection 2402
Kenalog-40 Injection 2403
Kenalog in Orabase 604
Kenalog Spray 2401
Mycolog II Cream and Ointment 2407
Mytrex Cream & Ointment 2080
Nasacort Nasal Inhaler 1844

Triamcinolone Diacetate (Decreased prothrombin time response). Products include:
Aristocort Suspension 1008

Triamcinolone Hexacetonide (Decreased prothrombin time response). Products include:
Aristospan Suspension 1011

Triamterene (Decreased or increased prothrombin time response). Products include:
Dyazide Capsules 2208
Dyrenium Capsules 2210
Maxzide 1215

Trimeprazine Tartrate (Decreased prothrombin time response). Products include:
Temaril Tablets, Syrup and Spansule Sustained Release Capsules 1085

Trimethoprim (Increased prothrombin time response). Products include:
Bactrim DS Tablets 1891
Bactrim I.V. Infusion 1889
Bactrim 1891
Proloprim Tablets 799
Septra 813
Septra I.V. Infusion 808
Septra I.V. Infusion ADD-Vantage Vials 810
Septra 813
Trimpex Tablets 1922

Tripelennamine Hydrochloride (Decreased prothrombin time response). Products include:
PBZ Tablets & Elixir 1037
PBZ-SR Tablets 1037

Triprolidine Hydrochloride (Decreased prothrombin time response). Products include:
Actidil ▣ 538
Actifed Capsules ▣ 539
Actifed Plus Caplets ▣ 539
Actifed Plus Tablets ▣ 540
Actifed with Codeine Cough Syrup 752
Actifed Syrup ▣ 540
Actifed Tablets ▣ 540
Actifed 12-Hour Capsules ▣ 539

Urokinase (Concurrent use is not recommended and may be hazardous). Products include:
Abbokinase 503
Abbokinase Open-Cath 505

Vitamin C (Decreased prothrombin time response). Products include:
Allbee with C Caplets ▣ 670
Allbee C-800 ▣ 670
Bromase Capsules 672
Bugs Bunny Children's Chewable Vitamins (Sugar Free) ▣ 625
Bugs Bunny With Extra C Children's Chewable Vitamins (Sugar Free) ▣ 626

Bugs Bunny Plus Iron Children's Chewable Vitamins (Sugar Free) ▣ 625
Cefol Filmtab ... 509
Centrum, Jr. (Children's Chewable) + Extra C ... ▣ 585
Cod Liver Oil Concentrate Tablets with Vitamin C ... ▣ 694
Ester-C Tablets ... ▣ 575
Ferancee Chewable Tablets ... 1155
Ferancee-HP Tablets ... 1155
Fero-Folic-500 Filmtab ... 527
Fero-Grad-500 Filmtab ... 528
Flintstones Children's Chewable Vitamins ... ▣ 625
Flintstones Children's Chewable Vitamins With Extra C ... ▣ 626
Flintstones Children's Chewable Vitamins Plus Iron ... ▣ 625
Halls Vitamin C Drops ... ▣ 742
Hyland's Vitamin C for Children ... ▣ 729
ICAPS Plus ... ⊙ 280
Mediatric Capsules ... 2476
Mol-Iron w/Vitamin C Tablets ... ▣ 703
Natalins Rx ... 1391
Natalins Tablets ... 1391
N'ICE Sugarless Vitamin C Drops .. ▣ 719
Niferex w/Vitamin C Tablets ... 847
Ocuvite Vitamin and Mineral Supplement ... ⊙ 312
One-A-Day Essential Vitamins ... ▣ 627
One-A-Day Maximum Formula Vitamins and Minerals ... ▣ 627
One-A-Day Plus Extra C Vitamins .. ▣ 627
Probec-T Tablets ... ▣ 581
Stressgard Stress Formula Vitamins ... ▣ 628
Stuart Prenatal Tablets ... ▣ 731
The Stuart Formula Tablets ... 1157
Stuartinic Tablets ... 1157
Sunkist Children's Chewable Multivitamins - Plus Extra C ... ▣ 553
Sunkist Vitamin C ... ▣ 553
Surbex with C ... ▣ 502
Trinsicon Capsules ... 2415
Tri-Vi-Flor 1.0 mg Vitamins with Fluoride Chewable Tablets ... 1400
Tri-Vi-Flor Drops ... 1400
Tri-Vi-Sol Vitamin Drops ... ▣ 614
Tri-Vi-Sol Vitamin Drops with Iron ▣ 614
Vicon Forte Capsules ... 2416
Vicon Plus ... ▣ 682
Vicon-C ... ▣ 682
Vi-Daylin ADC Vitamins Drops ... 1980
Vi-Daylin ADC Vitamins + Iron Drops ... 1980
Vi-Daylin/F ADC Vitamins Drops With Fluoride ... 1981
Vi-Daylin/F ADC Vitamins + Iron Drops With Fluoride ... 1981
Vi-Zac ... ▣ 682
Within Women's Formula Multivitamin with Calcium, Extra Iron and Zinc ... ▣ 628
Z-Bec Tablets ... ▣ 678

Food Interactions

Diet high in vitamin K (Decreased prothrombin time).

Vegetables, green leafy (Large amounts of green leafy vegetables may affect Coumadin therapy).

CREON CAPSULES
(Pancreatin, Amylase) ... 2245

Food Interactions

Food having a pH greater than 5.5 (Dissolves the protective enteric coating).

CRITIC-AID, ANTIMICROBIAL SKIN PASTE
(Zinc Oxide, Benzethonium Chloride) 2286
No interactions described in labeling.

CRUEX ANTIFUNGAL POWDER
(Calcium Undecylenate, Zinc Undecylenate, Undecylenic Acid) .... ▣ 560
No interactions described in labeling.

CRYSTODIGIN TABLETS
(Digitoxin) ... 1253
May interact with antihistamines, anticonvulsants, barbiturates, oral hypoglycemic agents, diuretics, and certain other agents. Compounds in these categories include:

Amphotericin B (Increased potassium excretion). Products include:
Fungizone Cream, Lotion and Ointment ... 2261
Fungizone Intravenous ... 2262

Aprobarbital (Digitoxin metabolism stimulated). Products include:
Alurate Elixir ... 1883

Astemizole (Digitoxin metabolism stimulated). Products include:
Hismanal Tablets ... 1138

Azatadine Maleate (Digitoxin metabolism stimulated). Products include:
Optimine Tablets ... 2115
Trinalin Repetabs Tablets ... 1170

Bendroflumethiazide (Hypokalemia). Products include:
Corzide Tablets ... 702
Naturetin Tablets ... 1789
Rauzide Tablets ... 1804

Bromodiphenhydramine Hydrochloride (Digitoxin metabolism stimulated).
No products indexed under this heading.

Brompheniramine Maleate (Digitoxin metabolism stimulated). Products include:
Alka Seltzer Plus Sinus Allergy Medicine ... ▣ 624
Atrohist Sprinkle Capsules ... 558
Bromfed Capsules (Timed Release) ... 1615
Bromfed Syrup ... ▣ 628
Bromfed ... 1615
Dimetane Decongestant ... ▣ 673
Dimetane ... ▣ 672
Dimetane-DC Cough Syrup ... 1857
Dimetane-DX Cough Syrup ... 1858
Dimetapp Elixir ... ▣ 673
Dimetapp DM Elixir ... ▣ 674
Dimetapp Extentabs ... ▣ 674
Dimetapp Plus Caplets ... ▣ 675
Dimetapp Tablets ... ▣ 675
Drixoral Antihistamine/Nasal Decongestant Syrup ... ▣ 698

Bumetanide (Hypokalemia). Products include:
Bumex ... 1895

Butabarbital (Digitoxin metabolism stimulated). Products include:
Pyridium Plus ... 1764

Butalbital (Digitoxin metabolism stimulated). Products include:
Esgic-Plus Tablets ... 1002
Esgic Tablets & Capsules ... 1001
Fioricet Tablets ... 2006
Fiorinal Capsules ... 2007
Fiorinal with Codeine Capsules ... 2008
Fiorinal Tablets ... 2007
Phrenilin ... 838
Sedapap Tablets 50 mg/650 mg .. 1360

Calcium, intravenous (Concurrent use is contraindicated).

Carbamazepine (Digitoxin metabolism stimulated). Products include:
Tegretol Chewable Tablets ... 654
Tegretol Suspension ... 656
Tegretol Tablets ... 654

Chlorothiazide (Hypokalemia). Products include:
Aldoclor Tablets ... 1413
Diupres Tablets ... 1461
Diuril Oral ... 1464

Chlorothiazide Sodium (Hypokalemia). Products include:
Diuril Sodium Intravenous ... 1463

Chlorpheniramine Maleate (Digitoxin metabolism stimulated). Products include:
A.R.M. Allergy Relief Medicine Caplets ... ▣ 615
Alka-Seltzer Plus Cold Medicine .... ▣ 623
Allerest ... ▣ 559
Ana-Kit Anaphylaxis Emergency Treatment Kit ... 1100
BC Cold Powder Multi-Symptom Formula ... ▣ 517
Brexin L.A. Capsules ... 2078
Cerose-DM ... 2443
Cheracol Plus Head Cold/Cough Formula ... ▣ 667
Chlor-Trimeton Allergy Syrup, Tablets & Long-Acting Repetabs Tablets ... ▣ 693
Chlor-Trimeton Decongestant ... ▣ 694
Comhist LA Capsules ... 1618
Allergy-Sinus Comtrex Multi-Symptom Allergy Sinus Formula Tablets & Caplets ... 746
Comtrex Multi-Symptom Cold Reliever Tablets/Caplets/Liqui-Gels/Liquid ... 745
Day-Night Comtrex ... 747
Contac Continuous Action Decongestant/Antihistamine Capsules ▣ 710
Contac Maximum Strength Continuous Action Decongestant/Antihistamine Caplets ... ▣ 709
Contac Severe Cold and Flu Formula Caplets ... ▣ 711
Coricidin 'D' Decongestant Tablets ... ▣ 695
Coricidin Demilets Tablets for Children ... ▣ 696
Coricidin Tablets ... ▣ 695
Deconamine ... 663
Demazin Nasal Decongestant/Antihistamine Repetabs Tablets & Syrup ... ▣ 697
Dorcol Children's Liquid Cold Formula ... ▣ 686
Dristan Decongestant/Antihistamine/ Analgesic Coated Caplets ... ▣ 749
Dristan Cold Nasal Decongestant/Antihistamine/ Analgesic Coated Tablets ... 2419
Dristan Advanced Formula Decongestant/Antihistamine/Analgesic Tablets ... ▣ 749
Extendryl ... 994
4-Way Cold Tablets ... 750
Fedahist Gyrocaps ... 2145
Fedahist Timecaps ... 2145
Hycomine Compound Tablets ... 929
Isoclor Timesule Capsules ... ▣ 561
Kronofed-A ... 970
Medi-Flu Caplet, Liquid ... ▣ 640
Naldecon Syrup, Tablets, Pediatric Drops and Pediatric Syrup ... 709
Nolamine Tablets ... 838
Novafed A Capsules ... 1342
Novahistine DH ... 1342
Novahistine Elixir ... ▣ 596
Ornade Spansule Capsules ... 2221
Orthoxicol Cough Syrup ... ▣ 668
PediaCare Allergy Relief Formula Liquid ... 1362
PediaCare Cough-Cold Formula Liquid ... 1362
PediaCare Night Rest Cough-Cold Formula Liquid ... 1362
PediaCare 6-12 Cough-Cold Formula Chewable Tablets ... 1362
Pyrroxate Capsules ... ▣ 669
Quelidrine Syrup ... 556
Ru-Tuss II Capsules ... 693
Ru-Tuss Tablets ... 693
Ryna ... ▣ 741
Sinarest Tablets & Extra Strength Tablets ... ▣ 562
Sine-Off Maximum Strength Allergy/Sinus Formula Caplets ... ▣ 721
Sine-Off Sinus Medicine Tablets-Aspirin Formula ... ▣ 722
Singlet Tablets ... ▣ 598
Sinulin ... 840
Sinutab Maximum Strength ... ▣ 641
St. Joseph Nighttime Cold Medicine ... ▣ 705
Sudafed Plus Liquid ... ▣ 544
Sudafed Plus Tablets ... ▣ 545
Teldrin Timed-Release Allergy Capsules, 12 mg ... 2192
TheraFlu Flu and Cold Medicine .... ▣ 687
Triaminic Allergy Tablets ... ▣ 688
Triaminic Chewables ... ▣ 688
Triaminic Cold Tablets ... ▣ 688
Triaminic Nite Light ... ▣ 689
Triaminic Syrup ... ▣ 689
Triaminic-12 Tablets ... ▣ 690
Triaminicin Tablets ... ▣ 690
Triaminicol Multi-Symptom Cold Tablets ... ▣ 691
Triaminicol Multi-Symptom Relief ▣ 691
Tylenol Allergy Sinus Medication Caplets and Gelcaps, Maximum Strength ... 1372
Children's Tylenol Cold Liquid Formula and Chewable Tablets 1368
Tylenol Cold & Flu Hot Medication, Packets ... 1369
Tylenol Cold Medication Caplets and Tablets ... 1370
Tylenol Cold Medication, Effervescent Tablets ... 1369
Vicks Children's NyQuil ... ▣ 664
Vicks Formula 44 Cough Medicine ... ▣ 661
Vicks Formula 44M Multi-Symptom Cough Medicine ... ▣ 662
Vicks Pediatric Formula 44m Multi-Symptom Cough & Cold Medicine ... ▣ 663

Chlorpheniramine Polistirex (Digitoxin metabolism stimulated). Products include:
Tussionex Extended-Release Suspension ... 988

Chlorpheniramine Tannate (Digitoxin metabolism stimulated). Products include:
Rynatan ... 2387
Rynatuss ... 2388

Chlorpropamide (Digitoxin metabolism stimulated). Products include:
Diabinese Tablets ... 1775

Chlorthalidone (Hypokalemia). Products include:
Combipres Tablets ... 678
Tenoretic Tablets ... 1105
Thalitone Tablets ... 687

Clemastine Fumarate (Digitoxin metabolism stimulated). Products include:
Tavist Syrup ... 2033
Tavist Tablets ... 2035
Tavist-D Tablets ... 2035

Cyproheptadine Hydrochloride (Digitoxin metabolism stimulated). Products include:
Periactin ... 1525

Dexchlorpheniramine Maleate (Digitoxin metabolism stimulated). Products include:
Polaramine ... 2116

Diphenhydramine Citrate (Digitoxin metabolism stimulated). Products include:
Alka-Seltzer Plus Night-Time Cold Medicine ... ▣ 623
Bufferin AF Nite Time Analgesic/Sleeping Aid Caplets ... 744
Excedrin P.M. Analgesic/Sleeping Aid Tablets, Caplets and Liquid 749

Diphenylpyraline Hydrochloride (Digitoxin metabolism stimulated).
No products indexed under this heading.

Divalproex Sodium (Digitoxin metabolism stimulated). Products include:
Depakote ... 512

Ethacrynic Acid (Hypokalemia). Products include:
Edecrin Tablets ... 1468

Ethosuximide (Digitoxin metabolism stimulated). Products include:
Zarontin Capsules ... 1768
Zarontin Syrup ... 1769

Ethotoin (Digitoxin metabolism stimulated). Products include:
Peganone Tablets ... 551

Furosemide (Hypokalemia). Products include:
Lasix ... 1093

Glipizide (Digitoxin metabolism stimulated). Products include:
Glucotrol ... 1952

Glyburide (Digitoxin metabolism stimulated). Products include:
DiaBeta ... 1091
Micronase Tablets ... 2350

Hydrochlorothiazide (Hypokalemia). Products include:
Aldactazide ... 2150
Aldoril Tablets ... 1418
Apresazide Capsules ... 854

Apresoline-Esidrix Tablets 857
Capozide 2258
Dyazide Capsules 2208
Esidrix Tablets 863
Esimil Tablets 864
HydroDIURIL Tablets 1484
Hydropres Tablets 1485
Inderide Tablets 2463
Inderide LA Long Acting Capsules .. 2465
Lopressor HCT Tablets 1034
Maxzide 1215
Moduretic Tablets 1510
Normozide Tablets 2112
Oretic Tablets 544
Oreticyl 545
Prinzide Tablets 1540
Ser-Ap-Es Tablets 881
Serpasil-Esidrix Tablets 886
Timolide Tablets 1547
Trandate HCT Tablets 579
Vaseretic Tablets 1559
Zestoretic 2274

Hydroflumethiazide (Hypokalemia). Products include:
Diucardin Tablets 2450
Saluron 718
Salutensin/Salutensin-Demi 719

Indapamide (Hypokalemia). Products include:
Lozol Tablets 1843

Mephenytoin (Digitoxin metabolism stimulated). Products include:
Mesantoin Tablets 2013

Mephobarbital (Digitoxin metabolism stimulated). Products include:
Mebaral Tablets 2061

Methdilazine Hydrochloride (Digitoxin metabolism stimulated). Products include:
Tacaryl Syrup & Tablets 2409

Methsuximide (Digitoxin metabolism stimulated). Products include:
Celontin 1692

Methyclothiazide (Hypokalemia). Products include:
Enduron Tablets 517
Enduronyl 518

Metolazone (Hypokalemia). Products include:
Diulo 2129
Mykrox ½ mg Tablets 984
Zaroxolyn Tablets 989

Paramethadione (Digitoxin metabolism stimulated). Products include:
Paradione Capsules 548

Pentobarbital Sodium (Digitoxin metabolism stimulated). Products include:
Nembutal Sodium Capsules 534
Nembutal Sodium Solution 536
Nembutal Sodium Suppositories 538

Phenacemide (Digitoxin metabolism stimulated). Products include:
Phenurone Tablets 552

Phenobarbital (Increases rate of metabolism of digitoxin). Products include:
Arco-Lase Plus Tablets 607
Bellergal-S Tablets 1998
Bronkolixir .... ▣ 761
Bronkotabs Tablets .... ▣ 762
Donnatal 1858
Donnatal Extentabs 1859
Donnatal Tablets 1858
Donnazyme Tablets 1860
Kinesed Tablets 2272
Phenobarbital Elixir and Tablets 1293
Primatene Tablets-P Formula 2421
Quadrinal Tablets 1183
Tedral SA 1765

Phensuximide (Digitoxin metabolism stimulated). Products include:
Milontin Kapseals 1741

Phenylbutazone (Increased rate of digitoxin metabolism). Products include:
Butazolidin Capsules & Tablets 1027

Phenytoin (Increased rate of digitoxin metabolism). Products include:
Dilantin Infatabs 1710
Dilantin-30 Pediatric/Dilantin-125 Suspension 1713

Phenytoin Sodium (Increased rate of digitoxin metabolism). Products include:
Dilantin Kapseals 1708
Dilantin Parenteral 1712
Dilantin with Phenobarbital Kapseals 1715

Polythiazide (Hypokalemia). Products include:
Minizide Capsules 1779
Renese Tablets 1785
Renese-R Tablets 1786

Prednisone (Increased potassium excretion). Products include:
Deltasone Tablets 2332

Primidone (Digitoxin metabolism stimulated). Products include:
Mysoline 2480

Promethazine Hydrochloride (Digitoxin metabolism stimulated). Products include:
Mepergan Injection 2479
Phenergan with Codeine 2497
Phenergan with Dextromethorphan 2499
Phenergan Injection 2493
Phenergan Suppositories 2496
Phenergan Syrup 2495
Phenergan Tablets 2496
Phenergan VC 2500
Phenergan VC with Codeine 2501

Pyrilamine Maleate (Digitoxin metabolism stimulated). Products include:
Codimal 846
4-Way Fast Acting Nasal Spray - Original Formula (regular & mentholated) & Metered Spray Pump (regular) 751
Maximum Strength Midol Multi-Symptom Menstrual Formula .... ▣ 571
Maximum Strength Midol PMS Premenstrual Syndrome Formula .... ▣ 570
Regular Strength Midol Multi-Symptom Menstrual Formula .... ▣ 570
Prefrin-A .... ⊙ 255
Prēmsyn PMS Capsules & Caplets ▣ 547
Primatene Tablets-M Formula 2421
Robitussin Night Relief .... ▣ 677
Ru-Tuss with Hydrocodone 694
Triaminic Expectorant DH 1995
Triaminic Oral Infant Drops 1996

Pyrilamine Tannate (Digitoxin metabolism stimulated). Products include:
Rynatan 2387

Secobarbital Sodium (Digitoxin metabolism stimulated). Products include:
Seconal Sodium Pulvules 1296

Terfenadine (Digitoxin metabolism stimulated). Products include:
Seldane Tablets 1349
Seldane-D Extended-Release Tablets 1350

Thiamylal Sodium (Digitoxin metabolism stimulated). Products include:
Surital Ampoules, Steri-Vials 1764

Tolazamide (Digitoxin metabolism stimulated). Products include:
Tolinase Tablets 2365

Tolbutamide (Digitoxin metabolism stimulated). Products include:
Orinase Tablets 2354

Trimeprazine Tartrate (Digitoxin metabolism stimulated). Products include:
Temaril Tablets, Syrup and Spansule Sustained Release Capsules 1085

Trimethadione (Digitoxin metabolism stimulated). Products include:
Tridione 557

Tripelennamine Hydrochloride (Digitoxin metabolism stimulated). Products include:
PBZ Tablets & Elixir 1037
PBZ-SR Tablets 1037

Triprolidine Hydrochloride (Digitoxin metabolism stimulated). Products include:
Actidil .... ▣ 538
Actifed Capsules .... ▣ 539
Actifed Plus Caplets .... ▣ 539
Actifed Plus Tablets .... ▣ 540
Actifed with Codeine Cough Syrup.. 752
Actifed Syrup .... ▣ 540
Actifed Tablets .... ▣ 540
Actifed 12-Hour Capsules .... ▣ 539

Valproic Acid (Digitoxin metabolism stimulated). Products include:
Depakene Capsules & Syrup 511

CUPRIMINE CAPSULES
(Penicillamine) 1442
May interact with cytotoxic drugs, antimalarials, and certain other agents. Compounds in these categories include:

Auranofin (Concurrent use not recommended). Products include:
Ridaura Capsules 2224

Aurothioglucose (Concurrent use not recommended). Products include:
Solganal Suspension 2122

Bleomycin Sulfate (Concurrent use not recommended). Products include:
Blenoxane 724

Chloroquine Hydrochloride (Concurrent use not recommended). Products include:
Aralen Hydrochloride Injection 2038

Chloroquine Phosphate (Concurrent use not recommended). Products include:
Aralen Phosphate with Primaquine Phosphate Tablets 2040
Aralen Phosphate Tablets 2039

Daunorubicin Hydrochloride (Concurrent use not recommended). Products include:
Cerubidine 2443

Doxorubicin Hydrochloride (Concurrent use not recommended). Products include:
Adriamycin PFS 561
Adriamycin RDF 562
Doxorubicin Hydrochloride for Injection, USP 622
Doxorubicin Hydrochloride Injection, USP 848
Rubex 739

Fluorouracil (Concurrent use not recommended). Products include:
Efudex 1880
Fluoroplex Topical Solution & Cream 1% 1082
Fluorouracil Injection 1897

Hydroxychloroquine Sulfate (Concurrent use not recommended). Products include:
Plaquenil Sulfate Tablets 2067

Hydroxyurea (Concurrent use not recommended). Products include:
Hydrea Capsules 728

Mefloquine Hydrochloride (Concurrent use not recommended). Products include:
Lariam Tablets 1904

Methotrexate Sodium (Concurrent use not recommended). Products include:
Methotrexate Tablets, Parenteral, LPF Parenteral 1217
Rheumatrex Methotrexate Dose Pack 1234

Mineral Supplements (Block response).

Mitotane (Concurrent use not recommended). Products include:
Lysodren 731

Mitoxantrone Hydrochloride (Concurrent use not recommended). Products include:
Novantrone for Injection Concentrate 1226

Oxyphenbutazone (Concurrent use not recommended).

Phenylbutazone (Concurrent use not recommended). Products include:
Butazolidin Capsules & Tablets 1027

Procarbazine Hydrochloride (Concurrent use not recommended). Products include:
Matulane Capsules 1907

Pyridoxine (Penicillamine increases pyridoxine requirement).

Pyrimethamine (Concurrent use not recommended). Products include:
Daraprim Tablets 761
Fansidar Tablets 1896

Tamoxifen Citrate (Concurrent use not recommended). Products include:
Nolvadex Tablets 1102

Vincristine Sulfate (Concurrent use not recommended). Products include:
Oncovin Solution Vials & Hyporets 1288

CUTIVATE CREAM 0.05%
(Fluticasone Propionate) 1054
No interactions described in labeling.

CUTIVATE OINTMENT 0.005%
(Fluticasone Propionate) 1054
No interactions described in labeling.

CYCLOCORT CREAM
(Amcinonide) 1198
No interactions described in labeling.

CYCLOCORT LOTION
(Amcinonide) 1198
No interactions described in labeling.

CYCLOCORT OINTMENT
(Amcinonide) 1198
No interactions described in labeling.

CYCLOGYL
(Cyclopentolate Hydrochloride) .... ⊙ 215
May interact with ophthalmic cholinesterase inhibitors and ophthalmic cholinergic miotics. Compounds in these categories include:

Carbachol (Cyclopentolate may interfere with antiglaucoma action of cholinergics). Products include:
Isopto Carbachol .... ⊙ 219
MIOSTAT .... ⊙ 233

Demecarium Bromide (Cyclopentolate may antagonize the antiglaucoma and miotic actions). Products include:
Humorsol Sterile Ophthalmic Solution 1475

Echothiophate Iodide (Cyclopentolate may antagonize the antiglaucoma and miotic actions). Products include:
Phospholine Iodide .... ⊙ 315

Isoflurophate (Cyclopentolate may antagonize the antiglaucoma and miotic actions). Products include:
Floropryl Sterile Ophthalmic Ointment 1473

Physostigmine Salicylate (Cyclopentolate may antagonize the antiglaucoma and miotic actions). Products include:
Antilirium Injectable 998

Pilocarpine (Cyclopentolate may interfere with antiglaucoma action of cholinergics). Products include:
Ocusert Pilo-20 and Pilo-40 Ocular Therapeutic Systems .... ⊙ 256

(▣ Described in PDR For Nonprescription Drugs) (⊙ Described in PDR For Ophthalmology)

Pilocarpine Hydrochloride (Cyclopentolate may interfere with antiglaucoma action of cholinergics). Products include:
Akarpine Ophthalmic Solution .... ◉ 201
Isopto Carpine .... ◉ 219
Pilocar .... ◉ 275
Pilopine HS Gel .... ◉ 227
Pilostat Sterile Ophthalmic Solution 0.5%, 1%, 2%, 3%, 4%, 5%, 6% .... ◉ 263
Pilocarpine Nitrate (Cyclopentolate may interfere with antiglaucoma action of cholinergics). Products include:
Pilagan .... ◉ 250

CYCLOMYDRIL
(Cyclopentolate Hydrochloride, Phenylephrine Hydrochloride) .... ◉ 216
No interactions described in labeling.

CYCRIN TABLETS
(Medroxyprogesterone Acetate) 2449
No interactions described in labeling.

CYKLOKAPRON TABLETS AND INJECTION
(Tranexamic Acid) 1159
No interactions described in labeling.

CYLERT CHEWABLE TABLETS
(Pemoline) 510
See **Cylert Tablets**

CYLERT TABLETS
(Pemoline) 510
May interact with anticonvulsants and central nervous system stimulants. Compounds in these categories include:

Amphetamine Resins (Effects not specified). Products include:
Biphetamine Capsules 973
Carbamazepine (Decreased seizure threshold). Products include:
Tegretol Chewable Tablets 654
Tegretol Suspension 656
Tegretol Tablets 654
Dextroamphetamine Sulfate (Effects not specified). Products include:
Dexedrine 2206
Divalproex Sodium (Decreased seizure threshold). Products include:
Depakote 512
Ethosuximide (Decreased seizure threshold). Products include:
Zarontin Capsules 1768
Zarontin Syrup 1769
Ethotoin (Decreased seizure threshold). Products include:
Peganone Tablets 551
Mephenytoin (Decreased seizure threshold). Products include:
Mesantoin Tablets 2013
Methamphetamine Hydrochloride (Effects not specified). Products include:
Desoxyn Gradumet Tablets 514
Methsuximide (Decreased seizure threshold). Products include:
Celontin 1692
Methylphenidate Hydrochloride (Effects not specified). Products include:
Ritalin 880
Paramethadione (Decreased seizure threshold). Products include:
Paradione Capsules 548
Phenacemide (Decreased seizure threshold). Products include:
Phenurone Tablets 552
Phenobarbital (Decreased seizure threshold). Products include:
Arco-Lase Plus Tablets 607
Bellergal-S Tablets 1998
Bronkolixir .... ᴺᴰ 761
Bronkotabs Tablets .... ᴺᴰ 762
Donnatal 1858
Donnatal Extentabs 1859
Donnatal Tablets 1858
Donnazyme Tablets 1860
Kinesed Tablets 2272
Phenobarbital Elixir and Tablets 1293
Primatene Tablets-P Formula 2421
Quadrinal Tablets 1183
Tedral SA 1765
Phensuximide (Decreased seizure threshold). Products include:
Milontin Kapseals 1741
Phenytoin (Decreased seizure threshold). Products include:
Dilantin Infatabs 1710
Dilantin-30 Pediatric/Dilantin-125 Suspension 1713
Phenytoin Sodium (Decreased seizure threshold). Products include:
Dilantin Kapseals 1708
Dilantin Parenteral 1712
Dilantin with Phenobarbital Kapseals 1715
Primidone (Decreased seizure threshold). Products include:
Mysoline 2480
Trimethadione (Decreased seizure threshold). Products include:
Tridione 557
Valproic Acid (Decreased seizure threshold). Products include:
Depakene Capsules & Syrup 511

CYSTOSPAZ TABLETS
(Hyoscyamine) 2395
No interactions described in labeling.

CYSTOSPAZ-M CAPSULES
(Hyoscyamine Sulfate) 2395
No interactions described in labeling.

CYTADREN TABLETS
(Aminoglutethimide) 861
May interact with oral anticoagulants and certain other agents. Compounds in these categories include:

Alcohol (Effects of alcohol potentiated).
Dexamethasone (Accelerates metabolism of dexamethasone). Products include:
AK-Trol Ointment & Suspension .... ◉ 207
Decadron Elixir 1445
Decadron Tablets 1447
Decaspray Topical Aerosol 1459
Dexacidin .... ◉ 272
Maxidex Sterile Ophthalmic Suspension .... ◉ 223
Maxitrol Ophthalmic Ointment/Suspension .... ◉ 223
TobraDex Ophthalmic Suspension and Ointment .... ◉ 228
Dexamethasone Acetate (Accelerates metabolism of dexamethasone). Products include:
Dalalone D.P. Injectable 999
Decadron-LA Sterile Suspension 1457
Dexamethasone Phosphate (Accelerates metabolism of dexamethasone).
No products indexed under this heading.
Dexamethasone Sodium Phosphate (Accelerates metabolism of dexamethasone). Products include:
AK-Dex .... ◉ 203
Decadron Phosphate Respihaler 1454
Decadron Phosphate Sterile Ophthalmic Ointment 1453
Decadron Phosphate Sterile Ophthalmic Solution 1453
Decadron Phosphate Topical Cream 1455
Decadron Phosphate Turbinaire 1456
Maxidex Sterile Ophthalmic Ointment .... ◉ 222
NeoDecadron Sterile Ophthalmic Ointment 1517
NeoDecadron Sterile Ophthalmic Solution 1518
NeoDecadron Topical Cream 1518
Dexamethasone Sodium Phosphate Injection (Accelerates metabolism of dexamethasone). Products include:
Decadron Phosphate Injection 1449
Decadron Phosphate with Xylocaine Injection, Sterile 1451
Dicumarol (Diminishes anticoagulant effect). Products include:
Dicumarol Tablets 516
Warfarin Sodium (Diminishes anticoagulant effect). Products include:
Coumadin Injection & Tablets 944
Panwarfin Tablets 547

CYTOGAM
(Cytomegalovirus Immune Globulin).. 891
May interact with:

Measles, Mumps & Rubella Virus Vaccine Live (May interfere with the immune response to live virus vaccine). Products include:
M-M-R II 1494

CYTOMEL TABLETS
(Sodium Liothyronine) 2203
May interact with oral anticoagulants, insulin, oral hypoglycemic agents, estrogens, oral contraceptives, tricyclic antidepressants, cardiac glycosides, and certain other agents. Compounds in these categories include:

Amitriptyline Hydrochloride (Enhanced antidepressant and thyroid activities). Products include:
Elavil 2269
Endep Tablets 1927
Etrafon 2087
Limbitrol 1933
Triavil Tablets 1556
Amoxapine (Enhanced antidepressant and thyroid activities). Products include:
Asendin Tablets 1196
Chlorpropamide (Possible increase in oral hypoglycemic requirements). Products include:
Diabinese Tablets 1775
Cholestyramine (Impaired absorption of T4 and T3). Products include:
Cholybar 1705
Questran Light 711
Questran Powder 710
Clomipramine Hydrochloride (Enhanced antidepressant and thyroid activities). Products include:
Anafranil Capsules 650
Desipramine Hydrochloride (Enhanced antidepressant and thyroid activities). Products include:
Norpramin Tablets 1340
Deslanoside (Toxic effects of digitalis glycosides potentiated).
No products indexed under this heading.
Dicumarol (Reduction of anticoagulant dosage may be necessary). Products include:
Dicumarol Tablets 516
Dienestrol (Increases thyroid requirements). Products include:
Ortho Dienestrol Cream 1664
Diethylstilbestrol (Increases thyroid requirements). Products include:
Diethylstilbestrol Tablets 1258
Digitoxin (Toxic effects of digitalis glycosides potentiated). Products include:
Crystodigin Tablets 1253
Digoxin (Toxic effects of digitalis glycosides potentiated). Products include:
Lanoxicaps 772
Lanoxin Elixir Pediatric 775
Lanoxin Injection 778
Lanoxin Injection Pediatric 781
Lanoxin Tablets 783
Doxepin Hydrochloride (Enhanced antidepressant and thyroid activities). Products include:
Sinequan 1960
Epinephrine (Increased adrenergic effect; increased risk of precipitating coronary insufficiency). Products include:
Ana-Kit Anaphylaxis Emergency Treatment Kit 1100
Bronkaid Mist .... ᴺᴰ 757
EpiPen 843
Marcaine Hydrochloride 0.5% with Epinephrine 1:200,000 (as bitartrate) 958
Marcaine Hydrochloride with Epinephrine 1:200,000 2055
Primatene Mist 2420
Sus-Phrine Injection 1006
Xylocaine with Epinephrine Injections 637
Epinephrine Bitartrate (Increased adrenergic effect; increased risk of precipitating coronary insufficiency). Products include:
AsthmaHaler Mist Epinephrine Bitartrate Bronchodilator .... ᴺᴰ 616
Bronkaid Mist Suspension .... ᴺᴰ 757
Primatene Mist Suspension 2421
Estradiol (Increases thyroid requirements). Products include:
Emcyt Capsules 1161
Estrace 1385
Estrace Vaginal Cream 1388
Estraderm Transdermal System 866
Estrogens, Conjugated (Increases thyroid requirements). Products include:
Mediatric Capsules 2476
PMB 200 and PMB 400 2504
Premarin Intravenous 2508
Premarin with Methyltestosterone 2515
Premarin Tablets 2510
Premarin Vaginal Cream 2512
Estrogens, Esterified (Increases thyroid requirements). Products include:
Estratest 2245
Menrium Tablets 1934
Estropipate (Increases thyroid requirements). Products include:
Ogen 540
Ethinyl Estradiol (Increases thyroid requirements). Products include:
Brevicon 2304
Demulen 2161
Estinyl Tablets 2085
Jenest-28 Tablets 1636
Levlen/Tri-Levlen 665
Lo/Ovral Tablets 2471
Lo/Ovral-28 Tablets 2476
Loestrin 1728
Modicon 1667
Nordette-21 Tablets 2481
Nordette-28 Tablets 2483
Norethin 2133
Norinyl 2304
Norlestrin 1746
Ortho-Cyclen Tablets 1658
Ortho-Novum 1667
Ovcon 1391
Ovral Tablets 2490
Ovral-28 Tablets 2491
Levlen/Tri-Levlen 665
Tri-Norinyl 2304
Triphasil-21 Tablets 2527
Triphasil-28 Tablets 2532
Ethynodiol Diacetate (Increases thyroid requirements). Products include:
Demulen 2161
Glipizide (Possible increase in oral hypoglycemic requirements). Products include:
Glucotrol 1952
Glyburide (Possible increase in oral hypoglycemic requirements). Products include:
DiaBeta 1091

Micronase Tablets 2350

Imipramine Hydrochloride (Enhanced antidepressant and thyroid activities). Products include:
- Tofranil Ampuls 1038
- Tofranil Tablets 1039

Imipramine Pamoate (Enhanced antidepressant and thyroid activities). Products include:
- Tofranil-PM Capsules 1041

Insulin, Human (Possible increase in insulin requirements).
No products indexed under this heading.

Insulin, Human Isophane Suspension (Possible increase in insulin requirements). Products include:
- Humulin N, 100 Units 1270

Insulin, Human NPH (Possible increase in insulin requirements). Products include:
- Insulatard NPH Human 1627
- Novolin N 1627
- Novolin N PenFill Cartridges 1628
- Novolin N Prefilled 1628

Insulin, Human Regular (Possible increase in insulin requirements). Products include:
- Humulin BR, 100 Units 1268
- Humulin R, 100 Units 1272
- Novolin R 1627
- Novolin R PenFill Cartridges 1628
- Novolin R Prefilled 1629
- Velosulin Human 1628

Insulin, Human, Zinc Suspension (Possible increase in insulin requirements). Products include:
- Humulin L, 100 Units 1268
- Humulin U, 100 Units 1272
- Novolin L 1627

Insulin, NPH (Possible increase in insulin requirements). Products include:
- NPH, 40 & 100 Units 1273
- Beef NPH, 100 Units 1274
- Pork NPH, 100 Units 1275
- Insulatard NPH 1626
- NPH Insulin 1626
- NPH Purified Pork Isophane Insulin 1626

Insulin, Regular (Possible increase in insulin requirements). Products include:
- Regular, 40 & 100 Units 1273
- Beef Regular, 100 Units 1275
- Pork Regular, 100 Units 1275
- Pork Regular (Concentrated), 500 Units 1276
- Regular Insulin 1625
- Regular Purified Pork Insulin 1626
- Velosulin 1627

Insulin, Zinc Crystals (Possible increase in insulin requirements). Products include:
- NPH, 40 & 100 Units 1273

Insulin, Zinc Suspension (Possible increase in insulin requirements). Products include:
- Lente, 40 & 100 Units 1272
- Protamine, Zinc, 40 & 100 Units 1273
- Lente Iletin I 1272
- Beef Lente, 100 Units 1274
- Beef Protamine Zinc, 100 Units 1274
- Pork Lente, 100 Units 1275
- Pork, Protamine, Zinc, 100 Units 1275
- Lente Insulin 1626
- Lente Purified Pork Insulin 1626
- Semilente Insulin 1625
- Ultralente Insulin 1626

Ketamine Hydrochloride (May cause hypertension, and tachycardia). Products include:
- Ketalar 1726

Levonorgestrel (Increases thyroid requirements). Products include:
- Levlen/Tri-Levlen 665
- Nordette-21 Tablets 2481
- Nordette-28 Tablets 2483
- Norplant System 2484
- Levlen/Tri-Levlen 665
- Triphasil-21 Tablets 2527
- Triphasil-28 Tablets 2532

Maprotiline Hydrochloride (Enhanced antidepressant and thyroid activities). Products include:
- Ludiomil Tablets 874

Mestranol (Increases thyroid requirements). Products include:
- Enovid 2161
- Norethin 2133
- Norinyl 2304
- Ortho-Novum 1667

Norepinephrine Bitartrate (Increased adrenergic effect; increased risk of precipitating coronary insufficiency). Products include:
- Levophed Bitartrate Injection 2054

Norethindrone (Increases thyroid requirements). Products include:
- Brevicon 2304
- Jenest-28 Tablets 1636
- Micronor Tablets 1667
- Modicon 1667
- Norethin 2133
- Norinyl 2304
- Norlutin 1755
- Nor-Q D Tablets 2304
- Ortho-Novum 1667
- Ovcon 1391
- Tri-Norinyl 2304

Norethynodrel (Increases thyroid requirements). Products include:
- Enovid 2161

Norgestimate (Increases thyroid requirements). Products include:
- Ortho-Cyclen Tablets 1658

Norgestrel (Increases thyroid requirements). Products include:
- Lo/Ovral Tablets 2471
- Lo/Ovral-28 Tablets 2476
- Ovral Tablets 2490
- Ovral-28 Tablets 2491
- Ovrette Tablets 2492

Nortriptyline Hydrochloride (Enhanced antidepressant and thyroid activities). Products include:
- Pamelor 2019

Polyestradiol Phosphate (Increases thyroid requirements). Products include:
- Estradurin 2452

Protriptyline Hydrochloride (Enhanced antidepressant and thyroid activities). Products include:
- Vivactil Tablets 1567

Quinestrol (Increases thyroid requirements). Products include:
- Estrovis 1721

Tolazamide (Possible increase in oral hypoglycemic requirements). Products include:
- Tolinase Tablets 2365

Tolbutamide (Possible increase in oral hypoglycemic requirements). Products include:
- Orinase Tablets 2354

Trimipramine Maleate (Enhanced antidepressant and thyroid activities). Products include:
- Surmontil Capsules 2524

Warfarin Sodium (Reduction of anticoagulant dosage may be necessary). Products include:
- Coumadin Injection & Tablets 944
- Panwarfin Tablets 547

CYTOSAR-U STERILE POWDER
(Cytarabine) 2329
May interact with:

Asparaginase (May result in acute pancreatitis). Products include:
- Elspar 1470

Cyclophosphamide (Increased cardiomyopathy). Products include:
- Cytoxan for Injection 726
- Neosar for Injection 566

Digoxin (A reversible decrease in steady-state plasma digoxin concentrations and renal glycoside excretion in patients receiving beta-acetyldigoxin and combination chemotherapy regimens). Products include:
- Lanoxicaps 772
- Lanoxin Elixir Pediatric 775
- Lanoxin Injection 778
- Lanoxin Injection Pediatric 781
- Lanoxin Tablets 783

Flucytosine (Possible inhibition of 5-fluorocytosine efficacy). Products include:
- Ancobon Capsules 1886

Gentamicin Sulfate (Possible lack of antibacterial therapeutic response). Products include:
- Garamycin Injectable 2093
- Garamycin Ophthalmic ..... ◉ 305
- Genoptic Liquifilm Sterile Ophthalmic Solution ..... ◉ 247
- Genoptic S.O.P. Sterile Ophthalmic Ointment ..... ◉ 247
- Gentacidin Ointment ..... ◉ 273
- Gentacidin Solution ..... ◉ 273
- Gentak Ointment & Solution ..... ◉ 208
- G-myticin Creme and Ointment 0.1% 1770
- Pred-G Liquifilm Sterile Ophthalmic Suspension ..... ◉ 252
- Pred-G S.O.P. Sterile Ophthalmic Ointment ..... ◉ 253

CYTOTEC
(Misoprostol) 2159
May interact with antacids containing aluminium, calcium and magnesium. Compounds in this category include:

Aluminum Carbonate Gel (Total availability of misoprostol is reduced by use of concomitant antacid). Products include:
- Basaljel 2438

Aluminum Hydroxide (Total availability of misoprostol is reduced by use of concomitant antacid). Products include:
- Cama Arthritis Pain Reliever ..... ◙ 685
- Gaviscon Extra Strength Relief Formula Liquid Antacid ..... ◙ 594
- Gaviscon Extra Strength Relief Formula Antacid Tablets ..... ◙ 594
- Gaviscon Liquid Antacid ..... ◙ 594
- Gelusil Liquid & Tablets ..... ◙ 639
- Extra Strength Maalox Plus Suspension 1850
- Maalox TC Suspension 1851
- Maalox Plus Tablets ..... ◙ 655
- Extra Strength Maalox Plus Tablets 1850
- Nephrox Suspension ..... ◙ 563
- WinGel Liquid & Tablets ..... ◙ 761

Aluminum Hydroxide Gel (Total availability of misoprostol is reduced by use of concomitant antacid). Products include:
- ALternaGEL Liquid 1154
- Aludrox Oral Suspension 2428
- Amphojel Suspension 2429
- Amphojel Suspension without Flavor 2429
- Mylanta Liquid 1155
- Mylanta Double Strength Liquid 1155

Aluminum Hydroxide Gel, Dried (Total availability of misoprostol is reduced by use of concomitant antacid). Products include:
- Alu-Tab/Alu-Cap 1309
- Amphojel Tablets 2429
- Ascriptin A/D Caplets 1850
- Regular Strength Ascriptin Tablets 1850
- Gaviscon Antacid Tablets ..... ◙ 593
- Gaviscon-2 Antacid Tablets ..... ◙ 594
- Mylanta Tablets 1155
- Mylanta Double Strength Tablets 1155

Dihydroxyaluminum Sodium Carbonate (Total availability of misoprostol is reduced by use of concomitant antacid). Products include:
- Rolaids ..... ◙ 743

Magaldrate (Avoid coadministration with magnesium containing antacids; total availability of misoprostol is reduced by use of concomitant antacid). Products include:
- Riopan Antacid Chew Tablets ..... ◙ 754
- Riopan Antacid Chew Tablets in Rollpacks ..... ◙ 754
- Riopan Antacid Suspension 2421
- Riopan Antacid Swallow Tablets 2421
- Riopan Plus Chew Tablets 2422
- Riopan Plus Chew Tablets in Rollpack 2422
- Riopan Plus 2 Chew Tablets, Mint Flavor, Cherry Flavor 2422
- Riopan Plus Suspension 2422
- Riopan Plus 2 Suspension, Mint Flavor, Cherry Flavor 2422

Magnesium Carbonate (Avoid coadministration with magnesium containing antacids). Products include:
- Bayer Plus Aspirin Tablets ..... ◙ 567
- Gaviscon Extra Strength Relief Formula Liquid Antacid ..... ◙ 594
- Gaviscon Extra Strength Relief Formula Antacid Tablets ..... ◙ 594
- Gaviscon Liquid Antacid ..... ◙ 594
- Marblen ..... ◙ 563
- Osti-Derm Lotion 1771

Magnesium Hydroxide (Avoid coadministration with magnesium containing antacids; total availability of misoprostol is reduced by use of concomitant antacid). Products include:
- Aludrox Oral Suspension 2428
- Ascriptin A/D Caplets 1850
- Regular Strength Ascriptin Tablets 1850
- Di-Gel Antacid/Anti-Gas ..... ◙ 697
- Gelusil Liquid & Tablets ..... ◙ 639
- Haley's M-O, Regular & Flavored ..... ◙ 569
- Extra Strength Maalox Plus Suspension 1850
- Maalox TC Suspension 1851
- Maalox Plus Tablets ..... ◙ 655
- Extra Strength Maalox Plus Tablets 1850
- Mylanta Liquid 1155
- Mylanta Tablets 1155
- Mylanta Double Strength Liquid 1155
- Mylanta Double Strength Tablets 1155
- Concentrated Phillips' Milk of Magnesia ..... ◙ 573
- Phillips' Milk of Magnesia Liquid ..... ◙ 572
- Phillips' Milk of Magnesia Tablets ◙ 573
- WinGel Liquid & Tablets ..... ◙ 761

Magnesium Oxide (Total availability of misoprostol is reduced by use of concomitant antacid). Products include:
- Bayer Plus Aspirin Tablets ..... ◙ 567
- Beelith Tablets 659
- Bufferin Analgesic Tablets and Caplets ..... ◙ 524
- Cama Arthritis Pain Reliever ..... ◙ 685
- Mag-Ox 400 673
- Uro-Mag 673

Food Interactions

Food, unspecified (Diminishes maximum plasma concentrations).

CYTOVENE STERILE POWDER
(Gancyclovir Sodium) 2292
May interact with drugs inhibiting replication of cell populations of bone marrow, spermatogonia, and germinal layers of skin and gi mucosa, inhibitors of renal tubular secretion or resorption, nucleoside analogues, and certain other agents. Compounds in these categories include:

Acyclovir (Potential for additive toxicity). Products include:
- Zovirax Capsules 824
- Zovirax Ointment 5% 827
- Zovirax 824

Acyclovir Sodium (Potential for additive toxicity). Products include:
- Zovirax Sterile Powder 828

Amphotericin B (Potential for additive toxicity). Products include:
- Fungizone Cream, Lotion and Ointment 2261
- Fungizone Intravenous 2262

Dapsone (Potential for additive toxicity). Products include:
- Dapsone USP 1130

Doxorubicin Hydrochloride (Potential for additive toxicity). Products include:
- Adriamycin PFS 561
- Adriamycin RDF 562
- Doxorubicin Hydrochloride for Injection, USP 622
- Doxorubicin Hydrochloride Injection, USP 848
- Rubex 739

Flucytosine (Potential for additive toxicity). Products include:
- Ancobon Capsules 1886

Imipenem-Cilastatin Sodium (Concomitant therapy may produce generalized seizures). Products include:
- Primaxin I.M. 1532
- Primaxin I.V. 1535

Pentamidine Isethionate (Potential for additive toxicity). Products include:
- NebuPent for Inhalation Solution 1017
- Pentam 300 Injection 1018

Probenecid (Reduces renal clearance of Cytovene). Products include:
- Benemid Tablets 1426
- ColBENEMID Tablets 1436
- Wycillin Injection and Probenecid Tablets 2539

Ribavirin (Potential for additive toxicity). Products include:
- Virazole 1126

Sulfamethoxazole (Potential for additive toxicity). Products include:
- Azo Gantanol Tablets 1887
- Bactrim DS Tablets 1891
- Bactrim I.V. Infusion 1889
- Bactrim 1891
- Gantanol 1899
- Septra 813
- Septra I.V. Infusion 808
- Septra I.V. Infusion ADD-Vantage Vials 810
- Septra 813

Sulfinpyrazone (Reduces renal clearance of Cytovene). Products include:
- Anturane 853

Trimethoprim (Potential for additive toxicity). Products include:
- Bactrim DS Tablets 1891
- Bactrim I.V. Infusion 1889
- Bactrim 1891
- Proloprim Tablets 799
- Septra 813
- Septra I.V. Infusion 808
- Septra I.V. Infusion ADD-Vantage Vials 810
- Septra 813
- Trimpex Tablets 1922

Vinblastine Sulfate (Potential for additive toxicity). Products include:
- Velban Vials 1305

Vincristine Sulfate (Potential for additive toxicity). Products include:
- Oncovin Solution Vials & Hyporets 1288

Zidovudine (Concomitant therapy is not recommended). Products include:
- Retrovir Capsules 802
- Retrovir I.V. Infusion 805
- Retrovir Syrup 802

CYTOXAN FOR INJECTION
(Cyclophosphamide) 726

May interact with cytotoxic drugs, general anesthetics, and certain other agents. Compounds in these categories include:

Bleomycin Sulfate (Concurrent use may require reduction in dose of Cytoxan as well as that of other cytotoxic drugs). Products include:
- Blenoxane 724

Daunorubicin Hydrochloride (Concurrent use may require reduction in dose of Cytoxan as well as that of other cytotoxic drugs). Products include:
- Cerubidine 2443

Doxorubicin Hydrochloride (Potentiation of doxorubicin-induced cardiotoxicity; concurrent use may require reduction in dose of Cytoxan as well as that of other cytotoxic drugs). Products include:
- Adriamycin PFS 561
- Adriamycin RDF 562
- Doxorubicin Hydrochloride for Injection, USP 622
- Doxorubicin Hydrochloride Injection, USP 848
- Rubex 739

Enflurane (Anesthesiologist should be alerted if patient has been treated with cyclophosphamide within 10 days). Products include:
- Ethrane 599

Fluorouracil (Concurrent use may require reduction in dose of Cytoxan as well as that of other cytotoxic drugs). Products include:
- Efudex 1880
- Fluoroplex Topical Solution & Cream 1% 1082
- Fluorouracil Injection 1897

Hydroxyurea (Concurrent use may require reduction in dose of Cytoxan as well as that of other cytotoxic drugs). Products include:
- Hydrea Capsules 728

Isoflurane (Anesthesiologist should be alerted if patient has been treated with cyclophosphamide within 10 days). Products include:
- Forane 600

Ketamine Hydrochloride (Anesthesiologist should be alerted if patient has been treated with cyclophosphamide within 10 days). Products include:
- Ketalar 1726

Methohexital Sodium (Anesthesiologist should be alerted if patient has been treated with cyclophosphamide within 10 days). Products include:
- Brevital Sodium Vials 1248

Methotrexate Sodium (Concurrent use may require reduction in dose of Cytoxan as well as that of other cytotoxic drugs). Products include:
- Methotrexate Tablets, Parenteral, LPF Parenteral 1217
- Rheumatrex Methotrexate Dose Pack 1234

Methoxyflurane (Anesthesiologist should be alerted if patient has been treated with cyclophosphamide within 10 days).
- No products indexed under this heading.

Mitotane (Concurrent use may require reduction in dose of Cytoxan as well as that of other cytotoxic drugs). Products include:
- Lysodren 731

Mitoxantrone Hydrochloride (Concurrent use may require reduction in dose of Cytoxan as well as that of other cytotoxic drugs). Products include:
- Novantrone for Injection Concentrate 1226

Phenobarbital (Increased rate of metabolism and leukopenic activity of cyclophosphamide). Products include:
- Arco-Lase Plus Tablets 607
- Bellergal-S Tablets 1998
- Bronkolixir .... ⊞ 761
- Bronkotabs Tablets .... ⊞ 762
- Donnatal 1858
- Donnatal Extentabs 1859
- Donnatal Tablets 1858
- Donnazyme Tablets 1860
- Kinesed Tablets 2272
- Phenobarbital Elixir and Tablets 1293
- Primatene Tablets-P Formula 2421
- Quadrinal Tablets 1183
- Tedral SA 1765

Procarbazine Hydrochloride (Concurrent use may require reduction in dose of Cytoxan as well as that of other cytotoxic drugs). Products include:
- Matulane Capsules 1907

Propofol (Anesthesiologist should be alerted if patient has been treated with cyclophosphamide within 10 days). Products include:
- Diprivan Injection 2267

Succinylcholine Chloride (Inhibition of cholinesterase activity and potentiation of succinylcholine chloride's effect). Products include:
- Anectine 755

Tamoxifen Citrate (Concurrent use may require reduction in dose of Cytoxan as well as that of other cytotoxic drugs). Products include:
- Nolvadex Tablets 1102

Vincristine Sulfate (Concurrent use may require reduction in dose of Cytoxan as well as that of other cytotoxic drugs). Products include:
- Oncovin Solution Vials & Hyporets 1288

DDAVP INJECTION
(Desmopressin Acetate) 1840

May interact with vasopressors. Compounds in this category include:

Dopamine Hydrochloride (Possible additive effects; use only with careful monitoring). Products include:
- Intropin Injection 930

Epinephrine Hydrochloride (Possible additive effects; use only with careful monitoring). Products include:
- Adrenalin Chloride Solution 1:100 & 1:1,000 1689
- Epifrin .... ◉ 244
- Glaucon .... ◉ 218

Metaraminol Bitartrate (Possible additive effects; use only with careful monitoring). Products include:
- Aramine Injection 1424

Methoxamine Hydrochloride (Possible additive effects; use only with careful monitoring). Products include:
- Vasoxyl Injection 819

Norepinephrine Bitartrate (Possible additive effects; use only with careful monitoring). Products include:
- Levophed Bitartrate Injection 2054

Phenylephrine Hydrochloride (Possible additive effects; use only with careful monitoring). Products include:
- AK-Dilate Solution 2.5% and 10% .... ◉ 203
- Atrohist Sprinkle Capsules 558
- Cerose-DM 2443
- Codimal 846
- Comhist LA Capsules 1618
- Congespirin For Children Aspirin Free Chewable Cold Tablets 748
- Cyclomydril .... ◉ 216
- Deconsal Sprinkle Capsules 559
- Dimetane Decongestant .... ⊞ 673
- Dristan Decongestant/Antihistamine/Analgesic Coated Caplets .... ⊞ 749
- Dristan Cold Nasal Decongestant/Antihistamine/ Analgesic Coated Tablets 2419
- Dristan Advanced Formula Decongestant/Antihistamine/Analgesic Tablets .... ⊞ 749
- Dristan Nasal Spray, Menthol 2419
- Dristan Nasal Spray, Regular and Regular with Metered Pump 2419
- Entex Capsules 1623
- Entex Liquid 1623
- Sinus Excedrin Analgesic, Decongestant Tablets & Caplets 750
- Extendryl 994
- 4-Way Fast Acting Nasal Spray - Original Formula (regular & mentholated) & Metered Spray Pump (regular) 751
- Hycomine Compound Tablets 929
- Murocoll-2 Sterile Ophthalmic Solution .... ◉ 261
- Mydfrin 2.5% .... ◉ 224
- Naldecon Syrup, Tablets, Pediatric Drops and Pediatric Syrup 709
- Neo-Synephrine Hydrochloride 1% Carpuject 2063
- Neo-Synephrine Hydrochloride 1% Injection 2063
- Neo-Synephrine Hydrochloride (Ophthalmic) 2064
- Neo-Synephrine .... ⊞ 759
- Nōstril Nasal Decongestant .... ⊞ 520
- Novahistine Elixir .... ⊞ 596
- Phenergan VC 2500
- Phenergan VC with Codeine 2501
- Prefrin Liquifilm Vasoconstrictor and Lubricant Eye Drops .... ◉ 254
- Prefrin-A .... ◉ 255
- Quelidrine Syrup 556
- Relief Vasoconstrictor and Lubricant Eye Drops .... ◉ 256
- Robitussin Night Relief .... ⊞ 677
- Ru-Tuss with Hydrocodone 694
- Ru-Tuss Tablets 693
- Vasosulf .... ◉ 279
- Vicks Sinex .... ⊞ 665
- Zincfrin .... ◉ 230

DDAVP NASAL SPRAY
(Desmopressin Acetate) 1841

See **DDAVP Rhinal Tube**

DDAVP RHINAL TUBE
(Desmopressin Acetate) 1841

May interact with vasopressors. Compounds in this category include:

Dopamine Hydrochloride (Possible additive effects; use only with careful monitoring). Products include:
- Intropin Injection 930

Epinephrine Hydrochloride (Possible additive effects; use only with careful monitoring). Products include:
- Adrenalin Chloride Solution 1:100 & 1:1,000 1689
- Epifrin .... ◉ 244
- Glaucon .... ◉ 218

Metaraminol Bitartrate (Possible additive effects; use only with careful monitoring). Products include:
- Aramine Injection 1424

Methoxamine Hydrochloride (Possible additive effects; use only with careful monitoring). Products include:
- Vasoxyl Injection 819

Norepinephrine Bitartrate (Possible additive effects; use only with careful monitoring). Products include:
- Levophed Bitartrate Injection 2054

Phenylephrine Hydrochloride (Possible additive effects; use only with careful monitoring). Products include:
- AK-Dilate Solution 2.5% and 10% .... ◉ 203
- Atrohist Sprinkle Capsules 558
- Cerose-DM 2443
- Codimal 846

Comhist LA Capsules 1618
Congespirin For Children Aspirin Free Chewable Cold Tablets 748
Cyclomydril ◎ 216
Deconsal Sprinkle Capsules 559
Dimetane Decongestant ▣ 673
Dristan Decongestant/Antihistamine/ Analgesic Coated Caplets ▣ 749
Dristan Cold Nasal Decongestant/ Antihistamine/ Analgesic Coated Tablets 2419
Dristan Advanced Formula Decongestant/Antihistamine/ Analgesic Tablets ▣ 749
Dristan Nasal Spray, Menthol 2419
Dristan Nasal Spray, Regular and Regular with Metered Pump 2419
Entex Capsules 1623
Entex Liquid 1623
Sinus Excedrin Analgesic, Decongestant Tablets & Caplets 750
Extendryl 994
4-Way Fast Acting Nasal Spray - Original Formula (regular & mentholated) & Metered Spray Pump (regular) 751
Hycomine Compound Tablets 929
Murocoll-2 Sterile Ophthalmic Solution ◎ 261
Mydfrin 2.5% ◎ 224
Naldecon Syrup, Tablets, Pediatric Drops and Pediatric Syrup 709
Neo-Synephrine Hydrochloride 1% Carpuject 2063
Neo-Synephrine Hydrochloride 1% Injection 2063
Neo-Synephrine Hydrochloride (Ophthalmic) 2064
Neo-Synephrine ▣ 759
Nōstril Nasal Decongestant ▣ 520
Novahistine Elixir ▣ 596
Phenergan VC 2500
Phenergan VC with Codeine 2501
Prefrin Liquifilm Vasoconstrictor and Lubricant Eye Drops ◎ 254
Prefrin-A ◎ 255
Quelidrine Syrup 556
Relief Vasoconstrictor and Lubricant Eye Drops ◎ 256
Robitussin Night Relief ▣ 677
Ru-Tuss with Hydrocodone 694
Ru-Tuss Tablets 693
Vasosulf ◎ 279
Vicks Sinex ▣ 665
Zincfrin ◎ 230

DDS-ACIDOPHILUS
(Lactobacillus Acidophilus) ▣ 735
No interactions described in labeling.

D.H.E. 45 INJECTION
(Dihydroergotamine Mesylate) 2003
No interactions described in labeling.

DHS CONDITIONING RINSE
(Cleanser) 1772
No interactions described in labeling.

DHS SHAMPOO
(Cleanser) 1772
No interactions described in labeling.

DHS CLEAR SHAMPOO
(Cleanser) 1772
No interactions described in labeling.

DHS TAR GEL SHAMPOO
(Coal Tar) 1772
No interactions described in labeling.

DHS TAR SHAMPOO
(Coal Tar) 1772
No interactions described in labeling.

DHS ZINC DANDRUFF SHAMPOO
(Zinc Pyrithione) 1772
No interactions described in labeling.

DHT (DIHYDROTACHYSTEROL) TABLETS & INTENSOL
(Dihydrotachysterol) 1984
May interact with thiazides. Compounds in this category include:

Bendroflumethiazide (May cause hypercalcemia in hypoparathyroid patients). Products include:
Corzide Tablets 702
Naturetin Tablets 1789
Rauzide Tablets 1804

Chlorothiazide (May cause hypercalcemia in hypoparathyroid patients). Products include:
Aldoclor Tablets 1413
Diupres Tablets 1461
Diuril Oral 1464

Chlorothiazide Sodium (May cause hypercalcemia in hypoparathyroid patients). Products include:
Diuril Sodium Intravenous 1463

Hydrochlorothiazide (May cause hypercalcemia in hypoparathyroid patients). Products include:
Aldactazide 2150
Aldoril Tablets 1418
Apresazide Capsules 854
Apresoline-Esidrix Tablets 857
Capozide 2258
Dyazide Capsules 2208
Esidrix Tablets 863
Esimil Tablets 864
HydroDIURIL Tablets 1484
Hydropres Tablets 1485
Inderide Tablets 2463
Inderide LA Long Acting Capsules 2465
Lopressor HCT Tablets 1034
Maxzide 1215
Moduretic Tablets 1510
Normozide Tablets 2112
Oretic Tablets 544
Oreticyl 545
Prinzide Tablets 1540
Ser-Ap-Es Tablets 881
Serpasil-Esidrix Tablets 886
Timolide Tablets 1547
Trandate HCT Tablets 579
Vaseretic Tablets 1559
Zestoretic 2274

Hydroflumethiazide (May cause hypercalcemia in hypoparathyroid patients). Products include:
Diucardin Tablets 2450
Saluron 718
Salutensin/Salutensin-Demi 719

Methyclothiazide (May cause hypercalcemia in hypoparathyroid patients). Products include:
Enduron Tablets 517
Enduronyl 518

Polythiazide (May cause hypercalcemia in hypoparathyroid patients). Products include:
Minizide Capsules 1779
Renese Tablets 1785
Renese-R Tablets 1786

DML FACIAL MOISTURIZER WITH SUNSCREEN
(Glycerin, Hyaluronic Acid, Octyl Methoxycinnamate, Oxybenzone) 1772
No interactions described in labeling.

DML FORTE CREAM
(Petrolatum) 1772
No interactions described in labeling.

DML MOISTURIZING LOTION
(Petrolatum) 1772
No interactions described in labeling.

DTIC-DOME
(Dacarbazine) 1595
May interact with antineoplastics. Compounds in this category include:

Altretamine (Hepatic toxicity). Products include:
Hexalen Capsules 2316

Asparaginase (Hepatic toxicity). Products include:
Elspar 1470

Bleomycin Sulfate (Hepatic toxicity). Products include:
Blenoxane 724

Busulfan (Hepatic toxicity). Products include:
Myleran Tablets 790

Carboplatin (Hepatic toxicity). Products include:
Paraplatin for Injection 735

Carmustine (BCNU) (Hepatic toxicity). Products include:
BiCNU 723

Chlorambucil (Hepatic toxicity). Products include:
Leukeran Tablets 788

Cisplatin (Hepatic toxicity). Products include:
Platinol 737
Platinol-AQ Injection 738

Cyclophosphamide (Hepatic toxicity). Products include:
Cytoxan for Injection 726
Neosar for Injection 566

Daunorubicin Hydrochloride (Hepatic toxicity). Products include:
Cerubidine 2443

Doxorubicin Hydrochloride (Hepatic toxicity). Products include:
Adriamycin PFS 561
Adriamycin RDF 562
Doxorubicin Hydrochloride for Injection, USP 622
Doxorubicin Hydrochloride Injection, USP 848
Rubex 739

Estramustine Phosphate Sodium (Hepatic toxicity). Products include:
Emcyt Capsules 1161

Etoposide (Hepatic toxicity). Products include:
VePesid Capsules and Injection 741

Floxuridine (Hepatic toxicity). Products include:
Sterile FUDR 1898

Fluorouracil (Hepatic toxicity). Products include:
Efudex 1880
Fluoroplex Topical Solution & Cream 1% 1082
Fluorouracil Injection 1897

Flutamide (Hepatic toxicity). Products include:
Eulexin Capsules 2089

Hydroxyurea (Hepatic toxicity). Products include:
Hydrea Capsules 728

Ifosfamide (Hepatic toxicity). Products include:
IFEX 729

Interferon alfa-2A, Recombinant (Hepatic toxicity). Products include:
Roferon-A Injection 1916

Interferon alfa-2B, Recombinant (Hepatic toxicity). Products include:
Intron A 2097

Levamisole Hydrochloride (Hepatic toxicity). Products include:
Ergamisol Tablets 1136

Lomustine (CCNU) (Hepatic toxicity). Products include:
CeeNU 725

Mechlorethamine Hydrochloride (Hepatic toxicity). Products include:
Mustargen 1514

Megestrol Acetate (Hepatic toxicity). Products include:
Megace Tablets 732

Melphalan (Hepatic toxicity). Products include:
Alkeran Tablets 754

Mercaptopurine (Hepatic toxicity). Products include:
Purinethol Tablets 800

Methotrexate Sodium (Hepatic toxicity). Products include:
Methotrexate Tablets, Parenteral, LPF Parenteral 1217
Rheumatrex Methotrexate Dose Pack 1234

Mitomycin (Mitomycin-C) (Hepatic toxicity). Products include:
Mutamycin 733

Mitotane (Hepatic toxicity). Products include:
Lysodren 731

Mitoxantrone Hydrochloride (Hepatic Toxicity). Products include:
Novantrone for Injection Concentrate 1226

Procarbazine Hydrochloride (Hepatic toxicity). Products include:
Matulane Capsules 1907

Streptozocin (Hepatic toxicity). Products include:
Zanosar Sterile Powder 2371

Tamoxifen Citrate (Hepatic toxicity). Products include:
Nolvadex Tablets 1102

Thioguanine (Hepatic toxicity). Products include:
Thioguanine Tablets, Tabloid Brand 815

Thiotepa (Hepatic toxicity). Products include:
Thiotepa Parenteral 1240

Vincristine Sulfate (Hepatic toxicity). Products include:
Oncovin Solution Vials & Hyporets 1288

DAISY 2 PREGNANCY TEST
(HCG Monoclonal Antibody) ▣ 773
No interactions described in labeling.

DALALONE D.P. INJECTABLE
(Dexamethasone Acetate) 999
May interact with oral anticoagulants and certain other agents. Compounds in these categories include:

Dicumarol (Corticosteroids may alter the response to this anticoagulant). Products include:
Dicumarol Tablets 516

Ephedrine (May alter cortisol metabolism).

Ephedrine Hydrochloride (May alter cortisol metabolism). Products include:
Amesec ▣ 682
Primatene Tablets-M Formula 2421
Primatene Tablets-P Formula 2421
Primatene Tablets-Regular Formula 2421
Quadrinal Tablets 1183
Quelidrine Syrup 556
Tedral SA 1765

Ephedrine Sulfate (May alter cortisol metabolism). Products include:
Bronkaid Tablets ▣ 757
Bronkolixir ▣ 761
Bronkotabs Tablets ▣ 762
Marax Tablets & DF Syrup 1954
Pazo Hemorrhoid Ointment & Suppositories 752
Vicks Vatronol Nose Drops ▣ 666

Ephedrine Tannate (May alter cortisol metabolism). Products include:
Rynatuss 2388

Flucytosine (Neurological complications and lack of antibody response). Products include:
Ancobon Capsules 1886

Phenobarbital (May alter cortisol metabolism). Products include:
Arco-Lase Plus Tablets 607
Bellergal-S Tablets 1998
Bronkolixir ⊡ 761
Bronkotabs Tablets ⊡ 762
Donnatal 1858
Donnatal Extentabs 1859
Donnatal Tablets 1858
Donnazyme Tablets 1860
Kinesed Tablets 2272
Phenobarbital Elixir and Tablets 1293
Primatene Tablets-P Formula 2421
Quadrinal Tablets 1183
Tedral SA 1765

Phenytoin (May alter cortisol metabolism). Products include:
Dilantin Infatabs 1710
Dilantin-30 Pediatric/Dilantin-125 Suspension 1713

Phenytoin Sodium (May alter cortisol metabolism). Products include:
Dilantin Kapseals 1708
Dilantin Parenteral 1712
Dilantin with Phenobarbital Kapseals 1715

Rifampin (May alter cortisol metabolism). Products include:
Rifadin 1345
Rifamate Capsules 1347
Rimactane Capsules 879

Smallpox Vaccine (Neurological complications and lack of antibody response).

Warfarin Sodium (Corticosteroids may alter the response to this anticoagulant). Products include:
Coumadin Injection & Tablets 944
Panwarfin Tablets 547

DALGAN INJECTION
(Dezocine) 620
May interact with central nervous system depressants, general anesthetics, hypnotics and sedatives, tranquilizers, narcotic analgesics, and certain other agents. Compounds in these categories include:

Alcohol (Concomitant administration may have an additive effect).

Alfentanil Hydrochloride (Concomitant administration may have an additive effect). Products include:
Alfenta Injection 1131

Alprazolam (Concomitant administration may have an additive effect). Products include:
Xanax Tablets 2367

Aprobarbital (Concomitant administration may have an additive effect). Products include:
Alurate Elixir 1883

Buprenorphine (Concomitant administration may have an additive effect).
No products indexed under this heading.

Buspirone Hydrochloride (Concomitant administration may have an additive effect). Products include:
BuSpar 1401

Butabarbital (Concomitant administration may have an additive effect). Products include:
Pyridium Plus 1764

Butalbital (Concomitant administration may have an additive effect). Products include:
Esgic-Plus Tablets 1002
Esgic Tablets & Capsules 1001
Fioricet Tablets 2006
Fiorinal Capsules 2007
Fiorinal with Codeine Capsules 2008
Fiorinal Tablets 2007
Phrenilin 838
Sedapap Tablets 50 mg/650 mg 1360

Chlordiazepoxide (Concomitant administration may have an additive effect). Products include:
Libritabs Tablets 1930
Limbitrol 1933
Menrium Tablets 1934

Chlordiazepoxide Hydrochloride (Concomitant administration may have an additive effect). Products include:
Librax Capsules 1929
Librium Capsules 1931
Librium Injectable 1932

Chlorpromazine (Concomitant administration may have an additive effect). Products include:
Thorazine 2234

Chlorprothixene (Concomitant administration may have an additive effect). Products include:
Taractan Tablets 1920

Chlorprothixene Hydrochloride (Concomitant administration may have an additive effect). Products include:
Taractan 1920

Clorazepate Dipotassium (Concomitant administration may have an additive effect). Products include:
Tranxene 556

Codeine (Concomitant administration may have an additive effect). Products include:
Calcidrine Syrup 506

Codeine Phosphate (Concomitant administration may have an additive effect). Products include:
Actifed with Codeine Cough Syrup 752
Cheracol Cough Syrup 1853
Codimal PH Syrup 846
Dimetane-DC Cough Syrup 1857
Empirin with Codeine Phosphate Nos. 2, 3 & 4 764
Fiorinal with Codeine Capsules 2008
Isoclor Expectorant 982
Naldecon CX Adult Liquid ⊡ 521
Novahistine DH 1342
Novahistine Expectorant 1343
Nucofed Capsules 2219
Nucofed Expectorant 2219
Nucofed Pediatric Expectorant 2220
Nucofed Syrup 2219
Phenaphen with Codeine Capsules 1865
Phenaphen-650 with Codeine Tablets 1866
Phenergan with Codeine 2497
Phenergan VC with Codeine 2501
Robitussin A-C Syrup 1875
Robitussin-DAC Syrup 1875
Ryna ⊡ 741
Soma Compound w/Codeine Tablets 2390
Triaminic Expectorant w/Codeine 1996
Tussi-Organidin Liquid 2391
Tylenol with Codeine 1381

Codeine Polistirex (Concomitant administration may have an additive effect).
No products indexed under this heading.

Diazepam (Concomitant administration may have an additive effect). Products include:
Valium Injectable 1937
Valium Tablets 1939
Valrelease Capsules 1923

Droperidol (Concomitant administration may have an additive effect). Products include:
Inapsine Injection 1140
Innovar Injection 1141

Enflurane (Concomitant administration may have an additive effect). Products include:
Ethrane 599

Estazolam (Concomitant administration may have an additive effect). Products include:
ProSom Tablets 554

Ethchlorvynol (Concomitant administration may have an additive effect). Products include:
Placidyl Capsules 553

Ethinamate (Concomitant administration may have an additive effect).
No products indexed under this heading.

Fentanyl (Concomitant administration may have an additive effect). Products include:
Duragesic Transdermal System 1133

Fentanyl Citrate (Concomitant administration may have an additive effect). Products include:
Innovar Injection 1141
Sublimaze Injection 1146

Fluphenazine Decanoate (Concomitant administration may have an additive effect). Products include:
Prolixin Decanoate 1795

Fluphenazine Enanthate (Concomitant administration may have an additive effect). Products include:
Prolixin Enanthate 1796

Fluphenazine Hydrochloride (Concomitant administration may have an additive effect). Products include:
Prolixin Elixir 1793
Prolixin Injection 1791
Prolixin Oral Concentrate 1792
Prolixin Tablets 1793

Flurazepam Hydrochloride (Concomitant administration may have an additive effect). Products include:
Dalmane Capsules 1927

Glutethimide (Concomitant administration may have an additive effect).
No products indexed under this heading.

Haloperidol (Concomitant administration may have an additive effect). Products include:
Haldol Injection, Tablets and Concentrate 1373

Haloperidol Decanoate (Concomitant administration may have an additive effect). Products include:
Haldol Decanoate 1375

Hydrocodone Bitartrate (Concomitant administration may have an additive effect). Products include:
Anexsia 5/500 Tablets 2196
Anexsia 7.5/650 Tablets 2197
Azdone Tablets 844
Codiclear DH Syrup 845
Codimal DH Syrup 846
Damason-P 1356
Hycodan Syrup, Tablets 927
Hycomine Compound Tablets 929
Hycomine Syrup 927
Hycotuss Expectorant Syrup 930
Hydrocet Capsules 835
Lortab ASA Tablets 2414
Lortab 2412
Ru-Tuss with Hydrocodone 694
Triaminic Expectorant DH 1995
Vicodin Tablets 1187
Vicodin ES Tablets 1189
Zydone Capsules 941

Hydrocodone Polistirex (Concomitant administration may have an additive effect), Products include:
Tussionex Extended-Release Suspension 988

Hydroxyzine Hydrochloride (Concomitant administration may have an additive effect). Products include:
Atarax Tablets & Syrup 1941
Marax Tablets & DF Syrup 1954
Vistaril Intramuscular Solution 1970

Isoflurane (Concomitant administration may have an additive effect). Products include:
Forane 600

Ketamine Hydrochloride (Concomitant administration may have an additive effect). Products include:
Ketalar 1726

Levorphanol Tartrate (Concomitant administration may have an additive effect). Products include:
Levo-Dromoran 1906

Lorazepam (Concomitant administration may have an additive effect). Products include:
Ativan Injection 2432
Ativan Tablets 2434

Loxapine Hydrochloride (Concomitant administration may have an additive effect). Products include:
Loxitane 1213

Loxapine Succinate (Concomitant administration may have an additive effect). Products include:
Loxitane Capsules 1213

Meperidine Hydrochloride (Concomitant administration may have an additive effect). Products include:
Demerol 2047
Mepergan Injection 2479

Mephobarbital (Concomitant administration may have an additive effect). Products include:
Mebaral Tablets 2061

Meprobamate (Concomitant administration may have an additive effect). Products include:
Deprol Tablets 2382
Equagesic Tablets 2451
Miltown Tablets 2386
PMB 200 and PMB 400 2504

Mesoridazine (Concomitant administration may have an additive effect). Products include:
Serentil 686

Methadone Hydrochloride (Concomitant administration may have an additive effect). Products include:
Dolophine Hydrochloride Ampoules & Vials 1260
Dolophine Hydrochloride Tablets 1261
Methadone Hydrochloride Diskets 1284
Methadone Hydrochloride Oral Solution & Tablets 1987

Methohexital Sodium (Concomitant administration may have an additive effect). Products include:
Brevital Sodium Vials 1248

Methoxyflurane (Concomitant administration may have an additive effect).
No products indexed under this heading.

Midazolam Hydrochloride (Concomitant administration may have an additive effect). Products include:
Versed Injection 1924

Molindone Hydrochloride (Concomitant administration may have an additive effect). Products include:
Moban Tablets & Concentrate 932

Morphine Sulfate (Concomitant administration may have an additive effect). Products include:
Astramorph/PF Injection, USP (Preservative-Free) 618
Duramorph 960
Infumorph 200 and Infumorph 500 Sterile Solutions 962
MS Contin Tablets 1814
MSIR 1817
Oramorph SR (Morphine Sulfate Sustained Release Tablets) 1988
Roxanol 1991

Opium Alkaloids (Concomitant administration may have an additive effect). Products include:
- B & O No. 15A & No. 16A Supprettes 2395
- Pantopon Injectable 1911

Oxazepam (Concomitant administration may have an additive effect). Products include:
- Serax Capsules 2522
- Serax Tablets 2522

Oxycodone Hydrochloride (Concomitant administration may have an additive effect). Products include:
- Percocet Tablets 950
- Percodan 951
- Roxicodone Tablets, Oral Solution & Intensol (Oxycodone) 1992
- Tylox Capsules 1382

Pentobarbital Sodium (Concomitant administration may have an additive effect). Products include:
- Nembutal Sodium Capsules 534
- Nembutal Sodium Solution 536
- Nembutal Sodium Suppositories 538

Perphenazine (Concomitant administration may have an additive effect). Products include:
- Etrafon 2087
- Triavil Tablets 1556
- Trilafon 2123

Phenobarbital (Concomitant administration may have an additive effect). Products include:
- Arco-Lase Plus Tablets 607
- Bellergal-S Tablets 1998
- Bronkolixir ..... ▣ 761
- Bronkotabs Tablets ..... ▣ 762
- Donnatal 1858
- Donnatal Extentabs 1859
- Donnatal Tablets 1858
- Donnazyme Tablets 1860
- Kinesed Tablets 2272
- Phenobarbital Elixir and Tablets 1293
- Primatene Tablets-P Formula 2421
- Quadrinal Tablets 1183
- Tedral SA 1765

Prazepam (Concomitant administration may have an additive effect). Products include:
- Centrax 1693

Prochlorperazine (Concomitant administration may have an additive effect). Products include:
- Compazine 2201

Promethazine Hydrochloride (Concomitant administration may have an additive effect). Products include:
- Mepergan Injection 2479
- Phenergan with Codeine 2497
- Phenergan with Dextromethorphan 2499
- Phenergan Injection 2493
- Phenergan Suppositories 2496
- Phenergan Syrup 2495
- Phenergan Tablets 2496
- Phenergan VC 2500
- Phenergan VC with Codeine 2501

Propofol (Concomitant administration may have an additive effect). Products include:
- Diprivan Injection 2267

Propoxyphene Hydrochloride (Concomitant administration may have an additive effect). Products include:
- Darvon 1256
- Wygesic Tablets 2540

Propoxyphene Napsylate (Concomitant administration may have an additive effect). Products include:
- Darvon-N/Darvocet-N 1254

Quazepam (Concomitant administration may have an additive effect). Products include:
- Doral Tablets 2383

Secobarbital Sodium (Concomitant administration may have an additive effect). Products include:
- Seconal Sodium Pulvules 1296

Sufentanil Citrate (Concomitant administration may have an additive effect). Products include:
- Sufenta Injection 1147

Temazepam (Concomitant administration may have an additive effect). Products include:
- Restoril Capsules 2023

Thiamylal Sodium (Concomitant administration may have an additive effect). Products include:
- Surital Ampoules, Steri-Vials 1764

Thioridazine Hydrochloride (Concomitant administration may have an additive effect). Products include:
- Mellaril 2011

Thiothixene (Concomitant administration may have an additive effect). Products include:
- Navane Capsules and Concentrate 1954
- Navane Intramuscular 1956

Triazolam (Concomitant administration may have an additive effect). Products include:
- Halcion Tablets 2340

Trifluoperazine Hydrochloride (Concomitant administration may have an additive effect). Products include:
- Stelazine 2226

DALMANE CAPSULES
(Flurazepam Hydrochloride) 1927
May interact with central nervous system depressants and certain other agents. Compounds in these categories include:

Alcohol (Additive effects; potential for continuation of interaction after discontinuance of flurazepam).

Alfentanil Hydrochloride (Additive effects). Products include:
- Alfenta Injection 1131

Alprazolam (Additive effects). Products include:
- Xanax Tablets 2367

Aprobarbital (Additive effects). Products include:
- Alurate Elixir 1883

Buprenorphine (Additive effects).
- No products indexed under this heading.

Buspirone Hydrochloride (Additive effects). Products include:
- BuSpar 1401

Butabarbital (Additive effects). Products include:
- Pyridium Plus 1764

Butalbital (Additive effects). Products include:
- Esgic-Plus Tablets 1002
- Esgic Tablets & Capsules 1001
- Fioricet Tablets 2006
- Fiorinal Capsules 2007
- Fiorinal with Codeine Capsules 2008
- Fiorinal Tablets 2007
- Phrenilin 838
- Sedapap Tablets 50 mg/650 mg .. 1360

Chlordiazepoxide (Additive effects). Products include:
- Libritabs Tablets 1930
- Limbitrol 1933
- Menrium Tablets 1934

Chlordiazepoxide Hydrochloride (Additive effects). Products include:
- Librax Capsules 1929
- Librium Capsules 1931
- Librium Injectable 1932

Chlorpromazine (Additive effects). Products include:
- Thorazine 2234

Chlorprothixene (Additive effects). Products include:
- Taractan Tablets 1920

Chlorprothixene Hydrochloride (Additive effects). Products include:
- Taractan 1920

Clorazepate Dipotassium (Additive effects). Products include:
- Tranxene 556

Codeine (Additive effects). Products include:
- Calcidrine Syrup 506

Codeine Phosphate (Additive effects). Products include:
- Actifed with Codeine Cough Syrup.. 752
- Cheracol Cough Syrup 1853
- Codimal PH Syrup 846
- Dimetane-DC Cough Syrup 1857
- Empirin with Codeine Phosphate Nos. 2, 3 & 4 764
- Fiorinal with Codeine Capsules 2008
- Isoclor Expectorant 982
- Naldecon CX Adult Liquid ..... ▣ 521
- Novahistine DH 1342
- Novahistine Expectorant 1343
- Nucofed Capsules 2219
- Nucofed Expectorant 2219
- Nucofed Pediatric Expectorant 2220
- Nucofed Syrup 2219
- Phenaphen with Codeine Capsules 1865
- Phenaphen-650 with Codeine Tablets 1866
- Phenergan with Codeine 2497
- Phenergan VC with Codeine 2501
- Robitussin A-C Syrup 1875
- Robitussin-DAC Syrup 1875
- Ryna ..... ▣ 741
- Soma Compound w/Codeine Tablets 2390
- Triaminic Expectorant w/Codeine .. 1996
- Tussi-Organidin Liquid 2391
- Tylenol with Codeine 1381

Codeine Polistirex (Additive effects).
- No products indexed under this heading.

Dezocine (Additive effects).

Diazepam (Additive effects). Products include:
- Valium Injectable 1937
- Valium Tablets 1939
- Valrelease Capsules 1923

Droperidol (Additive effects). Products include:
- Inapsine Injection 1140
- Innovar Injection 1141

Enflurane (Additive effects). Products include:
- Ethrane 599

Estazolam (Additive effects). Products include:
- ProSom Tablets 554

Ethchlorvynol (Additive effects). Products include:
- Placidyl Capsules 553

Ethinamate (Additive effects).
- No products indexed under this heading.

Fentanyl (Additive effects). Products include:
- Duragesic Transdermal System 1133

Fentanyl Citrate (Additive effects). Products include:
- Innovar Injection 1141
- Sublimaze Injection 1146

Fluphenazine Decanoate (Additive effects). Products include:
- Prolixin Decanoate 1795

Fluphenazine Enanthate (Additive effects). Products include:
- Prolixin Enanthate 1796

Fluphenazine Hydrochloride (Additive effects). Products include:
- Prolixin Elixir 1793
- Prolixin Injection 1791
- Prolixin Oral Concentrate 1792
- Prolixin Tablets 1793

Glutethimide (Additive effects).
- No products indexed under this heading.

Haloperidol (Additive effects). Products include:
- Haldol Injection, Tablets and Concentrate 1373

Haloperidol Decanoate (Additive effects). Products include:
- Haldol Decanoate 1375

Hydrocodone Bitartrate (Additive effects). Products include:
- Anexsia 5/500 Tablets 2196
- Anexsia 7.5/650 Tablets 2197
- Azdone Tablets 844
- Codiclear DH Syrup 845
- Codimal DH Syrup 846
- Damason-P 1356
- Hycodan Syrup, Tablets 927
- Hycomine Compound Tablets 929
- Hycomine Syrup 927
- Hycotuss Expectorant Syrup 930
- Hydrocet Capsules 835
- Lortab ASA Tablets 2414
- Lortab 2412
- Ru-Tuss with Hydrocodone 694
- Triaminic Expectorant DH 1995
- Vicodin Tablets 1187
- Vicodin ES Tablets 1189
- Zydone Capsules 941

Hydrocodone Polistirex (Additive effects). Products include:
- Tussionex Extended-Release Suspension 988

Hydroxyzine Hydrochloride (Additive effects). Products include:
- Atarax Tablets & Syrup 1941
- Marax Tablets & DF Syrup 1954
- Vistaril Intramuscular Solution 1970

Isoflurane (Additive effects). Products include:
- Forane 600

Ketamine Hydrochloride (Additive effects). Products include:
- Ketalar 1726

Levorphanol Tartrate (Additive effects). Products include:
- Levo-Dromoran 1906

Lorazepam (Additive effects). Products include:
- Ativan Injection 2432
- Ativan Tablets 2434

Loxapine Hydrochloride (Additive effects). Products include:
- Loxitane 1213

Loxapine Succinate (Additive effects). Products include:
- Loxitane Capsules 1213

Meperidine Hydrochloride (Additive effects). Products include:
- Demerol 2047
- Mepergan Injection 2479

Mephobarbital (Additive effects). Products include:
- Mebaral Tablets 2061

Meprobamate (Additive effects). Products include:
- Deprol Tablets 2382
- Equagesic Tablets 2451
- Miltown Tablets 2386
- PMB 200 and PMB 400 2504

Mesoridazine (Additive effects). Products include:
- Serentil 686

Methadone Hydrochloride (Additive effects). Products include:
- Dolophine Hydrochloride Ampoules & Vials 1260
- Dolophine Hydrochloride Tablets 1261
- Methadone Hydrochloride Diskets .. 1284
- Methadone Hydrochloride Oral Solution & Tablets 1987

Methohexital Sodium (Additive effects). Products include:
- Brevital Sodium Vials 1248

Methoxyflurane (Additive effects).
- No products indexed under this heading.

Midazolam Hydrochloride (Additive effects). Products include:
- Versed Injection 1924

Molindone Hydrochloride (Additive effects). Products include:
- Moban Tablets & Concentrate 932

Morphine Sulfate (Additive effects). Products include:
- Astramorph/PF Injection, USP (Preservative-Free) 618
- Duramorph 960
- Infumorph 200 and Infumorph 500 Sterile Solutions 962
- MS Contin Tablets 1814
- MSIR 1817
- Oramorph SR (Morphine Sulfate Sustained Release Tablets) 1988
- Roxanol 1991

Opium Alkaloids (Additive effects). Products include:
- B & O No. 15A & No. 16A Supprettes 2395
- Pantopon Injectable 1911

Oxazepam (Additive effects). Products include:
- Serax Capsules 2522
- Serax Tablets 2522

Oxycodone Hydrochloride (Additive effects). Products include:
- Percocet Tablets 950
- Percodan 951
- Roxicodone Tablets, Oral Solution & Intensol (Oxycodone) 1992
- Tylox Capsules 1382

Pentobarbital Sodium (Additive effects). Products include:
- Nembutal Sodium Capsules 534
- Nembutal Sodium Solution 536
- Nembutal Sodium Suppositories 538

Perphenazine (Additive effects). Products include:
- Etrafon 2087
- Triavil Tablets 1556
- Trilafon 2123

Phenobarbital (Additive effects). Products include:
- Arco-Lase Plus Tablets 607
- Bellergal-S Tablets 1998
- Bronkolixir .... ▣ 761
- Bronkotabs Tablets .... ▣ 762
- Donnatal 1858
- Donnatal Extentabs 1859
- Donnatal Tablets 1858
- Donnazyme Tablets 1860
- Kinesed Tablets 2272
- Phenobarbital Elixir and Tablets 1293
- Primatene Tablets-P Formula 2421
- Quadrinal Tablets 1183
- Tedral SA 1765

Prazepam (Additive effects). Products include:
- Centrax 1693

Prochlorperazine (Additive effects). Products include:
- Compazine 2201

Promethazine Hydrochloride (Additive effects). Products include:
- Mepergan Injection 2479
- Phenergan with Codeine 2497
- Phenergan with Dextromethorphan 2499
- Phenergan Injection 2493
- Phenergan Suppositories 2496
- Phenergan Syrup 2495
- Phenergan Tablets 2496
- Phenergan VC 2500
- Phenergan VC with Codeine 2501

Propofol (Additive effects). Products include:
- Diprivan Injection 2267

Propoxyphene Hydrochloride (Additive effects). Products include:
- Darvon 1256
- Wygesic Tablets 2540

Propoxyphene Napsylate (Additive effects). Products include:
- Darvon-N/Darvocet-N 1254

Quazepam (Additive effects). Products include:
- Doral Tablets 2383

Secobarbital Sodium (Additive effects). Products include:
- Seconal Sodium Pulvules 1296

Sufentanil Citrate (Additive effects). Products include:
- Sufenta Injection 1147

Temazepam (Additive effects). Products include:
- Restoril Capsules 2023

Thiamylal Sodium (Additive effects). Products include:
- Surital Ampoules, Steri-Vials 1764

Thioridazine Hydrochloride (Additive effects). Products include:
- Mellaril 2011

Thiothixene (Additive effects). Products include:
- Navane Capsules and Concentrate 1954
- Navane Intramuscular 1956

Triazolam (Additive effects). Products include:
- Halcion Tablets 2340

Trifluoperazine Hydrochloride (Additive effects). Products include:
- Stelazine 2226

DAMASON-P

(Hydrocodone Bitartrate, Aspirin) 1356
May interact with oral anticoagulants, antigout agents, narcotic analgesics, general anesthetics, tranquilizers, phenothiazines, hypnotics and sedatives, central nervous system depressants, oral hypoglycemic agents, insulin, anticholinergics, tricyclic antidepressants, monoamine oxidase inhibitors, barbiturates, corticosteroids, non-steroidal anti-inflammatory agents, and certain other agents. Compounds in these categories include:

Alcohol (Additive CNS depression).

Alfentanil Hydrochloride (Additive CNS depression). Products include:
- Alfenta Injection 1131

Allopurinol (Aspirin may inhibit uricosuric effects). Products include:
- Zyloprim Tablets 830

Alprazolam (Additive CNS depression). Products include:
- Xanax Tablets 2367

Amitriptyline Hydrochloride (Increased effects of either drug). Products include:
- Elavil 2269
- Endep Tablets 1927
- Etrafon 2087
- Limbitrol 1933
- Triavil Tablets 1556

Amoxapine (Increased effects of either drug). Products include:
- Asendin Tablets 1196

Aprobarbital (Additive CNS depression). Products include:
- Alurate Elixir 1883

Atropine Sulfate (May produce paralytic ileus). Products include:
- Arco-Lase Plus Tablets 607
- Atropine Sulfate Sterile Ophthalmic Solution and S.O.P. Sterile Ophthalmic Ointment .... ⊙ 239
- Donnagel .... ▣ 675
- Donnagel-PG 1858
- Donnatal 1858
- Donnatal Extentabs 1859
- Donnatal Tablets 1858
- Donnazyme Tablets 1860
- Isopto Atropine .... ⊙ 218
- Lomotil 2174
- Motofen Tablets 836
- Ru-Tuss Tablets 693
- Urised Tablets 2396

Belladonna Alkaloids (May produce paralytic ileus). Products include:
- Bellergal-S Tablets 1998
- Hyland's Bed Wetting Tablets .... ▣ 728
- Hyland's Teething Tablets .... ▣ 728
- Kinesed Tablets 2272

Benztropine Mesylate (May produce paralytic ileus). Products include:
- Cogentin 1435

Betamethasone Acetate (Enhanced corticosteroid effects). Products include:
- Celestone Soluspan Suspension 2081

Betamethasone Sodium Phosphate (Enhanced corticosteroid effects). Products include:
- Celestone Soluspan Suspension 2081

Biperiden (May produce paralytic ileus). Products include:
- Akineton 1171

Buprenorphine (Additive CNS depression).
- No products indexed under this heading.

Buspirone Hydrochloride (Additive CNS depression). Products include:
- BuSpar 1401

Butabarbital (Additive CNS depression). Products include:
- Pyridium Plus 1764

Butalbital (Additive CNS depression). Products include:
- Esgic-Plus Tablets 1002
- Esgic Tablets & Capsules 1001
- Fioricet Tablets 2006
- Fiorinal Capsules 2007
- Fiorinal with Codeine Capsules 2008
- Fiorinal Tablets 2007
- Phrenilin 838
- Sedapap Tablets 50 mg/650 mg .. 1360

Chlordiazepoxide (Additive CNS depression). Products include:
- Libritabs Tablets 1930
- Limbitrol 1933
- Menrium Tablets 1934

Chlordiazepoxide Hydrochloride (Additive CNS depression). Products include:
- Librax Capsules 1929
- Librium Capsules 1931
- Librium Injectable 1932

Chlorpromazine (Additive CNS depression). Products include:
- Thorazine 2234

Chlorpropamide (Enhanced effects of oral antidiabetic agents). Products include:
- Diabinese Tablets 1775

Chlorprothixene (Additive CNS depression). Products include:
- Taractan Tablets 1920

Chlorprothixene Hydrochloride (Additive CNS depression). Products include:
- Taractan 1920

Clidinium Bromide (May produce paralytic ileus). Products include:
- Librax Capsules 1929
- Quarzan Capsules 1937

Clomipramine Hydrochloride (Increased effects of either drug). Products include:
- Anafranil Capsules 650

Clorazepate Dipotassium (Additive CNS depression). Products include:
- Tranxene 556

Codeine (Additive CNS depression). Products include:
- Calcidrine Syrup 506

Codeine Phosphate (Additive CNS depression). Products include:
- Actifed with Codeine Cough Syrup .. 752
- Cheracol Cough Syrup 1853
- Codimal PH Syrup 846
- Dimetane-DC Cough Syrup 1857
- Empirin with Codeine Phosphate Nos. 2, 3 & 4 764
- Fiorinal with Codeine Capsules 2008
- Isoclor Expectorant 982
- Naldecon CX Adult Liquid .... ▣ 521
- Novahistine DH 1342
- Novahistine Expectorant 1343
- Nucofed Capsules 2219
- Nucofed Expectorant 2219
- Nucofed Pediatric Expectorant 2220
- Nucofed Syrup 2219
- Phenaphen with Codeine Capsules 1865
- Phenaphen-650 with Codeine Tablets 1866
- Phenergan with Codeine 2497
- Phenergan VC with Codeine 2501
- Robitussin A-C Syrup 1875
- Robitussin-DAC Syrup 1875
- Ryna .... ▣ 741
- Soma Compound w/Codeine Tablets 2390
- Triaminic Expectorant w/Codeine .. 1996
- Tussi-Organidin Liquid 2391
- Tylenol with Codeine 1381

Codeine Polistirex (Additive CNS depression).
- No products indexed under this heading.

Cortisone Acetate (Enhanced corticosteroid effects). Products include:
- Cortone Acetate Sterile Suspension 1437
- Cortone Acetate Tablets 1439

Desipramine Hydrochloride (Increased effects of either drug). Products include:
- Norpramin Tablets 1340

Dexamethasone (Enhanced corticosteroid effects). Products include:
- AK-Trol Ointment & Suspension .... ⊙ 207
- Decadron Elixir 1445
- Decadron Tablets 1447
- Decaspray Topical Aerosol 1459
- Dexacidin .... ⊙ 272
- Maxidex Sterile Ophthalmic Suspension .... ⊙ 223
- Maxitrol Ophthalmic Ointment/Suspension .... ⊙ 223
- TobraDex Ophthalmic Suspension and Ointment .... ⊙ 228

Dexamethasone Acetate (Enhanced corticosteroid effects). Products include:
- Dalalone D.P. Injectable 999
- Decadron-LA Sterile Suspension 1457

Dexamethasone Sodium Phosphate (Enhanced corticosteroid effects). Products include:
- AK-Dex .... ⊙ 203
- Decadron Phosphate Respihaler 1454
- Decadron Phosphate Sterile Ophthalmic Ointment 1453
- Decadron Phosphate Sterile Ophthalmic Solution 1453
- Decadron Phosphate Topical Cream 1455
- Decadron Phosphate Turbinaire 1456
- Maxidex Sterile Ophthalmic Ointment .... ⊙ 222
- NeoDecadron Sterile Ophthalmic Ointment 1517
- NeoDecadron Sterile Ophthalmic Solution 1518
- NeoDecadron Topical Cream 1518

Dezocine (Additive CNS depression).

Diazepam (Additive CNS depression). Products include:
- Valium Injectable 1937
- Valium Tablets 1939
- Valrelease Capsules 1923

Diclofenac Sodium (Increases the risk of peptic ulceration and bleeding). Products include:
- Voltaren Ophthalmic Sterile Ophthalmic Solution .... ⊙ 268
- Voltaren Tablets 1042

Dicumarol (Aspirin may enhance effects of dicumarol; concurrent use is contraindicated). Products include:
- Dicumarol Tablets 516

Dicyclomine Hydrochloride (May produce paralytic ileus). Products include:
- Bentyl 1322

Doxepin Hydrochloride (Increased effects of either drug). Products include:
- Sinequan 1960

Droperidol (Additive CNS depression). Products include:
- Inapsine Injection 1140
- Innovar Injection 1141

Enflurane (Additive CNS depression). Products include:
- Ethrane 599

Estazolam (Additive CNS depression). Products include:
- ProSom Tablets ... 554

Ethchlorvynol (Additive CNS depression). Products include:
- Placidyl Capsules ... 553

Ethinamate (Additive CNS depression).
- No products indexed under this heading.

Ethopropazine Hydrochloride (May produce paralytic ileus).

Etodolac (Increases the risk of peptic ulceration and bleeding). Products include:
- Lodine Capsules ... 2468

Fenoprofen Calcium (Increases the risk of peptic ulceration and bleeding). Products include:
- Nalfon Pulvules & Tablets ... 919

Fentanyl (Additive CNS depression). Products include:
- Duragesic Transdermal System ... 1133

Fentanyl Citrate (Additive CNS depression). Products include:
- Innovar Injection ... 1141
- Sublimaze Injection ... 1146

Fluphenazine Decanoate (Additive CNS depression). Products include:
- Prolixin Decanoate ... 1795

Fluphenazine Enanthate (Additive CNS depression). Products include:
- Prolixin Enanthate ... 1796

Fluphenazine Hydrochloride (Additive CNS depression). Products include:
- Prolixin Elixir ... 1793
- Prolixin Injection ... 1791
- Prolixin Oral Concentrate ... 1792
- Prolixin Tablets ... 1793

Flurazepam Hydrochloride (Additive CNS depression). Products include:
- Dalmane Capsules ... 1927

Flurbiprofen (Increases the risk of peptic ulceration and bleeding). Products include:
- Ansaid Tablets ... 2319

Furazolidone (Increased effects of either drug). Products include:
- Furoxone ... 1855

Glipizide (Enhanced effects of oral antidiabetic agents). Products include:
- Glucotrol ... 1952

Glutethimide (Additive CNS depression).
- No products indexed under this heading.

Glyburide (Enhanced effects of oral antidiabetic agents). Products include:
- DiaBeta ... 1091
- Micronase Tablets ... 2350

Glycopyrrolate (May produce paralytic ileus). Products include:
- Robinul Forte Tablets ... 1873
- Robinul Injectable ... 1873
- Robinul Tablets ... 1873

Haloperidol (Additive CNS depression). Products include:
- Haldol Injection, Tablets and Concentrate ... 1373

Haloperidol Decanoate (Additive CNS depression). Products include:
- Haldol Decanoate ... 1375

Hydrocodone Polistirex (Additive CNS depression). Products include:
- Tussionex Extended-Release Suspension ... 988

Hydrocortisone (Enhanced corticosteroid effects). Products include:
- AK-Spore H.C. ... ◉ 206
- Bactine Hydrocortisone Anti-Itch Cream ... ▣ 625
- CaldeCORT Anti-Itch Hydrocortisone Spray ... ▣ 560
- Carmol HC Cream 1% ... 2296
- Cortaid Spray ... ▣ 735
- Cortenema ... 2244
- Cortisporin Ointment ... 758
- Cortisporin Ophthalmic Ointment Sterile ... 758
- Cortisporin Ophthalmic Suspension Sterile ... 759
- Cortisporin Otic Solution Sterile ... 760
- Cortisporin Otic Suspension Sterile ... 760
- Cortizone-5 Creme & Ointment ... ▣ 732
- Dermolate Anti-Itch Cream ... ▣ 697
- Eldecort Cream 1.0% ... 1113
- Eldecort Cream 1.0% and 2.5% ... 1113
- Fungoid HC Creme ... 1770
- Hydrocortone Tablets ... 1482
- Hytone ... 909
- LazerSporin-C Solution ... 1770
- Massengill Medicated Soft Cloth Towelettes ... 2192
- Nutracort Cream & Lotion ... 1684
- PediOtic Suspension Sterile ... 797
- Synacort Creams 1%, 2.5% ... 2296
- Vanoxide-HC Acne Lotion ... 911
- Vioform-Hydrocortisone Cream and Mild Cream ... 889
- Vioform-Hydrocortisone Ointment ... 889
- VōSoL HC Otic Solution ... 2392
- Vytone Cream 1% ... 911

Hydrocortisone Acetate (Enhanced corticosteroid effects). Products include:
- Analpram-HC Rectal Cream 1% and 2.5% ... 970
- Anusol-HC Cream ... 1690
- Anusol-HC Suppositories ... 1691
- Caldecort ... ▣ 560
- Carmol HC Cream 1% ... 2296
- Chloromycetin Hydrocortisone Ophthalmic ... 1694
- Coly-Mycin S Otic w/Neomycin & Hydrocortisone ... 1708
- Cortaid ... ▣ 735
- Cortef Feminine Itch Cream ... ▣ 735
- Corticaine ... ▣ 682
- Cortifoam ... 1827
- Cortisporin Cream ... 757
- Epifoam ... 1828
- Gynecort 5 Creme ... ▣ 556
- Hydrocortone Acetate Sterile Suspension ... 1479
- Lanacort 5 Creme and Ointment ... ▣ 557
- Mantadil Cream ... 789
- Ophthocort ... ◉ 301
- Orabase HCA Oral Paste ... 890
- Pramosone Cream, Lotion & Ointment ... 971
- ProctoCream-HC ... 1834
- Proctofoam-HC ... 1835

Hydrocortisone Sodium Phosphate (Enhanced corticosteroid effects). Products include:
- Hydrocortone Phosphate Injection, Sterile ... 1481

Hydrocortisone Sodium Succinate (Enhanced corticosteroid effects). Products include:
- Solu-Cortef Sterile Powder ... 2361

Hydroxyzine Hydrochloride (Additive CNS depression). Products include:
- Atarax Tablets & Syrup ... 1941
- Marax Tablets & DF Syrup ... 1954
- Vistaril Intramuscular Solution ... 1970

Hyoscyamine (May produce paralytic ileus). Products include:
- Cystospaz Tablets ... 2395
- Urised Tablets ... 2396

Hyoscyamine Sulfate (May produce paralytic ileus). Products include:
- Arco-Lase Plus Tablets ... 607
- Cystospaz-M Capsules ... 2395
- Donnagel ... ▣ 675
- Donnagel-PG ... 1858
- Donnatal ... 1858
- Donnatal Extentabs ... 1859
- Donnatal Tablets ... 1858
- Donnazyme Tablets ... 1860
- Kutrase Capsules ... 2146
- Levsin/Levsinex ... 2147
- Ru-Tuss Tablets ... 693

Ibuprofen (Increases the risk of peptic ulceration and bleeding). Products include:
- Advil Cold & Sinus Caplets (formerly CoAdvil) ... 2416
- Advil Ibuprofen Tablets and Caplets ... 2416
- Children's Advil Suspension ... 2426
- CoAdvil ... ▣ 748
- Dristan Sinus Caplets ... 2419
- Haltran Tablets ... ▣ 668
- Ibuprofen ... ▣ 631
- Medipren ibuprofen Caplets and Tablets ... 1362
- Midol 200 Cramp Relief Formula ... ▣ 570
- Motrin Tablets ... 2351
- Motrin IB Caplets and Tablets ... ▣ 736
- Nuprin Ibuprofen/Analgesic Tablets & Caplets ... 752
- PediaProfen Suspension ... 1363
- Rufen Tablets ... 691
- Trendar Ibuprofen Tablets ... ▣ 756

Imipramine Hydrochloride (Increased effects of either drug). Products include:
- Tofranil Ampuls ... 1038
- Tofranil Tablets ... 1039

Imipramine Pamoate (Increased effects of either drug). Products include:
- Tofranil-PM Capsules ... 1041

Indomethacin (Increases the risk of peptic ulceration and bleeding). Products include:
- Indocin ... 1487

Indomethacin Sodium Trihydrate (Increases the risk of peptic ulceration and bleeding). Products include:
- Indocin I.V. ... 1490

Insulin, Human (Enhanced effects of insulin).
- No products indexed under this heading.

Insulin, Human Isophane Suspension (Enhanced effects of insulin). Products include:
- Humulin N, 100 Units ... 1270

Insulin, Human NPH (Enhanced effects of insulin). Products include:
- Insulatard NPH Human ... 1627
- Novolin N ... 1627
- Novolin N PenFill Cartridges ... 1628
- Novolin N Prefilled ... 1628

Insulin, Human Regular (Enhanced effects of insulin). Products include:
- Humulin BR, 100 Units ... 1268
- Humulin R, 100 Units ... 1272
- Novolin R ... 1627
- Novolin R PenFill Cartridges ... 1628
- Novolin R Prefilled ... 1629
- Velosulin Human ... 1628

Insulin, Human, Zinc Suspension (Enhanced effects of insulin). Products include:
- Humulin L, 100 Units ... 1268
- Humulin U, 100 Units ... 1272
- Novolin L ... 1627

Insulin, NPH (Enhanced effects of insulin). Products include:
- NPH, 40 & 100 Units ... 1273
- Beef NPH, 100 Units ... 1274
- Pork NPH, 100 Units ... 1275
- Insulatard NPH ... 1626
- NPH Insulin ... 1626
- NPH Purified Pork Isophane Insulin ... 1626

Insulin, Regular (Enhanced effects of insulin). Products include:
- Regular, 40 & 100 Units ... 1273
- Beef Regular, 100 Units ... 1275
- Pork Regular, 100 Units ... 1275
- Pork Regular (Concentrated), 500 Units ... 1276
- Regular Insulin ... 1625
- Regular Purified Pork Insulin ... 1626
- Velosulin ... 1627

Insulin, Zinc Crystals (Enhanced effects of insulin). Products include:
- NPH, 40 & 100 Units ... 1273

Insulin, Zinc Suspension (Enhanced effects of insulin). Products include:
- Lente, 40 & 100 Units ... 1272
- Protamine, Zinc, 40 & 100 Units ... 1273
- Lente Iletin I ... 1272
- Beef Lente, 100 Units ... 1274
- Beef Protamine Zinc, 100 Units ... 1274
- Pork Lente, 100 Units ... 1275
- Pork, Protamine, Zinc, 100 Units ... 1275
- Lente Insulin ... 1626
- Lente Purified Pork Insulin ... 1626
- Semilente Insulin ... 1625
- Ultralente Insulin ... 1626

Ipratropium Bromide (May produce paralytic ileus). Products include:
- Atrovent Inhalation Aerosol ... 675

Isocarboxazid (Increased effects of either drug). Products include:
- Marplan Tablets ... 1906

Isoflurane (Additive CNS depression). Products include:
- Forane ... 600

Ketamine Hydrochloride (Additive CNS depression). Products include:
- Ketalar ... 1726

Ketoprofen (Increases the risk of peptic ulceration and bleeding). Products include:
- Orudis Capsules ... 2488

Ketorolac Tromethamine (Increases the risk of peptic ulceration and bleeding). Products include:
- Toradol IM Injection ... 2302

Levorphanol Tartrate (Additive CNS depression). Products include:
- Levo-Dromoran ... 1906

Lorazepam (Additive CNS depression). Products include:
- Ativan Injection ... 2432
- Ativan Tablets ... 2434

Loxapine Hydrochloride (Additive CNS depression). Products include:
- Loxitane ... 1213

Loxapine Succinate (Additive CNS depression). Products include:
- Loxitane Capsules ... 1213

Maprotiline Hydrochloride (Increased effects of either drug). Products include:
- Ludiomil Tablets ... 874

Meclofenamate Sodium (Increases the risk of peptic ulceration and bleeding). Products include:
- Meclomen Capsules ... 1739

Mefenamic Acid (Increases the risk of peptic ulceration and bleeding). Products include:
- Ponstel ... 1758

Mepenzolate Bromide (May produce paralytic ileus). Products include:
- Cantil Tablets ... 1326

Meperidine Hydrochloride (Additive CNS depression). Products include:
- Demerol ... 2047
- Mepergan Injection ... 2479

Mephobarbital (Additive CNS depression). Products include:
- Mebaral Tablets ... 2061

Meprobamate (Additive CNS depression). Products include:
- Deprol Tablets ... 2382
- Equagesic Tablets ... 2451
- Miltown Tablets ... 2386
- PMB 200 and PMB 400 ... 2504

Mercaptopurine (Potential for bone marrow toxicity and blood dyscrasias). Products include:
- Purinethol Tablets ... 800

Mesoridazine (Additive CNS depression). Products include:
- Serentil ... 686

(▣ Described in PDR For Nonprescription Drugs) (◉ Described in PDR For Ophthalmology)

Methadone Hydrochloride (Additive CNS depression). Products include:
- Dolophine Hydrochloride Ampoules & Vials 1260
- Dolophine Hydrochloride Tablets 1261
- Methadone Hydrochloride Diskets .. 1284
- Methadone Hydrochloride Oral Solution & Tablets 1987

Methohexital Sodium (Additive CNS depression). Products include:
- Brevital Sodium Vials 1248

Methotrexate Sodium (Enhanced effects of methotrexate causing bone marrow toxicity and blood dyscrasias). Products include:
- Methotrexate Tablets, Parenteral, LPF Parenteral 1217
- Rheumatrex Methotrexate Dose Pack 1234

Methoxyflurane (Additive CNS depression).
- No products indexed under this heading.

Methylprednisolone Acetate (Enhanced corticosteroid effects). Products include:
- Depo-Medrol Sterile Aqueous Suspension 2334

Methylprednisolone Sodium Succinate (Enhanced corticosteroid effects). Products include:
- Solu-Medrol Sterile Powder 2363

Midazolam Hydrochloride (Additive CNS depression). Products include:
- Versed Injection 1924

Molindone Hydrochloride (Additive CNS depression). Products include:
- Moban Tablets & Concentrate 932

Morphine Sulfate (Additive CNS depression). Products include:
- Astramorph/PF Injection, USP (Preservative-Free) 618
- Duramorph 960
- Infumorph 200 and Infumorph 500 Sterile Solutions 962
- MS Contin Tablets 1814
- MSIR 1817
- Oramorph SR (Morphine Sulfate Sustained Release Tablets) 1988
- Roxanol 1991

Naproxen (Increases the risk of peptic ulceration and bleeding). Products include:
- Naprosyn 2297

Naproxen Sodium (Increases the risk of peptic ulceration and bleeding). Products include:
- Anaprox and Anaprox DS Tablets 2288

Nortriptyline Hydrochloride (Increased effects of either drug). Products include:
- Pamelor 2019

Opium Alkaloids (Additive CNS depression). Products include:
- B & O No. 15A & No. 16A Supprettes 2395
- Pantopon Injectable 1911

Oxazepam (Additive CNS depression). Products include:
- Serax Capsules 2522
- Serax Tablets 2522

Oxybutynin Chloride (May produce paralytic ileus). Products include:
- Ditropan 1332

Oxycodone Hydrochloride (Additive CNS depression). Products include:
- Percocet Tablets 950
- Percodan 951
- Roxicodone Tablets, Oral Solution & Intensol (Oxycodone) 1992
- Tylox Capsules 1382

Oxyphenonium Bromide (May produce paralytic ileus).

Pentobarbital Sodium (Additive CNS depression). Products include:
- Nembutal Sodium Capsules 534
- Nembutal Sodium Solution 536
- Nembutal Sodium Suppositories 538

Perphenazine (Additive CNS depression). Products include:
- Etrafon 2087
- Triavil Tablets 1556
- Trilafon 2123

Phenelzine Sulfate (Increased effects of either drug). Products include:
- Nardil 1742

Phenobarbital (Additive CNS depression). Products include:
- Arco-Lase Plus Tablets 607
- Bellergal-S Tablets 1998
- Bronkolixir .... ▣ 761
- Bronkotabs Tablets .... ▣ 762
- Donnatal 1858
- Donnatal Extentabs 1859
- Donnatal Tablets 1858
- Donnazyme Tablets 1860
- Kinesed Tablets 2272
- Phenobarbital Elixir and Tablets 1293
- Primatene Tablets-P Formula 2421
- Quadrinal Tablets 1183
- Tedral SA 1765

Phenylbutazone (Increases the risk of peptic ulceration and bleeding). Products include:
- Butazolidin Capsules & Tablets 1027

Piroxicam (Increases the risk of peptic ulceration and bleeding). Products include:
- Feldene Capsules 1777

Prazepam (Additive CNS depression). Products include:
- Centrax 1693

Prednisolone Acetate (Enhanced corticosteroid effects). Products include:
- AK-Cide Sterile Ophthalmic Ointment & Suspension .... ⊙ 202
- Blephamide Liquifilm Sterile Ophthalmic Suspension 586
- Blephamide S.O.P. Sterile Ophthalmic Ointment 586
- Cetapred Ointment .... ⊙ 220
- ⅛% Econopred & 1% Econopred Plus .... ⊙ 217
- Isopto Cetapred Suspension .... ⊙ 220
- Metimyd .... ⊙ 306
- Poly-Pred Liquifilm .... ⊙ 250
- Pred Forte .... ⊙ 252
- Pred Mild .... ⊙ 254
- Pred-G Liquifilm Sterile Ophthalmic Suspension .... ⊙ 252
- Pred-G S.O.P. Sterile Ophthalmic Ointment .... ⊙ 253
- Vasocidin Ointment .... ⊙ 275

Prednisolone Sodium Phosphate (Enhanced corticosteroid effects). Products include:
- AK-Pred .... ⊙ 205
- Hydeltrasol Injection, Sterile 1476
- Inflamase .... ⊙ 274
- Pediapred Oral Liquid 987
- Vasocidin Ophthalmic Solution .... ⊙ 276

Prednisolone Tebutate (Enhanced corticosteroid effects). Products include:
- Hydeltra-T.B.A. Sterile Suspension 1478

Prednisone (Enhanced corticosteroid effects). Products include:
- Deltasone Tablets 2332

Probenecid (Aspirin may inhibit uricosuric effects of probenecid). Products include:
- Benemid Tablets 1426
- ColBENEMID Tablets 1436
- Wycillin Injection and Probenecid Tablets 2539

Prochlorperazine (Additive CNS depression). Products include:
- Compazine 2201

Procyclidine Hydrochloride (May produce paralytic ileus). Products include:
- Kemadrin Tablets 771

Promethazine Hydrochloride (Additive CNS depression). Products include:
- Mepergan Injection 2479
- Phenergan with Codeine 2497
- Phenergan with Dextromethorphan 2499
- Phenergan Injection 2493
- Phenergan Suppositories 2496
- Phenergan Syrup 2495
- Phenergan Tablets 2496
- Phenergan VC 2500
- Phenergan VC with Codeine 2501

Propantheline Bromide (May produce paralytic ileus). Products include:
- Pro-Banthīne Tablets 2141

Propofol (Additive CNS depression). Products include:
- Diprivan Injection 2267

Propoxyphene Hydrochloride (Additive CNS depression). Products include:
- Darvon 1256
- Wygesic Tablets 2540

Propoxyphene Napsylate (Additive CNS depression). Products include:
- Darvon-N/Darvocet-N 1254

Protriptyline Hydrochloride (Increased effects of either drug). Products include:
- Vivactil Tablets 1567

Quazepam (Additive CNS depression). Products include:
- Doral Tablets 2383

Scopolamine Hydrobromide (May produce paralytic ileus). Products include:
- Donnagel .... ▣ 675
- Donnagel-PG 1858
- Donnatal 1858
- Donnatal Extentabs 1859
- Donnatal Tablets 1858
- Donnazyme Tablets 1860
- Isopto Hyoscine .... ⊙ 222
- Murocoll-2 Sterile Ophthalmic Solution .... ⊙ 261
- Ru-Tuss Tablets 693

Scopolamine Preparations (May produce paralytic ileus). Products include:
- Transderm Scōp Transdermal Therapeutic System 887

Secobarbital Sodium (Additive CNS depression). Products include:
- Seconal Sodium Pulvules 1296

Selegiline Hydrochloride (Increased effects of either drug). Products include:
- Eldepryl 2250

Sufentanil Citrate (Additive CNS depression). Products include:
- Sufenta Injection 1147

Sulfinpyrazone (Aspirin may inhibit uricosuric effects). Products include:
- Anturane 853

Sulindac (Increases the risk of peptic ulceration and bleeding). Products include:
- Clinoril Tablets 1433

Temazepam (Additive CNS depression). Products include:
- Restoril Capsules 2023

Thiamylal Sodium (Additive CNS depression). Products include:
- Surital Ampoules, Steri-Vials 1764

Thioridazine Hydrochloride (Additive CNS depression). Products include:
- Mellaril 2011

Thiothixene (Additive CNS depression). Products include:
- Navane Capsules and Concentrate 1954
- Navane Intramuscular 1956

Tolazamide (Enhanced effects of oral antidiabetic agents). Products include:
- Tolinase Tablets 2365

Tolbutamide (Enhanced effects of oral antidiabetic agents). Products include:
- Orinase Tablets 2354

Tolmetin Sodium (Increases the risk of peptic ulceration and bleeding). Products include:
- Tolectin (200, 400 and 600 mg) .. 1379

Tranylcypromine Sulfate (Increased effects of either drug). Products include:
- Parnate Tablets 2222

Triamcinolone (Enhanced corticosteroid effects).
- No products indexed under this heading.

Triamcinolone Acetonide (Enhanced corticosteroid effects). Products include:
- Aristocort A 1010
- Azmacort Inhaler 1837
- Kenalog Cream, Lotion & Ointment 2401
- Kenalog-10 Injection 2402
- Kenalog-40 Injection 2403
- Kenalog in Orabase 604
- Kenalog Spray 2401
- Mycolog II Cream and Ointment 2407
- Mytrex Cream & Ointment 2080
- Nasacort Nasal Inhaler 1844

Triamcinolone Diacetate (Enhanced corticosteroid effects). Products include:
- Aristocort Suspension 1008

Triamcinolone Hexacetonide (Enhanced corticosteroid effects). Products include:
- Aristospan Suspension 1011

Triazolam (Additive CNS depression). Products include:
- Halcion Tablets 2340

Tridihexethyl Chloride (May produce paralytic ileus).
- No products indexed under this heading.

Trifluoperazine Hydrochloride (Additive CNS depression). Products include:
- Stelazine 2226

Trihexyphenidyl Hydrochloride (May produce paralytic ileus). Products include:
- Artane 1195

Trimipramine Maleate (Increased effects of either drug). Products include:
- Surmontil Capsules 2524

Warfarin Sodium (Aspirin may enhance effects of warfarin; concurrent use is contraindicated). Products include:
- Coumadin Injection & Tablets 944
- Panwarfin Tablets 547

DANOCRINE CAPSULES
(Danazol) 2046
May interact with:

Carbamazepine (May result in increased carbamazepine levels). Products include:
- Tegretol Chewable Tablets 654
- Tegretol Suspension 656
- Tegretol Tablets 654

Warfarin Sodium (Prolongation of prothrombin time in patients stabilized on warfarin). Products include:
- Coumadin Injection & Tablets 944
- Panwarfin Tablets 547

DANTRIUM CAPSULES
(Dantrolene Sodium) 1619
May interact with estrogens, tranquilizers, and certain other agents. Compounds in these categories include:

Alprazolam (Caution should be exercised if administered concomitantly). Products include:
- Xanax Tablets 2367

(▣ Described in PDR For Nonprescription Drugs) (⊙ Described in PDR For Ophthalmology)

Buspirone Hydrochloride (Caution should be exercised if administered concomitantly). Products include:

BuSpar 1401

Chlordiazepoxide (Caution should be exercised if administered concomitantly). Products include:

Libritabs Tablets 1930
Limbitrol 1933
Menrium Tablets 1934

Chlordiazepoxide Hydrochloride (Caution should be exercised if administered concomitantly). Products include:

Librax Capsules 1929
Librium Capsules 1931
Librium Injectable 1932

Chlorotrianisene (Potential for hepatoxicity). Products include:

TACE 12 and 25 mg 1353

Chlorpromazine (Caution should be exercised if administered concomitantly). Products include:

Thorazine 2234

Chlorprothixene (Caution should be exercised if administered concomitantly). Products include:

Taractan Tablets 1920

Chlorprothixene Hydrochloride (Caution should be exercised if administered concomitantly). Products include:

Taractan 1920

Clorazepate Dipotassium (Caution should be exercised if administered concomitantly). Products include:

Tranxene 556

Diazepam (Caution should be exercised if administered concomitantly). Products include:

Valium Injectable 1937
Valium Tablets 1939
Valrelease Capsules 1923

Dienestrol (Potential for hepatoxicity). Products include:

Ortho Dienestrol Cream 1664

Diethylstilbestrol (Potential for hepatoxicity). Products include:

Diethylstilbestrol Tablets 1258

Droperidol (Caution should be exercised if administered concomitantly). Products include:

Inapsine Injection 1140
Innovar Injection 1141

Estradiol (Potential for hepatoxicity). Products include:

Emcyt Capsules 1161
Estrace 1385
Estrace Vaginal Cream 1388
Estraderm Transdermal System 866

Estrogens, Conjugated (Potential for hepatoxicity). Products include:

Mediatric Capsules 2476
PMB 200 and PMB 400 2504
Premarin Intravenous 2508
Premarin with Methyltestosterone 2515
Premarin Tablets 2510
Premarin Vaginal Cream 2512

Estrogens, Esterified (Potential for hepatoxicity). Products include:

Estratest 2245
Menrium Tablets 1934

Estropipate (Potential for hepatoxicity). Products include:

Ogen 540

Ethinyl Estradiol (Potential for hepatoxicity). Products include:

Brevicon 2304
Demulen 2161
Estinyl Tablets 2085
Jenest-28 Tablets 1636
Levlen/Tri-Levlen 665
Lo/Ovral Tablets 2471
Lo/Ovral-28 Tablets 2476
Loestrin 1728
Modicon 1667
Nordette-21 Tablets 2481
Nordette-28 Tablets 2483
Norethin 2133
Norinyl 2304
Norlestrin 1746
Ortho-Cyclen Tablets 1658
Ortho-Novum 1667
Ovcon 1391
Ovral Tablets 2490
Ovral-28 Tablets 2491
Levlen/Tri-Levlen 665
Tri-Norinyl 2304
Triphasil-21 Tablets 2527
Triphasil-28 Tablets 2532

Fluphenazine Decanoate (Caution should be exercised if administered concomitantly). Products include:

Prolixin Decanoate 1795

Fluphenazine Enanthate (Caution should be exercised if administered concomitantly). Products include:

Prolixin Enanthate 1796

Fluphenazine Hydrochloride (Caution should be exercised if administered concomitantly). Products include:

Prolixin Elixir 1793
Prolixin Injection 1791
Prolixin Oral Concentrate 1792
Prolixin Tablets 1793

Haloperidol (Caution should be exercised if administered concomitantly). Products include:

Haldol Injection, Tablets and Concentrate 1373

Haloperidol Decanoate (Caution should be exercised if administered concomitantly). Products include:

Haldol Decanoate 1375

Hydroxyzine Hydrochloride (Caution should be exercised if administered concomitantly). Products include:

Atarax Tablets & Syrup 1941
Marax Tablets & DF Syrup 1954
Vistaril Intramuscular Solution 1970

Lorazepam (Caution should be exercised if administered concomitantly). Products include:

Ativan Injection 2432
Ativan Tablets 2434

Loxapine Hydrochloride (Caution should be exercised if administered concomitantly). Products include:

Loxitane 1213

Loxapine Succinate (Caution should be exercised if administered concomitantly). Products include:

Loxitane Capsules 1213

Meprobamate (Caution should be exercised if administered concomitantly). Products include:

Deprol Tablets 2382
Equagesic Tablets 2451
Miltown Tablets 2386
PMB 200 and PMB 400 2504

Mesoridazine (Caution should be exercised if administered concomitantly). Products include:

Serentil 686

Molindone Hydrochloride (Caution should be exercised if administered concomitantly). Products include:

Moban Tablets & Concentrate 932

Oxazepam (Caution should be exercised if administered concomitantly). Products include:

Serax Capsules 2522
Serax Tablets 2522

Perphenazine (Caution should be exercised if administered concomitantly). Products include:

Etrafon 2087
Triavil Tablets 1556
Trilafon 2123

Polyestradiol Phosphate (Potential for hepatoxicity). Products include:

Estradurin 2452

Prazepam (Caution should be exercised if administered concomitantly). Products include:

Centrax 1693

Prochlorperazine (Caution should be exercised if administered concomitantly). Products include:

Compazine 2201

Promethazine Hydrochloride (Caution should be exercised if administered concomitantly). Products include:

Mepergan Injection 2479
Phenergan with Codeine 2497
Phenergan with Dextromethorphan 2499
Phenergan Injection 2493
Phenergan Suppositories 2496
Phenergan Syrup 2495
Phenergan Tablets 2496
Phenergan VC 2500
Phenergan VC with Codeine 2501

Quazepam (Caution should be exercised if administered concomitantly). Products include:

Doral Tablets 2383

Quinestrol (Potential for hepatoxicity). Products include:

Estrovis 1721

Thioridazine Hydrochloride (Caution should be exercised if administered concomitantly). Products include:

Mellaril 2011

Thiothixene (Caution should be exercised if administered concomitantly). Products include:

Navane Capsules and Concentrate 1954
Navane Intramuscular 1956

Trifluoperazine Hydrochloride (Caution should be exercised if administered concomitantly). Products include:

Stelazine 2226

Verapamil Hydrochloride (Concomitant administration may result in cardiovascular collapse). Products include:

Calan SR Caplets 2157
Calan Tablets 2155
Isoptin Injectable 1177
Isoptin Oral Tablets 1179
Isoptin SR Sustained Release Tablets 1181
Verelan Capsules 1243
Verelan Capsules 2535

DANTRIUM INTRAVENOUS
(Dantrolene Sodium) 1620
May interact with:

Clofibrate (Reduces binding of dantrolene to plasma proteins). Products include:

Atromid-S Capsules 2435

Tolbutamide (Increases binding of dantrolene to plasma proteins). Products include:

Orinase Tablets 2354

Verapamil Hydrochloride (Potential for ventricular fibrillation and cardiovascular collapse). Products include:

Calan SR Caplets 2157
Calan Tablets 2155
Isoptin Injectable 1177
Isoptin Oral Tablets 1179
Isoptin SR Sustained Release Tablets 1181
Verelan Capsules 1243
Verelan Capsules 2535

Warfarin Sodium (Reduces binding of dantrolene to plasma proteins). Products include:

Coumadin Injection & Tablets 944
Panwarfin Tablets 547

DAPSONE USP
(Dapsone) 1130
May interact with:

Pyrimethamine (Agranulocytosis; increased likelihood of hematological reactions). Products include:

Daraprim Tablets 761
Fansidar Tablets 1896

Rifampin (Lowered Dapsone levels). Products include:

Rifadin 1345
Rifamate Capsules 1347
Rimactane Capsules 879

DARANIDE TABLETS
(Dichlorphenamide) 1445
May interact with corticosteroids and certain other agents. Compounds in these categories include:

ACTH (Hypokalemia may develop).

Aspirin (Concomitant high-dose aspirin may produce anorexia, tachypnea, lethargy and coma). Products include:

Alka-Seltzer Effervescent Antacid and Pain Reliever 1568
Alka-Seltzer Extra Strength Effervescent Antacid and Pain Reliever 1570
Alka-Seltzer (Flavored) Effervescent Antacid and Pain Reliever 1569
Alka-Seltzer Plus Cold Medicine .... ⊞ 623
Alka-Seltzer Plus Night-Time Cold Medicine .... ⊞ 623
Alka Seltzer Plus Sinus Allergy Medicine .... ⊞ 624
Anacin Coated Analgesic Caplets 2417
Anacin Coated Analgesic Tablets 2417
Anacin Maximum Strength Analgesic Coated Tablets 2417
Maximum Strength Arthritis Pain Formula By the Makers of Anacin Analgesic Tablets and Caplets 2418
Arthritis Pain Formula by the Makers of Anacin Analgesic Tablets and Caplets .... ⊞ 747
Arthritis Strength BC Powder .... ⊞ 516
Ascriptin A/D Caplets 1850
Regular Strength Ascriptin Tablets 1850
Azdone Tablets 844
BC Powder .... ⊞ 517
BC Cold Powder .... ⊞ 517
Children's Bayer Chewable Aspirin .... ⊞ 564
Genuine Bayer Aspirin Tablets & Caplets .... ⊞ 564
Maximum Bayer Aspirin Tablets & Caplets .... ⊞ 566
Bayer Plus Aspirin Tablets .... ⊞ 567
Therapy Bayer Aspirin Caplets .... ⊞ 568
8 Hour Bayer Timed-Release Aspirin .... ⊞ 566
Arthritis Strength Bufferin Analgesic Caplets 744
Extra Strength Bufferin Analgesic Tablets 745
Bufferin Analgesic Tablets and Caplets 743
Cama Arthritis Pain Reliever .... ⊞ 685
Damason-P 1356
Easprin 1719
Ecotrin Enteric Coated Aspirin Maximum Strength Tablets and Caplets 2189
Ecotrin Enteric Coated Aspirin Regular Strength Tablets and Caplets 2189
Empirin Aspirin .... ⊞ 541
Empirin with Codeine Phosphate Nos. 2, 3 & 4 764
Equagesic Tablets 2451
Excedrin Extra-Strength Analgesic Tablets & Caplets 749
4-Way Cold Tablets 750
Fiorinal Capsules 2007
Fiorinal with Codeine Capsules 2008
Fiorinal Tablets 2007
Lortab ASA Tablets 2414
Momentum Muscular Backache Formula .... ⊞ 751
Norgesic 1314
Norwich Extra-Strength Aspirin .... ⊞ 546
Norwich Regular Strength Aspirin ⊞ 547
P-A-C Analgesic Tablets .... ⊞ 669
Percodan 951
Robaxisal Tablets 1872

Sine-Off Sinus Medicine Tablets-Aspirin Formula ▣ 722
Soma Compound w/Codeine Tablets 2390
Soma Compound Tablets 2389
St. Joseph Adult Chewable Aspirin (81 mg.) ▣ 703
Synalgos-DC Capsules 2525
Talwin Compound 2072
Ursinus Inlay-Tabs ▣ 691
Vanquish Analgesic Caplets ▣ 574
Zorprin Tablets 698

Aspirin, Enteric Coated (Concomitant high-dose aspirin may produce anorexia, tachypnea, lethargy and coma). Products include:
Therapy Bayer Aspirin Caplets ▣ 568
Ecotrin 2189

Betamethasone Acetate (Hypokalemia may develop). Products include:
Celestone Soluspan Suspension 2081

Betamethasone Sodium Phosphate (Hypokalemia may develop). Products include:
Celestone Soluspan Suspension 2081

Cortisone Acetate (Hypokalemia may develop). Products include:
Cortone Acetate Sterile Suspension 1437
Cortone Acetate Tablets 1439

Dexamethasone (Hypokalemia may develop). Products include:
AK-Trol Ointment & Suspension ◉ 207
Decadron Elixir 1445
Decadron Tablets 1447
Decaspray Topical Aerosol 1459
Dexacidin ◉ 272
Maxidex Sterile Ophthalmic Suspension ◉ 223
Maxitrol Ophthalmic Ointment/Suspension ◉ 223
TobraDex Ophthalmic Suspension and Ointment ◉ 228

Dexamethasone Acetate (Hypokalemia may develop). Products include:
Dalalone D.P. Injectable 999
Decadron-LA Sterile Suspension 1457

Dexamethasone Sodium Phosphate (Hypokalemia may develop). Products include:
AK-Dex ◉ 203
Decadron Phosphate Respihaler 1454
Decadron Phosphate Sterile Ophthalmic Ointment 1453
Decadron Phosphate Sterile Ophthalmic Solution 1453
Decadron Phosphate Topical Cream 1455
Decadron Phosphate Turbinaire 1456
Maxidex Sterile Ophthalmic Ointment ◉ 222
NeoDecadron Sterile Ophthalmic Ointment 1517
NeoDecadron Sterile Ophthalmic Solution 1518
NeoDecadron Topical Cream 1518

Hydrocortisone (Hypokalemia may develop). Products include:
AK-Spore H.C. ◉ 206
Bactine Hydrocortisone Anti-Itch Cream ▣ 625
CaldeCORT Anti-Itch Hydrocortisone Spray ▣ 560
Carmol HC Cream 1% 2296
Cortaid Spray ▣ 735
Cortenema 2244
Cortisporin Ointment 758
Cortisporin Ophthalmic Ointment Sterile 758
Cortisporin Ophthalmic Suspension Sterile 759
Cortisporin Otic Solution Sterile 760
Cortisporin Otic Suspension Sterile 760
Cortizone-5 Creme & Ointment ▣ 732
Dermolate Anti-Itch Cream ▣ 697
Eldecort Cream 1.0% 1113
Eldecort Cream 1.0% and 2.5% 1113
Fungoid HC Creme 1770
Hydrocortone Tablets 1482
Hytone 909
LazerSporin-C Solution 1770
Massengill Medicated Soft Cloth Towelettes 2192
Nutracort Cream & Lotion 1684
PediOtic Suspension Sterile 797
Synacort Creams 1%, 2.5% 2296
Vanoxide-HC Acne Lotion 911
Vioform-Hydrocortisone Cream and Mild Cream 889
Vioform-Hydrocortisone Ointment 889
VōSoL HC Otic Solution 2392
Vytone Cream 1% 911

Hydrocortisone Acetate (Hypokalemia may develop). Products include:
Analpram-HC Rectal Cream 1% and 2.5% 970
Anusol-HC Cream 1690
Anusol-HC Suppositories 1691
Caldecort ▣ 560
Carmol HC Cream 1% 2296
Chloromycetin Hydrocortisone Ophthalmic 1694
Coly-Mycin S Otic w/Neomycin & Hydrocortisone 1708
Cortaid ▣ 735
Cortef Feminine Itch Cream ▣ 735
Corticaine ▣ 682
Cortifoam 1827
Cortisporin Cream 757
Epifoam 1828
Gynecort 5 Creme ▣ 556
Hydrocortone Acetate Sterile Suspension 1479
Lanacort 5 Creme and Ointment ▣ 557
Mantadil Cream 789
Ophthocort ◉ 301
Orabase HCA Oral Paste 890
Pramosone Cream, Lotion & Ointment 971
ProctoCream-HC 1834
Proctofoam-HC 1835

Hydrocortisone Sodium Phosphate (Hypokalemia may develop). Products include:
Hydrocortone Phosphate Injection, Sterile 1481

Hydrocortisone Sodium Succinate (Hypokalemia may develop). Products include:
Solu-Cortef Sterile Powder 2361

Methylprednisolone Acetate (Hypokalemia may develop). Products include:
Depo-Medrol Sterile Aqueous Suspension 2334

Methylprednisolone Sodium Succinate (Hypokalemia may develop). Products include:
Solu-Medrol Sterile Powder 2363

Prednisolone Acetate (Hypokalemia may develop). Products include:
AK-Cide Sterile Ophthalmic Ointment & Suspension ◉ 202
Blephamide Liquifilm Sterile Ophthalmic Suspension 586
Blephamide S.O.P. Sterile Ophthalmic Ointment 586
Cetapred Ointment ◉ 220
⅛% Econopred & 1% Econopred Plus ◉ 217
Isopto Cetapred Suspension ◉ 220
Metimyd ◉ 306
Poly-Pred Liquifilm ◉ 250
Pred Forte ◉ 252
Pred Mild ◉ 254
Pred-G Liquifilm Sterile Ophthalmic Suspension ◉ 252
Pred-G S.O.P. Sterile Ophthalmic Ointment ◉ 253
Vasocidin Ointment ◉ 275

Prednisolone Sodium Phosphate (Hypokalemia may develop). Products include:
AK-Pred ◉ 205
Hydeltrasol Injection, Sterile 1476
Inflamase ◉ 274
Pediapred Oral Liquid 987
Vasocidin Ophthalmic Solution ◉ 276

Prednisolone Tebutate (Hypokalemia may develop). Products include:
Hydeltra-T.B.A. Sterile Suspension 1478

Prednisone (Hypokalemia may develop). Products include:
Deltasone Tablets 2332

Triamcinolone (Hypokalemia may develop).
No products indexed under this heading.

Triamcinolone Acetonide (Hypokalemia may develop). Products include:
Aristocort A 1010
Azmacort Inhaler 1837
Kenalog Cream, Lotion & Ointment 2401
Kenalog-10 Injection 2402
Kenalog-40 Injection 2403
Kenalog in Orabase 604
Kenalog Spray 2401
Mycolog II Cream and Ointment 2407
Mytrex Cream & Ointment 2080
Nasacort Nasal Inhaler 1844

Triamcinolone Diacetate (Hypokalemia may develop). Products include:
Aristocort Suspension 1008

Triamcinolone Hexacetonide (Hypokalemia may develop). Products include:
Aristospan Suspension 1011

DARAPRIM TABLETS
(Pyrimethamine) 761
May interact with sulfonamides and certain other agents. Compounds in these categories include:

Lorazepam (Concomitant therapy may result in mild hepatotoxicity). Products include:
Ativan Injection 2432
Ativan Tablets 2434

Phenytoin (Daraprim should be used with caution). Products include:
Dilantin Infatabs 1710
Dilantin-30 Pediatric/Dilantin-125 Suspension 1713

Phenytoin Sodium (Daraprim should be used with caution). Products include:
Dilantin Kapseals 1708
Dilantin Parenteral 1712
Dilantin with Phenobarbital Kapseals 1715

Sulfamethizole (Increased risk of bone marrow suppression and hypersensitivity reactions). Products include:
Thiosulfil Forte Tablets 2526
Urobiotic-250 Capsules 1968

Sulfamethoxazole (Increased risk of bone marrow suppression and hypersensitivity reactions). Products include:
Azo Gantanol Tablets 1887
Bactrim DS Tablets 1891
Bactrim I.V. Infusion 1889
Bactrim 1891
Gantanol 1899
Septra 813
Septra I.V. Infusion 808
Septra I.V. Infusion ADD-Vantage Vials 810
Septra 813

Sulfasalazine (Increased risk of bone marrow suppression and hypersensitivity reactions). Products include:
Azulfidine Tablets, EN-tabs, Oral Suspension 1157

Sulfinpyrazone (Increased risk of bone marrow suppression and hypersensitivity reactions). Products include:
Anturane 853

Sulfisoxazole (Increased risk of bone marrow suppression and hypersensitivity reactions). Products include:
Azo Gantrisin Tablets 1888
Gantrisin Tablets 1901
Pediazole 1973

Sulfisoxazole Diolamine (Increased risk of bone marrow suppression and hypersensitivity reactions). Products include:
Gantrisin Ophthalmic Ointment/Solution 1900

Trimethoprim (Increased risk of bone marrow suppression and hypersensitivity reactions). Products include:
Bactrim DS Tablets 1891
Bactrim I.V. Infusion 1889
Bactrim 1891
Proloprim Tablets 799
Septra 813
Septra I.V. Infusion 808
Septra I.V. Infusion ADD-Vantage Vials 810
Septra 813
Trimpex Tablets 1922

DARBID TABLETS
(Isopropamide Iodide) 2205
May interact with belladona products, anticholinergics, narcotic analgesics, cholinergic agents, corticosteroids, antihistamines, phenothiazines, tricyclic antidepressants, type 1 antiarrhythmic drugs, and certain other agents. Compounds in these categories include:

Alfentanil Hydrochloride (Concomitant administration may result in excessive cholinergic blockade). Products include:
Alfenta Injection 1131

Amitriptyline Hydrochloride (Concomitant administration may result in excessive cholinergic blockade). Products include:
Elavil 2269
Endep Tablets 1927
Etrafon 2087
Limbitrol 1933
Triavil Tablets 1556

Amoxapine (Concomitant administration may result in excessive cholinergic blockade). Products include:
Asendin Tablets 1196

Astemizole (Concomitant administration may result in excessive cholinergic blockade). Products include:
Hismanal Tablets 1138

Atropine Sulfate (Concurrent administration may result in excessive cholinergic blockade). Products include:
Arco-Lase Plus Tablets 607
Atropine Sulfate Sterile Ophthalmic Solution and S.O.P. Sterile Ophthalmic Ointment ◉ 239
Donnagel ▣ 675
Donnagel-PG 1858
Donnatal 1858
Donnatal Extentabs 1859
Donnatal Tablets 1858
Donnazyme Tablets 1860
Isopto Atropine ◉ 218
Lomotil 2174
Motofen Tablets 836
Ru-Tuss Tablets 693
Urised Tablets 2396

Azatadine Maleate (Concomitant administration may result in excessive cholinergic blockade). Products include:
Optimine Tablets 2115
Trinalin Repetabs Tablets 1170

Belladonna Alkaloids (Concurrent administration may result in excessive cholinergic blockade). Products include:
Bellergal-S Tablets 1998
Hyland's Bed Wetting Tablets ▣ 728
Hyland's Teething Tablets ▣ 728
Kinesed Tablets 2272

Benztropine Mesylate (Concurrent administration may result in excessive cholinergic blockade). Products include:
Cogentin 1435

Betamethasone Acetate (Increased intraocular pressure may result from concurrent administration). Products include:

Celestone Soluspan Suspension 2081

Betamethasone Sodium Phosphate (Increased intraocular pressure may result from concurrent administration). Products include:

Celestone Soluspan Suspension 2081

Biperiden (Concurrent administration may result in excessive cholinergic blockade). Products include:

Akineton 1171

Bromodiphenhydramine Hydrochloride (Concomitant administration may result in excessive cholinergic blockade).

No products indexed under this heading.

Brompheniramine Maleate (Concomitant administration may result in excessive cholinergic blockade). Products include:

Alka Seltzer Plus Sinus Allergy Medicine ...... ▣ 624
Atrohist Sprinkle Capsules 558
Bromfed Capsules (Timed Release) 1615
Bromfed Syrup ...... ▣ 628
Bromfed 1615
Dimetane Decongestant ...... ▣ 673
Dimetane ...... ▣ 672
Dimetane-DC Cough Syrup 1857
Dimetane-DX Cough Syrup 1858
Dimetapp Elixir ...... ▣ 673
Dimetapp DM Elixir ...... ▣ 674
Dimetapp Extentabs ...... ▣ 674
Dimetapp Plus Caplets ...... ▣ 675
Dimetapp Tablets ...... ▣ 675
Drixoral Antihistamine/Nasal Decongestant Syrup ...... ▣ 698

Buprenorphine (Concomitant administration may result in excessive cholinergic blockade).

No products indexed under this heading.

Chlorpheniramine Maleate (Concomitant administration may result in excessive cholinergic blockade). Products include:

A.R.M. Allergy Relief Medicine Caplets ...... ▣ 615
Alka-Seltzer Plus Cold Medicine ...... ▣ 623
Allerest ...... ▣ 559
Ana-Kit Anaphylaxis Emergency Treatment Kit 1100
BC Cold Powder Multi-Symptom Formula ...... ▣ 517
Brexin L.A. Capsules 2078
Cerose-DM 2443
Cheracol Plus Head Cold/Cough Formula ...... ▣ 667
Chlor-Trimeton Allergy Syrup, Tablets & Long-Acting Repetabs Tablets ...... ▣ 693
Chlor-Trimeton Decongestant ...... ▣ 694
Comhist LA Capsules 1618
Allergy-Sinus Comtrex Multi-Symptom Allergy Sinus Formula Tablets & Caplets 746
Comtrex Multi-Symptom Cold Reliever Tablets/Caplets/Liqui-Gels/Liquid 745
Day-Night Comtrex 747
Contac Continuous Action Decongestant/Antihistamine Capsules ▣ 710
Contac Maximum Strength Continuous Action Decongestant/Antihistamine Caplets ...... ▣ 709
Contac Severe Cold and Flu Formula Caplets ...... ▣ 711
Coricidin 'D' Decongestant Tablets ...... ▣ 695
Coricidin Demilets Tablets for Children ...... ▣ 696
Coricidin Tablets ...... ▣ 695
Deconamine 663
Demazin Nasal Decongestant/Antihistamine Repetabs Tablets & Syrup ...... ▣ 697
Dorcol Children's Liquid Cold Formula ...... ▣ 686
Dristan Decongestant/Antihistamine/Analgesic Coated Caplets ...... ▣ 749
Dristan Cold Nasal Decongestant/Antihistamine/ Analgesic Coated Tablets 2419
Dristan Advanced Formula Decongestant/Antihistamine/Analgesic Tablets ...... ▣ 749
Extendryl 994
4-Way Cold Tablets 750
Fedahist Gyrocaps 2145
Fedahist Timecaps 2145
Hycomine Compound Tablets 929
Isoclor Timesule Capsules ...... ▣ 561
Kronofed-A 970
Medi-Flu Caplet, Liquid ...... ▣ 640
Naldecon Syrup, Tablets, Pediatric Drops and Pediatric Syrup 709
Nolamine Tablets 838
Novafed A Capsules 1342
Novahistine DH 1342
Novahistine Elixir ...... ▣ 596
Ornade Spansule Capsules 2221
Orthoxicol Cough Syrup ...... ▣ 668
PediaCare Allergy Relief Formula Liquid 1362
PediaCare Cough-Cold Formula Liquid 1362
PediaCare Night Rest Cough-Cold Formula Liquid 1362
PediaCare 6-12 Cough-Cold Formula Chewable Tablets 1362
Pyrroxate Capsules ...... ▣ 669
Quelidrine Syrup 556
Ru-Tuss II Capsules 693
Ru-Tuss Tablets 693
Ryna ...... ▣ 741
Sinarest Tablets & Extra Strength Tablets ...... ▣ 562
Sine-Off Maximum Strength Allergy/Sinus Formula Caplets ...... ▣ 721
Sine-Off Sinus Medicine Tablets-Aspirin Formula ...... ▣ 722
Singlet Tablets ...... ▣ 598
Sinulin 840
Sinutab Maximum Strength ...... ▣ 641
St. Joseph Nighttime Cold Medicine ...... ▣ 705
Sudafed Plus Liquid ...... ▣ 544
Sudafed Plus Tablets ...... ▣ 545
Teldrin Timed-Release Allergy Capsules, 12 mg 2192
TheraFlu Flu and Cold Medicine ...... ▣ 687
Triaminic Allergy Tablets ...... ▣ 688
Triaminic Chewables ...... ▣ 688
Triaminic Cold Tablets ...... ▣ 688
Triaminic Nite Light ...... ▣ 689
Triaminic Syrup ...... ▣ 689
Triaminic-12 Tablets ...... ▣ 690
Triaminicin Tablets ...... ▣ 690
Triaminicol Multi-Symptom Cold Tablets ...... ▣ 691
Triaminicol Multi-Symptom Relief ▣ 691
Tylenol Allergy Sinus Medication Caplets and Gelcaps, Maximum Strength 1372
Children's Tylenol Cold Liquid Formula and Chewable Tablets 1368
Tylenol Cold & Flu Hot Medication, Packets 1369
Tylenol Cold Medication Caplets and Tablets 1370
Tylenol Cold Medication, Effervescent Tablets 1369
Vicks Children's NyQuil ...... ▣ 664
Vicks Formula 44 Cough Medicine ...... ▣ 661
Vicks Formula 44M Multi-Symptom Cough Medicine ...... ▣ 662
Vicks Pediatric Formula 44m Multi-Symptom Cough & Cold Medicine ...... ▣ 663

Chlorpheniramine Polistirex (Concomitant administration may result in excessive cholinergic blockade). Products include:

Tussionex Extended-Release Suspension 988

Chlorpheniramine Tannate (Concomitant administration may result in excessive cholinergic blockade). Products include:

Rynatan 2387
Rynatuss 2388

Chlorpromazine (Concomitant administration may result in excessive cholinergic blockade; potentiation of sedative effect of phenothiazines). Products include:

Thorazine 2234

Clemastine Fumarate (Concomitant administration may result in excessive cholinergic blockade). Products include:

Tavist Syrup 2033
Tavist Tablets 2035
Tavist-D Tablets 2035

Clidinium Bromide (Concurrent administration may result in excessive cholinergic blockade). Products include:

Librax Capsules 1929
Quarzan Capsules 1937

Clomipramine Hydrochloride (Concomitant administration may result in excessive cholinergic blockade). Products include:

Anafranil Capsules 650

Codeine (Concomitant administration may result in excessive cholinergic blockade). Products include:

Calcidrine Syrup 506

Codeine Phosphate (Concomitant administration may result in excessive cholinergic blockade). Products include:

Actifed with Codeine Cough Syrup.. 752
Cheracol Cough Syrup 1853
Codimal PH Syrup 846
Dimetane-DC Cough Syrup 1857
Empirin with Codeine Phosphate Nos. 2, 3 & 4 764
Fiorinal with Codeine Capsules 2008
Isoclor Expectorant 982
Naldecon CX Adult Liquid ...... ▣ 521
Novahistine DH 1342
Novahistine Expectorant 1343
Nucofed Capsules 2219
Nucofed Expectorant 2219
Nucofed Pediatric Expectorant 2220
Nucofed Syrup 2219
Phenaphen with Codeine Capsules 1865
Phenaphen-650 with Codeine Tablets 1866
Phenergan with Codeine 2497
Phenergan VC with Codeine 2501
Robitussin A-C Syrup 1875
Robitussin-DAC Syrup 1875
Ryna ...... ▣ 741
Soma Compound w/Codeine Tablets 2390
Triaminic Expectorant w/Codeine .. 1996
Tussi-Organidin Liquid 2391
Tylenol with Codeine 1381

Codeine Polistirex (Concomitant administration may result in excessive cholinergic blockade).

No products indexed under this heading.

Cortisone Acetate (Increased intraocular pressure may result from concurrent administration). Products include:

Cortone Acetate Sterile Suspension 1437
Cortone Acetate Tablets 1439

Cyproheptadine Hydrochloride (Concomitant administration may result in excessive cholinergic blockade). Products include:

Periactin 1525

Desipramine Hydrochloride (Concomitant administration may result in excessive cholinergic blockade). Products include:

Norpramin Tablets 1340

Dexamethasone (Increased intraocular pressure may result from concurrent administration). Products include:

AK-Trol Ointment & Suspension ...... ⊙ 207
Decadron Elixir 1445
Decadron Tablets 1447
Decaspray Topical Aerosol 1459
Dexacidin ...... ⊙ 272
Maxidex Sterile Ophthalmic Suspension ...... ⊙ 223
Maxitrol Ophthalmic Ointment/Suspension ...... ⊙ 223
TobraDex Ophthalmic Suspension and Ointment ...... ⊙ 228

Dexamethasone Acetate (Increased intraocular pressure may result from concurrent administration). Products include:

Dalalone D.P. Injectable 999
Decadron-LA Sterile Suspension 1457

Dexamethasone Sodium Phosphate (Increased intraocular pressure may result from concurrent administration). Products include:

AK-Dex ...... ⊙ 203
Decadron Phosphate Respihaler 1454
Decadron Phosphate Sterile Ophthalmic Ointment 1453
Decadron Phosphate Sterile Ophthalmic Solution 1453
Decadron Phosphate Topical Cream 1455
Decadron Phosphate Turbinaire 1456
Maxidex Sterile Ophthalmic Ointment ...... ⊙ 222
NeoDecadron Sterile Ophthalmic Ointment 1517
NeoDecadron Sterile Ophthalmic Solution 1518
NeoDecadron Topical Cream 1518

Dexchlorpheniramine Maleate (Concomitant administration may result in excessive cholinergic blockade). Products include:

Polaramine 2116

Dezocine (Concomitant administration may result in excessive cholinergic blockade).

Dicyclomine Hydrochloride (Concurrent administration may result in excessive cholinergic blockade). Products include:

Bentyl 1322

Diphenhydramine Citrate (Concomitant administration may result in excessive cholinergic blockade). Products include:

Alka-Seltzer Plus Night-Time Cold Medicine ...... ▣ 623
Bufferin AF Nite Time Analgesic/Sleeping Aid Caplets 744
Excedrin P.M. Analgesic/Sleeping Aid Tablets, Caplets and Liquid 749

Diphenhydramine Hydrochloride (Concomitant administration may result in excessive cholinergic blockade). Products include:

Benadryl Anti-Itch Cream ...... ▣ 635
Benadryl Capsules 1691
Benadryl Decongestant Elixir ...... ▣ 635
Benadryl Decongestant ...... ▣ 635
Benadryl Elixir ...... ▣ 636
Benadryl Kapseals 1691
Benadryl 25 Kapseals ...... ▣ 636
Benadryl Parenteral 1692
Benadryl Plus ...... ▣ 636
Benadryl Plus Nighttime ...... ▣ 637
Benadryl Spray, Maximum Strength ...... ▣ 637
Benadryl Spray, Regular Strength ▣ 637
Benadryl Steri-Vials, Ampoules, and Steri-Dose Syringe 1692
Benadryl 25 Tablets ...... ▣ 636
Benylin Cough Syrup ...... ▣ 637
Benylin Decongestant ...... ▣ 638
Caladryl Cream, Lotion, Spray ...... ▣ 638
Miles Nervine Nighttime Sleep-Aid ▣ 627
Nytol Tablets ...... ▣ 517
Sleep-ettes-D Tablets ...... ▣ 653
Sleep-eze 3 Tablets ...... ▣ 755
Sleepinal Night-time Sleep Aid Capsules ...... ▣ 734
Sominex Caplets and Tablets ...... ▣ 722
Sominex Liquid ...... ▣ 723
Sominex Pain Relief Formula ...... ▣ 723
Tylenol Cold Night Time Medication Liquid 1371
Tylenol PM, Extra Strength Caplets and Tablets 1368
Unisom Dual Relief Nighttime Sleep Aid/Analgesic 1774
Ziradryl Lotion ...... ▣ 643

Diphenylpyraline Hydrochloride (Concomitant administration may result in excessive cholinergic blockade).

No products indexed under this heading.

Disopyramide Phosphate (Concomitant administration may result in excessive cholinergic blockade). Products include:
- Norpace ... 2177

Doxepin Hydrochloride (Concomitant administration may result in excessive cholinergic blockade). Products include:
- Sinequan ... 1960

Edrophonium Chloride (Increased intraocular pressure may result from concurrent administration). Products include:
- Enlon Injection ... 598
- Tensilon Injectable ... 1123

Fentanyl (Concomitant administration may result in excessive cholinergic blockade). Products include:
- Duragesic Transdermal System ... 1133

Fentanyl Citrate (Concomitant administration may result in excessive cholinergic blockade). Products include:
- Innovar Injection ... 1141
- Sublimaze Injection ... 1146

Fluphenazine Decanoate (Concomitant administration may result in excessive cholinergic blockade; potentiation of sedative effect of phenothiazines). Products include:
- Prolixin Decanoate ... 1795

Fluphenazine Enanthate (Concomitant administration may result in excessive cholinergic blockade; potentiation of sedative effect of phenothiazines). Products include:
- Prolixin Enanthate ... 1796

Fluphenazine Hydrochloride (Concomitant administration may result in excessive cholinergic blockade; potentiation of sedative effect of phenothiazines). Products include:
- Prolixin Elixir ... 1793
- Prolixin Injection ... 1791
- Prolixin Oral Concentrate ... 1792
- Prolixin Tablets ... 1793

Glycopyrrolate (Concurrent administration may result in excessive cholinergic blockade). Products include:
- Robinul Forte Tablets ... 1873
- Robinul Injectable ... 1873
- Robinul Tablets ... 1873

Hydrocodone Bitartrate (Concomitant administration may result in excessive cholinergic blockade). Products include:
- Anexsia 5/500 Tablets ... 2196
- Anexsia 7.5/650 Tablets ... 2197
- Azdone Tablets ... 844
- Codiclear DH Syrup ... 845
- Codimal DH Syrup ... 846
- Damason-P ... 1356
- Hycodan Syrup, Tablets ... 927
- Hycomine Compound Tablets ... 929
- Hycomine Syrup ... 927
- Hycotuss Expectorant Syrup ... 930
- Hydrocet Capsules ... 835
- Lortab ASA Tablets ... 2414
- Lortab ... 2412
- Ru-Tuss with Hydrocodone ... 694
- Triaminic Expectorant DH ... 1995
- Vicodin Tablets ... 1187
- Vicodin ES Tablets ... 1189
- Zydone Capsules ... 941

Hydrocodone Polistirex (Concomitant administration may result in excessive cholinergic blockade). Products include:
- Tussionex Extended-Release Suspension ... 988

Hydrocortisone (Increased intraocular pressure may result from concurrent administration). Products include:
- AK-Spore H.C. ... ◉ 206
- Bactine Hydrocortisone Anti-Itch Cream ... ■ 625
- CaldeCORT Anti-Itch Hydrocortisone Spray ... ■ 560
- Carmol HC Cream 1% ... 2296
- Cortaid Spray ... ■ 735
- Cortenema ... 2244
- Cortisporin Ointment ... 758
- Cortisporin Ophthalmic Ointment Sterile ... 758
- Cortisporin Ophthalmic Suspension Sterile ... 759
- Cortisporin Otic Solution Sterile ... 760
- Cortisporin Otic Suspension Sterile ... 760
- Cortizone-5 Creme & Ointment ... ■ 732
- Dermolate Anti-Itch Cream ... ■ 697
- Eldecort Cream 1.0% ... 1113
- Eldecort Cream 1.0% and 2.5% ... 1113
- Fungoid HC Creme ... 1770
- Hydrocortone Tablets ... 1482
- Hytone ... 909
- LazerSporin-C Solution ... 1770
- Massengill Medicated Soft Cloth Towelettes ... 2192
- Nutracort Cream & Lotion ... 1684
- PediOtic Suspension Sterile ... 797
- Synacort Creams 1%, 2.5% ... 2296
- Vanoxide-HC Acne Lotion ... 911
- Vioform-Hydrocortisone Cream and Mild Cream ... 889
- Vioform-Hydrocortisone Ointment ... 889
- VōSoL HC Otic Solution ... 2392
- Vytone Cream 1% ... 911

Hydrocortisone Acetate (Increased intraocular pressure may result from concurrent administration). Products include:
- Analpram-HC Rectal Cream 1% and 2.5% ... 970
- Anusol-HC Cream ... 1690
- Anusol-HC Suppositories ... 1691
- Caldecort ... ■ 560
- Carmol HC Cream 1% ... 2296
- Chloromycetin Hydrocortisone Ophthalmic ... 1694
- Coly-Mycin S Otic w/Neomycin & Hydrocortisone ... 1708
- Cortaid ... ■ 735
- Cortef Feminine Itch Cream ... ■ 735
- Corticaine ... ■ 682
- Cortifoam ... 1827
- Cortisporin Cream ... 757
- Epifoam ... 1828
- Gynecort 5 Creme ... ■ 556
- Hydrocortone Acetate Sterile Suspension ... 1479
- Lanacort 5 Creme and Ointment ... ■ 557
- Mantadil Cream ... 789
- Ophthocort ... ◉ 301
- Orabase HCA Oral Paste ... 890
- Pramosone Cream, Lotion & Ointment ... 971
- ProctoCream-HC ... 1834
- Proctofoam-HC ... 1835

Hydrocortisone Sodium Phosphate (Increased intraocular pressure may result from concurrent administration). Products include:
- Hydrocortone Phosphate Injection, Sterile ... 1481

Hydrocortisone Sodium Succinate (Increased intraocular pressure may result from concurrent administration). Products include:
- Solu-Cortef Sterile Powder ... 2361

Hyoscyamine (Concurrent administration may result in excessive cholinergic blockade). Products include:
- Cystospaz Tablets ... 2395
- Urised Tablets ... 2396

Hyoscyamine Sulfate (Concurrent administration may result in excessive cholinergic blockade). Products include:
- Arco-Lase Plus Tablets ... 607
- Cystospaz-M Capsules ... 2395
- Donnagel ... ■ 675
- Donnagel-PG ... 1858
- Donnatal ... 1858
- Donnatal Extentabs ... 1859
- Donnatal Tablets ... 1858
- Donnazyme Tablets ... 1860
- Kutrase Capsules ... 2146
- Levsin/Levsinex ... 2147
- Ru-Tuss Tablets ... 693

Imipramine Hydrochloride (Concomitant administration may result in excessive cholinergic blockade). Products include:
- Tofranil Ampuls ... 1038
- Tofranil Tablets ... 1039

Imipramine Pamoate (Concomitant administration may result in excessive cholinergic blockade). Products include:
- Tofranil-PM Capsules ... 1041

Ipratropium Bromide (Concurrent administration may result in excessive cholinergic blockade). Products include:
- Atrovent Inhalation Aerosol ... 675

Isocarboxazid (Concurrent administration may result in excessive cholinergic blockage). Products include:
- Marplan Tablets ... 1906

Levorphanol Tartrate (Concomitant administration may result in excessive cholinergic blockade). Products include:
- Levo-Dromoran ... 1906

Maprotiline Hydrochloride (Concomitant administration may result in excessive cholinergic blockade). Products include:
- Ludiomil Tablets ... 874

Mepenzolate Bromide (Concurrent administration may result in excessive cholinergic blockade). Products include:
- Cantil Tablets ... 1326

Meperidine Hydrochloride (Concomitant administration may result in excessive cholinergic blockade). Products include:
- Demerol ... 2047
- Mepergan Injection ... 2479

Mesoridazine Besylate (Concomitant administration may result in excessive cholinergic blockade; potentiation of sedative effect of phenothiazines).

Methadone Hydrochloride (Concomitant administration may result in excessive cholinergic blockade). Products include:
- Dolophine Hydrochloride Ampoules & Vials ... 1260
- Dolophine Hydrochloride Tablets ... 1261
- Methadone Hydrochloride Diskets ... 1284
- Methadone Hydrochloride Oral Solution & Tablets ... 1987

Methdilazine Hydrochloride (Concomitant administration may result in excessive cholinergic blockade). Products include:
- Tacaryl Syrup & Tablets ... 2409

Methylprednisolone Acetate (Increased intraocular pressure may result from concurrent administration). Products include:
- Depo-Medrol Sterile Aqueous Suspension ... 2334

Methylprednisolone Sodium Succinate (Increased intraocular pressure may result from concurrent administration). Products include:
- Solu-Medrol Sterile Powder ... 2363

Moricizine Hydrochloride (Concomitant administration may result in excessive cholinergic blockade). Products include:
- Ethmozine Tablets ... 946

Morphine Sulfate (Concomitant administration may result in excessive cholinergic blockade). Products include:
- Astramorph/PF Injection, USP (Preservative-Free) ... 618
- Duramorph ... 960
- Infumorph 200 and Infumorph 500 Sterile Solutions ... 962
- MS Contin Tablets ... 1814
- MSIR ... 1817
- Oramorph SR (Morphine Sulfate Sustained Release Tablets) ... 1988
- Roxanol ... 1991

Neostigmine Bromide (Increased intraocular pressure may result from concurrent administration). Products include:
- Prostigmin Tablets ... 1121

Neostigmine Methylsulfate (Increased intraocular pressure may result from concurrent administration). Products include:
- Prostigmin Injectable ... 1120

Nortriptyline Hydrochloride (Concomitant administration may result in excessive cholinergic blockade). Products include:
- Pamelor ... 2019

Opium Alkaloids (Concomitant administration may result in excessive cholinergic blockade). Products include:
- B & O No. 15A & No. 16A Supprettes ... 2395
- Pantopon Injectable ... 1911

Oxybutynin Chloride (Concurrent administration may result in excessive cholinergic blockade). Products include:
- Ditropan ... 1332

Oxycodone Hydrochloride (Concomitant administration may result in excessive cholinergic blockade). Products include:
- Percocet Tablets ... 950
- Percodan ... 951
- Roxicodone Tablets, Oral Solution & Intensol (Oxycodone) ... 1992
- Tylox Capsules ... 1382

Perphenazine (Concomitant administration may result in excessive cholinergic blockade; potentiation of sedative effect of phenothiazines). Products include:
- Etrafon ... 2087
- Triavil Tablets ... 1556
- Trilafon ... 2123

Phenelzine Sulfate (Concomitant administration may result in excessive cholinergic blockade). Products include:
- Nardil ... 1742

Prednisolone Acetate (Increased intraocular pressure may result from concurrent administration). Products include:
- AK-Cide Sterile Ophthalmic Ointment & Suspension ... ◉ 202
- Blephamide Liquifilm Sterile Ophthalmic Suspension ... 586
- Blephamide S.O.P. Sterile Ophthalmic Ointment ... 586
- Cetapred Ointment ... ◉ 220
- ⅛% Econopred & 1% Econopred Plus ... ◉ 217
- Isopto Cetapred Suspension ... ◉ 220
- Metimyd ... ◉ 306
- Poly-Pred Liquifilm ... ◉ 250
- Pred Forte ... ◉ 252
- Pred Mild ... ◉ 254
- Pred-G Liquifilm Sterile Ophthalmic Suspension ... ◉ 252
- Pred-G S.O.P. Sterile Ophthalmic Ointment ... ◉ 253
- Vasocidin Ointment ... ◉ 275

Prednisolone Sodium Phosphate (Increased intraocular pressure may result from concurrent administration). Products include:
- AK-Pred ... ◉ 205
- Hydeltrasol Injection, Sterile ... 1476
- Inflamase ... ◉ 274
- Pediapred Oral Liquid ... 987
- Vasocidin Ophthalmic Solution ... ◉ 276

Prednisolone Tebutate (Increased intraocular pressure may result from concurrent administration). Products include:
- Hydeltra-T.B.A. Sterile Suspension ... 1478

Prednisone (Increased intraocular pressure may result from concurrent administration). Products include:
- Deltasone Tablets ... 2332

Prescription Drugs, unspecified (Anticholinergics may delay absorption of other drugs given concomitantly).

Procainamide Hydrochloride (Concomitant administration may result in excessive cholinergic blockade). Products include:
- Procan SR Tablets ... 1760
- Pronestyl Capsules and Tablets ... 1800
- Pronestyl Injection ... 1798
- Pronestyl-SR Tablets ... 1801

Prochlorperazine (Concomitant administration may result in excessive cholinergic blockade; potentiation of sedative effect of phenothiazines). Products include:
- Compazine ... 2201

Procyclidine Hydrochloride (Concurrent administration may result in excessive cholinergic blockade). Products include:
- Kemadrin Tablets ... 771

Promethazine Hydrochloride (Concomitant administration may result in excessive cholinergic blockade; potentiation of sedative effect of phenothiazines). Products include:
- Mepergan Injection ... 2479
- Phenergan with Codeine ... 2497
- Phenergan with Dextromethorphan 2499
- Phenergan Injection ... 2493
- Phenergan Suppositories ... 2496
- Phenergan Syrup ... 2495
- Phenergan Tablets ... 2496
- Phenergan VC ... 2500
- Phenergan VC with Codeine ... 2501

Propafenone Hydrochloride (Concomitant administration may result in excessive cholinergic blockade). Products include:
- Rythmol Tablets ... 1184

Propantheline Bromide (Concurrent administration may result in excessive cholinergic blockade). Products include:
- Pro-Banthīne Tablets ... 2141

Propoxyphene Hydrochloride (Concomitant administration may result in excessive cholinergic blockade). Products include:
- Darvon ... 1256
- Wygesic Tablets ... 2540

Propoxyphene Napsylate (Concomitant administration may result in excessive cholinergic blockade). Products include:
- Darvon-N/Darvocet-N ... 1254

Protriptyline Hydrochloride (Concomitant administration may result in excessive cholinergic blockade). Products include:
- Vivactil Tablets ... 1567

Pyridostigmine Bromide (Increased intraocular pressure may result from concurrent administration). Products include:
- Mestinon Injectable ... 1115
- Mestinon ... 1116

Pyrilamine Maleate (Concomitant administration may result in excessive cholinergic blockade). Products include:
- Codimal ... 846
- 4-Way Fast Acting Nasal Spray - Original Formula (regular & mentholated) & Metered Spray Pump (regular) ... 751
- Maximum Strength Midol Multi-Symptom Menstrual Formula ... ▣ 571
- Maximum Strength Midol PMS Premenstrual Syndrome Formula ... ▣ 570
- Regular Strength Midol Multi-Symptom Menstrual Formula ... ▣ 570
- Prefrin-A ... ◉ 255
- Prēmsyn PMS Capsules & Caplets ▣ 547
- Primatene Tablets-M Formula ... 2421
- Robitussin Night Relief ... ▣ 677
- Ru-Tuss with Hydrocodone ... 694
- Triaminic Expectorant DH ... 1995
- Triaminic Oral Infant Drops ... 1996

Pyrilamine Tannate (Concomitant administration may result in excessive cholinergic blockade). Products include:
- Rynatan ... 2387

Quinidine Gluconate (Concomitant administration may result in excessive cholinergic blockade). Products include:
- Quinaglute Dura-Tabs Tablets ... 663

Quinidine Polygalacturonate (Concomitant administration may result in excessive cholinergic blockade). Products include:
- Cardioquin Tablets ... 1812

Quinidine Sulfate (Concomitant administration may result in excessive cholinergic blockade). Products include:
- Quinidex Extentabs ... 1868

Scopolamine Hydrobromide (Concurrent administration may result in excessive cholinergic blockade). Products include:
- Donnagel ... ▣ 675
- Donnagel-PG ... 1858
- Donnatal ... 1858
- Donnatal Extentabs ... 1859
- Donnatal Tablets ... 1858
- Donnazyme Tablets ... 1860
- Isopto Hyoscine ... ◉ 222
- Murocoll-2 Sterile Ophthalmic Solution ... ◉ 261
- Ru-Tuss Tablets ... 693

Scopolamine Preparations (Concurrent administration may result in excessive cholinergic blockade). Products include:
- Transderm Scōp Transdermal Therapeutic System ... 887

Sufentanil Citrate (Concomitant administration may result in excessive cholinergic blockade). Products include:
- Sufenta Injection ... 1147

Terfenadine (Concomitant administration may result in excessive cholinergic blockade). Products include:
- Seldane Tablets ... 1349
- Seldane-D Extended-Release Tablets ... 1350

Thioridazine Hydrochloride (Concomitant administration may result in excessive cholinergic blockade; potentiation of sedative effect of phenothiazines). Products include:
- Mellaril ... 2011

Tranylcypromine Sulfate (Concomitant administration may result in excessive cholinergic blockade). Products include:
- Parnate Tablets ... 2222

Triamcinolone (Increased intraocular pressure may result from concurrent administration).
- No products indexed under this heading.

Triamcinolone Acetonide (Increased intraocular pressure may result from concurrent administration). Products include:
- Aristocort A ... 1010
- Azmacort Inhaler ... 1837
- Kenalog Cream, Lotion & Ointment 2401
- Kenalog-10 Injection ... 2402
- Kenalog-40 Injection ... 2403
- Kenalog in Orabase ... 604
- Kenalog Spray ... 2401
- Mycolog II Cream and Ointment ... 2407
- Mytrex Cream & Ointment ... 2080
- Nasacort Nasal Inhaler ... 1844

Triamcinolone Diacetate (Increased intraocular pressure may result from concurrent administration). Products include:
- Aristocort Suspension ... 1008

Triamcinolone Hexacetonide (Increased intraocular pressure may result from concurrent administration). Products include:
- Aristospan Suspension ... 1011

Tridihexethyl Chloride (Concurrent administration may result in excessive cholinergic blockade).
- No products indexed under this heading.

Trifluoperazine Hydrochloride (Concomitant administration may result in excessive cholinergic blockade; potentiation of sedative effect of phenothiazines). Products include:
- Stelazine ... 2226

Trihexyphenidyl Hydrochloride (Concurrent administration may result in excessive cholinergic blockade). Products include:
- Artane ... 1195

Trimeprazine Tartrate (Concomitant administration may result in excessive cholinergic blockade). Products include:
- Temaril Tablets, Syrup and Spansule Sustained Release Capsules 1085

Trimipramine Maleate (Concomitant administration may result in excessive cholinergic blockade). Products include:
- Surmontil Capsules ... 2524

Tripelennamine Hydrochloride (Concomitant administration may result in excessive cholinergic blockade). Products include:
- PBZ Tablets & Elixir ... 1037
- PBZ-SR Tablets ... 1037

Tripelennamine Preparations (Concomitant administration may result in excessive cholinergic blockade).

Triprolidine Hydrochloride (Concomitant administration may result in excessive cholinergic blockade). Products include:
- Actidil ... ▣ 538
- Actifed Capsules ... ▣ 539
- Actifed Plus Caplets ... ▣ 539
- Actifed Plus Tablets ... ▣ 540
- Actifed with Codeine Cough Syrup.. 752
- Actifed Syrup ... ▣ 540
- Actifed Tablets ... ▣ 540
- Actifed 12-Hour Capsules ... ▣ 539

DARVOCET-N 50 TABLETS

(Propoxyphene Napsylate, Acetaminophen) ... 1254

May interact with central nervous system depressants, tricyclic antidepressants, anticonvulsants, oral anticoagulants, and certain other agents. Compounds in these categories include:

Alcohol (Additive CNS depression).

Alfentanil Hydrochloride (Additive CNS depression). Products include:
- Alfenta Injection ... 1131

Alprazolam (Additive CNS depression). Products include:
- Xanax Tablets ... 2367

Amitriptyline Hydrochloride (Propoxyphene may slow metabolism). Products include:
- Elavil ... 2269
- Endep Tablets ... 1927
- Etrafon ... 2087
- Limbitrol ... 1933
- Triavil Tablets ... 1556

Amoxapine (Propoxyphene may slow metabolism). Products include:
- Asendin Tablets ... 1196

Aprobarbital (Additive CNS depression). Products include:
- Alurate Elixir ... 1883

Buprenorphine (Additive CNS depression).
- No products indexed under this heading.

Buspirone Hydrochloride (Additive CNS depression). Products include:
- BuSpar ... 1401

Butabarbital (Additive CNS depression). Products include:
- Pyridium Plus ... 1764

Butalbital (Additive CNS depression). Products include:
- Esgic-Plus Tablets ... 1002
- Esgic Tablets & Capsules ... 1001
- Fioricet Tablets ... 2006
- Fiorinal Capsules ... 2007
- Fiorinal with Codeine Capsules ... 2008
- Fiorinal Tablets ... 2007
- Phrenilin ... 838
- Sedapap Tablets 50 mg/650 mg .. 1360

Carbamazepine (Concurrent use may result in severe neurological signs, including coma). Products include:
- Tegretol Chewable Tablets ... 654
- Tegretol Suspension ... 656
- Tegretol Tablets ... 654

Chlordiazepoxide (Additive CNS depression). Products include:
- Libritabs Tablets ... 1930
- Limbitrol ... 1933
- Menrium Tablets ... 1934

Chlordiazepoxide Hydrochloride (Additive CNS depression). Products include:
- Librax Capsules ... 1929
- Librium Capsules ... 1931
- Librium Injectable ... 1932

Chlorpromazine (Additive CNS depression). Products include:
- Thorazine ... 2234

Chlorprothixene (Additive CNS depression). Products include:
- Taractan Tablets ... 1920

Chlorprothixene Hydrochloride (Additive CNS depression). Products include:
- Taractan ... 1920

Clomipramine Hydrochloride (Propoxyphene may slow metabolism). Products include:
- Anafranil Capsules ... 650

Clorazepate Dipotassium (Additive CNS depression). Products include:
- Tranxene ... 556

Codeine (Additive CNS depression). Products include:
- Calcidrine Syrup ... 506

Codeine Phosphate (Additive CNS depression). Products include:
- Actifed with Codeine Cough Syrup.. 752
- Cheracol Cough Syrup ... 1853
- Codimal PH Syrup ... 846
- Dimetane-DC Cough Syrup ... 1857
- Empirin with Codeine Phosphate Nos. 2, 3 & 4 ... 764
- Fiorinal with Codeine Capsules ... 2008
- Isoclor Expectorant ... 982
- Naldecon CX Adult Liquid ... ▣ 521
- Novahistine DH ... 1342
- Novahistine Expectorant ... 1343
- Nucofed Capsules ... 2219
- Nucofed Expectorant ... 2219
- Nucofed Pediatric Expectorant ... 2220
- Nucofed Syrup ... 2219
- Phenaphen with Codeine Capsules 1865
- Phenaphen-650 with Codeine Tablets ... 1866
- Phenergan with Codeine ... 2497
- Phenergan VC with Codeine ... 2501
- Robitussin A-C Syrup ... 1875
- Robitussin-DAC Syrup ... 1875
- Ryna ... ▣ 741
- Soma Compound w/Codeine Tablets ... 2390
- Triaminic Expectorant w/Codeine .. 1996
- Tussi-Organidin Liquid ... 2391

Tylenol with Codeine 1381

Codeine Polistirex (Additive CNS depression).
No products indexed under this heading.

Desipramine Hydrochloride (Propoxyphene may slow metabolism). Products include:
Norpramin Tablets 1340

Dezocine (Additive CNS depression).

Diazepam (Additive CNS depression). Products include:
Valium Injectable 1937
Valium Tablets 1939
Valrelease Capsules 1923

Dicumarol (Propoxyphene may slow metabolism). Products include:
Dicumarol Tablets 516

Divalproex Sodium (Propoxyphene may slow metabolism). Products include:
Depakote 512

Doxepin Hydrochloride (Propoxyphene may slow metabolism). Products include:
Sinequan 1960

Droperidol (Additive CNS depression). Products include:
Inapsine Injection 1140
Innovar Injection 1141

Enflurane (Additive CNS depression). Products include:
Ethrane 599

Estazolam (Additive CNS depression). Products include:
ProSom Tablets 554

Ethchlorvynol (Additive CNS depression). Products include:
Placidyl Capsules 553

Ethinamate (Additive CNS depression).
No products indexed under this heading.

Ethosuximide (Propoxyphene may slow metabolism). Products include:
Zarontin Capsules 1768
Zarontin Syrup 1769

Ethotoin (Propoxyphene may slow metabolism). Products include:
Peganone Tablets 551

Fentanyl (Additive CNS depression). Products include:
Duragesic Transdermal System 1133

Fentanyl Citrate (Additive CNS depression). Products include:
Innovar Injection 1141
Sublimaze Injection 1146

Fluphenazine Decanoate (Additive CNS depression). Products include:
Prolixin Decanoate 1795

Fluphenazine Enanthate (Additive CNS depression). Products include:
Prolixin Enanthate 1796

Fluphenazine Hydrochloride (Additive CNS depression). Products include:
Prolixin Elixir 1793
Prolixin Injection 1791
Prolixin Oral Concentrate 1792
Prolixin Tablets 1793

Flurazepam Hydrochloride (Additive CNS depression). Products include:
Dalmane Capsules 1927

Glutethimide (Additive CNS depression).
No products indexed under this heading.

Haloperidol (Additive CNS depression). Products include:
Haldol Injection, Tablets and Concentrate 1373

Haloperidol Decanoate (Additive CNS depression). Products include:
Haldol Decanoate 1375

Hydrocodone Bitartrate (Additive CNS depression). Products include:
Anexsia 5/500 Tablets 2196
Anexsia 7.5/650 Tablets 2197
Azdōne Tablets 844
Codiclear DH Syrup 845
Codimal DH Syrup 846
Damason-P 1356
Hycodan Syrup, Tablets 927
Hycomine Compound Tablets 929
Hycomine Syrup 927
Hycotuss Expectorant Syrup 930
Hydrocet Capsules 835
Lortab ASA Tablets 2414
Lortab 2412
Ru-Tuss with Hydrocodone 694
Triaminic Expectorant DH 1995
Vicodin Tablets 1187
Vicodin ES Tablets 1189
Zydone Capsules 941

Hydrocodone Polistirex (Additive CNS depression). Products include:
Tussionex Extended-Release Suspension 988

Hydroxyzine Hydrochloride (Additive CNS depression). Products include:
Atarax Tablets & Syrup 1941
Marax Tablets & DF Syrup 1954
Vistaril Intramuscular Solution 1970

Imipramine Hydrochloride (Propoxyphene may slow metabolism). Products include:
Tofranil Ampuls 1038
Tofranil Tablets 1039

Imipramine Pamoate (Propoxyphene may slow metabolism). Products include:
Tofranil-PM Capsules 1041

Isoflurane (Additive CNS depression). Products include:
Forane 600

Ketamine Hydrochloride (Additive CNS depression). Products include:
Ketalar 1726

Levorphanol Tartrate (Additive CNS depression). Products include:
Levo-Dromoran 1906

Lorazepam (Additive CNS depression). Products include:
Ativan Injection 2432
Ativan Tablets 2434

Loxapine Hydrochloride (Additive CNS depression). Products include:
Loxitane 1213

Loxapine Succinate (Additive CNS depression). Products include:
Loxitane Capsules 1213

Maprotiline Hydrochloride (Propoxyphene may slow metabolism). Products include:
Ludiomil Tablets 874

Meperidine Hydrochloride (Additive CNS depression). Products include:
Demerol 2047
Mepergan Injection 2479

Mephenytoin (Propoxyphene may slow metabolism). Products include:
Mesantoin Tablets 2013

Mephobarbital (Additive CNS depression). Products include:
Mebaral Tablets 2061

Meprobamate (Additive CNS depression). Products include:
Deprol Tablets 2382
Equagesic Tablets 2451
Miltown Tablets 2386
PMB 200 and PMB 400 2504

Mesoridazine (Additive CNS depression). Products include:
Serentil 686

Methadone Hydrochloride (Additive CNS depression). Products include:
Dolophine Hydrochloride Ampoules & Vials 1260
Dolophine Hydrochloride Tablets 1261
Methadone Hydrochloride Diskets 1284
Methadone Hydrochloride Oral Solution & Tablets 1987

Methohexital Sodium (Additive CNS depression). Products include:
Brevital Sodium Vials 1248

Methoxyflurane (Additive CNS depression).
No products indexed under this heading.

Methsuximide (Propoxyphene may slow metabolism). Products include:
Celontin 1692

Midazolam Hydrochloride (Additive CNS depression). Products include:
Versed Injection 1924

Molindone Hydrochloride (Additive CNS depression). Products include:
Moban Tablets & Concentrate 932

Morphine Sulfate (Additive CNS depression). Products include:
Astramorph/PF Injection, USP (Preservative-Free) 618
Duramorph 960
Infumorph 200 and Infumorph 500 Sterile Solutions 962
MS Contin Tablets 1814
MSIR 1817
Oramorph SR (Morphine Sulfate Sustained Release Tablets) 1988
Roxanol 1991

Nortriptyline Hydrochloride (Propoxyphene may slow metabolism). Products include:
Pamelor 2019

Opium Alkaloids (Additive CNS depression). Products include:
B & O No. 15A & No. 16A Supprettes 2395
Pantopon Injectable 1911

Oxazepam (Additive CNS depression). Products include:
Serax Capsules 2522
Serax Tablets 2522

Oxycodone Hydrochloride (Additive CNS depression). Products include:
Percocet Tablets 950
Percodan 951
Roxicodone Tablets, Oral Solution & Intensol (Oxycodone) 1992
Tylox Capsules 1382

Paramethadione (Propoxyphene may slow metabolism). Products include:
Paradione Capsules 548

Pentobarbital Sodium (Additive CNS depression). Products include:
Nembutal Sodium Capsules 534
Nembutal Sodium Solution 536
Nembutal Sodium Suppositories 538

Perphenazine (Additive CNS depression). Products include:
Etrafon 2087
Triavil Tablets 1556
Trilafon 2123

Phenacemide (Propoxyphene may slow metabolism). Products include:
Phenurone Tablets 552

Phenobarbital (Additive CNS depression; propoxyphene may slow metabolism). Products include:
Arco-Lase Plus Tablets 607
Bellergal-S Tablets 1998
Bronkolixir ◘ 761
Bronkotabs Tablets ◘ 762
Donnatal 1858
Donnatal Extentabs 1859
Donnatal Tablets 1858
Donnazyme Tablets 1860
Kinesed Tablets 2272
Phenobarbital Elixir and Tablets 1293
Primatene Tablets-P Formula 2421
Quadrinal Tablets 1183
Tedral SA 1765

Phensuximide (Propoxyphene may slow metabolism). Products include:
Milontin Kapseals 1741

Phenytoin (Propoxyphene may slow metabolism). Products include:
Dilantin Infatabs 1710
Dilantin-30 Pediatric/Dilantin-125 Suspension 1713

Phenytoin Sodium (Propoxyphene may slow metabolism). Products include:
Dilantin Kapseals 1708
Dilantin Parenteral 1712
Dilantin with Phenobarbital Kapseals 1715

Prazepam (Additive CNS depression). Products include:
Centrax 1693

Primidone (Propoxyphene may slow metabolism). Products include:
Mysoline 2480

Prochlorperazine (Additive CNS depression). Products include:
Compazine 2201

Promethazine Hydrochloride (Additive CNS depression). Products include:
Mepergan Injection 2479
Phenergan with Codeine 2497
Phenergan with Dextromethorphan 2499
Phenergan Injection 2493
Phenergan Suppositories 2496
Phenergan Syrup 2495
Phenergan Tablets 2496
Phenergan VC 2500
Phenergan VC with Codeine 2501

Propofol (Additive CNS depression). Products include:
Diprivan Injection 2267

Propoxyphene Hydrochloride (Additive CNS depression). Products include:
Darvon 1256
Wygesic Tablets 2540

Protriptyline Hydrochloride (Propoxyphene may slow metabolism). Products include:
Vivactil Tablets 1567

Quazepam (Additive CNS depression). Products include:
Doral Tablets 2383

Secobarbital Sodium (Additive CNS depression). Products include:
Seconal Sodium Pulvules 1296

Sufentanil Citrate (Additive CNS depression). Products include:
Sufenta Injection 1147

Temazepam (Additive CNS depression). Products include:
Restoril Capsules 2023

Thiamylal Sodium (Additive CNS depression). Products include:
Surital Ampoules, Steri-Vials 1764

Thioridazine Hydrochloride (Additive CNS depression). Products include:
Mellaril 2011

Thiothixene (Additive CNS depression). Products include:
Navane Capsules and Concentrate 1954
Navane Intramuscular 1956

Triazolam (Additive CNS depression). Products include:
Halcion Tablets 2340

Trifluoperazine Hydrochloride (Additive CNS depression). Products include:
Stelazine 2226

Trimethadione (Propoxyphene may slow metabolism). Products include:
Tridione 557

Trimipramine Maleate (Propoxyphene may slow metabolism). Products include:
Surmontil Capsules 2524

Valproic Acid (Propoxyphene may slow metabolism). Products include:
Depakene Capsules & Syrup 511

Warfarin Sodium (Propoxyphene may slow metabolism). Products include:
Coumadin Injection & Tablets 944
Panwarfin Tablets 547

DARVOCET-N 100 TABLETS
(Propoxyphene Napsylate, Acetaminophen) 1254
See **Darvocet-N 50 Tablets**

DARVON COMPOUND-65 PULVULES
(Propoxyphene Hydrochloride, Aspirin, Caffeine) 1256
May interact with central nervous system depressants, oral anticoagulants, antigout agents, antidepressant drugs, anticonvulsants, and certain other agents. Compounds in these categories include:

Alcohol (Additive CNS-depressant effect).

Alfentanil Hydrochloride (Additive CNS-depressant effect). Products include:
Alfenta Injection 1131

Allopurinol (Uricosuric effect inhibited). Products include:
Zyloprim Tablets 830

Alprazolam (Additive CNS-depressant effect). Products include:
Xanax Tablets 2367

Amitriptyline Hydrochloride (Propoxyphene slows the metabolism). Products include:
Elavil 2269
Endep Tablets 1927
Etrafon 2087
Limbitrol 1933
Triavil Tablets 1556

Amoxapine (Propoxyphene slows the metabolism). Products include:
Asendin Tablets 1196

Aprobarbital (Additive CNS-depressant effect). Products include:
Alurate Elixir 1883

Buprenorphine (Additive CNS-depressant effect).
No products indexed under this heading.

Bupropion Hydrochloride (Propoxyphene slows the metabolism). Products include:
Wellbutrin Tablets 821

Buspirone Hydrochloride (Additive CNS-depressant effect). Products include:
BuSpar 1401

Butabarbital (Additive CNS-depressant effect). Products include:
Pyridium Plus 1764

Butalbital (Additive CNS-depressant effect). Products include:
Esgic-Plus Tablets 1002
Esgic Tablets & Capsules 1001
Fioricet Tablets 2006
Fiorinal Capsules 2007
Fiorinal with Codeine Capsules 2008
Fiorinal Tablets 2007
Phrenilin 838
Sedapap Tablets 50 mg/650 mg 1360

Carbamazepine (Concurrent use may result in severe neurological signs, including coma). Products include:
Tegretol Chewable Tablets 654
Tegretol Suspension 656
Tegretol Tablets 654

Chlordiazepoxide (Additive CNS-depressant effect). Products include:
Libritabs Tablets 1930
Limbitrol 1933
Menrium Tablets 1934

Chlordiazepoxide Hydrochloride (Additive CNS-depressant effect). Products include:
Librax Capsules 1929
Librium Capsules 1931
Librium Injectable 1932

Chlorpromazine (Additive CNS-depressant effect). Products include:
Thorazine 2234

Chlorprothixene (Additive CNS-depressant effect). Products include:
Taractan Tablets 1920

Chlorprothixene Hydrochloride (Additive CNS-depressant effect). Products include:
Taractan 1920

Clorazepate Dipotassium (Additive CNS-depressant effect). Products include:
Tranxene 556

Codeine (Additive CNS-depressant effect). Products include:
Calcidrine Syrup 506

Codeine Phosphate (Additive CNS-depressant effect). Products include:
Actifed with Codeine Cough Syrup 752
Cheracol Cough Syrup 1853
Codimal PH Syrup 846
Dimetane-DC Cough Syrup 1857
Empirin with Codeine Phosphate Nos. 2, 3 & 4 764
Fiorinal with Codeine Capsules 2008
Isoclor Expectorant 982
Naldecon CX Adult Liquid ▣ 521
Novahistine DH 1342
Novahistine Expectorant 1343
Nucofed Capsules 2219
Nucofed Expectorant 2219
Nucofed Pediatric Expectorant 2220
Nucofed Syrup 2219
Phenaphen with Codeine Capsules 1865
Phenaphen-650 with Codeine Tablets 1866
Phenergan with Codeine 2497
Phenergan VC with Codeine 2501
Robitussin A-C Syrup 1875
Robitussin-DAC Syrup 1875
Ryna ▣ 741
Soma Compound w/Codeine Tablets 2390
Triaminic Expectorant w/Codeine 1996
Tussi-Organidin Liquid 2391
Tylenol with Codeine 1381

Codeine Polistirex (Additive CNS-depressant effect).
No products indexed under this heading.

Desipramine Hydrochloride (Propoxyphene slows the metabolism). Products include:
Norpramin Tablets 1340

Dezocine (Additive CNS-depressant effect).

Diazepam (Additive CNS-depressant effect). Products include:
Valium Injectable 1937
Valium Tablets 1939
Valrelease Capsules 1923

Dicumarol (Enhanced anticoagulant effect). Products include:
Dicumarol Tablets 516

Divalproex Sodium (Propoxyphene slows the metabolism). Products include:
Depakote 512

Doxepin Hydrochloride (Propoxyphene slows the metabolism). Products include:
Sinequan 1960

Droperidol (Additive CNS-depressant effect). Products include:
Inapsine Injection 1140
Innovar Injection 1141

Enflurane (Additive CNS-depressant effect). Products include:
Ethrane 599

Estazolam (Additive CNS-depressant effect). Products include:
ProSom Tablets 554

Ethchlorvynol (Additive CNS-depressant effect). Products include:
Placidyl Capsules 553

Ethinamate (Additive CNS-depressant effect).
No products indexed under this heading.

Ethosuximide (Propoxyphene slows the metabolism). Products include:
Zarontin Capsules 1768
Zarontin Syrup 1769

Ethotoin (Propoxyphene slows the metabolism). Products include:
Peganone Tablets 551

Fentanyl (Additive CNS-depressant effect). Products include:
Duragesic Transdermal System 1133

Fentanyl Citrate (Additive CNS-depressant effect). Products include:
Innovar Injection 1141
Sublimaze Injection 1146

Fluoxetine Hydrochloride (Propoxyphene slows the metabolism). Products include:
Prozac Pulvules 920

Fluphenazine Decanoate (Additive CNS-depressant effect). Products include:
Prolixin Decanoate 1795

Fluphenazine Enanthate (Additive CNS-depressant effect). Products include:
Prolixin Enanthate 1796

Fluphenazine Hydrochloride (Additive CNS-depressant effect). Products include:
Prolixin Elixir 1793
Prolixin Injection 1791
Prolixin Oral Concentrate 1792
Prolixin Tablets 1793

Flurazepam Hydrochloride (Additive CNS-depressant effect). Products include:
Dalmane Capsules 1927

Glutethimide (Additive CNS-depressant effect).
No products indexed under this heading.

Haloperidol (Additive CNS-depressant effect). Products include:
Haldol Injection, Tablets and Concentrate 1373

Haloperidol Decanoate (Additive CNS-depressant effect). Products include:
Haldol Decanoate 1375

Hydrocodone Bitartrate (Additive CNS-depressant effect). Products include:
Anexsia 5/500 Tablets 2196
Anexsia 7.5/650 Tablets 2197
Azdone Tablets 844
Codiclear DH Syrup 845
Codimal DH Syrup 846
Damason-P 1356
Hycodan Syrup, Tablets 927
Hycomine Compound Tablets 929
Hycomine Syrup 927
Hycotuss Expectorant Syrup 930
Hydrocet Capsules 835
Lortab ASA Tablets 2414
Lortab 2412
Ru-Tuss with Hydrocodone 694
Triaminic Expectorant DH 1995
Vicodin Tablets 1187
Vicodin ES Tablets 1189
Zydone Capsules 941

Hydrocodone Polistirex (Additive CNS-depressant effect). Products include:
Tussionex Extended-Release Suspension 988

Hydroxyzine Hydrochloride (Additive CNS-depressant effect). Products include:
Atarax Tablets & Syrup 1941
Marax Tablets & DF Syrup 1954
Vistaril Intramuscular Solution 1970

Imipramine Hydrochloride (Propoxyphene slows the metabolism). Products include:
Tofranil Ampuls 1038
Tofranil Tablets 1039

Imipramine Pamoate (Propoxyphene slows the metabolism). Products include:
Tofranil-PM Capsules 1041

Isocarboxazid (Propoxyphene slows the metabolism). Products include:
Marplan Tablets 1906

Isoflurane (Additive CNS-depressant effect). Products include:
Forane 600

Ketamine Hydrochloride (Additive CNS-depressant effect). Products include:
Ketalar 1726

Levorphanol Tartrate (Additive CNS-depressant effect). Products include:
Levo-Dromoran 1906

Lorazepam (Additive CNS-depressant effect). Products include:
Ativan Injection 2432
Ativan Tablets 2434

Loxapine Hydrochloride (Additive CNS-depressant effect). Products include:
Loxitane 1213

Loxapine Succinate (Additive CNS-depressant effect). Products include:
Loxitane Capsules 1213

Maprotiline Hydrochloride (Propoxyphen slows the metabolism). Products include:
Ludiomil Tablets 874

Meperidine Hydrochloride (Additive CNS-depressant effect). Products include:
Demerol 2047
Mepergan Injection 2479

Mephenytoin (Propoxyphene slows the metabolism). Products include:
Mesantoin Tablets 2013

Mephobarbital (Additive CNS-depressant effect). Products include:
Mebaral Tablets 2061

Meprobamate (Additive CNS-depressant effect). Products include:
Deprol Tablets 2382
Equagesic Tablets 2451
Miltown Tablets 2386
PMB 200 and PMB 400 2504

Mesoridazine (Additive CNS-depressant effect). Products include:
Serentil 686

Methadone Hydrochloride (Additive CNS-depressant effect). Products include:
Dolophine Hydrochloride Ampoules & Vials 1260
Dolophine Hydrochloride Tablets 1261
Methadone Hydrochloride Diskets 1284
Methadone Hydrochloride Oral Solution & Tablets 1987

Methohexital Sodium (Additive CNS-depressant effect). Products include:
Brevital Sodium Vials 1248

Methoxyflurane (Additive CNS-depressant effect).
No products indexed under this heading.

Methsuximide (Propoxyphene slows the metabolism). Products include:
Celontin 1692

Midazolam Hydrochloride (Additive CNS-depressant effect). Products include:
- Versed Injection 1924

Molindone Hydrochloride (Additive CNS-depressant effect). Products include:
- Moban Tablets & Concentrate 932

Morphine Sulfate (Additive CNS-depressant effect). Products include:
- Astramorph/PF Injection, USP (Preservative-Free) 618
- Duramorph 960
- Infumorph 200 and Infumorph 500 Sterile Solutions 962
- MS Contin Tablets 1814
- MSIR 1817
- Oramorph SR (Morphine Sulfate Sustained Release Tablets) 1988
- Roxanol 1991

Nortriptyline Hydrochloride (Propoxyphene slows the metabolism). Products include:
- Pamelor 2019

Opium Alkaloids (Additive CNS-depressant effect). Products include:
- B & O No. 15A & No. 16A Supprettes 2395
- Pantopon Injectable 1911

Oxazepam (Additive CNS-depressant effect). Products include:
- Serax Capsules 2522
- Serax Tablets 2522

Oxycodone Hydrochloride (Additive CNS-depressant effect). Products include:
- Percocet Tablets 950
- Percodan 951
- Roxicodone Tablets, Oral Solution & Intensol (Oxycodone) 1992
- Tylox Capsules 1382

Paramethadione (Propoxyphene slows the metabolism). Products include:
- Paradione Capsules 548

Pentobarbital Sodium (Additive CNS-depressant effect). Products include:
- Nembutal Sodium Capsules 534
- Nembutal Sodium Solution 536
- Nembutal Sodium Suppositories 538

Perphenazine (Additive CNS-depressant effect). Products include:
- Etrafon 2087
- Triavil Tablets 1556
- Trilafon 2123

Phenacemide (Propoxyphene slows the metabolism). Products include:
- Phenurone Tablets 552

Phenelzine Sulfate (Propoxyphene slows the metabolism). Products include:
- Nardil 1742

Phenobarbital (Propoxyphene slows the metabolism; additive CNS-depressant effect). Products include:
- Arco-Lase Plus Tablets 607
- Bellergal-S Tablets 1998
- Bronkolixir ..... ▣ 761
- Bronkotabs Tablets ..... ▣ 762
- Donnatal 1858
- Donnatal Extentabs 1859
- Donnatal Tablets 1858
- Donnazyme Tablets 1860
- Kinesed Tablets 2272
- Phenobarbital Elixir and Tablets 1293
- Primatene Tablets-P Formula 2421
- Quadrinal Tablets 1183
- Tedral SA 1765

Phensuximide (Propoxyphen slows the metabolism). Products include:
- Milontin Kapseals 1741

Phenytoin (Propoxyphene slows the metabolism). Products include:
- Dilantin Infatabs 1710
- Dilantin-30 Pediatric/Dilantin-125 Suspension 1713

Phenytoin Sodium (Propoxyphen slows the metabolism). Products include:
- Dilantin Kapseals 1708
- Dilantin Parenteral 1712
- Dilantin with Phenobarbital Kapseals 1715

Prazepam (Additive CNS-depressant effect). Products include:
- Centrax 1693

Primidone (Propoxyphen slows the metabolism). Products include:
- Mysoline 2480

Probenecid (Uricosuric effect inhibited). Products include:
- Benemid Tablets 1426
- ColBENEMID Tablets 1436
- Wycillin Injection and Probenecid Tablets 2539

Prochlorperazine (Additive CNS-depressant effect). Products include:
- Compazine 2201

Promethazine Hydrochloride (Additive CNS-depressant effect). Products include:
- Mepergan Injection 2479
- Phenergan with Codeine 2497
- Phenergan with Dextromethorphan 2499
- Phenergan Injection 2493
- Phenergan Suppositories 2496
- Phenergan Syrup 2495
- Phenergan Tablets 2496
- Phenergan VC 2500
- Phenergan VC with Codeine 2501

Propofol (Additive CNS-depressant effect). Products include:
- Diprivan Injection 2267

Propoxyphene Napsylate (Additive CNS-depressant effect). Products include:
- Darvon-N/Darvocet-N 1254

Protriptyline Hydrochloride (Propoxyphene slows the metabolism). Products include:
- Vivactil Tablets 1567

Quazepam (Additive CNS-depressant effect). Products include:
- Doral Tablets 2383

Secobarbital Sodium (Additive CNS-depressant effect). Products include:
- Seconal Sodium Pulvules 1296

Sufentanil Citrate (Additive CNS-depressant effect). Products include:
- Sufenta Injection 1147

Sulfinpyrazone (Uricosuric effect inhibited). Products include:
- Anturane 853

Temazepam (Additive CNS-depressant effect). Products include:
- Restoril Capsules 2023

Thiamylal Sodium (Additive CNS-depressant effect). Products include:
- Surital Ampoules, Steri-Vials 1764

Thioridazine Hydrochloride (Additive CNS-depressant effect). Products include:
- Mellaril 2011

Thiothixene (Additive CNS-depressant effect). Products include:
- Navane Capsules and Concentrate 1954
- Navane Intramuscular 1956

Tranylcypromine Sulfate (Propoxyphene slows the metabolism). Products include:
- Parnate Tablets 2222

Trazodone Hydrochloride (Propoxyphene slows the metabolism). Products include:
- Desyrel and Desyrel Dividose 1404

Triazolam (Additive CNS-depressant effect). Products include:
- Halcion Tablets 2340

Trifluoperazine Hydrochloride (Additive CNS-depressant effect). Products include:
- Stelazine 2226

Trimethadione (Propoxyphene slows the metabolism). Products include:
- Tridione 557

Trimipramine Maleate (Propoxyphene slows the metabolism). Products include:
- Surmontil Capsules 2524

Valproic Acid (Propoxyphene slows the metabolism). Products include:
- Depakene Capsules & Syrup 511

Warfarin Sodium (Enhanced anticoagulant effect). Products include:
- Coumadin Injection & Tablets 944
- Panwarfin Tablets 547

DARVON PULVULES
(Propoxyphene Hydrochloride) 1256
See **Darvocet-N 50 Tablets**

DARVON-N SUSPENSION & TABLETS
(Propoxyphene Napsylate) 1254
See **Darvocet-N 50 Tablets**

DATRIL EXTRA-STRENGTH ANALGESIC TABLETS
(Acetaminophen) 748
No interactions described in labeling.

DAYALETS FILMTAB
(Multivitamins) ..... ▣ 502
No interactions described in labeling.

DAYALETS PLUS IRON FILMTAB
(Vitamins with Iron) ..... ▣ 502
No interactions described in labeling.

DAYTO HIMBIN TABLETS AND LIQUID
(Yohimbine Hydrochloride) 905
No interactions described in labeling.

DEBRISAN WOUND CLEANING BEADS
(Polyethylene Glycol) 1150
No interactions described in labeling.

DEBRISAN WOUND CLEANING PASTE
(Polyethylene Glycol) 1150
No interactions described in labeling.

DEBROX DROPS
(Carbamide Peroxide) ..... ▣ 593
No interactions described in labeling.

DECADRON ELIXIR
(Dexamethasone) 1445
May interact with oral anticoagulants, potassium sparing diuretics, and certain other agents. Compounds in these categories include:

Amiloride Hydrochloride (Hypokalemia). Products include:
- Midamor Tablets 1508
- Moduretic Tablets 1510

Dicumarol (Response to dicumarol inhibited). Products include:
- Dicumarol Tablets 516

Ephedrine (Enhanced metabolic clearance of corticosteroids).

Ephedrine Hydrochloride (Enhanced metabolic clearance of corticosteroids). Products include:
- Amesec ..... ▣ 682
- Primatene Tablets-M Formula 2421
- Primatene Tablets-P Formula 2421
- Primatene Tablets-Regular Formula 2421
- Quadrinal Tablets 1183
- Quelidrine Syrup 556
- Tedral SA 1765

Ephedrine Sulfate (Enhanced metabolic clearance of corticosteroids). Products include:
- Bronkaid Tablets ..... ▣ 757
- Bronkolixir ..... ▣ 761
- Bronkotabs Tablets ..... ▣ 762
- Marax Tablets & DF Syrup 1954
- Pazo Hemorrhoid Ointment & Suppositories 752
- Vicks Vatronol Nose Drops ..... ▣ 666

Ephedrine Tannate (Enhanced metabolic clearance of corticosteroids). Products include:
- Rynatuss 2388

Live Virus Vaccines (Contraindicated).

Phenobarbital (Enhanced metabolic clearance of corticosteroids). Products include:
- Arco-Lase Plus Tablets 607
- Bellergal-S Tablets 1998
- Bronkolixir ..... ▣ 761
- Bronkotabs Tablets ..... ▣ 762
- Donnatal 1858
- Donnatal Extentabs 1859
- Donnatal Tablets 1858
- Donnazyme Tablets 1860
- Kinesed Tablets 2272
- Phenobarbital Elixir and Tablets 1293
- Primatene Tablets-P Formula 2421
- Quadrinal Tablets 1183
- Tedral SA 1765

Phenytoin (Enhanced metabolic clearance of corticosteroids). Products include:
- Dilantin Infatabs 1710
- Dilantin-30 Pediatric/Dilantin-125 Suspension 1713

Phenytoin Sodium (Enhanced metabolic clearance of corticosteroids). Products include:
- Dilantin Kapseals 1708
- Dilantin Parenteral 1712
- Dilantin with Phenobarbital Kapseals 1715

Rifampin (Enhanced metabolic clearance of corticosteroids). Products include:
- Rifadin 1345
- Rifamate Capsules 1347
- Rimactane Capsules 879

Spironolactone (Hypokalemia). Products include:
- Aldactazide 2150
- Aldactone 2152

Triamterene (Hypokalemia). Products include:
- Dyazide Capsules 2208
- Dyrenium Capsules 2210
- Maxzide 1215

Warfarin Sodium (Response to warfarin inhibited). Products include:
- Coumadin Injection & Tablets 944
- Panwarfin Tablets 547

DECADRON PHOSPHATE INJECTION
(Dexamethasone Sodium Phosphate) 1449
May interact with potassium sparing diuretics, oral anticoagulants, and certain other agents. Compounds in these categories include:

Amiloride Hydrochloride (Hypokalemia). Products include:
- Midamor Tablets 1508
- Moduretic Tablets 1510

Dicumarol (Response to dicumarol inhibited). Products include:
- Dicumarol Tablets 516

Ephedrine (Enhanced metabolic clearance of corticosteroids).

Ephedrine Hydrochloride (Enhanced metabolic clearance of corticosteroids). Products include:
- Amesec ..... ▣ 682
- Primatene Tablets-M Formula 2421
- Primatene Tablets-P Formula 2421
- Primatene Tablets-Regular Formula 2421
- Quadrinal Tablets 1183
- Quelidrine Syrup 556
- Tedral SA 1765

Ephedrine Sulfate (Enhanced metabolic clearance of corticosteroids). Products include:
- Bronkaid Tablets ⊞ 757
- Bronkolixir ⊞ 761
- Bronkotabs Tablets ⊞ 762
- Marax Tablets & DF Syrup 1954
- Pazo Hemorrhoid Ointment & Suppositories 752
- Vicks Vatronol Nose Drops ⊞ 666

Ephedrine Tannate (Enhanced metabolic clearance of corticosteroids). Products include:
- Rynatuss 2388

Live Virus Vaccines (Contraindicated).

Phenobarbital (Enhanced metabolic clearance of corticosteroids). Products include:
- Arco-Lase Plus Tablets 607
- Bellergal-S Tablets 1998
- Bronkolixir ⊞ 761
- Bronkotabs Tablets ⊞ 762
- Donnatal 1858
- Donnatal Extentabs 1859
- Donnatal Tablets 1858
- Donnazyme Tablets 1860
- Kinesed Tablets 2272
- Phenobarbital Elixir and Tablets 1293
- Primatene Tablets-P Formula 2421
- Quadrinal Tablets 1183
- Tedral SA 1765

Phenytoin (Enhanced metabolic clearance of corticosteroids). Products include:
- Dilantin Infatabs 1710
- Dilantin-30 Pediatric/Dilantin-125 Suspension 1713

Phenytoin Sodium (Enhanced metabolic clearance of corticosteroids). Products include:
- Dilantin Kapseals 1708
- Dilantin Parenteral 1712
- Dilantin with Phenobarbital Kapseals 1715

Rifampin (Enhanced metabolic clearance of corticosteroids). Products include:
- Rifadin 1345
- Rifamate Capsules 1347
- Rimactane Capsules 879

Spironolactone (Hypokalemia). Products include:
- Aldactazide 2150
- Aldactone 2152

Triamterene (Hypokalemia). Products include:
- Dyazide Capsules 2208
- Dyrenium Capsules 2210
- Maxzide 1215

Warfarin Sodium (Response to warfarin inhibited). Products include:
- Coumadin Injection & Tablets 944
- Panwarfin Tablets 547

DECADRON PHOSPHATE RESPIHALER

(Dexamethasone Sodium Phosphate) 1454
May interact with oral anticoagulants, potassium sparing diuretics, and certain other agents. Compounds in these categories include:

Amiloride Hydrochloride (Hypokalemia). Products include:
- Midamor Tablets 1508
- Moduretic Tablets 1510

Aspirin (Concomitant administration requires caution). Products include:
- Alka-Seltzer Effervescent Antacid and Pain Reliever 1568
- Alka-Seltzer Extra Strength Effervescent Antacid and Pain Reliever 1570
- Alka-Seltzer (Flavored) Effervescent Antacid and Pain Reliever 1569
- Alka-Seltzer Plus Cold Medicine ⊞ 623
- Alka-Seltzer Plus Night-Time Cold Medicine ⊞ 623
- Alka Seltzer Plus Sinus Allergy Medicine ⊞ 624
- Anacin Coated Analgesic Caplets 2417
- Anacin Coated Analgesic Tablets 2417
- Anacin Maximum Strength Analgesic Coated Tablets 2417
- Maximum Strength Arthritis Pain Formula By the Makers of Anacin Analgesic Tablets and Caplets 2418
- Arthritis Pain Formula by the Makers of Anacin Analgesic Tablets and Caplets ⊞ 747
- Arthritis Strength BC Powder ⊞ 516
- Ascriptin A/D Caplets 1850
- Regular Strength Ascriptin Tablets 1850
- Azdōne Tablets 844
- BC Powder ⊞ 517
- BC Cold Powder ⊞ 517
- Children's Bayer Chewable Aspirin ⊞ 564
- Genuine Bayer Aspirin Tablets & Caplets ⊞ 564
- Maximum Bayer Aspirin Tablets & Caplets ⊞ 566
- Bayer Plus Aspirin Tablets ⊞ 567
- Therapy Bayer Aspirin Caplets ⊞ 568
- 8 Hour Bayer Timed-Release Aspirin ⊞ 566
- Arthritis Strength Bufferin Analgesic Caplets 744
- Extra Strength Bufferin Analgesic Tablets 745
- Bufferin Analgesic Tablets and Caplets 743
- Cama Arthritis Pain Reliever ⊞ 685
- Damason-P 1356
- Easprin 1719
- Ecotrin Enteric Coated Aspirin Maximum Strength Tablets and Caplets 2189
- Ecotrin Enteric Coated Aspirin Regular Strength Tablets and Caplets 2189
- Empirin Aspirin ⊞ 541
- Empirin with Codeine Phosphate Nos. 2, 3 & 4 764
- Equagesic Tablets 2451
- Excedrin Extra-Strength Analgesic Tablets & Caplets 749
- 4-Way Cold Tablets 750
- Fiorinal Capsules 2007
- Fiorinal with Codeine Capsules 2008
- Fiorinal Tablets 2007
- Lortab ASA Tablets 2414
- Momentum Muscular Backache Formula ⊞ 751
- Norgesic 1314
- Norwich Extra-Strength Aspirin ⊞ 546
- Norwich Regular Strength Aspirin ⊞ 547
- P-A-C Analgesic Tablets ⊞ 669
- Percodan 951
- Robaxisal Tablets 1872
- Sine-Off Sinus Medicine Tablets-Aspirin Formula ⊞ 722
- Soma Compound w/Codeine Tablets 2390
- Soma Compound Tablets 2389
- St. Joseph Adult Chewable Aspirin (81 mg.) ⊞ 703
- Synalgos-DC Capsules 2525
- Talwin Compound 2072
- Ursinus Inlay-Tabs ⊞ 691
- Vanquish Analgesic Caplets ⊞ 574
- Zorprin Tablets 698

Aspirin, Enteric Coated (Concomitant administration requires caution). Products include:
- Therapy Bayer Aspirin Caplets ⊞ 568
- Ecotrin 2189

Dicumarol (Response to dicumarol inhibited). Products include:
- Dicumarol Tablets 516

Ephedrine (Enhanced metabolic clearance of corticosteroids).

Ephedrine Hydrochloride (Enhanced metabolic clearance of corticosteroids). Products include:
- Amesec ⊞ 682
- Primatene Tablets-M Formula 2421
- Primatene Tablets-P Formula 2421
- Primatene Tablets-Regular Formula 2421
- Quadrinal Tablets 1183
- Quelidrine Syrup 556
- Tedral SA 1765

Ephedrine Sulfate (Enhanced metabolic clearance of corticosteroids). Products include:
- Bronkaid Tablets ⊞ 757
- Bronkolixir ⊞ 761
- Bronkotabs Tablets ⊞ 762
- Marax Tablets & DF Syrup 1954
- Pazo Hemorrhoid Ointment & Suppositories 752
- Vicks Vatronol Nose Drops ⊞ 666

Ephedrine Tannate (Enhanced metabolic clearance of corticosteroids). Products include:
- Rynatuss 2388

Live Virus Vaccines (Contraindicated).

Phenobarbital (Enhanced metabolic clearance of corticosteroids). Products include:
- Arco-Lase Plus Tablets 607
- Bellergal-S Tablets 1998
- Bronkolixir ⊞ 761
- Bronkotabs Tablets ⊞ 762
- Donnatal 1858
- Donnatal Extentabs 1859
- Donnatal Tablets 1858
- Donnazyme Tablets 1860
- Kinesed Tablets 2272
- Phenobarbital Elixir and Tablets 1293
- Primatene Tablets-P Formula 2421
- Quadrinal Tablets 1183
- Tedral SA 1765

Phenytoin (Enhanced metabolic clearance of corticosteroids). Products include:
- Dilantin Infatabs 1710
- Dilantin-30 Pediatric/Dilantin-125 Suspension 1713

Phenytoin Sodium (Enhanced metabolic clearance of corticosteroids). Products include:
- Dilantin Kapseals 1708
- Dilantin Parenteral 1712
- Dilantin with Phenobarbital Kapseals 1715

Rifampin (Enhanced metabolic clearance of corticosteroids). Products include:
- Rifadin 1345
- Rifamate Capsules 1347
- Rimactane Capsules 879

Spironolactone (Hypokalemia). Products include:
- Aldactazide 2150
- Aldactone 2152

Triamterene (Hypokalemia). Products include:
- Dyazide Capsules 2208
- Dyrenium Capsules 2210
- Maxzide 1215

Warfarin Sodium (Response to warfarin inhibited). Products include:
- Coumadin Injection & Tablets 944
- Panwarfin Tablets 547

DECADRON PHOSPHATE STERILE OPHTHALMIC OINTMENT

(Dexamethasone Sodium Phosphate) 1453
No interactions described in labeling.

DECADRON PHOSPHATE STERILE OPHTHALMIC SOLUTION

(Dexamethasone Sodium Phosphate) 1453
No interactions described in labeling.

DECADRON PHOSPHATE TOPICAL CREAM

(Dexamethasone Sodium Phosphate) 1455
No interactions described in labeling.

DECADRON PHOSPHATE TURBINAIRE

(Dexamethasone Sodium Phosphate) 1456
May interact with potassium sparing diuretics, oral anticoagulants, and certain other agents. Compounds in these categories include:

Amiloride Hydrochloride (Hypokalemia). Products include:
- Midamor Tablets 1508
- Moduretic Tablets 1510

Aspirin (Concomitant administration requires caution). Products include:
- Alka-Seltzer Effervescent Antacid and Pain Reliever 1568
- Alka-Seltzer Extra Strength Effervescent Antacid and Pain Reliever 1570
- Alka-Seltzer (Flavored) Effervescent Antacid and Pain Reliever 1569
- Alka-Seltzer Plus Cold Medicine ⊞ 623
- Alka-Seltzer Plus Night-Time Cold Medicine ⊞ 623
- Alka Seltzer Plus Sinus Allergy Medicine ⊞ 624
- Anacin Coated Analgesic Caplets 2417
- Anacin Coated Analgesic Tablets 2417
- Anacin Maximum Strength Analgesic Coated Tablets 2417
- Maximum Strength Arthritis Pain Formula By the Makers of Anacin Analgesic Tablets and Caplets 2418
- Arthritis Pain Formula by the Makers of Anacin Analgesic Tablets and Caplets ⊞ 747
- Arthritis Strength BC Powder ⊞ 516
- Ascriptin A/D Caplets 1850
- Regular Strength Ascriptin Tablets 1850
- Azdōne Tablets 844
- BC Powder ⊞ 517
- BC Cold Powder ⊞ 517
- Children's Bayer Chewable Aspirin ⊞ 564
- Genuine Bayer Aspirin Tablets & Caplets ⊞ 564
- Maximum Bayer Aspirin Tablets & Caplets ⊞ 566
- Bayer Plus Aspirin Tablets ⊞ 567
- Therapy Bayer Aspirin Caplets ⊞ 568
- 8 Hour Bayer Timed-Release Aspirin ⊞ 566
- Arthritis Strength Bufferin Analgesic Caplets 744
- Extra Strength Bufferin Analgesic Tablets 745
- Bufferin Analgesic Tablets and Caplets 743
- Cama Arthritis Pain Reliever ⊞ 685
- Damason-P 1356
- Easprin 1719
- Ecotrin Enteric Coated Aspirin Maximum Strength Tablets and Caplets 2189
- Ecotrin Enteric Coated Aspirin Regular Strength Tablets and Caplets 2189
- Empirin Aspirin ⊞ 541
- Empirin with Codeine Phosphate Nos. 2, 3 & 4 764
- Equagesic Tablets 2451
- Excedrin Extra-Strength Analgesic Tablets & Caplets 749
- 4-Way Cold Tablets 750
- Fiorinal Capsules 2007
- Fiorinal with Codeine Capsules 2008
- Fiorinal Tablets 2007
- Lortab ASA Tablets 2414
- Momentum Muscular Backache Formula ⊞ 751
- Norgesic 1314
- Norwich Extra-Strength Aspirin ⊞ 546
- Norwich Regular Strength Aspirin ⊞ 547
- P-A-C Analgesic Tablets ⊞ 669
- Percodan 951
- Robaxisal Tablets 1872
- Sine-Off Sinus Medicine Tablets-Aspirin Formula ⊞ 722
- Soma Compound w/Codeine Tablets 2390
- Soma Compound Tablets 2389
- St. Joseph Adult Chewable Aspirin (81 mg.) ⊞ 703
- Synalgos-DC Capsules 2525
- Talwin Compound 2072
- Ursinus Inlay-Tabs ⊞ 691
- Vanquish Analgesic Caplets ⊞ 574
- Zorprin Tablets 698

Aspirin, Enteric Coated (Concomitant administration requires caution). Products include:
- Therapy Bayer Aspirin Caplets ⊞ 568
- Ecotrin 2189

Dicumarol (Response to dicumarol inhibited). Products include:
- Dicumarol Tablets 516

Ephedrine (Enhanced metabolic clearance of corticosteroids).

Ephedrine Hydrochloride (Enhanced metabolic clearance of corticosteroids). Products include:
Amesec ■ 682
Primatene Tablets-M Formula 2421
Primatene Tablets-P Formula 2421
Primatene Tablets-Regular Formula 2421
Quadrinal Tablets 1183
Quelidrine Syrup 556
Tedral SA 1765

Ephedrine Sulfate (Enhanced metabolic clearance of corticosteroids). Products include:
Bronkaid Tablets ■ 757
Bronkolixir ■ 761
Bronkotabs Tablets ■ 762
Marax Tablets & DF Syrup 1954
Pazo Hemorrhoid Ointment & Suppositories 752
Vicks Vatronol Nose Drops ■ 666

Ephedrine Tannate (Enhanced metabolic clearance of corticosteroids). Products include:
Rynatuss 2388

Live Virus Vaccines (Contraindicated).

Phenobarbital (Enhanced metabolic clearance of corticosteroids). Products include:
Arco-Lase Plus Tablets 607
Bellergal-S Tablets 1998
Bronkolixir ■ 761
Bronkotabs Tablets ■ 762
Donnatal 1858
Donnatal Extentabs 1859
Donnatal Tablets 1858
Donnazyme Tablets 1860
Kinesed Tablets 2272
Phenobarbital Elixir and Tablets 1293
Primatene Tablets-P Formula 2421
Quadrinal Tablets 1183
Tedral SA 1765

Phenytoin (Enhanced metabolic clearance of corticosteroids). Products include:
Dilantin Infatabs 1710
Dilantin-30 Pediatric/Dilantin-125 Suspension 1713

Phenytoin Sodium (Enhanced metabolic clearance of corticosteroids). Products include:
Dilantin Kapseals 1708
Dilantin Parenteral 1712
Dilantin with Phenobarbital Kapseals 1715

Rifampin (Enhanced metabolic clearance of corticosteroids). Products include:
Rifadin 1345
Rifamate Capsules 1347
Rimactane Capsules 879

Spironolactone (Hypokalemia). Products include:
Aldactazide 2150
Aldactone 2152

Triamterene (Hypokalemia). Products include:
Dyazide Capsules 2208
Dyrenium Capsules 2210
Maxzide 1215

Warfarin Sodium (Response to warfarin inhibited). Products include:
Coumadin Injection & Tablets 944
Panwarfin Tablets 547

DECADRON PHOSPHATE WITH XYLOCAINE INJECTION, STERILE
(Dexamethasone Sodium Phosphate, Lidocaine Hydrochloride) 1451
May interact with potassium sparing diuretics, oral anticoagulants, and certain other agents. Compounds in these categories include:

Amiloride Hydrochloride (Hypokalemia). Products include:
Midamor Tablets 1508
Moduretic Tablets 1510

Dicumarol (Response to dicumarol inhibited). Products include:
Dicumarol Tablets 516

Ephedrine Hydrochloride (Enhanced metabolic clearance of corticosteroids). Products include:
Amesec ■ 682
Primatene Tablets-M Formula 2421
Primatene Tablets-P Formula 2421
Primatene Tablets-Regular Formula 2421
Quadrinal Tablets 1183
Quelidrine Syrup 556
Tedral SA 1765

Ephedrine Sulfate (Enhanced metabolic clearance of corticosteroids). Products include:
Bronkaid Tablets ■ 757
Bronkolixir ■ 761
Bronkotabs Tablets ■ 762
Marax Tablets & DF Syrup 1954
Pazo Hemorrhoid Ointment & Suppositories 752
Vicks Vatronol Nose Drops ■ 666

Ephedrine Tannate (Enhanced metabolic clearance of corticosteroids). Products include:
Rynatuss 2388

Live Virus Vaccines (Contraindicated).

Phenobarbital (Enhanced metabolic clearance of corticosteroids). Products include:
Arco-Lase Plus Tablets 607
Bellergal-S Tablets 1998
Bronkolixir ■ 761
Bronkotabs Tablets ■ 762
Donnatal 1858
Donnatal Extentabs 1859
Donnatal Tablets 1858
Donnazyme Tablets 1860
Kinesed Tablets 2272
Phenobarbital Elixir and Tablets 1293
Primatene Tablets-P Formula 2421
Quadrinal Tablets 1183
Tedral SA 1765

Phenytoin (Enhanced metabolic clearance of corticosteroids). Products include:
Dilantin Infatabs 1710
Dilantin-30 Pediatric/Dilantin-125 Suspension 1713

Phenytoin Sodium (Enhanced metabolic clearance of corticosteroids). Products include:
Dilantin Kapseals 1708
Dilantin Parenteral 1712
Dilantin with Phenobarbital Kapseals 1715

Rifampin (Enhanced metabolic clearance of corticosteroids). Products include:
Rifadin 1345
Rifamate Capsules 1347
Rimactane Capsules 879

Spironolactone (Hypokalemia). Products include:
Aldactazide 2150
Aldactone 2152

Triamterene (Hypokalemia). Products include:
Dyazide Capsules 2208
Dyrenium Capsules 2210
Maxzide 1215

Warfarin Sodium (Response to warfarin inhibited). Products include:
Coumadin Injection & Tablets 944
Panwarfin Tablets 547

DECADRON TABLETS
(Dexamethasone) 1447
May interact with oral anticoagulants, potassium sparing diuretics, and certain other agents. Compounds in these categories include:

Amiloride Hydrochloride (Possible hypokalemia). Products include:
Midamor Tablets 1508
Moduretic Tablets 1510

Aspirin (Use cautiously with dexamethasome in hypoprothrombinemia). Products include:
Alka-Seltzer Effervescent Antacid and Pain Reliever 1568
Alka-Seltzer Extra Strength Effervescent Antacid and Pain Reliever 1570
Alka-Seltzer (Flavored) Effervescent Antacid and Pain Reliever 1569
Alka-Seltzer Plus Cold Medicine ■ 623
Alka-Seltzer Plus Night-Time Cold Medicine ■ 623
Alka Seltzer Plus Sinus Allergy Medicine ■ 624
Anacin Coated Analgesic Caplets 2417
Anacin Coated Analgesic Tablets 2417
Anacin Maximum Strength Analgesic Coated Tablets 2417
Maximum Strength Arthritis Pain Formula By the Makers of Anacin Analgesic Tablets and Caplets 2418
Arthritis Pain Formula by the Makers of Anacin Analgesic Tablets and Caplets ■ 747
Arthritis Strength BC Powder ■ 516
Ascriptin A/D Caplets 1850
Regular Strength Ascriptin Tablets 1850
Azdōne Tablets 844
BC Powder ■ 517
BC Cold Powder ■ 517
Children's Bayer Chewable Aspirin ■ 564
Genuine Bayer Aspirin Tablets & Caplets ■ 564
Maximum Bayer Aspirin Tablets & Caplets ■ 566
Bayer Plus Aspirin Tablets ■ 567
Therapy Bayer Aspirin Caplets ■ 568
8 Hour Bayer Timed-Release Aspirin ■ 566
Arthritis Strength Bufferin Analgesic Caplets 744
Extra Strength Bufferin Analgesic Tablets 745
Bufferin Analgesic Tablets and Caplets 743
Cama Arthritis Pain Reliever ■ 685
Damason-P 1356
Easprin 1719
Ecotrin Enteric Coated Aspirin Maximum Strength Tablets and Caplets 2189
Ecotrin Enteric Coated Aspirin Regular Strength Tablets and Caplets 2189
Empirin Aspirin ■ 541
Empirin with Codeine Phosphate Nos. 2, 3 & 4 764
Equagesic Tablets 2451
Excedrin Extra-Strength Analgesic Tablets & Caplets 749
4-Way Cold Tablets 750
Fiorinal Capsules 2007
Fiorinal with Codeine Capsules 2008
Fiorinal Tablets 2007
Lortab ASA Tablets 2414
Momentum Muscular Backache Formula ■ 751
Norgesic 1314
Norwich Extra-Strength Aspirin ■ 546
Norwich Regular Strength Aspirin ■ 547
P-A-C Analgesic Tablets ■ 669
Percodan 951
Robaxisal Tablets 1872
Sine-Off Sinus Medicine Tablets-Aspirin Formula ■ 722
Soma Compound w/Codeine Tablets 2390
Soma Compound Tablets 2389
St. Joseph Adult Chewable Aspirin (81 mg.) ■ 703
Synalgos-DC Capsules 2525
Talwin Compound 2072
Ursinus Inlay-Tabs ■ 691
Vanquish Analgesic Caplets ■ 574
Zorprin Tablets 698

Aspirin, Enteric Coated (Use cautiously with dexamethasone in hypoprothrombinemia). Products include:
Therapy Bayer Aspirin Caplets ■ 568
Ecotrin 2189

Dicumarol (Altered response to dicumarol). Products include:
Dicumarol Tablets 516

Ephedrine Hydrochloride (Decreases blood levels of dexamethasone). Products include:
Amesec ■ 682
Primatene Tablets-M Formula 2421
Primatene Tablets-P Formula 2421
Primatene Tablets-Regular Formula 2421
Quadrinal Tablets 1183
Quelidrine Syrup 556
Tedral SA 1765

Ephedrine Sulfate (Decreases blood levels of dexamethasone). Products include:
Bronkaid Tablets ■ 757
Bronkolixir ■ 761
Bronkotabs Tablets ■ 762
Marax Tablets & DF Syrup 1954
Pazo Hemorrhoid Ointment & Suppositories 752
Vicks Vatronol Nose Drops ■ 666

Ephedrine Tannate (Decreases blood levels of dexamethasone). Products include:
Rynatuss 2388

Live virus vaccines; smallpox (Contraindicated).

Phenobarbital (Decreases blood levels of dexamethasone). Products include:
Arco-Lase Plus Tablets 607
Bellergal-S Tablets 1998
Bronkolixir ■ 761
Bronkotabs Tablets ■ 762
Donnatal 1858
Donnatal Extentabs 1859
Donnatal Tablets 1858
Donnazyme Tablets 1860
Kinesed Tablets 2272
Phenobarbital Elixir and Tablets 1293
Primatene Tablets-P Formula 2421
Quadrinal Tablets 1183
Tedral SA 1765

Phenytoin (Decreases blood levels of dexamethasone). Products include:
Dilantin Infatabs 1710
Dilantin-30 Pediatric/Dilantin-125 Suspension 1713

Phenytoin Sodium (Decreases blood levels of dexamethasone). Products include:
Dilantin Kapseals 1708
Dilantin Parenteral 1712
Dilantin with Phenobarbital Kapseals 1715

Rifampin (Decreases blood levels of dexamethasone). Products include:
Rifadin 1345
Rifamate Capsules 1347
Rimactane Capsules 879

Spironolactone (Possible hypokalemia). Products include:
Aldactazide 2150
Aldactone 2152

Triamterene (Possible hypokalemia). Products include:
Dyazide Capsules 2208
Dyrenium Capsules 2210
Maxzide 1215

Warfarin Sodium (Altered response to warfarin). Products include:
Coumadin Injection & Tablets 944
Panwarfin Tablets 547

DECADRON-LA STERILE SUSPENSION
(Dexamethasone Acetate) 1457
May interact with oral anticoagulants, potassium sparing diuretics, and certain other agents. Compounds in these categories include:

Amiloride Hydrochloride (Possible hypokalemia). Products include:
Midamor Tablets 1508
Moduretic Tablets 1510

Aspirin (Use cautiously with dexamethasone in hypoprothrombinemia). Products include:
- Alka-Seltzer Effervescent Antacid and Pain Reliever ... 1568
- Alka-Seltzer Extra Strength Effervescent Antacid and Pain Reliever ... 1570
- Alka-Seltzer (Flavored) Effervescent Antacid and Pain Reliever ... 1569
- Alka-Seltzer Plus Cold Medicine ... ▣ 623
- Alka-Seltzer Plus Night-Time Cold Medicine ... ▣ 623
- Alka Seltzer Plus Sinus Allergy Medicine ... ▣ 624
- Anacin Coated Analgesic Caplets ... 2417
- Anacin Coated Analgesic Tablets ... 2417
- Anacin Maximum Strength Analgesic Coated Tablets ... 2417
- Maximum Strength Arthritis Pain Formula By the Makers of Anacin Analgesic Tablets and Caplets ... 2418
- Arthritis Pain Formula by the Makers of Anacin Analgesic Tablets and Caplets ... ▣ 747
- Arthritis Strength BC Powder ... ▣ 516
- Ascriptin A/D Caplets ... 1850
- Regular Strength Ascriptin Tablets 1850
- Azdone Tablets ... 844
- BC Powder ... ▣ 517
- BC Cold Powder ... ▣ 517
- Children's Bayer Chewable Aspirin ... ▣ 564
- Genuine Bayer Aspirin Tablets & Caplets ... ▣ 564
- Maximum Bayer Aspirin Tablets & Caplets ... ▣ 566
- Bayer Plus Aspirin Tablets ... ▣ 567
- Therapy Bayer Aspirin Caplets ... ▣ 568
- 8 Hour Bayer Timed-Release Aspirin ... ▣ 566
- Arthritis Strength Bufferin Analgesic Caplets ... 744
- Extra Strength Bufferin Analgesic Tablets ... 745
- Bufferin Analgesic Tablets and Caplets ... 743
- Cama Arthritis Pain Reliever ... ▣ 685
- Damason-P ... 1356
- Easprin ... 1719
- Ecotrin Enteric Coated Aspirin Maximum Strength Tablets and Caplets ... 2189
- Ecotrin Enteric Coated Aspirin Regular Strength Tablets and Caplets ... 2189
- Empirin Aspirin ... ▣ 541
- Empirin with Codeine Phosphate Nos. 2, 3 & 4 ... 764
- Equagesic Tablets ... 2451
- Excedrin Extra-Strength Analgesic Tablets & Caplets ... 749
- 4-Way Cold Tablets ... 750
- Fiorinal Capsules ... 2007
- Fiorinal with Codeine Capsules ... 2008
- Fiorinal Tablets ... 2007
- Lortab ASA Tablets ... 2414
- Momentum Muscular Backache Formula ... ▣ 751
- Norgesic ... 1314
- Norwich Extra-Strength Aspirin ... ▣ 546
- Norwich Regular Strength Aspirin ▣ 547
- P-A-C Analgesic Tablets ... ▣ 669
- Percodan ... 951
- Robaxisal Tablets ... 1872
- Sine-Off Sinus Medicine Tablets-Aspirin Formula ... ▣ 722
- Soma Compound w/Codeine Tablets ... 2390
- Soma Compound Tablets ... 2389
- St. Joseph Adult Chewable Aspirin (81 mg.) ... ▣ 703
- Synalgos-DC Capsules ... 2525
- Talwin Compound ... 2072
- Ursinus Inlay-Tabs ... ▣ 691
- Vanquish Analgesic Caplets ... ▣ 574
- Zorprin Tablets ... 698

Aspirin, Enteric Coated (Use cautiously with dexamethasone in hypoprothrombinemia). Products include:
- Therapy Bayer Aspirin Caplets ... ▣ 568
- Ecotrin ... 2189

Dicumarol (Altered response to dicumarol). Products include:
- Dicumarol Tablets ... 516

Ephedrine Hydrochloride (Decreases blood levels of dexamethasone). Products include:
- Amesec ... ▣ 682
- Primatene Tablets-M Formula ... 2421
- Primatene Tablets-P Formula ... 2421
- Primatene Tablets-Regular Formula ... 2421
- Quadrinal Tablets ... 1183
- Quelidrine Syrup ... 556
- Tedral SA ... 1765

Ephedrine Sulfate (Decreases blood levels of dexamethasone). Products include:
- Bronkaid Tablets ... ▣ 757
- Bronkolixir ... ▣ 761
- Bronkotabs Tablets ... ▣ 762
- Marax Tablets & DF Syrup ... 1954
- Pazo Hemorrhoid Ointment & Suppositories ... 752
- Vicks Vatronol Nose Drops ... ▣ 666

Ephedrine Tannate (Decreases blood levels of dexamethasone). Products include:
- Rynatuss ... 2388

Live virus vaccines; smallpox (Contraindicated).

Phenobarbital (Decreases blood levels of dexamethasone). Products include:
- Arco-Lase Plus Tablets ... 607
- Bellergal-S Tablets ... 1998
- Bronkolixir ... ▣ 761
- Bronkotabs Tablets ... ▣ 762
- Donnatal ... 1858
- Donnatal Extentabs ... 1859
- Donnatal Tablets ... 1858
- Donnazyme Tablets ... 1860
- Kinesed Tablets ... 2272
- Phenobarbital Elixir and Tablets ... 1293
- Primatene Tablets-P Formula ... 2421
- Quadrinal Tablets ... 1183
- Tedral SA ... 1765

Phenytoin (Decreases blood levels of dexamethasone). Products include:
- Dilantin Infatabs ... 1710
- Dilantin-30 Pediatric/Dilantin-125 Suspension ... 1713

Phenytoin Sodium (Decreases blood levels of dexamethasone). Products include:
- Dilantin Kapseals ... 1708
- Dilantin Parenteral ... 1712
- Dilantin with Phenobarbital Kapseals ... 1715

Rifampin (Decreases blood levels of dexamethasone). Products include:
- Rifadin ... 1345
- Rifamate Capsules ... 1347
- Rimactane Capsules ... 879

Spironolactone (Possible hypokalemia). Products include:
- Aldactazide ... 2150
- Aldactone ... 2152

Triamterene (Possible hypokalemia). Products include:
- Dyazide Capsules ... 2208
- Dyrenium Capsules ... 2210
- Maxzide ... 1215

Warfarin Sodium (Altered response to warfarin). Products include:
- Coumadin Injection & Tablets ... 944
- Panwarfin Tablets ... 547

DECASPRAY TOPICAL AEROSOL
(Dexamethasone) ... 1459
No interactions described in labeling.

DECLOMYCIN CAPSULES, TABLETS
(Demeclocycline Hydrochloride) ... 1199
May interact with anticoagulants, penicillins, antacids, oral contraceptives, and certain other agents. Compounds in these categories include:

Aluminum Carbonate Gel (Tetracycline absorption impaired). Products include:
- Basaljel ... 2438

Aluminum Hydroxide (Tetracycline absorption impaired). Products include:
- Cama Arthritis Pain Reliever ... ▣ 685
- Gaviscon Extra Strength Relief Formula Liquid Antacid ... ▣ 594
- Gaviscon Extra Strength Relief Formula Antacid Tablets ... ▣ 594
- Gaviscon Liquid Antacid ... ▣ 594
- Gelusil Liquid & Tablets ... ▣ 639
- Extra Strength Maalox Plus Suspension ... 1850
- Maalox TC Suspension ... 1851
- Maalox Plus Tablets ... ▣ 655
- Extra Strength Maalox Plus Tablets 1850
- Nephrox Suspension ... ▣ 563
- WinGel Liquid & Tablets ... ▣ 761

Aluminum Hydroxide Gel (Tetracycline absorption impaired). Products include:
- ALternaGEL Liquid ... 1154
- Aludrox Oral Suspension ... 2428
- Amphojel Suspension ... 2429
- Amphojel Suspension without Flavor ... 2429
- Mylanta Liquid ... 1155
- Mylanta Double Strength Liquid ... 1155

Aluminum Hydroxide Gel, Dried (Tetracycline absorption impaired). Products include:
- Alu-Tab/Alu-Cap ... 1309
- Amphojel Tablets ... 2429
- Ascriptin A/D Caplets ... 1850
- Regular Strength Ascriptin Tablets 1850
- Gaviscon Antacid Tablets ... ▣ 593
- Gaviscon-2 Antacid Tablets ... ▣ 594
- Mylanta Tablets ... 1155
- Mylanta Double Strength Tablets ... 1155

Amoxicillin (Interference with bactericidal action of penicillin). Products include:
- Amoxil ... 2193
- Augmentin Tablets, Powder for Oral Suspension, and Chewable Tablets ... 2198

Ampicillin Sodium (Interference with bactericidal action of penicillin). Products include:
- Unasyn ... 1965

Azlocillin Sodium (Interference with bactericidal action of penicillin).
- No products indexed under this heading.

Bacampicillin Hydrochloride (Interference with bactericidal action of penicillin). Products include:
- Spectrobid Tablets & Powder for Oral Suspension ... 1961

Carbenicillin Disodium (Interference with bactericidal action of penicillin).

Carbenicillin Indanyl Sodium (Interference with bactericidal action of penicillin). Products include:
- Geocillin Tablets ... 1951

Dicumarol (Plasma prothrombin activity depressed; downward adjustment of anticoagulant dosage may be necessary). Products include:
- Dicumarol Tablets ... 516

Dihydroxyaluminum Sodium Carbonate (Tetracycline absorption impaired). Products include:
- Rolaids ... ▣ 743

Ethinyl Estradiol (Reduced efficacy and increased breakthrough bleeding). Products include:
- Brevicon ... 2304
- Demulen ... 2161
- Estinyl Tablets ... 2085
- Jenest-28 Tablets ... 1636
- Levlen/Tri-Levlen ... 665
- Lo/Ovral Tablets ... 2471
- Lo/Ovral-28 Tablets ... 2476
- Loestrin ... 1728
- Modicon ... 1667
- Nordette-21 Tablets ... 2481
- Nordette-28 Tablets ... 2483
- Norethin ... 2133
- Norinyl ... 2304
- Norlestrin ... 1746
- Ortho-Cyclen Tablets ... 1658
- Ortho-Novum ... 1667
- Ovcon ... 1391
- Ovral Tablets ... 2490
- Ovral-28 Tablets ... 2491
- Levlen/Tri-Levlen ... 665
- Tri-Norinyl ... 2304
- Triphasil-21 Tablets ... 2527
- Triphasil-28 Tablets ... 2532

Ethynodiol Diacetate (Reduced efficacy and increased breakthrough bleeding). Products include:
- Demulen ... 2161

Heparin Calcium (Plasma prothrombin activity depressed; downward adjustment of anticoagulant dosage may be necessary). Products include:
- Calciparine Injection ... 925

Heparin Sodium (Plasma prothrombin activity depressed; downward adjustment of anticoagulant dosage may be necessary). Products include:
- Heparin Lock Flush Solution ... 2456
- Heparin Sodium Vials ... 1264
- Heparin Sodium Injection ... 2457
- Heparin Sodium Injection, USP, Sterile Solution ... 2342

Levonorgestrel (Reduced efficacy and increased breakthrough bleeding). Products include:
- Levlen/Tri-Levlen ... 665
- Nordette-21 Tablets ... 2481
- Nordette-28 Tablets ... 2483
- Norplant System ... 2484
- Levlen/Tri-Levlen ... 665
- Triphasil-21 Tablets ... 2527
- Triphasil-28 Tablets ... 2532

Magaldrate (Tetracycline absorption impaired). Products include:
- Riopan Antacid Chew Tablets ... ▣ 754
- Riopan Antacid Chew Tablets in Rollpacks ... ▣ 754
- Riopan Antacid Suspension ... 2421
- Riopan Antacid Swallow Tablets ... 2421
- Riopan Plus Chew Tablets ... 2422
- Riopan Plus Chew Tablets in Rollpack ... 2422
- Riopan Plus 2 Chew Tablets, Mint Flavor, Cherry Flavor ... 2422
- Riopan Plus Suspension ... 2422
- Riopan Plus 2 Suspension, Mint Flavor, Cherry Flavor ... 2422

Magnesium Hydroxide (Tetracycline absorption impaired). Products include:
- Aludrox Oral Suspension ... 2428
- Ascriptin A/D Caplets ... 1850
- Regular Strength Ascriptin Tablets 1850
- Di-Gel Antacid/Anti-Gas ... ▣ 697
- Gelusil Liquid & Tablets ... ▣ 639
- Haley's M-O, Regular & Flavored .. ▣ 569
- Extra Strength Maalox Plus Suspension ... 1850
- Maalox TC Suspension ... 1851
- Maalox Plus Tablets ... ▣ 655
- Extra Strength Maalox Plus Tablets 1850
- Mylanta Liquid ... 1155
- Mylanta Tablets ... 1155
- Mylanta Double Strength Liquid ... 1155
- Mylanta Double Strength Tablets ... 1155
- Concentrated Phillips' Milk of Magnesia ... ▣ 573
- Phillips' Milk of Magnesia Liquid ... ▣ 572
- Phillips' Milk of Magnesia Tablets ▣ 573
- WinGel Liquid & Tablets ... ▣ 761

Magnesium Oxide (Tetracycline absorption impaired). Products include:
- Bayer Plus Aspirin Tablets ... ▣ 567
- Beelith Tablets ... 659
- Bufferin Analgesic Tablets and Caplets ... ▣ 524
- Cama Arthritis Pain Reliever ... ▣ 685
- Mag-Ox 400 ... 673
- Uro-Mag ... 673

Mestranol (Reduced efficacy and increased breakthrough bleeding). Products include:
- Enovid ... 2161
- Norethin ... 2133
- Norinyl ... 2304
- Ortho-Novum ... 1667

Mezlocillin Sodium (Interference with bactericidal action of penicillin). Products include:
- Mezlin ... 1597
- Mezlin Pharmacy Bulk Package ... 1599

Nafcillin Sodium (Interference with bactericidal action of penicillin). Products include:
- Unipen ... 2533

Norethindrone (Reduced efficacy and increased breakthrough bleeding). Products include:
- Brevicon ... 2304
- Jenest-28 Tablets ... 1636
- Micronor Tablets ... 1667
- Modicon ... 1667
- Norethin ... 2133
- Norinyl ... 2304
- Norlutin ... 1755
- Nor-Q D Tablets ... 2304
- Ortho-Novum ... 1667
- Ovcon ... 1391
- Tri-Norinyl ... 2304

Norethynodrel (Reduced efficacy and increased breakthrough bleeding). Products include:
- Enovid ... 2161

Norgestimate (Reduced efficacy and increased breakthrough bleeding). Products include:
- Ortho-Cyclen Tablets ... 1658

Norgestrel (Reduced efficacy and increased breakthrough bleeding). Products include:
- Lo/Ovral Tablets ... 2471
- Lo/Ovral-28 Tablets ... 2476
- Ovral Tablets ... 2490
- Ovral-28 Tablets ... 2491
- Ovrette Tablets ... 2492

Penicillin G Potassium (Interference with bactericidal action of penicillin). Products include:
- Pfizerpen for Injection ... 1957

Penicillin G Procaine (Interference with bactericidal action of penicillin). Products include:
- Bicillin C-R Injection ... 2438
- Bicillin C-R 900/300 Injection ... 2440
- Pfizerpen-AS Aqueous Suspension ... 1959
- Wycillin Injection ... 2537
- Wycillin Injection and Probenecid Tablets ... 2539

Penicillin G, Benzathine (Interference with bactericidal action of penicillin). Products include:
- Bicillin C-R Injection ... 2438
- Bicillin C-R 900/300 Injection ... 2440
- Bicillin L-A Injection ... 2442

Penicillin V Potassium (Interference with bactericidal action of penicillin).
- No products indexed under this heading.

Ticarcillin Disodium (Interference with bactericidal action of penicillin). Products include:
- Ticar for Injection ... 2236
- Timentin for Injection ... 2239

Warfarin Sodium (Plasma prothrombin activity depressed; downward adjustment of anticoagulant dosage may be necessary). Products include:
- Coumadin Injection & Tablets ... 944
- Panwarfin Tablets ... 547

Food Interactions

Dairy products (Interferes with absorption).

Food, unspecified (Interferes with absorption).

DECONAMINE SR CAPSULES

(Chlorpheniramine Maleate, Pseudoephedrine Hydrochloride) ... 663

May interact with hypnotics and sedatives, tranquilizers, monoamine oxidase inhibitors, veratrum alkaloids, sympathomimetic aerosal brochodilators, and certain other agents. Compounds in these categories include:

Albuterol (Potentially harmful combined effect on cardiovascular system). Products include:
- Proventil Inhalation Aerosol ... 2117
- Ventolin Inhalation Aerosol and Refill ... 583

Albuterol Sulfate (Potentially harmful combined effect on cardiovascular system). Products include:
- Proventil Repetabs Tablets ... 2120
- Proventil Solutions for Inhalation 0.5% and 0.083% ... 2118
- Proventil Syrup ... 2119
- Proventil Tablets ... 2120
- Ventolin ... 583

Alcohol (Additive effects; potentiates the sedative effects of chlorpheniramine).

Alprazolam (Additive effects). Products include:
- Xanax Tablets ... 2367

Buspirone Hydrochloride (Additive effects). Products include:
- BuSpar ... 1401

Chlordiazepoxide (Additive effects). Products include:
- Libritabs Tablets ... 1930
- Limbitrol ... 1933
- Menrium Tablets ... 1934

Chlordiazepoxide Hydrochloride (Additive effects). Products include:
- Librax Capsules ... 1929
- Librium Capsules ... 1931
- Librium Injectable ... 1932

Chlorpromazine (Additive effects). Products include:
- Thorazine ... 2234

Clorazepate Dipotassium (Additive effects). Products include:
- Tranxene ... 556

Cryptenamine Preparations (Reduced antihypertensive effect of cryptenamine).

Diazepam (Additive effects). Products include:
- Valium Injectable ... 1937
- Valium Tablets ... 1939
- Valrelease Capsules ... 1923

Dobutamine Hydrochloride (Potentially harmful combined effect on cardiovascular system). Products include:
- Dobutrex Solution Vials ... 1259

Dopamine Hydrochloride (Potentially harmful combined effect on cardiovascular system). Products include:
- Intropin Injection ... 930

Droperidol (Additive effects). Products include:
- Inapsine Injection ... 1140
- Innovar Injection ... 1141

Ephedrine Hydrochloride (Potentially harmful combined effect on cardiovascular system). Products include:
- Amesec ... ⊞ 682
- Primatene Tablets-M Formula ... 2421
- Primatene Tablets-P Formula ... 2421
- Primatene Tablets-Regular Formula ... 2421
- Quadrinal Tablets ... 1183
- Quelidrine Syrup ... 556
- Tedral SA ... 1765

Ephedrine Sulfate (Potentially harmful combined effect on cardiovascular system). Products include:
- Bronkaid Tablets ... ⊞ 757
- Bronkolixir ... ⊞ 761
- Bronkotabs Tablets ... ⊞ 762
- Marax Tablets & DF Syrup ... 1954
- Pazo Hemorrhoid Ointment & Suppositories ... 752
- Vicks Vatronol Nose Drops ... ⊞ 666

Ephedrine Tannate (Potentially harmful combined effect on cardiovascular system). Products include:
- Rynatuss ... 2388

Epinephrine (Potentially harmful combined effect on cardiovascular system). Products include:
- Ana-Kit Anaphylaxis Emergency Treatment Kit ... 1100
- Bronkaid Mist ... ⊞ 757
- EpiPen ... 843
- Marcaine Hydrochloride 0.5% with Epinephrine 1:200,000 (as bitartrate) ... 958
- Marcaine Hydrochloride with Epinephrine 1:200,000 ... 2055
- Primatene Mist ... 2420
- Sus-Phrine Injection ... 1006
- Xylocaine with Epinephrine Injections ... 637

Epinephrine Bitartrate (Potentially harmful combined effect on cardiovascular system). Products include:
- AsthmaHaler Mist Epinephrine Bitartrate Bronchodilator ... ⊞ 616
- Bronkaid Mist Suspension ... ⊞ 757
- Primatene Mist Suspension ... 2421

Epinephrine Hydrochloride (Potentially harmful combined effect on cardiovascular system). Products include:
- Adrenalin Chloride Solution 1:100 & 1:1,000 ... 1689
- Epifrin ... ⊙ 244
- Glaucon ... ⊙ 218

Estazolam (Additive effects). Products include:
- ProSom Tablets ... 554

Ethchlorvynol (Additive effects). Products include:
- Placidyl Capsules ... 553

Ethinamate (Additive effects).
- No products indexed under this heading.

Fluphenazine Decanoate (Additive effects). Products include:
- Prolixin Decanoate ... 1795

Fluphenazine Enanthate (Additive effects). Products include:
- Prolixin Enanthate ... 1796

Fluphenazine Hydrochloride (Additive effects). Products include:
- Prolixin Elixir ... 1793
- Prolixin Injection ... 1791
- Prolixin Oral Concentrate ... 1792
- Prolixin Tablets ... 1793

Flurazepam Hydrochloride (Additive effects). Products include:
- Dalmane Capsules ... 1927

Furazolidone (May precipitate hypertensive crisis; prolong and intensify anticholinergic effects of antihistamines; contraindication). Products include:
- Furoxone ... 1855

Glutethimide (Additive effects).
- No products indexed under this heading.

Haloperidol (Additive effects). Products include:
- Haldol Injection, Tablets and Concentrate ... 1373

Haloperidol Decanoate (Additive effects). Products include:
- Haldol Decanoate ... 1375

Hydroxyzine Hydrochloride (Additive effects). Products include:
- Atarax Tablets & Syrup ... 1941
- Marax Tablets & DF Syrup ... 1954
- Vistaril Intramuscular Solution ... 1970

Isocarboxazid (May precipitate hypertensive crisis; prolong and intensify anticholinergic effects of antihistamines; contraindication). Products include:
- Marplan Tablets ... 1906

Isoproterenol Hydrochloride (Potentially harmful combined effect on cardiovascular system). Products include:
- Isuprel Hydrochloride Injection 1:5000 ... 2050
- Isuprel Hydrochloride Mistometer ... 2051
- Isuprel Hydrochloride Solution 1:200 & 1:100 ... 2052
- Norisodrine Aerotrol ... 540

Lorazepam (Additive effects). Products include:
- Ativan Injection ... 2432
- Ativan Tablets ... 2434

Loxapine Hydrochloride (Additive effects). Products include:
- Loxitane ... 1213

Mecamylamine Hydrochloride (Reduced antihypertensive effect of mecamylamine). Products include:
- Inversine Tablets ... 1492

Meprobamate (Additive effects). Products include:
- Deprol Tablets ... 2382
- Equagesic Tablets ... 2451
- Miltown Tablets ... 2386
- PMB 200 and PMB 400 ... 2504

Mesoridazine (Additive effects). Products include:
- Serentil ... 686

Metaproterenol Sulfate (Potentially harmful combined effect on cardiovascular system). Products include:
- Alupent ... 674
- Arm-a-Med Metaproterenol Sulfate Inhalation Solution, USP ... 617
- Metaprel Inhalation Aerosol Bronchodilator ... 2014
- Metaprel Inhalation Solution ... 2015
- Metaprel ... 2015
- Metaproterenol Sulfate Inhalation Solution, USP ... 912

Metaraminol Bitartrate (Potentially harmful combined effect on cardiovascular system). Products include:
- Aramine Injection ... 1424

Methoxamine Hydrochloride (Potentially harmful combined effect on cardiovascular system). Products include:
- Vasoxyl Injection ... 819

Methyldopa (Reduced antihypertensive effect of methyldopa). Products include:
- Aldoclor Tablets ... 1413
- Aldomet Oral ... 1415
- Aldoril Tablets ... 1418

Methyldopate Hydrochloride (Reduced antihypertensive effect of methyldopate hydrochloride). Products include:
- Aldomet Ester HCl Injection ... 1417

Midazolam Hydrochloride (Additive effects). Products include:
- Versed Injection ... 1924

Molindone Hydrochloride (Additive effects). Products include:
- Moban Tablets & Concentrate ... 932

Norepinephrine Bitartrate (Potentially harmful combined effect on cardiovascular system). Products include:
- Levophed Bitartrate Injection ... 2054

Oxazepam (Additive effects). Products include:
- Serax Capsules ... 2522
- Serax Tablets ... 2522

Perphenazine (Additive effects). Products include:
- Etrafon ... 2087
- Triavil Tablets ... 1556
- Trilafon ... 2123

Phenelzine Sulfate (May precipitate hypertensive crisis; prolong and intensify anticholinergic effects of antihistamines; contraindication). Products include:

Nardil 1742

Phenylephrine Hydrochloride (Potentially harmful combined effect on cardiovascular system). Products include:

AK-Dilate Solution 2.5% and 10% ⊙ 203
Atrohist Sprinkle Capsules 558
Cerose-DM 2443
Codimal 846
Comhist LA Capsules 1618
Congespirin For Children Aspirin Free Chewable Cold Tablets 748
Cyclomydril ⊙ 216
Deconsal Sprinkle Capsules 559
Dimetane Decongestant ■ 673
Dristan Decongestant/Antihistamine/Analgesic Coated Caplets ■ 749
Dristan Cold Nasal Decongestant/Antihistamine/ Analgesic Coated Tablets 2419
Dristan Advanced Formula Decongestant/Antihistamine/ Analgesic Tablets ■ 749
Dristan Nasal Spray, Menthol 2419
Dristan Nasal Spray, Regular and Regular with Metered Pump 2419
Entex Capsules 1623
Entex Liquid 1623
Sinus Excedrin Analgesic, Decongestant Tablets & Caplets 750
Extendryl 994
4-Way Fast Acting Nasal Spray - Original Formula (regular & mentholated) & Metered Spray Pump (regular) 751
Hycomine Compound Tablets 929
Murocoll-2 Sterile Ophthalmic Solution ⊙ 261
Mydfrin 2.5% ⊙ 224
Naldecon Syrup, Tablets, Pediatric Drops and Pediatric Syrup 709
Neo-Synephrine Hydrochloride 1% Carpuject 2063
Neo-Synephrine Hydrochloride 1% Injection 2063
Neo-Synephrine Hydrochloride (Ophthalmic) 2064
Neo-Synephrine ■ 759
Nōstril Nasal Decongestant ■ 520
Novahistine Elixir ■ 596
Phenergan VC 2500
Phenergan VC with Codeine 2501
Prefrin Liquifilm Vasoconstrictor and Lubricant Eye Drops ⊙ 254
Prefrin-A ⊙ 255
Quelidrine Syrup 556
Relief Vasoconstrictor and Lubricant Eye Drops ⊙ 256
Robitussin Night Relief ■ 677
Ru-Tuss with Hydrocodone 694
Ru-Tuss Tablets 693
Vasosulf ⊙ 279
Vicks Sinex ■ 665
Zincfrin ⊙ 230

Phenylephrine Tannate (Potentially harmful combined effect on cardiovascular system). Products include:

Rynatan 2387
Rynatuss 2388

Phenylpropanolamine Hydrochloride (Potentially harmful combined effect on cardiovascular system). Products include:

A.R.M. Allergy Relief Medicine Caplets ■ 615
Acutrim ■ 548
Allerest ■ 559
BC Cold Powder ■ 517
Cheracol Plus Head Cold/Cough Formula ■ 667
Codimal Expectorant 846
Comtrex Multi-Symptom Cold Reliever Tablets/Caplets/Liqui-Gels/Liquid 745
Contac Continuous Action Decongestant/Antihistamine Capsules ■ 710
Contac Maximum Strength Continuous Action Decongestant/Antihistamine Caplets ■ 709
Contac Severe Cold and Flu Formula Caplets ■ 711
Coricidin 'D' Decongestant Tablets ■ 695
Coricidin Demilets Tablets for Children ■ 696
Demazin Nasal Decongestant/Antihistamine Repetabs Tablets & Syrup ■ 697
Dexatrim ■ 733
Dimetane-DC Cough Syrup 1857
Dimetapp Elixir ■ 673
Dimetapp DM Elixir ■ 674
Dimetapp Extentabs ■ 674
Dimetapp Plus Caplets ■ 675
Dimetapp Tablets ■ 675
Entex Capsules 1623
Entex LA Tablets 1623
Entex Liquid 1623
4-Way Cold Tablets 750
Hycomine Syrup 927
Naldecon CX Adult Liquid ■ 521
Naldecon DX Adult Liquid ■ 521
Naldecon DX Children's Syrup ■ 522
Naldecon DX Pediatric Drops ■ 522
Naldecon EX Children's Syrup ■ 522
Naldecon EX Pediatric Drops ■ 523
Naldecon Syrup, Tablets, Pediatric Drops and Pediatric Syrup 709
Nolamine Tablets 838
Nolex LA Tablets 838
Ornade Spansule Capsules 2221
Orthoxicol Cough Syrup ■ 668
Propagest 839
Pyrroxate Capsules ■ 669
Robitussin-CF ■ 676
Ru-Tuss II Capsules 693
Ru-Tuss with Hydrocodone 694
Ru-Tuss Tablets 693
Sine-Off Sinus Medicine Tablets-Aspirin Formula ■ 722
Sinulin 840
St. Joseph Cold Tablets for Children ■ 704
Tavist-D Tablets 2035
Triaminic Allergy Tablets ■ 688
Triaminic Chewables ■ 688
Triaminic Cold Tablets ■ 688
Triaminic Expectorant ■ 688
Triaminic Expectorant w/Codeine 1996
Triaminic Expectorant DH 1995
Triaminic Oral Infant Drops 1996
Triaminic Syrup ■ 689
Triaminic-12 Tablets ■ 690
Triaminic-DM Syrup ■ 689
Triaminicin Tablets ■ 690
Triaminicol Multi-Symptom Cold Tablets ■ 691
Triaminicol Multi-Symptom Relief ■ 691
Tuss-Ornade Liquid 2242
Tuss-Ornade Spansule Capsules 2242
Tylenol Cold Medication, Effervescent Tablets 1369

Pirbuterol Acetate (Potentially harmful combined effect on cardiovascular system). Products include:

Maxair Inhaler 1311

Prazepam (Additive effects). Products include:

Centrax 1693

Prochlorperazine (Additive effects). Products include:

Compazine 2201

Promethazine Hydrochloride (Additive effects). Products include:

Mepergan Injection 2479
Phenergan with Codeine 2497
Phenergan with Dextromethorphan 2499
Phenergan Injection 2493
Phenergan Suppositories 2496
Phenergan Syrup 2495
Phenergan Tablets 2496
Phenergan VC 2500
Phenergan VC with Codeine 2501

Propofol (Additive effects). Products include:

Diprivan Injection 2267

Pseudoephedrine Sulfate (Potentially harmful combined effect on cardiovascular system). Products include:

Afrin Tablets ■ 693
Chlor-Trimeton Decongestant ■ 694
Disophrol Chronotab Sustained-Action Tablets ■ 698
Drixoral Antihistamine/Nasal Decongestant Syrup ■ 698
Drixoral Non-Drowsy Formula ■ 699
Drixoral Plus Extended-Release Tablets ■ 699
Drixoral Sinus ■ 700
Drixoral Sustained-Action Tablets ■ 698
Sinutab Allergy Formula Sustained Action Tablets ■ 640
Trinalin Repetabs Tablets 1170

Quazepam (Additive effects). Products include:

Doral Tablets 2383

Reserpine (Reduced antihypertensive effect of reserpine). Products include:

Diupres Tablets 1461
Hydromox R Tablets 1209
Hydropres Tablets 1485
Renese-R Tablets 1786
Salutensin/Salutensin-Demi 719
Ser-Ap-Es Tablets 881
Serpasil Tablets 883
Serpasil-Apresoline Tablets 884
Serpasil-Esidrix Tablets 886

Secobarbital Sodium (Additive effects). Products include:

Seconal Sodium Pulvules 1296

Selegiline Hydrochloride (May precipitate hypertensive crisis; prolong and intensify anticholinergic effects of antihistamines; contraindication). Products include:

Eldepryl 2250

Temazepam (Additive effects). Products include:

Restoril Capsules 2023

Terbutaline Sulfate (Potentially harmful combined effect on cardiovascular system). Products include:

Brethaire Inhaler 1024
Brethine Ampuls 1026
Brethine Tablets 1026
Bricanyl Injection 1324
Bricanyl Tablets 1325

Thioridazine Hydrochloride (Additive effects). Products include:

Mellaril 2011

Tranylcypromine Sulfate (May precipitate hypertensive crisis; prolong and intensify anticholinergic effects of antihistamines; contraindication). Products include:

Parnate Tablets 2222

Triazolam (Additive effects). Products include:

Halcion Tablets 2340

Trifluoperazine Hydrochloride (Additive effects). Products include:

Stelazine 2226

DECONAMINE SYRUP

(Chlorpheniramine Maleate, Pseudoephedrine Hydrochloride) 663
See **Deconamine SR Capsules**

DECONAMINE TABLETS

(Chlorpheniramine Maleate, Pseudoephedrine Hydrochloride) 663
See **Deconamine SR Capsules**

DECONSAL SPRINKLE CAPSULES

(Guaifenesin, Phenylephrine Hydrochloride) 559
See **Deconsal II Tablets**

DECONSAL II TABLETS

(Pseudoephedrine Hydrochloride, Guaifenesin) 559

May interact with monoamine oxidase inhibitors, beta blockers, cardiac glycosides, veratrum alkaloids, tricyclic antidepressants, catecholamine depleting drugs, and certain other agents. Compounds in these categories include:

Acebutolol Hydrochloride (Potentiates the pressor effect of sympathomimetic amines). Products include:

Sectral Capsules 2520

Amitriptyline Hydrochloride (Antagonizes the effects of sympathomimetic amines). Products include:

Elavil 2269
Endep Tablets 1927
Etrafon 2087
Limbitrol 1933
Triavil Tablets 1556

Amoxapine (Antagonizes the effects of sympathomimetic amines). Products include:

Asendin Tablets 1196

Atenolol (Potentiates the pressor effect of sympathomimetic amines). Products include:

Tenoretic Tablets 1105
Tenormin Tablets and I.V. Injection 1107

Betaxolol Hydrochloride (Potentiates the pressor effect of sympathomimetic amines). Products include:

Betoptic Sterile Ophthalmic Solution 569
Betoptic S Sterile Ophthalmic Suspension 570
Kerlone Tablets 2172

Carteolol Hydrochloride (Potentiates the pressor effect of sympathomimetic amines). Products include:

Cartrol Tablets 507

Clomipramine Hydrochloride (Antagonizes the effects of sympathomimetic amines). Products include:

Anafranil Capsules 650

Cryptenamine Preparations (Reduced hypotensive effect).

Deserpidine (Reduced hypotensive effect). Products include:

Enduronyl 518
Harmonyl Tablets 528
Oreticyl 545

Desipramine Hydrochloride (Antagonizes the effects of sympathomimetic amines). Products include:

Norpramin Tablets 1340

Deslanoside (Increased possibility of cardiac arrhythmias).

No products indexed under this heading.

Digitoxin (Increased possibility of cardiac arrhythmias). Products include:

Crystodigin Tablets 1253

Digoxin (Increased possibility of cardiac arrhythmias). Products include:

Lanoxicaps 772
Lanoxin Elixir Pediatric 775
Lanoxin Injection 778
Lanoxin Injection Pediatric 781
Lanoxin Tablets 783

Doxepin Hydrochloride (Antagonizes the effects of sympathomimetic amines). Products include:

Sinequan 1960

Esmolol Hydrochloride (Potentiates the pressor effect of sympathomimetic amines). Products include:

Brevibloc Injection 942

Furazolidone (Potentiates the pressor effect of sympathomimetic amines; concurrent use is contraindicated). Products include:

Furoxone 1855

Guanethidine Monosulfate (Reduced hypotensive effect). Products include:

Esimil Tablets 864
Ismelin Tablets 869

Imipramine Hydrochloride (Antagonizes the effects of sympathomimetic amines). Products include:

Tofranil Ampuls 1038
Tofranil Tablets 1039

(■ Described in PDR For Nonprescription Drugs)   (⊙ Described in PDR For Ophthalmology)

Imipramine Pamoate (Antagonizes the effects of sympathomimetic amines). Products include:
- Tofranil-PM Capsules ... 1041

Isocarboxazid (Potentiates the pressor effect of sympathomimetic amines; concurrent use is contraindicated). Products include:
- Marplan Tablets ... 1906

Labetalol Hydrochloride (Potentiates the pressor effect of sympathomimetic amines). Products include:
- Normodyne Injection ... 2108
- Normodyne Tablets ... 2110
- Normozide Tablets ... 2112
- Trandate HCT Tablets ... 579
- Trandate Injection ... 577
- Trandate Tablets ... 579

Maprotiline Hydrochloride (Antagonizes the effects of sympathomimetic amines). Products include:
- Ludiomil Tablets ... 874

Mecamylamine Hydrochloride (Reduced hypotensive effect). Products include:
- Inversine Tablets ... 1492

Methyldopa (Reduced hypotensive effect). Products include:
- Aldoclor Tablets ... 1413
- Aldomet Oral ... 1415
- Aldoril Tablets ... 1418

Methyldopate Hydrochloride (Reduced hypotensive effect). Products include:
- Aldomet Ester HCl Injection ... 1417

Metoprolol Tartrate (Potentiates the pressor effect of sympathomimetic amines). Products include:
- Lopressor Ampuls ... 1032
- Lopressor HCT Tablets ... 1034
- Lopressor Tablets ... 1032

Nadolol (Potentiates the pressor effect of sympathomimetic amines). Products include:
- Corgard Tablets ... 701
- Corzide Tablets ... 702

Nortriptyline Hydrochloride (Antagonizes the effects of sympathomimetic amines). Products include:
- Pamelor ... 2019

Penbutolol Sulfate (Potentiates the pressor effect of sympathomimetic amines). Products include:
- Levatol ... 1832

Phenelzine Sulfate (Potentiates the pressor effect of sympathomimetic amines; concurrent use is contraindicated). Products include:
- Nardil ... 1742

Pindolol (Potentiates the pressor effect of sympathomimetic amines). Products include:
- Visken Tablets ... 2036

Propranolol Hydrochloride (Potentiates the pressor effect of sympathomimetic amines). Products include:
- Inderal ... 2459
- Inderal LA Long Acting Capsules ... 2461
- Inderide Tablets ... 2463
- Inderide LA Long Acting Capsules ... 2465

Protriptyline Hydrochloride (Antagonizes the effects of sympathomimetic amines). Products include:
- Vivactil Tablets ... 1567

Rauwolfia Serpentina (Reduced hypotensive effect). Products include:
- Raudixin Tablets ... 1803
- Rauzide Tablets ... 1804

Rescinnamine (Reduced hypotensive effect).
No products indexed under this heading.

Reserpine (Reduced hypotensive effect). Products include:
- Diupres Tablets ... 1461
- Hydromox R Tablets ... 1209
- Hydropres Tablets ... 1485
- Renese-R Tablets ... 1786
- Salutensin/Salutensin-Demi ... 719
- Ser-Ap-Es Tablets ... 881
- Serpasil Tablets ... 883
- Serpasil-Apresoline Tablets ... 884
- Serpasil-Esidrix Tablets ... 886

Selegiline Hydrochloride (Potentiates the pressor effect of sympathomimetic amines; concurrent use is contraindicated). Products include:
- Eldepryl ... 2250

Timolol Maleate (Potentiates the pressor effect of sympathomimetic amines). Products include:
- Blocadren Tablets ... 1429
- Timolide Tablets ... 1547
- Timoptic in Ocudose ... 1552
- Timoptic Sterile Ophthalmic Solution ... 1550

Tranylcypromine Sulfate (Potentiates the pressor effect of sympathomimetic amines; concurrent use is contraindicated). Products include:
- Parnate Tablets ... 2222

Trimipramine Maleate (Antagonizes the effects of sympathomimetic amines). Products include:
- Surmontil Capsules ... 2524

DELFEN CONTRACEPTIVE FOAM
(Nonoxynol-9) ... ▣ 631
No interactions described in labeling.

DELSYM COUGH FORMULA
(Dextromethorphan Polistirex) ... ▣ 560
No interactions described in labeling.

DELTASONE TABLETS
(Prednisone) ... 2332
May interact with:

Aspirin (Use cautiously in hypoprothrombinemia). Products include:
- Alka-Seltzer Effervescent Antacid and Pain Reliever ... 1568
- Alka-Seltzer Extra Strength Effervescent Antacid and Pain Reliever ... 1570
- Alka-Seltzer (Flavored) Effervescent Antacid and Pain Reliever ... 1569
- Alka-Seltzer Plus Cold Medicine ... ▣ 623
- Alka-Seltzer Plus Night-Time Cold Medicine ... ▣ 623
- Alka Seltzer Plus Sinus Allergy Medicine ... ▣ 624
- Anacin Coated Analgesic Caplets ... 2417
- Anacin Coated Analgesic Tablets ... 2417
- Anacin Maximum Strength Analgesic Coated Tablets ... 2417
- Maximum Strength Arthritis Pain Formula By the Makers of Anacin Analgesic Tablets and Caplets ... 2418
- Arthritis Pain Formula by the Makers of Anacin Analgesic Tablets and Caplets ... ▣ 747
- Arthritis Strength BC Powder ... ▣ 516
- Ascriptin A/D Caplets ... 1850
- Regular Strength Ascriptin Tablets ... 1850
- Azdone Tablets ... 844
- BC Powder ... ▣ 517
- BC Cold Powder ... ▣ 517
- Children's Bayer Chewable Aspirin ... ▣ 564
- Genuine Bayer Aspirin Tablets & Caplets ... ▣ 564
- Maximum Bayer Aspirin Tablets & Caplets ... ▣ 566
- Bayer Plus Aspirin Tablets ... ▣ 567
- Therapy Bayer Aspirin Caplets ... ▣ 568
- 8 Hour Bayer Timed-Release Aspirin ... ▣ 566
- Arthritis Strength Bufferin Analgesic Caplets ... 744
- Extra Strength Bufferin Analgesic Tablets ... 745
- Bufferin Analgesic Tablets and Caplets ... 743
- Cama Arthritis Pain Reliever ... ▣ 685
- Damason-P ... 1356
- Easprin ... 1719
- Ecotrin Enteric Coated Aspirin Maximum Strength Tablets and Caplets ... 2189
- Ecotrin Enteric Coated Aspirin Regular Strength Tablets and Caplets ... 2189
- Empirin Aspirin ... ▣ 541
- Empirin with Codeine Phosphate Nos. 2, 3 & 4 ... 764
- Equagesic Tablets ... 2451
- Excedrin Extra-Strength Analgesic Tablets & Caplets ... 749
- 4-Way Cold Tablets ... 750
- Fiorinal Capsules ... 2007
- Fiorinal with Codeine Capsules ... 2008
- Fiorinal Tablets ... 2007
- Lortab ASA Tablets ... 2414
- Momentum Muscular Backache Formula ... ▣ 751
- Norgesic ... 1314
- Norwich Extra-Strength Aspirin ... ▣ 546
- Norwich Regular Strength Aspirin ... ▣ 547
- P-A-C Analgesic Tablets ... ▣ 669
- Percodan ... 951
- Robaxisal Tablets ... 1872
- Sine-Off Sinus Medicine Tablets-Aspirin Formula ... ▣ 722
- Soma Compound w/Codeine Tablets ... 2390
- Soma Compound Tablets ... 2389
- St. Joseph Adult Chewable Aspirin (81 mg.) ... ▣ 703
- Synalgos-DC Capsules ... 2525
- Talwin Compound ... 2072
- Ursinus Inlay-Tabs ... ▣ 691
- Vanquish Analgesic Caplets ... ▣ 574
- Zorprin Tablets ... 698

Cyclosporine (Potential for convulsions). Products include:
- Sandimmune ... 2024

Immunization (Neurological complications, lack of antibody response).

Smallpox Vaccine (Neurological complications, lack of antibody response).

DEMAZIN NASAL DECONGESTANT/ ANTIHISTAMINE REPETABS TABLETS & SYRUP
(Chlorpheniramine Maleate, Phenylpropanolamine Hydrochloride) ... ▣ 697
May interact with phenylpropanolamine containing anorectics, antihypertensives, antidepressant drugs, and certain other agents. Compounds in these categories include:

Acebutolol Hydrochloride (Effect not specified). Products include:
- Sectral Capsules ... 2520

Alcohol (Increases drowsiness effect).

Amitriptyline Hydrochloride (Effect not specified). Products include:
- Elavil ... 2269
- Endep Tablets ... 1927
- Etrafon ... 2087
- Limbitrol ... 1933
- Triavil Tablets ... 1556

Amoxapine (Effect not specified). Products include:
- Asendin Tablets ... 1196

Atenolol (Effect not specified). Products include:
- Tenoretic Tablets ... 1105
- Tenormin Tablets and I.V. Injection ... 1107

Benazepril Hydrochloride (Effect not specified). Products include:
- Lotensin Tablets ... 872

Bendroflumethiazide (Effect not specified). Products include:
- Corzide Tablets ... 702
- Naturetin Tablets ... 1789
- Rauzide Tablets ... 1804

Betaxolol Hydrochloride (Effect not specified). Products include:
- Betoptic Sterile Ophthalmic Solution ... 569
- Betoptic S Sterile Ophthalmic Suspension ... 570
- Kerlone Tablets ... 2172

Bupropion Hydrochloride (Effect not specified). Products include:
- Wellbutrin Tablets ... 821

Captopril (Effect not specified). Products include:
- Capoten ... 2255
- Capozide ... 2258

Carteolol Hydrochloride (Effect not specified). Products include:
- Cartrol Tablets ... 507

Chlorothiazide (Effect not specified). Products include:
- Aldoclor Tablets ... 1413
- Diupres Tablets ... 1461
- Diuril Oral ... 1464

Chlorothiazide Sodium (Effect not specified). Products include:
- Diuril Sodium Intravenous ... 1463

Chlorthalidone (Effect not specified). Products include:
- Combipres Tablets ... 678
- Tenoretic Tablets ... 1105
- Thalitone Tablets ... 687

Clonidine (Effect not specified). Products include:
- Catapres-TTS ... 677

Clonidine Hydrochloride (Effect not specified). Products include:
- Catapres Tablets ... 676
- Combipres Tablets ... 678

Deserpidine (Effect not specified). Products include:
- Enduronyl ... 518
- Harmonyl Tablets ... 528
- Oreticyl ... 545

Desipramine Hydrochloride (Effect not specified). Products include:
- Norpramin Tablets ... 1340

Diazoxide (Effect not specified). Products include:
- Hyperstat I.V. Injection ... 2095
- Proglycem ... 649

Doxazosin Mesylate (Effect not specified). Products include:
- Cardura Tablets ... 1941

Doxepin Hydrochloride (Effect not specified). Products include:
- Sinequan ... 1960

Enalapril Maleate (Effect not specified). Products include:
- Vaseretic Tablets ... 1559
- Vasotec Tablets ... 1564

Enalaprilat (Effect not specified). Products include:
- Vasotec I.V. ... 1562

Esmolol Hydrochloride (Effect not specified). Products include:
- Brevibloc Injection ... 942

Felodipine (Effect not specified). Products include:
- Plendil Extended-Release Tablets ... 1526

Fluoxetine Hydrochloride (Effect not specified). Products include:
- Prozac Pulvules ... 920

Fosinopril Sodium (Effect not specified). Products include:
- Monopril Tablets ... 1406

Furosemide (Effect not specified). Products include:
- Lasix ... 1093

Guanabenz Acetate (Effect not specified). Products include:
- Wytensin Tablets ... 2542

Guanethidine Monosulfate (Effect not specified). Products include:
- Esimil Tablets ... 864
- Ismelin Tablets ... 869

Hydralazine Hydrochloride (Effect not specified). Products include:
Apresazide Capsules 854
Apresoline Hydrochloride Parenteral (Ampuls) 856
Apresoline Hydrochloride Tablets 855
Apresoline-Esidrix Tablets 857
Ser-Ap-Es Tablets 881
Serpasil-Apresoline Tablets 884

Hydrochlorothiazide (Effect not specified). Products include:
Aldactazide 2150
Aldoril Tablets 1418
Apresazide Capsules 854
Apresoline-Esidrix Tablets 857
Capozide 2258
Dyazide Capsules 2208
Esidrix Tablets 863
Esimil Tablets 864
HydroDIURIL Tablets 1484
Hydropres Tablets 1485
Inderide Tablets 2463
Inderide LA Long Acting Capsules 2465
Lopressor HCT Tablets 1034
Maxzide 1215
Moduretic Tablets 1510
Normozide Tablets 2112
Oretic Tablets 544
Oreticyl 545
Prinzide Tablets 1540
Ser-Ap-Es Tablets 881
Serpasil-Esidrix Tablets 886
Timolide Tablets 1547
Trandate HCT Tablets 579
Vaseretic Tablets 1559
Zestoretic 2274

Hydroflumethiazide (Effect not specified). Products include:
Diucardin Tablets 2450
Saluron 718
Salutensin/Salutensin-Demi 719

Imipramine Hydrochloride (Effect not specified). Products include:
Tofranil Ampuls 1038
Tofranil Tablets 1039

Imipramine Pamoate (Effect not specified). Products include:
Tofranil-PM Capsules 1041

Indapamide (Effect not specified). Products include:
Lozol Tablets 1843

Isocarboxazid (Effect not specified). Products include:
Marplan Tablets 1906

Isradipine (Effect not specified). Products include:
DynaCirc Capsules 2004

Labetalol Hydrochloride (Effect not specified). Products include:
Normodyne Injection 2108
Normodyne Tablets 2110
Normozide Tablets 2112
Trandate HCT Tablets 579
Trandate Injection 577
Trandate Tablets 579

Lisinopril (Effect not specified). Products include:
Prinivil Tablets 1538
Prinzide Tablets 1540
Zestoretic 2274
Zestril Tablets 2277

Maprotiline Hydrochloride (Effect not specified). Products include:
Ludiomil Tablets 874

Mecamylamine Hydrochloride (Effect not specified). Products include:
Inversine Tablets 1492

Methyclothiazide (Effect not specified). Products include:
Enduron Tablets 517
Enduronyl 518

Methyldopa (Effect not specified). Products include:
Aldoclor Tablets 1413
Aldomet Oral 1415
Aldoril Tablets 1418

Methyldopate Hydrochloride (Effect not specified). Products include:
Aldomet Ester HCl Injection 1417

Metolazone (Effect not specified). Products include:
Diulo 2129
Mykrox ½ mg Tablets 984
Zaroxolyn Tablets 989

Metoprolol Tartrate (Effect not specified). Products include:
Lopressor Ampuls 1032
Lopressor HCT Tablets 1034
Lopressor Tablets 1032

Metyrosine (Effect not specified). Products include:
Demser Capsules 1460

Minoxidil (Effect not specified). Products include:
Loniten Tablets 2346
Rogaine Topical Solution 2357

Nadolol (Effect not specified). Products include:
Corgard Tablets 701
Corzide Tablets 702

Nicardipine Hydrochloride (Effect not specified). Products include:
Cardene Capsules 2290

Nitroglycerin (Effect not specified). Products include:
Deponit NTG Transdermal Delivery System 2143
Minitran Transdermal Delivery System 1312
Nitro-Bid Ointment 1339
Nitro-Bid Capsules 1338
Nitrodisc 2176
Nitro-Dur (nitroglycerin) Transdermal Infusion System 1164
Nitrogard Tablets 1004
Nitrolingual Spray 1846
Nitrostat Tablets 1743
Transderm-Nitro Transdermal Therapeutic System 2283

Nortriptyline Hydrochloride (Effect not specified). Products include:
Pamelor 2019

Penbutolol Sulfate (Effect not specified). Products include:
Levatol 1832

Phenelzine Sulfate (Effect not specified). Products include:
Nardil 1742

Phenoxybenzamine Hydrochloride (Effect not specified). Products include:
Dibenzyline Capsules 2207

Phentolamine Mesylate (Effect not specified). Products include:
Regitine 878

Phenylpropanolamine Containing Anorectics (Effect not specified).

Pindolol (Effect not specified). Products include:
Visken Tablets 2036

Polythiazide (Effect not specified). Products include:
Minizide Capsules 1779
Renese Tablets 1785
Renese-R Tablets 1786

Prazosin Hydrochloride (Effect not specified). Products include:
Minipress Capsules 1778
Minizide Capsules 1779

Propranolol Hydrochloride (Effect not specified). Products include:
Inderal 2459
Inderal LA Long Acting Capsules 2461
Inderide Tablets 2463
Inderide LA Long Acting Capsules 2465

Protriptyline Hydrochloride (Effect not specified). Products include:
Vivactil Tablets 1567

Ramipril (Effect not specified). Products include:
Altace Capsules 1086

Rauwolfia Serpentina (Effect not specified). Products include:
Raudixin Tablets 1803
Rauzide Tablets 1804

Rescinnamine (Effect not specified).
No products indexed under this heading.

Reserpine (Effect not specified). Products include:
Diupres Tablets 1461
Hydromox R Tablets 1209
Hydropres Tablets 1485
Renese-R Tablets 1786
Salutensin/Salutensin-Demi 719
Ser-Ap-Es Tablets 881
Serpasil Tablets 883
Serpasil-Apresoline Tablets 884
Serpasil-Esidrix Tablets 886

Sodium Nitroprusside (Effect not specified). Products include:
Nipride I.V. Infusion 1909

Terazosin Hydrochloride (Effect not specified). Products include:
Hytrin Tablets 529

Timolol Maleate (Effect not specified). Products include:
Blocadren Tablets 1429
Timolide Tablets 1547
Timoptic in Ocudose 1552
Timoptic Sterile Ophthalmic Solution 1550

Tranylcypromine Sulfate (Effect not specified). Products include:
Parnate Tablets 2222

Trazodone Hydrochloride (Effect not specified). Products include:
Desyrel and Desyrel Dividose 1404

Trimethaphan Camsylate (Effect not specified). Products include:
Arfonad Ampuls 1887

Trimipramine Maleate (Effect not specified). Products include:
Surmontil Capsules 2524

DEMEROL HYDROCHLORIDE CARPUJECT

(Meperidine Hydrochloride) 2047
May interact with narcotic analgesics, general anesthetics, phenothiazines, tranquilizers, hypnotics and sedatives, tricyclic antidepressants, central nervous system depressants, monoamine oxidase inhibitors, and certain other agents. Compounds in these categories include:

Alcohol (Respiratory depression, hypotension, profound sedation or coma).

Alfentanil Hydrochloride (Respiratory depression, hypotension, profound sedation or coma). Products include:
Alfenta Injection 1131

Alprazolam (Respiratory depression, hypotension, profound sedation or coma). Products include:
Xanax Tablets 2367

Amitriptyline Hydrochloride (Respiratory depression, hypotension, profound sedation or coma). Products include:
Elavil 2269
Endep Tablets 1927
Etrafon 2087
Limbitrol 1933
Triavil Tablets 1556

Amoxapine (Respiratory depression, hypotension, profound sedation or coma). Products include:
Asendin Tablets 1196

Aprobarbital (Respiratory depression, hypotension, profound sedation or coma). Products include:
Alurate Elixir 1883

Buprenorphine (Respiratory depression, hypotension, profound sedation or coma).
No products indexed under this heading.

Buspirone Hydrochloride (Respiratory depression, hypotension, profound sedation or coma). Products include:
BuSpar 1401

Butabarbital (Respiratory depression, hypotension, profound sedation or coma). Products include:
Pyridium Plus 1764

Butalbital (Respiratory depression, hypotension, profound sedation or coma). Products include:
Esgic-Plus Tablets 1002
Esgic Tablets & Capsules 1001
Fioricet Tablets 2006
Fiorinal Capsules 2007
Fiorinal with Codeine Capsules 2008
Fiorinal Tablets 2007
Phrenilin 838
Sedapap Tablets 50 mg/650 mg 1360

Chlordiazepoxide (Respiratory depression, hypotension, profound sedation or coma). Products include:
Libritabs Tablets 1930
Limbitrol 1933
Menrium Tablets 1934

Chlordiazepoxide Hydrochloride (Respiratory depression, hypotension, profound sedation or coma). Products include:
Librax Capsules 1929
Librium Capsules 1931
Librium Injectable 1932

Chlorpromazine (Respiratory depression, hypotension, profound sedation or coma). Products include:
Thorazine 2234

Chlorprothixene (Respiratory depression, hypotension, profound sedation or coma). Products include:
Taractan Tablets 1920

Chlorprothixene Hydrochloride (Respiratory depression, hypotension, profound sedation or coma). Products include:
Taractan 1920

Clomipramine Hydrochloride (Respiratory depression, hypotension, profound sedation or coma). Products include:
Anafranil Capsules 650

Clorazepate Dipotassium (Respiratory depression, hypotension, profound sedation or coma). Products include:
Tranxene 556

Codeine (Respiratory depression, hypotension, profound sedation or coma). Products include:
Calcidrine Syrup 506

Codeine Phosphate (Respiratory depression, hypotension, profound sedation or coma). Products include:
Actifed with Codeine Cough Syrup 752
Cheracol Cough Syrup 1853
Codimal PH Syrup 846
Dimetane-DC Cough Syrup 1857
Empirin with Codeine Phosphate Nos. 2, 3 & 4 764
Fiorinal with Codeine Capsules 2008
Isoclor Expectorant 982
Naldecon CX Adult Liquid ▣ 521
Novahistine DH 1342
Novahistine Expectorant 1343
Nucofed Capsules 2219
Nucofed Expectorant 2219
Nucofed Pediatric Expectorant 2220
Nucofed Syrup 2219
Phenaphen with Codeine Capsules 1865
Phenaphen-650 with Codeine Tablets 1866
Phenergan with Codeine 2497
Phenergan VC with Codeine 2501
Robitussin A-C Syrup 1875
Robitussin-DAC Syrup 1875
Ryna ▣ 741
Soma Compound w/Codeine Tablets 2390
Triaminic Expectorant w/Codeine 1996
Tussi-Organidin Liquid 2391
Tylenol with Codeine 1381

Codeine Polistirex (Respiratory depression, hypotension, profound sedation or coma).
No products indexed under this heading.

Desipramine Hydrochloride (Respiratory depression, hypotension, profound sedation or coma). Products include:
Norpramin Tablets ... 1340

Dezocine (Respiratory depression, hypotension, profound sedation or coma).

Diazepam (Respiratory depression, hypotension, profound sedation or coma). Products include:
Valium Injectable ... 1937
Valium Tablets ... 1939
Valrelease Capsules ... 1923

Doxepin Hydrochloride (Respiratory depression, hypotension, profound sedation or coma). Products include:
Sinequan ... 1960

Droperidol (Respiratory depression, hypotension, profound sedation or coma). Products include:
Inapsine Injection ... 1140
Innovar Injection ... 1141

Enflurane (Respiratory depression, hypotension, profound sedation or coma). Products include:
Ethrane ... 599

Estazolam (Respiratory depression, hypotension, profound sedation or coma). Products include:
ProSom Tablets ... 554

Ethchlorvynol (Respiratory depression, hypotension, profound sedation or coma). Products include:
Placidyl Capsules ... 553

Ethinamate (Respiratory depression, hypotension, profound sedation or coma).
No products indexed under this heading.

Fentanyl (Respiratory depression, hypotension, profound sedation or coma). Products include:
Duragesic Transdermal System ... 1133

Fentanyl Citrate (Respiratory depression, hypotension, profound sedation or coma). Products include:
Innovar Injection ... 1141
Sublimaze Injection ... 1146

Fluphenazine Decanoate (Respiratory depression, hypotension, profound sedation or coma). Products include:
Prolixin Decanoate ... 1795

Fluphenazine Enanthate (Respiratory depression, hypotension, profound sedation or coma). Products include:
Prolixin Enanthate ... 1796

Fluphenazine Hydrochloride (Respiratory depression, hypotension, profound sedation or coma). Products include:
Prolixin Elixir ... 1793
Prolixin Injection ... 1791
Prolixin Oral Concentrate ... 1792
Prolixin Tablets ... 1793

Flurazepam Hydrochloride (Respiratory depression, hypotension, profound sedation or coma). Products include:
Dalmane Capsules ... 1927

Furazolidone (Contraindicated: unpredictable, severe, and occasionally fatal reactions when given within 14 days). Products include:
Furoxone ... 1855

Glutethimide (Respiratory depression, hypotension, profound sedation or coma).
No products indexed under this heading.

Haloperidol (Respiratory depression, hypotension, profound sedation or coma). Products include:
Haldol Injection, Tablets and Concentrate ... 1373

Haloperidol Decanoate (Respiratory depression, hypotension, profound sedation or coma). Products include:
Haldol Decanoate ... 1375

Hydrocodone Bitartrate (Respiratory depression, hypotension, profound sedation or coma). Products include:
Anexsia 5/500 Tablets ... 2196
Anexsia 7.5/650 Tablets ... 2197
Azdone Tablets ... 844
Codiclear DH Syrup ... 845
Codimal DH Syrup ... 846
Damason-P ... 1356
Hycodan Syrup, Tablets ... 927
Hycomine Compound Tablets ... 929
Hycomine Syrup ... 927
Hycotuss Expectorant Syrup ... 930
Hydrocet Capsules ... 835
Lortab ASA Tablets ... 2414
Lortab ... 2412
Ru-Tuss with Hydrocodone ... 694
Triaminic Expectorant DH ... 1995
Vicodin Tablets ... 1187
Vicodin ES Tablets ... 1189
Zydone Capsules ... 941

Hydrocodone Polistirex (Respiratory depression, hypotension, profound sedation or coma). Products include:
Tussionex Extended-Release Suspension ... 988

Hydroxyzine Hydrochloride (Respiratory depression, hypotension, profound sedation or coma). Products include:
Atarax Tablets & Syrup ... 1941
Marax Tablets & DF Syrup ... 1954
Vistaril Intramuscular Solution ... 1970

Imipramine Hydrochloride (Respiratory depression, hypotension, profound sedation or coma). Products include:
Tofranil Ampuls ... 1038
Tofranil Tablets ... 1039

Imipramine Pamoate (Respiratory depression, hypotension, profound sedation or coma). Products include:
Tofranil-PM Capsules ... 1041

Isocarboxazid (Contraindicated: unpredictable, severe, and occasionally fatal reactions when given within 14 days). Products include:
Marplan Tablets ... 1906

Isoflurane (Respiratory depression, hypotension, profound sedation or coma). Products include:
Forane ... 600

Ketamine Hydrochloride (Respiratory depression, hypotension, profound sedation or coma). Products include:
Ketalar ... 1726

Levorphanol Tartrate (Respiratory depression, hypotension, profound sedation or coma). Products include:
Levo-Dromoran ... 1906

Lorazepam (Respiratory depression, hypotension, profound sedation or coma). Products include:
Ativan Injection ... 2432
Ativan Tablets ... 2434

Loxapine Hydrochloride (Respiratory depression, hypotension, profound sedation or coma). Products include:
Loxitane ... 1213

Loxapine Succinate (Respiratory depression, hypotension, profound sedation or coma). Products include:
Loxitane Capsules ... 1213

Maprotiline Hydrochloride (Respiratory depression, hypotension, profound sedation or coma). Products include:
Ludiomil Tablets ... 874

Mephobarbital (Respiratory depression, hypotension, profound sedation or coma). Products include:
Mebaral Tablets ... 2061

Meprobamate (Respiratory depression, hypotension, profound sedation or coma). Products include:
Deprol Tablets ... 2382
Equagesic Tablets ... 2451
Miltown Tablets ... 2386
PMB 200 and PMB 400 ... 2504

Mesoridazine (Respiratory depression, hypotension, profound sedation or coma). Products include:
Serentil ... 686

Methadone Hydrochloride (Respiratory depression, hypotension, profound sedation or coma). Products include:
Dolophine Hydrochloride Ampoules & Vials ... 1260
Dolophine Hydrochloride Tablets ... 1261
Methadone Hydrochloride Diskets ... 1284
Methadone Hydrochloride Oral Solution & Tablets ... 1987

Methohexital Sodium (Respiratory depression, hypotension, profound sedation or coma). Products include:
Brevital Sodium Vials ... 1248

Methoxyflurane (Respiratory depression, hypotension, profound sedation or coma).
No products indexed under this heading.

Midazolam Hydrochloride (Respiratory depression, hypotension, profound sedation or coma). Products include:
Versed Injection ... 1924

Molindone Hydrochloride (Respiratory depression, hypotension, profound sedation or coma). Products include:
Moban Tablets & Concentrate ... 932

Morphine Sulfate (Respiratory depression, hypotension, profound sedation or coma). Products include:
Astramorph/PF Injection, USP (Preservative-Free) ... 618
Duramorph ... 960
Infumorph 200 and Infumorph 500 Sterile Solutions ... 962
MS Contin Tablets ... 1814
MSIR ... 1817
Oramorph SR (Morphine Sulfate Sustained Release Tablets) ... 1988
Roxanol ... 1991

Nortriptyline Hydrochloride (Respiratory depression, hypotension, profound sedation or coma). Products include:
Pamelor ... 2019

Opium Alkaloids (Respiratory depression, hypotension, profound sedation or coma). Products include:
B & O No. 15A & No. 16A Supprettes ... 2395
Pantopon Injectable ... 1911

Oxazepam (Respiratory depression, hypotension, profound sedation or coma). Products include:
Serax Capsules ... 2522
Serax Tablets ... 2522

Oxycodone Hydrochloride (Respiratory depression, hypotension, profound sedation or coma). Products include:
Percocet Tablets ... 950
Percodan ... 951
Roxicodone Tablets, Oral Solution & Intensol (Oxycodone) ... 1992
Tylox Capsules ... 1382

Pentobarbital Sodium (Respiratory depression, hypotension, profound sedation or coma). Products include:
Nembutal Sodium Capsules ... 534
Nembutal Sodium Solution ... 536
Nembutal Sodium Suppositories ... 538

Perphenazine (Respiratory depression, hypotension, profound sedation or coma). Products include:
Etrafon ... 2087
Triavil Tablets ... 1556
Trilafon ... 2123

Phenelzine Sulfate (Contraindicated: unpredictable, severe, and occasionally fatal reactions when given within 14 days). Products include:
Nardil ... 1742

Phenobarbital (Respiratory depression, hypotension, profound sedation or coma). Products include:
Arco-Lase Plus Tablets ... 607
Bellergal-S Tablets ... 1998
Bronkolixir ... ▣ 761
Bronkotabs Tablets ... ▣ 762
Donnatal ... 1858
Donnatal Extentabs ... 1859
Donnatal Tablets ... 1858
Donnazyme Tablets ... 1860
Kinesed Tablets ... 2272
Phenobarbital Elixir and Tablets ... 1293
Primatene Tablets-P Formula ... 2421
Quadrinal Tablets ... 1183
Tedral SA ... 1765

Prazepam (Respiratory depression, hypotension, profound sedation or coma). Products include:
Centrax ... 1693

Prochlorperazine (Respiratory depression, hypotension, profound sedation or coma). Products include:
Compazine ... 2201

Promethazine Hydrochloride (Respiratory depression, hypotension, profound sedation or coma). Products include:
Mepergan Injection ... 2479
Phenergan with Codeine ... 2497
Phenergan with Dextromethorphan ... 2499
Phenergan Injection ... 2493
Phenergan Suppositories ... 2496
Phenergan Syrup ... 2495
Phenergan Tablets ... 2496
Phenergan VC ... 2500
Phenergan VC with Codeine ... 2501

Propofol (Respiratory depression, hypotension, profound sedation or coma). Products include:
Diprivan Injection ... 2267

Propoxyphene Hydrochloride (Respiratory depression, hypotension, profound sedation or coma). Products include:
Darvon ... 1256
Wygesic Tablets ... 2540

Propoxyphene Napsylate (Respiratory depression, hypotension, profound sedation or coma). Products include:
Darvon-N/Darvocet-N ... 1254

Protriptyline Hydrochloride (Respiratory depression, hypotension, profound sedation or coma). Products include:
Vivactil Tablets ... 1567

Quazepam (Respiratory depression, hypotension, profound sedation or coma). Products include:
Doral Tablets ... 2383

Secobarbital Sodium (Respiratory depression, hypotension, profound sedation or coma). Products include:
Seconal Sodium Pulvules ... 1296

Selegiline Hydrochloride (Contraindicated: unpredictable, severe, and occasionally fatal reactions when given within 14 days). Products include:
- Eldepryl ... 2250

Sufentanil Citrate (Respiratory depression, hypotension, profound sedation or coma). Products include:
- Sufenta Injection ... 1147

Temazepam (Respiratory depression, hypotension, profound sedation or coma). Products include:
- Restoril Capsules ... 2023

Thiamylal Sodium (Respiratory depression, hypotension, profound sedation or coma). Products include:
- Surital Ampoules, Steri-Vials ... 1764

Thioridazine Hydrochloride (Respiratory depression, hypotension, profound sedation or coma). Products include:
- Mellaril ... 2011

Thiothixene (Respiratory depression, hypotension, profound sedation or coma). Products include:
- Navane Capsules and Concentrate 1954
- Navane Intramuscular ... 1956

Tranylcypromine Sulfate (Contraindicated: unpredictable, severe, and occasionally fatal reactions when given within 14 days). Products include:
- Parnate Tablets ... 2222

Triazolam (Respiratory depression, hypotension, profound sedation or coma). Products include:
- Halcion Tablets ... 2340

Trifluoperazine Hydrochloride (Respiratory depression, hypotension, profound sedation or coma). Products include:
- Stelazine ... 2226

Trimipramine Maleate (Respiratory depression, hypotension, profound sedation or coma). Products include:
- Surmontil Capsules ... 2524

DEMEROL HYDROCHLORIDE INJECTION
(Meperidine Hydrochloride) ... 2047
See **Demerol Hydrochloride Carpuject**

DEMEROL HYDROCHLORIDE SYRUP
(Meperidine Hydrochloride) ... 2047
See **Demerol Hydrochloride Carpuject**

DEMEROL HYDROCHLORIDE TABLETS
(Meperidine Hydrochloride) ... 2047
See **Demerol Hydrochloride Carpuject**

DEMEROL HYDROCHLORIDE UNI-AMP
(Meperidine Hydrochloride) ... 2047
See **Demerol Hydrochloride Carpuject**

DEMSER CAPSULES
(Metyrosine) ... 1460
May interact with central nervous system depressants, phenothiazines, butyrophenones, and certain other agents. Compounds in these categories include:

Alcohol (Additive sedative effects).

Alfentanil Hydrochloride (Additive sedative effects). Products include:
- Alfenta Injection ... 1131

Alprazolam (Additive sedative effects). Products include:
- Xanax Tablets ... 2367

Aprobarbital (Additive sedative effects). Products include:
- Alurate Elixir ... 1883

Buprenorphine (Additive sedative effects).
- No products indexed under this heading.

Buspirone Hydrochloride (Additive sedative effects). Products include:
- BuSpar ... 1401

Butabarbital (Additive sedative effects). Products include:
- Pyridium Plus ... 1764

Butalbital (Additive sedative effects). Products include:
- Esgic-Plus Tablets ... 1002
- Esgic Tablets & Capsules ... 1001
- Fioricet Tablets ... 2006
- Fiorinal Capsules ... 2007
- Fiorinal with Codeine Capsules ... 2008
- Fiorinal Tablets ... 2007
- Phrenilin ... 838
- Sedapap Tablets 50 mg/650 mg .. 1360

Chlordiazepoxide (Additive sedative effects). Products include:
- Libritabs Tablets ... 1930
- Limbitrol ... 1933
- Menrium Tablets ... 1934

Chlordiazepoxide Hydrochloride (Additive sedative effects). Products include:
- Librax Capsules ... 1929
- Librium Capsules ... 1931
- Librium Injectable ... 1932

Chlorpromazine (Potentiation of extrapyramidal effects of chlorpromazine). Products include:
- Thorazine ... 2234

Chlorprothixene (Additive sedative effects). Products include:
- Taractan Tablets ... 1920

Chlorprothixene Hydrochloride (Additive sedative effects). Products include:
- Taractan ... 1920

Chlorprothixene Lactate (Additive sedative effects). Products include:
- Taractan Concentrate ... 1920

Clorazepate Dipotassium (Additive sedative effects). Products include:
- Tranxene ... 556

Codeine (Additive sedative effects). Products include:
- Calcidrine Syrup ... 506

Codeine Phosphate (Additive sedative effects). Products include:
- Actifed with Codeine Cough Syrup.. 752
- Cheracol Cough Syrup ... 1853
- Codimal PH Syrup ... 846
- Dimetane-DC Cough Syrup ... 1857
- Empirin with Codeine Phosphate Nos. 2, 3 & 4 ... 764
- Fiorinal with Codeine Capsules ... 2008
- Isoclor Expectorant ... 982
- Naldecon CX Adult Liquid ... ◘ 521
- Novahistine DH ... 1342
- Novahistine Expectorant ... 1343
- Nucofed Capsules ... 2219
- Nucofed Expectorant ... 2219
- Nucofed Pediatric Expectorant ... 2220
- Nucofed Syrup ... 2219
- Phenaphen with Codeine Capsules 1865
- Phenaphen-650 with Codeine Tablets ... 1866
- Phenergan with Codeine ... 2497
- Phenergan VC with Codeine ... 2501
- Robitussin A-C Syrup ... 1875
- Robitussin-DAC Syrup ... 1875
- Ryna ... ◘ 741
- Soma Compound w/Codeine Tablets ... 2390
- Triaminic Expectorant w/Codeine .. 1996
- Tussi-Organidin Liquid ... 2391
- Tylenol with Codeine ... 1381

Codeine Polistirex (Additive sedative effects).
- No products indexed under this heading.

Dezocine (Additive sedative effects).

Diazepam (Additive sedative effects). Products include:
- Valium Injectable ... 1937
- Valium Tablets ... 1939
- Valrelease Capsules ... 1923

Droperidol (Additive sedative effects). Products include:
- Inapsine Injection ... 1140
- Innovar Injection ... 1141

Enflurane (Additive sedative effects). Products include:
- Ethrane ... 599

Estazolam (Additive sedative effects). Products include:
- ProSom Tablets ... 554

Ethchlorvynol (Additive sedative effects). Products include:
- Placidyl Capsules ... 553

Ethinamate (Additive sedative effects).
- No products indexed under this heading.

Fentanyl (Additive sedative effects). Products include:
- Duragesic Transdermal System ... 1133

Fentanyl Citrate (Additive sedative effects). Products include:
- Innovar Injection ... 1141
- Sublimaze Injection ... 1146

Fluphenazine Decanoate (Potentiation of extrapyramidal effects of fluphenazine). Products include:
- Prolixin Decanoate ... 1795

Fluphenazine Enanthate (Potentiation of extrapyramidal effects of fluphenazine). Products include:
- Prolixin Enanthate ... 1796

Fluphenazine Hydrochloride (Potentiation of extrapyramidal effects of fluphenazine). Products include:
- Prolixin Elixir ... 1793
- Prolixin Injection ... 1791
- Prolixin Oral Concentrate ... 1792
- Prolixin Tablets ... 1793

Flurazepam Hydrochloride (Additive sedative effects). Products include:
- Dalmane Capsules ... 1927

Glutethimide (Additive sedative effects).
- No products indexed under this heading.

Haloperidol (Potentiation of extrapyramidal effects of haloperidol; additive sedative effects). Products include:
- Haldol Injection, Tablets and Concentrate ... 1373

Haloperidol Decanoate (Potentiation of extrapyramidal effects of haloperidol; additive sedative effects). Products include:
- Haldol Decanoate ... 1375

Hydrocodone Bitartrate (Additive sedative effects). Products include:
- Anexsia 5/500 Tablets ... 2196
- Anexsia 7.5/650 Tablets ... 2197
- Azdone Tablets ... 844
- Codiclear DH Syrup ... 845
- Codimal DH Syrup ... 846
- Damason-P ... 1356
- Hycodan Syrup, Tablets ... 927
- Hycomine Compound Tablets ... 929
- Hycomine Syrup ... 927
- Hycotuss Expectorant Syrup ... 930
- Hydrocet Capsules ... 835
- Lortab ASA Tablets ... 2414
- Lortab ... 2412
- Ru-Tuss with Hydrocodone ... 694
- Triaminic Expectorant DH ... 1995
- Vicodin Tablets ... 1187
- Vicodin ES Tablets ... 1189
- Zydone Capsules ... 941

Hydrocodone Polistirex (Additive sedative effects). Products include:
- Tussionex Extended-Release Suspension ... 988

Hydroxyzine Hydrochloride (Additive sedative effects). Products include:
- Atarax Tablets & Syrup ... 1941
- Marax Tablets & DF Syrup ... 1954
- Vistaril Intramuscular Solution ... 1970

Isoflurane (Additive sedative effects). Products include:
- Forane ... 600

Ketamine Hydrochloride (Additive sedative effects). Products include:
- Ketalar ... 1726

Levorphanol Tartrate (Additive sedative effects). Products include:
- Levo-Dromoran ... 1906

Lorazepam (Additive sedative effects). Products include:
- Ativan Injection ... 2432
- Ativan Tablets ... 2434

Loxapine Hydrochloride (Additive sedative effects). Products include:
- Loxitane ... 1213

Loxapine Succinate (Additive sedative effects). Products include:
- Loxitane Capsules ... 1213

Meperidine Hydrochloride (Additive sedative effects). Products include:
- Demerol ... 2047
- Mepergan Injection ... 2479

Mephobarbital (Additive sedative effects). Products include:
- Mebaral Tablets ... 2061

Meprobamate (Additive sedative effects). Products include:
- Deprol Tablets ... 2382
- Equagesic Tablets ... 2451
- Miltown Tablets ... 2386
- PMB 200 and PMB 400 ... 2504

Mesoridazine (Potentiation of extrapyramidal effects of mesoridazine). Products include:
- Serentil ... 686

Methadone Hydrochloride (Additive sedative effects). Products include:
- Dolophine Hydrochloride Ampoules & Vials ... 1260
- Dolophine Hydrochloride Tablets ... 1261
- Methadone Hydrochloride Diskets .. 1284
- Methadone Hydrochloride Oral Solution & Tablets ... 1987

Methohexital Sodium (Additive sedative effects). Products include:
- Brevital Sodium Vials ... 1248

Methoxyflurane (Additive sedative effects).
- No products indexed under this heading.

Midazolam Hydrochloride (Additive sedative effects). Products include:
- Versed Injection ... 1924

Molindone Hydrochloride (Additive sedative effects). Products include:
- Moban Tablets & Concentrate ... 932

Morphine Sulfate (Additive sedative effects). Products include:
- Astramorph/PF Injection, USP (Preservative-Free) ... 618
- Duramorph ... 960
- Infumorph 200 and Infumorph 500 Sterile Solutions ... 962
- MS Contin Tablets ... 1814
- MSIR ... 1817
- Oramorph SR (Morphine Sulfate Sustained Release Tablets) ... 1988
- Roxanol ... 1991

Opium Alkaloids (Additive sedative effects). Products include:
- B & O No. 15A & No. 16A Supprettes ... 2395
- Pantopon Injectable ... 1911

Oxazepam (Additive sedative effects). Products include:
- Serax Capsules ... 2522
- Serax Tablets ... 2522

Oxycodone Hydrochloride (Additive sedative effects). Products include:
- Percocet Tablets ... 950
- Percodan ... 951
- Roxicodone Tablets, Oral Solution & Intensol (Oxycodone) ... 1992
- Tylox Capsules ... 1382

Pentobarbital Sodium (Additive sedative effects). Products include:
- Nembutal Sodium Capsules ... 534
- Nembutal Sodium Solution ... 536
- Nembutal Sodium Suppositories ... 538

Perphenazine (Potentiation of extrapyramidal effects of perphenazine). Products include:
- Etrafon ... 2087
- Triavil Tablets ... 1556
- Trilafon ... 2123

Phenobarbital (Additive sedative effects). Products include:
- Arco-Lase Plus Tablets ... 607
- Bellergal-S Tablets ... 1998
- Bronkolixir ... ▣ 761
- Bronkotabs Tablets ... ▣ 762
- Donnatal ... 1858
- Donnatal Extentabs ... 1859
- Donnatal Tablets ... 1858
- Donnazyme Tablets ... 1860
- Kinesed Tablets ... 2272
- Phenobarbital Elixir and Tablets ... 1293
- Primatene Tablets-P Formula ... 2421
- Quadrinal Tablets ... 1183
- Tedral SA ... 1765

Prazepam (Additive sedative effects). Products include:
- Centrax ... 1693

Prochlorperazine (Potentiation of extrapyramidal effects of chlorpromazine). Products include:
- Compazine ... 2201

Promethazine Hydrochloride (Potentiation of extrapyramidal effects of promethazine). Products include:
- Mepergan Injection ... 2479
- Phenergan with Codeine ... 2497
- Phenergan with Dextromethorphan 2499
- Phenergan Injection ... 2493
- Phenergan Suppositories ... 2496
- Phenergan Syrup ... 2495
- Phenergan Tablets ... 2496
- Phenergan VC ... 2500
- Phenergan VC with Codeine ... 2501

Propofol (Additive sedative effects). Products include:
- Diprivan Injection ... 2267

Propoxyphene Hydrochloride (Additive sedative effects). Products include:
- Darvon ... 1256
- Wygesic Tablets ... 2540

Propoxyphene Napsylate (Additive sedative effects). Products include:
- Darvon-N/Darvocet-N ... 1254

Quazepam (Additive sedative effects). Products include:
- Doral Tablets ... 2383

Secobarbital Sodium (Additive sedative effects). Products include:
- Seconal Sodium Pulvules ... 1296

Sufentanil Citrate (Additive sedative effects). Products include:
- Sufenta Injection ... 1147

Temazepam (Additive sedative effects). Products include:
- Restoril Capsules ... 2023

Thiamylal Sodium (Additive sedative effects). Products include:
- Surital Ampoules, Steri-Vials ... 1764

Thioridazine Hydrochloride (Potentiation of extrapyramidal effects of thioridazine). Products include:
- Mellaril ... 2011

Thiothixene (Additive sedative effects). Products include:
- Navane Capsules and Concentrate 1954
- Navane Intramuscular ... 1956

Triazolam (Additive sedative effects). Products include:
- Halcion Tablets ... 2340

Trifluoperazine Hydrochloride (Potentiation of extrapyramidal effects of trifluoperazine). Products include:
- Stelazine ... 2226

DEMULEN 1/35-21

(Ethynodiol Diacetate, Ethinyl Estradiol) ... 2161

May interact with sulfonamides, barbiturates, tranquilizers, antimigraine drugs, oral anticoagulants, anticonvulsants, tricyclic antidepressants, oral hypoglycemic agents, corticosteroids, tetracyclines, and certain other agents. Compounds in these categories include:

Acetaminophen (Altered effectiveness of acetaminophen). Products include:
- Acetaminophen Uniserts Suppositories ... 2374
- Actifed Plus Caplets ... ▣ 539
- Actifed Plus Tablets ... ▣ 540
- Alka-Seltzer Advanced Formula Antacid & Non-Aspirin Pain Reliever ... ▣ 620
- Allerest ... ▣ 559
- Aspirin Free Anacin Maximum Strength Acetaminophen Film Coated Caplets ... 2417
- Aspirin Free Anacin Maximum Strength Acetaminophen Film Coated Tablets ... 2417
- Anacin-3 Regular Strength Acetaminophen Film Coated Tablets ▣ 746
- Anexsia 5/500 Tablets ... 2196
- Anexsia 7.5/650 Tablets ... 2197
- Benadryl Plus ... ▣ 636
- Benadryl Plus Nighttime ... ▣ 637
- Bufferin AF Nite Time Analgesic/Sleeping Aid Caplets ... 744
- Allergy-Sinus Comtrex Multi-Symptom Allergy Sinus Formula Tablets & Caplets ... 746
- Cough Formula Comtrex ... 746
- Comtrex Multi-Symptom Cold Reliever Tablets/Caplets/Liqui-Gels/Liquid ... 745
- Day-Night Comtrex ... 747
- Non-Drowsy Comtrex ... 747
- Congespirin For Children Aspirin Free Chewable Cold Tablets ... 748
- Contac Cough & Sore Throat Formula ... ▣ 712
- Contac Jr. Children's Cold Medicine ... ▣ 712
- Contac Nighttime Cold Medicine ... ▣ 713
- Contac Severe Cold and Flu Formula Caplets ... ▣ 711
- Contac Sinus Caplets Maximum Strength Non-Drowsy Formula ... ▣ 710
- Contac Sinus Tablets Maximum Strength Non-Drowsy Formula ... ▣ 710
- Coricidin 'D' Decongestant Tablets ... ▣ 695
- Coricidin Demilets Tablets for Children ... ▣ 696
- Coricidin Tablets ... ▣ 695
- Darvon-N/Darvocet-N ... 1254
- Datril Extra-Strength Analgesic Tablets ... 748
- Dimetapp Plus Caplets ... ▣ 675
- Dorcol Children's Fever & Pain Reducer ... ▣ 686
- Dristan Decongestant/Antihistamine/Analgesic Coated Caplets ... ▣ 749
- Dristan Cold Nasal Decongestant/Antihistamine/ Analgesic Coated Tablets ... 2419
- Dristan Advanced Formula Decongestant/Antihistamine/Analgesic Tablets ... ▣ 749
- Maximum Strength Dristan Decongestant/Analgesic Coated Caplets ... ▣ 750
- No Drowsiness Dristan Cold Nasal Decongestant/Analgesic Coated Caplets ... 2420
- Drixoral Plus Extended-Release Tablets ... ▣ 699
- Drixoral Sinus ... ▣ 700
- Esgic-Plus Tablets ... 1002
- Esgic Tablets & Capsules ... 1001
- Aspirin Free Excedrin Analgesic Caplets ... 748
- Excedrin Extra-Strength Analgesic Tablets & Caplets ... 749
- Excedrin P.M. Analgesic/Sleeping Aid Tablets, Caplets and Liquid ... 749
- Sinus Excedrin Analgesic, Decongestant Tablets & Caplets ... 750
- 4-Way Cold Tablets ... 750
- Feverall Sprinkle Caps ... 2374
- Feverall Suppositories ... 2374
- Fioricet Tablets ... 2006
- Hycomine Compound Tablets ... 929
- Hydrocet Capsules ... 835
- Isocom Capsules ... 1629
- Liquiprin ... ▣ 618
- Lortab ... 2412
- Lurline PMS Tablets ... 972
- Medi-Flu Caplet, Liquid ... ▣ 640
- Maximum Strength Midol Multi-Symptom Menstrual Formula ... ▣ 571
- Maximum Strength Midol PMS Premenstrual Syndrome Formula ... ▣ 570
- Regular Strength Midol Multi-Symptom Menstrual Formula ... ▣ 570
- Midrin Capsules ... 836
- Ornex Caplets ... ▣ 618
- Children's Panadol Chewable Tablets, Liquid, Infants' Drops ... ▣ 571
- Junior Strength Panadol ... ▣ 571
- Maximum Strength Panadol Tablets and Caplets ... ▣ 572
- Percocet Tablets ... 950
- Percogesic Analgesic Tablets ... ▣ 660
- Phenaphen with Codeine Capsules 1865
- Phenaphen-650 with Codeine Tablets ... 1866
- Phrenilin ... 838
- Prēmsyn PMS Capsules & Caplets ▣ 547
- Pyrroxate Capsules ... ▣ 669
- Robitussin Night Relief ... ▣ 677
- Sedapap Tablets 50 mg/650 mg .. 1360
- Sinarest ... ▣ 562
- Sine-Aid Maximum Strength Sinus Headache Caplets ... 1365
- Sine-Aid Maximum Strength Sinus Headache Tablets ... 1365
- Sine-Off Maximum Strength Allergy/Sinus Formula Caplets ... ▣ 721
- Sine-Off Maximum Strength No Drowsiness Formula Caplets ... ▣ 722
- Singlet Tablets ... ▣ 598
- Sinulin ... 840
- Sinutab Maximum Strength ... ▣ 641
- Sinutab Maximum Strength Without Drowsiness Tablets & Caplets ... ▣ 642
- Sinutab Regular Strength Without Drowsiness Formula ... ▣ 641
- Sominex Pain Relief Formula ... ▣ 723
- St. Joseph Aspirin-Free Fever Reducer for Children Chewable Tablets, Liquid & Infant Drops ... ▣ 704
- St. Joseph Cold Tablets for Children ... ▣ 704
- St. Joseph Nighttime Cold Medicine ... ▣ 705
- Sudafed Sinus Caplets ... ▣ 545
- Sudafed Sinus Tablets ... ▣ 545
- Talacen ... 2070
- Tempra, Acetaminophen ... ▣ 613
- TheraFlu Flu and Cold Medicine ... ▣ 687
- Triaminicin Tablets ... ▣ 690
- Tylenol acetaminophen Children's Chewable Tablets & Elixir ... 1366
- Tylenol Allergy Sinus Medication Caplets and Gelcaps, Maximum Strength ... 1372
- Tylenol with Codeine ... 1381
- Children's Tylenol Cold Liquid Formula and Chewable Tablets ... 1368
- Tylenol Cold & Flu Hot Medication, Packets ... 1369
- Tylenol Cold & Flu No Drowsiness Hot Medication, Packets ... 1371
- Tylenol Cold Medication Caplets and Tablets ... 1370
- Tylenol Cold Medication, Effervescent Tablets ... 1369
- Tylenol Cold Medication No Drowsiness Formula Caplets ... 1370
- Tylenol Cold Night Time Medication Liquid ... 1371
- Tylenol Cough Medication Liquid, Maximum Strength ... 1372
- Tylenol Cough Medication Liquid with Decongestant, Maximum Strength ... 1372
- Tylenol, Extra Strength, acetaminophen Adult Liquid Pain Reliever .. 1367
- Tylenol, Extra Strength, acetaminophen Gelcaps, Caplets, Tablets ... 1367
- Tylenol, Infants' Drops ... 1366
- Tylenol, Junior Strength, acetaminophen Coated Caplets, Grape and Fruit Chewable Tablets ... 1366
- Tylenol, Maximum Strength, Sinus Medication Gelcaps, Caplets and Tablets ... 1373
- Tylenol, Regular Strength, acetaminophen Tablets and Caplets ... 1367
- Tylenol PM, Extra Strength Caplets and Tablets ... 1368
- Tylox Capsules ... 1382
- Unisom Dual Relief Nighttime Sleep Aid/Analgesic ... 1774
- Vanquish Analgesic Caplets ... ▣ 574
- Vicks Daycare ... ▣ 660
- Vicks Formula 44M Multi-Symptom Cough Medicine ... ▣ 662
- Vicks NyQuil Nighttime Colds Medicine-Original & Cherry Flavor ... ▣ 664
- Vicodin Tablets ... 1187
- Vicodin ES Tablets ... 1189
- Wygesic Tablets ... 2540
- Zydone Capsules ... 941

Alprazolam (Reduces effectiveness and increased incidence of breakthrough bleeding). Products include:
- Xanax Tablets ... 2367

Aminophylline (Altered effectiveness of aminophylline). Products include:
- Amesec ... ▣ 682
- Aminophyllin Tablets ... 2153

Amitriptyline Hydrochloride (Altered effectiveness of tricyclic antidepressants). Products include:
- Elavil ... 2269
- Endep Tablets ... 1927
- Etrafon ... 2087
- Limbitrol ... 1933
- Triavil Tablets ... 1556

Amoxapine (Altered effectiveness of tricyclic antidepressants). Products include:
- Asendin Tablets ... 1196

Ampicillin Sodium (Reduces effectiveness and increased incidence of breakthrough bleeding). Products include:
- Unasyn ... 1965

Aprobarbital (Reduces effectiveness and increased incidence of breakthrough bleeding). Products include:
- Alurate Elixir ... 1883

Bendroflumethiazide (Reduces effectiveness and increased incidence of breakthrough bleeding). Products include:
- Corzide Tablets ... 702
- Naturetin Tablets ... 1789
- Rauzide Tablets ... 1804

Betamethasone Acetate (Altered effectiveness of glucocorticoids). Products include:
- Celestone Soluspan Suspension ... 2081

Betamethasone Sodium Phosphate (Altered effectiveness of glucocorticoids). Products include:
- Celestone Soluspan Suspension ... 2081

Buspirone Hydrochloride (Reduces effectiveness and increased incidence of breakthrough bleeding). Products include:
- BuSpar ... 1401

Butabarbital (Reduces effectiveness and increased incidence of breakthrough bleeding). Products include:
- Pyridium Plus ... 1764

Butalbital (Reduces effectiveness and increased incidence of breakthrough bleeding). Products include:
- Esgic-Plus Tablets ... 1002
- Esgic Tablets & Capsules ... 1001
- Fioricet Tablets ... 2006
- Fiorinal Capsules ... 2007
- Fiorinal with Codeine Capsules ... 2008
- Fiorinal Tablets ... 2007
- Phrenilin ... 838
- Sedapap Tablets 50 mg/650 mg ... 1360

Caffeine (Altered effectiveness of caffeine). Products include:
- Anacin Coated Analgesic Caplets ... 2417
- Anacin Coated Analgesic Tablets ... 2417
- Anacin Maximum Strength Analgesic Coated Tablets ... 2417
- Cafergot/Cafergot P-B ... 1999
- Esgic-Plus Tablets ... 1002
- Esgic Tablets & Capsules ... 1001
- Aspirin Free Excedrin Analgesic Caplets ... 748
- Excedrin Extra-Strength Analgesic Tablets & Caplets ... 749
- Fioricet Tablets ... 2006
- Fiorinal Capsules ... 2007
- Fiorinal with Codeine Capsules ... 2008
- Fiorinal Tablets ... 2007
- No Doz Fast Acting Alertness Aid Tablets ... 751
- No Doz Maximum Strength Caplets ... 751
- Norgesic ... 1314
- P-A-C Analgesic Tablets ... ▣ 669
- Synalgos-DC Capsules ... 2525
- Vanquish Analgesic Caplets ... ▣ 574
- Vivarin Stimulant Tablets ... ▣ 726
- Wigraine Tablets & Suppositories ... 1645

Captopril (Altered effectiveness of antihypertensives). Products include:
- Capoten ... 2255
- Capozide ... 2258

Carbamazepine (Reduces effectiveness and increased incidence of breakthrough bleeding). Products include:
- Tegretol Chewable Tablets ... 654
- Tegretol Suspension ... 656
- Tegretol Tablets ... 654

Chloramphenicol (Reduces effectiveness and increased incidence of breakthrough bleeding). Products include:
- AK-Chlor Sterile Ophthalmic Ointment & Solution ... ◉ 201
- Chloromycetin Cream, 1% ... 1694
- Chloromycetin Hydrocortisone Ophthalmic ... 1694
- Chloromycetin Kapseals ... 1695
- Chloromycetin Ophthalmic Ointment, 1% ... 1696
- Chloromycetin Ophthalmic Solution ... 1696
- Chloromycetin Otic ... 1697
- Chloroptic S.O.P. ... ◉ 243
- Chloroptic Sterile Ophthalmic Solution ... ◉ 243
- Ophthochlor Ophthalmic Solution ... ◉ 300
- Ophthocort ... ◉ 301

Chloramphenicol Palmitate (Reduces effectiveness and increased incidence of breakthrough bleeding). Products include:
- Chloromycetin Palmitate, Oral Suspension ... 1697

Chloramphenicol Sodium Succinate (Reduces effectiveness and increased incidence of breakthrough bleeding). Products include:
- Chloromycetin Sodium Succinate ... 1698

Chlordiazepoxide (Reduces effectiveness and increased incidence of breakthrough bleeding). Products include:
- Libritabs Tablets ... 1930
- Limbitrol ... 1933
- Menrium Tablets ... 1934

Chlordiazepoxide Hydrochloride (Reduces effectiveness and increased incidence of breakthrough bleeding). Products include:
- Librax Capsules ... 1929
- Librium Capsules ... 1931
- Librium Injectable ... 1932

Chlorothiazide (Reduces effectiveness and increased incidence of breakthrough bleeding). Products include:
- Aldoclor Tablets ... 1413
- Diupres Tablets ... 1461
- Diuril Oral ... 1464

Chlorothiazide Sodium (Reduces effectiveness and increased incidence of breakthrough bleeding). Products include:
- Diuril Sodium Intravenous ... 1463

Chlorpromazine (Reduces effectiveness and increased incidence of breakthrough bleeding). Products include:
- Thorazine ... 2234

Chlorpropamide (Reduces effectiveness and increased incidence of breakthrough bleeding). Products include:
- Diabinese Tablets ... 1775

Chlorprothixene (Reduces effectiveness and increased incidence of breakthrough bleeding). Products include:
- Taractan Tablets ... 1920

Chlorprothixene Hydrochloride (Reduces effectiveness and increased incidence of breakthrough bleeding). Products include:
- Taractan ... 1920

Clofibrate (Altered effectiveness of clofibrate). Products include:
- Atromid-S Capsules ... 2435

Clomipramine Hydrochloride (Altered effectiveness of tricyclic antidepressants). Products include:
- Anafranil Capsules ... 650

Clorazepate Dipotassium (Reduces effectiveness and increased incidence of breakthrough bleeding). Products include:
- Tranxene ... 556

Cortisone Acetate (Altered effectiveness of glucocorticoids). Products include:
- Cortone Acetate Sterile Suspension ... 1437
- Cortone Acetate Tablets ... 1439

Demeclocycline Hydrochloride (Reduces effectiveness and increased incidence of breakthrough bleeding). Products include:
- Declomycin Capsules, Tablets ... 1199

Deserpidine (Altered effectiveness of antihypertensives). Products include:
- Enduronyl ... 518
- Harmonyl Tablets ... 528
- Oreticyl ... 545

Desipramine Hydrochloride (Altered effectiveness of tricyclic antidepressants). Products include:
- Norpramin Tablets ... 1340

Dexamethasone Acetate (Altered effectiveness of glucocorticoids). Products include:
- Dalalone D.P. Injectable ... 999
- Decadron-LA Sterile Suspension ... 1457

Dexamethasone Sodium Phosphate (Altered effectiveness of glucocorticoids). Products include:
- AK-Dex ... ◉ 203
- Decadron Phosphate Respihaler ... 1454
- Decadron Phosphate Sterile Ophthalmic Ointment ... 1453
- Decadron Phosphate Sterile Ophthalmic Solution ... 1453
- Decadron Phosphate Topical Cream ... 1455
- Decadron Phosphate Turbinaire ... 1456
- Maxidex Sterile Ophthalmic Ointment ... ◉ 222
- NeoDecadron Sterile Ophthalmic Ointment ... 1517
- NeoDecadron Sterile Ophthalmic Solution ... 1518
- NeoDecadron Topical Cream ... 1518

Diazepam (Reduces effectiveness and increased incidence of breakthrough bleeding). Products include:
- Valium Injectable ... 1937
- Valium Tablets ... 1939
- Valrelease Capsules ... 1923

Dicumarol (Altered effectiveness of anticoagulants). Products include:
- Dicumarol Tablets ... 516

Dihydroergotamine Mesylate (Reduces effectiveness and increased incidence of breakthrough bleeding). Products include:
- D.H.E. 45 Injection ... 2003

Divalproex Sodium (Altered effectiveness of anticonvulsants). Products include:
- Depakote ... 512

Doxepin Hydrochloride (Altered effectiveness of tricyclic antidepressants). Products include:
- Sinequan ... 1960

Doxycycline Calcium (Reduces effectiveness and increased incidence of breakthrough bleeding).
- No products indexed under this heading.

Doxycycline Hyclate (Reduces effectiveness and increased incidence of breakthrough bleeding). Products include:
- Doryx Capsules ... 1717
- Vibramycin Hyclate Capsules ... 1787
- Vibramycin Hyclate Intravenous ... 1968
- Vibra-Tabs Film Coated Tablets ... 1787

Doxycycline Monohydrate (Reduces effectiveness and increased incidence of breakthrough bleeding). Products include:
- Monodox Capsules ... 1630
- Vibramycin Monohydrate for Oral Suspension ... 1787

Droperidol (Reduces effectiveness and increased incidence of breakthrough bleeding). Products include:
- Inapsine Injection ... 1140
- Innovar Injection ... 1141

Dyphylline (Altered effectiveness of dyphylline). Products include:
- Dilor ... 2079
- Dilor-G Tablets & Liquid ... 2079
- Lufyllin Elixir ... 2384
- Lufyllin & Lufyllin-400 Tablets ... 2384
- Lufyllin-GG Elixir & Tablets ... 2385

Ergotamine Tartrate (Reduces effectiveness and increased incidence of breakthrough bleeding). Products include:
- Bellergal-S Tablets ... 1998
- Cafergot/Cafergot P-B ... 1999
- Ergostat ... 1719
- Medihaler Ergotamine Aerosol ... 1312
- Wigraine Tablets & Suppositories ... 1645

Ethosuximide (Altered effectiveness of anticonvulsants). Products include:
- Zarontin Capsules ... 1768
- Zarontin Syrup ... 1769

Ethotoin (Altered effectiveness of anticonvulsants). Products include:
- Peganone Tablets ... 551

Fluphenazine Decanoate (Reduces effectiveness and increased incidence of breakthrough bleeding). Products include:
- Prolixin Decanoate ... 1795

Fluphenazine Enanthate (Reduces effectiveness and increased incidence of breakthrough bleeding). Products include:
- Prolixin Enanthate ... 1796

Fluphenazine Hydrochloride (Reduces effectiveness and increased incidence of breakthrough bleeding). Products include:
- Prolixin Elixir ... 1793
- Prolixin Injection ... 1791
- Prolixin Oral Concentrate ... 1792
- Prolixin Tablets ... 1793

Glipizide (Reduces effectiveness and increased incidence of breakthrough bleeding). Products include:
- Glucotrol ... 1952

Glyburide (Reduces effectiveness and increased incidence of breakthrough bleeding). Products include:
- DiaBeta ... 1091
- Micronase Tablets ... 2350

Griseofulvin (Reduces effectiveness and increased incidence of breakthrough bleeding). Products include:
- Fulvicin P/G Tablets ... 2090
- Fulvicin P/G 165 & 330 Tablets ... 2091
- Fulvicin-U/F Tablets ... 2092
- Grifulvin V (griseofulvin microsize) Tablets/Suspension ... 1678
- Grisactin ... 2454
- Grisactin Ultra Tablets ... 2455
- Gris-PEG Tablets, 125 mg & 250 mg ... 1083

Guanabenz Acetate (Altered effectiveness of antihypertensives). Products include:
- Wytensin Tablets ... 2542

Guanethidine Monosulfate (Altered effectiveness of antihypertensives). Products include:
- Esimil Tablets ... 864
- Ismelin Tablets ... 869

Haloperidol (Reduces effectiveness and increased incidence of breakthrough bleeding). Products include:
- Haldol Injection, Tablets and Concentrate ... 1373

Haloperidol Decanoate (Reduces effectiveness and increased incidence of breakthrough bleeding). Products include:
- Haldol Decanoate ... 1375

Hydralazine Hydrochloride (Altered effectiveness of antihypertensives). Products include:
- Apresazide Capsules ... 854
- Apresoline Hydrochloride Parenteral (Ampuls) ... 856
- Apresoline Hydrochloride Tablets ... 855
- Apresoline-Esidrix Tablets ... 857
- Ser-Ap-Es Tablets ... 881
- Serpasil-Apresoline Tablets ... 884

Hydrochlorothiazide (Reduces effectiveness and increased incidence of breakthrough bleeding). Products include:
- Aldactazide ... 2150
- Aldoril Tablets ... 1418
- Apresazide Capsules ... 854
- Apresoline-Esidrix Tablets ... 857
- Capozide ... 2258
- Dyazide Capsules ... 2208
- Esidrix Tablets ... 863
- Esimil Tablets ... 864
- HydroDIURIL Tablets ... 1484
- Hydropres Tablets ... 1485
- Inderide Tablets ... 2463
- Inderide LA Long Acting Capsules ... 2465
- Lopressor HCT Tablets ... 1034
- Maxzide ... 1215
- Moduretic Tablets ... 1510
- Normozide Tablets ... 2112
- Oretic Tablets ... 544
- Oreticyl ... 545
- Prinzide Tablets ... 1540
- Ser-Ap-Es Tablets ... 881
- Serpasil-Esidrix Tablets ... 886
- Timolide Tablets ... 1547
- Trandate HCT Tablets ... 579
- Vaseretic Tablets ... 1559
- Zestoretic ... 2274

Hydrocortisone (Altered effectiveness of glucocorticoids). Products include:
- AK-Spore H.C. ... ◉ 206

Bactine Hydrocortisone Anti-Itch Cream ▣ 625
CaldeCORT Anti-Itch Hydrocortisone Spray ▣ 560
Carmol HC Cream 1% 2296
Cortaid Spray ▣ 735
Cortenema 2244
Cortisporin Ointment 758
Cortisporin Ophthalmic Ointment Sterile 758
Cortisporin Ophthalmic Suspension Sterile 759
Cortisporin Otic Solution Sterile 760
Cortisporin Otic Suspension Sterile 760
Cortizone-5 Creme & Ointment ▣ 732
Dermolate Anti-Itch Cream ▣ 697
Eldecort Cream 1.0% 1113
Eldecort Cream 1.0% and 2.5% 1113
Fungoid HC Creme 1770
Hydrocortone Tablets 1482
Hytone 909
LazerSporin-C Solution 1770
Massengill Medicated Soft Cloth Towelettes 2192
Nutracort Cream & Lotion 1684
PediOtic Suspension Sterile 797
Synacort Creams 1%, 2.5% 2296
Vanoxide-HC Acne Lotion 911
Vioform-Hydrocortisone Cream and Mild Cream 889
Vioform-Hydrocortisone Ointment 889
VōSoL HC Otic Solution 2392
Vytone Cream 1% 911

Hydrocortisone Acetate (Altered effectiveness of glucocorticoids). Products include:
Analpram-HC Rectal Cream 1% and 2.5% 970
Anusol-HC Cream 1690
Anusol-HC Suppositories 1691
Caldecort ▣ 560
Carmol HC Cream 1% 2296
Chloromycetin Hydrocortisone Ophthalmic 1694
Coly-Mycin S Otic w/Neomycin & Hydrocortisone 1708
Cortaid ▣ 735
Cortef Feminine Itch Cream ▣ 735
Corticaine ▣ 682
Cortifoam 1827
Cortisporin Cream 757
Epifoam 1828
Gynecort 5 Creme ▣ 556
Hydrocortone Acetate Sterile Suspension 1479
Lanacort 5 Creme and Ointment ▣ 557
Mantadil Cream 789
Ophthocort ◉ 301
Orabase HCA Oral Paste 890
Pramosone Cream, Lotion & Ointment 971
ProctoCream-HC 1834
Proctofoam-HC 1835

Hydrocortisone Sodium Phosphate (Altered effectiveness of glucocorticoids). Products include:
Hydrocortone Phosphate Injection, Sterile 1481

Hydrocortisone Sodium Succinate (Altered effectiveness of glucocorticoids). Products include:
Solu-Cortef Sterile Powder 2361

Hydroflumethiazide (Reduces effectiveness and increased incidence of breakthrough bleeding). Products include:
Diucardin Tablets 2450
Saluron 718
Salutensin/Salutensin-Demi 719

Hydroxyzine Hydrochloride (Reduces effectiveness and increased incidence of breakthrough bleeding). Products include:
Atarax Tablets & Syrup 1941
Marax Tablets & DF Syrup 1954
Vistaril Intramuscular Solution 1970

Imipramine Hydrochloride (Altered effectiveness of tricyclic antidepressants). Products include:
Tofranil Ampuls 1038
Tofranil Tablets 1039

Imipramine Pamoate (Altered effectiveness of tricyclic antidepressants). Products include:
Tofranil-PM Capsules 1041

Isoniazid (Reduces effectiveness and increased incidence of breakthrough bleeding). Products include:
INH Tablets 868
Rifamate Capsules 1347

Lorazepam (Reduces effectiveness and increased incidence of breakthrough bleeding). Products include:
Ativan Injection 2432
Ativan Tablets 2434

Loxapine Hydrochloride (Reduces effectiveness and increased incidence of breakthrough bleeding). Products include:
Loxitane 1213

Loxapine Succinate (Reduces effectiveness and increased incidence of breakthrough bleeding). Products include:
Loxitane Capsules 1213

Maprotiline Hydrochloride (Altered effectiveness of tricyclic antidepressants). Products include:
Ludiomil Tablets 874

Mephenytoin (Altered effectiveness of anticonvulsants). Products include:
Mesantoin Tablets 2013

Mephobarbital (Reduces effectiveness and increased incidence of breakthrough bleeding). Products include:
Mebaral Tablets 2061

Meprobamate (Reduces effectiveness and increased incidence of breakthrough bleeding). Products include:
Deprol Tablets 2382
Equagesic Tablets 2451
Miltown Tablets 2386
PMB 200 and PMB 400 2504

Mesoridazine (Reduces effectiveness and increased incidence of breakthrough bleeding). Products include:
Serentil 686

Methacycline Hydrochloride (Reduces effectiveness and increased incidence of breakthrough bleeding).
No products indexed under this heading.

Methsuximide (Altered effectiveness of anticonvulsants). Products include:
Celontin 1692

Methyclothiazide (Reduces effectiveness and increased incidence of breakthrough bleeding). Products include:
Enduron Tablets 517
Enduronyl 518

Methylprednisolone Acetate (Altered effectiveness of glucocorticoids). Products include:
Depo-Medrol Sterile Aqueous Suspension 2334

Methylprednisolone Sodium Succinate (Altered effectiveness of glucocorticoids). Products include:
Solu-Medrol Sterile Powder 2363

Methysergide Maleate (Reduces effectiveness and increased incidence of breakthrough bleeding). Products include:
Sansert Tablets 2031

Metoclopramide Hydrochloride (Increased incidence of breakthrough bleeding). Products include:
Reglan 1869

Metolazone (Altered effectiveness of antihypertensives). Products include:
Diulo 2129
Mykrox ½ mg Tablets 984
Zaroxolyn Tablets 989

Minocycline Hydrochloride (Reduces effectiveness and increased incidence of breakthrough bleeding). Products include:
Minocin Intravenous 1221
Minocin Oral Suspension 1224
Minocin Pellet-Filled Capsules 1222

Molindone Hydrochloride (Reduces effectiveness and increased incidence of breakthrough bleeding). Products include:
Moban Tablets & Concentrate 932

Neomycin, oral (Reduces effectiveness and increased incidence of breakthrough bleeding).

Nitrofurantoin Macrocrystals (Reduces effectiveness and increased incidence of breakthrough bleeding). Products include:
Macrodantin Capsules 1624

Nortriptyline Hydrochloride (Altered effectiveness of tricyclic antidepressants). Products include:
Pamelor 2019

Oxazepam (Reduces effectiveness and increased incidence of breakthrough bleeding). Products include:
Serax Capsules 2522
Serax Tablets 2522

Oxytetracycline Hydrochloride (Reduces effectiveness and increased incidence of breakthrough bleeding). Products include:
Terra-Cortril Ophthalmic Suspension 1963
Terramycin Capsules 1786
Terramycin Intramuscular Solution 1964
Terramycin with Polymyxin B Sulfate Ophthalmic Ointment 1965

Paramethadione (Altered effectiveness of anticonvulsants). Products include:
Paradione Capsules 548

Penbutolol Sulfate (Altered effectiveness of antihypertensives). Products include:
Levatol 1832

Penicillin V Potassium (Reduces effectiveness and increased incidence of breakthrough bleeding).
No products indexed under this heading.

Pentobarbital Sodium (Reduces effectiveness and increased incidence of breakthrough bleeding). Products include:
Nembutal Sodium Capsules 534
Nembutal Sodium Solution 536
Nembutal Sodium Suppositories 538

Perphenazine (Reduces effectiveness and increased incidence of breakthrough bleeding). Products include:
Etrafon 2087
Triavil Tablets 1556
Trilafon 2123

Phenacemide (Altered effectiveness of anticonvulsants). Products include:
Phenurone Tablets 552

Phenobarbital (Reduces effectiveness and increased incidence of breakthrough bleeding). Products include:
Arco-Lase Plus Tablets 607
Bellergal-S Tablets 1998
Bronkolixir ▣ 761
Bronkotabs Tablets ▣ 762
Donnatal 1858
Donnatal Extentabs 1859
Donnatal Tablets 1858
Donnazyme Tablets 1860
Kinesed Tablets 2272
Phenobarbital Elixir and Tablets 1293
Primatene Tablets-P Formula 2421
Quadrinal Tablets 1183
Tedral SA 1765

Phenoxybenzamine Hydrochloride (Altered effectiveness of antihypertensives). Products include:
Dibenzyline Capsules 2207

Phensuximide (Altered effectiveness of anticonvulsants). Products include:
Milontin Kapseals 1741

Phentolamine Mesylate (Altered effectiveness of antihypertensives). Products include:
Regitine 878

Phenylbutazone (Reduces effectiveness and increased incidence of breakthrough bleeding). Products include:
Butazolidin Capsules & Tablets 1027

Phenytoin (Reduces effectiveness and increased incidence of breakthrough bleeding). Products include:
Dilantin Infatabs 1710
Dilantin-30 Pediatric/Dilantin-125 Suspension 1713

Phenytoin Sodium (Reduces effectiveness and increased incidence of breakthrough bleeding). Products include:
Dilantin Kapseals 1708
Dilantin Parenteral 1712
Dilantin with Phenobarbital Kapseals 1715

Polythiazide (Reduces effectiveness and increased incidence of breakthrough bleeding). Products include:
Minizide Capsules 1779
Renese Tablets 1785
Renese-R Tablets 1786

Prazepam (Reduces effectiveness and increased incidence of breakthrough bleeding). Products include:
Centrax 1693

Prazosin Hydrochloride (Altered effectiveness of antihypertensives). Products include:
Minipress Capsules 1778
Minizide Capsules 1779

Prednisolone Acetate (Altered effectiveness of glucocorticoids). Products include:
AK-Cide Sterile Ophthalmic Ointment & Suspension ◉ 202
Blephamide Liquifilm Sterile Ophthalmic Suspension 586
Blephamide S.O.P. Sterile Ophthalmic Ointment 586
Cetapred Ointment ◉ 220
⅛% Econopred & 1% Econopred Plus ◉ 217
Isopto Cetapred Suspension ◉ 220
Metimyd ◉ 306
Poly-Pred Liquifilm ◉ 250
Pred Forte ◉ 252
Pred Mild ◉ 254
Pred-G Liquifilm Sterile Ophthalmic Suspension ◉ 252
Pred-G S.O.P. Sterile Ophthalmic Ointment ◉ 253
Vasocidin Ointment ◉ 275

Prednisolone Sodium Phosphate (Altered effectiveness of glucocorticoids). Products include:
AK-Pred ◉ 205
Hydeltrasol Injection, Sterile 1476
Inflamase ◉ 274
Pediapred Oral Liquid 987
Vasocidin Ophthalmic Solution ◉ 276

Prednisolone Tebutate (Altered effectiveness of glucocorticoids). Products include:
Hydeltra-T.B.A. Sterile Suspension 1478

Prednisone (Altered effectiveness of glucocorticoids). Products include:
Deltasone Tablets 2332

Primidone (Reduces effectiveness and increased incidence of breakthrough bleeding). Products include:
Mysoline 2480

Prochlorperazine (Reduces effectiveness and increased incidence of breakthrough bleeding). Products include:
Compazine ... 2201
Promethazine Hydrochloride (Reduces effectiveness and increased incidence of breakthrough bleeding). Products include:
Mepergan Injection ... 2479
Phenergan with Codeine ... 2497
Phenergan with Dextromethorphan 2499
Phenergan Injection ... 2493
Phenergan Suppositories ... 2496
Phenergan Syrup ... 2495
Phenergan Tablets ... 2496
Phenergan VC ... 2500
Phenergan VC with Codeine ... 2501
Protriptyline Hydrochloride (Altered effectiveness of tricyclic antidepressants). Products include:
Vivactil Tablets ... 1567
Rifampin (Reduces effectiveness and increased incidence of breakthrough bleeding). Products include:
Rifadin ... 1345
Rifamate Capsules ... 1347
Rimactane Capsules ... 879
Secobarbital Sodium (Reduces effectiveness and increased incidence of breakthrough bleeding). Products include:
Seconal Sodium Pulvules ... 1296
Sulfamethizole (Reduces effectiveness and increased incidence of breakthrough bleeding). Products include:
Thiosulfil Forte Tablets ... 2526
Urobiotic-250 Capsules ... 1968
Sulfamethoxazole (Reduces effectiveness and increased incidence of breakthrough bleeding). Products include:
Azo Gantanol Tablets ... 1887
Bactrim DS Tablets ... 1891
Bactrim I.V. Infusion ... 1889
Bactrim ... 1891
Gantanol ... 1899
Septra ... 813
Septra I.V. Infusion ... 808
Septra I.V. Infusion ADD-Vantage Vials ... 810
Septra ... 813
Sulfasalazine (Reduces effectiveness and increased incidence of breakthrough bleeding). Products include:
Azulfidine Tablets, EN-tabs, Oral Suspension ... 1157
Sulfinpyrazone (Reduces effectiveness and increased incidence of breakthrough bleeding). Products include:
Anturane ... 853
Sulfisoxazole (Reduces effectiveness and increased incidence of breakthrough bleeding). Products include:
Azo Gantrisin Tablets ... 1888
Gantrisin Tablets ... 1901
Pediazole ... 1973
Sulfisoxazole Diolamine (Reduces effectiveness and increased incidence of breakthrough bleeding). Products include:
Gantrisin Ophthalmic Ointment/Solution ... 1900
Tetracycline Hydrochloride (Reduces effectiveness and increased incidence of breakthrough bleeding). Products include:
Achromycin V Capsules ... 1193
Achromycin Ophthalmic Ointment 1% ... ⊙ 307
Achromycin Ophthalmic Suspension 1% ... ⊙ 308
Topicycline for Topical Solution ... 1856
Theophylline (Altered effectiveness of theophylline). Products include:
Bronkaid Tablets ... ▣ 757
Bronkolixir ... ▣ 761
Bronkotabs Tablets ... ▣ 762
Constant-T Tablets ... 1029
Marax Tablets & DF Syrup ... 1954
Primatene Tablets ... 2421
Quibron Capsules ... 713
Quibron-T ... 714
Quibron-T/SR ... 716
Theolair Liquid ... 1317
Theo-Organidin Elixir ... 2391
Theophylline Anhydrous (Altered effectiveness of theophylline). Products include:
Aerolate ... 994
Primatene Tablets-M Formula ... ▣ 753
Primatene Tablets-Regular Formula ... 2421
Respbid Tablets ... 684
Slo-bid Gyrocaps ... 1847
T-PHYL (Uniphyl) 200 mg Tablets 1820
Tedral SA ... 1765
Theo-24 ... 2179
Theo-Dur Sprinkle ... 1168
Theo-Dur Extended-Release Tablets ... 1166
Theolair Tablets ... 1317
Theolair-SR Tablets ... 1319
TheoX Extended-Release Tablets ... 841
Uniphyl 400 mg Tablets ... 1823
Theophylline Calcium Salicylate (Altered effectiveness of theophylline). Products include:
Quadrinal Tablets ... 1183
Theophylline Sodium Glycinate (Altered effectiveness of theophylline). Products include:
Asbron G ... 1997
Thiamylal Sodium (Reduces effectiveness and increased incidence of breakthrough bleeding). Products include:
Surital Ampoules, Steri-Vials ... 1764
Thioridazine Hydrochloride (Reduces effectiveness and increased incidence of breakthrough bleeding). Products include:
Mellaril ... 2011
Thiothixene (Reduces effectiveness and increased incidence of breakthrough bleeding). Products include:
Navane Capsules and Concentrate 1954
Navane Intramuscular ... 1956
Tolazamide (Reduces effectiveness and increased incidence of breakthrough bleeding). Products include:
Tolinase Tablets ... 2365
Tolbutamide (Reduces effectiveness and increased incidence of breakthrough bleeding). Products include:
Orinase Tablets ... 2354
Triamcinolone (Altered effectiveness of glucocorticoids).
No products indexed under this heading.
Triamcinolone Acetonide (Altered effectiveness of glucocorticoids). Products include:
Aristocort A ... 1010
Azmacort Inhaler ... 1837
Kenalog Cream, Lotion & Ointment 2401
Kenalog-10 Injection ... 2402
Kenalog-40 Injection ... 2403
Kenalog in Orabase ... 604
Kenalog Spray ... 2401
Mycolog II Cream and Ointment ... 2407
Mytrex Cream & Ointment ... 2080
Nasacort Nasal Inhaler ... 1844
Triamcinolone Diacetate (Altered effectiveness of glucocorticoids). Products include:
Aristocort Suspension ... 1008
Triamcinolone Hexacetonide (Altered effectiveness of glucocorticoids). Products include:
Aristospan Suspension ... 1011
Trifluoperazine Hydrochloride (Reduces effectiveness and increased incidence of breakthrough bleeding). Products include:
Stelazine ... 2226
Trimethadione (Altered effectiveness of anticonvulsants). Products include:
Tridione ... 557
Trimipramine Maleate (Altered effectiveness of tricyclic antidepressants). Products include:
Surmontil Capsules ... 2524
Valproic Acid (Altered effectiveness of anticonvulsants). Products include:
Depakene Capsules & Syrup ... 511
Vitamins A & D (Altered effectiveness of vitamins).
Warfarin Sodium (Altered effectiveness of anticoagulants). Products include:
Coumadin Injection & Tablets ... 944
Panwarfin Tablets ... 547

DEMULEN 1/35-28
(Ethynodiol Diacetate, Ethinyl Estradiol) ... 2161
See **Demulen 1/35-21**

DEMULEN 1/50-21
(Ethynodiol Diacetate, Ethinyl Estradiol) ... 2161
See **Demulen 1/35-21**

DEMULEN 1/50-28
(Ethynodiol Diacetate, Ethinyl Estradiol) ... 2161
See **Demulen 1/35-21**

DENOREX MEDICATED SHAMPOO AND CONDITIONER
(Coal Tar, Menthol, Alcohol) ... 2418
No interactions described in labeling.

DENOREX MEDICATED SHAMPOO, EXTRA STRENGTH
(Coal Tar, Menthol) ... 2418
No interactions described in labeling.

DENOREX MEDICATED SHAMPOO, EXTRA STRENGTH WITH CONDITIONERS
(Coal Tar, Menthol) ... 2418
No interactions described in labeling.

DENOREX MEDICATED SHAMPOO, REGULAR & MOUNTAIN FRESH HERBAL SCENT
(Coal Tar, Menthol) ... 2418
No interactions described in labeling.

DENQUEL SENSITIVE TEETH TOOTHPASTE
(Potassium Nitrate) ... ▣ 648
No interactions described in labeling.

DEPAKENE CAPSULES & SYRUP
(Valproic Acid) ... 511
May interact with oral anticoagulants, oral contraceptives, and certain other agents. Compounds in these categories include:
Alcohol (Depakene may potentiate CNS depressant activity).
Aspirin (Altered serum drug levels). Products include:
Alka-Seltzer Effervescent Antacid and Pain Reliever ... 1568
Alka-Seltzer Extra Strength Effervescent Antacid and Pain Reliever ... 1570
Alka-Seltzer (Flavored) Effervescent Antacid and Pain Reliever ... 1569
Alka-Seltzer Plus Cold Medicine ... ▣ 623
Alka-Seltzer Plus Night-Time Cold Medicine ... ▣ 623
Alka Seltzer Plus Sinus Allergy Medicine ... ▣ 624
Anacin Coated Analgesic Caplets ... 2417
Anacin Coated Analgesic Tablets ... 2417
Anacin Maximum Strength Analgesic Coated Tablets ... 2417
Maximum Strength Arthritis Pain Formula By the Makers of Anacin Analgesic Tablets and Caplets ... 2418
Arthritis Pain Formula by the Makers of Anacin Analgesic Tablets and Caplets ... ▣ 747
Arthritis Strength BC Powder ... ▣ 516
Ascriptin A/D Caplets ... 1850
Regular Strength Ascriptin Tablets 1850
Azdōne Tablets ... 844
BC Powder ... ▣ 517
BC Cold Powder ... ▣ 517
Children's Bayer Chewable Aspirin ... ▣ 564
Genuine Bayer Aspirin Tablets & Caplets ... ▣ 564
Maximum Bayer Aspirin Tablets & Caplets ... ▣ 566
Bayer Plus Aspirin Tablets ... ▣ 567
Therapy Bayer Aspirin Caplets ... ▣ 568
8 Hour Bayer Timed-Release Aspirin ... ▣ 566
Arthritis Strength Bufferin Analgesic Caplets ... 744
Extra Strength Bufferin Analgesic Tablets ... 745
Bufferin Analgesic Tablets and Caplets ... 743
Cama Arthritis Pain Reliever ... ▣ 685
Damason-P ... 1356
Easprin ... 1719
Ecotrin Enteric Coated Aspirin Maximum Strength Tablets and Caplets ... 2189
Ecotrin Enteric Coated Aspirin Regular Strength Tablets and Caplets ... 2189
Empirin Aspirin ... ▣ 541
Empirin with Codeine Phosphate Nos. 2, 3 & 4 ... 764
Equagesic Tablets ... 2451
Excedrin Extra-Strength Analgesic Tablets & Caplets ... 749
4-Way Cold Tablets ... 750
Fiorinal Capsules ... 2007
Fiorinal with Codeine Capsules ... 2008
Fiorinal Tablets ... 2007
Lortab ASA Tablets ... 2414
Momentum Muscular Backache Formula ... ▣ 751
Norgesic ... 1314
Norwich Extra-Strength Aspirin ... ▣ 546
Norwich Regular Strength Aspirin ▣ 547
P-A-C Analgesic Tablets ... ▣ 669
Percodan ... 951
Robaxisal Tablets ... 1872
Sine-Off Sinus Medicine Tablets-Aspirin Formula ... ▣ 722
Soma Compound w/Codeine Tablets ... 2390
Soma Compound Tablets ... 2389
St. Joseph Adult Chewable Aspirin (81 mg.) ... ▣ 703
Synalgos-DC Capsules ... 2525
Talwin Compound ... 2072
Ursinus Inlay-Tabs ... ▣ 691
Vanquish Analgesic Caplets ... ▣ 574
Zorprin Tablets ... 698
Aspirin, Enteric Coated (Altered serum drug levels). Products include:
Therapy Bayer Aspirin Caplets ... ▣ 568
Ecotrin ... 2189
Carbamazepine (Altered serum drug levels). Products include:
Tegretol Chewable Tablets ... 654
Tegretol Suspension ... 656
Tegretol Tablets ... 654
Clonazepam (Concomitant use may produce absence status). Products include:
Klonopin Tablets ... 1902
Dicumarol (Altered serum drug levels). Products include:
Dicumarol Tablets ... 516

Ethinyl Estradiol (Possible oral contraceptive failure). Products include:
Brevicon 2304
Demulen 2161
Estinyl Tablets 2085
Jenest-28 Tablets 1636
Levlen/Tri-Levlen 665
Lo/Ovral Tablets 2471
Lo/Ovral-28 Tablets 2476
Loestrin 1728
Modicon 1667
Nordette-21 Tablets 2481
Nordette-28 Tablets 2483
Norethin 2133
Norinyl 2304
Norlestrin 1746
Ortho-Cyclen Tablets 1658
Ortho-Novum 1667
Ovcon 1391
Ovral Tablets 2490
Ovral-28 Tablets 2491
Levlen/Tri-Levlen 665
Tri-Norinyl 2304
Triphasil-21 Tablets 2527
Triphasil-28 Tablets 2532

Ethosuximide (Altered serum concentrations of both drugs). Products include:
Zarontin Capsules 1768
Zarontin Syrup 1769

Ethynodiol Diacetate (Possible oral contraceptive failure). Products include:
Demulen 2161

Levonorgestrel (Possible oral contraceptive failure). Products include:
Levlen/Tri-Levlen 665
Nordette-21 Tablets 2481
Nordette-28 Tablets 2483
Norplant System 2484
Levlen/Tri-Levlen 665
Triphasil-21 Tablets 2527
Triphasil-28 Tablets 2532

Mestranol (Possible oral contraceptive failure). Products include:
Enovid 2161
Norethin 2133
Norinyl 2304
Ortho-Novum 1667

Norethindrone (Possible oral contraceptive failure). Products include:
Brevicon 2304
Jenest-28 Tablets 1636
Micronor Tablets 1667
Modicon 1667
Norethin 2133
Norinyl 2304
Norlutin 1755
Nor-Q D Tablets 2304
Ortho-Novum 1667
Ovcon 1391
Tri-Norinyl 2304

Norethynodrel (Possible oral contraceptive failure). Products include:
Enovid 2161

Norgestimate (Possible oral contraceptive failure). Products include:
Ortho-Cyclen Tablets 1658

Norgestrel (Possible oral contraceptive failure). Products include:
Lo/Ovral Tablets 2471
Lo/Ovral-28 Tablets 2476
Ovral Tablets 2490
Ovral-28 Tablets 2491
Ovrette Tablets 2492

Phenobarbital (Increased serum phenobarbital levels; potential for increased CNS depression; monitor for neurological toxicity). Products include:
Arco-Lase Plus Tablets 607
Bellergal-S Tablets 1998
Bronkolixir ▣ 761
Bronkotabs Tablets ▣ 762
Donnatal 1858
Donnatal Extentabs 1859
Donnatal Tablets 1858
Donnazyme Tablets 1860
Kinesed Tablets 2272
Phenobarbital Elixir and Tablets 1293
Primatene Tablets-P Formula 2421
Quadrinal Tablets 1183
Tedral SA 1765

Phenytoin (Potential for breakthrough seizures; dosage of phenytoin should be adjusted). Products include:
Dilantin Infatabs 1710
Dilantin-30 Pediatric/Dilantin-125 Suspension 1713

Phenytoin Sodium (Potential for breakthrough seizures; dosage of phenytoin should be adjusted). Products include:
Dilantin Kapseals 1708
Dilantin Parenteral 1712
Dilantin with Phenobarbital Kapseals 1715

Primidone (Potential for neurological toxicity). Products include:
Mysoline 2480

Warfarin Sodium (Altered bleeding time). Products include:
Coumadin Injection & Tablets 944
Panwarfin Tablets 547

DEPAKOTE SPRINKLE CAPSULES
(Divalproex Sodium) 512
See **Depakote Tablets**

DEPAKOTE TABLETS
(Divalproex Sodium) 512
May interact with oral anticoagulants, oral contraceptives, and certain other agents. Compounds in these categories include:

Alcohol (Valproate may potentiate CNS depressant activity of alcohol).

Aspirin (Altered serum drug levels). Products include:
Alka-Seltzer Effervescent Antacid and Pain Reliever 1568
Alka-Seltzer Extra Strength Effervescent Antacid and Pain Reliever 1570
Alka-Seltzer (Flavored) Effervescent Antacid and Pain Reliever 1569
Alka-Seltzer Plus Cold Medicine ▣ 623
Alka-Seltzer Plus Night-Time Cold Medicine ▣ 623
Alka Seltzer Plus Sinus Allergy Medicine ▣ 624
Anacin Coated Analgesic Caplets 2417
Anacin Coated Analgesic Tablets 2417
Anacin Maximum Strength Analgesic Coated Tablets 2417
Maximum Strength Arthritis Pain Formula By the Makers of Anacin Analgesic Tablets and Caplets 2418
Arthritis Pain Formula by the Makers of Anacin Analgesic Tablets and Caplets ▣ 747
Arthritis Strength BC Powder ▣ 516
Ascriptin A/D Caplets 1850
Regular Strength Ascriptin Tablets 1850
Azdōne Tablets 844
BC Powder ▣ 517
BC Cold Powder ▣ 517
Children's Bayer Chewable Aspirin ▣ 564
Genuine Bayer Aspirin Tablets & Caplets ▣ 564
Maximum Bayer Aspirin Tablets & Caplets ▣ 566
Bayer Plus Aspirin Tablets ▣ 567
Therapy Bayer Aspirin Caplets ▣ 568
8 Hour Bayer Timed-Release Aspirin ▣ 566
Arthritis Strength Bufferin Analgesic Caplets 744
Extra Strength Bufferin Analgesic Tablets 745
Bufferin Analgesic Tablets and Caplets 743
Cama Arthritis Pain Reliever ▣ 685
Damason-P 1356
Easprin 1719
Ecotrin Enteric Coated Aspirin Maximum Strength Tablets and Caplets 2189
Ecotrin Enteric Coated Aspirin Regular Strength Tablets and Caplets 2189
Empirin Aspirin ▣ 541
Empirin with Codeine Phosphate Nos. 2, 3 & 4 764
Equagesic Tablets 2451
Excedrin Extra-Strength Analgesic Tablets & Caplets 749
4-Way Cold Tablets 750
Fiorinal Capsules 2007
Fiorinal with Codeine Capsules 2008
Fiorinal Tablets 2007
Lortab ASA Tablets 2414
Momentum Muscular Backache Formula ▣ 751
Norgesic 1314
Norwich Extra-Strength Aspirin ▣ 546
Norwich Regular Strength Aspirin ▣ 547
P-A-C Analgesic Tablets ▣ 669
Percodan 951
Robaxisal Tablets 1872
Sine-Off Sinus Medicine Tablets-Aspirin Formula ▣ 722
Soma Compound w/Codeine Tablets 2390
Soma Compound Tablets 2389
St. Joseph Adult Chewable Aspirin (81 mg.) ▣ 703
Synalgos-DC Capsules 2525
Talwin Compound 2072
Ursinus Inlay-Tabs ▣ 691
Vanquish Analgesic Caplets ▣ 574
Zorprin Tablets 698

Aspirin, Enteric Coated (Altered serum drug levels). Products include:
Therapy Bayer Aspirin Caplets ▣ 568
Ecotrin 2189

Carbamazepine (Altered serum drug levels). Products include:
Tegretol Chewable Tablets 654
Tegretol Suspension 656
Tegretol Tablets 654

Clonazepam (Concomitant use may produce absence status). Products include:
Klonopin Tablets 1902

Dicumarol (Altered serum drug levels). Products include:
Dicumarol Tablets 516

Ethinyl Estradiol (Possible oral contraceptive failure). Products include:
Brevicon 2304
Demulen 2161
Estinyl Tablets 2085
Jenest-28 Tablets 1636
Levlen/Tri-Levlen 665
Lo/Ovral Tablets 2471
Lo/Ovral-28 Tablets 2476
Loestrin 1728
Modicon 1667
Nordette-21 Tablets 2481
Nordette-28 Tablets 2483
Norethin 2133
Norinyl 2304
Norlestrin 1746
Ortho-Cyclen Tablets 1658
Ortho-Novum 1667
Ovcon 1391
Ovral Tablets 2490
Ovral-28 Tablets 2491
Levlen/Tri-Levlen 665
Tri-Norinyl 2304
Triphasil-21 Tablets 2527
Triphasil-28 Tablets 2532

Ethosuximide (Altered serum concentrations of both drugs). Products include:
Zarontin Capsules 1768
Zarontin Syrup 1769

Ethynodiol Diacetate (Possible oral contraceptive failure). Products include:
Demulen 2161

Levonorgestrel (Possible oral contraceptive failure). Products include:
Levlen/Tri-Levlen 665
Nordette-21 Tablets 2481
Nordette-28 Tablets 2483
Norplant System 2484
Levlen/Tri-Levlen 665
Triphasil-21 Tablets 2527
Triphasil-28 Tablets 2532

Mestranol (Possible oral contraceptive failure). Products include:
Enovid 2161
Norethin 2133
Norinyl 2304
Ortho-Novum 1667

Norethindrone (Possible oral contraceptive failure). Products include:
Brevicon 2304
Jenest-28 Tablets 1636
Micronor Tablets 1667
Modicon 1667
Norethin 2133
Norinyl 2304
Norlutin 1755
Nor-Q D Tablets 2304
Ortho-Novum 1667
Ovcon 1391
Tri-Norinyl 2304

Norethynodrel (Possible oral contraceptive failure). Products include:
Enovid 2161

Norgestimate (Possible oral contraceptive failure). Products include:
Ortho-Cyclen Tablets 1658

Norgestrel (Possible oral contraceptive failure). Products include:
Lo/Ovral Tablets 2471
Lo/Ovral-28 Tablets 2476
Ovral Tablets 2490
Ovral-28 Tablets 2491
Ovrette Tablets 2492

Phenobarbital (Increased serum phenobarbital levels; potential for increased CNS depression; monitor for neurological toxicity). Products include:
Arco-Lase Plus Tablets 607
Bellergal-S Tablets 1998
Bronkolixir ▣ 761
Bronkotabs Tablets ▣ 762
Donnatal 1858
Donnatal Extentabs 1859
Donnatal Tablets 1858
Donnazyme Tablets 1860
Kinesed Tablets 2272
Phenobarbital Elixir and Tablets 1293
Primatene Tablets-P Formula 2421
Quadrinal Tablets 1183
Tedral SA 1765

Phenytoin (Potential for breakthrough seizures; dosage of phenytoin should be adjusted). Products include:
Dilantin Infatabs 1710
Dilantin-30 Pediatric/Dilantin-125 Suspension 1713

Phenytoin Sodium (Potential for breakthrough seizures; dosage of phenytoin should be adjusted). Products include:
Dilantin Kapseals 1708
Dilantin Parenteral 1712
Dilantin with Phenobarbital Kapseals 1715

Primidone (Potential for neurological toxicity). Products include:
Mysoline 2480

Warfarin Sodium (Altered bleeding time). Products include:
Coumadin Injection & Tablets 944
Panwarfin Tablets 547

DEPEN TITRATABLE TABLETS
(Penicillamine) 2379
May interact with cytotoxic drugs, antimalarials, and certain other agents. Compounds in these categories include:

Auranofin (Serious hematologic and/or renal adverse reactions). Products include:
Ridaura Capsules 2224

Aurothioglucose (Serious hematologic and/or renal adverse reactions). Products include:
Solganal Suspension 2122

Bleomycin Sulfate (Hematologic and renal reactions). Products include:
Blenoxane 724

Chloroquine Hydrochloride (Serious hematologic and/or renal adverse reactions). Products include:
- Aralen Hydrochloride Injection 2038

Chloroquine Phosphate (Serious hematologic and/or renal adverse reactions). Products include:
- Aralen Phosphate with Primaquine Phosphate Tablets 2040
- Aralen Phosphate Tablets 2039

Daunorubicin Hydrochloride (Hematologic and renal reactions). Products include:
- Cerubidine 2443

Doxorubicin Hydrochloride (Hematologic and renal reactions). Products include:
- Adriamycin PFS 561
- Adriamycin RDF 562
- Doxorubicin Hydrochloride for Injection, USP 622
- Doxorubicin Hydrochloride Injection, USP 848
- Rubex 739

Fluorouracil (Hematologic and renal reactions). Products include:
- Efudex 1880
- Fluoroplex Topical Solution & Cream 1% 1082
- Fluorouracil Injection 1897

Gold Sodium Thiomalate (Serious hematologic and/or renal adverse reactions). Products include:
- Myochrysine Injection 1516

Hydroxyurea (Hematologic and renal reactions). Products include:
- Hydrea Capsules 728

Iron Supplements (Reduced effects of penicillamine with orally administered iron).

Mefloquine Hydrochloride (Serious hematologic and/or renal adverse reactions). Products include:
- Lariam Tablets 1904

Methotrexate Sodium (Hematologic and renal reactions). Products include:
- Methotrexate Tablets, Parenteral, LPF Parenteral 1217
- Rheumatrex Methotrexate Dose Pack 1234

Mineral Supplements (Blocked response to penicillamine).

Mitotane (Hematologic and renal reactions). Products include:
- Lysodren 731

Mitoxantrone Hydrochloride (Hematologic and renal reactions). Products include:
- Novantrone for Injection Concentrate 1226

Oxyphenbutazone (Hematologic and renal reactions).

Phenylbutazone (Hematologic and renal reactions). Products include:
- Butazolidin Capsules & Tablets 1027

Primaquine Phosphate (Serious hematologic and/or renal adverse reactions). Products include:
- Aralen Phosphate with Primaquine Phosphate Tablets 2040

Procarbazine Hydrochloride (Hematologic and renal reactions). Products include:
- Matulane Capsules 1907

Pyrimethamine (Serious hematologic and/or renal adverse reactions). Products include:
- Daraprim Tablets 761
- Fansidar Tablets 1896

Tamoxifen Citrate (Hematologic and renal reactions). Products include:
- Nolvadex Tablets 1102

Vincristine Sulfate (Hematologic and renal reactions). Products include:
- Oncovin Solution Vials & Hyporets 1288

DEPO-MEDROL STERILE AQUEOUS SUSPENSION
(Methylprednisolone Acetate) 2334
May interact with:

Aspirin (Aspirin should be used cautiously in conjunction with corticosteroids in hypoprothrombinemia). Products include:
- Alka-Seltzer Effervescent Antacid and Pain Reliever 1568
- Alka-Seltzer Extra Strength Effervescent Antacid and Pain Reliever 1570
- Alka-Seltzer (Flavored) Effervescent Antacid and Pain Reliever 1569
- Alka-Seltzer Plus Cold Medicine .... ⊞ 623
- Alka-Seltzer Plus Night-Time Cold Medicine .... ⊞ 623
- Alka Seltzer Plus Sinus Allergy Medicine .... ⊞ 624
- Anacin Coated Analgesic Caplets 2417
- Anacin Coated Analgesic Tablets 2417
- Anacin Maximum Strength Analgesic Coated Tablets 2417
- Maximum Strength Arthritis Pain Formula By the Makers of Anacin Analgesic Tablets and Caplets 2418
- Arthritis Pain Formula by the Makers of Anacin Analgesic Tablets and Caplets .... ⊞ 747
- Arthritis Strength BC Powder .... ⊞ 516
- Ascriptin A/D Caplets 1850
- Regular Strength Ascriptin Tablets 1850
- Azdone Tablets 844
- BC Powder .... ⊞ 517
- BC Cold Powder .... ⊞ 517
- Children's Bayer Chewable Aspirin .... ⊞ 564
- Genuine Bayer Aspirin Tablets & Caplets .... ⊞ 564
- Maximum Bayer Aspirin Tablets & Caplets .... ⊞ 566
- Bayer Plus Aspirin Tablets .... ⊞ 567
- Therapy Bayer Aspirin Caplets .... ⊞ 568
- 8 Hour Bayer Timed-Release Aspirin .... ⊞ 566
- Arthritis Strength Bufferin Analgesic Caplets 744
- Extra Strength Bufferin Analgesic Tablets 745
- Bufferin Analgesic Tablets and Caplets 743
- Cama Arthritis Pain Reliever .... ⊞ 685
- Damason-P 1356
- Easprin 1719
- Ecotrin Enteric Coated Aspirin Maximum Strength Tablets and Caplets 2189
- Ecotrin Enteric Coated Aspirin Regular Strength Tablets and Caplets 2189
- Empirin Aspirin .... ⊞ 541
- Empirin with Codeine Phosphate Nos. 2, 3 & 4 764
- Equagesic Tablets 2451
- Excedrin Extra-Strength Analgesic Tablets & Caplets 749
- 4-Way Cold Tablets 750
- Fiorinal Capsules 2007
- Fiorinal with Codeine Capsules 2008
- Fiorinal Tablets 2007
- Lortab ASA Tablets 2414
- Momentum Muscular Backache Formula .... ⊞ 751
- Norgesic 1314
- Norwich Extra-Strength Aspirin .... ⊞ 546
- Norwich Regular Strength Aspirin ⊞ 547
- P-A-C Analgesic Tablets .... ⊞ 669
- Percodan 951
- Robaxisal Tablets 1872
- Sine-Off Sinus Medicine Tablets-Aspirin Formula .... ⊞ 722
- Soma Compound w/Codeine Tablets 2390
- Soma Compound Tablets 2389
- St. Joseph Adult Chewable Aspirin (81 mg.) .... ⊞ 703
- Synalgos-DC Capsules 2525
- Talwin Compound 2072
- Ursinus Inlay-Tabs .... ⊞ 691
- Vanquish Analgesic Caplets .... ⊞ 574
- Zorprin Tablets 698

Cyclosporine (Potential for convulsions). Products include:
- Sandimmune 2024

Immunization (Possible neurological complications).

Smallpox Vaccine (Possible neurological complications).

DEPONIT NTG TRANSDERMAL DELIVERY SYSTEM
(Nitroglycerin) 2143
May interact with vasodilators and certain other agents. Compounds in these categories include:

Alcohol (Additive vasodilating effects).

Diazoxide (Additive vasodilating effects). Products include:
- Hyperstat I.V. Injection 2095
- Proglycem 649

Hydralazine Hydrochloride (Additive vasodilating effects). Products include:
- Apresazide Capsules 854
- Apresoline Hydrochloride Parenteral (Ampuls) 856
- Apresoline Hydrochloride Tablets .. 855
- Apresoline-Esidrix Tablets 857
- Ser-Ap-Es Tablets 881
- Serpasil-Apresoline Tablets 884

Minoxidil (Additive vasodilating effects). Products include:
- Loniten Tablets 2346
- Rogaine Topical Solution 2357

DEPO-PROVERA STERILE AQUEOUS SUSPENSION
(Medroxyprogesterone Acetate) 2336
May interact with:

Aminoglutethimide (Significantly depresses the bioavailability of Depo-Provera). Products include:
- Cytadren Tablets 861

DEPROL TABLETS
(Meprobamate, Benactyzine Hydrochloride) 2382
May interact with central nervous system depressants, neuromuscular blocking agents, and certain other agents. Compounds in these categories include:

Alcohol (Additive effects).

Alfentanil Hydrochloride (Additive effects). Products include:
- Alfenta Injection 1131

Alprazolam (Additive effects). Products include:
- Xanax Tablets 2367

Aprobarbital (Additive effects). Products include:
- Alurate Elixir 1883

Buprenorphine (Additive effects).
- No products indexed under this heading.

Buspirone Hydrochloride (Additive effects). Products include:
- BuSpar 1401

Butabarbital (Additive effects). Products include:
- Pyridium Plus 1764

Butalbital (Additive effects). Products include:
- Esgic-Plus Tablets 1002
- Esgic Tablets & Capsules 1001
- Fioricet Tablets 2006
- Fiorinal Capsules 2007
- Fiorinal with Codeine Capsules 2008
- Fiorinal Tablets 2007
- Phrenilin 838
- Sedapap Tablets 50 mg/650 mg .. 1360

Carisoprodol (Cross reaction). Products include:
- Soma Compound w/Codeine Tablets 2390
- Soma Compound Tablets 2389
- Soma Tablets 2388

Chlordiazepoxide (Additive effects). Products include:
- Libritabs Tablets 1930
- Limbitrol 1933
- Menrium Tablets 1934

Chlordiazepoxide Hydrochloride (Additive effects). Products include:
- Librax Capsules 1929
- Librium Capsules 1931
- Librium Injectable 1932

Chlorpromazine (Additive effects). Products include:
- Thorazine 2234

Chlorprothixene (Additive effects). Products include:
- Taractan Tablets 1920

Chlorprothixene Hydrochloride (Additive effects). Products include:
- Taractan 1920

Chlorprothixene Lactate (Additive effects). Products include:
- Taractan Concentrate 1920

Clorazepate Dipotassium (Additive effects). Products include:
- Tranxene 556

Clozapine (Additive effects). Products include:
- Clozaril Tablets 2000

Codeine (Additive effects). Products include:
- Calcidrine Syrup 506

Codeine Phosphate (Additive effects). Products include:
- Actifed with Codeine Cough Syrup.. 752
- Cheracol Cough Syrup 1853
- Codimal PH Syrup 846
- Dimetane-DC Cough Syrup 1857
- Empirin with Codeine Phosphate Nos. 2, 3 & 4 764
- Fiorinal with Codeine Capsules 2008
- Isoclor Expectorant 982
- Naldecon CX Adult Liquid .... ⊞ 521
- Novahistine DH 1342
- Novahistine Expectorant 1343
- Nucofed Capsules 2219
- Nucofed Expectorant 2219
- Nucofed Pediatric Expectorant 2220
- Nucofed Syrup 2219
- Phenaphen with Codeine Capsules 1865
- Phenaphen-650 with Codeine Tablets 1866
- Phenergan with Codeine 2497
- Phenergan VC with Codeine 2501
- Robitussin A-C Syrup 1875
- Robitussin-DAC Syrup 1875
- Ryna .... ⊞ 741
- Soma Compound w/Codeine Tablets 2390
- Triaminic Expectorant w/Codeine .. 1996
- Tussi-Organidin Liquid 2391
- Tylenol with Codeine 1381

Codeine Polistirex (Additive effects).
- No products indexed under this heading.

Dezocine (Additive effects).

Diazepam (Additive effects). Products include:
- Valium Injectable 1937
- Valium Tablets 1939
- Valrelease Capsules 1923

Droperidol (Additive effects). Products include:
- Inapsine Injection 1140
- Innovar Injection 1141

Enflurane (Additive effects). Products include:
- Ethrane 599

Estazolam (Additive effects). Products include:
- ProSom Tablets 554

Ethchlorvynol (Additive effects). Products include:
- Placidyl Capsules 553

Ethinamate (Additive effects).
- No products indexed under this heading.

Fentanyl (Additive effects). Products include:
- Duragesic Transdermal System 1133

Fentanyl Citrate (Additive effects). Products include:
- Innovar Injection 1141
- Sublimaze Injection 1146

Fluphenazine Decanoate (Additive effects). Products include:
- Prolixin Decanoate ... 1795

Fluphenazine Enanthate (Additive effects). Products include:
- Prolixin Enanthate ... 1796

Fluphenazine Hydrochloride (Additive effects). Products include:
- Prolixin Elixir ... 1793
- Prolixin Injection ... 1791
- Prolixin Oral Concentrate ... 1792
- Prolixin Tablets ... 1793

Flurazepam Hydrochloride (Additive effects). Products include:
- Dalmane Capsules ... 1927

Glutethimide (Additive effects).
- No products indexed under this heading.

Haloperidol (Additive effects). Products include:
- Haldol Injection, Tablets and Concentrate ... 1373

Haloperidol Decanoate (Additive effects). Products include:
- Haldol Decanoate ... 1375

Hydrocodone Bitartrate (Additive effects). Products include:
- Anexsia 5/500 Tablets ... 2196
- Anexsia 7.5/650 Tablets ... 2197
- Azdone Tablets ... 844
- Codiclear DH Syrup ... 845
- Codimal DH Syrup ... 846
- Damason-P ... 1356
- Hycodan Syrup, Tablets ... 927
- Hycomine Compound Tablets ... 929
- Hycomine Syrup ... 927
- Hycotuss Expectorant Syrup ... 930
- Hydrocet Capsules ... 835
- Lortab ASA Tablets ... 2414
- Lortab ... 2412
- Ru-Tuss with Hydrocodone ... 694
- Triaminic Expectorant DH ... 1995
- Vicodin Tablets ... 1187
- Vicodin ES Tablets ... 1189
- Zydone Capsules ... 941

Hydrocodone Polistirex (Additive effects). Products include:
- Tussionex Extended-Release Suspension ... 988

Hydroxyzine Hydrochloride (Additive effects). Products include:
- Atarax Tablets & Syrup ... 1941
- Marax Tablets & DF Syrup ... 1954
- Vistaril Intramuscular Solution ... 1970

Isoflurane (Additive effects). Products include:
- Forane ... 600

Ketamine Hydrochloride (Additive effects). Products include:
- Ketalar ... 1726

Levorphanol Tartrate (Additive effects). Products include:
- Levo-Dromoran ... 1906

Lithium Carbonate (Additive effects). Products include:
- Eskalith ... 2214
- Lithane Tablets ... 1596
- Lithium Carbonate Capsules & Tablets ... 1984
- Lithobid Tablets ... 870

Lithium Citrate (Additive effects). Products include:
- Cibalith-S ... 870

Lorazepam (Additive effects). Products include:
- Ativan Injection ... 2432
- Ativan Tablets ... 2434

Loxapine Hydrochloride (Additive effects). Products include:
- Loxitane ... 1213

Loxapine Succinate (Additive effects). Products include:
- Loxitane Capsules ... 1213

Meperidine Hydrochloride (Additive effects). Products include:
- Demerol ... 2047
- Mepergan Injection ... 2479

Mephobarbital (Additive effects). Products include:
- Mebaral Tablets ... 2061

Mesoridazine (Additive effects). Products include:
- Serentil ... 686

Methadone Hydrochloride (Additive effects). Products include:
- Dolophine Hydrochloride Ampoules & Vials ... 1260
- Dolophine Hydrochloride Tablets ... 1261
- Methadone Hydrochloride Diskets ... 1284
- Methadone Hydrochloride Oral Solution & Tablets ... 1987

Methohexital Sodium (Additive effects). Products include:
- Brevital Sodium Vials ... 1248

Methoxyflurane (Additive effects).
- No products indexed under this heading.

Midazolam Hydrochloride (Additive effects). Products include:
- Versed Injection ... 1924

Molindone Hydrochloride (Additive effects). Products include:
- Moban Tablets & Concentrate ... 932

Morphine Sulfate (Additive effects). Products include:
- Astramorph/PF Injection, USP (Preservative-Free) ... 618
- Duramorph ... 960
- Infumorph 200 and Infumorph 500 Sterile Solutions ... 962
- MS Contin Tablets ... 1814
- MSIR ... 1817
- Oramorph SR (Morphine Sulfate Sustained Release Tablets) ... 1988
- Roxanol ... 1991

Opium Alkaloids (Additive effects). Products include:
- B & O No. 15A & No. 16A Supprettes ... 2395
- Pantopon Injectable ... 1911

Oxazepam (Additive effects). Products include:
- Serax Capsules ... 2522
- Serax Tablets ... 2522

Oxycodone Hydrochloride (Additive effects). Products include:
- Percocet Tablets ... 950
- Percodan ... 951
- Roxicodone Tablets, Oral Solution & Intensol (Oxycodone) ... 1992
- Tylox Capsules ... 1382

Pentobarbital Sodium (Additive effects). Products include:
- Nembutal Sodium Capsules ... 534
- Nembutal Sodium Solution ... 536
- Nembutal Sodium Suppositories ... 538

Perphenazine (Additive effects). Products include:
- Etrafon ... 2087
- Triavil Tablets ... 1556
- Trilafon ... 2123

Phenobarbital (Additive effects). Products include:
- Arco-Lase Plus Tablets ... 607
- Bellergal-S Tablets ... 1998
- Bronkolixir ... ▣ 761
- Bronkotabs Tablets ... ▣ 762
- Donnatal ... 1858
- Donnatal Extentabs ... 1859
- Donnatal Tablets ... 1858
- Donnazyme Tablets ... 1860
- Kinesed Tablets ... 2272
- Phenobarbital Elixir and Tablets ... 1293
- Primatene Tablets-P Formula ... 2421
- Quadrinal Tablets ... 1183
- Tedral SA ... 1765

Pimozide (Additive effects). Products include:
- Orap Tablets ... 1020

Prazepam (Additive effects). Products include:
- Centrax ... 1693

Prednisolone (Bullous dermatitis).
- No products indexed under this heading.

Prednisolone Acetate (Bullous dermatitis). Products include:
- AK-Cide Sterile Ophthalmic Ointment & Suspension ... ◎ 202
- Blephamide Liquifilm Sterile Ophthalmic Suspension ... 586
- Blephamide S.O.P. Sterile Ophthalmic Ointment ... 586
- Cetapred Ointment ... ◎ 220
- ⅛% Econopred & 1% Econopred Plus ... ◎ 217
- Isopto Cetapred Suspension ... ◎ 220
- Metimyd ... ◎ 306
- Poly-Pred Liquifilm ... ◎ 250
- Pred Forte ... ◎ 252
- Pred Mild ... ◎ 254
- Pred-G Liquifilm Sterile Ophthalmic Suspension ... ◎ 252
- Pred-G S.O.P. Sterile Ophthalmic Ointment ... ◎ 253
- Vasocidin Ointment ... ◎ 275

Prednisolone Sodium Phosphate (Bullous dermatitis). Products include:
- AK-Pred ... ◎ 205
- Hydeltrasol Injection, Sterile ... 1476
- Inflamase ... ◎ 274
- Pediapred Oral Liquid ... 987
- Vasocidin Ophthalmic Solution ... ◎ 276

Prednisolone Tebutate (Bullous dermatitis). Products include:
- Hydeltra-T.B.A. Sterile Suspension 1478

Prochlorperazine (Additive effects). Products include:
- Compazine ... 2201

Promethazine Hydrochloride (Additive effects). Products include:
- Mepergan Injection ... 2479
- Phenergan with Codeine ... 2497
- Phenergan with Dextromethorphan 2499
- Phenergan Injection ... 2493
- Phenergan Suppositories ... 2496
- Phenergan Syrup ... 2495
- Phenergan Tablets ... 2496
- Phenergan VC ... 2500
- Phenergan VC with Codeine ... 2501

Propofol (Additive effects). Products include:
- Diprivan Injection ... 2267

Propoxyphene Hydrochloride (Additive effects). Products include:
- Darvon ... 1256
- Wygesic Tablets ... 2540

Propoxyphene Napsylate (Additive effects). Products include:
- Darvon-N/Darvocet-N ... 1254

Quazepam (Additive effects). Products include:
- Doral Tablets ... 2383

Secobarbital Sodium (Additive effects). Products include:
- Seconal Sodium Pulvules ... 1296

Sufentanil Citrate (Additive effects). Products include:
- Sufenta Injection ... 1147

Temazepam (Additive effects). Products include:
- Restoril Capsules ... 2023

Thiamylal Sodium (Additive effects). Products include:
- Surital Ampoules, Steri-Vials ... 1764

Thioridazine Hydrochloride (Additive effects). Products include:
- Mellaril ... 2011

Thiothixene (Additive effects). Products include:
- Navane Capsules and Concentrate 1954
- Navane Intramuscular ... 1956

Triazolam (Additive effects). Products include:
- Halcion Tablets ... 2340

Trifluoperazine Hydrochloride (Additive effects). Products include:
- Stelazine ... 2226

DERIFIL TABLETS
(Chlorophyllin Copper Complex) ... 1994
No interactions described in labeling.

DERMAIDE ALOE CREAM
(Aloe Vera) ... 906
No interactions described in labeling.

DERMOLATE ANTI-ITCH CREAM
(Hydrocortisone) ... ▣ 697
No interactions described in labeling.

DERMOPLAST ANESTHETIC PAIN RELIEF LOTION
(Benzocaine) ... 2418
No interactions described in labeling.

DERMOPLAST ANESTHETIC PAIN RELIEF SPRAY
(Benzocaine, Menthol) ... 2419
No interactions described in labeling.

DESENEX ANTIFUNGAL CREAM
(Undecylenic Acid, Zinc Undecylenate) ... ▣ 561
No interactions described in labeling.

DESENEX ANTIFUNGAL FOAM
(Undecylenic Acid) ... ▣ 561
No interactions described in labeling.

DESENEX ANTIFUNGAL OINTMENT
(Undecylenic Acid, Zinc Undecylenate) ... ▣ 561
No interactions described in labeling.

DESENEX ANTIFUNGAL POWDER
(Undecylenic Acid, Zinc Undecylenate) ... ▣ 561
No interactions described in labeling.

DESENEX ANTIFUNGAL SPRAY POWDER
(Undecylenic Acid, Zinc Undecylenate) ... ▣ 561
No interactions described in labeling.

DESENEX FOOT & SNEAKER DEODORANT SPRAY
(Aluminum Chlorohydrate) ... ▣ 561
No interactions described in labeling.

DESENEX SOAP
(Soap) ... ▣ 561
No interactions described in labeling.

DESFERAL VIALS
(Deferoxamine Mesylate) ... 862
No interactions described in labeling.

DESITIN OINTMENT
(Cod Liver Oil, Zinc Oxide) ... ▣ 644
No interactions described in labeling.

DESOWEN CREAM, OINTMENT AND LOTION
(Desonide) ... 1682
No interactions described in labeling.

DESOXYN GRADUMET TABLETS
(Methamphetamine Hydrochloride) .. 514
May interact with insulin, monoamine oxidase inhibitors, phenothiazines, tricyclic antidepressants, and certain other agents. Compounds in these categories include:

Amitriptyline Hydrochloride (Concurrent administration should be closely supervised and dosage carefully adjusted). Products include:
- Elavil ... 2269
- Endep Tablets ... 1927
- Etrafon ... 2087
- Limbitrol ... 1933
- Triavil Tablets ... 1556

Amoxapine (Concurrent administration should be closely supervised and dosage carefully adjusted). Products include:
- Asendin Tablets ... 1196

Chlorpromazine (May antagonize the CNS stimulant action of the amphetamine). Products include:
- Thorazine 2234

Clomipramine Hydrochloride (Concurrent administration should be closely supervised and dosage carefully adjusted). Products include:
- Anafranil Capsules 650

Desipramine Hydrochloride (Concurrent administration should be closely supervised and dosage carefully adjusted). Products include:
- Norpramin Tablets 1340

Doxepin Hydrochloride (Concurrent administration should be closely supervised and dosage carefully adjusted). Products include:
- Sinequan 1960

Fluphenazine Decanoate (May antagonize the CNS stimulant action of the amphetamine). Products include:
- Prolixin Decanoate 1795

Fluphenazine Enanthate (May antagonize the CNS stimulant action of the amphetamine). Products include:
- Prolixin Enanthate 1796

Fluphenazine Hydrochloride (May antagonize the CNS stimulant action of the amphetamine). Products include:
- Prolixin Elixir 1793
- Prolixin Injection 1791
- Prolixin Oral Concentrate 1792
- Prolixin Tablets 1793

Furazolidone (Concurrent or sequential administration is contraindicated). Products include:
- Furoxone 1855

Guanethidine Monosulfate (Decreased hypotensive effect). Products include:
- Esimil Tablets 864
- Ismelin Tablets 869

Imipramine Hydrochloride (Concurrent administration should be closely supervised and dosage carefully adjusted). Products include:
- Tofranil Ampuls 1038
- Tofranil Tablets 1039

Imipramine Pamoate (Concurrent administration should be closely supervised and dosage carefully adjusted). Products include:
- Tofranil-PM Capsules 1041

Insulin, Human (Insulin requirement in diabetics may be altered).
- No products indexed under this heading.

Insulin, Human Isophane Suspension (Insulin requirement in diabetics may be altered). Products include:
- Humulin N, 100 Units 1270

Insulin, Human NPH (Insulin requirement in diabetics may be altered). Products include:
- Insulatard NPH Human 1627
- Novolin N 1627
- Novolin N PenFill Cartridges 1628
- Novolin N Prefilled 1628

Insulin, Human Regular (Insulin requirement in diabetics may be altered). Products include:
- Humulin BR, 100 Units 1268
- Humulin R, 100 Units 1272
- Novolin R 1627
- Novolin R PenFill Cartridges 1628
- Novolin R Prefilled 1629
- Velosulin Human 1628

Insulin, Human, Zinc Suspension (Insulin requirement in diabetics may be altered). Products include:
- Humulin L, 100 Units 1268
- Humulin U, 100 Units 1272
- Novolin L 1627

Insulin, NPH (Insulin requirement in diabetics may be altered). Products include:
- NPH, 40 & 100 Units 1273
- Beef NPH, 100 Units 1274
- Pork NPH, 100 Units 1275
- Insulatard NPH 1626
- NPH Insulin 1626
- NPH Purified Pork Isophane Insulin 1626

Insulin, Regular (Insulin requirement in diabetics may be altered). Products include:
- Regular, 40 & 100 Units 1273
- Beef Regular, 100 Units 1275
- Pork Regular, 100 Units 1275
- Pork Regular (Concentrated), 500 Units 1276
- Regular Insulin 1625
- Regular Purified Pork Insulin 1626
- Velosulin 1627

Insulin, Zinc Crystals (Insulin requirement in diabetics may be altered). Products include:
- NPH, 40 & 100 Units 1273

Insulin, Zinc Suspension (Insulin requirement in diabetics may be altered). Products include:
- Lente, 40 & 100 Units 1272
- Protamine, Zinc, 40 & 100 Units 1273
- Lente Iletin I 1272
- Beef Lente, 100 Units 1274
- Beef Protamine Zinc, 100 Units 1274
- Pork Lente, 100 Units 1275
- Pork, Protamine, Zinc, 100 Units 1275
- Lente Insulin 1626
- Lente Purified Pork Insulin 1626
- Semilente Insulin 1625
- Ultralente Insulin 1626

Isocarboxazid (Concurrent or sequential administration is contraindicated). Products include:
- Marplan Tablets 1906

Maprotiline Hydrochloride (Concurrent administration should be closely supervised and dosage carefully adjusted). Products include:
- Ludiomil Tablets 874

Mesoridazine Besylate (May antagonize the CNS stimulant action of the amphetamine).

Nortriptyline Hydrochloride (Concurrent administration should be closely supervised and dosage carefully adjusted). Products include:
- Pamelor 2019

Perphenazine (May antagonize the CNS stimulant action of the amphetamine). Products include:
- Etrafon 2087
- Triavil Tablets 1556
- Trilafon 2123

Phenelzine Sulfate (Concurrent or sequential administration is contraindicated). Products include:
- Nardil 1742

Prochlorperazine (May antagonize the CNS stimulant action of the amphetamine). Products include:
- Compazine 2201

Promethazine Hydrochloride (May antagonize the CNS stimulant action of the amphetamine). Products include:
- Mepergan Injection 2479
- Phenergan with Codeine 2497
- Phenergan with Dextromethorphan 2499
- Phenergan Injection 2493
- Phenergan Suppositories 2496
- Phenergan Syrup 2495
- Phenergan Tablets 2496
- Phenergan VC 2500
- Phenergan VC with Codeine 2501

Protriptyline Hydrochloride (Concurrent administration should be closely supervised and dosage carefully adjusted). Products include:
- Vivactil Tablets 1567

Selegiline Hydrochloride (Concurrent or sequential administration is contraindicated). Products include:
- Eldepryl 2250

Thioridazine Hydrochloride (May antagonize the CNS stimulant action of the amphetamine). Products include:
- Mellaril 2011

Tranylcypromine Sulfate (Concurrent or sequential administration is contraindicated). Products include:
- Parnate Tablets 2222

Trifluoperazine Hydrochloride (May antagonize the CNS stimulant action of the amphetamine). Products include:
- Stelazine 2226

Trimipramine Maleate (Concurrent administration should be closely supervised and dosage carefully adjusted). Products include:
- Surmontil Capsules 2524

DESQUAM-E 2.5 EMOLLIENT GEL
(Benzoyl Peroxide) 2397
May interact with:

Octyl Dimethyl PABA (Concurrent use with PABA-containing sunscreens may result in transient discoloration of the skin). Products include:
- Herpecin-L Cold Sore Lip Balm 833
- PreSun 15 Facial Sunscreen .... ▣ 537
- PreSun 8, 15 and 39 Creamy Sunscreens .... ▣ 537
- PreSun 23 Spray Mist .... ▣ 537
- Solbar Plus 15 Cream 1772

DESQUAM-E 5 EMOLLIENT GEL
(Benzoyl Peroxide) 2397
See **Desquam-E 2.5 Emollient Gel**

DESQUAM-E 10 EMOLLIENT GEL
(Benzoyl Peroxide) 2397
See **Desquam-E 2.5 Emollient Gel**

DESQUAM-X 2.5 GEL
(Benzoyl Peroxide) 2397
See **Desquam-E 2.5 Emollient Gel**

DESQUAM-X 5 GEL
(Benzoyl Peroxide) 2397
See **Desquam-E 2.5 Emollient Gel**

DESQUAM-X 10 GEL
(Benzoyl Peroxide) 2397
See **Desquam-E 2.5 Emollient Gel**

DESQUAM-X 5 WASH
(Benzoyl Peroxide) 2397
See **Desquam-E 2.5 Emollient Gel**

DESQUAM-X 10 BAR
(Benzoyl Peroxide) 2397
See **Desquam-E 2.5 Emollient Gel**

DESQUAM-X 10 WASH
(Benzoyl Peroxide) 2397
See **Desquam-E 2.5 Emollient Gel**

DESYREL AND DESYREL DIVIDOSE
(Trazodone Hydrochloride) 1404
May interact with monoamine oxidase inhibitors, central nervous system depressants, antihypertensives, oral anticoagulants, and certain other agents. Compounds in these categories include:

Acebutolol Hydrochloride (Concomitant administration may require a reduction in the dose of the antihypertensives). Products include:
- Sectral Capsules 2520

Alcohol (Enhanced response to alcohol).

Alfentanil Hydrochloride (Enhanced response to CNS depressants). Products include:
- Alfenta Injection 1131

Alprazolam (Enhanced response to CNS depressants). Products include:
- Xanax Tablets 2367

Aprobarbital (Enhanced response to CNS depressants). Products include:
- Alurate Elixir 1883

Atenolol (Concomitant administration may require a reduction in the dose of the antihypertensives). Products include:
- Tenoretic Tablets 1105
- Tenormin Tablets and I.V. Injection 1107

Benazepril Hydrochloride (Concomitant administration may require a reduction in the dose of the antihypertensives). Products include:
- Lotensin Tablets 872

Bendroflumethiazide (Concomitant administration may require a reduction in the dose of the antihypertensives). Products include:
- Corzide Tablets 702
- Naturetin Tablets 1789
- Rauzide Tablets 1804

Betaxolol Hydrochloride (Concomitant administration may require a reduction in the dose of the antihypertensives). Products include:
- Betoptic Sterile Ophthalmic Solution 569
- Betoptic S Sterile Ophthalmic Suspension 570
- Kerlone Tablets 2172

Buprenorphine (Enhanced response to CNS depressants).
- No products indexed under this heading.

Buspirone Hydrochloride (Enhanced response to CNS depressants). Products include:
- BuSpar 1401

Butabarbital (Enhanced response to CNS depressants). Products include:
- Pyridium Plus 1764

Butalbital (Enhanced response to CNS depressants). Products include:
- Esgic-Plus Tablets 1002
- Esgic Tablets & Capsules 1001
- Fioricet Tablets 2006
- Fiorinal Capsules 2007
- Fiorinal with Codeine Capsules 2008
- Fiorinal Tablets 2007
- Phrenilin 838
- Sedapap Tablets 50 mg/650 mg . 1360

Captopril (Concomitant administration may require a reduction in the dose of the antihypertensives). Products include:
- Capoten 2255
- Capozide 2258

Carteolol Hydrochloride (Concomitant administration may require a reduction in the dose of the antihypertensives). Products include:
- Cartrol Tablets 507

Chlordiazepoxide (Enhanced response to CNS depressants). Products include:
- Libritabs Tablets 1930
- Limbitrol 1933
- Menrium Tablets 1934

Chlordiazepoxide Hydrochloride (Enhanced response to CNS depressants). Products include:
- Librax Capsules ... 1929
- Librium Capsules ... 1931
- Librium Injectable ... 1932

Chlorothiazide (Concomitant administration may require a reduction in the dose of the antihypertensives). Products include:
- Aldoclor Tablets ... 1413
- Diupres Tablets ... 1461
- Diuril Oral ... 1464

Chlorothiazide Sodium (Concomitant administration may require a reduction in the dose of the antihypertensives). Products include:
- Diuril Sodium Intravenous ... 1463

Chlorpromazine (Enhanced response to CNS depressants). Products include:
- Thorazine ... 2234

Chlorprothixene (Enhanced response to CNS depressants). Products include:
- Taractan Tablets ... 1920

Chlorprothixene Hydrochloride (Enhanced response to CNS depressants). Products include:
- Taractan ... 1920

Chlorthalidone (Concomitant administration may require a reduction in the dose of the antihypertensives). Products include:
- Combipres Tablets ... 678
- Tenoretic Tablets ... 1105
- Thalitone Tablets ... 687

Clonidine (Concomitant administration may require a reduction in the dose of the antihypertensives). Products include:
- Catapres-TTS ... 677

Clonidine Hydrochloride (Concomitant administration may require a reduction in the dose of the antihypertensives). Products include:
- Catapres Tablets ... 676
- Combipres Tablets ... 678

Clorazepate Dipotassium (Enhanced response to CNS depressants). Products include:
- Tranxene ... 556

Codeine (Enhanced response to CNS depressants). Products include:
- Calcidrine Syrup ... 506

Codeine Phosphate (Enhanced response to CNS depressants). Products include:
- Actifed with Codeine Cough Syrup ... 752
- Cheracol Cough Syrup ... 1853
- Codimal PH Syrup ... 846
- Dimetane-DC Cough Syrup ... 1857
- Empirin with Codeine Phosphate Nos. 2, 3 & 4 ... 764
- Fiorinal with Codeine Capsules ... 2008
- Isoclor Expectorant ... 982
- Naldecon CX Adult Liquid ... 521
- Novahistine DH ... 1342
- Novahistine Expectorant ... 1343
- Nucofed Capsules ... 2219
- Nucofed Expectorant ... 2219
- Nucofed Pediatric Expectorant ... 2220
- Nucofed Syrup ... 2219
- Phenaphen with Codeine Capsules 1865
- Phenaphen-650 with Codeine Tablets ... 1866
- Phenergan with Codeine ... 2497
- Phenergan VC with Codeine ... 2501
- Robitussin A-C Syrup ... 1875
- Robitussin-DAC Syrup ... 1875
- Ryna ... 741
- Soma Compound w/Codeine Tablets ... 2390
- Triaminic Expectorant w/Codeine ... 1996
- Tussi-Organidin Liquid ... 2391
- Tylenol with Codeine ... 1381

Codeine Polistirex (Enhanced response to CNS depressants).
- No products indexed under this heading.

Deserpidine (Concomitant administration may require a reduction in the dose of the antihypertensives). Products include:
- Enduronyl ... 518
- Harmonyl Tablets ... 528
- Oreticyl ... 545

Dezocine (Enhanced response to CNS depressants).

Diazepam (Enhanced response to CNS depressants). Products include:
- Valium Injectable ... 1937
- Valium Tablets ... 1939
- Valrelease Capsules ... 1923

Diazoxide (Concomitant administration may require a reduction in the dose of the antihypertensives). Products include:
- Hyperstat I.V. Injection ... 2095
- Proglycem ... 649

Dicumarol (Increased or decreased prothrombin time). Products include:
- Dicumarol Tablets ... 516

Digoxin (Increased serum levels of digoxin). Products include:
- Lanoxicaps ... 772
- Lanoxin Elixir Pediatric ... 775
- Lanoxin Injection ... 778
- Lanoxin Injection Pediatric ... 781
- Lanoxin Tablets ... 783

Doxazosin Mesylate (Concomitant administration may require a reduction in the dose of the antihypertensives). Products include:
- Cardura Tablets ... 1941

Droperidol (Enhanced response to CNS depressants). Products include:
- Inapsine Injection ... 1140
- Innovar Injection ... 1141

Enalapril Maleate (Concomitant administration may require a reduction in the dose of the antihypertensives). Products include:
- Vaseretic Tablets ... 1559
- Vasotec Tablets ... 1564

Enalaprilat (Concomitant administration may require a reduction in the dose of the antihypertensives). Products include:
- Vasotec I.V. ... 1562

Enflurane (Enhanced response to CNS depressants). Products include:
- Ethrane ... 599

Esmolol Hydrochloride (Concomitant administration may require a reduction in the dose of the antihypertensives). Products include:
- Brevibloc Injection ... 942

Estazolam (Enhanced response to CNS depressants). Products include:
- ProSom Tablets ... 554

Ethchlorvynol (Enhanced response to CNS depressants). Products include:
- Placidyl Capsules ... 553

Ethinamate (Enhanced response to CNS depressants).
- No products indexed under this heading.

Felodipine (Concomitant administration may require a reduction in the dose of the antihypertensives). Products include:
- Plendil Extended-Release Tablets ... 1526

Fentanyl (Enhanced response to CNS depressants). Products include:
- Duragesic Transdermal System ... 1133

Fentanyl Citrate (Enhanced response to CNS depressants). Products include:
- Innovar Injection ... 1141
- Sublimaze Injection ... 1146

Fluphenazine Decanoate (Enhanced response to CNS depressants). Products include:
- Prolixin Decanoate ... 1795

Fluphenazine Enanthate (Enhanced response to CNS depressants). Products include:
- Prolixin Enanthate ... 1796

Fluphenazine Hydrochloride (Enhanced response to CNS depressants). Products include:
- Prolixin Elixir ... 1793
- Prolixin Injection ... 1791
- Prolixin Oral Concentrate ... 1792
- Prolixin Tablets ... 1793

Flurazepam Hydrochloride (Enhanced response to CNS depressants). Products include:
- Dalmane Capsules ... 1927

Fosinopril Sodium (Concomitant administration may require a reduction in the dose of the antihypertensives). Products include:
- Monopril Tablets ... 1406

Furazolidone (Initiate Desyrel cautiously). Products include:
- Furoxone ... 1855

Furosemide (Concomitant administration may require a reduction in the dose of the antihypertensives). Products include:
- Lasix ... 1093

Glutethimide (Enhanced response to CNS depressants).
- No products indexed under this heading.

Guanabenz Acetate (Concomitant administration may require a reduction in the dose of the antihypertensives). Products include:
- Wytensin Tablets ... 2542

Guanethidine Monosulfate (Concomitant administration may require a reduction in the dose of the antihypertensives). Products include:
- Esimil Tablets ... 864
- Ismelin Tablets ... 869

Haloperidol (Enhanced response to CNS depressants). Products include:
- Haldol Injection, Tablets and Concentrate ... 1373

Haloperidol Decanoate (Enhanced response to CNS depressants). Products include:
- Haldol Decanoate ... 1375

Hydralazine Hydrochloride (Concomitant administration may require a reduction in the dose of the antihypertensives). Products include:
- Apresazide Capsules ... 854
- Apresoline Hydrochloride Parenteral (Ampuls) ... 856
- Apresoline Hydrochloride Tablets ... 855
- Apresoline-Esidrix Tablets ... 857
- Ser-Ap-Es Tablets ... 881
- Serpasil-Apresoline Tablets ... 884

Hydrochlorothiazide (Concomitant administration may require a reduction in the dose of the antihypertensives). Products include:
- Aldactazide ... 2150
- Aldoril Tablets ... 1418
- Apresazide Capsules ... 854
- Apresoline-Esidrix Tablets ... 857
- Capozide ... 2258
- Dyazide Capsules ... 2208
- Esidrix Tablets ... 863
- Esimil Tablets ... 864
- HydroDIURIL Tablets ... 1484
- Hydropres Tablets ... 1485
- Inderide Tablets ... 2463
- Inderide LA Long Acting Capsules ... 2465
- Lopressor HCT Tablets ... 1034
- Maxzide ... 1215
- Moduretic Tablets ... 1510
- Normozide Tablets ... 2112
- Oretic Tablets ... 544
- Oreticyl ... 545
- Prinzide Tablets ... 1540
- Ser-Ap-Es Tablets ... 881
- Serpasil-Esidrix Tablets ... 886
- Timolide Tablets ... 1547
- Trandate HCT Tablets ... 579
- Vaseretic Tablets ... 1559
- Zestoretic ... 2274

Hydrocodone Bitartrate (Enhanced response to CNS depressants). Products include:
- Anexsia 5/500 Tablets ... 2196
- Anexsia 7.5/650 Tablets ... 2197
- Azdone Tablets ... 844
- Codiclear DH Syrup ... 845
- Codimal DH Syrup ... 846
- Damason-P ... 1356
- Hycodan Syrup, Tablets ... 927
- Hycomine Compound Tablets ... 929
- Hycomine Syrup ... 927
- Hycotuss Expectorant Syrup ... 930
- Hydrocet Capsules ... 835
- Lortab ASA Tablets ... 2414
- Lortab ... 2412
- Ru-Tuss with Hydrocodone ... 694
- Triaminic Expectorant DH ... 1995
- Vicodin Tablets ... 1187
- Vicodin ES Tablets ... 1189
- Zydone Capsules ... 941

Hydrocodone Polistirex (Enhanced response to CNS depressants). Products include:
- Tussionex Extended-Release Suspension ... 988

Hydroflumethiazide (Concomitant administration may require a reduction in the dose of the antihypertensives). Products include:
- Diucardin Tablets ... 2450
- Saluron ... 718
- Salutensin/Salutensin-Demi ... 719

Hydroxyzine Hydrochloride (Enhanced response to CNS depressants). Products include:
- Atarax Tablets & Syrup ... 1941
- Marax Tablets & DF Syrup ... 1954
- Vistaril Intramuscular Solution ... 1970

Indapamide (Concomitant administration may require a reduction in the dose of the antihypertensives). Products include:
- Lozol Tablets ... 1843

Isocarboxazid (Initiate Desyrel cautiously). Products include:
- Marplan Tablets ... 1906

Isoflurane (Enhanced response to CNS depressants). Products include:
- Forane ... 600

Isradipine (Concomitant administration may require a reduction in the dose of the antihypertensives). Products include:
- DynaCirc Capsules ... 2004

Ketamine Hydrochloride (Enhanced response to CNS depressants). Products include:
- Ketalar ... 1726

Labetalol Hydrochloride (Concomitant administration may require a reduction in the dose of the antihypertensives). Products include:
- Normodyne Injection ... 2108
- Normodyne Tablets ... 2110
- Normozide Tablets ... 2112
- Trandate HCT Tablets ... 579
- Trandate Injection ... 577
- Trandate Tablets ... 579

Levorphanol Tartrate (Enhanced response to CNS depressants). Products include:
- Levo-Dromoran ... 1906

Lisinopril (Concomitant administration may require a reduction in the dose of the antihypertensives). Products include:
- Prinivil Tablets ... 1538
- Prinzide Tablets ... 1540
- Zestoretic ... 2274
- Zestril Tablets ... 2277

Lorazepam (Enhanced response to CNS depressants). Products include:
- Ativan Injection ... 2432
- Ativan Tablets ... 2434

Loxapine Hydrochloride (Enhanced response to CNS depressants). Products include:
- Loxitane ... 1213

Loxapine Succinate (Enhanced response to CNS depressants). Products include:
- Loxitane Capsules ... 1213

Mecamylamine Hydrochloride (Concomitant administration may require a reduction in the dose of the antihypertensives). Products include:
- Inversine Tablets ... 1492

Meperidine Hydrochloride (Enhanced response to CNS depressants). Products include:
- Demerol ... 2047
- Mepergan Injection ... 2479

Mephobarbital (Enhanced response to CNS depressants). Products include:
- Mebaral Tablets ... 2061

Meprobamate (Enhanced response to CNS depressants). Products include:
- Deprol Tablets ... 2382
- Equagesic Tablets ... 2451
- Miltown Tablets ... 2386
- PMB 200 and PMB 400 ... 2504

Mesoridazine (Enhanced response to CNS depressants). Products include:
- Serentil ... 686

Methadone Hydrochloride (Enhanced response to CNS depressants). Products include:
- Dolophine Hydrochloride Ampoules & Vials ... 1260
- Dolophine Hydrochloride Tablets ... 1261
- Methadone Hydrochloride Diskets ... 1284
- Methadone Hydrochloride Oral Solution & Tablets ... 1987

Methohexital Sodium (Enhanced response to CNS depressants). Products include:
- Brevital Sodium Vials ... 1248

Methoxyflurane (Enhanced response to CNS depressants).
- No products indexed under this heading.

Methyclothiazide (Concomitant administration may require a reduction in the dose of the antihypertensives). Products include:
- Enduron Tablets ... 517
- Enduronyl ... 518

Methyldopa (Concomitant administration may require a reduction in the dose of the antihypertensives). Products include:
- Aldoclor Tablets ... 1413
- Aldomet Oral ... 1415
- Aldoril Tablets ... 1418

Methyldopate Hydrochloride (Concomitant administration may require a reduction in the dose of the antihypertensives). Products include:
- Aldomet Ester HCl Injection ... 1417

Metolazone (Concomitant administration may require a reduction in the dose of the antihypertensives). Products include:
- Diulo ... 2129
- Mykrox ½ mg Tablets ... 984
- Zaroxolyn Tablets ... 989

Metoprolol Tartrate (Concomitant administration may require a reduction in the dose of the antihypertensives). Products include:
- Lopressor Ampuls ... 1032
- Lopressor HCT Tablets ... 1034
- Lopressor Tablets ... 1032

Metyrosine (Concomitant administration may require a reduction in the dose of the antihypertensives). Products include:
- Demser Capsules ... 1460

Midazolam Hydrochloride (Enhanced response to CNS depressants). Products include:
- Versed Injection ... 1924

Minoxidil (Concomitant administration may require a reduction in the dose of the antihypertensives). Products include:
- Loniten Tablets ... 2346
- Rogaine Topical Solution ... 2357

Molindone Hydrochloride (Enhanced response to CNS depressants). Products include:
- Moban Tablets & Concentrate ... 932

Morphine Sulfate (Enhanced response to CNS depressants). Products include:
- Astramorph/PF Injection, USP (Preservative-Free) ... 618
- Duramorph ... 960
- Infumorph 200 and Infumorph 500 Sterile Solutions ... 962
- MS Contin Tablets ... 1814
- MSIR ... 1817
- Oramorph SR (Morphine Sulfate Sustained Release Tablets) ... 1988
- Roxanol ... 1991

Nadolol (Concomitant administration may require a reduction in the dose of the antihypertensives). Products include:
- Corgard Tablets ... 701
- Corzide Tablets ... 702

Nicardipine Hydrochloride (Concomitant administration may require a reduction in the dose of the antihypertensives). Products include:
- Cardene Capsules ... 2290

Nitroglycerin (Concomitant administration may require a reduction in the dose of the antihypertensives). Products include:
- Deponit NTG Transdermal Delivery System ... 2143
- Minitran Transdermal Delivery System ... 1312
- Nitro-Bid Ointment ... 1339
- Nitro-Bid Capsules ... 1338
- Nitrodisc ... 2176
- Nitro-Dur (nitroglycerin) Transdermal Infusion System ... 1164
- Nitrogard Tablets ... 1004
- Nitrolingual Spray ... 1846
- Nitrostat Tablets ... 1743
- Transderm-Nitro Transdermal Therapeutic System ... 2283

Opium Alkaloids (Enhanced response to CNS depressants). Products include:
- B & O No. 15A & No. 16A Supprettes ... 2395
- Pantopon Injectable ... 1911

Oxazepam (Enhanced response to CNS depressants). Products include:
- Serax Capsules ... 2522
- Serax Tablets ... 2522

Oxycodone Hydrochloride (Enhanced response to CNS depressants). Products include:
- Percocet Tablets ... 950
- Percodan ... 951
- Roxicodone Tablets, Oral Solution & Intensol (Oxycodone) ... 1992
- Tylox Capsules ... 1382

Penbutolol Sulfate (Concomitant administration may require a reduction in the dose of the antihypertensives). Products include:
- Levatol ... 1832

Pentobarbital Sodium (Enhanced response to CNS depressants). Products include:
- Nembutal Sodium Capsules ... 534
- Nembutal Sodium Solution ... 536
- Nembutal Sodium Suppositories ... 538

Perphenazine (Enhanced response to CNS depressants). Products include:
- Etrafon ... 2087
- Triavil Tablets ... 1556
- Trilafon ... 2123

Phenelzine Sulfate (Initiate Desyrel cautiously). Products include:
- Nardil ... 1742

Phenobarbital (Enhanced response to CNS depressants). Products include:
- Arco-Lase Plus Tablets ... 607
- Bellergal-S Tablets ... 1998
- Bronkolixir ... ⊞ 761
- Bronkotabs Tablets ... ⊞ 762
- Donnatal ... 1858
- Donnatal Extentabs ... 1859
- Donnatal Tablets ... 1858
- Donnazyme Tablets ... 1860
- Kinesed Tablets ... 2272
- Phenobarbital Elixir and Tablets ... 1293
- Primatene Tablets-P Formula ... 2421
- Quadrinal Tablets ... 1183
- Tedral SA ... 1765

Phenoxybenzamine Hydrochloride (Concomitant administration may require a reduction in the dose of the antihypertensives). Products include:
- Dibenzyline Capsules ... 2207

Phentolamine Mesylate (Concomitant administration may require a reduction in the dose of the antihypertensives). Products include:
- Regitine ... 878

Phenytoin (Increased serum levels of phenytoin). Products include:
- Dilantin Infatabs ... 1710
- Dilantin-30 Pediatric/Dilantin-125 Suspension ... 1713

Phenytoin Sodium (Increased serum levels of phenytoin). Products include:
- Dilantin Kapseals ... 1708
- Dilantin Parenteral ... 1712
- Dilantin with Phenobarbital Kapseals ... 1715

Pindolol (Concomitant administration may require a reduction in the dose of the antihypertensives). Products include:
- Visken Tablets ... 2036

Polythiazide (Concomitant administration may require a reduction in the dose of the antihypertensives). Products include:
- Minizide Capsules ... 1779
- Renese Tablets ... 1785
- Renese-R Tablets ... 1786

Prazepam (Enhanced response to CNS depressants). Products include:
- Centrax ... 1693

Prazosin Hydrochloride (Concomitant administration may require a reduction in the dose of the antihypertensives). Products include:
- Minipress Capsules ... 1778
- Minizide Capsules ... 1779

Prochlorperazine (Enhanced response to CNS depressants). Products include:
- Compazine ... 2201

Promethazine Hydrochloride (Enhanced response to CNS depressants). Products include:
- Mepergan Injection ... 2479
- Phenergan with Codeine ... 2497
- Phenergan with Dextromethorphan ... 2499
- Phenergan Injection ... 2493
- Phenergan Suppositories ... 2496
- Phenergan Syrup ... 2495
- Phenergan Tablets ... 2496
- Phenergan VC ... 2500
- Phenergan VC with Codeine ... 2501

Propofol (Enhanced response to CNS depressants). Products include:
- Diprivan Injection ... 2267

Propoxyphene Hydrochloride (Enhanced response to CNS depressants). Products include:
- Darvon ... 1256
- Wygesic Tablets ... 2540

Propoxyphene Napsylate (Enhanced response to CNS depressants). Products include:
- Darvon-N/Darvocet-N ... 1254

Propranolol Hydrochloride (Concomitant administration may require a reduction in the dose of the antihypertensives). Products include:
- Inderal ... 2459
- Inderal LA Long Acting Capsules ... 2461
- Inderide Tablets ... 2463
- Inderide LA Long Acting Capsules ... 2465

Quazepam (Enhanced response to CNS depressants). Products include:
- Doral Tablets ... 2383

Ramipril (Concomitant administration may require a reduction in the dose of the antihypertensives). Products include:
- Altace Capsules ... 1086

Rauwolfia Serpentina (Concomitant administration may require a reduction in the dose of the antihypertensives). Products include:
- Raudixin Tablets ... 1803
- Rauzide Tablets ... 1804

Rescinnamine (Concomitant administration may require a reduction in the dose of the antihypertensives).
- No products indexed under this heading.

Reserpine (Concomitant administration may require a reduction in the dose of the antihypertensives). Products include:
- Diupres Tablets ... 1461
- Hydromox R Tablets ... 1209
- Hydropres Tablets ... 1485
- Renese-R Tablets ... 1786
- Salutensin/Salutensin-Demi ... 719
- Ser-Ap-Es Tablets ... 881
- Serpasil Tablets ... 883
- Serpasil-Apresoline Tablets ... 884
- Serpasil-Esidrix Tablets ... 886

Secobarbital Sodium (Enhanced response to CNS depressants). Products include:
- Seconal Sodium Pulvules ... 1296

Selegiline Hydrochloride (Initiate Desyrel cautiously). Products include:
- Eldepryl ... 2250

Sodium Nitroprusside (Concomitant administration may require a reduction in the dose of the antihypertensives). Products include:
- Nipride I.V. Infusion ... 1909

Sufentanil Citrate (Enhanced response to CNS depressants). Products include:
- Sufenta Injection ... 1147

Temazepam (Enhanced response to CNS depressants). Products include:
- Restoril Capsules ... 2023

Terazosin Hydrochloride (Concomitant administration may require a reduction in the dose of the antihypertensives). Products include:
- Hytrin Tablets ... 529

Thiamylal Sodium (Enhanced response to CNS depressants). Products include:
- Surital Ampoules, Steri-Vials ... 1764

Thioridazine Hydrochloride (Enhanced response to CNS depressants). Products include:
- Mellaril ... 2011

Thiothixene (Enhanced response to CNS depressants). Products include:
- Navane Capsules and Concentrate 1954
- Navane Intramuscular ... 1956

Timolol Maleate (Concomitant administration may require a reduction in the dose of the antihypertensives). Products include:
- Blocadren Tablets ... 1429
- Timolide Tablets ... 1547
- Timoptic in Ocudose ... 1552
- Timoptic Sterile Ophthalmic Solution ... 1550

Tranylcypromine Sulfate (Initiate Desyrel cautiously). Products include:
- Parnate Tablets ... 2222

Triazolam (Enhanced response to CNS depressants). Products include:
- Halcion Tablets ... 2340

Trifluoperazine Hydrochloride (Enhanced response to CNS depressants). Products include:
- Stelazine ... 2226

Trimethaphan Camsylate (Concomitant administration may require a reduction in the dose of the antihypertensives). Products include:
- Arfonad Ampuls ... 1887

Warfarin Sodium (Increased or decreased prothrombin time). Products include:
- Coumadin Injection & Tablets ... 944
- Panwarfin Tablets ... 547

Food Interactions

Food, unspecified (Food may affect the bioavailability including amount of drug absorbed and peak plasma levels).

DEXACIDIN OINTMENT

(Dexamethasone, Neomycin Sulfate, Polymyxin B Sulfate) ... ◉ 272
No interactions described in labeling.

DEXACIDIN SUSPENSION

(Dexamethasone, Neomycin Sulfate, Polymyxin B Sulfate) ... ◉ 272
No interactions described in labeling.

DEXATRIM CAPSULES

(Phenylpropanolamine Hydrochloride) ... ▣ 733
May interact with alpha adrenergic stimulants, antihypertensives, and antidepressant drugs. Compounds in these categories include:

Acebutolol Hydrochloride (Concurrent use not recommended). Products include:
- Sectral Capsules ... 2520

Amitriptyline Hydrochloride (Concurrent use not recommended). Products include:
- Elavil ... 2269
- Endep Tablets ... 1927
- Etrafon ... 2087
- Limbitrol ... 1933
- Triavil Tablets ... 1556

Amoxapine (Concurrent use not recommended). Products include:
- Asendin Tablets ... 1196

Atenolol (Concurrent use not recommended). Products include:
- Tenoretic Tablets ... 1105
- Tenormin Tablets and I.V. Injection 1107

Benazepril Hydrochloride (Concurrent use not recommended). Products include:
- Lotensin Tablets ... 872

Betaxolol Hydrochloride (Concurrent use not recommended). Products include:
- Betoptic Sterile Ophthalmic Solution ... 569
- Betoptic S Sterile Ophthalmic Suspension ... 570
- Kerlone Tablets ... 2172

Bupropion Hydrochloride (Concurrent use not recommended). Products include:
- Wellbutrin Tablets ... 821

Captopril (Concurrent use not recommended). Products include:
- Capoten ... 2255
- Capozide ... 2258

Carteolol Hydrochloride (Concurrent use not recommended). Products include:
- Cartrol Tablets ... 507

Clonidine (Concurrent use not recommended). Products include:
- Catapres-TTS ... 677

Clonidine Hydrochloride (Concurrent use not recommended). Products include:
- Catapres Tablets ... 676
- Combipres Tablets ... 678

Deserpidine (Concurrent use not recommended). Products include:
- Enduronyl ... 518
- Harmonyl Tablets ... 528
- Oreticyl ... 545

Desipramine Hydrochloride (Concurrent use not recommended). Products include:
- Norpramin Tablets ... 1340

Diazoxide (Concurrent use not recommended). Products include:
- Hyperstat I.V. Injection ... 2095
- Proglycem ... 649

Doxazosin Mesylate (Concurrent use not recommended). Products include:
- Cardura Tablets ... 1941

Doxepin Hydrochloride (Concurrent use not recommended). Products include:
- Sinequan ... 1960

Enalapril Maleate (Concurrent use not recommended). Products include:
- Vaseretic Tablets ... 1559
- Vasotec Tablets ... 1564

Enalaprilat (Concurrent use not recommended). Products include:
- Vasotec I.V. ... 1562

Esmolol Hydrochloride (Concurrent use not recommended). Products include:
- Brevibloc Injection ... 942

Felodipine (Concurrent use not recommended). Products include:
- Plendil Extended-Release Tablets ... 1526

Fluoxetine Hydrochloride (Concurrent use not recommended). Products include:
- Prozac Pulvules ... 920

Fosinopril Sodium (Concurrent use not recommended). Products include:
- Monopril Tablets ... 1406

Guanabenz Acetate (Concurrent use not recommended). Products include:
- Wytensin Tablets ... 2542

Guanethidine Monosulfate (Concurrent use not recommended). Products include:
- Esimil Tablets ... 864
- Ismelin Tablets ... 869

Hydralazine Hydrochloride (Concurrent use not recommended). Products include:
- Apresazide Capsules ... 854
- Apresoline Hydrochloride Parenteral (Ampuls) ... 856
- Apresoline Hydrochloride Tablets ... 855
- Apresoline-Esidrix Tablets ... 857
- Ser-Ap-Es Tablets ... 881
- Serpasil-Apresoline Tablets ... 884

Imipramine Hydrochloride (Concurrent use not recommended). Products include:
- Tofranil Ampuls ... 1038
- Tofranil Tablets ... 1039

Imipramine Pamoate (Concurrent use not recommended). Products include:
- Tofranil-PM Capsules ... 1041

Indapamide (Concurrent use not recommended). Products include:
- Lozol Tablets ... 1843

Isocarboxazid (Concurrent use not recommended). Products include:
- Marplan Tablets ... 1906

Isradipine (Concurrent use not recommended). Products include:
- DynaCirc Capsules ... 2004

Labetalol Hydrochloride (Concurrent use not recommended). Products include:
- Normodyne Injection ... 2108
- Normodyne Tablets ... 2110
- Normozide Tablets ... 2112
- Trandate HCT Tablets ... 579
- Trandate Injection ... 577
- Trandate Tablets ... 579

Lisinopril (Concurrent use not recommended). Products include:
- Prinivil Tablets ... 1538
- Prinzide Tablets ... 1540
- Zestoretic ... 2274
- Zestril Tablets ... 2277

Maprotiline Hydrochloride (Concurrent use not recommended). Products include:
- Ludiomil Tablets ... 874

Mecamylamine Hydrochloride (Concurrent use not recommended). Products include:
- Inversine Tablets ... 1492

Methyldopa (Concurrent use not recommended). Products include:
- Aldoclor Tablets ... 1413
- Aldomet Oral ... 1415
- Aldoril Tablets ... 1418

Methyldopate Hydrochloride (Concurrent use not recommended). Products include:
- Aldomet Ester HCl Injection ... 1417

Metoprolol Tartrate (Concurrent use not recommended). Products include:
- Lopressor Ampuls ... 1032
- Lopressor HCT Tablets ... 1034
- Lopressor Tablets ... 1032

Metyrosine (Concurrent use not recommended). Products include:
- Demser Capsules ... 1460

Minoxidil (Concurrent use not recommended). Products include:
- Loniten Tablets ... 2346
- Rogaine Topical Solution ... 2357

Nadolol (Concurrent use not recommended). Products include:
- Corgard Tablets ... 701
- Corzide Tablets ... 702

Naphazoline Hydrochloride (Effect not specified). Products include:
- AK-Con ... ◉ 202
- AK-Con-A ... ◉ 203
- Albalon Solution with Liquifilm ... ◉ 238
- Albalon-A Liquifilm ... ◉ 238
- Allergy Drops ... ◉ 258
- Clear Eyes ACR ... ◉ 305
- Clear Eyes Lubricating Eye Redness Reliever ... ◉ 304
- 4-Way Fast Acting Nasal Spray - Original Formula (regular & mentholated) & Metered Spray Pump (regular) ... 751
- Naphcon ... ◉ 226
- Naphcon Forte ... ◉ 226
- Naphcon-A Ophthalmic Solution ... 571
- Opcon-A Ophthalmic Solution ... ◉ 262
- Privine Nasal Solution ... ▣ 552
- Privine Nasal Solution ... 878
- Privine Nasal Spray ... ▣ 552
- Privine Nasal Spray ... 878
- Vasocon-A ... ◉ 278

Nicardipine Hydrochloride (Concurrent use not recommended). Products include:
- Cardene Capsules ... 2290

Nitroglycerin (Concurrent use not recommended). Products include:
- Deponit NTG Transdermal Delivery System ... 2143
- Minitran Transdermal Delivery System ... 1312
- Nitro-Bid Ointment ... 1339
- Nitro-Bid Capsules ... 1338
- Nitrodisc ... 2176
- Nitro-Dur (nitroglycerin) Transdermal Infusion System ... 1164
- Nitrogard Tablets ... 1004
- Nitrolingual Spray ... 1846
- Nitrostat Tablets ... 1743
- Transderm-Nitro Transdermal Therapeutic System ... 2283

Nortriptyline Hydrochloride (Concurrent use not recommended). Products include:
- Pamelor ... 2019

Oxymetazoline Hydrochloride (Effect not specified). Products include:
- Afrin ... ▣ 692
- Cheracol Nasal Spray Pump ... ▣ 667
- Dristan Long Lasting Menthol Nasal Spray ... 2419
- Dristan Long Lasting Nasal Spray, Regular and Regular with Metered Dose Pump ... 2419
- Duration Nasal Spray ... ▣ 700
- Duration 12 Hour Nasal Spray Pump ... ▣ 700
- 4-Way Long Lasting Nasal Spray & Metered Spray Pump ... 751
- NTZ Long Acting Nasal Spray & Drops 0.05% ... ▣ 760
- Neo-Synephrine Maximum Strength 12 Hour Nasal Spray ... ▣ 759
- Neo-Synephrine Maximum Strength 12 Hour Nasal Spray Pump ... ▣ 759
- Nōstrilla Long Acting Nasal Decongestant ... ▣ 520
- OcuClear Eye Drops ... ◉ 306
- Vicks Sinex Long Acting ... ▣ 665
- Visine L.R. Eye Drops ... ▣ 647
- Visine L.R. Eye Drope ... ◉ 303

Penbutolol Sulfate (Concurrent use not recommended). Products include:
- Levatol ... 1832

Phenelzine Sulfate (Concurrent use not recommended). Products include:
- Nardil ... 1742

Phenoxybenzamine Hydrochloride (Concurrent use not recommended). Products include:
- Dibenzyline Capsules ... 2207

Phentolamine Mesylate (Concurrent use not recommended). Products include:
- Regitine ... 878

Phenylephrine Hydrochloride (Effect not specified). Products include:
- AK-Dilate Solution 2.5% and 10% ... ◉ 203
- Atrohist Sprinkle Capsules ... 558
- Cerose-DM ... 2443
- Codimal ... 846
- Comhist LA Capsules ... 1618
- Congespirin For Children Aspirin Free Chewable Cold Tablets ... 748
- Cyclomydril ... ◉ 216
- Deconsal Sprinkle Capsules ... 559
- Dimetane Decongestant ... ▣ 673
- Dristan Decongestant/Antihistamine/Analgesic Coated Caplets ... ▣ 749
- Dristan Cold Nasal Decongestant/ Antihistamine/ Analgesic Coated Tablets ... 2419
- Dristan Advanced Formula Decongestant/Antihistamine/ Analgesic Tablets ... ▣ 749
- Dristan Nasal Spray, Menthol ... 2419
- Dristan Nasal Spray, Regular and Regular with Metered Pump ... 2419
- Entex Capsules ... 1623
- Entex Liquid ... 1623
- Sinus Excedrin Analgesic, Decongestant Tablets & Caplets ... 750
- Extendryl ... 994
- 4-Way Fast Acting Nasal Spray - Original Formula (regular & mentholated) & Metered Spray Pump (regular) ... 751
- Hycomine Compound Tablets ... 929
- Murocoll-2 Sterile Ophthalmic Solution ... ◉ 261
- Mydfrin 2.5% ... ◉ 224
- Naldecon Syrup, Tablets, Pediatric Drops and Pediatric Syrup ... 709
- Neo-Synephrine Hydrochloride 1% Carpuject ... 2063
- Neo-Synephrine Hydrochloride 1% Injection ... 2063

Neo-Synephrine Hydrochloride (Ophthalmic) 2064
Neo-Synephrine .... ND 759
Nöstril Nasal Decongestant .... ND 520
Novahistine Elixir .... ND 596
Phenergan VC 2500
Phenergan VC with Codeine 2501
Prefrin Liquifilm Vasoconstrictor and Lubricant Eye Drops .... ◉ 254
Prefrin-A .... ◉ 255
Quelidrine Syrup 556
Relief Vasoconstrictor and Lubricant Eye Drops .... ◉ 256
Robitussin Night Relief .... ND 677
Ru-Tuss with Hydrocodone 694
Ru-Tuss Tablets 693
Vasosulf .... ◉ 279
Vicks Sinex .... ND 665
Zincfrin .... ◉ 230

Phenylpropanolamine Containing Anorectics (Effect not specified).

Pindolol (Concurrent use not recommended). Products include:
Visken Tablets 2036

Prazosin Hydrochloride (Concurrent use not recommended). Products include:
Minipress Capsules 1778
Minizide Capsules 1779

Propranolol Hydrochloride (Concurrent use not recommended). Products include:
Inderal 2459
Inderal LA Long Acting Capsules 2461
Inderide Tablets 2463
Inderide LA Long Acting Capsules .. 2465

Protriptyline Hydrochloride (Concurrent use not recommended). Products include:
Vivactil Tablets 1567

Pseudoephedrine Hydrochloride (Effect not specified). Products include:
Actifed Capsules .... ND 539
Actifed Plus Caplets .... ND 539
Actifed Plus Tablets .... ND 540
Actifed with Codeine Cough Syrup.. 752
Actifed Syrup .... ND 540
Actifed Tablets .... ND 540
Actifed 12-Hour Capsules .... ND 539
Advil Cold & Sinus Caplets (formerly CoAdvil) 2416
Allerest .... ND 559
Anatuss LA Tablets 1359
Benadryl Decongestant Elixir .... ND 635
Benadryl Decongestant .... ND 635
Benadryl Plus .... ND 636
Benadryl Plus Nighttime .... ND 637
Benylin Decongestant .... ND 638
Brexin L.A. Capsules 2078
Bromfed Capsules (Timed Release) 1615
Bromfed Syrup .... ND 628
Bromfed 1615
CoAdvil .... ND 748
Allergy-Sinus Comtrex Multi-Symptom Allergy Sinus Formula Tablets & Caplets 746
Cough Formula Comtrex 746
Comtrex Multi-Symptom Cold Reliever Tablets/Caplets/Liqui-Gels/Liquid 745
Day-Night Comtrex 747
Non-Drowsy Comtrex 747
Congess 994
Congestac Caplets .... ND 617
Contac Jr. Children's Cold Medicine .... ND 712
Contac Nighttime Cold Medicine .... ND 713
Contac Sinus Caplets Maximum Strength Non-Drowsy Formula .... ND 710
Contac Sinus Tablets Maximum Strength Non-Drowsy Formula .... ND 710
Deconamine 663
Deconsal II Tablets 559
Dimacol Caplets .... ND 672
Dimetane-DX Cough Syrup 1858
Dorcol Children's Cough Syrup .... ND 685
Dorcol Children's Decongestant Liquid .... ND 685
Dorcol Children's Liquid Cold Formula .... ND 686
Maximum Strength Dristan Decongestant/Analgesic Coated Caplets .... ND 750
No Drowsiness Dristan Cold Nasal Decongestant/Analgesic Coated Caplets 2420
Dristan Sinus Caplets 2419
Sinus Excedrin Analgesic, Decongestant Tablets & Caplets .... ND 533
Fedahist Gyrocaps 2145
Fedahist Timecaps 2145
Guaifed 1615
Guaifed Syrup .... ND 629
Isoclor Expectorant 982
Isoclor Timesule Capsules .... ND 561
Kronofed-A 970
Medi-Flu Caplet, Liquid .... ND 640
Novafed A Capsules 1342
Novafed Capsules 1342
Novahistine DH 1342
Novahistine DMX .... ND 595
Novahistine Expectorant 1343
Nucofed Capsules 2219
Nucofed Expectorant 2219
Nucofed Pediatric Expectorant 2220
Nucofed Syrup 2219
Ornex Caplets .... ND 618
PediaCare Allergy Relief Formula Liquid 1362
PediaCare Cough-Cold Formula Liquid 1362
PediaCare Infants' Oral Decongestant Drops 1362
PediaCare Night Rest Cough-Cold Formula Liquid 1362
PediaCare 6-12 Cough-Cold Formula Chewable Tablets 1362
Robitussin-DAC Syrup 1875
Robitussin-PE .... ND 677
Rondec 1975
Rondec-DM 1976
Rondec-TR Tablet 1975
Ru-Tuss DE Tablets 694
Ryna .... ND 741
Seldane-D Extended-Release Tablets 1350
Sinarest .... ND 562
Sine-Aid Maximum Strength Sinus Headache Caplets 1365
Sine-Aid Maximum Strength Sinus Headache Tablets 1365
Sine-Off Maximum Strength Allergy/Sinus Formula Caplets .... ND 721
Sine-Off Maximum Strength No Drowsiness Formula Caplets .... ND 722
Singlet Tablets .... ND 598
Sinutab Maximum Strength .... ND 641
Sinutab Maximum Strength Without Drowsiness Tablets & Caplets .... ND 642
Sinutab Regular Strength Without Drowsiness Formula .... ND 641
St. Joseph Nighttime Cold Medicine .... ND 705
Sudafed Children's Liquid .... ND 543
Sudafed Cough Syrup .... ND 543
Sudafed Plus Liquid .... ND 544
Sudafed Plus Tablets .... ND 545
Sudafed Sinus Caplets .... ND 545
Sudafed Sinus Tablets .... ND 545
Sudafed Tablets, 30 mg .... ND 544
Sudafed Tablets, Adult Strength, 60 mg .... ND 544
Sudafed 12 Hour Capsules .... ND 545
TheraFlu Flu and Cold Medicine .... ND 687
Triaminic Nite Light .... ND 689
Tylenol Allergy Sinus Medication Caplets and Gelcaps, Maximum Strength 1372
Children's Tylenol Cold Liquid Formula and Chewable Tablets 1368
Tylenol Cold & Flu Hot Medication, Packets 1369
Tylenol Cold & Flu No Drowsiness Hot Medication, Packets 1371
Tylenol Cold Medication Caplets and Tablets 1370
Tylenol Cold Medication No Drowsiness Formula Caplets 1370
Tylenol Cold Night Time Medication Liquid 1371
Tylenol Cough Medication Liquid with Decongestant, Maximum Strength 1372
Tylenol, Maximum Strength, Sinus Medication Gelcaps, Caplets and Tablets 1373
Ursinus Inlay-Tabs .... ND 691
Vicks Children's NyQuil .... ND 664
Vicks Daycare .... ND 660
Vicks Formula 44D Decongestant Cough Medicine .... ND 662
Vicks Formula 44M Multi-Symptom Cough Medicine .... ND 662
Vicks NyQuil Nighttime Colds Medicine-Original & Cherry Flavor .... ND 664
Vicks Pediatric Formula 44 Cough & Congestion Medicine .... ND 663
Vicks Pediatric Formula 44m Multi-Symptom Cough & Cold Medicine .... ND 663

Ramipril (Concurrent use not recommended). Products include:
Altace Capsules 1086

Rauwolfia Serpentina (Concurrent use not recommended). Products include:
Raudixin Tablets 1803
Rauzide Tablets 1804

Rescinnamine (Concurrent use not recommended).
No products indexed under this heading.

Reserpine (Concurrent use not recommended). Products include:
Diupres Tablets 1461
Hydromox R Tablets 1209
Hydropres Tablets 1485
Renese-R Tablets 1786
Salutensin/Salutensin-Demi 719
Ser-Ap-Es Tablets 881
Serpasil Tablets 883
Serpasil-Apresoline Tablets 884
Serpasil-Esidrix Tablets 886

Sodium Nitroprusside (Concurrent use not recommended). Products include:
Nipride I.V. Infusion 1909

Terazosin Hydrochloride (Concurrent use not recommended). Products include:
Hytrin Tablets 529

Tetrahydrozoline Hydrochloride (Effect not specified). Products include:
Collyrium Fresh 2445
Murine Plus Lubricating Eye Redness Reliever .... ◉ 305
Visine A.C. Eye Drops .... ND 646
Visine A.C. Eye Drops .... ◉ 303
Visine EXTRA Eye Drops .... ND 647
Visine EXTRA Eye Drops .... ◉ 303
Visine Eye Drops .... ND 646
Visine Eye Drops .... ◉ 303

Timolol Maleate (Concurrent use not recommended). Products include:
Blocadren Tablets 1429
Timolide Tablets 1547
Timoptic in Ocudose 1552
Timoptic Sterile Ophthalmic Solution 1550

Tranylcypromine Sulfate (Concurrent use not recommended). Products include:
Parnate Tablets 2222

Trazodone Hydrochloride (Concurrent use not recommended). Products include:
Desyrel and Desyrel Dividose 1404

Trimethaphan Camsylate (Concurrent use not recommended). Products include:
Arfonad Ampuls 1887

Trimipramine Maleate (Concurrent use not recommended). Products include:
Surmontil Capsules 2524

DEXATRIM MAXIMUM STRENGTH CAFFEINE-FREE CAPLETS
(Phenylpropanolamine Hydrochloride) .... ND 733
See **Dexatrim Capsules**

DEXATRIM MAXIMUM STRENGTH CAFFEINE-FREE CAPSULES
(Phenylpropanolamine Hydrochloride) .... ND 733
See **Dexatrim Capsules**

DEXATRIM MAXIMUM STRENGTH PLUS VITAMIN C/ CAFFEINE-FREE CAPLETS
(Phenylpropanolamine Hydrochloride, Vitamin C) .... ND 733
See **Dexatrim Capsules**

DEXATRIM MAXIMUM STRENGTH PLUS VITAMIN C/CAFFEINE-FREE CAPSULES
(Phenylpropanolamine Hydrochloride, Vitamin C) .... ND 733
See **Dexatrim Capsules**

DEXATRIM MAXIMUM STRENGTH PRE-MEAL CAPLETS
(Phenylpropanolamine Hydrochloride) .... ND 733
See **Dexatrim Capsules**

DEXEDRINE ELIXIR
(Dextroamphetamine Sulfate) 2206
May interact with beta blockers, alpha adrenergic blockers, urinary alkalizing agents, tricyclic antidepressants, sympathomimetic aerosal brochodilators, monoamine oxidase inhibitors, antihistamines, veratrum alkaloids, antihypertensives, and certain other agents. Compounds in these categories include:

Acebutolol Hydrochloride (Inhibited by amphetamines). Products include:
Sectral Capsules 2520

Acetazolamide (Increases blood levels of amphetamines). Products include:
Diamox Parenteral 1200
Diamox Parenteral .... ◉ 308
Diamox Sequels (Sustained Release) 1201
Diamox Sequels (Sustained Release) .... ◉ 310
Diamox Tablets 1200
Diamox Tablets .... ◉ 308

Acidifying Agents (Urinary) (Lowers blood levels and efficacy of amphetamines).

Albuterol (Enhanced activity). Products include:
Proventil Inhalation Aerosol 2117
Ventolin Inhalation Aerosol and Refill 583

Albuterol Sulfate (Enhanced activity). Products include:
Proventil Repetabs Tablets 2120
Proventil Solutions for Inhalation 0.5% and 0.083% 2118
Proventil Syrup 2119
Proventil Tablets 2120
Ventolin 583

Amitriptyline Hydrochloride (Enhanced activity). Products include:
Elavil 2269
Endep Tablets 1927
Etrafon 2087
Limbitrol 1933
Triavil Tablets 1556

Ammonium Chloride (Lowers blood levels and efficacy of amphetamines). Products include:
Quelidrine Syrup 556

Amoxapine (Enhanced activity). Products include:
Asendin Tablets 1196

Astemizole (Sedative effects may be counteracted). Products include:
Hismanal Tablets 1138

Atenolol (Inhibited by amphetamines). Products include:
Tenoretic Tablets 1105
Tenormin Tablets and I.V. Injection 1107

Azatadine Maleate (Sedative effects may be counteracted). Products include:
- Optimine Tablets 2115
- Trinalin Repetabs Tablets 1170

Benazepril Hydrochloride (Antagonized). Products include:
- Lotensin Tablets 872

Bendroflumethiazide (Antagonized; increases blood levels of amphetamines). Products include:
- Corzide Tablets 702
- Naturetin Tablets 1789
- Rauzide Tablets 1804

Betaxolol Hydrochloride (Antagonized). Products include:
- Betoptic Sterile Ophthalmic Solution 569
- Betoptic S Sterile Ophthalmic Suspension 570
- Kerlone Tablets 2172

Bromodiphenhydramine Hydrochloride (Sedative effects may be counteracted).
- No products indexed under this heading.

Brompheniramine Maleate (Sedative effects of antihistamines may be counteracted). Products include:
- Alka Seltzer Plus Sinus Allergy Medicine ■ 624
- Atrohist Sprinkle Capsules 558
- Bromfed Capsules (Timed Release) 1615
- Bromfed Syrup ■ 628
- Bromfed 1615
- Dimetane Decongestant ■ 673
- Dimetane ■ 672
- Dimetane-DC Cough Syrup 1857
- Dimetane-DX Cough Syrup 1858
- Dimetapp Elixir ■ 673
- Dimetapp DM Elixir ■ 674
- Dimetapp Extentabs ■ 674
- Dimetapp Plus Caplets ■ 675
- Dimetapp Tablets ■ 675
- Drixoral Antihistamine/Nasal Decongestant Syrup ■ 698

Captopril (Antagonized). Products include:
- Capoten 2255
- Capozide 2258

Carteolol Hydrochloride (Inhibited by amphetamines; antagonized). Products include:
- Cartrol Tablets 507

Chlorothiazide (Antagonized; increases blood levels of amphetamines). Products include:
- Aldoclor Tablets 1413
- Diupres Tablets 1461
- Diuril Oral 1464

Chlorothiazide Sodium (Antagonized; increases blood levels of amphetamines). Products include:
- Diuril Sodium Intravenous 1463

Chlorpheniramine Maleate (Sedative effects may be counteracted). Products include:
- A.R.M. Allergy Relief Medicine Caplets ■ 615
- Alka-Seltzer Plus Cold Medicine ■ 623
- Allerest ■ 559
- Ana-Kit Anaphylaxis Emergency Treatment Kit 1100
- BC Cold Powder Multi-Symptom Formula ■ 517
- Brexin L.A. Capsules 2078
- Cerose-DM 2443
- Cheracol Plus Head Cold/Cough Formula ■ 667
- Chlor-Trimeton Allergy Syrup, Tablets & Long-Acting Repetabs Tablets ■ 693
- Chlor-Trimeton Decongestant ■ 694
- Comhist LA Capsules 1618
- Allergy-Sinus Comtrex Multi-Symptom Allergy Sinus Formula Tablets & Caplets 746
- Comtrex Multi-Symptom Cold Reliever Tablets/Caplets/Liqui-Gels/Liquid 745
- Day-Night Comtrex 747
- Contac Continuous Action Decongestant/Antihistamine Capsules ■ 710
- Contac Maximum Strength Continuous Action Decongestant/Antihistamine Caplets ■ 709
- Contac Severe Cold and Flu Formula Caplets ■ 711
- Coricidin 'D' Decongestant Tablets ■ 695
- Coricidin Demilets Tablets for Children ■ 696
- Coricidin Tablets ■ 695
- Deconamine 663
- Demazin Nasal Decongestant/Antihistamine Repetabs Tablets & Syrup ■ 697
- Dorcol Children's Liquid Cold Formula ■ 686
- Dristan Decongestant/Antihistamine/Analgesic Coated Caplets ■ 749
- Dristan Cold Nasal Decongestant/Antihistamine/Analgesic Coated Tablets 2419
- Dristan Advanced Formula Decongestant/Antihistamine/Analgesic Tablets ■ 749
- Extendryl 994
- 4-Way Cold Tablets 750
- Fedahist Gyrocaps 2145
- Fedahist Timecaps 2145
- Hycomine Compound Tablets 929
- Isoclor Timesule Capsules ■ 561
- Kronofed-A 970
- Medi-Flu Caplet, Liquid ■ 640
- Naldecon Syrup, Tablets, Pediatric Drops and Pediatric Syrup 709
- Nolamine Tablets 838
- Novafed A Capsules 1342
- Novahistine DH 1342
- Novahistine Elixir ■ 596
- Ornade Spansule Capsules 2221
- Orthoxicol Cough Syrup ■ 668
- PediaCare Allergy Relief Formula Liquid 1362
- PediaCare Cough-Cold Formula Liquid 1362
- PediaCare Night Rest Cough-Cold Formula Liquid 1362
- PediaCare 6-12 Cough-Cold Formula Chewable Tablets 1362
- Pyrroxate Capsules ■ 669
- Quelidrine Syrup 556
- Ru-Tuss II Capsules 693
- Ru-Tuss Tablets 693
- Ryna ■ 741
- Sinarest Tablets & Extra Strength Tablets ■ 562
- Sine-Off Maximum Strength Allergy/Sinus Formula Caplets ■ 721
- Sine-Off Sinus Medicine Tablets-Aspirin Formula ■ 722
- Singlet Tablets ■ 598
- Sinulin 840
- Sinutab Maximum Strength ■ 641
- St. Joseph Nighttime Cold Medicine ■ 705
- Sudafed Plus Liquid ■ 544
- Sudafed Plus Tablets ■ 545
- Teldrin Timed-Release Allergy Capsules, 12 mg 2192
- TheraFlu Flu and Cold Medicine ■ 687
- Triaminic Allergy Tablets ■ 688
- Triaminic Chewables ■ 688
- Triaminic Cold Tablets ■ 688
- Triaminic Nite Light ■ 689
- Triaminic Syrup ■ 689
- Triaminic-12 Tablets ■ 690
- Triaminicin Tablets ■ 690
- Triaminicol Multi-Symptom Cold Tablets ■ 691
- Triaminicol Multi-Symptom Relief ■ 691
- Tylenol Allergy Sinus Medication Caplets and Gelcaps, Maximum Strength 1372
- Children's Tylenol Cold Liquid Formula and Chewable Tablets 1368
- Tylenol Cold & Flu Hot Medication, Packets 1369
- Tylenol Cold Medication Caplets and Tablets 1370
- Tylenol Cold Medication, Effervescent Tablets 1369
- Vicks Children's NyQuil ■ 664
- Vicks Formula 44 Cough Medicine ■ 661
- Vicks Formula 44M Multi-Symptom Cough Medicine ■ 662
- Vicks Pediatric Formula 44m Multi-Symptom Cough & Cold Medicine ■ 663

Chlorpheniramine Polistirex (Sedative effects may be counteracted). Products include:
- Tussionex Extended-Release Suspension 988

Chlorpheniramine Tannate (Sedative effects may be counteracted). Products include:
- Rynatan 2387
- Rynatuss 2388

Chlorpromazine (Central stimulating effects of amphetamines inhibited). Products include:
- Thorazine 2234

Chlorthalidone (Inhibited by amphetamines). Products include:
- Combipres Tablets 678
- Tenoretic Tablets 1105
- Thalitone Tablets 687

Clemastine Fumarate (Sedative effects may be counteracted). Products include:
- Tavist Syrup 2033
- Tavist Tablets 2035
- Tavist-D Tablets 2035

Clomipramine Hydrochloride (Enhanced activity). Products include:
- Anafranil Capsules 650

Clonidine (Antagonized). Products include:
- Catapres-TTS 677

Clonidine Hydrochloride (Inhibited by amphetamines). Products include:
- Catapres Tablets 676
- Combipres Tablets 678

Cryptenamine Preparations (Hypotensive effects inhibited).

Cyproheptadine Hydrochloride (Sedative effects may be counteracted). Products include:
- Periactin 1525

Deserpidine (Antagonized). Products include:
- Enduronyl 518
- Harmonyl Tablets 528
- Oreticyl 545

Desipramine Hydrochloride (Potentiation of cardiovascular effects; enhanced activity). Products include:
- Norpramin Tablets 1340

Dexchlorpheniramine Maleate (Sedative effects may be counteracted). Products include:
- Polaramine 2116

Diazoxide (Inhibited by amphetamines). Products include:
- Hyperstat I.V. Injection 2095
- Proglycem 649

Diphenhydramine Citrate (Sedative effects may be counteracted). Products include:
- Alka-Seltzer Plus Night-Time Cold Medicine ■ 623
- Bufferin AF Nite Time Analgesic/Sleeping Aid Caplets 744
- Excedrin P.M. Analgesic/Sleeping Aid Tablets, Caplets and Liquid 749

Diphenylpyraline Hydrochloride (Sedative effects may be counteracted).
- No products indexed under this heading.

Dobutamine Hydrochloride (Enhanced activity). Products include:
- Dobutrex Solution Vials 1259

Dopamine Hydrochloride (Enhanced activity). Products include:
- Intropin Injection 930

Doxazosin Mesylate (Inhibited by amphetamines). Products include:
- Cardura Tablets 1941

Doxepin Hydrochloride (Enhanced activity). Products include:
- Sinequan 1960

Enalapril Maleate (Antagonized). Products include:
- Vaseretic Tablets 1559
- Vasotec Tablets 1564

Enalaprilat (Antagonized). Products include:
- Vasotec I.V. 1562

Ephedrine Hydrochloride (Enhanced activity). Products include:
- Amesec ■ 682
- Primatene Tablets-M Formula 2421
- Primatene Tablets-P Formula 2421
- Primatene Tablets-Regular Formula 2421
- Quadrinal Tablets 1183
- Quelidrine Syrup 556
- Tedral SA 1765

Ephedrine Sulfate (Enhanced activity). Products include:
- Bronkaid Tablets ■ 757
- Bronkolixir ■ 761
- Bronkotabs Tablets ■ 762
- Marax Tablets & DF Syrup 1954
- Pazo Hemorrhoid Ointment & Suppositories 752
- Vicks Vatronol Nose Drops ■ 666

Ephedrine Tannate (Enhanced activity). Products include:
- Rynatuss 2388

Epinephrine (Enhanced activity). Products include:
- Ana-Kit Anaphylaxis Emergency Treatment Kit 1100
- Bronkaid Mist ■ 757
- EpiPen 843
- Marcaine Hydrochloride 0.5% with Epinephrine 1:200,000 (as bitartrate) 958
- Marcaine Hydrochloride with Epinephrine 1:200,000 2055
- Primatene Mist 2420
- Sus-Phrine Injection 1006
- Xylocaine with Epinephrine Injections 637

Epinephrine Bitartrate (Enhanced activity). Products include:
- AsthmaHaler Mist Epinephrine Bitartrate Bronchodilator ■ 616
- Bronkaid Mist Suspension ■ 757
- Primatene Mist Suspension 2421

Epinephrine Hydrochloride (Enhanced activity). Products include:
- Adrenalin Chloride Solution 1:100 & 1:1,000 1689
- Epifrin ◉ 244
- Glaucon ◉ 218

Esmolol Hydrochloride (Inhibited by amphetamines). Products include:
- Brevibloc Injection 942

Ethosuximide (Intestinal absorption of ethosuximide may be delayed). Products include:
- Zarontin Capsules 1768
- Zarontin Syrup 1769

Felodipine (Antagonized). Products include:
- Plendil Extended-Release Tablets 1526

Fosinopril Sodium (Antagonized). Products include:
- Monopril Tablets 1406

Furazolidone (Potentiation of amphetamines; possibly fatal; concurrent use is contraindicated). Products include:
- Furoxone 1855

Furosemide (Antagonized). Products include:
- Lasix 1093

Glutamic Acid Hydrochloride (Lowers blood levels and efficacy of amphetamines).
- No products indexed under this heading.

Guanabenz Acetate (Antagonized). Products include:
- Wytensin Tablets 2542

(■ Described in PDR For Nonprescription Drugs) (◉ Described in PDR For Ophthalmology)

Guanethidine Monosulfate (Lowers blood levels and efficacy of amphetamines). Products include:
- Esimil Tablets ... 864
- Ismelin Tablets ... 869

Haloperidol (Central stimulant effects of amphetamines inhibited). Products include:
- Haldol Injection, Tablets and Concentrate ... 1373

Hydralazine Hydrochloride (Inhibited by amphetamines). Products include:
- Apresazide Capsules ... 854
- Apresoline Hydrochloride Parenteral (Ampuls) ... 856
- Apresoline Hydrochloride Tablets .. 855
- Apresoline-Esidrix Tablets ... 857
- Ser-Ap-Es Tablets ... 881
- Serpasil-Apresoline Tablets ... 884

Hydrochlorothiazide (Antagonized; increases blood levels of amphetamines). Products include:
- Aldactazide ... 2150
- Aldoril Tablets ... 1418
- Apresazide Capsules ... 854
- Apresoline-Esidrix Tablets ... 857
- Capozide ... 2258
- Dyazide Capsules ... 2208
- Esidrix Tablets ... 863
- Esimil Tablets ... 864
- HydroDIURIL Tablets ... 1484
- Hydropres Tablets ... 1485
- Inderide Tablets ... 2463
- Inderide LA Long Acting Capsules .. 2465
- Lopressor HCT Tablets ... 1034
- Maxzide ... 1215
- Moduretic Tablets ... 1510
- Normozide Tablets ... 2112
- Oretic Tablets ... 544
- Oreticyl ... 545
- Prinzide Tablets ... 1540
- Ser-Ap-Es Tablets ... 881
- Serpasil-Esidrix Tablets ... 886
- Timolide Tablets ... 1547
- Trandate HCT Tablets ... 579
- Vaseretic Tablets ... 1559
- Zestoretic ... 2274

Hydroflumethiazide (Antagonized; increases blood levels of amphetamines). Products include:
- Diucardin Tablets ... 2450
- Saluron ... 718
- Salutensin/Salutensin-Demi ... 719

Imipramine Hydrochloride (Enhanced activity). Products include:
- Tofranil Ampuls ... 1038
- Tofranil Tablets ... 1039

Imipramine Pamoate (Enhanced activity). Products include:
- Tofranil-PM Capsules ... 1041

Indapamide (Antagonized). Products include:
- Lozol Tablets ... 1843

Isocarboxazid (Potentiation of amphetamines; possibly fatal; concurrent use is contraindicated). Products include:
- Marplan Tablets ... 1906

Isoproterenol Hydrochloride (Enhanced activity). Products include:
- Isuprel Hydrochloride Injection 1:5000 ... 2050
- Isuprel Hydrochloride Mistometer .. 2051
- Isuprel Hydrochloride Solution 1:200 & 1:100 ... 2052
- Norisodrine Aerotrol ... 540

Isradipine (Antagonized). Products include:
- DynaCirc Capsules ... 2004

Labetalol Hydrochloride (Inhibited by amphetamines). Products include:
- Normodyne Injection ... 2108
- Normodyne Tablets ... 2110
- Normozide Tablets ... 2112
- Trandate HCT Tablets ... 579
- Trandate Injection ... 577
- Trandate Tablets ... 579

Lisinopril (Antagonized). Products include:
- Prinivil Tablets ... 1538
- Prinzide Tablets ... 1540
- Zestoretic ... 2274
- Zestril Tablets ... 2277

Lithium Carbonate (Antiobesity and stimulatory effects of amphetamines may be inhibited). Products include:
- Eskalith ... 2214
- Lithane Tablets ... 1596
- Lithium Carbonate Capsules & Tablets ... 1984
- Lithobid Tablets ... 870

Maprotiline Hydrochloride (Enhanced activity). Products include:
- Ludiomil Tablets ... 874

Mecamylamine Hydrochloride (Antagonized). Products include:
- Inversine Tablets ... 1492

Meperidine Hydrochloride (Analgesic effect potentiated). Products include:
- Demerol ... 2047
- Mepergan Injection ... 2479

Metaproterenol Sulfate (Enhanced activity). Products include:
- Alupent ... 674
- Arm-a-Med Metaproterenol Sulfate Inhalation Solution, USP ... 617
- Metaprel Inhalation Aerosol Bronchodilator ... 2014
- Metaprel Inhalation Solution ... 2015
- Metaprel ... 2015
- Metaproterenol Sulfate Inhalation Solution, USP ... 912

Metaraminol Bitartrate (Enhanced activity). Products include:
- Aramine Injection ... 1424

Methdilazine Hydrochloride (Sedative effects may be counteracted). Products include:
- Tacaryl Syrup & Tablets ... 2409

Methenamine (Increased urinary excretion of amphetamines; reduced efficacy). Products include:
- Urised Tablets ... 2396

Methoxamine Hydrochloride (Enhanced activity). Products include:
- Vasoxyl Injection ... 819

Methyclothiazide (Antagonized; increases blood levels of amphetamines). Products include:
- Enduron Tablets ... 517
- Enduronyl ... 518

Methyldopa (Antagonized). Products include:
- Aldoclor Tablets ... 1413
- Aldomet Oral ... 1415
- Aldoril Tablets ... 1418

Methyldopate Hydrochloride (Antagonized). Products include:
- Aldomet Ester HCl Injection ... 1417

Metolazone (Antagonized). Products include:
- Diulo ... 2129
- Mykrox ½ mg Tablets ... 984
- Zaroxolyn Tablets ... 989

Metoprolol Tartrate (Inhibited by amphetamines). Products include:
- Lopressor Ampuls ... 1032
- Lopressor HCT Tablets ... 1034
- Lopressor Tablets ... 1032

Metyrosine (Antagonized). Products include:
- Demser Capsules ... 1460

Minoxidil (Antagonized). Products include:
- Loniten Tablets ... 2346
- Rogaine Topical Solution ... 2357

Nadolol (Inhibited by amphetamines). Products include:
- Corgard Tablets ... 701
- Corzide Tablets ... 702

Nicardipine Hydrochloride (Inhibited by amphetamines). Products include:
- Cardene Capsules ... 2290

Nitroglycerin (Antagonized). Products include:
- Deponit NTG Transdermal Delivery System ... 2143
- Minitran Transdermal Delivery System ... 1312
- Nitro-Bid Ointment ... 1339
- Nitro-Bid Capsules ... 1338
- Nitrodisc ... 2176
- Nitro-Dur (nitroglycerin) Transdermal Infusion System ... 1164
- Nitrogard Tablets ... 1004
- Nitrolingual Spray ... 1846
- Nitrostat Tablets ... 1743
- Transderm-Nitro Transdermal Therapeutic System ... 2283

Norepinephrine Bitartrate (Enhanced adrenergic effect). Products include:
- Levophed Bitartrate Injection ... 2054

Nortriptyline Hydrochloride (Enhanced activity). Products include:
- Pamelor ... 2019

Penbutolol Sulfate (Inhibited by amphetamines; antagonized). Products include:
- Levatol ... 1832

Phenelzine Sulfate (Potentiation of amphetamines; possibly fatal; concurrent use is contraindicated). Products include:
- Nardil ... 1742

Phenobarbital (Delayed intestinal absorption of phenobarbital). Products include:
- Arco-Lase Plus Tablets ... 607
- Bellergal-S Tablets ... 1998
- Bronkolixir ... ▣ 761
- Bronkotabs Tablets ... ▣ 762
- Donnatal ... 1858
- Donnatal Extentabs ... 1859
- Donnatal Tablets ... 1858
- Donnazyme Tablets ... 1860
- Kinesed Tablets ... 2272
- Phenobarbital Elixir and Tablets ... 1293
- Primatene Tablets-P Formula ... 2421
- Quadrinal Tablets ... 1183
- Tedral SA ... 1765

Phenoxybenzamine Hydrochloride (Antagonized). Products include:
- Dibenzyline Capsules ... 2207

Phentolamine Mesylate (Antagonized). Products include:
- Regitine ... 878

Phenylephrine Bitartrate (Enhanced activity).
- No products indexed under this heading.

Phenylephrine Hydrochloride (Enhanced activity). Products include:
- AK-Dilate Solution 2.5% and 10% ... ⊙ 203
- Atrohist Sprinkle Capsules ... 558
- Cerose-DM ... 2443
- Codimal ... 846
- Comhist LA Capsules ... 1618
- Congespirin For Children Aspirin Free Chewable Cold Tablets ... 748
- Cyclomydril ... ⊙ 216
- Deconsal Sprinkle Capsules ... 559
- Dimetane Decongestant ... ▣ 673
- Dristan Decongestant/Antihistamine/Analgesic Coated Caplets ... ▣ 749
- Dristan Cold Nasal Decongestant/Antihistamine/ Analgesic Coated Tablets ... 2419
- Dristan Advanced Formula Decongestant/Antihistamine/Analgesic Tablets ... ▣ 749
- Dristan Nasal Spray, Menthol ... 2419
- Dristan Nasal Spray, Regular and Regular with Metered Pump ... 2419
- Entex Capsules ... 1623
- Entex Liquid ... 1623
- Sinus Excedrin Analgesic, Decongestant Tablets & Caplets ... 750
- Extendryl ... 994
- 4-Way Fast Acting Nasal Spray - Original Formula (regular & mentholated) & Metered Spray Pump (regular) ... 751
- Hycomine Compound Tablets ... 929
- Murocoll-2 Sterile Ophthalmic Solution ... ⊙ 261
- Mydfrin 2.5% ... ⊙ 224
- Naldecon Syrup, Tablets, Pediatric Drops and Pediatric Syrup ... 709
- Neo-Synephrine Hydrochloride 1% Carpuject ... 2063
- Neo-Synephrine Hydrochloride 1% Injection ... 2063
- Neo-Synephrine Hydrochloride (Ophthalmic) ... 2064
- Neo-Synephrine ... ▣ 759
- Nōstril Nasal Decongestant ... ▣ 520
- Novahistine Elixir ... ▣ 596
- Phenergan VC ... 2500
- Phenergan VC with Codeine ... 2501
- Prefrin Liquifilm Vasoconstrictor and Lubricant Eye Drops ... ⊙ 254
- Prefrin-A ... ⊙ 255
- Quelidrine Syrup ... 556
- Relief Vasoconstrictor and Lubricant Eye Drops ... ⊙ 256
- Robitussin Night Relief ... ▣ 677
- Ru-Tuss with Hydrocodone ... 694
- Ru-Tuss Tablets ... 693
- Vasosulf ... ⊙ 279
- Vicks Sinex ... ▣ 665
- Zincfrin ... ⊙ 230

Phenylephrine Tannate (Enhanced activity). Products include:
- Rynatan ... 2387
- Rynatuss ... 2388

Phenylpropanolamine Hydrochloride (Enhanced activity). Products include:
- A.R.M. Allergy Relief Medicine Caplets ... ▣ 615
- Acutrim ... ▣ 548
- Allerest ... ▣ 559
- BC Cold Powder ... ▣ 517
- Cheracol Plus Head Cold/Cough Formula ... ▣ 667
- Codimal Expectorant ... 846
- Comtrex Multi-Symptom Cold Reliever Tablets/Caplets/Liqui-Gels/Liquid ... 745
- Contac Continuous Action Decongestant/Antihistamine Capsules ▣ 710
- Contac Maximum Strength Continuous Action Decongestant/ Antihistamine Caplets ... ▣ 709
- Contac Severe Cold and Flu Formula Caplets ... ▣ 711
- Coricidin 'D' Decongestant Tablets ... ▣ 695
- Coricidin Demilets Tablets for Children ... ▣ 696
- Demazin Nasal Decongestant/ Antihistamine Repetabs Tablets & Syrup ... ▣ 697
- Dexatrim ... ▣ 733
- Dimetane-DC Cough Syrup ... 1857
- Dimetapp Elixir ... ▣ 673
- Dimetapp DM Elixir ... ▣ 674
- Dimetapp Extentabs ... ▣ 674
- Dimetapp Plus Caplets ... ▣ 675
- Dimetapp Tablets ... ▣ 675
- Entex Capsules ... 1623
- Entex LA Tablets ... 1623
- Entex Liquid ... 1623
- 4-Way Cold Tablets ... 750
- Hycomine Syrup ... 927
- Naldecon CX Adult Liquid ... ▣ 521
- Naldecon DX Adult Liquid ... ▣ 521
- Naldecon DX Children's Syrup ... ▣ 522
- Naldecon DX Pediatric Drops ... ▣ 522
- Naldecon EX Children's Syrup ... ▣ 522
- Naldecon EX Pediatric Drops ... ▣ 523
- Naldecon Syrup, Tablets, Pediatric Drops and Pediatric Syrup ... 709
- Nolamine Tablets ... 838
- Nolex LA Tablets ... 838
- Ornade Spansule Capsules ... 2221
- Orthoxicol Cough Syrup ... ▣ 668
- Propagest ... 839
- Pyrroxate Capsules ... ▣ 669
- Robitussin-CF ... ▣ 676
- Ru-Tuss II Capsules ... 693
- Ru-Tuss with Hydrocodone ... 694
- Ru-Tuss Tablets ... 693
- Sine-Off Sinus Medicine Tablets-Aspirin Formula ... ▣ 722
- Sinulin ... 840
- St. Joseph Cold Tablets for Children ... ▣ 704
- Tavist-D Tablets ... 2035
- Triaminic Allergy Tablets ... ▣ 688
- Triaminic Chewables ... ▣ 688
- Triaminic Cold Tablets ... ▣ 688

Triaminic Expectorant ▣ 688
Triaminic Expectorant w/Codeine .. 1996
Triaminic Expectorant DH 1995
Triaminic Oral Infant Drops 1996
Triaminic Syrup ▣ 689
Triaminic-12 Tablets ▣ 690
Triaminic-DM Syrup ▣ 689
Triaminicin Tablets ▣ 690
Triaminicol Multi-Symptom Cold Tablets ▣ 691
Triaminicol Multi-Symptom Relief ▣ 691
Tuss-Ornade Liquid 2242
Tuss-Ornade Spansule Capsules 2242
Tylenol Cold Medication, Effervescent Tablets 1369

Phenytoin (Delayed intestinal absorption of phenytoin). Products include:
Dilantin Infatabs 1710
Dilantin-30 Pediatric/Dilantin-125 Suspension 1713

Phenytoin Sodium (Delayed intestinal absorption of phenytoin). Products include:
Dilantin Kapseals 1708
Dilantin Parenteral 1712
Dilantin with Phenobarbital Kapseals 1715

Pindolol (Inhibited by amphetamines). Products include:
Visken Tablets 2036

Pirbuterol Acetate (Enhanced activity). Products include:
Maxair Inhaler 1311

Polythiazide (Antagonized; increases blood levels of amphetamines). Products include:
Minizide Capsules 1779
Renese Tablets 1785
Renese-R Tablets 1786

Potassium Citrate (Antagonized; increases blood levels of amphetamines). Products include:
Alka-Seltzer Effervescent Antacid .. 1570
K-Lyte 707
Polycitra Syrup 2424
Polycitra-K 2424
Polycitra-LC—Sugar-Free 2424
Ricelyte, Rice-Based Oral Electrolyte Maintenance Solution ▣ 613

Prazosin Hydrochloride (Inhibited by amphetamines). Products include:
Minipress Capsules 1778
Minizide Capsules 1779

Prochlorperazine (Central stimulating effects of amphetamines). Products include:
Compazine 2201

Promethazine Hydrochloride (Sedative effects may be counteracted). Products include:
Mepergan Injection 2479
Phenergan with Codeine 2497
Phenergan with Dextromethorphan 2499
Phenergan Injection 2493
Phenergan Suppositories 2496
Phenergan Syrup 2495
Phenergan Tablets 2496
Phenergan VC 2500
Phenergan VC with Codeine 2501

Propoxyphene Hydrochloride (Amphetamines' CNS stimulation potentiated in propoxyphene overdosage; fatal convulsions can occur). Products include:
Darvon 1256
Wygesic Tablets 2540

Propoxyphene Napsylate (Amphetamines' CNS stimulation potentiated in propoxyphene overdosage; fatal convulsions can occur). Products include:
Darvon-N/Darvocet-N 1254

Propranolol Hydrochloride (Inhibited by amphetamines). Products include:
Inderal 2459
Inderal LA Long Acting Capsules 2461
Inderide Tablets 2463
Inderide LA Long Acting Capsules .. 2465

Protriptyline Hydrochloride (Enhanced activity; potentiation of cardiovascular effects). Products include:
Vivactil Tablets 1567

Pseudoephedrine Hydrochloride (Enhanced activity). Products include:
Actifed Capsules ▣ 539
Actifed Plus Caplets ▣ 539
Actifed Plus Tablets ▣ 540
Actifed with Codeine Cough Syrup.. 752
Actifed Syrup ▣ 540
Actifed Tablets ▣ 540
Actifed 12-Hour Capsules ▣ 539
Advil Cold & Sinus Caplets (formerly CoAdvil) 2416
Allerest ▣ 559
Anatuss LA Tablets 1359
Benadryl Decongestant Elixir ▣ 635
Benadryl Decongestant ▣ 635
Benadryl Plus ▣ 636
Benadryl Plus Nighttime ▣ 637
Benylin Decongestant ▣ 638
Brexin L.A. Capsules 2078
Bromfed Capsules (Timed Release) 1615
Bromfed Syrup ▣ 628
Bromfed 1615
CoAdvil ▣ 748
Allergy-Sinus Comtrex Multi-Symptom Allergy Sinus Formula Tablets & Caplets 746
Cough Formula Comtrex 746
Comtrex Multi-Symptom Cold Reliever Tablets/Caplets/Liqui-Gels/Liquid 745
Day-Night Comtrex 747
Non-Drowsy Comtrex 747
Congess 994
Congestac Caplets ▣ 617
Contac Jr. Children's Cold Medicine ▣ 712
Contac Nighttime Cold Medicine ▣ 713
Contac Sinus Caplets Maximum Strength Non-Drowsy Formula ▣ 710
Contac Sinus Tablets Maximum Strength Non-Drowsy Formula ▣ 710
Deconamine 663
Deconsal II Tablets 559
Dimacol Caplets ▣ 672
Dimetane-DX Cough Syrup 1858
Dorcol Children's Cough Syrup ▣ 685
Dorcol Children's Decongestant Liquid ▣ 685
Dorcol Children's Liquid Cold Formula ▣ 686
Maximum Strength Dristan Decongestant/Analgesic Coated Caplets ▣ 750
No Drowsiness Dristan Cold Nasal Decongestant/Analgesic Coated Caplets 2420
Dristan Sinus Caplets 2419
Sinus Excedrin Analgesic, Decongestant Tablets & Caplets ▣ 533
Fedahist Gyrocaps 2145
Fedahist Timecaps 2145
Guaifed 1615
Guaifed Syrup ▣ 629
Isoclor Expectorant 982
Isoclor Timesule Capsules ▣ 561
Kronofed-A 970
Medi-Flu Caplet, Liquid ▣ 640
Novafed A Capsules 1342
Novafed Capsules 1342
Novahistine DH 1342
Novahistine DMX ▣ 595
Novahistine Expectorant 1343
Nucofed Capsules 2219
Nucofed Expectorant 2219
Nucofed Pediatric Expectorant 2220
Nucofed Syrup 2219
Ornex Caplets ▣ 618
PediaCare Allergy Relief Formula Liquid 1362
PediaCare Cough-Cold Formula Liquid 1362
PediaCare Infants' Oral Decongestant Drops 1362
PediaCare Night Rest Cough-Cold Formula Liquid 1362
PediaCare 6-12 Cough-Cold Formula Chewable Tablets 1362
Robitussin-DAC Syrup 1875
Robitussin-PE ▣ 677
Rondec 1975
Rondec-DM 1976
Rondec-TR Tablet 1975
Ru-Tuss DE Tablets 694
Ryna ▣ 741
Seldane-D Extended-Release Tablets 1350
Sinarest ▣ 562
Sine-Aid Maximum Strength Sinus Headache Caplets 1365
Sine-Aid Maximum Strength Sinus Headache Tablets 1365
Sine-Off Maximum Strength Allergy/Sinus Formula Caplets ▣ 721
Sine-Off Maximum Strength No Drowsiness Formula Caplets ▣ 722
Singlet Tablets ▣ 598
Sinutab Maximum Strength ▣ 641
Sinutab Maximum Strength Without Drowsiness Tablets & Caplets ▣ 642
Sinutab Regular Strength Without Drowsiness Formula ▣ 641
St. Joseph Nighttime Cold Medicine ▣ 705
Sudafed Children's Liquid ▣ 543
Sudafed Cough Syrup ▣ 543
Sudafed Plus Liquid ▣ 544
Sudafed Plus Tablets ▣ 545
Sudafed Sinus Caplets ▣ 545
Sudafed Sinus Tablets ▣ 545
Sudafed Tablets, 30 mg ▣ 544
Sudafed Tablets, Adult Strength, 60 mg ▣ 544
Sudafed 12 Hour Capsules ▣ 545
TheraFlu Flu and Cold Medicine ▣ 687
Triaminic Nite Light ▣ 689
Tylenol Allergy Sinus Medication Caplets and Gelcaps, Maximum Strength 1372
Children's Tylenol Cold Liquid Formula and Chewable Tablets 1368
Tylenol Cold & Flu Hot Medication, Packets 1369
Tylenol Cold & Flu No Drowsiness Hot Medication, Packets 1371
Tylenol Cold Medication Caplets and Tablets 1370
Tylenol Cold Medication No Drowsiness Formula Caplets 1370
Tylenol Cold Night Time Medication Liquid 1371
Tylenol Cough Medication Liquid with Decongestant, Maximum Strength 1372
Tylenol, Maximum Strength, Sinus Medication Gelcaps, Caplets and Tablets 1373
Ursinus Inlay-Tabs ▣ 691
Vicks Children's NyQuil ▣ 664
Vicks Daycare ▣ 660
Vicks Formula 44D Decongestant Cough Medicine ▣ 662
Vicks Formula 44M Multi-Symptom Cough Medicine ▣ 662
Vicks NyQuil Nighttime Colds Medicine-Original & Cherry Flavor ▣ 664
Vicks Pediatric Formula 44 Cough & Congestion Medicine ▣ 663
Vicks Pediatric Formula 44m Multi-Symptom Cough & Cold Medicine ▣ 663

Pseudoephedrine Sulfate (Enhanced activity). Products include:
Afrin Tablets ▣ 693
Chlor-Trimeton Decongestant ▣ 694
Disophrol Chronotab Sustained-Action Tablets ▣ 698
Drixoral Antihistamine/Nasal Decongestant Syrup ▣ 698
Drixoral Non-Drowsy Formula ▣ 699
Drixoral Plus Extended-Release Tablets ▣ 699
Drixoral Sinus ▣ 700
Drixoral Sustained-Action Tablets ▣ 698
Sinutab Allergy Formula Sustained Action Tablets ▣ 640
Trinalin Repetabs Tablets 1170

Pyrilamine Maleate (Sedative effects may be counteracted). Products include:
Codimal 846
4-Way Fast Acting Nasal Spray - Original Formula (regular & mentholated) & Metered Spray Pump (regular) 751
Maximum Strength Midol Multi-Symptom Menstrual Formula ▣ 571
Maximum Strength Midol PMS Premenstrual Syndrome Formula ▣ 570
Regular Strength Midol Multi-Symptom Menstrual Formula ▣ 570
Prefrin-A ⊙ 255
Prēmsyn PMS Capsules & Caplets ▣ 547
Primatene Tablets-M Formula 2421
Robitussin Night Relief ▣ 677
Ru-Tuss with Hydrocodone 694
Triaminic Expectorant DH 1995
Triaminic Oral Infant Drops 1996

Pyrilamine Tannate (Sedative effects may be counteracted). Products include:
Rynatan 2387

Ramipril (Antagonized). Products include:
Altace Capsules 1086

Rauwolfia Serpentina (Antagonized). Products include:
Raudixin Tablets 1803
Rauzide Tablets 1804

Rescinnamine (Antagonized).
No products indexed under this heading.

Reserpine (Lowers blood levels and efficacy of amphetamines). Products include:
Diupres Tablets 1461
Hydromox R Tablets 1209
Hydropres Tablets 1485
Renese-R Tablets 1786
Salutensin/Salutensin-Demi 719
Ser-Ap-Es Tablets 881
Serpasil Tablets 883
Serpasil-Apresoline Tablets 884
Serpasil-Esidrix Tablets 886

Selegiline Hydrochloride (Potentiation of amphetamines; possibly fatal; concurrent use is contraindicated). Products include:
Eldepryl 2250

Sodium Acid Phosphate (Lowers blood levels and efficacy of amphetamines). Products include:
K-Phos No. 2 Tablets 659
Uroqid-Acid 661

Sodium Nitroprusside (Antagonized). Products include:
Nipride I.V. Infusion 1909

Terazosin Hydrochloride (Inhibited by amphetamines). Products include:
Hytrin Tablets 529

Terbutaline Sulfate (Enhanced activity). Products include:
Brethaire Inhaler 1024
Brethine Ampuls 1026
Brethine Tablets 1026
Bricanyl Injection 1324
Bricanyl Tablets 1325

Terfenadine (Sedative effects may be counteracted). Products include:
Seldane Tablets 1349
Seldane-D Extended-Release Tablets 1350

Timolol Maleate (Inhibited by amphetamines). Products include:
Blocadren Tablets 1429
Timolide Tablets 1547
Timoptic in Ocudose 1552
Timoptic Sterile Ophthalmic Solution 1550

Tranylcypromine Sulfate (Potentiation of amphetamines; possibly fatal; concurrent use is contraindicated). Products include:
Parnate Tablets 2222

Trimeprazine Tartrate (Sedative effects may be counteracted). Products include:
Temaril Tablets, Syrup and Spansule Sustained Release Capsules 1085

Trimethaphan Camsylate (Antagonized). Products include:
Arfonad Ampuls 1887

Trimipramine Maleate (Enhanced activity). Products include:
Surmontil Capsules 2524

Tripelennamine Hydrochloride (Sedative effects may be counteracted). Products include:
PBZ Tablets & Elixir 1037

(▣ Described in PDR For Nonprescription Drugs) (⊙ Described in PDR For Ophthalmology)

PBZ-SR Tablets 1037

Tripelennamine Preparations (Sedative effects may be counteracted).

Triprolidine Hydrochloride (Sedative effects may be counteracted). Products include:

Actidil .... ■ 538
Actifed Capsules .... ■ 539
Actifed Plus Caplets .... ■ 539
Actifed Plus Tablets .... ■ 540
Actifed with Codeine Cough Syrup.. 752
Actifed Syrup .... ■ 540
Actifed Tablets .... ■ 540
Actifed 12-Hour Capsules .... ■ 539

Vitamin C (Lowers blood levels and efficacy). Products include:

Allbee with C Caplets .... ■ 670
Allbee C-800 .... ■ 670
Bromase Capsules 672
Bugs Bunny Children's Chewable Vitamins (Sugar Free) .... ■ 625
Bugs Bunny With Extra C Children's Chewable Vitamins (Sugar Free) .... ■ 626
Bugs Bunny Plus Iron Children's Chewable Vitamins (Sugar Free) ■ 625
Cefol Filmtab 509
Centrum, Jr. (Children's Chewable) + Extra C .... ■ 585
Cod Liver Oil Concentrate Tablets with Vitamin C .... ■ 694
Ester-C Tablets .... ■ 575
Ferancee Chewable Tablets 1155
Ferancee-HP Tablets 1155
Fero-Folic-500 Filmtab 527
Fero-Grad-500 Filmtab 528
Flintstones Children's Chewable Vitamins .... ■ 625
Flintstones Children's Chewable Vitamins With Extra C .... ■ 626
Flintstones Children's Chewable Vitamins Plus Iron .... ■ 625
Halls Vitamin C Drops .... ■ 742
Hyland's Vitamin C for Children .... ■ 729
ICAPS Plus .... ⊙ 280
Mediatric Capsules 2476
Mol-Iron w/Vitamin C Tablets .... ■ 703
Natalins Rx 1391
Natalins Tablets 1391
N'ICE Sugarless Vitamin C Drops .. ■ 719
Niferex w/Vitamin C Tablets 847
Ocuvite Vitamin and Mineral Supplement .... ⊙ 312
One-A-Day Essential Vitamins .... ■ 627
One-A-Day Maximum Formula Vitamins and Minerals .... ■ 627
One-A-Day Plus Extra C Vitamins .. ■ 627
Probec-T Tablets .... ■ 581
Stressgard Stress Formula Vitamins .... ■ 628
Stuart Prenatal Tablets .... ■ 731
The Stuart Formula Tablets 1157
Stuartinic Tablets 1157
Sunkist Children's Chewable Multivitamins - Plus Extra C .... ■ 553
Sunkist Vitamin C .... ■ 553
Surbex with C .... ■ 502
Trinsicon Capsules 2415
Tri-Vi-Flor 1.0 mg Vitamins with Fluoride Chewable Tablets 1400
Tri-Vi-Flor Drops 1400
Tri-Vi-Sol Vitamin Drops .... ■ 614
Tri-Vi-Sol Vitamin Drops with Iron ■ 614
Vicon Forte Capsules 2416
Vicon Plus .... ■ 682
Vicon-C .... ■ 682
Vi-Daylin ADC Vitamins Drops 1980
Vi-Daylin ADC Vitamins + Iron Drops 1980
Vi-Daylin/F ADC Vitamins Drops With Fluoride 1981
Vi-Daylin/F ADC Vitamins + Iron Drops With Fluoride 1981
Vi-Zac .... ■ 682
Within Women's Formula Multivitamins with Calcium, Extra Iron and Zinc .... ■ 628
Z-Bec Tablets .... ■ 678

Food Interactions

Fruit juices, unspecified (Lowers blood levels and efficacy).

DEXEDRINE SPANSULE CAPSULES
(Dextroamphetamine Sulfate) 2206
See **Dexedrine Elixir**

DEXEDRINE TABLETS
(Dextroamphetamine Sulfate) 2206
See **Dexedrine Elixir**

DIABETA
(Glyburide) 1091
May interact with salicylates, sulfonamides, oral anticoagulants, monoamine oxidase inhibitors, beta blockers, thiazides, diuretics, corticosteroids, phenothiazines, thyroid preparations, estrogens, oral contraceptives, sympathomimetic aerosal brochodilators, calcium channel blockers, non-steroidal anti-inflammatory agents, and certain other agents. Compounds in these categories include:

Acebutolol Hydrochloride (Potentiates hypoglycemic action). Products include:

Sectral Capsules 2520

Albuterol (Hyperglycemia; loss of control). Products include:

Proventil Inhalation Aerosol 2117
Ventolin Inhalation Aerosol and Refill 583

Albuterol Sulfate (Hyperglycemia; loss of control). Products include:

Proventil Repetabs Tablets 2120
Proventil Solutions for Inhalation 0.5% and 0.083% 2118
Proventil Syrup 2119
Proventil Tablets 2120
Ventolin 583

Amiloride Hydrochloride (Hyperglycemia; loss of control). Products include:

Midamor Tablets 1508
Moduretic Tablets 1510

Aspirin (Potentiates hypoglycemic action). Products include:

Alka-Seltzer Effervescent Antacid and Pain Reliever 1568
Alka-Seltzer Extra Strength Effervescent Antacid and Pain Reliever 1570
Alka-Seltzer (Flavored) Effervescent Antacid and Pain Reliever 1569
Alka-Seltzer Plus Cold Medicine .... ■ 623
Alka-Seltzer Plus Night-Time Cold Medicine .... ■ 623
Alka Seltzer Plus Sinus Allergy Medicine .... ■ 624
Anacin Coated Analgesic Caplets 2417
Anacin Coated Analgesic Tablets 2417
Anacin Maximum Strength Analgesic Coated Tablets 2417
Maximum Strength Arthritis Pain Formula By the Makers of Anacin Analgesic Tablets and Caplets 2418
Arthritis Pain Formula by the Makers of Anacin Analgesic Tablets and Caplets .... ■ 747
Arthritis Strength BC Powder .... ■ 516
Ascriptin A/D Caplets 1850
Regular Strength Ascriptin Tablets 1850
Azdone Tablets 844
BC Powder .... ■ 517
BC Cold Powder .... ■ 517
Children's Bayer Chewable Aspirin .... ■ 564
Genuine Bayer Aspirin Tablets & Caplets .... ■ 564
Maximum Bayer Aspirin Tablets & Caplets .... ■ 566
Bayer Plus Aspirin Tablets .... ■ 567
Therapy Bayer Aspirin Caplets .... ■ 568
8 Hour Bayer Timed-Release Aspirin .... ■ 566
Arthritis Strength Bufferin Analgesic Caplets 744
Extra Strength Bufferin Analgesic Tablets 745
Bufferin Analgesic Tablets and Caplets 743
Cama Arthritis Pain Reliever .... ■ 685
Damason-P 1356
Easprin 1719
Ecotrin Enteric Coated Aspirin Maximum Strength Tablets and Caplets 2189
Ecotrin Enteric Coated Aspirin Regular Strength Tablets and Caplets 2189
Empirin Aspirin .... ■ 541
Empirin with Codeine Phosphate Nos. 2, 3 & 4 764
Equagesic Tablets 2451
Excedrin Extra-Strength Analgesic Tablets & Caplets 749
4-Way Cold Tablets 750
Fiorinal Capsules 2007
Fiorinal with Codeine Capsules 2008
Fiorinal Tablets 2007
Lortab ASA Tablets 2414
Momentum Muscular Backache Formula .... ■ 751
Norgesic 1314
Norwich Extra-Strength Aspirin .... ■ 546
Norwich Regular Strength Aspirin ■ 547
P-A-C Analgesic Tablets .... ■ 669
Percodan 951
Robaxisal Tablets 1872
Sine-Off Sinus Medicine Tablets-Aspirin Formula .... ■ 722
Soma Compound w/Codeine Tablets 2390
Soma Compound Tablets 2389
St. Joseph Adult Chewable Aspirin (81 mg.) .... ■ 703
Synalgos-DC Capsules 2525
Talwin Compound 2072
Ursinus Inlay-Tabs .... ■ 691
Vanquish Analgesic Caplets .... ■ 574
Zorprin Tablets 698

Atenolol (Potentiates hypoglycemic action). Products include:

Tenoretic Tablets 1105
Tenormin Tablets and I.V. Injection 1107

Bendroflumethiazide (Hyperglycemia, loss of control). Products include:

Corzide Tablets 702
Naturetin Tablets 1789
Rauzide Tablets 1804

Bepridil Hydrochloride (Hyperglycemia; loss of control). Products include:

Vascor (200, 300 and 400 mg) Tablets 1383

Betamethasone Acetate (Hyperglycemia; loss of control). Products include:

Celestone Soluspan Suspension 2081

Betamethasone Sodium Phosphate (Hyperglycemia; loss of control). Products include:

Celestone Soluspan Suspension 2081

Betaxolol Hydrochloride (Potentiates hypoglycemic action). Products include:

Betoptic Sterile Ophthalmic Solution 569
Betoptic S Sterile Ophthalmic Suspension 570
Kerlone Tablets 2172

Bumetanide (Hyperglycemia; loss of control). Products include:

Bumex 1895

Carteolol Hydrochloride (Potentiates hypoglycemic action). Products include:

Cartrol Tablets 507

Chloramphenicol (Potentiates hypoglycemic action). Products include:

AK-Chlor Sterile Ophthalmic Ointment & Solution .... ⊙ 201
Chloromycetin Cream, 1% 1694
Chloromycetin Hydrocortisone Ophthalmic 1694
Chloromycetin Kapseals 1695
Chloromycetin Ophthalmic Ointment, 1% 1696
Chloromycetin Ophthalmic Solution 1696
Chloromycetin Otic 1697
Chloroptic S.O.P. .... ⊙ 243
Chloroptic Sterile Ophthalmic Solution .... ⊙ 243
Ophthochlor Ophthalmic Solution ⊙ 300
Ophthocort .... ⊙ 301

Chloramphenicol Palmitate (Potentiates hypoglycemic action). Products include:

Chloromycetin Palmitate, Oral Suspension 1697

Chloramphenicol Sodium Succinate (Potentiates hypoglycemic action). Products include:

Chloromycetin Sodium Succinate.... 1698

Chlorothiazide (Hyperglycemia, loss of control). Products include:

Aldoclor Tablets 1413
Diupres Tablets 1461
Diuril Oral 1464

Chlorothiazide Sodium (Hyperglycemia, loss of control). Products include:

Diuril Sodium Intravenous 1463

Chlorotrianisene (Hyperglycemia; loss of control). Products include:

TACE 12 and 25 mg 1353

Chlorpromazine (Hyperglycemia; loss of control). Products include:

Thorazine 2234

Chlorpropamide (Potentiates hypoglycemic action). Products include:

Diabinese Tablets 1775

Chlorthalidone (Hyperglycemia; loss of control). Products include:

Combipres Tablets 678
Tenoretic Tablets 1105
Thalitone Tablets 687

Choline Magnesium Trisalicylate (Potentiates hypoglycemic action). Products include:

Trilisate 1822

Cortisone Acetate (Hyperglycemia; loss of control). Products include:

Cortone Acetate Sterile Suspension 1437
Cortone Acetate Tablets 1439

Dexamethasone (Hyperglycemia; loss of control). Products include:

AK-Trol Ointment & Suspension .... ⊙ 207
Decadron Elixir 1445
Decadron Tablets 1447
Decaspray Topical Aerosol 1459
Dexacidin .... ⊙ 272
Maxidex Sterile Ophthalmic Suspension .... ⊙ 223
Maxitrol Ophthalmic Ointment/Suspension .... ⊙ 223
TobraDex Ophthalmic Suspension and Ointment .... ⊙ 228

Dexamethasone Acetate (Hyperglycemia; loss of control). Products include:

Dalalone D.P. Injectable 999
Decadron-LA Sterile Suspension 1457

Dexamethasone Sodium Phosphate (Hyperglycemia; loss of control). Products include:

AK-Dex .... ⊙ 203
Decadron Phosphate Respihaler 1454
Decadron Phosphate Sterile Ophthalmic Ointment 1453
Decadron Phosphate Sterile Ophthalmic Solution 1453
Decadron Phosphate Topical Cream 1455
Decadron Phosphate Turbinaire 1456
Maxidex Sterile Ophthalmic Ointment .... ⊙ 222
NeoDecadron Sterile Ophthalmic Ointment 1517
NeoDecadron Sterile Ophthalmic Solution 1518
NeoDecadron Topical Cream 1518

Diclofenac Sodium (Potentiates hypoglycemic effect of sulfonylureas). Products include:

Voltaren Ophthalmic Sterile Ophthalmic Solution .... ⊙ 268
Voltaren Tablets 1042

Dicumarol (Potentiates hypoglycemic action). Products include:

Dicumarol Tablets 516

Dienestrol (Hyperglycemia; loss of control). Products include:

Ortho Dienestrol Cream 1664

Diethylstilbestrol (Hyperglycemia; loss of control). Products include:

Diethylstilbestrol Tablets 1258

Diflunisal (Potentiates hypoglycemic action). Products include:
- Dolobid Tablets ... 1465

Diltiazem Hydrochloride (Hyperglycemia; loss of control). Products include:
- Cardizem Tablets-30 mg, 60 mg, 90 mg and 120 mg ... 1329
- Cardizem SR Capsules-60 mg, 90 mg and 120 mg ... 1327

Dobutamine Hydrochloride (Hyperglycemia; loss of control). Products include:
- Dobutrex Solution Vials ... 1259

Dopamine Hydrochloride (Hyperglycemia; loss of control). Products include:
- Intropin Injection ... 930

Ephedrine Hydrochloride (Hyperglycemia; loss of control). Products include:
- Amesec ... ▣ 682
- Primatene Tablets-M Formula ... 2421
- Primatene Tablets-P Formula ... 2421
- Primatene Tablets-Regular Formula ... 2421
- Quadrinal Tablets ... 1183
- Quelidrine Syrup ... 556
- Tedral SA ... 1765

Ephedrine Sulfate (Hyperglycemia; loss of control). Products include:
- Bronkaid Tablets ... ▣ 757
- Bronkolixir ... ▣ 761
- Bronkotabs Tablets ... ▣ 762
- Marax Tablets & DF Syrup ... 1954
- Pazo Hemorrhoid Ointment & Suppositories ... 752
- Vicks Vatronol Nose Drops ... ▣ 666

Ephedrine Tannate (Hyperglycemia; loss of control). Products include:
- Rynatuss ... 2388

Epinephrine (Hyperglycemia; loss of control). Products include:
- Ana-Kit Anaphylaxis Emergency Treatment Kit ... 1100
- Bronkaid Mist ... ▣ 757
- EpiPen ... 843
- Marcaine Hydrochloride 0.5% with Epinephrine 1:200,000 (as bitartrate) ... 958
- Marcaine Hydrochloride with Epinephrine 1:200,000 ... 2055
- Primatene Mist ... 2420
- Sus-Phrine Injection ... 1006
- Xylocaine with Epinephrine Injections ... 637

Epinephrine Bitartrate (Hyperglycemia; loss of control). Products include:
- AsthmaHaler Mist Epinephrine Bitartrate Bronchodilator ... ▣ 616
- Bronkaid Mist Suspension ... ▣ 757
- Primatene Mist Suspension ... 2421

Epinephrine Hydrochloride (Hyperglycemia; loss of control). Products include:
- Adrenalin Chloride Solution 1:100 & 1:1,000 ... 1689
- Epifrin ... ⊙ 244
- Glaucon ... ⊙ 218

Esmolol Hydrochloride (Potentiates hypoglycemic action). Products include:
- Brevibloc Injection ... 942

Estradiol (Hyperglycemia; loss of control). Products include:
- Emcyt Capsules ... 1161
- Estrace ... 1385
- Estrace Vaginal Cream ... 1388
- Estraderm Transdermal System ... 866

Estrogens, Conjugated (Hyperglycemia; loss of control). Products include:
- Mediatric Capsules ... 2476
- PMB 200 and PMB 400 ... 2504
- Premarin Intravenous ... 2508
- Premarin with Methyltestosterone ... 2515
- Premarin Tablets ... 2510
- Premarin Vaginal Cream ... 2512

Estrogens, Esterified (Hyperglycemia; loss of control). Products include:
- Estratest ... 2245
- Menrium Tablets ... 1934

Estropipate (Hyperglycemia; loss of control). Products include:
- Ogen ... 540

Ethacrynic Acid (Hyperglycemia; loss of control). Products include:
- Edecrin Tablets ... 1468

Ethinyl Estradiol (Hyperglycemia; loss of control). Products include:
- Brevicon ... 2304
- Demulen ... 2161
- Estinyl Tablets ... 2085
- Jenest-28 Tablets ... 1636
- Levlen/Tri-Levlen ... 665
- Lo/Ovral Tablets ... 2471
- Lo/Ovral-28 Tablets ... 2476
- Loestrin ... 1728
- Modicon ... 1667
- Nordette-21 Tablets ... 2481
- Nordette-28 Tablets ... 2483
- Norethin ... 2133
- Norinyl ... 2304
- Norlestrin ... 1746
- Ortho-Cyclen Tablets ... 1658
- Ortho-Novum ... 1667
- Ovcon ... 1391
- Ovral Tablets ... 2490
- Ovral-28 Tablets ... 2491
- Levlen/Tri-Levlen ... 665
- Tri-Norinyl ... 2304
- Triphasil-21 Tablets ... 2527
- Triphasil-28 Tablets ... 2532

Ethynodiol Diacetate (Hyperglycemia; loss of control). Products include:
- Demulen ... 2161

Etodolac (Potentiates hypoglycemic effect of sulfonylureas). Products include:
- Lodine Capsules ... 2468

Felodipine (Hyperglycemia; loss of control). Products include:
- Plendil Extended-Release Tablets ... 1526

Fenoprofen Calcium (Potentiates hypoglycemic effect of sulfonylureas). Products include:
- Nalfon Pulvules & Tablets ... 919

Fluphenazine Decanoate (Hyperglycemia; loss of control). Products include:
- Prolixin Decanoate ... 1795

Fluphenazine Enanthate (Hyperglycemia; loss of control). Products include:
- Prolixin Enanthate ... 1796

Fluphenazine Hydrochloride (Hyperglycemia; loss of control). Products include:
- Prolixin Elixir ... 1793
- Prolixin Injection ... 1791
- Prolixin Oral Concentrate ... 1792
- Prolixin Tablets ... 1793

Flurbiprofen (Potentiates hypoglycemic effect of sulfonylureas). Products include:
- Ansaid Tablets ... 2319

Furazolidone (Potentiates hypoglycemic action). Products include:
- Furoxone ... 1855

Furosemide (Hyperglycemia; loss of control). Products include:
- Lasix ... 1093

Glipizide (Potentiates hypoglycemic action). Products include:
- Glucotrol ... 1952

Hydrochlorothiazide (Hyperglycemia, loss of control). Products include:
- Aldactazide ... 2150
- Aldoril Tablets ... 1418
- Apresazide Capsules ... 854
- Apresoline-Esidrix Tablets ... 857
- Capozide ... 2258
- Dyazide Capsules ... 2208
- Esidrix Tablets ... 863
- Esimil Tablets ... 864
- HydroDIURIL Tablets ... 1484
- Hydropres Tablets ... 1485
- Inderide Tablets ... 2463
- Inderide LA Long Acting Capsules ... 2465
- Lopressor HCT Tablets ... 1034
- Maxzide ... 1215
- Moduretic Tablets ... 1510
- Normozide Tablets ... 2112
- Oretic Tablets ... 544
- Oreticyl ... 545
- Prinzide Tablets ... 1540
- Ser-Ap-Es Tablets ... 881
- Serpasil-Esidrix Tablets ... 886
- Timolide Tablets ... 1547
- Trandate HCT Tablets ... 579
- Vaseretic Tablets ... 1559
- Zestoretic ... 2274

Hydrocortisone (Hyperglycemia; loss of control). Products include:
- AK-Spore H.C. ... ⊙ 206
- Bactine Hydrocortisone Anti-Itch Cream ... ▣ 625
- CaldeCORT Anti-Itch Hydrocortisone Spray ... ▣ 560
- Carmol HC Cream 1% ... 2296
- Cortaid Spray ... ▣ 735
- Cortenema ... 2244
- Cortisporin Ointment ... 758
- Cortisporin Ophthalmic Ointment Sterile ... 758
- Cortisporin Ophthalmic Suspension Sterile ... 759
- Cortisporin Otic Solution Sterile ... 760
- Cortisporin Otic Suspension Sterile ... 760
- Cortizone-5 Creme & Ointment ... ▣ 732
- Dermolate Anti-Itch Cream ... ▣ 697
- Eldecort Cream 1.0% ... 1113
- Eldecort Cream 1.0% and 2.5% ... 1113
- Fungoid HC Creme ... 1770
- Hydrocortone Tablets ... 1482
- Hytone ... 909
- LazerSporin-C Solution ... 1770
- Massengill Medicated Soft Cloth Towelettes ... 2192
- Nutracort Cream & Lotion ... 1684
- PediOtic Suspension Sterile ... 797
- Synacort Creams 1%, 2.5% ... 2296
- Vanoxide-HC Acne Lotion ... 911
- Vioform-Hydrocortisone Cream and Mild Cream ... 889
- Vioform-Hydrocortisone Ointment ... 889
- VōSoL HC Otic Solution ... 2392
- Vytone Cream 1% ... 911

Hydrocortisone Acetate (Hyperglycemia; loss of control). Products include:
- Analpram-HC Rectal Cream 1% and 2.5% ... 970
- Anusol-HC Cream ... 1690
- Anusol-HC Suppositories ... 1691
- Caldecort ... ▣ 560
- Carmol HC Cream 1% ... 2296
- Chloromycetin Hydrocortisone Ophthalmic ... 1694
- Coly-Mycin S Otic w/Neomycin & Hydrocortisone ... 1708
- Cortaid ... ▣ 735
- Cortef Feminine Itch Cream ... ▣ 735
- Corticaine ... ▣ 682
- Cortifoam ... 1827
- Cortisporin Cream ... 757
- Epifoam ... 1828
- Gynecort 5 Creme ... ▣ 556
- Hydrocortone Acetate Sterile Suspension ... 1479
- Lanacort 5 Creme and Ointment ... ▣ 557
- Mantadil Cream ... 789
- Ophthocort ... ⊙ 301
- Orabase HCA Oral Paste ... 890
- Pramosone Cream, Lotion & Ointment ... 971
- ProctoCream-HC ... 1834
- Proctofoam-HC ... 1835

Hydrocortisone Sodium Phosphate (Hyperglycemia; loss of control). Products include:
- Hydrocortone Phosphate Injection, Sterile ... 1481

Hydrocortisone Sodium Succinate (Hyperglycemia; loss of control). Products include:
- Solu-Cortef Sterile Powder ... 2361

Hydroflumethiazide (Hyperglycemia, loss of control). Products include:
- Diucardin Tablets ... 2450
- Saluron ... 718
- Salutensin/Salutensin-Demi ... 719

Ibuprofen (Potentiates hypoglycemic effect of sulfonylureas). Products include:
- Advil Cold & Sinus Caplets (formerly CoAdvil) ... 2416
- Advil Ibuprofen Tablets and Caplets ... 2416
- Children's Advil Suspension ... 2426
- CoAdvil ... ▣ 748
- Dristan Sinus Caplets ... 2419
- Haltran Tablets ... ▣ 668
- Ibuprofen ... ▣ 631
- Medipren ibuprofen Caplets and Tablets ... 1362
- Midol 200 Cramp Relief Formula ... ▣ 570
- Motrin Tablets ... 2351
- Motrin IB Caplets and Tablets ... ▣ 736
- Nuprin Ibuprofen/Analgesic Tablets & Caplets ... 752
- PediaProfen Suspension ... 1363
- Rufen Tablets ... 691
- Trendar Ibuprofen Tablets ... ▣ 756

Indapamide (Hyperglycemia; loss of control). Products include:
- Lozol Tablets ... 1843

Indomethacin (Potentiates hypoglycemic effect of sulfonylureas). Products include:
- Indocin ... 1487

Indomethacin Sodium Trihydrate (Potentiates hypoglycemic effect of sulfonylureas). Products include:
- Indocin I.V. ... 1490

Isocarboxazid (Potentiates hypoglycemic action). Products include:
- Marplan Tablets ... 1906

Isoniazid (Hyperglycemia; loss of control). Products include:
- INH Tablets ... 868
- Rifamate Capsules ... 1347

Isoproterenol Hydrochloride (Hyperglycemia; loss of control). Products include:
- Isuprel Hydrochloride Injection 1:5000 ... 2050
- Isuprel Hydrochloride Mistometer ... 2051
- Isuprel Hydrochloride Solution 1:200 & 1:100 ... 2052
- Norisodrine Aerotrol ... 540

Isradipine (Hyperglycemia; loss of control). Products include:
- DynaCirc Capsules ... 2004

Ketoprofen (Potentiates hypoglycemic effect of sulfonylureas). Products include:
- Orudis Capsules ... 2488

Ketorolac Tromethamine (Potentiates hypoglycemic effect of sulfonylureas). Products include:
- Toradol IM Injection ... 2302

Labetalol Hydrochloride (Potentiates hypoglycemic action). Products include:
- Normodyne Injection ... 2108
- Normodyne Tablets ... 2110
- Normozide Tablets ... 2112
- Trandate HCT Tablets ... 579
- Trandate Injection ... 577
- Trandate Tablets ... 579

Levonorgestrel (Hyperglycemia; loss of control). Products include:
- Levlen/Tri-Levlen ... 665
- Nordette-21 Tablets ... 2481
- Nordette-28 Tablets ... 2483
- Norplant System ... 2484
- Levlen/Tri-Levlen ... 665
- Triphasil-21 Tablets ... 2527
- Triphasil-28 Tablets ... 2532

Levothyroxine Sodium (Hyperglycemia; loss of control). Products include:
- Levothroid Tablets ... 1003
- Levoxine Tablets ... 904
- Synthroid ... 695

Liothyronine Sodium (Hyperglycemia; loss of control). Products include:
- Cytomel Tablets ... 2203

Magnesium Salicylate (Potentiates hypoglycemic action). Products include:
Doan's - Extra-Strength Analgesic ■ 549
Doan's - Regular Strength Analgesic ■ 549
Mobigesic Analgesic Tablets ■ 507

Meclofenamate Sodium (Potentiates hypoglycemic effect of sulfonylureas). Products include:
Meclomen Capsules 1739

Mefenamic Acid (Potentiates hypoglycemic effect of sulfonylureas). Products include:
Ponstel 1758

Mesoridazine (Hyperglycemia; loss of control). Products include:
Serentil 686

Mestranol (Hyperglycemia; loss of control). Products include:
Enovid 2161
Norethin 2133
Norinyl 2304
Ortho-Novum 1667

Metaproterenol Sulfate (Hyperglycemia; loss of control). Products include:
Alupent 674
Arm-a-Med Metaproterenol Sulfate Inhalation Solution, USP 617
Metaprel Inhalation Aerosol Bronchodilator 2014
Metaprel Inhalation Solution 2015
Metaprel 2015
Metaproterenol Sulfate Inhalation Solution, USP 912

Metaraminol Bitartrate (Hyperglycemia; loss of control). Products include:
Aramine Injection 1424

Methoxamine Hydrochloride (Hyperglycemia; loss of control). Products include:
Vasoxyl Injection 819

Methyclothiazide (Hyperglycemia, loss of control). Products include:
Enduron Tablets 517
Enduronyl 518

Methylprednisolone Acetate (Hyperglycemia; loss of control). Products include:
Depo-Medrol Sterile Aqueous Suspension 2334

Methylprednisolone Sodium Succinate (Hyperglycemia; loss of control). Products include:
Solu-Medrol Sterile Powder 2363

Metolazone (Hyperglycemia; loss of control). Products include:
Diulo 2129
Mykrox ½ mg Tablets 984
Zaroxolyn Tablets 989

Metoprolol Tartrate (Potentiates hypoglycemic action). Products include:
Lopressor Ampuls 1032
Lopressor HCT Tablets 1034
Lopressor Tablets 1032

Miconazole (Severe hypoglycemia). Products include:
Monistat I.V. 1143

Nadolol (Potentiates hypoglycemic action). Products include:
Corgard Tablets 701
Corzide Tablets 702

Naproxen (Potentiates hypoglycemic effect of sulfonylureas). Products include:
Naprosyn 2297

Naproxen Sodium (Potentiates hypoglycemic effect of sulfonylureas). Products include:
Anaprox and Anaprox DS Tablets 2288

Nicardipine Hydrochloride (Hyperglycemia; loss of control). Products include:
Cardene Capsules 2290

Nicotinic Acid (Hyperglycemia; loss of control). Products include:
Niacor Tablets 2376
Nicobid 1846
Nicolar Tablets 1846
Nicotinex Elixir ■ 563
Slo-Niacin Tablets 2376

Nifedipine (Hyperglycemia; loss of control). Products include:
Adalat Capsules (10 mg and 20 mg) 1587
Procardia Capsules 1781
Procardia XL Tablets 1783

Nimodipine (Hyperglycemia; loss of control). Products include:
Nimotop Capsules 1607

Norepinephrine Bitartrate (Hyperglycemia; loss of control). Products include:
Levophed Bitartrate Injection 2054

Norethindrone (Hyperglycemia; loss of control). Products include:
Brevicon 2304
Jenest-28 Tablets 1636
Micronor Tablets 1667
Modicon 1667
Norethin 2133
Norinyl 2304
Norlutin 1755
Nor-Q D Tablets 2304
Ortho-Novum 1667
Ovcon 1391
Tri-Norinyl 2304

Norethynodrel (Hyperglycemia; loss of control). Products include:
Enovid 2161

Norgestimate (Hyperglycemia; loss of control). Products include:
Ortho-Cyclen Tablets 1658

Norgestrel (Hyperglycemia; loss of control). Products include:
Lo/Ovral Tablets 2471
Lo/Ovral-28 Tablets 2476
Ovral Tablets 2490
Ovral-28 Tablets 2491
Ovrette Tablets 2492

Penbutolol Sulfate (Potentiates hypoglycemic action). Products include:
Levatol 1832

Perphenazine (Hyperglycemia; loss of control). Products include:
Etrafon 2087
Triavil Tablets 1556
Trilafon 2123

Phenelzine Sulfate (Potentiates hypoglycemic action). Products include:
Nardil 1742

Phenylbutazone (Potentiates hypoglycemic effect of sulfonylureas). Products include:
Butazolidin Capsules & Tablets 1027

Phenylephrine Bitartrate (Hyperglycemia; loss of control).
No products indexed under this heading.

Phenylephrine Hydrochloride (Hyperglycemia; loss of control). Products include:
AK-Dilate Solution 2.5% and 10% ◉ 203
Atrohist Sprinkle Capsules 558
Cerose-DM 2443
Codimal 846
Comhist LA Capsules 1618
Congespirin For Children Aspirin Free Chewable Cold Tablets 748
Cyclomydril ◉ 216
Deconsal Sprinkle Capsules 559
Dimetane Decongestant ■ 673
Dristan Decongestant/Antihistamine/Analgesic Coated Caplets ■ 749
Dristan Cold Nasal Decongestant/Antihistamine/ Analgesic Coated Tablets 2419
Dristan Advanced Formula Decongestant/Antihistamine/ Analgesic Tablets ■ 749
Dristan Nasal Spray, Menthol 2419
Dristan Nasal Spray, Regular and Regular with Metered Pump 2419
Entex Capsules 1623
Entex Liquid 1623
Sinus Excedrin Analgesic, Decongestant Tablets & Caplets 750
Extendryl 994
4-Way Fast Acting Nasal Spray - Original Formula (regular & mentholated) & Metered Spray Pump (regular) 751
Hycomine Compound Tablets 929
Murocoll-2 Sterile Ophthalmic Solution ◉ 261
Mydfrin 2.5% ◉ 224
Naldecon Syrup, Tablets, Pediatric Drops and Pediatric Syrup 709
Neo-Synephrine Hydrochloride 1% Carpuject 2063
Neo-Synephrine Hydrochloride 1% Injection 2063
Neo-Synephrine Hydrochloride (Ophthalmic) 2064
Neo-Synephrine ■ 759
Nōstril Nasal Decongestant ■ 520
Novahistine Elixir ■ 596
Phenergan VC 2500
Phenergan VC with Codeine 2501
Prefrin Liquifilm Vasoconstrictor and Lubricant Eye Drops ◉ 254
Prefrin-A ◉ 255
Quelidrine Syrup 556
Relief Vasoconstrictor and Lubricant Eye Drops ◉ 256
Robitussin Night Relief ■ 677
Ru-Tuss with Hydrocodone 694
Ru-Tuss Tablets 693
Vasosulf ◉ 279
Vicks Sinex ■ 665
Zincfrin ◉ 230

Phenylephrine Tannate (Hyperglycemia; loss of control). Products include:
Rynatan 2387
Rynatuss 2388

Phenylpropanolamine Hydrochloride (Hyperglycemia; loss of control). Products include:
A.R.M. Allergy Relief Medicine Caplets ■ 615
Acutrim ■ 548
Allerest ■ 559
BC Cold Powder ■ 517
Cheracol Plus Head Cold/Cough Formula ■ 667
Codimal Expectorant 846
Comtrex Multi-Symptom Cold Reliever Tablets/Caplets/Liqui-Gels/Liquid 745
Contac Continuous Action Decongestant/Antihistamine Capsules ■ 710
Contac Maximum Strength Continuous Action Decongestant/ Antihistamine Caplets ■ 709
Contac Severe Cold and Flu Formula Caplets ■ 711
Coricidin 'D' Decongestant Tablets ■ 695
Coricidin Demilets Tablets for Children ■ 696
Demazin Nasal Decongestant/ Antihistamine Repetabs Tablets & Syrup ■ 697
Dexatrim ■ 733
Dimetane-DC Cough Syrup 1857
Dimetapp Elixir ■ 673
Dimetapp DM Elixir ■ 674
Dimetapp Extentabs ■ 674
Dimetapp Plus Caplets ■ 675
Dimetapp Tablets ■ 675
Entex Capsules 1623
Entex LA Tablets 1623
Entex Liquid 1623
4-Way Cold Tablets 750
Hycomine Syrup 927
Naldecon CX Adult Liquid ■ 521
Naldecon DX Adult Liquid ■ 521
Naldecon DX Children's Syrup ■ 522
Naldecon DX Pediatric Drops ■ 522
Naldecon EX Children's Syrup ■ 522
Naldecon EX Pediatric Drops ■ 523
Naldecon Syrup, Tablets, Pediatric Drops and Pediatric Syrup 709
Nolamine Tablets 838
Nolex LA Tablets 838
Ornade Spansule Capsules 2221
Orthoxicol Cough Syrup ■ 668
Propagest 839
Pyrroxate Capsules ■ 669
Robitussin-CF ■ 676
Ru-Tuss II Capsules 693
Ru-Tuss with Hydrocodone 694
Ru-Tuss Tablets 693
Sine-Off Sinus Medicine Tablets-Aspirin Formula ■ 722
Sinulin 840
St. Joseph Cold Tablets for Children ■ 704
Tavist-D Tablets 2035
Triaminic Allergy Tablets ■ 688
Triaminic Chewables ■ 688
Triaminic Cold Tablets ■ 688
Triaminic Expectorant ■ 688
Triaminic Expectorant w/Codeine 1996
Triaminic Expectorant DH 1995
Triaminic Oral Infant Drops 1996
Triaminic Syrup ■ 689
Triaminic-12 Tablets ■ 690
Triaminic-DM Syrup ■ 689
Triaminicin Tablets ■ 690
Triaminicol Multi-Symptom Cold Tablets ■ 691
Triaminicol Multi-Symptom Relief ■ 691
Tuss-Ornade Liquid 2242
Tuss-Ornade Spansule Capsules 2242
Tylenol Cold Medication, Effervescent Tablets 1369

Phenytoin (Hyperglycemia; loss of control). Products include:
Dilantin Infatabs 1710
Dilantin-30 Pediatric/Dilantin-125 Suspension 1713

Phenytoin Sodium (Hyperglycemia; loss of control). Products include:
Dilantin Kapseals 1708
Dilantin Parenteral 1712
Dilantin with Phenobarbital Kapseals 1715

Pindolol (Potentiates hypoglycemic action). Products include:
Visken Tablets 2036

Pirbuterol Acetate (Hyperglycemia; loss of control). Products include:
Maxair Inhaler 1311

Piroxicam (Potentiates hypoglycemic effect of sulfonylureas). Products include:
Feldene Capsules 1777

Polyestradiol Phosphate (Hyperglycemia; loss of control). Products include:
Estradurin 2452

Polythiazide (Hyperglycemia, loss of control). Products include:
Minizide Capsules 1779
Renese Tablets 1785
Renese-R Tablets 1786

Prednisolone Acetate (Hyperglycemia; loss of control). Products include:
AK-Cide Sterile Ophthalmic Ointment & Suspension ◉ 202
Blephamide Liquifilm Sterile Ophthalmic Suspension 586
Blephamide S.O.P. Sterile Ophthalmic Ointment 586
Cetapred Ointment ◉ 220
⅛% Econopred & 1% Econopred Plus ◉ 217
Isopto Cetapred Suspension ◉ 220
Metimyd ◉ 306
Poly-Pred Liquifilm ◉ 250
Pred Forte ◉ 252
Pred Mild ◉ 254
Pred-G Liquifilm Sterile Ophthalmic Suspension ◉ 252
Pred-G S.O.P. Sterile Ophthalmic Ointment ◉ 253
Vasocidin Ointment ◉ 275

Prednisolone Sodium Phosphate (Hyperglycemia; loss of control). Products include:
AK-Pred ◉ 205
Hydeltrasol Injection, Sterile 1476
Inflamase ◉ 274
Pediapred Oral Liquid 987
Vasocidin Ophthalmic Solution ◉ 276

Prednisolone Tebutate (Hyperglycemia; loss of control). Products include:
Hydeltra-T.B.A. Sterile Suspension 1478

Prednisone (Hyperglycemia; loss of control). Products include:
Deltasone Tablets 2332

Probenecid (Potentiates hypoglycemic action). Products include:
Benemid Tablets 1426
ColBENEMID Tablets 1436
Wycillin Injection and Probenecid Tablets 2539

Prochlorperazine (Hyperglycemia; loss of control). Products include:
Compazine 2201

Promethazine Hydrochloride (Hyperglycemia; loss of control). Products include:
Mepergan Injection 2479
Phenergan with Codeine 2497
Phenergan with Dextromethorphan 2499
Phenergan Injection 2493
Phenergan Suppositories 2496
Phenergan Syrup 2495
Phenergan Tablets 2496
Phenergan VC 2500
Phenergan VC with Codeine 2501

Propranolol Hydrochloride (Potentiates hypoglycemic action). Products include:
Inderal 2459
Inderal LA Long Acting Capsules 2461
Inderide Tablets 2463
Inderide LA Long Acting Capsules 2465

Pseudoephedrine Hydrochloride (Hyperglycemia; loss of control). Products include:
Actifed Capsules [BD] 539
Actifed Plus Caplets [BD] 539
Actifed Plus Tablets [BD] 540
Actifed with Codeine Cough Syrup 752
Actifed Syrup [BD] 540
Actifed Tablets [BD] 540
Actifed 12-Hour Capsules [BD] 539
Advil Cold & Sinus Caplets (formerly CoAdvil) 2416
Allerest [BD] 559
Anatuss LA Tablets 1359
Benadryl Decongestant Elixir [BD] 635
Benadryl Decongestant [BD] 635
Benadryl Plus [BD] 636
Benadryl Plus Nighttime [BD] 637
Benylin Decongestant [BD] 638
Brexin L.A. Capsules 2078
Bromfed Capsules (Timed Release) 1615
Bromfed Syrup [BD] 628
Bromfed 1615
CoAdvil [BD] 748
Allergy-Sinus Comtrex Multi-Symptom Allergy Sinus Formula Tablets & Caplets 746
Cough Formula Comtrex 746
Comtrex Multi-Symptom Cold Reliever Tablets/Caplets/Liqui-Gels/Liquid 745
Day-Night Comtrex 747
Non-Drowsy Comtrex 747
Congess 994
Congestac Caplets [BD] 617
Contac Jr. Children's Cold Medicine [BD] 712
Contac Nighttime Cold Medicine [BD] 713
Contac Sinus Caplets Maximum Strength Non-Drowsy Formula [BD] 710
Contac Sinus Tablets Maximum Strength Non-Drowsy Formula [BD] 710
Deconamine 663
Deconsal II Tablets 559
Dimacol Caplets [BD] 672
Dimetane-DX Cough Syrup 1858
Dorcol Children's Cough Syrup [BD] 685
Dorcol Children's Decongestant Liquid [BD] 685
Dorcol Children's Liquid Cold Formula [BD] 686
Maximum Strength Dristan Decongestant/Analgesic Coated Caplets [BD] 750
No Drowsiness Dristan Cold Nasal Decongestant/Analgesic Coated Caplets 2420
Dristan Sinus Caplets 2419
Sinus Excedrin Analgesic, Decongestant Tablets & Caplets [BD] 533
Fedahist Gyrocaps 2145
Fedahist Timecaps 2145
Guaifed 1615
Guaifed Syrup [BD] 629
Isoclor Expectorant 982
Isoclor Timesule Capsules [BD] 561
Kronofed-A 970
Medi-Flu Caplet, Liquid [BD] 640
Novafed A Capsules 1342
Novafed Capsules 1342
Novahistine DH 1342
Novahistine DMX [BD] 595
Novahistine Expectorant 1343
Nucofed Capsules 2219
Nucofed Expectorant 2219
Nucofed Pediatric Expectorant 2220
Nucofed Syrup 2219
Ornex Caplets [BD] 618
PediaCare Allergy Relief Formula Liquid 1362
PediaCare Cough-Cold Formula Liquid 1362
PediaCare Infants' Oral Decongestant Drops 1362
PediaCare Night Rest Cough-Cold Formula Liquid 1362
PediaCare 6-12 Cough-Cold Formula Chewable Tablets 1362
Robitussin-DAC Syrup 1875
Robitussin-PE [BD] 677
Rondec 1975
Rondec-DM 1976
Rondec-TR Tablet 1975
Ru-Tuss DE Tablets 694
Ryna [BD] 741
Seldane-D Extended-Release Tablets 1350
Sinarest [BD] 562
Sine-Aid Maximum Strength Sinus Headache Caplets 1365
Sine-Aid Maximum Strength Sinus Headache Tablets 1365
Sine-Off Maximum Strength Allergy/Sinus Formula Caplets [BD] 721
Sine-Off Maximum Strength No Drowsiness Formula Caplets [BD] 722
Singlet Tablets [BD] 598
Sinutab Maximum Strength [BD] 641
Sinutab Maximum Strength Without Drowsiness Tablets & Caplets [BD] 642
Sinutab Regular Strength Without Drowsiness Formula [BD] 641
St. Joseph Nighttime Cold Medicine [BD] 705
Sudafed Children's Liquid [BD] 543
Sudafed Cough Syrup [BD] 543
Sudafed Plus Liquid [BD] 544
Sudafed Plus Tablets [BD] 545
Sudafed Sinus Caplets [BD] 545
Sudafed Sinus Tablets [BD] 545
Sudafed Tablets, 30 mg [BD] 544
Sudafed Tablets, Adult Strength, 60 mg [BD] 544
Sudafed 12 Hour Capsules [BD] 545
TheraFlu Flu and Cold Medicine [BD] 687
Triaminic Nite Light [BD] 689
Tylenol Allergy Sinus Medication Caplets and Gelcaps, Maximum Strength 1372
Children's Tylenol Cold Liquid Formula and Chewable Tablets 1368
Tylenol Cold & Flu Hot Medication, Packets 1369
Tylenol Cold & Flu No Drowsiness Hot Medication, Packets 1371
Tylenol Cold Medication Caplets and Tablets 1370
Tylenol Cold Medication No Drowsiness Formula Caplets 1370
Tylenol Cold Night Time Medication Liquid 1371
Tylenol Cough Medication Liquid with Decongestant, Maximum Strength 1372
Tylenol, Maximum Strength, Sinus Medication Gelcaps, Caplets and Tablets 1373
Ursinus Inlay-Tabs [BD] 691
Vicks Children's NyQuil [BD] 664
Vicks Daycare [BD] 660
Vicks Formula 44D Decongestant Cough Medicine [BD] 662
Vicks Formula 44M Multi-Symptom Cough Medicine [BD] 662
Vicks NyQuil Nighttime Colds Medicine-Original & Cherry Flavor [BD] 664
Vicks Pediatric Formula 44 Cough & Congestion Medicine [BD] 663
Vicks Pediatric Formula 44m Multi-Symptom Cough & Cold Medicine [BD] 663

Pseudoephedrine Sulfate (Hyperglycemia; loss of control). Products include:
Afrin Tablets [BD] 693
Chlor-Trimeton Decongestant [BD] 694
Disophrol Chronotab Sustained-Action Tablets [BD] 698
Drixoral Antihistamine/Nasal Decongestant Syrup [BD] 698
Drixoral Non-Drowsy Formula [BD] 699
Drixoral Plus Extended-Release Tablets [BD] 699
Drixoral Sinus [BD] 700
Drixoral Sustained-Action Tablets [BD] 698
Sinutab Allergy Formula Sustained Action Tablets [BD] 640
Trinalin Repetabs Tablets 1170

Quinestrol (Hyperglycemia; loss of control). Products include:
Estrovis 1721

Salsalate (Potentiates hypoglycemic action). Products include:
Disalcid 1310
Mono-Gesic Tablets 846
Salflex 839

Selegiline Hydrochloride (Potentiates hypoglycemic action). Products include:
Eldepryl 2250

Spironolactone (Hyperglycemia; loss of control). Products include:
Aldactazide 2150
Aldactone 2152

Sulfamethizole (Potentiates hypoglycemic action). Products include:
Thiosulfil Forte Tablets 2526
Urobiotic-250 Capsules 1968

Sulfamethoxazole (Potentiates hypoglycemic action). Products include:
Azo Gantanol Tablets 1887
Bactrim DS Tablets 1891
Bactrim I.V. Infusion 1889
Bactrim 1891
Gantanol 1899
Septra 813
Septra I.V. Infusion 808
Septra I.V. Infusion ADD-Vantage Vials 810
Septra 813

Sulfasalazine (Potentiates hypoglycemic action). Products include:
Azulfidine Tablets, EN-tabs, Oral Suspension 1157

Sulfinpyrazone (Potentiates hypoglycemic action). Products include:
Anturane 853

Sulfisoxazole (Potentiates hypoglycemic action). Products include:
Azo Gantrisin Tablets 1888
Gantrisin Tablets 1901
Pediazole 1973

Sulfisoxazole Diolamine (Potentiates hypoglycemic action). Products include:
Gantrisin Ophthalmic Ointment/Solution 1900

Sulindac (Potentiates hypoglycemic effect of sulfonylureas). Products include:
Clinoril Tablets 1433

Terbutaline Sulfate (Hyperglycemia; loss of control). Products include:
Brethaire Inhaler 1024
Brethine Ampuls 1026
Brethine Tablets 1026
Bricanyl Injection 1324
Bricanyl Tablets 1325

Thioridazine Hydrochloride (Hyperglycemia; loss of control). Products include:
Mellaril 2011

Thyroid (Hyperglycemia; loss of control). Products include:
S-P-T "Liquid" Capsules 995

Thyroxine (Hyperglycemia; loss of control).
No products indexed under this heading.

Thyroxine Sodium (Hyperglycemia; loss of control).
No products indexed under this heading.

Timolol Maleate (Potentiates hypoglycemic action). Products include:
Blocadren Tablets 1429
Timolide Tablets 1547
Timoptic in Ocudose 1552
Timoptic Sterile Ophthalmic Solution 1550

Tolazamide (Potentiates hypoglycemic action). Products include:
Tolinase Tablets 2365

Tolbutamide (Potentiates hypoglycemic action). Products include:
Orinase Tablets 2354

Tolmetin Sodium (Potentiates hypoglycemic effect of sulfonylureas). Products include:
Tolectin (200, 400 and 600 mg) 1379

Tranylcypromine Sulfate (Potentiates hypoglycemic action). Products include:
Parnate Tablets 2222

Triamcinolone (Hyperglycemia; loss of control).
No products indexed under this heading.

Triamcinolone Acetonide (Hyperglycemia; loss of control). Products include:
Aristocort A 1010
Azmacort Inhaler 1837
Kenalog Cream, Lotion & Ointment 2401
Kenalog-10 Injection 2402
Kenalog-40 Injection 2403
Kenalog in Orabase 604
Kenalog Spray 2401
Mycolog II Cream and Ointment 2407
Mytrex Cream & Ointment 2080
Nasacort Nasal Inhaler 1844

Triamcinolone Diacetate (Hyperglycemia; loss of control). Products include:
Aristocort Suspension 1008

Triamcinolone Hexacetonide (Hyperglycemia; loss of control). Products include:
Aristospan Suspension 1011

Triamterene (Hyperglycemia; loss of control). Products include:
Dyazide Capsules 2208
Dyrenium Capsules 2210
Maxzide 1215

Trifluoperazine Hydrochloride (Hyperglycemia; loss of control). Products include:
Stelazine 2226

Verapamil Hydrochloride (Hyperglycemia; loss of control). Products include:
Calan SR Caplets 2157
Calan Tablets 2155
Isoptin Injectable 1177
Isoptin Oral Tablets 1179
Isoptin SR Sustained Release Tablets 1181
Verelan Capsules 1243
Verelan Capsules 2535

Warfarin Sodium (Potentiates hypoglycemic action). Products include:
Coumadin Injection & Tablets 944
Panwarfin Tablets 547

DIABINESE TABLETS (Chlorpropamide) 1775
May interact with sympathomimetic aerosal brochodilators, calcium channel blockers, barbiturates, nonsteroidal anti-inflammatory agents, salicylates, sulfonamides, oral anticoagulants, monoamine oxidase inhibitors, beta blockers, thiazides, diuretics, corticosteroids, phenothiazines, oral contraceptives, thyroid preparations, estrogens, and certain other agents. Compounds in these categories include:

Acebutolol Hydrochloride (Potentiation of hypoglycemic action). Products include:
Sectral Capsules 2520

Albuterol (Hyperglycemia). Products include:
- Proventil Inhalation Aerosol ... 2117
- Ventolin Inhalation Aerosol and Refill ... 583

Albuterol Sulfate (Hyperglycemia). Products include:
- Proventil Repetabs Tablets ... 2120
- Proventil Solutions for Inhalation 0.5% and 0.083% ... 2118
- Proventil Syrup ... 2119
- Proventil Tablets ... 2120
- Ventolin ... 583

Alcohol (Disulfiram-like reaction).

Amiloride Hydrochloride (Hyperglycemia). Products include:
- Midamor Tablets ... 1508
- Moduretic Tablets ... 1510

Aprobarbital (Prolonged barbiturate action). Products include:
- Alurate Elixir ... 1883

Aspirin (Potentiation of hypoglycemic action). Products include:
- Alka-Seltzer Effervescent Antacid and Pain Reliever ... 1568
- Alka-Seltzer Extra Strength Effervescent Antacid and Pain Reliever ... 1570
- Alka-Seltzer (Flavored) Effervescent Antacid and Pain Reliever ... 1569
- Alka-Seltzer Plus Cold Medicine ... ▣ 623
- Alka-Seltzer Plus Night-Time Cold Medicine ... ▣ 623
- Alka Seltzer Plus Sinus Allergy Medicine ... ▣ 624
- Anacin Coated Analgesic Caplets ... 2417
- Anacin Coated Analgesic Tablets ... 2417
- Anacin Maximum Strength Analgesic Coated Tablets ... 2417
- Maximum Strength Arthritis Pain Formula By the Makers of Anacin Analgesic Tablets and Caplets ... 2418
- Arthritis Pain Formula by the Makers of Anacin Analgesic Tablets and Caplets ... ▣ 747
- Arthritis Strength BC Powder ... ▣ 516
- Ascriptin A/D Caplets ... 1850
- Regular Strength Ascriptin Tablets 1850
- Azdōne Tablets ... 844
- BC Powder ... ▣ 517
- BC Cold Powder ... ▣ 517
- Children's Bayer Chewable Aspirin ... ▣ 564
- Genuine Bayer Aspirin Tablets & Caplets ... ▣ 564
- Maximum Bayer Aspirin Tablets & Caplets ... ▣ 566
- Bayer Plus Aspirin Tablets ... ▣ 567
- Therapy Bayer Aspirin Caplets ... ▣ 568
- 8 Hour Bayer Timed-Release Aspirin ... ▣ 566
- Arthritis Strength Bufferin Analgesic Caplets ... 744
- Extra Strength Bufferin Analgesic Tablets ... 745
- Bufferin Analgesic Tablets and Caplets ... 743
- Cama Arthritis Pain Reliever ... ▣ 685
- Damason-P ... 1356
- Easprin ... 1719
- Ecotrin Enteric Coated Aspirin Maximum Strength Tablets and Caplets ... 2189
- Ecotrin Enteric Coated Aspirin Regular Strength Tablets and Caplets ... 2189
- Empirin Aspirin ... ▣ 541
- Empirin with Codeine Phosphate Nos. 2, 3 & 4 ... 764
- Equagesic Tablets ... 2451
- Excedrin Extra-Strength Analgesic Tablets & Caplets ... 749
- 4-Way Cold Tablets ... 750
- Fiorinal Capsules ... 2007
- Fiorinal with Codeine Capsules ... 2008
- Fiorinal Tablets ... 2007
- Lortab ASA Tablets ... 2414
- Momentum Muscular Backache Formula ... ▣ 751
- Norgesic ... 1314
- Norwich Extra-Strength Aspirin ... ▣ 546
- Norwich Regular Strength Aspirin ▣ 547
- P-A-C Analgesic Tablets ... ▣ 669
- Percodan ... 951
- Robaxisal Tablets ... 1872
- Sine-Off Sinus Medicine Tablets-Aspirin Formula ... ▣ 722
- Soma Compound w/Codeine Tablets ... 2390
- Soma Compound Tablets ... 2389
- St. Joseph Adult Chewable Aspirin (81 mg.) ... ▣ 703
- Synalgos-DC Capsules ... 2525
- Talwin Compound ... 2072
- Ursinus Inlay-Tabs ... ▣ 691
- Vanquish Analgesic Caplets ... ▣ 574
- Zorprin Tablets ... 698

Atenolol (Potentiation of hypoglycemic action). Products include:
- Tenoretic Tablets ... 1105
- Tenormin Tablets and I.V. Injection 1107

Bendroflumethiazide (Hyperglycemia). Products include:
- Corzide Tablets ... 702
- Naturetin Tablets ... 1789
- Rauzide Tablets ... 1804

Bepridil Hydrochloride (Hyperglycemia). Products include:
- Vascor (200, 300 and 400 mg) Tablets ... 1383

Betamethasone Acetate (Hyperglycemia). Products include:
- Celestone Soluspan Suspension ... 2081

Betamethasone Sodium Phosphate (Hyperglycemia). Products include:
- Celestone Soluspan Suspension ... 2081

Betaxolol Hydrochloride (Potentiation of hypoglycemic action). Products include:
- Betoptic Sterile Ophthalmic Solution ... 569
- Betoptic S Sterile Ophthalmic Suspension ... 570
- Kerlone Tablets ... 2172

Bumetanide (Hyperglycemia). Products include:
- Bumex ... 1895

Butabarbital (Prolonged barbiturate action). Products include:
- Pyridium Plus ... 1764

Butalbital (Prolonged barbiturate action). Products include:
- Esgic-Plus Tablets ... 1002
- Esgic Tablets & Capsules ... 1001
- Fioricet Tablets ... 2006
- Fiorinal Capsules ... 2007
- Fiorinal with Codeine Capsules ... 2008
- Fiorinal Tablets ... 2007
- Phrenilin ... 838
- Sedapap Tablets 50 mg/650 mg ... 1360

Carteolol Hydrochloride (Potentiation of hypoglycemic action). Products include:
- Cartrol Tablets ... 507

Chloramphenicol (Potentiation of hypoglycemic action). Products include:
- AK-Chlor Sterile Ophthalmic Ointment & Solution ... ⊙ 201
- Chloromycetin Cream, 1% ... 1694
- Chloromycetin Hydrocortisone Ophthalmic ... 1694
- Chloromycetin Kapseals ... 1695
- Chloromycetin Ophthalmic Ointment, 1% ... 1696
- Chloromycetin Ophthalmic Solution ... 1696
- Chloromycetin Otic ... 1697
- Chloroptic S.O.P. ... ⊙ 243
- Chloroptic Sterile Ophthalmic Solution ... ⊙ 243
- Ophthochlor Ophthalmic Solution ⊙ 300
- Ophthocort ... ⊙ 301

Chloramphenicol Palmitate (Potentiation of hypoglycemic action). Products include:
- Chloromycetin Palmitate, Oral Suspension ... 1697

Chloramphenicol Sodium Succinate (Potentiation of hypoglycemic action). Products include:
- Chloromycetin Sodium Succinate ... 1698

Chlorothiazide (Hyperglycemia). Products include:
- Aldoclor Tablets ... 1413
- Diupres Tablets ... 1461
- Diuril Oral ... 1464

Chlorothiazide Sodium (Hyperglycemia). Products include:
- Diuril Sodium Intravenous ... 1463

Chlorotrianisene (Hyperglycemia). Products include:
- TACE 12 and 25 mg ... 1353

Chlorpromazine (Hyperglycemia). Products include:
- Thorazine ... 2234

Chlorthalidone (Hypergycemia). Products include:
- Combipres Tablets ... 678
- Tenoretic Tablets ... 1105
- Thalitone Tablets ... 687

Choline Magnesium Trisalicylate (Potentiation of hypoglycemic action). Products include:
- Trilisate ... 1822

Cortisone Acetate (Hyperglycemia). Products include:
- Cortone Acetate Sterile Suspension ... 1437
- Cortone Acetate Tablets ... 1439

Dexamethasone (Hyperglycemia). Products include:
- AK-Trol Ointment & Suspension ... ⊙ 207
- Decadron Elixir ... 1445
- Decadron Tablets ... 1447
- Decaspray Topical Aerosol ... 1459
- Dexacidin ... ⊙ 272
- Maxidex Sterile Ophthalmic Suspension ... ⊙ 223
- Maxitrol Ophthalmic Ointment/Suspension ... ⊙ 223
- TobraDex Ophthalmic Suspension and Ointment ... ⊙ 228

Dexamethasone Acetate (Hyperglycemia). Products include:
- Dalalone D.P. Injectable ... 999
- Decadron-LA Sterile Suspension ... 1457

Dexamethasone Sodium Phosphate (Hyperglycemia). Products include:
- AK-Dex ... ⊙ 203
- Decadron Phosphate Respihaler ... 1454
- Decadron Phosphate Sterile Ophthalmic Ointment ... 1453
- Decadron Phosphate Sterile Ophthalmic Solution ... 1453
- Decadron Phosphate Topical Cream ... 1455
- Decadron Phosphate Turbinaire ... 1456
- Maxidex Sterile Ophthalmic Ointment ... ⊙ 222
- NeoDecadron Sterile Ophthalmic Ointment ... 1517
- NeoDecadron Sterile Ophthalmic Solution ... 1518
- NeoDecadron Topical Cream ... 1518

Diclofenac Sodium (Potentiation of hypoglycemic action). Products include:
- Voltaren Ophthalmic Sterile Ophthalmic Solution ... ⊙ 268
- Voltaren Tablets ... 1042

Dicumarol (Potentiation of hypoglycemic action). Products include:
- Dicumarol Tablets ... 516

Dienestrol (Hyperglycemia). Products include:
- Ortho Dienestrol Cream ... 1664

Diethylstilbestrol (Hyperglycemia). Products include:
- Diethylstilbestrol Tablets ... 1258

Diflunisal (Potentiation of hypoglycemic action). Products include:
- Dolobid Tablets ... 1465

Diltiazem Hydrochloride (Hyperglycemia). Products include:
- Cardizem Tablets-30 mg, 60 mg, 90 mg and 120 mg ... 1329
- Cardizem SR Capsules-60 mg, 90 mg and 120 mg ... 1327

Dobutamine Hydrochloride (Hyperglycemia). Products include:
- Dobutrex Solution Vials ... 1259

Dopamine Hydrochloride (Hyperglycemia). Products include:
- Intropin Injection ... 930

Ephedrine Hydrochloride (Hyperglycemia). Products include:
- Amesec ... ▣ 682
- Primatene Tablets-M Formula ... 2421
- Primatene Tablets-P Formula ... 2421
- Primatene Tablets-Regular Formula ... 2421
- Quadrinal Tablets ... 1183
- Quelidrine Syrup ... 556
- Tedral SA ... 1765

Ephedrine Sulfate (Hyperglycemia). Products include:
- Bronkaid Tablets ... ▣ 757
- Bronkolixir ... ▣ 761
- Bronkotabs Tablets ... ▣ 762
- Marax Tablets & DF Syrup ... 1954
- Pazo Hemorrhoid Ointment & Suppositories ... 752
- Vicks Vatronol Nose Drops ... ▣ 666

Ephedrine Tannate (Hyperglycemia). Products include:
- Rynatuss ... 2388

Epinephrine (Hyperglycemia). Products include:
- Ana-Kit Anaphylaxis Emergency Treatment Kit ... 1100
- Bronkaid Mist ... ▣ 757
- EpiPen ... 843
- Marcaine Hydrochloride 0.5% with Epinephrine 1:200,000 (as bitartrate) ... 958
- Marcaine Hydrochloride with Epinephrine 1:200,000 ... 2055
- Primatene Mist ... 2420
- Sus-Phrine Injection ... 1006
- Xylocaine with Epinephrine Injections ... 637

Epinephrine Bitartrate (Hyperglycemia). Products include:
- AsthmaHaler Mist Epinephrine Bitartrate Bronchodilator ... ▣ 616
- Bronkaid Mist Suspension ... ▣ 757
- Primatene Mist Suspension ... 2421

Epinephrine Hydrochloride (Hyperglycemia). Products include:
- Adrenalin Chloride Solution 1:100 & 1:1,000 ... 1689
- Epifrin ... ⊙ 244
- Glaucon ... ⊙ 218

Esmolol Hydrochloride (Potentiation of hypoglycemic action). Products include:
- Brevibloc Injection ... 942

Estradiol (Hyperglycemia). Products include:
- Emcyt Capsules ... 1161
- Estrace ... 1385
- Estrace Vaginal Cream ... 1388
- Estraderm Transdermal System ... 866

Estrogens, Conjugated (Hyperglycemia). Products include:
- Mediatric Capsules ... 2476
- PMB 200 and PMB 400 ... 2504
- Premarin Intravenous ... 2508
- Premarin with Methyltestosterone ... 2515
- Premarin Tablets ... 2510
- Premarin Vaginal Cream ... 2512

Estrogens, Esterified (Hyperglycemia). Products include:
- Estratest ... 2245
- Menrium Tablets ... 1934

Estropipate (Hyperglycemia). Products include:
- Ogen ... 540

Ethacrynic Acid (Hyperglycemia). Products include:
- Edecrin Tablets ... 1468

Ethinyl Estradiol (Hyperglycemia). Products include:
- Brevicon ... 2304
- Demulen ... 2161
- Estinyl Tablets ... 2085
- Jenest-28 Tablets ... 1636
- Levlen/Tri-Levlen ... 665
- Lo/Ovral Tablets ... 2471
- Lo/Ovral-28 Tablets ... 2476
- Loestrin ... 1728
- Modicon ... 1667
- Nordette-21 Tablets ... 2481
- Nordette-28 Tablets ... 2483
- Norethin ... 2133
- Norinyl ... 2304
- Norlestrin ... 1746
- Ortho-Cyclen Tablets ... 1658

Ortho-Novum 1667
Ovcon 1391
Ovral Tablets 2490
Ovral-28 Tablets 2491
Levlen/Tri-Levlen 665
Tri-Norinyl 2304
Triphasil-21 Tablets 2527
Triphasil-28 Tablets 2532

Ethynodiol Diacetate (Hyperglycemia). Products include:
Demulen 2161

Etodolac (Potentiation of hypoglycemic action). Products include:
Lodine Capsules 2468

Felodipine (Hyperglycemia). Products include:
Plendil Extended-Release Tablets 1526

Fenoprofen Calcium (Potentiation of hypoglycemic action). Products include:
Nalfon Pulvules & Tablets 919

Fluphenazine Decanoate (Hyperglycemia). Products include:
Prolixin Decanoate 1795

Fluphenazine Enanthate (Hyperglycemia). Products include:
Prolixin Enanthate 1796

Fluphenazine Hydrochloride (Hyperglycemia). Products include:
Prolixin Elixir 1793
Prolixin Injection 1791
Prolixin Oral Concentrate 1792
Prolixin Tablets 1793

Flurbiprofen (Potentiation of hypoglycemic action). Products include:
Ansaid Tablets 2319

Furazolidone (Potentiation of hypoglycemic action). Products include:
Furoxone 1855

Furosemide (Hyperglycemia). Products include:
Lasix 1093

Glipizide (Potentiation of hypoglycemic action). Products include:
Glucotrol 1952

Glyburide (Potentiation of hypoglycemic action). Products include:
DiaBeta 1091
Micronase Tablets 2350

Hydrochlorothiazide (Hyperglycemia). Products include:
Aldactazide 2150
Aldoril Tablets 1418
Apresazide Capsules 854
Apresoline-Esidrix Tablets 857
Capozide 2258
Dyazide Capsules 2208
Esidrix Tablets 863
Esimil Tablets 864
HydroDIURIL Tablets 1484
Hydropres Tablets 1485
Inderide Tablets 2463
Inderide LA Long Acting Capsules 2465
Lopressor HCT Tablets 1034
Maxzide 1215
Moduretic Tablets 1510
Normozide Tablets 2112
Oretic Tablets 544
Oreticyl 545
Prinzide Tablets 1540
Ser-Ap-Es Tablets 881
Serpasil-Esidrix Tablets 886
Timolide Tablets 1547
Trandate HCT Tablets 579
Vaseretic Tablets 1559
Zestoretic 2274

Hydrocortisone (Hyperglycemia). Products include:
AK-Spore H.C. ◉ 206
Bactine Hydrocortisone Anti-Itch Cream ⊞ 625
CaldeCORT Anti-Itch Hydrocortisone Spray ⊞ 560
Carmol HC Cream 1% 2296
Cortaid Spray ⊞ 735
Cortenema 2244
Cortisporin Ointment 758
Cortisporin Ophthalmic Ointment Sterile 758
Cortisporin Ophthalmic Suspension Sterile 759
Cortisporin Otic Solution Sterile 760
Cortisporin Otic Suspension Sterile 760
Cortizone-5 Creme & Ointment ⊞ 732
Dermolate Anti-Itch Cream ⊞ 697
Eldecort Cream 1.0% 1113
Eldecort Cream 1.0% and 2.5% 1113
Fungoid HC Creme 1770
Hydrocortone Tablets 1482
Hytone 909
LazerSporin-C Solution 1770
Massengill Medicated Soft Cloth Towelettes 2192
Nutracort Cream & Lotion 1684
PediOtic Suspension Sterile 797
Synacort Creams 1%, 2.5% 2296
Vanoxide-HC Acne Lotion 911
Vioform-Hydrocortisone Cream and Mild Cream 889
Vioform-Hydrocortisone Ointment 889
VōSoL HC Otic Solution 2392
Vytone Cream 1% 911

Hydrocortisone Acetate (Hyperglycemia). Products include:
Analpram-HC Rectal Cream 1% and 2.5% 970
Anusol-HC Cream 1690
Anusol-HC Suppositories 1691
Caldecort ⊞ 560
Carmol HC Cream 1% 2296
Chloromycetin Hydrocortisone Ophthalmic 1694
Coly-Mycin S Otic w/Neomycin & Hydrocortisone 1708
Cortaid ⊞ 735
Cortef Feminine Itch Cream ⊞ 735
Corticaine ⊞ 682
Cortifoam 1827
Cortisporin Cream 757
Epifoam 1828
Gynecort 5 Creme ⊞ 556
Hydrocortone Acetate Sterile Suspension 1479
Lanacort 5 Creme and Ointment ⊞ 557
Mantadil Cream 789
Ophthocort ◉ 301
Orabase HCA Oral Paste 890
Pramosone Cream, Lotion & Ointment 971
ProctoCream-HC 1834
Proctofoam-HC 1835

Hydrocortisone Sodium Phosphate (Hyperglycemia). Products include:
Hydrocortone Phosphate Injection, Sterile 1481

Hydrocortisone Sodium Succinate (Hyperglycemia). Products include:
Solu-Cortef Sterile Powder 2361

Hydroflumethiazide (Hyperglycemia). Products include:
Diucardin Tablets 2450
Saluron 718
Salutensin/Salutensin-Demi 719

Ibuprofen (Potentiation of hypoglycemic action). Products include:
Advil Cold & Sinus Caplets (formerly CoAdvil) 2416
Advil Ibuprofen Tablets and Caplets 2416
Children's Advil Suspension 2426
CoAdvil ⊞ 748
Dristan Sinus Caplets 2419
Haltran Tablets ⊞ 668
Ibuprofen ⊞ 631
Medipren ibuprofen Caplets and Tablets 1362
Midol 200 Cramp Relief Formula ⊞ 570
Motrin Tablets 2351
Motrin IB Caplets and Tablets ⊞ 736
Nuprin Ibuprofen/Analgesic Tablets & Caplets 752
PediaProfen Suspension 1363
Rufen Tablets 691
Trendar Ibuprofen Tablets ⊞ 756

Indapamide (Hyperglycemia). Products include:
Lozol Tablets 1843

Indomethacin (Potentiation of hypoglycemic action). Products include:
Indocin 1487

Indomethacin Sodium Trihydrate (Potentiation of hypoglycemic action). Products include:
Indocin I.V. 1490

Isocarboxazid (Potentiation of hypoglycemic action). Products include:
Marplan Tablets 1906

Isoniazid (Hyperglycemia). Products include:
INH Tablets 868
Rifamate Capsules 1347

Isoproterenol Hydrochloride (Hyperglycemia). Products include:
Isuprel Hydrochloride Injection 1:5000 2050
Isuprel Hydrochloride Mistometer 2051
Isuprel Hydrochloride Solution 1:200 & 1:100 2052
Norisodrine Aerotrol 540

Isradipine (Hyperglycemia). Products include:
DynaCirc Capsules 2004

Ketoprofen (Potentiation of hypoglycemic action). Products include:
Orudis Capsules 2488

Ketorolac Tromethamine (Potentiation of hypoglycemic action). Products include:
Toradol IM Injection 2302

Labetalol Hydrochloride (Potentiation of hypoglycemic action). Products include:
Normodyne Injection 2108
Normodyne Tablets 2110
Normozide Tablets 2112
Trandate HCT Tablets 579
Trandate Injection 577
Trandate Tablets 579

Levonorgestrel (Hyperglycemia). Products include:
Levlen/Tri-Levlen 665
Nordette-21 Tablets 2481
Nordette-28 Tablets 2483
Norplant System 2484
Levlen/Tri-Levlen 665
Triphasil-21 Tablets 2527
Triphasil-28 Tablets 2532

Levothyroxine Sodium (Hyperglycemia). Products include:
Levothroid Tablets 1003
Levoxine Tablets 904
Synthroid 695

Liothyronine Sodium (Hyperglycemia). Products include:
Cytomel Tablets 2203

Magnesium Salicylate (Potentiation of hypoglycemic action). Products include:
Doan's - Extra-Strength Analgesic ⊞ 549
Doan's - Regular Strength Analgesic ⊞ 549
Mobigesic Analgesic Tablets ⊞ 507

Meclofenamate Sodium (Potentiation of hypoglycemic action). Products include:
Meclomen Capsules 1739

Mefenamic Acid (Potentiation of hypoglycemic action). Products include:
Ponstel 1758

Mephobarbital (Prolonged barbiturate action). Products include:
Mebaral Tablets 2061

Mesoridazine (Hyperglycemia). Products include:
Serentil 686

Mestranol (Hyperglycemia). Products include:
Enovid 2161
Norethin 2133
Norinyl 2304
Ortho-Novum 1667

Metaproterenol Sulfate (Hyperglycemia). Products include:
Alupent 674
Arm-a-Med Metaproterenol Sulfate Inhalation Solution, USP 617
Metaprel Inhalation Aerosol Bronchodilator 2014
Metaprel Inhalation Solution 2015
Metaprel 2015
Metaproterenol Sulfate Inhalation Solution, USP 912

Metaraminol Bitartrate (Hyperglycemia). Products include:
Aramine Injection 1424

Methoxamine Hydrochloride (Hyperglycemia). Products include:
Vasoxyl Injection 819

Methyclothiazide (Hyperglycemia). Products include:
Enduron Tablets 517
Enduronyl 518

Methylprednisolone (Hyperglycemia). Products include:
Medrol 2348

Methylprednisolone Acetate (Hyperglycemia). Products include:
Depo-Medrol Sterile Aqueous Suspension 2334

Methylprednisolone Sodium Succinate (Hyperglycemia). Products include:
Solu-Medrol Sterile Powder 2363

Metolazone (Hyperglycemia). Products include:
Diulo 2129
Mykrox ½ mg Tablets 984
Zaroxolyn Tablets 989

Metoprolol Tartrate (Potentiation of hypoglycemic action). Products include:
Lopressor Ampuls 1032
Lopressor HCT Tablets 1034
Lopressor Tablets 1032

Miconazole (Severe hypoglycemia). Products include:
Monistat I.V. 1143

Nadolol (Potentiation of hypoglycemic action). Products include:
Corgard Tablets 701
Corzide Tablets 702

Naproxen (Potentiation of hypoglycemic action). Products include:
Naprosyn 2297

Naproxen Sodium (Potentiation of hypoglycemic action). Products include:
Anaprox and Anaprox DS Tablets 2288

Nicardipine Hydrochloride (Hyperglycemia). Products include:
Cardene Capsules 2290

Nifedipine (Hyperglycemia). Products include:
Adalat Capsules (10 mg and 20 mg) 1587
Procardia Capsules 1781
Procardia XL Tablets 1783

Nimodipine (Hyperglycemia). Products include:
Nimotop Capsules 1607

Norepinephrine Bitartrate (Hyperglycemia). Products include:
Levophed Bitartrate Injection 2054

Norethindrone (Hyperglycemia). Products include:
Brevicon 2304
Jenest-28 Tablets 1636
Micronor Tablets 1667
Modicon 1667
Norethin 2133
Norinyl 2304
Norlutin 1755
Nor-Q D Tablets 2304
Ortho-Novum 1667
Ovcon 1391
Tri-Norinyl 2304

Norethynodrel (Hyperglycemia). Products include:
Enovid 2161

Norgestimate (Hyperglycemia). Products include:
Ortho-Cyclen Tablets 1658

Norgestrel (Hyperglycemia). Products include:
Lo/Ovral Tablets 2471
Lo/Ovral-28 Tablets 2476
Ovral Tablets 2490
Ovral-28 Tablets 2491
Ovrette Tablets 2492

(⊞ Described in PDR For Nonprescription Drugs) (◉ Described in PDR For Ophthalmology)

Penbutolol Sulfate (Potentiation of hypoglycemic action). Products include:
Levatol ... 1832

Pentobarbital Sodium (Prolonged barbiturate action). Products include:
Nembutal Sodium Capsules ... 534
Nembutal Sodium Solution ... 536
Nembutal Sodium Suppositories ... 538

Perphenazine (Hyperglycemia). Products include:
Etrafon ... 2087
Triavil Tablets ... 1556
Trilafon ... 2123

Phenelzine Sulfate (Potentiation of hypoglycemic action). Products include:
Nardil ... 1742

Phenobarbital (Prolonged barbiturate action). Products include:
Arco-Lase Plus Tablets ... 607
Bellergal-S Tablets ... 1998
Bronkolixir ... ◙ 761
Bronkotabs Tablets ... ◙ 762
Donnatal ... 1858
Donnatal Extentabs ... 1859
Donnatal Tablets ... 1858
Donnazyme Tablets ... 1860
Kinesed Tablets ... 2272
Phenobarbital Elixir and Tablets ... 1293
Primatene Tablets-P Formula ... 2421
Quadrinal Tablets ... 1183
Tedral SA ... 1765

Phenylbutazone (Potentiation of hypoglycemic action). Products include:
Butazolidin Capsules & Tablets ... 1027

Phenylephrine Bitartrate (Hyperglycemia).
No products indexed under this heading.

Phenylephrine Hydrochloride (Hyperglycemia). Products include:
AK-Dilate Solution 2.5% and 10% ... ⊙ 203
Atrohist Sprinkle Capsules ... 558
Cerose-DM ... 2443
Codimal ... 846
Comhist LA Capsules ... 1618
Congespirin For Children Aspirin Free Chewable Cold Tablets ... 748
Cyclomydril ... ⊙ 216
Deconsal Sprinkle Capsules ... 559
Dimetane Decongestant ... ◙ 673
Dristan Decongestant/Antihistamine/Analgesic Coated Caplets ... ◙ 749
Dristan Cold Nasal Decongestant/Antihistamine/ Analgesic Coated Tablets ... 2419
Dristan Advanced Formula Decongestant/Antihistamine/Analgesic Tablets ... ◙ 749
Dristan Nasal Spray, Menthol ... 2419
Dristan Nasal Spray, Regular and Regular with Metered Pump ... 2419
Entex Capsules ... 1623
Entex Liquid ... 1623
Sinus Excedrin Analgesic, Decongestant Tablets & Caplets ... 750
Extendryl ... 994
4-Way Fast Acting Nasal Spray - Original Formula (regular & mentholated) & Metered Spray Pump (regular) ... 751
Hycomine Compound Tablets ... 929
Murocoll-2 Sterile Ophthalmic Solution ... ⊙ 261
Mydfrin 2.5% ... ⊙ 224
Naldecon Syrup, Tablets, Pediatric Drops and Pediatric Syrup ... 709
Neo-Synephrine Hydrochloride 1% Carpuject ... 2063
Neo-Synephrine Hydrochloride 1% Injection ... 2063
Neo-Synephrine Hydrochloride (Ophthalmic) ... 2064
Neo-Synephrine ... ◙ 759
Nōstril Nasal Decongestant ... ◙ 520
Novahistine Elixir ... ◙ 596
Phenergan VC ... 2500
Phenergan VC with Codeine ... 2501
Prefrin Liquifilm Vasoconstrictor and Lubricant Eye Drops ... ⊙ 254
Prefrin-A ... ⊙ 255
Quelidrine Syrup ... 556
Relief Vasoconstrictor and Lubricant Eye Drops ... ⊙ 256
Robitussin Night Relief ... ◙ 677
Ru-Tuss with Hydrocodone ... 694
Ru-Tuss Tablets ... 693
Vasosulf ... ⊙ 279
Vicks Sinex ... ◙ 665
Zincfrin ... ⊙ 230

Phenylephrine Tannate (Hyperglycemia). Products include:
Rynatan ... 2387
Rynatuss ... 2388

Phenylpropanolamine Hydrochloride (Hyperglycemia). Products include:
A.R.M. Allergy Relief Medicine Caplets ... ◙ 615
Acutrim ... ◙ 548
Allerest ... ◙ 559
BC Cold Powder ... ◙ 517
Cheracol Plus Head Cold/Cough Formula ... ◙ 667
Codimal Expectorant ... 846
Comtrex Multi-Symptom Cold Reliever Tablets/Caplets/Liqui-Gels/Liquid ... 745
Contac Continuous Action Decongestant/Antihistamine Capsules ◙ 710
Contac Maximum Strength Continuous Action Decongestant/Antihistamine Caplets ... ◙ 709
Contac Severe Cold and Flu Formula Caplets ... ◙ 711
Coricidin 'D' Decongestant Tablets ... ◙ 695
Coricidin Demilets Tablets for Children ... ◙ 696
Demazin Nasal Decongestant/Antihistamine Repetabs Tablets & Syrup ... ◙ 697
Dexatrim ... ◙ 733
Dimetane-DC Cough Syrup ... 1857
Dimetapp Elixir ... ◙ 673
Dimetapp DM Elixir ... ◙ 674
Dimetapp Extentabs ... ◙ 674
Dimetapp Plus Caplets ... ◙ 675
Dimetapp Tablets ... ◙ 675
Entex Capsules ... 1623
Entex LA Tablets ... 1623
Entex Liquid ... 1623
4-Way Cold Tablets ... 750
Hycomine Syrup ... 927
Naldecon CX Adult Liquid ... ◙ 521
Naldecon DX Adult Liquid ... ◙ 521
Naldecon DX Children's Syrup ... ◙ 522
Naldecon DX Pediatric Drops ... ◙ 522
Naldecon EX Children's Syrup ... ◙ 522
Naldecon EX Pediatric Drops ... ◙ 523
Naldecon Syrup, Tablets, Pediatric Drops and Pediatric Syrup ... 709
Nolamine Tablets ... 838
Nolex LA Tablets ... 838
Ornade Spansule Capsules ... 2221
Orthoxicol Cough Syrup ... ◙ 668
Propagest ... 839
Pyrroxate Capsules ... ◙ 669
Robitussin-CF ... ◙ 676
Ru-Tuss II Capsules ... 693
Ru-Tuss with Hydrocodone ... 694
Ru-Tuss Tablets ... 693
Sine-Off Sinus Medicine Tablets-Aspirin Formula ... ◙ 722
Sinulin ... 840
St. Joseph Cold Tablets for Children ... ◙ 704
Tavist-D Tablets ... 2035
Triaminic Allergy Tablets ... ◙ 688
Triaminic Chewables ... ◙ 688
Triaminic Cold Tablets ... ◙ 688
Triaminic Expectorant ... ◙ 688
Triaminic Expectorant w/Codeine ... 1996
Triaminic Expectorant DH ... 1995
Triaminic Oral Infant Drops ... 1996
Triaminic Syrup ... ◙ 689
Triaminic-12 Tablets ... ◙ 690
Triaminic-DM Syrup ... ◙ 689
Triaminicin Tablets ... ◙ 690
Triaminicol Multi-Symptom Cold Tablets ... ◙ 691
Triaminicol Multi-Symptom Relief ◙ 691
Tuss-Ornade Liquid ... 2242
Tuss-Ornade Spansule Capsules ... 2242
Tylenol Cold Medication, Effervescent Tablets ... 1369

Phenytoin (Hyperglycemia). Products include:
Dilantin Infatabs ... 1710
Dilantin-30 Pediatric/Dilantin-125 Suspension ... 1713

Phenytoin Sodium (Hyperglycemia). Products include:
Dilantin Kapseals ... 1708
Dilantin Parenteral ... 1712
Dilantin with Phenobarbital Kapseals ... 1715

Pindolol (Potentiation of hypoglycemic action). Products include:
Visken Tablets ... 2036

Pirbuterol Acetate (Hyperglycemia). Products include:
Maxair Inhaler ... 1311

Piroxicam (Potentiation of hypoglycemic action). Products include:
Feldene Capsules ... 1777

Polyestradiol Phosphate (Hyperglycemia). Products include:
Estradurin ... 2452

Polythiazide (Hyperglycemia; potentiation of hypoglycemic action). Products include:
Minizide Capsules ... 1779
Renese Tablets ... 1785
Renese-R Tablets ... 1786

Prednisolone Acetate (Hyperglycemia). Products include:
AK-Cide Sterile Ophthalmic Ointment & Suspension ... ⊙ 202
Blephamide Liquifilm Sterile Ophthalmic Suspension ... 586
Blephamide S.O.P. Sterile Ophthalmic Ointment ... 586
Cetapred Ointment ... ⊙ 220
⅛% Econopred & 1% Econopred Plus ... ⊙ 217
Isopto Cetapred Suspension ... ⊙ 220
Metimyd ... ⊙ 306
Poly-Pred Liquifilm ... ⊙ 250
Pred Forte ... ⊙ 252
Pred Mild ... ⊙ 254
Pred-G Liquifilm Sterile Ophthalmic Suspension ... ⊙ 252
Pred-G S.O.P. Sterile Ophthalmic Ointment ... ⊙ 253
Vasocidin Ointment ... ⊙ 275

Prednisolone Sodium Phosphate (Hyperglycemia). Products include:
AK-Pred ... ⊙ 205
Hydeltrasol Injection, Sterile ... 1476
Inflamase ... ⊙ 274
Pediapred Oral Liquid ... 987
Vasocidin Ophthalmic Solution ... ⊙ 276

Prednisolone Tebutate (Hyperglycemia). Products include:
Hydeltra-T.B.A. Sterile Suspension 1478

Prednisone (Hyperglycemia). Products include:
Deltasone Tablets ... 2332

Probenecid (Potentiation of hypoglycemic action). Products include:
Benemid Tablets ... 1426
ColBENEMID Tablets ... 1436
Wycillin Injection and Probenecid Tablets ... 2539

Prochlorperazine (Hyperglycemia). Products include:
Compazine ... 2201

Promethazine Hydrochloride (Hyperglycemia). Products include:
Mepergan Injection ... 2479
Phenergan with Codeine ... 2497
Phenergan with Dextromethorphan 2499
Phenergan Injection ... 2493
Phenergan Suppositories ... 2496
Phenergan Syrup ... 2495
Phenergan Tablets ... 2496
Phenergan VC ... 2500
Phenergan VC with Codeine ... 2501

Propranolol Hydrochloride (Potentiation of hypoglycemic action). Products include:
Inderal ... 2459
Inderal LA Long Acting Capsules ... 2461
Inderide Tablets ... 2463
Inderide LA Long Acting Capsules .. 2465

Pseudoephedrine Hydrochloride (Hyperglycemia). Products include:
Actifed Capsules ... ◙ 539
Actifed Plus Caplets ... ◙ 539
Actifed Plus Tablets ... ◙ 540
Actifed with Codeine Cough Syrup .. 752
Actifed Syrup ... ◙ 540
Actifed Tablets ... ◙ 540
Actifed 12-Hour Capsules ... ◙ 539
Advil Cold & Sinus Caplets (formerly CoAdvil) ... 2416
Allerest ... ◙ 559
Anatuss LA Tablets ... 1359
Benadryl Decongestant Elixir ... ◙ 635
Benadryl Decongestant ... ◙ 635
Benadryl Plus ... ◙ 636
Benadryl Plus Nighttime ... ◙ 637
Benylin Decongestant ... ◙ 638
Brexin L.A. Capsules ... 2078
Bromfed Capsules (Timed Release) ... 1615
Bromfed Syrup ... ◙ 628
Bromfed ... 1615
CoAdvil ... ◙ 748
Allergy-Sinus Comtrex Multi-Symptom Allergy Sinus Formula Tablets & Caplets ... 746
Cough Formula Comtrex ... 746
Comtrex Multi-Symptom Cold Reliever Tablets/Caplets/Liqui-Gels/Liquid ... 745
Day-Night Comtrex ... 747
Non-Drowsy Comtrex ... 747
Congess ... 994
Congestac Caplets ... ◙ 617
Contac Jr. Children's Cold Medicine ... ◙ 712
Contac Nighttime Cold Medicine ... ◙ 713
Contac Sinus Caplets Maximum Strength Non-Drowsy Formula ... ◙ 710
Contac Sinus Tablets Maximum Strength Non-Drowsy Formula ... ◙ 710
Deconamine ... 663
Deconsal II Tablets ... 559
Dimacol Caplets ... ◙ 672
Dimetane-DX Cough Syrup ... 1858
Dorcol Children's Cough Syrup ... ◙ 685
Dorcol Children's Decongestant Liquid ... ◙ 685
Dorcol Children's Liquid Cold Formula ... ◙ 686
Maximum Strength Dristan Decongestant/Analgesic Coated Caplets ... ◙ 750
No Drowsiness Dristan Cold Nasal Decongestant/Analgesic Coated Caplets ... 2420
Dristan Sinus Caplets ... 2419
Sinus Excedrin Analgesic, Decongestant Tablets & Caplets ... ◙ 533
Fedahist Gyrocaps ... 2145
Fedahist Timecaps ... 2145
Guaifed ... 1615
Guaifed Syrup ... ◙ 629
Isoclor Expectorant ... 982
Isoclor Timesule Capsules ... ◙ 561
Kronofed-A ... 970
Medi-Flu Caplet, Liquid ... ◙ 640
Novafed A Capsules ... 1342
Novafed Capsules ... 1342
Novahistine DH ... 1342
Novahistine DMX ... ◙ 595
Novahistine Expectorant ... 1343
Nucofed Capsules ... 2219
Nucofed Expectorant ... 2219
Nucofed Pediatric Expectorant ... 2220
Nucofed Syrup ... 2219
Ornex Caplets ... ◙ 618
PediaCare Allergy Relief Formula Liquid ... 1362
PediaCare Cough-Cold Formula Liquid ... 1362
PediaCare Infants' Oral Decongestant Drops ... 1362
PediaCare Night Rest Cough-Cold Formula Liquid ... 1362
PediaCare 6-12 Cough-Cold Formula Chewable Tablets ... 1362
Robitussin-DAC Syrup ... 1875
Robitussin-PE ... ◙ 677
Rondec ... 1975
Rondec-DM ... 1976
Rondec-TR Tablet ... 1975
Ru-Tuss DE Tablets ... 694
Ryna ... ◙ 741
Seldane-D Extended-Release Tablets

1350
Sinarest ⊡ 562
Sine-Aid Maximum Strength Sinus Headache Caplets 1365
Sine-Aid Maximum Strength Sinus Headache Tablets 1365
Sine-Off Maximum Strength Allergy/Sinus Formula Caplets ⊡ 721
Sine-Off Maximum Strength No Drowsiness Formula Caplets ⊡ 722
Singlet Tablets ⊡ 598
Sinutab Maximum Strength ⊡ 641
Sinutab Maximum Strength Without Drowsiness Tablets & Caplets ⊡ 642
Sinutab Regular Strength Without Drowsiness Formula ⊡ 641
St. Joseph Nighttime Cold Medicine ⊡ 705
Sudafed Children's Liquid ⊡ 543
Sudafed Cough Syrup ⊡ 543
Sudafed Plus Liquid ⊡ 544
Sudafed Plus Tablets ⊡ 545
Sudafed Sinus Caplets ⊡ 545
Sudafed Sinus Tablets ⊡ 545
Sudafed Tablets, 30 mg ⊡ 544
Sudafed Tablets, Adult Strength, 60 mg ⊡ 544
Sudafed 12 Hour Capsules ⊡ 545
TheraFlu Flu and Cold Medicine ⊡ 687
Triaminic Nite Light ⊡ 689
Tylenol Allergy Sinus Medication Caplets and Gelcaps, Maximum Strength 1372
Children's Tylenol Cold Liquid Formula and Chewable Tablets 1368
Tylenol Cold & Flu Hot Medication, Packets 1369
Tylenol Cold & Flu No Drowsiness Hot Medication, Packets 1371
Tylenol Cold Medication Caplets and Tablets 1370
Tylenol Cold Medication No Drowsiness Formula Caplets 1370
Tylenol Cold Night Time Medication Liquid 1371
Tylenol Cough Medication Liquid with Decongestant, Maximum Strength 1372
Tylenol, Maximum Strength, Sinus Medication Gelcaps, Caplets and Tablets 1373
Ursinus Inlay-Tabs ⊡ 691
Vicks Children's NyQuil ⊡ 664
Vicks Daycare ⊡ 660
Vicks Formula 44D Decongestant Cough Medicine ⊡ 662
Vicks Formula 44M Multi-Symptom Cough Medicine ⊡ 662
Vicks NyQuil Nighttime Colds Medicine-Original & Cherry Flavor ⊡ 664
Vicks Pediatric Formula 44 Cough & Congestion Medicine ⊡ 663
Vicks Pediatric Formula 44m Multi-Symptom Cough & Cold Medicine ⊡ 663

Pseudoephedrine Sulfate (Hyperglycemia). Products include:
Afrin Tablets ⊡ 693
Chlor-Trimeton Decongestant ⊡ 694
Disophrol Chronotab Sustained-Action Tablets ⊡ 698
Drixoral Antihistamine/Nasal Decongestant Syrup ⊡ 698
Drixoral Non-Drowsy Formula ⊡ 699
Drixoral Plus Extended-Release Tablets ⊡ 699
Drixoral Sinus ⊡ 700
Drixoral Sustained-Action Tablets ⊡ 698
Sinutab Allergy Formula Sustained Action Tablets ⊡ 640
Trinalin Repetabs Tablets 1170

Quinestrol (Hyperglycemia). Products include:
Estrovis 1721

Salsalate (Potentiation of hypoglycemic action). Products include:
Disalcid 1310
Mono-Gesic Tablets 846
Salflex 839

Secobarbital Sodium (Prolonged barbiturate action). Products include:
Seconal Sodium Pulvules 1296

Selegiline Hydrochloride (Potentiation of hypoglycemic action). Products include:
Eldepryl 2250

Spironolactone (Hyperglycemia). Products include:
Aldactazide 2150
Aldactone 2152

Sulfamethizole (Potentiation of hypoglycemic action). Products include:
Thiosulfil Forte Tablets 2526
Urobiotic-250 Capsules 1968

Sulfamethoxazole (Potentiation of hypoglycemic action). Products include:
Azo Gantanol Tablets 1887
Bactrim DS Tablets 1891
Bactrim I.V. Infusion 1889
Bactrim 1891
Gantanol 1899
Septra 813
Septra I.V. Infusion 808
Septra I.V. Infusion ADD-Vantage Vials 810
Septra 813

Sulfasalazine (Potentiation of hypoglycemic action). Products include:
Azulfidine Tablets, EN-tabs, Oral Suspension 1157

Sulfinpyrazone (Potentiation of hypoglycemic action). Products include:
Anturane 853

Sulfisoxazole (Potentiation of hypoglycemic action). Products include:
Azo Gantrisin Tablets 1888
Gantrisin Tablets 1901
Pediazole 1973

Sulfisoxazole Diolamine (Potentiation of hypoglycemic action). Products include:
Gantrisin Ophthalmic Ointment/Solution 1900

Sulindac (Potentiation of hypoglycemic action). Products include:
Clinoril Tablets 1433

Terbutaline Sulfate (Hyperglycemia). Products include:
Brethaire Inhaler 1024
Brethine Ampuls 1026
Brethine Tablets 1026
Bricanyl Injection 1324
Bricanyl Tablets 1325

Thiamylal Sodium (Prolonged barbiturate action). Products include:
Surital Ampoules, Steri-Vials 1764

Thioridazine Hydrochloride (Hyperglycemia). Products include:
Mellaril 2011

Thyroid (Hyperglycemia). Products include:
S-P-T "Liquid" Capsules 995

Thyroxine (Hyperglycemia).
No products indexed under this heading.

Timolol Maleate (Potentiation of hypoglycemic action). Products include:
Blocadren Tablets 1429
Timolide Tablets 1547
Timoptic in Ocudose 1552
Timoptic Sterile Ophthalmic Solution 1550

Tolazamide (Potentiation of hypoglycemic action). Products include:
Tolinase Tablets 2365

Tolbutamide (Potentiation of hypoglycemic action). Products include:
Orinase Tablets 2354

Tolmetin Sodium (Potentiation of hypoglycemic action). Products include:
Tolectin (200, 400 and 600 mg) 1379

Tranylcypromine Sulfate (Potentiation of hypoglycemic action). Products include:
Parnate Tablets 2222

Triamcinolone (Hyperglycemia).
No products indexed under this heading.

Triamcinolone Acetonide (Hyperglycemia). Products include:
Aristocort A 1010
Azmacort Inhaler 1837
Kenalog Cream, Lotion & Ointment 2401
Kenalog-10 Injection 2402
Kenalog-40 Injection 2403
Kenalog in Orabase 604
Kenalog Spray 2401
Mycolog II Cream and Ointment 2407
Mytrex Cream & Ointment 2080
Nasacort Nasal Inhaler 1844

Triamcinolone Diacetate (Hyperglycemia). Products include:
Aristocort Suspension 1008

Triamcinolone Hexacetonide (Hyperglycemia). Products include:
Aristospan Suspension 1011

Triamterene (Hyperglycemia). Products include:
Dyazide Capsules 2208
Dyrenium Capsules 2210
Maxzide 1215

Trifluoperazine Hydrochloride (Hyperglycemia). Products include:
Stelazine 2226

Verapamil Hydrochloride (Hyperglycemia). Products include:
Calan SR Caplets 2157
Calan Tablets 2155
Isoptin Injectable 1177
Isoptin Oral Tablets 1179
Isoptin SR Sustained Release Tablets 1181
Verelan Capsules 1243
Verelan Capsules 2535

Warfarin Sodium (Potentiation of hypoglycemic action). Products include:
Coumadin Injection & Tablets 944
Panwarfin Tablets 547

DIALOSE TABLETS
(Docusate Sodium) 1154
May interact with:

Mineral Oil (Effect not specified). Products include:
AKWA Tears Ointment ◉ 208
Agoral ⊡ 634
Aqua Care Cream ⊡ 616
Aqua Care Lotion ⊡ 616
Aquaphor Antibiotic Formula 662
Aquaphor Healing Ointment, Original Formula 662
Aquaphor Natural Healing Formula 662
Complex 15 Hand & Body Moisturizing Cream ⊡ 694
Complex 15 Hand & Body Moisturizing Lotion ⊡ 695
Complex 15 Moisturizing Face Cream ⊡ 695
Duolube Eye Ointment ◉ 258
Duratears Naturale ◉ 216
Eucerin Dry Skin Care Lotion 662
Eucerin Moisturizing Creme (Unscented) 662
Eucerin Dry Skin Care Lotion (Fragrace-free) ⊡ 514
Fleet Mineral Oil Enema 992
Fleet Relief 993
Haley's M-O, Regular & Flavored ⊡ 569
Keri Lotion - Original Formula ⊡ 535
Lacri-Lube NP Lubricant Ophthalmic Ointment ◉ 249
Lacri-Lube S.O.P. Sterile Ophthalmic Ointment ◉ 249
Nephrox Suspension ⊡ 563
Nivea Bath Silk Bath Oil ⊡ 514
Nivea Bath Silk Bath & Shower Gel (Extra-Dry Skin) ⊡ 514
Nivea Moisturizing Creme ⊡ 514
Nivea Moisturizing Lotion (Original Formula) ⊡ 514
Nivea Moisturizing Oil ⊡ 515
Nivea Skin Oil ⊡ 515
Nivea Sun After Sun Lotion ⊡ 515
Nutraderm Cream & Lotion 1684
pHisoDerm For Baby ⊡ 761
pHisoDerm Skin Cleanser and Conditioner - Regular and Oily ⊡ 760
Refresh P.M. Lubricant Ophthalmic Ointment ◉ 256
Replens ⊡ 556
Tears Renewed Ointment ◉ 209
Theraplex ClearLotion 1410

Prescription Drugs, unspecified (Effect not specified).

DIALOSE PLUS TABLETS
(Docusate Sodium, Phenolphthalein, Yellow) 1154
May interact with:

Mineral Oil (Effect not specified). Products include:
AKWA Tears Ointment ◉ 208
Agoral ⊡ 634
Aqua Care Cream ⊡ 616
Aqua Care Lotion ⊡ 616
Aquaphor Antibiotic Formula 662
Aquaphor Healing Ointment, Original Formula 662
Aquaphor Natural Healing Formula 662
Complex 15 Hand & Body Moisturizing Cream ⊡ 694
Complex 15 Hand & Body Moisturizing Lotion ⊡ 695
Complex 15 Moisturizing Face Cream ⊡ 695
Duolube Eye Ointment ◉ 258
Duratears Naturale ◉ 216
Eucerin Dry Skin Care Lotion 662
Eucerin Moisturizing Creme (Unscented) 662
Eucerin Dry Skin Care Lotion (Fragrace-free) ⊡ 514
Fleet Mineral Oil Enema 992
Fleet Relief 993
Haley's M-O, Regular & Flavored ⊡ 569
Keri Lotion - Original Formula ⊡ 535
Lacri-Lube NP Lubricant Ophthalmic Ointment ◉ 249
Lacri-Lube S.O.P. Sterile Ophthalmic Ointment ◉ 249
Nephrox Suspension ⊡ 563
Nivea Bath Silk Bath Oil ⊡ 514
Nivea Bath Silk Bath & Shower Gel (Extra-Dry Skin) ⊡ 514
Nivea Moisturizing Creme ⊡ 514
Nivea Moisturizing Lotion (Original Formula) ⊡ 514
Nivea Moisturizing Oil ⊡ 515
Nivea Skin Oil ⊡ 515
Nivea Sun After Sun Lotion ⊡ 515
Nutraderm Cream & Lotion 1684
pHisoDerm For Baby ⊡ 761
pHisoDerm Skin Cleanser and Conditioner - Regular and Oily ⊡ 760
Refresh P.M. Lubricant Ophthalmic Ointment ◉ 256
Replens ⊡ 556
Tears Renewed Ointment ◉ 209
Theraplex ClearLotion 1410

Prescription Drugs, unspecified (Effect not specified).

DIAMOX PARENTERAL
(Acetazolamide) 1200
See **Diamox Tablets**

DIAMOX SEQUELS (SUSTAINED RELEASE)
(Acetazolamide) 1201
May interact with:

Aspirin (Concomitant administration with high-dose aspirin may result in anorexia, tachypnea, lethargy, coma and death). Products include:
Alka-Seltzer Effervescent Antacid and Pain Reliever 1568
Alka-Seltzer Extra Strength Effervescent Antacid and Pain Reliever 1570
Alka-Seltzer (Flavored) Effervescent Antacid and Pain Reliever 1569
Alka-Seltzer Plus Cold Medicine ⊡ 623
Alka-Seltzer Plus Night-Time Cold Medicine ⊡ 623
Alka Seltzer Plus Sinus Allergy Medicine ⊡ 624
Anacin Coated Analgesic Caplets 2417
Anacin Coated Analgesic Tablets 2417
Anacin Maximum Strength Analgesic Coated Tablets 2417

Maximum Strength Arthritis Pain Formula By the Makers of Anacin Analgesic Tablets and Caplets 2418
Arthritis Pain Formula by the Makers of Anacin Analgesic Tablets and Caplets ◙ 747
Arthritis Strength BC Powder ◙ 516
Ascriptin A/D Caplets 1850
Regular Strength Ascriptin Tablets 1850
Azdone Tablets 844
BC Powder ◙ 517
BC Cold Powder ◙ 517
Children's Bayer Chewable Aspirin ◙ 564
Genuine Bayer Aspirin Tablets & Caplets ◙ 564
Maximum Bayer Aspirin Tablets & Caplets ◙ 566
Bayer Plus Aspirin Tablets ◙ 567
Therapy Bayer Aspirin Caplets ◙ 568
8 Hour Bayer Timed-Release Aspirin ◙ 566
Arthritis Strength Bufferin Analgesic Caplets 744
Extra Strength Bufferin Analgesic Tablets 745
Bufferin Analgesic Tablets and Caplets 743
Cama Arthritis Pain Reliever ◙ 685
Damason-P 1356
Easprin 1719
Ecotrin Enteric Coated Aspirin Maximum Strength Tablets and Caplets 2189
Ecotrin Enteric Coated Aspirin Regular Strength Tablets and Caplets 2189
Empirin Aspirin ◙ 541
Empirin with Codeine Phosphate Nos. 2, 3 & 4 764
Equagesic Tablets 2451
Excedrin Extra-Strength Analgesic Tablets & Caplets 749
4-Way Cold Tablets 750
Fiorinal Capsules 2007
Fiorinal with Codeine Capsules 2008
Fiorinal Tablets 2007
Lortab ASA Tablets 2414
Momentum Muscular Backache Formula ◙ 751
Norgesic 1314
Norwich Extra-Strength Aspirin ◙ 546
Norwich Regular Strength Aspirin ◙ 547
P-A-C Analgesic Tablets ◙ 669
Percodan 951
Robaxisal Tablets 1872
Sine-Off Sinus Medicine Tablets-Aspirin Formula ◙ 722
Soma Compound w/Codeine Tablets 2390
Soma Compound Tablets 2389
St. Joseph Adult Chewable Aspirin (81 mg.) ◙ 703
Synalgos-DC Capsules 2525
Talwin Compound 2072
Ursinus Inlay-Tabs ◙ 691
Vanquish Analgesic Caplets ◙ 574
Zorprin Tablets 698

DIAMOX TABLETS

(Acetazolamide) 1200
May interact with:

Aspirin (Concomitant administration with high-dose aspirin may result in anorexia, tachypnea, lethargy, coma and death). Products include:

Alka-Seltzer Effervescent Antacid and Pain Reliever 1568
Alka-Seltzer Extra Strength Effervescent Antacid and Pain Reliever 1570
Alka-Seltzer (Flavored) Effervescent Antacid and Pain Reliever 1569
Alka-Seltzer Plus Cold Medicine ◙ 623
Alka-Seltzer Plus Night-Time Cold Medicine ◙ 623
Alka Seltzer Plus Sinus Allergy Medicine ◙ 624
Anacin Coated Analgesic Caplets 2417
Anacin Coated Analgesic Tablets 2417
Anacin Maximum Strength Analgesic Coated Tablets 2417
Maximum Strength Arthritis Pain Formula By the Makers of Anacin Analgesic Tablets and Caplets 2418
Arthritis Pain Formula by the Makers of Anacin Analgesic Tablets and Caplets ◙ 747
Arthritis Strength BC Powder ◙ 516
Ascriptin A/D Caplets 1850
Regular Strength Ascriptin Tablets 1850
Azdone Tablets 844
BC Powder ◙ 517
BC Cold Powder ◙ 517
Children's Bayer Chewable Aspirin ◙ 564
Genuine Bayer Aspirin Tablets & Caplets ◙ 564
Maximum Bayer Aspirin Tablets & Caplets ◙ 566
Bayer Plus Aspirin Tablets ◙ 567
Therapy Bayer Aspirin Caplets ◙ 568
8 Hour Bayer Timed-Release Aspirin ◙ 566
Arthritis Strength Bufferin Analgesic Caplets 744
Extra Strength Bufferin Analgesic Tablets 745
Bufferin Analgesic Tablets and Caplets 743
Cama Arthritis Pain Reliever ◙ 685
Damason-P 1356
Easprin 1719
Ecotrin Enteric Coated Aspirin Maximum Strength Tablets and Caplets 2189
Ecotrin Enteric Coated Aspirin Regular Strength Tablets and Caplets 2189
Empirin Aspirin ◙ 541
Empirin with Codeine Phosphate Nos. 2, 3 & 4 764
Equagesic Tablets 2451
Excedrin Extra-Strength Analgesic Tablets & Caplets 749
4-Way Cold Tablets 750
Fiorinal Capsules 2007
Fiorinal with Codeine Capsules 2008
Fiorinal Tablets 2007
Lortab ASA Tablets 2414
Momentum Muscular Backache Formula ◙ 751
Norgesic 1314
Norwich Extra-Strength Aspirin ◙ 546
Norwich Regular Strength Aspirin ◙ 547
P-A-C Analgesic Tablets ◙ 669
Percodan 951
Robaxisal Tablets 1872
Sine-Off Sinus Medicine Tablets-Aspirin Formula ◙ 722
Soma Compound w/Codeine Tablets 2390
Soma Compound Tablets 2389
St. Joseph Adult Chewable Aspirin (81 mg.) ◙ 703
Synalgos-DC Capsules 2525
Talwin Compound 2072
Ursinus Inlay-Tabs ◙ 691
Vanquish Analgesic Caplets ◙ 574
Zorprin Tablets 698

DIAPID NASAL SPRAY

(Lypressin) 2003
No interactions described in labeling.

DIASORB LIQUID

(Attapulgite, Nonfibrous Activated) ◙ 555
No interactions described in labeling.

DIASORB TABLETS

(Attapulgite, Nonfibrous Activated) ◙ 555
No interactions described in labeling.

DIBENZYLINE CAPSULES

(Phenoxybenzamine Hydrochloride) 2207
May interact with:

Alpha and Beta Adrenergic Stimulators (Exaggerated hypotensive response; tachycardia).

Epinephrine (Exaggerated hypotensive response; tachycardia). Products include:

Ana-Kit Anaphylaxis Emergency Treatment Kit 1100
Bronkaid Mist ◙ 757
EpiPen 843
Marcaine Hydrochloride 0.5% with Epinephrine 1:200,000 (as bitartrate) 958
Marcaine Hydrochloride with Epinephrine 1:200,000 2055
Primatene Mist 2420
Sus-Phrine Injection 1006
Xylocaine with Epinephrine Injections 637

Epinephrine Bitartrate (Exaggerated hypotensive response; tachycardia). Products include:

AsthmaHaler Mist Epinephrine Bitartrate Bronchodilator ◙ 616
Bronkaid Mist Suspension ◙ 757
Primatene Mist Suspension 2421

Norepinephrine Bitartrate (Hyperthermia production of levarterenol blocked by dibenzyline). Products include:

Levophed Bitartrate Injection 2054

Reserpine (Hypothermia production of reserpine blocked by dibenzyline). Products include:

Diupres Tablets 1461
Hydromox R Tablets 1209
Hydropres Tablets 1485
Renese-R Tablets 1786
Salutensin/Salutensin-Demi 719
Ser-Ap-Es Tablets 881
Serpasil Tablets 883
Serpasil-Apresoline Tablets 884
Serpasil-Esidrix Tablets 886

DICAL-D TABLETS & WAFERS

(Calcium Phosphate, Vitamin D) 515
No interactions described in labeling.

DICUMAROL TABLETS

(Dicumarol) 516
May interact with corticosteroids, antacids, antihistamines, barbiturates, narcotic analgesics, salicylates, sulfonamides, thyroid preparations, inhalant anesthetics, monoamine oxidase inhibitors, butyrophenones, oral contraceptives, oral hypoglycemic agents, anticonvulsants, diuretics, androgens, and certain other agents. Compounds in these categories include:

ACTH (Decreased prothrombin time).

Alcohol (Increased or decreased prothrombin times).

Alfentanil Hydrochloride (Increased prothrombin time). Products include:

Alfenta Injection 1131

Allopurinol (Increased prothrombin time). Products include:

Zyloprim Tablets 830

Aluminum Carbonate Gel (Decreased prothrombin time). Products include:

Basaljel 2438

Aluminum Hydroxide (Decreased prothrombin time). Products include:

Cama Arthritis Pain Reliever ◙ 685
Gaviscon Extra Strength Relief Formula Liquid Antacid ◙ 594
Gaviscon Extra Strength Relief Formula Antacid Tablets ◙ 594
Gaviscon Liquid Antacid ◙ 594
Gelusil Liquid & Tablets ◙ 639
Extra Strength Maalox Plus Suspension 1850
Maalox TC Suspension 1851
Maalox Plus Tablets ◙ 655
Extra Strength Maalox Plus Tablets 1850
Nephrox Suspension ◙ 563
WinGel Liquid & Tablets ◙ 761

Aluminum Hydroxide Gel (Decreased prothrombin time). Products include:

ALternaGEL Liquid 1154
Aludrox Oral Suspension 2428
Amphojel Suspension 2429
Amphojel Suspension without Flavor 2429
Mylanta Liquid 1155
Mylanta Double Strength Liquid 1155

Aluminum Hydroxide Gel, Dried (Decreased prothrombin time). Products include:

Alu-Tab/Alu-Cap 1309
Amphojel Tablets 2429
Ascriptin A/D Caplets 1850
Regular Strength Ascriptin Tablets 1850
Gaviscon Antacid Tablets ◙ 593
Gaviscon-2 Antacid Tablets ◙ 594
Mylanta Tablets 1155
Mylanta Double Strength Tablets 1155

Amiloride Hydrochloride (Increased or decreased prothrombin times). Products include:

Midamor Tablets 1508
Moduretic Tablets 1510

Aminosalicylic Acid (Increased prothrombin time).

Amiodarone Hydrochloride (Increased prothrombin time). Products include:

Cordarone Tablets 2446

Antibiotics, unspecified (Increased prothrombin time).

Aprobarbital (Decreased prothrombin time). Products include:

Alurate Elixir 1883

Aspirin (Increased prothrombin time). Products include:

Alka-Seltzer Effervescent Antacid and Pain Reliever 1568
Alka-Seltzer Extra Strength Effervescent Antacid and Pain Reliever 1570
Alka-Seltzer (Flavored) Effervescent Antacid and Pain Reliever 1569
Alka-Seltzer Plus Cold Medicine ◙ 623
Alka-Seltzer Plus Night-Time Cold Medicine ◙ 623
Alka Seltzer Plus Sinus Allergy Medicine ◙ 624
Anacin Coated Analgesic Caplets 2417
Anacin Coated Analgesic Tablets 2417
Anacin Maximum Strength Analgesic Coated Tablets 2417
Maximum Strength Arthritis Pain Formula By the Makers of Anacin Analgesic Tablets and Caplets 2418
Arthritis Pain Formula by the Makers of Anacin Analgesic Tablets and Caplets ◙ 747
Arthritis Strength BC Powder ◙ 516
Ascriptin A/D Caplets 1850
Regular Strength Ascriptin Tablets 1850
Azdone Tablets 844
BC Powder ◙ 517
BC Cold Powder ◙ 517
Children's Bayer Chewable Aspirin ◙ 564
Genuine Bayer Aspirin Tablets & Caplets ◙ 564
Maximum Bayer Aspirin Tablets & Caplets ◙ 566
Bayer Plus Aspirin Tablets ◙ 567
Therapy Bayer Aspirin Caplets ◙ 568
8 Hour Bayer Timed-Release Aspirin ◙ 566
Arthritis Strength Bufferin Analgesic Caplets 744
Extra Strength Bufferin Analgesic Tablets 745
Bufferin Analgesic Tablets and Caplets 743
Cama Arthritis Pain Reliever ◙ 685
Damason-P 1356
Easprin 1719
Ecotrin Enteric Coated Aspirin Maximum Strength Tablets and Caplets 2189
Ecotrin Enteric Coated Aspirin Regular Strength Tablets and Caplets 2189
Empirin Aspirin ◙ 541
Empirin with Codeine Phosphate Nos. 2, 3 & 4 764
Equagesic Tablets 2451
Excedrin Extra-Strength Analgesic Tablets & Caplets 749
4-Way Cold Tablets 750
Fiorinal Capsules 2007
Fiorinal with Codeine Capsules 2008
Fiorinal Tablets 2007
Lortab ASA Tablets 2414
Momentum Muscular Backache Formula ◙ 751
Norgesic 1314
Norwich Extra-Strength Aspirin ◙ 546
Norwich Regular Strength Aspirin ◙ 547
P-A-C Analgesic Tablets ◙ 669
Percodan 951
Robaxisal Tablets 1872
Sine-Off Sinus Medicine Tablets-Aspirin Formula ◙ 722
Soma Compound w/Codeine Tablets 2390
Soma Compound Tablets 2389

St. Joseph Adult Chewable Aspirin (81 mg.) ■ 703
Synalgos-DC Capsules 2525
Talwin Compound 2072
Ursinus Inlay-Tabs ■ 691
Vanquish Analgesic Caplets ■ 574
Zorprin Tablets 698

Astemizole (Decreased prothrombin time). Products include:
Hismanal Tablets 1138

Azatadine Maleate (Decreased prothrombin time). Products include:
Optimine Tablets 2115
Trinalin Repetabs Tablets 1170

Bendroflumethiazide (Increased or decreased prothrombin times). Products include:
Corzide Tablets 702
Naturetin Tablets 1789
Rauzide Tablets 1804

Betamethasone Acetate (Decreased prothrombin time). Products include:
Celestone Soluspan Suspension 2081

Betamethasone Sodium Phosphate (Decreased prothrombin time). Products include:
Celestone Soluspan Suspension 2081

Bromelains (Increased prothrombin time). Products include:
Bromase Capsules 672

Bromodiphenhydramine Hydrochloride (Decreased prothrombin time).
No products indexed under this heading.

Brompheniramine Maleate (Decreased prothrombin time). Products include:
Alka Seltzer Plus Sinus Allergy Medicine ■ 624
Atrohist Sprinkle Capsules 558
Bromfed Capsules (Timed Release) 1615
Bromfed Syrup ■ 628
Bromfed 1615
Dimetane Decongestant ■ 673
Dimetane ■ 672
Dimetane-DC Cough Syrup 1857
Dimetane-DX Cough Syrup 1858
Dimetapp Elixir ■ 673
Dimetapp DM Elixir ■ 674
Dimetapp Extentabs ■ 674
Dimetapp Plus Caplets ■ 675
Dimetapp Tablets ■ 675
Drixoral Antihistamine/Nasal Decongestant Syrup ■ 698

Bumetanide (Increased or decreased prothrombin times). Products include:
Bumex 1895

Buprenorphine (Increased prothrombin time).
No products indexed under this heading.

Butabarbital (Decreased prothrombin time). Products include:
Pyridium Plus 1764

Butalbital (Decreased prothrombin time). Products include:
Esgic-Plus Tablets 1002
Esgic Tablets & Capsules 1001
Fioricet Tablets 2006
Fiorinal Capsules 2007
Fiorinal with Codeine Capsules 2008
Fiorinal Tablets 2007
Phrenilin 838
Sedapap Tablets 50 mg/650 mg 1360

Carbamazepine (Decreased prothrombin time; possible accumulation of anticonvulsants). Products include:
Tegretol Chewable Tablets 654
Tegretol Suspension 656
Tegretol Tablets 654

Chloramphenicol (Increased prothrombin time). Products include:
AK-Chlor Sterile Ophthalmic Ointment & Solution ⊙ 201
Chloromycetin Cream, 1% 1694
Chloromycetin Hydrocortisone Ophthalmic 1694
Chloromycetin Kapseals 1695
Chloromycetin Ophthalmic Ointment, 1% 1696
Chloromycetin Ophthalmic Solution 1696
Chloromycetin Otic 1697
Chloroptic S.O.P. ⊙ 243
Chloroptic Sterile Ophthalmic Solution ⊙ 243
Ophthochlor Ophthalmic Solution ⊙ 300
Ophthocort ⊙ 301

Chloramphenicol Palmitate (Increased prothrombin time). Products include:
Chloromycetin Palmitate, Oral Suspension 1697

Chloramphenicol Sodium Succinate (Increased prothrombin time). Products include:
Chloromycetin Sodium Succinate 1698

Chlordiazepoxide (Decreased prothrombin time). Products include:
Libritabs Tablets 1930
Limbitrol 1933
Menrium Tablets 1934

Chlordiazepoxide Hydrochloride (Decreased prothrombin time). Products include:
Librax Capsules 1929
Librium Capsules 1931
Librium Injectable 1932

Chlorothiazide (Increased or decreased prothrombin times). Products include:
Aldoclor Tablets 1413
Diupres Tablets 1461
Diuril Oral 1464

Chlorothiazide Sodium (Increased or decreased prothrombin times). Products include:
Diuril Sodium Intravenous 1463

Chlorpheniramine Maleate (Decreased prothrombin time). Products include:
A.R.M. Allergy Relief Medicine Caplets ■ 615
Alka-Seltzer Plus Cold Medicine ■ 623
Allerest ■ 559
Ana-Kit Anaphylaxis Emergency Treatment Kit 1100
BC Cold Powder Multi-Symptom Formula ■ 517
Brexin L.A. Capsules 2078
Cerose-DM 2443
Cheracol Plus Head Cold/Cough Formula ■ 667
Chlor-Trimeton Allergy Syrup, Tablets & Long-Acting Repetabs Tablets ■ 693
Chlor-Trimeton Decongestant ■ 694
Comhist LA Capsules 1618
Allergy-Sinus Comtrex Multi-Symptom Allergy Sinus Formula Tablets & Caplets 746
Comtrex Multi-Symptom Cold Reliever Tablets/Caplets/Liqui-Gels/Liquid 745
Day-Night Comtrex 747
Contac Continuous Action Decongestant/Antihistamine Capsules ■ 710
Contac Maximum Strength Continuous Action Decongestant/Antihistamine Caplets ■ 709
Contac Severe Cold and Flu Formula Caplets ■ 711
Coricidin 'D' Decongestant Tablets ■ 695
Coricidin Demilets Tablets for Children ■ 696
Coricidin Tablets ■ 695
Deconamine 663
Demazin Nasal Decongestant/Antihistamine Repetabs Tablets & Syrup ■ 697
Dorcol Children's Liquid Cold Formula ■ 686
Dristan Decongestant/Antihistamine/ Analgesic Coated Caplets ■ 749
Dristan Cold Nasal Decongestant/Antihistamine/ Analgesic Coated Tablets 2419
Dristan Advanced Formula Decongestant/Antihistamine/Analgesic Tablets ■ 749
Extendryl 994
4-Way Cold Tablets 750
Fedahist Gyrocaps 2145
Fedahist Timecaps 2145
Hycomine Compound Tablets 929
Isoclor Timesule Capsules ■ 561
Kronofed-A 970
Medi-Flu Caplet, Liquid ■ 640
Naldecon Syrup, Tablets, Pediatric Drops and Pediatric Syrup 709
Nolamine Tablets 838
Novafed A Capsules 1342
Novahistine DH 1342
Novahistine Elixir ■ 596
Ornade Spansule Capsules 2221
Orthoxicol Cough Syrup ■ 668
PediaCare Allergy Relief Formula Liquid 1362
PediaCare Cough-Cold Formula Liquid 1362
PediaCare Night Rest Cough-Cold Formula Liquid 1362
PediaCare 6-12 Cough-Cold Formula Chewable Tablets 1362
Pyrroxate Capsules ■ 669
Quelidrine Syrup 556
Ru-Tuss II Capsules 693
Ru-Tuss Tablets 693
Ryna ■ 741
Sinarest Tablets & Extra Strength Tablets ■ 562
Sine-Off Maximum Strength Allergy/Sinus Formula Caplets ■ 721
Sine-Off Sinus Medicine Tablets-Aspirin Formula ■ 722
Singlet Tablets ■ 598
Sinulin 840
Sinutab Maximum Strength ■ 641
St. Joseph Nighttime Cold Medicine ■ 705
Sudafed Plus Liquid ■ 544
Sudafed Plus Tablets ■ 545
Teldrin Timed-Release Allergy Capsules, 12 mg 2192
TheraFlu Flu and Cold Medicine ■ 687
Triaminic Allergy Tablets ■ 688
Triaminic Chewables ■ 688
Triaminic Cold Tablets ■ 688
Triaminic Nite Light ■ 689
Triaminic Syrup ■ 689
Triaminic-12 Tablets ■ 690
Triaminicin Tablets ■ 690
Triaminicol Multi-Symptom Cold Tablets ■ 691
Triaminicol Multi-Symptom Relief ■ 691
Tylenol Allergy Sinus Medication Caplets and Gelcaps, Maximum Strength 1372
Children's Tylenol Cold Liquid Formula and Chewable Tablets 1368
Tylenol Cold & Flu Hot Medication, Packets 1369
Tylenol Cold Medication Caplets and Tablets 1370
Tylenol Cold Medication, Effervescent Tablets 1369
Vicks Children's NyQuil ■ 664
Vicks Formula 44 Cough Medicine ■ 661
Vicks Formula 44M Multi-Symptom Cough Medicine ■ 662
Vicks Pediatric Formula 44m Multi-Symptom Cough & Cold Medicine ■ 663

Chlorpheniramine Polistirex (Decreased prothrombin time). Products include:
Tussionex Extended-Release Suspension 988

Chlorpheniramine Tannate (Decreased prothrombin time). Products include:
Rynatan 2387
Rynatuss 2388

Chlorpropamide (Increased prothrombin time). Products include:
Diabinese Tablets 1775

Chlorthalidone (Increased or decreased prothrombin times). Products include:
Combipres Tablets 678
Tenoretic Tablets 1105
Thalitone Tablets 687

Cholestyramine (Decreased prothrombin time). Products include:
Cholybar 1705
Questran Light 711
Questran Powder 710

Choline Magnesium Trisalicylate (Increased prothrombin time). Products include:
Trilisate 1822

Chymotrypsin (Increased prothrombin time).
No products indexed under this heading.

Cimetidine (Increased prothrombin time). Products include:
Tagamet Tablets 2228

Cimetidine Hydrochloride (Increased prothrombin time). Products include:
Tagamet 2228

Cinchophen (Increased prothrombin time).

Clemastine Fumarate (Decreased prothrombin time). Products include:
Tavist Syrup 2033
Tavist Tablets 2035
Tavist-D Tablets 2035

Clofibrate (Increased prothrombin time). Products include:
Atromid-S Capsules 2435

Codeine (Increased prothrombin time). Products include:
Calcidrine Syrup 506

Codeine Phosphate (Increased prothrombin time). Products include:
Actifed with Codeine Cough Syrup 752
Cheracol Cough Syrup 1853
Codimal PH Syrup 846
Dimetane-DC Cough Syrup 1857
Empirin with Codeine Phosphate Nos. 2, 3 & 4 764
Fiorinal with Codeine Capsules 2008
Isoclor Expectorant 982
Naldecon CX Adult Liquid ■ 521
Novahistine DH 1342
Novahistine Expectorant 1343
Nucofed Capsules 2219
Nucofed Expectorant 2219
Nucofed Pediatric Expectorant 2220
Nucofed Syrup 2219
Phenaphen with Codeine Capsules 1865
Phenaphen-650 with Codeine Tablets 1866
Phenergan with Codeine 2497
Phenergan VC with Codeine 2501
Robitussin A-C Syrup 1875
Robitussin-DAC Syrup 1875
Ryna ■ 741
Soma Compound w/Codeine Tablets 2390
Triaminic Expectorant w/Codeine 1996
Tussi-Organidin Liquid 2391
Tylenol with Codeine 1381

Codeine Polistirex (Increased prothrombin time).
No products indexed under this heading.

Cortisone Acetate (Decreased prothrombin time). Products include:
Cortone Acetate Sterile Suspension 1437
Cortone Acetate Tablets 1439

Cyproheptadine Hydrochloride (Decreased prothrombin time). Products include:
Periactin 1525

Dexamethasone (Decreased prothrombin time). Products include:
AK-Trol Ointment & Suspension ⊙ 207
Decadron Elixir 1445
Decadron Tablets 1447
Decaspray Topical Aerosol 1459
Dexacidin ⊙ 272
Maxidex Sterile Ophthalmic Suspension ⊙ 223
Maxitrol Ophthalmic Ointment/Suspension ⊙ 223
TobraDex Ophthalmic Suspension and Ointment ⊙ 228

Dexamethasone Acetate (Decreased prothrombin time). Products include:
Dalalone D.P. Injectable 999
Decadron-LA Sterile Suspension 1457

(■ Described in PDR For Nonprescription Drugs) (⊙ Described in PDR For Ophthalmology)

Dexamethasone Sodium Phosphate (Decreased prothrombin time). Products include:
- AK-Dex ◉ 203
- Decadron Phosphate Respihaler 1454
- Decadron Phosphate Sterile Ophthalmic Ointment 1453
- Decadron Phosphate Sterile Ophthalmic Solution 1453
- Decadron Phosphate Topical Cream 1455
- Decadron Phosphate Turbinaire 1456
- Maxidex Sterile Ophthalmic Ointment ◉ 222
- NeoDecadron Sterile Ophthalmic Ointment 1517
- NeoDecadron Sterile Ophthalmic Solution 1518
- NeoDecadron Topical Cream 1518

Dexchlorpheniramine Maleate (Decreased prothrombin time). Products include:
- Polaramine 2116

Dextrothyroxine Sodium (Increased prothrombin time).
- No products indexed under this heading.

Dezocine (Increased prothrombin time).

Diazoxide (Increased prothrombin time). Products include:
- Hyperstat I.V. Injection 2095
- Proglycem 649

Diflunisal (Increased prothrombin time). Products include:
- Dolobid Tablets 1465

Dihydroxyaluminum Sodium Carbonate (Decreased prothrombin time). Products include:
- Rolaids ▣ 743

Diphenhydramine Citrate (Decreased prothrombin time). Products include:
- Alka-Seltzer Plus Night-Time Cold Medicine ▣ 623
- Bufferin AF Nite Time Analgesic/Sleeping Aid Caplets 744
- Excedrin P.M. Analgesic/Sleeping Aid Tablets, Caplets and Liquid 749

Diphenhydramine Hydrochloride (Decreased prothrombin time). Products include:
- Benadryl Anti-Itch Cream ▣ 635
- Benadryl Capsules 1691
- Benadryl Decongestant Elixir ▣ 635
- Benadryl Decongestant ▣ 635
- Benadryl Elixir ▣ 636
- Benadryl Kapseals 1691
- Benadryl 25 Kapseals ▣ 636
- Benadryl Parenteral 1692
- Benadryl Plus ▣ 636
- Benadryl Plus Nighttime ▣ 637
- Benadryl Spray, Maximum Strength ▣ 637
- Benadryl Spray, Regular Strength ▣ 637
- Benadryl Steri-Vials, Ampoules, and Steri-Dose Syringe 1692
- Benadryl 25 Tablets ▣ 636
- Benylin Cough Syrup ▣ 637
- Benylin Decongestant ▣ 638
- Caladryl Cream, Lotion, Spray ▣ 638
- Miles Nervine Nighttime Sleep-Aid ▣ 627
- Nytol Tablets ▣ 517
- Sleep-ettes-D Tablets ▣ 653
- Sleep-eze 3 Tablets ▣ 755
- Sleepinal Night-time Sleep Aid Capsules ▣ 734
- Sominex Caplets and Tablets ▣ 722
- Sominex Liquid ▣ 723
- Sominex Pain Relief Formula ▣ 723
- Tylenol Cold Night Time Medication Liquid 1371
- Tylenol PM, Extra Strength Caplets and Tablets 1368
- Unisom Dual Relief Nighttime Sleep Aid/Analgesic 1774
- Ziradryl Lotion ▣ 643

Disulfiram (Increased prothrombin time). Products include:
- Antabuse Tablets 2429

Divalproex Sodium (Possible accumulation of anticonvulsants). Products include:
- Depakote 512

Enflurane (Increased prothrombin time). Products include:
- Ethrane 599

Ethacrynic Acid (Increased or decreased prothrombin time). Products include:
- Edecrin Tablets 1468

Ethchlorvynol (Decreased prothrombin time). Products include:
- Placidyl Capsules 553

Ethinyl Estradiol (Decreased prothrombin time). Products include:
- Brevicon 2304
- Demulen 2161
- Estinyl Tablets 2085
- Jenest-28 Tablets 1636
- Levlen/Tri-Levlen 665
- Lo/Ovral Tablets 2471
- Lo/Ovral-28 Tablets 2476
- Loestrin 1728
- Modicon 1667
- Nordette-21 Tablets 2481
- Nordette-28 Tablets 2483
- Norethin 2133
- Norinyl 2304
- Norlestrin 1746
- Ortho-Cyclen Tablets 1658
- Ortho-Novum 1667
- Ovcon 1391
- Ovral Tablets 2490
- Ovral-28 Tablets 2491
- Levlen/Tri-Levlen 665
- Tri-Norinyl 2304
- Triphasil-21 Tablets 2527
- Triphasil-28 Tablets 2532

Ethosuximide (Possible accumulation of anticonvulsants). Products include:
- Zarontin Capsules 1768
- Zarontin Syrup 1769

Ethotoin (Possible accumulation of anticonvulsants). Products include:
- Peganone Tablets 551

Ethynodiol Diacetate (Decreased prothrombin time). Products include:
- Demulen 2161

Fenoprofen Calcium (Increased prothrombin time). Products include:
- Nalfon Pulvules & Tablets 919

Fentanyl (Increased prothrombin time). Products include:
- Duragesic Transdermal System 1133

Fentanyl Citrate (Increased prothrombin time). Products include:
- Innovar Injection 1141
- Sublimaze Injection 1146

Fluoxymesterone (Increased prothrombin time). Products include:
- Halotestin Tablets 2341

Furazolidone (Increased prothrombin time). Products include:
- Furoxone 1855

Furosemide (Increased or decreased prothrombin times). Products include:
- Lasix 1093

Glipizide (Increased prothrombin time). Products include:
- Glucotrol 1952

Glucagon (Increased prothrombin time). Products include:
- Glucagon for Injection Vials and Emergency Kit 1263

Glutethimide (Decreased prothrombin time).
- No products indexed under this heading.

Glyburide (Increased prothrombin time). Products include:
- DiaBeta 1091
- Micronase Tablets 2350

Griseofulvin (Decreased prothrombin time). Products include:
- Fulvicin P/G Tablets 2090
- Fulvicin P/G 165 & 330 Tablets 2091
- Fulvicin-U/F Tablets 2092
- Grifulvin V (griseofulvin microsize) Tablets/Suspension 1678
- Grisactin 2454
- Grisactin Ultra Tablets 2455
- Gris-PEG Tablets, 125 mg & 250 mg 1083

Haloperidol (Decreased prothrombin time). Products include:
- Haldol Injection, Tablets and Concentrate 1373

Haloperidol Decanoate (Decreased prothrombin time). Products include:
- Haldol Decanoate 1375

Halothane (Increased prothrombin time). Products include:
- Fluothane 2453

Hepatotoxic Drugs, unspecified (Increased prothrombin time).

Hydrochlorothiazide (Increased or decreased prothrombin times). Products include:
- Aldactazide 2150
- Aldoril Tablets 1418
- Apresazide Capsules 854
- Apresoline-Esidrix Tablets 857
- Capozide 2258
- Dyazide Capsules 2208
- Esidrix Tablets 863
- Esimil Tablets 864
- HydroDIURIL Tablets 1484
- Hydropres Tablets 1485
- Inderide Tablets 2463
- Inderide LA Long Acting Capsules 2465
- Lopressor HCT Tablets 1034
- Maxzide 1215
- Moduretic Tablets 1510
- Normozide Tablets 2112
- Oretic Tablets 544
- Oreticyl 545
- Prinzide Tablets 1540
- Ser-Ap-Es Tablets 881
- Serpasil-Esidrix Tablets 886
- Timolide Tablets 1547
- Trandate HCT Tablets 579
- Vaseretic Tablets 1559
- Zestoretic 2274

Hydrocodone Bitartrate (Increased prothrombin time). Products include:
- Anexsia 5/500 Tablets 2196
- Anexsia 7.5/650 Tablets 2197
- Azdone Tablets 844
- Codiclear DH Syrup 845
- Codimal DH Syrup 846
- Damason-P 1356
- Hycodan Syrup, Tablets 927
- Hycomine Compound Tablets 929
- Hycomine Syrup 927
- Hycotuss Expectorant Syrup 930
- Hydrocet Capsules 835
- Lortab ASA Tablets 2414
- Lortab 2412
- Ru-Tuss with Hydrocodone 694
- Triaminic Expectorant DH 1995
- Vicodin Tablets 1187
- Vicodin ES Tablets 1189
- Zydone Capsules 941

Hydrocodone Polistirex (Increased prothrombin time). Products include:
- Tussionex Extended-Release Suspension 988

Hydrocortisone Acetate (Decreased prothrombin time). Products include:
- Analpram-HC Rectal Cream 1% and 2.5% 970
- Anusol-HC Cream 1690
- Anusol-HC Suppositories 1691
- Caldecort ▣ 560
- Carmol HC Cream 1% 2296
- Chloromycetin Hydrocortisone Ophthalmic 1694
- Coly-Mycin S Otic w/Neomycin & Hydrocortisone 1708
- Cortaid ▣ 735
- Cortef Feminine Itch Cream ▣ 735
- Corticaine ▣ 682
- Cortifoam 1827
- Cortisporin Cream 757
- Epifoam 1828
- Gynecort 5 Creme ▣ 556
- Hydrocortone Acetate Sterile Suspension 1479
- Lanacort 5 Creme and Ointment ▣ 557
- Mantadil Cream 789
- Ophthocort ◉ 301
- Orabase HCA Oral Paste 890
- Pramosone Cream, Lotion & Ointment 971
- ProctoCream-HC 1834
- Proctofoam-HC 1835

Hydrocortisone Sodium Phosphate (Decreased prothrombin time). Products include:
- Hydrocortone Phosphate Injection, Sterile 1481

Hydrocortisone Sodium Succinate (Decreased prothrombin time). Products include:
- Solu-Cortef Sterile Powder 2361

Hydroflumethiazide (Increased or decreased prothrombin times). Products include:
- Diucardin Tablets 2450
- Saluron 718
- Salutensin/Salutensin-Demi 719

Ibuprofen (Increased prothrombin time). Products include:
- Advil Cold & Sinus Caplets (formerly CoAdvil) 2416
- Advil Ibuprofen Tablets and Caplets 2416
- Children's Advil Suspension 2426
- CoAdvil ▣ 748
- Dristan Sinus Caplets 2419
- Haltran Tablets ▣ 668
- Ibuprofen ▣ 631
- Medipren ibuprofen Caplets and Tablets 1362
- Midol 200 Cramp Relief Formula ▣ 570
- Motrin Tablets 2351
- Motrin IB Caplets and Tablets ▣ 736
- Nuprin Ibuprofen/Analgesic Tablets & Caplets 752
- PediaProfen Suspension 1363
- Rufen Tablets 691
- Trendar Ibuprofen Tablets ▣ 756

Indapamide (Increased or decreased prothrombin times). Products include:
- Lozol Tablets 1843

Indomethacin (Increased prothrombin time). Products include:
- Indocin 1487

Indomethacin Sodium Trihydrate (Increased prothrombin time). Products include:
- Indocin I.V. 1490

Influenza Virus Vaccine (Increased prothrombin time). Products include:
- Flu-Imune Influenza Virus Vaccine 1204

Isocarboxazid (Increased prothrombin time). Products include:
- Marplan Tablets 1906

Isoflurane (Increased prothrombin time). Products include:
- Forane 600

Levonorgestrel (Decreased prothrombin time). Products include:
- Levlen/Tri-Levlen 665
- Nordette-21 Tablets 2481
- Nordette-28 Tablets 2483
- Norplant System 2484
- Levlen/Tri-Levlen 665
- Triphasil-21 Tablets 2527
- Triphasil-28 Tablets 2532

Levorphanol Tartrate (Increased prothrombin time). Products include:
- Levo-Dromoran 1906

Levothyroxine Sodium (Increased prothrombin time). Products include:
- Levothroid Tablets 1003
- Levoxine Tablets 904
- Synthroid 695

Liothyronine Sodium (Increased prothrombin time). Products include:
- Cytomel Tablets 2203

Liotrix (Increased prothrombin time). Products include:
- Euthroid 1724

Magaldrate (Decreased prothrombin time). Products include:
- Riopan Antacid Chew Tablets ▣ 754
- Riopan Antacid Chew Tablets in Rollpacks ▣ 754
- Riopan Antacid Suspension 2421

(▣ Described in PDR For Nonprescription Drugs) (◉ Described in PDR For Ophthalmology)

Riopan Antacid Swallow Tablets 2421
Riopan Plus Chew Tablets 2422
Riopan Plus Chew Tablets in Roll-pack 2422
Riopan Plus 2 Chew Tablets, Mint Flavor, Cherry Flavor 2422
Riopan Plus Suspension 2422
Riopan Plus 2 Suspension, Mint Flavor, Cherry Flavor 2422

Magnesium Hydroxide (Decreased prothrombin time). Products include:
Aludrox Oral Suspension 2428
Ascriptin A/D Caplets 1850
Regular Strength Ascriptin Tablets 1850
Di-Gel Antacid/Anti-Gas ...... [ND] 697
Gelusil Liquid & Tablets ...... [ND] 639
Haley's M-O, Regular & Flavored .. [ND] 569
Extra Strength Maalox Plus Suspension 1850
Maalox TC Suspension 1851
Maalox Plus Tablets ...... [ND] 655
Extra Strength Maalox Plus Tablets 1850
Mylanta Liquid 1155
Mylanta Tablets 1155
Mylanta Double Strength Liquid 1155
Mylanta Double Strength Tablets 1155
Concentrated Phillips' Milk of Magnesia ...... [ND] 573
Phillips' Milk of Magnesia Liquid .... [ND] 572
Phillips' Milk of Magnesia Tablets [ND] 573
WinGel Liquid & Tablets ...... [ND] 761

Magnesium Oxide (Decreased prothrombin time). Products include:
Bayer Plus Aspirin Tablets ...... [ND] 567
Beelith Tablets 659
Bufferin Analgesic Tablets and Caplets ...... [ND] 524
Cama Arthritis Pain Reliever ...... [ND] 685
Mag-Ox 400 673
Uro-Mag 673

Magnesium Salicylate (Increased prothrombin time). Products include:
Doan's - Extra-Strength Analgesic [ND] 549
Doan's - Regular Strength Analgesic ...... [ND] 549
Mobigesic Analgesic Tablets ...... [ND] 507

Mefenamic Acid (Increased prothrombin time). Products include:
Ponstel 1758

Meperidine Hydrochloride (Increased prothrombin time). Products include:
Demerol 2047
Mepergan Injection 2479

Mephenytoin (Possible accumulation of anticonvulsants). Products include:
Mesantoin Tablets 2013

Mephobarbital (Decreased prothrombin time). Products include:
Mebaral Tablets 2061

Meprobamate (Decreased prothrombin time). Products include:
Deprol Tablets 2382
Equagesic Tablets 2451
Miltown Tablets 2386
PMB 200 and PMB 400 2504

Mestranol (Decreased prothrombin time). Products include:
Enovid 2161
Norethin 2133
Norinyl 2304
Ortho-Novum 1667

Methadone Hydrochloride (Increased prothrombin time). Products include:
Dolophine Hydrochloride Ampoules & Vials 1260
Dolophine Hydrochloride Tablets 1261
Methadone Hydrochloride Diskets .. 1284
Methadone Hydrochloride Oral Solution & Tablets 1987

Methdilazine Hydrochloride (Decreased prothrombin time). Products include:
Tacaryl Syrup & Tablets 2409

Methoxyflurane (Increased prothrombin time).
No products indexed under this heading.

Methsuximide (Possible accumulation of anticonvulsants). Products include:
Celontin 1692

Methyclothiazide (Increased or decreased prothrombin times). Products include:
Enduron Tablets 517
Enduronyl 518

Methyldopa (Increased prothrombin time). Products include:
Aldoclor Tablets 1413
Aldomet Oral 1415
Aldoril Tablets 1418

Methyldopate Hydrochloride (Increased prothrombin time). Products include:
Aldomet Ester HCl Injection 1417

Methylphenidate Hydrochloride (Increased prothrombin time). Products include:
Ritalin 880

Methylprednisolone (Decreased prothrombin time). Products include:
Medrol 2348

Methylprednisolone Acetate (Decreased prothrombin time). Products include:
Depo-Medrol Sterile Aqueous Suspension 2334

Methylprednisolone Sodium Succinate (Decreased prothrombin time). Products include:
Solu-Medrol Sterile Powder 2363

Methyltestosterone (Increased prothrombin time). Products include:
Android 1111
Estratest 2245
Mediatric Capsules 2476
Metandren Linguets and Tablets 875
Premarin with Methyltestosterone .. 2515
Testred Capsules 1124

Methylthiouracil (Increased prothrombin time).

Metolazone (Increased or decreased prothrombin times). Products include:
Diulo 2129
Mykrox ½ mg Tablets 984
Zaroxolyn Tablets 989

Metronidazole (Increased prothrombin time). Products include:
Flagyl I.V. RTU 2131
Flagyl Tablets 2170
MetroGel 903
Protostat Tablets 1674

Miconazole (Increased prothrombin time). Products include:
Monistat I.V. 1143

Morphine Sulfate (Increased prothrombin time). Products include:
Astramorph/PF Injection, USP (Preservative-Free) 618
Duramorph 960
Infumorph 200 and Infumorph 500 Sterile Solutions 962
MS Contin Tablets 1814
MSIR 1817
Oramorph SR (Morphine Sulfate Sustained Release Tablets) 1988
Roxanol 1991

Nalidixic Acid (Increased prothrombin time). Products include:
NegGram 2062

Naproxen (Increased prothrombin time). Products include:
Naprosyn 2297

Naproxen Sodium (Increased prothrombin time). Products include:
Anaprox and Anaprox DS Tablets 2288

Norethindrone (Decreased prothrombin time). Products include:
Brevicon 2304
Jenest-28 Tablets 1636
Micronor Tablets 1667
Modicon 1667
Norethin 2133
Norinyl 2304
Norlutin 1755
Nor-Q D Tablets 2304
Ortho-Novum 1667
Ovcon 1391
Tri-Norinyl 2304

Norethynodrel (Decreased prothrombin time). Products include:
Enovid 2161

Norgestimate (Decreased prothrombin time). Products include:
Ortho-Cyclen Tablets 1658

Norgestrel (Decreased prothrombin time). Products include:
Lo/Ovral Tablets 2471
Lo/Ovral-28 Tablets 2476
Ovral Tablets 2490
Ovral-28 Tablets 2491
Ovrette Tablets 2492

Nortriptyline Hydrochloride (Increased prothrombin time). Products include:
Pamelor 2019

Opium Alkaloids (Increased prothrombin time). Products include:
B & O No. 15A & No. 16A Supprettes 2395
Pantopon Injectable 1911

Oxandrolone (Increased prothrombin time).
No products indexed under this heading.

Oxolinic Acid (Increased prothrombin time).

Oxycodone Hydrochloride (Increased prothrombin time). Products include:
Percocet Tablets 950
Percodan 951
Roxicodone Tablets, Oral Solution & Intensol (Oxycodone) 1992
Tylox Capsules 1382

Oxymetholone (Increased prothrombin time). Products include:
Anadrol-50 Tablets 2287

Oxyphenbutazone (Increased prothrombin time).

Paramethadione (Possible accumulation of anticonvulsants). Products include:
Paradione Capsules 548

Pentobarbital Sodium (Decreased prothrombin time). Products include:
Nembutal Sodium Capsules 534
Nembutal Sodium Solution 536
Nembutal Sodium Suppositories 538

Pentoxifylline (Increased prothrombin time). Products include:
Trental 1099

Phenacemide (Possible accumulation of anticonvulsants). Products include:
Phenurone Tablets 552

Phenelzine Sulfate (Increased prothrombin time). Products include:
Nardil 1742

Phenobarbital (Decreased prothrombin time). Products include:
Arco-Lase Plus Tablets 607
Bellergal-S Tablets 1998
Bronkolixir ...... [ND] 761
Bronkotabs Tablets ...... [ND] 762
Donnatal 1858
Donnatal Extentabs 1859
Donnatal Tablets 1858
Donnazyme Tablets 1860
Kinesed Tablets 2272
Phenobarbital Elixir and Tablets 1293
Primatene Tablets-P Formula 2421
Quadrinal Tablets 1183
Tedral SA 1765

Phensuximide (Possible accumulation of anticonvulsants). Products include:
Milontin Kapseals 1741

Phenylbutazone (Increased prothrombin time). Products include:
Butazolidin Capsules & Tablets 1027

Phenyramidol (Increased prothrombin time).

Phenytoin (Possible accumulation of phenytoin). Products include:
Dilantin Infatabs 1710
Dilantin-30 Pediatric/Dilantin-125 Suspension 1713

Phenytoin Sodium (Possible accumulation of phenytoin). Products include:
Dilantin Kapseals 1708
Dilantin Parenteral 1712
Dilantin with Phenobarbital Kapseals 1715

Polythiazide (Increased or decreased prothrombin times). Products include:
Minizide Capsules 1779
Renese Tablets 1785
Renese-R Tablets 1786

Prednisolone Acetate (Decreased prothrombin time). Products include:
AK-Cide Sterile Ophthalmic Ointment & Suspension ...... ⊙ 202
Blephamide Liquifilm Sterile Ophthalmic Suspension 586
Blephamide S.O.P. Sterile Ophthalmic Ointment 586
Cetapred Ointment ...... ⊙ 220
⅛ % Econopred & 1 % Econopred Plus ...... ⊙ 217
Isopto Cetapred Suspension ...... ⊙ 220
Metimyd ...... ⊙ 306
Poly-Pred Liquifilm ...... ⊙ 250
Pred Forte ...... ⊙ 252
Pred Mild ...... ⊙ 254
Pred-G Liquifilm Sterile Ophthalmic Suspension ...... ⊙ 252
Pred-G S.O.P. Sterile Ophthalmic Ointment ...... ⊙ 253
Vasocidin Ointment ...... ⊙ 275

Prednisolone Sodium Phosphate (Decreased prothrombin time). Products include:
AK-Pred ...... ⊙ 205
Hydeltrasol Injection, Sterile 1476
Inflamase ...... ⊙ 274
Pediapred Oral Liquid 987
Vasocidin Ophthalmic Solution ...... ⊙ 276

Prednisolone Tebutate (Decreased prothrombin time). Products include:
Hydeltra-T.B.A. Sterile Suspension 1478

Prednisone (Decreased prothrombin time). Products include:
Deltasone Tablets 2332

Primidone (Decreased prothrombin time). Products include:
Mysoline 2480

Promethazine Hydrochloride (Decreased prothrombin time). Products include:
Mepergan Injection 2479
Phenergan with Codeine 2497
Phenergan with Dextromethorphan 2499
Phenergan Injection 2493
Phenergan Suppositories 2496
Phenergan Syrup 2495
Phenergan Tablets 2496
Phenergan VC 2500
Phenergan VC with Codeine 2501

Propoxyphene Hydrochloride (Increased prothrombin time). Products include:
Darvon 1256
Wygesic Tablets 2540

Propoxyphene Napsylate (Increased prothrombin time). Products include:
Darvon-N/Darvocet-N 1254

Propylthiouracil (Increased prothrombin time).
No products indexed under this heading.

Pyrazolones (Increased prothrombin time).

Pyrilamine Maleate (Decreased prothrombin time). Products include:
Codimal 846
4-Way Fast Acting Nasal Spray - Original Formula (regular & mentholated) & Metered Spray Pump (regular) 751

([ND] Described in PDR For Nonprescription Drugs)

(⊙ Described in PDR For Ophthalmology)

- Maximum Strength Midol Multi-Symptom Menstrual Formula ▣ 571
- Maximum Strength Midol PMS Premenstrual Syndrome Formula ▣ 570
- Regular Strength Midol Multi-Symptom Menstrual Formula ▣ 570
- Prefrin-A ⊙ 255
- Prēmsyn PMS Capsules & Caplets ▣ 547
- Primatene Tablets-M Formula 2421
- Robitussin Night Relief ▣ 677
- Ru-Tuss with Hydrocodone 694
- Triaminic Expectorant DH 1995
- Triaminic Oral Infant Drops 1996

Pyrilamine Tannate (Decreased prothrombin time). Products include:
- Rynatan 2387

Quinidine Gluconate (Increased prothrombin time). Products include:
- Quinaglute Dura-Tabs Tablets 663

Quinidine Polygalacturonate (Increased prothrombin time). Products include:
- Cardioquin Tablets 1812

Quinidine Sulfate (Increased prothrombin time). Products include:
- Quinidex Extentabs 1868

Quinine (Increased prothrombin time).

Ranitidine Hydrochloride (Increased or decreased prothrombin times). Products include:
- Zantac Injection and Zantac Injection Premixed 1063
- Zantac 1065

Rifampin (Decreased prothrombin time). Products include:
- Rifadin 1345
- Rifamate Capsules 1347
- Rimactane Capsules 879

Salsalate (Increased prothrombin time). Products include:
- Disalcid 1310
- Mono-Gesic Tablets 846
- Salflex 839

Secobarbital Sodium (Decreased prothrombin time). Products include:
- Seconal Sodium Pulvules 1296

Selegiline Hydrochloride (Increased prothrombin time). Products include:
- Eldepryl 2250

Sodium Bicarbonate (Decreased prothrombin time). Products include:
- Alka-Seltzer Advanced Formula Antacid & Non-Aspirin Pain Reliever ▣ 620
- Alka-Seltzer Effervescent Antacid ▣ 622
- Alka-Seltzer Effervescent Antacid and Pain Reliever 1568
- Alka-Seltzer Extra Strength Effervescent Antacid and Pain Reliever ▣ 623
- Alka-Seltzer (Flavored) Effervescent Antacid and Pain Reliever ▣ 621
- Arm & Hammer Pure Baking Soda ▣ 548
- Ceo-Two Rectal Suppositories 671
- Citrocarbonate Antacid ▣ 668
- Massengill Liquid Concentrate 2191
- NuLYTELY 699

Spironolactone (Increased or decreased prothrombin times). Products include:
- Aldactazide 2150
- Aldactone 2152

Stanozolol (Increased prothrombin time). Products include:
- Winstrol Tablets 2075

Streptokinase (Exercise caution; concomitant use may be hazardous). Products include:
- Kabikinase (Streptokinase) 1162
- Streptase for Infusion 635

Sufentanil Citrate (Increased prothrombin time). Products include:
- Sufenta Injection 1147

Sulfamethizole (Increased prothrombin time). Products include:
- Thiosulfil Forte Tablets 2526
- Urobiotic-250 Capsules 1968

Sulfamethoxazole (Increased prothrombin time). Products include:
- Azo Gantanol Tablets 1887
- Bactrim DS Tablets 1891
- Bactrim I.V. Infusion 1889
- Bactrim 1891
- Gantanol 1899
- Septra 813
- Septra I.V. Infusion 808
- Septra I.V. Infusion ADD-Vantage Vials 810
- Septra 813

Sulfasalazine (Increased prothrombin time). Products include:
- Azulfidine Tablets, EN-tabs, Oral Suspension 1157

Sulfinpyrazone (Increased prothrombin time). Products include:
- Anturane 853

Sulfisoxazole (Increased prothrombin time). Products include:
- Azo Gantrisin Tablets 1888
- Gantrisin Tablets 1901
- Pediazole 1973

Sulfisoxazole Diolamine (Increased prothrombin time). Products include:
- Gantrisin Ophthalmic Ointment/Solution 1900

Sulindac (Increased prothrombin time). Products include:
- Clinoril Tablets 1433

Terfenadine (Decreased prothrombin time). Products include:
- Seldane Tablets 1349
- Seldane-D Extended-Release Tablets 1350

Thiamylal Sodium (Decreased prothrombin time). Products include:
- Surital Ampoules, Steri-Vials 1764

Thyroglobulin (Increased prothrombin time). Products include:
- Proloid Tablets 1761

Thyroid (Increased prothrombin time). Products include:
- S-P-T "Liquid" Capsules 995

Tolazamide (Increased prothrombin time). Products include:
- Tolinase Tablets 2365

Tolbutamide (Increased prothrombin time). Products include:
- Orinase Tablets 2354

Tranylcypromine Sulfate (Increased prothrombin time). Products include:
- Parnate Tablets 2222

Triamcinolone (Decreased prothrombin time).
- No products indexed under this heading.

Triamcinolone Acetonide (Decreased prothrombin time). Products include:
- Aristocort A 1010
- Azmacort Inhaler 1837
- Kenalog Cream, Lotion & Ointment 2401
- Kenalog-10 Injection 2402
- Kenalog-40 Injection 2403
- Kenalog in Orabase 604
- Kenalog Spray 2401
- Mycolog II Cream and Ointment 2407
- Mytrex Cream & Ointment 2080
- Nasacort Nasal Inhaler 1844

Triamcinolone Diacetate (Decreased prothrombin time). Products include:
- Aristocort Suspension 1008

Triamcinolone Hexacetonide (Decreased prothrombin time). Products include:
- Aristospan Suspension 1011

Triamterene (Increased or decreased prothrombin times). Products include:
- Dyazide Capsules 2208
- Dyrenium Capsules 2210
- Maxzide 1215

Triclofos Sodium (Increased prothrombin time).

Trimeprazine Tartrate (Decreased prothrombin time). Products include:
- Temaril Tablets, Syrup and Spansule Sustained Release Capsules 1085

Trimethadione (Possible accumulation of anticonvulsants). Products include:
- Tridione 557

Tripelennamine Hydrochloride (Decreased prothrombin time). Products include:
- PBZ Tablets & Elixir 1037
- PBZ-SR Tablets 1037

Triprolidine Hydrochloride (Decreased prothrombin time). Products include:
- Actidil ▣ 538
- Actifed Capsules ▣ 539
- Actifed Plus Caplets ▣ 539
- Actifed Plus Tablets ▣ 540
- Actifed with Codeine Cough Syrup 752
- Actifed Syrup ▣ 540
- Actifed Tablets ▣ 540
- Actifed 12-Hour Capsules ▣ 539

Urokinase (Exercise caution-concomitant use may be hazardous). Products include:
- Abbokinase 503
- Abbokinase Open-Cath 505

Valproic Acid (Possible accumulation of anticonvulsants). Products include:
- Depakene Capsules & Syrup 511

Vitamin C (Decreased prothrombin time). Products include:
- Allbee with C Caplets ▣ 670
- Allbee C-800 ▣ 670
- Bromase Capsules 672
- Bugs Bunny Children's Chewable Vitamins (Sugar Free) ▣ 625
- Bugs Bunny With Extra C Children's Chewable Vitamins (Sugar Free) ▣ 626
- Bugs Bunny Plus Iron Children's Chewable Vitamins (Sugar Free) ▣ 625
- Cefol Filmtab 509
- Centrum, Jr. (Children's Chewable) + Extra C ▣ 585
- Cod Liver Oil Concentrate Tablets with Vitamin C ▣ 694
- Ester-C Tablets ▣ 575
- Ferancee Chewable Tablets 1155
- Ferancee-HP Tablets 1155
- Fero-Folic-500 Filmtab 527
- Fero-Grad-500 Filmtab 528
- Flintstones Children's Chewable Vitamins ▣ 625
- Flintstones Children's Chewable Vitamins With Extra C ▣ 626
- Flintstones Children's Chewable Vitamins Plus Iron ▣ 625
- Halls Vitamin C Drops ▣ 742
- Hyland's Vitamin C for Children ▣ 729
- ICAPS Plus ⊙ 280
- Mediatric Capsules 2476
- Mol-Iron w/Vitamin C Tablets ▣ 703
- Natalins Rx 1391
- Natalins Tablets 1391
- N'ICE Sugarless Vitamin C Drops ▣ 719
- Niferex w/Vitamin C Tablets 847
- Ocuvite Vitamin and Mineral Supplement ⊙ 312
- One-A-Day Essential Vitamins ▣ 627
- One-A-Day Maximum Formula Vitamins and Minerals ▣ 627
- One-A-Day Plus Extra C Vitamins ▣ 627
- Probec-T Tablets ▣ 581
- Stressgard Stress Formula Vitamins ▣ 628
- STUART PRENATAL Tablets ▣ 731
- The Stuart Formula Tablets 1157
- Stuartinic Tablets 1157
- Sunkist Children's Chewable Multivitamins - Plus Extra C ▣ 553
- Sunkist Vitamin C ▣ 553
- Surbex with C ▣ 502
- Trinsicon Capsules 2415
- Tri-Vi-Flor 1.0 mg Vitamins with Fluoride Chewable Tablets 1400
- Tri-Vi-Flor Drops 1400
- Tri-Vi-Sol Vitamin Drops ▣ 614
- Tri-Vi-Sol Vitamin Drops with Iron ▣ 614
- Vicon Forte Capsules 2416
- Vicon Plus ▣ 682
- Vicon-C ▣ 682
- Vi-Daylin ADC Vitamins Drops 1980
- Vi-Daylin ADC Vitamins + Iron Drops 1980
- Vi-Daylin/F ADC Vitamins Drops With Fluoride 1981
- Vi-Daylin/F ADC Vitamins + Iron Drops With Fluoride 1981
- Vi-Zac ▣ 682
- Within Women's Formula Multivitamin with Calcium, Extra Iron and Zinc ▣ 628
- Z-Bec Tablets ▣ 678

Vitamin K (Decreased prothrombin time). Products include:
- One-A-Day Maximum Formula Vitamins and Minerals ▣ 627
- Synkayvite Injection 1919
- Synkayvite Tablets 1920

Vitamin K_1 (Decreased prothrombin time). Products include:
- AquaMEPHYTON Injection 1422
- Konakion Injection 1903
- Mephyton Tablets 1503

Food Interactions

Diet high in vitamin K (Decreased prothrombin time response).

DIDREX TABLETS

(Benzphetamine Hydrochloride) 2338

May interact with monoamine oxidase inhibitors, central nervous system stimulants, tricyclic antidepressants, urinary alkalizing agents, antihypertensives, and insulin. Compounds in these categories include:

Acebutolol Hydrochloride (Decreased hypotensive effect). Products include:
- Sectral Capsules 2520

Acidifying Agents (Urinary) (Decreased amphetamine blood levels).

Amitriptyline Hydrochloride (Enhanced effects of tricyclic antidepressants). Products include:
- Elavil 2269
- Endep Tablets 1927
- Etrafon 2087
- Limbitrol 1933
- Triavil Tablets 1556

Amoxapine (Enhanced effects of tricyclic antidepressants). Products include:
- Asendin Tablets 1196

Amphetamine Resins (Contraindication). Products include:
- Biphetamine Capsules 973

Atenolol (Decreased hypotensive effect). Products include:
- Tenoretic Tablets 1105
- Tenormin Tablets and I.V. Injection 1107

Benazepril Hydrochloride (Decreased hypotensive effect). Products include:
- Lotensin Tablets 872

Bendroflumethiazide (Decreased hypotensive effect). Products include:
- Corzide Tablets 702
- Naturetin Tablets 1789
- Rauzide Tablets 1804

Betaxolol Hydrochloride (Decreased hypotensive effect). Products include:
- Betoptic Sterile Ophthalmic Solution 569
- Betoptic S Sterile Ophthalmic Suspension 570
- Kerlone Tablets 2172

Captopril (Decreased hypotensive effect). Products include:
- Capoten 2255
- Capozide 2258

Carteolol Hydrochloride (Decreased hypotensive effect). Products include:
- Cartrol Tablets 507

Chlorothiazide (Decreased hypotensive effect). Products include:
- Aldoclor Tablets 1413
- Diupres Tablets 1461

Diuril Oral ... 1464

Chlorothiazide Sodium (Decreased hypotensive effect). Products include:
Diuril Sodium Intravenous ... 1463

Chlorthalidone (Decreased hypotensive effect). Products include:
Combipres Tablets ... 678
Tenoretic Tablets ... 1105
Thalitone Tablets ... 687

Clomipramine Hydrochloride (Enhanced effects of tricyclic antidepressants). Products include:
Anafranil Capsules ... 650

Clonidine (Decreased hypotensive effect). Products include:
Catapres-TTS ... 677

Clonidine Hydrochloride (Decreased hypotensive effect). Products include:
Catapres Tablets ... 676
Combipres Tablets ... 678

Deserpidine (Decreased hypotensive effect). Products include:
Enduronyl ... 518
Harmonyl Tablets ... 528
Oreticyl ... 545

Desipramine Hydrochloride (Enhanced effects of tricyclic antidepressants). Products include:
Norpramin Tablets ... 1340

Dextroamphetamine Sulfate (Contraindication). Products include:
Dexedrine ... 2206

Diazoxide (Decreased hypotensive effect). Products include:
Hyperstat I.V. Injection ... 2095
Proglycem ... 649

Doxazosin Mesylate (Decreased hypotensive effect). Products include:
Cardura Tablets ... 1941

Doxepin Hydrochloride (Enhanced effects of tricyclic antidepressants). Products include:
Sinequan ... 1960

Enalapril Maleate (Decreased hypotensive effect). Products include:
Vaseretic Tablets ... 1559
Vasotec Tablets ... 1564

Enalaprilat (Decreased hypotensive effect). Products include:
Vasotec I.V. ... 1562

Esmolol Hydrochloride (Decreased hypotensive effect). Products include:
Brevibloc Injection ... 942

Felodipine (Decreased hypotensive effect). Products include:
Plendil Extended-Release Tablets ... 1526

Fosinopril Sodium (Decreased hypotensive effect). Products include:
Monopril Tablets ... 1406

Furazolidone (Contraindications; hypertensive crises). Products include:
Furoxone ... 1855

Furosemide (Decreased hypotensive effect). Products include:
Lasix ... 1093

Guanabenz Acetate (Decreased hypotensive effect). Products include:
Wytensin Tablets ... 2542

Guanethidine Monosulfate (Decreased hypotensive effect). Products include:
Esimil Tablets ... 864
Ismelin Tablets ... 869

Hydralazine Hydrochloride (Decreased hypotensive effect). Products include:
Apresazide Capsules ... 854
Apresoline Hydrochloride Parenteral (Ampuls) ... 856
Apresoline Hydrochloride Tablets ... 855
Apresoline-Esidrix Tablets ... 857
Ser-Ap-Es Tablets ... 881
Serpasil-Apresoline Tablets ... 884

Hydrochlorothiazide (Decreased hypotensive effect). Products include:
Aldactazide ... 2150
Aldoril Tablets ... 1418
Apresazide Capsules ... 854
Apresoline-Esidrix Tablets ... 857
Capozide ... 2258
Dyazide Capsules ... 2208
Esidrix Tablets ... 863
Esimil Tablets ... 864
HydroDIURIL Tablets ... 1484
Hydropres Tablets ... 1485
Inderide Tablets ... 2463
Inderide LA Long Acting Capsules ... 2465
Lopressor HCT Tablets ... 1034
Maxzide ... 1215
Moduretic Tablets ... 1510
Normozide Tablets ... 2112
Oretic Tablets ... 544
Oreticyl ... 545
Prinzide Tablets ... 1540
Ser-Ap-Es Tablets ... 881
Serpasil-Esidrix Tablets ... 886
Timolide Tablets ... 1547
Trandate HCT Tablets ... 579
Vaseretic Tablets ... 1559
Zestoretic ... 2274

Hydroflumethiazide (Decreased hypotensive effect). Products include:
Diucardin Tablets ... 2450
Saluron ... 718
Salutensin/Salutensin-Demi ... 719

Imipramine Hydrochloride (Enhanced effects of tricyclic antidepressants). Products include:
Tofranil Ampuls ... 1038
Tofranil Tablets ... 1039

Imipramine Pamoate (Enhanced effects of tricyclic antidepressants). Products include:
Tofranil-PM Capsules ... 1041

Indapamide (Decreased hypotensive effect). Products include:
Lozol Tablets ... 1843

Insulin, Human (Insulin requirements may be altered).
No products indexed under this heading.

Insulin, Human Isophane Suspension (Insulin requirements may be altered). Products include:
Humulin N, 100 Units ... 1270

Insulin, Human NPH (Insulin requirements may be altered). Products include:
Insulatard NPH Human ... 1627
Novolin N ... 1627
Novolin N PenFill Cartridges ... 1628
Novolin N Prefilled ... 1628

Insulin, Human Regular (Insulin requirements may be altered). Products include:
Humulin BR, 100 Units ... 1268
Humulin R, 100 Units ... 1272
Novolin R ... 1627
Novolin R PenFill Cartridges ... 1628
Novolin R Prefilled ... 1629
Velosulin Human ... 1628

Insulin, Human, Zinc Suspension (Insulin requirements may be altered). Products include:
Humulin L, 100 Units ... 1268
Humulin U, 100 Units ... 1272
Novolin L ... 1627

Insulin, NPH (Insulin requirements may be altered). Products include:
NPH, 40 & 100 Units ... 1273
Beef NPH, 100 Units ... 1274
Pork NPH, 100 Units ... 1275
Insulatard NPH ... 1626
NPH Insulin ... 1626
NPH Purified Pork Isophane Insulin ... 1626

Insulin, Regular (Insulin requirements may be altered). Products include:
Regular, 40 & 100 Units ... 1273
Beef Regular, 100 Units ... 1275
Pork Regular, 100 Units ... 1275
Pork Regular (Concentrated), 500 Units ... 1276
Regular Insulin ... 1625
Regular Purified Pork Insulin ... 1626
Velosulin ... 1627

Insulin, Zinc Crystals (Insulin requirements may be altered). Products include:
NPH, 40 & 100 Units ... 1273

Insulin, Zinc Suspension (Insulin requirements may be altered). Products include:
Lente, 40 & 100 Units ... 1272
Protamine, Zinc, 40 & 100 Units ... 1273
Lente Iletin I ... 1272
Beef Lente, 100 Units ... 1274
Beef Protamine Zinc, 100 Units ... 1274
Pork Lente, 100 Units ... 1275
Pork, Protamine, Zinc, 100 Units ... 1275
Lente Insulin ... 1626
Lente Purified Pork Insulin ... 1626
Semilente Insulin ... 1625
Ultralente Insulin ... 1626

Isocarboxazid (Contraindications; hypertensive crises). Products include:
Marplan Tablets ... 1906

Isradipine (Decreased hypotensive effect). Products include:
DynaCirc Capsules ... 2004

Labetalol Hydrochloride (Decreased hypotensive effect). Products include:
Normodyne Injection ... 2108
Normodyne Tablets ... 2110
Normozide Tablets ... 2112
Trandate HCT Tablets ... 579
Trandate Injection ... 577
Trandate Tablets ... 579

Lisinopril (Decreased hypotensive effect). Products include:
Prinivil Tablets ... 1538
Prinzide Tablets ... 1540
Zestoretic ... 2274
Zestril Tablets ... 2277

Maprotiline Hydrochloride (Enhanced effects of tricyclic antidepressants). Products include:
Ludiomil Tablets ... 874

Mecamylamine Hydrochloride (Decreased hypotensive effect). Products include:
Inversine Tablets ... 1492

Methamphetamine Hydrochloride (Contraindication). Products include:
Desoxyn Gradumet Tablets ... 514

Methyclothiazide (Decreased hypotensive effect). Products include:
Enduron Tablets ... 517
Enduronyl ... 518

Methyldopa (Decreased hypotensive effect). Products include:
Aldoclor Tablets ... 1413
Aldomet Oral ... 1415
Aldoril Tablets ... 1418

Methyldopate Hydrochloride (Decreased hypotensive effect). Products include:
Aldomet Ester HCl Injection ... 1417

Methylphenidate Hydrochloride (Contraindication). Products include:
Ritalin ... 880

Metolazone (Decreased hypotensive effect). Products include:
Diulo ... 2129
Mykrox ½ mg Tablets ... 984
Zaroxolyn Tablets ... 989

Metoprolol Tartrate (Decreased hypotensive effect). Products include:
Lopressor Ampuls ... 1032
Lopressor HCT Tablets ... 1034
Lopressor Tablets ... 1032

Metyrosine (Decreased hypotensive effect). Products include:
Demser Capsules ... 1460

Minoxidil (Decreased hypotensive effect). Products include:
Loniten Tablets ... 2346
Rogaine Topical Solution ... 2357

Nadolol (Decreased hypotensive effect). Products include:
Corgard Tablets ... 701
Corzide Tablets ... 702

Nicardipine Hydrochloride (Decreased hypotensive effect). Products include:
Cardene Capsules ... 2290

Nitroglycerin (Decreased hypotensive effect). Products include:
Deponit NTG Transdermal Delivery System ... 2143
Minitran Transdermal Delivery System ... 1312
Nitro-Bid Ointment ... 1339
Nitro-Bid Capsules ... 1338
Nitrodisc ... 2176
Nitro-Dur (nitroglycerin) Transdermal Infusion System ... 1164
Nitrogard Tablets ... 1004
Nitrolingual Spray ... 1846
Nitrostat Tablets ... 1743
Transderm-Nitro Transdermal Therapeutic System ... 2283

Nortriptyline Hydrochloride (Enhanced effects of tricyclic antidepressants). Products include:
Pamelor ... 2019

Pemoline (Contraindication). Products include:
Cylert Tablets ... 510

Penbutolol Sulfate (Decreased hypotensive effect). Products include:
Levatol ... 1832

Phenelzine Sulfate (Contraindication; hypertensive crises). Products include:
Nardil ... 1742

Phenoxybenzamine Hydrochloride (Decreased hypotensive effect). Products include:
Dibenzyline Capsules ... 2207

Phentolamine Mesylate (Decreased hypotensive effect). Products include:
Regitine ... 878

Pindolol (Decreased hypotensive effect). Products include:
Visken Tablets ... 2036

Polythiazide (Decreased hypotensive effect). Products include:
Minizide Capsules ... 1779
Renese Tablets ... 1785
Renese-R Tablets ... 1786

Potassium Citrate (Increased amphetamine blood levels). Products include:
Alka-Seltzer Effervescent Antacid ... 1570
K-Lyte ... 707
Polycitra Syrup ... 2424
Polycitra-K ... 2424
Polycitra-LC—Sugar-Free ... 2424
Ricelyte, Rice-Based Oral Electrolyte Maintenance Solution ... ▣ 613

Prazosin Hydrochloride (Decreased hypotensive effect). Products include:
Minipress Capsules ... 1778
Minizide Capsules ... 1779

Propranolol Hydrochloride (Decreased hypotensive effect). Products include:
Inderal ... 2459
Inderal LA Long Acting Capsules ... 2461
Inderide Tablets ... 2463
Inderide LA Long Acting Capsules ... 2465

Protriptyline Hydrochloride (Enhanced effects of tricyclic antidepressants). Products include:
Vivactil Tablets ... 1567

Ramipril (Decreased hypotensive effect). Products include:
Altace Capsules ... 1086

Rauwolfia Serpentina (Decreased hypotensive effect). Products include:

Raudixin Tablets 1803
Rauzide Tablets 1804

Rescinnamine (Decreased hypotensive effect).

No products indexed under this heading.

Reserpine (Decreased hypotensive effect). Products include:

Diupres Tablets 1461
Hydromox R Tablets 1209
Hydropres Tablets 1485
Renese-R Tablets 1786
Salutensin/Salutensin-Demi 719
Ser-Ap-Es Tablets 881
Serpasil Tablets 883
Serpasil-Apresoline Tablets 884
Serpasil-Esidrix Tablets 886

Selegiline Hydrochloride (Contraindications; hypertensive crises). Products include:

Eldepryl 2250

Sodium Citrate (Increased amphetamine blood levels). Products include:

Alka-Seltzer Effervescent Antacid .. 1570
Alka-Seltzer Extra Strength Effervescent Antacid and Pain Reliever 1570
Alka-Seltzer (Flavored) Effervescent Antacid and Pain Reliever 1569
Bicitra—Sugar-Free 2423
Citrocarbonate Antacid .... ⊞ 668
Polycitra 2424
Ricelyte, Rice-Based Oral Electrolyte Maintenance Solution .... ⊞ 613

Sodium Nitroprusside (Decreased hypotensive effect). Products include:

Nipride I.V. Infusion 1909

Terazosin Hydrochloride (Decreased hypotensive effect). Products include:

Hytrin Tablets 529

Timolol Maleate (Decreased hypotensive effect). Products include:

Blocadren Tablets 1429
Timolide Tablets 1547
Timoptic in Ocudose 1552
Timoptic Sterile Ophthalmic Solution 1550

Tranylcypromine Sulfate (Contraindication; hypertensive crises). Products include:

Parnate Tablets 2222

Trimethaphan Camsylate (Decreased hypotensive effect). Products include:

Arfonad Ampuls 1887

Trimipramine Maleate (Enhanced effects of tricyclic antidepressants). Products include:

Surmontil Capsules 2524

DIDRONEL I.V. INFUSION

(Etidronate Disodium (Diphosphonate)) 1307
May interact with:

Nephrotoxic Drugs (Potential for excessive depression of renal function).

DIDRONEL TABLETS

(Etidronate Disodium (Diphosphonate)) 1621
No interactions described in labeling.

DIETHYLSTILBESTROL TABLETS

(Diethylstilbestrol) 1258
No interactions described in labeling.

DIFLUCAN INJECTION AND TABLETS

(Fluconazole) 1948
May interact with oral contraceptives, oral hypoglycemic agents, oral anticoagulants, and certain other agents. Compounds in these categories include:

Chlorpropamide (Increased plasma concentrations and reduced metabolism of sulfonylurea oral hypoglycemics). Products include:

Diabinese Tablets 1775

Cimetidine (Concurrent administration may result in decreased AUC for cimetidine and reduced Cmax of fluconazole). Products include:

Tagamet Tablets 2228

Cimetidine Hydrochloride (Concurrent administration may result in decreased AUC for cimetidine and reduced Cmax of fluconazole). Products include:

Tagamet 2228

Cyclosporine (Increased plasma concentrations of cyclosporin; monitor plasma concentration of cyclosporin). Products include:

Sandimmune 2024

Dicumarol (Increased prothrombin time; monitoring of prothrombin time is recommended). Products include:

Dicumarol Tablets 516

Ethinyl Estradiol (Concurrent administration may result in decreased AUC for ethinyl estradiol). Products include:

Brevicon 2304
Demulen 2161
Estinyl Tablets 2085
Jenest-28 Tablets 1636
Levlen/Tri-Levlen 665
Lo/Ovral Tablets 2471
Lo/Ovral-28 Tablets 2476
Loestrin 1728
Modicon 1667
Nordette-21 Tablets 2481
Nordette-28 Tablets 2483
Norethin 2133
Norinyl 2304
Norlestrin 1746
Ortho-Cyclen Tablets 1658
Ortho-Novum 1667
Ovcon 1391
Ovral Tablets 2490
Ovral-28 Tablets 2491
Levlen/Tri-Levlen 665
Tri-Norinyl 2304
Triphasil-21 Tablets 2527
Triphasil-28 Tablets 2532

Ethynodiol Diacetate (Concurrent administration may result in decreased AUC for ethinyl estradiol). Products include:

Demulen 2161

Glipizide (Increased plasma concentrations and reduced metabolism of sulfonylurea oral hypoglycemics). Products include:

Glucotrol 1952

Glyburide (Increased plasma concentrations and reduced metabolism of sulfonylurea oral hypoglycemics). Products include:

DiaBeta 1091
Micronase Tablets 2350

Hydrochlorothiazide (Concurrent administration may result in increased AUC and Cmax of fluconazole). Products include:

Aldactazide 2150
Aldoril Tablets 1418
Apresazide Capsules 854
Apresoline-Esidrix Tablets 857
Capozide 2258
Dyazide Capsules 2208
Esidrix Tablets 863
Esimil Tablets 864
HydroDIURIL Tablets 1484
Hydropres Tablets 1485
Inderide Tablets 2463
Inderide LA Long Acting Capsules .. 2465
Lopressor HCT Tablets 1034
Maxzide 1215
Moduretic Tablets 1510
Normozide Tablets 2112
Oretic Tablets 544
Oreticyl 545
Prinzide Tablets 1540
Ser-Ap-Es Tablets 881
Serpasil-Esidrix Tablets 886
Timolide Tablets 1547
Trandate HCT Tablets 579
Vaseretic Tablets 1559
Zestoretic 2274

Mestranol (Concurrent administration may result in decreased AUC for ethinyl estradiol). Products include:

Enovid 2161
Norethin 2133
Norinyl 2304
Ortho-Novum 1667

Norethindrone (Concurrent administration may result in decreased AUC for ethinyl estradiol). Products include:

Brevicon 2304
Jenest-28 Tablets 1636
Micronor Tablets 1667
Modicon 1667
Norethin 2133
Norinyl 2304
Norlutin 1755
Nor-Q D Tablets 2304
Ortho-Novum 1667
Ovcon 1391
Tri-Norinyl 2304

Norethynodrel (Concurrent administration may result in decreased AUC for ethinyl estradiol). Products include:

Enovid 2161

Norgestimate (Concurrent administration may result in decreased AUC for ethinyl estradiol). Products include:

Ortho-Cyclen Tablets 1658

Norgestrel (Concurrent administration may result in decreased AUC for ethinyl estradiol). Products include:

Lo/Ovral Tablets 2471
Lo/Ovral-28 Tablets 2476
Ovral Tablets 2490
Ovral-28 Tablets 2491
Ovrette Tablets 2492

Phenytoin (Increased plasma concentrations of phenytoin; monitor phenytoin concentration). Products include:

Dilantin Infatabs 1710
Dilantin-30 Pediatric/Dilantin-125 Suspension 1713

Phenytoin Sodium (Increased plasma concentrations of phenytoin; monitor phenytoin concentration). Products include:

Dilantin Kapseals 1708
Dilantin Parenteral 1712
Dilantin with Phenobarbital Kapseals 1715

Rifampin (Enhances the metabolism of Diflucan). Products include:

Rifadin 1345
Rifamate Capsules 1347
Rimactane Capsules 879

Tolazamide (Increased plasma concentrations and reduced metabolism of sulfonylurea oral hypoglycemics). Products include:

Tolinase Tablets 2365

Tolbutamide (Increased plasma concentrations and reduced metabolism of sulfonylurea oral hypoglycemics). Products include:

Orinase Tablets 2354

Warfarin Sodium (Increased prothrombin time; monitoring of prothrombin time is recommended). Products include:

Coumadin Injection & Tablets 944
Panwarfin Tablets 547

DI-GEL ANTACID/ANTI-GAS

(Calcium Carbonate, Magnesium Hydroxide, Simethicone) .... ⊞ 697
May interact with tetracyclines. Compounds in this category include:

Demeclocycline Hydrochloride (Concurrent use with Di-Gel Liquid is not recommended). Products include:

Declomycin Capsules, Tablets 1199

Doxycycline Calcium (Concurrent use with Di-Gel Liquid is not recommended).

No products indexed under this heading.

Doxycycline Hyclate (Concurrent use with Di-Gel Liquid is not recommended). Products include:

Doryx Capsules 1717
Vibramycin Hyclate Capsules 1787
Vibramycin Hyclate Intravenous 1968
Vibra-Tabs Film Coated Tablets 1787

Doxycycline Monohydrate (Concurrent use with Di-Gel Liquid is not recommended). Products include:

Monodox Capsules 1630
Vibramycin Monohydrate for Oral Suspension 1787

Methacycline Hydrochloride (Concurrent use with Di-Gel Liquid is not recommended).

No products indexed under this heading.

Minocycline Hydrochloride (Concurrent use with Di-Gel Liquid is not recommended). Products include:

Minocin Intravenous 1221
Minocin Oral Suspension 1224
Minocin Pellet-Filled Capsules 1222

Oxytetracycline Hydrochloride (Concurrent use with Di-Gel Liquid is not recommended). Products include:

Terra-Cortril Ophthalmic Suspension 1963
Terramycin Capsules 1786
Terramycin Intramuscular Solution 1964
Terramycin with Polymyxin B Sulfate Ophthalmic Ointment 1965

Tetracycline Hydrochloride (Concurrent use with Di-Gel Liquid is not recommended). Products include:

Achromycin V Capsules 1193
Achromycin Ophthalmic Ointment 1% .... ◉ 307
Achromycin Ophthalmic Suspension 1% .... ◉ 308
Topicycline for Topical Solution 1856

DIGIBIND

(Digoxin Immune Fab (Ovine)) 762
No interactions described in labeling.

DILANTIN INFATABS

(Phenytoin Sodium) 1710
May interact with oral anticoagulants, corticosteroids, tricyclic antidepressants, oral contraceptives, salicylates, phenothiazines, estrogens, sulfonamides, histamine h2-receptor antagonists, succinimides, xanthine bronchodilators, and certain other agents. Compounds in these categories include:

Alcohol (Increased phenytoin serum levels with acute alcohol intake; decreased levels with chronic alcohol intake).

Aminophylline (Efficacy impaired by phenytoin). Products include:

Amesec .... ⊞ 682
Aminophyllin Tablets 2153

Amiodarone Hydrochloride (Increases phenytoin serum levels). Products include:

Cordarone Tablets 2446

Amitriptyline Hydrochloride (Tricyclic antidepressants may precipitate seizures in some patients; phenytoin dosage may need to be adjusted). Products include:

Elavil 2269
Endep Tablets 1927
Etrafon 2087
Limbitrol 1933
Triavil Tablets 1556

Amoxapine (Tricyclic antidepressants may precipitate seizures in some patients; phenytoin dosage may need to be adjusted). Products include:

Asendin Tablets 1196

Aspirin (Increased phenytoin levels). Products include:

Alka-Seltzer Effervescent Antacid and Pain Reliever 1568
Alka-Seltzer Extra Strength Effervescent Antacid and Pain Reliever 1570
Alka-Seltzer (Flavored) Effervescent Antacid and Pain Reliever 1569
Alka-Seltzer Plus Cold Medicine ▣ 623
Alka-Seltzer Plus Night-Time Cold Medicine ▣ 623
Alka Seltzer Plus Sinus Allergy Medicine ▣ 624
Anacin Coated Analgesic Caplets 2417
Anacin Coated Analgesic Tablets 2417
Anacin Maximum Strength Analgesic Coated Tablets 2417
Maximum Strength Arthritis Pain Formula By the Makers of Anacin Analgesic Tablets and Caplets 2418
Arthritis Pain Formula by the Makers of Anacin Analgesic Tablets and Caplets ▣ 747
Arthritis Strength BC Powder ▣ 516
Ascriptin A/D Caplets 1850
Regular Strength Ascriptin Tablets 1850
Azdōne Tablets 844
BC Powder ▣ 517
BC Cold Powder ▣ 517
Children's Bayer Chewable Aspirin ▣ 564
Genuine Bayer Aspirin Tablets & Caplets ▣ 564
Maximum Bayer Aspirin Tablets & Caplets ▣ 566
Bayer Plus Aspirin Tablets ▣ 567
Therapy Bayer Aspirin Caplets ▣ 568
8 Hour Bayer Timed-Release Aspirin ▣ 566
Arthritis Strength Bufferin Analgesic Caplets 744
Extra Strength Bufferin Analgesic Tablets 745
Bufferin Analgesic Tablets and Caplets 743
Cama Arthritis Pain Reliever ▣ 685
Damason-P 1356
Easprin 1719
Ecotrin Enteric Coated Aspirin Maximum Strength Tablets and Caplets 2189
Ecotrin Enteric Coated Aspirin Regular Strength Tablets and Caplets 2189
Empirin Aspirin ▣ 541
Empirin with Codeine Phosphate Nos. 2, 3 & 4 764
Equagesic Tablets 2451
Excedrin Extra-Strength Analgesic Tablets & Caplets 749
4-Way Cold Tablets 750
Fiorinal Capsules 2007
Fiorinal with Codeine Capsules 2008
Fiorinal Tablets 2007
Lortab ASA Tablets 2414
Momentum Muscular Backache Formula ▣ 751
Norgesic 1314
Norwich Extra-Strength Aspirin ▣ 546
Norwich Regular Strength Aspirin ▣ 547
P-A-C Analgesic Tablets ▣ 669
Percodan 951
Robaxisal Tablets 1872
Sine-Off Sinus Medicine Tablets-Aspirin Formula ▣ 722
Soma Compound w/Codeine Tablets 2390
Soma Compound Tablets 2389
St. Joseph Adult Chewable Aspirin (81 mg.) ▣ 703
Synalgos-DC Capsules 2525
Talwin Compound 2072
Ursinus Inlay-Tabs ▣ 691
Vanquish Analgesic Caplets ▣ 574
Zorprin Tablets 698

Bendroflumethiazide (Increased phenytoin levels). Products include:

Corzide Tablets 702
Naturetin Tablets 1789
Rauzide Tablets 1804

Betamethasone Acetate (Efficacy impaired by phenytoin). Products include:

Celestone Soluspan Suspension 2081

Betamethasone Sodium Phosphate (Efficacy impaired by phenytoin). Products include:

Celestone Soluspan Suspension 2081

Calcium Carbonate (Ingestion times of phenytoin and antacids containing calcium should be staggered to prevent absorption problems). Products include:

Alka-Mints Chewable Antacid ▣ 620
Alka-Seltzer Advanced Formula Antacid & Non-Aspirin Pain Reliever ▣ 620
Ascriptin A/D Caplets 1850
Regular Strength Ascriptin Tablets 1850
Balmex Baby Powder ▣ 590
Bayer Plus Aspirin Tablets ▣ 567
Biocal 500 mg Tablet Calcium Supplement ▣ 625
Bufferin Analgesic Tablets and Caplets ▣ 524
Caltrate 600 ▣ 583
Caltrate 600 + Iron ▣ 583
Caltrate 600 + Vitamin D ▣ 584
Caltrate, Jr. ▣ 583
Centrum, Jr. (Children's Chewable) + Extra Calcium ▣ 585
Di-Gel Antacid/Anti-Gas ▣ 697
Gerimed Tablets 972
Marblen ▣ 563
Natalins Rx 1391
Natalins Tablets 1391
Nephro-Calci Tablets 1826
Os-Cal 500 Chewable Tablets ▣ 596
Os-Cal 500 Tablets ▣ 597
Os-Cal 250+D Tablets ▣ 597
Os-Cal 500+D Tablets ▣ 597
Pramet FA 1974
Pramilet FA 1974
Rolaids (Calcium Rich/Sodium Free) ▣ 744
Extra Strength Rolaids ▣ 744
Thermotabs ▣ 619
Total Formula-2 (multivitamin/multimineral) 2377
Tums Liquid Extra ▣ 726
Zenate Tablets 2250

Calcium Carbonate, Precipitated (Ingestion times of phenytoin and antacids containing calcium should be staggered to prevent absorption problems). Products include:

Caltrate 600 Tablets 1197
Caltrate 600 + Iron & Vitamin D 1198
Caltrate 600 + Vitamin D 1197
Caltrate, Jr. Tablets 1198
Tums ▣ 725

Carbamazepine (Decreased phenytoin levels). Products include:

Tegretol Chewable Tablets 654
Tegretol Suspension 656
Tegretol Tablets 654

Chloramphenicol (Increased phenytoin levels). Products include:

AK-Chlor Sterile Ophthalmic Ointment & Solution ⊙ 201
Chloromycetin Cream, 1% 1694
Chloromycetin Hydrocortisone Ophthalmic 1694
Chloromycetin Kapseals 1695
Chloromycetin Ophthalmic Ointment, 1% 1696
Chloromycetin Ophthalmic Solution 1696
Chloromycetin Otic 1697
Chloroptic S.O.P. ⊙ 243
Chloroptic Sterile Ophthalmic Solution ⊙ 243
Ophthochlor Ophthalmic Solution ⊙ 300
Ophthocort ⊙ 301

Chloramphenicol Palmitate (Increased phenytoin levels). Products include:

Chloromycetin Palmitate, Oral Suspension 1697

Chloramphenicol Sodium Succinate (Increased phenytoin levels). Products include:

Chloromycetin Sodium Succinate 1698

Chlordiazepoxide (Increased phenytoin levels). Products include:

Libritabs Tablets 1930
Limbitrol 1933
Menrium Tablets 1934

Chlordiazepoxide Hydrochloride (Increased phenytoin levels). Products include:

Librax Capsules 1929
Librium Capsules 1931
Librium Injectable 1932

Chlorothiazide (Increased phenytoin levels). Products include:

Aldoclor Tablets 1413
Diupres Tablets 1461
Diuril Oral 1464

Chlorothiazide Sodium (Increased phenytoin levels). Products include:

Diuril Sodium Intravenous 1463

Chlorotrianisene (Increased phenytoin levels; efficacy impaired by phenytoin). Products include:

TACE 12 and 25 mg 1353

Chlorpromazine (Increased phenytoin levels). Products include:

Thorazine 2234

Chlorpropamide (Increased phenytoin levels). Products include:

Diabinese Tablets 1775

Choline Magnesium Trisalicylate (Increased phenytoin levels). Products include:

Trilisate 1822

Cimetidine (Increases phenytoin levels). Products include:

Tagamet Tablets 2228

Cimetidine Hydrochloride (Increases phenytoin serum levels). Products include:

Tagamet 2228

Clomipramine Hydrochloride (Tricyclic antidepressants may precipitate seizures in some patients; phenytoin dosage may need to be adjusted). Products include:

Anafranil Capsules 650

Cortisone Acetate (Efficacy impaired by phenytoin). Products include:

Cortone Acetate Sterile Suspension 1437
Cortone Acetate Tablets 1439

Desipramine Hydrochloride (Tricyclic antidepressants may precipitate seizures in some patients; phenytoin dosage may need to be adjusted). Products include:

Norpramin Tablets 1340

Dexamethasone (Efficacy impaired by phenytoin). Products include:

AK-Trol Ointment & Suspension ⊙ 207
Decadron Elixir 1445
Decadron Tablets 1447
Decaspray Topical Aerosol 1459
Dexacidin ⊙ 272
Maxidex Sterile Ophthalmic Suspension ⊙ 223
Maxitrol Ophthalmic Ointment/Suspension ⊙ 223
TobraDex Ophthalmic Suspension and Ointment ⊙ 228

Dexamethasone Acetate (Efficacy impaired by phenytoin). Products include:

Dalalone D.P. Injectable 999
Decadron-LA Sterile Suspension 1457

Dexamethasone Phosphate (Efficacy impaired by phenytoin).

No products indexed under this heading.

Dexamethasone Sodium Phosphate (Efficacy impaired by phenytoin). Products include:

AK-Dex ⊙ 203
Decadron Phosphate Respihaler 1454
Decadron Phosphate Sterile Ophthalmic Ointment 1453
Decadron Phosphate Sterile Ophthalmic Solution 1453
Decadron Phosphate Topical Cream 1455
Decadron Phosphate Turbinaire 1456
Maxidex Sterile Ophthalmic Ointment ⊙ 222
NeoDecadron Sterile Ophthalmic Ointment 1517
NeoDecadron Sterile Ophthalmic Solution 1518
NeoDecadron Topical Cream 1518

Diazepam (Increased phenytoin levels). Products include:

Valium Injectable 1937
Valium Tablets 1939
Valrelease Capsules 1923

Dicumarol (Efficacy impaired by phenytoin; increases phenytoin serum levels). Products include:

Dicumarol Tablets 516

Dienestrol (Increased phenytoin levels; efficacy impaired by phenytoin). Products include:

Ortho Dienestrol Cream 1664

Diethylstilbestrol (Increased phenytoin levels; efficacy impaired by phenytoin). Products include:

Diethylstilbestrol Tablets 1258

Diflunisal (Increased phenytoin levels). Products include:

Dolobid Tablets 1465

Digitoxin (Efficacy impaired by phenytoin). Products include:

Crystodigin Tablets 1253

Dihydroxyaluminum Sodium Carbonate (Interferes with absorption of phenytoin). Products include:

Rolaids ▣ 743

Disulfiram (Increased phenytoin levels). Products include:

Antabuse Tablets 2429

Divalproex Sodium (Increased or decreased phenytoin levels). Products include:

Depakote 512

Doxepin Hydrochloride (Tricyclic antidepressants may precipitate seizures in some patients; phenytoin dosage may need to be adjusted). Products include:

Sinequan 1960

Doxycycline Calcium (Efficacy impaired by phenytoin).

No products indexed under this heading.

Doxycycline Hyclate (Efficacy impaired by phenytoin). Products include:

Doryx Capsules 1717
Vibramycin Hyclate Capsules 1787
Vibramycin Hyclate Intravenous 1968
Vibra-Tabs Film Coated Tablets 1787

Doxycycline Monohydrate (Efficacy impaired by phenytoin). Products include:

Monodox Capsules 1630
Vibramycin Monohydrate for Oral Suspension 1787

Dyphylline (Efficacy impaired by phenytoin). Products include:

Dilor 2079
Dilor-G Tablets & Liquid 2079
Lufyllin Elixir 2384
Lufyllin & Lufyllin-400 Tablets 2384
Lufyllin-GG Elixir & Tablets 2385

Estradiol (Increased phenytoin levels; efficacy impaired by phenytoin). Products include:
- Emcyt Capsules ... 1161
- Estrace ... 1385
- Estrace Vaginal Cream ... 1388
- Estraderm Transdermal System ... 866

Estrogens, Conjugated (Increased phenytoin levels; efficacy impaired by phenytoin). Products include:
- Mediatric Capsules ... 2476
- PMB 200 and PMB 400 ... 2504
- Premarin Intravenous ... 2508
- Premarin with Methyltestosterone ... 2515
- Premarin Tablets ... 2510
- Premarin Vaginal Cream ... 2512

Estrogens, Esterified (Increased phenytoin levels; efficacy impaired by phenytoin). Products include:
- Estratest ... 2245
- Menrium Tablets ... 1934

Estropipate (Increased phenytoin levels; efficacy impaired by phenytoin). Products include:
- Ogen ... 540

Ethinyl Estradiol (Increased phenytoin levels; efficacy impaired by phenytoin). Products include:
- Brevicon ... 2304
- Demulen ... 2161
- Estinyl Tablets ... 2085
- Jenest-28 Tablets ... 1636
- Levlen/Tri-Levlen ... 665
- Lo/Ovral Tablets ... 2471
- Lo/Ovral-28 Tablets ... 2476
- Loestrin ... 1728
- Modicon ... 1667
- Nordette-21 Tablets ... 2481
- Nordette-28 Tablets ... 2483
- Norethin ... 2133
- Norinyl ... 2304
- Norlestrin ... 1746
- Ortho-Cyclen Tablets ... 1658
- Ortho-Novum ... 1667
- Ovcon ... 1391
- Ovral Tablets ... 2490
- Ovral-28 Tablets ... 2491
- Levlen/Tri-Levlen ... 665
- Tri-Norinyl ... 2304
- Triphasil-21 Tablets ... 2527
- Triphasil-28 Tablets ... 2532

Ethosuximide (Increases phenytoin levels). Products include:
- Zarontin Capsules ... 1768
- Zarontin Syrup ... 1769

Ethynodiol Diacetate (Efficacy impaired by phenytoin). Products include:
- Demulen ... 2161

Famotidine (Increases phenytoin serum levels). Products include:
- Pepcid ... 1524

Fluphenazine Enanthate (Increased phenytoin levels). Products include:
- Prolixin Enanthate ... 1796

Fluphenazine Hydrochloride (Increased phenytoin levels). Products include:
- Prolixin Elixir ... 1793
- Prolixin Injection ... 1791
- Prolixin Oral Concentrate ... 1792
- Prolixin Tablets ... 1793

Furosemide (Efficacy impaired by phenytoin). Products include:
- Lasix ... 1093

Glipizide (Increased phenytoin levels). Products include:
- Glucotrol ... 1952

Glyburide (Increased phenytoin levels). Products include:
- DiaBeta ... 1091
- Micronase Tablets ... 2350

Halothane (Increased phenytoin levels). Products include:
- Fluothane ... 2453

Hydrochlorothiazide (Increased phenytoin levels). Products include:
- Aldactazide ... 2150
- Aldoril Tablets ... 1418
- Apresazide Capsules ... 854
- Apresoline-Esidrix Tablets ... 857
- Capozide ... 2258
- Dyazide Capsules ... 2208
- Esidrix Tablets ... 863
- Esimil Tablets ... 864
- HydroDIURIL Tablets ... 1484
- Hydropres Tablets ... 1485
- Inderide Tablets ... 2463
- Inderide LA Long Acting Capsules ... 2465
- Lopressor HCT Tablets ... 1034
- Maxzide ... 1215
- Moduretic Tablets ... 1510
- Normozide Tablets ... 2112
- Oretic Tablets ... 544
- Oreticyl ... 545
- Prinzide Tablets ... 1540
- Ser-Ap-Es Tablets ... 881
- Serpasil-Esidrix Tablets ... 886
- Timolide Tablets ... 1547
- Trandate HCT Tablets ... 579
- Vaseretic Tablets ... 1559
- Zestoretic ... 2274

Hydrocortisone (Efficacy impaired by phenytoin). Products include:
- AK-Spore H.C. ... ⊙ 206
- Bactine Hydrocortisone Anti-Itch Cream ... ▣ 625
- CaldeCORT Anti-Itch Hydrocortisone Spray ... ▣ 560
- Carmol HC Cream 1% ... 2296
- Cortaid Spray ... ▣ 735
- Cortenema ... 2244
- Cortisporin Ointment ... 758
- Cortisporin Ophthalmic Ointment Sterile ... 758
- Cortisporin Ophthalmic Suspension Sterile ... 759
- Cortisporin Otic Solution Sterile ... 760
- Cortisporin Otic Suspension Sterile ... 760
- Cortizone-5 Creme & Ointment ... ▣ 732
- Dermolate Anti-Itch Cream ... ▣ 697
- Eldecort Cream 1.0% ... 1113
- Eldecort Cream 1.0% and 2.5% ... 1113
- Fungoid HC Creme ... 1770
- Hydrocortone Tablets ... 1482
- Hytone ... 909
- LazerSporin-C Solution ... 1770
- Massengill Medicated Soft Cloth Towelettes ... 2192
- Nutracort Cream & Lotion ... 1684
- PediOtic Suspension Sterile ... 797
- Synacort Creams 1%, 2.5% ... 2296
- Vanoxide-HC Acne Lotion ... 911
- Vioform-Hydrocortisone Cream and Mild Cream ... 889
- Vioform-Hydrocortisone Ointment ... 889
- VōSoL HC Otic Solution ... 2392
- Vytone Cream 1% ... 911

Hydrocortisone Acetate (Efficacy impaired by phenytoin). Products include:
- Analpram-HC Rectal Cream 1% and 2.5% ... 970
- Anusol-HC Cream ... 1690
- Anusol-HC Suppositories ... 1691
- Caldecort ... ▣ 560
- Carmol HC Cream 1% ... 2296
- Chloromycetin Hydrocortisone Ophthalmic ... 1694
- Coly-Mycin S Otic w/Neomycin & Hydrocortisone ... 1708
- Cortaid ... ▣ 735
- Cortef Feminine Itch Cream ... ▣ 735
- Corticaine ... ▣ 682
- Cortifoam ... 1827
- Cortisporin Cream ... 757
- Epifoam ... 1828
- Gynecort 5 Creme ... ▣ 556
- Hydrocortone Acetate Sterile Suspension ... 1479
- Lanacort 5 Creme and Ointment ... ▣ 557
- Mantadil Cream ... 789
- Ophthocort ... ⊙ 301
- Orabase HCA Oral Paste ... 890
- Pramosone Cream, Lotion & Ointment ... 971
- ProctoCream-HC ... 1834
- Proctofoam-HC ... 1835

Hydrocortisone Sodium Phosphate (Efficacy impaired by phenytoin). Products include:
- Hydrocortone Phosphate Injection, Sterile ... 1481

Hydrocortisone Sodium Succinate (Efficacy impaired by phenytoin). Products include:
- Solu-Cortef Sterile Powder ... 2361

Hydroflumethiazide (Increased phenytoin levels). Products include:
- Diucardin Tablets ... 2450
- Saluron ... 718
- Salutensin/Salutensin-Demi ... 719

Imipramine Hydrochloride (Tricyclic antidepressants may precipitate seizures in some patients; phenytoin dosage may need to be adjusted). Products include:
- Tofranil Ampuls ... 1038
- Tofranil Tablets ... 1039

Imipramine Pamoate (Tricyclic antidepressants may precipitate seizures in some patients; phenytoin dosage may need to be adjusted). Products include:
- Tofranil-PM Capsules ... 1041

Isoniazid (Increased phenytoin levels). Products include:
- INH Tablets ... 868
- Rifamate Capsules ... 1347

Levonorgestrel (Efficacy impaired by phenytoin). Products include:
- Levlen/Tri-Levlen ... 665
- Nordette-21 Tablets ... 2481
- Nordette-28 Tablets ... 2483
- Norplant System ... 2484
- Levlen/Tri-Levlen ... 665
- Triphasil-21 Tablets ... 2527
- Triphasil-28 Tablets ... 2532

Magnesium Salicylate (Increased phenytoin levels). Products include:
- Doan's - Extra-Strength Analgesic ... ▣ 549
- Doan's - Regular Strength Analgesic ... ▣ 549
- Mobigesic Analgesic Tablets ... ▣ 507

Maprotiline Hydrochloride (Tricyclic antidepressants may precipitate seizures in some patients; phenytoin dosage may need to be adjusted). Products include:
- Ludiomil Tablets ... 874

Mesoridazine (Increased phenytoin levels). Products include:
- Serentil ... 686

Mestranol (Efficacy impaired by phenytoin). Products include:
- Enovid ... 2161
- Norethin ... 2133
- Norinyl ... 2304
- Ortho-Novum ... 1667

Methsuximide (Increases phenytoin serum levels). Products include:
- Celontin ... 1692

Methyclothiazide (Increased phenytoin levels). Products include:
- Enduron Tablets ... 517
- Enduronyl ... 518

Methylphenidate Hydrochloride (Increased phenytoin levels). Products include:
- Ritalin ... 880

Methylprednisolone Acetate (Efficacy impaired by phenytoin). Products include:
- Depo-Medrol Sterile Aqueous Suspension ... 2334

Methylprednisolone Sodium Succinate (Efficacy impaired by phenytoin). Products include:
- Solu-Medrol Sterile Powder ... 2363

Molindone Hydrochloride (Interferes with absorption of phenytoin). Products include:
- Moban Tablets & Concentrate ... 932

Nizatidine (Increases phenytoin serum levels). Products include:
- Axid Pulvules ... 1246

Norethindrone (Efficacy impaired by phenytoin). Products include:
- Brevicon ... 2304
- Jenest-28 Tablets ... 1636
- Micronor Tablets ... 1667
- Modicon ... 1667
- Norethin ... 2133
- Norinyl ... 2304
- Norlutin ... 1755
- Nor-Q D Tablets ... 2304
- Ortho-Novum ... 1667
- Ovcon ... 1391
- Tri-Norinyl ... 2304

Norethynodrel (Efficacy impaired by phenytoin). Products include:
- Enovid ... 2161

Norgestimate (Increased phenytoin levels; efficacy impaired by phenytoin). Products include:
- Ortho-Cyclen Tablets ... 1658

Norgestrel (Efficacy impaired by phenytoin). Products include:
- Lo/Ovral Tablets ... 2471
- Lo/Ovral-28 Tablets ... 2476
- Ovral Tablets ... 2490
- Ovral-28 Tablets ... 2491
- Ovrette Tablets ... 2492

Nortriptyline Hydrochloride (Tricyclic antidepressants may precipitate seizures in some patients; phenytoin dosage may need to be adjusted). Products include:
- Pamelor ... 2019

Perphenazine (Increased phenytoin levels). Products include:
- Etrafon ... 2087
- Triavil Tablets ... 1556
- Trilafon ... 2123

Phenobarbital (Increased or decreased phenytoin levels). Products include:
- Arco-Lase Plus Tablets ... 607
- Bellergal-S Tablets ... 1998
- Bronkolixir ... ▣ 761
- Bronkotabs Tablets ... ▣ 762
- Donnatal ... 1858
- Donnatal Extentabs ... 1859
- Donnatal Tablets ... 1858
- Donnazyme Tablets ... 1860
- Kinesed Tablets ... 2272
- Phenobarbital Elixir and Tablets ... 1293
- Primatene Tablets-P Formula ... 2421
- Quadrinal Tablets ... 1183
- Tedral SA ... 1765

Phensuximide (Increases phenytoin serum levels). Products include:
- Milontin Kapseals ... 1741

Phenylbutazone (Increased phenytoin levels). Products include:
- Butazolidin Capsules & Tablets ... 1027

Polyestradiol Phosphate (Increased phenytoin levels; efficacy impaired by phenytoin). Products include:
- Estradurin ... 2452

Polythiazide (Increased phenytoin levels). Products include:
- Minizide Capsules ... 1779
- Renese Tablets ... 1785
- Renese-R Tablets ... 1786

Prednisolone (Efficacy impaired by phenytoin).
- No products indexed under this heading.

Prednisolone Acetate (Efficacy impaired by phenytoin). Products include:
- AK-Cide Sterile Ophthalmic Ointment & Suspension ... ⊙ 202
- Blephamide Liquifilm Sterile Ophthalmic Suspension ... 586
- Blephamide S.O.P. Sterile Ophthalmic Ointment ... 586
- Cetapred Ointment ... ⊙ 220
- ⅛% Econopred & 1% Econopred Plus ... ⊙ 217
- Isopto Cetapred Suspension ... ⊙ 220
- Metimyd ... ⊙ 306
- Poly-Pred Liquifilm ... ⊙ 250
- Pred Forte ... ⊙ 252
- Pred Mild ... ⊙ 254
- Pred-G Liquifilm Sterile Ophthalmic Suspension ... ⊙ 252
- Pred-G S.O.P. Sterile Ophthalmic Ointment ... ⊙ 253
- Vasocidin Ointment ... ⊙ 275

Prednisolone Sodium Phosphate (Efficacy impaired by phenytoin). Products include:
- AK-Pred ... ⊙ 205
- Hydeltrasol Injection, Sterile ... 1476
- Inflamase ... ⊙ 274
- Pediapred Oral Liquid ... 987
- Vasocidin Ophthalmic Solution ... ⊙ 276

Prednisolone Tebutate (Efficacy impaired by phenytoin). Products include:
Hydeltra-T.B.A. Sterile Suspension 1478

Prednisone (Efficacy impaired by phenytoin). Products include:
Deltasone Tablets 2332

Prochlorperazine (Increased phenytoin levels). Products include:
Compazine 2201

Promethazine Hydrochloride (Increased phenytoin levels). Products include:
Mepergan Injection 2479
Phenergan with Codeine 2497
Phenergan with Dextromethorphan 2499
Phenergan Injection 2493
Phenergan Suppositories 2496
Phenergan Syrup 2495
Phenergan Tablets 2496
Phenergan VC 2500
Phenergan VC with Codeine 2501

Protriptyline Hydrochloride (Tricyclic antidepressants may precipitate seizures in some patients; phenytoin dosage may need to be adjusted). Products include:
Vivactil Tablets 1567

Quinestrol (Increased phenytoin levels; efficacy impaired by phenytoin). Products include:
Estrovis 1721

Quinidine Gluconate (Efficacy impaired by phenytoin). Products include:
Quinaglute Dura-Tabs Tablets 663

Quinidine Polygalacturonate (Efficacy impaired by phenytoin). Products include:
Cardioquin Tablets 1812

Quinidine Sulfate (Efficacy impaired by phenytoin). Products include:
Quinidex Extentabs 1868

Ranitidine Hydrochloride (Increases phenytoin serum levels). Products include:
Zantac Injection and Zantac Injection Premixed 1063
Zantac 1065

Reserpine (Decreased phenytoin levels). Products include:
Diupres Tablets 1461
Hydromox R Tablets 1209
Hydropres Tablets 1485
Renese-R Tablets 1786
Salutensin/Salutensin-Demi 719
Ser-Ap-Es Tablets 881
Serpasil Tablets 883
Serpasil-Apresoline Tablets 884
Serpasil-Esidrix Tablets 886

Rifampin (Efficacy impaired by phenytoin). Products include:
Rifadin 1345
Rifamate Capsules 1347
Rimactane Capsules 879

Salsalate (Increased phenytoin levels). Products include:
Disalcid 1310
Mono-Gesic Tablets 846
Salflex 839

Sodium Valproate (Increased or decreased phenytoin levels).

Sucralfate (Decreases phenytoin serum levels). Products include:
Carafate Tablets 1326

Sulfamethizole (Increased phenytoin levels). Products include:
Thiosulfil Forte Tablets 2526
Urobiotic-250 Capsules 1968

Sulfamethoxazole (Increased phenytoin levels). Products include:
Azo Gantanol Tablets 1887
Bactrim DS Tablets 1891
Bactrim I.V. Infusion 1889
Bactrim 1891
Gantanol 1899
Septra 813
Septra I.V. Infusion 808
Septra I.V. Infusion ADD-Vantage Vials 810
Septra 813

Sulfasalazine (Increased phenytoin levels). Products include:
Azulfidine Tablets, EN-tabs, Oral Suspension 1157

Sulfinpyrazone (Increased phenytoin levels). Products include:
Anturane 853

Sulfisoxazole (Increased phenytoin levels). Products include:
Azo Gantrisin Tablets 1888
Gantrisin Tablets 1901
Pediazole 1973

Sulfisoxazole Diolamine (Increased phenytoin levels). Products include:
Gantrisin Ophthalmic Ointment/Solution 1900

Theophylline (Efficacy impaired by phenytoin). Products include:
Bronkaid Tablets ▣ 757
Bronkolixir ▣ 761
Bronkotabs Tablets ▣ 762
Constant-T Tablets 1029
Marax Tablets & DF Syrup 1954
Primatene Tablets 2421
Quibron Capsules 713
Quibron-T 714
Quibron-T/SR 716
Theolair Liquid 1317
Theo-Organidin Elixir 2391

Theophylline Anhydrous (Efficacy impaired by phenytoin). Products include:
Aerolate 994
Primatene Tablets-M Formula ▣ 753
Primatene Tablets-Regular Formula 2421
Respbid Tablets 684
Slo-bid Gyrocaps 1847
T-PHYL (Uniphyl) 200 mg Tablets 1820
Tedral SA 1765
Theo-24 2179
Theo-Dur Sprinkle 1168
Theo-Dur Extended-Release Tablets 1166
Theolair Tablets 1317
Theolair-SR Tablets 1319
TheoX Extended-Release Tablets 841
Uniphyl 400 mg Tablets 1823

Theophylline Calcium Salicylate (Efficacy impaired by phenytoin). Products include:
Quadrinal Tablets 1183

Theophylline Sodium Glycinate (Efficacy impaired by phenytoin). Products include:
Asbron G 1997

Thioridazine Hydrochloride (Increased phenytoin levels). Products include:
Mellaril 2011

Tolazamide (Increased phenytoin levels). Products include:
Tolinase Tablets 2365

Tolbutamide (Increased phenytoin levels). Products include:
Orinase Tablets 2354

Trazodone Hydrochloride (Increased phenytoin levels). Products include:
Desyrel and Desyrel Dividose 1404

Triamcinolone (Efficacy impaired by phenytoin).
No products indexed under this heading.

Triamcinolone Acetonide (Efficacy impaired by phenytoin). Products include:
Aristocort A 1010
Azmacort Inhaler 1837
Kenalog Cream, Lotion & Ointment 2401
Kenalog-10 Injection 2402
Kenalog-40 Injection 2403
Kenalog in Orabase 604
Kenalog Spray 2401
Mycolog II Cream and Ointment 2407
Mytrex Cream & Ointment 2080
Nasacort Nasal Inhaler 1844

Triamcinolone Diacetate (Efficacy impaired by phenytoin). Products include:
Aristocort Suspension 1008

Triamcinolone Hexacetonide (Efficacy impaired by phenytoin). Products include:
Aristospan Suspension 1011

Trifluoperazine Hydrochloride (Increased phenytoin levels). Products include:
Stelazine 2226

Trimipramine Maleate (Tricyclic antidepressants may precipitate seizures in some patients; phenytoin dosage may need to be adjusted). Products include:
Surmontil Capsules 2524

Valproic Acid (Increased or decreased phenytoin levels). Products include:
Depakene Capsules & Syrup 511

Vitamin D (Efficacy impaired by phenytoin). Products include:
Bugs Bunny Children's Chewable Vitamins (Sugar Free) ▣ 625
Bugs Bunny With Extra C Children's Chewable Vitamins (Sugar Free) ▣ 626
Bugs Bunny Plus Iron Children's Chewable Vitamins (Sugar Free) ▣ 625
Calderol Capsules 1635
Caltrate 600 + Iron & Vitamin D 1198
Caltrate 600 + Vitamin D 1197
Caltrate, Jr. Tablets 1198
Flintstones Children's Chewable Vitamins ▣ 625
Flintstones Children's Chewable Vitamins With Extra C ▣ 626
Flintstones Children's Chewable Vitamins Plus Iron ▣ 625
Natalins Rx 1391
Natalins Tablets 1391
One-A-Day Essential Vitamins ▣ 627
One-A-Day Maximum Formula Vitamins and Minerals ▣ 627
One-A-Day Plus Extra C Vitamins ▣ 627
Os-Cal 250+D Tablets ▣ 597
Os-Cal 500+D Tablets ▣ 597
Os-Cal Fortified Tablets ▣ 597
Os-Cal Plus Tablets ▣ 597
Posture-D 600 mg 2420
Stressgard Stress Formula Vitamins ▣ 628
Tri-Vi-Flor 1.0 mg Vitamins with Fluoride Chewable Tablets 1400
Tri-Vi-Flor Drops 1400
Tri-Vi-Sol Vitamin Drops ▣ 614
Tri-Vi-Sol Vitamin Drops with Iron ▣ 614
Vi-Daylin ADC Vitamins Drops 1980
Vi-Daylin ADC Vitamins + Iron Drops 1980
Vi-Daylin/F ADC Vitamins Drops With Fluoride 1981
Vi-Daylin/F ADC Vitamins + Iron Drops With Fluoride 1981
Within Women's Formula Multivitamin with Calcium, Extra Iron and Zinc ▣ 628
Zymacap Capsules ▣ 670

Warfarin Sodium (Efficacy impaired by phenytoin). Products include:
Coumadin Injection & Tablets 944
Panwarfin Tablets 547

DILANTIN KAPSEALS
(Phenytoin Sodium) 1708
May interact with oral anticoagulants, corticosteroids, oral contraceptives, salicylates, phenothiazines, estrogens, sulfonamides, tricyclic antidepressants, histamine h2-receptor antagonists, succinimides, xanthine bronchodilators, and certain other agents. Compounds in these categories include:

Alcohol (Increased phenytoin serum levels with acute alcohol intake; decreased levels with chronic alcohol intake).

Aminophylline (Efficacy impaired by phenytoin). Products include:
Amesec ▣ 682
Aminophyllin Tablets 2153

Amiodarone Hydrochloride (Increases phenytoin serum levels). Products include:
Cordarone Tablets 2446

Amitriptyline Hydrochloride (Tricyclic antidepressants may precipitate seizures in some patients; phenytoin dosage may need to be adjusted). Products include:
Elavil 2269
Endep Tablets 1927
Etrafon 2087
Limbitrol 1933
Triavil Tablets 1556

Amoxapine (Tricyclic antidepressants may precipitate seizures in some patients; phenytoin dosage may need to be adjusted). Products include:
Asendin Tablets 1196

Aspirin (Increased phenytoin serum levels). Products include:
Alka-Seltzer Effervescent Antacid and Pain Reliever 1568
Alka-Seltzer Extra Strength Effervescent Antacid and Pain Reliever 1570
Alka-Seltzer (Flavored) Effervescent Antacid and Pain Reliever 1569
Alka-Seltzer Plus Cold Medicine ▣ 623
Alka-Seltzer Plus Night-Time Cold Medicine ▣ 623
Alka Seltzer Plus Sinus Allergy Medicine ▣ 624
Anacin Coated Analgesic Caplets 2417
Anacin Coated Analgesic Tablets 2417
Anacin Maximum Strength Analgesic Coated Tablets 2417
Maximum Strength Arthritis Pain Formula By the Makers of Anacin Analgesic Tablets and Caplets 2418
Arthritis Pain Formula by the Makers of Anacin Analgesic Tablets and Caplets ▣ 747
Arthritis Strength BC Powder ▣ 516
Ascriptin A/D Caplets 1850
Regular Strength Ascriptin Tablets 1850
Azdōne Tablets 844
BC Powder ▣ 517
BC Cold Powder ▣ 517
Children's Bayer Chewable Aspirin ▣ 564
Genuine Bayer Aspirin Tablets & Caplets ▣ 564
Maximum Bayer Aspirin Tablets & Caplets ▣ 566
Bayer Plus Aspirin Tablets ▣ 567
Therapy Bayer Aspirin Caplets ▣ 568
8 Hour Bayer Timed-Release Aspirin ▣ 566
Arthritis Strength Bufferin Analgesic Caplets 744
Extra Strength Bufferin Analgesic Tablets 745
Bufferin Analgesic Tablets and Caplets 743
Cama Arthritis Pain Reliever ▣ 685
Damason-P 1356
Easprin 1719
Ecotrin Enteric Coated Aspirin Maximum Strength Tablets and Caplets 2189
Ecotrin Enteric Coated Aspirin Regular Strength Tablets and Caplets 2189
Empirin Aspirin ▣ 541
Empirin with Codeine Phosphate Nos. 2, 3 & 4 764
Equagesic Tablets 2451
Excedrin Extra-Strength Analgesic Tablets & Caplets 749
4-Way Cold Tablets 750
Fiorinal Capsules 2007
Fiorinal with Codeine Capsules 2008
Fiorinal Tablets 2007
Lortab ASA Tablets 2414
Momentum Muscular Backache Formula ▣ 751
Norgesic 1314
Norwich Extra-Strength Aspirin ▣ 546
Norwich Regular Strength Aspirin ▣ 547
P-A-C Analgesic Tablets ▣ 669
Percodan 951
Robaxisal Tablets 1872
Sine-Off Sinus Medicine Tablets-Aspirin Formula ▣ 722

Soma Compound w/Codeine Tablets ... 2390
Soma Compound Tablets ... 2389
St. Joseph Adult Chewable Aspirin (81 mg.) ... ▣ 703
Synalgos-DC Capsules ... 2525
Talwin Compound ... 2072
Ursinus Inlay-Tabs ... ▣ 691
Vanquish Analgesic Caplets ... ▣ 574
Zorprin Tablets ... 698

Bendroflumethiazide (Increased phenytoin serum levels). Products include:
Corzide Tablets ... 702
Naturetin Tablets ... 1789
Rauzide Tablets ... 1804

Betamethasone Acetate (Efficacy impaired by phenytoin). Products include:
Celestone Soluspan Suspension ... 2081

Betamethasone Sodium Phosphate (Efficacy impaired by phenytoin). Products include:
Celestone Soluspan Suspension ... 2081

Calcium Carbonate (Ingestion times of phenytoin and antacids containing calcium should be staggered to prevent absorption problems). Products include:
Alka-Mints Chewable Antacid ... ▣ 620
Alka-Seltzer Advanced Formula Antacid & Non-Aspirin Pain Reliever ... ▣ 620
Ascriptin A/D Caplets ... 1850
Regular Strength Ascriptin Tablets 1850
Balmex Baby Powder ... ▣ 590
Bayer Plus Aspirin Tablets ... ▣ 567
Biocal 500 mg Tablet Calcium Supplement ... ▣ 625
Bufferin Analgesic Tablets and Caplets ... ▣ 524
Caltrate 600 ... ▣ 583
Caltrate 600 + Iron ... ▣ 583
Caltrate 600 + Vitamin D ... ▣ 584
Caltrate, Jr. ... ▣ 583
Centrum, Jr. (Children's Chewable) + Extra Calcium ... ▣ 585
Di-Gel Antacid/Anti-Gas ... ▣ 697
Gerimed Tablets ... 972
Marblen ... ▣ 563
Natalins Rx ... 1391
Natalins Tablets ... 1391
Nephro-Calci Tablets ... 1826
Os-Cal 500 Chewable Tablets ... ▣ 596
Os-Cal 500 Tablets ... ▣ 597
Os-Cal 250+D Tablets ... ▣ 597
Os-Cal 500+D Tablets ... ▣ 597
Pramet FA ... 1974
Pramilet FA ... 1974
Rolaids (Calcium Rich/Sodium Free) ... ▣ 744
Extra Strength Rolaids ... ▣ 744
Thermotabs ... ▣ 619
Total Formula-2 (multivitamin/multimineral) ... 2377
Tums Liquid Extra ... ▣ 726
Zenate Tablets ... 2250

Calcium Carbonate, Precipitated (Ingestion times of phenytoin and antacids containing calcium should be staggered to prevent absorption problems). Products include:
Caltrate 600 Tablets ... 1197
Caltrate 600 + Iron & Vitamin D ... 1198
Caltrate 600 + Vitamin D ... 1197
Caltrate, Jr. Tablets ... 1198
Tums ... ▣ 725

Carbamazepine (Decreased phenytoin levels). Products include:
Tegretol Chewable Tablets ... 654
Tegretol Suspension ... 656
Tegretol Tablets ... 654

Chloramphenicol (Increased phenytoin serum levels). Products include:
AK-Chlor Sterile Ophthalmic Ointment & Solution ... ⊙ 201
Chloromycetin Cream, 1% ... 1694
Chloromycetin Hydrocortisone Ophthalmic ... 1694
Chloromycetin Kapseals ... 1695
Chloromycetin Ophthalmic Ointment, 1% ... 1696
Chloromycetin Ophthalmic Solution ... 1696
Chloromycetin Otic ... 1697
Chloroptic S.O.P. ... ⊙ 243
Chloroptic Sterile Ophthalmic Solution ... ⊙ 243
Ophthochlor Ophthalmic Solution ⊙ 300
Ophthocort ... ⊙ 301

Chloramphenicol Palmitate (Increased phenytoin serum levels). Products include:
Chloromycetin Palmitate, Oral Suspension ... 1697

Chloramphenicol Sodium Succinate (Increased phenytoin serum levels). Products include:
Chloromycetin Sodium Succinate ... 1698

Chlordiazepoxide (Increased phenytoin serum levels). Products include:
Libritabs Tablets ... 1930
Limbitrol ... 1933
Menrium Tablets ... 1934

Chlordiazepoxide Hydrochloride (Increased phenytoin serum levels). Products include:
Librax Capsules ... 1929
Librium Capsules ... 1931
Librium Injectable ... 1932

Chlorothiazide (Increased phenytoin serum levels). Products include:
Aldoclor Tablets ... 1413
Diupres Tablets ... 1461
Diuril Oral ... 1464

Chlorothiazide Sodium (Increased phenytoin serum levels). Products include:
Diuril Sodium Intravenous ... 1463

Chlorotrianisene (Increased phenytoin serum levels; efficacy impaired by phenytoin). Products include:
TACE 12 and 25 mg ... 1353

Chlorpromazine (Increased phenytoin serum levels). Products include:
Thorazine ... 2234

Chlorpropamide (Increased phenytoin serum levels). Products include:
Diabinese Tablets ... 1775

Choline Magnesium Trisalicylate (Increased phenytoin serum levels). Products include:
Trilisate ... 1822

Cimetidine (Increased phenytoin serum levels). Products include:
Tagamet Tablets ... 2228

Cimetidine Hydrochloride (Increases phenytoin serum levels). Products include:
Tagamet ... 2228

Clomipramine Hydrochloride (Tricyclic antidepressants may precipitate seizures in some patients; phenytoin dosage may need to be adjusted). Products include:
Anafranil Capsules ... 650

Cortisone Acetate (Efficacy impaired by phenytoin). Products include:
Cortone Acetate Sterile Suspension ... 1437
Cortone Acetate Tablets ... 1439

Desipramine Hydrochloride (Tricyclic antidepressants may precipitate seizures in some patients; phenytoin dosage may need to be adjusted). Products include:
Norpramin Tablets ... 1340

Dexamethasone (Efficacy impaired by phenytoin). Products include:
AK-Trol Ointment & Suspension ... ⊙ 207
Decadron Elixir ... 1445
Decadron Tablets ... 1447
Decaspray Topical Aerosol ... 1459
Dexacidin ... ⊙ 272
Maxidex Sterile Ophthalmic Suspension ... ⊙ 223
Maxitrol Ophthalmic Ointment/Suspension ... ⊙ 223
TobraDex Ophthalmic Suspension and Ointment ... ⊙ 228

Dexamethasone Acetate (Efficacy impaired by phenytoin). Products include:
Dalalone D.P. Injectable ... 999
Decadron-LA Sterile Suspension ... 1457

Dexamethasone Sodium Phosphate (Efficacy impaired by phenytoin). Products include:
AK-Dex ... ⊙ 203
Decadron Phosphate Respihaler ... 1454
Decadron Phosphate Sterile Ophthalmic Ointment ... 1453
Decadron Phosphate Sterile Ophthalmic Solution ... 1453
Decadron Phosphate Topical Cream ... 1455
Decadron Phosphate Turbinaire ... 1456
Maxidex Sterile Ophthalmic Ointment ... ⊙ 222
NeoDecadron Sterile Ophthalmic Ointment ... 1517
NeoDecadron Sterile Ophthalmic Solution ... 1518
NeoDecadron Topical Cream ... 1518

Diazepam (Increased phenytoin serum levels). Products include:
Valium Injectable ... 1937
Valium Tablets ... 1939
Valrelease Capsules ... 1923

Dicumarol (Efficacy impaired by phenytoin; increases phenytoin serum levels). Products include:
Dicumarol Tablets ... 516

Dienestrol (Increased phenytoin serum levels; efficacy impaired by phenytoin). Products include:
Ortho Dienestrol Cream ... 1664

Diethylstilbestrol (Increased phenytoin serum levels; efficacy impaired by phenytoin). Products include:
Diethylstilbestrol Tablets ... 1258

Diflunisal (Increased phenytoin serum levels). Products include:
Dolobid Tablets ... 1465

Digitoxin (Efficacy impaired by phenytoin). Products include:
Crystodigin Tablets ... 1253

Disulfiram (Increased phenytoin serum levels). Products include:
Antabuse Tablets ... 2429

Divalproex Sodium (Increased or decreased phenytoin serum levels). Products include:
Depakote ... 512

Doxepin Hydrochloride (Tricyclic antidepressants may precipitate seizures in some patients; phenytoin dosage may need to be adjusted). Products include:
Sinequan ... 1960

Doxycycline Calcium (Efficacy impaired by phenytoin).
No products indexed under this heading.

Doxycycline Hyclate (Efficacy impaired by phenytoin). Products include:
Doryx Capsules ... 1717
Vibramycin Hyclate Capsules ... 1787
Vibramycin Hyclate Intravenous ... 1968
Vibra-Tabs Film Coated Tablets ... 1787

Doxycycline Monohydrate (Efficacy impaired by phenytoin). Products include:
Monodox Capsules ... 1630
Vibramycin Monohydrate for Oral Suspension ... 1787

Dyphylline (Efficacy impaired by phenytoin). Products include:
Dilor ... 2079
Dilor-G Tablets & Liquid ... 2079
Lufyllin Elixir ... 2384
Lufyllin & Lufyllin-400 Tablets ... 2384
Lufyllin-GG Elixir & Tablets ... 2385

Estradiol (Increased phenytoin serum levels; efficacy impaired by phenytoin). Products include:
Emcyt Capsules ... 1161
Estrace ... 1385
Estrace Vaginal Cream ... 1388
Estraderm Transdermal System ... 866

Estrogens, Conjugated (Increased phenytoin serum levels; efficacy impaired by phenytoin). Products include:
Mediatric Capsules ... 2476
PMB 200 and PMB 400 ... 2504
Premarin Intravenous ... 2508
Premarin with Methyltestosterone .. 2515
Premarin Tablets ... 2510
Premarin Vaginal Cream ... 2512

Estrogens, Esterified (Increased phenytoin serum levels; efficacy impaired by phenytoin). Products include:
Estratest ... 2245
Menrium Tablets ... 1934

Estropipate (Increased phenytoin serum levels; efficacy impaired by phenytoin). Products include:
Ogen ... 540

Ethinyl Estradiol (Increased phenytoin serum levels; efficacy impaired by phenytoin). Products include:
Brevicon ... 2304
Demulen ... 2161
Estinyl Tablets ... 2085
Jenest-28 Tablets ... 1636
Levlen/Tri-Levlen ... 665
Lo/Ovral Tablets ... 2471
Lo/Ovral-28 Tablets ... 2476
Loestrin ... 1728
Modicon ... 1667
Nordette-21 Tablets ... 2481
Nordette-28 Tablets ... 2483
Norethin ... 2133
Norinyl ... 2304
Norlestrin ... 1746
Ortho-Cyclen Tablets ... 1658
Ortho-Novum ... 1667
Ovcon ... 1391
Ovral Tablets ... 2490
Ovral-28 Tablets ... 2491
Levlen/Tri-Levlen ... 665
Tri-Norinyl ... 2304
Triphasil-21 Tablets ... 2527
Triphasil-28 Tablets ... 2532

Ethosuximide (Increased phenytoin serum levels). Products include:
Zarontin Capsules ... 1768
Zarontin Syrup ... 1769

Ethynodiol Diacetate (Efficacy impaired by phenytoin). Products include:
Demulen ... 2161

Famotidine (Increases phenytoin serum levels). Products include:
Pepcid ... 1524

Fluphenazine Enanthate (Increased phenytoin serum levels). Products include:
Prolixin Enanthate ... 1796

Fluphenazine Hydrochloride (Increased phenytoin serum levels). Products include:
Prolixin Elixir ... 1793
Prolixin Injection ... 1791
Prolixin Oral Concentrate ... 1792
Prolixin Tablets ... 1793

Furosemide (Efficacy impaired by phenytoin). Products include:
Lasix ... 1093

Glipizide (Increased phenytoin serum levels). Products include:
Glucotrol ... 1952

Glyburide (Increased phenytoin serum levels). Products include:
DiaBeta ... 1091
Micronase Tablets ... 2350

Halothane (Increased phenytoin serum levels). Products include:
Fluothane ... 2453

Hydrochlorothiazide (Increased phenytoin serum levels). Products include:
Aldactazide 2150
Aldoril Tablets 1418
Apresazide Capsules 854
Apresoline-Esidrix Tablets 857
Capozide 2258
Dyazide Capsules 2208
Esidrix Tablets 863
Esimil Tablets 864
HydroDIURIL Tablets 1484
Hydropres Tablets 1485
Inderide Tablets 2463
Inderide LA Long Acting Capsules 2465
Lopressor HCT Tablets 1034
Maxzide 1215
Moduretic Tablets 1510
Normozide Tablets 2112
Oretic Tablets 544
Oreticyl 545
Prinzide Tablets 1540
Ser-Ap-Es Tablets 881
Serpasil-Esidrix Tablets 886
Timolide Tablets 1547
Trandate HCT Tablets 579
Vaseretic Tablets 1559
Zestoretic 2274

Hydrocortisone (Efficacy impaired by phenytoin). Products include:
AK-Spore H.C. ⊙ 206
Bactine Hydrocortisone Anti-Itch Cream ▣ 625
CaldeCORT Anti-Itch Hydrocortisone Spray ▣ 560
Carmol HC Cream 1% 2296
Cortaid Spray ▣ 735
Cortenema 2244
Cortisporin Ointment 758
Cortisporin Ophthalmic Ointment Sterile 758
Cortisporin Ophthalmic Suspension Sterile 759
Cortisporin Otic Solution Sterile 760
Cortisporin Otic Suspension Sterile 760
Cortizone-5 Creme & Ointment ▣ 732
Dermolate Anti-Itch Cream ▣ 697
Eldecort Cream 1.0% 1113
Eldecort Cream 1.0% and 2.5% 1113
Fungoid HC Creme 1770
Hydrocortone Tablets 1482
Hytone 909
LazerSporin-C Solution 1770
Massengill Medicated Soft Cloth Towelettes 2192
Nutracort Cream & Lotion 1684
PediOtic Suspension Sterile 797
Synacort Creams 1%, 2.5% 2296
Vanoxide-HC Acne Lotion 911
Vioform-Hydrocortisone Cream and Mild Cream 889
Vioform-Hydrocortisone Ointment 889
VōSoL HC Otic Solution 2392
Vytone Cream 1% 911

Hydrocortisone Acetate (Efficacy impaired by phenytoin). Products include:
Analpram-HC Rectal Cream 1% and 2.5% 970
Anusol-HC Cream 1690
Anusol-HC Suppositories 1691
Caldecort ▣ 560
Carmol HC Cream 1% 2296
Chloromycetin Hydrocortisone Ophthalmic 1694
Coly-Mycin S Otic w/Neomycin & Hydrocortisone 1708
Cortaid ▣ 735
Cortef Feminine Itch Cream ▣ 735
Corticaine ▣ 682
Cortifoam 1827
Cortisporin Cream 757
Epifoam 1828
Gynecort 5 Creme ▣ 556
Hydrocortone Acetate Sterile Suspension 1479
Lanacort 5 Creme and Ointment ▣ 557
Mantadil Cream 789
Ophthocort ⊙ 301
Orabase HCA Oral Paste 890
Pramosone Cream, Lotion & Ointment 971
ProctoCream-HC 1834
Proctofoam-HC 1835

Hydrocortisone Sodium Phosphate (Efficacy impaired by phenytoin). Products include:
Hydrocortone Phosphate Injection, Sterile 1481

Hydrocortisone Sodium Succinate (Efficacy impaired by phenytoin). Products include:
Solu-Cortef Sterile Powder 2361

Hydroflumethiazide (Increased phenytoin serum levels). Products include:
Diucardin Tablets 2450
Saluron 718
Salutensin/Salutensin-Demi 719

Imipramine Hydrochloride (Tricyclic antidepressants may precipitate seizures in some patients; phenytoin dosage may need to be adjusted). Products include:
Tofranil Ampuls 1038
Tofranil Tablets 1039

Imipramine Pamoate (Tricyclic antidepressants may precipitate seizures in some patients; phenytoin dosage may need to be adjusted). Products include:
Tofranil-PM Capsules 1041

Isoniazid (Increased phenytoin serum levels). Products include:
INH Tablets 868
Rifamate Capsules 1347

Levonorgestrel (Efficacy impaired by phenytoin). Products include:
Levlen/Tri-Levlen 665
Nordette-21 Tablets 2481
Nordette-28 Tablets 2483
Norplant System 2484
Levlen/Tri-Levlen 665
Triphasil-21 Tablets 2527
Triphasil-28 Tablets 2532

Magnesium Salicylate (Increased phenytoin serum levels). Products include:
Doan's - Extra-Strength Analgesic ▣ 549
Doan's - Regular Strength Analgesic ▣ 549
Mobigesic Analgesic Tablets ▣ 507

Maprotiline Hydrochloride (Tricyclic antidepressants may precipitate seizures in some patients; phenytoin dosage may need to be adjusted). Products include:
Ludiomil Tablets 874

Mesoridazine (Increased phenytoin serum levels). Products include:
Serentil 686

Mestranol (Efficacy impaired by phenytoin). Products include:
Enovid 2161
Norethin 2133
Norinyl 2304
Ortho-Novum 1667

Methsuximide (Increases phenytoin serum levels). Products include:
Celontin 1692

Methyclothiazide (Increased phenytoin serum levels). Products include:
Enduron Tablets 517
Enduronyl 518

Methylphenidate Hydrochloride (Increased phenytoin serum levels). Products include:
Ritalin 880

Methylprednisolone Acetate (Efficacy impaired by phenytoin). Products include:
Depo-Medrol Sterile Aqueous Suspension 2334

Methylprednisolone Sodium Succinate (Efficacy impaired by phenytoin). Products include:
Solu-Medrol Sterile Powder 2363

Molindone Hydrochloride (Interferes with absorption of phenytoin). Products include:
Moban Tablets & Concentrate 932

Nizatidine (Increases phenytoin serum levels). Products include:
Axid Pulvules 1246

Norethindrone (Efficacy impaired by phenytoin). Products include:
Brevicon 2304
Jenest-28 Tablets 1636
Micronor Tablets 1667
Modicon 1667
Norethin 2133
Norinyl 2304
Norlutin 1755
Nor-Q D Tablets 2304
Ortho-Novum 1667
Ovcon 1391
Tri-Norinyl 2304

Norethynodrel (Efficacy impaired by phenytoin). Products include:
Enovid 2161

Norgestimate (Increased phenytoin serum levels; efficacy impaired by phenytoin). Products include:
Ortho-Cyclen Tablets 1658

Norgestrel (Efficacy impaired by phenytoin). Products include:
Lo/Ovral Tablets 2471
Lo/Ovral-28 Tablets 2476
Ovral Tablets 2490
Ovral-28 Tablets 2491
Ovrette Tablets 2492

Nortriptyline Hydrochloride (Tricyclic antidepressants may precipitate seizures in some patients; phenytoin dosage may need to be adjusted). Products include:
Pamelor 2019

Perphenazine (Increased phenytoin serum levels). Products include:
Etrafon 2087
Triavil Tablets 1556
Trilafon 2123

Phenobarbital (Increased or decreased phenytoin serum levels). Products include:
Arco-Lase Plus Tablets 607
Bellergal-S Tablets 1998
Bronkolixir ▣ 761
Bronkotabs Tablets ▣ 762
Donnatal 1858
Donnatal Extentabs 1859
Donnatal Tablets 1858
Donnazyme Tablets 1860
Kinesed Tablets 2272
Phenobarbital Elixir and Tablets 1293
Primatene Tablets-P Formula 2421
Quadrinal Tablets 1183
Tedral SA 1765

Phensuximide (Increases phenytoin serum levels). Products include:
Milontin Kapseals 1741

Phenylbutazone (Increased phenytoin serum levels). Products include:
Butazolidin Capsules & Tablets 1027

Polyestradiol Phosphate (Increased phenytoin serum levels; efficacy impaired by phenytoin). Products include:
Estradurin 2452

Polythiazide (Increased phenytoin serum levels). Products include:
Minizide Capsules 1779
Renese Tablets 1785
Renese-R Tablets 1786

Prednisolone Acetate (Efficacy impaired by phenytoin). Products include:
AK-Cide Sterile Ophthalmic Ointment & Suspension ⊙ 202
Blephamide Liquifilm Sterile Ophthalmic Suspension 586
Blephamide S.O.P. Sterile Ophthalmic Ointment 586
Cetapred Ointment ⊙ 220
⅛% Econopred & 1% Econopred Plus ⊙ 217
Isopto Cetapred Suspension ⊙ 220
Metimyd ⊙ 306
Poly-Pred Liquifilm ⊙ 250
Pred Forte ⊙ 252
Pred Mild ⊙ 254
Pred-G Liquifilm Sterile Ophthalmic Suspension ⊙ 252
Pred-G S.O.P. Sterile Ophthalmic Ointment ⊙ 253
Vasocidin Ointment ⊙ 275

Prednisolone Sodium Phosphate (Efficacy impaired by phenytoin). Products include:
AK-Pred ⊙ 205
Hydeltrasol Injection, Sterile 1476
Inflamase ⊙ 274
Pediapred Oral Liquid 987
Vasocidin Ophthalmic Solution ⊙ 276

Prednisolone Tebutate (Efficacy impaired by phenytoin). Products include:
Hydeltra-T.B.A. Sterile Suspension 1478

Prednisone (Efficacy impaired by phenytoin). Products include:
Deltasone Tablets 2332

Prochlorperazine (Increased phenytoin serum levels). Products include:
Compazine 2201

Promethazine Hydrochloride (Increased phenytoin serum levels). Products include:
Mepergan Injection 2479
Phenergan with Codeine 2497
Phenergan with Dextromethorphan 2499
Phenergan Injection 2493
Phenergan Suppositories 2496
Phenergan Syrup 2495
Phenergan Tablets 2496
Phenergan VC 2500
Phenergan VC with Codeine 2501

Protriptyline Hydrochloride (Tricyclic antidepressants may precipitate seizures in some patients; phenytoin dosage may need to be adjusted). Products include:
Vivactil Tablets 1567

Quinestrol (Increased phenytoin serum levels; efficacy impaired by phenytoin). Products include:
Estrovis 1721

Quinidine Gluconate (Efficacy impaired by phenytoin). Products include:
Quinaglute Dura-Tabs Tablets 663

Quinidine Polygalacturonate (Efficacy impaired by phenytoin). Products include:
Cardioquin Tablets 1812

Quinidine Sulfate (Efficacy impaired by phenytoin). Products include:
Quinidex Extentabs 1868

Ranitidine Hydrochloride (Increases phenytoin serum levels). Products include:
Zantac Injection and Zantac Injection Premixed 1063
Zantac 1065

Reserpine (Decreased phenytoin levels). Products include:
Diupres Tablets 1461
Hydromox R Tablets 1209
Hydropres Tablets 1485
Renese-R Tablets 1786
Salutensin/Salutensin-Demi 719
Ser-Ap-Es Tablets 881
Serpasil Tablets 883
Serpasil-Apresoline Tablets 884
Serpasil-Esidrix Tablets 886

Rifampin (Efficacy impaired by phenytoin). Products include:
Rifadin 1345
Rifamate Capsules 1347
Rimactane Capsules 879

Salsalate (Increased phenytoin serum levels). Products include:
Disalcid 1310
Mono-Gesic Tablets 846
Salflex 839

Sodium Valproate (Increased or decreased phenytoin levels).

Sucralfate (Decreases phenytoin serum levels). Products include:
Carafate Tablets 1326

Sulfamethizole (Increased phenytoin serum levels). Products include:
- Thiosulfil Forte Tablets 2526
- Urobiotic-250 Capsules 1968

Sulfamethoxazole (Increased phenytoin serum levels). Products include:
- Azo Gantanol Tablets 1887
- Bactrim DS Tablets 1891
- Bactrim I.V. Infusion 1889
- Bactrim 1891
- Gantanol 1899
- Septra 813
- Septra I.V. Infusion 808
- Septra I.V. Infusion ADD-Vantage Vials 810
- Septra 813

Sulfasalazine (Increased phenytoin serum levels). Products include:
- Azulfidine Tablets, EN-tabs, Oral Suspension 1157

Sulfinpyrazone (Increased phenytoin serum levels). Products include:
- Anturane 853

Sulfisoxazole (Increased phenytoin serum levels). Products include:
- Azo Gantrisin Tablets 1888
- Gantrisin Tablets 1901
- Pediazole 1973

Sulfisoxazole Diolamine (Increased phenytoin serum levels). Products include:
- Gantrisin Ophthalmic Ointment/Solution 1900

Theophylline (Efficacy impaired by phenytoin). Products include:
- Bronkaid Tablets ■ 757
- Bronkolixir ■ 761
- Bronkotabs Tablets ■ 762
- Constant-T Tablets 1029
- Marax Tablets & DF Syrup 1954
- Primatene Tablets 2421
- Quibron Capsules 713
- Quibron-T 714
- Quibron-T/SR 716
- Theolair Liquid 1317
- Theo-Organidin Elixir 2391

Theophylline Anhydrous (Efficacy impaired by phenytoin). Products include:
- Aerolate 994
- Primatene Tablets-M Formula ■ 753
- Primatene Tablets-Regular Formula 2421
- Respbid Tablets 684
- Slo-bid Gyrocaps 1847
- T-PHYL (Uniphyl) 200 mg Tablets 1820
- Tedral SA 1765
- Theo-24 2179
- Theo-Dur Sprinkle 1168
- Theo-Dur Extended-Release Tablets 1166
- Theolair Tablets 1317
- Theolair-SR Tablets 1319
- TheoX Extended-Release Tablets 841
- Uniphyl 400 mg Tablets 1823

Theophylline Calcium Salicylate (Efficacy impaired by phenytoin). Products include:
- Quadrinal Tablets 1183

Theophylline Sodium Glycinate (Efficacy impaired by phenytoin). Products include:
- Asbron G 1997

Thioridazine Hydrochloride (Increased phenytoin serum levels). Products include:
- Mellaril 2011

Tolazamide (Increased phenytoin serum levels). Products include:
- Tolinase Tablets 2365

Tolbutamide (Increased phenytoin serum levels). Products include:
- Orinase Tablets 2354

Trazodone Hydrochloride (Increased phenytoin serum levels). Products include:
- Desyrel and Desyrel Dividose 1404

Triamcinolone (Efficacy impaired by phenytoin).
No products indexed under this heading.

Triamcinolone Acetonide (Efficacy impaired by phenytoin). Products include:
- Aristocort A 1010
- Azmacort Inhaler 1837
- Kenalog Cream, Lotion & Ointment 2401
- Kenalog-10 Injection 2402
- Kenalog-40 Injection 2403
- Kenalog in Orabase 604
- Kenalog Spray 2401
- Mycolog II Cream and Ointment 2407
- Mytrex Cream & Ointment 2080
- Nasacort Nasal Inhaler 1844

Triamcinolone Diacetate (Efficacy impaired by phenytoin). Products include:
- Aristocort Suspension 1008

Triamcinolone Hexacetonide (Efficacy impaired by phenytoin). Products include:
- Aristospan Suspension 1011

Trifluoperazine Hydrochloride (Increased phenytoin serum levels). Products include:
- Stelazine 2226

Trimipramine Maleate (Tricyclic antidepressants may precipitate seizures in some patients; phenytoin dosage may need to be adjusted). Products include:
- Surmontil Capsules 2524

Valproic Acid (Increased or decreased phenytoin serum levels). Products include:
- Depakene Capsules & Syrup 511

Vitamin D (Efficacy impaired by phenytoin). Products include:
- Bugs Bunny Children's Chewable Vitamins (Sugar Free) ■ 625
- Bugs Bunny With Extra C Children's Chewable Vitamins (Sugar Free) ■ 626
- Bugs Bunny Plus Iron Children's Chewable Vitamins (Sugar Free) ■ 625
- Calderol Capsules 1635
- Caltrate 600 + Iron & Vitamin D 1198
- Caltrate 600 + Vitamin D 1197
- Caltrate, Jr. Tablets 1198
- Flintstones Children's Chewable Vitamins ■ 625
- Flintstones Children's Chewable Vitamins With Extra C ■ 626
- Flintstones Children's Chewable Vitamins Plus Iron ■ 625
- Natalins Rx 1391
- Natalins Tablets 1391
- One-A-Day Essential Vitamins ■ 627
- One-A-Day Maximum Formula Vitamins and Minerals ■ 627
- One-A-Day Plus Extra C Vitamins ■ 627
- Os-Cal 250+D Tablets ■ 597
- Os-Cal 500+D Tablets ■ 597
- Os-Cal Fortified Tablets ■ 597
- Os-Cal Plus Tablets ■ 597
- Posture-D 600 mg 2420
- Stressgard Stress Formula Vitamins ■ 628
- Tri-Vi-Flor 1.0 mg Vitamins with Fluoride Chewable Tablets 1400
- Tri-Vi-Flor Drops 1400
- Tri-Vi-Sol Vitamin Drops ■ 614
- Tri-Vi-Sol Vitamin Drops with Iron ■ 614
- Vi-Daylin ADC Vitamins Drops 1980
- Vi-Daylin ADC Vitamins + Iron Drops 1980
- Vi-Daylin/F ADC Vitamins Drops With Fluoride 1981
- Vi-Daylin/F ADC Vitamins + Iron Drops With Fluoride 1981
- Within Women's Formula Multivitamin with Calcium, Extra Iron and Zinc ■ 628
- Zymacap Capsules ■ 670

Warfarin Sodium (Efficacy impaired by phenytoin). Products include:
- Coumadin Injection & Tablets 944
- Panwarfin Tablets 547

DILANTIN PARENTERAL

(Phenytoin Sodium) 1712

May interact with antacids containing aluminium, calcium and magnesium, oral anticoagulants, corticosteroids, salicylates, phenothiazines, estrogens, sulfonamides, and certain other agents. Compounds in these categories include:

Alcohol (Increased phenytoin levels).

Aluminum Carbonate Gel (Interferes with absorption of phenytoin). Products include:
- Basaljel 2438

Aluminum Hydroxide (Interferes with absorption of phenytoin). Products include:
- Cama Arthritis Pain Reliever ■ 685
- Gaviscon Extra Strength Relief Formula Liquid Antacid ■ 594
- Gaviscon Extra Strength Relief Formula Antacid Tablets ■ 594
- Gaviscon Liquid Antacid ■ 594
- Gelusil Liquid & Tablets ■ 639
- Extra Strength Maalox Plus Suspension 1850
- Maalox TC Suspension 1851
- Maalox Plus Tablets ■ 655
- Extra Strength Maalox Plus Tablets 1850
- Nephrox Suspension ■ 563
- WinGel Liquid & Tablets ■ 761

Aluminum Hydroxide Gel (Interferes with absorption of phenytoin). Products include:
- ALternaGEL Liquid 1154
- Aludrox Oral Suspension 2428
- Amphojel Suspension 2429
- Amphojel Suspension without Flavor 2429
- Mylanta Liquid 1155
- Mylanta Double Strength Liquid 1155

Aluminum Hydroxide Gel, Dried (Interferes with absorption of phenytoin). Products include:
- Alu-Tab/Alu-Cap 1309
- Amphojel Tablets 2429
- Ascriptin A/D Caplets 1850
- Regular Strength Ascriptin Tablets 1850
- Gaviscon Antacid Tablets ■ 593
- Gaviscon-2 Antacid Tablets ■ 594
- Mylanta Tablets 1155
- Mylanta Double Strength Tablets 1155

Aspirin (Increased phenytoin levels). Products include:
- Alka-Seltzer Effervescent Antacid and Pain Reliever 1568
- Alka-Seltzer Extra Strength Effervescent Antacid and Pain Reliever 1570
- Alka-Seltzer (Flavored) Effervescent Antacid and Pain Reliever 1569
- Alka-Seltzer Plus Cold Medicine ■ 623
- Alka-Seltzer Plus Night-Time Cold Medicine ■ 623
- Alka Seltzer Plus Sinus Allergy Medicine ■ 624
- Anacin Coated Analgesic Caplets 2417
- Anacin Coated Analgesic Tablets 2417
- Anacin Maximum Strength Analgesic Coated Tablets 2417
- Maximum Strength Arthritis Pain Formula By the Makers of Anacin Analgesic Tablets and Caplets 2418
- Arthritis Pain Formula by the Makers of Anacin Analgesic Tablets and Caplets ■ 747
- Arthritis Strength BC Powder ■ 516
- Ascriptin A/D Caplets 1850
- Regular Strength Ascriptin Tablets 1850
- Azdone Tablets 844
- BC Powder ■ 517
- BC Cold Powder ■ 517
- Children's Bayer Chewable Aspirin ■ 564
- Genuine Bayer Aspirin Tablets & Caplets ■ 564
- Maximum Bayer Aspirin Tablets & Caplets ■ 566
- Bayer Plus Aspirin Tablets ■ 567
- Therapy Bayer Aspirin Caplets ■ 568
- 8 Hour Bayer Timed-Release Aspirin ■ 566
- Arthritis Strength Bufferin Analgesic Caplets 744
- Extra Strength Bufferin Analgesic Tablets 745
- Bufferin Analgesic Tablets and Caplets 743
- Cama Arthritis Pain Reliever ■ 685
- Damason-P 1356
- Easprin 1719
- Ecotrin Enteric Coated Aspirin Maximum Strength Tablets and Caplets 2189
- Ecotrin Enteric Coated Aspirin Regular Strength Tablets and Caplets 2189
- Empirin Aspirin ■ 541
- Empirin with Codeine Phosphate Nos. 2, 3 & 4 764
- Equagesic Tablets 2451
- Excedrin Extra-Strength Analgesic Tablets & Caplets 749
- 4-Way Cold Tablets 750
- Fiorinal Capsules 2007
- Fiorinal with Codeine Capsules 2008
- Fiorinal Tablets 2007
- Lortab ASA Tablets 2414
- Momentum Muscular Backache Formula ■ 751
- Norgesic 1314
- Norwich Extra-Strength Aspirin ■ 546
- Norwich Regular Strength Aspirin ■ 547
- P-A-C Analgesic Tablets ■ 669
- Percodan 951
- Robaxisal Tablets 1872
- Sine-Off Sinus Medicine Tablets-Aspirin Formula ■ 722
- Soma Compound w/Codeine Tablets 2390
- Soma Compound Tablets 2389
- St. Joseph Adult Chewable Aspirin (81 mg.) ■ 703
- Synalgos-DC Capsules 2525
- Talwin Compound 2072
- Ursinus Inlay-Tabs ■ 691
- Vanquish Analgesic Caplets ■ 574
- Zorprin Tablets 698

Bendroflumethiazide (Increased phenytoin levels). Products include:
- Corzide Tablets 702
- Naturetin Tablets 1789
- Rauzide Tablets 1804

Betamethasone Acetate (Efficacy impaired by phenytoin). Products include:
- Celestone Soluspan Suspension 2081

Betamethasone Sodium Phosphate (Efficacy impaired by phenytoin). Products include:
- Celestone Soluspan Suspension 2081

Carbamazepine (Decreased phenytoin levels). Products include:
- Tegretol Chewable Tablets 654
- Tegretol Suspension 656
- Tegretol Tablets 654

Chloramphenicol (Increased phenytoin levels). Products include:
- AK-Chlor Sterile Ophthalmic Ointment & Solution ⊛ 201
- Chloromycetin Cream, 1% 1694
- Chloromycetin Hydrocortisone Ophthalmic 1694
- Chloromycetin Kapseals 1695
- Chloromycetin Ophthalmic Ointment, 1% 1696
- Chloromycetin Ophthalmic Solution 1696
- Chloromycetin Otic 1697
- Chloroptic S.O.P. ⊛ 243
- Chloroptic Sterile Ophthalmic Solution ⊛ 243
- Ophthochlor Ophthalmic Solution ⊛ 300
- Ophthocort ⊛ 301

Chloramphenicol Palmitate (Increased phenytoin levels). Products include:
- Chloromycetin Palmitate, Oral Suspension 1697

Chloramphenicol Sodium Succinate (Increased phenytoin levels). Products include:
- Chloromycetin Sodium Succinate 1698

Chlordiazepoxide (Increased phenytoin levels). Products include:
- Libritabs Tablets 1930
- Limbitrol 1933
- Menrium Tablets 1934

Chlordiazepoxide Hydrochloride (Increased phenytoin levels). Products include:
- Librax Capsules 1929
- Librium Capsules 1931
- Librium Injectable 1932

Chlorothiazide (Increased phenytoin levels). Products include:
- Aldoclor Tablets 1413
- Diupres Tablets 1461
- Diuril Oral 1464

Chlorothiazide Sodium (Increased phenytoin levels). Products include:
- Diuril Sodium Intravenous 1463

Chlorotrianisene (Increased phenytoin levels; efficacy impaired by phenytoin). Products include:
- TACE 12 and 25 mg 1353

Chlorpromazine (Increased phenytoin levels). Products include:
- Thorazine 2234

Chlorpropamide (Increased phenytoin levels). Products include:
- Diabinese Tablets 1775

Choline Magnesium Trisalicylate (Increased phenytoin levels). Products include:
- Trilisate 1822

Cimetidine (Increased phenytoin levels). Products include:
- Tagamet Tablets 2228

Cimetidine Hydrochloride (Increased phenytoin levels). Products include:
- Tagamet 2228

Cortisone Acetate (Efficacy impaired by phenytoin). Products include:
- Cortone Acetate Sterile Suspension 1437
- Cortone Acetate Tablets 1439

Dexamethasone (Efficacy impaired by phenytoin). Products include:
- AK-Trol Ointment & Suspension ⊙ 207
- Decadron Elixir 1445
- Decadron Tablets 1447
- Decaspray Topical Aerosol 1459
- Dexacidin ⊙ 272
- Maxidex Sterile Ophthalmic Suspension ⊙ 223
- Maxitrol Ophthalmic Ointment/Suspension ⊙ 223
- TobraDex Ophthalmic Suspension and Ointment ⊙ 228

Dexamethasone Acetate (Efficacy impaired by phenytoin). Products include:
- Dalalone D.P. Injectable 999
- Decadron-LA Sterile Suspension 1457

Dexamethasone Sodium Phosphate (Efficacy impaired by phenytoin). Products include:
- AK-Dex ⊙ 203
- Decadron Phosphate Respihaler 1454
- Decadron Phosphate Sterile Ophthalmic Ointment 1453
- Decadron Phosphate Sterile Ophthalmic Solution 1453
- Decadron Phosphate Topical Cream 1455
- Decadron Phosphate Turbinaire 1456
- Maxidex Sterile Ophthalmic Ointment ⊙ 222
- NeoDecadron Sterile Ophthalmic Ointment 1517
- NeoDecadron Sterile Ophthalmic Solution 1518
- NeoDecadron Topical Cream 1518

Diazepam (Increased phenytoin levels). Products include:
- Valium Injectable 1937
- Valium Tablets 1939
- Valrelease Capsules 1923

Dicumarol (Efficacy impaired by phenytoin). Products include:
- Dicumarol Tablets 516

Dienestrol (Increased phenytoin levels; efficacy impaired by phenytoin). Products include:
- Ortho Dienestrol Cream 1664

Diethylstilbestrol (Increased phenytoin levels; efficacy impaired by phenytoin). Products include:
- Diethylstilbestrol Tablets 1258

Diflunisal (Increased phenytoin levels). Products include:
- Dolobid Tablets 1465

Digitoxin (Efficacy impaired by phenytoin). Products include:
- Crystodigin Tablets 1253

Dihydroxyaluminum Sodium Carbonate (Interferes with absorption of phenytoin). Products include:
- Rolaids ■ 743

Disulfiram (Increased phenytoin levels). Products include:
- Antabuse Tablets 2429

Divalproex Sodium (Increased or decreased phenytoin serum levels). Products include:
- Depakote 512

Doxycycline Calcium (Efficacy impaired by phenytoin).
- No products indexed under this heading.

Doxycycline Hyclate (Efficacy impaired by phenytoin). Products include:
- Doryx Capsules 1717
- Vibramycin Hyclate Capsules 1787
- Vibramycin Hyclate Intravenous 1968
- Vibra-Tabs Film Coated Tablets 1787

Doxycycline Monohydrate (Efficacy impaired by phenytoin). Products include:
- Monodox Capsules 1630
- Vibramycin Monohydrate for Oral Suspension 1787

Estradiol (Increased phenytoin levels; efficacy impaired by phenytoin). Products include:
- Emcyt Capsules 1161
- Estrace 1385
- Estrace Vaginal Cream 1388
- Estraderm Transdermal System 866

Estrogens, Conjugated (Increased phenytoin levels; efficacy impaired by phenytoin). Products include:
- Mediatric Capsules 2476
- PMB 200 and PMB 400 2504
- Premarin Intravenous 2508
- Premarin with Methyltestosterone 2515
- Premarin Tablets 2510
- Premarin Vaginal Cream 2512

Estrogens, Esterified (Increased phenytoin levels; efficacy impaired by phenytoin). Products include:
- Estratest 2245
- Menrium Tablets 1934

Estropipate (Increased phenytoin levels; efficacy impaired by phenytoin). Products include:
- Ogen 540

Ethinyl Estradiol (Increased phenytoin levels; efficacy impaired by phenytoin). Products include:
- Brevicon 2304
- Demulen 2161
- Estinyl Tablets 2085
- Jenest-28 Tablets 1636
- Levlen/Tri-Levlen 665
- Lo/Ovral Tablets 2471
- Lo/Ovral-28 Tablets 2476
- Loestrin 1728
- Modicon 1667
- Nordette-21 Tablets 2481
- Nordette-28 Tablets 2483
- Norethin 2133
- Norinyl 2304
- Norlestrin 1746
- Ortho-Cyclen Tablets 1658
- Ortho-Novum 1667
- Ovcon 1391
- Ovral Tablets 2490
- Ovral-28 Tablets 2491
- Levlen/Tri-Levlen 665
- Tri-Norinyl 2304
- Triphasil-21 Tablets 2527
- Triphasil-28 Tablets 2532

Ethosuximide (Increased phenytoin levels). Products include:
- Zarontin Capsules 1768
- Zarontin Syrup 1769

Ethynodiol Diacetate (Efficacy impaired by phenytoin). Products include:
- Demulen 2161

Fluphenazine Enanthate (Increased phenytoin levels). Products include:
- Prolixin Enanthate 1796

Fluphenazine Hydrochloride (Increased phenytoin levels). Products include:
- Prolixin Elixir 1793
- Prolixin Injection 1791
- Prolixin Oral Concentrate 1792
- Prolixin Tablets 1793

Furosemide (Efficacy impaired by phenytoin). Products include:
- Lasix 1093

Glipizide (Increased phenytoin levels). Products include:
- Glucotrol 1952

Glyburide (Increased phenytoin levels). Products include:
- DiaBeta 1091
- Micronase Tablets 2350

Halothane (Increased phenytoin levels). Products include:
- Fluothane 2453

Hydrochlorothiazide (Increased phenytoin levels). Products include:
- Aldactazide 2150
- Aldoril Tablets 1418
- Apresazide Capsules 854
- Apresoline-Esidrix Tablets 857
- Capozide 2258
- Dyazide Capsules 2208
- Esidrix Tablets 863
- Esimil Tablets 864
- HydroDIURIL Tablets 1484
- Hydropres Tablets 1485
- Inderide Tablets 2463
- Inderide LA Long Acting Capsules 2465
- Lopressor HCT Tablets 1034
- Maxzide 1215
- Moduretic Tablets 1510
- Normozide Tablets 2112
- Oretic Tablets 544
- Oreticyl 545
- Prinzide Tablets 1540
- Ser-Ap-Es Tablets 881
- Serpasil-Esidrix Tablets 886
- Timolide Tablets 1547
- Trandate HCT Tablets 579
- Vaseretic Tablets 1559
- Zestoretic 2274

Hydrocortisone (Efficacy impaired by phenytoin). Products include:
- AK-Spore H.C. ⊙ 206
- Bactine Hydrocortisone Anti-Itch Cream ■ 625
- CaldeCORT Anti-Itch Hydrocortisone Spray ■ 560
- Carmol HC Cream 1% 2296
- Cortaid Spray ■ 735
- Cortenema 2244
- Cortisporin Ointment 758
- Cortisporin Ophthalmic Ointment Sterile 758
- Cortisporin Ophthalmic Suspension Sterile 759
- Cortisporin Otic Solution Sterile 760
- Cortisporin Otic Suspension Sterile 760
- Cortizone-5 Creme & Ointment ■ 732
- Dermolate Anti-Itch Cream ■ 697
- Eldecort Cream 1.0% 1113
- Eldecort Cream 1.0% and 2.5% 1113
- Fungoid HC Creme 1770
- Hydrocortone Tablets 1482
- Hytone 909
- LazerSporin-C Solution 1770
- Massengill Medicated Soft Cloth Towelettes 2192
- Nutracort Cream & Lotion 1684
- PediOtic Suspension Sterile 797
- Synacort Creams 1%, 2.5% 2296
- Vanoxide-HC Acne Lotion 911
- Vioform-Hydrocortisone Cream and Mild Cream 889
- Vioform-Hydrocortisone Ointment 889
- VōSoL HC Otic Solution 2392
- Vytone Cream 1% 911

Hydrocortisone Acetate (Efficacy impaired by phenytoin). Products include:
- Analpram-HC Rectal Cream 1% and 2.5% 970
- Anusol-HC Cream 1690
- Anusol-HC Suppositories 1691
- Caldecort ■ 560
- Carmol HC Cream 1% 2296
- Chloromycetin Hydrocortisone Ophthalmic 1694
- Coly-Mycin S Otic w/Neomycin & Hydrocortisone 1708
- Cortaid ■ 735
- Cortef Feminine Itch Cream ■ 735
- Corticaine ■ 682
- Cortifoam 1827
- Cortisporin Cream 757
- Epifoam 1828
- Gynecort 5 Creme ■ 556
- Hydrocortone Acetate Sterile Suspension 1479
- Lanacort 5 Creme and Ointment ■ 557
- Mantadil Cream 789
- Ophthocort ⊙ 301
- Orabase HCA Oral Paste 890
- Pramosone Cream, Lotion & Ointment 971
- ProctoCream-HC 1834
- Proctofoam-HC 1835

Hydrocortisone Sodium Phosphate (Efficacy impaired by phenytoin). Products include:
- Hydrocortone Phosphate Injection, Sterile 1481

Hydrocortisone Sodium Succinate (Efficacy impaired by phenytoin). Products include:
- Solu-Cortef Sterile Powder 2361

Hydroflumethiazide (Increased phenytoin levels). Products include:
- Diucardin Tablets 2450
- Saluron 718
- Salutensin/Salutensin-Demi 719

Isoniazid (Increased phenytoin levels). Products include:
- INH Tablets 868
- Rifamate Capsules 1347

Levonorgestrel (Efficacy impaired by phenytoin). Products include:
- Levlen/Tri-Levlen 665
- Nordette-21 Tablets 2481
- Nordette-28 Tablets 2483
- Norplant System 2484
- Levlen/Tri-Levlen 665
- Triphasil-21 Tablets 2527
- Triphasil-28 Tablets 2532

Magaldrate (Interferes with absorption of phenytoin). Products include:
- Riopan Antacid Chew Tablets ■ 754
- Riopan Antacid Chew Tablets in Rollpacks ■ 754
- Riopan Antacid Suspension 2421
- Riopan Antacid Swallow Tablets 2421
- Riopan Plus Chew Tablets 2422
- Riopan Plus Chew Tablets in Rollpack 2422
- Riopan Plus 2 Chew Tablets, Mint Flavor, Cherry Flavor 2422
- Riopan Plus Suspension 2422
- Riopan Plus 2 Suspension, Mint Flavor, Cherry Flavor 2422

Magnesium Hydroxide (Interferes with absorption of phenytoin). Products include:
- Aludrox Oral Suspension 2428
- Ascriptin A/D Caplets 1850
- Regular Strength Ascriptin Tablets 1850
- Di-Gel Antacid/Anti-Gas ■ 697
- Gelusil Liquid & Tablets ■ 639
- Haley's M-O, Regular & Flavored ■ 569
- Extra Strength Maalox Plus Suspension 1850
- Maalox TC Suspension 1851
- Maalox Plus Tablets ■ 655
- Extra Strength Maalox Plus Tablets 1850
- Mylanta Liquid 1155
- Mylanta Tablets 1155
- Mylanta Double Strength Liquid 1155
- Mylanta Double Strength Tablets 1155
- Concentrated Phillips' Milk of Magnesia ■ 573
- Phillips' Milk of Magnesia Liquid ■ 572
- Phillips' Milk of Magnesia Tablets ■ 573
- WinGel Liquid & Tablets ■ 761

Magnesium Oxide (Interferes with absorption of phenytoin). Products include:

- Bayer Plus Aspirin Tablets ▣ 567
- Beelith Tablets 659
- Bufferin Analgesic Tablets and Caplets ▣ 524
- Cama Arthritis Pain Reliever ▣ 685
- Mag-Ox 400 673
- Uro-Mag 673

Magnesium Salicylate (Increased phenytoin levels). Products include:

- Doan's - Extra-Strength Analgesic ▣ 549
- Doan's - Regular Strength Analgesic ▣ 549
- Mobigesic Analgesic Tablets ▣ 507

Mesoridazine (Increased phenytoin levels). Products include:

- Serentil 686

Mestranol (Efficacy impaired by phenytoin). Products include:

- Enovid 2161
- Norethin 2133
- Norinyl 2304
- Ortho-Novum 1667

Methyclothiazide (Increased phenytoin levels). Products include:

- Enduron Tablets 517
- Enduronyl 518

Methylphenidate Hydrochloride (Increased phenytoin levels). Products include:

- Ritalin 880

Methylprednisolone Acetate (Efficacy impaired by phenytoin). Products include:

- Depo-Medrol Sterile Aqueous Suspension 2334

Methylprednisolone Sodium Succinate (Efficacy impaired by phenytoin). Products include:

- Solu-Medrol Sterile Powder 2363

Molindone Hydrochloride (Moban brand interferes with absorption of phenytoin). Products include:

- Moban Tablets & Concentrate 932

Norethindrone (Efficacy impaired by phenytoin). Products include:

- Brevicon 2304
- Jenest-28 Tablets 1636
- Micronor Tablets 1667
- Modicon 1667
- Norethin 2133
- Norinyl 2304
- Norlutin 1755
- Nor-Q D Tablets 2304
- Ortho-Novum 1667
- Ovcon 1391
- Tri-Norinyl 2304

Norethynodrel (Efficacy impaired by phenytoin). Products include:

- Enovid 2161

Norgestimate (Increased phenytoin levels; efficacy impaired by phenytoin). Products include:

- Ortho-Cyclen Tablets 1658

Norgestrel (Efficacy impaired by phenytoin). Products include:

- Lo/Ovral Tablets 2471
- Lo/Ovral-28 Tablets 2476
- Ovral Tablets 2490
- Ovral-28 Tablets 2491
- Ovrette Tablets 2492

Perphenazine (Increased phenytoin levels). Products include:

- Etrafon 2087
- Triavil Tablets 1556
- Trilafon 2123

Phenobarbital (Increased or decreased phenytoin serum levels). Products include:

- Arco-Lase Plus Tablets 607
- Bellergal-S Tablets 1998
- Bronkolixir ▣ 761
- Bronkotabs Tablets ▣ 762
- Donnatal 1858
- Donnatal Extentabs 1859
- Donnatal Tablets 1858
- Donnazyme Tablets 1860
- Kinesed Tablets 2272
- Phenobarbital Elixir and Tablets 1293
- Primatene Tablets-P Formula 2421
- Quadrinal Tablets 1183
- Tedral SA 1765

Phenylbutazone (Increased phenytoin levels). Products include:

- Butazolidin Capsules & Tablets 1027

Polyestradiol Phosphate (Increased phenytoin levels; efficacy impaired by phenytoin). Products include:

- Estradurin 2452

Polythiazide (Increased phenytoin levels). Products include:

- Minizide Capsules 1779
- Renese Tablets 1785
- Renese-R Tablets 1786

Prednisolone Acetate (Efficacy impaired by phenytoin). Products include:

- AK-Cide Sterile Ophthalmic Ointment & Suspension ⊙ 202
- Blephamide Liquifilm Sterile Ophthalmic Suspension 586
- Blephamide S.O.P. Sterile Ophthalmic Ointment 586
- Cetapred Ointment ⊙ 220
- ⅛% Econopred & 1% Econopred Plus ⊙ 217
- Isopto Cetapred Suspension ⊙ 220
- Metimyd ⊙ 306
- Poly-Pred Liquifilm ⊙ 250
- Pred Forte ⊙ 252
- Pred Mild ⊙ 254
- Pred-G Liquifilm Sterile Ophthalmic Suspension ⊙ 252
- Pred-G S.O.P. Sterile Ophthalmic Ointment ⊙ 253
- Vasocidin Ointment ⊙ 275

Prednisolone Sodium Phosphate (Efficacy impaired by phenytoin). Products include:

- AK-Pred ⊙ 205
- Hydeltrasol Injection, Sterile 1476
- Inflamase ⊙ 274
- Pediapred Oral Liquid 987
- Vasocidin Ophthalmic Solution ⊙ 276

Prednisolone Tebutate (Efficacy impaired by phenytoin). Products include:

- Hydeltra-T.B.A. Sterile Suspension 1478

Prednisone (Efficacy impaired by phenytoin). Products include:

- Deltasone Tablets 2332

Prochlorperazine (Increased phenytoin levels). Products include:

- Compazine 2201

Promethazine Hydrochloride (Increased phenytoin levels). Products include:

- Mepergan Injection 2479
- Phenergan with Codeine 2497
- Phenergan with Dextromethorphan 2499
- Phenergan Injection 2493
- Phenergan Suppositories 2496
- Phenergan Syrup 2495
- Phenergan Tablets 2496
- Phenergan VC 2500
- Phenergan VC with Codeine 2501

Quinestrol (Increased phenytoin levels; efficacy impaired by phenytoin). Products include:

- Estrovis 1721

Quinidine Gluconate (Efficacy impaired by phenytoin). Products include:

- Quinaglute Dura-Tabs Tablets 663

Quinidine Polygalacturonate (Efficacy impaired by phenytoin). Products include:

- Cardioquin Tablets 1812

Quinidine Sulfate (Efficacy impaired by phenytoin). Products include:

- Quinidex Extentabs 1868

Reserpine (Decreased phenytoin levels). Products include:

- Diupres Tablets 1461
- Hydromox R Tablets 1209
- Hydropres Tablets 1485
- Renese-R Tablets 1786
- Salutensin/Salutensin-Demi 719
- Ser-Ap-Es Tablets 881
- Serpasil Tablets 883
- Serpasil-Apresoline Tablets 884
- Serpasil-Esidrix Tablets 886

Rifampin (Efficacy impaired by phenytoin). Products include:

- Rifadin 1345
- Rifamate Capsules 1347
- Rimactane Capsules 879

Salsalate (Increased phenytoin levels). Products include:

- Disalcid 1310
- Mono-Gesic Tablets 846
- Salflex 839

Sodium Valproate (Increased or decreased phenytoin levels).

Sulfamethizole (Increased phenytoin levels). Products include:

- Thiosulfil Forte Tablets 2526
- Urobiotic-250 Capsules 1968

Sulfamethoxazole (Increased phenytoin levels). Products include:

- Azo Gantanol Tablets 1887
- Bactrim DS Tablets 1891
- Bactrim I.V. Infusion 1889
- Bactrim 1891
- Gantanol 1899
- Septra 813
- Septra I.V. Infusion 808
- Septra I.V. Infusion ADD-Vantage Vials 810
- Septra 813

Sulfasalazine (Increased phenytoin levels). Products include:

- Azulfidine Tablets, EN-tabs, Oral Suspension 1157

Sulfinpyrazone (Increased phenytoin levels). Products include:

- Anturane 853

Sulfisoxazole (Increased phenytoin levels). Products include:

- Azo Gantrisin Tablets 1888
- Gantrisin Tablets 1901
- Pediazole 1973

Sulfisoxazole Diolamine (Increased phenytoin levels). Products include:

- Gantrisin Ophthalmic Ointment/Solution 1900

Thioridazine Hydrochloride (Increased phenytoin levels). Products include:

- Mellaril 2011

Tolazamide (Increased phenytoin levels). Products include:

- Tolinase Tablets 2365

Tolbutamide (Increased phenytoin levels). Products include:

- Orinase Tablets 2354

Trazodone Hydrochloride (Increased phenytoin levels). Products include:

- Desyrel and Desyrel Dividose 1404

Triamcinolone (Efficacy impaired by phenytoin).

- No products indexed under this heading.

Triamcinolone Acetonide (Efficacy impaired by phenytoin). Products include:

- Aristocort A 1010
- Azmacort Inhaler 1837
- Kenalog Cream, Lotion & Ointment 2401
- Kenalog-10 Injection 2402
- Kenalog-40 Injection 2403
- Kenalog in Orabase 604
- Kenalog Spray 2401
- Mycolog II Cream and Ointment 2407
- Mytrex Cream & Ointment 2080
- Nasacort Nasal Inhaler 1844

Triamcinolone Diacetate (Efficacy impaired by phenytoin). Products include:

- Aristocort Suspension 1008

Triamcinolone Hexacetonide (Efficacy impaired by phenytoin). Products include:

- Aristospan Suspension 1011

Trifluoperazine Hydrochloride (Increased phenytoin levels). Products include:

- Stelazine 2226

Valproic Acid (Increased or decreased phenytoin serum levels). Products include:

- Depakene Capsules & Syrup 511

Vitamin D (Efficacy impaired by phenytoin). Products include:

- Bugs Bunny Children's Chewable Vitamins (Sugar Free) ▣ 625
- Bugs Bunny With Extra C Children's Chewable Vitamins (Sugar Free) ▣ 626
- Bugs Bunny Plus Iron Children's Chewable Vitamins (Sugar Free) ▣ 625
- Calderol Capsules 1635
- Caltrate 600 + Iron & Vitamin D 1198
- Caltrate 600 + Vitamin D 1197
- Caltrate, Jr. Tablets 1198
- Flintstones Children's Chewable Vitamins ▣ 625
- Flintstones Children's Chewable Vitamins With Extra C ▣ 626
- Flintstones Children's Chewable Vitamins Plus Iron ▣ 625
- Natalins Rx 1391
- Natalins Tablets 1391
- One-A-Day Essential Vitamins ▣ 627
- One-A-Day Maximum Formula Vitamins and Minerals ▣ 627
- One-A-Day Plus Extra C Vitamins ▣ 627
- Os-Cal 250+D Tablets ▣ 597
- Os-Cal 500+D Tablets ▣ 597
- Os-Cal Fortified Tablets ▣ 597
- Os-Cal Plus Tablets ▣ 597
- Posture-D 600 mg 2420
- Stressgard Stress Formula Vitamins ▣ 628
- Tri-Vi-Flor 1.0 mg Vitamins with Fluoride Chewable Tablets 1400
- Tri-Vi-Flor Drops 1400
- Tri-Vi-Sol Vitamin Drops ▣ 614
- Tri-Vi-Sol Vitamin Drops with Iron ▣ 614
- Vi-Daylin ADC Vitamins Drops 1980
- Vi-Daylin ADC Vitamins + Iron Drops 1980
- Vi-Daylin/F ADC Vitamins Drops With Fluoride 1981
- Vi-Daylin/F ADC Vitamins + Iron Drops With Fluoride 1981
- Within Women's Formula Multivitamin with Calcium, Extra Iron and Zinc ▣ 628
- Zymacap Capsules ▣ 670

Warfarin Sodium (Efficacy impaired by phenytoin). Products include:

- Coumadin Injection & Tablets 944
- Panwarfin Tablets 547

DILANTIN-30 PEDIATRIC/DILANTIN-125 SUSPENSION

(Phenytoin) 1713

May interact with salicylates, phenothiazines, estrogens, sulfonamides, corticosteroids, oral anticoagulants, histamine h2-receptor antagonists, succinimides, tricyclic antidepressants, xanthine bronchodilators, oral contraceptives, and certain other agents. Compounds in these categories include:

Alcohol (Increased phenytoin serum levels with acute alcohol intake; decreased levels with chronic alcohol intake).

Aminophylline (Efficacy impaired by phenytoin). Products include:

- Amesec ▣ 682
- Aminophyllin Tablets 2153

Amiodarone Hydrochloride (Increases phenytoin serum levels). Products include:

- Cordarone Tablets 2446

Amitriptyline Hydrochloride (Tricyclic antidepressants may precipitate seizures in some patients; phenytoin dosage may need to be adjusted). Products include:

- Elavil 2269
- Endep Tablets 1927
- Etrafon 2087
- Limbitrol 1933
- Triavil Tablets 1556

(▣ Described in PDR For Nonprescription Drugs) (⊙ Described in PDR For Ophthalmology)

Amoxapine (Tricyclic antidepressants may precipitate seizures in some patients; phenytoin dosage may need to be adjusted). Products include:
- Asendin Tablets ... 1196

Aspirin (Increased phenytoin serum levels). Products include:
- Alka-Seltzer Effervescent Antacid and Pain Reliever ... 1568
- Alka-Seltzer Extra Strength Effervescent Antacid and Pain Reliever ... 1570
- Alka-Seltzer (Flavored) Effervescent Antacid and Pain Reliever ... 1569
- Alka-Seltzer Plus Cold Medicine ... ▣ 623
- Alka-Seltzer Plus Night-Time Cold Medicine ... ▣ 623
- Alka Seltzer Plus Sinus Allergy Medicine ... ▣ 624
- Anacin Coated Analgesic Caplets ... 2417
- Anacin Coated Analgesic Tablets ... 2417
- Anacin Maximum Strength Analgesic Coated Tablets ... 2417
- Maximum Strength Arthritis Pain Formula By the Makers of Anacin Analgesic Tablets and Caplets ... 2418
- Arthritis Pain Formula by the Makers of Anacin Analgesic Tablets and Caplets ... ▣ 747
- Arthritis Strength BC Powder ... ▣ 516
- Ascriptin A/D Caplets ... 1850
- Regular Strength Ascriptin Tablets 1850
- Azdone Tablets ... 844
- BC Powder ... ▣ 517
- BC Cold Powder ... ▣ 517
- Children's Bayer Chewable Aspirin ... ▣ 564
- Genuine Bayer Aspirin Tablets & Caplets ... ▣ 564
- Maximum Bayer Aspirin Tablets & Caplets ... ▣ 566
- Bayer Plus Aspirin Tablets ... ▣ 567
- Therapy Bayer Aspirin Caplets ... ▣ 568
- 8 Hour Bayer Timed-Release Aspirin ... ▣ 566
- Arthritis Strength Bufferin Analgesic Caplets ... 744
- Extra Strength Bufferin Analgesic Tablets ... 745
- Bufferin Analgesic Tablets and Caplets ... 743
- Cama Arthritis Pain Reliever ... ▣ 685
- Damason-P ... 1356
- Easprin ... 1719
- Ecotrin Enteric Coated Aspirin Maximum Strength Tablets and Caplets ... 2189
- Ecotrin Enteric Coated Aspirin Regular Strength Tablets and Caplets ... 2189
- Empirin Aspirin ... ▣ 541
- Empirin with Codeine Phosphate Nos. 2, 3 & 4 ... 764
- Equagesic Tablets ... 2451
- Excedrin Extra-Strength Analgesic Tablets & Caplets ... 749
- 4-Way Cold Tablets ... 750
- Fiorinal Capsules ... 2007
- Fiorinal with Codeine Capsules ... 2008
- Fiorinal Tablets ... 2007
- Lortab ASA Tablets ... 2414
- Momentum Muscular Backache Formula ... ▣ 751
- Norgesic ... 1314
- Norwich Extra-Strength Aspirin ... ▣ 546
- Norwich Regular Strength Aspirin ▣ 547
- P-A-C Analgesic Tablets ... ▣ 669
- Percodan ... 951
- Robaxisal Tablets ... 1872
- Sine-Off Sinus Medicine Tablets-Aspirin Formula ... ▣ 722
- Soma Compound w/Codeine Tablets ... 2390
- Soma Compound Tablets ... 2389
- St. Joseph Adult Chewable Aspirin (81 mg.) ... ▣ 703
- Synalgos-DC Capsules ... 2525
- Talwin Compound ... 2072
- Ursinus Inlay-Tabs ... ▣ 691
- Vanquish Analgesic Caplets ... ▣ 574
- Zorprin Tablets ... 698

Bendroflumethiazide (Increased phenytoin serum levels). Products include:
- Corzide Tablets ... 702
- Naturetin Tablets ... 1789
- Rauzide Tablets ... 1804

Betamethasone Acetate (Efficacy impaired by phenytoin). Products include:
- Celestone Soluspan Suspension ... 2081

Betamethasone Sodium Phosphate (Efficacy impaired by phenytoin). Products include:
- Celestone Soluspan Suspension ... 2081

Calcium Carbonate (Ingestion times of phenytoin and antacids containing calcium should be staggered to prevent absorption problems). Products include:
- Alka-Mints Chewable Antacid ... ▣ 620
- Alka-Seltzer Advanced Formula Antacid & Non-Aspirin Pain Reliever ... ▣ 620
- Ascriptin A/D Caplets ... 1850
- Regular Strength Ascriptin Tablets 1850
- Balmex Baby Powder ... ▣ 590
- Bayer Plus Aspirin Tablets ... ▣ 567
- Biocal 500 mg Tablet Calcium Supplement ... ▣ 625
- Bufferin Analgesic Tablets and Caplets ... ▣ 524
- Caltrate 600 ... ▣ 583
- Caltrate 600 + Iron ... ▣ 583
- Caltrate 600 + Vitamin D ... ▣ 584
- Caltrate, Jr. ... ▣ 583
- Centrum, Jr. (Children's Chewable) + Extra Calcium ... ▣ 585
- Di-Gel Antacid/Anti-Gas ... ▣ 697
- Gerimed Tablets ... 972
- Marblen ... ▣ 563
- Natalins Rx ... 1391
- Natalins Tablets ... 1391
- Nephro-Calci Tablets ... 1826
- Os-Cal 500 Chewable Tablets ... ▣ 596
- Os-Cal 500 Tablets ... ▣ 597
- Os-Cal 250+D Tablets ... ▣ 597
- Os-Cal 500+D Tablets ... ▣ 597
- Pramet FA ... 1974
- Pramilet FA ... 1974
- Rolaids (Calcium Rich/Sodium Free) ... ▣ 744
- Extra Strength Rolaids ... ▣ 744
- Thermotabs ... ▣ 619
- Total Formula-2 (multivitamin/multimineral) ... 2377
- Tums Liquid Extra ... ▣ 726
- Zenate Tablets ... 2250

Calcium Carbonate, Precipitated (Ingestion times of phenytoin and antacids containing calcium should be staggered to prevent absorption problems). Products include:
- Caltrate 600 Tablets ... 1197
- Caltrate 600 + Iron & Vitamin D ... 1198
- Caltrate 600 + Vitamin D ... 1197
- Caltrate, Jr. Tablets ... 1198
- Tums ... ▣ 725

Carbamazepine (Decreased phenytoin serum levels). Products include:
- Tegretol Chewable Tablets ... 654
- Tegretol Suspension ... 656
- Tegretol Tablets ... 654

Chloramphenicol (Increased phenytoin serum levels). Products include:
- AK-Chlor Sterile Ophthalmic Ointment & Solution ... ⊙ 201
- Chloromycetin Cream, 1% ... 1694
- Chloromycetin Hydrocortisone Ophthalmic ... 1694
- Chloromycetin Kapseals ... 1695
- Chloromycetin Ophthalmic Ointment, 1% ... 1696
- Chloromycetin Ophthalmic Solution ... 1696
- Chloromycetin Otic ... 1697
- Chloroptic S.O.P. ... ⊙ 243
- Chloroptic Sterile Ophthalmic Solution ... ⊙ 243
- Ophthochlor Ophthalmic Solution ⊙ 300
- Ophthocort ... ⊙ 301

Chloramphenicol Palmitate (Increased phenytoin serum levels). Products include:
- Chloromycetin Palmitate, Oral Suspension ... 1697

Chloramphenicol Sodium Succinate (Increased phenytoin serum levels). Products include:
- Chloromycetin Sodium Succinate ... 1698

Chlordiazepoxide (Increased phenytoin serum levels). Products include:
- Libritabs Tablets ... 1930
- Limbitrol ... 1933
- Menrium Tablets ... 1934

Chlordiazepoxide Hydrochloride (Increased phenytoin serum levels). Products include:
- Librax Capsules ... 1929
- Librium Capsules ... 1931
- Librium Injectable ... 1932

Chlorothiazide (Increased phenytoin serum levels). Products include:
- Aldoclor Tablets ... 1413
- Diupres Tablets ... 1461
- Diuril Oral ... 1464

Chlorothiazide Sodium (Increased phenytoin serum levels). Products include:
- Diuril Sodium Intravenous ... 1463

Chlorotrianisene (Increased phenytoin serum levels; efficacy impaired by phenytoin). Products include:
- TACE 12 and 25 mg ... 1353

Chlorpromazine (Increased phenytoin serum levels). Products include:
- Thorazine ... 2234

Chlorpropamide (Increased phenytoin serum levels). Products include:
- Diabinese Tablets ... 1775

Choline Magnesium Trisalicylate (Increased phenytoin serum levels). Products include:
- Trilisate ... 1822

Cimetidine (Increased phenytoin serum levels). Products include:
- Tagamet Tablets ... 2228

Cimetidine Hydrochloride (Increases phenytoin serum levels). Products include:
- Tagamet ... 2228

Clomipramine Hydrochloride (Tricyclic antidepressants may precipitate seizures in some patients; phenytoin dosage may need to be adjusted). Products include:
- Anafranil Capsules ... 650

Cortisone Acetate (Efficacy impaired by phenytoin). Products include:
- Cortone Acetate Sterile Suspension ... 1437
- Cortone Acetate Tablets ... 1439

Desipramine Hydrochloride (Tricyclic antidepressants may precipitate seizures in some patients; phenytoin dosage may need to be adjusted). Products include:
- Norpramin Tablets ... 1340

Dexamethasone (Efficacy impaired by phenytoin). Products include:
- AK-Trol Ointment & Suspension ... ⊙ 207
- Decadron Elixir ... 1445
- Decadron Tablets ... 1447
- Decaspray Topical Aerosol ... 1459
- Dexacidin ... ⊙ 272
- Maxidex Sterile Ophthalmic Suspension ... ⊙ 223
- Maxitrol Ophthalmic Ointment/Suspension ... ⊙ 223
- TobraDex Ophthalmic Suspension and Ointment ... ⊙ 228

Dexamethasone Acetate (Efficacy impaired by phenytoin). Products include:
- Dalalone D.P. Injectable ... 999
- Decadron-LA Sterile Suspension ... 1457

Dexamethasone Sodium Phosphate (Efficacy impaired by phenytoin). Products include:
- AK-Dex ... ⊙ 203
- Decadron Phosphate Respihaler ... 1454
- Decadron Phosphate Sterile Ophthalmic Ointment ... 1453
- Decadron Phosphate Sterile Ophthalmic Solution ... 1453
- Decadron Phosphate Topical Cream ... 1455
- Decadron Phosphate Turbinaire ... 1456
- Maxidex Sterile Ophthalmic Ointment ... ⊙ 222
- NeoDecadron Sterile Ophthalmic Ointment ... 1517
- NeoDecadron Sterile Ophthalmic Solution ... 1518
- NeoDecadron Topical Cream ... 1518

Diazepam (Increased phenytoin serum levels). Products include:
- Valium Injectable ... 1937
- Valium Tablets ... 1939
- Valrelease Capsules ... 1923

Dicumarol (Efficacy impaired by phenytoin; increases phenytoin serum levels). Products include:
- Dicumarol Tablets ... 516

Dienestrol (Increased phenytoin serum levels; efficacy impaired by phenytoin). Products include:
- Ortho Dienestrol Cream ... 1664

Diethylstilbestrol (Increased phenytoin serum levels; efficacy impaired by phenytoin). Products include:
- Diethylstilbestrol Tablets ... 1258

Diflunisal (Increased phenytoin serum levels). Products include:
- Dolobid Tablets ... 1465

Digitoxin (Efficacy impaired by phenytoin). Products include:
- Crystodigin Tablets ... 1253

Dihydroxyaluminum Sodium Carbonate (Interferes with absorption of phenytoin). Products include:
- Rolaids ... ▣ 743

Disulfiram (Increased phenytoin serum levels). Products include:
- Antabuse Tablets ... 2429

Divalproex Sodium (Increased or decreased phenytoin levels). Products include:
- Depakote ... 512

Doxepin Hydrochloride (Tricyclic antidepressants may precipitate seizures in some patients; phenytoin dosage may need to be adjusted). Products include:
- Sinequan ... 1960

Doxycycline Calcium (Efficacy impaired by phenytoin).
- No products indexed under this heading.

Doxycycline Hyclate (Efficacy impaired by phenytoin). Products include:
- Doryx Capsules ... 1717
- Vibramycin Hyclate Capsules ... 1787
- Vibramycin Hyclate Intravenous ... 1968
- Vibra-Tabs Film Coated Tablets ... 1787

Doxycycline Monohydrate (Efficacy impaired by phenytoin). Products include:
- Monodox Capsules ... 1630
- Vibramycin Monohydrate for Oral Suspension ... 1787

Dyphylline (Efficacy impaired by phenytoin). Products include:
- Dilor ... 2079
- Dilor-G Tablets & Liquid ... 2079
- Lufyllin Elixir ... 2384
- Lufyllin & Lufyllin-400 Tablets ... 2384
- Lufyllin-GG Elixir & Tablets ... 2385

Estradiol (Increased phenytoin serum levels; efficacy impaired by phenytoin). Products include:
- Emcyt Capsules ... 1161
- Estrace ... 1385
- Estrace Vaginal Cream ... 1388

Estraderm Transdermal System 866

Estrogens, Conjugated (Increased phenytoin serum levels; efficacy impaired by phenytoin). Products include:
- Mediatric Capsules 2476
- PMB 200 and PMB 400 2504
- Premarin Intravenous 2508
- Premarin with Methyltestosterone .. 2515
- Premarin Tablets 2510
- Premarin Vaginal Cream 2512

Estrogens, Esterified (Increased phenytoin serum levels; efficacy impaired by phenytoin). Products include:
- Estratest 2245
- Menrium Tablets 1934

Estropipate (Increased phenytoin serum levels; efficacy impaired by phenytoin). Products include:
- Ogen 540

Ethinyl Estradiol (Increased phenytoin serum levels; efficacy impaired by phenytoin). Products include:
- Brevicon 2304
- Demulen 2161
- Estinyl Tablets 2085
- Jenest-28 Tablets 1636
- Levlen/Tri-Levlen 665
- Lo/Ovral Tablets 2471
- Lo/Ovral-28 Tablets 2476
- Loestrin 1728
- Modicon 1667
- Nordette-21 Tablets 2481
- Nordette-28 Tablets 2483
- Norethin 2133
- Norinyl 2304
- Norlestrin 1746
- Ortho-Cyclen Tablets 1658
- Ortho-Novum 1667
- Ovcon 1391
- Ovral Tablets 2490
- Ovral-28 Tablets 2491
- Levlen/Tri-Levlen 665
- Tri-Norinyl 2304
- Triphasil-21 Tablets 2527
- Triphasil-28 Tablets 2532

Ethosuximide (Increased phenytoin serum levels). Products include:
- Zarontin Capsules 1768
- Zarontin Syrup 1769

Ethynodiol Diacetate (Efficacy impaired by phenytoin). Products include:
- Demulen 2161

Famotidine (Increases phenytoin serum levels). Products include:
- Pepcid 1524

Fluphenazine Enanthate (Increased phenytoin serum levels). Products include:
- Prolixin Enanthate 1796

Fluphenazine Hydrochloride (Increased phenytoin serum levels). Products include:
- Prolixin Elixir 1793
- Prolixin Injection 1791
- Prolixin Oral Concentrate 1792
- Prolixin Tablets 1793

Furosemide (Efficacy impaired by phenytoin). Products include:
- Lasix 1093

Glipizide (Increased phenytoin serum levels). Products include:
- Glucotrol 1952

Glyburide (Increased phenytoin serum levels). Products include:
- DiaBeta 1091
- Micronase Tablets 2350

Halothane (Increased phenytoin serum levels). Products include:
- Fluothane 2453

Hydrochlorothiazide (Increased phenytoin serum levels). Products include:
- Aldactazide 2150
- Aldoril Tablets 1418
- Apresazide Capsules 854
- Apresoline-Esidrix Tablets 857
- Capozide 2258
- Dyazide Capsules 2208
- Esidrix Tablets 863
- Esimil Tablets 864
- HydroDIURIL Tablets 1484
- Hydropres Tablets 1485
- Inderide Tablets 2463
- Inderide LA Long Acting Capsules .. 2465
- Lopressor HCT Tablets 1034
- Maxzide 1215
- Moduretic Tablets 1510
- Normozide Tablets 2112
- Oretic Tablets 544
- Oreticyl 545
- Prinzide Tablets 1540
- Ser-Ap-Es Tablets 881
- Serpasil-Esidrix Tablets 886
- Timolide Tablets 1547
- Trandate HCT Tablets 579
- Vaseretic Tablets 1559
- Zestoretic 2274

Hydrocortisone (Efficacy impaired by phenytoin). Products include:
- AK-Spore H.C. ...... ⊙ 206
- Bactine Hydrocortisone Anti-Itch Cream ...... ▣ 625
- CaldeCORT Anti-Itch Hydrocortisone Spray ...... ▣ 560
- Carmol HC Cream 1% 2296
- Cortaid Spray ...... ▣ 735
- Cortenema 2244
- Cortisporin Ointment 758
- Cortisporin Ophthalmic Ointment Sterile 758
- Cortisporin Ophthalmic Suspension Sterile 759
- Cortisporin Otic Solution Sterile 760
- Cortisporin Otic Suspension Sterile 760
- Cortizone-5 Creme & Ointment ...... ▣ 732
- Dermolate Anti-Itch Cream ...... ▣ 697
- Eldecort Cream 1.0% 1113
- Eldecort Cream 1.0% and 2.5% 1113
- Fungoid HC Creme 1770
- Hydrocortone Tablets 1482
- Hytone 909
- LazerSporin-C Solution 1770
- Massengill Medicated Soft Cloth Towelettes 2192
- Nutracort Cream & Lotion 1684
- PediOtic Suspension Sterile 797
- Synacort Creams 1%, 2.5% 2296
- Vanoxide-HC Acne Lotion 911
- Vioform-Hydrocortisone Cream and Mild Cream 889
- Vioform-Hydrocortisone Ointment .. 889
- VōSoL HC Otic Solution 2392
- Vytone Cream 1% 911

Hydrocortisone Acetate (Efficacy impaired by phenytoin). Products include:
- Analpram-HC Rectal Cream 1% and 2.5% 970
- Anusol-HC Cream 1690
- Anusol-HC Suppositories 1691
- Caldecort ...... ▣ 560
- Carmol HC Cream 1% 2296
- Chloromycetin Hydrocortisone Ophthalmic 1694
- Coly-Mycin S Otic w/Neomycin & Hydrocortisone 1708
- Cortaid ...... ▣ 735
- Cortef Feminine Itch Cream ...... ▣ 735
- Corticaine ...... ▣ 682
- Cortifoam 1827
- Cortisporin Cream 757
- Epifoam 1828
- Gynecort 5 Creme ...... ▣ 556
- Hydrocortone Acetate Sterile Suspension 1479
- Lanacort 5 Creme and Ointment .. ▣ 557
- Mantadil Cream 789
- Ophthocort ...... ⊙ 301
- Orabase HCA Oral Paste 890
- Pramosone Cream, Lotion & Ointment 971
- ProctoCream-HC 1834
- Proctofoam-HC 1835

Hydrocortisone Sodium Phosphate (Efficacy impaired by phenytoin). Products include:
- Hydrocortone Phosphate Injection, Sterile 1481

Hydrocortisone Sodium Succinate (Efficacy impaired by phenytoin). Products include:
- Solu-Cortef Sterile Powder 2361

Hydroflumethiazide (Increased phenytoin serum levels). Products include:
- Diucardin Tablets 2450
- Saluron 718
- Salutensin/Salutensin-Demi 719

Imipramine Hydrochloride (Tricyclic antidepressants may precipitate seizures in some patients; phenytoin dosage may need to be adjusted). Products include:
- Tofranil Ampuls 1038
- Tofranil Tablets 1039

Imipramine Pamoate (Tricyclic antidepressants may precipitate seizures in some patients; phenytoin dosage may need to be adjusted). Products include:
- Tofranil-PM Capsules 1041

Isoniazid (Increased phenytoin serum levels). Products include:
- INH Tablets 868
- Rifamate Capsules 1347

Levonorgestrel (Efficacy impaired by phenytoin). Products include:
- Levlen/Tri-Levlen 665
- Nordette-21 Tablets 2481
- Nordette-28 Tablets 2483
- Norplant System 2484
- Levlen/Tri-Levlen 665
- Triphasil-21 Tablets 2527
- Triphasil-28 Tablets 2532

Magnesium Salicylate (Increased phenytoin serum levels). Products include:
- Doan's - Extra-Strength Analgesic ▣ 549
- Doan's - Regular Strength Analgesic ...... ▣ 549
- Mobigesic Analgesic Tablets ...... ▣ 507

Maprotiline Hydrochloride (Tricyclic antidepressants may precipitate seizures in some patients; phenytoin dosage may need to be adjusted). Products include:
- Ludiomil Tablets 874

Mesoridazine (Increased phenytoin serum levels). Products include:
- Serentil 686

Mestranol (Efficacy impaired by phenytoin). Products include:
- Enovid 2161
- Norethin 2133
- Norinyl 2304
- Ortho-Novum 1667

Methsuximide (Increases phenytoin serum levels). Products include:
- Celontin 1692

Methyclothiazide (Increased phenytoin serum levels). Products include:
- Enduron Tablets 517
- Enduronyl 518

Methylphenidate Hydrochloride (Increased phenytoin serum levels). Products include:
- Ritalin 880

Methylprednisolone Acetate (Efficacy impaired by phenytoin). Products include:
- Depo-Medrol Sterile Aqueous Suspension 2334

Methylprednisolone Sodium Succinate (Efficacy impaired by phenytoin). Products include:
- Solu-Medrol Sterile Powder 2363

Molindone Hydrochloride (Interferes with absorption of phenytoin). Products include:
- Moban Tablets & Concentrate 932

Nizatidine (Increases phenytoin serum levels). Products include:
- Axid Pulvules 1246

Norethindrone (Efficacy impaired by phenytoin). Products include:
- Brevicon 2304
- Jenest-28 Tablets 1636
- Micronor Tablets 1667
- Modicon 1667
- Norethin 2133
- Norinyl 2304
- Norlutin 1755
- Nor-Q D Tablets 2304
- Ortho-Novum 1667
- Ovcon 1391
- Tri-Norinyl 2304

Norethynodrel (Efficacy impaired by phenytoin). Products include:
- Enovid 2161

Norgestimate (Increased phenytoin serum levels; efficacy impaired by phenytoin). Products include:
- Ortho-Cyclen Tablets 1658

Norgestrel (Efficacy impaired by phenytoin). Products include:
- Lo/Ovral Tablets 2471
- Lo/Ovral-28 Tablets 2476
- Ovral Tablets 2490
- Ovral-28 Tablets 2491
- Ovrette Tablets 2492

Nortriptyline Hydrochloride (Tricyclic antidepressants may precipitate seizures in some patients; phenytoin dosage may need to be adjusted). Products include:
- Pamelor 2019

Perphenazine (Increased phenytoin serum levels). Products include:
- Etrafon 2087
- Triavil Tablets 1556
- Trilafon 2123

Phenobarbital (Increased or decreased phenytoin levels). Products include:
- Arco-Lase Plus Tablets 607
- Bellergal-S Tablets 1998
- Bronkolixir ...... ▣ 761
- Bronkotabs Tablets ...... ▣ 762
- Donnatal 1858
- Donnatal Extentabs 1859
- Donnatal Tablets 1858
- Donnazyme Tablets 1860
- Kinesed Tablets 2272
- Phenobarbital Elixir and Tablets 1293
- Primatene Tablets-P Formula 2421
- Quadrinal Tablets 1183
- Tedral SA 1765

Phensuximide (Increases phenytoin serum levels). Products include:
- Milontin Kapseals 1741

Phenylbutazone (Increased phenytoin serum levels). Products include:
- Butazolidin Capsules & Tablets 1027

Polyestradiol Phosphate (Increased phenytoin serum levels; efficacy impaired by phenytoin). Products include:
- Estradurin 2452

Polythiazide (Increased phenytoin serum levels). Products include:
- Minizide Capsules 1779
- Renese Tablets 1785
- Renese-R Tablets 1786

Prednisolone Acetate (Efficacy impaired by phenytoin). Products include:
- AK-Cide Sterile Ophthalmic Ointment & Suspension ...... ⊙ 202
- Blephamide Liquifilm Sterile Ophthalmic Suspension 586
- Blephamide S.O.P. Sterile Ophthalmic Ointment 586
- Cetapred Ointment ...... ⊙ 220
- ⅛% Econopred & 1% Econopred Plus ...... ⊙ 217
- Isopto Cetapred Suspension ...... ⊙ 220
- Metimyd ...... ⊙ 306
- Poly-Pred Liquifilm ...... ⊙ 250
- Pred Forte ...... ⊙ 252
- Pred Mild ...... ⊙ 254
- Pred-G Liquifilm Sterile Ophthalmic Suspension ...... ⊙ 252
- Pred-G S.O.P. Sterile Ophthalmic Ointment ...... ⊙ 253
- Vasocidin Ointment ...... ⊙ 275

Prednisolone Sodium Phosphate (Efficacy impaired by phenytoin). Products include:
- AK-Pred ...... ⊙ 205
- Hydeltrasol Injection, Sterile 1476
- Inflamase ...... ⊙ 274
- Pediapred Oral Liquid 987
- Vasocidin Ophthalmic Solution ...... ⊙ 276

Prednisolone Tebutate (Efficacy impaired by phenytoin). Products include:
- Hydeltra-T.B.A. Sterile Suspension 1478

Prednisone (Efficacy impaired by phenytoin). Products include:
- Deltasone Tablets 2332

Prochlorperazine (Increased phenytoin levels). Products include:
- Compazine 2201

Promethazine Hydrochloride (Increased phenytoin serum levels). Products include:
- Mepergan Injection 2479
- Phenergan with Codeine 2497
- Phenergan with Dextromethorphan 2499
- Phenergan Injection 2493
- Phenergan Suppositories 2496
- Phenergan Syrup 2495
- Phenergan Tablets 2496
- Phenergan VC 2500
- Phenergan VC with Codeine 2501

Protriptyline Hydrochloride (Tricyclic antidepressants may precipitate seizures in some patients; phenytoin dosage may need to be adjusted). Products include:
- Vivactil Tablets 1567

Quinestrol (Increased phenytoin serum levels; efficacy impaired by phenytoin). Products include:
- Estrovis 1721

Quinidine Gluconate (Efficacy impaired by phenytoin). Products include:
- Quinaglute Dura-Tabs Tablets 663

Quinidine Polygalacturonate (Efficacy impaired by phenytoin). Products include:
- Cardioquin Tablets 1812

Quinidine Sulfate (Efficacy impaired by phenytoin). Products include:
- Quinidex Extentabs 1868

Ranitidine Hydrochloride (Increases phenytoin serum levels). Products include:
- Zantac Injection and Zantac Injection Premixed 1063
- Zantac 1065

Reserpine (Decreased phenytoin serum levels). Products include:
- Diupres Tablets 1461
- Hydromox R Tablets 1209
- Hydropres Tablets 1485
- Renese-R Tablets 1786
- Salutensin/Salutensin-Demi 719
- Ser-Ap-Es Tablets 881
- Serpasil Tablets 883
- Serpasil-Apresoline Tablets 884
- Serpasil-Esidrix Tablets 886

Rifampin (Efficacy impaired by phenytoin). Products include:
- Rifadin 1345
- Rifamate Capsules 1347
- Rimactane Capsules 879

Salsalate (Increased phenytoin serum levels). Products include:
- Disalcid 1310
- Mono-Gesic Tablets 846
- Salflex 839

Sodium Valproate (Increased or decreased phenytoin levels).

Sucralfate (Decreases phenytoin serum levels). Products include:
- Carafate Tablets 1326

Sulfamethizole (Increased phenytoin serum levels). Products include:
- Thiosulfil Forte Tablets 2526
- Urobiotic-250 Capsules 1968

Sulfamethoxazole (Increased phenytoin serum levels). Products include:
- Azo Gantanol Tablets 1887
- Bactrim DS Tablets 1891
- Bactrim I.V. Infusion 1889
- Bactrim 1891
- Gantanol 1899
- Septra 813
- Septra I.V. Infusion 808
- Septra I.V. Infusion ADD-Vantage Vials 810
- Septra 813

Sulfasalazine (Increased phenytoin serum levels). Products include:
- Azulfidine Tablets, EN-tabs, Oral Suspension 1157

Sulfinpyrazone (Increased phenytoin serum levels). Products include:
- Anturane 853

Sulfisoxazole (Increased phenytoin serum levels). Products include:
- Azo Gantrisin Tablets 1888
- Gantrisin Tablets 1901
- Pediazole 1973

Sulfisoxazole Diolamine (Increased phenytoin serum levels). Products include:
- Gantrisin Ophthalmic Ointment/Solution 1900

Theophylline (Efficacy impaired by phenytoin). Products include:
- Bronkaid Tablets 757
- Bronkolixir 761
- Bronkotabs Tablets 762
- Constant-T Tablets 1029
- Marax Tablets & DF Syrup 1954
- Primatene Tablets 2421
- Quibron Capsules 713
- Quibron-T 714
- Quibron-T/SR 716
- Theolair Liquid 1317
- Theo-Organidin Elixir 2391

Theophylline Anhydrous (Efficacy impaired by phenytoin). Products include:
- Aerolate 994
- Primatene Tablets-M Formula 753
- Primatene Tablets-Regular Formula 2421
- Respbid Tablets 684
- Slo-bid Gyrocaps 1847
- T-PHYL (Uniphyl) 200 mg Tablets 1820
- Tedral SA 1765
- Theo-24 2179
- Theo-Dur Sprinkle 1168
- Theo-Dur Extended-Release Tablets 1166
- Theolair Tablets 1317
- Theolair-SR Tablets 1319
- TheoX Extended-Release Tablets 841
- Uniphyl 400 mg Tablets 1823

Theophylline Calcium Salicylate (Efficacy impaired by phenytoin). Products include:
- Quadrinal Tablets 1183

Theophylline Sodium Glycinate (Efficacy impaired by phenytoin). Products include:
- Asbron G 1997

Thioridazine Hydrochloride (Increased phenytoin serum levels). Products include:
- Mellaril 2011

Tolazamide (Increased phenytoin serum levels). Products include:
- Tolinase Tablets 2365

Tolbutamide (Increased phenytoin serum levels). Products include:
- Orinase Tablets 2354

Trazodone Hydrochloride (Increased phenytoin serum levels). Products include:
- Desyrel and Desyrel Dividose 1404

Triamcinolone (Efficacy impaired by phenytoin).
- No products indexed under this heading.

Triamcinolone Acetonide (Efficacy impaired by phenytoin). Products include:
- Aristocort A 1010
- Azmacort Inhaler 1837
- Kenalog Cream, Lotion & Ointment 2401
- Kenalog-10 Injection 2402
- Kenalog-40 Injection 2403
- Kenalog in Orabase 604
- Kenalog Spray 2401
- Mycolog II Cream and Ointment 2407
- Mytrex Cream & Ointment 2080
- Nasacort Nasal Inhaler 1844

Triamcinolone Diacetate (Efficacy impaired by phenytoin). Products include:
- Aristocort Suspension 1008

Triamcinolone Hexacetonide (Efficacy impaired by phenytoin). Products include:
- Aristospan Suspension 1011

Trifluoperazine Hydrochloride (Increased phenytoin serum levels). Products include:
- Stelazine 2226

Trimipramine Maleate (Tricyclic antidepressants may precipitate seizures in some patients; phenytoin dosage may need to be adjusted). Products include:
- Surmontil Capsules 2524

Valproic Acid (Increased or decreased phenytoin levels). Products include:
- Depakene Capsules & Syrup 511

Vitamin D (Efficacy impaired by phenytoin). Products include:
- Bugs Bunny Children's Chewable Vitamins (Sugar Free) 625
- Bugs Bunny With Extra C Children's Chewable Vitamins (Sugar Free) 626
- Bugs Bunny Plus Iron Children's Chewable Vitamins (Sugar Free) 625
- Calderol Capsules 1635
- Caltrate 600 + Iron & Vitamin D 1198
- Caltrate 600 + Vitamin D 1197
- Caltrate, Jr. Tablets 1198
- Flintstones Children's Chewable Vitamins 625
- Flintstones Children's Chewable Vitamins With Extra C 626
- Flintstones Children's Chewable Vitamins Plus Iron 625
- Natalins Rx 1391
- Natalins Tablets 1391
- One-A-Day Essential Vitamins 627
- One-A-Day Maximum Formula Vitamins and Minerals 627
- One-A-Day Plus Extra C Vitamins 627
- Os-Cal 250+D Tablets 597
- Os-Cal 500+D Tablets 597
- Os-Cal Fortified Tablets 597
- Os-Cal Plus Tablets 597
- Posture-D 600 mg 2420
- Stressgard Stress Formula Vitamins 628
- Tri-Vi-Flor 1.0 mg Vitamins with Fluoride Chewable Tablets 1400
- Tri-Vi-Flor Drops 1400
- Tri-Vi-Sol Vitamin Drops 614
- Tri-Vi-Sol Vitamin Drops with Iron 614
- Vi-Daylin ADC Vitamins Drops 1980
- Vi-Daylin ADC Vitamins + Iron Drops 1980
- Vi-Daylin/F ADC Vitamins Drops With Fluoride 1981
- Vi-Daylin/F ADC Vitamins + Iron Drops With Fluoride 1981
- Within Women's Formula Multivitamin with Calcium, Extra Iron and Zinc 628
- Zymacap Capsules 670

Warfarin Sodium (Efficacy impaired by phenytoin). Products include:
- Coumadin Injection & Tablets 944
- Panwarfin Tablets 547

DILANTIN WITH PHENOBARBITAL KAPSEALS

(Phenytoin Sodium, Phenobarbital) ..1715

May interact with oral anticoagulants, corticosteroids, oral contraceptives, salicylates, phenothiazines, estrogens, tranquilizers, antihistamines, monoamine oxidase inhibitors, narcotic analgesics, sulfonamides, tricyclic antidepressants, histamine h2-receptor antagonists, succinimides, xanthine bronchodilators, and certain other agents. Compounds in these categories include:

Alcohol (Increased phenytoin serum levels with acute alcohol intake; decreased levels with chronic alcohol intake).

Alfentanil Hydrochloride (Increases phenobarbital effects). Products include:
- Alfenta Injection 1131

Alprazolam (Increases phenobarbital effects). Products include:
- Xanax Tablets 2367

Aminophylline (Efficacy impaired by phenytoin). Products include:
- Amesec 682
- Aminophyllin Tablets 2153

Amiodarone Hydrochloride (Increases phenytoin serum levels). Products include:
- Cordarone Tablets 2446

Amitriptyline Hydrochloride (Increases phenobarbital effects; tricyclic antidepressants may precipitate seizures in some patients; phenytoin dosage may need to be adjusted). Products include:
- Elavil 2269
- Endep Tablets 1927
- Etrafon 2087
- Limbitrol 1933
- Triavil Tablets 1556

Amoxapine (Tricyclic antidepressants may precipitate seizures in some patients; phenytoin dosage may need to be adjusted). Products include:
- Asendin Tablets 1196

Aspirin (Increased phenytoin levels). Products include:
- Alka-Seltzer Effervescent Antacid and Pain Reliever 1568
- Alka-Seltzer Extra Strength Effervescent Antacid and Pain Reliever 1570
- Alka-Seltzer (Flavored) Effervescent Antacid and Pain Reliever 1569
- Alka-Seltzer Plus Cold Medicine 623
- Alka-Seltzer Plus Night-Time Cold Medicine 623
- Alka Seltzer Plus Sinus Allergy Medicine 624
- Anacin Coated Analgesic Caplets 2417
- Anacin Coated Analgesic Tablets 2417
- Anacin Maximum Strength Analgesic Coated Tablets 2417
- Maximum Strength Arthritis Pain Formula By the Makers of Anacin Analgesic Tablets and Caplets 2418
- Arthritis Pain Formula by the Makers of Anacin Analgesic Tablets and Caplets 747
- Arthritis Strength BC Powder 516
- Ascriptin A/D Caplets 1850
- Regular Strength Ascriptin Tablets 1850
- Azdōne Tablets 844
- BC Powder 517
- BC Cold Powder 517
- Children's Bayer Chewable Aspirin 564
- Genuine Bayer Aspirin Tablets & Caplets 564
- Maximum Bayer Aspirin Tablets & Caplets 566
- Bayer Plus Aspirin Tablets 567
- Therapy Bayer Aspirin Caplets 568
- 8 Hour Bayer Timed-Release Aspirin 566
- Arthritis Strength Bufferin Analgesic Caplets 744
- Extra Strength Bufferin Analgesic Tablets 745
- Bufferin Analgesic Tablets and Caplets 743
- Cama Arthritis Pain Reliever 685
- Damason-P 1356
- Easprin 1719
- Ecotrin Enteric Coated Aspirin Maximum Strength Tablets and Caplets 2189
- Ecotrin Enteric Coated Aspirin Regular Strength Tablets and Caplets 2189
- Empirin Aspirin 541
- Empirin with Codeine Phosphate Nos. 2, 3 & 4 764
- Equagesic Tablets 2451
- Excedrin Extra-Strength Analgesic Tablets & Caplets 749
- 4-Way Cold Tablets 750

Fiorinal Capsules ... 2007
Fiorinal with Codeine Capsules ... 2008
Fiorinal Tablets ... 2007
Lortab ASA Tablets ... 2414
Momentum Muscular Backache Formula ... ▣ 751
Norgesic ... 1314
Norwich Extra-Strength Aspirin ... ▣ 546
Norwich Regular Strength Aspirin ▣ 547
P-A-C Analgesic Tablets ... ▣ 669
Percodan ... 951
Robaxisal Tablets ... 1872
Sine-Off Sinus Medicine Tablets-Aspirin Formula ... ▣ 722
Soma Compound w/Codeine Tablets ... 2390
Soma Compound Tablets ... 2389
St. Joseph Adult Chewable Aspirin (81 mg.) ... ▣ 703
Synalgos-DC Capsules ... 2525
Talwin Compound ... 2072
Ursinus Inlay-Tabs ... ▣ 691
Vanquish Analgesic Caplets ... ▣ 574
Zorprin Tablets ... 698

Astemizole (Increases phenobarbital effects). Products include:
Hismanal Tablets ... 1138

Azatadine Maleate (Increases phenobarbital effects). Products include:
Optimine Tablets ... 2115
Trinalin Repetabs Tablets ... 1170

Bendroflumethiazide (Increased phenytoin serum levels). Products include:
Corzide Tablets ... 702
Naturetin Tablets ... 1789
Rauzide Tablets ... 1804

Betamethasone Acetate (Efficacy impaired by phenytoin; increases phenobarbital effects). Products include:
Celestone Soluspan Suspension ... 2081

Betamethasone Sodium Phosphate (Efficacy impaired by phenytoin; increases phenobarbital effects). Products include:
Celestone Soluspan Suspension ... 2081

Bromodiphenhydramine Hydrochloride (Increases phenobarbital effects).
No products indexed under this heading.

Brompheniramine Maleate (Increases phenobarbital effects). Products include:
Alka Seltzer Plus Sinus Allergy Medicine ... ▣ 624
Atrohist Sprinkle Capsules ... 558
Bromfed Capsules (Timed Release) ... 1615
Bromfed Syrup ... ▣ 628
Bromfed ... 1615
Dimetane Decongestant ... ▣ 673
Dimetane ... ▣ 672
Dimetane-DC Cough Syrup ... 1857
Dimetane-DX Cough Syrup ... 1858
Dimetapp Elixir ... ▣ 673
Dimetapp DM Elixir ... ▣ 674
Dimetapp Extentabs ... ▣ 674
Dimetapp Plus Caplets ... ▣ 675
Dimetapp Tablets ... ▣ 675
Drixoral Antihistamine/Nasal Decongestant Syrup ... ▣ 698

Buprenorphine (Increases phenobarbital effects).
No products indexed under this heading.

Buspirone Hydrochloride (Increases phenobarbital effects). Products include:
BuSpar ... 1401

Calcium Carbonate (Ingestion times of phenytoin and antacids containing calcium should be staggered to prevent absorption problems). Products include:
Alka-Mints Chewable Antacid ... ▣ 620
Alka-Seltzer Advanced Formula Antacid & Non-Aspirin Pain Reliever ... ▣ 620
Ascriptin A/D Caplets ... 1850
Regular Strength Ascriptin Tablets 1850
Balmex Baby Powder ... ▣ 590
Bayer Plus Aspirin Tablets ... ▣ 567
Biocal 500 mg Tablet Calcium Supplement ... ▣ 625
Bufferin Analgesic Tablets and Caplets ... ▣ 524
Caltrate 600 ... ▣ 583
Caltrate 600 + Iron ... ▣ 583
Caltrate 600 + Vitamin D ... ▣ 584
Caltrate, Jr. ... ▣ 583
Centrum, Jr. (Children's Chewable) + Extra Calcium ... ▣ 585
Di-Gel Antacid/Anti-Gas ... ▣ 697
Gerimed Tablets ... 972
Marblen ... ▣ 563
Natalins Rx ... 1391
Natalins Tablets ... 1391
Nephro-Calci Tablets ... 1826
Os-Cal 500 Chewable Tablets ... ▣ 596
Os-Cal 500 Tablets ... ▣ 597
Os-Cal 250+D Tablets ... ▣ 597
Os-Cal 500+D Tablets ... ▣ 597
Pramet FA ... 1974
Pramilet FA ... 1974
Rolaids (Calcium Rich/Sodium Free) ... ▣ 744
Extra Strength Rolaids ... ▣ 744
Thermotabs ... ▣ 619
Total Formula-2 (multivitamin/multimineral) ... 2377
Tums Liquid Extra ... ▣ 726
Zenate Tablets ... 2250

Calcium Carbonate, Precipitated (Ingestion times of phenytoin and antacids containing calcium should be staggered to prevent absorption problems). Products include:
Caltrate 600 Tablets ... 1197
Caltrate 600 + Iron & Vitamin D ... 1198
Caltrate 600 + Vitamin D ... 1197
Caltrate, Jr. Tablets ... 1198
Tums ... ▣ 725

Carbamazepine (Decreased phenytoin serum levels). Products include:
Tegretol Chewable Tablets ... 654
Tegretol Suspension ... 656
Tegretol Tablets ... 654

Chloramphenicol (Increased phenytoin levels). Products include:
AK-Chlor Sterile Ophthalmic Ointment & Solution ... ⊙ 201
Chloromycetin Cream, 1% ... 1694
Chloromycetin Hydrocortisone Ophthalmic ... 1694
Chloromycetin Kapseals ... 1695
Chloromycetin Ophthalmic Ointment, 1% ... 1696
Chloromycetin Ophthalmic Solution ... 1696
Chloromycetin Otic ... 1697
Chloroptic S.O.P. ... ⊙ 243
Chloroptic Sterile Ophthalmic Solution ... ⊙ 243
Ophthochlor Ophthalmic Solution ⊙ 300
Ophthocort ... ⊙ 301

Chloramphenicol Palmitate (Increased phenytoin levels). Products include:
Chloromycetin Palmitate, Oral Suspension ... 1697

Chloramphenicol Sodium Succinate (Increased phenytoin levels). Products include:
Chloromycetin Sodium Succinate ... 1698

Chlordiazepoxide (Increased phenytoin levels; increases phenobarbital effects). Products include:
Libritabs Tablets ... 1930
Limbitrol ... 1933
Menrium Tablets ... 1934

Chlordiazepoxide Hydrochloride (Increased phenytoin levels; increases phenobarbital effects). Products include:
Librax Capsules ... 1929
Librium Capsules ... 1931
Librium Injectable ... 1932

Chlorothiazide (Increased phenytoin serum levels). Products include:
Aldoclor Tablets ... 1413
Diupres Tablets ... 1461
Diuril Oral ... 1464

Chlorothiazide Sodium (Increased phenytoin serum levels). Products include:
Diuril Sodium Intravenous ... 1463

Chlorotrianisene (Increased phenytoin levels; efficacy impaired by phenytoin). Products include:
TACE 12 and 25 mg ... 1353

Chlorpheniramine Maleate (Increases phenobarbital effects). Products include:
A.R.M. Allergy Relief Medicine Caplets ... ▣ 615
Alka-Seltzer Plus Cold Medicine ... ▣ 623
Allerest ... ▣ 559
Ana-Kit Anaphylaxis Emergency Treatment Kit ... 1100
BC Cold Powder Multi-Symptom Formula ... ▣ 517
Brexin L.A. Capsules ... 2078
Cerose-DM ... 2443
Cheracol Plus Head Cold/Cough Formula ... ▣ 667
Chlor-Trimeton Allergy Syrup, Tablets & Long-Acting Repetabs Tablets ... ▣ 693
Chlor-Trimeton Decongestant ... ▣ 694
Comhist LA Capsules ... 1618
Allergy-Sinus Comtrex Multi-Symptom Allergy Sinus Formula Tablets & Caplets ... 746
Comtrex Multi-Symptom Cold Reliever Tablets/Caplets/Liqui-Gels/Liquid ... 745
Day-Night Comtrex ... 747
Contac Continuous Action Decongestant/Antihistamine Capsules ▣ 710
Contac Maximum Strength Continuous Action Decongestant/Antihistamine Caplets ... ▣ 709
Contac Severe Cold and Flu Formula Caplets ... ▣ 711
Coricidin 'D' Decongestant Tablets ... ▣ 695
Coricidin Demilets Tablets for Children ... ▣ 696
Coricidin Tablets ... ▣ 695
Deconamine ... 663
Demazin Nasal Decongestant/Antihistamine Repetabs Tablets & Syrup ... ▣ 697
Dorcol Children's Liquid Cold Formula ... ▣ 686
Dristan Decongestant/Antihistamine/Analgesic Coated Caplets ... ▣ 749
Dristan Cold Nasal Decongestant/Antihistamine/ Analgesic Coated Tablets ... 2419
Dristan Advanced Formula Decongestant/Antihistamine/Analgesic Tablets ... ▣ 749
Extendryl ... 994
4-Way Cold Tablets ... 750
Fedahist Gyrocaps ... 2145
Fedahist Timecaps ... 2145
Hycomine Compound Tablets ... 929
Isoclor Timesule Capsules ... ▣ 561
Kronofed-A ... 970
Medi-Flu Caplet, Liquid ... ▣ 640
Naldecon Syrup, Tablets, Pediatric Drops and Pediatric Syrup ... 709
Nolamine Tablets ... 838
Novafed A Capsules ... 1342
Novahistine DH ... 1342
Novahistine Elixir ... ▣ 596
Ornade Spansule Capsules ... 2221
Orthoxicol Cough Syrup ... ▣ 668
PediaCare Allergy Relief Formula Liquid ... 1362
PediaCare Cough-Cold Formula Liquid ... 1362
PediaCare Night Rest Cough-Cold Formula Liquid ... 1362
PediaCare 6-12 Cough-Cold Formula Chewable Tablets ... 1362
Pyrroxate Capsules ... ▣ 669
Quelidrine Syrup ... 556
Ru-Tuss II Capsules ... 693
Ru-Tuss Tablets ... 693
Ryna ... ▣ 741
Sinarest Tablets & Extra Strength Tablets ... ▣ 562
Sine-Off Maximum Strength Allergy/Sinus Formula Caplets ... ▣ 721
Sine-Off Sinus Medicine Tablets-Aspirin Formula ... ▣ 722
Singlet Tablets ... ▣ 598
Sinulin ... 840
Sinutab Maximum Strength ... ▣ 641
St. Joseph Nighttime Cold Medicine ... ▣ 705
Sudafed Plus Liquid ... ▣ 544
Sudafed Plus Tablets ... ▣ 545
Teldrin Timed-Release Allergy Capsules, 12 mg ... 2192
TheraFlu Flu and Cold Medicine ... ▣ 687
Triaminic Allergy Tablets ... ▣ 688
Triaminic Chewables ... ▣ 688
Triaminic Cold Tablets ... ▣ 688
Triaminic Nite Light ... ▣ 689
Triaminic Syrup ... ▣ 689
Triaminic-12 Tablets ... ▣ 690
Triaminicin Tablets ... ▣ 690
Triaminicol Multi-Symptom Cold Tablets ... ▣ 691
Triaminicol Multi-Symptom Relief ▣ 691
Tylenol Allergy Sinus Medication Caplets and Gelcaps, Maximum Strength ... 1372
Children's Tylenol Cold Liquid Formula and Chewable Tablets ... 1368
Tylenol Cold & Flu Hot Medication, Packets ... 1369
Tylenol Cold Medication Caplets and Tablets ... 1370
Tylenol Cold Medication, Effervescent Tablets ... 1369
Vicks Children's NyQuil ... ▣ 664
Vicks Formula 44 Cough Medicine ... ▣ 661
Vicks Formula 44M Multi-Symptom Cough Medicine ... ▣ 662
Vicks Pediatric Formula 44m Multi-Symptom Cough & Cold Medicine ... ▣ 663

Chlorpheniramine Polistirex (Increases phenobarbital effects). Products include:
Tussionex Extended-Release Suspension ... 988

Chlorpheniramine Tannate (Increases phenobarbital effects). Products include:
Rynatan ... 2387
Rynatuss ... 2388

Chlorpromazine (Increased phenytoin levels; increases phenobarbital effects). Products include:
Thorazine ... 2234

Chlorpropamide (Increased phenytoin serum levels). Products include:
Diabinese Tablets ... 1775

Chlorprothixene (Increases phenobarbital effects). Products include:
Taractan Tablets ... 1920

Chlorprothixene Hydrochloride (Increases phenobarbital effects). Products include:
Taractan ... 1920

Choline Magnesium Trisalicylate (Increased phenytoin levels). Products include:
Trilisate ... 1822

Cimetidine (Increases phenytoin serum levels). Products include:
Tagamet Tablets ... 2228

Cimetidine Hydrochloride (Increases phenytoin serum levels). Products include:
Tagamet ... 2228

Clemastine Fumarate (Increases phenobarbital effects). Products include:
Tavist Syrup ... 2033
Tavist Tablets ... 2035
Tavist-D Tablets ... 2035

Clomipramine Hydrochloride (Tricyclic antidepressants may precipitate seizures in some patients; phenytoin dosage may need to be adjusted). Products include:
Anafranil Capsules ... 650

Clorazepate Dipotassium (Increases phenobarbital effects). Products include:
Tranxene ... 556

Codeine (Increases phenobarbital effects). Products include:
Calcidrine Syrup ... 506

Codeine Phosphate (Increases phenobarbital effects). Products include:
- Actifed with Codeine Cough Syrup.. 752
- Cheracol Cough Syrup 1853
- Codimal PH Syrup 846
- Dimetane-DC Cough Syrup 1857
- Empirin with Codeine Phosphate Nos. 2, 3 & 4 764
- Fiorinal with Codeine Capsules 2008
- Isoclor Expectorant 982
- Naldecon CX Adult Liquid ▣ 521
- Novahistine DH 1342
- Novahistine Expectorant 1343
- Nucofed Capsules 2219
- Nucofed Expectorant 2219
- Nucofed Pediatric Expectorant 2220
- Nucofed Syrup 2219
- Phenaphen with Codeine Capsules 1865
- Phenaphen-650 with Codeine Tablets 1866
- Phenergan with Codeine 2497
- Phenergan VC with Codeine 2501
- Robitussin A-C Syrup 1875
- Robitussin-DAC Syrup 1875
- Ryna ▣ 741
- Soma Compound w/Codeine Tablets 2390
- Triaminic Expectorant w/Codeine .. 1996
- Tussi-Organidin Liquid 2391
- Tylenol with Codeine 1381

Codeine Polistirex (Increases phenobarbital effects).
- No products indexed under this heading.

Cortisone Acetate (Efficacy impaired by phenytoin; increases phenobarbital effects). Products include:
- Cortone Acetate Sterile Suspension 1437
- Cortone Acetate Tablets 1439

Cyproheptadine Hydrochloride (Increases phenobarbital effects). Products include:
- Periactin 1525

Deserpidine (Increases phenobarbital effects). Products include:
- Enduronyl 518
- Harmonyl Tablets 528
- Oreticyl 545

Desipramine Hydrochloride (Tricyclic antidepressants may precipitate seizures in some patients; phenytoin dosage may need to be adjusted). Products include:
- Norpramin Tablets 1340

Dexamethasone (Efficacy impaired by phenytoin; increases phenobarbital effects). Products include:
- AK-Trol Ointment & Suspension .... ⊙ 207
- Decadron Elixir 1445
- Decadron Tablets 1447
- Decaspray Topical Aerosol 1459
- Dexacidin ⊙ 272
- Maxidex Sterile Ophthalmic Suspension ⊙ 223
- Maxitrol Ophthalmic Ointment/Suspension ⊙ 223
- TobraDex Ophthalmic Suspension and Ointment ⊙ 228

Dexamethasone Acetate (Efficacy impaired by phenytoin; increases phenobarbital effects). Products include:
- Dalalone D.P. Injectable 999
- Decadron-LA Sterile Suspension 1457

Dexamethasone Sodium Phosphate (Efficacy impaired by phenytoin; increases phenobarbital effects). Products include:
- AK-Dex ⊙ 203
- Decadron Phosphate Respihaler 1454
- Decadron Phosphate Sterile Ophthalmic Ointment 1453
- Decadron Phosphate Sterile Ophthalmic Solution 1453
- Decadron Phosphate Topical Cream 1455
- Decadron Phosphate Turbinaire 1456
- Maxidex Sterile Ophthalmic Ointment ⊙ 222
- NeoDecadron Sterile Ophthalmic Ointment 1517
- NeoDecadron Sterile Ophthalmic Solution 1518
- NeoDecadron Topical Cream 1518

Dexchlorpheniramine Maleate (Increases phenobarbital effects). Products include:
- Polaramine 2116

Dezocine (Increases phenobarbital effects).

Diazepam (Increased phenytoin levels; increases phenobarbital effects). Products include:
- Valium Injectable 1937
- Valium Tablets 1939
- Valrelease Capsules 1923

Dicumarol (Efficacy impaired by phenytoin; increases phenytoin serum levels). Products include:
- Dicumarol Tablets 516

Dienestrol (Increased phenytoin levels; efficacy impaired by phenytoin). Products include:
- Ortho Dienestrol Cream 1664

Diethylstilbestrol (Increased phenytoin levels; efficacy impaired by phenytoin). Products include:
- Diethylstilbestrol Tablets 1258

Diflunisal (Increased phenytoin levels). Products include:
- Dolobid Tablets 1465

Digitoxin (Efficacy impaired by phenytoin). Products include:
- Crystodigin Tablets 1253

Diphenhydramine Citrate (Increases phenobarbital effects). Products include:
- Alka-Seltzer Plus Night-Time Cold Medicine ▣ 623
- Bufferin AF Nite Time Analgesic/Sleeping Aid Caplets 744
- Excedrin P.M. Analgesic/Sleeping Aid Tablets, Caplets and Liquid.... 749

Diphenhydramine Hydrochloride (Increases phenobarbital effects). Products include:
- Benadryl Anti-Itch Cream ▣ 635
- Benadryl Capsules 1691
- Benadryl Decongestant Elixir ▣ 635
- Benadryl Decongestant ▣ 635
- Benadryl Elixir ▣ 636
- Benadryl Kapseals 1691
- Benadryl 25 Kapseals ▣ 636
- Benadryl Parenteral 1692
- Benadryl Plus ▣ 636
- Benadryl Plus Nighttime ▣ 637
- Benadryl Spray, Maximum Strength ▣ 637
- Benadryl Spray, Regular Strength ▣ 637
- Benadryl Steri-Vials, Ampoules, and Steri-Dose Syringe 1692
- Benadryl 25 Tablets ▣ 636
- Benylin Cough Syrup ▣ 637
- Benylin Decongestant ▣ 638
- Caladryl Cream, Lotion, Spray ▣ 638
- Miles Nervine Nighttime Sleep-Aid ▣ 627
- Nytol Tablets ▣ 517
- Sleep-ettes-D Tablets ▣ 653
- Sleep-eze 3 Tablets ▣ 755
- Sleepinal Night-time Sleep Aid Capsules ▣ 734
- Sominex Caplets and Tablets ▣ 722
- Sominex Liquid ▣ 723
- Sominex Pain Relief Formula ▣ 723
- Tylenol Cold Night Time Medication Liquid 1371
- Tylenol PM, Extra Strength Caplets and Tablets 1368
- Unisom Dual Relief Nighttime Sleep Aid/Analgesic 1774
- Ziradryl Lotion ▣ 643

Diphenylpyraline Hydrochloride (Increases phenobarbital effects).
- No products indexed under this heading.

Disulfiram (Increased phenytoin levels). Products include:
- Antabuse Tablets 2429

Divalproex Sodium (Increased or decreased phenytoin levels). Products include:
- Depakote 512

Doxepin Hydrochloride (Tricyclic antidepressants may precipitate seizures in some patients; phenytoin dosage may need to be adjusted). Products include:
- Sinequan 1960

Doxycycline Calcium (Efficacy impaired by phenytoin).
- No products indexed under this heading.

Doxycycline Hyclate (Efficacy impaired by phenytoin). Products include:
- Doryx Capsules 1717
- Vibramycin Hyclate Capsules 1787
- Vibramycin Hyclate Intravenous 1968
- Vibra-Tabs Film Coated Tablets 1787

Doxycycline Monohydrate (Efficacy impaired by phenytoin). Products include:
- Monodox Capsules 1630
- Vibramycin Monohydrate for Oral Suspension 1787

Droperidol (Increases phenobarbital effects). Products include:
- Inapsine Injection 1140
- Innovar Injection 1141

Dyphylline (Efficacy impaired by phenytoin). Products include:
- Dilor 2079
- Dilor-G Tablets & Liquid 2079
- Lufyllin Elixir 2384
- Lufyllin & Lufyllin-400 Tablets 2384
- Lufyllin-GG Elixir & Tablets 2385

Estradiol (Increased phenytoin levels; efficacy impaired by phenytoin). Products include:
- Emcyt Capsules 1161
- Estrace 1385
- Estrace Vaginal Cream 1388
- Estraderm Transdermal System 866

Estrogens, Conjugated (Increased phenytoin levels; efficacy impaired by phenytoin). Products include:
- Mediatric Capsules 2476
- PMB 200 and PMB 400 2504
- Premarin Intravenous 2508
- Premarin with Methyltestosterone .. 2515
- Premarin Tablets 2510
- Premarin Vaginal Cream 2512

Estrogens, Esterified (Increased phenytoin levels; efficacy impaired by phenytoin). Products include:
- Estratest 2245
- Menrium Tablets 1934

Estropipate (Increased phenytoin levels; efficacy impaired by phenytoin). Products include:
- Ogen 540

Ethinyl Estradiol (Increased phenytoin levels; efficacy impaired by phenytoin). Products include:
- Brevicon 2304
- Demulen 2161
- Estinyl Tablets 2085
- Jenest-28 Tablets 1636
- Levlen/Tri-Levlen 665
- Lo/Ovral Tablets 2471
- Lo/Ovral-28 Tablets 2476
- Loestrin 1728
- Modicon 1667
- Nordette-21 Tablets 2481
- Nordette-28 Tablets 2483
- Norethin 2133
- Norinyl 2304
- Norlestrin 1746
- Ortho-Cyclen Tablets 1658
- Ortho-Novum 1667
- Ovcon 1391
- Ovral Tablets 2490
- Ovral-28 Tablets 2491
- Levlen/Tri-Levlen 665
- Tri-Norinyl 2304
- Triphasil-21 Tablets 2527
- Triphasil-28 Tablets 2532

Ethosuximide (Increases phenytoin serum levels). Products include:
- Zarontin Capsules 1768
- Zarontin Syrup 1769

Ethynodiol Diacetate (Efficacy impaired by phenytoin). Products include:
- Demulen 2161

Famotidine (Increases phenytoin serum levels). Products include:
- Pepcid 1524

Fentanyl (Increases phenobarbital effects). Products include:
- Duragesic Transdermal System 1133

Fentanyl Citrate (Increases phenobarbital effects). Products include:
- Innovar Injection 1141
- Sublimaze Injection 1146

Fluphenazine Decanoate (Increases phenobarbital effects). Products include:
- Prolixin Decanoate 1795

Fluphenazine Enanthate (Increased phenytoin levels; increases phenobarbital effects). Products include:
- Prolixin Enanthate 1796

Fluphenazine Hydrochloride (Increased phenytoin levels; increases phenobarbital effects). Products include:
- Prolixin Elixir 1793
- Prolixin Injection 1791
- Prolixin Oral Concentrate 1792
- Prolixin Tablets 1793

Furazolidone (Increases phenobarbital effects). Products include:
- Furoxone 1855

Furosemide (Efficacy impaired by phenytoin). Products include:
- Lasix 1093

Glipizide (Increased phenytoin serum levels). Products include:
- Glucotrol 1952

Glyburide (Increased phenytoin serum levels). Products include:
- DiaBeta 1091
- Micronase Tablets 2350

Haloperidol (Increases phenobarbital effects). Products include:
- Haldol Injection, Tablets and Concentrate 1373

Haloperidol Decanoate (Increases phenobarbital effects). Products include:
- Haldol Decanoate 1375

Halothane (Increased phenytoin levels). Products include:
- Fluothane 2453

Hydrochlorothiazide (Increased phenytoin serum levels). Products include:
- Aldactazide 2150
- Aldoril Tablets 1418
- Apresazide Capsules 854
- Apresoline-Esidrix Tablets 857
- Capozide 2258
- Dyazide Capsules 2208
- Esidrix Tablets 863
- Esimil Tablets 864
- HydroDIURIL Tablets 1484
- Hydropres Tablets 1485
- Inderide Tablets 2463
- Inderide LA Long Acting Capsules .. 2465
- Lopressor HCT Tablets 1034
- Maxzide 1215
- Moduretic Tablets 1510
- Normozide Tablets 2112
- Oretic Tablets 544
- Oreticyl 545
- Prinzide Tablets 1540
- Ser-Ap-Es Tablets 881
- Serpasil-Esidrix Tablets 886
- Timolide Tablets 1547
- Trandate HCT Tablets 579
- Vaseretic Tablets 1559
- Zestoretic 2274

Hydrocodone Bitartrate (Increases phenobarbital effects). Products include:
- Anexsia 5/500 Tablets 2196
- Anexsia 7.5/650 Tablets 2197
- Azdone Tablets 844
- Codiclear DH Syrup 845
- Codimal DH Syrup 846

- Damason-P ... 1356
- Hycodan Syrup, Tablets ... 927
- Hycomine Compound Tablets ... 929
- Hycomine Syrup ... 927
- Hycotuss Expectorant Syrup ... 930
- Hydrocet Capsules ... 835
- Lortab ASA Tablets ... 2414
- Lortab ... 2412
- Ru-Tuss with Hydrocodone ... 694
- Triaminic Expectorant DH ... 1995
- Vicodin Tablets ... 1187
- Vicodin ES Tablets ... 1189
- Zydone Capsules ... 941

Hydrocodone Polistirex (Increases phenobarbital effects). Products include:

- Tussionex Extended-Release Suspension ... 988

Hydrocortisone (Efficacy impaired by phenytoin; increases phenobarbital effects). Products include:

- AK-Spore H.C. ... ⊙ 206
- Bactine Hydrocortisone Anti-Itch Cream ... ▣ 625
- CaldeCORT Anti-Itch Hydrocortisone Spray ... ▣ 560
- Carmol HC Cream 1% ... 2296
- Cortaid Spray ... ▣ 735
- Cortenema ... 2244
- Cortisporin Ointment ... 758
- Cortisporin Ophthalmic Ointment Sterile ... 758
- Cortisporin Ophthalmic Suspension Sterile ... 759
- Cortisporin Otic Solution Sterile ... 760
- Cortisporin Otic Suspension Sterile ... 760
- Cortizone-5 Creme & Ointment ... ▣ 732
- Dermolate Anti-Itch Cream ... ▣ 697
- Eldecort Cream 1.0% ... 1113
- Eldecort Cream 1.0% and 2.5% ... 1113
- Fungoid HC Creme ... 1770
- Hydrocortone Tablets ... 1482
- Hytone ... 909
- LazerSporin-C Solution ... 1770
- Massengill Medicated Soft Cloth Towelettes ... 2192
- Nutracort Cream & Lotion ... 1684
- PediOtic Suspension Sterile ... 797
- Synacort Creams 1%, 2.5% ... 2296
- Vanoxide-HC Acne Lotion ... 911
- Vioform-Hydrocortisone Cream and Mild Cream ... 889
- Vioform-Hydrocortisone Ointment ... 889
- VōSoL HC Otic Solution ... 2392
- Vytone Cream 1% ... 911

Hydrocortisone Acetate (Efficacy impaired by phenytoin; increases phenobarbital effects). Products include:

- Analpram-HC Rectal Cream 1% and 2.5% ... 970
- Anusol-HC Cream ... 1690
- Anusol-HC Suppositories ... 1691
- Caldecort ... ▣ 560
- Carmol HC Cream 1% ... 2296
- Chloromycetin Hydrocortisone Ophthalmic ... 1694
- Coly-Mycin S Otic w/Neomycin & Hydrocortisone ... 1708
- Cortaid ... ▣ 735
- Cortef Feminine Itch Cream ... ▣ 735
- Corticaine ... ▣ 682
- Cortifoam ... 1827
- Cortisporin Cream ... 757
- Epifoam ... 1828
- Gynecort 5 Creme ... ▣ 556
- Hydrocortone Acetate Sterile Suspension ... 1479
- Lanacort 5 Creme and Ointment ... ▣ 557
- Mantadil Cream ... 789
- Ophthocort ... ⊙ 301
- Orabase HCA Oral Paste ... 890
- Pramosone Cream, Lotion & Ointment ... 971
- ProctoCream-HC ... 1834
- Proctofoam-HC ... 1835

Hydrocortisone Sodium Phosphate (Efficacy impaired by phenytoin; increases phenobarbital effects). Products include:

- Hydrocortone Phosphate Injection, Sterile ... 1481

Hydrocortisone Sodium Succinate (Efficacy impaired by phenytoin; increases phenobarbital effects). Products include:

- Solu-Cortef Sterile Powder ... 2361

Hydroflumethiazide (Increased phenytoin serum levels). Products include:

- Diucardin Tablets ... 2450
- Saluron ... 718
- Salutensin/Salutensin-Demi ... 719

Hydroxyzine Hydrochloride (Increases phenobarbital effects). Products include:

- Atarax Tablets & Syrup ... 1941
- Marax Tablets & DF Syrup ... 1954
- Vistaril Intramuscular Solution ... 1970

Imipramine Hydrochloride (Increases phenobarbital effects; tricyclic antidepressants may precipitate seizures in some patients; phenytoin dosage may need to be adjusted). Products include:

- Tofranil Ampuls ... 1038
- Tofranil Tablets ... 1039

Imipramine Pamoate (Increases phenobarbital effects; tricyclic antidepressants may precipitate seizures in some patients; phenytoin dosage may need to be adjusted). Products include:

- Tofranil-PM Capsules ... 1041

Isocarboxazid (Increases phenobarbital effects). Products include:

- Marplan Tablets ... 1906

Isoniazid (Increased phenytoin levels). Products include:

- INH Tablets ... 868
- Rifamate Capsules ... 1347

Levonorgestrel (Efficacy impaired by phenytoin). Products include:

- Levlen/Tri-Levlen ... 665
- Nordette-21 Tablets ... 2481
- Nordette-28 Tablets ... 2483
- Norplant System ... 2484
- Levlen/Tri-Levlen ... 665
- Triphasil-21 Tablets ... 2527
- Triphasil-28 Tablets ... 2532

Levorphanol Tartrate (Increases phenobarbital effects). Products include:

- Levo-Dromoran ... 1906

Lorazepam (Increases phenobarbital effects). Products include:

- Ativan Injection ... 2432
- Ativan Tablets ... 2434

Loxapine Hydrochloride (Increases phenobarbital effects). Products include:

- Loxitane ... 1213

Loxapine Succinate (Increases phenobarbital effects). Products include:

- Loxitane Capsules ... 1213

Magnesium Salicylate (Increased phenytoin levels). Products include:

- Doan's - Extra-Strength Analgesic ... ▣ 549
- Doan's - Regular Strength Analgesic ... ▣ 549
- Mobigesic Analgesic Tablets ... ▣ 507

Maprotiline Hydrochloride (Tricyclic antidepressants may precipitate seizures in some patients; phenytoin dosage may need to be adjusted). Products include:

- Ludiomil Tablets ... 874

Meperidine Hydrochloride (Increases phenobarbital effects). Products include:

- Demerol ... 2047
- Mepergan Injection ... 2479

Meprobamate (Increases phenobarbital effects). Products include:

- Deprol Tablets ... 2382
- Equagesic Tablets ... 2451
- Miltown Tablets ... 2386
- PMB 200 and PMB 400 ... 2504

Mesoridazine (Increased phenytoin levels; increases phenobarbital effects). Products include:

- Serentil ... 686

Mestranol (Efficacy impaired by phenytoin). Products include:

- Enovid ... 2161
- Norethin ... 2133
- Norinyl ... 2304
- Ortho-Novum ... 1667

Methadone Hydrochloride (Increases phenobarbital effects). Products include:

- Dolophine Hydrochloride Ampoules & Vials ... 1260
- Dolophine Hydrochloride Tablets ... 1261
- Methadone Hydrochloride Diskets ... 1284
- Methadone Hydrochloride Oral Solution & Tablets ... 1987

Methdilazine Hydrochloride (Increases phenobarbital effects). Products include:

- Tacaryl Syrup & Tablets ... 2409

Methsuximide (Increases phenytoin serum levels). Products include:

- Celontin ... 1692

Methyclothiazide (Increased phenytoin serum levels). Products include:

- Enduron Tablets ... 517
- Enduronyl ... 518

Methylphenidate Hydrochloride (Increased phenytoin serum levels). Products include:

- Ritalin ... 880

Methylprednisolone Acetate (Efficacy impaired by phenytoin; increases phenobarbital effects). Products include:

- Depo-Medrol Sterile Aqueous Suspension ... 2334

Methylprednisolone Sodium Succinate (Efficacy impaired by phenytoin; increases phenobarbital effects). Products include:

- Solu-Medrol Sterile Powder ... 2363

Molindone Hydrochloride (Interferes with absorption of phenytoin; increases phenobarbital effects). Products include:

- Moban Tablets & Concentrate ... 932

Morphine Sulfate (Increases phenobarbital effects). Products include:

- Astramorph/PF Injection, USP (Preservative-Free) ... 618
- Duramorph ... 960
- Infumorph 200 and Infumorph 500 Sterile Solutions ... 962
- MS Contin Tablets ... 1814
- MSIR ... 1817
- Oramorph SR (Morphine Sulfate Sustained Release Tablets) ... 1988
- Roxanol ... 1991

Nizatidine (Increases phenytoin serum levels). Products include:

- Axid Pulvules ... 1246

Norethindrone (Efficacy impaired by phenytoin). Products include:

- Brevicon ... 2304
- Jenest-28 Tablets ... 1636
- Micronor Tablets ... 1667
- Modicon ... 1667
- Norethin ... 2133
- Norinyl ... 2304
- Norlutin ... 1755
- Nor-Q D Tablets ... 2304
- Ortho-Novum ... 1667
- Ovcon ... 1391
- Tri-Norinyl ... 2304

Norethynodrel (Efficacy impaired by phenytoin). Products include:

- Enovid ... 2161

Norgestimate (Increased phenytoin levels; efficacy impaired by phenytoin). Products include:

- Ortho-Cyclen Tablets ... 1658

Norgestrel (Efficacy impaired by phenytoin). Products include:

- Lo/Ovral Tablets ... 2471
- Lo/Ovral-28 Tablets ... 2476
- Ovral Tablets ... 2490
- Ovral-28 Tablets ... 2491
- Ovrette Tablets ... 2492

Nortriptyline Hydrochloride (Tricyclic antidepressants may precipitate seizures in some patients; phenytoin dosage may need to be adjusted). Products include:

- Pamelor ... 2019

Opium Alkaloids (Increases phenobarbital effects). Products include:

- B & O No. 15A & No. 16A Supprettes ... 2395
- Pantopon Injectable ... 1911

Oxazepam (Increases phenobarbital effects). Products include:

- Serax Capsules ... 2522
- Serax Tablets ... 2522

Oxycodone Hydrochloride (Increases phenobarbital effects). Products include:

- Percocet Tablets ... 950
- Percodan ... 951
- Roxicodone Tablets, Oral Solution & Intensol (Oxycodone) ... 1992
- Tylox Capsules ... 1382

Perphenazine (Increased phenytoin levels; increases phenobarbital effects). Products include:

- Etrafon ... 2087
- Triavil Tablets ... 1556
- Trilafon ... 2123

Phenelzine Sulfate (Increases phenobarbital effects). Products include:

- Nardil ... 1742

Phensuximide (Increases phenytoin serum levels). Products include:

- Milontin Kapseals ... 1741

Phenylbutazone (Increased phenytoin levels). Products include:

- Butazolidin Capsules & Tablets ... 1027

Polyestradiol Phosphate (Increased phenytoin levels; efficacy impaired by phenytoin). Products include:

- Estradurin ... 2452

Polythiazide (Increased phenytoin serum levels). Products include:

- Minizide Capsules ... 1779
- Renese Tablets ... 1785
- Renese-R Tablets ... 1786

Prazepam (Increases phenobarbital effects). Products include:

- Centrax ... 1693

Prednisolone Acetate (Efficacy impaired by phenytoin; increases phenobarbital effects). Products include:

- AK-Cide Sterile Ophthalmic Ointment & Suspension ... ⊙ 202
- Blephamide Liquifilm Sterile Ophthalmic Suspension ... 586
- Blephamide S.O.P. Sterile Ophthalmic Ointment ... 586
- Cetapred Ointment ... ⊙ 220
- ⅛% Econopred & 1% Econopred Plus ... ⊙ 217
- Isopto Cetapred Suspension ... ⊙ 220
- Metimyd ... ⊙ 306
- Poly-Pred Liquifilm ... ⊙ 250
- Pred Forte ... ⊙ 252
- Pred Mild ... ⊙ 254
- Pred-G Liquifilm Sterile Ophthalmic Suspension ... ⊙ 252
- Pred-G S.O.P. Sterile Ophthalmic Ointment ... ⊙ 253
- Vasocidin Ointment ... ⊙ 275

Prednisolone Sodium Phosphate (Efficacy impaired by phenytoin; increases phenobarbital effects). Products include:

- AK-Pred ... ⊙ 205
- Hydeltrasol Injection, Sterile ... 1476
- Inflamase ... ⊙ 274
- Pediapred Oral Liquid ... 987
- Vasocidin Ophthalmic Solution ... ⊙ 276

Prednisolone Tebutate (Efficacy impaired by phenytoin; increases phenobarbital effects). Products include:

- Hydeltra-T.B.A. Sterile Suspension 1478

Prednisone (Efficacy impaired by phenytoin; increases phenobarbital effects). Products include:
- Deltasone Tablets ... 2332

Prochlorperazine (Increased phenytoin levels; increases phenobarbital effects). Products include:
- Compazine ... 2201

Promethazine Hydrochloride (Increased phenytoin levels; increases phenobarbital effects). Products include:
- Mepergan Injection ... 2479
- Phenergan with Codeine ... 2497
- Phenergan with Dextromethorphan 2499
- Phenergan Injection ... 2493
- Phenergan Suppositories ... 2496
- Phenergan Syrup ... 2495
- Phenergan Tablets ... 2496
- Phenergan VC ... 2500
- Phenergan VC with Codeine ... 2501

Propoxyphene Hydrochloride (Increases phenobarbital effects). Products include:
- Darvon ... 1256
- Wygesic Tablets ... 2540

Propoxyphene Napsylate (Increases phenobarbital effects). Products include:
- Darvon-N/Darvocet-N ... 1254

Protriptyline Hydrochloride (Tricyclic antidepressants may precipitate seizures in some patients; phenytoin dosage may need to be adjusted). Products include:
- Vivactil Tablets ... 1567

Pyrilamine Maleate (Increases phenobarbital effects). Products include:
- Codimal ... 846
- 4-Way Fast Acting Nasal Spray - Original Formula (regular & mentholated) & Metered Spray Pump (regular) ... 751
- Maximum Strength Midol Multi-Symptom Menstrual Formula ... ▣ 571
- Maximum Strength Midol PMS Premenstrual Syndrome Formula ... ▣ 570
- Regular Strength Midol Multi-Symptom Menstrual Formula ... ▣ 570
- Prefrin-A ... ⊙ 255
- Prēmsyn PMS Capsules & Caplets ▣ 547
- Primatene Tablets-M Formula ... 2421
- Robitussin Night Relief ... ▣ 677
- Ru-Tuss with Hydrocodone ... 694
- Triaminic Expectorant DH ... 1995
- Triaminic Oral Infant Drops ... 1996

Pyrilamine Tannate (Increases phenobarbital effects). Products include:
- Rynatan ... 2387

Quinestrol (Increased phenytoin levels; efficacy impaired by phenytoin). Products include:
- Estrovis ... 1721

Quinidine Gluconate (Efficacy impaired by phenytoin). Products include:
- Quinaglute Dura-Tabs Tablets ... 663

Quinidine Polygalacturonate (Efficacy impaired by phenytoin). Products include:
- Cardioquin Tablets ... 1812

Quinidine Sulfate (Efficacy impaired by phenytoin). Products include:
- Quinidex Extentabs ... 1868

Ranitidine Hydrochloride (Increases phenytoin serum levels). Products include:
- Zantac Injection and Zantac Injection Premixed ... 1063
- Zantac ... 1065

Rauwolfia Serpentina (Increases phenobarbital effects). Products include:
- Raudixin Tablets ... 1803
- Rauzide Tablets ... 1804

Rescinnamine (Increases phenobarbital effects).
- No products indexed under this heading.

Reserpine (Increases phenobarbital effects). Products include:
- Diupres Tablets ... 1461
- Hydromox R Tablets ... 1209
- Hydropres Tablets ... 1485
- Renese-R Tablets ... 1786
- Salutensin/Salutensin-Demi ... 719
- Ser-Ap-Es Tablets ... 881
- Serpasil Tablets ... 883
- Serpasil-Apresoline Tablets ... 884
- Serpasil-Esidrix Tablets ... 886

Rifampin (Efficacy impaired by phenytoin). Products include:
- Rifadin ... 1345
- Rifamate Capsules ... 1347
- Rimactane Capsules ... 879

Salsalate (Increased phenytoin levels). Products include:
- Disalcid ... 1310
- Mono-Gesic Tablets ... 846
- Salflex ... 839

Selegiline Hydrochloride (Increases phenobarbital effects). Products include:
- Eldepryl ... 2250

Sodium Valproate (Increased or decreased phenytoin levels).

Sucralfate (Decreases phenytoin serum levels). Products include:
- Carafate Tablets ... 1326

Sufentanil Citrate (Increases phenobarbital effects). Products include:
- Sufenta Injection ... 1147

Sulfamethizole (Increased phenytoin serum levels). Products include:
- Thiosulfil Forte Tablets ... 2526
- Urobiotic-250 Capsules ... 1968

Sulfamethoxazole (Increased phenytoin serum levels). Products include:
- Azo Gantanol Tablets ... 1887
- Bactrim DS Tablets ... 1891
- Bactrim I.V. Infusion ... 1889
- Bactrim ... 1891
- Gantanol ... 1899
- Septra ... 813
- Septra I.V. Infusion ... 808
- Septra I.V. Infusion ADD-Vantage Vials ... 810
- Septra ... 813

Sulfasalazine (Increased phenytoin serum levels). Products include:
- Azulfidine Tablets, EN-tabs, Oral Suspension ... 1157

Sulfinpyrazone (Increased phenytoin serum levels). Products include:
- Anturane ... 853

Sulfisoxazole (Increased phenytoin serum levels). Products include:
- Azo Gantrisin Tablets ... 1888
- Gantrisin Tablets ... 1901
- Pediazole ... 1973

Sulfisoxazole Diolamine (Increased phenytoin serum levels). Products include:
- Gantrisin Ophthalmic Ointment/Solution ... 1900

Terfenadine (Increases phenobarbital effects). Products include:
- Seldane Tablets ... 1349
- Seldane-D Extended-Release Tablets ... 1350

Theophylline (Efficacy impaired by phenytoin). Products include:
- Bronkaid Tablets ... ▣ 757
- Bronkolixir ... ▣ 761
- Bronkotabs Tablets ... ▣ 762
- Constant-T Tablets ... 1029
- Marax Tablets & DF Syrup ... 1954
- Primatene Tablets ... 2421
- Quibron Capsules ... 713
- Quibron-T ... 714
- Quibron-T/SR ... 716
- Theolair Liquid ... 1317
- Theo-Organidin Elixir ... 2391

Theophylline Anhydrous (Efficacy impaired by phenytoin). Products include:
- Aerolate ... 994
- Primatene Tablets-M Formula ... ▣ 753
- Primatene Tablets-Regular Formula ... 2421
- Respbid Tablets ... 684
- Slo-bid Gyrocaps ... 1847
- T-PHYL (Uniphyl) 200 mg Tablets 1820
- Tedral SA ... 1765
- Theo-24 ... 2179
- Theo-Dur Sprinkle ... 1168
- Theo-Dur Extended-Release Tablets ... 1166
- Theolair Tablets ... 1317
- Theolair-SR Tablets ... 1319
- TheoX Extended-Release Tablets ... 841
- Uniphyl 400 mg Tablets ... 1823

Theophylline Calcium Salicylate (Efficacy impaired by phenytoin). Products include:
- Quadrinal Tablets ... 1183

Theophylline Sodium Glycinate (Efficacy impaired by phenytoin). Products include:
- Asbron G ... 1997

Thioridazine Hydrochloride (Increased phenytoin levels; increases phenobarbital effects). Products include:
- Mellaril ... 2011

Thiothixene (Increases phenobarbital effects). Products include:
- Navane Capsules and Concentrate 1954
- Navane Intramuscular ... 1956

Tolazamide (Increased phenytoin serum levels). Products include:
- Tolinase Tablets ... 2365

Tolbutamide (Increased phenytoin serum levels; increased phenytoin levels). Products include:
- Orinase Tablets ... 2354

Tranylcypromine Sulfate (Increases phenobarbital effects). Products include:
- Parnate Tablets ... 2222

Trazodone Hydrochloride (Increased phenytoin serum levels). Products include:
- Desyrel and Desyrel Dividose ... 1404

Triamcinolone (Efficacy impaired by phenytoin; increases phenobarbital effects).
- No products indexed under this heading.

Triamcinolone Acetonide (Efficacy impaired by phenytoin; increases phenobarbital effects). Products include:
- Aristocort A ... 1010
- Azmacort Inhaler ... 1837
- Kenalog Cream, Lotion & Ointment 2401
- Kenalog-10 Injection ... 2402
- Kenalog-40 Injection ... 2403
- Kenalog in Orabase ... 604
- Kenalog Spray ... 2401
- Mycolog II Cream and Ointment ... 2407
- Mytrex Cream & Ointment ... 2080
- Nasacort Nasal Inhaler ... 1844

Triamcinolone Diacetate (Efficacy impaired by phenytoin; increases phenobarbital effects). Products include:
- Aristocort Suspension ... 1008

Triamcinolone Hexacetonide (Efficacy impaired by phenytoin; increases phenobarbital effects). Products include:
- Aristospan Suspension ... 1011

Trifluoperazine Hydrochloride (Increased phenytoin levels; increases phenobarbital effects). Products include:
- Stelazine ... 2226

Trimeprazine Tartrate (Increases phenobarbital effects). Products include:
- Temaril Tablets, Syrup and Spansule Sustained Release Capsules 1085

Trimipramine Maleate (Tricyclic antidepressants may precipitate seizures in some patients; phenytoin dosage may need to be adjusted). Products include:
- Surmontil Capsules ... 2524

Tripelennamine Hydrochloride (Increases phenobarbital effects). Products include:
- PBZ Tablets & Elixir ... 1037
- PBZ-SR Tablets ... 1037

Triprolidine Hydrochloride (Increases phenobarbital effects). Products include:
- Actidil ... ▣ 538
- Actifed Capsules ... ▣ 539
- Actifed Plus Caplets ... ▣ 539
- Actifed Plus Tablets ... ▣ 540
- Actifed with Codeine Cough Syrup .. 752
- Actifed Syrup ... ▣ 540
- Actifed Tablets ... ▣ 540
- Actifed 12-Hour Capsules ... ▣ 539

Valproic Acid (Increased or decreased phenytoin levels). Products include:
- Depakene Capsules & Syrup ... 511

Vitamin D (Efficacy impaired by phenytoin). Products include:
- Bugs Bunny Children's Chewable Vitamins (Sugar Free) ... ▣ 625
- Bugs Bunny With Extra C Children's Chewable Vitamins (Sugar Free) ... ▣ 626
- Bugs Bunny Plus Iron Children's Chewable Vitamins (Sugar Free) ▣ 625
- Calderol Capsules ... 1635
- Caltrate 600 + Iron & Vitamin D ... 1198
- Caltrate 600 + Vitamin D ... 1197
- Caltrate, Jr. Tablets ... 1198
- Flintstones Children's Chewable Vitamins ... ▣ 625
- Flintstones Children's Chewable Vitamins With Extra C ... ▣ 626
- Flintstones Children's Chewable Vitamins Plus Iron ... ▣ 625
- Natalins Rx ... 1391
- Natalins Tablets ... 1391
- One-A-Day Essential Vitamins ... ▣ 627
- One-A-Day Maximum Formula Vitamins and Minerals ... ▣ 627
- One-A-Day Plus Extra C Vitamins .. ▣ 627
- Os-Cal 250+D Tablets ... ▣ 597
- Os-Cal 500+D Tablets ... ▣ 597
- Os-Cal Fortified Tablets ... ▣ 597
- Os-Cal Plus Tablets ... ▣ 597
- Posture-D 600 mg ... 2420
- Stressgard Stress Formula Vitamins ... ▣ 628
- Tri-Vi-Flor 1.0 mg Vitamins with Fluoride Chewable Tablets ... 1400
- Tri-Vi-Flor Drops ... 1400
- Tri-Vi-Sol Vitamin Drops ... ▣ 614
- Tri-Vi-Sol Vitamin Drops with Iron ▣ 614
- Vi-Daylin ADC Vitamins Drops ... 1980
- Vi-Daylin ADC Vitamins + Iron Drops ... 1980
- Vi-Daylin/F ADC Vitamins Drops With Fluoride ... 1981
- Vi-Daylin/F ADC Vitamins + Iron Drops With Fluoride ... 1981
- Within Women's Formula Multivitamin with Calcium, Extra Iron and Zinc ... ▣ 628
- Zymacap Capsules ... ▣ 670

Warfarin Sodium (Efficacy impaired by phenytoin). Products include:
- Coumadin Injection & Tablets ... 944
- Panwarfin Tablets ... 547

DILATRATE-SR
(Isosorbide Dinitrate) ... 1827

May interact with calcium channel blockers and certain other agents. Compounds in these categories include:

Alcohol (Enhanced hypotensive effects).

Bepridil Hydrochloride (Marked orthostatic hypotension). Products include:
- Vascor (200, 300 and 400 mg) Tablets ... 1383

(▣ Described in PDR For Nonprescription Drugs) (⊙ Described in PDR For Ophthalmology)

Diltiazem Hydrochloride (Marked orthostatic hypotension). Products include:
Cardizem Tablets-30 mg, 60 mg, 90 mg and 120 mg 1329
Cardizem SR Capsules-60 mg, 90 mg and 120 mg 1327

Felodipine (Marked orthostatic hypotension). Products include:
Plendil Extended-Release Tablets 1526

Isradipine (Marked orthostatic hypotension). Products include:
DynaCirc Capsules 2004

Nicardipine Hydrochloride (Marked orthostatic hypotension). Products include:
Cardene Capsules 2290

Nifedipine (Marked orthostatic hypotension). Products include:
Adalat Capsules (10 mg and 20 mg) 1587
Procardia Capsules 1781
Procardia XL Tablets 1783

Nimodipine (Marked orthostatic hypotension). Products include:
Nimotop Capsules 1607

Verapamil Hydrochloride (Marked orthostatic hypotension). Products include:
Calan SR Caplets 2157
Calan Tablets 2155
Isoptin Injectable 1177
Isoptin Oral Tablets 1179
Isoptin SR Sustained Release Tablets 1181
Verelan Capsules 1243
Verelan Capsules 2535

DILAUDID COUGH SYRUP
(Hydromorphone Hydrochloride) 1174
May interact with central nervous system depressants, tricyclic antidepressants, and certain other agents. Compounds in these categories include:

Alcohol (Additive CNS depression).

Alfentanil Hydrochloride (Additive CNS depression). Products include:
Alfenta Injection 1131

Alprazolam (Additive CNS depression). Products include:
Xanax Tablets 2367

Amitriptyline Hydrochloride (Additive CNS depression). Products include:
Elavil 2269
Endep Tablets 1927
Etrafon 2087
Limbitrol 1933
Triavil Tablets 1556

Amoxapine (Additive CNS depression). Products include:
Asendin Tablets 1196

Aprobarbital (Additive CNS depression). Products include:
Alurate Elixir 1883

Buprenorphine (Additive CNS depression).
No products indexed under this heading.

Buspirone Hydrochloride (Additive CNS depression). Products include:
BuSpar 1401

Butabarbital (Additive CNS depression). Products include:
Pyridium Plus 1764

Butalbital (Additive CNS depression). Products include:
Esgic-Plus Tablets 1002
Esgic Tablets & Capsules 1001
Fioricet Tablets 2006
Fiorinal Capsules 2007
Fiorinal with Codeine Capsules 2008
Fiorinal Tablets 2007
Phrenilin 838
Sedapap Tablets 50 mg/650 mg 1360

Chlordiazepoxide (Additive CNS depression). Products include:
Libritabs Tablets 1930
Limbitrol 1933
Menrium Tablets 1934

Chlordiazepoxide Hydrochloride (Additive CNS depression). Products include:
Librax Capsules 1929
Librium Capsules 1931
Librium Injectable 1932

Chlorpromazine (Additive CNS depression). Products include:
Thorazine 2234

Chlorprothixene (Additive CNS depression). Products include:
Taractan Tablets 1920

Chlorprothixene Hydrochloride (Additive CNS depression). Products include:
Taractan 1920

Chlorprothixene Lactate (Additive CNS depression). Products include:
Taractan Concentrate 1920

Clomipramine Hydrochloride (Additive CNS depression). Products include:
Anafranil Capsules 650

Clorazepate Dipotassium (Additive CNS depression). Products include:
Tranxene 556

Codeine (Additive CNS depression). Products include:
Calcidrine Syrup 506

Codeine Phosphate (Additive CNS depression). Products include:
Actifed with Codeine Cough Syrup 752
Cheracol Cough Syrup 1853
Codimal PH Syrup 846
Dimetane-DC Cough Syrup 1857
Empirin with Codeine Phosphate Nos. 2, 3 & 4 764
Fiorinal with Codeine Capsules 2008
Isoclor Expectorant 982
Naldecon CX Adult Liquid 521
Novahistine DH 1342
Novahistine Expectorant 1343
Nucofed Capsules 2219
Nucofed Expectorant 2219
Nucofed Pediatric Expectorant 2220
Nucofed Syrup 2219
Phenaphen with Codeine Capsules 1865
Phenaphen-650 with Codeine Tablets 1866
Phenergan with Codeine 2497
Phenergan VC with Codeine 2501
Robitussin A-C Syrup 1875
Robitussin-DAC Syrup 1875
Ryna 741
Soma Compound w/Codeine Tablets 2390
Triaminic Expectorant w/Codeine 1996
Tussi-Organidin Liquid 2391
Tylenol with Codeine 1381

Codeine Polistirex (Additive CNS depression).
No products indexed under this heading.

Desipramine Hydrochloride (Additive CNS depression). Products include:
Norpramin Tablets 1340

Dezocine (Additive CNS depression).

Diazepam (Additive CNS depression). Products include:
Valium Injectable 1937
Valium Tablets 1939
Valrelease Capsules 1923

Doxepin Hydrochloride (Additive CNS depression). Products include:
Sinequan 1960

Droperidol (Additive CNS depression). Products include:
Inapsine Injection 1140
Innovar Injection 1141

Enflurane (Additive CNS depression). Products include:
Ethrane 599

Estazolam (Additive CNS depression). Products include:
ProSom Tablets 554

Ethchlorvynol (Additive CNS depression). Products include:
Placidyl Capsules 553

Ethinamate (Additive CNS depression).
No products indexed under this heading.

Fentanyl (Additive CNS depression). Products include:
Duragesic Transdermal System 1133

Fentanyl Citrate (Additive CNS depression). Products include:
Innovar Injection 1141
Sublimaze Injection 1146

Fluphenazine Decanoate (Additive CNS depression). Products include:
Prolixin Decanoate 1795

Fluphenazine Enanthate (Additive CNS depression). Products include:
Prolixin Enanthate 1796

Fluphenazine Hydrochloride (Additive CNS depression). Products include:
Prolixin Elixir 1793
Prolixin Injection 1791
Prolixin Oral Concentrate 1792
Prolixin Tablets 1793

Flurazepam Hydrochloride (Additive CNS depression). Products include:
Dalmane Capsules 1927

Glutethimide (Additive CNS depression).
No products indexed under this heading.

Haloperidol (Additive CNS depression). Products include:
Haldol Injection, Tablets and Concentrate 1373

Haloperidol Decanoate (Additive CNS depression). Products include:
Haldol Decanoate 1375

Hydrocodone Bitartrate (Additive CNS depression). Products include:
Anexsia 5/500 Tablets 2196
Anexsia 7.5/650 Tablets 2197
Azdöne Tablets 844
Codiclear DH Syrup 845
Codimal DH Syrup 846
Damason-P 1356
Hycodan Syrup, Tablets 927
Hycomine Compound Tablets 929
Hycomine Syrup 927
Hycotuss Expectorant Syrup 930
Hydrocet Capsules 835
Lortab ASA Tablets 2414
Lortab 2412
Ru-Tuss with Hydrocodone 694
Triaminic Expectorant DH 1995
Vicodin Tablets 1187
Vicodin ES Tablets 1189
Zydone Capsules 941

Hydrocodone Polistirex (Additive CNS depression). Products include:
Tussionex Extended-Release Suspension 988

Hydroxyzine Hydrochloride (Additive CNS depression). Products include:
Atarax Tablets & Syrup 1941
Marax Tablets & DF Syrup 1954
Vistaril Intramuscular Solution 1970

Imipramine Hydrochloride (Additive CNS depression). Products include:
Tofranil Ampuls 1038
Tofranil Tablets 1039

Imipramine Pamoate (Additive CNS depression). Products include:
Tofranil-PM Capsules 1041

Isoflurane (Additive CNS depression). Products include:
Forane 600

Ketamine Hydrochloride (Additive CNS depression). Products include:
Ketalar 1726

Levorphanol Tartrate (Additive CNS depression). Products include:
Levo-Dromoran 1906

Lorazepam (Additive CNS depression). Products include:
Ativan Injection 2432
Ativan Tablets 2434

Loxapine Hydrochloride (Additive CNS depression). Products include:
Loxitane 1213

Loxapine Succinate (Additive CNS depression). Products include:
Loxitane Capsules 1213

Maprotiline Hydrochloride (Additive CNS depression). Products include:
Ludiomil Tablets 874

Meperidine Hydrochloride (Additive CNS depression). Products include:
Demerol 2047
Mepergan Injection 2479

Mephobarbital (Additive CNS depression). Products include:
Mebaral Tablets 2061

Meprobamate (Additive CNS depression). Products include:
Deprol Tablets 2382
Equagesic Tablets 2451
Miltown Tablets 2386
PMB 200 and PMB 400 2504

Mesoridazine (Additive CNS depression). Products include:
Serentil 686

Methadone Hydrochloride (Additive CNS depression). Products include:
Dolophine Hydrochloride Ampoules & Vials 1260
Dolophine Hydrochloride Tablets 1261
Methadone Hydrochloride Diskets 1284
Methadone Hydrochloride Oral Solution & Tablets 1987

Methohexital Sodium (Additive CNS depression). Products include:
Brevital Sodium Vials 1248

Methoxyflurane (Additive CNS depression).
No products indexed under this heading.

Midazolam Hydrochloride (Additive CNS depression). Products include:
Versed Injection 1924

Molindone Hydrochloride (Additive CNS depression). Products include:
Moban Tablets & Concentrate 932

Morphine Sulfate (Additive CNS depression). Products include:
Astramorph/PF Injection, USP (Preservative-Free) 618
Duramorph 960
Infumorph 200 and Infumorph 500 Sterile Solutions 962
MS Contin Tablets 1814
MSIR 1817
Oramorph SR (Morphine Sulfate Sustained Release Tablets) 1988
Roxanol 1991

Nortriptyline Hydrochloride (Additive CNS depression). Products include:
Pamelor 2019

Opium Alkaloids (Additive CNS depression). Products include:
B & O No. 15A & No. 16A Supprettes 2395
Pantopon Injectable 1911

Oxazepam (Additive CNS depression). Products include:
Serax Capsules 2522
Serax Tablets 2522

Oxycodone Hydrochloride (Additive CNS depression). Products include:
- Percocet Tablets ... 950
- Percodan ... 951
- Roxicodone Tablets, Oral Solution & Intensol (Oxycodone) ... 1992
- Tylox Capsules ... 1382

Pentobarbital Sodium (Additive CNS depression). Products include:
- Nembutal Sodium Capsules ... 534
- Nembutal Sodium Solution ... 536
- Nembutal Sodium Suppositories ... 538

Perphenazine (Additive CNS depression). Products include:
- Etrafon ... 2087
- Triavil Tablets ... 1556
- Trilafon ... 2123

Phenobarbital (Additive CNS depression). Products include:
- Arco-Lase Plus Tablets ... 607
- Bellergal-S Tablets ... 1998
- Bronkolixir ... 761
- Bronkotabs Tablets ... 762
- Donnatal ... 1858
- Donnatal Extentabs ... 1859
- Donnatal Tablets ... 1858
- Donnazyme Tablets ... 1860
- Kinesed Tablets ... 2272
- Phenobarbital Elixir and Tablets ... 1293
- Primatene Tablets-P Formula ... 2421
- Quadrinal Tablets ... 1183
- Tedral SA ... 1765

Prazepam (Additive CNS depression). Products include:
- Centrax ... 1693

Prochlorperazine (Additive CNS depression). Products include:
- Compazine ... 2201

Promethazine Hydrochloride (Additive CNS depression). Products include:
- Mepergan Injection ... 2479
- Phenergan with Codeine ... 2497
- Phenergan with Dextromethorphan 2499
- Phenergan Injection ... 2493
- Phenergan Suppositories ... 2496
- Phenergan Syrup ... 2495
- Phenergan Tablets ... 2496
- Phenergan VC ... 2500
- Phenergan VC with Codeine ... 2501

Propofol (Additive CNS depression). Products include:
- Diprivan Injection ... 2267

Propoxyphene Hydrochloride (Additive CNS depression). Products include:
- Darvon ... 1256
- Wygesic Tablets ... 2540

Propoxyphene Napsylate (Additive CNS depression). Products include:
- Darvon-N/Darvocet-N ... 1254

Protriptyline Hydrochloride (Additive CNS depression). Products include:
- Vivactil Tablets ... 1567

Quazepam (Additive CNS depression). Products include:
- Doral Tablets ... 2383

Secobarbital Sodium (Additive CNS depression). Products include:
- Seconal Sodium Pulvules ... 1296

Sufentanil Citrate (Additive CNS depression). Products include:
- Sufenta Injection ... 1147

Temazepam (Additive CNS depression). Products include:
- Restoril Capsules ... 2023

Thiamylal Sodium (Additive CNS depression). Products include:
- Surital Ampoules, Steri-Vials ... 1764

Thioridazine Hydrochloride (Additive CNS depression). Products include:
- Mellaril ... 2011

Thiothixene (Additive CNS depression). Products include:
- Navane Capsules and Concentrate 1954
- Navane Intramuscular ... 1956

Triazolam (Additive CNS depression). Products include:
- Halcion Tablets ... 2340

Trifluoperazine Hydrochloride (Additive CNS depression). Products include:
- Stelazine ... 2226

Trimipramine Maleate (Additive CNS depression). Products include:
- Surmontil Capsules ... 2524

DILAUDID HYDROCHLORIDE AMPULES
(Hydromorphone Hydrochloride) ...1173
May interact with central nervous system depressants, tricyclic antidepressants, and certain other agents. Compounds in these categories include:

Alcohol (Additive CNS depression).

Alfentanil Hydrochloride (Additive CNS depression). Products include:
- Alfenta Injection ... 1131

Alprazolam (Additive CNS depression). Products include:
- Xanax Tablets ... 2367

Amitriptyline Hydrochloride (Additive CNS depression). Products include:
- Elavil ... 2269
- Endep Tablets ... 1927
- Etrafon ... 2087
- Limbitrol ... 1933
- Triavil Tablets ... 1556

Amoxapine (Additive CNS depression). Products include:
- Asendin Tablets ... 1196

Aprobarbital (Additive CNS depression). Products include:
- Alurate Elixir ... 1883

Buprenorphine (Additive CNS depression).
- No products indexed under this heading.

Buspirone Hydrochloride (Additive CNS depression). Products include:
- BuSpar ... 1401

Butabarbital (Additive CNS depression). Products include:
- Pyridium Plus ... 1764

Butalbital (Additive CNS depression). Products include:
- Esgic-Plus Tablets ... 1002
- Esgic Tablets & Capsules ... 1001
- Fioricet Tablets ... 2006
- Fiorinal Capsules ... 2007
- Fiorinal with Codeine Capsules ... 2008
- Fiorinal Tablets ... 2007
- Phrenilin ... 838
- Sedapap Tablets 50 mg/650 mg .. 1360

Chlordiazepoxide (Additive CNS depression). Products include:
- Libritabs Tablets ... 1930
- Limbitrol ... 1933
- Menrium Tablets ... 1934

Chlordiazepoxide Hydrochloride (Additive CNS depression). Products include:
- Librax Capsules ... 1929
- Librium Capsules ... 1931
- Librium Injectable ... 1932

Chlorpromazine (Additive CNS depression). Products include:
- Thorazine ... 2234

Chlorprothixene (Additive CNS depression). Products include:
- Taractan Tablets ... 1920

Chlorprothixene Hydrochloride (Additive CNS depression). Products include:
- Taractan ... 1920

Chlorprothixene Lactate (Additive CNS depression). Products include:
- Taractan Concentrate ... 1920

Clomipramine Hydrochloride (Additive CNS depression). Products include:
- Anafranil Capsules ... 650

Clorazepate Dipotassium (Additive CNS depression). Products include:
- Tranxene ... 556

Codeine (Additive CNS depression). Products include:
- Calcidrine Syrup ... 506

Codeine Phosphate (Additive CNS depression). Products include:
- Actifed with Codeine Cough Syrup.. 752
- Cheracol Cough Syrup ... 1853
- Codimal PH Syrup ... 846
- Dimetane-DC Cough Syrup ... 1857
- Empirin with Codeine Phosphate Nos. 2, 3 & 4 ... 764
- Fiorinal with Codeine Capsules ... 2008
- Isoclor Expectorant ... 982
- Naldecon CX Adult Liquid ... 521
- Novahistine DH ... 1342
- Novahistine Expectorant ... 1343
- Nucofed Capsules ... 2219
- Nucofed Expectorant ... 2219
- Nucofed Pediatric Expectorant ... 2220
- Nucofed Syrup ... 2219
- Phenaphen with Codeine Capsules 1865
- Phenaphen-650 with Codeine Tablets ... 1866
- Phenergan with Codeine ... 2497
- Phenergan VC with Codeine ... 2501
- Robitussin A-C Syrup ... 1875
- Robitussin-DAC Syrup ... 1875
- Ryna ... 741
- Soma Compound w/Codeine Tablets ... 2390
- Triaminic Expectorant w/Codeine .. 1996
- Tussi-Organidin Liquid ... 2391
- Tylenol with Codeine ... 1381

Codeine Polistirex (Additive CNS depression).
- No products indexed under this heading.

Desipramine Hydrochloride (Additive CNS depression). Products include:
- Norpramin Tablets ... 1340

Dezocine (Additive CNS depression).

Diazepam (Additive CNS depression). Products include:
- Valium Injectable ... 1937
- Valium Tablets ... 1939
- Valrelease Capsules ... 1923

Doxepin Hydrochloride (Additive CNS depression). Products include:
- Sinequan ... 1960

Droperidol (Additive CNS depression). Products include:
- Inapsine Injection ... 1140
- Innovar Injection ... 1141

Enflurane (Additive CNS depression). Products include:
- Ethrane ... 599

Estazolam (Additive CNS depression). Products include:
- ProSom Tablets ... 554

Ethchlorvynol (Additive CNS depression). Products include:
- Placidyl Capsules ... 553

Ethinamate (Additive CNS depression).
- No products indexed under this heading.

Fentanyl (Additive CNS depression). Products include:
- Duragesic Transdermal System ... 1133

Fentanyl Citrate (Additive CNS depression). Products include:
- Innovar Injection ... 1141
- Sublimaze Injection ... 1146

Fluphenazine Decanoate (Additive CNS depression). Products include:
- Prolixin Decanoate ... 1795

Fluphenazine Enanthate (Additive CNS depression). Products include:
- Prolixin Enanthate ... 1796

Fluphenazine Hydrochloride (Additive CNS depression). Products include:
- Prolixin Elixir ... 1793
- Prolixin Injection ... 1791
- Prolixin Oral Concentrate ... 1792
- Prolixin Tablets ... 1793

Flurazepam Hydrochloride (Additive CNS depression). Products include:
- Dalmane Capsules ... 1927

Glutethimide (Additive CNS depression).
- No products indexed under this heading.

Haloperidol (Additive CNS depression). Products include:
- Haldol Injection, Tablets and Concentrate ... 1373

Haloperidol Decanoate (Additive CNS depression). Products include:
- Haldol Decanoate ... 1375

Hydrocodone Bitartrate (Additive CNS depression). Products include:
- Anexsia 5/500 Tablets ... 2196
- Anexsia 7.5/650 Tablets ... 2197
- Azdōne Tablets ... 844
- Codiclear DH Syrup ... 845
- Codimal DH Syrup ... 846
- Damason-P ... 1356
- Hycodan Syrup, Tablets ... 927
- Hycomine Compound Tablets ... 929
- Hycomine Syrup ... 927
- Hycotuss Expectorant Syrup ... 930
- Hydrocet Capsules ... 835
- Lortab ASA Tablets ... 2414
- Lortab ... 2412
- Ru-Tuss with Hydrocodone ... 694
- Triaminic Expectorant DH ... 1995
- Vicodin Tablets ... 1187
- Vicodin ES Tablets ... 1189
- Zydone Capsules ... 941

Hydrocodone Polistirex (Additive CNS depression). Products include:
- Tussionex Extended-Release Suspension ... 988

Hydroxyzine Hydrochloride (Additive CNS depression). Products include:
- Atarax Tablets & Syrup ... 1941
- Marax Tablets & DF Syrup ... 1954
- Vistaril Intramuscular Solution ... 1970

Imipramine Hydrochloride (Additive CNS depression). Products include:
- Tofranil Ampuls ... 1038
- Tofranil Tablets ... 1039

Imipramine Pamoate (Additive CNS depression). Products include:
- Tofranil-PM Capsules ... 1041

Isoflurane (Additive CNS depression). Products include:
- Forane ... 600

Ketamine Hydrochloride (Additive CNS depression). Products include:
- Ketalar ... 1726

Levorphanol Tartrate (Additive CNS depression). Products include:
- Levo-Dromoran ... 1906

Lorazepam (Additive CNS depression). Products include:
- Ativan Injection ... 2432
- Ativan Tablets ... 2434

Loxapine Hydrochloride (Additive CNS depression). Products include:
- Loxitane ... 1213

Loxapine Succinate (Additive CNS depression). Products include:
- Loxitane Capsules ... 1213

Maprotiline Hydrochloride (Additive CNS depression). Products include:
- Ludiomil Tablets ... 874

Meperidine Hydrochloride (Additive CNS depression). Products include:
Demerol 2047
Mepergan Injection 2479

Mephobarbital (Additive CNS depression). Products include:
Mebaral Tablets 2061

Meprobamate (Additive CNS depression). Products include:
Deprol Tablets 2382
Equagesic Tablets 2451
Miltown Tablets 2386
PMB 200 and PMB 400 2504

Mesoridazine (Additive CNS depression). Products include:
Serentil 686

Methadone Hydrochloride (Additive CNS depression). Products include:
Dolophine Hydrochloride Ampoules & Vials 1260
Dolophine Hydrochloride Tablets 1261
Methadone Hydrochloride Diskets 1284
Methadone Hydrochloride Oral Solution & Tablets 1987

Methohexital Sodium (Additive CNS depression). Products include:
Brevital Sodium Vials 1248

Methoxyflurane (Additive CNS depression).
No products indexed under this heading.

Midazolam Hydrochloride (Additive CNS depression). Products include:
Versed Injection 1924

Molindone Hydrochloride (Additive CNS depression). Products include:
Moban Tablets & Concentrate 932

Morphine Sulfate (Additive CNS depression). Products include:
Astramorph/PF Injection, USP (Preservative-Free) 618
Duramorph 960
Infumorph 200 and Infumorph 500 Sterile Solutions 962
MS Contin Tablets 1814
MSIR 1817
Oramorph SR (Morphine Sulfate Sustained Release Tablets) 1988
Roxanol 1991

Nortriptyline Hydrochloride (Additive CNS depression). Products include:
Pamelor 2019

Opium Alkaloids (Additive CNS depression). Products include:
B & O No. 15A & No. 16A Supprettes 2395
Pantopon Injectable 1911

Oxazepam (Additive CNS depression). Products include:
Serax Capsules 2522
Serax Tablets 2522

Oxycodone Hydrochloride (Additive CNS depression). Products include:
Percocet Tablets 950
Percodan 951
Roxicodone Tablets, Oral Solution & Intensol (Oxycodone) 1992
Tylox Capsules 1382

Pentobarbital Sodium (Additive CNS depression). Products include:
Nembutal Sodium Capsules 534
Nembutal Sodium Solution 536
Nembutal Sodium Suppositories 538

Perphenazine (Additive CNS depression). Products include:
Etrafon 2087
Triavil Tablets 1556
Trilafon 2123

Phenobarbital (Additive CNS depression). Products include:
Arco-Lase Plus Tablets 607
Bellergal-S Tablets 1998
Bronkolixir ⓑⓓ 761
Bronkotabs Tablets ⓑⓓ 762
Donnatal 1858
Donnatal Extentabs 1859
Donnatal Tablets 1858
Donnazyme Tablets 1860
Kinesed Tablets 2272
Phenobarbital Elixir and Tablets 1293
Primatene Tablets-P Formula 2421
Quadrinal Tablets 1183
Tedral SA 1765

Prazepam (Additive CNS depression). Products include:
Centrax 1693

Prochlorperazine (Additive CNS depression). Products include:
Compazine 2201

Promethazine Hydrochloride (Additive CNS depression). Products include:
Mepergan Injection 2479
Phenergan with Codeine 2497
Phenergan with Dextromethorphan 2499
Phenergan Injection 2493
Phenergan Suppositories 2496
Phenergan Syrup 2495
Phenergan Tablets 2496
Phenergan VC 2500
Phenergan VC with Codeine 2501

Propofol (Additive CNS depression). Products include:
Diprivan Injection 2267

Propoxyphene Hydrochloride (Additive CNS depression). Products include:
Darvon 1256
Wygesic Tablets 2540

Propoxyphene Napsylate (Additive CNS depression). Products include:
Darvon-N/Darvocet-N 1254

Protriptyline Hydrochloride (Additive CNS depression). Products include:
Vivactil Tablets 1567

Quazepam (Additive CNS depression). Products include:
Doral Tablets 2383

Secobarbital Sodium (Additive CNS depression). Products include:
Seconal Sodium Pulvules 1296

Sufentanil Citrate (Additive CNS depression). Products include:
Sufenta Injection 1147

Temazepam (Additive CNS depression). Products include:
Restoril Capsules 2023

Thiamylal Sodium (Additive CNS depression). Products include:
Surital Ampoules, Steri-Vials 1764

Thioridazine Hydrochloride (Additive CNS depression). Products include:
Mellaril 2011

Thiothixene (Additive CNS depression). Products include:
Navane Capsules and Concentrate 1954
Navane Intramuscular 1956

Triazolam (Additive CNS depression). Products include:
Halcion Tablets 2340

Trifluoperazine Hydrochloride (Additive CNS depression). Products include:
Stelazine 2226

Trimipramine Maleate (Additive CNS depression). Products include:
Surmontil Capsules 2524

DILAUDID INJECTION
(Hydromorphone Hydrochloride) 1173
See **Dilaudid Hydrochloride Ampules**

DILAUDID MULTIPLE DOSE VIALS (STERILE SOLUTION)
(Hydromorphone Hydrochloride) 1173
See **Dilaudid Hydrochloride Ampules**

DILAUDID POWDER
(Hydromorphone Hydrochloride) 1173
See **Dilaudid Hydrochloride Ampules**

DILAUDID RECTAL SUPPOSITORIES
(Hydromorphone Hydrochloride) 1173
See **Dilaudid Hydrochloride Ampules**

DILAUDID TABLETS
(Hydromorphone Hydrochloride) 1173
See **Dilaudid Hydrochloride Ampules**

DILAUDID-HP INJECTION
(Hydromorphone Hydrochloride) 1175
May interact with central nervous system depressants, nondepolarizing neuromuscular blocking agents, and certain other agents. Compounds in these categories include:

Alcohol (Additive depressant effects).

Alfentanil Hydrochloride (Additive depressant effects). Products include:
Alfenta Injection 1131

Alprazolam (Additive depressant effects). Products include:
Xanax Tablets 2367

Aprobarbital (Additive depressant effects). Products include:
Alurate Elixir 1883

Atracurium Besylate (Increased respiratory depression; enhanced action of neuromuscular blocking agents). Products include:
Tracrium Injection 817

Buprenorphine (Additive depressant effects).
No products indexed under this heading.

Buspirone Hydrochloride (Additive depressant effects). Products include:
BuSpar 1401

Butabarbital (Additive depressant effects). Products include:
Pyridium Plus 1764

Butalbital (Additive depressant effects). Products include:
Esgic-Plus Tablets 1002
Esgic Tablets & Capsules 1001
Fioricet Tablets 2006
Fiorinal Capsules 2007
Fiorinal with Codeine Capsules 2008
Fiorinal Tablets 2007
Phrenilin 838
Sedapap Tablets 50 mg/650 mg 1360

Chlordiazepoxide (Additive depressant effects). Products include:
Libritabs Tablets 1930
Limbitrol 1933
Menrium Tablets 1934

Chlordiazepoxide Hydrochloride (Additive depressant effects). Products include:
Librax Capsules 1929
Librium Capsules 1931
Librium Injectable 1932

Chlorpromazine (Additive depressant effects). Products include:
Thorazine 2234

Chlorprothixene (Additive depressant effects). Products include:
Taractan Tablets 1920

Chlorprothixene Hydrochloride (Additive depressant effects). Products include:
Taractan 1920

Chlorprothixene Lactate (Additive depressant effects). Products include:
Taractan Concentrate 1920

Clorazepate Dipotassium (Additive depressant effects). Products include:
Tranxene 556

Codeine (Additive depressant effects). Products include:
Calcidrine Syrup 506

Codeine Phosphate (Additive depressant effects). Products include:
Actifed with Codeine Cough Syrup 752
Cheracol Cough Syrup 1853
Codimal PH Syrup 846
Dimetane-DC Cough Syrup 1857
Empirin with Codeine Phosphate Nos. 2, 3 & 4 764
Fiorinal with Codeine Capsules 2008
Isoclor Expectorant 982
Naldecon CX Adult Liquid ⓑⓓ 521
Novahistine DH 1342
Novahistine Expectorant 1343
Nucofed Capsules 2219
Nucofed Expectorant 2219
Nucofed Pediatric Expectorant 2220
Nucofed Syrup 2219
Phenaphen with Codeine Capsules 1865
Phenaphen-650 with Codeine Tablets 1866
Phenergan with Codeine 2497
Phenergan VC with Codeine 2501
Robitussin A-C Syrup 1875
Robitussin-DAC Syrup 1875
Ryna ⓑⓓ 741
Soma Compound w/Codeine Tablets 2390
Triaminic Expectorant w/Codeine 1996
Tussi-Organidin Liquid 2391
Tylenol with Codeine 1381

Codeine Polistirex (Additive depressant effects).
No products indexed under this heading.

Dezocine (Additive depressant effects).

Diazepam (Additive depressant effects). Products include:
Valium Injectable 1937
Valium Tablets 1939
Valrelease Capsules 1923

Droperidol (Additive depressant effects). Products include:
Inapsine Injection 1140
Innovar Injection 1141

Enflurane (Additive depressant effects). Products include:
Ethrane 599

Estazolam (Additive depressant effects). Products include:
ProSom Tablets 554

Ethchlorvynol (Additive depressant effects). Products include:
Placidyl Capsules 553

Ethinamate (Additive depressant effects).
No products indexed under this heading.

Fentanyl (Additive depressant effects). Products include:
Duragesic Transdermal System 1133

Fentanyl Citrate (Additive depressant effects). Products include:
Innovar Injection 1141
Sublimaze Injection 1146

Fluphenazine Decanoate (Additive depressant effects). Products include:
Prolixin Decanoate 1795

Fluphenazine Enanthate (Additive depressant effects). Products include:
Prolixin Enanthate 1796

Fluphenazine Hydrochloride (Additive depressant effects). Products include:
Prolixin Elixir 1793
Prolixin Injection 1791
Prolixin Oral Concentrate 1792
Prolixin Tablets 1793

Flurazepam Hydrochloride (Additive depressant effects). Products include:
Dalmane Capsules ... 1927

Glutethimide (Additive depressant effects).
No products indexed under this heading.

Haloperidol (Additive depressant effects). Products include:
Haldol Injection, Tablets and Concentrate ... 1373

Haloperidol Decanoate (Additive depressant effects). Products include:
Haldol Decanoate ... 1375

Hydrocodone Bitartrate (Additive depressant effects). Products include:
Anexsia 5/500 Tablets ... 2196
Anexsia 7.5/650 Tablets ... 2197
Azdōne Tablets ... 844
Codiclear DH Syrup ... 845
Codimal DH Syrup ... 846
Damason-P ... 1356
Hycodan Syrup, Tablets ... 927
Hycomine Compound Tablets ... 929
Hycomine Syrup ... 927
Hycotuss Expectorant Syrup ... 930
Hydrocet Capsules ... 835
Lortab ASA Tablets ... 2414
Lortab ... 2412
Ru-Tuss with Hydrocodone ... 694
Triaminic Expectorant DH ... 1995
Vicodin Tablets ... 1187
Vicodin ES Tablets ... 1189
Zydone Capsules ... 941

Hydrocodone Polistirex (Additive depressant effects). Products include:
Tussionex Extended-Release Suspension ... 988

Hydroxyzine Hydrochloride (Additive depressant effects). Products include:
Atarax Tablets & Syrup ... 1941
Marax Tablets & DF Syrup ... 1954
Vistaril Intramuscular Solution ... 1970

Isoflurane (Additive depressant effects). Products include:
Forane ... 600

Ketamine Hydrochloride (Additive depressant effects). Products include:
Ketalar ... 1726

Levorphanol Tartrate (Additive depressant effects). Products include:
Levo-Dromoran ... 1906

Lorazepam (Additive depressant effects). Products include:
Ativan Injection ... 2432
Ativan Tablets ... 2434

Loxapine Hydrochloride (Additive depressant effects). Products include:
Loxitane ... 1213

Loxapine Succinate (Additive depressant effects). Products include:
Loxitane Capsules ... 1213

Meperidine Hydrochloride (Additive depressant effects). Products include:
Demerol ... 2047
Mepergan Injection ... 2479

Mephobarbital (Additive depressant effects). Products include:
Mebaral Tablets ... 2061

Meprobamate (Additive depressant effects). Products include:
Deprol Tablets ... 2382
Equagesic Tablets ... 2451
Miltown Tablets ... 2386
PMB 200 and PMB 400 ... 2504

Mesoridazine (Additive depressant effects). Products include:
Serentil ... 686

Methadone Hydrochloride (Additive depressant effects). Products include:
Dolophine Hydrochloride Ampoules & Vials ... 1260
Dolophine Hydrochloride Tablets ... 1261
Methadone Hydrochloride Diskets ... 1284
Methadone Hydrochloride Oral Solution & Tablets ... 1987

Methohexital Sodium (Additive depressant effects). Products include:
Brevital Sodium Vials ... 1248

Methoxyflurane (Additive depressant effects).
No products indexed under this heading.

Metocurine Iodide (Increased respiratory depression; enhanced action of neuromuscular blocking agents). Products include:
Metubine Iodide Vials ... 1285

Midazolam Hydrochloride (Additive depressant effects). Products include:
Versed Injection ... 1924

Molindone Hydrochloride (Additive depressant effects). Products include:
Moban Tablets & Concentrate ... 932

Morphine Sulfate (Additive depressant effects). Products include:
Astramorph/PF Injection, USP (Preservative-Free) ... 618
Duramorph ... 960
Infumorph 200 and Infumorph 500 Sterile Solutions ... 962
MS Contin Tablets ... 1814
MSIR ... 1817
Oramorph SR (Morphine Sulfate Sustained Release Tablets) ... 1988
Roxanol ... 1991

Opium Alkaloids (Additive depressant effects). Products include:
B & O No. 15A & No. 16A Supprettes ... 2395
Pantopon Injectable ... 1911

Oxazepam (Additive depressant effects). Products include:
Serax Capsules ... 2522
Serax Tablets ... 2522

Oxycodone Hydrochloride (Additive depressant effects). Products include:
Percocet Tablets ... 950
Percodan ... 951
Roxicodone Tablets, Oral Solution & Intensol (Oxycodone) ... 1992
Tylox Capsules ... 1382

Pancuronium Bromide Injection (Increased respiratory depression; enhanced action of neuromuscular blocking agents).
No products indexed under this heading.

Pentobarbital Sodium (Additive depressant effects). Products include:
Nembutal Sodium Capsules ... 534
Nembutal Sodium Solution ... 536
Nembutal Sodium Suppositories ... 538

Perphenazine (Additive depressant effects). Products include:
Etrafon ... 2087
Triavil Tablets ... 1556
Trilafon ... 2123

Phenobarbital (Additive depressant effects). Products include:
Arco-Lase Plus Tablets ... 607
Bellergal-S Tablets ... 1998
Bronkolixir ... 761
Bronkotabs Tablets ... 762
Donnatal ... 1858
Donnatal Extentabs ... 1859
Donnatal Tablets ... 1858
Donnazyme Tablets ... 1860
Kinesed Tablets ... 2272
Phenobarbital Elixir and Tablets ... 1293
Primatene Tablets-P Formula ... 2421
Quadrinal Tablets ... 1183
Tedral SA ... 1765

Prazepam (Additive depressant effects). Products include:
Centrax ... 1693

Prochlorperazine (Additive depressant effects). Products include:
Compazine ... 2201

Promethazine Hydrochloride (Additive depressant effects). Products include:
Mepergan Injection ... 2479
Phenergan with Codeine ... 2497
Phenergan with Dextromethorphan ... 2499
Phenergan Injection ... 2493
Phenergan Suppositories ... 2496
Phenergan Syrup ... 2495
Phenergan Tablets ... 2496
Phenergan VC ... 2500
Phenergan VC with Codeine ... 2501

Propofol (Additive depressant effects). Products include:
Diprivan Injection ... 2267

Propoxyphene Hydrochloride (Additive depressant effects). Products include:
Darvon ... 1256
Wygesic Tablets ... 2540

Propoxyphene Napsylate (Additive depressant effects). Products include:
Darvon-N/Darvocet-N ... 1254

Quazepam (Additive depressant effects). Products include:
Doral Tablets ... 2383

Secobarbital Sodium (Additive depressant effects). Products include:
Seconal Sodium Pulvules ... 1296

Sufentanil Citrate (Additive depressant effects). Products include:
Sufenta Injection ... 1147

Temazepam (Additive depressant effects). Products include:
Restoril Capsules ... 2023

Thiamylal Sodium (Additive depressant effects). Products include:
Surital Ampoules, Steri-Vials ... 1764

Thioridazine Hydrochloride (Additive depressant effects). Products include:
Mellaril ... 2011

Thiothixene (Additive depressant effects). Products include:
Navane Capsules and Concentrate ... 1954
Navane Intramuscular ... 1956

Triazolam (Additive depressant effects). Products include:
Halcion Tablets ... 2340

Trifluoperazine Hydrochloride (Additive depressant effects). Products include:
Stelazine ... 2226

Vecuronium Bromide (Increased respiratory depression; enhanced action of neuromuscular blocking agents). Products include:
Norcuron ... 1642

DILOR-200 TABLETS
(Dyphylline) ... 2079
May interact with xanthine bronchodilators. Compounds in this category include:

Aminophylline (Contraindicated). Products include:
Amesec ... 682
Aminophyllin Tablets ... 2153

Theophylline (Contraindicated). Products include:
Bronkaid Tablets ... 757
Bronkolixir ... 761
Bronkotabs Tablets ... 762
Constant-T Tablets ... 1029
Marax Tablets & DF Syrup ... 1954
Primatene Tablets ... 2421
Quibron Capsules ... 713
Quibron-T ... 714
Quibron-T/SR ... 716
Theolair Liquid ... 1317
Theo-Organidin Elixir ... 2391

Theophylline Anhydrous (Contraindicated). Products include:
Aerolate ... 994
Primatene Tablets-M Formula ... 753
Primatene Tablets-Regular Formula ... 2421
Respbid Tablets ... 684
Slo-bid Gyrocaps ... 1847
T-PHYL (Uniphyl) 200 mg Tablets ... 1820
Tedral SA ... 1765
Theo-24 ... 2179
Theo-Dur Sprinkle ... 1168
Theo-Dur Extended-Release Tablets ... 1166
Theolair Tablets ... 1317
Theolair-SR Tablets ... 1319
TheoX Extended-Release Tablets ... 841
Uniphyl 400 mg Tablets ... 1823

Theophylline Calcium Salicylate (Contraindicated). Products include:
Quadrinal Tablets ... 1183

Theophylline Sodium Glycinate (Contraindicated). Products include:
Asbron G ... 1997

DILOR-400 TABLETS
(Dyphylline) ... 2079
See **Dilor-200 Tablets**

DILOR-G TABLETS & LIQUID
(Dyphylline, Guaifenesin) ... 2079
May interact with sympathomimetic aerosal brochodilators. Compounds in this category include:

Albuterol (Potential for excessive CNS stimulation). Products include:
Proventil Inhalation Aerosol ... 2117
Ventolin Inhalation Aerosol and Refill ... 583

Albuterol Sulfate (Potential for excessive CNS stimulation). Products include:
Proventil Repetabs Tablets ... 2120
Proventil Solutions for Inhalation 0.5% and 0.083% ... 2118
Proventil Syrup ... 2119
Proventil Tablets ... 2120
Ventolin ... 583

Dobutamine Hydrochloride (Potential for excessive CNS stimulation). Products include:
Dobutrex Solution Vials ... 1259

Dopamine Hydrochloride (Potential for excessive CNS stimulation). Products include:
Intropin Injection ... 930

Ephedrine Hydrochloride (Potential for excessive CNS stimulation). Products include:
Amesec ... 682
Primatene Tablets-M Formula ... 2421
Primatene Tablets-P Formula ... 2421
Primatene Tablets-Regular Formula ... 2421
Quadrinal Tablets ... 1183
Quelidrine Syrup ... 556
Tedral SA ... 1765

Ephedrine Sulfate (Potential for excessive CNS stimulation). Products include:
Bronkaid Tablets ... 757
Bronkolixir ... 761
Bronkotabs Tablets ... 762
Marax Tablets & DF Syrup ... 1954
Pazo Hemorrhoid Ointment & Suppositories ... 752
Vicks Vatronol Nose Drops ... 666

Ephedrine Tannate (Potential for excessive CNS stimulation). Products include:
Rynatuss ... 2388

Epinephrine (Potential for excessive CNS stimulation). Products include:
Ana-Kit Anaphylaxis Emergency Treatment Kit ... 1100
Bronkaid Mist ... 757
EpiPen ... 843

Marcaine Hydrochloride 0.5% with Epinephrine 1:200,000 (as bitartrate) 958
Marcaine Hydrochloride with Epinephrine 1:200,000 2055
Primatene Mist 2420
Sus-Phrine Injection 1006
Xylocaine with Epinephrine Injections 637

Epinephrine Bitartrate (Potential for excessive CNS stimulation). Products include:
AsthmaHaler Mist Epinephrine Bitartrate Bronchodilator ▣ 616
Bronkaid Mist Suspension ▣ 757
Primatene Mist Suspension 2421

Epinephrine Hydrochloride (Potential for excessive CNS stimulation). Products include:
Adrenalin Chloride Solution 1:100 & 1:1,000 1689
Epifrin ⊙ 244
Glaucon ⊙ 218

Isoproterenol Hydrochloride (Potential for excessive CNS stimulation). Products include:
Isuprel Hydrochloride Injection 1:5000 2050
Isuprel Hydrochloride Mistometer 2051
Isuprel Hydrochloride Solution 1:200 & 1:100 2052
Norisodrine Aerotrol 540

Metaproterenol Sulfate (Potential for excessive CNS stimulation). Products include:
Alupent 674
Arm-a-Med Metaproterenol Sulfate Inhalation Solution, USP 617
Metaprel Inhalation Aerosol Bronchodilator 2014
Metaprel Inhalation Solution 2015
Metaprel 2015
Metaproterenol Sulfate Inhalation Solution, USP 912

Metaraminol Bitartrate (Potential for excessive CNS stimulation). Products include:
Aramine Injection 1424

Methoxamine Hydrochloride (Potential for excessive CNS stimulation). Products include:
Vasoxyl Injection 819

Norepinephrine Bitartrate (Potential for excessive CNS stimulation). Products include:
Levophed Bitartrate Injection 2054

Phenylephrine Bitartrate (Potential for excessive CNS stimulation).
No products indexed under this heading.

Phenylephrine Hydrochloride (Potential for excessive CNS stimulation). Products include:
AK-Dilate Solution 2.5% and 10% ⊙ 203
Atrohist Sprinkle Capsules 558
Cerose-DM 2443
Codimal 846
Comhist LA Capsules 1618
Congespirin For Children Aspirin Free Chewable Cold Tablets 748
Cyclomydril ⊙ 216
Deconsal Sprinkle Capsules 559
Dimetane Decongestant ▣ 673
Dristan Decongestant/Antihistamine/ Analgesic Coated Caplets ▣ 749
Dristan Cold Nasal Decongestant/ Antihistamine/ Analgesic Coated Tablets 2419
Dristan Advanced Formula Decongestant/Antihistamine/ Analgesic Tablets ▣ 749
Dristan Nasal Spray, Menthol 2419
Dristan Nasal Spray, Regular and Regular with Metered Pump 2419
Entex Capsules 1623
Entex Liquid 1623
Sinus Excedrin Analgesic, Decongestant Tablets & Caplets 750
Extendryl 994
4-Way Fast Acting Nasal Spray - Original Formula (regular & mentholated) & Metered Spray Pump (regular) 751
Hycomine Compound Tablets 929
Murocoll-2 Sterile Ophthalmic Solution ⊙ 261
Mydfrin 2.5% ⊙ 224
Naldecon Syrup, Tablets, Pediatric Drops and Pediatric Syrup 709
Neo-Synephrine Hydrochloride 1% Carpuject 2063
Neo-Synephrine Hydrochloride 1% Injection 2063
Neo-Synephrine Hydrochloride (Ophthalmic) 2064
Neo-Synephrine ▣ 759
Nōstril Nasal Decongestant ▣ 520
Novahistine Elixir ▣ 596
Phenergan VC 2500
Phenergan VC with Codeine 2501
Prefrin Liquifilm Vasoconstrictor and Lubricant Eye Drops ⊙ 254
Prefrin-A ⊙ 255
Quelidrine Syrup 556
Relief Vasoconstrictor and Lubricant Eye Drops ⊙ 256
Robitussin Night Relief ▣ 677
Ru-Tuss with Hydrocodone 694
Ru-Tuss Tablets 693
Vasosulf ⊙ 279
Vicks Sinex ▣ 665
Zincfrin ⊙ 230

Phenylephrine Tannate (Potential for excessive CNS stimulation). Products include:
Rynatan 2387
Rynatuss 2388

Phenylpropanolamine Hydrochloride (Potential for excessive CNS stimulation). Products include:
A.R.M. Allergy Relief Medicine Caplets ▣ 615
Acutrim ▣ 548
Allerest ▣ 559
BC Cold Powder ▣ 517
Cheracol Plus Head Cold/Cough Formula ▣ 667
Codimal Expectorant 846
Comtrex Multi-Symptom Cold Reliever Tablets/Caplets/Liqui-Gels/Liquid 745
Contac Continuous Action Decongestant/Antihistamine Capsules ▣ 710
Contac Maximum Strength Continuous Action Decongestant/ Antihistamine Caplets ▣ 709
Contac Severe Cold and Flu Formula Caplets ▣ 711
Coricidin 'D' Decongestant Tablets ▣ 695
Coricidin Demilets Tablets for Children ▣ 696
Demazin Nasal Decongestant/ Antihistamine Repetabs Tablets & Syrup ▣ 697
Dexatrim ▣ 733
Dimetane-DC Cough Syrup 1857
Dimetapp Elixir ▣ 673
Dimetapp DM Elixir ▣ 674
Dimetapp Extentabs ▣ 674
Dimetapp Plus Caplets ▣ 675
Dimetapp Tablets ▣ 675
Entex Capsules 1623
Entex LA Tablets 1623
Entex Liquid 1623
4-Way Cold Tablets 750
Hycomine Syrup 927
Naldecon CX Adult Liquid ▣ 521
Naldecon DX Adult Liquid ▣ 521
Naldecon DX Children's Syrup ▣ 522
Naldecon DX Pediatric Drops ▣ 522
Naldecon EX Children's Syrup ▣ 522
Naldecon EX Pediatric Drops ▣ 523
Naldecon Syrup, Tablets, Pediatric Drops and Pediatric Syrup 709
Nolamine Tablets 838
Nolex LA Tablets 838
Ornade Spansule Capsules 2221
Orthoxicol Cough Syrup ▣ 668
Propagest 839
Pyrroxate Capsules ▣ 669
Robitussin-CF ▣ 676
Ru-Tuss II Capsules 693
Ru-Tuss with Hydrocodone 694
Ru-Tuss Tablets 693
Sine-Off Sinus Medicine Tablets-Aspirin Formula ▣ 722
Sinulin 840
St. Joseph Cold Tablets for Children ▣ 704
Tavist-D Tablets 2035
Triaminic Allergy Tablets ▣ 688
Triaminic Chewables ▣ 688
Triaminic Cold Tablets ▣ 688
Triaminic Expectorant ▣ 688
Triaminic Expectorant w/Codeine 1996
Triaminic Expectorant DH 1995
Triaminic Oral Infant Drops 1996
Triaminic Syrup ▣ 689
Triaminic-12 Tablets ▣ 690
Triaminic-DM Syrup ▣ 689
Triaminicin Tablets ▣ 690
Triaminicol Multi-Symptom Cold Tablets ▣ 691
Triaminicol Multi-Symptom Relief ▣ 691
Tuss-Ornade Liquid 2242
Tuss-Ornade Spansule Capsules 2242
Tylenol Cold Medication, Effervescent Tablets 1369

Pirbuterol Acetate (Potential for excessive CNS stimulation). Products include:
Maxair Inhaler 1311

Pseudoephedrine Hydrochloride (Potential for excessive CNS stimulation). Products include:
Actifed Capsules ▣ 539
Actifed Plus Caplets ▣ 539
Actifed Plus Tablets ▣ 540
Actifed with Codeine Cough Syrup 752
Actifed Syrup ▣ 540
Actifed Tablets ▣ 540
Actifed 12-Hour Capsules ▣ 539
Advil Cold & Sinus Caplets (formerly CoAdvil) 2416
Allerest ▣ 559
Anatuss LA Tablets 1359
Benadryl Decongestant Elixir ▣ 635
Benadryl Decongestant ▣ 635
Benadryl Plus ▣ 636
Benadryl Plus Nighttime ▣ 637
Benylin Decongestant ▣ 638
Brexin L.A. Capsules 2078
Bromfed Capsules (Timed Release) 1615
Bromfed Syrup ▣ 628
Bromfed 1615
CoAdvil ▣ 748
Allergy-Sinus Comtrex Multi-Symptom Allergy Sinus Formula Tablets & Caplets 746
Cough Formula Comtrex 746
Comtrex Multi-Symptom Cold Reliever Tablets/Caplets/Liqui-Gels/Liquid 745
Day-Night Comtrex 747
Non-Drowsy Comtrex 747
Congess 994
Congestac Caplets ▣ 617
Contac Jr. Children's Cold Medicine ▣ 712
Contac Nighttime Cold Medicine ▣ 713
Contac Sinus Caplets Maximum Strength Non-Drowsy Formula ▣ 710
Contac Sinus Tablets Maximum Strength Non-Drowsy Formula ▣ 710
Deconamine 663
Deconsal II Tablets 559
Dimacol Caplets ▣ 672
Dimetane-DX Cough Syrup 1858
Dorcol Children's Cough Syrup ▣ 685
Dorcol Children's Decongestant Liquid ▣ 685
Dorcol Children's Liquid Cold Formula ▣ 686
Maximum Strength Dristan Decongestant/Analgesic Coated Caplets ▣ 750
No Drowsiness Dristan Cold Nasal Decongestant/Analgesic Coated Caplets 2420
Dristan Sinus Caplets 2419
Sinus Excedrin Analgesic, Decongestant Tablets & Caplets ▣ 533
Fedahist Gyrocaps 2145
Fedahist Timecaps 2145
Guaifed 1615
Guaifed Syrup ▣ 629
Isoclor Expectorant 982
Isoclor Timesule Capsules ▣ 561
Kronofed-A 970
Medi-Flu Caplet, Liquid ▣ 640
Novafed A Capsules 1342
Novafed Capsules 1342
Novahistine DH 1342
Novahistine DMX ▣ 595
Novahistine Expectorant 1343
Nucofed Capsules 2219
Nucofed Expectorant 2219
Nucofed Pediatric Expectorant 2220
Nucofed Syrup 2219
Ornex Caplets ▣ 618
PediaCare Allergy Relief Formula Liquid 1362
PediaCare Cough-Cold Formula Liquid 1362
PediaCare Infants' Oral Decongestant Drops 1362
PediaCare Night Rest Cough-Cold Formula Liquid 1362
PediaCare 6-12 Cough-Cold Formula Chewable Tablets 1362
Robitussin-DAC Syrup 1875
Robitussin-PE ▣ 677
Rondec 1975
Rondec-DM 1976
Rondec-TR Tablet 1975
Ru-Tuss DE Tablets 694
Ryna ▣ 741
Seldane-D Extended-Release Tablets 1350
Sinarest ▣ 562
Sine-Aid Maximum Strength Sinus Headache Caplets 1365
Sine-Aid Maximum Strength Sinus Headache Tablets 1365
Sine-Off Maximum Strength Allergy/Sinus Formula Caplets ▣ 721
Sine-Off Maximum Strength No Drowsiness Formula Caplets ▣ 722
Singlet Tablets ▣ 598
Sinutab Maximum Strength ▣ 641
Sinutab Maximum Strength Without Drowsiness Tablets & Caplets ▣ 642
Sinutab Regular Strength Without Drowsiness Formula ▣ 641
St. Joseph Nighttime Cold Medicine ▣ 705
Sudafed Children's Liquid ▣ 543
Sudafed Cough Syrup ▣ 543
Sudafed Plus Liquid ▣ 544
Sudafed Plus Tablets ▣ 545
Sudafed Sinus Caplets ▣ 545
Sudafed Sinus Tablets ▣ 545
Sudafed Tablets, 30 mg ▣ 544
Sudafed Tablets, Adult Strength, 60 mg ▣ 544
Sudafed 12 Hour Capsules ▣ 545
TheraFlu Flu and Cold Medicine ▣ 687
Triaminic Nite Light ▣ 689
Tylenol Allergy Sinus Medication Caplets and Gelcaps, Maximum Strength 1372
Children's Tylenol Cold Liquid Formula and Chewable Tablets 1368
Tylenol Cold & Flu Hot Medication, Packets 1369
Tylenol Cold & Flu No Drowsiness Hot Medication, Packets 1371
Tylenol Cold Medication Caplets and Tablets 1370
Tylenol Cold Medication No Drowsiness Formula Caplets 1370
Tylenol Cold Night Time Medication Liquid 1371
Tylenol Cough Medication Liquid with Decongestant, Maximum Strength 1372
Tylenol, Maximum Strength, Sinus Medication Gelcaps, Caplets and Tablets 1373
Ursinus Inlay-Tabs ▣ 691
Vicks Children's NyQuil ▣ 664
Vicks Daycare ▣ 660
Vicks Formula 44D Decongestant Cough Medicine ▣ 662
Vicks Formula 44M Multi-Symptom Cough Medicine ▣ 662
Vicks NyQuil Nighttime Colds Medicine-Original & Cherry Flavor ▣ 664
Vicks Pediatric Formula 44 Cough & Congestion Medicine ▣ 663
Vicks Pediatric Formula 44m Multi-Symptom Cough & Cold Medicine ▣ 663

Pseudoephedrine Sulfate (Potential for excessive CNS stimulation). Products include:
Afrin Tablets ▣ 693
Chlor-Trimeton Decongestant ▣ 694
Disophrol Chronotab Sustained-Action Tablets ▣ 698
Drixoral Antihistamine/Nasal Decongestant Syrup ▣ 698
Drixoral Non-Drowsy Formula ▣ 699
Drixoral Plus Extended-Release Tablets ▣ 699
Drixoral Sinus ▣ 700
Drixoral Sustained-Action Tablets ▣ 698
Sinutab Allergy Formula Sustained Action Tablets ▣ 640

Trinalin Repetabs Tablets 1170

Terbutaline Sulfate (Potential for excessive CNS stimulation). Products include:

Brethaire Inhaler 1024
Brethine Ampuls 1026
Brethine Tablets 1026
Bricanyl Injection 1324
Bricanyl Tablets 1325

DIMACOL CAPLETS
(Dextromethorphan Hydrobromide, Guaifenesin, Pseudoephedrine Hydrochloride) ◘ 672
May interact with monoamine oxidase inhibitors, sympathomimetic aerosal brochodilators, and certain other agents. Compounds in these categories include:

Albuterol (May produce additive effects and increased toxicity). Products include:

Proventil Inhalation Aerosol 2117
Ventolin Inhalation Aerosol and Refill 583

Albuterol Sulfate (May produce additive effects and increased toxicity). Products include:

Proventil Repetabs Tablets 2120
Proventil Solutions for Inhalation 0.5% and 0.083% 2118
Proventil Syrup 2119
Proventil Tablets 2120
Ventolin 583

Blood Pressure Medications, unspecified (Diminished antihypertensive effects).

No products indexed under this heading.

Dobutamine Hydrochloride (May produce additive effects and increased toxicity). Products include:

Dobutrex Solution Vials 1259

Dopamine Hydrochloride (May produce additive effects and increased toxicity). Products include:

Intropin Injection 930

Ephedrine Hydrochloride (May produce additive effects and increased toxicity). Products include:

Amesec ◘ 682
Primatene Tablets-M Formula 2421
Primatene Tablets-P Formula 2421
Primatene Tablets-Regular Formula 2421
Quadrinal Tablets 1183
Quelidrine Syrup 556
Tedral SA 1765

Ephedrine Sulfate (May produce additive effects and increased toxicity). Products include:

Bronkaid Tablets ◘ 757
Bronkolixir ◘ 761
Bronkotabs Tablets ◘ 762
Marax Tablets & DF Syrup 1954
Pazo Hemorrhoid Ointment & Suppositories 752
Vicks Vatronol Nose Drops ◘ 666

Ephedrine Tannate (May produce additive effects and increased toxicity). Products include:

Rynatuss 2388

Epinephrine (May produce additive effects and increased toxicity). Products include:

Ana-Kit Anaphylaxis Emergency Treatment Kit 1100
Bronkaid Mist ◘ 757
EpiPen 843
Marcaine Hydrochloride 0.5% with Epinephrine 1:200,000 (as bitartrate) 958
Marcaine Hydrochloride with Epinephrine 1:200,000 2055
Primatene Mist 2420
Sus-Phrine Injection 1006
Xylocaine with Epinephrine Injections 637

Epinephrine Bitartrate (May produce additive effects and increased toxicity). Products include:

AsthmaHaler Mist Epinephrine Bitartrate Bronchodilator ◘ 616
Bronkaid Mist Suspension ◘ 757
Primatene Mist Suspension 2421

Epinephrine Hydrochloride (May produce additive effects and increased toxicity). Products include:

Adrenalin Chloride Solution 1:100 & 1:1,000 1689
Epifrin ⊙ 244
Glaucon ⊙ 218

Furazolidone (May produce hypertensive crisis and serious toxicity). Products include:

Furoxone 1855

Isocarboxazid (May produce hypertensive crisis and serious toxicity). Products include:

Marplan Tablets 1906

Metaproterenol Sulfate (May produce additive effects and increased toxicity). Products include:

Alupent 674
Arm-a-Med Metaproterenol Sulfate Inhalation Solution, USP 617
Metaprel Inhalation Aerosol Bronchodilator 2014
Metaprel Inhalation Solution 2015
Metaprel 2015
Metaproterenol Sulfate Inhalation Solution, USP 912

Metaraminol Bitartrate (May produce additive effects and increased toxicity). Products include:

Aramine Injection 1424

Methoxamine Hydrochloride (May produce additive effects and increased toxicity). Products include:

Vasoxyl Injection 819

Norepinephrine Bitartrate (May produce additive effects and increased toxicity). Products include:

Levophed Bitartrate Injection 2054

Phenelzine Sulfate (May produce hypertensive crisis and serious toxicity). Products include:

Nardil 1742

Phentolamine Mesylate (Diminished antihypertensive effects). Products include:

Regitine 878

Phenylephrine Bitartrate (May produce additive effects and increased toxicity).

No products indexed under this heading.

Phenylephrine Hydrochloride (May produce additive effects and increased toxicity). Products include:

AK-Dilate Solution 2.5% and 10% ⊙ 203
Atrohist Sprinkle Capsules 558
Cerose-DM 2443
Codimal 846
Comhist LA Capsules 1618
Congespirin For Children Aspirin Free Chewable Cold Tablets 748
Cyclomydril ⊙ 216
Deconsal Sprinkle Capsules 559
Dimetane Decongestant ◘ 673
Dristan Decongestant/Antihistamine/ Analgesic Coated Caplets ◘ 749
Dristan Cold Nasal Decongestant/ Antihistamine/ Analgesic Coated Tablets 2419
Dristan Advanced Formula Decongestant/Antihistamine/ Analgesic Tablets ◘ 749
Dristan Nasal Spray, Menthol 2419
Dristan Nasal Spray, Regular and Regular with Metered Pump 2419
Entex Capsules 1623
Entex Liquid 1623
Sinus Excedrin Analgesic, Decongestant Tablets & Caplets 750
Extendryl 994
4-Way Fast Acting Nasal Spray - Original Formula (regular & mentholated) & Metered Spray Pump (regular) 751
Hycomine Compound Tablets 929
Murocoll-2 Sterile Ophthalmic Solution ⊙ 261
Mydfrin 2.5% ⊙ 224
Naldecon Syrup, Tablets, Pediatric Drops and Pediatric Syrup 709
Neo-Synephrine Hydrochloride 1% Carpuject 2063
Neo-Synephrine Hydrochloride 1% Injection 2063
Neo-Synephrine Hydrochloride (Ophthalmic) 2064
Neo-Synephrine ◘ 759
Nōstril Nasal Decongestant ◘ 520
Novahistine Elixir ◘ 596
Phenergan VC 2500
Phenergan VC with Codeine 2501
Prefrin Liquifilm Vasoconstrictor and Lubricant Eye Drops ⊙ 254
Prefrin-A ⊙ 255
Quelidrine Syrup 556
Relief Vasoconstrictor and Lubricant Eye Drops ⊙ 256
Robitussin Night Relief ◘ 677
Ru-Tuss with Hydrocodone 694
Ru-Tuss Tablets 693
Vasosulf ⊙ 279
Vicks Sinex ◘ 665
Zincfrin ⊙ 230

Phenylephrine Tannate (May produce additive effects and increased toxicity). Products include:

Rynatan 2387
Rynatuss 2388

Phenylpropanolamine Hydrochloride (May produce additive effects and increased toxicity). Products include:

A.R.M. Allergy Relief Medicine Caplets ◘ 615
Acutrim ◘ 548
Allerest ◘ 559
BC Cold Powder ◘ 517
Cheracol Plus Head Cold/Cough Formula ◘ 667
Codimal Expectorant 846
Comtrex Multi-Symptom Cold Reliever Tablets/Caplets/Liqui-Gels/Liquid 745
Contac Continuous Action Decongestant/Antihistamine Capsules ◘ 710
Contac Maximum Strength Continuous Action Decongestant/ Antihistamine Caplets ◘ 709
Contac Severe Cold and Flu Formula Caplets ◘ 711
Coricidin 'D' Decongestant Tablets ◘ 695
Coricidin Demilets Tablets for Children ◘ 696
Demazin Nasal Decongestant/ Antihistamine Repetabs Tablets & Syrup ◘ 697
Dexatrim ◘ 733
Dimetane-DC Cough Syrup 1857
Dimetapp Elixir ◘ 673
Dimetapp DM Elixir ◘ 674
Dimetapp Extentabs ◘ 674
Dimetapp Plus Caplets ◘ 675
Dimetapp Tablets ◘ 675
Entex Capsules 1623
Entex LA Tablets 1623
Entex Liquid 1623
4-Way Cold Tablets 750
Hycomine Syrup 927
Naldecon CX Adult Liquid ◘ 521
Naldecon DX Adult Liquid ◘ 521
Naldecon DX Children's Syrup ◘ 522
Naldecon DX Pediatric Drops ◘ 522
Naldecon EX Children's Syrup ◘ 522
Naldecon EX Pediatric Drops ◘ 523
Naldecon Syrup, Tablets, Pediatric Drops and Pediatric Syrup 709
Nolamine Tablets 838
Nolex LA Tablets 838
Ornade Spansule Capsules 2221
Orthoxicol Cough Syrup ◘ 668
Propagest 839
Pyrroxate Capsules ◘ 669
Robitussin-CF ◘ 676
Ru-Tuss II Capsules 693
Ru-Tuss with Hydrocodone 694
Ru-Tuss Tablets 693
Sine-Off Sinus Medicine Tablets-Aspirin Formula ◘ 722
Sinulin 840
St. Joseph Cold Tablets for Children ◘ 704
Tavist-D Tablets 2035
Triaminic Allergy Tablets ◘ 688
Triaminic Chewables ◘ 688
Triaminic Cold Tablets ◘ 688
Triaminic Expectorant ◘ 688
Triaminic Expectorant w/Codeine 1996
Triaminic Expectorant DH 1995
Triaminic Oral Infant Drops 1996
Triaminic Syrup ◘ 689
Triaminic-12 Tablets ◘ 690
Triaminic-DM Syrup ◘ 689
Triaminicin Tablets ◘ 690
Triaminicol Multi-Symptom Cold Tablets ◘ 691
Triaminicol Multi-Symptom Relief ◘ 691
Tuss-Ornade Liquid 2242
Tuss-Ornade Spansule Capsules 2242
Tylenol Cold Medication, Effervescent Tablets 1369

Pirbuterol Acetate (May produce additive effects and increased toxicity). Products include:

Maxair Inhaler 1311

Pseudoephedrine Sulfate (May produce additive effects and increased toxicity). Products include:

Afrin Tablets ◘ 693
Chlor-Trimeton Decongestant ◘ 694
Disophrol Chronotab Sustained-Action Tablets ◘ 698
Drixoral Antihistamine/Nasal Decongestant Syrup ◘ 698
Drixoral Non-Drowsy Formula ◘ 699
Drixoral Plus Extended-Release Tablets ◘ 699
Drixoral Sinus ◘ 700
Drixoral Sustained-Action Tablets ◘ 698
Sinutab Allergy Formula Sustained Action Tablets ◘ 640
Trinalin Repetabs Tablets 1170

Selegiline Hydrochloride (May produce hypertensive crisis and serious toxicity). Products include:

Eldepryl 2250

Terbutaline Sulfate (May produce additive effects and increased toxicity). Products include:

Brethaire Inhaler 1024
Brethine Ampuls 1026
Brethine Tablets 1026
Bricanyl Injection 1324
Bricanyl Tablets 1325

Tranylcypromine Sulfate (May produce hypertensive crisis and serious toxicity). Products include:

Parnate Tablets 2222

Trimethaphan Camsylate (Diminished antihypertensive effects). Products include:

Arfonad Ampuls 1887

DIMETANE DECONGESTANT CAPLETS
(Brompheniramine Maleate, Phenylephrine Hydrochloride) ◘ 673
May interact with monoamine oxidase inhibitors, sympathomimetic aerosal brochodilators, and certain other agents. Compounds in these categories include:

Albuterol (May produce additive effects). Products include:

Proventil Inhalation Aerosol 2117
Ventolin Inhalation Aerosol and Refill 583

Albuterol Sulfate (May produce additive effects). Products include:

Proventil Repetabs Tablets 2120
Proventil Solutions for Inhalation 0.5% and 0.083% 2118
Proventil Syrup 2119
Proventil Tablets 2120
Ventolin 583

Alcohol (Do not use concomitantly).

Blood Pressure Medications, unspecified (Diminished antihypertensive effect).

No products indexed under this heading.

Dobutamine Hydrochloride (May produce additive effects). Products include:

- Dobutrex Solution Vials 1259

Dopamine Hydrochloride (May produce additive effects). Products include:

- Intropin Injection 930

Ephedrine Hydrochloride (May produce additive effects). Products include:

- Amesec .... ▣ 682
- Primatene Tablets-M Formula 2421
- Primatene Tablets-P Formula 2421
- Primatene Tablets-Regular Formula 2421
- Quadrinal Tablets 1183
- Quelidrine Syrup 556
- Tedral SA 1765

Ephedrine Sulfate (May produce additive effects). Products include:

- Bronkaid Tablets .... ▣ 757
- Bronkolixir .... ▣ 761
- Bronkotabs Tablets .... ▣ 762
- Marax Tablets & DF Syrup 1954
- Pazo Hemorrhoid Ointment & Suppositories 752
- Vicks Vatronol Nose Drops .... ▣ 666

Ephedrine Tannate (May produce additive effects). Products include:

- Rynatuss 2388

Epinephrine (May produce additive effects). Products include:

- Ana-Kit Anaphylaxis Emergency Treatment Kit 1100
- Bronkaid Mist .... ▣ 757
- EpiPen 843
- Marcaine Hydrochloride 0.5% with Epinephrine 1:200,000 (as bitartrate) 958
- Marcaine Hydrochloride with Epinephrine 1:200,000 2055
- Primatene Mist 2420
- Sus-Phrine Injection 1006
- Xylocaine with Epinephrine Injections 637

Epinephrine Bitartrate (May produce additive effects). Products include:

- AsthmaHaler Mist Epinephrine Bitartrate Bronchodilator .... ▣ 616
- Bronkaid Mist Suspension .... ▣ 757
- Primatene Mist Suspension 2421

Epinephrine Hydrochloride (May produce additive effects). Products include:

- Adrenalin Chloride Solution 1:100 & 1:1,000 1689
- Epifrin .... ⊙ 244
- Glaucon .... ⊙ 218

Furazolidone (May produce hypertensive crisis). Products include:

- Furoxone 1855

Isocarboxazid (May produce hypertensive crisis). Products include:

- Marplan Tablets 1906

Isoproterenol Hydrochloride (May produce additive effects). Products include:

- Isuprel Hydrochloride Injection 1:5000 2050
- Isuprel Hydrochloride Mistometer .. 2051
- Isuprel Hydrochloride Solution 1:200 & 1:100 2052
- Norisodrine Aerotrol 540

Metaproterenol Sulfate (May produce additive effects). Products include:

- Alupent 674
- Arm-a-Med Metaproterenol Sulfate Inhalation Solution, USP 617
- Metaprel Inhalation Aerosol Bronchodilator 2014
- Metaprel Inhalation Solution 2015
- Metaprel 2015
- Metaproterenol Sulfate Inhalation Solution, USP 912

Metaraminol Bitartrate (May produce additive effects). Products include:

- Aramine Injection 1424

Methoxamine Hydrochloride (May produce additive effects). Products include:

- Vasoxyl Injection 819

Norepinephrine Bitartrate (May produce additive effects). Products include:

- Levophed Bitartrate Injection 2054

Phenelzine Sulfate (May produce hypertensive crisis). Products include:

- Nardil 1742

Phenylephrine Bitartrate (May produce additive effects).

- No products indexed under this heading.

Phenylephrine Tannate (May produce additive effects). Products include:

- Rynatan 2387
- Rynatuss 2388

Phenylpropanolamine Hydrochloride (May produce additive effects). Products include:

- A.R.M. Allergy Relief Medicine Caplets .... ▣ 615
- Acutrim .... ▣ 548
- Allerest .... ▣ 559
- BC Cold Powder .... ▣ 517
- Cheracol Plus Head Cold/Cough Formula .... ▣ 667
- Codimal Expectorant 846
- Comtrex Multi-Symptom Cold Reliever Tablets/Caplets/Liqui-Gels/Liquid 745
- Contac Continuous Action Decongestant/Antihistamine Capsules ▣ 710
- Contac Maximum Strength Continuous Action Decongestant/Antihistamine Caplets .... ▣ 709
- Contac Severe Cold and Flu Formula Caplets .... ▣ 711
- Coricidin 'D' Decongestant Tablets .... ▣ 695
- Coricidin Demilets Tablets for Children .... ▣ 696
- Demazin Nasal Decongestant/Antihistamine Repetabs Tablets & Syrup .... ▣ 697
- Dexatrim .... ▣ 733
- Dimetane-DC Cough Syrup 1857
- Dimetapp Elixir .... ▣ 673
- Dimetapp DM Elixir .... ▣ 674
- Dimetapp Extentabs .... ▣ 674
- Dimetapp Plus Caplets .... ▣ 675
- Dimetapp Tablets .... ▣ 675
- Entex Capsules 1623
- Entex LA Tablets 1623
- Entex Liquid 1623
- 4-Way Cold Tablets 750
- Hycomine Syrup 927
- Naldecon CX Adult Liquid .... ▣ 521
- Naldecon DX Adult Liquid .... ▣ 521
- Naldecon DX Children's Syrup .... ▣ 522
- Naldecon DX Pediatric Drops .... ▣ 522
- Naldecon EX Children's Syrup .... ▣ 522
- Naldecon EX Pediatric Drops .... ▣ 523
- Naldecon Syrup, Tablets, Pediatric Drops and Pediatric Syrup 709
- Nolamine Tablets 838
- Nolex LA Tablets 838
- Ornade Spansule Capsules 2221
- Orthoxicol Cough Syrup .... ▣ 668
- Propagest 839
- Pyrroxate Capsules .... ▣ 669
- Robitussin-CF .... ▣ 676
- Ru-Tuss II Capsules 693
- Ru-Tuss with Hydrocodone 694
- Ru-Tuss Tablets 693
- Sine-Off Sinus Medicine Tablets-Aspirin Formula .... ▣ 722
- Sinulin 840
- St. Joseph Cold Tablets for Children .... ▣ 704
- Tavist-D Tablets 2035
- Triaminic Allergy Tablets .... ▣ 688
- Triaminic Chewables .... ▣ 688
- Triaminic Cold Tablets .... ▣ 688
- Triaminic Expectorant .... ▣ 688
- Triaminic Expectorant w/Codeine .. 1996
- Triaminic Expectorant DH 1995
- Triaminic Oral Infant Drops 1996
- Triaminic Syrup .... ▣ 689
- Triaminic-12 Tablets .... ▣ 690
- Triaminic-DM Syrup .... ▣ 689
- Triaminicin Tablets .... ▣ 690
- Triaminicol Multi-Symptom Cold Tablets .... ▣ 691
- Triaminicol Multi-Symptom Relief ▣ 691
- Tuss-Ornade Liquid 2242
- Tuss-Ornade Spansule Capsules 2242
- Tylenol Cold Medication, Effervescent Tablets 1369

Pirbuterol Acetate (May produce additive effects). Products include:

- Maxair Inhaler 1311

Pseudoephedrine Hydrochloride (May produce additive effects). Products include:

- Actifed Capsules .... ▣ 539
- Actifed Plus Caplets .... ▣ 539
- Actifed Plus Tablets .... ▣ 540
- Actifed with Codeine Cough Syrup.. 752
- Actifed Syrup .... ▣ 540
- Actifed Tablets .... ▣ 540
- Actifed 12-Hour Capsules .... ▣ 539
- Advil Cold & Sinus Caplets (formerly CoAdvil) 2416
- Allerest .... ▣ 559
- Anatuss LA Tablets 1359
- Benadryl Decongestant Elixir .... ▣ 635
- Benadryl Decongestant .... ▣ 635
- Benadryl Plus .... ▣ 636
- Benadryl Plus Nighttime .... ▣ 637
- Benylin Decongestant .... ▣ 638
- Brexin L.A. Capsules 2078
- Bromfed Capsules (Timed Release) 1615
- Bromfed Syrup .... ▣ 628
- Bromfed 1615
- CoAdvil .... ▣ 748
- Allergy-Sinus Comtrex Multi-Symptom Allergy Sinus Formula Tablets & Caplets 746
- Cough Formula Comtrex 746
- Comtrex Multi-Symptom Cold Reliever Tablets/Caplets/Liqui-Gels/Liquid 745
- Day-Night Comtrex 747
- Non-Drowsy Comtrex 747
- Congess 994
- Congestac Caplets .... ▣ 617
- Contac Jr. Children's Cold Medicine .... ▣ 712
- Contac Nighttime Cold Medicine .... ▣ 713
- Contac Sinus Caplets Maximum Strength Non-Drowsy Formula .... ▣ 710
- Contac Sinus Tablets Maximum Strength Non-Drowsy Formula .... ▣ 710
- Deconamine 663
- Deconsal II Tablets 559
- Dimacol Caplets .... ▣ 672
- Dimetane-DX Cough Syrup 1858
- Dorcol Children's Cough Syrup .... ▣ 685
- Dorcol Children's Decongestant Liquid .... ▣ 685
- Dorcol Children's Liquid Cold Formula .... ▣ 686
- Maximum Strength Dristan Decongestant/Analgesic Coated Caplets .... ▣ 750
- No Drowsiness Dristan Cold Nasal Decongestant/Analgesic Coated Caplets 2420
- Dristan Sinus Caplets 2419
- Sinus Excedrin Analgesic, Decongestant Tablets & Caplets .... ▣ 533
- Fedahist Gyrocaps 2145
- Fedahist Timecaps 2145
- Guaifed 1615
- Guaifed Syrup .... ▣ 629
- Isoclor Expectorant 982
- Isoclor Timesule Capsules .... ▣ 561
- Kronofed-A 970
- Medi-Flu Caplet, Liquid .... ▣ 640
- Novafed A Capsules 1342
- Novafed Capsules 1342
- Novahistine DH 1342
- Novahistine DMX .... ▣ 595
- Novahistine Expectorant 1343
- Nucofed Capsules 2219
- Nucofed Expectorant 2219
- Nucofed Pediatric Expectorant 2220
- Nucofed Syrup 2219
- Ornex Caplets .... ▣ 618
- PediaCare Allergy Relief Formula Liquid 1362
- PediaCare Cough-Cold Formula Liquid 1362
- PediaCare Infants' Oral Decongestant Drops 1362
- PediaCare Night Rest Cough-Cold Formula Liquid 1362
- PediaCare 6-12 Cough-Cold Formula Chewable Tablets 1362
- Robitussin-DAC Syrup 1875
- Robitussin-PE .... ▣ 677
- Rondec 1975
- Rondec-DM 1976
- Rondec-TR Tablet 1975
- Ru-Tuss DE Tablets 694
- Ryna .... ▣ 741
- Seldane-D Extended-Release Tablets 1350
- Sinarest .... ▣ 562
- Sine-Aid Maximum Strength Sinus Headache Caplets 1365
- Sine-Aid Maximum Strength Sinus Headache Tablets 1365
- Sine-Off Maximum Strength Allergy/Sinus Formula Caplets .... ▣ 721
- Sine-Off Maximum Strength No Drowsiness Formula Caplets .... ▣ 722
- Singlet Tablets .... ▣ 598
- Sinutab Maximum Strength .... ▣ 641
- Sinutab Maximum Strength Without Drowsiness Tablets & Caplets .... ▣ 642
- Sinutab Regular Strength Without Drowsiness Formula .... ▣ 641
- St. Joseph Nighttime Cold Medicine .... ▣ 705
- Sudafed Children's Liquid .... ▣ 543
- Sudafed Cough Syrup .... ▣ 543
- Sudafed Plus Liquid .... ▣ 544
- Sudafed Plus Tablets .... ▣ 545
- Sudafed Sinus Caplets .... ▣ 545
- Sudafed Sinus Tablets .... ▣ 545
- Sudafed Tablets, 30 mg .... ▣ 544
- Sudafed Tablets, Adult Strength, 60 mg .... ▣ 544
- Sudafed 12 Hour Capsules .... ▣ 545
- TheraFlu Flu and Cold Medicine .... ▣ 687
- Triaminic Nite Light .... ▣ 689
- Tylenol Allergy Sinus Medication Caplets and Gelcaps, Maximum Strength 1372
- Children's Tylenol Cold Liquid Formula and Chewable Tablets 1368
- Tylenol Cold & Flu Hot Medication, Packets 1369
- Tylenol Cold & Flu No Drowsiness Hot Medication, Packets 1371
- Tylenol Cold Medication Caplets and Tablets 1370
- Tylenol Cold Medication No Drowsiness Formula Caplets 1370
- Tylenol Cold Night Time Medication Liquid 1371
- Tylenol Cough Medication Liquid with Decongestant, Maximum Strength 1372
- Tylenol, Maximum Strength, Sinus Medication Gelcaps, Caplets and Tablets 1373
- Ursinus Inlay-Tabs .... ▣ 691
- Vicks Children's NyQuil .... ▣ 664
- Vicks Daycare .... ▣ 660
- Vicks Formula 44D Decongestant Cough Medicine .... ▣ 662
- Vicks Formula 44M Multi-Symptom Cough Medicine .... ▣ 662
- Vicks NyQuil Nighttime Colds Medicine-Original & Cherry Flavor .... ▣ 664
- Vicks Pediatric Formula 44 Cough & Congestion Medicine .... ▣ 663
- Vicks Pediatric Formula 44m Multi-Symptom Cough & Cold Medicine .... ▣ 663

Pseudoephedrine Sulfate (May produce additive effects). Products include:

- Afrin Tablets .... ▣ 693
- Chlor-Trimeton Decongestant .... ▣ 694
- Disophrol Chronotab Sustained-Action Tablets .... ▣ 698
- Drixoral Antihistamine/Nasal Decongestant Syrup .... ▣ 698
- Drixoral Non-Drowsy Formula .... ▣ 699
- Drixoral Plus Extended-Release Tablets .... ▣ 699
- Drixoral Sinus .... ▣ 700
- Drixoral Sustained-Action Tablets ▣ 698
- Sinutab Allergy Formula Sustained Action Tablets .... ▣ 640
- Trinalin Repetabs Tablets 1170

Selegiline Hydrochloride (May produce hypertensive crisis). Products include:

- Eldepryl 2250

Terbutaline Sulfate (May produce additive effects). Products include:
- Brethaire Inhaler ... 1024
- Brethine Ampuls ... 1026
- Brethine Tablets ... 1026
- Bricanyl Injection ... 1324
- Bricanyl Tablets ... 1325

Tranylcypromine Sulfate (May produce hypertensive crisis). Products include:
- Parnate Tablets ... 2222

DIMETANE DECONGESTANT ELIXIR
(Brompheniramine Maleate, Phenylephrine Hydrochloride) ... ◘ 673
See **Dimetane Decongestant Caplets**

DIMETANE ELIXIR
(Brompheniramine Maleate) ... ◘ 672
May interact with:

Alcohol (Do not use concomitantly).

DIMETANE EXTENTABS 8 MG
(Brompheniramine Maleate) ... ◘ 672
See **Dimetane Elixir**

DIMETANE EXTENTABS 12 MG
(Brompheniramine Maleate) ... ◘ 672
See **Dimetane Elixir**

DIMETANE TABLETS
(Brompheniramine Maleate) ... ◘ 672
See **Dimetane Elixir**

DIMETANE-DC COUGH SYRUP
(Brompheniramine Maleate, Phenylpropanolamine Hydrochloride, Codeine Phosphate) ... 1857
May interact with hypnotics and sedatives, tranquilizers, benzodiazepines, monoamine oxidase inhibitors, antihypertensives, central nervous system depressants, and certain other agents. Compounds in these categories include:

Acebutolol Hydrochloride (Reduced antihypertensive effects). Products include:
- Sectral Capsules ... 2520

Alcohol (Additive effects).

Alfentanil Hydrochloride (Additive effects). Products include:
- Alfenta Injection ... 1131

Alprazolam (Additive effects). Products include:
- Xanax Tablets ... 2367

Aprobarbital (Additive effects). Products include:
- Alurate Elixir ... 1883

Atenolol (Reduced antihypertensive effects). Products include:
- Tenoretic Tablets ... 1105
- Tenormin Tablets and I.V. Injection 1107

Benazepril Hydrochloride (Reduced antihypertensive effects). Products include:
- Lotensin Tablets ... 872

Bendroflumethiazide (Reduced antihypertensive effects). Products include:
- Corzide Tablets ... 702
- Naturetin Tablets ... 1789
- Rauzide Tablets ... 1804

Betaxolol Hydrochloride (Reduced antihypertensive effects). Products include:
- Betoptic Sterile Ophthalmic Solution ... 569
- Betoptic S Sterile Ophthalmic Suspension ... 570
- Kerlone Tablets ... 2172

Buprenorphine (Additive effects).
No products indexed under this heading.

Buspirone Hydrochloride (Additive effects). Products include:
- BuSpar ... 1401

Butabarbital (Additive effects). Products include:
- Pyridium Plus ... 1764

Butalbital (Additive effects). Products include:
- Esgic-Plus Tablets ... 1002
- Esgic Tablets & Capsules ... 1001
- Fioricet Tablets ... 2006
- Fiorinal Capsules ... 2007
- Fiorinal with Codeine Capsules ... 2008
- Fiorinal Tablets ... 2007
- Phrenilin ... 838
- Sedapap Tablets 50 mg/650 mg .. 1360

Captopril (Reduced antihypertensive effects). Products include:
- Capoten ... 2255
- Capozide ... 2258

Carteolol Hydrochloride (Reduced antihypertensive effects). Products include:
- Cartrol Tablets ... 507

Chlordiazepoxide (Additive effects). Products include:
- Libritabs Tablets ... 1930
- Limbitrol ... 1933
- Menrium Tablets ... 1934

Chlordiazepoxide Hydrochloride (Additive effects). Products include:
- Librax Capsules ... 1929
- Librium Capsules ... 1931
- Librium Injectable ... 1932

Chlorothiazide (Reduced antihypertensive effects). Products include:
- Aldoclor Tablets ... 1413
- Diupres Tablets ... 1461
- Diuril Oral ... 1464

Chlorothiazide Sodium (Reduced antihypertensive effects). Products include:
- Diuril Sodium Intravenous ... 1463

Chlorpromazine (Additive effects). Products include:
- Thorazine ... 2234

Chlorprothixene (Additive effects). Products include:
- Taractan Tablets ... 1920

Chlorprothixene Hydrochloride (Additive effects). Products include:
- Taractan ... 1920

Chlorthalidone (Reduced antihypertensive effects). Products include:
- Combipres Tablets ... 678
- Tenoretic Tablets ... 1105
- Thalitone Tablets ... 687

Clonidine (Reduced antihypertensive effects). Products include:
- Catapres-TTS ... 677

Clonidine Hydrochloride (Additive effects; reduced antihypertensive effects). Products include:
- Catapres Tablets ... 676
- Combipres Tablets ... 678

Clorazepate Dipotassium (Additive effects). Products include:
- Tranxene ... 556

Codeine (Additive effects). Products include:
- Calcidrine Syrup ... 506

Codeine Polistirex (Additive effects).
No products indexed under this heading.

Deserpidine (Reduced antihypertensive effects). Products include:
- Enduronyl ... 518
- Harmonyl Tablets ... 528
- Oreticyl ... 545

Dezocine (Additive effects).

Diazepam (Additive effects). Products include:
- Valium Injectable ... 1937
- Valium Tablets ... 1939
- Valrelease Capsules ... 1923

Diazoxide (Reduced antihypertensive effects). Products include:
- Hyperstat I.V. Injection ... 2095
- Proglycem ... 649

Doxazosin Mesylate (Reduced antihypertensive effects). Products include:
- Cardura Tablets ... 1941

Droperidol (Additive effects). Products include:
- Inapsine Injection ... 1140
- Innovar Injection ... 1141

Enalapril Maleate (Reduced antihypertensive effects). Products include:
- Vaseretic Tablets ... 1559
- Vasotec Tablets ... 1564

Enalaprilat (Reduced antihypertensive effects). Products include:
- Vasotec I.V. ... 1562

Enflurane (Additive effects). Products include:
- Ethrane ... 599

Esmolol Hydrochloride (Reduced antihypertensive effects). Products include:
- Brevibloc Injection ... 942

Estazolam (Additive effects). Products include:
- ProSom Tablets ... 554

Ethchlorvynol (Additive effects). Products include:
- Placidyl Capsules ... 553

Ethinamate (Additive effects).
No products indexed under this heading.

Felodipine (Reduced antihypertensive effects). Products include:
- Plendil Extended-Release Tablets ... 1526

Fentanyl (Additive effects). Products include:
- Duragesic Transdermal System ... 1133

Fentanyl Citrate (Additive effects). Products include:
- Innovar Injection ... 1141
- Sublimaze Injection ... 1146

Fluphenazine Decanoate (Additive effects). Products include:
- Prolixin Decanoate ... 1795

Fluphenazine Enanthate (Additive effects). Products include:
- Prolixin Enanthate ... 1796

Fluphenazine Hydrochloride (Additive effects). Products include:
- Prolixin Elixir ... 1793
- Prolixin Injection ... 1791
- Prolixin Oral Concentrate ... 1792
- Prolixin Tablets ... 1793

Flurazepam Hydrochloride (Additive effects). Products include:
- Dalmane Capsules ... 1927

Fosinopril Sodium (Reduced antihypertensive effects). Products include:
- Monopril Tablets ... 1406

Furazolidone (Enhances phenylpropanolamine's effect and anticholinergic effects of antihistamines). Products include:
- Furoxone ... 1855

Furosemide (Reduced antihypertensive effects). Products include:
- Lasix ... 1093

Glutethimide (Additive effects).
No products indexed under this heading.

Guanabenz Acetate (Reduced antihypertensive effects). Products include:
- Wytensin Tablets ... 2542

Guanethidine Monosulfate (Reduced antihypertensive effects). Products include:
- Esimil Tablets ... 864
- Ismelin Tablets ... 869

Haloperidol (Additive effects). Products include:
- Haldol Injection, Tablets and Concentrate ... 1373

Haloperidol Decanoate (Additive effects). Products include:
- Haldol Decanoate ... 1375

Hydralazine Hydrochloride (Reduced antihypertensive effects). Products include:
- Apresazide Capsules ... 854
- Apresoline Hydrochloride Parenteral (Ampuls) ... 856
- Apresoline Hydrochloride Tablets .. 855
- Apresoline-Esidrix Tablets ... 857
- Ser-Ap-Es Tablets ... 881
- Serpasil-Apresoline Tablets ... 884

Hydrochlorothiazide (Reduced antihypertensive effects). Products include:
- Aldactazide ... 2150
- Aldoril Tablets ... 1418
- Apresazide Capsules ... 854
- Apresoline-Esidrix Tablets ... 857
- Capozide ... 2258
- Dyazide Capsules ... 2208
- Esidrix Tablets ... 863
- Esimil Tablets ... 864
- HydroDIURIL Tablets ... 1484
- Hydropres Tablets ... 1485
- Inderide Tablets ... 2463
- Inderide LA Long Acting Capsules .. 2465
- Lopressor HCT Tablets ... 1034
- Maxzide ... 1215
- Moduretic Tablets ... 1510
- Normozide Tablets ... 2112
- Oretic Tablets ... 544
- Oreticyl ... 545
- Prinzide Tablets ... 1540
- Ser-Ap-Es Tablets ... 881
- Serpasil-Esidrix Tablets ... 886
- Timolide Tablets ... 1547
- Trandate HCT Tablets ... 579
- Vaseretic Tablets ... 1559
- Zestoretic ... 2274

Hydrocodone Bitartrate (Additive effects). Products include:
- Anexsia 5/500 Tablets ... 2196
- Anexsia 7.5/650 Tablets ... 2197
- Azdōne Tablets ... 844
- Codiclear DH Syrup ... 845
- Codimal DH Syrup ... 846
- Damason-P ... 1356
- Hycodan Syrup, Tablets ... 927
- Hycomine Compound Tablets ... 929
- Hycomine Syrup ... 927
- Hycotuss Expectorant Syrup ... 930
- Hydrocet Capsules ... 835
- Lortab ASA Tablets ... 2414
- Lortab ... 2412
- Ru-Tuss with Hydrocodone ... 694
- Triaminic Expectorant DH ... 1995
- Vicodin Tablets ... 1187
- Vicodin ES Tablets ... 1189
- Zydone Capsules ... 941

Hydrocodone Polistirex (Additive effects). Products include:
- Tussionex Extended-Release Suspension ... 988

Hydroflumethiazide (Reduced antihypertensive effects). Products include:
- Diucardin Tablets ... 2450
- Saluron ... 718
- Salutensin/Salutensin-Demi ... 719

Hydroxyzine Hydrochloride (Additive effects). Products include:
- Atarax Tablets & Syrup ... 1941
- Marax Tablets & DF Syrup ... 1954
- Vistaril Intramuscular Solution ... 1970

Indapamide (Reduced antihypertensive effects). Products include:
- Lozol Tablets ... 1843

Isocarboxazid (Enhances phenylpropanolamine's effect and anticholinergic effects of antihistamines). Products include:
- Marplan Tablets ... 1906

Isoflurane (Additive effects). Products include:
Forane 600
Isoproterenol Hydrochloride (Reduced effects of antihypertensive drugs). Products include:
Isuprel Hydrochloride Injection 1:5000 2050
Isuprel Hydrochloride Mistometer 2051
Isuprel Hydrochloride Solution 1:200 & 1:100 2052
Norisodrine Aerotrol 540
Isoproterenol Sulfate (Reduced effects of antihypeertensive drugs).
No products indexed under this heading.
Isradipine (Reduced antihypertensive effects). Products include:
DynaCirc Capsules 2004
Ketamine Hydrochloride (Additive effects). Products include:
Ketalar 1726
Labetalol Hydrochloride (Reduced antihypertensive effects). Products include:
Normodyne Injection 2108
Normodyne Tablets 2110
Normozide Tablets 2112
Trandate HCT Tablets 579
Trandate Injection 577
Trandate Tablets 579
Levorphanol Tartrate (Additive effects). Products include:
Levo-Dromoran 1906
Lisinopril (Reduced antihypertensive effects). Products include:
Prinivil Tablets 1538
Prinzide Tablets 1540
Zestoretic 2274
Zestril Tablets 2277
Lorazepam (Additive effects). Products include:
Ativan Injection 2432
Ativan Tablets 2434
Loxapine Hydrochloride (Additive effects). Products include:
Loxitane 1213
Loxapine Succinate (Additive effects). Products include:
Loxitane Capsules 1213
Mecamylamine Hydrochloride (Reduced antihypertensive effects). Products include:
Inversine Tablets 1492
Meperidine Hydrochloride (Additive effects). Products include:
Demerol 2047
Mepergan Injection 2479
Mephobarbital (Additive effects). Products include:
Mebaral Tablets 2061
Meprobamate (Additive effects). Products include:
Deprol Tablets 2382
Equagesic Tablets 2451
Miltown Tablets 2386
PMB 200 and PMB 400 2504
Mesoridazine (Additive effects). Products include:
Serentil 686
Methadone Hydrochloride (Additive effects). Products include:
Dolophine Hydrochloride Ampoules & Vials 1260
Dolophine Hydrochloride Tablets 1261
Methadone Hydrochloride Diskets 1284
Methadone Hydrochloride Oral Solution & Tablets 1987
Methohexital Sodium (Additive effects). Products include:
Brevital Sodium Vials 1248
Methoxyflurane (Additive effects).
No products indexed under this heading.
Methyclothiazide (Reduced antihypertensive effects). Products include:
Enduron Tablets 517
Enduronyl 518
Methyldopa (Reduced antihypertensive effects). Products include:
Aldoclor Tablets 1413
Aldomet Oral 1415
Aldoril Tablets 1418
Methyldopate Hydrochloride (Reduced antihypertensive effects). Products include:
Aldomet Ester HCl Injection 1417
Metolazone (Reduced antihypertensive effects). Products include:
Diulo 2129
Mykrox ½ mg Tablets 984
Zaroxolyn Tablets 989
Metoprolol Tartrate (Reduced antihypertensive effects). Products include:
Lopressor Ampuls 1032
Lopressor HCT Tablets 1034
Lopressor Tablets 1032
Midazolam Hydrochloride (Additive effects). Products include:
Versed Injection 1924
Minoxidil (Reduced antihypertensive effects). Products include:
Loniten Tablets 2346
Rogaine Topical Solution 2357
Molindone Hydrochloride (Additive effects). Products include:
Moban Tablets & Concentrate 932
Morphine Sulfate (Additive effects). Products include:
Astramorph/PF Injection, USP (Preservative-Free) 618
Duramorph 960
Infumorph 200 and Infumorph 500 Sterile Solutions 962
MS Contin Tablets 1814
MSIR 1817
Oramorph SR (Morphine Sulfate Sustained Release Tablets) 1988
Roxanol 1991
Nadolol (Reduced antihypertensive effects). Products include:
Corgard Tablets 701
Corzide Tablets 702
Nicardipine Hydrochloride (Reduced antihypertensive effects). Products include:
Cardene Capsules 2290
Nitroglycerin (Reduced antihypertensive effects). Products include:
Deponit NTG Transdermal Delivery System 2143
Minitran Transdermal Delivery System 1312
Nitro-Bid Ointment 1339
Nitro-Bid Capsules 1338
Nitrodisc 2176
Nitro-Dur (nitroglycerin) Transdermal Infusion System 1164
Nitrogard Tablets 1004
Nitrolingual Spray 1846
Nitrostat Tablets 1743
Transderm-Nitro Transdermal Therapeutic System 2283
Opium Alkaloids (Additive effects). Products include:
B & O No. 15A & No. 16A Supprettes 2395
Pantopon Injectable 1911
Oxazepam (Additive effects). Products include:
Serax Capsules 2522
Serax Tablets 2522
Oxycodone Hydrochloride (Additive effects). Products include:
Percocet Tablets 950
Percodan 951
Roxicodone Tablets, Oral Solution & Intensol (Oxycodone) 1992
Tylox Capsules 1382
Penbutolol Sulfate (Reduced antihypertensive effects). Products include:
Levatol 1832
Pentobarbital Sodium (Additive effects). Products include:
Nembutal Sodium Capsules 534
Nembutal Sodium Solution 536
Nembutal Sodium Suppositories 538
Perphenazine (Additive effects). Products include:
Etrafon 2087
Triavil Tablets 1556
Trilafon 2123
Phenelzine Sulfate (Enhances phenylpropanolamine's effect and anticholinergic effects of antihistamines). Products include:
Nardil 1742
Phenobarbital (Additive effects). Products include:
Arco-Lase Plus Tablets 607
Bellergal-S Tablets 1998
Bronkolixir 761
Bronkotabs Tablets 762
Donnatal 1858
Donnatal Extentabs 1859
Donnatal Tablets 1858
Donnazyme Tablets 1860
Kinesed Tablets 2272
Phenobarbital Elixir and Tablets 1293
Primatene Tablets-P Formula 2421
Quadrinal Tablets 1183
Tedral SA 1765
Phenoxybenzamine Hydrochloride (Reduced antihypertensive effects). Products include:
Dibenzyline Capsules 2207
Phentolamine Mesylate (Reduced antihypertensive effects). Products include:
Regitine 878
Pindolol (Reduced antihypertensive effects). Products include:
Visken Tablets 2036
Polythiazide (Reduced antihypertensive effects). Products include:
Minizide Capsules 1779
Renese Tablets 1785
Renese-R Tablets 1786
Prazepam (Additive effects). Products include:
Centrax 1693
Prazosin Hydrochloride (Reduced antihypertensive effects). Products include:
Minipress Capsules 1778
Minizide Capsules 1779
Prochlorperazine (Additive effects). Products include:
Compazine 2201
Promethazine Hydrochloride (Additive effects). Products include:
Mepergan Injection 2479
Phenergan with Codeine 2497
Phenergan with Dextromethorphan 2499
Phenergan Injection 2493
Phenergan Suppositories 2496
Phenergan Syrup 2495
Phenergan Tablets 2496
Phenergan VC 2500
Phenergan VC with Codeine 2501
Propofol (Additive effects). Products include:
Diprivan Injection 2267
Propoxyphene Hydrochloride (Additive effects). Products include:
Darvon 1256
Wygesic Tablets 2540
Propoxyphene Napsylate (Additive effects). Products include:
Darvon-N/Darvocet-N 1254
Propranolol Hydrochloride (Reduced antihypertensive effects). Products include:
Inderal 2459
Inderal LA Long Acting Capsules 2461
Inderide Tablets 2463
Inderide LA Long Acting Capsules 2465
Quazepam (Additive effects). Products include:
Doral Tablets 2383
Ramipril (Reduced antihypertensive effects). Products include:
Altace Capsules 1086
Rauwolfia Serpentina (Reduced antihypertensive effects). Products include:
Raudixin Tablets 1803
Rauzide Tablets 1804
Rescinnamine (Reduced antihypertensive effects).
No products indexed under this heading.
Reserpine (Reduced antihypertensive effects). Products include:
Diupres Tablets 1461
Hydromox R Tablets 1209
Hydropres Tablets 1485
Renese-R Tablets 1786
Salutensin/Salutensin-Demi 719
Ser-Ap-Es Tablets 881
Serpasil Tablets 883
Serpasil-Apresoline Tablets 884
Serpasil-Esidrix Tablets 886
Secobarbital Sodium (Additive effects). Products include:
Seconal Sodium Pulvules 1296
Selegiline Hydrochloride (Enhances phenylpropanolamine's effect and anticholinergic effects of antihistamines). Products include:
Eldepryl 2250
Sodium Nitroprusside (Reduced antihypertensive effects). Products include:
Nipride I.V. Infusion 1909
Sufentanil Citrate (Additive effects). Products include:
Sufenta Injection 1147
Temazepam (Additive effects). Products include:
Restoril Capsules 2023
Terazosin Hydrochloride (Reduced antihypertensive effects). Products include:
Hytrin Tablets 529
Thiamylal Sodium (Additive effects). Products include:
Surital Ampoules, Steri-Vials 1764
Thioridazine Hydrochloride (Additive effects). Products include:
Mellaril 2011
Thiothixene (Additive effects). Products include:
Navane Capsules and Concentrate 1954
Navane Intramuscular 1956
Timolol Maleate (Reduced antihypertensive effects). Products include:
Blocadren Tablets 1429
Timolide Tablets 1547
Timoptic in Ocudose 1552
Timoptic Sterile Ophthalmic Solution 1550
Tranylcypromine Sulfate (Enhances phenylpropanolamine's effect and anticholinergic effects of antihistamines). Products include:
Parnate Tablets 2222
Triazolam (Additive effects). Products include:
Halcion Tablets 2340
Trifluoperazine Hydrochloride (Additive effects). Products include:
Stelazine 2226
Trimethaphan Camsylate (Reduced antihypertensive effects). Products include:
Arfonad Ampuls 1887

DIMETANE-DX COUGH SYRUP
(Brompheniramine Maleate, Pseudoephedrine Hydrochloride, Dextromethorphan) 1858
May interact with monoamine oxidase inhibitors, central nervous system depressants, and antihypertensives. Compounds in these categories include:

Acebutolol Hydrochloride (Decreased antihypertensive effect). Products include:
Sectral Capsules 2520
Alcohol (Additive effect).

Alfentanil Hydrochloride (Additive effect). Products include:
Alfenta Injection 1131
Alprazolam (Additive effect). Products include:
Xanax Tablets 2367
Aprobarbital (Additive effect). Products include:
Alurate Elixir 1883
Atenolol (Decreased antihypertensive effect). Products include:
Tenoretic Tablets 1105
Tenormin Tablets and I.V. Injection 1107
Benazepril Hydrochloride (Decreased antihypertensive effect). Products include:
Lotensin Tablets 872
Bendroflumethiazide (Decreased antihypertensive effect). Products include:
Corzide Tablets 702
Naturetin Tablets 1789
Rauzide Tablets 1804
Betaxolol Hydrochloride (Decreased antihypertensive effect). Products include:
Betoptic Sterile Ophthalmic Solution 569
Betoptic S Sterile Ophthalmic Suspension 570
Kerlone Tablets 2172
Buprenorphine (Additive effect).
No products indexed under this heading.
Buspirone Hydrochloride (Additive effect). Products include:
BuSpar 1401
Butabarbital (Additive effect). Products include:
Pyridium Plus 1764
Butalbital (Additive effect). Products include:
Esgic-Plus Tablets 1002
Esgic Tablets & Capsules 1001
Fioricet Tablets 2006
Fiorinal Capsules 2007
Fiorinal with Codeine Capsules 2008
Fiorinal Tablets 2007
Phrenilin 838
Sedapap Tablets 50 mg/650 mg 1360
Captopril (Decreased antihypertensive effect). Products include:
Capoten 2255
Capozide 2258
Carteolol Hydrochloride (Decreased antihypertensive effect). Products include:
Cartrol Tablets 507
Chlordiazepoxide (Additive effect). Products include:
Libritabs Tablets 1930
Limbitrol 1933
Menrium Tablets 1934
Chlordiazepoxide Hydrochloride (Additive effect). Products include:
Librax Capsules 1929
Librium Capsules 1931
Librium Injectable 1932
Chlorothiazide (Decreased antihypertensive effect). Products include:
Aldoclor Tablets 1413
Diupres Tablets 1461
Diuril Oral 1464
Chlorothiazide Sodium (Decreased antihypertensive effect). Products include:
Diuril Sodium Intravenous 1463
Chlorpromazine (Additive effect). Products include:
Thorazine 2234
Chlorprothixene (Additive effect). Products include:
Taractan Tablets 1920
Chlorprothixene Hydrochloride (Additive effect). Products include:
Taractan 1920
Chlorthalidone (Decreased antihypertensive effect). Products include:
Combipres Tablets 678
Tenoretic Tablets 1105
Thalitone Tablets 687
Clonidine (Decreased antihypertensive effect). Products include:
Catapres-TTS 677
Clonidine Hydrochloride (Decreased antihypertensive effect). Products include:
Catapres Tablets 676
Combipres Tablets 678
Clorazepate Dipotassium (Additive effect). Products include:
Tranxene 556
Codeine (Additive effect). Products include:
Calcidrine Syrup 506
Codeine Phosphate (Additive effect). Products include:
Actifed with Codeine Cough Syrup 752
Cheracol Cough Syrup 1853
Codimal PH Syrup 846
Dimetane-DC Cough Syrup 1857
Empirin with Codeine Phosphate Nos. 2, 3 & 4 764
Fiorinal with Codeine Capsules 2008
Isoclor Expectorant 982
Naldecon CX Adult Liquid ▣ 521
Novahistine DH 1342
Novahistine Expectorant 1343
Nucofed Capsules 2219
Nucofed Expectorant 2219
Nucofed Pediatric Expectorant 2220
Nucofed Syrup 2219
Phenaphen with Codeine Capsules 1865
Phenaphen-650 with Codeine Tablets 1866
Phenergan with Codeine 2497
Phenergan VC with Codeine 2501
Robitussin A-C Syrup 1875
Robitussin-DAC Syrup 1875
Ryna ▣ 741
Soma Compound w/Codeine Tablets 2390
Triaminic Expectorant w/Codeine 1996
Tussi-Organidin Liquid 2391
Tylenol with Codeine 1381
Codeine Polistirex (Additive effect).
No products indexed under this heading.
Deserpidine (Decreased antihypertensive effect). Products include:
Enduronyl 518
Harmonyl Tablets 528
Oreticyl 545
Dezocine (Additive effect).
Diazepam (Additive effect). Products include:
Valium Injectable 1937
Valium Tablets 1939
Valrelease Capsules 1923
Diazoxide (Decreased antihypertensive effect). Products include:
Hyperstat I.V. Injection 2095
Proglycem 649
Doxazosin Mesylate (Decreased antihypertensive effect). Products include:
Cardura Tablets 1941
Droperidol (Additive effect). Products include:
Inapsine Injection 1140
Innovar Injection 1141
Enalapril Maleate (Decreased antihypertensive effect). Products include:
Vaseretic Tablets 1559
Vasotec Tablets 1564
Enalaprilat (Decreased antihypertensive effect). Products include:
Vasotec I.V. 1562
Enflurane (Additive effect). Products include:
Ethrane 599
Esmolol Hydrochloride (Decreased antihypertensive effect). Products include:
Brevibloc Injection 942
Estazolam (Additive effect). Products include:
ProSom Tablets 554
Ethchlorvynol (Additive effect). Products include:
Placidyl Capsules 553
Ethinamate (Additive effect).
No products indexed under this heading.
Felodipine (Decreased antihypertensive effect). Products include:
Plendil Extended-Release Tablets 1526
Fentanyl (Additive effect). Products include:
Duragesic Transdermal System 1133
Fentanyl Citrate (Additive effect). Products include:
Innovar Injection 1141
Sublimaze Injection 1146
Fluphenazine Decanoate (Additive effect). Products include:
Prolixin Decanoate 1795
Fluphenazine Enanthate (Additive effect). Products include:
Prolixin Enanthate 1796
Fluphenazine Hydrochloride (Additive effect). Products include:
Prolixin Elixir 1793
Prolixin Injection 1791
Prolixin Oral Concentrate 1792
Prolixin Tablets 1793
Flurazepam Hydrochloride (Additive effect). Products include:
Dalmane Capsules 1927
Fosinopril Sodium (Decreased antihypertensive effect). Products include:
Monopril Tablets 1406
Furazolidone (Prolonged anticholinergic effect). Products include:
Furoxone 1855
Furosemide (Decreased antihypertensive effect). Products include:
Lasix 1093
Glutethimide (Additive effect).
No products indexed under this heading.
Guanabenz Acetate (Decreased antihypertensive effect). Products include:
Wytensin Tablets 2542
Guanethidine Monosulfate (Decreased antihypertensive effect). Products include:
Esimil Tablets 864
Ismelin Tablets 869
Haloperidol (Additive effect). Products include:
Haldol Injection, Tablets and Concentrate 1373
Haloperidol Decanoate (Additive effect). Products include:
Haldol Decanoate 1375
Hydralazine Hydrochloride (Decreased antihypertensive effect). Products include:
Apresazide Capsules 854
Apresoline Hydrochloride Parenteral (Ampuls) 856
Apresoline Hydrochloride Tablets 855
Apresoline-Esidrix Tablets 857
Ser-Ap-Es Tablets 881
Serpasil-Apresoline Tablets 884
Hydrochlorothiazide (Decreased antihypertensive effect). Products include:
Aldactazide 2150
Aldoril Tablets 1418
Apresazide Capsules 854
Apresoline-Esidrix Tablets 857
Capozide 2258
Dyazide Capsules 2208
Esidrix Tablets 863
Esimil Tablets 864
HydroDIURIL Tablets 1484
Hydropres Tablets 1485
Inderide Tablets 2463
Inderide LA Long Acting Capsules 2465
Lopressor HCT Tablets 1034
Maxzide 1215
Moduretic Tablets 1510
Normozide Tablets 2112
Oretic Tablets 544
Oreticyl 545
Prinzide Tablets 1540
Ser-Ap-Es Tablets 881
Serpasil-Esidrix Tablets 886
Timolide Tablets 1547
Trandate HCT Tablets 579
Vaseretic Tablets 1559
Zestoretic 2274
Hydrocodone Bitartrate (Additive effect). Products include:
Anexsia 5/500 Tablets 2196
Anexsia 7.5/650 Tablets 2197
Azdone Tablets 844
Codiclear DH Syrup 845
Codimal DH Syrup 846
Damason-P 1356
Hycodan Syrup, Tablets 927
Hycomine Compound Tablets 929
Hycomine Syrup 927
Hycotuss Expectorant Syrup 930
Hydrocet Capsules 835
Lortab ASA Tablets 2414
Lortab 2412
Ru-Tuss with Hydrocodone 694
Triaminic Expectorant DH 1995
Vicodin Tablets 1187
Vicodin ES Tablets 1189
Zydone Capsules 941
Hydrocodone Polistirex (Additive effect). Products include:
Tussionex Extended-Release Suspension 988
Hydroflumethiazide (Decreased antihypertensive effect). Products include:
Diucardin Tablets 2450
Saluron 718
Salutensin/Salutensin-Demi 719
Hydroxyzine Hydrochloride (Additive effect). Products include:
Atarax Tablets & Syrup 1941
Marax Tablets & DF Syrup 1954
Vistaril Intramuscular Solution 1970
Indapamide (Decreased antihypertensive effect). Products include:
Lozol Tablets 1843
Isocarboxazid (Prolonged anticholinergic effect). Products include:
Marplan Tablets 1906
Isoflurane (Additive effect). Products include:
Forane 600
Isradipine (Decreased antihypertensive effect). Products include:
DynaCirc Capsules 2004
Ketamine Hydrochloride (Additive effect). Products include:
Ketalar 1726
Labetalol Hydrochloride (Decreased antihypertensive effect). Products include:
Normodyne Injection 2108
Normodyne Tablets 2110
Normozide Tablets 2112
Trandate HCT Tablets 579
Trandate Injection 577
Trandate Tablets 579
Levorphanol Tartrate (Additive effect). Products include:
Levo-Dromoran 1906
Lisinopril (Decreased antihypertensive effect). Products include:
Prinivil Tablets 1538
Prinzide Tablets 1540
Zestoretic 2274
Zestril Tablets 2277
Lorazepam (Additive effect). Products include:
Ativan Injection 2432
Ativan Tablets 2434
Loxapine Hydrochloride (Additive effect). Products include:
Loxitane 1213
Loxapine Succinate (Additive effect). Products include:
Loxitane Capsules 1213

Mecamylamine Hydrochloride (Decreased antihypertensive effect). Products include:
- Inversine Tablets ... 1492

Meperidine Hydrochloride (Additive effect). Products include:
- Demerol ... 2047
- Mepergan Injection ... 2479

Mephobarbital (Additive effect). Products include:
- Mebaral Tablets ... 2061

Meprobamate (Additive effect). Products include:
- Deprol Tablets ... 2382
- Equagesic Tablets ... 2451
- Miltown Tablets ... 2386
- PMB 200 and PMB 400 ... 2504

Mesoridazine (Additive effect). Products include:
- Serentil ... 686

Methadone Hydrochloride (Additive effect). Products include:
- Dolophine Hydrochloride Ampoules & Vials ... 1260
- Dolophine Hydrochloride Tablets ... 1261
- Methadone Hydrochloride Diskets ... 1284
- Methadone Hydrochloride Oral Solution & Tablets ... 1987

Methohexital Sodium (Additive effect). Products include:
- Brevital Sodium Vials ... 1248

Methoxyflurane (Additive effect).
- No products indexed under this heading.

Methyclothiazide (Decreased antihypertensive effect). Products include:
- Enduron Tablets ... 517
- Enduronyl ... 518

Methyldopa (Decreased antihypertensive effect). Products include:
- Aldoclor Tablets ... 1413
- Aldomet Oral ... 1415
- Aldoril Tablets ... 1418

Methyldopate Hydrochloride (Decreased antihypertensive effect). Products include:
- Aldomet Ester HCl Injection ... 1417

Metolazone (Decreased antihypertensive effect). Products include:
- Diulo ... 2129
- Mykrox ½ mg Tablets ... 984
- Zaroxolyn Tablets ... 989

Metoprolol Tartrate (Decreased antihypertensive effect). Products include:
- Lopressor Ampuls ... 1032
- Lopressor HCT Tablets ... 1034
- Lopressor Tablets ... 1032

Metyrosine (Decreased antihypertensive effect). Products include:
- Demser Capsules ... 1460

Midazolam Hydrochloride (Additive effect). Products include:
- Versed Injection ... 1924

Minoxidil (Decreased antihypertensive effect). Products include:
- Loniten Tablets ... 2346
- Rogaine Topical Solution ... 2357

Molindone Hydrochloride (Additive effect). Products include:
- Moban Tablets & Concentrate ... 932

Morphine Sulfate (Additive effect). Products include:
- Astramorph/PF Injection, USP (Preservative-Free) ... 618
- Duramorph ... 960
- Infumorph 200 and Infumorph 500 Sterile Solutions ... 962
- MS Contin Tablets ... 1814
- MSIR ... 1817
- Oramorph SR (Morphine Sulfate Sustained Release Tablets) ... 1988
- Roxanol ... 1991

Nadolol (Decreased antihypertensive effect). Products include:
- Corgard Tablets ... 701
- Corzide Tablets ... 702

Nicardipine Hydrochloride (Decreased antihypertensive effect). Products include:
- Cardene Capsules ... 2290

Nitroglycerin (Decreased antihypertensive effect). Products include:
- Deponit NTG Transdermal Delivery System ... 2143
- Minitran Transdermal Delivery System ... 1312
- Nitro-Bid Ointment ... 1339
- Nitro-Bid Capsules ... 1338
- Nitrodisc ... 2176
- Nitro-Dur (nitroglycerin) Transdermal Infusion System ... 1164
- Nitrogard Tablets ... 1004
- Nitrolingual Spray ... 1846
- Nitrostat Tablets ... 1743
- Transderm-Nitro Transdermal Therapeutic System ... 2283

Opium Alkaloids (Additive effect). Products include:
- B & O No. 15A & No. 16A Supprettes ... 2395
- Pantopon Injectable ... 1911

Oxazepam (Additive effect). Products include:
- Serax Capsules ... 2522
- Serax Tablets ... 2522

Oxycodone Hydrochloride (Additive effect). Products include:
- Percocet Tablets ... 950
- Percodan ... 951
- Roxicodone Tablets, Oral Solution & Intensol (Oxycodone) ... 1992
- Tylox Capsules ... 1382

Penbutolol Sulfate (Decreased antihypertensive effect). Products include:
- Levatol ... 1832

Pentobarbital Sodium (Additive effect). Products include:
- Nembutal Sodium Capsules ... 534
- Nembutal Sodium Solution ... 536
- Nembutal Sodium Suppositories ... 538

Perphenazine (Additive effect). Products include:
- Etrafon ... 2087
- Triavil Tablets ... 1556
- Trilafon ... 2123

Phenelzine Sulfate (Prolonged anticholinergic effect). Products include:
- Nardil ... 1742

Phenobarbital (Additive effect). Products include:
- Arco-Lase Plus Tablets ... 607
- Bellergal-S Tablets ... 1998
- Bronkolixir ... ◘ 761
- Bronkotabs Tablets ... ◘ 762
- Donnatal ... 1858
- Donnatal Extentabs ... 1859
- Donnatal Tablets ... 1858
- Donnazyme Tablets ... 1860
- Kinesed Tablets ... 2272
- Phenobarbital Elixir and Tablets ... 1293
- Primatene Tablets-P Formula ... 2421
- Quadrinal Tablets ... 1183
- Tedral SA ... 1765

Phenoxybenzamine Hydrochloride (Decreased antihypertensive effect). Products include:
- Dibenzyline Capsules ... 2207

Phentolamine Mesylate (Decreased antihypertensive effect). Products include:
- Regitine ... 878

Pindolol (Decreased antihypertensive effect). Products include:
- Visken Tablets ... 2036

Polythiazide (Decreased antihypertensive effect). Products include:
- Minizide Capsules ... 1779
- Renese Tablets ... 1785
- Renese-R Tablets ... 1786

Prazepam (Additive effect). Products include:
- Centrax ... 1693

Prazosin Hydrochloride (Decreased antihypertensive effect). Products include:
- Minipress Capsules ... 1778
- Minizide Capsules ... 1779

Prochlorperazine (Additive effect). Products include:
- Compazine ... 2201

Promethazine Hydrochloride (Additive effect). Products include:
- Mepergan Injection ... 2479
- Phenergan with Codeine ... 2497
- Phenergan with Dextromethorphan ... 2499
- Phenergan Injection ... 2493
- Phenergan Suppositories ... 2496
- Phenergan Syrup ... 2495
- Phenergan Tablets ... 2496
- Phenergan VC ... 2500
- Phenergan VC with Codeine ... 2501

Propofol (Additive effect). Products include:
- Diprivan Injection ... 2267

Propoxyphene Hydrochloride (Additive effect). Products include:
- Darvon ... 1256
- Wygesic Tablets ... 2540

Propoxyphene Napsylate (Additive effect). Products include:
- Darvon-N/Darvocet-N ... 1254

Propranolol Hydrochloride (Decreased antihypertensive effect). Products include:
- Inderal ... 2459
- Inderal LA Long Acting Capsules ... 2461
- Inderide Tablets ... 2463
- Inderide LA Long Acting Capsules ... 2465

Quazepam (Additive effect). Products include:
- Doral Tablets ... 2383

Ramipril (Decreased antihypertensive effect). Products include:
- Altace Capsules ... 1086

Rauwolfia Serpentina (Decreased antihypertensive effect). Products include:
- Raudixin Tablets ... 1803
- Rauzide Tablets ... 1804

Rescinnamine (Decreased antihypertensive effect).
- No products indexed under this heading.

Reserpine (Decreased antihypertensive effect). Products include:
- Diupres Tablets ... 1461
- Hydromox R Tablets ... 1209
- Hydropres Tablets ... 1485
- Renese-R Tablets ... 1786
- Salutensin/Salutensin-Demi ... 719
- Ser-Ap-Es Tablets ... 881
- Serpasil Tablets ... 883
- Serpasil-Apresoline Tablets ... 884
- Serpasil-Esidrix Tablets ... 886

Secobarbital Sodium (Additive effect). Products include:
- Seconal Sodium Pulvules ... 1296

Selegiline Hydrochloride (Prolonged anticholinergic effect). Products include:
- Eldepryl ... 2250

Sodium Nitroprusside (Decreased antihypertensive effect). Products include:
- Nipride I.V. Infusion ... 1909

Sufentanil Citrate (Additive effect). Products include:
- Sufenta Injection ... 1147

Temazepam (Additive effect). Products include:
- Restoril Capsules ... 2023

Terazosin Hydrochloride (Decreased antihypertensive effect). Products include:
- Hytrin Tablets ... 529

Thiamylal Sodium (Additive effect). Products include:
- Surital Ampoules, Steri-Vials ... 1764

Thioridazine Hydrochloride (Additive effect). Products include:
- Mellaril ... 2011

Thiothixene (Additive effect). Products include:
- Navane Capsules and Concentrate ... 1954
- Navane Intramuscular ... 1956

Timolol Maleate (Decreased antihypertensive effect). Products include:
- Blocadren Tablets ... 1429
- Timolide Tablets ... 1547
- Timoptic in Ocudose ... 1552
- Timoptic Sterile Ophthalmic Solution ... 1550

Tranylcypromine Sulfate (Prolonged anticholinergic effect). Products include:
- Parnate Tablets ... 2222

Triazolam (Additive effect). Products include:
- Halcion Tablets ... 2340

Trifluoperazine Hydrochloride (Additive effect). Products include:
- Stelazine ... 2226

Trimethaphan Camsylate (Decreased antihypertensive effect). Products include:
- Arfonad Ampuls ... 1887

DIMETAPP ELIXIR
(Brompheniramine Maleate, Phenylpropanolamine Hydrochloride) ... ◘ 673
May interact with monoamine oxidase inhibitors, sympathomimetic aerosal brochodilators, and certain other agents. Compounds in these categories include:

Albuterol (Results in additive effects). Products include:
- Proventil Inhalation Aerosol ... 2117
- Ventolin Inhalation Aerosol and Refill ... 583

Albuterol Sulfate (Results in additive effects). Products include:
- Proventil Repetabs Tablets ... 2120
- Proventil Solutions for Inhalation 0.5% and 0.083% ... 2118
- Proventil Syrup ... 2119
- Proventil Tablets ... 2120
- Ventolin ... 583

Alcohol (Do not use concomitantly).

Antihypertensive agents, unspecified (Diminished antihypertensive effect).

Dobutamine Hydrochloride (Results in additive effects). Products include:
- Dobutrex Solution Vials ... 1259

Dopamine Hydrochloride (Results in additive effects). Products include:
- Intropin Injection ... 930

Ephedrine Hydrochloride (Results in additive effects). Products include:
- Amesec ... ◘ 682
- Primatene Tablets-M Formula ... 2421
- Primatene Tablets-P Formula ... 2421
- Primatene Tablets-Regular Formula ... 2421
- Quadrinal Tablets ... 1183
- Quelidrine Syrup ... 556
- Tedral SA ... 1765

Ephedrine Sulfate (Results in additive effects). Products include:
- Bronkaid Tablets ... ◘ 757
- Bronkolixir ... ◘ 761
- Bronkotabs Tablets ... ◘ 762
- Marax Tablets & DF Syrup ... 1954
- Pazo Hemorrhoid Ointment & Suppositories ... 752
- Vicks Vatronol Nose Drops ... ◘ 666

Ephedrine Tannate (Results in additive effects). Products include:
- Rynatuss ... 2388

Epinephrine (Results in additive effects). Products include:
- Ana-Kit Anaphylaxis Emergency Treatment Kit ... 1100
- Bronkaid Mist ... ◘ 757

EpiPen 843
Marcaine Hydrochloride 0.5% with Epinephrine 1:200,000 (as bitartrate) 958
Marcaine Hydrochloride with Epinephrine 1:200,000 2055
Primatene Mist 2420
Sus-Phrine Injection 1006
Xylocaine with Epinephrine Injections 637

Epinephrine Bitartrate (Results in additive effects). Products include:
AsthmaHaler Mist Epinephrine Bitartrate Bronchodilator ▣ 616
Bronkaid Mist Suspension ▣ 757
Primatene Mist Suspension 2421

Epinephrine Hydrochloride (Results in additive effects). Products include:
Adrenalin Chloride Solution 1:100 & 1:1,000 1689
Epifrin ⊙ 244
Glaucon ⊙ 218

Furazolidone (Results in hypertensive crisis). Products include:
Furoxone 1855

Isocarboxazid (Results in hypertensive crisis). Products include:
Marplan Tablets 1906

Isoproterenol Hydrochloride (Results in additive effects). Products include:
Isuprel Hydrochloride Injection 1:5000 2050
Isuprel Hydrochloride Mistometer 2051
Isuprel Hydrochloride Solution 1:200 & 1:100 2052
Norisodrine Aerotrol 540

Metaproterenol Sulfate (Results in additive effects). Products include:
Alupent 674
Arm-a-Med Metaproterenol Sulfate Inhalation Solution, USP 617
Metaprel Inhalation Aerosol Bronchodilator 2014
Metaprel Inhalation Solution 2015
Metaprel 2015
Metaproterenol Sulfate Inhalation Solution, USP 912

Metaraminol Bitartrate (Results in additive effects). Products include:
Aramine Injection 1424

Methoxamine Hydrochloride (Results in additive effects). Products include:
Vasoxyl Injection 819

Norepinephrine Bitartrate (Results in additive effects). Products include:
Levophed Bitartrate Injection 2054

Phenelzine Sulfate (Results in hypertensive crisis). Products include:
Nardil 1742

Phenylephrine Bitartrate (Results in additive effects).
No products indexed under this heading.

Phenylephrine Hydrochloride (Results in additive effects). Products include:
AK-Dilate Solution 2.5% and 10% ⊙ 203
Atrohist Sprinkle Capsules 558
Cerose-DM 2443
Codimal 846
Comhist LA Capsules 1618
Congespirin For Children Aspirin Free Chewable Cold Tablets 748
Cyclomydril ⊙ 216
Deconsal Sprinkle Capsules 559
Dimetane Decongestant ▣ 673
Dristan Decongestant/Antihistamine/ Analgesic Coated Caplets ▣ 749
Dristan Cold Nasal Decongestant/ Antihistamine/ Analgesic Coated Tablets 2419
Dristan Advanced Formula Decongestant/Antihistamine/ Analgesic Tablets ▣ 749
Dristan Nasal Spray, Menthol 2419
Dristan Nasal Spray, Regular and Regular with Metered Pump 2419
Entex Capsules 1623
Entex Liquid 1623
Sinus Excedrin Analgesic, Decongestant Tablets & Caplets 750
Extendryl 994
4-Way Fast Acting Nasal Spray - Original Formula (regular & mentholated) & Metered Spray Pump (regular) 751
Hycomine Compound Tablets 929
Murocoll-2 Sterile Ophthalmic Solution ⊙ 261
Mydfrin 2.5% ⊙ 224
Naldecon Syrup, Tablets, Pediatric Drops and Pediatric Syrup 709
Neo-Synephrine Hydrochloride 1% Carpuject 2063
Neo-Synephrine Hydrochloride 1% Injection 2063
Neo-Synephrine Hydrochloride (Ophthalmic) 2064
Neo-Synephrine ▣ 759
Nōstril Nasal Decongestant ▣ 520
Novahistine Elixir ▣ 596
Phenergan VC 2500
Phenergan VC with Codeine 2501
Prefrin Liquifilm Vasoconstrictor and Lubricant Eye Drops ⊙ 254
Prefrin-A ⊙ 255
Quelidrine Syrup 556
Relief Vasoconstrictor and Lubricant Eye Drops ⊙ 256
Robitussin Night Relief ▣ 677
Ru-Tuss with Hydrocodone 694
Ru-Tuss Tablets 693
Vasosulf ⊙ 279
Vicks Sinex ▣ 665
Zincfrin ⊙ 230

Phenylephrine Tannate (Results in additive effects). Products include:
Rynatan 2387
Rynatuss 2388

Pirbuterol Acetate (Results in additive effects). Products include:
Maxair Inhaler 1311

Pseudoephedrine Hydrochloride (Results in additive effects). Products include:
Actifed Capsules ▣ 539
Actifed Plus Caplets ▣ 539
Actifed Plus Tablets ▣ 540
Actifed with Codeine Cough Syrup 752
Actifed Syrup ▣ 540
Actifed Tablets ▣ 540
Actifed 12-Hour Capsules ▣ 539
Advil Cold & Sinus Caplets (formerly CoAdvil) 2416
Allerest ▣ 559
Anatuss LA Tablets 1359
Benadryl Decongestant Elixir ▣ 635
Benadryl Decongestant ▣ 635
Benadryl Plus ▣ 636
Benadryl Plus Nighttime ▣ 637
Benylin Decongestant ▣ 638
Brexin L.A. Capsules 2078
Bromfed Capsules (Timed Release) 1615
Bromfed Syrup ▣ 628
Bromfed 1615
CoAdvil ▣ 748
Allergy-Sinus Comtrex Multi-Symptom Allergy Sinus Formula Tablets & Caplets 746
Cough Formula Comtrex 746
Comtrex Multi-Symptom Cold Reliever Tablets/Caplets/Liqui-Gels/Liquid 745
Day-Night Comtrex 747
Non-Drowsy Comtrex 747
Congess 994
Congestac Caplets ▣ 617
Contac Jr. Children's Cold Medicine ▣ 712
Contac Nighttime Cold Medicine ▣ 713
Contac Sinus Caplets Maximum Strength Non-Drowsy Formula ▣ 710
Contac Sinus Tablets Maximum Strength Non-Drowsy Formula ▣ 710
Deconamine 663
Deconsal II Tablets 559
Dimacol Caplets ▣ 672
Dimetane-DX Cough Syrup 1858
Dorcol Children's Cough Syrup ▣ 685
Dorcol Children's Decongestant Liquid ▣ 685
Dorcol Children's Liquid Cold Formula ▣ 686
Maximum Strength Dristan Decongestant/Analgesic Coated Caplets ▣ 750
No Drowsiness Dristan Cold Nasal Decongestant/Analgesic Coated Caplets 2420
Dristan Sinus Caplets 2419
Sinus Excedrin Analgesic, Decongestant Tablets & Caplets ▣ 533
Fedahist Gyrocaps 2145
Fedahist Timecaps 2145
Guaifed 1615
Guaifed Syrup ▣ 629
Isoclor Expectorant 982
Isoclor Timesule Capsules ▣ 561
Kronofed-A 970
Medi-Flu Caplet, Liquid ▣ 640
Novafed A Capsules 1342
Novafed Capsules 1342
Novahistine DH 1342
Novahistine DMX ▣ 595
Novahistine Expectorant 1343
Nucofed Capsules 2219
Nucofed Expectorant 2219
Nucofed Pediatric Expectorant 2220
Nucofed Syrup 2219
Ornex Caplets ▣ 618
PediaCare Allergy Relief Formula Liquid 1362
PediaCare Cough-Cold Formula Liquid 1362
PediaCare Infants' Oral Decongestant Drops 1362
PediaCare Night Rest Cough-Cold Formula Liquid 1362
PediaCare 6-12 Cough-Cold Formula Chewable Tablets 1362
Robitussin-DAC Syrup 1875
Robitussin-PE ▣ 677
Rondec 1975
Rondec-DM 1976
Rondec-TR Tablet 1975
Ru-Tuss DE Tablets 694
Ryna ▣ 741
Seldane-D Extended-Release Tablets 1350
Sinarest ▣ 562
Sine-Aid Maximum Strength Sinus Headache Caplets 1365
Sine-Aid Maximum Strength Sinus Headache Tablets 1365
Sine-Off Maximum Strength Allergy/Sinus Formula Caplets ▣ 721
Sine-Off Maximum Strength No Drowsiness Formula Caplets ▣ 722
Singlet Tablets ▣ 598
Sinutab Maximum Strength ▣ 641
Sinutab Maximum Strength Without Drowsiness Tablets & Caplets ▣ 642
Sinutab Regular Strength Without Drowsiness Formula ▣ 641
St. Joseph Nighttime Cold Medicine ▣ 705
Sudafed Children's Liquid ▣ 543
Sudafed Cough Syrup ▣ 543
Sudafed Plus Liquid ▣ 544
Sudafed Plus Tablets ▣ 545
Sudafed Sinus Caplets ▣ 545
Sudafed Sinus Tablets ▣ 545
Sudafed Tablets, 30 mg ▣ 544
Sudafed Tablets, Adult Strength, 60 mg ▣ 544
Sudafed 12 Hour Capsules ▣ 545
TheraFlu Flu and Cold Medicine ▣ 687
Triaminic Nite Light ▣ 689
Tylenol Allergy Sinus Medication Caplets and Gelcaps, Maximum Strength 1372
Children's Tylenol Cold Liquid Formula and Chewable Tablets 1368
Tylenol Cold & Flu Hot Medication, Packets 1369
Tylenol Cold & Flu No Drowsiness Hot Medication, Packets 1371
Tylenol Cold Medication Caplets and Tablets 1370
Tylenol Cold Medication No Drowsiness Formula Caplets 1370
Tylenol Cold Night Time Medication Liquid 1371
Tylenol Cough Medication Liquid with Decongestant, Maximum Strength 1372
Tylenol, Maximum Strength, Sinus Medication Gelcaps, Caplets and Tablets 1373
Ursinus Inlay-Tabs ▣ 691
Vicks Children's NyQuil ▣ 664
Vicks Daycare ▣ 660
Vicks Formula 44D Decongestant Cough Medicine ▣ 662
Vicks Formula 44M Multi-Symptom Cough Medicine ▣ 662
Vicks NyQuil Nighttime Colds Medicine-Original & Cherry Flavor ▣ 664
Vicks Pediatric Formula 44 Cough & Congestion Medicine ▣ 663
Vicks Pediatric Formula 44m Multi-Symptom Cough & Cold Medicine ▣ 663

Pseudoephedrine Sulfate (Results in additive effects). Products include:
Afrin Tablets ▣ 693
Chlor-Trimeton Decongestant ▣ 694
Disophrol Chronotab Sustained-Action Tablets ▣ 698
Drixoral Antihistamine/Nasal Decongestant Syrup ▣ 698
Drixoral Non-Drowsy Formula ▣ 699
Drixoral Plus Extended-Release Tablets ▣ 699
Drixoral Sinus ▣ 700
Drixoral Sustained-Action Tablets ▣ 698
Sinutab Allergy Formula Sustained Action Tablets ▣ 640
Trinalin Repetabs Tablets 1170

Selegiline Hydrochloride (Results in hypertensive crisis). Products include:
Eldepryl 2250

Terbutaline Sulfate (Results in additive effects). Products include:
Brethaire Inhaler 1024
Brethine Ampuls 1026
Brethine Tablets 1026
Bricanyl Injection 1324
Bricanyl Tablets 1325

Tranylcypromine Sulfate (Results in hypertensive crisis). Products include:
Parnate Tablets 2222

DIMETAPP DM ELIXIR
(Brompheniramine Maleate, Dextromethorphan Hydrobromide) ▣ 674
May interact with monoamine oxidase inhibitors, sympathomimetic aerosal brochodilators, and certain other agents. Compounds in these categories include:

Albuterol (Produces additive effects and increased toxicity). Products include:
Proventil Inhalation Aerosol 2117
Ventolin Inhalation Aerosol and Refill 583

Albuterol Sulfate (Produces additive effects and increased toxicity). Products include:
Proventil Repetabs Tablets 2120
Proventil Solutions for Inhalation 0.5% and 0.083% 2118
Proventil Syrup 2119
Proventil Tablets 2120
Ventolin 583

Antihypertensive agents, unspecified (Diminished antihypertensive effect).

Dobutamine Hydrochloride (Produces additive effects and increased toxicity). Products include:
Dobutrex Solution Vials 1259

Dopamine Hydrochloride (Produces additive effects and increased toxicity). Products include:
Intropin Injection 930

Ephedrine Hydrochloride (Produces additive effects and increased toxicity). Products include:
Amesec ▣ 682
Primatene Tablets-M Formula 2421
Primatene Tablets-P Formula 2421
Primatene Tablets-Regular Formula 2421
Quadrinal Tablets 1183
Quelidrine Syrup 556
Tedral SA 1765

Ephedrine Sulfate (Produces additive effects and increased toxicity). Products include:

- Bronkaid Tablets ■ 757
- Bronkolixir ■ 761
- Bronkotabs Tablets ■ 762
- Marax Tablets & DF Syrup 1954
- Pazo Hemorrhoid Ointment & Suppositories 752
- Vicks Vatronol Nose Drops ■ 666

Ephedrine Tannate (Produces additive effects and increased toxicity). Products include:

- Rynatuss 2388

Epinephrine (Produces additive effects and increased toxicity). Products include:

- Ana-Kit Anaphylaxis Emergency Treatment Kit 1100
- Bronkaid Mist ■ 757
- EpiPen 843
- Marcaine Hydrochloride 0.5% with Epinephrine 1:200,000 (as bitartrate) 958
- Marcaine Hydrochloride with Epinephrine 1:200,000 2055
- Primatene Mist 2420
- Sus-Phrine Injection 1006
- Xylocaine with Epinephrine Injections 637

Epinephrine Bitartrate (Produces additive effects and increased toxicity). Products include:

- AsthmaHaler Mist Epinephrine Bitartrate Bronchodilator ■ 616
- Bronkaid Mist Suspension ■ 757
- Primatene Mist Suspension 2421

Epinephrine Hydrochloride (Produces additive effects and increased toxicity). Products include:

- Adrenalin Chloride Solution 1:100 & 1:1,000 1689
- Epifrin ⊙ 244
- Glaucon ⊙ 218

Furazolidone (Produces a hypertensive crisis and may result in serious toxicity). Products include:

- Furoxone 1855

Isocarboxazid (Produces a hypertensive crisis and may result in serious toxicity). Products include:

- Marplan Tablets 1906

Isoproterenol Hydrochloride (Produces additive effects and increased toxicity). Products include:

- Isuprel Hydrochloride Injection 1:5000 2050
- Isuprel Hydrochloride Mistometer 2051
- Isuprel Hydrochloride Solution 1:200 & 1:100 2052
- Norisodrine Aerotrol 540

Metaproterenol Sulfate (Produces additive effects and increased toxicity). Products include:

- Alupent 674
- Arm-a-Med Metaproterenol Sulfate Inhalation Solution, USP 617
- Metaprel Inhalation Aerosol Bronchodilator 2014
- Metaprel Inhalation Solution 2015
- Metaprel 2015
- Metaproterenol Sulfate Inhalation Solution, USP 912

Metaraminol Bitartrate (Produces additive effects and increased toxicity). Products include:

- Aramine Injection 1424

Methoxamine Hydrochloride (Produces additive effects and increased toxicity). Products include:

- Vasoxyl Injection 819

Norepinephrine Bitartrate (Produces additive effects and increased toxicity). Products include:

- Levophed Bitartrate Injection 2054

Phenelzine Sulfate (Produces a hypertensive crisis and may result in serious toxicity). Products include:

- Nardil 1742

Phenylephrine Bitartrate (Produces additive effects and increased toxicity).

- No products indexed under this heading.

Phenylephrine Hydrochloride (Produces additive effects and increased toxicity). Products include:

- AK-Dilate Solution 2.5% and 10% ⊙ 203
- Atrohist Sprinkle Capsules 558
- Cerose-DM 2443
- Codimal 846
- Comhist LA Capsules 1618
- Congespirin For Children Aspirin Free Chewable Cold Tablets 748
- Cyclomydril ⊙ 216
- Deconsal Sprinkle Capsules 559
- Dimetane Decongestant ■ 673
- Dristan Decongestant/Antihistamine/ Analgesic Coated Caplets ■ 749
- Dristan Cold Nasal Decongestant/ Antihistamine/ Analgesic Coated Tablets 2419
- Dristan Advanced Formula Decongestant/Antihistamine/ Analgesic Tablets ■ 749
- Dristan Nasal Spray, Menthol 2419
- Dristan Nasal Spray, Regular and Regular with Metered Pump 2419
- Entex Capsules 1623
- Entex Liquid 1623
- Sinus Excedrin Analgesic, Decongestant Tablets & Caplets 750
- Extendryl 994
- 4-Way Fast Acting Nasal Spray - Original Formula (regular & mentholated) & Metered Spray Pump (regular) 751
- Hycomine Compound Tablets 929
- Murocoll-2 Sterile Ophthalmic Solution ⊙ 261
- Mydfrin 2.5% ⊙ 224
- Naldecon Syrup, Tablets, Pediatric Drops and Pediatric Syrup 709
- Neo-Synephrine Hydrochloride 1% Carpuject 2063
- Neo-Synephrine Hydrochloride 1% Injection 2063
- Neo-Synephrine Hydrochloride (Ophthalmic) 2064
- Neo-Synephrine ■ 759
- Nōstril Nasal Decongestant ■ 520
- Novahistine Elixir ■ 596
- Phenergan VC 2500
- Phenergan VC with Codeine 2501
- Prefrin Liquifilm Vasoconstrictor and Lubricant Eye Drops ⊙ 254
- Prefrin-A ⊙ 255
- Quelidrine Syrup 556
- Relief Vasoconstrictor and Lubricant Eye Drops ⊙ 256
- Robitussin Night Relief ■ 677
- Ru-Tuss with Hydrocodone 694
- Ru-Tuss Tablets 693
- Vasosulf ⊙ 279
- Vicks Sinex ■ 665
- Zincfrin ⊙ 230

Phenylephrine Tannate (Produces additive effects and increased toxicity). Products include:

- Rynatan 2387
- Rynatuss 2388

Phenylpropanolamine Hydrochloride (Produces additive effects and increased toxicity). Products include:

- A.R.M. Allergy Relief Medicine Caplets ■ 615
- Acutrim ■ 548
- Allerest ■ 559
- BC Cold Powder ■ 517
- Cheracol Plus Head Cold/Cough Formula ■ 667
- Codimal Expectorant 846
- Comtrex Multi-Symptom Cold Reliever Tablets/Caplets/Liqui-Gels/Liquid 745
- Contac Continuous Action Decongestant/Antihistamine Capsules ■ 710
- Contac Maximum Strength Continuous Action Decongestant/ Antihistamine Caplets ■ 709
- Contac Severe Cold and Flu Formula Caplets ■ 711
- Coricidin 'D' Decongestant Tablets ■ 695
- Coricidin Demilets Tablets for Children ■ 696
- Demazin Nasal Decongestant/ Antihistamine Repetabs Tablets & Syrup ■ 697
- Dexatrim ■ 733
- Dimetane-DC Cough Syrup 1857
- Dimetapp Elixir ■ 673
- Dimetapp DM Elixir ■ 674
- Dimetapp Extentabs ■ 674
- Dimetapp Plus Caplets ■ 675
- Dimetapp Tablets ■ 675
- Entex Capsules 1623
- Entex LA Tablets 1623
- Entex Liquid 1623
- 4-Way Cold Tablets 750
- Hycomine Syrup 927
- Naldecon CX Adult Liquid ■ 521
- Naldecon DX Adult Liquid ■ 521
- Naldecon DX Children's Syrup ■ 522
- Naldecon DX Pediatric Drops ■ 522
- Naldecon EX Children's Syrup ■ 522
- Naldecon EX Pediatric Drops ■ 523
- Naldecon Syrup, Tablets, Pediatric Drops and Pediatric Syrup 709
- Nolamine Tablets 838
- Nolex LA Tablets 838
- Ornade Spansule Capsules 2221
- Orthoxicol Cough Syrup ■ 668
- Propagest 839
- Pyrroxate Capsules ■ 669
- Robitussin-CF ■ 676
- Ru-Tuss II Capsules 693
- Ru-Tuss with Hydrocodone 694
- Ru-Tuss Tablets 693
- Sine-Off Sinus Medicine Tablets-Aspirin Formula ■ 722
- Sinulin 840
- St. Joseph Cold Tablets for Children ■ 704
- Tavist-D Tablets 2035
- Triaminic Allergy Tablets ■ 688
- Triaminic Chewables ■ 688
- Triaminic Cold Tablets ■ 688
- Triaminic Expectorant ■ 688
- Triaminic Expectorant w/Codeine 1996
- Triaminic Expectorant DH 1995
- Triaminic Oral Infant Drops 1996
- Triaminic Syrup ■ 689
- Triaminic-12 Tablets ■ 690
- Triaminic-DM Syrup ■ 689
- Triaminicin Tablets ■ 690
- Triaminicol Multi-Symptom Cold Tablets ■ 691
- Triaminicol Multi-Symptom Relief ■ 691
- Tuss-Ornade Liquid 2242
- Tuss-Ornade Spansule Capsules 2242
- Tylenol Cold Medication, Effervescent Tablets 1369

Pirbuterol Acetate (Produces additive effects and increased toxicity). Products include:

- Maxair Inhaler 1311

Pseudoephedrine Hydrochloride (Produces additive effects and increased toxicity). Products include:

- Actifed Capsules ■ 539
- Actifed Plus Caplets ■ 539
- Actifed Plus Tablets ■ 540
- Actifed with Codeine Cough Syrup 752
- Actifed Syrup ■ 540
- Actifed Tablets ■ 540
- Actifed 12-Hour Capsules ■ 539
- Advil Cold & Sinus Caplets (formerly CoAdvil) 2416
- Allerest ■ 559
- Anatuss LA Tablets 1359
- Benadryl Decongestant Elixir ■ 635
- Benadryl Decongestant ■ 635
- Benadryl Plus ■ 636
- Benadryl Plus Nighttime ■ 637
- Benylin Decongestant ■ 638
- Brexin L.A. Capsules 2078
- Bromfed Capsules (Timed Release) 1615
- Bromfed Syrup ■ 628
- Bromfed 1615
- CoAdvil ■ 748
- Allergy-Sinus Comtrex Multi-Symptom Allergy Sinus Formula Tablets & Caplets 746
- Cough Formula Comtrex 746
- Comtrex Multi-Symptom Cold Reliever Tablets/Caplets/Liqui-Gels/Liquid 745
- Day-Night Comtrex 747
- Non-Drowsy Comtrex 747
- Congess 994
- Congestac Caplets ■ 617
- Contac Jr. Children's Cold Medicine ■ 712
- Contac Nighttime Cold Medicine ■ 713
- Contac Sinus Caplets Maximum Strength Non-Drowsy Formula ■ 710
- Contac Sinus Tablets Maximum Strength Non-Drowsy Formula ■ 710
- Deconamine 663
- Deconsal II Tablets 559
- Dimacol Caplets ■ 672
- Dimetane-DX Cough Syrup 1858
- Dorcol Children's Cough Syrup ■ 685
- Dorcol Children's Decongestant Liquid ■ 685
- Dorcol Children's Liquid Cold Formula ■ 686
- Maximum Strength Dristan Decongestant/Analgesic Coated Caplets ■ 750
- No Drowsiness Dristan Cold Nasal Decongestant/Analgesic Coated Caplets 2420
- Dristan Sinus Caplets 2419
- Sinus Excedrin Analgesic, Decongestant Tablets & Caplets ■ 533
- Fedahist Gyrocaps 2145
- Fedahist Timecaps 2145
- Guaifed 1615
- Guaifed Syrup ■ 629
- Isoclor Expectorant 982
- Isoclor Timesule Capsules ■ 561
- Kronofed-A 970
- Medi-Flu Caplet, Liquid ■ 640
- Novafed A Capsules 1342
- Novafed Capsules 1342
- Novahistine DH 1342
- Novahistine DMX ■ 595
- Novahistine Expectorant 1343
- Nucofed Capsules 2219
- Nucofed Expectorant 2219
- Nucofed Pediatric Expectorant 2220
- Nucofed Syrup 2219
- Ornex Caplets ■ 618
- PediaCare Allergy Relief Formula Liquid 1362
- PediaCare Cough-Cold Formula Liquid 1362
- PediaCare Infants' Oral Decongestant Drops 1362
- PediaCare Night Rest Cough-Cold Formula Liquid 1362
- PediaCare 6-12 Cough-Cold Formula Chewable Tablets 1362
- Robitussin-DAC Syrup 1875
- Robitussin-PE ■ 677
- Rondec 1975
- Rondec-DM 1976
- Rondec-TR Tablet 1975
- Ru-Tuss DE Tablets 694
- Ryna ■ 741
- Seldane-D Extended-Release Tablets 1350
- Sinarest ■ 562
- Sine-Aid Maximum Strength Sinus Headache Caplets 1365
- Sine-Aid Maximum Strength Sinus Headache Tablets 1365
- Sine-Off Maximum Strength Allergy/Sinus Formula Caplets ■ 721
- Sine-Off Maximum Strength No Drowsiness Formula Caplets ■ 722
- Singlet Tablets ■ 598
- Sinutab Maximum Strength ■ 641
- Sinutab Maximum Strength Without Drowsiness Tablets & Caplets ■ 642
- Sinutab Regular Strength Without Drowsiness Formula ■ 641
- St. Joseph Nighttime Cold Medicine ■ 705
- Sudafed Children's Liquid ■ 543
- Sudafed Cough Syrup ■ 543
- Sudafed Plus Liquid ■ 544
- Sudafed Plus Tablets ■ 545
- Sudafed Sinus Caplets ■ 545
- Sudafed Sinus Tablets ■ 545
- Sudafed Tablets, 30 mg ■ 544
- Sudafed Tablets, Adult Strength, 60 mg ■ 544
- Sudafed 12 Hour Capsules ■ 545
- TheraFlu Flu and Cold Medicine ■ 687
- Triaminic Nite Light ■ 689
- Tylenol Allergy Sinus Medication Caplets and Gelcaps, Maximum Strength 1372
- Children's Tylenol Cold Liquid Formula and Chewable Tablets 1368
- Tylenol Cold & Flu Hot Medication, Packets 1369

Tylenol Cold & Flu No Drowsiness Hot Medication, Packets 1371
Tylenol Cold Medication Caplets and Tablets 1370
Tylenol Cold Medication No Drowsiness Formula Caplets 1370
Tylenol Cold Night Time Medication Liquid 1371
Tylenol Cough Medication Liquid with Decongestant, Maximum Strength 1372
Tylenol, Maximum Strength, Sinus Medication Gelcaps, Caplets and Tablets 1373
Ursinus Inlay-Tabs ▣ 691
Vicks Children's NyQuil ▣ 664
Vicks Daycare ▣ 660
Vicks Formula 44D Decongestant Cough Medicine ▣ 662
Vicks Formula 44M Multi-Symptom Cough Medicine ▣ 662
Vicks NyQuil Nighttime Colds Medicine-Original & Cherry Flavor ▣ 664
Vicks Pediatric Formula 44 Cough & Congestion Medicine ▣ 663
Vicks Pediatric Formula 44m Multi-Symptom Cough & Cold Medicine ▣ 663

Pseudoephedrine Sulfate (Produces additive effects and increased toxicity). Products include:
Afrin Tablets ▣ 693
Chlor-Trimeton Decongestant ▣ 694
Disophrol Chronotab Sustained-Action Tablets ▣ 698
Drixoral Antihistamine/Nasal Decongestant Syrup ▣ 698
Drixoral Non-Drowsy Formula ▣ 699
Drixoral Plus Extended-Release Tablets ▣ 699
Drixoral Sinus ▣ 700
Drixoral Sustained-Action Tablets ▣ 698
Sinutab Allergy Formula Sustained Action Tablets ▣ 640
Trinalin Repetabs Tablets 1170

Selegiline Hydrochloride (Produces a hypertensive crisis and may result in serious toxicity). Products include:
Eldepryl 2250

Terbutaline Sulfate (Produces additive effects and increased toxicity). Products include:
Brethaire Inhaler 1024
Brethine Ampuls 1026
Brethine Tablets 1026
Bricanyl Injection 1324
Bricanyl Tablets 1325

Tranylcypromine Sulfate (Produces a hypertensive crisis and may result in serious toxicity). Products include:
Parnate Tablets 2222

DIMETAPP EXTENTABS
(Brompheniramine Maleate, Phenylpropanolamine Hydrochloride) ▣ 674
May interact with sympathomimetic aerosal brochodilators, monoamine oxidase inhibitors, and certain other agents. Compounds in these categories include:

Albuterol (May produce additive effects). Products include:
Proventil Inhalation Aerosol 2117
Ventolin Inhalation Aerosol and Refill 583

Albuterol Sulfate (May produce additive effects). Products include:
Proventil Repetabs Tablets 2120
Proventil Solutions for Inhalation 0.5% and 0.083% 2118
Proventil Syrup 2119
Proventil Tablets 2120
Ventolin 583

Alcohol (Do not use concomitantly).

Antihypertensive agents, unspecified (Diminished antihypertensive effect).

Dobutamine Hydrochloride (May produce additive effects). Products include:
Dobutrex Solution Vials 1259

Dopamine Hydrochloride (May produce additive effects). Products include:
Intropin Injection 930

Ephedrine Hydrochloride (May produce additive effects). Products include:
Amesec ▣ 682
Primatene Tablets-M Formula 2421
Primatene Tablets-P Formula 2421
Primatene Tablets-Regular Formula 2421
Quadrinal Tablets 1183
Quelidrine Syrup 556
Tedral SA 1765

Ephedrine Sulfate (May produce additive effects). Products include:
Bronkaid Tablets ▣ 757
Bronkolixir ▣ 761
Bronkotabs Tablets ▣ 762
Marax Tablets & DF Syrup 1954
Pazo Hemorrhoid Ointment & Suppositories 752
Vicks Vatronol Nose Drops ▣ 666

Ephedrine Tannate (May produce additive effects). Products include:
Rynatuss 2388

Epinephrine (May produce additive effects). Products include:
Ana-Kit Anaphylaxis Emergency Treatment Kit 1100
Bronkaid Mist ▣ 757
EpiPen 843
Marcaine Hydrochloride 0.5% with Epinephrine 1:200,000 (as bitartrate) 958
Marcaine Hydrochloride with Epinephrine 1:200,000 2055
Primatene Mist 2420
Sus-Phrine Injection 1006
Xylocaine with Epinephrine Injections 637

Epinephrine Bitartrate (May produce additive effects). Products include:
AsthmaHaler Mist Epinephrine Bitartrate Bronchodilator ▣ 616
Bronkaid Mist Suspension ▣ 757
Primatene Mist Suspension 2421

Epinephrine Hydrochloride (May produce additive effects). Products include:
Adrenalin Chloride Solution 1:100 & 1:1,000 1689
Epifrin ⊙ 244
Glaucon ⊙ 218

Furazolidone (May produce hypertensive crisis). Products include:
Furoxone 1855

Isocarboxazid (May produce hypertensive crisis). Products include:
Marplan Tablets 1906

Isoproterenol Hydrochloride (May produce additive effects). Products include:
Isuprel Hydrochloride Injection 1:5000 2050
Isuprel Hydrochloride Mistometer 2051
Isuprel Hydrochloride Solution 1:200 & 1:100 2052
Norisodrine Aerotrol 540

Metaproterenol Sulfate (May produce additive effects). Products include:
Alupent 674
Arm-a-Med Metaproterenol Sulfate Inhalation Solution, USP 617
Metaprel Inhalation Aerosol Bronchodilator 2014
Metaprel Inhalation Solution 2015
Metaprel 2015
Metaproterenol Sulfate Inhalation Solution, USP 912

Metaraminol Bitartrate (May produce additive effects). Products include:
Aramine Injection 1424

Methoxamine Hydrochloride (May produce additive effects). Products include:
Vasoxyl Injection 819

Norepinephrine Bitartrate (May produce additive effects). Products include:
Levophed Bitartrate Injection 2054

Phenelzine Sulfate (May produce hypertensive crisis). Products include:
Nardil 1742

Phenylephrine Bitartrate (May produce additive effects).
No products indexed under this heading.

Phenylephrine Hydrochloride (May produce additive effects). Products include:
AK-Dilate Solution 2.5% and 10% ⊙ 203
Atrohist Sprinkle Capsules 558
Cerose-DM 2443
Codimal 846
Comhist LA Capsules 1618
Congespirin For Children Aspirin Free Chewable Cold Tablets 748
Cyclomydril ⊙ 216
Deconsal Sprinkle Capsules 559
Dimetane Decongestant ▣ 673
Dristan Decongestant/Antihistamine/ Analgesic Coated Caplets ▣ 749
Dristan Cold Nasal Decongestant/ Antihistamine/ Analgesic Coated Tablets 2419
Dristan Advanced Formula Decongestant/Antihistamine/ Analgesic Tablets ▣ 749
Dristan Nasal Spray, Menthol 2419
Dristan Nasal Spray, Regular and Regular with Metered Pump 2419
Entex Capsules 1623
Entex Liquid 1623
Sinus Excedrin Analgesic, Decongestant Tablets & Caplets 750
Extendryl 994
4-Way Fast Acting Nasal Spray - Original Formula (regular & mentholated) & Metered Spray Pump (regular) 751
Hycomine Compound Tablets 929
Murocoll-2 Sterile Ophthalmic Solution ⊙ 261
Mydfrin 2.5% ⊙ 224
Naldecon Syrup, Tablets, Pediatric Drops and Pediatric Syrup 709
Neo-Synephrine Hydrochloride 1% Carpuject 2063
Neo-Synephrine Hydrochloride 1% Injection 2063
Neo-Synephrine Hydrochloride (Ophthalmic) 2064
Neo-Synephrine ▣ 759
Nōstril Nasal Decongestant ▣ 520
Novahistine Elixir ▣ 596
Phenergan VC 2500
Phenergan VC with Codeine 2501
Prefrin Liquifilm Vasoconstrictor and Lubricant Eye Drops ⊙ 254
Prefrin-A ⊙ 255
Quelidrine Syrup 556
Relief Vasoconstrictor and Lubricant Eye Drops ⊙ 256
Robitussin Night Relief ▣ 677
Ru-Tuss with Hydrocodone 694
Ru-Tuss Tablets 693
Vasosulf ⊙ 279
Vicks Sinex ▣ 665
Zincfrin ⊙ 230

Phenylephrine Tannate (May produce additive effects). Products include:
Rynatan 2387
Rynatuss 2388

Pirbuterol Acetate (May produce additive effects). Products include:
Maxair Inhaler 1311

Pseudoephedrine Hydrochloride (May produce additive effects). Products include:
Actifed Capsules ▣ 539
Actifed Plus Caplets ▣ 539
Actifed Plus Tablets ▣ 540
Actifed with Codeine Cough Syrup 752
Actifed Syrup ▣ 540
Actifed Tablets ▣ 540
Actifed 12-Hour Capsules ▣ 539
Advil Cold & Sinus Caplets (formerly CoAdvil) 2416
Allerest ▣ 559
Anatuss LA Tablets 1359
Benadryl Decongestant Elixir ▣ 635
Benadryl Decongestant ▣ 635
Benadryl Plus ▣ 636
Benadryl Plus Nighttime ▣ 637
Benylin Decongestant ▣ 638
Brexin L.A. Capsules 2078
Bromfed Capsules (Timed Release) 1615
Bromfed Syrup ▣ 628
Bromfed 1615
CoAdvil ▣ 748
Allergy-Sinus Comtrex Multi-Symptom Allergy Sinus Formula Tablets & Caplets 746
Cough Formula Comtrex 746
Comtrex Multi-Symptom Cold Reliever Tablets/Caplets/Liqui-Gels/Liquid 745
Day-Night Comtrex 747
Non-Drowsy Comtrex 747
Congess 994
Congestac Caplets ▣ 617
Contac Jr. Children's Cold Medicine ▣ 712
Contac Nighttime Cold Medicine ▣ 713
Contac Sinus Caplets Maximum Strength Non-Drowsy Formula ▣ 710
Contac Sinus Tablets Maximum Strength Non-Drowsy Formula ▣ 710
Deconamine 663
Deconsal II Tablets 559
Dimacol Caplets ▣ 672
Dimetane-DX Cough Syrup 1858
Dorcol Children's Cough Syrup ▣ 685
Dorcol Children's Decongestant Liquid ▣ 685
Dorcol Children's Liquid Cold Formula ▣ 686
Maximum Strength Dristan Decongestant/Analgesic Coated Caplets ▣ 750
No Drowsiness Dristan Cold Nasal Decongestant/Analgesic Coated Caplets 2420
Dristan Sinus Caplets 2419
Sinus Excedrin Analgesic, Decongestant Tablets & Caplets ▣ 533
Fedahist Gyrocaps 2145
Fedahist Timecaps 2145
Guaifed 1615
Guaifed Syrup ▣ 629
Isoclor Expectorant 982
Isoclor Timesule Capsules ▣ 561
Kronofed-A 970
Medi-Flu Caplet, Liquid ▣ 640
Novafed A Capsules 1342
Novafed Capsules 1342
Novahistine DH 1342
Novahistine DMX ▣ 595
Novahistine Expectorant 1343
Nucofed Capsules 2219
Nucofed Expectorant 2219
Nucofed Pediatric Expectorant 2220
Nucofed Syrup 2219
Ornex Caplets ▣ 618
PediaCare Allergy Relief Formula Liquid 1362
PediaCare Cough-Cold Formula Liquid 1362
PediaCare Infants' Oral Decongestant Drops 1362
PediaCare Night Rest Cough-Cold Formula Liquid 1362
PediaCare 6-12 Cough-Cold Formula Chewable Tablets 1362
Robitussin-DAC Syrup 1875
Robitussin-PE ▣ 677
Rondec 1975
Rondec-DM 1976
Rondec-TR Tablet 1975
Ru-Tuss DE Tablets 694
Ryna ▣ 741
Seldane-D Extended-Release Tablets 1350
Sinarest ▣ 562
Sine-Aid Maximum Strength Sinus Headache Caplets 1365
Sine-Aid Maximum Strength Sinus Headache Tablets 1365
Sine-Off Maximum Strength Allergy/Sinus Formula Caplets ▣ 721
Sine-Off Maximum Strength No Drowsiness Formula Caplets ▣ 722
Singlet Tablets ▣ 598

- Sinutab Maximum Strength ⊡ 641
- Sinutab Maximum Strength Without Drowsiness Tablets & Caplets ⊡ 642
- Sinutab Regular Strength Without Drowsiness Formula ⊡ 641
- St. Joseph Nighttime Cold Medicine ⊡ 705
- Sudafed Children's Liquid ⊡ 543
- Sudafed Cough Syrup ⊡ 543
- Sudafed Plus Liquid ⊡ 544
- Sudafed Plus Tablets ⊡ 545
- Sudafed Sinus Caplets ⊡ 545
- Sudafed Sinus Tablets ⊡ 545
- Sudafed Tablets, 30 mg ⊡ 544
- Sudafed Tablets, Adult Strength, 60 mg ⊡ 544
- Sudafed 12 Hour Capsules ⊡ 545
- TheraFlu Flu and Cold Medicine ⊡ 687
- Triaminic Nite Light ⊡ 689
- Tylenol Allergy Sinus Medication Caplets and Gelcaps, Maximum Strength 1372
- Children's Tylenol Cold Liquid Formula and Chewable Tablets 1368
- Tylenol Cold & Flu Hot Medication, Packets 1369
- Tylenol Cold & Flu No Drowsiness Hot Medication, Packets 1371
- Tylenol Cold Medication Caplets and Tablets 1370
- Tylenol Cold Medication No Drowsiness Formula Caplets 1370
- Tylenol Cold Night Time Medication Liquid 1371
- Tylenol Cough Medication Liquid with Decongestant, Maximum Strength 1372
- Tylenol, Maximum Strength, Sinus Medication Gelcaps, Caplets and Tablets 1373
- Ursinus Inlay-Tabs ⊡ 691
- Vicks Children's NyQuil ⊡ 664
- Vicks Daycare ⊡ 660
- Vicks Formula 44D Decongestant Cough Medicine ⊡ 662
- Vicks Formula 44M Multi-Symptom Cough Medicine ⊡ 662
- Vicks NyQuil Nighttime Colds Medicine-Original & Cherry Flavor ⊡ 664
- Vicks Pediatric Formula 44 Cough & Congestion Medicine ⊡ 663
- Vicks Pediatric Formula 44m Multi-Symptom Cough & Cold Medicine ⊡ 663

Pseudoephedrine Sulfate (May produce additive effects). Products include:
- Afrin Tablets ⊡ 693
- Chlor-Trimeton Decongestant ⊡ 694
- Disophrol Chronotab Sustained-Action Tablets ⊡ 698
- Drixoral Antihistamine/Nasal Decongestant Syrup ⊡ 698
- Drixoral Non-Drowsy Formula ⊡ 699
- Drixoral Plus Extended-Release Tablets ⊡ 699
- Drixoral Sinus ⊡ 700
- Drixoral Sustained-Action Tablets ⊡ 698
- Sinutab Allergy Formula Sustained Action Tablets ⊡ 640
- Trinalin Repetabs Tablets 1170

Selegiline Hydrochloride (May produce hypertensive crisis). Products include:
- Eldepryl 2250

Terbutaline Sulfate (May produce additive effects). Products include:
- Brethaire Inhaler 1024
- Brethine Ampuls 1026
- Brethine Tablets 1026
- Bricanyl Injection 1324
- Bricanyl Tablets 1325

Tranylcypromine Sulfate (May produce hypertensive crisis). Products include:
- Parnate Tablets 2222

DIMETAPP PLUS CAPLETS
(Acetaminophen, Brompheniramine Maleate, Phenylpropanolamine Hydrochloride) ⊡ 675
May interact with monoamine oxidase inhibitors, sympathomimetic aerosal brochodilators, and certain other agents. Compounds in these categories include:

Albuterol (May produce additive effects and increased toxicity). Products include:
- Proventil Inhalation Aerosol 2117
- Ventolin Inhalation Aerosol and Refill 583

Albuterol Sulfate (May produce additive effects and increased toxicity). Products include:
- Proventil Repetabs Tablets 2120
- Proventil Solutions for Inhalation 0.5% and 0.083% 2118
- Proventil Syrup 2119
- Proventil Tablets 2120
- Ventolin 583

Alcohol (Concurrent use not recommended).

Antihypertensive agents, unspecified (Diminished antihypertensive effect).

Dobutamine Hydrochloride (May produce additive effects and increased toxicity). Products include:
- Dobutrex Solution Vials 1259

Dopamine Hydrochloride (May produce additive effects and increased toxicity). Products include:
- Intropin Injection 930

Ephedrine Hydrochloride (May produce additive effects and increased toxicity). Products include:
- Amesec ⊡ 682
- Primatene Tablets-M Formula 2421
- Primatene Tablets-P Formula 2421
- Primatene Tablets-Regular Formula 2421
- Quadrinal Tablets 1183
- Quelidrine Syrup 556
- Tedral SA 1765

Ephedrine Sulfate (May produce additive effects and increased toxicity). Products include:
- Bronkaid Tablets ⊡ 757
- Bronkolixir ⊡ 761
- Bronkotabs Tablets ⊡ 762
- Marax Tablets & DF Syrup 1954
- Pazo Hemorrhoid Ointment & Suppositories 752
- Vicks Vatronol Nose Drops ⊡ 666

Ephedrine Tannate (May produce additive effects and increased toxicity). Products include:
- Rynatuss 2388

Epinephrine (May produce additive effects and increased toxicity). Products include:
- Ana-Kit Anaphylaxis Emergency Treatment Kit 1100
- Bronkaid Mist ⊡ 757
- EpiPen 843
- Marcaine Hydrochloride 0.5% with Epinephrine 1:200,000 (as bitartrate) 958
- Marcaine Hydrochloride with Epinephrine 1:200,000 2055
- Primatene Mist 2420
- Sus-Phrine Injection 1006
- Xylocaine with Epinephrine Injections 637

Epinephrine Bitartrate (May produce additive effects and increased toxicity). Products include:
- AsthmaHaler Mist Epinephrine Bitartrate Bronchodilator ⊡ 616
- Bronkaid Mist Suspension ⊡ 757
- Primatene Mist Suspension 2421

Epinephrine Hydrochloride (May produce additive effects and increased toxicity). Products include:
- Adrenalin Chloride Solution 1:100 & 1:1,000 1689
- Epifrin ⊙ 244
- Glaucon ⊙ 218

Furazolidone (May produce hypertensive crisis). Products include:
- Furoxone 1855

Isocarboxazid (May produce hypertensive crisis). Products include:
- Marplan Tablets 1906

Isoproterenol Hydrochloride (May produce additive effects and increased toxicity). Products include:
- Isuprel Hydrochloride Injection 1:5000 2050
- Isuprel Hydrochloride Mistometer 2051
- Isuprel Hydrochloride Solution 1:200 & 1:100 2052
- Norisodrine Aerotrol 540

Metaproterenol Sulfate (May produce additive effects and increased toxicity). Products include:
- Alupent 674
- Arm-a-Med Metaproterenol Sulfate Inhalation Solution, USP 617
- Metaprel Inhalation Aerosol Bronchodilator 2014
- Metaprel Inhalation Solution 2015
- Metaprel 2015
- Metaproterenol Sulfate Inhalation Solution, USP 912

Metaraminol Bitartrate (May produce additive effects and increased toxicity). Products include:
- Aramine Injection 1424

Methoxamine Hydrochloride (May produce additive effects and increased toxicity). Products include:
- Vasoxyl Injection 819

Norepinephrine Bitartrate (May produce additive effects and increased toxicity). Products include:
- Levophed Bitartrate Injection 2054

Phenelzine Sulfate (May produce hypertensive crisis). Products include:
- Nardil 1742

Phenylephrine Bitartrate (May produce additive effects and increased toxicity).
- No products indexed under this heading.

Phenylephrine Hydrochloride (May produce additive effects and increased toxicity). Products include:
- AK-Dilate Solution 2.5% and 10% ⊙ 203
- Atrohist Sprinkle Capsules 558
- Cerose-DM 2443
- Codimal 846
- Comhist LA Capsules 1618
- Congespirin For Children Aspirin Free Chewable Cold Tablets 748
- Cyclomydril ⊙ 216
- Deconsal Sprinkle Capsules 559
- Dimetane Decongestant ⊡ 673
- Dristan Decongestant/Antihistamine/ Analgesic Coated Caplets ⊡ 749
- Dristan Cold Nasal Decongestant/ Antihistamine/ Analgesic Coated Tablets 2419
- Dristan Advanced Formula Decongestant/Antihistamine/ Analgesic Tablets ⊡ 749
- Dristan Nasal Spray, Menthol 2419
- Dristan Nasal Spray, Regular and Regular with Metered Pump 2419
- Entex Capsules 1623
- Entex Liquid 1623
- Sinus Excedrin Analgesic, Decongestant Tablets & Caplets 750
- Extendryl 994
- 4-Way Fast Acting Nasal Spray - Original Formula (regular & mentholated) & Metered Spray Pump (regular) 751
- Hycomine Compound Tablets 929
- Murocoll-2 Sterile Ophthalmic Solution ⊙ 261
- Mydfrin 2.5% ⊙ 224
- Naldecon Syrup, Tablets, Pediatric Drops and Pediatric Syrup 709
- Neo-Synephrine Hydrochloride 1% Carpuject 2063
- Neo-Synephrine Hydrochloride 1% Injection 2063
- Neo-Synephrine Hydrochloride (Ophthalmic) 2064
- Neo-Synephrine ⊡ 759
- Nōstril Nasal Decongestant ⊡ 520
- Novahistine Elixir ⊡ 596
- Phenergan VC 2500
- Phenergan VC with Codeine 2501
- Prefrin Liquifilm Vasoconstrictor and Lubricant Eye Drops ⊙ 254
- Prefrin-A ⊙ 255
- Quelidrine Syrup 556
- Relief Vasoconstrictor and Lubricant Eye Drops ⊙ 256
- Robitussin Night Relief ⊡ 677
- Ru-Tuss with Hydrocodone 694
- Ru-Tuss Tablets 693
- Vasosulf ⊙ 279
- Vicks Sinex ⊡ 665
- Zincfrin ⊙ 230

Phenylephrine Tannate (May produce additive effects and increased toxicity). Products include:
- Rynatan 2387
- Rynatuss 2388

Pseudoephedrine Hydrochloride (May produce additive effects and increased toxicity). Products include:
- Actifed Capsules ⊡ 539
- Actifed Plus Caplets ⊡ 539
- Actifed Plus Tablets ⊡ 540
- Actifed with Codeine Cough Syrup 752
- Actifed Syrup ⊡ 540
- Actifed Tablets ⊡ 540
- Actifed 12-Hour Capsules ⊡ 539
- Advil Cold & Sinus Caplets (formerly CoAdvil) 2416
- Allerest ⊡ 559
- Anatuss LA Tablets 1359
- Benadryl Decongestant Elixir ⊡ 635
- Benadryl Decongestant ⊡ 635
- Benadryl Plus ⊡ 636
- Benadryl Plus Nighttime ⊡ 637
- Benylin Decongestant ⊡ 638
- Brexin L.A. Capsules 2078
- Bromfed Capsules (Timed Release) 1615
- Bromfed Syrup ⊡ 628
- Bromfed 1615
- CoAdvil ⊡ 748
- Allergy-Sinus Comtrex Multi-Symptom Allergy Sinus Formula Tablets & Caplets 746
- Cough Formula Comtrex 746
- Comtrex Multi-Symptom Cold Reliever Tablets/Caplets/Liqui-Gels/Liquid 745
- Day-Night Comtrex 747
- Non-Drowsy Comtrex 747
- Congess 994
- Congestac Caplets ⊡ 617
- Contac Jr. Children's Cold Medicine ⊡ 712
- Contac Nighttime Cold Medicine ⊡ 713
- Contac Sinus Caplets Maximum Strength Non-Drowsy Formula ⊡ 710
- Contac Sinus Tablets Maximum Strength Non-Drowsy Formula ⊡ 710
- Deconamine 663
- Deconsal II Tablets 559
- Dimacol Caplets ⊡ 672
- Dimetane-DX Cough Syrup 1858
- Dorcol Children's Cough Syrup ⊡ 685
- Dorcol Children's Decongestant Liquid ⊡ 685
- Dorcol Children's Liquid Cold Formula ⊡ 686
- Maximum Strength Dristan Decongestant/Analgesic Coated Caplets ⊡ 750
- No Drowsiness Dristan Cold Nasal Decongestant/Analgesic Coated Caplets 2420
- Dristan Sinus Caplets 2419
- Sinus Excedrin Analgesic, Decongestant Tablets & Caplets ⊡ 533
- Fedahist Gyrocaps 2145
- Fedahist Timecaps 2145
- Guaifed 1615
- Guaifed Syrup ⊡ 629
- Isoclor Expectorant 982
- Isoclor Timesule Capsules ⊡ 561
- Kronofed-A 970
- Medi-Flu Caplet, Liquid ⊡ 640
- Novafed A Capsules 1342
- Novafed Capsules 1342
- Novahistine DH 1342
- Novahistine DMX ⊡ 595
- Novahistine Expectorant 1343
- Nucofed Capsules 2219
- Nucofed Expectorant 2219
- Nucofed Pediatric Expectorant 2220
- Nucofed Syrup 2219
- Ornex Caplets ⊡ 618
- PediaCare Allergy Relief Formula Liquid 1362
- PediaCare Cough-Cold Formula Liquid 1362

PediaCare Infants' Oral Decongestant Drops ... 1362
PediaCare Night Rest Cough-Cold Formula Liquid ... 1362
PediaCare 6-12 Cough-Cold Formula Chewable Tablets ... 1362
Robitussin-DAC Syrup ... 1875
Robitussin-PE ... ▣ 677
Rondec ... 1975
Rondec-DM ... 1976
Rondec-TR Tablet ... 1975
Ru-Tuss DE Tablets ... 694
Ryna ... ▣ 741
Seldane-D Extended-Release Tablets ... 1350
Sinarest ... ▣ 562
Sine-Aid Maximum Strength Sinus Headache Caplets ... 1365
Sine-Aid Maximum Strength Sinus Headache Tablets ... 1365
Sine-Off Maximum Strength Allergy/Sinus Formula Caplets ... ▣ 721
Sine-Off Maximum Strength No Drowsiness Formula Caplets ... ▣ 722
Singlet Tablets ... ▣ 598
Sinutab Maximum Strength ... ▣ 641
Sinutab Maximum Strength Without Drowsiness Tablets & Caplets ... ▣ 642
Sinutab Regular Strength Without Drowsiness Formula ... ▣ 641
St. Joseph Nighttime Cold Medicine ... ▣ 705
Sudafed Children's Liquid ... ▣ 543
Sudafed Cough Syrup ... ▣ 543
Sudafed Plus Liquid ... ▣ 544
Sudafed Plus Tablets ... ▣ 545
Sudafed Sinus Caplets ... ▣ 545
Sudafed Sinus Tablets ... ▣ 545
Sudafed Tablets, 30 mg ... ▣ 544
Sudafed Tablets, Adult Strength, 60 mg ... ▣ 544
Sudafed 12 Hour Capsules ... ▣ 545
TheraFlu Flu and Cold Medicine ... ▣ 687
Triaminic Nite Light ... ▣ 689
Tylenol Allergy Sinus Medication Caplets and Gelcaps, Maximum Strength ... 1372
Children's Tylenol Cold Liquid Formula and Chewable Tablets ... 1368
Tylenol Cold & Flu Hot Medication, Packets ... 1369
Tylenol Cold & Flu No Drowsiness Hot Medication, Packets ... 1371
Tylenol Cold Medication Caplets and Tablets ... 1370
Tylenol Cold Medication No Drowsiness Formula Caplets ... 1370
Tylenol Cold Night Time Medication Liquid ... 1371
Tylenol Cough Medication Liquid with Decongestant, Maximum Strength ... 1372
Tylenol, Maximum Strength, Sinus Medication Gelcaps, Caplets and Tablets ... 1373
Ursinus Inlay-Tabs ... ▣ 691
Vicks Children's NyQuil ... ▣ 664
Vicks Daycare ... ▣ 660
Vicks Formula 44D Decongestant Cough Medicine ... ▣ 662
Vicks Formula 44M Multi-Symptom Cough Medicine ... ▣ 662
Vicks NyQuil Nighttime Colds Medicine-Original & Cherry Flavor ... ▣ 664
Vicks Pediatric Formula 44 Cough & Congestion Medicine ... ▣ 663
Vicks Pediatric Formula 44m Multi-Symptom Cough & Cold Medicine ... ▣ 663

Pseudoephedrine Sulfate (May produce additive effects and increased toxicity). Products include:
Afrin Tablets ... ▣ 693
Chlor-Trimeton Decongestant ... ▣ 694
Disophrol Chronotab Sustained-Action Tablets ... ▣ 698
Drixoral Antihistamine/Nasal Decongestant Syrup ... ▣ 698
Drixoral Non-Drowsy Formula ... ▣ 699
Drixoral Plus Extended-Release Tablets ... ▣ 699
Drixoral Sinus ... ▣ 700
Drixoral Sustained-Action Tablets ... ▣ 698
Sinutab Allergy Formula Sustained Action Tablets ... ▣ 640
Trinalin Repetabs Tablets ... 1170

Selegiline Hydrochloride (May produce hypertensive crisis). Products include:
Eldepryl ... 2250

Terbutaline Sulfate (May produce additive effects and increased toxicity). Products include:
Brethaire Inhaler ... 1024
Brethine Ampuls ... 1026
Brethine Tablets ... 1026
Bricanyl Injection ... 1324
Bricanyl Tablets ... 1325

Tranylcypromine Sulfate (May produce hypertensive crisis). Products include:
Parnate Tablets ... 2222

DIMETAPP TABLETS

(Brompheniramine Maleate, Phenylpropanolamine Hydrochloride) ... ▣ 675

May interact with sympathomimetic aerosal brochodilators, monoamine oxidase inhibitors, and certain other agents. Compounds in these categories include:

Albuterol (May produce additive effects). Products include:
Proventil Inhalation Aerosol ... 2117
Ventolin Inhalation Aerosol and Refill ... 583

Albuterol Sulfate (May produce additive effects). Products include:
Proventil Repetabs Tablets ... 2120
Proventil Solutions for Inhalation 0.5% and 0.083% ... 2118
Proventil Syrup ... 2119
Proventil Tablets ... 2120
Ventolin ... 583

Alcohol (Do not use concomitantly).

Antihypertensive agents, unspecified (Diminished antihypertensive effect).

Dobutamine Hydrochloride (May produce additive effects). Products include:
Dobutrex Solution Vials ... 1259

Dopamine Hydrochloride (May produce additive effects). Products include:
Intropin Injection ... 930

Ephedrine Hydrochloride (May produce additive effects). Products include:
Amesec ... ▣ 682
Primatene Tablets-M Formula ... 2421
Primatene Tablets-P Formula ... 2421
Primatene Tablets-Regular Formula ... 2421
Quadrinal Tablets ... 1183
Quelidrine Syrup ... 556
Tedral SA ... 1765

Ephedrine Sulfate (May produce additive effects). Products include:
Bronkaid Tablets ... ▣ 757
Bronkolixir ... ▣ 761
Bronkotabs Tablets ... ▣ 762
Marax Tablets & DF Syrup ... 1954
Pazo Hemorrhoid Ointment & Suppositories ... 752
Vicks Vatronol Nose Drops ... ▣ 666

Ephedrine Tannate (May produce additive effects). Products include:
Rynatuss ... 2388

Epinephrine (May produce additive effects). Products include:
Ana-Kit Anaphylaxis Emergency Treatment Kit ... 1100
Bronkaid Mist ... ▣ 757
EpiPen ... 843
Marcaine Hydrochloride 0.5% with Epinephrine 1:200,000 (as bitartrate) ... 958
Marcaine Hydrochloride with Epinephrine 1:200,000 ... 2055
Primatene Mist ... 2420
Sus-Phrine Injection ... 1006
Xylocaine with Epinephrine Injections ... 637

Epinephrine Bitartrate (May produce additive effects). Products include:
AsthmaHaler Mist Epinephrine Bitartrate Bronchodilator ... ▣ 616
Bronkaid Mist Suspension ... ▣ 757
Primatene Mist Suspension ... 2421

Epinephrine Hydrochloride (May produce additive effects). Products include:
Adrenalin Chloride Solution 1:100 & 1:1,000 ... 1689
Epifrin ... ◉ 244
Glaucon ... ◉ 218

Furazolidone (May produce hypertensive crisis). Products include:
Furoxone ... 1855

Isocarboxazid (May produce hypertensive crisis). Products include:
Marplan Tablets ... 1906

Isoproterenol Hydrochloride (May produce additive effects). Products include:
Isuprel Hydrochloride Injection 1:5000 ... 2050
Isuprel Hydrochloride Mistometer .. 2051
Isuprel Hydrochloride Solution 1:200 & 1:100 ... 2052
Norisodrine Aerotrol ... 540

Metaproterenol Sulfate (May produce additive effects). Products include:
Alupent ... 674
Arm-a-Med Metaproterenol Sulfate Inhalation Solution, USP ... 617
Metaprel Inhalation Aerosol Bronchodilator ... 2014
Metaprel Inhalation Solution ... 2015
Metaprel ... 2015
Metaproterenol Sulfate Inhalation Solution, USP ... 912

Metaraminol Bitartrate (May produce additive effects). Products include:
Aramine Injection ... 1424

Methoxamine Hydrochloride (May produce additive effects). Products include:
Vasoxyl Injection ... 819

Norepinephrine Bitartrate (May produce additive effects). Products include:
Levophed Bitartrate Injection ... 2054

Phenelzine Sulfate (May produce hypertensive crisis). Products include:
Nardil ... 1742

Phenylephrine Bitartrate (May produce additive effects).
No products indexed under this heading.

Phenylephrine Hydrochloride (May produce additive effects). Products include:
AK-Dilate Solution 2.5% and 10% ... ◉ 203
Atrohist Sprinkle Capsules ... 558
Cerose-DM ... 2443
Codimal ... 846
Comhist LA Capsules ... 1618
Congespirin For Children Aspirin Free Chewable Cold Tablets ... 748
Cyclomydril ... ◉ 216
Deconsal Sprinkle Capsules ... 559
Dimetane Decongestant ... ▣ 673
Dristan Decongestant/Antihistamine/ Analgesic Coated Caplets ... ▣ 749
Dristan Cold Nasal Decongestant/ Antihistamine/ Analgesic Coated Tablets ... 2419
Dristan Advanced Formula Decongestant/Antihistamine/ Analgesic Tablets ... ▣ 749
Dristan Nasal Spray, Menthol ... 2419
Dristan Nasal Spray, Regular and Regular with Metered Pump ... 2419
Entex Capsules ... 1623
Entex Liquid ... 1623
Sinus Excedrin Analgesic, Decongestant Tablets & Caplets ... 750
Extendryl ... 994
4-Way Fast Acting Nasal Spray - Original Formula (regular & mentholated) & Metered Spray Pump (regular) ... 751
Hycomine Compound Tablets ... 929
Murocoll-2 Sterile Ophthalmic Solution ... ◉ 261
Mydfrin 2.5% ... ◉ 224
Naldecon Syrup, Tablets, Pediatric Drops and Pediatric Syrup ... 709
Neo-Synephrine Hydrochloride 1% Carpuject ... 2063
Neo-Synephrine Hydrochloride 1% Injection ... 2063
Neo-Synephrine Hydrochloride (Ophthalmic) ... 2064
Neo-Synephrine ... ▣ 759
Nōstril Nasal Decongestant ... ▣ 520
Novahistine Elixir ... ▣ 596
Phenergan VC ... 2500
Phenergan VC with Codeine ... 2501
Prefrin Liquifilm Vasoconstrictor and Lubricant Eye Drops ... ◉ 254
Prefrin-A ... ◉ 255
Quelidrine Syrup ... 556
Relief Vasoconstrictor and Lubricant Eye Drops ... ◉ 256
Robitussin Night Relief ... ▣ 677
Ru-Tuss with Hydrocodone ... 694
Ru-Tuss Tablets ... 693
Vasosulf ... ◉ 279
Vicks Sinex ... ▣ 665
Zincfrin ... ◉ 230

Phenylephrine Tannate (May produce additive effects). Products include:
Rynatan ... 2387
Rynatuss ... 2388

Pindolol (Diminished antihypertensive effect). Products include:
Visken Tablets ... 2036

Pirbuterol Acetate (May produce additive effects). Products include:
Maxair Inhaler ... 1311

Pseudoephedrine Hydrochloride (May produce additive effects). Products include:
Actifed Capsules ... ▣ 539
Actifed Plus Caplets ... ▣ 539
Actifed Plus Tablets ... ▣ 540
Actifed with Codeine Cough Syrup .. 752
Actifed Syrup ... ▣ 540
Actifed Tablets ... ▣ 540
Actifed 12-Hour Capsules ... ▣ 539
Advil Cold & Sinus Caplets (formerly CoAdvil) ... 2416
Allerest ... ▣ 559
Anatuss LA Tablets ... 1359
Benadryl Decongestant Elixir ... ▣ 635
Benadryl Decongestant ... ▣ 635
Benadryl Plus ... ▣ 636
Benadryl Plus Nighttime ... ▣ 637
Benylin Decongestant ... ▣ 638
Brexin L.A. Capsules ... 2078
Bromfed Capsules (Timed Release) ... 1615
Bromfed Syrup ... ▣ 628
Bromfed ... 1615
CoAdvil ... ▣ 748
Allergy-Sinus Comtrex Multi-Symptom Allergy Sinus Formula Tablets & Caplets ... 746
Cough Formula Comtrex ... 746
Comtrex Multi-Symptom Cold Reliever Tablets/Caplets/Liqui-Gels/Liquid ... 745
Day-Night Comtrex ... 747
Non-Drowsy Comtrex ... 747
Congess ... 994
Congestac Caplets ... ▣ 617
Contac Jr. Children's Cold Medicine ... ▣ 712
Contac Nighttime Cold Medicine ... ▣ 713
Contac Sinus Caplets Maximum Strength Non-Drowsy Formula ... ▣ 710
Contac Sinus Tablets Maximum Strength Non-Drowsy Formula ... ▣ 710
Deconamine ... 663
Deconsal II Tablets ... 559
Dimacol Caplets ... ▣ 672
Dimetane-DX Cough Syrup ... 1858
Dorcol Children's Cough Syrup ... ▣ 685
Dorcol Children's Decongestant Liquid ... ▣ 685
Dorcol Children's Liquid Cold Formula ... ▣ 686
Maximum Strength Dristan Decongestant/Analgesic Coated Caplets ... ▣ 750

No Drowsiness Dristan Cold Nasal Decongestant/Analgesic Coated Caplets 2420
Dristan Sinus Caplets 2419
Sinus Excedrin Analgesic, Decongestant Tablets & Caplets ▣ 533
Fedahist Gyrocaps 2145
Fedahist Timecaps 2145
Guaifed 1615
Guaifed Syrup ▣ 629
Isoclor Expectorant 982
Isoclor Timesule Capsules ▣ 561
Kronofed-A 970
Medi-Flu Caplet, Liquid ▣ 640
Novafed A Capsules 1342
Novafed Capsules 1342
Novahistine DH 1342
Novahistine DMX ▣ 595
Novahistine Expectorant 1343
Nucofed Capsules 2219
Nucofed Expectorant 2219
Nucofed Pediatric Expectorant 2220
Nucofed Syrup 2219
Ornex Caplets ▣ 618
PediaCare Allergy Relief Formula Liquid 1362
PediaCare Cough-Cold Formula Liquid 1362
PediaCare Infants' Oral Decongestant Drops 1362
PediaCare Night Rest Cough-Cold Formula Liquid 1362
PediaCare 6-12 Cough-Cold Formula Chewable Tablets 1362
Robitussin-DAC Syrup 1875
Robitussin-PE ▣ 677
Rondec 1975
Rondec-DM 1976
Rondec-TR Tablet 1975
Ru-Tuss DE Tablets 694
Ryna ▣ 741
Seldane-D Extended-Release Tablets 1350
Sinarest ▣ 562
Sine-Aid Maximum Strength Sinus Headache Caplets 1365
Sine-Aid Maximum Strength Sinus Headache Tablets 1365
Sine-Off Maximum Strength Allergy/Sinus Formula Caplets ▣ 721
Sine-Off Maximum Strength No Drowsiness Formula Caplets ▣ 722
Singlet Tablets ▣ 598
Sinutab Maximum Strength ▣ 641
Sinutab Maximum Strength Without Drowsiness Tablets & Caplets ▣ 642
Sinutab Regular Strength Without Drowsiness Formula ▣ 641
St. Joseph Nighttime Cold Medicine ▣ 705
Sudafed Children's Liquid ▣ 543
Sudafed Cough Syrup ▣ 543
Sudafed Plus Liquid ▣ 544
Sudafed Plus Tablets ▣ 545
Sudafed Sinus Caplets ▣ 545
Sudafed Sinus Tablets ▣ 545
Sudafed Tablets, 30 mg ▣ 544
Sudafed Tablets, Adult Strength, 60 mg ▣ 544
Sudafed 12 Hour Capsules ▣ 545
TheraFlu Flu and Cold Medicine ▣ 687
Triaminic Nite Light ▣ 689
Tylenol Allergy Sinus Medication Caplets and Gelcaps, Maximum Strength 1372
Children's Tylenol Cold Liquid Formula and Chewable Tablets 1368
Tylenol Cold & Flu Hot Medication, Packets 1369
Tylenol Cold & Flu No Drowsiness Hot Medication, Packets 1371
Tylenol Cold Medication Caplets and Tablets 1370
Tylenol Cold Medication No Drowsiness Formula Caplets 1370
Tylenol Cold Night Time Medication Liquid 1371
Tylenol Cough Medication Liquid with Decongestant, Maximum Strength 1372
Tylenol, Maximum Strength, Sinus Medication Gelcaps, Caplets and Tablets 1373
Ursinus Inlay-Tabs ▣ 691
Vicks Children's NyQuil ▣ 664
Vicks Daycare ▣ 660
Vicks Formula 44D Decongestant Cough Medicine ▣ 662
Vicks Formula 44M Multi-Symptom Cough Medicine ▣ 662
Vicks NyQuil Nighttime Colds Medicine-Original & Cherry Flavor ▣ 664
Vicks Pediatric Formula 44 Cough & Congestion Medicine ▣ 663
Vicks Pediatric Formula 44m Multi-Symptom Cough & Cold Medicine ▣ 663

Pseudoephedrine Sulfate (May produce additive effects). Products include:
Afrin Tablets ▣ 693
Chlor-Trimeton Decongestant ▣ 694
Disophrol Chronotab Sustained-Action Tablets ▣ 698
Drixoral Antihistamine/Nasal Decongestant Syrup ▣ 698
Drixoral Non-Drowsy Formula ▣ 699
Drixoral Plus Extended-Release Tablets ▣ 699
Drixoral Sinus ▣ 700
Drixoral Sustained-Action Tablets ▣ 698
Sinutab Allergy Formula Sustained Action Tablets ▣ 640
Trinalin Repetabs Tablets 1170

Selegiline Hydrochloride (May produce hypertensive crisis). Products include:
Eldepryl 2250

Terbutaline Sulfate (May produce additive effects). Products include:
Brethaire Inhaler 1024
Brethine Ampuls 1026
Brethine Tablets 1026
Bricanyl Injection 1324
Bricanyl Tablets 1325

Tranylcypromine Sulfate (May produce hypertensive crisis). Products include:
Parnate Tablets 2222

DIPENTUM CAPSULES
(Olsalarine) 1160
No interactions described in labeling.

DIPHTHERIA & TETANUS TOXOIDS, ADSORBED PUROGENATED
(Diphtheria & Tetanus Toxoids Adsorbed, (For Pediatric Use)) 1202
No interactions described in labeling.

DIPHTHERIA AND TETANUS TOXOIDS AND PERTUSSIS VACCINE ADSORBED USP (FOR PEDIATRIC USE)
(Diphtheria & Tetanus Toxoids w/Pertussis Vaccine Combined, Aluminum Potassium Sulfate Adsorbed) 892
May interact with immunosuppressive agents, corticosteroids, antineoplastics, and cytotoxic drugs. Compounds in these categories include:

Altretamine (May reduce immune response to vaccines). Products include:
Hexalen Capsules 2316

Asparaginase (May reduce immune response to vaccines). Products include:
Elspar 1470

Azathioprine (May reduce immune response to vaccines). Products include:
Imuran 768

Betamethasone Acetate (May reduce immune response to vaccines). Products include:
Celestone Soluspan Suspension 2081

Betamethasone Sodium Phosphate (May reduce immune response to vaccines). Products include:
Celestone Soluspan Suspension 2081

Bleomycin Sulfate (May reduce immune response to vaccines). Products include:
Blenoxane 724

Busulfan (May reduce immune response to vaccines). Products include:
Myleran Tablets 790

Carboplatin (May reduce immune response to vaccines). Products include:
Paraplatin for Injection 735

Carmustine (BCNU) (May reduce immune response to vaccines). Products include:
BiCNU 723

Chlorambucil (May reduce immune response to vaccines). Products include:
Leukeran Tablets 788

Cisplatin (May reduce immune response to vaccines). Products include:
Platinol 737
Platinol-AQ Injection 738

Cortisone Acetate (May reduce immune response to vaccines). Products include:
Cortone Acetate Sterile Suspension 1437
Cortone Acetate Tablets 1439

Cyclophosphamide (May reduce immune response to vaccines). Products include:
Cytoxan for Injection 726
Neosar for Injection 566

Cyclosporine (May reduce immune response to vaccines). Products include:
Sandimmune 2024

Dacarbazine (May reduce immune response to vaccines). Products include:
DTIC-Dome 1595

Daunorubicin Hydrochloride (May reduce immune response to vaccines). Products include:
Cerubidine 2443

Dexamethasone (May reduce immune response to vaccines). Products include:
AK-Trol Ointment & Suspension ⊙ 207
Decadron Elixir 1445
Decadron Tablets 1447
Decaspray Topical Aerosol 1459
Dexacidin ⊙ 272
Maxidex Sterile Ophthalmic Suspension ⊙ 223
Maxitrol Ophthalmic Ointment/Suspension ⊙ 223
TobraDex Ophthalmic Suspension and Ointment ⊙ 228

Dexamethasone Acetate (May reduce immune response to vaccines). Products include:
Dalalone D.P. Injectable 999
Decadron-LA Sterile Suspension 1457

Dexamethasone Sodium Phosphate (May reduce immune response to vaccines). Products include:
AK-Dex ⊙ 203
Decadron Phosphate Respihaler 1454
Decadron Phosphate Sterile Ophthalmic Ointment 1453
Decadron Phosphate Sterile Ophthalmic Solution 1453
Decadron Phosphate Topical Cream 1455
Decadron Phosphate Turbinaire 1456
Maxidex Sterile Ophthalmic Ointment ⊙ 222
NeoDecadron Sterile Ophthalmic Ointment 1517
NeoDecadron Sterile Ophthalmic Solution 1518
NeoDecadron Topical Cream 1518

Doxorubicin Hydrochloride (May reduce immune response to vaccines). Products include:
Adriamycin PFS 561
Adriamycin RDF 562
Doxorubicin Hydrochloride for Injection, USP 622
Doxorubicin Hydrochloride Injection, USP 848
Rubex 739

Estramustine Phosphate Sodium (May reduce immune response to vaccines). Products include:
Emcyt Capsules 1161

Etoposide (May reduce immune response to vaccines). Products include:
VePesid Capsules and Injection 741

Floxuridine (May reduce immune response to vaccines). Products include:
Sterile FUDR 1898

Fluorouracil (May reduce immune response to vaccines). Products include:
Efudex 1880
Fluoroplex Topical Solution & Cream 1% 1082
Fluorouracil Injection 1897

Flutamide (May reduce immune response to vaccines). Products include:
Eulexin Capsules 2089

Hydrocortisone (May reduce immune response to vaccines). Products include:
AK-Spore H.C. ⊙ 206
Bactine Hydrocortisone Anti-Itch Cream ▣ 625
CaldeCORT Anti-Itch Hydrocortisone Spray ▣ 560
Carmol HC Cream 1% 2296
Cortaid Spray ▣ 735
Cortenema 2244
Cortisporin Ointment 758
Cortisporin Ophthalmic Ointment Sterile 758
Cortisporin Ophthalmic Suspension Sterile 759
Cortisporin Otic Solution Sterile 760
Cortisporin Otic Suspension Sterile 760
Cortizone-5 Creme & Ointment ▣ 732
Dermolate Anti-Itch Cream ▣ 697
Eldecort Cream 1.0% 1113
Eldecort Cream 1.0% and 2.5% 1113
Fungoid HC Creme 1770
Hydrocortone Tablets 1482
Hytone 909
LazerSporin-C Solution 1770
Massengill Medicated Soft Cloth Towelettes 2192
Nutracort Cream & Lotion 1684
PediOtic Suspension Sterile 797
Synacort Creams 1%, 2.5% 2296
Vanoxide-HC Acne Lotion 911
Vioform-Hydrocortisone Cream and Mild Cream 889
Vioform-Hydrocortisone Ointment 889
VōSoL HC Otic Solution 2392
Vytone Cream 1% 911

Hydrocortisone Acetate (May reduce immune response to vaccines). Products include:
Analpram-HC Rectal Cream 1% and 2.5% 970
Anusol-HC Cream 1690
Anusol-HC Suppositories 1691
Caldecort ▣ 560
Carmol HC Cream 1% 2296
Chloromycetin Hydrocortisone Ophthalmic 1694
Coly-Mycin S Otic w/Neomycin & Hydrocortisone 1708
Cortaid ▣ 735
Cortef Feminine Itch Cream ▣ 735
Corticaine ▣ 682
Cortifoam 1827
Cortisporin Cream 757
Epifoam 1828
Gynecort 5 Creme ▣ 556
Hydrocortone Acetate Sterile Suspension 1479
Lanacort 5 Creme and Ointment ▣ 557
Mantadil Cream 789
Ophthocort ⊙ 301
Orabase HCA Oral Paste 890
Pramosone Cream, Lotion & Ointment 971
ProctoCream-HC 1834

Proctofoam-HC ... 1835

Hydrocortisone Sodium Phosphate (May reduce immune response to vaccines). Products include:

Hydrocortone Phosphate Injection, Sterile ... 1481

Hydrocortisone Sodium Succinate (May reduce immune response to vaccines). Products include:

Solu-Cortef Sterile Powder ... 2361

Hydroxyurea (May reduce immune response to vaccines). Products include:

Hydrea Capsules ... 728

Ifosfamide (May reduce immune response to vaccines). Products include:

IFEX ... 729

Immune Globulin (Human) (May reduce immune response to vaccines). Products include:

MICRhoGAM Rh_o(D) Immune Globulin (Human) ... 1650
RhoGAM Rh_o(D) Immune Globulin (Human) ... 1651

Immune Globulin Intravenous (Human) (May reduce immune response to vaccines). Products include:

Gamimune N Immune Globulin Intravenous (Human) ... 1572
Gammagard Immune Globulin, Intravenous (Human) ... 658
Iveegam ... 1129
Sandoglobulin I.V. ... 2027

Interferon alfa-2A, Recombinant (May reduce immune response to vaccines). Products include:

Roferon-A Injection ... 1916

Interferon alfa-2B, Recombinant (May reduce immune response to vaccines). Products include:

Intron A ... 2097

Levamisole Hydrochloride (May reduce immune response to vaccines). Products include:

Ergamisol Tablets ... 1136

Lomustine (CCNU) (May reduce immune response to vaccines). Products include:

CeeNU ... 725

Mechlorethamine Hydrochloride (May reduce immune response to vaccines). Products include:

Mustargen ... 1514

Megestrol Acetate (May reduce immune response to vaccines). Products include:

Megace Tablets ... 732

Melphalan (May reduce immune response to vaccines). Products include:

Alkeran Tablets ... 754

Mercaptopurine (May reduce immune response to vaccines). Products include:

Purinethol Tablets ... 800

Methotrexate Sodium (May reduce immune response to vaccines). Products include:

Methotrexate Tablets, Parenteral, LPF Parenteral ... 1217
Rheumatrex Methotrexate Dose Pack ... 1234

Methylprednisolone Acetate (May reduce immune response to vaccines). Products include:

Depo-Medrol Sterile Aqueous Suspension ... 2334

Methylprednisolone Sodium Succinate (May reduce immune response to vaccines). Products include:

Solu-Medrol Sterile Powder ... 2363

Mitomycin (Mitomycin-C) (May reduce immune response to vaccines). Products include:

Mutamycin ... 733

Mitotane (May reduce immune response to vaccines). Products include:

Lysodren ... 731

Mitoxantrone Hydrochloride (May reduce immune response to vaccines). Products include:

Novantrone for Injection Concentrate ... 1226

Muromonab-CD3 (May reduce immune response to vaccines). Products include:

Orthoclone OKT3 Sterile Solution .. 1645

Prednisolone Acetate (May reduce immune response to vaccines). Products include:

AK-Cide Sterile Ophthalmic Ointment & Suspension ... ◉ 202
Blephamide Liquifilm Sterile Ophthalmic Suspension ... 586
Blephamide S.O.P. Sterile Ophthalmic Ointment ... 586
Cetapred Ointment ... ◉ 220
⅛% Econopred & 1% Econopred Plus ... ◉ 217
Isopto Cetapred Suspension ... ◉ 220
Metimyd ... ◉ 306
Poly-Pred Liquifilm ... ◉ 250
Pred Forte ... ◉ 252
Pred Mild ... ◉ 254
Pred-G Liquifilm Sterile Ophthalmic Suspension ... ◉ 252
Pred-G S.O.P. Sterile Ophthalmic Ointment ... ◉ 253
Vasocidin Ointment ... ◉ 275

Prednisolone Sodium Phosphate (May reduce immune response to vaccines). Products include:

AK-Pred ... ◉ 205
Hydeltrasol Injection, Sterile ... 1476
Inflamase ... ◉ 274
Pediapred Oral Liquid ... 987
Vasocidin Ophthalmic Solution ... ◉ 276

Prednisolone Tebutate (May reduce immune response to vaccines). Products include:

Hydeltra-T.B.A. Sterile Suspension 1478

Prednisone (May reduce immune response to vaccines). Products include:

Deltasone Tablets ... 2332

Procarbazine Hydrochloride (May reduce immune response to vaccines). Products include:

Matulane Capsules ... 1907

Streptozocin (May reduce immune response to vaccines). Products include:

Zanosar Sterile Powder ... 2371

Tamoxifen Citrate (May reduce immune response to vaccines). Products include:

Nolvadex Tablets ... 1102

Thioguanine (May reduce immune response to vaccines). Products include:

Thioguanine Tablets, Tabloid Brand ... 815

Thiotepa (May reduce immune response to vaccines). Products include:

Thiotepa Parenteral ... 1240

Triamcinolone (May reduce immune response to vaccines).

No products indexed under this heading.

Triamcinolone Acetonide (May reduce immune response to vaccines). Products include:

Aristocort A ... 1010
Azmacort Inhaler ... 1837
Kenalog Cream, Lotion & Ointment 2401
Kenalog-10 Injection ... 2402
Kenalog-40 Injection ... 2403
Kenalog in Orabase ... 604
Kenalog Spray ... 2401
Mycolog II Cream and Ointment ... 2407
Mytrex Cream & Ointment ... 2080
Nasacort Nasal Inhaler ... 1844

Triamcinolone Diacetate (May reduce immune response to vaccines). Products include:

Aristocort Suspension ... 1008

Triamcinolone Hexacetonide (May reduce immune response to vaccines). Products include:

Aristospan Suspension ... 1011

Vincristine Sulfate (May reduce immune response to vaccines). Products include:

Oncovin Solution Vials & Hyporets 1288

DIPRIVAN INJECTION
(Propofol) ... 2267
May interact with narcotic analgesics, hypnotics and sedatives, benzodiazepines, barbiturates, inhalant anesthetics, and certain other agents. Compounds in these categories include:

Alfentanil Hydrochloride (Increases anesthetic effects; may also result in pronounced decrease in cardiac output and blood pressure). Products include:

Alfenta Injection ... 1131

Alprazolam (Increases anesthetic effects; may also result in pronounced decrease in cardiac output and blood pressure). Products include:

Xanax Tablets ... 2367

Aprobarbital (Increases anesthetic effects; may also result in pronounced decrease in cardiac output and blood pressure). Products include:

Alurate Elixir ... 1883

Buprenorphine (Increases anesthetic effects; may also result in pronounced decrease in cardiac output and blood pressure).

No products indexed under this heading.

Butabarbital (Increases anesthetic effects; may also result in pronounced decrease in cardiac output and blood pressure). Products include:

Pyridium Plus ... 1764

Butalbital (Increases anesthetic effects; may also result in pronounced decrease in cardiac output and blood pressure). Products include:

Esgic-Plus Tablets ... 1002
Esgic Tablets & Capsules ... 1001
Fioricet Tablets ... 2006
Fiorinal Capsules ... 2007
Fiorinal with Codeine Capsules ... 2008
Fiorinal Tablets ... 2007
Phrenilin ... 838
Sedapap Tablets 50 mg/650 mg .. 1360

Chlordiazepoxide (Increases anesthetic effects; may also result in pronounced decrease in cardiac output and blood pressure). Products include:

Libritabs Tablets ... 1930
Limbitrol ... 1933
Menrium Tablets ... 1934

Chlordiazepoxide Hydrochloride (Increases anesthetic effects; may also result in pronounced decrease in cardiac output and blood pressure). Products include:

Librax Capsules ... 1929
Librium Capsules ... 1931
Librium Injectable ... 1932

Clorazepate Dipotassium (Increases anesthetic effects; may also result in pronounced decrease in cardiac output and blood pressure). Products include:

Tranxene ... 556

Codeine (Increases anesthetic effects; may also result in pronounced decrease in cardiac output and blood pressure). Products include:

Calcidrine Syrup ... 506

Codeine Phosphate (Increases anesthetic effects; may also result in pronounced decrease in cardiac output and blood pressure). Products include:

Actifed with Codeine Cough Syrup.. 752
Cheracol Cough Syrup ... 1853
Codimal PH Syrup ... 846
Dimetane-DC Cough Syrup ... 1857
Empirin with Codeine Phosphate Nos. 2, 3 & 4 ... 764
Fiorinal with Codeine Capsules ... 2008
Isoclor Expectorant ... 982
Naldecon CX Adult Liquid ... ▣ 521
Novahistine DH ... 1342
Novahistine Expectorant ... 1343
Nucofed Capsules ... 2219
Nucofed Expectorant ... 2219
Nucofed Pediatric Expectorant ... 2220
Nucofed Syrup ... 2219
Phenaphen with Codeine Capsules 1865
Phenaphen-650 with Codeine Tablets ... 1866
Phenergan with Codeine ... 2497
Phenergan VC with Codeine ... 2501
Robitussin A-C Syrup ... 1875
Robitussin-DAC Syrup ... 1875
Ryna ... ▣ 741
Soma Compound w/Codeine Tablets ... 2390
Triaminic Expectorant w/Codeine .. 1996
Tussi-Organidin Liquid ... 2391
Tylenol with Codeine ... 1381

Codeine Polistirex (Increases anesthetic effects; may also result in pronounced decrease in cardiac output and blood pressure).

No products indexed under this heading.

Dezocine (Increases anesthetic effects; may also result in pronounced decrease in cardiac output and blood pressure).

Diazepam (Increases anesthetic effects; may also result in pronounced decrease in cardiac output and blood pressure). Products include:

Valium Injectable ... 1937
Valium Tablets ... 1939
Valrelease Capsules ... 1923

Droperidol (Increases anesthetic effects; may also result in pronounced decrease in cardiac output and blood pressure). Products include:

Inapsine Injection ... 1140
Innovar Injection ... 1141

Enflurane (Increases anesthetic and cardiorespiratory effects). Products include:

Ethrane ... 599

Estazolam (Increases anesthetic effects; may also result in pronounced decrease in cardiac output and blood pressure). Products include:

ProSom Tablets ... 554

Ethchlorvynol (Increases anesthetic effects; may also result in pronounced decrease in cardiac output and blood pressure). Products include:

Placidyl Capsules ... 553

Ethinamate (Increases anesthetic effects; may also result in pronounced decrease in cardiac output and blood pressure).

No products indexed under this heading.

Fentanyl (Increases anesthetic effects; may also result in pronounced decrease in cardiac output and blood pressure). Products include:

- Duragesic Transdermal System 1133

Fentanyl Citrate (Increases anesthetic effects; may also result in pronounced decrease in cardiac output and blood pressure). Products include:

- Innovar Injection 1141
- Sublimaze Injection 1146

Flurazepam Hydrochloride (Increases anesthetic effects; may also result in pronounced decrease in cardiac output and blood pressure). Products include:

- Dalmane Capsules 1927

Glutethimide (Increases anesthetic effects; may also result in pronounced decrease in cardiac output and blood pressure).

- No products indexed under this heading.

Halothane (Increases anesthetic and cardiorespiratory effects). Products include:

- Fluothane 2453

Hydrocodone Bitartrate (Increases anesthetic effects; may also result in pronounced decrease in cardiac output and blood pressure). Products include:

- Anexsia 5/500 Tablets 2196
- Anexsia 7.5/650 Tablets 2197
- Azdōne Tablets 844
- Codiclear DH Syrup 845
- Codimal DH Syrup 846
- Damason-P 1356
- Hycodan Syrup, Tablets 927
- Hycomine Compound Tablets 929
- Hycomine Syrup 927
- Hycotuss Expectorant Syrup 930
- Hydrocet Capsules 835
- Lortab ASA Tablets 2414
- Lortab 2412
- Ru-Tuss with Hydrocodone 694
- Triaminic Expectorant DH 1995
- Vicodin Tablets 1187
- Vicodin ES Tablets 1189
- Zydone Capsules 941

Hydrocodone Polistirex (Increases anesthetic effects; may also result in pronounced decrease in cardiac output and blood pressure). Products include:

- Tussionex Extended-Release Suspension 988

Isoflurane (Increases anesthetic and cardiorespiratory effects). Products include:

- Forane 600

Levorphanol Tartrate (Increases anesthetic effects; may also result in pronounced decrease in cardiac output and blood pressure). Products include:

- Levo-Dromoran 1906

Lorazepam (Increases anesthetic effects; may also result in pronounced decrease in cardiac output and blood pressure). Products include:

- Ativan Injection 2432
- Ativan Tablets 2434

Meperidine Hydrochloride (Increases anesthetic effects; may also result in pronounced decrease in cardiac output and blood pressure). Products include:

- Demerol 2047
- Mepergan Injection 2479

Mephobarbital (Increases anesthetic effects; may also result in pronounced decrease in cardiac output and blood pressure). Products include:

- Mebaral Tablets 2061

Methadone Hydrochloride (Increases anesthetic effects; may also result in pronounced decrease in cardiac output and blood pressure). Products include:

- Dolophine Hydrochloride Ampoules & Vials 1260
- Dolophine Hydrochloride Tablets 1261
- Methadone Hydrochloride Diskets 1284
- Methadone Hydrochloride Oral Solution & Tablets 1987

Methoxyflurane (Increases anesthetic and cardiorespiratory effects).

- No products indexed under this heading.

Midazolam Hydrochloride (Increases anesthetic effects; may also result in pronounced decrease in cardiac output and blood pressure). Products include:

- Versed Injection 1924

Morphine Sulfate (Increases anesthetic effects; may also result in pronounced decrease in cardiac output and blood pressure). Products include:

- Astramorph/PF Injection, USP (Preservative-Free) 618
- Duramorph 960
- Infumorph 200 and Infumorph 500 Sterile Solutions 962
- MS Contin Tablets 1814
- MSIR 1817
- Oramorph SR (Morphine Sulfate Sustained Release Tablets) 1988
- Roxanol 1991

Opium Alkaloids (Increases anesthetic effects; may also result in pronounced decrease in cardiac output and blood pressure). Products include:

- B & O No. 15A & No. 16A Supprettes 2395
- Pantopon Injectable 1911

Oxazepam (Increases anesthetic effects; may also result in pronounced decrease in cardiac output and blood pressure). Products include:

- Serax Capsules 2522
- Serax Tablets 2522

Oxycodone Hydrochloride (Increases anesthetic effects; may also result in pronounced decrease in cardiac output and blood pressure). Products include:

- Percocet Tablets 950
- Percodan 951
- Roxicodone Tablets, Oral Solution & Intensol (Oxycodone) 1992
- Tylox Capsules 1382

Pentobarbital Sodium (Increases anesthetic effects; may also result in pronounced decrease in cardiac output and blood pressure). Products include:

- Nembutal Sodium Capsules 534
- Nembutal Sodium Solution 536
- Nembutal Sodium Suppositories 538

Phenobarbital (Increases anesthetic effects; may also result in pronounced decrease in cardiac output and blood pressure). Products include:

- Arco-Lase Plus Tablets 607
- Bellergal-S Tablets 1998
- Bronkolixir .... ◘ 761
- Bronkotabs Tablets .... ◘ 762
- Donnatal 1858
- Donnatal Extentabs 1859
- Donnatal Tablets 1858
- Donnazyme Tablets 1860
- Kinesed Tablets 2272
- Phenobarbital Elixir and Tablets 1293
- Primatene Tablets-P Formula 2421
- Quadrinal Tablets 1183
- Tedral SA 1765

Prazepam (Increases anesthetic effects; may also result in pronounced decrease in cardiac output and blood pressure). Products include:

- Centrax 1693

Propoxyphene Hydrochloride (Increases anesthetic effects; may also result in pronounced decrease in cardiac output and blood pressure). Products include:

- Darvon 1256
- Wygesic Tablets 2540

Propoxyphene Napsylate (Increases anesthetic effects; may also result in pronounced decrease in cardiac output and blood pressure). Products include:

- Darvon-N/Darvocet-N 1254

Quazepam (Increases anesthetic effects; may also result in pronounced decrease in cardiac output and blood pressure). Products include:

- Doral Tablets 2383

Secobarbital Sodium (Increases anesthetic effects; may also result in pronounced decrease in cardiac output and blood pressure). Products include:

- Seconal Sodium Pulvules 1296

Sufentanil Citrate (Increases anesthetic effects; may also result in pronounced decrease in cardiac output and blood pressure). Products include:

- Sufenta Injection 1147

Temazepam (Increases anesthetic effects; may also result in pronounced decrease in cardiac output and blood pressure). Products include:

- Restoril Capsules 2023

Thiamylal Sodium (Increases anesthetic effects; may also result in pronounced decrease in cardiac output and blood pressure). Products include:

- Surital Ampoules, Steri-Vials 1764

Triazolam (Increases anesthetic effects; may also result in pronounced decrease in cardiac output and blood pressure). Products include:

- Halcion Tablets 2340

DIPROLENE AF CREAM

(Betamethasone Dipropionate) 2083
No interactions described in labeling.

DIPROLENE CREAM 0.05%

(Betamethasone Dipropionate) 2083
No interactions described in labeling.

DIPROLENE LOTION 0.05%

(Betamethasone Dipropionate) 2083
No interactions described in labeling.

DIPROLENE OINTMENT 0.05%

(Betamethasone Dipropionate) 2083
No interactions described in labeling.

DISALCID CAPSULES

(Salsalate) 1310
May interact with antigout agents, salicylates, anticoagulants, oral hypoglycemic agents, penicillins, corticosteroids, and certain other agents. Compounds in these categories include:

Allopurinol (Uricosuric action antagonized). Products include:

- Zyloprim Tablets 830

Amoxicillin (Competition for protein binding sites). Products include:

- Amoxil 2193
- Augmentin Tablets, Powder for Oral Suspension, and Chewable Tablets 2198

Ampicillin Sodium (Competition for protein binding sites). Products include:

- Unasyn 1965

Aspirin (Additive effect; potentially toxic concentrations of salicylic acid). Products include:

- Alka-Seltzer Effervescent Antacid and Pain Reliever 1568
- Alka-Seltzer Extra Strength Effervescent Antacid and Pain Reliever 1570
- Alka-Seltzer (Flavored) Effervescent Antacid and Pain Reliever 1569
- Alka-Seltzer Plus Cold Medicine .... ◘ 623
- Alka-Seltzer Plus Night-Time Cold Medicine .... ◘ 623
- Alka Seltzer Plus Sinus Allergy Medicine .... ◘ 624
- Anacin Coated Analgesic Caplets 2417
- Anacin Coated Analgesic Tablets 2417
- Anacin Maximum Strength Analgesic Coated Tablets 2417
- Maximum Strength Arthritis Pain Formula By the Makers of Anacin Analgesic Tablets and Caplets 2418
- Arthritis Pain Formula by the Makers of Anacin Analgesic Tablets and Caplets .... ◘ 747
- Arthritis Strength BC Powder .... ◘ 516
- Ascriptin A/D Caplets 1850
- Regular Strength Ascriptin Tablets 1850
- Azdōne Tablets 844
- BC Powder .... ◘ 517
- BC Cold Powder .... ◘ 517
- Children's Bayer Chewable Aspirin .... ◘ 564
- Genuine Bayer Aspirin Tablets & Caplets .... ◘ 564
- Maximum Bayer Aspirin Tablets & Caplets .... ◘ 566
- Bayer Plus Aspirin Tablets .... ◘ 567
- Therapy Bayer Aspirin Caplets .... ◘ 568
- 8 Hour Bayer Timed-Release Aspirin .... ◘ 566
- Arthritis Strength Bufferin Analgesic Caplets 744
- Extra Strength Bufferin Analgesic Tablets 745
- Bufferin Analgesic Tablets and Caplets 743
- Cama Arthritis Pain Reliever .... ◘ 685
- Damason-P 1356
- Easprin 1719
- Ecotrin Enteric Coated Aspirin Maximum Strength Tablets and Caplets 2189
- Ecotrin Enteric Coated Aspirin Regular Strength Tablets and Caplets 2189
- Empirin Aspirin .... ◘ 541
- Empirin with Codeine Phosphate Nos. 2, 3 & 4 764
- Equagesic Tablets 2451
- Excedrin Extra-Strength Analgesic Tablets & Caplets 749
- 4-Way Cold Tablets 750
- Fiorinal Capsules 2007
- Fiorinal with Codeine Capsules 2008
- Fiorinal Tablets 2007
- Lortab ASA Tablets 2414
- Momentum Muscular Backache Formula .... ◘ 751
- Norgesic 1314
- Norwich Extra-Strength Aspirin .... ◘ 546
- Norwich Regular Strength Aspirin ◘ 547
- P-A-C Analgesic Tablets .... ◘ 669
- Percodan 951
- Robaxisal Tablets 1872
- Sine-Off Sinus Medicine Tablets-Aspirin Formula .... ◘ 722
- Soma Compound w/Codeine Tablets 2390
- Soma Compound Tablets 2389
- St. Joseph Adult Chewable Aspirin (81 mg.) .... ◘ 703
- Synalgos-DC Capsules 2525
- Talwin Compound 2072
- Ursinus Inlay-Tabs .... ◘ 691
- Vanquish Analgesic Caplets .... ◘ 574
- Zorprin Tablets 698

Azlocillin Sodium (Competition for protein binding sites).
- No products indexed under this heading.

Bacampicillin Hydrochloride (Competition for protein binding sites). Products include:
- Spectrobid Tablets & Powder for Oral Suspension 1961

Betamethasone Acetate (Competition for protein binding sites). Products include:
- Celestone Soluspan Suspension 2081

Betamethasone Sodium Phosphate (Competition for protein binding sites). Products include:
- Celestone Soluspan Suspension 2081

Carbenicillin Disodium (Competition for protein binding sites).

Carbenicillin Indanyl Sodium (Competition for protein binding sites). Products include:
- Geocillin Tablets 1951

Chlorpropamide (Enhanced hypoglycemic effect). Products include:
- Diabinese Tablets 1775

Choline Magnesium Trisalicylate (Additive effect; potentially toxic concentrations of salicylic acid). Products include:
- Trilisate 1822

Cortisone Acetate (Competition for protein binding sites). Products include:
- Cortone Acetate Sterile Suspension 1437
- Cortone Acetate Tablets 1439

Dexamethasone (Competition for protein binding sites). Products include:
- AK-Trol Ointment & Suspension ..... ⊙ 207
- Decadron Elixir 1445
- Decadron Tablets 1447
- Decaspray Topical Aerosol 1459
- Dexacidin ..... ⊙ 272
- Maxidex Sterile Ophthalmic Suspension ..... ⊙ 223
- Maxitrol Ophthalmic Ointment/ Suspension ..... ⊙ 223
- TobraDex Ophthalmic Suspension and Ointment ..... ⊙ 228

Dexamethasone Acetate (Competition for protein binding sites). Products include:
- Dalalone D.P. Injectable 999
- Decadron-LA Sterile Suspension 1457

Dexamethasone Sodium Phosphate (Competition for protein binding sites). Products include:
- AK-Dex ..... ⊙ 203
- Decadron Phosphate Respihaler 1454
- Decadron Phosphate Sterile Ophthalmic Ointment 1453
- Decadron Phosphate Sterile Ophthalmic Solution 1453
- Decadron Phosphate Topical Cream 1455
- Decadron Phosphate Turbinaire 1456
- Maxidex Sterile Ophthalmic Ointment ..... ⊙ 222
- NeoDecadron Sterile Ophthalmic Ointment 1517
- NeoDecadron Sterile Ophthalmic Solution 1518
- NeoDecadron Topical Cream 1518

Dicumarol (Concomitant anticoagulant drugs may predispose to systemic bleeding). Products include:
- Dicumarol Tablets 516

Diflunisal (Additive effect; potentially toxic concentrations of salicylic acid). Products include:
- Dolobid Tablets 1465

Glipizide (Enhanced hypoglycemic effect). Products include:
- Glucotrol 1952

Glyburide (Enhanced hypoglycemic effect). Products include:
- DiaBeta 1091
- Micronase Tablets 2350

Heparin Calcium (Concomitant anticoagulant drugs may predispose to systemic bleeding). Products include:
- Calciparine Injection 925

Heparin Sodium (Concomitant anticoagulant drugs may predispose to systemic bleeding). Products include:
- Heparin Lock Flush Solution 2456
- Heparin Sodium Vials 1264
- Heparin Sodium Injection 2457
- Heparin Sodium Injection, USP, Sterile Solution 2342

Hydrocortisone (Competition for protein binding sites). Products include:
- AK-Spore H.C. ..... ⊙ 206
- Bactine Hydrocortisone Anti-Itch Cream ..... ▣ 625
- CaldeCORT Anti-Itch Hydrocortisone Spray ..... ▣ 560
- Carmol HC Cream 1% 2296
- Cortaid Spray ..... ▣ 735
- Cortenema 2244
- Cortisporin Ointment 758
- Cortisporin Ophthalmic Ointment Sterile 758
- Cortisporin Ophthalmic Suspension Sterile 759
- Cortisporin Otic Solution Sterile 760
- Cortisporin Otic Suspension Sterile 760
- Cortizone-5 Creme & Ointment ..... ▣ 732
- Dermolate Anti-Itch Cream ..... ▣ 697
- Eldecort Cream 1.0% 1113
- Eldecort Cream 1.0% and 2.5% 1113
- Fungoid HC Creme 1770
- Hydrocortone Tablets 1482
- Hytone 909
- LazerSporin-C Solution 1770
- Massengill Medicated Soft Cloth Towelettes 2192
- Nutracort Cream & Lotion 1684
- PediOtic Suspension Sterile 797
- Synacort Creams 1%, 2.5% 2296
- Vanoxide-HC Acne Lotion 911
- Vioform-Hydrocortisone Cream and Mild Cream 889
- Vioform-Hydrocortisone Ointment 889
- VōSoL HC Otic Solution 2392
- Vytone Cream 1% 911

Hydrocortisone Acetate (Competition for protein binding sites). Products include:
- Analpram-HC Rectal Cream 1% and 2.5% 970
- Anusol-HC Cream 1690
- Anusol-HC Suppositories 1691
- Caldecort ..... ▣ 560
- Carmol HC Cream 1% 2296
- Chloromycetin Hydrocortisone Ophthalmic 1694
- Coly-Mycin S Otic w/Neomycin & Hydrocortisone 1708
- Cortaid ..... ▣ 735
- Cortef Feminine Itch Cream ..... ▣ 735
- Corticaine ..... ▣ 682
- Cortifoam 1827
- Cortisporin Cream 757
- Epifoam 1828
- Gynecort 5 Creme ..... ▣ 556
- Hydrocortone Acetate Sterile Suspension 1479
- Lanacort 5 Creme and Ointment ..... ▣ 557
- Mantadil Cream 789
- Ophthocort ..... ⊙ 301
- Orabase HCA Oral Paste 890
- Pramosone Cream, Lotion & Ointment 971
- ProctoCream-HC 1834
- Proctofoam-HC 1835

Hydrocortisone Sodium Phosphate (Competition for protein binding sites). Products include:
- Hydrocortone Phosphate Injection, Sterile 1481

Hydrocortisone Sodium Succinate (Competition for protein binding sites). Products include:
- Solu-Cortef Sterile Powder 2361

Magnesium Salicylate (Additive effect; potentially toxic concentrations of salicylic acid). Products include:
- Doan's - Extra-Strength Analgesic ..... ▣ 549
- Doan's - Regular Strength Analgesic ..... ▣ 549
- Mobigesic Analgesic Tablets ..... ▣ 507

Methotrexate Sodium (Competition for protein binding sites). Products include:
- Methotrexate Tablets, Parenteral, LPF Parenteral 1217
- Rheumatrex Methotrexate Dose Pack 1234

Methylprednisolone (Competition for protein binding sites). Products include:
- Medrol 2348

Methylprednisolone Acetate (Competition for protein binding sites). Products include:
- Depo-Medrol Sterile Aqueous Suspension 2334

Methylprednisolone Sodium Succinate (Competition for protein binding sites). Products include:
- Solu-Medrol Sterile Powder 2363

Mezlocillin Sodium (Competition for protein binding sites). Products include:
- Mezlin 1597
- Mezlin Pharmacy Bulk Package 1599

Nafcillin Sodium (Competition for protein binding sites). Products include:
- Unipen 2533

Naproxen (Competition for protein binding sites). Products include:
- Naprosyn 2297

Naproxen Sodium (Competition for protein binding sites). Products include:
- Anaprox and Anaprox DS Tablets 2288

Penicillin G Potassium (Competition for protein binding sites). Products include:
- Pfizerpen for Injection 1957

Penicillin G Procaine (Competition for protein binding sites). Products include:
- Bicillin C-R Injection 2438
- Bicillin C-R 900/300 Injection 2440
- Pfizerpen-AS Aqueous Suspension 1959
- Wycillin Injection 2537
- Wycillin Injection and Probenecid Tablets 2539

Penicillin G Sodium (Competition for protein binding sites).
- No products indexed under this heading.

Penicillin G, Benzathine (Competition for protein binding sites). Products include:
- Bicillin C-R Injection 2438
- Bicillin C-R 900/300 Injection 2440
- Bicillin L-A Injection 2442

Penicillin V Potassium (Competition for protein binding sites).
- No products indexed under this heading.

Phenytoin (Competition for protein binding sites). Products include:
- Dilantin Infatabs 1710
- Dilantin-30 Pediatric/Dilantin-125 Suspension 1713

Phenytoin Sodium (Competition for protein binding sites). Products include:
- Dilantin Kapseals 1708
- Dilantin Parenteral 1712
- Dilantin with Phenobarbital Kapseals 1715

Prednisolone Acetate (Competition for protein binding sites). Products include:
- AK-Cide Sterile Ophthalmic Ointment & Suspension ..... ⊙ 202
- Blephamide Liquifilm Sterile Ophthalmic Suspension 586
- Blephamide S.O.P. Sterile Ophthalmic Ointment 586
- Cetapred Ointment ..... ⊙ 220
- ⅛% Econopred & 1% Econopred Plus ..... ⊙ 217
- Isopto Cetapred Suspension ..... ⊙ 220
- Metimyd ..... ⊙ 306
- Poly-Pred Liquifilm ..... ⊙ 250
- Pred Forte ..... ⊙ 252
- Pred Mild ..... ⊙ 254
- Pred-G Liquifilm Sterile Ophthalmic Suspension ..... ⊙ 252
- Pred-G S.O.P. Sterile Ophthalmic Ointment ..... ⊙ 253
- Vasocidin Ointment ..... ⊙ 275

Prednisolone Sodium Phosphate (Competition for protein binding sites). Products include:
- AK-Pred ..... ⊙ 205
- Hydeltrasol Injection, Sterile 1476
- Inflamase ..... ⊙ 274
- Pediapred Oral Liquid 987
- Vasocidin Ophthalmic Solution ..... ⊙ 276

Prednisolone Tebutate (Competition for protein binding sites). Products include:
- Hydeltra-T.B.A. Sterile Suspension 1478

Prednisone (Competition for protein binding sites). Products include:
- Deltasone Tablets 2332

Probenecid (Uricosuric action antagonized). Products include:
- Benemid Tablets 1426
- ColBENEMID Tablets 1436
- Wycillin Injection and Probenecid Tablets 2539

Sulfinpyrazone (Uricosuric action antagonized). Products include:
- Anturane 853

Thyroxine (Competition for protein binding sites).
- No products indexed under this heading.

Ticarcillin Disodium (Competition for protein binding sites). Products include:
- Ticar for Injection 2236
- Timentin for Injection 2239

Tolazamide (Enhanced hypoglycemic effect). Products include:
- Tolinase Tablets 2365

Tolbutamide (Enhanced hypoglycemic effect). Products include:
- Orinase Tablets 2354

Triamcinolone (Competition for protein binding sites).
- No products indexed under this heading.

Triamcinolone Acetonide (Competition for protein binding sites). Products include:
- Aristocort A 1010
- Azmacort Inhaler 1837
- Kenalog Cream, Lotion & Ointment 2401
- Kenalog-10 Injection 2402
- Kenalog-40 Injection 2403
- Kenalog in Orabase 604
- Kenalog Spray 2401
- Mycolog II Cream and Ointment 2407
- Mytrex Cream & Ointment 2080
- Nasacort Nasal Inhaler 1844

Triamcinolone Diacetate (Competition for protein binding sites). Products include:
- Aristocort Suspension 1008

Triamcinolone Hexacetonide (Competition for protein binding sites). Products include:
- Aristospan Suspension 1011

l-Triiodothyronine (Competition for protein binding sites).

Warfarin Sodium (Concomitant anticoagulant drugs may predispose to systemic bleeding). Products include:
- Coumadin Injection & Tablets 944
- Panwarfin Tablets 547

Food Interactions

Food that lowers urinary pH (Decreases urinary excretion and increases plasma levels).

Food that raises urinary pH (Increases renal clearance and urinary excretion of salicylic acid).

DISALCID TABLETS
(Salsalate) 1310
See **Disalcid Capsules**

DISOPHROL CHRONOTAB SUSTAINED-ACTION TABLETS
(Dexbrompheniramine Maleate, Pseudoephedrine Sulfate) .... ■ 698
May interact with antihypertensives, antidepressant drugs, and certain other agents. Compounds in these categories include:

Acebutolol Hydrochloride (Concurrent use is not recommended). Products include:
Sectral Capsules 2520

Alcohol (Increases the drowsiness effect).

Amitriptyline Hydrochloride (Concurrent use is not recommended). Products include:
Elavil 2269
Endep Tablets 1927
Etrafon 2087
Limbitrol 1933
Triavil Tablets 1556

Amoxapine (Concurrent use is not recommended). Products include:
Asendin Tablets 1196

Atenolol (Concurrent use is not recommended). Products include:
Tenoretic Tablets 1105
Tenormin Tablets and I.V. Injection 1107

Benazepril Hydrochloride (Concurrent use is not recommended). Products include:
Lotensin Tablets 872

Bendroflumethiazide (Concurrent use is not recommended). Products include:
Corzide Tablets 702
Naturetin Tablets 1789
Rauzide Tablets 1804

Betaxolol Hydrochloride (Concurrent use is not recommended). Products include:
Betoptic Sterile Ophthalmic Solution 569
Betoptic S Sterile Ophthalmic Suspension 570
Kerlone Tablets 2172

Bupropion Hydrochloride (Concurrent use is not recommended). Products include:
Wellbutrin Tablets 821

Captopril (Concurrent use is not recommended). Products include:
Capoten 2255
Capozide 2258

Carteolol Hydrochloride (Concurrent use is not recommended). Products include:
Cartrol Tablets 507

Chlorothiazide (Concurrent use is not recommended). Products include:
Aldoclor Tablets 1413
Diupres Tablets 1461
Diuril Oral 1464

Chlorothiazide Sodium (Concurrent use is not recommended). Products include:
Diuril Sodium Intravenous 1463

Chlorthalidone (Concurrent use is not recommended). Products include:
Combipres Tablets 678
Tenoretic Tablets 1105
Thalitone Tablets 687

Clonidine (Concurrent use is not recommended). Products include:
Catapres-TTS 677

Clonidine Hydrochloride (Concurrent use is not recommended). Products include:
Catapres Tablets 676
Combipres Tablets 678

Deserpidine (Concurrent use is not recommended). Products include:
Enduronyl 518
Harmonyl Tablets 528
Oreticyl 545

Desipramine Hydrochloride (Concurrent use is not recommended). Products include:
Norpramin Tablets 1340

Diazoxide (Concurrent use is not recommended). Products include:
Hyperstat I.V. Injection 2095
Proglycem 649

Doxazosin Mesylate (Concurrent use is not recommended). Products include:
Cardura Tablets 1941

Doxepin Hydrochloride (Concurrent use is not recommended). Products include:
Sinequan 1960

Enalapril Maleate (Concurrent use is not recommended). Products include:
Vaseretic Tablets 1559
Vasotec Tablets 1564

Enalaprilat (Concurrent use is not recommended). Products include:
Vasotec I.V. 1562

Esmolol Hydrochloride (Concurrent use is not recommended). Products include:
Brevibloc Injection 942

Felodipine (Concurrent use is not recommended). Products include:
Plendil Extended-Release Tablets 1526

Fluoxetine Hydrochloride (Concurrent use is not recommended). Products include:
Prozac Pulvules 920

Fosinopril Sodium (Concurrent use is not recommended). Products include:
Monopril Tablets 1406

Furosemide (Concurrent use is not recommended). Products include:
Lasix 1093

Guanabenz Acetate (Concurrent use is not recommended). Products include:
Wytensin Tablets 2542

Guanethidine Monosulfate (Concurrent use is not recommended). Products include:
Esimil Tablets 864
Ismelin Tablets 869

Hydralazine Hydrochloride (Concurrent use is not recommended). Products include:
Apresazide Capsules 854
Apresoline Hydrochloride Parenteral (Ampuls) 856
Apresoline Hydrochloride Tablets .. 855
Apresoline-Esidrix Tablets 857
Ser-Ap-Es Tablets 881
Serpasil-Apresoline Tablets 884

Hydrochlorothiazide (Concurrent use is not recommended). Products include:
Aldactazide 2150
Aldoril Tablets 1418
Apresazide Capsules 854
Apresoline-Esidrix Tablets 857
Capozide 2258
Dyazide Capsules 2208
Esidrix Tablets 863
Esimil Tablets 864
HydroDIURIL Tablets 1484
Hydropres Tablets 1485
Inderide Tablets 2463
Inderide LA Long Acting Capsules .. 2465
Lopressor HCT Tablets 1034
Maxzide 1215
Moduretic Tablets 1510
Normozide Tablets 2112
Oretic Tablets 544
Oreticyl 545
Prinzide Tablets 1540
Ser-Ap-Es Tablets 881
Serpasil-Esidrix Tablets 886
Timolide Tablets 1547
Trandate HCT Tablets 579
Vaseretic Tablets 1559
Zestoretic 2274

Hydroflumethiazide (Concurrent use is not recommended). Products include:
Diucardin Tablets 2450
Saluron 718
Salutensin/Salutensin-Demi 719

Imipramine Hydrochloride (Concurrent use is not recommended). Products include:
Tofranil Ampuls 1038
Tofranil Tablets 1039

Imipramine Pamoate (Concurrent use is not recommended). Products include:
Tofranil-PM Capsules 1041

Indapamide (Concurrent use is not recommended). Products include:
Lozol Tablets 1843

Isocarboxazid (Concurrent use is not recommended). Products include:
Marplan Tablets 1906

Isradipine (Concurrent use is not recommended). Products include:
DynaCirc Capsules 2004

Labetalol Hydrochloride (Concurrent use is not recommended). Products include:
Normodyne Injection 2108
Normodyne Tablets 2110
Normozide Tablets 2112
Trandate HCT Tablets 579
Trandate Injection 577
Trandate Tablets 579

Lisinopril (Concurrent use is not recommended). Products include:
Prinivil Tablets 1538
Prinzide Tablets 1540
Zestoretic 2274
Zestril Tablets 2277

Maprotiline Hydrochloride (Concurrent use is not recommended). Products include:
Ludiomil Tablets 874

Mecamylamine Hydrochloride (Concurrent use is not recommended). Products include:
Inversine Tablets 1492

Methyclothiazide (Concurrent use is not recommended). Products include:
Enduron Tablets 517
Enduronyl 518

Methyldopa (Concurrent use is not recommended). Products include:
Aldoclor Tablets 1413
Aldomet Oral 1415
Aldoril Tablets 1418

Methyldopate Hydrochloride (Concurrent use is not recommended). Products include:
Aldomet Ester HCl Injection 1417

Metolazone (Concurrent use is not recommended). Products include:
Diulo 2129
Mykrox ½ mg Tablets 984
Zaroxolyn Tablets 989

Metoprolol Tartrate (Concurrent use is not recommended). Products include:
Lopressor Ampuls 1032
Lopressor HCT Tablets 1034
Lopressor Tablets 1032

Metyrosine (Concurrent use is not recommended). Products include:
Demser Capsules 1460

Minoxidil (Concurrent use is not recommended). Products include:
Loniten Tablets 2346
Rogaine Topical Solution 2357

Nadolol (Concurrent use is not recommended). Products include:
Corgard Tablets 701
Corzide Tablets 702

Nicardipine Hydrochloride (Concurrent use is not recommended). Products include:
Cardene Capsules 2290

Nitroglycerin (Concurrent use is not recommended). Products include:
Deponit NTG Transdermal Delivery System 2143
Minitran Transdermal Delivery System 1312
Nitro-Bid Ointment 1339
Nitro-Bid Capsules 1338
Nitrodisc 2176
Nitro-Dur (nitroglycerin) Transdermal Infusion System 1164
Nitrogard Tablets 1004
Nitrolingual Spray 1846
Nitrostat Tablets 1743
Transderm-Nitro Transdermal Therapeutic System 2283

Nortriptyline Hydrochloride (Concurrent use is not recommended). Products include:
Pamelor 2019

Penbutolol Sulfate (Concurrent use is not recommended). Products include:
Levatol 1832

Phenelzine Sulfate (Concurrent use is not recommended). Products include:
Nardil 1742

Phenoxybenzamine Hydrochloride (Concurrent use is not recommended). Products include:
Dibenzyline Capsules 2207

Phentolamine Mesylate (Concurrent use is not recommended). Products include:
Regitine 878

Pindolol (Concurrent use is not recommended). Products include:
Visken Tablets 2036

Polythiazide (Concurrent use is not recommended). Products include:
Minizide Capsules 1779
Renese Tablets 1785
Renese-R Tablets 1786

Prazosin Hydrochloride (Concurrent use is not recommended). Products include:
Minipress Capsules 1778
Minizide Capsules 1779

Propranolol Hydrochloride (Concurrent use is not recommended). Products include:
Inderal 2459
Inderal LA Long Acting Capsules 2461
Inderide Tablets 2463
Inderide LA Long Acting Capsules .. 2465

Protriptyline Hydrochloride (Concurrent use is not recommended). Products include:
Vivactil Tablets 1567

Ramipril (Concurrent use is not recommended). Products include:
Altace Capsules 1086

Rauwolfia Serpentina (Concurrent use is not recommended). Products include:
Raudixin Tablets 1803
Rauzide Tablets 1804

Rescinnamine (Concurrent use is not recommended).
No products indexed under this heading.

Reserpine (Concurrent use is not recommended). Products include:
Diupres Tablets 1461
Hydromox R Tablets 1209
Hydropres Tablets 1485
Renese-R Tablets 1786
Salutensin/Salutensin-Demi 719
Ser-Ap-Es Tablets 881
Serpasil Tablets 883
Serpasil-Apresoline Tablets 884
Serpasil-Esidrix Tablets 886

Sodium Nitroprusside (Concurrent use is not recommended). Products include:
- Nipride I.V. Infusion ... 1909

Terazosin Hydrochloride (Concurrent use is not recommended). Products include:
- Hytrin Tablets ... 529

Timolol Maleate (Concurrent use is not recommended). Products include:
- Blocadren Tablets ... 1429
- Timolide Tablets ... 1547
- Timoptic in Ocudose ... 1552
- Timoptic Sterile Ophthalmic Solution ... 1550

Tranylcypromine Sulfate (Concurrent use is not recommended). Products include:
- Parnate Tablets ... 2222

Trazodone Hydrochloride (Concurrent use is not recommended). Products include:
- Desyrel and Desyrel Dividose ... 1404

Trimethaphan Camsylate (Concurrent use is not recommended). Products include:
- Arfonad Ampuls ... 1887

Trimipramine Maleate (Concurrent use is not recommended). Products include:
- Surmontil Capsules ... 2524

DITROPAN SYRUP
(Oxybutynin Chloride) ... 1332
See **Ditropan Tablets**

DITROPAN TABLETS
(Oxybutynin Chloride) ... 1332
May interact with hypnotics and sedatives and certain other agents. Compounds in these categories include:

Alcohol (Enhances the drowsiness effect).

Estazolam (Enhances the drowsiness effect). Products include:
- ProSom Tablets ... 554

Ethchlorvynol (Enhances the drowsiness effect). Products include:
- Placidyl Capsules ... 553

Ethinamate (Enhances the drowsiness effect).
- No products indexed under this heading.

Flurazepam Hydrochloride (Enhances the drowsiness effect). Products include:
- Dalmane Capsules ... 1927

Glutethimide (Enhances the drowsiness effect).
- No products indexed under this heading.

Lorazepam (Enhances the drowsiness effect). Products include:
- Ativan Injection ... 2432
- Ativan Tablets ... 2434

Midazolam Hydrochloride (Enhances the drowsiness effect). Products include:
- Versed Injection ... 1924

Propofol (Enhances the drowsiness effect). Products include:
- Diprivan Injection ... 2267

Quazepam (Enhances the drowsiness effect). Products include:
- Doral Tablets ... 2383

Secobarbital Sodium (Enhances the drowsiness effect). Products include:
- Seconal Sodium Pulvules ... 1296

Temazepam (Enhances the drowsiness effect). Products include:
- Restoril Capsules ... 2023

Triazolam (Enhances the drowsiness effect). Products include:
- Halcion Tablets ... 2340

DIUCARDIN TABLETS
(Hydroflumethiazide) ... 2450
May interact with antihypertensives, corticosteroids, insulin, lithium preparations, general anesthetics, preanesthetic medications, nondepolarizing neuromuscular blocking agents, cardiac glycosides, oral hypoglycemic agents, oral anticoagulants, barbiturates, narcotic analgesics, and certain other agents. Compounds in these categories include:

Acebutolol Hydrochloride (Effects may be potentiated when used concurrently with thiazide diuretics). Products include:
- Sectral Capsules ... 2520

ACTH (Concurrent use with thiazide diuretics may intensify electrolyte imbalance, particularly hypokalemia).
- No products indexed under this heading.

Alfentanil Hydrochloride (Orthostatic hypotension may be aggravated). Products include:
- Alfenta Injection ... 1131

Allopurinol (Thiazide diuretics may raise the level of blood uric acid). Products include:
- Zyloprim Tablets ... 830

Amphotericin B (Concurrent use with thiazide diuretics may intensify electrolyte imbalance, particularly hypokalemia). Products include:
- Fungizone Cream, Lotion and Ointment ... 2261
- Fungizone Intravenous ... 2262

Aprobarbital (Orthostatic hypotension may be aggravated). Products include:
- Alurate Elixir ... 1883

Atenolol (Effects may be potentiated when used concurrently with thiazide diuretics). Products include:
- Tenoretic Tablets ... 1105
- Tenormin Tablets and I.V. Injection ... 1107

Atracurium Besylate (Effects may be potentiated when used concurrently with thiazide diuretics). Products include:
- Tracrium Injection ... 817

Benazepril Hydrochloride (Effects may be potentiated when used concurrently with thiazide diuretics). Products include:
- Lotensin Tablets ... 872

Bendroflumethiazide (Effects may be potentiated when used concurrently with thiazide diuretics). Products include:
- Corzide Tablets ... 702
- Naturetin Tablets ... 1789
- Rauzide Tablets ... 1804

Betamethasone Acetate (Concurrent use with thiazide diuretics may intensify electrolyte imbalance, particularly hypokalemia). Products include:
- Celestone Soluspan Suspension ... 2081

Betamethasone Sodium Phosphate (Concurrent use with thiazide diuretics may intensify electrolyte imbalance, particularly hypokalemia). Products include:
- Celestone Soluspan Suspension ... 2081

Betaxolol Hydrochloride (Effects may be potentiated when used concurrently with thiazide diuretics). Products include:
- Betoptic Sterile Ophthalmic Solution ... 569
- Betoptic S Sterile Ophthalmic Suspension ... 570
- Kerlone Tablets ... 2172

Buprenorphine (Orthostatic hypotension may be aggravated).
- No products indexed under this heading.

Butabarbital (Orthostatic hypotension may be aggravated). Products include:
- Pyridium Plus ... 1764

Butalbital (Orthostatic hypotension may be aggravated). Products include:
- Esgic-Plus Tablets ... 1002
- Esgic Tablets & Capsules ... 1001
- Fioricet Tablets ... 2006
- Fiorinal Capsules ... 2007
- Fiorinal with Codeine Capsules ... 2008
- Fiorinal Tablets ... 2007
- Phrenilin ... 838
- Sedapap Tablets 50 mg/650 mg ... 1360

Captopril (Effects may be potentiated when used concurrently with thiazide diuretics). Products include:
- Capoten ... 2255
- Capozide ... 2258

Carteolol Hydrochloride (Effects may be potentiated when used concurrently with thiazide diuretics). Products include:
- Cartrol Tablets ... 507

Chlorothiazide (Effects may be potentiated when used concurrently with thiazide diuretics). Products include:
- Aldoclor Tablets ... 1413
- Diupres Tablets ... 1461
- Diuril Oral ... 1464

Chlorothiazide Sodium (Effects may be potentiated when used concurrently with thiazide diuretics). Products include:
- Diuril Sodium Intravenous ... 1463

Chlorpropamide (Thiazides may raise blood glucose levels). Products include:
- Diabinese Tablets ... 1775

Chlorthalidone (Effects may be potentiated when used concurrently with thiazide diuretics). Products include:
- Combipres Tablets ... 678
- Tenoretic Tablets ... 1105
- Thalitone Tablets ... 687

Clonidine (Effects may be potentiated when used concurrently with thiazide diuretics). Products include:
- Catapres-TTS ... 677

Clonidine Hydrochloride (Effects may be potentiated when used concurrently with thiazide diuretics). Products include:
- Catapres Tablets ... 676
- Combipres Tablets ... 678

Codeine (Orthostatic hypotension may be aggravated). Products include:
- Calcidrine Syrup ... 506

Codeine Phosphate (Orthostatic hypotension may be aggravated). Products include:
- Actifed with Codeine Cough Syrup ... 752
- Cheracol Cough Syrup ... 1853
- Codimal PH Syrup ... 846
- Dimetane-DC Cough Syrup ... 1857
- Empirin with Codeine Phosphate Nos. 2, 3 & 4 ... 764
- Fiorinal with Codeine Capsules ... 2008
- Isoclor Expectorant ... 982
- Naldecon CX Adult Liquid ... ▣ 521
- Novahistine DH ... 1342
- Novahistine Expectorant ... 1343
- Nucofed Capsules ... 2219
- Nucofed Expectorant ... 2219
- Nucofed Pediatric Expectorant ... 2220
- Nucofed Syrup ... 2219
- Phenaphen with Codeine Capsules ... 1865
- Phenaphen-650 with Codeine Tablets ... 1866
- Phenergan with Codeine ... 2497
- Phenergan VC with Codeine ... 2501
- Robitussin A-C Syrup ... 1875
- Robitussin-DAC Syrup ... 1875
- Ryna ... ▣ 741
- Soma Compound w/Codeine Tablets ... 2390
- Triaminic Expectorant w/Codeine ... 1996
- Tussi-Organidin Liquid ... 2391
- Tylenol with Codeine ... 1381

Codeine Polistirex (Orthostatic hypotension may be aggravated).
- No products indexed under this heading.

Colestipol Hydrochloride (May inhibit gastrointestinal absorption of the thiazide diuretics). Products include:
- Colestid Granules ... 2328

Cortisone Acetate (Concurrent use with thiazide diuretics may intensify electrolyte imbalance, particularly hypokalemia). Products include:
- Cortone Acetate Sterile Suspension ... 1437
- Cortone Acetate Tablets ... 1439

Deserpidine (Effects may be potentiated when used concurrently with thiazide diuretics). Products include:
- Enduronyl ... 518
- Harmonyl Tablets ... 528
- Oreticyl ... 545

Deslanoside (Enhanced possibility of digitalis toxicity associated with hypokalemia).
- No products indexed under this heading.

Dexamethasone (Concurrent use with thiazide diuretics may intensify electrolyte imbalance, particularly hypokalemia). Products include:
- AK-Trol Ointment & Suspension ... ⊚ 207
- Decadron Elixir ... 1445
- Decadron Tablets ... 1447
- Decaspray Topical Aerosol ... 1459
- Dexacidin ... ⊚ 272
- Maxidex Sterile Ophthalmic Suspension ... ⊚ 223
- Maxitrol Ophthalmic Ointment/Suspension ... ⊚ 223
- TobraDex Ophthalmic Suspension and Ointment ... ⊚ 228

Dexamethasone Acetate (Concurrent use with thiazide diuretics may intensify electrolyte imbalance, particularly hypokalemia). Products include:
- Dalalone D.P. Injectable ... 999
- Decadron-LA Sterile Suspension ... 1457

Dexamethasone Sodium Phosphate (Concurrent use with thiazide diuretics may intensify electrolyte imbalance, particularly hypokalemia). Products include:
- AK-Dex ... ⊚ 203
- Decadron Phosphate Respihaler ... 1454
- Decadron Phosphate Sterile Ophthalmic Ointment ... 1453
- Decadron Phosphate Sterile Ophthalmic Solution ... 1453
- Decadron Phosphate Topical Cream ... 1455
- Decadron Phosphate Turbinaire ... 1456
- Maxidex Sterile Ophthalmic Ointment ... ⊚ 222
- NeoDecadron Sterile Ophthalmic Ointment ... 1517
- NeoDecadron Sterile Ophthalmic Solution ... 1518
- NeoDecadron Topical Cream ... 1518

Dezocine (Orthostatic hypotension may be aggravated).

Diazepam (Effects may be potentiated when used concurrently with thiazide diuretics). Products include:
- Valium Injectable ... 1937
- Valium Tablets ... 1939
- Valrelease Capsules ... 1923

Diazoxide (Effects may be potentiated when used concurrently with thiazide diuretics). Products include:
- Hyperstat I.V. Injection ... 2095
- Proglycem ... 649

Dicumarol (Effects may be decreased when used concurrently with thiazide diuretics; dosage adjustment may be necessary). Products include:
Dicumarol Tablets 516

Digitoxin (Enhanced possibility of digitalis toxicity associated with hypokalemia). Products include:
Crystodigin Tablets 1253

Digoxin (Enhanced possibility of digitalis toxicity associated with hypokalemia). Products include:
Lanoxicaps 772
Lanoxin Elixir Pediatric 775
Lanoxin Injection 778
Lanoxin Injection Pediatric 781
Lanoxin Tablets 783

Doxazosin Mesylate (Effects may be potentiated when used concurrently with thiazide diuretics). Products include:
Cardura Tablets 1941

Droperidol (Effects may be potentiated when used concurrently with thiazide diuretics). Products include:
Inapsine Injection 1140
Innovar Injection 1141

Enalapril Maleate (Effects may be potentiated when used concurrently with thiazide diuretics). Products include:
Vaseretic Tablets 1559
Vasotec Tablets 1564

Enalaprilat (Effects may be potentiated when used concurrently with thiazide diuretics). Products include:
Vasotec I.V. 1562

Enflurane (Effects may be potentiated when used concurrently with thiazide diuretics). Products include:
Ethrane 599

Esmolol Hydrochloride (Effects may be potentiated when used concurrently with thiazide diuretics). Products include:
Brevibloc Injection 942

Felodipine (Effects may be potentiated when used concurrently with thiazide diuretics). Products include:
Plendil Extended-Release Tablets 1526

Fentanyl (Orthostatic hypotension may be aggravated). Products include:
Duragesic Transdermal System 1133

Fentanyl Citrate (Effects may be potentiated when used concurrently with thiazide diuretics; orthostatic hypotension may be aggravated). Products include:
Innovar Injection 1141
Sublimaze Injection 1146

Fosinopril Sodium (Effects may be potentiated when used concurrently with thiazide diuretics). Products include:
Monopril Tablets 1406

Furosemide (Effects may be potentiated when used concurrently with thiazide diuretics). Products include:
Lasix 1093

Glipizide (Thiazides may raise blood glucose levels). Products include:
Glucotrol 1952

Glyburide (Thiazides may raise blood glucose levels). Products include:
DiaBeta 1091
Micronase Tablets 2350

Guanabenz Acetate (Effects may be potentiated when used concurrently with thiazide diuretics). Products include:
Wytensin Tablets 2542

Guanethidine Monosulfate (Effects may be potentiated when used concurrently with thiazide diuretics). Products include:
Esimil Tablets 864
Ismelin Tablets 869

Hydralazine Hydrochloride (Effects may be potentiated when used concurrently with thiazide diuretics). Products include:
Apresazide Capsules 854
Apresoline Hydrochloride Parenteral (Ampuls) 856
Apresoline Hydrochloride Tablets 855
Apresoline-Esidrix Tablets 857
Ser-Ap-Es Tablets 881
Serpasil-Apresoline Tablets 884

Hydrochlorothiazide (Effects may be potentiated when used concurrently with thiazide diuretics). Products include:
Aldactazide 2150
Aldoril Tablets 1418
Apresazide Capsules 854
Apresoline-Esidrix Tablets 857
Capozide 2258
Dyazide Capsules 2208
Esidrix Tablets 863
Esimil Tablets 864
HydroDIURIL Tablets 1484
Hydropres Tablets 1485
Inderide Tablets 2463
Inderide LA Long Acting Capsules 2465
Lopressor HCT Tablets 1034
Maxzide 1215
Moduretic Tablets 1510
Normozide Tablets 2112
Oretic Tablets 544
Oreticyl 545
Prinzide Tablets 1540
Ser-Ap-Es Tablets 881
Serpasil-Esidrix Tablets 886
Timolide Tablets 1547
Trandate HCT Tablets 579
Vaseretic Tablets 1559
Zestoretic 2274

Hydrocodone Bitartrate (Orthostatic hypotension may be aggravated). Products include:
Anexsia 5/500 Tablets 2196
Anexsia 7.5/650 Tablets 2197
Azdone Tablets 844
Codiclear DH Syrup 845
Codimal DH Syrup 846
Damason-P 1356
Hycodan Syrup, Tablets 927
Hycomine Compound Tablets 929
Hycomine Syrup 927
Hycotuss Expectorant Syrup 930
Hydrocet Capsules 835
Lortab ASA Tablets 2414
Lortab 2412
Ru-Tuss with Hydrocodone 694
Triaminic Expectorant DH 1995
Vicodin Tablets 1187
Vicodin ES Tablets 1189
Zydone Capsules 941

Hydrocodone Polistirex (Orthostatic hypotension may be aggravated). Products include:
Tussionex Extended-Release Suspension 988

Hydrocortisone (Concurrent use with thiazide diuretics may intensify electrolyte imbalance, particularly hypokalemia). Products include:
AK-Spore H.C. ⊙ 206
Bactine Hydrocortisone Anti-Itch Cream ▣ 625
CaldeCORT Anti-Itch Hydrocortisone Spray ▣ 560
Carmol HC Cream 1% 2296
Cortaid Spray ▣ 735
Cortenema 2244
Cortisporin Ointment 758
Cortisporin Ophthalmic Ointment Sterile 758
Cortisporin Ophthalmic Suspension Sterile 759
Cortisporin Otic Solution Sterile 760
Cortisporin Otic Suspension Sterile 760
Cortizone-5 Creme & Ointment ▣ 732
Dermolate Anti-Itch Cream ▣ 697
Eldecort Cream 1.0% 1113
Eldecort Cream 1.0% and 2.5% 1113
Fungoid HC Creme 1770
Hydrocortone Tablets 1482
Hytone 909
LazerSporin-C Solution 1770
Massengill Medicated Soft Cloth Towelettes 2192
Nutracort Cream & Lotion 1684
PediOtic Suspension Sterile 797
Synacort Creams 1%, 2.5% 2296
Vanoxide-HC Acne Lotion 911
Vioform-Hydrocortisone Cream and Mild Cream 889
Vioform-Hydrocortisone Ointment 889
VōSoL HC Otic Solution 2392
Vytone Cream 1% 911

Hydrocortisone Acetate (Concurrent use with thiazide diuretics may intensify electrolyte imbalance, particularly hypokalemia). Products include:
Analpram-HC Rectal Cream 1% and 2.5% 970
Anusol-HC Cream 1690
Anusol-HC Suppositories 1691
Caldecort ▣ 560
Carmol HC Cream 1% 2296
Chloromycetin Hydrocortisone Ophthalmic 1694
Coly-Mycin S Otic w/Neomycin & Hydrocortisone 1708
Cortaid ▣ 735
Cortef Feminine Itch Cream ▣ 735
Corticaine ▣ 682
Cortifoam 1827
Cortisporin Cream 757
Epifoam 1828
Gynecort 5 Creme ▣ 556
Hydrocortone Acetate Sterile Suspension 1479
Lanacort 5 Creme and Ointment ▣ 557
Mantadil Cream 789
Ophthocort ⊙ 301
Orabase HCA Oral Paste 890
Pramosone Cream, Lotion & Ointment 971
ProctoCream-HC 1834
Proctofoam-HC 1835

Hydrocortisone Sodium Phosphate (Concurrent use with thiazide diuretics may intensify electrolyte imbalance, particularly hypokalemia). Products include:
Hydrocortone Phosphate Injection, Sterile 1481

Hydrocortisone Sodium Succinate (Concurrent use with thiazide diuretics may intensify electrolyte imbalance, particularly hypokalemia). Products include:
Solu-Cortef Sterile Powder 2361

Hydroxyzine Hydrochloride (Effects may be potentiated when used concurrently with thiazide diuretics). Products include:
Atarax Tablets & Syrup 1941
Marax Tablets & DF Syrup 1954
Vistaril Intramuscular Solution 1970

Indapamide (Effects may be potentiated when used concurrently with thiazide diuretics). Products include:
Lozol Tablets 1843

Insulin, Human (Insulin requirements may be increased, decreased, or unchanged).
No products indexed under this heading.

Insulin, Human Isophane Suspension (Insulin requirements may be increased, decreased, or unchanged). Products include:
Humulin N, 100 Units 1270

Insulin, Human NPH (Insulin requirements may be increased, decreased, or unchanged). Products include:
Insulatard NPH Human 1627
Novolin N 1627
Novolin N PenFill Cartridges 1628
Novolin N Prefilled 1628

Insulin, Human Regular (Insulin requirements may be increased, decreased, or unchanged). Products include:
Humulin BR, 100 Units 1268
Humulin R, 100 Units 1272
Novolin R 1627
Novolin R PenFill Cartridges 1628
Novolin R Prefilled 1629
Velosulin Human 1628

Insulin, Human, Zinc Suspension (Insulin requirements may be increased, decreased, or unchanged). Products include:
Humulin L, 100 Units 1268
Humulin U, 100 Units 1272
Novolin L 1627

Insulin, NPH (Insulin requirements may be increased, decreased, or unchanged). Products include:
NPH, 40 & 100 Units 1273
Beef NPH, 100 Units 1274
Pork NPH, 100 Units 1275
Insulatard NPH 1626
NPH Insulin 1626
NPH Purified Pork Isophane Insulin 1626

Insulin, Regular (Insulin requirements may be increased, decreased, or unchanged). Products include:
Regular, 40 & 100 Units 1273
Beef Regular, 100 Units 1275
Pork Regular, 100 Units 1275
Pork Regular (Concentrated), 500 Units 1276
Regular Insulin 1625
Regular Purified Pork Insulin 1626
Velosulin 1627

Insulin, Zinc Crystals (Insulin requirements may be increased, decreased, or unchanged). Products include:
NPH, 40 & 100 Units 1273

Insulin, Zinc Suspension (Insulin requirements may be increased, decreased, or unchanged). Products include:
Lente, 40 & 100 Units 1272
Protamine, Zinc, 40 & 100 Units 1273
Lente Iletin I 1272
Beef Lente, 100 Units 1274
Beef Protamine Zinc, 100 Units 1274
Pork Lente, 100 Units 1275
Pork, Protamine, Zinc, 100 Units 1275
Lente Insulin 1626
Lente Purified Pork Insulin 1626
Semilente Insulin 1625
Ultralente Insulin 1626

Isoflurane (Effects may be potentiated when used concurrently with thiazide diuretics). Products include:
Forane 600

Isradipine (Effects may be potentiated when used concurrently with thiazide diuretics). Products include:
DynaCirc Capsules 2004

Ketamine Hydrochloride (Effects may be potentiated when used concurrently with thiazide diuretics). Products include:
Ketalar 1726

Labetalol Hydrochloride (Effects may be potentiated when used concurrently with thiazide diuretics). Products include:
Normodyne Injection 2108
Normodyne Tablets 2110
Normozide Tablets 2112
Trandate HCT Tablets 579
Trandate Injection 577
Trandate Tablets 579

Levorphanol Tartrate (Orthostatic hypotension may be aggravated). Products include:
Levo-Dromoran 1906

Lisinopril (Effects may be potentiated when used concurrently with thiazide diuretics). Products include:
Prinivil Tablets 1538
Prinzide Tablets 1540
Zestoretic 2274
Zestril Tablets 2277

Lithium Carbonate (Potential for lithium toxicity because of reduced renal clearance). Products include:
Eskalith 2214
Lithane Tablets 1596

Lithium Carbonate Capsules & Tablets ... 1984
Lithobid Tablets ... 870

Lithium Citrate (Potential for lithium toxicity because of reduced renal clearance). Products include:
Cibalith-S ... 870

Lorazepam (Effects may be potentiated when used concurrently with thiazide diuretics). Products include:
Ativan Injection ... 2432
Ativan Tablets ... 2434

Mecamylamine Hydrochloride (Effects may be potentiated when used concurrently with thiazide diuretics). Products include:
Inversine Tablets ... 1492

Meperidine Hydrochloride (Effects may be potentiated when used concurrently with thiazide diuretics; orthostatic hypotension may be aggravated). Products include:
Demerol ... 2047
Mepergan Injection ... 2479

Mephobarbital (Orthostatic hypotension may be aggravated). Products include:
Mebaral Tablets ... 2061

Methadone Hydrochloride (Orthostatic hypotension may be aggravated). Products include:
Dolophine Hydrochloride Ampoules & Vials ... 1260
Dolophine Hydrochloride Tablets ... 1261
Methadone Hydrochloride Diskets ... 1284
Methadone Hydrochloride Oral Solution & Tablets ... 1987

Methenamine (Reduced effectiveness because of alkalinization of urine). Products include:
Urised Tablets ... 2396

Methenamine Hippurate (Reduced effectiveness because of alkalinization of urine). Products include:
Hiprex Tablets ... 1333
Urex Tablets ... 1321

Methenamine Mandelate (Reduced effectiveness because of alkalinization of urine). Products include:
Mandelamine ... 1738
Uroqid-Acid ... 661

Methohexital Sodium (Effects may be potentiated when used concurrently with thiazide diuretics). Products include:
Brevital Sodium Vials ... 1248

Methoxyflurane (Effects may be potentiated when used concurrently with thiazide diuretics).
No products indexed under this heading.

Methyclothiazide (Effects may be potentiated when used concurrently with thiazide diuretics). Products include:
Enduron Tablets ... 517
Enduronyl ... 518

Methyldopa (Effects may be potentiated when used concurrently with thiazide diuretics). Products include:
Aldoclor Tablets ... 1413
Aldomet Oral ... 1415
Aldoril Tablets ... 1418

Methyldopate Hydrochloride (Effects may be potentiated when used concurrently with thiazide diuretics). Products include:
Aldomet Ester HCl Injection ... 1417

Methylprednisolone Acetate (Concurrent use with thiazide diuretics may intensify electrolyte imbalance, particularly hypokalemia). Products include:
Depo-Medrol Sterile Aqueous Suspension ... 2334

Methylprednisolone Sodium Succinate (Concurrent use with thiazide diuretics may intensify electrolyte imbalance, particularly hypokalemia). Products include:
Solu-Medrol Sterile Powder ... 2363

Metocurine Iodide (Effects may be potentiated when used concurrently with thiazide diuretics). Products include:
Metubine Iodide Vials ... 1285

Metolazone (Effects may be potentiated when used concurrently with thiazide diuretics). Products include:
Diulo ... 2129
Mykrox ½ mg Tablets ... 984
Zaroxolyn Tablets ... 989

Metoprolol Tartrate (Effects may be potentiated when used concurrently with thiazide diuretics). Products include:
Lopressor Ampuls ... 1032
Lopressor HCT Tablets ... 1034
Lopressor Tablets ... 1032

Metyrosine (Effects may be potentiated when used concurrently with thiazide diuretics). Products include:
Demser Capsules ... 1460

Minoxidil (Effects may be potentiated when used concurrently with thiazide diuretics). Products include:
Loniten Tablets ... 2346
Rogaine Topical Solution ... 2357

Morphine Sulfate (Effects may be potentiated when used concurrently with thiazide diuretics; orthostatic hypotension may be aggravated). Products include:
Astramorph/PF Injection, USP (Preservative-Free) ... 618
Duramorph ... 960
Infumorph 200 and Infumorph 500 Sterile Solutions ... 962
MS Contin Tablets ... 1814
MSIR ... 1817
Oramorph SR (Morphine Sulfate Sustained Release Tablets) ... 1988
Roxanol ... 1991

Nadolol (Effects may be potentiated when used concurrently with thiazide diuretics). Products include:
Corgard Tablets ... 701
Corzide Tablets ... 702

Nicardipine Hydrochloride (Effects may be potentiated when used concurrently with thiazide diuretics). Products include:
Cardene Capsules ... 2290

Nitroglycerin (Effects may be potentiated when used concurrently with thiazide diuretics). Products include:
Deponit NTG Transdermal Delivery System ... 2143
Minitran Transdermal Delivery System ... 1312
Nitro-Bid Ointment ... 1339
Nitro-Bid Capsules ... 1338
Nitrodisc ... 2176
Nitro-Dur (nitroglycerin) Transdermal Infusion System ... 1164
Nitrogard Tablets ... 1004
Nitrolingual Spray ... 1846
Nitrostat Tablets ... 1743
Transderm-Nitro Transdermal Therapeutic System ... 2283

Opium Alkaloids (Orthostatic hypotension may be aggravated). Products include:
B & O No. 15A & No. 16A Supprettes ... 2395
Pantopon Injectable ... 1911

Oxycodone Hydrochloride (Orthostatic hypotension may be aggravated). Products include:
Percocet Tablets ... 950
Percodan ... 951
Roxicodone Tablets, Oral Solution & Intensol (Oxycodone) ... 1992
Tylox Capsules ... 1382

Pancuronium Bromide Injection (Effects may be potentiated when used concurrently with thiazide diuretics).
No products indexed under this heading.

Penbutolol Sulfate (Effects may be potentiated when used concurrently with thiazide diuretics). Products include:
Levatol ... 1832

Pentobarbital Sodium (Effects may be potentiated when used concurrently with thiazide diuretics; orthostatic hypotension may be aggravated). Products include:
Nembutal Sodium Capsules ... 534
Nembutal Sodium Solution ... 536
Nembutal Sodium Suppositories ... 538

Phenobarbital (Orthostatic hypotension may be aggravated). Products include:
Arco-Lase Plus Tablets ... 607
Bellergal-S Tablets ... 1998
Bronkolixir ... ▣ 761
Bronkotabs Tablets ... ▣ 762
Donnatal ... 1858
Donnatal Extentabs ... 1859
Donnatal Tablets ... 1858
Donnazyme Tablets ... 1860
Kinesed Tablets ... 2272
Phenobarbital Elixir and Tablets ... 1293
Primatene Tablets-P Formula ... 2421
Quadrinal Tablets ... 1183
Tedral SA ... 1765

Phenoxybenzamine Hydrochloride (Effects may be potentiated when used concurrently with thiazide diuretics). Products include:
Dibenzyline Capsules ... 2207

Phentolamine Mesylate (Effects may be potentiated when used concurrently with thiazide diuretics). Products include:
Regitine ... 878

Pindolol (Effects may be potentiated when used concurrently with thiazide diuretics). Products include:
Visken Tablets ... 2036

Polythiazide (Effects may be potentiated when used concurrently with thiazide diuretics). Products include:
Minizide Capsules ... 1779
Renese Tablets ... 1785
Renese-R Tablets ... 1786

Prazosin Hydrochloride (Effects may be potentiated when used concurrently with thiazide diuretics). Products include:
Minipress Capsules ... 1778
Minizide Capsules ... 1779

Prednisolone Acetate (Concurrent use with thiazide diuretics may intensify electrolyte imbalance, particularly hypokalemia). Products include:
AK-Cide Sterile Ophthalmic Ointment & Suspension ... ⊚ 202
Blephamide Liquifilm Sterile Ophthalmic Suspension ... 586
Blephamide S.O.P. Sterile Ophthalmic Ointment ... 586
Cetapred Ointment ... ⊚ 220
⅛ % Econopred & 1 % Econopred Plus ... ⊚ 217
Isopto Cetapred Suspension ... ⊚ 220
Metimyd ... ⊚ 306
Poly-Pred Liquifilm ... ⊚ 250
Pred Forte ... ⊚ 252
Pred Mild ... ⊚ 254
Pred-G Liquifilm Sterile Ophthalmic Suspension ... ⊚ 252
Pred-G S.O.P. Sterile Ophthalmic Ointment ... ⊚ 253
Vasocidin Ointment ... ⊚ 275

Prednisolone Sodium Phosphate (Concurrent use with thiazide diuretics may intensify electrolyte imbalance, particularly hypokalemia). Products include:
AK-Pred ... ⊚ 205
Hydeltrasol Injection, Sterile ... 1476
Inflamase ... ⊚ 274
Pediapred Oral Liquid ... 987
Vasocidin Ophthalmic Solution ... ⊚ 276

Prednisolone Tebutate (Concurrent use with thiazide diuretics may intensify electrolyte imbalance, particularly hypokalemia). Products include:
Hydeltra-T.B.A. Sterile Suspension 1478

Prednisone (Concurrent use with thiazide diuretics may intensify electrolyte imbalance, particularly hypokalemia). Products include:
Deltasone Tablets ... 2332

Probenecid (Thiazide diuretics may raise the level of blood uric acid). Products include:
Benemid Tablets ... 1426
ColBENEMID Tablets ... 1436
Wycillin Injection and Probenecid Tablets ... 2539

Promethazine Hydrochloride (Effects may be potentiated when used concurrently with thiazide diuretics). Products include:
Mepergan Injection ... 2479
Phenergan with Codeine ... 2497
Phenergan with Dextromethorphan 2499
Phenergan Injection ... 2493
Phenergan Suppositories ... 2496
Phenergan Syrup ... 2495
Phenergan Tablets ... 2496
Phenergan VC ... 2500
Phenergan VC with Codeine ... 2501

Propofol (Effects may be potentiated when used concurrently with thiazide diuretics). Products include:
Diprivan Injection ... 2267

Propoxyphene Hydrochloride (Orthostatic hypotension may be aggravated). Products include:
Darvon ... 1256
Wygesic Tablets ... 2540

Propoxyphene Napsylate (Orthostatic hypotension may be aggravated). Products include:
Darvon-N/Darvocet-N ... 1254

Propranolol Hydrochloride (Effects may be potentiated when used concurrently with thiazide diuretics). Products include:
Inderal ... 2459
Inderal LA Long Acting Capsules ... 2461
Inderide Tablets ... 2463
Inderide LA Long Acting Capsules ... 2465

Ramipril (Effects may be potentiated when used concurrently with thiazide diuretics). Products include:
Altace Capsules ... 1086

Rauwolfia Serpentina (Effects may be potentiated when used concurrently with thiazide diuretics). Products include:
Raudixin Tablets ... 1803
Rauzide Tablets ... 1804

Rescinnamine (Effects may be potentiated when used concurrently with thiazide diuretics).
No products indexed under this heading.

Reserpine (Effects may be potentiated when used concurrently with thiazide diuretics). Products include:
Diupres Tablets ... 1461
Hydromox R Tablets ... 1209
Hydropres Tablets ... 1485
Renese-R Tablets ... 1786
Salutensin/Salutensin-Demi ... 719
Ser-Ap-Es Tablets ... 881
Serpasil Tablets ... 883
Serpasil-Apresoline Tablets ... 884
Serpasil-Esidrix Tablets ... 886

Secobarbital Sodium (Orthostatic hypotension may be aggravated). Products include:
Seconal Sodium Pulvules ... 1296

Sodium Nitroprusside (Effects may be potentiated when used concurrently with thiazide diuretics). Products include:
- Nipride I.V. Infusion 1909

Sufentanil Citrate (Orthostatic hypotension may be aggravated). Products include:
- Sufenta Injection 1147

Sulfinpyrazone (Thiazide diuretics may raise the level of blood uric acid). Products include:
- Anturane 853

Terazosin Hydrochloride (Effects may be potentiated when used concurrently with thiazide diuretics). Products include:
- Hytrin Tablets 529

Thiamylal Sodium (Orthostatic hypotension may be aggravated). Products include:
- Surital Ampoules, Steri-Vials 1764

Timolol Maleate (Effects may be potentiated when used concurrently with thiazide diuretics). Products include:
- Blocadren Tablets 1429
- Timolide Tablets 1547
- Timoptic in Ocudose 1552
- Timoptic Sterile Ophthalmic Solution 1550

Tolazamide (Thiazides may raise blood glucose levels). Products include:
- Tolinase Tablets 2365

Tolbutamide (Thiazides may raise blood glucose levels). Products include:
- Orinase Tablets 2354

Triamcinolone (Concurrent use with thiazide diuretics may intensify electrolyte imbalance, particularly hypokalemia).
- No products indexed under this heading.

Triamcinolone Acetonide (Concurrent use with thiazide diuretics may intensify electrolyte imbalance, particularly hypokalemia). Products include:
- Aristocort A 1010
- Azmacort Inhaler 1837
- Kenalog Cream, Lotion & Ointment 2401
- Kenalog-10 Injection 2402
- Kenalog-40 Injection 2403
- Kenalog in Orabase 604
- Kenalog Spray 2401
- Mycolog II Cream and Ointment 2407
- Mytrex Cream & Ointment 2080
- Nasacort Nasal Inhaler 1844

Triamcinolone Diacetate (Concurrent use with thiazide diuretics may intensify electrolyte imbalance, particularly hypokalemia). Products include:
- Aristocort Suspension 1008

Triamcinolone Hexacetonide (Concurrent use with thiazide diuretics may intensify electrolyte imbalance, particularly hypokalemia). Products include:
- Aristospan Suspension 1011

Trimethaphan Camsylate (Effects may be potentiated when used concurrently with thiazide diuretics). Products include:
- Arfonad Ampuls 1887

Tubocurarine Chloride (Increased responsiveness to tubocurarine).
- No products indexed under this heading.

Vecuronium Bromide (Effects may be potentiated when used concurrently with thiazide diuretics). Products include:
- Norcuron 1642

Warfarin Sodium (Effects may be decreased when used concurrently with thiazide diuretics; dosage adjustment may be necessary). Products include:
- Coumadin Injection & Tablets 944
- Panwarfin Tablets 547

DIULO
(Metolazone) 2129
May interact with antihypertensives, barbiturates, narcotic analgesics, corticosteroids, loop diuretics, cardiac glycosides, oral hypoglycemic agents, insulin, non-steroidal anti-inflammatory agents, salicylates, lithium preparations, and certain other agents. Compounds in these categories include:

Acebutolol Hydrochloride (Dosage adjustments of other antihypertensives may be necessary). Products include:
- Sectral Capsules 2520

ACTH (May increase the risk of hypokalemia and increase salt and water retention).
- No products indexed under this heading.

Alcohol (Potentiation of hypotensive effects by metolazone-induced volume contraction).

Alfentanil Hydrochloride (Potentiation of hypotensive effects by metolazone-induced volume contraction). Products include:
- Alfenta Injection 1131

Aprobarbital (Potentiation of hypotensive effects by metolazone-induced volume contraction). Products include:
- Alurate Elixir 1883

Aspirin (Reduces antihypertensive effects). Products include:
- Alka-Seltzer Effervescent Antacid and Pain Reliever 1568
- Alka-Seltzer Extra Strength Effervescent Antacid and Pain Reliever 1570
- Alka-Seltzer (Flavored) Effervescent Antacid and Pain Reliever 1569
- Alka-Seltzer Plus Cold Medicine .... ◘ 623
- Alka-Seltzer Plus Night-Time Cold Medicine .... ◘ 623
- Alka Seltzer Plus Sinus Allergy Medicine .... ◘ 624
- Anacin Coated Analgesic Caplets 2417
- Anacin Coated Analgesic Tablets 2417
- Anacin Maximum Strength Analgesic Coated Tablets 2417
- Maximum Strength Arthritis Pain Formula By the Makers of Anacin Analgesic Tablets and Caplets 2418
- Arthritis Pain Formula by the Makers of Anacin Analgesic Tablets and Caplets .... ◘ 747
- Arthritis Strength BC Powder .... ◘ 516
- Ascriptin A/D Caplets 1850
- Regular Strength Ascriptin Tablets 1850
- Azdone Tablets 844
- BC Powder .... ◘ 517
- BC Cold Powder .... ◘ 517
- Children's Bayer Chewable Aspirin .... ◘ 564
- Genuine Bayer Aspirin Tablets & Caplets .... ◘ 564
- Maximum Bayer Aspirin Tablets & Caplets .... ◘ 566
- Bayer Plus Aspirin Tablets .... ◘ 567
- Therapy Bayer Aspirin Caplets .... ◘ 568
- 8 Hour Bayer Timed-Release Aspirin .... ◘ 566
- Arthritis Strength Bufferin Analgesic Caplets 744
- Extra Strength Bufferin Analgesic Tablets 745
- Bufferin Analgesic Tablets and Caplets 743
- Cama Arthritis Pain Reliever .... ◘ 685
- Damason-P 1356
- Easprin 1719
- Ecotrin Enteric Coated Aspirin Maximum Strength Tablets and Caplets 2189
- Ecotrin Enteric Coated Aspirin Regular Strength Tablets and Caplets 2189
- Empirin Aspirin .... ◘ 541
- Empirin with Codeine Phosphate Nos. 2, 3 & 4 764
- Equagesic Tablets 2451
- Excedrin Extra-Strength Analgesic Tablets & Caplets 749
- 4-Way Cold Tablets 750
- Fiorinal Capsules 2007
- Fiorinal with Codeine Capsules 2008
- Fiorinal Tablets 2007
- Lortab ASA Tablets 2414
- Momentum Muscular Backache Formula .... ◘ 751
- Norgesic 1314
- Norwich Extra-Strength Aspirin .... ◘ 546
- Norwich Regular Strength Aspirin .... ◘ 547
- P-A-C Analgesic Tablets .... ◘ 669
- Percodan 951
- Robaxisal Tablets 1872
- Sine-Off Sinus Medicine Tablets-Aspirin Formula .... ◘ 722
- Soma Compound w/Codeine Tablets 2390
- Soma Compound Tablets 2389
- St. Joseph Adult Chewable Aspirin (81 mg.) .... ◘ 703
- Synalgos-DC Capsules 2525
- Talwin Compound 2072
- Ursinus Inlay-Tabs .... ◘ 691
- Vanquish Analgesic Caplets .... ◘ 574
- Zorprin Tablets 698

Atenolol (Dosage adjustments of other antihypertensives may be necessary). Products include:
- Tenoretic Tablets 1105
- Tenormin Tablets and I.V. Injection 1107

Benazepril Hydrochloride (Dosage adjustments of other antihypertensives may be necessary). Products include:
- Lotensin Tablets 872

Bendroflumethiazide (Dosage adjustments of other antihypertensives may be necessary). Products include:
- Corzide Tablets 702
- Naturetin Tablets 1789
- Rauzide Tablets 1804

Betamethasone Acetate (May increase the risk of hypokalemia and increase salt and water retention). Products include:
- Celestone Soluspan Suspension 2081

Betamethasone Sodium Phosphate (May increase the risk of hypokalemia and increase salt and water retention). Products include:
- Celestone Soluspan Suspension 2081

Betaxolol Hydrochloride (Dosage adjustments of other antihypertensives may be necessary). Products include:
- Betoptic Sterile Ophthalmic Solution 569
- Betoptic S Sterile Ophthalmic Suspension 570
- Kerlone Tablets 2172

Bumetanide (Concomitant administration may result in prolonged or large losses of fluid and electrolytes). Products include:
- Bumex 1895

Buprenorphine (Potentiation of hypotensive effects by metolazone-induced volume contraction).
- No products indexed under this heading.

Butabarbital (Potentiation of hypotensive effects by metolazone-induced volume contraction). Products include:
- Pyridium Plus 1764

Butalbital (Potentiation of hypotensive effects by metolazone-induced volume contraction). Products include:
- Esgic-Plus Tablets 1002
- Esgic Tablets & Capsules 1001
- Fioricet Tablets 2006
- Fiorinal Capsules 2007
- Fiorinal with Codeine Capsules 2008
- Fiorinal Tablets 2007
- Phrenilin 838
- Sedapap Tablets 50 mg/650 mg 1360

Captopril (Dosage adjustments of other antihypertensives may be necessary). Products include:
- Capoten 2255
- Capozide 2258

Carteolol Hydrochloride (Dosage adjustments of other antihypertensives may be necessary). Products include:
- Cartrol Tablets 507

Chlorothiazide (Dosage adjustments of other antihypertensives may be necessary). Products include:
- Aldoclor Tablets 1413
- Diupres Tablets 1461
- Diuril Oral 1464

Chlorothiazide Sodium (Dosage adjustments of other antihypertensives may be necessary). Products include:
- Diuril Sodium Intravenous 1463

Chlorpropamide (Metolazone elevates blood glucose levels; dosage adjustment of antidiabetic agent may be required). Products include:
- Diabinese Tablets 1775

Chlorthalidone (Dosage adjustments of other antihypertensives may be necessary). Products include:
- Combipres Tablets 678
- Tenoretic Tablets 1105
- Thalitone Tablets 687

Choline Magnesium Trisalicylate (Reduces antihypertensive effects). Products include:
- Trilisate 1822

Clonidine (Dosage adjustments of other antihypertensives may be necessary). Products include:
- Catapres-TTS 677

Clonidine Hydrochloride (Dosage adjustments of other antihypertensives may be necessary). Products include:
- Catapres Tablets 676
- Combipres Tablets 678

Codeine (Potentiation of hypotensive effects by metolazone-induced volume contraction). Products include:
- Calcidrine Syrup 506

Codeine Phosphate (Potentiation of hypotensive effects by metolazone-induced volume contraction). Products include:
- Actifed with Codeine Cough Syrup 752
- Cheracol Cough Syrup 1853
- Codimal PH Syrup 846
- Dimetane-DC Cough Syrup 1857
- Empirin with Codeine Phosphate Nos. 2, 3 & 4 764
- Fiorinal with Codeine Capsules 2008
- Isoclor Expectorant 982
- Naldecon CX Adult Liquid .... ◘ 521
- Novahistine DH 1342
- Novahistine Expectorant 1343
- Nucofed Capsules 2219
- Nucofed Expectorant 2219
- Nucofed Pediatric Expectorant 2220
- Nucofed Syrup 2219
- Phenaphen with Codeine Capsules 1865
- Phenaphen-650 with Codeine Tablets 1866
- Phenergan with Codeine 2497
- Phenergan VC with Codeine 2501
- Robitussin A-C Syrup 1875
- Robitussin-DAC Syrup 1875
- Ryna .... ◘ 741
- Soma Compound w/Codeine Tablets 2390
- Triaminic Expectorant w/Codeine 1996
- Tussi-Organidin Liquid 2391
- Tylenol with Codeine 1381

Codeine Polistirex (Potentiation of hypotensive effects by metolazone-induced volume contraction).
No products indexed under this heading.

Cortisone Acetate (May increase the risk of hypokalemia and increase salt and water retention). Products include:
Cortone Acetate Sterile Suspension ... 1437
Cortone Acetate Tablets ... 1439

Deserpidine (Dosage adjustments of other antihypertensives may be necessary). Products include:
Enduronyl ... 518
Harmonyl Tablets ... 528
Oreticyl ... 545

Deslanoside (Enhanced possibility of digitalis toxicity associated with hypokalemia).
No products indexed under this heading.

Dexamethasone (May increase the risk of hypokalemia and increase salt and water retention). Products include:
AK-Trol Ointment & Suspension ... ⊙ 207
Decadron Elixir ... 1445
Decadron Tablets ... 1447
Decaspray Topical Aerosol ... 1459
Dexacidin ... ⊙ 272
Maxidex Sterile Ophthalmic Suspension ... ⊙ 223
Maxitrol Ophthalmic Ointment/Suspension ... ⊙ 223
TobraDex Ophthalmic Suspension and Ointment ... ⊙ 228

Dexamethasone Acetate (May increase the risk of hypokalemia and increase salt and water retention). Products include:
Dalalone D.P. Injectable ... 999
Decadron-LA Sterile Suspension ... 1457

Dexamethasone Sodium Phosphate (May increase the risk of hypokalemia and increase salt and water retention). Products include:
AK-Dex ... ⊙ 203
Decadron Phosphate Respihaler ... 1454
Decadron Phosphate Sterile Ophthalmic Ointment ... 1453
Decadron Phosphate Sterile Ophthalmic Solution ... 1453
Decadron Phosphate Topical Cream ... 1455
Decadron Phosphate Turbinaire ... 1456
Maxidex Sterile Ophthalmic Ointment ... ⊙ 222
NeoDecadron Sterile Ophthalmic Ointment ... 1517
NeoDecadron Sterile Ophthalmic Solution ... 1518
NeoDecadron Topical Cream ... 1518

Dezocine (Potentiation of hypotensive effects by metolazone-induced volume contraction).

Diazoxide (Dosage adjustments of other antihypertensives may be necessary). Products include:
Hyperstat I.V. Injection ... 2095
Proglycem ... 649

Diclofenac Sodium (Reduces antihypertensive effects). Products include:
Voltaren Ophthalmic Sterile Ophthalmic Solution ... ⊙ 268
Voltaren Tablets ... 1042

Diflunisal (Reduces antihypertensive effects). Products include:
Dolobid Tablets ... 1465

Digitoxin (Enhanced possibility of digitalis toxicity associated with hypokalemia). Products include:
Crystodigin Tablets ... 1253

Digoxin (Enhanced possibility of digitalis toxicity associated with hypokalemia). Products include:
Lanoxicaps ... 772
Lanoxin Elixir Pediatric ... 775
Lanoxin Injection ... 778
Lanoxin Injection Pediatric ... 781
Lanoxin Tablets ... 783

Doxazosin Mesylate (Dosage adjustments of other antihypertensives may be necessary). Products include:
Cardura Tablets ... 1941

Enalapril Maleate (Dosage adjustments of other antihypertensives may be necessary). Products include:
Vaseretic Tablets ... 1559
Vasotec Tablets ... 1564

Enalaprilat (Dosage adjustments of other antihypertensives may be necessary). Products include:
Vasotec I.V. ... 1562

Esmolol Hydrochloride (Dosage adjustments of other antihypertensives may be necessary). Products include:
Brevibloc Injection ... 942

Ethacrynic Acid (Concomitant administration may result in prolonged or large losses of fluid and electrolytes). Products include:
Edecrin Tablets ... 1468

Etodolac (Reduces antihypertensive effects). Products include:
Lodine Capsules ... 2468

Felodipine (Dosage adjustments of other antihypertensives may be necessary). Products include:
Plendil Extended-Release Tablets ... 1526

Fenoprofen Calcium (Reduces antihypertensive effects). Products include:
Nalfon Pulvules & Tablets ... 919

Fentanyl (Potentiation of hypotensive effects by metolazone-induced volume contraction). Products include:
Duragesic Transdermal System ... 1133

Fentanyl Citrate (Potentiation of hypotensive effects by metolazone-induced volume contraction). Products include:
Innovar Injection ... 1141
Sublimaze Injection ... 1146

Flurbiprofen (Reduces antihypertensive effects). Products include:
Ansaid Tablets ... 2319

Fosinopril Sodium (Dosage adjustments of other antihypertensives may be necessary). Products include:
Monopril Tablets ... 1406

Furosemide (Concomitant administration may result in prolonged or large losses of fluid and electrolytes). Products include:
Lasix ... 1093

Glipizide (Metolazone elevates blood glucose levels; dosage adjustment of antidiabetic agent may be required). Products include:
Glucotrol ... 1952

Glyburide (Metolazone elevates blood glucose levels; dosage adjustment of antidiabetic agent may be required). Products include:
DiaBeta ... 1091
Micronase Tablets ... 2350

Guanabenz Acetate (Dosage adjustments of other antihypertensives may be necessary). Products include:
Wytensin Tablets ... 2542

Guanethidine Monosulfate (Dosage adjustments of other antihypertensives may be necessary). Products include:
Esimil Tablets ... 864
Ismelin Tablets ... 869

Hydralazine Hydrochloride (Dosage adjustments of other antihypertensives may be necessary). Products include:
Apresazide Capsules ... 854
Apresoline Hydrochloride Parenteral (Ampuls) ... 856
Apresoline Hydrochloride Tablets ... 855
Apresoline-Esidrix Tablets ... 857
Ser-Ap-Es Tablets ... 881
Serpasil-Apresoline Tablets ... 884

Hydrochlorothiazide (Dosage adjustments of other antihypertensives may be necessary). Products include:
Aldactazide ... 2150
Aldoril Tablets ... 1418
Apresazide Capsules ... 854
Apresoline-Esidrix Tablets ... 857
Capozide ... 2258
Dyazide Capsules ... 2208
Esidrix Tablets ... 863
Esimil Tablets ... 864
HydroDIURIL Tablets ... 1484
Hydropres Tablets ... 1485
Inderide Tablets ... 2463
Inderide LA Long Acting Capsules ... 2465
Lopressor HCT Tablets ... 1034
Maxzide ... 1215
Moduretic Tablets ... 1510
Normozide Tablets ... 2112
Oretic Tablets ... 544
Oreticyl ... 545
Prinzide Tablets ... 1540
Ser-Ap-Es Tablets ... 881
Serpasil-Esidrix Tablets ... 886
Timolide Tablets ... 1547
Trandate HCT Tablets ... 579
Vaseretic Tablets ... 1559
Zestoretic ... 2274

Hydrocodone Bitartrate (Potentiation of hypotensive effects by metolazone-induced volume contraction). Products include:
Anexsia 5/500 Tablets ... 2196
Anexsia 7.5/650 Tablets ... 2197
Azdōne Tablets ... 844
Codiclear DH Syrup ... 845
Codimal DH Syrup ... 846
Damason-P ... 1356
Hycodan Syrup, Tablets ... 927
Hycomine Compound Tablets ... 929
Hycomine Syrup ... 927
Hycotuss Expectorant Syrup ... 930
Hydrocet Capsules ... 835
Lortab ASA Tablets ... 2414
Lortab ... 2412
Ru-Tuss with Hydrocodone ... 694
Triaminic Expectorant DH ... 1995
Vicodin Tablets ... 1187
Vicodin ES Tablets ... 1189
Zydone Capsules ... 941

Hydrocodone Polistirex (Potentiation of hypotensive effects by metolazone-induced volume contraction). Products include:
Tussionex Extended-Release Suspension ... 988

Hydrocortisone (May increase the risk of hypokalemia and increase salt and water retention). Products include:
AK-Spore H.C. ... ⊙ 206
Bactine Hydrocortisone Anti-Itch Cream ... ■ 625
CaldeCORT Anti-Itch Hydrocortisone Spray ... ■ 560
Carmol HC Cream 1% ... 2296
Cortaid Spray ... ■ 735
Cortenema ... 2244
Cortisporin Ointment ... 758
Cortisporin Ophthalmic Ointment Sterile ... 758
Cortisporin Ophthalmic Suspension Sterile ... 759
Cortisporin Otic Solution Sterile ... 760
Cortisporin Otic Suspension Sterile 760
Cortizone-5 Creme & Ointment ... ■ 732
Dermolate Anti-Itch Cream ... ■ 697
Eldecort Cream 1.0% ... 1113
Eldecort Cream 1.0% and 2.5% ... 1113
Fungoid HC Creme ... 1770
Hydrocortone Tablets ... 1482
Hytone ... 909
LazerSporin-C Solution ... 1770
Massengill Medicated Soft Cloth Towelettes ... 2192
Nutracort Cream & Lotion ... 1684
PediOtic Suspension Sterile ... 797
Synacort Creams 1%, 2.5% ... 2296
Vanoxide-HC Acne Lotion ... 911
Vioform-Hydrocortisone Cream and Mild Cream ... 889
Vioform-Hydrocortisone Ointment ... 889
VōSoL HC Otic Solution ... 2392
Vytone Cream 1% ... 911

Hydrocortisone Acetate (May increase the risk of hypokalemia and increase salt and water retention). Products include:
Analpram-HC Rectal Cream 1% and 2.5% ... 970
Anusol-HC Cream ... 1690
Anusol-HC Suppositories ... 1691
Caldecort ... ■ 560
Carmol HC Cream 1% ... 2296
Chloromycetin Hydrocortisone Ophthalmic ... 1694
Coly-Mycin S Otic w/Neomycin & Hydrocortisone ... 1708
Cortaid ... ■ 735
Cortef Feminine Itch Cream ... ■ 735
Corticaine ... ■ 682
Cortifoam ... 1827
Cortisporin Cream ... 757
Epifoam ... 1828
Gynecort 5 Creme ... ■ 556
Hydrocortone Acetate Sterile Suspension ... 1479
Lanacort 5 Creme and Ointment ... ■ 557
Mantadil Cream ... 789
Ophthocort ... ⊙ 301
Orabase HCA Oral Paste ... 890
Pramosone Cream, Lotion & Ointment ... 971
ProctoCream-HC ... 1834
Proctofoam-HC ... 1835

Hydrocortisone Sodium Phosphate (May increase the risk of hypokalemia and increase salt and water retention). Products include:
Hydrocortone Phosphate Injection, Sterile ... 1481

Hydrocortisone Sodium Succinate (May increase the risk of hypokalemia and increase salt and water retention). Products include:
Solu-Cortef Sterile Powder ... 2361

Hydroflumethiazide (Dosage adjustments of other antihypertensives may be necessary). Products include:
Diucardin Tablets ... 2450
Saluron ... 718
Salutensin/Salutensin-Demi ... 719

Ibuprofen (Reduces antihypertensive effects). Products include:
Advil Cold & Sinus Caplets (formerly CoAdvil) ... 2416
Advil Ibuprofen Tablets and Caplets ... 2416
Children's Advil Suspension ... 2426
CoAdvil ... ■ 748
Dristan Sinus Caplets ... 2419
Haltran Tablets ... ■ 668
Ibuprofen ... ■ 631
Medipren ibuprofen Caplets and Tablets ... 1362
Midol 200 Cramp Relief Formula ... ■ 570
Motrin Tablets ... 2351
Motrin IB Caplets and Tablets ... ■ 736
Nuprin Ibuprofen/Analgesic Tablets & Caplets ... 752
PediaProfen Suspension ... 1363
Rufen Tablets ... 691
Trendar Ibuprofen Tablets ... ■ 756

Indapamide (Dosage adjustments of other antihypertensives may be necessary). Products include:
Lozol Tablets ... 1843

Indomethacin (Reduces antihypertensive effects). Products include:
Indocin ... 1487

Indomethacin Sodium Trihydrate (Reduces antihypertensive effects). Products include:
Indocin I.V. ... 1490

Insulin, Human (Metolazone elevates blood glucose levels; dosage adjustment of antidiabetic agent may be required).
No products indexed under this heading.

Insulin, Human Isophane Suspension (Metolazone elevates blood glucose levels; dosage adjustment of antidiabetic agent may be required). Products include:
Humulin N, 100 Units 1270

Insulin, Human NPH (Metolazone elevates blood glucose levels; dosage adjustment of antidiabetic agent may be required). Products include:
Insulatard NPH Human 1627
Novolin N 1627
Novolin N PenFill Cartridges 1628
Novolin N Prefilled 1628

Insulin, Human Regular (Metolazone elevates blood glucose levels; dosage adjustment of antidiabetic agent may be required). Products include:
Humulin BR, 100 Units 1268
Humulin R, 100 Units 1272
Novolin R 1627
Novolin R PenFill Cartridges 1628
Novolin R Prefilled 1629
Velosulin Human 1628

Insulin, Human, Zinc Suspension (Metolazone elevates blood glucose levels; dosage adjustment of antidiabetic agent may be required). Products include:
Humulin L, 100 Units 1268
Humulin U, 100 Units 1272
Novolin L 1627

Insulin, NPH (Metolazone elevates blood glucose levels; dosage adjustment of antidiabetic agent may be required). Products include:
NPH, 40 & 100 Units 1273
Beef NPH, 100 Units 1274
Pork NPH, 100 Units 1275
Insulatard NPH 1626
NPH Insulin 1626
NPH Purified Pork Isophane Insulin 1626

Insulin, Regular (Metolazone elevates blood glucose levels; dosage adjustment of antidiabetic agent may be required). Products include:
Regular, 40 & 100 Units 1273
Beef Regular, 100 Units 1275
Pork Regular, 100 Units 1275
Pork Regular (Concentrated), 500 Units 1276
Regular Insulin 1625
Regular Purified Pork Insulin 1626
Velosulin 1627

Insulin, Zinc Crystals (Metolazone elevates blood glucose levels; dosage adjustment of antidiabetic agent may be required). Products include:
NPH, 40 & 100 Units 1273

Insulin, Zinc Suspension (Metolazone elevates blood glucose levels; dosage adjustment of antidiabetic agent may be required). Products include:
Lente, 40 & 100 Units 1272
Protamine, Zinc, 40 & 100 Units 1273
Lente Iletin I 1272
Beef Lente, 100 Units 1274
Beef Protamine Zinc, 100 Units 1274
Pork Lente, 100 Units 1275
Pork, Protamine, Zinc, 100 Units 1275
Lente Insulin 1626
Lente Purified Pork Insulin 1626
Semilente Insulin 1625
Ultralente Insulin 1626

Isradipine (Dosage adjustments of other antihypertensives may be necessary). Products include:
DynaCirc Capsules 2004

Ketoprofen (Reduces antihypertensive effects). Products include:
Orudis Capsules 2488

Ketorolac Tromethamine (Reduces antihypertensive effects). Products include:
Toradol IM Injection 2302

Labetalol Hydrochloride (Dosage adjustments of other antihypertensives may be necessary). Products include:
Normodyne Injection 2108
Normodyne Tablets 2110
Normozide Tablets 2112
Trandate HCT Tablets 579
Trandate Injection 577
Trandate Tablets 579

Levorphanol Tartrate (Potentiation of hypotensive effects by metolazone-induced volume contraction). Products include:
Levo-Dromoran 1906

Lisinopril (Dosage adjustments of other antihypertensives may be necessary). Products include:
Prinivil Tablets 1538
Prinzide Tablets 1540
Zestoretic 2274
Zestril Tablets 2277

Lithium Carbonate (Enhanced lithium toxicity due to reduced renal clearance; avoid concurrent use). Products include:
Eskalith 2214
Lithane Tablets 1596
Lithium Carbonate Capsules & Tablets 1984
Lithobid Tablets 870

Lithium Citrate (Enhanced lithium toxicity due to reduced renal clearance; avoid concurrent use). Products include:
Cibalith-S 870

Magnesium Salicylate (Reduces antihypertensive effects). Products include:
Doan's - Extra-Strength Analgesic ▣ 549
Doan's - Regular Strength Analgesic .... ▣ 549
Mobigesic Analgesic Tablets .... ▣ 507

Mecamylamine Hydrochloride (Dosage adjustments of other antihypertensives may be necessary). Products include:
Inversine Tablets 1492

Meclofenamate Sodium (Reduces antihypertensive effects). Products include:
Meclomen Capsules 1739

Mefenamic Acid (Reduces antihypertensive effects). Products include:
Ponstel 1758

Meperidine Hydrochloride (Potentiation of hypotensive effects by metolazone-induced volume contraction). Products include:
Demerol 2047
Mepergan Injection 2479

Mephobarbital (Potentiation of hypotensive effects by metolazone-induced volume contraction). Products include:
Mebaral Tablets 2061

Methadone Hydrochloride (Potentiation of hypotensive effects by metolazone-induced volume contraction). Products include:
Dolophine Hydrochloride Ampoules & Vials 1260
Dolophine Hydrochloride Tablets 1261
Methadone Hydrochloride Diskets 1284
Methadone Hydrochloride Oral Solution & Tablets 1987

Methenamine (Possible decreased effectiveness due to alkalinization of urine). Products include:
Urised Tablets 2396

Methenamine Hippurate (Possible decreased effectiveness due to alkalinization of urine). Products include:
Hiprex Tablets 1333
Urex Tablets 1321

Methenamine Mandelate (Possible decreased effectiveness due to alkalinization of urine). Products include:
Mandelamine 1738
Uroqid-Acid 661

Methyclothiazide (Dosage adjustments of other antihypertensives may be necessary). Products include:
Enduron Tablets 517
Enduronyl 518

Methyldopa (Dosage adjustments of other antihypertensives may be necessary). Products include:
Aldoclor Tablets 1413
Aldomet Oral 1415
Aldoril Tablets 1418

Methyldopate Hydrochloride (Dosage adjustments of other antihypertensives may be necessary). Products include:
Aldomet Ester HCl Injection 1417

Methylprednisolone Acetate (May increase the risk of hypokalemia and increase salt and water retention). Products include:
Depo-Medrol Sterile Aqueous Suspension 2334

Methylprednisolone Sodium Succinate (May increase the risk of hypokalemia and increase salt and water retention). Products include:
Solu-Medrol Sterile Powder 2363

Metoprolol Tartrate (Dosage adjustments of other antihypertensives may be necessary). Products include:
Lopressor Ampuls 1032
Lopressor HCT Tablets 1034
Lopressor Tablets 1032

Metyrosine (Dosage adjustments of other antihypertensives may be necessary). Products include:
Demser Capsules 1460

Minoxidil (Dosage adjustments of other antihypertensives may be necessary). Products include:
Loniten Tablets 2346
Rogaine Topical Solution 2357

Morphine Sulfate (Potentiation of hypotensive effects by metolazone-induced volume contraction). Products include:
Astramorph/PF Injection, USP (Preservative-Free) 618
Duramorph 960
Infumorph 200 and Infumorph 500 Sterile Solutions 962
MS Contin Tablets 1814
MSIR 1817
Oramorph SR (Morphine Sulfate Sustained Release Tablets) 1988
Roxanol 1991

Nadolol (Dosage adjustments of other antihypertensives may be necessary). Products include:
Corgard Tablets 701
Corzide Tablets 702

Naproxen (Reduces antihypertensive effects). Products include:
Naprosyn 2297

Naproxen Sodium (Reduces antihypertensive effects). Products include:
Anaprox and Anaprox DS Tablets 2288

Nicardipine Hydrochloride (Dosage adjustments of other antihypertensives may be necessary). Products include:
Cardene Capsules 2290

Nitroglycerin (Dosage adjustments of other antihypertensives may be necessary). Products include:
Deponit NTG Transdermal Delivery System 2143
Minitran Transdermal Delivery System 1312
Nitro-Bid Ointment 1339
Nitro-Bid Capsules 1338
Nitrodisc 2176
Nitro-Dur (nitroglycerin) Transdermal Infusion System 1164
Nitrogard Tablets 1004
Nitrolingual Spray 1846
Nitrostat Tablets 1743
Transderm-Nitro Transdermal Therapeutic System 2283

Norepinephrine Bitartrate (Decreased arterial responsiveness). Products include:
Levophed Bitartrate Injection 2054

Opium Alkaloids (Potentiation of hypotensive effects by metolazone-induced volume contraction). Products include:
B & O No. 15A & No. 16A Supprettes 2395
Pantopon Injectable 1911

Oxycodone Hydrochloride (Potentiation of hypotensive effects by metolazone-induced volume contraction). Products include:
Percocet Tablets 950
Percodan 951
Roxicodone Tablets, Oral Solution & Intensol (Oxycodone) 1992
Tylox Capsules 1382

Penbutolol Sulfate (Dosage adjustments of other antihypertensives may be necessary). Products include:
Levatol 1832

Pentobarbital Sodium (Potentiation of hypotensive effects by metolazone-induced volume contraction). Products include:
Nembutal Sodium Capsules 534
Nembutal Sodium Solution 536
Nembutal Sodium Suppositories 538

Phenobarbital (Potentiation of hypotensive effects by metolazone-induced volume contraction). Products include:
Arco-Lase Plus Tablets 607
Bellergal-S Tablets 1998
Bronkolixir .... ▣ 761
Bronkotabs Tablets .... ▣ 762
Donnatal 1858
Donnatal Extentabs 1859
Donnatal Tablets 1858
Donnazyme Tablets 1860
Kinesed Tablets 2272
Phenobarbital Elixir and Tablets 1293
Primatene Tablets-P Formula 2421
Quadrinal Tablets 1183
Tedral SA 1765

Phenoxybenzamine Hydrochloride (Dosage adjustments of other antihypertensives may be necessary). Products include:
Dibenzyline Capsules 2207

Phentolamine Mesylate (Dosage adjustments of other antihypertensives may be necessary). Products include:
Regitine 878

Phenylbutazone (Reduces antihypertensive effects). Products include:
Butazolidin Capsules & Tablets 1027

Pindolol (Dosage adjustments of other antihypertensives may be necessary). Products include:
Visken Tablets 2036

Piroxicam (Reduces antihypertensive effects). Products include:
Feldene Capsules 1777

Polythiazide (Dosage adjustments of other antihypertensives may be necessary). Products include:
Minizide Capsules 1779
Renese Tablets 1785
Renese-R Tablets 1786

Prazosin Hydrochloride (Dosage adjustments of other antihypertensives may be necessary). Products include:
Minipress Capsules 1778

Minizide Capsules 1779

Prednisolone Acetate (May increase the risk of hypokalemia and increase salt and water retention). Products include:

AK-Cide Sterile Ophthalmic Ointment & Suspension .... ◎ 202
Blephamide Liquifilm Sterile Ophthalmic Suspension 586
Blephamide S.O.P. Sterile Ophthalmic Ointment 586
Cetapred Ointment .... ◎ 220
⅛% Econopred & 1% Econopred Plus .... ◎ 217
Isopto Cetapred Suspension .... ◎ 220
Metimyd .... ◎ 306
Poly-Pred Liquifilm .... ◎ 250
Pred Forte .... ◎ 252
Pred Mild .... ◎ 254
Pred-G Liquifilm Sterile Ophthalmic Suspension .... ◎ 252
Pred-G S.O.P. Sterile Ophthalmic Ointment .... ◎ 253
Vasocidin Ointment .... ◎ 275

Prednisolone Sodium Phosphate (May increase the risk of hypokalemia and increase salt and water retention). Products include:

AK-Pred .... ◎ 205
Hydeltrasol Injection, Sterile 1476
Inflamase .... ◎ 274
Pediapred Oral Liquid 987
Vasocidin Ophthalmic Solution .... ◎ 276

Prednisolone Tebutate (May increase the risk of hypokalemia and increase salt and water retention). Products include:

Hydeltra-T.B.A. Sterile Suspension 1478

Prednisone (May increase the risk of hypokalemia and increase salt and water retention). Products include:

Deltasone Tablets 2332

Propoxyphene Hydrochloride (Potentiation of hypotensive effects by metolazone-induced volume contraction). Products include:

Darvon 1256
Wygesic Tablets 2540

Propoxyphene Napsylate (Potentiation of hypotensive effects by metolazone-induced volume contraction). Products include:

Darvon-N/Darvocet-N 1254

Propranolol Hydrochloride (Dosage adjustments of other antihypertensives may be necessary). Products include:

Inderal 2459
Inderal LA Long Acting Capsules 2461
Inderide Tablets 2463
Inderide LA Long Acting Capsules .. 2465

Ramipril (Dosage adjustments of other antihypertensives may be necessary). Products include:

Altace Capsules 1086

Rauwolfia Serpentina (Dosage adjustments of other antihypertensives may be necessary). Products include:

Raudixin Tablets 1803
Rauzide Tablets 1804

Rescinnamine (Dosage adjustments of other antihypertensives may be necessary).

No products indexed under this heading.

Reserpine (Dosage adjustments of other antihypertensives may be necessary). Products include:

Diupres Tablets 1461
Hydromox R Tablets 1209
Hydropres Tablets 1485
Renese-R Tablets 1786
Salutensin/Salutensin-Demi 719
Ser-Ap-Es Tablets 881
Serpasil Tablets 883
Serpasil-Apresoline Tablets 884
Serpasil-Esidrix Tablets 886

Salsalate (Reduces antihypertensive effects). Products include:

Disalcid 1310

Mono-Gesic Tablets 846
Salflex 839

Secobarbital Sodium (Potentiation of hypotensive effects by metolazone-induced volume contraction). Products include:

Seconal Sodium Pulvules 1296

Sodium Nitroprusside (Dosage adjustments of other antihypertensives may be necessary). Products include:

Nipride I.V. Infusion 1909

Sufentanil Citrate (Potentiation of hypotensive effects by metolazone-induced volume contraction). Products include:

Sufenta Injection 1147

Sulindac (Reduces antihypertensive effects). Products include:

Clinoril Tablets 1433

Terazosin Hydrochloride (Dosage adjustments of other antihypertensives may be necessary). Products include:

Hytrin Tablets 529

Thiamylal Sodium (Potentiation of hypotensive effects by metolazone-induced volume contraction). Products include:

Surital Ampoules, Steri-Vials 1764

Timolol Maleate (Dosage adjustments of other antihypertensives may be necessary). Products include:

Blocadren Tablets 1429
Timolide Tablets 1547
Timoptic in Ocudose 1552
Timoptic Sterile Ophthalmic Solution 1550

Tolazamide (Metolazone elevates blood glucose levels; dosage adjustment of antidiabetic agent may be required). Products include:

Tolinase Tablets 2365

Tolbutamide (Metolazone elevates blood glucose levels; dosage adjustment of antidiabetic agent may be required). Products include:

Orinase Tablets 2354

Tolmetin Sodium (Reduces antihypertensive effects). Products include:

Tolectin (200, 400 and 600 mg) .. 1379

Triamcinolone (May increase the risk of hypokalemia and increase salt and water retention).

No products indexed under this heading.

Triamcinolone Acetonide (May increase the risk of hypokalemia and increase salt and water retention). Products include:

Aristocort A 1010
Azmacort Inhaler 1837
Kenalog Cream, Lotion & Ointment 2401
Kenalog-10 Injection 2402
Kenalog-40 Injection 2403
Kenalog in Orabase 604
Kenalog Spray 2401
Mycolog II Cream and Ointment 2407
Mytrex Cream & Ointment 2080
Nasacort Nasal Inhaler 1844

Triamcinolone Diacetate (May increase the risk of hypokalemia and increase salt and water retention). Products include:

Aristocort Suspension 1008

Triamcinolone Hexacetonide (May increase the risk of hypokalemia and increase salt and water retention). Products include:

Aristospan Suspension 1011

Trimethaphan Camsylate (Dosage adjustments of other antihypertensives may be necessary). Products include:

Arfonad Ampuls 1887

Tubocurarine Chloride (Diuretic-induced hypokalemia may enhance neuromuscular blockade).

No products indexed under this heading.

DIUPRES TABLETS
(Reserpine, Chlorothiazide) 1461
May interact with antihypertensives, lithium preparations, cardiac glycosides, corticosteroids, insulin, non-steroidal anti-inflammatory agents, barbiturates, narcotic analgesics, oral hypoglycemic agents, general anesthetics, and certain other agents. Compounds in these categories include:

Acebutolol Hydrochloride (Potentiated; additive effects). Products include:

Sectral Capsules 2520

ACTH (Hypokalemia).

No products indexed under this heading.

Alcohol (Orthostatic hypotension may be aggravated).

Alfentanil Hydrochloride (Orthostatic hypotension may be aggravated). Products include:

Alfenta Injection 1131

Aprobarbital (Orthostatic hypotension may be aggravated). Products include:

Alurate Elixir 1883

Atenolol (Potentiated; additive effects). Products include:

Tenoretic Tablets 1105
Tenormin Tablets and I.V. Injection 1107

Benazepril Hydrochloride (Potentiated; additive effects). Products include:

Lotensin Tablets 872

Bendroflumethiazide (Potentiated; additive effects). Products include:

Corzide Tablets 702
Naturetin Tablets 1789
Rauzide Tablets 1804

Betamethasone Acetate (Hypokalemia). Products include:

Celestone Soluspan Suspension 2081

Betamethasone Sodium Phosphate (Hypokalemia). Products include:

Celestone Soluspan Suspension 2081

Betaxolol Hydrochloride (Potentiated; additive effects). Products include:

Betoptic Sterile Ophthalmic Solution 569
Betoptic S Sterile Ophthalmic Suspension 570
Kerlone Tablets 2172

Buprenorphine (Orthostatic hypotension may be aggravated).

No products indexed under this heading.

Butabarbital (Orthostatic hypotension may be aggravated). Products include:

Pyridium Plus 1764

Butalbital (Orthostatic hypotension may be aggravated). Products include:

Esgic-Plus Tablets 1002
Esgic Tablets & Capsules 1001
Fioricet Tablets 2006
Fiorinal Capsules 2007
Fiorinal with Codeine Capsules 2008
Fiorinal Tablets 2007
Phrenilin 838
Sedapap Tablets 50 mg/650 mg .. 1360

Captopril (Potentiated; additive effects). Products include:

Capoten 2255
Capozide 2258

Carteolol Hydrochloride (Potentiated; additive effects). Products include:

Cartrol Tablets 507

Chlorothiazide Sodium (Potentiated; additive effects). Products include:

Diuril Sodium Intravenous 1463

Chlorpropamide (Dosage adjustment of the antidiabetic drug may be required). Products include:

Diabinese Tablets 1775

Chlorthalidone (Potentiated; additive effects). Products include:

Combipres Tablets 678
Tenoretic Tablets 1105
Thalitone Tablets 687

Clonidine (Potentiated; additive effects). Products include:

Catapres-TTS 677

Clonidine Hydrochloride (Potentiated; additive effects). Products include:

Catapres Tablets 676
Combipres Tablets 678

Codeine (Orthostatic hypotension may be aggravated). Products include:

Calcidrine Syrup 506

Codeine Phosphate (Orthostatic hypotension may be aggravated). Products include:

Actifed with Codeine Cough Syrup.. 752
Cheracol Cough Syrup 1853
Codimal PH Syrup 846
Dimetane-DC Cough Syrup 1857
Empirin with Codeine Phosphate Nos. 2, 3 & 4 764
Fiorinal with Codeine Capsules 2008
Isoclor Expectorant 982
Naldecon CX Adult Liquid .... ▣ 521
Novahistine DH 1342
Novahistine Expectorant 1343
Nucofed Capsules 2219
Nucofed Expectorant 2219
Nucofed Pediatric Expectorant 2220
Nucofed Syrup 2219
Phenaphen with Codeine Capsules 1865
Phenaphen-650 with Codeine Tablets 1866
Phenergan with Codeine 2497
Phenergan VC with Codeine 2501
Robitussin A-C Syrup 1875
Robitussin-DAC Syrup 1875
Ryna .... ▣ 741
Soma Compound w/Codeine Tablets 2390
Triaminic Expectorant w/Codeine .. 1996
Tussi-Organidin Liquid 2391
Tylenol with Codeine 1381

Codeine Polistirex (Orthostatic hypotension may be aggravated).

No products indexed under this heading.

Cortisone Acetate (Hypokalemia). Products include:

Cortone Acetate Sterile Suspension 1437
Cortone Acetate Tablets 1439

Deserpidine (Potentiated; additive effects). Products include:

Enduronyl 518
Harmonyl Tablets 528
Oreticyl 545

Deslanoside (Cardiac arrhythmias; increased ventricular irritability).

No products indexed under this heading.

Dexamethasone (Hypokalemia). Products include:

AK-Trol Ointment & Suspension .... ◎ 207
Decadron Elixir 1445
Decadron Tablets 1447
Decaspray Topical Aerosol 1459
Dexacidin .... ◎ 272
Maxidex Sterile Ophthalmic Suspension .... ◎ 223
Maxitrol Ophthalmic Ointment/Suspension .... ◎ 223
TobraDex Ophthalmic Suspension and Ointment .... ◎ 228

Dexamethasone Acetate (Hypokalemia). Products include:
- Dalalone D.P. Injectable ... 999
- Decadron-LA Sterile Suspension ... 1457

Dexamethasone Sodium Phosphate (Hypokalemia). Products include:
- AK-Dex ... ◉ 203
- Decadron Phosphate Respihaler ... 1454
- Decadron Phosphate Sterile Ophthalmic Ointment ... 1453
- Decadron Phosphate Sterile Ophthalmic Solution ... 1453
- Decadron Phosphate Topical Cream ... 1455
- Decadron Phosphate Turbinaire ... 1456
- Maxidex Sterile Ophthalmic Ointment ... ◉ 222
- NeoDecadron Sterile Ophthalmic Ointment ... 1517
- NeoDecadron Sterile Ophthalmic Solution ... 1518
- NeoDecadron Topical Cream ... 1518

Dezocine (Orthostatic hypotension may be aggravated).

Diazoxide (Potentiated; additive effects). Products include:
- Hyperstat I.V. Injection ... 2095
- Proglycem ... 649

Diclofenac Sodium (Reduced diuretic, natriuretic, and antihypertensive effects of chlorothiazide). Products include:
- Voltaren Ophthalmic Sterile Ophthalmic Solution ... ◉ 268
- Voltaren Tablets ... 1042

Digitoxin (Cardiac arrhythmias; increased ventricular irritability). Products include:
- Crystodigin Tablets ... 1253

Digoxin (Cardiac arrhythmias; increased ventricular irritability). Products include:
- Lanoxicaps ... 772
- Lanoxin Elixir Pediatric ... 775
- Lanoxin Injection ... 778
- Lanoxin Injection Pediatric ... 781
- Lanoxin Tablets ... 783

Doxazosin Mesylate (Potentiated; additive effects). Products include:
- Cardura Tablets ... 1941

Enalapril Maleate (Potentiated; additive effects). Products include:
- Vaseretic Tablets ... 1559
- Vasotec Tablets ... 1564

Enalaprilat (Potentiation of antihypertensive effect). Products include:
- Vasotec I.V. ... 1562

Enflurane (Significant hypotension; bradycardia). Products include:
- Ethrane ... 599

Esmolol Hydrochloride (Potentiated; additive effects). Products include:
- Brevibloc Injection ... 942

Etodolac (Reduced diuretic, natriuretic, and antihypertensive effects of chlorothiazide). Products include:
- Lodine Capsules ... 2468

Felodipine (Potentiated; additive effects). Products include:
- Plendil Extended-Release Tablets ... 1526

Fenoprofen Calcium (Reduced diuretic, natriuretic, and antihypertensive effects of chlorothiazide). Products include:
- Nalfon Pulvules & Tablets ... 919

Fentanyl (Orthostatic hypotension may be aggravated). Products include:
- Duragesic Transdermal System ... 1133

Fentanyl Citrate (Orthostatic hypotension may be aggravated). Products include:
- Innovar Injection ... 1141
- Sublimaze Injection ... 1146

Flurbiprofen (Reduced diuretic, natriuretic, and antihypertensive effects of chlorothiazide). Products include:
- Ansaid Tablets ... 2319

Fosinopril Sodium (Potentiated; additive effects). Products include:
- Monopril Tablets ... 1406

Furosemide (Potentiated; additive effects). Products include:
- Lasix ... 1093

Glipizide (Dosage adjustment of the antidiabetic drug may be required). Products include:
- Glucotrol ... 1952

Glyburide (Dosage adjustment of the antidiabetic drug may be required). Products include:
- DiaBeta ... 1091
- Micronase Tablets ... 2350

Guanabenz Acetate (Potentiated; additive effects). Products include:
- Wytensin Tablets ... 2542

Guanethidine Monosulfate (Potentiated; additive effects). Products include:
- Esimil Tablets ... 864
- Ismelin Tablets ... 869

Hydralazine Hydrochloride (Potentiated; additive effects). Products include:
- Apresazide Capsules ... 854
- Apresoline Hydrochloride Parenteral (Ampuls) ... 856
- Apresoline Hydrochloride Tablets ... 855
- Apresoline-Esidrix Tablets ... 857
- Ser-Ap-Es Tablets ... 881
- Serpasil-Apresoline Tablets ... 884

Hydrochlorothiazide (Potentiated; additive effects). Products include:
- Aldactazide ... 2150
- Aldoril Tablets ... 1418
- Apresazide Capsules ... 854
- Apresoline-Esidrix Tablets ... 857
- Capozide ... 2258
- Dyazide Capsules ... 2208
- Esidrix Tablets ... 863
- Esimil Tablets ... 864
- HydroDIURIL Tablets ... 1484
- Hydropres Tablets ... 1485
- Inderide Tablets ... 2463
- Inderide LA Long Acting Capsules ... 2465
- Lopressor HCT Tablets ... 1034
- Maxzide ... 1215
- Moduretic Tablets ... 1510
- Normozide Tablets ... 2112
- Oretic Tablets ... 544
- Oreticyl ... 545
- Prinzide Tablets ... 1540
- Ser-Ap-Es Tablets ... 881
- Serpasil-Esidrix Tablets ... 886
- Timolide Tablets ... 1547
- Trandate HCT Tablets ... 579
- Vaseretic Tablets ... 1559
- Zestoretic ... 2274

Hydrocodone Bitartrate (Orthostatic hypotension may be aggravated). Products include:
- Anexsia 5/500 Tablets ... 2196
- Anexsia 7.5/650 Tablets ... 2197
- Azdone Tablets ... 844
- Codiclear DH Syrup ... 845
- Codimal DH Syrup ... 846
- Damason-P ... 1356
- Hycodan Syrup, Tablets ... 927
- Hycomine Compound Tablets ... 929
- Hycomine Syrup ... 927
- Hycotuss Expectorant Syrup ... 930
- Hydrocet Capsules ... 835
- Lortab ASA Tablets ... 2414
- Lortab ... 2412
- Ru-Tuss with Hydrocodone ... 694
- Triaminic Expectorant DH ... 1995
- Vicodin Tablets ... 1187
- Vicodin ES Tablets ... 1189
- Zydone Capsules ... 941

Hydrocodone Polistirex (Orthostatic hypotension may be aggravated). Products include:
- Tussionex Extended-Release Suspension ... 988

Hydrocortisone (Hypokalemia). Products include:
- AK-Spore H.C. ... ◉ 206
- Bactine Hydrocortisone Anti-Itch Cream ... ▣ 625
- CaldeCORT Anti-Itch Hydrocortisone Spray ... ▣ 560
- Carmol HC Cream 1% ... 2296
- Cortaid Spray ... ▣ 735
- Cortenema ... 2244
- Cortisporin Ointment ... 758
- Cortisporin Ophthalmic Ointment Sterile ... 758
- Cortisporin Ophthalmic Suspension Sterile ... 759
- Cortisporin Otic Solution Sterile ... 760
- Cortisporin Otic Suspension Sterile ... 760
- Cortizone-5 Creme & Ointment ... ▣ 732
- Dermolate Anti-Itch Cream ... ▣ 697
- Eldecort Cream 1.0% ... 1113
- Eldecort Cream 1.0% and 2.5% ... 1113
- Fungoid HC Creme ... 1770
- Hydrocortone Tablets ... 1482
- Hytone ... 909
- LazerSporin-C Solution ... 1770
- Massengill Medicated Soft Cloth Towelettes ... 2192
- Nutracort Cream & Lotion ... 1684
- PediOtic Suspension Sterile ... 797
- Synacort Creams 1%, 2.5% ... 2296
- Vanoxide-HC Acne Lotion ... 911
- Vioform-Hydrocortisone Cream and Mild Cream ... 889
- Vioform-Hydrocortisone Ointment ... 889
- VōSoL HC Otic Solution ... 2392
- Vytone Cream 1% ... 911

Hydrocortisone Acetate (Hypokalemia). Products include:
- Analpram-HC Rectal Cream 1% and 2.5% ... 970
- Anusol-HC Cream ... 1690
- Anusol-HC Suppositories ... 1691
- Caldecort ... ▣ 560
- Carmol HC Cream 1% ... 2296
- Chloromycetin Hydrocortisone Ophthalmic ... 1694
- Coly-Mycin S Otic w/Neomycin & Hydrocortisone ... 1708
- Cortaid ... ▣ 735
- Cortef Feminine Itch Cream ... ▣ 735
- Corticaine ... ▣ 682
- Cortifoam ... 1827
- Cortisporin Cream ... 757
- Epifoam ... 1828
- Gynecort 5 Creme ... ▣ 556
- Hydrocortone Acetate Sterile Suspension ... 1479
- Lanacort 5 Creme and Ointment ... ▣ 557
- Mantadil Cream ... 789
- Ophthocort ... ◉ 301
- Orabase HCA Oral Paste ... 890
- Pramosone Cream, Lotion & Ointment ... 971
- ProctoCream-HC ... 1834
- Proctofoam-HC ... 1835

Hydrocortisone Sodium Phosphate (Hypokalemia). Products include:
- Hydrocortone Phosphate Injection, Sterile ... 1481

Hydrocortisone Sodium Succinate (Hypokalemia). Products include:
- Solu-Cortef Sterile Powder ... 2361

Hydroflumethiazide (Potentiated; additive effects). Products include:
- Diucardin Tablets ... 2450
- Saluron ... 718
- Salutensin/Salutensin-Demi ... 719

Ibuprofen (Reduced diuretic, natriuretic, and antihypertensive effects of chlorothiazide). Products include:
- Advil Cold & Sinus Caplets (formerly CoAdvil) ... 2416
- Advil Ibuprofen Tablets and Caplets ... 2416
- Children's Advil Suspension ... 2426
- CoAdvil ... ▣ 748
- Dristan Sinus Caplets ... 2419
- Haltran Tablets ... ▣ 668
- Ibuprofen ... ▣ 631
- Medipren ibuprofen Caplets and Tablets ... 1362
- Midol 200 Cramp Relief Formula ... ▣ 570
- Motrin Tablets ... 2351
- Motrin IB Caplets and Tablets ... ▣ 736
- Nuprin Ibuprofen/Analgesic Tablets & Caplets ... 752
- PediaProfen Suspension ... 1363
- Rufen Tablets ... 691
- Trendar Ibuprofen Tablets ... ▣ 756

Indapamide (Potentiated; additive effects). Products include:
- Lozol Tablets ... 1843

Indomethacin (Reduced diuretic, natriuretic, and antihypertensive effects of chlorothiazide). Products include:
- Indocin ... 1487

Indomethacin Sodium Trihydrate (Reduced diuretic, natriuretic, and antihypertensive effects of chlorothiazide). Products include:
- Indocin I.V. ... 1490

Insulin, Human (Insulin requirements may be altered).
- No products indexed under this heading.

Insulin, Human Isophane Suspension (Insulin requirements may be altered). Products include:
- Humulin N, 100 Units ... 1270

Insulin, Human NPH (Insulin requirements may be altered). Products include:
- Insulatard NPH Human ... 1627
- Novolin N ... 1627
- Novolin N PenFill Cartridges ... 1628
- Novolin N Prefilled ... 1628

Insulin, Human Regular (Insulin requirements may be altered). Products include:
- Humulin BR, 100 Units ... 1268
- Humulin R, 100 Units ... 1272
- Novolin R ... 1627
- Novolin R PenFill Cartridges ... 1628
- Novolin R Prefilled ... 1629
- Velosulin Human ... 1628

Insulin, Human, Zinc Suspension (Insulin requirements may be altered). Products include:
- Humulin L, 100 Units ... 1268
- Humulin U, 100 Units ... 1272
- Novolin L ... 1627

Insulin, NPH (Insulin requirements may be altered). Products include:
- NPH, 40 & 100 Units ... 1273
- Beef NPH, 100 Units ... 1274
- Pork NPH, 100 Units ... 1275
- Insulatard NPH ... 1626
- NPH Insulin ... 1626
- NPH Purified Pork Isophane Insulin ... 1626

Insulin, Regular (Insulin requirements may be altered). Products include:
- Regular, 40 & 100 Units ... 1273
- Beef Regular, 100 Units ... 1275
- Pork Regular, 100 Units ... 1275
- Pork Regular (Concentrated), 500 Units ... 1276
- Regular Insulin ... 1625
- Regular Purified Pork Insulin ... 1626
- Velosulin ... 1627

Insulin, Zinc Crystals (Insulin requirements may be altered). Products include:
- NPH, 40 & 100 Units ... 1273

Insulin, Zinc Suspension (Insulin requirements may be altered). Products include:
- Lente, 40 & 100 Units ... 1272
- Protamine, Zinc, 40 & 100 Units ... 1273
- Lente Iletin I ... 1272
- Beef Lente, 100 Units ... 1274
- Beef Protamine Zinc, 100 Units ... 1274
- Pork Lente, 100 Units ... 1275
- Pork, Protamine, Zinc, 100 Units ... 1275
- Lente Insulin ... 1626
- Lente Purified Pork Insulin ... 1626
- Semilente Insulin ... 1625
- Ultralente Insulin ... 1626

Isoflurane (Significant hypotension; bradycardia). Products include:
- Forane ... 600

Isradipine (Potentiated; additive effects). Products include:
- DynaCirc Capsules ... 2004

Ketamine Hydrochloride (May require reduced dose of anesthetics). Products include:
- Ketalar ... 1726

Ketoprofen (Reduced diuretic, natriuretic, and antihypertensive effects of chlorothiazide). Products include:
- Orudis Capsules ... 2488

Ketorolac Tromethamine (Reduced diuretic, natriuretic, and antihypertensive effects of chlorothiazide). Products include:
- Toradol IM Injection ... 2302

Labetalol Hydrochloride (Potentiated; additive effects). Products include:
- Normodyne Injection ... 2108
- Normodyne Tablets ... 2110
- Normozide Tablets ... 2112
- Trandate HCT Tablets ... 579
- Trandate Injection ... 577
- Trandate Tablets ... 579

Levorphanol Tartrate (Orthostatic hypotension may be aggravated). Products include:
- Levo-Dromoran ... 1906

Lisinopril (Potentiation of antihypertensive effect). Products include:
- Prinivil Tablets ... 1538
- Prinzide Tablets ... 1540
- Zestoretic ... 2274
- Zestril Tablets ... 2277

Lithium Carbonate (High risk of lithium toxicity). Products include:
- Eskalith ... 2214
- Lithane Tablets ... 1596
- Lithium Carbonate Capsules & Tablets ... 1984
- Lithobid Tablets ... 870

Lithium Citrate (High risk of lithium toxicity). Products include:
- Cibalith-S ... 870

Mecamylamine Hydrochloride (Potentiated; additive effects). Products include:
- Inversine Tablets ... 1492

Meclofenamate Sodium (Reduced diuretic, natriuretic, and antihypertensive effects of chlorothiazide). Products include:
- Meclomen Capsules ... 1739

Mefenamic Acid (Reduced diuretic, natriuretic, and antihypertensive effects of chlorothiazide). Products include:
- Ponstel ... 1758

Meperidine Hydrochloride (Orthostatic hypotension may be aggravated). Products include:
- Demerol ... 2047
- Mepergan Injection ... 2479

Mephobarbital (Orthostatic hypotension may be aggravated). Products include:
- Mebaral Tablets ... 2061

Methadone Hydrochloride (Orthostatic hypotension may be aggravated). Products include:
- Dolophine Hydrochloride Ampoules & Vials ... 1260
- Dolophine Hydrochloride Tablets ... 1261
- Methadone Hydrochloride Diskets ... 1284
- Methadone Hydrochloride Oral Solution & Tablets ... 1987

Methohexital Sodium (Significant hypotension; bradycardia). Products include:
- Brevital Sodium Vials ... 1248

Methoxyflurane (Significant hypotension; bradycardia).
- No products indexed under this heading.

Methyclothiazide (Potentiated; additive effects). Products include:
- Enduron Tablets ... 517
- Enduronyl ... 518

Methyldopa (Potentiated; additive effects). Products include:
- Aldoclor Tablets ... 1413
- Aldomet Oral ... 1415
- Aldoril Tablets ... 1418

Methyldopate Hydrochloride (Potentiated; additive effects). Products include:
- Aldomet Ester HCl Injection ... 1417

Methylprednisolone Acetate (Hypokalemia). Products include:
- Depo-Medrol Sterile Aqueous Suspension ... 2334

Methylprednisolone Sodium Succinate (Hypokalemia). Products include:
- Solu-Medrol Sterile Powder ... 2363

Metolazone (Potentiated; additive effects). Products include:
- Diulo ... 2129
- Mykrox ½ mg Tablets ... 984
- Zaroxolyn Tablets ... 989

Metoprolol Tartrate (Potentiated; additive effects). Products include:
- Lopressor Ampuls ... 1032
- Lopressor HCT Tablets ... 1034
- Lopressor Tablets ... 1032

Metyrosine (Potentiated; additive effects). Products include:
- Demser Capsules ... 1460

Minoxidil (Potentiated; additive effects). Products include:
- Loniten Tablets ... 2346
- Rogaine Topical Solution ... 2357

Morphine Sulfate (Orthostatic hypotension may be aggravated). Products include:
- Astramorph/PF Injection, USP (Preservative-Free) ... 618
- Duramorph ... 960
- Infumorph 200 and Infumorph 500 Sterile Solutions ... 962
- MS Contin Tablets ... 1814
- MSIR ... 1817
- Oramorph SR (Morphine Sulfate Sustained Release Tablets) ... 1988
- Roxanol ... 1991

Nadolol (Potentiated; additive effects). Products include:
- Corgard Tablets ... 701
- Corzide Tablets ... 702

Naproxen (Reduced diuretic natriuretic, and antihypertensive effects of chlorothiazide). Products include:
- Naprosyn ... 2297

Naproxen Sodium (Reduced diuretic, natriuretic, and antihypertensive effects of chlorothiazide). Products include:
- Anaprox and Anaprox DS Tablets ... 2288

Nicardipine Hydrochloride (Potentiated; additive effects). Products include:
- Cardene Capsules ... 2290

Nitroglycerin (Potentiated; additive effects). Products include:
- Deponit NTG Transdermal Delivery System ... 2143
- Minitran Transdermal Delivery System ... 1312
- Nitro-Bid Ointment ... 1339
- Nitro-Bid Capsules ... 1338
- Nitrodisc ... 2176
- Nitro-Dur (nitroglycerin) Transdermal Infusion System ... 1164
- Nitrogard Tablets ... 1004
- Nitrolingual Spray ... 1846
- Nitrostat Tablets ... 1743
- Transderm-Nitro Transdermal Therapeutic System ... 2283

Norepinephrine Bitartrate (Decreased arterial responsiveness to norepinephrine). Products include:
- Levophed Bitartrate Injection ... 2054

Opium Alkaloids (Orthostatic hypotension may be aggravated). Products include:
- B & O No. 15A & No. 16A Supprettes ... 2395
- Pantopon Injectable ... 1911

Oxycodone Hydrochloride (Orthostatic hypotension may be aggravated). Products include:
- Percocet Tablets ... 950
- Percodan ... 951
- Roxicodone Tablets, Oral Solution & Intensol (Oxycodone) ... 1992
- Tylox Capsules ... 1382

Penbutolol Sulfate (Potentiated; additive effects). Products include:
- Levatol ... 1832

Pentobarbital Sodium (Orthostatic hypotension may be aggravated). Products include:
- Nembutal Sodium Capsules ... 534
- Nembutal Sodium Solution ... 536
- Nembutal Sodium Suppositories ... 538

Phenobarbital (Orthostatic hypotension may be aggravated). Products include:
- Arco-Lase Plus Tablets ... 607
- Bellergal-S Tablets ... 1998
- Bronkolixir ... ▣ 761
- Bronkotabs Tablets ... ▣ 762
- Donnatal ... 1858
- Donnatal Extentabs ... 1859
- Donnatal Tablets ... 1858
- Donnazyme Tablets ... 1860
- Kinesed Tablets ... 2272
- Phenobarbital Elixir and Tablets ... 1293
- Primatene Tablets-P Formula ... 2421
- Quadrinal Tablets ... 1183
- Tedral SA ... 1765

Phenoxybenzamine Hydrochloride (Potentiated; additive effects). Products include:
- Dibenzyline Capsules ... 2207

Phentolamine Mesylate (Potentiated; additive effects). Products include:
- Regitine ... 878

Phenylbutazone (Reduced diuretic, natriuretic, and antihypertensive effects of chlorothiazide). Products include:
- Butazolidin Capsules & Tablets ... 1027

Pindolol (Potentiated; additive effects). Products include:
- Visken Tablets ... 2036

Piroxicam (Reduced diuretic, natriuretic, and antihypertensive effects of chlorothiazide). Products include:
- Feldene Capsules ... 1777

Polythiazide (Potentiated; additive effects). Products include:
- Minizide Capsules ... 1779
- Renese Tablets ... 1785
- Renese-R Tablets ... 1786

Prazosin Hydrochloride (Potentiated; additive effects). Products include:
- Minipress Capsules ... 1778
- Minizide Capsules ... 1779

Prednisolone Acetate (Hypokalemia). Products include:
- AK-Cide Sterile Ophthalmic Ointment & Suspension ... ⊙ 202
- Blephamide Liquifilm Sterile Ophthalmic Suspension ... 586
- Blephamide S.O.P. Sterile Ophthalmic Ointment ... 586
- Cetapred Ointment ... ⊙ 220
- ⅛% Econopred & 1% Econopred Plus ... ⊙ 217
- Isopto Cetapred Suspension ... ⊙ 220
- Metimyd ... ⊙ 306
- Poly-Pred Liquifilm ... ⊙ 250
- Pred Forte ... ⊙ 252
- Pred Mild ... ⊙ 254
- Pred-G Liquifilm Sterile Ophthalmic Suspension ... ⊙ 252
- Pred-G S.O.P. Sterile Ophthalmic Ointment ... ⊙ 253
- Vasocidin Ointment ... ⊙ 275

Prednisolone Sodium Phosphate (Hypokalemia). Products include:
- AK-Pred ... ⊙ 205
- Hydeltrasol Injection, Sterile ... 1476
- Inflamase ... ⊙ 274
- Pediapred Oral Liquid ... 987
- Vasocidin Ophthalmic Solution ... ⊙ 276

Prednisolone Tebutate (Hypokalemia). Products include:
- Hydeltra-T.B.A. Sterile Suspension 1478

Prednisone (Hypokalemia). Products include:
- Deltasone Tablets ... 2332

Propofol (Significant hypotension; bradycardia). Products include:
- Diprivan Injection ... 2267

Propoxyphene Hydrochloride (Orthostatic hypotension may be aggravated). Products include:
- Darvon ... 1256
- Wygesic Tablets ... 2540

Propoxyphene Napsylate (Orthostatic hypotension may be aggravated). Products include:
- Darvon-N/Darvocet-N ... 1254

Propranolol Hydrochloride (Potentiated; additive effects). Products include:
- Inderal ... 2459
- Inderal LA Long Acting Capsules ... 2461
- Inderide Tablets ... 2463
- Inderide LA Long Acting Capsules ... 2465

Quinidine Gluconate (Cardiac arrhythmias). Products include:
- Quinaglute Dura-Tabs Tablets ... 663

Quinidine Polygalacturonate (Cardiac arrhythmias). Products include:
- Cardioquin Tablets ... 1812

Quinidine Sulfate (Cardiac arrhythmias). Products include:
- Quinidex Extentabs ... 1868

Ramipril (Potentiated; additive effects). Products include:
- Altace Capsules ... 1086

Rauwolfia Serpentina (Potentiated; additive effects). Products include:
- Raudixin Tablets ... 1803
- Rauzide Tablets ... 1804

Rescinnamine (Potentiated; additive effects).
- No products indexed under this heading.

Secobarbital Sodium (Orthostatic hypotension may be aggravated). Products include:
- Seconal Sodium Pulvules ... 1296

Sodium Nitroprusside (Potentiated; additive effects). Products include:
- Nipride I.V. Infusion ... 1909

Sufentanil Citrate (Orthostatic hypotension may be aggravated). Products include:
- Sufenta Injection ... 1147

Sulindac (Reduced diuretic, natriuretic, and antihypertensive effects of chlorothiazide). Products include:
- Clinoril Tablets ... 1433

Terazosin Hydrochloride (Potentiated; additive effects). Products include:
- Hytrin Tablets ... 529

Thiamylal Sodium (Orthostatic hypotension may be aggravated). Products include:
- Surital Ampoules, Steri-Vials ... 1764

Timolol Maleate (Potentiated; additive effects). Products include:
- Blocadren Tablets ... 1429
- Timolide Tablets ... 1547
- Timoptic in Ocudose ... 1552
- Timoptic Sterile Ophthalmic Solution ... 1550

Tolazamide (Dosage adjustment of the antidiabetic drug may be required). Products include:
- Tolinase Tablets ... 2365

Tolbutamide (Dosage adjustment of the antidiabetic drug may be required). Products include:
- Orinase Tablets ... 2354

Tolmetin Sodium (Reduced diuretic, natriuretic, and antihypertensive effects of chlorothiazide). Products include:
Tolectin (200, 400 and 600 mg) .. 1379

Triamcinolone (Hypokalemia).
No products indexed under this heading.

Triamcinolone Acetonide (Hypokalemia). Products include:
Aristocort A 1010
Azmacort Inhaler 1837
Kenalog Cream, Lotion & Ointment 2401
Kenalog-10 Injection 2402
Kenalog-40 Injection 2403
Kenalog in Orabase 604
Kenalog Spray 2401
Mycolog II Cream and Ointment 2407
Mytrex Cream & Ointment 2080
Nasacort Nasal Inhaler 1844

Triamcinolone Diacetate (Hypokalemia). Products include:
Aristocort Suspension 1008

Triamcinolone Hexacetonide (Hypokalemia). Products include:
Aristospan Suspension 1011

Trimethaphan Camsylate (Potentiated; additive effects). Products include:
Arfonad Ampuls 1887

Tubocurarine Chloride (Increased responsiveness to tubocurarine).
No products indexed under this heading.

DIURIL ORAL SUSPENSION
(Chlorothiazide) 1464
May interact with lithium preparations, corticosteroids, insulin, nonsteroidal anti-inflammatory agents, barbiturates, narcotic analgesics, cardiac glycosides, antihypertensives, oral hypoglycemic agents, and certain other agents. Compounds in these categories include:

Acebutolol Hydrochloride (Potentiated or additive effects). Products include:
Sectral Capsules 2520

ACTH (Hypokalemia).
No products indexed under this heading.

Alcohol (Orthostatic hypotension may be aggravated).

Alfentanil Hydrochloride (Orthostatic hypotension may be aggravated). Products include:
Alfenta Injection 1131

Aprobarbital (Orthostatic hypotension may be aggravated). Products include:
Alurate Elixir 1883

Atenolol (Potentiated or additive effects). Products include:
Tenoretic Tablets 1105
Tenormin Tablets and I.V. Injection 1107

Benazepril Hydrochloride (Potentiated or additive effects). Products include:
Lotensin Tablets 872

Bendroflumethiazide (Potentiated or additive effects). Products include:
Corzide Tablets 702
Naturetin Tablets 1789
Rauzide Tablets 1804

Betamethasone Acetate (Hypokalemia). Products include:
Celestone Soluspan Suspension 2081

Betamethasone Sodium Phosphate (Hypokalemia). Products include:
Celestone Soluspan Suspension 2081

Betaxolol Hydrochloride (Potentiated or additive effects). Products include:
Betoptic Sterile Ophthalmic Solution 569
Betoptic S Sterile Ophthalmic Suspension 570
Kerlone Tablets 2172

Buprenorphine (Orthostatic hypotension may be aggravated).
No products indexed under this heading.

Butabarbital (Orthostatic hypotension may be aggravated). Products include:
Pyridium Plus 1764

Butalbital (Orthostatic hypotension may be aggravated). Products include:
Esgic-Plus Tablets 1002
Esgic Tablets & Capsules 1001
Fioricet Tablets 2006
Fiorinal Capsules 2007
Fiorinal with Codeine Capsules 2008
Fiorinal Tablets 2007
Phrenilin 838
Sedapap Tablets 50 mg/650 mg .. 1360

Captopril (Potentiated or additive effects). Products include:
Capoten 2255
Capozide 2258

Carteolol Hydrochloride (Potentiated or additive effects). Products include:
Cartrol Tablets 507

Chlorothiazide Sodium (Potentiated or additive effects). Products include:
Diuril Sodium Intravenous 1463

Chlorpropamide (Dosage adjustment of the antidiabetic drug may be required). Products include:
Diabinese Tablets 1775

Chlorthalidone (Potentiated or additive effects). Products include:
Combipres Tablets 678
Tenoretic Tablets 1105
Thalitone Tablets 687

Clonidine (Potentiated or additive effects). Products include:
Catapres-TTS 677

Clonidine Hydrochloride (Potentiated or additive effects). Products include:
Catapres Tablets 676
Combipres Tablets 678

Codeine (Orthostatic hypotension may be aggravated). Products include:
Calcidrine Syrup 506

Codeine Phosphate (Orthostatic hypotension may be aggravated). Products include:
Actifed with Codeine Cough Syrup .. 752
Cheracol Cough Syrup 1853
Codimal PH Syrup 846
Dimetane-DC Cough Syrup 1857
Empirin with Codeine Phosphate Nos. 2, 3 & 4 764
Fiorinal with Codeine Capsules 2008
Isoclor Expectorant 982
Naldecon CX Adult Liquid .... ▣ 521
Novahistine DH 1342
Novahistine Expectorant 1343
Nucofed Capsules 2219
Nucofed Expectorant 2219
Nucofed Pediatric Expectorant 2220
Nucofed Syrup 2219
Phenaphen with Codeine Capsules 1865
Phenaphen-650 with Codeine Tablets 1866
Phenergan with Codeine 2497
Phenergan VC with Codeine 2501
Robitussin A-C Syrup 1875
Robitussin-DAC Syrup 1875
Ryna .... ▣ 741
Soma Compound w/Codeine Tablets 2390
Triaminic Expectorant w/Codeine .. 1996
Tussi-Organidin Liquid 2391
Tylenol with Codeine 1381

Codeine Polistirex (Orthostatic hypotension may be aggravated).
No products indexed under this heading.

Cortisone Acetate (Hypokalemia). Products include:
Cortone Acetate Sterile Suspension 1437
Cortone Acetate Tablets 1439

Deserpidine (Potentiated or additive effects). Products include:
Enduronyl 518
Harmonyl Tablets 528
Oreticyl 545

Deslanoside (Increased ventricular irritability).
No products indexed under this heading.

Dexamethasone (Hypokalemia). Products include:
AK-Trol Ointment & Suspension .... ⊙ 207
Decadron Elixir 1445
Decadron Tablets 1447
Decaspray Topical Aerosol 1459
Dexacidin .... ⊙ 272
Maxidex Sterile Ophthalmic Suspension .... ⊙ 223
Maxitrol Ophthalmic Ointment/Suspension .... ⊙ 223
TobraDex Ophthalmic Suspension and Ointment .... ⊙ 228

Dexamethasone Acetate (Hypokalemia). Products include:
Dalalone D.P. Injectable 999
Decadron-LA Sterile Suspension 1457

Dexamethasone Sodium Phosphate (Hypokalemia). Products include:
AK-Dex .... ⊙ 203
Decadron Phosphate Respihaler 1454
Decadron Phosphate Sterile Ophthalmic Ointment 1453
Decadron Phosphate Sterile Ophthalmic Solution 1453
Decadron Phosphate Topical Cream 1455
Decadron Phosphate Turbinaire 1456
Maxidex Sterile Ophthalmic Ointment .... ⊙ 222
NeoDecadron Sterile Ophthalmic Ointment 1517
NeoDecadron Sterile Ophthalmic Solution 1518
NeoDecadron Topical Cream 1518

Dezocine (Orthostatic hypotension may be aggravated).

Diazoxide (Potentiated or additive effects). Products include:
Hyperstat I.V. Injection 2095
Proglycem 649

Diclofenac Sodium (Reduces diuretic, natriuretic, and antihypertensive effects). Products include:
Voltaren Ophthalmic Sterile Ophthalmic Solution .... ⊙ 268
Voltaren Tablets 1042

Digitoxin (Increased ventricular irritability). Products include:
Crystodigin Tablets 1253

Digoxin (Increased ventricular irritability). Products include:
Lanoxicaps 772
Lanoxin Elixir Pediatric 775
Lanoxin Injection 778
Lanoxin Injection Pediatric 781
Lanoxin Tablets 783

Doxazosin Mesylate (Potentiated or additive effects). Products include:
Cardura Tablets 1941

Enalapril Maleate (Potentiated or additive effects). Products include:
Vaseretic Tablets 1559
Vasotec Tablets 1564

Enalaprilat (Potentiation of antihypertensive effect). Products include:
Vasotec I.V. 1562

Esmolol Hydrochloride (Potentiated or additive effects). Products include:
Brevibloc Injection 942

Etodolac (Reduces diuretic, natriuretic, and antihypertensive effects). Products include:
Lodine Capsules 2468

Felodipine (Potentiated or additive effects). Products include:
Plendil Extended-Release Tablets 1526

Fenoprofen Calcium (Reduces diuretic, natriuretic, and antihypertensive effects). Products include:
Nalfon Pulvules & Tablets 919

Fentanyl (Orthostatic hypotension may be aggravated). Products include:
Duragesic Transdermal System 1133

Fentanyl Citrate (Orthostatic hypotension may be aggravated). Products include:
Innovar Injection 1141
Sublimaze Injection 1146

Flurbiprofen (Reduces diuretic, natriuretic, and antihypertensive effects). Products include:
Ansaid Tablets 2319

Fosinopril Sodium (Potentiated or additive effects). Products include:
Monopril Tablets 1406

Furosemide (Potentiated or additive effects). Products include:
Lasix 1093

Glipizide (Dosage adjustment of the antidiabetic drug may be required). Products include:
Glucotrol 1952

Glyburide (Dosage adjustment of the antidiabetic drug may be required). Products include:
DiaBeta 1091
Micronase Tablets 2350

Guanabenz Acetate (Potentiated or additive effects). Products include:
Wytensin Tablets 2542

Guanethidine Monosulfate (Potentiated or additive effects). Products include:
Esimil Tablets 864
Ismelin Tablets 869

Hydralazine Hydrochloride (Potentiated or additive effects). Products include:
Apresazide Capsules 854
Apresoline Hydrochloride Parenteral (Ampuls) 856
Apresoline Hydrochloride Tablets .. 855
Apresoline-Esidrix Tablets 857
Ser-Ap-Es Tablets 881
Serpasil-Apresoline Tablets 884

Hydrochlorothiazide (Potentiated or additive effects). Products include:
Aldactazide 2150
Aldoril Tablets 1418
Apresazide Capsules 854
Apresoline-Esidrix Tablets 857
Capozide 2258
Dyazide Capsules 2208
Esidrix Tablets 863
Esimil Tablets 864
HydroDIURIL Tablets 1484
Hydropres Tablets 1485
Inderide Tablets 2463
Inderide LA Long Acting Capsules .. 2465
Lopressor HCT Tablets 1034
Maxzide 1215
Moduretic Tablets 1510
Normozide Tablets 2112
Oretic Tablets 544
Oreticyl 545
Prinzide Tablets 1540
Ser-Ap-Es Tablets 881
Serpasil-Esidrix Tablets 886
Timolide Tablets 1547
Trandate HCT Tablets 579
Vaseretic Tablets 1559
Zestoretic 2274

Hydrocodone Bitartrate (Orthostatic hypotension may be aggravated). Products include:
Anexsia 5/500 Tablets 2196
Anexsia 7.5/650 Tablets 2197
Azdōne Tablets 844
Codiclear DH Syrup 845
Codimal DH Syrup 846
Damason-P 1356

(▣ Described in PDR For Nonprescription Drugs) (⊙ Described in PDR For Ophthalmology)

Hycodan Syrup, Tablets 927
Hycomine Compound Tablets 929
Hycomine Syrup 927
Hycotuss Expectorant Syrup 930
Hydrocet Capsules 835
Lortab ASA Tablets 2414
Lortab 2412
Ru-Tuss with Hydrocodone 694
Triaminic Expectorant DH 1995
Vicodin Tablets 1187
Vicodin ES Tablets 1189
Zydone Capsules 941

Hydrocodone Polistirex (Orthostatic hypotension may be aggravated). Products include:

Tussionex Extended-Release Suspension 988

Hydrocortisone (Hypokalemia). Products include:

AK-Spore H.C. .... ⊙ 206
Bactine Hydrocortisone Anti-Itch Cream .... ▣ 625
CaldeCORT Anti-Itch Hydrocortisone Spray .... ▣ 560
Carmol HC Cream 1% 2296
Cortaid Spray .... ▣ 735
Cortenema 2244
Cortisporin Ointment 758
Cortisporin Ophthalmic Ointment Sterile 758
Cortisporin Ophthalmic Suspension Sterile 759
Cortisporin Otic Solution Sterile 760
Cortisporin Otic Suspension Sterile 760
Cortizone-5 Creme & Ointment .... ▣ 732
Dermolate Anti-Itch Cream .... ▣ 697
Eldecort Cream 1.0% 1113
Eldecort Cream 1.0% and 2.5% 1113
Fungoid HC Creme 1770
Hydrocortone Tablets 1482
Hytone 909
LazerSporin-C Solution 1770
Massengill Medicated Soft Cloth Towelettes 2192
Nutracort Cream & Lotion 1684
PediOtic Suspension Sterile 797
Synacort Creams 1%, 2.5% 2296
Vanoxide-HC Acne Lotion 911
Vioform-Hydrocortisone Cream and Mild Cream 889
Vioform-Hydrocortisone Ointment 889
VōSoL HC Otic Solution 2392
Vytone Cream 1% 911

Hydrocortisone Acetate (Hypokalemia). Products include:

Analpram-HC Rectal Cream 1% and 2.5% 970
Anusol-HC Cream 1690
Anusol-HC Suppositories 1691
Caldecort .... ▣ 560
Carmol HC Cream 1% 2296
Chloromycetin Hydrocortisone Ophthalmic 1694
Coly-Mycin S Otic w/Neomycin & Hydrocortisone 1708
Cortaid .... ▣ 735
Cortef Feminine Itch Cream .... ▣ 735
Corticaine .... ▣ 682
Cortifoam 1827
Cortisporin Cream 757
Epifoam 1828
Gynecort 5 Creme .... ▣ 556
Hydrocortone Acetate Sterile Suspension 1479
Lanacort 5 Creme and Ointment .... ▣ 557
Mantadil Cream 789
Ophthocort .... ⊙ 301
Orabase HCA Oral Paste 890
Pramosone Cream, Lotion & Ointment 971
ProctoCream-HC 1834
Proctofoam-HC 1835

Hydrocortisone Sodium Phosphate (Hypokalemia). Products include:

Hydrocortone Phosphate Injection, Sterile 1481

Hydrocortisone Sodium Succinate (Hypokalemia). Products include:

Solu-Cortef Sterile Powder 2361

Hydroflumethiazide (Potentiated or additive effects). Products include:

Diucardin Tablets 2450
Saluron 718
Salutensin/Salutensin-Demi 719

Ibuprofen (Reduces diuretic, natriuretic, and antihypertensive effects). Products include:

Advil Cold & Sinus Caplets (formerly CoAdvil) 2416
Advil Ibuprofen Tablets and Caplets 2416
Children's Advil Suspension 2426
CoAdvil .... ▣ 748
Dristan Sinus Caplets 2419
Haltran Tablets .... ▣ 668
Ibuprofen .... ▣ 631
Medipren ibuprofen Caplets and Tablets 1362
Midol 200 Cramp Relief Formula .... ▣ 570
Motrin Tablets 2351
Motrin IB Caplets and Tablets .... ▣ 736
Nuprin Ibuprofen/Analgesic Tablets & Caplets 752
PediaProfen Suspension 1363
Rufen Tablets 691
Trendar Ibuprofen Tablets .... ▣ 756

Indapamide (Potentiated or additive effects). Products include:

Lozol Tablets 1843

Indomethacin (Reduces diuretic, natriuretic, and antihypertensive effects). Products include:

Indocin 1487

Indomethacin Sodium Trihydrate (Reduces diuretic, natriuretic, and antihypertensive effects). Products include:

Indocin I.V. 1490

Insulin, Human (Altered insulin requirements).

No products indexed under this heading.

Insulin, Human Isophane Suspension (Altered insulin requirements). Products include:

Humulin N, 100 Units 1270

Insulin, Human NPH (Altered insulin requirements). Products include:

Insulatard NPH Human 1627
Novolin N 1627
Novolin N PenFill Cartridges 1628
Novolin N Prefilled 1628

Insulin, Human Regular (Altered insulin requirements). Products include:

Humulin BR, 100 Units 1268
Humulin R, 100 Units 1272
Novolin R 1627
Novolin R PenFill Cartridges 1628
Novolin R Prefilled 1629
Velosulin Human 1628

Insulin, Human, Zinc Suspension (Altered insulin requirements). Products include:

Humulin L, 100 Units 1268
Humulin U, 100 Units 1272
Novolin L 1627

Insulin, NPH (Altered insulin requirements). Products include:

NPH, 40 & 100 Units 1273
Beef NPH, 100 Units 1274
Pork NPH, 100 Units 1275
Insulatard NPH 1626
NPH Insulin 1626
NPH Purified Pork Isophane Insulin 1626

Insulin, Regular (Altered insulin requirements). Products include:

Regular, 40 & 100 Units 1273
Beef Regular, 100 Units 1275
Pork Regular, 100 Units 1275
Pork Regular (Concentrated), 500 Units 1276
Regular Insulin 1625
Regular Purified Pork Insulin 1626
Velosulin 1627

Insulin, Zinc Crystals (Altered insulin requirements). Products include:

NPH, 40 & 100 Units 1273

Insulin, Zinc Suspension (Altered insulin requirements). Products include:

Lente, 40 & 100 Units 1272
Protamine, Zinc, 40 & 100 Units 1273
Lente Iletin I 1272
Beef Lente, 100 Units 1274
Beef Protamine Zinc, 100 Units 1274
Pork Lente, 100 Units 1275
Pork, Protamine, Zinc, 100 Units 1275
Lente Insulin 1626
Lente Purified Pork Insulin 1626
Semilente Insulin 1625
Ultralente Insulin 1626

Isradipine (Potentiated or additive effects). Products include:

DynaCirc Capsules 2004

Ketoprofen (Reduces diuretic, natriuretic, and antihypertensive effects). Products include:

Orudis Capsules 2488

Ketorolac Tromethamine (Reduces diuretic, natriuretic, and antihypertensive effects). Products include:

Toradol IM Injection 2302

Labetalol Hydrochloride (Potentiated or additive effects). Products include:

Normodyne Injection 2108
Normodyne Tablets 2110
Normozide Tablets 2112
Trandate HCT Tablets 579
Trandate Injection 577
Trandate Tablets 579

Levorphanol Tartrate (Orthostatic hypotension may be aggravated). Products include:

Levo-Dromoran 1906

Lisinopril (Potentiation of antihypertensive effect). Products include:

Prinivil Tablets 1538
Prinzide Tablets 1540
Zestoretic 2274
Zestril Tablets 2277

Lithium Carbonate (High risk of lithium toxicity). Products include:

Eskalith 2214
Lithane Tablets 1596
Lithium Carbonate Capsules & Tablets 1984
Lithobid Tablets 870

Lithium Citrate (High risk of lithium toxicity). Products include:

Cibalith-S 870

Mecamylamine Hydrochloride (Potentiated or additive effects). Products include:

Inversine Tablets 1492

Meclofenamate Sodium (Reduced diuretic, natriuretic, and antihypertensive effects of chlorothiazide). Products include:

Meclomen Capsules 1739

Mefenamic Acid (Reduced diuretic, natriuretic, and antihypertensive effects of chlorothiazide). Products include:

Ponstel 1758

Meperidine Hydrochloride (Orthostatic hypotension may be aggravated). Products include:

Demerol 2047
Mepergan Injection 2479

Mephobarbital (Orthostatic hypotension may be aggravated). Products include:

Mebaral Tablets 2061

Methadone Hydrochloride (Orthostatic hypotension may be aggravated). Products include:

Dolophine Hydrochloride Ampoules & Vials 1260
Dolophine Hydrochloride Tablets 1261
Methadone Hydrochloride Diskets 1284
Methadone Hydrochloride Oral Solution & Tablets 1987

Methyclothiazide (Potentiated or additive effects). Products include:

Enduron Tablets 517
Enduronyl 518

Methyldopa (Potentiated or additive effects). Products include:

Aldoclor Tablets 1413
Aldomet Oral 1415
Aldoril Tablets 1418

Methyldopate Hydrochloride (Potentiated or additive effects). Products include:

Aldomet Ester HCl Injection 1417

Methylprednisolone (Hypokalemia). Products include:

Medrol 2348

Methylprednisolone Acetate (Hypokalemia). Products include:

Depo-Medrol Sterile Aqueous Suspension 2334

Methylprednisolone Sodium Succinate (Hypokalemia). Products include:

Solu-Medrol Sterile Powder 2363

Metolazone (Potentiated or additive effects). Products include:

Diulo 2129
Mykrox ½ mg Tablets 984
Zaroxolyn Tablets 989

Metoprolol Tartrate (Potentiated or additive effects). Products include:

Lopressor Ampuls 1032
Lopressor HCT Tablets 1034
Lopressor Tablets 1032

Metyrosine (Potentiated or additive effects). Products include:

Demser Capsules 1460

Minoxidil (Potentiated or additive effects). Products include:

Loniten Tablets 2346
Rogaine Topical Solution 2357

Morphine Sulfate (Orthostatic hypotension may be aggravated). Products include:

Astramorph/PF Injection, USP (Preservative-Free) 618
Duramorph 960
Infumorph 200 and Infumorph 500 Sterile Solutions 962
MS Contin Tablets 1814
MSIR 1817
Oramorph SR (Morphine Sulfate Sustained Release Tablets) 1988
Roxanol 1991

Nadolol (Potentiated or additive effects). Products include:

Corgard Tablets 701
Corzide Tablets 702

Naproxen (Reduces diuretic, natriuretic, and antihypertensive effects). Products include:

Naprosyn 2297

Naproxen Sodium (Reduces diuretic, natriuretic, and antihypertensive effects). Products include:

Anaprox and Anaprox DS Tablets 2288

Nicardipine Hydrochloride (Potentiated or additive effects). Products include:

Cardene Capsules 2290

Nitroglycerin (Potentiated or additive effects). Products include:

Deponit NTG Transdermal Delivery System 2143
Minitran Transdermal Delivery System 1312
Nitro-Bid Ointment 1339
Nitro-Bid Capsules 1338
Nitrodisc 2176
Nitro-Dur (nitroglycerin) Transdermal Infusion System 1164
Nitrogard Tablets 1004
Nitrolingual Spray 1846
Nitrostat Tablets 1743
Transderm-Nitro Transdermal Therapeutic System 2283

Norepinephrine Bitartrate (Decreased arterial responsiveness to norepinephrine). Products include:

Levophed Bitartrate Injection 2054

Opium Alkaloids (Orthostatic hypotension may be aggravated). Products include:

B & O No. 15A & No. 16A Supprettes 2395
Pantopon Injectable 1911

Oxycodone Hydrochloride (Orthostatic hypotension may be aggravated). Products include:
- Percocet Tablets ... 950
- Percodan ... 951
- Roxicodone Tablets, Oral Solution & Intensol (Oxycodone) ... 1992
- Tylox Capsules ... 1382

Penbutolol Sulfate (Potentiated or additive effects). Products include:
- Levatol ... 1832

Pentobarbital Sodium (Orthostatic hypotension may be aggravated). Products include:
- Nembutal Sodium Capsules ... 534
- Nembutal Sodium Solution ... 536
- Nembutal Sodium Suppositories ... 538

Phenobarbital (Orthostatic hypotension may be aggravated). Products include:
- Arco-Lase Plus Tablets ... 607
- Bellergal-S Tablets ... 1998
- Bronkolixir ... ▣ 761
- Bronkotabs Tablets ... ▣ 762
- Donnatal ... 1858
- Donnatal Extentabs ... 1859
- Donnatal Tablets ... 1858
- Donnazyme Tablets ... 1860
- Kinesed Tablets ... 2272
- Phenobarbital Elixir and Tablets ... 1293
- Primatene Tablets-P Formula ... 2421
- Quadrinal Tablets ... 1183
- Tedral SA ... 1765

Phenoxybenzamine Hydrochloride (Potentiated or additive effects). Products include:
- Dibenzyline Capsules ... 2207

Phentolamine Mesylate (Potentiated or additive effects). Products include:
- Regitine ... 878

Phenylbutazone (Reduces diuretic, natriuretic, and antihypertensive effects). Products include:
- Butazolidin Capsules & Tablets ... 1027

Pindolol (Potentiated or additive effects). Products include:
- Visken Tablets ... 2036

Piroxicam (Reduces diuretic, natriuretic, and antihypertensive effects). Products include:
- Feldene Capsules ... 1777

Polythiazide (Potentiated or additive effects). Products include:
- Minizide Capsules ... 1779
- Renese Tablets ... 1785
- Renese-R Tablets ... 1786

Prazosin Hydrochloride (Potentiated or additive effects). Products include:
- Minipress Capsules ... 1778
- Minizide Capsules ... 1779

Prednisolone Acetate (Hypokalemia). Products include:
- AK-Cide Sterile Ophthalmic Ointment & Suspension ... ⊙ 202
- Blephamide Liquifilm Sterile Ophthalmic Suspension ... 586
- Blephamide S.O.P. Sterile Ophthalmic Ointment ... 586
- Cetapred Ointment ... ⊙ 220
- ⅛% Econopred & 1% Econopred Plus ... ⊙ 217
- Isopto Cetapred Suspension ... ⊙ 220
- Metimyd ... ⊙ 306
- Poly-Pred Liquifilm ... ⊙ 250
- Pred Forte ... ⊙ 252
- Pred Mild ... ⊙ 254
- Pred-G Liquifilm Sterile Ophthalmic Suspension ... ⊙ 252
- Pred-G S.O.P. Sterile Ophthalmic Ointment ... ⊙ 253
- Vasocidin Ointment ... ⊙ 275

Prednisolone Sodium Phosphate (Hypokalemia). Products include:
- AK-Pred ... ⊙ 205
- Hydeltrasol Injection, Sterile ... 1476
- Inflamase ... ⊙ 274
- Pediapred Oral Liquid ... 987
- Vasocidin Ophthalmic Solution ... ⊙ 276

Prednisolone Tebutate (Hypokalemia). Products include:
- Hydeltra-T.B.A. Sterile Suspension 1478

Prednisone (Hypokalemia). Products include:
- Deltasone Tablets ... 2332

Propoxyphene Hydrochloride (Orthostatic hypotension may be aggravated). Products include:
- Darvon ... 1256
- Wygesic Tablets ... 2540

Propoxyphene Napsylate (Orthostatic hypotension may be aggravated). Products include:
- Darvon-N/Darvocet-N ... 1254

Propranolol Hydrochloride (Potentiated or additive effects). Products include:
- Inderal ... 2459
- Inderal LA Long Acting Capsules ... 2461
- Inderide Tablets ... 2463
- Inderide LA Long Acting Capsules .. 2465

Ramipril (Potentiated or additive effects). Products include:
- Altace Capsules ... 1086

Rauwolfia Serpentina (Potentiated or additive effects). Products include:
- Raudixin Tablets ... 1803
- Rauzide Tablets ... 1804

Rescinnamine (Potentiated or additive effects).
- No products indexed under this heading.

Reserpine (Potentiated or additive effects). Products include:
- Diupres Tablets ... 1461
- Hydromox R Tablets ... 1209
- Hydropres Tablets ... 1485
- Renese-R Tablets ... 1786
- Salutensin/Salutensin-Demi ... 719
- Ser-Ap-Es Tablets ... 881
- Serpasil Tablets ... 883
- Serpasil-Apresoline Tablets ... 884
- Serpasil-Esidrix Tablets ... 886

Secobarbital Sodium (Orthostatic hypotension may be aggravated). Products include:
- Seconal Sodium Pulvules ... 1296

Sodium Nitroprusside (Potentiated or additive effects). Products include:
- Nipride I.V. Infusion ... 1909

Sufentanil Citrate (Orthostatic hypotension may be aggravated). Products include:
- Sufenta Injection ... 1147

Sulindac (Reduces diuretic, natriuretic, and antihypertensive effects). Products include:
- Clinoril Tablets ... 1433

Terazosin Hydrochloride (Potentiated or additive effects). Products include:
- Hytrin Tablets ... 529

Thiamylal Sodium (Orthostatic hypotension may be aggravated). Products include:
- Surital Ampoules, Steri-Vials ... 1764

Timolol Maleate (Potentiated or additive effects). Products include:
- Blocadren Tablets ... 1429
- Timolide Tablets ... 1547
- Timoptic in Ocudose ... 1552
- Timoptic Sterile Ophthalmic Solution ... 1550

Tolazamide (Dosage adjustment of the antidiabetic drug may be required). Products include:
- Tolinase Tablets ... 2365

Tolbutamide (Dosage adjustment of the antidiabetic drug may be required). Products include:
- Orinase Tablets ... 2354

Tolmetin Sodium (Reduces diuretic, natriuretic, and antihypertensive effects). Products include:
- Tolectin (200, 400 and 600 mg) .. 1379

Triamcinolone (Hypokalemia).
- No products indexed under this heading.

Triamcinolone Acetonide (Hypokalemia). Products include:
- Aristocort A ... 1010
- Azmacort Inhaler ... 1837
- Kenalog Cream, Lotion & Ointment 2401
- Kenalog-10 Injection ... 2402
- Kenalog-40 Injection ... 2403
- Kenalog in Orabase ... 604
- Kenalog Spray ... 2401
- Mycolog II Cream and Ointment ... 2407
- Mytrex Cream & Ointment ... 2080
- Nasacort Nasal Inhaler ... 1844

Triamcinolone Diacetate (Hypokalemia). Products include:
- Aristocort Suspension ... 1008

Triamcinolone Hexacetonide (Hypokalemia). Products include:
- Aristospan Suspension ... 1011

Trimethaphan Camsylate (Potentiated or additive effects). Products include:
- Arfonad Ampuls ... 1887

Tubocurarine Chloride (Increased responsiveness to tubocurarine).
- No products indexed under this heading.

DIURIL SODIUM INTRAVENOUS

(Chlorothiazide Sodium) ... 1463

May interact with lithium preparations, corticosteroids, insulin, nonsteroidal anti-inflammatory agents, barbiturates, narcotic analgesics, cardiac glycosides, antihypertensives, oral hypoglycemic agents, and certain other agents. Compounds in these categories include:

Acebutolol Hydrochloride (Potentiated or additive effects). Products include:
- Sectral Capsules ... 2520

ACTH (Hypokalemia).
- No products indexed under this heading.

Alcohol (Potentiation of orthostatic hypotension).

Alfentanil Hydrochloride (Potentiation of orthostatic hypotension). Products include:
- Alfenta Injection ... 1131

Aprobarbital (Potentiation of orthostatic hypotension). Products include:
- Alurate Elixir ... 1883

Atenolol (Potentiated or additive effects). Products include:
- Tenoretic Tablets ... 1105
- Tenormin Tablets and I.V. Injection 1107

Benazepril Hydrochloride (Potentiated or additive effects). Products include:
- Lotensin Tablets ... 872

Bendroflumethiazide (Potentiated or additive effects). Products include:
- Corzide Tablets ... 702
- Naturetin Tablets ... 1789
- Rauzide Tablets ... 1804

Betamethasone Acetate (Hypokalemia). Products include:
- Celestone Soluspan Suspension ... 2081

Betamethasone Sodium Phosphate (Hypokalemia). Products include:
- Celestone Soluspan Suspension ... 2081

Betaxolol Hydrochloride (Potentiated or additive effects). Products include:
- Betoptic Sterile Ophthalmic Solution ... 569
- Betoptic S Sterile Ophthalmic Suspension ... 570
- Kerlone Tablets ... 2172

Buprenorphine (Potentiation of orthostatic hypotension).
- No products indexed under this heading.

Butabarbital (Potentiation of orthostatic hypotension). Products include:
- Pyridium Plus ... 1764

Butalbital (Potentiation of orthostatic hypotension aggravated). Products include:
- Esgic-Plus Tablets ... 1002
- Esgic Tablets & Capsules ... 1001
- Fioricet Tablets ... 2006
- Fiorinal Capsules ... 2007
- Fiorinal with Codeine Capsules ... 2008
- Fiorinal Tablets ... 2007
- Phrenilin ... 838
- Sedapap Tablets 50 mg/650 mg .. 1360

Captopril (Potentiated or additive effects). Products include:
- Capoten ... 2255
- Capozide ... 2258

Carteolol Hydrochloride (Potentiated or additive effects). Products include:
- Cartrol Tablets ... 507

Chlorpropamide (Dosage adjustment of oral hypoglycemic agent may be necessary). Products include:
- Diabinese Tablets ... 1775

Chlorthalidone (Potentiated or additive effects). Products include:
- Combipres Tablets ... 678
- Tenoretic Tablets ... 1105
- Thalitone Tablets ... 687

Clonidine (Potentiated or additive effects). Products include:
- Catapres-TTS ... 677

Clonidine Hydrochloride (Potentiated or additive effects). Products include:
- Catapres Tablets ... 676
- Combipres Tablets ... 678

Codeine (Potentiation of orthostatic hypotension). Products include:
- Calcidrine Syrup ... 506

Codeine Phosphate (Potentiation of orthostatic hypotension). Products include:
- Actifed with Codeine Cough Syrup.. 752
- Cheracol Cough Syrup ... 1853
- Codimal PH Syrup ... 846
- Dimetane-DC Cough Syrup ... 1857
- Empirin with Codeine Phosphate Nos. 2, 3 & 4 ... 764
- Fiorinal with Codeine Capsules ... 2008
- Isoclor Expectorant ... 982
- Naldecon CX Adult Liquid ... ▣ 521
- Novahistine DH ... 1342
- Novahistine Expectorant ... 1343
- Nucofed Capsules ... 2219
- Nucofed Expectorant ... 2219
- Nucofed Pediatric Expectorant ... 2220
- Nucofed Syrup ... 2219
- Phenaphen with Codeine Capsules 1865
- Phenaphen-650 with Codeine Tablets ... 1866
- Phenergan with Codeine ... 2497
- Phenergan VC with Codeine ... 2501
- Robitussin A-C Syrup ... 1875
- Robitussin-DAC Syrup ... 1875
- Ryna ... ▣ 741
- Soma Compound w/Codeine Tablets ... 2390
- Triaminic Expectorant w/Codeine .. 1996
- Tussi-Organidin Liquid ... 2391
- Tylenol with Codeine ... 1381

Codeine Polistirex (Potentiation of orthostatic hypotension).
- No products indexed under this heading.

Cortisone Acetate (Hypokalemia). Products include:
- Cortone Acetate Sterile Suspension ... 1437
- Cortone Acetate Tablets ... 1439

Deserpidine (Potentiated or additive effects). Products include:
- Enduronyl ... 518

Harmonyl Tablets 528
Oreticyl 545

Deslanoside (Increased ventricular irritability).
No products indexed under this heading.

Dexamethasone (Hypokalemia). Products include:
AK-Trol Ointment & Suspension .... ⊙ 207
Decadron Elixir 1445
Decadron Tablets 1447
Decaspray Topical Aerosol 1459
Dexacidin .... ⊙ 272
Maxidex Sterile Ophthalmic Suspension .... ⊙ 223
Maxitrol Ophthalmic Ointment/Suspension .... ⊙ 223
TobraDex Ophthalmic Suspension and Ointment .... ⊙ 228

Dexamethasone Acetate (Hypokalemia). Products include:
Dalalone D.P. Injectable 999
Decadron-LA Sterile Suspension 1457

Dexamethasone Sodium Phosphate (Hypokalemia). Products include:
AK-Dex .... ⊙ 203
Decadron Phosphate Respihaler 1454
Decadron Phosphate Sterile Ophthalmic Ointment 1453
Decadron Phosphate Sterile Ophthalmic Solution 1453
Decadron Phosphate Topical Cream 1455
Decadron Phosphate Turbinaire 1456
Maxidex Sterile Ophthalmic Ointment .... ⊙ 222
NeoDecadron Sterile Ophthalmic Ointment 1517
NeoDecadron Sterile Ophthalmic Solution 1518
NeoDecadron Topical Cream 1518

Dezocine (Potentiation of orthostatic hypotension).

Diazoxide (Potentiated or additive effects). Products include:
Hyperstat I.V. Injection 2095
Proglycem 649

Diclofenac Sodium (Reduces diuretic, natriuretic, and antihypertensive effects). Products include:
Voltaren Ophthalmic Sterile Ophthalmic Solution .... ⊙ 268
Voltaren Tablets 1042

Digitoxin (Increased ventricular irritability). Products include:
Crystodigin Tablets 1253

Digoxin (Increased ventricular irritability). Products include:
Lanoxicaps 772
Lanoxin Elixir Pediatric 775
Lanoxin Injection 778
Lanoxin Injection Pediatric 781
Lanoxin Tablets 783

Doxazosin Mesylate (Potentiated or additive effects). Products include:
Cardura Tablets 1941

Enalapril Maleate (Potentiated or additive effects). Products include:
Vaseretic Tablets 1559
Vasotec Tablets 1564

Enalaprilat (Potentiated or additive effects). Products include:
Vasotec I.V. 1562

Esmolol Hydrochloride (Potentiated or additive effects). Products include:
Brevibloc Injection 942

Etodolac (Reduces diuretic, natriuretic, and antihypertensive effects). Products include:
Lodine Capsules 2468

Felodipine (Potentiated or additive effects). Products include:
Plendil Extended-Release Tablets 1526

Fenoprofen Calcium (Reduces diuretic, natriuretic, and antihypertensive effects). Products include:
Nalfon Pulvules & Tablets 919

Fentanyl (Potentiation of orthostatic hypotension). Products include:
Duragesic Transdermal System 1133

Fentanyl Citrate (Potentiation of orthostatic hypotension). Products include:
Innovar Injection 1141
Sublimaze Injection 1146

Flurbiprofen (Reduces diuretic, natriuretic, and antihypertensive effects). Products include:
Ansaid Tablets 2319

Fosinopril Sodium (Potentiated or additive effects). Products include:
Monopril Tablets 1406

Furosemide (Potentiated or additive effects). Products include:
Lasix 1093

Glipizide (Dosage adjustment of oral hypoglycemic agent may be necessary). Products include:
Glucotrol 1952

Glyburide (Dosage adjustment of oral hypoglycemic agent may be necessary). Products include:
DiaBeta 1091
Micronase Tablets 2350

Guanabenz Acetate (Potentiated or additive effects). Products include:
Wytensin Tablets 2542

Guanethidine Monosulfate (Potentiated or additive effects). Products include:
Esimil Tablets 864
Ismelin Tablets 869

Hydralazine Hydrochloride (Potentiated or additive effects). Products include:
Apresazide Capsules 854
Apresoline Hydrochloride Parenteral (Ampuls) 856
Apresoline Hydrochloride Tablets 855
Apresoline-Esidrix Tablets 857
Ser-Ap-Es Tablets 881
Serpasil-Apresoline Tablets 884

Hydrochlorothiazide (Potentiated or additive effects). Products include:
Aldactazide 2150
Aldoril Tablets 1418
Apresazide Capsules 854
Apresoline-Esidrix Tablets 857
Capozide 2258
Dyazide Capsules 2208
Esidrix Tablets 863
Esimil Tablets 864
HydroDIURIL Tablets 1484
Hydropres Tablets 1485
Inderide Tablets 2463
Inderide LA Long Acting Capsules 2465
Lopressor HCT Tablets 1034
Maxzide 1215
Moduretic Tablets 1510
Normozide Tablets 2112
Oretic Tablets 544
Oreticyl 545
Prinzide Tablets 1540
Ser-Ap-Es Tablets 881
Serpasil-Esidrix Tablets 886
Timolide Tablets 1547
Trandate HCT Tablets 579
Vaseretic Tablets 1559
Zestoretic 2274

Hydrocodone Bitartrate (Potentiation of orthostatic hypotension). Products include:
Anexsia 5/500 Tablets 2196
Anexsia 7.5/650 Tablets 2197
Azdone Tablets 844
Codiclear DH Syrup 845
Codimal DH Syrup 846
Damason-P 1356
Hycodan Syrup, Tablets 927
Hycomine Compound Tablets 929
Hycomine Syrup 927
Hycotuss Expectorant Syrup 930
Hydrocet Capsules 835
Lortab ASA Tablets 2414
Lortab 2412
Ru-Tuss with Hydrocodone 694
Triaminic Expectorant DH 1995
Vicodin Tablets 1187
Vicodin ES Tablets 1189
Zydone Capsules 941

Hydrocodone Polistirex (Potentiation of orthostatic hypotension). Products include:
Tussionex Extended-Release Suspension 988

Hydrocortisone (Hypokalemia). Products include:
AK-Spore H.C. .... ⊙ 206
Bactine Hydrocortisone Anti-Itch Cream .... ▣ 625
CaldeCORT Anti-Itch Hydrocortisone Spray .... ▣ 560
Carmol HC Cream 1% 2296
Cortaid Spray .... ▣ 735
Cortenema 2244
Cortisporin Ointment 758
Cortisporin Ophthalmic Ointment Sterile 758
Cortisporin Ophthalmic Suspension Sterile 759
Cortisporin Otic Solution Sterile 760
Cortisporin Otic Suspension Sterile 760
Cortizone-5 Creme & Ointment .... ▣ 732
Dermolate Anti-Itch Cream .... ▣ 697
Eldecort Cream 1.0% 1113
Eldecort Cream 1.0% and 2.5% 1113
Fungoid HC Creme 1770
Hydrocortone Tablets 1482
Hytone 909
LazerSporin-C Solution 1770
Massengill Medicated Soft Cloth Towelettes 2192
Nutracort Cream & Lotion 1684
PediOtic Suspension Sterile 797
Synacort Creams 1%, 2.5% 2296
Vanoxide-HC Acne Lotion 911
Vioform-Hydrocortisone Cream and Mild Cream 889
Vioform-Hydrocortisone Ointment 889
VōSoL HC Otic Solution 2392
Vytone Cream 1% 911

Hydrocortisone Acetate (Hypokalemia). Products include:
Analpram-HC Rectal Cream 1% and 2.5% 970
Anusol-HC Cream 1690
Anusol-HC Suppositories 1691
Caldecort .... ▣ 560
Carmol HC Cream 1% 2296
Chloromycetin Hydrocortisone Ophthalmic 1694
Coly-Mycin S Otic w/Neomycin & Hydrocortisone 1708
Cortaid .... ▣ 735
Cortef Feminine Itch Cream .... ▣ 735
Corticaine .... ▣ 682
Cortifoam 1827
Cortisporin Cream 757
Epifoam 1828
Gynecort 5 Creme .... ▣ 556
Hydrocortone Acetate Sterile Suspension 1479
Lanacort 5 Creme and Ointment .... ▣ 557
Mantadil Cream 789
Ophthocort .... ⊙ 301
Orabase HCA Oral Paste 890
Pramosone Cream, Lotion & Ointment 971
ProctoCream-HC 1834
Proctofoam-HC 1835

Hydrocortisone Sodium Phosphate (Hypokalemia). Products include:
Hydrocortone Phosphate Injection, Sterile 1481

Hydrocortisone Sodium Succinate (Hypokalemia). Products include:
Solu-Cortef Sterile Powder 2361

Hydroflumethiazide (Potentiated or additive effects). Products include:
Diucardin Tablets 2450
Saluron 718
Salutensin/Salutensin-Demi 719

Ibuprofen (Reduces diuretic, natriuretic, and antihypertensive effects). Products include:
Advil Cold & Sinus Caplets (formerly CoAdvil) 2416
Advil Ibuprofen Tablets and Caplets 2416
Children's Advil Suspension 2426
CoAdvil .... ▣ 748
Dristan Sinus Caplets 2419
Haltran Tablets .... ▣ 668
Ibuprofen .... ▣ 631
Medipren ibuprofen Caplets and Tablets 1362
Midol 200 Cramp Relief Formula .... ▣ 570
Motrin Tablets 2351
Motrin IB Caplets and Tablets .... ▣ 736
Nuprin Ibuprofen/Analgesic Tablets & Caplets 752
PediaProfen Suspension 1363
Rufen Tablets 691
Trendar Ibuprofen Tablets .... ▣ 756

Indapamide (Potentiated or additive effects). Products include:
Lozol Tablets 1843

Indomethacin (Reduces diuretic, natriuretic, and antihypertensive effects). Products include:
Indocin 1487

Indomethacin Sodium Trihydrate (Reduces diuretic, natriuretic, and antihypertensive effects). Products include:
Indocin I.V. 1490

Insulin, Human (Altered insulin requirements).
No products indexed under this heading.

Insulin, Human Isophane Suspension (Altered insulin requirements). Products include:
Humulin N, 100 Units 1270

Insulin, Human NPH (Altered insulin requirements). Products include:
Insulatard NPH Human 1627
Novolin N 1627
Novolin N PenFill Cartridges 1628
Novolin N Prefilled 1628

Insulin, Human Regular (Altered insulin requirements). Products include:
Humulin BR, 100 Units 1268
Humulin R, 100 Units 1272
Novolin R 1627
Novolin R PenFill Cartridges 1628
Novolin R Prefilled 1629
Velosulin Human 1628

Insulin, Human, Zinc Suspension (Altered insulin requirements). Products include:
Humulin L, 100 Units 1268
Humulin U, 100 Units 1272
Novolin L 1627

Insulin, NPH (Altered insulin requirements). Products include:
NPH, 40 & 100 Units 1273
Beef NPH, 100 Units 1274
Pork NPH, 100 Units 1275
Insulatard NPH 1626
NPH Insulin 1626
NPH Purified Pork Isophane Insulin 1626

Insulin, Regular (Altered insulin requirements). Products include:
Regular, 40 & 100 Units 1273
Beef Regular, 100 Units 1275
Pork Regular, 100 Units 1275
Pork Regular (Concentrated), 500 Units 1276
Regular Insulin 1625
Regular Purified Pork Insulin 1626
Velosulin 1627

Insulin, Zinc Crystals (Altered insulin requirements). Products include:
NPH, 40 & 100 Units 1273

Insulin, Zinc Suspension (Altered insulin requirements). Products include:
Lente, 40 & 100 Units 1272
Protamine, Zinc, 40 & 100 Units 1273
Lente Iletin I 1272
Beef Lente, 100 Units 1274
Beef Protamine Zinc, 100 Units 1274
Pork Lente, 100 Units 1275
Pork, Protamine, Zinc, 100 Units 1275
Lente Insulin 1626
Lente Purified Pork Insulin 1626
Semilente Insulin 1625
Ultralente Insulin 1626

Isradipine (Potentiated or additive effects). Products include:
- DynaCirc Capsules 2004

Ketoprofen (Reduces diuretic, natriuretic, and antihypertensive effects). Products include:
- Orudis Capsules 2488

Ketorolac Tromethamine (Reduces diuretic, natriuretic, and antihypertensive effects). Products include:
- Toradol IM Injection 2302

Labetalol Hydrochloride (Potentiated or additive effects). Products include:
- Normodyne Injection 2108
- Normodyne Tablets 2110
- Normozide Tablets 2112
- Trandate HCT Tablets 579
- Trandate Injection 577
- Trandate Tablets 579

Levorphanol Tartrate (Potentiation of orthostatic hypotension). Products include:
- Levo-Dromoran 1906

Lisinopril (Potentiated or additive effects). Products include:
- Prinivil Tablets 1538
- Prinzide Tablets 1540
- Zestoretic 2274
- Zestril Tablets 2277

Lithium Carbonate (High risk of lithium toxicity). Products include:
- Eskalith 2214
- Lithane Tablets 1596
- Lithium Carbonate Capsules & Tablets 1984
- Lithobid Tablets 870

Lithium Citrate (High risk of lithium toxicity). Products include:
- Cibalith-S 870

Mecamylamine Hydrochloride (Potentiated or additive effects). Products include:
- Inversine Tablets 1492

Meclofenamate Sodium (Reduces diuretic, natriuretic, and antihypertensive effects). Products include:
- Meclomen Capsules 1739

Mefenamic Acid (Reduces diuretic, natriuretic, and antihypertensive effects). Products include:
- Ponstel 1758

Meperidine Hydrochloride (Potentiation of orthostatic hypotension). Products include:
- Demerol 2047
- Mepergan Injection 2479

Mephobarbital (Potentiation of orthostatic hypotension). Products include:
- Mebaral Tablets 2061

Methadone Hydrochloride (Potentiation of orthostatic hypotension). Products include:
- Dolophine Hydrochloride Ampoules & Vials 1260
- Dolophine Hydrochloride Tablets 1261
- Methadone Hydrochloride Diskets 1284
- Methadone Hydrochloride Oral Solution & Tablets 1987

Methyclothiazide (Potentiated or additive effects). Products include:
- Enduron Tablets 517
- Enduronyl 518

Methyldopa (Potentiated or additive effects). Products include:
- Aldoclor Tablets 1413
- Aldomet Oral 1415
- Aldoril Tablets 1418

Methyldopate Hydrochloride (Potentiated or additive effects). Products include:
- Aldomet Ester HCl Injection 1417

Methylprednisolone Acetate (Hypokalemia). Products include:
- Depo-Medrol Sterile Aqueous Suspension 2334

Methylprednisolone Sodium Succinate (Hypokalemia). Products include:
- Solu-Medrol Sterile Powder 2363

Metolazone (Potentiated or additive effects). Products include:
- Diulo 2129
- Mykrox ½ mg Tablets 984
- Zaroxolyn Tablets 989

Metoprolol Tartrate (Potentiated or additive effects). Products include:
- Lopressor Ampuls 1032
- Lopressor HCT Tablets 1034
- Lopressor Tablets 1032

Metyrosine (Potentiated or additive effects). Products include:
- Demser Capsules 1460

Minoxidil (Potentiated or additive effects). Products include:
- Loniten Tablets 2346
- Rogaine Topical Solution 2357

Morphine Sulfate (Potentiation of orthostatic hypotension). Products include:
- Astramorph/PF Injection, USP (Preservative-Free) 618
- Duramorph 960
- Infumorph 200 and Infumorph 500 Sterile Solutions 962
- MS Contin Tablets 1814
- MSIR 1817
- Oramorph SR (Morphine Sulfate Sustained Release Tablets) 1988
- Roxanol 1991

Nadolol (Potentiated or additive effects). Products include:
- Corgard Tablets 701
- Corzide Tablets 702

Naproxen (Reduces diuretic, natriuretic, and antihypertensive effects). Products include:
- Naprosyn 2297

Naproxen Sodium (Reduces diuretic, natriuretic, and antihypertensive effects). Products include:
- Anaprox and Anaprox DS Tablets 2288

Nicardipine Hydrochloride (Potentiated or additive effects). Products include:
- Cardene Capsules 2290

Nitroglycerin (Potentiated or additive effects). Products include:
- Deponit NTG Transdermal Delivery System 2143
- Minitran Transdermal Delivery System 1312
- Nitro-Bid Ointment 1339
- Nitro-Bid Capsules 1338
- Nitrodisc 2176
- Nitro-Dur (nitroglycerin) Transdermal Infusion System 1164
- Nitrogard Tablets 1004
- Nitrolingual Spray 1846
- Nitrostat Tablets 1743
- Transderm-Nitro Transdermal Therapeutic System 2283

Norepinephrine Bitartrate (Decreased arterial responsiveness to norepinephrine). Products include:
- Levophed Bitartrate Injection 2054

Opium Alkaloids (Potentiation of orthostatic hypotension). Products include:
- B & O No. 15A & No. 16A Supprettes 2395
- Pantopon Injectable 1911

Oxycodone Hydrochloride (Potentiation of orthostatic hypotension). Products include:
- Percocet Tablets 950
- Percodan 951
- Roxicodone Tablets, Oral Solution & Intensol (Oxycodone) 1992
- Tylox Capsules 1382

Penbutolol Sulfate (Potentiated or additive effects). Products include:
- Levatol 1832

Pentobarbital Sodium (Potentiation of orthostatic hypotension). Products include:
- Nembutal Sodium Capsules 534
- Nembutal Sodium Solution 536
- Nembutal Sodium Suppositories 538

Phenobarbital (Potentiation of orthostatic hypotension). Products include:
- Arco-Lase Plus Tablets 607
- Bellergal-S Tablets 1998
- Bronkolixir .... ◘ 761
- Bronkotabs Tablets .... ◘ 762
- Donnatal 1858
- Donnatal Extentabs 1859
- Donnatal Tablets 1858
- Donnazyme Tablets 1860
- Kinesed Tablets 2272
- Phenobarbital Elixir and Tablets 1293
- Primatene Tablets-P Formula 2421
- Quadrinal Tablets 1183
- Tedral SA 1765

Phenoxybenzamine Hydrochloride (Potentiated or additive effects). Products include:
- Dibenzyline Capsules 2207

Phentolamine Mesylate (Potentiated or additive effects). Products include:
- Regitine 878

Phenylbutazone (Reduces diuretic, natriuretic, and antihypertensive effects). Products include:
- Butazolidin Capsules & Tablets 1027

Pindolol (Potentiated or additive effects). Products include:
- Visken Tablets 2036

Piroxicam (Reduces diuretic, natriuretic, and antihypertensive effects). Products include:
- Feldene Capsules 1777

Polythiazide (Potentiated or additive effects). Products include:
- Minizide Capsules 1779
- Renese Tablets 1785
- Renese-R Tablets 1786

Prazosin Hydrochloride (Potentiated or additive effects). Products include:
- Minipress Capsules 1778
- Minizide Capsules 1779

Prednisolone Acetate (Hypokalemia). Products include:
- AK-Cide Sterile Ophthalmic Ointment & Suspension .... ⊙ 202
- Blephamide Liquifilm Sterile Ophthalmic Suspension 586
- Blephamide S.O.P. Sterile Ophthalmic Ointment 586
- Cetapred Ointment .... ⊙ 220
- ⅛% Econopred & 1% Econopred Plus .... ⊙ 217
- Isopto Cetapred Suspension .... ⊙ 220
- Metimyd .... ⊙ 306
- Poly-Pred Liquifilm .... ⊙ 250
- Pred Forte .... ⊙ 252
- Pred Mild .... ⊙ 254
- Pred-G Liquifilm Sterile Ophthalmic Suspension .... ⊙ 252
- Pred-G S.O.P. Sterile Ophthalmic Ointment .... ⊙ 253
- Vasocidin Ointment .... ⊙ 275

Prednisolone Sodium Phosphate (Hypokalemia). Products include:
- AK-Pred .... ⊙ 205
- Hydeltrasol Injection, Sterile 1476
- Inflamase .... ⊙ 274
- Pediapred Oral Liquid 987
- Vasocidin Ophthalmic Solution .... ⊙ 276

Prednisolone Tebutate (Hypokalemia). Products include:
- Hydeltra-T.B.A. Sterile Suspension 1478

Prednisone (Hypokalemia). Products include:
- Deltasone Tablets 2332

Propoxyphene Hydrochloride (Potentiation of orthostatic hypotension). Products include:
- Darvon 1256
- Wygesic Tablets 2540

Propoxyphene Napsylate (Potentiation of orthostatic hypotension). Products include:
- Darvon-N/Darvocet-N 1254

Propranolol Hydrochloride (Potentiated or additive effects). Products include:
- Inderal 2459
- Inderal LA Long Acting Capsules 2461
- Inderide Tablets 2463
- Inderide LA Long Acting Capsules 2465

Ramipril (Potentiated or additive effects). Products include:
- Altace Capsules 1086

Rauwolfia Serpentina (Potentiated or additive effects). Products include:
- Raudixin Tablets 1803
- Rauzide Tablets 1804

Rescinnamine (Potentiated or additive effects).
- No products indexed under this heading.

Reserpine (Potentiated or additive effects). Products include:
- Diupres Tablets 1461
- Hydromox R Tablets 1209
- Hydropres Tablets 1485
- Renese-R Tablets 1786
- Salutensin/Salutensin-Demi 719
- Ser-Ap-Es Tablets 881
- Serpasil Tablets 883
- Serpasil-Apresoline Tablets 884
- Serpasil-Esidrix Tablets 886

Secobarbital Sodium (Potentiation of orthostatic hypotension). Products include:
- Seconal Sodium Pulvules 1296

Sodium Nitroprusside (Potentiated or additive effects). Products include:
- Nipride I.V. Infusion 1909

Sufentanil Citrate (Potentiation of orthostatic hypotension). Products include:
- Sufenta Injection 1147

Sulindac (Reduces diuretic, natriuretic, and antihypertensive effects). Products include:
- Clinoril Tablets 1433

Terazosin Hydrochloride (Potentiated or additive effects). Products include:
- Hytrin Tablets 529

Thiamylal Sodium (Potentiation of orthostatic hypotension). Products include:
- Surital Ampoules, Steri-Vials 1764

Timolol Maleate (Potentiated or additive effects). Products include:
- Blocadren Tablets 1429
- Timolide Tablets 1547
- Timoptic in Ocudose 1552
- Timoptic Sterile Ophthalmic Solution 1550

Tolazamide (Dosage adjustment of oral hypoglycemic agent may be necessary). Products include:
- Tolinase Tablets 2365

Tolbutamide (Dosage adjustment of oral hypoglycemic agent may be necessary). Products include:
- Orinase Tablets 2354

Tolmetin Sodium (Reduces diuretic, natriuretic, and antihypertensive effects). Products include:
- Tolectin (200, 400 and 600 mg) 1379

Triamcinolone (Hypokalemia).
- No products indexed under this heading.

Triamcinolone Acetonide (Hypokalemia). Products include:
- Aristocort A 1010
- Azmacort Inhaler 1837
- Kenalog Cream, Lotion & Ointment 2401
- Kenalog-10 Injection 2402
- Kenalog-40 Injection 2403
- Kenalog in Orabase 604
- Kenalog Spray 2401
- Mycolog II Cream and Ointment 2407

Mytrex Cream & Ointment 2080
Nasacort Nasal Inhaler 1844

Triamcinolone Diacetate (Hypokalemia). Products include:
Aristocort Suspension 1008

Triamcinolone Hexacetonide (Hypokalemia). Products include:
Aristospan Suspension 1011

Trimethaphan Camsylate (Potentiated or additive effects). Products include:
Arfonad Ampuls 1887

Tubocurarine Chloride (Increased responsiveness to tubocurarine).
No products indexed under this heading.

DIURIL TABLETS
(Chlorothiazide) **1464**
See **Diuril Oral Suspension**

DOAN'S - EXTRA-STRENGTH ANALGESIC
(Magnesium Salicylate) .... ⊞ **549**
No interactions described in labeling.

DOAN'S - REGULAR STRENGTH ANALGESIC
(Magnesium Salicylate) .... ⊞ **549**
No interactions described in labeling.

DOBUTREX SOLUTION VIALS
(Dobutamine Hydrochloride) **1259**
May interact with beta blockers and certain other agents. Compounds in these categories include:

Acebutolol Hydrochloride (Increased peripheral-vascular resistance in patient who has recently received beta blocker). Products include:
Sectral Capsules 2520

Atenolol (Increased peripheral-vascular resistance in patient who has recently received beta blocker). Products include:
Tenoretic Tablets 1105
Tenormin Tablets and I.V. Injection 1107

Betaxolol Hydrochloride (Increased peripheral-vascular resistance in patient who has recently received beta blocker). Products include:
Betoptic Sterile Ophthalmic Solution 569
Betoptic S Sterile Ophthalmic Suspension 570
Kerlone Tablets 2172

Carteolol Hydrochloride (Increased peripheral-vascular resistance in patient who has recently received beta blocker). Products include:
Cartrol Tablets 507

Esmolol Hydrochloride (Increased peripheral-vascular resistance in patient who has recently received beta blocker). Products include:
Brevibloc Injection 942

Labetalol Hydrochloride (Increased peripheral-vascular resistance in patient who has recently received beta blocker). Products include:
Normodyne Injection 2108
Normodyne Tablets 2110
Normozide Tablets 2112
Trandate HCT Tablets 579
Trandate Injection 577
Trandate Tablets 579

Metoprolol Tartrate (Increased peripheral-vascular resistance in patient who has recently received beta blocker). Products include:
Lopressor Ampuls 1032
Lopressor HCT Tablets 1034
Lopressor Tablets 1032

Nadolol (Increased peripheral-vascular resistance in patient who has recently received beta blocker). Products include:
Corgard Tablets 701
Corzide Tablets 702

Penbutolol Sulfate (Increased peripheral-vascular resistance in patient who has recently received beta blocker). Products include:
Levatol 1832

Pindolol (Increased peripheral-vascular resistance in patient who has recently received beta blocker). Products include:
Visken Tablets 2036

Propranolol Hydrochloride (Increased peripheral-vascular resistance in patient who has recently received beta blocker). Products include:
Inderal 2459
Inderal LA Long Acting Capsules 2461
Inderide Tablets 2463
Inderide LA Long Acting Capsules 2465

Sodium Nitroprusside (Concomitant use results in a higher cardiac output and, usually, a lower pulmonary wedge pressure). Products include:
Nipride I.V. Infusion 1909

Timolol Maleate (Increased peripheral-vascular resistance in patient who has recently received beta blocker). Products include:
Blocadren Tablets 1429
Timolide Tablets 1547
Timoptic in Ocudose 1552
Timoptic Sterile Ophthalmic Solution 1550

DOCTAR GEL
(Coal Tar) **2079**
No interactions described in labeling.

DOLOBID TABLETS
(Diflunisal) **1465**
May interact with oral anticoagulants, antacids, and certain other agents. Compounds in these categories include:

Acetaminophen (Increased plasma levels of acetaminophen). Products include:
Acetaminophen Uniserts Suppositories 2374
Actifed Plus Caplets .... ⊞ 539
Actifed Plus Tablets .... ⊞ 540
Alka-Seltzer Advanced Formula Antacid & Non-Aspirin Pain Reliever .... ⊞ 620
Allerest .... ⊞ 559
Aspirin Free Anacin Maximum Strength Acetaminophen Film Coated Caplets 2417
Aspirin Free Anacin Maximum Strength Acetaminophen Film Coated Tablets 2417
Anacin-3 Regular Strength Acetaminophen Film Coated Tablets ⊞ 746
Anexsia 5/500 Tablets 2196
Anexsia 7.5/650 Tablets 2197
Benadryl Plus .... ⊞ 636
Benadryl Plus Nighttime .... ⊞ 637
Bufferin AF Nite Time Analgesic/Sleeping Aid Caplets 744
Allergy-Sinus Comtrex Multi-Symptom Allergy Sinus Formula Tablets & Caplets 746
Cough Formula Comtrex 746
Comtrex Multi-Symptom Cold Reliever Tablets/Caplets/Liqui-Gels/Liquid 745
Day-Night Comtrex 747
Non-Drowsy Comtrex 747
Congespirin For Children Aspirin Free Chewable Cold Tablets 748
Contac Cough & Sore Throat Formula .... ⊞ 712
Contac Jr. Children's Cold Medicine .... ⊞ 712
Contac Nighttime Cold Medicine .... ⊞ 713
Contac Severe Cold and Flu Formula Caplets .... ⊞ 711
Contac Sinus Caplets Maximum Strength Non-Drowsy Formula .... ⊞ 710
Contac Sinus Tablets Maximum Strength Non-Drowsy Formula .... ⊞ 710
Coricidin 'D' Decongestant Tablets .... ⊞ 695
Coricidin Demilets Tablets for Children .... ⊞ 696
Coricidin Tablets .... ⊞ 695
Darvon-N/Darvocet-N 1254
Datril Extra-Strength Analgesic Tablets 748
Dimetapp Plus Caplets .... ⊞ 675
Dorcol Children's Fever & Pain Reducer .... ⊞ 686
Dristan Decongestant/Antihistamine/ Analgesic Coated Caplets .... ⊞ 749
Dristan Cold Nasal Decongestant/ Antihistamine/ Analgesic Coated Tablets 2419
Dristan Advanced Formula Decongestant/Antihistamine/ Analgesic Tablets .... ⊞ 749
Maximum Strength Dristan Decongestant/Analgesic Coated Caplets .... ⊞ 750
No Drowsiness Dristan Cold Nasal Decongestant/Analgesic Coated Caplets 2420
Drixoral Plus Extended-Release Tablets .... ⊞ 699
Drixoral Sinus .... ⊞ 700
Esgic-Plus Tablets 1002
Esgic Tablets & Capsules 1001
Aspirin Free Excedrin Analgesic Caplets 748
Excedrin Extra-Strength Analgesic Tablets & Caplets 749
Excedrin P.M. Analgesic/Sleeping Aid Tablets, Caplets and Liquid 749
Sinus Excedrin Analgesic, Decongestant Tablets & Caplets 750
4-Way Cold Tablets 750
Feverall Sprinkle Caps 2374
Feverall Suppositories 2374
Fioricet Tablets 2006
Hycomine Compound Tablets 929
Hydrocet Capsules 835
Isocom Capsules 1629
Liquiprin .... ⊞ 618
Lortab 2412
Lurline PMS Tablets 972
Medi-Flu Caplet, Liquid .... ⊞ 640
Maximum Strength Midol Multi-Symptom Menstrual Formula .... ⊞ 571
Maximum Strength Midol PMS Premenstrual Syndrome Formula .... ⊞ 570
Regular Strength Midol Multi-Symptom Menstrual Formula .... ⊞ 570
Midrin Capsules 836
Ornex Caplets .... ⊞ 618
Children's Panadol Chewable Tablets, Liquid, Infants' Drops .... ⊞ 571
Junior Strength Panadol .... ⊞ 571
Maximum Strength Panadol Tablets and Caplets .... ⊞ 572
Percocet Tablets 950
Percogesic Analgesic Tablets .... ⊞ 660
Phenaphen with Codeine Capsules 1865
Phenaphen-650 with Codeine Tablets 1866
Phrenilin 838
Prēmsyn PMS Capsules & Caplets ⊞ 547
Pyrroxate Capsules .... ⊞ 669
Robitussin Night Relief .... ⊞ 677
Sedapap Tablets 50 mg/650 mg 1360
Sinarest .... ⊞ 562
Sine-Aid Maximum Strength Sinus Headache Caplets 1365
Sine-Aid Maximum Strength Sinus Headache Tablets 1365
Sine-Off Maximum Strength Allergy/Sinus Formula Caplets .... ⊞ 721
Sine-Off Maximum Strength No Drowsiness Formula Caplets .... ⊞ 722
Singlet Tablets .... ⊞ 598
Sinulin 840
Sinutab Maximum Strength .... ⊞ 641
Sinutab Maximum Strength Without Drowsiness Tablets & Caplets .... ⊞ 642
Sinutab Regular Strength Without Drowsiness Formula .... ⊞ 641
Sominex Pain Relief Formula .... ⊞ 723
St. Joseph Aspirin-Free Fever Reducer for Children Chewable Tablets, Liquid & Infant Drops .... ⊞ 704
St. Joseph Cold Tablets for Children .... ⊞ 704
St. Joseph Nighttime Cold Medicine .... ⊞ 705
Sudafed Sinus Caplets .... ⊞ 545
Sudafed Sinus Tablets .... ⊞ 545
Talacen 2070
Tempra, Acetaminophen .... ⊞ 613
TheraFlu Flu and Cold Medicine .... ⊞ 687
Triaminicin Tablets .... ⊞ 690
Tylenol acetaminophen Children's Chewable Tablets & Elixir 1366
Tylenol Allergy Sinus Medication Caplets and Gelcaps, Maximum Strength 1372
Tylenol with Codeine 1381
Children's Tylenol Cold Liquid Formula and Chewable Tablets 1368
Tylenol Cold & Flu Hot Medication, Packets 1369
Tylenol Cold & Flu No Drowsiness Hot Medication, Packets 1371
Tylenol Cold Medication Caplets and Tablets 1370
Tylenol Cold Medication, Effervescent Tablets 1369
Tylenol Cold Medication No Drowsiness Formula Caplets 1370
Tylenol Cold Night Time Medication Liquid 1371
Tylenol Cough Medication Liquid, Maximum Strength 1372
Tylenol Cough Medication Liquid with Decongestant, Maximum Strength 1372
Tylenol, Extra Strength, acetaminophen Adult Liquid Pain Reliever 1367
Tylenol, Extra Strength, acetaminophen Gelcaps, Caplets, Tablets 1367
Tylenol, Infants' Drops 1366
Tylenol, Junior Strength, acetaminophen Coated Caplets, Grape and Fruit Chewable Tablets 1366
Tylenol, Maximum Strength, Sinus Medication Gelcaps, Caplets and Tablets 1373
Tylenol, Regular Strength, acetaminophen Tablets and Caplets 1367
Tylenol PM, Extra Strength Caplets and Tablets 1368
Tylox Capsules 1382
Unisom Dual Relief Nighttime Sleep Aid/Analgesic 1774
Vanquish Analgesic Caplets .... ⊞ 574
Vicks Daycare .... ⊞ 660
Vicks Formula 44M Multi-Symptom Cough Medicine .... ⊞ 662
Vicks NyQuil Nighttime Colds Medicine-Original & Cherry Flavor .... ⊞ 664
Vicodin Tablets 1187
Vicodin ES Tablets 1189
Wygesic Tablets 2540
Zydone Capsules 941

Aluminum Carbonate Gel (Reduced plasma levels of Dolobid). Products include:
Basaljel 2438

Aluminum Hydroxide (Reduced plasma levels of Dolobid). Products include:
Cama Arthritis Pain Reliever .... ⊞ 685
Gaviscon Extra Strength Relief Formula Liquid Antacid .... ⊞ 594
Gaviscon Extra Strength Relief Formula Antacid Tablets .... ⊞ 594
Gaviscon Liquid Antacid .... ⊞ 594
Gelusil Liquid & Tablets .... ⊞ 639
Extra Strength Maalox Plus Suspension 1850
Maalox TC Suspension 1851
Maalox Plus Tablets .... ⊞ 655
Extra Strength Maalox Plus Tablets 1850
Nephrox Suspension .... ⊞ 563
WinGel Liquid & Tablets .... ⊞ 761

Aluminum Hydroxide Gel (Reduced plasma levels of Dolobid). Products include:
ALternaGEL Liquid 1154
Aludrox Oral Suspension 2428

Amphojel Suspension 2429
Amphojel Suspension without Flavor 2429
Mylanta Liquid 1155
Mylanta Double Strength Liquid 1155

Aluminum Hydroxide Gel, Dried (Reduced plasma levels of Dolobid). Products include:
Alu-Tab/Alu-Cap 1309
Amphojel Tablets 2429
Ascriptin A/D Caplets 1850
Regular Strength Ascriptin Tablets 1850
Gaviscon Antacid Tablets .... ▣ 593
Gaviscon-2 Antacid Tablets .... ▣ 594
Mylanta Tablets 1155
Mylanta Double Strength Tablets 1155

Aspirin (Small decrease in diflunisal levels). Products include:
Alka-Seltzer Effervescent Antacid and Pain Reliever 1568
Alka-Seltzer Extra Strength Effervescent Antacid and Pain Reliever 1570
Alka-Seltzer (Flavored) Effervescent Antacid and Pain Reliever 1569
Alka-Seltzer Plus Cold Medicine .... ▣ 623
Alka-Seltzer Plus Night-Time Cold Medicine .... ▣ 623
Alka Seltzer Plus Sinus Allergy Medicine .... ▣ 624
Anacin Coated Analgesic Caplets 2417
Anacin Coated Analgesic Tablets 2417
Anacin Maximum Strength Analgesic Coated Tablets 2417
Maximum Strength Arthritis Pain Formula By the Makers of Anacin Analgesic Tablets and Caplets 2418
Arthritis Pain Formula by the Makers of Anacin Analgesic Tablets and Caplets .... ▣ 747
Arthritis Strength BC Powder .... ▣ 516
Ascriptin A/D Caplets 1850
Regular Strength Ascriptin Tablets 1850
Azdone Tablets 844
BC Powder .... ▣ 517
BC Cold Powder .... ▣ 517
Children's Bayer Chewable Aspirin .... ▣ 564
Genuine Bayer Aspirin Tablets & Caplets .... ▣ 564
Maximum Bayer Aspirin Tablets & Caplets .... ▣ 566
Bayer Plus Aspirin Tablets .... ▣ 567
Therapy Bayer Aspirin Caplets .... ▣ 568
8 Hour Bayer Timed-Release Aspirin .... ▣ 566
Arthritis Strength Bufferin Analgesic Caplets 744
Extra Strength Bufferin Analgesic Tablets 745
Bufferin Analgesic Tablets and Caplets 743
Cama Arthritis Pain Reliever .... ▣ 685
Damason-P 1356
Easprin 1719
Ecotrin Enteric Coated Aspirin Maximum Strength Tablets and Caplets 2189
Ecotrin Enteric Coated Aspirin Regular Strength Tablets and Caplets 2189
Empirin Aspirin .... ▣ 541
Empirin with Codeine Phosphate Nos. 2, 3 & 4 764
Equagesic Tablets 2451
Excedrin Extra-Strength Analgesic Tablets & Caplets 749
4-Way Cold Tablets 750
Fiorinal Capsules 2007
Fiorinal with Codeine Capsules 2008
Fiorinal Tablets 2007
Lortab ASA Tablets 2414
Momentum Muscular Backache Formula .... ▣ 751
Norgesic 1314
Norwich Extra-Strength Aspirin .... ▣ 546
Norwich Regular Strength Aspirin ▣ 547
P-A-C Analgesic Tablets .... ▣ 669
Percodan 951
Robaxisal Tablets 1872
Sine-Off Sinus Medicine Tablets-Aspirin Formula .... ▣ 722
Soma Compound w/Codeine Tablets 2390
Soma Compound Tablets 2389
St. Joseph Adult Chewable Aspirin (81 mg.) .... ▣ 703
Synalgos-DC Capsules 2525
Talwin Compound 2072
Ursinus Inlay-Tabs .... ▣ 691
Vanquish Analgesic Caplets .... ▣ 574
Zorprin Tablets 698

Cyclosporine (Increased cyclosporine-induced toxicity). Products include:
Sandimmune 2024

Dicumarol (Prolonged prothrombin time; adjustment of dosage of oral anticoagulants may be required). Products include:
Dicumarol Tablets 516

Dihydroxyaluminum Sodium Carbonate (Reduced plasma levels of Dolobid). Products include:
Rolaids .... ▣ 743

Furosemide (Decreased hyperuricemic effect). Products include:
Lasix 1093

Hydrochlorothiazide (Decreased hyperuricemic effect; increased plasma levels). Products include:
Aldactazide 2150
Aldoril Tablets 1418
Apresazide Capsules 854
Apresoline-Esidrix Tablets 857
Capozide 2258
Dyazide Capsules 2208
Esidrix Tablets 863
Esimil Tablets 864
HydroDIURIL Tablets 1484
Hydropres Tablets 1485
Inderide Tablets 2463
Inderide LA Long Acting Capsules 2465
Lopressor HCT Tablets 1034
Maxzide 1215
Moduretic Tablets 1510
Normozide Tablets 2112
Oretic Tablets 544
Oreticyl 545
Prinzide Tablets 1540
Ser-Ap-Es Tablets 881
Serpasil-Esidrix Tablets 886
Timolide Tablets 1547
Trandate HCT Tablets 579
Vaseretic Tablets 1559
Zestoretic 2274

Indomethacin (Fatal gastrointestinal hemorrhage; concomitant use is not recommended). Products include:
Indocin 1487

Indomethacin Sodium Trihydrate (Fatal gastrointestinal hemorrhage; concomitant use is not recommended). Products include:
Indocin I.V. 1490

Magaldrate (Reduced plasma levels of Dolobid). Products include:
Riopan Antacid Chew Tablets .... ▣ 754
Riopan Antacid Chew Tablets in Rollpacks .... ▣ 754
Riopan Antacid Suspension 2421
Riopan Antacid Swallow Tablets 2421
Riopan Plus Chew Tablets 2422
Riopan Plus Chew Tablets in Rollpack 2422
Riopan Plus 2 Chew Tablets, Mint Flavor, Cherry Flavor 2422
Riopan Plus Suspension 2422
Riopan Plus 2 Suspension, Mint Flavor, Cherry Flavor 2422

Magnesium Hydroxide (Reduced plasma levels of Dolobid). Products include:
Aludrox Oral Suspension 2428
Ascriptin A/D Caplets 1850
Regular Strength Ascriptin Tablets 1850
Di-Gel Antacid/Anti-Gas .... ▣ 697
Gelusil Liquid & Tablets .... ▣ 639
Haley's M-O, Regular & Flavored .... ▣ 569
Extra Strength Maalox Plus Suspension 1850
Maalox TC Suspension 1851
Maalox Plus Tablets .... ▣ 655
Extra Strength Maalox Plus Tablets 1850
Mylanta Liquid 1155
Mylanta Tablets 1155
Mylanta Double Strength Liquid 1155
Mylanta Double Strength Tablets 1155
Concentrated Phillips' Milk of Magnesia .... ▣ 573
Phillips' Milk of Magnesia Liquid .... ▣ 572
Phillips' Milk of Magnesia Tablets ▣ 573
WinGel Liquid & Tablets .... ▣ 761

Magnesium Oxide (Reduced plasma levels of Dolobid). Products include:
Bayer Plus Aspirin Tablets .... ▣ 567
Beelith Tablets 659
Bufferin Analgesic Tablets and Caplets .... ▣ 524
Cama Arthritis Pain Reliever .... ▣ 685
Mag-Ox 400 673
Uro-Mag 673

Methotrexate Sodium (Decreased tubular secretion of methotrexate and potentiation of its toxicity). Products include:
Methotrexate Tablets, Parenteral, LPF Parenteral 1217
Rheumatrex Methotrexate Dose Pack 1234

Naproxen (Decreased urinary excretion of naproxen and its glucuronide metabolite). Products include:
Naprosyn 2297

Naproxen Sodium (Decreased urinary excretion of naproxen and its glucoronide metabolite). Products include:
Anaprox and Anaprox DS Tablets 2288

Nephrotoxic Drugs (Overt renal decompensation).

Phenprocoumon (Prolonged prothrombin time).

Sulindac (Decreased plasma levels of active sulindac sulfide metabolite). Products include:
Clinoril Tablets 1433

Warfarin Sodium (Prolonged prothrombin time; adjustment of dosage of oral anticoagulants may be required). Products include:
Coumadin Injection & Tablets 944
Panwarfin Tablets 547

DOLOPHINE HYDROCHLORIDE AMPOULES & VIALS
(Methadone Hydrochloride) 1260
May interact with central nervous system depressants, tricyclic antidepressants, and certain other agents. Compounds in these categories include:

Alcohol (Respiratory depression, hypotension, profound sedation, or coma).

Alfentanil Hydrochloride (Respiratory depression, hypotension, profound sedation, or coma). Products include:
Alfenta Injection 1131

Alprazolam (Respiratory depression, hypotension, profound sedation, or coma). Products include:
Xanax Tablets 2367

Amitriptyline Hydrochloride (Respiratory depression, hypotension, profound sedation, or coma). Products include:
Elavil 2269
Endep Tablets 1927
Etrafon 2087
Limbitrol 1933
Triavil Tablets 1556

Amoxapine (Respiratory depression, hypotension, profound sedation, or coma). Products include:
Asendin Tablets 1196

Aprobarbital (Respiratory depression, hypotension, profound sedation, or coma). Products include:
Alurate Elixir 1883

Buprenorphine (Respiratory depression, hypotension, profound sedation, or coma).
No products indexed under this heading.

Buspirone Hydrochloride (Respiratory depression, hypotension, profound sedation, or coma). Products include:
BuSpar 1401

Butabarbital (Respiratory depression, hypotension, profound sedation, or coma). Products include:
Pyridium Plus 1764

Butalbital (Respiratory depression, hypotension, profound sedation, or coma). Products include:
Esgic-Plus Tablets 1002
Esgic Tablets & Capsules 1001
Fioricet Tablets 2006
Fiorinal Capsules 2007
Fiorinal with Codeine Capsules 2008
Fiorinal Tablets 2007
Phrenilin 838
Sedapap Tablets 50 mg/650 mg 1360

Chlordiazepoxide (Respiratory depression, hypotension, profound sedation, or coma). Products include:
Libritabs Tablets 1930
Limbitrol 1933
Menrium Tablets 1934

Chlordiazepoxide Hydrochloride (Respiratory depression, hypotension, profound sedation, or coma). Products include:
Librax Capsules 1929
Librium Capsules 1931
Librium Injectable 1932

Chlorpromazine (Respiratory depression, hypotension, profound sedation, or coma). Products include:
Thorazine 2234

Chlorprothixene (Respiratory depression, hypotension, profound sedation, or coma). Products include:
Taractan Tablets 1920

Chlorprothixene Hydrochloride (Respiratory depression, hypotension, profound sedation, or coma). Products include:
Taractan 1920

Clomipramine Hydrochloride (Respiratory depression, hypotension, profound sedation, or coma). Products include:
Anafranil Capsules 650

Clorazepate Dipotassium (Respiratory depression, hypotension, profound sedation, or coma). Products include:
Tranxene 556

Codeine (Respiratory depression, hypotension, profound sedation, or coma). Products include:
Calcidrine Syrup 506

Codeine Phosphate (Respiratory depression, hypotension, profound sedation, or coma). Products include:
Actifed with Codeine Cough Syrup 752
Cheracol Cough Syrup 1853
Codimal PH Syrup 846
Dimetane-DC Cough Syrup 1857
Empirin with Codeine Phosphate Nos. 2, 3 & 4 764
Fiorinal with Codeine Capsules 2008
Isoclor Expectorant 982
Naldecon CX Adult Liquid .... ▣ 521
Novahistine DH 1342
Novahistine Expectorant 1343
Nucofed Capsules 2219
Nucofed Expectorant 2219
Nucofed Pediatric Expectorant 2220
Nucofed Syrup 2219
Phenaphen with Codeine Capsules 1865
Phenaphen-650 with Codeine Tablets 1866
Phenergan with Codeine 2497
Phenergan VC with Codeine 2501
Robitussin A-C Syrup 1875
Robitussin-DAC Syrup 1875
Ryna .... ▣ 741
Soma Compound w/Codeine Tablets 2390

Triaminic Expectorant w/Codeine .. 1996
Tussi-Organidin Liquid 2391
Tylenol with Codeine 1381

Codeine Polistirex (Respiratory depression, hypotension, profound sedation, or coma).
No products indexed under this heading.

Desipramine Hydrochloride (Increased blood levels of desipramine with concurrent therapy). Products include:
Norpramin Tablets 1340

Dezocine (Respiratory depression, hypotension, profound sedation, or coma).

Diazepam (Respiratory depression, hypotension, profound sedation, or coma). Products include:
Valium Injectable 1937
Valium Tablets 1939
Valrelease Capsules 1923

Doxepin Hydrochloride (Respiratory depression, hypotension, profound sedation, or coma). Products include:
Sinequan 1960

Droperidol (Respiratory depression, hypotension, profound sedation, or coma). Products include:
Inapsine Injection 1140
Innovar Injection 1141

Enflurane (Respiratory depression, hypotension, profound sedation, or coma). Products include:
Ethrane 599

Estazolam (Respiratory depression, hypotension, profound sedation, or coma). Products include:
ProSom Tablets 554

Ethchlorvynol (Respiratory depression, hypotension, profound sedation, or coma). Products include:
Placidyl Capsules 553

Ethinamate (Respiratory depression, hypotension, profound sedation, or coma).
No products indexed under this heading.

Fentanyl (Respiratory depression, hypotension, profound sedation, or coma). Products include:
Duragesic Transdermal System........ 1133

Fentanyl Citrate (Respiratory depression, hypotension, profound sedation, or coma). Products include:
Innovar Injection 1141
Sublimaze Injection 1146

Fluphenazine Decanoate (Respiratory depression, hypotension, profound sedation, or coma). Products include:
Prolixin Decanoate 1795

Fluphenazine Enanthate (Respiratory depression, hypotension, profound sedation, or coma). Products include:
Prolixin Enanthate 1796

Fluphenazine Hydrochloride (Respiratory depression, hypotension, profound sedation, or coma). Products include:
Prolixin Elixir 1793
Prolixin Injection 1791
Prolixin Oral Concentrate 1792
Prolixin Tablets 1793

Flurazepam Hydrochloride (Respiratory depression, hypotension, profound sedation, or coma). Products include:
Dalmane Capsules 1927

Glutethimide (Respiratory depression, hypotension, profound sedation, or coma).
No products indexed under this heading.

Haloperidol (Respiratory depression, hypotension, profound sedation, or coma). Products include:
Haldol Injection, Tablets and Concentrate 1373

Haloperidol Decanoate (Respiratory depression, hypotension, profound sedation, or coma). Products include:
Haldol Decanoate 1375

Hydrocodone Bitartrate (Respiratory depression, hypotension, profound sedation, or coma). Products include:
Anexsia 5/500 Tablets 2196
Anexsia 7.5/650 Tablets 2197
Azdone Tablets 844
Codiclear DH Syrup 845
Codimal DH Syrup 846
Damason-P 1356
Hycodan Syrup, Tablets 927
Hycomine Compound Tablets 929
Hycomine Syrup 927
Hycotuss Expectorant Syrup 930
Hydrocet Capsules 835
Lortab ASA Tablets 2414
Lortab 2412
Ru-Tuss with Hydrocodone 694
Triaminic Expectorant DH 1995
Vicodin Tablets 1187
Vicodin ES Tablets 1189
Zydone Capsules 941

Hydrocodone Polistirex (Respiratory depression, hypotension, profound sedation, or coma). Products include:
Tussionex Extended-Release Suspension 988

Hydroxyzine Hydrochloride (Respiratory depression, hypotension, profound sedation, or coma). Products include:
Atarax Tablets & Syrup 1941
Marax Tablets & DF Syrup 1954
Vistaril Intramuscular Solution 1970

Imipramine Hydrochloride (Respiratory depression, hypotension, profound sedation, or coma). Products include:
Tofranil Ampuls 1038
Tofranil Tablets 1039

Imipramine Pamoate (Respiratory depression, hypotension, profound sedation, or coma). Products include:
Tofranil-PM Capsules 1041

Isoflurane (Respiratory depression, hypotension, profound sedation, or coma). Products include:
Forane 600

Ketamine Hydrochloride (Respiratory depression, hypotension, profound sedation, or coma). Products include:
Ketalar 1726

Levorphanol Tartrate (Respiratory depression, hypotension, profound sedation, or coma). Products include:
Levo-Dromoran 1906

Lorazepam (Respiratory depression, hypotension, profound sedation, or coma). Products include:
Ativan Injection 2432
Ativan Tablets 2434

Loxapine Hydrochloride (Respiratory depression, hypotension, profound sedation, or coma). Products include:
Loxitane 1213

Loxapine Succinate (Respiratory depression, hypotension, profound sedation, or coma). Products include:
Loxitane Capsules 1213

Maprotiline Hydrochloride (Respiratory depression, hypotension, profound sedation, or coma). Products include:
Ludiomil Tablets 874

Meperidine Hydrochloride (Respiratory depression, hypotension, profound sedation, or coma). Products include:
Demerol 2047
Mepergan Injection 2479

Mephobarbital (Respiratory depression, hypotension, profound sedation, or coma). Products include:
Mebaral Tablets 2061

Meprobamate (Respiratory depression, hypotension, profound sedation, or coma). Products include:
Deprol Tablets 2382
Equagesic Tablets 2451
Miltown Tablets 2386
PMB 200 and PMB 400 2504

Mesoridazine (Respiratory depression, hypotension, profound sedation, or coma). Products include:
Serentil 686

Methohexital Sodium (Respiratory depression, hypotension, profound sedation, or coma). Products include:
Brevital Sodium Vials 1248

Methoxyflurane (Respiratory depression, hypotension, profound sedation, or coma).
No products indexed under this heading.

Midazolam Hydrochloride (Respiratory depression, hypotension, profound sedation, or coma). Products include:
Versed Injection 1924

Molindone Hydrochloride (Respiratory depression, hypotension, profound sedation, or coma). Products include:
Moban Tablets & Concentrate 932

Morphine Sulfate (Respiratory depression, hypotension, profound sedation, or coma). Products include:
Astramorph/PF Injection, USP (Preservative-Free) 618
Duramorph 960
Infumorph 200 and Infumorph 500 Sterile Solutions 962
MS Contin Tablets 1814
MSIR 1817
Oramorph SR (Morphine Sulfate Sustained Release Tablets) 1988
Roxanol 1991

Nortriptyline Hydrochloride (Respiratory depression, hypotension, profound sedation, or coma). Products include:
Pamelor 2019

Opium Alkaloids (Respiratory depression, hypotension, profound sedation or coma). Products include:
B & O No. 15A & No. 16A Supprettes 2395
Pantopon Injectable 1911

Oxazepam (Respiratory depression, hypotension, profound sedation, or coma). Products include:
Serax Capsules 2522
Serax Tablets 2522

Oxycodone Hydrochloride (Respiratory depression, hypotension, profound sedation, or coma). Products include:
Percocet Tablets 950
Percodan 951
Roxicodone Tablets, Oral Solution & Intensol (Oxycodone) 1992
Tylox Capsules 1382

Pentazocine Hydrochloride (Withdrawal symptoms). Products include:
Talacen 2070
Talwin Compound 2072
Talwin Nx 2073

Pentazocine Lactate (Withdrawal symptoms). Products include:
Talwin Injection 2071

Pentobarbital Sodium (Respiratory depression, hypotension, profound sedation, or coma). Products include:
Nembutal Sodium Capsules 534
Nembutal Sodium Solution 536
Nembutal Sodium Suppositories 538

Perphenazine (Respiratory depression, hypotension, profound sedation, or coma). Products include:
Etrafon 2087
Triavil Tablets 1556
Trilafon 2123

Phenobarbital (Respiratory depression, hypotension, profound sedation, or coma). Products include:
Arco-Lase Plus Tablets 607
Bellergal-S Tablets 1998
Bronkolixir .... ◙ 761
Bronkotabs Tablets .... ◙ 762
Donnatal 1858
Donnatal Extentabs 1859
Donnatal Tablets 1858
Donnazyme Tablets 1860
Kinesed Tablets 2272
Phenobarbital Elixir and Tablets 1293
Primatene Tablets-P Formula 2421
Quadrinal Tablets 1183
Tedral SA 1765

Phenoxybenzamine Hydrochloride (Respiratory depression, hypotension, profound sedation, or coma). Products include:
Dibenzyline Capsules 2207

Prazepam (Respiratory depression, hypotension, profound sedation, or coma). Products include:
Centrax 1693

Prochlorperazine (Respiratory depression, hypotension, profound sedation, or coma). Products include:
Compazine 2201

Promethazine Hydrochloride (Respiratory depression, hypotension, profound sedation, or coma). Products include:
Mepergan Injection 2479
Phenergan with Codeine 2497
Phenergan with Dextromethorphan 2499
Phenergan Injection 2493
Phenergan Suppositories 2496
Phenergan Syrup 2495
Phenergan Tablets 2496
Phenergan VC 2500
Phenergan VC with Codeine 2501

Propofol (Respiratory depression, hypotension, profound sedation, or coma). Products include:
Diprivan Injection 2267

Propoxyphene Hydrochloride (Respiratory depression, hypotension, profound sedation, or coma). Products include:
Darvon 1256
Wygesic Tablets 2540

Propoxyphene Napsylate (Respiratory depression, hypotension, profound sedation, or coma). Products include:
Darvon-N/Darvocet-N 1254

Protriptyline Hydrochloride (Respiratory depression, hypotension, profound sedation, or coma). Products include:
Vivactil Tablets 1567

Quazepam (Respiratory depression, hypotension, profound sedation, or coma). Products include:
Doral Tablets 2383

Rifampin (Withdrawal symptoms). Products include:
Rifadin 1345
Rifamate Capsules 1347
Rimactane Capsules 879

Secobarbital Sodium (Respiratory depression, hypotension, profound sedation, or coma). Products include:
Seconal Sodium Pulvules 1296

Sufentanil Citrate (Respiratory depression, hypotension, profound sedation, or coma). Products include:
Sufenta Injection 1147

Temazepam (Respiratory depression, hypotension, profound sedation, or coma). Products include:
Restoril Capsules 2023

Thiamylal Sodium (Respiratory depression, hypotension, profound sedation, or coma). Products include:
Surital Ampoules, Steri-Vials 1764

Thioridazine Hydrochloride (Respiratory depression, hypotension, profound sedation, or coma). Products include:
Mellaril 2011

Thiothixene (Respiratory depression, hypotension, profound sedation, or coma). Products include:
Navane Capsules and Concentrate 1954
Navane Intramuscular 1956

Triazolam (Respiratory depression, hypotension, profound sedation, or coma). Products include:
Halcion Tablets 2340

Trifluoperazine Hydrochloride (Respiratory depression, hypotension, profound sedation, or coma). Products include:
Stelazine 2226

Trimipramine Maleate (Respiratory depression, hypotension, profound sedation, or coma). Products include:
Surmontil Capsules 2524

DOLOPHINE HYDROCHLORIDE TABLETS

(Methadone Hydrochloride) 1261
May interact with central nervous system depressants, narcotic analgesics, general anesthetics, hypnotics and sedatives, tricyclic antidepressants, phenothiazines, tranquilizers, monoamine oxidase inhibitors, and certain other agents. Compounds in these categories include:

Alcohol (May result in respiratory depression, hypotension, profound sedation or coma).

Alfentanil Hydrochloride (May result in respiratory depression, hypotension, profound sedation or coma). Products include:
Alfenta Injection 1131

Alprazolam (May result in respiratory depression, hypotension, profound sedation or coma). Products include:
Xanax Tablets 2367

Amitriptyline Hydrochloride (May result in respiratory depression, hypotension, profound sedation or coma). Products include:
Elavil 2269
Endep Tablets 1927
Etrafon 2087
Limbitrol 1933
Triavil Tablets 1556

Amoxapine (May result in respiratory depression, hypotension, profound sedation or coma). Products include:
Asendin Tablets 1196

Aprobarbital (May result in respiratory depression, hypotension, profound sedation or coma). Products include:
Alurate Elixir 1883

Buprenorphine (May result in respiratory depression, hypotension, profound sedation or coma).
No products indexed under this heading.

Buspirone Hydrochloride (May result in respiratory depression, hypotension, profound sedation or coma). Products include:
BuSpar 1401

Butabarbital (May result in respiratory depression, hypotension, profound sedation or coma). Products include:
Pyridium Plus 1764

Butalbital (May result in respiratory depression, hypotension, profound sedation or coma). Products include:
Esgic-Plus Tablets 1002
Esgic Tablets & Capsules 1001
Fioricet Tablets 2006
Fiorinal Capsules 2007
Fiorinal with Codeine Capsules 2008
Fiorinal Tablets 2007
Phrenilin 838
Sedapap Tablets 50 mg/650 mg .. 1360

Chlordiazepoxide (May result in respiratory depression, hypotension, profound sedation or coma). Products include:
Libritabs Tablets 1930
Limbitrol 1933
Menrium Tablets 1934

Chlordiazepoxide Hydrochloride (May result in respiratory depression, hypotension, profound sedation or coma). Products include:
Librax Capsules 1929
Librium Capsules 1931
Librium Injectable 1932

Chlorpromazine (May result in respiratory depression, hypotension, profound sedation or coma). Products include:
Thorazine 2234

Chlorprothixene (May result in respiratory depression, hypotension, profound sedation or coma). Products include:
Taractan Tablets 1920

Chlorprothixene Hydrochloride (May result in respiratory depression, hypotension, profound sedation or coma). Products include:
Taractan 1920

Clomipramine Hydrochloride (May result in respiratory depression, hypotension, profound sedation or coma). Products include:
Anafranil Capsules 650

Clorazepate Dipotassium (May result in respiratory depression, hypotension, profound sedation or coma). Products include:
Tranxene 556

Codeine (May result in respiratory depression, hypotension, profound sedation or coma). Products include:
Calcidrine Syrup 506

Codeine Phosphate (May result in respiratory depression, hypotension, profound sedation or coma). Products include:
Actifed with Codeine Cough Syrup.. 752
Cheracol Cough Syrup 1853
Codimal PH Syrup 846
Dimetane-DC Cough Syrup 1857
Empirin with Codeine Phosphate Nos. 2, 3 & 4 764
Fiorinal with Codeine Capsules 2008
Isoclor Expectorant 982
Naldecon CX Adult Liquid ..... ▣ 521
Novahistine DH 1342
Novahistine Expectorant 1343
Nucofed Capsules 2219
Nucofed Expectorant 2219
Nucofed Pediatric Expectorant 2220
Nucofed Syrup 2219
Phenaphen with Codeine Capsules 1865
Phenaphen-650 with Codeine Tablets 1866
Phenergan with Codeine 2497
Phenergan VC with Codeine 2501
Robitussin A-C Syrup 1875
Robitussin-DAC Syrup 1875
Ryna ..... ▣ 741
Soma Compound w/Codeine Tablets 2390
Triaminic Expectorant w/Codeine .. 1996
Tussi-Organidin Liquid 2391
Tylenol with Codeine 1381

Codeine Polistirex (May result in respiratory depression, hypotension, profound sedation or coma).
No products indexed under this heading.

Desipramine Hydrochloride (Increased blood levels of desipramine with concurrent therapy; may result in respiratory depression, hypotension, profound sedation or coma). Products include:
Norpramin Tablets 1340

Dezocine (May result in respiratory depression, hypotension, profound sedation or coma).

Diazepam (May result in respiratory depression, hypotension, profound sedation or coma). Products include:
Valium Injectable 1937
Valium Tablets 1939
Valrelease Capsules 1923

Doxepin Hydrochloride (May result in respiratory depression, hypotension, profound sedation or coma). Products include:
Sinequan 1960

Droperidol (May result in respiratory depression, hypotension, profound sedation or coma). Products include:
Inapsine Injection 1140
Innovar Injection 1141

Enflurane (May result in respiratory depression, hypotension, profound sedation or coma). Products include:
Ethrane 599

Estazolam (May result in respiratory depression, hypotension, profound sedation or coma). Products include:
ProSom Tablets 554

Ethchlorvynol (May result in respiratory depression, hypotension, profound sedation or coma). Products include:
Placidyl Capsules 553

Ethinamate (May result in respiratory depression, hypotension, profound sedation or coma).
No products indexed under this heading.

Fentanyl (May result in respiratory depression, hypotension, profound sedation or coma). Products include:
Duragesic Transdermal System 1133

Fentanyl Citrate (May result in respiratory depression, hypotension, profound sedation or coma). Products include:
Innovar Injection 1141
Sublimaze Injection 1146

Fluphenazine Decanoate (May result in respiratory depression, hypotension, profound sedation or coma). Products include:
Prolixin Decanoate 1795

Fluphenazine Enanthate (May result in respiratory depression, hypotension, profound sedation or coma). Products include:
Prolixin Enanthate 1796

Fluphenazine Hydrochloride (May result in respiratory depression, hypotension, profound sedation or coma). Products include:
Prolixin Elixir 1793
Prolixin Injection 1791
Prolixin Oral Concentrate 1792
Prolixin Tablets 1793

Flurazepam Hydrochloride (May result in respiratory depression, hypotension, profound sedation or coma). Products include:
Dalmane Capsules 1927

Furazolidone (Potential for meperidine-MAOI-type reactions exists). Products include:
Furoxone 1855

Glutethimide (May result in respiratory depression, hypotension, profound sedation or coma).
No products indexed under this heading.

Haloperidol (May result in respiratory depression, hypotension, profound sedation or coma). Products include:
Haldol Injection, Tablets and Concentrate 1373

Haloperidol Decanoate (May result in respiratory depression, hypotension, profound sedation or coma). Products include:
Haldol Decanoate 1375

Hydrocodone Bitartrate (May result in respiratory depression, hypotension, profound sedation or coma). Products include:
Anexsia 5/500 Tablets 2196
Anexsia 7.5/650 Tablets 2197
Azdōne Tablets 844
Codiclear DH Syrup 845
Codimal DH Syrup 846
Damason-P 1356
Hycodan Syrup, Tablets 927
Hycomine Compound Tablets 929
Hycomine Syrup 927
Hycotuss Expectorant Syrup 930
Hydrocet Capsules 835
Lortab ASA Tablets 2414
Lortab 2412
Ru-Tuss with Hydrocodone 694
Triaminic Expectorant DH 1995
Vicodin Tablets 1187
Vicodin ES Tablets 1189
Zydone Capsules 941

Hydrocodone Polistirex (May result in respiratory depression, hypotension, profound sedation or coma). Products include:
Tussionex Extended-Release Suspension 988

Hydroxyzine Hydrochloride (May result in respiratory depression, hypotension, profound sedation or coma). Products include:
Atarax Tablets & Syrup 1941
Marax Tablets & DF Syrup 1954
Vistaril Intramuscular Solution 1970

Imipramine Hydrochloride (May result in respiratory depression, hypotension, profound sedation or coma). Products include:
Tofranil Ampuls 1038
Tofranil Tablets 1039

Imipramine Pamoate (May result in respiratory depression, hypotension, profound sedation or coma). Products include:
Tofranil-PM Capsules 1041

Isocarboxazid (Potential for meperidine-MAOI-type reactions exists). Products include:
Marplan Tablets 1906

Isoflurane (May result in respiratory depression, hypotension, profound sedation or coma). Products include:
Forane 600

(▣ Described in PDR For Nonprescription Drugs) (◉ Described in PDR For Ophthalmology)

Ketamine Hydrochloride (May result in respiratory depression, hypotension, profound sedation or coma). Products include:
Ketalar 1726
Levorphanol Tartrate (May result in respiratory depression, hypotension, profound sedation or coma). Products include:
Levo-Dromoran 1906
Lorazepam (May result in respiratory depression, hypotension, profound sedation or coma). Products include:
Ativan Injection 2432
Ativan Tablets 2434
Loxapine Hydrochloride (May result in respiratory depression, hypotension, profound sedation or coma). Products include:
Loxitane 1213
Loxapine Succinate (May result in respiratory depression, hypotension, profound sedation or coma). Products include:
Loxitane Capsules 1213
Maprotiline Hydrochloride (May result in respiratory depression, hypotension, profound sedation or coma). Products include:
Ludiomil Tablets 874
Meperidine Hydrochloride (May result in respiratory depression, hypotension, profound sedation or coma). Products include:
Demerol 2047
Mepergan Injection 2479
Mephobarbital (May result in respiratory depression, hypotension, profound sedation or coma). Products include:
Mebaral Tablets 2061
Meprobamate (May result in respiratory depression, hypotension, profound sedation or coma). Products include:
Deprol Tablets 2382
Equagesic Tablets 2451
Miltown Tablets 2386
PMB 200 and PMB 400 2504
Mesoridazine (May result in respiratory depression, hypotension, profound sedation or coma). Products include:
Serentil 686
Mesoridazine Besylate (May result in respiratory depression, hypotension, profound sedation or coma).
Methohexital Sodium (May result in respiratory depression, hypotension, profound sedation or coma). Products include:
Brevital Sodium Vials 1248
Methoxyflurane (May result in respiratory depression, hypotension, profound sedation or coma).
No products indexed under this heading.
Midazolam Hydrochloride (May result in respiratory depression, hypotension, profound sedation or coma). Products include:
Versed Injection 1924
Molindone Hydrochloride (May result in respiratory depression, hypotension, profound sedation or coma). Products include:
Moban Tablets & Concentrate 932
Morphine Sulfate (May result in respiratory depression, hypotension, profound sedation or coma). Products include:
Astramorph/PF Injection, USP (Preservative-Free) 618
Duramorph 960
Infumorph 200 and Infumorph 500 Sterile Solutions 962
MS Contin Tablets 1814
MSIR 1817
Oramorph SR (Morphine Sulfate Sustained Release Tablets) 1988
Roxanol 1991
Nortriptyline Hydrochloride (May result in respiratory depression, hypotension, profound sedation or coma). Products include:
Pamelor 2019
Opium Alkaloids (May result in respiratory depression, hypotension, profound sedation or coma). Products include:
B & O No. 15A & No. 16A Supprettes 2395
Pantopon Injectable 1911
Oxazepam (May result in respiratory depression, hypotension, profound sedation or coma). Products include:
Serax Capsules 2522
Serax Tablets 2522
Oxycodone Hydrochloride (May result in respiratory depression, hypotension, profound sedation or coma). Products include:
Percocet Tablets 950
Percodan 951
Roxicodone Tablets, Oral Solution & Intensol (Oxycodone) 1992
Tylox Capsules 1382
Pentazocine Hydrochloride (Potential for withdrawal symptoms, reduces the blood concentration of methadone to produce withdrawal symptoms). Products include:
Talacen 2070
Talwin Compound 2072
Talwin Nx 2073
Pentazocine Lactate (Potential for withdrawal symptoms, reduces the blood concentration of methadone to produce withdrawal symptoms). Products include:
Talwin Injection 2071
Pentobarbital Sodium (May result in respiratory depression, hypotension, profound sedation or coma). Products include:
Nembutal Sodium Capsules 534
Nembutal Sodium Solution 536
Nembutal Sodium Suppositories 538
Perphenazine (May result in respiratory depression, hypotension, profound sedation or coma). Products include:
Etrafon 2087
Triavil Tablets 1556
Trilafon 2123
Phenelzine Sulfate (Potential for meperidine-MAOI-type reactions exists). Products include:
Nardil 1742
Phenobarbital (May result in respiratory depression, hypotension, profound sedation or coma). Products include:
Arco-Lase Plus Tablets 607
Bellergal-S Tablets 1998
Bronkolixir .... ▣ 761
Bronkotabs Tablets .... ▣ 762
Donnatal 1858
Donnatal Extentabs 1859
Donnatal Tablets 1858
Donnazyme Tablets 1860
Kinesed Tablets 2272
Phenobarbital Elixir and Tablets 1293
Primatene Tablets-P Formula 2421
Quadrinal Tablets 1183
Tedral SA 1765
Prazepam (May result in respiratory depression, hypotension, profound sedation or coma). Products include:
Centrax 1693
Prochlorperazine (May result in respiratory depression, hypotension, profound sedation or coma). Products include:
Compazine 2201
Promethazine Hydrochloride (May result in respiratory depression, hypotension, profound sedation or coma). Products include:
Mepergan Injection 2479
Phenergan with Codeine 2497
Phenergan with Dextromethorphan 2499
Phenergan Injection 2493
Phenergan Suppositories 2496
Phenergan Syrup 2495
Phenergan Tablets 2496
Phenergan VC 2500
Phenergan VC with Codeine 2501
Propofol (May result in respiratory depression, hypotension, profound sedation or coma). Products include:
Diprivan Injection 2267
Propoxyphene Hydrochloride (May result in respiratory depression, hypotension, profound sedation or coma). Products include:
Darvon 1256
Wygesic Tablets 2540
Propoxyphene Napsylate (May result in respiratory depression, hypotension, profound sedation or coma). Products include:
Darvon-N/Darvocet-N 1254
Protriptyline Hydrochloride (May result in respiratory depression, hypotension, profound sedation or coma). Products include:
Vivactil Tablets 1567
Quazepam (May result in respiratory depression, hypotension, profound sedation or coma). Products include:
Doral Tablets 2383
Secobarbital Sodium (May result in respiratory depression, hypotension, profound sedation or coma). Products include:
Seconal Sodium Pulvules 1296
Selegiline Hydrochloride (Potential for meperidine-MAOI-type reactions exists). Products include:
Eldepryl 2250
Sufentanil Citrate (May result in respiratory depression, hypotension, profound sedation or coma). Products include:
Sufenta Injection 1147
Temazepam (May result in respiratory depression, hypotension, profound sedation or coma). Products include:
Restoril Capsules 2023
Thiamylal Sodium (May result in respiratory depression, hypotension, profound sedation or coma). Products include:
Surital Ampoules, Steri-Vials 1764
Thioridazine Hydrochloride (May result in respiratory depression, hypotension, profound sedation or coma). Products include:
Mellaril 2011
Thiothixene (May result in respiratory depression, hypotension, profound sedation or coma). Products include:
Navane Capsules and Concentrate 1954
Navane Intramuscular 1956
Tranylcypromine Sulfate (Potential for meperidine-MAOI-type reactions exists). Products include:
Parnate Tablets 2222
Triazolam (May result in respiratory depression, hypotension, profound sedation or coma). Products include:
Halcion Tablets 2340
Trifluoperazine Hydrochloride (May result in respiratory depression, hypotension, profound sedation or coma). Products include:
Stelazine 2226
Trimipramine Maleate (May result in respiratory depression, hypotension, profound sedation or coma). Products include:
Surmontil Capsules 2524

DOMEBORO ASTRINGENT SOLUTION EFFERVESCENT TABLETS
(Aluminum Sulfate, Calcium Acetate) .... ▣ 626
No interactions described in labeling.

DOMEBORO ASTRINGENT SOLUTION POWDER PACKETS
(Aluminum Sulfate, Calcium Acetate) .... ▣ 626
No interactions described in labeling.

DONNAGEL
(Atropine Sulfate, Hyoscyamine Sulfate, Kaolin, Pectin, Scopolamine Hydrobromide) .... ▣ 675
No interactions described in labeling.

DONNAGEL-PG
(Belladonna Alkaloids, Opium Preparations) 1858
No interactions described in labeling.

DONNATAL CAPSULES
(Phenobarbital, Belladonna Alkaloids) 1858
May interact with oral anticoagulants. Compounds in this category include:
Dicumarol (Decreased phenobarbital effect). Products include:
Dicumarol Tablets 516
Warfarin Sodium (Decreased phenobarbital effect). Products include:
Coumadin Injection & Tablets 944
Panwarfin Tablets 547

DONNATAL ELIXIR
(Phenobarbital, Belladonna Alkaloids) 1858
See **Donnatal Capsules**

DONNATAL EXTENTABS
(Phenobarbital, Belladonna Alkaloids) 1859
May interact with oral anticoagulants. Compounds in this category include:
Dicumarol (Decreased phenobarbital effect). Products include:
Dicumarol Tablets 516
Warfarin Sodium (Decreased phenobarbital effect). Products include:
Coumadin Injection & Tablets 944
Panwarfin Tablets 547

DONNATAL TABLETS
(Phenobarbital, Belladonna Alkaloids) 1858
See **Donnatal Capsules**

DONNAZYME TABLETS
(Phenobarbital, Belladonna Alkaloids) 1860
May interact with oral anticoagulants. Compounds in this category include:
Dicumarol (Decreased anticoagulant effect). Products include:
Dicumarol Tablets 516
Warfarin Sodium (Decreased anticoagulant effect). Products include:
Coumadin Injection & Tablets 944
Panwarfin Tablets 547

DOPRAM INJECTABLE
(Doxapram Hydrochloride) 1860
May interact with sympathomimetic aerosal brochodilators, monoamine oxidase inhibitors, muscle relaxants, inhalant anesthetics, and certain other agents. Compounds in these categories include:

Albuterol (Additive pressor effect). Products include:
Proventil Inhalation Aerosol 2117
Ventolin Inhalation Aerosol and Refill 583

Albuterol Sulfate (Additive pressor effect). Products include:
Proventil Repetabs Tablets 2120
Proventil Solutions for Inhalation 0.5% and 0.083% 2118
Proventil Syrup 2119
Proventil Tablets 2120
Ventolin 583

Atracurium Besylate (Residual effects masked by Dopram). Products include:
Tracrium Injection 817

Baclofen (Residual effects masked by Dopram). Products include:
Lioresal Tablets 1031

Carisoprodol (Residual effects masked by Dopram). Products include:
Soma Compound w/Codeine Tablets 2390
Soma Compound Tablets 2389
Soma Tablets 2388

Chlorzoxazone (Residual effects masked by Dopram). Products include:
Paraflex Caplets 1378
Parafon Forte DSC Caplets 1379

Cyclobenzaprine Hydrochloride (Residual effects masked by Dopram). Products include:
Flexeril Tablets 1471

Dantrolene Sodium (Residual effects masked by Dopram). Products include:
Dantrium Capsules 1619
Dantrium Intravenous 1620

Dobutamine Hydrochloride (Additive pressor effect). Products include:
Dobutrex Solution Vials 1259

Dopamine Hydrochloride (Additive pressor effect). Products include:
Intropin Injection 930

Doxacurium Chloride (Residual effects masked by Dopram). Products include:
Nuromax Injection 794

Enflurane (Increased epinephrine release). Products include:
Ethrane 599

Ephedrine Hydrochloride (Additive pressor effect). Products include:
Amesec .... ▣ 682
Primatene Tablets-M Formula 2421
Primatene Tablets-P Formula 2421
Primatene Tablets-Regular Formula 2421
Quadrinal Tablets 1183
Quelidrine Syrup 556
Tedral SA 1765

Ephedrine Sulfate (Additive pressor effect). Products include:
Bronkaid Tablets .... ▣ 757
Bronkolixir .... ▣ 761
Bronkotabs Tablets .... ▣ 762
Marax Tablets & DF Syrup 1954
Pazo Hemorrhoid Ointment & Suppositories 752
Vicks Vatronol Nose Drops .... ▣ 666

Ephedrine Tannate (Additive pressor effect). Products include:
Rynatuss 2388

Epinephrine (Additive pressor effect). Products include:
Ana-Kit Anaphylaxis Emergency Treatment Kit 1100
Bronkaid Mist .... ▣ 757
EpiPen 843
Marcaine Hydrochloride 0.5% with Epinephrine 1:200,000 (as bitartrate) 958
Marcaine Hydrochloride with Epinephrine 1:200,000 2055
Primatene Mist 2420
Sus-Phrine Injection 1006
Xylocaine with Epinephrine Injections 637

Epinephrine Bitartrate (Additive pressor effect). Products include:
AsthmaHaler Mist Epinephrine Bitartrate Bronchodilator .... ▣ 616
Bronkaid Mist Suspension .... ▣ 757
Primatene Mist Suspension 2421

Epinephrine Hydrochloride (Additive pressor effect). Products include:
Adrenalin Chloride Solution 1:100 & 1:1,000 1689
Epifrin .... ⊙ 244
Glaucon .... ⊙ 218

Furazolidone (Additive pressor effect). Products include:
Furoxone 1855

Halothane (Increased epinephrine release). Products include:
Fluothane 2453

Isocarboxazid (Additive pressor effect). Products include:
Marplan Tablets 1906

Isoflurane (Increased epinephrine release). Products include:
Forane 600

Isoproterenol Hydrochloride (Additive pressor effect). Products include:
Isuprel Hydrochloride Injection 1:5000 2050
Isuprel Hydrochloride Mistometer .. 2051
Isuprel Hydrochloride Solution 1:200 & 1:100 2052
Norisodrine Aerotrol 540

Metaproterenol Sulfate (Additive pressor effect). Products include:
Alupent 674
Arm-a-Med Metaproterenol Sulfate Inhalation Solution, USP 617
Metaprel Inhalation Aerosol Bronchodilator 2014
Metaprel Inhalation Solution 2015
Metaprel 2015
Metaproterenol Sulfate Inhalation Solution, USP 912

Metaraminol Bitartrate (Additive pressor effect). Products include:
Aramine Injection 1424

Metaxalone (Residual effects masked by Dopram). Products include:
Skelaxin 840

Methocarbamol (Residual effects masked by Dopram). Products include:
Robaxin Injectable 1871
Robaxin Tablets 1872
Robaxisal Tablets 1872

Methoxamine Hydrochloride (Additive pressor effect). Products include:
Vasoxyl Injection 819

Methoxyflurane (Increased epinephrine release).
No products indexed under this heading.

Metocurine Iodide (Residual effects masked by Dopram). Products include:
Metubine Iodide Vials 1285

Norepinephrine Bitartrate (Additive pressor effect). Products include:
Levophed Bitartrate Injection 2054

Orphenadrine Citrate (Residual effects masked by Dopram). Products include:
Norflex 1314
Norgesic 1314

Pancuronium Bromide Injection (Residual effects masked by Dopram).
No products indexed under this heading.

Phenelzine Sulfate (Additive pressor effect). Products include:
Nardil 1742

Phenylephrine Bitartrate (Additive pressor effect).
No products indexed under this heading.

Phenylephrine Hydrochloride (Additive pressor effect). Products include:
AK-Dilate Solution 2.5% and 10% .... ⊙ 203
Atrohist Sprinkle Capsules 558
Cerose-DM 2443
Codimal 846
Comhist LA Capsules 1618
Congespirin For Children Aspirin Free Chewable Cold Tablets 748
Cyclomydril .... ⊙ 216
Deconsal Sprinkle Capsules 559
Dimetane Decongestant .... ▣ 673
Dristan Decongestant/Antihistamine/ Analgesic Coated Caplets .... ▣ 749
Dristan Cold Nasal Decongestant/ Antihistamine/ Analgesic Coated Tablets 2419
Dristan Advanced Formula Decongestant/Antihistamine/ Analgesic Tablets .... ▣ 749
Dristan Nasal Spray, Menthol 2419
Dristan Nasal Spray, Regular and Regular with Metered Pump 2419
Entex Capsules 1623
Entex Liquid 1623
Sinus Excedrin Analgesic, Decongestant Tablets & Caplets 750
Extendryl 994
4-Way Fast Acting Nasal Spray - Original Formula (regular & mentholated) & Metered Spray Pump (regular) 751
Hycomine Compound Tablets 929
Murocoll-2 Sterile Ophthalmic Solution .... ⊙ 261
Mydfrin 2.5% .... ⊙ 224
Naldecon Syrup, Tablets, Pediatric Drops and Pediatric Syrup 709
Neo-Synephrine Hydrochloride 1% Carpuject 2063
Neo-Synephrine Hydrochloride 1% Injection 2063
Neo-Synephrine Hydrochloride (Ophthalmic) 2064
Neo-Synephrine .... ▣ 759
Nōstril Nasal Decongestant .... ▣ 520
Novahistine Elixir .... ▣ 596
Phenergan VC 2500
Phenergan VC with Codeine 2501
Prefrin Liquifilm Vasoconstrictor and Lubricant Eye Drops .... ⊙ 254
Prefrin-A .... ⊙ 255
Quelidrine Syrup 556
Relief Vasoconstrictor and Lubricant Eye Drops .... ⊙ 256
Robitussin Night Relief .... ▣ 677
Ru-Tuss with Hydrocodone 694
Ru-Tuss Tablets 693
Vasosulf .... ⊙ 279
Vicks Sinex .... ▣ 665
Zincfrin .... ⊙ 230

Phenylephrine Tannate (Additive pressor effect). Products include:
Rynatan 2387
Rynatuss 2388

Phenylpropanolamine Hydrochloride (Additive pressor effect). Products include:
A.R.M. Allergy Relief Medicine Caplets .... ▣ 615
Acutrim .... ▣ 548
Allerest .... ▣ 559
BC Cold Powder .... ▣ 517
Cheracol Plus Head Cold/Cough Formula .... ▣ 667
Codimal Expectorant 846
Comtrex Multi-Symptom Cold Reliever Tablets/Caplets/Liqui-Gels/Liquid 745
Contac Continuous Action Decongestant/Antihistamine Capsules ▣ 710
Contac Maximum Strength Continuous Action Decongestant/ Antihistamine Caplets .... ▣ 709
Contac Severe Cold and Flu Formula Caplets .... ▣ 711
Coricidin 'D' Decongestant Tablets .... ▣ 695
Coricidin Demilets Tablets for Children .... ▣ 696
Demazin Nasal Decongestant/ Antihistamine Repetabs Tablets & Syrup .... ▣ 697
Dexatrim .... ▣ 733
Dimetane-DC Cough Syrup 1857
Dimetapp Elixir .... ▣ 673
Dimetapp DM Elixir .... ▣ 674
Dimetapp Extentabs .... ▣ 674
Dimetapp Plus Caplets .... ▣ 675
Dimetapp Tablets .... ▣ 675
Entex Capsules 1623
Entex LA Tablets 1623
Entex Liquid 1623
4-Way Cold Tablets 750
Hycomine Syrup 927
Naldecon CX Adult Liquid .... ▣ 521
Naldecon DX Adult Liquid .... ▣ 521
Naldecon DX Children's Syrup .... ▣ 522
Naldecon DX Pediatric Drops .... ▣ 522
Naldecon EX Children's Syrup .... ▣ 522
Naldecon EX Pediatric Drops .... ▣ 523
Naldecon Syrup, Tablets, Pediatric Drops and Pediatric Syrup 709
Nolamine Tablets 838
Nolex LA Tablets 838
Ornade Spansule Capsules 2221
Orthoxicol Cough Syrup .... ▣ 668
Propagest 839
Pyrroxate Capsules .... ▣ 669
Robitussin-CF .... ▣ 676
Ru-Tuss II Capsules 693
Ru-Tuss with Hydrocodone 694
Ru-Tuss Tablets 693
Sine-Off Sinus Medicine Tablets-Aspirin Formula .... ▣ 722
Sinulin 840
St. Joseph Cold Tablets for Children .... ▣ 704
Tavist-D Tablets 2035
Triaminic Allergy Tablets .... ▣ 688
Triaminic Chewables .... ▣ 688
Triaminic Cold Tablets .... ▣ 688
Triaminic Expectorant .... ▣ 688
Triaminic Expectorant w/Codeine .. 1996
Triaminic Expectorant DH 1995
Triaminic Oral Infant Drops 1996
Triaminic Syrup .... ▣ 689
Triaminic-12 Tablets .... ▣ 690
Triaminic-DM Syrup .... ▣ 689
Triaminicin Tablets .... ▣ 690
Triaminicol Multi-Symptom Cold Tablets .... ▣ 691
Triaminicol Multi-Symptom Relief ▣ 691
Tuss-Ornade Liquid 2242
Tuss-Ornade Spansule Capsules 2242
Tylenol Cold Medication, Effervescent Tablets 1369

Pirbuterol Acetate (Additive pressor effect). Products include:
Maxair Inhaler 1311

Pseudoephedrine Hydrochloride (Additive pressor effect). Products include:
Actifed Capsules .... ▣ 539
Actifed Plus Caplets .... ▣ 539
Actifed Plus Tablets .... ▣ 540
Actifed with Codeine Cough Syrup .. 752
Actifed Syrup .... ▣ 540
Actifed Tablets .... ▣ 540
Actifed 12-Hour Capsules .... ▣ 539
Advil Cold & Sinus Caplets (formerly CoAdvil) 2416
Allerest .... ▣ 559
Anatuss LA Tablets 1359
Benadryl Decongestant Elixir .... ▣ 635
Benadryl Decongestant .... ▣ 635
Benadryl Plus .... ▣ 636
Benadryl Plus Nighttime .... ▣ 637
Benylin Decongestant .... ▣ 638
Brexin L.A. Capsules 2078
Bromfed Capsules (Timed Release) 1615
Bromfed Syrup .... ▣ 628
Bromfed 1615
CoAdvil .... ▣ 748

Allergy-Sinus Comtrex Multi-Symptom Allergy Sinus Formula Tablets & Caplets 746
Cough Formula Comtrex 746
Comtrex Multi-Symptom Cold Reliever Tablets/Caplets/Liqui-Gels/Liquid 745
Day-Night Comtrex 747
Non-Drowsy Comtrex 747
Congess 994
Congestac Caplets ..... ▣ 617
Contac Jr. Children's Cold Medicine ..... ▣ 712
Contac Nighttime Cold Medicine ..... ▣ 713
Contac Sinus Caplets Maximum Strength Non-Drowsy Formula ..... ▣ 710
Contac Sinus Tablets Maximum Strength Non-Drowsy Formula ..... ▣ 710
Deconamine 663
Deconsal II Tablets 559
Dimacol Caplets ..... ▣ 672
Dimetane-DX Cough Syrup 1858
Dorcol Children's Cough Syrup ..... ▣ 685
Dorcol Children's Decongestant Liquid ..... ▣ 685
Dorcol Children's Liquid Cold Formula ..... ▣ 686
Maximum Strength Dristan Decongestant/Analgesic Coated Caplets ..... ▣ 750
No Drowsiness Dristan Cold Nasal Decongestant/Analgesic Coated Caplets 2420
Dristan Sinus Caplets 2419
Sinus Excedrin Analgesic, Decongestant Tablets & Caplets ..... ▣ 533
Fedahist Gyrocaps 2145
Fedahist Timecaps 2145
Guaifed 1615
Guaifed Syrup ..... ▣ 629
Isoclor Expectorant 982
Isoclor Timesule Capsules ..... ▣ 561
Kronofed-A 970
Medi-Flu Caplet, Liquid ..... ▣ 640
Novafed A Capsules 1342
Novafed Capsules 1342
Novahistine DH 1342
Novahistine DMX ..... ▣ 595
Novahistine Expectorant 1343
Nucofed Capsules 2219
Nucofed Expectorant 2219
Nucofed Pediatric Expectorant 2220
Nucofed Syrup 2219
Ornex Caplets ..... ▣ 618
PediaCare Allergy Relief Formula Liquid 1362
PediaCare Cough-Cold Formula Liquid 1362
PediaCare Infants' Oral Decongestant Drops 1362
PediaCare Night Rest Cough-Cold Formula Liquid 1362
PediaCare 6-12 Cough-Cold Formula Chewable Tablets 1362
Robitussin-DAC Syrup 1875
Robitussin-PE ..... ▣ 677
Rondec 1975
Rondec-DM 1976
Rondec-TR Tablet 1975
Ru-Tuss DE Tablets 694
Ryna ..... ▣ 741
Seldane-D Extended-Release Tablets 1350
Sinarest ..... ▣ 562
Sine-Aid Maximum Strength Sinus Headache Caplets 1365
Sine-Aid Maximum Strength Sinus Headache Tablets 1365
Sine-Off Maximum Strength Allergy/Sinus Formula Caplets ..... ▣ 721
Sine-Off Maximum Strength No Drowsiness Formula Caplets ..... ▣ 722
Singlet Tablets ..... ▣ 598
Sinutab Maximum Strength ..... ▣ 641
Sinutab Maximum Strength Without Drowsiness Tablets & Caplets ..... ▣ 642
Sinutab Regular Strength Without Drowsiness Formula ..... ▣ 641
St. Joseph Nighttime Cold Medicine ..... ▣ 705
Sudafed Children's Liquid ..... ▣ 543
Sudafed Cough Syrup ..... ▣ 543
Sudafed Plus Liquid ..... ▣ 544
Sudafed Plus Tablets ..... ▣ 545
Sudafed Sinus Caplets ..... ▣ 545
Sudafed Sinus Tablets ..... ▣ 545
Sudafed Tablets, 30 mg ..... ▣ 544
Sudafed Tablets, Adult Strength, 60 mg ..... ▣ 544
Sudafed 12 Hour Capsules ..... ▣ 545
TheraFlu Flu and Cold Medicine ..... ▣ 687
Triaminic Nite Light ..... ▣ 689
Tylenol Allergy Sinus Medication Caplets and Gelcaps, Maximum Strength 1372
Children's Tylenol Cold Liquid Formula and Chewable Tablets 1368
Tylenol Cold & Flu Hot Medication, Packets 1369
Tylenol Cold & Flu No Drowsiness Hot Medication, Packets 1371
Tylenol Cold Medication Caplets and Tablets 1370
Tylenol Cold Medication No Drowsiness Formula Caplets 1370
Tylenol Cold Night Time Medication Liquid 1371
Tylenol Cough Medication Liquid with Decongestant, Maximum Strength 1372
Tylenol, Maximum Strength, Sinus Medication Gelcaps, Caplets and Tablets 1373
Ursinus Inlay-Tabs ..... ▣ 691
Vicks Children's NyQuil ..... ▣ 664
Vicks Daycare ..... ▣ 660
Vicks Formula 44D Decongestant Cough Medicine ..... ▣ 662
Vicks Formula 44M Multi-Symptom Cough Medicine ..... ▣ 662
Vicks NyQuil Nighttime Colds Medicine-Original & Cherry Flavor ..... ▣ 664
Vicks Pediatric Formula 44 Cough & Congestion Medicine ..... ▣ 663
Vicks Pediatric Formula 44m Multi-Symptom Cough & Cold Medicine ..... ▣ 663

Pseudoephedrine Sulfate (Additive pressor effect). Products include:
Afrin Tablets ..... ▣ 693
Chlor-Trimeton Decongestant ..... ▣ 694
Disophrol Chronotab Sustained-Action Tablets ..... ▣ 698
Drixoral Antihistamine/Nasal Decongestant Syrup ..... ▣ 698
Drixoral Non-Drowsy Formula ..... ▣ 699
Drixoral Plus Extended-Release Tablets ..... ▣ 699
Drixoral Sinus ..... ▣ 700
Drixoral Sustained-Action Tablets ..... ▣ 698
Sinutab Allergy Formula Sustained Action Tablets ..... ▣ 640
Trinalin Repetabs Tablets 1170

Selegiline Hydrochloride (Additive pressor effect). Products include:
Eldepryl 2250

Succinylcholine Chloride (Residual effects masked by Dopram). Products include:
Anectine 755

Terbutaline Sulfate (Additive pressor effect). Products include:
Brethaire Inhaler 1024
Brethine Ampuls 1026
Brethine Tablets 1026
Bricanyl Injection 1324
Bricanyl Tablets 1325

Tranylcypromine Sulfate (Additive pressor effect). Products include:
Parnate Tablets 2222

Vecuronium Bromide (Residual effects masked by Dopram). Products include:
Norcuron 1642

DORAL TABLETS
(Quazepam) 2383
May interact with central nervous system depressants, anticonvulsants, psychotropics, and certain other agents. Compounds in these categories include:

Alcohol (Additive CNS depressant effects).

Alfentanil Hydrochloride (Additive CNS depressant effects). Products include:
Alfenta Injection 1131

Alprazolam (Additive CNS depressant effects). Products include:
Xanax Tablets 2367

Amitriptyline Hydrochloride (Additive CNS depressant effects). Products include:
Elavil 2269
Endep Tablets 1927
Etrafon 2087
Limbitrol 1933
Triavil Tablets 1556

Amoxapine (Additive CNS depressant effects). Products include:
Asendin Tablets 1196

Aprobarbital (Additive CNS depressant effects). Products include:
Alurate Elixir 1883

Buprenorphine (Additive CNS depressant effects).
No products indexed under this heading.

Buspirone Hydrochloride (Additive CNS depressant effects). Products include:
BuSpar 1401

Butabarbital (Additive CNS depressant effects). Products include:
Pyridium Plus 1764

Butalbital (Additive CNS depressant effects). Products include:
Esgic-Plus Tablets 1002
Esgic Tablets & Capsules 1001
Fioricet Tablets 2006
Fiorinal Capsules 2007
Fiorinal with Codeine Capsules 2008
Fiorinal Tablets 2007
Phrenilin 838
Sedapap Tablets 50 mg/650 mg .. 1360

Carbamazepine (Additive CNS depressant effects). Products include:
Tegretol Chewable Tablets 654
Tegretol Suspension 656
Tegretol Tablets 654

Chlordiazepoxide (Additive CNS depressant effects). Products include:
Libritabs Tablets 1930
Limbitrol 1933
Menrium Tablets 1934

Chlordiazepoxide Hydrochloride (Additive CNS depressant effects). Products include:
Librax Capsules 1929
Librium Capsules 1931
Librium Injectable 1932

Chlorpromazine (Additive CNS depressant effects). Products include:
Thorazine 2234

Chlorprothixene (Additive CNS depressant effects). Products include:
Taractan Tablets 1920

Chlorprothixene Hydrochloride (Additive CNS depressant effects). Products include:
Taractan 1920

Clorazepate Dipotassium (Additive CNS depressant effects). Products include:
Tranxene 556

Codeine (Additive CNS depressant effects). Products include:
Calcidrine Syrup 506

Codeine Phosphate (Additive CNS depressant effects). Products include:
Actifed with Codeine Cough Syrup .. 752
Cheracol Cough Syrup 1853
Codimal PH Syrup 846
Dimetane-DC Cough Syrup 1857
Empirin with Codeine Phosphate Nos. 2, 3 & 4 764
Fiorinal with Codeine Capsules 2008
Isoclor Expectorant 982
Naldecon CX Adult Liquid ..... ▣ 521
Novahistine DH 1342
Novahistine Expectorant 1343
Nucofed Capsules 2219
Nucofed Expectorant 2219
Nucofed Pediatric Expectorant 2220
Nucofed Syrup 2219
Phenaphen with Codeine Capsules 1865
Phenaphen-650 with Codeine Tablets 1866
Phenergan with Codeine 2497
Phenergan VC with Codeine 2501
Robitussin A-C Syrup 1875
Robitussin-DAC Syrup 1875
Ryna ..... ▣ 741
Soma Compound w/Codeine Tablets 2390
Triaminic Expectorant w/Codeine .. 1996
Tussi-Organidin Liquid 2391
Tylenol with Codeine 1381

Codeine Polistirex (Additive CNS depressant effects).
No products indexed under this heading.

Desipramine Hydrochloride (Additive CNS depressant effects). Products include:
Norpramin Tablets 1340

Dezocine (Additive CNS depressant effects).

Diazepam (Additive CNS depressant effects). Products include:
Valium Injectable 1937
Valium Tablets 1939
Valrelease Capsules 1923

Divalproex Sodium (Additive CNS depressant effects). Products include:
Depakote 512

Doxepin Hydrochloride (Additive CNS depressant effects). Products include:
Sinequan 1960

Droperidol (Additive CNS depressant effects). Products include:
Inapsine Injection 1140
Innovar Injection 1141

Enflurane (Additive CNS depressant effects). Products include:
Ethrane 599

Estazolam (Additive CNS depressant effects). Products include:
ProSom Tablets 554

Ethchlorvynol (Additive CNS depressant effects). Products include:
Placidyl Capsules 553

Ethinamate (Additive CNS depressant effects).
No products indexed under this heading.

Ethosuximide (Additive CNS depressant effects). Products include:
Zarontin Capsules 1768
Zarontin Syrup 1769

Ethotoin (Additive CNS depressant effects). Products include:
Peganone Tablets 551

Fentanyl (Additive CNS depressant effects). Products include:
Duragesic Transdermal System 1133

Fentanyl Citrate (Additive CNS depressant effects). Products include:
Innovar Injection 1141
Sublimaze Injection 1146

Fluphenazine Decanoate (Additive CNS depressant effects). Products include:
Prolixin Decanoate 1795

Fluphenazine Enanthate (Additive CNS depressant effects). Products include:
Prolixin Enanthate 1796

Fluphenazine Hydrochloride (Additive CNS depressant effects). Products include:
Prolixin Elixir 1793
Prolixin Injection 1791
Prolixin Oral Concentrate 1792
Prolixin Tablets 1793

Flurazepam Hydrochloride (Additive CNS depressant effects). Products include:
Dalmane Capsules 1927

Glutethimide (Additive CNS depressant effects).
No products indexed under this heading.

Haloperidol (Additive CNS depressant effects). Products include:
Haldol Injection, Tablets and Concentrate 1373

Haloperidol Decanoate (Additive CNS depressant effects). Products include:
Haldol Decanoate 1375

Hydrocodone Bitartrate (Additive CNS depressant effects). Products include:
Anexsia 5/500 Tablets 2196
Anexsia 7.5/650 Tablets 2197
Azdōne Tablets 844
Codiclear DH Syrup 845
Codimal DH Syrup 846
Damason-P 1356
Hycodan Syrup, Tablets 927
Hycomine Compound Tablets 929
Hycomine Syrup 927
Hycotuss Expectorant Syrup 930
Hydrocet Capsules 835
Lortab ASA Tablets 2414
Lortab 2412
Ru-Tuss with Hydrocodone 694
Triaminic Expectorant DH 1995
Vicodin Tablets 1187
Vicodin ES Tablets 1189
Zydone Capsules 941

Hydrocodone Polistirex (Additive CNS depressant effects). Products include:
Tussionex Extended-Release Suspension 988

Hydroxyzine Hydrochloride (Additive CNS depressant effects). Products include:
Atarax Tablets & Syrup 1941
Marax Tablets & DF Syrup 1954
Vistaril Intramuscular Solution 1970

Imipramine Hydrochloride (Additive CNS depressant effects). Products include:
Tofranil Ampuls 1038
Tofranil Tablets 1039

Imipramine Pamoate (Additive CNS depressant effects). Products include:
Tofranil-PM Capsules 1041

Isocarboxazid (Additive CNS depressant effects). Products include:
Marplan Tablets 1906

Isoflurane (Additive CNS depressant effects). Products include:
Forane 600

Ketamine Hydrochloride (Additive CNS depressant effects). Products include:
Ketalar 1726

Levorphanol Tartrate (Additive CNS depressant effects). Products include:
Levo-Dromoran 1906

Lithium Carbonate (Additive CNS depressant effects). Products include:
Eskalith 2214
Lithane Tablets 1596
Lithium Carbonate Capsules & Tablets 1984
Lithobid Tablets 870

Lithium Citrate (Additive CNS depressant effects). Products include:
Cibalith-S 870

Lorazepam (Additive CNS depressant effects). Products include:
Ativan Injection 2432
Ativan Tablets 2434

Loxapine Hydrochloride (Additive CNS depressant effects). Products include:
Loxitane 1213

Loxapine Succinate (Additive CNS depressant effects). Products include:
Loxitane Capsules 1213

Maprotiline Hydrochloride (Additive CNS depressant effects). Products include:
Ludiomil Tablets 874

Meperidine Hydrochloride (Additive CNS depressant effects). Products include:
Demerol 2047
Mepergan Injection 2479

Mephenytoin (Additive CNS depressant effects). Products include:
Mesantoin Tablets 2013

Mephobarbital (Additive CNS depressant effects). Products include:
Mebaral Tablets 2061

Meprobamate (Additive CNS depressant effects). Products include:
Deprol Tablets 2382
Equagesic Tablets 2451
Miltown Tablets 2386
PMB 200 and PMB 400 2504

Mesoridazine (Additive CNS depressant effects). Products include:
Serentil 686

Methadone Hydrochloride (Additive CNS depressant effects). Products include:
Dolophine Hydrochloride Ampoules & Vials 1260
Dolophine Hydrochloride Tablets 1261
Methadone Hydrochloride Diskets 1284
Methadone Hydrochloride Oral Solution & Tablets 1987

Methohexital Sodium (Additive CNS depressant effects). Products include:
Brevital Sodium Vials 1248

Methoxyflurane (Additive CNS depressant effects).
No products indexed under this heading.

Methsuximide (Additive CNS depressant effects). Products include:
Celontin 1692

Midazolam Hydrochloride (Additive CNS depressant effects). Products include:
Versed Injection 1924

Molindone Hydrochloride (Additive CNS depressant effects). Products include:
Moban Tablets & Concentrate 932

Morphine Sulfate (Additive CNS depressant effects). Products include:
Astramorph/PF Injection, USP (Preservative-Free) 618
Duramorph 960
Infumorph 200 and Infumorph 500 Sterile Solutions 962
MS Contin Tablets 1814
MSIR 1817
Oramorph SR (Morphine Sulfate Sustained Release Tablets) 1988
Roxanol 1991

Nortriptyline Hydrochloride (Additive CNS depressant effects). Products include:
Pamelor 2019

Opium Alkaloids (Additive CNS depressant effects). Products include:
B & O No. 15A & No. 16A Supprettes 2395
Pantopon Injectable 1911

Oxazepam (Additive CNS depressant effects). Products include:
Serax Capsules 2522
Serax Tablets 2522

Oxycodone Hydrochloride (Additive CNS depressant effects). Products include:
Percocet Tablets 950
Percodan 951
Roxicodone Tablets, Oral Solution & Intensol (Oxycodone) 1992
Tylox Capsules 1382

Paramethadione (Additive CNS depressant effects). Products include:
Paradione Capsules 548

Pentobarbital Sodium (Additive CNS depressant effects). Products include:
Nembutal Sodium Capsules 534
Nembutal Sodium Solution 536
Nembutal Sodium Suppositories 538

Perphenazine (Additive CNS depressant effects). Products include:
Etrafon 2087
Triavil Tablets 1556
Trilafon 2123

Phenacemide (Additive CNS depressant effects). Products include:
Phenurone Tablets 552

Phenelzine Sulfate (Additive CNS depressant effects). Products include:
Nardil 1742

Phenobarbital (Additive CNS depressant effects). Products include:
Arco-Lase Plus Tablets 607
Bellergal-S Tablets 1998
Bronkolixir .... ■ 761
Bronkotabs Tablets .... ■ 762
Donnatal 1858
Donnatal Extentabs 1859
Donnatal Tablets 1858
Donnazyme Tablets 1860
Kinesed Tablets 2272
Phenobarbital Elixir and Tablets 1293
Primatene Tablets-P Formula 2421
Quadrinal Tablets 1183
Tedral SA 1765

Phensuximide (Additive CNS depressant effects). Products include:
Milontin Kapseals 1741

Phenytoin (Additive CNS depressant effects). Products include:
Dilantin Infatabs 1710
Dilantin-30 Pediatric/Dilantin-125 Suspension 1713

Phenytoin Sodium (Additive CNS depressant effects). Products include:
Dilantin Kapseals 1708
Dilantin Parenteral 1712
Dilantin with Phenobarbital Kapseals 1715

Prazepam (Additive CNS depressant effects). Products include:
Centrax 1693

Primidone (Additive CNS depressant effects). Products include:
Mysoline 2480

Prochlorperazine (Additive CNS depressant effects). Products include:
Compazine 2201

Promethazine Hydrochloride (Additive CNS depressant effects). Products include:
Mepergan Injection 2479
Phenergan with Codeine 2497
Phenergan with Dextromethorphan 2499
Phenergan Injection 2493
Phenergan Suppositories 2496
Phenergan Syrup 2495
Phenergan Tablets 2496
Phenergan VC 2500
Phenergan VC with Codeine 2501

Propofol (Additive CNS depressant effects). Products include:
Diprivan Injection 2267

Propoxyphene Hydrochloride (Additive CNS depressant effects). Products include:
Darvon 1256
Wygesic Tablets 2540

Propoxyphene Napsylate (Additive CNS depressant effects). Products include:
Darvon-N/Darvocet-N 1254

Protriptyline Hydrochloride (Additive CNS depressant effects). Products include:
Vivactil Tablets 1567

Secobarbital Sodium (Additive CNS depressant effects). Products include:
Seconal Sodium Pulvules 1296

Sufentanil Citrate (Additive CNS depressant effects). Products include:
Sufenta Injection 1147

Temazepam (Additive CNS depressant effects). Products include:
Restoril Capsules 2023

Thiamylal Sodium (Additive CNS depressant effects). Products include:
Surital Ampoules, Steri-Vials 1764

Thioridazine Hydrochloride (Additive CNS depressant effects). Products include:
Mellaril 2011

Thiothixene (Additive CNS depressant effects). Products include:
Navane Capsules and Concentrate 1954
Navane Intramuscular 1956

Tranylcypromine Sulfate (Additive CNS depressant effects). Products include:
Parnate Tablets 2222

Triazolam (Additive CNS depressant effects). Products include:
Halcion Tablets 2340

Trifluoperazine Hydrochloride (Additive CNS depressant effects). Products include:
Stelazine 2226

Trimethadione (Additive CNS depressant effects). Products include:
Tridione 557

Trimipramine Maleate (Additive CNS depressant effects). Products include:
Surmontil Capsules 2524

Valproic Acid (Additive CNS depressant effects). Products include:
Depakene Capsules & Syrup 511

DORCOL CHILDREN'S COUGH SYRUP
(Pseudoephedrine Hydrochloride, Guaifenesin, Dextromethorphan Hydrobromide) .... ■ 685
May interact with monoamine oxidase inhibitors. Compounds in this category include:

Furazolidone (Contraindicated). Products include:
Furoxone 1855

Isocarboxazid (Contraindicated). Products include:
Marplan Tablets 1906

Phenelzine Sulfate (Contraindicated). Products include:
Nardil 1742

Selegiline Hydrochloride (Contraindicated). Products include:
Eldepryl 2250

Tranylcypromine Sulfate (Contraindicated). Products include:
Parnate Tablets 2222

DORCOL CHILDREN'S DECONGESTANT LIQUID
(Pseudoephedrine Hydrochloride, Guaifenesin, Dextromethorphan Hydrobromide) .... ■ 685
May interact with monoamine oxidase inhibitors. Compounds in this category include:

Furazolidone (Contraindicated). Products include:
Furoxone 1855

Isocarboxazid (Contraindicated). Products include:
- Marplan Tablets ... 1906

Phenelzine Sulfate (Contraindicated). Products include:
- Nardil ... 1742

Selegiline Hydrochloride (Contraindicated). Products include:
- Eldepryl ... 2250

Tranylcypromine Sulfate (Contraindicated). Products include:
- Parnate Tablets ... 2222

DORCOL CHILDREN'S FEVER & PAIN REDUCER
(Acetaminophen) ... ◘ 686
No interactions described in labeling.

DORCOL CHILDREN'S LIQUID COLD FORMULA
(Pseudoephedrine Hydrochloride, Chlorpheniramine Maleate) ... ◘ 686
May interact with monoamine oxidase inhibitors. Compounds in this category include:

Furazolidone (Contraindicated). Products include:
- Furoxone ... 1855

Isocarboxazid (Contraindicated). Products include:
- Marplan Tablets ... 1906

Phenelzine Sulfate (Contraindicated). Products include:
- Nardil ... 1742

Selegiline Hydrochloride (Contraindicated). Products include:
- Eldepryl ... 2250

Tranylcypromine Sulfate (Contraindicated). Products include:
- Parnate Tablets ... 2222

DORYX CAPSULES
(Doxycycline Hyclate) ... 1717
May interact with penicillins, antacids, anticoagulants, and certain other agents. Compounds in these categories include:

Aluminum Carbonate Gel (Should not be given concurrently). Products include:
- Basaljel ... 2438

Aluminum Hydroxide (Should not be given concurrently). Products include:
- Cama Arthritis Pain Reliever ... ◘ 685
- Gaviscon Extra Strength Relief Formula Liquid Antacid ... ◘ 594
- Gaviscon Extra Strength Relief Formula Antacid Tablets ... ◘ 594
- Gaviscon Liquid Antacid ... ◘ 594
- Gelusil Liquid & Tablets ... ◘ 639
- Extra Strength Maalox Plus Suspension ... 1850
- Maalox TC Suspension ... 1851
- Maalox Plus Tablets ... ◘ 655
- Extra Strength Maalox Plus Tablets 1850
- Nephrox Suspension ... ◘ 563
- WinGel Liquid & Tablets ... ◘ 761

Aluminum Hydroxide Gel (Should not be given concurrently). Products include:
- ALternaGEL Liquid ... 1154
- Aludrox Oral Suspension ... 2428
- Amphojel Suspension ... 2429
- Amphojel Suspension without Flavor ... 2429
- Mylanta Liquid ... 1155
- Mylanta Double Strength Liquid ... 1155

Aluminum Hydroxide Gel, Dried (Should not be given concurrently). Products include:
- Alu-Tab/Alu-Cap ... 1309
- Amphojel Tablets ... 2429
- Ascriptin A/D Caplets ... 1850
- Regular Strength Ascriptin Tablets 1850
- Gaviscon Antacid Tablets ... ◘ 593
- Gaviscon-2 Antacid Tablets ... ◘ 594
- Mylanta Tablets ... 1155
- Mylanta Double Strength Tablets ... 1155

Amoxicillin (Interference with bactericidal action of penicillins). Products include:
- Amoxil ... 2193
- Augmentin Tablets, Powder for Oral Suspension, and Chewable Tablets ... 2198

Ampicillin Sodium (Interference with bactericidal action of penicillins). Products include:
- Unasyn ... 1965

Azlocillin Sodium (Interference with bactericidal action of penicillins).
- No products indexed under this heading.

Bacampicillin Hydrochloride (Interference with bactericidal action of penicillins). Products include:
- Spectrobid Tablets & Powder for Oral Suspension ... 1961

Carbenicillin Disodium (Interference with bactericidal action of penicillins).

Carbenicillin Indanyl Sodium (Interference with bactericidal action of penicillins). Products include:
- Geocillin Tablets ... 1951

Dicumarol (Downward adjustment of anticoagulant dosage may be necessary). Products include:
- Dicumarol Tablets ... 516

Dihydroxyaluminum Sodium Carbonate (Should not be given concurrently). Products include:
- Rolaids ... ◘ 743

Heparin Calcium (Downward adjustment of anticoagulant dosage may be necessary). Products include:
- Calciparine Injection ... 925

Heparin Sodium (Downward adjustment of anticoagulant dosage may be necessary). Products include:
- Heparin Lock Flush Solution ... 2456
- Heparin Sodium Vials ... 1264
- Heparin Sodium Injection ... 2457
- Heparin Sodium Injection, USP, Sterile Solution ... 2342

Iron Preparations (Should not be given concurrently). Products include:
- Allbee C-800 Plus Iron Tablets ... ◘ 670
- Bugs Bunny Children's Chewable Vitamins + Minerals with Iron and Calcium (Sugar Free) ... ◘ 626
- Bugs Bunny Plus Iron Children's Chewable Vitamins (Sugar Free) ◘ 625
- FemIron Multi-Vitamins and Iron ... ◘ 617
- Ferancee Chewable Tablets ... 1155
- Ferancee-HP Tablets ... 1155
- Fergon ... ◘ 758
- Fero-Folic-500 Filmtab ... 527
- Fero-Grad-500 Filmtab ... 528
- Fero-Gradumet Filmtab ... 528
- Ferro-Sequels ... 1203
- Flintstones Children's Chewable Vitamins Plus Iron ... ◘ 625
- Flintstones Complete With Calcium, Iron & Minerals Children's Chewable Vitamins ... ◘ 626
- Geritol Extend Tablets and Caplets ... ◘ 717
- Geritol Liquid - High Potency Iron & Vitamin Tonic ... ◘ 717
- Iberet Tablets ... 531
- Iberet-500 Liquid ... 531
- Iberet-Folic-500 Filmtab ... 527
- Iberet-Liquid ... 531
- Incremin w/Iron Syrup ... ◘ 588
- Irospan ... 972
- Mol-Iron ... ◘ 703
- Niferex ... 847
- Niferex-150 Forte Capsules ... 847
- Niferex Forte Elixir ... 847
- Niferex ... 847
- Niferex-PN Tablets ... 847
- One-A-Day Maximum Formula Vitamins and Minerals ... ◘ 627
- Peritinic Tablets ... ◘ 589
- Poly-Vi-Flor with Iron ... 1399
- Poly-Vi-Flor with Iron Drops ... 1399
- Poly-Vi-Sol Vitamins with Iron, Chewable Tablets and Circus Shapes Chewable ... ◘ 612
- Poly-Vi-Sol Vitamins with Iron, Drops ... ◘ 612
- SMA Iron Fortified Infant Formula, Concentrated, Ready-to-Feed and Powder ... ◘ 767
- Slow Fe Tablets ... ◘ 552
- The Stuart Formula Tablets ... ◘ 581
- Stuartinic Tablets ... 1157
- Surbex-750 with Iron ... ◘ 503
- Tri-Vi-Flor 0.25 mg Vitamins with Iron and Fluoride Drops ... 1401
- Unicap Plus Iron Vitamin Formula Tablets ... ◘ 738
- Vi-Daylin ADC Vitamins + Iron Drops ... 1980
- Vi-Daylin Multivitamin + Iron Drops ... 1981
- Vi-Daylin/F ADC Vitamins + Iron Drops With Fluoride ... 1981
- Vi-Daylin/F Multivitamin + Iron Drops With Fluoride ... 1981
- Vi-Daylin Multivitamin + Iron Chewable Tablets ... 1982
- Vi-Daylin/F Multivitamin + Iron Chewable Tablets With Fluoride .. 1982
- Vi-Daylin Multivitamin + Iron Liquid ... 1983

Magaldrate (Should not be given concurrently). Products include:
- Riopan Antacid Chew Tablets ... ◘ 754
- Riopan Antacid Chew Tablets in Rollpacks ... ◘ 754
- Riopan Antacid Suspension ... 2421
- Riopan Antacid Swallow Tablets ... 2421
- Riopan Plus Chew Tablets ... 2422
- Riopan Plus Chew Tablets in Rollpack ... 2422
- Riopan Plus 2 Chew Tablets, Mint Flavor, Cherry Flavor ... 2422
- Riopan Plus Suspension ... 2422
- Riopan Plus 2 Suspension, Mint Flavor, Cherry Flavor ... 2422

Magnesium Hydroxide (Should not be given concurrently). Products include:
- Aludrox Oral Suspension ... 2428
- Ascriptin A/D Caplets ... 1850
- Regular Strength Ascriptin Tablets 1850
- Di-Gel Antacid/Anti-Gas ... ◘ 697
- Gelusil Liquid & Tablets ... ◘ 639
- Haley's M-O, Regular & Flavored .. ◘ 569
- Extra Strength Maalox Plus Suspension ... 1850
- Maalox TC Suspension ... 1851
- Maalox Plus Tablets ... ◘ 655
- Extra Strength Maalox Plus Tablets 1850
- Mylanta Liquid ... 1155
- Mylanta Tablets ... 1155
- Mylanta Double Strength Liquid ... 1155
- Mylanta Double Strength Tablets ... 1155
- Concentrated Phillips' Milk of Magnesia ... ◘ 573
- Phillips' Milk of Magnesia Liquid ... ◘ 572
- Phillips' Milk of Magnesia Tablets ◘ 573
- WinGel Liquid & Tablets ... ◘ 761

Magnesium Oxide (Should not be given concurrently). Products include:
- Bayer Plus Aspirin Tablets ... ◘ 567
- Beelith Tablets ... 659
- Bufferin Analgesic Tablets and Caplets ... ◘ 524
- Cama Arthritis Pain Reliever ... ◘ 685
- Mag-Ox 400 ... 673
- Uro-Mag ... 673

Mezlocillin Sodium (Interference with bactericidal action of penicillins). Products include:
- Mezlin ... 1597
- Mezlin Pharmacy Bulk Package ... 1599

Nafcillin Sodium (Interference with bactericidal action of penicillins). Products include:
- Unipen ... 2533

Penicillin G Potassium (Interference with bactericidal action of penicillin). Products include:
- Pfizerpen for Injection ... 1957

Penicillin G Procaine (Interference with bactericidal action of penicillin). Products include:
- Bicillin C-R Injection ... 2438
- Bicillin C-R 900/300 Injection ... 2440
- Pfizerpen-AS Aqueous Suspension 1959
- Wycillin Injection ... 2537
- Wycillin Injection and Probenecid Tablets ... 2539

Penicillin G Sodium (Interference with bactericidal action of penicillin).
- No products indexed under this heading.

Penicillin G, Benzathine (Interference with bactericidal action of penicillin). Products include:
- Bicillin C-R Injection ... 2438
- Bicillin C-R 900/300 Injection ... 2440
- Bicillin L-A Injection ... 2442

Penicillin V Potassium (Interference with bactericidal action of penicillin).
- No products indexed under this heading.

Ticarcillin Disodium (Interference with bactericidal action of penicillins). Products include:
- Ticar for Injection ... 2236
- Timentin for Injection ... 2239

Warfarin Sodium (Downward adjustment of anticoagulant dosage may be necessary). Products include:
- Coumadin Injection & Tablets ... 944
- Panwarfin Tablets ... 547

DOXIDAN CAPSULES
(Docusate Calcium, Phenolphthalein) ... ◘ 736
No interactions described in labeling.

DOXORUBICIN HYDROCHLORIDE FOR INJECTION, USP
(Doxorubicin Hydrochloride) ... 622
May interact with antineoplastics and certain other agents. Compounds in these categories include:

Altretamine (Toxicity of other anticancer therapies potentiated). Products include:
- Hexalen Capsules ... 2316

Asparaginase (Toxicity of other anticancer therapies potentiated). Products include:
- Elspar ... 1470

Bleomycin Sulfate (Toxicity of other anticancer therapies potentiated). Products include:
- Blenoxane ... 724

Busulfan (Toxicity of other anticancer therapies potentiated). Products include:
- Myleran Tablets ... 790

Carboplatin (Toxicity of other anticancer therapies potentiated). Products include:
- Paraplatin for Injection ... 735

Carmustine (BCNU) (Toxicity of other anticancer therapies potentiated). Products include:
- BiCNU ... 723

Chlorambucil (Toxicity of other anticancer therapies potentiated). Products include:
- Leukeran Tablets ... 788

Cisplatin (Toxicity of other anticancer therapies potentiated). Products include:
- Platinol ... 737
- Platinol-AQ Injection ... 738

Cyclophosphamide (Toxicity of other anticancer therapies potentiated; exacerbation of cyclophosphamide induced hemorrhagic cystitis). Products include:
- Cytoxan for Injection ... 726
- Neosar for Injection ... 566

Dacarbazine (Toxicity of other anticancer therapies potentiated). Products include:
- DTIC-Dome ... 1595

Daunorubicin Hydrochloride (Toxicity of other anticancer therapies potentiated). Products include:
Cerubidine ... 2443
Estramustine Phosphate Sodium (Toxicity of other anticancer therapies potentiated). Products include:
Emcyt Capsules ... 1161
Etoposide (Toxicity of other anticancer therapies potentiated). Products include:
VePesid Capsules and Injection ... 741
Floxuridine (Toxicity of other anticancer therapies potentiated). Products include:
Sterile FUDR ... 1898
Fluorouracil (Toxicity of other anticancer therapies potentiated). Products include:
Efudex ... 1880
Fluoroplex Topical Solution & Cream 1% ... 1082
Fluorouracil Injection ... 1897
Flutamide (Toxicity of other anticancer therapies potentiated). Products include:
Eulexin Capsules ... 2089
Hydroxyurea (Toxicity of other anticancer therapies potentiated). Products include:
Hydrea Capsules ... 728
Ifosfamide (Toxicity of other anticancer therapies potentiated). Products include:
IFEX ... 729
Interferon alfa-2A, Recombinant (Toxicity of other anticancer therapies potentiated). Products include:
Roferon-A Injection ... 1916
Interferon alfa-2B, Recombinant (Toxicity of other anticancer therapies potentiated). Products include:
Intron A ... 2097
Levamisole Hydrochloride (Toxicity of other anticancer therapies potentiated). Products include:
Ergamisol Tablets ... 1136
Lomustine (CCNU) (Toxicity of other anticancer therapies potentiated). Products include:
CeeNU ... 725
Mechlorethamine Hydrochloride (Toxicity of other anticancer therapies potentiated). Products include:
Mustargen ... 1514
Megestrol Acetate (Toxicity of other anticancer therapies potentiated). Products include:
Megace Tablets ... 732
Melphalan (Toxicity of other anticancer therapies potentiated). Products include:
Alkeran Tablets ... 754
Mercaptopurine (Toxicity of other anticancer therapies potentiated; enhancement of the hepatotoxicity of 6-mercaptopurine). Products include:
Purinethol Tablets ... 800
Methotrexate Sodium (Toxicity of other anticancer therapies potentiated). Products include:
Methotrexate Tablets, Parenteral, LPF Parenteral ... 1217
Rheumatrex Methotrexate Dose Pack ... 1234
Mitomycin (Mitomycin-C) (Toxicity of other anticancer therapies potentiated). Products include:
Mutamycin ... 733
Mitotane (Toxicity of other anticancer therapies potentiated). Products include:
Lysodren ... 731
Mitoxantrone Hydrochloride (Toxicity of other anticancer therapies potentiated). Products include:
Novantrone for Injection Concentrate ... 1226
Procarbazine Hydrochloride (Toxicity of other anticancer therapies potentiated). Products include:
Matulane Capsules ... 1907
Streptozocin (Toxicity of other anticancer therapies potentiated). Products include:
Zanosar Sterile Powder ... 2371
Tamoxifen Citrate (Toxicity of other anticancer therapies potentiated). Products include:
Nolvadex Tablets ... 1102
Thioguanine (Toxicity of other anticancer therapies potentiated). Products include:
Thioguanine Tablets, Tabloid Brand ... 815
Thiotepa (Toxicity of other anticancer therapies potentiated). Products include:
Thiotepa Parenteral ... 1240
Vincristine Sulfate (Toxicity of other anticancer therapies potentiated). Products include:
Oncovin Solution Vials & Hyporets 1288

DOXORUBICIN HYDROCHLORIDE INJECTION, USP
(Doxorubicin Hydrochloride) ... 848
May interact with antineoplastics and certain other agents. Compounds in these categories include:

Altretamine (Concomitant administration may potentiate toxicity). Products include:
Hexalen Capsules ... 2316
Asparaginase (Concomitant administration may potentiate toxicity). Products include:
Elspar ... 1470
Bleomycin Sulfate (Concomitant administration may potentiate toxicity). Products include:
Blenoxane ... 724
Busulfan (Concomitant administration may potentiate toxicity). Products include:
Myleran Tablets ... 790
Carboplatin (Concomitant administration may potentiate toxicity). Products include:
Paraplatin for Injection ... 735
Carmustine (BCNU) (Concomitant administration may potentiate toxicity). Products include:
BiCNU ... 723
Chlorambucil (Concomitant administration may potentiate toxicity). Products include:
Leukeran Tablets ... 788
Cisplatin (Concomitant administration may potentiate toxicity). Products include:
Platinol ... 737
Platinol-AQ Injection ... 738
Cyclophosphamide (Concomitant administration may potentiate toxicity). Products include:
Cytoxan for Injection ... 726
Neosar for Injection ... 566
Cytarabine (Combination therapy may result in necrotizing colitis and fatal infections). Products include:
Cytosar-U Sterile Powder ... 2329
Dacarbazine (Concomitant administration may potentiate toxicity). Products include:
DTIC-Dome ... 1595
Daunorubicin Hydrochloride (Concomitant administration may potentiate toxicity). Products include:
Cerubidine ... 2443
Estramustine Phosphate Sodium (Concomitant administration may potentiate toxicity). Products include:
Emcyt Capsules ... 1161
Etoposide (Concomitant administration may potentiate toxicity). Products include:
VePesid Capsules and Injection ... 741
Floxuridine (Concomitant administration may potentiate toxicity). Products include:
Sterile FUDR ... 1898
Fluorouracil (Concomitant administration may potentiate toxicity). Products include:
Efudex ... 1880
Fluoroplex Topical Solution & Cream 1% ... 1082
Fluorouracil Injection ... 1897
Flutamide (Concomitant administration may potentiate toxicity). Products include:
Eulexin Capsules ... 2089
Hydroxyurea (Concomitant administration may potentiate toxicity). Products include:
Hydrea Capsules ... 728
Ifosfamide (Concomitant administration may potentiate toxicity). Products include:
IFEX ... 729
Interferon alfa-2A, Recombinant (Concomitant administration may potentiate toxicity). Products include:
Roferon-A Injection ... 1916
Interferon alfa-2B, Recombinant (Concomitant administration may potentiate toxicity). Products include:
Intron A ... 2097
Levamisole Hydrochloride (Concomitant administration may potentiate toxicity). Products include:
Ergamisol Tablets ... 1136
Lomustine (CCNU) (Concomitant administration may potentiate toxicity). Products include:
CeeNU ... 725
Mechlorethamine Hydrochloride (Concomitant administration may potentiate toxicity). Products include:
Mustargen ... 1514
Megestrol Acetate (Concomitant administration may potentiate toxicity). Products include:
Megace Tablets ... 732
Melphalan (Concomitant administration may potentiate toxicity). Products include:
Alkeran Tablets ... 754
Mercaptopurine (Concomitant administration may potentiate toxicity). Products include:
Purinethol Tablets ... 800
Methotrexate Sodium (Concomitant administration may potentiate toxicity). Products include:
Methotrexate Tablets, Parenteral, LPF Parenteral ... 1217
Rheumatrex Methotrexate Dose Pack ... 1234
Mitomycin (Mitomycin-C) (Concomitant administration may potentiate toxicity). Products include:
Mutamycin ... 733
Mitotane (Concomitant administration may potentiate toxicity). Products include:
Lysodren ... 731
Mitoxantrone Hydrochloride (Concomitant administration may potentiate toxicity). Products include:
Novantrone for Injection Concentrate ... 1226
Procarbazine Hydrochloride (Concomitant administration may potentiate toxicity). Products include:
Matulane Capsules ... 1907
Streptozocin (Concomitant administration may potentiate toxicity). Products include:
Zanosar Sterile Powder ... 2371
Tamoxifen Citrate (Concomitant administration may potentiate toxicity). Products include:
Nolvadex Tablets ... 1102
Thioguanine (Concomitant administration may potentiate toxicity). Products include:
Thioguanine Tablets, Tabloid Brand ... 815
Thiotepa (Concomitant administration may potentiate toxicity). Products include:
Thiotepa Parenteral ... 1240
Vincristine Sulfate (Concomitant administration may potentiate toxicity). Products include:
Oncovin Solution Vials & Hyporets 1288

DRISDOL
(Vitamin D) ... ⊞ 762
No interactions described in labeling.

DRISTAN COLD NASAL DECONGESTANT/ ANTIHISTAMINE/ ANALGESIC COATED TABLETS
(Phenylephrine Hydrochloride, Chlorpheniramine Maleate, Acetaminophen) ... 2419
May interact with antidepressant drugs and certain other agents. Compounds in these categories include:

Alcohol (Concurrent use should be avoided).
Amitriptyline Hydrochloride (Effect not specified). Products include:
Elavil ... 2269
Endep Tablets ... 1927
Etrafon ... 2087
Limbitrol ... 1933
Triavil Tablets ... 1556
Amoxapine (Effect not specified). Products include:
Asendin Tablets ... 1196
Bupropion Hydrochloride (Effect not specified). Products include:
Wellbutrin Tablets ... 821
Desipramine Hydrochloride (Effect not specified). Products include:
Norpramin Tablets ... 1340
Doxepin Hydrochloride (Effect not specified). Products include:
Sinequan ... 1960
Fluoxetine Hydrochloride (Effect not specified). Products include:
Prozac Pulvules ... 920
Imipramine Hydrochloride (Effect not specified). Products include:
Tofranil Ampuls ... 1038
Tofranil Tablets ... 1039

Imipramine Pamoate (Effect not specified). Products include:
Tofranil-PM Capsules 1041
Isocarboxazid (Effect not specified). Products include:
Marplan Tablets 1906
Maprotiline Hydrochloride (Effect not specified). Products include:
Ludiomil Tablets 874
Nortriptyline Hydrochloride (Effect not specified). Products include:
Pamelor 2019
Phenelzine Sulfate (Effect not specified). Products include:
Nardil 1742
Protriptyline Hydrochloride (Effect not specified). Products include:
Vivactil Tablets 1567
Tranylcypromine Sulfate (Effect not specified). Products include:
Parnate Tablets 2222
Trazodone Hydrochloride (Effect not specified). Products include:
Desyrel and Desyrel Dividose 1404
Trimipramine Maleate (Effect not specified). Products include:
Surmontil Capsules 2524

DRISTAN LONG LASTING MENTHOL NASAL SPRAY
(Oxymetazoline Hydrochloride) 2419
No interactions described in labeling.

DRISTAN LONG LASTING NASAL SPRAY, REGULAR AND REGULAR WITH METERED DOSE PUMP
(Oxymetazoline Hydrochloride) 2419
No interactions described in labeling.

DRISTAN NASAL SPRAY, MENTHOL
(Phenylephrine Hydrochloride, Pheniramine Maleate) 2419
No interactions described in labeling.

DRISTAN NASAL SPRAY, REGULAR AND REGULAR WITH METERED PUMP
(Phenylephrine Hydrochloride, Pheniramine Maleate) 2419
No interactions described in labeling.

NO DROWSINESS DRISTAN COLD NASAL DECONGESTANT/ANALGESIC COATED CAPLETS
(Acetaminophen, Pseudoephedrine Hydrochloride) 2420
May interact with antidepressant drugs. Compounds in this category include:

Amitriptyline Hydrochloride (Concurrent use is recommended only under physician's supervision). Products include:
Elavil 2269
Endep Tablets 1927
Etrafon 2087
Limbitrol 1933
Triavil Tablets 1556
Amoxapine (Concurrent use is recommended only under physician's supervision). Products include:
Asendin Tablets 1196
Bupropion Hydrochloride (Concurrent use is recommended only under physician's supervision). Products include:
Wellbutrin Tablets 821
Desipramine Hydrochloride (Concurrent use is recommended only under physician's supervision). Products include:
Norpramin Tablets 1340
Doxepin Hydrochloride (Concurrent use is recommended only under physician's supervision). Products include:
Sinequan 1960
Fluoxetine Hydrochloride (Concurrent use is recommended only under physician's supervision). Products include:
Prozac Pulvules 920
Imipramine Hydrochloride (Concurrent use is recommended only under physician's supervision). Products include:
Tofranil Ampuls 1038
Tofranil Tablets 1039
Imipramine Pamoate (Concurrent use is recommended only under physician's supervision). Products include:
Tofranil-PM Capsules 1041
Isocarboxazid (Concurrent use is recommended only under physician's supervision). Products include:
Marplan Tablets 1906
Maprotiline Hydrochloride (Concurrent use is recommended only under physician's supervision). Products include:
Ludiomil Tablets 874
Nortriptyline Hydrochloride (Concurrent use is recommended only under physician's supervision). Products include:
Pamelor 2019
Phenelzine Sulfate (Concurrent use is recommended only under physician's supervision). Products include:
Nardil 1742
Protriptyline Hydrochloride (Concurrent use is recommended only under physician's supervision). Products include:
Vivactil Tablets 1567
Tranylcypromine Sulfate (Concurrent use is recommended only under physician's supervision). Products include:
Parnate Tablets 2222
Trazodone Hydrochloride (Concurrent use is recommended only under physician's supervision). Products include:
Desyrel and Desyrel Dividose 1404
Trimipramine Maleate (Concurrent use is recommended only under physician's supervision). Products include:
Surmontil Capsules 2524

DRISTAN SINUS CAPLETS
(Ibuprofen, Pseudoephedrine Hydrochloride) 2419
May interact with antihypertensives, antidepressant drugs, and certain other agents. Compounds in these categories include:

Acebutolol Hydrochloride (Effect not specified). Products include:
Sectral Capsules 2520
Amitriptyline Hydrochloride (Effect not specified). Products include:
Elavil 2269
Endep Tablets 1927
Etrafon 2087
Limbitrol 1933
Triavil Tablets 1556
Amoxapine (Effect not specified). Products include:
Asendin Tablets 1196
Analgesics, unspecified (Effect not specified).
Atenolol (Effect not specified). Products include:
Tenoretic Tablets 1105
Tenormin Tablets and I.V. Injection 1107
Benazepril Hydrochloride (Effect not specified). Products include:
Lotensin Tablets 872
Betaxolol Hydrochloride (Effect not specified). Products include:
Betoptic Sterile Ophthalmic Solution 569
Betoptic S Sterile Ophthalmic Suspension 570
Kerlone Tablets 2172
Bupropion Hydrochloride (Effect not specified). Products include:
Wellbutrin Tablets 821
Captopril (Effect not specified). Products include:
Capoten 2255
Capozide 2258
Carteolol Hydrochloride (Effect not specified). Products include:
Cartrol Tablets 507
Clonidine (Effect not specified). Products include:
Catapres-TTS 677
Clonidine Hydrochloride (Effect not specified). Products include:
Catapres Tablets 676
Combipres Tablets 678
Deserpidine (Effect not specified). Products include:
Enduronyl 518
Harmonyl Tablets 528
Oreticyl 545
Desipramine Hydrochloride (Effect not specified). Products include:
Norpramin Tablets 1340
Diazoxide (Effect not specified). Products include:
Hyperstat I.V. Injection 2095
Proglycem 649
Doxazosin Mesylate (Effect not specified). Products include:
Cardura Tablets 1941
Doxepin Hydrochloride (Effect not specified). Products include:
Sinequan 1960
Enalapril Maleate (Effect not specified). Products include:
Vaseretic Tablets 1559
Vasotec Tablets 1564
Enalaprilat (Effect not specified). Products include:
Vasotec I.V. 1562
Esmolol Hydrochloride (Effect not specified). Products include:
Brevibloc Injection 942
Felodipine (Effect not specified). Products include:
Plendil Extended-Release Tablets 1526
Fluoxetine Hydrochloride (Effect not specified). Products include:
Prozac Pulvules 920
Fosinopril Sodium (Effect not specified). Products include:
Monopril Tablets 1406
Guanabenz Acetate (Effect not specified). Products include:
Wytensin Tablets 2542
Guanethidine Monosulfate (Effect not specified). Products include:
Esimil Tablets 864
Ismelin Tablets 869
Hydralazine Hydrochloride (Effect not specified). Products include:
Apresazide Capsules 854
Apresoline Hydrochloride Parenteral (Ampuls) 856
Apresoline Hydrochloride Tablets .. 855
Apresoline-Esidrix Tablets 857
Ser-Ap-Es Tablets 881
Serpasil-Apresoline Tablets 884
Imipramine Hydrochloride (Effect not specified). Products include:
Tofranil Ampuls 1038
Tofranil Tablets 1039
Imipramine Pamoate (Effect not specified). Products include:
Tofranil-PM Capsules 1041
Isocarboxazid (Effect not specified). Products include:
Marplan Tablets 1906
Isradipine (Effect not specified). Products include:
DynaCirc Capsules 2004
Labetalol Hydrochloride (Effect not specified). Products include:
Normodyne Injection 2108
Normodyne Tablets 2110
Normozide Tablets 2112
Trandate HCT Tablets 579
Trandate Injection 577
Trandate Tablets 579
Lisinopril (Effect not specified). Products include:
Prinivil Tablets 1538
Prinzide Tablets 1540
Zestoretic 2274
Zestril Tablets 2277
Maprotiline Hydrochloride (Effect not specified). Products include:
Ludiomil Tablets 874
Mecamylamine Hydrochloride (Effect not specified). Products include:
Inversine Tablets 1492
Methyldopa (Effect not specified). Products include:
Aldoclor Tablets 1413
Aldomet Oral 1415
Aldoril Tablets 1418
Metoprolol Tartrate (Effect not specified). Products include:
Lopressor Ampuls 1032
Lopressor HCT Tablets 1034
Lopressor Tablets 1032
Metyrosine (Effect not specified). Products include:
Demser Capsules 1460
Minoxidil (Effect not specified). Products include:
Loniten Tablets 2346
Rogaine Topical Solution 2357
Nadolol (Effect not specified). Products include:
Corgard Tablets 701
Corzide Tablets 702
Nicardipine Hydrochloride (Effect not specified). Products include:
Cardene Capsules 2290
Nitroglycerin (Effect not specified). Products include:
Deponit NTG Transdermal Delivery System 2143
Minitran Transdermal Delivery System 1312
Nitro-Bid Ointment 1339
Nitro-Bid Capsules 1338
Nitrodisc 2176
Nitro-Dur (nitroglycerin) Transdermal Infusion System 1164
Nitrogard Tablets 1004
Nitrolingual Spray 1846
Nitrostat Tablets 1743
Transderm-Nitro Transdermal Therapeutic System 2283
Nortriptyline Hydrochloride (Effect not specified). Products include:
Pamelor 2019
Penbutolol Sulfate (Effect not specified). Products include:
Levatol 1832
Phenelzine Sulfate (Effect not specified). Products include:
Nardil 1742
Phenoxybenzamine Hydrochloride (Effect not specified). Products include:
Dibenzyline Capsules 2207

Phentolamine Mesylate (Effect not specified). Products include:
- Regitine 878

Pindolol (Effect not specified). Products include:
- Visken Tablets 2036

Prazosin Hydrochloride (Effect not specified). Products include:
- Minipress Capsules 1778
- Minizide Capsules 1779

Propranolol Hydrochloride (Effect not specified). Products include:
- Inderal 2459
- Inderal LA Long Acting Capsules 2461
- Inderide Tablets 2463
- Inderide LA Long Acting Capsules 2465

Protriptyline Hydrochloride (Effect not specified). Products include:
- Vivactil Tablets 1567

Ramipril (Effect not specified). Products include:
- Altace Capsules 1086

Rauwolfia Serpentina (Effect not specified). Products include:
- Raudixin Tablets 1803
- Rauzide Tablets 1804

Rescinnamine (Effect not specified).
- No products indexed under this heading.

Reserpine (Effect not specified). Products include:
- Diupres Tablets 1461
- Hydromox R Tablets 1209
- Hydropres Tablets 1485
- Renese-R Tablets 1786
- Salutensin/Salutensin-Demi 719
- Ser-Ap-Es Tablets 881
- Serpasil Tablets 883
- Serpasil-Apresoline Tablets 884
- Serpasil-Esidrix Tablets 886

Sodium Nitroprusside (Effect not specified). Products include:
- Nipride I.V. Infusion 1909

Terazosin Hydrochloride (Effect not specified). Products include:
- Hytrin Tablets 529

Timolol Maleate (Effect not specified). Products include:
- Blocadren Tablets 1429
- Timolide Tablets 1547
- Timoptic in Ocudose 1552
- Timoptic Sterile Ophthalmic Solution 1550

Tranylcypromine Sulfate (Effect not specified). Products include:
- Parnate Tablets 2222

Trazodone Hydrochloride (Effect not specified). Products include:
- Desyrel and Desyrel Dividose 1404

Trimethaphan Camsylate (Effect not specified). Products include:
- Arfonad Ampuls 1887

Trimipramine Maleate (Effect not specified). Products include:
- Surmontil Capsules 2524

DRITHOCREME
(Anthralin) 590
No interactions described in labeling.

DRITHO-SCALP
(Anthralin) 591
No interactions described in labeling.

DRIXORAL ANTIHISTAMINE/NASAL DECONGESTANT SYRUP
(Brompheniramine Maleate, Pseudoephedrine Sulfate) .... ⊞ 698
May interact with antihypertensives, antidepressant drugs, and certain other agents. Compounds in these categories include:

Acebutolol Hydrochloride (Concurrent use is not recommended). Products include:
- Sectral Capsules 2520

Alcohol (Increases drowsiness effect).

Amitriptyline Hydrochloride (Concurrent use is not recommended). Products include:
- Elavil 2269
- Endep Tablets 1927
- Etrafon 2087
- Limbitrol 1933
- Triavil Tablets 1556

Amoxapine (Concurrent use is not recommended). Products include:
- Asendin Tablets 1196

Atenolol (Concurrent use is not recommended). Products include:
- Tenoretic Tablets 1105
- Tenormin Tablets and I.V. Injection 1107

Benazepril Hydrochloride (Concurrent use is not recommended). Products include:
- Lotensin Tablets 872

Bendroflumethiazide (Concurrent use is not recommended). Products include:
- Corzide Tablets 702
- Naturetin Tablets 1789
- Rauzide Tablets 1804

Betaxolol Hydrochloride (Concurrent use is not recommended). Products include:
- Betoptic Sterile Ophthalmic Solution 569
- Betoptic S Sterile Ophthalmic Suspension 570
- Kerlone Tablets 2172

Bupropion Hydrochloride (Concurrent use is not recommended). Products include:
- Wellbutrin Tablets 821

Captopril (Concurrent use is not recommended). Products include:
- Capoten 2255
- Capozide 2258

Carteolol Hydrochloride (Concurrent use is not recommended). Products include:
- Cartrol Tablets 507

Chlorothiazide (Concurrent use is not recommended). Products include:
- Aldoclor Tablets 1413
- Diupres Tablets 1461
- Diuril Oral 1464

Chlorothiazide Sodium (Concurrent use is not recommended). Products include:
- Diuril Sodium Intravenous 1463

Chlorthalidone (Concurrent use is not recommended). Products include:
- Combipres Tablets 678
- Tenoretic Tablets 1105
- Thalitone Tablets 687

Clonidine (Concurrent use is not recommended). Products include:
- Catapres-TTS 677

Clonidine Hydrochloride (Concurrent use is not recommended). Products include:
- Catapres Tablets 676
- Combipres Tablets 678

Deserpidine (Concurrent use is not recommended). Products include:
- Enduronyl 518
- Harmonyl Tablets 528
- Oreticyl 545

Desipramine Hydrochloride (Concurrent use is not recommended). Products include:
- Norpramin Tablets 1340

Diazoxide (Concurrent use is not recommended). Products include:
- Hyperstat I.V. Injection 2095
- Proglycem 649

Doxazosin Mesylate (Concurrent use is not recommended). Products include:
- Cardura Tablets 1941

Doxepin Hydrochloride (Concurrent use is not recommended). Products include:
- Sinequan 1960

Enalapril Maleate (Concurrent use is not recommended). Products include:
- Vaseretic Tablets 1559
- Vasotec Tablets 1564

Enalaprilat (Concurrent use is not recommended). Products include:
- Vasotec I.V. 1562

Esmolol Hydrochloride (Concurrent use is not recommended). Products include:
- Brevibloc Injection 942

Felodipine (Concurrent use is not recommended). Products include:
- Plendil Extended-Release Tablets 1526

Fluoxetine Hydrochloride (Concurrent use is not recommended). Products include:
- Prozac Pulvules 920

Fosinopril Sodium (Concurrent use is not recommended). Products include:
- Monopril Tablets 1406

Furosemide (Concurrent use is not recommended). Products include:
- Lasix 1093

Guanabenz Acetate (Concurrent use is not recommended). Products include:
- Wytensin Tablets 2542

Guanethidine Monosulfate (Concurrent use is not recommended). Products include:
- Esimil Tablets 864
- Ismelin Tablets 869

Hydralazine Hydrochloride (Concurrent use is not recommended). Products include:
- Apresazide Capsules 854
- Apresoline Hydrochloride Parenteral (Ampuls) 856
- Apresoline Hydrochloride Tablets 855
- Apresoline-Esidrix Tablets 857
- Ser-Ap-Es Tablets 881
- Serpasil-Apresoline Tablets 884

Hydrochlorothiazide (Concurrent use is not recommended). Products include:
- Aldactazide 2150
- Aldoril Tablets 1418
- Apresazide Capsules 854
- Apresoline-Esidrix Tablets 857
- Capozide 2258
- Dyazide Capsules 2208
- Esidrix Tablets 863
- Esimil Tablets 864
- HydroDIURIL Tablets 1484
- Hydropres Tablets 1485
- Inderide Tablets 2463
- Inderide LA Long Acting Capsules 2465
- Lopressor HCT Tablets 1034
- Maxzide 1215
- Moduretic Tablets 1510
- Normozide Tablets 2112
- Oretic Tablets 544
- Oreticyl 545
- Prinzide Tablets 1540
- Ser-Ap-Es Tablets 881
- Serpasil-Esidrix Tablets 886
- Timolide Tablets 1547
- Trandate HCT Tablets 579
- Vaseretic Tablets 1559
- Zestoretic 2274

Hydroflumethiazide (Concurrent use is not recommended). Products include:
- Diucardin Tablets 2450
- Saluron 718
- Salutensin/Salutensin-Demi 719

Imipramine Hydrochloride (Concurrent use is not recommended). Products include:
- Tofranil Ampuls 1038
- Tofranil Tablets 1039

Imipramine Pamoate (Concurrent use is not recommended). Products include:
- Tofranil-PM Capsules 1041

Indapamide (Concurrent use is not recommended). Products include:
- Lozol Tablets 1843

Isocarboxazid (Concurrent use is not recommended). Products include:
- Marplan Tablets 1906

Isradipine (Concurrent use is not recommended). Products include:
- DynaCirc Capsules 2004

Labetalol Hydrochloride (Concurrent use is not recommended). Products include:
- Normodyne Injection 2108
- Normodyne Tablets 2110
- Normozide Tablets 2112
- Trandate HCT Tablets 579
- Trandate Injection 577
- Trandate Tablets 579

Lisinopril (Concurrent use is not recommended). Products include:
- Prinivil Tablets 1538
- Prinzide Tablets 1540
- Zestoretic 2274
- Zestril Tablets 2277

Maprotiline Hydrochloride (Concurrent use is not recommended). Products include:
- Ludiomil Tablets 874

Mecamylamine Hydrochloride (Concurrent use is not recommended). Products include:
- Inversine Tablets 1492

Methyclothiazide (Concurrent use is not recommended). Products include:
- Enduron Tablets 517
- Enduronyl 518

Methyldopa (Concurrent use is not recommended). Products include:
- Aldoclor Tablets 1413
- Aldomet Oral 1415
- Aldoril Tablets 1418

Methyldopate Hydrochloride (Concurrent use is not recommended). Products include:
- Aldomet Ester HCl Injection 1417

Metolazone (Concurrent use is not recommended). Products include:
- Diulo 2129
- Mykrox ½ mg Tablets 984
- Zaroxolyn Tablets 989

Metoprolol Tartrate (Concurrent use is not recommended). Products include:
- Lopressor Ampuls 1032
- Lopressor HCT Tablets 1034
- Lopressor Tablets 1032

Metyrosine (Concurrent use is not recommended). Products include:
- Demser Capsules 1460

Minoxidil (Concurrent use is not recommended). Products include:
- Loniten Tablets 2346
- Rogaine Topical Solution 2357

Nadolol (Concurrent use is not recommended). Products include:
- Corgard Tablets 701
- Corzide Tablets 702

Nicardipine Hydrochloride (Concurrent use is not recommended). Products include:
- Cardene Capsules 2290

Nitroglycerin (Concurrent use is not recommended). Products include:
- Deponit NTG Transdermal Delivery System 2143
- Minitran Transdermal Delivery System 1312
- Nitro-Bid Ointment 1339

Nitro-Bid Capsules 1338
Nitrodisc 2176
Nitro-Dur (nitroglycerin) Transdermal Infusion System 1164
Nitrogard Tablets 1004
Nitrolingual Spray 1846
Nitrostat Tablets 1743
Transderm-Nitro Transdermal Therapeutic System 2283

Nortriptyline Hydrochloride (Concurrent use is not recommended). Products include:
Pamelor 2019

Penbutolol Sulfate (Concurrent use is not recommended). Products include:
Levatol 1832

Phenelzine Sulfate (Concurrent use is not recommended). Products include:
Nardil 1742

Phenoxybenzamine Hydrochloride (Concurrent use is not recommended). Products include:
Dibenzyline Capsules 2207

Phentolamine Mesylate (Concurrent use is not recommended). Products include:
Regitine 878

Pindolol (Concurrent use is not recommended). Products include:
Visken Tablets 2036

Polythiazide (Concurrent use is not recommended). Products include:
Minizide Capsules 1779
Renese Tablets 1785
Renese-R Tablets 1786

Prazosin Hydrochloride (Concurrent use is not recommended). Products include:
Minipress Capsules 1778
Minizide Capsules 1779

Propranolol Hydrochloride (Concurrent use is not recommended). Products include:
Inderal 2459
Inderal LA Long Acting Capsules 2461
Inderide Tablets 2463
Inderide LA Long Acting Capsules 2465

Protriptyline Hydrochloride (Concurrent use is not recommended). Products include:
Vivactil Tablets 1567

Ramipril (Concurrent use is not recommended). Products include:
Altace Capsules 1086

Rauwolfia Serpentina (Concurrent use is not recommended). Products include:
Raudixin Tablets 1803
Rauzide Tablets 1804

Rescinnamine (Concurrent use is not recommended).
No products indexed under this heading.

Reserpine (Concurrent use is not recommended). Products include:
Diupres Tablets 1461
Hydromox R Tablets 1209
Hydropres Tablets 1485
Renese-R Tablets 1786
Salutensin/Salutensin-Demi 719
Ser-Ap-Es Tablets 881
Serpasil Tablets 883
Serpasil-Apresoline Tablets 884
Serpasil-Esidrix Tablets 886

Sodium Nitroprusside (Concurrent use is not recommended). Products include:
Nipride I.V. Infusion 1909

Terazosin Hydrochloride (Concurrent use is not recommended). Products include:
Hytrin Tablets 529

Timolol Maleate (Concurrent use is not recommended). Products include:
Blocadren Tablets 1429
Timolide Tablets 1547
Timoptic in Ocudose 1552
Timoptic Sterile Ophthalmic Solution 1550

Tranylcypromine Sulfate (Concurrent use is not recommended). Products include:
Parnate Tablets 2222

Trazodone Hydrochloride (Concurrent use is not recommended). Products include:
Desyrel and Desyrel Dividose 1404

Trimethaphan Camsylate (Concurrent use is not recommended). Products include:
Arfonad Ampuls 1887

Trimipramine Maleate (Concurrent use is not recommended). Products include:
Surmontil Capsules 2524

DRIXORAL NON-DROWSY FORMULA
(Pseudoephedrine Sulfate) .... ▣ 699
May interact with:

Antidepressant Medications, unspecified (Effects not specified).

Blood Pressure Medications, unspecified (Effects not specified).
No products indexed under this heading.

DRIXORAL PLUS EXTENDED-RELEASE TABLETS
(Acetaminophen, Dexbrompheniramine Maleate, Pseudoephedrine Sulfate) .... ▣ 699
May interact with antihypertensives, antidepressant drugs, hypnotics and sedatives, tranquilizers, and certain other agents. Compounds in these categories include:

Acebutolol Hydrochloride (Concurrent use is not recommended). Products include:
Sectral Capsules 2520

Alcohol (Increases drowsiness effect).

Alprazolam (Concurrent use is not recommended). Products include:
Xanax Tablets 2367

Amitriptyline Hydrochloride (Concurrent use is not recommended). Products include:
Elavil 2269
Endep Tablets 1927
Etrafon 2087
Limbitrol 1933
Triavil Tablets 1556

Amoxapine (Concurrent use is not recommended). Products include:
Asendin Tablets 1196

Atenolol (Concurrent use is not recommended). Products include:
Tenoretic Tablets 1105
Tenormin Tablets and I.V. Injection 1107

Benazepril Hydrochloride (Concurrent use is not recommended). Products include:
Lotensin Tablets 872

Bendroflumethiazide (Concurrent use is not recommended). Products include:
Corzide Tablets 702
Naturetin Tablets 1789
Rauzide Tablets 1804

Betaxolol Hydrochloride (Concurrent use is not recommended). Products include:
Betoptic Sterile Ophthalmic Solution 569
Betoptic S Sterile Ophthalmic Suspension 570
Kerlone Tablets 2172

Bupropion Hydrochloride (Concurrent use is not recommended). Products include:
Wellbutrin Tablets 821

Buspirone Hydrochloride (Concurrent use is not recommended). Products include:
BuSpar 1401

Captopril (Concurrent use is not recommended). Products include:
Capoten 2255
Capozide 2258

Carteolol Hydrochloride (Concurrent use is not recommended). Products include:
Cartrol Tablets 507

Chlordiazepoxide (Concurrent use is not recommended). Products include:
Libritabs Tablets 1930
Limbitrol 1933
Menrium Tablets 1934

Chlordiazepoxide Hydrochloride (Concurrent use is not recommended). Products include:
Librax Capsules 1929
Librium Capsules 1931
Librium Injectable 1932

Chlorothiazide (Concurrent use is not recommended). Products include:
Aldoclor Tablets 1413
Diupres Tablets 1461
Diuril Oral 1464

Chlorothiazide Sodium (Concurrent use is not recommended). Products include:
Diuril Sodium Intravenous 1463

Chlorpromazine (Concurrent use is not recommended). Products include:
Thorazine 2234

Chlorprothixene (Concurrent use is not recommended). Products include:
Taractan Tablets 1920

Chlorprothixene Hydrochloride (Concurrent use is not recommended). Products include:
Taractan 1920

Chlorthalidone (Concurrent use is not recommended). Products include:
Combipres Tablets 678
Tenoretic Tablets 1105
Thalitone Tablets 687

Clonidine (Concurrent use is not recommended). Products include:
Catapres-TTS 677

Clonidine Hydrochloride (Concurrent use is not recommended). Products include:
Catapres Tablets 676
Combipres Tablets 678

Clorazepate Dipotassium (Concurrent use is not recommended). Products include:
Tranxene 556

Deserpidine (Concurrent use is not recommended). Products include:
Enduronyl 518
Harmonyl Tablets 528
Oreticyl 545

Desipramine Hydrochloride (Concurrent use is not recommended). Products include:
Norpramin Tablets 1340

Diazepam (Concurrent use is not recommended). Products include:
Valium Injectable 1937
Valium Tablets 1939
Valrelease Capsules 1923

Diazoxide (Concurrent use is not recommended). Products include:
Hyperstat I.V. Injection 2095
Proglycem 649

Doxazosin Mesylate (Concurrent use is not recommended). Products include:
Cardura Tablets 1941

Doxepin Hydrochloride (Concurrent use is not recommended). Products include:
Sinequan 1960

Droperidol (Concurrent use is not recommended). Products include:
Inapsine Injection 1140
Innovar Injection 1141

Enalapril Maleate (Concurrent use is not recommended). Products include:
Vaseretic Tablets 1559
Vasotec Tablets 1564

Enalaprilat (Concurrent use is not recommended). Products include:
Vasotec I.V. 1562

Esmolol Hydrochloride (Concurrent use is not recommended). Products include:
Brevibloc Injection 942

Estazolam (Concurrent use is not recommended). Products include:
ProSom Tablets 554

Ethchlorvynol (Concurrent use is not recommended). Products include:
Placidyl Capsules 553

Ethinamate (Concurrent use is not recommended).
No products indexed under this heading.

Felodipine (Concurrent use is not recommended). Products include:
Plendil Extended-Release Tablets 1526

Fluoxetine Hydrochloride (Concurrent use is not recommended). Products include:
Prozac Pulvules 920

Fluphenazine Decanoate (Concurrent use is not recommended). Products include:
Prolixin Decanoate 1795

Fluphenazine Enanthate (Concurrent use is not recommended). Products include:
Prolixin Enanthate 1796

Fluphenazine Hydrochloride (Concurrent use is not recommended). Products include:
Prolixin Elixir 1793
Prolixin Injection 1791
Prolixin Oral Concentrate 1792
Prolixin Tablets 1793

Flurazepam Hydrochloride (Concurrent use is not recommended). Products include:
Dalmane Capsules 1927

Fosinopril Sodium (Concurrent use is not recommended). Products include:
Monopril Tablets 1406

Furosemide (Concurrent use is not recommended). Products include:
Lasix 1093

Glutethimide (Concurrent use is not recommended).
No products indexed under this heading.

Guanabenz Acetate (Concurrent use is not recommended). Products include:
Wytensin Tablets 2542

Guanethidine Monosulfate (Concurrent use is not recommended). Products include:
Esimil Tablets 864
Ismelin Tablets 869

Haloperidol (Concurrent use is not recommended). Products include:
Haldol Injection, Tablets and Concentrate 1373

Haloperidol Decanoate (Concurrent use is not recommended). Products include:
Haldol Decanoate 1375

Hydralazine Hydrochloride (Concurrent use is not recommended). Products include:
Apresazide Capsules ... 854
Apresoline Hydrochloride Parenteral (Ampuls) ... 856
Apresoline Hydrochloride Tablets .. 855
Apresoline-Esidrix Tablets ... 857
Ser-Ap-Es Tablets ... 881
Serpasil-Apresoline Tablets ... 884

Hydrochlorothiazide (Concurrent use is not recommended). Products include:
Aldactazide ... 2150
Aldoril Tablets ... 1418
Apresazide Capsules ... 854
Apresoline-Esidrix Tablets ... 857
Capozide ... 2258
Dyazide Capsules ... 2208
Esidrix Tablets ... 863
Esimil Tablets ... 864
HydroDIURIL Tablets ... 1484
Hydropres Tablets ... 1485
Inderide Tablets ... 2463
Inderide LA Long Acting Capsules .. 2465
Lopressor HCT Tablets ... 1034
Maxzide ... 1215
Moduretic Tablets ... 1510
Normozide Tablets ... 2112
Oretic Tablets ... 544
Oreticyl ... 545
Prinzide Tablets ... 1540
Ser-Ap-Es Tablets ... 881
Serpasil-Esidrix Tablets ... 886
Timolide Tablets ... 1547
Trandate HCT Tablets ... 579
Vaseretic Tablets ... 1559
Zestoretic ... 2274

Hydroflumethiazide (Concurrent use is not recommended). Products include:
Diucardin Tablets ... 2450
Saluron ... 718
Salutensin/Salutensin-Demi ... 719

Hydroxyzine Hydrochloride (Concurrent use is not recommended). Products include:
Atarax Tablets & Syrup ... 1941
Marax Tablets & DF Syrup ... 1954
Vistaril Intramuscular Solution ... 1970

Imipramine Hydrochloride (Concurrent use is not recommended). Products include:
Tofranil Ampuls ... 1038
Tofranil Tablets ... 1039

Imipramine Pamoate (Concurrent use is not recommended). Products include:
Tofranil-PM Capsules ... 1041

Indapamide (Concurrent use is not recommended). Products include:
Lozol Tablets ... 1843

Isocarboxazid (Concurrent use is not recommended). Products include:
Marplan Tablets ... 1906

Isradipine (Concurrent use is not recommended). Products include:
DynaCirc Capsules ... 2004

Labetalol Hydrochloride (Concurrent use is not recommended). Products include:
Normodyne Injection ... 2108
Normodyne Tablets ... 2110
Normozide Tablets ... 2112
Trandate HCT Tablets ... 579
Trandate Injection ... 577
Trandate Tablets ... 579

Lisinopril (Concurrent use is not recommended). Products include:
Prinivil Tablets ... 1538
Prinzide Tablets ... 1540
Zestoretic ... 2274
Zestril Tablets ... 2277

Lorazepam (Concurrent use is not recommended). Products include:
Ativan Injection ... 2432
Ativan Tablets ... 2434

Loxapine Hydrochloride (Concurrent use is not recommended). Products include:
Loxitane ... 1213

Loxapine Succinate (Concurrent use is not recommended). Products include:
Loxitane Capsules ... 1213

Maprotiline Hydrochloride (Concurrent use is not recommended). Products include:
Ludiomil Tablets ... 874

Mecamylamine Hydrochloride (Concurrent use is not recommended). Products include:
Inversine Tablets ... 1492

Meprobamate (Concurrent use is not recommended). Products include:
Deprol Tablets ... 2382
Equagesic Tablets ... 2451
Miltown Tablets ... 2386
PMB 200 and PMB 400 ... 2504

Mesoridazine Besylate (Concurrent use is not recommended).

Methyclothiazide (Concurrent use is not recommended). Products include:
Enduron Tablets ... 517
Enduronyl ... 518

Methyldopa (Concurrent use is not recommended). Products include:
Aldoclor Tablets ... 1413
Aldomet Oral ... 1415
Aldoril Tablets ... 1418

Methyldopate Hydrochloride (Concurrent use is not recommended). Products include:
Aldomet Ester HCl Injection ... 1417

Metolazone (Concurrent use is not recommended). Products include:
Diulo ... 2129
Mykrox ½ mg Tablets ... 984
Zaroxolyn Tablets ... 989

Metoprolol Tartrate (Concurrent use is not recommended). Products include:
Lopressor Ampuls ... 1032
Lopressor HCT Tablets ... 1034
Lopressor Tablets ... 1032

Metyrosine (Concurrent use is not recommended). Products include:
Demser Capsules ... 1460

Midazolam Hydrochloride (Concurrent use is not recommended). Products include:
Versed Injection ... 1924

Minoxidil (Concurrent use is not recommended). Products include:
Loniten Tablets ... 2346
Rogaine Topical Solution ... 2357

Molindone Hydrochloride (Concurrent use is not recommended). Products include:
Moban Tablets & Concentrate ... 932

Nadolol (Concurrent use is not recommended). Products include:
Corgard Tablets ... 701
Corzide Tablets ... 702

Nicardipine Hydrochloride (Concurrent use is not recommended). Products include:
Cardene Capsules ... 2290

Nitroglycerin (Concurrent use is not recommended). Products include:
Deponit NTG Transdermal Delivery System ... 2143
Minitran Transdermal Delivery System ... 1312
Nitro-Bid Ointment ... 1339
Nitro-Bid Capsules ... 1338
Nitrodisc ... 2176
Nitro-Dur (nitroglycerin) Transdermal Infusion System ... 1164
Nitrogard Tablets ... 1004
Nitrolingual Spray ... 1846
Nitrostat Tablets ... 1743
Transderm-Nitro Transdermal Therapeutic System ... 2283

Nortriptyline Hydrochloride (Concurrent use is not recommended). Products include:
Pamelor ... 2019

Oxazepam (Concurrent use is not recommended). Products include:
Serax Capsules ... 2522
Serax Tablets ... 2522

Penbutolol Sulfate (Concurrent use is not recommended). Products include:
Levatol ... 1832

Perphenazine (Concurrent use is not recommended). Products include:
Etrafon ... 2087
Triavil Tablets ... 1556
Trilafon ... 2123

Phenelzine Sulfate (Concurrent use is not recommended). Products include:
Nardil ... 1742

Phenoxybenzamine Hydrochloride (Concurrent use is not recommended). Products include:
Dibenzyline Capsules ... 2207

Phentolamine Mesylate (Concurrent use is not recommended). Products include:
Regitine ... 878

Pindolol (Concurrent use is not recommended). Products include:
Visken Tablets ... 2036

Polythiazide (Concurrent use is not recommended). Products include:
Minizide Capsules ... 1779
Renese Tablets ... 1785
Renese-R Tablets ... 1786

Prazepam (Concurrent use is not recommended). Products include:
Centrax ... 1693

Prazosin Hydrochloride (Concurrent use is not recommended). Products include:
Minipress Capsules ... 1778
Minizide Capsules ... 1779

Prochlorperazine (Concurrent use is not recommended). Products include:
Compazine ... 2201

Promethazine Hydrochloride (Concurrent use is not recommended). Products include:
Mepergan Injection ... 2479
Phenergan with Codeine ... 2497
Phenergan with Dextromethorphan 2499
Phenergan Injection ... 2493
Phenergan Suppositories ... 2496
Phenergan Syrup ... 2495
Phenergan Tablets ... 2496
Phenergan VC ... 2500
Phenergan VC with Codeine ... 2501

Propofol (Concurrent use is not recommended). Products include:
Diprivan Injection ... 2267

Propranolol Hydrochloride (Concurrent use is not recommended). Products include:
Inderal ... 2459
Inderal LA Long Acting Capsules ... 2461
Inderide Tablets ... 2463
Inderide LA Long Acting Capsules .. 2465

Protriptyline Hydrochloride (Concurrent use is not recommended). Products include:
Vivactil Tablets ... 1567

Quazepam (Concurrent use is not recommended). Products include:
Doral Tablets ... 2383

Ramipril (Concurrent use is not recommended). Products include:
Altace Capsules ... 1086

Rauwolfia Serpentina (Concurrent use is not recommended). Products include:
Raudixin Tablets ... 1803
Rauzide Tablets ... 1804

Rescinnamine (Concurrent use is not recommended).
No products indexed under this heading.

Reserpine (Concurrent use is not recommended). Products include:
Diupres Tablets ... 1461
Hydromox R Tablets ... 1209
Hydropres Tablets ... 1485
Renese-R Tablets ... 1786
Salutensin/Salutensin-Demi ... 719
Ser-Ap-Es Tablets ... 881
Serpasil Tablets ... 883
Serpasil-Apresoline Tablets ... 884
Serpasil-Esidrix Tablets ... 886

Secobarbital Sodium (Concurrent use is not recommended). Products include:
Seconal Sodium Pulvules ... 1296

Sodium Nitroprusside (Concurrent use is not recommended). Products include:
Nipride I.V. Infusion ... 1909

Temazepam (Concurrent use is not recommended). Products include:
Restoril Capsules ... 2023

Terazosin Hydrochloride (Concurrent use is not recommended). Products include:
Hytrin Tablets ... 529

Thioridazine Hydrochloride (Concurrent use is not recommended). Products include:
Mellaril ... 2011

Thiothixene (Concurrent use is not recommended). Products include:
Navane Capsules and Concentrate 1954
Navane Intramuscular ... 1956

Timolol Maleate (Concurrent use is not recommended). Products include:
Blocadren Tablets ... 1429
Timolide Tablets ... 1547
Timoptic in Ocudose ... 1552
Timoptic Sterile Ophthalmic Solution ... 1550

Tranylcypromine Sulfate (Concurrent use is not recommended). Products include:
Parnate Tablets ... 2222

Trazodone Hydrochloride (Concurrent use is not recommended). Products include:
Desyrel and Desyrel Dividose ... 1404

Triazolam (Concurrent use is not recommended). Products include:
Halcion Tablets ... 2340

Trifluoperazine Hydrochloride (Concurrent use is not recommended). Products include:
Stelazine ... 2226

Trimethaphan Camsylate (Concurrent use is not recommended). Products include:
Arfonad Ampuls ... 1887

Trimipramine Maleate (Concurrent use is not recommended). Products include:
Surmontil Capsules ... 2524

DRIXORAL SINUS
(Pseudoephedrine Sulfate, Brompheniramine Maleate, Acetaminophen) ... ◘ 700
May interact with hypnotics and sedatives, tranquilizers, antidepressant drugs, antihypertensives, and certain other agents. Compounds in these categories include:

Acebutolol Hydrochloride (Effect not specified). Products include:
Sectral Capsules ... 2520

Alcohol (May increase the drowsiness effect).

Alprazolam (May increase the drowsiness effect). Products include:
Xanax Tablets ... 2367

Amitriptyline Hydrochloride (Effect not specified). Products include:
Elavil ... 2269
Endep Tablets ... 1927

Etrafon ... 2087
Limbitrol ... 1933
Triavil Tablets ... 1556

Amoxapine (Effect not specified). Products include:
Asendin Tablets ... 1196

Atenolol (Effect not specified). Products include:
Tenoretic Tablets ... 1105
Tenormin Tablets and I.V. Injection 1107

Benazepril Hydrochloride (Effect not specified). Products include:
Lotensin Tablets ... 872

Bendroflumethiazide (Effect not specified). Products include:
Corzide Tablets ... 702
Naturetin Tablets ... 1789
Rauzide Tablets ... 1804

Betaxolol Hydrochloride (Effect not specified). Products include:
Betoptic Sterile Ophthalmic Solution ... 569
Betoptic S Sterile Ophthalmic Suspension ... 570
Kerlone Tablets ... 2172

Bupropion Hydrochloride (Effect not specified). Products include:
Wellbutrin Tablets ... 821

Buspirone Hydrochloride (May increase the drowsiness effect). Products include:
BuSpar ... 1401

Captopril (Effect not specified). Products include:
Capoten ... 2255
Capozide ... 2258

Carteolol Hydrochloride (Effect not specified). Products include:
Cartrol Tablets ... 507

Chlordiazepoxide (May increase the drowsiness effect). Products include:
Libritabs Tablets ... 1930
Limbitrol ... 1933
Menrium Tablets ... 1934

Chlordiazepoxide Hydrochloride (May increase the drowsiness effect). Products include:
Librax Capsules ... 1929
Librium Capsules ... 1931
Librium Injectable ... 1932

Chlorothiazide (Effect not specified). Products include:
Aldoclor Tablets ... 1413
Diupres Tablets ... 1461
Diuril Oral ... 1464

Chlorothiazide Sodium (Effect not specified). Products include:
Diuril Sodium Intravenous ... 1463

Chlorpromazine (May increase the drowsiness effect). Products include:
Thorazine ... 2234

Chlorprothixene (May increase the drowsiness effect). Products include:
Taractan Tablets ... 1920

Chlorprothixene Hydrochloride (May increase the drowsiness effect). Products include:
Taractan ... 1920

Chlorthalidone (Effect not specified). Products include:
Combipres Tablets ... 678
Tenoretic Tablets ... 1105
Thalitone Tablets ... 687

Clonidine (Effect not specified). Products include:
Catapres-TTS ... 677

Clonidine Hydrochloride (Effect not specified). Products include:
Catapres Tablets ... 676
Combipres Tablets ... 678

Clorazepate Dipotassium (May increase the drowsiness effect). Products include:
Tranxene ... 556

Deserpidine (Effect not specified). Products include:
Enduronyl ... 518
Harmonyl Tablets ... 528
Oreticyl ... 545

Desipramine Hydrochloride (Effect not specified). Products include:
Norpramin Tablets ... 1340

Diazepam (May increase the drowsiness effect). Products include:
Valium Injectable ... 1937
Valium Tablets ... 1939
Valrelease Capsules ... 1923

Diazoxide (Effect not specified). Products include:
Hyperstat I.V. Injection ... 2095
Proglycem ... 649

Doxazosin Mesylate (Effect not specified). Products include:
Cardura Tablets ... 1941

Doxepin Hydrochloride (Effect not specified). Products include:
Sinequan ... 1960

Droperidol (May increase the drowsiness effect). Products include:
Inapsine Injection ... 1140
Innovar Injection ... 1141

Enalapril Maleate (Effect not specified). Products include:
Vaseretic Tablets ... 1559
Vasotec Tablets ... 1564

Enalaprilat (Effect not specified). Products include:
Vasotec I.V. ... 1562

Esmolol Hydrochloride (Effect not specified). Products include:
Brevibloc Injection ... 942

Estazolam (May increase the drowsiness effect). Products include:
ProSom Tablets ... 554

Ethchlorvynol (May increase the drowsiness effect). Products include:
Placidyl Capsules ... 553

Ethinamate (May increase the drowsiness effect).
No products indexed under this heading.

Felodipine (Effect not specified). Products include:
Plendil Extended-Release Tablets ... 1526

Fluoxetine Hydrochloride (Effect not specified). Products include:
Prozac Pulvules ... 920

Fluphenazine Decanoate (May increase the drowsiness effect). Products include:
Prolixin Decanoate ... 1795

Fluphenazine Enanthate (May increase the drowsiness effect). Products include:
Prolixin Enanthate ... 1796

Fluphenazine Hydrochloride (May increase the drowsiness effect). Products include:
Prolixin Elixir ... 1793
Prolixin Injection ... 1791
Prolixin Oral Concentrate ... 1792
Prolixin Tablets ... 1793

Flurazepam Hydrochloride (May increase the drowsiness effect). Products include:
Dalmane Capsules ... 1927

Fosinopril Sodium (Effect not specified). Products include:
Monopril Tablets ... 1406

Furosemide (Effect not specified). Products include:
Lasix ... 1093

Glutethimide (May increase the drowsiness effect).
No products indexed under this heading.

Guanabenz Acetate (Effect not specified). Products include:
Wytensin Tablets ... 2542

Guanethidine Monosulfate (Effect not specified). Products include:
Esimil Tablets ... 864
Ismelin Tablets ... 869

Haloperidol (May increase the drowsiness effect). Products include:
Haldol Injection, Tablets and Concentrate ... 1373

Haloperidol Decanoate (May increase the drowsiness effect). Products include:
Haldol Decanoate ... 1375

Hydralazine Hydrochloride (Effect not specified). Products include:
Apresazide Capsules ... 854
Apresoline Hydrochloride Parenteral (Ampuls) ... 856
Apresoline Hydrochloride Tablets ... 855
Apresoline-Esidrix Tablets ... 857
Ser-Ap-Es Tablets ... 881
Serpasil-Apresoline Tablets ... 884

Hydrochlorothiazide (Effect not specified). Products include:
Aldactazide ... 2150
Aldoril Tablets ... 1418
Apresazide Capsules ... 854
Apresoline-Esidrix Tablets ... 857
Capozide ... 2258
Dyazide Capsules ... 2208
Esidrix Tablets ... 863
Esimil Tablets ... 864
HydroDIURIL Tablets ... 1484
Hydropres Tablets ... 1485
Inderide Tablets ... 2463
Inderide LA Long Acting Capsules ... 2465
Lopressor HCT Tablets ... 1034
Maxzide ... 1215
Moduretic Tablets ... 1510
Normozide Tablets ... 2112
Oretic Tablets ... 544
Oreticyl ... 545
Prinzide Tablets ... 1540
Ser-Ap-Es Tablets ... 881
Serpasil-Esidrix Tablets ... 886
Timolide Tablets ... 1547
Trandate HCT Tablets ... 579
Vaseretic Tablets ... 1559
Zestoretic ... 2274

Hydroflumethiazide (Effect not specified). Products include:
Diucardin Tablets ... 2450
Saluron ... 718
Salutensin/Salutensin-Demi ... 719

Hydroxyzine Hydrochloride (May increase the drowsiness effect). Products include:
Atarax Tablets & Syrup ... 1941
Marax Tablets & DF Syrup ... 1954
Vistaril Intramuscular Solution ... 1970

Imipramine Hydrochloride (Effect not specified). Products include:
Tofranil Ampuls ... 1038
Tofranil Tablets ... 1039

Imipramine Pamoate (Effect not specified). Products include:
Tofranil-PM Capsules ... 1041

Indapamide (Effect not specified). Products include:
Lozol Tablets ... 1843

Isocarboxazid (Effect not specified). Products include:
Marplan Tablets ... 1906

Isradipine (Effect not specified). Products include:
DynaCirc Capsules ... 2004

Labetalol Hydrochloride (Effect not specified). Products include:
Normodyne Injection ... 2108
Normodyne Tablets ... 2110
Normozide Tablets ... 2112
Trandate HCT Tablets ... 579
Trandate Injection ... 577
Trandate Tablets ... 579

Lisinopril (Effect not specified). Products include:
Prinivil Tablets ... 1538
Prinzide Tablets ... 1540
Zestoretic ... 2274
Zestril Tablets ... 2277

Lorazepam (May increase the drowsiness effect). Products include:
Ativan Injection ... 2432
Ativan Tablets ... 2434

Loxapine Hydrochloride (May increase the drowsiness effect). Products include:
Loxitane ... 1213

Loxapine Succinate (May increase the drowsiness effect). Products include:
Loxitane Capsules ... 1213

Maprotiline Hydrochloride (Effect not specified). Products include:
Ludiomil Tablets ... 874

Mecamylamine Hydrochloride (Effect not specified). Products include:
Inversine Tablets ... 1492

Meprobamate (May increase the drowsiness effect). Products include:
Deprol Tablets ... 2382
Equagesic Tablets ... 2451
Miltown Tablets ... 2386
PMB 200 and PMB 400 ... 2504

Mesoridazine (May increase the drowsiness effect). Products include:
Serentil ... 686

Methyclothiazide (Effect not specified). Products include:
Enduron Tablets ... 517
Enduronyl ... 518

Methyldopa (Effect not specified). Products include:
Aldoclor Tablets ... 1413
Aldomet Oral ... 1415
Aldoril Tablets ... 1418

Methyldopate Hydrochloride (Effect not specified). Products include:
Aldomet Ester HCl Injection ... 1417

Metolazone (Effect not specified). Products include:
Diulo ... 2129
Mykrox ½ mg Tablets ... 984
Zaroxolyn Tablets ... 989

Metoprolol Tartrate (Effect not specified). Products include:
Lopressor Ampuls ... 1032
Lopressor HCT Tablets ... 1034
Lopressor Tablets ... 1032

Metyrosine (Effect not specified). Products include:
Demser Capsules ... 1460

Midazolam Hydrochloride (May increase the drowsiness effect). Products include:
Versed Injection ... 1924

Minoxidil (Effect not specified). Products include:
Loniten Tablets ... 2346
Rogaine Topical Solution ... 2357

Molindone Hydrochloride (May increase the drowsiness effect). Products include:
Moban Tablets & Concentrate ... 932

Nadolol (Effect not specified). Products include:
Corgard Tablets ... 701
Corzide Tablets ... 702

Nicardipine Hydrochloride (Effect not specified). Products include:
Cardene Capsules ... 2290

Nitroglycerin (Effect not specified). Products include:
Deponit NTG Transdermal Delivery System ... 2143
Minitran Transdermal Delivery System ... 1312
Nitro-Bid Ointment ... 1339
Nitro-Bid Capsules ... 1338
Nitrodisc ... 2176
Nitro-Dur (nitroglycerin) Transdermal Infusion System ... 1164
Nitrogard Tablets ... 1004
Nitrolingual Spray ... 1846
Nitrostat Tablets ... 1743
Transderm-Nitro Transdermal Therapeutic System ... 2283

Nortriptyline Hydrochloride (Effect not specified). Products include:
Pamelor ... 2019

Oxazepam (May increase the drowsiness effect). Products include:
Serax Capsules ... 2522
Serax Tablets ... 2522

Penbutolol Sulfate (Effect not specified). Products include:
Levatol ... 1832

Perphenazine (May increase the drowsiness effect). Products include:
Etrafon ... 2087
Triavil Tablets ... 1556
Trilafon ... 2123

Phenelzine Sulfate (Effect not specified). Products include:
Nardil ... 1742

Phenoxybenzamine Hydrochloride (Effect not specified). Products include:
Dibenzyline Capsules ... 2207

Phentolamine Mesylate (Effect not specified). Products include:
Regitine ... 878

Pindolol (Effect not specified). Products include:
Visken Tablets ... 2036

Polythiazide (Effect not specified). Products include:
Minizide Capsules ... 1779
Renese Tablets ... 1785
Renese-R Tablets ... 1786

Prazepam (May increase the drowsiness effect). Products include:
Centrax ... 1693

Prazosin Hydrochloride (Effect not specified). Products include:
Minipress Capsules ... 1778
Minizide Capsules ... 1779

Prochlorperazine (May increase the drowsiness effect). Products include:
Compazine ... 2201

Promethazine Hydrochloride (May increase the drowsiness effect). Products include:
Mepergan Injection ... 2479
Phenergan with Codeine ... 2497
Phenergan with Dextromethorphan 2499
Phenergan Injection ... 2493
Phenergan Suppositories ... 2496
Phenergan Syrup ... 2495
Phenergan Tablets ... 2496
Phenergan VC ... 2500
Phenergan VC with Codeine ... 2501

Propofol (May increase the drowsiness effect). Products include:
Diprivan Injection ... 2267

Propranolol Hydrochloride (Effect not specified). Products include:
Inderal ... 2459
Inderal LA Long Acting Capsules ... 2461
Inderide Tablets ... 2463
Inderide LA Long Acting Capsules .. 2465

Protriptyline Hydrochloride (Effect not specified). Products include:
Vivactil Tablets ... 1567

Quazepam (May increase the drowsiness effect). Products include:
Doral Tablets ... 2383

Ramipril (Effect not specified). Products include:
Altace Capsules ... 1086

Rauwolfia Serpentina (Effect not specified). Products include:
Raudixin Tablets ... 1803
Rauzide Tablets ... 1804

Rescinnamine (Effect not specified).
No products indexed under this heading.

Reserpine (Effect not specified). Products include:
Diupres Tablets ... 1461
Hydromox R Tablets ... 1209
Hydropres Tablets ... 1485
Renese-R Tablets ... 1786
Salutensin/Salutensin-Demi ... 719
Ser-Ap-Es Tablets ... 881
Serpasil Tablets ... 883
Serpasil-Apresoline Tablets ... 884
Serpasil-Esidrix Tablets ... 886

Secobarbital Sodium (May increase the drowsiness effect). Products include:
Seconal Sodium Pulvules ... 1296

Sodium Nitroprusside (Effect not specified). Products include:
Nipride I.V. Infusion ... 1909

Temazepam (May increase the drowsiness effect). Products include:
Restoril Capsules ... 2023

Terazosin Hydrochloride (Effect not specified). Products include:
Hytrin Tablets ... 529

Thioridazine Hydrochloride (May increase the drowsiness effect). Products include:
Mellaril ... 2011

Thiothixene (May increase the drowsiness effect). Products include:
Navane Capsules and Concentrate 1954
Navane Intramuscular ... 1956

Timolol Maleate (Effect not specified). Products include:
Blocadren Tablets ... 1429
Timolide Tablets ... 1547
Timoptic in Ocudose ... 1552
Timoptic Sterile Ophthalmic Solution ... 1550

Tranylcypromine Sulfate (Effect not specified). Products include:
Parnate Tablets ... 2222

Trazodone Hydrochloride (Effect not specified). Products include:
Desyrel and Desyrel Dividose ... 1404

Triazolam (May increase the drowsiness effect). Products include:
Halcion Tablets ... 2340

Trifluoperazine Hydrochloride (May increase the drowsiness effect). Products include:
Stelazine ... 2226

Trimethaphan Camsylate (Effect not specified). Products include:
Arfonad Ampuls ... 1887

Trimipramine Maleate (Effect not specified). Products include:
Surmontil Capsules ... 2524

DRIXORAL SUSTAINED-ACTION TABLETS
(Dexbrompheniramine Maleate, Pseudoephedrine Sulfate) ... 698
May interact with antihypertensives, antidepressant drugs, and certain other agents. Compounds in these categories include:

Acebutolol Hydrochloride (Concurrent use is not recommended). Products include:
Sectral Capsules ... 2520

Alcohol (Increases drowsiness effect).

Amitriptyline Hydrochloride (Concurrent use is not recommended). Products include:
Elavil ... 2269
Endep Tablets ... 1927
Etrafon ... 2087
Limbitrol ... 1933
Triavil Tablets ... 1556

Amoxapine (Concurrent use is not recommended). Products include:
Asendin Tablets ... 1196

Atenolol (Concurrent use is not recommended). Products include:
Tenoretic Tablets ... 1105
Tenormin Tablets and I.V. Injection 1107

Benazepril Hydrochloride (Concurrent use is not recommended). Products include:
Lotensin Tablets ... 872

Bendroflumethiazide (Concurrent use is not recommended). Products include:
Corzide Tablets ... 702
Naturetin Tablets ... 1789
Rauzide Tablets ... 1804

Betaxolol Hydrochloride (Concurrent use is not recommended). Products include:
Betoptic Sterile Ophthalmic Solution ... 569
Betoptic S Sterile Ophthalmic Suspension ... 570
Kerlone Tablets ... 2172

Bupropion Hydrochloride (Concurrent use is not recommended). Products include:
Wellbutrin Tablets ... 821

Captopril (Concurrent use is not recommended). Products include:
Capoten ... 2255
Capozide ... 2258

Carteolol Hydrochloride (Concurrent use is not recommended). Products include:
Cartrol Tablets ... 507

Chlorothiazide (Concurrent use is not recommended). Products include:
Aldoclor Tablets ... 1413
Diupres Tablets ... 1461
Diuril Oral ... 1464

Chlorothiazide Sodium (Concurrent use is not recommended). Products include:
Diuril Sodium Intravenous ... 1463

Chlorthalidone (Concurrent use is not recommended). Products include:
Combipres Tablets ... 678
Tenoretic Tablets ... 1105
Thalitone Tablets ... 687

Clonidine (Concurrent use is not recommended). Products include:
Catapres-TTS ... 677

Clonidine Hydrochloride (Concurrent use is not recommended). Products include:
Catapres Tablets ... 676
Combipres Tablets ... 678

Deserpidine (Concurrent use is not recommended). Products include:
Enduronyl ... 518
Harmonyl Tablets ... 528
Oreticyl ... 545

Desipramine Hydrochloride (Concurrent use is not recommended). Products include:
Norpramin Tablets ... 1340

Diazoxide (Concurrent use is not recommended). Products include:
Hyperstat I.V. Injection ... 2095
Proglycem ... 649

Doxazosin Mesylate (Concurrent use is not recommended). Products include:
Cardura Tablets ... 1941

Doxepin Hydrochloride (Concurrent use is not recommended). Products include:
Sinequan ... 1960

Enalapril Maleate (Concurrent use is not recommended). Products include:
Vaseretic Tablets ... 1559
Vasotec Tablets ... 1564

Enalaprilat (Concurrent use is not recommended). Products include:
Vasotec I.V. ... 1562

Esmolol Hydrochloride (Concurrent use is not recommended). Products include:
Brevibloc Injection ... 942

Felodipine (Concurrent use is not recommended). Products include:
Plendil Extended-Release Tablets 1526

Fluoxetine Hydrochloride (Concurrent use is not recommended). Products include:
Prozac Pulvules ... 920

Fosinopril Sodium (Concurrent use is not recommended). Products include:
Monopril Tablets ... 1406

Furosemide (Concurrent use is not recommended). Products include:
Lasix ... 1093

Guanabenz Acetate (Concurrent use is not recommended). Products include:
Wytensin Tablets ... 2542

Guanethidine Monosulfate (Concurrent use is not recommended). Products include:
Esimil Tablets ... 864
Ismelin Tablets ... 869

Hydralazine Hydrochloride (Concurrent use is not recommended). Products include:
Apresazide Capsules ... 854
Apresoline Hydrochloride Parenteral (Ampuls) ... 856
Apresoline Hydrochloride Tablets .. 855
Apresoline-Esidrix Tablets ... 857
Ser-Ap-Es Tablets ... 881
Serpasil-Apresoline Tablets ... 884

Hydrochlorothiazide (Concurrent use is not recommended). Products include:
Aldactazide ... 2150
Aldoril Tablets ... 1418
Apresazide Capsules ... 854
Apresoline-Esidrix Tablets ... 857
Capozide ... 2258
Dyazide Capsules ... 2208
Esidrix Tablets ... 863
Esimil Tablets ... 864
HydroDIURIL Tablets ... 1484
Hydropres Tablets ... 1485
Inderide Tablets ... 2463
Inderide LA Long Acting Capsules .. 2465
Lopressor HCT Tablets ... 1034
Maxzide ... 1215
Moduretic Tablets ... 1510
Normozide Tablets ... 2112
Oretic Tablets ... 544
Oreticyl ... 545
Prinzide Tablets ... 1540
Ser-Ap-Es Tablets ... 881
Serpasil-Esidrix Tablets ... 886
Timolide Tablets ... 1547
Trandate HCT Tablets ... 579
Vaseretic Tablets ... 1559
Zestoretic ... 2274

Hydroflumethiazide (Concurrent use is not recommended). Products include:
Diucardin Tablets ... 2450
Saluron ... 718
Salutensin/Salutensin-Demi ... 719

Imipramine Hydrochloride (Concurrent use is not recommended). Products include:
Tofranil Ampuls ... 1038
Tofranil Tablets ... 1039

Imipramine Pamoate (Concurrent use is not recommended). Products include:
Tofranil-PM Capsules ... 1041

Indapamide (Concurrent use is not recommended). Products include:
Lozol Tablets ... 1843

Isocarboxazid (Concurrent use is not recommended). Products include:
Marplan Tablets ... 1906

Isradipine (Concurrent use is not recommended). Products include:
DynaCirc Capsules ... 2004

Labetalol Hydrochloride (Concurrent use is not recommended). Products include:
Normodyne Injection ... 2108
Normodyne Tablets ... 2110
Normozide Tablets ... 2112
Trandate HCT Tablets ... 579
Trandate Injection ... 577
Trandate Tablets ... 579

Lisinopril (Concurrent use is not recommended). Products include:
Prinivil Tablets ... 1538
Prinzide Tablets ... 1540

Zestoretic ... 2274
Zestril Tablets ... 2277

Maprotiline Hydrochloride (Concurrent use is not recommended). Products include:
Ludiomil Tablets ... 874

Mecamylamine Hydrochloride (Concurrent use is not recommended). Products include:
Inversine Tablets ... 1492

Methyclothiazide (Concurrent use is not recommended). Products include:
Enduron Tablets ... 517
Enduronyl ... 518

Methyldopa (Concurrent use is not recommended). Products include:
Aldoclor Tablets ... 1413
Aldomet Oral ... 1415
Aldoril Tablets ... 1418

Methyldopate Hydrochloride (Concurrent use is not recommended). Products include:
Aldomet Ester HCl Injection ... 1417

Metolazone (Concurrent use is not recommended). Products include:
Diulo ... 2129
Mykrox ½ mg Tablets ... 984
Zaroxolyn Tablets ... 989

Metoprolol Tartrate (Concurrent use is not recommended). Products include:
Lopressor Ampuls ... 1032
Lopressor HCT Tablets ... 1034
Lopressor Tablets ... 1032

Metyrosine (Concurrent use is not recommended). Products include:
Demser Capsules ... 1460

Minoxidil (Concurrent use is not recommended). Products include:
Loniten Tablets ... 2346
Rogaine Topical Solution ... 2357

Nadolol (Concurrent use is not recommended). Products include:
Corgard Tablets ... 701
Corzide Tablets ... 702

Nicardipine Hydrochloride (Concurrent use is not recommended). Products include:
Cardene Capsules ... 2290

Nitroglycerin (Concurrent use is not recommended). Products include:
Deponit NTG Transdermal Delivery System ... 2143
Minitran Transdermal Delivery System ... 1312
Nitro-Bid Ointment ... 1339
Nitro-Bid Capsules ... 1338
Nitrodisc ... 2176
Nitro-Dur (nitroglycerin) Transdermal Infusion System ... 1164
Nitrogard Tablets ... 1004
Nitrolingual Spray ... 1846
Nitrostat Tablets ... 1743
Transderm-Nitro Transdermal Therapeutic System ... 2283

Nortriptyline Hydrochloride (Concurrent use is not recommended). Products include:
Pamelor ... 2019

Penbutolol Sulfate (Concurrent use is not recommended). Products include:
Levatol ... 1832

Phenelzine Sulfate (Concurrent use is not recommended). Products include:
Nardil ... 1742

Phenoxybenzamine Hydrochloride (Concurrent use is not recommended). Products include:
Dibenzyline Capsules ... 2207

Phentolamine Mesylate (Concurrent use is not recommended). Products include:
Regitine ... 878

Pindolol (Concurrent use is not recommended). Products include:
Visken Tablets ... 2036

Polythiazide (Concurrent use is not recommended). Products include:
Minizide Capsules ... 1779
Renese Tablets ... 1785
Renese-R Tablets ... 1786

Prazosin Hydrochloride (Concurrent use is not recommended). Products include:
Minipress Capsules ... 1778
Minizide Capsules ... 1779

Propranolol Hydrochloride (Concurrent use is not recommended). Products include:
Inderal ... 2459
Inderal LA Long Acting Capsules ... 2461
Inderide Tablets ... 2463
Inderide LA Long Acting Capsules ... 2465

Protriptyline Hydrochloride (Concurrent use is not recommended). Products include:
Vivactil Tablets ... 1567

Ramipril (Concurrent use is not recommended). Products include:
Altace Capsules ... 1086

Rauwolfia Serpentina (Concurrent use is not recommended). Products include:
Raudixin Tablets ... 1803
Rauzide Tablets ... 1804

Rescinnamine (Concurrent use is not recommended).
No products indexed under this heading.

Reserpine (Concurrent use is not recommended). Products include:
Diupres Tablets ... 1461
Hydromox R Tablets ... 1209
Hydropres Tablets ... 1485
Renese-R Tablets ... 1786
Salutensin/Salutensin-Demi ... 719
Ser-Ap-Es Tablets ... 881
Serpasil Tablets ... 883
Serpasil-Apresoline Tablets ... 884
Serpasil-Esidrix Tablets ... 886

Sodium Nitroprusside (Concurrent use is not recommended). Products include:
Nipride I.V. Infusion ... 1909

Terazosin Hydrochloride (Concurrent use is not recommended). Products include:
Hytrin Tablets ... 529

Timolol Maleate (Concurrent use is not recommended). Products include:
Blocadren Tablets ... 1429
Timolide Tablets ... 1547
Timoptic in Ocudose ... 1552
Timoptic Sterile Ophthalmic Solution ... 1550

Tranylcypromine Sulfate (Concurrent use is not recommended). Products include:
Parnate Tablets ... 2222

Trazodone Hydrochloride (Concurrent use is not recommended). Products include:
Desyrel and Desyrel Dividose ... 1404

Trimethaphan Camsylate (Concurrent use is not recommended). Products include:
Arfonad Ampuls ... 1887

Trimipramine Maleate (Concurrent use is not recommended). Products include:
Surmontil Capsules ... 2524

DRY EYE THERAPY
(Glycerin) ... ⊙ 258
No interactions described in labeling.

DRYSOL
(Aluminum Chloride) ... 1772
No interactions described in labeling.

DUOBAR
(Dietary Supplement) ... 2149
No interactions described in labeling.

DUOCAL
(Dietary Supplement) ... 2150
No interactions described in labeling.

DUODERM ADHESIVE COMPRESSION BANDAGE
(Hydrocolloid Adhesive Layer) ... 900
No interactions described in labeling.

DUODERM CGF (CONTROL GEL FORMULA DRESSING)
(Control Gel Formula Dressing) ... 901
No interactions described in labeling.

DUODERM CGF BORDER
(Control Gel Formula Dressing) ... 902
No interactions described in labeling.

DUODERM EXTRA THIN CGF DRESSING
(Control Gel Formula Dressing) ... 902
No interactions described in labeling.

DUODERM HYDROACTIVE DRESSING
(Hydrocolloid Adhesive Layer) ... 901
No interactions described in labeling.

DUODERM HYDROACTIVE GRANULES
(Hydrocolloids) ... 901
No interactions described in labeling.

DUODERM HYDROACTIVE PASTE
(Hydrocolloids) ... 902
No interactions described in labeling.

DUOLUBE EYE OINTMENT
(Mineral Oil, Petrolatum, White) ... ⊙ 258
No interactions described in labeling.

DURAGESIC TRANSDERMAL SYSTEM
(Fentanyl) ... 1133
May interact with central nervous system depressants, narcotic analgesics, hypnotics and sedatives, tranquilizers, phenothiazines, antihistamines, and certain other agents. Compounds in these categories include:

Alcohol (May produce additive depressant effects).

Alfentanil Hydrochloride (May produce additive depressant effects, hypoventilation, hypotension and profound sedation or coma may occur). Products include:
Alfenta Injection ... 1131

Alprazolam (May produce additive depressant effects, hypoventilation, hypotension and profound sedation or coma may occur). Products include:
Xanax Tablets ... 2367

Aprobarbital (May produce additive depressant effects, hypoventilation, hypotension and profound sedation or coma may occur). Products include:
Alurate Elixir ... 1883

Astemizole (May produce additive depressant effects, hypoventilation, hypotension and profound sedation or coma may occur). Products include:
Hismanal Tablets ... 1138

Azatadine Maleate (May produce additive depressant effects, hypoventilation, hypotension and profound sedation or coma may occur). Products include:
Optimine Tablets ... 2115
Trinalin Repetabs Tablets ... 1170

Bromodiphenhydramine Hydrochloride (May produce additive depressant effects, hypoventilation, hypotension and profound sedation or coma may occur).
No products indexed under this heading.

Brompheniramine Maleate (May produce additive depressant effects, hypoventilation, hypotension and profound sedation or coma may occur). Products include:
Alka Seltzer Plus Sinus Allergy Medicine ... ■ 624
Atrohist Sprinkle Capsules ... 558
Bromfed Capsules (Timed Release) ... 1615
Bromfed Syrup ... ■ 628
Bromfed ... 1615
Dimetane Decongestant ... ■ 673
Dimetane ... ■ 672
Dimetane-DC Cough Syrup ... 1857
Dimetane-DX Cough Syrup ... 1858
Dimetapp Elixir ... ■ 673
Dimetapp DM Elixir ... ■ 674
Dimetapp Extentabs ... ■ 674
Dimetapp Plus Caplets ... ■ 675
Dimetapp Tablets ... ■ 675
Drixoral Antihistamine/Nasal Decongestant Syrup ... ■ 698

Buprenorphine (May produce additive depressant effects, hypoventilation, hypotension and profound sedation or coma may occur).
No products indexed under this heading.

Buspirone Hydrochloride (May produce additive depressant effects, hypoventilation, hypotension and profound sedation or coma may occur). Products include:
BuSpar ... 1401

Butabarbital (May produce additive depressant effects, hypoventilation, hypotension and profound sedation or coma may occur). Products include:
Pyridium Plus ... 1764

Butalbital (May produce additive depressant effects, hypoventilation, hypotension and profound sedation or coma may occur). Products include:
Esgic-Plus Tablets ... 1002
Esgic Tablets & Capsules ... 1001
Fioricet Tablets ... 2006
Fiorinal Capsules ... 2007
Fiorinal with Codeine Capsules ... 2008
Fiorinal Tablets ... 2007
Phrenilin ... 838
Sedapap Tablets 50 mg/650 mg ... 1360

Chlordiazepoxide (May produce additive depressant effects, hypoventilation, hypotension and profound sedation or coma may occur). Products include:
Libritabs Tablets ... 1930
Limbitrol ... 1933
Menrium Tablets ... 1934

Chlordiazepoxide Hydrochloride (May produce additive depressant effects, hypoventilation, hypotension and profound sedation or coma may occur). Products include:
Librax Capsules ... 1929
Librium Capsules ... 1931
Librium Injectable ... 1932

Chlorpheniramine Maleate (May produce additive depressant effects, hypoventilation, hypotension and profound sedation or coma may occur). Products include:
A.R.M. Allergy Relief Medicine Caplets ... ■ 615
Alka-Seltzer Plus Cold Medicine ... ■ 623
Allerest ... ■ 559
Ana-Kit Anaphylaxis Emergency Treatment Kit ... 1100
BC Cold Powder Multi-Symptom Formula ... ■ 517
Brexin L.A. Capsules ... 2078
Cerose-DM ... 2443

Cheracol Plus Head Cold/Cough Formula 667
Chlor-Trimeton Allergy Syrup, Tablets & Long-Acting Repetabs Tablets 693
Chlor-Trimeton Decongestant 694
Comhist LA Capsules 1618
Allergy-Sinus Comtrex Multi-Symptom Allergy Sinus Formula Tablets & Caplets 746
Comtrex Multi-Symptom Cold Reliever Tablets/Caplets/Liqui-Gels/Liquid 745
Day-Night Comtrex 747
Contac Continuous Action Decongestant/Antihistamine Capsules 710
Contac Maximum Strength Continuous Action Decongestant/Antihistamine Caplets 709
Contac Severe Cold and Flu Formula Caplets 711
Coricidin 'D' Decongestant Tablets 695
Coricidin Demilets Tablets for Children 696
Coricidin Tablets 695
Deconamine 663
Demazin Nasal Decongestant/Antihistamine Repetabs Tablets & Syrup 697
Dorcol Children's Liquid Cold Formula 686
Dristan Decongestant/Antihistamine/Analgesic Coated Caplets 749
Dristan Cold Nasal Decongestant/Antihistamine/Analgesic Coated Tablets 2419
Dristan Advanced Formula Decongestant/Antihistamine/Analgesic Tablets 749
Extendryl 994
4-Way Cold Tablets 750
Fedahist Gyrocaps 2145
Fedahist Timecaps 2145
Hycomine Compound Tablets 929
Isoclor Timesule Capsules 561
Kronofed-A 970
Medi-Flu Caplet, Liquid 640
Naldecon Syrup, Tablets, Pediatric Drops and Pediatric Syrup 709
Nolamine Tablets 838
Novafed A Capsules 1342
Novahistine DH 1342
Novahistine Elixir 596
Ornade Spansule Capsules 2221
Orthoxicol Cough Syrup 668
PediaCare Allergy Relief Formula Liquid 1362
PediaCare Cough-Cold Formula Liquid 1362
PediaCare Night Rest Cough-Cold Formula Liquid 1362
PediaCare 6-12 Cough-Cold Formula Chewable Tablets 1362
Pyrroxate Capsules 669
Quelidrine Syrup 556
Ru-Tuss II Capsules 693
Ru-Tuss Tablets 693
Ryna 741
Sinarest Tablets & Extra Strength Tablets 562
Sine-Off Maximum Strength Allergy/Sinus Formula Caplets 721
Sine-Off Sinus Medicine Tablets-Aspirin Formula 722
Singlet Tablets 598
Sinulin 840
Sinutab Maximum Strength 641
St. Joseph Nighttime Cold Medicine 705
Sudafed Plus Liquid 544
Sudafed Plus Tablets 545
Teldrin Timed-Release Allergy Capsules, 12 mg 2192
TheraFlu Flu and Cold Medicine 687
Triaminic Allergy Tablets 688
Triaminic Chewables 688
Triaminic Cold Tablets 688
Triaminic Nite Light 689
Triaminic Syrup 689
Triaminic-12 Tablets 690
Triaminicin Tablets 690
Triaminicol Multi-Symptom Cold Tablets 691
Triaminicol Multi-Symptom Relief 691
Tylenol Allergy Sinus Medication Caplets and Gelcaps, Maximum Strength 1372
Children's Tylenol Cold Liquid Formula and Chewable Tablets 1368
Tylenol Cold & Flu Hot Medication, Packets 1369
Tylenol Cold Medication Caplets and Tablets 1370
Tylenol Cold Medication, Effervescent Tablets 1369
Vicks Children's NyQuil 664
Vicks Formula 44 Cough Medicine 661
Vicks Formula 44M Multi-Symptom Cough Medicine 662
Vicks Pediatric Formula 44m Multi-Symptom Cough & Cold Medicine 663

Chlorpheniramine Polistirex (May produce additive depressant effects, hypoventilation, hypotension and profound sedation or coma may occur). Products include:
Tussionex Extended-Release Suspension 988

Chlorpheniramine Tannate (May produce additive depressant effects, hypoventilation, hypotension and profound sedation or coma may occur). Products include:
Rynatan 2387
Rynatuss 2388

Chlorpromazine (May produce additive depressant effects, hypoventilation, hypotension and profound sedation or coma may occur). Products include:
Thorazine 2234

Chlorprothixene (May produce additive depressant effects, hypoventilation, hypotension and profound sedation or coma may occur). Products include:
Taractan Tablets 1920

Chlorprothixene Hydrochloride (May produce additive depressant effects, hypoventilation, hypotension and profound sedation or coma may occur). Products include:
Taractan 1920

Clemastine Fumarate (May produce additive depressant effects, hypoventilation, hypotension and profound sedation or coma may occur). Products include:
Tavist Syrup 2033
Tavist Tablets 2035
Tavist-D Tablets 2035

Clorazepate Dipotassium (May produce additive depressant effects, hypoventilation, hypotension and profound sedation or coma may occur). Products include:
Tranxene 556

Codeine (May produce additive depressant effects, hypoventilation, hypotension and profound sedation or coma may occur). Products include:
Calcidrine Syrup 506

Codeine Phosphate (May produce additive depressant effects, hypoventilation, hypotension and profound sedation or coma may occur). Products include:
Actifed with Codeine Cough Syrup 752
Cheracol Cough Syrup 1853
Codimal PH Syrup 846
Dimetane-DC Cough Syrup 1857
Empirin with Codeine Phosphate Nos. 2, 3 & 4 764
Fiorinal with Codeine Capsules 2008
Isoclor Expectorant 982
Naldecon CX Adult Liquid 521
Novahistine DH 1342
Novahistine Expectorant 1343
Nucofed Capsules 2219
Nucofed Expectorant 2219
Nucofed Pediatric Expectorant 2220
Nucofed Syrup 2219
Phenaphen with Codeine Capsules 1865
Phenaphen-650 with Codeine Tablets 1866
Phenergan with Codeine 2497
Phenergan VC with Codeine 2501
Robitussin A-C Syrup 1875
Robitussin-DAC Syrup 1875
Ryna 741
Soma Compound w/Codeine Tablets 2390
Triaminic Expectorant w/Codeine 1996
Tussi-Organidin Liquid 2391
Tylenol with Codeine 1381

Codeine Polistirex (May produce additive depressant effects, hypoventilation, hypotension and profound sedation or coma may occur).
No products indexed under this heading.

Cyproheptadine Hydrochloride (May produce additive depressant effects, hypoventilation, hypotension and profound sedation or coma may occur). Products include:
Periactin 1525

Dexchlorpheniramine Maleate (May produce additive depressant effects, hypoventilation, hypotension and profound sedation or coma may occur). Products include:
Polaramine 2116

Dezocine (May produce additive depressant effects, hypoventilation, hypotension and profound sedation or coma may occur).

Diazepam (May produce additive depressant effects, hypoventilation, hypotension and profound sedation or coma may occur). Products include:
Valium Injectable 1937
Valium Tablets 1939
Valrelease Capsules 1923

Diphenhydramine Citrate (May produce additive depressant effects, hypoventilation, hypotension and profound sedation or coma may occur). Products include:
Alka-Seltzer Plus Night-Time Cold Medicine 623
Bufferin AF Nite Time Analgesic/Sleeping Aid Caplets 744
Excedrin P.M. Analgesic/Sleeping Aid Tablets, Caplets and Liquid 749

Diphenhydramine Hydrochloride (May produce additive depressant effects, hypoventilation, hypotension and profound sedation or coma may occur). Products include:
Benadryl Anti-Itch Cream 635
Benadryl Capsules 1691
Benadryl Decongestant Elixir 635
Benadryl Decongestant 635
Benadryl Elixir 636
Benadryl Kapseals 1691
Benadryl 25 Kapseals 636
Benadryl Parenteral 1692
Benadryl Plus 636
Benadryl Plus Nighttime 637
Benadryl Spray, Maximum Strength 637
Benadryl Spray, Regular Strength 637
Benadryl Steri-Vials, Ampoules, and Steri-Dose Syringe 1692
Benadryl 25 Tablets 636
Benylin Cough Syrup 637
Benylin Decongestant 638
Caladryl Cream, Lotion, Spray 638
Miles Nervine Nighttime Sleep-Aid 627
Nytol Tablets 517
Sleep-ettes-D Tablets 653
Sleep-eze 3 Tablets 755
Sleepinal Night-time Sleep Aid Capsules 734
Sominex Caplets and Tablets 722
Sominex Liquid 723
Sominex Pain Relief Formula 723
Tylenol Cold Night Time Medication Liquid 1371
Tylenol PM, Extra Strength Caplets and Tablets 1368
Unisom Dual Relief Nighttime Sleep Aid/Analgesic 1774
Ziradryl Lotion 643

Droperidol (May produce additive depressant effects, hypoventilation, hypotension and profound sedation or coma may occur). Products include:
Inapsine Injection 1140
Innovar Injection 1141

Enflurane (May produce additive depressant effects, hypoventilation, hypotension and profound sedation or coma may occur). Products include:
Ethrane 599

Estazolam (May produce additive depressant effects, hypoventilation, hypotension and profound sedation or coma may occur). Products include:
ProSom Tablets 554

Ethchlorvynol (May produce additive depressant effects, hypoventilation, hypotension and profound sedation or coma may occur). Products include:
Placidyl Capsules 553

Ethinamate (May produce additive depressant effects, hypoventilation, hypotension and profound sedation or coma may occur).
No products indexed under this heading.

Fentanyl Citrate (May produce additive depressant effects, hypoventilation, hypotension and profound sedation or coma may occur). Products include:
Innovar Injection 1141
Sublimaze Injection 1146

Fluphenazine Decanoate (May produce additive depressant effects, hypoventilation, hypotension and profound sedation or coma may occur). Products include:
Prolixin Decanoate 1795

Fluphenazine Enanthate (May produce additive depressant effects, hypoventilation, hypotension and profound sedation or coma may occur). Products include:
Prolixin Enanthate 1796

Fluphenazine Hydrochloride (May produce additive depressant effects, hypoventilation, hypotension and profound sedation or coma may occur). Products include:
Prolixin Elixir 1793
Prolixin Injection 1791
Prolixin Oral Concentrate 1792
Prolixin Tablets 1793

Flurazepam Hydrochloride (May produce additive depressant effects, hypoventilation, hypotension and profound sedation or coma may occur). Products include:
Dalmane Capsules 1927

Glutethimide (May produce additive depressant effects, hypoventilation, hypotension and profound sedation or coma may occur).
No products indexed under this heading.

Haloperidol (May produce additive depressant effects, hypoventilation, hypotension and profound sedation or coma may occur). Products include:
Haldol Injection, Tablets and Concentrate 1373

Haloperidol Decanoate (May produce additive depressant effects, hypoventilation, hypotension and profound sedation or coma may occur). Products include:
Haldol Decanoate 1375

Hydrocodone Bitartrate (May produce additive depressant effects, hypoventilation, hypotension and profound sedation or coma may occur). Products include:
Anexsia 5/500 Tablets 2196
Anexsia 7.5/650 Tablets 2197
Azdone Tablets 844
Codiclear DH Syrup 845
Codimal DH Syrup 846
Damason-P 1356
Hycodan Syrup, Tablets 927

Hycomine Compound Tablets 929
Hycomine Syrup 927
Hycotuss Expectorant Syrup 930
Hydrocet Capsules 835
Lortab ASA Tablets 2414
Lortab 2412
Ru-Tuss with Hydrocodone 694
Triaminic Expectorant DH 1995
Vicodin Tablets 1187
Vicodin ES Tablets 1189
Zydone Capsules 941

Hydrocodone Polistirex (May produce additive depressant effects, hypoventilation, hypotension and profound sedation or coma may occur). Products include:

Tussionex Extended-Release Suspension 988

Hydroxyzine Hydrochloride (May produce additive depressant effects, hypoventilation, hypotension and profound sedation or coma may occur). Products include:

Atarax Tablets & Syrup 1941
Marax Tablets & DF Syrup 1954
Vistaril Intramuscular Solution 1970

Isoflurane (May produce additive depressant effects, hypoventilation, hypotension and profound sedation or coma may occur). Products include:

Forane 600

Ketamine Hydrochloride (May produce additive depressant effects, hypoventilation, hypotension and profound sedation or coma may occur). Products include:

Ketalar 1726

Levorphanol Tartrate (May produce additive depressant effects, hypoventilation, hypotension and profound sedation or coma may occur). Products include:

Levo-Dromoran 1906

Lorazepam (May produce additive depressant effects, hypoventilation, hypotension and profound sedation or coma may occur). Products include:

Ativan Injection 2432
Ativan Tablets 2434

Loxapine Hydrochloride (May produce additive depressant effects, hypoventilation, hypotension and profound sedation or coma may occur). Products include:

Loxitane 1213

Loxapine Succinate (May produce additive depressant effects, hypoventilation, hypotension and profound sedation or coma may occur). Products include:

Loxitane Capsules 1213

Meperidine Hydrochloride (May produce additive depressant effects, hypoventilation, hypotension and profound sedation or coma may occur). Products include:

Demerol 2047
Mepergan Injection 2479

Mephobarbital (May produce additive depressant effects, hypoventilation, hypotension and profound sedation or coma may occur). Products include:

Mebaral Tablets 2061

Meprobamate (May produce additive depressant effects, hypoventilation, hypotension and profound sedation or coma may occur). Products include:

Deprol Tablets 2382
Equagesic Tablets 2451
Miltown Tablets 2386
PMB 200 and PMB 400 2504

Mesoridazine (May produce additive depressant effects, hypoventilation, hypotension and profound sedation or coma may occur). Products include:

Serentil 686

Methadone Hydrochloride (May produce additive depressant effects, hypoventilation, hypotension and profound sedation or coma may occur). Products include:

Dolophine Hydrochloride Ampoules & Vials 1260
Dolophine Hydrochloride Tablets 1261
Methadone Hydrochloride Diskets 1284
Methadone Hydrochloride Oral Solution & Tablets 1987

Methdilazine Hydrochloride (May produce additive depressant effects, hypoventilation, hypotension and profound sedation or coma may occur). Products include:

Tacaryl Syrup & Tablets 2409

Methohexital Sodium (May produce additive depressant effects, hypoventilation, hypotension and profound sedation or coma may occur). Products include:

Brevital Sodium Vials 1248

Methoxyflurane (May produce additive depressant effects, hypoventilation, hypotension and profound sedation or coma may occur).

No products indexed under this heading.

Midazolam Hydrochloride (May produce additive depressant effects, hypoventilation, hypotension and profound sedation or coma may occur). Products include:

Versed Injection 1924

Molindone Hydrochloride (May produce additive depressant effects, hypoventilation, hypotension and profound sedation or coma may occur). Products include:

Moban Tablets & Concentrate 932

Morphine Sulfate (May produce additive depressant effects, hypoventilation, hypotension and profound sedation or coma may occur). Products include:

Astramorph/PF Injection, USP (Preservative-Free) 618
Duramorph 960
Infumorph 200 and Infumorph 500 Sterile Solutions 962
MS Contin Tablets 1814
MSIR 1817
Oramorph SR (Morphine Sulfate Sustained Release Tablets) 1988
Roxanol 1991

Opium Alkaloids (May produce additive depressant effects, hypoventilation, hypotension and profound sedation or coma may occur). Products include:

B & O No. 15A & No. 16A Supprettes 2395
Pantopon Injectable 1911

Oxazepam (May produce additive depressant effects, hypoventilation, hypotension and profound sedation or coma may occur). Products include:

Serax Capsules 2522
Serax Tablets 2522

Oxycodone Hydrochloride (May produce additive depressant effects, hypoventilation, hypotension and profound sedation or coma may occur). Products include:

Percocet Tablets 950
Percodan 951
Roxicodone Tablets, Oral Solution & Intensol (Oxycodone) 1992
Tylox Capsules 1382

Pentobarbital Sodium (May produce additive depressant effects, hypoventilation, hypotension and profound sedation or coma may occur). Products include:

Nembutal Sodium Capsules 534
Nembutal Sodium Solution 536
Nembutal Sodium Suppositories 538

Perphenazine (May produce additive depressant effects, hypoventilation, hypotension and profound sedation or coma may occur). Products include:

Etrafon 2087
Triavil Tablets 1556
Trilafon 2123

Phenobarbital (May produce additive depressant effects, hypoventilation, hypotension and profound sedation or coma may occur). Products include:

Arco-Lase Plus Tablets 607
Bellergal-S Tablets 1998
Bronkolixir .... ▣ 761
Bronkotabs Tablets .... ▣ 762
Donnatal 1858
Donnatal Extentabs 1859
Donnatal Tablets 1858
Donnazyme Tablets 1860
Kinesed Tablets 2272
Phenobarbital Elixir and Tablets 1293
Primatene Tablets-P Formula 2421
Quadrinal Tablets 1183
Tedral SA 1765

Prazepam (May produce additive depressant effects, hypoventilation, hypotension and profound sedation or coma may occur). Products include:

Centrax 1693

Prochlorperazine (May produce additive depressant effects, hypoventilation, hypotension and profound sedation or coma may occur). Products include:

Compazine 2201

Promethazine Hydrochloride (May produce additive depressant effects, hypoventilation, hypotension and profound sedation or coma may occur). Products include:

Mepergan Injection 2479
Phenergan with Codeine 2497
Phenergan with Dextromethorphan 2499
Phenergan Injection 2493
Phenergan Suppositories 2496
Phenergan Syrup 2495
Phenergan Tablets 2496
Phenergan VC 2500
Phenergan VC with Codeine 2501

Propofol (May produce additive depressant effects, hypoventilation, hypotension and profound sedation or coma may occur). Products include:

Diprivan Injection 2267

Propoxyphene Hydrochloride (May produce additive depressant effects, hypoventilation, hypotension and profound sedation or coma may occur). Products include:

Darvon 1256
Wygesic Tablets 2540

Propoxyphene Napsylate (May produce additive depressant effects, hypoventilation, hypotension and profound sedation or coma may occur). Products include:

Darvon-N/Darvocet-N 1254

Pyrilamine Maleate (May produce additive depressant effects, hypoventilation, hypotension and profound sedation or coma may occur). Products include:

Codimal 846
4-Way Fast Acting Nasal Spray - Original Formula (regular & mentholated) & Metered Spray Pump (regular) 751
Maximum Strength Midol Multi-Symptom Menstrual Formula .... ▣ 571
Maximum Strength Midol PMS Premenstrual Syndrome Formula .... ▣ 570
Regular Strength Midol Multi-Symptom Menstrual Formula .... ▣ 570
Prefrin-A .... ◉ 255
Prēmsyn PMS Capsules & Caplets ▣ 547
Primatene Tablets-M Formula 2421
Robitussin Night Relief .... ▣ 677
Ru-Tuss with Hydrocodone 694
Triaminic Expectorant DH 1995
Triaminic Oral Infant Drops 1996

Pyrilamine Tannate (May produce additive depressant effects, hypoventilation, hypotension and profound sedation or coma may occur). Products include:

Rynatan 2387

Quazepam (May produce additive depressant effects, hypoventilation, hypotension and profound sedation or coma may occur). Products include:

Doral Tablets 2383

Secobarbital Sodium (May produce additive depressant effects, hypoventilation, hypotension and profound sedation or coma may occur). Products include:

Seconal Sodium Pulvules 1296

Sufentanil Citrate (May produce additive depressant effects, hypoventilation, hypotension and profound sedation or coma may occur). Products include:

Sufenta Injection 1147

Temazepam (May produce additive depressant effects, hypoventilation, hypotension and profound sedation or coma may occur). Products include:

Restoril Capsules 2023

Terfenadine (May produce additive depressant effects, hypoventilation, hypotension and profound sedation or coma may occur). Products include:

Seldane Tablets 1349
Seldane-D Extended-Release Tablets 1350

Thiamylal Sodium (May produce additive depressant effects, hypoventilation, hypotension and profound sedation or coma may occur). Products include:

Surital Ampoules, Steri-Vials 1764

Thioridazine Hydrochloride (May produce additive depressant effects, hypoventilation, hypotension and profound sedation or coma may occur). Products include:

Mellaril 2011

Thiothixene (May produce additive depressant effects, hypoventilation, hypotension and profound sedation or coma may occur). Products include:

Navane Capsules and Concentrate 1954
Navane Intramuscular 1956

Triazolam (May produce additive depressant effects, hypoventilation, hypotension and profound sedation or coma may occur). Products include:

Halcion Tablets 2340

Trifluoperazine Hydrochloride (May produce additive depressant effects, hypoventilation, hypotension and profound sedation or coma may occur). Products include:

Stelazine 2226

Trimeprazine Tartrate (May produce additive depressant effects, hypoventilation, hypotension and profound sedation or coma may occur). Products include:

Temaril Tablets, Syrup and Spansule Sustained Release Capsules 1085

Tripelennamine Hydrochloride (May produce additive depressant effects, hypoventilation, hypotension and profound sedation or coma may occur). Products include:

PBZ Tablets & Elixir ... 1037
PBZ-SR Tablets ... 1037

Triprolidine Hydrochloride (May produce additive depressant effects, hypoventilation, hypotension and profound sedation or coma may occur). Products include:

Actidil ... ND 538
Actifed Capsules ... ND 539
Actifed Plus Caplets ... ND 539
Actifed Plus Tablets ... ND 540
Actifed with Codeine Cough Syrup.. 752
Actifed Syrup ... ND 540
Actifed Tablets ... ND 540
Actifed 12-Hour Capsules ... ND 539

DURAMORPH

(Morphine Sulfate) ... 960

May interact with hypnotics and sedatives, monoamine oxidase inhibitors, tricyclic antidepressants, butyrophenones, corticosteroids, anticoagulants, antihistamines, psychotropics, phenothiazines, neuromuscular blocking agents, and certain other agents. Compounds in these categories include:

Alcohol (Potentiation of depressant effect).

Alfentanil Hydrochloride (Potentiation of depressant effect). Products include:

Alfenta Injection ... 1131

Alprazolam (Potentiation of depressant effect). Products include:

Xanax Tablets ... 2367

Amitriptyline Hydrochloride (Potentiation of depressant effect). Products include:

Elavil ... 2269
Endep Tablets ... 1927
Etrafon ... 2087
Limbitrol ... 1933
Triavil Tablets ... 1556

Amoxapine (Potentiation of depressant effect). Products include:

Asendin Tablets ... 1196

Aprobarbital (Potentiation of depressant effect). Products include:

Alurate Elixir ... 1883

Astemizole (Potentiation of depressant effect). Products include:

Hismanal Tablets ... 1138

Azatadine Maleate (Potentiation of depressant effect). Products include:

Optimine Tablets ... 2115
Trinalin Repetabs Tablets ... 1170

Betamethasone Acetate (Concurrent use by epidural or intrathecal route is contraindicated with parenteral corticosteroids). Products include:

Celestone Soluspan Suspension ... 2081

Betamethasone Sodium Phosphate (Concurrent use by epidural or intrathecal route is contraindicated with parenteral corticosteroids). Products include:

Celestone Soluspan Suspension ... 2081

Bromodiphenhydramine Hydrochloride (Potentiation of depressant effect).

No products indexed under this heading.

Brompheniramine Maleate (Potentiation of depressant effect). Products include:

Alka Seltzer Plus Sinus Allergy Medicine ... ND 624
Atrohist Sprinkle Capsules ... 558
Bromfed Capsules (Timed Release) ... 1615
Bromfed Syrup ... ND 628
Bromfed ... 1615
Dimetane Decongestant ... ND 673
Dimetane ... ND 672
Dimetane-DC Cough Syrup ... 1857
Dimetane-DX Cough Syrup ... 1858
Dimetapp Elixir ... ND 673
Dimetapp DM Elixir ... ND 674
Dimetapp Extentabs ... ND 674
Dimetapp Plus Caplets ... ND 675
Dimetapp Tablets ... ND 675
Drixoral Antihistamine/Nasal Decongestant Syrup ... ND 698

Buprenorphine (Potentiation of depressant effect).

No products indexed under this heading.

Buspirone Hydrochloride (Potentiation of depressant effect). Products include:

BuSpar ... 1401

Butabarbital (Potentiation of depressant effect). Products include:

Pyridium Plus ... 1764

Butalbital (Potentiation of depressant effect). Products include:

Esgic-Plus Tablets ... 1002
Esgic Tablets & Capsules ... 1001
Fioricet Tablets ... 2006
Fiorinal Capsules ... 2007
Fiorinal with Codeine Capsules ... 2008
Fiorinal Tablets ... 2007
Phrenilin ... 838
Sedapap Tablets 50 mg/650 mg .. 1360

Chlordiazepoxide (Potentiation of depressant effect). Products include:

Libritabs Tablets ... 1930
Limbitrol ... 1933
Menrium Tablets ... 1934

Chlordiazepoxide Hydrochloride (Potentiation of depressant effect). Products include:

Librax Capsules ... 1929
Librium Capsules ... 1931
Librium Injectable ... 1932

Chlorpheniramine Maleate (Potentiation of depressant effect). Products include:

A.R.M. Allergy Relief Medicine Caplets ... ND 615
Alka-Seltzer Plus Cold Medicine ... ND 623
Allerest ... ND 559
Ana-Kit Anaphylaxis Emergency Treatment Kit ... 1100
BC Cold Powder Multi-Symptom Formula ... ND 517
Brexin L.A. Capsules ... 2078
Cerose-DM ... 2443
Cheracol Plus Head Cold/Cough Formula ... ND 667
Chlor-Trimeton Allergy Syrup, Tablets & Long-Acting Repetabs Tablets ... ND 693
Chlor-Trimeton Decongestant ... ND 694
Comhist LA Capsules ... 1618
Allergy-Sinus Comtrex Multi-Symptom Allergy Sinus Formula Tablets & Caplets ... 746
Comtrex Multi-Symptom Cold Reliever Tablets/Caplets/Liqui-Gels/Liquid ... 745
Day-Night Comtrex ... 747
Contac Continuous Action Decongestant/Antihistamine Capsules ND 710
Contac Maximum Strength Continuous Action Decongestant/ Antihistamine Caplets ... ND 709
Contac Severe Cold and Flu Formula Caplets ... ND 711
Coricidin 'D' Decongestant Tablets ... ND 695
Coricidin Demilets Tablets for Children ... ND 696
Coricidin Tablets ... ND 695
Deconamine ... 663
Demazin Nasal Decongestant/ Antihistamine Repetabs Tablets & Syrup ... ND 697
Dorcol Children's Liquid Cold Formula ... ND 686
Dristan Decongestant/Antihistamine/ Analgesic Coated Caplets ... ND 749
Dristan Cold Nasal Decongestant/ Antihistamine/ Analgesic Coated Tablets ... 2419
Dristan Advanced Formula Decongestant/Antihistamine/ Analgesic Tablets ... ND 749
Extendryl ... 994
4-Way Cold Tablets ... 750
Fedahist Gyrocaps ... 2145
Fedahist Timecaps ... 2145
Hycomine Compound Tablets ... 929
Isoclor Timesule Capsules ... ND 561
Kronofed-A ... 970
Medi-Flu Caplet, Liquid ... ND 640
Naldecon Syrup, Tablets, Pediatric Drops and Pediatric Syrup ... 709
Nolamine Tablets ... 838
Novafed A Capsules ... 1342
Novahistine DH ... 1342
Novahistine Elixir ... ND 596
Ornade Spansule Capsules ... 2221
Orthoxicol Cough Syrup ... ND 668
PediaCare Allergy Relief Formula Liquid ... 1362
PediaCare Cough-Cold Formula Liquid ... 1362
PediaCare Night Rest Cough-Cold Formula Liquid ... 1362
PediaCare 6-12 Cough-Cold Formula Chewable Tablets ... 1362
Pyrroxate Capsules ... ND 669
Quelidrine Syrup ... 556
Ru-Tuss II Capsules ... 693
Ru-Tuss Tablets ... 693
Ryna ... ND 741
Sinarest Tablets & Extra Strength Tablets ... ND 562
Sine-Off Maximum Strength Allergy/Sinus Formula Caplets ... ND 721
Sine-Off Sinus Medicine Tablets-Aspirin Formula ... ND 722
Singlet Tablets ... ND 598
Sinulin ... 840
Sinutab Maximum Strength ... ND 641
St. Joseph Nighttime Cold Medicine ... ND 705
Sudafed Plus Liquid ... ND 544
Sudafed Plus Tablets ... ND 545
Teldrin Timed-Release Allergy Capsules, 12 mg ... 2192
TheraFlu Flu and Cold Medicine ... ND 687
Triaminic Allergy Tablets ... ND 688
Triaminic Chewables ... ND 688
Triaminic Cold Tablets ... ND 688
Triaminic Nite Light ... ND 689
Triaminic Syrup ... ND 689
Triaminic-12 Tablets ... ND 690
Triaminicin Tablets ... ND 690
Triaminicol Multi-Symptom Cold Tablets ... ND 691
Triaminicol Multi-Symptom Relief ND 691
Tylenol Allergy Sinus Medication Caplets and Gelcaps, Maximum Strength ... 1372
Children's Tylenol Cold Liquid Formula and Chewable Tablets ... 1368
Tylenol Cold & Flu Hot Medication, Packets ... 1369
Tylenol Cold Medication Caplets and Tablets ... 1370
Tylenol Cold Medication, Effervescent Tablets ... 1369
Vicks Children's NyQuil ... ND 664
Vicks Formula 44 Cough Medicine ... ND 661
Vicks Formula 44M Multi-Symptom Cough Medicine ... ND 662
Vicks Pediatric Formula 44m Multi-Symptom Cough & Cold Medicine ... ND 663

Chlorpheniramine Polistirex (Potentiation of depressant effect). Products include:

Tussionex Extended-Release Suspension ... 988

Chlorpheniramine Tannate (Potentiation of depressant effect). Products include:

Rynatan ... 2387
Rynatuss ... 2388

Chlorpromazine (Potentiation of depressant effect; increased risk of respiratory depression). Products include:

Thorazine ... 2234

Chlorprothixene (Potentiation of depressant effect; increased risk of respiratory depression). Products include:

Taractan Tablets ... 1920

Chlorprothixene Hydrochloride (Potentiation of depressant effect; increased risk of respiratory depression). Products include:

Taractan ... 1920

Clemastine Fumarate (Potentiation of depressant effect). Products include:

Tavist Syrup ... 2033
Tavist Tablets ... 2035
Tavist-D Tablets ... 2035

Clomipramine Hydrochloride (Potentiation of depressant effect). Products include:

Anafranil Capsules ... 650

Clorazepate Dipotassium (Potentiation of depressant effect). Products include:

Tranxene ... 556

Clozapine (Potentiation of depressant effect; increased risk of respiratory depression). Products include:

Clozaril Tablets ... 2000

Codeine (Potentiation of depressant effect). Products include:

Calcidrine Syrup ... 506

Codeine Phosphate (Potentiation of depressant effect). Products include:

Actifed with Codeine Cough Syrup.. 752
Cheracol Cough Syrup ... 1853
Codimal PH Syrup ... 846
Dimetane-DC Cough Syrup ... 1857
Empirin with Codeine Phosphate Nos. 2, 3 & 4 ... 764
Fiorinal with Codeine Capsules ... 2008
Isoclor Expectorant ... 982
Naldecon CX Adult Liquid ... ND 521
Novahistine DH ... 1342
Novahistine Expectorant ... 1343
Nucofed Capsules ... 2219
Nucofed Expectorant ... 2219
Nucofed Pediatric Expectorant ... 2220
Nucofed Syrup ... 2219
Phenaphen with Codeine Capsules 1865
Phenaphen-650 with Codeine Tablets ... 1866
Phenergan with Codeine ... 2497
Phenergan VC with Codeine ... 2501
Robitussin A-C Syrup ... 1875
Robitussin-DAC Syrup ... 1875
Ryna ... ND 741
Soma Compound w/Codeine Tablets ... 2390
Triaminic Expectorant w/Codeine .. 1996
Tussi-Organidin Liquid ... 2391
Tylenol with Codeine ... 1381

Codeine Polistirex (Potentiation of depressant effect).

No products indexed under this heading.

Cortisone Acetate (Concurrent use by epidural or intrathecal route is contraindicated with parenteral corticosteroids). Products include:

Cortone Acetate Sterile Suspension ... 1437
Cortone Acetate Tablets ... 1439

Cyproheptadine Hydrochloride (Potentiation of depressant effect). Products include:

Periactin ... 1525

Desipramine Hydrochloride (Potentiation of depressant effect). Products include:

Norpramin Tablets ... 1340

Dexamethasone (Concurrent use by epidural or intrathecal route is contraindicated with parenteral corticosteroids). Products include:

AK-Trol Ointment & Suspension ... ⊙ 207
Decadron Elixir ... 1445
Decadron Tablets ... 1447
Decaspray Topical Aerosol ... 1459
Dexacidin ... ⊙ 272
Maxidex Sterile Ophthalmic Suspension ... ⊙ 223
Maxitrol Ophthalmic Ointment/ Suspension ... ⊙ 223
TobraDex Ophthalmic Suspension and Ointment ... ⊙ 228

Dexamethasone Acetate (Concurrent use by epidural or intrathecal route is contraindicated with parenteral corticosteroids). Products include:
- Dalalone D.P. Injectable ... 999
- Decadron-LA Sterile Suspension ... 1457

Dexamethasone Sodium Phosphate (Concurrent use by epidural or intrathecal route is contraindicated with parenteral corticosteroids). Products include:
- AK-Dex ... ◉ 203
- Decadron Phosphate Respihaler ... 1454
- Decadron Phosphate Sterile Ophthalmic Ointment ... 1453
- Decadron Phosphate Sterile Ophthalmic Solution ... 1453
- Decadron Phosphate Topical Cream ... 1455
- Decadron Phosphate Turbinaire ... 1456
- Maxidex Sterile Ophthalmic Ointment ... ◉ 222
- NeoDecadron Sterile Ophthalmic Ointment ... 1517
- NeoDecadron Sterile Ophthalmic Solution ... 1518
- NeoDecadron Topical Cream ... 1518

Dexchlorpheniramine Maleate (Potentiation of depressant effect). Products include:
- Polaramine ... 2116

Diazepam (Potentiation of depressant effect). Products include:
- Valium Injectable ... 1937
- Valium Tablets ... 1939
- Valrelease Capsules ... 1923

Dicumarol (Concurrent use by epidural or intrathecal route is contraindicated with anticoagulant therapy). Products include:
- Dicumarol Tablets ... 516

Diphenhydramine Citrate (Potentiation of depressant effect). Products include:
- Alka-Seltzer Plus Night-Time Cold Medicine ... ▣ 623
- Bufferin AF Nite Time Analgesic/Sleeping Aid Caplets ... 744
- Excedrin P.M. Analgesic/Sleeping Aid Tablets, Caplets and Liquid ... 749

Diphenhydramine Hydrochloride (Potentiation of depressant effect). Products include:
- Benadryl Anti-Itch Cream ... ▣ 635
- Benadryl Capsules ... 1691
- Benadryl Decongestant Elixir ... ▣ 635
- Benadryl Decongestant ... ▣ 635
- Benadryl Elixir ... ▣ 636
- Benadryl Kapseals ... 1691
- Benadryl 25 Kapseals ... ▣ 636
- Benadryl Parenteral ... 1692
- Benadryl Plus ... ▣ 636
- Benadryl Plus Nighttime ... ▣ 637
- Benadryl Spray, Maximum Strength ... ▣ 637
- Benadryl Spray, Regular Strength ▣ 637
- Benadryl Steri-Vials, Ampoules, and Steri-Dose Syringe ... 1692
- Benadryl 25 Tablets ... ▣ 636
- Benylin Cough Syrup ... ▣ 637
- Benylin Decongestant ... ▣ 638
- Caladryl Cream, Lotion, Spray ... ▣ 638
- Miles Nervine Nighttime Sleep-Aid ▣ 627
- Nytol Tablets ... ▣ 517
- Sleep-ettes-D Tablets ... ▣ 653
- Sleep-eze 3 Tablets ... ▣ 755
- Sleepinal Night-time Sleep Aid Capsules ... ▣ 734
- Sominex Caplets and Tablets ... ▣ 722
- Sominex Liquid ... ▣ 723
- Sominex Pain Relief Formula ... ▣ 723
- Tylenol Cold Night Time Medication Liquid ... 1371
- Tylenol PM, Extra Strength Caplets and Tablets ... 1368
- Unisom Dual Relief Nighttime Sleep Aid/Analgesic ... 1774
- Ziradryl Lotion ... ▣ 643

Diphenylpyraline Hydrochloride (Potentiation of depressant effect).
- No products indexed under this heading.

Doxepin Hydrochloride (Potentiation of depressant effect). Products include:
- Sinequan ... 1960

Droperidol (Potentiation of depressant effect). Products include:
- Inapsine Injection ... 1140
- Innovar Injection ... 1141

Enflurane (Potentiation of depressant effect). Products include:
- Ethrane ... 599

Estazolam (Potentiation of depressant effect). Products include:
- ProSom Tablets ... 554

Ethchlorvynol (Potentiation of depressant effect). Products include:
- Placidyl Capsules ... 553

Ethinamate (Potentiation of depressant effect).
- No products indexed under this heading.

Fentanyl Citrate (Potentiation of depressant effect). Products include:
- Innovar Injection ... 1141
- Sublimaze Injection ... 1146

Fluphenazine Decanoate (Potentiation of depressant effect; increased risk of respiratory depression). Products include:
- Prolixin Decanoate ... 1795

Fluphenazine Enanthate (Potentiation of depressant effect; increased risk of respiratory depression). Products include:
- Prolixin Enanthate ... 1796

Fluphenazine Hydrochloride (Potentiation of depressant effect; increased risk of respiratory depression). Products include:
- Prolixin Elixir ... 1793
- Prolixin Injection ... 1791
- Prolixin Oral Concentrate ... 1792
- Prolixin Tablets ... 1793

Flurazepam Hydrochloride (Potentiation of depressant effect). Products include:
- Dalmane Capsules ... 1927

Furazolidone (Potentiation of depressant effect). Products include:
- Furoxone ... 1855

Glutethimide (Potentiation of depressant effect).
- No products indexed under this heading.

Haloperidol (Potentiation of depressant effect; increased risk of respiratory depression). Products include:
- Haldol Injection, Tablets and Concentrate ... 1373

Haloperidol Decanoate (Potentiation of depressant effect; increased risk of respiratory depression). Products include:
- Haldol Decanoate ... 1375

Heparin Calcium (Concurrent use by epidural or intrathecal route is contraindicated with anticoagulant therapy). Products include:
- Calciparine Injection ... 925

Heparin Sodium (Concurrent use by epidural or intrathecal route is contraindicated with anticoagulant therapy). Products include:
- Heparin Lock Flush Solution ... 2456
- Heparin Sodium Vials ... 1264
- Heparin Sodium Injection ... 2457
- Heparin Sodium Injection, USP, Sterile Solution ... 2342

Hydrocodone Bitartrate (Potentiation of depressant effect). Products include:
- Anexsia 5/500 Tablets ... 2196
- Anexsia 7.5/650 Tablets ... 2197
- Azdōne Tablets ... 844
- Codiclear DH Syrup ... 845
- Codimal DH Syrup ... 846
- Damason-P ... 1356
- Hycodan Syrup, Tablets ... 927
- Hycomine Compound Tablets ... 929
- Hycomine Syrup ... 927
- Hycotuss Expectorant Syrup ... 930
- Hydrocet Capsules ... 835
- Lortab ASA Tablets ... 2414
- Lortab ... 2412
- Ru-Tuss with Hydrocodone ... 694
- Triaminic Expectorant DH ... 1995
- Vicodin Tablets ... 1187
- Vicodin ES Tablets ... 1189
- Zydone Capsules ... 941

Hydrocodone Polistirex (Potentiation of depressant effect). Products include:
- Tussionex Extended-Release Suspension ... 988

Hydrocortisone (Concurrent use by epidural or intrathecal route is contraindicated with parenteral corticosteroids). Products include:
- AK-Spore H.C. ... ◉ 206
- Bactine Hydrocortisone Anti-Itch Cream ... ▣ 625
- CaldeCORT Anti-Itch Hydrocortisone Spray ... ▣ 560
- Carmol HC Cream 1% ... 2296
- Cortaid Spray ... ▣ 735
- Cortenema ... 2244
- Cortisporin Ointment ... 758
- Cortisporin Ophthalmic Ointment Sterile ... 758
- Cortisporin Ophthalmic Suspension Sterile ... 759
- Cortisporin Otic Solution Sterile ... 760
- Cortisporin Otic Suspension Sterile 760
- Cortizone-5 Creme & Ointment ... ▣ 732
- Dermolate Anti-Itch Cream ... ▣ 697
- Eldecort Cream 1.0% ... 1113
- Eldecort Cream 1.0% and 2.5% ... 1113
- Fungoid HC Creme ... 1770
- Hydrocortone Tablets ... 1482
- Hytone ... 909
- LazerSporin-C Solution ... 1770
- Massengill Medicated Soft Cloth Towelettes ... 2192
- Nutracort Cream & Lotion ... 1684
- PediOtic Suspension Sterile ... 797
- Synacort Creams 1%, 2.5% ... 2296
- Vanoxide-HC Acne Lotion ... 911
- Vioform-Hydrocortisone Cream and Mild Cream ... 889
- Vioform-Hydrocortisone Ointment ... 889
- VōSoL HC Otic Solution ... 2392
- Vytone Cream 1% ... 911

Hydrocortisone Acetate (Concurrent use by epidural or intrathecal route is contraindicated with parenteral corticosteroids). Products include:
- Analpram-HC Rectal Cream 1% and 2.5% ... 970
- Anusol-HC Cream ... 1690
- Anusol-HC Suppositories ... 1691
- Caldecort ... ▣ 560
- Carmol HC Cream 1% ... 2296
- Chloromycetin Hydrocortisone Ophthalmic ... 1694
- Coly-Mycin S Otic w/Neomycin & Hydrocortisone ... 1708
- Cortaid ... ▣ 735
- Cortef Feminine Itch Cream ... ▣ 735
- Corticaine ... ▣ 682
- Cortifoam ... 1827
- Cortisporin Cream ... 757
- Epifoam ... 1828
- Gynecort 5 Creme ... ▣ 556
- Hydrocortone Acetate Sterile Suspension ... 1479
- Lanacort 5 Creme and Ointment ... ▣ 557
- Mantadil Cream ... 789
- Ophthocort ... ◉ 301
- Orabase HCA Oral Paste ... 890
- Pramosone Cream, Lotion & Ointment ... 971
- ProctoCream-HC ... 1834
- Proctofoam-HC ... 1835

Hydrocortisone Sodium Phosphate (Concurrent use by epidural or intrathecal route is contraindicated with parenteral corticosteroids). Products include:
- Hydrocortone Phosphate Injection, Sterile ... 1481

Hydrocortisone Sodium Succinate (Concurrent use by epidural or intrathecal route is contraindicated with parenteral corticosteroids). Products include:
- Solu-Cortef Sterile Powder ... 2361

Hydroxyzine Hydrochloride (Potentiation of depressant effect). Products include:
- Atarax Tablets & Syrup ... 1941
- Marax Tablets & DF Syrup ... 1954
- Vistaril Intramuscular Solution ... 1970

Imipramine Hydrochloride (Potentiation of depressant effect). Products include:
- Tofranil Ampuls ... 1038
- Tofranil Tablets ... 1039

Imipramine Pamoate (Potentiation of depressant effect). Products include:
- Tofranil-PM Capsules ... 1041

Isocarboxazid (Potentiation of depressant effect). Products include:
- Marplan Tablets ... 1906

Isoflurane (Potentiation of depressant effect). Products include:
- Forane ... 600

Ketamine Hydrochloride (Potentiation of depressant effect). Products include:
- Ketalar ... 1726

Levorphanol Tartrate (Potentiation of depressant effect). Products include:
- Levo-Dromoran ... 1906

Lithium Carbonate (Potentiation of depressant effect; increased risk of respiratory depression). Products include:
- Eskalith ... 2214
- Lithane Tablets ... 1596
- Lithium Carbonate Capsules & Tablets ... 1984
- Lithobid Tablets ... 870

Lithium Citrate (Potentiation of depressant effect; increased risk of respiratory depression). Products include:
- Cibalith-S ... 870

Lorazepam (Potentiation of depressant effect). Products include:
- Ativan Injection ... 2432
- Ativan Tablets ... 2434

Loxapine Hydrochloride (Potentiation of depressant effect; increased risk of respiratory depression). Products include:
- Loxitane ... 1213

Loxapine Succinate (Potentiation of depressant effect; increased risk of respiratory depression). Products include:
- Loxitane Capsules ... 1213

Maprotiline Hydrochloride (Potentiation of depressant effect). Products include:
- Ludiomil Tablets ... 874

Meperidine Hydrochloride (Potentiation of depressant effect). Products include:
- Demerol ... 2047
- Mepergan Injection ... 2479

Mephobarbital (Potentiation of depressant effect). Products include:
- Mebaral Tablets ... 2061

Meprobamate (Potentiation of depressant effect). Products include:
- Deprol Tablets ... 2382
- Equagesic Tablets ... 2451
- Miltown Tablets ... 2386
- PMB 200 and PMB 400 ... 2504

Mesoridazine (Potentiation of depressant effect; increased risk of respiratory depression). Products include:
- Serentil ... 686

Methadone Hydrochloride (Potentiation of depressant effect). Products include:
- Dolophine Hydrochloride Ampoules & Vials 1260
- Dolophine Hydrochloride Tablets 1261
- Methadone Hydrochloride Diskets .. 1284
- Methadone Hydrochloride Oral Solution & Tablets 1987

Methdilazine Hydrochloride (Potentiation of depressant effect). Products include:
- Tacaryl Syrup & Tablets 2409

Methohexital Sodium (Potentiation of depressant effect). Products include:
- Brevital Sodium Vials 1248

Methoxyflurane (Potentiation of depressant effect).
- No products indexed under this heading.

Methylprednisolone Acetate (Concurrent use by epidural or intrathecal route is contraindicated with parenteral corticosteroids). Products include:
- Depo-Medrol Sterile Aqueous Suspension 2334

Methylprednisolone Sodium Succinate (Concurrent use by epidural or intrathecal route is contraindicated with parenteral corticosteroids). Products include:
- Solu-Medrol Sterile Powder 2363

Midazolam Hydrochloride (Potentiation of depressant effect). Products include:
- Versed Injection 1924

Molindone Hydrochloride (Potentiation of depressant effect; increased risk of respiratory depression). Products include:
- Moban Tablets & Concentrate 932

Nortriptyline Hydrochloride (Potentiation of depressant effect). Products include:
- Pamelor 2019

Opium Alkaloids (Potentiation of depressant effect). Products include:
- B & O No. 15A & No. 16A Supprettes 2395
- Pantopon Injectable 1911

Oxazepam (Potentiation of depressant effect). Products include:
- Serax Capsules 2522
- Serax Tablets 2522

Oxycodone Hydrochloride (Potentiation of depressant effect). Products include:
- Percocet Tablets 950
- Percodan 951
- Roxicodone Tablets, Oral Solution & Intensol (Oxycodone) 1992
- Tylox Capsules 1382

Pentobarbital Sodium (Potentiation of depressant effect). Products include:
- Nembutal Sodium Capsules 534
- Nembutal Sodium Solution 536
- Nembutal Sodium Suppositories 538

Perphenazine (Potentiation of depressant effect; increased risk of respiratory depression). Products include:
- Etrafon 2087
- Triavil Tablets 1556
- Trilafon 2123

Phenelzine Sulfate (Potentiation of depressant effect). Products include:
- Nardil 1742

Phenobarbital (Potentiation of depressant effect). Products include:
- Arco-Lase Plus Tablets 607
- Bellergal-S Tablets 1998
- Bronkolixir .... ▣ 761
- Bronkotabs Tablets .... ▣ 762
- Donnatal 1858
- Donnatal Extentabs 1859
- Donnatal Tablets 1858
- Donnazyme Tablets 1860
- Kinesed Tablets 2272
- Phenobarbital Elixir and Tablets 1293
- Primatene Tablets-P Formula 2421
- Quadrinal Tablets 1183
- Tedral SA 1765

Pimozide (Potentiation of depressant effect; increased risk of respiratory depression). Products include:
- Orap Tablets 1020

Prazepam (Potentiation of depressant effect). Products include:
- Centrax 1693

Prednisolone Acetate (Concurrent use by epidural or intrathecal route is contraindicated with parenteral corticosteroids). Products include:
- AK-Cide Sterile Ophthalmic Ointment & Suspension .... ⊙ 202
- Blephamide Liquifilm Sterile Ophthalmic Suspension 586
- Blephamide S.O.P. Sterile Ophthalmic Ointment 586
- Cetapred Ointment .... ⊙ 220
- ⅛% Econopred & 1% Econopred Plus .... ⊙ 217
- Isopto Cetapred Suspension .... ⊙ 220
- Metimyd .... ⊙ 306
- Poly-Pred Liquifilm .... ⊙ 250
- Pred Forte .... ⊙ 252
- Pred Mild .... ⊙ 254
- Pred-G Liquifilm Sterile Ophthalmic Suspension .... ⊙ 252
- Pred-G S.O.P. Sterile Ophthalmic Ointment .... ⊙ 253
- Vasocidin Ointment .... ⊙ 275

Prednisolone Sodium Phosphate (Concurrent use by epidural or intrathecal route is contraindicated with parenteral corticosteroids). Products include:
- AK-Pred .... ⊙ 205
- Hydeltrasol Injection, Sterile 1476
- Inflamase .... ⊙ 274
- Pediapred Oral Liquid 987
- Vasocidin Ophthalmic Solution .... ⊙ 276

Prednisolone Tebutate (Concurrent use by epidural or intrathecal route is contraindicated with parenteral corticosteroids). Products include:
- Hydeltra-T.B.A. Sterile Suspension 1478

Prednisone (Concurrent use by epidural or intrathecal route is contraindicated with parenteral corticosteroids). Products include:
- Deltasone Tablets 2332

Prochlorperazine (Potentiation of depressant effect; increased risk of respiratory depression). Products include:
- Compazine 2201

Promethazine Hydrochloride (Potentiation of depressant effect; increased risk of respiratory depression). Products include:
- Mepergan Injection 2479
- Phenergan with Codeine 2497
- Phenergan with Dextromethorphan 2499
- Phenergan Injection 2493
- Phenergan Suppositories 2496
- Phenergan Syrup 2495
- Phenergan Tablets 2496
- Phenergan VC 2500
- Phenergan VC with Codeine 2501

Propofol (Potentiation of depressant effect). Products include:
- Diprivan Injection 2267

Propoxyphene Hydrochloride (Potentiation of depressant effect). Products include:
- Darvon 1256
- Wygesic Tablets 2540

Propoxyphene Napsylate (Potentiation of depressant effect). Products include:
- Darvon-N/Darvocet-N 1254

Protriptyline Hydrochloride (Potentiation of depressant effect). Products include:
- Vivactil Tablets 1567

Pyrilamine Maleate (Potentiation of depressant effect). Products include:
- Codimal 846
- 4-Way Fast Acting Nasal Spray - Original Formula (regular & mentholated) & Metered Spray Pump (regular) 751
- Maximum Strength Midol Multi-Symptom Menstrual Formula .... ▣ 571
- Maximum Strength Midol PMS Premenstrual Syndrome Formula .... ▣ 570
- Regular Strength Midol Multi-Symptom Menstrual Formula .... ▣ 570
- Prefrin-A .... ⊙ 255
- Prēmsyn PMS Capsules & Caplets ▣ 547
- Primatene Tablets-M Formula 2421
- Robitussin Night Relief .... ▣ 677
- Ru-Tuss with Hydrocodone 694
- Triaminic Expectorant DH 1995
- Triaminic Oral Infant Drops 1996

Pyrilamine Tannate (Potentiation of depressant effect). Products include:
- Rynatan 2387

Quazepam (Potentiation of depressant effect). Products include:
- Doral Tablets 2383

Secobarbital Sodium (Potentiation of depressant effect). Products include:
- Seconal Sodium Pulvules 1296

Selegiline Hydrochloride (Potentiation of depressant effect). Products include:
- Eldepryl 2250

Sufentanil Citrate (Potentiation of depressant effect). Products include:
- Sufenta Injection 1147

Temazepam (Potentiation of depressant effect). Products include:
- Restoril Capsules 2023

Terfenadine (Potentiation of depressant effect). Products include:
- Seldane Tablets 1349
- Seldane-D Extended-Release Tablets 1350

Thiamylal Sodium (Potentiation of depressant effect). Products include:
- Surital Ampoules, Steri-Vials 1764

Thioridazine Hydrochloride (Potentiation of depressant effect; increased risk of respiratory depression). Products include:
- Mellaril 2011

Thiothixene (Potentiation of depressant effect; increased risk of respiratory depression). Products include:
- Navane Capsules and Concentrate 1954
- Navane Intramuscular 1956

Tranylcypromine Sulfate (Potentiation of depressant effect). Products include:
- Parnate Tablets 2222

Triamcinolone (Concurrent use by epidural or intrathecal route is contraindicated with parenteral corticosteroids).
- No products indexed under this heading.

Triamcinolone Acetonide (Concurrent use by epidural or intrathecal route is contraindicated with parenteral corticosteroids). Products include:
- Aristocort A 1010
- Azmacort Inhaler 1837
- Kenalog Cream, Lotion & Ointment 2401
- Kenalog-10 Injection 2402
- Kenalog-40 Injection 2403
- Kenalog in Orabase 604
- Kenalog Spray 2401
- Mycolog II Cream and Ointment 2407
- Mytrex Cream & Ointment 2080
- Nasacort Nasal Inhaler 1844

Triamcinolone Diacetate (Concurrent use by epidural or intrathecal route is contraindicated with parenteral corticosteroids). Products include:
- Aristocort Suspension 1008

Triamcinolone Hexacetonide (Concurrent use by epidural or intrathecal route is contraindicated with parenteral corticosteroids). Products include:
- Aristospan Suspension 1011

Triazolam (Potentiation of depressant effect). Products include:
- Halcion Tablets 2340

Trifluoperazine Hydrochloride (Potentiation of depressant effect; increased risk of respiratory depression). Products include:
- Stelazine 2226

Trimeprazine Tartrate (Potentiation of depressant effect). Products include:
- Temaril Tablets, Syrup and Spansule Sustained Release Capsules 1085

Trimipramine Maleate (Potentiation of depressant effect). Products include:
- Surmontil Capsules 2524

Tripelennamine Hydrochloride (Potentiation of depressant effect). Products include:
- PBZ Tablets & Elixir 1037
- PBZ-SR Tablets 1037

Triprolidine Hydrochloride (Potentiation of depressant effect). Products include:
- Actidil .... ▣ 538
- Actifed Capsules .... ▣ 539
- Actifed Plus Caplets .... ▣ 539
- Actifed Plus Tablets .... ▣ 540
- Actifed with Codeine Cough Syrup.. 752
- Actifed Syrup .... ▣ 540
- Actifed Tablets .... ▣ 540
- Actifed 12-Hour Capsules .... ▣ 539

Warfarin Sodium (Concurrent use by epidural or intrathecal route is contraindicated with anticoagulant therapy). Products include:
- Coumadin Injection & Tablets 944
- Panwarfin Tablets 547

DURANEST INJECTIONS
(Etidocaine Hydrochloride) 624
May interact with (with epinephrine solutions only), monoamine oxidase inhibitors, tricyclic antidepressants, phenothiazines, vasopressors, and certain other agents. Compounds in these categories include:

Amitriptyline Hydrochloride (Severe, prolonged hypotension or hypertension). Products include:
- Elavil 2269
- Endep Tablets 1927
- Etrafon 2087
- Limbitrol 1933
- Triavil Tablets 1556

Amoxapine (Severe, prolonged hypotension or hypertension). Products include:
- Asendin Tablets 1196

Chlorpromazine (Severe, prolonged hypotension or hypertension). Products include:
- Thorazine 2234

Clomipramine Hydrochloride (Severe, prolonged hypotension or hypertension). Products include:
- Anafranil Capsules 650

Desipramine Hydrochloride (Severe, prolonged hypotension or hypertension). Products include:
- Norpramin Tablets 1340

Dopamine Hydrochloride (Severe, persistent hypertension or cerebrovascular accidents). Products include:
- Intropin Injection 930

Doxepin Hydrochloride (Severe prolonged hypotension or hypertension). Products include:
- Sinequan 1960

Epinephrine Bitartrate (Severe, persistent hypertension or cerebrovascular accidents). Products include:
- AsthmaHaler Mist Epinephrine Bitartrate Bronchodilator .... ▣ 616
- Bronkaid Mist Suspension .... ▣ 757
- Primatene Mist Suspension 2421

Epinephrine Hydrochloride (Severe, persistent hypertension or cerebrovascular accidents). Products include:
- Adrenalin Chloride Solution 1:100 & 1:1,000 1689
- Epifrin .... ◉ 244
- Glaucon .... ◉ 218

Ergonovine Maleate (Severe, persistent hypertension or cerebrovascular accident).

Fluphenazine Decanoate (Severe, prolonged hypotension or hypertension). Products include:
- Prolixin Decanoate 1795

Fluphenazine Enanthate (Severe, prolonged hypotension or hypertension). Products include:
- Prolixin Enanthate 1796

Fluphenazine Hydrochloride (Severe, prolonged hypotension or hypertension). Products include:
- Prolixin Elixir 1793
- Prolixin Injection 1791
- Prolixin Oral Concentrate 1792
- Prolixin Tablets 1793

Furazolidone (Severe, prolonged hypotension or hypertension). Products include:
- Furoxone 1855

Imipramine Hydrochloride (Severe, prolonged hypotension or hypertension). Products include:
- Tofranil Ampuls 1038
- Tofranil Tablets 1039

Imipramine Pamoate (Severe, prolonged hypotension or hypertension). Products include:
- Tofranil-PM Capsules 1041

Isocarboxazid (Severe, prolonged hypotension or hypertension). Products include:
- Marplan Tablets 1906

Maprotiline Hydrochloride (Severe, prolonged hypotension or hypertension). Products include:
- Ludiomil Tablets 874

Mesoridazine (Severe, prolonged hypotension or hypertension). Products include:
- Serentil 686

Metaraminol Bitartrate (Severe, persistent hypertension or cerebrovascular accidents). Products include:
- Aramine Injection 1424

Methoxamine Hydrochloride (Severe, persistent hypertension or cerebrovascular accidents). Products include:
- Vasoxyl Injection 819

Methylergonovine Maleate (Severe, persistent hypertension or cerebrovascular accidents). Products include:
- Methergine 2016

Norepinephrine Bitartrate (Severe, persistent hypertension or cerebrovascular accidents). Products include:
- Levophed Bitartrate Injection 2054

Nortriptyline Hydrochloride (Severe, prolonged hypotension or hypertension). Products include:
- Pamelor 2019

Perphenazine (Severe, prolonged hypotension or hypertension). Products include:
- Etrafon 2087
- Triavil Tablets 1556
- Trilafon 2123

Phenelzine Sulfate (Severe, prolonged hypotension or hypertension). Products include:
- Nardil 1742

Phenylephrine Hydrochloride (Severe, persistent hypertension or cerebrovascular accidents). Products include:
- AK-Dilate Solution 2.5% and 10% .... ◉ 203
- Atrohist Sprinkle Capsules 558
- Cerose-DM 2443
- Codimal 846
- Comhist LA Capsules 1618
- Congespirin For Children Aspirin Free Chewable Cold Tablets 748
- Cyclomydril .... ◉ 216
- Deconsal Sprinkle Capsules 559
- Dimetane Decongestant .... ▣ 673
- Dristan Decongestant/Antihistamine/ Analgesic Coated Caplets .... ▣ 749
- Dristan Cold Nasal Decongestant/ Antihistamine/ Analgesic Coated Tablets 2419
- Dristan Advanced Formula Decongestant/Antihistamine/ Analgesic Tablets .... ▣ 749
- Dristan Nasal Spray, Menthol 2419
- Dristan Nasal Spray, Regular and Regular with Metered Pump 2419
- Entex Capsules 1623
- Entex Liquid 1623
- Sinus Excedrin Analgesic, Decongestant Tablets & Caplets 750
- Extendryl 994
- 4-Way Fast Acting Nasal Spray - Original Formula (regular & mentholated) & Metered Spray Pump (regular) 751
- Hycomine Compound Tablets 929
- Murocoll-2 Sterile Ophthalmic Solution .... ◉ 261
- Mydfrin 2.5% .... ◉ 224
- Naldecon Syrup, Tablets, Pediatric Drops and Pediatric Syrup 709
- Neo-Synephrine Hydrochloride 1% Carpuject 2063
- Neo-Synephrine Hydrochloride 1% Injection 2063
- Neo-Synephrine Hydrochloride (Ophthalmic) 2064
- Neo-Synephrine .... ▣ 759
- Nōstril Nasal Decongestant .... ▣ 520
- Novahistine Elixir .... ▣ 596
- Phenergan VC 2500
- Phenergan VC with Codeine 2501
- Prefrin Liquifilm Vasoconstrictor and Lubricant Eye Drops .... ◉ 254
- Prefrin-A .... ◉ 255
- Quelidrine Syrup 556
- Relief Vasoconstrictor and Lubricant Eye Drops .... ◉ 256
- Robitussin Night Relief .... ▣ 677
- Ru-Tuss with Hydrocodone 694
- Ru-Tuss Tablets 693
- Vasosulf .... ◉ 279
- Vicks Sinex .... ▣ 665
- Zincfrin .... ◉ 230

Prochlorperazine (Severe, prolonged hypotension or hypertension). Products include:
- Compazine 2201

Promethazine Hydrochloride (Severe, prolonged hypotension or hypertension). Products include:
- Mepergan Injection 2479
- Phenergan with Codeine 2497
- Phenergan with Dextromethorphan 2499
- Phenergan Injection 2493
- Phenergan Suppositories 2496
- Phenergan Syrup 2495
- Phenergan Tablets 2496
- Phenergan VC 2500
- Phenergan VC with Codeine 2501

Protriptyline Hydrochloride (Severe, prolonged hypotension or hypertension). Products include:
- Vivactil Tablets 1567

Selegiline Hydrochloride (Severe, prolonged hypotension or hypertension). Products include:
- Eldepryl 2250

Thioridazine Hydrochloride (Severe, prolonged hypotension or hypertension). Products include:
- Mellaril 2011

Tranylcypromine Sulfate (Severe, prolonged hypotension or hypertension). Products include:
- Parnate Tablets 2222

Trifluoperazine Hydrochloride (Severe, prolonged hypotension or hypertension). Products include:
- Stelazine 2226

Trimipramine Maleate (Severe, prolonged hypotension or hypertension). Products include:
- Surmontil Capsules 2524

DURATEARS NATURALE
(Mineral Oil, Petrolatum, White) .... ◉ 216
No interactions described in labeling.

DURATION 12 HOUR MENTHOLATED NASAL SPRAY
(Oxymetazoline Hydrochloride) .... ▣ 700
No interactions described in labeling.

DURATION 12 HOUR NASAL SPRAY
(Oxymetazoline Hydrochloride) .... ▣ 700
No interactions described in labeling.

DURATION 12 HOUR NASAL SPRAY PUMP
(Oxymetazoline Hydrochloride) .... ▣ 700
No interactions described in labeling.

DURICEF
(Cefadroxil Monohydrate) 1405
No interactions described in labeling.

DUVOID TABLETS
(Bethanechol Chloride) 1853
May interact with ganglionic blocking agents. Compounds in this category include:

Mecamylamine Hydrochloride (Potential for critical fall in blood pressure). Products include:
- Inversine Tablets 1492

Trimethaphan Camsylate (Potential for critical fall in blood pressure). Products include:
- Arfonad Ampuls 1887

DYAZIDE CAPSULES
(Hydrochlorothiazide, Triamterene) .. 2208
May interact with potassium sparing diuretics, lithium preparations, corticosteroids, oral anticoagulants, nonsteroidal anti-inflammatory agents, antihypertensives, ACE inhibitors, oral hypoglycemic agents, antigout agents, potassium-depleting corticosteroids, nondepolarizing neuromuscular blocking agents, and certain other agents. Compounds in these categories include:

Acebutolol Hydrochloride (Additive or potentiated action). Products include:
- Sectral Capsules 2520

ACTH (May intensify electrolyte imbalance, particularly hypokalemia).
- No products indexed under this heading.

Allopurinol (Dyazide may raise the level of blood uric acid). Products include:
- Zyloprim Tablets 830

Amiloride Hydrochloride (Contraindicated). Products include:
- Midamor Tablets 1508
- Moduretic Tablets 1510

Amphotericin B (May intensify electrolyte imbalance, particularly hypokalemia). Products include:
- Fungizone Cream, Lotion and Ointment 2261
- Fungizone Intravenous 2262

Atenolol (Additive or potentiated action). Products include:
- Tenoretic Tablets 1105
- Tenormin Tablets and I.V. Injection 1107

Atracurium Besylate (Increased paralyzing effects). Products include:
- Tracrium Injection 817

Benazepril Hydrochloride (Increased risk of hyperkalemia and additive antihypertensive effects). Products include:
- Lotensin Tablets 872

Bendroflumethiazide (Additive or potentiated action). Products include:
- Corzide Tablets 702
- Naturetin Tablets 1789
- Rauzide Tablets 1804

Betamethasone Acetate (May intensify electrolyte imbalance, particularly hypokalemia). Products include:
- Celestone Soluspan Suspension 2081

Betamethasone Sodium Phosphate (May intensify electrolyte imbalance, particularly hypokalemia). Products include:
- Celestone Soluspan Suspension 2081

Betaxolol Hydrochloride (Increased risk of hyperkalemia and additive antihypertensive effects). Products include:
- Betoptic Sterile Ophthalmic Solution 569
- Betoptic S Sterile Ophthalmic Suspension 570
- Kerlone Tablets 2172

Captopril (Increased risk of hyperkalemia and additive antihypertensive effects). Products include:
- Capoten 2255
- Capozide 2258

Carteolol Hydrochloride (Additive or potentiated action). Products include:
- Cartrol Tablets 507

Chlorothiazide (Additive or potentiated action). Products include:
- Aldoclor Tablets 1413
- Diupres Tablets 1461
- Diuril Oral 1464

Chlorothiazide Sodium (Additive or potentiated action). Products include:
- Diuril Sodium Intravenous 1463

Chlorpropamide (Increased risk of severe hyponatremia). Products include:
- Diabinese Tablets 1775

Chlorthalidone (Additive or potentiated action; contraindicated). Products include:
- Combipres Tablets 678
- Tenoretic Tablets 1105
- Thalitone Tablets 687

Clonidine (Additive or potentiated action). Products include:
- Catapres-TTS 677

Clonidine Hydrochloride (Additive or potentiated action). Products include:
- Catapres Tablets 676
- Combipres Tablets 678

Cortisone Acetate (May intensify electrolyte imbalance, particularly hypokalemia). Products include:
- Cortone Acetate Sterile Suspension 1437
- Cortone Acetate Tablets 1439

Deserpidine (Additive or potentiated action). Products include:
- Enduronyl 518

(▣ Described in PDR For Nonprescription Drugs) (◉ Described in PDR For Ophthalmology)

Harmonyl Tablets 528
Oreticyl 545

Dexamethasone (May intensify electrolyte imbalance, particularly hypokalemia). Products include:
AK-Trol Ointment & Suspension ⊙ 207
Decadron Elixir 1445
Decadron Tablets 1447
Decaspray Topical Aerosol 1459
Dexacidin ⊙ 272
Maxidex Sterile Ophthalmic Suspension ⊙ 223
Maxitrol Ophthalmic Ointment/Suspension ⊙ 223
TobraDex Ophthalmic Suspension and Ointment ⊙ 228

Dexamethasone Acetate (May intensify electrolyte imbalance, particularly hypokalemia). Products include:
Dalalone D.P. Injectable 999
Decadron-LA Sterile Suspension 1457

Dexamethasone Sodium Phosphate (May intensify electrolyte imbalance, particularly hypokalemia). Products include:
AK-Dex ⊙ 203
Decadron Phosphate Respihaler 1454
Decadron Phosphate Sterile Ophthalmic Ointment 1453
Decadron Phosphate Sterile Ophthalmic Solution 1453
Decadron Phosphate Topical Cream 1455
Decadron Phosphate Turbinaire 1456
Maxidex Sterile Ophthalmic Ointment ⊙ 222
NeoDecadron Sterile Ophthalmic Ointment 1517
NeoDecadron Sterile Ophthalmic Solution 1518
NeoDecadron Topical Cream 1518

Diazoxide (Additive or potentiated action). Products include:
Hyperstat I.V. Injection 2095
Proglycem 649

Diclofenac Sodium (Potential for acute renal failure). Products include:
Voltaren Ophthalmic Sterile Ophthalmic Solution ⊙ 268
Voltaren Tablets 1042

Dicumarol (Effects of oral anticoagulants may be decreased). Products include:
Dicumarol Tablets 516

Doxazosin Mesylate (Increased risk of hyperkalemia and additive antihypertensive effects). Products include:
Cardura Tablets 1941

Enalapril Maleate (Increased risk of hyperkalemia and additive antihypertensive effects). Products include:
Vaseretic Tablets 1559
Vasotec Tablets 1564

Enalaprilat (Increased risk of hyperkalemia and additive antihypertensive effects). Products include:
Vasotec I.V. 1562

Esmolol Hydrochloride (Additive or potentiated action). Products include:
Brevibloc Injection 942

Etodolac (Potential for acute renal failure). Products include:
Lodine Capsules 2468

Felodipine (Increased risk of hyperkalemia and additive antihypertensive effects). Products include:
Plendil Extended-Release Tablets 1526

Fenoprofen Calcium (Potential for acute renal failure). Products include:
Nalfon Pulvules & Tablets 919

Flurbiprofen (Potential for acute renal failure). Products include:
Ansaid Tablets 2319

Fosinopril Sodium (Increased risk of hyperkalemia and additive antihypertensive effects). Products include:
Monopril Tablets 1406

Furosemide (Additive or potentiated action). Products include:
Lasix 1093

Glipizide (Increased risk of severe hyponatremia). Products include:
Glucotrol 1952

Glyburide (Increased risk of severe hyponatremia). Products include:
DiaBeta 1091
Micronase Tablets 2350

Guanabenz Acetate (Additive or potentiated action). Products include:
Wytensin Tablets 2542

Guanethidine Monosulfate (Additive or potentiated action). Products include:
Esimil Tablets 864
Ismelin Tablets 869

Hydralazine Hydrochloride (Additive or potentiated action). Products include:
Apresazide Capsules 854
Apresoline Hydrochloride Parenteral (Ampuls) 856
Apresoline Hydrochloride Tablets 855
Apresoline-Esidrix Tablets 857
Ser-Ap-Es Tablets 881
Serpasil-Apresoline Tablets 884

Hydrocortisone (May intensify electrolyte imbalance, particularly hypokalemia). Products include:
AK-Spore H.C. ⊙ 206
Bactine Hydrocortisone Anti-Itch Cream ▣ 625
CaldeCORT Anti-Itch Hydrocortisone Spray ▣ 560
Carmol HC Cream 1% 2296
Cortaid Spray ▣ 735
Cortenema 2244
Cortisporin Ointment 758
Cortisporin Ophthalmic Ointment Sterile 758
Cortisporin Ophthalmic Suspension Sterile 759
Cortisporin Otic Solution Sterile 760
Cortisporin Otic Suspension Sterile 760
Cortizone-5 Creme & Ointment ▣ 732
Dermolate Anti-Itch Cream ▣ 697
Eldecort Cream 1.0% 1113
Eldecort Cream 1.0% and 2.5% 1113
Fungoid HC Creme 1770
Hydrocortone Tablets 1482
Hytone 909
LazerSporin-C Solution 1770
Massengill Medicated Soft Cloth Towelettes 2192
Nutracort Cream & Lotion 1684
PediOtic Suspension Sterile 797
Synacort Creams 1%, 2.5% 2296
Vanoxide-HC Acne Lotion 911
Vioform-Hydrocortisone Cream and Mild Cream 889
Vioform-Hydrocortisone Ointment 889
VōSoL HC Otic Solution 2392
Vytone Cream 1% 911

Hydrocortisone Acetate (May intensify electrolyte imbalance, particularly hypokalemia). Products include:
Analpram-HC Rectal Cream 1% and 2.5% 970
Anusol-HC Cream 1690
Anusol-HC Suppositories 1691
Caldecort ▣ 560
Carmol HC Cream 1% 2296
Chloromycetin Hydrocortisone Ophthalmic 1694
Coly-Mycin S Otic w/Neomycin & Hydrocortisone 1708
Cortaid ▣ 735
Cortef Feminine Itch Cream ▣ 735
Corticaine ▣ 682
Cortifoam 1827
Cortisporin Cream 757
Epifoam 1828
Gynecort 5 Creme ▣ 556
Hydrocortone Acetate Sterile Suspension 1479
Lanacort 5 Creme and Ointment ▣ 557
Mantadil Cream 789
Ophthocort ⊙ 301
Orabase HCA Oral Paste 890
Pramosone Cream, Lotion & Ointment 971
ProctoCream-HC 1834
Proctofoam-HC 1835

Hydrocortisone Sodium Phosphate (May intensify electrolyte imbalance, particularly hypokalemia). Products include:
Hydrocortone Phosphate Injection, Sterile 1481

Hydrocortisone Sodium Succinate (May intensify electrolyte imbalance, particularly hypokalemia). Products include:
Solu-Cortef Sterile Powder 2361

Hydroflumethiazide (Additive or potentiated action). Products include:
Diucardin Tablets 2450
Saluron 718
Salutensin/Salutensin-Demi 719

Ibuprofen (Potential for acute renal failure). Products include:
Advil Cold & Sinus Caplets (formerly CoAdvil) 2416
Advil Ibuprofen Tablets and Caplets 2416
Children's Advil Suspension 2426
CoAdvil ▣ 748
Dristan Sinus Caplets 2419
Haltran Tablets ▣ 668
Ibuprofen ▣ 631
Medipren ibuprofen Caplets and Tablets 1362
Midol 200 Cramp Relief Formula ▣ 570
Motrin Tablets 2351
Motrin IB Caplets and Tablets ▣ 736
Nuprin Ibuprofen/Analgesic Tablets & Caplets 752
PediaProfen Suspension 1363
Rufen Tablets 691
Trendar Ibuprofen Tablets ▣ 756

Indapamide (Additive or potentiated action). Products include:
Lozol Tablets 1843

Indomethacin (Potential for acute renal failure). Products include:
Indocin 1487

Indomethacin Sodium Trihydrate (Potential for acute renal failure). Products include:
Indocin I.V. 1490

Isradipine (Increased risk of hyperkalemia and additive antihypertensive effects). Products include:
DynaCirc Capsules 2004

Ketoprofen (Potential for acute renal failure). Products include:
Orudis Capsules 2488

Ketorolac Tromethamine (Potential for acute renal failure). Products include:
Toradol IM Injection 2302

Labetalol Hydrochloride (Additive or potentiated action). Products include:
Normodyne Injection 2108
Normodyne Tablets 2110
Normozide Tablets 2112
Trandate HCT Tablets 579
Trandate Injection 577
Trandate Tablets 579

Levorphanol Tartrate (May aggravate postural hypotension). Products include:
Levo-Dromoran 1906

Lisinopril (Increased risk of hyperkalemia and additive antihypertensive effects). Products include:
Prinivil Tablets 1538
Prinzide Tablets 1540
Zestoretic 2274
Zestril Tablets 2277

Lithium Carbonate (Reduced renal clearance of lithium; increased risk of lithium toxicity). Products include:
Eskalith 2214
Lithane Tablets 1596
Lithium Carbonate Capsules & Tablets 1984
Lithobid Tablets 870

Lithium Citrate (Reduced renal clearance of lithium; increased risk of lithium toxicity). Products include:
Cibalith-S 870

Mecamylamine Hydrochloride (Additive or potentiated action). Products include:
Inversine Tablets 1492

Meclofenamate Sodium (Potential for acute renal failure). Products include:
Meclomen Capsules 1739

Mefenamic Acid (Potential for acute renal failure). Products include:
Ponstel 1758

Methenamine (Decreased effectiveness due to alkalinization of urine). Products include:
Urised Tablets 2396

Methenamine Hippurate (Decreased effectiveness due to alkalinization of urine). Products include:
Hiprex Tablets 1333
Urex Tablets 1321

Methenamine Mandelate (Decreased effectiveness due to alkalinization of urine). Products include:
Mandelamine 1738
Uroqid-Acid 661

Methyclothiazide (Additive or potentiated action). Products include:
Enduron Tablets 517
Enduronyl 518

Methyldopa (Additive or potentiated action). Products include:
Aldoclor Tablets 1413
Aldomet Oral 1415
Aldoril Tablets 1418

Methyldopate Hydrochloride (Additive or potentiated action effects). Products include:
Aldomet Ester HCl Injection 1417

Methylprednisolone Acetate (May intensify electrolyte imbalance, particularly hypokalemia). Products include:
Depo-Medrol Sterile Aqueous Suspension 2334

Methylprednisolone Sodium Succinate (May intensify electrolyte imbalance, particularly hypokalemia). Products include:
Solu-Medrol Sterile Powder 2363

Metocurine Iodide (Increased paralyzing effects). Products include:
Metubine Iodide Vials 1285

Metolazone (Additive or potentiated action). Products include:
Diulo 2129
Mykrox ½ mg Tablets 984
Zaroxolyn Tablets 989

Metoprolol Tartrate (Additive or potentiated action). Products include:
Lopressor Ampuls 1032
Lopressor HCT Tablets 1034
Lopressor Tablets 1032

Metyrosine (Additive or potentiated action). Products include:
Demser Capsules 1460

Minoxidil (Additive or potentiated action). Products include:
Loniten Tablets 2346
Rogaine Topical Solution 2357

Nadolol (Additive or potentiated action). Products include:
Corgard Tablets 701
Corzide Tablets 702

Naproxen (Potential for acute renal failure). Products include:
Naprosyn 2297

Naproxen Sodium (Potential for acute renal failure). Products include:
- Anaprox and Anaprox DS Tablets.... 2288

Nicardipine Hydrochloride (Additive or potentiated action). Products include:
- Cardene Capsules 2290

Nitroglycerin (Additive or potentiated action). Products include:
- Deponit NTG Transdermal Delivery System 2143
- Minitran Transdermal Delivery System 1312
- Nitro-Bid Ointment 1339
- Nitro-Bid Capsules 1338
- Nitrodisc 2176
- Nitro-Dur (nitroglycerin) Transdermal Infusion System 1164
- Nitrogard Tablets 1004
- Nitrolingual Spray 1846
- Nitrostat Tablets 1743
- Transderm-Nitro Transdermal Therapeutic System 2283

Norepinephrine Bitartrate (Decreased arterial responsiveness to norepinephrine). Products include:
- Levophed Bitartrate Injection 2054

Pancuronium Bromide Injection (Increased paralyzing effects).
- No products indexed under this heading.

Penbutolol Sulfate (Additive or potentiated action). Products include:
- Levatol 1832

Phenoxybenzamine Hydrochloride (Additive or potentiated action). Products include:
- Dibenzyline Capsules 2207

Phentolamine Mesylate (Additive or potentiated action). Products include:
- Regitine 878

Phenylbutazone (Potential for acute renal failure). Products include:
- Butazolidin Capsules & Tablets 1027

Pindolol (Additive or potentiated action). Products include:
- Visken Tablets 2036

Piroxicam (Potential for acute renal failure). Products include:
- Feldene Capsules 1777

Polythiazide (Additive or potentiated action). Products include:
- Minizide Capsules 1779
- Renese Tablets 1785
- Renese-R Tablets 1786

Potassium Acid Phosphate (Potential for hyperkalemia). Products include:
- K-Phos M.F. Tablets 659
- K-Phos Original Formula 'Sodium Free' Tablets 660
- K-Phos No. 2 Tablets 659

Potassium Bicarbonate (Potential for hyperkalemia). Products include:
- Alka-Seltzer Advanced Formula Antacid & Non-Aspirin Pain Reliever .... ▣ 620
- Alka-Seltzer Effervescent Antacid ▣ 622
- K-Lyte 707
- Klorvess Effervescent Granules 2010
- Klorvess Effervescent Tablets 2011

Potassium Chloride (Potential for hyperkalemia). Products include:
- Chlor-3 Condiment 994
- K-Dur Microburst Release System (potassium chloride, USP) E.R. Tablets 1163
- K-Lor Powder Packets 531
- K-Lyte 707
- K-Norm Capsules 982
- K-Tab Filmtab 532
- Kato Potassium Supplement 1114
- Klor-Con 8/Klor-Con 10 Extended-release Tablets 2374
- Klorvess Effervescent Granules 2010
- Klorvess Effervescent Tablets 2011
- Klorvess 10% Liquid 2010
- Klotrix 708
- Kolyum Liquid 983
- Micro-K 1863
- Micro-K LS Packets 1864
- NuLYTELY 699
- Oral Rehydration Salts, Citrate 1150
- Rum-K Syrup 995
- Slow-K Tablets 2281
- Ten-K Controlled-Release Tablets 2282
- Thermotabs .... ▣ 619

Potassium Citrate (Potential for hyperkalemia). Products include:
- Alka-Seltzer Effervescent Antacid .. 1570
- K-Lyte 707
- Polycitra Syrup 2424
- Polycitra-K 2424
- Polycitra-LC—Sugar-Free 2424
- Ricelyte, Rice-Based Oral Electrolyte Maintenance Solution .... ▣ 613

Potassium Gluconate (Potential for hyperkalemia). Products include:
- Kolyum Liquid 983

Potassium Phosphate, Dibasic (Potential for hyperkalemia). Products include:
- Neutra-Phos 2423

Potassium Phosphate, Monobasic (Potential for hyperkalemia). Products include:
- K-Phos M.F. Tablets 659
- K-Phos Neutral Tablets 660
- Neutra-Phos 2423

Prazosin Hydrochloride (Additive or potentiated action). Products include:
- Minipress Capsules 1778
- Minizide Capsules 1779

Prednisolone Acetate (May intensify electrolyte imbalance). Products include:
- AK-Cide Sterile Ophthalmic Ointment & Suspension .... ⊙ 202
- Blephamide Liquifilm Sterile Ophthalmic Suspension 586
- Blephamide S.O.P. Sterile Ophthalmic Ointment 586
- Cetapred Ointment .... ⊙ 220
- ⅛% Econopred & 1% Econopred Plus .... ⊙ 217
- Isopto Cetapred Suspension .... ⊙ 220
- Metimyd .... ⊙ 306
- Poly-Pred Liquifilm .... ⊙ 250
- Pred Forte .... ⊙ 252
- Pred Mild .... ⊙ 254
- Pred-G Liquifilm Sterile Ophthalmic Suspension .... ⊙ 252
- Pred-G S.O.P. Sterile Ophthalmic Ointment .... ⊙ 253
- Vasocidin Ointment .... ⊙ 275

Prednisolone Sodium Phosphate (May intensify electrolyte imbalance, particularly hypokalemia). Products include:
- AK-Pred .... ⊙ 205
- Hydeltrasol Injection, Sterile 1476
- Inflamase .... ⊙ 274
- Pediapred Oral Liquid 987
- Vasocidin Ophthalmic Solution .... ⊙ 276

Prednisolone Tebutate (May intensify electrolyte imbalance, particularly hypokalemia). Products include:
- Hydeltra-T.B.A. Sterile Suspension 1478

Prednisone (May intensify electrolyte imbalance, particularly hypokalemia). Products include:
- Deltasone Tablets 2332

Probenecid (Dyazide may raise the level of blood uric acid). Products include:
- Benemid Tablets 1426
- ColBENEMID Tablets 1436
- Wycillin Injection and Probenecid Tablets 2539

Propranolol Hydrochloride (Additive or potentiated action). Products include:
- Inderal 2459
- Inderal LA Long Acting Capsules 2461
- Inderide Tablets 2463
- Inderide LA Long Acting Capsules .. 2465

Ramipril (Increased risk of hyperkalemia and additive antihypertensive effects). Products include:
- Altace Capsules 1086

Rauwolfia Serpentina (Additive or potentiated action). Products include:
- Raudixin Tablets 1803
- Rauzide Tablets 1804

Rescinnamine (Additive or potentiated action).
- No products indexed under this heading.

Reserpine (Additive or potentiated action). Products include:
- Diupres Tablets 1461
- Hydromox R Tablets 1209
- Hydropres Tablets 1485
- Renese-R Tablets 1786
- Salutensin/Salutensin-Demi 719
- Ser-Ap-Es Tablets 881
- Serpasil Tablets 883
- Serpasil-Apresoline Tablets 884
- Serpasil-Esidrix Tablets 886

Sodium Nitroprusside (Additive or potentiated action). Products include:
- Nipride I.V. Infusion 1909

Sodium Polystyrene Sulfonate (May result in fluid retention). Products include:
- Kayexalate 2053
- Sodium Polystyrene Sulfonate Suspension 1993

Spironolactone (Contraindicated). Products include:
- Aldactazide 2150
- Aldactone 2152

Sulfinpyrazone (Dyazide may raise the level of blood uric acid). Products include:
- Anturane 853

Sulindac (Potential for acute renal failure). Products include:
- Clinoril Tablets 1433

Terazosin Hydrochloride (Additive or potentiated action). Products include:
- Hytrin Tablets 529

Timolol Maleate (Additive or potentiated action). Products include:
- Blocadren Tablets 1429
- Timolide Tablets 1547
- Timoptic in Ocudose 1552
- Timoptic Sterile Ophthalmic Solution 1550

Tolazamide (Increased risk of severe hyponatremia). Products include:
- Tolinase Tablets 2365

Tolbutamide (Increased risk of severe hyponatremia). Products include:
- Orinase Tablets 2354

Tolmetin Sodium (Potential for acute renal failure). Products include:
- Tolectin (200, 400 and 600 mg) .. 1379

Triamcinolone (May intensify electrolyte imbalance, particularly hypokalemia).
- No products indexed under this heading.

Triamcinolone Acetonide (May intensify electrolyte imbalance, particularly hypokalemia). Products include:
- Aristocort A 1010
- Azmacort Inhaler 1837
- Kenalog Cream, Lotion & Ointment 2401
- Kenalog-10 Injection 2402
- Kenalog-40 Injection 2403
- Kenalog in Orabase 604
- Kenalog Spray 2401
- Mycolog II Cream and Ointment 2407
- Mytrex Cream & Ointment 2080
- Nasacort Nasal Inhaler 1844

Triamcinolone Diacetate (May intensify electrolyte imbalance, particularly hypokalemia). Products include:
- Aristocort Suspension 1008

Triamcinolone Hexacetonide (May intensify electrolyte imbalance, particularly hypokalemia). Products include:
- Aristospan Suspension 1011

Trimethaphan Camsylate (Additive or potentiated action). Products include:
- Arfonad Ampuls 1887

Tubocurarine Chloride (Increased paralyzing effect).
- No products indexed under this heading.

Vecuronium Bromide (Increased paralyzing effects). Products include:
- Norcuron 1642

Warfarin Sodium (Effects of oral anticoagulants may be decreased). Products include:
- Coumadin Injection & Tablets 944
- Panwarfin Tablets 547

DYCLONE 0.5% AND 1% TOPICAL SOLUTIONS, USP
(Dyclonine Hydrochloride) 626

Food Interactions

Food, unspecified (Topical anesthesia may impair swallowing and thus enhance the danger of aspiration; food should not be ingested for 60 minutes).

DYNACIRC CAPSULES
(Isradipine) 2004
May interact with:

Fentanyl (Severe hypotension has been reported during fentanyl anesthesia with concomitant use of beta blocker and calcium channel blocker). Products include:
- Duragesic Transdermal System 1133

Fentanyl Citrate (Severe hypotension has been reported during fentanyl anesthesia with concomitant use of beta blocker and calcium channel blocker). Products include:
- Innovar Injection 1141
- Sublimaze Injection 1146

Hydrochlorothiazide (Potential for additive antihypertensive effect). Products include:
- Aldactazide 2150
- Aldoril Tablets 1418
- Apresazide Capsules 854
- Apresoline-Esidrix Tablets 857
- Capozide 2258
- Dyazide Capsules 2208
- Esidrix Tablets 863
- Esimil Tablets 864
- HydroDIURIL Tablets 1484
- Hydropres Tablets 1485
- Inderide Tablets 2463
- Inderide LA Long Acting Capsules .. 2465
- Lopressor HCT Tablets 1034
- Maxzide 1215
- Moduretic Tablets 1510
- Normozide Tablets 2112
- Oretic Tablets 544
- Oreticyl 545
- Prinzide Tablets 1540
- Ser-Ap-Es Tablets 881
- Serpasil-Esidrix Tablets 886
- Timolide Tablets 1547
- Trandate HCT Tablets 579
- Vaseretic Tablets 1559
- Zestoretic 2274

Propranolol Hydrochloride (Coadministration of DynaCirc resulted in significant increases in AUC and C_{max} and decreases in t_{max} of propranolol). Products include:
- Inderal 2459
- Inderal LA Long Acting Capsules 2461
- Inderide Tablets 2463
- Inderide LA Long Acting Capsules .. 2465

Food Interactions

Food, unspecified (Coadministration significantly increases the time to peak by about an hour with no effect on AUC).

DYRENIUM CAPSULES
(Triamterene) 2210
May interact with potassium-depleting corticosteroids, lithium preparations, non-steroidal anti-inflammatory agents, antihypertensives, diuretics, preanesthetic medications, general anesthetics, nondepolarizing neuromuscular blocking agents, ACE inhibitors, oral hypoglycemic agents, potassium sparing diuretics, and certain other agents. Compounds in these categories include:

Acebutolol Hydrochloride (Potentiated). Products include:
- Sectral Capsules 2520

Amiloride Hydrochloride (Contraindicated). Products include:
- Midamor Tablets 1508
- Moduretic Tablets 1510

Atenolol (Potentiated). Products include:
- Tenoretic Tablets 1105
- Tenormin Tablets and I.V. Injection 1107

Atracurium Besylate (Potentiated). Products include:
- Tracrium Injection 817

Benazepril Hydrochloride (Increased risk of hyperkalemia). Products include:
- Lotensin Tablets 872

Bendroflumethiazide (Potentiated). Products include:
- Corzide Tablets 702
- Naturetin Tablets 1789
- Rauzide Tablets 1804

Betaxolol Hydrochloride (Increased risk of hyperkalemia). Products include:
- Betoptic Sterile Ophthalmic Solution 569
- Betoptic S Sterile Ophthalmic Suspension 570
- Kerlone Tablets 2172

Bumetanide (Potentiated). Products include:
- Bumex 1895

Captopril (Increased risk of hyperkalemia). Products include:
- Capoten 2255
- Capozide 2258

Carteolol Hydrochloride (Potentiated). Products include:
- Cartrol Tablets 507

Chlorothiazide (Potentiated). Products include:
- Aldoclor Tablets 1413
- Diupres Tablets 1461
- Diuril Oral 1464

Chlorothiazide Sodium (Potentiated). Products include:
- Diuril Sodium Intravenous 1463

Chlorpropamide (Increased risk of severe hyponatremia). Products include:
- Diabinese Tablets 1775

Chlorthalidone (Potentiated; contraindicated). Products include:
- Combipres Tablets 678
- Tenoretic Tablets 1105
- Thalitone Tablets 687

Clonidine (Potentiated). Products include:
- Catapres-TTS 677

Clonidine Hydrochloride (Potentiated). Products include:
- Catapres Tablets 676
- Combipres Tablets 678

Deserpidine (Potentiated). Products include:
- Enduronyl 518
- Harmonyl Tablets 528
- Oreticyl 545

Diazepam (Potentiated). Products include:
- Valium Injectable 1937
- Valium Tablets 1939
- Valrelease Capsules 1923

Diazoxide (Potentiated). Products include:
- Hyperstat I.V. Injection 2095
- Proglycem 649

Diclofenac Sodium (Possibility of acute renal failure). Products include:
- Voltaren Ophthalmic Sterile Ophthalmic Solution .... ◉ 268
- Voltaren Tablets 1042

Doxazosin Mesylate (Increased risk of hyperkalemia). Products include:
- Cardura Tablets 1941

Droperidol (Potentiated). Products include:
- Inapsine Injection 1140
- Innovar Injection 1141

Enalapril Maleate (Increased risk of hyperkalemia). Products include:
- Vaseretic Tablets 1559
- Vasotec Tablets 1564

Enalaprilat (Increased risk of hyperkalemia). Products include:
- Vasotec I.V. 1562

Enflurane (Potentiated). Products include:
- Ethrane 599

Esmolol Hydrochloride (Potentiated). Products include:
- Brevibloc Injection 942

Ethacrynic Acid (Potentiated). Products include:
- Edecrin Tablets 1468

Etodolac (Possibility of acute renal failure). Products include:
- Lodine Capsules 2468

Felodipine (Increased risk of hyperkalemia). Products include:
- Plendil Extended-Release Tablets 1526

Fenoprofen Calcium (Possibility of acute renal failure). Products include:
- Nalfon Pulvules & Tablets 919

Fentanyl Citrate (Potentiated). Products include:
- Innovar Injection 1141
- Sublimaze Injection 1146

Flurbiprofen (Possibility of acute renal failure). Products include:
- Ansaid Tablets 2319

Fosinopril Sodium (Increased risk of hyperkalemia). Products include:
- Monopril Tablets 1406

Furosemide (Potentiated). Products include:
- Lasix 1093

Glipizide (Dosage adjustments of hypoglycemics may be necessary). Products include:
- Glucotrol 1952

Glyburide (Dosage adjustments of hypoglycemics may be necessary). Products include:
- DiaBeta 1091
- Micronase Tablets 2350

Guanabenz Acetate (Potentiated). Products include:
- Wytensin Tablets 2542

Guanethidine Monosulfate (Potentiated). Products include:
- Esimil Tablets 864
- Ismelin Tablets 869

Hydralazine Hydrochloride (Potentiated). Products include:
- Apresazide Capsules 854
- Apresoline Hydrochloride Parenteral (Ampuls) 856
- Apresoline Hydrochloride Tablets .. 855
- Apresoline-Esidrix Tablets 857
- Ser-Ap-Es Tablets 881
- Serpasil-Apresoline Tablets 884

Hydrochlorothiazide (Potentiated). Products include:
- Aldactazide 2150
- Aldoril Tablets 1418
- Apresazide Capsules 854
- Apresoline-Esidrix Tablets 857
- Capozide 2258
- Dyazide Capsules 2208
- Esidrix Tablets 863
- Esimil Tablets 864
- HydroDIURIL Tablets 1484
- Hydropres Tablets 1485
- Inderide Tablets 2463
- Inderide LA Long Acting Capsules .. 2465
- Lopressor HCT Tablets 1034
- Maxzide 1215
- Moduretic Tablets 1510
- Normozide Tablets 2112
- Oretic Tablets 544
- Oreticyl 545
- Prinzide Tablets 1540
- Ser-Ap-Es Tablets 881
- Serpasil-Esidrix Tablets 886
- Timolide Tablets 1547
- Trandate HCT Tablets 579
- Vaseretic Tablets 1559
- Zestoretic 2274

Hydroflumethiazide (Potentiated). Products include:
- Diucardin Tablets 2450
- Saluron 718
- Salutensin/Salutensin-Demi 719

Hydroxyzine Hydrochloride (Potentiated). Products include:
- Atarax Tablets & Syrup 1941
- Marax Tablets & DF Syrup 1954
- Vistaril Intramuscular Solution 1970

Ibuprofen (Possibility of acute renal failure). Products include:
- Advil Cold & Sinus Caplets (formerly CoAdvil) 2416
- Advil Ibuprofen Tablets and Caplets 2416
- Children's Advil Suspension 2426
- CoAdvil .... ▣ 748
- Dristan Sinus Caplets 2419
- Haltran Tablets .... ▣ 668
- Ibuprofen .... ▣ 631
- Medipren ibuprofen Caplets and Tablets 1362
- Midol 200 Cramp Relief Formula .. ▣ 570
- Motrin Tablets 2351
- Motrin IB Caplets and Tablets .... ▣ 736
- Nuprin Ibuprofen/Analgesic Tablets & Caplets 752
- PediaProfen Suspension 1363
- Rufen Tablets 691
- Trendar Ibuprofen Tablets .... ▣ 756

Indapamide (Potentiated). Products include:
- Lozol Tablets 1843

Indomethacin (Possibility of acute renal failure). Products include:
- Indocin 1487

Indomethacin Sodium Trihydrate (Possibility of acute renal failure). Products include:
- Indocin I.V. 1490

Isoflurane (Potentiated). Products include:
- Forane 600

Isradipine (Increased risk of hyperkalemia). Products include:
- DynaCirc Capsules 2004

Ketamine Hydrochloride (Potentiated). Products include:
- Ketalar 1726

Ketoprofen (Possibility of acute renal failure). Products include:
- Orudis Capsules 2488

Ketorolac Tromethamine (Possibility of acute renal failure). Products include:
- Toradol IM Injection 2302

Labetalol Hydrochloride (Potentiated). Products include:
- Normodyne Injection 2108
- Normodyne Tablets 2110
- Normozide Tablets 2112
- Trandate HCT Tablets 579
- Trandate Injection 577
- Trandate Tablets 579

Lisinopril (Increased risk of hyperkalemia). Products include:
- Prinivil Tablets 1538
- Prinzide Tablets 1540
- Zestoretic 2274
- Zestril Tablets 2277

Lithium Carbonate (Reduced renal clearance of lithium; increased risk of lithium toxicity). Products include:
- Eskalith 2214
- Lithane Tablets 1596
- Lithium Carbonate Capsules & Tablets 1984
- Lithobid Tablets 870

Lithium Citrate (Reduced renal clearance of lithium; increased risk of lithium toxicity). Products include:
- Cibalith-S 870

Lorazepam (Potentiated). Products include:
- Ativan Injection 2432
- Ativan Tablets 2434

Mecamylamine Hydrochloride (Potentiated). Products include:
- Inversine Tablets 1492

Meclofenamate Sodium (Possibility of acute renal failure). Products include:
- Meclomen Capsules 1739

Mefenamic Acid (Possibility of acute renal failure). Products include:
- Ponstel 1758

Meperidine Hydrochloride (Potentiated). Products include:
- Demerol 2047
- Mepergan Injection 2479

Methohexital Sodium (Potentiated). Products include:
- Brevital Sodium Vials 1248

Methoxyflurane (Potentiated).
- No products indexed under this heading.

Methyclothiazide (Potentiated). Products include:
- Enduron Tablets 517
- Enduronyl 518

Methyldopa (Potentiated). Products include:
- Aldoclor Tablets 1413
- Aldomet Oral 1415
- Aldoril Tablets 1418

Methyldopate Hydrochloride (Potentiated). Products include:
- Aldomet Ester HCl Injection 1417

Metocurine Iodide (Potentiated). Products include:
- Metubine Iodide Vials 1285

Metolazone (Potentiated). Products include:
- Diulo 2129
- Mykrox ½ mg Tablets 984
- Zaroxolyn Tablets 989

Metoprolol Tartrate (Potentiated). Products include:
- Lopressor Ampuls 1032
- Lopressor HCT Tablets 1034
- Lopressor Tablets 1032

Metyrosine (Potentiated). Products include:
- Demser Capsules 1460

Minoxidil (Potentiated). Products include:
- Loniten Tablets 2346
- Rogaine Topical Solution 2357

Morphine Sulfate (Potentiated). Products include:
- Astramorph/PF Injection, USP (Preservative-Free) 618
- Duramorph 960
- Infumorph 200 and Infumorph 500 Sterile Solutions 962
- MS Contin Tablets 1814
- MSIR 1817
- Oramorph SR (Morphine Sulfate Sustained Release Tablets) 1988
- Roxanol 1991

Nadolol (Potentiated). Products include:
Corgard Tablets ... 701
Corzide Tablets ... 702

Naproxen (Possibility of acute renal failure). Products include:
Naprosyn ... 2297

Naproxen Sodium (Possibility of acute renal failure). Products include:
Anaprox and Anaprox DS Tablets ... 2288

Nicardipine Hydrochloride (Potentiated). Products include:
Cardene Capsules ... 2290

Nitroglycerin (Potentiated). Products include:
Deponit NTG Transdermal Delivery System ... 2143
Minitran Transdermal Delivery System ... 1312
Nitro-Bid Ointment ... 1339
Nitro-Bid Capsules ... 1338
Nitrodisc ... 2176
Nitro-Dur (nitroglycerin) Transdermal Infusion System ... 1164
Nitrogard Tablets ... 1004
Nitrolingual Spray ... 1846
Nitrostat Tablets ... 1743
Transderm-Nitro Transdermal Therapeutic System ... 2283

Opium Alkaloids (Potentiated). Products include:
B & O No. 15A & No. 16A Supprettes ... 2395
Pantopon Injectable ... 1911

Pancuronium Bromide Injection (Potentiated).
No products indexed under this heading.

Penbutolol Sulfate (Potentiated). Products include:
Levatol ... 1832

Penicillin G Potassium (Hyperkalemia). Products include:
Pfizerpen for Injection ... 1957

Pentobarbital Sodium (Potentiated). Products include:
Nembutal Sodium Capsules ... 534
Nembutal Sodium Solution ... 536
Nembutal Sodium Suppositories ... 538

Phenoxybenzamine Hydrochloride (Potentiated). Products include:
Dibenzyline Capsules ... 2207

Phentolamine Mesylate (Potentiated). Products include:
Regitine ... 878

Phenylbutazone (Possibility of acute renal failure). Products include:
Butazolidin Capsules & Tablets ... 1027

Pindolol (Potentiated). Products include:
Visken Tablets ... 2036

Piroxicam (Possibility of acute renal failure). Products include:
Feldene Capsules ... 1777

Polythiazide (Potentiated). Products include:
Minizide Capsules ... 1779
Renese Tablets ... 1785
Renese-R Tablets ... 1786

Potassium Acid Phosphate (Contraindicated). Products include:
K-Phos M.F. Tablets ... 659
K-Phos Original Formula 'Sodium Free' Tablets ... 660
K-Phos No. 2 Tablets ... 659

Potassium Bicarbonate (Contraindicated). Products include:
Alka-Seltzer Advanced Formula Antacid & Non-Aspirin Pain Reliever ... ◘ 620
Alka-Seltzer Effervescent Antacid ◘ 622
K-Lyte ... 707
Klorvess Effervescent Granules ... 2010
Klorvess Effervescent Tablets ... 2011

Potassium Chloride (Contraindicated). Products include:
Chlor-3 Condiment ... 994
K-Dur Microburst Release System (potassium chloride, USP) E.R. Tablets ... 1163
K-Lor Powder Packets ... 531
K-Lyte ... 707
K-Norm Capsules ... 982
K-Tab Filmtab ... 532
Kato Potassium Supplement ... 1114
Klor-Con 8/Klor-Con 10 Extended-release Tablets ... 2374
Klorvess Effervescent Granules ... 2010
Klorvess Effervescent Tablets ... 2011
Klorvess 10% Liquid ... 2010
Klotrix ... 708
Kolyum Liquid ... 983
Micro-K ... 1863
Micro-K LS Packets ... 1864
NuLYTELY ... 699
Oral Rehydration Salts, Citrate ... 1150
Rum-K Syrup ... 995
Slow-K Tablets ... 2281
Ten-K Controlled-Release Tablets ... 2282
Thermotabs ... ◘ 619

Potassium Citrate (Contraindicated). Products include:
Alka-Seltzer Effervescent Antacid .. 1570
K-Lyte ... 707
Polycitra Syrup ... 2424
Polycitra-K ... 2424
Polycitra-LC—Sugar-Free ... 2424
Ricelyte, Rice-Based Oral Electrolyte Maintenance Solution ... ◘ 613

Potassium Gluconate (Contraindicated). Products include:
Kolyum Liquid ... 983

Potassium Phosphate, Dibasic (Contraindicated). Products include:
Neutra-Phos ... 2423

Potassium Phosphate, Monobasic (Contraindicated). Products include:
K-Phos M.F. Tablets ... 659
K-Phos Neutral Tablets ... 660
Neutra-Phos ... 2423

Prazosin Hydrochloride (Potentiated). Products include:
Minipress Capsules ... 1778
Minizide Capsules ... 1779

Promethazine (Potentiated).

Promethazine Hydrochloride (Potentiated). Products include:
Mepergan Injection ... 2479
Phenergan with Codeine ... 2497
Phenergan with Dextromethorphan 2499
Phenergan Injection ... 2493
Phenergan Suppositories ... 2496
Phenergan Syrup ... 2495
Phenergan Tablets ... 2496
Phenergan VC ... 2500
Phenergan VC with Codeine ... 2501

Propofol (Potentiated). Products include:
Diprivan Injection ... 2267

Propranolol Hydrochloride (Potentiated). Products include:
Inderal ... 2459
Inderal LA Long Acting Capsules ... 2461
Inderide Tablets ... 2463
Inderide LA Long Acting Capsules .. 2465

Ramipril (Increased risk of hyperkalemia). Products include:
Altace Capsules ... 1086

Rauwolfia Serpentina (Potentiated). Products include:
Raudixin Tablets ... 1803
Rauzide Tablets ... 1804

Rescinnamine (Potentiated).
No products indexed under this heading.

Reserpine (Potentiated). Products include:
Diupres Tablets ... 1461
Hydromox R Tablets ... 1209
Hydropres Tablets ... 1485
Renese-R Tablets ... 1786
Salutensin/Salutensin-Demi ... 719
Ser-Ap-Es Tablets ... 881
Serpasil Tablets ... 883
Serpasil-Apresoline Tablets ... 884
Serpasil-Esidrix Tablets ... 886

Secobarbital Sodium (Potentiated). Products include:
Seconal Sodium Pulvules ... 1296

Sodium Nitroprusside (Potentiated). Products include:
Nipride I.V. Infusion ... 1909

Spironolactone (Contraindicated). Products include:
Aldactazide ... 2150
Aldactone ... 2152

Sulindac (Possibility of acute renal failure). Products include:
Clinoril Tablets ... 1433

Terazosin Hydrochloride (Potentiated). Products include:
Hytrin Tablets ... 529

Timolol Maleate (Potentiated). Products include:
Blocadren Tablets ... 1429
Timolide Tablets ... 1547
Timoptic in Ocudose ... 1552
Timoptic Sterile Ophthalmic Solution ... 1550

Tolazamide (Dosage adjustments of hypoglycemics may be necessary). Products include:
Tolinase Tablets ... 2365

Tolbutamide (Dosage adjustments of hypoglycemics may be necessary). Products include:
Orinase Tablets ... 2354

Tolmetin Sodium (Possibility of acute renal failure). Products include:
Tolectin (200, 400 and 600 mg) .. 1379

Trimethaphan Camsylate (Potentiated). Products include:
Arfonad Ampuls ... 1887

Vecuronium Bromide (Potentiated). Products include:
Norcuron ... 1642

E.E.S. 400 FILMTAB
(Erythromycin Ethylsuccinate) ... 522
May interact with xanthine bronchodilators, oral anticoagulants, and certain other agents. Compounds in these categories include:

Aminophylline (Concomitant administration with high doses of theophylline may be associated with increased theophylline levels and potential toxicity). Products include:
Amesec ... ◘ 682
Aminophyllin Tablets ... 2153

Carbamazepine (Elevations in serum erythromycin and carbamazepine concentration). Products include:
Tegretol Chewable Tablets ... 654
Tegretol Suspension ... 656
Tegretol Tablets ... 654

Cyclosporine (Elevations in serum erythromycin and cyclosporine concentration). Products include:
Sandimmune ... 2024

Dicumarol (Increased anticoagulant effects). Products include:
Dicumarol Tablets ... 516

Digoxin (Elevated digoxin serum levels). Products include:
Lanoxicaps ... 772
Lanoxin Elixir Pediatric ... 775
Lanoxin Injection ... 778
Lanoxin Injection Pediatric ... 781
Lanoxin Tablets ... 783

Dihydroergotamine Mesylate (Potential for acute ergot toxicity characterized by severe peripheral vasospasm and dysesthesia). Products include:
D.H.E. 45 Injection ... 2003

Dyphylline (Concomitant administration with high doses of theophylline may be associated with increased theophylline levels and potential toxicity). Products include:
Dilor ... 2079
Dilor-G Tablets & Liquid ... 2079
Lufyllin Elixir ... 2384
Lufyllin & Lufyllin-400 Tablets ... 2384
Lufyllin-GG Elixir & Tablets ... 2385

Ergotamine Tartrate (Potential for acute ergot toxicity characterized by severe peripheral vasospasm and dysesthesia). Products include:
Bellergal-S Tablets ... 1998
Cafergot/Cafergot P-B ... 1999
Ergostat ... 1719
Medihaler Ergotamine Aerosol ... 1312
Wigraine Tablets & Suppositories .. 1645

Hexobarbital (Elevations in serum erythromycin and hexobarbital concentration).

Lovastatin (Potential for rhabdomyolysis in seriously ill patients). Products include:
Mevacor Tablets ... 1505

Phenytoin (Elevations in serum erythromycin and phenytoin concentration). Products include:
Dilantin Infatabs ... 1710
Dilantin-30 Pediatric/Dilantin-125 Suspension ... 1713

Phenytoin Sodium (Elevations in serum erythromycin and phenytoin concentration). Products include:
Dilantin Kapseals ... 1708
Dilantin Parenteral ... 1712
Dilantin with Phenobarbital Kapseals ... 1715

Terfenadine (Potential for altered terfenadine metabolism). Products include:
Seldane Tablets ... 1349
Seldane-D Extended-Release Tablets ... 1350

Theophylline (Concomitant administration with high doses of theophylline may be associated with increased theophylline levels and potential toxicity). Products include:
Bronkaid Tablets ... ◘ 757
Bronkolixir ... ◘ 761
Bronkotabs Tablets ... ◘ 762
Constant-T Tablets ... 1029
Marax Tablets & DF Syrup ... 1954
Primatene Tablets ... 2421
Quibron Capsules ... 713
Quibron-T ... 714
Quibron-T/SR ... 716
Theolair Liquid ... 1317
Theo-Organidin Elixir ... 2391

Theophylline Anhydrous (Concomitant administration with high doses of theophylline may be associated with increased theophylline levels and potential toxicity). Products include:
Aerolate ... 994
Primatene Tablets-M Formula ... ◘ 753
Primatene Tablets-Regular Formula ... 2421
Respbid Tablets ... 684
Slo-bid Gyrocaps ... 1847
T-PHYL (Uniphyl) 200 mg Tablets 1820
Tedral SA ... 1765
Theo-24 ... 2179
Theo-Dur Sprinkle ... 1168
Theo-Dur Extended-Release Tablets ... 1166
Theolair Tablets ... 1317
Theolair-SR Tablets ... 1319
TheoX Extended-Release Tablets ... 841
Uniphyl 400 mg Tablets ... 1823

Theophylline Calcium Salicylate (Concomitant administration with high doses of theophylline may be associated with increased theophylline levels and potential toxicity). Products include:
Quadrinal Tablets ... 1183

Theophylline Sodium Glycinate (Concomitant administration with high doses of theophylline may be associated with increased theophylline levels and potential toxicity). Products include:
Asbron G ... 1997

Triazolam (Decreased clearance of triazolam and increased the pharmacologic effect of triazolam). Products include:
Halcion Tablets ... 2340

Warfarin Sodium (Increased anticoagulant effects). Products include:
Coumadin Injection & Tablets ... 944
Panwarfin Tablets ... 547

E.E.S. GRANULES
(Erythromycin Ethylsuccinate) ... 522
See **E.E.S. 400 Filmtab**

E.E.S. 200 LIQUID
(Erythromycin Ethylsuccinate) ... 522
See **E.E.S. 400 Filmtab**

E.E.S. 400 LIQUID
(Erythromycin Ethylsuccinate) ... 522
See **E.E.S. 400 Filmtab**

E-MYCIN TABLETS
(Erythromycin) ... 688
May interact with xanthine bronchodilators and certain other agents. Compounds in these categories include:

Aminophylline (Potential theophylline toxicity). Products include:
Amesec ... ■ 682
Aminophyllin Tablets ... 2153

Carbamazepine (Increased blood levels of carbamazepine). Products include:
Tegretol Chewable Tablets ... 654
Tegretol Suspension ... 656
Tegretol Tablets ... 654

Cyclosporine (Increased cyclosporine blood levels). Products include:
Sandimmune ... 2024

Dihydroergotamine Mesylate (Increased vasospasm). Products include:
D.H.E. 45 Injection ... 2003

Dyphylline (Potential theophylline toxicity). Products include:
Dilor ... 2079
Dilor-G Tablets & Liquid ... 2079
Lufyllin Elixir ... 2384
Lufyllin & Lufyllin-400 Tablets ... 2384
Lufyllin-GG Elixir & Tablets ... 2385

Ergotamine Tartrate (Increased vasospasm). Products include:
Bellergal-S Tablets ... 1998
Cafergot/Cafergot P-B ... 1999
Ergostat ... 1719
Medihaler Ergotamine Aerosol ... 1312
Wigraine Tablets & Suppositories ... 1645

Theophylline (Potential theophylline toxicity). Products include:
Bronkaid Tablets ... ■ 757
Bronkolixir ... ■ 761
Bronkotabs Tablets ... ■ 762
Constant-T Tablets ... 1029
Marax Tablets & DF Syrup ... 1954
Primatene Tablets ... 2421
Quibron Capsules ... 713
Quibron-T ... 714
Quibron-T/SR ... 716
Theolair Liquid ... 1317
Theo-Organidin Elixir ... 2391

Theophylline Anhydrous (Potential theophylline toxicity). Products include:
Aerolate ... 994
Primatene Tablets-M Formula ... ■ 753
Primatene Tablets-Regular Formula ... 2421
Respbid Tablets ... 684
Slo-bid Gyrocaps ... 1847
T-PHYL (Uniphyl) 200 mg Tablets ... 1820
Tedral SA ... 1765
Theo-24 ... 2179
Theo-Dur Sprinkle ... 1168
Theo-Dur Extended-Release Tablets ... 1166
Theolair Tablets ... 1317
Theolair-SR Tablets ... 1319
TheoX Extended-Release Tablets ... 841
Uniphyl 400 mg Tablets ... 1823

Theophylline Calcium Salicylate (Potential theophylline toxicity). Products include:
Quadrinal Tablets ... 1183

Theophylline Sodium Glycinate (Potential theophylline toxicity). Products include:
Asbron G ... 1997

Triazolam (Decreased triazolam clearance; pharmacologic effect of triazolam may be increased). Products include:
Halcion Tablets ... 2340

Warfarin Sodium (Decreased warfarin clearance; hypoprothrombinemic effect potentiated). Products include:
Coumadin Injection & Tablets ... 944
Panwarfin Tablets ... 547

E.P.T. EARLY PREGNANCY TEST
(HCG Monoclonal Antibody) ... ■ 774
No interactions described in labeling.

ETS-2%
(Erythromycin) ... 1685
May interact with:

Concomitant Topical Acne Therapy (Irritation).

EASPRIN
(Aspirin, Enteric Coated) ... 1719
May interact with anticoagulants, oral hypoglycemic agents, antigout agents, corticosteroids, insulin, urinary alkalizing agents, antacids, pyrazolon derivatives, and certain other agents. Compounds in these categories include:

Alcohol (Synergism; gastrointestinal bleeding).

Aluminum Carbonate Gel (Increases stomach pH; affects enteric coating of tablets). Products include:
Basaljel ... 2438

Aluminum Hydroxide (Increases stomach pH; affects enteric coating of tablets). Products include:
Cama Arthritis Pain Reliever ... ■ 685
Gaviscon Extra Strength Relief Formula Liquid Antacid ... ■ 594
Gaviscon Extra Strength Relief Formula Antacid Tablets ... ■ 594
Gaviscon Liquid Antacid ... ■ 594
Gelusil Liquid & Tablets ... ■ 639
Extra Strength Maalox Plus Suspension ... 1850
Maalox TC Suspension ... 1851
Maalox Plus Tablets ... ■ 655
Extra Strength Maalox Plus Tablets 1850
Nephrox Suspension ... ■ 563
WinGel Liquid & Tablets ... ■ 761

Aluminum Hydroxide Gel (Increases stomach pH; affects enteric coating of tablets). Products include:
ALternaGEL Liquid ... 1154
Aludrox Oral Suspension ... 2428
Amphojel Suspension ... 2429
Amphojel Suspension without Flavor ... 2429
Mylanta Liquid ... 1155
Mylanta Double Strength Liquid ... 1155

Aluminum Hydroxide Gel, Dried (Increases stomach pH; affects enteric coating of tablets). Products include:
Alu-Tab/Alu-Cap ... 1309
Amphojel Tablets ... 2429
Ascriptin A/D Caplets ... 1850
Regular Strength Ascriptin Tablets 1850
Gaviscon Antacid Tablets ... ■ 593
Gaviscon-2 Antacid Tablets ... ■ 594
Mylanta Tablets ... 1155
Mylanta Double Strength Tablets ... 1155

Antipyrine (Increased risk of gastrointestinal ulceration). Products include:
Auralgan Otic Solution ... 2437

Betamethasone Acetate (Increased risk of gastrointestinal ulceration; may reduce serum salicylate levels). Products include:
Celestone Soluspan Suspension ... 2081

Betamethasone Sodium Phosphate (Increased risk of gastrointestinal ulceration; may reduce serum salicylate levels). Products include:
Celestone Soluspan Suspension ... 2081

Chlorpropamide (Enhanced effect of hypoglycemics). Products include:
Diabinese Tablets ... 1775

Cortisone Acetate (Increased risk of gastrointestinal ulceration; may reduce serum salicylate levels). Products include:
Cortone Acetate Sterile Suspension ... 1437
Cortone Acetate Tablets ... 1439

Dexamethasone (Increased risk of gastrointestinal ulceration; may reduce serum salicylate levels). Products include:
AK-Trol Ointment & Suspension ... ◉ 207
Decadron Elixir ... 1445
Decadron Tablets ... 1447
Decaspray Topical Aerosol ... 1459
Dexacidin ... ◉ 272
Maxidex Sterile Ophthalmic Suspension ... ◉ 223
Maxitrol Ophthalmic Ointment/Suspension ... ◉ 223
TobraDex Ophthalmic Suspension and Ointment ... ◉ 228

Dexamethasone Acetate (Increased risk of gastrointestinal ulceration; may reduce serum salicylate levels). Products include:
Dalalone D.P. Injectable ... 999
Decadron-LA Sterile Suspension ... 1457

Dexamethasone Sodium Phosphate (Increased risk of gastrointestinal ulceration; may reduce serum salicylate levels). Products include:
AK-Dex ... ◉ 203
Decadron Phosphate Respihaler ... 1454
Decadron Phosphate Sterile Ophthalmic Ointment ... 1453
Decadron Phosphate Sterile Ophthalmic Solution ... 1453
Decadron Phosphate Topical Cream ... 1455
Decadron Phosphate Turbinaire ... 1456
Maxidex Sterile Ophthalmic Ointment ... ◉ 222
NeoDecadron Sterile Ophthalmic Ointment ... 1517
NeoDecadron Sterile Ophthalmic Solution ... 1518
NeoDecadron Topical Cream ... 1518

Dicumarol (Increased bleeding time). Products include:
Dicumarol Tablets ... 516

Dihydroxyaluminum Sodium Carbonate (Increases stomach pH; affects enteric coating of tablets). Products include:
Rolaids ... ■ 743

Dipyrone (Possible increase in gastrointestinal ulceration).

Glipizide (Enhanced effect of hypoglycemics). Products include:
Glucotrol ... 1952

Glyburide (Enhanced effect of hypoglycemics). Products include:
DiaBeta ... 1091
Micronase Tablets ... 2350

Heparin Calcium (Increased bleeding time). Products include:
Calciparine Injection ... 925

Heparin Sodium (Increased bleeding time). Products include:
Heparin Lock Flush Solution ... 2456
Heparin Sodium Vials ... 1264
Heparin Sodium Injection ... 2457
Heparin Sodium Injection, USP, Sterile Solution ... 2342

Hydrocortisone (Increased risk of gastrointestinal ulceration; may reduce serum salicylate levels). Products include:
AK-Spore H.C. ... ◉ 206
Bactine Hydrocortisone Anti-Itch Cream ... ■ 625
CaldeCORT Anti-Itch Hydrocortisone Spray ... ■ 560
Carmol HC Cream 1% ... 2296
Cortaid Spray ... ■ 735
Cortenema ... 2244
Cortisporin Ointment ... 758
Cortisporin Ophthalmic Ointment Sterile ... 758
Cortisporin Ophthalmic Suspension Sterile ... 759
Cortisporin Otic Solution Sterile ... 760
Cortisporin Otic Suspension Sterile 760
Cortizone-5 Creme & Ointment ... ■ 732
Dermolate Anti-Itch Cream ... ■ 697
Eldecort Cream 1.0% ... 1113
Eldecort Cream 1.0% and 2.5% ... 1113
Fungoid HC Creme ... 1770
Hydrocortone Tablets ... 1482
Hytone ... 909
LazerSporin-C Solution ... 1770
Massengill Medicated Soft Cloth Towelettes ... 2192
Nutracort Cream & Lotion ... 1684
PediOtic Suspension Sterile ... 797
Synacort Creams 1%, 2.5% ... 2296
Vanoxide-HC Acne Lotion ... 911
Vioform-Hydrocortisone Cream and Mild Cream ... 889
Vioform-Hydrocortisone Ointment ... 889
VōSoL HC Otic Solution ... 2392
Vytone Cream 1% ... 911

Hydrocortisone Acetate (Increased risk of gastrointestinal ulceration; may reduce serum salicylate levels). Products include:
Analpram-HC Rectal Cream 1% and 2.5% ... 970
Anusol-HC Cream ... 1690
Anusol-HC Suppositories ... 1691
Caldecort ... ■ 560
Carmol HC Cream 1% ... 2296
Chloromycetin Hydrocortisone Ophthalmic ... 1694
Coly-Mycin S Otic w/Neomycin & Hydrocortisone ... 1708
Cortaid ... ■ 735
Cortef Feminine Itch Cream ... ■ 735
Corticaine ... ■ 682
Cortifoam ... 1827
Cortisporin Cream ... 757
Epifoam ... 1828
Gynecort 5 Creme ... ■ 556
Hydrocortone Acetate Sterile Suspension ... 1479
Lanacort 5 Creme and Ointment ... ■ 557
Mantadil Cream ... 789
Ophthocort ... ◉ 301
Orabase HCA Oral Paste ... 890
Pramosone Cream, Lotion & Ointment ... 971
ProctoCream-HC ... 1834
Proctofoam-HC ... 1835

Hydrocortisone Sodium Phosphate (Increased risk of gastrointestinal ulceration; may reduce serum salicylate levels). Products include:
Hydrocortone Phosphate Injection, Sterile ... 1481

Hydrocortisone Sodium Succinate (Increased risk of gastrointestinal ulceration; may reduce serum salicylate levels). Products include:
Solu-Cortef Sterile Powder ... 2361

Hydrocortisone Valerate (Increased risk of gastrointestinal ulceration). Products include:
Westcort ... 2411

Insulin, Human (Altered insulin requirements).
No products indexed under this heading.

Insulin, Human Isophane Suspension (Altered insulin requirements). Products include:
Humulin N, 100 Units ... 1270

Insulin, Human NPH (Altered insulin requirements). Products include:
Insulatard NPH Human 1627
Novolin N 1627
Novolin N PenFill Cartridges 1628
Novolin N Prefilled 1628
Insulin, Human Regular (Altered insulin requirements). Products include:
Humulin BR, 100 Units 1268
Humulin R, 100 Units 1272
Novolin R 1627
Novolin R PenFill Cartridges 1628
Novolin R Prefilled 1629
Velosulin Human 1628
Insulin, Human, Zinc Suspension (Altered insulin requirements). Products include:
Humulin L, 100 Units 1268
Humulin U, 100 Units 1272
Novolin L 1627
Insulin, NPH (Altered insulin requirements). Products include:
NPH, 40 & 100 Units 1273
Beef NPH, 100 Units 1274
Pork NPH, 100 Units 1275
Insulatard NPH 1626
NPH Insulin 1626
NPH Purified Pork Isophane Insulin 1626
Insulin, Regular (Altered insulin requirements). Products include:
Regular, 40 & 100 Units 1273
Beef Regular, 100 Units 1275
Pork Regular, 100 Units 1275
Pork Regular (Concentrated), 500 Units 1276
Regular Insulin 1625
Regular Purified Pork Insulin 1626
Velosulin 1627
Insulin, Zinc Crystals (Altered insulin requirements). Products include:
NPH, 40 & 100 Units 1273
Insulin, Zinc Suspension (Altered insulin requirements). Products include:
Lente, 40 & 100 Units 1272
Protamine, Zinc, 40 & 100 Units 1273
Lente Iletin I 1272
Beef Lente, 100 Units 1274
Beef Protamine Zinc, 100 Units 1274
Pork Lente, 100 Units 1275
Pork, Protamine, Zinc, 100 Units 1275
Lente Insulin 1626
Lente Purified Pork Insulin 1626
Semilente Insulin 1625
Ultralente Insulin 1626
Magaldrate (Increases stomach pH; affects enteric coating of tablets). Products include:
Riopan Antacid Chew Tablets ▣ 754
Riopan Antacid Chew Tablets in Rollpacks ▣ 754
Riopan Antacid Suspension 2421
Riopan Antacid Swallow Tablets 2421
Riopan Plus Chew Tablets 2422
Riopan Plus Chew Tablets in Rollpack 2422
Riopan Plus 2 Chew Tablets, Mint Flavor, Cherry Flavor 2422
Riopan Plus Suspension 2422
Riopan Plus 2 Suspension, Mint Flavor, Cherry Flavor 2422
Magnesium Hydroxide (Increases stomach pH; affects enteric coating of tablets). Products include:
Aludrox Oral Suspension 2428
Ascriptin A/D Caplets 1850
Regular Strength Ascriptin Tablets 1850
Di-Gel Antacid/Anti-Gas ▣ 697
Gelusil Liquid & Tablets ▣ 639
Haley's M-O, Regular & Flavored ▣ 569
Extra Strength Maalox Plus Suspension 1850
Maalox TC Suspension 1851
Maalox Plus Tablets ▣ 655
Extra Strength Maalox Plus Tablets 1850
Mylanta Liquid 1155
Mylanta Tablets 1155
Mylanta Double Strength Liquid 1155
Mylanta Double Strength Tablets 1155
Concentrated Phillips' Milk of Magnesia ▣ 573
Phillips' Milk of Magnesia Liquid ▣ 572
Phillips' Milk of Magnesia Tablets ▣ 573
WinGel Liquid & Tablets ▣ 761
Magnesium Oxide (Increases stomach pH; affects enteric coating of tablets). Products include:
Bayer Plus Aspirin Tablets ▣ 567
Beelith Tablets 659
Bufferin Analgesic Tablets and Caplets ▣ 524
Cama Arthritis Pain Reliever ▣ 685
Mag-Ox 400 673
Uro-Mag 673
Methylprednisolone (Increased risk of gastrointestinal ulceration). Products include:
Medrol 2348
Methylprednisolone Acetate (Increased risk of gastrointestinal ulceration; may reduce serum salicylate levels). Products include:
Depo-Medrol Sterile Aqueous Suspension 2334
Methylprednisolone Sodium Succinate (Increased risk of gastrointestinal ulceration; may reduce serum salicylate levels). Products include:
Solu-Medrol Sterile Powder 2363
Oxyphenbutazone (Increased risk of gastrointestinal ulceration).
Phenobarbital (Decreases aspirin effectiveness). Products include:
Arco-Lase Plus Tablets 607
Bellergal-S Tablets 1998
Bronkolixir ▣ 761
Bronkotabs Tablets ▣ 762
Donnatal 1858
Donnatal Extentabs 1859
Donnatal Tablets 1858
Donnazyme Tablets 1860
Kinesed Tablets 2272
Phenobarbital Elixir and Tablets 1293
Primatene Tablets-P Formula 2421
Quadrinal Tablets 1183
Tedral SA 1765
Phenylbutazone (Decreased effects of phenylbutazone; increased risk of gastrointestinal ulceration). Products include:
Butazolidin Capsules & Tablets 1027
Phenytoin (Increased serum phenytoin levels). Products include:
Dilantin Infatabs 1710
Dilantin-30 Pediatric/Dilantin-125 Suspension 1713
Phenytoin Sodium (Increased phenytoin levels). Products include:
Dilantin Kapseals 1708
Dilantin Parenteral 1712
Dilantin with Phenobarbital Kapseals 1715
Potassium Citrate (Decreases aspirin effectiveness). Products include:
Alka-Seltzer Effervescent Antacid 1570
K-Lyte 707
Polycitra Syrup 2424
Polycitra-K 2424
Polycitra-LC—Sugar-Free 2424
Ricelyte, Rice-Based Oral Electrolyte Maintenance Solution ▣ 613
Prednisolone Acetate (Increased risk of gastrointestinal ulceration; may reduce serum salicylate levels). Products include:
AK-Cide Sterile Ophthalmic Ointment & Suspension ⊚ 202
Blephamide Liquifilm Sterile Ophthalmic Suspension 586
Blephamide S.O.P. Sterile Ophthalmic Ointment 586
Cetapred Ointment ⊚ 220
⅛% Econopred & 1% Econopred Plus ⊚ 217
Isopto Cetapred Suspension ⊚ 220
Metimyd ⊚ 306
Poly-Pred Liquifilm ⊚ 250
Pred Forte ⊚ 252
Pred Mild ⊚ 254
Pred-G Liquifilm Sterile Ophthalmic Suspension ⊚ 252
Pred-G S.O.P. Sterile Ophthalmic Ointment ⊚ 253
Vasocidin Ointment ⊚ 275
Prednisolone Sodium Phosphate (Increased risk of gastrointestinal ulceration; may reduce serum salicylate levels). Products include:
AK-Pred ⊚ 205
Hydeltrasol Injection, Sterile 1476
Inflamase ⊚ 274
Pediapred Oral Liquid 987
Vasocidin Ophthalmic Solution ⊚ 276
Prednisolone Tebutate (Increased risk of gastrointestinal ulceration; may reduce serum salicylate levels). Products include:
Hydeltra-T.B.A. Sterile Suspension 1478
Prednisone (Increased risk of gastrointestinal ulceration; may reduce serum salicylate levels). Products include:
Deltasone Tablets 2332
Probenecid (Decreased effects of probenecid). Products include:
Benemid Tablets 1426
ColBENEMID Tablets 1436
Wycillin Injection and Probenecid Tablets 2539
Propranolol Hydrochloride (Decreases antiinflammatory action of aspirin). Products include:
Inderal 2459
Inderal LA Long Acting Capsules 2461
Inderide Tablets 2463
Inderide LA Long Acting Capsules 2465
Sodium Bicarbonate (Increases stomach pH affects enteric coating of tablets). Products include:
Alka-Seltzer Advanced Formula Antacid & Non-Aspirin Pain Reliever ▣ 620
Alka-Seltzer Effervescent Antacid ▣ 622
Alka-Seltzer Effervescent Antacid and Pain Reliever 1568
Alka-Seltzer Extra Strength Effervescent Antacid and Pain Reliever ▣ 623
Alka-Seltzer (Flavored) Effervescent Antacid and Pain Reliever ▣ 621
Arm & Hammer Pure Baking Soda ▣ 548
Ceo-Two Rectal Suppositories 671
Citrocarbonate Antacid ▣ 668
Massengill Liquid Concentrate 2191
NuLYTELY 699
Sodium Citrate (Decreases aspirin effectiveness). Products include:
Alka-Seltzer Effervescent Antacid 1570
Alka-Seltzer Extra Strength Effervescent Antacid and Pain Reliever 1570
Alka-Seltzer (Flavored) Effervescent Antacid and Pain Reliever 1569
Bicitra—Sugar-Free 2423
Citrocarbonate Antacid ▣ 668
Polycitra 2424
Ricelyte, Rice-Based Oral Electrolyte Maintenance Solution ▣ 613
Spironolactone (Decreased sodium excretion). Products include:
Aldactazide 2150
Aldactone 2152
Sulfinpyrazone (Decreased effects of sulfinpyrazone). Products include:
Anturane 853
Tolazamide (Enhanced effect of hypoglycemics). Products include:
Tolinase Tablets 2365
Tolbutamide (Enhanced effect of hypoglycemics). Products include:
Orinase Tablets 2354
Triamcinolone (Increased risk of gastrointestinal ulceration; may reduce serum salicylate levels).
No products indexed under this heading.
Triamcinolone Acetonide (Increased risk of gastrointestinal ulceration; may reduce serum salicylate levels). Products include:
Aristocort A 1010
Azmacort Inhaler 1837
Kenalog Cream, Lotion & Ointment 2401
Kenalog-10 Injection 2402
Kenalog-40 Injection 2403
Kenalog in Orabase 604
Kenalog Spray 2401
Mycolog II Cream and Ointment 2407
Mytrex Cream & Ointment 2080
Nasacort Nasal Inhaler 1844
Triamcinolone Diacetate (Increased risk of gastrointestinal ulceration; may reduce serum salicylate levels). Products include:
Aristocort Suspension 1008
Triamcinolone Hexacetonide (Increased risk of gastrointestinal ulceration; may reduce serum salicylate levels). Products include:
Aristospan Suspension 1011
Warfarin Sodium (Increased bleeding time). Products include:
Coumadin Injection & Tablets 944
Panwarfin Tablets 547

⅛% ECONOPRED & 1% ECONOPRED PLUS
(Prednisolone Acetate) ⊚ 217
No interactions described in labeling.

ECOTRIN ENTERIC COATED ASPIRIN MAXIMUM STRENGTH TABLETS AND CAPLETS
(Aspirin, Enteric Coated) 2189
May interact with antacids containing aluminum, calcium and magnesium and certain other agents. Compounds in these categories include:

Aluminum Carbonate Gel (Concurrent administration of nonabsorbable antacids may alter the rate of absorption of aspirin). Products include:
Basaljel 2438
Aluminum Hydroxide (Concurrent administration of nonabsorbable antacids may alter the rate of absorption of aspirin). Products include:
Cama Arthritis Pain Reliever ▣ 685
Gaviscon Extra Strength Relief Formula Liquid Antacid ▣ 594
Gaviscon Extra Strength Relief Formula Antacid Tablets ▣ 594
Gaviscon Liquid Antacid ▣ 594
Gelusil Liquid & Tablets ▣ 639
Extra Strength Maalox Plus Suspension 1850
Maalox TC Suspension 1851
Maalox Plus Tablets ▣ 655
Extra Strength Maalox Plus Tablets 1850
Nephrox Suspension ▣ 563
WinGel Liquid & Tablets ▣ 761
Aluminum Hydroxide Gel (Concurrent administration of nonabsorbable antacids may alter the rate of absorption of aspirin). Products include:
ALternaGEL Liquid 1154
Aludrox Oral Suspension 2428
Amphojel Suspension 2429
Amphojel Suspension without Flavor 2429
Mylanta Liquid 1155
Mylanta Double Strength Liquid 1155
Aluminum Hydroxide Gel, Dried (Concurrent administration of nonabsorbable antacids may alter the rate of absorption of aspirin). Products include:
Alu-Tab/Alu-Cap 1309
Amphojel Tablets 2429
Ascriptin A/D Caplets 1850
Regular Strength Ascriptin Tablets 1850
Gaviscon Antacid Tablets ▣ 593
Gaviscon-2 Antacid Tablets ▣ 594
Mylanta Tablets 1155
Mylanta Double Strength Tablets 1155
Antiarthritic Drugs, unspecified (Effect not specified).
Anticoagulant Drugs, unspecified (Effect not specified).

Antidiabetic Drugs, unspecified (Effect not specified).

Antigout Drugs, unspecified (Effect not specified).

Dihydroxyaluminum Sodium Carbonate (Concurrent administration of nonabsorbable antacids may alter the rate of absorption of aspirin). Products include:

- Rolaids ▣ 743

Magaldrate (Concurrent administration of nonabsorbable antacids may alter the rate of absorption of aspirin). Products include:

- Riopan Antacid Chew Tablets ▣ 754
- Riopan Antacid Chew Tablets in Rollpacks ▣ 754
- Riopan Antacid Suspension 2421
- Riopan Antacid Swallow Tablets 2421
- Riopan Plus Chew Tablets 2422
- Riopan Plus Chew Tablets in Rollpack 2422
- Riopan Plus 2 Chew Tablets, Mint Flavor, Cherry Flavor 2422
- Riopan Plus Suspension 2422
- Riopan Plus 2 Suspension, Mint Flavor, Cherry Flavor 2422

Magnesium Hydroxide (Concurrent administration of nonabsorbable antacids may alter the rate of absorption of aspirin). Products include:

- Aludrox Oral Suspension 2428
- Ascriptin A/D Caplets 1850
- Regular Strength Ascriptin Tablets 1850
- Di-Gel Antacid/Anti-Gas ▣ 697
- Gelusil Liquid & Tablets ▣ 639
- Haley's M-O, Regular & Flavored .. ▣ 569
- Extra Strength Maalox Plus Suspension 1850
- Maalox TC Suspension 1851
- Maalox Plus Tablets ▣ 655
- Extra Strength Maalox Plus Tablets 1850
- Mylanta Liquid 1155
- Mylanta Tablets 1155
- Mylanta Double Strength Liquid 1155
- Mylanta Double Strength Tablets 1155
- Concentrated Phillips' Milk of Magnesia ▣ 573
- Phillips' Milk of Magnesia Liquid ▣ 572
- Phillips' Milk of Magnesia Tablets ▣ 573
- WinGel Liquid & Tablets ▣ 761

Magnesium Oxide (Concurrent administration of nonabsorbable antacids may alter the rate of absorption of aspirin). Products include:

- Bayer Plus Aspirin Tablets ▣ 567
- Beelith Tablets 659
- Bufferin Analgesic Tablets and Caplets ▣ 524
- Cama Arthritis Pain Reliever ▣ 685
- Mag-Ox 400 673
- Uro-Mag 673

Sodium Bicarbonate (Concurrent administration with absorbable antacids may increase the clearance of salicylates). Products include:

- Alka-Seltzer Advanced Formula Antacid & Non-Aspirin Pain Reliever ▣ 620
- Alka-Seltzer Effervescent Antacid ▣ 622
- Alka-Seltzer Effervescent Antacid and Pain Reliever 1568
- Alka-Seltzer Extra Strength Effervescent Antacid and Pain Reliever ▣ 623
- Alka-Seltzer (Flavored) Effervescent Antacid and Pain Reliever .. ▣ 621
- Arm & Hammer Pure Baking Soda ▣ 548
- Ceo-Two Rectal Suppositories 671
- Citrocarbonate Antacid ▣ 668
- Massengill Liquid Concentrate 2191
- NuLYTELY 699

ECOTRIN ENTERIC COATED ASPIRIN REGULAR STRENGTH TABLETS AND CAPLETS

(Aspirin, Enteric Coated) 2189

See **Ecotrin Enteric Coated Aspirin Maximum Strength Tablets and Caplets**

EDECRIN SODIUM INTRAVENOUS

(Ethacrynate Sodium) 1468

May interact with aminoglycosides, cephalosporins, non-steroidal anti-inflammatory agents, cardiac glycosides, and certain other agents. Compounds in these categories include:

Amikacin Sulfate (Increased ototoxic potential of aminoglycosides). Products include:

- Amikin Injectable 602

Cefaclor (Increased ototoxic potential of cephalosporins). Products include:

- Ceclor Pulvules & Suspension 1251

Cefadroxil Monohydrate (Increased ototoxic potential of cephalosporins). Products include:

- Duricef 1405
- Ultracef Capsules, Tablets & Oral Suspension 722

Cefamandole Nafate (Increased ototoxic potential of cephalosporins). Products include:

- Mandol Vials, Faspak & ADD-Vantage 1281

Cefazolin Sodium (Increased ototoxic potential of cephalosporins). Products include:

- Ancef Injection 2194
- Kefzol Vials, Faspak & ADD-Vantage 1279

Cefixime (Increased ototoxic potential of cephalosporins). Products include:

- Suprax 1235

Cefmetazole Sodium (Increased ototoxic potential of cephalosporins). Products include:

- Zefazone Sterile Powder 2372

Cefonicid Sodium (Increased ototoxic potential of cephalosporins). Products include:

- Monocid Injection 2217

Cefoperazone Sodium (Increased ototoxic potential of cephalosporins). Products include:

- Cefobid Intravenous/Intramuscular 1943
- Cefobid Pharmacy Bulk Package - Not for Direct Infusion 1945

Ceforanide (Increased ototoxic potential of cephalosporins).

- No products indexed under this heading.

Cefotaxime Sodium (Increased ototoxic potential of cephalosporins). Products include:

- Claforan Sterile Injection 1089

Cefotetan (Increased ototoxic potential of cephalosporins). Products include:

- Cefotan 2265

Cefoxitin Sodium (Increased ototoxic potential of cephalosporins). Products include:

- Mefoxin 1498
- Mefoxin Premixed Intravenous Solution 1500

Ceftazidime (Increased ototoxic potential of cephalosporins). Products include:

- Ceptaz for Injection 1057
- Fortaz 1060
- Tazicef for Injection 2231
- Tazidime Vials, Faspak & ADD-Vantage 1299

Ceftizoxime Sodium (Increased ototoxic potential of cephalosporins). Products include:

- Cefizox Injection 1012

Ceftriaxone Sodium (Increased ototoxic potential of cephalosporins). Products include:

- Rocephin Injectable Vials, ADD-Vantage 1914

Cefuroxime Axetil (Increased ototoxic potential of cephalosporins). Products include:

- Ceftin Tablets 575

Cefuroxime Sodium (Increased ototoxic potential of cephalosporins). Products include:

- Kefurox Vials, Faspak & ADD-Vantage 1277
- Zinacef 1066

Cephalexin (Increased ototoxic potential of cephalosporins). Products include:

- Keflex Pulvules, Oral Suspension & Pediatric Drops 916

Cephalothin Sodium (Increased ototoxic potential of cephalosporins).

Cephapirin Sodium (Increased ototoxic potential of cephalosporins).

- No products indexed under this heading.

Cephradine (Increased ototoxic potential of cephalosporins). Products include:

- Velosef Capsules and for Oral Suspension 606

Deslanoside (Excessive potassium loss may precipitate digitalis toxicity).

- No products indexed under this heading.

Diclofenac Sodium (Reduces diuretic, natriuretic, and antihypertensive effects). Products include:

- Voltaren Ophthalmic Sterile Ophthalmic Solution ⊙ 268
- Voltaren Tablets 1042

Digitoxin (Excessive potassium loss may precipitate digitalis toxicity). Products include:

- Crystodigin Tablets 1253

Digoxin (Excessive potassium loss may precipitate digitalis toxicity). Products include:

- Lanoxicaps 772
- Lanoxin Elixir Pediatric 775
- Lanoxin Injection 778
- Lanoxin Injection Pediatric 781
- Lanoxin Tablets 783

Etodolac (Reduces diuretic, natriuretic, and antihypertensive effects). Products include:

- Lodine Capsules 2468

Fenoprofen Calcium (Reduces diuretic, natriuretic, and antihypertensive effects). Products include:

- Nalfon Pulvules & Tablets 919

Flurbiprofen (Reduces diuretic, natriuretic, and antihypertensive effects). Products include:

- Ansaid Tablets 2319

Gentamicin Sulfate (Increased ototoxic potential of aminoglycosides). Products include:

- Garamycin Injectable 2093
- Garamycin Ophthalmic ⊙ 305
- Genoptic Liquifilm Sterile Ophthalmic Solution ⊙ 247
- Genoptic S.O.P. Sterile Ophthalmic Ointment ⊙ 247
- Gentacidin Ointment ⊙ 273
- Gentacidin Solution ⊙ 273
- Gentak Ointment & Solution ⊙ 208
- G-myticin Creme and Ointment 0.1% 1770
- Pred-G Liquifilm Sterile Ophthalmic Suspension ⊙ 252
- Pred-G S.O.P. Sterile Ophthalmic Ointment ⊙ 253

Ibuprofen (Reduces diuretic, natriuretic, and antihypertensive effects). Products include:

- Advil Cold & Sinus Caplets (formerly CoAdvil) 2416
- Advil Ibuprofen Tablets and Caplets 2416
- Children's Advil Suspension 2426
- CoAdvil ▣ 748
- Dristan Sinus Caplets 2419
- Haltran Tablets ▣ 668
- Ibuprofen ▣ 631
- Medipren ibuprofen Caplets and Tablets 1362
- Midol 200 Cramp Relief Formula .. ▣ 570
- Motrin Tablets 2351
- Motrin IB Caplets and Tablets ▣ 736
- Nuprin Ibuprofen/Analgesic Tablets & Caplets 752
- PediaProfen Suspension 1363
- Rufen Tablets 691
- Trendar Ibuprofen Tablets ▣ 756

Indomethacin (Reduces diuretic, natriuretic, and antihypertensive effects). Products include:

- Indocin 1487

Indomethacin Sodium Trihydrate (Reduces diuretic, natriuretic, and antihypertensive effects). Products include:

- Indocin I.V. 1490

Isoproterenol Hydrochloride (Careful adjustment of dosages required). Products include:

- Isuprel Hydrochloride Injection 1:5000 2050
- Isuprel Hydrochloride Mistometer .. 2051
- Isuprel Hydrochloride Solution 1:200 & 1:100 2052
- Norisodrine Aerotrol 540

Kanamycin Sulfate (Increased ototoxic potential of aminoglycosides). Products include:

- Kantrex Injection 601
- Kantrex Pediatric Injection 601

Ketoprofen (Reduces diuretic, natriuretic, and antihypertensive effects). Products include:

- Orudis Capsules 2488

Ketorolac Tromethamine (Reduces diuretic, natriuretic, and antihypertensive effects). Products include:

- Toradol IM Injection 2302

Lithium Carbonate (High risk of lithium toxicity). Products include:

- Eskalith 2214
- Lithane Tablets 1596
- Lithium Carbonate Capsules & Tablets 1984
- Lithobid Tablets 870

Lithium Citrate (High risk of lithium toxicity). Products include:

- Cibalith-S 870

Meclofenamate Sodium (Reduces diuretic, natriuretic, and antihypertensive effects). Products include:

- Meclomen Capsules 1739

Mefenamic Acid (Reduces diuretic, natriuretic, and antihypertensive effects). Products include:

- Ponstel 1758

Naproxen (Reduces diuretic, natriuretic, and antihypertensive effects). Products include:

- Naprosyn 2297

Naproxen Sodium (Reduces diuretic, natriuretic, and antihypertensive effects). Products include:

- Anaprox and Anaprox DS Tablets 2288

Phenylbutazone (Reduces diuretic, natriuretic, and antihypertensive effects). Products include:

- Butazolidin Capsules & Tablets 1027

Piroxicam (Reduces diuretic, natriuretic, and antihypertensive effects). Products include:

- Feldene Capsules 1777

Streptomycin Sulfate (Increased ototoxic potential of aminoglycosides).

- No products indexed under this heading.

Sulindac (Reduces diuretic, natriuretic, and antihypertensive effects). Products include:

- Clinoril Tablets 1433

Tobramycin Sulfate (Increased ototoxic potential of aminoglycosides). Products include:
- Nebcin Vials, Hyporets & ADD-Vantage ... 1286

Tolmetin Sodium (Reduces diuretic, natriuretic, and antihypertensive effects). Products include:
- Tolectin (200, 400 and 600 mg) .. 1379

Warfarin Sodium (Warfarin displaced from plasma protein; reduction in warfarin dosage may be required). Products include:
- Coumadin Injection & Tablets ... 944
- Panwarfin Tablets ... 547

EDECRIN TABLETS
(Ethacrynic Acid) ... 1468
See **Edecrin Sodium Intravenous**

PROFESSIONAL STRENGTH EFFERDENT
(Denture Cleanser) ... ▣ 742
No interactions described in labeling.

EFFER-SYLLIUM NATURAL FIBER BULKING AGENT
(Psyllium Preparations) ... 1154
No interactions described in labeling.

EFUDEX CREAM
(Fluorouracil) ... 1880
No interactions described in labeling.

EFUDEX SOLUTIONS
(Fluorouracil) ... 1880
No interactions described in labeling.

ELASE OINTMENT
(Desoxyribonuclease, Fibrinolysin) ... 1015
No interactions described in labeling.

ELASE VIALS
(Fibrinolysin, Desoxyribonuclease) ... 1015
No interactions described in labeling.

ELASE-CHLOROMYCETIN OINTMENT
(Fibrinolysin, Desoxyribonuclease, Chloramphenicol) ... 1015
No interactions described in labeling.

ELAVIL INJECTION
(Amitriptyline Hydrochloride) ... 2269
May interact with barbiturates, central nervous system depressants, anticholinergics, sympathomimetic aerosal brochodilators, neuromuscular blocking agents, and certain other agents. Compounds in these categories include:

Albuterol (Careful adjustment of dosages required). Products include:
- Proventil Inhalation Aerosol ... 2117
- Ventolin Inhalation Aerosol and Refill ... 583

Albuterol Sulfate (Careful adjustment of dosages required). Products include:
- Proventil Repetabs Tablets ... 2120
- Proventil Solutions for Inhalation 0.5% and 0.083% ... 2118
- Proventil Syrup ... 2119
- Proventil Tablets ... 2120
- Ventolin ... 583

Alcohol (Enhanced response to alcohol).

Alfentanil Hydrochloride (Enhanced effects of CNS depressants). Products include:
- Alfenta Injection ... 1131

Alprazolam (Enhanced effects of CNS depressants). Products include:
- Xanax Tablets ... 2367

Aprobarbital (Enhanced effects of CNS depressants). Products include:
- Alurate Elixir ... 1883

Atropine Sulfate (Hyperpyrexia; paralytic ileus; careful adjustment of dosages required). Products include:
- Arco-Lase Plus Tablets ... 607
- Atropine Sulfate Sterile Ophthalmic Solution and S.O.P. Sterile Ophthalmic Ointment ... ◉ 239
- Donnagel ... ▣ 675
- Donnagel-PG ... 1858
- Donnatal ... 1858
- Donnatal Extentabs ... 1859
- Donnatal Tablets ... 1858
- Donnazyme Tablets ... 1860
- Isopto Atropine ... ◉ 218
- Lomotil ... 2174
- Motofen Tablets ... 836
- Ru-Tuss Tablets ... 693
- Urised Tablets ... 2396

Belladonna Alkaloids (Hyperpyrexia; paralytic ileus; careful adjustment of dosages required). Products include:
- Bellergal-S Tablets ... 1998
- Hyland's Bed Wetting Tablets ... ▣ 728
- Hyland's Teething Tablets ... ▣ 728
- Kinesed Tablets ... 2272

Benztropine Mesylate (Hyperpyrexia; paralytic ileus; careful adjustment of dosages required). Products include:
- Cogentin ... 1435

Biperiden (Hyperpyrexia; paralytic ileus; careful adjustment of dosages required). Products include:
- Akineton ... 1171

Buprenorphine (Enhanced effects of CNS depressants).
No products indexed under this heading.

Buspirone Hydrochloride (Enhanced effects of CNS depressants). Products include:
- BuSpar ... 1401

Butabarbital (Enhanced effects of CNS depressants). Products include:
- Pyridium Plus ... 1764

Butalbital (Enhanced effects of CNS depressants). Products include:
- Esgic-Plus Tablets ... 1002
- Esgic Tablets & Capsules ... 1001
- Fioricet Tablets ... 2006
- Fiorinal Capsules ... 2007
- Fiorinal with Codeine Capsules ... 2008
- Fiorinal Tablets ... 2007
- Phrenilin ... 838
- Sedapap Tablets 50 mg/650 mg .. 1360

Chlordiazepoxide (Enhanced effects of CNS depressants). Products include:
- Libritabs Tablets ... 1930
- Limbitrol ... 1933
- Menrium Tablets ... 1934

Chlordiazepoxide Hydrochloride (Enhanced effects of CNS depressants). Products include:
- Librax Capsules ... 1929
- Librium Capsules ... 1931
- Librium Injectable ... 1932

Chlorpromazine (Enhanced effects of CNS depressants; hyperpyrexia). Products include:
- Thorazine ... 2234

Chlorprothixene (Enhanced effects of CNS depressants; hyperpyrexia). Products include:
- Taractan Tablets ... 1920

Chlorprothixene Hydrochloride (Enhanced effects of CNS depressants; hyperpyrexia). Products include:
- Taractan ... 1920

Cimetidine (Increased frequency and severity of antidepressant's side effects). Products include:
- Tagamet Tablets ... 2228

Cimetidine Hydrochloride (Increased frequency and severity of antidepressant's side effects). Products include:
- Tagamet ... 2228

Clidinium Bromide (Hyperpyrexia; paralytic ileus; careful adjustment of dosages required). Products include:
- Librax Capsules ... 1929
- Quarzan Capsules ... 1937

Clorazepate Dipotassium (Enhanced effects of CNS depressants). Products include:
- Tranxene ... 556

Clozapine (Enhanced effects of CNS depressants; hyperpyrexia). Products include:
- Clozaril Tablets ... 2000

Codeine (Enhanced effects of CNS depressants). Products include:
- Calcidrine Syrup ... 506

Codeine Phosphate (Enhanced effects of CNS depressants). Products include:
- Actifed with Codeine Cough Syrup.. 752
- Cheracol Cough Syrup ... 1853
- Codimal PH Syrup ... 846
- Dimetane-DC Cough Syrup ... 1857
- Empirin with Codeine Phosphate Nos. 2, 3 & 4 ... 764
- Fiorinal with Codeine Capsules ... 2008
- Isoclor Expectorant ... 982
- Naldecon CX Adult Liquid ... ▣ 521
- Novahistine DH ... 1342
- Novahistine Expectorant ... 1343
- Nucofed Capsules ... 2219
- Nucofed Expectorant ... 2219
- Nucofed Pediatric Expectorant ... 2220
- Nucofed Syrup ... 2219
- Phenaphen with Codeine Capsules 1865
- Phenaphen-650 with Codeine Tablets ... 1866
- Phenergan with Codeine ... 2497
- Phenergan VC with Codeine ... 2501
- Robitussin A-C Syrup ... 1875
- Robitussin-DAC Syrup ... 1875
- Ryna ... ▣ 741
- Soma Compound w/Codeine Tablets ... 2390
- Triaminic Expectorant w/Codeine .. 1996
- Tussi-Organidin Liquid ... 2391
- Tylenol with Codeine ... 1381

Codeine Polistirex (Enhanced effects of CNS depressants).
No products indexed under this heading.

Dezocine (Enhanced effects of CNS depressants).

Diazepam (Enhanced effects of CNS depressants). Products include:
- Valium Injectable ... 1937
- Valium Tablets ... 1939
- Valrelease Capsules ... 1923

Dicyclomine Hydrochloride (Hyperpyrexia; paralytic ileus; careful adjustment of dosage required). Products include:
- Bentyl ... 1322

Disulfiram (Delirium). Products include:
- Antabuse Tablets ... 2429

Dobutamine Hydrochloride (Careful adjustment of dosages required). Products include:
- Dobutrex Solution Vials ... 1259

Dopamine Hydrochloride (Careful adjustment of dosages required). Products include:
- Intropin Injection ... 930

Droperidol (Enhanced effects of CNS depressants). Products include:
- Inapsine Injection ... 1140
- Innovar Injection ... 1141

Enflurane (Enhanced effects of CNS depressants). Products include:
- Ethrane ... 599

Ephedrine Hydrochloride (Careful adjustment of dosages required). Products include:
- Amesec ... ▣ 682
- Primatene Tablets-M Formula ... 2421
- Primatene Tablets-P Formula ... 2421
- Primatene Tablets-Regular Formula ... 2421
- Quadrinal Tablets ... 1183
- Quelidrine Syrup ... 556
- Tedral SA ... 1765

Ephedrine Sulfate (Careful adjustment of dosages required). Products include:
- Bronkaid Tablets ... ▣ 757
- Bronkolixir ... ▣ 761
- Bronkotabs Tablets ... ▣ 762
- Marax Tablets & DF Syrup ... 1954
- Pazo Hemorrhoid Ointment & Suppositories ... 752
- Vicks Vatronol Nose Drops ... ▣ 666

Ephedrine Tannate (Careful adjustment of dosages required). Products include:
- Rynatuss ... 2388

Epinephrine (Careful adjustment of dosages required). Products include:
- Ana-Kit Anaphylaxis Emergency Treatment Kit ... 1100
- Bronkaid Mist ... ▣ 757
- EpiPen ... 843
- Marcaine Hydrochloride 0.5% with Epinephrine 1:200,000 (as bitartrate) ... 958
- Marcaine Hydrochloride with Epinephrine 1:200,000 ... 2055
- Primatene Mist ... 2420
- Sus-Phrine Injection ... 1006
- Xylocaine with Epinephrine Injections ... 637

Epinephrine Bitartrate (Careful adjustment of dosages required). Products include:
- AsthmaHaler Mist Epinephrine Bitartrate Bronchodilator ... ▣ 616
- Bronkaid Mist Suspension ... ▣ 757
- Primatene Mist Suspension ... 2421

Epinephrine Hydrochloride (Careful adjustment of dosages required). Products include:
- Adrenalin Chloride Solution 1:100 & 1:1,000 ... 1689
- Epifrin ... ◉ 244
- Glaucon ... ◉ 218

Estazolam (Enhanced effects of CNS depressants). Products include:
- ProSom Tablets ... 554

Ethchlorvynol (Transient delirium effects; enhanced effects of CNS depressants). Products include:
- Placidyl Capsules ... 553

Ethinamate (Enhanced effects of CNS depressants).
No products indexed under this heading.

Fentanyl (Enhanced effects of CNS depressants). Products include:
- Duragesic Transdermal System ... 1133

Fentanyl Citrate (Enhanced effects of CNS depressants). Products include:
- Innovar Injection ... 1141
- Sublimaze Injection ... 1146

Fluphenazine Decanoate (Enhanced effects of CNS depressants; hyperpyrexia). Products include:
- Prolixin Decanoate ... 1795

Fluphenazine Enanthate (Enhanced effects of CNS depressants; hyperpyrexia). Products include:
- Prolixin Enanthate ... 1796

Fluphenazine Hydrochloride (Enhanced effects of CNS depressants; hyperpyrexia). Products include:
- Prolixin Elixir ... 1793
- Prolixin Injection ... 1791
- Prolixin Oral Concentrate ... 1792
- Prolixin Tablets ... 1793

Flurazepam Hydrochloride (Enhanced effects of CNS depressants). Products include:
- Dalmane Capsules ... 1927

Glutethimide (Enhanced effects of CNS depressants).
No products indexed under this heading.

Glycopyrrolate (Hyperpyrexia; paralytic ileus; careful adjustment of dosage required). Products include:
- Robinul Forte Tablets 1873
- Robinul Injectable 1873
- Robinul Tablets 1873

Guanethidine Monosulfate (Antihypertensive action blocked). Products include:
- Esimil Tablets 864
- Ismelin Tablets 869

Haloperidol (Enhanced effects of CNS depressants; hyperpyrexia). Products include:
- Haldol Injection, Tablets and Concentrate 1373

Haloperidol Decanoate (Enhanced effects of CNS depressants; hyperpyrexia). Products include:
- Haldol Decanoate 1375

Hydrocodone Bitartrate (Enhanced effects of CNS depressants). Products include:
- Anexsia 5/500 Tablets 2196
- Anexsia 7.5/650 Tablets 2197
- Azdone Tablets 844
- Codiclear DH Syrup 845
- Codimal DH Syrup 846
- Damason-P 1356
- Hycodan Syrup, Tablets 927
- Hycomine Compound Tablets 929
- Hycomine Syrup 927
- Hycotuss Expectorant Syrup 930
- Hydrocet Capsules 835
- Lortab ASA Tablets 2414
- Lortab 2412
- Ru-Tuss with Hydrocodone 694
- Triaminic Expectorant DH 1995
- Vicodin Tablets 1187
- Vicodin ES Tablets 1189
- Zydone Capsules 941

Hydrocodone Polistirex (Enhanced effects of CNS depressants). Products include:
- Tussionex Extended-Release Suspension 988

Hydroxyzine Hydrochloride (Enhanced effects of CNS depressants). Products include:
- Atarax Tablets & Syrup 1941
- Marax Tablets & DF Syrup 1954
- Vistaril Intramuscular Solution 1970

Hyoscyamine (Hyperpyrexia; paralytic ileus; careful adjustment of dosage required). Products include:
- Cystospaz Tablets 2395
- Urised Tablets 2396

Hyoscyamine Sulfate (Hyperpyrexia; paralytic ileus; careful adjustment of dosage required). Products include:
- Arco-Lase Plus Tablets 607
- Cystospaz-M Capsules 2395
- Donnagel .... ▣ 675
- Donnagel-PG 1858
- Donnatal 1858
- Donnatal Extentabs 1859
- Donnatal Tablets 1858
- Donnazyme Tablets 1860
- Kutrase Capsules 2146
- Levsin/Levsinex 2147
- Ru-Tuss Tablets 693

Ipratropium Bromide (Hyperpyrexia; paralytic ileus; careful adjustment of dosage required). Products include:
- Atrovent Inhalation Aerosol 675

Isocarboxazid (Contraindication; hyperpyretic crises; severe convulsions; death). Products include:
- Marplan Tablets 1906

Isoflurane (Enhanced effects of CNS depressants). Products include:
- Forane 600

Isoproterenol Hydrochloride (Careful adjustment of dosages required). Products include:
- Isuprel Hydrochloride Injection 1:5000 2050
- Isuprel Hydrochloride Mistometer 2051
- Isuprel Hydrochloride Solution 1:200 & 1:100 2052
- Norisodrine Aerotrol 540

Ketamine Hydrochloride (Enhanced effects of CNS depressants). Products include:
- Ketalar 1726

Levorphanol Tartrate (Enhanced effects of CNS depressants). Products include:
- Levo-Dromoran 1906

Levothyroxine Sodium (Close supervision required). Products include:
- Levothroid Tablets 1003
- Levoxine Tablets 904
- Synthroid 695

Liothyronine Sodium (Close supervision required). Products include:
- Cytomel Tablets 2203

Liotrix (Close supervision required). Products include:
- Euthroid 1724

Lithium Carbonate (Hyperpyrexia). Products include:
- Eskalith 2214
- Lithane Tablets 1596
- Lithium Carbonate Capsules & Tablets 1984
- Lithobid Tablets 870

Lithium Citrate (Hyperpyrexia). Products include:
- Cibalith-S 870

Lorazepam (Enhanced effects of CNS depressants). Products include:
- Ativan Injection 2432
- Ativan Tablets 2434

Loxapine Hydrochloride (Enhanced effects of CNS depressants; hyperpyrexia). Products include:
- Loxitane 1213

Loxapine Succinate (Enhanced effects of CNS depressants; hyperpyrexia). Products include:
- Loxitane Capsules 1213

Mepenzolate Bromide (Hyperpyrexia; paralytic ileus; careful adjustment of dosage required). Products include:
- Cantil Tablets 1326

Meperidine Hydrochloride (Enhanced effects of CNS depressants). Products include:
- Demerol 2047
- Mepergan Injection 2479

Mephobarbital (Enhanced effects of CNS depressants). Products include:
- Mebaral Tablets 2061

Meprobamate (Enhanced effects of CNS depressants). Products include:
- Deprol Tablets 2382
- Equagesic Tablets 2451
- Miltown Tablets 2386
- PMB 200 and PMB 400 2504

Mesoridazine (Enhanced effects of CNS depressants; hyperpyrexia). Products include:
- Serentil 686

Metaproterenol Sulfate (Careful adjustment of dosages required). Products include:
- Alupent 674
- Arm-a-Med Metaproterenol Sulfate Inhalation Solution, USP 617
- Metaprel Inhalation Aerosol Bronchodilator 2014
- Metaprel Inhalation Solution 2015
- Metaprel 2015
- Metaproterenol Sulfate Inhalation Solution, USP 912

Metaraminol Bitartrate (Careful adjustment of dosages required). Products include:
- Aramine Injection 1424

Methadone Hydrochloride (Enhanced effects of CNS depressants). Products include:
- Dolophine Hydrochloride Ampoules & Vials 1260
- Dolophine Hydrochloride Tablets 1261
- Methadone Hydrochloride Diskets 1284
- Methadone Hydrochloride Oral Solution & Tablets 1987

Methohexital Sodium (Enhanced effects of CNS depressants). Products include:
- Brevital Sodium Vials 1248

Methoxyflurane (Enhanced effects of CNS depressants).
- No products indexed under this heading.

Methyldopate Hydrochloride (Potentiated or additive effects). Products include:
- Aldomet Ester HCl Injection 1417

Midazolam Hydrochloride (Enhanced effects of CNS depressants). Products include:
- Versed Injection 1924

Molindone Hydrochloride (Enhanced effects of CNS depressants; hyperpyrexia). Products include:
- Moban Tablets & Concentrate 932

Morphine Sulfate (Enhanced effects of CNS depressants). Products include:
- Astramorph/PF Injection, USP (Preservative-Free) 618
- Duramorph 960
- Infumorph 200 and Infumorph 500 Sterile Solutions 962
- MS Contin Tablets 1814
- MSIR 1817
- Oramorph SR (Morphine Sulfate Sustained Release Tablets) 1988
- Roxanol 1991

Norepinephrine Bitartrate (Careful adjustment of dosages required). Products include:
- Levophed Bitartrate Injection 2054

Opium Alkaloids (Enhanced effects of CNS depressants). Products include:
- B & O No. 15A & No. 16A Supprettes 2395
- Pantopon Injectable 1911

Oxazepam (Enhanced effects of CNS depressants). Products include:
- Serax Capsules 2522
- Serax Tablets 2522

Oxybutynin Chloride (Hyperpyrexia; paralytic ileus; careful adjustment of dosages required). Products include:
- Ditropan 1332

Oxycodone Hydrochloride (Enhanced effects of CNS depressants). Products include:
- Percocet Tablets 950
- Percodan 951
- Roxicodone Tablets, Oral Solution & Intensol (Oxycodone) 1992
- Tylox Capsules 1382

Pargyline Hydrochloride (Contraindication; hyperpyretic crises; severe convulsions; death).
- No products indexed under this heading.

Pentobarbital Sodium (Enhanced effects of CNS depressants). Products include:
- Nembutal Sodium Capsules 534
- Nembutal Sodium Solution 536
- Nembutal Sodium Suppositories 538

Perphenazine (Enhanced effects of CNS depressants; hyperpyrexia). Products include:
- Etrafon 2087
- Triavil Tablets 1556
- Trilafon 2123

Phenelzine Sulfate (Contraindication; hyperpyretic crises; severe convulsions; death). Products include:
- Nardil 1742

Phenobarbital (Enhanced effects of CNS depressants). Products include:
- Arco-Lase Plus Tablets 607
- Bellergal-S Tablets 1998
- Bronkolixir .... ▣ 761
- Bronkotabs Tablets .... ▣ 762
- Donnatal 1858
- Donnatal Extentabs 1859
- Donnatal Tablets 1858
- Donnazyme Tablets 1860
- Kinesed Tablets 2272
- Phenobarbital Elixir and Tablets 1293
- Primatene Tablets-P Formula 2421
- Quadrinal Tablets 1183
- Tedral SA 1765

Phenylephrine Bitartrate (Careful adjustment of dosages required).
- No products indexed under this heading.

Phenylephrine Hydrochloride (Careful adjustment of dosages required). Products include:
- AK-Dilate Solution 2.5% and 10% .... ⊙ 203
- Atrohist Sprinkle Capsules 558
- Cerose-DM 2443
- Codimal 846
- Comhist LA Capsules 1618
- Congespirin For Children Aspirin Free Chewable Cold Tablets 748
- Cyclomydril .... ⊙ 216
- Deconsal Sprinkle Capsules 559
- Dimetane Decongestant .... ▣ 673
- Dristan Decongestant/Antihistamine/ Analgesic Coated Caplets .... ▣ 749
- Dristan Cold Nasal Decongestant/ Antihistamine/ Analgesic Coated Tablets 2419
- Dristan Advanced Formula Decongestant/Antihistamine/ Analgesic Tablets .... ▣ 749
- Dristan Nasal Spray, Menthol 2419
- Dristan Nasal Spray, Regular and Regular with Metered Pump 2419
- Entex Capsules 1623
- Entex Liquid 1623
- Sinus Excedrin Analgesic, Decongestant Tablets & Caplets 750
- Extendryl 994
- 4-Way Fast Acting Nasal Spray - Original Formula (regular & mentholated) & Metered Spray Pump (regular) 751
- Hycomine Compound Tablets 929
- Murocoll-2 Sterile Ophthalmic Solution .... ⊙ 261
- Mydfrin 2.5% .... ⊙ 224
- Naldecon Syrup, Tablets, Pediatric Drops and Pediatric Syrup 709
- Neo-Synephrine Hydrochloride 1% Carpuject 2063
- Neo-Synephrine Hydrochloride 1% Injection 2063
- Neo-Synephrine Hydrochloride (Ophthalmic) 2064
- Neo-Synephrine .... ▣ 759
- Nōstril Nasal Decongestant .... ▣ 520
- Novahistine Elixir .... ▣ 596
- Phenergan VC 2500
- Phenergan VC with Codeine 2501
- Prefrin Liquifilm Vasoconstrictor and Lubricant Eye Drops .... ⊙ 254
- Prefrin-A .... ⊙ 255
- Quelidrine Syrup 556
- Relief Vasoconstrictor and Lubricant Eye Drops .... ⊙ 256
- Robitussin Night Relief .... ▣ 677
- Ru-Tuss with Hydrocodone 694
- Ru-Tuss Tablets 693
- Vasosulf .... ⊙ 279
- Vicks Sinex .... ▣ 665
- Zincfrin .... ⊙ 230

Phenylephrine Tannate (Careful adjustment of dosages required). Products include:
- Rynatan 2387
- Rynatuss 2388

(▣ Described in PDR For Nonprescription Drugs) (⊙ Described in PDR For Ophthalmology)

Phenylpropanolamine Hydrochloride (Careful adjustment of dosages required). Products include:
A.R.M. Allergy Relief Medicine Caplets ▣ 615
Acutrim ▣ 548
Allerest ▣ 559
BC Cold Powder ▣ 517
Cheracol Plus Head Cold/Cough Formula ▣ 667
Codimal Expectorant 846
Comtrex Multi-Symptom Cold Reliever Tablets/Caplets/Liqui-Gels/Liquid 745
Contac Continuous Action Decongestant/Antihistamine Capsules ▣ 710
Contac Maximum Strength Continuous Action Decongestant/Antihistamine Caplets ▣ 709
Contac Severe Cold and Flu Formula Caplets ▣ 711
Coricidin 'D' Decongestant Tablets ▣ 695
Coricidin Demilets Tablets for Children ▣ 696
Demazin Nasal Decongestant/Antihistamine Repetabs Tablets & Syrup ▣ 697
Dexatrim ▣ 733
Dimetane-DC Cough Syrup 1857
Dimetapp Elixir ▣ 673
Dimetapp DM Elixir ▣ 674
Dimetapp Extentabs ▣ 674
Dimetapp Plus Caplets ▣ 675
Dimetapp Tablets ▣ 675
Entex Capsules 1623
Entex LA Tablets 1623
Entex Liquid 1623
4-Way Cold Tablets 750
Hycomine Syrup 927
Naldecon CX Adult Liquid ▣ 521
Naldecon DX Adult Liquid ▣ 521
Naldecon DX Children's Syrup ▣ 522
Naldecon DX Pediatric Drops ▣ 522
Naldecon EX Children's Syrup ▣ 522
Naldecon EX Pediatric Drops ▣ 523
Naldecon Syrup, Tablets, Pediatric Drops and Pediatric Syrup 709
Nolamine Tablets 838
Nolex LA Tablets 838
Ornade Spansule Capsules 2221
Orthoxicol Cough Syrup ▣ 668
Propagest 839
Pyrroxate Capsules ▣ 669
Robitussin-CF ▣ 676
Ru-Tuss II Capsules 693
Ru-Tuss with Hydrocodone 694
Ru-Tuss Tablets 693
Sine-Off Sinus Medicine Tablets-Aspirin Formula ▣ 722
Sinulin 840
St. Joseph Cold Tablets for Children ▣ 704
Tavist-D Tablets 2035
Triaminic Allergy Tablets ▣ 688
Triaminic Chewables ▣ 688
Triaminic Cold Tablets ▣ 688
Triaminic Expectorant ▣ 688
Triaminic Expectorant w/Codeine 1996
Triaminic Expectorant DH 1995
Triaminic Oral Infant Drops 1996
Triaminic Syrup ▣ 689
Triaminic-12 Tablets ▣ 690
Triaminic-DM Syrup ▣ 689
Triaminicin Tablets ▣ 690
Triaminicol Multi-Symptom Cold Tablets ▣ 691
Triaminicol Multi-Symptom Relief ▣ 691
Tuss-Ornade Liquid 2242
Tuss-Ornade Spansule Capsules 2242
Tylenol Cold Medication, Effervescent Tablets 1369

Pimozide (Hyperpyrexia). Products include:
Orap Tablets 1020

Pirbuterol Acetate (Careful adjustment of dosages required). Products include:
Maxair Inhaler 1311

Prazepam (Enhanced effects of CNS depressants). Products include:
Centrax 1693

Prochlorperazine (Enhanced effects of CNS depressants; hyperpyrexia). Products include:
Compazine 2201

Procyclidine Hydrochloride (Hyperpyrexia; paralytic ileus; careful adjustment of dosages required). Products include:
Kemadrin Tablets 771

Promethazine Hydrochloride (Enhanced effects of CNS depressants; hyperpyrexia). Products include:
Mepergan Injection 2479
Phenergan with Codeine 2497
Phenergan with Dextromethorphan 2499
Phenergan Injection 2493
Phenergan Suppositories 2496
Phenergan Syrup 2495
Phenergan Tablets 2496
Phenergan VC 2500
Phenergan VC with Codeine 2501

Propantheline Bromide (Hyperpyrexia; paralytic ileus; careful adjustment of dosages required). Products include:
Pro-Banthīne Tablets 2141

Propofol (Enhanced effects of CNS depressants). Products include:
Diprivan Injection 2267

Propoxyphene Hydrochloride (Enhanced effects of CNS depressants). Products include:
Darvon 1256
Wygesic Tablets 2540

Propoxyphene Napsylate (Enhanced effects of CNS depressants). Products include:
Darvon-N/Darvocet-N 1254

Pseudoephedrine Hydrochloride (Careful adjustment of dosages required). Products include:
Actifed Capsules ▣ 539
Actifed Plus Caplets ▣ 539
Actifed Plus Tablets ▣ 540
Actifed with Codeine Cough Syrup 752
Actifed Syrup ▣ 540
Actifed Tablets ▣ 540
Actifed 12-Hour Capsules ▣ 539
Advil Cold & Sinus Caplets (formerly CoAdvil) 2416
Allerest ▣ 559
Anatuss LA Tablets 1359
Benadryl Decongestant Elixir ▣ 635
Benadryl Decongestant ▣ 635
Benadryl Plus ▣ 636
Benadryl Plus Nighttime ▣ 637
Benylin Decongestant ▣ 638
Brexin L.A. Capsules 2078
Bromfed Capsules (Timed Release) 1615
Bromfed Syrup ▣ 628
Bromfed 1615
CoAdvil ▣ 748
Allergy-Sinus Comtrex Multi-Symptom Allergy Sinus Formula Tablets & Caplets 746
Cough Formula Comtrex 746
Comtrex Multi-Symptom Cold Reliever Tablets/Caplets/Liqui-Gels/Liquid 745
Day-Night Comtrex 747
Non-Drowsy Comtrex 747
Congess 994
Congestac Caplets ▣ 617
Contac Jr. Children's Cold Medicine ▣ 712
Contac Nighttime Cold Medicine ▣ 713
Contac Sinus Caplets Maximum Strength Non-Drowsy Formula ▣ 710
Contac Sinus Tablets Maximum Strength Non-Drowsy Formula ▣ 710
Deconamine 663
Deconsal II Tablets 559
Dimacol Caplets ▣ 672
Dimetane-DX Cough Syrup 1858
Dorcol Children's Cough Syrup ▣ 685
Dorcol Children's Decongestant Liquid ▣ 685
Dorcol Children's Liquid Cold Formula ▣ 686
Maximum Strength Dristan Decongestant/Analgesic Coated Caplets ▣ 750
No Drowsiness Dristan Cold Nasal Decongestant/Analgesic Coated Caplets 2420
Dristan Sinus Caplets 2419
Sinus Excedrin Analgesic, Decongestant Tablets & Caplets ▣ 533
Fedahist Gyrocaps 2145
Fedahist Timecaps 2145
Guaifed 1615
Guaifed Syrup ▣ 629
Isoclor Expectorant 982
Isoclor Timesule Capsules ▣ 561
Kronofed-A 970
Medi-Flu Caplet, Liquid ▣ 640
Novafed A Capsules 1342
Novafed Capsules 1342
Novahistine DH 1342
Novahistine DMX ▣ 595
Novahistine Expectorant 1343
Nucofed Capsules 2219
Nucofed Expectorant 2219
Nucofed Pediatric Expectorant 2220
Nucofed Syrup 2219
Ornex Caplets ▣ 618
PediaCare Allergy Relief Formula Liquid 1362
PediaCare Cough-Cold Formula Liquid 1362
PediaCare Infants' Oral Decongestant Drops 1362
PediaCare Night Rest Cough-Cold Formula Liquid 1362
PediaCare 6-12 Cough-Cold Formula Chewable Tablets 1362
Robitussin-DAC Syrup 1875
Robitussin-PE ▣ 677
Rondec 1975
Rondec-DM 1976
Rondec-TR Tablet 1975
Ru-Tuss DE Tablets 694
Ryna ▣ 741
Seldane-D Extended-Release Tablets 1350
Sinarest ▣ 562
Sine-Aid Maximum Strength Sinus Headache Caplets 1365
Sine-Aid Maximum Strength Sinus Headache Tablets 1365
Sine-Off Maximum Strength Allergy/Sinus Formula Caplets ▣ 721
Sine-Off Maximum Strength No Drowsiness Formula Caplets ▣ 722
Singlet Tablets ▣ 598
Sinutab Maximum Strength ▣ 641
Sinutab Maximum Strength Without Drowsiness Tablets & Caplets ▣ 642
Sinutab Regular Strength Without Drowsiness Formula ▣ 641
St. Joseph Nighttime Cold Medicine ▣ 705
Sudafed Children's Liquid ▣ 543
Sudafed Cough Syrup ▣ 543
Sudafed Plus Liquid ▣ 544
Sudafed Plus Tablets ▣ 545
Sudafed Sinus Caplets ▣ 545
Sudafed Sinus Tablets ▣ 545
Sudafed Tablets, 30 mg ▣ 544
Sudafed Tablets, Adult Strength, 60 mg ▣ 544
Sudafed 12 Hour Capsules ▣ 545
TheraFlu Flu and Cold Medicine ▣ 687
Triaminic Nite Light ▣ 689
Tylenol Allergy Sinus Medication Caplets and Gelcaps, Maximum Strength 1372
Children's Tylenol Cold Liquid Formula and Chewable Tablets 1368
Tylenol Cold & Flu Hot Medication, Packets 1369
Tylenol Cold & Flu No Drowsiness Hot Medication, Packets 1371
Tylenol Cold Medication Caplets and Tablets 1370
Tylenol Cold Medication No Drowsiness Formula Caplets 1370
Tylenol Cold Night Time Medication Liquid 1371
Tylenol Cough Medication Liquid with Decongestant, Maximum Strength 1372
Tylenol, Maximum Strength, Sinus Medication Gelcaps, Caplets and Tablets 1373
Ursinus Inlay-Tabs ▣ 691
Vicks Children's NyQuil ▣ 664
Vicks Daycare ▣ 660
Vicks Formula 44D Decongestant Cough Medicine ▣ 662
Vicks Formula 44M Multi-Symptom Cough Medicine ▣ 662
Vicks NyQuil Nighttime Colds Medicine-Original & Cherry Flavor ▣ 664
Vicks Pediatric Formula 44 Cough & Congestion Medicine ▣ 663
Vicks Pediatric Formula 44m Multi-Symptom Cough & Cold Medicine ▣ 663

Pseudoephedrine Sulfate (Careful adjustment of dosages required). Products include:
Afrin Tablets ▣ 693
Chlor-Trimeton Decongestant ▣ 694
Disophrol Chronotab Sustained-Action Tablets ▣ 698
Drixoral Antihistamine/Nasal Decongestant Syrup ▣ 698
Drixoral Non-Drowsy Formula ▣ 699
Drixoral Plus Extended-Release Tablets ▣ 699
Drixoral Sinus ▣ 700
Drixoral Sustained-Action Tablets ▣ 698
Sinutab Allergy Formula Sustained Action Tablets ▣ 640
Trinalin Repetabs Tablets 1170

Quazepam (Enhanced effects of CNS depressants). Products include:
Doral Tablets 2383

Scopolamine Hydrobromide (Hyperpyrexia; paralytic ileus; careful adjustment of dosages required). Products include:
Donnagel ▣ 675
Donnagel-PG 1858
Donnatal 1858
Donnatal Extentabs 1859
Donnatal Tablets 1858
Donnazyme Tablets 1860
Isopto Hyoscine ⊙ 222
Murocoll-2 Sterile Ophthalmic Solution ⊙ 261
Ru-Tuss Tablets 693

Scopolamine Preparations (Hyperpyrexia; paralytic ileus; careful adjustment of dosages required). Products include:
Transderm Scōp Transdermal Therapeutic System 887

Secobarbital Sodium (Enhanced effects of CNS depressants). Products include:
Seconal Sodium Pulvules 1296

Sufentanil Citrate (Enhanced effects of CNS depressants). Products include:
Sufenta Injection 1147

Temazepam (Enhanced effects of CNS depressants). Products include:
Restoril Capsules 2023

Terbutaline Sulfate (Careful adjustment of dosages required). Products include:
Brethaire Inhaler 1024
Brethine Ampuls 1026
Brethine Tablets 1026
Bricanyl Injection 1324
Bricanyl Tablets 1325

Thiamylal Sodium (Enhanced effects of CNS depressants). Products include:
Surital Ampoules, Steri-Vials 1764

Thioridazine Hydrochloride (Enhanced effects of CNS depressants; hyperpyrexia). Products include:
Mellaril 2011

Thiothixene (Enhanced effects of CNS depressants; hyperpyrexia). Products include:
Navane Capsules and Concentrate 1954
Navane Intramuscular 1956

Thyroglobulin (Close supervision required). Products include:
Proloid Tablets 1761

Thyroid (Close supervision required). Products include:
S-P-T "Liquid" Capsules 995

Thyroxine (Close supervision required).
No products indexed under this heading.

Thyroxine Sodium (Close supervision required).
No products indexed under this heading.

Tranylcypromine Sulfate (Contraindication; hyperpyretic crises; severe convulsions; death). Products include:
Parnate Tablets 2222

Triazolam (Enhanced effects of CNS depressants). Products include:
Halcion Tablets 2340

Tridihexethyl Chloride (Hyperpyrexia; paralytic ileus; careful adjustment of dosages required).
No products indexed under this heading.

Trifluoperazine Hydrochloride (Enhanced effects of CNS depressants; hyperpyrexia). Products include:
Stelazine 2226

Trihexyphenidyl Hydrochloride (Hyperpyrexia; paralytic ileus; careful adjustment of dosages required). Products include:
Artane 1195

ELAVIL TABLETS
(Amitriptyline Hydrochloride) 2269
See **Elavil Injection**

ELDECORT CREAM 1.0%
(Hydrocortisone) 1113
No interactions described in labeling.

ELDECORT CREAM 1.0% AND 2.5%
(Hydrocortisone) 1113
No interactions described in labeling.

ELDEPRYL
(Selegiline Hydrochloride) 2250
May interact with narcotic analgesics, tricyclic antidepressants, and certain other agents. Compounds in these categories include:

Alfentanil Hydrochloride (Contraindication warning for meperidine is extended to other opiods). Products include:
Alfenta Injection 1131

Amitriptyline Hydrochloride (Concurrent use should be avoided). Products include:
Elavil 2269
Endep Tablets 1927
Etrafon 2087
Limbitrol 1933
Triavil Tablets 1556

Amoxapine (Concurrent use should be avoided). Products include:
Asendin Tablets 1196

Buprenorphine (Contraindication warning for meperidine is extended to other opiods).
No products indexed under this heading.

Clomipramine Hydrochloride (Concurrent use should be avoided). Products include:
Anafranil Capsules 650

Codeine (Contraindication warning for meperidine is extended to other opiods). Products include:
Calcidrine Syrup 506

Codeine Phosphate (Contraindication warning for meperidine is extended to other opiods). Products include:
Actifed with Codeine Cough Syrup 752
Cheracol Cough Syrup 1853
Codimal PH Syrup 846
Dimetane-DC Cough Syrup 1857
Empirin with Codeine Phosphate Nos. 2, 3 & 4 764
Fiorinal with Codeine Capsules 2008
Isoclor Expectorant 982
Naldecon CX Adult Liquid .... ▣ 521
Novahistine DH 1342
Novahistine Expectorant 1343
Nucofed Capsules 2219
Nucofed Expectorant 2219
Nucofed Pediatric Expectorant 2220
Nucofed Syrup 2219
Phenaphen with Codeine Capsules 1865
Phenaphen-650 with Codeine Tablets 1866
Phenergan with Codeine 2497
Phenergan VC with Codeine 2501
Robitussin A-C Syrup 1875
Robitussin-DAC Syrup 1875
Ryna .... ▣ 741
Soma Compound w/Codeine Tablets 2390
Triaminic Expectorant w/Codeine .. 1996
Tussi-Organidin Liquid 2391
Tylenol with Codeine 1381

Codeine Polistirex (Contraindication warning for meperidine is extended to other opiods).
No products indexed under this heading.

Desipramine Hydrochloride (Concurrent use should be avoided). Products include:
Norpramin Tablets 1340

Dezocine (Contraindication warning for meperidine is extended to other opiods).

Doxepin Hydrochloride (Concurrent use should be avoided). Products include:
Sinequan 1960

Fentanyl (Contraindication warning for meperidine is extended to other opiods). Products include:
Duragesic Transdermal System 1133

Fentanyl Citrate (Contraindication warning for meperidine is extended to other opiods). Products include:
Innovar Injection 1141
Sublimaze Injection 1146

Fluoxetine Hydrochloride (Potential for fatal reaction; at least 14 days should elapse between discontinuation of MAOI and initiation of treatment with fluoxetine). Products include:
Prozac Pulvules 920

Hydrocodone Bitartrate (Contraindication warning for meperidine is extended to other opiods). Products include:
Anexsia 5/500 Tablets 2196
Anexsia 7.5/650 Tablets 2197
Azdone Tablets 844
Codiclear DH Syrup 845
Codimal DH Syrup 846
Damason-P 1356
Hycodan Syrup, Tablets 927
Hycomine Compound Tablets 929
Hycomine Syrup 927
Hycotuss Expectorant Syrup 930
Hydrocet Capsules 835
Lortab ASA Tablets 2414
Lortab 2412
Ru-Tuss with Hydrocodone 694
Triaminic Expectorant DH 1995
Vicodin Tablets 1187
Vicodin ES Tablets 1189
Zydone Capsules 941

Hydrocodone Polistirex (Contraindication warning for meperidine is extended to other opiods). Products include:
Tussionex Extended-Release Suspension 988

Imipramine Hydrochloride (Concurrent use should be avoided). Products include:
Tofranil Ampuls 1038
Tofranil Tablets 1039

Imipramine Pamoate (Concurrent use should be avoided). Products include:
Tofranil-PM Capsules 1041

Levodopa (Potential exacerbation of levodopa associated side effects). Products include:
Larodopa Tablets 1905
Sinemet Tablets 952
Sinemet CR Tablets 953

Levorphanol Tartrate (Contraindication warning for meperidine is extended to other opiods). Products include:
Levo-Dromoran 1906

Maprotiline Hydrochloride (Concurrent use should be avoided). Products include:
Ludiomil Tablets 874

Meperidine Hydrochloride (Concurrent use is contraindicated; potential for muscular rigidity, stupor, severe agitation, and elevated temperature). Products include:
Demerol 2047
Mepergan Injection 2479

Methadone Hydrochloride (Contraindication warning for meperidine is extended to other opiods). Products include:
Dolophine Hydrochloride Ampoules & Vials 1260
Dolophine Hydrochloride Tablets 1261
Methadone Hydrochloride Diskets .. 1284
Methadone Hydrochloride Oral Solution & Tablets 1987

Morphine Sulfate (Contraindication warning for meperidine is extended to other opiods). Products include:
Astramorph/PF Injection, USP (Preservative-Free) 618
Duramorph 960
Infumorph 200 and Infumorph 500 Sterile Solutions 962
MS Contin Tablets 1814
MSIR 1817
Oramorph SR (Morphine Sulfate Sustained Release Tablets) 1988
Roxanol 1991

Nortriptyline Hydrochloride (Concurrent use should be avoided). Products include:
Pamelor 2019

Opium Alkaloids (Contraindication warning for meperidine is extended to other opiods). Products include:
B & O No. 15A & No. 16A Supprettes 2395
Pantopon Injectable 1911

Oxycodone Hydrochloride (Contraindication warning for meperidine is extended to other opiods). Products include:
Percocet Tablets 950
Percodan 951
Roxicodone Tablets, Oral Solution & Intensol (Oxycodone) 1992
Tylox Capsules 1382

Propoxyphene Hydrochloride (Contraindication warning for meperidine is extended to other opiods). Products include:
Darvon 1256
Wygesic Tablets 2540

Propoxyphene Napsylate (Contraindication warning for meperidine is extended to other opiods). Products include:
Darvon-N/Darvocet-N 1254

Protriptyline Hydrochloride (Concurrent use should be avoided). Products include:
Vivactil Tablets 1567

Sufentanil Citrate (Contraindication warning for meperidine is extended to other opiods). Products include:
Sufenta Injection 1147

Trimipramine Maleate (Concurrent use should be avoided). Products include:
Surmontil Capsules 2524

Food Interactions

Food with high concentration of tyramine (Potential for "cheese reaction" if attention is not paid to the dose dependent nature of selegine's selectivity).

ELDERTONIC
(Vitamins with Minerals) 1359
No interactions described in labeling.

ELDOPAQUE FORTE 4% CREAM
(Hydroquinone) 1114
No interactions described in labeling.

ELDOQUIN FORTE 4% CREAM
(Hydroquinone) 1114
No interactions described in labeling.

ELEMENTAL 028
(Dietary Supplement) 2149
No interactions described in labeling.

ELIMITE (PERMETHRIN) 5% CREAM
(Permethrin) 1082
No interactions described in labeling.

ELOCON CREAM 0.1%
(Mometasone Furoate) 2084
No interactions described in labeling.

ELOCON LOTION 0.1%
(Mometasone Furoate) 2084
No interactions described in labeling.

ELOCON OINTMENT 0.1%
(Mometasone Furoate) 2084
No interactions described in labeling.

ELSPAR
(Asparaginase) 1470
May interact with:

Methotrexate Sodium (Diminished or abolished effect of methotrexate on malignant cells). Products include:
Methotrexate Tablets, Parenteral, LPF Parenteral 1217
Rheumatrex Methotrexate Dose Pack 1234

Prednisone (Increased toxicity). Products include:
Deltasone Tablets 2332

Vincristine Sulfate (Increased toxicity). Products include:
Oncovin Solution Vials & Hyporets 1288

EMCYT CAPSULES
(Estramustine Phosphate Sodium) 1161
May interact with calcium preparations. Compounds in this category include:

Calcium Carbonate (Impaired absorption of Emcyt). Products include:
Alka-Mints Chewable Antacid .... ▣ 620
Alka-Seltzer Advanced Formula Antacid & Non-Aspirin Pain Reliever .... ▣ 620
Ascriptin A/D Caplets 1850
Regular Strength Ascriptin Tablets 1850
Balmex Baby Powder .... ▣ 590
Bayer Plus Aspirin Tablets .... ▣ 567
Biocal 500 mg Tablet Calcium Supplement .... ▣ 625
Bufferin Analgesic Tablets and Caplets .... ▣ 524
Caltrate 600 .... ▣ 583
Caltrate 600 + Iron .... ▣ 583
Caltrate 600 + Vitamin D .... ▣ 584
Caltrate, Jr. .... ▣ 583
Centrum, Jr. (Children's Chewable) + Extra Calcium .... ▣ 585
Di-Gel Antacid/Anti-Gas .... ▣ 697
Gerimed Tablets 972
Marblen .... ▣ 563
Natalins Rx 1391
Natalins Tablets 1391
Nephro-Calci Tablets 1826
Os-Cal 500 Chewable Tablets .... ▣ 596
Os-Cal 500 Tablets .... ▣ 597
Os-Cal 250+D Tablets .... ▣ 597
Os-Cal 500+D Tablets .... ▣ 597
Pramet FA 1974
Pramilet FA 1974

Rolaids (Calcium Rich/Sodium Free) ▣ 744
Extra Strength Rolaids ▣ 744
Thermotabs ▣ 619
Total Formula-2 (multivitamin/multimineral) 2377
Tums Liquid Extra ▣ 726
Zenate Tablets 2250

Calcium Chloride (Impaired absorption of Emcyt).
No products indexed under this heading.

Calcium Citrate (Impaired absorption of Emcyt). Products include:
Citracal Liquitab 1613
Total Formula-2 (multivitamin/multimineral) 2377

Calcium Glubionate (Impaired absorption of Emcyt). Products include:
Neo-Calglucon Syrup 2018

Food Interactions

Dairy products (Impairs the absorption of Emcyt).

Food, calcium-rich (Impairs the absorption of Emcyt).

EMETE-CON INTRAMUSCULAR/INTRAVENOUS

(Benzquinamide Hydrochloride) 1950
May interact with preanesthetic medications, vasopressors, and sympathomimetic aerosal brochodilators. Compounds in these categories include:

Albuterol (In simultaneous use, benzquinamide should be decreased). Products include:
Proventil Inhalation Aerosol 2117
Ventolin Inhalation Aerosol and Refill 583

Albuterol Sulfate (In simultaneous use, benzquinamide should be decreased). Products include:
Proventil Repetabs Tablets 2120
Proventil Solutions for Inhalation 0.5% and 0.083% 2118
Proventil Syrup 2119
Proventil Tablets 2120
Ventolin 583

Diazepam (Do not administer benzquinamide by IV route). Products include:
Valium Injectable 1937
Valium Tablets 1939
Valrelease Capsules 1923

Dobutamine Hydrochloride (In simultaneous use, benzquinamide should be decreased). Products include:
Dobutrex Solution Vials 1259

Dopamine Hydrochloride (In simultaneous use, benzquinamide should be decreased). Products include:
Intropin Injection 930

Droperidol (Do not administer benzquinamide by IV route). Products include:
Inapsine Injection 1140
Innovar Injection 1141

Ephedrine Hydrochloride (In simultaneous use, benzquinamide should be decreased). Products include:
Amesec ▣ 682
Primatene Tablets-M Formula 2421
Primatene Tablets-P Formula 2421
Primatene Tablets-Regular Formula 2421
Quadrinal Tablets 1183
Quelidrine Syrup 556
Tedral SA 1765

Ephedrine Sulfate (In simultaneous use, benzquinamide should be decreased). Products include:
Bronkaid Tablets ▣ 757
Bronkolixir ▣ 761
Bronkotabs Tablets ▣ 762
Marax Tablets & DF Syrup 1954
Pazo Hemorrhoid Ointment & Suppositories 752
Vicks Vatronol Nose Drops ▣ 666

Ephedrine Tannate (In simultaneous use, benzquinamide should be decreased). Products include:
Rynatuss 2388

Epinephrine Bitartrate (In simultaneous use, benzquinamide should be decreased). Products include:
AsthmaHaler Mist Epinephrine Bitartrate Bronchodilator ▣ 616
Bronkaid Mist Suspension ▣ 757
Primatene Mist Suspension 2421

Epinephrine Hydrochloride (In simultaneous use, benzquinamide should be decreased). Products include:
Adrenalin Chloride Solution 1:100 & 1:1,000 1689
Epifrin ⊚ 244
Glaucon ⊚ 218

Fentanyl Citrate (Do not administer benzquinamide by IV route). Products include:
Innovar Injection 1141
Sublimaze Injection 1146

Hydroxyzine Hydrochloride (Do not administer benzquinamide by IV route). Products include:
Atarax Tablets & Syrup 1941
Marax Tablets & DF Syrup 1954
Vistaril Intramuscular Solution 1970

Isoproterenol Hydrochloride (In simultaneous use, benzquinamide should be decreased; careful dosage adjustment required). Products include:
Isuprel Hydrochloride Injection 1:5000 2050
Isuprel Hydrochloride Mistometer 2051
Isuprel Hydrochloride Solution 1:200 & 1:100 2052
Norisodrine Aerotrol 540

Lorazepam (Do not administer benzquinamide by IV route). Products include:
Ativan Injection 2432
Ativan Tablets 2434

Meperidine Hydrochloride (Do not administer benzquinamide by IV route). Products include:
Demerol 2047
Mepergan Injection 2479

Metaproterenol Sulfate (In simultaneous use, benzquinamide should be decreased). Products include:
Alupent 674
Arm-a-Med Metaproterenol Sulfate Inhalation Solution, USP 617
Metaprel Inhalation Aerosol Bronchodilator 2014
Metaprel Inhalation Solution 2015
Metaprel 2015
Metaproterenol Sulfate Inhalation Solution, USP 912

Metaraminol Bitartrate (In simultaneous use, benzquinamide should be decreased). Products include:
Aramine Injection 1424

Methoxamine Hydrochloride (In simultaneous use, benzquinamide should be decreased). Products include:
Vasoxyl Injection 819

Morphine Sulfate (Do not administer benzquinamide by IV route). Products include:
Astramorph/PF Injection, USP (Preservative-Free) 618
Duramorph 960
Infumorph 200 and Infumorph 500 Sterile Solutions 962
MS Contin Tablets 1814
MSIR 1817
Oramorph SR (Morphine Sulfate Sustained Release Tablets) 1988
Roxanol 1991

Norepinephrine Bitartrate (I.V. use not with cardiovascular drugs; in simultaneous use, benzquinamide should be decreased). Products include:
Levophed Bitartrate Injection 2054

Pentobarbital Sodium (Do not administer benzquinamide by IV route). Products include:
Nembutal Sodium Capsules 534
Nembutal Sodium Solution 536
Nembutal Sodium Suppositories 538

Phenylephrine Bitartrate (In simultaneous use, benzquinamide should be decreased).
No products indexed under this heading.

Phenylephrine Hydrochloride (In simultaneous use, benzquinamide should be decreased). Products include:
AK-Dilate Solution 2.5% and 10% ⊚ 203
Atrohist Sprinkle Capsules 558
Cerose-DM 2443
Codimal 846
Comhist LA Capsules 1618
Congespirin For Children Aspirin Free Chewable Cold Tablets 748
Cyclomydril ⊚ 216
Deconsal Sprinkle Capsules 559
Dimetane Decongestant ▣ 673
Dristan Decongestant/Antihistamine/ Analgesic Coated Caplets ▣ 749
Dristan Cold Nasal Decongestant/ Antihistamine/ Analgesic Coated Tablets 2419
Dristan Advanced Formula Decongestant/Antihistamine/ Analgesic Tablets ▣ 749
Dristan Nasal Spray, Menthol 2419
Dristan Nasal Spray, Regular and Regular with Metered Pump 2419
Entex Capsules 1623
Entex Liquid 1623
Sinus Excedrin Analgesic, Decongestant Tablets & Caplets 750
Extendryl 994
4-Way Fast Acting Nasal Spray - Original Formula (regular & mentholated) & Metered Spray Pump (regular) 751
Hycomine Compound Tablets 929
Murocoll-2 Sterile Ophthalmic Solution ⊚ 261
Mydfrin 2.5% ⊚ 224
Naldecon Syrup, Tablets, Pediatric Drops and Pediatric Syrup 709
Neo-Synephrine Hydrochloride 1% Carpuject 2063
Neo-Synephrine Hydrochloride 1% Injection 2063
Neo-Synephrine Hydrochloride (Ophthalmic) 2064
Neo-Synephrine ▣ 759
Nöstril Nasal Decongestant ▣ 520
Novahistine Elixir ▣ 596
Phenergan VC 2500
Phenergan VC with Codeine 2501
Prefrin Liquifilm Vasoconstrictor and Lubricant Eye Drops ⊚ 254
Prefrin-A ⊚ 255
Quelidrine Syrup 556
Relief Vasoconstrictor and Lubricant Eye Drops ⊚ 256
Robitussin Night Relief ▣ 677
Ru-Tuss with Hydrocodone 694
Ru-Tuss Tablets 693
Vasosulf ⊚ 279
Vicks Sinex ▣ 665
Zincfrin ⊚ 230

Phenylephrine Tannate (In simultaneous use, benzquinamide should be decreased). Products include:
Rynatan 2387
Rynatuss 2388

Phenylpropanolamine Hydrochloride (In simultaneous use, benzquinamide should be decreased). Products include:
A.R.M. Allergy Relief Medicine Caplets ▣ 615
Acutrim ▣ 548
Allerest ▣ 559
BC Cold Powder ▣ 517
Cheracol Plus Head Cold/Cough Formula ▣ 667
Codimal Expectorant 846
Comtrex Multi-Symptom Cold Reliever Tablets/Caplets/Liqui-Gels/Liquid 745
Contac Continuous Action Decongestant/Antihistamine Capsules ▣ 710
Contac Maximum Strength Continuous Action Decongestant/ Antihistamine Caplets ▣ 709
Contac Severe Cold and Flu Formula Caplets ▣ 711
Coricidin 'D' Decongestant Tablets ▣ 695
Coricidin Demilets Tablets for Children ▣ 696
Demazin Nasal Decongestant/ Antihistamine Repetabs Tablets & Syrup ▣ 697
Dexatrim ▣ 733
Dimetane-DC Cough Syrup 1857
Dimetapp Elixir ▣ 673
Dimetapp DM Elixir ▣ 674
Dimetapp Extentabs ▣ 674
Dimetapp Plus Caplets ▣ 675
Dimetapp Tablets ▣ 675
Entex Capsules 1623
Entex LA Tablets 1623
Entex Liquid 1623
4-Way Cold Tablets 750
Hycomine Syrup 927
Naldecon CX Adult Liquid ▣ 521
Naldecon DX Adult Liquid ▣ 521
Naldecon DX Children's Syrup ▣ 522
Naldecon DX Pediatric Drops ▣ 522
Naldecon EX Children's Syrup ▣ 522
Naldecon EX Pediatric Drops ▣ 523
Naldecon Syrup, Tablets, Pediatric Drops and Pediatric Syrup 709
Nolamine Tablets 838
Nolex LA Tablets 838
Ornade Spansule Capsules 2221
Orthoxicol Cough Syrup ▣ 668
Propagest 839
Pyrroxate Capsules ▣ 669
Robitussin-CF ▣ 676
Ru-Tuss II Capsules 693
Ru-Tuss with Hydrocodone 694
Ru-Tuss Tablets 693
Sine-Off Sinus Medicine Tablets-Aspirin Formula ▣ 722
Sinulin 840
St. Joseph Cold Tablets for Children ▣ 704
Tavist-D Tablets 2035
Triaminic Allergy Tablets ▣ 688
Triaminic Chewables ▣ 688
Triaminic Cold Tablets ▣ 688
Triaminic Expectorant ▣ 688
Triaminic Expectorant w/Codeine 1996
Triaminic Expectorant DH 1995
Triaminic Oral Infant Drops 1996
Triaminic Syrup ▣ 689
Triaminic-12 Tablets ▣ 690
Triaminic-DM Syrup ▣ 689
Triaminicin Tablets ▣ 690
Triaminicol Multi-Symptom Cold Tablets ▣ 691
Triaminicol Multi-Symptom Relief ▣ 691
Tuss-Ornade Liquid 2242
Tuss-Ornade Spansule Capsules 2242
Tylenol Cold Medication, Effervescent Tablets 1369

Pirbuterol Acetate (In simultaneous use, benzquinamide should be decreased). Products include:
Maxair Inhaler 1311

Promethazine (Do not administer benzquinamide by IV route).

Promethazine Hydrochloride (Do not administer benzquinamide by IV route). Products include:
Mepergan Injection 2479
Phenergan with Codeine 2497
Phenergan with Dextromethorphan 2499
Phenergan Injection 2493
Phenergan Suppositories 2496
Phenergan Syrup 2495
Phenergan Tablets 2496
Phenergan VC 2500
Phenergan VC with Codeine 2501

Pseudoephedrine Hydrochloride (In simultaneous use, benzquinamide should be decreased). Products include:
Actifed Capsules ▣ 539
Actifed Plus Caplets ▣ 539

Actifed Plus Tablets ■ 540
Actifed with Codeine Cough Syrup 752
Actifed Syrup ■ 540
Actifed Tablets ■ 540
Actifed 12-Hour Capsules ■ 539
Advil Cold & Sinus Caplets (formerly CoAdvil) 2416
Allerest ■ 559
Anatuss LA Tablets 1359
Benadryl Decongestant Elixir ■ 635
Benadryl Decongestant ■ 635
Benadryl Plus ■ 636
Benadryl Plus Nighttime ■ 637
Benylin Decongestant ■ 638
Brexin L.A. Capsules 2078
Bromfed Capsules (Timed Release) 1615
Bromfed Syrup ■ 628
Bromfed 1615
CoAdvil ■ 748
Allergy-Sinus Comtrex Multi-Symptom Allergy Sinus Formula Tablets & Caplets 746
Cough Formula Comtrex 746
Comtrex Multi-Symptom Cold Reliever Tablets/Caplets/Liqui-Gels/Liquid 745
Day-Night Comtrex 747
Non-Drowsy Comtrex 747
Congess 994
Congestac Caplets ■ 617
Contac Jr. Children's Cold Medicine ■ 712
Contac Nighttime Cold Medicine ■ 713
Contac Sinus Caplets Maximum Strength Non-Drowsy Formula ■ 710
Contac Sinus Tablets Maximum Strength Non-Drowsy Formula ■ 710
Deconamine 663
Deconsal II Tablets 559
Dimacol Caplets ■ 672
Dimetane-DX Cough Syrup 1858
Dorcol Children's Cough Syrup ■ 685
Dorcol Children's Decongestant Liquid ■ 685
Dorcol Children's Liquid Cold Formula ■ 686
Maximum Strength Dristan Decongestant/Analgesic Coated Caplets ■ 750
No Drowsiness Dristan Cold Nasal Decongestant/Analgesic Coated Caplets 2420
Dristan Sinus Caplets 2419
Sinus Excedrin Analgesic, Decongestant Tablets & Caplets ■ 533
Fedahist Gyrocaps 2145
Fedahist Timecaps 2145
Guaifed 1615
Guaifed Syrup ■ 629
Isoclor Expectorant 982
Isoclor Timesule Capsules ■ 561
Kronofed-A 970
Medi-Flu Caplet, Liquid ■ 640
Novafed A Capsules 1342
Novafed Capsules 1342
Novahistine DH 1342
Novahistine DMX ■ 595
Novahistine Expectorant 1343
Nucofed Capsules 2219
Nucofed Expectorant 2219
Nucofed Pediatric Expectorant 2220
Nucofed Syrup 2219
Ornex Caplets ■ 618
PediaCare Allergy Relief Formula Liquid 1362
PediaCare Cough-Cold Formula Liquid 1362
PediaCare Infants' Oral Decongestant Drops 1362
PediaCare Night Rest Cough-Cold Formula Liquid 1362
PediaCare 6-12 Cough-Cold Formula Chewable Tablets 1362
Robitussin-DAC Syrup 1875
Robitussin-PE ■ 677
Rondec 1975
Rondec-DM 1976
Rondec-TR Tablet 1975
Ru-Tuss DE Tablets 694
Ryna ■ 741
Seldane-D Extended-Release Tablets 1350
Sinarest ■ 562
Sine-Aid Maximum Strength Sinus Headache Caplets 1365
Sine-Aid Maximum Strength Sinus Headache Tablets 1365
Sine-Off Maximum Strength Allergy/Sinus Formula Caplets ■ 721
Sine-Off Maximum Strength No Drowsiness Formula Caplets ■ 722
Singlet Tablets ■ 598
Sinutab Maximum Strength ■ 641
Sinutab Maximum Strength Without Drowsiness Tablets & Caplets ■ 642
Sinutab Regular Strength Without Drowsiness Formula ■ 641
St. Joseph Nighttime Cold Medicine ■ 705
Sudafed Children's Liquid ■ 543
Sudafed Cough Syrup ■ 543
Sudafed Plus Liquid ■ 544
Sudafed Plus Tablets ■ 545
Sudafed Sinus Caplets ■ 545
Sudafed Sinus Tablets ■ 545
Sudafed Tablets, 30 mg ■ 544
Sudafed Tablets, Adult Strength, 60 mg ■ 544
Sudafed 12 Hour Capsules ■ 545
TheraFlu Flu and Cold Medicine ■ 687
Triaminic Nite Light ■ 689
Tylenol Allergy Sinus Medication Caplets and Gelcaps, Maximum Strength 1372
Children's Tylenol Cold Liquid Formula and Chewable Tablets 1368
Tylenol Cold & Flu Hot Medication, Packets 1369
Tylenol Cold & Flu No Drowsiness Hot Medication, Packets 1371
Tylenol Cold Medication Caplets and Tablets 1370
Tylenol Cold Medication No Drowsiness Formula Caplets 1370
Tylenol Cold Night Time Medication Liquid 1371
Tylenol Cough Medication Liquid with Decongestant, Maximum Strength 1372
Tylenol, Maximum Strength, Sinus Medication Gelcaps, Caplets and Tablets 1373
Ursinus Inlay-Tabs ■ 691
Vicks Children's NyQuil ■ 664
Vicks Daycare ■ 660
Vicks Formula 44D Decongestant Cough Medicine ■ 662
Vicks Formula 44M Multi-Symptom Cough Medicine ■ 662
Vicks NyQuil Nighttime Colds Medicine-Original & Cherry Flavor ■ 664
Vicks Pediatric Formula 44 Cough & Congestion Medicine ■ 663
Vicks Pediatric Formula 44m Multi-Symptom Cough & Cold Medicine ■ 663

Pseudoephedrine Sulfate (In simultaneous use, benzquinamide should be decreased). Products include:
Afrin Tablets ■ 693
Chlor-Trimeton Decongestant ■ 694
Disophrol Chronotab Sustained-Action Tablets ■ 698
Drixoral Antihistamine/Nasal Decongestant Syrup ■ 698
Drixoral Non-Drowsy Formula ■ 699
Drixoral Plus Extended-Release Tablets ■ 699
Drixoral Sinus ■ 700
Drixoral Sustained-Action Tablets ■ 698
Sinutab Allergy Formula Sustained Action Tablets ■ 640
Trinalin Repetabs Tablets 1170

Secobarbital Sodium (Do not administer benzquinamide by IV route). Products include:
Seconal Sodium Pulvules 1296

Terbutaline Sulfate (In simultaneous use, benzquinamide should be decreased). Products include:
Brethaire Inhaler 1024
Brethine Ampuls 1026
Brethine Tablets 1026
Bricanyl Injection 1324
Bricanyl Tablets 1325

EMETROL
(Phosphorated Carbohydrate Solution) 564
No interactions described in labeling.

EMINASE
(Anistreplase) 2211
May interact with anticoagulants, platelet inhibitors, and certain other agents. Compounds in these categories include:

Aspirin (Increases risk of bleeding and bleeding events). Products include:
Alka-Seltzer Effervescent Antacid and Pain Reliever 1568
Alka-Seltzer Extra Strength Effervescent Antacid and Pain Reliever 1570
Alka-Seltzer (Flavored) Effervescent Antacid and Pain Reliever 1569
Alka-Seltzer Plus Cold Medicine ■ 623
Alka-Seltzer Plus Night-Time Cold Medicine ■ 623
Alka Seltzer Plus Sinus Allergy Medicine ■ 624
Anacin Coated Analgesic Caplets 2417
Anacin Coated Analgesic Tablets 2417
Anacin Maximum Strength Analgesic Coated Tablets 2417
Maximum Strength Arthritis Pain Formula By the Makers of Anacin Analgesic Tablets and Caplets 2418
Arthritis Pain Formula by the Makers of Anacin Analgesic Tablets and Caplets ■ 747
Arthritis Strength BC Powder ■ 516
Ascriptin A/D Caplets 1850
Regular Strength Ascriptin Tablets 1850
Azdōne Tablets 844
BC Powder ■ 517
BC Cold Powder ■ 517
Children's Bayer Chewable Aspirin ■ 564
Genuine Bayer Aspirin Tablets & Caplets ■ 564
Maximum Bayer Aspirin Tablets & Caplets ■ 566
Bayer Plus Aspirin Tablets ■ 567
Therapy Bayer Aspirin Caplets ■ 568
8 Hour Bayer Timed-Release Aspirin ■ 566
Arthritis Strength Bufferin Analgesic Caplets 744
Extra Strength Bufferin Analgesic Tablets 745
Bufferin Analgesic Tablets and Caplets 743
Cama Arthritis Pain Reliever ■ 685
Damason-P 1356
Easprin 1719
Ecotrin Enteric Coated Aspirin Maximum Strength Tablets and Caplets 2189
Ecotrin Enteric Coated Aspirin Regular Strength Tablets and Caplets 2189
Empirin Aspirin ■ 541
Empirin with Codeine Phosphate Nos. 2, 3 & 4 764
Equagesic Tablets 2451
Excedrin Extra-Strength Analgesic Tablets & Caplets 749
4-Way Cold Tablets 750
Fiorinal Capsules 2007
Fiorinal with Codeine Capsules 2008
Fiorinal Tablets 2007
Lortab ASA Tablets 2414
Momentum Muscular Backache Formula ■ 751
Norgesic 1314
Norwich Extra-Strength Aspirin ■ 546
Norwich Regular Strength Aspirin ■ 547
P-A-C Analgesic Tablets ■ 669
Percodan 951
Robaxisal Tablets 1872
Sine-Off Sinus Medicine Tablets-Aspirin Formula ■ 722
Soma Compound w/Codeine Tablets 2390
Soma Compound Tablets 2389
St. Joseph Adult Chewable Aspirin (81 mg.) ■ 703
Synalgos-DC Capsules 2525
Talwin Compound 2072
Ursinus Inlay-Tabs ■ 691
Vanquish Analgesic Caplets ■ 574
Zorprin Tablets 698

Azlocillin Sodium (Increases risk of bleeding and bleeding events).
No products indexed under this heading.

Carbenicillin Indanyl Sodium (Increases risk of bleeding and bleeding events). Products include:
Geocillin Tablets 1951

Choline Magnesium Trisalicylate (Increases risk of bleeding and bleeding events). Products include:
Trilisate 1822

Diclofenac Sodium (Increases risk of bleeding and bleeding events). Products include:
Voltaren Ophthalmic Sterile Ophthalmic Solution ⊙ 268
Voltaren Tablets 1042

Dicumarol (Potential for bleeding and bleeding complications). Products include:
Dicumarol Tablets 516

Diflunisal (Increases risk of bleeding and bleeding events). Products include:
Dolobid Tablets 1465

Dipyridamole (Increases risk of bleeding and bleeding events). Products include:
Persantine Tablets 683

Fenoprofen Calcium (Increases risk of bleeding and bleeding events). Products include:
Nalfon Pulvules & Tablets 919

Flurbiprofen (Increases risk of bleeding and bleeding events). Products include:
Ansaid Tablets 2319

Heparin Calcium (Potential for bleeding and bleeding complications). Products include:
Calciparine Injection 925

Heparin Sodium (Potential for bleeding and bleeding complications). Products include:
Heparin Lock Flush Solution 2456
Heparin Sodium Vials 1264
Heparin Sodium Injection 2457
Heparin Sodium Injection, USP, Sterile Solution 2342

Ibuprofen (Increases risk of bleeding and bleeding events). Products include:
Advil Cold & Sinus Caplets (formerly CoAdvil) 2416
Advil Ibuprofen Tablets and Caplets 2416
Children's Advil Suspension 2426
CoAdvil ■ 748
Dristan Sinus Caplets 2419
Haltran Tablets ■ 668
Ibuprofen ■ 631
Medipren ibuprofen Caplets and Tablets 1362
Midol 200 Cramp Relief Formula ■ 570
Motrin Tablets 2351
Motrin IB Caplets and Tablets ■ 736
Nuprin Ibuprofen/Analgesic Tablets & Caplets 752
PediaProfen Suspension 1363
Rufen Tablets 691
Trendar Ibuprofen Tablets ■ 756

Indomethacin (Increases risk of bleeding and bleeding events). Products include:
Indocin 1487

Indomethacin Sodium Trihydrate (Increases risk of bleeding and bleeding events). Products include:
Indocin I.V. 1490

Ketoprofen (Increases risk of bleeding and bleeding events). Products include:
Orudis Capsules 2488

Magnesium Salicylate (Increases risk of bleeding and bleeding events). Products include:
Doan's - Extra-Strength Analgesic ■ 549
Doan's - Regular Strength Analgesic ■ 549
Mobigesic Analgesic Tablets ■ 507

Meclofenamate Sodium (Increases risk of bleeding and bleeding events). Products include:
Meclomen Capsules 1739

Mefenamic Acid (Increases risk of bleeding and bleeding events). Products include:
- Ponstel 1758

Mezlocillin Sodium (Increases risk of bleeding and bleeding events). Products include:
- Mezlin 1597
- Mezlin Pharmacy Bulk Package 1599

Nafcillin Sodium (Increases risk of bleeding and bleeding events). Products include:
- Unipen 2533

Naproxen (Increases risk of bleeding and bleeding events). Products include:
- Naprosyn 2297

Naproxen Sodium (Increases risk of bleeding and bleeding events). Products include:
- Anaprox and Anaprox DS Tablets 2288

Penicillin G Procaine (Increases risk of bleeding and bleeding events). Products include:
- Bicillin C-R Injection 2438
- Bicillin C-R 900/300 Injection 2440
- Pfizerpen-AS Aqueous Suspension 1959
- Wycillin Injection 2537
- Wycillin Injection and Probenecid Tablets 2539

Penicillin G, Benzathine (Increases risk of bleeding and bleeding events). Products include:
- Bicillin C-R Injection 2438
- Bicillin C-R 900/300 Injection 2440
- Bicillin L-A Injection 2442

Phenylbutazone (Increases risk of bleeding and bleeding events). Products include:
- Butazolidin Capsules & Tablets 1027

Piroxicam (Increases risk of bleeding and bleeding events). Products include:
- Feldene Capsules 1777

Salsalate (Increases risk of bleeding and bleeding events). Products include:
- Disalcid 1310
- Mono-Gesic Tablets 846
- Salflex 839

Sulindac (Increases risk of bleeding and bleeding events). Products include:
- Clinoril Tablets 1433

Ticarcillin Disodium (Increases risk of bleeding and bleeding events). Products include:
- Ticar for Injection 2236
- Timentin for Injection 2239

Tolmetin Sodium (Increases risk of bleeding and bleeding events). Products include:
- Tolectin (200, 400 and 600 mg) 1379

Warfarin Sodium (Potential for bleeding and bleeding complications). Products include:
- Coumadin Injection & Tablets 944
- Panwarfin Tablets 547

EMKO BECAUSE CONTRACEPTOR VAGINAL CONTRACEPTIVE FOAM
(Nonoxynol-9) ▣ 700
No interactions described in labeling.

EMKO VAGINAL CONTRACEPTIVE FOAM
(Nonoxynol-9) ▣ 701
No interactions described in labeling.

EMPIRIN ASPIRIN
(Aspirin) ▣ 541
May interact with oral anticoagulants. Compounds in this category include:

Dicumarol (Concurrent administration is not recommended). Products include:
- Dicumarol Tablets 516

Warfarin Sodium (Concurrent administration is not recommended). Products include:
- Coumadin Injection & Tablets 944
- Panwarfin Tablets 547

EMPIRIN WITH CODEINE PHOSPHATE NOS. 2, 3 & 4
(Aspirin, Codeine Phosphate) 764
May interact with central nervous system depressants, monoamine oxidase inhibitors, oral anticoagulants, oral hypoglycemic agents, penicillins, sulfonamides, non-steroidal anti-inflammatory agents, narcotic analgesics, general anesthetics, tranquilizers, corticosteroids, hypnotics and sedatives, and certain other agents. Compounds in these categories include:

Alcohol (Increased CNS depressant).

Alfentanil Hydrochloride (Increased CNS depression). Products include:
- Alfenta Injection 1131

Alprazolam (Increased CNS depression). Products include:
- Xanax Tablets 2367

Amoxicillin (Enhanced effect). Products include:
- Amoxil 2193
- Augmentin Tablets, Powder for Oral Suspension, and Chewable Tablets 2198

Ampicillin Sodium (Enhanced effect). Products include:
- Unasyn 1965

Aprobarbital (Increased CNS depression). Products include:
- Alurate Elixir 1883

Azlocillin Sodium (Enhanced effect).
- No products indexed under this heading.

Bacampicillin Hydrochloride (Enhanced effect). Products include:
- Spectrobid Tablets & Powder for Oral Suspension 1961

Betamethasone Acetate (Steroid effects potentiated). Products include:
- Celestone Soluspan Suspension 2081

Betamethasone Sodium Phosphate (Steroid effects potentiated). Products include:
- Celestone Soluspan Suspension 2081

Buprenorphine (Increased CNS depression).
- No products indexed under this heading.

Buspirone Hydrochloride (Increased CNS depression). Products include:
- BuSpar 1401

Butabarbital (Increased CNS depression). Products include:
- Pyridium Plus 1764

Butalbital (Increased CNS depression). Products include:
- Esgic-Plus Tablets 1002
- Esgic Tablets & Capsules 1001
- Fioricet Tablets 2006
- Fiorinal Capsules 2007
- Fiorinal with Codeine Capsules 2008
- Fiorinal Tablets 2007
- Phrenilin 838
- Sedapap Tablets 50 mg/650 mg 1360

Carbenicillin Disodium (Enhanced effect).

Carbenicillin Indanyl Sodium (Enhanced effect). Products include:
- Geocillin Tablets 1951

Chlordiazepoxide (Increased CNS depression). Products include:
- Libritabs Tablets 1930
- Limbitrol 1933
- Menrium Tablets 1934

Chlordiazepoxide Hydrochloride (Increased CNS depression). Products include:
- Librax Capsules 1929
- Librium Capsules 1931
- Librium Injectable 1932

Chlorpromazine (Increased CNS depression). Products include:
- Thorazine 2234

Chlorpropamide (May result in hypoglycemia). Products include:
- Diabinese Tablets 1775

Chlorprothixene (Increased CNS depression). Products include:
- Taractan Tablets 1920

Chlorprothixene Hydrochloride (Increased CNS depression). Products include:
- Taractan 1920

Chlorprothixene Lactate (Increased CNS depression). Products include:
- Taractan Concentrate 1920

Clorazepate Dipotassium (Increased CNS depression). Products include:
- Tranxene 556

Codeine (Increased CNS depression). Products include:
- Calcidrine Syrup 506

Codeine Polistirex (Increased CNS depression).
- No products indexed under this heading.

Colchicine (Diminished uricosoric effect). Products include:
- ColBENEMID Tablets 1436
- Colchicine Ampoules 1252

Cortisone Acetate (Steroid effects potentiated). Products include:
- Cortone Acetate Sterile Suspension 1437
- Cortone Acetate Tablets 1439

Dexamethasone (Steroid effects potentiated). Products include:
- AK-Trol Ointment & Suspension ◉ 207
- Decadron Elixir 1445
- Decadron Tablets 1447
- Decaspray Topical Aerosol 1459
- Dexacidin ◉ 272
- Maxidex Sterile Ophthalmic Suspension ◉ 223
- Maxitrol Ophthalmic Ointment/Suspension ◉ 223
- TobraDex Ophthalmic Suspension and Ointment ◉ 228

Dexamethasone Acetate (Steroid effects potentiated). Products include:
- Dalalone D.P. Injectable 999
- Decadron-LA Sterile Suspension 1457

Dexamethasone Sodium Phosphate (Steroid effects potentiated). Products include:
- AK-Dex ◉ 203
- Decadron Phosphate Respihaler 1454
- Decadron Phosphate Sterile Ophthalmic Ointment 1453
- Decadron Phosphate Sterile Ophthalmic Solution 1453
- Decadron Phosphate Topical Cream 1455
- Decadron Phosphate Turbinaire 1456
- Maxidex Sterile Ophthalmic Ointment ◉ 222
- NeoDecadron Sterile Ophthalmic Ointment 1517
- NeoDecadron Sterile Ophthalmic Solution 1518
- NeoDecadron Topical Cream 1518

Dezocine (Increased CNS depression).

Diazepam (Increased CNS depression). Products include:
- Valium Injectable 1937
- Valium Tablets 1939
- Valrelease Capsules 1923

Diclofenac Sodium (Enhanced effect of NSAID). Products include:
- Voltaren Ophthalmic Sterile Ophthalmic Solution ◉ 268
- Voltaren Tablets 1042

Dicumarol (Enhanced effect, bleeding). Products include:
- Dicumarol Tablets 516

Droperidol (Increased CNS depression). Products include:
- Inapsine Injection 1140
- Innovar Injection 1141

Enflurane (Increased CNS depression). Products include:
- Ethrane 599

Estazolam (Increased CNS depression). Products include:
- ProSom Tablets 554

Ethchlorvynol (Increased CNS depression). Products include:
- Placidyl Capsules 553

Ethinamate (Increased CNS depression).
- No products indexed under this heading.

Etodolac (Enhanced effect of NSAID). Products include:
- Lodine Capsules 2468

Fenoprofen Calcium (Enhanced effect of NSAID). Products include:
- Nalfon Pulvules & Tablets 919

Fentanyl (Increased CNS depression). Products include:
- Duragesic Transdermal System 1133

Fentanyl Citrate (Increased CNS depression). Products include:
- Innovar Injection 1141
- Sublimaze Injection 1146

Fluphenazine Decanoate (Increased CNS depression). Products include:
- Prolixin Decanoate 1795

Fluphenazine Enanthate (Increased CNS depression). Products include:
- Prolixin Enanthate 1796

Fluphenazine Hydrochloride (Increased CNS depression). Products include:
- Prolixin Elixir 1793
- Prolixin Injection 1791
- Prolixin Oral Concentrate 1792
- Prolixin Tablets 1793

Flurazepam Hydrochloride (Increased CNS depression). Products include:
- Dalmane Capsules 1927

Flurbiprofen (Enhanced effect of NSAID). Products include:
- Ansaid Tablets 2319

Furazolidone (Enhanced effect). Products include:
- Furoxone 1855

Furosemide (Causes aspirin accumulation). Products include:
- Lasix 1093

Glipizide (May result in hypoglycemia). Products include:
- Glucotrol 1952

Glutethimide (Increased CNS depression).
- No products indexed under this heading.

Glyburide (May result in hypoglycemia). Products include:
- DiaBeta 1091
- Micronase Tablets 2350

Haloperidol (Increased CNS depression). Products include:
- Haldol Injection, Tablets and Concentrate 1373

Haloperidol Decanoate (Increased CNS depression). Products include:
- Haldol Decanoate ... 1375

Hydrocodone Bitartrate (Increased CNS depression). Products include:
- Anexsia 5/500 Tablets ... 2196
- Anexsia 7.5/650 Tablets ... 2197
- Azdone Tablets ... 844
- Codiclear DH Syrup ... 845
- Codimal DH Syrup ... 846
- Damason-P ... 1356
- Hycodan Syrup, Tablets ... 927
- Hycomine Compound Tablets ... 929
- Hycomine Syrup ... 927
- Hycotuss Expectorant Syrup ... 930
- Hydrocet Capsules ... 835
- Lortab ASA Tablets ... 2414
- Lortab ... 2412
- Ru-Tuss with Hydrocodone ... 694
- Triaminic Expectorant DH ... 1995
- Vicodin Tablets ... 1187
- Vicodin ES Tablets ... 1189
- Zydone Capsules ... 941

Hydrocodone Polistirex (Increased CNS depression). Products include:
- Tussionex Extended-Release Suspension ... 988

Hydrocortisone Acetate (Steroid effects potentiated). Products include:
- Analpram-HC Rectal Cream 1% and 2.5% ... 970
- Anusol-HC Cream ... 1690
- Anusol-HC Suppositories ... 1691
- Caldecort ... ⊡ 560
- Carmol HC Cream 1% ... 2296
- Chloromycetin Hydrocortisone Ophthalmic ... 1694
- Coly-Mycin S Otic w/Neomycin & Hydrocortisone ... 1708
- Cortaid ... ⊡ 735
- Cortef Feminine Itch Cream ... ⊡ 735
- Corticaine ... ⊡ 682
- Cortifoam ... 1827
- Cortisporin Cream ... 757
- Epifoam ... 1828
- Gynecort 5 Creme ... ⊡ 556
- Hydrocortone Acetate Sterile Suspension ... 1479
- Lanacort 5 Creme and Ointment .. ⊡ 557
- Mantadil Cream ... 789
- Ophthocort ... ⊙ 301
- Orabase HCA Oral Paste ... 890
- Pramosone Cream, Lotion & Ointment ... 971
- ProctoCream-HC ... 1834
- Proctofoam-HC ... 1835

Hydrocortisone Sodium Phosphate (Steroid effects potentiated). Products include:
- Hydrocortone Phosphate Injection, Sterile ... 1481

Hydrocortisone Sodium Succinate (Steroid effects potentiated). Products include:
- Solu-Cortef Sterile Powder ... 2361

Hydroxyzine Hydrochloride (Increased CNS depression). Products include:
- Atarax Tablets & Syrup ... 1941
- Marax Tablets & DF Syrup ... 1954
- Vistaril Intramuscular Solution ... 1970

Ibuprofen (Enhanced effect of NSAID). Products include:
- Advil Cold & Sinus Caplets (formerly CoAdvil) ... 2416
- Advil Ibuprofen Tablets and Caplets ... 2416
- Children's Advil Suspension ... 2426
- CoAdvil ... ⊡ 748
- Dristan Sinus Caplets ... 2419
- Haltran Tablets ... ⊡ 668
- Ibuprofen ... ⊡ 631
- Medipren ibuprofen Caplets and Tablets ... 1362
- Midol 200 Cramp Relief Formula .. ⊡ 570
- Motrin Tablets ... 2351
- Motrin IB Caplets and Tablets ... ⊡ 736
- Nuprin Ibuprofen/Analgesic Tablets & Caplets ... 752
- PediaProfen Suspension ... 1363
- Rufen Tablets ... 691
- Trendar Ibuprofen Tablets ... ⊡ 756

Indomethacin (Enhanced effect of NSAID). Products include:
- Indocin ... 1487

Indomethacin Sodium Trihydrate (Enhanced effect of NSAID). Products include:
- Indocin I.V. ... 1490

Isocarboxazid (Enhanced effect). Products include:
- Marplan Tablets ... 1906

Isoflurane (Increased CNS depression). Products include:
- Forane ... 600

Ketamine Hydrochloride (Increased CNS depression). Products include:
- Ketalar ... 1726

Ketoprofen (Enhanced effect of NSAID). Products include:
- Orudis Capsules ... 2488

Ketorolac Tromethamine (Enhanced effect of NSAID). Products include:
- Toradol IM Injection ... 2302

Levorphanol Tartrate (Increased CNS depression). Products include:
- Levo-Dromoran ... 1906

Lorazepam (Increased CNS depression). Products include:
- Ativan Injection ... 2432
- Ativan Tablets ... 2434

Loxapine Hydrochloride (Increased CNS depression). Products include:
- Loxitane ... 1213

Loxapine Succinate (Increased CNS depression). Products include:
- Loxitane Capsules ... 1213

Meclofenamate Sodium (Enhanced effect of NSAID). Products include:
- Meclomen Capsules ... 1739

Mefenamic Acid (Enhanced effect of NSAIDS). Products include:
- Ponstel ... 1758

Meperidine Hydrochloride (Increased CNS depression). Products include:
- Demerol ... 2047
- Mepergan Injection ... 2479

Mephobarbital (Increased CNS depression). Products include:
- Mebaral Tablets ... 2061

Meprobamate (Increased CNS depression). Products include:
- Deprol Tablets ... 2382
- Equagesic Tablets ... 2451
- Miltown Tablets ... 2386
- PMB 200 and PMB 400 ... 2504

Mercaptopurine (Enhanced bone marrow toxicity and blood dyscrasias). Products include:
- Purinethol Tablets ... 800

Mesoridazine (Increased CNS depression). Products include:
- Serentil ... 686

Methadone Hydrochloride (Increased CNS depression). Products include:
- Dolophine Hydrochloride Ampoules & Vials ... 1260
- Dolophine Hydrochloride Tablets ... 1261
- Methadone Hydrochloride Diskets .. 1284
- Methadone Hydrochloride Oral Solution & Tablets ... 1987

Methohexital Sodium (Increased CNS depression). Products include:
- Brevital Sodium Vials ... 1248

Methoxyflurane (Increased CNS depression).
- No products indexed under this heading.

Methylprednisolone (Steroid effects potentiated). Products include:
- Medrol ... 2348

Methylprednisolone Acetate (Steroid effects potentiated). Products include:
- Depo-Medrol Sterile Aqueous Suspension ... 2334

Methylprednisolone Sodium Succinate (Steroid effects potentiated). Products include:
- Solu-Medrol Sterile Powder ... 2363

Mezlocillin Sodium (Enhanced effect). Products include:
- Mezlin ... 1597
- Mezlin Pharmacy Bulk Package ... 1599

Midazolam Hydrochloride (Increased CNS depression). Products include:
- Versed Injection ... 1924

Molindone Hydrochloride (Increased CNS depression). Products include:
- Moban Tablets & Concentrate ... 932

Morphine Sulfate (Increased CNS depression). Products include:
- Astramorph/PF Injection, USP (Preservative-Free) ... 618
- Duramorph ... 960
- Infumorph 200 and Infumorph 500 Sterile Solutions ... 962
- MS Contin Tablets ... 1814
- MSIR ... 1817
- Oramorph SR (Morphine Sulfate Sustained Release Tablets) ... 1988
- Roxanol ... 1991

Nafcillin Sodium (Enhanced effect). Products include:
- Unipen ... 2533

Naproxen (Enhanced effect of NSAID). Products include:
- Naprosyn ... 2297

Naproxen Sodium (Enhanced effect of NSAID). Products include:
- Anaprox and Anaprox DS Tablets 2288

Opium Alkaloids (Increased CNS depression). Products include:
- B & O No. 15A & No. 16A Supprettes ... 2395
- Pantopon Injectable ... 1911

Oxazepam (Increased CNS depression). Products include:
- Serax Capsules ... 2522
- Serax Tablets ... 2522

Oxycodone Hydrochloride (Increased CNS depression). Products include:
- Percocet Tablets ... 950
- Percodan ... 951
- Roxicodone Tablets, Oral Solution & Intensol (Oxycodone) ... 1992
- Tylox Capsules ... 1382

Penicillin G Potassium (Enhanced effect). Products include:
- Pfizerpen for Injection ... 1957

Penicillin G Procaine (Enhanced effect). Products include:
- Bicillin C-R Injection ... 2438
- Bicillin C-R 900/300 Injection ... 2440
- Pfizerpen-AS Aqueous Suspension 1959
- Wycillin Injection ... 2537
- Wycillin Injection and Probenecid Tablets ... 2539

Penicillin G Sodium (Enhanced effect).
- No products indexed under this heading.

Penicillin G, Benzathine (Enhanced effect). Products include:
- Bicillin C-R Injection ... 2438
- Bicillin C-R 900/300 Injection ... 2440
- Bicillin L-A Injection ... 2442

Penicillin V Potassium (Enhanced effect).
- No products indexed under this heading.

Pentobarbital Sodium (Increased CNS depression). Products include:
- Nembutal Sodium Capsules ... 534
- Nembutal Sodium Solution ... 536
- Nembutal Sodium Suppositories ... 538

Perphenazine (Increased CNS depression). Products include:
- Etrafon ... 2087
- Triavil Tablets ... 1556
- Trilafon ... 2123

Phenelzine Sulfate (Enhanced effect). Products include:
- Nardil ... 1742

Phenobarbital (Increased CNS depression). Products include:
- Arco-Lase Plus Tablets ... 607
- Bellergal-S Tablets ... 1998
- Bronkolixir ... ⊡ 761
- Bronkotabs Tablets ... ⊡ 762
- Donnatal ... 1858
- Donnatal Extentabs ... 1859
- Donnatal Tablets ... 1858
- Donnazyme Tablets ... 1860
- Kinesed Tablets ... 2272
- Phenobarbital Elixir and Tablets ... 1293
- Primatene Tablets-P Formula ... 2421
- Quadrinal Tablets ... 1183
- Tedral SA ... 1765

Phenylbutazone (Enhanced effect of NSAID). Products include:
- Butazolidin Capsules & Tablets ... 1027

Piroxicam (Enhanced effect of NSAID). Products include:
- Feldene Capsules ... 1777

Prazepam (Increased CNS depression). Products include:
- Centrax ... 1693

Prednisolone Acetate (Steroid effects potentiated). Products include:
- AK-Cide Sterile Ophthalmic Ointment & Suspension ... ⊙ 202
- Blephamide Liquifilm Sterile Ophthalmic Suspension ... 586
- Blephamide S.O.P. Sterile Ophthalmic Ointment ... 586
- Cetapred Ointment ... ⊙ 220
- ⅛% Econopred & 1% Econopred Plus ... ⊙ 217
- Isopto Cetapred Suspension ... ⊙ 220
- Metimyd ... ⊙ 306
- Poly-Pred Liquifilm ... ⊙ 250
- Pred Forte ... ⊙ 252
- Pred Mild ... ⊙ 254
- Pred-G Liquifilm Sterile Ophthalmic Suspension ... ⊙ 252
- Pred-G S.O.P. Sterile Ophthalmic Ointment ... ⊙ 253
- Vasocidin Ointment ... ⊙ 275

Prednisolone Sodium Phosphate (Steroid effects potentiated). Products include:
- AK-Pred ... ⊙ 205
- Hydeltrasol Injection, Sterile ... 1476
- Inflamase ... ⊙ 274
- Pediapred Oral Liquid ... 987
- Vasocidin Ophthalmic Solution ... ⊙ 276

Prednisolone Tebutate (Steroid effects potentiated). Products include:
- Hydeltra-T.B.A. Sterile Suspension 1478

Prednisone (Steroid effects potentiated). Products include:
- Deltasone Tablets ... 2332

Probenecid (Diminished uricosuric effect). Products include:
- Benemid Tablets ... 1426
- ColBENEMID Tablets ... 1436
- Wycillin Injection and Probenecid Tablets ... 2539

Prochlorperazine (Increased CNS depression). Products include:
- Compazine ... 2201

Promethazine Hydrochloride (Increased CNS depression). Products include:
- Mepergan Injection ... 2479
- Phenergan with Codeine ... 2497
- Phenergan with Dextromethorphan 2499
- Phenergan Injection ... 2493
- Phenergan Suppositories ... 2496
- Phenergan Syrup ... 2495
- Phenergan Tablets ... 2496
- Phenergan VC ... 2500
- Phenergan VC with Codeine ... 2501

Propofol (Increased CNS depression). Products include:
- Diprivan Injection ... 2267

Propoxyphene Hydrochloride (Increased CNS depression). Products include:
- Darvon ... 1256
- Wygesic Tablets ... 2540

Propoxyphene Napsylate (Increased CNS depression). Products include:
- Darvon-N/Darvocet-N ... 1254

Quazepam (Increased CNS depression). Products include:
- Doral Tablets ... 2383

Secobarbital Sodium (Increased CNS depression). Products include:
- Seconal Sodium Pulvules ... 1296

Selegiline Hydrochloride (Enhanced effect). Products include:
- Eldepryl ... 2250

Sufentanil Citrate (Increased CNS depression). Products include:
- Sufenta Injection ... 1147

Sulfamethizole (Enhanced effect of sulfonamides). Products include:
- Thiosulfil Forte Tablets ... 2526
- Urobiotic-250 Capsules ... 1968

Sulfamethoxazole (Enhanced effect of sulfonamides). Products include:
- Azo Gantanol Tablets ... 1887
- Bactrim DS Tablets ... 1891
- Bactrim I.V. Infusion ... 1889
- Bactrim ... 1891
- Gantanol ... 1899
- Septra ... 813
- Septra I.V. Infusion ... 808
- Septra I.V. Infusion ADD-Vantage Vials ... 810
- Septra ... 813

Sulfasalazine (Enhanced effect of sulfonamides). Products include:
- Azulfidine Tablets, EN-tabs, Oral Suspension ... 1157

Sulfinpyrazone (Diminished uricosuric effect). Products include:
- Anturane ... 853

Sulfisoxazole (Enhanced effect of sulfonamides). Products include:
- Azo Gantrisin Tablets ... 1888
- Gantrisin Tablets ... 1901
- Pediazole ... 1973

Sulfisoxazole Diolamine (Enhanced effect of sulfonamides). Products include:
- Gantrisin Ophthalmic Ointment/Solution ... 1900

Sulindac (Enhanced effect of NSAID). Products include:
- Clinoril Tablets ... 1433

Temazepam (Increased CNS depression). Products include:
- Restoril Capsules ... 2023

Thiamylal Sodium (Increased CNS depression). Products include:
- Surital Ampoules, Steri-Vials ... 1764

Thioridazine Hydrochloride (Increased CNS depression). Products include:
- Mellaril ... 2011

Thiothixene (Increased CNS depression). Products include:
- Navane Capsules and Concentrate 1954
- Navane Intramuscular ... 1956

Ticarcillin Disodium (Enhanced effect). Products include:
- Ticar for Injection ... 2236
- Timentin for Injection ... 2239

Tolazamide (May result in hypoglycemia). Products include:
- Tolinase Tablets ... 2365

Tolbutamide (May result in hypoglycemia). Products include:
- Orinase Tablets ... 2354

Tolmetin Sodium (Enhanced effect of NSAID). Products include:
- Tolectin (200, 400 and 600 mg) .. 1379

Tranylcypromine Sulfate (Enhanced effect). Products include:
- Parnate Tablets ... 2222

Triamcinolone (Steroid effects potentiated).
- No products indexed under this heading.

Triamcinolone Acetonide (Steroid effects potentiated). Products include:
- Aristocort A ... 1010
- Azmacort Inhaler ... 1837
- Kenalog Cream, Lotion & Ointment 2401
- Kenalog-10 Injection ... 2402
- Kenalog-40 Injection ... 2403
- Kenalog in Orabase ... 604
- Kenalog Spray ... 2401
- Mycolog II Cream and Ointment ... 2407
- Mytrex Cream & Ointment ... 2080
- Nasacort Nasal Inhaler ... 1844

Triamcinolone Diacetate (Steroid effects potentiated). Products include:
- Aristocort Suspension ... 1008

Triamcinolone Hexacetonide (Steroid effects potentiated). Products include:
- Aristospan Suspension ... 1011

Triazolam (Increased CNS depression). Products include:
- Halcion Tablets ... 2340

Trifluoperazine Hydrochloride (Increased CNS depression). Products include:
- Stelazine ... 2226

Vitamin C (Causes aspirin accumulation). Products include:
- Allbee with C Caplets ... ▣ 670
- Allbee C-800 ... ▣ 670
- Bromase Capsules ... 672
- Bugs Bunny Children's Chewable Vitamins (Sugar Free) ... ▣ 625
- Bugs Bunny With Extra C Children's Chewable Vitamins (Sugar Free) ... ▣ 626
- Bugs Bunny Plus Iron Children's Chewable Vitamins (Sugar Free) ▣ 625
- Cefol Filmtab ... 509
- Centrum, Jr. (Children's Chewable) + Extra C ... ▣ 585
- Cod Liver Oil Concentrate Tablets with Vitamin C ... ▣ 694
- Ester-C Tablets ... ▣ 575
- Ferancee Chewable Tablets ... 1155
- Ferancee-HP Tablets ... 1155
- Fero-Folic-500 Filmtab ... 527
- Fero-Grad-500 Filmtab ... 528
- Flintstones Children's Chewable Vitamins ... ▣ 625
- Flintstones Children's Chewable Vitamins With Extra C ... ▣ 626
- Flintstones Children's Chewable Vitamins Plus Iron ... ▣ 625
- Halls Vitamin C Drops ... ▣ 742
- Hyland's Vitamin C for Children ... ▣ 729
- ICAPS Plus ... ⊙ 280
- Mediatric Capsules ... 2476
- Mol-Iron w/Vitamin C Tablets ... ▣ 703
- Natalins Rx ... 1391
- Natalins Tablets ... 1391
- N'ICE Sugarless Vitamin C Drops .. ▣ 719
- Niferex w/Vitamin C Tablets ... 847
- Ocuvite Vitamin and Mineral Supplement ... ⊙ 312
- One-A-Day Essential Vitamins ... ▣ 627
- One-A-Day Maximum Formula Vitamins and Minerals ... ▣ 627
- One-A-Day Plus Extra C Vitamins .. ▣ 627
- Probec-T Tablets ... ▣ 581
- Stressgard Stress Formula Vitamins ... ▣ 628
- Stuart Prenatal Tablets ... ▣ 731
- The Stuart Formula Tablets ... 1157
- Stuartinic Tablets ... 1157
- Sunkist Children's Chewable Multivitamins - Plus Extra C ... ▣ 553
- Sunkist Vitamin C ... ▣ 553
- Surbex with C ... ▣ 502
- Trinsicon Capsules ... 2415
- Tri-Vi-Flor 1.0 mg Vitamins with Fluoride Chewable Tablets ... 1400
- Tri-Vi-Flor Drops ... 1400
- Tri-Vi-Sol Vitamin Drops ... ▣ 614
- Tri-Vi-Sol Vitamin Drops with Iron ▣ 614
- Vicon Forte Capsules ... 2416
- Vicon Plus ... ▣ 682
- Vicon-C ... ▣ 682
- Vi-Daylin ADC Vitamins Drops ... 1980
- Vi-Daylin ADC Vitamins + Iron Drops ... 1980
- Vi-Daylin/F ADC Vitamins Drops With Fluoride ... 1981
- Vi-Daylin/F ADC Vitamins + Iron Drops With Fluoride ... 1981
- Vi-Zac ... ▣ 682
- Within Women's Formula Multivitamin with Calcium, Extra Iron and Zinc ... ▣ 628
- Z-Bec Tablets ... ▣ 678

Warfarin Sodium (Enhanced effect, bleeding). Products include:
- Coumadin Injection & Tablets ... 944
- Panwarfin Tablets ... 547

Food Interactions

Food, unspecified (The presence of food slightly delays absorption).

EMULSOIL

(Castor Oil) ... ▣ 633
No interactions described in labeling.

ENCARE VAGINAL CONTRACEPTIVE SUPPOSITORIES

(Nonoxynol-9) ... ▣ 733
No interactions described in labeling.

ENDEP TABLETS

(Amitriptyline Hydrochloride) ... 1927
May interact with monoamine oxidase inhibitors, central nervous system depressants, anticholinergics, sympathomimetic aerosal bronchodilators, thyroid preparations, and certain other agents. Compounds in these categories include:

Albuterol (Careful dosage adjustments required). Products include:
- Proventil Inhalation Aerosol ... 2117
- Ventolin Inhalation Aerosol and Refill ... 583

Albuterol Sulfate (Careful dosage adjustments required). Products include:
- Proventil Repetabs Tablets ... 2120
- Proventil Solutions for Inhalation 0.5% and 0.083% ... 2118
- Proventil Syrup ... 2119
- Proventil Tablets ... 2120
- Ventolin ... 583

Alcohol (Increased response).

Alfentanil Hydrochloride (Increased response to the effects of CNS depressants). Products include:
- Alfenta Injection ... 1131

Alprazolam (Increased response to the effects of CNS depressants). Products include:
- Xanax Tablets ... 2367

Aprobarbital (Increased response to the effects of CNS depressants). Products include:
- Alurate Elixir ... 1883

Atropine Sulfate (Paralytic ileus). Products include:
- Arco-Lase Plus Tablets ... 607
- Atropine Sulfate Sterile Ophthalmic Solution and S.O.P. Sterile Ophthalmic Ointment ... ⊙ 239
- Donnagel ... ▣ 675
- Donnagel-PG ... 1858
- Donnatal ... 1858
- Donnatal Extentabs ... 1859
- Donnatal Tablets ... 1858
- Donnazyme Tablets ... 1860
- Isopto Atropine ... ⊙ 218
- Lomotil ... 2174
- Motofen Tablets ... 836
- Ru-Tuss Tablets ... 693
- Urised Tablets ... 2396

Belladonna Alkaloids (Paralytic ileus). Products include:
- Bellergal-S Tablets ... 1998
- Hyland's Bed Wetting Tablets ... ▣ 728
- Hyland's Teething Tablets ... ▣ 728
- Kinesed Tablets ... 2272

Benztropine Mesylate (Paralytic ileus). Products include:
- Cogentin ... 1435

Biperiden (Paralytic ileus). Products include:
- Akineton ... 1171

Buprenorphine (Increased response to the effects of CNS depressants).
- No products indexed under this heading.

Buspirone Hydrochloride (Increased response to the effects of CNS depressants). Products include:
- BuSpar ... 1401

Butabarbital (Increased response to the effects of CNS depressants). Products include:
- Pyridium Plus ... 1764

Butalbital (Increased response to the effects of CNS depressants). Products include:
- Esgic-Plus Tablets ... 1002
- Esgic Tablets & Capsules ... 1001
- Fioricet Tablets ... 2006
- Fiorinal Capsules ... 2007
- Fiorinal with Codeine Capsules ... 2008
- Fiorinal Tablets ... 2007
- Phrenilin ... 838
- Sedapap Tablets 50 mg/650 mg .. 1360

Chlordiazepoxide (Increased response to the effects of CNS depressants). Products include:
- Libritabs Tablets ... 1930
- Limbitrol ... 1933
- Menrium Tablets ... 1934

Chlordiazepoxide Hydrochloride (Increased response to the effects of CNS depressants). Products include:
- Librax Capsules ... 1929
- Librium Capsules ... 1931
- Librium Injectable ... 1932

Chlorpromazine (Increased response to the effects of CNS depressants). Products include:
- Thorazine ... 2234

Chlorprothixene (Increased response to the effects of CNS depressants). Products include:
- Taractan Tablets ... 1920

Chlorprothixene Hydrochloride (Increased response to the effects of CNS depressants). Products include:
- Taractan ... 1920

Cimetidine (Increased plasma levels of tricyclic antidepressants; increased frequency of anticholinergic side effects). Products include:
- Tagamet Tablets ... 2228

Cimetidine Hydrochloride (Increased plasma levels of tricyclic antidepressants; increased frequency of anticholinergic side effects). Products include:
- Tagamet ... 2228

Clidinium Bromide (Paralytic ileus). Products include:
- Librax Capsules ... 1929
- Quarzan Capsules ... 1937

Clorazepate Dipotassium (Increased response to the effects of CNS depressants). Products include:
- Tranxene ... 556

Codeine (Increased response to the effects of CNS depressants). Products include:
- Calcidrine Syrup ... 506

Codeine Phosphate (Increased response to the effects of CNS depressants). Products include:
- Actifed with Codeine Cough Syrup .. 752
- Cheracol Cough Syrup ... 1853
- Codimal PH Syrup ... 846
- Dimetane-DC Cough Syrup ... 1857
- Empirin with Codeine Phosphate Nos. 2, 3 & 4 ... 764
- Fiorinal with Codeine Capsules ... 2008
- Isoclor Expectorant ... 982
- Naldecon CX Adult Liquid ... ▣ 521
- Novahistine DH ... 1342
- Novahistine Expectorant ... 1343
- Nucofed Capsules ... 2219

Nucofed Expectorant 2219
Nucofed Pediatric Expectorant 2220
Nucofed Syrup 2219
Phenaphen with Codeine Capsules 1865
Phenaphen-650 with Codeine Tablets 1866
Phenergan with Codeine 2497
Phenergan VC with Codeine 2501
Robitussin A-C Syrup 1875
Robitussin-DAC Syrup 1875
Ryna .... ▣ 741
Soma Compound w/Codeine Tablets 2390
Triaminic Expectorant w/Codeine .. 1996
Tussi-Organidin Liquid 2391
Tylenol with Codeine 1381

Codeine Polistirex (Increased response to the effects of CNS depressants).
No products indexed under this heading.

Dezocine (Increased response to the effects of CNS depressants).

Diazepam (Increased response to the effects of CNS depressants). Products include:
Valium Injectable 1937
Valium Tablets 1939
Valrelease Capsules 1923

Dicyclomine Hydrochloride (Paralytic ileus). Products include:
Bentyl 1322

Disulfiram (Delirium may result). Products include:
Antabuse Tablets 2429

Dobutamine Hydrochloride (Careful dosage adjustments required). Products include:
Dobutrex Solution Vials 1259

Dopamine Hydrochloride (Careful dosage adjustments required). Products include:
Intropin Injection 930

Droperidol (Increased response to the effects of CNS depressants). Products include:
Inapsine Injection 1140
Innovar Injection 1141

Enflurane (Increased response to the effects of CNS depressants). Products include:
Ethrane 599

Ephedrine Hydrochloride (Careful dosage adjustments required). Products include:
Amesec .... ▣ 682
Primatene Tablets-M Formula 2421
Primatene Tablets-P Formula 2421
Primatene Tablets-Regular Formula 2421
Quadrinal Tablets 1183
Quelidrine Syrup 556
Tedral SA 1765

Ephedrine Sulfate (Careful dosage adjustments required). Products include:
Bronkaid Tablets .... ▣ 757
Bronkolixir .... ▣ 761
Bronkotabs Tablets .... ▣ 762
Marax Tablets & DF Syrup 1954
Pazo Hemorrhoid Ointment & Suppositories 752
Vicks Vatronol Nose Drops .... ▣ 666

Ephedrine Tannate (Careful dosage adjustments required). Products include:
Rynatuss 2388

Epinephrine (Careful dosage adjustments required). Products include:
Ana-Kit Anaphylaxis Emergency Treatment Kit 1100
Bronkaid Mist .... ▣ 757
EpiPen 843
Marcaine Hydrochloride 0.5% with Epinephrine 1:200,000 (as bitartrate) 958
Marcaine Hydrochloride with Epinephrine 1:200,000 2055
Primatene Mist 2420
Sus-Phrine Injection 1006
Xylocaine with Epinephrine Injections 637

Epinephrine Bitartrate (Careful dosage adjustments required). Products include:
AsthmaHaler Mist Epinephrine Bitartrate Bronchodilator .... ▣ 616
Bronkaid Mist Suspension .... ▣ 757
Primatene Mist Suspension 2421

Epinephrine Hydrochloride (Careful dosage adjustments required). Products include:
Adrenalin Chloride Solution 1:100 & 1:1,000 1689
Epifrin .... ⊙ 244
Glaucon .... ⊙ 218

Estazolam (Increased response to the effects of CNS depressants). Products include:
ProSom Tablets 554

Ethchlorvynol (Transient delirium; increased response to the effects of CNS depressants). Products include:
Placidyl Capsules 553

Ethinamate (Increased response to the effects of CNS depressants).
No products indexed under this heading.

Fentanyl (Increased response to the effects of CNS depressants). Products include:
Duragesic Transdermal System 1133

Fentanyl Citrate (Increased response to the effects of CNS depressants). Products include:
Innovar Injection 1141
Sublimaze Injection 1146

Fluphenazine Decanoate (Increased response to the effects of CNS depressants). Products include:
Prolixin Decanoate 1795

Fluphenazine Enanthate (Increased response to the effects of CNS depressants). Products include:
Prolixin Enanthate 1796

Fluphenazine Hydrochloride (Increased response to the effects of CNS depressants). Products include:
Prolixin Elixir 1793
Prolixin Injection 1791
Prolixin Oral Concentrate 1792
Prolixin Tablets 1793

Flurazepam Hydrochloride (Increased response to the effects of CNS depressants). Products include:
Dalmane Capsules 1927

Furazolidone (Hyperpyretic crisis; concurrent or sequential use within 14 days is contraindicated). Products include:
Furoxone 1855

Glutethimide (Increased response to the effects of CNS depressants).
No products indexed under this heading.

Glycopyrrolate (Paralytic ileus). Products include:
Robinul Forte Tablets 1873
Robinul Injectable 1873
Robinul Tablets 1873

Guanethidine Sulfate (Decreased antihypertensive action of guanethidine).

Haloperidol (Increased response to the effects of CNS depressants). Products include:
Haldol Injection, Tablets and Concentrate 1373

Haloperidol Decanoate (Increased response to the effects of CNS depressants). Products include:
Haldol Decanoate 1375

Hydrocodone Bitartrate (Increased response to the effects of CNS depressants). Products include:
Anexsia 5/500 Tablets 2196
Anexsia 7.5/650 Tablets 2197
Azdone Tablets 844
Codiclear DH Syrup 845
Codimal DH Syrup 846
Damason-P 1356
Hycodan Syrup, Tablets 927
Hycomine Compound Tablets 929
Hycomine Syrup 927
Hycotuss Expectorant Syrup 930
Hydrocet Capsules 835
Lortab ASA Tablets 2414
Lortab 2412
Ru-Tuss with Hydrocodone 694
Triaminic Expectorant DH 1995
Vicodin Tablets 1187
Vicodin ES Tablets 1189
Zydone Capsules 941

Hydrocodone Polistirex (Increased response to the effects of CNS depressants). Products include:
Tussionex Extended-Release Suspension 988

Hydroxyzine Hydrochloride (Increased response to the effects of CNS depressants). Products include:
Atarax Tablets & Syrup 1941
Marax Tablets & DF Syrup 1954
Vistaril Intramuscular Solution 1970

Hyoscyamine (Paralytic ileus). Products include:
Cystospaz Tablets 2395
Urised Tablets 2396

Hyoscyamine Sulfate (Paralytic ileus). Products include:
Arco-Lase Plus Tablets 607
Cystospaz-M Capsules 2395
Donnagel .... ▣ 675
Donnagel-PG 1858
Donnatal 1858
Donnatal Extentabs 1859
Donnatal Tablets 1858
Donnazyme Tablets 1860
Kutrase Capsules 2146
Levsin/Levsinex 2147
Ru-Tuss Tablets 693

Ipratropium Bromide (Paralytic ileus). Products include:
Atrovent Inhalation Aerosol 675

Isocarboxazid (Hyperpyretic crisis; concurrent or sequential use within 14 days is contraindicated). Products include:
Marplan Tablets 1906

Isoflurane (Increased response to the effects of CNS depressants). Products include:
Forane 600

Isoproterenol Hydrochloride (Careful dosage adjustments required). Products include:
Isuprel Hydrochloride Injection 1:5000 2050
Isuprel Hydrochloride Mistometer .. 2051
Isuprel Hydrochloride Solution 1:200 & 1:100 2052
Norisodrine Aerotrol 540

Ketamine Hydrochloride (Increased response to the effects of CNS depressants). Products include:
Ketalar 1726

Levorphanol Tartrate (Increased response to the effects of CNS depressants). Products include:
Levo-Dromoran 1906

Levothyroxine Sodium (Careful dosage adjustments required). Products include:
Levothroid Tablets 1003
Levoxine Tablets 904
Synthroid 695

Liothyronine Sodium (Careful dosage adjustments required). Products include:
Cytomel Tablets 2203

Liotrix (Careful dosage adjustments required). Products include:
Euthroid 1724

Lorazepam (Increased response to the effects of CNS depressants). Products include:
Ativan Injection 2432
Ativan Tablets 2434

Loxapine Hydrochloride (Increased response to the effects of CNS depressants). Products include:
Loxitane 1213

Loxapine Succinate (Increased response to the effects of CNS depressants). Products include:
Loxitane Capsules 1213

Mepenzolate Bromide (Paralytic ileus). Products include:
Cantil Tablets 1326

Meperidine Hydrochloride (Increased response to the effects of CNS depressants). Products include:
Demerol 2047
Mepergan Injection 2479

Mephobarbital (Increased response to the effects of CNS depressants). Products include:
Mebaral Tablets 2061

Meprobamate (Increased response to the effects of CNS depressants). Products include:
Deprol Tablets 2382
Equagesic Tablets 2451
Miltown Tablets 2386
PMB 200 and PMB 400 2504

Mesoridazine (Increased response to the effects of CNS depressants). Products include:
Serentil 686

Metaproterenol Sulfate (Careful dosage adjustments required). Products include:
Alupent 674
Arm-a-Med Metaproterenol Sulfate Inhalation Solution, USP 617
Metaprel Inhalation Aerosol Bronchodilator 2014
Metaprel Inhalation Solution 2015
Metaprel 2015
Metaproterenol Sulfate Inhalation Solution, USP 912

Metaraminol Bitartrate (Careful dosage adjustments required). Products include:
Aramine Injection 1424

Methadone Hydrochloride (Increased response to the effects of CNS depressants). Products include:
Dolophine Hydrochloride Ampoules & Vials 1260
Dolophine Hydrochloride Tablets 1261
Methadone Hydrochloride Diskets .. 1284
Methadone Hydrochloride Oral Solution & Tablets 1987

Methohexital Sodium (Increased response to the effects of CNS depressants). Products include:
Brevital Sodium Vials 1248

Methoxamine Hydrochloride (Careful dosage adjustments required). Products include:
Vasoxyl Injection 819

Methoxyflurane (Increased response to the effects of CNS depressants).
No products indexed under this heading.

Midazolam Hydrochloride (Increased response to the effects of CNS depressants). Products include:
Versed Injection 1924

Molindone Hydrochloride (Increased response to the effects of CNS depressants). Products include:
Moban Tablets & Concentrate 932

Morphine Sulfate (Increased response to the effects of CNS depressants). Products include:
Astramorph/PF Injection, USP (Preservative-Free) 618
Duramorph 960
Infumorph 200 and Infumorph 500 Sterile Solutions 962
MS Contin Tablets 1814
MSIR 1817
Oramorph SR (Morphine Sulfate Sustained Release Tablets) 1988
Roxanol 1991

Norepinephrine Bitartrate (Careful dosage adjustments required). Products include:
Levophed Bitartrate Injection 2054

Opium Alkaloids (Increased response to the effects of CNS depressants). Products include:
B & O No. 15A & No. 16A Supprettes ... 2395
Pantopon Injectable ... 1911

Oxazepam (Increased response to the effects of CNS depressants). Products include:
Serax Capsules ... 2522
Serax Tablets ... 2522

Oxycodone Hydrochloride (Increased response to the effects of CNS depressants). Products include:
Percocet Tablets ... 950
Percodan ... 951
Roxicodone Tablets, Oral Solution & Intensol (Oxycodone) ... 1992
Tylox Capsules ... 1382

Oxyphenonium Bromide (Paralytic ileus).

Pentobarbital Sodium (Increased response to the effects of CNS depressants). Products include:
Nembutal Sodium Capsules ... 534
Nembutal Sodium Solution ... 536
Nembutal Sodium Suppositories ... 538

Perphenazine (Increased response to the effects of CNS depressants). Products include:
Etrafon ... 2087
Triavil Tablets ... 1556
Trilafon ... 2123

Phenelzine Sulfate (Hyperpyretic crisis; concurrent or sequential use within 14 days is contraindicated). Products include:
Nardil ... 1742

Phenobarbital (Increased response to the effects of CNS depressants). Products include:
Arco-Lase Plus Tablets ... 607
Bellergal-S Tablets ... 1998
Bronkolixir ... ▣ 761
Bronkotabs Tablets ... ▣ 762
Donnatal ... 1858
Donnatal Extentabs ... 1859
Donnatal Tablets ... 1858
Donnazyme Tablets ... 1860
Kinesed Tablets ... 2272
Phenobarbital Elixir and Tablets ... 1293
Primatene Tablets-P Formula ... 2421
Quadrinal Tablets ... 1183
Tedral SA ... 1765

Phenylephrine Bitartrate (Careful dosage adjustments required).
No products indexed under this heading.

Phenylephrine Hydrochloride (Careful dosage adjustments required). Products include:
AK-Dilate Solution 2.5% and 10% ... ⊙ 203
Atrohist Sprinkle Capsules ... 558
Cerose-DM ... 2443
Codimal ... 846
Comhist LA Capsules ... 1618
Congespirin For Children Aspirin Free Chewable Cold Tablets ... 748
Cyclomydril ... ⊙ 216
Deconsal Sprinkle Capsules ... 559
Dimetane Decongestant ... ▣ 673
Dristan Decongestant/Antihistamine/ Analgesic Coated Caplets ... ▣ 749
Dristan Cold Nasal Decongestant/ Antihistamine/ Analgesic Coated Tablets ... 2419
Dristan Advanced Formula Decongestant/Antihistamine/ Analgesic Tablets ... ▣ 749
Dristan Nasal Spray, Menthol ... 2419
Dristan Nasal Spray, Regular and Regular with Metered Pump ... 2419
Entex Capsules ... 1623
Entex Liquid ... 1623
Sinus Excedrin Analgesic, Decongestant Tablets & Caplets ... 750
Extendryl ... 994
4-Way Fast Acting Nasal Spray - Original Formula (regular & mentholated) & Metered Spray Pump (regular) ... 751
Hycomine Compound Tablets ... 929
Murocoll-2 Sterile Ophthalmic Solution ... ⊙ 261
Mydfrin 2.5% ... ⊙ 224
Naldecon Syrup, Tablets, Pediatric Drops and Pediatric Syrup ... 709
Neo-Synephrine Hydrochloride 1% Carpuject ... 2063
Neo-Synephrine Hydrochloride 1% Injection ... 2063
Neo-Synephrine Hydrochloride (Ophthalmic) ... 2064
Neo-Synephrine ... ▣ 759
Nōstril Nasal Decongestant ... ▣ 520
Novahistine Elixir ... ▣ 596
Phenergan VC ... 2500
Phenergan VC with Codeine ... 2501
Prefrin Liquifilm Vasoconstrictor and Lubricant Eye Drops ... ⊙ 254
Prefrin-A ... ⊙ 255
Quelidrine Syrup ... 556
Relief Vasoconstrictor and Lubricant Eye Drops ... ⊙ 256
Robitussin Night Relief ... ▣ 677
Ru-Tuss with Hydrocodone ... 694
Ru-Tuss Tablets ... 693
Vasosulf ... ⊙ 279
Vicks Sinex ... ▣ 665
Zincfrin ... ⊙ 230

Phenylephrine Tannate (Careful dosage adjustments required). Products include:
Rynatan ... 2387
Rynatuss ... 2388

Phenylpropanolamine Hydrochloride (Careful dosage adjustments required). Products include:
A.R.M. Allergy Relief Medicine Caplets ... ▣ 615
Acutrim ... ▣ 548
Allerest ... ▣ 559
BC Cold Powder ... ▣ 517
Cheracol Plus Head Cold/Cough Formula ... ▣ 667
Codimal Expectorant ... 846
Comtrex Multi-Symptom Cold Reliever Tablets/Caplets/Liqui-Gels/Liquid ... 745
Contac Continuous Action Decongestant/Antihistamine Capsules ▣ 710
Contac Maximum Strength Continuous Action Decongestant/ Antihistamine Caplets ... ▣ 709
Contac Severe Cold and Flu Formula Caplets ... ▣ 711
Coricidin 'D' Decongestant Tablets ... ▣ 695
Coricidin Demilets Tablets for Children ... ▣ 696
Demazin Nasal Decongestant/ Antihistamine Repetabs Tablets & Syrup ... ▣ 697
Dexatrim ... ▣ 733
Dimetane-DC Cough Syrup ... 1857
Dimetapp Elixir ... ▣ 673
Dimetapp DM Elixir ... ▣ 674
Dimetapp Extentabs ... ▣ 674
Dimetapp Plus Caplets ... ▣ 675
Dimetapp Tablets ... ▣ 675
Entex Capsules ... 1623
Entex LA Tablets ... 1623
Entex Liquid ... 1623
4-Way Cold Tablets ... 750
Hycomine Syrup ... 927
Naldecon CX Adult Liquid ... ▣ 521
Naldecon DX Adult Liquid ... ▣ 521
Naldecon DX Children's Syrup ... ▣ 522
Naldecon DX Pediatric Drops ... ▣ 522
Naldecon EX Children's Syrup ... ▣ 522
Naldecon EX Pediatric Drops ... ▣ 523
Naldecon Syrup, Tablets, Pediatric Drops and Pediatric Syrup ... 709
Nolamine Tablets ... 838
Nolex LA Tablets ... 838
Ornade Spansule Capsules ... 2221
Orthoxicol Cough Syrup ... ▣ 668
Propagest ... 839
Pyrroxate Capsules ... ▣ 669
Robitussin-CF ... ▣ 676
Ru-Tuss II Capsules ... 693
Ru-Tuss with Hydrocodone ... 694
Ru-Tuss Tablets ... 693
Sine-Off Sinus Medicine Tablets-Aspirin Formula ... ▣ 722
Sinulin ... 840
St. Joseph Cold Tablets for Children ... ▣ 704
Tavist-D Tablets ... 2035
Triaminic Allergy Tablets ... ▣ 688
Triaminic Chewables ... ▣ 688
Triaminic Cold Tablets ... ▣ 688
Triaminic Expectorant ... ▣ 688
Triaminic Expectorant w/Codeine .. 1996
Triaminic Expectorant DH ... 1995
Triaminic Oral Infant Drops ... 1996
Triaminic Syrup ... ▣ 689
Triaminic-12 Tablets ... ▣ 690
Triaminic-DM Syrup ... ▣ 689
Triaminicin Tablets ... ▣ 690
Triaminicol Multi-Symptom Cold Tablets ... ▣ 691
Triaminicol Multi-Symptom Relief ▣ 691
Tuss-Ornade Liquid ... 2242
Tuss-Ornade Spansule Capsules ... 2242
Tylenol Cold Medication, Effervescent Tablets ... 1369

Pirbuterol Acetate (Careful dosage adjustments required). Products include:
Maxair Inhaler ... 1311

Prazepam (Increased response to the effects of CNS depressants). Products include:
Centrax ... 1693

Prochlorperazine (Increased response to the effects of CNS depressants). Products include:
Compazine ... 2201

Procyclidine Hydrochloride (Paralytic ileus). Products include:
Kemadrin Tablets ... 771

Promethazine Hydrochloride (Increased response to the effects of CNS depressants). Products include:
Mepergan Injection ... 2479
Phenergan with Codeine ... 2497
Phenergan with Dextromethorphan 2499
Phenergan Injection ... 2493
Phenergan Suppositories ... 2496
Phenergan Syrup ... 2495
Phenergan Tablets ... 2496
Phenergan VC ... 2500
Phenergan VC with Codeine ... 2501

Propantheline Bromide (Paralytic ileus). Products include:
Pro-Banthīne Tablets ... 2141

Propofol (Increased response to the effects of CNS depressants). Products include:
Diprivan Injection ... 2267

Propoxyphene Hydrochloride (Increased response to the effects of CNS depressants). Products include:
Darvon ... 1256
Wygesic Tablets ... 2540

Propoxyphene Napsylate (Increased response to the effects of CNS depressants). Products include:
Darvon-N/Darvocet-N ... 1254

Pseudoephedrine Hydrochloride (Careful dosage adjustments required). Products include:
Actifed Capsules ... ▣ 539
Actifed Plus Caplets ... ▣ 539
Actifed Plus Tablets ... ▣ 540
Actifed with Codeine Cough Syrup.. 752
Actifed Syrup ... ▣ 540
Actifed Tablets ... ▣ 540
Actifed 12-Hour Capsules ... ▣ 539
Advil Cold & Sinus Caplets (formerly CoAdvil) ... 2416
Allerest ... ▣ 559
Anatuss LA Tablets ... 1359
Benadryl Decongestant Elixir ... ▣ 635
Benadryl Decongestant ... ▣ 635
Benadryl Plus ... ▣ 636
Benadryl Plus Nighttime ... ▣ 637
Benylin Decongestant ... ▣ 638
Brexin L.A. Capsules ... 2078
Bromfed Capsules (Timed Release) ... 1615
Bromfed Syrup ... ▣ 628
Bromfed ... 1615
CoAdvil ... ▣ 748
Allergy-Sinus Comtrex Multi-Symptom Allergy Sinus Formula Tablets & Caplets ... 746
Cough Formula Comtrex ... 746
Comtrex Multi-Symptom Cold Reliever Tablets/Caplets/Liqui-Gels/Liquid ... 745
Day-Night Comtrex ... 747
Non-Drowsy Comtrex ... 747
Congess ... 994
Congestac Caplets ... ▣ 617
Contac Jr. Children's Cold Medicine ... ▣ 712
Contac Nighttime Cold Medicine ... ▣ 713
Contac Sinus Caplets Maximum Strength Non-Drowsy Formula ... ▣ 710
Contac Sinus Tablets Maximum Strength Non-Drowsy Formula ... ▣ 710
Deconamine ... 663
Deconsal II Tablets ... 559
Dimacol Caplets ... ▣ 672
Dimetane-DX Cough Syrup ... 1858
Dorcol Children's Cough Syrup ... ▣ 685
Dorcol Children's Decongestant Liquid ... ▣ 685
Dorcol Children's Liquid Cold Formula ... ▣ 686
Maximum Strength Dristan Decongestant/Analgesic Coated Caplets ... ▣ 750
No Drowsiness Dristan Cold Nasal Decongestant/Analgesic Coated Caplets ... 2420
Dristan Sinus Caplets ... 2419
Sinus Excedrin Analgesic, Decongestant Tablets & Caplets ... ▣ 533
Fedahist Gyrocaps ... 2145
Fedahist Timecaps ... 2145
Guaifed ... 1615
Guaifed Syrup ... ▣ 629
Isoclor Expectorant ... 982
Isoclor Timesule Capsules ... ▣ 561
Kronofed-A ... 970
Medi-Flu Caplet, Liquid ... ▣ 640
Novafed A Capsules ... 1342
Novafed Capsules ... 1342
Novahistine DH ... 1342
Novahistine DMX ... ▣ 595
Novahistine Expectorant ... 1343
Nucofed Capsules ... 2219
Nucofed Expectorant ... 2219
Nucofed Pediatric Expectorant ... 2220
Nucofed Syrup ... 2219
Ornex Caplets ... ▣ 618
PediaCare Allergy Relief Formula Liquid ... 1362
PediaCare Cough-Cold Formula Liquid ... 1362
PediaCare Infants' Oral Decongestant Drops ... 1362
PediaCare Night Rest Cough-Cold Formula Liquid ... 1362
PediaCare 6-12 Cough-Cold Formula Chewable Tablets ... 1362
Robitussin-DAC Syrup ... 1875
Robitussin-PE ... ▣ 677
Rondec ... 1975
Rondec-DM ... 1976
Rondec-TR Tablet ... 1975
Ru-Tuss DE Tablets ... 694
Ryna ... ▣ 741
Seldane-D Extended-Release Tablets ... 1350
Sinarest ... ▣ 562
Sine-Aid Maximum Strength Sinus Headache Caplets ... 1365
Sine-Aid Maximum Strength Sinus Headache Tablets ... 1365
Sine-Off Maximum Strength Allergy/Sinus Formula Caplets ... ▣ 721
Sine-Off Maximum Strength No Drowsiness Formula Caplets ... ▣ 722
Singlet Tablets ... ▣ 598
Sinutab Maximum Strength ... ▣ 641
Sinutab Maximum Strength Without Drowsiness Tablets & Caplets ... ▣ 642
Sinutab Regular Strength Without Drowsiness Formula ... ▣ 641
St. Joseph Nighttime Cold Medicine ... ▣ 705
Sudafed Children's Liquid ... ▣ 543
Sudafed Cough Syrup ... ▣ 543
Sudafed Plus Liquid ... ▣ 544
Sudafed Plus Tablets ... ▣ 545
Sudafed Sinus Caplets ... ▣ 545
Sudafed Sinus Tablets ... ▣ 545
Sudafed Tablets, 30 mg ... ▣ 544
Sudafed Tablets, Adult Strength, 60 mg ... ▣ 544
Sudafed 12 Hour Capsules ... ▣ 545
TheraFlu Flu and Cold Medicine ... ▣ 687
Triaminic Nite Light ... ▣ 689
Tylenol Allergy Sinus Medication Caplets and Gelcaps, Maximum Strength ... 1372
Children's Tylenol Cold Liquid Formula and Chewable Tablets ... 1368
Tylenol Cold & Flu Hot Medication, Packets ... 1369

Tylenol Cold & Flu No Drowsiness Hot Medication, Packets 1371
Tylenol Cold Medication Caplets and Tablets 1370
Tylenol Cold Medication No Drowsiness Formula Caplets 1370
Tylenol Cold Night Time Medication Liquid 1371
Tylenol Cough Medication Liquid with Decongestant, Maximum Strength 1372
Tylenol, Maximum Strength, Sinus Medication Gelcaps, Caplets and Tablets 1373
Ursinus Inlay-Tabs ..... ▣ 691
Vicks Children's NyQuil ..... ▣ 664
Vicks Daycare ..... ▣ 660
Vicks Formula 44D Decongestant Cough Medicine ..... ▣ 662
Vicks Formula 44M Multi-Symptom Cough Medicine ..... ▣ 662
Vicks NyQuil Nighttime Colds Medicine-Original & Cherry Flavor ..... ▣ 664
Vicks Pediatric Formula 44 Cough & Congestion Medicine ..... ▣ 663
Vicks Pediatric Formula 44m Multi-Symptom Cough & Cold Medicine ..... ▣ 663

Pseudoephedrine Sulfate (Careful dosage adjustments required). Products include:
Afrin Tablets ..... ▣ 693
Chlor-Trimeton Decongestant ..... ▣ 694
Disophrol Chronotab Sustained-Action Tablets ..... ▣ 698
Drixoral Antihistamine/Nasal Decongestant Syrup ..... ▣ 698
Drixoral Non-Drowsy Formula ..... ▣ 699
Drixoral Plus Extended-Release Tablets ..... ▣ 699
Drixoral Sinus ..... ▣ 700
Drixoral Sustained-Action Tablets ▣ 698
Sinutab Allergy Formula Sustained Action Tablets ..... ▣ 640
Trinalin Repetabs Tablets 1170

Quazepam (Increased response to the effects of CNS depressants). Products include:
Doral Tablets 2383

Scopolamine Hydrobromide (Paralytic ileus). Products include:
Donnagel ..... ▣ 675
Donnagel-PG 1858
Donnatal 1858
Donnatal Extentabs 1859
Donnatal Tablets 1858
Donnazyme Tablets 1860
Isopto Hyoscine ..... ◉ 222
Murocoll-2 Sterile Ophthalmic Solution ..... ◉ 261
Ru-Tuss Tablets 693

Scopolamine Preparations (Paralytic ileus). Products include:
Transderm Scōp Transdermal Therapeutic System 887

Secobarbital Sodium (Increased response to the effects of CNS depressants). Products include:
Seconal Sodium Pulvules 1296

Selegiline Hydrochloride (Hyperpyretic crisis; concurrent or sequential use within 14 days is contraindicated). Products include:
Eldepryl 2250

Sufentanil Citrate (Increased response to the effects of CNS depressants). Products include:
Sufenta Injection 1147

Temazepam (Increased response to the effects of CNS depressants). Products include:
Restoril Capsules 2023

Terbutaline Sulfate (Careful dosage adjustments required). Products include:
Brethaire Inhaler 1024
Brethine Ampuls 1026
Brethine Tablets 1026
Bricanyl Injection 1324
Bricanyl Tablets 1325

Thiamylal Sodium (Increased response to the effects of CNS depressants). Products include:
Surital Ampoules, Steri-Vials 1764

Thioridazine Hydrochloride (Increased response to the effects of CNS depressants). Products include:
Mellaril 2011

Thiothixene (Increased response to the effects of CNS depressants). Products include:
Navane Capsules and Concentrate 1954
Navane Intramuscular 1956

Thyroglobulin (Careful dosage adjustments required). Products include:
Proloid Tablets 1761

Thyroid (Careful dosage adjustments required). Products include:
S-P-T "Liquid" Capsules 995

Thyroxine (Careful dosage adjustments required).
No products indexed under this heading.

Tranylcypromine Sulfate (Hyperpyretic crisis; concurrent or sequential use within 14 days is contraindicated). Products include:
Parnate Tablets 2222

Triazolam (Increased response to the effects of CNS depressants). Products include:
Halcion Tablets 2340

Tridihexethyl Chloride (Paralytic ileus).
No products indexed under this heading.

Trifluoperazine Hydrochloride (Increased response to the effects of CNS depressants). Products include:
Stelazine 2226

Trihexyphenidyl Hydrochloride (Paralytic ileus). Products include:
Artane 1195

ENDURON TABLETS
(Methyclothiazide) 517
May interact with antihypertensives, beta blockers , corticosteroids, insulin, barbiturates, narcotic analgesics, cardiac glycosides, lithium preparations, and certain other agents. Compounds in these categories include:

Acebutolol Hydrochloride (Additive action). Products include:
Sectral Capsules 2520

ACTH (Hypokalemia).
No products indexed under this heading.

Alcohol (Potentiates orthostatic hypotension).

Alfentanil Hydrochloride (Potentiates orthostatic hypotension). Products include:
Alfenta Injection 1131

Aprobarbital (Potentiates orthostatic hypotension). Products include:
Alurate Elixir 1883

Atenolol (Additive action). Products include:
Tenoretic Tablets 1105
Tenormin Tablets and I.V. Injection 1107

Benazepril Hydrochloride (Additive action). Products include:
Lotensin Tablets 872

Bendroflumethiazide (Additive action). Products include:
Corzide Tablets 702
Naturetin Tablets 1789
Rauzide Tablets 1804

Betamethasone Acetate (Hypokalemia). Products include:
Celestone Soluspan Suspension 2081

Betamethasone Sodium Phosphate (Hypokalemia). Products include:
Celestone Soluspan Suspension 2081

Betaxolol Hydrochloride (Additive action). Products include:
Betoptic Sterile Ophthalmic Solution 569
Betoptic S Sterile Ophthalmic Suspension 570
Kerlone Tablets 2172

Buprenorphine (Potentiates orthostatic hypotension).
No products indexed under this heading.

Butabarbital (Potentiates orthostatic hypotension). Products include:
Pyridium Plus 1764

Butalbital (Potentiates orthostatic hypotension). Products include:
Esgic-Plus Tablets 1002
Esgic Tablets & Capsules 1001
Fioricet Tablets 2006
Fiorinal Capsules 2007
Fiorinal with Codeine Capsules 2008
Fiorinal Tablets 2007
Phrenilin 838
Sedapap Tablets 50 mg/650 mg .. 1360

Captopril (Additive action). Products include:
Capoten 2255
Capozide 2258

Carteolol Hydrochloride (Additive action). Products include:
Cartrol Tablets 507

Chlorothiazide (Additive action). Products include:
Aldoclor Tablets 1413
Diupres Tablets 1461
Diuril Oral 1464

Chlorothiazide Sodium (Additive action). Products include:
Diuril Sodium Intravenous 1463

Chlorthalidone (Additive action). Products include:
Combipres Tablets 678
Tenoretic Tablets 1105
Thalitone Tablets 687

Clonidine (Additive action). Products include:
Catapres-TTS 677

Clonidine Hydrochloride (Additive action). Products include:
Catapres Tablets 676
Combipres Tablets 678

Codeine (Potentiates orthostatic hypotension). Products include:
Calcidrine Syrup 506

Codeine Phosphate (Potentiates orthostatic hypotension). Products include:
Actifed with Codeine Cough Syrup.. 752
Cheracol Cough Syrup 1853
Codimal PH Syrup 846
Dimetane-DC Cough Syrup 1857
Empirin with Codeine Phosphate Nos. 2, 3 & 4 764
Fiorinal with Codeine Capsules 2008
Isoclor Expectorant 982
Naldecon CX Adult Liquid ..... ▣ 521
Novahistine DH 1342
Novahistine Expectorant 1343
Nucofed Capsules 2219
Nucofed Expectorant 2219
Nucofed Pediatric Expectorant 2220
Nucofed Syrup 2219
Phenaphen with Codeine Capsules 1865
Phenaphen-650 with Codeine Tablets 1866
Phenergan with Codeine 2497
Phenergan VC with Codeine 2501
Robitussin A-C Syrup 1875
Robitussin-DAC Syrup 1875
Ryna ..... ▣ 741
Soma Compound w/Codeine Tablets 2390
Triaminic Expectorant w/Codeine .. 1996
Tussi-Organidin Liquid 2391
Tylenol with Codeine 1381

Codeine Polistirex (Potentiates orthostatic hypotension).
No products indexed under this heading.

Cortisone Acetate (Hypokalemia). Products include:
Cortone Acetate Sterile Suspension 1437
Cortone Acetate Tablets 1439

Deserpidine (Additive or potentiative action). Products include:
Enduronyl 518
Harmonyl Tablets 528
Oreticyl 545

Deslanoside (Thiazide-induced hypokalemia may exaggerate the response of the heart to the toxic effects of digitalis).
No products indexed under this heading.

Dexamethasone (Hypokalemia). Products include:
AK-Trol Ointment & Suspension ..... ◉ 207
Decadron Elixir 1445
Decadron Tablets 1447
Decaspray Topical Aerosol 1459
Dexacidin ..... ◉ 272
Maxidex Sterile Ophthalmic Suspension ..... ◉ 223
Maxitrol Ophthalmic Ointment/Suspension ..... ◉ 223
TobraDex Ophthalmic Suspension and Ointment ..... ◉ 228

Dexamethasone Acetate (Hypokalemia). Products include:
Dalalone D.P. Injectable 999
Decadron-LA Sterile Suspension 1457

Dexamethasone Sodium Phosphate (Hypokalemia). Products include:
AK-Dex ..... ◉ 203
Decadron Phosphate Respihaler 1454
Decadron Phosphate Sterile Ophthalmic Ointment 1453
Decadron Phosphate Sterile Ophthalmic Solution 1453
Decadron Phosphate Topical Cream 1455
Decadron Phosphate Turbinaire 1456
Maxidex Sterile Ophthalmic Ointment ..... ◉ 222
NeoDecadron Sterile Ophthalmic Ointment 1517
NeoDecadron Sterile Ophthalmic Solution 1518
NeoDecadron Topical Cream 1518

Dezocine (Potentiates orthostatic hypotension).

Diazoxide (Additive action). Products include:
Hyperstat I.V. Injection 2095
Proglycem 649

Digitoxin (Thiazide-induced hypokalemia may exaggerate the response of the heart to the toxic effects of digitalis). Products include:
Crystodigin Tablets 1253

Digoxin (Thiazide-induced hypokalemia may exaggerate the response of the heart to the toxic effects of digitalis). Products include:
Lanoxicaps 772
Lanoxin Elixir Pediatric 775
Lanoxin Injection 778
Lanoxin Injection Pediatric 781
Lanoxin Tablets 783

Doxazosin Mesylate (Additive action). Products include:
Cardura Tablets 1941

Enalapril Maleate (Additive action). Products include:
Vaseretic Tablets 1559
Vasotec Tablets 1564

Enalaprilat (Additive action). Products include:
Vasotec I.V. 1562

Esmolol Hydrochloride (Additive action). Products include:
Brevibloc Injection 942

Felodipine (Additive action). Products include:
Plendil Extended-Release Tablets 1526

Fentanyl (Potentiates orthostatic hypotension). Products include:
Duragesic Transdermal System 1133

(▣ Described in PDR For Nonprescription Drugs) (◉ Described in PDR For Ophthalmology)

Fentanyl Citrate (Potentiates orthostatic hypotension). Products include:
- Innovar Injection 1141
- Sublimaze Injection 1146

Fosinopril Sodium (Additive action). Products include:
- Monopril Tablets 1406

Furosemide (Additive action). Products include:
- Lasix 1093

Guanabenz Acetate (Additive action). Products include:
- Wytensin Tablets 2542

Guanethidine Monosulfate (Additive or potentiative action). Products include:
- Esimil Tablets 864
- Ismelin Tablets 869

Hydralazine Hydrochloride (Additive action). Products include:
- Apresazide Capsules 854
- Apresoline Hydrochloride Parenteral (Ampuls) 856
- Apresoline Hydrochloride Tablets .. 855
- Apresoline-Esidrix Tablets 857
- Ser-Ap-Es Tablets 881
- Serpasil-Apresoline Tablets 884

Hydrochlorothiazide (Additive action). Products include:
- Aldactazide 2150
- Aldoril Tablets 1418
- Apresazide Capsules 854
- Apresoline-Esidrix Tablets 857
- Capozide 2258
- Dyazide Capsules 2208
- Esidrix Tablets 863
- Esimil Tablets 864
- HydroDIURIL Tablets 1484
- Hydropres Tablets 1485
- Inderide Tablets 2463
- Inderide LA Long Acting Capsules .. 2465
- Lopressor HCT Tablets 1034
- Maxzide 1215
- Moduretic Tablets 1510
- Normozide Tablets 2112
- Oretic Tablets 544
- Oreticyl 545
- Prinzide Tablets 1540
- Ser-Ap-Es Tablets 881
- Serpasil-Esidrix Tablets 886
- Timolide Tablets 1547
- Trandate HCT Tablets 579
- Vaseretic Tablets 1559
- Zestoretic 2274

Hydrocodone Bitartrate (Potentiates orthostatic hypotension). Products include:
- Anexsia 5/500 Tablets 2196
- Anexsia 7.5/650 Tablets 2197
- Azdone Tablets 844
- Codiclear DH Syrup 845
- Codimal DH Syrup 846
- Damason-P 1356
- Hycodan Syrup, Tablets 927
- Hycomine Compound Tablets 929
- Hycomine Syrup 927
- Hycotuss Expectorant Syrup 930
- Hydrocet Capsules 835
- Lortab ASA Tablets 2414
- Lortab 2412
- Ru-Tuss with Hydrocodone 694
- Triaminic Expectorant DH 1995
- Vicodin Tablets 1187
- Vicodin ES Tablets 1189
- Zydone Capsules 941

Hydrocodone Polistirex (Potentiates orthostatic hypotension). Products include:
- Tussionex Extended-Release Suspension 988

Hydrocortisone (Hypokalemia). Products include:
- AK-Spore H.C. .... ◉ 206
- Bactine Hydrocortisone Anti-Itch Cream .... ▣ 625
- CaldeCORT Anti-Itch Hydrocortisone Spray .... ▣ 560
- Carmol HC Cream 1% 2296
- Cortaid Spray .... ▣ 735
- Cortenema 2244
- Cortisporin Ointment 758
- Cortisporin Ophthalmic Ointment Sterile 758
- Cortisporin Ophthalmic Suspension Sterile 759
- Cortisporin Otic Solution Sterile 760
- Cortisporin Otic Suspension Sterile 760
- Cortizone-5 Creme & Ointment .... ▣ 732
- Dermolate Anti-Itch Cream .... ▣ 697
- Eldecort Cream 1.0% 1113
- Eldecort Cream 1.0% and 2.5% 1113
- Fungoid HC Creme 1770
- Hydrocortone Tablets 1482
- Hytone 909
- LazerSporin-C Solution 1770
- Massengill Medicated Soft Cloth Towelettes 2192
- Nutracort Cream & Lotion 1684
- PediOtic Suspension Sterile 797
- Synacort Creams 1%, 2.5% 2296
- Vanoxide-HC Acne Lotion 911
- Vioform-Hydrocortisone Cream and Mild Cream 889
- Vioform-Hydrocortisone Ointment .. 889
- VōSoL HC Otic Solution 2392
- Vytone Cream 1% 911

Hydrocortisone Acetate (Hypokalemia). Products include:
- Analpram-HC Rectal Cream 1% and 2.5% 970
- Anusol-HC Cream 1690
- Anusol-HC Suppositories 1691
- Caldecort .... ▣ 560
- Carmol HC Cream 1% 2296
- Chloromycetin Hydrocortisone Ophthalmic 1694
- Coly-Mycin S Otic w/Neomycin & Hydrocortisone 1708
- Cortaid .... ▣ 735
- Cortef Feminine Itch Cream .... ▣ 735
- Corticaine .... ▣ 682
- Cortifoam 1827
- Cortisporin Cream 757
- Epifoam 1828
- Gynecort 5 Creme .... ▣ 556
- Hydrocortone Acetate Sterile Suspension 1479
- Lanacort 5 Creme and Ointment .. ▣ 557
- Mantadil Cream 789
- Ophthocort .... ◉ 301
- Orabase HCA Oral Paste 890
- Pramosone Cream, Lotion & Ointment 971
- ProctoCream-HC 1834
- Proctofoam-HC 1835

Hydrocortisone Sodium Phosphate (Hypokalemia). Products include:
- Hydrocortone Phosphate Injection, Sterile 1481

Hydrocortisone Sodium Succinate (Hypokalemia). Products include:
- Solu-Cortef Sterile Powder 2361

Hydroflumethiazide (Additive action). Products include:
- Diucardin Tablets 2450
- Saluron 718
- Salutensin/Salutensin-Demi 719

Indapamide (Additive action). Products include:
- Lozol Tablets 1843

Insulin, Human (Changes in insulin requirements).
- No products indexed under this heading.

Insulin, Human Isophane Suspension (Changes in insulin requirements). Products include:
- Humulin N, 100 Units 1270

Insulin, Human NPH (Changes in insulin requirements). Products include:
- Insulatard NPH Human 1627
- Novolin N 1627
- Novolin N PenFill Cartridges 1628
- Novolin N Prefilled 1628

Insulin, Human Regular (Changes in insulin requirements). Products include:
- Humulin BR, 100 Units 1268
- Humulin R, 100 Units 1272
- Novolin R 1627
- Novolin R PenFill Cartridges 1628
- Novolin R Prefilled 1629
- Velosulin Human 1628

Insulin, Human, Zinc Suspension (Changes in insulin requirements). Products include:
- Humulin L, 100 Units 1268
- Humulin U, 100 Units 1272
- Novolin L 1627

Insulin, NPH (Changes in insulin requirements). Products include:
- NPH, 40 & 100 Units 1273
- Beef NPH, 100 Units 1274
- Pork NPH, 100 Units 1275
- Insulatard NPH 1626
- NPH Insulin 1626
- NPH Purified Pork Isophane Insulin 1626

Insulin, Regular (Changes in insulin requirements). Products include:
- Regular, 40 & 100 Units 1273
- Beef Regular, 100 Units 1275
- Pork Regular, 100 Units 1275
- Pork Regular (Concentrated), 500 Units 1276
- Regular Insulin 1625
- Regular Purified Pork Insulin 1626
- Velosulin 1627

Insulin, Zinc Crystals (Changes in insulin requirements). Products include:
- NPH, 40 & 100 Units 1273

Insulin, Zinc Suspension (Changes in insulin requirements). Products include:
- Lente, 40 & 100 Units 1272
- Protamine, Zinc, 40 & 100 Units 1273
- Lente Iletin I 1272
- Beef Lente, 100 Units 1274
- Beef Protamine Zinc, 100 Units 1274
- Pork Lente, 100 Units 1275
- Pork, Protamine, Zinc, 100 Units 1275
- Lente Insulin 1626
- Lente Purified Pork Insulin 1626
- Semilente Insulin 1625
- Ultralente Insulin 1626

Isradipine (Additive action). Products include:
- DynaCirc Capsules 2004

Labetalol Hydrochloride (Additive action). Products include:
- Normodyne Injection 2108
- Normodyne Tablets 2110
- Normozide Tablets 2112
- Trandate HCT Tablets 579
- Trandate Injection 577
- Trandate Tablets 579

Levorphanol Tartrate (Potentiates orthostatic hypotension). Products include:
- Levo-Dromoran 1906

Lisinopril (Additive action). Products include:
- Prinivil Tablets 1538
- Prinzide Tablets 1540
- Zestoretic 2274
- Zestril Tablets 2277

Lithium Carbonate (Increased risk of lithium toxicity). Products include:
- Eskalith 2214
- Lithane Tablets 1596
- Lithium Carbonate Capsules & Tablets 1984
- Lithobid Tablets 870

Lithium Citrate (Increased risk of lithium toxicity). Products include:
- Cibalith-S 870

Mecamylamine Hydrochloride (Additive or potentiative action). Products include:
- Inversine Tablets 1492

Meperidine Hydrochloride (Potentiates orthostatic hypotension). Products include:
- Demerol 2047
- Mepergan Injection 2479

Mephobarbital (Potentiates orthostatic hypotension). Products include:
- Mebaral Tablets 2061

Methadone Hydrochloride (Potentiates orthostatic hypotension). Products include:
- Dolophine Hydrochloride Ampoules & Vials 1260
- Dolophine Hydrochloride Tablets 1261
- Methadone Hydrochloride Diskets .. 1284
- Methadone Hydrochloride Oral Solution & Tablets 1987

Methyldopa (Additive action). Products include:
- Aldoclor Tablets 1413
- Aldomet Oral 1415
- Aldoril Tablets 1418

Methyldopate Hydrochloride (Additive action). Products include:
- Aldomet Ester HCl Injection 1417

Methylprednisolone (Hypokalemia). Products include:
- Medrol 2348

Methylprednisolone Acetate (Hypokalemia). Products include:
- Depo-Medrol Sterile Aqueous Suspension 2334

Methylprednisolone Sodium Succinate (Hypokalemia). Products include:
- Solu-Medrol Sterile Powder 2363

Metolazone (Additive action). Products include:
- Diulo 2129
- Mykrox ½ mg Tablets 984
- Zaroxolyn Tablets 989

Metoprolol Tartrate (Additive action). Products include:
- Lopressor Ampuls 1032
- Lopressor HCT Tablets 1034
- Lopressor Tablets 1032

Metyrosine (Additive action). Products include:
- Demser Capsules 1460

Minoxidil (Additive action). Products include:
- Loniten Tablets 2346
- Rogaine Topical Solution 2357

Morphine Sulfate (Potentiates orthostatic hypotension). Products include:
- Astramorph/PF Injection, USP (Preservative-Free) 618
- Duramorph 960
- Infumorph 200 and Infumorph 500 Sterile Solutions 962
- MS Contin Tablets 1814
- MSIR 1817
- Oramorph SR (Morphine Sulfate Sustained Release Tablets) 1988
- Roxanol 1991

Nadolol (Additive action). Products include:
- Corgard Tablets 701
- Corzide Tablets 702

Nicardipine Hydrochloride (Additive action). Products include:
- Cardene Capsules 2290

Nitroglycerin (Additive action). Products include:
- Deponit NTG Transdermal Delivery System 2143
- Minitran Transdermal Delivery System 1312
- Nitro-Bid Ointment 1339
- Nitro-Bid Capsules 1338
- Nitrodisc 2176
- Nitro-Dur (nitroglycerin) Transdermal Infusion System 1164
- Nitrogard Tablets 1004
- Nitrolingual Spray 1846
- Nitrostat Tablets 1743
- Transderm-Nitro Transdermal Therapeutic System 2283

Norepinephrine Bitartrate (Decreased arterial responsiveness). Products include:
- Levophed Bitartrate Injection 2054

Opium Alkaloids (Potentiates orthostatic hypotension). Products include:
- B & O No. 15A & No. 16A Supprettes 2395
- Pantopon Injectable 1911

Oxycodone Hydrochloride (Potentiates orthostatic hypotension). Products include:
- Percocet Tablets ... 950
- Percodan ... 951
- Roxicodone Tablets, Oral Solution & Intensol (Oxycodone) ... 1992
- Tylox Capsules ... 1382

Pancuronium Bromide Injection (Decreased serum levels).
- No products indexed under this heading.

Penbutolol Sulfate (Additive action). Products include:
- Levatol ... 1832

Pentobarbital Sodium (Potentiates orthostatic hypotension). Products include:
- Nembutal Sodium Capsules ... 534
- Nembutal Sodium Solution ... 536
- Nembutal Sodium Suppositories ... 538

Phenobarbital (Potentiates orthostatic hypotension). Products include:
- Arco-Lase Plus Tablets ... 607
- Bellergal-S Tablets ... 1998
- Bronkolixir ... ▣ 761
- Bronkotabs Tablets ... ▣ 762
- Donnatal ... 1858
- Donnatal Extentabs ... 1859
- Donnatal Tablets ... 1858
- Donnazyme Tablets ... 1860
- Kinesed Tablets ... 2272
- Phenobarbital Elixir and Tablets ... 1293
- Primatene Tablets-P Formula ... 2421
- Quadrinal Tablets ... 1183
- Tedral SA ... 1765

Phenoxybenzamine Hydrochloride (Additive action). Products include:
- Dibenzyline Capsules ... 2207

Phentolamine Mesylate (Additive action). Products include:
- Regitine ... 878

Pindolol (Additive action). Products include:
- Visken Tablets ... 2036

Polythiazide (Additive action). Products include:
- Minizide Capsules ... 1779
- Renese Tablets ... 1785
- Renese-R Tablets ... 1786

Prazosin Hydrochloride (Additive or potentiative action). Products include:
- Minipress Capsules ... 1778
- Minizide Capsules ... 1779

Prednisolone Acetate (Hypokalemia). Products include:
- AK-Cide Sterile Ophthalmic Ointment & Suspension ... ⊙ 202
- Blephamide Liquifilm Sterile Ophthalmic Suspension ... 586
- Blephamide S.O.P. Sterile Ophthalmic Ointment ... 586
- Cetapred Ointment ... ⊙ 220
- ⅛% Econopred & 1% Econopred Plus ... ⊙ 217
- Isopto Cetapred Suspension ... ⊙ 220
- Metimyd ... ⊙ 306
- Poly-Pred Liquifilm ... ⊙ 250
- Pred Forte ... ⊙ 252
- Pred Mild ... ⊙ 254
- Pred-G Liquifilm Sterile Ophthalmic Suspension ... ⊙ 252
- Pred-G S.O.P. Sterile Ophthalmic Ointment ... ⊙ 253
- Vasocidin Ointment ... ⊙ 275

Prednisolone Sodium Phosphate (Hypokalemia). Products include:
- AK-Pred ... ⊙ 205
- Hydeltrasol Injection, Sterile ... 1476
- Inflamase ... ⊙ 274
- Pediapred Oral Liquid ... 987
- Vasocidin Ophthalmic Solution ... ⊙ 276

Prednisolone Tebutate (Hypokalemia). Products include:
- Hydeltra-T.B.A. Sterile Suspension 1478

Prednisone (Hypokalemia). Products include:
- Deltasone Tablets ... 2332

Propoxyphene Hydrochloride (Potentiates orthostatic hypotension). Products include:
- Darvon ... 1256
- Wygesic Tablets ... 2540

Propoxyphene Napsylate (Potentiates orthostatic hypotension). Products include:
- Darvon-N/Darvocet-N ... 1254

Propranolol Hydrochloride (Additive action). Products include:
- Inderal ... 2459
- Inderal LA Long Acting Capsules ... 2461
- Inderide Tablets ... 2463
- Inderide LA Long Acting Capsules ... 2465

Ramipril (Additive action). Products include:
- Altace Capsules ... 1086

Rauwolfia Serpentina (Additive or potentiative action). Products include:
- Raudixin Tablets ... 1803
- Rauzide Tablets ... 1804

Rescinnamine (Additive or potentiative action).
- No products indexed under this heading.

Reserpine (Additive or potentiative action). Products include:
- Diupres Tablets ... 1461
- Hydromox R Tablets ... 1209
- Hydropres Tablets ... 1485
- Renese-R Tablets ... 1786
- Salutensin/Salutensin-Demi ... 719
- Ser-Ap-Es Tablets ... 881
- Serpasil Tablets ... 883
- Serpasil-Apresoline Tablets ... 884
- Serpasil-Esidrix Tablets ... 886

Secobarbital Sodium (Potentiates orthostatic hypotension). Products include:
- Seconal Sodium Pulvules ... 1296

Sodium Nitroprusside (Additive action). Products include:
- Nipride I.V. Infusion ... 1909

Sufentanil Citrate (Potentiates orthostatic hypotension). Products include:
- Sufenta Injection ... 1147

Terazosin Hydrochloride (Additive or potentiative action). Products include:
- Hytrin Tablets ... 529

Thiamylal Sodium (Potentiates orthostatic hypotension). Products include:
- Surital Ampoules, Steri-Vials ... 1764

Timolol Maleate (Additive action). Products include:
- Blocadren Tablets ... 1429
- Timolide Tablets ... 1547
- Timoptic in Ocudose ... 1552
- Timoptic Sterile Ophthalmic Solution ... 1550

Triamcinolone Acetonide (Hypokalemia). Products include:
- Aristocort A ... 1010
- Azmacort Inhaler ... 1837
- Kenalog Cream, Lotion & Ointment 2401
- Kenalog-10 Injection ... 2402
- Kenalog-40 Injection ... 2403
- Kenalog in Orabase ... 604
- Kenalog Spray ... 2401
- Mycolog II Cream and Ointment ... 2407
- Mytrex Cream & Ointment ... 2080
- Nasacort Nasal Inhaler ... 1844

Triamcinolone Diacetate (Hypokalemia). Products include:
- Aristocort Suspension ... 1008

Triamcinolone Hexacetonide (Hypokalemia). Products include:
- Aristospan Suspension ... 1011

Trimethaphan Camsylate (Additive or potentiative action). Products include:
- Arfonad Ampuls ... 1887

Tubocurarine Chloride (Increase responsiveness).
- No products indexed under this heading.

ENDURONYL FORTE TABLETS
(Methyclothiazide, Deserpidine) ... 518
May interact with antihypertensives, beta blockers, corticosteroids, insulin, and certain other agents. Compounds in these categories include:

Acebutolol Hydrochloride (Potentiates action). Products include:
- Sectral Capsules ... 2520

ACTH (Hypokalemia).
- No products indexed under this heading.

Atenolol (Potentiates action). Products include:
- Tenoretic Tablets ... 1105
- Tenormin Tablets and I.V. Injection 1107

Benazepril Hydrochloride (Potentiates action). Products include:
- Lotensin Tablets ... 872

Bendroflumethiazide (Potentiates action). Products include:
- Corzide Tablets ... 702
- Naturetin Tablets ... 1789
- Rauzide Tablets ... 1804

Betamethasone Acetate (Hypokalemia). Products include:
- Celestone Soluspan Suspension ... 2081

Betamethasone Sodium Phosphate (Hypokalemia). Products include:
- Celestone Soluspan Suspension ... 2081

Betaxolol Hydrochloride (Potentiates action). Products include:
- Betoptic Sterile Ophthalmic Solution ... 569
- Betoptic S Sterile Ophthalmic Suspension ... 570
- Kerlone Tablets ... 2172

Captopril (Potentiates action). Products include:
- Capoten ... 2255
- Capozide ... 2258

Carteolol Hydrochloride (Potentiates action). Products include:
- Cartrol Tablets ... 507

Chlorothiazide (Potentiates action). Products include:
- Aldoclor Tablets ... 1413
- Diupres Tablets ... 1461
- Diuril Oral ... 1464

Chlorothiazide Sodium (Potentiates action). Products include:
- Diuril Sodium Intravenous ... 1463

Chlorthalidone (Potentiates action). Products include:
- Combipres Tablets ... 678
- Tenoretic Tablets ... 1105
- Thalitone Tablets ... 687

Clonidine (Potentiates action). Products include:
- Catapres-TTS ... 677

Clonidine Hydrochloride (Potentiates action). Products include:
- Catapres Tablets ... 676
- Combipres Tablets ... 678

Cortisone Acetate (Hypokalemia). Products include:
- Cortone Acetate Sterile Suspension ... 1437
- Cortone Acetate Tablets ... 1439

Dexamethasone (Hypokalemia). Products include:
- AK-Trol Ointment & Suspension ... ⊙ 207
- Decadron Elixir ... 1445
- Decadron Tablets ... 1447
- Decaspray Topical Aerosol ... 1459
- Dexacidin ... ⊙ 272
- Maxidex Sterile Ophthalmic Suspension ... ⊙ 223
- Maxitrol Ophthalmic Ointment/Suspension ... ⊙ 223
- TobraDex Ophthalmic Suspension and Ointment ... ⊙ 228

Dexamethasone Acetate (Hypokalemia). Products include:
- Dalalone D.P. Injectable ... 999
- Decadron-LA Sterile Suspension ... 1457

Dexamethasone Sodium Phosphate (Hypokalemia). Products include:
- AK-Dex ... ⊙ 203
- Decadron Phosphate Respihaler ... 1454
- Decadron Phosphate Sterile Ophthalmic Ointment ... 1453
- Decadron Phosphate Sterile Ophthalmic Solution ... 1453
- Decadron Phosphate Topical Cream ... 1455
- Decadron Phosphate Turbinaire ... 1456
- Maxidex Sterile Ophthalmic Ointment ... ⊙ 222
- NeoDecadron Sterile Ophthalmic Ointment ... 1517
- NeoDecadron Sterile Ophthalmic Solution ... 1518
- NeoDecadron Topical Cream ... 1518

Diazoxide (Potentiates action). Products include:
- Hyperstat I.V. Injection ... 2095
- Proglycem ... 649

Doxazosin Mesylate (Potentiates action). Products include:
- Cardura Tablets ... 1941

Enalapril Maleate (Potentiates action). Products include:
- Vaseretic Tablets ... 1559
- Vasotec Tablets ... 1564

Enalaprilat (Potentiates action). Products include:
- Vasotec I.V. ... 1562

Esmolol Hydrochloride (Potentiates action). Products include:
- Brevibloc Injection ... 942

Felodipine (Potentiates action). Products include:
- Plendil Extended-Release Tablets ... 1526

Fosinopril Sodium (Potentiates action). Products include:
- Monopril Tablets ... 1406

Furosemide (Potentiates action). Products include:
- Lasix ... 1093

Guanabenz Acetate (Potentiates action). Products include:
- Wytensin Tablets ... 2542

Guanethidine Monosulfate (Potentiates action). Products include:
- Esimil Tablets ... 864
- Ismelin Tablets ... 869

Hydralazine Hydrochloride (Potentiates action). Products include:
- Apresazide Capsules ... 854
- Apresoline Hydrochloride Parenteral (Ampuls) ... 856
- Apresoline Hydrochloride Tablets ... 855
- Apresoline-Esidrix Tablets ... 857
- Ser-Ap-Es Tablets ... 881
- Serpasil-Apresoline Tablets ... 884

Hydrochlorothiazide (Potentiates action). Products include:
- Aldactazide ... 2150
- Aldoril Tablets ... 1418
- Apresazide Capsules ... 854
- Apresoline-Esidrix Tablets ... 857
- Capozide ... 2258
- Dyazide Capsules ... 2208
- Esidrix Tablets ... 863
- Esimil Tablets ... 864
- HydroDIURIL Tablets ... 1484
- Hydropres Tablets ... 1485
- Inderide Tablets ... 2463
- Inderide LA Long Acting Capsules ... 2465
- Lopressor HCT Tablets ... 1034
- Maxzide ... 1215
- Moduretic Tablets ... 1510
- Normozide Tablets ... 2112
- Oretic Tablets ... 544
- Oreticyl ... 545
- Prinzide Tablets ... 1540
- Ser-Ap-Es Tablets ... 881
- Serpasil-Esidrix Tablets ... 886
- Timolide Tablets ... 1547
- Trandate HCT Tablets ... 579
- Vaseretic Tablets ... 1559
- Zestoretic ... 2274

Hydrocortisone (Hypokalemia). Products include:
- AK-Spore H.C. ... ⊙ 206

Bactine Hydrocortisone Anti-Itch Cream ▣ 625
CaldeCORT Anti-Itch Hydrocortisone Spray ▣ 560
Carmol HC Cream 1% 2296
Cortaid Spray ▣ 735
Cortenema 2244
Cortisporin Ointment 758
Cortisporin Ophthalmic Ointment Sterile 758
Cortisporin Ophthalmic Suspension Sterile 759
Cortisporin Otic Solution Sterile 760
Cortisporin Otic Suspension Sterile 760
Cortizone-5 Creme & Ointment ▣ 732
Dermolate Anti-Itch Cream ▣ 697
Eldecort Cream 1.0% 1113
Eldecort Cream 1.0% and 2.5% 1113
Fungoid HC Creme 1770
Hydrocortone Tablets 1482
Hytone 909
LazerSporin-C Solution 1770
Massengill Medicated Soft Cloth Towelettes 2192
Nutracort Cream & Lotion 1684
PediOtic Suspension Sterile 797
Synacort Creams 1%, 2.5% 2296
Vanoxide-HC Acne Lotion 911
Vioform-Hydrocortisone Cream and Mild Cream 889
Vioform-Hydrocortisone Ointment 889
VōSoL HC Otic Solution 2392
Vytone Cream 1% 911

Hydrocortisone Acetate (Hypokalemia). Products include:
Analpram-HC Rectal Cream 1% and 2.5% 970
Anusol-HC Cream 1690
Anusol-HC Suppositories 1691
Caldecort ▣ 560
Carmol HC Cream 1% 2296
Chloromycetin Hydrocortisone Ophthalmic 1694
Coly-Mycin S Otic w/Neomycin & Hydrocortisone 1708
Cortaid ▣ 735
Cortef Feminine Itch Cream ▣ 735
Corticaine ▣ 682
Cortifoam 1827
Cortisporin Cream 757
Epifoam 1828
Gynecort 5 Creme ▣ 556
Hydrocortone Acetate Sterile Suspension 1479
Lanacort 5 Creme and Ointment ▣ 557
Mantadil Cream 789
Ophthocort ⊙ 301
Orabase HCA Oral Paste 890
Pramosone Cream, Lotion & Ointment 971
ProctoCream-HC 1834
Proctofoam-HC 1835

Hydrocortisone Sodium Phosphate (Hypokalemia). Products include:
Hydrocortone Phosphate Injection, Sterile 1481

Hydrocortisone Sodium Succinate (Hypokalemia). Products include:
Solu-Cortef Sterile Powder 2361

Hydroflumethiazide (Potentiates action). Products include:
Diucardin Tablets 2450
Saluron 718
Salutensin/Salutensin-Demi 719

Indapamide (Potentiates action). Products include:
Lozol Tablets 1843

Insulin, Human (Changes in insulin requirements).
No products indexed under this heading.

Insulin, Human Isophane Suspension (Changes in insulin requirements). Products include:
Humulin N, 100 Units 1270

Insulin, Human NPH (Changes in insulin requirements). Products include:
Insulatard NPH Human 1627
Novolin N 1627
Novolin N PenFill Cartridges 1628
Novolin N Prefilled 1628

Insulin, Human Regular (Changes in insulin requirements). Products include:
Humulin BR, 100 Units 1268
Humulin R, 100 Units 1272
Novolin R 1627
Novolin R PenFill Cartridges 1628
Novolin R Prefilled 1629
Velosulin Human 1628

Insulin, Human, Zinc Suspension (Changes in insulin requirements). Products include:
Humulin L, 100 Units 1268
Humulin U, 100 Units 1272
Novolin L 1627

Insulin, NPH (Changes in insulin requirements). Products include:
NPH, 40 & 100 Units 1273
Beef NPH, 100 Units 1274
Pork NPH, 100 Units 1275
Insulatard NPH 1626
NPH Insulin 1626
NPH Purified Pork Isophane Insulin 1626

Insulin, Regular (Changes in insulin requirements). Products include:
Regular, 40 & 100 Units 1273
Beef Regular, 100 Units 1275
Pork Regular, 100 Units 1275
Pork Regular (Concentrated), 500 Units 1276
Regular Insulin 1625
Regular Purified Pork Insulin 1626
Velosulin 1627

Insulin, Zinc Crystals (Changes in insulin requirements). Products include:
NPH, 40 & 100 Units 1273

Insulin, Zinc Suspension (Changes in insulin requirements). Products include:
Lente, 40 & 100 Units 1272
Protamine, Zinc, 40 & 100 Units 1273
Lente Iletin I 1272
Beef Lente, 100 Units 1274
Beef Protamine Zinc, 100 Units 1274
Pork Lente, 100 Units 1275
Pork, Protamine, Zinc, 100 Units 1275
Lente Insulin 1626
Lente Purified Pork Insulin 1626
Semilente Insulin 1625
Ultralente Insulin 1626

Isradipine (Potentiates action). Products include:
DynaCirc Capsules 2004

Labetalol Hydrochloride (Potentiates action). Products include:
Normodyne Injection 2108
Normodyne Tablets 2110
Normozide Tablets 2112
Trandate HCT Tablets 579
Trandate Injection 577
Trandate Tablets 579

Lisinopril (Potentiates action). Products include:
Prinivil Tablets 1538
Prinzide Tablets 1540
Zestoretic 2274
Zestril Tablets 2277

Mecamylamine Hydrochloride (Potentiates action). Products include:
Inversine Tablets 1492

Methyldopa (Potentiates action or additive). Products include:
Aldoclor Tablets 1413
Aldomet Oral 1415
Aldoril Tablets 1418

Methyldopate Hydrochloride (Potentiates action). Products include:
Aldomet Ester HCl Injection 1417

Methylprednisolone (Hypokalemia). Products include:
Medrol 2348

Methylprednisolone Acetate (Hypokalemia). Products include:
Depo-Medrol Sterile Aqueous Suspension 2334

Methylprednisolone Sodium Succinate (Hypokalemia). Products include:
Solu-Medrol Sterile Powder 2363

Metolazone (Potentiates action). Products include:
Diulo 2129
Mykrox ½ mg Tablets 984
Zaroxolyn Tablets 989

Metoprolol Tartrate (Potentiates action). Products include:
Lopressor Ampuls 1032
Lopressor HCT Tablets 1034
Lopressor Tablets 1032

Metyrosine (Potentiates action). Products include:
Demser Capsules 1460

Minoxidil (Potentiates action). Products include:
Loniten Tablets 2346
Rogaine Topical Solution 2357

Nadolol (Potentiates action). Products include:
Corgard Tablets 701
Corzide Tablets 702

Nicardipine Hydrochloride (Potentiates action). Products include:
Cardene Capsules 2290

Nitroglycerin (Potentiates action). Products include:
Deponit NTG Transdermal Delivery System 2143
Minitran Transdermal Delivery System 1312
Nitro-Bid Ointment 1339
Nitro-Bid Capsules 1338
Nitrodisc 2176
Nitro-Dur (nitroglycerin) Transdermal Infusion System 1164
Nitrogard Tablets 1004
Nitrolingual Spray 1846
Nitrostat Tablets 1743
Transderm-Nitro Transdermal Therapeutic System 2283

Norepinephrine Bitartrate (Decreased arterial responsiveness). Products include:
Levophed Bitartrate Injection 2054

Pancuronium Bromide Injection (Decreased serum levels).
No products indexed under this heading.

Penbutolol Sulfate (Potentiates action). Products include:
Levatol 1832

Phenoxybenzamine Hydrochloride (Potentiates action). Products include:
Dibenzyline Capsules 2207

Phentolamine Mesylate (Potentiates action). Products include:
Regitine 878

Pindolol (Potentiates action). Products include:
Visken Tablets 2036

Polythiazide (Potentiates action). Products include:
Minizide Capsules 1779
Renese Tablets 1785
Renese-R Tablets 1786

Prazosin Hydrochloride (Potentiates action). Products include:
Minipress Capsules 1778
Minizide Capsules 1779

Prednisolone Acetate (Hypokalemia). Products include:
AK-Cide Sterile Ophthalmic Ointment & Suspension ⊙ 202
Blephamide Liquifilm Sterile Ophthalmic Suspension 586
Blephamide S.O.P. Sterile Ophthalmic Ointment 586
Cetapred Ointment ⊙ 220
⅛% Econopred & 1% Econopred Plus ⊙ 217
Isopto Cetapred Suspension ⊙ 220
Metimyd ⊙ 306
Poly-Pred Liquifilm ⊙ 250
Pred Forte ⊙ 252
Pred Mild ⊙ 254
Pred-G Liquifilm Sterile Ophthalmic Suspension ⊙ 252
Pred-G S.O.P. Sterile Ophthalmic Ointment ⊙ 253
Vasocidin Ointment ⊙ 275

Prednisolone Sodium Phosphate (Hypokalemia). Products include:
AK-Pred ⊙ 205
Hydeltrasol Injection, Sterile 1476
Inflamase ⊙ 274
Pediapred Oral Liquid 987
Vasocidin Ophthalmic Solution ⊙ 276

Prednisolone Tebutate (Hypokalemia). Products include:
Hydeltra-T.B.A. Sterile Suspension 1478

Prednisone (Hypokalemia). Products include:
Deltasone Tablets 2332

Propranolol Hydrochloride (Potentiates action). Products include:
Inderal 2459
Inderal LA Long Acting Capsules 2461
Inderide Tablets 2463
Inderide LA Long Acting Capsules 2465

Quinidine Gluconate (Cardiac arrhythmias). Products include:
Quinaglute Dura-Tabs Tablets 663

Quinidine Polygalacturonate (Cardiac arrhythmias). Products include:
Cardioquin Tablets 1812

Quinidine Sulfate (Cardiac arrhythmias). Products include:
Quinidex Extentabs 1868

Ramipril (Potentiates action). Products include:
Altace Capsules 1086

Rauwolfia Serpentina (Potentiates action). Products include:
Raudixin Tablets 1803
Rauzide Tablets 1804

Rescinnamine (Potentiates action).
No products indexed under this heading.

Reserpine (Potentiates action). Products include:
Diupres Tablets 1461
Hydromox R Tablets 1209
Hydropres Tablets 1485
Renese-R Tablets 1786
Salutensin/Salutensin-Demi 719
Ser-Ap-Es Tablets 881
Serpasil Tablets 883
Serpasil-Apresoline Tablets 884
Serpasil-Esidrix Tablets 886

Sodium Nitroprusside (Potentiates action). Products include:
Nipride I.V. Infusion 1909

Terazosin Hydrochloride (Potentiates action). Products include:
Hytrin Tablets 529

Timolol Maleate (Potentiates action). Products include:
Blocadren Tablets 1429
Timolide Tablets 1547
Timoptic in Ocudose 1552
Timoptic Sterile Ophthalmic Solution 1550

Triamcinolone (Hypokalemia).
No products indexed under this heading.

Triamcinolone Acetonide (Hypokalemia). Products include:
Aristocort A 1010
Azmacort Inhaler 1837
Kenalog Cream, Lotion & Ointment 2401
Kenalog-10 Injection 2402
Kenalog-40 Injection 2403
Kenalog in Orabase 604
Kenalog Spray 2401
Mycolog II Cream and Ointment 2407
Mytrex Cream & Ointment 2080
Nasacort Nasal Inhaler 1844

Triamcinolone Diacetate (Hypokalemia). Products include:
Aristocort Suspension 1008

Triamcinolone Hexacetonide (Hypokalemia). Products include:
Aristospan Suspension 1011

Trimethaphan Camsylate (Potentiates action). Products include:
Arfonad Ampuls 1887

Tubocurarine Chloride (Increased responsiveness).
No products indexed under this heading.

ENDURONYL TABLETS
(Methyclothiazide, Deserpidine) 518
See **Enduronyl Forte Tablets**

ENER-B VITAMIN B_{12} NASAL GEL DIETARY SUPPLEMENT
(Vitamin B_{12}, Nasal Delivery) 1617
No interactions described in labeling.

ENGERIX-B UNIT-DOSE VIALS
(Hepatitis B Vaccine) 2213
No interactions described in labeling.

ENLON INJECTION
(Edrophonium Chloride) 598
May interact with nondepolarizing neuromuscular blocking agents and cholinergic agents. Compounds in these categories include:

Atracurium Besylate (Do not administer Enlon prior to this compound). Products include:
Tracrium Injection 817

Metocurine Iodide (Do not administer Enlon prior to this compound). Products include:
Metubine Iodide Vials 1285

Neostigmine Bromide (Administer Enlon cautiously to myasthenic patients on anticholinesterase drugs). Products include:
Prostigmin Tablets 1121

Neostigmine Methylsulfate (Administer Enlon cautiously to myasthenic patients on anticholinesterase drugs). Products include:
Prostigmin Injectable 1120

Pancuronium Bromide Injection (Do not administer Enlon prior to this compound).
No products indexed under this heading.

Pyridostigmine Bromide (Administer Enlon cautiously to myasthenic patients on anticholinesterase drugs). Products include:
Mestinon Injectable 1115
Mestinon 1116

Vecuronium Bromide (Do not administer Enlon prior to this compound). Products include:
Norcuron 1642

ENOVID 5 MG
(Norethynodrel, Mestranol) 2161
See **Demulen 1/35-21**

ENOVID 10 MG
(Norethynodrel, Mestranol) 2161
See **Demulen 1/35-21**

ENRICH LIQUID NUTRITION WITH FIBER
(Nutritional Supplement) 1971
No interactions described in labeling.

ENSURE LIQUID NUTRITION
(Nutritional Supplement) 1971
No interactions described in labeling.

ENSURE PLUS HIGH CALORIE LIQUID NUTRITION
(Nutritional Supplement) 1971
No interactions described in labeling.

ENTEX CAPSULES
(Phenylephrine Hydrochloride, Phenylpropanolamine Hydrochloride, Guaifenesin) 1623
May interact with monoamine oxidase inhibitors and sympathomimetic aerosal brochodilators. Compounds in these categories include:

Albuterol (Entex usage not recommended). Products include:
Proventil Inhalation Aerosol 2117
Ventolin Inhalation Aerosol and Refill 583

Albuterol Sulfate (Entex usage not recommended). Products include:
Proventil Repetabs Tablets 2120
Proventil Solutions for Inhalation 0.5% and 0.083% 2118
Proventil Syrup 2119
Proventil Tablets 2120
Ventolin 583

Dobutamine Hydrochloride (Entex usage not recommended). Products include:
Dobutrex Solution Vials 1259

Dopamine Hydrochloride (Entex usage not recommended). Products include:
Intropin Injection 930

Ephedrine Hydrochloride (Entex usage not recommended). Products include:
Amesec .... ▣ 682
Primatene Tablets-M Formula 2421
Primatene Tablets-P Formula 2421
Primatene Tablets-Regular Formula 2421
Quadrinal Tablets 1183
Quelidrine Syrup 556
Tedral SA 1765

Ephedrine Sulfate (Entex usage not recommended). Products include:
Bronkaid Tablets .... ▣ 757
Bronkolixir .... ▣ 761
Bronkotabs Tablets .... ▣ 762
Marax Tablets & DF Syrup 1954
Pazo Hemorrhoid Ointment & Suppositories 752
Vicks Vatronol Nose Drops .... ▣ 666

Ephedrine Tannate (Entex usage not recommended). Products include:
Rynatuss 2388

Epinephrine (Entex usage not recommended). Products include:
Ana-Kit Anaphylaxis Emergency Treatment Kit 1100
Bronkaid Mist .... ▣ 757
EpiPen 843
Marcaine Hydrochloride 0.5% with Epinephrine 1:200,000 (as bitartrate) 958
Marcaine Hydrochloride with Epinephrine 1:200,000 2055
Primatene Mist 2420
Sus-Phrine Injection 1006
Xylocaine with Epinephrine Injections 637

Epinephrine Bitartrate (Entex usage not recommended). Products include:
AsthmaHaler Mist Epinephrine Bitartrate Bronchodilator .... ▣ 616
Bronkaid Mist Suspension .... ▣ 757
Primatene Mist Suspension 2421

Epinephrine Hydrochloride (Entex usage not recommended). Products include:
Adrenalin Chloride Solution 1:100 & 1:1,000 1689
Epifrin .... ⊙ 244
Glaucon .... ⊙ 218

Furazolidone (Entex usage not recommended). Products include:
Furoxone 1855

Isocarboxazid (Entex usage not recommended). Products include:
Marplan Tablets 1906

Isoproterenol Hydrochloride (Entex usage not recommended). Products include:
Isuprel Hydrochloride Injection 1:5000 2050
Isuprel Hydrochloride Mistometer .. 2051
Isuprel Hydrochloride Solution 1:200 & 1:100 2052
Norisodrine Aerotrol 540

Metaproterenol Sulfate (Entex usage not recommended). Products include:
Alupent 674
Arm-a-Med Metaproterenol Sulfate Inhalation Solution, USP 617
Metaprel Inhalation Aerosol Bronchodilator 2014
Metaprel Inhalation Solution 2015
Metaprel 2015
Metaproterenol Sulfate Inhalation Solution, USP 912

Metaraminol Bitartrate (Entex usage not recommended). Products include:
Aramine Injection 1424

Methoxamine Hydrochloride (Entex usage not recommended). Products include:
Vasoxyl Injection 819

Norepinephrine Bitartrate (Entex usage not recommended). Products include:
Levophed Bitartrate Injection 2054

Phenelzine Sulfate (Entex usage not recommended). Products include:
Nardil 1742

Phenylephrine Bitartrate (Entex usage not recommended).
No products indexed under this heading.

Phenylephrine Tannate (Entex usage not recommended). Products include:
Rynatan 2387
Rynatuss 2388

Pirbuterol Acetate (Entex usage not recommended). Products include:
Maxair Inhaler 1311

Pseudoephedrine Hydrochloride (Entex usage not recommended). Products include:
Actifed Capsules .... ▣ 539
Actifed Plus Caplets .... ▣ 539
Actifed Plus Tablets .... ▣ 540
Actifed with Codeine Cough Syrup .. 752
Actifed Syrup .... ▣ 540
Actifed Tablets .... ▣ 540
Actifed 12-Hour Capsules .... ▣ 539
Advil Cold & Sinus Caplets (formerly CoAdvil) 2416
Allerest .... ▣ 559
Anatuss LA Tablets 1359
Benadryl Decongestant Elixir .... ▣ 635
Benadryl Decongestant .... ▣ 635
Benadryl Plus .... ▣ 636
Benadryl Plus Nighttime .... ▣ 637
Benylin Decongestant .... ▣ 638
Brexin L.A. Capsules 2078
Bromfed Capsules (Timed Release) 1615
Bromfed Syrup .... ▣ 628
Bromfed 1615
CoAdvil .... ▣ 748
Allergy-Sinus Comtrex Multi-Symptom Allergy Sinus Formula Tablets & Caplets 746
Cough Formula Comtrex 746
Comtrex Multi-Symptom Cold Reliever Tablets/Caplets/Liqui-Gels/Liquid 745
Day-Night Comtrex 747
Non-Drowsy Comtrex 747
Congess 994
Congestac Caplets .... ▣ 617
Contac Jr. Children's Cold Medicine .... ▣ 712
Contac Nighttime Cold Medicine .... ▣ 713
Contac Sinus Caplets Maximum Strength Non-Drowsy Formula .... ▣ 710
Contac Sinus Tablets Maximum Strength Non-Drowsy Formula .... ▣ 710
Deconamine 663
Deconsal II Tablets 559
Dimacol Caplets .... ▣ 672
Dimetane-DX Cough Syrup 1858
Dorcol Children's Cough Syrup .... ▣ 685
Dorcol Children's Decongestant Liquid .... ▣ 685
Dorcol Children's Liquid Cold Formula .... ▣ 686
Maximum Strength Dristan Decongestant/Analgesic Coated Caplets .... ▣ 750
No Drowsiness Dristan Cold Nasal Decongestant/Analgesic Coated Caplets 2420
Dristan Sinus Caplets 2419
Sinus Excedrin Analgesic, Decongestant Tablets & Caplets .... ▣ 533
Fedahist Gyrocaps 2145
Fedahist Timecaps 2145
Guaifed 1615
Guaifed Syrup .... ▣ 629
Isoclor Expectorant 982
Isoclor Timesule Capsules .... ▣ 561
Kronofed-A 970
Medi-Flu Caplet, Liquid .... ▣ 640
Novafed A Capsules 1342
Novafed Capsules 1342
Novahistine DH 1342
Novahistine DMX .... ▣ 595
Novahistine Expectorant 1343
Nucofed Capsules 2219
Nucofed Expectorant 2219
Nucofed Pediatric Expectorant 2220
Nucofed Syrup 2219
Ornex Caplets .... ▣ 618
PediaCare Allergy Relief Formula Liquid 1362
PediaCare Cough-Cold Formula Liquid 1362
PediaCare Infants' Oral Decongestant Drops 1362
PediaCare Night Rest Cough-Cold Formula Liquid 1362
PediaCare 6-12 Cough-Cold Formula Chewable Tablets 1362
Robitussin-DAC Syrup 1875
Robitussin-PE .... ▣ 677
Rondec 1975
Rondec-DM 1976
Rondec-TR Tablet 1975
Ru-Tuss DE Tablets 694
Ryna .... ▣ 741
Seldane-D Extended-Release Tablets 1350
Sinarest .... ▣ 562
Sine-Aid Maximum Strength Sinus Headache Caplets 1365
Sine-Aid Maximum Strength Sinus Headache Tablets 1365
Sine-Off Maximum Strength Allergy/Sinus Formula Caplets .... ▣ 721
Sine-Off Maximum Strength No Drowsiness Formula Caplets .... ▣ 722
Singlet Tablets .... ▣ 598
Sinutab Maximum Strength .... ▣ 641
Sinutab Maximum Strength Without Drowsiness Tablets & Caplets .... ▣ 642
Sinutab Regular Strength Without Drowsiness Formula .... ▣ 641
St. Joseph Nighttime Cold Medicine .... ▣ 705
Sudafed Children's Liquid .... ▣ 543
Sudafed Cough Syrup .... ▣ 543
Sudafed Plus Liquid .... ▣ 544
Sudafed Plus Tablets .... ▣ 545
Sudafed Sinus Caplets .... ▣ 545
Sudafed Sinus Tablets .... ▣ 545
Sudafed Tablets, 30 mg .... ▣ 544
Sudafed Tablets, Adult Strength, 60 mg .... ▣ 544
Sudafed 12 Hour Capsules .... ▣ 545
TheraFlu Flu and Cold Medicine .... ▣ 687
Triaminic Nite Light .... ▣ 689
Tylenol Allergy Sinus Medication Caplets and Gelcaps, Maximum Strength 1372
Children's Tylenol Cold Liquid Formula and Chewable Tablets 1368
Tylenol Cold & Flu Hot Medication, Packets 1369
Tylenol Cold & Flu No Drowsiness Hot Medication, Packets 1371
Tylenol Cold Medication Caplets and Tablets 1370
Tylenol Cold Medication No Drowsiness Formula Caplets 1370
Tylenol Cold Night Time Medication Liquid 1371

Tylenol Cough Medication Liquid with Decongestant, Maximum Strength ... 1372
Tylenol, Maximum Strength, Sinus Medication Gelcaps, Caplets and Tablets ... 1373
Ursinus Inlay-Tabs ... ■ 691
Vicks Children's NyQuil ... ■ 664
Vicks Daycare ... ■ 660
Vicks Formula 44D Decongestant Cough Medicine ... ■ 662
Vicks Formula 44M Multi-Symptom Cough Medicine ... ■ 662
Vicks NyQuil Nighttime Colds Medicine-Original & Cherry Flavor ... ■ 664
Vicks Pediatric Formula 44 Cough & Congestion Medicine ... ■ 663
Vicks Pediatric Formula 44m Multi-Symptom Cough & Cold Medicine ... ■ 663

Pseudoephedrine Sulfate (Entex usage not recommended). Products include:
Afrin Tablets ... ■ 693
Chlor-Trimeton Decongestant ... ■ 694
Disophrol Chronotab Sustained-Action Tablets ... ■ 698
Drixoral Antihistamine/Nasal Decongestant Syrup ... ■ 698
Drixoral Non-Drowsy Formula ... ■ 699
Drixoral Plus Extended-Release Tablets ... ■ 699
Drixoral Sinus ... ■ 700
Drixoral Sustained-Action Tablets ■ 698
Sinutab Allergy Formula Sustained Action Tablets ... ■ 640
Trinalin Repetabs Tablets ... 1170

Selegiline Hydrochloride (Entex usage not recommended). Products include:
Eldepryl ... 2250

Terbutaline Sulfate (Entex usage not recommended). Products include:
Brethaire Inhaler ... 1024
Brethine Ampuls ... 1026
Brethine Tablets ... 1026
Bricanyl Injection ... 1324
Bricanyl Tablets ... 1325

Tranylcypromine Sulfate (Entex usage not recommended). Products include:
Parnate Tablets ... 2222

ENTEX LA TABLETS

(Phenylpropanolamine Hydrochloride, Guaifenesin) ... 1623
May interact with monoamine oxidase inhibitors and sympathomimetic aerosal brochodilators. Compounds in these categories include:

Albuterol (Entex LA usage not recommended). Products include:
Proventil Inhalation Aerosol ... 2117
Ventolin Inhalation Aerosol and Refill ... 583

Albuterol Sulfate (Entex LA usage not recommended). Products include:
Proventil Repetabs Tablets ... 2120
Proventil Solutions for Inhalation 0.5% and 0.083% ... 2118
Proventil Syrup ... 2119
Proventil Tablets ... 2120
Ventolin ... 583

Dobutamine Hydrochloride (Entex LA usage not recommended). Products include:
Dobutrex Solution Vials ... 1259

Dopamine Hydrochloride (Entex LA usage not recommended). Products include:
Intropin Injection ... 930

Ephedrine Hydrochloride (Entex LA usage not recommended). Products include:
Amesec ... ■ 682
Primatene Tablets-M Formula ... 2421
Primatene Tablets-P Formula ... 2421
Primatene Tablets-Regular Formula ... 2421
Quadrinal Tablets ... 1183
Quelidrine Syrup ... 556
Tedral SA ... 1765

Ephedrine Sulfate (Entex LA usage not recommended). Products include:
Bronkaid Tablets ... ■ 757
Bronkolixir ... ■ 761
Bronkotabs Tablets ... ■ 762
Marax Tablets & DF Syrup ... 1954
Pazo Hemorrhoid Ointment & Suppositories ... 752
Vicks Vatronol Nose Drops ... ■ 666

Ephedrine Tannate (Entex LA usage not recommended). Products include:
Rynatuss ... 2388

Epinephrine (Entex LA usage not recommended). Products include:
Ana-Kit Anaphylaxis Emergency Treatment Kit ... 1100
Bronkaid Mist ... ■ 757
EpiPen ... 843
Marcaine Hydrochloride 0.5% with Epinephrine 1:200,000 (as bitartrate) ... 958
Marcaine Hydrochloride with Epinephrine 1:200,000 ... 2055
Primatene Mist ... 2420
Sus-Phrine Injection ... 1006
Xylocaine with Epinephrine Injections ... 637

Epinephrine Bitartrate (Entex LA usage not recommended). Products include:
AsthmaHaler Mist Epinephrine Bitartrate Bronchodilator ... ■ 616
Bronkaid Mist Suspension ... ■ 757
Primatene Mist Suspension ... 2421

Epinephrine Hydrochloride (Entex LA usage not recommended). Products include:
Adrenalin Chloride Solution 1:100 & 1:1,000 ... 1689
Epifrin ... ⊙ 244
Glaucon ... ⊙ 218

Furazolidone (Entex LA usage not recommended). Products include:
Furoxone ... 1855

Isocarboxazid (Entex LA usage not recommended). Products include:
Marplan Tablets ... 1906

Isoproterenol Hydrochloride (Entex LA usage not recommended). Products include:
Isuprel Hydrochloride Injection 1:5000 ... 2050
Isuprel Hydrochloride Mistometer .. 2051
Isuprel Hydrochloride Solution 1:200 & 1:100 ... 2052
Norisodrine Aerotrol ... 540

Metaproterenol Sulfate (Entex LA usage not recommended). Products include:
Alupent ... 674
Arm-a-Med Metaproterenol Sulfate Inhalation Solution, USP ... 617
Metaprel Inhalation Aerosol Bronchodilator ... 2014
Metaprel Inhalation Solution ... 2015
Metaprel ... 2015
Metaproterenol Sulfate Inhalation Solution, USP ... 912

Metaraminol Bitartrate (Entex LA usage not recommended). Products include:
Aramine Injection ... 1424

Methoxamine Hydrochloride (Entex LA usage not recommended). Products include:
Vasoxyl Injection ... 819

Norepinephrine Bitartrate (Entex LA usage not recommended). Products include:
Levophed Bitartrate Injection ... 2054

Phenelzine Sulfate (Entex LA usage not recommended). Products include:
Nardil ... 1742

Phenylephrine Bitartrate (Entex LA usage not recommended).
No products indexed under this heading.

Phenylephrine Hydrochloride (Entex LA usage not recommended). Products include:
AK-Dilate Solution 2.5% and 10% ... ⊙ 203
Atrohist Sprinkle Capsules ... 558
Cerose-DM ... 2443
Codimal ... 846
Comhist LA Capsules ... 1618
Congespirin For Children Aspirin Free Chewable Cold Tablets ... 748
Cyclomydril ... ⊙ 216
Deconsal Sprinkle Capsules ... 559
Dimetane Decongestant ... ■ 673
Dristan Decongestant/Antihistamine/ Analgesic Coated Caplets ... ■ 749
Dristan Cold Nasal Decongestant/ Antihistamine/ Analgesic Coated Tablets ... 2419
Dristan Advanced Formula Decongestant/Antihistamine/ Analgesic Tablets ... ■ 749
Dristan Nasal Spray, Menthol ... 2419
Dristan Nasal Spray, Regular and Regular with Metered Pump ... 2419
Entex Capsules ... 1623
Entex Liquid ... 1623
Sinus Excedrin Analgesic, Decongestant Tablets & Caplets ... 750
Extendryl ... 994
4-Way Fast Acting Nasal Spray - Original Formula (regular & mentholated) & Metered Spray Pump (regular) ... 751
Hycomine Compound Tablets ... 929
Murocoll-2 Sterile Ophthalmic Solution ... ⊙ 261
Mydfrin 2.5% ... ⊙ 224
Naldecon Syrup, Tablets, Pediatric Drops and Pediatric Syrup ... 709
Neo-Synephrine Hydrochloride 1% Carpuject ... 2063
Neo-Synephrine Hydrochloride 1% Injection ... 2063
Neo-Synephrine Hydrochloride (Ophthalmic) ... 2064
Neo-Synephrine ... ■ 759
Nōstril Nasal Decongestant ... ■ 520
Novahistine Elixir ... ■ 596
Phenergan VC ... 2500
Phenergan VC with Codeine ... 2501
Prefrin Liquifilm Vasoconstrictor and Lubricant Eye Drops ... ⊙ 254
Prefrin-A ... ⊙ 255
Quelidrine Syrup ... 556
Relief Vasoconstrictor and Lubricant Eye Drops ... ⊙ 256
Robitussin Night Relief ... ■ 677
Ru-Tuss with Hydrocodone ... 694
Ru-Tuss Tablets ... 693
Vasosulf ... ⊙ 279
Vicks Sinex ... ■ 665
Zincfrin ... ⊙ 230

Phenylephrine Tannate (Entex LA usage not recommended). Products include:
Rynatan ... 2387
Rynatuss ... 2388

Pirbuterol Acetate (Entex LA usage not recommended). Products include:
Maxair Inhaler ... 1311

Pseudoephedrine Hydrochloride (Entex LA usage not recommended). Products include:
Actifed Capsules ... ■ 539
Actifed Plus Caplets ... ■ 539
Actifed Plus Tablets ... ■ 540
Actifed with Codeine Cough Syrup .. 752
Actifed Syrup ... ■ 540
Actifed Tablets ... ■ 540
Actifed 12-Hour Capsules ... ■ 539
Advil Cold & Sinus Caplets (formerly CoAdvil) ... 2416
Allerest ... ■ 559
Anatuss LA Tablets ... 1359
Benadryl Decongestant Elixir ... ■ 635
Benadryl Decongestant ... ■ 635
Benadryl Plus ... ■ 636
Benadryl Plus Nighttime ... ■ 637
Benylin Decongestant ... ■ 638
Brexin L.A. Capsules ... 2078
Bromfed Capsules (Timed Release) ... 1615
Bromfed Syrup ... ■ 628
Bromfed ... 1615
CoAdvil ... ■ 748
Allergy-Sinus Comtrex Multi-Symptom Allergy Sinus Formula Tablets & Caplets ... 746
Cough Formula Comtrex ... 746
Comtrex Multi-Symptom Cold Reliever Tablets/Caplets/Liqui-Gels/Liquid ... 745
Day-Night Comtrex ... 747
Non-Drowsy Comtrex ... 747
Congess ... 994
Congestac Caplets ... ■ 617
Contac Jr. Children's Cold Medicine ... ■ 712
Contac Nighttime Cold Medicine ... ■ 713
Contac Sinus Caplets Maximum Strength Non-Drowsy Formula ... ■ 710
Contac Sinus Tablets Maximum Strength Non-Drowsy Formula ... ■ 710
Deconamine ... 663
Deconsal II Tablets ... 559
Dimacol Caplets ... ■ 672
Dimetane-DX Cough Syrup ... 1858
Dorcol Children's Cough Syrup ... ■ 685
Dorcol Children's Decongestant Liquid ... ■ 685
Dorcol Children's Liquid Cold Formula ... ■ 686
Maximum Strength Dristan Decongestant/Analgesic Coated Caplets ... ■ 750
No Drowsiness Dristan Cold Nasal Decongestant/Analgesic Coated Caplets ... 2420
Dristan Sinus Caplets ... 2419
Sinus Excedrin Analgesic, Decongestant Tablets & Caplets ... ■ 533
Fedahist Gyrocaps ... 2145
Fedahist Timecaps ... 2145
Guaifed ... 1615
Guaifed Syrup ... ■ 629
Isoclor Expectorant ... 982
Isoclor Timesule Capsules ... ■ 561
Kronofed-A ... 970
Medi-Flu Caplet, Liquid ... ■ 640
Novafed A Capsules ... 1342
Novafed Capsules ... 1342
Novahistine DH ... 1342
Novahistine DMX ... ■ 595
Novahistine Expectorant ... 1343
Nucofed Capsules ... 2219
Nucofed Expectorant ... 2219
Nucofed Pediatric Expectorant ... 2220
Nucofed Syrup ... 2219
Ornex Caplets ... ■ 618
PediaCare Allergy Relief Formula Liquid ... 1362
PediaCare Cough-Cold Formula Liquid ... 1362
PediaCare Infants' Oral Decongestant Drops ... 1362
PediaCare Night Rest Cough-Cold Formula Liquid ... 1362
PediaCare 6-12 Cough-Cold Formula Chewable Tablets ... 1362
Robitussin-DAC Syrup ... 1875
Robitussin-PE ... ■ 677
Rondec ... 1975
Rondec-DM ... 1976
Rondec-TR Tablet ... 1975
Ru-Tuss DE Tablets ... 694
Ryna ... ■ 741
Seldane-D Extended-Release Tablets ... 1350
Sinarest ... ■ 562
Sine-Aid Maximum Strength Sinus Headache Caplets ... 1365
Sine-Aid Maximum Strength Sinus Headache Tablets ... 1365
Sine-Off Maximum Strength Allergy/Sinus Formula Caplets ... ■ 721
Sine-Off Maximum Strength No Drowsiness Formula Caplets ... ■ 722
Singlet Tablets ... ■ 598
Sinutab Maximum Strength ... ■ 641
Sinutab Maximum Strength Without Drowsiness Tablets & Caplets ... ■ 642
Sinutab Regular Strength Without Drowsiness Formula ... ■ 641
St. Joseph Nighttime Cold Medicine ... ■ 705
Sudafed Children's Liquid ... ■ 543
Sudafed Cough Syrup ... ■ 543
Sudafed Plus Liquid ... ■ 544
Sudafed Plus Tablets ... ■ 545
Sudafed Sinus Caplets ... ■ 545
Sudafed Sinus Tablets ... ■ 545
Sudafed Tablets, 30 mg ... ■ 544
Sudafed Tablets, Adult Strength, 60 mg ... ■ 544

Sudafed 12 Hour Capsules ▣ 545
TheraFlu Flu and Cold Medicine ▣ 687
Triaminic Nite Light ▣ 689
Tylenol Allergy Sinus Medication Caplets and Gelcaps, Maximum Strength 1372
Children's Tylenol Cold Liquid Formula and Chewable Tablets 1368
Tylenol Cold & Flu Hot Medication, Packets 1369
Tylenol Cold & Flu No Drowsiness Hot Medication, Packets 1371
Tylenol Cold Medication Caplets and Tablets 1370
Tylenol Cold Medication No Drowsiness Formula Caplets 1370
Tylenol Cold Night Time Medication Liquid 1371
Tylenol Cough Medication Liquid with Decongestant, Maximum Strength 1372
Tylenol, Maximum Strength, Sinus Medication Gelcaps, Caplets and Tablets 1373
Ursinus Inlay-Tabs ▣ 691
Vicks Children's NyQuil ▣ 664
Vicks Daycare ▣ 660
Vicks Formula 44D Decongestant Cough Medicine ▣ 662
Vicks Formula 44M Multi-Symptom Cough Medicine ▣ 662
Vicks NyQuil Nighttime Colds Medicine-Original & Cherry Flavor ▣ 664
Vicks Pediatric Formula 44 Cough & Congestion Medicine ▣ 663
Vicks Pediatric Formula 44m Multi-Symptom Cough & Cold Medicine ▣ 663

Pseudoephedrine Sulfate (Entex LA usage not recommended). Products include:
Afrin Tablets ▣ 693
Chlor-Trimeton Decongestant ▣ 694
Disophrol Chronotab Sustained-Action Tablets ▣ 698
Drixoral Antihistamine/Nasal Decongestant Syrup ▣ 698
Drixoral Non-Drowsy Formula ▣ 699
Drixoral Plus Extended-Release Tablets ▣ 699
Drixoral Sinus ▣ 700
Drixoral Sustained-Action Tablets ▣ 698
Sinutab Allergy Formula Sustained Action Tablets ▣ 640
Trinalin Repetabs Tablets 1170

Selegiline Hydrochloride (Entex LA usage not recommended). Products include:
Eldepryl 2250

Terbutaline Sulfate (Entex LA usage not recommended). Products include:
Brethaire Inhaler 1024
Brethine Ampuls 1026
Brethine Tablets 1026
Bricanyl Injection 1324
Bricanyl Tablets 1325

Tranylcypromine Sulfate (Entex LA usage not recommended). Products include:
Parnate Tablets 2222

ENTEX LIQUID
(Phenylephrine Hydrochloride, Phenylpropanolamine Hydrochloride, Guaifenesin) 1623
May interact with monoamine oxidase inhibitors and sympathomimetic aerosal brochodilators. Compounds in these categories include:

Albuterol (Entex usage not recommended). Products include:
Proventil Inhalation Aerosol 2117
Ventolin Inhalation Aerosol and Refill 583

Albuterol Sulfate (Entex usage not recommended). Products include:
Proventil Repetabs Tablets 2120
Proventil Solutions for Inhalation 0.5% and 0.083% 2118
Proventil Syrup 2119
Proventil Tablets 2120
Ventolin 583

Dobutamine Hydrochloride (Entex usage not recommended). Products include:
Dobutrex Solution Vials 1259

Dopamine Hydrochloride (Entex usage not recommended). Products include:
Intropin Injection 930

Ephedrine Hydrochloride (Entex usage not recommended). Products include:
Amesec ▣ 682
Primatene Tablets-M Formula 2421
Primatene Tablets-P Formula 2421
Primatene Tablets-Regular Formula 2421
Quadrinal Tablets 1183
Quelidrine Syrup 556
Tedral SA 1765

Ephedrine Sulfate (Entex usage not recommended). Products include:
Bronkaid Tablets ▣ 757
Bronkolixir ▣ 761
Bronkotabs Tablets ▣ 762
Marax Tablets & DF Syrup 1954
Pazo Hemorrhoid Ointment & Suppositories 752
Vicks Vatronol Nose Drops ▣ 666

Ephedrine Tannate (Entex usage not recommended). Products include:
Rynatuss 2388

Epinephrine (Entex usage not recommended). Products include:
Ana-Kit Anaphylaxis Emergency Treatment Kit 1100
Bronkaid Mist ▣ 757
EpiPen 843
Marcaine Hydrochloride 0.5% with Epinephrine 1:200,000 (as bitartrate) 958
Marcaine Hydrochloride with Epinephrine 1:200,000 2055
Primatene Mist 2420
Sus-Phrine Injection 1006
Xylocaine with Epinephrine Injections 637

Epinephrine Bitartrate (Entex usage not recommended). Products include:
AsthmaHaler Mist Epinephrine Bitartrate Bronchodilator ▣ 616
Bronkaid Mist Suspension ▣ 757
Primatene Mist Suspension 2421

Epinephrine Hydrochloride (Entex usage not recommended). Products include:
Adrenalin Chloride Solution 1:100 & 1:1,000 1689
Epifrin ⊙ 244
Glaucon ⊙ 218

Furazolidone (Entex usage not recommended). Products include:
Furoxone 1855

Isocarboxazid (Entex usage not recommended). Products include:
Marplan Tablets 1906

Isoproterenol Hydrochloride (Entex usage not recommended). Products include:
Isuprel Hydrochloride Injection 1:5000 2050
Isuprel Hydrochloride Mistometer 2051
Isuprel Hydrochloride Solution 1:200 & 1:100 2052
Norisodrine Aerotrol 540

Metaproterenol Sulfate (Entex usage not recommended). Products include:
Alupent 674
Arm-a-Med Metaproterenol Sulfate Inhalation Solution, USP 617
Metaprel Inhalation Aerosol Bronchodilator 2014
Metaprel Inhalation Solution 2015
Metaprel 2015
Metaproterenol Sulfate Inhalation Solution, USP 912

Metaraminol Bitartrate (Entex usage not recommended). Products include:
Aramine Injection 1424

Methoxamine Hydrochloride (Entex usage not recommended). Products include:
Vasoxyl Injection 819

Norepinephrine Bitartrate (Entex usage not recommended). Products include:
Levophed Bitartrate Injection 2054

Phenelzine Sulfate (Entex usage not recommended). Products include:
Nardil 1742

Phenylephrine Bitartrate (Entex usage not recommended).
No products indexed under this heading.

Phenylephrine Tannate (Entex usage not recommended). Products include:
Rynatan 2387
Rynatuss 2388

Pirbuterol Acetate (Entex usage not recommended). Products include:
Maxair Inhaler 1311

Pseudoephedrine Hydrochloride (Entex usage not recommended). Products include:
Actifed Capsules ▣ 539
Actifed Plus Caplets ▣ 539
Actifed Plus Tablets ▣ 540
Actifed with Codeine Cough Syrup 752
Actifed Syrup ▣ 540
Actifed Tablets ▣ 540
Actifed 12-Hour Capsules ▣ 539
Advil Cold & Sinus Caplets (formerly CoAdvil) 2416
Allerest ▣ 559
Anatuss LA Tablets 1359
Benadryl Decongestant Elixir ▣ 635
Benadryl Decongestant ▣ 635
Benadryl Plus ▣ 636
Benadryl Plus Nighttime ▣ 637
Benylin Decongestant ▣ 638
Brexin L.A. Capsules 2078
Bromfed Capsules (Timed Release) 1615
Bromfed Syrup ▣ 628
Bromfed 1615
CoAdvil ▣ 748
Allergy-Sinus Comtrex Multi-Symptom Allergy Sinus Formula Tablets & Caplets 746
Cough Formula Comtrex 746
Comtrex Multi-Symptom Cold Reliever Tablets/Caplets/Liqui-Gels/Liquid 745
Day-Night Comtrex 747
Non-Drowsy Comtrex 747
Congess 994
Congestac Caplets ▣ 617
Contac Jr. Children's Cold Medicine ▣ 712
Contac Nighttime Cold Medicine ▣ 713
Contac Sinus Caplets Maximum Strength Non-Drowsy Formula ▣ 710
Contac Sinus Tablets Maximum Strength Non-Drowsy Formula ▣ 710
Deconamine 663
Deconsal II Tablets 559
Dimacol Caplets ▣ 672
Dimetane-DX Cough Syrup 1858
Dorcol Children's Cough Syrup ▣ 685
Dorcol Children's Decongestant Liquid ▣ 685
Dorcol Children's Liquid Cold Formula ▣ 686
Maximum Strength Dristan Decongestant/Analgesic Coated Caplets ▣ 750
No Drowsiness Dristan Cold Nasal Decongestant/Analgesic Coated Caplets 2420
Dristan Sinus Caplets 2419
Sinus Excedrin Analgesic, Decongestant Tablets & Caplets ▣ 533
Fedahist Gyrocaps 2145
Fedahist Timecaps 2145
Guaifed 1615
Guaifed Syrup ▣ 629
Isoclor Expectorant 982
Isoclor Timesule Capsules ▣ 561
Kronofed-A 970
Medi-Flu Caplet, Liquid ▣ 640
Novafed A Capsules 1342
Novafed Capsules 1342
Novahistine DH 1342
Novahistine DMX ▣ 595
Novahistine Expectorant 1343
Nucofed Capsules 2219
Nucofed Expectorant 2219
Nucofed Pediatric Expectorant 2220
Nucofed Syrup 2219
Ornex Caplets ▣ 618
PediaCare Allergy Relief Formula Liquid 1362
PediaCare Cough-Cold Formula Liquid 1362
PediaCare Infants' Oral Decongestant Drops 1362
PediaCare Night Rest Cough-Cold Formula Liquid 1362
PediaCare 6-12 Cough-Cold Formula Chewable Tablets 1362
Robitussin-DAC Syrup 1875
Robitussin-PE ▣ 677
Rondec 1975
Rondec-DM 1976
Rondec-TR Tablet 1975
Ru-Tuss DE Tablets 694
Ryna ▣ 741
Seldane-D Extended-Release Tablets 1350
Sinarest ▣ 562
Sine-Aid Maximum Strength Sinus Headache Caplets 1365
Sine-Aid Maximum Strength Sinus Headache Tablets 1365
Sine-Off Maximum Strength Allergy/Sinus Formula Caplets ▣ 721
Sine-Off Maximum Strength No Drowsiness Formula Caplets ▣ 722
Singlet Tablets ▣ 598
Sinutab Maximum Strength ▣ 641
Sinutab Maximum Strength Without Drowsiness Tablets & Caplets ▣ 642
Sinutab Regular Strength Without Drowsiness Formula ▣ 641
St. Joseph Nighttime Cold Medicine ▣ 705
Sudafed Children's Liquid ▣ 543
Sudafed Cough Syrup ▣ 543
Sudafed Plus Liquid ▣ 544
Sudafed Plus Tablets ▣ 545
Sudafed Sinus Caplets ▣ 545
Sudafed Sinus Tablets ▣ 545
Sudafed Tablets, 30 mg ▣ 544
Sudafed Tablets, Adult Strength, 60 mg ▣ 544
Sudafed 12 Hour Capsules ▣ 545
TheraFlu Flu and Cold Medicine ▣ 687
Triaminic Nite Light ▣ 689
Tylenol Allergy Sinus Medication Caplets and Gelcaps, Maximum Strength 1372
Children's Tylenol Cold Liquid Formula and Chewable Tablets 1368
Tylenol Cold & Flu Hot Medication, Packets 1369
Tylenol Cold & Flu No Drowsiness Hot Medication, Packets 1371
Tylenol Cold Medication Caplets and Tablets 1370
Tylenol Cold Medication No Drowsiness Formula Caplets 1370
Tylenol Cold Night Time Medication Liquid 1371
Tylenol Cough Medication Liquid with Decongestant, Maximum Strength 1372
Tylenol, Maximum Strength, Sinus Medication Gelcaps, Caplets and Tablets 1373
Ursinus Inlay-Tabs ▣ 691
Vicks Children's NyQuil ▣ 664
Vicks Daycare ▣ 660
Vicks Formula 44D Decongestant Cough Medicine ▣ 662
Vicks Formula 44M Multi-Symptom Cough Medicine ▣ 662
Vicks NyQuil Nighttime Colds Medicine-Original & Cherry Flavor ▣ 664
Vicks Pediatric Formula 44 Cough & Congestion Medicine ▣ 663
Vicks Pediatric Formula 44m Multi-Symptom Cough & Cold Medicine ▣ 663

Pseudoephedrine Sulfate (Entex usage not recommended). Products include:
Afrin Tablets ▣ 693
Chlor-Trimeton Decongestant ▣ 694
Disophrol Chronotab Sustained-Action Tablets ▣ 698

Drixoral Antihistamine/Nasal Decongestant Syrup ▣ 698
Drixoral Non-Drowsy Formula ▣ 699
Drixoral Plus Extended-Release Tablets ▣ 699
Drixoral Sinus ▣ 700
Drixoral Sustained-Action Tablets ▣ 698
Sinutab Allergy Formula Sustained Action Tablets ▣ 640
Trinalin Repetabs Tablets 1170

Selegiline Hydrochloride (Entex usage not recommended). Products include:
Eldepryl 2250

Terbutaline Sulfate (Entex usage not recommended). Products include:
Brethaire Inhaler 1024
Brethine Ampuls 1026
Brethine Tablets 1026
Bricanyl Injection 1324
Bricanyl Tablets 1325

Tranylcypromine Sulfate (Entex usage not recommended). Products include:
Parnate Tablets 2222

ENTOZYME TABLETS
(Enzymes, Digestive) 1862
No interactions described in labeling.

ENUCLENE
(Benzalkonium Chloride, Tyloxapol) ⊙ 232
No interactions described in labeling.

EPIFOAM
(Hydrocortisone Acetate, Pramoxine Hydrochloride) 1828
No interactions described in labeling.

EPIFRIN
(Epinephrine) ⊙ 244
No interactions described in labeling.

EPIPEN JR.
(Epinephrine) 843
See **EpiPen—Epinephrine Auto-Injector**

EPIPEN—EPINEPHRINE AUTO-INJECTOR
(Epinephrine) 843
May interact with tricyclic antidepressants, monoamine oxidase inhibitors, cardiac glycosides, and certain other agents. Compounds in these categories include:

Amitriptyline Hydrochloride (Potentiation of epinephrine). Products include:
Elavil 2269
Endep Tablets 1927
Etrafon 2087
Limbitrol 1933
Triavil Tablets 1556

Amoxapine (Potentiation of epinephrine). Products include:
Asendin Tablets 1196

Clomipramine Hydrochloride (Potentiation of epinephrine). Products include:
Anafranil Capsules 650

Desipramine Hydrochloride (Potentiation of epinephrine). Products include:
Norpramin Tablets 1340

Deslanoside (Concurrent use is not recommended).
No products indexed under this heading.

Digitoxin (Concurrent use is not recommended). Products include:
Crystodigin Tablets 1253

Digoxin (Concurrent use is not recommended). Products include:
Lanoxicaps 772
Lanoxin Elixir Pediatric 775
Lanoxin Injection 778
Lanoxin Injection Pediatric 781
Lanoxin Tablets 783

Doxepin Hydrochloride (Potentiation of epinephrine). Products include:
Sinequan 1960

Furazolidone (Potentiation of epinephrine). Products include:
Furoxone 1855

Imipramine Hydrochloride (Potentiation of epinephrine). Products include:
Tofranil Ampuls 1038
Tofranil Tablets 1039

Imipramine Pamoate (Potentiation of epinephrine). Products include:
Tofranil-PM Capsules 1041

Isocarboxazid (Potentiation of epinephrine). Products include:
Marplan Tablets 1906

Maprotiline Hydrochloride (Potentiation of epinephrine). Products include:
Ludiomil Tablets 874

Nortriptyline Hydrochloride (Potentiation of epinephrine). Products include:
Pamelor 2019

Phenelzine Sulfate (Potentiation of epinephrine). Products include:
Nardil 1742

Protriptyline Hydrochloride (Potentiation of epinephrine). Products include:
Vivactil Tablets 1567

Quinidine Gluconate (Concurrent use is not recommended). Products include:
Quinaglute Dura-Tabs Tablets 663

Quinidine Polygalacturonate (Concurrent use is not recommended). Products include:
Cardioquin Tablets 1812

Quinidine Sulfate (Concurrent use is not recommended). Products include:
Quinidex Extentabs 1868

Selegiline Hydrochloride (Potentiation of epinephrine). Products include:
Eldepryl 2250

Tranylcypromine Sulfate (Potentiation of epinephrine). Products include:
Parnate Tablets 2222

Trimipramine Maleate (Potentiation of epinephrine). Products include:
Surmontil Capsules 2524

EPOGEN FOR INJECTION
(Epoetin Alfa) 591
No interactions described in labeling.

EQUAGESIC TABLETS
(Meprobamate, Aspirin) 2451
May interact with oral hypoglycemic agents, psychotropics, and certain other agents. Compounds in these categories include:

Alcohol (Additive CNS-suppressant effects).

Alprazolam (Additive CNS-suppressant effects). Products include:
Xanax Tablets 2367

Amitriptyline Hydrochloride (Additive CNS-suppressant effects). Products include:
Elavil 2269
Endep Tablets 1927
Etrafon 2087
Limbitrol 1933
Triavil Tablets 1556

Amoxapine (Additive CNS-suppressant effects). Products include:
Asendin Tablets 1196

Buspirone Hydrochloride (Additive CNS-suppressant effects). Products include:
BuSpar 1401

Chlordiazepoxide (Additive CNS-suppressant effects). Products include:
Libritabs Tablets 1930
Limbitrol 1933
Menrium Tablets 1934

Chlordiazepoxide Hydrochloride (Additive CNS-suppressant effects). Products include:
Librax Capsules 1929
Librium Capsules 1931
Librium Injectable 1932

Chlorpromazine (Additive CNS-suppressant effects). Products include:
Thorazine 2234

Chlorpropamide (Hypoglycemic effect enhanced). Products include:
Diabinese Tablets 1775

Chlorprothixene (Additive CNS-suppressant effects). Products include:
Taractan Tablets 1920

Chlorprothixene Hydrochloride (Additive CNS-suppressant effects). Products include:
Taractan 1920

Clorazepate Dipotassium (Additive CNS-suppressant effects). Products include:
Tranxene 556

Desipramine Hydrochloride (Additive CNS-suppressant effects). Products include:
Norpramin Tablets 1340

Diazepam (Additive CNS-suppressant effects). Products include:
Valium Injectable 1937
Valium Tablets 1939
Valrelease Capsules 1923

Doxepin Hydrochloride (Additive CNS-suppressant effects). Products include:
Sinequan 1960

Droperidol (Additive CNS-suppressant effects). Products include:
Inapsine Injection 1140
Innovar Injection 1141

Fluphenazine Decanoate (Additive CNS-suppressant effects). Products include:
Prolixin Decanoate 1795

Fluphenazine Enanthate (Additive CNS-suppressant effects). Products include:
Prolixin Enanthate 1796

Fluphenazine Hydrochloride (Additive CNS-suppressant effects). Products include:
Prolixin Elixir 1793
Prolixin Injection 1791
Prolixin Oral Concentrate 1792
Prolixin Tablets 1793

Glipizide (Hypoglycemic effect enhanced). Products include:
Glucotrol 1952

Glyburide (Hypoglycemic effect enhanced). Products include:
DiaBeta 1091
Micronase Tablets 2350

Haloperidol (Additive CNS-suppressant effects). Products include:
Haldol Injection, Tablets and Concentrate 1373

Haloperidol Decanoate (Additive CNS-suppressant effects). Products include:
Haldol Decanoate 1375

Hydroxyzine Hydrochloride (Additive CNS-suppressant effects). Products include:
Atarax Tablets & Syrup 1941
Marax Tablets & DF Syrup 1954
Vistaril Intramuscular Solution 1970

Imipramine Hydrochloride (Additive CNS-suppressant effects). Products include:
Tofranil Ampuls 1038
Tofranil Tablets 1039

Imipramine Pamoate (Additive CNS-suppressant effects). Products include:
Tofranil-PM Capsules 1041

Isocarboxazid (Additive CNS-suppressant effects). Products include:
Marplan Tablets 1906

Lithium Carbonate (Additive CNS-suppressant effects). Products include:
Eskalith 2214
Lithane Tablets 1596
Lithium Carbonate Capsules & Tablets 1984
Lithobid Tablets 870

Lithium Citrate (Additive CNS-suppressant effects). Products include:
Cibalith-S 870

Lorazepam (Additive CNS-suppressant effects). Products include:
Ativan Injection 2432
Ativan Tablets 2434

Loxapine Hydrochloride (Additive CNS-suppressant effects). Products include:
Loxitane 1213

Loxapine Succinate (Additive CNS-suppressant effects). Products include:
Loxitane Capsules 1213

Maprotiline Hydrochloride (Additive CNS-suppressant effects). Products include:
Ludiomil Tablets 874

Mesoridazine (Additive CNS-suppressant effects). Products include:
Serentil 686

Midazolam Hydrochloride (Additive CNS-suppressant effects). Products include:
Versed Injection 1924

Molindone Hydrochloride (Additive CNS-suppressant effects). Products include:
Moban Tablets & Concentrate 932

Nortriptyline Hydrochloride (Additive CNS-suppressant effects). Products include:
Pamelor 2019

Oxazepam (Additive CNS-suppressant effects). Products include:
Serax Capsules 2522
Serax Tablets 2522

Perphenazine (Additive CNS-suppressant effects). Products include:
Etrafon 2087
Triavil Tablets 1556
Trilafon 2123

Phenelzine Sulfate (Additive CNS-suppressant effects). Products include:
Nardil 1742

Prazepam (Additive CNS-suppressant effects). Products include:
Centrax 1693

Probenecid (Uricosuric activity antagonized). Products include:
Benemid Tablets 1426
ColBENEMID Tablets 1436
Wycillin Injection and Probenecid Tablets 2539

Prochlorperazine (Additive CNS-suppressant effects). Products include:
Compazine 2201

Promethazine Hydrochloride (Additive CNS-suppressant effects). Products include:
Mepergan Injection 2479
Phenergan with Codeine 2497
Phenergan with Dextromethorphan 2499
Phenergan Injection 2493

Phenergan Suppositories 2496
Phenergan Syrup 2495
Phenergan Tablets 2496
Phenergan VC 2500
Phenergan VC with Codeine 2501

Protriptyline Hydrochloride (Additive CNS-suppressant effects). Products include:
Vivactil Tablets 1567

Sulfinpyrazone (Uricosuric activity antagonized). Products include:
Anturane 853

Thioridazine Hydrochloride (Additive CNS-suppressant effects). Products include:
Mellaril 2011

Thiothixene (Additive CNS-suppressant effects). Products include:
Navane Capsules and Concentrate 1954
Navane Intramuscular 1956

Tolazamide (Hypoglycemic effect enhanced). Products include:
Tolinase Tablets 2365

Tolbutamide (Hypoglycemic effect enhanced). Products include:
Orinase Tablets 2354

Tranylcypromine Sulfate (Additive CNS-suppressant effects). Products include:
Parnate Tablets 2222

Trifluoperazine Hydrochloride (Additive CNS-suppressant effects). Products include:
Stelazine 2226

Trimipramine Maleate (Additive CNS-suppressant effects). Products include:
Surmontil Capsules 2524

ERGAMISOL TABLETS

(Levamisole Hydrochloride) 1136
May interact with oral anticoagulants and certain other agents. Compounds in these categories include:

Alcohol (May result in ANTABUSE -like side effects).

Dicumarol (Prolongs prothrombin time; dose of coumarin adjusted accordingly). Products include:
Dicumarol Tablets 516

Phenytoin (Concomitant administration of phenytoin and Ergamisol plus fluorouracil has led to increased plasma levels of phenytoin). Products include:
Dilantin Infatabs 1710
Dilantin-30 Pediatric/Dilantin-125 Suspension 1713

Phenytoin Sodium (Concomitant administration of phenytoin and Ergamisol plus fluorouracil has led to increased plasma levels of phenytoin). Products include:
Dilantin Kapseals 1708
Dilantin Parenteral 1712
Dilantin with Phenobarbital Kapseals 1715

Warfarin Sodium (Prolongs prothrombin time; dose of coumarin adjusted accordingly). Products include:
Coumadin Injection & Tablets 944
Panwarfin Tablets 547

ERGOSTAT

(Ergotamine Tartrate) 1719
May interact with vasopressors and certain other agents. Compounds in these categories include:

Dopamine Hydrochloride (Hypertension). Products include:
Intropin Injection 930

Epinephrine Hydrochloride (Hypertension). Products include:
Adrenalin Chloride Solution 1:100 & 1:1,000 1689
Epifrin .... ⊙ 244
Glaucon .... ⊙ 218

Metaraminol Bitartrate (Hypertension). Products include:
Aramine Injection 1424

Methoxamine Hydrochloride (Hypertension). Products include:
Vasoxyl Injection 819

Norepinephrine Bitartrate (Hypertension). Products include:
Levophed Bitartrate Injection 2054

Phenylephrine Hydrochloride (Hypertension). Products include:
AK-Dilate Solution 2.5% and 10% .... ⊙ 203
Atrohist Sprinkle Capsules 558
Cerose-DM 2443
Codimal 846
Comhist LA Capsules 1618
Congespirin For Children Aspirin Free Chewable Cold Tablets 748
Cyclomydril .... ⊙ 216
Deconsal Sprinkle Capsules 559
Dimetane Decongestant .... ■ 673
Dristan Decongestant/Antihistamine/ Analgesic Coated Caplets .... ■ 749
Dristan Cold Nasal Decongestant/ Antihistamine/ Analgesic Coated Tablets 2419
Dristan Advanced Formula Decongestant/Antihistamine/ Analgesic Tablets .... ■ 749
Dristan Nasal Spray, Menthol 2419
Dristan Nasal Spray, Regular and Regular with Metered Pump 2419
Entex Capsules 1623
Entex Liquid 1623
Sinus Excedrin Analgesic, Decongestant Tablets & Caplets 750
Extendryl 994
4-Way Fast Acting Nasal Spray - Original Formula (regular & mentholated) & Metered Spray Pump (regular) 751
Hycomine Compound Tablets 929
Murocoll-2 Sterile Ophthalmic Solution .... ⊙ 261
Mydfrin 2.5% .... ⊙ 224
Naldecon Syrup, Tablets, Pediatric Drops and Pediatric Syrup 709
Neo-Synephrine Hydrochloride 1% Carpuject 2063
Neo-Synephrine Hydrochloride 1% Injection 2063
Neo-Synephrine Hydrochloride (Ophthalmic) 2064
Neo-Synephrine .... ■ 759
Nōstril Nasal Decongestant .... ■ 520
Novahistine Elixir .... ■ 596
Phenergan VC 2500
Phenergan VC with Codeine 2501
Prefrin Liquifilm Vasoconstrictor and Lubricant Eye Drops .... ⊙ 254
Prefrin-A .... ⊙ 255
Quelidrine Syrup 556
Relief Vasoconstrictor and Lubricant Eye Drops .... ⊙ 256
Robitussin Night Relief .... ■ 677
Ru-Tuss with Hydrocodone 694
Ru-Tuss Tablets 693
Vasosulf .... ⊙ 279
Vicks Sinex .... ■ 665
Zincfrin .... ⊙ 230

Troleandomycin (Potentiates ergotamine). Products include:
Tao Capsules 1963

ERGOTRATE MALEATE AMPOULES

(Ergonovine Maleate) 1263
No interactions described in labeling.

ERYC

(Erythromycin) 1720
May interact with xanthine bronchodilators, oral anticoagulants, and certain other agents. Compounds in these categories include:

Aminophylline (Increased serum theophylline levels). Products include:
Amesec .... ■ 682
Aminophyllin Tablets 2153

Carbamazepine (Increased blood levels of carbamazepine in children). Products include:
Tegretol Chewable Tablets 654
Tegretol Suspension 656
Tegretol Tablets 654

Cyclosporine (Decreased clearance and increased cyclosporine levels). Products include:
Sandimmune 2024

Dicumarol (Increased anticoagulant effect). Products include:
Dicumarol Tablets 516

Digoxin (Elevated digoxin serum levels). Products include:
Lanoxicaps 772
Lanoxin Elixir Pediatric 775
Lanoxin Injection 778
Lanoxin Injection Pediatric 781
Lanoxin Tablets 783

Dyphylline (Increased serum theophylline levels). Products include:
Dilor 2079
Dilor-G Tablets & Liquid 2079
Lufyllin Elixir 2384
Lufyllin & Lufyllin-400 Tablets 2384
Lufyllin-GG Elixir & Tablets 2385

Ergotamine Tartrate (Increased vasospasm associated with ergotamine). Products include:
Bellergal-S Tablets 1998
Cafergot/Cafergot P-B 1999
Ergostat 1719
Medihaler Ergotamine Aerosol 1312
Wigraine Tablets & Suppositories .. 1645

Theophylline (Increased serum theophylline levels). Products include:
Bronkaid Tablets .... ■ 757
Bronkolixir .... ■ 761
Bronkotabs Tablets .... ■ 762
Constant-T Tablets 1029
Marax Tablets & DF Syrup 1954
Primatene Tablets 2421
Quibron Capsules 713
Quibron-T 714
Quibron-T/SR 716
Theolair Liquid 1317
Theo-Organidin Elixir 2391

Theophylline Anhydrous (Increased serum theophylline levels). Products include:
Aerolate 994
Primatene Tablets-M Formula .... ■ 753
Primatene Tablets-Regular Formula 2421
Respbid Tablets 684
Slo-bid Gyrocaps 1847
T-PHYL (Uniphyl) 200 mg Tablets 1820
Tedral SA 1765
Theo-24 2179
Theo-Dur Sprinkle 1168
Theo-Dur Extended-Release Tablets 1166
Theolair Tablets 1317
Theolair-SR Tablets 1319
TheoX Extended-Release Tablets 841
Uniphyl 400 mg Tablets 1823

Theophylline Calcium Salicylate (Increased serum theophylline levels). Products include:
Quadrinal Tablets 1183

Theophylline Sodium Glycinate (Increased serum theophylline levels). Products include:
Asbron G 1997

Triazolam (Decreased clearance and increased pharmacologic effect of triazolam). Products include:
Halcion Tablets 2340

Warfarin Sodium (Increased anticoagulant effect). Products include:
Coumadin Injection & Tablets 944
Panwarfin Tablets 547

Food Interactions

Meal, unspecified (Optimum blood levels are obtained on a fasting stomach; administration is preferable one-half hour pre- or two hours post-meal).

ERYCETTE (ERYTHROMYCIN 2%) TOPICAL SOLUTION

(Erythromycin) 1678
No interactions described in labeling.

ERYPED DROPS AND CHEWABLE TABLETS

(Erythromycin Ethylsuccinate) 519
May interact with xanthine bronchodilators, oral anticoagulants, and certain other agents. Compounds in these categories include:

Aminophylline (Concomitant administration with high doses of theophylline may be associated with increased theophylline levels and potential toxicity). Products include:
Amesec .... ■ 682
Aminophyllin Tablets 2153

Carbamazepine (Elevations in serum erythromycin and carbamazepine concentration). Products include:
Tegretol Chewable Tablets 654
Tegretol Suspension 656
Tegretol Tablets 654

Cyclosporine (Elevations in serum erythromycin and cyclosporine concentration). Products include:
Sandimmune 2024

Dicumarol (Increased anticoagulant effects). Products include:
Dicumarol Tablets 516

Digoxin (Elevated digoxin serum levels). Products include:
Lanoxicaps 772
Lanoxin Elixir Pediatric 775
Lanoxin Injection 778
Lanoxin Injection Pediatric 781
Lanoxin Tablets 783

Dihydroergotamine Mesylate (Potential for acute ergot toxicity characterized by severe peripheral vasospasm and dysesthesia). Products include:
D.H.E. 45 Injection 2003

Dyphylline (Concomitant administration with high doses of theophylline may be associated with increased theophylline levels and potential toxicity). Products include:
Dilor 2079
Dilor-G Tablets & Liquid 2079
Lufyllin Elixir 2384
Lufyllin & Lufyllin-400 Tablets 2384
Lufyllin-GG Elixir & Tablets 2385

Ergotamine Tartrate (Potential for acute ergot toxicity characterized by severe peripheral vasospasm and dysesthesia). Products include:
Bellergal-S Tablets 1998
Cafergot/Cafergot P-B 1999
Ergostat 1719
Medihaler Ergotamine Aerosol 1312
Wigraine Tablets & Suppositories .. 1645

Hexobarbital (Elevations in serum erythromycin and hexobarbital concentration).

Lovastatin (Potential for rhabdomyolysis in seriously ill patients). Products include:
Mevacor Tablets 1505

Phenytoin (Elevations in serum erythromycin and phenytoin concentration). Products include:
Dilantin Infatabs 1710
Dilantin-30 Pediatric/Dilantin-125 Suspension 1713

Phenytoin Sodium (Elevations in serum erythromycin and phenytoin concentration). Products include:
Dilantin Kapseals 1708
Dilantin Parenteral 1712
Dilantin with Phenobarbital Kapseals 1715

Terfenadine (Potential for altered terfenadine metabolism). Products include:
- Seldane Tablets ... 1349
- Seldane-D Extended-Release Tablets ... 1350

Theophylline (Concomitant administration with high doses of theophylline may be associated with increased theophylline levels and potential toxicity). Products include:
- Bronkaid Tablets ... ■ 757
- Bronkolixir ... ■ 761
- Bronkotabs Tablets ... ■ 762
- Constant-T Tablets ... 1029
- Marax Tablets & DF Syrup ... 1954
- Primatene Tablets ... 2421
- Quibron Capsules ... 713
- Quibron-T ... 714
- Quibron-T/SR ... 716
- Theolair Liquid ... 1317
- Theo-Organidin Elixir ... 2391

Theophylline Anhydrous (Concomitant administration with high doses of theophylline may be associated with increased theophylline levels and potential toxicity). Products include:
- Aerolate ... 994
- Primatene Tablets-M Formula ... ■ 753
- Primatene Tablets-Regular Formula ... 2421
- Respbid Tablets ... 684
- Slo-bid Gyrocaps ... 1847
- T-PHYL (Uniphyl) 200 mg Tablets 1820
- Tedral SA ... 1765
- Theo-24 ... 2179
- Theo-Dur Sprinkle ... 1168
- Theo-Dur Extended-Release Tablets ... 1166
- Theolair Tablets ... 1317
- Theolair-SR Tablets ... 1319
- TheoX Extended-Release Tablets ... 841
- Uniphyl 400 mg Tablets ... 1823

Theophylline Calcium Salicylate (Concomitant administration with high doses of theophylline may be associated with increased theophylline levels and potential toxicity). Products include:
- Quadrinal Tablets ... 1183

Theophylline Sodium Glycinate (Concomitant administration with high doses of theophylline may be associated with increased theophylline levels and potential toxicity). Products include:
- Asbron G ... 1997

Triazolam (Decreased clearance of triazolam and increased the pharmacologic effect of triazolam). Products include:
- Halcion Tablets ... 2340

Warfarin Sodium (Increased anticoagulant effects). Products include:
- Coumadin Injection & Tablets ... 944
- Panwarfin Tablets ... 547

ERYPED 200 & ERYPED 400 GRANULES
(Erythromycin Ethylsuccinate) ... 519
- See **EryPed Drops and Chewable Tablets**

ERY-TAB TABLETS
(Erythromycin) ... 521
May interact with xanthine bronchodilators, oral anticoagulants, and certain other agents. Compounds in these categories include:

Aminophylline (Concomitant administration with high doses of theophylline may be associated with increased theophylline levels and potential toxicity). Products include:
- Amesec ... ■ 682
- Aminophyllin Tablets ... 2153

Carbamazepine (Elevations in serum erythromycin and carbamazepine concentration). Products include:
- Tegretol Chewable Tablets ... 654
- Tegretol Suspension ... 656
- Tegretol Tablets ... 654

Cyclosporine (Elevations in serum erythromycin and cyclosporine concentration). Products include:
- Sandimmune ... 2024

Dicumarol (Increased anticoagulant effects). Products include:
- Dicumarol Tablets ... 516

Digoxin (Elevated digoxin serum levels). Products include:
- Lanoxicaps ... 772
- Lanoxin Elixir Pediatric ... 775
- Lanoxin Injection ... 778
- Lanoxin Injection Pediatric ... 781
- Lanoxin Tablets ... 783

Dihydroergotamine Mesylate (Potential for acute ergot toxicity characterized by severe peripheral vasospasm and dysesthesia). Products include:
- D.H.E. 45 Injection ... 2003

Dyphylline (Concomitant administration with high doses of theophylline may be associated with increased theophylline levels and potential toxicity). Products include:
- Dilor ... 2079
- Dilor-G Tablets & Liquid ... 2079
- Lufyllin Elixir ... 2384
- Lufyllin & Lufyllin-400 Tablets ... 2384
- Lufyllin-GG Elixir & Tablets ... 2385

Ergotamine Tartrate (Potential for acute ergot toxicity characterized by severe peripheral vasospasm and dysesthesia). Products include:
- Bellergal-S Tablets ... 1998
- Cafergot/Cafergot P-B ... 1999
- Ergostat ... 1719
- Medihaler Ergotamine Aerosol ... 1312
- Wigraine Tablets & Suppositories .. 1645

Hexobarbital (Elevations in serum erythromycin and hexobarbital concentration).

Lovastatin (Potential for rhabdomyolysis in seriously ill patients). Products include:
- Mevacor Tablets ... 1505

Phenytoin (Elevations in serum erythromycin and phenytoin concentration). Products include:
- Dilantin Infatabs ... 1710
- Dilantin-30 Pediatric/Dilantin-125 Suspension ... 1713

Phenytoin Sodium (Elevations in serum erythromycin and phenytoin concentration). Products include:
- Dilantin Kapseals ... 1708
- Dilantin Parenteral ... 1712
- Dilantin with Phenobarbital Kapseals ... 1715

Terfenadine (Potential for altered terfenadine metabolism). Products include:
- Seldane Tablets ... 1349
- Seldane-D Extended-Release Tablets ... 1350

Theophylline (Concomitant administration with high doses of theophylline may be associated with increased theophylline levels and potential toxicity). Products include:
- Bronkaid Tablets ... ■ 757
- Bronkolixir ... ■ 761
- Bronkotabs Tablets ... ■ 762
- Constant-T Tablets ... 1029
- Marax Tablets & DF Syrup ... 1954
- Primatene Tablets ... 2421
- Quibron Capsules ... 713
- Quibron-T ... 714
- Quibron-T/SR ... 716
- Theolair Liquid ... 1317
- Theo-Organidin Elixir ... 2391

Theophylline Anhydrous (Concomitant administration with high doses of theophylline may be associated with increased theophylline levels and potential toxicity). Products include:
- Aerolate ... 994
- Primatene Tablets-M Formula ... ■ 753
- Primatene Tablets-Regular Formula ... 2421
- Respbid Tablets ... 684
- Slo-bid Gyrocaps ... 1847
- T-PHYL (Uniphyl) 200 mg Tablets 1820
- Tedral SA ... 1765
- Theo-24 ... 2179
- Theo-Dur Sprinkle ... 1168
- Theo-Dur Extended-Release Tablets ... 1166
- Theolair Tablets ... 1317
- Theolair-SR Tablets ... 1319
- TheoX Extended-Release Tablets ... 841
- Uniphyl 400 mg Tablets ... 1823

Theophylline Calcium Salicylate (Concomitant administration with high doses of theophylline may be associated with increased theophylline levels and potential toxicity). Products include:
- Quadrinal Tablets ... 1183

Theophylline Sodium Glycinate (Concomitant administration with high doses of theophylline may be associated with increased theophylline levels and potential toxicity). Products include:
- Asbron G ... 1997

Triazolam (Decreased clearance of triazolam and increased the pharmacologic effect of triazolam). Products include:
- Halcion Tablets ... 2340

Warfarin Sodium (Increased anticoagulant effects). Products include:
- Coumadin Injection & Tablets ... 944
- Panwarfin Tablets ... 547

ERYTHROCIN STEARATE FILMTAB
(Erythromycin Stearate) ... 523
May interact with xanthine bronchodilators, oral anticoagulants, and certain other agents. Compounds in these categories include:

Aminophylline (Concomitant administration with high doses of theophylline may be associated with increased theophylline levels and potential toxicity). Products include:
- Amesec ... ■ 682
- Aminophyllin Tablets ... 2153

Carbamazepine (Elevations in serum erythromycin and carbamazepine concentration). Products include:
- Tegretol Chewable Tablets ... 654
- Tegretol Suspension ... 656
- Tegretol Tablets ... 654

Cyclosporine (Elevations in serum erythromycin and cyclosporine concentration). Products include:
- Sandimmune ... 2024

Dicumarol (Increased anticoagulant effects). Products include:
- Dicumarol Tablets ... 516

Digoxin (Elevated digoxin serum levels). Products include:
- Lanoxicaps ... 772
- Lanoxin Elixir Pediatric ... 775
- Lanoxin Injection ... 778
- Lanoxin Injection Pediatric ... 781
- Lanoxin Tablets ... 783

Dihydroergotamine Mesylate (Potential for acute ergot toxicity characterized by severe peripheral vasospasm and dysesthesia). Products include:
- D.H.E. 45 Injection ... 2003

Dyphylline (Concomitant administration with high doses of theophylline may be associated with increased theophylline levels and potential toxicity). Products include:
- Dilor ... 2079
- Dilor-G Tablets & Liquid ... 2079
- Lufyllin Elixir ... 2384
- Lufyllin & Lufyllin-400 Tablets ... 2384
- Lufyllin-GG Elixir & Tablets ... 2385

Ergotamine Tartrate (Potential for acute ergot toxicity characterized by severe peripheral vasospasm and dysesthesia). Products include:
- Bellergal-S Tablets ... 1998
- Cafergot/Cafergot P-B ... 1999
- Ergostat ... 1719
- Medihaler Ergotamine Aerosol ... 1312
- Wigraine Tablets & Suppositories .. 1645

Hexobarbital (Elevations in serum erythromycin and hexobarbital concentration).

Lovastatin (Potential for rhabdomyolysis in seriously ill patients). Products include:
- Mevacor Tablets ... 1505

Phenytoin (Elevations in serum erythromycin and phenytoin concentration). Products include:
- Dilantin Infatabs ... 1710
- Dilantin-30 Pediatric/Dilantin-125 Suspension ... 1713

Phenytoin Sodium (Elevations in serum erythromycin and phenytoin concentration). Products include:
- Dilantin Kapseals ... 1708
- Dilantin Parenteral ... 1712
- Dilantin with Phenobarbital Kapseals ... 1715

Terfenadine (Potential for altered terfenadine metabolism). Products include:
- Seldane Tablets ... 1349
- Seldane-D Extended-Release Tablets ... 1350

Theophylline (Concomitant administration with high doses of theophylline may be associated with increased theophylline levels and potential toxicity). Products include:
- Bronkaid Tablets ... ■ 757
- Bronkolixir ... ■ 761
- Bronkotabs Tablets ... ■ 762
- Constant-T Tablets ... 1029
- Marax Tablets & DF Syrup ... 1954
- Primatene Tablets ... 2421
- Quibron Capsules ... 713
- Quibron-T ... 714
- Quibron-T/SR ... 716
- Theolair Liquid ... 1317
- Theo-Organidin Elixir ... 2391

Theophylline Anhydrous (Concomitant administration with high doses of theophylline may be associated with increased theophylline levels and potential toxicity). Products include:
- Aerolate ... 994
- Primatene Tablets-M Formula ... ■ 753
- Primatene Tablets-Regular Formula ... 2421
- Respbid Tablets ... 684
- Slo-bid Gyrocaps ... 1847
- T-PHYL (Uniphyl) 200 mg Tablets 1820
- Tedral SA ... 1765
- Theo-24 ... 2179
- Theo-Dur Sprinkle ... 1168
- Theo-Dur Extended-Release Tablets ... 1166
- Theolair Tablets ... 1317
- Theolair-SR Tablets ... 1319
- TheoX Extended-Release Tablets ... 841
- Uniphyl 400 mg Tablets ... 1823

Theophylline Calcium Salicylate (Concomitant administration with high doses of theophylline may be associated with increased theophylline levels and potential toxicity). Products include:
- Quadrinal Tablets ... 1183

Theophylline Sodium Glycinate (Concomitant administration with high doses of theophylline may be associated with increased theophylline levels and potential toxicity). Products include:
- Asbron G 1997

Triazolam (Decreased clearance of triazolam and increased the pharmacologic effect of triazolam). Products include:
- Halcion Tablets 2340

Warfarin Sodium (Increased anticoagulant effects). Products include:
- Coumadin Injection & Tablets 944
- Panwarfin Tablets 547

ERYTHROMYCIN BASE FILMTAB

(Erythromycin) 525

May interact with xanthine bronchodilators, oral anticoagulants, and certain other agents. Compounds in these categories include:

Aminophylline (Concomitant administration with high doses of theophylline may be associated with increased theophylline levels and potential toxicity). Products include:
- Amesec .... ◘ 682
- Aminophyllin Tablets 2153

Carbamazepine (Elevations in serum erythromycin and carbamazepine concentration). Products include:
- Tegretol Chewable Tablets 654
- Tegretol Suspension 656
- Tegretol Tablets 654

Cyclosporine (Elevations in serum erythromycin and cyclosporine concentration). Products include:
- Sandimmune 2024

Dicumarol (Increased anticoagulant effects). Products include:
- Dicumarol Tablets 516

Digoxin (Elevated digoxin serum levels). Products include:
- Lanoxicaps 772
- Lanoxin Elixir Pediatric 775
- Lanoxin Injection 778
- Lanoxin Injection Pediatric 781
- Lanoxin Tablets 783

Dihydroergotamine Mesylate (Potential for acute ergot toxicity characterized by severe peripheral vasospasm and dysesthesia). Products include:
- D.H.E. 45 Injection 2003

Dyphylline (Concomitant administration with high doses of theophylline may be associated with increased theophylline levels and potential toxicity). Products include:
- Dilor 2079
- Dilor-G Tablets & Liquid 2079
- Lufyllin Elixir 2384
- Lufyllin & Lufyllin-400 Tablets 2384
- Lufyllin-GG Elixir & Tablets 2385

Ergotamine Tartrate (Potential for acute ergot toxicity characterized by severe peripheral vasospasm and dysesthesia). Products include:
- Bellergal-S Tablets 1998
- Cafergot/Cafergot P-B 1999
- Ergostat 1719
- Medihaler Ergotamine Aerosol 1312
- Wigraine Tablets & Suppositories 1645

Hexobarbital (Elevations in serum erythromycin and hexobarbital concentration).

Lovastatin (Potential for rhabdomyolysis in seriously ill patients). Products include:
- Mevacor Tablets 1505

Phenytoin (Elevations in serum erythromycin and phenytoin concentration). Products include:
- Dilantin Infatabs 1710
- Dilantin-30 Pediatric/Dilantin-125 Suspension 1713

Phenytoin Sodium (Elevations in serum erythromycin and phenytoin concentration). Products include:
- Dilantin Kapseals 1708
- Dilantin Parenteral 1712
- Dilantin with Phenobarbital Kapseals 1715

Terfenadine (Potential for altered terfenadine metabolism). Products include:
- Seldane Tablets 1349
- Seldane-D Extended-Release Tablets 1350

Theophylline (Concomitant administration with high doses of theophylline may be associated with increased theophylline levels and potential toxicity). Products include:
- Bronkaid Tablets .... ◘ 757
- Bronkolixir .... ◘ 761
- Bronkotabs Tablets .... ◘ 762
- Constant-T Tablets 1029
- Marax Tablets & DF Syrup 1954
- Primatene Tablets 2421
- Quibron Capsules 713
- Quibron-T 714
- Quibron-T/SR 716
- Theolair Liquid 1317
- Theo-Organidin Elixir 2391

Theophylline Anhydrous (Concomitant administration with high doses of theophylline may be associated with increased theophylline levels and potential toxicity). Products include:
- Aerolate 994
- Primatene Tablets-M Formula .... ◘ 753
- Primatene Tablets-Regular Formula 2421
- Respbid Tablets 684
- Slo-bid Gyrocaps 1847
- T-PHYL (Uniphyl) 200 mg Tablets 1820
- Tedral SA 1765
- Theo-24 2179
- Theo-Dur Sprinkle 1168
- Theo-Dur Extended-Release Tablets 1166
- Theolair Tablets 1317
- Theolair-SR Tablets 1319
- TheoX Extended-Release Tablets 841
- Uniphyl 400 mg Tablets 1823

Theophylline Calcium Salicylate (Concomitant administration with high doses of theophylline may be associated with increased theophylline levels and potential toxicity). Products include:
- Quadrinal Tablets 1183

Theophylline Sodium Glycinate (Concomitant administration with high doses of theophylline may be associated with increased theophylline levels and potential toxicity). Products include:
- Asbron G 1997

Triazolam (Decreased clearance of triazolam and increased the pharmacologic effect of triazolam). Products include:
- Halcion Tablets 2340

Warfarin Sodium (Increased anticoagulant effects). Products include:
- Coumadin Injection & Tablets 944
- Panwarfin Tablets 547

ERYTHROMYCIN DELAYED-RELEASE CAPSULES, USP

(Erythromycin) 526

May interact with xanthine bronchodilators, oral anticoagulants, and certain other agents. Compounds in these categories include:

Aminophylline (Concomitant administration with high doses of theophylline may be associated with increased theophylline levels and potential toxicity). Products include:
- Amesec .... ◘ 682
- Aminophyllin Tablets 2153

Carbamazepine (Elevations in serum erythromycin and carbamazepine concentration). Products include:
- Tegretol Chewable Tablets 654
- Tegretol Suspension 656
- Tegretol Tablets 654

Cyclosporine (Elevations in serum erythromycin and cyclosporine concentration). Products include:
- Sandimmune 2024

Dicumarol (Increased anticoagulant effects). Products include:
- Dicumarol Tablets 516

Digoxin (Elevated digoxin serum levels). Products include:
- Lanoxicaps 772
- Lanoxin Elixir Pediatric 775
- Lanoxin Injection 778
- Lanoxin Injection Pediatric 781
- Lanoxin Tablets 783

Dihydroergotamine Mesylate (Potential for acute ergot toxicity characterized by severe peripheral vasospasm and dysesthesia). Products include:
- D.H.E. 45 Injection 2003

Drugs which undergo biotransformation by cytochrome P-450 mixed function oxidase (Potential for elevation in serum levels).

Dyphylline (Concomitant administration with high doses of theophylline may be associated with increased theophylline levels and potential toxicity). Products include:
- Dilor 2079
- Dilor-G Tablets & Liquid 2079
- Lufyllin Elixir 2384
- Lufyllin & Lufyllin-400 Tablets 2384
- Lufyllin-GG Elixir & Tablets 2385

Ergotamine Tartrate (Potential for acute ergot toxicity characterized by severe peripheral vasospasm and dysesthesia). Products include:
- Bellergal-S Tablets 1998
- Cafergot/Cafergot P-B 1999
- Ergostat 1719
- Medihaler Ergotamine Aerosol 1312
- Wigraine Tablets & Suppositories 1645

Hexobarbital (Elevations in serum erythromycin and hexobarbital concentration).

Lovastatin (Potential for rhabdomyolysis in seriously ill patients). Products include:
- Mevacor Tablets 1505

Phenytoin (Elevations in serum erythromycin and phenytoin concentration). Products include:
- Dilantin Infatabs 1710
- Dilantin-30 Pediatric/Dilantin-125 Suspension 1713

Phenytoin Sodium (Elevations in serum erythromycin and phenytoin concentration). Products include:
- Dilantin Kapseals 1708
- Dilantin Parenteral 1712
- Dilantin with Phenobarbital Kapseals 1715

Terfenadine (Potential for altered terfenadine metabolism). Products include:
- Seldane Tablets 1349
- Seldane-D Extended-Release Tablets 1350

Theophylline (Concomitant administration with high doses of theophylline may be associated with increased theophylline levels and potential toxicity). Products include:
- Bronkaid Tablets .... ◘ 757
- Bronkolixir .... ◘ 761
- Bronkotabs Tablets .... ◘ 762
- Constant-T Tablets 1029
- Marax Tablets & DF Syrup 1954
- Primatene Tablets 2421
- Quibron Capsules 713
- Quibron-T 714
- Quibron-T/SR 716
- Theolair Liquid 1317
- Theo-Organidin Elixir 2391

Theophylline Anhydrous (Concomitant administration with high doses of theophylline may be associated with increased theophylline levels and potential toxicity). Products include:
- Aerolate 994
- Primatene Tablets-M Formula .... ◘ 753
- Primatene Tablets-Regular Formula 2421
- Respbid Tablets 684
- Slo-bid Gyrocaps 1847
- T-PHYL (Uniphyl) 200 mg Tablets 1820
- Tedral SA 1765
- Theo-24 2179
- Theo-Dur Sprinkle 1168
- Theo-Dur Extended-Release Tablets 1166
- Theolair Tablets 1317
- Theolair-SR Tablets 1319
- TheoX Extended-Release Tablets 841
- Uniphyl 400 mg Tablets 1823

Theophylline Calcium Salicylate (Concomitant administration with high doses of theophylline may be associated with increased theophylline levels and potential toxicity). Products include:
- Quadrinal Tablets 1183

Theophylline Sodium Glycinate (Concomitant administration with high doses of theophylline may be associated with increased theophylline levels and potential toxicity). Products include:
- Asbron G 1997

Triazolam (Decreased clearance of triazolam and increased the pharmacologic effect of triazolam). Products include:
- Halcion Tablets 2340

Warfarin Sodium (Increased anticoagulant effects). Products include:
- Coumadin Injection & Tablets 944
- Panwarfin Tablets 547

Food Interactions

Food, unspecified (Lowers the blood levels of systemically available erythromycin).

ESGIC-PLUS TABLETS

(Butalbital, Acetaminophen, Caffeine) 1002

May interact with oral anticoagulants, barbiturates, benzodiazepines, hypnotics and sedatives, central nervous system depressants, narcotic analgesics, tricyclic antidepressants, antihistamines, tranquilizers, and certain other agents. Compounds in these categories include:

Alcohol (May exhibit additive CNS depressant effects).

Alfentanil Hydrochloride (May exhibit additive CNS depressant effects). Products include:
- Alfenta Injection 1131

Alprazolam (May exhibit additive CNS depressant effects). Products include:
- Xanax Tablets 2367

Amitriptyline Hydrochloride (May exhibit additive CNS depressant effects; decreased blood levels of the antidepressant). Products include:
- Elavil 2269
- Endep Tablets 1927
- Etrafon 2087
- Limbitrol 1933
- Triavil Tablets 1556

Amoxapine (May exhibit additive CNS depressant effects; decreased blood levels of the antidepressant). Products include:
- Asendin Tablets 1196

Aprobarbital (May exhibit additive CNS depressant effects). Products include:
- Alurate Elixir ... 1883

Astemizole (May exhibit additive CNS depressant effects). Products include:
- Hismanal Tablets ... 1138

Azatadine Maleate (May exhibit additive CNS depressant effects). Products include:
- Optimine Tablets ... 2115
- Trinalin Repetabs Tablets ... 1170

Bromodiphenhydramine Hydrochloride (May exhibit additive CNS depressant effects).
- No products indexed under this heading.

Brompheniramine Maleate (May exhibit additive CNS depressant effects). Products include:
- Alka Seltzer Plus Sinus Allergy Medicine ... ▣ 624
- Atrohist Sprinkle Capsules ... 558
- Bromfed Capsules (Timed Release) ... 1615
- Bromfed Syrup ... ▣ 628
- Bromfed ... 1615
- Dimetane Decongestant ... ▣ 673
- Dimetane ... ▣ 672
- Dimetane-DC Cough Syrup ... 1857
- Dimetane-DX Cough Syrup ... 1858
- Dimetapp Elixir ... ▣ 673
- Dimetapp DM Elixir ... ▣ 674
- Dimetapp Extentabs ... ▣ 674
- Dimetapp Plus Caplets ... ▣ 675
- Dimetapp Tablets ... ▣ 675
- Drixoral Antihistamine/Nasal Decongestant Syrup ... ▣ 698

Buprenorphine (May exhibit additive CNS depressant effects).
- No products indexed under this heading.

Buspirone Hydrochloride (May exhibit additive CNS depressant effects). Products include:
- BuSpar ... 1401

Butabarbital (May exhibit additive CNS depressant effects). Products include:
- Pyridium Plus ... 1764

Chlordiazepoxide (May exhibit additive CNS depressant effects). Products include:
- Libritabs Tablets ... 1930
- Limbitrol ... 1933
- Menrium Tablets ... 1934

Chlordiazepoxide Hydrochloride (May exhibit additive CNS depressant effects). Products include:
- Librax Capsules ... 1929
- Librium Capsules ... 1931
- Librium Injectable ... 1932

Chlorpheniramine Maleate (May exhibit additive CNS depressant effects). Products include:
- A.R.M. Allergy Relief Medicine Caplets ... ▣ 615
- Alka-Seltzer Plus Cold Medicine ... ▣ 623
- Allerest ... ▣ 559
- Ana-Kit Anaphylaxis Emergency Treatment Kit ... 1100
- BC Cold Powder Multi-Symptom Formula ... ▣ 517
- Brexin L.A. Capsules ... 2078
- Cerose-DM ... 2443
- Cheracol Plus Head Cold/Cough Formula ... ▣ 667
- Chlor-Trimeton Allergy Syrup, Tablets & Long-Acting Repetabs Tablets ... ▣ 693
- Chlor-Trimeton Decongestant ... ▣ 694
- Comhist LA Capsules ... 1618
- Allergy-Sinus Comtrex Multi-Symptom Allergy Sinus Formula Tablets & Caplets ... 746
- Comtrex Multi-Symptom Cold Reliever Tablets/Caplets/Liqui-Gels/Liquid ... 745
- Day-Night Comtrex ... 747
- Contac Continuous Action Decongestant/Antihistamine Capsules ▣ 710
- Contac Maximum Strength Continuous Action Decongestant/Antihistamine Caplets ... ▣ 709
- Contac Severe Cold and Flu Formula Caplets ... ▣ 711
- Coricidin 'D' Decongestant Tablets ... ▣ 695
- Coricidin Demilets Tablets for Children ... ▣ 696
- Coricidin Tablets ... ▣ 695
- Deconamine ... 663
- Demazin Nasal Decongestant/Antihistamine Repetabs Tablets & Syrup ... ▣ 697
- Dorcol Children's Liquid Cold Formula ... ▣ 686
- Dristan Decongestant/Antihistamine/ Analgesic Coated Caplets ... ▣ 749
- Dristan Cold Nasal Decongestant/Antihistamine/ Analgesic Coated Tablets ... 2419
- Dristan Advanced Formula Decongestant/Antihistamine/Analgesic Tablets ... ▣ 749
- Extendryl ... 994
- 4-Way Cold Tablets ... 750
- Fedahist Gyrocaps ... 2145
- Fedahist Timecaps ... 2145
- Hycomine Compound Tablets ... 929
- Isoclor Timesule Capsules ... ▣ 561
- Kronofed-A ... 970
- Medi-Flu Caplet, Liquid ... ▣ 640
- Naldecon Syrup, Tablets, Pediatric Drops and Pediatric Syrup ... 709
- Nolamine Tablets ... 838
- Novafed A Capsules ... 1342
- Novahistine DH ... 1342
- Novahistine Elixir ... ▣ 596
- Ornade Spansule Capsules ... 2221
- Orthoxicol Cough Syrup ... ▣ 668
- PediaCare Allergy Relief Formula Liquid ... 1362
- PediaCare Cough-Cold Formula Liquid ... 1362
- PediaCare Night Rest Cough-Cold Formula Liquid ... 1362
- PediaCare 6-12 Cough-Cold Formula Chewable Tablets ... 1362
- Pyrroxate Capsules ... ▣ 669
- Quelidrine Syrup ... 556
- Ru-Tuss II Capsules ... 693
- Ru-Tuss Tablets ... 693
- Ryna ... ▣ 741
- Sinarest Tablets & Extra Strength Tablets ... ▣ 562
- Sine-Off Maximum Strength Allergy/Sinus Formula Caplets ... ▣ 721
- Sine-Off Sinus Medicine Tablets-Aspirin Formula ... ▣ 722
- Singlet Tablets ... ▣ 598
- Sinulin ... 840
- Sinutab Maximum Strength ... ▣ 641
- St. Joseph Nighttime Cold Medicine ... ▣ 705
- Sudafed Plus Liquid ... ▣ 544
- Sudafed Plus Tablets ... ▣ 545
- Teldrin Timed-Release Allergy Capsules, 12 mg ... 2192
- TheraFlu Flu and Cold Medicine ... ▣ 687
- Triaminic Allergy Tablets ... ▣ 688
- Triaminic Chewables ... ▣ 688
- Triaminic Cold Tablets ... ▣ 688
- Triaminic Nite Light ... ▣ 689
- Triaminic Syrup ... ▣ 689
- Triaminic-12 Tablets ... ▣ 690
- Triaminicin Tablets ... ▣ 690
- Triaminicol Multi-Symptom Cold Tablets ... ▣ 691
- Triaminicol Multi-Symptom Relief ▣ 691
- Tylenol Allergy Sinus Medication Caplets and Gelcaps, Maximum Strength ... 1372
- Children's Tylenol Cold Liquid Formula and Chewable Tablets ... 1368
- Tylenol Cold & Flu Hot Medication, Packets ... 1369
- Tylenol Cold Medication Caplets and Tablets ... 1370
- Tylenol Cold Medication, Effervescent Tablets ... 1369
- Vicks Children's NyQuil ... ▣ 664
- Vicks Formula 44 Cough Medicine ... ▣ 661
- Vicks Formula 44M Multi-Symptom Cough Medicine ... ▣ 662
- Vicks Pediatric Formula 44m Multi-Symptom Cough & Cold Medicine ... ▣ 663

Chlorpheniramine Polistirex (May exhibit additive CNS depressant effects). Products include:
- Tussionex Extended-Release Suspension ... 988

Chlorpheniramine Tannate (May exhibit additive CNS depressant effects). Products include:
- Rynatan ... 2387
- Rynatuss ... 2388

Chlorpromazine (May exhibit additive CNS depressant effects). Products include:
- Thorazine ... 2234

Chlorprothixene (May exhibit additive CNS depressant effects). Products include:
- Taractan Tablets ... 1920

Chlorprothixene Hydrochloride (May exhibit additive CNS depressant effects). Products include:
- Taractan ... 1920

Chlorprothixene Lactate (May exhibit additive CNS depressant effects). Products include:
- Taractan Concentrate ... 1920

Clemastine Fumarate (May exhibit additive CNS depressant effects). Products include:
- Tavist Syrup ... 2033
- Tavist Tablets ... 2035
- Tavist-D Tablets ... 2035

Clomipramine Hydrochloride (May exhibit additive CNS depressant effects; decreased blood levels of the antidepressant). Products include:
- Anafranil Capsules ... 650

Clorazepate Dipotassium (May exhibit additive CNS depressant effects). Products include:
- Tranxene ... 556

Codeine (May exhibit additive CNS depressant effects). Products include:
- Calcidrine Syrup ... 506

Codeine Phosphate (May exhibit additive CNS depressant effects). Products include:
- Actifed with Codeine Cough Syrup ... 752
- Cheracol Cough Syrup ... 1853
- Codimal PH Syrup ... 846
- Dimetane-DC Cough Syrup ... 1857
- Empirin with Codeine Phosphate Nos. 2, 3 & 4 ... 764
- Fiorinal with Codeine Capsules ... 2008
- Isoclor Expectorant ... 982
- Naldecon CX Adult Liquid ... ▣ 521
- Novahistine DH ... 1342
- Novahistine Expectorant ... 1343
- Nucofed Capsules ... 2219
- Nucofed Expectorant ... 2219
- Nucofed Pediatric Expectorant ... 2220
- Nucofed Syrup ... 2219
- Phenaphen with Codeine Capsules 1865
- Phenaphen-650 with Codeine Tablets ... 1866
- Phenergan with Codeine ... 2497
- Phenergan VC with Codeine ... 2501
- Robitussin A-C Syrup ... 1875
- Robitussin-DAC Syrup ... 1875
- Ryna ... ▣ 741
- Soma Compound w/Codeine Tablets ... 2390
- Triaminic Expectorant w/Codeine ... 1996
- Tussi-Organidin Liquid ... 2391
- Tylenol with Codeine ... 1381

Codeine Polistirex (May exhibit additive CNS depressant effects).
- No products indexed under this heading.

Cyproheptadine Hydrochloride (May exhibit additive CNS depressant effects). Products include:
- Periactin ... 1525

Desipramine Hydrochloride (May exhibit additive CNS depressant effects; decreased blood levels of the antidepressant). Products include:
- Norpramin Tablets ... 1340

Dexchlorpheniramine Maleate (May exhibit additive CNS depressant effects). Products include:
- Polaramine ... 2116

Dezocine (May exhibit additive CNS depressant effects).

Diazepam (May exhibit additive CNS depressant effects). Products include:
- Valium Injectable ... 1937
- Valium Tablets ... 1939
- Valrelease Capsules ... 1923

Dicumarol (Decreased effect of anticoagulant). Products include:
- Dicumarol Tablets ... 516

Diphenhydramine Citrate (May exhibit additive CNS depressant effects). Products include:
- Alka-Seltzer Plus Night-Time Cold Medicine ... ▣ 623
- Bufferin AF Nite Time Analgesic/Sleeping Aid Caplets ... 744
- Excedrin P.M. Analgesic/Sleeping Aid Tablets, Caplets and Liquid ... 749

Diphenhydramine Hydrochloride (May exhibit additive CNS depressant effects). Products include:
- Benadryl Anti-Itch Cream ... ▣ 635
- Benadryl Capsules ... 1691
- Benadryl Decongestant Elixir ... ▣ 635
- Benadryl Decongestant ... ▣ 635
- Benadryl Elixir ... ▣ 636
- Benadryl Kapseals ... 1691
- Benadryl 25 Kapseals ... ▣ 636
- Benadryl Parenteral ... 1692
- Benadryl Plus ... ▣ 636
- Benadryl Plus Nighttime ... ▣ 637
- Benadryl Spray, Maximum Strength ... ▣ 637
- Benadryl Spray, Regular Strength ▣ 637
- Benadryl Steri-Vials, Ampoules, and Steri-Dose Syringe ... 1692
- Benadryl 25 Tablets ... ▣ 636
- Benylin Cough Syrup ... ▣ 637
- Benylin Decongestant ... ▣ 638
- Caladryl Cream, Lotion, Spray ... ▣ 638
- Miles Nervine Nighttime Sleep-Aid ▣ 627
- Nytol Tablets ... ▣ 517
- Sleep-ettes-D Tablets ... ▣ 653
- Sleep-eze 3 Tablets ... ▣ 755
- Sleepinal Night-time Sleep Aid Capsules ... ▣ 734
- Sominex Caplets and Tablets ... ▣ 722
- Sominex Liquid ... ▣ 723
- Sominex Pain Relief Formula ... ▣ 723
- Tylenol Cold Night Time Medication Liquid ... 1371
- Tylenol PM, Extra Strength Caplets and Tablets ... 1368
- Unisom Dual Relief Nighttime Sleep Aid/Analgesic ... 1774
- Ziradryl Lotion ... ▣ 643

Diphenylpyraline Hydrochloride (May exhibit additive CNS depressant effects).
- No products indexed under this heading.

Doxepin Hydrochloride (May exhibit additive CNS depressant effects; decreased blood levels of the antidepressant). Products include:
- Sinequan ... 1960

Droperidol (May exhibit additive CNS depressant effects). Products include:
- Inapsine Injection ... 1140
- Innovar Injection ... 1141

Enflurane (May exhibit additive CNS depressant effects). Products include:
- Ethrane ... 599

Estazolam (May exhibit additive CNS depressant effects). Products include:
- ProSom Tablets ... 554

Ethchlorvynol (May exhibit additive CNS depressant effects). Products include:
- Placidyl Capsules ... 553

Ethinamate (May exhibit additive CNS depressant effects).
- No products indexed under this heading.

Fentanyl (May exhibit additive CNS depressant effects). Products include:
- Duragesic Transdermal System........ 1133

Fentanyl Citrate (May exhibit additive CNS depressant effects). Products include:
- Innovar Injection........ 1141
- Sublimaze Injection........ 1146

Fluphenazine Decanoate (May exhibit additive CNS depressant effects). Products include:
- Prolixin Decanoate........ 1795

Fluphenazine Enanthate (May exhibit additive CNS depressant effects). Products include:
- Prolixin Enanthate........ 1796

Fluphenazine Hydrochloride (May exhibit additive CNS depressant effects). Products include:
- Prolixin Elixir........ 1793
- Prolixin Injection........ 1791
- Prolixin Oral Concentrate........ 1792
- Prolixin Tablets........ 1793

Flurazepam Hydrochloride (May exhibit additive CNS depressant effects). Products include:
- Dalmane Capsules........ 1927

Glutethimide (May exhibit additive CNS depressant effects).
- No products indexed under this heading.

Haloperidol (May exhibit additive CNS depressant effects). Products include:
- Haldol Injection, Tablets and Concentrate........ 1373

Haloperidol Decanoate (May exhibit additive CNS depressant effects). Products include:
- Haldol Decanoate........ 1375

Hydrocodone Bitartrate (May exhibit additive CNS depressant effects). Products include:
- Anexsia 5/500 Tablets........ 2196
- Anexsia 7.5/650 Tablets........ 2197
- Azdōne Tablets........ 844
- Codiclear DH Syrup........ 845
- Codimal DH Syrup........ 846
- Damason-P........ 1356
- Hycodan Syrup, Tablets........ 927
- Hycomine Compound Tablets........ 929
- Hycomine Syrup........ 927
- Hycotuss Expectorant Syrup........ 930
- Hydrocet Capsules........ 835
- Lortab ASA Tablets........ 2414
- Lortab........ 2412
- Ru-Tuss with Hydrocodone........ 694
- Triaminic Expectorant DH........ 1995
- Vicodin Tablets........ 1187
- Vicodin ES Tablets........ 1189
- Zydone Capsules........ 941

Hydrocodone Polistirex (May exhibit additive CNS depressant effects). Products include:
- Tussionex Extended-Release Suspension........ 988

Hydroxyzine Hydrochloride (May exhibit additive CNS depressant effects). Products include:
- Atarax Tablets & Syrup........ 1941
- Marax Tablets & DF Syrup........ 1954
- Vistaril Intramuscular Solution........ 1970

Imipramine Hydrochloride (May exhibit additive CNS depressant effects; decreased blood levels of the antidepressant). Products include:
- Tofranil Ampuls........ 1038
- Tofranil Tablets........ 1039

Imipramine Pamoate (May exhibit additive CNS depressant effects; decreased blood levels of the antidepressant). Products include:
- Tofranil-PM Capsules........ 1041

Isoflurane (May exhibit additive CNS depressant effects). Products include:
- Forane........ 600

Ketamine Hydrochloride (May exhibit additive CNS depressant effects). Products include:
- Ketalar........ 1726

Levorphanol Tartrate (May exhibit additive CNS depressant effects). Products include:
- Levo-Dromoran........ 1906

Lorazepam (May exhibit additive CNS depressant effects). Products include:
- Ativan Injection........ 2432
- Ativan Tablets........ 2434

Loxapine Hydrochloride (May exhibit additive CNS depressant effects). Products include:
- Loxitane........ 1213

Loxapine Succinate (May exhibit additive CNS depressant effects). Products include:
- Loxitane Capsules........ 1213

Maprotiline Hydrochloride (May exhibit additive CNS depressant effects; decreased blood levels of the antidepressant). Products include:
- Ludiomil Tablets........ 874

Meperidine Hydrochloride (May exhibit additive CNS depressant effects). Products include:
- Demerol........ 2047
- Mepergan Injection........ 2479

Mephobarbital (May exhibit additive CNS depressant effects). Products include:
- Mebaral Tablets........ 2061

Meprobamate (May exhibit additive CNS depressant effects). Products include:
- Deprol Tablets........ 2382
- Equagesic Tablets........ 2451
- Miltown Tablets........ 2386
- PMB 200 and PMB 400........ 2504

Mesoridazine (May exhibit additive CNS depressant effects). Products include:
- Serentil........ 686

Methadone Hydrochloride (May exhibit additive CNS depressant effects). Products include:
- Dolophine Hydrochloride Ampoules & Vials........ 1260
- Dolophine Hydrochloride Tablets........ 1261
- Methadone Hydrochloride Diskets........ 1284
- Methadone Hydrochloride Oral Solution & Tablets........ 1987

Methdilazine Hydrochloride (May exhibit additive CNS depressant effects). Products include:
- Tacaryl Syrup & Tablets........ 2409

Methohexital Sodium (May exhibit additive CNS depressant effects). Products include:
- Brevital Sodium Vials........ 1248

Methoxyflurane (May exhibit additive CNS depressant effects).
- No products indexed under this heading.

Midazolam Hydrochloride (May exhibit additive CNS depressant effects). Products include:
- Versed Injection........ 1924

Molindone Hydrochloride (May exhibit additive CNS depressant effects). Products include:
- Moban Tablets & Concentrate........ 932

Morphine Sulfate (May exhibit additive CNS depressant effects). Products include:
- Astramorph/PF Injection, USP (Preservative-Free)........ 618
- Duramorph........ 960
- Infumorph 200 and Infumorph 500 Sterile Solutions........ 962
- MS Contin Tablets........ 1814
- MSIR........ 1817
- Oramorph SR (Morphine Sulfate Sustained Release Tablets)........ 1988
- Roxanol........ 1991

Nortriptyline Hydrochloride (May exhibit additive CNS depressant effects; decreased blood levels of the antidepressant). Products include:
- Pamelor........ 2019

Opium Alkaloids (May exhibit additive CNS depressant effects). Products include:
- B & O No. 15A & No. 16A Supprettes........ 2395
- Pantopon Injectable........ 1911

Oxazepam (May exhibit additive CNS depressant effects). Products include:
- Serax Capsules........ 2522
- Serax Tablets........ 2522

Oxycodone Hydrochloride (May exhibit additive CNS depressant effects). Products include:
- Percocet Tablets........ 950
- Percodan........ 951
- Roxicodone Tablets, Oral Solution & Intensol (Oxycodone)........ 1992
- Tylox Capsules........ 1382

Pentobarbital Sodium (May exhibit additive CNS depressant effects). Products include:
- Nembutal Sodium Capsules........ 534
- Nembutal Sodium Solution........ 536
- Nembutal Sodium Suppositories........ 538

Perphenazine (May exhibit additive CNS depressant effects). Products include:
- Etrafon........ 2087
- Triavil Tablets........ 1556
- Trilafon........ 2123

Phenobarbital (May exhibit additive CNS depressant effects). Products include:
- Arco-Lase Plus Tablets........ 607
- Bellergal-S Tablets........ 1998
- Bronkolixir........ ■ 761
- Bronkotabs Tablets........ ■ 762
- Donnatal........ 1858
- Donnatal Extentabs........ 1859
- Donnatal Tablets........ 1858
- Donnazyme Tablets........ 1860
- Kinesed Tablets........ 2272
- Phenobarbital Elixir and Tablets........ 1293
- Primatene Tablets-P Formula........ 2421
- Quadrinal Tablets........ 1183
- Tedral SA........ 1765

Prazepam (May exhibit additive CNS depressant effects). Products include:
- Centrax........ 1693

Prochlorperazine (May exhibit additive CNS depressant effects). Products include:
- Compazine........ 2201

Promethazine Hydrochloride (May exhibit additive CNS depressant effects). Products include:
- Mepergan Injection........ 2479
- Phenergan with Codeine........ 2497
- Phenergan with Dextromethorphan 2499
- Phenergan Injection........ 2493
- Phenergan Suppositories........ 2496
- Phenergan Syrup........ 2495
- Phenergan Tablets........ 2496
- Phenergan VC........ 2500
- Phenergan VC with Codeine........ 2501

Propofol (May exhibit additive CNS depressant effects). Products include:
- Diprivan Injection........ 2267

Propoxyphene Hydrochloride (May exhibit additive CNS depressant effects). Products include:
- Darvon........ 1256
- Wygesic Tablets........ 2540

Propoxyphene Napsylate (May exhibit additive CNS depressant effects). Products include:
- Darvon-N/Darvocet-N........ 1254

Protriptyline Hydrochloride (May exhibit additive CNS depressant effects; decreased blood levels of the antidepressant). Products include:
- Vivactil Tablets........ 1567

Pyrilamine Maleate (May exhibit additive CNS depressant effects). Products include:
- Codimal........ 846
- 4-Way Fast Acting Nasal Spray - Original Formula (regular & mentholated) & Metered Spray Pump (regular)........ 751
- Maximum Strength Midol Multi-Symptom Menstrual Formula........ ■ 571
- Maximum Strength Midol PMS Premenstrual Syndrome Formula........ ■ 570
- Regular Strength Midol Multi-Symptom Menstrual Formula........ ■ 570
- Prefrin-A........ ⊙ 255
- Prēmsyn PMS Capsules & Caplets ■ 547
- Primatene Tablets-M Formula........ 2421
- Robitussin Night Relief........ ■ 677
- Ru-Tuss with Hydrocodone........ 694
- Triaminic Expectorant DH........ 1995
- Triaminic Oral Infant Drops........ 1996

Pyrilamine Tannate (May exhibit additive CNS depressant effects). Products include:
- Rynatan........ 2387

Quazepam (May exhibit additive CNS depressant effects). Products include:
- Doral Tablets........ 2383

Secobarbital Sodium (May exhibit additive CNS depressant effects). Products include:
- Seconal Sodium Pulvules........ 1296

Sufentanil Citrate (May exhibit additive CNS depressant effects). Products include:
- Sufenta Injection........ 1147

Temazepam (May exhibit additive CNS depressant effects). Products include:
- Restoril Capsules........ 2023

Terfenadine (May exhibit additive CNS depressant effects). Products include:
- Seldane Tablets........ 1349
- Seldane-D Extended-Release Tablets........ 1350

Thiamylal Sodium (May exhibit additive CNS depressant effects). Products include:
- Surital Ampoules, Steri-Vials........ 1764

Thioridazine Hydrochloride (May exhibit additive CNS depressant effects). Products include:
- Mellaril........ 2011

Thiothixene (May exhibit additive CNS depressant effects). Products include:
- Navane Capsules and Concentrate 1954
- Navane Intramuscular........ 1956

Triazolam (May exhibit additive CNS depressant effects). Products include:
- Halcion Tablets........ 2340

Trifluoperazine Hydrochloride (May exhibit additive CNS depressant effects). Products include:
- Stelazine........ 2226

Trimeprazine Tartrate (May exhibit additive CNS depressant effects). Products include:
- Temaril Tablets, Syrup and Spansule Sustained Release Capsules 1085

Trimipramine Maleate (May exhibit additive CNS depressant effects; decreased blood levels of the antidepressant). Products include:
- Surmontil Capsules........ 2524

Tripelennamine Hydrochloride (May exhibit additive CNS depressant effects). Products include:
- PBZ Tablets & Elixir........ 1037
- PBZ-SR Tablets........ 1037

Triprolidine Hydrochloride (May exhibit additive CNS depressant effects). Products include:
- Actidil ■D 538
- Actifed Capsules ■D 539
- Actifed Plus Caplets ■D 539
- Actifed Plus Tablets ■D 540
- Actifed with Codeine Cough Syrup 752
- Actifed Syrup ■D 540
- Actifed Tablets ■D 540
- Actifed 12-Hour Capsules ■D 539

Warfarin Sodium (Decreased effect of anticoagulant). Products include:
- Coumadin Injection & Tablets 944
- Panwarfin Tablets 547

ESGIC TABLETS & CAPSULES

(Butalbital, Acetaminophen) 1001

May interact with oral anticoagulants, tricyclic antidepressants, narcotic analgesics, central nervous system depressants, and certain other agents. Compounds in these categories include:

Alcohol (May exhibit additive CNS depressant effects).

Alfentanil Hydrochloride (May exhibit additive CNS depressant effects). Products include:
- Alfenta Injection 1131

Alprazolam (May exhibit additive CNS depressant effects). Products include:
- Xanax Tablets 2367

Amitriptyline Hydrochloride (Decreased blood levels of the antidepressant). Products include:
- Elavil 2269
- Endep Tablets 1927
- Etrafon 2087
- Limbitrol 1933
- Triavil Tablets 1556

Amoxapine (Decreased blood levels of the antidepressant). Products include:
- Asendin Tablets 1196

Aprobarbital (May exhibit additive CNS depressant effects). Products include:
- Alurate Elixir 1883

Buprenorphine (May exhibit additive CNS depressant effects).
- No products indexed under this heading.

Buspirone Hydrochloride (May exhibit additive CNS depressant effects). Products include:
- BuSpar 1401

Butabarbital (May exhibit additive CNS depressant effects). Products include:
- Pyridium Plus 1764

Chlordiazepoxide (May exhibit additive CNS depressant effects). Products include:
- Libritabs Tablets 1930
- Limbitrol 1933
- Menrium Tablets 1934

Chlordiazepoxide Hydrochloride (May exhibit additive CNS depressant effects). Products include:
- Librax Capsules 1929
- Librium Capsules 1931
- Librium Injectable 1932

Chlorpromazine (May exhibit additive CNS depressant effects). Products include:
- Thorazine 2234

Chlorprothixene (May exhibit additive CNS depressant effects). Products include:
- Taractan Tablets 1920

Chlorprothixene Hydrochloride (May exhibit additive CNS depressant effects). Products include:
- Taractan 1920

Clomipramine Hydrochloride (Decreased blood levels of the antidepressant). Products include:
- Anafranil Capsules 650

Clorazepate Dipotassium (May exhibit additive CNS depressant effects). Products include:
- Tranxene 556

Codeine (May exhibit additive CNS depressant effects). Products include:
- Calcidrine Syrup 506

Codeine Phosphate (May exhibit additive CNS depressant effects). Products include:
- Actifed with Codeine Cough Syrup 752
- Cheracol Cough Syrup 1853
- Codimal PH Syrup 846
- Dimetane-DC Cough Syrup 1857
- Empirin with Codeine Phosphate Nos. 2, 3 & 4 764
- Fiorinal with Codeine Capsules 2008
- Isoclor Expectorant 982
- Naldecon CX Adult Liquid ■D 521
- Novahistine DH 1342
- Novahistine Expectorant 1343
- Nucofed Capsules 2219
- Nucofed Expectorant 2219
- Nucofed Pediatric Expectorant 2220
- Nucofed Syrup 2219
- Phenaphen with Codeine Capsules 1865
- Phenaphen-650 with Codeine Tablets 1866
- Phenergan with Codeine 2497
- Phenergan VC with Codeine 2501
- Robitussin A-C Syrup 1875
- Robitussin-DAC Syrup 1875
- Ryna ■D 741
- Soma Compound w/Codeine Tablets 2390
- Triaminic Expectorant w/Codeine 1996
- Tussi-Organidin Liquid 2391
- Tylenol with Codeine 1381

Codeine Polistirex (May exhibit additive CNS depressant effects).
- No products indexed under this heading.

Desipramine Hydrochloride (Decreased blood levels of the antidepressant). Products include:
- Norpramin Tablets 1340

Dezocine (May exhibit additive CNS depressant effects).

Diazepam (May exhibit additive CNS depressant effects). Products include:
- Valium Injectable 1937
- Valium Tablets 1939
- Valrelease Capsules 1923

Dicumarol (Decreased effect of anticoagulant). Products include:
- Dicumarol Tablets 516

Doxepin Hydrochloride (Decreased blood levels of the antidepressant). Products include:
- Sinequan 1960

Droperidol (May exhibit additive CNS depressant effects). Products include:
- Inapsine Injection 1140
- Innovar Injection 1141

Enflurane (May exhibit additive CNS depressant effects). Products include:
- Ethrane 599

Estazolam (May exhibit additive CNS depressant effects). Products include:
- ProSom Tablets 554

Ethchlorvynol (May exhibit additive CNS depressant effects). Products include:
- Placidyl Capsules 553

Ethinamate (May exhibit additive CNS depressant effects).
- No products indexed under this heading.

Fentanyl (May exhibit additive CNS depressant effects). Products include:
- Duragesic Transdermal System 1133

Fentanyl Citrate (May exhibit additive CNS depressant effects). Products include:
- Innovar Injection 1141
- Sublimaze Injection 1146

Fluphenazine Decanoate (May exhibit additive CNS depressant effects). Products include:
- Prolixin Decanoate 1795

Fluphenazine Enanthate (May exhibit additive CNS depressant effects). Products include:
- Prolixin Enanthate 1796

Fluphenazine Hydrochloride (May exhibit additive CNS depressant effects). Products include:
- Prolixin Elixir 1793
- Prolixin Injection 1791
- Prolixin Oral Concentrate 1792
- Prolixin Tablets 1793

Flurazepam Hydrochloride (May exhibit additive CNS depressant effects). Products include:
- Dalmane Capsules 1927

Glutethimide (May exhibit additive CNS depressant effects).
- No products indexed under this heading.

Haloperidol (May exhibit additive CNS depressant effects). Products include:
- Haldol Injection, Tablets and Concentrate 1373

Haloperidol Decanoate (May exhibit additive CNS depressant effects). Products include:
- Haldol Decanoate 1375

Hydrocodone Bitartrate (May exhibit additive CNS depressant effects). Products include:
- Anexsia 5/500 Tablets 2196
- Anexsia 7.5/650 Tablets 2197
- Azdone Tablets 844
- Codiclear DH Syrup 845
- Codimal DH Syrup 846
- Damason-P 1356
- Hycodan Syrup, Tablets 927
- Hycomine Compound Tablets 929
- Hycomine Syrup 927
- Hycotuss Expectorant Syrup 930
- Hydrocet Capsules 835
- Lortab ASA Tablets 2414
- Lortab 2412
- Ru-Tuss with Hydrocodone 694
- Triaminic Expectorant DH 1995
- Vicodin Tablets 1187
- Vicodin ES Tablets 1189
- Zydone Capsules 941

Hydrocodone Polistirex (May exhibit additive CNS depressant effects). Products include:
- Tussionex Extended-Release Suspension 988

Hydroxyzine Hydrochloride (May exhibit additive CNS depressant effects). Products include:
- Atarax Tablets & Syrup 1941
- Marax Tablets & DF Syrup 1954
- Vistaril Intramuscular Solution 1970

Imipramine Hydrochloride (Decreased blood levels of the antidepressant). Products include:
- Tofranil Ampuls 1038
- Tofranil Tablets 1039

Imipramine Pamoate (Decreased blood levels of the antidepressant). Products include:
- Tofranil-PM Capsules 1041

Isoflurane (May exhibit additive CNS depressant effects). Products include:
- Forane 600

Ketamine Hydrochloride (May exhibit additive CNS depressant effects). Products include:
- Ketalar 1726

Levorphanol Tartrate (May exhibit additive CNS depressant effects). Products include:
- Levo-Dromoran 1906

Lorazepam (May exhibit additive CNS depressant effects). Products include:
- Ativan Injection 2432
- Ativan Tablets 2434

Loxapine Hydrochloride (May exhibit additive CNS depressant effects). Products include:
- Loxitane 1213

Loxapine Succinate (May exhibit additive CNS depressant effects). Products include:
- Loxitane Capsules 1213

Maprotiline Hydrochloride (Decreased blood levels of the antidepressant). Products include:
- Ludiomil Tablets 874

Meperidine Hydrochloride (May exhibit additive CNS depressant effects). Products include:
- Demerol 2047
- Mepergan Injection 2479

Mephobarbital (May exhibit additive CNS depressant effects). Products include:
- Mebaral Tablets 2061

Meprobamate (May exhibit additive CNS depressant effects). Products include:
- Deprol Tablets 2382
- Equagesic Tablets 2451
- Miltown Tablets 2386
- PMB 200 and PMB 400 2504

Mesoridazine (May exhibit additive CNS depressant effects). Products include:
- Serentil 686

Methadone Hydrochloride (May exhibit additive CNS depressant effects). Products include:
- Dolophine Hydrochloride Ampoules & Vials 1260
- Dolophine Hydrochloride Tablets 1261
- Methadone Hydrochloride Diskets 1284
- Methadone Hydrochloride Oral Solution & Tablets 1987

Methohexital Sodium (May exhibit additive CNS depressant effects). Products include:
- Brevital Sodium Vials 1248

Methoxyflurane (May exhibit additive CNS depressant effects).
- No products indexed under this heading.

Midazolam Hydrochloride (May exhibit additive CNS depressant effects). Products include:
- Versed Injection 1924

Molindone Hydrochloride (May exhibit additive CNS depressant effects). Products include:
- Moban Tablets & Concentrate 932

Morphine Sulfate (May exhibit additive CNS depressant effects). Products include:
- Astramorph/PF Injection, USP (Preservative-Free) 618
- Duramorph 960
- Infumorph 200 and Infumorph 500 Sterile Solutions 962
- MS Contin Tablets 1814
- MSIR 1817
- Oramorph SR (Morphine Sulfate Sustained Release Tablets) 1988
- Roxanol 1991

Nortriptyline Hydrochloride (Decreased blood levels of the antidepressant). Products include:
- Pamelor 2019

Opium Alkaloids (May exhibit additive CNS depressant effects). Products include:
- B & O No. 15A & No. 16A Supprettes 2395
- Pantopon Injectable 1911

Oxazepam (May exhibit additive CNS depressant effects). Products include:
- Serax Capsules 2522
- Serax Tablets 2522

Oxycodone Hydrochloride (May exhibit additive CNS depressant effects). Products include:
- Percocet Tablets 950
- Percodan 951
- Roxicodone Tablets, Oral Solution & Intensol (Oxycodone) 1992
- Tylox Capsules 1382

Pentobarbital Sodium (May exhibit additive CNS depressant effects). Products include:
- Nembutal Sodium Capsules 534
- Nembutal Sodium Solution 536
- Nembutal Sodium Suppositories 538

Perphenazine (May exhibit additive CNS depressant effects). Products include:
- Etrafon 2087
- Triavil Tablets 1556
- Trilafon 2123

Phenobarbital (May exhibit additive CNS depressant effects). Products include:
- Arco-Lase Plus Tablets 607
- Bellergal-S Tablets 1998
- Bronkolixir .... ▣ 761
- Bronkotabs Tablets .... ▣ 762
- Donnatal 1858
- Donnatal Extentabs 1859
- Donnatal Tablets 1858
- Donnazyme Tablets 1860
- Kinesed Tablets 2272
- Phenobarbital Elixir and Tablets 1293
- Primatene Tablets-P Formula 2421
- Quadrinal Tablets 1183
- Tedral SA 1765

Prazepam (May exhibit additive CNS depressant effects). Products include:
- Centrax 1693

Prochlorperazine (May exhibit additive CNS depressant effects). Products include:
- Compazine 2201

Promethazine Hydrochloride (May exhibit additive CNS depressant effects). Products include:
- Mepergan Injection 2479
- Phenergan with Codeine 2497
- Phenergan with Dextromethorphan 2499
- Phenergan Injection 2493
- Phenergan Suppositories 2496
- Phenergan Syrup 2495
- Phenergan Tablets 2496
- Phenergan VC 2500
- Phenergan VC with Codeine 2501

Propofol (May exhibit additive CNS depressant effects). Products include:
- Diprivan Injection 2267

Propoxyphene Hydrochloride (May exhibit additive CNS depressant effects). Products include:
- Darvon 1256
- Wygesic Tablets 2540

Propoxyphene Napsylate (May exhibit additive CNS depressant effects). Products include:
- Darvon-N/Darvocet-N 1254

Protriptyline Hydrochloride (Decreased blood levels of the antidepressant). Products include:
- Vivactil Tablets 1567

Quazepam (May exhibit additive CNS depressant effects). Products include:
- Doral Tablets 2383

Secobarbital Sodium (May exhibit additive CNS depressant effects). Products include:
- Seconal Sodium Pulvules 1296

Sufentanil Citrate (May exhibit additive CNS depressant effects). Products include:
- Sufenta Injection 1147

Temazepam (May exhibit additive CNS depressant effects). Products include:
- Restoril Capsules 2023

Thiamylal Sodium (May exhibit additive CNS depressant effects). Products include:
- Surital Ampoules, Steri-Vials 1764

Thioridazine Hydrochloride (May exhibit additive CNS depressant effects). Products include:
- Mellaril 2011

Thiothixene (May exhibit additive CNS depressant effects). Products include:
- Navane Capsules and Concentrate 1954
- Navane Intramuscular 1956

Triazolam (May exhibit additive CNS depressant effects). Products include:
- Halcion Tablets 2340

Trifluoperazine Hydrochloride (May exhibit additive CNS depressant effects). Products include:
- Stelazine 2226

Trimipramine Maleate (Decreased blood levels of the antidepressant). Products include:
- Surmontil Capsules 2524

Warfarin Sodium (Decreased effect of anticoagulant). Products include:
- Coumadin Injection & Tablets 944
- Panwarfin Tablets 547

ESIDRIX TABLETS (Hydrochlorothiazide) 863
May interact with corticosteroids, insulin, antihypertensives, barbiturates, cardiac glycosides, lithium preparations, narcotic analgesics, non-steroidal anti-inflammatory agents, and certain other agents. Compounds in these categories include:

Acebutolol Hydrochloride (Additive or potentiated action). Products include:
- Sectral Capsules 2520

ACTH (Hypokalemia).
No products indexed under this heading.

Alcohol (May potentiate orthostatic hypotension).

Alfentanil Hydrochloride (May potentiate orthostatic hypotension). Products include:
- Alfenta Injection 1131

Aprobarbital (May potentiate orthostatic hypotension). Products include:
- Alurate Elixir 1883

Atenolol (Additive or potentiated action). Products include:
- Tenoretic Tablets 1105
- Tenormin Tablets and I.V. Injection 1107

Benazepril Hydrochloride (Additive or potentiated action). Products include:
- Lotensin Tablets 872

Bendroflumethiazide (Additive or potentiated action). Products include:
- Corzide Tablets 702
- Naturetin Tablets 1789
- Rauzide Tablets 1804

Betamethasone Acetate (Hypokalemia). Products include:
- Celestone Soluspan Suspension 2081

Betamethasone Sodium Phosphate (Hypokalemia). Products include:
- Celestone Soluspan Suspension 2081

Betaxolol Hydrochloride (Additive or potentiated action). Products include:
- Betoptic Sterile Ophthalmic Solution 569
- Betoptic S Sterile Ophthalmic Suspension 570
- Kerlone Tablets 2172

Buprenorphine (May potentiate orthostatic hypotension).
No products indexed under this heading.

Butabarbital (May potentiate orthostatic hypotension). Products include:
- Pyridium Plus 1764

Butalbital (May potentiate orthostatic hypotension). Products include:
- Esgic-Plus Tablets 1002
- Esgic Tablets & Capsules 1001
- Fioricet Tablets 2006
- Fiorinal Capsules 2007
- Fiorinal with Codeine Capsules 2008
- Fiorinal Tablets 2007
- Phrenilin 838
- Sedapap Tablets 50 mg/650 mg .. 1360

Captopril (Additive or potentiated action). Products include:
- Capoten 2255
- Capozide 2258

Carteolol Hydrochloride (Additive or potentiated action). Products include:
- Cartrol Tablets 507

Chlorothiazide (Additive or potentiated action). Products include:
- Aldoclor Tablets 1413
- Diupres Tablets 1461
- Diuril Oral 1464

Chlorothiazide Sodium (Additive or potentiated action). Products include:
- Diuril Sodium Intravenous 1463

Chlorthalidone (Additive or potentiated action). Products include:
- Combipres Tablets 678
- Tenoretic Tablets 1105
- Thalitone Tablets 687

Clonidine (Additive or potentiated action). Products include:
- Catapres-TTS 677

Clonidine Hydrochloride (Additive or potentiated action). Products include:
- Catapres Tablets 676
- Combipres Tablets 678

Codeine (May potentiate orthostatic hypotension). Products include:
- Calcidrine Syrup 506

Codeine Phosphate (May potentiate orthostatic hypotension). Products include:
- Actifed with Codeine Cough Syrup .. 752
- Cheracol Cough Syrup 1853
- Codimal PH Syrup 846
- Dimetane-DC Cough Syrup 1857
- Empirin with Codeine Phosphate Nos. 2, 3 & 4 764
- Fiorinal with Codeine Capsules 2008
- Isoclor Expectorant 982
- Naldecon CX Adult Liquid .... ▣ 521
- Novahistine DH 1342
- Novahistine Expectorant 1343
- Nucofed Capsules 2219
- Nucofed Expectorant 2219
- Nucofed Pediatric Expectorant 2220
- Nucofed Syrup 2219
- Phenaphen with Codeine Capsules 1865
- Phenaphen-650 with Codeine Tablets 1866
- Phenergan with Codeine 2497
- Phenergan VC with Codeine 2501
- Robitussin A-C Syrup 1875
- Robitussin-DAC Syrup 1875
- Ryna .... ▣ 741
- Soma Compound w/Codeine Tablets 2390
- Triaminic Expectorant w/Codeine .. 1996
- Tussi-Organidin Liquid 2391
- Tylenol with Codeine 1381

Codeine Polistirex (May potentiate orthostatic hypotension).
No products indexed under this heading.

Cortisone Acetate (Hypokalemia). Products include:
- Cortone Acetate Sterile Suspension 1437
- Cortone Acetate Tablets 1439

Deserpidine (Additive or potentiated action). Products include:
- Enduronyl 518
- Harmonyl Tablets 528
- Oreticyl 545

Deslanoside (Increased ventricular irritability).
No products indexed under this heading.

Dexamethasone (Hypokalemia). Products include:
- AK-Trol Ointment & Suspension .... ◉ 207
- Decadron Elixir 1445
- Decadron Tablets 1447
- Decaspray Topical Aerosol 1459
- Dexacidin .... ◉ 272
- Maxidex Sterile Ophthalmic Suspension .... ◉ 223
- Maxitrol Ophthalmic Ointment/Suspension .... ◉ 223
- TobraDex Ophthalmic Suspension and Ointment .... ◉ 228

Dexamethasone Acetate (Hypokalemia). Products include:
- Dalalone D.P. Injectable 999
- Decadron-LA Sterile Suspension 1457

Dexamethasone Sodium Phosphate (Hypokalemia). Products include:
- AK-Dex .... ◉ 203
- Decadron Phosphate Respihaler 1454
- Decadron Phosphate Sterile Ophthalmic Ointment 1453
- Decadron Phosphate Sterile Ophthalmic Solution 1453
- Decadron Phosphate Topical Cream 1455
- Decadron Phosphate Turbinaire 1456
- Maxidex Sterile Ophthalmic Ointment .... ◉ 222
- NeoDecadron Sterile Ophthalmic Ointment 1517
- NeoDecadron Sterile Ophthalmic Solution 1518
- NeoDecadron Topical Cream 1518

Dezocine (May potentiate orthostatic hypotension).

Diazoxide (Additive or potentiated action). Products include:
- Hyperstat I.V. Injection 2095
- Proglycem 649

Diclofenac Sodium (May reduce diuretic, natriuretic, and antihypertensive effects of thiazide diuretics). Products include:
- Voltaren Ophthalmic Sterile Ophthalmic Solution .... ◉ 268
- Voltaren Tablets 1042

Digitoxin (Increased ventricular irritability). Products include:
- Crystodigin Tablets 1253

Digoxin (Increased ventricular irritability). Products include:
- Lanoxicaps 772
- Lanoxin Elixir Pediatric 775
- Lanoxin Injection 778
- Lanoxin Injection Pediatric 781
- Lanoxin Tablets 783

Doxazosin Mesylate (Additive or potentiated action). Products include:
- Cardura Tablets 1941

Enalapril Maleate (Additive or potentiated action). Products include:
- Vaseretic Tablets 1559
- Vasotec Tablets 1564

Enalaprilat (Additive or potentiated action). Products include:
- Vasotec I.V. 1562

Esmolol Hydrochloride (Additive or potentiated action). Products include:
- Brevibloc Injection 942

Etodolac (May reduce diuretic, natriuretic, and antihypertensive effects of thiazide diuretics). Products include:
- Lodine Capsules 2468

Felodipine (Additive or potentiated action). Products include:
Plendil Extended-Release Tablets.... 1526

Fenoprofen Calcium (May reduce diuretic, natriuretic, and antihypertensive effects of thiazide diuretics). Products include:
Nalfon Pulvules & Tablets 919

Fentanyl (May potentiate orthostatic hypotension). Products include:
Duragesic Transdermal System...... 1133

Fentanyl Citrate (May potentiate orthostatic hypotension). Products include:
Innovar Injection.......... 1141
Sublimaze Injection.......... 1146

Flurbiprofen (May reduce diuretic, natriuretic, and antihypertensive effects of thiazide diuretics). Products include:
Ansaid Tablets 2319

Fosinopril Sodium (Additive or potentiated action). Products include:
Monopril Tablets 1406

Furosemide (Additive or potentiated action). Products include:
Lasix 1093

Guanabenz Acetate (Additive or potentiated action). Products include:
Wytensin Tablets 2542

Guanethidine Monosulfate (Additive or potentiated action). Products include:
Esimil Tablets 864
Ismelin Tablets 869

Hydralazine Hydrochloride (Additive or potentiated action). Products include:
Apresazide Capsules 854
Apresoline Hydrochloride Parenteral (Ampuls).......... 856
Apresoline Hydrochloride Tablets .. 855
Apresoline-Esidrix Tablets 857
Ser-Ap-Es Tablets 881
Serpasil-Apresoline Tablets.......... 884

Hydrocodone Bitartrate (May potentiate orthostatic hypotension). Products include:
Anexsia 5/500 Tablets.......... 2196
Anexsia 7.5/650 Tablets 2197
Azdone Tablets.......... 844
Codiclear DH Syrup 845
Codimal DH Syrup.......... 846
Damason-P.......... 1356
Hycodan Syrup, Tablets 927
Hycomine Compound Tablets 929
Hycomine Syrup.......... 927
Hycotuss Expectorant Syrup 930
Hydrocet Capsules 835
Lortab ASA Tablets.......... 2414
Lortab.......... 2412
Ru-Tuss with Hydrocodone 694
Triaminic Expectorant DH 1995
Vicodin Tablets.......... 1187
Vicodin ES Tablets 1189
Zydone Capsules 941

Hydrocodone Polistirex (May potentiate orthostatic hypotension). Products include:
Tussionex Extended-Release Suspension.......... 988

Hydrocortisone (Hypokalemia). Products include:
AK-Spore H.C. .... ⊙ 206
Bactine Hydrocortisone Anti-Itch Cream.......... ▣ 625
CaldeCORT Anti-Itch Hydrocortisone Spray .... ▣ 560
Carmol HC Cream 1% 2296
Cortaid Spray .... ▣ 735
Cortenema 2244
Cortisporin Ointment.......... 758
Cortisporin Ophthalmic Ointment Sterile 758
Cortisporin Ophthalmic Suspension Sterile 759
Cortisporin Otic Solution Sterile 760
Cortisporin Otic Suspension Sterile 760
Cortizone-5 Creme & Ointment...... ▣ 732
Dermolate Anti-Itch Cream .... ▣ 697
Eldecort Cream 1.0% 1113
Eldecort Cream 1.0% and 2.5% 1113
Fungoid HC Creme 1770
Hydrocortone Tablets 1482
Hytone 909
LazerSporin-C Solution 1770
Massengill Medicated Soft Cloth Towelettes.......... 2192
Nutracort Cream & Lotion.......... 1684
PediOtic Suspension Sterile 797
Synacort Creams 1%, 2.5% 2296
Vanoxide-HC Acne Lotion.......... 911
Vioform-Hydrocortisone Cream and Mild Cream 889
Vioform-Hydrocortisone Ointment.. 889
VōSoL HC Otic Solution.......... 2392
Vytone Cream 1%.......... 911

Hydrocortisone Acetate (Hypokalemia). Products include:
Analpram-HC Rectal Cream 1% and 2.5% 970
Anusol-HC Cream 1690
Anusol-HC Suppositories 1691
Caldecort.......... ▣ 560
Carmol HC Cream 1% 2296
Chloromycetin Hydrocortisone Ophthalmic.......... 1694
Coly-Mycin S Otic w/Neomycin & Hydrocortisone.......... 1708
Cortaid .... ▣ 735
Cortef Feminine Itch Cream .... ▣ 735
Corticaine .... ▣ 682
Cortifoam 1827
Cortisporin Cream.......... 757
Epifoam 1828
Gynecort 5 Creme.......... ▣ 556
Hydrocortone Acetate Sterile Suspension.......... 1479
Lanacort 5 Creme and Ointment .. ▣ 557
Mantadil Cream 789
Ophthocort .... ⊙ 301
Orabase HCA Oral Paste 890
Pramosone Cream, Lotion & Ointment 971
ProctoCream-HC 1834
Proctofoam-HC.......... 1835

Hydrocortisone Sodium Phosphate (Hypokalemia). Products include:
Hydrocortone Phosphate Injection, Sterile 1481

Hydrocortisone Sodium Succinate (Hypokalemia). Products include:
Solu-Cortef Sterile Powder.......... 2361

Hydroflumethiazide (Additive or potentiated action). Products include:
Diucardin Tablets.......... 2450
Saluron.......... 718
Salutensin/Salutensin-Demi 719

Ibuprofen (May reduce diuretic, natriuretic, and antihypertensive effects of thiazide diuretics). Products include:
Advil Cold & Sinus Caplets (formerly CoAdvil) 2416
Advil Ibuprofen Tablets and Caplets 2416
Children's Advil Suspension 2426
CoAdvil.......... ▣ 748
Dristan Sinus Caplets.......... 2419
Haltran Tablets.......... ▣ 668
Ibuprofen.......... ▣ 631
Medipren ibuprofen Caplets and Tablets 1362
Midol 200 Cramp Relief Formula.. ▣ 570
Motrin Tablets.......... 2351
Motrin IB Caplets and Tablets .... ▣ 736
Nuprin Ibuprofen/Analgesic Tablets & Caplets 752
PediaProfen Suspension.......... 1363
Rufen Tablets 691
Trendar Ibuprofen Tablets.......... ▣ 756

Indapamide (Additive or potentiated action). Products include:
Lozol Tablets 1843

Indomethacin (May reduce diuretic, natriuretic, and antihypertensive effects of thiazide diuretics). Products include:
Indocin 1487

Indomethacin Sodium Trihydrate (May reduce diuretic, natriuretic, and antihypertensive effects of thiazide diuretics). Products include:
Indocin I.V. 1490

Insulin, Human (Insulin requirements may be altered).
No products indexed under this heading.

Insulin, Human Isophane Suspension (Insulin requirements may be altered). Products include:
Humulin N, 100 Units 1270

Insulin, Human NPH (Insulin requirements may be altered). Products include:
Insulatard NPH Human.......... 1627
Novolin N.......... 1627
Novolin N PenFill Cartridges.......... 1628
Novolin N Prefilled 1628

Insulin, Human Regular (Insulin requirements may be altered). Products include:
Humulin BR, 100 Units 1268
Humulin R, 100 Units 1272
Novolin R.......... 1627
Novolin R PenFill Cartridges.......... 1628
Novolin R Prefilled.......... 1629
Velosulin Human 1628

Insulin, Human, Zinc Suspension (Insulin requirements may be altered). Products include:
Humulin L, 100 Units 1268
Humulin U, 100 Units 1272
Novolin L 1627

Insulin, NPH (Insulin requirements may be altered). Products include:
NPH, 40 & 100 Units 1273
Beef NPH, 100 Units.......... 1274
Pork NPH, 100 Units.......... 1275
Insulatard NPH 1626
NPH Insulin 1626
NPH Purified Pork Isophane Insulin 1626

Insulin, Regular (Insulin requirements may be altered). Products include:
Regular, 40 & 100 Units 1273
Beef Regular, 100 Units.......... 1275
Pork Regular, 100 Units 1275
Pork Regular (Concentrated), 500 Units 1276
Regular Insulin 1625
Regular Purified Pork Insulin 1626
Velosulin 1627

Insulin, Zinc Crystals (Insulin requirements may be altered). Products include:
NPH, 40 & 100 Units 1273

Insulin, Zinc Suspension (Insulin requirements may be altered). Products include:
Lente, 40 & 100 Units 1272
Protamine, Zinc, 40 & 100 Units.... 1273
Lente Iletin I 1272
Beef Lente, 100 Units.......... 1274
Beef Protamine Zinc, 100 Units...... 1274
Pork Lente, 100 Units.......... 1275
Pork, Protamine, Zinc, 100 Units.... 1275
Lente Insulin.......... 1626
Lente Purified Pork Insulin 1626
Semilente Insulin 1625
Ultralente Insulin 1626

Isradipine (Additive or potentiated action). Products include:
DynaCirc Capsules 2004

Ketoprofen (May reduce diuretic, natriuretic, and antihypertensive effects of thiazide diuretics). Products include:
Orudis Capsules.......... 2488

Ketorolac Tromethamine (May reduce diuretic, natriuretic, and antihypertensive effects of thiazide diuretics). Products include:
Toradol IM Injection 2302

Labetalol Hydrochloride (Additive or potentiated action). Products include:
Normodyne Injection 2108
Normodyne Tablets 2110
Normozide Tablets 2112
Trandate HCT Tablets.......... 579
Trandate Injection 577
Trandate Tablets 579

Levorphanol Tartrate (May potentiate orthostatic hypotension). Products include:
Levo-Dromoran.......... 1906

Lisinopril (Additive or potentiated action). Products include:
Prinivil Tablets 1538
Prinzide Tablets 1540
Zestoretic 2274
Zestril Tablets 2277

Lithium Carbonate (Increased risk of lithium toxicity). Products include:
Eskalith 2214
Lithane Tablets.......... 1596
Lithium Carbonate Capsules & Tablets 1984
Lithobid Tablets 870

Lithium Citrate (Increased risk of lithium toxicity). Products include:
Cibalith-S.......... 870

Mecamylamine Hydrochloride (Additive or potentiated action). Products include:
Inversine Tablets 1492

Meclofenamate Sodium (May reduce diuretic, natriuretic, and antihypertensive effects of thiazide diuretics). Products include:
Meclomen Capsules 1739

Mefenamic Acid (May reduce diuretic, natriuretic, and antihypertensive effects of thiazide diuretics). Products include:
Ponstel 1758

Meperidine Hydrochloride (May potentiate orthostatic hypotension). Products include:
Demerol 2047
Mepergan Injection 2479

Mephobarbital (May potentiate orthostatic hypotension). Products include:
Mebaral Tablets 2061

Methadone Hydrochloride (May potentiate orthostatic hypotension). Products include:
Dolophine Hydrochloride Ampoules & Vials 1260
Dolophine Hydrochloride Tablets 1261
Methadone Hydrochloride Diskets .. 1284
Methadone Hydrochloride Oral Solution & Tablets.......... 1987

Methyclothiazide (Additive or potentiated action). Products include:
Enduron Tablets.......... 517
Enduronyl 518

Methyldopa (Additive or potentiated action; hemolytic anemia). Products include:
Aldoclor Tablets.......... 1413
Aldomet Oral 1415
Aldoril Tablets.......... 1418

Methyldopate Hydrochloride (Additive or potentiated action). Products include:
Aldomet Ester HCl Injection 1417

Methylprednisolone (Hypokalemia). Products include:
Medrol 2348

Methylprednisolone Acetate (Hypokalemia). Products include:
Depo-Medrol Sterile Aqueous Suspension.......... 2334

Methylprednisolone Sodium Succinate (Hypokalemia). Products include:
Solu-Medrol Sterile Powder.......... 2363

Metolazone (Additive or potentiated action). Products include:
Diulo 2129
Mykrox ½ mg Tablets 984
Zaroxolyn Tablets 989

Metoprolol Tartrate (Additive or potentiated action). Products include:
- Lopressor Ampuls ... 1032
- Lopressor HCT Tablets ... 1034
- Lopressor Tablets ... 1032

Metyrosine (Additive or potentiated action). Products include:
- Demser Capsules ... 1460

Minoxidil (Additive or potentiated action). Products include:
- Loniten Tablets ... 2346
- Rogaine Topical Solution ... 2357

Morphine Sulfate (May potentiate orthostatic hypotension). Products include:
- Astramorph/PF Injection, USP (Preservative-Free) ... 618
- Duramorph ... 960
- Infumorph 200 and Infumorph 500 Sterile Solutions ... 962
- MS Contin Tablets ... 1814
- MSIR ... 1817
- Oramorph SR (Morphine Sulfate Sustained Release Tablets) ... 1988
- Roxanol ... 1991

Nadolol (Additive or potentiated action). Products include:
- Corgard Tablets ... 701
- Corzide Tablets ... 702

Naproxen (May reduce diuretic, natriuretic, and antihypertensive effects of thiazide diuretics). Products include:
- Naprosyn ... 2297

Naproxen Sodium (May reduce diuretic, natriuretic, and antihypertensive effects of thiazide diuretics). Products include:
- Anaprox and Anaprox DS Tablets ... 2288

Nicardipine Hydrochloride (Additive or potentiated action). Products include:
- Cardene Capsules ... 2290

Nitroglycerin (Additive or potentiated action). Products include:
- Deponit NTG Transdermal Delivery System ... 2143
- Minitran Transdermal Delivery System ... 1312
- Nitro-Bid Ointment ... 1339
- Nitro-Bid Capsules ... 1338
- Nitrodisc ... 2176
- Nitro-Dur (nitroglycerin) Transdermal Infusion System ... 1164
- Nitrogard Tablets ... 1004
- Nitrolingual Spray ... 1846
- Nitrostat Tablets ... 1743
- Transderm-Nitro Transdermal Therapeutic System ... 2283

Norepinephrine Bitartrate (Decreased arterial response to norepinephrine). Products include:
- Levophed Bitartrate Injection ... 2054

Opium Alkaloids (May potentiate orthostatic hypotension). Products include:
- B & O No. 15A & No. 16A Supprettes ... 2395
- Pantopon Injectable ... 1911

Oxycodone Hydrochloride (May potentiate orthostatic hypotension). Products include:
- Percocet Tablets ... 950
- Percodan ... 951
- Roxicodone Tablets, Oral Solution & Intensol (Oxycodone) ... 1992
- Tylox Capsules ... 1382

Penbutolol Sulfate (Additive or potentiated action). Products include:
- Levatol ... 1832

Pentobarbital Sodium (May potentiate orthostatic hypotension). Products include:
- Nembutal Sodium Capsules ... 534
- Nembutal Sodium Solution ... 536
- Nembutal Sodium Suppositories ... 538

Phenobarbital (May potentiate orthostatic hypotension). Products include:
- Arco-Lase Plus Tablets ... 607
- Bellergal-S Tablets ... 1998
- Bronkolixir ... ⊞ 761
- Bronkotabs Tablets ... ⊞ 762
- Donnatal ... 1858
- Donnatal Extentabs ... 1859
- Donnatal Tablets ... 1858
- Donnazyme Tablets ... 1860
- Kinesed Tablets ... 2272
- Phenobarbital Elixir and Tablets ... 1293
- Primatene Tablets-P Formula ... 2421
- Quadrinal Tablets ... 1183
- Tedral SA ... 1765

Phenoxybenzamine Hydrochloride (Additive or potentiated action). Products include:
- Dibenzyline Capsules ... 2207

Phentolamine Mesylate (Additive or potentiated action). Products include:
- Regitine ... 878

Phenylbutazone (May reduce diuretic, natriuretic, and antihypertensive effects of thiazide diuretics). Products include:
- Butazolidin Capsules & Tablets ... 1027

Pindolol (Additive or potentiated action). Products include:
- Visken Tablets ... 2036

Piroxicam (May reduce diuretic, natriuretic, and antihypertensive effects of thiazide diuretics). Products include:
- Feldene Capsules ... 1777

Polythiazide (Additive or potentiated action). Products include:
- Minizide Capsules ... 1779
- Renese Tablets ... 1785
- Renese-R Tablets ... 1786

Prazosin Hydrochloride (Additive or potentiated action). Products include:
- Minipress Capsules ... 1778
- Minizide Capsules ... 1779

Prednisolone Acetate (Hypokalemia). Products include:
- AK-Cide Sterile Ophthalmic Ointment & Suspension ... ◉ 202
- Blephamide Liquifilm Sterile Ophthalmic Suspension ... 586
- Blephamide S.O.P. Sterile Ophthalmic Ointment ... 586
- Cetapred Ointment ... ◉ 220
- ⅛% Econopred & 1% Econopred Plus ... ◉ 217
- Isopto Cetapred Suspension ... ◉ 220
- Metimyd ... ◉ 306
- Poly-Pred Liquifilm ... ◉ 250
- Pred Forte ... ◉ 252
- Pred Mild ... ◉ 254
- Pred-G Liquifilm Sterile Ophthalmic Suspension ... ◉ 252
- Pred-G S.O.P. Sterile Ophthalmic Ointment ... ◉ 253
- Vasocidin Ointment ... ◉ 275

Prednisolone Sodium Phosphate (Hypokalemia). Products include:
- AK-Pred ... ◉ 205
- Hydeltrasol Injection, Sterile ... 1476
- Inflamase ... ◉ 274
- Pediapred Oral Liquid ... 987
- Vasocidin Ophthalmic Solution ... ◉ 276

Prednisolone Tebutate (Hypokalemia). Products include:
- Hydeltra-T.B.A. Sterile Suspension 1478

Prednisone (Hypokalemia). Products include:
- Deltasone Tablets ... 2332

Propoxyphene Hydrochloride (May potentiate orthostatic hypotension). Products include:
- Darvon ... 1256
- Wygesic Tablets ... 2540

Propoxyphene Napsylate (May potentiate orthostatic hypotension). Products include:
- Darvon-N/Darvocet-N ... 1254

Propranolol Hydrochloride (Additive or potentiated action). Products include:
- Inderal ... 2459
- Inderal LA Long Acting Capsules ... 2461
- Inderide Tablets ... 2463
- Inderide LA Long Acting Capsules .. 2465

Ramipril (Additive or potentiated action). Products include:
- Altace Capsules ... 1086

Rauwolfia Serpentina (Additive or potentiated action). Products include:
- Raudixin Tablets ... 1803
- Rauzide Tablets ... 1804

Rescinnamine (Additive or potentiated action).
- No products indexed under this heading.

Reserpine (Additive or potentiated action). Products include:
- Diupres Tablets ... 1461
- Hydromox R Tablets ... 1209
- Hydropres Tablets ... 1485
- Renese-R Tablets ... 1786
- Salutensin/Salutensin-Demi ... 719
- Ser-Ap-Es Tablets ... 881
- Serpasil Tablets ... 883
- Serpasil-Apresoline Tablets ... 884
- Serpasil-Esidrix Tablets ... 886

Secobarbital Sodium (May potentiate orthostatic hypotension). Products include:
- Seconal Sodium Pulvules ... 1296

Sodium Nitroprusside (Additive or potentiated action). Products include:
- Nipride I.V. Infusion ... 1909

Sufentanil Citrate (May potentiate orthostatic hypotension). Products include:
- Sufenta Injection ... 1147

Sulindac (May reduce diuretic, natriuretic, and antihypertensive effects of thiazide diuretics). Products include:
- Clinoril Tablets ... 1433

Terazosin Hydrochloride (Additive or potentiated action). Products include:
- Hytrin Tablets ... 529

Thiamylal Sodium (May potentiate orthostatic hypotension). Products include:
- Surital Ampoules, Steri-Vials ... 1764

Timolol Maleate (Additive or potentiated action). Products include:
- Blocadren Tablets ... 1429
- Timolide Tablets ... 1547
- Timoptic in Ocudose ... 1552
- Timoptic Sterile Ophthalmic Solution ... 1550

Tolmetin Sodium (May reduce diuretic, natriuretic, and antihypertensive effects of thiazide diuretics). Products include:
- Tolectin (200, 400 and 600 mg) .. 1379

Triamcinolone (Hypokalemia).
- No products indexed under this heading.

Triamcinolone Acetonide (Hypokalemia). Products include:
- Aristocort A ... 1010
- Azmacort Inhaler ... 1837
- Kenalog Cream, Lotion & Ointment 2401
- Kenalog-10 Injection ... 2402
- Kenalog-40 Injection ... 2403
- Kenalog in Orabase ... 604
- Kenalog Spray ... 2401
- Mycolog II Cream and Ointment ... 2407
- Mytrex Cream & Ointment ... 2080
- Nasacort Nasal Inhaler ... 1844

Triamcinolone Diacetate (Hypokalemia). Products include:
- Aristocort Suspension ... 1008

Triamcinolone Hexacetonide (Hypokalemia). Products include:
- Aristospan Suspension ... 1011

Trimethaphan Camsylate (Additive or potentiated action). Products include:
- Arfonad Ampuls ... 1887

Tubocurarine Chloride (Increased responsiveness to tubocurarine).
- No products indexed under this heading.

ESIMIL TABLETS (Guanethidine Monosulfate, Hydrochlorothiazide) ... 864
May interact with monoamine oxidase inhibitors, tricyclic antidepressants, phenothiazines, estrogens, corticosteroids, lithium preparations, insulin, non-steroidal anti-inflammatory agents, antihypertensives, oral contraceptives, cardiac glycosides, barbiturates, narcotic analgesics, and certain other agents. Compounds in these categories include:

Acebutolol Hydrochloride (Additive or potentiated action). Products include:
- Sectral Capsules ... 2520

ACTH (Hypokalemia).
- No products indexed under this heading.

Alcohol (Orthostatic hypotension aggravated).

Alfentanil Hydrochloride (May potentiate orthostatic hypotension). Products include:
- Alfenta Injection ... 1131

Amitriptyline Hydrochloride (Reduces hypotensive effect). Products include:
- Elavil ... 2269
- Endep Tablets ... 1927
- Etrafon ... 2087
- Limbitrol ... 1933
- Triavil Tablets ... 1556

Amoxapine (Reduces hypotensive effect). Products include:
- Asendin Tablets ... 1196

Aprobarbital (May potentiate orthostatic hypotension). Products include:
- Alurate Elixir ... 1883

Atenolol (Additive or potentiated action). Products include:
- Tenoretic Tablets ... 1105
- Tenormin Tablets and I.V. Injection 1107

Benazepril Hydrochloride (Additive or potentiated action). Products include:
- Lotensin Tablets ... 872

Bendroflumethiazide (Additive or potentiated action). Products include:
- Corzide Tablets ... 702
- Naturetin Tablets ... 1789
- Rauzide Tablets ... 1804

Betamethasone Acetate (Hypokalemia). Products include:
- Celestone Soluspan Suspension ... 2081

Betamethasone Dipropionate (Hypokalemia). Products include:
- Alphatrex Cream, Ointment & Lotion ... 2076
- Diprolene ... 2083
- Lotrisone Cream ... 2103
- Maxivate Cream, Lotion & Ointment 0.05% ... 2406
- Psorion Cream 0.05% ... 1121

Betamethasone Sodium Phosphate (Hypokalemia). Products include:
- Celestone Soluspan Suspension ... 2081

Betaxolol Hydrochloride (Additive or potentiated action). Products include:
- Betoptic Sterile Ophthalmic Solution ... 569
- Betoptic S Sterile Ophthalmic Suspension ... 570
- Kerlone Tablets ... 2172

(⊞ Described in PDR For Nonprescription Drugs) (◉ Described in PDR For Ophthalmology)

Buprenorphine (May potentiate orthostatic hypotension).
- No products indexed under this heading.

Butabarbital (May potentiate orthostatic hypotension). Products include:
- Pyridium Plus 1764

Butalbital (May potentiate orthostatic hypotension). Products include:
- Esgic-Plus Tablets 1002
- Esgic Tablets & Capsules 1001
- Fioricet Tablets 2006
- Fiorinal Capsules 2007
- Fiorinal with Codeine Capsules 2008
- Fiorinal Tablets 2007
- Phrenilin 838
- Sedapap Tablets 50 mg/650 mg .. 1360

Captopril (Additive or potentiated action). Products include:
- Capoten 2255
- Capozide 2258

Carteolol Hydrochloride (Additive or potentiated action). Products include:
- Cartrol Tablets 507

Chlorothiazide (Additive or potentiated action). Products include:
- Aldoclor Tablets 1413
- Diupres Tablets 1461
- Diuril Oral 1464

Chlorothiazide Sodium (Additive or potentiated action). Products include:
- Diuril Sodium Intravenous 1463

Chlorotrianisene (Reduces hypotensive effect). Products include:
- TACE 12 and 25 mg 1353

Chlorpromazine (Reduces hypotensive effect). Products include:
- Thorazine 2234

Chlorthalidone (Additive or potentiated action). Products include:
- Combipres Tablets 678
- Tenoretic Tablets 1105
- Thalitone Tablets 687

Clomipramine Hydrochloride (Reduces hypotensive effect). Products include:
- Anafranil Capsules 650

Clonidine (Additive or potentiated action). Products include:
- Catapres-TTS 677

Clonidine Hydrochloride (Additive or potentiated action). Products include:
- Catapres Tablets 676
- Combipres Tablets 678

Codeine (May potentiate orthostatic hypotension). Products include:
- Calcidrine Syrup 506

Codeine Phosphate (May potentiate orthostatic hypotension). Products include:
- Actifed with Codeine Cough Syrup.. 752
- Cheracol Cough Syrup 1853
- Codimal PH Syrup 846
- Dimetane-DC Cough Syrup 1857
- Empirin with Codeine Phosphate Nos. 2, 3 & 4 764
- Fiorinal with Codeine Capsules 2008
- Isoclor Expectorant 982
- Naldecon CX Adult Liquid .... ▣ 521
- Novahistine DH 1342
- Novahistine Expectorant 1343
- Nucofed Capsules 2219
- Nucofed Expectorant 2219
- Nucofed Pediatric Expectorant 2220
- Nucofed Syrup 2219
- Phenaphen with Codeine Capsules 1865
- Phenaphen-650 with Codeine Tablets 1866
- Phenergan with Codeine 2497
- Phenergan VC with Codeine 2501
- Robitussin A-C Syrup 1875
- Robitussin-DAC Syrup 1875
- Ryna .... ▣ 741
- Soma Compound w/Codeine Tablets 2390
- Triaminic Expectorant w/Codeine .. 1996
- Tussi-Organidin Liquid 2391
- Tylenol with Codeine 1381

Codeine Polistirex (May potentiate orthostatic hypotension).
- No products indexed under this heading.

Cortisone Acetate (Hypokalemia). Products include:
- Cortone Acetate Sterile Suspension 1437
- Cortone Acetate Tablets 1439

Deserpidine (May result in excessive postural hypotension, bradycardia and mental depression). Products include:
- Enduronyl 518
- Harmonyl Tablets 528
- Oreticyl 545

Desipramine Hydrochloride (Reduces hypotensive effect). Products include:
- Norpramin Tablets 1340

Deslanoside (Increased ventricular irritability; slow heart).
- No products indexed under this heading.

Dexamethasone Acetate (Hypokalemia). Products include:
- Dalalone D.P. Injectable 999
- Decadron-LA Sterile Suspension 1457

Dexamethasone Sodium Phosphate (Hypokalemia). Products include:
- AK-Dex .... ⊙ 203
- Decadron Phosphate Respihaler 1454
- Decadron Phosphate Sterile Ophthalmic Ointment 1453
- Decadron Phosphate Sterile Ophthalmic Solution 1453
- Decadron Phosphate Topical Cream 1455
- Decadron Phosphate Turbinaire 1456
- Maxidex Sterile Ophthalmic Ointment .... ⊙ 222
- NeoDecadron Sterile Ophthalmic Ointment 1517
- NeoDecadron Sterile Ophthalmic Solution 1518
- NeoDecadron Topical Cream 1518

Dezocine (May potentiate orthostatic hypotension).

Diazoxide (Additive or potentiated action). Products include:
- Hyperstat I.V. Injection 2095
- Proglycem 649

Diclofenac Sodium (May reduce diuretic, natriuretic, and antihypertensive effects of thiazide diuretics). Products include:
- Voltaren Ophthalmic Sterile Ophthalmic Solution .... ⊙ 268
- Voltaren Tablets 1042

Dienestrol (Reduces hypotensive effect). Products include:
- Ortho Dienestrol Cream 1664

Diethylstilbestrol (Reduces hypotensive effect). Products include:
- Diethylstilbestrol Tablets 1258

Digitoxin (Increased ventricular irritability; slow heart). Products include:
- Crystodigin Tablets 1253

Digoxin (Increased ventricular irritability; slow heart). Products include:
- Lanoxicaps 772
- Lanoxin Elixir Pediatric 775
- Lanoxin Injection 778
- Lanoxin Injection Pediatric 781
- Lanoxin Tablets 783

Doxazosin Mesylate (Additive or potentiated action). Products include:
- Cardura Tablets 1941

Doxepin Hydrochloride (Reduces hypotensive effect). Products include:
- Sinequan 1960

Enalapril Maleate (Additive or potentiated action). Products include:
- Vaseretic Tablets 1559
- Vasotec Tablets 1564

Enalaprilat (Additive or potentiated action). Products include:
- Vasotec I.V. 1562

Ephedrine Hydrochloride (Reduces hypotensive effect). Products include:
- Amesec .... ▣ 682
- Primatene Tablets-M Formula 2421
- Primatene Tablets-P Formula 2421
- Primatene Tablets-Regular Formula 2421
- Quadrinal Tablets 1183
- Quelidrine Syrup 556
- Tedral SA 1765

Ephedrine Sulfate (Reduces hypotensive effect). Products include:
- Bronkaid Tablets .... ▣ 757
- Bronkolixir .... ▣ 761
- Bronkotabs Tablets .... ▣ 762
- Marax Tablets & DF Syrup 1954
- Pazo Hemorrhoid Ointment & Suppositories 752
- Vicks Vatronol Nose Drops .... ▣ 666

Ephedrine Tannate (Reduces hypotensive effect). Products include:
- Rynatuss 2388

Esmolol Hydrochloride (Additive or potentiated action). Products include:
- Brevibloc Injection 942

Estradiol (Reduces hypotensive effect). Products include:
- Emcyt Capsules 1161
- Estrace 1385
- Estrace Vaginal Cream 1388
- Estraderm Transdermal System 866

Estrogens, Conjugated (Reduces hypotensive effect). Products include:
- Mediatric Capsules 2476
- PMB 200 and PMB 400 2504
- Premarin Intravenous 2508
- Premarin with Methyltestosterone .. 2515
- Premarin Tablets 2510
- Premarin Vaginal Cream 2512

Estrogens, Esterified (Reduces hypotensive effect). Products include:
- Estratest 2245
- Menrium Tablets 1934

Estropipate (Reduces hypotensive effect). Products include:
- Ogen 540

Ethinyl Estradiol (Reduces hypotensive effect). Products include:
- Brevicon 2304
- Demulen 2161
- Estinyl Tablets 2085
- Jenest-28 Tablets 1636
- Levlen/Tri-Levlen 665
- Lo/Ovral Tablets 2471
- Lo/Ovral-28 Tablets 2476
- Loestrin 1728
- Modicon 1667
- Nordette-21 Tablets 2481
- Nordette-28 Tablets 2483
- Norethin 2133
- Norinyl 2304
- Norlestrin 1746
- Ortho-Cyclen Tablets 1658
- Ortho-Novum 1667
- Ovcon 1391
- Ovral Tablets 2490
- Ovral-28 Tablets 2491
- Levlen/Tri-Levlen 665
- Tri-Norinyl 2304
- Triphasil-21 Tablets 2527
- Triphasil-28 Tablets 2532

Ethynodiol Diacetate (Reduces hypotensive effect). Products include:
- Demulen 2161

Etodolac (May reduce diuretic, natriuretic, and antihypertensive effects of thiazide diuretics). Products include:
- Lodine Capsules 2468

Felodipine (Additive or potentiated action). Products include:
- Plendil Extended-Release Tablets 1526

Fenoprofen Calcium (May reduce the diuretic, natriuretic, and antihypertensive effects of thiazide diuretics). Products include:
- Nalfon Pulvules & Tablets 919

Fentanyl (May potentiate orthostatic hypotension). Products include:
- Duragesic Transdermal System 1133

Fentanyl Citrate (May potentiate orthostatic hypotension). Products include:
- Innovar Injection 1141
- Sublimaze Injection 1146

Fluphenazine Decanoate (Reduces hypotensive effect). Products include:
- Prolixin Decanoate 1795

Fluphenazine Enanthate (Reduces hypotensive effect). Products include:
- Prolixin Enanthate 1796

Fluphenazine Hydrochloride (Reduces hypotensive effect). Products include:
- Prolixin Elixir 1793
- Prolixin Injection 1791
- Prolixin Oral Concentrate 1792
- Prolixin Tablets 1793

Flurbiprofen (May reduce diuretic, natriuretic, and antihypertensive effects of thiazide diuretics). Products include:
- Ansaid Tablets 2319

Fosinopril Sodium (Additive or potentiated action). Products include:
- Monopril Tablets 1406

Furazolidone (Concurrent use contraindicated). Products include:
- Furoxone 1855

Furosemide (Additive or potentiated action). Products include:
- Lasix 1093

Guanabenz Acetate (Additive or potentiated action). Products include:
- Wytensin Tablets 2542

Hydralazine Hydrochloride (Additive or potentiated action). Products include:
- Apresazide Capsules 854
- Apresoline Hydrochloride Parenteral (Ampuls) 856
- Apresoline Hydrochloride Tablets .. 855
- Apresoline-Esidrix Tablets 857
- Ser-Ap-Es Tablets 881
- Serpasil-Apresoline Tablets 884

Hydrocodone Bitartrate (May potentiate orthostatic hypotension). Products include:
- Anexsia 5/500 Tablets 2196
- Anexsia 7.5/650 Tablets 2197
- Azdone Tablets 844
- Codiclear DH Syrup 845
- Codimal DH Syrup 846
- Damason-P 1356
- Hycodan Syrup, Tablets 927
- Hycomine Compound Tablets 929
- Hycomine Syrup 927
- Hycotuss Expectorant Syrup 930
- Hydrocet Capsules 835
- Lortab ASA Tablets 2414
- Lortab 2412
- Ru-Tuss with Hydrocodone 694
- Triaminic Expectorant DH 1995
- Vicodin Tablets 1187
- Vicodin ES Tablets 1189
- Zydone Capsules 941

Hydrocodone Polistirex (May potentiate orthostatic hypotension). Products include:
- Tussionex Extended-Release Suspension 988

Hydrocortisone (Hypokalemia). Products include:
- AK-Spore H.C. .... ⊙ 206

Bactine Hydrocortisone Anti-Itch Cream ⊞ 625
CaldeCORT Anti-Itch Hydrocortisone Spray ⊞ 560
Carmol HC Cream 1% 2296
Cortaid Spray ⊞ 735
Cortenema 2244
Cortisporin Ointment 758
Cortisporin Ophthalmic Ointment Sterile 758
Cortisporin Ophthalmic Suspension Sterile 759
Cortisporin Otic Solution Sterile 760
Cortisporin Otic Suspension Sterile 760
Cortizone-5 Creme & Ointment ⊞ 732
Dermolate Anti-Itch Cream ⊞ 697
Eldecort Cream 1.0% 1113
Eldecort Cream 1.0% and 2.5% 1113
Fungoid HC Creme 1770
Hydrocortone Tablets 1482
Hytone 909
LazerSporin-C Solution 1770
Massengill Medicated Soft Cloth Towelettes 2192
Nutracort Cream & Lotion 1684
PediOtic Suspension Sterile 797
Synacort Creams 1%, 2.5% 2296
Vanoxide-HC Acne Lotion 911
Vioform-Hydrocortisone Cream and Mild Cream 889
Vioform-Hydrocortisone Ointment 889
VōSoL HC Otic Solution 2392
Vytone Cream 1% 911

Hydrocortisone Acetate (Hypokalemia). Products include:
Analpram-HC Rectal Cream 1% and 2.5% 970
Anusol-HC Cream 1690
Anusol-HC Suppositories 1691
Caldecort ⊞ 560
Carmol HC Cream 1% 2296
Chloromycetin Hydrocortisone Ophthalmic 1694
Coly-Mycin S Otic w/Neomycin & Hydrocortisone 1708
Cortaid ⊞ 735
Cortef Feminine Itch Cream ⊞ 735
Corticaine ⊞ 682
Cortifoam 1827
Cortisporin Cream 757
Epifoam 1828
Gynecort 5 Creme ⊞ 556
Hydrocortone Acetate Sterile Suspension 1479
Lanacort 5 Creme and Ointment ⊞ 557
Mantadil Cream 789
Ophthocort ⊙ 301
Orabase HCA Oral Paste 890
Pramosone Cream, Lotion & Ointment 971
ProctoCream-HC 1834
Proctofoam-HC 1835

Hydrocortisone Sodium Phosphate (Hypokalemia). Products include:
Hydrocortone Phosphate Injection, Sterile 1481

Hydrocortisone Sodium Succinate (Hypokalemia). Products include:
Solu-Cortef Sterile Powder 2361

Hydroflumethiazide (Additive or potentiated action). Products include:
Diucardin Tablets 2450
Saluron 718
Salutensin/Salutensin-Demi 719

Ibuprofen (May reduce the diuretic, natriuretic, and antihypertensive effects of thiazide diuretics). Products include:
Advil Cold & Sinus Caplets (formerly CoAdvil) 2416
Advil Ibuprofen Tablets and Caplets 2416
Children's Advil Suspension 2426
CoAdvil ⊞ 748
Dristan Sinus Caplets 2419
Haltran Tablets ⊞ 668
Ibuprofen ⊞ 631
Medipren ibuprofen Caplets and Tablets 1362
Midol 200 Cramp Relief Formula ⊞ 570
Motrin Tablets 2351
Motrin IB Caplets and Tablets ⊞ 736
Nuprin Ibuprofen/Analgesic Tablets & Caplets 752
PediaProfen Suspension 1363
Rufen Tablets 691
Trendar Ibuprofen Tablets ⊞ 756

Imipramine Hydrochloride (Reduces hypotensive effect). Products include:
Tofranil Ampuls 1038
Tofranil Tablets 1039

Imipramine Pamoate (Reduces hypotensive effect). Products include:
Tofranil-PM Capsules 1041

Indapamide (Additive or potentiated action). Products include:
Lozol Tablets 1843

Indomethacin (May reduce the diuretic, natriuretic, and antihypertensive effects of thiazide diuretics). Products include:
Indocin 1487

Indomethacin Sodium Trihydrate (May reduce the diuretic, natriuretic, and antihypertensive effects of thiazide diuretics). Products include:
Indocin I.V. 1490

Insulin, Human (Insulin requirements may be altered).
No products indexed under this heading.

Insulin, Human Isophane Suspension (Insulin requirements may be altered). Products include:
Humulin N, 100 Units 1270

Insulin, Human NPH (Insulin requirements may be altered). Products include:
Insulatard NPH Human 1627
Novolin N 1627
Novolin N PenFill Cartridges 1628
Novolin N Prefilled 1628

Insulin, Human Regular (Insulin requirements may be altered). Products include:
Humulin BR, 100 Units 1268
Humulin R, 100 Units 1272
Novolin R 1627
Novolin R PenFill Cartridges 1628
Novolin R Prefilled 1629
Velosulin Human 1628

Insulin, Human, Zinc Suspension (Insulin requirements may be altered). Products include:
Humulin L, 100 Units 1268
Humulin U, 100 Units 1272
Novolin L 1627

Insulin, NPH (Insulin requirements may be altered). Products include:
NPH, 40 & 100 Units 1273
Beef NPH, 100 Units 1274
Pork NPH, 100 Units 1275
Insulatard NPH 1626
NPH Insulin 1626
NPH Purified Pork Isophane Insulin 1626

Insulin, Regular (Insulin requirements may be altered). Products include:
Regular, 40 & 100 Units 1273
Beef Regular, 100 Units 1275
Pork Regular, 100 Units 1275
Pork Regular (Concentrated), 500 Units 1276
Regular Insulin 1625
Regular Purified Pork Insulin 1626
Velosulin 1627

Insulin, Zinc Crystals (Insulin requirements may be altered). Products include:
NPH, 40 & 100 Units 1273

Insulin, Zinc Suspension (Insulin requirements may be altered). Products include:
Lente, 40 & 100 Units 1272
Protamine, Zinc, 40 & 100 Units 1273
Lente Iletin I 1272
Beef Lente, 100 Units 1274
Beef Protamine Zinc, 100 Units 1274
Pork Lente, 100 Units 1275
Pork, Protamine, Zinc, 100 Units 1275
Lente Insulin 1626
Lente Purified Pork Insulin 1626
Semilente Insulin 1625
Ultralente Insulin 1626

Isocarboxazid (Concurrent use contraindicated). Products include:
Marplan Tablets 1906

Isradipine (Additive or potentiated action). Products include:
DynaCirc Capsules 2004

Ketoprofen (May reduce the diuretic, natriuretic, and antihypertensive effects of thiazide diuretics). Products include:
Orudis Capsules 2488

Ketorolac Tromethamine (May reduce diuretic, natriuretic, and antihypertensive effects of thiazide diuretics). Products include:
Toradol IM Injection 2302

Labetalol Hydrochloride (Additive or potentiated action). Products include:
Normodyne Injection 2108
Normodyne Tablets 2110
Normozide Tablets 2112
Trandate HCT Tablets 579
Trandate Injection 577
Trandate Tablets 579

Levonorgestrel (Reduces hypotensive effect). Products include:
Levlen/Tri-Levlen 665
Nordette-21 Tablets 2481
Nordette-28 Tablets 2483
Norplant System 2484
Levlen/Tri-Levlen 665
Triphasil-21 Tablets 2527
Triphasil-28 Tablets 2532

Levorphanol Tartrate (May potentiate orthostatic hypotension). Products include:
Levo-Dromoran 1906

Lisinopril (Additive or potentiated action). Products include:
Prinivil Tablets 1538
Prinzide Tablets 1540
Zestoretic 2274
Zestril Tablets 2277

Lithium Carbonate (Increased risk of lithium toxicity). Products include:
Eskalith 2214
Lithane Tablets 1596
Lithium Carbonate Capsules & Tablets 1984
Lithobid Tablets 870

Lithium Citrate (Increases risk of lithium toxicity). Products include:
Cibalith-S 870

Maprotiline Hydrochloride (Reduces hypotensive effect). Products include:
Ludiomil Tablets 874

Mecamylamine Hydrochloride (Additive or potentiated action). Products include:
Inversine Tablets 1492

Meclofenamate Sodium (May reduce the diuretic, natriuretic, and antihypertensive effects of thiazide diuretics). Products include:
Meclomen Capsules 1739

Mefenamic Acid (May reduce the diuretic, natriuretic, and antihypertensive effects of thiazide diuretics). Products include:
Ponstel 1758

Meperidine Hydrochloride (May potentiate orthostatic hypotension). Products include:
Demerol 2047
Mepergan Injection 2479

Mephobarbital (May potentiate orthostatic hypotension). Products include:
Mebaral Tablets 2061

Mesoridazine (Reduces hypotensive effect). Products include:
Serentil 686

Mestranol (Reduces hypotensive effect). Products include:
Enovid 2161
Norethin 2133
Norinyl 2304
Ortho-Novum 1667

Methadone Hydrochloride (May potentiate orthostatic hypotension). Products include:
Dolophine Hydrochloride Ampoules & Vials 1260
Dolophine Hydrochloride Tablets 1261
Methadone Hydrochloride Diskets 1284
Methadone Hydrochloride Oral Solution & Tablets 1987

Methyclothiazide (Additive or potentiated action). Products include:
Enduron Tablets 517
Enduronyl 518

Methyldopa (Additive or potentiated action; hemolytic anemia). Products include:
Aldoclor Tablets 1413
Aldomet Oral 1415
Aldoril Tablets 1418

Methyldopate Hydrochloride (Additive or potentiated action; hemolytic anemia). Products include:
Aldomet Ester HCl Injection 1417

Methylphenidate Hydrochloride (Reduces hypotensive effect). Products include:
Ritalin 880

Methylprednisolone (Hypokalemia). Products include:
Medrol 2348

Methylprednisolone Acetate (Hypokalemia). Products include:
Depo-Medrol Sterile Aqueous Suspension 2334

Methylprednisolone Sodium Succinate (Hypokalemia). Products include:
Solu-Medrol Sterile Powder 2363

Metolazone (Additive or potentiated action). Products include:
Diulo 2129
Mykrox ½ mg Tablets 984
Zaroxolyn Tablets 989

Metoprolol Tartrate (Additive or potentiated action). Products include:
Lopressor Ampuls 1032
Lopressor HCT Tablets 1034
Lopressor Tablets 1032

Metyrosine (Additive or potentiated action). Products include:
Demser Capsules 1460

Minoxidil (Additive or potentiated action). Products include:
Loniten Tablets 2346
Rogaine Topical Solution 2357

Morphine Sulfate (May potentiate orthostatic hypotension). Products include:
Astramorph/PF Injection, USP (Preservative-Free) 618
Duramorph 960
Infumorph 200 and Infumorph 500 Sterile Solutions 962
MS Contin Tablets 1814
MSIR 1817
Oramorph SR (Morphine Sulfate Sustained Release Tablets) 1988
Roxanol 1991

Nadolol (Additive or potentiated action). Products include:
Corgard Tablets 701
Corzide Tablets 702

Naproxen (May reduce the diuretic, natriuretic, and antihypertensive effects of thiazide diuretics). Products include:
Naprosyn 2297

Naproxen Sodium (May reduce the diuretic, natriuretic, and antihypertensive effects of thiazide diuretics). Products include:
Anaprox and Anaprox DS Tablets 2288

Nicardipine Hydrochloride (Additive or potentiated action). Products include:
Cardene Capsules ... 2290

Nitroglycerin (Additive or potentiated action). Products include:
Deponit NTG Transdermal Delivery System ... 2143
Minitran Transdermal Delivery System ... 1312
Nitro-Bid Ointment ... 1339
Nitro-Bid Capsules ... 1338
Nitrodisc ... 2176
Nitro-Dur (nitroglycerin) Transdermal Infusion System ... 1164
Nitrogard Tablets ... 1004
Nitrolingual Spray ... 1846
Nitrostat Tablets ... 1743
Transderm-Nitro Transdermal Therapeutic System ... 2283

Norepinephrine Bitartrate (Decreased arterial response to norepinephrine). Products include:
Levophed Bitartrate Injection ... 2054

Norethindrone (Reduces hypotensive effect). Products include:
Brevicon ... 2304
Jenest-28 Tablets ... 1636
Micronor Tablets ... 1667
Modicon ... 1667
Norethin ... 2133
Norinyl ... 2304
Norlutin ... 1755
Nor-Q D Tablets ... 2304
Ortho-Novum ... 1667
Ovcon ... 1391
Tri-Norinyl ... 2304

Norethynodrel (Reduces hypotensive effect). Products include:
Enovid ... 2161

Norgestimate (Reduces hypotensive effect). Products include:
Ortho-Cyclen Tablets ... 1658

Norgestrel (Reduces hypotensive effect). Products include:
Lo/Ovral Tablets ... 2471
Lo/Ovral-28 Tablets ... 2476
Ovral Tablets ... 2490
Ovral-28 Tablets ... 2491
Ovrette Tablets ... 2492

Nortriptyline Hydrochloride (Reduces hypotensive effect). Products include:
Pamelor ... 2019

Opium Alkaloids (May potentiate orthostatic hypotension). Products include:
B & O No. 15A & No. 16A Supprettes ... 2395
Pantopon Injectable ... 1911

Oxycodone Hydrochloride (May potentiate orthostatic hypotension). Products include:
Percocet Tablets ... 950
Percodan ... 951
Roxicodone Tablets, Oral Solution & Intensol (Oxycodone) ... 1992
Tylox Capsules ... 1382

Penbutolol Sulfate (Additive or potentiated action). Products include:
Levatol ... 1832

Pentobarbital Sodium (May potentiate orthostatic hypotension). Products include:
Nembutal Sodium Capsules ... 534
Nembutal Sodium Solution ... 536
Nembutal Sodium Suppositories ... 538

Perphenazine (Reduces hypotensive effect). Products include:
Etrafon ... 2087
Triavil Tablets ... 1556
Trilafon ... 2123

Phenelzine Sulfate (Concurrent use contraindicated). Products include:
Nardil ... 1742

Phenobarbital (May potentiate orthostatic hypotension). Products include:
Arco-Lase Plus Tablets ... 607
Bellergal-S Tablets ... 1998
Bronkolixir ... ▣ 761
Bronkotabs Tablets ... ▣ 762
Donnatal ... 1858
Donnatal Extentabs ... 1859
Donnatal Tablets ... 1858
Donnazyme Tablets ... 1860
Kinesed Tablets ... 2272
Phenobarbital Elixir and Tablets ... 1293
Primatene Tablets-P Formula ... 2421
Quadrinal Tablets ... 1183
Tedral SA ... 1765

Phenoxybenzamine Hydrochloride (Additive or potentiated action). Products include:
Dibenzyline Capsules ... 2207

Phentolamine Mesylate (Additive or potentiated action). Products include:
Regitine ... 878

Phenylbutazone (May reduce the diuretic, natriuretic, and antihypertensive effects of thiazide diuretics). Products include:
Butazolidin Capsules & Tablets ... 1027

Pindolol (Additive or potentiated action). Products include:
Visken Tablets ... 2036

Piroxicam (May reduce the diuretic, natriuretic, and antihypertensive effects of thiazide diuretics). Products include:
Feldene Capsules ... 1777

Polythiazide (Additive or potentiated action). Products include:
Minizide Capsules ... 1779
Renese Tablets ... 1785
Renese-R Tablets ... 1786

Prazosin Hydrochloride (Additive or potentiated action). Products include:
Minipress Capsules ... 1778
Minizide Capsules ... 1779

Prednisolone Acetate (Hypokalemia). Products include:
AK-Cide Sterile Ophthalmic Ointment & Suspension ... ◉ 202
Blephamide Liquifilm Sterile Ophthalmic Suspension ... 586
Blephamide S.O.P. Sterile Ophthalmic Ointment ... 586
Cetapred Ointment ... ◉ 220
⅛% Econopred & 1% Econopred Plus ... ◉ 217
Isopto Cetapred Suspension ... ◉ 220
Metimyd ... ◉ 306
Poly-Pred Liquifilm ... ◉ 250
Pred Forte ... ◉ 252
Pred Mild ... ◉ 254
Pred-G Liquifilm Sterile Ophthalmic Suspension ... ◉ 252
Pred-G S.O.P. Sterile Ophthalmic Ointment ... ◉ 253
Vasocidin Ointment ... ◉ 275

Prednisolone Sodium Phosphate (Hypokalemia). Products include:
AK-Pred ... ◉ 205
Hydeltrasol Injection, Sterile ... 1476
Inflamase ... ◉ 274
Pediapred Oral Liquid ... 987
Vasocidin Ophthalmic Solution ... ◉ 276

Prednisolone Tebutate (Hypokalemia). Products include:
Hydeltra-T.B.A. Sterile Suspension 1478

Prednisone (Hypokalemia). Products include:
Deltasone Tablets ... 2332

Prochlorperazine (Reduced hypotensive effect). Products include:
Compazine ... 2201

Promethazine Hydrochloride (Reduces hypotensive effect). Products include:
Mepergan Injection ... 2479
Phenergan with Codeine ... 2497
Phenergan with Dextromethorphan 2499
Phenergan Injection ... 2493
Phenergan Suppositories ... 2496
Phenergan Syrup ... 2495
Phenergan Tablets ... 2496
Phenergan VC ... 2500
Phenergan VC with Codeine ... 2501

Propoxyphene Hydrochloride (May potentiate orthostatic hypotension). Products include:
Darvon ... 1256
Wygesic Tablets ... 2540

Propoxyphene Napsylate (May potentiate orthostatic hypotension). Products include:
Darvon-N/Darvocet-N ... 1254

Propranolol Hydrochloride (Additive or potentiated action). Products include:
Inderal ... 2459
Inderal LA Long Acting Capsules ... 2461
Inderide Tablets ... 2463
Inderide LA Long Acting Capsules .. 2465

Protriptyline Hydrochloride (Reduces hypotensive effect). Products include:
Vivactil Tablets ... 1567

Quinestrol (Reduces hypotensive effect). Products include:
Estrovis ... 1721

Ramipril (Additive or potentiated action). Products include:
Altace Capsules ... 1086

Rauwolfia Serpentina (May result in excessive postural hypotension, bradycardia and mental depression). Products include:
Raudixin Tablets ... 1803
Rauzide Tablets ... 1804

Rescinnamine (May result in excessive postural hypotension, bradycardia and mental depression).
No products indexed under this heading.

Reserpine (May result in excessive postural hypotension, bradycardia and mental depression). Products include:
Diupres Tablets ... 1461
Hydromox R Tablets ... 1209
Hydropres Tablets ... 1485
Renese-R Tablets ... 1786
Salutensin/Salutensin-Demi ... 719
Ser-Ap-Es Tablets ... 881
Serpasil Tablets ... 883
Serpasil-Apresoline Tablets ... 884
Serpasil-Esidrix Tablets ... 886

Secobarbital Sodium (May potentiate orthostatic hypotension). Products include:
Seconal Sodium Pulvules ... 1296

Selegiline Hydrochloride (Concurrent use contraindicated). Products include:
Eldepryl ... 2250

Sodium Nitroprusside (Additive or potentiated action). Products include:
Nipride I.V. Infusion ... 1909

Sufentanil Citrate (May potentiate orthostatic hypotension). Products include:
Sufenta Injection ... 1147

Sulindac (May reduce the diuretic, natriuretic, and antihypertensive effects of thiazide diuretics). Products include:
Clinoril Tablets ... 1433

Terazosin Hydrochloride (Additive or potentiated action). Products include:
Hytrin Tablets ... 529

Thiamylal Sodium (May potentiate orthostatic hypotension). Products include:
Surital Ampoules, Steri-Vials ... 1764

Thioridazine Hydrochloride (Reduces hypotensive effect). Products include:
Mellaril ... 2011

Timolol Maleate (Additive or potentiated action). Products include:
Blocadren Tablets ... 1429
Timolide Tablets ... 1547
Timoptic in Ocudose ... 1552
Timoptic Sterile Ophthalmic Solution ... 1550

Tolmetin Sodium (May reduce the diuretic, natriuretic, and antihypertensive effects of thiazide diuretics). Products include:
Tolectin (200, 400 and 600 mg) .. 1379

Tranylcypromine Sulfate (Concurrent use contraindicated). Products include:
Parnate Tablets ... 2222

Triamcinolone (Hypokalemia).
No products indexed under this heading.

Triamcinolone Acetonide (Hypokalemia). Products include:
Aristocort A ... 1010
Azmacort Inhaler ... 1837
Kenalog Cream, Lotion & Ointment 2401
Kenalog-10 Injection ... 2402
Kenalog-40 Injection ... 2403
Kenalog in Orabase ... 604
Kenalog Spray ... 2401
Mycolog II Cream and Ointment ... 2407
Mytrex Cream & Ointment ... 2080
Nasacort Nasal Inhaler ... 1844

Triamcinolone Diacetate (Hypokalemia). Products include:
Aristocort Suspension ... 1008

Triamcinolone Hexacetonide (Hypokalemia). Products include:
Aristospan Suspension ... 1011

Trifluoperazine Hydrochloride (Reduces hypotensive effect). Products include:
Stelazine ... 2226

Trimethaphan Camsylate (Additive or potentiated action). Products include:
Arfonad Ampuls ... 1887

Trimipramine Maleate (Reduces hypotensive effect). Products include:
Surmontil Capsules ... 2524

Tubocurarine Chloride (Increased response to tubocurarine).
No products indexed under this heading.

Food Interactions

Food, unspecified (Enhances gastrointestinal absorption of hydrochlorothiazide).

ESKALITH CAPSULES

(Lithium Carbonate) ... 2214
May interact with nondepolarizing neuromuscular blocking agents, diuretics, urinary alkalizing agents, xanthine bronchodilators, neuromuscular blocking agents, non-steroidal anti-inflammatory agents, and certain other agents. Compounds in these categories include:

Acetazolamide (Increases urinary lithium excretion). Products include:
Diamox Parenteral ... 1200
Diamox Parenteral ... ◉ 308
Diamox Sequels (Sustained Release) ... 1201
Diamox Sequels (Sustained Release) ... ◉ 310
Diamox Tablets ... 1200
Diamox Tablets ... ◉ 308

Amiloride Hydrochloride (Increased risk of lithium toxicity). Products include:
Midamor Tablets ... 1508
Moduretic Tablets ... 1510

Aminophylline (Lowers serum lithium concentrations). Products include:
Amesec ... ▣ 682
Aminophyllin Tablets ... 2153

Atracurium Besylate (Effects may be prolonged). Products include:
Tracrium Injection ... 817

Bendroflumethiazide (Increased risk of lithium toxicity). Products include:
- Corzide Tablets ... 702
- Naturetin Tablets ... 1789
- Rauzide Tablets ... 1804

Bumetanide (Increases risk of lithium toxicity). Products include:
- Bumex ... 1895

Chlorothiazide (Increases risk of lithium toxicity). Products include:
- Aldoclor Tablets ... 1413
- Diupres Tablets ... 1461
- Diuril Oral ... 1464

Chlorothiazide Sodium (Increases risk of lithium toxicity). Products include:
- Diuril Sodium Intravenous ... 1463

Chlorpromazine (Neurologic toxicity). Products include:
- Thorazine ... 2234

Chlorprothixene (Neurologic toxicity). Products include:
- Taractan Tablets ... 1920

Chlorprothixene Hydrochloride (Neurological toxicity). Products include:
- Taractan ... 1920

Chlorthalidone (Increased risk of lithium toxicity). Products include:
- Combipres Tablets ... 678
- Tenoretic Tablets ... 1105
- Thalitone Tablets ... 687

Clozapine (Neurologic toxicity). Products include:
- Clozaril Tablets ... 2000

Diclofenac Sodium (Increases lithium toxicity). Products include:
- Voltaren Ophthalmic Sterile Ophthalmic Solution ... ⊙ 268
- Voltaren Tablets ... 1042

Dyphylline (Lowers serum lithium concentrations). Products include:
- Dilor ... 2079
- Dilor-G Tablets & Liquid ... 2079
- Lufyllin Elixir ... 2384
- Lufyllin & Lufyllin-400 Tablets ... 2384
- Lufyllin-GG Elixir & Tablets ... 2385

Ethacrynic Acid (Increases risk of lithium toxicity). Products include:
- Edecrin Tablets ... 1468

Etodolac (Increases lithium toxicity). Products include:
- Lodine Capsules ... 2468

Fenoprofen Calcium (Increases lithium toxicity). Products include:
- Nalfon Pulvules & Tablets ... 919

Fluphenazine Decanoate (Neurologic toxicity). Products include:
- Prolixin Decanoate ... 1795

Fluphenazine Enanthate (Neurologic toxicity). Products include:
- Prolixin Enanthate ... 1796

Fluphenazine Hydrochloride (Neurologic toxicity). Products include:
- Prolixin Elixir ... 1793
- Prolixin Injection ... 1791
- Prolixin Oral Concentrate ... 1792
- Prolixin Tablets ... 1793

Flurbiprofen (Increases lithium toxicity). Products include:
- Ansaid Tablets ... 2319

Furosemide (Increases risk of lithium toxicity). Products include:
- Lasix ... 1093

Haloperidol (Neurologic toxicity). Products include:
- Haldol Injection, Tablets and Concentrate ... 1373

Haloperidol Decanoate (Neurologic toxicity). Products include:
- Haldol Decanoate ... 1375

Hydrochlorothiazide (Increases risk of lithium toxicity). Products include:
- Aldactazide ... 2150
- Aldoril Tablets ... 1418
- Apresazide Capsules ... 854
- Apresoline-Esidrix Tablets ... 857
- Capozide ... 2258
- Dyazide Capsules ... 2208
- Esidrix Tablets ... 863
- Esimil Tablets ... 864
- HydroDIURIL Tablets ... 1484
- Hydropres Tablets ... 1485
- Inderide Tablets ... 2463
- Inderide LA Long Acting Capsules ... 2465
- Lopressor HCT Tablets ... 1034
- Maxzide ... 1215
- Moduretic Tablets ... 1510
- Normozide Tablets ... 2112
- Oretic Tablets ... 544
- Oreticyl ... 545
- Prinzide Tablets ... 1540
- Ser-Ap-Es Tablets ... 881
- Serpasil-Esidrix Tablets ... 886
- Timolide Tablets ... 1547
- Trandate HCT Tablets ... 579
- Vaseretic Tablets ... 1559
- Zestoretic ... 2274

Hydroflumethiazide (Increases risk of lithium toxicity). Products include:
- Diucardin Tablets ... 2450
- Saluron ... 718
- Salutensin/Salutensin-Demi ... 719

Ibuprofen (Increases lithium toxicity). Products include:
- Advil Cold & Sinus Caplets (formerly CoAdvil) ... 2416
- Advil Ibuprofen Tablets and Caplets ... 2416
- Children's Advil Suspension ... 2426
- CoAdvil ... ▣ 748
- Dristan Sinus Caplets ... 2419
- Haltran Tablets ... ▣ 668
- Ibuprofen ... ▣ 631
- Medipren ibuprofen Caplets and Tablets ... 1362
- Midol 200 Cramp Relief Formula ... ▣ 570
- Motrin Tablets ... 2351
- Motrin IB Caplets and Tablets ... ▣ 736
- Nuprin Ibuprofen/Analgesic Tablets & Caplets ... 752
- PediaProfen Suspension ... 1363
- Rufen Tablets ... 691
- Trendar Ibuprofen Tablets ... ▣ 756

Indapamide (Increases risk of lithium toxicity). Products include:
- Lozol Tablets ... 1843

Indomethacin (Increases lithium toxicity). Products include:
- Indocin ... 1487

Indomethacin Sodium Trihydrate (Increases lithium toxicity). Products include:
- Indocin I.V. ... 1490

Ketoprofen (Increases lithium toxicity). Products include:
- Orudis Capsules ... 2488

Ketorolac Tromethamine (Increases lithium toxicity). Products include:
- Toradol IM Injection ... 2302

Loxapine Hydrochloride (Neurologic toxicity). Products include:
- Loxitane ... 1213

Loxapine Succinate (Neurologic toxicity). Products include:
- Loxitane Capsules ... 1213

Meclofenamate Sodium (Increases lithium toxicity). Products include:
- Meclomen Capsules ... 1739

Mefenamic Acid (Increases lithium toxicity). Products include:
- Ponstel ... 1758

Mesoridazine (Neurologic toxicity). Products include:
- Serentil ... 686

Methyclothiazide (Increases risk of lithium toxicity). Products include:
- Enduron Tablets ... 517
- Enduronyl ... 518

Metocurine Iodide (Effects of neuromuscular blockers may be prolonged). Products include:
- Metubine Iodide Vials ... 1285

Metolazone (Increases risk of lithium toxicity). Products include:
- Diulo ... 2129
- Mykrox ½ mg Tablets ... 984
- Zaroxolyn Tablets ... 989

Metronidazole (May provoke lithium toxicity due to reduced renal clearance). Products include:
- Flagyl I.V. RTU ... 2131
- Flagyl Tablets ... 2170
- MetroGel ... 903
- Protostat Tablets ... 1674

Metronidazole Hydrochloride (May provoke lithium toxicity due to reduced renal clearance). Products include:
- Flagyl I.V. ... 2131

Molindone Hydrochloride (Neurologic toxicity). Products include:
- Moban Tablets & Concentrate ... 932

Naproxen (Increases lithium toxicity). Products include:
- Naprosyn ... 2297

Naproxen Sodium (Increases lithium toxicity). Products include:
- Anaprox and Anaprox DS Tablets ... 2288

Pancuronium Bromide Injection (Effects of neuromuscular blockers may be prolonged).
- No products indexed under this heading.

Perphenazine (Neurologic toxicity). Products include:
- Etrafon ... 2087
- Triavil Tablets ... 1556
- Trilafon ... 2123

Phenylbutazone (Increases lithium toxicity). Products include:
- Butazolidin Capsules & Tablets ... 1027

Pimozide (Neurologic toxicity). Products include:
- Orap Tablets ... 1020

Piroxicam (Increases lithium toxicity). Products include:
- Feldene Capsules ... 1777

Polythiazide (Increases risk of lithium toxicity). Products include:
- Minizide Capsules ... 1779
- Renese Tablets ... 1785
- Renese-R Tablets ... 1786

Potassium Citrate (Increases urinary lithium excretion). Products include:
- Alka-Seltzer Effervescent Antacid ... 1570
- K-Lyte ... 707
- Polycitra Syrup ... 2424
- Polycitra-K ... 2424
- Polycitra-LC—Sugar-Free ... 2424
- Ricelyte, Rice-Based Oral Electrolyte Maintenance Solution ... ▣ 613

Prochlorperazine (Neurologic toxicity). Products include:
- Compazine ... 2201

Promethazine Hydrochloride (Neurologic toxicity). Products include:
- Mepergan Injection ... 2479
- Phenergan with Codeine ... 2497
- Phenergan with Dextromethorphan ... 2499
- Phenergan Injection ... 2493
- Phenergan Suppositories ... 2496
- Phenergan Syrup ... 2495
- Phenergan Tablets ... 2496
- Phenergan VC ... 2500
- Phenergan VC with Codeine ... 2501

Sodium Bicarbonate (Increases urinary lithium excretion). Products include:
- Alka-Seltzer Advanced Formula Antacid & Non-Aspirin Pain Reliever ... ▣ 620
- Alka-Seltzer Effervescent Antacid ... ▣ 622
- Alka-Seltzer Effervescent Antacid and Pain Reliever ... 1568
- Alka-Seltzer Extra Strength Effervescent Antacid and Pain Reliever ... ▣ 623
- Alka-Seltzer (Flavored) Effervescent Antacid and Pain Reliever ... ▣ 621
- Arm & Hammer Pure Baking Soda ... ▣ 548
- Ceo-Two Rectal Suppositories ... 671
- Citrocarbonate Antacid ... ▣ 668
- Massengill Liquid Concentrate ... 2191
- NuLYTELY ... 699

Sodium Citrate (Increases urinary lithium excretion). Products include:
- Alka-Seltzer Effervescent Antacid ... 1570
- Alka-Seltzer Extra Strength Effervescent Antacid and Pain Reliever ... 1570
- Alka-Seltzer (Flavored) Effervescent Antacid and Pain Reliever ... 1569
- Bicitra—Sugar-Free ... 2423
- Citrocarbonate Antacid ... ▣ 668
- Polycitra ... 2424
- Ricelyte, Rice-Based Oral Electrolyte Maintenance Solution ... ▣ 613

Spironolactone (Increases risk of lithium toxicity). Products include:
- Aldactazide ... 2150
- Aldactone ... 2152

Sulindac (Increases lithium toxicity). Products include:
- Clinoril Tablets ... 1433

Theophylline (Lowers serum lithium concentrations). Products include:
- Bronkaid Tablets ... ▣ 757
- Bronkolixir ... ▣ 761
- Bronkotabs Tablets ... ▣ 762
- Constant-T Tablets ... 1029
- Marax Tablets & DF Syrup ... 1954
- Primatene Tablets ... 2421
- Quibron Capsules ... 713
- Quibron-T ... 714
- Quibron-T/SR ... 716
- Theolair Liquid ... 1317
- Theo-Organidin Elixir ... 2391

Theophylline Anhydrous (Lowers serum lithium concentrations). Products include:
- Aerolate ... 994
- Primatene Tablets-M Formula ... ▣ 753
- Primatene Tablets-Regular Formula ... 2421
- Respbid Tablets ... 684
- Slo-bid Gyrocaps ... 1847
- T-PHYL (Uniphyl) 200 mg Tablets ... 1820
- Tedral SA ... 1765
- Theo-24 ... 2179
- Theo-Dur Sprinkle ... 1168
- Theo-Dur Extended-Release Tablets ... 1166
- Theolair Tablets ... 1317
- Theolair-SR Tablets ... 1319
- TheoX Extended-Release Tablets ... 841
- Uniphyl 400 mg Tablets ... 1823

Theophylline Calcium Salicylate (Lowers serum lithium concentrations). Products include:
- Quadrinal Tablets ... 1183

Theophylline Sodium Glycinate (Lowers serum lithium concentrations). Products include:
- Asbron G ... 1997

Thioridazine Hydrochloride (Neurologic toxicity). Products include:
- Mellaril ... 2011

Thiothixene (Neurologic toxicity). Products include:
- Navane Capsules and Concentrate ... 1954
- Navane Intramuscular ... 1956

Tolmetin Sodium (Increases lithium toxicity). Products include:
- Tolectin (200, 400 and 600 mg) ... 1379

Triamterene (Increases risk of lithium toxicity). Products include:
- Dyazide Capsules ... 2208
- Dyrenium Capsules ... 2210
- Maxzide ... 1215

Trifluoperazine Hydrochloride (Neurologic toxicity). Products include:
- Stelazine ... 2226

Urea Preparations (Lowers serum lithium concentrations).

Vecuronium Bromide (Effects of neuromuscular blockers may be prolonged). Products include:
- Norcuron ... 1642

ESKALITH CR CONTROLLED RELEASE TABLETS
(Lithium Carbonate) 2214
See **Eskalith Capsules**

ESKALITH TABLETS
(Lithium Carbonate) 2214
See **Eskalith Capsules**

ESOTÉRICA MEDICATED FADE CREAM
(Hydroquinone) .... ▣ 715
No interactions described in labeling.

ESTER-C TABLETS
(Calcium Ascorbate) .... ▣ 575
May interact with oral anticoagulants and cardiac glycosides. Compounds in these categories include:

Deslanoside (Concurrent use requires caution).

Dicumarol (Vitamin C may influence the intensity and duration of action). Products include:
- Dicumarol Tablets 516

Digitoxin (Concurrent use requires caution). Products include:
- Crystodigin Tablets 1253

Digoxin (Concurrent use requires caution). Products include:
- Lanoxicaps 772
- Lanoxin Elixir Pediatric 775
- Lanoxin Injection 778
- Lanoxin Injection Pediatric 781
- Lanoxin Tablets 783

Warfarin Sodium (Vitamin C may influence the intensity and duration of action). Products include:
- Coumadin Injection & Tablets 944
- Panwarfin Tablets 547

ESTINYL TABLETS
(Ethinyl Estradiol) 2085
No interactions described in labeling.

ESTRACE
(Estradiol) 1385
No interactions described in labeling.

ESTRACE VAGINAL CREAM
(Estradiol) 1388
No interactions described in labeling.

ESTRADERM TRANSDERMAL SYSTEM
(Estradiol) 866
May interact with progestins. Compounds in this category include:

Medroxyprogesterone Acetate (Potential for adverse effects on carbohydrate and lipid metabolism). Products include:
- Amen 833
- Cycrin Tablets 2449
- Depo-Provera Sterile Aqueous Suspension 2336
- Provera Tablets 2356

Megestrol Acetate (Potential for adverse effects on carbohydrate and lipid metabolism). Products include:
- Megace Tablets 732

Norgestimate (Potential for adverse effects on carbohydrate and lipid metabolism). Products include:
- Ortho-Cyclen Tablets 1658

ESTRADURIN
(Polyestradiol Phosphate) 2452
No interactions described in labeling.

ESTRATEST TABLETS
(Estrogens, Esterified, Methyltestosterone) 2245
See **Estratest H.S. Tablets**

ESTRATEST H.S. TABLETS
(Estrogens, Esterified, Methyltestosterone) 2245
May interact with oral anticoagulants, insulin, and certain other agents. Compounds in these categories include:

Dicumarol (Decreased anticoagulant requirements). Products include:
- Dicumarol Tablets 516

Insulin, Human (Decreased blood glucose and insulin requirements).
No products indexed under this heading.

Insulin, Human Isophane Suspension (Decreased blood glucose and insulin requirements). Products include:
- Humulin N, 100 Units 1270

Insulin, Human NPH (Decreased blood glucose and insulin requirements). Products include:
- Insulatard NPH Human 1627
- Novolin N 1627
- Novolin N PenFill Cartridges 1628
- Novolin N Prefilled 1628

Insulin, Human Regular (Decreased blood glucose and insulin requirements). Products include:
- Humulin BR, 100 Units 1268
- Humulin R, 100 Units 1272
- Novolin R 1627
- Novolin R PenFill Cartridges 1628
- Novolin R Prefilled 1629
- Velosulin Human 1628

Insulin, Human, Zinc Suspension (Decreased blood glucose and insulin requirements). Products include:
- Humulin L, 100 Units 1268
- Humulin U, 100 Units 1272
- Novolin L 1627

Insulin, NPH (Decreased blood glucose and insulin requirements). Products include:
- NPH, 40 & 100 Units 1273
- Beef NPH, 100 Units 1274
- Pork NPH, 100 Units 1275
- Insulatard NPH 1626
- NPH Insulin 1626
- NPH Purified Pork Isophane Insulin 1626

Insulin, Regular (Decreased blood glucose and insulin requirements). Products include:
- Regular, 40 & 100 Units 1273
- Beef Regular, 100 Units 1275
- Pork Regular, 100 Units 1275
- Pork Regular (Concentrated), 500 Units 1276
- Regular Insulin 1625
- Regular Purified Pork Insulin 1626
- Velosulin 1627

Insulin, Zinc Crystals (Decreased blood glucose and insulin requirements). Products include:
- NPH, 40 & 100 Units 1273

Insulin, Zinc Suspension (Decreased blood glucose and insulin requirements). Products include:
- Lente, 40 & 100 Units 1272
- Protamine, Zinc, 40 & 100 Units 1273
- Lente Iletin I 1272
- Beef Lente, 100 Units 1274
- Beef Protamine Zinc, 100 Units 1274
- Pork Lente, 100 Units 1275
- Pork, Protamine, Zinc, 100 Units 1275
- Lente Insulin 1626
- Lente Purified Pork Insulin 1626
- Semilente Insulin 1625
- Ultralente Insulin 1626

Oxyphenbutazone (Concurrent use may result in elevated serum levels of oxyphenbutazone).

Warfarin Sodium (Decreased anticoagulant requirements). Products include:
- Coumadin Injection & Tablets 944
- Panwarfin Tablets 547

ESTROVIS
(Quinestrol) 1721
May interact with progestins. Compounds in this category include:

Medroxyprogesterone Acetate (Potential for adverse effects on carbohydrate and lipid metabolism). Products include:
- Amen 833
- Cycrin Tablets 2449
- Depo-Provera Sterile Aqueous Suspension 2336
- Provera Tablets 2356

Megestrol Acetate (Potential for adverse effects on carbohydrate and lipid metabolism). Products include:
- Megace Tablets 732

Norgestimate (Potential for adverse effects on carbohydrate and lipid metabolism). Products include:
- Ortho-Cyclen Tablets 1658

ETHAMOLIN
(Ethanolamine Oleate) 1829
No interactions described in labeling.

ETHMOZINE TABLETS
(Moricizine Hydrochloride) 946
May interact with xanthine bronchodilators and certain other agents. Compounds in these categories include:

Aminophylline (Theophylline clearance and plasma half-life significantly affected). Products include:
- Amesec .... ▣ 682
- Aminophyllin Tablets 2153

Cimetidine (Concomitant use results in a decrease in Ethmozine clearance of 49% and a 1.4 fold increase in plasma levels). Products include:
- Tagamet Tablets 2228

Cimetidine Hydrochloride (Concomitant use results in a decrease in Ethmozine clearance of 49% and a 1.4 fold increase in plasma levels). Products include:
- Tagamet 2228

Digoxin (Potential for additive prolongation of the PR interval). Products include:
- Lanoxicaps 772
- Lanoxin Elixir Pediatric 775
- Lanoxin Injection 778
- Lanoxin Injection Pediatric 781
- Lanoxin Tablets 783

Dyphylline (Theophylline clearance and plasma half-life significantly affected). Products include:
- Dilor 2079
- Dilor-G Tablets & Liquid 2079
- Lufyllin Elixir 2384
- Lufyllin & Lufyllin-400 Tablets 2384
- Lufyllin-GG Elixir & Tablets 2385

Propranolol Hydrochloride (Small additive increase in the PR interval). Products include:
- Inderal 2459
- Inderal LA Long Acting Capsules 2461
- Inderide Tablets 2463
- Inderide LA Long Acting Capsules 2465

Theophylline (Theophylline clearance and plasma half-life significantly affected). Products include:
- Bronkaid Tablets .... ▣ 757
- Bronkolixir .... ▣ 761
- Bronkotabs Tablets .... ▣ 762
- Constant-T Tablets 1029
- Marax Tablets & DF Syrup 1954
- Primatene Tablets 2421
- Quibron Capsules 713
- Quibron-T 714
- Quibron-T/SR 716
- Theolair Liquid 1317
- Theo-Organidin Elixir 2391

Theophylline Anhydrous (Theophylline clearance and plasma half-life significantly affected). Products include:
- Aerolate 994
- Primatene Tablets-M Formula .... ▣ 753
- Primatene Tablets-Regular Formula 2421
- Respbid Tablets 684
- Slo-bid Gyrocaps 1847
- T-PHYL (Uniphyl) 200 mg Tablets 1820
- Tedral SA 1765
- Theo-24 2179
- Theo-Dur Sprinkle 1168
- Theo-Dur Extended-Release Tablets 1166
- Theolair Tablets 1317
- Theolair-SR Tablets 1319
- TheoX Extended-Release Tablets 841
- Uniphyl 400 mg Tablets 1823

Theophylline Calcium Salicylate (Theophylline clearance and plasma half-life significantly affected). Products include:
- Quadrinal Tablets 1183

Theophylline Sodium Glycinate (Theophylline clearance and plasma half-life significantly affected). Products include:
- Asbron G 1997

Food Interactions

Meal, unspecified (Administration 30 minutes after a meal delays the rate of absorption but the extent of absorption is not altered).

ETHRANE
(Enflurane) 599
May interact with nondepolarizing neuromuscular blocking agents. Compounds in this category include:

Atracurium Besylate (Action augmented; longer time for recovery from neuromuscular blockade; use lower dosages). Products include:
- Tracrium Injection 817

Metocurine Iodide (Action augmented; longer time for recovery from neuromuscular blockade; use lower dosages). Products include:
- Metubine Iodide Vials 1285

Pancuronium Bromide Injection (Action augmented; longer time for recovery from neuromuscular blockade; use lower dosages).
No products indexed under this heading.

Vecuronium Bromide (Action augmented; longer time for recovery from neuromuscular blockade; use lower dosages). Products include:
- Norcuron 1642

ETHYL CHLORIDE, U.S.P.
(Chloroethane, Ethyl Chloride) 1022
No interactions described in labeling.

ETRAFON FORTE TABLETS (4-25)
(Perphenazine, Amitriptyline Hydrochloride) 2087
See **Etrafon-A Tablets (4-10)**

ETRAFON 2-10 TABLETS (2-10)
(Perphenazine, Amitriptyline Hydrochloride) 2087
See **Etrafon-A Tablets (4-10)**

ETRAFON TABLETS (2-25)
(Perphenazine, Amitriptyline Hydrochloride) 2087
See **Etrafon-A Tablets (4-10)**

ETRAFON-A TABLETS (4-10)
(Perphenazine, Amitriptyline Hydrochloride) 2087
May interact with central nervous

system depressants, barbiturates, narcotic analgesics, antihistamines, monoamine oxidase inhibitors, thyroid preparations, anticholinergics, sympathomimetic aerosol bronchodilators, and certain other agents. Compounds in these categories include:

Albuterol (Use with caution). Products include:
Proventil Inhalation Aerosol 2117
Ventolin Inhalation Aerosol and Refill 583

Albuterol Sulfate (Use with caution). Products include:
Proventil Repetabs Tablets 2120
Proventil Solutions for Inhalation 0.5% and 0.083% 2118
Proventil Syrup 2119
Proventil Tablets 2120
Ventolin 583

Alcohol (Potentiation; hypotension).

Alfentanil Hydrochloride (Potentiation of both drugs). Products include:
Alfenta Injection 1131

Alprazolam (Potentiation of both drugs). Products include:
Xanax Tablets 2367

Aprobarbital (Potentiation of both drugs). Products include:
Alurate Elixir 1883

Astemizole (Potentiation of both drugs). Products include:
Hismanal Tablets 1138

Atropine Derivatives (Additive anticholinergic effects).

Atropine Sulfate (Additive anticholinergic effects). Products include:
Arco-Lase Plus Tablets 607
Atropine Sulfate Sterile Ophthalmic Solution and S.O.P. Sterile Ophthalmic Ointment .... ⊙ 239
Donnagel .... ■ 675
Donnagel-PG 1858
Donnatal 1858
Donnatal Extentabs 1859
Donnatal Tablets 1858
Donnazyme Tablets 1860
Isopto Atropine .... ⊙ 218
Lomotil 2174
Motofen Tablets 836
Ru-Tuss Tablets 693
Urised Tablets 2396

Azatadine Maleate (Potentiation of both drugs). Products include:
Optimine Tablets 2115
Trinalin Repetabs Tablets 1170

Belladonna Alkaloids (Additive anticholinergic effects). Products include:
Bellergal-S Tablets 1998
Hyland's Bed Wetting Tablets .... ■ 728
Hyland's Teething Tablets .... ■ 728
Kinesed Tablets 2272

Benztropine Mesylate (Additive anticholinergic effects). Products include:
Cogentin 1435

Biperiden (Additive anticholinergic effects). Products include:
Akineton 1171

Bromodiphenhydramine Hydrochloride (Potentiation of both drugs).
No products indexed under this heading.

Brompheniramine Maleate (Potentiation of both drugs). Products include:
Alka Seltzer Plus Sinus Allergy Medicine .... ■ 624
Atrohist Sprinkle Capsules 558
Bromfed Capsules (Timed Release) 1615
Bromfed Syrup .... ■ 628
Bromfed 1615
Dimetane Decongestant .... ■ 673
Dimetane .... ■ 672
Dimetane-DC Cough Syrup 1857
Dimetane-DX Cough Syrup 1858
Dimetapp Elixir .... ■ 673
Dimetapp DM Elixir .... ■ 674
Dimetapp Extentabs .... ■ 674
Dimetapp Plus Caplets .... ■ 675
Dimetapp Tablets .... ■ 675
Drixoral Antihistamine/Nasal Decongestant Syrup .... ■ 698

Buprenorphine (Potentiation of both drugs).
No products indexed under this heading.

Buspirone Hydrochloride (Potentiation of both drugs). Products include:
BuSpar 1401

Butabarbital (Potentiation of both drugs). Products include:
Pyridium Plus 1764

Butalbital (Potentiation of both drugs). Products include:
Esgic-Plus Tablets 1002
Esgic Tablets & Capsules 1001
Fioricet Tablets 2006
Fiorinal Capsules 2007
Fiorinal with Codeine Capsules 2008
Fiorinal Tablets 2007
Phrenilin 838
Sedapap Tablets 50 mg/650 mg 1360

Chlordiazepoxide (Potentiation of both drugs). Products include:
Libritabs Tablets 1930
Limbitrol 1933
Menrium Tablets 1934

Chlordiazepoxide Hydrochloride (Potentiation of both drugs). Products include:
Librax Capsules 1929
Librium Capsules 1931
Librium Injectable 1932

Chlorpheniramine Maleate (Potentiation of both drugs). Products include:
A.R.M. Allergy Relief Medicine Caplets .... ■ 615
Alka-Seltzer Plus Cold Medicine .... ■ 623
Allerest .... ■ 559
Ana-Kit Anaphylaxis Emergency Treatment Kit 1100
BC Cold Powder Multi-Symptom Formula .... ■ 517
Brexin L.A. Capsules 2078
Cerose-DM 2443
Cheracol Plus Head Cold/Cough Formula .... ■ 667
Chlor-Trimeton Allergy Syrup, Tablets & Long-Acting Repetabs Tablets .... ■ 693
Chlor-Trimeton Decongestant .... ■ 694
Comhist LA Capsules 1618
Allergy-Sinus Comtrex Multi-Symptom Allergy Sinus Formula Tablets & Caplets 746
Comtrex Multi-Symptom Cold Reliever Tablets/Caplets/Liqui-Gels/Liquid 745
Day-Night Comtrex 747
Contac Continuous Action Decongestant/Antihistamine Capsules ■ 710
Contac Maximum Strength Continuous Action Decongestant/Antihistamine Caplets .... ■ 709
Contac Severe Cold and Flu Formula Caplets .... ■ 711
Coricidin 'D' Decongestant Tablets .... ■ 695
Coricidin Demilets Tablets for Children .... ■ 696
Coricidin Tablets .... ■ 695
Deconamine 663
Demazin Nasal Decongestant/Antihistamine Repetabs Tablets & Syrup .... ■ 697
Dorcol Children's Liquid Cold Formula .... ■ 686
Dristan Decongestant/Antihistamine/ Analgesic Coated Caplets .... ■ 749
Dristan Cold Nasal Decongestant/Antihistamine/ Analgesic Coated Tablets 2419
Dristan Advanced Formula Decongestant/Antihistamine/ Analgesic Tablets .... ■ 749
Extendryl 994
4-Way Cold Tablets 750
Fedahist Gyrocaps 2145
Fedahist Timecaps 2145
Hycomine Compound Tablets 929
Isoclor Timesule Capsules .... ■ 561
Kronofed-A 970
Medi-Flu Caplet, Liquid .... ■ 640
Naldecon Syrup, Tablets, Pediatric Drops and Pediatric Syrup 709
Nolamine Tablets 838
Novafed A Capsules 1342
Novahistine DH 1342
Novahistine Elixir .... ■ 596
Ornade Spansule Capsules 2221
Orthoxicol Cough Syrup .... ■ 668
PediaCare Allergy Relief Formula Liquid 1362
PediaCare Cough-Cold Formula Liquid 1362
PediaCare Night Rest Cough-Cold Formula Liquid 1362
PediaCare 6-12 Cough-Cold Formula Chewable Tablets 1362
Pyrroxate Capsules .... ■ 669
Quelidrine Syrup 556
Ru-Tuss II Capsules 693
Ru-Tuss Tablets 693
Ryna .... ■ 741
Sinarest Tablets & Extra Strength Tablets .... ■ 562
Sine-Off Maximum Strength Allergy/Sinus Formula Caplets .... ■ 721
Sine-Off Sinus Medicine Tablets-Aspirin Formula .... ■ 722
Singlet Tablets .... ■ 598
Sinulin 840
Sinutab Maximum Strength .... ■ 641
St. Joseph Nighttime Cold Medicine .... ■ 705
Sudafed Plus Liquid .... ■ 544
Sudafed Plus Tablets .... ■ 545
Teldrin Timed-Release Allergy Capsules, 12 mg 2192
TheraFlu Flu and Cold Medicine .... ■ 687
Triaminic Allergy Tablets .... ■ 688
Triaminic Chewables .... ■ 688
Triaminic Cold Tablets .... ■ 688
Triaminic Nite Light .... ■ 689
Triaminic Syrup .... ■ 689
Triaminic-12 Tablets .... ■ 690
Triaminicin Tablets .... ■ 690
Triaminicol Multi-Symptom Cold Tablets .... ■ 691
Triaminicol Multi-Symptom Relief ■ 691
Tylenol Allergy Sinus Medication Caplets and Gelcaps, Maximum Strength 1372
Children's Tylenol Cold Liquid Formula and Chewable Tablets 1368
Tylenol Cold & Flu Hot Medication, Packets 1369
Tylenol Cold Medication Caplets and Tablets 1370
Tylenol Cold Medication, Effervescent Tablets 1369
Vicks Children's NyQuil .... ■ 664
Vicks Formula 44 Cough Medicine .... ■ 661
Vicks Formula 44M Multi-Symptom Cough Medicine .... ■ 662
Vicks Pediatric Formula 44m Multi-Symptom Cough & Cold Medicine .... ■ 663

Chlorpheniramine Polistirex (Potentiation of both drugs). Products include:
Tussionex Extended-Release Suspension 988

Chlorpheniramine Tannate (Potentiation of both drugs). Products include:
Rynatan 2387
Rynatuss 2388

Chlorpromazine (Potentiation of both drugs). Products include:
Thorazine 2234

Chlorprothixene (Potentiation of both drugs). Products include:
Taractan Tablets 1920

Chlorprothixene Hydrochloride (Potentiation of both drugs). Products include:
Taractan 1920

Cimetidine (Increased plasma concentrations of tricyclic antidepressant). Products include:
Tagamet Tablets 2228

Cimetidine Hydrochloride (Increased plasma concentrations of tricyclic antidepressant). Products include:
Tagamet 2228

Clemastine Fumarate (Potentiation of both drugs). Products include:
Tavist Syrup 2033
Tavist Tablets 2035
Tavist-D Tablets 2035

Clidinium Bromide (Additive anticholinergic effects). Products include:
Librax Capsules 1929
Quarzan Capsules 1937

Clorazepate Dipotassium (Potentiation of both drugs). Products include:
Tranxene 556

Codeine (Potentiation of both drugs). Products include:
Calcidrine Syrup 506

Codeine Phosphate (Potentiation of both drugs). Products include:
Actifed with Codeine Cough Syrup.. 752
Cheracol Cough Syrup 1853
Codimal PH Syrup 846
Dimetane-DC Cough Syrup 1857
Empirin with Codeine Phosphate Nos. 2, 3 & 4 764
Fiorinal with Codeine Capsules 2008
Isoclor Expectorant 982
Naldecon CX Adult Liquid .... ■ 521
Novahistine DH 1342
Novahistine Expectorant 1343
Nucofed Capsules 2219
Nucofed Expectorant 2219
Nucofed Pediatric Expectorant 2220
Nucofed Syrup 2219
Phenaphen with Codeine Capsules 1865
Phenaphen-650 with Codeine Tablets 1866
Phenergan with Codeine 2497
Phenergan VC with Codeine 2501
Robitussin A-C Syrup 1875
Robitussin-DAC Syrup 1875
Ryna .... ■ 741
Soma Compound w/Codeine Tablets 2390
Triaminic Expectorant w/Codeine .. 1996
Tussi-Organidin Liquid 2391
Tylenol with Codeine 1381

Codeine Polistirex (Potentiation of both drugs).
No products indexed under this heading.

Cyproheptadine Hydrochloride (Potentiation of both drugs). Products include:
Periactin 1525

Dexchlorpheniramine Maleate (Potentiation of both drugs). Products include:
Polaramine 2116

Dezocine (Potentiation of both drugs).

Diazepam (Potentiation of both drugs). Products include:
Valium Injectable 1937
Valium Tablets 1939
Valrelease Capsules 1923

Dicyclomine Hydrochloride (Additive anticholinergic effects). Products include:
Bentyl 1322

Diphenhydramine Citrate (Potentiation of both drugs). Products include:
Alka-Seltzer Plus Night-Time Cold Medicine .... ■ 623
Bufferin AF Nite Time Analgesic/Sleeping Aid Caplets 744
Excedrin P.M. Analgesic/Sleeping Aid Tablets, Caplets and Liquid 749

Dobutamine Hydrochloride (Use with caution). Products include:
Dobutrex Solution Vials 1259

Dopamine Hydrochloride (Use with caution). Products include:
Intropin Injection 930

Droperidol (Potentiation of both drugs). Products include:
- Inapsine Injection 1140
- Innovar Injection 1141

Enflurane (Potentiation of both drugs). Products include:
- Ethrane 599

Ephedrine Hydrochloride (Use with caution). Products include:
- Amesec .... ▣ 682
- Primatene Tablets-M Formula 2421
- Primatene Tablets-P Formula 2421
- Primatene Tablets-Regular Formula 2421
- Quadrinal Tablets 1183
- Quelidrine Syrup 556
- Tedral SA 1765

Ephedrine Sulfate (Use with caution). Products include:
- Bronkaid Tablets .... ▣ 757
- Bronkolixir .... ▣ 761
- Bronkotabs Tablets .... ▣ 762
- Marax Tablets & DF Syrup 1954
- Pazo Hemorrhoid Ointment & Suppositories 752
- Vicks Vatronol Nose Drops .... ▣ 666

Ephedrine Tannate (Use with caution). Products include:
- Rynatuss 2388

Epinephrine (Use with caution). Products include:
- Ana-Kit Anaphylaxis Emergency Treatment Kit 1100
- Bronkaid Mist .... ▣ 757
- EpiPen 843
- Marcaine Hydrochloride 0.5% with Epinephrine 1:200,000 (as bitartrate) 958
- Marcaine Hydrochloride with Epinephrine 1:200,000 2055
- Primatene Mist 2420
- Sus-Phrine Injection 1006
- Xylocaine with Epinephrine Injections 637

Epinephrine Bitartrate (Use with caution). Products include:
- AsthmaHaler Mist Epinephrine Bitartrate Bronchodilator .... ▣ 616
- Bronkaid Mist Suspension .... ▣ 757
- Primatene Mist Suspension 2421

Epinephrine Hydrochloride (Use with caution). Products include:
- Adrenalin Chloride Solution 1:100 & 1:1,000 1689
- Epifrin .... ⊙ 244
- Glaucon .... ⊙ 218

Estazolam (Potentiation of both drugs). Products include:
- ProSom Tablets 554

Ethchlorvynol (Delirium; potentiation of both drugs). Products include:
- Placidyl Capsules 553

Ethinamate (Potentiation of both drugs).
- No products indexed under this heading.

Fentanyl (Potentiation of both drugs). Products include:
- Duragesic Transdermal System 1133

Fentanyl Citrate (Potentiation of both drugs). Products include:
- Innovar Injection 1141
- Sublimaze Injection 1146

Fluphenazine Decanoate (Potentiation of both drugs). Products include:
- Prolixin Decanoate 1795

Fluphenazine Enanthate (Potentiation of both drugs). Products include:
- Prolixin Enanthate 1796

Fluphenazine Hydrochloride (Potentiation of both drugs). Products include:
- Prolixin Elixir 1793
- Prolixin Injection 1791
- Prolixin Oral Concentrate 1792
- Prolixin Tablets 1793

Flurazepam Hydrochloride (Potentiation of both drugs). Products include:
- Dalmane Capsules 1927

Furazolidone (Convulsions, hyperpyretic crises; contraindicated). Products include:
- Furoxone 1855

Glutethimide (Potentiation of both drugs).
- No products indexed under this heading.

Glycopyrrolate (Additive anticholinergic effects). Products include:
- Robinul Forte Tablets 1873
- Robinul Injectable 1873
- Robinul Tablets 1873

Guanethidine Monosulfate (Antihypertensive effects of guanethidine blocked). Products include:
- Esimil Tablets 864
- Ismelin Tablets 869

Haloperidol (Potentiation of both drugs). Products include:
- Haldol Injection, Tablets and Concentrate 1373

Haloperidol Decanoate (Potentiation of both drugs). Products include:
- Haldol Decanoate 1375

Hydrocodone Bitartrate (Potentiation of both drugs). Products include:
- Anexsia 5/500 Tablets 2196
- Anexsia 7.5/650 Tablets 2197
- Azdone Tablets 844
- Codiclear DH Syrup 845
- Codimal DH Syrup 846
- Damason-P 1356
- Hycodan Syrup, Tablets 927
- Hycomine Compound Tablets 929
- Hycomine Syrup 927
- Hycotuss Expectorant Syrup 930
- Hydrocet Capsules 835
- Lortab ASA Tablets 2414
- Lortab 2412
- Ru-Tuss with Hydrocodone 694
- Triaminic Expectorant DH 1995
- Vicodin Tablets 1187
- Vicodin ES Tablets 1189
- Zydone Capsules 941

Hydrocodone Polistirex (Potentiation of both drugs). Products include:
- Tussionex Extended-Release Suspension 988

Hydroxyzine Hydrochloride (Potentiation of both drugs). Products include:
- Atarax Tablets & Syrup 1941
- Marax Tablets & DF Syrup 1954
- Vistaril Intramuscular Solution 1970

Hyoscyamine (Additive anticholinergic effects). Products include:
- Cystospaz Tablets 2395
- Urised Tablets 2396

Hyoscyamine Sulfate (Additive anticholinergic effects). Products include:
- Arco-Lase Plus Tablets 607
- Cystospaz-M Capsules 2395
- Donnagel .... ▣ 675
- Donnagel-PG 1858
- Donnatal 1858
- Donnatal Extentabs 1859
- Donnatal Tablets 1858
- Donnazyme Tablets 1860
- Kutrase Capsules 2146
- Levsin/Levsinex 2147
- Ru-Tuss Tablets 693

Ipratropium Bromide (Additive anticholinergic effects). Products include:
- Atrovent Inhalation Aerosol 675

Isocarboxazid (Convulsions, hyperpyretic crises; contraindicated). Products include:
- Marplan Tablets 1906

Isoflurane (Potentiation of both drugs). Products include:
- Forane 600

Isoproterenol Hydrochloride (Use with caution). Products include:
- Isuprel Hydrochloride Injection 1:5000 2050
- Isuprel Hydrochloride Mistometer 2051
- Isuprel Hydrochloride Solution 1:200 & 1:100 2052
- Norisodrine Aerotrol 540

Ketamine Hydrochloride (Potentiation of both drugs). Products include:
- Ketalar 1726

Levorphanol Tartrate (Potentiation of both drugs). Products include:
- Levo-Dromoran 1906

Levothyroxine Sodium (Use with caution). Products include:
- Levothroid Tablets 1003
- Levoxine Tablets 904
- Synthroid 695

Liothyronine Sodium (Use with caution). Products include:
- Cytomel Tablets 2203

Liotrix (Use with caution). Products include:
- Euthroid 1724

Lorazepam (Potentiation of both drugs). Products include:
- Ativan Injection 2432
- Ativan Tablets 2434

Loxapine Hydrochloride (Potentiation of both drugs). Products include:
- Loxitane 1213

Loxapine Succinate (Potentiation of both drugs). Products include:
- Loxitane Capsules 1213

Mepenzolate Bromide (Additive anticholinergic effects). Products include:
- Cantil Tablets 1326

Meperidine Hydrochloride (Potentiation of both drugs). Products include:
- Demerol 2047
- Mepergan Injection 2479

Mephobarbital (Potentiation of both drugs). Products include:
- Mebaral Tablets 2061

Meprobamate (Potentiation of both drugs). Products include:
- Deprol Tablets 2382
- Equagesic Tablets 2451
- Miltown Tablets 2386
- PMB 200 and PMB 400 2504

Mesoridazine (Potentiation of both drugs). Products include:
- Serentil 686

Metaproterenol Sulfate (Use with caution). Products include:
- Alupent 674
- Arm-a-Med Metaproterenol Sulfate Inhalation Solution, USP 617
- Metaprel Inhalation Aerosol Bronchodilator 2014
- Metaprel Inhalation Solution 2015
- Metaprel 2015
- Metaproterenol Sulfate Inhalation Solution, USP 912

Metaraminol Bitartrate (Use with caution). Products include:
- Aramine Injection 1424

Methadone Hydrochloride (Potentiation of both drugs). Products include:
- Dolophine Hydrochloride Ampoules & Vials 1260
- Dolophine Hydrochloride Tablets 1261
- Methadone Hydrochloride Diskets 1284
- Methadone Hydrochloride Oral Solution & Tablets 1987

Methdilazine Hydrochloride (Potentiation of both drugs). Products include:
- Tacaryl Syrup & Tablets 2409

Methohexital Sodium (Potentiation of both drugs). Products include:
- Brevital Sodium Vials 1248

Methoxamine Hydrochloride (Use with caution). Products include:
- Vasoxyl Injection 819

Methoxyflurane (Potentiation of both drugs).
- No products indexed under this heading.

Midazolam Hydrochloride (Potentiation of both drugs). Products include:
- Versed Injection 1924

Molindone Hydrochloride (Potentiation of both drugs). Products include:
- Moban Tablets & Concentrate 932

Morphine Sulfate (Potentiation of both drugs). Products include:
- Astramorph/PF Injection, USP (Preservative-Free) 618
- Duramorph 960
- Infumorph 200 and Infumorph 500 Sterile Solutions 962
- MS Contin Tablets 1814
- MSIR 1817
- Oramorph SR (Morphine Sulfate Sustained Release Tablets) 1988
- Roxanol 1991

Norepinephrine Bitartrate (Use with caution). Products include:
- Levophed Bitartrate Injection 2054

Opium Alkaloids (Potentiation of both drugs). Products include:
- B & O No. 15A & No. 16A Supprettes 2395
- Pantopon Injectable 1911

Oxazepam (Potentiation of both drugs). Products include:
- Serax Capsules 2522
- Serax Tablets 2522

Oxycodone Hydrochloride (Potentiation of both drugs). Products include:
- Percocet Tablets 950
- Percodan 951
- Roxicodone Tablets, Oral Solution & Intensol (Oxycodone) 1992
- Tylox Capsules 1382

Pentobarbital Sodium (Potentiation of both drugs). Products include:
- Nembutal Sodium Capsules 534
- Nembutal Sodium Solution 536
- Nembutal Sodium Suppositories 538

Phenelzine Sulfate (Convulsions, hyperpyretic crises; contraindicated). Products include:
- Nardil 1742

Phenobarbital (Potentiation of both drugs). Products include:
- Arco-Lase Plus Tablets 607
- Bellergal-S Tablets 1998
- Bronkolixir .... ▣ 761
- Bronkotabs Tablets .... ▣ 762
- Donnatal 1858
- Donnatal Extentabs 1859
- Donnatal Tablets 1858
- Donnazyme Tablets 1860
- Kinesed Tablets 2272
- Phenobarbital Elixir and Tablets 1293
- Primatene Tablets-P Formula 2421
- Quadrinal Tablets 1183
- Tedral SA 1765

Phenylephrine Hydrochloride (Use with caution). Products include:
- AK-Dilate Solution 2.5% and 10% .... ⊙ 203
- Atrohist Sprinkle Capsules 558
- Cerose-DM 2443
- Codimal 846
- Comhist LA Capsules 1618
- Congespirin For Children Aspirin Free Chewable Cold Tablets 748
- Cyclomydril .... ⊙ 216
- Deconsal Sprinkle Capsules 559
- Dimetane Decongestant .... ▣ 673
- Dristan Decongestant/Antihistamine/ Analgesic Coated Caplets .... ▣ 749
- Dristan Cold Nasal Decongestant/ Antihistamine/Analgesic Coated Tablets 2419
- Dristan Advanced Formula Decongestant/Antihistamine/ Analgesic Tablets .... ▣ 749

Dristan Nasal Spray, Menthol 2419
Dristan Nasal Spray, Regular and Regular with Metered Pump 2419
Entex Capsules 1623
Entex Liquid 1623
Sinus Excedrin Analgesic, Decongestant Tablets & Caplets 750
Extendryl 994
4-Way Fast Acting Nasal Spray - Original Formula (regular & mentholated) & Metered Spray Pump (regular) 751
Hycomine Compound Tablets 929
Murocoll-2 Sterile Ophthalmic Solution ◉ 261
Mydfrin 2.5% ◉ 224
Naldecon Syrup, Tablets, Pediatric Drops and Pediatric Syrup 709
Neo-Synephrine Hydrochloride 1% Carpuject 2063
Neo-Synephrine Hydrochloride 1% Injection 2063
Neo-Synephrine Hydrochloride (Ophthalmic) 2064
Neo-Synephrine [ND] 759
Nōstril Nasal Decongestant [ND] 520
Novahistine Elixir [ND] 596
Phenergan VC 2500
Phenergan VC with Codeine 2501
Prefrin Liquifilm Vasoconstrictor and Lubricant Eye Drops ◉ 254
Prefrin-A ◉ 255
Quelidrine Syrup 556
Relief Vasoconstrictor and Lubricant Eye Drops ◉ 256
Robitussin Night Relief [ND] 677
Ru-Tuss with Hydrocodone 694
Ru-Tuss Tablets 693
Vasosulf ◉ 279
Vicks Sinex [ND] 665
Zincfrin ◉ 230

Phenylephrine Tannate (Use with caution). Products include:

Rynatan 2387
Rynatuss 2388

Phenylpropanolamine Hydrochloride (Use with caution). Products include:

A.R.M. Allergy Relief Medicine Caplets [ND] 615
Acutrim [ND] 548
Allerest [ND] 559
BC Cold Powder [ND] 517
Cheracol Plus Head Cold/Cough Formula [ND] 667
Codimal Expectorant 846
Comtrex Multi-Symptom Cold Reliever Tablets/Caplets/Liqui-Gels/Liquid 745
Contac Continuous Action Decongestant/Antihistamine Capsules [ND] 710
Contac Maximum Strength Continuous Action Decongestant/Antihistamine Caplets [ND] 709
Contac Severe Cold and Flu Formula Caplets [ND] 711
Coricidin 'D' Decongestant Tablets [ND] 695
Coricidin Demilets Tablets for Children [ND] 696
Demazin Nasal Decongestant/Antihistamine Repetabs Tablets & Syrup [ND] 697
Dexatrim [ND] 733
Dimetane-DC Cough Syrup 1857
Dimetapp Elixir [ND] 673
Dimetapp DM Elixir [ND] 674
Dimetapp Extentabs [ND] 674
Dimetapp Plus Caplets [ND] 675
Dimetapp Tablets [ND] 675
Entex Capsules 1623
Entex LA Tablets 1623
Entex Liquid 1623
4-Way Cold Tablets 750
Hycomine Syrup 927
Naldecon CX Adult Liquid [ND] 521
Naldecon DX Adult Liquid [ND] 521
Naldecon DX Children's Syrup [ND] 522
Naldecon DX Pediatric Drops [ND] 522
Naldecon EX Children's Syrup [ND] 522
Naldecon EX Pediatric Drops [ND] 523
Naldecon Syrup, Tablets, Pediatric Drops and Pediatric Syrup 709
Nolamine Tablets 838
Nolex LA Tablets 838
Ornade Spansule Capsules 2221
Orthoxicol Cough Syrup [ND] 668
Propagest 839
Pyrroxate Capsules [ND] 669
Robitussin-CF [ND] 676
Ru-Tuss II Capsules 693
Ru-Tuss with Hydrocodone 694
Ru-Tuss Tablets 693
Sine-Off Sinus Medicine Tablets-Aspirin Formula [ND] 722
Sinulin 840
St. Joseph Cold Tablets for Children [ND] 704
Tavist-D Tablets 2035
Triaminic Allergy Tablets [ND] 688
Triaminic Chewables [ND] 688
Triaminic Cold Tablets [ND] 688
Triaminic Expectorant [ND] 688
Triaminic Expectorant w/Codeine 1996
Triaminic Expectorant DH 1995
Triaminic Oral Infant Drops 1996
Triaminic Syrup [ND] 689
Triaminic-12 Tablets [ND] 690
Triaminic-DM Syrup [ND] 689
Triaminicin Tablets [ND] 690
Triaminicol Multi-Symptom Cold Tablets [ND] 691
Triaminicol Multi-Symptom Relief [ND] 691
Tuss-Ornade Liquid 2242
Tuss-Ornade Spansule Capsules 2242
Tylenol Cold Medication, Effervescent Tablets 1369

Pirbuterol Acetate (Use with caution). Products include:

Maxair Inhaler 1311

Prazepam (Potentiation of both drugs). Products include:

Centrax 1693

Prochlorperazine (Potentiation of both drugs). Products include:

Compazine 2201

Procyclidine Hydrochloride (Additive anticholinergic effects). Products include:

Kemadrin Tablets 771

Promethazine Hydrochloride (Potentiation of both drugs). Products include:

Mepergan Injection 2479
Phenergan with Codeine 2497
Phenergan with Dextromethorphan 2499
Phenergan Injection 2493
Phenergan Suppositories 2496
Phenergan Syrup 2495
Phenergan Tablets 2496
Phenergan VC 2500
Phenergan VC with Codeine 2501

Propantheline Bromide (Additive anticholinergic effects). Products include:

Pro-Banthīne Tablets 2141

Propofol (Potentiation of both drugs). Products include:

Diprivan Injection 2267

Propoxyphene Hydrochloride (Potentiation of both drugs). Products include:

Darvon 1256
Wygesic Tablets 2540

Propoxyphene Napsylate (Potentiation of both drugs). Products include:

Darvon-N/Darvocet-N 1254

Pseudoephedrine Hydrochloride (Use with caution). Products include:

Actifed Capsules [ND] 539
Actifed Plus Caplets [ND] 539
Actifed Plus Tablets [ND] 540
Actifed with Codeine Cough Syrup 752
Actifed Syrup [ND] 540
Actifed Tablets [ND] 540
Actifed 12-Hour Capsules [ND] 539
Advil Cold & Sinus Caplets (formerly CoAdvil) 2416
Allerest [ND] 559
Anatuss LA Tablets 1359
Benadryl Decongestant Elixir [ND] 635
Benadryl Decongestant [ND] 635
Benadryl Plus [ND] 636
Benadryl Plus Nighttime [ND] 637
Benylin Decongestant [ND] 638
Brexin L.A. Capsules 2078
Bromfed Capsules (Timed Release) 1615
Bromfed Syrup [ND] 628
Bromfed 1615
CoAdvil [ND] 748
Allergy-Sinus Comtrex Multi-Symptom Allergy Sinus Formula Tablets & Caplets 746
Cough Formula Comtrex 746
Comtrex Multi-Symptom Cold Reliever Tablets/Caplets/Liqui-Gels/Liquid 745
Day-Night Comtrex 747
Non-Drowsy Comtrex 747
Congess 994
Congestac Caplets [ND] 617
Contac Jr. Children's Cold Medicine [ND] 712
Contac Nighttime Cold Medicine [ND] 713
Contac Sinus Caplets Maximum Strength Non-Drowsy Formula [ND] 710
Contac Sinus Tablets Maximum Strength Non-Drowsy Formula [ND] 710
Deconamine 663
Deconsal II Tablets 559
Dimacol Caplets [ND] 672
Dimetane-DX Cough Syrup 1858
Dorcol Children's Cough Syrup [ND] 685
Dorcol Children's Decongestant Liquid [ND] 685
Dorcol Children's Liquid Cold Formula [ND] 686
Maximum Strength Dristan Decongestant/Analgesic Coated Caplets [ND] 750
No Drowsiness Dristan Cold Nasal Decongestant/Analgesic Coated Caplets 2420
Dristan Sinus Caplets 2419
Sinus Excedrin Analgesic, Decongestant Tablets & Caplets [ND] 533
Fedahist Gyrocaps 2145
Fedahist Timecaps 2145
Guaifed 1615
Guaifed Syrup [ND] 629
Isoclor Expectorant 982
Isoclor Timesule Capsules [ND] 561
Kronofed-A 970
Medi-Flu Caplet, Liquid [ND] 640
Novafed A Capsules 1342
Novafed Capsules 1342
Novahistine DH 1342
Novahistine DMX [ND] 595
Novahistine Expectorant 1343
Nucofed Capsules 2219
Nucofed Expectorant 2219
Nucofed Pediatric Expectorant 2220
Nucofed Syrup 2219
Ornex Caplets [ND] 618
PediaCare Allergy Relief Formula Liquid 1362
PediaCare Cough-Cold Formula Liquid 1362
PediaCare Infants' Oral Decongestant Drops 1362
PediaCare Night Rest Cough-Cold Formula Liquid 1362
PediaCare 6-12 Cough-Cold Formula Chewable Tablets 1362
Robitussin-DAC Syrup 1875
Robitussin-PE [ND] 677
Rondec 1975
Rondec-DM 1976
Rondec-TR Tablet 1975
Ru-Tuss DE Tablets 694
Ryna [ND] 741
Seldane-D Extended-Release Tablets 1350
Sinarest [ND] 562
Sine-Aid Maximum Strength Sinus Headache Caplets 1365
Sine-Aid Maximum Strength Sinus Headache Tablets 1365
Sine-Off Maximum Strength Allergy/Sinus Formula Caplets [ND] 721
Sine-Off Maximum Strength No Drowsiness Formula Caplets [ND] 722
Singlet Tablets [ND] 598
Sinutab Maximum Strength [ND] 641
Sinutab Maximum Strength Without Drowsiness Tablets & Caplets [ND] 642
Sinutab Regular Strength Without Drowsiness Formula [ND] 641
St. Joseph Nighttime Cold Medicine [ND] 705
Sudafed Children's Liquid [ND] 543
Sudafed Cough Syrup [ND] 543
Sudafed Plus Liquid [ND] 544
Sudafed Plus Tablets [ND] 545
Sudafed Sinus Caplets [ND] 545
Sudafed Sinus Tablets [ND] 545
Sudafed Tablets, 30 mg [ND] 544
Sudafed Tablets, Adult Strength, 60 mg [ND] 544
Sudafed 12 Hour Capsules [ND] 545
TheraFlu Flu and Cold Medicine [ND] 687
Triaminic Nite Light [ND] 689
Tylenol Allergy Sinus Medication Caplets and Gelcaps, Maximum Strength 1372
Children's Tylenol Cold Liquid Formula and Chewable Tablets 1368
Tylenol Cold & Flu Hot Medication, Packets 1369
Tylenol Cold & Flu No Drowsiness Hot Medication, Packets 1371
Tylenol Cold Medication Caplets and Tablets 1370
Tylenol Cold Medication No Drowsiness Formula Caplets 1370
Tylenol Cold Night Time Medication Liquid 1371
Tylenol Cough Medication Liquid with Decongestant, Maximum Strength 1372
Tylenol, Maximum Strength, Sinus Medication Gelcaps, Caplets and Tablets 1373
Ursinus Inlay-Tabs [ND] 691
Vicks Children's NyQuil [ND] 664
Vicks Daycare [ND] 660
Vicks Formula 44D Decongestant Cough Medicine [ND] 662
Vicks Formula 44M Multi-Symptom Cough Medicine [ND] 662
Vicks NyQuil Nighttime Colds Medicine-Original & Cherry Flavor [ND] 664
Vicks Pediatric Formula 44 Cough & Congestion Medicine [ND] 663
Vicks Pediatric Formula 44m Multi-Symptom Cough & Cold Medicine [ND] 663

Pseudoephedrine Sulfate (Use with caution). Products include:

Afrin Tablets [ND] 693
Chlor-Trimeton Decongestant [ND] 694
Disophrol Chronotab Sustained-Action Tablets [ND] 698
Drixoral Antihistamine/Nasal Decongestant Syrup [ND] 698
Drixoral Non-Drowsy Formula [ND] 699
Drixoral Plus Extended-Release Tablets [ND] 699
Drixoral Sinus [ND] 700
Drixoral Sustained-Action Tablets [ND] 698
Sinutab Allergy Formula Sustained Action Tablets [ND] 640
Trinalin Repetabs Tablets 1170

Pyrilamine Maleate (Potentiation of both drugs). Products include:

Codimal 846
4-Way Fast Acting Nasal Spray - Original Formula (regular & mentholated) & Metered Spray Pump (regular) 751
Maximum Strength Midol Multi-Symptom Menstrual Formula [ND] 571
Maximum Strength Midol PMS Premenstrual Syndrome Formula [ND] 570
Regular Strength Midol Multi-Symptom Menstrual Formula [ND] 570
Prefrin-A ◉ 255
Prēmsyn PMS Capsules & Caplets [ND] 547
Primatene Tablets-M Formula 2421
Robitussin Night Relief [ND] 677
Ru-Tuss with Hydrocodone 694
Triaminic Expectorant DH 1995
Triaminic Oral Infant Drops 1996

Pyrilamine Tannate (Potentiation of both drugs). Products include:

Rynatan 2387

Quazepam (Potentiation of both drugs). Products include:

Doral Tablets 2383

Scopolamine Hydrobromide (Additive anticholinergic effects). Products include:

Donnagel [ND] 675
Donnagel-PG 1858
Donnatal 1858
Donnatal Extentabs 1859
Donnatal Tablets 1858
Donnazyme Tablets 1860
Isopto Hyoscine ◉ 222
Murocoll-2 Sterile Ophthalmic Solution ◉ 261

Ru-Tuss Tablets 693

Scopolamine Preparations (Additive anticholinergic effects). Products include:
Transderm Scōp Transdermal Therapeutic System 887

Secobarbital Sodium (Potentiation of both drugs). Products include:
Seconal Sodium Pulvules 1296

Selegiline Hydrochloride (Convulsions, hyperpyretic crises; contraindicated). Products include:
Eldepryl 2250

Sufentanil Citrate (Potentiation of both drugs). Products include:
Sufenta Injection 1147

Temazepam (Potentiation of both drugs). Products include:
Restoril Capsules 2023

Terbutaline Sulfate (Use with caution). Products include:
Brethaire Inhaler 1024
Brethine Ampuls 1026
Brethine Tablets 1026
Bricanyl Injection 1324
Bricanyl Tablets 1325

Terfenadine (Potentiation of both drugs). Products include:
Seldane Tablets 1349
Seldane-D Extended-Release Tablets 1350

Thiamylal Sodium (Potentiation of both drugs). Products include:
Surital Ampoules, Steri-Vials 1764

Thioridazine Hydrochloride (Potentiation of both drugs). Products include:
Mellaril 2011

Thiothixene (Potentiation of both drugs). Products include:
Navane Capsules and Concentrate 1954
Navane Intramuscular 1956

Thyroglobulin (Use with caution). Products include:
Proloid Tablets 1761

Thyroid (Use with caution). Products include:
S-P-T "Liquid" Capsules 995

Thyroxine (Use with caution).
No products indexed under this heading.

Tranylcypromine Sulfate (Convulsions, hyperpyretic crises; contraindicated). Products include:
Parnate Tablets 2222

Triazolam (Potentiation of both drugs). Products include:
Halcion Tablets 2340

Tridihexethyl Chloride (Additive anticholinergic effects).
No products indexed under this heading.

Trifluoperazine Hydrochloride (Potentiation of both drugs). Products include:
Stelazine 2226

Trihexyphenidyl Hydrochloride (Additive anticholinergic effects). Products include:
Artane 1195

Trimeprazine Tartrate (Potentiation of both drugs). Products include:
Temaril Tablets, Syrup and Spansule Sustained Release Capsules 1085

Tripelennamine Hydrochloride (Potentiation of both drugs). Products include:
PBZ Tablets & Elixir 1037
PBZ-SR Tablets 1037

Triprolidine Hydrochloride (Potentiation of both drugs). Products include:
Actidil .... ■ 538
Actifed Capsules .... ■ 539
Actifed Plus Caplets .... ■ 539
Actifed Plus Tablets .... ■ 540
Actifed with Codeine Cough Syrup.. 752
Actifed Syrup .... ■ 540
Actifed Tablets .... ■ 540
Actifed 12-Hour Capsules .... ■ 539

EUCALYPTAMINT 100% ALL NATURAL OINTMENT
(Menthol) .... ■ 549
No interactions described in labeling.

EUCERIN DRY SKIN CARE CLEANSING BAR
(Moisturizing formula) 662
No interactions described in labeling.

EUCERIN CLEANSING LOTION (DRY SKIN CARE)
(Eucerite) 662
No interactions described in labeling.

EUCERIN DAILY FACIAL LOTION
(Octyl Methoxycinnamate) 662
No interactions described in labeling.

EUCERIN DRY SKIN CARE LOTION
(Moisturizing formula) 662
No interactions described in labeling.

EUCERIN MOISTURIZING CREME (UNSCENTED)
(Moisturizing formula) 662
No interactions described in labeling.

EULEXIN CAPSULES
(Flutamide) 2089
May interact with:

Warfarin Sodium (Increases in prothrombin time have been noted in patients receiving long-term warfarin therapy after flutamide was initiated). Products include:
Coumadin Injection & Tablets 944
Panwarfin Tablets 547

EURAX CREAM & LOTION
(Crotamiton) 2398
No interactions described in labeling.

EUTHROID
(Liotrix) 1724
May interact with oral anticoagulants, estrogens, oral hypoglycemic agents, insulin, oral contraceptives, and certain other agents. Compounds in these categories include:

Chlorotrianisene (Increased thyroid requirements). Products include:
TACE 12 and 25 mg 1353

Chlorpropamide (Increased oral hypoglycemic requirements). Products include:
Diabinese Tablets 1775

Cholestyramine (Impaired absorption of thyroid hormones). Products include:
Cholybar 1705
Questran Light 711
Questran Powder 710

Dicumarol (Increased catabolism of Vitamin K-dependent clotting factors). Products include:
Dicumarol Tablets 516

Dienestrol (Increased thyroid requirements). Products include:
Ortho Dienestrol Cream 1664

Diethylstilbestrol (Increased thyroid requirements). Products include:
Diethylstilbestrol Tablets 1258

Estradiol (Increased thyroid requirements). Products include:
Emcyt Capsules 1161
Estrace 1385
Estrace Vaginal Cream 1388
Estraderm Transdermal System 866

Estrogens, Conjugated (Increased thyroid requirements). Products include:
Mediatric Capsules 2476
PMB 200 and PMB 400 2504
Premarin Intravenous 2508
Premarin with Methyltestosterone .. 2515
Premarin Tablets 2510
Premarin Vaginal Cream 2512

Estrogens, Esterified (Increased thyroid requirements). Products include:
Estratest 2245
Menrium Tablets 1934

Estropipate (Increased thyroid requirements). Products include:
Ogen 540

Ethinyl Estradiol (Increased thyroid requirements). Products include:
Brevicon 2304
Demulen 2161
Estinyl Tablets 2085
Jenest-28 Tablets 1636
Levlen/Tri-Levlen 665
Lo/Ovral Tablets 2471
Lo/Ovral-28 Tablets 2476
Loestrin 1728
Modicon 1667
Nordette-21 Tablets 2481
Nordette-28 Tablets 2483
Norethin 2133
Norinyl 2304
Norlestrin 1746
Ortho-Cyclen Tablets 1658
Ortho-Novum 1667
Ovcon 1391
Ovral Tablets 2490
Ovral-28 Tablets 2491
Levlen/Tri-Levlen 665
Tri-Norinyl 2304
Triphasil-21 Tablets 2527
Triphasil-28 Tablets 2532

Ethynodiol Diacetate (Increased thyroid requirements). Products include:
Demulen 2161

Glipizide (Increased oral hypoglycemic requirements). Products include:
Glucotrol 1952

Glyburide (Increased oral hypoglycemic requirements). Products include:
DiaBeta 1091
Micronase Tablets 2350

Insulin, Human (Increased insulin requirements).
No products indexed under this heading.

Insulin, Human Isophane Suspension (Increased insulin requirements). Products include:
Humulin N, 100 Units 1270

Insulin, Human NPH (Increased insulin requirements). Products include:
Insulatard NPH Human 1627
Novolin N 1627
Novolin N PenFill Cartridges 1628
Novolin N Prefilled 1628

Insulin, Human Regular (Increased insulin requirements). Products include:
Humulin BR, 100 Units 1268
Humulin R, 100 Units 1272
Novolin R 1627
Novolin R PenFill Cartridges 1628
Novolin R Prefilled 1629
Velosulin Human 1628

Insulin, Human, Zinc Suspension (Increased insulin requirements). Products include:
Humulin L, 100 Units 1268
Humulin U, 100 Units 1272
Novolin L 1627

Insulin, NPH (Increased insulin requirements). Products include:
NPH, 40 & 100 Units 1273
Beef NPH, 100 Units 1274
Pork NPH, 100 Units 1275
Insulatard NPH 1626
NPH Insulin 1626
NPH Purified Pork Isophane Insulin 1626

Insulin, Regular (Increased insulin requirements). Products include:
Regular, 40 & 100 Units 1273
Beef Regular, 100 Units 1275
Pork Regular, 100 Units 1275
Pork Regular (Concentrated), 500 Units 1276
Regular Insulin 1625
Regular Purified Pork Insulin 1626
Velosulin 1627

Insulin, Zinc Crystals (Increased insulin requirements). Products include:
NPH, 40 & 100 Units 1273

Insulin, Zinc Suspension (Increased insulin requirements). Products include:
Lente, 40 & 100 Units 1272
Protamine, Zinc, 40 & 100 Units 1273
Lente Iletin I 1272
Beef Lente, 100 Units 1274
Beef Protamine Zinc, 100 Units 1274
Pork Lente, 100 Units 1275
Pork, Protamine, Zinc, 100 Units 1275
Lente Insulin 1626
Lente Purified Pork Insulin 1626
Semilente Insulin 1625
Ultralente Insulin 1626

Levonorgestrel (Increased thyroid requirements). Products include:
Levlen/Tri-Levlen 665
Nordette-21 Tablets 2481
Nordette-28 Tablets 2483
Norplant System 2484
Levlen/Tri-Levlen 665
Triphasil-21 Tablets 2527
Triphasil-28 Tablets 2532

Mestranol (Increased thyroid requirements). Products include:
Enovid 2161
Norethin 2133
Norinyl 2304
Ortho-Novum 1667

Norethindrone (Increased thyroid requirements). Products include:
Brevicon 2304
Jenest-28 Tablets 1636
Micronor Tablets 1667
Modicon 1667
Norethin 2133
Norinyl 2304
Norlutin 1755
Nor-Q D Tablets 2304
Ortho-Novum 1667
Ovcon 1391
Tri-Norinyl 2304

Norethynodrel (Increased thyroid requirements). Products include:
Enovid 2161

Norgestimate (Increased thyroid requirements). Products include:
Ortho-Cyclen Tablets 1658

Norgestrel (Increased thyroid requirements). Products include:
Lo/Ovral Tablets 2471
Lo/Ovral-28 Tablets 2476
Ovral Tablets 2490
Ovral-28 Tablets 2491
Ovrette Tablets 2492

Polyestradiol Phosphate (Increased thyroid requirements). Products include:
Estradurin 2452

Quinestrol (Increased thyroid requirements). Products include:
Estrovis 1721

Tolazamide (Increased oral hypoglycemic requirements). Products include:
Tolinase Tablets 2365

Tolbutamide (Increased oral hypoglycemic requirements). Products include:
Orinase Tablets 2354

Warfarin Sodium (Increased catabolism of Vitamin K-dependent clotting factors). Products include:
Coumadin Injection & Tablets 944
Panwarfin Tablets 547

Food Interactions

Soybean formula, children's (May cause excessive fecal loss).

EVAC-U-GEN MILD LAXATIVE
(Phenolphthalein, Yellow) .... ▣ 739
No interactions described in labeling.

ASPIRIN FREE EXCEDRIN ANALGESIC CAPLETS
(Acetaminophen, Caffeine)................. 748
No interactions described in labeling.

EXCEDRIN EXTRA-STRENGTH ANALGESIC TABLETS & CAPLETS
(Acetaminophen, Aspirin, Caffeine) .. 749
May interact with:

Antiarthritic Drugs, unspecified (Effect not specified).
Anticoagulant Drugs, unspecified (Effect not specified).
Antidiabetic Drugs, unspecified (Effect not specified).
Antigout Drugs, unspecified (Effect not specified).

EXCEDRIN P.M. ANALGESIC/SLEEPING AID TABLETS, CAPLETS AND LIQUID
(Acetaminophen, Diphenhydramine Citrate) 749
May interact with hypnotics and sedatives, tranquilizers, and certain other agents. Compounds in these categories include:

Alcohol (Effect not specified).
Alprazolam (Effect not specified). Products include:
Xanax Tablets 2367
Buspirone Hydrochloride (Effect not specified). Products include:
BuSpar 1401
Chlordiazepoxide (Effect not specified). Products include:
Libritabs Tablets 1930
Limbitrol 1933
Menrium Tablets 1934
Chlordiazepoxide Hydrochloride (Effect not specified). Products include:
Librax Capsules 1929
Librium Capsules 1931
Librium Injectable 1932
Chlorpromazine (Effect not specified). Products include:
Thorazine 2234
Chlorprothixene (Effect not specified). Products include:
Taractan Tablets 1920
Chlorprothixene Hydrochloride (Effect not specified). Products include:
Taractan 1920
Clorazepate Dipotassium (Effect not specified). Products include:
Tranxene 556
Diazepam (Effect not specified). Products include:
Valium Injectable 1937
Valium Tablets 1939
Valrelease Capsules 1923
Droperidol (Effect not specified). Products include:
Inapsine Injection 1140
Innovar Injection 1141
Estazolam (Effect not specified). Products include:
ProSom Tablets 554
Ethchlorvynol (Effect not specified). Products include:
Placidyl Capsules 553
Ethinamate (Effect not specified).
No products indexed under this heading.
Fluphenazine Decanoate (Effect not specified). Products include:
Prolixin Decanoate 1795
Fluphenazine Enanthate (Effect not specified). Products include:
Prolixin Enanthate 1796
Fluphenazine Hydrochloride (Effect not specified). Products include:
Prolixin Elixir 1793
Prolixin Injection 1791
Prolixin Oral Concentrate 1792
Prolixin Tablets 1793
Flurazepam Hydrochloride (Effect not specified). Products include:
Dalmane Capsules 1927
Glutethimide (Effect not specified).
No products indexed under this heading.
Haloperidol (Effect not specified). Products include:
Haldol Injection, Tablets and Concentrate 1373
Haloperidol Decanoate (Effect not specified). Products include:
Haldol Decanoate 1375
Hydroxyzine Hydrochloride (Effect not specified). Products include:
Atarax Tablets & Syrup 1941
Marax Tablets & DF Syrup 1954
Vistaril Intramuscular Solution 1970
Lorazepam (Effect not specified). Products include:
Ativan Injection 2432
Ativan Tablets 2434
Loxapine Hydrochloride (Effect not specified). Products include:
Loxitane 1213
Loxapine Succinate (Effect not specified). Products include:
Loxitane Capsules 1213
Meprobamate (Effect not specified). Products include:
Deprol Tablets 2382
Equagesic Tablets 2451
Miltown Tablets 2386
PMB 200 and PMB 400 2504
Mesoridazine Besylate (Effect not specified).
Midazolam Hydrochloride (Effect not specified). Products include:
Versed Injection 1924
Molindone Hydrochloride (Effect not specified). Products include:
Moban Tablets & Concentrate 932
Oxazepam (Effect not specified). Products include:
Serax Capsules 2522
Serax Tablets 2522
Perphenazine (Effect not specified). Products include:
Etrafon 2087
Triavil Tablets 1556
Trilafon 2123
Prazepam (Effect not specified). Products include:
Centrax 1693
Prochlorperazine (Effect not specified). Products include:
Compazine 2201
Promethazine Hydrochloride (Effect not specified). Products include:
Mepergan Injection 2479
Phenergan with Codeine 2497
Phenergan with Dextromethorphan 2499
Phenergan Injection 2493
Phenergan Suppositories 2496
Phenergan Syrup 2495
Phenergan Tablets 2496
Phenergan VC 2500
Phenergan VC with Codeine 2501
Propofol (Effect not specified). Products include:
Diprivan Injection 2267
Quazepam (Effect not specified). Products include:
Doral Tablets 2383
Secobarbital Sodium (Effect not specified). Products include:
Seconal Sodium Pulvules 1296
Temazepam (Effect not specified). Products include:
Restoril Capsules 2023
Thioridazine Hydrochloride (Effect not specified). Products include:
Mellaril 2011
Thiothixene (Effect not specified). Products include:
Navane Capsules and Concentrate 1954
Navane Intramuscular 1956
Triazolam (Effect not specified). Products include:
Halcion Tablets 2340
Trifluoperazine Hydrochloride (Effect not specified). Products include:
Stelazine 2226

SINUS EXCEDRIN ANALGESIC, DECONGESTANT TABLETS & CAPLETS
(Acetaminophen, Pseudoephedrine Hydrochloride) 750
May interact with antihypertensives and antidepressant drugs. Compounds in these categories include:

Acebutolol Hydrochloride (Effect not specified). Products include:
Sectral Capsules 2520
Amitriptyline Hydrochloride (Effect not specified). Products include:
Elavil 2269
Endep Tablets 1927
Etrafon 2087
Limbitrol 1933
Triavil Tablets 1556
Amoxapine (Effect not specified). Products include:
Asendin Tablets 1196
Atenolol (Effect not specified). Products include:
Tenoretic Tablets 1105
Tenormin Tablets and I.V. Injection 1107
Benazepril Hydrochloride (Effect not specified). Products include:
Lotensin Tablets 872
Betaxolol Hydrochloride (Effect not specified). Products include:
Betoptic Sterile Ophthalmic Solution .... ◉ 569
Betoptic S Sterile Ophthalmic Suspension .... ◉ 570
Kerlone Tablets 2172
Bupropion Hydrochloride (Effect not specified). Products include:
Wellbutrin Tablets 821
Captopril (Effect not specified). Products include:
Capoten 2255
Capozide 2258
Carteolol Hydrochloride (Effect not specified). Products include:
Cartrol Tablets 507
Clonidine (Effect not specified). Products include:
Catapres-TTS 677
Clonidine Hydrochloride (Effect not specified). Products include:
Catapres Tablets 676
Combipres Tablets 678
Deserpidine (Effect not specified). Products include:
Enduronyl 518
Harmonyl Tablets 528
Oreticyl 545
Desipramine Hydrochloride (Effect not specified). Products include:
Norpramin Tablets 1340
Diazoxide (Effect not specified). Products include:
Hyperstat I.V. Injection 2095
Proglycem 649
Doxazosin Mesylate (Effect not specified). Products include:
Cardura Tablets 1941
Doxepin Hydrochloride (Effect not specified). Products include:
Sinequan 1960
Enalapril Maleate (Effect not specified). Products include:
Vaseretic Tablets 1559
Vasotec Tablets 1564
Enalaprilat (Effect not specified). Products include:
Vasotec I.V. 1562
Esmolol Hydrochloride (Effect not specified). Products include:
Brevibloc Injection 942
Felodipine (Effect not specified). Products include:
Plendil Extended-Release Tablets 1526
Fluoxetine Hydrochloride (Effect not specified). Products include:
Prozac Pulvules 920
Fosinopril Sodium (Effect not specified). Products include:
Monopril Tablets 1406
Guanabenz Acetate (Effect not specified). Products include:
Wytensin Tablets 2542
Guanethidine Monosulfate (Effect not specified). Products include:
Esimil Tablets 864
Ismelin Tablets 869
Hydralazine Hydrochloride (Effect not specified). Products include:
Apresazide Capsules 854
Apresoline Hydrochloride Parenteral (Ampuls) 856
Apresoline Hydrochloride Tablets .. 855
Apresoline-Esidrix Tablets 857
Ser-Ap-Es Tablets 881
Serpasil-Apresoline Tablets 884
Imipramine Hydrochloride (Effect not specified). Products include:
Tofranil Ampuls 1038
Tofranil Tablets 1039
Imipramine Pamoate (Effect not specified). Products include:
Tofranil-PM Capsules 1041
Isocarboxazid (Effect not specified). Products include:
Marplan Tablets 1906
Isradipine (Effect not specified). Products include:
DynaCirc Capsules 2004
Labetalol Hydrochloride (Effect not specified). Products include:
Normodyne Injection 2108
Normodyne Tablets 2110
Normozide Tablets 2112
Trandate HCT Tablets 579
Trandate Injection 577
Trandate Tablets 579
Lisinopril (Effect not specified). Products include:
Prinivil Tablets 1538
Prinzide Tablets 1540
Zestoretic 2274
Zestril Tablets 2277
Maprotiline Hydrochloride (Effect not specified). Products include:
Ludiomil Tablets 874
Mecamylamine Hydrochloride (Effect not specified). Products include:
Inversine Tablets 1492
Methyldopa (Effect not specified). Products include:
Aldoclor Tablets 1413
Aldomet Oral 1415
Aldoril Tablets 1418

Methyldopate Hydrochloride (Effect not specified). Products include:
- Aldomet Ester HCl Injection ... 1417

Metoprolol Tartrate (Effect not specified). Products include:
- Lopressor Ampuls ... 1032
- Lopressor HCT Tablets ... 1034
- Lopressor Tablets ... 1032

Metyrosine (Effect not specified). Products include:
- Demser Capsules ... 1460

Minoxidil (Effect not specified). Products include:
- Loniten Tablets ... 2346
- Rogaine Topical Solution ... 2357

Nadolol (Effect not specified). Products include:
- Corgard Tablets ... 701
- Corzide Tablets ... 702

Nicardipine Hydrochloride (Effect not specified). Products include:
- Cardene Capsules ... 2290

Nitroglycerin (Effect not specified). Products include:
- Deponit NTG Transdermal Delivery System ... 2143
- Minitran Transdermal Delivery System ... 1312
- Nitro-Bid Ointment ... 1339
- Nitro-Bid Capsules ... 1338
- Nitrodisc ... 2176
- Nitro-Dur (nitroglycerin) Transdermal Infusion System ... 1164
- Nitrogard Tablets ... 1004
- Nitrolingual Spray ... 1846
- Nitrostat Tablets ... 1743
- Transderm-Nitro Transdermal Therapeutic System ... 2283

Nortriptyline Hydrochloride (Effect not specified). Products include:
- Pamelor ... 2019

Penbutolol Sulfate (Effect not specified). Products include:
- Levatol ... 1832

Phenelzine Sulfate (Effect not specified). Products include:
- Nardil ... 1742

Phenoxybenzamine Hydrochloride (Effect not specified). Products include:
- Dibenzyline Capsules ... 2207

Phentolamine Mesylate (Effect not specified). Products include:
- Regitine ... 878

Pindolol (Effect not specified). Products include:
- Visken Tablets ... 2036

Prazosin Hydrochloride (Effect not specified). Products include:
- Minipress Capsules ... 1778
- Minizide Capsules ... 1779

Propranolol Hydrochloride (Effect not specified). Products include:
- Inderal ... 2459
- Inderal LA Long Acting Capsules ... 2461
- Inderide Tablets ... 2463
- Inderide LA Long Acting Capsules ... 2465

Protriptyline Hydrochloride (Effect not specified). Products include:
- Vivactil Tablets ... 1567

Ramipril (Effect not specified). Products include:
- Altace Capsules ... 1086

Rauwolfia Serpentina (Effect not specified). Products include:
- Raudixin Tablets ... 1803
- Rauzide Tablets ... 1804

Rescinnamine (Effect not specified).
- No products indexed under this heading.

Reserpine (Effect not specified). Products include:
- Diupres Tablets ... 1461
- Hydromox R Tablets ... 1209
- Hydropres Tablets ... 1485
- Renese-R Tablets ... 1786
- Salutensin/Salutensin-Demi ... 719
- Ser-Ap-Es Tablets ... 881
- Serpasil Tablets ... 883
- Serpasil-Apresoline Tablets ... 884
- Serpasil-Esidrix Tablets ... 886

Sodium Nitroprusside (Effect not specified). Products include:
- Nipride I.V. Infusion ... 1909

Terazosin Hydrochloride (Effect not specified). Products include:
- Hytrin Tablets ... 529

Timolol Maleate (Effect not specified). Products include:
- Blocadren Tablets ... 1429
- Timolide Tablets ... 1547
- Timoptic in Ocudose ... 1552
- Timoptic Sterile Ophthalmic Solution ... 1550

Tranylcypromine Sulfate (Effect not specified). Products include:
- Parnate Tablets ... 2222

Trazodone Hydrochloride (Effect not specified). Products include:
- Desyrel and Desyrel Dividose ... 1404

Trimethaphan Camsylate (Effect not specified). Products include:
- Arfonad Ampuls ... 1887

Trimipramine Maleate (Effect not specified). Products include:
- Surmontil Capsules ... 2524

EXELDERM CREAM 1.0%
(Sulconazole Nitrate) ... 2398
No interactions described in labeling.

EXELDERM SOLUTION 1.0%
(Sulconazole Nitrate) ... 2399
No interactions described in labeling.

EX-LAX CHOCOLATED LAXATIVE
(Phenolphthalein, Yellow) ... ▣ 686
No interactions described in labeling.

EX-LAX PILLS, UNFLAVORED
(Phenolphthalein, Yellow) ... ▣ 686
No interactions described in labeling.

EXTRA GENTLE EX-LAX
(Docusate Sodium, Phenolphthalein, Yellow) ... ▣ 687
May interact with:

Mineral Oil (Concurrent use with systemic mineral oil is not recommended). Products include:
- AKWA Tears Ointment ... ◉ 208
- Agoral ... ▣ 634
- Aqua Care Cream ... ▣ 616
- Aqua Care Lotion ... ▣ 616
- Aquaphor Antibiotic Formula ... 662
- Aquaphor Healing Ointment, Original Formula ... 662
- Aquaphor Natural Healing Formula ... 662
- Complex 15 Hand & Body Moisturizing Cream ... ▣ 694
- Complex 15 Hand & Body Moisturizing Lotion ... ▣ 695
- Complex 15 Moisturizing Face Cream ... ▣ 695
- Duolube Eye Ointment ... ◉ 258
- Duratears Naturale ... ◉ 216
- Eucerin Dry Skin Care Lotion ... 662
- Eucerin Moisturizing Creme (Unscented) ... 662
- Eucerin Dry Skin Care Lotion (Fragrance-free) ... ▣ 514
- Fleet Mineral Oil Enema ... 992
- Fleet Relief ... 993
- Haley's M-O, Regular & Flavored ... ▣ 569
- Keri Lotion - Original Formula ... ▣ 535
- Lacri-Lube NP Lubricant Ophthalmic Ointment ... ◉ 249
- Lacri-Lube S.O.P. Sterile Ophthalmic Ointment ... ◉ 249
- Nephrox Suspension ... ▣ 563
- Nivea Bath Silk Bath Oil ... ▣ 514
- Nivea Bath Silk Bath & Shower Gel (Extra-Dry Skin) ... ▣ 514
- Nivea Moisturizing Creme ... ▣ 514
- Nivea Moisturizing Lotion (Original Formula) ... ▣ 514
- Nivea Moisturizing Oil ... ▣ 515
- Nivea Skin Oil ... ▣ 515
- Nivea Sun After Sun Lotion ... ▣ 515
- Nutraderm Cream & Lotion ... 1684
- pHisoDerm For Baby ... ▣ 761
- pHisoDerm Skin Cleanser and Conditioner - Regular and Oily ... ▣ 760
- Refresh P.M. Lubricant Ophthalmic Ointment ... ◉ 256
- Replens ... ▣ 556
- Tears Renewed Ointment ... ◉ 209
- Theraplex ClearLotion ... 1410

EXNA TABLETS
(Benzthiazide) ... 1862
May interact with antihypertensives, ganglionic blocking agents, para-aminobenzoic acid based local anesthetics, cardiac glycosides, insulin, barbiturates, narcotic analgesics, and certain other agents. Compounds in these categories include:

Acebutolol Hydrochloride (Additive or potentiated action). Products include:
- Sectral Capsules ... 2520

Alcohol (Aggravates orthostatic hypotension).

Alfentanil Hydrochloride (Aggravates orthostatic hypotension). Products include:
- Alfenta Injection ... 1131

Aprobarbital (Aggravates orthostatic hypotension). Products include:
- Alurate Elixir ... 1883

Atenolol (Additive or potentiated action). Products include:
- Tenoretic Tablets ... 1105
- Tenormin Tablets and I.V. Injection ... 1107

Benazepril Hydrochloride (Additive or potentiated action). Products include:
- Lotensin Tablets ... 872

Bendroflumethiazide (Additive or potentiated action). Products include:
- Corzide Tablets ... 702
- Naturetin Tablets ... 1789
- Rauzide Tablets ... 1804

Betaxolol Hydrochloride (Additive or potentiated action). Products include:
- Betoptic Sterile Ophthalmic Solution ... 569
- Betoptic S Sterile Ophthalmic Suspension ... 570
- Kerlone Tablets ... 2172

Buprenorphine (Aggravates orthostatic hypotension).
- No products indexed under this heading.

Butabarbital (Aggravates orthostatic hypotension). Products include:
- Pyridium Plus ... 1764

Butalbital (Aggravates orthostatic hypotension). Products include:
- Esgic-Plus Tablets ... 1002
- Esgic Tablets & Capsules ... 1001
- Fioricet Tablets ... 2006
- Fiorinal Capsules ... 2007
- Fiorinal with Codeine Capsules ... 2008
- Fiorinal Tablets ... 2007
- Phrenilin ... 838
- Sedapap Tablets 50 mg/650 mg ... 1360

Captopril (Additive or potentiated action). Products include:
- Capoten ... 2255
- Capozide ... 2258

Carteolol Hydrochloride (Additive or potentiated action). Products include:
- Cartrol Tablets ... 507

Chlorothiazide (Additive or potentiated action). Products include:
- Aldoclor Tablets ... 1413
- Diupres Tablets ... 1461
- Diuril Oral ... 1464

Chlorothiazide Sodium (Additive or potentiated action). Products include:
- Diuril Sodium Intravenous ... 1463

Chlorthalidone (Additive or potentiated action). Products include:
- Combipres Tablets ... 678
- Tenoretic Tablets ... 1105
- Thalitone Tablets ... 687

Clonidine (Additive or potentiated action). Products include:
- Catapres-TTS ... 677

Clonidine Hydrochloride (Additive or potentiated action). Products include:
- Catapres Tablets ... 676
- Combipres Tablets ... 678

Codeine (Aggravates orthostatic hypotension). Products include:
- Calcidrine Syrup ... 506

Codeine Phosphate (Aggravates orthostatic hypotension). Products include:
- Actifed with Codeine Cough Syrup ... 752
- Cheracol Cough Syrup ... 1853
- Codimal PH Syrup ... 846
- Dimetane-DC Cough Syrup ... 1857
- Empirin with Codeine Phosphate Nos. 2, 3 & 4 ... 764
- Fiorinal with Codeine Capsules ... 2008
- Isoclor Expectorant ... 982
- Naldecon CX Adult Liquid ... ▣ 521
- Novahistine DH ... 1342
- Novahistine Expectorant ... 1343
- Nucofed Capsules ... 2219
- Nucofed Expectorant ... 2219
- Nucofed Pediatric Expectorant ... 2220
- Nucofed Syrup ... 2219
- Phenaphen with Codeine Capsules ... 1865
- Phenaphen-650 with Codeine Tablets ... 1866
- Phenergan with Codeine ... 2497
- Phenergan VC with Codeine ... 2501
- Robitussin A-C Syrup ... 1875
- Robitussin-DAC Syrup ... 1875
- Ryna ... ▣ 741
- Soma Compound w/Codeine Tablets ... 2390
- Triaminic Expectorant w/Codeine ... 1996
- Tussi-Organidin Liquid ... 2391
- Tylenol with Codeine ... 1381

Codeine Polistirex (Aggravates orthostatic hypotension).
- No products indexed under this heading.

Deserpidine (Increased hypotensive effect). Products include:
- Enduronyl ... 518
- Harmonyl Tablets ... 528
- Oreticyl ... 545

Deslanoside (Increased hypokalemia).
- No products indexed under this heading.

Dezocine (Aggravates orthostatic hypotension).

Diazoxide (Additive or potentiated action). Products include:
- Hyperstat I.V. Injection ... 2095
- Proglycem ... 649

Digitoxin (Increased hypokalemia). Products include:
- Crystodigin Tablets ... 1253

Digoxin (Increased hypokalemia). Products include:
- Lanoxicaps ... 772
- Lanoxin Elixir Pediatric ... 775
- Lanoxin Injection ... 778
- Lanoxin Injection Pediatric ... 781
- Lanoxin Tablets ... 783

Doxazosin Mesylate (Additive or potentiated action). Products include:
- Cardura Tablets ... 1941

Enalapril Maleate (Additive or potentiated action). Products include:

Vaseretic Tablets ... 1559
Vasotec Tablets ... 1564

Enalaprilat (Additive or potentiated action). Products include:
Vasotec I.V. ... 1562

Esmolol Hydrochloride (Additive or potentiated action). Products include:
Brevibloc Injection ... 942

Felodipine (Additive or potentiated action). Products include:
Plendil Extended-Release Tablets ... 1526

Fentanyl (Aggravates orthostatic hypotension). Products include:
Duragesic Transdermal System ... 1133

Fentanyl Citrate (Aggravates orthostatic hypotension). Products include:
Innovar Injection ... 1141
Sublimaze Injection ... 1146

Fosinopril Sodium (Additive or potentiated action). Products include:
Monopril Tablets ... 1406

Furosemide (Additive or potentiated action). Products include:
Lasix ... 1093

Guanabenz Acetate (Additive or potentiated action). Products include:
Wytensin Tablets ... 2542

Guanethidine Monosulfate (Increased hypotensive effect). Products include:
Esimil Tablets ... 864
Ismelin Tablets ... 869

Hydralazine Hydrochloride (Additive or potentiated action). Products include:
Apresazide Capsules ... 854
Apresoline Hydrochloride Parenteral (Ampuls) ... 856
Apresoline Hydrochloride Tablets ... 855
Apresoline-Esidrix Tablets ... 857
Ser-Ap-Es Tablets ... 881
Serpasil-Apresoline Tablets ... 884

Hydrochlorothiazide (Additive or potentiated action). Products include:
Aldactazide ... 2150
Aldoril Tablets ... 1418
Apresazide Capsules ... 854
Apresoline-Esidrix Tablets ... 857
Capozide ... 2258
Dyazide Capsules ... 2208
Esidrix Tablets ... 863
Esimil Tablets ... 864
HydroDIURIL Tablets ... 1484
Hydropres Tablets ... 1485
Inderide Tablets ... 2463
Inderide LA Long Acting Capsules ... 2465
Lopressor HCT Tablets ... 1034
Maxzide ... 1215
Moduretic Tablets ... 1510
Normozide Tablets ... 2112
Oretic Tablets ... 544
Oreticyl ... 545
Prinzide Tablets ... 1540
Ser-Ap-Es Tablets ... 881
Serpasil-Esidrix Tablets ... 886
Timolide Tablets ... 1547
Trandate HCT Tablets ... 579
Vaseretic Tablets ... 1559
Zestoretic ... 2274

Hydrocodone Bitartrate (Aggravates orthostatic hypotension). Products include:
Anexsia 5/500 Tablets ... 2196
Anexsia 7.5/650 Tablets ... 2197
Azdone Tablets ... 844
Codiclear DH Syrup ... 845
Codimal DH Syrup ... 846
Damason-P ... 1356
Hycodan Syrup, Tablets ... 927
Hycomine Compound Tablets ... 929
Hycomine Syrup ... 927
Hycotuss Expectorant Syrup ... 930
Hydrocet Capsules ... 835
Lortab ASA Tablets ... 2414
Lortab ... 2412
Ru-Tuss with Hydrocodone ... 694
Triaminic Expectorant DH ... 1995
Vicodin Tablets ... 1187
Vicodin ES Tablets ... 1189
Zydone Capsules ... 941

Hydrocodone Polistirex (Aggravates orthostatic hypotension). Products include:
Tussionex Extended-Release Suspension ... 988

Hydroflumethiazide (Additive or potentiated action). Products include:
Diucardin Tablets ... 2450
Saluron ... 718
Salutensin/Salutensin-Demi ... 719

Indapamide (Additive or potentiated action). Products include:
Lozol Tablets ... 1843

Insulin, Human (Increased, decreased or unchanged insulin requirement).
No products indexed under this heading.

Insulin, Human Isophane Suspension (Increased, decreased or unchanged insulin requirement). Products include:
Humulin N, 100 Units ... 1270

Insulin, Human NPH (Increased, decreased or unchanged insulin requirement). Products include:
Insulatard NPH Human ... 1627
Novolin N ... 1627
Novolin N PenFill Cartridges ... 1628
Novolin N Prefilled ... 1628

Insulin, Human Regular (Increased, decreased or unchanged insulin requirement). Products include:
Humulin BR, 100 Units ... 1268
Humulin R, 100 Units ... 1272
Novolin R ... 1627
Novolin R PenFill Cartridges ... 1628
Novolin R Prefilled ... 1629
Velosulin Human ... 1628

Insulin, Human, Zinc Suspension (Increased, decreased or unchanged insulin requirement). Products include:
Humulin L, 100 Units ... 1268
Humulin U, 100 Units ... 1272
Novolin L ... 1627

Insulin, NPH (Increased, decreased or unchanged insulin requirement). Products include:
NPH, 40 & 100 Units ... 1273
Beef NPH, 100 Units ... 1274
Pork NPH, 100 Units ... 1275
Insulatard NPH ... 1626
NPH Insulin ... 1626
NPH Purified Pork Isophane Insulin ... 1626

Insulin, Regular (Increased, decreased or unchanged insulin requirement). Products include:
Regular, 40 & 100 Units ... 1273
Beef Regular, 100 Units ... 1275
Pork Regular, 100 Units ... 1275
Pork Regular (Concentrated), 500 Units ... 1276
Regular Insulin ... 1625
Regular Purified Pork Insulin ... 1626
Velosulin ... 1627

Insulin, Zinc Crystals (Increased, decreased or unchanged insulin requirement). Products include:
NPH, 40 & 100 Units ... 1273

Insulin, Zinc Suspension (Increased, decreased or unchanged insulin requirement). Products include:
Lente, 40 & 100 Units ... 1272
Protamine, Zinc, 40 & 100 Units ... 1273
Lente Iletin I ... 1272
Beef Lente, 100 Units ... 1274
Beef Protamine Zinc, 100 Units ... 1274
Pork Lente, 100 Units ... 1275
Pork, Protamine, Zinc, 100 Units ... 1275
Lente Insulin ... 1626
Lente Purified Pork Insulin ... 1626
Semilente Insulin ... 1625
Ultralente Insulin ... 1626

Isradipine (Additive or potentiated action). Products include:
DynaCirc Capsules ... 2004

Labetalol Hydrochloride (Additive or potentiated action). Products include:
Normodyne Injection ... 2108
Normodyne Tablets ... 2110
Normozide Tablets ... 2112
Trandate HCT Tablets ... 579
Trandate Injection ... 577
Trandate Tablets ... 579

Levorphanol Tartrate (Aggravates orthostatic hypotension). Products include:
Levo-Dromoran ... 1906

Lisinopril (Additive or potentiated action). Products include:
Prinivil Tablets ... 1538
Prinzide Tablets ... 1540
Zestoretic ... 2274
Zestril Tablets ... 2277

Mecamylamine Hydrochloride (Increased hypotensive effect). Products include:
Inversine Tablets ... 1492

Meperidine Hydrochloride (Aggravates orthostatic hypotension). Products include:
Demerol ... 2047
Mepergan Injection ... 2479

Mephobarbital (Aggravates orthostatic hypotension). Products include:
Mebaral Tablets ... 2061

Methadone Hydrochloride (Aggravates orthostatic hypotension). Products include:
Dolophine Hydrochloride Ampoules & Vials ... 1260
Dolophine Hydrochloride Tablets ... 1261
Methadone Hydrochloride Diskets ... 1284
Methadone Hydrochloride Oral Solution & Tablets ... 1987

Methyclothiazide (Additive or potentiated action). Products include:
Enduron Tablets ... 517
Enduronyl ... 518

Methyldopa (Additive or potentiated action). Products include:
Aldoclor Tablets ... 1413
Aldomet Oral ... 1415
Aldoril Tablets ... 1418

Methyldopate Hydrochloride (Additive or potentiated action). Products include:
Aldomet Ester HCl Injection ... 1417

Metolazone (Additive or potentiated action). Products include:
Diulo ... 2129
Mykrox ½ mg Tablets ... 984
Zaroxolyn Tablets ... 989

Metoprolol Tartrate (Additive or potentiated action). Products include:
Lopressor Ampuls ... 1032
Lopressor HCT Tablets ... 1034
Lopressor Tablets ... 1032

Metyrosine (Additive or potentiated action). Products include:
Demser Capsules ... 1460

Minoxidil (Additive or potentiated action). Products include:
Loniten Tablets ... 2346
Rogaine Topical Solution ... 2357

Morphine Sulfate (Aggravates orthostatic hypotension). Products include:
Astramorph/PF Injection, USP (Preservative-Free) ... 618
Duramorph ... 960
Infumorph 200 and Infumorph 500 Sterile Solutions ... 962
MS Contin Tablets ... 1814
MSIR ... 1817
Oramorph SR (Morphine Sulfate Sustained Release Tablets) ... 1988
Roxanol ... 1991

Nadolol (Additive or potentiated action). Products include:
Corgard Tablets ... 701
Corzide Tablets ... 702

Nicardipine Hydrochloride (Additive or potentiated action). Products include:
Cardene Capsules ... 2290

Nitroglycerin (Additive or potentiated action). Products include:
Deponit NTG Transdermal Delivery System ... 2143
Minitran Transdermal Delivery System ... 1312
Nitro-Bid Ointment ... 1339
Nitro-Bid Capsules ... 1338
Nitrodisc ... 2176
Nitro-Dur (nitroglycerin) Transdermal Infusion System ... 1164
Nitrogard Tablets ... 1004
Nitrolingual Spray ... 1846
Nitrostat Tablets ... 1743
Transderm-Nitro Transdermal Therapeutic System ... 2283

Norepinephrine Bitartrate (Decreased arterial response to norepinephrine). Products include:
Levophed Bitartrate Injection ... 2054

Opium Alkaloids (Aggravates orthostatic hypotension). Products include:
B & O No. 15A & No. 16A Supprettes ... 2395
Pantopon Injectable ... 1911

Oxycodone Hydrochloride (Aggravates orthostatic hypotension). Products include:
Percocet Tablets ... 950
Percodan ... 951
Roxicodone Tablets, Oral Solution & Intensol (Oxycodone) ... 1992
Tylox Capsules ... 1382

Penbutolol Sulfate (Additive or potentiated action). Products include:
Levatol ... 1832

Pentobarbital Sodium (Aggravates orthostatic hypotension). Products include:
Nembutal Sodium Capsules ... 534
Nembutal Sodium Solution ... 536
Nembutal Sodium Suppositories ... 538

Phenobarbital (Aggravates orthostatic hypotension). Products include:
Arco-Lase Plus Tablets ... 607
Bellergal-S Tablets ... 1998
Bronkolixir ... ▣ 761
Bronkotabs Tablets ... ▣ 762
Donnatal ... 1858
Donnatal Extentabs ... 1859
Donnatal Tablets ... 1858
Donnazyme Tablets ... 1860
Kinesed Tablets ... 2272
Phenobarbital Elixir and Tablets ... 1293
Primatene Tablets-P Formula ... 2421
Quadrinal Tablets ... 1183
Tedral SA ... 1765

Phenoxybenzamine Hydrochloride (Additive or potentiated action). Products include:
Dibenzyline Capsules ... 2207

Phentolamine Mesylate (Additive or potentiated action). Products include:
Regitine ... 878

Pindolol (Additive or potentiated action). Products include:
Visken Tablets ... 2036

Polythiazide (Additive or potentiated action). Products include:
Minizide Capsules ... 1779
Renese Tablets ... 1785
Renese-R Tablets ... 1786

Prazosin Hydrochloride (Increased hypotensive effect). Products include:
Minipress Capsules ... 1778
Minizide Capsules ... 1779

Propoxyphene Hydrochloride (Aggravates orthostatic hypotension). Products include:
Darvon ... 1256
Wygesic Tablets ... 2540

Propoxyphene Napsylate (Aggravates orthostatic hypotension). Products include:
- Darvon-N/Darvocet-N 1254

Propranolol Hydrochloride (Additive or potentiated action). Products include:
- Inderal 2459
- Inderal LA Long Acting Capsules 2461
- Inderide Tablets 2463
- Inderide LA Long Acting Capsules .. 2465

Ramipril (Additive or potentiated action). Products include:
- Altace Capsules 1086

Rauwolfia Serpentina (Increased hypotensive effect). Products include:
- Raudixin Tablets 1803
- Rauzide Tablets 1804

Rescinnamine (Increased hypotensive effect).
- No products indexed under this heading.

Reserpine (Increased hypotensive effect). Products include:
- Diupres Tablets 1461
- Hydromox R Tablets 1209
- Hydropres Tablets 1485
- Renese-R Tablets 1786
- Salutensin/Salutensin-Demi 719
- Ser-Ap-Es Tablets 881
- Serpasil Tablets 883
- Serpasil-Apresoline Tablets 884
- Serpasil-Esidrix Tablets 886

Secobarbital Sodium (Aggravates orthostatic hypotension). Products include:
- Seconal Sodium Pulvules 1296

Sodium Nitroprusside (Additive or potentiated action). Products include:
- Nipride I.V. Infusion 1909

Sufentanil Citrate (Aggravates orthostatic hypotension). Products include:
- Sufenta Injection 1147

Terazosin Hydrochloride (Additive or potentiated action). Products include:
- Hytrin Tablets 529

Thiamylal Sodium (Aggravates orthostatic hypotension). Products include:
- Surital Ampoules, Steri-Vials........ 1764

Timolol Maleate (Additive or potentiated action). Products include:
- Blocadren Tablets 1429
- Timolide Tablets 1547
- Timoptic in Ocudose 1552
- Timoptic Sterile Ophthalmic Solution 1550

Trimethaphan Camsylate (Increased hypotensive effect). Products include:
- Arfonad Ampuls 1887

Tubocurarine Chloride (Increased response to tubocurarine).
- No products indexed under this heading.

EXOSURF NEONATAL FOR INTRATRACHEAL SUSPENSION
(Colfosceril Palmitate)........ 765
No interactions described in labeling.

EXTENDRYL CHEWABLE TABLETS
(Allergy remedy) 994
No interactions described in labeling.

EXTENDRYL SR. & JR. T.D. CAPSULES
(Allergy remedy) 994
No interactions described in labeling.

EXTENDRYL SYRUP
(Allergy remedy) 994
No interactions described in labeling.

EYESCRUB EYELID CLEANSER
(Disodium Laureth Sulfosuccinate, PEG-200 Glyceryl Tallowate) .... ⊙ 269
No interactions described in labeling.

EYE-STREAM
(Balanced Salt Solution) 571
No interactions described in labeling.

EYE WASH
(Isotonic Solution)........ ▣ 511
No interactions described in labeling.

4-WAY COLD TABLETS
(Acetaminophen, Chlorpheniramine Maleate, Phenylpropanolamine Hydrochloride) 750
May interact with antihypertensives and antidepressant drugs. Compounds in these categories include:

Acebutolol Hydrochloride (Concurrent use is not recommended). Products include:
- Sectral Capsules 2520

Alcohol (Increases drowsiness effect).

Amitriptyline Hydrochloride (Concurrent use is not recommended). Products include:
- Elavil 2269
- Endep Tablets 1927
- Etrafon 2087
- Limbitrol 1933
- Triavil Tablets 1556

Amoxapine (Concurrent use is not recommended). Products include:
- Asendin Tablets 1196

Atenolol (Concurrent use is not recommended). Products include:
- Tenoretic Tablets 1105
- Tenormin Tablets and I.V. Injection 1107

Benazepril Hydrochloride (Concurrent use is not recommended). Products include:
- Lotensin Tablets 872

Betaxolol Hydrochloride (Concurrent use is not recommended). Products include:
- Betoptic Sterile Ophthalmic Solution 569
- Betoptic S Sterile Ophthalmic Suspension 570
- Kerlone Tablets 2172

Bupropion Hydrochloride (Concurrent use is not recommended). Products include:
- Wellbutrin Tablets 821

Captopril (Concurrent use is not recommended). Products include:
- Capoten 2255
- Capozide 2258

Carteolol Hydrochloride (Concurrent use is not recommended). Products include:
- Cartrol Tablets 507

Clonidine (Concurrent use is not recommended). Products include:
- Catapres-TTS 677

Clonidine Hydrochloride (Concurrent use is not recommended). Products include:
- Catapres Tablets 676
- Combipres Tablets 678

Deserpidine (Concurrent use is not recommended). Products include:
- Enduronyl 518
- Harmonyl Tablets 528
- Oreticyl 545

Desipramine Hydrochloride (Concurrent use is not recommended). Products include:
- Norpramin Tablets 1340

Diazoxide (Concurrent use is not recommended). Products include:
- Hyperstat I.V. Injection 2095
- Proglycem 649

Doxazosin Mesylate (Concurrent use is not recommended). Products include:
- Cardura Tablets 1941

Doxepin Hydrochloride (Concurrent use is not recommended). Products include:
- Sinequan 1960

Enalapril Maleate (Concurrent use is not recommended). Products include:
- Vaseretic Tablets 1559
- Vasotec Tablets 1564

Enalaprilat (Concurrent use is not recommended). Products include:
- Vasotec I.V. 1562

Esmolol Hydrochloride (Concurrent use is not recommended). Products include:
- Brevibloc Injection 942

Felodipine (Concurrent use is not recommended). Products include:
- Plendil Extended-Release Tablets 1526

Fluoxetine Hydrochloride (Concurrent use is not recommended). Products include:
- Prozac Pulvules 920

Fosinopril Sodium (Concurrent use is not recommended). Products include:
- Monopril Tablets 1406

Guanabenz Acetate (Concurrent use is not recommended). Products include:
- Wytensin Tablets 2542

Guanethidine Monosulfate (Concurrent use is not recommended). Products include:
- Esimil Tablets 864
- Ismelin Tablets 869

Hydralazine Hydrochloride (Concurrent use is not recommended). Products include:
- Apresazide Capsules 854
- Apresoline Hydrochloride Parenteral (Ampuls) 856
- Apresoline Hydrochloride Tablets .. 855
- Apresoline-Esidrix Tablets 857
- Ser-Ap-Es Tablets 881
- Serpasil-Apresoline Tablets 884

Imipramine Hydrochloride (Concurrent use is not recommended). Products include:
- Tofranil Ampuls 1038
- Tofranil Tablets 1039

Imipramine Pamoate (Concurrent use is not recommended). Products include:
- Tofranil-PM Capsules 1041

Isocarboxazid (Concurrent use is not recommended). Products include:
- Marplan Tablets 1906

Isradipine (Concurrent use is not recommended). Products include:
- DynaCirc Capsules 2004

Labetalol Hydrochloride (Concurrent use is not recommended). Products include:
- Normodyne Injection 2108
- Normodyne Tablets 2110
- Normozide Tablets 2112
- Trandate HCT Tablets 579
- Trandate Injection 577
- Trandate Tablets 579

Lisinopril (Concurrent use is not recommended). Products include:
- Prinivil Tablets 1538
- Prinzide Tablets 1540
- Zestoretic 2274
- Zestril Tablets 2277

Maprotiline Hydrochloride (Concurrent use is not recommended). Products include:
- Ludiomil Tablets 874

Mecamylamine Hydrochloride (Concurrent use is not recommended). Products include:
- Inversine Tablets 1492

Methyldopa (Concurrent use is not recommended). Products include:
- Aldoclor Tablets 1413
- Aldomet Oral 1415
- Aldoril Tablets 1418

Methyldopate Hydrochloride (Concurrent use is not recommended). Products include:
- Aldomet Ester HCl Injection 1417

Metoprolol Tartrate (Concurrent use is not recommended). Products include:
- Lopressor Ampuls 1032
- Lopressor HCT Tablets 1034
- Lopressor Tablets 1032

Metyrosine (Concurrent use is not recommended). Products include:
- Demser Capsules 1460

Minoxidil (Concurrent use is not recommended). Products include:
- Loniten Tablets 2346
- Rogaine Topical Solution 2357

Nadolol (Concurrent use is not recommended). Products include:
- Corgard Tablets 701
- Corzide Tablets 702

Nicardipine Hydrochloride (Concurrent use is not recommended). Products include:
- Cardene Capsules 2290

Nitroglycerin (Concurrent use is not recommended). Products include:
- Deponit NTG Transdermal Delivery System 2143
- Minitran Transdermal Delivery System 1312
- Nitro-Bid Ointment 1339
- Nitro-Bid Capsules 1338
- Nitrodisc 2176
- Nitro-Dur (nitroglycerin) Transdermal Infusion System 1164
- Nitrogard Tablets 1004
- Nitrolingual Spray 1846
- Nitrostat Tablets 1743
- Transderm-Nitro Transdermal Therapeutic System 2283

Nortriptyline Hydrochloride (Concurrent use is not recommended). Products include:
- Pamelor 2019

Penbutolol Sulfate (Concurrent use is not recommended). Products include:
- Levatol 1832

Phenelzine Sulfate (Concurrent use is not recommended). Products include:
- Nardil 1742

Phenoxybenzamine Hydrochloride (Concurrent use is not recommended). Products include:
- Dibenzyline Capsules 2207

Phentolamine Mesylate (Concurrent use is not recommended). Products include:
- Regitine 878

Pindolol (Concurrent use is not recommended). Products include:
- Visken Tablets 2036

Prazosin Hydrochloride (Concurrent use is not recommended). Products include:
- Minipress Capsules 1778
- Minizide Capsules 1779

Propranolol Hydrochloride (Concurrent use is not recommended). Products include:
- Inderal 2459
- Inderal LA Long Acting Capsules 2461
- Inderide Tablets 2463
- Inderide LA Long Acting Capsules .. 2465

Protriptyline Hydrochloride (Concurrent use is not recommended). Products include:
- Vivactil Tablets 1567

Ramipril (Concurrent use is not recommended). Products include:
- Altace Capsules ... 1086

Rauwolfia Serpentina (Concurrent use is not recommended). Products include:
- Raudixin Tablets ... 1803
- Rauzide Tablets ... 1804

Rescinnamine (Concurrent use is not recommended).
- No products indexed under this heading.

Reserpine (Concurrent use is not recommended). Products include:
- Diupres Tablets ... 1461
- Hydromox R Tablets ... 1209
- Hydropres Tablets ... 1485
- Renese-R Tablets ... 1786
- Salutensin/Salutensin-Demi ... 719
- Ser-Ap-Es Tablets ... 881
- Serpasil Tablets ... 883
- Serpasil-Apresoline Tablets ... 884
- Serpasil-Esidrix Tablets ... 886

Sodium Nitroprusside (Concurrent use is not recommended). Products include:
- Nipride I.V. Infusion ... 1909

Terazosin Hydrochloride (Concurrent use is not recommended). Products include:
- Hytrin Tablets ... 529

Timolol Maleate (Concurrent use is not recommended). Products include:
- Blocadren Tablets ... 1429
- Timolide Tablets ... 1547
- Timoptic in Ocudose ... 1552
- Timoptic Sterile Ophthalmic Solution ... 1550

Tranylcypromine Sulfate (Concurrent use is not recommended). Products include:
- Parnate Tablets ... 2222

Trazodone Hydrochloride (Concurrent use is not recommended). Products include:
- Desyrel and Desyrel Dividose ... 1404

Trimethaphan Camsylate (Concurrent use is not recommended). Products include:
- Arfonad Ampuls ... 1887

Trimipramine Maleate (Concurrent use is not recommended). Products include:
- Surmontil Capsules ... 2524

4-WAY FAST ACTING NASAL SPRAY - ORIGINAL FORMULA (REGULAR & MENTHOLATED) & METERED SPRAY PUMP (REGULAR)
(Naphazoline Hydrochloride, Phenylephrine Hydrochloride, Pyrilamine Maleate) ... 751
No interactions described in labeling.

4-WAY LONG LASTING NASAL SPRAY & METERED SPRAY PUMP
(Oxymetazoline Hydrochloride) ... 751
No interactions described in labeling.

FML FORTE LIQUIFILM
(Fluorometholone) ... ⊙ 245
No interactions described in labeling.

FML LIQUIFILM
(Fluorometholone) ... ⊙ 244
No interactions described in labeling.

FML S.O.P.
(Fluorometholone) ... ⊙ 245
No interactions described in labeling.

FML-S STERILE OPHTHALMIC SUSPENSION
(Sulfacetamide Sodium, Fluorometholone) ... ⊙ 246
May interact with silver preparations. Compounds in this category include:

Silver Nitrate (Physical incompatibility).

STERILE FUDR
(Floxuridine) ... 1898
May interact with alkylating agents and bone marrow depressants. Compounds in these categories include:

Bone Marrow Depressants, unspecified (Increased toxicity of FUDR).

Busulfan (FUDR should be used with extreme caution in patients with previous use of alkylating agents). Products include:
- Myleran Tablets ... 790

Carmustine (BCNU) (FUDR should be used with extreme caution in patients with previous use of alkylating agents). Products include:
- BiCNU ... 723

Chlorambucil (FUDR should be used with extreme caution in patients with previous use of alkylating agents). Products include:
- Leukeran Tablets ... 788

Cyclophosphamide (FUDR should be used with extreme caution in patients with previous use of alkylating agents). Products include:
- Cytoxan for Injection ... 726
- Neosar for Injection ... 566

Dacarbazine (FUDR should be used with extreme caution in patients with previous use of alkylating agents). Products include:
- DTIC-Dome ... 1595

Lomustine (CCNU) (FUDR should be used with extreme caution in patients with previous use of alkylating agents). Products include:
- CeeNU ... 725

Mechlorethamine Hydrochloride (FUDR should be used with extreme caution in patients with previous use of alkylating agents). Products include:
- Mustargen ... 1514

Melphalan (FUDR should be used with extreme caution in patients with previous use of alkylating agents). Products include:
- Alkeran Tablets ... 754

Thiotepa (FUDR should be used with extreme caution in patients with previous use of alkylating agents). Products include:
- Thiotepa Parenteral ... 1240

FACT PLUS PREGNANCY TEST
(HCG Monoclonal Antibody) ... ▣ 773
No interactions described in labeling.

FACTREL
(Gonadorelin Hydrochloride) ... 2561
May interact with androgens, estrogens, progestins, corticosteroids, oral contraceptives, phenothiazines, dopamine antagonists, and certain other agents. Compounds in these categories include:

Betamethasone (Pituitary secretion of gonadotropins affected).

Betamethasone Acetate (Pituitary secretion of gonadotropins affected). Products include:
- Celestone Soluspan Suspension ... 2081

Betamethasone Sodium Phosphate (Pituitary secretion of gonadotropins affected). Products include:
- Celestone Soluspan Suspension ... 2081

Chlorotrianisene (Pituitary secretion of gonadotropins affected). Products include:
- TACE 12 and 25 mg ... 1353

Chlorpromazine (Rise in prolactin; response to Factrel may be blunted). Products include:
- Thorazine ... 2234

Clozapine (Rise in prolactin; response to Factrel may be blunted). Products include:
- Clozaril Tablets ... 2000

Cortisone Acetate (Pituitary secretion of gonadotropins affected). Products include:
- Cortone Acetate Sterile Suspension ... 1437
- Cortone Acetate Tablets ... 1439

Dexamethasone (Pituitary secretion of gonadotropins affected). Products include:
- AK-Trol Ointment & Suspension ... ⊙ 207
- Decadron Elixir ... 1445
- Decadron Tablets ... 1447
- Decaspray Topical Aerosol ... 1459
- Dexacidin ... ⊙ 272
- Maxidex Sterile Ophthalmic Suspension ... ⊙ 223
- Maxitrol Ophthalmic Ointment/Suspension ... ⊙ 223
- TobraDex Ophthalmic Suspension and Ointment ... ⊙ 228

Dexamethasone Sodium Phosphate (Pituitary secretion of gonadotropins affected). Products include:
- AK-Dex ... ⊙ 203
- Decadron Phosphate Respihaler ... 1454
- Decadron Phosphate Sterile Ophthalmic Ointment ... 1453
- Decadron Phosphate Sterile Ophthalmic Solution ... 1453
- Decadron Phosphate Topical Cream ... 1455
- Decadron Phosphate Turbinaire ... 1456
- Maxidex Sterile Ophthalmic Ointment ... ⊙ 222
- NeoDecadron Sterile Ophthalmic Ointment ... 1517
- NeoDecadron Sterile Ophthalmic Solution ... 1518
- NeoDecadron Topical Cream ... 1518

Dienestrol (Pituitary secretion of gonadotropins affected). Products include:
- Ortho Dienestrol Cream ... 1664

Diethylstilbestrol (Pituitary secretion of gonadotropins affected). Products include:
- Diethylstilbestrol Tablets ... 1258

Digitoxin (Gonadotropin levels suppressed). Products include:
- Crystodigin Tablets ... 1253

Digoxin (Gonadotropin levels suppressed). Products include:
- Lanoxicaps ... 772
- Lanoxin Elixir Pediatric ... 775
- Lanoxin Injection ... 778
- Lanoxin Injection Pediatric ... 781
- Lanoxin Tablets ... 783

Estradiol (Pituitary secretion of gonadotropins affected). Products include:
- Emcyt Capsules ... 1161
- Estrace ... 1385
- Estrace Vaginal Cream ... 1388
- Estraderm Transdermal System ... 866

Estrogens, Conjugated (Pituitary secretion of gonadotropins affected). Products include:
- Mediatric Capsules ... 2476
- PMB 200 and PMB 400 ... 2504
- Premarin Intravenous ... 2508
- Premarin with Methyltestosterone ... 2515
- Premarin Tablets ... 2510
- Premarin Vaginal Cream ... 2512

Estrogens, Esterified (Pituitary secretion of gonadotropins affected). Products include:
- Estratest ... 2245
- Menrium Tablets ... 1934

Estropipate (Pituitary secretion of gonadotropins affected). Products include:
- Ogen ... 540

Ethinyl Estradiol (Pituitary secretion of gonadotropins affected; gonadotropin levels suppressed). Products include:
- Brevicon ... 2304
- Demulen ... 2161
- Estinyl Tablets ... 2085
- Jenest-28 Tablets ... 1636
- Levlen/Tri-Levlen ... 665
- Lo/Ovral Tablets ... 2471
- Lo/Ovral-28 Tablets ... 2476
- Loestrin ... 1728
- Modicon ... 1667
- Nordette-21 Tablets ... 2481
- Nordette-28 Tablets ... 2483
- Norethin ... 2133
- Norinyl ... 2304
- Norlestrin ... 1746
- Ortho-Cyclen Tablets ... 1658
- Ortho-Novum ... 1667
- Ovcon ... 1391
- Ovral Tablets ... 2490
- Ovral-28 Tablets ... 2491
- Levlen/Tri-Levlen ... 665
- Tri-Norinyl ... 2304
- Triphasil-21 Tablets ... 2527
- Triphasil-28 Tablets ... 2532

Ethynodiol Diacetate (Gonadotropin levels suppressed). Products include:
- Demulen ... 2161

Fluoxymesterone (Pituitary secretion of gonadotropins affected). Products include:
- Halotestin Tablets ... 2341

Fluphenazine Decanoate (Rise in prolactin; response to Factrel may be blunted). Products include:
- Prolixin Decanoate ... 1795

Fluphenazine Enanthate (Rise in prolactin; response to Factrel may be blunted). Products include:
- Prolixin Enanthate ... 1796

Fluphenazine Hydrochloride (Rise in prolactin; response to Factrel may be blunted). Products include:
- Prolixin Elixir ... 1793
- Prolixin Injection ... 1791
- Prolixin Oral Concentrate ... 1792
- Prolixin Tablets ... 1793

Haloperidol (Rise in prolactin; response to Factrel may be blunted). Products include:
- Haldol Injection, Tablets and Concentrate ... 1373

Haloperidol Decanoate (Rise in prolactin; response to Factrel may be blunted). Products include:
- Haldol Decanoate ... 1375

Hydrocortisone (Pituitary secretion of gonadotropins affected). Products include:
- AK-Spore H.C. ... ⊙ 206
- Bactine Hydrocortisone Anti-Itch Cream ... ▣ 625
- CaldeCORT Anti-Itch Hydrocortisone Spray ... ▣ 560
- Carmol HC Cream 1% ... 2296
- Cortaid Spray ... ▣ 735
- Cortenema ... 2244
- Cortisporin Ointment ... 758
- Cortisporin Ophthalmic Ointment Sterile ... 758
- Cortisporin Ophthalmic Suspension Sterile ... 759
- Cortisporin Otic Solution Sterile ... 760
- Cortisporin Otic Suspension Sterile ... 760
- Cortizone-5 Creme & Ointment ... ▣ 732
- Dermolate Anti-Itch Cream ... ▣ 697
- Eldecort Cream 1.0% ... 1113
- Eldecort Cream 1.0% and 2.5% ... 1113
- Fungoid HC Creme ... 1770
- Hydrocortone Tablets ... 1482

- Hytone 909
- LazerSporin-C Solution 1770
- Massengill Medicated Soft Cloth Towelettes 2192
- Nutracort Cream & Lotion 1684
- PediOtic Suspension Sterile 797
- Synacort Creams 1%, 2.5% 2296
- Vanoxide-HC Acne Lotion 911
- Vioform-Hydrocortisone Cream and Mild Cream 889
- Vioform-Hydrocortisone Ointment 889
- VōSoL HC Otic Solution 2392
- Vytone Cream 1% 911

Hydrocortisone Acetate (Pituitary secretion of gonadotropins affected). Products include:
- Analpram-HC Rectal Cream 1% and 2.5% 970
- Anusol-HC Cream 1690
- Anusol-HC Suppositories 1691
- Caldecort ⊡ 560
- Carmol HC Cream 1% 2296
- Chloromycetin Hydrocortisone Ophthalmic 1694
- Coly-Mycin S Otic w/Neomycin & Hydrocortisone 1708
- Cortaid ⊡ 735
- Cortef Feminine Itch Cream ⊡ 735
- Corticaine ⊡ 682
- Cortifoam 1827
- Cortisporin Cream 757
- Epifoam 1828
- Gynecort 5 Creme ⊡ 556
- Hydrocortone Acetate Sterile Suspension 1479
- Lanacort 5 Creme and Ointment ⊡ 557
- Mantadil Cream 789
- Ophthocort ⊙ 301
- Orabase HCA Oral Paste 890
- Pramosone Cream, Lotion & Ointment 971
- ProctoCream-HC 1834
- Proctofoam-HC 1835

Hydrocortisone Sodium Phosphate (Pituitary secretion of gonadotropins affected). Products include:
- Hydrocortone Phosphate Injection, Sterile 1481

Hydrocortisone Sodium Succinate (Pituitary secretion of gonadotropins affected). Products include:
- Solu-Cortef Sterile Powder 2361

Levodopa (Minimal elevation of gonadotropin levels). Products include:
- Larodopa Tablets 1905
- Sinemet Tablets 952
- Sinemet CR Tablets 953

Levonorgestrel (Gonadotropin levels suppressed). Products include:
- Levlen/Tri-Levlen 665
- Nordette-21 Tablets 2481
- Nordette-28 Tablets 2483
- Norplant System 2484
- Levlen/Tri-Levlen 665
- Triphasil-21 Tablets 2527
- Triphasil-28 Tablets 2532

Medroxyprogesterone Acetate (Pituitary secretion of gonadotropins affected). Products include:
- Amen 833
- Cycrin Tablets 2449
- Depo-Provera Sterile Aqueous Suspension 2336
- Provera Tablets 2356

Megestrol Acetate (Pituitary secretion of gonadotropins affected). Products include:
- Megace Tablets 732

Mesoridazine Besylate (Rise in prolactin; response to Factrel may be blunted).

Mestranol (Gonadotropin levels suppressed). Products include:
- Enovid 2161
- Norethin 2133
- Norinyl 2304
- Ortho-Novum 1667

Methylprednisolone Acetate (Pituitary secretion of gonadotropins affected). Products include:
- Depo-Medrol Sterile Aqueous Suspension 2334

Methylprednisolone Sodium Succinate (Pituitary secretion of gonadotropins affected). Products include:
- Solu-Medrol Sterile Powder 2363

Methyltestosterone (Pituitary secretion of gonadotropins affected). Products include:
- Android 1111
- Estratest 2245
- Mediatric Capsules 2476
- Metandren Linguets and Tablets 875
- Premarin with Methyltestosterone 2515
- Tested Capsules 1124

Norethindrone (Gonadotropin levels suppressed). Products include:
- Brevicon 2304
- Jenest-28 Tablets 1636
- Micronor Tablets 1667
- Modicon 1667
- Norethin 2133
- Norinyl 2304
- Norlutin 1755
- Nor-Q D Tablets 2304
- Ortho-Novum 1667
- Ovcon 1391
- Tri-Norinyl 2304

Norethynodrel (Gonadotropin levels suppressed). Products include:
- Enovid 2161

Norgestimate (Pituitary secretion of gonadotropins affected; gonadotropin levels suppressed). Products include:
- Ortho-Cyclen Tablets 1658

Norgestrel (Gonadotropin levels suppressed). Products include:
- Lo/Ovral Tablets 2471
- Lo/Ovral-28 Tablets 2476
- Ovral Tablets 2490
- Ovral-28 Tablets 2491
- Ovrette Tablets 2492

Oxandrolone (Pituitary secretion of gonadotropins affected).
- No products indexed under this heading.

Oxymetholone (Pituitary secretion of gonadotropins affected). Products include:
- Anadrol-50 Tablets 2287

Perphenazine (Rise in prolactin; response to Factrel may be blunted). Products include:
- Etrafon 2087
- Triavil Tablets 1556
- Trilafon 2123

Pimozide (Rise in prolactin; response to Factrel may be blunted). Products include:
- Orap Tablets 1020

Polyestradiol Phosphate (Pituitary secretion of gonadotropins affected). Products include:
- Estradurin 2452

Prednisolone Acetate (Pituitary secretion of gonadotropins affected). Products include:
- AK-Cide Sterile Ophthalmic Ointment & Suspension ⊙ 202
- Blephamide Liquifilm Sterile Ophthalmic Suspension 586
- Blephamide S.O.P. Sterile Ophthalmic Ointment 586
- Cetapred Ointment ⊙ 220
- ⅛% Econopred & 1% Econopred Plus ⊙ 217
- Isopto Cetapred Suspension ⊙ 220
- Metimyd ⊙ 306
- Poly-Pred Liquifilm ⊙ 250
- Pred Forte ⊙ 252
- Pred Mild ⊙ 254
- Pred-G Liquifilm Sterile Ophthalmic Suspension ⊙ 252
- Pred-G S.O.P. Sterile Ophthalmic Ointment ⊙ 253
- Vasocidin Ointment ⊙ 275

Prednisolone Sodium Phosphate (Pituitary secretion of gonadotropins affected). Products include:
- AK-Pred ⊙ 205
- Hydeltrasol Injection, Sterile 1476
- Inflamase ⊙ 274
- Pediapred Oral Liquid 987
- Vasocidin Ophthalmic Solution ⊙ 276

Prednisolone Tebutate (Pituitary secretion of gonadotropins affected). Products include:
- Hydeltra-T.B.A. Sterile Suspension 1478

Prednisone (Pituitary secretion of gonadotropins affected). Products include:
- Deltasone Tablets 2332

Prochlorperazine (Rise in prolactin; response to Factrel may be blunted). Products include:
- Compazine 2201

Promethazine Hydrochloride (Rise in prolactin; response to Factrel may be blunted). Products include:
- Mepergan Injection 2479
- Phenergan with Codeine 2497
- Phenergan with Dextromethorphan 2499
- Phenergan Injection 2493
- Phenergan Suppositories 2496
- Phenergan Syrup 2495
- Phenergan Tablets 2496
- Phenergan VC 2500
- Phenergan VC with Codeine 2501

Quinestrol (Pituitary secretion of gonadotropins affected). Products include:
- Estrovis 1721

Spironolactone (Gonadotropin levels transiently elevated). Products include:
- Aldactazide 2150
- Aldactone 2152

Stanozolol (Pituitary secretion of gonadotropins affected). Products include:
- Winstrol Tablets 2075

Thioridazine Hydrochloride (Rise in prolactin; response to Factrel may be blunted). Products include:
- Mellaril 2011

Triamcinolone (Pituitary secretion of gonadotropins affected).
- No products indexed under this heading.

Triamcinolone Acetonide (Pituitary secretion of gonadotropins affected). Products include:
- Aristocort A 1010
- Azmacort Inhaler 1837
- Kenalog Cream, Lotion & Ointment 2401
- Kenalog-10 Injection 2402
- Kenalog-40 Injection 2403
- Kenalog in Orabase 604
- Kenalog Spray 2401
- Mycolog II Cream and Ointment 2407
- Mytrex Cream & Ointment 2080
- Nasacort Nasal Inhaler 1844

Triamcinolone Diacetate (Pituitary secretion of gonadotropins affected). Products include:
- Aristocort Suspension 1008

Triamcinolone Hexacetonide (Pituitary secretion of gonadotropins affected). Products include:
- Aristospan Suspension 1011

Trifluoperazine Hydrochloride (Rise in prolactin; response to Factrel may be blunted). Products include:
- Stelazine 2226

FANSIDAR TABLETS
(Sulfadoxine, Pyrimethamine) 1896
May interact with sulfonamides and certain other agents. Compounds in these categories include:

Chloroquine (Increased incidence and severity of adverse reactions).

Sulfamethizole (Interferes with antimalarial prophylaxis). Products include:
- Thiosulfil Forte Tablets 2526
- Urobiotic-250 Capsules 1968

Sulfamethoxazole (Interferes with antimalarial prophylaxis). Products include:
- Azo Gantanol Tablets 1887
- Bactrim DS Tablets 1891
- Bactrim I.V. Infusion 1889
- Bactrim 1891
- Gantanol 1899
- Septra 813
- Septra I.V. Infusion 808
- Septra I.V. Infusion ADD-Vantage Vials 810
- Septra 813

Sulfasalazine (Interferes with antimalarial prophylaxis). Products include:
- Azulfidine Tablets, EN-tabs, Oral Suspension 1157

Sulfinpyrazone (Interferes with antimalarial prophylaxis). Products include:
- Anturane 853

Sulfisoxazole (Interferes with antimalarial prophylaxis). Products include:
- Azo Gantrisin Tablets 1888
- Gantrisin Tablets 1901
- Pediazole 1973

Sulfisoxazole Diolamine (Interferes with antimalarial prophylaxis). Products include:
- Gantrisin Ophthalmic Ointment/Solution 1900

FASTIN CAPSULES
(Phentermine Hydrochloride) 2216
May interact with monoamine oxidase inhibitors, insulin, and certain other agents. Compounds in these categories include:

Alcohol (Concomitant use may result in adverse drug interaction).

Furazolidone (Hypertensive crises may result). Products include:
- Furoxone 1855

Guanethidine Monosulfate (May decrease hypotensive effect of guanethidine). Products include:
- Esimil Tablets 864
- Ismelin Tablets 869

Insulin, Human (Insulin requirements may be altered).
- No products indexed under this heading.

Insulin, Human Isophane Suspension (Insulin requirements may be altered). Products include:
- Humulin N, 100 Units 1270

Insulin, Human NPH (Insulin requirements may be altered). Products include:
- Insulatard NPH Human 1627
- Novolin N 1627
- Novolin N PenFill Cartridges 1628
- Novolin N Prefilled 1628

Insulin, Human Regular (Insulin requirements may be altered). Products include:
- Humulin BR, 100 Units 1268
- Humulin R, 100 Units 1272
- Novolin R 1627
- Novolin R PenFill Cartridges 1628
- Novolin R Prefilled 1629
- Velosulin Human 1628

Insulin, Human, Zinc Suspension (Insulin requirements may be altered). Products include:
- Humulin L, 100 Units 1268
- Humulin U, 100 Units 1272
- Novolin L 1627

Insulin, NPH (Insulin requirements may be altered). Products include:
- NPH, 40 & 100 Units 1273
- Beef NPH, 100 Units 1274
- Pork NPH, 100 Units 1275

Insulatard NPH 1626
NPH Insulin 1626
NPH Purified Pork Isophane Insulin 1626

Insulin, Regular (Insulin requirements may be altered). Products include:
Regular, 40 & 100 Units 1273
Beef Regular, 100 Units 1275
Pork Regular, 100 Units 1275
Pork Regular (Concentrated), 500 Units 1276
Regular Insulin 1625
Regular Purified Pork Insulin 1626
Velosulin 1627

Insulin, Zinc Crystals (Insulin requirements may be altered). Products include:
NPH, 40 & 100 Units 1273

Insulin, Zinc Suspension (Insulin requirements may be altered). Products include:
Lente, 40 & 100 Units 1272
Protamine, Zinc, 40 & 100 Units 1273
Lente Iletin I 1272
Beef Lente, 100 Units 1274
Beef Protamine Zinc, 100 Units 1274
Pork Lente, 100 Units 1275
Pork, Protamine, Zinc, 100 Units 1275
Lente Insulin 1626
Lente Purified Pork Insulin 1626
Semilente Insulin 1625
Ultralente Insulin 1626

Isocarboxazid (Hypertensive crises may result). Products include:
Marplan Tablets 1906

Phenelzine Sulfate (Hypertensive crises may result). Products include:
Nardil 1742

Selegiline Hydrochloride (Hypertensive crises may result). Products include:
Eldepryl 2250

Tranylcypromine Sulfate (Hypertensive crises may result). Products include:
Parnate Tablets 2222

FEDAHIST GYROCAPS
(Pseudoephedrine Hydrochloride, Chlorpheniramine Maleate) 2145
May interact with monoamine oxidase inhibitors, beta blockers, veratrum alkaloids, tricyclic antidepressants, barbiturates, central nervous system depressants, and certain other agents. Compounds in these categories include:

Acebutolol Hydrochloride (Increases the effect of sympathomimetics). Products include:
Sectral Capsules 2520

Alcohol (May have an additive CNS depressant effect).

Alfentanil Hydrochloride (May have an additive CNS depressant effect). Products include:
Alfenta Injection 1131

Alprazolam (May have an additive CNS depressant effect). Products include:
Xanax Tablets 2367

Amitriptyline Hydrochloride (May have an additive CNS depressant effect). Products include:
Elavil 2269
Endep Tablets 1927
Etrafon 2087
Limbitrol 1933
Triavil Tablets 1556

Amoxapine (May have an additive CNS depressant effect). Products include:
Asendin Tablets 1196

Aprobarbital (May have an additive CNS depressant effect). Products include:
Alurate Elixir 1883

Atenolol (Increases the effect of sympathomimetics). Products include:
Tenoretic Tablets 1105
Tenormin Tablets and I.V. Injection 1107

Betaxolol Hydrochloride (Increases the effect of sympathomimetics). Products include:
Betoptic Sterile Ophthalmic Solution 569
Betoptic S Sterile Ophthalmic Suspension 570
Kerlone Tablets 2172

Buprenorphine (May have an additive CNS depressant effect).
No products indexed under this heading.

Buspirone Hydrochloride (May have an additive CNS depressant effect). Products include:
BuSpar 1401

Butabarbital (May have an additive CNS depressant effect). Products include:
Pyridium Plus 1764

Butalbital (May have an additive CNS depressant effect). Products include:
Esgic-Plus Tablets 1002
Esgic Tablets & Capsules 1001
Fioricet Tablets 2006
Fiorinal Capsules 2007
Fiorinal with Codeine Capsules 2008
Fiorinal Tablets 2007
Phrenilin 838
Sedapap Tablets 50 mg/650 mg 1360

Carteolol Hydrochloride (Increases the effect of sympathomimetics). Products include:
Cartrol Tablets 507

Chlordiazepoxide (May have an additive CNS depressant effect). Products include:
Libritabs Tablets 1930
Limbitrol 1933
Menrium Tablets 1934

Chlordiazepoxide Hydrochloride (May have an additive CNS depressant effect). Products include:
Librax Capsules 1929
Librium Capsules 1931
Librium Injectable 1932

Chlorpromazine (May have an additive CNS depressant effect). Products include:
Thorazine 2234

Chlorprothixene (May have an additive CNS depressant effect). Products include:
Taractan Tablets 1920

Chlorprothixene Hydrochloride (May have an additive CNS depressant effect). Products include:
Taractan 1920

Clomipramine Hydrochloride (May have an additive CNS depressant effect). Products include:
Anafranil Capsules 650

Clorazepate Dipotassium (May have an additive CNS depressant effect). Products include:
Tranxene 556

Codeine (May have an additive CNS depressant effect). Products include:
Calcidrine Syrup 506

Codeine Phosphate (May have an additive CNS depressant effect). Products include:
Actifed with Codeine Cough Syrup 752
Cheracol Cough Syrup 1853
Codimal PH Syrup 846
Dimetane-DC Cough Syrup 1857
Empirin with Codeine Phosphate Nos. 2, 3 & 4 764
Fiorinal with Codeine Capsules 2008
Isoclor Expectorant 982
Naldecon CX Adult Liquid 521
Novahistine DH 1342
Novahistine Expectorant 1343
Nucofed Capsules 2219
Nucofed Expectorant 2219
Nucofed Pediatric Expectorant 2220
Nucofed Syrup 2219
Phenaphen with Codeine Capsules 1865
Phenaphen-650 with Codeine Tablets 1866
Phenergan with Codeine 2497
Phenergan VC with Codeine 2501
Robitussin A-C Syrup 1875
Robitussin-DAC Syrup 1875
Ryna 741
Soma Compound w/Codeine Tablets 2390
Triaminic Expectorant w/Codeine 1996
Tussi-Organidin Liquid 2391
Tylenol with Codeine 1381

Codeine Polistirex (May have an additive CNS depressant effect).
No products indexed under this heading.

Cryptenamine Preparations (Reduced antihypertensive effect).

Desipramine Hydrochloride (May have an additive CNS depressant effect). Products include:
Norpramin Tablets 1340

Dezocine (May have an additive CNS depressant effect).

Diazepam (May have an additive CNS depressant effect). Products include:
Valium Injectable 1937
Valium Tablets 1939
Valrelease Capsules 1923

Doxepin Hydrochloride (May have an additive CNS depressant effect). Products include:
Sinequan 1960

Droperidol (May have an additive CNS depressant effect). Products include:
Inapsine Injection 1140
Innovar Injection 1141

Enflurane (May have an additive CNS depressant effect). Products include:
Ethrane 599

Esmolol Hydrochloride (Increases the effect of sympathomimetics). Products include:
Brevibloc Injection 942

Estazolam (May have an additive CNS depressant effect). Products include:
ProSom Tablets 554

Ethchlorvynol (May have an additive CNS depressant effect). Products include:
Placidyl Capsules 553

Ethinamate (May have an additive CNS depressant effect).
No products indexed under this heading.

Fentanyl (May have an additive CNS depressant effect). Products include:
Duragesic Transdermal System 1133

Fentanyl Citrate (May have an additive CNS depressant effect). Products include:
Innovar Injection 1141
Sublimaze Injection 1146

Fluphenazine Decanoate (May have an additive CNS depressant effect). Products include:
Prolixin Decanoate 1795

Fluphenazine Enanthate (May have an additive CNS depressant effect). Products include:
Prolixin Enanthate 1796

Fluphenazine Hydrochloride (May have an additive CNS depressant effect). Products include:
Prolixin Elixir 1793
Prolixin Injection 1791
Prolixin Oral Concentrate 1792
Prolixin Tablets 1793

Flurazepam Hydrochloride (May have an additive CNS depressant effect). Products include:
Dalmane Capsules 1927

Furazolidone (Increases the effect of sympathomimetics; concurrent use is contraindicated). Products include:
Furoxone 1855

Glutethimide (May have an additive CNS depressant effect).
No products indexed under this heading.

Haloperidol (May have an additive CNS depressant effect). Products include:
Haldol Injection, Tablets and Concentrate 1373

Haloperidol Decanoate (May have an additive CNS depressant effect). Products include:
Haldol Decanoate 1375

Hydrocodone Bitartrate (May have an additive CNS depressant effect). Products include:
Anexsia 5/500 Tablets 2196
Anexsia 7.5/650 Tablets 2197
Azdōne Tablets 844
Codiclear DH Syrup 845
Codimal DH Syrup 846
Damason-P 1356
Hycodan Syrup, Tablets 927
Hycomine Compound Tablets 929
Hycomine Syrup 927
Hycotuss Expectorant Syrup 930
Hydrocet Capsules 835
Lortab ASA Tablets 2414
Lortab 2412
Ru-Tuss with Hydrocodone 694
Triaminic Expectorant DH 1995
Vicodin Tablets 1187
Vicodin ES Tablets 1189
Zydone Capsules 941

Hydrocodone Polistirex (May have an additive CNS depressant effect). Products include:
Tussionex Extended-Release Suspension 988

Hydroxyzine Hydrochloride (May have an additive CNS depressant effect). Products include:
Atarax Tablets & Syrup 1941
Marax Tablets & DF Syrup 1954
Vistaril Intramuscular Solution 1970

Imipramine Hydrochloride (May have an additive CNS depressant effect). Products include:
Tofranil Ampuls 1038
Tofranil Tablets 1039

Imipramine Pamoate (May have an additive CNS depressant effect). Products include:
Tofranil-PM Capsules 1041

Isocarboxazid (Increases the effect of sympathomimetics; concurrent use is contraindicated). Products include:
Marplan Tablets 1906

Isoflurane (May have an additive CNS depressant effect). Products include:
Forane 600

Ketamine Hydrochloride (May have an additive CNS depressant effect). Products include:
Ketalar 1726

Labetalol Hydrochloride (Increases the effect of sympathomimetics). Products include:
Normodyne Injection 2108
Normodyne Tablets 2110
Normozide Tablets 2112
Trandate HCT Tablets 579
Trandate Injection 577
Trandate Tablets 579

Levorphanol Tartrate (May have an additive CNS depressant effect). Products include:
Levo-Dromoran 1906

Lorazepam (May have an additive CNS depressant effect). Products include:
- Ativan Injection 2432
- Ativan Tablets 2434

Loxapine Hydrochloride (May have an additive CNS depressant effect). Products include:
- Loxitane 1213

Loxapine Succinate (May have an additive CNS depressant effect). Products include:
- Loxitane Capsules 1213

Maprotiline Hydrochloride (May have an additive CNS depressant effect). Products include:
- Ludiomil Tablets 874

Mecamylamine Hydrochloride (Reduced antihypertensive effect). Products include:
- Inversine Tablets 1492

Meperidine Hydrochloride (May have an additive CNS depressant effect). Products include:
- Demerol 2047
- Mepergan Injection 2479

Mephobarbital (May have an additive CNS depressant effect). Products include:
- Mebaral Tablets 2061

Meprobamate (May have an additive CNS depressant effect). Products include:
- Deprol Tablets 2382
- Equagesic Tablets 2451
- Miltown Tablets 2386
- PMB 200 and PMB 400 2504

Mesoridazine (May have an additive CNS depressant effect). Products include:
- Serentil 686

Methadone Hydrochloride (May have an additive CNS depressant effect). Products include:
- Dolophine Hydrochloride Ampoules & Vials 1260
- Dolophine Hydrochloride Tablets ... 1261
- Methadone Hydrochloride Diskets .. 1284
- Methadone Hydrochloride Oral Solution & Tablets 1987

Methohexital Sodium (May have an additive CNS depressant effect). Products include:
- Brevital Sodium Vials 1248

Methoxyflurane (May have an additive CNS depressant effect).
- No products indexed under this heading.

Methyldopa (Reduced antihypertensive effect). Products include:
- Aldoclor Tablets 1413
- Aldomet Oral 1415
- Aldoril Tablets 1418

Methyldopate Hydrochloride (Reduced antihypertensive effect). Products include:
- Aldomet Ester HCl Injection 1417

Metoprolol Tartrate (Increases the effect of sympathomimetics). Products include:
- Lopressor Ampuls 1032
- Lopressor HCT Tablets 1034
- Lopressor Tablets 1032

Midazolam Hydrochloride (May have an additive CNS depressant effect). Products include:
- Versed Injection 1924

Molindone Hydrochloride (May have an additive CNS depressant effect). Products include:
- Moban Tablets & Concentrate 932

Morphine Sulfate (May have an additive CNS depressant effect). Products include:
- Astramorph/PF Injection, USP (Preservative-Free) 618
- Duramorph 960
- Infumorph 200 and Infumorph 500 Sterile Solutions 962
- MS Contin Tablets 1814
- MSIR 1817
- Oramorph SR (Morphine Sulfate Sustained Release Tablets) 1988
- Roxanol 1991

Nadolol (Increases the effect of sympathomimetics). Products include:
- Corgard Tablets 701
- Corzide Tablets 702

Nortriptyline Hydrochloride (May have an additive CNS depressant effect). Products include:
- Pamelor 2019

Opium Alkaloids (May have an additive CNS depressant effect). Products include:
- B & O No. 15A & No. 16A Supprettes 2395
- Pantopon Injectable 1911

Oxazepam (May have an additive CNS depressant effect). Products include:
- Serax Capsules 2522
- Serax Tablets 2522

Oxycodone Hydrochloride (May have an additive CNS depressant effect). Products include:
- Percocet Tablets 950
- Percodan 951
- Roxicodone Tablets, Oral Solution & Intensol (Oxycodone) 1992
- Tylox Capsules 1382

Penbutolol Sulfate (Increases the effect of sympathomimetics). Products include:
- Levatol 1832

Pentobarbital Sodium (May have an additive CNS depressant effect). Products include:
- Nembutal Sodium Capsules 534
- Nembutal Sodium Solution 536
- Nembutal Sodium Suppositories 538

Perphenazine (May have an additive CNS depressant effect). Products include:
- Etrafon 2087
- Triavil Tablets 1556
- Trilafon 2123

Phenelzine Sulfate (Increases the effect of sympathomimetics; concurrent use is contraindicated). Products include:
- Nardil 1742

Phenobarbital (May have an additive CNS depressant effect). Products include:
- Arco-Lase Plus Tablets 607
- Bellergal-S Tablets 1998
- Bronkolixir .... ▣ 761
- Bronkotabs Tablets .... ▣ 762
- Donnatal 1858
- Donnatal Extentabs 1859
- Donnatal Tablets 1858
- Donnazyme Tablets 1860
- Kinesed Tablets 2272
- Phenobarbital Elixir and Tablets 1293
- Primatene Tablets-P Formula 2421
- Quadrinal Tablets 1183
- Tedral SA 1765

Pindolol (Increases the effect of sympathomimetics). Products include:
- Visken Tablets 2036

Prazepam (May have an additive CNS depressant effect). Products include:
- Centrax 1693

Prochlorperazine (May have an additive CNS depressant effect). Products include:
- Compazine 2201

Promethazine Hydrochloride (May have an additive CNS depressant effect). Products include:
- Mepergan Injection 2479
- Phenergan with Codeine 2497
- Phenergan with Dextromethorphan 2499
- Phenergan Injection 2493
- Phenergan Suppositories 2496
- Phenergan Syrup 2495
- Phenergan Tablets 2496
- Phenergan VC 2500
- Phenergan VC with Codeine 2501

Propofol (May have an additive CNS depressant effect). Products include:
- Diprivan Injection 2267

Propoxyphene Hydrochloride (May have an additive CNS depressant effect). Products include:
- Darvon 1256
- Wygesic Tablets 2540

Propoxyphene Napsylate (May have an additive CNS depressant effect). Products include:
- Darvon-N/Darvocet-N 1254

Propranolol Hydrochloride (Increases the effect of sympathomimetics). Products include:
- Inderal 2459
- Inderal LA Long Acting Capsules 2461
- Inderide Tablets 2463
- Inderide LA Long Acting Capsules .. 2465

Protriptyline Hydrochloride (May have an additive CNS depressant effect). Products include:
- Vivactil Tablets 1567

Quazepam (May have an additive CNS depressant effect). Products include:
- Doral Tablets 2383

Rauwolfia Serpentina (Reduced antihypertensive effect). Products include:
- Raudixin Tablets 1803
- Rauzide Tablets 1804

Reserpine (Reduced antihypertensive effect). Products include:
- Diupres Tablets 1461
- Hydromox R Tablets 1209
- Hydropres Tablets 1485
- Renese-R Tablets 1786
- Salutensin/Salutensin-Demi 719
- Ser-Ap-Es Tablets 881
- Serpasil Tablets 883
- Serpasil-Apresoline Tablets 884
- Serpasil-Esidrix Tablets 886

Secobarbital Sodium (May have an additive CNS depressant effect). Products include:
- Seconal Sodium Pulvules 1296

Selegiline Hydrochloride (Increases the effect of sympathomimetics; concurrent use is contraindicated). Products include:
- Eldepryl 2250

Sufentanil Citrate (May have an additive CNS depressant effect). Products include:
- Sufenta Injection 1147

Temazepam (May have an additive CNS depressant effect). Products include:
- Restoril Capsules 2023

Thiamylal Sodium (May have an additive CNS depressant effect). Products include:
- Surital Ampoules, Steri-Vials 1764

Thioridazine Hydrochloride (May have an additive CNS depressant effect). Products include:
- Mellaril 2011

Thiothixene (May have an additive CNS depressant effect). Products include:
- Navane Capsules and Concentrate 1954
- Navane Intramuscular 1956

Timolol Maleate (Increases the effect of sympathomimetics). Products include:
- Blocadren Tablets 1429
- Timolide Tablets 1547
- Timoptic in Ocudose 1552
- Timoptic Sterile Ophthalmic Solution 1550

Tranylcypromine Sulfate (Increases the effect of sympathomimetics; concurrent use is contraindicated). Products include:
- Parnate Tablets 2222

Triazolam (May have an additive CNS depressant effect). Products include:
- Halcion Tablets 2340

Trifluoperazine Hydrochloride (May have an additive CNS depressant effect). Products include:
- Stelazine 2226

Trimipramine Maleate (May have an additive CNS depressant effect). Products include:
- Surmontil Capsules 2524

FEDAHIST TIMECAPS
(Pseudoephedrine Hydrochloride, Chlorpheniramine Maleate) 2145
See **Fedahist Gyrocaps**

FEEN-A-MINT GUM
(Phenolphthalein, Yellow) .... ▣ 702
No interactions described in labeling.

FEEN-A-MINT LAXATIVE PILLS AND CHOCOLATED MINT TABLETS
(Phenolphthalein, Yellow, Docusate Sodium) .... ▣ 702
No interactions described in labeling.

FELDENE CAPSULES
(Piroxicam) 1777
May interact with oral anticoagulants, lithium preparations, highly protein bound drugs (selected), and certain other agents. Compounds in these categories include:

Amiodarone Hydrochloride (Feldene might displace other highly protein bound drugs). Products include:
- Cordarone Tablets 2446

Amitriptyline Hydrochloride (Feldene might displace other highly protein bound drugs). Products include:
- Elavil 2269
- Endep Tablets 1927
- Etrafon 2087
- Limbitrol 1933
- Triavil Tablets 1556

Aspirin (Aspirin (3900 mg/day) depresses plasma levels of piroxicam). Products include:
- Alka-Seltzer Effervescent Antacid and Pain Reliever 1568
- Alka-Seltzer Extra Strength Effervescent Antacid and Pain Reliever 1570
- Alka-Seltzer (Flavored) Effervescent Antacid and Pain Reliever 1569
- Alka-Seltzer Plus Cold Medicine .... ▣ 623
- Alka-Seltzer Plus Night-Time Cold Medicine .... ▣ 623
- Alka Seltzer Plus Sinus Allergy Medicine .... ▣ 624
- Anacin Coated Analgesic Caplets 2417
- Anacin Coated Analgesic Tablets 2417
- Anacin Maximum Strength Analgesic Coated Tablets 2417
- Maximum Strength Arthritis Pain Formula By the Makers of Anacin Analgesic Tablets and Caplets 2418
- Arthritis Pain Formula by the Makers of Anacin Analgesic Tablets and Caplets .... ▣ 747
- Arthritis Strength BC Powder .... ▣ 516
- Ascriptin A/D Caplets 1850
- Regular Strength Ascriptin Tablets 1850
- Azdōne Tablets 844
- BC Powder .... ▣ 517
- BC Cold Powder .... ▣ 517
- Children's Bayer Chewable Aspirin .... ▣ 564
- Genuine Bayer Aspirin Tablets & Caplets .... ▣ 564
- Maximum Bayer Aspirin Tablets & Caplets .... ▣ 566
- Bayer Plus Aspirin Tablets .... ▣ 567
- Therapy Bayer Aspirin Caplets .... ▣ 568
- 8 Hour Bayer Timed-Release Aspirin .... ▣ 566
- Arthritis Strength Bufferin Analgesic Caplets 744

Extra Strength Bufferin Analgesic Tablets ... 745
Bufferin Analgesic Tablets and Caplets ... 743
Cama Arthritis Pain Reliever ... ■ 685
Damason-P ... 1356
Easprin ... 1719
Ecotrin Enteric Coated Aspirin Maximum Strength Tablets and Caplets ... 2189
Ecotrin Enteric Coated Aspirin Regular Strength Tablets and Caplets ... 2189
Empirin Aspirin ... ■ 541
Empirin with Codeine Phosphate Nos. 2, 3 & 4 ... 764
Equagesic Tablets ... 2451
Excedrin Extra-Strength Analgesic Tablets & Caplets ... 749
4-Way Cold Tablets ... 750
Fiorinal Capsules ... 2007
Fiorinal with Codeine Capsules ... 2008
Fiorinal Tablets ... 2007
Lortab ASA Tablets ... 2414
Momentum Muscular Backache Formula ... ■ 751
Norgesic ... 1314
Norwich Extra-Strength Aspirin ... ■ 546
Norwich Regular Strength Aspirin ■ 547
P-A-C Analgesic Tablets ... ■ 669
Percodan ... 951
Robaxisal Tablets ... 1872
Sine-Off Sinus Medicine Tablets-Aspirin Formula ... ■ 722
Soma Compound w/Codeine Tablets ... 2390
Soma Compound Tablets ... 2389
St. Joseph Adult Chewable Aspirin (81 mg.) ... ■ 703
Synalgos-DC Capsules ... 2525
Talwin Compound ... 2072
Ursinus Inlay-Tabs ... ■ 691
Vanquish Analgesic Caplets ... ■ 574
Zorprin Tablets ... 698

Aspirin, Enteric Coated (Aspirin (3900 mg/day) depresses plasma levels of piroxicam). Products include:
Therapy Bayer Aspirin Caplets ... ■ 568
Ecotrin ... 2189

Cefonicid Sodium (Feldene might displace other highly protein bound drugs). Products include:
Monocid Injection ... 2217

Chlordiazepoxide (Feldene might displace other highly protein bound drugs). Products include:
Libritabs Tablets ... 1930
Limbitrol ... 1933
Menrium Tablets ... 1934

Chlordiazepoxide Hydrochloride (Feldene might displace other highly protein bound drugs). Products include:
Librax Capsules ... 1929
Librium Capsules ... 1931
Librium Injectable ... 1932

Chlorpromazine (Feldene might displace other highly protein bound drugs). Products include:
Thorazine ... 2234

Clomipramine Hydrochloride (Feldene might displace other highly protein bound drugs). Products include:
Anafranil Capsules ... 650

Clozapine (Feldene might displace other highly protein bound drugs). Products include:
Clozaril Tablets ... 2000

Cyclosporine (Feldene might displace other highly protein bound drugs). Products include:
Sandimmune ... 2024

Diazepam (Feldene might displace other highly protein bound drugs). Products include:
Valium Injectable ... 1937
Valium Tablets ... 1939
Valrelease Capsules ... 1923

Diclofenac Sodium (Feldene might displace other highly protein bound drugs). Products include:
Voltaren Ophthalmic Sterile Ophthalmic Solution ... ⊙ 268
Voltaren Tablets ... 1042

Dicumarol (Altered dosage requirements). Products include:
Dicumarol Tablets ... 516

Dipyridamole (Feldene might displace other highly protein bound drugs). Products include:
Persantine Tablets ... 683

Fenoprofen Calcium (Feldene might displace other highly protein bound drugs). Products include:
Nalfon Pulvules & Tablets ... 919

Flurazepam Hydrochloride (Feldene might displace other highly protein bound drugs). Products include:
Dalmane Capsules ... 1927

Flurbiprofen (Feldene might displace other highly protein bound drugs). Products include:
Ansaid Tablets ... 2319

Glipizide (Feldene might displace other highly protein bound drugs). Products include:
Glucotrol ... 1952

Ibuprofen (Feldene might displace other highly protein bound drugs). Products include:
Advil Cold & Sinus Caplets (formerly CoAdvil) ... 2416
Advil Ibuprofen Tablets and Caplets ... 2416
Children's Advil Suspension ... 2426
CoAdvil ... ■ 748
Dristan Sinus Caplets ... 2419
Haltran Tablets ... ■ 668
Ibuprofen ... ■ 631
Medipren ibuprofen Caplets and Tablets ... 1362
Midol 200 Cramp Relief Formula .. ■ 570
Motrin Tablets ... 2351
Motrin IB Caplets and Tablets ... ■ 736
Nuprin Ibuprofen/Analgesic Tablets & Caplets ... 752
PediaProfen Suspension ... 1363
Rufen Tablets ... 691
Trendar Ibuprofen Tablets ... ■ 756

Imipramine Hydrochloride (Feldene might displace other highly protein bound drugs). Products include:
Tofranil Ampuls ... 1038
Tofranil Tablets ... 1039

Imipramine Pamoate (Feldene might displace other highly protein bound drugs). Products include:
Tofranil-PM Capsules ... 1041

Indomethacin (Feldene might displace other highly protein bound drugs). Products include:
Indocin ... 1487

Indomethacin Sodium Trihydrate (Feldene might displace other highly protein bound drugs). Products include:
Indocin I.V. ... 1490

Ketoprofen (Feldene might displace other highly protein bound drugs). Products include:
Orudis Capsules ... 2488

Ketorolac Tromethamine (Feldene might displace other highly protein bound drugs). Products include:
Toradol IM Injection ... 2302

Lithium Carbonate (Increased plasma lithium levels). Products include:
Eskalith ... 2214
Lithane Tablets ... 1596
Lithium Carbonate Capsules & Tablets ... 1984
Lithobid Tablets ... 870

Lithium Citrate (Increased plasma lithium levels). Products include:
Cibalith-S ... 870

Meclofenamate Sodium (Feldene might displace other highly protein bound drugs). Products include:
Meclomen Capsules ... 1739

Mefenamic Acid (Feldene might displace other highly protein bound drugs). Products include:
Ponstel ... 1758

Midazolam Hydrochloride (Feldene might displace other highly protein bound drugs). Products include:
Versed Injection ... 1924

Naproxen (Feldene might displace other highly protein bound drugs). Products include:
Naprosyn ... 2297

Naproxen Sodium (Feldene might displace other highly protein bound drugs). Products include:
Anaprox and Anaprox DS Tablets ... 2288

Nortriptyline Hydrochloride (Feldene might displace other highly protein bound drugs). Products include:
Pamelor ... 2019

Oxazepam (Feldene might displace other highly protein bound drugs). Products include:
Serax Capsules ... 2522
Serax Tablets ... 2522

Phenylbutazone (Feldene might displace other highly protein bound drugs). Products include:
Butazolidin Capsules & Tablets ... 1027

Propranolol Hydrochloride (Feldene might displace other highly protein bound drugs). Products include:
Inderal ... 2459
Inderal LA Long Acting Capsules ... 2461
Inderide Tablets ... 2463
Inderide LA Long Acting Capsules .. 2465

Sulindac (Feldene might displace other highly protein bound drugs). Products include:
Clinoril Tablets ... 1433

Temazepam (Feldene might displace other highly protein bound drugs). Products include:
Restoril Capsules ... 2023

Tolbutamide (Feldene might displace other highly protein bound drugs). Products include:
Orinase Tablets ... 2354

Tolmetin Sodium (Feldene might displace other highly protein bound drugs). Products include:
Tolectin (200, 400 and 600 mg) .. 1379

Trimipramine Maleate (Feldene might displace other highly protein bound drugs). Products include:
Surmontil Capsules ... 2524

Warfarin Sodium (Altered dosage requirements; Feldene might displace other highly protein bound drugs). Products include:
Coumadin Injection & Tablets ... 944
Panwarfin Tablets ... 547

FEMININE GOLD
(Camphor, Menthol) ... ■ 509
No interactions described in labeling.

FEMIRON MULTI-VITAMINS AND IRON
(Ferrous Fumarate, Multivitamins) .. ■ 617
May interact with:

Alcohol (Enhances iron absorption with the potential for iron overload).

FEMSTAT PREFILL VAGINAL CREAM 2%
(Butoconazole Nitrate) ... 2295
No interactions described in labeling.

FEMSTAT VAGINAL CREAM 2%
(Butoconazole Nitrate) ... 2295
No interactions described in labeling.

FEOSOL CAPSULES
(Ferrous Sulfate) ... 2191
May interact with tetracyclines. Compounds in this category include:

Demeclocycline Hydrochloride (Interference with absorption of oral tetracycline products). Products include:
Declomycin Capsules, Tablets ... 1199

Doxycycline Calcium (Interference with absorption of oral tetracycline products).
No products indexed under this heading.

Doxycycline Hyclate (Interference with absorption of oral tetracycline products). Products include:
Doryx Capsules ... 1717
Vibramycin Hyclate Capsules ... 1787
Vibramycin Hyclate Intravenous ... 1968
Vibra-Tabs Film Coated Tablets ... 1787

Doxycycline Monohydrate (Interference with absorption of oral tetracycline products). Products include:
Monodox Capsules ... 1630
Vibramycin Monohydrate for Oral Suspension ... 1787

Methacycline Hydrochloride (Interference with absorption of oral tetracycline products).
No products indexed under this heading.

Minocycline Hydrochloride (Interference with absorption of oral tetracycline products). Products include:
Minocin Intravenous ... 1221
Minocin Oral Suspension ... 1224
Minocin Pellet-Filled Capsules ... 1222

Oxytetracycline (Interference with absorption of oral tetracycline products). Products include:
Terramycin Intramuscular Solution 1964
Urobiotic-250 Capsules ... 1968

Oxytetracycline Hydrochloride (Interference with absorption of oral tetracycline products). Products include:
Terra-Cortril Ophthalmic Suspension ... 1963
Terramycin Capsules ... 1786
Terramycin Intramuscular Solution 1964
Terramycin with Polymyxin B Sulfate Ophthalmic Ointment ... 1965

Tetracycline Hydrochloride (Interference with absorption of oral tetracycline products). Products include:
Achromycin V Capsules ... 1193
Achromycin Ophthalmic Ointment 1% ... ⊙ 307
Achromycin Ophthalmic Suspension 1% ... ⊙ 308
Topicycline for Topical Solution ... 1856

FEOSOL ELIXIR
(Ferrous Sulfate) ... 2191
May interact with tetracyclines. Compounds in this category include:

Demeclocycline Hydrochloride (Interference with absorption of oral tetracycline products). Products include:
Declomycin Capsules, Tablets ... 1199

Doxycycline Calcium (Interference with absorption of oral tetracycline products).
No products indexed under this heading.

Doxycycline Hyclate (Interference with absorption of oral tetracycline products). Products include:
- Doryx Capsules 1717
- Vibramycin Hyclate Capsules 1787
- Vibramycin Hyclate Intravenous 1968
- Vibra-Tabs Film Coated Tablets 1787

Doxycycline Monohydrate (Interference with absorption of oral tetracycline products). Products include:
- Monodox Capsules 1630
- Vibramycin Monohydrate for Oral Suspension 1787

Methacycline Hydrochloride (Interference with absorption of oral tetracycline products).
No products indexed under this heading.

Minocycline Hydrochloride (Interference with absorption of oral tetracycline products). Products include:
- Minocin Intravenous 1221
- Minocin Oral Suspension 1224
- Minocin Pellet-Filled Capsules 1222

Oxytetracycline (Interference with absorption of oral tetracycline products). Products include:
- Terramycin Intramuscular Solution 1964
- Urobiotic-250 Capsules 1968

Oxytetracycline Hydrochloride (Interference with absorption of oral tetracycline products). Products include:
- Terra-Cortril Ophthalmic Suspension 1963
- Terramycin Capsules 1786
- Terramycin Intramuscular Solution 1964
- Terramycin with Polymyxin B Sulfate Ophthalmic Ointment 1965

Tetracycline Hydrochloride (Interference with absorption of oral tetracycline products). Products include:
- Achromycin V Capsules 1193
- Achromycin Ophthalmic Ointment 1% .... ⊚ 307
- Achromycin Ophthalmic Suspension 1% .... ⊚ 308
- Topicycline for Topical Solution 1856

FEOSOL TABLETS
(Ferrous Sulfate) 2191
May interact with tetracyclines. Compounds in this category include:

Demeclocycline Hydrochloride (Interference with absorption of oral tetracycline products). Products include:
- Declomycin Capsules, Tablets 1199

Doxycycline Calcium (Interference with absorption of oral tetracycline products).
No products indexed under this heading.

Doxycycline Hyclate (Interference with absorption of oral tetracycline products). Products include:
- Doryx Capsules 1717
- Vibramycin Hyclate Capsules 1787
- Vibramycin Hyclate Intravenous 1968
- Vibra-Tabs Film Coated Tablets 1787

Doxycycline Monohydrate (Interference with absorption of oral tetracycline products). Products include:
- Monodox Capsules 1630
- Vibramycin Monohydrate for Oral Suspension 1787

Methacycline Hydrochloride (Interference with absorption of oral tetracycline products).
No products indexed under this heading.

Minocycline Hydrochloride (Interference with absorption of oral tetracycline products). Products include:
- Minocin Intravenous 1221
- Minocin Oral Suspension 1224
- Minocin Pellet-Filled Capsules 1222

Oxytetracycline (Interference with absorption of oral tetracycline). Products include:
- Terramycin Intramuscular Solution 1964
- Urobiotic-250 Capsules 1968

Oxytetracycline Hydrochloride (Interference with absorption of oral tetracycline products). Products include:
- Terra-Cortril Ophthalmic Suspension 1963
- Terramycin Capsules 1786
- Terramycin Intramuscular Solution 1964
- Terramycin with Polymyxin B Sulfate Ophthalmic Ointment 1965

Tetracycline Hydrochloride (Interference with absorption of oral tetracycline products). Products include:
- Achromycin V Capsules 1193
- Achromycin Ophthalmic Ointment 1% .... ⊚ 307
- Achromycin Ophthalmic Suspension 1% .... ⊚ 308
- Topicycline for Topical Solution 1856

FERANCEE CHEWABLE TABLETS
(Ferrous Fumarate, Vitamin C, Sodium Ascorbate) 1155
No interactions described in labeling.

FERANCEE-HP TABLETS
(Ferrous Fumarate, Vitamin C, Sodium Ascorbate) 1155
No interactions described in labeling.

FERGON ELIXIR
(Ferrous Gluconate) .... ▣ 758
May interact with tetracyclines. Compounds in this category include:

Demeclocycline Hydrochloride (Oral iron products interfere with absorption of oral tetracyclines). Products include:
- Declomycin Capsules, Tablets 1199

Doxycycline Calcium (Oral iron products interfere with absorption of oral tetracyclines).
No products indexed under this heading.

Doxycycline Hyclate (Oral iron products interfere with absorption of oral tetracyclines). Products include:
- Doryx Capsules 1717
- Vibramycin Hyclate Capsules 1787
- Vibramycin Hyclate Intravenous 1968
- Vibra-Tabs Film Coated Tablets 1787

Doxycycline Monohydrate (Oral iron products interfere with absorption of oral tetracyclines). Products include:
- Monodox Capsules 1630
- Vibramycin Monohydrate for Oral Suspension 1787

Methacycline Hydrochloride (Oral iron products interfere with absorption of oral tetracyclines).
No products indexed under this heading.

Minocycline Hydrochloride (Oral iron products interfere with absorption of oral tetracyclines). Products include:
- Minocin Intravenous 1221
- Minocin Oral Suspension 1224
- Minocin Pellet-Filled Capsules 1222

Oxytetracycline Hydrochloride (Oral iron products interfere with absorption of oral tetracyclines). Products include:
- Terra-Cortril Ophthalmic Suspension 1963
- Terramycin Capsules 1786
- Terramycin Intramuscular Solution 1964
- Terramycin with Polymyxin B Sulfate Ophthalmic Ointment 1965

Tetracycline Hydrochloride (Oral iron products interfere with absorption of oral tetracyclines). Products include:
- Achromycin V Capsules 1193
- Achromycin Ophthalmic Ointment 1% .... ⊚ 307
- Achromycin Ophthalmic Suspension 1% .... ⊚ 308
- Topicycline for Topical Solution 1856

FERGON TABLETS
(Ferrous Gluconate) .... ▣ 758
See **Fergon Elixir**

FERO-FOLIC-500 FILMTAB
(Ferrous Sulfate, Folic Acid, Vitamin C) 527
May interact with tetracyclines and certain other agents. Compounds in these categories include:

Calcium Carbonate (Inhibits iron absorption). Products include:
- Alka-Mints Chewable Antacid .... ▣ 620
- Alka-Seltzer Advanced Formula Antacid & Non-Aspirin Pain Reliever .... ▣ 620
- Ascriptin A/D Caplets 1850
- Regular Strength Ascriptin Tablets 1850
- Balmex Baby Powder .... ▣ 590
- Bayer Plus Aspirin Tablets .... ▣ 567
- Biocal 500 mg Tablet Calcium Supplement .... ▣ 625
- Bufferin Analgesic Tablets and Caplets .... ▣ 524
- Caltrate 600 .... ▣ 583
- Caltrate 600 + Iron .... ▣ 583
- Caltrate 600 + Vitamin D .... ▣ 584
- Caltrate, Jr. .... ▣ 583
- Centrum, Jr. (Children's Chewable) + Extra Calcium .... ▣ 585
- Di-Gel Antacid/Anti-Gas .... ▣ 697
- Gerimed Tablets 972
- Marblen .... ▣ 563
- Natalins Rx 1391
- Natalins Tablets 1391
- Nephro-Calci Tablets 1826
- Os-Cal 500 Chewable Tablets .... ▣ 596
- Os-Cal 500 Tablets .... ▣ 597
- Os-Cal 250+D Tablets .... ▣ 597
- Os-Cal 500+D Tablets .... ▣ 597
- Pramet FA 1974
- Pramilet FA 1974
- Rolaids (Calcium Rich/Sodium Free) .... ▣ 744
- Extra Strength Rolaids .... ▣ 744
- Thermotabs .... ▣ 619
- Total Formula-2 (multivitamin/multimineral) 2377
- Tums Liquid Extra .... ▣ 726
- Zenate Tablets 2250

Demeclocycline Hydrochloride (Ferrous sulfate may interfere with absorption of tetracycline). Products include:
- Declomycin Capsules, Tablets 1199

Doxycycline Calcium (Ferrous sulfate may interfere with absorption of tetracycline).
No products indexed under this heading.

Doxycycline Hyclate (Ferrous sulfate may interfere with absorption of tetracycline). Products include:
- Doryx Capsules 1717
- Vibramycin Hyclate Capsules 1787
- Vibramycin Hyclate Intravenous 1968
- Vibra-Tabs Film Coated Tablets 1787

Doxycycline Monohydrate (Ferrous sulfate may interfere with absorption of tetracycline). Products include:
- Monodox Capsules 1630
- Vibramycin Monohydrate for Oral Suspension 1787

Levodopa (Antiparkinsonism effects of levodopa may be reversed by pyridoxine). Products include:
- Larodopa Tablets 1905
- Sinemet Tablets 952
- Sinemet CR Tablets 953

Magnesium Trisilicate (Inhibits absorption of iron). Products include:
- Gaviscon Antacid Tablets .... ▣ 593
- Gaviscon-2 Antacid Tablets .... ▣ 594

Methacycline Hydrochloride (Ferrous sulfate may interfere with absorption of tetracycline).
No products indexed under this heading.

Minocycline Hydrochloride (Ferrous sulfate may interfere with absorption of tetracycline). Products include:
- Minocin Intravenous 1221
- Minocin Oral Suspension 1224
- Minocin Pellet-Filled Capsules 1222

Oxytetracycline (Ferrous sulfate may interfere with absorption of tetracycline). Products include:
- Terramycin Intramuscular Solution 1964
- Urobiotic-250 Capsules 1968

Oxytetracycline Hydrochloride (Ferrous sulfate may interfere with absorption of tetracycline). Products include:
- Terra-Cortril Ophthalmic Suspension 1963
- Terramycin Capsules 1786
- Terramycin Intramuscular Solution 1964
- Terramycin with Polymyxin B Sulfate Ophthalmic Ointment 1965

Sodium Bicarbonate (Inhibits iron absorption). Products include:
- Alka-Seltzer Advanced Formula Antacid & Non-Aspirin Pain Reliever .... ▣ 620
- Alka-Seltzer Effervescent Antacid ▣ 622
- Alka-Seltzer Effervescent Antacid and Pain Reliever 1568
- Alka-Seltzer Extra Strength Effervescent Antacid and Pain Reliever .... ▣ 623
- Alka-Seltzer (Flavored) Effervescent Antacid and Pain Reliever .. ▣ 621
- Arm & Hammer Pure Baking Soda .... ▣ 548
- Ceo-Two Rectal Suppositories 671
- Citrocarbonate Antacid .... ▣ 668
- Massengill Liquid Concentrate 2191
- NuLYTELY 699

Tetracycline Hydrochloride (Ferrous sulfate may interfere with absorption of tetracycline). Products include:
- Achromycin V Capsules 1193
- Achromycin Ophthalmic Ointment 1% .... ⊚ 307
- Achromycin Ophthalmic Suspension 1% .... ⊚ 308
- Topicycline for Topical Solution 1856

Food Interactions

Dairy products (Ingestion of milk inhibits its iron absorption).

Eggs (Ingestion of eggs inhibits iron absorption).

FERO-GRAD-500 FILMTAB
(Ferrous Sulfate, Vitamin C) 528
No interactions described in labeling.

FERO-GRADUMET FILMTAB
(Ferrous Sulfate) 528
No interactions described in labeling.

FERRO-SEQUELS
(Ferrous Fumarate) 1203
No interactions described in labeling.

FESTAL II DIGESTIVE AID
(Amylase, Lipase, Protease) .... ▣ 574
No interactions described in labeling.

FEVERALL SPRINKLE CAPS
(Acetaminophen) 2374
No interactions described in labeling.

FEVERALL SUPPOSITORIES
(Acetaminophen) 2374
No interactions described in labeling.

FIBERALL CHEWABLE TABLETS, LEMON CREME FLAVOR
(Polycarbophil) 851
May interact with:

Oxytetracycline (Give 1 hour before or 2 to 3 hours after Fiberall). Products include:
- Terramycin Intramuscular Solution 1964
- Urobiotic-250 Capsules 1968

Oxytetracycline Hydrochloride (Give 1 hour before or 2 to 3 hours after Fiberall). Products include:
- Terra-Cortril Ophthalmic Suspension 1963
- Terramycin Capsules 1786
- Terramycin Intramuscular Solution 1964
- Terramycin with Polymyxin B Sulfate Ophthalmic Ointment 1965

Tetracycline Hydrochloride (Give 1 hour before or 2 to 3 hours after Fiberall). Products include:
- Achromycin V Capsules 1193
- Achromycin Ophthalmic Ointment 1% .... ⊙ 307
- Achromycin Ophthalmic Suspension 1% .... ⊙ 308
- Topicycline for Topical Solution 1856

FIBERALL FIBER WAFERS-FRUIT & NUT
(Psyllium Preparations) 851
No interactions described in labeling.

FIBERALL FIBER WAFERS - OATMEAL RAISIN
(Psyllium Preparations) 851
No interactions described in labeling.

FIBERALL POWDER, NATURAL FLAVOR
(Hydrophilic mucilloid) 851
No interactions described in labeling.

FIBERALL POWDER, ORANGE FLAVOR
(Hydrophilic mucilloid) 851
No interactions described in labeling.

FIBERCON TABLETS
(Calcium Polycarbophil) 1204
May interact with tetracyclines. Compounds in this category include:

Demeclocycline Hydrochloride (Concurrent administration with any form of oral tetracycline must be avoided). Products include:
- Declomycin Capsules, Tablets 1199

Doxycycline Calcium (Concurrent administration with any form of oral tetracycline must be avoided).
- No products indexed under this heading.

Doxycycline Hyclate (Concurrent administration with any form of oral tetracycline must be avoided). Products include:
- Doryx Capsules 1717
- Vibramycin Hyclate Capsules 1787
- Vibramycin Hyclate Intravenous 1968
- Vibra-Tabs Film Coated Tablets 1787

Doxycycline Monohydrate (Concurrent administration with any form of oral tetracycline must be avoided). Products include:
- Monodox Capsules 1630
- Vibramycin Monohydrate for Oral Suspension 1787

Methacycline Hydrochloride (Concurrent administration with any form of oral tetracycline must be avoided).
- No products indexed under this heading.

Minocycline Hydrochloride (Concurrent administration with any form of oral tetracycline must be avoided). Products include:
- Minocin Intravenous 1221
- Minocin Oral Suspension 1224
- Minocin Pellet-Filled Capsules 1222

Oxytetracycline Hydrochloride (Concurrent administration with any form of oral tetracycline must be avoided). Products include:
- Terra-Cortril Ophthalmic Suspension 1963
- Terramycin Capsules 1786
- Terramycin Intramuscular Solution 1964
- Terramycin with Polymyxin B Sulfate Ophthalmic Ointment 1965

Tetracycline Hydrochloride (Concurrent administration with any form of oral tetracycline must be avoided). Products include:
- Achromycin V Capsules 1193
- Achromycin Ophthalmic Ointment 1% .... ⊙ 307
- Achromycin Ophthalmic Suspension 1% .... ⊙ 308
- Topicycline for Topical Solution 1856

FIBER-MALT
(Malt Extract) 1190
No interactions described in labeling.

FIBERMED HIGH FIBER SUPPLEMENTS
(Fiber Supplement) 1814
No interactions described in labeling.

FIBERMED MINIATURES
(Fiber Supplement) 1814
No interactions described in labeling.

FILTERAY BROAD SPECTRUM SUNSCREEN LOTION
(Avobenzone, Padimate O (Octyl Dimethyl Paba)) .... ▣ 541
No interactions described in labeling.

FIORICET TABLETS
(Butalbital, Acetaminophen, Caffeine) 2006
May interact with narcotic analgesics, antihistamines, tranquilizers, central nervous system depressants, neuromuscular blocking agents, tricyclic antidepressants, oral anticoagulants, and certain other agents. Compounds in these categories include:

Alcohol (Additive CNS depressant effects).

Alfentanil Hydrochloride (Additive CNS depressant effects). Products include:
- Alfenta Injection 1131

Alprazolam (Additive CNS depressant effects). Products include:
- Xanax Tablets 2367

Amitriptyline Hydrochloride (Decreased blood levels of depressant). Products include:
- Elavil 2269
- Endep Tablets 1927
- Etrafon 2087
- Limbitrol 1933
- Triavil Tablets 1556

Amoxapine (Decreased blood levels of depressant). Products include:
- Asendin Tablets 1196

Aprobarbital (Additive CNS depressant effects). Products include:
- Alurate Elixir 1883

Astemizole (Additive CNS depressant effects). Products include:
- Hismanal Tablets 1138

Azatadine Maleate (Additive CNS depressant effects). Products include:
- Optimine Tablets 2115
- Trinalin Repetabs Tablets 1170

Bromodiphenhydramine Hydrochloride (Additive CNS depressant effects).
- No products indexed under this heading.

Brompheniramine Maleate (Additive CNS depressant effects). Products include:
- Alka Seltzer Plus Sinus Allergy Medicine .... ▣ 624
- Atrohist Sprinkle Capsules 558
- Bromfed Capsules (Timed Release) 1615
- Bromfed Syrup .... ▣ 628
- Bromfed 1615
- Dimetane Decongestant .... ▣ 673
- Dimetane .... ▣ 672
- Dimetane-DC Cough Syrup 1857
- Dimetane-DX Cough Syrup 1858
- Dimetapp Elixir .... ▣ 673
- Dimetapp DM Elixir .... ▣ 674
- Dimetapp Extentabs .... ▣ 674
- Dimetapp Plus Caplets .... ▣ 675
- Dimetapp Tablets .... ▣ 675
- Drixoral Antihistamine/Nasal Decongestant Syrup .... ▣ 698

Buprenorphine (Additive CNS depressant effects).
- No products indexed under this heading.

Buspirone Hydrochloride (Additive CNS depressant effects). Products include:
- BuSpar 1401

Butabarbital (Additive CNS depressant effects). Products include:
- Pyridium Plus 1764

Chlordiazepoxide (Additive CNS depressant effects). Products include:
- Libritabs Tablets 1930
- Limbitrol 1933
- Menrium Tablets 1934

Chlordiazepoxide Hydrochloride (Additive CNS depressant effects). Products include:
- Librax Capsules 1929
- Librium Capsules 1931
- Librium Injectable 1932

Chlorpheniramine Maleate (Additive CNS depressant effects). Products include:
- A.R.M. Allergy Relief Medicine Caplets .... ▣ 615
- Alka-Seltzer Plus Cold Medicine .... ▣ 623
- Allerest .... ▣ 559
- Ana-Kit Anaphylaxis Emergency Treatment Kit 1100
- BC Cold Powder Multi-Symptom Formula .... ▣ 517
- Brexin L.A. Capsules 2078
- Cerose-DM 2443
- Cheracol Plus Head Cold/Cough Formula .... ▣ 667
- Chlor-Trimeton Allergy Syrup, Tablets & Long-Acting Repetabs Tablets .... ▣ 693
- Chlor-Trimeton Decongestant .... ▣ 694
- Comhist LA Capsules 1618
- Allergy-Sinus Comtrex Multi-Symptom Allergy Sinus Formula Tablets & Caplets 746
- Comtrex Multi-Symptom Cold Reliever Tablets/Caplets/Liqui-Gels/Liquid 745
- Day-Night Comtrex 747
- Contac Continuous Action Decongestant/Antihistamine Capsules ▣ 710
- Contac Maximum Strength Continuous Action Decongestant/Antihistamine Caplets .... ▣ 709
- Contac Severe Cold and Flu Formula Caplets .... ▣ 711
- Coricidin 'D' Decongestant Tablets .... ▣ 695
- Coricidin Demilets Tablets for Children .... ▣ 696
- Coricidin Tablets .... ▣ 695
- Deconamine 663
- Demazin Nasal Decongestant/Antihistamine Repetabs Tablets & Syrup .... ▣ 697
- Dorcol Children's Liquid Cold Formula .... ▣ 686
- Dristan Decongestant/Antihistamine/ Analgesic Coated Caplets .... ▣ 749
- Dristan Cold Nasal Decongestant/Antihistamine/ Analgesic Coated Tablets 2419
- Dristan Advanced Formula Decongestant/Antihistamine/Analgesic Tablets .... ▣ 749
- Extendryl 994
- 4-Way Cold Tablets 750
- Fedahist Gyrocaps 2145
- Fedahist Timecaps 2145
- Hycomine Compound Tablets 929
- Isoclor Timesule Capsules .... ▣ 561
- Kronofed-A 970
- Medi-Flu Caplet, Liquid .... ▣ 640
- Naldecon Syrup, Tablets, Pediatric Drops and Pediatric Syrup 709
- Nolamine Tablets 838
- Novafed A Capsules 1342
- Novahistine DH 1342
- Novahistine Elixir .... ▣ 596
- Ornade Spansule Capsules 2221
- Orthoxicol Cough Syrup .... ▣ 668
- PediaCare Allergy Relief Formula Liquid 1362
- PediaCare Cough-Cold Formula Liquid 1362
- PediaCare Night Rest Cough-Cold Formula Liquid 1362
- PediaCare 6-12 Cough-Cold Formula Chewable Tablets 1362
- Pyrroxate Capsules .... ▣ 669
- Quelidrine Syrup 556
- Ru-Tuss II Capsules 693
- Ru-Tuss Tablets 693
- Ryna .... ▣ 741
- Sinarest Tablets & Extra Strength Tablets .... ▣ 562
- Sine-Off Maximum Strength Allergy/Sinus Formula Caplets .... ▣ 721
- Sine-Off Sinus Medicine Tablets-Aspirin Formula .... ▣ 722
- Singlet Tablets .... ▣ 598
- Sinulin 840
- Sinutab Maximum Strength .... ▣ 641
- St. Joseph Nighttime Cold Medicine .... ▣ 705
- Sudafed Plus Liquid .... ▣ 544
- Sudafed Plus Tablets .... ▣ 545
- Teldrin Timed-Release Allergy Capsules, 12 mg 2192
- TheraFlu Flu and Cold Medicine .... ▣ 687
- Triaminic Allergy Tablets .... ▣ 688
- Triaminic Chewables .... ▣ 688
- Triaminic Cold Tablets .... ▣ 688
- Triaminic Nite Light .... ▣ 689
- Triaminic Syrup .... ▣ 689
- Triaminic-12 Tablets .... ▣ 690
- Triaminicin Tablets .... ▣ 690
- Triaminicol Multi-Symptom Cold Tablets .... ▣ 691
- Triaminicol Multi-Symptom Relief ▣ 691
- Tylenol Allergy Sinus Medication Caplets and Gelcaps, Maximum Strength 1372
- Children's Tylenol Cold Liquid Formula and Chewable Tablets 1368
- Tylenol Cold & Flu Hot Medication, Packets 1369
- Tylenol Cold Medication Caplets and Tablets 1370
- Tylenol Cold Medication, Effervescent Tablets 1369
- Vicks Children's NyQuil .... ▣ 664
- Vicks Formula 44 Cough Medicine .... ▣ 661
- Vicks Formula 44M Multi-Symptom Cough Medicine .... ▣ 662
- Vicks Pediatric Formula 44m Multi-Symptom Cough & Cold Medicine .... ▣ 663

Chlorpheniramine Polistirex (Additive CNS depressant effects). Products include:
- Tussionex Extended-Release Suspension 988

Chlorpheniramine Tannate (Additive CNS depressant effects). Products include:
- Rynatan 2387
- Rynatuss 2388

Chlorpromazine (Additive CNS depressant effects). Products include:
- Thorazine ... 2234

Chlorprothixene (Additive CNS depressant effects). Products include:
- Taractan Tablets ... 1920

Chlorprothixene Hydrochloride (Additive CNS depressant effects). Products include:
- Taractan ... 1920

Clemastine Fumarate (Additive CNS depressant effects). Products include:
- Tavist Syrup ... 2033
- Tavist Tablets ... 2035
- Tavist-D Tablets ... 2035

Clomipramine Hydrochloride (Decreased blood levels of depressant). Products include:
- Anafranil Capsules ... 650

Clorazepate Dipotassium (Additive CNS depressant effects). Products include:
- Tranxene ... 556

Clozapine (Additive CNS depressant effects). Products include:
- Clozaril Tablets ... 2000

Codeine (Additive CNS depressant effects). Products include:
- Calcidrine Syrup ... 506

Codeine Phosphate (Additive CNS depressant effects). Products include:
- Actifed with Codeine Cough Syrup ... 752
- Cheracol Cough Syrup ... 1853
- Codimal PH Syrup ... 846
- Dimetane-DC Cough Syrup ... 1857
- Empirin with Codeine Phosphate Nos. 2, 3 & 4 ... 764
- Fiorinal with Codeine Capsules ... 2008
- Isoclor Expectorant ... 982
- Naldecon CX Adult Liquid ... ▣ 521
- Novahistine DH ... 1342
- Novahistine Expectorant ... 1343
- Nucofed Capsules ... 2219
- Nucofed Expectorant ... 2219
- Nucofed Pediatric Expectorant ... 2220
- Nucofed Syrup ... 2219
- Phenaphen with Codeine Capsules 1865
- Phenaphen-650 with Codeine Tablets ... 1866
- Phenergan with Codeine ... 2497
- Phenergan VC with Codeine ... 2501
- Robitussin A-C Syrup ... 1875
- Robitussin-DAC Syrup ... 1875
- Ryna ... ▣ 741
- Soma Compound w/Codeine Tablets ... 2390
- Triaminic Expectorant w/Codeine ... 1996
- Tussi-Organidin Liquid ... 2391
- Tylenol with Codeine ... 1381

Codeine Polistirex (Additive CNS depressant effects).
- No products indexed under this heading.

Cyproheptadine Hydrochloride (Additive CNS depressant effects). Products include:
- Periactin ... 1525

Desipramine Hydrochloride (Decreased blood levels of depressant). Products include:
- Norpramin Tablets ... 1340

Dexchlorpheniramine Maleate (Additive CNS depressant effects). Products include:
- Polaramine ... 2116

Dezocine (Additive CNS depressant effects).

Diazepam (Additive CNS depressant effects). Products include:
- Valium Injectable ... 1937
- Valium Tablets ... 1939
- Valrelease Capsules ... 1923

Dicumarol (Decreased anticoagulant effect). Products include:
- Dicumarol Tablets ... 516

Diphenhydramine Citrate (Additive CNS depressant effects). Products include:
- Alka-Seltzer Plus Night-Time Cold Medicine ... ▣ 623
- Bufferin AF Nite Time Analgesic/Sleeping Aid Caplets ... 744
- Excedrin P.M. Analgesic/Sleeping Aid Tablets, Caplets and Liquid ... 749

Diphenylpyraline Hydrochloride (Additive CNS depressant effects).
- No products indexed under this heading.

Doxepin Hydrochloride (Decreased blood levels of depressant). Products include:
- Sinequan ... 1960

Droperidol (Additive CNS depressant effects). Products include:
- Inapsine Injection ... 1140
- Innovar Injection ... 1141

Enflurane (Additive CNS depressant effects). Products include:
- Ethrane ... 599

Estazolam (Additive CNS depressant effects). Products include:
- ProSom Tablets ... 554

Ethchlorvynol (Additive CNS depressant effects). Products include:
- Placidyl Capsules ... 553

Ethinamate (Additive CNS depressant effects).
- No products indexed under this heading.

Fentanyl (Additive CNS depressant effects). Products include:
- Duragesic Transdermal System ... 1133

Fentanyl Citrate (Additive CNS depressant effects). Products include:
- Innovar Injection ... 1141
- Sublimaze Injection ... 1146

Fluphenazine Decanoate (Additive CNS depressant effects). Products include:
- Prolixin Decanoate ... 1795

Fluphenazine Enanthate (Additive CNS depressant effects). Products include:
- Prolixin Enanthate ... 1796

Fluphenazine Hydrochloride (Additive CNS depressant effects). Products include:
- Prolixin Elixir ... 1793
- Prolixin Injection ... 1791
- Prolixin Oral Concentrate ... 1792
- Prolixin Tablets ... 1793

Flurazepam Hydrochloride (Additive CNS depressant effects). Products include:
- Dalmane Capsules ... 1927

Glutethimide (Additive CNS depressant effects).
- No products indexed under this heading.

Haloperidol (Additive CNS depressant effects). Products include:
- Haldol Injection, Tablets and Concentrate ... 1373

Haloperidol Decanoate (Additive CNS depressant effects). Products include:
- Haldol Decanoate ... 1375

Hydrocodone Bitartrate (Additive CNS depressant effects). Products include:
- Anexsia 5/500 Tablets ... 2196
- Anexsia 7.5/650 Tablets ... 2197
- Azdone Tablets ... 844
- Codiclear DH Syrup ... 845
- Codimal DH Syrup ... 846
- Damason-P ... 1356
- Hycodan Syrup, Tablets ... 927
- Hycomine Compound Tablets ... 929
- Hycomine Syrup ... 927
- Hycotuss Expectorant Syrup ... 930
- Hydrocet Capsules ... 835
- Lortab ASA Tablets ... 2414
- Lortab ... 2412
- Ru-Tuss with Hydrocodone ... 694
- Triaminic Expectorant DH ... 1995
- Vicodin Tablets ... 1187
- Vicodin ES Tablets ... 1189
- Zydone Capsules ... 941

Hydrocodone Polistirex (Additive CNS depressant effects). Products include:
- Tussionex Extended-Release Suspension ... 988

Hydroxyzine Hydrochloride (Additive CNS depressant effects). Products include:
- Atarax Tablets & Syrup ... 1941
- Marax Tablets & DF Syrup ... 1954
- Vistaril Intramuscular Solution ... 1970

Imipramine Hydrochloride (Decreased blood levels of depressant). Products include:
- Tofranil Ampuls ... 1038
- Tofranil Tablets ... 1039

Imipramine Pamoate (Decreased blood levels of depressant). Products include:
- Tofranil-PM Capsules ... 1041

Isocarboxazid (Additive CNS depressant effects). Products include:
- Marplan Tablets ... 1906

Isoflurane (Additive CNS depressant effects). Products include:
- Forane ... 600

Ketamine Hydrochloride (Additive CNS depressant effects). Products include:
- Ketalar ... 1726

Levorphanol Tartrate (Additive CNS depressant effects). Products include:
- Levo-Dromoran ... 1906

Lithium Carbonate (Additive CNS depressant effects). Products include:
- Eskalith ... 2214
- Lithane Tablets ... 1596
- Lithium Carbonate Capsules & Tablets ... 1984
- Lithobid Tablets ... 870

Lithium Citrate (Additive CNS depressant effects). Products include:
- Cibalith-S ... 870

Lorazepam (Additive CNS depressant effects). Products include:
- Ativan Injection ... 2432
- Ativan Tablets ... 2434

Loxapine Hydrochloride (Additive CNS depressant effects). Products include:
- Loxitane ... 1213

Loxapine Succinate (Additive CNS depressant effects). Products include:
- Loxitane Capsules ... 1213

Maprotiline Hydrochloride (Decreased blood levels of depressant). Products include:
- Ludiomil Tablets ... 874

Meperidine Hydrochloride (Additive CNS depressant effects). Products include:
- Demerol ... 2047
- Mepergan Injection ... 2479

Mephobarbital (Additive CNS depressant effects). Products include:
- Mebaral Tablets ... 2061

Meprobamate (Additive CNS depressant effects). Products include:
- Deprol Tablets ... 2382
- Equagesic Tablets ... 2451
- Miltown Tablets ... 2386
- PMB 200 and PMB 400 ... 2504

Mesoridazine (Additive CNS depressant effects). Products include:
- Serentil ... 686

Methadone Hydrochloride (Additive CNS depressant effects). Products include:
- Dolophine Hydrochloride Ampoules & Vials ... 1260
- Dolophine Hydrochloride Tablets ... 1261
- Methadone Hydrochloride Diskets ... 1284
- Methadone Hydrochloride Oral Solution & Tablets ... 1987

Methdilazine Hydrochloride (Additive CNS depressant effects). Products include:
- Tacaryl Syrup & Tablets ... 2409

Methohexital Sodium (Additive CNS depressant effects). Products include:
- Brevital Sodium Vials ... 1248

Methoxyflurane (Additive CNS depressant effects).
- No products indexed under this heading.

Midazolam Hydrochloride (Additive CNS depressant effects). Products include:
- Versed Injection ... 1924

Molindone Hydrochloride (Additive CNS depressant effects). Products include:
- Moban Tablets & Concentrate ... 932

Morphine Sulfate (Additive CNS depressant effects). Products include:
- Astramorph/PF Injection, USP (Preservative-Free) ... 618
- Duramorph ... 960
- Infumorph 200 and Infumorph 500 Sterile Solutions ... 962
- MS Contin Tablets ... 1814
- MSIR ... 1817
- Oramorph SR (Morphine Sulfate Sustained Release Tablets) ... 1988
- Roxanol ... 1991

Nortriptyline Hydrochloride (Decreased blood levels of depressant). Products include:
- Pamelor ... 2019

Opium Alkaloids (Additive CNS depressant effects). Products include:
- B & O No. 15A & No. 16A Supprettes ... 2395
- Pantopon Injectable ... 1911

Oxazepam (Additive CNS depressant effects). Products include:
- Serax Capsules ... 2522
- Serax Tablets ... 2522

Oxycodone Hydrochloride (Additive CNS depressant effects). Products include:
- Percocet Tablets ... 950
- Percodan ... 951
- Roxicodone Tablets, Oral Solution & Intensol (Oxycodone) ... 1992
- Tylox Capsules ... 1382

Pargyline Hydrochloride (Additive CNS depressant effects).
- No products indexed under this heading.

Pentobarbital Sodium (Additive CNS depressant effects). Products include:
- Nembutal Sodium Capsules ... 534
- Nembutal Sodium Solution ... 536
- Nembutal Sodium Suppositories ... 538

Perphenazine (Additive CNS depressant effects). Products include:
- Etrafon ... 2087
- Triavil Tablets ... 1556
- Trilafon ... 2123

Phenelzine Sulfate (Additive CNS depressant effects). Products include:
- Nardil ... 1742

Phenobarbital (Additive CNS depressant effects). Products include:
- Arco-Lase Plus Tablets ... 607
- Bellergal-S Tablets ... 1998
- Bronkolixir ... ▣ 761
- Bronkotabs Tablets ... ▣ 762
- Donnatal ... 1858
- Donnatal Extentabs ... 1859

Donnatal Tablets ... 1858
Donnazyme Tablets ... 1860
Kinesed Tablets ... 2272
Phenobarbital Elixir and Tablets ... 1293
Primatene Tablets-P Formula ... 2421
Quadrinal Tablets ... 1183
Tedral SA ... 1765

Prazepam (Additive CNS depressant effects). Products include:
Centrax ... 1693

Prochlorperazine (Additive CNS depressant effects). Products include:
Compazine ... 2201

Promethazine Hydrochloride (Additive CNS depressant effects). Products include:
Mepergan Injection ... 2479
Phenergan with Codeine ... 2497
Phenergan with Dextromethorphan 2499
Phenergan Injection ... 2493
Phenergan Suppositories ... 2496
Phenergan Syrup ... 2495
Phenergan Tablets ... 2496
Phenergan VC ... 2500
Phenergan VC with Codeine ... 2501

Propofol (Additive CNS depressant effects). Products include:
Diprivan Injection ... 2267

Propoxyphene Hydrochloride (Additive CNS depressant effects). Products include:
Darvon ... 1256
Wygesic Tablets ... 2540

Propoxyphene Napsylate (Additive CNS depressant effects). Products include:
Darvon-N/Darvocet-N ... 1254

Protriptyline Hydrochloride (Decreased blood levels of depressant). Products include:
Vivactil Tablets ... 1567

Pyrilamine Maleate (Additive CNS depressant effects). Products include:
Codimal ... 846
4-Way Fast Acting Nasal Spray - Original Formula (regular & mentholated) & Metered Spray Pump (regular) ... 751
Maximum Strength Midol Multi-Symptom Menstrual Formula ... ▣ 571
Maximum Strength Midol PMS Premenstrual Syndrome Formula ... ▣ 570
Regular Strength Midol Multi-Symptom Menstrual Formula ... ▣ 570
Prefrin-A ... ◉ 255
Prēmsyn PMS Capsules & Caplets ▣ 547
Primatene Tablets-M Formula ... 2421
Robitussin Night Relief ... ▣ 677
Ru-Tuss with Hydrocodone ... 694
Triaminic Expectorant DH ... 1995
Triaminic Oral Infant Drops ... 1996

Pyrilamine Tannate (Additive CNS depressant effects). Products include:
Rynatan ... 2387

Quazepam (Additive CNS depressant effects). Products include:
Doral Tablets ... 2383

Secobarbital Sodium (Additive CNS depressant effects). Products include:
Seconal Sodium Pulvules ... 1296

Sufentanil Citrate (Additive CNS depressant effects). Products include:
Sufenta Injection ... 1147

Temazepam (Additive CNS depressant effects). Products include:
Restoril Capsules ... 2023

Terfenadine (Additive CNS depressant effects). Products include:
Seldane Tablets ... 1349
Seldane-D Extended-Release Tablets ... 1350

Thiamylal Sodium (Additive CNS depressant effects). Products include:
Surital Ampoules, Steri-Vials ... 1764

Thioridazine Hydrochloride (Additive CNS depressant effects). Products include:
Mellaril ... 2011

Thiothixene (Additive CNS depressant effects). Products include:
Navane Capsules and Concentrate 1954
Navane Intramuscular ... 1956

Tranylcypromine Sulfate (Additive CNS depressant effects). Products include:
Parnate Tablets ... 2222

Triazolam (Additive CNS depressant effects). Products include:
Halcion Tablets ... 2340

Trifluoperazine Hydrochloride (Additive CNS depressant effects). Products include:
Stelazine ... 2226

Trimeprazine Tartrate (Additive CNS depressant effects). Products include:
Temaril Tablets, Syrup and Spansule Sustained Release Capsules 1085

Trimipramine Maleate (Decreased blood levels of depressant). Products include:
Surmontil Capsules ... 2524

Tripelennamine Hydrochloride (Additive CNS depressant effects). Products include:
PBZ Tablets & Elixir ... 1037
PBZ-SR Tablets ... 1037

Triprolidine Hydrochloride (Additive CNS depressant effects). Products include:
Actidil ... ▣ 538
Actifed Capsules ... ▣ 539
Actifed Plus Caplets ... ▣ 539
Actifed Plus Tablets ... ▣ 540
Actifed with Codeine Cough Syrup .. 752
Actifed Syrup ... ▣ 540
Actifed Tablets ... ▣ 540
Actifed 12-Hour Capsules ... ▣ 539

Warfarin Sodium (Decreased anticoagulant effect). Products include:
Coumadin Injection & Tablets ... 944
Panwarfin Tablets ... 547

FIORINAL CAPSULES
(Butalbital, Aspirin) ... 2007
May interact with central nervous system depressants, hypnotics and sedatives, and certain other agents. Compounds in these categories include:

Alcohol (Additive effects).

Alfentanil Hydrochloride (Additive effects). Products include:
Alfenta Injection ... 1131

Alprazolam (Additive effects). Products include:
Xanax Tablets ... 2367

Aprobarbital (Additive effects). Products include:
Alurate Elixir ... 1883

Buprenorphine (Additive effects).
No products indexed under this heading.

Buspirone Hydrochloride (Additive effects). Products include:
BuSpar ... 1401

Butabarbital (Additive effects). Products include:
Pyridium Plus ... 1764

Chlordiazepoxide (Additive effects). Products include:
Libritabs Tablets ... 1930
Limbitrol ... 1933
Menrium Tablets ... 1934

Chlordiazepoxide Hydrochloride (Additive effects). Products include:
Librax Capsules ... 1929
Librium Capsules ... 1931
Librium Injectable ... 1932

Chlorpromazine (Additive effects). Products include:
Thorazine ... 2234

Chlorprothixene (Additive effects). Products include:
Taractan Tablets ... 1920

Chlorprothixene Hydrochloride (Additive effects). Products include:
Taractan ... 1920

Clorazepate Dipotassium (Additive effects). Products include:
Tranxene ... 556

Codeine (Additive effects). Products include:
Calcidrine Syrup ... 506

Codeine Phosphate (Additive effects). Products include:
Actifed with Codeine Cough Syrup.. 752
Cheracol Cough Syrup ... 1853
Codimal PH Syrup ... 846
Dimetane-DC Cough Syrup ... 1857
Empirin with Codeine Phosphate Nos. 2, 3 & 4 ... 764
Fiorinal with Codeine Capsules ... 2008
Isoclor Expectorant ... 982
Naldecon CX Adult Liquid ... ▣ 521
Novahistine DH ... 1342
Novahistine Expectorant ... 1343
Nucofed Capsules ... 2219
Nucofed Expectorant ... 2219
Nucofed Pediatric Expectorant ... 2220
Nucofed Syrup ... 2219
Phenaphen with Codeine Capsules 1865
Phenaphen-650 with Codeine Tablets ... 1866
Phenergan with Codeine ... 2497
Phenergan VC with Codeine ... 2501
Robitussin A-C Syrup ... 1875
Robitussin-DAC Syrup ... 1875
Ryna ... ▣ 741
Soma Compound w/Codeine Tablets ... 2390
Triaminic Expectorant w/Codeine .. 1996
Tussi-Organidin Liquid ... 2391
Tylenol with Codeine ... 1381

Codeine Polistirex (Additive effects).
No products indexed under this heading.

Dezocine (Additive effects).

Diazepam (Additive effects). Products include:
Valium Injectable ... 1937
Valium Tablets ... 1939
Valrelease Capsules ... 1923

Droperidol (Additive effects). Products include:
Inapsine Injection ... 1140
Innovar Injection ... 1141

Enflurane (Additive effects). Products include:
Ethrane ... 599

Estazolam (Additive effects). Products include:
ProSom Tablets ... 554

Ethchlorvynol (Additive effects). Products include:
Placidyl Capsules ... 553

Ethinamate (Additive effects).
No products indexed under this heading.

Fentanyl (Additive effects). Products include:
Duragesic Transdermal System ... 1133

Fentanyl Citrate (Additive effects). Products include:
Innovar Injection ... 1141
Sublimaze Injection ... 1146

Fluphenazine Decanoate (Additive effects). Products include:
Prolixin Decanoate ... 1795

Fluphenazine Enanthate (Additive effects). Products include:
Prolixin Enanthate ... 1796

Fluphenazine Hydrochloride (Additive effects). Products include:
Prolixin Elixir ... 1793
Prolixin Injection ... 1791
Prolixin Oral Concentrate ... 1792
Prolixin Tablets ... 1793

Flurazepam Hydrochloride (Additive effects). Products include:
Dalmane Capsules ... 1927

Glutethimide (Additive effects).
No products indexed under this heading.

Haloperidol (Additive effects). Products include:
Haldol Injection, Tablets and Concentrate ... 1373

Haloperidol Decanoate (Additive effects). Products include:
Haldol Decanoate ... 1375

Hydrocodone Bitartrate (Additive effects). Products include:
Anexsia 5/500 Tablets ... 2196
Anexsia 7.5/650 Tablets ... 2197
Azdōne Tablets ... 844
Codiclear DH Syrup ... 845
Codimal DH Syrup ... 846
Damason-P ... 1356
Hycodan Syrup, Tablets ... 927
Hycomine Compound Tablets ... 929
Hycomine Syrup ... 927
Hycotuss Expectorant Syrup ... 930
Hydrocet Capsules ... 835
Lortab ASA Tablets ... 2414
Lortab ... 2412
Ru-Tuss with Hydrocodone ... 694
Triaminic Expectorant DH ... 1995
Vicodin Tablets ... 1187
Vicodin ES Tablets ... 1189
Zydone Capsules ... 941

Hydrocodone Polistirex (Additive effects). Products include:
Tussionex Extended-Release Suspension ... 988

Hydroxyzine Hydrochloride (Additive effects). Products include:
Atarax Tablets & Syrup ... 1941
Marax Tablets & DF Syrup ... 1954
Vistaril Intramuscular Solution ... 1970

Isoflurane (Additive effects). Products include:
Forane ... 600

Ketamine Hydrochloride (Additive effects). Products include:
Ketalar ... 1726

Levorphanol Tartrate (Additive effects). Products include:
Levo-Dromoran ... 1906

Lorazepam (Additive effects). Products include:
Ativan Injection ... 2432
Ativan Tablets ... 2434

Loxapine Hydrochloride (Additive effects). Products include:
Loxitane ... 1213

Loxapine Succinate (Additive effects). Products include:
Loxitane Capsules ... 1213

Meperidine Hydrochloride (Additive effects). Products include:
Demerol ... 2047
Mepergan Injection ... 2479

Mephobarbital (Additive effects). Products include:
Mebaral Tablets ... 2061

Meprobamate (Additive effects). Products include:
Deprol Tablets ... 2382
Equagesic Tablets ... 2451
Miltown Tablets ... 2386
PMB 200 and PMB 400 ... 2504

Mesoridazine (Additive effects). Products include:
Serentil ... 686

Methadone Hydrochloride (Additive effects). Products include:
Dolophine Hydrochloride Ampoules & Vials ... 1260
Dolophine Hydrochloride Tablets ... 1261
Methadone Hydrochloride Diskets .. 1284
Methadone Hydrochloride Oral Solution & Tablets ... 1987

Methohexital Sodium (Additive effects). Products include:
Brevital Sodium Vials ... 1248

Methoxyflurane (Additive effects).
No products indexed under this heading.

Midazolam Hydrochloride (Additive effects). Products include:
Versed Injection 1924

Molindone Hydrochloride (Additive effects). Products include:
Moban Tablets & Concentrate 932

Morphine Sulfate (Additive effects). Products include:
Astramorph/PF Injection, USP (Preservative-Free) 618
Duramorph 960
Infumorph 200 and Infumorph 500 Sterile Solutions 962
MS Contin Tablets 1814
MSIR 1817
Oramorph SR (Morphine Sulfate Sustained Release Tablets) 1988
Roxanol 1991

Opium Alkaloids (Additive effects). Products include:
B & O No. 15A & No. 16A Supprettes 2395
Pantopon Injectable 1911

Oxazepam (Additive effects). Products include:
Serax Capsules 2522
Serax Tablets 2522

Oxycodone Hydrochloride (Additive effects). Products include:
Percocet Tablets 950
Percodan 951
Roxicodone Tablets, Oral Solution & Intensol (Oxycodone) 1992
Tylox Capsules 1382

Pentobarbital Sodium (Additive effects). Products include:
Nembutal Sodium Capsules 534
Nembutal Sodium Solution 536
Nembutal Sodium Suppositories 538

Perphenazine (Additive effects). Products include:
Etrafon 2087
Triavil Tablets 1556
Trilafon 2123

Phenobarbital (Additive effects). Products include:
Arco-Lase Plus Tablets 607
Bellergal-S Tablets 1998
Bronkolixir .... ▣ 761
Bronkotabs Tablets .... ▣ 762
Donnatal 1858
Donnatal Extentabs 1859
Donnatal Tablets 1858
Donnazyme Tablets 1860
Kinesed Tablets 2272
Phenobarbital Elixir and Tablets 1293
Primatene Tablets-P Formula 2421
Quadrinal Tablets 1183
Tedral SA 1765

Prazepam (Additive effects). Products include:
Centrax 1693

Prochlorperazine (Additive effects). Products include:
Compazine 2201

Promethazine Hydrochloride (Additive effects). Products include:
Mepergan Injection 2479
Phenergan with Codeine 2497
Phenergan with Dextromethorphan 2499
Phenergan Injection 2493
Phenergan Suppositories 2496
Phenergan Syrup 2495
Phenergan Tablets 2496
Phenergan VC 2500
Phenergan VC with Codeine 2501

Propofol (Additive effects). Products include:
Diprivan Injection 2267

Propoxyphene Hydrochloride (Additive effects). Products include:
Darvon 1256
Wygesic Tablets 2540

Propoxyphene Napsylate (Additive effects). Products include:
Darvon-N/Darvocet-N 1254

Quazepam (Additive effects). Products include:
Doral Tablets 2383

Secobarbital Sodium (Additive effects). Products include:
Seconal Sodium Pulvules 1296

Sufentanil Citrate (Additive effects). Products include:
Sufenta Injection 1147

Temazepam (Additive effects). Products include:
Restoril Capsules 2023

Thiamylal Sodium (Additive effects). Products include:
Surital Ampoules, Steri-Vials 1764

Thioridazine Hydrochloride (Additive effects). Products include:
Mellaril 2011

Thiothixene (Additive effects). Products include:
Navane Capsules and Concentrate 1954
Navane Intramuscular 1956

Triazolam (Additive effects). Products include:
Halcion Tablets 2340

Trifluoperazine Hydrochloride (Additive effects). Products include:
Stelazine 2226

FIORINAL WITH CODEINE CAPSULES
(Codeine Phosphate, Butalbital, Caffeine, Aspirin) 2008
May interact with central nervous system depressants, hypnotics and sedatives, monoamine oxidase inhibitors, corticosteroids, oral anticoagulants, oral hypoglycemic agents, insulin, tranquilizers, narcotic analgesics, non-steroidal anti-inflammatory agents, general anesthetics, and certain other agents. Compounds in these categories include:

Alcohol (Increased CNS depression).

Alfentanil Hydrochloride (Increased CNS depression). Products include:
Alfenta Injection 1131

Alprazolam (Increased CNS depression). Products include:
Xanax Tablets 2367

Aprobarbital (Increased CNS depression). Products include:
Alurate Elixir 1883

Betamethasone Acetate (Potential for salicylism when corticosteroid therapy is stopped). Products include:
Celestone Soluspan Suspension 2081

Betamethasone Sodium Phosphate (Potential for salicylism when corticosteroid therapy is stopped). Products include:
Celestone Soluspan Suspension 2081

Buprenorphine (Increased CNS depression).
No products indexed under this heading.

Buspirone Hydrochloride (Increased CNS depression). Products include:
BuSpar 1401

Butabarbital (Increased CNS depression). Products include:
Pyridium Plus 1764

Chlordiazepoxide (Increased CNS depression). Products include:
Libritabs Tablets 1930
Limbitrol 1933
Menrium Tablets 1934

Chlordiazepoxide Hydrochloride (Increased CNS depression). Products include:
Librax Capsules 1929
Librium Capsules 1931
Librium Injectable 1932

Chlorpromazine (Increased CNS depression). Products include:
Thorazine 2234

Chlorpropamide (Potential for hypoglycemia). Products include:
Diabinese Tablets 1775

Chlorprothixene (Increased CNS depression). Products include:
Taractan Tablets 1920

Chlorprothixene Hydrochloride (Increased CNS depression). Products include:
Taractan 1920

Clorazepate Dipotassium (Increased CNS depression). Products include:
Tranxene 556

Codeine (Increased CNS depression). Products include:
Calcidrine Syrup 506

Codeine Polistirex (Increased CNS depression).
No products indexed under this heading.

Cortisone Acetate (Potential for salicylism when corticosteroid therapy is stopped). Products include:
Cortone Acetate Sterile Suspension 1437
Cortone Acetate Tablets 1439

Dexamethasone (Potential for salicylism when corticosteroid therapy is stopped). Products include:
AK-Trol Ointment & Suspension .... ⊚ 207
Decadron Elixir 1445
Decadron Tablets 1447
Decaspray Topical Aerosol 1459
Dexacidin .... ⊚ 272
Maxidex Sterile Ophthalmic Suspension .... ⊚ 223
Maxitrol Ophthalmic Ointment/Suspension .... ⊚ 223
TobraDex Ophthalmic Suspension and Ointment .... ⊚ 228

Dexamethasone Acetate (Potential for salicylism when corticosteroid therapy is stopped). Products include:
Dalalone D.P. Injectable 999
Decadron-LA Sterile Suspension 1457

Dexamethasone Sodium Phosphate (Potential for salicylism when corticosteroid therapy is stopped). Products include:
AK-Dex .... ⊚ 203
Decadron Phosphate Respihaler 1454
Decadron Phosphate Sterile Ophthalmic Ointment 1453
Decadron Phosphate Sterile Ophthalmic Solution 1453
Decadron Phosphate Topical Cream 1455
Decadron Phosphate Turbinaire 1456
Maxidex Sterile Ophthalmic Ointment .... ⊚ 222
NeoDecadron Sterile Ophthalmic Ointment 1517
NeoDecadron Sterile Ophthalmic Solution 1518
NeoDecadron Topical Cream 1518

Dezocine (Increased CNS depression).

Diazepam (Increased CNS depression). Products include:
Valium Injectable 1937
Valium Tablets 1939
Valrelease Capsules 1923

Diclofenac Sodium (Increased risk of peptic ulceration and bleeding). Products include:
Voltaren Ophthalmic Sterile Ophthalmic Solution .... ⊚ 268
Voltaren Tablets 1042

Dicumarol (Enhanced effects of anticoagulants). Products include:
Dicumarol Tablets 516

Droperidol (Increased CNS depression). Products include:
Inapsine Injection 1140
Innovar Injection 1141

Enflurane (Increased CNS depression). Products include:
Ethrane 599

Estazolam (Increased CNS depression). Products include:
ProSom Tablets 554

Ethchlorvynol (Increased CNS depression). Products include:
Placidyl Capsules 553

Ethinamate (Increased CNS depression).
No products indexed under this heading.

Etodolac (Increased risk of peptic ulceration and bleeding). Products include:
Lodine Capsules 2468

Fenoprofen Calcium (Increased risk of peptic ulceration and bleeding). Products include:
Nalfon Pulvules & Tablets 919

Fentanyl (Increased CNS depression). Products include:
Duragesic Transdermal System 1133

Fentanyl Citrate (Increased CNS depression). Products include:
Innovar Injection 1141
Sublimaze Injection 1146

Fluphenazine Decanoate (Increased CNS depression). Products include:
Prolixin Decanoate 1795

Fluphenazine Enanthate (Increased CNS depression). Products include:
Prolixin Enanthate 1796

Fluphenazine Hydrochloride (Increased CNS depression). Products include:
Prolixin Elixir 1793
Prolixin Injection 1791
Prolixin Oral Concentrate 1792
Prolixin Tablets 1793

Flurazepam Hydrochloride (Increased CNS depression). Products include:
Dalmane Capsules 1927

Flurbiprofen (Increased risk of peptic ulceration and bleeding). Products include:
Ansaid Tablets 2319

Furazolidone (Enhances CNS effects of butalbital). Products include:
Furoxone 1855

Glipizide (Potential for hypoglycemia). Products include:
Glucotrol 1952

Glutethimide (Increased CNS depression).
No products indexed under this heading.

Glyburide (Potential for hypoglycemia). Products include:
DiaBeta 1091
Micronase Tablets 2350

Haloperidol (Increased CNS depression). Products include:
Haldol Injection, Tablets and Concentrate 1373

Haloperidol Decanoate (Increased CNS depression). Products include:
Haldol Decanoate 1375

Hydrocodone Bitartrate (Increased CNS depression). Products include:
Anexsia 5/500 Tablets 2196
Anexsia 7.5/650 Tablets 2197
Azdone Tablets 844
Codiclear DH Syrup 845
Codimal DH Syrup 846
Damason-P 1356
Hycodan Syrup, Tablets 927
Hycomine Compound Tablets 929
Hycomine Syrup 927
Hycotuss Expectorant Syrup 930
Hydrocet Capsules 835
Lortab ASA Tablets 2414
Lortab 2412
Ru-Tuss with Hydrocodone 694
Triaminic Expectorant DH 1995
Vicodin Tablets 1187

Vicodin ES Tablets ... 1189
Zydone Capsules ... 941

Hydrocodone Polistirex (Increased CNS depression). Products include:
Tussionex Extended-Release Suspension ... 988

Hydrocortisone (Potential for salicylism when corticosteroid therapy is stopped). Products include:
AK-Spore H.C. ... ⊙ 206
Bactine Hydrocortisone Anti-Itch Cream ... ◙ 625
CaldeCORT Anti-Itch Hydrocortisone Spray ... ◙ 560
Carmol HC Cream 1% ... 2296
Cortaid Spray ... ◙ 735
Cortenema ... 2244
Cortisporin Ointment ... 758
Cortisporin Ophthalmic Ointment Sterile ... 758
Cortisporin Ophthalmic Suspension Sterile ... 759
Cortisporin Otic Solution Sterile ... 760
Cortisporin Otic Suspension Sterile 760
Cortizone-5 Creme & Ointment ... ◙ 732
Dermolate Anti-Itch Cream ... ◙ 697
Eldecort Cream 1.0% ... 1113
Eldecort Cream 1.0% and 2.5% ... 1113
Fungoid HC Creme ... 1770
Hydrocortone Tablets ... 1482
Hytone ... 909
LazerSporin-C Solution ... 1770
Massengill Medicated Soft Cloth Towelettes ... 2192
Nutracort Cream & Lotion ... 1684
PediOtic Suspension Sterile ... 797
Synacort Creams 1%, 2.5% ... 2296
Vanoxide-HC Acne Lotion ... 911
Vioform-Hydrocortisone Cream and Mild Cream ... 889
Vioform-Hydrocortisone Ointment ... 889
VōSoL HC Otic Solution ... 2392
Vytone Cream 1% ... 911

Hydrocortisone Acetate (Potential for salicylism when corticosteroid therapy is stopped). Products include:
Analpram-HC Rectal Cream 1% and 2.5% ... 970
Anusol-HC Cream ... 1690
Anusol-HC Suppositories ... 1691
Caldecort ... ◙ 560
Carmol HC Cream 1% ... 2296
Chloromycetin Hydrocortisone Ophthalmic ... 1694
Coly-Mycin S Otic w/Neomycin & Hydrocortisone ... 1708
Cortaid ... ◙ 735
Cortef Feminine Itch Cream ... ◙ 735
Corticaine ... ◙ 682
Cortifoam ... 1827
Cortisporin Cream ... 757
Epifoam ... 1828
Gynecort 5 Creme ... ◙ 556
Hydrocortone Acetate Sterile Suspension ... 1479
Lanacort 5 Creme and Ointment ... ◙ 557
Mantadil Cream ... 789
Ophthocort ... ⊙ 301
Orabase HCA Oral Paste ... 890
Pramosone Cream, Lotion & Ointment ... 971
ProctoCream-HC ... 1834
Proctofoam-HC ... 1835

Hydrocortisone Sodium Phosphate (Potential for salicylism when corticosteroid therapy is stopped). Products include:
Hydrocortone Phosphate Injection, Sterile ... 1481

Hydrocortisone Sodium Succinate (Potential for salicylism when corticosteroid therapy is stopped). Products include:
Solu-Cortef Sterile Powder ... 2361

Hydroxyzine Hydrochloride (Increased CNS depression). Products include:
Atarax Tablets & Syrup ... 1941
Marax Tablets & DF Syrup ... 1954
Vistaril Intramuscular Solution ... 1970

Ibuprofen (Increased risk of peptic ulceration and bleeding). Products include:
Advil Cold & Sinus Caplets (formerly CoAdvil) ... 2416
Advil Ibuprofen Tablets and Caplets ... 2416
Children's Advil Suspension ... 2426
CoAdvil ... ◙ 748
Dristan Sinus Caplets ... 2419
Haltran Tablets ... ◙ 668
Ibuprofen ... ◙ 631
Medipren ibuprofen Caplets and Tablets ... 1362
Midol 200 Cramp Relief Formula ... ◙ 570
Motrin Tablets ... 2351
Motrin IB Caplets and Tablets ... ◙ 736
Nuprin Ibuprofen/Analgesic Tablets & Caplets ... 752
PediaProfen Suspension ... 1363
Rufen Tablets ... 691
Trendar Ibuprofen Tablets ... ◙ 756

Indomethacin (Increased risk of peptic ulceration and bleeding). Products include:
Indocin ... 1487

Indomethacin Sodium Trihydrate (Increased risk of peptic ulceration and bleeding). Products include:
Indocin I.V. ... 1490

Insulin, Human (Potential for hypoglycemia).
No products indexed under this heading.

Insulin, Human Isophane Suspension (Potential for hypoglycemia). Products include:
Humulin N, 100 Units ... 1270

Insulin, Human NPH (Potential for hypoglycemia). Products include:
Insulatard NPH Human ... 1627
Novolin N ... 1627
Novolin N PenFill Cartridges ... 1628
Novolin N Prefilled ... 1628

Insulin, Human Regular (Potential for hypoglycemia). Products include:
Humulin BR, 100 Units ... 1268
Humulin R, 100 Units ... 1272
Novolin R ... 1627
Novolin R PenFill Cartridges ... 1628
Novolin R Prefilled ... 1629
Velosulin Human ... 1628

Insulin, Human, Zinc Suspension (Potential for hypoglycemia). Products include:
Humulin L, 100 Units ... 1268
Humulin U, 100 Units ... 1272
Novolin L ... 1627

Insulin, NPH (Potential for hypoglycemia). Products include:
NPH, 40 & 100 Units ... 1273
Beef NPH, 100 Units ... 1274
Pork NPH, 100 Units ... 1275
Insulatard NPH ... 1626
NPH Insulin ... 1626
NPH Purified Pork Isophane Insulin ... 1626

Insulin, Regular (Potential for hypoglycemia). Products include:
Regular, 40 & 100 Units ... 1273
Beef Regular, 100 Units ... 1275
Pork Regular, 100 Units ... 1275
Pork Regular (Concentrated), 500 Units ... 1276
Regular Insulin ... 1625
Regular Purified Pork Insulin ... 1626
Velosulin ... 1627

Insulin, Zinc Crystals (Potential for hypoglycemia). Products include:
NPH, 40 & 100 Units ... 1273

Insulin, Zinc Suspension (Potential for hypoglycemia). Products include:
Lente, 40 & 100 Units ... 1272
Protamine, Zinc, 40 & 100 Units ... 1273
Lente Iletin I ... 1272
Beef Lente, 100 Units ... 1274
Beef Protamine Zinc, 100 Units ... 1274
Pork Lente, 100 Units ... 1275
Pork, Protamine, Zinc, 100 Units ... 1275
Lente Insulin ... 1626
Lente Purified Pork Insulin ... 1626
Semilente Insulin ... 1625
Ultralente Insulin ... 1626

Isocarboxazid (Enhances CNS effects of butalbital). Products include:
Marplan Tablets ... 1906

Isoflurane (Increased CNS depression). Products include:
Forane ... 600

Ketamine Hydrochloride (Increased CNS depression). Products include:
Ketalar ... 1726

Ketoprofen (Increased risk of peptic ulceration and bleeding). Products include:
Orudis Capsules ... 2488

Ketorolac Tromethamine (Increased risk of peptic ulceration and bleeding). Products include:
Toradol IM Injection ... 2302

Levorphanol Tartrate (Increased CNS depression). Products include:
Levo-Dromoran ... 1906

Lorazepam (Increased CNS depression). Products include:
Ativan Injection ... 2432
Ativan Tablets ... 2434

Loxapine Hydrochloride (Increased CNS depression). Products include:
Loxitane ... 1213

Loxapine Succinate (Increased CNS depression). Products include:
Loxitane Capsules ... 1213

Meclofenamate Sodium (Increased risk of peptic ulceration and bleeding). Products include:
Meclomen Capsules ... 1739

Mefenamic Acid (Increased risk of peptic ulceration and bleeding). Products include:
Ponstel ... 1758

Meperidine Hydrochloride (Increased CNS depression). Products include:
Demerol ... 2047
Mepergan Injection ... 2479

Mephobarbital (Increased CNS depression). Products include:
Mebaral Tablets ... 2061

Meprobamate (Increased CNS depression). Products include:
Deprol Tablets ... 2382
Equagesic Tablets ... 2451
Miltown Tablets ... 2386
PMB 200 and PMB 400 ... 2504

Mercaptopurine (Enhanced effects of 6-mercaptopurine and potential for bone marrow toxicity and blood dyscrasias). Products include:
Purinethol Tablets ... 800

Mesoridazine (Increased CNS depression). Products include:
Serentil ... 686

Mesoridazine Besylate (Increased CNS depression).

Methadone Hydrochloride (Increased CNS depression). Products include:
Dolophine Hydrochloride Ampoules & Vials ... 1260
Dolophine Hydrochloride Tablets ... 1261
Methadone Hydrochloride Diskets ... 1284
Methadone Hydrochloride Oral Solution & Tablets ... 1987

Methohexital Sodium (Increased CNS depression). Products include:
Brevital Sodium Vials ... 1248

Methotrexate Sodium (Enhanced effects of methotrexate and potential for bone marrow toxicity and blood dyscrasias). Products include:
Methotrexate Tablets, Parenteral, LPF Parenteral ... 1217
Rheumatrex Methotrexate Dose Pack ... 1234

Methoxyflurane (Increased CNS depression).
No products indexed under this heading.

Methylprednisolone Acetate (Potential for salicylism when corticosteroid therapy is stopped). Products include:
Depo-Medrol Sterile Aqueous Suspension ... 2334

Methylprednisolone Sodium Succinate (Potential for salicylism when corticosteroid therapy is stopped). Products include:
Solu-Medrol Sterile Powder ... 2363

Midazolam Hydrochloride (Increased CNS depression). Products include:
Versed Injection ... 1924

Molindone Hydrochloride (Increased CNS depression). Products include:
Moban Tablets & Concentrate ... 932

Morphine Sulfate (Increased CNS depression). Products include:
Astramorph/PF Injection, USP (Preservative-Free) ... 618
Duramorph ... 960
Infumorph 200 and Infumorph 500 Sterile Solutions ... 962
MS Contin Tablets ... 1814
MSIR ... 1817
Oramorph SR (Morphine Sulfate Sustained Release Tablets) ... 1988
Roxanol ... 1991

Naproxen (Increased risk of peptic ulceration and bleeding). Products include:
Naprosyn ... 2297

Naproxen Sodium (Increased risk of peptic ulceration and bleeding). Products include:
Anaprox and Anaprox DS Tablets ... 2288

Opium Alkaloids (Increased CNS depression). Products include:
B & O No. 15A & No. 16A Supprettes ... 2395
Pantopon Injectable ... 1911

Oxazepam (Increased CNS depression). Products include:
Serax Capsules ... 2522
Serax Tablets ... 2522

Oxycodone Hydrochloride (Increased CNS depression). Products include:
Percocet Tablets ... 950
Percodan ... 951
Roxicodone Tablets, Oral Solution & Intensol (Oxycodone) ... 1992
Tylox Capsules ... 1382

Pentobarbital Sodium (Increased CNS depression). Products include:
Nembutal Sodium Capsules ... 534
Nembutal Sodium Solution ... 536
Nembutal Sodium Suppositories ... 538

Perphenazine (Increased CNS depression). Products include:
Etrafon ... 2087
Triavil Tablets ... 1556
Trilafon ... 2123

Phenelzine Sulfate (Enhances CNS effects of butalbital). Products include:
Nardil ... 1742

Phenobarbital (Increased CNS depression). Products include:
Arco-Lase Plus Tablets ... 607
Bellergal-S Tablets ... 1998
Bronkolixir ... ◙ 761
Bronkotabs Tablets ... ◙ 762
Donnatal ... 1858
Donnatal Extentabs ... 1859
Donnatal Tablets ... 1858
Donnazyme Tablets ... 1860
Kinesed Tablets ... 2272
Phenobarbital Elixir and Tablets ... 1293
Primatene Tablets-P Formula ... 2421
Quadrinal Tablets ... 1183
Tedral SA ... 1765

Phenylbutazone (Increased risk of peptic ulceration and bleeding). Products include:
- Butazolidin Capsules & Tablets 1027

Piroxicam (Increased risk of peptic ulceration and bleeding). Products include:
- Feldene Capsules 1777

Prazepam (Increased CNS depression). Products include:
- Centrax 1693

Prednisolone Acetate (Potential for salicylism when corticosteroid therapy is stopped). Products include:
- AK-Cide Sterile Ophthalmic Ointment & Suspension .... ⊚ 202
- Blephamide Liquifilm Sterile Ophthalmic Suspension 586
- Blephamide S.O.P. Sterile Ophthalmic Ointment 586
- Cetapred Ointment .... ⊚ 220
- ⅛ % Econopred & 1 % Econopred Plus .... ⊚ 217
- Isopto Cetapred Suspension .... ⊚ 220
- Metimyd .... ⊚ 306
- Poly-Pred Liquifilm .... ⊚ 250
- Pred Forte .... ⊚ 252
- Pred Mild .... ⊚ 254
- Pred-G Liquifilm Sterile Ophthalmic Suspension .... ⊚ 252
- Pred-G S.O.P. Sterile Ophthalmic Ointment .... ⊚ 253
- Vasocidin Ointment .... ⊚ 275

Prednisolone Sodium Phosphate (Potential for salicylism when corticosteroid therapy is stopped). Products include:
- AK-Pred .... ⊚ 205
- Hydeltrasol Injection, Sterile 1476
- Inflamase .... ⊚ 274
- Pediapred Oral Liquid 987
- Vasocidin Ophthalmic Solution .... ⊚ 276

Prednisolone Tebutate (Potential for salicylism when corticosteroid therapy is stopped). Products include:
- Hydeltra-T.B.A. Sterile Suspension 1478

Prednisone (Potential for salicylism when corticosteroid therapy is stopped). Products include:
- Deltasone Tablets 2332

Probenecid (Reduced uricosuric effects). Products include:
- Benemid Tablets 1426
- ColBENEMID Tablets 1436
- Wycillin Injection and Probenecid Tablets 2539

Prochlorperazine (Increased CNS depression). Products include:
- Compazine 2201

Promethazine Hydrochloride (Increased CNS depression). Products include:
- Mepergan Injection 2479
- Phenergan with Codeine 2497
- Phenergan with Dextromethorphan 2499
- Phenergan Injection 2493
- Phenergan Suppositories 2496
- Phenergan Syrup 2495
- Phenergan Tablets 2496
- Phenergan VC 2500
- Phenergan VC with Codeine 2501

Propofol (Increased CNS depression). Products include:
- Diprivan Injection 2267

Propoxyphene Hydrochloride (Increased CNS depression). Products include:
- Darvon 1256
- Wygesic Tablets 2540

Propoxyphene Napsylate (Increased CNS depression). Products include:
- Darvon-N/Darvocet-N 1254

Quazepam (Increased CNS depression). Products include:
- Doral Tablets 2383

Secobarbital Sodium (Increased CNS depression). Products include:
- Seconal Sodium Pulvules 1296

Selegiline Hydrochloride (Enhances CNS effects of butalbital). Products include:
- Eldepryl 2250

Sufentanil Citrate (Increased CNS depression). Products include:
- Sufenta Injection 1147

Sulfinpyrazone (Reduced uricosuric effects). Products include:
- Anturane 853

Sulindac (Increased risk of peptic ulceration and bleeding). Products include:
- Clinoril Tablets 1433

Temazepam (Increased CNS depression). Products include:
- Restoril Capsules 2023

Thiamylal Sodium (Increased CNS depression). Products include:
- Surital Ampoules, Steri-Vials 1764

Thioridazine Hydrochloride (Increased CNS depression). Products include:
- Mellaril 2011

Thiothixene (Increased CNS depression). Products include:
- Navane Capsules and Concentrate 1954
- Navane Intramuscular 1956

Tolazamide (Potential for hypoglycemia). Products include:
- Tolinase Tablets 2365

Tolbutamide (Potential for hypoglycemia). Products include:
- Orinase Tablets 2354

Tolmetin Sodium (Increased risk of peptic ulceration and bleeding). Products include:
- Tolectin (200, 400 and 600 mg) .. 1379

Tranylcypromine Sulfate (Enhances CNS effects of butalbital). Products include:
- Parnate Tablets 2222

Triamcinolone (Potential for salicylism when corticosteroids therapy is stopped).
- No products indexed under this heading.

Triamcinolone Acetonide (Potential for salicylism when corticosteroids therapy is stopped). Products include:
- Aristocort A 1010
- Azmacort Inhaler 1837
- Kenalog Cream, Lotion & Ointment 2401
- Kenalog-10 Injection 2402
- Kenalog-40 Injection 2403
- Kenalog in Orabase 604
- Kenalog Spray 2401
- Mycolog II Cream and Ointment 2407
- Mytrex Cream & Ointment 2080
- Nasacort Nasal Inhaler 1844

Triamcinolone Diacetate (Potential for salicylism when corticosteroids therapy is stopped). Products include:
- Aristocort Suspension 1008

Triamcinolone Hexacetonide (Potential for salicylism when corticosteroids therapy is stopped). Products include:
- Aristospan Suspension 1011

Triazolam (Increased CNS depression). Products include:
- Halcion Tablets 2340

Trifluoperazine Hydrochloride (Increased CNS depression). Products include:
- Stelazine 2226

Warfarin Sodium (Enhanced effects of anticoagulants). Products include:
- Coumadin Injection & Tablets 944
- Panwarfin Tablets 547

FIORINAL TABLETS
(Butalbital, Aspirin) 2007
See **Fiorinal Capsules**

FLAGYL I.V.
(Metronidazole Hydrochloride) 2131
May interact with oral anticoagulants and certain other agents. Compounds in these categories include:

Alcohol (Potential gastrointestinal side effects).

Cimetidine (Decreases plasma clearance of metronidazole). Products include:
- Tagamet Tablets 2228

Cimetidine Hydrochloride (Decreases plasma clearance of metronidazole). Products include:
- Tagamet 2228

Dicumarol (Potentiation of anticoagulant effect). Products include:
- Dicumarol Tablets 516

Disulfiram (Psychotic reactions have been reported in alcoholic patients who are using metronidazole and disulfiram concurrently). Products include:
- Antabuse Tablets 2429

Phenobarbital (Reduces metronidazole plasma levels). Products include:
- Arco-Lase Plus Tablets 607
- Bellergal-S Tablets 1998
- Bronkolixir .... ▣ 761
- Bronkotabs Tablets .... ▣ 762
- Donnatal 1858
- Donnatal Extentabs 1859
- Donnatal Tablets 1858
- Donnazyme Tablets 1860
- Kinesed Tablets 2272
- Phenobarbital Elixir and Tablets 1293
- Primatene Tablets-P Formula 2421
- Quadrinal Tablets 1183
- Tedral SA 1765

Phenytoin (Reduces metronidazole plasma levels; impaired clearance of phenytoin). Products include:
- Dilantin Infatabs 1710
- Dilantin-30 Pediatric/Dilantin-125 Suspension 1713

Phenytoin Sodium (Reduces metronidazole plasma levels; impaired clearance of phenytoin). Products include:
- Dilantin Kapseals 1708
- Dilantin Parenteral 1712
- Dilantin with Phenobarbital Kapseals 1715

Warfarin Sodium (Potentiation of anticoagulant effect). Products include:
- Coumadin Injection & Tablets 944
- Panwarfin Tablets 547

FLAGYL I.V. RTU
(Metronidazole Hydrochloride) 2131
See **Flagyl I.V.**

FLAGYL TABLETS
(Metronidazole) 2170
May interact with oral anticoagulants, lithium preparations, and certain other agents. Compounds in these categories include:

Alcohol (Abdominal cramps, nausea, vomiting, headaches and flushing may occur).

Cimetidine (Decrease in plasma clearance of metronidazole). Products include:
- Tagamet Tablets 2228

Cimetidine Hydrochloride (Decrease in plasma clearance of metronidazole). Products include:
- Tagamet 2228

Dicumarol (Potentiation of anticoagulant effect). Products include:
- Dicumarol Tablets 516

Disulfiram (Psychotic reactions have been reported in alcoholic patients who are using metronidazole and disulfiram concurrently). Products include:
- Antabuse Tablets 2429

Lithium Carbonate (Potential for lithium toxicity in patients stabilized on high doses of lithium, who are on short-term Flagyl therapy). Products include:
- Eskalith 2214
- Lithane Tablets 1596
- Lithium Carbonate Capsules & Tablets 1984
- Lithobid Tablets 870

Lithium Citrate (Potential for lithium toxicity in patients stabilized on high doses of lithium, who are on short-term Flagyl therapy). Products include:
- Cibalith-S 870

Phenobarbital (Reduces metronidazole plasma levels). Products include:
- Arco-Lase Plus Tablets 607
- Bellergal-S Tablets 1998
- Bronkolixir .... ▣ 761
- Bronkotabs Tablets .... ▣ 762
- Donnatal 1858
- Donnatal Extentabs 1859
- Donnatal Tablets 1858
- Donnazyme Tablets 1860
- Kinesed Tablets 2272
- Phenobarbital Elixir and Tablets 1293
- Primatene Tablets-P Formula 2421
- Quadrinal Tablets 1183
- Tedral SA 1765

Phenytoin (Reduces metronidazole plasma levels). Products include:
- Dilantin Infatabs 1710
- Dilantin-30 Pediatric/Dilantin-125 Suspension 1713

Phenytoin Sodium (Reduces metronidazole plasma levels). Products include:
- Dilantin Kapseals 1708
- Dilantin Parenteral 1712
- Dilantin with Phenobarbital Kapseals 1715

Warfarin Sodium (Potentiation of anticoagulant effect). Products include:
- Coumadin Injection & Tablets 944
- Panwarfin Tablets 547

FLATULEX TABLETS
(Simethicone, Charcoal, Activated) 905

May absorb medication(s) while in the digestive tract.

FLEET BABYLAX
(Glycerin) 991
No interactions described in labeling.

FLEET BISACODYL ENEMA
(Bisacodyl) 991
No interactions described in labeling.

FLEET CHILDREN'S ENEMA
(Sodium Biphosphate, Sodium Phosphate) 991
No interactions described in labeling.

FLEET ENEMA
(Sodium Biphosphate, Sodium Phosphate) 991
No interactions described in labeling.

FLEET FLAVORED CASTOR OIL EMULSION
(Castor Oil) 993
No interactions described in labeling.

FLEET MINERAL OIL ENEMA
(Mineral Oil) 992
No interactions described in labeling.

FLEET PHOSPHO-SODA
(Sodium Phosphate, Dibasic, Sodium Phosphate, Monobasic) 992
No interactions described in labeling.

FLEET PREP KITS
(Sodium Biphosphate, Sodium Phosphate, Bisacodyl) 993
No interactions described in labeling.

FLEET RELIEF
(Zinc Oxide, Mineral Oil, Petrolatum, White) 993
No interactions described in labeling.

FLEX-ALL 454 PAIN RELIEVING GEL
(Menthol) .... ▣ 546
No interactions described in labeling.

FLEXERIL TABLETS
(Cyclobenzaprine Hydrochloride) 1471
May interact with central nervous system depressants, anticholinergics, monoamine oxidase inhibitors, barbiturates, and certain other agents. Compounds in these categories include:

Alcohol (Enhanced effect of alcohol).

Alfentanil Hydrochloride (Enhanced effect of CNS depressants). Products include:
- Alfenta Injection 1131

Alprazolam (Enhanced effect of CNS depressants). Products include:
- Xanax Tablets 2367

Aprobarbital (Enhanced effect of barbiturates). Products include:
- Alurate Elixir 1883

Atropine Sulfate (Use cyclobenzaprine with caution). Products include:
- Arco-Lase Plus Tablets 607
- Atropine Sulfate Sterile Ophthalmic Solution and S.O.P. Sterile Ophthalmic Ointment .... ⊙ 239
- Donnagel .... ▣ 675
- Donnagel-PG 1858
- Donnatal 1858
- Donnatal Extentabs 1859
- Donnatal Tablets 1858
- Donnazyme Tablets 1860
- Isopto Atropine .... ⊙ 218
- Lomotil 2174
- Motofen Tablets 836
- Ru-Tuss Tablets 693
- Urised Tablets 2396

Belladonna Alkaloids (Use cyclobenzaprine with caution). Products include:
- Bellergal-S Tablets 1998
- Hyland's Bed Wetting Tablets .... ▣ 728
- Hyland's Teething Tablets .... ▣ 728
- Kinesed Tablets 2272

Benztropine Mesylate (Use cyclobenzaprine with caution). Products include:
- Cogentin 1435

Biperiden (Use cyclobenzaprine with caution). Products include:
- Akineton 1171

Buprenorphine (Enhanced effect of CNS depressants).
- No products indexed under this heading.

Buspirone Hydrochloride (Enhanced effect of CNS depressants). Products include:
- BuSpar 1401

Butabarbital (Enhanced effect of barbiturates). Products include:
- Pyridium Plus 1764

Butalbital (Enhanced effect of barbiturates). Products include:
- Esgic-Plus Tablets 1002
- Esgic Tablets & Capsules 1001
- Fioricet Tablets 2006
- Fiorinal Capsules 2007
- Fiorinal with Codeine Capsules 2008
- Fiorinal Tablets 2007
- Phrenilin 838
- Sedapap Tablets 50 mg/650 mg .. 1360

Chlordiazepoxide (Enhanced effect of CNS depressants). Products include:
- Libritabs Tablets 1930
- Limbitrol 1933
- Menrium Tablets 1934

Chlordiazepoxide Hydrochloride (Enhanced effect of CNS depressants). Products include:
- Librax Capsules 1929
- Librium Capsules 1931
- Librium Injectable 1932

Chlorpromazine (Enhanced effect of CNS depressants). Products include:
- Thorazine 2234

Chlorprothixene (Enhanced effect of CNS depressants). Products include:
- Taractan Tablets 1920

Chlorprothixene Hydrochloride (Enhanced effect of CNS depressants). Products include:
- Taractan 1920

Clidinium Bromide (Use cyclobenzaprine with caution). Products include:
- Librax Capsules 1929
- Quarzan Capsules 1937

Clorazepate Dipotassium (Enhanced effect of CNS depressants). Products include:
- Tranxene 556

Codeine (Enhanced effect of CNS depressants). Products include:
- Calcidrine Syrup 506

Codeine Phosphate (Enhanced effect of CNS depressants). Products include:
- Actifed with Codeine Cough Syrup.. 752
- Cheracol Cough Syrup 1853
- Codimal PH Syrup 846
- Dimetane-DC Cough Syrup 1857
- Empirin with Codeine Phosphate Nos. 2, 3 & 4 764
- Fiorinal with Codeine Capsules 2008
- Isoclor Expectorant 982
- Naldecon CX Adult Liquid .... ▣ 521
- Novahistine DH 1342
- Novahistine Expectorant 1343
- Nucofed Capsules 2219
- Nucofed Expectorant 2219
- Nucofed Pediatric Expectorant 2220
- Nucofed Syrup 2219
- Phenaphen with Codeine Capsules 1865
- Phenaphen-650 with Codeine Tablets 1866
- Phenergan with Codeine 2497
- Phenergan VC with Codeine 2501
- Robitussin A-C Syrup 1875
- Robitussin-DAC Syrup 1875
- Ryna .... ▣ 741
- Soma Compound w/Codeine Tablets 2390
- Triaminic Expectorant w/Codeine .. 1996
- Tussi-Organidin Liquid 2391
- Tylenol with Codeine 1381

Codeine Polistirex (Enhanced effect of CNS depressants).
- No products indexed under this heading.

Dezocine (Enhanced effect of CNS depressants).

Diazepam (Enhanced effect of CNS depressants). Products include:
- Valium Injectable 1937
- Valium Tablets 1939
- Valrelease Capsules 1923

Dicyclomine Hydrochloride (Use cyclobenzaprine with caution). Products include:
- Bentyl 1322

Droperidol (Enhanced effect of CNS depressants). Products include:
- Inapsine Injection 1140
- Innovar Injection 1141

Enflurane (Enhanced effect of CNS depressants). Products include:
- Ethrane 599

Estazolam (Enhanced effect of CNS depressants). Products include:
- ProSom Tablets 554

Ethchlorvynol (Enhanced effect of CNS depressants). Products include:
- Placidyl Capsules 553

Ethinamate (Enhanced effect of CNS depressants).
- No products indexed under this heading.

Fentanyl (Enhanced effect of CNS depressants). Products include:
- Duragesic Transdermal System 1133

Fentanyl Citrate (Enhanced effect of CNS depressants). Products include:
- Innovar Injection 1141
- Sublimaze Injection 1146

Fluphenazine Decanoate (Enhanced effect of CNS depressants). Products include:
- Prolixin Decanoate 1795

Fluphenazine Enanthate (Enhanced effect of CNS depressants). Products include:
- Prolixin Enanthate 1796

Fluphenazine Hydrochloride (Enhanced effect of CNS depressants). Products include:
- Prolixin Elixir 1793
- Prolixin Injection 1791
- Prolixin Oral Concentrate 1792
- Prolixin Tablets 1793

Flurazepam Hydrochloride (Enhanced effect of CNS depressants). Products include:
- Dalmane Capsules 1927

Furazolidone (Contraindication; hyperpyretic crisis; severe convulsions; death). Products include:
- Furoxone 1855

Glutethimide (Enhanced effect of CNS depressants).
- No products indexed under this heading.

Glycopyrrolate (Use cyclobenzaprine with caution). Products include:
- Robinul Forte Tablets 1873
- Robinul Injectable 1873
- Robinul Tablets 1873

Guanethidine Monosulfate (Antihypertensive action of guanethidine blocked). Products include:
- Esimil Tablets 864
- Ismelin Tablets 869

Haloperidol (Enhanced effect of CNS depressants). Products include:
- Haldol Injection, Tablets and Concentrate 1373

Haloperidol Decanoate (Enhanced effect of CNS depressants). Products include:
- Haldol Decanoate 1375

Hydrocodone Bitartrate (Enhanced effect of CNS depressants). Products include:
- Anexsia 5/500 Tablets 2196
- Anexsia 7.5/650 Tablets 2197
- Azdone Tablets 844
- Codiclear DH Syrup 845
- Codimal DH Syrup 846
- Damason-P 1356
- Hycodan Syrup, Tablets 927
- Hycomine Compound Tablets 929
- Hycomine Syrup 927
- Hycotuss Expectorant Syrup 930
- Hydrocet Capsules 835
- Lortab ASA Tablets 2414
- Lortab 2412
- Ru-Tuss with Hydrocodone 694
- Triaminic Expectorant DH 1995
- Vicodin Tablets 1187
- Vicodin ES Tablets 1189
- Zydone Capsules 941

Hydrocodone Polistirex (Enhanced effect of CNS depressants). Products include:
- Tussionex Extended-Release Suspension 988

Hydroxyzine Hydrochloride (Enhanced effect of CNS depressants). Products include:
- Atarax Tablets & Syrup 1941
- Marax Tablets & DF Syrup 1954
- Vistaril Intramuscular Solution 1970

Hyoscyamine (Use cyclobenzaprine with caution). Products include:
- Cystospaz Tablets 2395
- Urised Tablets 2396

Hyoscyamine Sulfate (Use cyclobenzaprine with caution). Products include:
- Arco-Lase Plus Tablets 607
- Cystospaz-M Capsules 2395
- Donnagel .... ▣ 675
- Donnagel-PG 1858
- Donnatal 1858
- Donnatal Extentabs 1859
- Donnatal Tablets 1858
- Donnazyme Tablets 1860
- Kutrase Capsules 2146
- Levsin/Levsinex 2147
- Ru-Tuss Tablets 693

Ipratropium Bromide (Use cyclobenzaprine with caution). Products include:
- Atrovent Inhalation Aerosol 675

Isocarboxazid (Contraindication; hyperpyretic crisis; severe convulsions; death). Products include:
- Marplan Tablets 1906

Isoflurane (Enhanced effect of CNS depressants). Products include:
- Forane 600

Ketamine Hydrochloride (Enhanced effect of CNS depressants). Products include:
- Ketalar 1726

Levorphanol Tartrate (Enhanced effect of CNS depressants). Products include:
- Levo-Dromoran 1906

Lorazepam (Enhanced effect of CNS depressants). Products include:
- Ativan Injection 2432
- Ativan Tablets 2434

Loxapine Hydrochloride (Enhanced effect of CNS depressants). Products include:
- Loxitane 1213

Loxapine Succinate (Enhanced effect of CNS depressants). Products include:
- Loxitane Capsules 1213

Mepenzolate Bromide (Use cyclobenzaprine with caution). Products include:
- Cantil Tablets 1326

Meperidine Hydrochloride (Enhanced effect of CNS depressants). Products include:
- Demerol 2047
- Mepergan Injection 2479

Mephobarbital (Enhanced effect of barbiturates). Products include:
- Mebaral Tablets 2061

Meprobamate (Enhanced effect of CNS depressants). Products include:
- Deprol Tablets 2382
- Equagesic Tablets 2451
- Miltown Tablets 2386
- PMB 200 and PMB 400 2504

Mesoridazine (Enhanced effect of CNS depressants). Products include:
- Serentil 686

Methadone Hydrochloride (Enhanced effect of CNS depressants). Products include:
- Dolophine Hydrochloride Ampoules & Vials 1260
- Dolophine Hydrochloride Tablets 1261
- Methadone Hydrochloride Diskets .. 1284
- Methadone Hydrochloride Oral Solution & Tablets 1987

(▣ Described in PDR For Nonprescription Drugs) (⊙ Described in PDR For Ophthalmology)

Methohexital Sodium (Enhanced effect of CNS depressants). Products include:
- Brevital Sodium Vials 1248

Methoxyflurane (Enhanced effect of CNS depressants).
- No products indexed under this heading.

Midazolam Hydrochloride (Enhanced effect of CNS depressants). Products include:
- Versed Injection 1924

Molindone Hydrochloride (Enhanced effect of CNS depressants). Products include:
- Moban Tablets & Concentrate 932

Morphine Sulfate (Enhanced effect of CNS depressants). Products include:
- Astramorph/PF Injection, USP (Preservative-Free) 618
- Duramorph 960
- Infumorph 200 and Infumorph 500 Sterile Solutions 962
- MS Contin Tablets 1814
- MSIR 1817
- Oramorph SR (Morphine Sulfate Sustained Release Tablets) 1988
- Roxanol 1991

Opium Alkaloids (Enhanced effect of CNS depressants). Products include:
- B & O No. 15A & No. 16A Supprettes 2395
- Pantopon Injectable 1911

Oxazepam (Enhanced effect of CNS depressants). Products include:
- Serax Capsules 2522
- Serax Tablets 2522

Oxybutynin Chloride (Use cyclobenzaprine with caution). Products include:
- Ditropan 1332

Oxycodone Hydrochloride (Enhanced effect of CNS depressants). Products include:
- Percocet Tablets 950
- Percodan 951
- Roxicodone Tablets, Oral Solution & Intensol (Oxycodone) 1992
- Tylox Capsules 1382

Oxyphenonium Bromide (Use cyclobenzaprine with caution).

Pentobarbital Sodium (Enhanced effect of barbiturates). Products include:
- Nembutal Sodium Capsules 534
- Nembutal Sodium Solution 536
- Nembutal Sodium Suppositories 538

Perphenazine (Enhanced effect of CNS depressants). Products include:
- Etrafon 2087
- Triavil Tablets 1556
- Trilafon 2123

Phenelzine Sulfate (Contraindication; hyperpyretic crisis; severe convulsions; death). Products include:
- Nardil 1742

Phenobarbital (Enhanced effect of barbiturates). Products include:
- Arco-Lase Plus Tablets 607
- Bellergal-S Tablets 1998
- Bronkolixir .... ▣ 761
- Bronkotabs Tablets .... ▣ 762
- Donnatal 1858
- Donnatal Extentabs 1859
- Donnatal Tablets 1858
- Donnazyme Tablets 1860
- Kinesed Tablets 2272
- Phenobarbital Elixir and Tablets 1293
- Primatene Tablets-P Formula 2421
- Quadrinal Tablets 1183
- Tedral SA 1765

Prazepam (Enhanced effect of CNS depressants). Products include:
- Centrax 1693

Prochlorperazine (Enhanced effects of CNS depressants). Products include:
- Compazine 2201

Procyclidine Hydrochloride (Use cyclobenzaprine with caution). Products include:
- Kemadrin Tablets 771

Promethazine Hydrochloride (Enhanced effect of CNS depressants). Products include:
- Mepergan Injection 2479
- Phenergan with Codeine 2497
- Phenergan with Dextromethorphan 2499
- Phenergan Injection 2493
- Phenergan Suppositories 2496
- Phenergan Syrup 2495
- Phenergan Tablets 2496
- Phenergan VC 2500
- Phenergan VC with Codeine 2501

Propantheline Bromide (Use cyclobenzaprine with caution). Products include:
- Pro-Banthīne Tablets 2141

Propofol (Enhanced effect of CNS depressants). Products include:
- Diprivan Injection 2267

Propoxyphene Hydrochloride (Enhanced effect of CNS depressants). Products include:
- Darvon 1256
- Wygesic Tablets 2540

Propoxyphene Napsylate (Enhanced effect of CNS depressants). Products include:
- Darvon-N/Darvocet-N 1254

Quazepam (Enhanced effect of CNS depressants). Products include:
- Doral Tablets 2383

Scopolamine Hydrobromide (Use cyclobenzaprine with caution). Products include:
- Donnagel .... ▣ 675
- Donnagel-PG 1858
- Donnatal 1858
- Donnatal Extentabs 1859
- Donnatal Tablets 1858
- Donnazyme Tablets 1860
- Isopto Hyoscine .... ⊙ 222
- Murocoll-2 Sterile Ophthalmic Solution .... ⊙ 261
- Ru-Tuss Tablets 693

Scopolamine Preparations (Use cyclobenzaprine with caution). Products include:
- Transderm Scōp Transdermal Therapeutic System 887

Secobarbital Sodium (Enhanced effect of barbiturates). Products include:
- Seconal Sodium Pulvules 1296

Selegiline Hydrochloride (Contraindication; hyperpyretic crisis; severe convulsions; death). Products include:
- Eldepryl 2250

Sufentanil Citrate (Enhanced effect of CNS depressants). Products include:
- Sufenta Injection 1147

Temazepam (Enhanced effect of CNS depressants). Products include:
- Restoril Capsules 2023

Thiamylal Sodium (Enhanced effect of barbiturates). Products include:
- Surital Ampoules, Steri-Vials 1764

Thioridazine Hydrochloride (Enhanced effect of CNS depressants). Products include:
- Mellaril 2011

Thiothixene (Enhanced effect of CNS depressants). Products include:
- Navane Capsules and Concentrate 1954
- Navane Intramuscular 1956

Tranylcypromine Sulfate (Contraindication; hyperpyretic crisis; severe convulsions; death). Products include:
- Parnate Tablets 2222

Triazolam (Enhanced effect of CNS depressants). Products include:
- Halcion Tablets 2340

Tridihexethyl Chloride (Use cyclobenzaprine with caution).
- No products indexed under this heading.

Trifluoperazine Hydrochloride (Enhanced effect of CNS depressants). Products include:
- Stelazine 2226

Trihexyphenidyl Hydrochloride (Use cyclobenzaprine with caution). Products include:
- Artane 1195

FLINTSTONES CHILDREN'S CHEWABLE VITAMINS
(Multivitamins) .... ▣ 625
No interactions described in labeling.

FLINTSTONES CHILDREN'S CHEWABLE VITAMINS WITH EXTRA C
(Multivitamins) .... ▣ 626
No interactions described in labeling.

FLINTSTONES CHILDREN'S CHEWABLE VITAMINS PLUS IRON
(Vitamins with Iron) .... ▣ 625
No interactions described in labeling.

FLINTSTONES COMPLETE WITH CALCIUM, IRON & MINERALS CHILDREN'S CHEWABLE VITAMINS
(Vitamins with Minerals) .... ▣ 626
No interactions described in labeling.

FLORONE CREAM 0.05%
(Diflorasone Diacetate) 908
No interactions described in labeling.

FLORONE E EMOLLIENT CREAM 0.05%
(Diflorasone Diacetate) 908
No interactions described in labeling.

FLORONE OINTMENT 0.05%
(Diflorasone Diacetate) 908
No interactions described in labeling.

FLOROPRYL STERILE OPHTHALMIC OINTMENT
(Isoflurophate) 1473
May interact with cholinergic agents and certain other agents. Compounds in these categories include:

Edrophonium Chloride (Additive adverse effects). Products include:
- Enlon Injection 598
- Tensilon Injectable 1123

Neostigmine Bromide (Additive adverse effects). Products include:
- Prostigmin Tablets 1121

Neostigmine Methylsulfate (Additive adverse effects). Products include:
- Prostigmin Injectable 1120

Pyridostigmine Bromide (Additive adverse effects). Products include:
- Mestinon Injectable 1115
- Mestinon 1116

Succinylcholine Chloride (Possible respiratory and cardiovascular collapse). Products include:
- Anectine 755

FLOXIN TABLETS
(Ofloxacin) 1652
May interact with xanthine bronchodilators, antacids containing aluminium, calcium and magnesium, and certain other agents. Compounds in these categories include:

Aluminum Carbonate Gel (May substantially interfere with the absorption of quinolones). Products include:
- Basaljel 2438

Aluminum Hydroxide (May substantially interfere with the absorption of quinolones). Products include:
- Cama Arthritis Pain Reliever .... ▣ 685
- Gaviscon Extra Strength Relief Formula Liquid Antacid .... ▣ 594
- Gaviscon Extra Strength Relief Formula Antacid Tablets .... ▣ 594
- Gaviscon Liquid Antacid .... ▣ 594
- Gelusil Liquid & Tablets .... ▣ 639
- Extra Strength Maalox Plus Suspension 1850
- Maalox TC Suspension 1851
- Maalox Plus Tablets .... ▣ 655
- Extra Strength Maalox Plus Tablets 1850
- Nephrox Suspension .... ▣ 563
- WinGel Liquid & Tablets .... ▣ 761

Aluminum Hydroxide Gel (May substantially interfere with the absorption of quinolones). Products include:
- ALternaGEL Liquid 1154
- Aludrox Oral Suspension 2428
- Amphojel Suspension 2429
- Amphojel Suspension without Flavor 2429
- Mylanta Liquid 1155
- Mylanta Double Strength Liquid 1155

Aluminum Hydroxide Gel, Dried (May substantially interfere with the absorption of quinolones). Products include:
- Alu-Tab/Alu-Cap 1309
- Amphojel Tablets 2429
- Ascriptin A/D Caplets 1850
- Regular Strength Ascriptin Tablets 1850
- Gaviscon Antacid Tablets .... ▣ 593
- Gaviscon-2 Antacid Tablets .... ▣ 594
- Mylanta Tablets 1155
- Mylanta Double Strength Tablets 1155

Aminophylline (Increased steady-state theophylline levels). Products include:
- Amesec .... ▣ 682
- Aminophyllin Tablets 2153

Dihydroxyaluminum Sodium Carbonate (May substantially interfere with the absorption of quinolones). Products include:
- Rolaids .... ▣ 743

Dyphylline (Increased steady-state theophylline levels). Products include:
- Dilor 2079
- Dilor-G Tablets & Liquid 2079
- Lufyllin Elixir 2384
- Lufyllin & Lufyllin-400 Tablets 2384
- Lufyllin-GG Elixir & Tablets 2385

Iron Preparations (May substantially interfere with the absorption of quinolones). Products include:
- Allbee C-800 Plus Iron Tablets .... ▣ 670
- Bugs Bunny Children's Chewable Vitamins + Minerals with Iron and Calcium (Sugar Free) .... ▣ 626
- Bugs Bunny Plus Iron Children's Chewable Vitamins (Sugar Free) ▣ 625
- Femlron Multi-Vitamins and Iron .... ▣ 617
- Ferancee Chewable Tablets 1155
- Ferancee-HP Tablets 1155
- Fergon .... ▣ 758
- Fero-Folic-500 Filmtab 527
- Fero-Grad-500 Filmtab 528
- Fero-Gradumet Filmtab 528
- Ferro-Sequels 1203
- Flintstones Children's Chewable Vitamins Plus Iron .... ▣ 625
- Flintstones Complete With Calcium, Iron & Minerals Children's Chewable Vitamins .... ▣ 626
- Geritol Extend Tablets and Caplets .... ▣ 717
- Geritol Liquid - High Potency Iron & Vitamin Tonic .... ▣ 717
- Iberet Tablets 531
- Iberet-500 Liquid 531

Iberet-Folic-500 Filmtab 527
Iberet-Liquid 531
Incremin w/Iron Syrup ..... ◘ 588
Irospan 972
Mol-Iron ..... ◘ 703
Niferex 847
Niferex-150 Forte Capsules 847
Niferex Forte Elixir 847
Niferex 847
Niferex-PN Tablets 847
One-A-Day Maximum Formula Vitamins and Minerals ..... ◘ 627
Peritinic Tablets ..... ◘ 589
Poly-Vi-Flor with Iron 1399
Poly-Vi-Flor with Iron Drops 1399
Poly-Vi-Sol Vitamins with Iron, Chewable Tablets and Circus Shapes Chewable ..... ◘ 612
Poly-Vi-Sol Vitamins with Iron, Drops ..... ◘ 612
SMA Iron Fortified Infant Formula, Concentrated, Ready-to-Feed and Powder ..... ◘ 767
Slow Fe Tablets ..... ◘ 552
The Stuart Formula Tablets ..... ◘ 581
Stuartinic Tablets 1157
Surbex-750 with Iron ..... ◘ 503
Tri-Vi-Flor 0.25 mg Vitamins with Iron and Fluoride Drops 1401
Unicap Plus Iron Vitamin Formula Tablets ..... ◘ 738
Vi-Daylin ADC Vitamins + Iron Drops 1980
Vi-Daylin Multivitamin + Iron Drops 1981
Vi-Daylin/F ADC Vitamins + Iron Drops With Fluoride 1981
Vi-Daylin/F Multivitamin + Iron Drops With Fluoride 1981
Vi-Daylin Multivitamin + Iron Chewable Tablets 1982
Vi-Daylin/F Multivitamin + Iron Chewable Tablets With Fluoride .. 1982
Vi-Daylin Multivitamin + Iron Liquid 1983

Magaldrate (May substantially interfere with the absorption of quinolones). Products include:
Riopan Antacid Chew Tablets ..... ◘ 754
Riopan Antacid Chew Tablets in Rollpacks ..... ◘ 754
Riopan Antacid Suspension 2421
Riopan Antacid Swallow Tablets 2421
Riopan Plus Chew Tablets 2422
Riopan Plus Chew Tablets in Rollpack 2422
Riopan Plus 2 Chew Tablets, Mint Flavor, Cherry Flavor 2422
Riopan Plus Suspension 2422
Riopan Plus 2 Suspension, Mint Flavor, Cherry Flavor 2422

Magnesium Hydroxide (May substantially interfere with the absorption of quinolones). Products include:
Aludrox Oral Suspension 2428
Ascriptin A/D Caplets 1850
Regular Strength Ascriptin Tablets 1850
Di-Gel Antacid/Anti-Gas ..... ◘ 697
Gelusil Liquid & Tablets ..... ◘ 639
Haley's M-O, Regular & Flavored .. ◘ 569
Extra Strength Maalox Plus Suspension 1850
Maalox TC Suspension 1851
Maalox Plus Tablets ..... ◘ 655
Extra Strength Maalox Plus Tablets 1850
Mylanta Liquid 1155
Mylanta Tablets 1155
Mylanta Double Strength Liquid 1155
Mylanta Double Strength Tablets 1155
Concentrated Phillips' Milk of Magnesia ..... ◘ 573
Phillips' Milk of Magnesia Liquid .... ◘ 572
Phillips' Milk of Magnesia Tablets ◘ 573
WinGel Liquid & Tablets ..... ◘ 761

Magnesium Oxide (May substantially interfere with the absorption of quinolones). Products include:
Bayer Plus Aspirin Tablets ..... ◘ 567
Beelith Tablets 659
Bufferin Analgesic Tablets and Caplets ..... ◘ 524
Cama Arthritis Pain Reliever ..... ◘ 685
Mag-Ox 400 673
Uro-Mag 673

Sucralfate (May substantially interfere with the absorption of quinolones). Products include:
Carafate Tablets 1326

Theophylline (Increased steady-state theophylline levels). Products include:
Bronkaid Tablets ..... ◘ 757
Bronkolixir ..... ◘ 761
Bronkotabs Tablets ..... ◘ 762
Constant-T Tablets 1029
Marax Tablets & DF Syrup 1954
Primatene Tablets 2421
Quibron Capsules 713
Quibron-T 714
Quibron-T/SR 716
Theolair Liquid 1317
Theo-Organidin Elixir 2391

Theophylline Anhydrous (Increased steady-state theophylline levels). Products include:
Aerolate 994
Primatene Tablets-M Formula ..... ◘ 753
Primatene Tablets-Regular Formula 2421
Respbid Tablets 684
Slo-bid Gyrocaps 1847
T-PHYL (Uniphyl) 200 mg Tablets 1820
Tedral SA 1765
Theo-24 2179
Theo-Dur Sprinkle 1168
Theo-Dur Extended-Release Tablets 1166
Theolair Tablets 1317
Theolair-SR Tablets 1319
TheoX Extended-Release Tablets 841
Uniphyl 400 mg Tablets 1823

Theophylline Calcium Salicylate (Increased steady-state theophylline levels). Products include:
Quadrinal Tablets 1183

Theophylline Sodium Glycinate (Increased steady-state theophylline levels). Products include:
Asbron G 1997

Zinc Sulfate (May substantially interfere with the absorption of quinolones). Products include:
Clear Eyes ACR ..... ⊙ 305
Eldertonic 1359
Surbex-750 with Zinc ..... ◘ 503
Vicon Forte Capsules 2416
Visine A.C. Eye Drops ..... ◘ 646
Visine A.C. Eye Drops ..... ⊙ 303
Zincfrin ..... ⊙ 230

Food Interactions

Food, unspecified (Concurrent intake should be avoided).

FLU-IMUNE INFLUENZA VIRUS VACCINE
(Influenza Virus Vaccine) 1204
May interact with xanthine bronchodilators, corticosteroids, immunosuppressive agents, alkylating agents, cytotoxic drugs, and certain other agents. Compounds in these categories include:

Aminophylline (Influenza immunization can inhibit the clearance of theophylline). Products include:
Amesec ..... ◘ 682
Aminophyllin Tablets 2153

Azathioprine (Reduces antibody response). Products include:
Imuran 768

Betamethasone Acetate (Reduces antibody response). Products include:
Celestone Soluspan Suspension 2081

Betamethasone Sodium Phosphate (Reduces antibody response). Products include:
Celestone Soluspan Suspension 2081

Bleomycin Sulfate (Reduces antibody response). Products include:
Blenoxane 724

Busulfan (Reduces antibody response). Products include:
Myleran Tablets 790

Carmustine (BCNU) (Reduces antibody response). Products include:
BiCNU 723

Chlorambucil (Reduces antibody response). Products include:
Leukeran Tablets 788

Cortisone Acetate (Reduces antibody response). Products include:
Cortone Acetate Sterile Suspension 1437
Cortone Acetate Tablets 1439

Cyclophosphamide (Reduces antibody responses). Products include:
Cytoxan for Injection 726
Neosar for Injection 566

Cyclosporine (Reduces antibody response). Products include:
Sandimmune 2024

Dacarbazine (Reduces antibody response). Products include:
DTIC-Dome 1595

Daunorubicin Hydrochloride (Reduces antibody response). Products include:
Cerubidine 2443

Dexamethasone (Reduces antibody response). Products include:
AK-Trol Ointment & Suspension ..... ⊙ 207
Decadron Elixir 1445
Decadron Tablets 1447
Decaspray Topical Aerosol 1459
Dexacidin ..... ⊙ 272
Maxidex Sterile Ophthalmic Suspension ..... ⊙ 223
Maxitrol Ophthalmic Ointment/Suspension ..... ⊙ 223
TobraDex Ophthalmic Suspension and Ointment ..... ⊙ 228

Dexamethasone Acetate (Reduces antibody response). Products include:
Dalalone D.P. Injectable 999
Decadron-LA Sterile Suspension 1457

Dexamethasone Sodium Phosphate (Reduces antibody response). Products include:
AK-Dex ..... ⊙ 203
Decadron Phosphate Respihaler 1454
Decadron Phosphate Sterile Ophthalmic Ointment 1453
Decadron Phosphate Sterile Ophthalmic Solution 1453
Decadron Phosphate Topical Cream 1455
Decadron Phosphate Turbinaire 1456
Maxidex Sterile Ophthalmic Ointment ..... ⊙ 222
NeoDecadron Sterile Ophthalmic Ointment 1517
NeoDecadron Sterile Ophthalmic Solution 1518
NeoDecadron Topical Cream 1518

Doxorubicin Hydrochloride (Reduces antibody response). Products include:
Adriamycin PFS 561
Adriamycin RDF 562
Doxorubicin Hydrochloride for Injection, USP 622
Doxorubicin Hydrochloride Injection, USP 848
Rubex 739

Dyphylline (Influenza immunization can inhibit the clearance of theophylline). Products include:
Dilor 2079
Dilor-G Tablets & Liquid 2079
Lufyllin Elixir 2384
Lufyllin & Lufyllin-400 Tablets 2384
Lufyllin-GG Elixir & Tablets 2385

Fluorouracil (Reduces antibody response). Products include:
Efudex 1880
Fluoroplex Topical Solution & Cream 1% 1082
Fluorouracil Injection 1897

Hydrocortisone (Reduces antibody response). Products include:
AK-Spore H.C. ..... ⊙ 206
Bactine Hydrocortisone Anti-Itch Cream ..... ◘ 625
CaldeCORT Anti-Itch Hydrocortisone Spray ..... ◘ 560
Carmol HC Cream 1% 2296
Cortaid Spray ..... ◘ 735
Cortenema 2244
Cortisporin Ointment 758
Cortisporin Ophthalmic Ointment Sterile 758
Cortisporin Ophthalmic Suspension Sterile 759
Cortisporin Otic Solution Sterile 760
Cortisporin Otic Suspension Sterile 760
Cortizone-5 Creme & Ointment ..... ◘ 732
Dermolate Anti-Itch Cream ..... ◘ 697
Eldecort Cream 1.0% 1113
Eldecort Cream 1.0% and 2.5% 1113
Fungoid HC Creme 1770
Hydrocortone Tablets 1482
Hytone 909
LazerSporin-C Solution 1770
Massengill Medicated Soft Cloth Towelettes 2192
Nutracort Cream & Lotion 1684
PediOtic Suspension Sterile 797
Synacort Creams 1%, 2.5% 2296
Vanoxide-HC Acne Lotion 911
Vioform-Hydrocortisone Cream and Mild Cream 889
Vioform-Hydrocortisone Ointment .. 889
VōSoL HC Otic Solution 2392
Vytone Cream 1% 911

Hydrocortisone Acetate (Reduces antibody response). Products include:
Analpram-HC Rectal Cream 1% and 2.5% 970
Anusol-HC Cream 1690
Anusol-HC Suppositories 1691
Caldecort ..... ◘ 560
Carmol HC Cream 1% 2296
Chloromycetin Hydrocortisone Ophthalmic 1694
Coly-Mycin S Otic w/Neomycin & Hydrocortisone 1708
Cortaid ..... ◘ 735
Cortef Feminine Itch Cream ..... ◘ 735
Corticaine ..... ◘ 682
Cortifoam 1827
Cortisporin Cream 757
Epifoam 1828
Gynecort 5 Creme ..... ◘ 556
Hydrocortone Acetate Sterile Suspension 1479
Lanacort 5 Creme and Ointment .. ◘ 557
Mantadil Cream 789
Ophthocort ..... ⊙ 301
Orabase HCA Oral Paste 890
Pramosone Cream, Lotion & Ointment 971
ProctoCream-HC 1834
Proctofoam-HC 1835

Hydrocortisone Sodium Phosphate (Reduces antibody response). Products include:
Hydrocortone Phosphate Injection, Sterile 1481

Hydrocortisone Sodium Succinate (Reduces antibody response). Products include:
Solu-Cortef Sterile Powder 2361

Hydroxyurea (Reduces antibody response). Products include:
Hydrea Capsules 728

Immune Globulin (Human) (Reduces antibody response). Products include:
MICRhoGAM $Rh_0(D)$ Immune Globulin (Human) 1650
RhoGAM $Rh_0(D)$ Immune Globulin (Human) 1651

Immune Globulin Intravenous (Human) (Reduces antibody response). Products include:
Gamimune N Immune Globulin Intravenous (Human) 1572
Gammagard Immune Globulin, Intravenous (Human) 658
Iveegam 1129
Sandoglobulin I.V. 2027

Lomustine (CCNU) (Reduces antibody response). Products include:
CeeNU 725

Mechlorethamine Hydrochloride (Reduces antibody response). Products include:
Mustargen 1514

Melphalan (Reduces antibody response). Products include:
Alkeran Tablets 754

Methotrexate Sodium (Reduces antibody response). Products include:
Methotrexate Tablets, Parenteral, LPF Parenteral 1217
Rheumatrex Methotrexate Dose Pack 1234

Methylprednisolone Acetate (Reduces antibody response). Products include:
Depo-Medrol Sterile Aqueous Suspension 2334

Methylprednisolone Sodium Succinate (Reduces antibody response). Products include:
Solu-Medrol Sterile Powder 2363

Mitotane (Reduces antibody response). Products include:
Lysodren 731

Mitoxantrone Hydrochloride (Reduces antibody response). Products include:
Novantrone for Injection Concentrate 1226

Muromonab-CD3 (Reduces antibody response). Products include:
Orthoclone OKT3 Sterile Solution .. 1645

Prednisolone Acetate (Reduces antibody response). Products include:
AK-Cide Sterile Ophthalmic Ointment & Suspension .... ⊙ 202
Blephamide Liquifilm Sterile Ophthalmic Suspension 586
Blephamide S.O.P. Sterile Ophthalmic Ointment 586
Cetapred Ointment .... ⊙ 220
⅛% Econopred & 1% Econopred Plus .... ⊙ 217
Isopto Cetapred Suspension .... ⊙ 220
Metimyd .... ⊙ 306
Poly-Pred Liquifilm .... ⊙ 250
Pred Forte .... ⊙ 252
Pred Mild .... ⊙ 254
Pred-G Liquifilm Sterile Ophthalmic Suspension .... ⊙ 252
Pred-G S.O.P. Sterile Ophthalmic Ointment .... ⊙ 253
Vasocidin Ointment .... ⊙ 275

Prednisolone Sodium Phosphate (Reduces antibody response). Products include:
AK-Pred .... ⊙ 205
Hydeltrasol Injection, Sterile 1476
Inflamase .... ⊙ 274
Pediapred Oral Liquid 987
Vasocidin Ophthalmic Solution .... ⊙ 276

Prednisolone Tebutate (Reduces antibody response). Products include:
Hydeltra-T.B.A. Sterile Suspension 1478

Prednisone (Reduces antibody response). Products include:
Deltasone Tablets 2332

Procarbazine Hydrochloride (Reduces antibody response). Products include:
Matulane Capsules 1907

Tamoxifen Citrate (Reduces antibody response). Products include:
Nolvadex Tablets 1102

Theophylline (Influenza immunization can inhibit the clearance of theophylline). Products include:
Bronkaid Tablets .... ▣ 757
Bronkolixir .... ▣ 761
Bronkotabs Tablets .... ▣ 762
Constant-T Tablets 1029
Marax Tablets & DF Syrup 1954
Primatene Tablets 2421
Quibron Capsules 713
Quibron-T 714
Quibron-T/SR 716
Theolair Liquid 1317
Theo-Organidin Elixir 2391

Theophylline Anhydrous (Influenza immunization can inhibit the clearance of theophylline). Products include:
Aerolate 994
Primatene Tablets-M Formula .... ▣ 753
Primatene Tablets-Regular Formula 2421
Respbid Tablets 684
Slo-bid Gyrocaps 1847
T-PHYL (Uniphyl) 200 mg Tablets 1820
Tedral SA 1765
Theo-24 2179
Theo-Dur Sprinkle 1168
Theo-Dur Extended-Release Tablets 1166
Theolair Tablets 1317
Theolair-SR Tablets 1319
TheoX Extended-Release Tablets 841
Uniphyl 400 mg Tablets 1823

Theophylline Calcium Salicylate (Influenza immunization can inhibit the clearance of theophylline). Products include:
Quadrinal Tablets 1183

Theophylline Sodium Glycinate (Influenza immunization can inhibit the clearance of theophylline). Products include:
Asbron G 1997

Thiotepa (Reduces antibody response). Products include:
Thiotepa Parenteral 1240

Triamcinolone (Reduces antibody response).
No products indexed under this heading.

Triamcinolone Acetonide (Reduces antibody response). Products include:
Aristocort A 1010
Azmacort Inhaler 1837
Kenalog Cream, Lotion & Ointment 2401
Kenalog-10 Injection 2402
Kenalog-40 Injection 2403
Kenalog in Orabase 604
Kenalog Spray 2401
Mycolog II Cream and Ointment 2407
Mytrex Cream & Ointment 2080
Nasacort Nasal Inhaler 1844

Triamcinolone Diacetate (Reduces antibody response). Products include:
Aristocort Suspension 1008

Triamcinolone Hexacetonide (Reduces antibody response). Products include:
Aristospan Suspension 1011

Vincristine Sulfate (Reduces antibody response). Products include:
Oncovin Solution Vials & Hyporets 1288

Warfarin Sodium (Influenza immunization can inhibit the clearance of warfarin). Products include:
Coumadin Injection & Tablets 944
Panwarfin Tablets 547

FLUORACAINE
(Fluorescein Sodium, Proparacaine Hydrochloride) .... ⊙ 208
No interactions described in labeling.

FLUORESCITE INJECTION
(Fluorescein Sodium) .... ⊙ 217
No interactions described in labeling.

FLUORESCITE SYRINGE
(Fluorescein Sodium) .... ⊙ 217
No interactions described in labeling.

FLUORETS OPHTHALMIC STRIPS
(Fluorescein Sodium) .... ⊙ 208
No interactions described in labeling.

FLUORIGARD ANTI-CAVITY FLUORIDE RINSE
(Sodium Fluoride) .... ▣ 555
No interactions described in labeling.

FLUORI-METHANE
(Dichlorodifluoromethane, Trichloromonofluoromethane) 1022
No interactions described in labeling.

FLUOR-I-STRIP
(Fluorescein Sodium) .... ⊙ 314
No interactions described in labeling.

FLUOR-I-STRIP A.T.
(Fluorescein Sodium) .... ⊙ 314
No interactions described in labeling.

FLUORITAB LIQUID
(Sodium Fluoride) 995
No interactions described in labeling.

FLUORITAB TABLETS
(Sodium Fluoride) 995
No interactions described in labeling.

FLUOR-OP OPHTHALMIC SUSPENSION
(Fluorometholone) .... ⊙ 272
No interactions described in labeling.

FLUOROPLEX TOPICAL SOLUTION & CREAM 1%
(Fluorouracil) 1082
No interactions described in labeling.

FLUOROURACIL INJECTION
(Fluorouracil) 1897
May interact with alkylating agents and certain other agents. Compounds in these categories include:

Busulfan (Fluorouracil should be used with extreme caution in patients with previous use of alkylating agents). Products include:
Myleran Tablets 790

Carmustine (BCNU) (Fluorouracil should be used with extreme caution in patients with previous use of alkylating agents). Products include:
BiCNU 723

Chlorambucil (Fluorouracil should be used with extreme caution in patients with previous use of alkylating agents). Products include:
Leukeran Tablets 788

Cyclophosphamide (Fluorouracil should be used with extreme caution in patients with previous use of alkylating agents). Products include:
Cytoxan for Injection 726
Neosar for Injection 566

Dacarbazine (Fluorouracil should be used with extreme caution in patients with previous use of alkylating agents). Products include:
DTIC-Dome 1595

Leucovorin Calcium (Increased toxicity of fluorouracil). Products include:
Leucovorin Calcium for Injection, Wellcovorin Brand 786
Leucovorin Calcium Injection 1210
Leucovorin Calcium Tablets, Wellcovorin Brand 787
Leucovorin Calcium Tablets 1212

Lomustine (CCNU) (Fluorouracil should be used with extreme caution in patients with previous use of alkylating agents). Products include:
CeeNU 725

Mechlorethamine Hydrochloride (Fluorouracil should be used with extreme caution in patients with previous use of alkylating agents). Products include:
Mustargen 1514

Melphalan (Fluorouracil should be used with extreme caution in patients with previous use of alkylating agents). Products include:
Alkeran Tablets 754

Thiotepa (Fluorouracil should be used with extreme caution in patients with previous use of alkylating agents). Products include:
Thiotepa Parenteral 1240

FLUOTHANE
(Halothane) 2453
May interact with nondepolarizing neuromuscular blocking agents, ganglionic blocking agents, and certain other agents. Compounds in these categories include:

Atracurium Besylate (Actions augmented by Fluothane). Products include:
Tracrium Injection 817

Epinephrine Hydrochloride (Simultaneous use may induce ventricular tachycardia or fibrillation). Products include:
Adrenalin Chloride Solution 1:100 & 1:1,000 1689
Epifrin .... ⊙ 244
Glaucon .... ⊙ 218

Guanethidine Monosulfate (Actions augmented by Fluothane). Products include:
Esimil Tablets 864
Ismelin Tablets 869

Mecamylamine Hydrochloride (Actions augmented by Fluothane). Products include:
Inversine Tablets 1492

Metocurine Iodide (Actions augmented by Fluothane). Products include:
Metubine Iodide Vials 1285

Norepinephrine Bitartrate (Simultaneous use may induce ventricular tachycardia or fibrillation). Products include:
Levophed Bitartrate Injection 2054

Pancuronium Bromide Injection (Actions augmented by Fluothane).
No products indexed under this heading.

Succinylcholine Chloride (Malignant hyperthermic crisis may be triggered in genetically susceptible individuals). Products include:
Anectine 755

Trimethaphan Camsylate (Actions augmented by Fluothane). Products include:
Arfonad Ampuls 1887

Vecuronium Bromide (Actions augmented by Fluothane). Products include:
Norcuron 1642

FLURO-ETHYL
(Dichlorotetrafluoroethane, Ethyl Chloride) 1023
No interactions described in labeling.

FORANE
(Isoflurane) 600
May interact with muscle relaxants, nondepolarizing neuromuscular blocking agents, and certain other agents. Compounds in these categories include:

Atracurium Besylate (Relaxant effect potentiated). Products include:
Tracrium Injection 817

Baclofen (Relaxant effect potentiated). Products include:
Lioresal Tablets 1031

Carisoprodol (Relaxant effect potentiated). Products include:
Soma Compound w/Codeine Tablets 2390
Soma Compound Tablets 2389
Soma Tablets 2388

Chlorzoxazone (Relaxant effect potentiated). Products include:
Paraflex Caplets 1378
Parafon Forte DSC Caplets 1379

Cyclobenzaprine Hydrochloride (Relaxant effect potentiated). Products include:
Flexeril Tablets 1471

Dantrolene Sodium (Relaxant effect potentiated). Products include:
Dantrium Capsules 1619
Dantrium Intravenous 1620

Doxacurium Chloride (Relaxant effect potentiated). Products include:
Nuromax Injection 794

Metaxalone (Relaxant effect potentiated). Products include:
Skelaxin 840

Methocarbamol (Relaxant effect potentiated). Products include:
Robaxin Injectable 1871
Robaxin Tablets 1872
Robaxisal Tablets 1872

Metocurine Iodide (Relaxant effect potentiated). Products include:
Metubine Iodide Vials 1285

Nitrous Oxide (Minimum alveolar concentration reduced).

Orphenadrine Citrate (Relaxant effect potentiated). Products include:
Norflex 1314
Norgesic 1314

Pancuronium Bromide Injection (Relaxant effect potentiated).
No products indexed under this heading.

Succinylcholine Chloride (Relaxant effect potentiated). Products include:
Anectine 755

Vecuronium Bromide (Relaxant effect potentiated). Products include:
Norcuron 1642

FORMALYDE-10 SPRAY
(Formaldehyde) 1769
No interactions described in labeling.

FORTAZ
(Ceftazidime) 1060
May interact with aminoglycosides and certain other agents. Compounds in these categories include:

Amikacin Sulfate (Potential for nephrotoxicity following concomitant administration). Products include:
Amikin Injectable 602

Furosemide (Potential for nephrotoxicity following concomitant administration). Products include:
Lasix 1093

Gentamicin Sulfate (Potential for nephrotoxicity following concomitant administration). Products include:
Garamycin Injectable 2093
Garamycin Ophthalmic .... ⊙ 305
Genoptic Liquifilm Sterile Ophthalmic Solution .... ⊙ 247
Genoptic S.O.P. Sterile Ophthalmic Ointment .... ⊙ 247
Gentacidin Ointment .... ⊙ 273
Gentacidin Solution .... ⊙ 273
Gentak Ointment & Solution .... ⊙ 208
G-myticin Creme and Ointment 0.1% 1770
Pred-G Liquifilm Sterile Ophthalmic Suspension .... ⊙ 252
Pred-G S.O.P. Sterile Ophthalmic Ointment .... ⊙ 253

Kanamycin Sulfate (Potential for nephrotoxicity following concomitant administration). Products include:
Kantrex Injection 601
Kantrex Pediatric Injection 601

Streptomycin Sulfate (Potential for nephrotoxicity following concomitant administration).
No products indexed under this heading.

Tobramycin Sulfate (Potential for nephrotoxicity following concomitant administration). Products include:
Nebcin Vials, Hyporets & ADD-Vantage 1286

FREEZONE SOLUTION
(Salicylic Acid) .... ⊞ 751
No interactions described in labeling.

FULVICIN P/G TABLETS
(Griseofulvin) 2090
May interact with barbiturates, oral anticoagulants, oral contraceptives, and certain other agents. Compounds in these categories include:

Alcohol (Potentiation of effects).

Aprobarbital (Depresses griseofulvin activity). Products include:
Alurate Elixir 1883

Butabarbital (Depresses griseofulvin activity). Products include:
Pyridium Plus 1764

Butalbital (Depresses griseofulvin activity). Products include:
Esgic-Plus Tablets 1002
Esgic Tablets & Capsules 1001
Fioricet Tablets 2006
Fiorinal Capsules 2007
Fiorinal with Codeine Capsules 2008
Fiorinal Tablets 2007
Phrenilin 838
Sedapap Tablets 50 mg/650 mg 1360

Dicumarol (Decreased anticoagulant effects). Products include:
Dicumarol Tablets 516

Ethinyl Estradiol (Decreased contraceptive effects). Products include:
Brevicon 2304
Demulen 2161
Estinyl Tablets 2085
Jenest-28 Tablets 1636
Levlen/Tri-Levlen 665
Lo/Ovral Tablets 2471
Lo/Ovral-28 Tablets 2476
Loestrin 1728
Modicon 1667
Nordette-21 Tablets 2481
Nordette-28 Tablets 2483
Norethin 2133
Norinyl 2304
Norlestrin 1746
Ortho-Cyclen Tablets 1658
Ortho-Novum 1667
Ovcon 1391
Ovral Tablets 2490
Ovral-28 Tablets 2491
Levlen/Tri-Levlen 665
Tri-Norinyl 2304
Triphasil-21 Tablets 2527
Triphasil-28 Tablets 2532

Ethynodiol Diacetate (Decreased contraceptive effects). Products include:
Demulen 2161

Levonorgestrel (Decreased contraceptive effects). Products include:
Levlen/Tri-Levlen 665
Nordette-21 Tablets 2481
Nordette-28 Tablets 2483
Norplant System 2484
Levlen/Tri-Levlen 665
Triphasil-21 Tablets 2527
Triphasil-28 Tablets 2532

Mephobarbital (Depresses griseofulvin activity). Products include:
Mebaral Tablets 2061

Mestranol (Decreased contraceptive effects). Products include:
Enovid 2161
Norethin 2133
Norinyl 2304
Ortho-Novum 1667

Norethindrone (Decreased contraceptive effects). Products include:
Brevicon 2304
Jenest-28 Tablets 1636
Micronor Tablets 1667
Modicon 1667
Norethin 2133
Norinyl 2304
Norlutin 1755
Nor-Q D Tablets 2304
Ortho-Novum 1667
Ovcon 1391
Tri-Norinyl 2304

Norethynodrel (Decreased contraceptive effects). Products include:
Enovid 2161

Norgestimate (Decreased contraceptive effects). Products include:
Ortho-Cyclen Tablets 1658

Norgestrel (Decreased contraceptive effects). Products include:
Lo/Ovral Tablets 2471
Lo/Ovral-28 Tablets 2476
Ovral Tablets 2490
Ovral-28 Tablets 2491
Ovrette Tablets 2492

Pentobarbital Sodium (Depresses griseofulvin activity). Products include:
Nembutal Sodium Capsules 534
Nembutal Sodium Solution 536
Nembutal Sodium Suppositories 538

Phenobarbital (Depresses griseofulvin activity). Products include:
Arco-Lase Plus Tablets 607
Bellergal-S Tablets 1998
Bronkolixir .... ⊞ 761
Bronkotabs Tablets .... ⊞ 762
Donnatal 1858
Donnatal Extentabs 1859
Donnatal Tablets 1858
Donnazyme Tablets 1860
Kinesed Tablets 2272
Phenobarbital Elixir and Tablets 1293
Primatene Tablets-P Formula 2421
Quadrinal Tablets 1183
Tedral SA 1765

Secobarbital Sodium (Depresses griseofulvin activity). Products include:
Seconal Sodium Pulvules 1296

Thiamylal Sodium (Depresses griseofulvin activity). Products include:
Surital Ampoules, Steri-Vials 1764

Warfarin Sodium (Depresses anticoagulant effects). Products include:
Coumadin Injection & Tablets 944
Panwarfin Tablets 547

FULVICIN P/G 165 & 330 TABLETS
(Griseofulvin) 2091
May interact with oral anticoagulants, barbiturates, oral contraceptives, and certain other agents. Compounds in these categories include:

Alcohol (Potentiation of effects).

Aprobarbital (Depresses griseofulvin activity). Products include:
Alurate Elixir 1883

Butabarbital (Depresses griseofulvin activity). Products include:
Pyridium Plus 1764

Butalbital (Depresses griseofulvin activity). Products include:
Esgic-Plus Tablets 1002
Esgic Tablets & Capsules 1001
Fioricet Tablets 2006
Fiorinal Capsules 2007
Fiorinal with Codeine Capsules 2008
Fiorinal Tablets 2007
Phrenilin 838
Sedapap Tablets 50 mg/650 mg 1360

Dicumarol (Decreased anticoagulant effect). Products include:
Dicumarol Tablets 516

Ethinyl Estradiol (Decreased contraceptive effects). Products include:
Brevicon 2304
Demulen 2161
Estinyl Tablets 2085
Jenest-28 Tablets 1636
Levlen/Tri-Levlen 665
Lo/Ovral Tablets 2471
Lo/Ovral-28 Tablets 2476
Loestrin 1728
Modicon 1667
Nordette-21 Tablets 2481
Nordette-28 Tablets 2483
Norethin 2133
Norinyl 2304
Norlestrin 1746
Ortho-Cyclen Tablets 1658
Ortho-Novum 1667
Ovcon 1391
Ovral Tablets 2490
Ovral-28 Tablets 2491
Levlen/Tri-Levlen 665
Tri-Norinyl 2304
Triphasil-21 Tablets 2527
Triphasil-28 Tablets 2532

Ethynodiol Diacetate (Decreased contraceptive effects). Products include:
Demulen 2161

Levonorgestrel (Decreased contraceptive effects). Products include:
Levlen/Tri-Levlen 665
Nordette-21 Tablets 2481
Nordette-28 Tablets 2483
Norplant System 2484
Levlen/Tri-Levlen 665
Triphasil-21 Tablets 2527
Triphasil-28 Tablets 2532

Mephobarbital (Depresses griseofulvin activity). Products include:
Mebaral Tablets 2061

Mestranol (Decreased contraceptive effects). Products include:
Enovid 2161
Norethin 2133
Norinyl 2304
Ortho-Novum 1667

Norethindrone (Decreased contraceptive effects). Products include:
Brevicon 2304
Jenest-28 Tablets 1636
Micronor Tablets 1667
Modicon 1667
Norethin 2133
Norinyl 2304
Norlutin 1755
Nor-Q D Tablets 2304
Ortho-Novum 1667
Ovcon 1391
Tri-Norinyl 2304

Norethynodrel (Decreased contraceptive effects). Products include:
Enovid 2161

Norgestimate (Decreased contraceptive effects). Products include:
Ortho-Cyclen Tablets 1658

Norgestrel (Decreased contraceptive effects). Products include:
Lo/Ovral Tablets 2471
Lo/Ovral-28 Tablets 2476
Ovral Tablets 2490
Ovral-28 Tablets 2491
Ovrette Tablets 2492

Pentobarbital Sodium (Depresses griseofulvin activity). Products include:
Nembutal Sodium Capsules 534
Nembutal Sodium Solution 536
Nembutal Sodium Suppositories 538

Phenobarbital (Depresses griseofulvin activity). Products include:
Arco-Lase Plus Tablets 607
Bellergal-S Tablets 1998
Bronkolixir .... ⊞ 761
Bronkotabs Tablets .... ⊞ 762
Donnatal 1858
Donnatal Extentabs 1859
Donnatal Tablets 1858
Donnazyme Tablets 1860
Kinesed Tablets 2272
Phenobarbital Elixir and Tablets 1293
Primatene Tablets-P Formula 2421
Quadrinal Tablets 1183
Tedral SA 1765

Secobarbital Sodium (Depresses griseofulvin activity). Products include:
Seconal Sodium Pulvules 1296

Thiamylal Sodium (Depresses griseofulvin activity). Products include:
- Surital Ampoules, Steri-Vials 1764

Warfarin Sodium (Decreased anticoagulant effect). Products include:
- Coumadin Injection & Tablets 944
- Panwarfin Tablets 547

FULVICIN-U/F TABLETS
(Griseofulvin) 2092
May interact with oral anticoagulants, barbiturates, oral contraceptives, and certain other agents. Compounds in these categories include:

Alcohol (Potentiation of effects).

Aprobarbital (Depresses griseofulvin activity). Products include:
- Alurate Elixir 1883

Butabarbital (Depresses griseofulvin activity). Products include:
- Pyridium Plus 1764

Butalbital (Depresses griseofulvin activity). Products include:
- Esgic-Plus Tablets 1002
- Esgic Tablets & Capsules 1001
- Fioricet Tablets 2006
- Fiorinal Capsules 2007
- Fiorinal with Codeine Capsules 2008
- Fiorinal Tablets 2007
- Phrenilin 838
- Sedapap Tablets 50 mg/650 mg .. 1360

Dicumarol (Decreased anticoagulant activity). Products include:
- Dicumarol Tablets 516

Ethinyl Estradiol (Decreased contraceptive effects). Products include:
- Brevicon 2304
- Demulen 2161
- Estinyl Tablets 2085
- Jenest-28 Tablets 1636
- Levlen/Tri-Levlen 665
- Lo/Ovral Tablets 2471
- Lo/Ovral-28 Tablets 2476
- Loestrin 1728
- Modicon 1667
- Nordette-21 Tablets 2481
- Nordette-28 Tablets 2483
- Norethin 2133
- Norinyl 2304
- Norlestrin 1746
- Ortho-Cyclen Tablets 1658
- Ortho-Novum 1667
- Ovcon 1391
- Ovral Tablets 2490
- Ovral-28 Tablets 2491
- Levlen/Tri-Levlen 665
- Tri-Norinyl 2304
- Triphasil-21 Tablets 2527
- Triphasil-28 Tablets 2532

Ethynodiol Diacetate (Decreased contraceptive effects). Products include:
- Demulen 2161

Levonorgestrel (Decreased contraceptive effects). Products include:
- Levlen/Tri-Levlen 665
- Nordette-21 Tablets 2481
- Nordette-28 Tablets 2483
- Norplant System 2484
- Levlen/Tri-Levlen 665
- Triphasil-21 Tablets 2527
- Triphasil-28 Tablets 2532

Mephobarbital (Depresses griseofulvin activity). Products include:
- Mebaral Tablets 2061

Mestranol (Decreased contraceptive effects). Products include:
- Enovid 2161
- Norethin 2133
- Norinyl 2304
- Ortho-Novum 1667

Norethindrone (Decreased contraceptive effects). Products include:
- Brevicon 2304
- Jenest-28 Tablets 1636
- Micronor Tablets 1667
- Modicon 1667
- Norethin 2133
- Norinyl 2304
- Norlutin 1755
- Nor-Q D Tablets 2304
- Ortho-Novum 1667
- Ovcon 1391
- Tri-Norinyl 2304

Norethynodrel (Decreased contraceptive effects). Products include:
- Enovid 2161

Norgestimate (Decreased contraceptive effects). Products include:
- Ortho-Cyclen Tablets 1658

Norgestrel (Decreased contraceptive effects). Products include:
- Lo/Ovral Tablets 2471
- Lo/Ovral-28 Tablets 2476
- Ovral Tablets 2490
- Ovral-28 Tablets 2491
- Ovrette Tablets 2492

Pentobarbital Sodium (Depresses griseofulvin activity). Products include:
- Nembutal Sodium Capsules 534
- Nembutal Sodium Solution 536
- Nembutal Sodium Suppositories 538

Phenobarbital (Depresses griseofulvin activity). Products include:
- Arco-Lase Plus Tablets 607
- Bellergal-S Tablets 1998
- Bronkolixir .... ▣ 761
- Bronkotabs Tablets .... ▣ 762
- Donnatal 1858
- Donnatal Extentabs 1859
- Donnatal Tablets 1858
- Donnazyme Tablets 1860
- Kinesed Tablets 2272
- Phenobarbital Elixir and Tablets 1293
- Primatene Tablets-P Formula 2421
- Quadrinal Tablets 1183
- Tedral SA 1765

Secobarbital Sodium (Depresses griseofulvin activity). Products include:
- Seconal Sodium Pulvules 1296

Thiamylal Sodium (Depresses griseofulvin activity). Products include:
- Surital Ampoules, Steri-Vials 1764

Warfarin Sodium (Decreased anticoagulant activity). Products include:
- Coumadin Injection & Tablets 944
- Panwarfin Tablets 547

FUNGI-NAIL TINCTURE
(Salicylic Acid, Undecylenic Acid) 1190
No interactions described in labeling.

FUNGIZONE CREAM, LOTION AND OINTMENT
(Amphotericin B) 2261
No interactions described in labeling.

FUNGIZONE INTRAVENOUS
(Amphotericin B) 2262
May interact with corticosteroids, antineoplastics, cardiac glycosides, nephrotoxic drugs, muscle relaxants, imidazoles, aminoglycosides, and certain other agents. Compounds in these categories include:

ACTH (Potentiates amphotericin B-induced hypokalemia).

Altretamine (May enhance potential for renal toxicity, bronchospasm and hypotension). Products include:
- Hexalen Capsules 2316

Amikacin Sulfate (May enhance the potential for renal toxicity). Products include:
- Amikin Injectable 602

Asparaginase (May enhance potential for renal toxicity, bronchospasm and hypotension). Products include:
- Elspar 1470

Atracurium Besylate (Amphotericin B-induced hypokalemia may enhance curariform effect). Products include:
- Tracrium Injection 817

Baclofen (Amphotericin B-induced hypokalemia may enhance curariform effect). Products include:
- Lioresal Tablets 1031

Betamethasone Acetate (Potentiates amphotericin B-induced hypokalemia). Products include:
- Celestone Soluspan Suspension 2081

Betamethasone Sodium Phosphate (Potentiates amphotericin B-induced hypokalemia). Products include:
- Celestone Soluspan Suspension 2081

Bleomycin Sulfate (May enhance potential for renal toxicity, bronchospasm and hypotension). Products include:
- Blenoxane 724

Busulfan (May enhance potential for renal toxicity, bronchospasm and hypotension). Products include:
- Myleran Tablets 790

Carboplatin (May enhance potential for renal toxicity, bronchospasm and hypotension). Products include:
- Paraplatin for Injection 735

Carisoprodol (Amphotericin B-induced hypokalemia may enhance curariform effect). Products include:
- Soma Compound w/Codeine Tablets 2390
- Soma Compound Tablets 2389
- Soma Tablets 2388

Carmustine (BCNU) (May enhance potential for renal toxicity, bronchospasm and hypotension). Products include:
- BiCNU 723

Chlorambucil (May enhance potential for renal toxicity, bronchospasm and hypotension). Products include:
- Leukeran Tablets 788

Chlorzoxazone (Amphotericin B-induced hypokalemia may enhance curariform effect). Products include:
- Paraflex Caplets 1378
- Parafon Forte DSC Caplets 1379

Cisplatin (May enhance potential for renal toxicity, bronchospasm and hypotension). Products include:
- Platinol 737
- Platinol-AQ Injection 738

Clotrimazole (Imidazoles may induce fungal resistance to amphotericin). Products include:
- Gyne-Lotrimin Vaginal Cream Antifungal .... ▣ 702
- Gyne-Lotrimin Vaginal Inserts .... ▣ 702
- Lotrimin 2102
- Lotrimin AF Antifungal Cream, Lotion and Solution .... ▣ 702
- Lotrisone Cream 2103
- Mycelex 1% Cream and Topical Solution 1% 1604
- Mycelex OTC Antifungal Cream and Solution 1571
- Mycelex Troches 1605
- Mycelex-G 1% Vaginal Cream 1605
- Mycelex-G 100 mg Vaginal Tablets 1606
- Mycelex-G 500 mg Vaginal Tablets 1606

Cortisone Acetate (Potentiates amphotericin B-induced hypokalemia). Products include:
- Cortone Acetate Sterile Suspension 1437
- Cortone Acetate Tablets 1439

Cyclobenzaprine Hydrochloride (Amphotericin B-induced hypokalemia may enhance curariform effect). Products include:
- Flexeril Tablets 1471

Cyclophosphamide (May enhance potential for renal toxicity, bronchospasm and hypotension). Products include:
- Cytoxan for Injection 726
- Neosar for Injection 566

Cyclosporine (May enhance the potential for renal toxicity). Products include:
- Sandimmune 2024

Dacarbazine (May enhance potential for renal toxicity, bronchospasm and hypotension). Products include:
- DTIC-Dome 1595

Dantrolene Sodium (Amphotericin B-induced hypokalemia may enhance curariform effect). Products include:
- Dantrium Capsules 1619
- Dantrium Intravenous 1620

Daunorubicin Hydrochloride (May enhance potential for renal toxicity, bronchospasm and hypotension). Products include:
- Cerubidine 2443

Deslanoside (Amphotericin B-induced hypokalemia may potentiate digitalis toxicity, avoid concomitant use).
- No products indexed under this heading.

Dexamethasone (Potentiates amphotericin B-induced hypokalemia). Products include:
- AK-Trol Ointment & Suspension .... ⊙ 207
- Decadron Elixir 1445
- Decadron Tablets 1447
- Decaspray Topical Aerosol 1459
- Dexacidin .... ⊙ 272
- Maxidex Sterile Ophthalmic Suspension .... ⊙ 223
- Maxitrol Ophthalmic Ointment/Suspension .... ⊙ 223
- TobraDex Ophthalmic Suspension and Ointment .... ⊙ 228

Dexamethasone Acetate (Potentiates amphotericin B-induced hypokalemia). Products include:
- Dalalone D.P. Injectable 999
- Decadron-LA Sterile Suspension 1457

Dexamethasone Sodium Phosphate (Potentiates amphotericin B-induced hypokalemia). Products include:
- AK-Dex .... ⊙ 203
- Decadron Phosphate Respihaler 1454
- Decadron Phosphate Sterile Ophthalmic Ointment 1453
- Decadron Phosphate Sterile Ophthalmic Solution 1453
- Decadron Phosphate Topical Cream 1455
- Decadron Phosphate Turbinaire 1456
- Maxidex Sterile Ophthalmic Ointment .... ⊙ 222
- NeoDecadron Sterile Ophthalmic Ointment 1517
- NeoDecadron Sterile Ophthalmic Solution 1518
- NeoDecadron Topical Cream 1518

Digitoxin (Amphotericin B-induced hypokalemia may potentiate digitalis toxicity, avoid concomitant use). Products include:
- Crystodigin Tablets 1253

Digoxin (Amphotericin B-induced hypokalemia may potentiate digitalis toxicity, avoid concomitant use). Products include:
- Lanoxicaps 772
- Lanoxin Elixir Pediatric 775
- Lanoxin Injection 778
- Lanoxin Injection Pediatric 781
- Lanoxin Tablets 783

Doxacurium Chloride (Amphotericin B-induced hypokalemia may enhance curariform effect). Products include:
- Nuromax Injection 794

Doxorubicin Hydrochloride (May enhance potential for renal toxicity, bronchospasm and hypotension). Products include:
- Adriamycin PFS 561
- Adriamycin RDF 562
- Doxorubicin Hydrochloride for Injection, USP 622

Doxorubicin Hydrochloride Injection, USP ... 848
Rubex ... 739

Estramustine Phosphate Sodium (May enhance potential for renal toxicity, bronchospasm and hypotension). Products include:
Emcyt Capsules ... 1161

Etoposide (May enhance potential for renal toxicity, bronchospasm and hypotension). Products include:
VePesid Capsules and Injection ... 741

Floxuridine (May enhance potential for renal toxicity, bronchospasm and hypotension). Products include:
Sterile FUDR ... 1898

Fluconazole (Imidazoles may induce fungal resistance to amphotericin). Products include:
Diflucan Injection and Tablets ... 1948

Flucytosine (Amphotericin B may increase toxicity of flucytosine). Products include:
Ancobon Capsules ... 1886

Fluorouracil (May enhance potential for renal toxicity, bronchospasm and hypotension). Products include:
Efudex ... 1880
Fluoroplex Topical Solution & Cream 1% ... 1082
Fluorouracil Injection ... 1897

Flutamide (May enhance potential for renal toxicity, bronchospasm and hypotension). Products include:
Eulexin Capsules ... 2089

Gentamicin Sulfate (May enhance the potential for renal toxicity). Products include:
Garamycin Injectable ... 2093
Garamycin Ophthalmic ... ◉ 305
Genoptic Liquifilm Sterile Ophthalmic Solution ... ◉ 247
Genoptic S.O.P. Sterile Ophthalmic Ointment ... ◉ 247
Gentacidin Ointment ... ◉ 273
Gentacidin Solution ... ◉ 273
Gentak Ointment & Solution ... ◉ 208
G-myticin Creme and Ointment 0.1% ... 1770
Pred-G Liquifilm Sterile Ophthalmic Suspension ... ◉ 252
Pred-G S.O.P. Sterile Ophthalmic Ointment ... ◉ 253

Hydrocortisone (Potentiates amphotericin B-induced hypokalemia). Products include:
AK-Spore H.C. ... ◉ 206
Bactine Hydrocortisone Anti-Itch Cream ... ■ 625
CaldeCORT Anti-Itch Hydrocortisone Spray ... ■ 560
Carmol HC Cream 1% ... 2296
Cortaid Spray ... ■ 735
Cortenema ... 2244
Cortisporin Ointment ... 758
Cortisporin Ophthalmic Ointment Sterile ... 758
Cortisporin Ophthalmic Suspension Sterile ... 759
Cortisporin Otic Solution Sterile ... 760
Cortisporin Otic Suspension Sterile 760
Cortizone-5 Creme & Ointment ... ■ 732
Dermolate Anti-Itch Cream ... ■ 697
Eldecort Cream 1.0% ... 1113
Eldecort Cream 1.0% and 2.5% ... 1113
Fungoid HC Creme ... 1770
Hydrocortone Tablets ... 1482
Hytone ... 909
LazerSporin-C Solution ... 1770
Massengill Medicated Soft Cloth Towelettes ... 2192
Nutracort Cream & Lotion ... 1684
PediOtic Suspension Sterile ... 797
Synacort Creams 1%, 2.5% ... 2296
Vanoxide-HC Acne Lotion ... 911
Vioform-Hydrocortisone Cream and Mild Cream ... 889
Vioform-Hydrocortisone Ointment ... 889
VōSoL HC Otic Solution ... 2392
Vytone Cream 1% ... 911

Hydrocortisone Acetate (Potentiates amphotericin B-induced hypokalemia). Products include:
Analpram-HC Rectal Cream 1% and 2.5% ... 970
Anusol-HC Cream ... 1690
Anusol-HC Suppositories ... 1691
Caldecort ... ■ 560
Carmol HC Cream 1% ... 2296
Chloromycetin Hydrocortisone Ophthalmic ... 1694
Coly-Mycin S Otic w/Neomycin & Hydrocortisone ... 1708
Cortaid ... ■ 735
Cortef Feminine Itch Cream ... ■ 735
Corticaine ... ■ 682
Cortifoam ... 1827
Cortisporin Cream ... 757
Epifoam ... 1828
Gynecort 5 Creme ... ■ 556
Hydrocortone Acetate Sterile Suspension ... 1479
Lanacort 5 Creme and Ointment ... ■ 557
Mantadil Cream ... 789
Ophthocort ... ◉ 301
Orabase HCA Oral Paste ... 890
Pramosone Cream, Lotion & Ointment ... 971
ProctoCream-HC ... 1834
Proctofoam-HC ... 1835

Hydrocortisone Sodium Phosphate (Potentiates amphotericin B-induced hypokalemia). Products include:
Hydrocortone Phosphate Injection, Sterile ... 1481

Hydrocortisone Sodium Succinate (Potentiates amphotericin B-induced hypokalemia). Products include:
Solu-Cortef Sterile Powder ... 2361

Hydroxyurea (May enhance potential for renal toxicity, bronchospasm and hypotension). Products include:
Hydrea Capsules ... 728

Ifosfamide (May enhance potential for renal toxicity, bronchospasm and hypotension). Products include:
IFEX ... 729

Interferon alfa-2A, Recombinant (May enhance potential for renal toxicity, bronchospasm and hypotension). Products include:
Roferon-A Injection ... 1916

Interferon alfa-2B, Recombinant (May enhance potential for renal toxicity, bronchospasm and hypotension). Products include:
Intron A ... 2097

Kanamycin Sulfate (May enhance the potential for renal toxicity). Products include:
Kantrex Injection ... 601
Kantrex Pediatric Injection ... 601

Ketoconazole (Imidazoles may induce fungal resistance to amphotericin). Products include:
Nizoral 2% Cream ... 1143
Nizoral 2% Shampoo ... 1144
Nizoral Tablets ... 1145

Levamisole Hydrochloride (May enhance potential for renal toxicity, bronchospasm and hypotension). Products include:
Ergamisol Tablets ... 1136

Lomustine (CCNU) (May enhance potential for renal toxicity, bronchospasm and hypotension). Products include:
CeeNU ... 725

Mechlorethamine Hydrochloride (May enhance potential for renal toxicity, bronchospasm and hypotension). Products include:
Mustargen ... 1514

Megestrol Acetate (May enhance potential for renal toxicity, bronchospasm and hypotension). Products include:
Megace Tablets ... 732

Melphalan (May enhance potential for renal toxicity, bronchospasm and hypotension). Products include:
Alkeran Tablets ... 754

Mercaptopurine (May enhance potential for renal toxicity, bronchospasm and hypotension). Products include:
Purinethol Tablets ... 800

Metaxalone (Amphotericin B-induced hypokalemia may enhance curariform effect). Products include:
Skelaxin ... 840

Methocarbamol (Amphotericin B-induced hypokalemia may enhance curariform effect). Products include:
Robaxin Injectable ... 1871
Robaxin Tablets ... 1872
Robaxisal Tablets ... 1872

Methotrexate Sodium (May enhance potential for renal toxicity, bronchospasm and hypotension). Products include:
Methotrexate Tablets, Parenteral, LPF Parenteral ... 1217
Rheumatrex Methotrexate Dose Pack ... 1234

Methylprednisolone Acetate (Potentiates amphotericin B-induced hypokalemia). Products include:
Depo-Medrol Sterile Aqueous Suspension ... 2334

Methylprednisolone Sodium Succinate (Potentiates amphotericin B-induced hypokalemia). Products include:
Solu-Medrol Sterile Powder ... 2363

Metocurine Iodide (Amphotericin B-induced hypokalemia may enhance curariform effect). Products include:
Metubine Iodide Vials ... 1285

Miconazole (Imidazoles may induce fungal resistance to amphotericin). Products include:
Monistat I.V. ... 1143

Miconazole Nitrate (Imidazoles may induce fungal resistance to amphotericin). Products include:
Micatin ... ■ 632
Micatin for Jock Itch ... ■ 633
Monistat Dual-Pak ... 1657
Monistat 3 Vaginal Suppositories ... 1657
Monistat-Derm (miconazole nitrate) Cream ... 1679

Mitomycin (Mitomycin-C) (May enhance potential for renal toxicity, bronchospasm and hypotension). Products include:
Mutamycin ... 733

Mitotane (May enhance potential for renal toxicity, bronchospasm and hypotension). Products include:
Lysodren ... 731

Mitoxantrone Hydrochloride (May enhance potential for renal toxicity, bronchospasm and hypotension). Products include:
Novantrone for Injection Concentrate ... 1226

Nephrotoxic Drugs (May enhance potential for renal toxicity).

Orphenadrine Citrate (Amphotericin B-induced hypokalemia may enhance curariform effect). Products include:
Norflex ... 1314
Norgesic ... 1314

Pancuronium Bromide Injection (Amphotericin B-induced hypokalemia may enhance curariform effect).
No products indexed under this heading.

Pentamidine Isethionate (May enhance the potential for renal toxicity). Products include:
NebuPent for Inhalation Solution ... 1017
Pentam 300 Injection ... 1018

Prednisolone Acetate (Potentiates amphotericin B-induced hypokalemia). Products include:
AK-Cide Sterile Ophthalmic Ointment & Suspension ... ◉ 202
Blephamide Liquifilm Sterile Ophthalmic Suspension ... 586
Blephamide S.O.P. Sterile Ophthalmic Ointment ... 586
Cetapred Ointment ... ◉ 220
⅛% Econopred & 1% Econopred Plus ... ◉ 217
Isopto Cetapred Suspension ... ◉ 220
Metimyd ... ◉ 306
Poly-Pred Liquifilm ... ◉ 250
Pred Forte ... ◉ 252
Pred Mild ... ◉ 254
Pred-G Liquifilm Sterile Ophthalmic Suspension ... ◉ 252
Pred-G S.O.P. Sterile Ophthalmic Ointment ... ◉ 253
Vasocidin Ointment ... ◉ 275

Prednisolone Sodium Phosphate (Potentiates amphotericin B-induced hypokalemia). Products include:
AK-Pred ... ◉ 205
Hydeltrasol Injection, Sterile ... 1476
Inflamase ... ◉ 274
Pediapred Oral Liquid ... 987
Vasocidin Ophthalmic Solution ... ◉ 276

Prednisolone Tebutate (Potentiates amphotericin B-induced hypokalemia). Products include:
Hydeltra-T.B.A. Sterile Suspension 1478

Prednisone (Potentiates amphotericin B-induced hypokalemia). Products include:
Deltasone Tablets ... 2332

Procarbazine Hydrochloride (May enhance potential for renal toxicity, bronchospasm and hypotension). Products include:
Matulane Capsules ... 1907

Streptomycin Sulfate (May enhance the potential for renal toxicity).
No products indexed under this heading.

Streptozocin (May enhance potential for renal toxicity, bronchospasm and hypotension). Products include:
Zanosar Sterile Powder ... 2371

Succinylcholine Chloride (Amphotericin B-induced hypokalemia may enhance curariform effect). Products include:
Anectine ... 755

Tamoxifen Citrate (May enhance potential for renal toxicity, bronchospasm and hypotension). Products include:
Nolvadex Tablets ... 1102

Thioguanine (May enhance potential for renal toxicity, bronchospasm and hypotension). Products include:
Thioguanine Tablets, Tabloid Brand ... 815

Thiotepa (May enhance potential for renal toxicity, bronchospasm and hypotension). Products include:
Thiotepa Parenteral ... 1240

Tobramycin (May enhance the potential for renal toxicity). Products include:
TobraDex Ophthalmic Suspension and Ointment ... ◉ 228
Tobrex Ophthalmic Ointment and Solution ... 572

Tobramycin Sulfate (May enhance the potential for renal toxicity). Products include:
Nebcin Vials, Hyporets & ADD-Vantage ... 1286

Triamcinolone (Potentiates amphotericin B-induced hypokalemia).
No products indexed under this heading.

Triamcinolone Acetonide (Potentiates amphotericin B-induced hypokalemia). Products include:
Aristocort A ... 1010
Azmacort Inhaler ... 1837
Kenalog Cream, Lotion & Ointment 2401
Kenalog-10 Injection ... 2402
Kenalog-40 Injection ... 2403
Kenalog in Orabase ... 604
Kenalog Spray ... 2401
Mycolog II Cream and Ointment ... 2407
Mytrex Cream & Ointment ... 2080
Nasacort Nasal Inhaler ... 1844

Triamcinolone Diacetate (Potentiates amphotericin B-induced hypokalemia). Products include:
Aristocort Suspension ... 1008

Triamcinolone Hexacetonide (Potentiates amphotericin B-induced hypokalemia). Products include:
Aristospan Suspension ... 1011

Tubocurarine Chloride (Amphotericin B-induced hypokalemia may enhance curariform effect).
No products indexed under this heading.

Vecuronium Bromide (Amphotericin B-induced hypokalemia may enhance curariform effect). Products include:
Norcuron ... 1642

Vincristine Sulfate (May enhance potential for renal toxicity, bronchospasm and hypotension). Products include:
Oncovin Solution Vials & Hyporets 1288

FUNGOID CREME & SOLUTION
(Cetylpyridinium Chloride, Triacetin) 1770
No interactions described in labeling.

FUNGOID HC CREME
(Hydrocortisone, Cetylpyridinium Chloride, Triacetin) ... 1770
No interactions described in labeling.

FUNGOID TINCTURE
(Cetylpyridinium Chloride, Triacetin) 1770
No interactions described in labeling.

FURACIN SOLUBLE DRESSING
(Nitrofurazone) ... 1854
No interactions described in labeling.

FURACIN TOPICAL CREAM
(Nitrofurazone) ... 1854
No interactions described in labeling.

FURACIN TOPICAL SOLUTION 0.2%
(Nitrofurazone) ... 1855
No interactions described in labeling.

FUROXONE ORAL SUSPENSION
(Furazolidone) ... 1855
May interact with anorexiants, monoamine oxidase inhibitors, antihistamines, hypnotics and sedatives, narcotic analgesics, tranquilizers, indirect-acting sympathomimetic amines, and certain other agents. Compounds in these categories include:

Alcohol (Possible disulfiram-like reaction may occur; alcohol intake should be avoided).

Alfentanil Hydrochloride (Use with caution at reduced dosages). Products include:
Alfenta Injection ... 1131

Alprazolam (Use with caution at reduced dosages). Products include:
Xanax Tablets ... 2367

Amphetamine Resins (Concurrent administration is contraindicated). Products include:
Biphetamine Capsules ... 973

Astemizole (Use with caution at reduced dosages). Products include:
Hismanal Tablets ... 1138

Azatadine Maleate (Use with caution at reduced dosages). Products include:
Optimine Tablets ... 2115
Trinalin Repetabs Tablets ... 1170

Benzphetamine Hydrochloride (Concurrent administration is contraindicated). Products include:
Didrex Tablets ... 2338

Bromodiphenhydramine Hydrochloride (Use with caution at reduced dosages).
No products indexed under this heading.

Brompheniramine Maleate (Use with caution at reduced dosages). Products include:
Alka Seltzer Plus Sinus Allergy Medicine ... 624
Atrohist Sprinkle Capsules ... 558
Bromfed Capsules (Timed Release) ... 1615
Bromfed Syrup ... 628
Bromfed ... 1615
Dimetane Decongestant ... 673
Dimetane ... 672
Dimetane-DC Cough Syrup ... 1857
Dimetane-DX Cough Syrup ... 1858
Dimetapp Elixir ... 673
Dimetapp DM Elixir ... 674
Dimetapp Extentabs ... 674
Dimetapp Plus Caplets ... 675
Dimetapp Tablets ... 675
Drixoral Antihistamine/Nasal Decongestant Syrup ... 698

Buprenorphine (Use with caution at reduced dosages).
No products indexed under this heading.

Buspirone Hydrochloride (Use with caution at reduced dosages). Products include:
BuSpar ... 1401

Chlordiazepoxide (Use with caution at reduced dosages). Products include:
Libritabs Tablets ... 1930
Limbitrol ... 1933
Menrium Tablets ... 1934

Chlordiazepoxide Hydrochloride (Use with caution at reduced dosages). Products include:
Librax Capsules ... 1929
Librium Capsules ... 1931
Librium Injectable ... 1932

Chlorpheniramine Maleate (Use with caution at reduced dosages). Products include:
A.R.M. Allergy Relief Medicine Caplets ... 615
Alka-Seltzer Plus Cold Medicine ... 623
Allerest ... 559
Ana-Kit Anaphylaxis Emergency Treatment Kit ... 1100
BC Cold Powder Multi-Symptom Formula ... 517
Brexin L.A. Capsules ... 2078
Cerose-DM ... 2443
Cheracol Plus Head Cold/Cough Formula ... 667
Chlor-Trimeton Allergy Syrup, Tablets & Long-Acting Repetabs Tablets ... 693
Chlor-Trimeton Decongestant ... 694
Comhist LA Capsules ... 1618
Allergy-Sinus Comtrex Multi-Symptom Allergy Sinus Formula Tablets & Caplets ... 746
Comtrex Multi-Symptom Cold Reliever Tablets/Caplets/Liqui-Gels/Liquid ... 745
Day-Night Comtrex ... 747
Contac Continuous Action Decongestant/Antihistamine Capsules ... 710
Contac Maximum Strength Continuous Action Decongestant/Antihistamine Caplets ... 709
Contac Severe Cold and Flu Formula Caplets ... 711
Coricidin 'D' Decongestant Tablets ... 695
Coricidin Demilets Tablets for Children ... 696
Coricidin Tablets ... 695
Deconamine ... 663
Demazin Nasal Decongestant/Antihistamine Repetabs Tablets & Syrup ... 697
Dorcol Children's Liquid Cold Formula ... 686
Dristan Decongestant/Antihistamine/ Analgesic Coated Caplets ... 749
Dristan Cold Nasal Decongestant/Antihistamine/ Analgesic Coated Tablets ... 2419
Dristan Advanced Formula Decongestant/Antihistamine/ Analgesic Tablets ... 749
Extendryl ... 994
4-Way Cold Tablets ... 750
Fedahist Gyrocaps ... 2145
Fedahist Timecaps ... 2145
Hycomine Compound Tablets ... 929
Isoclor Timesule Capsules ... 561
Kronofed-A ... 970
Medi-Flu Caplet, Liquid ... 640
Naldecon Syrup, Tablets, Pediatric Drops and Pediatric Syrup ... 709
Nolamine Tablets ... 838
Novafed A Capsules ... 1342
Novahistine DH ... 1342
Novahistine Elixir ... 596
Ornade Spansule Capsules ... 2221
Orthoxicol Cough Syrup ... 668
PediaCare Allergy Relief Formula Liquid ... 1362
PediaCare Cough-Cold Formula Liquid ... 1362
PediaCare Night Rest Cough-Cold Formula Liquid ... 1362
PediaCare 6-12 Cough-Cold Formula Chewable Tablets ... 1362
Pyrroxate Capsules ... 669
Quelidrine Syrup ... 556
Ru-Tuss II Capsules ... 693
Ru-Tuss Tablets ... 693
Ryna ... 741
Sinarest Tablets & Extra Strength Tablets ... 562
Sine-Off Maximum Strength Allergy/Sinus Formula Caplets ... 721
Sine-Off Sinus Medicine Tablets-Aspirin Formula ... 722
Singlet Tablets ... 598
Sinulin ... 840
Sinutab Maximum Strength ... 641
St. Joseph Nighttime Cold Medicine ... 705
Sudafed Plus Liquid ... 544
Sudafed Plus Tablets ... 545
Teldrin Timed-Release Allergy Capsules, 12 mg ... 2192
TheraFlu Flu and Cold Medicine ... 687
Triaminic Allergy Tablets ... 688
Triaminic Chewables ... 688
Triaminic Cold Tablets ... 688
Triaminic Nite Light ... 689
Triaminic Syrup ... 689
Triaminic-12 Tablets ... 690
Triaminicin Tablets ... 690
Triaminicol Multi-Symptom Cold Tablets ... 691
Triaminicol Multi-Symptom Relief ... 691
Tylenol Allergy Sinus Medication Caplets and Gelcaps, Maximum Strength ... 1372
Children's Tylenol Cold Liquid Formula and Chewable Tablets ... 1368
Tylenol Cold & Flu Hot Medication, Packets ... 1369
Tylenol Cold Medication Caplets and Tablets ... 1370
Tylenol Cold Medication, Effervescent Tablets ... 1369
Vicks Children's NyQuil ... 664
Vicks Formula 44 Cough Medicine ... 661
Vicks Formula 44M Multi-Symptom Cough Medicine ... 662
Vicks Pediatric Formula 44m Multi-Symptom Cough & Cold Medicine ... 663

Chlorpheniramine Polistirex (Use with caution at reduced dosages). Products include:
Tussionex Extended-Release Suspension ... 988

Chlorpheniramine Tannate (Use with caution at reduced dosages). Products include:
Rynatan ... 2387
Rynatuss ... 2388

Chlorpromazine (Use with caution at reduced dosages). Products include:
Thorazine ... 2234

Chlorprothixene (Use with caution at reduced dosages). Products include:
Taractan Tablets ... 1920

Chlorprothixene Hydrochloride (Use with caution at reduced dosages). Products include:
Taractan ... 1920

Clemastine Fumarate (Use with caution at reduced dosages). Products include:
Tavist Syrup ... 2033
Tavist Tablets ... 2035
Tavist-D Tablets ... 2035

Clorazepate Dipotassium (Use with caution at reduced dosages). Products include:
Tranxene ... 556

Codeine (Use with caution at reduced dosages). Products include:
Calcidrine Syrup ... 506

Codeine Phosphate (Use with caution at reduced dosages). Products include:
Actifed with Codeine Cough Syrup .. 752
Cheracol Cough Syrup ... 1853
Codimal PH Syrup ... 846
Dimetane-DC Cough Syrup ... 1857
Empirin with Codeine Phosphate Nos. 2, 3 & 4 ... 764
Fiorinal with Codeine Capsules ... 2008
Isoclor Expectorant ... 982
Naldecon CX Adult Liquid ... 521
Novahistine DH ... 1342
Novahistine Expectorant ... 1343
Nucofed Capsules ... 2219
Nucofed Expectorant ... 2219
Nucofed Pediatric Expectorant ... 2220
Nucofed Syrup ... 2219
Phenaphen with Codeine Capsules 1865
Phenaphen-650 with Codeine Tablets ... 1866
Phenergan with Codeine ... 2497
Phenergan VC with Codeine ... 2501
Robitussin A-C Syrup ... 1875
Robitussin-DAC Syrup ... 1875
Ryna ... 741
Soma Compound w/Codeine Tablets ... 2390
Triaminic Expectorant w/Codeine .. 1996
Tussi-Organidin Liquid ... 2391
Tylenol with Codeine ... 1381

Codeine Polistirex (Use with caution at reduced dosages).
No products indexed under this heading.

Cyproheptadine Hydrochloride (Use with caution at reduced dosages). Products include:
Periactin ... 1525

Dexchlorpheniramine Maleate (Use with caution at reduced dosages). Products include:
Polaramine ... 2116

Dextroamphetamine Sulfate (Concurrent administration is contraindicated). Products include:
Dexedrine ... 2206

Dezocine (Use with caution at reduced dosages).

Diazepam (Use with caution at reduced dosages). Products include:
Valium Injectable ... 1937
Valium Tablets ... 1939
Valrelease Capsules ... 1923

Diethylpropion Hydrochloride (Concurrent administration is contraindicated). Products include:
Tenuate ... 1354

Diphenhydramine Citrate (Use with caution at reduced dosages). Products include:

- Alka-Seltzer Plus Night-Time Cold Medicine ⊡ 623
- Bufferin AF Nite Time Analgesic/ Sleeping Aid Caplets 744
- Excedrin P.M. Analgesic/Sleeping Aid Tablets, Caplets and Liquid 749

Diphenhydramine Hydrochloride (Use with caution at reduced dosages). Products include:

- Benadryl Anti-Itch Cream ⊡ 635
- Benadryl Capsules 1691
- Benadryl Decongestant Elixir ⊡ 635
- Benadryl Decongestant ⊡ 635
- Benadryl Elixir ⊡ 636
- Benadryl Kapseals 1691
- Benadryl 25 Kapseals ⊡ 636
- Benadryl Parenteral 1692
- Benadryl Plus ⊡ 636
- Benadryl Plus Nighttime ⊡ 637
- Benadryl Spray, Maximum Strength ⊡ 637
- Benadryl Spray, Regular Strength ⊡ 637
- Benadryl Steri-Vials, Ampoules, and Steri-Dose Syringe 1692
- Benadryl 25 Tablets ⊡ 636
- Benylin Cough Syrup ⊡ 637
- Benylin Decongestant ⊡ 638
- Caladryl Cream, Lotion, Spray ⊡ 638
- Miles Nervine Nighttime Sleep-Aid ⊡ 627
- Nytol Tablets ⊡ 517
- Sleep-ettes-D Tablets ⊡ 653
- Sleep-eze 3 Tablets ⊡ 755
- Sleepinal Night-time Sleep Aid Capsules ⊡ 734
- Sominex Caplets and Tablets ⊡ 722
- Sominex Liquid ⊡ 723
- Sominex Pain Relief Formula ⊡ 723
- Tylenol Cold Night Time Medication Liquid 1371
- Tylenol PM, Extra Strength Caplets and Tablets 1368
- Unisom Dual Relief Nighttime Sleep Aid/Analgesic 1774
- Ziradryl Lotion ⊡ 643

Diphenylpyraline Hydrochloride (Use with caution at reduced dosages).

- No products indexed under this heading.

Droperidol (Use with caution at reduced dosages). Products include:

- Inapsine Injection 1140
- Innovar Injection 1141

Ephedrine Hydrochloride (Concurrent administration is contraindicated). Products include:

- Amesec ⊡ 682
- Primatene Tablets-M Formula 2421
- Primatene Tablets-P Formula 2421
- Primatene Tablets-Regular Formula 2421
- Quadrinal Tablets 1183
- Quelidrine Syrup 556
- Tedral SA 1765

Ephedrine Sulfate (Concurrent administration is contraindicated). Products include:

- Bronkaid Tablets ⊡ 757
- Bronkolixir ⊡ 761
- Bronkotabs Tablets ⊡ 762
- Marax Tablets & DF Syrup 1954
- Pazo Hemorrhoid Ointment & Suppositories 752
- Vicks Vatronol Nose Drops ⊡ 666

Ephedrine Tannate (Concurrent administration is contraindicated). Products include:

- Rynatuss 2388

Estazolam (Use with caution at reduced dosages). Products include:

- ProSom Tablets 554

Ethchlorvynol (Use with caution at reduced dosages). Products include:

- Placidyl Capsules 553

Ethinamate (Use with caution at reduced dosages).

- No products indexed under this heading.

Fenfluramine Hydrochloride (Concurrent administration is contraindicated). Products include:

- Pondimin Tablets 1867

Fentanyl (Use with caution at reduced dosages). Products include:

- Duragesic Transdermal System 1133

Fentanyl Citrate (Use with caution at reduced dosages). Products include:

- Innovar Injection 1141
- Sublimaze Injection 1146

Fluphenazine Decanoate (Use with caution at reduced dosages). Products include:

- Prolixin Decanoate 1795

Fluphenazine Enanthate (Use with caution at reduced dosages). Products include:

- Prolixin Enanthate 1796

Fluphenazine Hydrochloride (Use with caution at reduced dosages). Products include:

- Prolixin Elixir 1793
- Prolixin Injection 1791
- Prolixin Oral Concentrate 1792
- Prolixin Tablets 1793

Flurazepam Hydrochloride (Use with caution at reduced dosages). Products include:

- Dalmane Capsules 1927

Glutethimide (Use with caution at reduced dosages).

- No products indexed under this heading.

Haloperidol (Use with caution at reduced dosages). Products include:

- Haldol Injection, Tablets and Concentrate 1373

Haloperidol Decanoate (Use with caution at reduced dosages). Products include:

- Haldol Decanoate 1375

Hydrocodone Bitartrate (Use with caution at reduced dosages). Products include:

- Anexsia 5/500 Tablets 2196
- Anexsia 7.5/650 Tablets 2197
- Azdone Tablets 844
- Codiclear DH Syrup 845
- Codimal DH Syrup 846
- Damason-P 1356
- Hycodan Syrup, Tablets 927
- Hycomine Compound Tablets 929
- Hycomine Syrup 927
- Hycotuss Expectorant Syrup 930
- Hydrocet Capsules 835
- Lortab ASA Tablets 2414
- Lortab 2412
- Ru-Tuss with Hydrocodone 694
- Triaminic Expectorant DH 1995
- Vicodin Tablets 1187
- Vicodin ES Tablets 1189
- Zydone Capsules 941

Hydrocodone Polistirex (Use with caution at reduced dosages). Products include:

- Tussionex Extended-Release Suspension 988

Hydroxyzine Hydrochloride (Use with caution at reduced dosages). Products include:

- Atarax Tablets & Syrup 1941
- Marax Tablets & DF Syrup 1954
- Vistaril Intramuscular Solution 1970

Isocarboxazid (Concurrent administration is contraindicated). Products include:

- Marplan Tablets 1906

Levorphanol Tartrate (Use with caution at reduced dosages). Products include:

- Levo-Dromoran 1906

Lorazepam (Use with caution at reduced dosages). Products include:

- Ativan Injection 2432
- Ativan Tablets 2434

Loxapine Hydrochloride (Use with caution at reduced dosages). Products include:

- Loxitane 1213

Loxapine Succinate (Use with caution at reduced dosages). Products include:

- Loxitane Capsules 1213

Mazindol (Concurrent administration is contraindicated). Products include:

- Sanorex Tablets 2030

Meperidine Hydrochloride (Use with caution at reduced dosages). Products include:

- Demerol 2047
- Mepergan Injection 2479

Meprobamate (Use with caution at reduced dosages). Products include:

- Deprol Tablets 2382
- Equagesic Tablets 2451
- Miltown Tablets 2386
- PMB 200 and PMB 400 2504

Mesoridazine (Use with caution at reduced dosages). Products include:

- Serentil 686

Methadone Hydrochloride (Use with caution at reduced dosages). Products include:

- Dolophine Hydrochloride Ampoules & Vials 1260
- Dolophine Hydrochloride Tablets 1261
- Methadone Hydrochloride Diskets 1284
- Methadone Hydrochloride Oral Solution & Tablets 1987

Methamphetamine Hydrochloride (Concurrent administration is contraindicated). Products include:

- Desoxyn Gradumet Tablets 514

Methdilazine Hydrochloride (Use with caution at reduced dosages). Products include:

- Tacaryl Syrup & Tablets 2409

Midazolam Hydrochloride (Use with caution at reduced dosages). Products include:

- Versed Injection 1924

Molindone Hydrochloride (Use with caution at reduced dosages). Products include:

- Moban Tablets & Concentrate 932

Morphine Sulfate (Use with caution at reduced dosages). Products include:

- Astramorph/PF Injection, USP (Preservative-Free) 618
- Duramorph 960
- Infumorph 200 and Infumorph 500 Sterile Solutions 962
- MS Contin Tablets 1814
- MSIR 1817
- Oramorph SR (Morphine Sulfate Sustained Release Tablets) 1988
- Roxanol 1991

Naphazoline Hydrochloride (Concurrent administration is contraindicated). Products include:

- AK-Con ⊙ 202
- AK-Con-A ⊙ 203
- Albalon Solution with Liquifilm ⊙ 238
- Albalon-A Liquifilm ⊙ 238
- Allergy Drops ⊙ 258
- Clear Eyes ACR ⊙ 305
- Clear Eyes Lubricating Eye Redness Reliever ⊙ 304
- 4-Way Fast Acting Nasal Spray - Original Formula (regular & mentholated) & Metered Spray Pump (regular) 751
- Naphcon ⊙ 226
- Naphcon Forte ⊙ 226
- Naphcon-A Ophthalmic Solution 571
- Opcon-A Ophthalmic Solution ⊙ 262
- Privine Nasal Solution ⊡ 552
- Privine Nasal Solution 878
- Privine Nasal Spray ⊡ 552
- Privine Nasal Spray 878
- Vasocon-A ⊙ 278

Opium Alkaloids (Use with caution at reduced dosages). Products include:

- B & O No. 15A & No. 16A Supprettes 2395
- Pantopon Injectable 1911

Oxazepam (Use with caution at reduced dosages). Products include:

- Serax Capsules 2522
- Serax Tablets 2522

Oxycodone Hydrochloride (Use with caution at reduced dosages). Products include:

- Percocet Tablets 950
- Percodan 951
- Roxicodone Tablets, Oral Solution & Intensol (Oxycodone) 1992
- Tylox Capsules 1382

Oxymetazoline Hydrochloride (Concurrent administration is contraindicated). Products include:

- Afrin ⊡ 692
- Cheracol Nasal Spray Pump ⊡ 667
- Dristan Long Lasting Menthol Nasal Spray 2419
- Dristan Long Lasting Nasal Spray, Regular and Regular with Metered Dose Pump 2419
- Duration Nasal Spray ⊡ 700
- Duration 12 Hour Nasal Spray Pump ⊡ 700
- 4-Way Long Lasting Nasal Spray & Metered Spray Pump 751
- NTZ Long Acting Nasal Spray & Drops 0.05% ⊡ 760
- Neo-Synephrine Maximum Strength 12 Hour Nasal Spray ⊡ 759
- Neo-Synephrine Maximum Strength 12 Hour Nasal Spray Pump ⊡ 759
- Nōstrilla Long Acting Nasal Decongestant ⊡ 520
- OcuClear Eye Drops ⊙ 306
- Vicks Sinex Long Acting ⊡ 665
- Visine L.R. Eye Drops ⊡ 647
- Visine L.R. Eye Drops ⊙ 303

Perphenazine (Use with caution at reduced dosages). Products include:

- Etrafon 2087
- Triavil Tablets 1556
- Trilafon 2123

Phendimetrazine Tartrate (Concurrent administration is contraindicated). Products include:

- Bontril Slow-Release 834
- Plegine Tablets 2504
- Prelu-2 Capsules 683

Phenelzine Sulfate (Concurrent administration is contraindicated). Products include:

- Nardil 1742

Phenmetrazine Hydrochloride (Concurrent administration is contraindicated).

- No products indexed under this heading.

Phenylephrine Hydrochloride (Concurrent administration is contraindicated). Products include:

- AK-Dilate Solution 2.5% and 10% ⊙ 203
- Atrohist Sprinkle Capsules 558
- Cerose-DM 2443
- Codimal 846
- Comhist LA Capsules 1618
- Congespirin For Children Aspirin Free Chewable Cold Tablets 748
- Cyclomydril ⊙ 216
- Deconsal Sprinkle Capsules 559
- Dimetane Decongestant ⊡ 673
- Dristan Decongestant/Antihistamine/ Analgesic Coated Caplets ⊡ 749
- Dristan Cold Nasal Decongestant/ Antihistamine/ Analgesic Coated Tablets 2419
- Dristan Advanced Formula Decongestant/Antihistamine/ Analgesic Tablets ⊡ 749
- Dristan Nasal Spray, Menthol 2419
- Dristan Nasal Spray, Regular and Regular with Metered Pump 2419
- Entex Capsules 1623
- Entex Liquid 1623
- Sinus Excedrin Analgesic, Decongestant Tablets & Caplets 750

Extendryl 994
4-Way Fast Acting Nasal Spray - Original Formula (regular & mentholated) & Metered Spray Pump (regular) 751
Hycomine Compound Tablets 929
Murocoll-2 Sterile Ophthalmic Solution ⊙ 261
Mydfrin 2.5% ⊙ 224
Naldecon Syrup, Tablets, Pediatric Drops and Pediatric Syrup 709
Neo-Synephrine Hydrochloride 1% Carpuject 2063
Neo-Synephrine Hydrochloride 1% Injection 2063
Neo-Synephrine Hydrochloride (Ophthalmic) 2064
Neo-Synephrine ■ 759
Nōstril Nasal Decongestant ■ 520
Novahistine Elixir ■ 596
Phenergan VC 2500
Phenergan VC with Codeine 2501
Prefrin Liquifilm Vasoconstrictor and Lubricant Eye Drops ⊙ 254
Prefrin-A ⊙ 255
Quelidrine Syrup 556
Relief Vasoconstrictor and Lubricant Eye Drops ⊙ 256
Robitussin Night Relief ■ 677
Ru-Tuss with Hydrocodone 694
Ru-Tuss Tablets 693
Vasosulf ⊙ 279
Vicks Sinex ■ 665
Zincfrin ⊙ 230

Phenylpropanolamine Hydrochloride (Concurrent administration is contraindicated). Products include:

A.R.M. Allergy Relief Medicine Caplets ■ 615
Acutrim ■ 548
Allerest ■ 559
BC Cold Powder ■ 517
Cheracol Plus Head Cold/Cough Formula ■ 667
Codimal Expectorant 846
Comtrex Multi-Symptom Cold Reliever Tablets/Caplets/Liqui-Gels/Liquid 745
Contac Continuous Action Decongestant/Antihistamine Capsules ■ 710
Contac Maximum Strength Continuous Action Decongestant/Antihistamine Caplets ■ 709
Contac Severe Cold and Flu Formula Caplets ■ 711
Coricidin 'D' Decongestant Tablets ■ 695
Coricidin Demilets Tablets for Children ■ 696
Demazin Nasal Decongestant/Antihistamine Repetabs Tablets & Syrup ■ 697
Dexatrim ■ 733
Dimetane-DC Cough Syrup 1857
Dimetapp Elixir ■ 673
Dimetapp DM Elixir ■ 674
Dimetapp Extentabs ■ 674
Dimetapp Plus Caplets ■ 675
Dimetapp Tablets ■ 675
Entex Capsules 1623
Entex LA Tablets 1623
Entex Liquid 1623
4-Way Cold Tablets 750
Hycomine Syrup 927
Naldecon CX Adult Liquid ■ 521
Naldecon DX Adult Liquid ■ 521
Naldecon DX Children's Syrup ■ 522
Naldecon DX Pediatric Drops ■ 522
Naldecon EX Children's Syrup ■ 522
Naldecon EX Pediatric Drops ■ 523
Naldecon Syrup, Tablets, Pediatric Drops and Pediatric Syrup 709
Nolamine Tablets 838
Nolex LA Tablets 838
Ornade Spansule Capsules 2221
Orthoxicol Cough Syrup ■ 668
Propagest 839
Pyrroxate Capsules ■ 669
Robitussin-CF ■ 676
Ru-Tuss II Capsules 693
Ru-Tuss with Hydrocodone 694
Ru-Tuss Tablets 693
Sine-Off Sinus Medicine Tablets-Aspirin Formula ■ 722
Sinulin 840
St. Joseph Cold Tablets for Children ■ 704
Tavist-D Tablets 2035
Triaminic Allergy Tablets ■ 688
Triaminic Chewables ■ 688
Triaminic Cold Tablets ■ 688
Triaminic Expectorant ■ 688
Triaminic Expectorant w/Codeine 1996
Triaminic Expectorant DH 1995
Triaminic Oral Infant Drops 1996
Triaminic Syrup ■ 689
Triaminic-12 Tablets ■ 690
Triaminic-DM Syrup ■ 689
Triaminicin Tablets ■ 690
Triaminicol Multi-Symptom Cold Tablets ■ 691
Triaminicol Multi-Symptom Relief ■ 691
Tuss-Ornade Liquid 2242
Tuss-Ornade Spansule Capsules 2242
Tylenol Cold Medication, Effervescent Tablets 1369

Prazepam (Use with caution at reduced dosages). Products include:

Centrax 1693

Prochlorperazine (Use with caution at reduced dosages). Products include:

Compazine 2201

Promethazine Hydrochloride (Use with caution at reduced dosages). Products include:

Mepergan Injection 2479
Phenergan with Codeine 2497
Phenergan with Dextromethorphan 2499
Phenergan Injection 2493
Phenergan Suppositories 2496
Phenergan Syrup 2495
Phenergan Tablets 2496
Phenergan VC 2500
Phenergan VC with Codeine 2501

Propofol (Use with caution at reduced dosages). Products include:

Diprivan Injection 2267

Propoxyphene Hydrochloride (Use with caution at reduced dosages). Products include:

Darvon 1256
Wygesic Tablets 2540

Propoxyphene Napsylate (Use with caution at reduced dosages). Products include:

Darvon-N/Darvocet-N 1254

Pseudoephedrine Hydrochloride (Concurrent administration is contraindicated). Products include:

Actifed Capsules ■ 539
Actifed Plus Caplets ■ 539
Actifed Plus Tablets ■ 540
Actifed with Codeine Cough Syrup 752
Actifed Syrup ■ 540
Actifed Tablets ■ 540
Actifed 12-Hour Capsules ■ 539
Advil Cold & Sinus Caplets (formerly CoAdvil) 2416
Allerest ■ 559
Anatuss LA Tablets 1359
Benadryl Decongestant Elixir ■ 635
Benadryl Decongestant ■ 635
Benadryl Plus ■ 636
Benadryl Plus Nighttime ■ 637
Benylin Decongestant ■ 638
Brexin L.A. Capsules 2078
Bromfed Capsules (Timed Release) 1615
Bromfed Syrup ■ 628
Bromfed 1615
CoAdvil ■ 748
Allergy-Sinus Comtrex Multi-Symptom Allergy Sinus Formula Tablets & Caplets 746
Cough Formula Comtrex 746
Comtrex Multi-Symptom Cold Reliever Tablets/Caplets/Liqui-Gels/Liquid 745
Day-Night Comtrex 747
Non-Drowsy Comtrex 747
Congess 994
Congestac Caplets ■ 617
Contac Jr. Children's Cold Medicine ■ 712
Contac Nighttime Cold Medicine ■ 713
Contac Sinus Caplets Maximum Strength Non-Drowsy Formula ■ 710
Contac Sinus Tablets Maximum Strength Non-Drowsy Formula ■ 710
Deconamine 663
Deconsal II Tablets 559
Dimacol Caplets ■ 672
Dimetane-DX Cough Syrup 1858
Dorcol Children's Cough Syrup ■ 685
Dorcol Children's Decongestant Liquid ■ 685
Dorcol Children's Liquid Cold Formula ■ 686
Maximum Strength Dristan Decongestant/Analgesic Coated Caplets ■ 750
No Drowsiness Dristan Cold Nasal Decongestant/Analgesic Coated Caplets 2420
Dristan Sinus Caplets 2419
Sinus Excedrin Analgesic, Decongestant Tablets & Caplets ■ 533
Fedahist Gyrocaps 2145
Fedahist Timecaps 2145
Guaifed 1615
Guaifed Syrup ■ 629
Isoclor Expectorant 982
Isoclor Timesule Capsules ■ 561
Kronofed-A 970
Medi-Flu Caplet, Liquid ■ 640
Novafed A Capsules 1342
Novafed Capsules 1342
Novahistine DH 1342
Novahistine DMX ■ 595
Novahistine Expectorant 1343
Nucofed Capsules 2219
Nucofed Expectorant 2219
Nucofed Pediatric Expectorant 2220
Nucofed Syrup 2219
Ornex Caplets ■ 618
PediaCare Allergy Relief Formula Liquid 1362
PediaCare Cough-Cold Formula Liquid 1362
PediaCare Infants' Oral Decongestant Drops 1362
PediaCare Night Rest Cough-Cold Formula Liquid 1362
PediaCare 6-12 Cough-Cold Formula Chewable Tablets 1362
Robitussin-DAC Syrup 1875
Robitussin-PE ■ 677
Rondec 1975
Rondec-DM 1976
Rondec-TR Tablet 1975
Ru-Tuss DE Tablets 694
Ryna ■ 741
Seldane-D Extended-Release Tablets 1350
Sinarest ■ 562
Sine-Aid Maximum Strength Sinus Headache Caplets 1365
Sine-Aid Maximum Strength Sinus Headache Tablets 1365
Sine-Off Maximum Strength Allergy/Sinus Formula Caplets ■ 721
Sine-Off Maximum Strength No Drowsiness Formula Caplets ■ 722
Singlet Tablets ■ 598
Sinutab Maximum Strength ■ 641
Sinutab Maximum Strength Without Drowsiness Tablets & Caplets ■ 642
Sinutab Regular Strength Without Drowsiness Formula ■ 641
St. Joseph Nighttime Cold Medicine ■ 705
Sudafed Children's Liquid ■ 543
Sudafed Cough Syrup ■ 543
Sudafed Plus Liquid ■ 544
Sudafed Plus Tablets ■ 545
Sudafed Sinus Caplets ■ 545
Sudafed Sinus Tablets ■ 545
Sudafed Tablets, 30 mg ■ 544
Sudafed Tablets, Adult Strength, 60 mg ■ 544
Sudafed 12 Hour Capsules ■ 545
TheraFlu Flu and Cold Medicine ■ 687
Triaminic Nite Light ■ 689
Tylenol Allergy Sinus Medication Caplets and Gelcaps, Maximum Strength 1372
Children's Tylenol Cold Liquid Formula and Chewable Tablets 1368
Tylenol Cold & Flu Hot Medication, Packets 1369
Tylenol Cold & Flu No Drowsiness Hot Medication, Packets 1371
Tylenol Cold Medication Caplets and Tablets 1370
Tylenol Cold Medication No Drowsiness Formula Caplets 1370
Tylenol Cold Night Time Medication Liquid 1371
Tylenol Cough Medication Liquid with Decongestant, Maximum Strength 1372
Tylenol, Maximum Strength, Sinus Medication Gelcaps, Caplets and Tablets 1373
Ursinus Inlay-Tabs ■ 691
Vicks Children's NyQuil ■ 664
Vicks Daycare ■ 660
Vicks Formula 44D Decongestant Cough Medicine ■ 662
Vicks Formula 44M Multi-Symptom Cough Medicine ■ 662
Vicks NyQuil Nighttime Colds Medicine-Original & Cherry Flavor ■ 664
Vicks Pediatric Formula 44 Cough & Congestion Medicine ■ 663
Vicks Pediatric Formula 44m Multi-Symptom Cough & Cold Medicine ■ 663

Pyrilamine Maleate (Use with caution at reduced dosages). Products include:

Codimal 846
4-Way Fast Acting Nasal Spray - Original Formula (regular & mentholated) & Metered Spray Pump (regular) 751
Maximum Strength Midol Multi-Symptom Menstrual Formula ■ 571
Maximum Strength Midol PMS Premenstrual Syndrome Formula ■ 570
Regular Strength Midol Multi-Symptom Menstrual Formula ■ 570
Prefrin-A ⊙ 255
Prēmsyn PMS Capsules & Caplets ■ 547
Primatene Tablets-M Formula 2421
Robitussin Night Relief ■ 677
Ru-Tuss with Hydrocodone 694
Triaminic Expectorant DH 1995
Triaminic Oral Infant Drops 1996

Pyrilamine Tannate (Use with caution at reduced dosages). Products include:

Rynatan 2387

Quazepam (Use with caution at reduced dosages). Products include:

Doral Tablets 2383

Secobarbital Sodium (Use with caution at reduced dosages). Products include:

Seconal Sodium Pulvules 1296

Selegiline Hydrochloride (Concurrent administration is contraindicated). Products include:

Eldepryl 2250

Sufentanil Citrate (Use with caution at reduced dosages). Products include:

Sufenta Injection 1147

Temazepam (Use with caution at reduced dosages). Products include:

Restoril Capsules 2023

Terfenadine (Use with caution at reduced dosages). Products include:

Seldane Tablets 1349
Seldane-D Extended-Release Tablets 1350

Tetrahydrozoline Hydrochloride (Concurrent administration is contraindicated). Products include:

Collyrium Fresh 2445
Murine Plus Lubricating Eye Redness Reliever ⊙ 305
Visine A.C. Eye Drops ■ 646
Visine A.C. Eye Drops ⊙ 303
Visine EXTRA Eye Drops ■ 647
Visine EXTRA Eye Drops ⊙ 303
Visine Eye Drops ■ 646
Visine Eye Drops ⊙ 303

Thioridazine Hydrochloride (Use with caution at reduced dosages). Products include:

Mellaril 2011

Thiothixene (Use with caution at reduced dosages). Products include:

Navane Capsules and Concentrate 1954
Navane Intramuscular 1956

Tranylcypromine Sulfate (Concurrent administration is contraindicated). Products include:

Parnate Tablets 2222

Triazolam (Use with caution at reduced dosages). Products include:

Halcion Tablets 2340

(■ Described in PDR For Nonprescription Drugs) (⊙ Described in PDR For Ophthalmology)

Trifluoperazine Hydrochloride (Use with caution at reduced dosages). Products include:
- Stelazine ... 2226

Trimeprazine Tartrate (Use with caution at reduced dosages). Products include:
- Temaril Tablets, Syrup and Spansule Sustained Release Capsules 1085

Tripelennamine Hydrochloride (Use with caution at reduced dosages). Products include:
- PBZ Tablets & Elixir ... 1037
- PBZ-SR Tablets ... 1037

Triprolidine Hydrochloride (Use with caution at reduced dosages). Products include:
- Actidil ... ▣ 538
- Actifed Capsules ... ▣ 539
- Actifed Plus Caplets ... ▣ 539
- Actifed Plus Tablets ... ▣ 540
- Actifed with Codeine Cough Syrup .. 752
- Actifed Syrup ... ▣ 540
- Actifed Tablets ... ▣ 540
- Actifed 12-Hour Capsules ... ▣ 539

Tyramine (Concurrent administration is contraindicated).

Food Interactions

Beans, broad (Concurrent and/or sequential intake must be avoided).

Beans, Fava (Concurrent and/or sequential intake must be avoided).

Beer, unspecified (Concurrent and/or sequential intake must be avoided).

Cheese, strong, unpasteurized (Concurrent and/or sequential intake must be avoided).

Food with high concentration of dopamine (Concurrent and/or sequential intake must be avoided).

Food with high concentration of tyramine (Concurrent and/or sequential intake must be avoided).

Herring, pickled (Concurrent and/or sequential intake must be avoided).

Liver, chicken (Concurrent and/or sequential intake must be avoided).

Wine, unspecified (Concurrent and/or sequential intake must be avoided).

Yeast extract (Concurrent and/or sequential intake must be avoided).

FUROXONE TABLETS

(Furazolidone) ... 1855
See **Furoxone Oral Suspension**

GAMIMUNE N IMMUNE GLOBULIN INTRAVENOUS (HUMAN)

(Immune Globulin Intravenous (Human)) ... 1572
No interactions described in labeling.

GAMMAGARD IMMUNE GLOBULIN, INTRAVENOUS (HUMAN)

(Globulin, Immune (Human)) ... 658
No interactions described in labeling.

GAMMAR, IMMUNE GLOBULIN (HUMAN) U.S.P.

(Immune Globulin (Human)) ... 609
May interact with:

Measles Virus Vaccine Live (Interference with the response to live viral vaccines). Products include:
- Attenuvax ... 1424

Measles & Rubella Virus Vaccine Live (Interference with the response to live viral vaccines). Products include:
- M-R-VAX II ... 1496

Measles, Mumps & Rubella Virus Vaccine Live (Interference with the response to live viral vaccines). Products include:
- M-M-R II ... 1494

GAMMAR-IV, IMMUNE GLOBULIN INTRAVENOUS (HUMAN)

(Immune Globulin Intravenous (Human)) ... 610
No interactions described in labeling.

GAMULIN RH, $RH_0(D)$ IMMUNE GLOBULIN (HUMAN)

($Rh_0(D)$ Immune Globulin (Human)) .. 610
No interactions described in labeling.

GANITE INJECTION

(Gallium Nitrate) ... 1016
May interact with aminoglycosides and certain other agents. Compounds in these categories include:

Amikacin Sulfate (May increase the risk for developing renal insufficiency). Products include:
- Amikin Injectable ... 602

Amphotericin B (May increase the risk for developing renal insufficiency). Products include:
- Fungizone Cream, Lotion and Ointment ... 2261
- Fungizone Intravenous ... 2262

Gentamicin Sulfate (May increase the risk for developing renal insufficiency). Products include:
- Garamycin Injectable ... 2093
- Garamycin Ophthalmic ... ⊙ 305
- Genoptic Liquifilm Sterile Ophthalmic Solution ... ⊙ 247
- Genoptic S.O.P. Sterile Ophthalmic Ointment ... ⊙ 247
- Gentacidin Ointment ... ⊙ 273
- Gentacidin Solution ... ⊙ 273
- Gentak Ointment & Solution ... ⊙ 208
- G-myticin Creme and Ointment 0.1% ... 1770
- Pred-G Liquifilm Sterile Ophthalmic Suspension ... ⊙ 252
- Pred-G S.O.P. Sterile Ophthalmic Ointment ... ⊙ 253

Kanamycin Sulfate (May increase the risk for developing renal insufficiency). Products include:
- Kantrex Injection ... 601
- Kantrex Pediatric Injection ... 601

Nephrotoxic Drugs (May increase the risk for developing renal insufficiency).

Streptomycin Sulfate (May increase the risk for developing renal insufficiency).
- No products indexed under this heading.

Tobramycin (May increase the risk for developing renal insufficiency). Products include:
- TobraDex Ophthalmic Suspension and Ointment ... ⊙ 228
- Tobrex Ophthalmic Ointment and Solution ... 572

Tobramycin Sulfate (May increase the risk for developing renal insufficiency). Products include:
- Nebcin Vials, Hyporets & ADD-Vantage ... 1286

GANTANOL SUSPENSION

(Sulfamethoxazole) ... 1899
May interact with thiazides, oral anticoagulants, and certain other agents. Compounds in these categories include:

Bendroflumethiazide (Increased incidence of thrombopenia with purpura in elderly). Products include:
- Corzide Tablets ... 702
- Naturetin Tablets ... 1789
- Rauzide Tablets ... 1804

Chlorothiazide (Increased incidence of thrombopenia with purpura in elderly). Products include:
- Aldoclor Tablets ... 1413
- Diupres Tablets ... 1461
- Diuril Oral ... 1464

Chlorothiazide Sodium (Increased incidence of thrombopenia with purpura in elderly). Products include:
- Diuril Sodium Intravenous ... 1463

Dicumarol (Increased prothrombin time). Products include:
- Dicumarol Tablets ... 516

Hydrochlorothiazide (Increased incidence of thrombopenia with purpura in elderly). Products include:
- Aldactazide ... 2150
- Aldoril Tablets ... 1418
- Apresazide Capsules ... 854
- Apresoline-Esidrix Tablets ... 857
- Capozide ... 2258
- Dyazide Capsules ... 2208
- Esidrix Tablets ... 863
- Esimil Tablets ... 864
- HydroDIURIL Tablets ... 1484
- Hydropres Tablets ... 1485
- Inderide Tablets ... 2463
- Inderide LA Long Acting Capsules .. 2465
- Lopressor HCT Tablets ... 1034
- Maxzide ... 1215
- Moduretic Tablets ... 1510
- Normozide Tablets ... 2112
- Oretic Tablets ... 544
- Oreticyl ... 545
- Prinzide Tablets ... 1540
- Ser-Ap-Es Tablets ... 881
- Serpasil-Esidrix Tablets ... 886
- Timolide Tablets ... 1547
- Trandate HCT Tablets ... 579
- Vaseretic Tablets ... 1559
- Zestoretic ... 2274

Hydroflumethiazide (Increased incidence of thrombopenia with purpura in elderly). Products include:
- Diucardin Tablets ... 2450
- Saluron ... 718
- Salutensin/Salutensin-Demi ... 719

Methotrexate Sodium (May be displaced from protein-binding sites). Products include:
- Methotrexate Tablets, Parenteral, LPF Parenteral ... 1217
- Rheumatrex Methotrexate Dose Pack ... 1234

Methyclothiazide (Increased incidence of thrombopenia with purpura in elderly). Products include:
- Enduron Tablets ... 517
- Enduronyl ... 518

Phenytoin (May inhibit hepatic metabolism; possible excessive phenytoin effect). Products include:
- Dilantin Infatabs ... 1710
- Dilantin-30 Pediatric/Dilantin-125 Suspension ... 1713

Phenytoin Sodium (May inhibit hepatic metabolism; possible excessive phenytoin effect). Products include:
- Dilantin Kapseals ... 1708
- Dilantin Parenteral ... 1712
- Dilantin with Phenobarbital Kapseals ... 1715

Polythiazide (Increased incidence of thrombopenia with purpura in elderly). Products include:
- Minizide Capsules ... 1779
- Renese Tablets ... 1785
- Renese-R Tablets ... 1786

Warfarin Sodium (Increased prothrombin time). Products include:
- Coumadin Injection & Tablets ... 944
- Panwarfin Tablets ... 547

GANTANOL TABLETS

(Sulfamethoxazole) ... 1899
See **Gantanol Suspension**

GANTRISIN OPHTHALMIC OINTMENT/SOLUTION

(Sulfisoxazole Diolamine) ... 1900
May interact with silver preparations and certain other agents. Compounds in these categories include:

Gentamicin Sulfate (In vitro antagonism has been reported). Products include:
- Garamycin Injectable ... 2093
- Garamycin Ophthalmic ... ⊙ 305
- Genoptic Liquifilm Sterile Ophthalmic Solution ... ⊙ 247
- Genoptic S.O.P. Sterile Ophthalmic Ointment ... ⊙ 247
- Gentacidin Ointment ... ⊙ 273
- Gentacidin Solution ... ⊙ 273
- Gentak Ointment & Solution ... ⊙ 208
- G-myticin Creme and Ointment 0.1% ... 1770
- Pred-G Liquifilm Sterile Ophthalmic Suspension ... ⊙ 252
- Pred-G S.O.P. Sterile Ophthalmic Ointment ... ⊙ 253

Silver Nitrate (Incompatible).
- No products indexed under this heading.

GANTRISIN PEDIATRIC SUSPENSION

(Acetyl Sulfisoxazole) ... 1901
May interact with oral anticoagulants, barbiturates, oral hypoglycemic agents, and certain other agents. Compounds in these categories include:

Aprobarbital (Competes for plasma protein binding). Products include:
- Alurate Elixir ... 1883

Butabarbital (Competes for plasma protein binding). Products include:
- Pyridium Plus ... 1764

Butalbital (Competes for plasma protein binding). Products include:
- Esgic-Plus Tablets ... 1002
- Esgic Tablets & Capsules ... 1001
- Fioricet Tablets ... 2006
- Fiorinal Capsules ... 2007
- Fiorinal with Codeine Capsules ... 2008
- Fiorinal Tablets ... 2007
- Phrenilin ... 838
- Sedapap Tablets 50 mg/650 mg .. 1360

Chlorpropamide (Potentiated blood sugar lowering activity). Products include:
- Diabinese Tablets ... 1775

Dicumarol (Prolonged prothrombin time). Products include:
- Dicumarol Tablets ... 516

Glipizide (Potentiated blood sugar lowering activity). Products include:
- Glucotrol ... 1952

Glyburide (Potentiated blood sugar lowering activity). Products include:
- DiaBeta ... 1091
- Micronase Tablets ... 2350

Mephobarbital (Competes for plasma protein binding). Products include:
- Mebaral Tablets ... 2061

Methotrexate Sodium (Displaced from plasma protein-binding sites). Products include:
- Methotrexate Tablets, Parenteral, LPF Parenteral ... 1217
- Rheumatrex Methotrexate Dose Pack ... 1234

Pentobarbital Sodium (Competes for plasma protein binding). Products include:
- Nembutal Sodium Capsules ... 534
- Nembutal Sodium Solution ... 536
- Nembutal Sodium Suppositories ... 538

Phenobarbital (Competes for plasma protein binding). Products include:
- Arco-Lase Plus Tablets ... 607
- Bellergal-S Tablets ... 1998

Bronkolixir ▣ 761
Bronkotabs Tablets ▣ 762
Donnatal 1858
Donnatal Extentabs 1859
Donnatal Tablets 1858
Donnazyme Tablets 1860
Kinesed Tablets 2272
Phenobarbital Elixir and Tablets 1293
Primatene Tablets-P Formula 2421
Quadrinal Tablets 1183
Tedral SA 1765

Secobarbital Sodium (Competes for plasma protein binding). Products include:
Seconal Sodium Pulvules 1296

Thiamylal Sodium (Competes for plasma protein binding). Products include:
Surital Ampoules, Steri-Vials 1764

Tolazamide (Potentiated blood sugar lowering activity). Products include:
Tolinase Tablets 2365

Tolbutamide (Potentiated blood sugar lowering activity). Products include:
Orinase Tablets 2354

Warfarin Sodium (Prolonged prothrombin time). Products include:
Coumadin Injection & Tablets 944
Panwarfin Tablets 547

GANTRISIN SYRUP
(Acetyl Sulfisoxazole) 1901
See **Gantrisin Pediatric Suspension**

GANTRISIN TABLETS
(Sulfisoxazole) 1901
See **Gantrisin Pediatric Suspension**

GARAMYCIN INJECTABLE
(Gentamicin Sulfate) 2093
May interact with cephalosporins, nondepolarizing neuromuscular blocking agents, and certain other agents. Compounds in these categories include:

Amikacin Sulfate (Increased nephrotoxicity). Products include:
Amikin Injectable 602

Atracurium Besylate (Enhanced neuromuscular blockade and respiratory paralysis). Products include:
Tracrium Injection 817

Carbenicillin Disodium (Decreased effects of gentamicin).

Carbenicillin Indanyl Sodium (Decreases effects). Products include:
Geocillin Tablets 1951

Cefaclor (Increased nephrotoxicity). Products include:
Ceclor Pulvules & Suspension 1251

Cefadroxil Monohydrate (Increased nephrotoxicity). Products include:
Duricef 1405
Ultracef Capsules, Tablets & Oral Suspension 722

Cefamandole Nafate (Increased nephrotoxicity). Products include:
Mandol Vials, Faspak & ADD-Vantage 1281

Cefazolin Sodium (Increased nephrotoxicity). Products include:
Ancef Injection 2194
Kefzol Vials, Faspak & ADD-Vantage 1279

Cefixime (Increased nephrotoxicity). Products include:
Suprax 1235

Cefmetazole Sodium (Increased nephrotoxicity). Products include:
Zefazone Sterile Powder 2372

Cefonicid Sodium (Increased nephrotoxicity). Products include:
Monocid Injection 2217

Cefoperazone Sodium (Increased nephrotoxicity). Products include:
Cefobid Intravenous/Intramuscular 1943
Cefobid Pharmacy Bulk Package - Not for Direct Infusion 1945

Ceforanide (Increased nephrotoxicity).
No products indexed under this heading.

Cefotaxime Sodium (Increased nephrotoxicity). Products include:
Claforan Sterile Injection 1089

Cefotetan (Increased nephrotoxicity). Products include:
Cefotan 2265

Cefoxitin Sodium (Increased nephrotoxicity). Products include:
Mefoxin 1498
Mefoxin Premixed Intravenous Solution 1500

Ceftazidime (Increased nephrotoxicity). Products include:
Ceptaz for Injection 1057
Fortaz 1060
Tazicef for Injection 2231
Tazidime Vials, Faspak & ADD-Vantage 1299

Ceftizoxime Sodium (Increased nephrotoxicity). Products include:
Cefizox Injection 1012

Ceftriaxone Sodium (Increased nephrotoxicity). Products include:
Rocephin Injectable Vials, ADD-Vantage 1914

Cefuroxime Axetil (Increased nephrotoxicity). Products include:
Ceftin Tablets 575

Cefuroxime Sodium (Increased nephrotoxicity). Products include:
Kefurox Vials, Faspak & ADD-Vantage 1277
Zinacef 1066

Cephalexin (Increased nephrotoxicity). Products include:
Keflex Pulvules, Oral Suspension & Pediatric Drops 916

Cephalothin Sodium (Increased nephrotoxicity).

Cephapirin Sodium (Increased nephrotoxicity).
No products indexed under this heading.

Cephradine (Increased nephrotoxicity). Products include:
Velosef Capsules and for Oral Suspension 606

Cisplatin (Increased nephrotoxicity). Products include:
Platinol 737
Platinol-AQ Injection 738

Colistin Sulfate (Increased nephrotoxicity). Products include:
Coly-Mycin S For Oral Suspension 1708
Coly-Mycin S Otic w/Neomycin & Hydrocortisone 1708

Decamethonium (Enhanced neuromuscular blockade and respiratory paralysis).

Ethacrynic Acid (Increased ototoxicity). Products include:
Edecrin Tablets 1468

Furosemide (Increased ototoxicity). Products include:
Lasix 1093

Kanamycin Sulfate (Increased nephrotoxicity). Products include:
Kantrex Injection 601
Kantrex Pediatric Injection 601

Metocurine Iodide (Enhanced neuromuscular blockade and respiratory paralysis). Products include:
Metubine Iodide Vials 1285

Neomycin Sulfate (Increased nephrotoxicity). Products include:
AK-Spore H.C. ⊙ 206
AK-Spore ⊙ 205
AK-Trol Ointment & Suspension ⊙ 207
Bactine First Aid Antibiotic Ointment ▣ 625
Campho-Phenique Triple Antibiotic Ointment Plus Pain Reliever ▣ 758
Coly-Mycin S Otic w/Neomycin & Hydrocortisone 1708
Cortisporin Cream 757
Cortisporin Ointment 758
Cortisporin Ophthalmic Ointment Sterile 758
Cortisporin Ophthalmic Suspension Sterile 759
Cortisporin Otic Solution Sterile 760
Cortisporin Otic Suspension Sterile 760
Dexacidin ⊙ 272
Lanabiotic Ointment ▣ 556
LazerSporin-C Solution 1770
Maxitrol Ophthalmic Ointment/Suspension ⊙ 223
Myciguent Antibiotic Ointment ▣ 737
Mycitracin ▣ 737
NeoDecadron Sterile Ophthalmic Ointment 1517
NeoDecadron Sterile Ophthalmic Solution 1518
NeoDecadron Topical Cream 1518
Neosporin Cream 792
Neosporin G.U. Irrigant Sterile 793
Neosporin Ointment 793
Maximum Strength Neosporin Ointment 793
Neosporin Ophthalmic Ointment Sterile 793
Neosporin Ophthalmic Solution Sterile 794
Neo-Synalar Cream 2296
PediOtic Suspension Sterile 797
Poly-Pred Liquifilm ⊙ 250

Pancuronium Bromide Injection (Enhanced neuromuscular blockade and respiratory paralysis).
No products indexed under this heading.

Paromomycin Sulfate (Increased nephrotoxicity). Products include:
Humatin Capsules 1726

Polymyxin B Sulfate (Increased nephrotoxicity). Products include:
AK-Poly-Bac Ointment ⊙ 205
AK-Spore H.C. ⊙ 206
AK-Spore ⊙ 205
AK-Trol Ointment & Suspension ⊙ 207
Aquaphor Antibiotic Formula 662
Bactine First Aid Antibiotic Ointment ▣ 625
Campho-Phenique Triple Antibiotic Ointment Plus Pain Reliever ▣ 758
Cortisporin Cream 757
Cortisporin Ointment 758
Cortisporin Ophthalmic Ointment Sterile 758
Cortisporin Ophthalmic Suspension Sterile 759
Cortisporin Otic Solution Sterile 760
Cortisporin Otic Suspension Sterile 760
Dexacidin ⊙ 272
Lanabiotic Ointment ▣ 556
LazerSporin-C Solution 1770
Maxitrol Ophthalmic Ointment/Suspension ⊙ 223
Mycitracin ▣ 737
Neosporin Cream 792
Neosporin G.U. Irrigant Sterile 793
Neosporin Ointment 793
Maximum Strength Neosporin Ointment 793
Neosporin Ophthalmic Ointment Sterile 793
Neosporin Ophthalmic Solution Sterile 794
Ophthocort ⊙ 301
PediOtic Suspension Sterile 797
Polymyxin B Sulfate, Aerosporin Brand Sterile Powder 798
Poly-Pred Liquifilm ⊙ 250
Polysporin Ointment ▣ 543
Polysporin Ophthalmic Ointment Sterile 798
Polysporin Powder ▣ 543
Polysporin Spray ▣ 543
Polytrim Ophthalmic Solution Sterile 588
Terramycin with Polymyxin B Sulfate Ophthalmic Ointment 1965

Streptomycin Sulfate (Increased nephrotoxicity).
No products indexed under this heading.

Succinylcholine Chloride (Enhanced neuromuscular blockade and respiratory paralysis). Products include:
Anectine 755

Tobramycin Sulfate (Increased nephrotoxicity). Products include:
Nebcin Vials, Hyporets & ADD-Vantage 1286

Vancomycin Hydrochloride (Increased nephrotoxicity). Products include:
Vancocin HCl, Oral Solution & Pulvules 1304
Vancocin HCl, Vials & ADD-Vantage 1302

Vecuronium Bromide (Enhanced neuromuscular blockade and respiratory paralysis). Products include:
Norcuron 1642

Viomycin (Increased nephrotoxicity).

GARAMYCIN OPHTHALMIC OINTMENT—STERILE
(Gentamicin Sulfate) ⊙ 305
No interactions described in labeling.

GARAMYCIN OPHTHALMIC SOLUTION—STERILE
(Gentamicin Sulfate) ⊙ 305
No interactions described in labeling.

GASTROCROM CAPSULES
(Cromolyn Sodium) 974
May interact with:

Isoproterenol Hydrochloride (Concurrent use at extremely high doses of both drugs appears to have increased resorptions and malformations in animal studies). Products include:
Isuprel Hydrochloride Injection 1:5000 2050
Isuprel Hydrochloride Mistometer 2051
Isuprel Hydrochloride Solution 1:200 & 1:100 2052
Norisodrine Aerotrol 540

GAS-X TABLETS
(Simethicone) ▣ 687
No interactions described in labeling.

EXTRA STRENGTH GAS-X TABLETS
(Simethicone) ▣ 687
No interactions described in labeling.

GAVISCON ANTACID TABLETS
(Aluminum Hydroxide Gel, Dried, Magnesium Trisilicate) ▣ 593
May interact with tetracyclines. Compounds in this category include:

Demeclocycline Hydrochloride (Gaviscon contraindicated). Products include:
Declomycin Capsules, Tablets 1199

Doxycycline Calcium (Gaviscon contraindicated).
No products indexed under this heading.

Doxycycline Hyclate (Gaviscon contraindicated). Products include:
Doryx Capsules 1717
Vibramycin Hyclate Capsules 1787
Vibramycin Hyclate Intravenous 1968
Vibra-Tabs Film Coated Tablets 1787

Doxycycline Monohydrate (Gaviscon contraindicated). Products include:
Monodox Capsules 1630
Vibramycin Monohydrate for Oral Suspension 1787

Methacycline Hydrochloride (Gaviscon contraindicated).
No products indexed under this heading.

Minocycline Hydrochloride (Gaviscon contraindicated). Products include:
- Minocin Intravenous ... 1221
- Minocin Oral Suspension ... 1224
- Minocin Pellet-Filled Capsules ... 1222

Oxytetracycline (Gaviscon contraindicated). Products include:
- Terramycin Intramuscular Solution 1964
- Urobiotic-250 Capsules ... 1968

Oxytetracycline Hydrochloride (Gaviscon contraindicated). Products include:
- Terra-Cortril Ophthalmic Suspension ... 1963
- Terramycin Capsules ... 1786
- Terramycin Intramuscular Solution 1964
- Terramycin with Polymyxin B Sulfate Ophthalmic Ointment ... 1965

Tetracycline Hydrochloride (Gaviscon contraindicated). Products include:
- Achromycin V Capsules ... 1193
- Achromycin Ophthalmic Ointment 1% ... ⊙ 307
- Achromycin Ophthalmic Suspension 1% ... ⊙ 308
- Topicycline for Topical Solution ... 1856

GAVISCON-2 ANTACID TABLETS

(Aluminum Hydroxide Gel, Dried, Magnesium Trisilicate) ... ⊡ 594
May interact with tetracyclines. Compounds in this category include:

Demeclocycline Hydrochloride (Concurrent oral use not recommended). Products include:
- Declomycin Capsules, Tablets ... 1199

Doxycycline Calcium (Concurrent oral use not recommended).
- No products indexed under this heading.

Doxycycline Hyclate (Concurrent oral use not recommended). Products include:
- Doryx Capsules ... 1717
- Vibramycin Hyclate Capsules ... 1787
- Vibramycin Hyclate Intravenous ... 1968
- Vibra-Tabs Film Coated Tablets ... 1787

Doxycycline Monohydrate (Concurrent oral use not recommended). Products include:
- Monodox Capsules ... 1630
- Vibramycin Monohydrate for Oral Suspension ... 1787

Methacycline Hydrochloride (Concurrent oral use not recommended).
- No products indexed under this heading.

Minocycline Hydrochloride (Concurrent oral use not recommended). Products include:
- Minocin Intravenous ... 1221
- Minocin Oral Suspension ... 1224
- Minocin Pellet-Filled Capsules ... 1222

Oxytetracycline Hydrochloride (Concurrent oral use not recommended). Products include:
- Terra-Cortril Ophthalmic Suspension ... 1963
- Terramycin Capsules ... 1786
- Terramycin Intramuscular Solution 1964
- Terramycin with Polymyxin B Sulfate Ophthalmic Ointment ... 1965

Tetracycline Hydrochloride (Concurrent oral use not recommended). Products include:
- Achromycin V Capsules ... 1193
- Achromycin Ophthalmic Ointment 1% ... ⊙ 307
- Achromycin Ophthalmic Suspension 1% ... ⊙ 308
- Topicycline for Topical Solution ... 1856

GAVISCON EXTRA STRENGTH RELIEF FORMULA LIQUID ANTACID

(Aluminum Hydroxide, Magnesium Carbonate) ... ⊡ 594
May interact with tetracyclines. Compounds in this category include:

Demeclocycline Hydrochloride (Concurrent oral administration is not recommended). Products include:
- Declomycin Capsules, Tablets ... 1199

Doxycycline Calcium (Concurrent oral administration is not recommended).
- No products indexed under this heading.

Doxycycline Hyclate (Concurrent oral administration is not recommended). Products include:
- Doryx Capsules ... 1717
- Vibramycin Hyclate Capsules ... 1787
- Vibramycin Hyclate Intravenous ... 1968
- Vibra-Tabs Film Coated Tablets ... 1787

Doxycycline Monohydrate (Concurrent oral administration is not recommended). Products include:
- Monodox Capsules ... 1630
- Vibramycin Monohydrate for Oral Suspension ... 1787

Methacycline Hydrochloride (Concurrent oral administration is not recommended).
- No products indexed under this heading.

Minocycline Hydrochloride (Concurrent oral administration is not recommended). Products include:
- Minocin Intravenous ... 1221
- Minocin Oral Suspension ... 1224
- Minocin Pellet-Filled Capsules ... 1222

Oxytetracycline Hydrochloride (Concurrent oral administration is not recommended). Products include:
- Terra-Cortril Ophthalmic Suspension ... 1963
- Terramycin Capsules ... 1786
- Terramycin Intramuscular Solution 1964
- Terramycin with Polymyxin B Sulfate Ophthalmic Ointment ... 1965

Tetracycline Hydrochloride (Concurrent oral administration is not recommended). Products include:
- Achromycin V Capsules ... 1193
- Achromycin Ophthalmic Ointment 1% ... ⊙ 307
- Achromycin Ophthalmic Suspension 1% ... ⊙ 308
- Topicycline for Topical Solution ... 1856

GAVISCON EXTRA STRENGTH RELIEF FORMULA ANTACID TABLETS

(Aluminum Hydroxide, Magnesium Carbonate) ... ⊡ 594
May interact with tetracyclines. Compounds in this category include:

Demeclocycline Hydrochloride (Concurrent administration is not recommended). Products include:
- Declomycin Capsules, Tablets ... 1199

Doxycycline Calcium (Concurrent administration is not recommended).
- No products indexed under this heading.

Doxycycline Hyclate (Concurrent administration is not recommended). Products include:
- Doryx Capsules ... 1717
- Vibramycin Hyclate Capsules ... 1787
- Vibramycin Hyclate Intravenous ... 1968
- Vibra-Tabs Film Coated Tablets ... 1787

Doxycycline Monohydrate (Concurrent oral administration is not recommended). Products include:
- Monodox Capsules ... 1630
- Vibramycin Monohydrate for Oral Suspension ... 1787

Methacycline Hydrochloride (Concurrent administration is not recommended).
- No products indexed under this heading.

Minocycline Hydrochloride (Concurrent administration is not recommended). Products include:
- Minocin Intravenous ... 1221
- Minocin Oral Suspension ... 1224
- Minocin Pellet-Filled Capsules ... 1222

Oxytetracycline Hydrochloride (Concurrent administration is not recommended). Products include:
- Terra-Cortril Ophthalmic Suspension ... 1963
- Terramycin Capsules ... 1786
- Terramycin Intramuscular Solution 1964
- Terramycin with Polymyxin B Sulfate Ophthalmic Ointment ... 1965

Tetracycline Hydrochloride (Concurrent administration is not recommended). Products include:
- Achromycin V Capsules ... 1193
- Achromycin Ophthalmic Ointment 1% ... ⊙ 307
- Achromycin Ophthalmic Suspension 1% ... ⊙ 308
- Topicycline for Topical Solution ... 1856

GAVISCON LIQUID ANTACID

(Aluminum Hydroxide, Magnesium Carbonate) ... ⊡ 594
May interact with tetracyclines. Compounds in this category include:

Demeclocycline Hydrochloride (Gaviscon contraindicated). Products include:
- Declomycin Capsules, Tablets ... 1199

Doxycycline Calcium (Gaviscon contraindicated).
- No products indexed under this heading.

Doxycycline Hyclate (Gaviscon contraindicated). Products include:
- Doryx Capsules ... 1717
- Vibramycin Hyclate Capsules ... 1787
- Vibramycin Hyclate Intravenous ... 1968
- Vibra-Tabs Film Coated Tablets ... 1787

Doxycycline Monohydrate (Gaviscon contraindicated). Products include:
- Monodox Capsules ... 1630
- Vibramycin Monohydrate for Oral Suspension ... 1787

Methacycline Hydrochloride (Gaviscon contraindicated).
- No products indexed under this heading.

Minocycline Hydrochloride (Gaviscon contraindicated). Products include:
- Minocin Intravenous ... 1221
- Minocin Oral Suspension ... 1224
- Minocin Pellet-Filled Capsules ... 1222

Oxytetracycline (Gaviscon contraindicated). Products include:
- Terramycin Intramuscular Solution 1964
- Urobiotic-250 Capsules ... 1968

Oxytetracycline Hydrochloride (Gaviscon contraindicated). Products include:
- Terra-Cortril Ophthalmic Suspension ... 1963
- Terramycin Capsules ... 1786
- Terramycin Intramuscular Solution 1964
- Terramycin with Polymyxin B Sulfate Ophthalmic Ointment ... 1965

Tetracycline Hydrochloride (Gaviscon contraindicated). Products include:
- Achromycin V Capsules ... 1193
- Achromycin Ophthalmic Ointment 1% ... ⊙ 307
- Achromycin Ophthalmic Suspension 1% ... ⊙ 308
- Topicycline for Topical Solution ... 1856

GELFOAM STERILE SPONGE

(Gelatin Preparations) ... 2338
No interactions described in labeling.

GELUSIL LIQUID & TABLETS

(Aluminum Hydroxide, Magnesium Hydroxide, Simethicone) ... ⊡ 639
May interact with tetracyclines. Compounds in this category include:

Demeclocycline Hydrochloride (Do not use concomitantly). Products include:
- Declomycin Capsules, Tablets ... 1199

Doxycycline Calcium (Do not use concomitantly).
- No products indexed under this heading.

Doxycycline Hyclate (Do not use concomitantly). Products include:
- Doryx Capsules ... 1717
- Vibramycin Hyclate Capsules ... 1787
- Vibramycin Hyclate Intravenous ... 1968
- Vibra-Tabs Film Coated Tablets ... 1787

Doxycycline Monohydrate (Do not use concomitantly). Products include:
- Monodox Capsules ... 1630
- Vibramycin Monohydrate for Oral Suspension ... 1787

Methacycline Hydrochloride (Do not use concomitantly).
- No products indexed under this heading.

Minocycline Hydrochloride (Do not use concomitantly). Products include:
- Minocin Intravenous ... 1221
- Minocin Oral Suspension ... 1224
- Minocin Pellet-Filled Capsules ... 1222

Oxytetracycline Hydrochloride (Do not use concomitantly). Products include:
- Terra-Cortril Ophthalmic Suspension ... 1963
- Terramycin Capsules ... 1786
- Terramycin Intramuscular Solution 1964
- Terramycin with Polymyxin B Sulfate Ophthalmic Ointment ... 1965

Tetracycline Hydrochloride (Do not use concomitantly). Products include:
- Achromycin V Capsules ... 1193
- Achromycin Ophthalmic Ointment 1% ... ⊙ 307
- Achromycin Ophthalmic Suspension 1% ... ⊙ 308
- Topicycline for Topical Solution ... 1856

GENOPTIC LIQUIFILM STERILE OPHTHALMIC SOLUTION

(Gentamicin Sulfate) ... ⊙ 247
No interactions described in labeling.

GENOPTIC S.O.P. STERILE OPHTHALMIC OINTMENT

(Gentamicin Sulfate) ... ⊙ 247
No interactions described in labeling.

GENTACIDIN OINTMENT

(Gentamicin Sulfate) ... ⊙ 273
No interactions described in labeling.

GENTACIDIN SOLUTION

(Gentamicin Sulfate) ... ⊙ 273
No interactions described in labeling.

GENTAK OINTMENT & SOLUTION

(Gentamicin Sulfate) ... ⊙ 208
No interactions described in labeling.

GENTLE NATURE NATURAL VEGETABLE LAXATIVE
(Sennosides (A & B)) ■D 687
No interactions described in labeling.

GEOCILLIN TABLETS
(Carbenicillin Indanyl Sodium) 1951
May interact with:

Probenecid (Geocillin blood levels may be increased and prolonged). Products include:
- Benemid Tablets 1426
- ColBENEMID Tablets 1436
- Wycillin Injection and Probenecid Tablets 2539

GEREF (SERMORELIN ACETATE FOR INJECTION)
(Sermorelin Acetate) 2560
May interact with drugs directly affecting the pituitary secretion of somatotropin, cyclooxygenase inhibitors, antimuscarinic drugs, antithyroid agents, and certain other agents. Compounds in these categories include:

Aspirin (The Geref test should not be conducted in the presence of this drug). Products include:
- Alka-Seltzer Effervescent Antacid and Pain Reliever 1568
- Alka-Seltzer Extra Strength Effervescent Antacid and Pain Reliever 1570
- Alka-Seltzer (Flavored) Effervescent Antacid and Pain Reliever 1569
- Alka-Seltzer Plus Cold Medicine ■D 623
- Alka-Seltzer Plus Night-Time Cold Medicine ■D 623
- Alka Seltzer Plus Sinus Allergy Medicine ■D 624
- Anacin Coated Analgesic Caplets 2417
- Anacin Coated Analgesic Tablets 2417
- Anacin Maximum Strength Analgesic Coated Tablets 2417
- Maximum Strength Arthritis Pain Formula By the Makers of Anacin Analgesic Tablets and Caplets 2418
- Arthritis Pain Formula by the Makers of Anacin Analgesic Tablets and Caplets ■D 747
- Arthritis Strength BC Powder ■D 516
- Ascriptin A/D Caplets 1850
- Regular Strength Ascriptin Tablets 1850
- Azdōne Tablets 844
- BC Powder ■D 517
- BC Cold Powder ■D 517
- Children's Bayer Chewable Aspirin ■D 564
- Genuine Bayer Aspirin Tablets & Caplets ■D 564
- Maximum Bayer Aspirin Tablets & Caplets ■D 566
- Bayer Plus Aspirin Tablets ■D 567
- Therapy Bayer Aspirin Caplets ■D 568
- 8 Hour Bayer Timed-Release Aspirin ■D 566
- Arthritis Strength Bufferin Analgesic Caplets 744
- Extra Strength Bufferin Analgesic Tablets 745
- Bufferin Analgesic Tablets and Caplets 743
- Cama Arthritis Pain Reliever ■D 685
- Damason-P 1356
- Easprin 1719
- Ecotrin Enteric Coated Aspirin Maximum Strength Tablets and Caplets 2189
- Ecotrin Enteric Coated Aspirin Regular Strength Tablets and Caplets 2189
- Empirin Aspirin ■D 541
- Empirin with Codeine Phosphate Nos. 2, 3 & 4 764
- Equagesic Tablets 2451
- Excedrin Extra-Strength Analgesic Tablets & Caplets 749
- 4-Way Cold Tablets 750
- Fiorinal Capsules 2007
- Fiorinal with Codeine Capsules 2008
- Fiorinal Tablets 2007
- Lortab ASA Tablets 2414
- Momentum Muscular Backache Formula ■D 751
- Norgesic 1314
- Norwich Extra-Strength Aspirin ■D 546
- Norwich Regular Strength Aspirin ■D 547
- P-A-C Analgesic Tablets ■D 669
- Percodan 951
- Robaxisal Tablets 1872
- Sine-Off Sinus Medicine Tablets-Aspirin Formula ■D 722
- Soma Compound w/Codeine Tablets 2390
- Soma Compound Tablets 2389
- St. Joseph Adult Chewable Aspirin (81 mg.) ■D 703
- Synalgos-DC Capsules 2525
- Talwin Compound 2072
- Ursinus Inlay-Tabs ■D 691
- Vanquish Analgesic Caplets ■D 574
- Zorprin Tablets 698

Atropine Sulfate (Response to Geref may be blunted). Products include:
- Arco-Lase Plus Tablets 607
- Atropine Sulfate Sterile Ophthalmic Solution and S.O.P. Sterile Ophthalmic Ointment ⊙ 239
- Donnagel ■D 675
- Donnagel-PG 1858
- Donnatal 1858
- Donnatal Extentabs 1859
- Donnatal Tablets 1858
- Donnazyme Tablets 1860
- Isopto Atropine ⊙ 218
- Lomotil 2174
- Motofen Tablets 836
- Ru-Tuss Tablets 693
- Urised Tablets 2396

Belladonna Alkaloids (Response to Geref may be blunted). Products include:
- Bellergal-S Tablets 1998
- Hyland's Bed Wetting Tablets ■D 728
- Hyland's Teething Tablets ■D 728
- Kinesed Tablets 2272

Betamethasone Acetate (The Geref test should not be conducted in the presence of this drug). Products include:
- Celestone Soluspan Suspension 2081

Betamethasone Sodium Phosphate (The Geref test should not be conducted in the presence of this drug). Products include:
- Celestone Soluspan Suspension 2081

Clidinium Bromide (Response to Geref may be blunted). Products include:
- Librax Capsules 1929
- Quarzan Capsules 1937

Cortisone Acetate (The Geref test should not be conducted in the presence of this drug). Products include:
- Cortone Acetate Sterile Suspension 1437
- Cortone Acetate Tablets 1439

Dexamethasone (The Geref test should not be conducted in the presence of this drug). Products include:
- AK-Trol Ointment & Suspension ⊙ 207
- Decadron Elixir 1445
- Decadron Tablets 1447
- Decaspray Topical Aerosol 1459
- Dexacidin ⊙ 272
- Maxidex Sterile Ophthalmic Suspension ⊙ 223
- Maxitrol Ophthalmic Ointment/Suspension ⊙ 223
- TobraDex Ophthalmic Suspension and Ointment ⊙ 228

Dexamethasone Acetate (The Geref test should not be conducted in the presence of this drug). Products include:
- Dalalone D.P. Injectable 999
- Decadron-LA Sterile Suspension 1457

Dexamethasone Sodium Phosphate (The Geref test should not be conducted in the presence of this drug). Products include:
- AK-Dex ⊙ 203
- Decadron Phosphate Respihaler 1454
- Decadron Phosphate Sterile Ophthalmic Ointment 1453
- Decadron Phosphate Sterile Ophthalmic Solution 1453
- Decadron Phosphate Topical Cream 1455
- Decadron Phosphate Turbinaire 1456
- Maxidex Sterile Ophthalmic Ointment ⊙ 222
- NeoDecadron Sterile Ophthalmic Ointment 1517
- NeoDecadron Sterile Ophthalmic Solution 1518
- NeoDecadron Topical Cream 1518

Dicyclomine Hydrochloride (Response to Geref may be blunted). Products include:
- Bentyl 1322

Glycopyrrolate (Response to Geref may be blunted). Products include:
- Robinul Forte Tablets 1873
- Robinul Injectable 1873
- Robinul Tablets 1873

Hydrocortisone (The Geref test should not be conducted in the presence of this drug). Products include:
- AK-Spore H.C. ⊙ 206
- Bactine Hydrocortisone Anti-Itch Cream ■D 625
- CaldeCORT Anti-Itch Hydrocortisone Spray ■D 560
- Carmol HC Cream 1% 2296
- Cortaid Spray ■D 735
- Cortenema 2244
- Cortisporin Ointment 758
- Cortisporin Ophthalmic Ointment Sterile 758
- Cortisporin Ophthalmic Suspension Sterile 759
- Cortisporin Otic Solution Sterile 760
- Cortisporin Otic Suspension Sterile 760
- Cortizone-5 Creme & Ointment ■D 732
- Dermolate Anti-Itch Cream ■D 697
- Eldecort Cream 1.0% 1113
- Eldecort Cream 1.0% and 2.5% 1113
- Fungoid HC Creme 1770
- Hydrocortone Tablets 1482
- Hytone 909
- LazerSporin-C Solution 1770
- Massengill Medicated Soft Cloth Towelettes 2192
- Nutracort Cream & Lotion 1684
- PediOtic Suspension Sterile 797
- Synacort Creams 1%, 2.5% 2296
- Vanoxide-HC Acne Lotion 911
- Vioform-Hydrocortisone Cream and Mild Cream 889
- Vioform-Hydrocortisone Ointment 889
- VōSoL HC Otic Solution 2392
- Vytone Cream 1% 911

Hydrocortisone Acetate (The Geref test should not be conducted in the presence of this drug). Products include:
- Analpram-HC Rectal Cream 1% and 2.5% 970
- Anusol-HC Cream 1690
- Anusol-HC Suppositories 1691
- Caldecort ■D 560
- Carmol HC Cream 1% 2296
- Chloromycetin Hydrocortisone Ophthalmic 1694
- Coly-Mycin S Otic w/Neomycin & Hydrocortisone 1708
- Cortaid ■D 735
- Cortef Feminine Itch Cream ■D 735
- Corticaine ■D 682
- Cortifoam 1827
- Cortisporin Cream 757
- Epifoam 1828
- Gynecort 5 Creme ■D 556
- Hydrocortone Acetate Sterile Suspension 1479
- Lanacort 5 Creme and Ointment ■D 557
- Mantadil Cream 789
- Ophthocort ⊙ 301
- Orabase HCA Oral Paste 890
- Pramosone Cream, Lotion & Ointment 971
- ProctoCream-HC 1834
- Proctofoam-HC 1835

Hydrocortisone Sodium Phosphate (The Geref test should not be conducted in the presence of this drug). Products include:
- Hydrocortone Phosphate Injection, Sterile 1481

Hydrocortisone Sodium Succinate (The Geref test should not be conducted in the presence of this drug). Products include:
- Solu-Cortef Sterile Powder 2361

Hyoscyamine (Response to Geref may be blunted). Products include:
- Cystospaz Tablets 2395
- Urised Tablets 2396

Hyoscyamine Sulfate (Response to Geref may be blunted). Products include:
- Arco-Lase Plus Tablets 607
- Cystospaz-M Capsules 2395
- Donnagel ■D 675
- Donnagel-PG 1858
- Donnatal 1858
- Donnatal Extentabs 1859
- Donnatal Tablets 1858
- Donnazyme Tablets 1860
- Kutrase Capsules 2146
- Levsin/Levsinex 2147
- Ru-Tuss Tablets 693

Indomethacin (The Geref test should not be conducted in the presence of this drug). Products include:
- Indocin 1487

Indomethacin Sodium Trihydrate (The Geref test should not be conducted in the presence of this drug). Products include:
- Indocin I.V. 1490

Insulin, Human (The Geref test should not be conducted in the presence of this drug).
- No products indexed under this heading.

Insulin, Human Isophane Suspension (The Geref test should not be conducted in the presence of this drug). Products include:
- Humulin N, 100 Units 1270

Insulin, Human NPH (The Geref test should not be conducted in the presence of this drug). Products include:
- Insulatard NPH Human 1627
- Novolin N 1627
- Novolin N PenFill Cartridges 1628
- Novolin N Prefilled 1628

Insulin, Human Regular (The Geref test should not be conducted in the presence of this drug). Products include:
- Humulin BR, 100 Units 1268
- Humulin R, 100 Units 1272
- Novolin R 1627
- Novolin R PenFill Cartridges 1628
- Novolin R Prefilled 1629
- Velosulin Human 1628

Insulin, Human, Zinc Suspension (The Geref test should not be conducted in the presence of this drug). Products include:
- Humulin L, 100 Units 1268
- Humulin U, 100 Units 1272
- Novolin L 1627

Insulin, NPH (The Geref test should not be conducted in the presence of this drug). Products include:
- NPH, 40 & 100 Units 1273
- Beef NPH, 100 Units 1274
- Pork NPH, 100 Units 1275
- Insulatard NPH 1626
- NPH Insulin 1626
- NPH Purified Pork Isophane Insulin 1626

Insulin, Regular (The Geref test should not be conducted in the presence of this drug). Products include:
- Regular, 40 & 100 Units 1273
- Beef Regular, 100 Units 1275
- Pork Regular, 100 Units 1275
- Pork Regular (Concentrated), 500 Units 1276
- Regular Insulin 1625
- Regular Purified Pork Insulin 1626
- Velosulin 1627

Insulin, Zinc Crystals (The Geref test should not be conducted in the presence of this drug). Products include:
NPH, 40 & 100 Units ... 1273
Insulin, Zinc Suspension (The Geref test should not be conducted in the presence of this drug). Products include:
Lente, 40 & 100 Units ... 1272
Protamine, Zinc, 40 & 100 Units ... 1273
Lente Iletin I ... 1272
Beef Lente, 100 Units ... 1274
Beef Protamine Zinc, 100 Units ... 1274
Pork Lente, 100 Units ... 1275
Pork, Protamine, Zinc, 100 Units ... 1275
Lente Insulin ... 1626
Lente Purified Pork Insulin ... 1626
Semilente Insulin ... 1625
Ultralente Insulin ... 1626
Ipratropium Bromide (Response to Geref may be blunted). Products include:
Atrovent Inhalation Aerosol ... 675
Levodopa (Somatropin levels may be transiently elevated by levodopa). Products include:
Larodopa Tablets ... 1905
Sinemet Tablets ... 952
Sinemet CR Tablets ... 953
Mepenzolate Bromide (Response to Geref may be blunted). Products include:
Cantil Tablets ... 1326
Methimazole (Response to Geref may be blunted). Products include:
Tapazole Tablets ... 1298
Methylprednisolone Acetate (The Geref test should not be conducted in the presence of this drug). Products include:
Depo-Medrol Sterile Aqueous Suspension ... 2334
Methylprednisolone Sodium Succinate (The Geref test should not be conducted in the presence of this drug). Products include:
Solu-Medrol Sterile Powder ... 2363
Oxyphenonium Bromide (Response to Geref may be blunted).
Prednisolone Acetate (The Geref test should not be conducted in the presence of this drug). Products include:
AK-Cide Sterile Ophthalmic Ointment & Suspension ... ⊙ 202
Blephamide Liquifilm Sterile Ophthalmic Suspension ... 586
Blephamide S.O.P. Sterile Ophthalmic Ointment ... 586
Cetapred Ointment ... ⊙ 220
⅛% Econopred & 1% Econopred Plus ... ⊙ 217
Isopto Cetapred Suspension ... ⊙ 220
Metimyd ... ⊙ 306
Poly-Pred Liquifilm ... ⊙ 250
Pred Forte ... ⊙ 252
Pred Mild ... ⊙ 254
Pred-G Liquifilm Sterile Ophthalmic Suspension ... ⊙ 252
Pred-G S.O.P. Sterile Ophthalmic Ointment ... ⊙ 253
Vasocidin Ointment ... ⊙ 275
Prednisolone Sodium Phosphate (The Geref test should not be conducted in the presence of this drug). Products include:
AK-Pred ... ⊙ 205
Hydeltrasol Injection, Sterile ... 1476
Inflamase ... ⊙ 274
Pediapred Oral Liquid ... 987
Vasocidin Ophthalmic Solution ... ⊙ 276
Prednisolone Tebutate (The Geref test should not be conducted in the presence of this drug). Products include:
Hydeltra-T.B.A. Sterile Suspension 1478
Prednisone (The Geref test should not be conducted in the presence of this drug). Products include:
Deltasone Tablets ... 2332
Propantheline Bromide (Response to Geref may be blunted). Products include:
Pro-Banthīne Tablets ... 2141
Propylthiouracil (Response to Geref may be blunted).
No products indexed under this heading.
Scopolamine Hydrobromide (Response to Geref may be blunted). Products include:
Donnagel ... ▣ 675
Donnagel-PG ... 1858
Donnatal ... 1858
Donnatal Extentabs ... 1859
Donnatal Tablets ... 1858
Donnazyme Tablets ... 1860
Isopto Hyoscine ... ⊙ 222
Murocoll-2 Sterile Ophthalmic Solution ... ⊙ 261
Ru-Tuss Tablets ... 693
Scopolamine Preparations (Response to Geref may be blunted). Products include:
Transderm Scōp Transdermal Therapeutic System ... 887
Triamcinolone (The Geref test should not be conducted in the presence of this drug).
No products indexed under this heading.
Triamcinolone Acetonide (The Geref test should not be conducted in the presence of this drug). Products include:
Aristocort A ... 1010
Azmacort Inhaler ... 1837
Kenalog Cream, Lotion & Ointment 2401
Kenalog-10 Injection ... 2402
Kenalog-40 Injection ... 2403
Kenalog in Orabase ... 604
Kenalog Spray ... 2401
Mycolog II Cream and Ointment ... 2407
Mytrex Cream & Ointment ... 2080
Nasacort Nasal Inhaler ... 1844
Triamcinolone Diacetate (The Geref test should not be conducted in the presence of this drug). Products include:
Aristocort Suspension ... 1008
Triamcinolone Hexacetonide (The Geref test should not be conducted in the presence of this drug). Products include:
Aristospan Suspension ... 1011
Tridihexethyl Chloride (Response to Geref may be blunted).
No products indexed under this heading.

GERIMED TABLETS
(Vitamins with Minerals) ... 972
No interactions described in labeling.

GERIPLEX-FS KAPSEALS
(Vitamins with Minerals, Docusate Sodium) ... ▣ 639
No interactions described in labeling.

GERIPLEX-FS LIQUID
(Vitamins with Iron) ... ▣ 639
No interactions described in labeling.

GERITOL COMPLETE TABLETS
(Vitamins with Minerals) ... ▣ 717
May interact with:
Alcohol (Enhances iron absorption with the potential for iron overload).

GERITOL EXTEND TABLETS AND CAPLETS
(Vitamins, Multiple) ... ▣ 717
No interactions described in labeling.

GERITOL LIQUID-HIGH POTENCY IRON & VITAMIN TONIC
(Vitamins with Iron) ... ▣ 717
May interact with:
Alcohol (Accelerates absorption of ferric ion).

GEVRABON LIQUID
(Vitamins with Minerals) ... ▣ 587
No interactions described in labeling.

GEVRAL TABLETS
(Vitamins with Minerals) ... ▣ 588
No interactions described in labeling.

GEVRAL T TABLETS
(Vitamins with Minerals) ... ▣ 588
No interactions described in labeling.

GLANDOSANE SYNTHETIC SALIVA
(Carboxymethylcellulose Sodium) ... 2314
No interactions described in labeling.

GLAUCON
(Epinephrine Hydrochloride) ... ⊙ 218
No interactions described in labeling.

GLUCAGON FOR INJECTION VIALS AND EMERGENCY KIT
(Glucagon) ... 1263
No interactions described in labeling.

GLUCERNA SPECIALIZED NUTRITION WITH FIBER FOR PATIENTS WITH ABNORMAL GLUCOSE TOLERANCE
(Nutritional Supplement) ... 1971
No interactions described in labeling.

GLUCOTROL
(Glipizide) ... 1952
May interact with non-steroidal anti-inflammatory agents, salicylates, sulfonamides, oral anticoagulants, monoamine oxidase inhibitors, beta blockers, thiazides, diuretics, corticosteroids, phenothiazines, thyroid preparations, estrogens, sympathomimetic aerosol bronchodilators, calcium channel blockers, oral contraceptives, and certain other agents. Compounds in these categories include:

Acebutolol Hydrochloride (Increased hypoglycemic action). Products include:
Sectral Capsules ... 2520
Albuterol (Hyperglycemic effect). Products include:
Proventil Inhalation Aerosol ... 2117
Ventolin Inhalation Aerosol and Refill ... 583
Albuterol Sulfate (Hyperglycemic effect). Products include:
Proventil Repetabs Tablets ... 2120
Proventil Solutions for Inhalation 0.5% and 0.083% ... 2118
Proventil Syrup ... 2119
Proventil Tablets ... 2120
Ventolin ... 583
Amiloride Hydrochloride (Hyperglycemic effect). Products include:
Midamor Tablets ... 1508
Moduretic Tablets ... 1510
Aspirin (Increased hypoglycemic action). Products include:
Alka-Seltzer Effervescent Antacid and Pain Reliever ... 1568
Alka-Seltzer Extra Strength Effervescent Antacid and Pain Reliever ... 1570
Alka-Seltzer (Flavored) Effervescent Antacid and Pain Reliever ... 1569
Alka-Seltzer Plus Cold Medicine ... ▣ 623
Alka-Seltzer Plus Night-Time Cold Medicine ... ▣ 623
Alka Seltzer Plus Sinus Allergy Medicine ... ▣ 624
Anacin Coated Analgesic Caplets ... 2417
Anacin Coated Analgesic Tablets ... 2417
Anacin Maximum Strength Analgesic Coated Tablets ... 2417
Maximum Strength Arthritis Pain Formula By the Makers of Anacin Analgesic Tablets and Caplets ... 2418
Arthritis Pain Formula by the Makers of Anacin Analgesic Tablets and Caplets ... ▣ 747
Arthritis Strength BC Powder ... ▣ 516
Ascriptin A/D Caplets ... 1850
Regular Strength Ascriptin Tablets 1850
Azdōne Tablets ... 844
BC Powder ... ▣ 517
BC Cold Powder ... ▣ 517
Children's Bayer Chewable Aspirin ... ▣ 564
Genuine Bayer Aspirin Tablets & Caplets ... ▣ 564
Maximum Bayer Aspirin Tablets & Caplets ... ▣ 566
Bayer Plus Aspirin Tablets ... ▣ 567
Therapy Bayer Aspirin Caplets ... ▣ 568
8 Hour Bayer Timed-Release Aspirin ... ▣ 566
Arthritis Strength Bufferin Analgesic Caplets ... 744
Extra Strength Bufferin Analgesic Tablets ... 745
Bufferin Analgesic Tablets and Caplets ... 743
Cama Arthritis Pain Reliever ... ▣ 685
Damason-P ... 1356
Easprin ... 1719
Ecotrin Enteric Coated Aspirin Maximum Strength Tablets and Caplets ... 2189
Ecotrin Enteric Coated Aspirin Regular Strength Tablets and Caplets ... 2189
Empirin Aspirin ... ▣ 541
Empirin with Codeine Phosphate Nos. 2, 3 & 4 ... 764
Equagesic Tablets ... 2451
Excedrin Extra-Strength Analgesic Tablets & Caplets ... 749
4-Way Cold Tablets ... 750
Fiorinal Capsules ... 2007
Fiorinal with Codeine Capsules ... 2008
Fiorinal Tablets ... 2007
Lortab ASA Tablets ... 2414
Momentum Muscular Backache Formula ... ▣ 751
Norgesic ... 1314
Norwich Extra-Strength Aspirin ... ▣ 546
Norwich Regular Strength Aspirin ▣ 547
P-A-C Analgesic Tablets ... ▣ 669
Percodan ... 951
Robaxisal Tablets ... 1872
Sine-Off Sinus Medicine Tablets-Aspirin Formula ... ▣ 722
Soma Compound w/Codeine Tablets ... 2390
Soma Compound Tablets ... 2389
St. Joseph Adult Chewable Aspirin (81 mg.) ... ▣ 703
Synalgos-DC Capsules ... 2525
Talwin Compound ... 2072
Ursinus Inlay-Tabs ... ▣ 691
Vanquish Analgesic Caplets ... ▣ 574
Zorprin Tablets ... 698
Atenolol (Increased hypoglycemic action). Products include:
Tenoretic Tablets ... 1105
Tenormin Tablets and I.V. Injection 1107
Bendroflumethiazide (Hyperglycemic effect). Products include:
Corzide Tablets ... 702
Naturetin Tablets ... 1789
Rauzide Tablets ... 1804
Bepridil Hydrochloride (Hyperglycemic effect). Products include:
Vascor (200, 300 and 400 mg) Tablets ... 1383
Betamethasone Acetate (Hyperglycemic effect). Products include:
Celestone Soluspan Suspension ... 2081
Betamethasone Sodium Phosphate (Hyperglycemic effect). Products include:
Celestone Soluspan Suspension ... 2081

Betaxolol Hydrochloride (Increased hypoglycemic action). Products include:
- Betoptic Sterile Ophthalmic Solution ... 569
- Betoptic S Sterile Ophthalmic Suspension ... 570
- Kerlone Tablets ... 2172

Bumetanide (Hyperglycemic effect). Products include:
- Bumex ... 1895

Carteolol Hydrochloride (Increased hypoglycemic action). Products include:
- Cartrol Tablets ... 507

Chloramphenicol (Increased hypoglycemic action). Products include:
- AK-Chlor Sterile Ophthalmic Ointment & Solution ... ⊙ 201
- Chloromycetin Cream, 1% ... 1694
- Chloromycetin Hydrocortisone Ophthalmic ... 1694
- Chloromycetin Kapseals ... 1695
- Chloromycetin Ophthalmic Ointment, 1% ... 1696
- Chloromycetin Ophthalmic Solution ... 1696
- Chloromycetin Otic ... 1697
- Chloroptic S.O.P. ... ⊙ 243
- Chloroptic Sterile Ophthalmic Solution ... ⊙ 243
- Ophthochlor Ophthalmic Solution ... ⊙ 300
- Ophthocort ... ⊙ 301

Chloramphenicol Palmitate (Increased hypoglycemic action). Products include:
- Chloromycetin Palmitate, Oral Suspension ... 1697

Chloramphenicol Sodium Succinate (Increased hypoglycemic action). Products include:
- Chloromycetin Sodium Succinate ... 1698

Chlorothiazide (Hyperglycemic effect). Products include:
- Aldoclor Tablets ... 1413
- Diupres Tablets ... 1461
- Diuril Oral ... 1464

Chlorothiazide Sodium (Hyperglycemic effect). Products include:
- Diuril Sodium Intravenous ... 1463

Chlorotrianisene (Hyperglycemic effect). Products include:
- TACE 12 and 25 mg ... 1353

Chlorpromazine (Hyperglycemic effect). Products include:
- Thorazine ... 2234

Chlorpropamide (Increased hypoglycemic action). Products include:
- Diabinese Tablets ... 1775

Chlorthalidone (Hyperglycemic effect). Products include:
- Combipres Tablets ... 678
- Tenoretic Tablets ... 1105
- Thalitone Tablets ... 687

Choline Magnesium Trisalicylate (Increased hypoglycemic action). Products include:
- Trilisate ... 1822

Cortisone Acetate (Hyperglycemic effect). Products include:
- Cortone Acetate Sterile Suspension ... 1437
- Cortone Acetate Tablets ... 1439

Dexamethasone (Hyperglycemic effect). Products include:
- AK-Trol Ointment & Suspension ... ⊙ 207
- Decadron Elixir ... 1445
- Decadron Tablets ... 1447
- Decaspray Topical Aerosol ... 1459
- Dexacidin ... ⊙ 272
- Maxidex Sterile Ophthalmic Suspension ... ⊙ 223
- Maxitrol Ophthalmic Ointment/Suspension ... ⊙ 223
- TobraDex Ophthalmic Suspension and Ointment ... ⊙ 228

Dexamethasone Acetate (Hyperglycemic effect). Products include:
- Dalalone D.P. Injectable ... 999
- Decadron-LA Sterile Suspension ... 1457

Dexamethasone Sodium Phosphate (Hyperglycemic effect). Products include:
- AK-Dex ... ⊙ 203
- Decadron Phosphate Respihaler ... 1454
- Decadron Phosphate Sterile Ophthalmic Ointment ... 1453
- Decadron Phosphate Sterile Ophthalmic Solution ... 1453
- Decadron Phosphate Topical Cream ... 1455
- Decadron Phosphate Turbinaire ... 1456
- Maxidex Sterile Ophthalmic Ointment ... ⊙ 222
- NeoDecadron Sterile Ophthalmic Ointment ... 1517
- NeoDecadron Sterile Ophthalmic Solution ... 1518
- NeoDecadron Topical Cream ... 1518

Diclofenac Sodium (Increased hypoglycemic action). Products include:
- Voltaren Ophthalmic Sterile Ophthalmic Solution ... ⊙ 268
- Voltaren Tablets ... 1042

Dienestrol (Hyperglycemic effect). Products include:
- Ortho Dienestrol Cream ... 1664

Diethylstilbestrol (Hyperglycemic effect). Products include:
- Diethylstilbestrol Tablets ... 1258

Diflunisal (Increased hypoglycemic action). Products include:
- Dolobid Tablets ... 1465

Diltiazem Hydrochloride (Hyperglycemic effect). Products include:
- Cardizem Tablets-30 mg, 60 mg, 90 mg and 120 mg ... 1329
- Cardizem SR Capsules-60 mg, 90 mg and 120 mg ... 1327

Dobutamine Hydrochloride (Hyperglycemic effect). Products include:
- Dobutrex Solution Vials ... 1259

Dopamine Hydrochloride (Hyperglycemic effect). Products include:
- Intropin Injection ... 930

Ephedrine Hydrochloride (Hyperglycemic effect). Products include:
- Amesec ... ▣ 682
- Primatene Tablets-M Formula ... 2421
- Primatene Tablets-P Formula ... 2421
- Primatene Tablets-Regular Formula ... 2421
- Quadrinal Tablets ... 1183
- Quelidrine Syrup ... 556
- Tedral SA ... 1765

Ephedrine Sulfate (Hyperglycemic effect). Products include:
- Bronkaid Tablets ... ▣ 757
- Bronkolixir ... ▣ 761
- Bronkotabs Tablets ... ▣ 762
- Marax Tablets & DF Syrup ... 1954
- Pazo Hemorrhoid Ointment & Suppositories ... 752
- Vicks Vatronol Nose Drops ... ▣ 666

Ephedrine Tannate (Hyperglycemic effect). Products include:
- Rynatuss ... 2388

Epinephrine (Hyperglycemic effect). Products include:
- Ana-Kit Anaphylaxis Emergency Treatment Kit ... 1100
- Bronkaid Mist ... ▣ 757
- EpiPen ... 843
- Marcaine Hydrochloride 0.5% with Epinephrine 1:200,000 (as bitartrate) ... 958
- Marcaine Hydrochloride with Epinephrine 1:200,000 ... 2055
- Primatene Mist ... 2420
- Sus-Phrine Injection ... 1006
- Xylocaine with Epinephrine Injections ... 637

Epinephrine Bitartrate (Hyperglycemic effect). Products include:
- AsthmaHaler Mist Epinephrine Bitartrate Bronchodilator ... ▣ 616
- Bronkaid Mist Suspension ... ▣ 757
- Primatene Mist Suspension ... 2421

Epinephrine Hydrochloride (Hyperglycemic effect). Products include:
- Adrenalin Chloride Solution 1:100 & 1:1,000 ... 1689
- Epifrin ... ⊙ 244
- Glaucon ... ⊙ 218

Esmolol Hydrochloride (Increased hypoglycemic action). Products include:
- Brevibloc Injection ... 942

Estradiol (Hyperglycemic effect). Products include:
- Emcyt Capsules ... 1161
- Estrace ... 1385
- Estrace Vaginal Cream ... 1388
- Estraderm Transdermal System ... 866

Estrogens, Conjugated (Hyperglycemic effect). Products include:
- Mediatric Capsules ... 2476
- PMB 200 and PMB 400 ... 2504
- Premarin Intravenous ... 2508
- Premarin with Methyltestosterone ... 2515
- Premarin Tablets ... 2510
- Premarin Vaginal Cream ... 2512

Estrogens, Esterified (Hyperglycemic effect). Products include:
- Estratest ... 2245
- Menrium Tablets ... 1934

Estropipate (Hyperglycemic effect). Products include:
- Ogen ... 540

Ethacrynic Acid (Hyperglycemic effect). Products include:
- Edecrin Tablets ... 1468

Ethinyl Estradiol (Hyperglycemic effect). Products include:
- Brevicon ... 2304
- Demulen ... 2161
- Estinyl Tablets ... 2085
- Jenest-28 Tablets ... 1636
- Levlen/Tri-Levlen ... 665
- Lo/Ovral Tablets ... 2471
- Lo/Ovral-28 Tablets ... 2476
- Loestrin ... 1728
- Modicon ... 1667
- Nordette-21 Tablets ... 2481
- Nordette-28 Tablets ... 2483
- Norethin ... 2133
- Norinyl ... 2304
- Norlestrin ... 1746
- Ortho-Cyclen Tablets ... 1658
- Ortho-Novum ... 1667
- Ovcon ... 1391
- Ovral Tablets ... 2490
- Ovral-28 Tablets ... 2491
- Levlen/Tri-Levlen ... 665
- Tri-Norinyl ... 2304
- Triphasil-21 Tablets ... 2527
- Triphasil-28 Tablets ... 2532

Ethynodiol Diacetate (Hyperglycemic effect). Products include:
- Demulen ... 2161

Etodolac (Increased hypoglycemic action). Products include:
- Lodine Capsules ... 2468

Felodipine (Hyperglycemic effect). Products include:
- Plendil Extended-Release Tablets ... 1526

Fenoprofen Calcium (Increased hypoglycemic action). Products include:
- Nalfon Pulvules & Tablets ... 919

Fluphenazine Decanoate (Hyperglycemic effect). Products include:
- Prolixin Decanoate ... 1795

Fluphenazine Enanthate (Hyperglycemic effect). Products include:
- Prolixin Enanthate ... 1796

Fluphenazine Hydrochloride (Hyperglycemic effect). Products include:
- Prolixin Elixir ... 1793
- Prolixin Injection ... 1791
- Prolixin Oral Concentrate ... 1792
- Prolixin Tablets ... 1793

Flurbiprofen (Increased hypoglycemic action). Products include:
- Ansaid Tablets ... 2319

Furazolidone (Increased hypoglycemic action). Products include:
- Furoxone ... 1855

Furosemide (Hyperglycemic effect). Products include:
- Lasix ... 1093

Glyburide (Increased hypoglycemic action). Products include:
- DiaBeta ... 1091
- Micronase Tablets ... 2350

Hydrochlorothiazide (Hyperglycemic effect). Products include:
- Aldactazide ... 2150
- Aldoril Tablets ... 1418
- Apresazide Capsules ... 854
- Apresoline-Esidrix Tablets ... 857
- Capozide ... 2258
- Dyazide Capsules ... 2208
- Esidrix Tablets ... 863
- Esimil Tablets ... 864
- HydroDIURIL Tablets ... 1484
- Hydropres Tablets ... 1485
- Inderide Tablets ... 2463
- Inderide LA Long Acting Capsules ... 2465
- Lopressor HCT Tablets ... 1034
- Maxzide ... 1215
- Moduretic Tablets ... 1510
- Normozide Tablets ... 2112
- Oretic Tablets ... 544
- Oreticyl ... 545
- Prinzide Tablets ... 1540
- Ser-Ap-Es Tablets ... 881
- Serpasil-Esidrix Tablets ... 886
- Timolide Tablets ... 1547
- Trandate HCT Tablets ... 579
- Vaseretic Tablets ... 1559
- Zestoretic ... 2274

Hydrocortisone (Hyperglycemic effect). Products include:
- AK-Spore H.C. ... ⊙ 206
- Bactine Hydrocortisone Anti-Itch Cream ... ▣ 625
- CaldeCORT Anti-Itch Hydrocortisone Spray ... ▣ 560
- Carmol HC Cream 1% ... 2296
- Cortaid Spray ... ▣ 735
- Cortenema ... 2244
- Cortisporin Ointment ... 758
- Cortisporin Ophthalmic Ointment Sterile ... 758
- Cortisporin Ophthalmic Suspension Sterile ... 759
- Cortisporin Otic Solution Sterile ... 760
- Cortisporin Otic Suspension Sterile ... 760
- Cortizone-5 Creme & Ointment ... ▣ 732
- Dermolate Anti-Itch Cream ... ▣ 697
- Eldecort Cream 1.0% ... 1113
- Eldecort Cream 1.0% and 2.5% ... 1113
- Fungoid HC Creme ... 1770
- Hydrocortone Tablets ... 1482
- Hytone ... 909
- LazerSporin-C Solution ... 1770
- Massengill Medicated Soft Cloth Towelettes ... 2192
- Nutracort Cream & Lotion ... 1684
- PediOtic Suspension Sterile ... 797
- Synacort Creams 1%, 2.5% ... 2296
- Vanoxide-HC Acne Lotion ... 911
- Vioform-Hydrocortisone Cream and Mild Cream ... 889
- Vioform-Hydrocortisone Ointment ... 889
- VōSoL HC Otic Solution ... 2392
- Vytone Cream 1% ... 911

Hydrocortisone Acetate (Hyperglycemic effect). Products include:
- Analpram-HC Rectal Cream 1% and 2.5% ... 970
- Anusol-HC Cream ... 1690
- Anusol-HC Suppositories ... 1691
- Caldecort ... ▣ 560
- Carmol HC Cream 1% ... 2296
- Chloromycetin Hydrocortisone Ophthalmic ... 1694
- Coly-Mycin S Otic w/Neomycin & Hydrocortisone ... 1708
- Cortaid ... ▣ 735
- Cortef Feminine Itch Cream ... ▣ 735
- Corticaine ... ▣ 682
- Cortifoam ... 1827
- Cortisporin Cream ... 757
- Epifoam ... 1828
- Gynecort 5 Creme ... ▣ 556
- Hydrocortone Acetate Sterile Suspension ... 1479
- Lanacort 5 Creme and Ointment ... ▣ 557
- Mantadil Cream ... 789
- Ophthocort ... ⊙ 301
- Orabase HCA Oral Paste ... 890

(▣ Described in PDR For Nonprescription Drugs) (⊙ Described in PDR For Ophthalmology)

Pramosone Cream, Lotion & Ointment ... 971
ProctoCream-HC ... 1834
Proctofoam-HC ... 1835

Hydrocortisone Sodium Phosphate (Hyperglycemic effect). Products include:
Hydrocortone Phosphate Injection, Sterile ... 1481

Hydrocortisone Sodium Succinate (Hyperglycemic effect). Products include:
Solu-Cortef Sterile Powder ... 2361

Hydroflumethiazide (Hyperglycemic effect). Products include:
Diucardin Tablets ... 2450
Saluron ... 718
Salutensin/Salutensin-Demi ... 719

Ibuprofen (Increased hypoglycemic action). Products include:
Advil Cold & Sinus Caplets (formerly CoAdvil) ... 2416
Advil Ibuprofen Tablets and Caplets ... 2416
Children's Advil Suspension ... 2426
CoAdvil ... ▣ 748
Dristan Sinus Caplets ... 2419
Haltran Tablets ... ▣ 668
Ibuprofen ... ▣ 631
Medipren ibuprofen Caplets and Tablets ... 1362
Midol 200 Cramp Relief Formula ... ▣ 570
Motrin Tablets ... 2351
Motrin IB Caplets and Tablets ... ▣ 736
Nuprin Ibuprofen/Analgesic Tablets & Caplets ... 752
PediaProfen Suspension ... 1363
Rufen Tablets ... 691
Trendar Ibuprofen Tablets ... ▣ 756

Indapamide (Hyperglycemic effect). Products include:
Lozol Tablets ... 1843

Indomethacin (Increased hypoglycemic action). Products include:
Indocin ... 1487

Indomethacin Sodium Trihydrate (Increased hypoglycemic action). Products include:
Indocin I.V. ... 1490

Isocarboxazid (Increased hypoglycemic action). Products include:
Marplan Tablets ... 1906

Isoniazid (Hyperglycemic effect). Products include:
INH Tablets ... 868
Rifamate Capsules ... 1347

Isoproterenol Hydrochloride (Hyperglycemic effect). Products include:
Isuprel Hydrochloride Injection 1:5000 ... 2050
Isuprel Hydrochloride Mistometer ... 2051
Isuprel Hydrochloride Solution 1:200 & 1:100 ... 2052
Norisodrine Aerotrol ... 540

Isradipine (Hyperglycemic effect). Products include:
DynaCirc Capsules ... 2004

Ketoprofen (Increased hypoglycemic action). Products include:
Orudis Capsules ... 2488

Ketorolac Tromethamine (Increased hypoglycemic action). Products include:
Toradol IM Injection ... 2302

Labetalol Hydrochloride (Increased hypoglycemic action). Products include:
Normodyne Injection ... 2108
Normodyne Tablets ... 2110
Normozide Tablets ... 2112
Trandate HCT Tablets ... 579
Trandate Injection ... 577
Trandate Tablets ... 579

Levonorgestrel (Hyperglycemic effect). Products include:
Levlen/Tri-Levlen ... 665
Nordette-21 Tablets ... 2481
Nordette-28 Tablets ... 2483
Norplant System ... 2484
Levlen/Tri-Levlen ... 665
Triphasil-21 Tablets ... 2527
Triphasil-28 Tablets ... 2532

Levothyroxine Sodium (Hyperglycemic effect). Products include:
Levothroid Tablets ... 1003
Levoxine Tablets ... 904
Synthroid ... 695

Liothyronine Sodium (Hyperglycemic effect). Products include:
Cytomel Tablets ... 2203

Magnesium Salicylate (Increased hypoglycemic action). Products include:
Doan's - Extra-Strength Analgesic ... ▣ 549
Doan's - Regular Strength Analgesic ... ▣ 549
Mobigesic Analgesic Tablets ... ▣ 507

Meclofenamate Sodium (Increased hypoglycemic action). Products include:
Meclomen Capsules ... 1739

Mefenamic Acid (Increased hypoglycemic action). Products include:
Ponstel ... 1758

Mesoridazine (Hyperglycemic effect). Products include:
Serentil ... 686

Mestranol (Hyperglycemic effect). Products include:
Enovid ... 2161
Norethin ... 2133
Norinyl ... 2304
Ortho-Novum ... 1667

Metaproterenol Sulfate (Hyperglycemic effect). Products include:
Alupent ... 674
Arm-a-Med Metaproterenol Sulfate Inhalation Solution, USP ... 617
Metaprel Inhalation Aerosol Bronchodilator ... 2014
Metaprel Inhalation Solution ... 2015
Metaprel ... 2015
Metaproterenol Sulfate Inhalation Solution, USP ... 912

Metaraminol Bitartrate (Hyperglycemic effect). Products include:
Aramine Injection ... 1424

Methoxamine Hydrochloride (Hyperglycemic effect). Products include:
Vasoxyl Injection ... 819

Methyclothiazide (Hyperglycemic effect). Products include:
Enduron Tablets ... 517
Enduronyl ... 518

Methylprednisolone Acetate (Hyperglycemic effect). Products include:
Depo-Medrol Sterile Aqueous Suspension ... 2334

Methylprednisolone Sodium Succinate (Hyperglycemic effect). Products include:
Solu-Medrol Sterile Powder ... 2363

Metolazone (Hyperglycemic effect). Products include:
Diulo ... 2129
Mykrox ½ mg Tablets ... 984
Zaroxolyn Tablets ... 989

Metoprolol Tartrate (Increased hypoglycemic action). Products include:
Lopressor Ampuls ... 1032
Lopressor HCT Tablets ... 1034
Lopressor Tablets ... 1032

Miconazole (Increased hypoglycemic effect). Products include:
Monistat I.V. ... 1143

Nadolol (Increased hypoglycemic action). Products include:
Corgard Tablets ... 701
Corzide Tablets ... 702

Naproxen (Increased hypoglycemic action). Products include:
Naprosyn ... 2297

Naproxen Sodium (Increased hypoglycemic action). Products include:
Anaprox and Anaprox DS Tablets ... 2288

Nicardipine Hydrochloride (Hyperglycemic effect). Products include:
Cardene Capsules ... 2290

Nicotinic Acid (Hyperglycemic effect). Products include:
Niacor Tablets ... 2376
Nicobid ... 1846
Nicolar Tablets ... 1846
Nicotinex Elixir ... ▣ 563
Slo-Niacin Tablets ... 2376

Nifedipine (Hyperglycemic effect). Products include:
Adalat Capsules (10 mg and 20 mg) ... 1587
Procardia Capsules ... 1781
Procardia XL Tablets ... 1783

Nimodipine (Hyperglycemic effect). Products include:
Nimotop Capsules ... 1607

Norepinephrine Bitartrate (Hyperglycemic effect). Products include:
Levophed Bitartrate Injection ... 2054

Norethindrone (Hyperglycemic effect). Products include:
Brevicon ... 2304
Jenest-28 Tablets ... 1636
Micronor Tablets ... 1667
Modicon ... 1667
Norethin ... 2133
Norinyl ... 2304
Norlutin ... 1755
Nor-Q D Tablets ... 2304
Ortho-Novum ... 1667
Ovcon ... 1391
Tri-Norinyl ... 2304

Norethynodrel (Hyperglycemic effect). Products include:
Enovid ... 2161

Norgestimate (Hyperglycemic effect). Products include:
Ortho-Cyclen Tablets ... 1658

Norgestrel (Hyperglycemic effect). Products include:
Lo/Ovral Tablets ... 2471
Lo/Ovral-28 Tablets ... 2476
Ovral Tablets ... 2490
Ovral-28 Tablets ... 2491
Ovrette Tablets ... 2492

Penbutolol Sulfate (Increased hypoglycemic action). Products include:
Levatol ... 1832

Perphenazine (Hyperglycemic effect). Products include:
Etrafon ... 2087
Triavil Tablets ... 1556
Trilafon ... 2123

Phenelzine Sulfate (Increased hypoglycemic action). Products include:
Nardil ... 1742

Phenylbutazone (Increased hypoglycemic action). Products include:
Butazolidin Capsules & Tablets ... 1027

Phenylephrine Bitartrate (Hyperglycemic effect).
No products indexed under this heading.

Phenylephrine Hydrochloride (Hyperglycemic effect). Products include:
AK-Dilate Solution 2.5% and 10% ... ⊙ 203
Atrohist Sprinkle Capsules ... 558
Cerose-DM ... 2443
Codimal ... 846
Comhist LA Capsules ... 1618
Congespirin For Children Aspirin Free Chewable Cold Tablets ... 748
Cyclomydril ... ⊙ 216
Deconsal Sprinkle Capsules ... 559
Dimetane Decongestant ... ▣ 673
Dristan Decongestant/Antihistamine/ Analgesic Coated Caplets ... ▣ 749
Dristan Cold Nasal Decongestant/ Antihistamine/ Analgesic Coated Tablets ... 2419
Dristan Advanced Formula Decongestant/Antihistamine/ Analgesic Tablets ... ▣ 749
Dristan Nasal Spray, Menthol ... 2419
Dristan Nasal Spray, Regular and Regular with Metered Pump ... 2419
Entex Capsules ... 1623
Entex Liquid ... 1623
Sinus Excedrin Analgesic, Decongestant Tablets & Caplets ... 750
Extendryl ... 994
4-Way Fast Acting Nasal Spray - Original Formula (regular & mentholated) & Metered Spray Pump (regular) ... 751
Hycomine Compound Tablets ... 929
Murocoll-2 Sterile Ophthalmic Solution ... ⊙ 261
Mydfrin 2.5% ... ⊙ 224
Naldecon Syrup, Tablets, Pediatric Drops and Pediatric Syrup ... 709
Neo-Synephrine Hydrochloride 1% Carpuject ... 2063
Neo-Synephrine Hydrochloride 1% Injection ... 2063
Neo-Synephrine Hydrochloride (Ophthalmic) ... 2064
Neo-Synephrine ... ▣ 759
Nōstril Nasal Decongestant ... ▣ 520
Novahistine Elixir ... ▣ 596
Phenergan VC ... 2500
Phenergan VC with Codeine ... 2501
Prefrin Liquifilm Vasoconstrictor and Lubricant Eye Drops ... ⊙ 254
Prefrin-A ... ⊙ 255
Quelidrine Syrup ... 556
Relief Vasoconstrictor and Lubricant Eye Drops ... ⊙ 256
Robitussin Night Relief ... ▣ 677
Ru-Tuss with Hydrocodone ... 694
Ru-Tuss Tablets ... 693
Vasosulf ... ⊙ 279
Vicks Sinex ... ▣ 665
Zincfrin ... ⊙ 230

Phenylephrine Tannate (Hyperglycemic effect). Products include:
Rynatan ... 2387
Rynatuss ... 2388

Phenylpropanolamine Hydrochloride (Hyperglycemic effect). Products include:
A.R.M. Allergy Relief Medicine Caplets ... ▣ 615
Acutrim ... ▣ 548
Allerest ... ▣ 559
BC Cold Powder ... ▣ 517
Cheracol Plus Head Cold/Cough Formula ... ▣ 667
Codimal Expectorant ... 846
Comtrex Multi-Symptom Cold Reliever Tablets/Caplets/Liqui-Gels/Liquid ... 745
Contac Continuous Action Decongestant/Antihistamine Capsules ▣ 710
Contac Maximum Strength Continuous Action Decongestant/ Antihistamine Caplets ... ▣ 709
Contac Severe Cold and Flu Formula Caplets ... ▣ 711
Coricidin 'D' Decongestant Tablets ... ▣ 695
Coricidin Demilets Tablets for Children ... ▣ 696
Demazin Nasal Decongestant/ Antihistamine Repetabs Tablets & Syrup ... ▣ 697
Dexatrim ... ▣ 733
Dimetane-DC Cough Syrup ... 1857
Dimetapp Elixir ... ▣ 673
Dimetapp DM Elixir ... ▣ 674
Dimetapp Extentabs ... ▣ 674
Dimetapp Plus Caplets ... ▣ 675
Dimetapp Tablets ... ▣ 675
Entex Capsules ... 1623
Entex LA Tablets ... 1623
Entex Liquid ... 1623
4-Way Cold Tablets ... 750
Hycomine Syrup ... 927
Naldecon CX Adult Liquid ... ▣ 521
Naldecon DX Adult Liquid ... ▣ 521
Naldecon DX Children's Syrup ... ▣ 522
Naldecon DX Pediatric Drops ... ▣ 522
Naldecon EX Children's Syrup ... ▣ 522
Naldecon EX Pediatric Drops ... ▣ 523
Naldecon Syrup, Tablets, Pediatric Drops and Pediatric Syrup ... 709
Nolamine Tablets ... 838
Nolex LA Tablets ... 838
Ornade Spansule Capsules ... 2221
Orthoxicol Cough Syrup ... ▣ 668

Propagest ... 839
Pyrroxate Capsules ... ▣ 669
Robitussin-CF ... ▣ 676
Ru-Tuss II Capsules ... 693
Ru-Tuss with Hydrocodone ... 694
Ru-Tuss Tablets ... 693
Sine-Off Sinus Medicine Tablets-Aspirin Formula ... ▣ 722
Sinulin ... 840
St. Joseph Cold Tablets for Children ... ▣ 704
Tavist-D Tablets ... 2035
Triaminic Allergy Tablets ... ▣ 688
Triaminic Chewables ... ▣ 688
Triaminic Cold Tablets ... ▣ 688
Triaminic Expectorant ... ▣ 688
Triaminic Expectorant w/Codeine ... 1996
Triaminic Expectorant DH ... 1995
Triaminic Oral Infant Drops ... 1996
Triaminic Syrup ... ▣ 689
Triaminic-12 Tablets ... ▣ 690
Triaminic-DM Syrup ... ▣ 689
Triaminicin Tablets ... ▣ 690
Triaminicol Multi-Symptom Cold Tablets ... ▣ 691
Triaminicol Multi-Symptom Relief ▣ 691
Tuss-Ornade Liquid ... 2242
Tuss-Ornade Spansule Capsules ... 2242
Tylenol Cold Medication, Effervescent Tablets ... 1369

Phenytoin (Hyperglycemic effect). Products include:
Dilantin Infatabs ... 1710
Dilantin-30 Pediatric/Dilantin-125 Suspension ... 1713

Phenytoin Sodium (Hyperglycemic effect). Products include:
Dilantin Kapseals ... 1708
Dilantin Parenteral ... 1712
Dilantin with Phenobarbital Kapseals ... 1715

Pindolol (Increased hypoglycemic action). Products include:
Visken Tablets ... 2036

Pirbuterol Acetate (Hyperglycemic effect). Products include:
Maxair Inhaler ... 1311

Piroxicam (Increased hypoglycemic action). Products include:
Feldene Capsules ... 1777

Polyestradiol Phosphate (Hyperglycemic effect). Products include:
Estradurin ... 2452

Polythiazide (Hyperglycemic effect). Products include:
Minizide Capsules ... 1779
Renese Tablets ... 1785
Renese-R Tablets ... 1786

Prednisolone Acetate (Hyperglycemic effect). Products include:
AK-Cide Sterile Ophthalmic Ointment & Suspension ... ⊙ 202
Blephamide Liquifilm Sterile Ophthalmic Suspension ... 586
Blephamide S.O.P. Sterile Ophthalmic Ointment ... 586
Cetapred Ointment ... ⊙ 220
⅛% Econopred & 1% Econopred Plus ... ⊙ 217
Isopto Cetapred Suspension ... ⊙ 220
Metimyd ... ⊙ 306
Poly-Pred Liquifilm ... ⊙ 250
Pred Forte ... ⊙ 252
Pred Mild ... ⊙ 254
Pred-G Liquifilm Sterile Ophthalmic Suspension ... ⊙ 252
Pred-G S.O.P. Sterile Ophthalmic Ointment ... ⊙ 253
Vasocidin Ointment ... ⊙ 275

Prednisolone Sodium Phosphate (Hyperglycemic effect). Products include:
AK-Pred ... ⊙ 205
Hydeltrasol Injection, Sterile ... 1476
Inflamase ... ⊙ 274
Pediapred Oral Liquid ... 987
Vasocidin Ophthalmic Solution ... ⊙ 276

Prednisolone Tebutate (Hyperglycemic effect). Products include:
Hydeltra-T.B.A. Sterile Suspension 1478

Prednisone (Hyperglycemic effect). Products include:
Deltasone Tablets ... 2332

Probenecid (Increased hypoglycemic action). Products include:
Benemid Tablets ... 1426
ColBENEMID Tablets ... 1436
Wycillin Injection and Probenecid Tablets ... 2539

Prochlorperazine (Hyperglycemic effect). Products include:
Compazine ... 2201

Promethazine Hydrochloride (Hyperglycemic effect). Products include:
Mepergan Injection ... 2479
Phenergan with Codeine ... 2497
Phenergan with Dextromethorphan 2499
Phenergan Injection ... 2493
Phenergan Suppositories ... 2496
Phenergan Syrup ... 2495
Phenergan Tablets ... 2496
Phenergan VC ... 2500
Phenergan VC with Codeine ... 2501

Propranolol Hydrochloride (Increased hypoglycemic action). Products include:
Inderal ... 2459
Inderal LA Long Acting Capsules ... 2461
Inderide Tablets ... 2463
Inderide LA Long Acting Capsules ... 2465

Pseudoephedrine Hydrochloride (Hyperglycemic effect). Products include:
Actifed Capsules ... ▣ 539
Actifed Plus Caplets ... ▣ 539
Actifed Plus Tablets ... ▣ 540
Actifed with Codeine Cough Syrup... 752
Actifed Syrup ... ▣ 540
Actifed Tablets ... ▣ 540
Actifed 12-Hour Capsules ... ▣ 539
Advil Cold & Sinus Caplets (formerly CoAdvil) ... 2416
Allerest ... ▣ 559
Anatuss LA Tablets ... 1359
Benadryl Decongestant Elixir ... ▣ 635
Benadryl Decongestant ... ▣ 635
Benadryl Plus ... ▣ 636
Benadryl Plus Nighttime ... ▣ 637
Benylin Decongestant ... ▣ 638
Brexin L.A. Capsules ... 2078
Bromfed Capsules (Timed Release) ... 1615
Bromfed Syrup ... ▣ 628
Bromfed ... 1615
CoAdvil ... ▣ 748
Allergy-Sinus Comtrex Multi-Symptom Allergy Sinus Formula Tablets & Caplets ... 746
Cough Formula Comtrex ... 746
Comtrex Multi-Symptom Cold Reliever Tablets/Caplets/Liqui-Gels/Liquid ... 745
Day-Night Comtrex ... 747
Non-Drowsy Comtrex ... 747
Congess ... 994
Congestac Caplets ... ▣ 617
Contac Jr. Children's Cold Medicine ... ▣ 712
Contac Nighttime Cold Medicine ... ▣ 713
Contac Sinus Caplets Maximum Strength Non-Drowsy Formula ... ▣ 710
Contac Sinus Tablets Maximum Strength Non-Drowsy Formula ... ▣ 710
Deconamine ... 663
Deconsal II Tablets ... 559
Dimacol Caplets ... ▣ 672
Dimetane-DX Cough Syrup ... 1858
Dorcol Children's Cough Syrup ... ▣ 685
Dorcol Children's Decongestant Liquid ... ▣ 685
Dorcol Children's Liquid Cold Formula ... ▣ 686
Maximum Strength Dristan Decongestant/Analgesic Coated Caplets ... ▣ 750
No Drowsiness Dristan Cold Nasal Decongestant/Analgesic Coated Caplets ... 2420
Dristan Sinus Caplets ... 2419
Sinus Excedrin Analgesic, Decongestant Tablets & Caplets ... ▣ 533
Fedahist Gyrocaps ... 2145
Fedahist Timecaps ... 2145
Guaifed ... 1615
Guaifed Syrup ... ▣ 629
Isoclor Expectorant ... 982
Isoclor Timesule Capsules ... ▣ 561
Kronofed-A ... 970
Medi-Flu Caplet, Liquid ... ▣ 640
Novafed A Capsules ... 1342
Novafed Capsules ... 1342
Novahistine DH ... 1342
Novahistine DMX ... ▣ 595
Novahistine Expectorant ... 1343
Nucofed Capsules ... 2219
Nucofed Expectorant ... 2219
Nucofed Pediatric Expectorant ... 2220
Nucofed Syrup ... 2219
Ornex Caplets ... ▣ 618
PediaCare Allergy Relief Formula Liquid ... 1362
PediaCare Cough-Cold Formula Liquid ... 1362
PediaCare Infants' Oral Decongestant Drops ... 1362
PediaCare Night Rest Cough-Cold Formula Liquid ... 1362
PediaCare 6-12 Cough-Cold Formula Chewable Tablets ... 1362
Robitussin-DAC Syrup ... 1875
Robitussin-PE ... ▣ 677
Rondec ... 1975
Rondec-DM ... 1976
Rondec-TR Tablet ... 1975
Ru-Tuss DE Tablets ... 694
Ryna ... ▣ 741
Seldane-D Extended-Release Tablets ... 1350
Sinarest ... ▣ 562
Sine-Aid Maximum Strength Sinus Headache Caplets ... 1365
Sine-Aid Maximum Strength Sinus Headache Tablets ... 1365
Sine-Off Maximum Strength Allergy/Sinus Formula Caplets ... ▣ 721
Sine-Off Maximum Strength No Drowsiness Formula Caplets ... ▣ 722
Singlet Tablets ... ▣ 598
Sinutab Maximum Strength ... ▣ 641
Sinutab Maximum Strength Without Drowsiness Tablets & Caplets ... ▣ 642
Sinutab Regular Strength Without Drowsiness Formula ... ▣ 641
St. Joseph Nighttime Cold Medicine ... ▣ 705
Sudafed Children's Liquid ... ▣ 543
Sudafed Cough Syrup ... ▣ 543
Sudafed Plus Liquid ... ▣ 544
Sudafed Plus Tablets ... ▣ 545
Sudafed Sinus Caplets ... ▣ 545
Sudafed Sinus Tablets ... ▣ 545
Sudafed Tablets, 30 mg ... ▣ 544
Sudafed Tablets, Adult Strength, 60 mg ... ▣ 544
Sudafed 12 Hour Capsules ... ▣ 545
TheraFlu Flu and Cold Medicine ... ▣ 687
Triaminic Nite Light ... ▣ 689
Tylenol Allergy Sinus Medication Caplets and Gelcaps, Maximum Strength ... 1372
Children's Tylenol Cold Liquid Formula and Chewable Tablets ... 1368
Tylenol Cold & Flu Hot Medication, Packets ... 1369
Tylenol Cold & Flu No Drowsiness Hot Medication, Packets ... 1371
Tylenol Cold Medication Caplets and Tablets ... 1370
Tylenol Cold Medication No Drowsiness Formula Caplets ... 1370
Tylenol Cold Night Time Medication Liquid ... 1371
Tylenol Cough Medication Liquid with Decongestant, Maximum Strength ... 1372
Tylenol, Maximum Strength, Sinus Medication Gelcaps, Caplets and Tablets ... 1373
Ursinus Inlay-Tabs ... ▣ 691
Vicks Children's NyQuil ... ▣ 664
Vicks Daycare ... ▣ 660
Vicks Formula 44D Decongestant Cough Medicine ... ▣ 662
Vicks Formula 44M Multi-Symptom Cough Medicine ... ▣ 662
Vicks NyQuil Nighttime Colds Medicine-Original & Cherry Flavor ... ▣ 664
Vicks Pediatric Formula 44 Cough & Congestion Medicine ... ▣ 663
Vicks Pediatric Formula 44m Multi-Symptom Cough & Cold Medicine ... ▣ 663

Pseudoephedrine Sulfate (Hyperglycemic effect). Products include:
Afrin Tablets ... ▣ 693
Chlor-Trimeton Decongestant ... ▣ 694
Disophrol Chronotab Sustained-Action Tablets ... ▣ 698
Drixoral Antihistamine/Nasal Decongestant Syrup ... ▣ 698
Drixoral Non-Drowsy Formula ... ▣ 699
Drixoral Plus Extended-Release Tablets ... ▣ 699
Drixoral Sinus ... ▣ 700
Drixoral Sustained-Action Tablets ▣ 698
Sinutab Allergy Formula Sustained Action Tablets ... ▣ 640
Trinalin Repetabs Tablets ... 1170

Quinestrol (Hyperglycemic effect). Products include:
Estrovis ... 1721

Salsalate (Increased hypoglycemic action). Products include:
Disalcid ... 1310
Mono-Gesic Tablets ... 846
Salflex ... 839

Selegiline Hydrochloride (Increased hypoglycemic action). Products include:
Eldepryl ... 2250

Spironolactone (Hyperglycemic effect). Products include:
Aldactazide ... 2150
Aldactone ... 2152

Sulfamethizole (Increased hypoglycemic action). Products include:
Thiosulfil Forte Tablets ... 2526
Urobiotic-250 Capsules ... 1968

Sulfamethoxazole (Increased hypoglycemic action). Products include:
Azo Gantanol Tablets ... 1887
Bactrim DS Tablets ... 1891
Bactrim I.V. Infusion ... 1889
Bactrim ... 1891
Gantanol ... 1899
Septra ... 813
Septra I.V. Infusion ... 808
Septra I.V. Infusion ADD-Vantage Vials ... 810
Septra ... 813

Sulfasalazine (Increased hypoglycemic action). Products include:
Azulfidine Tablets, EN-tabs, Oral Suspension ... 1157

Sulfinpyrazone (Increased hypoglycemic action). Products include:
Anturane ... 853

Sulfisoxazole (Increased hypoglycemic action). Products include:
Azo Gantrisin Tablets ... 1888
Gantrisin Tablets ... 1901
Pediazole ... 1973

Sulfisoxazole Diolamine (Increased hypoglycemic action). Products include:
Gantrisin Ophthalmic Ointment/Solution ... 1900

Sulindac (Increased hypoglycemic action). Products include:
Clinoril Tablets ... 1433

Terbutaline Sulfate (Hyperglycemic effect). Products include:
Brethaire Inhaler ... 1024
Brethine Ampuls ... 1026
Brethine Tablets ... 1026
Bricanyl Injection ... 1324
Bricanyl Tablets ... 1325

Thioridazine Hydrochloride (Hyperglycemic effect). Products include:
Mellaril ... 2011

Thyroid (Hyperglycemic effect). Products include:
S-P-T "Liquid" Capsules ... 995

Thyroxine Sodium (Hyperglycemic effect).
No products indexed under this heading.

Timolol Maleate (Increased hypoglycemic action). Products include:
Blocadren Tablets ... 1429
Timolide Tablets ... 1547
Timoptic in Ocudose ... 1552
Timoptic Sterile Ophthalmic Solution ... 1550

(▣ Described in PDR For Nonprescription Drugs) (⊙ Described in PDR For Ophthalmology)

Tolazamide (Increased hypoglycemic action). Products include:
Tolinase Tablets ... 2365
Tolbutamide (Increased hypoglycemic action). Products include:
Orinase Tablets ... 2354
Tolmetin Sodium (Increased hypoglycemic action). Products include:
Tolectin (200, 400 and 600 mg) .. 1379
Tranylcypromine Sulfate (Increased hypoglycemic action). Products include:
Parnate Tablets ... 2222
Triamcinolone (Hyperglycemic effect).
No products indexed under this heading.
Triamcinolone Acetonide (Hyperglycemic effect). Products include:
Aristocort A ... 1010
Azmacort Inhaler ... 1837
Kenalog Cream, Lotion & Ointment 2401
Kenalog-10 Injection ... 2402
Kenalog-40 Injection ... 2403
Kenalog in Orabase ... 604
Kenalog Spray ... 2401
Mycolog II Cream and Ointment ... 2407
Mytrex Cream & Ointment ... 2080
Nasacort Nasal Inhaler ... 1844
Triamcinolone Diacetate (Hyperglycemic effect). Products include:
Aristocort Suspension ... 1008
Triamcinolone Hexacetonide (Hyperglycemic effect). Products include:
Aristospan Suspension ... 1011
Triamterene (Hyperglycemic effect). Products include:
Dyazide Capsules ... 2208
Dyrenium Capsules ... 2210
Maxzide ... 1215
Trifluoperazine Hydrochloride (Hyperglycemic effect). Products include:
Stelazine ... 2226
Verapamil Hydrochloride (Hyperglycemic effect). Products include:
Calan SR Caplets ... 2157
Calan Tablets ... 2155
Isoptin Injectable ... 1177
Isoptin Oral Tablets ... 1179
Isoptin SR Sustained Release Tablets ... 1181
Verelan Capsules ... 1243
Verelan Capsules ... 2535
Warfarin Sodium (Increased hypoglycemic action). Products include:
Coumadin Injection & Tablets ... 944
Panwarfin Tablets ... 547

Food Interactions

Food, unspecified (Delays absorption by about 40 minutes).

GLUTOSE
(Dextrose) ... ▣ 633
No interactions described in labeling.

GLY-OXIDE LIQUID
(Carbamide Peroxide) ... ▣ 595
No interactions described in labeling.

G-MYTICIN CREME AND OINTMENT 0.1%
(Gentamicin Sulfate) ... 1770
No interactions described in labeling.

GOLD PLUS - THE GOLD LOTION
(Methyl Salicylate, Menthol, Camphor) ... ▣ 508
No interactions described in labeling.

GOLYTELY
(Polyethylene Glycol) ... 699
May interact with:

Oral Medications (Those administered within one hour of GoLYTELY usage may be flushed from the gastrointestinal tract and not absorbed).

Food Interactions

Food, unspecified (For best results, no solid food should be consumed during 3 to 4 hour period before drinking solution).

GONAK OPHTHALMIC DEMULCENT SOLUTION
(Hydroxypropyl Methylcellulose) .... ◉ 209
No interactions described in labeling.

GONIOSCOPIC PRISM SOLUTION
(Hydroxyethyl Cellulose) ... ◉ 218
No interactions described in labeling.

GORDOCHOM SOLUTION
(Chloroxylenol, Undecylenic Acid) ... 1072
No interactions described in labeling.

GRANULEX
(Trypsin, Balsam Peru, Castor Oil) 1086
No interactions described in labeling.

GRIFULVIN V (GRISEOFULVIN MICROSIZE) TABLETS/SUSPENSION
(Griseofulvin) ... 1678
May interact with oral anticoagulants, barbiturates, and oral contraceptives. Compounds in these categories include:

Aprobarbital (Usually depresses griseofulvin activity; may necessitate dosage increase). Products include:
Alurate Elixir ... 1883
Butabarbital (Usually depresses griseofulvin activity; may necessitate dosage increase). Products include:
Pyridium Plus ... 1764
Butalbital (Usually depresses griseofulvin activity; may necessitate dosage increase). Products include:
Esgic-Plus Tablets ... 1002
Esgic Tablets & Capsules ... 1001
Fioricet Tablets ... 2006
Fiorinal Capsules ... 2007
Fiorinal with Codeine Capsules ... 2008
Fiorinal Tablets ... 2007
Phrenilin ... 838
Sedapap Tablets 50 mg/650 mg .. 1360
Dicumarol (Dosage adjustment of anticoagulant may be necessary). Products include:
Dicumarol Tablets ... 516
Ethinyl Estradiol (Reduced contraceptive efficacy; increased incidence of breakthrough bleeding). Products include:
Brevicon ... 2304
Demulen ... 2161
Estinyl Tablets ... 2085
Jenest-28 Tablets ... 1636
Levlen/Tri-Levlen ... 665
Lo/Ovral Tablets ... 2471
Lo/Ovral-28 Tablets ... 2476
Loestrin ... 1728
Modicon ... 1667
Nordette-21 Tablets ... 2481
Nordette-28 Tablets ... 2483
Norethin ... 2133
Norinyl ... 2304
Norlestrin ... 1746
Ortho-Cyclen Tablets ... 1658
Ortho-Novum ... 1667
Ovcon ... 1391
Ovral Tablets ... 2490
Ovral-28 Tablets ... 2491
Levlen/Tri-Levlen ... 665
Tri-Norinyl ... 2304
Triphasil-21 Tablets ... 2527
Triphasil-28 Tablets ... 2532
Ethynodiol Diacetate (Reduced contraceptive efficacy; increased incidence of breakthrough bleeding). Products include:
Demulen ... 2161
Levonorgestrel (Reduced contraceptive efficacy; increased incidence of breakthrough bleeding). Products include:
Levlen/Tri-Levlen ... 665
Nordette-21 Tablets ... 2481
Nordette-28 Tablets ... 2483
Norplant System ... 2484
Levlen/Tri-Levlen ... 665
Triphasil-21 Tablets ... 2527
Triphasil-28 Tablets ... 2532
Mephobarbital (Usually depresses griseofulvin activity; may necessitate dosage increase). Products include:
Mebaral Tablets ... 2061
Mestranol (Reduced contraceptive efficacy; increased incidence of breakthrough bleeding). Products include:
Enovid ... 2161
Norethin ... 2133
Norinyl ... 2304
Ortho-Novum ... 1667
Norethindrone (Reduced contraceptive efficacy; increased incidence of breakthrough bleeding). Products include:
Brevicon ... 2304
Jenest-28 Tablets ... 1636
Micronor Tablets ... 1667
Modicon ... 1667
Norethin ... 2133
Norinyl ... 2304
Norlutin ... 1755
Nor-Q D Tablets ... 2304
Ortho-Novum ... 1667
Ovcon ... 1391
Tri-Norinyl ... 2304
Norethynodrel (Reduced contraceptive efficacy; increased incidence of breakthrough bleeding). Products include:
Enovid ... 2161
Norgestimate (Reduced contraceptive efficacy; increased incidence of breakthrough bleeding). Products include:
Ortho-Cyclen Tablets ... 1658
Norgestrel (Reduced contraceptive efficacy; increased incidence of breakthrough bleeding). Products include:
Lo/Ovral Tablets ... 2471
Lo/Ovral-28 Tablets ... 2476
Ovral Tablets ... 2490
Ovral-28 Tablets ... 2491
Ovrette Tablets ... 2492
Pentobarbital Sodium (Usually depresses griseofulvin activity; may necessitate dosage increase). Products include:
Nembutal Sodium Capsules ... 534
Nembutal Sodium Solution ... 536
Nembutal Sodium Suppositories ... 538
Phenobarbital (Usually depresses griseofulvin activity; may necessitate dosage increase). Products include:
Arco-Lase Plus Tablets ... 607
Bellergal-S Tablets ... 1998
Bronkolixir ... ▣ 761
Bronkotabs Tablets ... ▣ 762
Donnatal ... 1858
Donnatal Extentabs ... 1859
Donnatal Tablets ... 1858
Donnazyme Tablets ... 1860
Kinesed Tablets ... 2272
Phenobarbital Elixir and Tablets ... 1293
Primatene Tablets-P Formula ... 2421
Quadrinal Tablets ... 1183
Tedral SA ... 1765
Secobarbital Sodium (Usually depresses griseofulvin activity; may necessitate dosage increase). Products include:
Seconal Sodium Pulvules ... 1296
Thiamylal Sodium (Usually depresses griseofulvin activity; may necessitate dosage increase). Products include:
Surital Ampoules, Steri-Vials ... 1764
Warfarin Sodium (Dosage adjustment of anticoagulant may be necessary). Products include:
Coumadin Injection & Tablets ... 944
Panwarfin Tablets ... 547

GRISACTIN CAPSULES
(Griseofulvin) ... 2454
May interact with oral anticoagulants, barbiturates, and certain other agents. Compounds in these categories include:

Alcohol (Potentiation; tachycardia and flushing may result).
Aprobarbital (Depressed griseofulvin activity). Products include:
Alurate Elixir ... 1883
Butabarbital (Depressed griseofulvin activity). Products include:
Pyridium Plus ... 1764
Butalbital (Depressed griseofulvin activity). Products include:
Esgic-Plus Tablets ... 1002
Esgic Tablets & Capsules ... 1001
Fioricet Tablets ... 2006
Fiorinal Capsules ... 2007
Fiorinal with Codeine Capsules ... 2008
Fiorinal Tablets ... 2007
Phrenilin ... 838
Sedapap Tablets 50 mg/650 mg .. 1360
Dicumarol (Decreased anticoagulant activity). Products include:
Dicumarol Tablets ... 516
Mephobarbital (Depressed griseofulvin activity). Products include:
Mebaral Tablets ... 2061
Pentobarbital Sodium (Depressed griseofulvin activity). Products include:
Nembutal Sodium Capsules ... 534
Nembutal Sodium Solution ... 536
Nembutal Sodium Suppositories ... 538
Phenobarbital (Depressed griseofulvin activity). Products include:
Arco-Lase Plus Tablets ... 607
Bellergal-S Tablets ... 1998
Bronkolixir ... ▣ 761
Bronkotabs Tablets ... ▣ 762
Donnatal ... 1858
Donnatal Extentabs ... 1859
Donnatal Tablets ... 1858
Donnazyme Tablets ... 1860
Kinesed Tablets ... 2272
Phenobarbital Elixir and Tablets ... 1293
Primatene Tablets-P Formula ... 2421
Quadrinal Tablets ... 1183
Tedral SA ... 1765
Secobarbital Sodium (Depressed griseofulvin activity). Products include:
Seconal Sodium Pulvules ... 1296
Thiamylal Sodium (Depressed griseofulvin activity). Products include:
Surital Ampoules, Steri-Vials ... 1764
Warfarin Sodium (Decreased anticoagulant activity). Products include:
Coumadin Injection & Tablets ... 944
Panwarfin Tablets ... 547

GRISACTIN TABLETS
(Griseofulvin) ... 2454

See **Grisactin Capsules**

GRISACTIN ULTRA TABLETS
(Griseofulvin) ... 2455
May interact with oral anticoagulants, barbiturates, and certain other

agents. Compounds in these categories include:

Alcohol (Potentiation of the effects of alcohol resulting in tachycardia and flushing).

Aprobarbital (Depresses griseofulvin activity). Products include:
Alurate Elixir ... 1883

Butabarbital (Depresses griseofulvin activity). Products include:
Pyridium Plus ... 1764

Butalbital (Depresses griseofulvin activity). Products include:
Esgic-Plus Tablets ... 1002
Esgic Tablets & Capsules ... 1001
Fioricet Tablets ... 2006
Fiorinal Capsules ... 2007
Fiorinal with Codeine Capsules ... 2008
Fiorinal Tablets ... 2007
Phrenilin ... 838
Sedapap Tablets 50 mg/650 mg ... 1360

Dicumarol (Decreased anticoagulant activity). Products include:
Dicumarol Tablets ... 516

Mephobarbital (Depresses griseofulvin activity). Products include:
Mebaral Tablets ... 2061

Pentobarbital Sodium (Depresses griseofulvin activity). Products include:
Nembutal Sodium Capsules ... 534
Nembutal Sodium Solution ... 536
Nembutal Sodium Suppositories ... 538

Phenobarbital (Depresses griseofulvin activity). Products include:
Arco-Lase Plus Tablets ... 607
Bellergal-S Tablets ... 1998
Bronkolixir ... ⊞ 761
Bronkotabs Tablets ... ⊞ 762
Donnatal ... 1858
Donnatal Extentabs ... 1859
Donnatal Tablets ... 1858
Donnazyme Tablets ... 1860
Kinesed Tablets ... 2272
Phenobarbital Elixir and Tablets ... 1293
Primatene Tablets-P Formula ... 2421
Quadrinal Tablets ... 1183
Tedral SA ... 1765

Secobarbital Sodium (Depresses griseofulvin activity). Products include:
Seconal Sodium Pulvules ... 1296

Thiamylal Sodium (Depresses griseofulvin activity). Products include:
Surital Ampoules, Steri-Vials ... 1764

Warfarin Sodium (Decreased anticoagulant activity). Products include:
Coumadin Injection & Tablets ... 944
Panwarfin Tablets ... 547

GRIS-PEG TABLETS, 125 MG & 250 MG
(Griseofulvin) ... 1083
May interact with oral anticoagulants, barbiturates, oral contraceptives, and certain other agents. Compounds in these categories include:

Alcohol (The effect of alcohol may be potentiated).

Aprobarbital (Depresses griseofulvin activity). Products include:
Alurate Elixir ... 1883

Butabarbital (Depresses griseofulvin activity). Products include:
Pyridium Plus ... 1764

Butalbital (Depresses griseofulvin activity). Products include:
Esgic-Plus Tablets ... 1002
Esgic Tablets & Capsules ... 1001
Fioricet Tablets ... 2006
Fiorinal Capsules ... 2007
Fiorinal with Codeine Capsules ... 2008
Fiorinal Tablets ... 2007
Phrenilin ... 838
Sedapap Tablets 50 mg/650 mg ... 1360

Dicumarol (Decreased activity of anticoagulants; dosage adjustment may be required). Products include:
Dicumarol Tablets ... 516

Ethinyl Estradiol (Effects not specified). Products include:
Brevicon ... 2304
Demulen ... 2161
Estinyl Tablets ... 2085
Jenest-28 Tablets ... 1636
Levlen/Tri-Levlen ... 665
Lo/Ovral Tablets ... 2471
Lo/Ovral-28 Tablets ... 2476
Loestrin ... 1728
Modicon ... 1667
Nordette-21 Tablets ... 2481
Nordette-28 Tablets ... 2483
Norethin ... 2133
Norinyl ... 2304
Norlestrin ... 1746
Ortho-Cyclen Tablets ... 1658
Ortho-Novum ... 1667
Ovcon ... 1391
Ovral Tablets ... 2490
Ovral-28 Tablets ... 2491
Levlen/Tri-Levlen ... 665
Tri-Norinyl ... 2304
Triphasil-21 Tablets ... 2527
Triphasil-28 Tablets ... 2532

Ethynodiol Diacetate (Effects not specified). Products include:
Demulen ... 2161

Levonorgestrel (Effects not specified). Products include:
Levlen/Tri-Levlen ... 665
Nordette-21 Tablets ... 2481
Nordette-28 Tablets ... 2483
Norplant System ... 2484
Levlen/Tri-Levlen ... 665
Triphasil-21 Tablets ... 2527
Triphasil-28 Tablets ... 2532

Mephobarbital (Depresses griseofulvin activity). Products include:
Mebaral Tablets ... 2061

Mestranol (Effects not specified). Products include:
Enovid ... 2161
Norethin ... 2133
Norinyl ... 2304
Ortho-Novum ... 1667

Norethindrone (Effects not specified). Products include:
Brevicon ... 2304
Jenest-28 Tablets ... 1636
Micronor Tablets ... 1667
Modicon ... 1667
Norethin ... 2133
Norinyl ... 2304
Norlutin ... 1755
Nor-Q D Tablets ... 2304
Ortho-Novum ... 1667
Ovcon ... 1391
Tri-Norinyl ... 2304

Norethynodrel (Effects not specified). Products include:
Enovid ... 2161

Norgestimate (Effects not specified). Products include:
Ortho-Cyclen Tablets ... 1658

Norgestrel (Effects not specified). Products include:
Lo/Ovral Tablets ... 2471
Lo/Ovral-28 Tablets ... 2476
Ovral Tablets ... 2490
Ovral-28 Tablets ... 2491
Ovrette Tablets ... 2492

Pentobarbital Sodium (Depresses griseofulvin activity). Products include:
Nembutal Sodium Capsules ... 534
Nembutal Sodium Solution ... 536
Nembutal Sodium Suppositories ... 538

Phenobarbital (Depresses griseofulvin activity). Products include:
Arco-Lase Plus Tablets ... 607
Bellergal-S Tablets ... 1998
Bronkolixir ... ⊞ 761
Bronkotabs Tablets ... ⊞ 762
Donnatal ... 1858
Donnatal Extentabs ... 1859
Donnatal Tablets ... 1858
Donnazyme Tablets ... 1860
Kinesed Tablets ... 2272
Phenobarbital Elixir and Tablets ... 1293
Primatene Tablets-P Formula ... 2421
Quadrinal Tablets ... 1183
Tedral SA ... 1765

Secobarbital Sodium (Depresses griseofulvin activity). Products include:
Seconal Sodium Pulvules ... 1296

Thiamylal Sodium (Depresses griseofulvin activity). Products include:
Surital Ampoules, Steri-Vials ... 1764

Warfarin Sodium (Decreased activity of anticoagulants; dosage adjustment may be required). Products include:
Coumadin Injection & Tablets ... 944
Panwarfin Tablets ... 547

GUAIFED CAPSULES (TIMED RELEASE)
(Guaifenesin, Pseudoephedrine Hydrochloride) ... 1615
May interact with monoamine oxidase inhibitors, beta blockers, veratrum alkaloids, cardiac glycosides, and certain other agents. Compounds in these categories include:

Acebutolol Hydrochloride (Increased effect of sympathomimetic). Products include:
Sectral Capsules ... 2520

Antidepressant Medications, unspecified (Effect not specified).

Atenolol (Increased effect of sympathomimetic). Products include:
Tenoretic Tablets ... 1105
Tenormin Tablets and I.V. Injection 1107

Betaxolol Hydrochloride (Increased effect of sympathomimetic). Products include:
Betoptic Sterile Ophthalmic Solution ... 569
Betoptic S Sterile Ophthalmic Suspension ... 570
Kerlone Tablets ... 2172

Blood Pressure Medications, unspecified (Effect not specified).
No products indexed under this heading.

Carteolol Hydrochloride (Increased effect of sympathomimetic). Products include:
Cartrol Tablets ... 507

Cryptenamine Preparations (Reduced antihypertensive effects).

Deslanoside (Increased possibility of cardiac arrhythmias).
No products indexed under this heading.

Digitoxin (Increased possibility of cardiac arrhythmias). Products include:
Crystodigin Tablets ... 1253

Digoxin (Increased possibility of cardiac arrhythmias). Products include:
Lanoxicaps ... 772
Lanoxin Elixir Pediatric ... 775
Lanoxin Injection ... 778
Lanoxin Injection Pediatric ... 781
Lanoxin Tablets ... 783

Esmolol Hydrochloride (Increased effect of sympathomimetic). Products include:
Brevibloc Injection ... 942

Furazolidone (Increased effect of sympathomimetic; concurrent therapy is contraindicated). Products include:
Furoxone ... 1855

Isocarboxazid (Increased effect of sympathomimetic; concurrent therapy is contraindicated). Products include:
Marplan Tablets ... 1906

Labetalol Hydrochloride (Increased effect of sympathomimetic). Products include:
Normodyne Injection ... 2108
Normodyne Tablets ... 2110
Normozide Tablets ... 2112
Trandate HCT Tablets ... 579
Trandate Injection ... 577
Trandate Tablets ... 579

Mecamylamine Hydrochloride (Reduced antihypertensive effects). Products include:
Inversine Tablets ... 1492

Methyldopa (Reduced antihypertensive effects). Products include:
Aldoclor Tablets ... 1413
Aldomet Oral ... 1415
Aldoril Tablets ... 1418

Methyldopate Hydrochloride (Reduced antihypertensive effects). Products include:
Aldomet Ester HCl Injection ... 1417

Metoprolol Tartrate (Increased effect of sympathomimetic). Products include:
Lopressor Ampuls ... 1032
Lopressor HCT Tablets ... 1034
Lopressor Tablets ... 1032

Nadolol (Increased effect of sympathomimetic). Products include:
Corgard Tablets ... 701
Corzide Tablets ... 702

Penbutolol Sulfate (Increased effect of sympathomimetic). Products include:
Levatol ... 1832

Phenelzine Sulfate (Increased effect of sympathomimetic; concurrent therapy is contraindicated). Products include:
Nardil ... 1742

Pindolol (Increased effect of sympathomimetic). Products include:
Visken Tablets ... 2036

Propranolol Hydrochloride (Increased effect of sympathomimetic). Products include:
Inderal ... 2459
Inderal LA Long Acting Capsules ... 2461
Inderide Tablets ... 2463
Inderide LA Long Acting Capsules .. 2465

Reserpine (Reduced antihypertensive effects). Products include:
Diupres Tablets ... 1461
Hydromox R Tablets ... 1209
Hydropres Tablets ... 1485
Renese-R Tablets ... 1786
Salutensin/Salutensin-Demi ... 719
Ser-Ap-Es Tablets ... 881
Serpasil Tablets ... 883
Serpasil-Apresoline Tablets ... 884
Serpasil-Esidrix Tablets ... 886

Selegiline Hydrochloride (Increased effect of sympathomimetic; concurrent therapy is contraindicated). Products include:
Eldepryl ... 2250

Timolol Maleate (Increased effect of sympathomimetic). Products include:
Blocadren Tablets ... 1429
Timolide Tablets ... 1547
Timoptic in Ocudose ... 1552
Timoptic Sterile Ophthalmic Solution ... 1550

Tranylcypromine Sulfate (Increased effect of sympathomimetic; concurrent therapy is contraindicated). Products include:
Parnate Tablets ... 2222

GUAIFED-PD CAPSULES (TIMED RELEASE)
(Guaifenesin, Pseudoephedrine Hydrochloride) ... 1615
See **Guaifed Capsules (Timed Release)**

GUAIFED SYRUP
(Guaifenesin, Pseudoephedrine Hydrochloride)........ND 629
May interact with monoamine oxidase inhibitors. Compounds in this category include:

Furazolidone (Concurrent use is contraindicated). Products include:
Furoxone........1855

Isocarboxazid (Concurrent use is contraindicated). Products include:
Marplan Tablets........1906

Phenelzine Sulfate (Concurrent use is contraindicated). Products include:
Nardil........1742

Selegiline Hydrochloride (Concurrent use is contraindicated). Products include:
Eldepryl........2250

Tranylcypromine Sulfate (Concurrent use is contraindicated). Products include:
Parnate Tablets........2222

GYNECORT 5 CREME
(Hydrocortisone)........ND 556
No interactions described in labeling.

GYNE-LOTRIMIN VAGINAL INSERTS
(Clotrimazole)........ND 702
No interactions described in labeling.

GYNOL II EXTRA STRENGTH CONTRACEPTIVE JELLY
(Nonoxynol-9)........ND 632
No interactions described in labeling.

GYNOL II ORIGINAL FORMULA CONTRACEPTIVE JELLY
(Nonoxynol-9)........ND 632
No interactions described in labeling.

HMS LIQUIFILM
(Medrysone)........⊙ 247
No interactions described in labeling.

HALCION TABLETS
(Triazolam)........2340
May interact with benzodiazepines, psychotropics, anticonvulsants, antihistamines, central nervous system depressants, and certain other agents. Compounds in these categories include:

Alcohol (Additive CNS depressant effects).

Alfentanil Hydrochloride (Additive CNS depressant effects). Products include:
Alfenta Injection........1131

Alprazolam (Additive CNS depressant effects). Products include:
Xanax Tablets........2367

Amitriptyline Hydrochloride (Additive CNS depressant effects). Products include:
Elavil........2269
Endep Tablets........1927
Etrafon........2087
Limbitrol........1933
Triavil Tablets........1556

Amoxapine (Additive CNS depressant effects). Products include:
Asendin Tablets........1196

Aprobarbital (Additive CNS depressant effects). Products include:
Alurate Elixir........1883

Astemizole (Additive CNS depressant effects). Products include:
Hismanal Tablets........1138

Azatadine Maleate (Additive CNS depressant effects). Products include:
Optimine Tablets........2115
Trinalin Repetabs Tablets........1170

Bromodiphenhydramine Hydrochloride (Additive CNS depressant effects).
No products indexed under this heading.

Brompheniramine Maleate (Additive CNS depressant effects). Products include:
Alka Seltzer Plus Sinus Allergy Medicine........ND 624
Atrohist Sprinkle Capsules........558
Bromfed Capsules (Timed Release)........1615
Bromfed Syrup........ND 628
Bromfed........1615
Dimetane Decongestant........ND 673
Dimetane........ND 672
Dimetane-DC Cough Syrup........1857
Dimetane-DX Cough Syrup........1858
Dimetapp Elixir........ND 673
Dimetapp DM Elixir........ND 674
Dimetapp Extentabs........ND 674
Dimetapp Plus Caplets........ND 675
Dimetapp Tablets........ND 675
Drixoral Antihistamine/Nasal Decongestant Syrup........ND 698

Buprenorphine (Additive CNS depressant effects).
No products indexed under this heading.

Buspirone Hydrochloride (Additive CNS depressant effects). Products include:
BuSpar........1401

Butabarbital (Additive CNS depressant effects). Products include:
Pyridium Plus........1764

Butalbital (Additive CNS depressant effects). Products include:
Esgic-Plus Tablets........1002
Esgic Tablets & Capsules........1001
Fioricet Tablets........2006
Fiorinal Capsules........2007
Fiorinal with Codeine Capsules........2008
Fiorinal Tablets........2007
Phrenilin........838
Sedapap Tablets 50 mg/650 mg..1360

Carbamazepine (Additive CNS depressant effects). Products include:
Tegretol Chewable Tablets........654
Tegretol Suspension........656
Tegretol Tablets........654

Chlordiazepoxide (Additive CNS depressant effects). Products include:
Libritabs Tablets........1930
Limbitrol........1933
Menrium Tablets........1934

Chlordiazepoxide Hydrochloride (Additive CNS depressant effects). Products include:
Librax Capsules........1929
Librium Capsules........1931
Librium Injectable........1932

Chlorpheniramine Maleate (Additive CNS depressant effects). Products include:
A.R.M. Allergy Relief Medicine Caplets........ND 615
Alka-Seltzer Plus Cold Medicine........ND 623
Allerest........ND 559
Ana-Kit Anaphylaxis Emergency Treatment Kit........1100
BC Cold Powder Multi-Symptom Formula........ND 517
Brexin L.A. Capsules........2078
Cerose-DM........2443
Cheracol Plus Head Cold/Cough Formula........ND 667
Chlor-Trimeton Allergy Syrup, Tablets & Long-Acting Repetabs Tablets........ND 693
Chlor-Trimeton Decongestant........ND 694
Comhist LA Capsules........1618
Allergy-Sinus Comtrex Multi-Symptom Allergy Sinus Formula Tablets & Caplets........746
Comtrex Multi-Symptom Cold Reliever Tablets/Caplets/Liqui-Gels/Liquid........745
Day-Night Comtrex........747
Contac Continuous Action Decongestant/Antihistamine Capsules ND 710
Contac Maximum Strength Continuous Action Decongestant/Antihistamine Caplets........ND 709
Contac Severe Cold and Flu Formula Caplets........ND 711
Coricidin 'D' Decongestant Tablets........ND 695
Coricidin Demilets Tablets for Children........ND 696
Coricidin Tablets........ND 695
Deconamine........663
Demazin Nasal Decongestant/Antihistamine Repetabs Tablets & Syrup........ND 697
Dorcol Children's Liquid Cold Formula........ND 686
Dristan Decongestant/Antihistamine/ Analgesic Coated Caplets........ND 749
Dristan Cold Nasal Decongestant/Antihistamine/ Analgesic Coated Tablets........2419
Dristan Advanced Formula Decongestant/Antihistamine/Analgesic Tablets........ND 749
Extendryl........994
4-Way Cold Tablets........750
Fedahist Gyrocaps........2145
Fedahist Timecaps........2145
Hycomine Compound Tablets........929
Isoclor Timesule Capsules........ND 561
Kronofed-A........970
Medi-Flu Caplet, Liquid........ND 640
Naldecon Syrup, Tablets, Pediatric Drops and Pediatric Syrup........709
Nolamine Tablets........838
Novafed A Capsules........1342
Novahistine DH........1342
Novahistine Elixir........ND 596
Ornade Spansule Capsules........2221
Orthoxicol Cough Syrup........ND 668
PediaCare Allergy Relief Formula Liquid........1362
PediaCare Cough-Cold Formula Liquid........1362
PediaCare Night Rest Cough-Cold Formula Liquid........1362
PediaCare 6-12 Cough-Cold Formula Chewable Tablets........1362
Pyrroxate Capsules........ND 669
Quelidrine Syrup........556
Ru-Tuss II Capsules........693
Ru-Tuss Tablets........693
Ryna........ND 741
Sinarest Tablets & Extra Strength Tablets........ND 562
Sine-Off Maximum Strength Allergy/Sinus Formula Caplets........ND 721
Sine-Off Sinus Medicine Tablets-Aspirin Formula........ND 722
Singlet Tablets........ND 598
Sinulin........840
Sinutab Maximum Strength........ND 641
St. Joseph Nighttime Cold Medicine........ND 705
Sudafed Plus Liquid........ND 544
Sudafed Plus Tablets........ND 545
Teldrin Timed-Release Allergy Capsules, 12 mg........2192
TheraFlu Flu and Cold Medicine........ND 687
Triaminic Allergy Tablets........ND 688
Triaminic Chewables........ND 688
Triaminic Cold Tablets........ND 688
Triaminic Nite Light........ND 689
Triaminic Syrup........ND 689
Triaminic-12 Tablets........ND 690
Triaminicin Tablets........ND 690
Triaminicol Multi-Symptom Cold Tablets........ND 691
Triaminicol Multi-Symptom Relief ND 691
Tylenol Allergy Sinus Medication Caplets and Gelcaps, Maximum Strength........1372
Children's Tylenol Cold Liquid Formula and Chewable Tablets........1368
Tylenol Cold & Flu Hot Medication, Packets........1369
Tylenol Cold Medication Caplets and Tablets........1370
Tylenol Cold Medication, Effervescent Tablets........1369
Vicks Children's NyQuil........ND 664
Vicks Formula 44 Cough Medicine........ND 661
Vicks Formula 44M Multi-Symptom Cough Medicine........ND 662
Vicks Pediatric Formula 44m Multi-Symptom Cough & Cold Medicine........ND 663

Chlorpheniramine Polistirex (Additive CNS depressant effects). Products include:
Tussionex Extended-Release Suspension........988

Chlorpheniramine Tannate (Additive CNS depressant effects). Products include:
Rynatan........2387
Rynatuss........2388

Chlorpromazine (Additive CNS depressant effects). Products include:
Thorazine........2234

Chlorprothixene (Additive CNS depressant effects). Products include:
Taractan Tablets........1920

Chlorprothixene Hydrochloride (Additive CNS depressant effects). Products include:
Taractan........1920

Cimetidine (Plasma levels and elimination half-life of triazolam doubled). Products include:
Tagamet Tablets........2228

Cimetidine Hydrochloride (Plasma levels and elimination half-life of triazolam doubled). Products include:
Tagamet........2228

Clemastine Fumarate (Additive CNS depressant effects). Products include:
Tavist Syrup........2033
Tavist Tablets........2035
Tavist-D Tablets........2035

Clorazepate Dipotassium (Additive CNS depressant effects). Products include:
Tranxene........556

Codeine (Additive CNS depressant effects). Products include:
Calcidrine Syrup........506

Codeine Phosphate (Additive CNS depressant effects). Products include:
Actifed with Codeine Cough Syrup..752
Cheracol Cough Syrup........1853
Codimal PH Syrup........846
Dimetane-DC Cough Syrup........1857
Empirin with Codeine Phosphate Nos. 2, 3 & 4........764
Fiorinal with Codeine Capsules........2008
Isoclor Expectorant........982
Naldecon CX Adult Liquid........ND 521
Novahistine DH........1342
Novahistine Expectorant........1343
Nucofed Capsules........2219
Nucofed Expectorant........2219
Nucofed Pediatric Expectorant........2220
Nucofed Syrup........2219
Phenaphen with Codeine Capsules 1865
Phenaphen-650 with Codeine Tablets........1866
Phenergan with Codeine........2497
Phenergan VC with Codeine........2501
Robitussin A-C Syrup........1875
Robitussin-DAC Syrup........1875
Ryna........ND 741
Soma Compound w/Codeine Tablets........2390
Triaminic Expectorant w/Codeine..1996
Tussi-Organidin Liquid........2391
Tylenol with Codeine........1381

Codeine Polistirex (Additive CNS depressant effects).
No products indexed under this heading.

Cyproheptadine Hydrochloride (Additive CNS depressant effects). Products include:
Periactin........1525

Desipramine Hydrochloride (Additive CNS depressant effects). Products include:
Norpramin Tablets........1340

Dexchlorpheniramine Maleate (Additive CNS depressant effects). Products include:
- Polaramine ... 2116

Dezocine (Additive CNS depressant effects).

Diazepam (Additive CNS depressant effects). Products include:
- Valium Injectable ... 1937
- Valium Tablets ... 1939
- Valrelease Capsules ... 1923

Diphenhydramine Hydrochloride (Additive CNS depressant effects). Products include:
- Benadryl Anti-Itch Cream ... ▣ 635
- Benadryl Capsules ... 1691
- Benadryl Decongestant Elixir ... ▣ 635
- Benadryl Decongestant ... ▣ 635
- Benadryl Elixir ... ▣ 636
- Benadryl Kapseals ... 1691
- Benadryl 25 Kapseals ... ▣ 636
- Benadryl Parenteral ... 1692
- Benadryl Plus ... ▣ 636
- Benadryl Plus Nighttime ... ▣ 637
- Benadryl Spray, Maximum Strength ... ▣ 637
- Benadryl Spray, Regular Strength ▣ 637
- Benadryl Steri-Vials, Ampoules, and Steri-Dose Syringe ... 1692
- Benadryl 25 Tablets ... ▣ 636
- Benylin Cough Syrup ... ▣ 637
- Benylin Decongestant ... ▣ 638
- Caladryl Cream, Lotion, Spray ... ▣ 638
- Miles Nervine Nighttime Sleep-Aid ▣ 627
- Nytol Tablets ... ▣ 517
- Sleep-ettes-D Tablets ... ▣ 653
- Sleep-eze 3 Tablets ... ▣ 755
- Sleepinal Night-time Sleep Aid Capsules ... ▣ 734
- Sominex Caplets and Tablets ... ▣ 722
- Sominex Liquid ... ▣ 723
- Sominex Pain Relief Formula ... ▣ 723
- Tylenol Cold Night Time Medication Liquid ... 1371
- Tylenol PM, Extra Strength Caplets and Tablets ... 1368
- Unisom Dual Relief Nighttime Sleep Aid/Analgesic ... 1774
- Ziradryl Lotion ... ▣ 643

Diphenylpyraline Hydrochloride (Additive CNS depressant effects).
- No products indexed under this heading.

Divalproex Sodium (Additive CNS depressant effects). Products include:
- Depakote ... 512

Doxepin Hydrochloride (Additive CNS depressant effects). Products include:
- Sinequan ... 1960

Droperidol (Additive CNS depressant effects). Products include:
- Inapsine Injection ... 1140
- Innovar Injection ... 1141

Enflurane (Additive CNS depressant effects). Products include:
- Ethrane ... 599

Erythromycin (Plasma levels and elimination half-life of triazolam doubled). Products include:
- A/T/S Topical Gel and Topical Solution ... 1089
- AK-Mycin Ointment ... ◉ 204
- Benzamycin Topical Gel ... 907
- E-Mycin Tablets ... 688
- ETS-2% ... 1685
- ERYC ... 1720
- Erycette (erythromycin 2%) Topical Solution ... 1678
- Ery-Tab Tablets ... 521
- Erythromycin Base Filmtab ... 525
- Erythromycin Delayed-Release Capsules, USP ... 526
- Ilotycin Ophthalmic Ointment ... 915
- PCE Dispertab Tablets ... 549
- Pediazole ... 1973
- T-Stat 2.0% Topical Solution and Pads ... 2409
- Theramycin Z Topical Solution 2% 1410

Erythromycin Estolate (Plasma levels and elimination half-life of triazolam doubled). Products include:
- Ilosone ... 913

Erythromycin Ethylsuccinate (Plasma levels and elimination half-life of triazolam doubled). Products include:
- E.E.S. ... 522
- EryPed ... 519
- Pediazole ... 1973

Erythromycin Gluceptate (Plasma levels and elimination half-life of triazolam doubled). Products include:
- Ilotycin Gluceptate, IV, Vials ... 915

Erythromycin Stearate (Plasma levels and elimination half-life of triazolam doubled). Products include:
- Erythrocin Stearate Filmtab ... 523

Estazolam (Additive CNS depressant effects). Products include:
- ProSom Tablets ... 554

Ethchlorvynol (Additive CNS depressant effects). Products include:
- Placidyl Capsules ... 553

Ethinamate (Additive CNS depressant effects).
- No products indexed under this heading.

Ethosuximide (Additive CNS depressant effects). Products include:
- Zarontin Capsules ... 1768
- Zarontin Syrup ... 1769

Ethotoin (Additive CNS depressant effects). Products include:
- Peganone Tablets ... 551

Fentanyl (Additive CNS depressant effects). Products include:
- Duragesic Transdermal System ... 1133

Fentanyl Citrate (Additive CNS depressant effects). Products include:
- Innovar Injection ... 1141
- Sublimaze Injection ... 1146

Fluphenazine Decanoate (Additive CNS depressant effects). Products include:
- Prolixin Decanoate ... 1795

Fluphenazine Enanthate (Additive CNS depressant effects). Products include:
- Prolixin Enanthate ... 1796

Fluphenazine Hydrochloride (Additive CNS depressant effects). Products include:
- Prolixin Elixir ... 1793
- Prolixin Injection ... 1791
- Prolixin Oral Concentrate ... 1792
- Prolixin Tablets ... 1793

Flurazepam Hydrochloride (Additive CNS depressant effects). Products include:
- Dalmane Capsules ... 1927

Glutethimide (Additive CNS depressant effects).
- No products indexed under this heading.

Haloperidol (Additive CNS depressant effects). Products include:
- Haldol Injection, Tablets and Concentrate ... 1373

Haloperidol Decanoate (Additive CNS depressant effects). Products include:
- Haldol Decanoate ... 1375

Hydrocodone Bitartrate (Additive CNS depressant effects). Products include:
- Anexsia 5/500 Tablets ... 2196
- Anexsia 7.5/650 Tablets ... 2197
- Azdone Tablets ... 844
- Codiclear DH Syrup ... 845
- Codimal DH Syrup ... 846
- Damason-P ... 1356
- Hycodan Syrup, Tablets ... 927
- Hycomine Compound Tablets ... 929
- Hycomine Syrup ... 927
- Hycotuss Expectorant Syrup ... 930
- Hydrocet Capsules ... 835
- Lortab ASA Tablets ... 2414
- Lortab ... 2412
- Ru-Tuss with Hydrocodone ... 694
- Triaminic Expectorant DH ... 1995
- Vicodin Tablets ... 1187
- Vicodin ES Tablets ... 1189
- Zydone Capsules ... 941

Hydrocodone Polistirex (Additive CNS depressant effects). Products include:
- Tussionex Extended-Release Suspension ... 988

Hydroxyzine Hydrochloride (Additive CNS depressant effects). Products include:
- Atarax Tablets & Syrup ... 1941
- Marax Tablets & DF Syrup ... 1954
- Vistaril Intramuscular Solution ... 1970

Imipramine Hydrochloride (Additive CNS depressant effects). Products include:
- Tofranil Ampuls ... 1038
- Tofranil Tablets ... 1039

Imipramine Pamoate (Additive CNS depressant effects). Products include:
- Tofranil-PM Capsules ... 1041

Isocarboxazid (Additive CNS depressant effects). Products include:
- Marplan Tablets ... 1906

Isoflurane (Additive CNS depressant effects). Products include:
- Forane ... 600

Ketamine Hydrochloride (Additive CNS depressant effects). Products include:
- Ketalar ... 1726

Levorphanol Tartrate (Additive CNS depressant effects). Products include:
- Levo-Dromoran ... 1906

Lithium Carbonate (Additive CNS depressant effects). Products include:
- Eskalith ... 2214
- Lithane Tablets ... 1596
- Lithium Carbonate Capsules & Tablets ... 1984
- Lithobid Tablets ... 870

Lithium Citrate (Additive CNS depressant effects). Products include:
- Cibalith-S ... 870

Lorazepam (Additive CNS depressant effects). Products include:
- Ativan Injection ... 2432
- Ativan Tablets ... 2434

Loxapine Hydrochloride (Additive CNS depressant effects). Products include:
- Loxitane ... 1213

Loxapine Succinate (Additive CNS depressant effects). Products include:
- Loxitane Capsules ... 1213

Maprotiline Hydrochloride (Additive CNS depressant effects). Products include:
- Ludiomil Tablets ... 874

Meperidine Hydrochloride (Additive CNS depressant effects). Products include:
- Demerol ... 2047
- Mepergan Injection ... 2479

Mephenytoin (Additive CNS depressant effects). Products include:
- Mesantoin Tablets ... 2013

Mephobarbital (Additive CNS depressant effects). Products include:
- Mebaral Tablets ... 2061

Meprobamate (Additive CNS depressant effects). Products include:
- Deprol Tablets ... 2382
- Equagesic Tablets ... 2451
- Miltown Tablets ... 2386
- PMB 200 and PMB 400 ... 2504

Mesoridazine (Additive CNS depressant effects). Products include:
- Serentil ... 686

Methadone Hydrochloride (Additive CNS depressant effects). Products include:
- Dolophine Hydrochloride Ampoules & Vials ... 1260
- Dolophine Hydrochloride Tablets ... 1261
- Methadone Hydrochloride Diskets .. 1284
- Methadone Hydrochloride Oral Solution & Tablets ... 1987

Methdilazine Hydrochloride (Additive CNS depressant effects). Products include:
- Tacaryl Syrup & Tablets ... 2409

Methohexital Sodium (Additive CNS depressant effects). Products include:
- Brevital Sodium Vials ... 1248

Methoxyflurane (Additive CNS depressant effects).
- No products indexed under this heading.

Methsuximide (Additive CNS depressant effects). Products include:
- Celontin ... 1692

Midazolam Hydrochloride (Additive CNS depressant effects). Products include:
- Versed Injection ... 1924

Molindone Hydrochloride (Additive CNS depressant effects). Products include:
- Moban Tablets & Concentrate ... 932

Morphine Sulfate (Additive CNS depressant effects). Products include:
- Astramorph/PF Injection, USP (Preservative-Free) ... 618
- Duramorph ... 960
- Infumorph 200 and Infumorph 500 Sterile Solutions ... 962
- MS Contin Tablets ... 1814
- MSIR ... 1817
- Oramorph SR (Morphine Sulfate Sustained Release Tablets) ... 1988
- Roxanol ... 1991

Nortriptyline Hydrochloride (Additive CNS depressant effects). Products include:
- Pamelor ... 2019

Opium Alkaloids (Additive CNS depressant effects). Products include:
- B & O No. 15A & No. 16A Supprettes ... 2395
- Pantopon Injectable ... 1911

Oxazepam (Additive CNS depressant effects). Products include:
- Serax Capsules ... 2522
- Serax Tablets ... 2522

Oxycodone Hydrochloride (Additive CNS depressant effects). Products include:
- Percocet Tablets ... 950
- Percodan ... 951
- Roxicodone Tablets, Oral Solution & Intensol (Oxycodone) ... 1992
- Tylox Capsules ... 1382

Paramethadione (Additive CNS depressant effects). Products include:
- Paradione Capsules ... 548

Pentobarbital Sodium (Additive CNS depressant effects). Products include:
- Nembutal Sodium Capsules ... 534
- Nembutal Sodium Solution ... 536
- Nembutal Sodium Suppositories ... 538

Perphenazine (Additive CNS depressant effects). Products include:
- Etrafon ... 2087
- Triavil Tablets ... 1556
- Trilafon ... 2123

Phenacemide (Additive CNS depressant effects). Products include:
- Phenurone Tablets ... 552

(▣ Described in PDR For Nonprescription Drugs)

(◉ Described in PDR For Ophthalmology)

Phenelzine Sulfate (Additive CNS depressant effects). Products include:
Nardil 1742

Phenobarbital (Additive CNS depressant effects). Products include:
Arco-Lase Plus Tablets 607
Bellergal-S Tablets 1998
Bronkolixir ..... ▣ 761
Bronkotabs Tablets ..... ▣ 762
Donnatal 1858
Donnatal Extentabs 1859
Donnatal Tablets 1858
Donnazyme Tablets 1860
Kinesed Tablets 2272
Phenobarbital Elixir and Tablets 1293
Primatene Tablets-P Formula 2421
Quadrinal Tablets 1183
Tedral SA 1765

Phensuximide (Additive CNS depressant effects). Products include:
Milontin Kapseals 1741

Phenytoin (Additive CNS depressant effects). Products include:
Dilantin Infatabs 1710
Dilantin-30 Pediatric/Dilantin-125 Suspension 1713

Phenytoin Sodium (Additive CNS depressant effects). Products include:
Dilantin Kapseals 1708
Dilantin Parenteral 1712
Dilantin with Phenobarbital Kapseals 1715

Prazepam (Additive CNS depressant effects). Products include:
Centrax 1693

Primidone (Additive CNS depressant effects). Products include:
Mysoline 2480

Prochlorperazine (Additive CNS depressant effects). Products include:
Compazine 2201

Promethazine Hydrochloride (Additive CNS depressant effects). Products include:
Mepergan Injection 2479
Phenergan with Codeine 2497
Phenergan with Dextromethorphan 2499
Phenergan Injection 2493
Phenergan Suppositories 2496
Phenergan Syrup 2495
Phenergan Tablets 2496
Phenergan VC 2500
Phenergan VC with Codeine 2501

Propofol (Additive CNS depressant effects). Products include:
Diprivan Injection 2267

Propoxyphene Hydrochloride (Additive CNS depressant effects). Products include:
Darvon 1256
Wygesic Tablets 2540

Propoxyphene Napsylate (Additive CNS depressant effects). Products include:
Darvon-N/Darvocet-N 1254

Protriptyline Hydrochloride (Additive CNS depressant effects). Products include:
Vivactil Tablets 1567

Pyrilamine Maleate (Additive CNS depressant effects). Products include:
Codimal 846
4-Way Fast Acting Nasal Spray - Original Formula (regular & mentholated) & Metered Spray Pump (regular) 751
Maximum Strength Midol Multi-Symptom Menstrual Formula ..... ▣ 571
Maximum Strength Midol PMS Premenstrual Syndrome Formula ..... ▣ 570
Regular Strength Midol Multi-Symptom Menstrual Formula ..... ▣ 570
Prefrin-A ..... ⊙ 255
Prēmsyn PMS Capsules & Caplets ▣ 547
Primatene Tablets-M Formula 2421
Robitussin Night Relief ..... ▣ 677
Ru-Tuss with Hydrocodone 694
Triaminic Expectorant DH 1995
Triaminic Oral Infant Drops 1996

Pyrilamine Tannate (Additive CNS depressant effects). Products include:
Rynatan 2387

Quazepam (Additive CNS depressant effects). Products include:
Doral Tablets 2383

Secobarbital Sodium (Additive CNS depressant effects). Products include:
Seconal Sodium Pulvules 1296

Sufentanil Citrate (Additive CNS depressant effects). Products include:
Sufenta Injection 1147

Temazepam (Additive CNS depressant effects). Products include:
Restoril Capsules 2023

Terfenadine (Additive CNS depressant effects). Products include:
Seldane Tablets 1349
Seldane-D Extended-Release Tablets 1350

Thiamylal Sodium (Additive CNS depressant effects). Products include:
Surital Ampoules, Steri-Vials 1764

Thioridazine Hydrochloride (Additive CNS depressant effects). Products include:
Mellaril 2011

Thiothixene (Additive CNS depressant effects). Products include:
Navane Capsules and Concentrate 1954
Navane Intramuscular 1956

Tranylcypromine Sulfate (Additive CNS depressant effects). Products include:
Parnate Tablets 2222

Trifluoperazine Hydrochloride (Additive CNS depressant effects). Products include:
Stelazine 2226

Trimeprazine Tartrate (Additive CNS depressant effects). Products include:
Temaril Tablets, Syrup and Spansule Sustained Release Capsules 1085

Trimethadione (Additive CNS depressant effects). Products include:
Tridione 557

Trimipramine Maleate (Additive CNS depressant effects). Products include:
Surmontil Capsules 2524

Tripelennamine Hydrochloride (Additive CNS depressant effects). Products include:
PBZ Tablets & Elixir 1037
PBZ-SR Tablets 1037

Triprolidine Hydrochloride (Additive CNS depressant effects). Products include:
Actidil ..... ▣ 538
Actifed Capsules ..... ▣ 539
Actifed Plus Caplets ..... ▣ 539
Actifed Plus Tablets ..... ▣ 540
Actifed with Codeine Cough Syrup .. 752
Actifed Syrup ..... ▣ 540
Actifed Tablets ..... ▣ 540
Actifed 12-Hour Capsules ..... ▣ 539

Valproic Acid (Additive CNS depressant effects). Products include:
Depakene Capsules & Syrup 511

HALDOL DECANOATE 50 (50 MG/ML) INJECTION

(Haloperidol Decanoate) 1375

May interact with narcotic analgesics, general anesthetics, oral anticoagulants, lithium preparations, central nervous system depressants, anticonvulsants, and certain other agents. Compounds in these categories include:

Alcohol (CNS depressant potentiated).

Alfentanil Hydrochloride (CNS depressant potentiated). Products include:
Alfenta Injection 1131

Alprazolam (CNS depressant potentiated). Products include:
Xanax Tablets 2367

Aprobarbital (CNS depressant potentiated). Products include:
Alurate Elixir 1883

Buprenorphine (CNS depressant potentiated).
No products indexed under this heading.

Buspirone Hydrochloride (CNS depressant potentiated). Products include:
BuSpar 1401

Butabarbital (CNS depressant potentiated). Products include:
Pyridium Plus 1764

Butalbital (CNS depressant potentiated). Products include:
Esgic-Plus Tablets 1002
Esgic Tablets & Capsules 1001
Fioricet Tablets 2006
Fiorinal Capsules 2007
Fiorinal with Codeine Capsules 2008
Fiorinal Tablets 2007
Phrenilin 838
Sedapap Tablets 50 mg/650 mg .. 1360

Carbamazepine (Haldol lowers the convulsive threshold). Products include:
Tegretol Chewable Tablets 654
Tegretol Suspension 656
Tegretol Tablets 654

Chlordiazepoxide (CNS depressant potentiated). Products include:
Libritabs Tablets 1930
Limbitrol 1933
Menrium Tablets 1934

Chlordiazepoxide Hydrochloride (CNS depressant potentiated). Products include:
Librax Capsules 1929
Librium Capsules 1931
Librium Injectable 1932

Chlorpromazine (CNS depressant potentiated). Products include:
Thorazine 2234

Chlorprothixene (CNS depressant potentiated). Products include:
Taractan Tablets 1920

Chlorprothixene Hydrochloride (CNS depressant potentiated). Products include:
Taractan 1920

Clorazepate Dipotassium (CNS depressant potentiated). Products include:
Tranxene 556

Codeine (CNS depressant potentiated). Products include:
Calcidrine Syrup 506

Codeine Phosphate (CNS depressant potentiated). Products include:
Actifed with Codeine Cough Syrup .. 752
Cheracol Cough Syrup 1853
Codimal PH Syrup 846
Dimetane-DC Cough Syrup 1857
Empirin with Codeine Phosphate Nos. 2, 3 & 4 764
Fiorinal with Codeine Capsules 2008
Isoclor Expectorant 982
Naldecon CX Adult Liquid ..... ▣ 521
Novahistine DH 1342
Novahistine Expectorant 1343
Nucofed Capsules 2219
Nucofed Expectorant 2219
Nucofed Pediatric Expectorant 2220
Nucofed Syrup 2219
Phenaphen with Codeine Capsules 1865
Phenaphen-650 with Codeine Tablets 1866
Phenergan with Codeine 2497
Phenergan VC with Codeine 2501
Robitussin A-C Syrup 1875
Robitussin-DAC Syrup 1875
Ryna ..... ▣ 741
Soma Compound w/Codeine Tablets 2390
Triaminic Expectorant w/Codeine .. 1996
Tussi-Organidin Liquid 2391
Tylenol with Codeine 1381

Codeine Polistirex (CNS depressant potentiated).
No products indexed under this heading.

Dezocine (CNS depressant potentiated).

Diazepam (CNS depressant potentiated). Products include:
Valium Injectable 1937
Valium Tablets 1939
Valrelease Capsules 1923

Dicumarol (Potential interference with anticoagulant activity). Products include:
Dicumarol Tablets 516

Divalproex Sodium (Haldol lowers the convulsive threshold). Products include:
Depakote 512

Droperidol (CNS depressant potentiated). Products include:
Inapsine Injection 1140
Innovar Injection 1141

Enflurane (CNS depressant potentiated). Products include:
Ethrane 599

Epinephrine Hydrochloride (Haloperidol may block vasopressor activity of epinephrine). Products include:
Adrenalin Chloride Solution 1:100 & 1:1,000 1689
Epifrin ..... ⊙ 244
Glaucon ..... ⊙ 218

Estazolam (CNS depressant potentiated). Products include:
ProSom Tablets 554

Ethchlorvynol (CNS depressant potentiated). Products include:
Placidyl Capsules 553

Ethinamate (CNS depressant potentiated).
No products indexed under this heading.

Ethosuximide (Haldol lowers the convulsive threshold). Products include:
Zarontin Capsules 1768
Zarontin Syrup 1769

Ethotoin (Haldol lowers the convulsive threshold). Products include:
Peganone Tablets 551

Fentanyl (CNS depressant potentiated). Products include:
Duragesic Transdermal System 1133

Fentanyl Citrate (CNS depressant potentiated). Products include:
Innovar Injection 1141
Sublimaze Injection 1146

Fluphenazine Decanoate (CNS depressant potentiated). Products include:
Prolixin Decanoate 1795

Fluphenazine Enanthate (CNS depressant potentiated). Products include:
Prolixin Enanthate 1796

Fluphenazine Hydrochloride (CNS depressant potentiated). Products include:
Prolixin Elixir 1793
Prolixin Injection 1791
Prolixin Oral Concentrate 1792
Prolixin Tablets 1793

Flurazepam Hydrochloride (CNS depressant potentiated). Products include:
Dalmane Capsules 1927

Glutethimide (CNS depressant potentiated).
No products indexed under this heading.

Haloperidol (CNS depressant potentiated). Products include:
Haldol Injection, Tablets and Concentrate ... 1373

Hydrocodone Bitartrate (CNS depressant potentiated). Products include:
Anexsia 5/500 Tablets ... 2196
Anexsia 7.5/650 Tablets ... 2197
Azdone Tablets ... 844
Codiclear DH Syrup ... 845
Codimal DH Syrup ... 846
Damason-P ... 1356
Hycodan Syrup, Tablets ... 927
Hycomine Compound Tablets ... 929
Hycomine Syrup ... 927
Hycotuss Expectorant Syrup ... 930
Hydrocet Capsules ... 835
Lortab ASA Tablets ... 2414
Lortab ... 2412
Ru-Tuss with Hydrocodone ... 694
Triaminic Expectorant DH ... 1995
Vicodin Tablets ... 1187
Vicodin ES Tablets ... 1189
Zydone Capsules ... 941

Hydrocodone Polistirex (CNS depressant potentiated). Products include:
Tussionex Extended-Release Suspension ... 988

Hydroxyzine Hydrochloride (CNS depressant potentiated). Products include:
Atarax Tablets & Syrup ... 1941
Marax Tablets & DF Syrup ... 1954
Vistaril Intramuscular Solution ... 1970

Isoflurane (CNS depressant potentiated). Products include:
Forane ... 600

Ketamine Hydrochloride (CNS depressant potentiated). Products include:
Ketalar ... 1726

Levorphanol Tartrate (CNS depressant potentiated). Products include:
Levo-Dromoran ... 1906

Lithium Carbonate (Potential for an encephalopathic syndrome followed by irreversible brain damage). Products include:
Eskalith ... 2214
Lithane Tablets ... 1596
Lithium Carbonate Capsules & Tablets ... 1984
Lithobid Tablets ... 870

Lithium Citrate (Potential for an encephalopathic syndrome followed by irreversible brain damage). Products include:
Cibalith-S ... 870

Lorazepam (CNS depressant potentiated). Products include:
Ativan Injection ... 2432
Ativan Tablets ... 2434

Loxapine Hydrochloride (CNS depressant potentiated). Products include:
Loxitane ... 1213

Loxapine Succinate (CNS depressant potentiated). Products include:
Loxitane Capsules ... 1213

Meperidine Hydrochloride (CNS depressant potentiated). Products include:
Demerol ... 2047
Mepergan Injection ... 2479

Mephenytoin (Haldol lowers the convulsive threshold). Products include:
Mesantoin Tablets ... 2013

Mephobarbital (CNS depressant potentiated). Products include:
Mebaral Tablets ... 2061

Meprobamate (CNS depressant potentiated). Products include:
Deprol Tablets ... 2382
Equagesic Tablets ... 2451
Miltown Tablets ... 2386
PMB 200 and PMB 400 ... 2504

Mesoridazine (CNS depressant potentiated). Products include:
Serentil ... 686

Methadone Hydrochloride (CNS depressant potentiated). Products include:
Dolophine Hydrochloride Ampoules & Vials ... 1260
Dolophine Hydrochloride Tablets ... 1261
Methadone Hydrochloride Diskets ... 1284
Methadone Hydrochloride Oral Solution & Tablets ... 1987

Methohexital Sodium (CNS depressant potentiated). Products include:
Brevital Sodium Vials ... 1248

Methoxyflurane (CNS depressant potentiated).
No products indexed under this heading.

Methsuximide (Haldol lowers the convulsive threshold). Products include:
Celontin ... 1692

Midazolam Hydrochloride (CNS depressant potentiated). Products include:
Versed Injection ... 1924

Molindone Hydrochloride (CNS depressant potentiated). Products include:
Moban Tablets & Concentrate ... 932

Morphine Sulfate (CNS depressant potentiated). Products include:
Astramorph/PF Injection, USP (Preservative-Free) ... 618
Duramorph ... 960
Infumorph 200 and Infumorph 500 Sterile Solutions ... 962
MS Contin Tablets ... 1814
MSIR ... 1817
Oramorph SR (Morphine Sulfate Sustained Release Tablets) ... 1988
Roxanol ... 1991

Opium Alkaloids (CNS depressant potentiated). Products include:
B & O No. 15A & No. 16A Supprettes ... 2395
Pantopon Injectable ... 1911

Oxazepam (CNS depressant potentiated). Products include:
Serax Capsules ... 2522
Serax Tablets ... 2522

Oxycodone Hydrochloride (CNS depressant potentiated). Products include:
Percocet Tablets ... 950
Percodan ... 951
Roxicodone Tablets, Oral Solution & Intensol (Oxycodone) ... 1992
Tylox Capsules ... 1382

Paramethadione (Haldol lowers the convulsive threshold). Products include:
Paradione Capsules ... 548

Pentobarbital Sodium (CNS depressant potentiated). Products include:
Nembutal Sodium Capsules ... 534
Nembutal Sodium Solution ... 536
Nembutal Sodium Suppositories ... 538

Perphenazine (CNS depressant potentiated). Products include:
Etrafon ... 2087
Triavil Tablets ... 1556
Trilafon ... 2123

Phenacemide (Haldol lowers the convulsive threshold). Products include:
Phenurone Tablets ... 552

Phenobarbital (Haldol lowers the convulsive threshold). Products include:
Arco-Lase Plus Tablets ... 607
Bellergal-S Tablets ... 1998
Bronkolixir ... ⊞ 761
Bronkotabs Tablets ... ⊞ 762
Donnatal ... 1858
Donnatal Extentabs ... 1859
Donnatal Tablets ... 1858
Donnazyme Tablets ... 1860
Kinesed Tablets ... 2272
Phenobarbital Elixir and Tablets ... 1293
Primatene Tablets-P Formula ... 2421
Quadrinal Tablets ... 1183
Tedral SA ... 1765

Phensuximide (Haldol lowers the convulsive threshold). Products include:
Milontin Kapseals ... 1741

Phenytoin (Haldol lowers the convulsive threshold). Products include:
Dilantin Infatabs ... 1710
Dilantin-30 Pediatric/Dilantin-125 Suspension ... 1713

Phenytoin Sodium (Haldol lowers the convulsive threshold). Products include:
Dilantin Kapseals ... 1708
Dilantin Parenteral ... 1712
Dilantin with Phenobarbital Kapseals ... 1715

Prazepam (CNS depressant potentiated). Products include:
Centrax ... 1693

Primidone (Haldol lowers the convulsive threshold). Products include:
Mysoline ... 2480

Prochlorperazine (CNS depressant potentiated). Products include:
Compazine ... 2201

Promethazine Hydrochloride (CNS depressant potentiated). Products include:
Mepergan Injection ... 2479
Phenergan with Codeine ... 2497
Phenergan with Dextromethorphan ... 2499
Phenergan Injection ... 2493
Phenergan Suppositories ... 2496
Phenergan Syrup ... 2495
Phenergan Tablets ... 2496
Phenergan VC ... 2500
Phenergan VC with Codeine ... 2501

Propofol (CNS depressant potentiated). Products include:
Diprivan Injection ... 2267

Propoxyphene Hydrochloride (CNS depressant potentiated). Products include:
Darvon ... 1256
Wygesic Tablets ... 2540

Propoxyphene Napsylate (CNS depressant potentiated). Products include:
Darvon-N/Darvocet-N ... 1254

Quazepam (CNS depressant potentiated). Products include:
Doral Tablets ... 2383

Secobarbital Sodium (CNS depressant potentiated). Products include:
Seconal Sodium Pulvules ... 1296

Sufentanil Citrate (CNS depressant potentiated). Products include:
Sufenta Injection ... 1147

Temazepam (CNS depressant potentiated). Products include:
Restoril Capsules ... 2023

Thiamylal Sodium (CNS depressant potentiated). Products include:
Surital Ampoules, Steri-Vials ... 1764

Thioridazine Hydrochloride (CNS depressant potentiated). Products include:
Mellaril ... 2011

Thiothixene (CNS depressant potentiated). Products include:
Navane Capsules and Concentrate ... 1954
Navane Intramuscular ... 1956

Triazolam (CNS depressant potentiated). Products include:
Halcion Tablets ... 2340

Tridihexethyl Chloride (Possible increase in intraocular pressure).
No products indexed under this heading.

Trifluoperazine Hydrochloride (CNS depressant potentiated). Products include:
Stelazine ... 2226

Trihexyphenidyl Hydrochloride (Possible increase in intraocular pressure). Products include:
Artane ... 1195

Trimethadione (Haldol lowers the convulsive threshold). Products include:
Tridione ... 557

Valproic Acid (Haldol lowers the convulsive threshold). Products include:
Depakene Capsules & Syrup ... 511

Warfarin Sodium (Potential interference with anticoagulant activity). Products include:
Coumadin Injection & Tablets ... 944
Panwarfin Tablets ... 547

HALDOL DECANOATE 100 (100 MG/ML) INJECTION
(Haloperidol Decanoate) ... 1375
See **Haldol Decanoate 50 (50 mg/mL) Injection**

HALDOL INJECTION, TABLETS AND CONCENTRATE
(Haloperidol) ... 1373
May interact with general anesthetics, narcotic analgesics, anticholinergics, and certain other agents. Compounds in these categories include:

Alcohol (CNS depressant potentiated).

Alfentanil Hydrochloride (CNS depressant potentiated). Products include:
Alfenta Injection ... 1131

Atropine Sulfate (Possible increase in intraocular pressure). Products include:
Arco-Lase Plus Tablets ... 607
Atropine Sulfate Sterile Ophthalmic Solution and S.O.P. Sterile Ophthalmic Ointment ... ⊙ 239
Donnagel ... ⊞ 675
Donnagel-PG ... 1858
Donnatal ... 1858
Donnatal Extentabs ... 1859
Donnatal Tablets ... 1858
Donnazyme Tablets ... 1860
Isopto Atropine ... ⊙ 218
Lomotil ... 2174
Motofen Tablets ... 836
Ru-Tuss Tablets ... 693
Urised Tablets ... 2396

Belladonna Alkaloids (Possible increase in intraocular pressure). Products include:
Bellergal-S Tablets ... 1998
Hyland's Bed Wetting Tablets ... ⊞ 728
Hyland's Teething Tablets ... ⊞ 728
Kinesed Tablets ... 2272

Benztropine Mesylate (Possible increase in intraocular pressure). Products include:
Cogentin ... 1435

Biperiden (Possible increase in intraocular pressure). Products include:
Akineton ... 1171

Buprenorphine (CNS depressant potentiated).
No products indexed under this heading.

Clidinium Bromide (Possible increase in intraocular pressure). Products include:
Librax Capsules ... 1929
Quarzan Capsules ... 1937

(⊞ Described in PDR For Nonprescription Drugs) (⊙ Described in PDR For Ophthalmology)

Codeine (CNS depressant potentiated). Products include:
- Calcidrine Syrup 506

Codeine Phosphate (CNS depressant potentiated). Products include:
- Actifed with Codeine Cough Syrup .. 752
- Cheracol Cough Syrup 1853
- Codimal PH Syrup 846
- Dimetane-DC Cough Syrup 1857
- Empirin with Codeine Phosphate Nos. 2, 3 & 4 764
- Fiorinal with Codeine Capsules 2008
- Isoclor Expectorant 982
- Naldecon CX Adult Liquid .... ▣ 521
- Novahistine DH 1342
- Novahistine Expectorant 1343
- Nucofed Capsules 2219
- Nucofed Expectorant 2219
- Nucofed Pediatric Expectorant 2220
- Nucofed Syrup 2219
- Phenaphen with Codeine Capsules 1865
- Phenaphen-650 with Codeine Tablets 1866
- Phenergan with Codeine 2497
- Phenergan VC with Codeine 2501
- Robitussin A-C Syrup 1875
- Robitussin-DAC Syrup 1875
- Ryna .... ▣ 741
- Soma Compound w/Codeine Tablets 2390
- Triaminic Expectorant w/Codeine .. 1996
- Tussi-Organidin Liquid 2391
- Tylenol with Codeine 1381

Codeine Polistirex (CNS depressant potentiated).
- No products indexed under this heading.

Dezocine (CNS depressant potentiated).

Dicyclomine Hydrochloride (Possible increase in intraocular pressure). Products include:
- Bentyl 1322

Enflurane (CNS depressant potentiated). Products include:
- Ethrane 599

Epinephrine Hydrochloride (Haloperidol may block vasopressor activity of epinephrine). Products include:
- Adrenalin Chloride Solution 1:100 & 1:1,000 1689
- Epifrin .... ◉ 244
- Glaucon .... ◉ 218

Ethopropazine Hydrochloride (Possible increase in intraocular pressure).

Fentanyl (CNS depressant potentiated). Products include:
- Duragesic Transdermal System 1133

Fentanyl Citrate (CNS depressant potentiated). Products include:
- Innovar Injection 1141
- Sublimaze Injection 1146

Glycopyrrolate (Possible increase in intraocular pressure). Products include:
- Robinul Forte Tablets 1873
- Robinul Injectable 1873
- Robinul Tablets 1873

Hydrocodone Bitartrate (CNS depressant potentiated). Products include:
- Anexsia 5/500 Tablets 2196
- Anexsia 7.5/650 Tablets 2197
- Azdōne Tablets 844
- Codiclear DH Syrup 845
- Codimal DH Syrup 846
- Damason-P 1356
- Hycodan Syrup, Tablets 927
- Hycomine Compound Tablets 929
- Hycomine Syrup 927
- Hycotuss Expectorant Syrup 930
- Hydrocet Capsules 835
- Lortab ASA Tablets 2414
- Lortab 2412
- Ru-Tuss with Hydrocodone 694
- Triaminic Expectorant DH 1995
- Vicodin Tablets 1187
- Vicodin ES Tablets 1189
- Zydone Capsules 941

Hydrocodone Polistirex (CNS depressant potentiated). Products include:
- Tussionex Extended-Release Suspension 988

Hyoscyamine (Possible increase in intraocular pressure). Products include:
- Cystospaz Tablets 2395
- Urised Tablets 2396

Hyoscyamine Sulfate (Possible increase in intraocular pressure). Products include:
- Arco-Lase Plus Tablets 607
- Cystospaz-M Capsules 2395
- Donnagel .... ▣ 675
- Donnagel-PG 1858
- Donnatal 1858
- Donnatal Extentabs 1859
- Donnatal Tablets 1858
- Donnazyme Tablets 1860
- Kutrase Capsules 2146
- Levsin/Levsinex 2147
- Ru-Tuss Tablets 693

Ipratropium Bromide (Possible increase in intraocular pressure). Products include:
- Atrovent Inhalation Aerosol 675

Isoflurane (CNS depressant potentiated). Products include:
- Forane 600

Levorphanol Tartrate (CNS depressant potentiated). Products include:
- Levo-Dromoran 1906

Lithium Carbonate (May produce neurotoxicity). Products include:
- Eskalith 2214
- Lithane Tablets 1596
- Lithium Carbonate Capsules & Tablets 1984
- Lithobid Tablets 870

Lithium Citrate (May produce neurotoxicity). Products include:
- Cibalith-S 870

Mepenzolate Bromide (Possible increase in intraocular pressure). Products include:
- Cantil Tablets 1326

Meperidine Hydrochloride (CNS depressant potentiated). Products include:
- Demerol 2047
- Mepergan Injection 2479

Methadone Hydrochloride (CNS depressant potentiated). Products include:
- Dolophine Hydrochloride Ampoules & Vials 1260
- Dolophine Hydrochloride Tablets 1261
- Methadone Hydrochloride Diskets .. 1284
- Methadone Hydrochloride Oral Solution & Tablets 1987

Methohexital Sodium (CNS depressant potentiated). Products include:
- Brevital Sodium Vials 1248

Methoxyflurane (CNS depressant potentiated).
- No products indexed under this heading.

Morphine Sulfate (CNS depressant potentiated). Products include:
- Astramorph/PF Injection, USP (Preservative-Free) 618
- Duramorph 960
- Infumorph 200 and Infumorph 500 Sterile Solutions 962
- MS Contin Tablets 1814
- MSIR 1817
- Oramorph SR (Morphine Sulfate Sustained Release Tablets) 1988
- Roxanol 1991

Opium Alkaloids (CNS depressant potentiated). Products include:
- B & O No. 15A & No. 16A Supprettes 2395
- Pantopon Injectable 1911

Oxybutynin Chloride (Possible increase in intraocular pressure). Products include:
- Ditropan 1332

Oxycodone Hydrochloride (CNS depressant potentiated). Products include:
- Percocet Tablets 950
- Percodan 951
- Roxicodone Tablets, Oral Solution & Intensol (Oxycodone) 1992
- Tylox Capsules 1382

Oxyphenonium Bromide (Possible increase in intraocular pressure).

Procyclidine Hydrochloride (Possible increase in intraocular pressure). Products include:
- Kemadrin Tablets 771

Propantheline Bromide (Possible increase in intraocular pressure). Products include:
- Pro-Banthine Tablets 2141

Propofol (CNS depressant potentiated). Products include:
- Diprivan Injection 2267

Propoxyphene Hydrochloride (CNS depressant potentiated). Products include:
- Darvon 1256
- Wygesic Tablets 2540

Propoxyphene Napsylate (CNS depressant potentiated). Products include:
- Darvon-N/Darvocet-N 1254

Scopolamine Hydrobromide (Possible increase in intraocular pressure). Products include:
- Donnagel .... ▣ 675
- Donnagel-PG 1858
- Donnatal 1858
- Donnatal Extentabs 1859
- Donnatal Tablets 1858
- Donnazyme Tablets 1860
- Isopto Hyoscine .... ◉ 222
- Murocoll-2 Sterile Ophthalmic Solution .... ◉ 261
- Ru-Tuss Tablets 693

Scopolamine Preparations (Possible increase in intraocular pressure). Products include:
- Transderm Scōp Transdermal Therapeutic System 887

Sufentanil Citrate (CNS depressant potentiated). Products include:
- Sufenta Injection 1147

Tridihexethyl Chloride (Possible increase in intraocular pressure).
- No products indexed under this heading.

Trihexyphenidyl Hydrochloride (Possible increase in intraocular pressure). Products include:
- Artane 1195

HALEY'S M-O, REGULAR & FLAVORED
(Magnesium Hydroxide, Mineral Oil) .... ▣ 569
May interact with stool softener laxatives. Compounds in this category include:

Docusate Calcium (Concurrent use is not recommended). Products include:
- Doxidan Capsules .... ▣ 736
- Surfak Capsules .... ▣ 737

Docusate Potassium (Concurrent use is not recommended). Products include:
- Dialose Capsules .... ▣ 577
- Dialose Plus Capsules .... ▣ 577
- Kasof Capsules .... ▣ 579

Docusate Sodium (Concurrent use is not recommended). Products include:
- Anticon .... ▣ 629
- Colace 1403
- Correctol Laxative Tablets .... ▣ 696
- Dialose Tablets 1154
- Dialose Plus Tablets 1154
- Extra Gentle Ex-Lax .... ▣ 687
- Feen-A-Mint Laxative Pills and Chocolated Mint Tablets .... ▣ 702
- Ferro-Sequels 1203
- Geriplex-FS Kapseals .... ▣ 639
- Geriplex-FS Liquid .... ▣ 639
- Modane Plus Tablets .... ▣ 504
- Peri-Colace 1409
- Peritinic Tablets .... ▣ 589
- Phillips' LaxCaps .... ▣ 572
- Senokot-S Tablets 1820

HALLS MENTHO-LYPTUS COUGH SUPPRESSANT TABLETS
(Eucalyptus, Oil of, Menthol) .... ▣ 742
No interactions described in labeling.

HALLS PLUS COUGH SUPPRESSANT TABLETS
(Menthol, Eucalyptus, Oil of) .... ▣ 742
No interactions described in labeling.

HALLS VITAMIN C DROPS
(Vitamin C) .... ▣ 742
No interactions described in labeling.

HALOG CREAM, OINTMENT & SOLUTION
(Halcinonide) 2399
No interactions described in labeling.

HALOG-E CREAM
(Halcinonide) 2399
No interactions described in labeling.

HALOTESTIN TABLETS
(Fluoxymesterone) 2341
May interact with oral anticoagulants, insulin, and certain other agents. Compounds in these categories include:

Dicumarol (Increased sensitivity to dicumarol). Products include:
- Dicumarol Tablets 516

Insulin, Human (Insulin requirements may be decreased).
- No products indexed under this heading.

Insulin, Human Isophane Suspension (Insulin requirements may be decreased). Products include:
- Humulin N, 100 Units 1270

Insulin, Human NPH (Insulin requirements may be decreased). Products include:
- Insulatard NPH Human 1627
- Novolin N 1627
- Novolin N PenFill Cartridges 1628
- Novolin N Prefilled 1628

Insulin, Human Regular (Insulin requirements may be decreased). Products include:
- Humulin BR, 100 Units 1268
- Humulin R, 100 Units 1272
- Novolin R 1627
- Novolin R PenFill Cartridges 1628
- Novolin R Prefilled 1629
- Velosulin Human 1628

Insulin, Human, Zinc Suspension (Insulin requirements may be decreased). Products include:
- Humulin L, 100 Units 1268
- Humulin U, 100 Units 1272
- Novolin L 1627

Insulin, NPH (Insulin requirements may be decreased). Products include:
- NPH, 40 & 100 Units 1273
- Beef NPH, 100 Units 1274
- Pork NPH, 100 Units 1275
- Insulatard NPH 1626
- NPH Insulin 1626
- NPH Purified Pork Isophane Insulin 1626

Insulin, Regular (Insulin requirements may be decreased). Products include:
- Regular, 40 & 100 Units 1273
- Beef Regular, 100 Units 1275
- Pork Regular, 100 Units 1275

Pork Regular (Concentrated), 500 Units 1276
Regular Insulin 1625
Regular Purified Pork Insulin 1626
Velosulin 1627

Insulin, Zinc Crystals (Insulin requirements may be decreased). Products include:
NPH, 40 & 100 Units 1273

Insulin, Zinc Suspension (Insulin requirements may be decreased). Products include:
Lente, 40 & 100 Units 1272
Protamine, Zinc, 40 & 100 Units 1273
Lente Iletin I 1272
Beef Lente, 100 Units 1274
Beef Protamine Zinc, 100 Units 1274
Pork Lente, 100 Units 1275
Pork, Protamine, Zinc, 100 Units 1275
Lente Insulin 1626
Lente Purified Pork Insulin 1626
Semilente Insulin 1625
Ultralente Insulin 1626

Oxyphenbutazone (Elevated serum levels of oxyphenbutazone).

Warfarin Sodium (Increased sensitivity to warfarin). Products include:
Coumadin Injection & Tablets 944
Panwarfin Tablets 547

HALOTEX CREAM & SOLUTION
(Haloprogin) 2400
No interactions described in labeling.

HALTRAN TABLETS
(Ibuprofen) .... ▣ 668
May interact with aspirin and acetaminophen containing products. Compounds in this category include:

Acetaminophen (Effect not specified). Products include:
Acetaminophen Uniserts Suppositories 2374
Actifed Plus Caplets .... ▣ 539
Actifed Plus Tablets .... ▣ 540
Alka-Seltzer Advanced Formula Antacid & Non-Aspirin Pain Reliever .... ▣ 620
Allerest .... ▣ 559
Aspirin Free Anacin Maximum Strength Acetaminophen Film Coated Caplets 2417
Aspirin Free Anacin Maximum Strength Acetaminophen Film Coated Tablets 2417
Anacin-3 Regular Strength Acetaminophen Film Coated Tablets ▣ 746
Anexsia 5/500 Tablets 2196
Anexsia 7.5/650 Tablets 2197
Benadryl Plus .... ▣ 636
Benadryl Plus Nighttime .... ▣ 637
Bufferin AF Nite Time Analgesic/Sleeping Aid Caplets 744
Allergy-Sinus Comtrex Multi-Symptom Allergy Sinus Formula Tablets & Caplets 746
Cough Formula Comtrex 746
Comtrex Multi-Symptom Cold Reliever Tablets/Caplets/Liqui-Gels/Liquid 745
Day-Night Comtrex 747
Non-Drowsy Comtrex 747
Congespirin For Children Aspirin Free Chewable Cold Tablets 748
Contac Cough & Sore Throat Formula .... ▣ 712
Contac Jr. Children's Cold Medicine .... ▣ 712
Contac Nighttime Cold Medicine .... ▣ 713
Contac Severe Cold and Flu Formula Caplets .... ▣ 711
Contac Sinus Caplets Maximum Strength Non-Drowsy Formula .... ▣ 710
Contac Sinus Tablets Maximum Strength Non-Drowsy Formula .... ▣ 710
Coricidin 'D' Decongestant Tablets .... ▣ 695
Coricidin Demilets Tablets for Children .... ▣ 696
Coricidin Tablets .... ▣ 695
Darvon-N/Darvocet-N 1254
Datril Extra-Strength Analgesic Tablets 748
Dimetapp Plus Caplets .... ▣ 675
Dorcol Children's Fever & Pain Reducer .... ▣ 686
Dristan Decongestant/Antihistamine/ Analgesic Coated Caplets .... ▣ 749
Dristan Cold Nasal Decongestant/ Antihistamine/ Analgesic Coated Tablets 2419
Dristan Advanced Formula Decongestant/Antihistamine/ Analgesic Tablets .... ▣ 749
Maximum Strength Dristan Decongestant/Analgesic Coated Caplets .... ▣ 750
No Drowsiness Dristan Cold Nasal Decongestant/Analgesic Coated Caplets 2420
Drixoral Plus Extended-Release Tablets .... ▣ 699
Drixoral Sinus .... ▣ 700
Esgic-Plus Tablets 1002
Esgic Tablets & Capsules 1001
Aspirin Free Excedrin Analgesic Caplets 748
Excedrin Extra-Strength Analgesic Tablets & Caplets 749
Excedrin P.M. Analgesic/Sleeping Aid Tablets, Caplets and Liquid 749
Sinus Excedrin Analgesic, Decongestant Tablets & Caplets 750
4-Way Cold Tablets 750
Feverall Sprinkle Caps 2374
Feverall Suppositories 2374
Fioricet Tablets 2006
Hycomine Compound Tablets 929
Hydrocet Capsules 835
Isocom Capsules 1629
Liquiprin .... ▣ 618
Lortab 2412
Lurline PMS Tablets 972
Medi-Flu Caplet, Liquid .... ▣ 640
Maximum Strength Midol Multi-Symptom Menstrual Formula .... ▣ 571
Maximum Strength Midol PMS Premenstrual Syndrome Formula .... ▣ 570
Regular Strength Midol Multi-Symptom Menstrual Formula .... ▣ 570
Midrin Capsules 836
Ornex Caplets .... ▣ 618
Children's Panadol Chewable Tablets, Liquid, Infants' Drops .... ▣ 571
Junior Strength Panadol .... ▣ 571
Maximum Strength Panadol Tablets and Caplets .... ▣ 572
Percocet Tablets 950
Percogesic Analgesic Tablets .... ▣ 660
Phenaphen with Codeine Capsules 1865
Phenaphen-650 with Codeine Tablets 1866
Phrenilin 838
Prēmsyn PMS Capsules & Caplets ▣ 547
Pyrroxate Capsules .... ▣ 669
Robitussin Night Relief .... ▣ 677
Sedapap Tablets 50 mg/650 mg .. 1360
Sinarest .... ▣ 562
Sine-Aid Maximum Strength Sinus Headache Caplets 1365
Sine-Aid Maximum Strength Sinus Headache Tablets 1365
Sine-Off Maximum Strength Allergy/Sinus Formula Caplets .... ▣ 721
Sine-Off Maximum Strength No Drowsiness Formula Caplets .... ▣ 722
Singlet Tablets .... ▣ 598
Sinulin 840
Sinutab Maximum Strength .... ▣ 641
Sinutab Maximum Strength Without Drowsiness Tablets & Caplets .... ▣ 642
Sinutab Regular Strength Without Drowsiness Formula .... ▣ 641
Sominex Pain Relief Formula .... ▣ 723
St. Joseph Aspirin-Free Fever Reducer for Children Chewable Tablets, Liquid & Infant Drops .... ▣ 704
St. Joseph Cold Tablets for Children .... ▣ 704
St. Joseph Nighttime Cold Medicine .... ▣ 705
Sudafed Sinus Caplets .... ▣ 545
Sudafed Sinus Tablets .... ▣ 545
Talacen 2070
Tempra, Acetaminophen .... ▣ 613
TheraFlu Flu and Cold Medicine .... ▣ 687
Triaminicin Tablets .... ▣ 690
Tylenol acetaminophen Children's Chewable Tablets & Elixir 1366
Tylenol Allergy Sinus Medication Caplets and Gelcaps, Maximum Strength 1372
Tylenol with Codeine 1381
Children's Tylenol Cold Liquid Formula and Chewable Tablets 1368
Tylenol Cold & Flu Hot Medication, Packets 1369
Tylenol Cold & Flu No Drowsiness Hot Medication, Packets 1371
Tylenol Cold Medication Caplets and Tablets 1370
Tylenol Cold Medication, Effervescent Tablets 1369
Tylenol Cold Medication No Drowsiness Formula Caplets 1370
Tylenol Cold Night Time Medication Liquid 1371
Tylenol Cough Medication Liquid, Maximum Strength 1372
Tylenol Cough Medication Liquid with Decongestant, Maximum Strength 1372
Tylenol, Extra Strength, acetaminophen Adult Liquid Pain Reliever .. 1367
Tylenol, Extra Strength, acetaminophen Gelcaps, Caplets, Tablets 1367
Tylenol, Infants' Drops 1366
Tylenol, Junior Strength, acetaminophen Coated Caplets, Grape and Fruit Chewable Tablets 1366
Tylenol, Maximum Strength, Sinus Medication Gelcaps, Caplets and Tablets 1373
Tylenol, Regular Strength, acetaminophen Tablets and Caplets 1367
Tylenol PM, Extra Strength Caplets and Tablets 1368
Tylox Capsules 1382
Unisom Dual Relief Nighttime Sleep Aid/Analgesic 1774
Vanquish Analgesic Caplets .... ▣ 574
Vicks Daycare .... ▣ 660
Vicks Formula 44M Multi-Symptom Cough Medicine .... ▣ 662
Vicks NyQuil Nighttime Colds Medicine-Original & Cherry Flavor .... ▣ 664
Vicodin Tablets 1187
Vicodin ES Tablets 1189
Wygesic Tablets 2540
Zydone Capsules 941

Aspirin (Effect not specified). Products include:
Alka-Seltzer Effervescent Antacid and Pain Reliever 1568
Alka-Seltzer Extra Strength Effervescent Antacid and Pain Reliever 1570
Alka-Seltzer (Flavored) Effervescent Antacid and Pain Reliever 1569
Alka-Seltzer Plus Cold Medicine .... ▣ 623
Alka-Seltzer Plus Night-Time Cold Medicine .... ▣ 623
Alka Seltzer Plus Sinus Allergy Medicine .... ▣ 624
Anacin Coated Analgesic Caplets 2417
Anacin Coated Analgesic Tablets 2417
Anacin Maximum Strength Analgesic Coated Tablets 2417
Maximum Strength Arthritis Pain Formula By the Makers of Anacin Analgesic Tablets and Caplets 2418
Arthritis Pain Formula by the Makers of Anacin Analgesic Tablets and Caplets .... ▣ 747
Arthritis Strength BC Powder .... ▣ 516
Ascriptin A/D Caplets 1850
Regular Strength Ascriptin Tablets 1850
Azdōne Tablets 844
BC Powder .... ▣ 517
BC Cold Powder .... ▣ 517
Children's Bayer Chewable Aspirin .... ▣ 564
Genuine Bayer Aspirin Tablets & Caplets .... ▣ 564
Maximum Bayer Aspirin Tablets & Caplets .... ▣ 566
Bayer Plus Aspirin Tablets .... ▣ 567
Therapy Bayer Aspirin Caplets .... ▣ 568
8 Hour Bayer Timed-Release Aspirin .... ▣ 566
Arthritis Strength Bufferin Analgesic Caplets 744
Extra Strength Bufferin Analgesic Tablets 745
Bufferin Analgesic Tablets and Caplets 743
Cama Arthritis Pain Reliever .... ▣ 685
Damason-P 1356
Easprin 1719
Ecotrin Enteric Coated Aspirin Maximum Strength Tablets and Caplets 2189
Ecotrin Enteric Coated Aspirin Regular Strength Tablets and Caplets 2189
Empirin Aspirin .... ▣ 541
Empirin with Codeine Phosphate Nos. 2, 3 & 4 764
Equagesic Tablets 2451
Excedrin Extra-Strength Analgesic Tablets & Caplets 749
4-Way Cold Tablets 750
Fiorinal Capsules 2007
Fiorinal with Codeine Capsules 2008
Fiorinal Tablets 2007
Lortab ASA Tablets 2414
Momentum Muscular Backache Formula .... ▣ 751
Norgesic 1314
Norwich Extra-Strength Aspirin .... ▣ 546
Norwich Regular Strength Aspirin ▣ 547
P-A-C Analgesic Tablets .... ▣ 669
Percodan 951
Robaxisal Tablets 1872
Sine-Off Sinus Medicine Tablets-Aspirin Formula .... ▣ 722
Soma Compound w/Codeine Tablets 2390
Soma Compound Tablets 2389
St. Joseph Adult Chewable Aspirin (81 mg.) .... ▣ 703
Synalgos-DC Capsules 2525
Talwin Compound 2072
Ursinus Inlay-Tabs .... ▣ 691
Vanquish Analgesic Caplets .... ▣ 574
Zorprin Tablets 698

HARMONYL TABLETS
(Deserpidine) 528
May interact with cardiac glycosides and certain other agents. Compounds in these categories include:

Deslanoside (Potential for cardiac arrhythmias).

Digitoxin (Potential for cardiac arrhythmias). Products include:
Crystodigin Tablets 1253

Digoxin (Potential for cardiac arrhythmias). Products include:
Lanoxicaps 772
Lanoxin Elixir Pediatric 775
Lanoxin Injection 778
Lanoxin Injection Pediatric 781
Lanoxin Tablets 783

Quinidine Gluconate (Potential for cardiac arrhythmias). Products include:
Quinaglute Dura-Tabs Tablets 663

Quinidine Polygalacturonate (Potential for cardiac arrhythmias). Products include:
Cardioquin Tablets 1812

Quinidine Sulfate (Potential for cardiac arrhythmias). Products include:
Quinidex Extentabs 1868

HEAD & SHOULDERS ANTIDANDRUFF SHAMPOO
(Pyrithione Zinc) .... ▣ 648
No interactions described in labeling.

HEAD & SHOULDERS DRY SCALP SHAMPOO
(Zinc Pyrithione) .... ▣ 648
No interactions described in labeling.

HEAD & SHOULDERS INTENSIVE TREATMENT DANDRUFF SHAMPOO
(Selenium Sulfide) .... ▣ 648
No interactions described in labeling.

HEALON
(Sodium Hyaluronate) .... ⊙ 279
No interactions described in labeling.

(▣ Described in PDR For Nonprescription Drugs)

(⊙ Described in PDR For Ophthalmology)

HEMOPAD ABSORBABLE COLLAGEN HEMOSTAT
(Collagen) 627
No interactions described in labeling.

HEPARIN LOCK FLUSH SOLUTION
(Heparin Sodium) 2456
May interact with cardiac glycosides, antihistamines, tetracyclines, non-steroidal anti-inflammatory agents, platelet inhibitors, and certain other agents. Compounds in these categories include:

Aspirin (Interferes with platelet-aggregation reactions and may induce bleeding). Products include:
- Alka-Seltzer Effervescent Antacid and Pain Reliever 1568
- Alka-Seltzer Extra Strength Effervescent Antacid and Pain Reliever 1570
- Alka-Seltzer (Flavored) Effervescent Antacid and Pain Reliever 1569
- Alka-Seltzer Plus Cold Medicine .... ⊞ 623
- Alka-Seltzer Plus Night-Time Cold Medicine .... ⊞ 623
- Alka Seltzer Plus Sinus Allergy Medicine .... ⊞ 624
- Anacin Coated Analgesic Caplets 2417
- Anacin Coated Analgesic Tablets 2417
- Anacin Maximum Strength Analgesic Coated Tablets 2417
- Maximum Strength Arthritis Pain Formula By the Makers of Anacin Analgesic Tablets and Caplets 2418
- Arthritis Pain Formula by the Makers of Anacin Analgesic Tablets and Caplets .... ⊞ 747
- Arthritis Strength BC Powder .... ⊞ 516
- Ascriptin A/D Caplets 1850
- Regular Strength Ascriptin Tablets 1850
- Azdōne Tablets 844
- BC Powder .... ⊞ 517
- BC Cold Powder .... ⊞ 517
- Children's Bayer Chewable Aspirin .... ⊞ 564
- Genuine Bayer Aspirin Tablets & Caplets .... ⊞ 564
- Maximum Bayer Aspirin Tablets & Caplets .... ⊞ 566
- Bayer Plus Aspirin Tablets .... ⊞ 567
- Therapy Bayer Aspirin Caplets .... ⊞ 568
- 8 Hour Bayer Timed-Release Aspirin .... ⊞ 566
- Arthritis Strength Bufferin Analgesic Caplets 744
- Extra Strength Bufferin Analgesic Tablets 745
- Bufferin Analgesic Tablets and Caplets 743
- Cama Arthritis Pain Reliever .... ⊞ 685
- Damason-P 1356
- Easprin 1719
- Ecotrin Enteric Coated Aspirin Maximum Strength Tablets and Caplets 2189
- Ecotrin Enteric Coated Aspirin Regular Strength Tablets and Caplets 2189
- Empirin Aspirin .... ⊞ 541
- Empirin with Codeine Phosphate Nos. 2, 3 & 4 764
- Equagesic Tablets 2451
- Excedrin Extra-Strength Analgesic Tablets & Caplets 749
- 4-Way Cold Tablets 750
- Fiorinal Capsules 2007
- Fiorinal with Codeine Capsules 2008
- Fiorinal Tablets 2007
- Lortab ASA Tablets 2414
- Momentum Muscular Backache Formula .... ⊞ 751
- Norgesic 1314
- Norwich Extra-Strength Aspirin .... ⊞ 546
- Norwich Regular Strength Aspirin .... ⊞ 547
- P-A-C Analgesic Tablets .... ⊞ 669
- Percodan 951
- Robaxisal Tablets 1872
- Sine-Off Sinus Medicine Tablets-Aspirin Formula .... ⊞ 722
- Soma Compound w/Codeine Tablets 2390
- Soma Compound Tablets 2389
- St. Joseph Adult Chewable Aspirin (81 mg.) .... ⊞ 703
- Synalgos-DC Capsules 2525
- Talwin Compound 2072
- Ursinus Inlay-Tabs .... ⊞ 691
- Vanquish Analgesic Caplets .... ⊞ 574
- Zorprin Tablets 698

Astemizole (Anticoagulant action partially counteracted). Products include:
- Hismanal Tablets 1138

Azatadine Maleate (Anticoagulant action partially counteracted). Products include:
- Optimine Tablets 2115
- Trinalin Repetabs Tablets 1170

Azlocillin Sodium (Interferes with platelet-aggregation reactions and may induce bleeding).
- No products indexed under this heading.

Bromodiphenhydramine Hydrochloride (Anticoagulant action partially counteracted).
- No products indexed under this heading.

Brompheniramine Maleate (Anticoagulant action partially counteracted). Products include:
- Alka Seltzer Plus Sinus Allergy Medicine .... ⊞ 624
- Atrohist Sprinkle Capsules 558
- Bromfed Capsules (Timed Release) 1615
- Bromfed Syrup .... ⊞ 628
- Bromfed 1615
- Dimetane Decongestant .... ⊞ 673
- Dimetane .... ⊞ 672
- Dimetane-DC Cough Syrup 1857
- Dimetane-DX Cough Syrup 1858
- Dimetapp Elixir .... ⊞ 673
- Dimetapp DM Elixir .... ⊞ 674
- Dimetapp Extentabs .... ⊞ 674
- Dimetapp Plus Caplets .... ⊞ 675
- Dimetapp Tablets .... ⊞ 675
- Drixoral Antihistamine/Nasal Decongestant Syrup .... ⊞ 698

Carbenicillin Indanyl Sodium (Interferes with platelet-aggregation reactions and may induce bleeding). Products include:
- Geocillin Tablets 1951

Chlorpheniramine Maleate (Anticoagulant action partially counteracted). Products include:
- A.R.M. Allergy Relief Medicine Caplets .... ⊞ 615
- Alka-Seltzer Plus Cold Medicine .... ⊞ 623
- Allerest .... ⊞ 559
- Ana-Kit Anaphylaxis Emergency Treatment Kit 1100
- BC Cold Powder Multi-Symptom Formula .... ⊞ 517
- Brexin L.A. Capsules 2078
- Cerose-DM 2443
- Cheracol Plus Head Cold/Cough Formula .... ⊞ 667
- Chlor-Trimeton Allergy Syrup, Tablets & Long-Acting Repetabs Tablets .... ⊞ 693
- Chlor-Trimeton Decongestant .... ⊞ 694
- Comhist LA Capsules 1618
- Allergy-Sinus Comtrex Multi-Symptom Allergy Sinus Formula Tablets & Caplets 746
- Comtrex Multi-Symptom Cold Reliever Tablets/Caplets/Liqui-Gels/Liquid 745
- Day-Night Comtrex 747
- Contac Continuous Action Decongestant/Antihistamine Capsules ⊞ 710
- Contac Maximum Strength Continuous Action Decongestant/Antihistamine Caplets .... ⊞ 709
- Contac Severe Cold and Flu Formula Caplets .... ⊞ 711
- Coricidin 'D' Decongestant Tablets .... ⊞ 695
- Coricidin Demilets Tablets for Children .... ⊞ 696
- Coricidin Tablets .... ⊞ 695
- Deconamine 663
- Demazin Nasal Decongestant/Antihistamine Repetabs Tablets & Syrup .... ⊞ 697
- Dorcol Children's Liquid Cold Formula .... ⊞ 686
- Dristan Decongestant/Antihistamine/ Analgesic Coated Caplets .... ⊞ 749
- Dristan Cold Nasal Decongestant/ Antihistamine/ Analgesic Coated Tablets 2419
- Dristan Advanced Formula Decongestant/Antihistamine/ Analgesic Tablets .... ⊞ 749
- Extendryl 994
- 4-Way Cold Tablets 750
- Fedahist Gyrocaps 2145
- Fedahist Timecaps 2145
- Hycomine Compound Tablets 929
- Isoclor Timesule Capsules .... ⊞ 561
- Kronofed-A 970
- Medi-Flu Caplet, Liquid .... ⊞ 640
- Naldecon Syrup, Tablets, Pediatric Drops and Pediatric Syrup 709
- Nolamine Tablets 838
- Novafed A Capsules 1342
- Novahistine DH 1342
- Novahistine Elixir .... ⊞ 596
- Ornade Spansule Capsules 2221
- Orthoxicol Cough Syrup .... ⊞ 668
- PediaCare Allergy Relief Formula Liquid 1362
- PediaCare Cough-Cold Formula Liquid 1362
- PediaCare Night Rest Cough-Cold Formula Liquid 1362
- PediaCare 6-12 Cough-Cold Formula Chewable Tablets 1362
- Pyrroxate Capsules .... ⊞ 669
- Quelidrine Syrup 556
- Ru-Tuss II Capsules 693
- Ru-Tuss Tablets 693
- Ryna .... ⊞ 741
- Sinarest Tablets & Extra Strength Tablets .... ⊞ 562
- Sine-Off Maximum Strength Allergy/Sinus Formula Caplets .... ⊞ 721
- Sine-Off Sinus Medicine Tablets-Aspirin Formula .... ⊞ 722
- Singlet Tablets .... ⊞ 598
- Sinulin 840
- Sinutab Maximum Strength .... ⊞ 641
- St. Joseph Nighttime Cold Medicine .... ⊞ 705
- Sudafed Plus Liquid .... ⊞ 544
- Sudafed Plus Tablets .... ⊞ 545
- Teldrin Timed-Release Allergy Capsules, 12 mg. 2192
- TheraFlu Flu and Cold Medicine .... ⊞ 687
- Triaminic Allergy Tablets .... ⊞ 688
- Triaminic Chewables .... ⊞ 688
- Triaminic Cold Tablets .... ⊞ 688
- Triaminic Nite Light .... ⊞ 689
- Triaminic Syrup .... ⊞ 689
- Triaminic-12 Tablets .... ⊞ 690
- Triaminicin Tablets .... ⊞ 690
- Triaminicol Multi-Symptom Cold Tablets .... ⊞ 691
- Triaminicol Multi-Symptom Relief ⊞ 691
- Tylenol Allergy Sinus Medication Caplets and Gelcaps, Maximum Strength 1372
- Children's Tylenol Cold Liquid Formula and Chewable Tablets 1368
- Tylenol Cold & Flu Hot Medication, Packets 1369
- Tylenol Cold Medication Caplets and Tablets 1370
- Tylenol Cold Medication, Effervescent Tablets 1369
- Vicks Children's NyQuil .... ⊞ 664
- Vicks Formula 44 Cough Medicine .... ⊞ 661
- Vicks Formula 44M Multi-Symptom Cough Medicine .... ⊞ 662
- Vicks Pediatric Formula 44m Multi-Symptom Cough & Cold Medicine .... ⊞ 663

Chlorpheniramine Polistirex (Anticoagulant action partially counteracted). Products include:
- Tussionex Extended-Release Suspension 988

Chlorpheniramine Tannate (Anticoagulant action partially counteracted). Products include:
- Rynatan 2387
- Rynatuss 2388

Choline Magnesium Trisalicylate (Interferes with platelet-aggregation reactions and may induce bleeding). Products include:
- Trilisate 1822

Clemastine Fumarate (Anticoagulant action partially counteracted). Products include:
- Tavist Syrup 2033
- Tavist Tablets 2035
- Tavist-D Tablets 2035

Cyproheptadine Hydrochloride (Anticoagulant action partially counteracted). Products include:
- Periactin 1525

Demeclocycline Hydrochloride (Anticoagulant action partially counteracted). Products include:
- Declomycin Capsules, Tablets 1199

Deslanoside (Anticoagulant action partially counteracted).
- No products indexed under this heading.

Dexchlorpheniramine Maleate (Anticoagulant action partially counteracted). Products include:
- Polaramine 2116

Dextran 40 (Interferes with platelet-aggregation reactions and may induce bleeding).
- No products indexed under this heading.

Diclofenac Sodium (Interferes with platelet-aggregation reactions and may induce bleeding). Products include:
- Voltaren Ophthalmic Sterile Ophthalmic Solution .... ⊙ 268
- Voltaren Tablets 1042

Diflunisal (Interferes with platelet-aggregation reactions and may induce bleeding). Products include:
- Dolobid Tablets 1465

Digitoxin (Anticoagulant action partially counteracted). Products include:
- Crystodigin Tablets 1253

Digoxin (Anticoagulant action partially counteracted). Products include:
- Lanoxicaps 772
- Lanoxin Elixir Pediatric 775
- Lanoxin Injection 778
- Lanoxin Injection Pediatric 781
- Lanoxin Tablets 783

Diphenhydramine Citrate (Anticoagulant action partially counteracted). Products include:
- Alka-Seltzer Plus Night-Time Cold Medicine .... ⊞ 623
- Bufferin AF Nite Time Analgesic/ Sleeping Aid Caplets 744
- Excedrin P.M. Analgesic/Sleeping Aid Tablets, Caplets and Liquid 749

Diphenylpyraline Hydrochloride (Anticoagulant action partially counteracted).
- No products indexed under this heading.

Dipyridamole (Interferes with platelet-aggregation reactions and may induce bleeding). Products include:
- Persantine Tablets 683

Doxycycline Calcium (Anticoagulant action partially counteracted).
- No products indexed under this heading.

Doxycycline Hyclate (Anticoagulant action partially counteracted). Products include:
- Doryx Capsules 1717
- Vibramycin Hyclate Capsules 1787
- Vibramycin Hyclate Intravenous 1968
- Vibra-Tabs Film Coated Tablets 1787

Doxycycline Monohydrate (Anticoagulant action partially counteracted). Products include:
- Monodox Capsules 1630
- Vibramycin Monohydrate for Oral Suspension 1787

Etodolac (Interferes with platelet-aggregation reactions and may induce bleeding). Products include:
- Lodine Capsules 2468

(⊞ Described in PDR For Nonprescription Drugs)

(⊙ Described in PDR For Ophthalmology)

Fenoprofen Calcium (Interferes with platelet-aggregation ractions and may induce bleeding). Products include:
Nalfon Pulvules & Tablets 919

Flurbiprofen (Interferes with platelet-aggregation reactions and may induce bleeding). Products include:
Ansaid Tablets 2319

Hydroxychloroquine Sulfate (Interferes with platelet-aggregation reactions and may induce bleeding). Products include:
Plaquenil Sulfate Tablets 2067

Ibuprofen (Interferes with platelet-aggregation reactions and may induce bleeding). Products include:
Advil Cold & Sinus Caplets (formerly CoAdvil) 2416
Advil Ibuprofen Tablets and Caplets 2416
Children's Advil Suspension 2426
CoAdvil .... ▣ 748
Dristan Sinus Caplets 2419
Haltran Tablets .... ▣ 668
Ibuprofen .... ▣ 631
Medipren ibuprofen Caplets and Tablets 1362
Midol 200 Cramp Relief Formula .... ▣ 570
Motrin Tablets 2351
Motrin IB Caplets and Tablets .... ▣ 736
Nuprin Ibuprofen/Analgesic Tablets & Caplets 752
PediaProfen Suspension 1363
Rufen Tablets 691
Trendar Ibuprofen Tablets .... ▣ 756

Indomethacin (Interferes with platelet-aggregation reactions and may induce bleeding). Products include:
Indocin 1487

Indomethacin Sodium Trihydrate (Interferes with platelet-aggregation reactions and may induce bleeding). Products include:
Indocin I.V. 1490

Ketoprofen (Interferes with platelet-aggregation reactions and may induce bleeding). Products include:
Orudis Capsules 2488

Ketorolac Tromethamine (Interferes with platelet-aggregation reactions and may induce bleeding). Products include:
Toradol IM Injection 2302

Magnesium Salicylate (Interferes with platelet-aggregation reactions and may induce bleeding). Products include:
Doan's - Extra-Strength Analgesic ▣ 549
Doan's - Regular Strength Analgesic .... ▣ 549
Mobigesic Analgesic Tablets .... ▣ 507

Meclofenamate Sodium (Interferes with platelet-aggregation reactions and may induce bleeding). Products include:
Meclomen Capsules 1739

Mefenamic Acid (Interferes with platelet-aggregation reactions and may induce bleeding). Products include:
Ponstel 1758

Methacycline Hydrochloride (Anticoagulant action partially counteracted).
No products indexed under this heading.

Methdilazine Hydrochloride (Anticoagulant action partially counteracted). Products include:
Tacaryl Syrup & Tablets 2409

Mezlocillin Sodium (Interferes with platelet-aggregation reactions and may induce bleeding). Products include:
Mezlin 1597
Mezlin Pharmacy Bulk Package 1599

Minocycline Hydrochloride (Anticoagulant action partially counteracted). Products include:
Minocin Intravenous 1221
Minocin Oral Suspension 1224
Minocin Pellet-Filled Capsules 1222

Nafcillin Sodium (Interferes with platelet-aggregation reactions and may induce bleeding). Products include:
Unipen 2533

Naproxen (Interferes with platelet-aggregation reactions and may induce bleeding). Products include:
Naprosyn 2297

Naproxen Sodium (Interferes with platelet-aggregation reactions and may induce bleeding). Products include:
Anaprox and Anaprox DS Tablets 2288

Nicotine Polacrilex (Anticoagulant action partially counteracted). Products include:
Nicorette 1335

Oxytetracycline (Anticoagulant action partially counteracted). Products include:
Terramycin Intramuscular Solution 1964
Urobiotic-250 Capsules 1968

Oxytetracycline Hydrochloride (Anticoagulant action partially counteracted). Products include:
Terra-Cortril Ophthalmic Suspension 1963
Terramycin Capsules 1786
Terramycin Intramuscular Solution 1964
Terramycin with Polymyxin B Sulfate Ophthalmic Ointment 1965

Penicillin G Procaine (Interferes with platelet-aggregation reactions and may induce bleeding). Products include:
Bicillin C-R Injection 2438
Bicillin C-R 900/300 Injection 2440
Pfizerpen-AS Aqueous Suspension 1959
Wycillin Injection 2537
Wycillin Injection and Probenecid Tablets 2539

Penicillin G, Benzathine (Interferes with platelet-aggregation reactions and may induce bleeding). Products include:
Bicillin C-R Injection 2438
Bicillin C-R 900/300 Injection 2440
Bicillin L-A Injection 2442

Phenylbutazone (Interferes with platelet-aggregation reactions and may induce bleeding). Products include:
Butazolidin Capsules & Tablets 1027

Piroxicam (Interferes with platelet-aggregation reactions and may induce bleeding). Products include:
Feldene Capsules 1777

Promethazine Hydrochloride (Anticoagulant action partially counteracted). Products include:
Mepergan Injection 2479
Phenergan with Codeine 2497
Phenergan with Dextromethorphan 2499
Phenergan Injection 2493
Phenergan Suppositories 2496
Phenergan Syrup 2495
Phenergan Tablets 2496
Phenergan VC 2500
Phenergan VC with Codeine 2501

Pyrilamine Maleate (Anticoagulant action partially counteracted). Products include:
Codimal 846
4-Way Fast Acting Nasal Spray - Original Formula (regular & mentholated) & Metered Spray Pump (regular) 751
Maximum Strength Midol Multi-Symptom Menstrual Formula .... ▣ 571
Maximum Strength Midol PMS Premenstrual Syndrome Formula .... ▣ 570
Regular Strength Midol Multi-Symptom Menstrual Formula .... ▣ 570
Prefrin-A .... ⊙ 255
Prēmsyn PMS Capsules & Caplets ▣ 547
Primatene Tablets-M Formula 2421
Robitussin Night Relief .... ▣ 677
Ru-Tuss with Hydrocodone 694
Triaminic Expectorant DH 1995
Triaminic Oral Infant Drops 1996

Pyrilamine Tannate (Anticoagulant action partially counteracted). Products include:
Rynatan 2387

Salsalate (Interferes with platelet-aggregation reactions and may induce bleeding). Products include:
Disalcid 1310
Mono-Gesic Tablets 846
Salflex 839

Sulindac (Interferes with platelet-aggregation reactions and may induce bleeding). Products include:
Clinoril Tablets 1433

Terfenadine (Anticoagulant action partially counteracted). Products include:
Seldane Tablets 1349
Seldane-D Extended-Release Tablets 1350

Tetracycline Hydrochloride (Anticoagulant action partially counteracted). Products include:
Achromycin V Capsules 1193
Achromycin Ophthalmic Ointment 1% .... ⊙ 307
Achromycin Ophthalmic Suspension 1% .... ⊙ 308
Topicycline for Topical Solution 1856

Ticarcillin Disodium (Interferes with platelet-aggregation reactions and may induce bleeding). Products include:
Ticar for Injection 2236
Timentin for Injection 2239

Tolmetin Sodium (Interferes with platelet-aggregation reactions and may induce bleeding). Products include:
Tolectin (200, 400 and 600 mg) .. 1379

Trimeprazine Tartrate (Anticoagulant action partially counteracted). Products include:
Temaril Tablets, Syrup and Spansule Sustained Release Capsules 1085

Tripelennamine Hydrochloride (Anticoagulant action partially counteracted). Products include:
PBZ Tablets & Elixir 1037
PBZ-SR Tablets 1037

Triprolidine Hydrochloride (Anticoagulant action partially counteracted). Products include:
Actidil .... ▣ 538
Actifed Capsules .... ▣ 539
Actifed Plus Caplets .... ▣ 539
Actifed Plus Tablets .... ▣ 540
Actifed with Codeine Cough Syrup .. 752
Actifed Syrup .... ▣ 540
Actifed Tablets .... ▣ 540
Actifed 12-Hour Capsules .... ▣ 539

HEPARIN SODIUM VIALS
(Heparin Sodium) 1264
May interact with oral anticoagulants, non-steroidal anti-inflammatory agents, salicylates, cardiac glycosides, high doses of parenteral penicillins, phenothiazines, tetracyclines, antihistamines, platelet inhibitors, cephalosporins with methylthiotetrazole side chains, macrolide antibiotics, and certain other agents. Compounds in these categories include:

Aspirin (Coadministration may result in an additive or synergistic activity and can result in an increased risk of bleeding). Products include:
Alka-Seltzer Effervescent Antacid and Pain Reliever 1568
Alka-Seltzer Extra Strength Effervescent Antacid and Pain Reliever 1570
Alka-Seltzer (Flavored) Effervescent Antacid and Pain Reliever 1569
Alka-Seltzer Plus Cold Medicine .... ▣ 623
Alka-Seltzer Plus Night-Time Cold Medicine .... ▣ 623
Alka Seltzer Plus Sinus Allergy Medicine .... ▣ 624
Anacin Coated Analgesic Caplets 2417
Anacin Coated Analgesic Tablets 2417
Anacin Maximum Strength Analgesic Coated Tablets 2417
Maximum Strength Arthritis Pain Formula By the Makers of Anacin Analgesic Tablets and Caplets 2418
Arthritis Pain Formula by the Makers of Anacin Analgesic Tablets and Caplets .... ▣ 747
Arthritis Strength BC Powder .... ▣ 516
Ascriptin A/D Caplets 1850
Regular Strength Ascriptin Tablets 1850
Azdone Tablets 844
BC Powder .... ▣ 517
BC Cold Powder .... ▣ 517
Children's Bayer Chewable Aspirin .... ▣ 564
Genuine Bayer Aspirin Tablets & Caplets .... ▣ 564
Maximum Bayer Aspirin Tablets & Caplets .... ▣ 566
Bayer Plus Aspirin Tablets .... ▣ 567
Therapy Bayer Aspirin Caplets .... ▣ 568
8 Hour Bayer Timed-Release Aspirin .... ▣ 566
Arthritis Strength Bufferin Analgesic Caplets 744
Extra Strength Bufferin Analgesic Tablets 745
Bufferin Analgesic Tablets and Caplets 743
Cama Arthritis Pain Reliever .... ▣ 685
Damason-P 1356
Easprin 1719
Ecotrin Enteric Coated Aspirin Maximum Strength Tablets and Caplets 2189
Ecotrin Enteric Coated Aspirin Regular Strength Tablets and Caplets 2189
Empirin Aspirin .... ▣ 541
Empirin with Codeine Phosphate Nos. 2, 3 & 4 764
Equagesic Tablets 2451
Excedrin Extra-Strength Analgesic Tablets & Caplets 749
4-Way Cold Tablets 750
Fiorinal Capsules 2007
Fiorinal with Codeine Capsules 2008
Fiorinal Tablets 2007
Lortab ASA Tablets 2414
Momentum Muscular Backache Formula .... ▣ 751
Norgesic 1314
Norwich Extra-Strength Aspirin .... ▣ 546
Norwich Regular Strength Aspirin ▣ 547
P-A-C Analgesic Tablets .... ▣ 669
Percodan 951
Robaxisal Tablets 1872
Sine-Off Sinus Medicine Tablets-Aspirin Formula .... ▣ 722
Soma Compound w/Codeine Tablets 2390
Soma Compound Tablets 2389
St. Joseph Adult Chewable Aspirin (81 mg.) .... ▣ 703
Synalgos-DC Capsules 2525
Talwin Compound 2072
Ursinus Inlay-Tabs .... ▣ 691
Vanquish Analgesic Caplets .... ▣ 574
Zorprin Tablets 698

Astemizole (Antagonizes the antithrombotic activity of heparin). Products include:
Hismanal Tablets 1138

Azatadine Maleate (Antagonizes the antithrombotic activity of heparin). Products include:
Optimine Tablets 2115
Trinalin Repetabs Tablets 1170

Azlocillin Sodium (Coadministration may result in an additive or synergistic activity and can result in an increased risk of bleeding).
No products indexed under this heading.

Bromodiphenhydramine Hydrochloride (Antagonizes the antithrombotic activity of heparin).
No products indexed under this heading.

Brompheniramine Maleate (Antagonizes the antithrombotic activity of heparin). Products include:
Alka Seltzer Plus Sinus Allergy Medicine ▣ 624
Atrohist Sprinkle Capsules 558
Bromfed Capsules (Timed Release) 1615
Bromfed Syrup ▣ 628
Bromfed 1615
Dimetane Decongestant ▣ 673
Dimetane ▣ 672
Dimetane-DC Cough Syrup 1857
Dimetane-DX Cough Syrup 1858
Dimetapp Elixir ▣ 673
Dimetapp DM Elixir ▣ 674
Dimetapp Extentabs ▣ 674
Dimetapp Plus Caplets ▣ 675
Dimetapp Tablets ▣ 675
Drixoral Antihistamine/Nasal Decongestant Syrup ▣ 698

Carbenicillin Indanyl Sodium (Coadministration may result in an additive or synergistic activity and can result in an increased risk of bleeding). Products include:
Geocillin Tablets 1951

Cefamandole Nafate (Coadministration may result in an additive or synergistic activity and can result in an increased risk of bleeding). Products include:
Mandol Vials, Faspak & ADD-Vantage 1281

Cefmetazole Sodium (Coadministration may result in an additive or synergistic activity and can result in an increased risk of bleeding). Products include:
Zefazone Sterile Powder 2372

Cefoperazone Sodium (Coadministration may result in an additive or synergistic activity and can result in an increased risk of bleeding). Products include:
Cefobid Intravenous/Intramuscular 1943
Cefobid Pharmacy Bulk Package - Not for Direct Infusion 1945

Cefotetan (Coadministration may result in an additive or synergistic activity and can result in an increased risk of bleeding). Products include:
Cefotan 2265

Chlorpheniramine Maleate (Antagonizes the antithrombotic activity of heparin). Products include:
A.R.M. Allergy Relief Medicine Caplets ▣ 615
Alka-Seltzer Plus Cold Medicine ▣ 623
Allerest ▣ 559
Ana-Kit Anaphylaxis Emergency Treatment Kit 1100
BC Cold Powder Multi-Symptom Formula ▣ 517
Brexin L.A. Capsules 2078
Cerose-DM 2443
Cheracol Plus Head Cold/Cough Formula ▣ 667
Chlor-Trimeton Allergy Syrup, Tablets & Long-Acting Repetabs Tablets ▣ 693
Chlor-Trimeton Decongestant ▣ 694
Comhist LA Capsules 1618
Allergy-Sinus Comtrex Multi-Symptom Allergy Sinus Formula Tablets & Caplets 746
Comtrex Multi-Symptom Cold Reliever Tablets/Caplets/Liqui-Gels/Liquid 745
Day-Night Comtrex 747
Contac Continuous Action Decongestant/Antihistamine Capsules ▣ 710
Contac Maximum Strength Continuous Action Decongestant/Antihistamine Caplets ▣ 709
Contac Severe Cold and Flu Formula Caplets ▣ 711
Coricidin 'D' Decongestant Tablets ▣ 695
Coricidin Demilets Tablets for Children ▣ 696
Coricidin Tablets ▣ 695
Deconamine 663
Demazin Nasal Decongestant/Antihistamine Repetabs Tablets & Syrup ▣ 697
Dorcol Children's Liquid Cold Formula ▣ 686
Dristan Decongestant/Antihistamine/ Analgesic Coated Caplets ▣ 749
Dristan Cold Nasal Decongestant/Antihistamine/ Analgesic Coated Tablets 2419
Dristan Advanced Formula Decongestant/Antihistamine/ Analgesic Tablets ▣ 749
Extendryl 994
4-Way Cold Tablets 750
Fedahist Gyrocaps 2145
Fedahist Timecaps 2145
Hycomine Compound Tablets 929
Isoclor Timesule Capsules ▣ 561
Kronofed-A 970
Medi-Flu Caplet, Liquid ▣ 640
Naldecon Syrup, Tablets, Pediatric Drops and Pediatric Syrup 709
Nolamine Tablets 838
Novafed A Capsules 1342
Novahistine DH 1342
Novahistine Elixir ▣ 596
Ornade Spansule Capsules 2221
Orthoxicol Cough Syrup ▣ 668
PediaCare Allergy Relief Formula Liquid 1362
PediaCare Cough-Cold Formula Liquid 1362
PediaCare Night Rest Cough-Cold Formula Liquid 1362
PediaCare 6-12 Cough-Cold Formula Chewable Tablets 1362
Pyrroxate Capsules ▣ 669
Quelidrine Syrup 556
Ru-Tuss II Capsules 693
Ru-Tuss Tablets 693
Ryna ▣ 741
Sinarest Tablets & Extra Strength Tablets ▣ 562
Sine-Off Maximum Strength Allergy/Sinus Formula Caplets ▣ 721
Sine-Off Sinus Medicine Tablets-Aspirin Formula ▣ 722
Singlet Tablets ▣ 598
Sinulin 840
Sinutab Maximum Strength ▣ 641
St. Joseph Nighttime Cold Medicine ▣ 705
Sudafed Plus Liquid ▣ 544
Sudafed Plus Tablets ▣ 545
Teldrin Timed-Release Allergy Capsules, 12 mg 2192
TheraFlu Flu and Cold Medicine ▣ 687
Triaminic Allergy Tablets ▣ 688
Triaminic Chewables ▣ 688
Triaminic Cold Tablets ▣ 688
Triaminic Nite Light ▣ 689
Triaminic Syrup ▣ 689
Triaminic-12 Tablets ▣ 690
Triaminicin Tablets ▣ 690
Triaminicol Multi-Symptom Cold Tablets ▣ 691
Triaminicol Multi-Symptom Relief ▣ 691
Tylenol Allergy Sinus Medication Caplets and Gelcaps, Maximum Strength 1372
Children's Tylenol Cold Liquid Formula and Chewable Tablets 1368
Tylenol Cold & Flu Hot Medication, Packets 1369
Tylenol Cold Medication Caplets and Tablets 1370
Tylenol Cold Medication, Effervescent Tablets 1369
Vicks Children's NyQuil ▣ 664
Vicks Formula 44 Cough Medicine ▣ 661
Vicks Formula 44M Multi-Symptom Cough Medicine ▣ 662
Vicks Pediatric Formula 44m Multi-Symptom Cough & Cold Medicine ▣ 663

Chlorpheniramine Polistirex (Antagonizes the antithrombotic activity of heparin). Products include:
Tussionex Extended-Release Suspension 988

Chlorpheniramine Tannate (Antagonizes the antithrombotic activity of heparin). Products include:
Rynatan 2387
Rynatuss 2388

Chlorpromazine (Antagonizes the antithrombotic activity of heparin). Products include:
Thorazine 2234

Choline Magnesium Trisalicylate (Coadministration may result in an additive or synergistic activity and can result in an increased risk of bleeding). Products include:
Trilisate 1822

Clemastine Fumarate (Antagonizes the antithrombotic activity of heparin). Products include:
Tavist Syrup 2033
Tavist Tablets 2035
Tavist-D Tablets 2035

Cyproheptadine Hydrochloride (Antagonizes the antithrombotic activity of heparin). Products include:
Periactin 1525

Demeclocycline Hydrochloride (Loss of pharmacological activity of either or both drugs). Products include:
Declomycin Capsules, Tablets 1199

Deslanoside (Antagonizes the antithrombotic activity of heparin).
No products indexed under this heading.

Dexchlorpheniramine Maleate (Antagonizes the antithrombotic activity of heparin). Products include:
Polaramine 2116

Dextran 40 (Interferes with platelet aggregation reactions).
No products indexed under this heading.

Dextran 70 (Interferes with platelet aggregation reactions). Products include:
Hyskon Hysteroscopy Fluid 1162
Moisture Drops ⊙ 258
Tears Naturale II 572

Diclofenac Sodium (Coadministration may result in an additive or synergistic activity and can result in an increased risk of bleeding). Products include:
Voltaren Ophthalmic Sterile Ophthalmic Solution ⊙ 268
Voltaren Tablets 1042

Dicumarol (One-stage prothrombin time prolonged). Products include:
Dicumarol Tablets 516

Diflunisal (Coadministration may result in an additive or synergistic activity and can result in an increased risk of bleeding). Products include:
Dolobid Tablets 1465

Digitoxin (Antagonizes the antithrombotic activity of heparin). Products include:
Crystodigin Tablets 1253

Digoxin (Antagonizes the antithrombotic activity of heparin). Products include:
Lanoxicaps 772
Lanoxin Elixir Pediatric 775
Lanoxin Injection 778
Lanoxin Injection Pediatric 781
Lanoxin Tablets 783

Diphenhydramine Citrate (Antagonizes the antithrombotic activity of heparin). Products include:
Alka-Seltzer Plus Night-Time Cold Medicine ▣ 623
Bufferin AF Nite Time Analgesic/Sleeping Aid Caplets 744
Excedrin P.M. Analgesic/Sleeping Aid Tablets, Caplets and Liquid 749

Diphenhydramine Hydrochloride (Antagonizes the antithrombotic activity of heparin). Products include:
Benadryl Anti-Itch Cream ▣ 635
Benadryl Capsules 1691
Benadryl Decongestant Elixir ▣ 635
Benadryl Decongestant ▣ 635
Benadryl Elixir ▣ 636
Benadryl Kapseals 1691
Benadryl 25 Kapseals ▣ 636
Benadryl Parenteral 1692
Benadryl Plus ▣ 636
Benadryl Plus Nighttime ▣ 637
Benadryl Spray, Maximum Strength ▣ 637
Benadryl Spray, Regular Strength ▣ 637
Benadryl Steri-Vials, Ampoules, and Steri-Dose Syringe 1692
Benadryl 25 Tablets ▣ 636
Benylin Cough Syrup ▣ 637
Benylin Decongestant ▣ 638
Caladryl Cream, Lotion, Spray ▣ 638
Miles Nervine Nighttime Sleep-Aid ▣ 627
Nytol Tablets ▣ 517
Sleep-ettes-D Tablets ▣ 653
Sleep-eze 3 Tablets ▣ 755
Sleepinal Night-time Sleep Aid Capsules ▣ 734
Sominex Caplets and Tablets ▣ 722
Sominex Liquid ▣ 723
Sominex Pain Relief Formula ▣ 723
Tylenol Cold Night Time Medication Liquid 1371
Tylenol PM, Extra Strength Caplets and Tablets 1368
Unisom Dual Relief Nighttime Sleep Aid/Analgesic 1774
Ziradryl Lotion ▣ 643

Diphenylpyraline Hydrochloride (Antagonizes the antithrombotic activity of heparin).
No products indexed under this heading.

Dipyridamole (Coadministration may result in an additive or synergistic activity and can result in an increased risk of bleeding). Products include:
Persantine Tablets 683

Doxycycline Calcium (Loss of pharmacological activity of either or both drugs).
No products indexed under this heading.

Doxycycline Hyclate (Loss of pharmacological activity of either or both drugs). Products include:
Doryx Capsules 1717
Vibramycin Hyclate Capsules 1787
Vibramycin Hyclate Intravenous 1968
Vibra-Tabs Film Coated Tablets 1787

Doxycycline Monohydrate (Loss of pharmacological activity of either or both drugs). Products include:
Monodox Capsules 1630
Vibramycin Monohydrate for Oral Suspension 1787

Erythromycin (Loss of pharmacological activity of either or both drugs). Products include:
A/T/S Topical Gel and Topical Solution 1089
AK-Mycin Ointment ⊙ 204
Benzamycin Topical Gel 907
E-Mycin Tablets 688
ETS-2% 1685
ERYC 1720
Erycette (erythromycin 2%) Topical Solution 1678
Ery-Tab Tablets 521
Erythromycin Base Filmtab 525
Erythromycin Delayed-Release Capsules, USP 526
Ilotycin Ophthalmic Ointment 915
PCE Dispertab Tablets 549

Pediazole 1973
T-Stat 2.0% Topical Solution and Pads 2409
Theramycin Z Topical Solution 2% 1410

Erythromycin Estolate (Loss of pharmacological activity of either or both drugs). Products include:
Ilosone 913

Erythromycin Ethylsuccinate (Loss of pharmacological activity of either or both drugs). Products include:
E.E.S. 522
EryPed 519
Pediazole 1973

Erythromycin Gluceptate (Loss of pharmacological activity of either or both drugs). Products include:
Ilotycin Gluceptate, IV, Vials 915

Erythromycin Stearate (Loss of pharmacological activity of either or both drugs). Products include:
Erythrocin Stearate Filmtab 523

Etodolac (Coadministration may result in an additive or synergistic activity and can result in an increased risk of bleeding). Products include:
Lodine Capsules 2468

Fenoprofen Calcium (Coadministration may result in an additive or synergistic activity and can result in an increased risk of bleeding). Products include:
Nalfon Pulvules & Tablets 919

Fluphenazine Decanoate (Antagonizes the antithrombotic activity of heparin). Products include:
Prolixin Decanoate 1795

Fluphenazine Enanthate (Antagonizes the antithrombotic activity of heparin). Products include:
Prolixin Enanthate 1796

Fluphenazine Hydrochloride (Antagonizes the antithrombotic activity of heparin). Products include:
Prolixin Elixir 1793
Prolixin Injection 1791
Prolixin Oral Concentrate 1792
Prolixin Tablets 1793

Flurbiprofen (Coadministration may result in an additive or synergistic activity and can result in an increased risk of bleeding). Products include:
Ansaid Tablets 2319

Gentamicin Sulfate (Loss of pharmacological activity of either or both drugs). Products include:
Garamycin Injectable 2093
Garamycin Ophthalmic .... ◉ 305
Genoptic Liquifilm Sterile Ophthalmic Solution .... ◉ 247
Genoptic S.O.P. Sterile Ophthalmic Ointment .... ◉ 247
Gentacidin Ointment .... ◉ 273
Gentacidin Solution .... ◉ 273
Gentak Ointment & Solution .... ◉ 208
G-myticin Creme and Ointment 0.1% 1770
Pred-G Liquifilm Sterile Ophthalmic Suspension .... ◉ 252
Pred-G S.O.P. Sterile Ophthalmic Ointment .... ◉ 253

Ibuprofen (Coadministration may result in an additive or synergistic activity and can result in an increased risk of bleeding). Products include:
Advil Cold & Sinus Caplets (formerly CoAdvil) 2416
Advil Ibuprofen Tablets and Caplets 2416
Children's Advil Suspension 2426
CoAdvil .... ▣ 748
Dristan Sinus Caplets 2419
Haltran Tablets .... ▣ 668
Ibuprofen .... ▣ 631
Medipren ibuprofen Caplets and Tablets 1362
Midol 200 Cramp Relief Formula .. ▣ 570
Motrin Tablets 2351
Motrin IB Caplets and Tablets .... ▣ 736
Nuprin Ibuprofen/Analgesic Tablets & Caplets 752
PediaProfen Suspension 1363
Rufen Tablets 691
Trendar Ibuprofen Tablets .... ▣ 756

Indomethacin (Coadministration may result in an additive or synergistic activity and can result in an increased risk of bleeding). Products include:
Indocin 1487

Indomethacin Sodium Trihydrate (Coadministration may result in an additive or synergistic activity and can result in an increased risk of bleeding). Products include:
Indocin I.V. 1490

Ketoprofen (Coadministration may result in an additive or synergistic activity and can result in an increased risk of bleeding). Products include:
Orudis Capsules 2488

Ketorolac Tromethamine (Coadministration may result in an additive or synergistic activity and can result in an increased risk of bleeding). Products include:
Toradol IM Injection 2302

Magnesium Salicylate (Coadministration may result in an additive or synergistic activity and can result in an increased risk of bleeding). Products include:
Doan's - Extra-Strength Analgesic ▣ 549
Doan's - Regular Strength Analgesic .... ▣ 549
Mobigesic Analgesic Tablets .... ▣ 507

Meclofenamate Sodium (Coadministration may result in an additive or synergistic activity and can result in an increased risk of bleeding). Products include:
Meclomen Capsules 1739

Mefenamic Acid (Coadministration may result in an additive or synergistic activity and can result in an increased risk of bleeding). Products include:
Ponstel 1758

Mesoridazine (Antagonizes the antithrombotic activity of heparin). Products include:
Serentil 686

Methacycline Hydrochloride (Loss of pharmacological activity of either or both drugs).
No products indexed under this heading.

Methdilazine Hydrochloride (Antagonizes the antithrombotic activity of heparin). Products include:
Tacaryl Syrup & Tablets 2409

Mezlocillin Sodium (Coadministration may result in an additive or synergistic activity and can result in an increased risk of bleeding). Products include:
Mezlin 1597
Mezlin Pharmacy Bulk Package 1599

Minocycline Hydrochloride (Loss of pharmacological activity of either or both drugs). Products include:
Minocin Intravenous 1221
Minocin Oral Suspension 1224
Minocin Pellet-Filled Capsules 1222

Moxalactam Disodium (Coadministration may result in an additive or synergistic activity and can result in an increased risk of bleeding).

Nafcillin Sodium (Coadministration may result in an additive or synergistic activity and can result in an increased risk of bleeding). Products include:
Unipen 2533

Naproxen (Coadministration may result in an additive or synergistic activity and can result in an increased risk of bleeding). Products include:
Naprosyn 2297

Naproxen Sodium (Coadministration may result in an additive or synergistic activity and can result in an increased risk of bleeding). Products include:
Anaprox and Anaprox DS Tablets 2288

Neomycin, oral (Loss of pharmacological activity of either or both drugs).

Nicotine Polacrilex (Antagonizes the antithrombotic activity of heparin). Products include:
Nicorette 1335

Nitroglycerin Intravenous (May require higher doses of heparin; close monitoring of the partial thromboplastin time is required). Products include:
Nitro-Bid IV 1338
Nitrostat IV 1744
Tridil Ampuls & Vials 939

Oxytetracycline Hydrochloride (Loss of pharmacological activity of either or both drugs). Products include:
Terra-Cortril Ophthalmic Suspension 1963
Terramycin Capsules 1786
Terramycin Intramuscular Solution 1964
Terramycin with Polymyxin B Sulfate Ophthalmic Ointment 1965

Penicillin G Procaine (Coadministration may result in an additive or synergistic activity and can result in an increased risk of bleeding). Products include:
Bicillin C-R Injection 2438
Bicillin C-R 900/300 Injection 2440
Pfizerpen-AS Aqueous Suspension 1959
Wycillin Injection 2537
Wycillin Injection and Probenecid Tablets 2539

Penicillin G, Benzathine (Coadministration may result in an additive or synergistic activity and can result in an increased risk of bleeding). Products include:
Bicillin C-R Injection 2438
Bicillin C-R 900/300 Injection 2440
Bicillin L-A Injection 2442

Perphenazine (Antagonizes the antithrombotic activity of heparin). Products include:
Etrafon 2087
Triavil Tablets 1556
Trilafon 2123

Phenylbutazone (Coadministration may result in an additive or synergistic activity and can result in an increased risk of bleeding). Products include:
Butazolidin Capsules & Tablets 1027

Piroxicam (Coadministration may result in an additive or synergistic activity and can result in an increased risk of bleeding). Products include:
Feldene Capsules 1777

Polymyxin B Sulfate (Loss of pharmacological activity of either or both drugs). Products include:
AK-Poly-Bac Ointment .... ◉ 205
AK-Spore H.C. .... ◉ 206
AK-Spore .... ◉ 205
AK-Trol Ointment & Suspension .... ◉ 207
Aquaphor Antibiotic Formula 662
Bactine First Aid Antibiotic Ointment .... ▣ 625
Campho-Phenique Triple Antibiotic Ointment Plus Pain Reliever ▣ 758
Cortisporin Cream 757
Cortisporin Ointment 758
Cortisporin Ophthalmic Ointment Sterile 758
Cortisporin Ophthalmic Suspension Sterile 759
Cortisporin Otic Solution Sterile 760
Cortisporin Otic Suspension Sterile 760
Dexacidin .... ◉ 272
Lanabiotic Ointment .... ▣ 556
LazerSporin-C Solution 1770
Maxitrol Ophthalmic Ointment/Suspension .... ◉ 223
Mycitracin .... ▣ 737
Neosporin Cream 792
Neosporin G.U. Irrigant Sterile 793
Neosporin Ointment 793
Maximum Strength Neosporin Ointment 793
Neosporin Ophthalmic Ointment Sterile 793
Neosporin Ophthalmic Solution Sterile 794
Ophthocort .... ◉ 301
PediOtic Suspension Sterile 797
Polymyxin B Sulfate, Aerosporin Brand Sterile Powder 798
Poly-Pred Liquifilm .... ◉ 250
Polysporin Ointment .... ▣ 543
Polysporin Ophthalmic Ointment Sterile 798
Polysporin Powder .... ▣ 543
Polysporin Spray .... ▣ 543
Polytrim Ophthalmic Solution Sterile 588
Terramycin with Polymyxin B Sulfate Ophthalmic Ointment 1965

Prochlorperazine (Antagonizes the antithrombotic activity of heparin). Products include:
Compazine 2201

Promethazine Hydrochloride (Antagonizes the antithrombotic activity of heparin). Products include:
Mepergan Injection 2479
Phenergan with Codeine 2497
Phenergan with Dextromethorphan 2499
Phenergan Injection 2493
Phenergan Suppositories 2496
Phenergan Syrup 2495
Phenergan Tablets 2496
Phenergan VC 2500
Phenergan VC with Codeine 2501

Pyrilamine Maleate (Antagonizes the antithrombotic activity of heparin). Products include:
Codimal 846
4-Way Fast Acting Nasal Spray - Original Formula (regular & mentholated) & Metered Spray Pump (regular) 751
Maximum Strength Midol Multi-Symptom Menstrual Formula .... ▣ 571
Maximum Strength Midol PMS Premenstrual Syndrome Formula .... ▣ 570
Regular Strength Midol Multi-Symptom Menstrual Formula .... ▣ 570
Prefrin-A .... ◉ 255
Prēmsyn PMS Capsules & Caplets ▣ 547
Primatene Tablets-M Formula 2421
Robitussin Night Relief .... ▣ 677
Ru-Tuss with Hydrocodone 694
Triaminic Expectorant DH 1995
Triaminic Oral Infant Drops 1996

Pyrilamine Tannate (Antagonizes the antithrombotic activity of heparin). Products include:
Rynatan 2387

Salsalate (Coadministration may result in an additive or synergistic activity and can result in an increased risk of bleeding). Products include:
Disalcid 1310
Mono-Gesic Tablets 846
Salflex 839

Streptomycin Sulfate (Loss of pharmacological activity of either or both drugs).
No products indexed under this heading.

Sulindac (Coadministration may result in an additive or synergistic activity and can result in an increased risk of bleeding). Products include:

Clinoril Tablets ... 1433

Terfenadine (Antagonizes the antithrombotic activity of heparin). Products include:

Seldane Tablets ... 1349
Seldane-D Extended-Release Tablets ... 1350

Tetracycline Hydrochloride (Loss of pharmacological activity of either or both drugs). Products include:

Achromycin V Capsules ... 1193
Achromycin Ophthalmic Ointment 1% ... ◉ 307
Achromycin Ophthalmic Suspension 1% ... ◉ 308
Topicycline for Topical Solution ... 1856

Thioridazine Hydrochloride (Antagonizes the antithrombotic activity of heparin). Products include:

Mellaril ... 2011

Ticarcillin Disodium (Coadministration may result in an additive or synergistic activity and can result in an increased risk of bleeding). Products include:

Ticar for Injection ... 2236
Timentin for Injection ... 2239

Tolmetin Sodium (Coadministration may result in an additive or synergistic activity and can result in an increased risk of bleeding). Products include:

Tolectin (200, 400 and 600 mg) .. 1379

Trifluoperazine Hydrochloride (Antagonizes the antithrombotic activity of heparin). Products include:

Stelazine ... 2226

Trimeprazine Tartrate (Antagonizes the antithrombotic activity of heparin). Products include:

Temaril Tablets, Syrup and Spansule Sustained Release Capsules 1085

Tripelennamine Hydrochloride (Antagonizes the antithrombotic activity of heparin). Products include:

PBZ Tablets & Elixir ... 1037
PBZ-SR Tablets ... 1037

Triprolidine Hydrochloride (Antagonizes the antithrombotic activity of heparin). Products include:

Actidil ... ⊞ 538
Actifed Capsules ... ⊞ 539
Actifed Plus Caplets ... ⊞ 539
Actifed Plus Tablets ... ⊞ 540
Actifed with Codeine Cough Syrup.. 752
Actifed Syrup ... ⊞ 540
Actifed Tablets ... ⊞ 540
Actifed 12-Hour Capsules ... ⊞ 539

Troleandomycin (Loss of pharmacological activity of either or both drugs). Products include:

Tao Capsules ... 1963

Vitamin C (Antagonizes the antithrombotic activity of heparin). Products include:

Allbee with C Caplets ... ⊞ 670
Allbee C-800 ... ⊞ 670
Bromase Capsules ... 672
Bugs Bunny Children's Chewable Vitamins (Sugar Free) ... ⊞ 625
Bugs Bunny With Extra C Children's Chewable Vitamins (Sugar Free) ... ⊞ 626
Bugs Bunny Plus Iron Children's Chewable Vitamins (Sugar Free) ⊞ 625
Cefol Filmtab ... 509
Centrum, Jr. (Children's Chewable) + Extra C ... ⊞ 585
Cod Liver Oil Concentrate Tablets with Vitamin C ... ⊞ 694
Ester-C Tablets ... ⊞ 575
Ferancee Chewable Tablets ... 1155
Ferancee-HP Tablets ... 1155
Fero-Folic-500 Filmtab ... 527
Fero-Grad-500 Filmtab ... 528
Flintstones Children's Chewable Vitamins ... ⊞ 625
Flintstones Children's Chewable Vitamins With Extra C ... ⊞ 626
Flintstones Children's Chewable Vitamins Plus Iron ... ⊞ 625
Halls Vitamin C Drops ... ⊞ 742
Hyland's Vitamin C for Children ... ⊞ 729
ICAPS Plus ... ◉ 280
Mediatric Capsules ... 2476
Mol-Iron w/Vitamin C Tablets ... ⊞ 703
Natalins Rx ... 1391
Natalins Tablets ... 1391
N'ICE Sugarless Vitamin C Drops .. ⊞ 719
Niferex w/Vitamin C Tablets ... 847
Ocuvite Vitamin and Mineral Supplement ... ◉ 312
One-A-Day Essential Vitamins ... ⊞ 627
One-A-Day Maximum Formula Vitamins and Minerals ... ⊞ 627
One-A-Day Plus Extra C Vitamins .. ⊞ 627
Probec-T Tablets ... ⊞ 581
Stressgard Stress Formula Vitamins ... ⊞ 628
STUART PRENATAL Tablets ... ⊞ 731
The Stuart Formula Tablets ... 1157
Stuartinic Tablets ... 1157
Sunkist Children's Chewable Multivitamins - Plus Extra C ... ⊞ 553
Sunkist Vitamin C ... ⊞ 553
Surbex with C ... ⊞ 502
Trinsicon Capsules ... 2415
Tri-Vi-Flor 1.0 mg Vitamins with Fluoride Chewable Tablets ... 1400
Tri-Vi-Flor Drops ... 1400
Tri-Vi-Sol Vitamin Drops ... ⊞ 614
Tri-Vi-Sol Vitamin Drops with Iron ⊞ 614
Vicon Forte Capsules ... 2416
Vicon Plus ... ⊞ 682
Vicon-C ... ⊞ 682
Vi-Daylin ADC Vitamins Drops ... 1980
Vi-Daylin ADC Vitamins + Iron Drops ... 1980
Vi-Daylin/F ADC Vitamins Drops With Fluoride ... 1981
Vi-Daylin/F ADC Vitamins + Iron Drops With Fluoride ... 1981
Vi-Zac ... ⊞ 682
Within Women's Formula Multivitamin with Calcium, Extra Iron and Zinc ... ⊞ 628
Z-Bec Tablets ... ⊞ 678

Warfarin Sodium (One-stage prothrombin time prolonged). Products include:

Coumadin Injection & Tablets ... 944
Panwarfin Tablets ... 547

HEPARIN SODIUM INJECTION
(Heparin Sodium) ... 2457
May interact with cardiac glycosides, antihistamines, oral anticoagulants, tetracyclines, non-steroidal anti-inflammatory agents, platelet inhibitors, and certain other agents. Compounds in these categories include:

Aspirin (Interferes with platelet-aggregation reactions and may induce bleeding). Products include:

Alka-Seltzer Effervescent Antacid and Pain Reliever ... 1568
Alka-Seltzer Extra Strength Effervescent Antacid and Pain Reliever ... 1570
Alka-Seltzer (Flavored) Effervescent Antacid and Pain Reliever ... 1569
Alka-Seltzer Plus Cold Medicine ... ⊞ 623
Alka-Seltzer Plus Night-Time Cold Medicine ... ⊞ 623
Alka Seltzer Plus Sinus Allergy Medicine ... ⊞ 624
Anacin Coated Analgesic Caplets ... 2417
Anacin Coated Analgesic Tablets ... 2417
Anacin Maximum Strength Analgesic Coated Tablets ... 2417
Maximum Strength Arthritis Pain Formula By the Makers of Anacin Analgesic Tablets and Caplets ... 2418
Arthritis Pain Formula by the Makers of Anacin Analgesic Tablets and Caplets ... ⊞ 747
Arthritis Strength BC Powder ... ⊞ 516
Ascriptin A/D Caplets ... 1850
Regular Strength Ascriptin Tablets 1850
Azdōne Tablets ... 844
BC Powder ... ⊞ 517
BC Cold Powder ... ⊞ 517
Children's Bayer Chewable Aspirin ... ⊞ 564
Genuine Bayer Aspirin Tablets & Caplets ... ⊞ 564
Maximum Bayer Aspirin Tablets & Caplets ... ⊞ 566
Bayer Plus Aspirin Tablets ... ⊞ 567
Therapy Bayer Aspirin Caplets ... ⊞ 568
8 Hour Bayer Timed-Release Aspirin ... ⊞ 566
Arthritis Strength Bufferin Analgesic Caplets ... 744
Extra Strength Bufferin Analgesic Tablets ... 745
Bufferin Analgesic Tablets and Caplets ... 743
Cama Arthritis Pain Reliever ... ⊞ 685
Damason-P ... 1356
Easprin ... 1719
Ecotrin Enteric Coated Aspirin Maximum Strength Tablets and Caplets ... 2189
Ecotrin Enteric Coated Aspirin Regular Strength Tablets and Caplets ... 2189
Empirin Aspirin ... ⊞ 541
Empirin with Codeine Phosphate Nos. 2, 3 & 4 ... 764
Equagesic Tablets ... 2451
Excedrin Extra-Strength Analgesic Tablets & Caplets ... 749
4-Way Cold Tablets ... 750
Fiorinal Capsules ... 2007
Fiorinal with Codeine Capsules ... 2008
Fiorinal Tablets ... 2007
Lortab ASA Tablets ... 2414
Momentum Muscular Backache Formula ... ⊞ 751
Norgesic ... 1314
Norwich Extra-Strength Aspirin ... ⊞ 546
Norwich Regular Strength Aspirin ⊞ 547
P-A-C Analgesic Tablets ... ⊞ 669
Percodan ... 951
Robaxisal Tablets ... 1872
Sine-Off Sinus Medicine Tablets-Aspirin Formula ... ⊞ 722
Soma Compound w/Codeine Tablets ... 2390
Soma Compound Tablets ... 2389
St. Joseph Adult Chewable Aspirin (81 mg.) ... ⊞ 703
Synalgos-DC Capsules ... 2525
Talwin Compound ... 2072
Ursinus Inlay-Tabs ... ⊞ 691
Vanquish Analgesic Caplets ... ⊞ 574
Zorprin Tablets ... 698

Astemizole (Anticoagulant action partially counteracted). Products include:

Hismanal Tablets ... 1138

Azatadine Maleate (Anticoagulant action partially counteracted). Products include:

Optimine Tablets ... 2115
Trinalin Repetabs Tablets ... 1170

Azlocillin Sodium (Interferes with platelet-aggregation reactions and may induce bleeding).

No products indexed under this heading.

Bromodiphenhydramine Hydrochloride (Anticoagulant action partially counteracted).

No products indexed under this heading.

Brompheniramine Maleate (Anticoagulant action partially counteracted). Products include:

Alka Seltzer Plus Sinus Allergy Medicine ... ⊞ 624
Atrohist Sprinkle Capsules ... 558
Bromfed Capsules (Timed Release) ... 1615
Bromfed Syrup ... ⊞ 628
Bromfed ... 1615
Dimetane Decongestant ... ⊞ 673
Dimetane ... ⊞ 672
Dimetane-DC Cough Syrup ... 1857
Dimetane-DX Cough Syrup ... 1858
Dimetapp Elixir ... ⊞ 673
Dimetapp DM Elixir ... ⊞ 674
Dimetapp Extentabs ... ⊞ 674
Dimetapp Plus Caplets ... ⊞ 675
Dimetapp Tablets ... ⊞ 675
Drixoral Antihistamine/Nasal Decongestant Syrup ... ⊞ 698

Carbenicillin Indanyl Sodium (Interferes with platelet-aggregation reactions and may induce bleeding). Products include:

Geocillin Tablets ... 1951

Chlorpheniramine Maleate (Anticoagulant action partially counteracted). Products include:

A.R.M. Allergy Relief Medicine Caplets ... ⊞ 615
Alka-Seltzer Plus Cold Medicine ... ⊞ 623
Allerest ... ⊞ 559
Ana-Kit Anaphylaxis Emergency Treatment Kit ... 1100
BC Cold Powder Multi-Symptom Formula ... ⊞ 517
Brexin L.A. Capsules ... 2078
Cerose-DM ... 2443
Cheracol Plus Head Cold/Cough Formula ... ⊞ 667
Chlor-Trimeton Allergy Syrup, Tablets & Long-Acting Repetabs Tablets ... ⊞ 693
Chlor-Trimeton Decongestant ... ⊞ 694
Comhist LA Capsules ... 1618
Allergy-Sinus Comtrex Multi-Symptom Allergy Sinus Formula Tablets & Caplets ... 746
Comtrex Multi-Symptom Cold Reliever Tablets/Caplets/Liqui-Gels/Liquid ... 745
Day-Night Comtrex ... 747
Contac Continuous Action Decongestant/Antihistamine Capsules ⊞ 710
Contac Maximum Strength Continuous Action Decongestant/Antihistamine Caplets ... ⊞ 709
Contac Severe Cold and Flu Formula Caplets ... ⊞ 711
Coricidin 'D' Decongestant Tablets ... ⊞ 695
Coricidin Demilets Tablets for Children ... ⊞ 696
Coricidin Tablets ... ⊞ 695
Deconamine ... 663
Demazin Nasal Decongestant/Antihistamine Repetabs Tablets & Syrup ... ⊞ 697
Dorcol Children's Liquid Cold Formula ... ⊞ 686
Dristan Decongestant/Antihistamine/ Analgesic Coated Caplets ... ⊞ 749
Dristan Cold Nasal Decongestant/Antihistamine/ Analgesic Coated Tablets ... 2419
Dristan Advanced Formula Decongestant/Antihistamine/ Analgesic Tablets ... ⊞ 749
Extendryl ... 994
4-Way Cold Tablets ... 750
Fedahist Gyrocaps ... 2145
Fedahist Timecaps ... 2145
Hycomine Compound Tablets ... 929
Isoclor Timesule Capsules ... ⊞ 561
Kronofed-A ... 970
Medi-Flu Caplet, Liquid ... ⊞ 640
Naldecon Syrup, Tablets, Pediatric Drops and Pediatric Syrup ... 709
Nolamine Tablets ... 838
Novafed A Capsules ... 1342
Novahistine DH ... 1342
Novahistine Elixir ... ⊞ 596
Ornade Spansule Capsules ... 2221
Orthoxicol Cough Syrup ... ⊞ 668
PediaCare Allergy Relief Formula Liquid ... 1362
PediaCare Cough-Cold Formula Liquid ... 1362
PediaCare Night Rest Cough-Cold Formula Liquid ... 1362
PediaCare 6-12 Cough-Cold Formula Chewable Tablets ... 1362
Pyrroxate Capsules ... ⊞ 669
Quelidrine Syrup ... 556
Ru-Tuss II Capsules ... 693
Ru-Tuss Tablets ... 693
Ryna ... ⊞ 741
Sinarest Tablets & Extra Strength Tablets ... ⊞ 562
Sine-Off Maximum Strength Allergy/Sinus Formula Caplets ... ⊞ 721
Sine-Off Sinus Medicine Tablets-Aspirin Formula ... ⊞ 722
Singlet Tablets ... ⊞ 598
Sinulin ... 840
Sinutab Maximum Strength ... ⊞ 641
St. Joseph Nighttime Cold Medicine ... ⊞ 705
Sudafed Plus Liquid ... ⊞ 544

Sudafed Plus Tablets ▣ 545
Teldrin Timed-Release Allergy Capsules, 12 mg 2192
TheraFlu Flu and Cold Medicine ▣ 687
Triaminic Allergy Tablets ▣ 688
Triaminic Chewables ▣ 688
Triaminic Cold Tablets ▣ 688
Triaminic Nite Light ▣ 689
Triaminic Syrup ▣ 689
Triaminic-12 Tablets ▣ 690
Triaminicin Tablets ▣ 690
Triaminicol Multi-Symptom Cold Tablets ▣ 691
Triaminicol Multi-Symptom Relief ▣ 691
Tylenol Allergy Sinus Medication Caplets and Gelcaps, Maximum Strength 1372
Children's Tylenol Cold Liquid Formula and Chewable Tablets 1368
Tylenol Cold & Flu Hot Medication, Packets 1369
Tylenol Cold Medication Caplets and Tablets 1370
Tylenol Cold Medication, Effervescent Tablets 1369
Vicks Children's NyQuil ▣ 664
Vicks Formula 44 Cough Medicine ▣ 661
Vicks Formula 44M Multi-Symptom Cough Medicine ▣ 662
Vicks Pediatric Formula 44m Multi-Symptom Cough & Cold Medicine ▣ 663

Chlorpheniramine Polistirex (Anticoagulant action partially counteracted). Products include:
Tussionex Extended-Release Suspension 988

Chlorpheniramine Tannate (Anticoagulant action partially counteracted). Products include:
Rynatan 2387
Rynatuss 2388

Choline Magnesium Trisalicylate (Interferes with platelet-aggregation reactions and may induce bleeding). Products include:
Trilisate 1822

Clemastine Fumarate (Anticoagulant action partially counteracted). Products include:
Tavist Syrup 2033
Tavist Tablets 2035
Tavist-D Tablets 2035

Cyproheptadine Hydrochloride (Anticoagulant action partially counteracted). Products include:
Periactin 1525

Demeclocycline Hydrochloride (Anticoagulant action partially counteracted). Products include:
Declomycin Capsules, Tablets 1199

Deslanoside (Anticoagulant action partially counteracted).
No products indexed under this heading.

Dexchlorpheniramine Maleate (Anticoagulant action partially counteracted). Products include:
Polaramine 2116

Dextran 40 (Interferes with platelet-aggregation reactions and may induce bleeding).
No products indexed under this heading.

Diclofenac Sodium (Interferes with platelet-aggregation reactions and may induce bleeding). Products include:
Voltaren Ophthalmic Sterile Ophthalmic Solution ◎ 268
Voltaren Tablets 1042

Dicumarol (Prolonged prothrombin time). Products include:
Dicumarol Tablets 516

Diflunisal (Interferes with platelet-aggregation reactions and may induce bleeding). Products include:
Dolobid Tablets 1465

Digitoxin (Anticoagulant action partially counteracted). Products include:
Crystodigin Tablets 1253

Digoxin (Anticoagulant action partially counteracted). Products include:
Lanoxicaps 772
Lanoxin Elixir Pediatric 775
Lanoxin Injection 778
Lanoxin Injection Pediatric 781
Lanoxin Tablets 783

Diphenhydramine Citrate (Anticoagulant action partially counteracted). Products include:
Alka-Seltzer Plus Night-Time Cold Medicine ▣ 623
Bufferin AF Nite Time Analgesic/Sleeping Aid Caplets 744
Excedrin P.M. Analgesic/Sleeping Aid Tablets, Caplets and Liquid 749

Diphenhydramine Hydrochloride (Anticoagulant action partially counteracted). Products include:
Benadryl Anti-Itch Cream ▣ 635
Benadryl Capsules 1691
Benadryl Decongestant Elixir ▣ 635
Benadryl Decongestant ▣ 635
Benadryl Elixir ▣ 636
Benadryl Kapseals 1691
Benadryl 25 Kapseals ▣ 636
Benadryl Parenteral 1692
Benadryl Plus ▣ 636
Benadryl Plus Nighttime ▣ 637
Benadryl Spray, Maximum Strength ▣ 637
Benadryl Spray, Regular Strength ▣ 637
Benadryl Steri-Vials, Ampoules, and Steri-Dose Syringe 1692
Benadryl 25 Tablets ▣ 636
Benylin Cough Syrup ▣ 637
Benylin Decongestant ▣ 638
Caladryl Cream, Lotion, Spray ▣ 638
Miles Nervine Nighttime Sleep-Aid ▣ 627
Nytol Tablets ▣ 517
Sleep-ettes-D Tablets ▣ 653
Sleep-eze 3 Tablets ▣ 755
Sleepinal Night-time Sleep Aid Capsules ▣ 734
Sominex Caplets and Tablets ▣ 722
Sominex Liquid ▣ 723
Sominex Pain Relief Formula ▣ 723
Tylenol Cold Night Time Medication Liquid 1371
Tylenol PM, Extra Strength Caplets and Tablets 1368
Unisom Dual Relief Nighttime Sleep Aid/Analgesic 1774
Ziradryl Lotion ▣ 643

Diphenylpyraline Hydrochloride (Anticoagulant action partially counteracted).
No products indexed under this heading.

Dipyridamole (Interferes with platelet-aggregation reactions and may induce bleeding). Products include:
Persantine Tablets 683

Doxycycline Calcium (Anticoagulant action partially counteracted).
No products indexed under this heading.

Doxycycline Hyclate (Anticoagulant action partially counteracted). Products include:
Doryx Capsules 1717
Vibramycin Hyclate Capsules 1787
Vibramycin Hyclate Intravenous 1968
Vibra-Tabs Film Coated Tablets 1787

Doxycycline Monohydrate (Anticoagulant action partially counteracted). Products include:
Monodox Capsules 1630
Vibramycin Monohydrate for Oral Suspension 1787

Etodolac (Interferes with platelet-aggregation reactions and may induce bleeding). Products include:
Lodine Capsules 2468

Fenoprofen Calcium (Interferes with platelet-aggregation reactions and may induce bleeding). Products include:
Nalfon Pulvules & Tablets 919

Flurbiprofen (Interferes with platelet-aggregation reactions and may induce bleeding). Products include:
Ansaid Tablets 2319

Hydroxychloroquine Sulfate (Interferes with platelet-aggregation reactions and may induce bleeding). Products include:
Plaquenil Sulfate Tablets 2067

Ibuprofen (Interferes with platelet-aggregation reactions and may induce bleeding). Products include:
Advil Cold & Sinus Caplets (formerly CoAdvil) 2416
Advil Ibuprofen Tablets and Caplets 2416
Children's Advil Suspension 2426
CoAdvil ▣ 748
Dristan Sinus Caplets 2419
Haltran Tablets ▣ 668
Ibuprofen ▣ 631
Medipren ibuprofen Caplets and Tablets 1362
Midol 200 Cramp Relief Formula ▣ 570
Motrin Tablets 2351
Motrin IB Caplets and Tablets ▣ 736
Nuprin Ibuprofen/Analgesic Tablets & Caplets 752
PediaProfen Suspension 1363
Rufen Tablets 691
Trendar Ibuprofen Tablets ▣ 756

Indomethacin (Interferes with platelet-aggregation reactions and may induce bleeding). Products include:
Indocin 1487

Indomethacin Sodium Trihydrate (Interferes with platelet-aggregation reactions and may induce bleeding). Products include:
Indocin I.V. 1490

Ketoprofen (Interferes with platelet-aggregation reactions and may induce bleeding). Products include:
Orudis Capsules 2488

Ketorolac Tromethamine (Interferes with platelet-aggregation reactions and may induce bleeding). Products include:
Toradol IM Injection 2302

Magnesium Salicylate (Interferes with platelet-aggregation reactions and may induce bleeding). Products include:
Doan's - Extra-Strength Analgesic ▣ 549
Doan's - Regular Strength Analgesic ▣ 549
Mobigesic Analgesic Tablets ▣ 507

Meclofenamate Sodium (Interferes with platelet-aggregation reactions and may induce bleeding). Products include:
Meclomen Capsules 1739

Mefenamic Acid (Interferes with platelet-aggregation reactions and may induce bleeding). Products include:
Ponstel 1758

Methacycline Hydrochloride (Anticoagulant action partially counteracted).
No products indexed under this heading.

Methdilazine Hydrochloride (Anticoagulant action partially counteracted). Products include:
Tacaryl Syrup & Tablets 2409

Mezlocillin Sodium (Interferes with platelet-aggregation reactions and may induce bleeding). Products include:
Mezlin 1597
Mezlin Pharmacy Bulk Package 1599

Minocycline Hydrochloride (Anticoagulant action partially counteracted). Products include:
Minocin Intravenous 1221
Minocin Oral Suspension 1224
Minocin Pellet-Filled Capsules 1222

Nafcillin Sodium (Interferes with platelet-aggregation reactions and may induce bleeding). Products include:
Unipen 2533

Naproxen (Interferes with platelet-aggregation reactions and may induce bleeding). Products include:
Naprosyn 2297

Naproxen Sodium (Interferes with platelet-aggregation reactions and may induce bleeding). Products include:
Anaprox and Anaprox DS Tablets 2288

Nicotine Polacrilex (Anticoagulant action partially counteracted). Products include:
Nicorette 1335

Oxytetracycline (Anticoagulant action partially counteracted). Products include:
Terramycin Intramuscular Solution 1964
Urobiotic-250 Capsules 1968

Oxytetracycline Hydrochloride (Anticoagulant action partially counteracted). Products include:
Terra-Cortril Ophthalmic Suspension 1963
Terramycin Capsules 1786
Terramycin Intramuscular Solution 1964
Terramycin with Polymyxin B Sulfate Ophthalmic Ointment 1965

Penicillin G Procaine (Interferes with platelet-aggregation reactions and may induce bleeding). Products include:
Bicillin C-R Injection 2438
Bicillin C-R 900/300 Injection 2440
Pfizerpen-AS Aqueous Suspension 1959
Wycillin Injection 2537
Wycillin Injection and Probenecid Tablets 2539

Penicillin G, Benzathine (Interferes with platelet-aggregation reactions and may induce bleeding). Products include:
Bicillin C-R Injection 2438
Bicillin C-R 900/300 Injection 2440
Bicillin L-A Injection 2442

Phenylbutazone (Interferes with platelet-aggregation reactions and may induce bleeding). Products include:
Butazolidin Capsules & Tablets 1027

Piroxicam (Interferes with platelet-aggregation reactions and may induce bleeding). Products include:
Feldene Capsules 1777

Promethazine Hydrochloride (Anticoagulant action partially counteracted). Products include:
Mepergan Injection 2479
Phenergan with Codeine 2497
Phenergan with Dextromethorphan 2499
Phenergan Injection 2493
Phenergan Suppositories 2496
Phenergan Syrup 2495
Phenergan Tablets 2496
Phenergan VC 2500
Phenergan VC with Codeine 2501

Pyrilamine Maleate (Anticoagulant action partially counteracted). Products include:
Codimal 846
4-Way Fast Acting Nasal Spray - Original Formula (regular & mentholated) & Metered Spray Pump (regular) 751
Maximum Strength Midol Multi-Symptom Menstrual Formula ▣ 571
Maximum Strength Midol PMS Premenstrual Syndrome Formula ▣ 570
Regular Strength Midol Multi-Symptom Menstrual Formula ▣ 570
Prefrin-A ◎ 255
Prēmsyn PMS Capsules & Caplets ▣ 547
Primatene Tablets-M Formula 2421
Robitussin Night Relief ▣ 677
Ru-Tuss with Hydrocodone 694
Triaminic Expectorant DH 1995
Triaminic Oral Infant Drops 1996

Pyrilamine Tannate (Anticoagulant action partially counteracted). Products include:

Rynatan ... 2387

Salsalate (Interferes with platelet-aggregation reactions and may induce bleeding). Products include:

Disalcid ... 1310
Mono-Gesic Tablets ... 846
Salflex ... 839

Sulindac (Interferes with platelet-aggregation reactions and may induce bleeding). Products include:

Clinoril Tablets ... 1433

Terfenadine (Anticoagulant action partially counteracted). Products include:

Seldane Tablets ... 1349
Seldane-D Extended-Release Tablets ... 1350

Tetracycline Hydrochloride (Anticoagulant action partially counteracted). Products include:

Achromycin V Capsules ... 1193
Achromycin Ophthalmic Ointment 1% ... ⊙ 307
Achromycin Ophthalmic Suspension 1% ... ⊙ 308
Topicycline for Topical Solution ... 1856

Ticarcillin Disodium (Interferes with platelet-aggregation reactions and may induce bleeding). Products include:

Ticar for Injection ... 2236
Timentin for Injection ... 2239

Tolmetin Sodium (Interferes with platelet-aggregation reactions and may induce bleeding). Products include:

Tolectin (200, 400 and 600 mg) ... 1379

Trimeprazine Tartrate (Anticoagulant action partially counteracted). Products include:

Temaril Tablets, Syrup and Spansule Sustained Release Capsules 1085

Tripelennamine Hydrochloride (Anticoagulant action partially counteracted). Products include:

PBZ Tablets & Elixir ... 1037
PBZ-SR Tablets ... 1037

Triprolidine Hydrochloride (Anticoagulant action partially counteracted). Products include:

Actidil ... ■ 538
Actifed Capsules ... ■ 539
Actifed Plus Caplets ... ■ 539
Actifed Plus Tablets ... ■ 540
Actifed with Codeine Cough Syrup ... 752
Actifed Syrup ... ■ 540
Actifed Tablets ... ■ 540
Actifed 12-Hour Capsules ... ■ 539

Warfarin Sodium (Prolonged prothrombin time). Products include:

Coumadin Injection & Tablets ... 944
Panwarfin Tablets ... 547

HEPARIN SODIUM INJECTION, USP, STERILE SOLUTION

(Heparin Sodium) ... 2342

May interact with oral anticoagulants, antihistamines, salicylates, cardiac glycosides, tetracyclines, non-steroidal anti-inflammatory agents, and certain other agents. Compounds in these categories include:

Aspirin (May induce bleeding). Products include:

Alka-Seltzer Effervescent Antacid and Pain Reliever ... 1568
Alka-Seltzer Extra Strength Effervescent Antacid and Pain Reliever ... 1570
Alka-Seltzer (Flavored) Effervescent Antacid and Pain Reliever ... 1569
Alka-Seltzer Plus Cold Medicine ... ■ 623
Alka-Seltzer Plus Night-Time Cold Medicine ... ■ 623
Alka Seltzer Plus Sinus Allergy Medicine ... ■ 624
Anacin Coated Analgesic Caplets ... 2417
Anacin Coated Analgesic Tablets ... 2417
Anacin Maximum Strength Analgesic Coated Tablets ... 2417
Maximum Strength Arthritis Pain Formula By the Makers of Anacin Analgesic Tablets and Caplets ... 2418
Arthritis Pain Formula by the Makers of Anacin Analgesic Tablets and Caplets ... ■ 747
Arthritis Strength BC Powder ... ■ 516
Ascriptin A/D Caplets ... 1850
Regular Strength Ascriptin Tablets 1850
Azdone Tablets ... 844
BC Powder ... ■ 517
BC Cold Powder ... ■ 517
Children's Bayer Chewable Aspirin ... ■ 564
Genuine Bayer Aspirin Tablets & Caplets ... ■ 564
Maximum Bayer Aspirin Tablets & Caplets ... ■ 566
Bayer Plus Aspirin Tablets ... ■ 567
Therapy Bayer Aspirin Caplets ... ■ 568
8 Hour Bayer Timed-Release Aspirin ... ■ 566
Arthritis Strength Bufferin Analgesic Caplets ... 744
Extra Strength Bufferin Analgesic Tablets ... 745
Bufferin Analgesic Tablets and Caplets ... 743
Cama Arthritis Pain Reliever ... ■ 685
Damason-P ... 1356
Easprin ... 1719
Ecotrin Enteric Coated Aspirin Maximum Strength Tablets and Caplets ... 2189
Ecotrin Enteric Coated Aspirin Regular Strength Tablets and Caplets ... 2189
Empirin Aspirin ... ■ 541
Empirin with Codeine Phosphate Nos. 2, 3 & 4 ... 764
Equagesic Tablets ... 2451
Excedrin Extra-Strength Analgesic Tablets & Caplets ... 749
4-Way Cold Tablets ... 750
Fiorinal Capsules ... 2007
Fiorinal with Codeine Capsules ... 2008
Fiorinal Tablets ... 2007
Lortab ASA Tablets ... 2414
Momentum Muscular Backache Formula ... ■ 751
Norgesic ... 1314
Norwich Extra-Strength Aspirin ... ■ 546
Norwich Regular Strength Aspirin ■ 547
P-A-C Analgesic Tablets ... ■ 669
Percodan ... 951
Robaxisal Tablets ... 1872
Sine-Off Sinus Medicine Tablets-Aspirin Formula ... ■ 722
Soma Compound w/Codeine Tablets ... 2390
Soma Compound Tablets ... 2389
St. Joseph Adult Chewable Aspirin (81 mg.) ... ■ 703
Synalgos-DC Capsules ... 2525
Talwin Compound ... 2072
Ursinus Inlay-Tabs ... ■ 691
Vanquish Analgesic Caplets ... ■ 574
Zorprin Tablets ... 698

Astemizole (May partially counteract anticoagulant effect of Heparin). Products include:

Hismanal Tablets ... 1138

Azatadine Maleate (May partially counteract anticoagulant effect of Heparin). Products include:

Optimine Tablets ... 2115
Trinalin Repetabs Tablets ... 1170

Bromodiphenhydramine Hydrochloride (May partially counteract anticoagulant effect of Heparin).

No products indexed under this heading.

Brompheniramine Maleate (May partially counteract anticoagulant effect of Heparin). Products include:

Alka Seltzer Plus Sinus Allergy Medicine ... ■ 624
Atrohist Sprinkle Capsules ... 558
Bromfed Capsules (Timed Release) ... 1615
Bromfed Syrup ... ■ 628
Bromfed ... 1615
Dimetane Decongestant ... ■ 673
Dimetane ... ■ 672
Dimetane-DC Cough Syrup ... 1857
Dimetane-DX Cough Syrup ... 1858
Dimetapp Elixir ... ■ 673
Dimetapp DM Elixir ... ■ 674
Dimetapp Extentabs ... ■ 674
Dimetapp Plus Caplets ... ■ 675
Dimetapp Tablets ... ■ 675
Drixoral Antihistamine/Nasal Decongestant Syrup ... ■ 698

Chlorpheniramine Maleate (May partially counteract anticoagulant effect of Heparin). Products include:

A.R.M. Allergy Relief Medicine Caplets ... ■ 615
Alka-Seltzer Plus Cold Medicine ... ■ 623
Allerest ... ■ 559
Ana-Kit Anaphylaxis Emergency Treatment Kit ... 1100
BC Cold Powder Multi-Symptom Formula ... ■ 517
Brexin L.A. Capsules ... 2078
Cerose-DM ... 2443
Cheracol Plus Head Cold/Cough Formula ... ■ 667
Chlor-Trimeton Allergy Syrup, Tablets & Long-Acting Repetabs Tablets ... ■ 693
Chlor-Trimeton Decongestant ... ■ 694
Comhist LA Capsules ... 1618
Allergy-Sinus Comtrex Multi-Symptom Allergy Sinus Formula Tablets & Caplets ... 746
Comtrex Multi-Symptom Cold Reliever Tablets/Caplets/Liqui-Gels/Liquid ... 745
Day-Night Comtrex ... 747
Contac Continuous Action Decongestant/Antihistamine Capsules ■ 710
Contac Maximum Strength Continuous Action Decongestant/Antihistamine Caplets ... ■ 709
Contac Severe Cold and Flu Formula Caplets ... ■ 711
Coricidin 'D' Decongestant Tablets ... ■ 695
Coricidin Demilets Tablets for Children ... ■ 696
Coricidin Tablets ... ■ 695
Deconamine ... 663
Demazin Nasal Decongestant/Antihistamine Repetabs Tablets & Syrup ... ■ 697
Dorcol Children's Liquid Cold Formula ... ■ 686
Dristan Decongestant/Antihistamine/ Analgesic Coated Caplets ... ■ 749
Dristan Cold Nasal Decongestant/Antihistamine/ Analgesic Coated Tablets ... 2419
Dristan Advanced Formula Decongestant/Antihistamine/Analgesic Tablets ... ■ 749
Extendryl ... 994
4-Way Cold Tablets ... 750
Fedahist Gyrocaps ... 2145
Fedahist Timecaps ... 2145
Hycomine Compound Tablets ... 929
Isoclor Timesule Capsules ... ■ 561
Kronofed-A ... 970
Medi-Flu Caplet, Liquid ... ■ 640
Naldecon Syrup, Tablets, Pediatric Drops and Pediatric Syrup ... 709
Nolamine Tablets ... 838
Novafed A Capsules ... 1342
Novahistine DH ... 1342
Novahistine Elixir ... ■ 596
Ornade Spansule Capsules ... 2221
Orthoxicol Cough Syrup ... ■ 668
PediaCare Allergy Relief Formula Liquid ... 1362
PediaCare Cough-Cold Formula Liquid ... 1362
PediaCare Night Rest Cough-Cold Formula Liquid ... 1362
PediaCare 6-12 Cough-Cold Formula Chewable Tablets ... 1362
Pyrroxate Capsules ... ■ 669
Quelidrine Syrup ... 556
Ru-Tuss II Capsules ... 693
Ru-Tuss Tablets ... 693
Ryna ... ■ 741
Sinarest Tablets & Extra Strength Tablets ... ■ 562
Sine-Off Maximum Strength Allergy/Sinus Formula Caplets ... ■ 721
Sine-Off Sinus Medicine Tablets-Aspirin Formula ... ■ 722
Singlet Tablets ... ■ 598
Sinulin ... 840
Sinutab Maximum Strength ... ■ 641
St. Joseph Nighttime Cold Medicine ... ■ 705
Sudafed Plus Liquid ... ■ 544
Sudafed Plus Tablets ... ■ 545
Teldrin Timed-Release Allergy Capsules, 12 mg. ... 2192
TheraFlu Flu and Cold Medicine ... ■ 687
Triaminic Allergy Tablets ... ■ 688
Triaminic Chewables ... ■ 688
Triaminic Cold Tablets ... ■ 688
Triaminic Nite Light ... ■ 689
Triaminic Syrup ... ■ 689
Triaminic-12 Tablets ... ■ 690
Triaminicin Tablets ... ■ 690
Triaminicol Multi-Symptom Cold Tablets ... ■ 691
Triaminicol Multi-Symptom Relief ■ 691
Tylenol Allergy Sinus Medication Caplets and Gelcaps, Maximum Strength ... 1372
Children's Tylenol Cold Liquid Formula and Chewable Tablets ... 1368
Tylenol Cold & Flu Hot Medication, Packets ... 1369
Tylenol Cold Medication Caplets and Tablets ... 1370
Tylenol Cold Medication, Effervescent Tablets ... 1369
Vicks Children's NyQuil ... ■ 664
Vicks Formula 44 Cough Medicine ... ■ 661
Vicks Formula 44M Multi-Symptom Cough Medicine ... ■ 662
Vicks Pediatric Formula 44m Multi-Symptom Cough & Cold Medicine ... ■ 663

Chlorpheniramine Polistirex (May partially counteract anticoagulant effect of Heparin). Products include:

Tussionex Extended-Release Suspension ... 988

Chlorpheniramine Tannate (May partially counteract anticoagulant effect of Heparin). Products include:

Rynatan ... 2387
Rynatuss ... 2388

Choline Magnesium Trisalicylate (May induce bleeding). Products include:

Trilisate ... 1822

Clemastine Fumarate (May partially counteract anticoagulant effect of Heparin). Products include:

Tavist Syrup ... 2033
Tavist Tablets ... 2035
Tavist-D Tablets ... 2035

Cyproheptadine Hydrochloride (May partially counteract anticoagulant effect of Heparin). Products include:

Periactin ... 1525

Demeclocycline Hydrochloride (May partially counteract anticoagulant effect of Heparin). Products include:

Declomycin Capsules, Tablets ... 1199

Deslanoside (May partially counteract anticoagulant effect of Heparin).

No products indexed under this heading.

Dexchlorpheniramine Maleate (May partially counteract anticoagulant effect of Heparin). Products include:

Polaramine ... 2116

Dextrans (Low Molecular Weight) (May induce bleeding).

No products indexed under this heading.

Diclofenac Sodium (May induce bleeding). Products include:

Voltaren Ophthalmic Sterile Ophthalmic Solution ... ⊙ 268
Voltaren Tablets ... 1042

Dicumarol (Prolonged prothrombin time). Products include:

Dicumarol Tablets ... 516

Diflunisal (May induce bleeding). Products include:
- Dolobid Tablets ... 1465

Digitoxin (Counteract anticoagulant action). Products include:
- Crystodigin Tablets ... 1253

Digoxin (May partially counteract anticoagulant effect of Heparin). Products include:
- Lanoxicaps ... 772
- Lanoxin Elixir Pediatric ... 775
- Lanoxin Injection ... 778
- Lanoxin Injection Pediatric ... 781
- Lanoxin Tablets ... 783

Diphenhydramine Citrate (May partially counteract anticoagulant effect of Heparin). Products include:
- Alka-Seltzer Plus Night-Time Cold Medicine ... ■ 623
- Bufferin AF Nite Time Analgesic/Sleeping Aid Caplets ... 744
- Excedrin P.M. Analgesic/Sleeping Aid Tablets, Caplets and Liquid ... 749

Diphenylpyraline Hydrochloride (May partially counteract anticoagulant effect of Heparin).
- No products indexed under this heading.

Dipyridamole (May induce bleeding). Products include:
- Persantine Tablets ... 683

Doxycycline Calcium (May partially counteract anticoagulant effect of Heparin).
- No products indexed under this heading.

Doxycycline Hyclate (May partially counteract anticoagulant effect of Heparin). Products include:
- Doryx Capsules ... 1717
- Vibramycin Hyclate Capsules ... 1787
- Vibramycin Hyclate Intravenous ... 1968
- Vibra-Tabs Film Coated Tablets ... 1787

Doxycycline Monohydrate (May partially counteract anticoagulant effect of Heparin). Products include:
- Monodox Capsules ... 1630
- Vibramycin Monohydrate for Oral Suspension ... 1787

Etodolac (May induce bleeding). Products include:
- Lodine Capsules ... 2468

Fenoprofen Calcium (May induce bleeding). Products include:
- Nalfon Pulvules & Tablets ... 919

Flurbiprofen (May induce bleeding). Products include:
- Ansaid Tablets ... 2319

Hydroxychloroquine Sulfate (May induce bleeding). Products include:
- Plaquenil Sulfate Tablets ... 2067

Ibuprofen (May induce bleeding). Products include:
- Advil Cold & Sinus Caplets (formerly CoAdvil) ... 2416
- Advil Ibuprofen Tablets and Caplets ... 2416
- Children's Advil Suspension ... 2426
- CoAdvil ... ■ 748
- Dristan Sinus Caplets ... 2419
- Haltran Tablets ... ■ 668
- Ibuprofen ... ■ 631
- Medipren ibuprofen Caplets and Tablets ... 1362
- Midol 200 Cramp Relief Formula ... ■ 570
- Motrin Tablets ... 2351
- Motrin IB Caplets and Tablets ... ■ 736
- Nuprin Ibuprofen/Analgesic Tablets & Caplets ... 752
- PediaProfen Suspension ... 1363
- Rufen Tablets ... 691
- Trendar Ibuprofen Tablets ... ■ 756

Indomethacin (May induce bleeding). Products include:
- Indocin ... 1487

Indomethacin Sodium Trihydrate (May induce bleeding). Products include:
- Indocin I.V. ... 1490

Ketoprofen (May induce bleeding). Products include:
- Orudis Capsules ... 2488

Ketorolac Tromethamine (May induce bleeding). Products include:
- Toradol IM Injection ... 2302

Magnesium Salicylate (May induce bleeding). Products include:
- Doan's - Extra-Strength Analgesic ■ 549
- Doan's - Regular Strength Analgesic ... ■ 549
- Mobigesic Analgesic Tablets ... ■ 507

Meclofenamate Sodium (May induce bleeding). Products include:
- Meclomen Capsules ... 1739

Mefenamic Acid (May induce bleeding). Products include:
- Ponstel ... 1758

Methacycline Hydrochloride (May partially counteract anticoagulant effect of Heparin).
- No products indexed under this heading.

Methdilazine Hydrochloride (May partially counteract anticoagulant effect of Heparin). Products include:
- Tacaryl Syrup & Tablets ... 2409

Minocycline Hydrochloride (May partially counteract anticoagulant effect of Heparin). Products include:
- Minocin Intravenous ... 1221
- Minocin Oral Suspension ... 1224
- Minocin Pellet-Filled Capsules ... 1222

Naproxen (May induce bleeding). Products include:
- Naprosyn ... 2297

Naproxen Sodium (May induce bleeding). Products include:
- Anaprox and Anaprox DS Tablets ... 2288

Nicotine Polacrilex (May partially counteract anticoagulant effect of Heparin). Products include:
- Nicorette ... 1335

Oxytetracycline (May partially counteract anticoagulant effect). Products include:
- Terramycin Intramuscular Solution 1964
- Urobiotic-250 Capsules ... 1968

Oxytetracycline Hydrochloride (May partially counteract anticoagulant effect). Products include:
- Terra-Cortril Ophthalmic Suspension ... 1963
- Terramycin Capsules ... 1786
- Terramycin Intramuscular Solution 1964
- Terramycin with Polymyxin B Sulfate Ophthalmic Ointment ... 1965

Phenylbutazone (May induce bleeding). Products include:
- Butazolidin Capsules & Tablets ... 1027

Piroxicam (May induce bleeding). Products include:
- Feldene Capsules ... 1777

Promethazine Hydrochloride (May partially counteract anticoagulant effect of Heparin). Products include:
- Mepergan Injection ... 2479
- Phenergan with Codeine ... 2497
- Phenergan with Dextromethorphan 2499
- Phenergan Injection ... 2493
- Phenergan Suppositories ... 2496
- Phenergan Syrup ... 2495
- Phenergan Tablets ... 2496
- Phenergan VC ... 2500
- Phenergan VC with Codeine ... 2501

Pyrilamine Maleate (May partially counteract anticoagulant effect of Heparin). Products include:
- Codimal ... 846
- 4-Way Fast Acting Nasal Spray - Original Formula (regular & mentholated) & Metered Spray Pump (regular) ... 751
- Maximum Strength Midol Multi-Symptom Menstrual Formula ... ■ 571
- Maximum Strength Midol PMS Premenstrual Syndrome Formula ... ■ 570
- Regular Strength Midol Multi-Symptom Menstrual Formula ... ■ 570
- Prefrin-A ... ⊙ 255
- Prēmsyn PMS Capsules & Caplets ■ 547
- Primatene Tablets-M Formula ... 2421
- Robitussin Night Relief ... ■ 677
- Ru-Tuss with Hydrocodone ... 694
- Triaminic Expectorant DH ... 1995
- Triaminic Oral Infant Drops ... 1996

Pyrilamine Tannate (May partially counteract anticoagulant effect of Heparin). Products include:
- Rynatan ... 2387

Salsalate (May induce bleeding). Products include:
- Disalcid ... 1310
- Mono-Gesic Tablets ... 846
- Salflex ... 839

Sulindac (May induce bleeding). Products include:
- Clinoril Tablets ... 1433

Terfenadine (May partially counteract anticoagulant effect of Heparin). Products include:
- Seldane Tablets ... 1349
- Seldane-D Extended-Release Tablets ... 1350

Tetracycline Hydrochloride (May partially counteract anticoagulant effect of Heparin). Products include:
- Achromycin V Capsules ... 1193
- Achromycin Ophthalmic Ointment 1% ... ⊙ 307
- Achromycin Ophthalmic Suspension 1% ... ⊙ 308
- Topicycline for Topical Solution ... 1856

Tolmetin Sodium (May induce bleeding). Products include:
- Tolectin (200, 400 and 600 mg) .. 1379

Trimeprazine Tartrate (May partially counteract anticoagulant effect of Heparin). Products include:
- Temaril Tablets, Syrup and Spansule Sustained Release Capsules 1085

Tripelennamine Hydrochloride (May partially counteract anticoagulant effect of Heparin). Products include:
- PBZ Tablets & Elixir ... 1037
- PBZ-SR Tablets ... 1037

Triprolidine Hydrochloride (May partially counteract anticoagulant effect of Heparin). Products include:
- Actidil ... ■ 538
- Actifed Capsules ... ■ 539
- Actifed Plus Caplets ... ■ 539
- Actifed Plus Tablets ... ■ 540
- Actifed with Codeine Cough Syrup .. 752
- Actifed Syrup ... ■ 540
- Actifed Tablets ... ■ 540
- Actifed 12-Hour Capsules ... ■ 539

Warfarin Sodium (Prolonged prothrombin time). Products include:
- Coumadin Injection & Tablets ... 944
- Panwarfin Tablets ... 547

HEP-B-GAMMAGEE
(Hepatitis B Immune Globulin (Human)) ... 1474
May interact with:

Measles Virus Vaccine Live (Interference with immune response to live virus vaccines). Products include:
- Attenuvax ... 1424

Measles & Rubella Virus Vaccine Live (Interference with immune response to live virus vaccines). Products include:
- M-R-VAX II ... 1496

Measles, Mumps & Rubella Virus Vaccine Live (Interference with immune response to live virus vaccines). Products include:
- M-M-R II ... 1494

Rubella Virus Vaccine Live (Interference with immune response to live virus vaccines). Products include:
- Meruvax II ... 1503

Rubella & Mumps Virus Vaccine Live (Interference with immune response to live virus vaccines). Products include:
- Biavax II ... 1427

HEP-FORTE CAPSULES
(Vitamins with Minerals) ... 1356
No interactions described in labeling.

HERPECIN-L COLD SORE LIP BALM
(Allantoin) ... 833
No interactions described in labeling.

HERPLEX LIQUIFILM
(Idoxuridine) ... ⊙ 248
May interact with:

Boric Acid (Concurrent administration is not recommended). Products include:
- Borofax Ointment ... ■ 541
- Clear Eyes ACR ... ⊙ 305
- Collyrium for Fresh Eyes ... 2445
- Collyrium Fresh ... 2445
- Eye Wash ... ⊙ 258
- Star-Otic Ear Solution ... ■ 729

HESPAN INJECTION
(Hetastarch) ... 948
No interactions described in labeling.

HEXALEN CAPSULES
(Altretamine) ... 2316
May interact with monoamine oxidase inhibitors and certain other agents. Compounds in these categories include:

Cimetidine (Increases altretamine's half-life and toxicity in a rat model). Products include:
- Tagamet Tablets ... 2228

Cimetidine Hydrochloride (Increases altretamine's half-life and toxicity in a rat model). Products include:
- Tagamet ... 2228

Furazolidone (Potential for severe orthostatic hypotension). Products include:
- Furoxone ... 1855

Isocarboxazid (Potential for severe orthostatic hypotension). Products include:
- Marplan Tablets ... 1906

Phenelzine Sulfate (Potential for severe orthostatic hypotension). Products include:
- Nardil ... 1742

Selegiline Hydrochloride (Potential for severe orthostatic hypotension). Products include:
- Eldepryl ... 2250

Tranylcypromine Sulfate (Potential for severe orthostatic hypotension). Products include:
- Parnate Tablets ... 2222

HIBICLENS ANTIMICROBIAL SKIN CLEANSER
(Chlorhexidine Gluconate) ... 2271
No interactions described in labeling.

HIBISTAT GERMICIDAL HAND RINSE
(Chlorhexidine Gluconate) ... 2272
No interactions described in labeling.

HIBISTAT TOWELETTE
(Chlorhexidine Gluconate) ... 2272
No interactions described in labeling.

HIBTITER
(Haemophilus B Conjugate Vaccine)..1206
May interact with immunosuppressive agents. Compounds in this category include:

Azathioprine (The expected immune response may not be obtained). Products include:
Imuran 768

Cyclosporine (The expected immune response may not be obtained). Products include:
Sandimmune 2024

Immune Globulin (Human) (The expected immune response may not be obtained). Products include:
MICRhoGAM Rh$_0$(D) Immune Globulin (Human) 1650
RhoGAM Rh$_0$(D) Immune Globulin (Human) 1651

Immune Globulin Intravenous (Human) (The expected immune response may not be obtained). Products include:
Gamimune N Immune Globulin Intravenous (Human) 1572
Gammagard Immune Globulin, Intravenous (Human) 658
Iveegam 1129
Sandoglobulin I.V. 2027

Muromonab-CD3 (The expected immune response may not be obtained). Products include:
Orthoclone OKT3 Sterile Solution 1645

HIPREX TABLETS
(Methenamine Hippurate) 1333
May interact with sulfonamides. Compounds in this category include:

Sulfamethizole (Concurrent use is contraindicated; may form an insoluble precipitate with formaldehyde in urine). Products include:
Thiosulfil Forte Tablets 2526
Urobiotic-250 Capsules 1968

Sulfamethoxazole (Concurrent use is contraindicated; may form an insoluble precipitate with formaldehyde in urine). Products include:
Azo Gantanol Tablets 1887
Bactrim DS Tablets 1891
Bactrim I.V. Infusion 1889
Bactrim 1891
Gantanol 1899
Septra 813
Septra I.V. Infusion 808
Septra I.V. Infusion ADD-Vantage Vials 810
Septra 813

Sulfasalazine (Concurrent use is contraindicated; may form an insoluble precipitate with formaldehyde in urine). Products include:
Azulfidine Tablets, EN-tabs, Oral Suspension 1157

Sulfinpyrazone (Concurrent use is contraindicated; may form an insoluble precipitate with formaldehyde in urine). Products include:
Anturane 853

Sulfisoxazole (Concurrent use is contraindicated; may form an insoluble precipitate with formaldehyde in urine). Products include:
Azo Gantrisin Tablets 1888
Gantrisin Tablets 1901
Pediazole 1973

Sulfisoxazole Diolamine (Concurrent use is contraindicated; may form an insoluble precipitate with formaldehyde in urine). Products include:
Gantrisin Ophthalmic Ointment/Solution 1900

HISMANAL TABLETS
(Astemizole) 1138

Food Interactions

Meal, unspecified (Reduces the absorption by 60%).

HOLD COUGH SUPPRESSANT LOZENGE
(Dextromethorphan Hydrobromide) ◘ 617
No interactions described in labeling.

HUMATIN CAPSULES
(Paromomycin Sulfate) 1726
No interactions described in labeling.

HUMATROPE VIALS
(Somatropin) 1266
May interact with glucocorticoids. Compounds in this category include:

Betamethasone Acetate (Excessive glucocorticoid therapy will inhibit the growth promoting effect of somatropin). Products include:
Celestone Soluspan Suspension 2081

Betamethasone Sodium Phosphate (Excessive glucocorticoid therapy will inhibit the growth promoting effect of somatropin). Products include:
Celestone Soluspan Suspension 2081

Cortisone Acetate (Excessive glucocorticoid therapy will inhibit the growth promoting effect of somatropin). Products include:
Cortone Acetate Sterile Suspension 1437
Cortone Acetate Tablets 1439

Dexamethasone (Excessive glucocorticoid therapy will inhibit the growth promoting effect of somatropin). Products include:
AK-Trol Ointment & Suspension ⊙ 207
Decadron Elixir 1445
Decadron Tablets 1447
Decaspray Topical Aerosol 1459
Dexacidin ⊙ 272
Maxidex Sterile Ophthalmic Suspension ⊙ 223
Maxitrol Ophthalmic Ointment/Suspension ⊙ 223
TobraDex Ophthalmic Suspension and Ointment ⊙ 228

Dexamethasone Acetate (Excessive glucocorticoid therapy will inhibit the growth promoting effect of somatropin). Products include:
Dalalone D.P. Injectable 999
Decadron-LA Sterile Suspension 1457

Dexamethasone Sodium Phosphate (Excessive glucocorticoid therapy will inhibit the growth promoting effect of somatropin). Products include:
AK-Dex ⊙ 203
Decadron Phosphate Respihaler 1454
Decadron Phosphate Sterile Ophthalmic Ointment 1453
Decadron Phosphate Sterile Ophthalmic Solution 1453
Decadron Phosphate Topical Cream 1455
Decadron Phosphate Turbinaire 1456
Maxidex Sterile Ophthalmic Ointment ⊙ 222
NeoDecadron Sterile Ophthalmic Ointment 1517
NeoDecadron Sterile Ophthalmic Solution 1518
NeoDecadron Topical Cream 1518

Hydrocortisone (Excessive glucocorticoid therapy will inhibit the growth promoting effect of somatropin). Products include:
AK-Spore H.C. ⊙ 206
Bactine Hydrocortisone Anti-Itch Cream ◘ 625
CaldeCORT Anti-Itch Hydrocortisone Spray ◘ 560
Carmol HC Cream 1% 2296
Cortaid Spray ◘ 735
Cortenema 2244
Cortisporin Ointment 758
Cortisporin Ophthalmic Ointment Sterile 758
Cortisporin Ophthalmic Suspension Sterile 759
Cortisporin Otic Solution Sterile 760
Cortisporin Otic Suspension Sterile 760
Cortizone-5 Creme & Ointment ◘ 732
Dermolate Anti-Itch Cream ◘ 697
Eldecort Cream 1.0% 1113
Eldecort Cream 1.0% and 2.5% 1113
Fungoid HC Creme 1770
Hydrocortone Tablets 1482
Hytone 909
LazerSporin-C Solution 1770
Massengill Medicated Soft Cloth Towelettes 2192
Nutracort Cream & Lotion 1684
PediOtic Suspension Sterile 797
Synacort Creams 1%, 2.5% 2296
Vanoxide-HC Acne Lotion 911
Vioform-Hydrocortisone Cream and Mild Cream 889
Vioform-Hydrocortisone Ointment 889
VōSoL HC Otic Solution 2392
Vytone Cream 1% 911

Hydrocortisone Acetate (Excessive glucocorticoid therapy will inhibit the growth promoting effect of somatropin). Products include:
Analpram-HC Rectal Cream 1% and 2.5% 970
Anusol-HC Cream 1690
Anusol-HC Suppositories 1691
Caldecort ◘ 560
Carmol HC Cream 1% 2296
Chloromycetin Hydrocortisone Ophthalmic 1694
Coly-Mycin S Otic w/Neomycin & Hydrocortisone 1708
Cortaid ◘ 735
Cortef Feminine Itch Cream ◘ 735
Corticaine ◘ 682
Cortifoam 1827
Cortisporin Cream 757
Epifoam 1828
Gynecort 5 Creme ◘ 556
Hydrocortone Acetate Sterile Suspension 1479
Lanacort 5 Creme and Ointment ◘ 557
Mantadil Cream 789
Ophthocort ⊙ 301
Orabase HCA Oral Paste 890
Pramosone Cream, Lotion & Ointment 971
ProctoCream-HC 1834
Proctofoam-HC 1835

Hydrocortisone Sodium Phosphate (Excessive glucocorticoid therapy will inhibit the growth promoting effect of somatropin). Products include:
Hydrocortone Phosphate Injection, Sterile 1481

Hydrocortisone Sodium Succinate (Excessive glucocorticoid therapy will inhibit the growth promoting effect of somatropin). Products include:
Solu-Cortef Sterile Powder 2361

Methylprednisolone Acetate (Excessive glucocorticoid therapy will inhibit the growth promoting effect of somatropin). Products include:
Depo-Medrol Sterile Aqueous Suspension 2334

Methylprednisolone Sodium Succinate (Excessive glucocorticoid therapy will inhibit the growth promoting effect of somatropin). Products include:
Solu-Medrol Sterile Powder 2363

Prednisolone Acetate (Excessive glucocorticoid therapy will inhibit the growth promoting effect of somatropin). Products include:
AK-Cide Sterile Ophthalmic Ointment & Suspension ⊙ 202
Blephamide Liquifilm Sterile Ophthalmic Suspension 586
Blephamide S.O.P. Sterile Ophthalmic Ointment 586
Cetapred Ointment ⊙ 220
⅛% Econopred & 1% Econopred Plus ⊙ 217
Isopto Cetapred Suspension ⊙ 220
Metimyd ⊙ 306
Poly-Pred Liquifilm ⊙ 250
Pred Forte ⊙ 252
Pred Mild ⊙ 254
Pred-G Liquifilm Sterile Ophthalmic Suspension ⊙ 252
Pred-G S.O.P. Sterile Ophthalmic Ointment ⊙ 253
Vasocidin Ointment ⊙ 275

Prednisolone Sodium Phosphate (Excessive glucocorticoid therapy will inhibit the growth promoting effect of somatropin). Products include:
AK-Pred ⊙ 205
Hydeltrasol Injection, Sterile 1476
Inflamase ⊙ 274
Pediapred Oral Liquid 987
Vasocidin Ophthalmic Solution ⊙ 276

Prednisolone Tebutate (Excessive glucocorticoid therapy will inhibit the growth promoting effect of somatropin). Products include:
Hydeltra-T.B.A. Sterile Suspension 1478

Prednisone (Excessive glucocorticoid therapy will inhibit the growth promoting effect of somatropin). Products include:
Deltasone Tablets 2332

Triamcinolone (Excessive glucocorticoid therapy will inhibit the growth promoting effect of somatropin).
No products indexed under this heading.

Triamcinolone Acetonide (Excessive glucocorticoid therapy will inhibit the growth promoting effect of somatropin). Products include:
Aristocort A 1010
Azmacort Inhaler 1837
Kenalog Cream, Lotion & Ointment 2401
Kenalog-10 Injection 2402
Kenalog-40 Injection 2403
Kenalog in Orabase 604
Kenalog Spray 2401
Mycolog II Cream and Ointment 2407
Mytrex Cream & Ointment 2080
Nasacort Nasal Inhaler 1844

Triamcinolone Diacetate (Excessive glucocorticoid therapy will inhibit the growth promoting effect of somatropin). Products include:
Aristocort Suspension 1008

Triamcinolone Hexacetonide (Excessive glucocorticoid therapy will inhibit the growth promoting effect of somatropin). Products include:
Aristospan Suspension 1011

HUMIBID DM TABLETS
(Guaifenesin, Dextromethorphan Hydrobromide) 560
May interact with monoamine oxidase inhibitors. Compounds in this category include:

Furazolidone (Concurrent therapy should be avoided). Products include:
Furoxone 1855

Isocarboxazid (Concurrent therapy should be avoided). Products include:
Marplan Tablets 1906

Phenelzine Sulfate (Concurrent therapy should be avoided). Products include:
Nardil 1742

Selegiline Hydrochloride (Concurrent therapy should be avoided). Products include:
Eldepryl 2250

Tranylcypromine Sulfate (Concurrent therapy should be avoided). Products include:
Parnate Tablets 2222

HUMIBID L.A. TABLETS
(Guaifenesin) 560
No interactions described in labeling.

HUMIBID SPRINKLE CAPSULES
(Guaifenesin) 560
No interactions described in labeling.

HUMORSOL STERILE OPHTHALMIC SOLUTION
(Demecarium Bromide) 1475
May interact with cholinergic agents and certain other agents. Compounds in these categories include:

Edrophonium Chloride (Additive adverse effects). Products include:
- Enlon Injection 598
- Tensilon Injectable 1123

Neostigmine Bromide (Additive adverse effects). Products include:
- Prostigmin Tablets 1121

Neostigmine Methylsulfate (Additive adverse effects). Products include:
- Prostigmin Injectable 1120

Pyridostigmine Bromide (Additive adverse effects). Products include:
- Mestinon Injectable 1115
- Mestinon 1116

Succinylcholine Chloride (Possible respiratory and cardiovascular collapse). Products include:
- Anectine 755

HUMULIN 70/30, 100 UNITS
(Insulin, Human) 1267
No interactions described in labeling.

HUMULIN BR, 100 UNITS
(Insulin, Human Regular) 1268
No interactions described in labeling.

HUMULIN L, 100 UNITS
(Insulin, Human, Zinc Suspension) 1268
No interactions described in labeling.

HUMULIN N, 100 UNITS
(Insulin, Human Isophane Suspension) 1270
No interactions described in labeling.

HUMULIN R, 100 UNITS
(Insulin, Human) 1272
No interactions described in labeling.

HUMULIN U, 100 UNITS
(Insulin, Human, Zinc Suspension) 1272
No interactions described in labeling.

HURRICAINE TOPICAL ANESTHETIC AEROSOL SPRAY, 2 OZ
(Benzocaine) 672
No interactions described in labeling.

HURRICAINE TOPICAL ANESTHETIC GEL, 1 OZ ORIGINAL AND PINA COLADA, ⅛ OZ ORIGINAL AND PINA COLADA
(Benzocaine) 672
No interactions described in labeling.

HURRICAINE TOPICAL ANESTHETIC LIQUID, 1 OZ ORIGINAL AND PINA COLADA ⅛ OZ ORIGINAL AND PINA COLADA
(Benzocaine) 672
No interactions described in labeling.

HURRICAINE TOPICAL ANESTHETIC SPRAY KIT
(Benzocaine) 672
No interactions described in labeling.

HYCODAN SYRUP, TABLETS
(Hydrocodone Bitartrate, Homatropine Methylbromide) 927
May interact with narcotic analgesics, phenothiazines, hypnotics and sedatives, tranquilizers, central nervous system depressants, antihistamines, tricyclic antidepressants, monoamine oxidase inhibitors, and certain other agents. Compounds in these categories include:

Alcohol (Additive CNS depression).

Alfentanil Hydrochloride (Additive CNS depression). Products include:
- Alfenta Injection 1131

Alprazolam (Additive CNS depression). Products include:
- Xanax Tablets 2367

Amitriptyline Hydrochloride (Increased effect of either drug). Products include:
- Elavil 2269
- Endep Tablets 1927
- Etrafon 2087
- Limbitrol 1933
- Triavil Tablets 1556

Amoxapine (Increased effect of either drug). Products include:
- Asendin Tablets 1196

Aprobarbital (Additive CNS depression). Products include:
- Alurate Elixir 1883

Astemizole (Additive CNS depression). Products include:
- Hismanal Tablets 1138

Azatadine Maleate (Additive CNS depression). Products include:
- Optimine Tablets 2115
- Trinalin Repetabs Tablets 1170

Bromodiphenhydramine Hydrochloride (Additive CNS depression).
- No products indexed under this heading.

Brompheniramine Maleate (Additive CNS depression). Products include:
- Alka Seltzer Plus Sinus Allergy Medicine .... ◘ 624
- Atrohist Sprinkle Capsules 558
- Bromfed Capsules (Timed Release) 1615
- Bromfed Syrup .... ◘ 628
- Bromfed 1615
- Dimetane Decongestant .... ◘ 673
- Dimetane .... ◘ 672
- Dimetane-DC Cough Syrup 1857
- Dimetane-DX Cough Syrup 1858
- Dimetapp Elixir .... ◘ 673
- Dimetapp DM Elixir .... ◘ 674
- Dimetapp Extentabs .... ◘ 674
- Dimetapp Plus Caplets .... ◘ 675
- Dimetapp Tablets .... ◘ 675
- Drixoral Antihistamine/Nasal Decongestant Syrup .... ◘ 698

Buprenorphine (Additive CNS depression).
- No products indexed under this heading.

Buspirone Hydrochloride (Additive CNS depression). Products include:
- BuSpar 1401

Butabarbital (Additive CNS depression). Products include:
- Pyridium Plus 1764

Butalbital (Additive CNS depression). Products include:
- Esgic-Plus Tablets 1002
- Esgic Tablets & Capsules 1001
- Fioricet Tablets 2006
- Fiorinal Capsules 2007
- Fiorinal with Codeine Capsules 2008
- Fiorinal Tablets 2007
- Phrenilin 838
- Sedapap Tablets 50 mg/650 mg 1360

Chlordiazepoxide (Additive CNS depression). Products include:
- Libritabs Tablets 1930
- Limbitrol 1933
- Menrium Tablets 1934

Chlordiazepoxide Hydrochloride (Additive CNS depression). Products include:
- Librax Capsules 1929
- Librium Capsules 1931
- Librium Injectable 1932

Chlorpheniramine Maleate (Additive CNS depression). Products include:
- A.R.M. Allergy Relief Medicine Caplets .... ◘ 615
- Alka-Seltzer Plus Cold Medicine .... ◘ 623
- Allerest .... ◘ 559
- Ana-Kit Anaphylaxis Emergency Treatment Kit 1100
- BC Cold Powder Multi-Symptom Formula .... ◘ 517
- Brexin L.A. Capsules 2078
- Cerose-DM 2443
- Cheracol Plus Head Cold/Cough Formula .... ◘ 667
- Chlor-Trimeton Allergy Syrup, Tablets & Long-Acting Repetabs Tablets .... ◘ 693
- Chlor-Trimeton Decongestant .... ◘ 694
- Comhist LA Capsules 1618
- Allergy-Sinus Comtrex Multi-Symptom Allergy Sinus Formula Tablets & Caplets 746
- Comtrex Multi-Symptom Cold Reliever Tablets/Caplets/Liqui-Gels/Liquid 745
- Day-Night Comtrex 747
- Contac Continuous Action Decongestant/Antihistamine Capsules .... ◘ 710
- Contac Maximum Strength Continuous Action Decongestant/Antihistamine Caplets .... ◘ 709
- Contac Severe Cold and Flu Formula Caplets .... ◘ 711
- Coricidin 'D' Decongestant Tablets .... ◘ 695
- Coricidin Demilets Tablets for Children .... ◘ 696
- Coricidin Tablets .... ◘ 695
- Deconamine 663
- Demazin Nasal Decongestant/Antihistamine Repetabs Tablets & Syrup .... ◘ 697
- Dorcol Children's Liquid Cold Formula .... ◘ 686
- Dristan Decongestant/Antihistamine/ Analgesic Coated Caplets .... ◘ 749
- Dristan Cold Nasal Decongestant/ Antihistamine/ Analgesic Coated Tablets 2419
- Dristan Advanced Formula Decongestant/Antihistamine/ Analgesic Tablets .... ◘ 749
- Extendryl 994
- 4-Way Cold Tablets 750
- Fedahist Gyrocaps 2145
- Fedahist Timecaps 2145
- Hycomine Compound Tablets 929
- Isoclor Timesule Capsules .... ◘ 561
- Kronofed-A 970
- Medi-Flu Caplet, Liquid .... ◘ 640
- Naldecon Syrup, Tablets, Pediatric Drops and Pediatric Syrup 709
- Nolamine Tablets 838
- Novafed A Capsules 1342
- Novahistine DH 1342
- Novahistine Elixir .... ◘ 596
- Ornade Spansule Capsules 2221
- Orthoxicol Cough Syrup .... ◘ 668
- PediaCare Allergy Relief Formula Liquid 1362
- PediaCare Cough-Cold Formula Liquid 1362
- PediaCare Night Rest Cough-Cold Formula Liquid 1362
- PediaCare 6-12 Cough-Cold Formula Chewable Tablets 1362
- Pyrroxate Capsules .... ◘ 669
- Quelidrine Syrup 556
- Ru-Tuss II Capsules 693
- Ru-Tuss Tablets 693
- Ryna .... ◘ 741
- Sinarest Tablets & Extra Strength Tablets .... ◘ 562
- Sine-Off Maximum Strength Allergy/Sinus Formula Caplets .... ◘ 721
- Sine-Off Sinus Medicine Tablets-Aspirin Formula .... ◘ 722
- Singlet Tablets .... ◘ 598
- Sinulin 840
- Sinutab Maximum Strength .... ◘ 641
- St. Joseph Nighttime Cold Medicine .... ◘ 705
- Sudafed Plus Liquid .... ◘ 544
- Sudafed Plus Tablets .... ◘ 545
- Teldrin Timed-Release Allergy Capsules, 12 mg 2192
- TheraFlu Flu and Cold Medicine .... ◘ 687
- Triaminic Allergy Tablets .... ◘ 688
- Triaminic Chewables .... ◘ 688
- Triaminic Cold Tablets .... ◘ 688
- Triaminic Nite Light .... ◘ 689
- Triaminic Syrup .... ◘ 689
- Triaminic-12 Tablets .... ◘ 690
- Triaminicin Tablets .... ◘ 690
- Triaminicol Multi-Symptom Cold Tablets .... ◘ 691
- Triaminicol Multi-Symptom Relief .... ◘ 691
- Tylenol Allergy Sinus Medication Caplets and Gelcaps, Maximum Strength 1372
- Children's Tylenol Cold Liquid Formula and Chewable Tablets 1368
- Tylenol Cold & Flu Hot Medication, Packets 1369
- Tylenol Cold Medication Caplets and Tablets 1370
- Tylenol Cold Medication, Effervescent Tablets 1369
- Vicks Children's NyQuil .... ◘ 664
- Vicks Formula 44 Cough Medicine .... ◘ 661
- Vicks Formula 44M Multi-Symptom Cough Medicine .... ◘ 662
- Vicks Pediatric Formula 44m Multi-Symptom Cough & Cold Medicine .... ◘ 663

Chlorpheniramine Polistirex (Additive CNS depression). Products include:
- Tussionex Extended-Release Suspension 988

Chlorpheniramine Tannate (Additive CNS depression). Products include:
- Rynatan 2387
- Rynatuss 2388

Chlorpromazine (Additive CNS depression). Products include:
- Thorazine 2234

Chlorprothixene (Additive CNS depression). Products include:
- Taractan Tablets 1920

Chlorprothixene Hydrochloride (Additive CNS depression). Products include:
- Taractan 1920

Clemastine Fumarate (Additive CNS depression). Products include:
- Tavist Syrup 2033
- Tavist Tablets 2035
- Tavist-D Tablets 2035

Clomipramine Hydrochloride (Increased effect of either drug). Products include:
- Anafranil Capsules 650

Clorazepate Dipotassium (Additive CNS depression). Products include:
- Tranxene 556

Codeine (Additive CNS depression). Products include:
- Calcidrine Syrup 506

Codeine Phosphate (Additive CNS depression). Products include:
- Actifed with Codeine Cough Syrup 752
- Cheracol Cough Syrup 1853
- Codimal PH Syrup 846
- Dimetane-DC Cough Syrup 1857
- Empirin with Codeine Phosphate Nos. 2, 3 & 4 764
- Fiorinal with Codeine Capsules 2008
- Isoclor Expectorant 982
- Naldecon CX Adult Liquid .... ◘ 521
- Novahistine DH 1342
- Novahistine Expectorant 1343
- Nucofed Capsules 2219
- Nucofed Expectorant 2219
- Nucofed Pediatric Expectorant 2220
- Nucofed Syrup 2219
- Phenaphen with Codeine Capsules 1865

Phenaphen-650 with Codeine Tablets ... 1866
Phenergan with Codeine ... 2497
Phenergan VC with Codeine ... 2501
Robitussin A-C Syrup ... 1875
Robitussin-DAC Syrup ... 1875
Ryna ... ▣ 741
Soma Compound w/Codeine Tablets ... 2390
Triaminic Expectorant w/Codeine .. 1996
Tussi-Organidin Liquid ... 2391
Tylenol with Codeine ... 1381

Codeine Polistirex (Additive CNS depression).
No products indexed under this heading.

Cyproheptadine Hydrochloride (Additive CNS depression). Products include:
Periactin ... 1525

Desipramine Hydrochloride (Increased effect of either drug). Products include:
Norpramin Tablets ... 1340

Dexchlorpheniramine Maleate (Additive CNS depression). Products include:
Polaramine ... 2116

Dezocine (Additive CNS depression).

Diazepam (Additive CNS depression). Products include:
Valium Injectable ... 1937
Valium Tablets ... 1939
Valrelease Capsules ... 1923

Diphenhydramine Citrate (Additive CNS depression). Products include:
Alka-Seltzer Plus Night-Time Cold Medicine ... ▣ 623
Bufferin AF Nite Time Analgesic/Sleeping Aid Caplets ... 744
Excedrin P.M. Analgesic/Sleeping Aid Tablets, Caplets and Liquid ... 749

Diphenhydramine Hydrochloride (Additive CNS depression). Products include:
Benadryl Anti-Itch Cream ... ▣ 635
Benadryl Capsules ... 1691
Benadryl Decongestant Elixir ... ▣ 635
Benadryl Decongestant ... ▣ 635
Benadryl Elixir ... ▣ 636
Benadryl Kapseals ... 1691
Benadryl 25 Kapseals ... ▣ 636
Benadryl Parenteral ... 1692
Benadryl Plus ... ▣ 636
Benadryl Plus Nighttime ... ▣ 637
Benadryl Spray, Maximum Strength ... ▣ 637
Benadryl Spray, Regular Strength ▣ 637
Benadryl Steri-Vials, Ampoules, and Steri-Dose Syringe ... 1692
Benadryl 25 Tablets ... ▣ 636
Benylin Cough Syrup ... ▣ 637
Benylin Decongestant ... ▣ 638
Caladryl Cream, Lotion, Spray ... ▣ 638
Miles Nervine Nighttime Sleep-Aid ▣ 627
Nytol Tablets ... ▣ 517
Sleep-ettes-D Tablets ... ▣ 653
Sleep-eze 3 Tablets ... ▣ 755
Sleepinal Night-time Sleep Aid Capsules ... ▣ 734
Sominex Caplets and Tablets ... ▣ 722
Sominex Liquid ... ▣ 723
Sominex Pain Relief Formula ... ▣ 723
Tylenol Cold Night Time Medication Liquid ... 1371
Tylenol PM, Extra Strength Caplets and Tablets ... 1368
Unisom Dual Relief Nighttime Sleep Aid/Analgesic ... 1774
Ziradryl Lotion ... ▣ 643

Diphenylpyraline Hydrochloride (Additive CNS depression).
No products indexed under this heading.

Doxepin Hydrochloride (Increased effect of either drug). Products include:
Sinequan ... 1960

Droperidol (Additive CNS depression). Products include:
Inapsine Injection ... 1140
Innovar Injection ... 1141

Enflurane (Additive CNS depression). Products include:
Ethrane ... 599

Estazolam (Additive CNS depression). Products include:
ProSom Tablets ... 554

Ethchlorvynol (Additive CNS depression). Products include:
Placidyl Capsules ... 553

Ethinamate (Additive CNS depression).
No products indexed under this heading.

Fentanyl (Additive CNS depression). Products include:
Duragesic Transdermal System ... 1133

Fentanyl Citrate (Additive CNS depression). Products include:
Innovar Injection ... 1141
Sublimaze Injection ... 1146

Fluphenazine Decanoate (Additive CNS depression). Products include:
Prolixin Decanoate ... 1795

Fluphenazine Enanthate (Additive CNS depression). Products include:
Prolixin Enanthate ... 1796

Fluphenazine Hydrochloride (Additive CNS depression). Products include:
Prolixin Elixir ... 1793
Prolixin Injection ... 1791
Prolixin Oral Concentrate ... 1792
Prolixin Tablets ... 1793

Flurazepam Hydrochloride (Additive CNS depression). Products include:
Dalmane Capsules ... 1927

Furazolidone (Increased effect of either drug). Products include:
Furoxone ... 1855

Glutethimide (Additive CNS depression).
No products indexed under this heading.

Haloperidol (Additive CNS depression). Products include:
Haldol Injection, Tablets and Concentrate ... 1373

Haloperidol Decanoate (Additive CNS depression). Products include:
Haldol Decanoate ... 1375

Hydrocodone Polistirex (Additive CNS depression). Products include:
Tussionex Extended-Release Suspension ... 988

Hydroxyzine Hydrochloride (Additive CNS depression). Products include:
Atarax Tablets & Syrup ... 1941
Marax Tablets & DF Syrup ... 1954
Vistaril Intramuscular Solution ... 1970

Imipramine Hydrochloride (Increased effect of either drug). Products include:
Tofranil Ampuls ... 1038
Tofranil Tablets ... 1039

Imipramine Pamoate (Increased effect of either drug). Products include:
Tofranil-PM Capsules ... 1041

Isocarboxazid (Increased effect of either drug). Products include:
Marplan Tablets ... 1906

Isoflurane (Additive CNS depression). Products include:
Forane ... 600

Ketamine Hydrochloride (Additive CNS depression). Products include:
Ketalar ... 1726

Levorphanol Tartrate (Additive CNS depression). Products include:
Levo-Dromoran ... 1906

Lorazepam (Additive CNS depression). Products include:
Ativan Injection ... 2432
Ativan Tablets ... 2434

Loxapine Hydrochloride (Additive CNS depression). Products include:
Loxitane ... 1213

Loxapine Succinate (Additive CNS depression). Products include:
Loxitane Capsules ... 1213

Maprotiline Hydrochloride (Increased effect of either drug). Products include:
Ludiomil Tablets ... 874

Meperidine Hydrochloride (Additive CNS depression). Products include:
Demerol ... 2047
Mepergan Injection ... 2479

Mephobarbital (Additive CNS depression). Products include:
Mebaral Tablets ... 2061

Meprobamate (Additive CNS depression). Products include:
Deprol Tablets ... 2382
Equagesic Tablets ... 2451
Miltown Tablets ... 2386
PMB 200 and PMB 400 ... 2504

Mesoridazine (Additive CNS depression). Products include:
Serentil ... 686

Methadone Hydrochloride (Additive CNS depression). Products include:
Dolophine Hydrochloride Ampoules & Vials ... 1260
Dolophine Hydrochloride Tablets ... 1261
Methadone Hydrochloride Diskets .. 1284
Methadone Hydrochloride Oral Solution & Tablets ... 1987

Methdilazine Hydrochloride (Additive CNS depression). Products include:
Tacaryl Syrup & Tablets ... 2409

Methohexital Sodium (Additive CNS depression). Products include:
Brevital Sodium Vials ... 1248

Methoxyflurane (Additive CNS depression).
No products indexed under this heading.

Midazolam Hydrochloride (Additive CNS depression). Products include:
Versed Injection ... 1924

Molindone Hydrochloride (Additive CNS depression). Products include:
Moban Tablets & Concentrate ... 932

Morphine Sulfate (Additive CNS depression). Products include:
Astramorph/PF Injection, USP (Preservative-Free) ... 618
Duramorph ... 960
Infumorph 200 and Infumorph 500 Sterile Solutions ... 962
MS Contin Tablets ... 1814
MSIR ... 1817
Oramorph SR (Morphine Sulfate Sustained Release Tablets) ... 1988
Roxanol ... 1991

Nortriptyline Hydrochloride (Increased effect of either drug). Products include:
Pamelor ... 2019

Opium Alkaloids (Additive CNS depression). Products include:
B & O No. 15A & No. 16A Supprettes ... 2395
Pantopon Injectable ... 1911

Oxazepam (Additive CNS depression). Products include:
Serax Capsules ... 2522
Serax Tablets ... 2522

Oxycodone Hydrochloride (Additive CNS depression). Products include:
Percocet Tablets ... 950
Percodan ... 951
Roxicodone Tablets, Oral Solution & Intensol (Oxycodone) ... 1992
Tylox Capsules ... 1382

Pentobarbital Sodium (Additive CNS depression). Products include:
Nembutal Sodium Capsules ... 534
Nembutal Sodium Solution ... 536
Nembutal Sodium Suppositories ... 538

Perphenazine (Additive CNS depression). Products include:
Etrafon ... 2087
Triavil Tablets ... 1556
Trilafon ... 2123

Phenelzine Sulfate (Increased effect of either drug). Products include:
Nardil ... 1742

Phenobarbital (Additive CNS depression). Products include:
Arco-Lase Plus Tablets ... 607
Bellergal-S Tablets ... 1998
Bronkolixir ... ▣ 761
Bronkotabs Tablets ... ▣ 762
Donnatal ... 1858
Donnatal Extentabs ... 1859
Donnatal Tablets ... 1858
Donnazyme Tablets ... 1860
Kinesed Tablets ... 2272
Phenobarbital Elixir and Tablets ... 1293
Primatene Tablets-P Formula ... 2421
Quadrinal Tablets ... 1183
Tedral SA ... 1765

Prazepam (Additive CNS depression). Products include:
Centrax ... 1693

Prochlorperazine (Additive CNS depression). Products include:
Compazine ... 2201

Promethazine Hydrochloride (Additive CNS depression). Products include:
Mepergan Injection ... 2479
Phenergan with Codeine ... 2497
Phenergan with Dextromethorphan 2499
Phenergan Injection ... 2493
Phenergan Suppositories ... 2496
Phenergan Syrup ... 2495
Phenergan Tablets ... 2496
Phenergan VC ... 2500
Phenergan VC with Codeine ... 2501

Propofol (Additive CNS depression). Products include:
Diprivan Injection ... 2267

Propoxyphene Hydrochloride (Additive CNS depression). Products include:
Darvon ... 1256
Wygesic Tablets ... 2540

Propoxyphene Napsylate (Additive CNS depression). Products include:
Darvon-N/Darvocet-N ... 1254

Protriptyline Hydrochloride (Increased effect of either drug). Products include:
Vivactil Tablets ... 1567

Pyrilamine Maleate (Additive CNS depression). Products include:
Codimal ... 846
4-Way Fast Acting Nasal Spray - Original Formula (regular & mentholated) & Metered Spray Pump (regular) ... 751
Maximum Strength Midol Multi-Symptom Menstrual Formula ... ▣ 571
Maximum Strength Midol PMS Premenstrual Syndrome Formula ... ▣ 570
Regular Strength Midol Multi-Symptom Menstrual Formula ... ▣ 570
Prefrin-A ... ⊙ 255
Prēmsyn PMS Capsules & Caplets ▣ 547
Primatene Tablets-M Formula ... 2421
Robitussin Night Relief ... ▣ 677
Ru-Tuss with Hydrocodone ... 694
Triaminic Expectorant DH ... 1995
Triaminic Oral Infant Drops ... 1996

Pyrilamine Tannate (Additive CNS depression). Products include:
Rynatan ... 2387

Quazepam (Additive CNS depression). Products include:
Doral Tablets ... 2383

Secobarbital Sodium (Additive CNS depression). Products include:
Seconal Sodium Pulvules 1296

Selegiline Hydrochloride (Increased effect of either drug). Products include:
Eldepryl 2250

Sufentanil Citrate (Additive CNS depression). Products include:
Sufenta Injection 1147

Temazepam (Additive CNS depression). Products include:
Restoril Capsules 2023

Terfenadine (Additive CNS depression). Products include:
Seldane Tablets 1349
Seldane-D Extended-Release Tablets 1350

Thiamylal Sodium (Additive CNS depression). Products include:
Surital Ampoules, Steri-Vials 1764

Thioridazine Hydrochloride (Additive CNS depression). Products include:
Mellaril 2011

Thiothixene (Additive CNS depression). Products include:
Navane Capsules and Concentrate 1954
Navane Intramuscular 1956

Tranylcypromine Sulfate (Increased effect of either drug). Products include:
Parnate Tablets 2222

Triazolam (Additive CNS depression). Products include:
Halcion Tablets 2340

Trifluoperazine Hydrochloride (Additive CNS depression). Products include:
Stelazine 2226

Trimeprazine Tartrate (Additive CNS depression). Products include:
Temaril Tablets, Syrup and Spansule Sustained Release Capsules 1085

Trimipramine Maleate (Increased effect of either drug). Products include:
Surmontil Capsules 2524

Tripelennamine Hydrochloride (Additive CNS depression). Products include:
PBZ Tablets & Elixir 1037
PBZ-SR Tablets 1037

Tripelennamine Preparations (Additive CNS depression).

Triprolidine Hydrochloride (Additive CNS depression). Products include:
Actidil .... ▣ 538
Actifed Capsules .... ▣ 539
Actifed Plus Caplets .... ▣ 539
Actifed Plus Tablets .... ▣ 540
Actifed with Codeine Cough Syrup.. 752
Actifed Syrup .... ▣ 540
Actifed Tablets .... ▣ 540
Actifed 12-Hour Capsules .... ▣ 539

HYCOMINE COMPOUND TABLETS

(Hydrocodone Bitartrate, Chlorpheniramine Maleate, Phenylephrine Hydrochloride, Acetaminophen) 929

May interact with narcotic analgesics, phenothiazines, hypnotics and sedatives, sympathomimetic aerosol bronchodilators, monoamine oxidase inhibitors, and certain other agents. Compounds in these categories include:

Albuterol (Additive hypertension). Products include:
Proventil Inhalation Aerosol 2117
Ventolin Inhalation Aerosol and Refill 583

Albuterol Sulfate (Additive hypertension). Products include:
Proventil Repetabs Tablets 2120
Proventil Solutions for Inhalation 0.5% and 0.083% 2118
Proventil Syrup 2119
Proventil Tablets 2120
Ventolin 583

Alcohol (Additive CNS depression).

Alfentanil Hydrochloride (Additive CNS depression). Products include:
Alfenta Injection 1131

Buprenorphine (Additive CNS depression).
No products indexed under this heading.

Chlorpromazine (Additive CNS depression). Products include:
Thorazine 2234

Codeine (Additive CNS depression). Products include:
Calcidrine Syrup 506

Codeine Phosphate (Additive CNS depression). Products include:
Actifed with Codeine Cough Syrup.. 752
Cheracol Cough Syrup 1853
Codimal PH Syrup 846
Dimetane-DC Cough Syrup 1857
Empirin with Codeine Phosphate Nos. 2, 3 & 4 764
Fiorinal with Codeine Capsules 2008
Isoclor Expectorant 982
Naldecon CX Adult Liquid .... ▣ 521
Novahistine DH 1342
Novahistine Expectorant 1343
Nucofed Capsules 2219
Nucofed Expectorant 2219
Nucofed Pediatric Expectorant 2220
Nucofed Syrup 2219
Phenaphen with Codeine Capsules 1865
Phenaphen-650 with Codeine Tablets 1866
Phenergan with Codeine 2497
Phenergan VC with Codeine 2501
Robitussin A-C Syrup 1875
Robitussin-DAC Syrup 1875
Ryna .... ▣ 741
Soma Compound w/Codeine Tablets 2390
Triaminic Expectorant w/Codeine .. 1996
Tussi-Organidin Liquid 2391
Tylenol with Codeine 1381

Codeine Polistirex (Additive CNS depression).
No products indexed under this heading.

Dezocine (Additive CNS depression).

Dobutamine Hydrochloride (Additive hypertension). Products include:
Dobutrex Solution Vials 1259

Dopamine Hydrochloride (Additive hypertension). Products include:
Intropin Injection 930

Ephedrine Hydrochloride (Additive hypertension). Products include:
Amesec .... ▣ 682
Primatene Tablets-M Formula 2421
Primatene Tablets-P Formula 2421
Primatene Tablets-Regular Formula 2421
Quadrinal Tablets 1183
Quelidrine Syrup 556
Tedral SA 1765

Ephedrine Sulfate (Additive hypertension). Products include:
Bronkaid Tablets .... ▣ 757
Bronkolixir .... ▣ 761
Bronkotabs Tablets .... ▣ 762
Marax Tablets & DF Syrup 1954
Pazo Hemorrhoid Ointment & Suppositories 752
Vicks Vatronol Nose Drops .... ▣ 666

Ephedrine Tannate (Additive hypertension). Products include:
Rynatuss 2388

Epinephrine (Additive hypertension). Products include:
Ana-Kit Anaphylaxis Emergency Treatment Kit 1100
Bronkaid Mist .... ▣ 757
EpiPen 843
Marcaine Hydrochloride 0.5% with Epinephrine 1:200,000 (as bitartrate) 958
Marcaine Hydrochloride with Epinephrine 1:200,000 2055
Primatene Mist 2420
Sus-Phrine Injection 1006
Xylocaine with Epinephrine Injections 637

Epinephrine Bitartrate (Additive hypertension). Products include:
AsthmaHaler Mist Epinephrine Bitartrate Bronchodilator .... ▣ 616
Bronkaid Mist Suspension .... ▣ 757
Primatene Mist Suspension 2421

Epinephrine Hydrochloride (Additive hypertension). Products include:
Adrenalin Chloride Solution 1:100 & 1:1,000 1689
Epifrin .... ⊙ 244
Glaucon .... ⊙ 218

Estazolam (Additive CNS depression). Products include:
ProSom Tablets 554

Ethchlorvynol (Additive CNS depression). Products include:
Placidyl Capsules 553

Ethinamate (Additive CNS depression).
No products indexed under this heading.

Fentanyl (Additive CNS depression). Products include:
Duragesic Transdermal System 1133

Fentanyl Citrate (Additive CNS depression). Products include:
Innovar Injection 1141
Sublimaze Injection 1146

Fluphenazine Decanoate (Additive CNS depression). Products include:
Prolixin Decanoate 1795

Fluphenazine Enanthate (Additive CNS depression). Products include:
Prolixin Enanthate 1796

Fluphenazine Hydrochloride (Additive CNS depression). Products include:
Prolixin Elixir 1793
Prolixin Injection 1791
Prolixin Oral Concentrate 1792
Prolixin Tablets 1793

Flurazepam Hydrochloride (Additive CNS depression). Products include:
Dalmane Capsules 1927

Furazolidone (Hypertensive crisis). Products include:
Furoxone 1855

Glutethimide (Additive CNS depression).
No products indexed under this heading.

Hydrocodone Polistirex (Additive CNS depression). Products include:
Tussionex Extended-Release Suspension 988

Isocarboxazid (Hypertensive crisis). Products include:
Marplan Tablets 1906

Isoproterenol Hydrochloride (Additive hypertension). Products include:
Isuprel Hydrochloride Injection 1:5000 2050
Isuprel Hydrochloride Mistometer .. 2051
Isuprel Hydrochloride Solution 1:200 & 1:100 2052
Norisodrine Aerotrol 540

Levorphanol Tartrate (Additive CNS depression). Products include:
Levo-Dromoran 1906

Lorazepam (Additive CNS depression). Products include:
Ativan Injection 2432
Ativan Tablets 2434

Meperidine Hydrochloride (Additive CNS depression). Products include:
Demerol 2047
Mepergan Injection 2479

Mesoridazine (Additive CNS depression). Products include:
Serentil 686

Metaproterenol Sulfate (Additive hypertension). Products include:
Alupent 674
Arm-a-Med Metaproterenol Sulfate Inhalation Solution, USP 617
Metaprel Inhalation Aerosol Bronchodilator 2014
Metaprel Inhalation Solution 2015
Metaprel 2015
Metaproterenol Sulfate Inhalation Solution, USP 912

Metaraminol Bitartrate (Additive hypertension). Products include:
Aramine Injection 1424

Methadone Hydrochloride (Additive CNS depression). Products include:
Dolophine Hydrochloride Ampoules & Vials 1260
Dolophine Hydrochloride Tablets 1261
Methadone Hydrochloride Diskets .. 1284
Methadone Hydrochloride Oral Solution & Tablets 1987

Methoxamine Hydrochloride (Additive hypertension). Products include:
Vasoxyl Injection 819

Midazolam Hydrochloride (Additive CNS depression). Products include:
Versed Injection 1924

Morphine Sulfate (Additive CNS depression). Products include:
Astramorph/PF Injection, USP (Preservative-Free) 618
Duramorph 960
Infumorph 200 and Infumorph 500 Sterile Solutions 962
MS Contin Tablets 1814
MSIR 1817
Oramorph SR (Morphine Sulfate Sustained Release Tablets) 1988
Roxanol 1991

Norepinephrine Bitartrate (Additive hypertension). Products include:
Levophed Bitartrate Injection 2054

Opium Alkaloids (Additive CNS depression). Products include:
B & O No. 15A & No. 16A Supprettes 2395
Pantopon Injectable 1911

Oxycodone Hydrochloride (Additive CNS depression). Products include:
Percocet Tablets 950
Percodan 951
Roxicodone Tablets, Oral Solution & Intensol (Oxycodone) 1992
Tylox Capsules 1382

Perphenazine (Additive CNS depression). Products include:
Etrafon 2087
Triavil Tablets 1556
Trilafon 2123

Phenelzine Sulfate (Hypertensive crisis). Products include:
Nardil 1742

Phenylephrine Bitartrate (Additive hypertension).
No products indexed under this heading.

Phenylephrine Tannate (Additive hypertension). Products include:
Rynatan 2387
Rynatuss 2388

Phenylpropanolamine Hydrochloride (Additive hypertension). Products include:
A.R.M. Allergy Relief Medicine Caplets .... ▣ 615
Acutrim .... ▣ 548
Allerest .... ▣ 559

BC Cold Powder ▣ 517
Cheracol Plus Head Cold/Cough Formula ▣ 667
Codimal Expectorant 846
Comtrex Multi-Symptom Cold Reliever Tablets/Caplets/Liqui-Gels/Liquid 745
Contac Continuous Action Decongestant/Antihistamine Capsules ▣ 710
Contac Maximum Strength Continuous Action Decongestant/Antihistamine Caplets ▣ 709
Contac Severe Cold and Flu Formula Caplets ▣ 711
Coricidin 'D' Decongestant Tablets ▣ 695
Coricidin Demilets Tablets for Children ▣ 696
Demazin Nasal Decongestant/Antihistamine Repetabs Tablets & Syrup ▣ 697
Dexatrim ▣ 733
Dimetane-DC Cough Syrup 1857
Dimetapp Elixir ▣ 673
Dimetapp DM Elixir ▣ 674
Dimetapp Extentabs ▣ 674
Dimetapp Plus Caplets ▣ 675
Dimetapp Tablets ▣ 675
Entex Capsules 1623
Entex LA Tablets 1623
Entex Liquid 1623
4-Way Cold Tablets 750
Hycomine Syrup 927
Naldecon CX Adult Liquid ▣ 521
Naldecon DX Adult Liquid ▣ 521
Naldecon DX Children's Syrup ▣ 522
Naldecon DX Pediatric Drops ▣ 522
Naldecon EX Children's Syrup ▣ 522
Naldecon EX Pediatric Drops ▣ 523
Naldecon Syrup, Tablets, Pediatric Drops and Pediatric Syrup 709
Nolamine Tablets 838
Nolex LA Tablets 838
Ornade Spansule Capsules 2221
Orthoxicol Cough Syrup ▣ 668
Propagest 839
Pyrroxate Capsules ▣ 669
Robitussin-CF ▣ 676
Ru-Tuss II Capsules 693
Ru-Tuss with Hydrocodone 694
Ru-Tuss Tablets 693
Sine-Off Sinus Medicine Tablets-Aspirin Formula ▣ 722
Sinulin 840
St. Joseph Cold Tablets for Children ▣ 704
Tavist-D Tablets 2035
Triaminic Allergy Tablets ▣ 688
Triaminic Chewables ▣ 688
Triaminic Cold Tablets ▣ 688
Triaminic Expectorant ▣ 688
Triaminic Expectorant w/Codeine 1996
Triaminic Expectorant DH 1995
Triaminic Oral Infant Drops 1996
Triaminic Syrup ▣ 689
Triaminic-12 Tablets ▣ 690
Triaminic-DM Syrup ▣ 689
Triaminicin Tablets ▣ 690
Triaminicol Multi-Symptom Cold Tablets ▣ 691
Triaminicol Multi-Symptom Relief ▣ 691
Tuss-Ornade Liquid 2242
Tuss-Ornade Spansule Capsules 2242
Tylenol Cold Medication, Effervescent Tablets 1369

Pirbuterol Acetate (Additive hypertension). Products include:
Maxair Inhaler 1311

Prochlorperazine (Additive CNS depression). Products include:
Compazine 2201

Promethazine Hydrochloride (Additive CNS depression). Products include:
Meperigan Injection 2479
Phenergan with Codeine 2497
Phenergan with Dextromethorphan 2499
Phenergan Injection 2493
Phenergan Suppositories 2496
Phenergan Syrup 2495
Phenergan Tablets 2496
Phenergan VC 2500
Phenergan VC with Codeine 2501

Propofol (Additive CNS depression). Products include:
Diprivan Injection 2267

Propoxyphene Hydrochloride (Additive CNS depression). Products include:
Darvon 1256
Wygesic Tablets 2540

Propoxyphene Napsylate (Additive CNS depression). Products include:
Darvon-N/Darvocet-N 1254

Pseudoephedrine Hydrochloride (Additive hypertension). Products include:
Actifed Capsules ▣ 539
Actifed Plus Caplets ▣ 539
Actifed Plus Tablets ▣ 540
Actifed with Codeine Cough Syrup 752
Actifed Syrup ▣ 540
Actifed Tablets ▣ 540
Actifed 12-Hour Capsules ▣ 539
Advil Cold & Sinus Caplets (formerly CoAdvil) 2416
Allerest ▣ 559
Anatuss LA Tablets 1359
Benadryl Decongestant Elixir ▣ 635
Benadryl Decongestant ▣ 635
Benadryl Plus ▣ 636
Benadryl Plus Nighttime ▣ 637
Benylin Decongestant ▣ 638
Brexin L.A. Capsules 2078
Bromfed Capsules (Timed Release) 1615
Bromfed Syrup ▣ 628
Bromfed 1615
CoAdvil ▣ 748
Allergy-Sinus Comtrex Multi-Symptom Allergy Sinus Formula Tablets & Caplets 746
Cough Formula Comtrex 746
Comtrex Multi-Symptom Cold Reliever Tablets/Caplets/Liqui-Gels/Liquid 745
Day-Night Comtrex 747
Non-Drowsy Comtrex 747
Congess 994
Congestac Caplets ▣ 617
Contac Jr. Children's Cold Medicine ▣ 712
Contac Nighttime Cold Medicine ▣ 713
Contac Sinus Caplets Maximum Strength Non-Drowsy Formula ▣ 710
Contac Sinus Tablets Maximum Strength Non-Drowsy Formula ▣ 710
Deconamine 663
Deconsal II Tablets 559
Dimacol Caplets ▣ 672
Dimetane-DX Cough Syrup 1858
Dorcol Children's Cough Syrup ▣ 685
Dorcol Children's Decongestant Liquid ▣ 685
Dorcol Children's Liquid Cold Formula ▣ 686
Maximum Strength Dristan Decongestant/Analgesic Coated Caplets ▣ 750
No Drowsiness Dristan Cold Nasal Decongestant/Analgesic Coated Caplets 2420
Dristan Sinus Caplets 2419
Sinus Excedrin Analgesic, Decongestant Tablets & Caplets ▣ 533
Fedahist Gyrocaps 2145
Fedahist Timecaps 2145
Guaifed 1615
Guaifed Syrup ▣ 629
Isoclor Expectorant 982
Isoclor Timesule Capsules ▣ 561
Kronofed-A 970
Medi-Flu Caplet, Liquid ▣ 640
Novafed A Capsules 1342
Novafed Capsules 1342
Novahistine DH 1342
Novahistine DMX ▣ 595
Novahistine Expectorant 1343
Nucofed Capsules 2219
Nucofed Expectorant 2219
Nucofed Pediatric Expectorant 2220
Nucofed Syrup 2219
Ornex Caplets ▣ 618
PediaCare Allergy Relief Formula Liquid 1362
PediaCare Cough-Cold Formula Liquid 1362
PediaCare Infants' Oral Decongestant Drops 1362
PediaCare Night Rest Cough-Cold Formula Liquid 1362
PediaCare 6-12 Cough-Cold Formula Chewable Tablets 1362
Robitussin-DAC Syrup 1875
Robitussin-PE ▣ 677
Rondec 1975
Rondec-DM 1976
Rondec-TR Tablet 1975
Ru-Tuss DE Tablets 694
Ryna ▣ 741
Seldane-D Extended-Release Tablets 1350
Sinarest ▣ 562
Sine-Aid Maximum Strength Sinus Headache Caplets 1365
Sine-Aid Maximum Strength Sinus Headache Tablets 1365
Sine-Off Maximum Strength Allergy/Sinus Formula Caplets ▣ 721
Sine-Off Maximum Strength No Drowsiness Formula Caplets ▣ 722
Singlet Tablets ▣ 598
Sinutab Maximum Strength ▣ 641
Sinutab Maximum Strength Without Drowsiness Tablets & Caplets ▣ 642
Sinutab Regular Strength Without Drowsiness Formula ▣ 641
St. Joseph Nighttime Cold Medicine ▣ 705
Sudafed Children's Liquid ▣ 543
Sudafed Cough Syrup ▣ 543
Sudafed Plus Liquid ▣ 544
Sudafed Plus Tablets ▣ 545
Sudafed Sinus Caplets ▣ 545
Sudafed Sinus Tablets ▣ 545
Sudafed Tablets, 30 mg ▣ 544
Sudafed Tablets, Adult Strength, 60 mg ▣ 544
Sudafed 12 Hour Capsules ▣ 545
TheraFlu Flu and Cold Medicine ▣ 687
Triaminic Nite Light ▣ 689
Tylenol Allergy Sinus Medication Caplets and Gelcaps, Maximum Strength 1372
Children's Tylenol Cold Liquid Formula and Chewable Tablets 1368
Tylenol Cold & Flu Hot Medication, Packets 1369
Tylenol Cold & Flu No Drowsiness Hot Medication, Packets 1371
Tylenol Cold Medication Caplets and Tablets 1370
Tylenol Cold Medication No Drowsiness Formula Caplets 1370
Tylenol Cold Night Time Medication Liquid 1371
Tylenol Cough Medication Liquid with Decongestant, Maximum Strength 1372
Tylenol, Maximum Strength, Sinus Medication Gelcaps, Caplets and Tablets 1373
Ursinus Inlay-Tabs ▣ 691
Vicks Children's NyQuil ▣ 664
Vicks Daycare ▣ 660
Vicks Formula 44D Decongestant Cough Medicine ▣ 662
Vicks Formula 44M Multi-Symptom Cough Medicine ▣ 662
Vicks NyQuil Nighttime Colds Medicine-Original & Cherry Flavor ▣ 664
Vicks Pediatric Formula 44 Cough & Congestion Medicine ▣ 663
Vicks Pediatric Formula 44m Multi-Symptom Cough & Cold Medicine ▣ 663

Pseudoephedrine Sulfate (Additive hypertension). Products include:
Afrin Tablets ▣ 693
Chlor-Trimeton Decongestant ▣ 694
Disophrol Chronotab Sustained-Action Tablets ▣ 698
Drixoral Antihistamine/Nasal Decongestant Syrup ▣ 698
Drixoral Non-Drowsy Formula ▣ 699
Drixoral Plus Extended-Release Tablets ▣ 699
Drixoral Sinus ▣ 700
Drixoral Sustained-Action Tablets ▣ 698
Sinutab Allergy Formula Sustained Action Tablets ▣ 640
Trinalin Repetabs Tablets 1170

Quazepam (Additive CNS depression). Products include:
Doral Tablets 2383

Secobarbital Sodium (Additive CNS depression). Products include:
Seconal Sodium Pulvules 1296

Selegiline Hydrochloride (Hypertensive crisis). Products include:
Eldepryl 2250

Sufentanil Citrate (Additive CNS depression). Products include:
Sufenta Injection 1147

Temazepam (Additive CNS depression). Products include:
Restoril Capsules 2023

Terbutaline Sulfate (Additive hypertension). Products include:
Brethaire Inhaler 1024
Brethine Ampuls 1026
Brethine Tablets 1026
Bricanyl Injection 1324
Bricanyl Tablets 1325

Thioridazine Hydrochloride (Additive CNS depression). Products include:
Mellaril 2011

Tranylcypromine Sulfate (Hypertensive crisis). Products include:
Parnate Tablets 2222

Triazolam (Additive CNS depression). Products include:
Halcion Tablets 2340

Trifluoperazine Hydrochloride (Additive CNS depression). Products include:
Stelazine 2226

HYCOMINE PEDIATRIC SYRUP

(Hydrocodone Bitartrate, Phenylpropanolamine Hydrochloride) 927

May interact with narcotic analgesics, phenothiazines, hypnotics and sedatives, monoamine oxidase inhibitors, sympathomimetic aerosol bronchodilators, general anesthetics, tranquilizers, central nervous system depressants, and certain other agents. Compounds in these categories include:

Albuterol (Additive hypertension). Products include:
Proventil Inhalation Aerosol 2117
Ventolin Inhalation Aerosol and Refill 583

Albuterol Sulfate (Additive hypertension). Products include:
Proventil Repetabs Tablets 2120
Proventil Solutions for Inhalation 0.5% and 0.083% 2118
Proventil Syrup 2119
Proventil Tablets 2120
Ventolin 583

Alcohol (Additive CNS depression).

Alfentanil Hydrochloride (Additive CNS depression). Products include:
Alfenta Injection 1131

Alprazolam (Additive CNS depression). Products include:
Xanax Tablets 2367

Aprobarbital (Additive CNS depression). Products include:
Alurate Elixir 1883

Buprenorphine (Additive CNS depression).
No products indexed under this heading.

Buspirone Hydrochloride (Additive CNS depression). Products include:
BuSpar 1401

Butabarbital (Additive CNS depression). Products include:
Pyridium Plus 1764

Butalbital (Additive CNS depression). Products include:
Esgic-Plus Tablets 1002
Esgic Tablets & Capsules 1001
Fioricet Tablets 2006
Fiorinal Capsules 2007
Fiorinal with Codeine Capsules 2008
Fiorinal Tablets 2007
Phrenilin 838

Sedapap Tablets 50 mg/650 mg .. 1360

Chlordiazepoxide (Additive CNS depression). Products include:
Libritabs Tablets ... 1930
Limbitrol ... 1933
Menrium Tablets ... 1934

Chlordiazepoxide Hydrochloride (Additive CNS depression). Products include:
Librax Capsules ... 1929
Librium Capsules ... 1931
Librium Injectable ... 1932

Chlorpromazine (Additive CNS depression). Products include:
Thorazine ... 2234

Chlorprothixene (Additive CNS depression). Products include:
Taractan Tablets ... 1920

Chlorprothixene Hydrochloride (Additive CNS depression). Products include:
Taractan ... 1920

Clorazepate Dipotassium (Additive CNS depression). Products include:
Tranxene ... 556

Codeine (Additive CNS depression). Products include:
Calcidrine Syrup ... 506

Codeine Phosphate (Additive CNS depression). Products include:
Actifed with Codeine Cough Syrup.. 752
Cheracol Cough Syrup ... 1853
Codimal PH Syrup ... 846
Dimetane-DC Cough Syrup ... 1857
Empirin with Codeine Phosphate Nos. 2, 3 & 4 ... 764
Fiorinal with Codeine Capsules ... 2008
Isoclor Expectorant ... 982
Naldecon CX Adult Liquid ... ▣ 521
Novahistine DH ... 1342
Novahistine Expectorant ... 1343
Nucofed Capsules ... 2219
Nucofed Expectorant ... 2219
Nucofed Pediatric Expectorant ... 2220
Nucofed Syrup ... 2219
Phenaphen with Codeine Capsules 1865
Phenaphen-650 with Codeine Tablets ... 1866
Phenergan with Codeine ... 2497
Phenergan VC with Codeine ... 2501
Robitussin A-C Syrup ... 1875
Robitussin-DAC Syrup ... 1875
Ryna ... ▣ 741
Soma Compound w/Codeine Tablets ... 2390
Triaminic Expectorant w/Codeine .. 1996
Tussi-Organidin Liquid ... 2391
Tylenol with Codeine ... 1381

Codeine Polistirex (Additive CNS depression).
No products indexed under this heading.

Dezocine (Additive CNS depression).

Diazepam (Additive CNS depression). Products include:
Valium Injectable ... 1937
Valium Tablets ... 1939
Valrelease Capsules ... 1923

Dobutamine Hydrochloride (Additive hypertension). Products include:
Dobutrex Solution Vials ... 1259

Dopamine Hydrochloride (Additive hypertension). Products include:
Intropin Injection ... 930

Droperidol (Additive CNS depression). Products include:
Inapsine Injection ... 1140
Innovar Injection ... 1141

Enflurane (Additive CNS depression). Products include:
Ethrane ... 599

Ephedrine Hydrochloride (Additive hypertension). Products include:
Amesec ... ▣ 682
Primatene Tablets-M Formula ... 2421
Primatene Tablets-P Formula ... 2421
Primatene Tablets-Regular Formula ... 2421
Quadrinal Tablets ... 1183
Quelidrine Syrup ... 556
Tedral SA ... 1765

Ephedrine Sulfate (Additive hypertension). Products include:
Bronkaid Tablets ... ▣ 757
Bronkolixir ... ▣ 761
Bronkotabs Tablets ... ▣ 762
Marax Tablets & DF Syrup ... 1954
Pazo Hemorrhoid Ointment & Suppositories ... 752
Vicks Vatronol Nose Drops ... ▣ 666

Ephedrine Tannate (Additive hypertension). Products include:
Rynatuss ... 2388

Epinephrine (Additive hypertension). Products include:
Ana-Kit Anaphylaxis Emergency Treatment Kit ... 1100
Bronkaid Mist ... ▣ 757
EpiPen ... 843
Marcaine Hydrochloride 0.5% with Epinephrine 1:200,000 (as bitartrate) ... 958
Marcaine Hydrochloride with Epinephrine 1:200,000 ... 2055
Primatene Mist ... 2420
Sus-Phrine Injection ... 1006
Xylocaine with Epinephrine Injections ... 637

Epinephrine Bitartrate (Additive hypertension). Products include:
AsthmaHaler Mist Epinephrine Bitartrate Bronchodilator ... ▣ 616
Bronkaid Mist Suspension ... ▣ 757
Primatene Mist Suspension ... 2421

Epinephrine Hydrochloride (Additive hypertension). Products include:
Adrenalin Chloride Solution 1:100 & 1:1,000 ... 1689
Epifrin ... ⊙ 244
Glaucon ... ⊙ 218

Estazolam (Additive CNS depression). Products include:
ProSom Tablets ... 554

Ethchlorvynol (Additive CNS depression). Products include:
Placidyl Capsules ... 553

Ethinamate (Additive CNS depression).
No products indexed under this heading.

Fentanyl (Additive CNS depression). Products include:
Duragesic Transdermal System ... 1133

Fentanyl Citrate (Additive CNS depression). Products include:
Innovar Injection ... 1141
Sublimaze Injection ... 1146

Fluphenazine Decanoate (Additive CNS depression). Products include:
Prolixin Decanoate ... 1795

Fluphenazine Enanthate (Additive CNS depression). Products include:
Prolixin Enanthate ... 1796

Fluphenazine Hydrochloride (Additive CNS depression). Products include:
Prolixin Elixir ... 1793
Prolixin Injection ... 1791
Prolixin Oral Concentrate ... 1792
Prolixin Tablets ... 1793

Flurazepam Hydrochloride (Additive CNS depression). Products include:
Dalmane Capsules ... 1927

Furazolidone (Hypertensive crisis; concurrent use is contraindicated). Products include:
Furoxone ... 1855

Glutethimide (Additive CNS depression).
No products indexed under this heading.

Haloperidol (Additive CNS depression). Products include:
Haldol Injection, Tablets and Concentrate ... 1373

Haloperidol Decanoate (Additive CNS depression). Products include:
Haldol Decanoate ... 1375

Hydrocodone Polistirex (Additive CNS depression). Products include:
Tussionex Extended-Release Suspension ... 988

Hydroxyzine Hydrochloride (Additive CNS depression). Products include:
Atarax Tablets & Syrup ... 1941
Marax Tablets & DF Syrup ... 1954
Vistaril Intramuscular Solution ... 1970

Isocarboxazid (Hypertensive crisis; concurrent use is contraindicated). Products include:
Marplan Tablets ... 1906

Isoflurane (Additive CNS depression). Products include:
Forane ... 600

Isoproterenol Hydrochloride (Additive hypertension). Products include:
Isuprel Hydrochloride Injection 1:5000 ... 2050
Isuprel Hydrochloride Mistometer .. 2051
Isuprel Hydrochloride Solution 1:200 & 1:100 ... 2052
Norisodrine Aerotrol ... 540

Ketamine Hydrochloride (Additive CNS depression). Products include:
Ketalar ... 1726

Levorphanol Tartrate (Additive CNS depression). Products include:
Levo-Dromoran ... 1906

Lorazepam (Additive CNS depression). Products include:
Ativan Injection ... 2432
Ativan Tablets ... 2434

Loxapine Hydrochloride (Additive CNS depression). Products include:
Loxitane ... 1213

Loxapine Succinate (Additive CNS depression). Products include:
Loxitane Capsules ... 1213

Meperidine Hydrochloride (Additive CNS depression). Products include:
Demerol ... 2047
Mepergan Injection ... 2479

Mephobarbital (Additive CNS depression). Products include:
Mebaral Tablets ... 2061

Meprobamate (Additive CNS depression). Products include:
Deprol Tablets ... 2382
Equagesic Tablets ... 2451
Miltown Tablets ... 2386
PMB 200 and PMB 400 ... 2504

Mesoridazine (Additive CNS depression). Products include:
Serentil ... 686

Mesoridazine Besylate (Additive CNS depression).

Metaproterenol Sulfate (Additive hypertension). Products include:
Alupent ... 674
Arm-a-Med Metaproterenol Sulfate Inhalation Solution, USP ... 617
Metaprel Inhalation Aerosol Bronchodilator ... 2014
Metaprel Inhalation Solution ... 2015
Metaprel ... 2015
Metaproterenol Sulfate Inhalation Solution, USP ... 912

Metaraminol Bitartrate (Additive hypertension). Products include:
Aramine Injection ... 1424

Methadone Hydrochloride (Additive CNS depression). Products include:
Dolophine Hydrochloride Ampoules & Vials ... 1260
Dolophine Hydrochloride Tablets ... 1261
Methadone Hydrochloride Diskets .. 1284
Methadone Hydrochloride Oral Solution & Tablets ... 1987

Methohexital Sodium (Additive CNS depression). Products include:
Brevital Sodium Vials ... 1248

Methoxamine Hydrochloride (Additive hypertension). Products include:
Vasoxyl Injection ... 819

Methoxyflurane (Additive CNS depression).
No products indexed under this heading.

Midazolam Hydrochloride (Additive CNS depression). Products include:
Versed Injection ... 1924

Molindone Hydrochloride (Additive CNS depression). Products include:
Moban Tablets & Concentrate ... 932

Morphine Sulfate (Additive CNS depression). Products include:
Astramorph/PF Injection, USP (Preservative-Free) ... 618
Duramorph ... 960
Infumorph 200 and Infumorph 500 Sterile Solutions ... 962
MS Contin Tablets ... 1814
MSIR ... 1817
Oramorph SR (Morphine Sulfate Sustained Release Tablets) ... 1988
Roxanol ... 1991

Norepinephrine Bitartrate (Additive hypertension). Products include:
Levophed Bitartrate Injection ... 2054

Opium Alkaloids (Additive CNS depression). Products include:
B & O No. 15A & No. 16A Supprettes ... 2395
Pantopon Injectable ... 1911

Oxazepam (Additive CNS depression). Products include:
Serax Capsules ... 2522
Serax Tablets ... 2522

Oxycodone Hydrochloride (Additive CNS depression). Products include:
Percocet Tablets ... 950
Percodan ... 951
Roxicodone Tablets, Oral Solution & Intensol (Oxycodone) ... 1992
Tylox Capsules ... 1382

Pentobarbital Sodium (Additive CNS depression). Products include:
Nembutal Sodium Capsules ... 534
Nembutal Sodium Solution ... 536
Nembutal Sodium Suppositories ... 538

Perphenazine (Additive CNS depression). Products include:
Etrafon ... 2087
Triavil Tablets ... 1556
Trilafon ... 2123

Phenelzine Sulfate (Hypertensive crisis; concurrent use is contraindicated). Products include:
Nardil ... 1742

Phenobarbital (Additive CNS depression). Products include:
Arco-Lase Plus Tablets ... 607
Bellergal-S Tablets ... 1998
Bronkolixir ... ▣ 761
Bronkotabs Tablets ... ▣ 762
Donnatal ... 1858
Donnatal Extentabs ... 1859
Donnatal Tablets ... 1858
Donnazyme Tablets ... 1860
Kinesed Tablets ... 2272
Phenobarbital Elixir and Tablets ... 1293
Primatene Tablets-P Formula ... 2421
Quadrinal Tablets ... 1183
Tedral SA ... 1765

Phenylephrine Bitartrate (Additive hypertension).
No products indexed under this heading.

Phenylephrine Hydrochloride (Additive hypertension). Products include:
AK-Dilate Solution 2.5% and 10% ... ⊙ 203
Atrohist Sprinkle Capsules ... 558
Cerose-DM ... 2443

Codimal 846
Comhist LA Capsules 1618
Congespirin For Children Aspirin Free Chewable Cold Tablets 748
Cyclomydril ◉ 216
Deconsal Sprinkle Capsules 559
Dimetane Decongestant ▣ 673
Dristan Decongestant/Antihistamine/ Analgesic Coated Caplets ▣ 749
Dristan Cold Nasal Decongestant/ Antihistamine/ Analgesic Coated Tablets 2419
Dristan Advanced Formula Decongestant/Antihistamine/ Analgesic Tablets ▣ 749
Dristan Nasal Spray, Menthol 2419
Dristan Nasal Spray, Regular and Regular with Metered Pump 2419
Entex Capsules 1623
Entex Liquid 1623
Sinus Excedrin Analgesic, Decongestant Tablets & Caplets 750
Extendryl 994
4-Way Fast Acting Nasal Spray - Original Formula (regular & mentholated) & Metered Spray Pump (regular) 751
Hycomine Compound Tablets 929
Murocoll-2 Sterile Ophthalmic Solution ◉ 261
Mydfrin 2.5% ◉ 224
Naldecon Syrup, Tablets, Pediatric Drops and Pediatric Syrup 709
Neo-Synephrine Hydrochloride 1% Carpuject 2063
Neo-Synephrine Hydrochloride 1% Injection 2063
Neo-Synephrine Hydrochloride (Ophthalmic) 2064
Neo-Synephrine ▣ 759
Nōstril Nasal Decongestant ▣ 520
Novahistine Elixir ▣ 596
Phenergan VC 2500
Phenergan VC with Codeine 2501
Prefrin Liquifilm Vasoconstrictor and Lubricant Eye Drops ◉ 254
Prefrin-A ◉ 255
Quelidrine Syrup 556
Relief Vasoconstrictor and Lubricant Eye Drops ◉ 256
Robitussin Night Relief ▣ 677
Ru-Tuss with Hydrocodone 694
Ru-Tuss Tablets 693
Vasosulf ◉ 279
Vicks Sinex ▣ 665
Zincfrin ◉ 230

Phenylephrine Tannate (Additive hypertension). Products include:
Rynatan 2387
Rynatuss 2388

Pirbuterol Acetate (Additive hypertension). Products include:
Maxair Inhaler 1311

Prazepam (Additive CNS depression). Products include:
Centrax 1693

Prochlorperazine (Additive CNS depression). Products include:
Compazine 2201

Promethazine Hydrochloride (Additive CNS depression). Products include:
Mepergan Injection 2479
Phenergan with Codeine 2497
Phenergan with Dextromethorphan 2499
Phenergan Injection 2493
Phenergan Suppositories 2496
Phenergan Syrup 2495
Phenergan Tablets 2496
Phenergan VC 2500
Phenergan VC with Codeine 2501

Propofol (Additive CNS depression). Products include:
Diprivan Injection 2267

Propoxyphene Hydrochloride (Additive CNS depression). Products include:
Darvon 1256
Wygesic Tablets 2540

Propoxyphene Napsylate (Additive CNS depression). Products include:
Darvon-N/Darvocet-N 1254

Pseudoephedrine Hydrochloride (Additive hypertension). Products include:
Actifed Capsules ▣ 539
Actifed Plus Caplets ▣ 539
Actifed Plus Tablets ▣ 540
Actifed with Codeine Cough Syrup 752
Actifed Syrup ▣ 540
Actifed Tablets ▣ 540
Actifed 12-Hour Capsules ▣ 539
Advil Cold & Sinus Caplets (formerly CoAdvil) 2416
Allerest ▣ 559
Anatuss LA Tablets 1359
Benadryl Decongestant Elixir ▣ 635
Benadryl Decongestant ▣ 635
Benadryl Plus ▣ 636
Benadryl Plus Nighttime ▣ 637
Benylin Decongestant ▣ 638
Brexin L.A. Capsules 2078
Bromfed Capsules (Timed Release) 1615
Bromfed Syrup ▣ 628
Bromfed 1615
CoAdvil ▣ 748
Allergy-Sinus Comtrex Multi-Symptom Allergy Sinus Formula Tablets & Caplets 746
Cough Formula Comtrex 746
Comtrex Multi-Symptom Cold Reliever Tablets/Caplets/Liqui-Gels/Liquid 745
Day-Night Comtrex 747
Non-Drowsy Comtrex 747
Congess 994
Congestac Caplets ▣ 617
Contac Jr. Children's Cold Medicine ▣ 712
Contac Nighttime Cold Medicine ▣ 713
Contac Sinus Caplets Maximum Strength Non-Drowsy Formula ▣ 710
Contac Sinus Tablets Maximum Strength Non-Drowsy Formula ▣ 710
Deconamine 663
Deconsal II Tablets 559
Dimacol Caplets ▣ 672
Dimetane-DX Cough Syrup 1858
Dorcol Children's Cough Syrup ▣ 685
Dorcol Children's Decongestant Liquid ▣ 685
Dorcol Children's Liquid Cold Formula ▣ 686
Maximum Strength Dristan Decongestant/Analgesic Coated Caplets ▣ 750
No Drowsiness Dristan Cold Nasal Decongestant/Analgesic Coated Caplets 2420
Dristan Sinus Caplets 2419
Sinus Excedrin Analgesic, Decongestant Tablets & Caplets ▣ 533
Fedahist Gyrocaps 2145
Fedahist Timecaps 2145
Guaifed 1615
Guaifed Syrup ▣ 629
Isoclor Expectorant 982
Isoclor Timesule Capsules ▣ 561
Kronofed-A 970
Medi-Flu Caplet, Liquid ▣ 640
Novafed A Capsules 1342
Novafed Capsules 1342
Novahistine DH 1342
Novahistine DMX ▣ 595
Novahistine Expectorant 1343
Nucofed Capsules 2219
Nucofed Expectorant 2219
Nucofed Pediatric Expectorant 2220
Nucofed Syrup 2219
Ornex Caplets ▣ 618
PediaCare Allergy Relief Formula Liquid 1362
PediaCare Cough-Cold Formula Liquid 1362
PediaCare Infants' Oral Decongestant Drops 1362
PediaCare Night Rest Cough-Cold Formula Liquid 1362
PediaCare 6-12 Cough-Cold Formula Chewable Tablets 1362
Robitussin-DAC Syrup 1875
Robitussin-PE ▣ 677
Rondec 1975
Rondec-DM 1976
Rondec-TR Tablet 1975
Ru-Tuss DE Tablets 694
Ryna ▣ 741
Seldane-D Extended-Release Tablets 1350
Sinarest ▣ 562
Sine-Aid Maximum Strength Sinus Headache Caplets 1365
Sine-Aid Maximum Strength Sinus Headache Tablets 1365
Sine-Off Maximum Strength Allergy/Sinus Formula Caplets ▣ 721
Sine-Off Maximum Strength No Drowsiness Formula Caplets ▣ 722
Singlet Tablets ▣ 598
Sinutab Maximum Strength ▣ 641
Sinutab Maximum Strength Without Drowsiness Tablets & Caplets ▣ 642
Sinutab Regular Strength Without Drowsiness Formula ▣ 641
St. Joseph Nighttime Cold Medicine ▣ 705
Sudafed Children's Liquid ▣ 543
Sudafed Cough Syrup ▣ 543
Sudafed Plus Liquid ▣ 544
Sudafed Plus Tablets ▣ 545
Sudafed Sinus Caplets ▣ 545
Sudafed Sinus Tablets ▣ 545
Sudafed Tablets, 30 mg ▣ 544
Sudafed Tablets, Adult Strength, 60 mg ▣ 544
Sudafed 12 Hour Capsules ▣ 545
TheraFlu Flu and Cold Medicine ▣ 687
Triaminic Nite Light ▣ 689
Tylenol Allergy Sinus Medication Caplets and Gelcaps, Maximum Strength 1372
Children's Tylenol Cold Liquid Formula and Chewable Tablets 1368
Tylenol Cold & Flu Hot Medication, Packets 1369
Tylenol Cold & Flu No Drowsiness Hot Medication, Packets 1371
Tylenol Cold Medication Caplets and Tablets 1370
Tylenol Cold Medication No Drowsiness Formula Caplets 1370
Tylenol Cold Night Time Medication Liquid 1371
Tylenol Cough Medication Liquid with Decongestant, Maximum Strength 1372
Tylenol, Maximum Strength, Sinus Medication Gelcaps, Caplets and Tablets 1373
Ursinus Inlay-Tabs ▣ 691
Vicks Children's NyQuil ▣ 664
Vicks Daycare ▣ 660
Vicks Formula 44D Decongestant Cough Medicine ▣ 662
Vicks Formula 44M Multi-Symptom Cough Medicine ▣ 662
Vicks NyQuil Nighttime Colds Medicine-Original & Cherry Flavor ▣ 664
Vicks Pediatric Formula 44 Cough & Congestion Medicine ▣ 663
Vicks Pediatric Formula 44m Multi-Symptom Cough & Cold Medicine ▣ 663

Pseudoephedrine Sulfate (Additive hypertension). Products include:
Afrin Tablets ▣ 693
Chlor-Trimeton Decongestant ▣ 694
Disophrol Chronotab Sustained-Action Tablets ▣ 698
Drixoral Antihistamine/Nasal Decongestant Syrup ▣ 698
Drixoral Non-Drowsy Formula ▣ 699
Drixoral Plus Extended-Release Tablets ▣ 699
Drixoral Sinus ▣ 700
Drixoral Sustained-Action Tablets ▣ 698
Sinutab Allergy Formula Sustained Action Tablets ▣ 640
Trinalin Repetabs Tablets 1170

Quazepam (Additive CNS depression). Products include:
Doral Tablets 2383

Secobarbital Sodium (Additive CNS depression). Products include:
Seconal Sodium Pulvules 1296

Selegiline Hydrochloride (Hypertensive crisis; concurrent use is contraindicated). Products include:
Eldepryl 2250

Sufentanil Citrate (Additive CNS depression). Products include:
Sufenta Injection 1147

Temazepam (Additive CNS depression). Products include:
Restoril Capsules 2023

Terbutaline Sulfate (Additive hypertension). Products include:
Brethaire Inhaler 1024
Brethine Ampuls 1026
Brethine Tablets 1026
Bricanyl Injection 1324
Bricanyl Tablets 1325

Thiamylal Sodium (Additive CNS depression). Products include:
Surital Ampoules, Steri-Vials 1764

Thioridazine Hydrochloride (Additive CNS depression). Products include:
Mellaril 2011

Thiothixene (Additive CNS depression). Products include:
Navane Capsules and Concentrate 1954
Navane Intramuscular 1956

Tranylcypromine Sulfate (Hypertensive crisis; concurrent use is contraindicated). Products include:
Parnate Tablets 2222

Triazolam (Additive CNS depression). Products include:
Halcion Tablets 2340

Trifluoperazine Hydrochloride (Additive CNS depression). Products include:
Stelazine 2226

HYCOMINE SYRUP

(Hydrocodone Bitartrate, Phenylpropanolamine Hydrochloride) 927
See **Hycomine Pediatric Syrup**

HYCOTUSS EXPECTORANT SYRUP

(Hydrocodone Bitartrate, Guaifenesin) 930
May interact with narcotic analgesics, general anesthetics, tranquilizers, hypnotics and sedatives, phenothiazines, and certain other agents. Compounds in these categories include:

Alcohol (Additive CNS depression).

Alfentanil Hydrochloride (Additive CNS depression). Products include:
Alfenta Injection 1131

Alprazolam (Additive CNS depression). Products include:
Xanax Tablets 2367

Buprenorphine (Additive CNS depression).
No products indexed under this heading.

Buspirone Hydrochloride (Additive CNS depression). Products include:
BuSpar 1401

Chlordiazepoxide (Additive CNS depression). Products include:
Libritabs Tablets 1930
Limbitrol 1933
Menrium Tablets 1934

Chlordiazepoxide Hydrochloride (Additive CNS depression). Products include:
Librax Capsules 1929
Librium Capsules 1931
Librium Injectable 1932

Chlorpromazine (Additive CNS depression). Products include:
Thorazine 2234

Clorazepate Dipotassium (Additive CNS depression). Products include:
Tranxene 556

Codeine (Additive CNS depression). Products include:
Calcidrine Syrup 506

Codeine Phosphate (Additive CNS depression). Products include:
Actifed with Codeine Cough Syrup 752
Cheracol Cough Syrup 1853
Codimal PH Syrup 846
Dimetane-DC Cough Syrup 1857

(▣ Described in PDR For Nonprescription Drugs) (◉ Described in PDR For Ophthalmology)

Empirin with Codeine Phosphate Nos. 2, 3 & 4 764
Fiorinal with Codeine Capsules 2008
Isoclor Expectorant 982
Naldecon CX Adult Liquid ◘ 521
Novahistine DH 1342
Novahistine Expectorant 1343
Nucofed Capsules 2219
Nucofed Expectorant 2219
Nucofed Pediatric Expectorant 2220
Nucofed Syrup 2219
Phenaphen with Codeine Capsules 1865
Phenaphen-650 with Codeine Tablets 1866
Phenergan with Codeine 2497
Phenergan VC with Codeine 2501
Robitussin A-C Syrup 1875
Robitussin-DAC Syrup 1875
Ryna ◘ 741
Soma Compound w/Codeine Tablets 2390
Triaminic Expectorant w/Codeine 1996
Tussi-Organidin Liquid 2391
Tylenol with Codeine 1381

Codeine Polistirex (Additive CNS depression).
No products indexed under this heading.

Dezocine (Additive CNS depression).

Diazepam (Additive CNS depression). Products include:
Valium Injectable 1937
Valium Tablets 1939
Valrelease Capsules 1923

Droperidol (Additive CNS depression). Products include:
Inapsine Injection 1140
Innovar Injection 1141

Enflurane (Additive CNS depression). Products include:
Ethrane 599

Estazolam (Additive CNS depression). Products include:
ProSom Tablets 554

Ethchlorvynol (Additive CNS depression). Products include:
Placidyl Capsules 553

Ethinamate (Additive CNS depression).
No products indexed under this heading.

Fentanyl (Additive CNS depression). Products include:
Duragesic Transdermal System 1133

Fentanyl Citrate (Additive CNS depression). Products include:
Innovar Injection 1141
Sublimaze Injection 1146

Fluphenazine Decanoate (Additive CNS depression). Products include:
Prolixin Decanoate 1795

Fluphenazine Enanthate (Additive CNS depression). Products include:
Prolixin Enanthate 1796

Fluphenazine Hydrochloride (Additive CNS depression). Products include:
Prolixin Elixir 1793
Prolixin Injection 1791
Prolixin Oral Concentrate 1792
Prolixin Tablets 1793

Flurazepam Hydrochloride (Additive CNS depression). Products include:
Dalmane Capsules 1927

Glutethimide (Additive CNS depression).
No products indexed under this heading.

Haloperidol (Additive CNS depression). Products include:
Haldol Injection, Tablets and Concentrate 1373

Haloperidol Decanoate (Additive CNS depression). Products include:
Haldol Decanoate 1375

Hydrocodone Polistirex (Additive CNS depression). Products include:
Tussionex Extended-Release Suspension 988

Hydroxyzine Hydrochloride (Additive CNS depression). Products include:
Atarax Tablets & Syrup 1941
Marax Tablets & DF Syrup 1954
Vistaril Intramuscular Solution 1970

Isoflurane (Additive CNS depression). Products include:
Forane 600

Levorphanol Tartrate (Additive CNS depression). Products include:
Levo-Dromoran 1906

Lorazepam (Additive CNS depression). Products include:
Ativan Injection 2432
Ativan Tablets 2434

Loxapine Hydrochloride (Additive CNS depression). Products include:
Loxitane 1213

Meperidine Hydrochloride (Additive CNS depression). Products include:
Demerol 2047
Mepergan Injection 2479

Meprobamate (Additive CNS depression). Products include:
Deprol Tablets 2382
Equagesic Tablets 2451
Miltown Tablets 2386
PMB 200 and PMB 400 2504

Mesoridazine (Additive CNS depression). Products include:
Serentil 686

Methadone Hydrochloride (Additive CNS depression). Products include:
Dolophine Hydrochloride Ampoules & Vials 1260
Dolophine Hydrochloride Tablets 1261
Methadone Hydrochloride Diskets 1284
Methadone Hydrochloride Oral Solution & Tablets 1987

Methohexital Sodium (Additive CNS depression). Products include:
Brevital Sodium Vials 1248

Methoxyflurane (Additive CNS depression).
No products indexed under this heading.

Midazolam Hydrochloride (Additive CNS depression). Products include:
Versed Injection 1924

Molindone Hydrochloride (Additive CNS depression). Products include:
Moban Tablets & Concentrate 932

Morphine Sulfate (Additive CNS depression). Products include:
Astramorph/PF Injection, USP (Preservative-Free) 618
Duramorph 960
Infumorph 200 and Infumorph 500 Sterile Solutions 962
MS Contin Tablets 1814
MSIR 1817
Oramorph SR (Morphine Sulfate Sustained Release Tablets) 1988
Roxanol 1991

Opium Alkaloids (Additive CNS depression). Products include:
B & O No. 15A & No. 16A Supprettes 2395
Pantopon Injectable 1911

Oxazepam (Additive CNS depression). Products include:
Serax Capsules 2522
Serax Tablets 2522

Oxycodone Hydrochloride (Additive CNS depression). Products include:
Percocet Tablets 950
Percodan 951
Roxicodone Tablets, Oral Solution & Intensol (Oxycodone) 1992
Tylox Capsules 1382

Perphenazine (Additive CNS depression). Products include:
Etrafon 2087
Triavil Tablets 1556
Trilafon 2123

Prazepam (Additive CNS depression). Products include:
Centrax 1693

Prochlorperazine (Additive CNS depression). Products include:
Compazine 2201

Promethazine Hydrochloride (Additive CNS depression). Products include:
Mepergan Injection 2479
Phenergan with Codeine 2497
Phenergan with Dextromethorphan 2499
Phenergan Injection 2493
Phenergan Suppositories 2496
Phenergan Syrup 2495
Phenergan Tablets 2496
Phenergan VC 2500
Phenergan VC with Codeine 2501

Propofol (Additive CNS depression). Products include:
Diprivan Injection 2267

Propoxyphene Hydrochloride (Additive CNS depression). Products include:
Darvon 1256
Wygesic Tablets 2540

Propoxyphene Napsylate (Additive CNS depression). Products include:
Darvon-N/Darvocet-N 1254

Quazepam (Additive CNS depression). Products include:
Doral Tablets 2383

Secobarbital Sodium (Additive CNS depression). Products include:
Seconal Sodium Pulvules 1296

Sufentanil Citrate (Additive CNS depression). Products include:
Sufenta Injection 1147

Temazepam (Additive CNS depression). Products include:
Restoril Capsules 2023

Thioridazine Hydrochloride (Additive CNS depression). Products include:
Mellaril 2011

Triazolam (Additive CNS depression). Products include:
Halcion Tablets 2340

Trifluoperazine Hydrochloride (Additive CNS depression). Products include:
Stelazine 2226

HYDELTRASOL INJECTION, STERILE
(Prednisolone Sodium Phosphate) 1476
May interact with oral anticoagulants, potassium sparing diuretics, and certain other agents. Compounds in these categories include:

Amiloride Hydrochloride (Hypokalemia). Products include:
Midamor Tablets 1508
Moduretic Tablets 1510

Aspirin (Use cautiously). Products include:
Alka-Seltzer Effervescent Antacid and Pain Reliever 1568
Alka-Seltzer Extra Strength Effervescent Antacid and Pain Reliever 1570
Alka-Seltzer (Flavored) Effervescent Antacid and Pain Reliever 1569
Alka-Seltzer Plus Cold Medicine ◘ 623
Alka-Seltzer Plus Night-Time Cold Medicine ◘ 623
Alka Seltzer Plus Sinus Allergy Medicine ◘ 624
Anacin Coated Analgesic Caplets 2417
Anacin Coated Analgesic Tablets 2417
Anacin Maximum Strength Analgesic Coated Tablets 2417
Maximum Strength Arthritis Pain Formula By the Makers of Anacin Analgesic Tablets and Caplets 2418
Arthritis Pain Formula by the Makers of Anacin Analgesic Tablets and Caplets ◘ 747
Arthritis Strength BC Powder ◘ 516
Ascriptin A/D Caplets 1850
Regular Strength Ascriptin Tablets 1850
Azdone Tablets 844
BC Powder ◘ 517
BC Cold Powder ◘ 517
Children's Bayer Chewable Aspirin ◘ 564
Genuine Bayer Aspirin Tablets & Caplets ◘ 564
Maximum Bayer Aspirin Tablets & Caplets ◘ 566
Bayer Plus Aspirin Tablets ◘ 567
Therapy Bayer Aspirin Caplets ◘ 568
8 Hour Bayer Timed-Release Aspirin ◘ 566
Arthritis Strength Bufferin Analgesic Caplets 744
Extra Strength Bufferin Analgesic Tablets 745
Bufferin Analgesic Tablets and Caplets 743
Cama Arthritis Pain Reliever ◘ 685
Damason-P 1356
Easprin 1719
Ecotrin Enteric Coated Aspirin Maximum Strength Tablets and Caplets 2189
Ecotrin Enteric Coated Aspirin Regular Strength Tablets and Caplets 2189
Empirin Aspirin ◘ 541
Empirin with Codeine Phosphate Nos. 2, 3 & 4 764
Equagesic Tablets 2451
Excedrin Extra-Strength Analgesic Tablets & Caplets 749
4-Way Cold Tablets 750
Fiorinal Capsules 2007
Fiorinal with Codeine Capsules 2008
Fiorinal Tablets 2007
Lortab ASA Tablets 2414
Momentum Muscular Backache Formula ◘ 751
Norgesic 1314
Norwich Extra-Strength Aspirin ◘ 546
Norwich Regular Strength Aspirin ◘ 547
P-A-C Analgesic Tablets ◘ 669
Percodan 951
Robaxisal Tablets 1872
Sine-Off Sinus Medicine Tablets-Aspirin Formula ◘ 722
Soma Compound w/Codeine Tablets 2390
Soma Compound Tablets 2389
St. Joseph Adult Chewable Aspirin (81 mg.) ◘ 703
Synalgos-DC Capsules 2525
Talwin Compound 2072
Ursinus Inlay-Tabs ◘ 691
Vanquish Analgesic Caplets ◘ 574
Zorprin Tablets 698

Aspirin, Enteric Coated (Use cautiously). Products include:
Therapy Bayer Aspirin Caplets ◘ 568
Ecotrin 2189

Dicumarol (Inhibited response to coumarins). Products include:
Dicumarol Tablets 516

Ephedrine Hydrochloride (Lessened physiologic activity of corticosteroids). Products include:
Amesec ◘ 682
Primatene Tablets-M Formula 2421
Primatene Tablets-P Formula 2421
Primatene Tablets-Regular Formula 2421
Quadrinal Tablets 1183
Quelidrine Syrup 556
Tedral SA 1765

Ephedrine Sulfate (Lessened physiologic activity of corticosteroids). Products include:
Bronkaid Tablets ◘ 757
Bronkolixir ◘ 761
Bronkotabs Tablets ◘ 762
Marax Tablets & DF Syrup 1954
Pazo Hemorrhoid Ointment & Suppositories 752
Vicks Vatronol Nose Drops ◘ 666

Ephedrine Tannate (Lessened physiologic activity to corticosteroids). Products include:
- Rynatuss ... 2388

Live virus vaccines; smallpox (Contraindicated).

Phenobarbital (Lessened physiologic activity of corticosteroids). Products include:
- Arco-Lase Plus Tablets ... 607
- Bellergal-S Tablets ... 1998
- Bronkolixir ... ■ 761
- Bronkotabs Tablets ... ■ 762
- Donnatal ... 1858
- Donnatal Extentabs ... 1859
- Donnatal Tablets ... 1858
- Donnazyme Tablets ... 1860
- Kinesed Tablets ... 2272
- Phenobarbital Elixir and Tablets ... 1293
- Primatene Tablets-P Formula ... 2421
- Quadrinal Tablets ... 1183
- Tedral SA ... 1765

Phenytoin (Lessened physiologic activity of corticosteroids). Products include:
- Dilantin Infatabs ... 1710
- Dilantin-30 Pediatric/Dilantin-125 Suspension ... 1713

Phenytoin Sodium (Lessened physiologic activity of corticosteroids). Products include:
- Dilantin Kapseals ... 1708
- Dilantin Parenteral ... 1712
- Dilantin with Phenobarbital Kapseals ... 1715

Rifampin (Lessened physiologic activity of corticosteroids). Products include:
- Rifadin ... 1345
- Rifamate Capsules ... 1347
- Rimactane Capsules ... 879

Spironolactone (Hypokalemia). Products include:
- Aldactazide ... 2150
- Aldactone ... 2152

Triamterene (Hypokalemia). Products include:
- Dyazide Capsules ... 2208
- Dyrenium Capsules ... 2210
- Maxzide ... 1215

Warfarin Sodium (Inhibited response to coumarins). Products include:
- Coumadin Injection & Tablets ... 944
- Panwarfin Tablets ... 547

HYDELTRA-T.B.A. STERILE SUSPENSION

(Prednisolone Tebutate) ... 1478

May interact with oral anticoagulants, potassium sparing diuretics, and certain other agents. Compounds in these categories include:

Amiloride Hydrochloride (Hypokalemia). Products include:
- Midamor Tablets ... 1508
- Moduretic Tablets ... 1510

Aspirin (Use cautiously). Products include:
- Alka-Seltzer Effervescent Antacid and Pain Reliever ... 1568
- Alka-Seltzer Extra Strength Effervescent Antacid and Pain Reliever ... 1570
- Alka-Seltzer (Flavored) Effervescent Antacid and Pain Reliever ... 1569
- Alka-Seltzer Plus Cold Medicine ... ■ 623
- Alka-Seltzer Plus Night-Time Cold Medicine ... ■ 623
- Alka Seltzer Plus Sinus Allergy Medicine ... ■ 624
- Anacin Coated Analgesic Caplets ... 2417
- Anacin Coated Analgesic Tablets ... 2417
- Anacin Maximum Strength Analgesic Coated Tablets ... 2417
- Maximum Strength Arthritis Pain Formula By the Makers of Anacin Analgesic Tablets and Caplets ... 2418
- Arthritis Pain Formula by the Makers of Anacin Analgesic Tablets and Caplets ... ■ 747
- Arthritis Strength BC Powder ... ■ 516
- Ascriptin A/D Caplets ... 1850
- Regular Strength Ascriptin Tablets 1850
- Azdöne Tablets ... 844
- BC Powder ... ■ 517
- BC Cold Powder ... ■ 517
- Children's Bayer Chewable Aspirin ... ■ 564
- Genuine Bayer Aspirin Tablets & Caplets ... ■ 564
- Maximum Bayer Aspirin Tablets & Caplets ... ■ 566
- Bayer Plus Aspirin Tablets ... ■ 567
- Therapy Bayer Aspirin Caplets ... ■ 568
- 8 Hour Bayer Timed-Release Aspirin ... ■ 566
- Arthritis Strength Bufferin Analgesic Caplets ... 744
- Extra Strength Bufferin Analgesic Tablets ... 745
- Bufferin Analgesic Tablets and Caplets ... 743
- Cama Arthritis Pain Reliever ... ■ 685
- Damason-P ... 1356
- Easprin ... 1719
- Ecotrin Enteric Coated Aspirin Maximum Strength Tablets and Caplets ... 2189
- Ecotrin Enteric Coated Aspirin Regular Strength Tablets and Caplets ... 2189
- Empirin Aspirin ... ■ 541
- Empirin with Codeine Phosphate Nos. 2, 3 & 4 ... 764
- Equagesic Tablets ... 2451
- Excedrin Extra-Strength Analgesic Tablets & Caplets ... 749
- 4-Way Cold Tablets ... 750
- Fiorinal Capsules ... 2007
- Fiorinal with Codeine Capsules ... 2008
- Fiorinal Tablets ... 2007
- Lortab ASA Tablets ... 2414
- Momentum Muscular Backache Formula ... ■ 751
- Norgesic ... 1314
- Norwich Extra-Strength Aspirin ... ■ 546
- Norwich Regular Strength Aspirin ■ 547
- P-A-C Analgesic Tablets ... ■ 669
- Percodan ... 951
- Robaxisal Tablets ... 1872
- Sine-Off Sinus Medicine Tablets-Aspirin Formula ... ■ 722
- Soma Compound w/Codeine Tablets ... 2390
- Soma Compound Tablets ... 2389
- St. Joseph Adult Chewable Aspirin (81 mg.) ... ■ 703
- Synalgos-DC Capsules ... 2525
- Talwin Compound ... 2072
- Ursinus Inlay-Tabs ... ■ 691
- Vanquish Analgesic Caplets ... ■ 574
- Zorprin Tablets ... 698

Aspirin, Enteric Coated (Use cautiously). Products include:
- Therapy Bayer Aspirin Caplets ... ■ 568
- Ecotrin ... 2189

Dicumarol (Inhibited response to coumarins). Products include:
- Dicumarol Tablets ... 516

Ephedrine Hydrochloride (Lessened physiologic activity of corticosteroids). Products include:
- Amesec ... ■ 682
- Primatene Tablets-M Formula ... 2421
- Primatene Tablets-P Formula ... 2421
- Primatene Tablets-Regular Formula ... 2421
- Quadrinal Tablets ... 1183
- Quelidrine Syrup ... 556
- Tedral SA ... 1765

Ephedrine Sulfate (Lessened physiologic activity of corticosteroids). Products include:
- Bronkaid Tablets ... ■ 757
- Bronkolixir ... ■ 761
- Bronkotabs Tablets ... ■ 762
- Marax Tablets & DF Syrup ... 1954
- Pazo Hemorrhoid Ointment & Suppositories ... 752
- Vicks Vatronol Nose Drops ... ■ 666

Ephedrine Tannate (Lessened physiologic activity of corticosteroids). Products include:
- Rynatuss ... 2388

Phenobarbital (Lessened physiologic activity of corticosteroids). Products include:
- Arco-Lase Plus Tablets ... 607
- Bellergal-S Tablets ... 1998
- Bronkolixir ... ■ 761
- Bronkotabs Tablets ... ■ 762
- Donnatal ... 1858
- Donnatal Extentabs ... 1859
- Donnatal Tablets ... 1858
- Donnazyme Tablets ... 1860
- Kinesed Tablets ... 2272
- Phenobarbital Elixir and Tablets ... 1293
- Primatene Tablets-P Formula ... 2421
- Quadrinal Tablets ... 1183
- Tedral SA ... 1765

Phenytoin (Lessened physiologic activity of corticosteroids). Products include:
- Dilantin Infatabs ... 1710
- Dilantin-30 Pediatric/Dilantin-125 Suspension ... 1713

Phenytoin Sodium (Lessened physiologic activity of corticosteroids). Products include:
- Dilantin Kapseals ... 1708
- Dilantin Parenteral ... 1712
- Dilantin with Phenobarbital Kapseals ... 1715

Rifampin (Lessened physiologic activity of corticosteroids). Products include:
- Rifadin ... 1345
- Rifamate Capsules ... 1347
- Rimactane Capsules ... 879

Spironolactone (Hypokalemia). Products include:
- Aldactazide ... 2150
- Aldactone ... 2152

Triamterene (Hypokalemia). Products include:
- Dyazide Capsules ... 2208
- Dyrenium Capsules ... 2210
- Maxzide ... 1215

Warfarin Sodium (Inhibited response to coumarins). Products include:
- Coumadin Injection & Tablets ... 944
- Panwarfin Tablets ... 547

HYDERGINE LIQUID

(Ergoloid Mesylates) ... 2010

No interactions described in labeling.

HYDERGINE LC LIQUID CAPSULES

(Ergoloid Mesylates) ... 2010

No interactions described in labeling.

HYDERGINE ORAL TABLETS

(Ergoloid Mesylates) ... 2010

No interactions described in labeling.

HYDERGINE SUBLINGUAL TABLETS

(Ergoloid Mesylates) ... 2010

No interactions described in labeling.

HYDREA CAPSULES

(Hydroxyurea) ... 728

No interactions described in labeling.

HYDRISALIC GEL

(Salicylic Acid) ... 1770

No interactions described in labeling.

HYDRISINOL CREME & LOTION

(Hydrogenated Vegetable Oil) ... 1770

No interactions described in labeling.

HYDROCET CAPSULES

(Acetaminophen, Hydrocodone Bitartrate) ... 835

May interact with monoamine oxidase inhibitors, tricyclic antidepressants, anticholinergics, central nervous system depressants, neuromuscular blocking agents, narcotic analgesics, and certain other agents. Compounds in these categories include:

Alcohol (Additive CNS depression).

Alfentanil Hydrochloride (Additive CNS depression). Products include:
- Alfenta Injection ... 1131

Alprazolam (Additive CNS depression). Products include:
- Xanax Tablets ... 2367

Amitriptyline Hydrochloride (Enhanced effect of either/both drugs). Products include:
- Elavil ... 2269
- Endep Tablets ... 1927
- Etrafon ... 2087
- Limbitrol ... 1933
- Triavil Tablets ... 1556

Amoxapine (Enhanced effect of either/both drugs). Products include:
- Asendin Tablets ... 1196

Aprobarbital (Additive CNS depression). Products include:
- Alurate Elixir ... 1883

Atropine Sulfate (Paralytic ileus). Products include:
- Arco-Lase Plus Tablets ... 607
- Atropine Sulfate Sterile Ophthalmic Solution and S.O.P. Sterile Ophthalmic Ointment ... ◉ 239
- Donnagel ... ■ 675
- Donnagel-PG ... 1858
- Donnatal ... 1858
- Donnatal Extentabs ... 1859
- Donnatal Tablets ... 1858
- Donnazyme Tablets ... 1860
- Isopto Atropine ... ◉ 218
- Lomotil ... 2174
- Motofen Tablets ... 836
- Ru-Tuss Tablets ... 693
- Urised Tablets ... 2396

Belladonna Alkaloids (Paralytic ileus). Products include:
- Bellergal-S Tablets ... 1998
- Hyland's Bed Wetting Tablets ... ■ 728
- Hyland's Teething Tablets ... ■ 728
- Kinesed Tablets ... 2272

Benztropine Mesylate (Paralytic ileus). Products include:
- Cogentin ... 1435

Biperiden (Paralytic ileus). Products include:
- Akineton ... 1171

Buprenorphine (Additive CNS depression).
- No products indexed under this heading.

Buspirone Hydrochloride (Additive CNS depression). Products include:
- BuSpar ... 1401

Butabarbital (Additive CNS depression). Products include:
- Pyridium Plus ... 1764

Butalbital (Additive CNS depression). Products include:
- Esgic-Plus Tablets ... 1002
- Esgic Tablets & Capsules ... 1001
- Fioricet Tablets ... 2006
- Fiorinal Capsules ... 2007
- Fiorinal with Codeine Capsules ... 2008
- Fiorinal Tablets ... 2007
- Phrenilin ... 838
- Sedapap Tablets 50 mg/650 mg .. 1360

Chlordiazepoxide (Additive CNS depression). Products include:
- Libritabs Tablets ... 1930
- Limbitrol ... 1933
- Menrium Tablets ... 1934

Chlordiazepoxide Hydrochloride (Additive CNS depression). Products include:
- Librax Capsules ... 1929
- Librium Capsules ... 1931
- Librium Injectable ... 1932

Chlorpromazine (Additive CNS depression). Products include:
- Thorazine ... 2234

Chlorprothixene (Additive CNS depression). Products include:
- Taractan Tablets ... 1920

Chlorprothixene Hydrochloride (Additive CNS depression). Products include:
- Taractan 1920

Chlorprothixene Lactate (Additive CNS depression). Products include:
- Taractan Concentrate 1920

Clidinium Bromide (Paralytic ileus). Products include:
- Librax Capsules 1929
- Quarzan Capsules 1937

Clomipramine Hydrochloride (Enhanced effect of either/both drugs). Products include:
- Anafranil Capsules 650

Clorazepate Dipotassium (Additive CNS depression). Products include:
- Tranxene 556

Clozapine (Additive CNS depression). Products include:
- Clozaril Tablets 2000

Codeine (Additive CNS depression). Products include:
- Calcidrine Syrup 506

Codeine Phosphate (Additive CNS depression). Products include:
- Actifed with Codeine Cough Syrup.. 752
- Cheracol Cough Syrup 1853
- Codimal PH Syrup 846
- Dimetane-DC Cough Syrup 1857
- Empirin with Codeine Phosphate Nos. 2, 3 & 4 764
- Fiorinal with Codeine Capsules 2008
- Isoclor Expectorant 982
- Naldecon CX Adult Liquid ..... ◘ 521
- Novahistine DH 1342
- Novahistine Expectorant 1343
- Nucofed Capsules 2219
- Nucofed Expectorant 2219
- Nucofed Pediatric Expectorant 2220
- Nucofed Syrup 2219
- Phenaphen with Codeine Capsules 1865
- Phenaphen-650 with Codeine Tablets 1866
- Phenergan with Codeine 2497
- Phenergan VC with Codeine 2501
- Robitussin A-C Syrup 1875
- Robitussin-DAC Syrup 1875
- Ryna ..... ◘ 741
- Soma Compound w/Codeine Tablets 2390
- Triaminic Expectorant w/Codeine .. 1996
- Tussi-Organidin Liquid 2391
- Tylenol with Codeine 1381

Codeine Polistirex (Additive CNS depression).
- No products indexed under this heading.

Desipramine Hydrochloride (Enhanced effect of either/both drugs). Products include:
- Norpramin Tablets 1340

Dezocine (Additive CNS depression).

Diazepam (Additive CNS depression). Products include:
- Valium Injectable 1937
- Valium Tablets 1939
- Valrelease Capsules 1923

Dicyclomine Hydrochloride (Paralytic ileus). Products include:
- Bentyl 1322

Doxepin Hydrochloride (Enhanced effect of either/both drugs). Products include:
- Sinequan 1960

Droperidol (Additive CNS depression). Products include:
- Inapsine Injection 1140
- Innovar Injection 1141

Enflurane (Additive CNS depression). Products include:
- Ethrane 599

Estazolam (Additive CNS depression). Products include:
- ProSom Tablets 554

Ethchlorvynol (Additive CNS depression). Products include:
- Placidyl Capsules 553

Ethinamate (Additive CNS depression).
- No products indexed under this heading.

Ethopropazine Hydrochloride (Paralytic ileus).

Ethyl Alcohol (Additive CNS depression). Products include:
- Anbesol Gel Antiseptic-Anesthetic .. 2417
- Anbesol Gel Antiseptic-Anesthetic - Maximum Strength 2417
- Anbesol Liquid Antiseptic-Anesthetic 2417
- Anbesol Liquid Antiseptic-Anesthetic - Maximum Strength 2417
- P & S Plus Tar Gel ..... ◘ 510
- X-Seb T Shampoo ..... ◘ 510
- X-Seb T Plus Conditioning Shampoo ..... ◘ 510

Fentanyl (Additive CNS depression). Products include:
- Duragesic Transdermal System 1133

Fentanyl Citrate (Additive CNS depression). Products include:
- Innovar Injection 1141
- Sublimaze Injection 1146

Fluphenazine Decanoate (Additive CNS depression). Products include:
- Prolixin Decanoate 1795

Fluphenazine Enanthate (Additive CNS depression). Products include:
- Prolixin Enanthate 1796

Fluphenazine Hydrochloride (Additive CNS depression). Products include:
- Prolixin Elixir 1793
- Prolixin Injection 1791
- Prolixin Oral Concentrate 1792
- Prolixin Tablets 1793

Flurazepam Hydrochloride (Additive CNS depression). Products include:
- Dalmane Capsules 1927

Furazolidone (Enhanced effect of either/both drugs). Products include:
- Furoxone 1855

Glutethimide (Additive CNS depression).
- No products indexed under this heading.

Glycopyrrolate (Paralytic ileus). Products include:
- Robinul Forte Tablets 1873
- Robinul Injectable 1873
- Robinul Tablets 1873

Haloperidol (Additive CNS depression). Products include:
- Haldol Injection, Tablets and Concentrate 1373

Haloperidol Decanoate (Additive CNS depression). Products include:
- Haldol Decanoate 1375

Hydrocodone Polistirex (Additive CNS depression). Products include:
- Tussionex Extended-Release Suspension 988

Hydroxyzine Hydrochloride (Additive CNS depression). Products include:
- Atarax Tablets & Syrup 1941
- Marax Tablets & DF Syrup 1954
- Vistaril Intramuscular Solution 1970

Hyoscyamine (Paralytic ileus). Products include:
- Cystospaz Tablets 2395
- Urised Tablets 2396

Hyoscyamine Sulfate (Paralytic ileus). Products include:
- Arco-Lase Plus Tablets 607
- Cystospaz-M Capsules 2395
- Donnagel ..... ◘ 675
- Donnagel-PG 1858
- Donnatal 1858
- Donnatal Extentabs 1859
- Donnatal Tablets 1858
- Donnazyme Tablets 1860
- Kutrase Capsules 2146
- Levsin/Levsinex 2147
- Ru-Tuss Tablets 693

Imipramine Hydrochloride (Enhanced effect of either/both drugs). Products include:
- Tofranil Ampuls 1038
- Tofranil Tablets 1039

Imipramine Pamoate (Enhanced effect of either/both drugs). Products include:
- Tofranil-PM Capsules 1041

Ipratropium Bromide (Paralytic ileus). Products include:
- Atrovent Inhalation Aerosol 675

Isocarboxazid (Enhanced effect of either/both drugs). Products include:
- Marplan Tablets 1906

Isoflurane (Additive CNS depression). Products include:
- Forane 600

Ketamine Hydrochloride (Additive CNS depression). Products include:
- Ketalar 1726

Levorphanol Tartrate (Additive CNS depression). Products include:
- Levo-Dromoran 1906

Lithium Carbonate (Additive CNS depression). Products include:
- Eskalith 2214
- Lithane Tablets 1596
- Lithium Carbonate Capsules & Tablets 1984
- Lithobid Tablets 870

Lithium Citrate (Additive CNS depression). Products include:
- Cibalith-S 870

Lorazepam (Additive CNS depression). Products include:
- Ativan Injection 2432
- Ativan Tablets 2434

Loxapine Hydrochloride (Additive CNS depression). Products include:
- Loxitane 1213

Loxapine Succinate (Additive CNS depression). Products include:
- Loxitane Capsules 1213

Maprotiline Hydrochloride (Enhanced effect of either/both drugs). Products include:
- Ludiomil Tablets 874

Mepenzolate Bromide (Paralytic ileus). Products include:
- Cantil Tablets 1326

Meperidine Hydrochloride (Additive CNS depression). Products include:
- Demerol 2047
- Mepergan Injection 2479

Mephobarbital (Additive CNS depression). Products include:
- Mebaral Tablets 2061

Meprobamate (Additive CNS depression). Products include:
- Deprol Tablets 2382
- Equagesic Tablets 2451
- Miltown Tablets 2386
- PMB 200 and PMB 400 2504

Mesoridazine (Additive CNS depression). Products include:
- Serentil 686

Methadone Hydrochloride (Additive CNS depression). Products include:
- Dolophine Hydrochloride Ampoules & Vials 1260
- Dolophine Hydrochloride Tablets 1261
- Methadone Hydrochloride Diskets .. 1284
- Methadone Hydrochloride Oral Solution & Tablets 1987

Methohexital Sodium (Additive CNS depression). Products include:
- Brevital Sodium Vials 1248

Methoxyflurane (Additive CNS depression).
- No products indexed under this heading.

Midazolam Hydrochloride (Additive CNS depression). Products include:
- Versed Injection 1924

Molindone Hydrochloride (Additive CNS depression). Products include:
- Moban Tablets & Concentrate 932

Morphine Sulfate (Additive CNS depression). Products include:
- Astramorph/PF Injection, USP (Preservative-Free) 618
- Duramorph 960
- Infumorph 200 and Infumorph 500 Sterile Solutions 962
- MS Contin Tablets 1814
- MSIR 1817
- Oramorph SR (Morphine Sulfate Sustained Release Tablets) 1988
- Roxanol 1991

Nortriptyline Hydrochloride (Enhanced effect of either/both drugs). Products include:
- Pamelor 2019

Opium Alkaloids (Additive CNS depression). Products include:
- B & O No. 15A & No. 16A Supprettes 2395
- Pantopon Injectable 1911

Oxazepam (Additive CNS depression). Products include:
- Serax Capsules 2522
- Serax Tablets 2522

Oxybutynin Chloride (Paralytic ileus). Products include:
- Ditropan 1332

Oxycodone Hydrochloride (Additive CNS depression). Products include:
- Percocet Tablets 950
- Percodan 951
- Roxicodone Tablets, Oral Solution & Intensol (Oxycodone) 1992
- Tylox Capsules 1382

Oxyphenonium Bromide (Paralytic ileus).

Pentobarbital Sodium (Additive CNS depression). Products include:
- Nembutal Sodium Capsules 534
- Nembutal Sodium Solution 536
- Nembutal Sodium Suppositories 538

Perphenazine (Additive CNS depression). Products include:
- Etrafon 2087
- Triavil Tablets 1556
- Trilafon 2123

Phenelzine Sulfate (Enhanced effect of either/both drugs). Products include:
- Nardil 1742

Phenobarbital (Additive CNS depression). Products include:
- Arco-Lase Plus Tablets 607
- Bellergal-S Tablets 1998
- Bronkolixir ..... ◘ 761
- Bronkotabs Tablets ..... ◘ 762
- Donnatal 1858
- Donnatal Extentabs 1859
- Donnatal Tablets 1858
- Donnazyme Tablets 1860
- Kinesed Tablets 2272
- Phenobarbital Elixir and Tablets 1293
- Primatene Tablets-P Formula 2421
- Quadrinal Tablets 1183
- Tedral SA 1765

Pimozide (Additive CNS depression). Products include:
- Orap Tablets 1020

Prazepam (Additive CNS depression). Products include:
- Centrax 1693

Prochlorperazine (Additive CNS depression). Products include:
- Compazine 2201

Procyclidine Hydrochloride (Paralytic ileus). Products include:
- Kemadrin Tablets 771

Promethazine Hydrochloride (Additive CNS depression). Products include:

- Mepergan Injection 2479
- Phenergan with Codeine 2497
- Phenergan with Dextromethorphan 2499
- Phenergan Injection 2493
- Phenergan Suppositories 2496
- Phenergan Syrup 2495
- Phenergan Tablets 2496
- Phenergan VC 2500
- Phenergan VC with Codeine 2501

Propantheline Bromide (Paralytic ileus). Products include:

- Pro-Banthīne Tablets 2141

Propofol (Additive CNS depression). Products include:

- Diprivan Injection 2267

Propoxyphene Hydrochloride (Additive CNS depression). Products include:

- Darvon 1256
- Wygesic Tablets 2540

Propoxyphene Napsylate (Additive CNS depression). Products include:

- Darvon-N/Darvocet-N 1254

Protriptyline Hydrochloride (Enhanced effect of either/both drugs). Products include:

- Vivactil Tablets 1567

Quazepam (Additive CNS depression). Products include:

- Doral Tablets 2383

Scopolamine Hydrobromide (Paralytic ileus). Products include:

- Donnagel ▣ 675
- Donnagel-PG 1858
- Donnatal 1858
- Donnatal Extentabs 1859
- Donnatal Tablets 1858
- Donnazyme Tablets 1860
- Isopto Hyoscine ⊙ 222
- Murocoll-2 Sterile Ophthalmic Solution ⊙ 261
- Ru-Tuss Tablets 693

Scopolamine Preparations (Paralytic ileus). Products include:

- Transderm Scōp Transdermal Therapeutic System 887

Secobarbital Sodium (Additive CNS depression). Products include:

- Seconal Sodium Pulvules 1296

Selegiline Hydrochloride (Enhanced effect of either/both drugs). Products include:

- Eldepryl 2250

Sufentanil Citrate (Additive CNS depression). Products include:

- Sufenta Injection 1147

Temazepam (Additive CNS depression). Products include:

- Restoril Capsules 2023

Thiamylal Sodium (Additive CNS depression). Products include:

- Surital Ampoules, Steri-Vials 1764

Thioridazine Hydrochloride (Additive CNS depression). Products include:

- Mellaril 2011

Thiothixene (Additive CNS depression). Products include:

- Navane Capsules and Concentrate 1954
- Navane Intramuscular 1956

Tranylcypromine Sulfate (Enhanced effect of either/both drugs). Products include:

- Parnate Tablets 2222

Triazolam (Additive CNS depression). Products include:

- Halcion Tablets 2340

Tridihexethyl Chloride (Paralytic ileus).

- No products indexed under this heading.

Trifluoperazine Hydrochloride (Additive CNS depression). Products include:

- Stelazine 2226

Trihexyphenidyl Hydrochloride (Paralytic ileus). Products include:

- Artane 1195

Trimipramine Maleate (Enhanced effect of either/both drugs). Products include:

- Surmontil Capsules 2524

HYDROCORTONE ACETATE STERILE SUSPENSION

(Hydrocortisone Acetate) 1479

May interact with oral anticoagulants, potassium sparing diuretics, and certain other agents. Compounds in these categories include:

Amiloride Hydrochloride (Hypokalemia). Products include:

- Midamor Tablets 1508
- Moduretic Tablets 1510

Aspirin (Use cautiously). Products include:

- Alka-Seltzer Effervescent Antacid and Pain Reliever 1568
- Alka-Seltzer Extra Strength Effervescent Antacid and Pain Reliever 1570
- Alka-Seltzer (Flavored) Effervescent Antacid and Pain Reliever 1569
- Alka-Seltzer Plus Cold Medicine ▣ 623
- Alka-Seltzer Plus Night-Time Cold Medicine ▣ 623
- Alka Seltzer Plus Sinus Allergy Medicine ▣ 624
- Anacin Coated Analgesic Caplets 2417
- Anacin Coated Analgesic Tablets 2417
- Anacin Maximum Strength Analgesic Coated Tablets 2417
- Maximum Strength Arthritis Pain Formula By the Makers of Anacin Analgesic Tablets and Caplets 2418
- Arthritis Pain Formula by the Makers of Anacin Analgesic Tablets and Caplets ▣ 747
- Arthritis Strength BC Powder ▣ 516
- Ascriptin A/D Caplets 1850
- Regular Strength Ascriptin Tablets 1850
- Azdōne Tablets 844
- BC Powder ▣ 517
- BC Cold Powder ▣ 517
- Children's Bayer Chewable Aspirin ▣ 564
- Genuine Bayer Aspirin Tablets & Caplets ▣ 564
- Maximum Bayer Aspirin Tablets & Caplets ▣ 566
- Bayer Plus Aspirin Tablets ▣ 567
- Therapy Bayer Aspirin Caplets ▣ 568
- 8 Hour Bayer Timed-Release Aspirin ▣ 566
- Arthritis Strength Bufferin Analgesic Caplets 744
- Extra Strength Bufferin Analgesic Tablets 745
- Bufferin Analgesic Tablets and Caplets 743
- Cama Arthritis Pain Reliever ▣ 685
- Damason-P 1356
- Easprin 1719
- Ecotrin Enteric Coated Aspirin Maximum Strength Tablets and Caplets 2189
- Ecotrin Enteric Coated Aspirin Regular Strength Tablets and Caplets 2189
- Empirin Aspirin ▣ 541
- Empirin with Codeine Phosphate Nos. 2, 3 & 4 764
- Equagesic Tablets 2451
- Excedrin Extra-Strength Analgesic Tablets & Caplets 749
- 4-Way Cold Tablets 750
- Fiorinal Capsules 2007
- Fiorinal with Codeine Capsules 2008
- Fiorinal Tablets 2007
- Lortab ASA Tablets 2414
- Momentum Muscular Backache Formula ▣ 751
- Norgesic 1314
- Norwich Extra-Strength Aspirin ▣ 546
- Norwich Regular Strength Aspirin ▣ 547
- P-A-C Analgesic Tablets ▣ 669
- Percodan 951
- Robaxisal Tablets 1872
- Sine-Off Sinus Medicine Tablets-Aspirin Formula ▣ 722
- Soma Compound w/Codeine Tablets 2390
- Soma Compound Tablets 2389
- St. Joseph Adult Chewable Aspirin (81 mg.) ▣ 703
- Synalgos-DC Capsules 2525
- Talwin Compound 2072
- Ursinus Inlay-Tabs ▣ 691
- Vanquish Analgesic Caplets ▣ 574
- Zorprin Tablets 698

Aspirin, Enteric Coated (Use cautiously). Products include:

- Therapy Bayer Aspirin Caplets ▣ 568
- Ecotrin 2189

Dicumarol (Inhibited response to coumarins). Products include:

- Dicumarol Tablets 516

Ephedrine Hydrochloride (Lessened physiologic activity of corticosteroids). Products include:

- Amesec ▣ 682
- Primatene Tablets-M Formula 2421
- Primatene Tablets-P Formula 2421
- Primatene Tablets-Regular Formula 2421
- Quadrinal Tablets 1183
- Quelidrine Syrup 556
- Tedral SA 1765

Ephedrine Sulfate (Lessened physiologic activity of corticosteroids). Products include:

- Bronkaid Tablets ▣ 757
- Bronkolixir ▣ 761
- Bronkotabs Tablets ▣ 762
- Marax Tablets & DF Syrup 1954
- Pazo Hemorrhoid Ointment & Suppositories 752
- Vicks Vatronol Nose Drops ▣ 666

Ephedrine Tannate (Lessened physiologic activity of corticosteroids). Products include:

- Rynatuss 2388

Live virus vaccines; smallpox (Contraindicated).

Phenobarbital (Lessened physiologic activity of corticosteroids). Products include:

- Arco-Lase Plus Tablets 607
- Bellergal-S Tablets 1998
- Bronkolixir ▣ 761
- Bronkotabs Tablets ▣ 762
- Donnatal 1858
- Donnatal Extentabs 1859
- Donnatal Tablets 1858
- Donnazyme Tablets 1860
- Kinesed Tablets 2272
- Phenobarbital Elixir and Tablets 1293
- Primatene Tablets-P Formula 2421
- Quadrinal Tablets 1183
- Tedral SA 1765

Phenytoin (Lessened physiologic activity of corticosteroids). Products include:

- Dilantin Infatabs 1710
- Dilantin-30 Pediatric/Dilantin-125 Suspension 1713

Phenytoin Sodium (Lessened physiologic activity of corticosteroids). Products include:

- Dilantin Kapseals 1708
- Dilantin Parenteral 1712
- Dilantin with Phenobarbital Kapseals 1715

Rifampin (Lessened physiologic activity of corticosteroids). Products include:

- Rifadin 1345
- Rifamate Capsules 1347
- Rimactane Capsules 879

Spironolactone (Hypokalemia). Products include:

- Aldactazide 2150
- Aldactone 2152

Triamterene (Hypokalemia). Products include:

- Dyazide Capsules 2208
- Dyrenium Capsules 2210
- Maxzide 1215

Warfarin Sodium (Inhibited response to coumarins). Products include:

- Coumadin Injection & Tablets 944
- Panwarfin Tablets 547

HYDROCORTONE PHOSPHATE INJECTION, STERILE

(Hydrocortisone Sodium Phosphate) 1481

May interact with oral anticoagulants, potassium sparing diuretics, and certain other agents. Compounds in these categories include:

Amiloride Hydrochloride (Hypokalemia). Products include:

- Midamor Tablets 1508
- Moduretic Tablets 1510

Amphotericin B (Cardiac enlargement and congestive failure). Products include:

- Fungizone Cream, Lotion and Ointment 2261
- Fungizone Intravenous 2262

Aspirin (Use cautiously). Products include:

- Alka-Seltzer Effervescent Antacid and Pain Reliever 1568
- Alka-Seltzer Extra Strength Effervescent Antacid and Pain Reliever 1570
- Alka-Seltzer (Flavored) Effervescent Antacid and Pain Reliever 1569
- Alka-Seltzer Plus Cold Medicine ▣ 623
- Alka-Seltzer Plus Night-Time Cold Medicine ▣ 623
- Alka Seltzer Plus Sinus Allergy Medicine ▣ 624
- Anacin Coated Analgesic Caplets 2417
- Anacin Coated Analgesic Tablets 2417
- Anacin Maximum Strength Analgesic Coated Tablets 2417
- Maximum Strength Arthritis Pain Formula By the Makers of Anacin Analgesic Tablets and Caplets 2418
- Arthritis Pain Formula by the Makers of Anacin Analgesic Tablets and Caplets ▣ 747
- Arthritis Strength BC Powder ▣ 516
- Ascriptin A/D Caplets 1850
- Regular Strength Ascriptin Tablets 1850
- Azdōne Tablets 844
- BC Powder ▣ 517
- BC Cold Powder ▣ 517
- Children's Bayer Chewable Aspirin ▣ 564
- Genuine Bayer Aspirin Tablets & Caplets ▣ 564
- Maximum Bayer Aspirin Tablets & Caplets ▣ 566
- Bayer Plus Aspirin Tablets ▣ 567
- Therapy Bayer Aspirin Caplets ▣ 568
- 8 Hour Bayer Timed-Release Aspirin ▣ 566
- Arthritis Strength Bufferin Analgesic Caplets 744
- Extra Strength Bufferin Analgesic Tablets 745
- Bufferin Analgesic Tablets and Caplets 743
- Cama Arthritis Pain Reliever ▣ 685
- Damason-P 1356
- Easprin 1719
- Ecotrin Enteric Coated Aspirin Maximum Strength Tablets and Caplets 2189
- Ecotrin Enteric Coated Aspirin Regular Strength Tablets and Caplets 2189
- Empirin Aspirin ▣ 541
- Empirin with Codeine Phosphate Nos. 2, 3 & 4 764
- Equagesic Tablets 2451
- Excedrin Extra-Strength Analgesic Tablets & Caplets 749
- 4-Way Cold Tablets 750
- Fiorinal Capsules 2007
- Fiorinal with Codeine Capsules 2008
- Fiorinal Tablets 2007
- Lortab ASA Tablets 2414
- Momentum Muscular Backache Formula ▣ 751
- Norgesic 1314
- Norwich Extra-Strength Aspirin ▣ 546
- Norwich Regular Strength Aspirin ▣ 547
- P-A-C Analgesic Tablets ▣ 669
- Percodan 951
- Robaxisal Tablets 1872
- Sine-Off Sinus Medicine Tablets-Aspirin Formula ▣ 722
- Soma Compound w/Codeine Tablets 2390
- Soma Compound Tablets 2389

- St. Joseph Adult Chewable Aspirin (81 mg.) ⊞ 703
- Synalgos-DC Capsules 2525
- Talwin Compound 2072
- Ursinus Inlay-Tabs ⊞ 691
- Vanquish Analgesic Caplets ⊞ 574
- Zorprin Tablets 698

Aspirin, Enteric Coated (Use cautiously). Products include:

- Therapy Bayer Aspirin Caplets ⊞ 568
- Ecotrin 2189

Dicumarol (Inhibited of response to coumarins). Products include:

- Dicumarol Tablets 516

Ephedrine Hydrochloride (Lessened physiologic activity of corticosteroids). Products include:

- Amesec ⊞ 682
- Primatene Tablets-M Formula 2421
- Primatene Tablets-P Formula 2421
- Primatene Tablets-Regular Formula 2421
- Quadrinal Tablets 1183
- Quelidrine Syrup 556
- Tedral SA 1765

Ephedrine Sulfate (Lessened physiologic activity of corticosteroids). Products include:

- Bronkaid Tablets ⊞ 757
- Bronkolixir ⊞ 761
- Bronkotabs Tablets ⊞ 762
- Marax Tablets & DF Syrup 1954
- Pazo Hemorrhoid Ointment & Suppositories 752
- Vicks Vatronol Nose Drops ⊞ 666

Ephedrine Tannate (Lessened physiologic activity of corticosteroids). Products include:

- Rynatuss 2388

Live Virus Vaccines (Contraindicated).

Phenobarbital (Lessened physiologic activity of corticosteroids). Products include:

- Arco-Lase Plus Tablets 607
- Bellergal-S Tablets 1998
- Bronkolixir ⊞ 761
- Bronkotabs Tablets ⊞ 762
- Donnatal 1858
- Donnatal Extentabs 1859
- Donnatal Tablets 1858
- Donnazyme Tablets 1860
- Kinesed Tablets 2272
- Phenobarbital Elixir and Tablets 1293
- Primatene Tablets-P Formula 2421
- Quadrinal Tablets 1183
- Tedral SA 1765

Phenytoin (Lessened physiologic activity of corticosteroids). Products include:

- Dilantin Infatabs 1710
- Dilantin-30 Pediatric/Dilantin-125 Suspension 1713

Phenytoin Sodium (Lessened physiologic activity of corticosteroids). Products include:

- Dilantin Kapseals 1708
- Dilantin Parenteral 1712
- Dilantin with Phenobarbital Kapseals 1715

Rifampin (Lessened physiologic activity of corticosteroids). Products include:

- Rifadin 1345
- Rifamate Capsules 1347
- Rimactane Capsules 879

Spironolactone (Hypokalemia). Products include:

- Aldactazide 2150
- Aldactone 2152

Triamterene (Hypokalemia). Products include:

- Dyazide Capsules 2208
- Dyrenium Capsules 2210
- Maxzide 1215

Warfarin Sodium (Inhibited of response to coumarins). Products include:

- Coumadin Injection & Tablets 944
- Panwarfin Tablets 547

HYDROCORTONE TABLETS

(Hydrocortisone) 1482

May interact with oral anticoagulants, potassium sparing diuretics, oral hypoglycemic agents, insulin, and certain other agents. Compounds in these categories include:

Amiloride Hydrochloride (Hypokalemia). Products include:

- Midamor Tablets 1508
- Moduretic Tablets 1510

Aspirin (Use cautiously). Products include:

- Alka-Seltzer Effervescent Antacid and Pain Reliever 1568
- Alka-Seltzer Extra Strength Effervescent Antacid and Pain Reliever 1570
- Alka-Seltzer (Flavored) Effervescent Antacid and Pain Reliever 1569
- Alka-Seltzer Plus Cold Medicine ⊞ 623
- Alka-Seltzer Plus Night-Time Cold Medicine ⊞ 623
- Alka Seltzer Plus Sinus Allergy Medicine ⊞ 624
- Anacin Coated Analgesic Caplets 2417
- Anacin Coated Analgesic Tablets 2417
- Anacin Maximum Strength Analgesic Coated Tablets 2417
- Maximum Strength Arthritis Pain Formula By the Makers of Anacin Analgesic Tablets and Caplets 2418
- Arthritis Pain Formula by the Makers of Anacin Analgesic Tablets and Caplets ⊞ 747
- Arthritis Strength BC Powder ⊞ 516
- Ascriptin A/D Caplets 1850
- Regular Strength Ascriptin Tablets 1850
- Azdōne Tablets 844
- BC Powder ⊞ 517
- BC Cold Powder ⊞ 517
- Children's Bayer Chewable Aspirin ⊞ 564
- Genuine Bayer Aspirin Tablets & Caplets ⊞ 564
- Maximum Bayer Aspirin Tablets & Caplets ⊞ 566
- Bayer Plus Aspirin Tablets ⊞ 567
- Therapy Bayer Aspirin Caplets ⊞ 568
- 8 Hour Bayer Timed-Release Aspirin ⊞ 566
- Arthritis Strength Bufferin Analgesic Caplets 744
- Extra Strength Bufferin Analgesic Tablets 745
- Bufferin Analgesic Tablets and Caplets 743
- Cama Arthritis Pain Reliever ⊞ 685
- Damason-P 1356
- Easprin 1719
- Ecotrin Enteric Coated Aspirin Maximum Strength Tablets and Caplets 2189
- Ecotrin Enteric Coated Aspirin Regular Strength Tablets and Caplets 2189
- Empirin Aspirin ⊞ 541
- Empirin with Codeine Phosphate Nos. 2, 3 & 4 764
- Equagesic Tablets 2451
- Excedrin Extra-Strength Analgesic Tablets & Caplets 749
- 4-Way Cold Tablets 750
- Fiorinal Capsules 2007
- Fiorinal with Codeine Capsules 2008
- Fiorinal Tablets 2007
- Lortab ASA Tablets 2414
- Momentum Muscular Backache Formula ⊞ 751
- Norgesic 1314
- Norwich Extra-Strength Aspirin ⊞ 546
- Norwich Regular Strength Aspirin ⊞ 547
- P-A-C Analgesic Tablets ⊞ 669
- Percodan 951
- Robaxisal Tablets 1872
- Sine-Off Sinus Medicine Tablets-Aspirin Formula ⊞ 722
- Soma Compound w/Codeine Tablets 2390
- Soma Compound Tablets 2389
- St. Joseph Adult Chewable Aspirin (81 mg.) ⊞ 703
- Synalgos-DC Capsules 2525
- Talwin Compound 2072
- Ursinus Inlay-Tabs ⊞ 691
- Vanquish Analgesic Caplets ⊞ 574
- Zorprin Tablets 698

Aspirin, Enteric Coated (Use cautiously). Products include:

- Therapy Bayer Aspirin Caplets ⊞ 568
- Ecotrin 2189

Chlorpropamide (Increased requirements for hypoglycemic agents in diabetics). Products include:

- Diabinese Tablets 1775

Dicumarol (Inhibited response to coumarins). Products include:

- Dicumarol Tablets 516

Ephedrine Hydrochloride (Reduces physiologic activity of corticosteroids). Products include:

- Amesec ⊞ 682
- Primatene Tablets-M Formula 2421
- Primatene Tablets-P Formula 2421
- Primatene Tablets-Regular Formula 2421
- Quadrinal Tablets 1183
- Quelidrine Syrup 556
- Tedral SA 1765

Glipizide (Increased requirements for hypoglycemic agents in diabetics). Products include:

- Glucotrol 1952

Glyburide (Increased requirements for hypoglycemic agents in diabetics). Products include:

- DiaBeta 1091
- Micronase Tablets 2350

Insulin, Human (Increased requirements for insulin in diabetics).

No products indexed under this heading.

Insulin, Human Isophane Suspension (Increased requirements for insulin in diabetics). Products include:

- Humulin N, 100 Units 1270

Insulin, Human NPH (Increased requirements for insulin in diabetics). Products include:

- Insulatard NPH Human 1627
- Novolin N 1627
- Novolin N PenFill Cartridges 1628
- Novolin N Prefilled 1628

Insulin, Human Regular (Increased requirements for insulin in diabetics). Products include:

- Humulin BR, 100 Units 1268
- Humulin R, 100 Units 1272
- Novolin R 1627
- Novolin R PenFill Cartridges 1628
- Novolin R Prefilled 1629
- Velosulin Human 1628

Insulin, Human, Zinc Suspension (Increased requirements for insulin in diabetics). Products include:

- Humulin L, 100 Units 1268
- Humulin U, 100 Units 1272
- Novolin L 1627

Insulin, NPH (Increased requirements for insulin in diabetics). Products include:

- NPH, 40 & 100 Units 1273
- Beef NPH, 100 Units 1274
- Pork NPH, 100 Units 1275
- Insulatard NPH 1626
- NPH Insulin 1626
- NPH Purified Pork Isophane Insulin 1626

Insulin, Regular (Increased requirements for insulin in diabetics). Products include:

- Regular, 40 & 100 Units 1273
- Beef Regular, 100 Units 1275
- Pork Regular, 100 Units 1275
- Pork Regular (Concentrated), 500 Units 1276
- Regular Insulin 1625
- Regular Purified Pork Insulin 1626
- Velosulin 1627

Insulin, Zinc Crystals (Increased requirements for insulin in diabetics). Products include:

- NPH, 40 & 100 Units 1273

Insulin, Zinc Suspension (Increased requirements for insulin in diabetics). Products include:

- Lente, 40 & 100 Units 1272
- Protamine, Zinc, 40 & 100 Units 1273
- Lente Iletin I 1272
- Beef Lente, 100 Units 1274
- Beef Protamine Zinc, 100 Units 1274
- Pork Lente, 100 Units 1275
- Pork, Protamine, Zinc, 100 Units 1275
- Lente Insulin 1626
- Lente Purified Pork Insulin 1626
- Semilente Insulin 1625
- Ultralente Insulin 1626

Phenobarbital (Lessened physiologic activity of corticosteroids). Products include:

- Arco-Lase Plus Tablets 607
- Bellergal-S Tablets 1998
- Bronkolixir ⊞ 761
- Bronkotabs Tablets ⊞ 762
- Donnatal 1858
- Donnatal Extentabs 1859
- Donnatal Tablets 1858
- Donnazyme Tablets 1860
- Kinesed Tablets 2272
- Phenobarbital Elixir and Tablets 1293
- Primatene Tablets-P Formula 2421
- Quadrinal Tablets 1183
- Tedral SA 1765

Phenytoin (Lessened physiologic activity of corticosteroids). Products include:

- Dilantin Infatabs 1710
- Dilantin-30 Pediatric/Dilantin-125 Suspension 1713

Phenytoin Sodium (Lessened physiologic activity of corticosteroids). Products include:

- Dilantin Kapseals 1708
- Dilantin Parenteral 1712
- Dilantin with Phenobarbital Kapseals 1715

Rifampin (Lessened physiologic activity of corticosteroids). Products include:

- Rifadin 1345
- Rifamate Capsules 1347
- Rimactane Capsules 879

Spironolactone (Hypokalemia). Products include:

- Aldactazide 2150
- Aldactone 2152

Tolazamide (Increased requirements for hypoglycemic agents in diabetics). Products include:

- Tolinase Tablets 2365

Tolbutamide (Increased requirements for hypoglycemic agents in diabetics). Products include:

- Orinase Tablets 2354

Triamterene (Hypokalemia). Products include:

- Dyazide Capsules 2208
- Dyrenium Capsules 2210
- Maxzide 1215

Warfarin Sodium (Inhibited response to coumarins). Products include:

- Coumadin Injection & Tablets 944
- Panwarfin Tablets 547

HYDRODIURIL TABLETS

(Hydrochlorothiazide) 1484

May interact with antihypertensives, lithium preparations, corticosteroids, cardiac glycosides, insulin, non-steroidal anti-inflammatory agents, barbiturates, narcotic analgesics, oral hypoglycemic agents, and certain other agents. Compounds in these categories include:

Acebutolol Hydrochloride (Potentiation of antihypertensive drugs). Products include:

- Sectral Capsules 2520

ACTH (Hypokalemia).

No products indexed under this heading.

Alcohol (Potentiation of orthostatic hypotension).

Alfentanil Hydrochloride (Potentiation of orthostatic hypotension). Products include:
- Alfenta Injection ... 1131

Aprobarbital (Potentiation of orthostatic hypotension). Products include:
- Alurate Elixir ... 1883

Atenolol (Potentiation of antihypertensive drugs). Products include:
- Tenoretic Tablets ... 1105
- Tenormin Tablets and I.V. Injection 1107

Benazepril Hydrochloride (Potentiation of antihypertensive drugs). Products include:
- Lotensin Tablets ... 872

Bendroflumethiazide (Potentiation of antihypertensive drugs). Products include:
- Corzide Tablets ... 702
- Naturetin Tablets ... 1789
- Rauzide Tablets ... 1804

Betamethasone Acetate (Hypokalemia). Products include:
- Celestone Soluspan Suspension ... 2081

Betamethasone Sodium Phosphate (Hypokalemia). Products include:
- Celestone Soluspan Suspension ... 2081

Betaxolol Hydrochloride (Potentiation of antihypertensive drugs). Products include:
- Betoptic Sterile Ophthalmic Solution ... 569
- Betoptic S Sterile Ophthalmic Suspension ... 570
- Kerlone Tablets ... 2172

Buprenorphine (Potentiation of orthostatic hypotension).
- No products indexed under this heading.

Butabarbital (Potentiation of orthostatic hypotension). Products include:
- Pyridium Plus ... 1764

Butalbital (Potentiation of orthostatic hypotension). Products include:
- Esgic-Plus Tablets ... 1002
- Esgic Tablets & Capsules ... 1001
- Fioricet Tablets ... 2006
- Fiorinal Capsules ... 2007
- Fiorinal with Codeine Capsules ... 2008
- Fiorinal Tablets ... 2007
- Phrenilin ... 838
- Sedapap Tablets 50 mg/650 mg .. 1360

Captopril (Potentiation of antihypertensive drugs). Products include:
- Capoten ... 2255
- Capozide ... 2258

Carteolol Hydrochloride (Potentiation of antihypertensive drugs). Products include:
- Cartrol Tablets ... 507

Chlorothiazide (Potentiation of antihypertensive drugs). Products include:
- Aldoclor Tablets ... 1413
- Diupres Tablets ... 1461
- Diuril Oral ... 1464

Chlorothiazide Sodium (Potentiation of antihypertensive drugs). Products include:
- Diuril Sodium Intravenous ... 1463

Chlorpropamide (Dosage adjustment of oral hypoglycemic may be necessary). Products include:
- Diabinese Tablets ... 1775

Chlorthalidone (Potentiation of antihypertensive drugs). Products include:
- Combipres Tablets ... 678
- Tenoretic Tablets ... 1105
- Thalitone Tablets ... 687

Clonidine (Potentiation of antihypertensive drugs). Products include:
- Catapres-TTS ... 677

Clonidine Hydrochloride (Potentiation of antihypertensive drugs). Products include:
- Catapres Tablets ... 676
- Combipres Tablets ... 678

Codeine (Potentiation of orthostatic hypotension). Products include:
- Calcidrine Syrup ... 506

Codeine Phosphate (Potentiation of orthostatic hypotension). Products include:
- Actifed with Codeine Cough Syrup.. 752
- Cheracol Cough Syrup ... 1853
- Codimal PH Syrup ... 846
- Dimetane-DC Cough Syrup ... 1857
- Empirin with Codeine Phosphate Nos. 2, 3 & 4 ... 764
- Fiorinal with Codeine Capsules ... 2008
- Isoclor Expectorant ... 982
- Naldecon CX Adult Liquid ... ■ 521
- Novahistine DH ... 1342
- Novahistine Expectorant ... 1343
- Nucofed Capsules ... 2219
- Nucofed Expectorant ... 2219
- Nucofed Pediatric Expectorant ... 2220
- Nucofed Syrup ... 2219
- Phenaphen with Codeine Capsules 1865
- Phenaphen-650 with Codeine Tablets ... 1866
- Phenergan with Codeine ... 2497
- Phenergan VC with Codeine ... 2501
- Robitussin A-C Syrup ... 1875
- Robitussin-DAC Syrup ... 1875
- Ryna ... ■ 741
- Soma Compound w/Codeine Tablets ... 2390
- Triaminic Expectorant w/Codeine .. 1996
- Tussi-Organidin Liquid ... 2391
- Tylenol with Codeine ... 1381

Codeine Polistirex (Potentiation of orthostatic hypotension).
- No products indexed under this heading.

Cortisone Acetate (Hypokalemia). Products include:
- Cortone Acetate Sterile Suspension ... 1437
- Cortone Acetate Tablets ... 1439

Deserpidine (Potentiation of antihypertensive drugs). Products include:
- Enduronyl ... 518
- Harmonyl Tablets ... 528
- Oreticyl ... 545

Deslanoside (Resultant hypokalemia may exaggerate cardiac toxicity of digitalis).
- No products indexed under this heading.

Dexamethasone (Hypokalemia). Products include:
- AK-Trol Ointment & Suspension ... ⊙ 207
- Decadron Elixir ... 1445
- Decadron Tablets ... 1447
- Decaspray Topical Aerosol ... 1459
- Dexacidin ... ⊙ 272
- Maxidex Sterile Ophthalmic Suspension ... ⊙ 223
- Maxitrol Ophthalmic Ointment/Suspension ... ⊙ 223
- TobraDex Ophthalmic Suspension and Ointment ... ⊙ 228

Dexamethasone Acetate (Hypokalemia). Products include:
- Dalalone D.P. Injectable ... 999
- Decadron-LA Sterile Suspension ... 1457

Dexamethasone Sodium Phosphate (Hypokalemia). Products include:
- AK-Dex ... ⊙ 203
- Decadron Phosphate Respihaler ... 1454
- Decadron Phosphate Sterile Ophthalmic Ointment ... 1453
- Decadron Phosphate Sterile Ophthalmic Solution ... 1453
- Decadron Phosphate Topical Cream ... 1455
- Decadron Phosphate Turbinaire ... 1456
- Maxidex Sterile Ophthalmic Ointment ... ⊙ 222
- NeoDecadron Sterile Ophthalmic Ointment ... 1517
- NeoDecadron Sterile Ophthalmic Solution ... 1518
- NeoDecadron Topical Cream ... 1518

Dezocine (Potentiation of orthostatic hypotension).

Diazoxide (Potentiation of antihypertensive drugs). Products include:
- Hyperstat I.V. Injection ... 2095
- Proglycem ... 649

Diclofenac Sodium (Reduced diuretic, natriuretic, and antihypertensive effects). Products include:
- Voltaren Ophthalmic Sterile Ophthalmic Solution ... ⊙ 268
- Voltaren Tablets ... 1042

Digitoxin (Resultant hypokalemia may exaggerate cardiac toxicity of digitalis). Products include:
- Crystodigin Tablets ... 1253

Digoxin (Resultant hypokalemia may exaggerate cardiac toxicity of digitalis). Products include:
- Lanoxicaps ... 772
- Lanoxin Elixir Pediatric ... 775
- Lanoxin Injection ... 778
- Lanoxin Injection Pediatric ... 781
- Lanoxin Tablets ... 783

Doxazosin Mesylate (Potentiation of antihypertensive drugs). Products include:
- Cardura Tablets ... 1941

Enalapril Maleate (Potentiation of antihypertensive drugs). Products include:
- Vaseretic Tablets ... 1559
- Vasotec Tablets ... 1564

Enalaprilat (Potentiation of antihypertensive drugs). Products include:
- Vasotec I.V. ... 1562

Esmolol Hydrochloride (Potentiation of antihypertensive drugs). Products include:
- Brevibloc Injection ... 942

Etodolac (Reduced diuretic, natriuretic, and antihypertensive effects). Products include:
- Lodine Capsules ... 2468

Felodipine (Potentiation of antihypertensive drugs). Products include:
- Plendil Extended-Release Tablets ... 1526

Fenoprofen Calcium (Reduced diuretic, natriuretic, and antihypertensive effects). Products include:
- Nalfon Pulvules & Tablets ... 919

Fentanyl (Potentiation of orthostatic hypotension). Products include:
- Duragesic Transdermal System ... 1133

Fentanyl Citrate (Potentiation of orthostatic hypotension). Products include:
- Innovar Injection ... 1141
- Sublimaze Injection ... 1146

Flurbiprofen (Reduced diuretic, natriuretic, and antihypertensive effects). Products include:
- Ansaid Tablets ... 2319

Fosinopril Sodium (Potentiation of antihypertensive drugs). Products include:
- Monopril Tablets ... 1406

Furosemide (Potentiation of antihypertensive drugs). Products include:
- Lasix ... 1093

Glipizide (Dosage adjustment of oral hypoglycemic may be necessary). Products include:
- Glucotrol ... 1952

Glyburide (Dosage adjustment of oral hypoglycemic may be necessary). Products include:
- DiaBeta ... 1091
- Micronase Tablets ... 2350

Guanabenz Acetate (Potentiation of antihypertensive drugs). Products include:
- Wytensin Tablets ... 2542

Guanethidine Monosulfate (Potentiation of antihypertensive drugs). Products include:
- Esimil Tablets ... 864
- Ismelin Tablets ... 869

Hydralazine Hydrochloride (Potentiation of antihypertensive drugs). Products include:
- Apresazide Capsules ... 854
- Apresoline Hydrochloride Parenteral (Ampuls) ... 856
- Apresoline Hydrochloride Tablets .. 855
- Apresoline-Esidrix Tablets ... 857
- Ser-Ap-Es Tablets ... 881
- Serpasil-Apresoline Tablets ... 884

Hydrocodone Bitartrate (Potentiation of orthostatic hypotension). Products include:
- Anexsia 5/500 Tablets ... 2196
- Anexsia 7.5/650 Tablets ... 2197
- Azdōne Tablets ... 844
- Codiclear DH Syrup ... 845
- Codimal DH Syrup ... 846
- Damason-P ... 1356
- Hycodan Syrup, Tablets ... 927
- Hycomine Compound Tablets ... 929
- Hycomine Syrup ... 927
- Hycotuss Expectorant Syrup ... 930
- Hydrocet Capsules ... 835
- Lortab ASA Tablets ... 2414
- Lortab ... 2412
- Ru-Tuss with Hydrocodone ... 694
- Triaminic Expectorant DH ... 1995
- Vicodin Tablets ... 1187
- Vicodin ES Tablets ... 1189
- Zydone Capsules ... 941

Hydrocodone Polistirex (Potentiation of orthostatic hypotension). Products include:
- Tussionex Extended-Release Suspension ... 988

Hydrocortisone (Hypokalemia). Products include:
- AK-Spore H.C. ... ⊙ 206
- Bactine Hydrocortisone Anti-Itch Cream ... ■ 625
- CaldeCORT Anti-Itch Hydrocortisone Spray ... ■ 560
- Carmol HC Cream 1% ... 2296
- Cortaid Spray ... ■ 735
- Cortenema ... 2244
- Cortisporin Ointment ... 758
- Cortisporin Ophthalmic Ointment Sterile ... 758
- Cortisporin Ophthalmic Suspension Sterile ... 759
- Cortisporin Otic Solution Sterile ... 760
- Cortisporin Otic Suspension Sterile 760
- Cortizone-5 Creme & Ointment ... ■ 732
- Dermolate Anti-Itch Cream ... ■ 697
- Eldecort Cream 1.0% ... 1113
- Eldecort Cream 1.0% and 2.5% ... 1113
- Fungoid HC Creme ... 1770
- Hydrocortone Tablets ... 1482
- Hytone ... 909
- LazerSporin-C Solution ... 1770
- Massengill Medicated Soft Cloth Towelettes ... 2192
- Nutracort Cream & Lotion ... 1684
- PediOtic Suspension Sterile ... 797
- Synacort Creams 1%, 2.5% ... 2296
- Vanoxide-HC Acne Lotion ... 911
- Vioform-Hydrocortisone Cream and Mild Cream ... 889
- Vioform-Hydrocortisone Ointment .. 889
- VōSoL HC Otic Solution ... 2392
- Vytone Cream 1% ... 911

Hydrocortisone Acetate (Hypokalemia). Products include:
- Analpram-HC Rectal Cream 1% and 2.5% ... 970
- Anusol-HC Cream ... 1690
- Anusol-HC Suppositories ... 1691
- Caldecort ... ■ 560
- Carmol HC Cream 1% ... 2296
- Chloromycetin Hydrocortisone Ophthalmic ... 1694
- Coly-Mycin S Otic w/Neomycin & Hydrocortisone ... 1708
- Cortaid ... ■ 735
- Cortef Feminine Itch Cream ... ■ 735
- Corticaine ... ■ 682
- Cortifoam ... 1827
- Cortisporin Cream ... 757
- Epifoam ... 1828
- Gynecort 5 Creme ... ■ 556
- Hydrocortone Acetate Sterile Suspension ... 1479

(■ Described in PDR For Nonprescription Drugs) (⊙ Described in PDR For Ophthalmology)

Lanacort 5 Creme and Ointment .. ■ 557
Mantadil Cream ... 789
Ophthocort ... ◉ 301
Orabase HCA Oral Paste ... 890
Pramosone Cream, Lotion & Ointment ... 971
ProctoCream-HC ... 1834
Proctofoam-HC ... 1835

Hydrocortisone Sodium Phosphate (Hypokalemia). Products include:
Hydrocortone Phosphate Injection, Sterile ... 1481

Hydrocortisone Sodium Succinate (Hypokalemia). Products include:
Solu-Cortef Sterile Powder ... 2361

Hydroflumethiazide (Potentiation of antihypertensive drugs). Products include:
Diucardin Tablets ... 2450
Saluron ... 718
Salutensin/Salutensin-Demi ... 719

Ibuprofen (Reduced diuretic, natriuretic, and antihypertensive effects). Products include:
Advil Cold & Sinus Caplets (formerly CoAdvil) ... 2416
Advil Ibuprofen Tablets and Caplets ... 2416
Children's Advil Suspension ... 2426
CoAdvil ... ■ 748
Dristan Sinus Caplets ... 2419
Haltran Tablets ... ■ 668
Ibuprofen ... ■ 631
Medipren ibuprofen Caplets and Tablets ... 1362
Midol 200 Cramp Relief Formula .. ■ 570
Motrin Tablets ... 2351
Motrin IB Caplets and Tablets ... ■ 736
Nuprin Ibuprofen/Analgesic Tablets & Caplets ... 752
PediaProfen Suspension ... 1363
Rufen Tablets ... 691
Trendar Ibuprofen Tablets ... ■ 756

Indapamide (Potentiation of antihypertensive drugs). Products include:
Lozol Tablets ... 1843

Indomethacin (Reducted diuretic, natriuretic, and antihypertensive effects). Products include:
Indocin ... 1487

Indomethacin Sodium Trihydrate (Reduced diuretic, natriuretic, and antihypertensive effects). Products include:
Indocin I.V. ... 1490

Insulin, Human (Altered insulin requirements).
No products indexed under this heading.

Insulin, Human Isophane Suspension (Altered insulin requirements). Products include:
Humulin N, 100 Units ... 1270

Insulin, Human NPH (Altered insulin requirements). Products include:
Insulatard NPH Human ... 1627
Novolin N ... 1627
Novolin N PenFill Cartridges ... 1628
Novolin N Prefilled ... 1628

Insulin, Human Regular (Altered insulin requirements). Products include:
Humulin BR, 100 Units ... 1268
Humulin R, 100 Units ... 1272
Novolin R ... 1627
Novolin R PenFill Cartridges ... 1628
Novolin R Prefilled ... 1629
Velosulin Human ... 1628

Insulin, Human, Zinc Suspension (Altered insulin requirements). Products include:
Humulin L, 100 Units ... 1268
Humulin U, 100 Units ... 1272
Novolin L ... 1627

Insulin, NPH (Altered insulin requirements). Products include:
NPH, 40 & 100 Units ... 1273
Beef NPH, 100 Units ... 1274
Pork NPH, 100 Units ... 1275
Insulatard NPH ... 1626
NPH Insulin ... 1626
NPH Purified Pork Isophane Insulin ... 1626

Insulin, Regular (Altered insulin requirements). Products include:
Regular, 40 & 100 Units ... 1273
Beef Regular, 100 Units ... 1275
Pork Regular, 100 Units ... 1275
Pork Regular (Concentrated), 500 Units ... 1276
Regular Insulin ... 1625
Regular Purified Pork Insulin ... 1626
Velosulin ... 1627

Insulin, Zinc Crystals (Altered insulin requirements). Products include:
NPH, 40 & 100 Units ... 1273

Insulin, Zinc Suspension (Altered insulin requirements). Products include:
Lente, 40 & 100 Units ... 1272
Protamine, Zinc, 40 & 100 Units ... 1273
Lente Iletin I ... 1272
Beef Lente, 100 Units ... 1274
Beef Protamine Zinc, 100 Units ... 1274
Pork Lente, 100 Units ... 1275
Pork, Protamine, Zinc, 100 Units ... 1275
Lente Insulin ... 1626
Lente Purified Pork Insulin ... 1626
Semilente Insulin ... 1625
Ultralente Insulin ... 1626

Isradipine (Potentiation of antihypertensive drugs). Products include:
DynaCirc Capsules ... 2004

Ketoprofen (Reduced diuretic, natriuretic, antihypertensive effects). Products include:
Orudis Capsules ... 2488

Ketorolac Tromethamine (Reduced diuretic, natriuretic, and antihypertensive effects). Products include:
Toradol IM Injection ... 2302

Labetalol Hydrochloride (Potentiation of antihypertensive drugs). Products include:
Normodyne Injection ... 2108
Normodyne Tablets ... 2110
Normozide Tablets ... 2112
Trandate HCT Tablets ... 579
Trandate Injection ... 577
Trandate Tablets ... 579

Levorphanol Tartrate (Potentiation of orthostatic hypotension). Products include:
Levo-Dromoran ... 1906

Lisinopril (Potentiation of antihypertensive drugs). Products include:
Prinivil Tablets ... 1538
Prinzide Tablets ... 1540
Zestoretic ... 2274
Zestril Tablets ... 2277

Lithium Carbonate (High risk of lithium toxicity). Products include:
Eskalith ... 2214
Lithane Tablets ... 1596
Lithium Carbonate Capsules & Tablets ... 1984
Lithobid Tablets ... 870

Lithium Citrate (High risk of lithium toxicity). Products include:
Cibalith-S ... 870

Mecamylamine Hydrochloride (Potentiation of antihypertensive drugs). Products include:
Inversine Tablets ... 1492

Meclofenamate Sodium (Reduced diuretic, natriuretic, and antihypertensive effects). Products include:
Meclomen Capsules ... 1739

Mefenamic Acid (Reduced diuretic, natriuretic, and antihypertensive effects). Products include:
Ponstel ... 1758

Meperidine Hydrochloride (Potentiation of orthostatic hypotension). Products include:
Demerol ... 2047
Mepergan Injection ... 2479

Mephobarbital (Potentiation of orthostatic hypotension). Products include:
Mebaral Tablets ... 2061

Methadone Hydrochloride (Potentiation of orthostatic hypotension). Products include:
Dolophine Hydrochloride Ampoules & Vials ... 1260
Dolophine Hydrochloride Tablets ... 1261
Methadone Hydrochloride Diskets .. 1284
Methadone Hydrochloride Oral Solution & Tablets ... 1987

Methyclothiazide (Potentiation of antihypertensive drugs). Products include:
Enduron Tablets ... 517
Enduronyl ... 518

Methyldopa (Potentiation of antihypertensive drugs). Products include:
Aldoclor Tablets ... 1413
Aldomet Oral ... 1415
Aldoril Tablets ... 1418

Methyldopate Hydrochloride (Potentiation of antihypertensive drugs). Products include:
Aldomet Ester HCl Injection ... 1417

Methylprednisolone (Hypokalemia). Products include:
Medrol ... 2348

Methylprednisolone Acetate (Hypokalemia). Products include:
Depo-Medrol Sterile Aqueous Suspension ... 2334

Methylprednisolone Sodium Succinate (Hypokalemia). Products include:
Solu-Medrol Sterile Powder ... 2363

Metolazone (Potentiation of antihypertensive drugs). Products include:
Diulo ... 2129
Mykrox ½ mg Tablets ... 984
Zaroxolyn Tablets ... 989

Metoprolol Tartrate (Potentiation of antihypertensive drugs). Products include:
Lopressor Ampuls ... 1032
Lopressor HCT Tablets ... 1034
Lopressor Tablets ... 1032

Metyrosine (Potentiation of antihypertensive drugs). Products include:
Demser Capsules ... 1460

Minoxidil (Potentiation of antihypertensive drugs). Products include:
Loniten Tablets ... 2346
Rogaine Topical Solution ... 2357

Morphine Sulfate (Potentiation of orthostatic hypotension). Products include:
Astramorph/PF Injection, USP (Preservative-Free) ... 618
Duramorph ... 960
Infumorph 200 and Infumorph 500 Sterile Solutions ... 962
MS Contin Tablets ... 1814
MSIR ... 1817
Oramorph SR (Morphine Sulfate Sustained Release Tablets) ... 1988
Roxanol ... 1991

Nadolol (Potentiation of antihypertensive drugs). Products include:
Corgard Tablets ... 701
Corzide Tablets ... 702

Naproxen (Reduced diuretic, natriuretic, and antihypertensive effects). Products include:
Naprosyn ... 2297

Naproxen Sodium (Reduced diuretic, natriuretic, and antihypertensive effects). Products include:
Anaprox and Anaprox DS Tablets ... 2288

Nicardipine Hydrochloride (Potentiation of ahtihypertensive drugs). Products include:
Cardene Capsules ... 2290

Nitroglycerin (Potentiation of antihypertensive drugs). Products include:
Deponit NTG Transdermal Delivery System ... 2143
Minitran Transdermal Delivery System ... 1312
Nitro-Bid Ointment ... 1339
Nitro-Bid Capsules ... 1338
Nitrodisc ... 2176
Nitro-Dur (nitroglycerin) Transdermal Infusion System ... 1164
Nitrogard Tablets ... 1004
Nitrolingual Spray ... 1846
Nitrostat Tablets ... 1743
Transderm-Nitro Transdermal Therapeutic System ... 2283

Norepinephrine Bitartrate (Decreased arterial responsiveness to norepinephrine). Products include:
Levophed Bitartrate Injection ... 2054

Opium Alkaloids (Potentiation of orthostatic hypotension). Products include:
B & O No. 15A & No. 16A Supprettes ... 2395
Pantopon Injectable ... 1911

Oxycodone Hydrochloride (Potentiation of orthostatic hypotension). Products include:
Percocet Tablets ... 950
Percodan ... 951
Roxicodone Tablets, Oral Solution & Intensol (Oxycodone) ... 1992
Tylox Capsules ... 1382

Penbutolol Sulfate (Potentiation of antihypertensive drugs). Products include:
Levatol ... 1832

Pentobarbital Sodium (Potentiation of orthostatic hypotension). Products include:
Nembutal Sodium Capsules ... 534
Nembutal Sodium Solution ... 536
Nembutal Sodium Suppositories ... 538

Phenobarbital (Potentiation of orthostatic hypotension). Products include:
Arco-Lase Plus Tablets ... 607
Bellergal-S Tablets ... 1998
Bronkolixir ... ■ 761
Bronkotabs Tablets ... ■ 762
Donnatal ... 1858
Donnatal Extentabs ... 1859
Donnatal Tablets ... 1858
Donnazyme Tablets ... 1860
Kinesed Tablets ... 2272
Phenobarbital Elixir and Tablets ... 1293
Primatene Tablets-P Formula ... 2421
Quadrinal Tablets ... 1183
Tedral SA ... 1765

Phenoxybenzamine Hydrochloride (Potentiation of antihypertensive drugs). Products include:
Dibenzyline Capsules ... 2207

Phentolamine Mesylate (Potentiation of antihypertensive drugs). Products include:
Regitine ... 878

Phenylbutazone (Reduced diuretic, natriuretic, and antihypertensive effects). Products include:
Butazolidin Capsules & Tablets ... 1027

Pindolol (Potentiation of antihypertensive drugs). Products include:
Visken Tablets ... 2036

Piroxicam (Reduced diuretic, natriuretic, and antihypertensive effects). Products include:
Feldene Capsules ... 1777

Polythiazide (Potentiation of antihypertensive drugs). Products include:
Minizide Capsules ... 1779
Renese Tablets ... 1785
Renese-R Tablets ... 1786

Prazosin Hydrochloride (Potentiation of antihypertensive drugs). Products include:
Minipress Capsules ... 1778
Minizide Capsules ... 1779

Prednisolone Acetate (Hypokalemia). Products include:
- AK-Cide Sterile Ophthalmic Ointment & Suspension ◉ 202
- Blephamide Liquifilm Sterile Ophthalmic Suspension 586
- Blephamide S.O.P. Sterile Ophthalmic Ointment 586
- Cetapred Ointment ◉ 220
- ⅛% Econopred & 1% Econopred Plus ◉ 217
- Isopto Cetapred Suspension ◉ 220
- Metimyd ◉ 306
- Poly-Pred Liquifilm ◉ 250
- Pred Forte ◉ 252
- Pred Mild ◉ 254
- Pred-G Liquifilm Sterile Ophthalmic Suspension ◉ 252
- Pred-G S.O.P. Sterile Ophthalmic Ointment ◉ 253
- Vasocidin Ointment ◉ 275

Prednisolone Sodium Phosphate (Hypokalemia). Products include:
- AK-Pred ◉ 205
- Hydeltrasol Injection, Sterile 1476
- Inflamase ◉ 274
- Pediapred Oral Liquid 987
- Vasocidin Ophthalmic Solution ◉ 276

Prednisolone Tebutate (Hypokalemia). Products include:
- Hydeltra-T.B.A. Sterile Suspension 1478

Prednisone (Hypokalemia). Products include:
- Deltasone Tablets 2332

Propoxyphene Hydrochloride (Potentiation of orthostatic hypotension). Products include:
- Darvon 1256
- Wygesic Tablets 2540

Propoxyphene Napsylate (Potentiation of orthostatic hypotension). Products include:
- Darvon-N/Darvocet-N 1254

Propranolol Hydrochloride (Potentiation of antihypertensive drugs). Products include:
- Inderal 2459
- Inderal LA Long Acting Capsules 2461
- Inderide Tablets 2463
- Inderide LA Long Acting Capsules 2465

Ramipril (Potentiation of antihypertensive drugs). Products include:
- Altace Capsules 1086

Rauwolfia Serpentina (Potentiation of antihypertensive drugs). Products include:
- Raudixin Tablets 1803
- Rauzide Tablets 1804

Rescinnamine (Potentiation of antihypertensive drugs).
- No products indexed under this heading.

Reserpine (Potentiation of antihypertensive drugs). Products include:
- Diupres Tablets 1461
- Hydromox R Tablets 1209
- Hydropres Tablets 1485
- Renese-R Tablets 1786
- Salutensin/Salutensin-Demi 719
- Ser-Ap-Es Tablets 881
- Serpasil Tablets 883
- Serpasil-Apresoline Tablets 884
- Serpasil-Esidrix Tablets 886

Secobarbital Sodium (Potentiation of orthostatic hypotension). Products include:
- Seconal Sodium Pulvules 1296

Sodium Nitroprusside (Potentiation of antihypertensive drugs). Products include:
- Nipride I.V. Infusion 1909

Sufentanil Citrate (Potentiation of orthostatic hypotension). Products include:
- Sufenta Injection 1147

Sulindac (Reduced diuretic, natriuretic, and antihypertensive effects). Products include:
- Clinoril Tablets 1433

Terazosin Hydrochloride (Potentiation of antihypertensive drugs). Products include:
- Hytrin Tablets 529

Thiamylal Sodium (Potentiation of orthostatic hypotension). Products include:
- Surital Ampoules, Steri-Vials 1764

Timolol Maleate (Potentiation of antihypertensive drugs). Products include:
- Blocadren Tablets 1429
- Timolide Tablets 1547
- Timoptic in Ocudose 1552
- Timoptic Sterile Ophthalmic Solution 1550

Tolazamide (Dosage adjustment of oral hypoglycemic may be necessary). Products include:
- Tolinase Tablets 2365

Tolbutamide (Dosage adjustment of oral hypoglycemic may be necessary). Products include:
- Orinase Tablets 2354

Tolmetin Sodium (Reduced diuretic, natriuretic, and antihypertensive effects). Products include:
- Tolectin (200, 400 and 600 mg) 1379

Triamcinolone (Hypokalemia).
- No products indexed under this heading.

Triamcinolone Acetonide (Hypokalemia). Products include:
- Aristocort A 1010
- Azmacort Inhaler 1837
- Kenalog Cream, Lotion & Ointment 2401
- Kenalog-10 Injection 2402
- Kenalog-40 Injection 2403
- Kenalog in Orabase 604
- Kenalog Spray 2401
- Mycolog II Cream and Ointment 2407
- Mytrex Cream & Ointment 2080
- Nasacort Nasal Inhaler 1844

Triamcinolone Diacetate (Hypokalemia). Products include:
- Aristocort Suspension 1008

Triamcinolone Hexacetonide (Hypokalemia). Products include:
- Aristospan Suspension 1011

Trimethaphan Camsylate (Potentiation of antihypertensive drugs). Products include:
- Arfonad Ampuls 1887

Tubocurarine Chloride (Increased responsiveness to tubocurarine).
- No products indexed under this heading.

HYDROMOX R TABLETS

(Quinethazone, Reserpine) 1209

May interact with para-aminobenzoic acid based local anesthetics, ganglionic blocking agents, antihypertensives, corticosteroids, barbiturates, narcotic analgesics, cardiac glycosides, and certain other agents. Compounds in these categories include:

Acebutolol Hydrochloride (Potentiated). Products include:
- Sectral Capsules 2520

ACTH (Electrolyte abnormalities aggravated).
- No products indexed under this heading.

Alcohol (May potentiate orthostatic hypotension).

Alfentanil Hydrochloride (May potentiate orthostatic hypotension). Products include:
- Alfenta Injection 1131

Aprobarbital (May potentiate orthostatic hypotension). Products include:
- Alurate Elixir 1883

Atenolol (Potentiated). Products include:
- Tenoretic Tablets 1105
- Tenormin Tablets and I.V. Injection 1107

Benazepril Hydrochloride (Potentiated). Products include:
- Lotensin Tablets 872

Bendroflumethiazide (Potentiated). Products include:
- Corzide Tablets 702
- Naturetin Tablets 1789
- Rauzide Tablets 1804

Betamethasone Acetate (Electrolyte abnormalities aggravated). Products include:
- Celestone Soluspan Suspension 2081

Betamethasone Sodium Phosphate (Electrolyte abnormalities aggravated). Products include:
- Celestone Soluspan Suspension 2081

Betaxolol Hydrochloride (Potentiated). Products include:
- Betoptic Sterile Ophthalmic Solution 569
- Betoptic S Sterile Ophthalmic Suspension 570
- Kerlone Tablets 2172

Buprenorphine (May potentiate orthostatic hypotension).
- No products indexed under this heading.

Butabarbital (May potentiate orthostatic hypotension). Products include:
- Pyridium Plus 1764

Butalbital (May potentiate orthostatic hypotension). Products include:
- Esgic-Plus Tablets 1002
- Esgic Tablets & Capsules 1001
- Fioricet Tablets 2006
- Fiorinal Capsules 2007
- Fiorinal with Codeine Capsules 2008
- Fiorinal Tablets 2007
- Phrenilin 838
- Sedapap Tablets 50 mg/650 mg 1360

Captopril (Potentiated). Products include:
- Capoten 2255
- Capozide 2258

Carteolol Hydrochloride (Potentiated). Products include:
- Cartrol Tablets 507

Chlorothiazide (Potentiated). Products include:
- Aldoclor Tablets 1413
- Diupres Tablets 1461
- Diuril Oral 1464

Chlorothiazide Sodium (Potentiated). Products include:
- Diuril Sodium Intravenous 1463

Chlorthalidone (Potentiated). Products include:
- Combipres Tablets 678
- Tenoretic Tablets 1105
- Thalitone Tablets 687

Clonidine (Potentiated). Products include:
- Catapres-TTS 677

Clonidine Hydrochloride (Potentiated). Products include:
- Catapres Tablets 676
- Combipres Tablets 678

Codeine (May potentiate orthostatic hypotension). Products include:
- Calcidrine Syrup 506

Codeine Phosphate (May potentiate orthostatic hypotension). Products include:
- Actifed with Codeine Cough Syrup 752
- Cheracol Cough Syrup 1853
- Codimal PH Syrup 846
- Dimetane-DC Cough Syrup 1857
- Empirin with Codeine Phosphate Nos. 2, 3 & 4 764
- Fiorinal with Codeine Capsules 2008
- Isoclor Expectorant 982
- Naldecon CX Adult Liquid ▣ 521
- Novahistine DH 1342
- Novahistine Expectorant 1343
- Nucofed Capsules 2219
- Nucofed Expectorant 2219
- Nucofed Pediatric Expectorant 2220
- Nucofed Syrup 2219
- Phenaphen with Codeine Capsules 1865
- Phenaphen-650 with Codeine Tablets 1866
- Phenergan with Codeine 2497
- Phenergan VC with Codeine 2501
- Robitussin A-C Syrup 1875
- Robitussin-DAC Syrup 1875
- Ryna ▣ 741
- Soma Compound w/Codeine Tablets 2390
- Triaminic Expectorant w/Codeine 1996
- Tussi-Organidin Liquid 2391
- Tylenol with Codeine 1381

Codeine Polistirex (May potentiate orthostatic hypotension).
- No products indexed under this heading.

Cortisone Acetate (Electrolyte abnormalities aggravated). Products include:
- Cortone Acetate Sterile Suspension 1437
- Cortone Acetate Tablets 1439

Deserpidine (Potentiated). Products include:
- Enduronyl 518
- Harmonyl Tablets 528
- Oreticyl 545

Deslanoside (Potential for increased digitalis cardiac toxicity).
- No products indexed under this heading.

Dexamethasone (Electrolyte abnormalities aggravated). Products include:
- AK-Trol Ointment & Suspension ◉ 207
- Decadron Elixir 1445
- Decadron Tablets 1447
- Decaspray Topical Aerosol 1459
- Dexacidin ◉ 272
- Maxidex Sterile Ophthalmic Suspension ◉ 223
- Maxitrol Ophthalmic Ointment/Suspension ◉ 223
- TobraDex Ophthalmic Suspension and Ointment ◉ 228

Dexamethasone Acetate (Electrolyte abnormalities aggravated). Products include:
- Dalalone D.P. Injectable 999
- Decadron-LA Sterile Suspension 1457

Dexamethasone Sodium Phosphate (Electrolyte abnormalities aggravated). Products include:
- AK-Dex ◉ 203
- Decadron Phosphate Respihaler 1454
- Decadron Phosphate Sterile Ophthalmic Ointment 1453
- Decadron Phosphate Sterile Ophthalmic Solution 1453
- Decadron Phosphate Topical Cream 1455
- Decadron Phosphate Turbinaire 1456
- Maxidex Sterile Ophthalmic Ointment ◉ 222
- NeoDecadron Sterile Ophthalmic Ointment 1517
- NeoDecadron Sterile Ophthalmic Solution 1518
- NeoDecadron Topical Cream 1518

Dezocine (May potentiate orthostatic hypotension).

Diazoxide (Potentiated). Products include:
- Hyperstat I.V. Injection 2095
- Proglycem 649

Digitoxin (Potential for increased digitalis cardiac toxicity). Products include:
- Crystodigin Tablets 1253

Digoxin (Potential for increased digitalis cardiac toxicity). Products include:
- Lanoxicaps 772
- Lanoxin Elixir Pediatric 775
- Lanoxin Injection 778
- Lanoxin Injection Pediatric 781
- Lanoxin Tablets 783

Doxazosin Mesylate (Potentiated). Products include:
- Cardura Tablets 1941

Enalapril Maleate (Potentiated). Products include:
- Vaseretic Tablets 1559
- Vasotec Tablets 1564

Enalaprilat (Potentiated). Products include:
- Vasotec I.V. 1562

Esmolol Hydrochloride (Potentiated). Products include:
- Brevibloc Injection 942

Felodipine (Potentiated). Products include:
- Plendil Extended-Release Tablets 1526

Fentanyl (May potentiate orthostatic hypotension). Products include:
- Duragesic Transdermal System 1133

Fentanyl Citrate (May potentiate orthostatic hypotension). Products include:
- Innovar Injection 1141
- Sublimaze Injection 1146

Fosinopril Sodium (Potentiated). Products include:
- Monopril Tablets 1406

Furosemide (Potentiated). Products include:
- Lasix 1093

Guanabenz Acetate (Potentiated). Products include:
- Wytensin Tablets 2542

Guanethidine Monosulfate (Potentiated). Products include:
- Esimil Tablets 864
- Ismelin Tablets 869

Hydralazine Hydrochloride (Potentiated). Products include:
- Apresazide Capsules 854
- Apresoline Hydrochloride Parenteral (Ampuls) 856
- Apresoline Hydrochloride Tablets 855
- Apresoline-Esidrix Tablets 857
- Ser-Ap-Es Tablets 881
- Serpasil-Apresoline Tablets 884

Hydrochlorothiazide (Potentiated). Products include:
- Aldactazide 2150
- Aldoril Tablets 1418
- Apresazide Capsules 854
- Apresoline-Esidrix Tablets 857
- Capozide 2258
- Dyazide Capsules 2208
- Esidrix Tablets 863
- Esimil Tablets 864
- HydroDIURIL Tablets 1484
- Hydropres Tablets 1485
- Inderide Tablets 2463
- Inderide LA Long Acting Capsules 2465
- Lopressor HCT Tablets 1034
- Maxzide 1215
- Moduretic Tablets 1510
- Normozide Tablets 2112
- Oretic Tablets 544
- Oreticyl 545
- Prinzide Tablets 1540
- Ser-Ap-Es Tablets 881
- Serpasil-Esidrix Tablets 886
- Timolide Tablets 1547
- Trandate HCT Tablets 579
- Vaseretic Tablets 1559
- Zestoretic 2274

Hydrocodone Bitartrate (May potentiate orthostatic hypotension). Products include:
- Anexsia 5/500 Tablets 2196
- Anexsia 7.5/650 Tablets 2197
- Azdone Tablets 844
- Codiclear DH Syrup 845
- Codimal DH Syrup 846
- Damason-P 1356
- Hycodan Syrup, Tablets 927
- Hycomine Compound Tablets 929
- Hycomine Syrup 927
- Hycotuss Expectorant Syrup 930
- Hydrocet Capsules 835
- Lortab ASA Tablets 2414
- Lortab 2412
- Ru-Tuss with Hydrocodone 694
- Triaminic Expectorant DH 1995
- Vicodin Tablets 1187
- Vicodin ES Tablets 1189
- Zydone Capsules 941

Hydrocodone Polistirex (May potentiate orthostatic hypotension). Products include:
- Tussionex Extended-Release Suspension 988

Hydrocortisone (Electrolyte abnormalities aggravated). Products include:
- AK-Spore H.C. ⊙ 206
- Bactine Hydrocortisone Anti-Itch Cream ■ 625
- CaldeCORT Anti-Itch Hydrocortisone Spray ■ 560
- Carmol HC Cream 1% 2296
- Cortaid Spray ■ 735
- Cortenema 2244
- Cortisporin Ointment 758
- Cortisporin Ophthalmic Ointment Sterile 758
- Cortisporin Ophthalmic Suspension Sterile 759
- Cortisporin Otic Solution Sterile 760
- Cortisporin Otic Suspension Sterile 760
- Cortizone-5 Creme & Ointment ■ 732
- Dermolate Anti-Itch Cream ■ 697
- Eldecort Cream 1.0% 1113
- Eldecort Cream 1.0% and 2.5% 1113
- Fungoid HC Creme 1770
- Hydrocortone Tablets 1482
- Hytone 909
- LazerSporin-C Solution 1770
- Massengill Medicated Soft Cloth Towelettes 2192
- Nutracort Cream & Lotion 1684
- PediOtic Suspension Sterile 797
- Synacort Creams 1%, 2.5% 2296
- Vanoxide-HC Acne Lotion 911
- Vioform-Hydrocortisone Cream and Mild Cream 889
- Vioform-Hydrocortisone Ointment 889
- VōSoL HC Otic Solution 2392
- Vytone Cream 1% 911

Hydrocortisone Acetate (Electrolyte abnormalities aggravated). Products include:
- Analpram-HC Rectal Cream 1% and 2.5% 970
- Anusol-HC Cream 1690
- Anusol-HC Suppositories 1691
- Caldecort ■ 560
- Carmol HC Cream 1% 2296
- Chloromycetin Hydrocortisone Ophthalmic 1694
- Coly-Mycin S Otic w/Neomycin & Hydrocortisone 1708
- Cortaid ■ 735
- Cortef Feminine Itch Cream ■ 735
- Corticaine ■ 682
- Cortifoam 1827
- Cortisporin Cream 757
- Epifoam 1828
- Gynecort 5 Creme ■ 556
- Hydrocortone Acetate Sterile Suspension 1479
- Lanacort 5 Creme and Ointment ■ 557
- Mantadil Cream 789
- Ophthocort ⊙ 301
- Orabase HCA Oral Paste 890
- Pramosone Cream, Lotion & Ointment 971
- ProctoCream-HC 1834
- Proctofoam-HC 1835

Hydrocortisone Sodium Phosphate (Electrolyte abnormalities aggravated). Products include:
- Hydrocortone Phosphate Injection, Sterile 1481

Hydrocortisone Sodium Succinate (Electrolyte abnormalities aggravated). Products include:
- Solu-Cortef Sterile Powder 2361

Hydroflumethiazide (Potentiated). Products include:
- Diucardin Tablets 2450
- Saluron 718
- Salutensin/Salutensin-Demi 719

Indapamide (Potentiated). Products include:
- Lozol Tablets 1843

Isradipine (Potentiated). Products include:
- DynaCirc Capsules 2004

Labetalol Hydrochloride (Potentiated). Products include:
- Normodyne Injection 2108
- Normodyne Tablets 2110
- Normozide Tablets 2112
- Trandate HCT Tablets 579
- Trandate Injection 577
- Trandate Tablets 579

Levorphanol Tartrate (May potentiate orthostatic hypotension). Products include:
- Levo-Dromoran 1906

Lisinopril (Potentiated). Products include:
- Prinivil Tablets 1538
- Prinzide Tablets 1540
- Zestoretic 2274
- Zestril Tablets 2277

Mecamylamine Hydrochloride (Potentiated). Products include:
- Inversine Tablets 1492

Meperidine Hydrochloride (May potentiate orthostatic hypotension). Products include:
- Demerol 2047
- Mepergan Injection 2479

Mephobarbital (May potentiate orthostatic hypotension). Products include:
- Mebaral Tablets 2061

Methadone Hydrochloride (May potentiate orthostatic hypotension). Products include:
- Dolophine Hydrochloride Ampoules & Vials 1260
- Dolophine Hydrochloride Tablets 1261
- Methadone Hydrochloride Diskets 1284
- Methadone Hydrochloride Oral Solution & Tablets 1987

Methyclothiazide (Potentiated). Products include:
- Enduron Tablets 517
- Enduronyl 518

Methyldopa (Potentiated). Products include:
- Aldoclor Tablets 1413
- Aldomet Oral 1415
- Aldoril Tablets 1418

Methyldopate Hydrochloride (Potentiated). Products include:
- Aldomet Ester HCl Injection 1417

Methylprednisolone Acetate (Electrolyte abnormalities aggravated). Products include:
- Depo-Medrol Sterile Aqueous Suspension 2334

Methylprednisolone Sodium Succinate (Electrolyte abnormalities aggravated). Products include:
- Solu-Medrol Sterile Powder 2363

Metolazone (Potentiated). Products include:
- Diulo 2129
- Mykrox ½ mg Tablets 984
- Zaroxolyn Tablets 989

Metoprolol Tartrate (Potentiated). Products include:
- Lopressor Ampuls 1032
- Lopressor HCT Tablets 1034
- Lopressor Tablets 1032

Metyrosine (Potentiated). Products include:
- Demser Capsules 1460

Minoxidil (Potentiated). Products include:
- Loniten Tablets 2346
- Rogaine Topical Solution 2357

Morphine Sulfate (May potentiate orthostatic hypotension). Products include:
- Astramorph/PF Injection, USP (Preservative-Free) 618
- Duramorph 960
- Infumorph 200 and Infumorph 500 Sterile Solutions 962
- MS Contin Tablets 1814
- MSIR 1817
- Oramorph SR (Morphine Sulfate Sustained Release Tablets) 1988
- Roxanol 1991

Nadolol (Potentiated). Products include:
- Corgard Tablets 701
- Corzide Tablets 702

Nicardipine Hydrochloride (Potentiated). Products include:
- Cardene Capsules 2290

Nitroglycerin (Potentiated). Products include:
- Deponit NTG Transdermal Delivery System 2143
- Minitran Transdermal Delivery System 1312
- Nitro-Bid Ointment 1339
- Nitro-Bid Capsules 1338
- Nitrodisc 2176
- Nitro-Dur (nitroglycerin) Transdermal Infusion System 1164
- Nitrogard Tablets 1004
- Nitrolingual Spray 1846
- Nitrostat Tablets 1743
- Transderm-Nitro Transdermal Therapeutic System 2283

Norepinephrine Bitartrate (Decreased arterial responsiveness to norepinephrine). Products include:
- Levophed Bitartrate Injection 2054

Opium Alkaloids (May potentiate orthostatic hypotension). Products include:
- B & O No. 15A & No. 16A Supprettes 2395
- Pantopon Injectable 1911

Oxycodone Hydrochloride (May potentiate orthostatic hypotension). Products include:
- Percocet Tablets 950
- Percodan 951
- Roxicodone Tablets, Oral Solution & Intensol (Oxycodone) 1992
- Tylox Capsules 1382

Penbutolol Sulfate (Potentiated). Products include:
- Levatol 1832

Pentobarbital Sodium (May potentiate orthostatic hypotension). Products include:
- Nembutal Sodium Capsules 534
- Nembutal Sodium Solution 536
- Nembutal Sodium Suppositories 538

Phenobarbital (May potentiate orthostatic hypotension). Products include:
- Arco-Lase Plus Tablets 607
- Bellergal-S Tablets 1998
- Bronkolixir ■ 761
- Bronkotabs Tablets ■ 762
- Donnatal 1858
- Donnatal Extentabs 1859
- Donnatal Tablets 1858
- Donnazyme Tablets 1860
- Kinesed Tablets 2272
- Phenobarbital Elixir and Tablets 1293
- Primatene Tablets-P Formula 2421
- Quadrinal Tablets 1183
- Tedral SA 1765

Phenoxybenzamine Hydrochloride (Potentiated). Products include:
- Dibenzyline Capsules 2207

Phentolamine Mesylate (Potentiated). Products include:
- Regitine 878

Pindolol (Potentiated). Products include:
- Visken Tablets 2036

Polythiazide (Potentiated). Products include:
- Minizide Capsules 1779
- Renese Tablets 1785
- Renese-R Tablets 1786

Prazosin Hydrochloride (Potentiated). Products include:
- Minipress Capsules 1778
- Minizide Capsules 1779

Prednisolone Acetate (Electrolyte abnormalities aggravated). Products include:
- AK-Cide Sterile Ophthalmic Ointment & Suspension ⊙ 202
- Blephamide Liquifilm Sterile Ophthalmic Suspension 586
- Blephamide S.O.P. Sterile Ophthalmic Ointment 586
- Cetapred Ointment ⊙ 220
- ⅛% Econopred & 1% Econopred Plus ⊙ 217
- Isopto Cetapred Suspension ⊙ 220

Metimyd ⊙ 306
Poly-Pred Liquifilm ⊙ 250
Pred Forte ⊙ 252
Pred Mild ⊙ 254
Pred-G Liquifilm Sterile Ophthalmic Suspension ⊙ 252
Pred-G S.O.P. Sterile Ophthalmic Ointment ⊙ 253
Vasocidin Ointment ⊙ 275

Prednisolone Sodium Phosphate (Electrolyte abnormalities aggravated). Products include:
AK-Pred ⊙ 205
Hydeltrasol Injection, Sterile 1476
Inflamase ⊙ 274
Pediapred Oral Liquid 987
Vasocidin Ophthalmic Solution ⊙ 276

Prednisolone Tebutate (Electrolyte abnormalities aggravated). Products include:
Hydeltra-T.B.A. Sterile Suspension 1478

Prednisone (Electrolyte abnormalities aggravated). Products include:
Deltasone Tablets 2332

Propoxyphene Hydrochloride (May potentiate orthostatic hypotension). Products include:
Darvon 1256
Wygesic Tablets 2540

Propoxyphene Napsylate (May potentiate orthostatic hypotension). Products include:
Darvon-N/Darvocet-N 1254

Propranolol Hydrochloride (Potentiated). Products include:
Inderal 2459
Inderal LA Long Acting Capsules 2461
Inderide Tablets 2463
Inderide LA Long Acting Capsules 2465

Ramipril (Potentiated). Products include:
Altace Capsules 1086

Rauwolfia Serpentina (Potentiated). Products include:
Raudixin Tablets 1803
Rauzide Tablets 1804

Rescinnamine (Potentiated).
No products indexed under this heading.

Secobarbital Sodium (May potentiate orthostatic hypotension). Products include:
Seconal Sodium Pulvules 1296

Sodium Nitroprusside (Potentiated). Products include:
Nipride I.V. Infusion 1909

Sufentanil Citrate (May potentiate orthostatic hypotension). Products include:
Sufenta Injection 1147

Terazosin Hydrochloride (Potentiated). Products include:
Hytrin Tablets 529

Thiamylal Sodium (May potentiate orthostatic hypotension). Products include:
Surital Ampoules, Steri-Vials 1764

Timolol Maleate (Potentiated). Products include:
Blocadren Tablets 1429
Timolide Tablets 1547
Timoptic in Ocudose 1552
Timoptic Sterile Ophthalmic Solution 1550

Triamcinolone (Electrolyte abnormalities aggravated).
No products indexed under this heading.

Triamcinolone Acetonide (Electrolyte abnormalities aggravated). Products include:
Aristocort A 1010
Azmacort Inhaler 1837
Kenalog Cream, Lotion & Ointment 2401
Kenalog-10 Injection 2402
Kenalog-40 Injection 2403
Kenalog in Orabase 604
Kenalog Spray 2401
Mycolog II Cream and Ointment 2407
Mytrex Cream & Ointment 2080
Nasacort Nasal Inhaler 1844

Triamcinolone Diacetate (Electrolyte abnormalities aggravated). Products include:
Aristocort Suspension 1008

Triamcinolone Hexacetonide (Electrolyte abnormalities aggravated). Products include:
Aristospan Suspension 1011

Trimethaphan Camsylate (Potentiated). Products include:
Arfonad Ampuls 1887

Tubocurarine Chloride (Increased responsiveness to tubocurarine).
No products indexed under this heading.

HYDROMOX TABLETS
(Quinethazone) 1208
May interact with antihypertensives, ganglionic blocking agents, para-aminobenzoic acid based local anesthetics, corticosteroids, barbiturates, narcotic analgesics, cardiac glycosides, and certain other agents. Compounds in these categories include:

Acebutolol Hydrochloride (Potentiated). Products include:
Sectral Capsules 2520

ACTH (Electrolyte abnormalities aggravated).
No products indexed under this heading.

Alcohol (May potentiate orthostatic hypotension).

Alfentanil Hydrochloride (May potentiate orthostatic hypotension). Products include:
Alfenta Injection 1131

Aprobarbital (May potentiate orthostatic hypotension). Products include:
Alurate Elixir 1883

Atenolol (Potentiated). Products include:
Tenoretic Tablets 1105
Tenormin Tablets and I.V. Injection 1107

Benazepril Hydrochloride (Potentiated). Products include:
Lotensin Tablets 872

Bendroflumethiazide (Potentiated). Products include:
Corzide Tablets 702
Naturetin Tablets 1789
Rauzide Tablets 1804

Betamethasone Acetate (Electrolyte abnormalities aggravated). Products include:
Celestone Soluspan Suspension 2081

Betaxolol Hydrochloride (Potentiated). Products include:
Betoptic Sterile Ophthalmic Solution 569
Betoptic S Sterile Ophthalmic Suspension 570
Kerlone Tablets 2172

Buprenorphine (May potentiate orthostatic hypotension).
No products indexed under this heading.

Butabarbital (May potentiate orthostatic hypotension). Products include:
Pyridium Plus 1764

Butalbital (May potentiate orthostatic hypotension). Products include:
Esgic-Plus Tablets 1002
Esgic Tablets & Capsules 1001
Fioricet Tablets 2006
Fiorinal Capsules 2007
Fiorinal with Codeine Capsules 2008
Fiorinal Tablets 2007
Phrenilin 838
Sedapap Tablets 50 mg/650 mg 1360

Captopril (Potentiated). Products include:
Capoten 2255
Capozide 2258

Carteolol Hydrochloride (Potentiated). Products include:
Cartrol Tablets 507

Chlorothiazide (Potentiated). Products include:
Aldoclor Tablets 1413
Diupres Tablets 1461
Diuril Oral 1464

Chlorothiazide Sodium (Potentiated). Products include:
Diuril Sodium Intravenous 1463

Chlorthalidone (Potentiated). Products include:
Combipres Tablets 678
Tenoretic Tablets 1105
Thalitone Tablets 687

Clonidine (Potentiated). Products include:
Catapres-TTS 677

Clonidine Hydrochloride (Potentiated). Products include:
Catapres Tablets 676
Combipres Tablets 678

Codeine (May potentiate orthostatic hypotension). Products include:
Calcidrine Syrup 506

Codeine Phosphate (May potentiate orthostatic hypotension). Products include:
Actifed with Codeine Cough Syrup 752
Cheracol Cough Syrup 1853
Codimal PH Syrup 846
Dimetane-DC Cough Syrup 1857
Empirin with Codeine Phosphate Nos. 2, 3 & 4 764
Fiorinal with Codeine Capsules 2008
Isoclor Expectorant 982
Naldecon CX Adult Liquid ▣ 521
Novahistine DH 1342
Novahistine Expectorant 1343
Nucofed Capsules 2219
Nucofed Expectorant 2219
Nucofed Pediatric Expectorant 2220
Nucofed Syrup 2219
Phenaphen with Codeine Capsules 1865
Phenaphen-650 with Codeine Tablets 1866
Phenergan with Codeine 2497
Phenergan VC with Codeine 2501
Robitussin A-C Syrup 1875
Robitussin-DAC Syrup 1875
Ryna ▣ 741
Soma Compound w/Codeine Tablets 2390
Triaminic Expectorant w/Codeine 1996
Tussi-Organidin Liquid 2391
Tylenol with Codeine 1381

Codeine Polistirex (May potentiate orthostatic hypotension).
No products indexed under this heading.

Cortisone Acetate (Electrolyte abnormalities aggravated). Products include:
Cortone Acetate Sterile Suspension 1437
Cortone Acetate Tablets 1439

Deserpidine (Potentiated). Products include:
Enduronyl 518
Harmonyl Tablets 528
Oreticyl 545

Deslanoside (Hypokalemia and its toxic sequelae must be kept in mind in patients receiving digitalis).
No products indexed under this heading.

Dexamethasone (Electrolyte abnormalities aggravated). Products include:
AK-Trol Ointment & Suspension ⊙ 207
Decadron Elixir 1445
Decadron Tablets 1447
Decaspray Topical Aerosol 1459
Dexacidin ⊙ 272
Maxidex Sterile Ophthalmic Suspension ⊙ 223
Maxitrol Ophthalmic Ointment/Suspension ⊙ 223
TobraDex Ophthalmic Suspension and Ointment ⊙ 228

Dexamethasone Acetate (Electrolyte abnormalities aggravated). Products include:
Dalalone D.P. Injectable 999
Decadron-LA Sterile Suspension 1457

Dexamethasone Sodium Phosphate (Electrolyte abnormalities aggravated). Products include:
AK-Dex ⊙ 203
Decadron Phosphate Respihaler 1454
Decadron Phosphate Sterile Ophthalmic Ointment 1453
Decadron Phosphate Sterile Ophthalmic Solution 1453
Decadron Phosphate Topical Cream 1455
Decadron Phosphate Turbinaire 1456
Maxidex Sterile Ophthalmic Ointment ⊙ 222
NeoDecadron Sterile Ophthalmic Ointment 1517
NeoDecadron Sterile Ophthalmic Solution 1518
NeoDecadron Topical Cream 1518

Dezocine (May potentiate orthostatic hypotension).

Diazoxide (Potentiated). Products include:
Hyperstat I.V. Injection 2095
Proglycem 649

Digitoxin (Hypokalemia and its toxic sequelae must be kept in mind in patients receiving digitalis). Products include:
Crystodigin Tablets 1253

Digoxin (Hypokalemia and its toxic sequelae must be kept in mind in patients receiving digitalis). Products include:
Lanoxicaps 772
Lanoxin Elixir Pediatric 775
Lanoxin Injection 778
Lanoxin Injection Pediatric 781
Lanoxin Tablets 783

Doxazosin Mesylate (Potentiated). Products include:
Cardura Tablets 1941

Enalapril Maleate (Potentiated). Products include:
Vaseretic Tablets 1559
Vasotec Tablets 1564

Enalaprilat (Potentiated). Products include:
Vasotec I.V. 1562

Esmolol Hydrochloride (Potentiated). Products include:
Brevibloc Injection 942

Felodipine (Potentiated). Products include:
Plendil Extended-Release Tablets 1526

Fentanyl (May potentiate orthostatic hypotension). Products include:
Duragesic Transdermal System 1133

Fentanyl Citrate (May potentiate orthostatic hypotension). Products include:
Innovar Injection 1141
Sublimaze Injection 1146

Fosinopril Sodium (Potentiated). Products include:
Monopril Tablets 1406

Furosemide (Potentiated). Products include:
Lasix 1093

Guanabenz Acetate (Potentiated). Products include:
Wytensin Tablets 2542

Guanethidine Monosulfate (Potentiated). Products include:
Esimil Tablets 864
Ismelin Tablets 869

Hydralazine Hydrochloride (Potentiated). Products include:
Apresazide Capsules 854
Apresoline Hydrochloride Parenteral (Ampuls) 856
Apresoline Hydrochloride Tablets 855
Apresoline-Esidrix Tablets 857
Ser-Ap-Es Tablets 881

Serpasil-Apresoline Tablets ... 884

Hydrochlorothiazide (Potentiated). Products include:
Aldactazide ... 2150
Aldoril Tablets ... 1418
Apresazide Capsules ... 854
Apresoline-Esidrix Tablets ... 857
Capozide ... 2258
Dyazide Capsules ... 2208
Esidrix Tablets ... 863
Esimil Tablets ... 864
HydroDIURIL Tablets ... 1484
Hydropres Tablets ... 1485
Inderide Tablets ... 2463
Inderide LA Long Acting Capsules ... 2465
Lopressor HCT Tablets ... 1034
Maxzide ... 1215
Moduretic Tablets ... 1510
Normozide Tablets ... 2112
Oretic Tablets ... 544
Oreticyl ... 545
Prinzide Tablets ... 1540
Ser-Ap-Es Tablets ... 881
Serpasil-Esidrix Tablets ... 886
Timolide Tablets ... 1547
Trandate HCT Tablets ... 579
Vaseretic Tablets ... 1559
Zestoretic ... 2274

Hydrocodone Bitartrate (May potentiate orthostatic hypotension). Products include:
Anexsia 5/500 Tablets ... 2196
Anexsia 7.5/650 Tablets ... 2197
Azdone Tablets ... 844
Codiclear DH Syrup ... 845
Codimal DH Syrup ... 846
Damason-P ... 1356
Hycodan Syrup, Tablets ... 927
Hycomine Compound Tablets ... 929
Hycomine Syrup ... 927
Hycotuss Expectorant Syrup ... 930
Hydrocet Capsules ... 835
Lortab ASA Tablets ... 2414
Lortab ... 2412
Ru-Tuss with Hydrocodone ... 694
Triaminic Expectorant DH ... 1995
Vicodin Tablets ... 1187
Vicodin ES Tablets ... 1189
Zydone Capsules ... 941

Hydrocodone Polistirex (May potentiate orthostatic hypotension). Products include:
Tussionex Extended-Release Suspension ... 988

Hydrocortisone (Electrolyte abnormalities aggravated). Products include:
AK-Spore H.C. ... ◉ 206
Bactine Hydrocortisone Anti-Itch Cream ... ⊞ 625
CaldeCORT Anti-Itch Hydrocortisone Spray ... ⊞ 560
Carmol HC Cream 1% ... 2296
Cortaid Spray ... ⊞ 735
Cortenema ... 2244
Cortisporin Ointment ... 758
Cortisporin Ophthalmic Ointment Sterile ... 758
Cortisporin Ophthalmic Suspension Sterile ... 759
Cortisporin Otic Solution Sterile ... 760
Cortisporin Otic Suspension Sterile ... 760
Cortizone-5 Creme & Ointment ... ⊞ 732
Dermolate Anti-Itch Cream ... ⊞ 697
Eldecort Cream 1.0% ... 1113
Eldecort Cream 1.0% and 2.5% ... 1113
Fungoid HC Creme ... 1770
Hydrocortone Tablets ... 1482
Hytone ... 909
LazerSporin-C Solution ... 1770
Massengill Medicated Soft Cloth Towelettes ... 2192
Nutracort Cream & Lotion ... 1684
PediOtic Suspension Sterile ... 797
Synacort Creams 1%, 2.5% ... 2296
Vanoxide-HC Acne Lotion ... 911
Vioform-Hydrocortisone Cream and Mild Cream ... 889
Vioform-Hydrocortisone Ointment ... 889
VōSoL HC Otic Solution ... 2392
Vytone Cream 1% ... 911

Hydrocortisone Acetate (Electrolyte abnormalities aggravated). Products include:
Analpram-HC Rectal Cream 1% and 2.5% ... 970
Anusol-HC Cream ... 1690
Anusol-HC Suppositories ... 1691
Caldecort ... ⊞ 560
Carmol HC Cream 1% ... 2296
Chloromycetin Hydrocortisone Ophthalmic ... 1694
Coly-Mycin S Otic w/Neomycin & Hydrocortisone ... 1708
Cortaid ... ⊞ 735
Cortef Feminine Itch Cream ... ⊞ 735
Corticaine ... ⊞ 682
Cortifoam ... 1827
Cortisporin Cream ... 757
Epifoam ... 1828
Gynecort 5 Creme ... ⊞ 556
Hydrocortone Acetate Sterile Suspension ... 1479
Lanacort 5 Creme and Ointment ... ⊞ 557
Mantadil Cream ... 789
Ophthocort ... ◉ 301
Orabase HCA Oral Paste ... 890
Pramosone Cream, Lotion & Ointment ... 971
ProctoCream-HC ... 1834
Proctofoam-HC ... 1835

Hydrocortisone Sodium Phosphate (Electrolyte abnormalities aggravated). Products include:
Hydrocortone Phosphate Injection, Sterile ... 1481

Hydrocortisone Sodium Succinate (Electrolyte abnormalities aggravated). Products include:
Solu-Cortef Sterile Powder ... 2361

Hydroflumethiazide (Potentiated). Products include:
Diucardin Tablets ... 2450
Saluron ... 718
Salutensin/Salutensin-Demi ... 719

Indapamide (Potentiated). Products include:
Lozol Tablets ... 1843

Isradipine (Potentiated). Products include:
DynaCirc Capsules ... 2004

Labetalol Hydrochloride (Potentiated). Products include:
Normodyne Injection ... 2108
Normodyne Tablets ... 2110
Normozide Tablets ... 2112
Trandate HCT Tablets ... 579
Trandate Injection ... 577
Trandate Tablets ... 579

Levorphanol Tartrate (May potentiate orthostatic hypotension). Products include:
Levo-Dromoran ... 1906

Lisinopril (Potentiated). Products include:
Prinivil Tablets ... 1538
Prinzide Tablets ... 1540
Zestoretic ... 2274
Zestril Tablets ... 2277

Mecamylamine Hydrochloride (Potentiated). Products include:
Inversine Tablets ... 1492

Meperidine Hydrochloride (May potentiate orthostatic hypotension). Products include:
Demerol ... 2047
Mepergan Injection ... 2479

Mephobarbital (May potentiate orthostatic hypotension). Products include:
Mebaral Tablets ... 2061

Methadone Hydrochloride (May potentiate orthostatic hypotension). Products include:
Dolophine Hydrochloride Ampoules & Vials ... 1260
Dolophine Hydrochloride Tablets ... 1261
Methadone Hydrochloride Diskets ... 1284
Methadone Hydrochloride Oral Solution & Tablets ... 1987

Methyclothiazide (Potentiated). Products include:
Enduron Tablets ... 517
Enduronyl ... 518

Methyldopa (Potentiated). Products include:
Aldoclor Tablets ... 1413
Aldomet Oral ... 1415
Aldoril Tablets ... 1418

Methyldopate Hydrochloride (Potentiated). Products include:
Aldomet Ester HCl Injection ... 1417

Methylprednisolone Acetate (Electrolyte abnormalities aggravated). Products include:
Depo-Medrol Sterile Aqueous Suspension ... 2334

Methylprednisolone Sodium Succinate (Electrolyte abnormalities aggravated). Products include:
Solu-Medrol Sterile Powder ... 2363

Metolazone (Potentiated). Products include:
Diulo ... 2129
Mykrox ½ mg Tablets ... 984
Zaroxolyn Tablets ... 989

Metoprolol Tartrate (Potentiated). Products include:
Lopressor Ampuls ... 1032
Lopressor HCT Tablets ... 1034
Lopressor Tablets ... 1032

Metyrosine (Potentiated). Products include:
Demser Capsules ... 1460

Minoxidil (Potentiated). Products include:
Loniten Tablets ... 2346
Rogaine Topical Solution ... 2357

Morphine Sulfate (May potentiate orthostatic hypotension). Products include:
Astramorph/PF Injection, USP (Preservative-Free) ... 618
Duramorph ... 960
Infumorph 200 and Infumorph 500 Sterile Solutions ... 962
MS Contin Tablets ... 1814
MSIR ... 1817
Oramorph SR (Morphine Sulfate Sustained Release Tablets) ... 1988
Roxanol ... 1991

Nadolol (Potentiated). Products include:
Corgard Tablets ... 701
Corzide Tablets ... 702

Nicardipine Hydrochloride (Potentiated). Products include:
Cardene Capsules ... 2290

Nitroglycerin (Potentiated). Products include:
Deponit NTG Transdermal Delivery System ... 2143
Minitran Transdermal Delivery System ... 1312
Nitro-Bid Ointment ... 1339
Nitro-Bid Capsules ... 1338
Nitrodisc ... 2176
Nitro-Dur (nitroglycerin) Transdermal Infusion System ... 1164
Nitrogard Tablets ... 1004
Nitrolingual Spray ... 1846
Nitrostat Tablets ... 1743
Transderm-Nitro Transdermal Therapeutic System ... 2283

Norepinephrine Bitartrate (Decreased arterial responsiveness to norepinephrine). Products include:
Levophed Bitartrate Injection ... 2054

Opium Alkaloids (May potentiate orthostatic hypotension). Products include:
B & O No. 15A & No. 16A Supprettes ... 2395
Pantopon Injectable ... 1911

Oxycodone Hydrochloride (May potentiate orthostatic hypotension). Products include:
Percocet Tablets ... 950
Percodan ... 951
Roxicodone Tablets, Oral Solution & Intensol (Oxycodone) ... 1992
Tylox Capsules ... 1382

Penbutolol Sulfate (Potentiated). Products include:
Levatol ... 1832

Pentobarbital Sodium (May potentiate orthostatic hypotension). Products include:
Nembutal Sodium Capsules ... 534
Nembutal Sodium Solution ... 536
Nembutal Sodium Suppositories ... 538

Phenobarbital (May potentiate orthostatic hypotension). Products include:
Arco-Lase Plus Tablets ... 607
Bellergal-S Tablets ... 1998
Bronkolixir ... ⊞ 761
Bronkotabs Tablets ... ⊞ 762
Donnatal ... 1858
Donnatal Extentabs ... 1859
Donnatal Tablets ... 1858
Donnazyme Tablets ... 1860
Kinesed Tablets ... 2272
Phenobarbital Elixir and Tablets ... 1293
Primatene Tablets-P Formula ... 2421
Quadrinal Tablets ... 1183
Tedral SA ... 1765

Phenoxybenzamine Hydrochloride (Potentiated). Products include:
Dibenzyline Capsules ... 2207

Phentolamine Mesylate (Potentiated). Products include:
Regitine ... 878

Pindolol (Potentiated). Products include:
Visken Tablets ... 2036

Polythiazide (Potentiated). Products include:
Minizide Capsules ... 1779
Renese Tablets ... 1785
Renese-R Tablets ... 1786

Prazosin Hydrochloride (Potentiated). Products include:
Minipress Capsules ... 1778
Minizide Capsules ... 1779

Prednisolone Acetate (Electrolyte abnormalities aggravated). Products include:
AK-Cide Sterile Ophthalmic Ointment & Suspension ... ◉ 202
Blephamide Liquifilm Sterile Ophthalmic Suspension ... 586
Blephamide S.O.P. Sterile Ophthalmic Ointment ... 586
Cetapred Ointment ... ◉ 220
⅛% Econopred & 1% Econopred Plus ... ◉ 217
Isopto Cetapred Suspension ... ◉ 220
Metimyd ... ◉ 306
Poly-Pred Liquifilm ... ◉ 250
Pred Forte ... ◉ 252
Pred Mild ... ◉ 254
Pred-G Liquifilm Sterile Ophthalmic Suspension ... ◉ 252
Pred-G S.O.P. Sterile Ophthalmic Ointment ... ◉ 253
Vasocidin Ointment ... ◉ 275

Prednisolone Sodium Phosphate (Electrolyte abnormalities aggravated). Products include:
AK-Pred ... ◉ 205
Hydeltrasol Injection, Sterile ... 1476
Inflamase ... ◉ 274
Pediapred Oral Liquid ... 987
Vasocidin Ophthalmic Solution ... ◉ 276

Prednisolone Tebutate (Electrolyte abnormalities aggravated). Products include:
Hydeltra-T.B.A. Sterile Suspension 1478

Prednisone (Electrolyte abnormalities aggravated). Products include:
Deltasone Tablets ... 2332

Propoxyphene Hydrochloride (May potentiate orthostatic hypotension). Products include:
Darvon ... 1256
Wygesic Tablets ... 2540

Propoxyphene Napsylate (May potentiate orthostatic hypotension). Products include:
Darvon-N/Darvocet-N ... 1254

Propranolol Hydrochloride (Potentiated). Products include:
Inderal ... 2459
Inderal LA Long Acting Capsules ... 2461
Inderide Tablets ... 2463
Inderide LA Long Acting Capsules ... 2465

Ramipril (Potentiated). Products include:
Altace Capsules ... 1086

Rauwolfia Serpentina (Potentiated). Products include:
Raudixin Tablets ... 1803

Rauzide Tablets 1804

Rescinnamine (Potentiated).
No products indexed under this heading.

Secobarbital Sodium (May potentiate orthostatic hypotension). Products include:
Seconal Sodium Pulvules 1296

Sodium Nitroprusside (Potentiated). Products include:
Nipride I.V. Infusion 1909

Sufentanil Citrate (May potentiate orthostatic hypotension). Products include:
Sufenta Injection 1147

Terazosin Hydrochloride (Potentiated). Products include:
Hytrin Tablets 529

Thiamylal Sodium (May potentiate orthostatic hypotension). Products include:
Surital Ampoules, Steri-Vials 1764

Timolol Maleate (Potentiated). Products include:
Blocadren Tablets 1429
Timolide Tablets 1547
Timoptic in Ocudose 1552
Timoptic Sterile Ophthalmic Solution 1550

Triamcinolone (Electrolyte abnormalities aggravated).
No products indexed under this heading.

Triamcinolone Acetonide (Electrolyte abnormalities aggravated). Products include:
Aristocort A 1010
Azmacort Inhaler 1837
Kenalog Cream, Lotion & Ointment 2401
Kenalog-10 Injection 2402
Kenalog-40 Injection 2403
Kenalog in Orabase 604
Kenalog Spray 2401
Mycolog II Cream and Ointment 2407
Mytrex Cream & Ointment 2080
Nasacort Nasal Inhaler 1844

Triamcinolone Diacetate (Electrolyte abnormalities aggravated). Products include:
Aristocort Suspension 1008

Triamcinolone Hexacetonide (Electrolyte abnormalities aggravated). Products include:
Aristospan Suspension 1011

Trimethaphan Camsylate (Potentiated). Products include:
Arfonad Ampuls 1887

Tubocurarine Chloride (Increased responsiveness to tubocurarine).
No products indexed under this heading.

HYDROPRES TABLETS

(Reserpine, Hydrochlorothiazide) 1485
May interact with antihypertensives, lithium preparations, corticosteroids, insulin, non-steroidal anti-inflammatory agents, barbiturates, narcotic analgesics, oral hypoglycemic agents, cardiac glycosides, and certain other agents. Compounds in these categories include:

Acebutolol Hydrochloride (Potentiation of antihypertensive drugs). Products include:
Sectral Capsules 2520

ACTH (Hypokalemia).
No products indexed under this heading.

Alcohol (Potentiation of orthostatic hypotension).

Alfentanil Hydrochloride (Potentiation of orthostatic hypotension; enhanced CNS depressant effects of reserpine). Products include:
Alfenta Injection 1131

Aprobarbital (Potentiation of orthostatic hypotension; enhanced CNS depressant effects of reserpine). Products include:
Alurate Elixir 1883

Atenolol (Potentiation of antihypertensive drugs). Products include:
Tenoretic Tablets 1105
Tenormin Tablets and I.V. Injection 1107

Benazepril Hydrochloride (Potentiation of antihypertensive drugs). Products include:
Lotensin Tablets 872

Bendroflumethiazide (Potentiation of antihypertensive drugs). Products include:
Corzide Tablets 702
Naturetin Tablets 1789
Rauzide Tablets 1804

Betamethasone Acetate (Hypokalemia). Products include:
Celestone Soluspan Suspension 2081

Betamethasone Sodium Phosphate (Hypokalemia). Products include:
Celestone Soluspan Suspension 2081

Betaxolol Hydrochloride (Potentiation of antihypertensive drugs). Products include:
Betoptic Sterile Ophthalmic Solution 569
Betoptic S Sterile Ophthalmic Suspension 570
Kerlone Tablets 2172

Buprenorphine (Potentiation of orthostatic hypotension; enhanced CNS depressant effects of reserpine).
No products indexed under this heading.

Butabarbital (Potentiation of orthostatic hypotension; enhanced CNS depressant effects of reserpine). Products include:
Pyridium Plus 1764

Butalbital (Potentiation of orthostatic hypotension; enhanced CNS depressant effects of reserpine). Products include:
Esgic-Plus Tablets 1002
Esgic Tablets & Capsules 1001
Fioricet Tablets 2006
Fiorinal Capsules 2007
Fiorinal with Codeine Capsules 2008
Fiorinal Tablets 2007
Phrenilin 838
Sedapap Tablets 50 mg/650 mg .. 1360

Captopril (Potentiation of antihypertensive drugs). Products include:
Capoten 2255
Capozide 2258

Carteolol Hydrochloride (Potentiation of antihypertensive drugs). Products include:
Cartrol Tablets 507

Chlorothiazide (Potentiation of antihypertensive drugs). Products include:
Aldoclor Tablets 1413
Diupres Tablets 1461
Diuril Oral 1464

Chlorothiazide Sodium (Potentiation of antihypertensive drugs). Products include:
Diuril Sodium Intravenous 1463

Chlorpropamide (Dosage adjustment of the antidiabetic drug may be required). Products include:
Diabinese Tablets 1775

Chlorthalidone (Potentiation of antihypertensive drugs). Products include:
Combipres Tablets 678
Tenoretic Tablets 1105
Thalitone Tablets 687

Clobetasol Propionate (Hypokalemia). Products include:
Temovate 1056

Clonidine (Potentiation of antihypertensive drugs). Products include:
Catapres-TTS 677

Clonidine Hydrochloride (Potentiation of antihypertensive drugs). Products include:
Catapres Tablets 676
Combipres Tablets 678

Codeine (Potentiation of orthostatic hypotension; enhanced CNS depressant effects of reserpine). Products include:
Calcidrine Syrup 506

Codeine Phosphate (Potentiation of orthostatic hypotension; enhanced CNS depressant effects of reserpine). Products include:
Actifed with Codeine Cough Syrup.. 752
Cheracol Cough Syrup 1853
Codimal PH Syrup 846
Dimetane-DC Cough Syrup 1857
Empirin with Codeine Phosphate Nos. 2, 3 & 4 764
Fiorinal with Codeine Capsules 2008
Isoclor Expectorant 982
Naldecon CX Adult Liquid .... ▣ 521
Novahistine DH 1342
Novahistine Expectorant 1343
Nucofed Capsules 2219
Nucofed Expectorant 2219
Nucofed Pediatric Expectorant 2220
Nucofed Syrup 2219
Phenaphen with Codeine Capsules 1865
Phenaphen-650 with Codeine Tablets 1866
Phenergan with Codeine 2497
Phenergan VC with Codeine 2501
Robitussin A-C Syrup 1875
Robitussin-DAC Syrup 1875
Ryna .... ▣ 741
Soma Compound w/Codeine Tablets 2390
Triaminic Expectorant w/Codeine .. 1996
Tussi-Organidin Liquid 2391
Tylenol with Codeine 1381

Codeine Polistirex (Potentiation of orthostatic hypotension; enhanced CNS depressant effects of reserpine).
No products indexed under this heading.

Cortisone Acetate (Hypokalemia). Products include:
Cortone Acetate Sterile Suspension 1437
Cortone Acetate Tablets 1439

Deserpidine (Potentiation of antihypertensive drugs). Products include:
Enduronyl 518
Harmonyl Tablets 528
Oreticyl 545

Deslanoside (Use cautiously; cardiac arrhythmias have occurred with reserpine).
No products indexed under this heading.

Dexamethasone (Hypokalemia). Products include:
AK-Trol Ointment & Suspension .... ◉ 207
Decadron Elixir 1445
Decadron Tablets 1447
Decaspray Topical Aerosol 1459
Dexacidin .... ◉ 272
Maxidex Sterile Ophthalmic Suspension .... ◉ 223
Maxitrol Ophthalmic Ointment/ Suspension .... ◉ 223
TobraDex Ophthalmic Suspension and Ointment .... ◉ 228

Dexamethasone Acetate (Hypokalemia). Products include:
Dalalone D.P. Injectable 999
Decadron-LA Sterile Suspension 1457

Dexamethasone Sodium Phosphate (Hypokalemia). Products include:
AK-Dex .... ◉ 203
Decadron Phosphate Respihaler 1454
Decadron Phosphate Sterile Ophthalmic Ointment 1453
Decadron Phosphate Sterile Ophthalmic Solution 1453
Decadron Phosphate Topical Cream 1455
Decadron Phosphate Turbinaire 1456
Maxidex Sterile Ophthalmic Ointment .... ◉ 222
NeoDecadron Sterile Ophthalmic Ointment 1517
NeoDecadron Sterile Ophthalmic Solution 1518
NeoDecadron Topical Cream 1518

Dezocine (Potentiation of orthostatic hypotension; enhanced CNS depressant effects of reserpine).

Diazoxide (Potentiation of antihypertensive drugs). Products include:
Hyperstat I.V. Injection 2095
Proglycem 649

Diclofenac Sodium (Reduced diuretic, natriuretic, and antihypertensive effects). Products include:
Voltaren Ophthalmic Sterile Ophthalmic Solution .... ◉ 268
Voltaren Tablets 1042

Digitoxin (Use cautiously; cardiac arrhythmias have occurred with reserpine). Products include:
Crystodigin Tablets 1253

Digoxin (Use cautiously; cardiac arrhythmias have occurred with reserpine). Products include:
Lanoxicaps 772
Lanoxin Elixir Pediatric 775
Lanoxin Injection 778
Lanoxin Injection Pediatric 781
Lanoxin Tablets 783

Doxazosin Mesylate (Potentiation of antihypertensive drugs). Products include:
Cardura Tablets 1941

Enalapril Maleate (Potentiation of antihypertensive drugs). Products include:
Vaseretic Tablets 1559
Vasotec Tablets 1564

Enalaprilat (Potentiation of antihypertensive drugs). Products include:
Vasotec I.V. 1562

Esmolol Hydrochloride (Potentiation of antihypertensive drugs). Products include:
Brevibloc Injection 942

Etodolac (Reduced diuretic, natriuretic, and antihypertensive effects). Products include:
Lodine Capsules 2468

Felodipine (Potentiation of antihypertensive drugs). Products include:
Plendil Extended-Release Tablets.... 1526

Fenoprofen Calcium (Reduced diuretic, natriuretic, and antihypertensive effects). Products include:
Nalfon Pulvules & Tablets 919

Fentanyl (Potentiation of orthostatic hypotension; enhanced CNS depressant effects of reserpine). Products include:
Duragesic Transdermal System 1133

Fentanyl Citrate (Potentiation of orthostatic hypotension; enhanced CNS depressant effects of reserpine). Products include:
Innovar Injection 1141
Sublimaze Injection 1146

Flurbiprofen (Reduced diuretic, natriuretic, and antihypertensive effects). Products include:
Ansaid Tablets 2319

Fosinopril Sodium (Potentiation of antihypertensive drugs). Products include:
Monopril Tablets 1406

Furosemide (Potentiation of antihypertensive drugs). Products include:
Lasix 1093

Glipizide (Dosage adjustment of the antidiabetic drug may be required). Products include:
Glucotrol 1952

Glyburide (Dosage adjustment of the antidiabetic drug may be required). Products include:
- DiaBeta 1091
- Micronase Tablets 2350

Guanabenz Acetate (Potentiation of antihypertensive drugs). Products include:
- Wytensin Tablets 2542

Guanethidine Monosulfate (Potentiation of antihypertensive drugs). Products include:
- Esimil Tablets 864
- Ismelin Tablets 869

Hydralazine Hydrochloride (Potentiation of antihypertensive drugs). Products include:
- Apresazide Capsules 854
- Apresoline Hydrochloride Parenteral (Ampuls) 856
- Apresoline Hydrochloride Tablets .. 855
- Apresoline-Esidrix Tablets 857
- Ser-Ap-Es Tablets 881
- Serpasil-Apresoline Tablets 884

Hydrocodone Bitartrate (Potentiation of orthostatic hypotension; enhanced CNS depressant effects of reserpine). Products include:
- Anexsia 5/500 Tablets 2196
- Anexsia 7.5/650 Tablets 2197
- Azdone Tablets 844
- Codiclear DH Syrup 845
- Codimal DH Syrup 846
- Damason-P 1356
- Hycodan Syrup, Tablets 927
- Hycomine Compound Tablets 929
- Hycomine Syrup 927
- Hycotuss Expectorant Syrup 930
- Hydrocet Capsules 835
- Lortab ASA Tablets 2414
- Lortab 2412
- Ru-Tuss with Hydrocodone 694
- Triaminic Expectorant DH 1995
- Vicodin Tablets 1187
- Vicodin ES Tablets 1189
- Zydone Capsules 941

Hydrocodone Polistirex (Potentiation of orthostatic hypotension; enhanced CNS depressant effects of reserpine). Products include:
- Tussionex Extended-Release Suspension 988

Hydrocortisone (Hypokalemia). Products include:
- AK-Spore H.C. .... ⊙ 206
- Bactine Hydrocortisone Anti-Itch Cream .... ▣ 625
- CaldeCORT Anti-Itch Hydrocortisone Spray .... ▣ 560
- Carmol HC Cream 1% 2296
- Cortaid Spray .... ▣ 735
- Cortenema 2244
- Cortisporin Ointment 758
- Cortisporin Ophthalmic Ointment Sterile 758
- Cortisporin Ophthalmic Suspension Sterile 759
- Cortisporin Otic Solution Sterile 760
- Cortisporin Otic Suspension Sterile 760
- Cortizone-5 Creme & Ointment .... ▣ 732
- Dermolate Anti-Itch Cream .... ▣ 697
- Eldecort Cream 1.0% 1113
- Eldecort Cream 1.0% and 2.5% 1113
- Fungoid HC Creme 1770
- Hydrocortone Tablets 1482
- Hytone 909
- LazerSporin-C Solution 1770
- Massengill Medicated Soft Cloth Towelettes 2192
- Nutracort Cream & Lotion 1684
- PediOtic Suspension Sterile 797
- Synacort Creams 1%, 2.5% 2296
- Vanoxide-HC Acne Lotion 911
- Vioform-Hydrocortisone Cream and Mild Cream 889
- Vioform-Hydrocortisone Ointment .. 889
- VōSoL HC Otic Solution 2392
- Vytone Cream 1% 911

Hydrocortisone Acetate (Hypokalemia). Products include:
- Analpram-HC Rectal Cream 1% and 2.5% 970
- Anusol-HC Cream 1690
- Anusol-HC Suppositories 1691
- Caldecort .... ▣ 560
- Carmol HC Cream 1% 2296
- Chloromycetin Hydrocortisone Ophthalmic 1694
- Coly-Mycin S Otic w/Neomycin & Hydrocortisone 1708
- Cortaid .... ▣ 735
- Cortef Feminine Itch Cream .... ▣ 735
- Corticaine .... ▣ 682
- Cortifoam 1827
- Cortisporin Cream 757
- Epifoam 1828
- Gynecort 5 Creme .... ▣ 556
- Hydrocortone Acetate Sterile Suspension 1479
- Lanacort 5 Creme and Ointment .. ▣ 557
- Mantadil Cream 789
- Ophthocort .... ⊙ 301
- Orabase HCA Oral Paste 890
- Pramosone Cream, Lotion & Ointment 971
- ProctoCream-HC 1834
- Proctofoam-HC 1835

Hydrocortisone Sodium Phosphate (Hypokalemia). Products include:
- Hydrocortone Phosphate Injection, Sterile 1481

Hydrocortisone Sodium Succinate (Hypokalemia). Products include:
- Solu-Cortef Sterile Powder 2361

Hydroflumethiazide (Potentiation of antihypertensive drugs). Products include:
- Diucardin Tablets 2450
- Saluron 718
- Salutensin/Salutensin-Demi 719

Ibuprofen (Reduced diuretic, natriuretic, and antihypertensive effects). Products include:
- Advil Cold & Sinus Caplets (formerly CoAdvil) 2416
- Advil Ibuprofen Tablets and Caplets 2416
- Children's Advil Suspension 2426
- CoAdvil .... ▣ 748
- Dristan Sinus Caplets 2419
- Haltran Tablets .... ▣ 668
- Ibuprofen .... ▣ 631
- Medipren ibuprofen Caplets and Tablets 1362
- Midol 200 Cramp Relief Formula .. ▣ 570
- Motrin Tablets 2351
- Motrin IB Caplets and Tablets .... ▣ 736
- Nuprin Ibuprofen/Analgesic Tablets & Caplets 752
- PediaProfen Suspension 1363
- Rufen Tablets 691
- Trendar Ibuprofen Tablets .... ▣ 756

Indapamide (Potentiation of antihypertensive drugs). Products include:
- Lozol Tablets 1843

Indomethacin (Reduced diuretic, natriuretic, and antihypertensive effects). Products include:
- Indocin 1487

Indomethacin Sodium Trihydrate (Reduced diuretic, natriuretic, and antihypertensive effects). Products include:
- Indocin I.V. 1490

Insulin, Human (Altered insulin requirements).
- No products indexed under this heading.

Insulin, Human Isophane Suspension (Altered insulin requirements). Products include:
- Humulin N, 100 Units 1270

Insulin, Human NPH (Altered insulin requirements). Products include:
- Insulatard NPH Human 1627
- Novolin N 1627
- Novolin N PenFill Cartridges 1628
- Novolin N Prefilled 1628

Insulin, Human Regular (Altered insulin requirements). Products include:
- Humulin BR, 100 Units 1268
- Humulin R, 100 Units 1272
- Novolin R 1627
- Novolin R PenFill Cartridges 1628
- Novolin R Prefilled 1629
- Velosulin Human 1628

Insulin, Human, Zinc Suspension (Altered insulin requirements). Products include:
- Humulin L, 100 Units 1268
- Humulin U, 100 Units 1272
- Novolin L 1627

Insulin, NPH (Altered insulin requirements). Products include:
- NPH, 40 & 100 Units 1273
- Beef NPH, 100 Units 1274
- Pork NPH, 100 Units 1275
- Insulatard NPH 1626
- NPH Insulin 1626
- NPH Purified Pork Isophane Insulin 1626

Insulin, Regular (Altered insulin requirements). Products include:
- Regular, 40 & 100 Units 1273
- Beef Regular, 100 Units 1275
- Pork Regular, 100 Units 1275
- Pork Regular (Concentrated), 500 Units 1276
- Regular Insulin 1625
- Regular Purified Pork Insulin 1626
- Velosulin 1627

Insulin, Zinc Crystals (Altered insulin requirements). Products include:
- NPH, 40 & 100 Units 1273

Insulin, Zinc Suspension (Altered insulin requirements). Products include:
- Lente, 40 & 100 Units 1272
- Protamine, Zinc, 40 & 100 Units 1273
- Lente Iletin I 1272
- Beef Lente, 100 Units 1274
- Beef Protamine Zinc, 100 Units 1274
- Pork Lente, 100 Units 1275
- Pork, Protamine, Zinc, 100 Units 1275
- Lente Insulin 1626
- Lente Purified Pork Insulin 1626
- Semilente Insulin 1625
- Ultralente Insulin 1626

Isradipine (Potentiation of antihypertensive drugs). Products include:
- DynaCirc Capsules 2004

Ketoprofen (Reduced diuretic, natriuretic, and antihypertensive effects). Products include:
- Orudis Capsules 2488

Ketorolac Tromethamine (Reduced diuretic, natriuretic, and antihypertensive effects). Products include:
- Toradol IM Injection 2302

Labetalol Hydrochloride (Potentiation of antihypertensive drugs). Products include:
- Normodyne Injection 2108
- Normodyne Tablets 2110
- Normozide Tablets 2112
- Trandate HCT Tablets 579
- Trandate Injection 577
- Trandate Tablets 579

Levorphanol Tartrate (Potentiation of orthostatic hypotension; enhanced CNS depressant effects of reserpine). Products include:
- Levo-Dromoran 1906

Lisinopril (Potentiation of antihypertensive drugs). Products include:
- Prinivil Tablets 1538
- Prinzide Tablets 1540
- Zestoretic 2274
- Zestril Tablets 2277

Lithium Carbonate (High risk of lithium toxicity). Products include:
- Eskalith 2214
- Lithane Tablets 1596
- Lithium Carbonate Capsules & Tablets 1984
- Lithobid Tablets 870

Lithium Citrate (High risk of lithium toxicity). Products include:
- Cibalith-S 870

Mecamylamine Hydrochloride (Potentiation of antihypertensive drugs). Products include:
- Inversine Tablets 1492

Meclofenamate Sodium (Reduced diuretic, natriuretic, and antihypertensive effects). Products include:
- Meclomen Capsules 1739

Mefenamic Acid (Reduced diuretic, natriuretic, and antihypertensive effects). Products include:
- Ponstel 1758

Meperidine Hydrochloride (Potentiation of orthostatic hypotension; enhanced CNS depressant effects of reserpine). Products include:
- Demerol 2047
- Mepergan Injection 2479

Mephobarbital (Potentiation of orthostatic hypotension; enhanced CNS depressant effects of reserpine). Products include:
- Mebaral Tablets 2061

Methadone Hydrochloride (Potentiation of orthostatic hypotension; enhanced CNS depressant effects of reserpine). Products include:
- Dolophine Hydrochloride Ampoules & Vials 1260
- Dolophine Hydrochloride Tablets 1261
- Methadone Hydrochloride Diskets .. 1284
- Methadone Hydrochloride Oral Solution & Tablets 1987

Methyclothiazide (Potentiation of antihypertensive drugs). Products include:
- Enduron Tablets 517
- Enduronyl 518

Methyldopa (Potentiation of antihypertensive drugs). Products include:
- Aldoclor Tablets 1413
- Aldomet Oral 1415
- Aldoril Tablets 1418

Methyldopate Hydrochloride (Potentiation of antihypertensive drugs). Products include:
- Aldomet Ester HCl Injection 1417

Methylprednisolone Acetate (Hypokalemia). Products include:
- Depo-Medrol Sterile Aqueous Suspension 2334

Methylprednisolone Sodium Succinate (Hypokalemia). Products include:
- Solu-Medrol Sterile Powder 2363

Metolazone (Potentiation of antihypertensive drugs). Products include:
- Diulo 2129
- Mykrox ½ mg Tablets 984
- Zaroxolyn Tablets 989

Metoprolol Tartrate (Potentiation of antihypertensive drugs). Products include:
- Lopressor Ampuls 1032
- Lopressor HCT Tablets 1034
- Lopressor Tablets 1032

Metyrosine (Potentiation of antihypertensive drugs). Products include:
- Demser Capsules 1460

Minoxidil (Potentiation of antihypertensive drugs). Products include:
- Loniten Tablets 2346
- Rogaine Topical Solution 2357

Morphine Sulfate (Potentiation of orthostatic hypotension; enhanced CNS depressant effects of reserpine). Products include:
- Astramorph/PF Injection, USP (Preservative-Free) 618
- Duramorph 960
- Infumorph 200 and Infumorph 500 Sterile Solutions 962
- MS Contin Tablets 1814
- MSIR 1817
- Oramorph SR (Morphine Sulfate Sustained Release Tablets) 1988
- Roxanol 1991

Nadolol (Potentiation of antihypertensive drugs). Products include:
- Corgard Tablets 701
- Corzide Tablets 702

Naproxen (Reduced diuretic, natriuretic, and antihypertensive effects). Products include:
- Naprosyn 2297

Naproxen Sodium (Reduced diuretic, natriuretic, and antihypertensive effects). Products include:
- Anaprox and Anaprox DS Tablets.... 2288

Nicardipine Hydrochloride (Potentiation of antihypertensive drugs). Products include:
- Cardene Capsules 2290

Nitroglycerin (Potentiation of antihypertensive drugs). Products include:
- Deponit NTG Transdermal Delivery System 2143
- Minitran Transdermal Delivery System 1312
- Nitro-Bid Ointment 1339
- Nitro-Bid Capsules 1338
- Nitrodisc 2176
- Nitro-Dur (nitroglycerin) Transdermal Infusion System 1164
- Nitrogard Tablets.......... 1004
- Nitrolingual Spray 1846
- Nitrostat Tablets 1743
- Transderm-Nitro Transdermal Therapeutic System 2283

Norepinephrine Bitartrate (Decreased arterial responsiveness to norepinephrine). Products include:
- Levophed Bitartrate Injection.......... 2054

Opium Alkaloids (Potentiation of orthostatic hypotension; enhanced CNS depressant effects of reserpine). Products include:
- B & O No. 15A & No. 16A Supprettes 2395
- Pantopon Injectable 1911

Oxycodone Hydrochloride (Potentiation of orthostatic hypotension; enhanced CNS depressant effects of reserpine). Products include:
- Percocet Tablets 950
- Percodan.......... 951
- Roxicodone Tablets, Oral Solution & Intensol (Oxycodone) 1992
- Tylox Capsules 1382

Penbutolol Sulfate (Potentiation of antihypertensive drugs). Products include:
- Levatol 1832

Pentobarbital Sodium (Potentiation of orthostatic hypotension; enhanced CNS depressant effects of reserpine). Products include:
- Nembutal Sodium Capsules 534
- Nembutal Sodium Solution 536
- Nembutal Sodium Suppositories...... 538

Phenobarbital (Potentiation of orthostatic hypotension; enhanced CNS depressant effects of reserpine). Products include:
- Arco-Lase Plus Tablets 607
- Bellergal-S Tablets 1998
- Bronkolixir .... ▣ 761
- Bronkotabs Tablets.......... ▣ 762
- Donnatal 1858
- Donnatal Extentabs.......... 1859
- Donnatal Tablets 1858
- Donnazyme Tablets 1860
- Kinesed Tablets 2272
- Phenobarbital Elixir and Tablets...... 1293
- Primatene Tablets-P Formula.......... 2421
- Quadrinal Tablets 1183
- Tedral SA 1765

Phenoxybenzamine Hydrochloride (Potentiation of antihypertensive drugs). Products include:
- Dibenzyline Capsules 2207

Phentolamine Mesylate (Potentiation of antihypertensive drugs). Products include:
- Regitine 878

Phenylbutazone (Reduced diuretic, natriuretic, and antihypertensive effects). Products include:
- Butazolidin Capsules & Tablets....... 1027

Pindolol (Potentiation of antihypertensive drugs). Products include:
- Visken Tablets.......... 2036

Piroxicam (Reduced diuretic, natriuretic, and antihypertensive effects). Products include:
- Feldene Capsules 1777

Polythiazide (Potentiation of antihypertensive drugs). Products include:
- Minizide Capsules 1779
- Renese Tablets 1785
- Renese-R Tablets.......... 1786

Prazosin Hydrochloride (Potentiation of antihypertensive drugs). Products include:
- Minipress Capsules.......... 1778
- Minizide Capsules 1779

Prednisolone Acetate (Hypokalemia). Products include:
- AK-Cide Sterile Ophthalmic Ointment & Suspension.......... ◉ 202
- Blephamide Liquifilm Sterile Ophthalmic Suspension.......... 586
- Blephamide S.O.P. Sterile Ophthalmic Ointment.......... 586
- Cetapred Ointment .... ◉ 220
- ⅛% Econopred & 1% Econopred Plus .... ◉ 217
- Isopto Cetapred Suspension.......... ◉ 220
- Metimyd.......... ◉ 306
- Poly-Pred Liquifilm .... ◉ 250
- Pred Forte.......... ◉ 252
- Pred Mild.......... ◉ 254
- Pred-G Liquifilm Sterile Ophthalmic Suspension .... ◉ 252
- Pred-G S.O.P. Sterile Ophthalmic Ointment .... ◉ 253
- Vasocidin Ointment .... ◉ 275

Prednisolone Sodium Phosphate (Hypokalemia). Products include:
- AK-Pred .... ◉ 205
- Hydeltrasol Injection, Sterile.......... 1476
- Inflamase.......... ◉ 274
- Pediapred Oral Liquid 987
- Vasocidin Ophthalmic Solution ...... ◉ 276

Prednisolone Tebutate (Hypokalemia). Products include:
- Hydeltra-T.B.A. Sterile Suspension 1478

Prednisone (Hypokalemia). Products include:
- Deltasone Tablets 2332

Propoxyphene Hydrochloride (Potentiation of orthostatic hypotension; enhanced CNS depressant effects of reserpine). Products include:
- Darvon 1256
- Wygesic Tablets 2540

Propoxyphene Napsylate (Potentiation of orthostatic hypotension; enhanced CNS depressant effects of reserpine). Products include:
- Darvon-N/Darvocet-N 1254

Propranolol Hydrochloride (Potentiation of antihypertensive drugs). Products include:
- Inderal 2459
- Inderal LA Long Acting Capsules 2461
- Inderide Tablets 2463
- Inderide LA Long Acting Capsules .. 2465

Quinidine Gluconate (Use cautiously; cardiac arrhythmias have occurred with reserpine). Products include:
- Quinaglute Dura-Tabs Tablets 663

Quinidine Polygalacturonate (Use cautiously; cardiac arrhythmias have occurred with reserpine). Products include:
- Cardioquin Tablets 1812

Quinidine Sulfate (Use cautiously; cardiac arrhythmias have occurred with reserpine). Products include:
- Quinidex Extentabs.......... 1868

Ramipril (Potentiation of antihypertensive drugs). Products include:
- Altace Capsules 1086

Rauwolfia Serpentina (Potentiation of antihypertensive drugs). Products include:
- Raudixin Tablets.......... 1803
- Rauzide Tablets 1804

Rescinnamine (Potentiation of antihypertensive drugs).
- No products indexed under this heading.

Secobarbital Sodium (Potentiation of orthostatic hypotension; enhanced CNS depressant effects of reserpine). Products include:
- Seconal Sodium Pulvules 1296

Sodium Nitroprusside (Potentiation of antihypertensive drugs). Products include:
- Nipride I.V. Infusion 1909

Sufentanil Citrate (Potentiation of orthostatic hypotension; enhanced CNS depressant effects of reserpine). Products include:
- Sufenta Injection 1147

Sulindac (Reduced diuretic, natriuretic, and antihypertensive effects). Products include:
- Clinoril Tablets 1433

Terazosin Hydrochloride (Potentiation of antihypertensive drugs). Products include:
- Hytrin Tablets 529

Thiamylal Sodium (Potentiation of orthostatic hypotension; enhanced CNS depressant effects of reserpine). Products include:
- Surital Ampoules, Steri-Vials.......... 1764

Timolol Maleate (Potentiation of antihypertensive drugs). Products include:
- Blocadren Tablets 1429
- Timolide Tablets.......... 1547
- Timoptic in Ocudose 1552
- Timoptic Sterile Ophthalmic Solution.......... 1550

Tolazamide (Dosage adjustment of the antidiabetic drug may be required). Products include:
- Tolinase Tablets 2365

Tolbutamide (Dosage adjustment of the antidiabetic drug may be required). Products include:
- Orinase Tablets 2354

Tolmetin Sodium (Reduced diuretic, natriuretic, and antihypertensive effects). Products include:
- Tolectin (200, 400 and 600 mg) .. 1379

Triamcinolone (Hypokalemia).
- No products indexed under this heading.

Triamcinolone Acetonide (Hypokalemia). Products include:
- Aristocort A 1010
- Azmacort Inhaler 1837
- Kenalog Cream, Lotion & Ointment 2401
- Kenalog-10 Injection 2402
- Kenalog-40 Injection 2403
- Kenalog in Orabase.......... 604
- Kenalog Spray.......... 2401
- Mycolog II Cream and Ointment 2407
- Mytrex Cream & Ointment.......... 2080
- Nasacort Nasal Inhaler 1844

Triamcinolone Diacetate (Hypokalemia). Products include:
- Aristocort Suspension 1008

Triamcinolone Hexacetonide (Hypokalemia). Products include:
- Aristospan Suspension 1011

Trimethaphan Camsylate (Potentiation of antihypertensive drugs). Products include:
- Arfonad Ampuls.......... 1887

Tubocurarine Chloride (Increased responsiveness to tubocurarine).
- No products indexed under this heading.

HYLAND'S BED WETTING TABLETS
(Homeopathic Medications) .... ▣ 728
No interactions described in labeling.

HYLAND'S CALMS FORTÉ TABLETS
(Homeopathic Medications) .... ▣ 728
No interactions described in labeling.

HYLAND'S COLIC TABLETS
(Homeopathic Medications) .... ▣ 728
No interactions described in labeling.

HYLAND'S COUGH SYRUP WITH HONEY
(Ipecac).......... ▣ 728
No interactions described in labeling.

HYLAND'S C-PLUS COLD TABLETS
(Homeopathic Medications) .... ▣ 728
No interactions described in labeling.

HYLAND'S TEETHING TABLETS
(Calcium Phosphate, Homeopathic Medications) .... ▣ 728
No interactions described in labeling.

HYLAND'S VITAMIN C FOR CHILDREN
(Vitamin C).......... ▣ 729
No interactions described in labeling.

HYLOREL TABLETS
(Guanadrel Sulfate) 975
May interact with monoamine oxidase inhibitors, phenothiazines, tricyclic antidepressants, vasodilators, sympathomimetic bronchodilators, alpha adrenergic blockers, direct-acting sympathomimetic amines, indirect-acting sympathomimetic amines, beta blockers, catecholamine depleting drugs, and certain other agents. Compounds in these categories include:

Acebutolol Hydrochloride (May cause excessive postural hypotension and bradycardia). Products include:
- Sectral Capsules 2520

Albuterol (May interfere with the hypotensive effect). Products include:
- Proventil Inhalation Aerosol 2117
- Ventolin Inhalation Aerosol and Refill 583

Albuterol Sulfate (May interfere with the hypotensive effect). Products include:
- Proventil Repetabs Tablets 2120
- Proventil Solutions for Inhalation 0.5% and 0.083%.......... 2118
- Proventil Syrup.......... 2119
- Proventil Tablets 2120
- Ventolin 583

Alcohol (Exaggerates postural hypotension).

Amitriptyline Hydrochloride (Possible reversal of the effects of guanadrel). Products include:
- Elavil 2269
- Endep Tablets.......... 1927
- Etrafon.......... 2087
- Limbitrol 1933
- Triavil Tablets 1556

Amoxapine (Possible reversal of the effects of guanadrel). Products include:
- Asendin Tablets 1196

Amphetamine Resins (May reverse the effects of neuronal blocking agents). Products include:
- Biphetamine Capsules.......... 973

Atenolol (May cause excessive postural hypotension and bradycardia). Products include:
- Tenoretic Tablets 1105
- Tenormin Tablets and I.V. Injection 1107

Betaxolol Hydrochloride (May cause excessive postural hypotension and bradycardia). Products include:
- Betoptic Sterile Ophthalmic Solution 569
- Betoptic S Sterile Ophthalmic Suspension 570
- Kerlone Tablets 2172

Bitolterol Mesylate (May interfere with the hypotensive effect). Products include:
- Tornalate 2074

Carteolol Hydrochloride (May cause excessive postural hypotension and bradycardia). Products include:
- Cartrol Tablets 507

Chlorpromazine (Possible reversal of the effects of guanadrel). Products include:
- Thorazine 2234

Clomipramine Hydrochloride (Possible reversal of the effects of guanadrel). Products include:
- Anafranil Capsules 650

Deserpidine (May cause excessive postural hypotension and bradycardia). Products include:
- Enduronyl 518
- Harmonyl Tablets 528
- Oreticyl 545

Desipramine Hydrochloride (Possible reversal of the effects of guanadrel). Products include:
- Norpramin Tablets 1340

Dextroamphetamine Sulfate (May reverse the effects of neuronal blocking agents). Products include:
- Dexedrine 2206

Diazoxide (Comcomitant use may increase the potential for symptomatic or orthostatic hypotension). Products include:
- Hyperstat I.V. Injection 2095
- Proglycem 649

Doxazosin Mesylate (May cause excessive postural hypotension and bradycardia). Products include:
- Cardura Tablets 1941

Doxepin Hydrochloride (Possible reversal of the effects of guanadrel). Products include:
- Sinequan 1960

Ephedrine Hydrochloride (May interfere with the hypotensive effect; may reverse the effects of neuronal blocking agents). Products include:
- Amesec .... ▣ 682
- Primatene Tablets-M Formula 2421
- Primatene Tablets-P Formula 2421
- Primatene Tablets-Regular Formula 2421
- Quadrinal Tablets 1183
- Quelidrine Syrup 556
- Tedral SA 1765

Ephedrine Sulfate (May interfere with the hypotensive effect; may reverse the effects of neuronal blocking agents). Products include:
- Bronkaid Tablets .... ▣ 757
- Bronkolixir .... ▣ 761
- Bronkotabs Tablets .... ▣ 762
- Marax Tablets & DF Syrup 1954
- Pazo Hemorrhoid Ointment & Suppositories 752
- Vicks Vatronol Nose Drops .... ▣ 666

Ephedrine Tannate (May interfere with the hypotensive effect; may reverse the effects of neuronal blocking agents). Products include:
- Rynatuss 2388

Epinephrine (May interfere with the hypotensive effect). Products include:
- Ana-Kit Anaphylaxis Emergency Treatment Kit 1100
- Bronkaid Mist .... ▣ 757
- EpiPen 843
- Marcaine Hydrochloride 0.5% with Epinephrine 1:200,000 (as bitartrate) 958
- Marcaine Hydrochloride with Epinephrine 1:200,000 2055
- Primatene Mist 2420
- Sus-Phrine Injection 1006
- Xylocaine with Epinephrine Injections 637

Epinephrine Hydrochloride (May interfere with the hypotensive effect; enhances the activity of direct acting sympathomimetic amines). Products include:
- Adrenalin Chloride Solution 1:100 & 1:1,000 1689
- Epifrin .... ⊙ 244
- Glaucon .... ⊙ 218

Esmolol Hydrochloride (May cause excessive postural hypotension and bradycardia). Products include:
- Brevibloc Injection 942

Ethylnorepinephrine Hydrochloride (May interfere with the hypotensive effect). Products include:
- Bronkephrine Injection 2042

Fluphenazine Decanoate (Possible reversal of the effects of guanadrel). Products include:
- Prolixin Decanoate 1795

Fluphenazine Enanthate (Possible reversal of the effects of guanadrel). Products include:
- Prolixin Enanthate 1796

Fluphenazine Hydrochloride (Possible reversal of the effects of guanadrel). Products include:
- Prolixin Elixir 1793
- Prolixin Injection 1791
- Prolixin Oral Concentrate 1792
- Prolixin Tablets 1793

Furazolidone (Concurrent or sequential use with MAO inhibitor is contraindicated). Products include:
- Furoxone 1855

Hydralazine Hydrochloride (Comcomitant use may increase the potential for symptomatic or orthostatic hypotension). Products include:
- Apresazide Capsules 854
- Apresoline Hydrochloride Parenteral (Ampuls) 856
- Apresoline Hydrochloride Tablets .. 855
- Apresoline-Esidrix Tablets 857
- Ser-Ap-Es Tablets 881
- Serpasil-Apresoline Tablets 884

Imipramine Hydrochloride (Possible reversal of the effects of guanadrel). Products include:
- Tofranil Ampuls 1038
- Tofranil Tablets 1039

Imipramine Pamoate (Possible reversal of the effects of guanadrel). Products include:
- Tofranil-PM Capsules 1041

Isocarboxazid (Concurrent or sequential use with MAO inhibitor is contraindicated). Products include:
- Marplan Tablets 1906

Isoetharine (May interfere with the hypotensive effect). Products include:
- Arm-a-Med Isoetharine Inhalation Solution, USP 616
- Bronkometer Aerosol 2042
- Bronkosol Solution 2042

Isoproterenol Hydrochloride (May interfere with the hypotensive effect; enhances the activity of direct acting sympathomimetic amines). Products include:
- Isuprel Hydrochloride Injection 1:5000 2050
- Isuprel Hydrochloride Mistometer .. 2051
- Isuprel Hydrochloride Solution 1:200 & 1:100 2052
- Norisodrine Aerotrol 540

Labetalol Hydrochloride (May cause excessive postural hypotension and bradycardia). Products include:
- Normodyne Injection 2108
- Normodyne Tablets 2110
- Normozide Tablets 2112
- Trandate HCT Tablets 579
- Trandate Injection 577
- Trandate Tablets 579

Maprotiline Hydrochloride (Possible reversal of the effects of guanadrel). Products include:
- Ludiomil Tablets 874

Mesoridazine (Possible reversal of the effects of guanadrel). Products include:
- Serentil 686

Metaproterenol Sulfate (May interfere with the hypotensive effect). Products include:
- Alupent 674
- Arm-a-Med Metaproterenol Sulfate Inhalation Solution, USP 617
- Metaprel Inhalation Aerosol Bronchodilator 2014
- Metaprel Inhalation Solution 2015
- Metaprel 2015
- Metaproterenol Sulfate Inhalation Solution, USP 912

Metaraminol Bitartrate (Enhances the activity of direct acting sympathomimetic amines). Products include:
- Aramine Injection 1424

Metoprolol Tartrate (May cause excessive postural hypotension and bradycardia). Products include:
- Lopressor Ampuls 1032
- Lopressor HCT Tablets 1034
- Lopressor Tablets 1032

Minoxidil (Comcomitant use may increase the potential for symptomatic or orthostatic hypotension). Products include:
- Loniten Tablets 2346
- Rogaine Topical Solution 2357

Nadolol (May cause excessive postural hypotension and bradycardia). Products include:
- Corgard Tablets 701
- Corzide Tablets 702

Norepinephrine Bitartrate (Enhanced effect of norepinephrine). Products include:
- Levophed Bitartrate Injection 2054

Norepinephrine Hydrochloride (Enhances the activity of direct acting sympathomimetic amines).

Nortriptyline Hydrochloride (Possible reversal of the effects of guanadrel). Products include:
- Pamelor 2019

Penbutolol Sulfate (May cause excessive postural hypotension and bradycardia). Products include:
- Levatol 1832

Perphenazine (Possible reversal of the effects of guanadrel). Products include:
- Etrafon 2087
- Triavil Tablets 1556
- Trilafon 2123

Phenelzine Sulfate (Concurrent or sequential use with MAO inhibitor is contraindicated). Products include:
- Nardil 1742

Phenylephrine Hydrochloride (Enhances the activity of direct acting sympathomimetic amines). Products include:
- AK-Dilate Solution 2.5% and 10% .... ⊙ 203
- Atrohist Sprinkle Capsules 558
- Cerose-DM 2443
- Codimal 846
- Comhist LA Capsules 1618
- Congespirin For Children Aspirin Free Chewable Cold Tablets 748
- Cyclomydril .... ⊙ 216
- Deconsal Sprinkle Capsules 559
- Dimetane Decongestant .... ▣ 673
- Dristan Decongestant/Antihistamine/ Analgesic Coated Caplets .... ▣ 749
- Dristan Cold Nasal Decongestant/ Antihistamine/ Analgesic Coated Tablets 2419
- Dristan Advanced Formula Decongestant/Antihistamine/ Analgesic Tablets .... ▣ 749
- Dristan Nasal Spray, Menthol 2419
- Dristan Nasal Spray, Regular and Regular with Metered Pump 2419
- Entex Capsules 1623
- Entex Liquid 1623
- Sinus Excedrin Analgesic, Decongestant Tablets & Caplets 750
- Extendryl 994
- 4-Way Fast Acting Nasal Spray - Original Formula (regular & mentholated) & Metered Spray Pump (regular) 751
- Hycomine Compound Tablets 929
- Murocoll-2 Sterile Ophthalmic Solution .... ⊙ 261
- Mydfrin 2.5% .... ⊙ 224
- Naldecon Syrup, Tablets, Pediatric Drops and Pediatric Syrup 709
- Neo-Synephrine Hydrochloride 1% Carpuject 2063
- Neo-Synephrine Hydrochloride 1% Injection 2063
- Neo-Synephrine Hydrochloride (Ophthalmic) 2064
- Neo-Synephrine .... ▣ 759
- Nōstril Nasal Decongestant .... ▣ 520
- Novahistine Elixir .... ▣ 596
- Phenergan VC 2500
- Phenergan VC with Codeine 2501
- Prefrin Liquifilm Vasoconstrictor and Lubricant Eye Drops .... ⊙ 254
- Prefrin-A .... ⊙ 255
- Quelidrine Syrup 556
- Relief Vasoconstrictor and Lubricant Eye Drops .... ⊙ 256
- Robitussin Night Relief .... ▣ 677
- Ru-Tuss with Hydrocodone 694
- Ru-Tuss Tablets 693
- Vasosulf .... ⊙ 279
- Vicks Sinex .... ▣ 665
- Zincfrin .... ⊙ 230

Phenylephrine Tannate (Enhances the activity of direct acting sympathomimetic amines). Products include:
- Rynatan 2387
- Rynatuss 2388

Phenylpropanolamine Hydrochloride (May reverse the effects of neuronal blocking agents). Products include:
- A.R.M. Allergy Relief Medicine Caplets .... ▣ 615
- Acutrim .... ▣ 548
- Allerest .... ▣ 559
- BC Cold Powder .... ▣ 517
- Cheracol Plus Head Cold/Cough Formula .... ▣ 667
- Codimal Expectorant 846
- Comtrex Multi-Symptom Cold Reliever Tablets/Caplets/Liqui-Gels/Liquid 745
- Contac Continuous Action Decongestant/Antihistamine Capsules ▣ 710
- Contac Maximum Strength Continuous Action Decongestant/ Antihistamine Caplets .... ▣ 709
- Contac Severe Cold and Flu Formula Caplets .... ▣ 711
- Coricidin 'D' Decongestant Tablets .... ▣ 695
- Coricidin Demilets Tablets for Children .... ▣ 696

- Demazin Nasal Decongestant/ Antihistamine Repetabs Tablets & Syrup ▣ 697
- Dexatrim ▣ 733
- Dimetane-DC Cough Syrup 1857
- Dimetapp Elixir ▣ 673
- Dimetapp DM Elixir ▣ 674
- Dimetapp Extentabs ▣ 674
- Dimetapp Plus Caplets ▣ 675
- Dimetapp Tablets ▣ 675
- Entex Capsules 1623
- Entex LA Tablets 1623
- Entex Liquid 1623
- 4-Way Cold Tablets 750
- Hycomine Syrup 927
- Naldecon CX Adult Liquid ▣ 521
- Naldecon DX Adult Liquid ▣ 521
- Naldecon DX Children's Syrup ▣ 522
- Naldecon DX Pediatric Drops ▣ 522
- Naldecon EX Children's Syrup ▣ 522
- Naldecon EX Pediatric Drops ▣ 523
- Naldecon Syrup, Tablets, Pediatric Drops and Pediatric Syrup 709
- Nolamine Tablets 838
- Nolex LA Tablets 838
- Ornade Spansule Capsules 2221
- Orthoxicol Cough Syrup ▣ 668
- Propagest 839
- Pyrroxate Capsules ▣ 669
- Robitussin-CF ▣ 676
- Ru-Tuss II Capsules 693
- Ru-Tuss with Hydrocodone 694
- Ru-Tuss Tablets 693
- Sine-Off Sinus Medicine Tablets-Aspirin Formula ▣ 722
- Sinulin 840
- St. Joseph Cold Tablets for Children ▣ 704
- Tavist-D Tablets 2035
- Triaminic Allergy Tablets ▣ 688
- Triaminic Chewables ▣ 688
- Triaminic Cold Tablets ▣ 688
- Triaminic Expectorant ▣ 688
- Triaminic Expectorant w/Codeine 1996
- Triaminic Expectorant DH 1995
- Triaminic Oral Infant Drops 1996
- Triaminic Syrup ▣ 689
- Triaminic-12 Tablets ▣ 690
- Triaminic-DM Syrup ▣ 689
- Triaminicin Tablets ▣ 690
- Triaminicol Multi-Symptom Cold Tablets ▣ 691
- Triaminicol Multi-Symptom Relief ▣ 691
- Tuss-Ornade Liquid 2242
- Tuss-Ornade Spansule Capsules 2242
- Tylenol Cold Medication, Effervescent Tablets 1369

Pindolol (May cause excessive postural hypotension and bradycardia). Products include:
- Visken Tablets 2036

Pirbuterol Acetate (May interfere with the hypotensive effect). Products include:
- Maxair Inhaler 1311

Prazosin Hydrochloride (May cause excessive postural hypotension and bradycardia). Products include:
- Minipress Capsules 1778
- Minizide Capsules 1779

Prochlorperazine (Possible reversal of the effects of guanadrel). Products include:
- Compazine 2201

Promethazine Hydrochloride (Possible reversal of the effects of guanadrel). Products include:
- Mepergan Injection 2479
- Phenergan with Codeine 2497
- Phenergan with Dextromethorphan 2499
- Phenergan Injection 2493
- Phenergan Suppositories 2496
- Phenergan Syrup 2495
- Phenergan Tablets 2496
- Phenergan VC 2500
- Phenergan VC with Codeine 2501

Propranolol Hydrochloride (May cause excessive postural hypotension and bradycardia). Products include:
- Inderal 2459
- Inderal LA Long Acting Capsules 2461
- Inderide Tablets 2463
- Inderide LA Long Acting Capsules 2465

Protriptyline Hydrochloride (Possible reversal of the effects of guanadrel). Products include:
- Vivactil Tablets 1567

Rauwolfia Serpentina (May cause excessive postural hypotension and bradycardia). Products include:
- Raudixin Tablets 1803
- Rauzide Tablets 1804

Rescinnamine (May cause excessive postural hypotension and bradycardia).
- No products indexed under this heading.

Reserpine (May cause excessive postural hypotension and bradycardia). Products include:
- Diupres Tablets 1461
- Hydromox R Tablets 1209
- Hydropres Tablets 1485
- Renese-R Tablets 1786
- Salutensin/Salutensin-Demi 719
- Ser-Ap-Es Tablets 881
- Serpasil Tablets 883
- Serpasil-Apresoline Tablets 884
- Serpasil-Esidrix Tablets 886

Selegiline Hydrochloride (Concurrent or sequential use with MAO inhibitor is contraindicated). Products include:
- Eldepryl 2250

Terazosin Hydrochloride (May cause excessive postural hypotension and bradycardia). Products include:
- Hytrin Tablets 529

Terbutaline Sulfate (May interfere with the hypotensive effect). Products include:
- Brethaire Inhaler 1024
- Brethine Ampuls 1026
- Brethine Tablets 1026
- Bricanyl Injection 1324
- Bricanyl Tablets 1325

Thioridazine Hydrochloride (Possible reversal of the effects of guanadrel). Products include:
- Mellaril 2011

Timolol Maleate (May cause excessive postural hypotension and bradycardia). Products include:
- Blocadren Tablets 1429
- Timolide Tablets 1547
- Timoptic in Ocudose 1552
- Timoptic Sterile Ophthalmic Solution 1550

Tranylcypromine Sulfate (Concurrent or sequential use with MAO inhibitor is contraindicated). Products include:
- Parnate Tablets 2222

Trifluoperazine Hydrochloride (Possible reversal of the effects of guanadrel). Products include:
- Stelazine 2226

Trimipramine Maleate (Possible reversal of the effects of guanadrel). Products include:
- Surmontil Capsules 2524

HYPERAB RABIES IMMUNE GLOBULIN (HUMAN)

(Rabies Immune Globulin (Human)) 1574

May interact with:

Measles Virus Vaccine Live (Interference with the response to live viral vaccines). Products include:
- Attenuvax 1424

Measles & Rubella Virus Vaccine Live (Interference with the response to live viral vaccines). Products include:
- M-R-VAX || 1496

Measles, Mumps & Rubella Virus Vaccine Live (Interference with the response to live viral vaccines). Products include:
- M-M-R || 1494

Mumps Virus Vaccine, Live (Interference with the response to live viral vaccines). Products include:
- Mumpsvax 1513

Poliovirus Vaccine, Live, Oral, Trivalent, Types 1,2,3 (Sabin) (Interference with the response to live viral vaccines). Products include:
- Orimune Poliovirus Vaccine Live Oral Trivalent 1228

Rubella Virus Vaccine Live (Interference with the response to live viral vaccines). Products include:
- Meruvax II 1503

Rubella & Mumps Virus Vaccine Live (Interference with the response to live viral vaccines). Products include:
- Biavax || 1427

HYPERHEP HEPATITIS B IMMUNE GLOBULIN (HUMAN)

(Hepatitis B Immune Globulin (Human)) 1575

May interact with:

Vaccines (Live) (May interfere with response. Use should be deferred for 3 months after administration of HyperHep). Products include:
- Attenuvax 1424
- Biavax || 1427
- M-M-R || 1494
- M-R-VAX || 1496
- Meruvax II 1503
- Mumpsvax 1513

HYPERSTAT I.V. INJECTION

(Diazoxide) 2095

May interact with oral anticoagulants, antihypertensives, beta blockers, thiazides, diuretics, and certain other agents. Compounds in these categories include:

Acebutolol Hydrochloride (Potentiation of effects of diazoxide; hypotension). Products include:
- Sectral Capsules 2520

Alphaprodine Hydrochloride (Potentiation of effects of diazoxide).

Atenolol (Potentiation of effects of diazoxide; hypotension). Products include:
- Tenoretic Tablets 1105
- Tenormin Tablets and I.V. Injection 1107

Benazepril Hydrochloride (Hypotension). Products include:
- Lotensin Tablets 872

Bendroflumethiazide (Potentiation of effects of diazoxide; hypotension). Products include:
- Corzide Tablets 702
- Naturetin Tablets 1789
- Rauzide Tablets 1804

Betaxolol Hydrochloride (Hypotension). Products include:
- Betoptic Sterile Ophthalmic Solution ⊙ 569
- Betoptic S Sterile Ophthalmic Suspension ⊙ 570
- Kerlone Tablets 2172

Captopril (Hypotension). Products include:
- Capoten 2255
- Capozide 2258

Carteolol Hydrochloride (Potentiation of effects of diazoxide; hypotension). Products include:
- Cartrol Tablets 507

Chlorothiazide (Potentiation of effects of diazoxide; hypotension). Products include:
- Aldoclor Tablets 1413
- Diupres Tablets 1461
- Diuril Oral 1464

Chlorothiazide Sodium (Potentiation of effects of diazoxide; hypotension). Products include:
- Diuril Sodium Intravenous 1463

Chlorthalidone (Potentiation of effects of diazoxide; hypotension). Products include:
- Combipres Tablets 678
- Tenoretic Tablets 1105
- Thalitone Tablets 687

Clonidine (Hypotension). Products include:
- Catapres-TTS 677

Clonidine Hydrochloride (Hypotension; potentiation of effects of diazoxide). Products include:
- Catapres Tablets 676
- Combipres Tablets 678

Deserpidine (Hypotension). Products include:
- Enduronyl 518
- Harmonyl Tablets 528
- Oreticyl 545

Dicumarol (Increased blood levels). Products include:
- Dicumarol Tablets 516

Doxazosin Mesylate (Hypotension). Products include:
- Cardura Tablets 1941

Enalapril Maleate (Hypotension). Products include:
- Vaseretic Tablets 1559
- Vasotec Tablets 1564

Enalaprilat (Potentiation of effects of diazoxide; hypotension). Products include:
- Vasotec I.V. 1562

Esmolol Hydrochloride (Potentiation of effects of diazoxide; hypotension). Products include:
- Brevibloc Injection 942

Felodipine (Hypotension). Products include:
- Plendil Extended-Release Tablets 1526

Fosinopril Sodium (Hypotension). Products include:
- Monopril Tablets 1406

Furosemide (Hypotension). Products include:
- Lasix 1093

Guanabenz Acetate (Hypotension). Products include:
- Wytensin Tablets 2542

Guanethidine Monosulfate (Hypotension). Products include:
- Esimil Tablets 864
- Ismelin Tablets 869

Hydralazine Hydrochloride (Potentiation of effects of diazoxide; hypotension). Products include:
- Apresazide Capsules 854
- Apresoline Hydrochloride Parenteral (Ampuls) 856
- Apresoline Hydrochloride Tablets 855
- Apresoline-Esidrix Tablets 857
- Ser-Ap-Es Tablets 881
- Serpasil-Apresoline Tablets 884

Hydrochlorothiazide (Potentiation of effects of diazoxide; hypotension). Products include:
- Aldactazide 2150
- Aldoril Tablets 1418
- Apresazide Capsules 854
- Apresoline-Esidrix Tablets 857
- Capozide 2258
- Dyazide Capsules 2208
- Esidrix Tablets 863
- Esimil Tablets 864
- HydroDIURIL Tablets 1484
- Hydropres Tablets 1485
- Inderide Tablets 2463
- Inderide LA Long Acting Capsules 2465
- Lopressor HCT Tablets 1034
- Maxzide 1215

Moduretic Tablets 1510
Normozide Tablets 2112
Oretic Tablets 544
Oreticyl 545
Prinzide Tablets 1540
Ser-Ap-Es Tablets 881
Serpasil-Esidrix Tablets 886
Timolide Tablets 1547
Trandate HCT Tablets 579
Vaseretic Tablets 1559
Zestoretic 2274

Hydroflumethiazide (Potentiation of effects of diazoxide; hypotension). Products include:
Diucardin Tablets 2450
Saluron 718
Salutensin/Salutensin-Demi 719

Indapamide (Hypotension). Products include:
Lozol Tablets 1843

Isradipine (Hypotension). Products include:
DynaCirc Capsules 2004

Labetalol Hydrochloride (Potentiation of effects of diazoxide; hypotension). Products include:
Normodyne Injection 2108
Normodyne Tablets 2110
Normozide Tablets 2112
Trandate HCT Tablets 579
Trandate Injection 577
Trandate Tablets 579

Lisinopril (Potentiation of effects of diazoxide; hypotension). Products include:
Prinivil Tablets 1538
Prinzide Tablets 1540
Zestoretic 2274
Zestril Tablets 2277

Mecamylamine Hydrochloride (Hypotension). Products include:
Inversine Tablets 1492

Methyclothiazide (Potentiation of effects of diazoxide; hypotension). Products include:
Enduron Tablets 517
Enduronyl 518

Methyldopa (Hypotension). Products include:
Aldoclor Tablets 1413
Aldomet Oral 1415
Aldoril Tablets 1418

Methyldopate Hydrochloride (Hypotension). Products include:
Aldomet Ester HCl Injection 1417

Metolazone (Hypotension). Products include:
Diulo 2129
Mykrox ½ mg Tablets 984
Zaroxolyn Tablets 989

Metoprolol Tartrate (Potentiation of effects of diazoxide; hypotension). Products include:
Lopressor Ampuls 1032
Lopressor HCT Tablets 1034
Lopressor Tablets 1032

Metyrosine (Hypotension). Products include:
Demser Capsules 1460

Minoxidil (Potentiation of effects of diazoxide; hypotension). Products include:
Loniten Tablets 2346
Rogaine Topical Solution 2357

Nadolol (Potentiation of effects of diazoxide; hypotension). Products include:
Corgard Tablets 701
Corzide Tablets 702

Nicardipine Hydrochloride (Potentiation of effects of diazoxide; hypotension). Products include:
Cardene Capsules 2290

Nitroglycerin (Hypotension). Products include:
Deponit NTG Transdermal Delivery System 2143
Minitran Transdermal Delivery System 1312
Nitro-Bid Ointment 1339
Nitro-Bid Capsules 1338
Nitrodisc 2176
Nitro-Dur (nitroglycerin) Transdermal Infusion System 1164
Nitrogard Tablets 1004
Nitrolingual Spray 1846
Nitrostat Tablets 1743
Transderm-Nitro Transdermal Therapeutic System 2283

Papaverine Hydrochloride (Potentiation of effects of diazoxide). Products include:
Papaverine Hydrochloride Vials and Ampoules 1290
Pavabid Capsules 1344
Pavabid HP Capsulets 1344

Penbutolol Sulfate (Potentiation of effects of diazoxide; hypotension). Products include:
Levatol 1832

Phenoxybenzamine Hydrochloride (Hypotension). Products include:
Dibenzyline Capsules 2207

Phentolamine Mesylate (Hypotension). Products include:
Regitine 878

Pindolol (Potentiation of effects of diazoxide; hypotension). Products include:
Visken Tablets 2036

Polythiazide (Potentiation of effects of diazoxide; hypotension). Products include:
Minizide Capsules 1779
Renese Tablets 1785
Renese-R Tablets 1786

Prazosin Hydrochloride (Potentiation of effects of diazoxide; hypotension). Products include:
Minipress Capsules 1778
Minizide Capsules 1779

Propranolol Hydrochloride (Potentiation of effects of diazoxide; hypotension). Products include:
Inderal 2459
Inderal LA Long Acting Capsules 2461
Inderide Tablets 2463
Inderide LA Long Acting Capsules 2465

Ramipril (Hypotension). Products include:
Altace Capsules 1086

Rauwolfia Serpentina (Hypotension). Products include:
Raudixin Tablets 1803
Rauzide Tablets 1804

Rescinnamine (Hypotension).
No products indexed under this heading.

Reserpine (Hypotension). Products include:
Diupres Tablets 1461
Hydromox R Tablets 1209
Hydropres Tablets 1485
Renese-R Tablets 1786
Salutensin/Salutensin-Demi 719
Ser-Ap-Es Tablets 881
Serpasil Tablets 883
Serpasil-Apresoline Tablets 884
Serpasil-Esidrix Tablets 886

Sodium Nitroprusside (Hypotension). Products include:
Nipride I.V. Infusion 1909

Terazosin Hydrochloride (Hypotension). Products include:
Hytrin Tablets 529

Timolol Maleate (Potentiation of effects of diazoxide; hypotension). Products include:
Blocadren Tablets 1429
Timolide Tablets 1547
Timoptic in Ocudose 1552
Timoptic Sterile Ophthalmic Solution 1550

Trimethaphan Camsylate (Hypotension). Products include:
Arfonad Ampuls 1887

Warfarin Sodium (Increased blood levels). Products include:
Coumadin Injection & Tablets 944
Panwarfin Tablets 547

HYPER-TET TETANUS IMMUNE GLOBULIN (HUMAN)
(Tetanus Immune Globulin (Human)) 1576
May interact with:

Vaccines (Live) (May interfere with response. Use should be deferred for 3 months). Products include:
Attenuvax 1424
Biavax II 1427
M-M-R II 1494
M-R-VAX II 1496
Meruvax II 1503
Mumpsvax 1513

HYPOTEARS LUBRICATING EYE DROPS
(Polyvinyl Alcohol) .... ⊙ 273
No interactions described in labeling.

HYPOTEARS OINTMENT
(Petrolatum, White) .... ⊙ 273
No interactions described in labeling.

HYPOTEARS PF PRESERVATIVE-FREE LUBRICATING EYE DROPS
(Polyvinyl Alcohol) .... ⊙ 273
No interactions described in labeling.

HYPRHO-D RH₀-D IMMUNE GLOBULIN (HUMAN)
(Immune Globulin (Human)) 1578
May interact with:

Measles Virus Vaccine Live (Interference with response to live vaccines). Products include:
Attenuvax 1424

Measles & Rubella Virus Vaccine Live (Interference with response to live vaccines). Products include:
M-R-VAX II 1496

Measles, Mumps & Rubella Virus Vaccine Live (Interference with response to live vaccines). Products include:
M-M-R II 1494

Rubella Virus Vaccine Live (Intereference with response to live vaccines). Products include:
Meruvax II 1503

Rubella & Mumps Virus Vaccine Live (Interference with response to live vaccines). Products include:
Biavax II 1427

HYPRHO-D MINI-DOSE RH₀-D IMMUNE GLOBULIN (HUMAN)
(Immune Globulin (Human)) 1578
May interact with:

Measles Virus Vaccine Live (Interference with response to live vaccines). Products include:
Attenuvax 1424

Measles & Rubella Virus Vaccine Live (Interference with response to live vaccines). Products include:
M-R-VAX II 1496

Measles, Mumps & Rubella Virus Vaccine Live (Interference with response to live vaccines). Products include:
M-M-R II 1494

Rubella Virus Vaccine Live (Interference with response to live vaccines). Products include:
Meruvax II 1503

Rubella & Mumps Virus Vaccine Live (Interference with response to live vaccines). Products include:
Biavax II 1427

HYSKON HYSTEROSCOPY FLUID
(Dextran 70) 1162
No interactions described in labeling.

HYTONE CREAM 1%, 2 ½%
(Hydrocortisone) 909
No interactions described in labeling.

HYTONE LOTION 1%, 2 ½%
(Hydrocortisone) 909
No interactions described in labeling.

HYTONE OINTMENT 1%, 2 ½%
(Hydrocortisone) 909
No interactions described in labeling.

HYTRIN TABLETS
(Terazosin Hydrochloride) 529
May interact with antihypertensives. Compounds in this category include:

Acebutolol Hydrochloride (Possibility of significant hypotension; dosage reduction and retitration may be necessary). Products include:
Sectral Capsules 2520

Atenolol (Possibility of significant hypotension; dosage reduction and retitration may be necessary). Products include:
Tenoretic Tablets 1105
Tenormin Tablets and I.V. Injection 1107

Benazepril Hydrochloride (Possibility of significant hypotension; dosage reduction and retitration may be necessary). Products include:
Lotensin Tablets 872

Bendroflumethiazide (Possibility of significant hypotension; dosage reduction and retitration may be necessary). Products include:
Corzide Tablets 702
Naturetin Tablets 1789
Rauzide Tablets 1804

Betaxolol Hydrochloride (Possibility of significant hypotension; dosage reduction and retitration may be necessary). Products include:
Betoptic Sterile Ophthalmic Solution 569
Betoptic S Sterile Ophthalmic Suspension 570
Kerlone Tablets 2172

Captopril (Possibility of significant hypotension; dosage reduction and retitration may be necessary). Products include:
Capoten 2255
Capozide 2258

Carteolol Hydrochloride (Possibility of significant hypotension; dosage reduction and retitration may be necessary). Products include:
Cartrol Tablets 507

Chlorothiazide (Possibility of significant hypotension; dosage reduction and retitration may be necessary). Products include:
Aldoclor Tablets 1413
Diupres Tablets 1461
Diuril Oral 1464

Chlorothiazide Sodium (Possibility of significant hypotension; dosage reduction and retitration may be necessary). Products include:
Diuril Sodium Intravenous 1463

Chlorthalidone (Possibility of significant hypotension; dosage reduction and retitration may be necessary). Products include:
Combipres Tablets 678
Tenoretic Tablets 1105
Thalitone Tablets 687

Clonidine (Possibility of significant hypotension; dosage reduction and retitration may be necessary). Products include:
Catapres-TTS 677

Clonidine Hydrochloride (Possibility of significant hypotension; dosage reduction and retitration may be necessary). Products include:
Catapres Tablets 676
Combipres Tablets 678

Deserpidine (Possibility of significant hypotension; dosage reduction and retitration may be necessary). Products include:
Enduronyl 518
Harmonyl Tablets 528
Oreticyl 545

Diazoxide (Possibility of significant hypotension; dosage reduction and retitration may be necessary). Products include:
Hyperstat I.V. Injection 2095
Proglycem 649

Doxazosin Mesylate (Possibility of significant hypotension; dosage reduction and retitration may be necessary). Products include:
Cardura Tablets 1941

Enalapril Maleate (Possibility of significant hypotension; dosage reduction and retitration may be necessary). Products include:
Vaseretic Tablets 1559
Vasotec Tablets 1564

Enalaprilat (Possibility of significant hypotension; dosage reduction and retitration may be necessary). Products include:
Vasotec I.V. 1562

Esmolol Hydrochloride (Possibility of significant hypotension; dosage reduction and retitration may be necessary). Products include:
Brevibloc Injection 942

Felodipine (Possibility of significant hypotension; dosage reduction and retitration may be necessary). Products include:
Plendil Extended-Release Tablets 1526

Fosinopril Sodium (Possibility of significant hypotension; dosage reduction and retitration may be necessary). Products include:
Monopril Tablets 1406

Furosemide (Possibility of significant hypotension; dosage reduction and retitration may be necessary). Products include:
Lasix 1093

Guanabenz Acetate (Possibility of significant hypotension; dosage reduction and retitration may be necessary). Products include:
Wytensin Tablets 2542

Guanethidine Monosulfate (Possibility of significant hypotension; dosage reduction and retitration may be necessary). Products include:
Esimil Tablets 864
Ismelin Tablets 869

Hydralazine Hydrochloride (Possibility of significant hypotension; dosage reduction and retitration may be necessary). Products include:
Apresazide Capsules 854
Apresoline Hydrochloride Parenteral (Ampuls) 856
Apresoline Hydrochloride Tablets 855
Apresoline-Esidrix Tablets 857
Ser-Ap-Es Tablets 881
Serpasil-Apresoline Tablets 884

Hydrochlorothiazide (Possibility of significant hypotension; dosage reduction and retitration may be necessary). Products include:
Aldactazide 2150
Aldoril Tablets 1418
Apresazide Capsules 854
Apresoline-Esidrix Tablets 857
Capozide 2258
Dyazide Capsules 2208
Esidrix Tablets 863
Esimil Tablets 864
HydroDIURIL Tablets 1484
Hydropres Tablets 1485
Inderide Tablets 2463
Inderide LA Long Acting Capsules 2465
Lopressor HCT Tablets 1034
Maxzide 1215
Moduretic Tablets 1510
Normozide Tablets 2112
Oretic Tablets 544
Oreticyl 545
Prinzide Tablets 1540
Ser-Ap-Es Tablets 881
Serpasil-Esidrix Tablets 886
Timolide Tablets 1547
Trandate HCT Tablets 579
Vaseretic Tablets 1559
Zestoretic 2274

Hydroflumethiazide (Possibility of significant hypotension; dosage reduction and retitration may be necessary). Products include:
Diucardin Tablets 2450
Saluron 718
Salutensin/Salutensin-Demi 719

Indapamide (Possibility of significant hypotension; dosage reduction and retitration may be necessary). Products include:
Lozol Tablets 1843

Isradipine (Possibility of significant hypotension; dosage reduction and retitration may be necessary). Products include:
DynaCirc Capsules 2004

Labetalol Hydrochloride (Possibility of significant hypotension; dosage reduction and retitration may be necessary). Products include:
Normodyne Injection 2108
Normodyne Tablets 2110
Normozide Tablets 2112
Trandate HCT Tablets 579
Trandate Injection 577
Trandate Tablets 579

Lisinopril (Possibility of significant hypotension; dosage reduction and retitration may be necessary). Products include:
Prinivil Tablets 1538
Prinzide Tablets 1540
Zestoretic 2274
Zestril Tablets 2277

Mecamylamine Hydrochloride (Possibility of significant hypotension; dosage reduction and retitration may be necessary). Products include:
Inversine Tablets 1492

Methyclothiazide (Possibility of significant hypotension; dosage reduction and retitration may be necessary). Products include:
Enduron Tablets 517
Enduronyl 518

Methyldopa (Possibility of significant hypotension; dosage reduction and retitration may be necessary). Products include:
Aldoclor Tablets 1413
Aldomet Oral 1415
Aldoril Tablets 1418

Methyldopate Hydrochloride (Possibility of significant hypotension; dosage reduction and retitration may be necessary). Products include:
Aldomet Ester HCl Injection 1417

Metolazone (Possibility of significant hypotension; dosage reduction and retitration may be necessary). Products include:
Diulo 2129
Mykrox ½ mg Tablets 984
Zaroxolyn Tablets 989

Metoprolol Tartrate (Possibility of significant hypotension; dosage reduction and retitration may be necessary). Products include:
Lopressor Ampuls 1032
Lopressor HCT Tablets 1034
Lopressor Tablets 1032

Metyrosine (Possibility of significant hypotension; dosage reduction and retitration may be necessary). Products include:
Demser Capsules 1460

Minoxidil (Possibility of significant hypotension; dosage reduction and retitration may be necessary). Products include:
Loniten Tablets 2346
Rogaine Topical Solution 2357

Nadolol (Possibility of significant hypotension; dosage reduction and retitration may be necessary). Products include:
Corgard Tablets 701
Corzide Tablets 702

Nicardipine Hydrochloride (Possibility of significant hypotension; dosage reduction and retitration may be necessary). Products include:
Cardene Capsules 2290

Nitroglycerin (Possibility of significant hypotension; dosage reduction and retitration may be necessary). Products include:
Deponit NTG Transdermal Delivery System 2143
Minitran Transdermal Delivery System 1312
Nitro-Bid Ointment 1339
Nitro-Bid Capsules 1338
Nitrodisc 2176
Nitro-Dur (nitroglycerin) Transdermal Infusion System 1164
Nitrogard Tablets 1004
Nitrolingual Spray 1846
Nitrostat Tablets 1743
Transderm-Nitro Transdermal Therapeutic System 2283

Penbutolol Sulfate (Possibility of significant hypotension; dosage reduction and retitration may be necessary). Products include:
Levatol 1832

Phenoxybenzamine Hydrochloride (Possibility of significant hypotension; dosage reduction and retitration may be necessary). Products include:
Dibenzyline Capsules 2207

Phentolamine Mesylate (Possibility of significant hypotension; dosage reduction and retitration may be necessary). Products include:
Regitine 878

Pindolol (Possibility of significant hypotension; dosage reduction and retitration may be necessary). Products include:
Visken Tablets 2036

Polythiazide (Possibility of significant hypotension; dosage reduction and retitration may be necessary). Products include:
Minizide Capsules 1779
Renese Tablets 1785
Renese-R Tablets 1786

Prazosin Hydrochloride (Possibility of significant hypotension; dosage reduction and retitration may be necessary). Products include:
Minipress Capsules 1778
Minizide Capsules 1779

Propranolol Hydrochloride (Possibility of significant hypotension; dosage reduction and retitration may be necessary). Products include:
Inderal 2459
Inderal LA Long Acting Capsules 2461
Inderide Tablets 2463
Inderide LA Long Acting Capsules 2465

Ramipril (Possibility of significant hypotension; dosage reduction and retitration may be necessary). Products include:
Altace Capsules 1086

Rauwolfia Serpentina (Possibility of significant hypotension; dosage reduction and retitration may be necessary). Products include:
Raudixin Tablets 1803
Rauzide Tablets 1804

Rescinnamine (Possibility of significant hypotension; dosage reduction and retitration may be necessary).
No products indexed under this heading.

Reserpine (Possibility of significant hypotension; dosage reduction and retitration may be necessary). Products include:
Diupres Tablets 1461
Hydromox R Tablets 1209
Hydropres Tablets 1485
Renese-R Tablets 1786
Salutensin/Salutensin-Demi 719
Ser-Ap-Es Tablets 881
Serpasil Tablets 883
Serpasil-Apresoline Tablets 884
Serpasil-Esidrix Tablets 886

Sodium Nitroprusside (Possibility of significant hypotension; dosage reduction and retitration may be necessary). Products include:
Nipride I.V. Infusion 1909

Timolol Maleate (Possibility of significant hypotension; dosage reduction and retitration may be necessary). Products include:
Blocadren Tablets 1429
Timolide Tablets 1547
Timoptic in Ocudose 1552
Timoptic Sterile Ophthalmic Solution 1550

Trimethaphan Camsylate (Possibility of significant hypotension; dosage reduction and retitration may be necessary). Products include:
Arfonad Ampuls 1887

ICAPS PLUS
(Vitamins with Minerals) ◉ 280
No interactions described in labeling.

INH TABLETS
(Isoniazid) 868
May interact with:

Alcohol (Higher incidence of isoniazide hepatitis).

Phenytoin (Enhancement of phenytoin effects). Products include:
Dilantin Infatabs 1710
Dilantin-30 Pediatric/Dilantin-125 Suspension 1713

Phenytoin Sodium (Enhancement of phenytoin effects). Products include:
Dilantin Kapseals 1708
Dilantin Parenteral 1712
Dilantin with Phenobarbital Kapseals 1715

IBERET FILMTAB
(Vitamin B Complex With Vitamin C, Ferrous Sulfate) 531
No interactions described in labeling.

IBERET-500 FILMTAB
(Vitamin B Complex With Vitamin C, Ferrous Sulfate) 531
No interactions described in labeling.

IBERET-500 LIQUID
(Vitamin B Complex With Vitamin C, Ferrous Sulfate) 531
No interactions described in labeling.

IBERET-FOLIC-500 FILMTAB
(Vitamin B Complex With Vitamin C, Ferrous Sulfate) 527
See **Fero-Folic-500 Filmtab**

IBERET-LIQUID
(Vitamin B Complex With Vitamin C, Ferrous Sulfate) 531
No interactions described in labeling.

IBUPROHM IBUPROFEN CAPLETS
(Ibuprofen) .... ■ 631
May interact with aspirin and acetaminophen containing products. Compounds in this category include:

Acetaminophen (Concurrent use not recommended). Products include:
- Acetaminophen Uniserts Suppositories 2374
- Actifed Plus Caplets .... ■ 539
- Actifed Plus Tablets .... ■ 540
- Alka-Seltzer Advanced Formula Antacid & Non-Aspirin Pain Reliever .... ■ 620
- Allerest .... ■ 559
- Aspirin Free Anacin Maximum Strength Acetaminophen Film Coated Caplets 2417
- Aspirin Free Anacin Maximum Strength Acetaminophen Film Coated Tablets 2417
- Anacin-3 Regular Strength Acetaminophen Film Coated Tablets ■ 746
- Anexsia 5/500 Tablets 2196
- Anexsia 7.5/650 Tablets 2197
- Benadryl Plus .... ■ 636
- Benadryl Plus Nighttime .... ■ 637
- Bufferin AF Nite Time Analgesic/Sleeping Aid Caplets 744
- Allergy-Sinus Comtrex Multi-Symptom Allergy Sinus Formula Tablets & Caplets 746
- Cough Formula Comtrex 746
- Comtrex Multi-Symptom Cold Reliever Tablets/Caplets/Liqui-Gels/Liquid 745
- Day-Night Comtrex 747
- Non-Drowsy Comtrex 747
- Congespirin For Children Aspirin Free Chewable Cold Tablets 748
- Contac Cough & Sore Throat Formula .... ■ 712
- Contac Jr. Children's Cold Medicine .... ■ 712
- Contac Nighttime Cold Medicine .... ■ 713
- Contac Severe Cold and Flu Formula Caplets .... ■ 711
- Contac Sinus Caplets Maximum Strength Non-Drowsy Formula .... ■ 710
- Contac Sinus Tablets Maximum Strength Non-Drowsy Formula .... ■ 710
- Coricidin 'D' Decongestant Tablets .... ■ 695
- Coricidin Demilets Tablets for Children .... ■ 696
- Coricidin Tablets .... ■ 695
- Darvon-N/Darvocet-N 1254
- Datril Extra-Strength Analgesic Tablets 748
- Dimetapp Plus Caplets .... ■ 675
- Dorcol Children's Fever & Pain Reducer .... ■ 686
- Dristan Decongestant/Antihistamine/Analgesic Coated Caplets .... ■ 749
- Dristan Cold Nasal Decongestant/Antihistamine/Analgesic Coated Tablets 2419
- Dristan Advanced Formula Decongestant/Antihistamine/Analgesic Tablets .... ■ 749
- Maximum Strength Dristan Decongestant/Analgesic Coated Caplets .... ■ 750
- No Drowsiness Dristan Cold Nasal Decongestant/Analgesic Coated Caplets 2420
- Drixoral Plus Extended-Release Tablets .... ■ 699
- Drixoral Sinus .... ■ 700
- Esgic-Plus Tablets 1002
- Esgic Tablets & Capsules 1001
- Aspirin Free Excedrin Analgesic Caplets 748
- Excedrin Extra-Strength Analgesic Tablets & Caplets 749
- Excedrin P.M. Analgesic/Sleeping Aid Tablets, Caplets and Liquid 749
- Sinus Excedrin Analgesic, Decongestant Tablets & Caplets 750
- 4-Way Cold Tablets 750
- Feverall Sprinkle Caps 2374
- Feverall Suppositories 2374
- Fioricet Tablets 2006
- Hycomine Compound Tablets 929
- Hydrocet Capsules 835
- Isocom Capsules 1629
- Liquiprin .... ■ 618
- Lortab 2412
- Lurline PMS Tablets 972
- Medi-Flu Caplet, Liquid .... ■ 640
- Maximum Strength Midol Multi-Symptom Menstrual Formula .... ■ 571
- Maximum Strength Midol PMS Premenstrual Syndrome Formula .... ■ 570
- Regular Strength Midol Multi-Symptom Menstrual Formula .... ■ 570
- Midrin Capsules 836
- Ornex Caplets .... ■ 618
- Children's Panadol Chewable Tablets, Liquid, Infants' Drops .... ■ 571
- Junior Strength Panadol .... ■ 571
- Maximum Strength Panadol Tablets and Caplets .... ■ 572
- Percocet Tablets 950
- Percogesic Analgesic Tablets .... ■ 660
- Phenaphen with Codeine Capsules 1865
- Phenaphen-650 with Codeine Tablets 1866
- Phrenilin 838
- Prēmsyn PMS Capsules & Caplets ■ 547
- Pyrroxate Capsules .... ■ 669
- Robitussin Night Relief .... ■ 677
- Sedapap Tablets 50 mg/650 mg .. 1360
- Sinarest .... ■ 562
- Sine-Aid Maximum Strength Sinus Headache Caplets 1365
- Sine-Aid Maximum Strength Sinus Headache Tablets 1365
- Sine-Off Maximum Strength Allergy/Sinus Formula Caplets .... ■ 721
- Sine-Off Maximum Strength No Drowsiness Formula Caplets .... ■ 722
- Singlet Tablets .... ■ 598
- Sinulin 840
- Sinutab Maximum Strength .... ■ 641
- Sinutab Maximum Strength Without Drowsiness Tablets & Caplets .... ■ 642
- Sinutab Regular Strength Without Drowsiness Formula .... ■ 641
- Sominex Pain Relief Formula .... ■ 723
- St. Joseph Aspirin-Free Fever Reducer for Children Chewable Tablets, Liquid & Infant Drops .... ■ 704
- St. Joseph Cold Tablets for Children .... ■ 704
- St. Joseph Nighttime Cold Medicine .... ■ 705
- Sudafed Sinus Caplets .... ■ 545
- Sudafed Sinus Tablets .... ■ 545
- Talacen 2070
- Tempra, Acetaminophen .... ■ 613
- TheraFlu Flu and Cold Medicine .... ■ 687
- Triaminicin Tablets .... ■ 690
- Tylenol acetaminophen Children's Chewable Tablets & Elixir 1366
- Tylenol Allergy Sinus Medication Caplets and Gelcaps, Maximum Strength 1372
- Tylenol with Codeine 1381
- Children's Tylenol Cold Liquid Formula and Chewable Tablets 1368
- Tylenol Cold & Flu Hot Medication, Packets 1369
- Tylenol Cold & Flu No Drowsiness Hot Medication, Packets 1371
- Tylenol Cold Medication Caplets and Tablets 1370
- Tylenol Cold Medication, Effervescent Tablets 1369
- Tylenol Cold Medication No Drowsiness Formula Caplets 1370
- Tylenol Cold Night Time Medication Liquid 1371
- Tylenol Cough Medication Liquid, Maximum Strength 1372
- Tylenol Cough Medication Liquid with Decongestant, Maximum Strength 1372
- Tylenol, Extra Strength, acetaminophen Adult Liquid Pain Reliever .. 1367
- Tylenol, Extra Strength, acetaminophen Gelcaps, Caplets, Tablets 1367
- Tylenol, Infants' Drops 1366
- Tylenol, Junior Strength, acetaminophen Coated Caplets, Grape and Fruit Chewable Tablets 1366
- Tylenol, Maximum Strength, Sinus Medication Gelcaps, Caplets and Tablets 1373
- Tylenol, Regular Strength, acetaminophen Tablets and Caplets 1367
- Tylenol PM, Extra Strength Caplets and Tablets 1368
- Tylox Capsules 1382
- Unisom Dual Relief Nighttime Sleep Aid/Analgesic 1774
- Vanquish Analgesic Caplets .... ■ 574
- Vicks Daycare .... ■ 660
- Vicks Formula 44M Multi-Symptom Cough Medicine .... ■ 662
- Vicks NyQuil Nighttime Colds Medicine-Original & Cherry Flavor .... ■ 664
- Vicodin Tablets 1187
- Vicodin ES Tablets 1189
- Wygesic Tablets 2540
- Zydone Capsules 941

Aspirin (Concurrent use not recommended). Products include:
- Alka-Seltzer Effervescent Antacid and Pain Reliever 1568
- Alka-Seltzer Extra Strength Effervescent Antacid and Pain Reliever 1570
- Alka-Seltzer (Flavored) Effervescent Antacid and Pain Reliever 1569
- Alka-Seltzer Plus Cold Medicine .... ■ 623
- Alka-Seltzer Plus Night-Time Cold Medicine .... ■ 623
- Alka Seltzer Plus Sinus Allergy Medicine .... ■ 624
- Anacin Coated Analgesic Caplets 2417
- Anacin Coated Analgesic Tablets 2417
- Anacin Maximum Strength Analgesic Coated Tablets 2417
- Maximum Strength Arthritis Pain Formula By the Makers of Anacin Analgesic Tablets and Caplets 2418
- Arthritis Pain Formula by the Makers of Anacin Analgesic Tablets and Caplets .... ■ 747
- Arthritis Strength BC Powder .... ■ 516
- Ascriptin A/D Caplets 1850
- Regular Strength Ascriptin Tablets 1850
- Azdōne Tablets 844
- BC Powder .... ■ 517
- BC Cold Powder .... ■ 517
- Children's Bayer Chewable Aspirin .... ■ 564
- Genuine Bayer Aspirin Tablets & Caplets .... ■ 564
- Maximum Bayer Aspirin Tablets & Caplets .... ■ 566
- Bayer Plus Aspirin Tablets .... ■ 567
- Therapy Bayer Aspirin Caplets .... ■ 568
- 8 Hour Bayer Timed-Release Aspirin .... ■ 566
- Arthritis Strength Bufferin Analgesic Caplets 744
- Extra Strength Bufferin Analgesic Tablets 745
- Bufferin Analgesic Tablets and Caplets 743
- Cama Arthritis Pain Reliever .... ■ 685
- Damason-P 1356
- Easprin 1719
- Ecotrin Enteric Coated Aspirin Maximum Strength Tablets and Caplets 2189
- Ecotrin Enteric Coated Aspirin Regular Strength Tablets and Caplets 2189
- Empirin Aspirin .... ■ 541
- Empirin with Codeine Phosphate Nos. 2, 3 & 4 764
- Equagesic Tablets 2451
- Excedrin Extra-Strength Analgesic Tablets & Caplets 749
- 4-Way Cold Tablets 750
- Fiorinal Capsules 2007
- Fiorinal with Codeine Capsules 2008
- Fiorinal Tablets 2007
- Lortab ASA Tablets 2414
- Momentum Muscular Backache Formula .... ■ 751
- Norgesic 1314
- Norwich Extra-Strength Aspirin .... ■ 546
- Norwich Regular Strength Aspirin ■ 547
- P-A-C Analgesic Tablets .... ■ 669
- Percodan 951
- Robaxisal Tablets 1872
- Sine-Off Sinus Medicine Tablets-Aspirin Formula .... ■ 722
- Soma Compound w/Codeine Tablets 2390
- Soma Compound Tablets 2389
- St. Joseph Adult Chewable Aspirin (81 mg.) .... ■ 703
- Synalgos-DC Capsules 2525
- Talwin Compound 2072
- Ursinus Inlay-Tabs .... ■ 691
- Vanquish Analgesic Caplets .... ■ 574
- Zorprin Tablets 698

IBUPROHM IBUPROFEN TABLETS
(Ibuprofen) .... ■ 631
See **Ibuprohm Ibuprofen Caplets**

ICY HOT BALM
(Menthol, Methyl Salicylate) .... ■ 659
No interactions described in labeling.

ICY HOT CREAM
(Menthol, Methyl Salicylate) .... ■ 659
No interactions described in labeling.

ICY HOT STICK
(Menthol, Methyl Salicylate) .... ■ 659
No interactions described in labeling.

IDAMYCIN FOR INJECTION
(Idarubicin Hydrochloride) 564
May interact with anthracyclines. Compounds in this category include:

Daunorubicin Hydrochloride (Previous therapy with anthracyclines is co-factor for increased cardiac toxicity). Products include:
- Cerubidine 2443

Doxorubicin Hydrochloride (Previous therapy with anthracyclines is co-factor for increased cardiac toxicity). Products include:
- Adriamycin PFS 561
- Adriamycin RDF 562
- Doxorubicin Hydrochloride for Injection, USP 622
- Doxorubicin Hydrochloride Injection, USP 848
- Rubex 739

IFEX
(Ifosfamide) 729
May interact with:

Bone Marrow Depressants, unspecified (Adjustments in dosing may be necessary).

ILETIN I
(Insulin, Zinc Suspension) 1272
No interactions described in labeling.

LENTE, 40 & 100 UNITS
(Insulin, Zinc Suspension) 1272
No interactions described in labeling.

NPH, 40 & 100 UNITS
(Insulin, NPH) 1273
No interactions described in labeling.

PROTAMINE, ZINC, 40 & 100 UNITS
(Insulin, Zinc Suspension) 1273
No interactions described in labeling.

REGULAR, 40 & 100 UNITS
(Insulin, Zinc Crystals) 1273
No interactions described in labeling.

SEMILENTE, 40 & 100 UNITS
(Insulin, Zinc Suspension) 1272
No interactions described in labeling.

ULTRALENTE, 40 & 100 UNITS
(Insulin, Zinc Suspension)....................1272
No interactions described in labeling.

ILETIN II
(Insulin, Zinc Suspension)....................1274
No interactions described in labeling.

BEEF LENTE, 100 UNITS
(Insulin, Zinc Suspension)....................1274
No interactions described in labeling.

BEEF NPH, 100 UNITS
(Insulin, NPH)..1274
No interactions described in labeling.

BEEF PROTAMINE ZINC, 100 UNITS
(Insulin, Zinc Suspension)....................1274
No interactions described in labeling.

BEEF REGULAR, 100 UNITS
(Insulin, Regular) 1275
May interact with oral hypoglycemic agents. Compounds in this category include:

Chlorpropamide (The concurrent use of oral hypoglycemic agents with Iletin II, U-500 is not recommended). Products include:
Diabinese Tablets 1775

Glipizide (The concurrent use of oral hypoglycemic agents with Iletin II, U-500 is not recommended). Products include:
Glucotrol 1952

Glyburide (The concurrent use of oral hypoglycemic agents with Iletin II, U-500 is not recommended). Products include:
DiaBeta.. 1091
Micronase Tablets 2350

Tolazamide (The concurrent use of oral hypoglycemic agents with Iletin II, U-500 is not recommended). Products include:
Tolinase Tablets 2365

Tolbutamide (The concurrent use of oral hypoglycemic agents with Iletin II, U-500 is not recommended). Products include:
Orinase Tablets 2354

PORK LENTE, 100 UNITS
(Insulin, Zinc Suspension)....................1275
No interactions described in labeling.

PORK NPH, 100 UNITS
(Insulin, Zinc Suspension)....................1275
No interactions described in labeling.

PORK, PROTAMINE, ZINC, 100 UNITS
(Insulin, Zinc Suspension)....................1275
No interactions described in labeling.

PORK REGULAR, 100 UNITS
(Insulin, Regular) 1275
No interactions described in labeling.

PORK REGULAR (CONCENTRATED), 500 UNITS
(Insulin, Regular) 1276
No interactions described in labeling.

ILOSONE LIQUID, ORAL SUSPENSIONS
(Erythromycin Estolate) 913
See **Ilosone Pulvules & Tablets**

ILOSONE PULVULES & TABLETS
(Erythromycin Estolate) 913
May interact with drugs which undergo biotransformation by cytochrome p-450 mixed function oxidase, oral anticoagulants, and certain other agents. Compounds in these categories include:

Alfentanil Hydrochloride (Elevated serum concentrations of alfentanil). Products include:
Alfenta Injection 1131

Aminophylline (Concurrent use with high dose of theophylline may result in increased potential for theophylline toxicity). Products include:
Amesec .... ▣ 682
Aminophyllin Tablets 2153

Bromocriptine Mesylate (Elevated serum concentrations of bromocriptine). Products include:
Parlodel 2020

Carbamazepine (Elevated serum concentrations of carbamacepine). Products include:
Tegretol Chewable Tablets 654
Tegretol Suspension.......................... 656
Tegretol Tablets 654

Clindamycin Hydrochloride (Antagonistic under some conditions). Products include:
Cleocin HCl Capsules........................ 2322

Clindamycin Palmitate Hydrochloride (Antagonistic under some conditions). Products include:
Cleocin Pediatric Flavored Granules 2324

Cyclosporine (Elevated serum concentrations of cyclosporine). Products include:
Sandimmune 2024

Dicumarol (Increased anticoagulant effects). Products include:
Dicumarol Tablets 516

Digoxin (Concomitant administration results in elevated digoxin levels). Products include:
Lanoxicaps 772
Lanoxin Elixir Pediatric 775
Lanoxin Injection 778
Lanoxin Injection Pediatric.................. 781
Lanoxin Tablets 783

Dihydroergotamine Mesylate (Potential for acute ergot toxicity). Products include:
D.H.E. 45 Injection 2003

Disopyramide Phosphate (Elevated serum concentrations). Products include:
Norpace 2177

Drugs which undergo biotransformation by cytochrome P-450 mixed function oxidase (Elevated serum concentrations).

Dyphylline (Concurrent use with high dose of theophylline may result in increased potential for theophylline toxicity). Products include:
Dilor 2079
Dilor-G Tablets & Liquid 2079
Lufyllin Elixir 2384
Lufyllin & Lufyllin-400 Tablets 2384
Lufyllin-GG Elixir & Tablets 2385

Ergotamine Tartrate (Potential for acute ergot toxicity). Products include:
Bellergal-S Tablets 1998
Cafergot/Cafergot P-B 1999
Ergostat 1719
Medihaler Ergotamine Aerosol........... 1312
Wigraine Tablets & Suppositories .. 1645

Hexobarbital (Elevated serum concentrations of hexobarbital).

Lincomycin Hydrochloride Monohydrate (Antagonistic under some conditions).
No products indexed under this heading.

Lovastatin (Elevated serum concentrations of lovastatin). Products include:
Mevacor Tablets 1505

Phenytoin (Elevated serum concentrations of phenytoin). Products include:
Dilantin Infatabs 1710
Dilantin-30 Pediatric/Dilantin-125 Suspension 1713

Phenytoin Sodium (Elevated serum concentrations of phenytoin). Products include:
Dilantin Kapseals 1708
Dilantin Parenteral 1712
Dilantin with Phenobarbital Kapseals 1715

Probenecid (Inhibits tubular reabsorption of erythromycin). Products include:
Benemid Tablets 1426
ColBENEMID Tablets 1436
Wycillin Injection and Probenecid Tablets 2539

Theophylline (Concurrent use with high dose of theophylline may result in increased potential for theophylline toxicity). Products include:
Bronkaid Tablets .... ▣ 757
Bronkolixir .... ▣ 761
Bronkotabs Tablets........................... ▣ 762
Constant-T Tablets 1029
Marax Tablets & DF Syrup.................. 1954
Primatene Tablets............................... 2421
Quibron Capsules 713
Quibron-T 714
Quibron-T/SR 716
Theolair Liquid 1317
Theo-Organidin Elixir 2391

Theophylline Anhydrous (Concurrent use with high dose of theophylline may result in increased potential for theophylline toxicity). Products include:
Aerolate 994
Primatene Tablets-M Formula .... ▣ 753
Primatene Tablets-Regular Formula 2421
Respbid Tablets 684
Slo-bid Gyrocaps 1847
T-PHYL (Uniphyl) 200 mg Tablets 1820
Tedral SA 1765
Theo-24... 2179
Theo-Dur Sprinkle 1168
Theo-Dur Extended-Release Tablets 1166
Theolair Tablets 1317
Theolair-SR Tablets............................. 1319
TheoX Extended-Release Tablets 841
Uniphyl 400 mg Tablets...................... 1823

Theophylline Calcium Salicylate (Concurrent use with high dose of theophylline may result in increased potential for theophylline toxicity). Products include:
Quadrinal Tablets 1183

Theophylline Sodium Glycinate (Concurrent use with high dose of theophylline may result in increased potential for theophylline toxicity). Products include:
Asbron G 1997

Triazolam (Decreased clearance of triazolam). Products include:
Halcion Tablets.................................... 2340

Warfarin Sodium (Increased anticoagulant effects). Products include:
Coumadin Injection & Tablets 944
Panwarfin Tablets 547

ILOTYCIN GLUCEPTATE, IV, VIALS
(Erythromycin Gluceptate) 915
May interact with oral anticoagulants, drugs which undergo biotransformation by cytochrome p-450 mixed function oxidase, and certain other agents. Compounds in these categories include:

Alfentanil Hydrochloride (Elevated serum levels). Products include:
Alfenta Injection 1131

Aminophylline (Concomitant administration with high doses of theophylline may be associated with increased theophylline levels and potential toxicity). Products include:
Amesec .... ▣ 682
Aminophyllin Tablets 2153

Bromocriptine Mesylate (Elevated bromocriptine serum levels). Products include:
Parlodel 2020

Carbamazepine (Elevations in serum erythromycin and carbamazepine concentration). Products include:
Tegretol Chewable Tablets 654
Tegretol Suspension.......................... 656
Tegretol Tablets 654

Cyclosporine (Elevations in serum erythromycin and cyclosporine concentration). Products include:
Sandimmune 2024

Dicumarol (Increased anticoagulant effects). Products include:
Dicumarol Tablets 516

Digoxin (Elevated digoxin serum levels). Products include:
Lanoxicaps 772
Lanoxin Elixir Pediatric 775
Lanoxin Injection 778
Lanoxin Injection Pediatric.................. 781
Lanoxin Tablets 783

Dihydroergotamine Mesylate (Potential for acute ergot toxicity characterized by severe peripheral vasospasm and dysesthesia). Products include:
D.H.E. 45 Injection 2003

Disopyramide Phosphate (Elevated serum levels). Products include:
Norpace 2177

Drugs which undergo biotransformation by cytochrome P-450 mixed function oxidase (Elevated serum levels).

Dyphylline (Concomitant administration with high doses of theophylline may be associated with increased theophylline levels and potential toxicity). Products include:
Dilor 2079
Dilor-G Tablets & Liquid 2079
Lufyllin Elixir 2384
Lufyllin & Lufyllin-400 Tablets 2384
Lufyllin-GG Elixir & Tablets 2385

Ergotamine Tartrate (Potential for acute ergot toxicity characterized by severe peripheral vasospasm and dysesthesia). Products include:
Bellergal-S Tablets 1998
Cafergot/Cafergot P-B 1999
Ergostat 1719
Medihaler Ergotamine Aerosol........... 1312
Wigraine Tablets & Suppositories .. 1645

Hexobarbital (Elevations in serum erythromycin and hexobarbital concentration).

Lovastatin (Potential for rhabdomyolysis in seriously ill patients). Products include:
Mevacor Tablets 1505

Phenytoin (Elevations in serum erythromycin and phenytoin concentration). Products include:
Dilantin Infatabs 1710
Dilantin-30 Pediatric/Dilantin-125 Suspension 1713

Phenytoin Sodium (Elevations in serum erythromycin and phenytoin concentration). Products include:
Dilantin Kapseals 1708

- Dilantin Parenteral ... 1712
- Dilantin with Phenobarbital Kapseals ... 1715

Terfenadine (Potential for altered terfenadine metabolism). Products include:
- Seldane Tablets ... 1349
- Seldane-D Extended-Release Tablets ... 1350

Theophylline (Concomitant administration with high doses of theophylline may be associated with increased theophylline levels and potential toxicity). Products include:
- Bronkaid Tablets ... ▣ 757
- Bronkolixir ... ▣ 761
- Bronkotabs Tablets ... ▣ 762
- Constant-T Tablets ... 1029
- Marax Tablets & DF Syrup ... 1954
- Primatene Tablets ... 2421
- Quibron Capsules ... 713
- Quibron-T ... 714
- Quibron-T/SR ... 716
- Theolair Liquid ... 1317
- Theo-Organidin Elixir ... 2391

Theophylline Anhydrous (Concomitant administration with high doses of theophylline may be associated with increased theophylline levels and potential toxicity). Products include:
- Aerolate ... 994
- Primatene Tablets-M Formula ... ▣ 753
- Primatene Tablets-Regular Formula ... 2421
- Respbid Tablets ... 684
- Slo-bid Gyrocaps ... 1847
- T-PHYL (Uniphyl) 200 mg Tablets 1820
- Tedral SA ... 1765
- Theo-24 ... 2179
- Theo-Dur Sprinkle ... 1168
- Theo-Dur Extended-Release Tablets ... 1166
- Theolair Tablets ... 1317
- Theolair-SR Tablets ... 1319
- TheoX Extended-Release Tablets ... 841
- Uniphyl 400 mg Tablets ... 1823

Theophylline Calcium Salicylate (Concomitant administration with high doses of theophylline may be associated with increased theophylline levels and potential toxicity). Products include:
- Quadrinal Tablets ... 1183

Theophylline Sodium Glycinate (Concomitant administration with high doses of theophylline may be associated with increased theophylline levels and potential toxicity). Products include:
- Asbron G ... 1997

Triazolam (Decreased clearance of triazolam and increased the pharmacologic effect of triazolam). Products include:
- Halcion Tablets ... 2340

Warfarin Sodium (Increased anticoagulant effects). Products include:
- Coumadin Injection & Tablets ... 944
- Panwarfin Tablets ... 547

ILOTYCIN OPHTHALMIC OINTMENT
(Erythromycin) ... 915
No interactions described in labeling.

IMFERON
(Iron Dextran) ... 976
No interactions described in labeling.

IMODIUM A-D CAPLETS AND LIQUID
(Loperamide Hydrochloride) ... 1362
No interactions described in labeling.

IMODIUM CAPSULES
(Loperamide Hydrochloride) ... 1139
No interactions described in labeling.

IMPREGON CONCENTRATE
(Tetrachlorosalicylanilide) ... 994
No interactions described in labeling.

IMURAN INJECTION
(Azathioprine Sodium) ... 768
See **Imuran Tablets**

IMURAN TABLETS
(Azathioprine) ... 768
May interact with ACE inhibitors and certain other agents. Compounds in these categories include:

Allopurinol (Inhibition of degradative pathway of azathioprine; reduce Imuran dosage by 1/3 to 1/4 the usual dose). Products include:
- Zyloprim Tablets ... 830

Benazepril Hydrochloride (Potential for severe leukopenia). Products include:
- Lotensin Tablets ... 872

Captopril (Potential for severe leukopenia). Products include:
- Capoten ... 2255
- Capozide ... 2258

Enalapril Maleate (Potential for severe leukopenia). Products include:
- Vaseretic Tablets ... 1559
- Vasotec Tablets ... 1564

Enalaprilat (Potential for severe leukopenia). Products include:
- Vasotec I.V. ... 1562

Fosinopril Sodium (Potential for severe leukopenia). Products include:
- Monopril Tablets ... 1406

Lisinopril (Potential for severe leukopenia). Products include:
- Prinivil Tablets ... 1538
- Prinzide Tablets ... 1540
- Zestoretic ... 2274
- Zestril Tablets ... 2277

Ramipril (Potential for severe leukopenia). Products include:
- Altace Capsules ... 1086

Sulfamethoxazole (Potential for exaggerated leukopenia). Products include:
- Azo Gantanol Tablets ... 1887
- Bactrim DS Tablets ... 1891
- Bactrim I.V. Infusion ... 1889
- Bactrim ... 1891
- Gantanol ... 1899
- Septra ... 813
- Septra I.V. Infusion ... 808
- Septra I.V. Infusion ADD-Vantage Vials ... 810
- Septra ... 813

Trimethoprim (Potential for exaggerated leukopenia). Products include:
- Bactrim DS Tablets ... 1891
- Bactrim I.V. Infusion ... 1889
- Bactrim ... 1891
- Proloprim Tablets ... 799
- Septra ... 813
- Septra I.V. Infusion ... 808
- Septra I.V. Infusion ADD-Vantage Vials ... 810
- Septra ... 813
- Trimpex Tablets ... 1922

INAPSINE INJECTION
(Droperidol) ... 1140
May interact with central nervous system depressants and certain other agents. Compounds in these categories include:

Alfentanil Hydrochloride (Additive or potentiating effects). Products include:
- Alfenta Injection ... 1131

Alprazolam (Additive or potentiating effects). Products include:
- Xanax Tablets ... 2367

Aprobarbital (Additive or potentiating effects). Products include:
- Alurate Elixir ... 1883

Buprenorphine (Additive or potentiating effects).
No products indexed under this heading.

Buspirone Hydrochloride (Additive or potentiating effects). Products include:
- BuSpar ... 1401

Butabarbital (Additive or potentiating effects). Products include:
- Pyridium Plus ... 1764

Butalbital (Additive or potentiating effects). Products include:
- Esgic-Plus Tablets ... 1002
- Esgic Tablets & Capsules ... 1001
- Fioricet Tablets ... 2006
- Fiorinal Capsules ... 2007
- Fiorinal with Codeine Capsules ... 2008
- Fiorinal Tablets ... 2007
- Phrenilin ... 838
- Sedapap Tablets 50 mg/650 mg ... 1360

Chlordiazepoxide (Additive or potentiating effects). Products include:
- Libritabs Tablets ... 1930
- Limbitrol ... 1933
- Menrium Tablets ... 1934

Chlordiazepoxide Hydrochloride (Additive or potentiating effects). Products include:
- Librax Capsules ... 1929
- Librium Capsules ... 1931
- Librium Injectable ... 1932

Chlorpromazine (Additive or potentiating effects). Products include:
- Thorazine ... 2234

Chlorprothixene (Additive or potentiating effects). Products include:
- Taractan Tablets ... 1920

Chlorprothixene Hydrochloride (Additive or potentiating effects). Products include:
- Taractan ... 1920

Clorazepate Dipotassium (Additive or potentiating effects). Products include:
- Tranxene ... 556

Codeine (Additive or potentiating effects). Products include:
- Calcidrine Syrup ... 506

Codeine Phosphate (Additive or potentiating effects). Products include:
- Actifed with Codeine Cough Syrup ... 752
- Cheracol Cough Syrup ... 1853
- Codimal PH Syrup ... 846
- Dimetane-DC Cough Syrup ... 1857
- Empirin with Codeine Phosphate Nos. 2, 3 & 4 ... 764
- Fiorinal with Codeine Capsules ... 2008
- Isoclor Expectorant ... 982
- Naldecon CX Adult Liquid ... ▣ 521
- Novahistine DH ... 1342
- Novahistine Expectorant ... 1343
- Nucofed Capsules ... 2219
- Nucofed Expectorant ... 2219
- Nucofed Pediatric Expectorant ... 2220
- Nucofed Syrup ... 2219
- Phenaphen with Codeine Capsules 1865
- Phenaphen-650 with Codeine Tablets ... 1866
- Phenergan with Codeine ... 2497
- Phenergan VC with Codeine ... 2501
- Robitussin A-C Syrup ... 1875
- Robitussin-DAC Syrup ... 1875
- Ryna ... ▣ 741
- Soma Compound w/Codeine Tablets ... 2390
- Triaminic Expectorant w/Codeine ... 1996
- Tussi-Organidin Liquid ... 2391
- Tylenol with Codeine ... 1381

Codeine Polistirex (Additive or potentiating effects).
No products indexed under this heading.

Dezocine (Additive or potentiating effects).

Diazepam (Additive or potentiating effects). Products include:
- Valium Injectable ... 1937
- Valium Tablets ... 1939
- Valrelease Capsules ... 1923

Enflurane (Additive or potentiating effects). Products include:
- Ethrane ... 599

Epinephrine (Epinephrine may cause paradoxical hypotension due to alpha blockade produced by Inapsine). Products include:
- Ana-Kit Anaphylaxis Emergency Treatment Kit ... 1100
- Bronkaid Mist ... ▣ 757
- EpiPen ... 843
- Marcaine Hydrochloride 0.5% with Epinephrine 1:200,000 (as bitartrate) ... 958
- Marcaine Hydrochloride with Epinephrine 1:200,000 ... 2055
- Primatene Mist ... 2420
- Sus-Phrine Injection ... 1006
- Xylocaine with Epinephrine Injections ... 637

Estazolam (Additive or potentiating effects). Products include:
- ProSom Tablets ... 554

Ethchlorvynol (Additive or potentiating effects). Products include:
- Placidyl Capsules ... 553

Ethinamate (Additive or potentiating effects).
No products indexed under this heading.

Fentanyl (Additive or potentiating effects). Products include:
- Duragesic Transdermal System ... 1133

Fentanyl Citrate (Additive or potentiating effects). Products include:
- Innovar Injection ... 1141
- Sublimaze Injection ... 1146

Fluphenazine Decanoate (Additive or potentiating effects). Products include:
- Prolixin Decanoate ... 1795

Fluphenazine Enanthate (Additive or potentiating effects). Products include:
- Prolixin Enanthate ... 1796

Fluphenazine Hydrochloride (Additive or potentiating effects). Products include:
- Prolixin Elixir ... 1793
- Prolixin Injection ... 1791
- Prolixin Oral Concentrate ... 1792
- Prolixin Tablets ... 1793

Flurazepam Hydrochloride (Additive or potentiating effects). Products include:
- Dalmane Capsules ... 1927

Glutethimide (Additive or potentiating effects).
No products indexed under this heading.

Haloperidol (Additive or potentiating effects). Products include:
- Haldol Injection, Tablets and Concentrate ... 1373

Haloperidol Decanoate (Additive or potentiating effects). Products include:
- Haldol Decanoate ... 1375

Hydrocodone Bitartrate (Additive or potentiating effects). Products include:
- Anexsia 5/500 Tablets ... 2196
- Anexsia 7.5/650 Tablets ... 2197
- Azdone Tablets ... 844
- Codiclear DH Syrup ... 845
- Codimal DH Syrup ... 846
- Damason-P ... 1356
- Hycodan Syrup, Tablets ... 927
- Hycomine Compound Tablets ... 929
- Hycomine Syrup ... 927
- Hycotuss Expectorant Syrup ... 930
- Hydrocet Capsules ... 835
- Lortab ASA Tablets ... 2414
- Lortab ... 2412
- Ru-Tuss with Hydrocodone ... 694
- Triaminic Expectorant DH ... 1995

Vicodin Tablets 1187
Vicodin ES Tablets 1189
Zydone Capsules 941

Hydrocodone Polistirex (Additive or potentiating effects). Products include:
Tussionex Extended-Release Suspension 988

Hydroxyzine Hydrochloride (Additive or potentiating effects). Products include:
Atarax Tablets & Syrup 1941
Marax Tablets & DF Syrup 1954
Vistaril Intramuscular Solution 1970

Isoflurane (Additive or potentiating effects). Products include:
Forane 600

Ketamine Hydrochloride (Additive or potentiating effects). Products include:
Ketalar 1726

Levorphanol Tartrate (Additive or potentiating effects). Products include:
Levo-Dromoran 1906

Lorazepam (Additive or potentiating effects). Products include:
Ativan Injection 2432
Ativan Tablets 2434

Loxapine Hydrochloride (Additive or potentiating effects). Products include:
Loxitane 1213

Loxapine Succinate (Additive or potentiating effects). Products include:
Loxitane Capsules 1213

Meperidine Hydrochloride (Additive or potentiating effects). Products include:
Demerol 2047
Mepergan Injection 2479

Mephobarbital (Additive or potentiating effects). Products include:
Mebaral Tablets 2061

Meprobamate (Additive or potentiating effects). Products include:
Deprol Tablets 2382
Equagesic Tablets 2451
Miltown Tablets 2386
PMB 200 and PMB 400 2504

Mesoridazine (Additive or potentiating effects). Products include:
Serentil 686

Methadone Hydrochloride (Additive or potentiating effects). Products include:
Dolophine Hydrochloride Ampoules & Vials 1260
Dolophine Hydrochloride Tablets 1261
Methadone Hydrochloride Diskets 1284
Methadone Hydrochloride Oral Solution & Tablets 1987

Methohexital Sodium (Additive or potentiating effects). Products include:
Brevital Sodium Vials 1248

Methoxyflurane (Additive or potentiating effects).
No products indexed under this heading.

Midazolam Hydrochloride (Additive or potentiating effects). Products include:
Versed Injection 1924

Molindone Hydrochloride (Additive or potentiating effects). Products include:
Moban Tablets & Concentrate 932

Morphine Sulfate (Additive or potentiating effects). Products include:
Astramorph/PF Injection, USP (Preservative-Free) 618
Duramorph 960
Infumorph 200 and Infumorph 500 Sterile Solutions 962
MS Contin Tablets 1814
MSIR 1817
Oramorph SR (Morphine Sulfate Sustained Release Tablets) 1988
Roxanol 1991

Opium Alkaloids (Additive or potentiating effects). Products include:
B & O No. 15A & No. 16A Supprettes 2395
Pantopon Injectable 1911

Oxazepam (Additive or potentiating effects). Products include:
Serax Capsules 2522
Serax Tablets 2522

Oxycodone Hydrochloride (Additive or potentiating effects). Products include:
Percocet Tablets 950
Percodan 951
Roxicodone Tablets, Oral Solution & Intensol (Oxycodone) 1992
Tylox Capsules 1382

Pentobarbital Sodium (Additive or potentiating effects). Products include:
Nembutal Sodium Capsules 534
Nembutal Sodium Solution 536
Nembutal Sodium Suppositories 538

Perphenazine (Additive or potentiating effects). Products include:
Etrafon 2087
Triavil Tablets 1556
Trilafon 2123

Phenobarbital (Additive or potentiating effects). Products include:
Arco-Lase Plus Tablets 607
Bellergal-S Tablets 1998
Bronkolixir .... ▣ 761
Bronkotabs Tablets .... ▣ 762
Donnatal 1858
Donnatal Extentabs 1859
Donnatal Tablets 1858
Donnazyme Tablets 1860
Kinesed Tablets 2272
Phenobarbital Elixir and Tablets 1293
Primatene Tablets-P Formula 2421
Quadrinal Tablets 1183
Tedral SA 1765

Prazepam (Additive or potentiating effects). Products include:
Centrax 1693

Prochlorperazine (Additive or potentiating effects). Products include:
Compazine 2201

Promethazine Hydrochloride (Additive or potentiating effects). Products include:
Mepergan Injection 2479
Phenergan with Codeine 2497
Phenergan with Dextromethorphan 2499
Phenergan Injection 2493
Phenergan Suppositories 2496
Phenergan Syrup 2495
Phenergan Tablets 2496
Phenergan VC 2500
Phenergan VC with Codeine 2501

Propofol (Additive or potentiating effects). Products include:
Diprivan Injection 2267

Propoxyphene Hydrochloride (Additive or potentiating effects). Products include:
Darvon 1256
Wygesic Tablets 2540

Propoxyphene Napsylate (Additive or potentiating effects). Products include:
Darvon-N/Darvocet-N 1254

Quazepam (Additive or potentiating effects). Products include:
Doral Tablets 2383

Secobarbital Sodium (Additive or potentiating effects). Products include:
Seconal Sodium Pulvules 1296

Sufentanil Citrate (Additive or potentiating effects). Products include:
Sufenta Injection 1147

Temazepam (Additive or potentiating effects). Products include:
Restoril Capsules 2023

Thiamylal Sodium (Additive or potentiating effects). Products include:
Surital Ampoules, Steri-Vials 1764

Thioridazine Hydrochloride (Additive or potentiating effects). Products include:
Mellaril 2011

Thiothixene (Additive or potentiating effects). Products include:
Navane Capsules and Concentrate 1954
Navane Intramuscular 1956

Triazolam (Additive or potentiating effects). Products include:
Halcion Tablets 2340

Trifluoperazine Hydrochloride (Additive or potentiating effects). Products include:
Stelazine 2226

INCREMIN W/IRON SYRUP

(L-Lysine, Vitamins with Iron) .... ▣ 588
No interactions described in labeling.

INDERAL INJECTABLE

(Propranolol Hydrochloride) 2459
May interact with insulin, catecholamine depleting drugs, calcium channel blockers, non-steroidal anti-inflammatory agents, and certain other agents. Compounds in these categories include:

Alcohol (Slows the rate of absorption of propranolol).

Aluminum Hydroxide (Greatly reduces intestinal absorption of propranolol). Products include:
Cama Arthritis Pain Reliever .... ▣ 685
Gaviscon Extra Strength Relief Formula Liquid Antacid .... ▣ 594
Gaviscon Extra Strength Relief Formula Antacid Tablets .... ▣ 594
Gaviscon Liquid Antacid .... ▣ 594
Gelusil Liquid & Tablets .... ▣ 639
Extra Strength Maalox Plus Suspension 1850
Maalox TC Suspension 1851
Maalox Plus Tablets .... ▣ 655
Extra Strength Maalox Plus Tablets 1850
Nephrox Suspension .... ▣ 563
WinGel Liquid & Tablets .... ▣ 761

Aluminum Hydroxide Gel (Greatly reduces intestinal absorption of propranolol). Products include:
ALternaGEL Liquid 1154
Aludrox Oral Suspension 2428
Amphojel Suspension 2429
Amphojel Suspension without Flavor 2429
Mylanta Liquid 1155
Mylanta Double Strength Liquid 1155

Aluminum Hydroxide Gel, Dried (Greatly reduces intestinal absorption of propranolol). Products include:
Alu-Tab/Alu-Cap 1309
Amphojel Tablets 2429
Ascriptin A/D Caplets 1850
Regular Strength Ascriptin Tablets 1850
Gaviscon Antacid Tablets .... ▣ 593
Gaviscon-2 Antacid Tablets .... ▣ 594
Mylanta Tablets 1155
Mylanta Double Strength Tablets 1155

Aminophylline (Reduced theophylline clearance). Products include:
Amesec .... ▣ 682
Aminophyllin Tablets 2153

Antipyrine (Reduced clearance of antipyrine). Products include:
Auralgan Otic Solution 2437

Bepridil Hydrochloride (Both agents may depress myocardial contractility or AV conduction resulting in increased adverse reactions). Products include:
Vascor (200, 300 and 400 mg) Tablets 1383

Chlorpromazine (Increased plasma levels of both drugs). Products include:
Thorazine 2234

Cimetidine (Decreases hepatic metabolism of propranolol resulting in increased blood levels). Products include:
Tagamet Tablets 2228

Cimetidine Hydrochloride (Decreases hepatic metabolism of propranolol resulting in increased blood levels). Products include:
Tagamet 2228

Deserpidine (May produce an excessive hypotension with bradycardia and orthostatic effects). Products include:
Enduronyl 518
Harmonyl Tablets 528
Oreticyl 545

Diclofenac Sodium (Blunts antihypertensive effect of beta blocker). Products include:
Voltaren Ophthalmic Sterile Ophthalmic Solution .... ◉ 268
Voltaren Tablets 1042

Diltiazem Hydrochloride (Both agents may depress myocardial contractility or AV conduction resulting in increased adverse reactions). Products include:
Cardizem Tablets-30 mg, 60 mg, 90 mg and 120 mg 1329
Cardizem SR Capsules-60 mg, 90 mg and 120 mg 1327

Dobutamine Hydrochloride (Reversed effects of propranolol). Products include:
Dobutrex Solution Vials 1259

Dyphylline (Reduced theophylline clearance). Products include:
Dilor 2079
Dilor-G Tablets & Liquid 2079
Lufyllin Elixir 2384
Lufyllin & Lufyllin-400 Tablets 2384
Lufyllin-GG Elixir & Tablets 2385

Etodolac (Blunts antihypertensive effect of beta blocker). Products include:
Lodine Capsules 2468

Felodipine (Both agents may depress myocardial contractility or AV conduction resulting in increased adverse reactions). Products include:
Plendil Extended-Release Tablets 1526

Fenoprofen Calcium (Blunts antihypertensive effect of beta blocker). Products include:
Nalfon Pulvules & Tablets 919

Flurbiprofen (Blunts antihypertensive effect of beta blocker). Products include:
Ansaid Tablets 2319

Haloperidol (Hypotension and cardiac arrest have been reported with the concomitant use of propranolol and haloperidol). Products include:
Haldol Injection, Tablets and Concentrate 1373

Haloperidol Decanoate (Hypotension and cardiac arrest have been reported with the concomitant use of propranolol and haloperidol). Products include:
Haldol Decanoate 1375

Ibuprofen (Blunts antihypertensive effect of beta blocker). Products include:
Advil Cold & Sinus Caplets (formerly CoAdvil) 2416
Advil Ibuprofen Tablets and Caplets 2416
Children's Advil Suspension 2426
CoAdvil .... ▣ 748
Dristan Sinus Caplets 2419
Haltran Tablets .... ▣ 668
Ibuprofen .... ▣ 631

Medipren ibuprofen Caplets and Tablets 1362
Midol 200 Cramp Relief Formula.. ⊞ 570
Motrin Tablets 2351
Motrin IB Caplets and Tablets ..... ⊞ 736
Nuprin Ibuprofen/Analgesic Tablets & Caplets 752
PediaProfen Suspension 1363
Rufen Tablets 691
Trendar Ibuprofen Tablets ..... ⊞ 756

Indomethacin (Blunts antihypertensive effect of beta blocker). Products include:
Indocin 1487

Indomethacin Sodium Trihydrate (Blunts antihypertensive effect of beta blocker). Products include:
Indocin I.V. 1490

Insulin, Human (Delayed recovery of blood glucose to normal levels following insulin-induced hypoglycemia).
No products indexed under this heading.

Insulin, Human Isophane Suspension (Delayed recovery of blood glucose to normal levels following insulin-induced hypoglycemia). Products include:
Humulin N, 100 Units 1270

Insulin, Human NPH (Delayed recovery of blood glucose to normal levels following insulin-induced hypoglycemia). Products include:
Insulatard NPH Human 1627
Novolin N 1627
Novolin N PenFill Cartridges 1628
Novolin N Prefilled 1628

Insulin, Human Regular (Delayed recovery of blood glucose to normal levels following insulin-induced hypoglycemia). Products include:
Humulin BR, 100 Units 1268
Humulin R, 100 Units 1272
Novolin R 1627
Novolin R PenFill Cartridges 1628
Novolin R Prefilled 1629
Velosulin Human 1628

Insulin, Human, Zinc Suspension (Delayed recovery of blood glucose to normal levels following insulin-induced hypoglycemia). Products include:
Humulin L, 100 Units 1268
Humulin U, 100 Units 1272
Novolin L 1627

Insulin, NPH (Delayed recovery of blood glucose to normal levels following insulin-induced hypoglycemia). Products include:
NPH, 40 & 100 Units 1273
Beef NPH, 100 Units 1274
Pork NPH, 100 Units 1275
Insulatard NPH 1626
NPH Insulin 1626
NPH Purified Pork Isophane Insulin 1626

Insulin, Regular (Delayed recovery of blood glucose to normal levels following insulin-induced hypoglycemia). Products include:
Regular, 40 & 100 Units 1273
Beef Regular, 100 Units 1275
Pork Regular, 100 Units 1275
Pork Regular (Concentrated), 500 Units 1276
Regular Insulin 1625
Regular Purified Pork Insulin 1626
Velosulin 1627

Insulin, Zinc Crystals (Delayed recovery of blood glucose to normal levels following insulin-induced hypoglycemia). Products include:
NPH, 40 & 100 Units 1273

Insulin, Zinc Suspension (Delayed recovery of blood glucose to normal levels following insulin-induced hypoglycemia). Products include:
Lente, 40 & 100 Units 1272
Protamine, Zinc, 40 & 100 Units 1273
Lente Iletin I 1272
Beef Lente, 100 Units 1274
Beef Protamine Zinc, 100 Units 1274
Pork Lente, 100 Units 1275
Pork, Protamine, Zinc, 100 Units 1275
Lente Insulin 1626
Lente Purified Pork Insulin 1626
Semilente Insulin 1625
Ultralente Insulin 1626

Isoproterenol Hydrochloride (Reversed effects of propranolol). Products include:
Isuprel Hydrochloride Injection 1:5000 2050
Isuprel Hydrochloride Mistometer .. 2051
Isuprel Hydrochloride Solution 1:200 & 1:100 2052
Norisodrine Aerotrol 540

Isoproterenol Sulfate (Reversed effects of propranolol).
No products indexed under this heading.

Isradipine (Both agents may depress myocardial contractility or AV conduction resulting in increased adverse reactions). Products include:
DynaCirc Capsules 2004

Ketoprofen (Blunts antihypertensive effect of beta blocker). Products include:
Orudis Capsules 2488

Ketorolac Tromethamine (Blunts antihypertensive effect of beta blocker). Products include:
Toradol IM Injection 2302

Lidocaine Hydrochloride (Reduced clearance of lidocaine). Products include:
Anestacon Solution 2394
Bactine Antiseptic/Anesthetic First Aid Spray ..... ⊞ 624
Decadron Phosphate with Xylocaine Injection, Sterile 1451
Xylocaine Injections 637
Xylocaine Injections for Ventricular Arrhythmias 639
Xylocaine 2% Jelly 643
4% Xylocaine-MPF Sterile Solution 641
Xylocaine 2% Viscous Solution 646

Meclofenamate Sodium (Blunts antihypertensive effect of beta blocker). Products include:
Meclomen Capsules 1739

Mefenamic Acid (Blunts antihypertensive effect of beta blocker). Products include:
Ponstel 1758

Naproxen (Blunts antihypertensive effect of beta blocker). Products include:
Naprosyn 2297

Naproxen Sodium (Blunts antihypertensive effect of beta blocker). Products include:
Anaprox and Anaprox DS Tablets 2288

Nicardipine Hydrochloride (Both agents may depress myocardial contractility or AV conduction resulting in increased adverse reactions). Products include:
Cardene Capsules 2290

Nifedipine (Both agents may depress myocardial contractility or AV conduction resulting in increased adverse reactions). Products include:
Adalat Capsules (10 mg and 20 mg) 1587
Procardia Capsules 1781
Procardia XL Tablets 1783

Nimodipine (Both agents may depress myocardial contractility or AV conduction resulting in increased adverse reactions). Products include:
Nimotop Capsules 1607

Phenobarbital (Accelerates propranolol clearance). Products include:
Arco-Lase Plus Tablets 607
Bellergal-S Tablets 1998
Bronkolixir ..... ⊞ 761
Bronkotabs Tablets ..... ⊞ 762
Donnatal 1858
Donnatal Extentabs 1859
Donnatal Tablets 1858
Donnazyme Tablets 1860
Kinesed Tablets 2272
Phenobarbital Elixir and Tablets 1293
Primatene Tablets-P Formula 2421
Quadrinal Tablets 1183
Tedral SA 1765

Phenylbutazone (Blunts antihypertensive effect of beta blocker). Products include:
Butazolidin Capsules & Tablets 1027

Phenytoin (Accelerates propranolol clearance). Products include:
Dilantin Infatabs 1710
Dilantin-30 Pediatric/Dilantin-125 Suspension 1713

Phenytoin Sodium (Accelerates propranolol clearance). Products include:
Dilantin Kapseals 1708
Dilantin Parenteral 1712
Dilantin with Phenobarbital Kapseals 1715

Piroxicam (Blunts antihypertensive effect of beta blocker). Products include:
Feldene Capsules 1777

Rauwolfia Serpentina (May produce an excessive hypotension with bradycardia and orthostatic effects). Products include:
Raudixin Tablets 1803
Rauzide Tablets 1804

Rescinnamine (May produce an excessive hypotension with bradycardia and orthostatic effects).
No products indexed under this heading.

Reserpine (May produce an excessive hypotension with bradycardia and orthostatic effects). Products include:
Diupres Tablets 1461
Hydromox R Tablets 1209
Hydropres Tablets 1485
Renese-R Tablets 1786
Salutensin/Salutensin-Demi 719
Ser-Ap-Es Tablets 881
Serpasil Tablets 883
Serpasil-Apresoline Tablets 884
Serpasil-Esidrix Tablets 886

Rifampin (Accelerates propranolol clearance). Products include:
Rifadin 1345
Rifamate Capsules 1347
Rimactane Capsules 879

Sulindac (Blunts antihypertensive effect of beta blocker). Products include:
Clinoril Tablets 1433

Theophylline (Reduced theophylline clearance). Products include:
Bronkaid Tablets ..... ⊞ 757
Bronkolixir ..... ⊞ 761
Bronkotabs Tablets ..... ⊞ 762
Constant-T Tablets 1029
Marax Tablets & DF Syrup 1954
Primatene Tablets 2421
Quibron Capsules 713
Quibron-T 714
Quibron-T/SR 716
Theolair Liquid 1317
Theo-Organidin Elixir 2391

Theophylline Anhydrous (Reduced theophylline clearance). Products include:
Aerolate 994
Primatene Tablets-M Formula ..... ⊞ 753
Primatene Tablets-Regular Formula 2421
Respbid Tablets 684
Slo-bid Gyrocaps 1847
T-PHYL (Uniphyl) 200 mg Tablets 1820
Tedral SA 1765
Theo-24 2179
Theo-Dur Sprinkle 1168
Theo-Dur Extended-Release Tablets 1166
Theolair Tablets 1317
Theolair-SR Tablets 1319
TheoX Extended-Release Tablets 841
Uniphyl 400 mg Tablets 1823

Theophylline Calcium Salicylate (Reduced theophylline clearance). Products include:
Quadrinal Tablets 1183

Theophylline Sodium Glycinate (Reduced theophylline clearance). Products include:
Asbron G 1997

Thyroxine (Lower than expected T3 concentration).
No products indexed under this heading.

Thyroxine Sodium (Lower than expected T3 concentration).
No products indexed under this heading.

Tolmetin Sodium (Blunts antihypertensive effect of beta blocker). Products include:
Tolectin (200, 400 and 600 mg) .. 1379

Verapamil Hydrochloride (Both agents may depress myocardial contractility or AV conduction resulting in increased adverse reactions). Products include:
Calan SR Caplets 2157
Calan Tablets 2155
Isoptin Injectable 1177
Isoptin Oral Tablets 1179
Isoptin SR Sustained Release Tablets 1181
Verelan Capsules 1243
Verelan Capsules 2535

INDERAL TABLETS
(Propranolol Hydrochloride) 2459
See **Inderal Injectable**

INDERAL LA LONG ACTING CAPSULES
(Propranolol Hydrochloride) 2461
May interact with catecholamine depleting drugs, calcium channel blockers, insulin, and certain other agents. Compounds in these categories include:

Alcohol (Absorption rate of propranolol slowed).

Aluminum Hydroxide Gel (Intestinal absorption of propranolol greatly reduced). Products include:
ALternaGEL Liquid 1154
Aludrox Oral Suspension 2428
Amphojel Suspension 2429
Amphojel Suspension without Flavor 2429
Mylanta Liquid 1155
Mylanta Double Strength Liquid 1155

Antipyrine (Reduced clearance of antipyrine). Products include:
Auralgan Otic Solution 2437

Bepridil Hydrochloride (Caution should be exercised when administered concomitantly). Products include:
Vascor (200, 300 and 400 mg) Tablets 1383

Chlorpromazine (Increased plasma levels of both drugs). Products include:
Thorazine 2234

Cimetidine (Delayed elimination and increased blood levels of propranolol). Products include:
Tagamet Tablets 2228

Cimetidine Hydrochloride (Delayed elimination and increased blood levels of propranolol). Products include:
Tagamet 2228

Deserpidine (May produce excessive hypotension with bradycardia and orthostatic effects). Products include:
Enduronyl 518
Harmonyl Tablets 528
Oreticyl 545

Diltiazem Hydrochloride (Caution should be exercised when administered concomitantly). Products include:
- Cardizem Tablets-30 mg, 60 mg, 90 mg and 120 mg ... 1329
- Cardizem SR Capsules-60 mg, 90 mg and 120 mg ... 1327

Felodipine (Caution should be exercised when administered concomitantly). Products include:
- Plendil Extended-Release Tablets ... 1526

Insulin, Human (Delayed recovery of blood glucose to normal levels following insulin-induced hypoglycemia).
- No products indexed under this heading.

Insulin, Human Isophane Suspension (Delayed recovery of blood glucose to normal levels following insulin-induced hypoglycemia). Products include:
- Humulin N, 100 Units ... 1270

Insulin, Human NPH (Delayed recovery of blood glucose to normal levels following insulin-induced hypoglycemia). Products include:
- Insulatard NPH Human ... 1627
- Novolin N ... 1627
- Novolin N PenFill Cartridges ... 1628
- Novolin N Prefilled ... 1628

Insulin, Human Regular (Delayed recovery of blood glucose to normal levels following insulin-induced hypoglycemia). Products include:
- Humulin BR, 100 Units ... 1268
- Humulin R, 100 Units ... 1272
- Novolin R ... 1627
- Novolin R PenFill Cartridges ... 1628
- Novolin R Prefilled ... 1629
- Velosulin Human ... 1628

Insulin, Human, Zinc Suspension (Delayed recovery of blood glucose to normal levels following insulin-induced hypoglycemia). Products include:
- Humulin L, 100 Units ... 1268
- Humulin U, 100 Units ... 1272
- Novolin L ... 1627

Insulin, NPH (Delayed recovery of blood glucose to normal levels following insulin-induced hypoglycemia). Products include:
- NPH, 40 & 100 Units ... 1273
- Beef NPH, 100 Units ... 1274
- Pork NPH, 100 Units ... 1275
- Insulatard NPH ... 1626
- NPH Insulin ... 1626
- NPH Purified Pork Isophane Insulin ... 1626

Insulin, Regular (Delayed recovery of blood glucose to normal levels following insulin-induced hypoglycemia). Products include:
- Regular, 40 & 100 Units ... 1273
- Beef Regular, 100 Units ... 1275
- Pork Regular, 100 Units ... 1275
- Pork Regular (Concentrated), 500 Units ... 1276
- Regular Insulin ... 1625
- Regular Purified Pork Insulin ... 1626
- Velosulin ... 1627

Insulin, Zinc Crystals (Delayed recovery of blood glucose to normal levels following insulin-induced hypoglycemia). Products include:
- NPH, 40 & 100 Units ... 1273

Insulin, Zinc Suspension (Delayed recovery of blood glucose to normal levels following insulin-induced hypoglycemia). Products include:
- Lente, 40 & 100 Units ... 1272
- Protamine, Zinc, 40 & 100 Units ... 1273
- Lente Iletin I ... 1272
- Beef Lente, 100 Units ... 1274
- Beef Protamine Zinc, 100 Units ... 1274
- Pork Lente, 100 Units ... 1275
- Pork, Protamine, Zinc, 100 Units ... 1275
- Lente Insulin ... 1626
- Lente Purified Pork Insulin ... 1626
- Semilente Insulin ... 1625
- Ultralente Insulin ... 1626

Isradipine (Caution should be exercised when administered concomitantly). Products include:
- DynaCirc Capsules ... 2004

Lidocaine Hydrochloride (Reduced clearance of lidocaine). Products include:
- Anestacon Solution ... 2394
- Bactine Antiseptic/Anesthetic First Aid Spray ... ◘ 624
- Decadron Phosphate with Xylocaine Injection, Sterile ... 1451
- Xylocaine Injections ... 637
- Xylocaine Injections for Ventricular Arrhythmias ... 639
- Xylocaine 2% Jelly ... 643
- 4% Xylocaine-MPF Sterile Solution ... 641
- Xylocaine 2% Viscous Solution ... 646

Nicardipine Hydrochloride (Caution should be exercised when administered concomitantly). Products include:
- Cardene Capsules ... 2290

Nifedipine (Caution should be exercised when administered concomitantly). Products include:
- Adalat Capsules (10 mg and 20 mg) ... 1587
- Procardia Capsules ... 1781
- Procardia XL Tablets ... 1783

Nimodipine (Caution should be exercised when administered concomitantly). Products include:
- Nimotop Capsules ... 1607

Phenobarbital (Propranolol clearance accelerated). Products include:
- Arco-Lase Plus Tablets ... 607
- Bellergal-S Tablets ... 1998
- Bronkolixir ... ◘ 761
- Bronkotabs Tablets ... ◘ 762
- Donnatal ... 1858
- Donnatal Extentabs ... 1859
- Donnatal Tablets ... 1858
- Donnazyme Tablets ... 1860
- Kinesed Tablets ... 2272
- Phenobarbital Elixir and Tablets ... 1293
- Primatene Tablets-P Formula ... 2421
- Quadrinal Tablets ... 1183
- Tedral SA ... 1765

Phenytoin (Propranolol clearance accelerated). Products include:
- Dilantin Infatabs ... 1710
- Dilantin-30 Pediatric/Dilantin-125 Suspension ... 1713

Phenytoin Sodium (Propranolol clearance accelerated). Products include:
- Dilantin Kapseals ... 1708
- Dilantin Parenteral ... 1712
- Dilantin with Phenobarbital Kapseals ... 1715

Rauwolfia Serpentina (May produce excessive hypotension with bradycardia and orthostatic effects). Products include:
- Raudixin Tablets ... 1803
- Rauzide Tablets ... 1804

Rescinnamine (May produce excessive hypotension with bradycardia and orthostatic effects).
- No products indexed under this heading.

Reserpine (May produce excessive hypotension with bradycardia and orthostatic effects). Products include:
- Diupres Tablets ... 1461
- Hydromox R Tablets ... 1209
- Hydropres Tablets ... 1485
- Renese-R Tablets ... 1786
- Salutensin/Salutensin-Demi ... 719
- Ser-Ap-Es Tablets ... 881
- Serpasil Tablets ... 883
- Serpasil-Apresoline Tablets ... 884
- Serpasil-Esidrix Tablets ... 886

Rifampin (Propranolol clearance accelerated). Products include:
- Rifadin ... 1345
- Rifamate Capsules ... 1347
- Rimactane Capsules ... 879

Theophylline (Reduced theophylline clearance). Products include:
- Bronkaid Tablets ... ◘ 757
- Bronkolixir ... ◘ 761
- Bronkotabs Tablets ... ◘ 762
- Constant-T Tablets ... 1029
- Marax Tablets & DF Syrup ... 1954
- Primatene Tablets ... 2421
- Quibron Capsules ... 713
- Quibron-T ... 714
- Quibron-T/SR ... 716
- Theolair Liquid ... 1317
- Theo-Organidin Elixir ... 2391

Theophylline Anhydrous (Reduced theophylline clearance). Products include:
- Aerolate ... 994
- Primatene Tablets-M Formula ... ◘ 753
- Primatene Tablets-Regular Formula ... 2421
- Respbid Tablets ... 684
- Slo-bid Gyrocaps ... 1847
- T-PHYL (Uniphyl) 200 mg Tablets ... 1820
- Tedral SA ... 1765
- Theo-24 ... 2179
- Theo-Dur Sprinkle ... 1168
- Theo-Dur Extended-Release Tablets ... 1166
- Theolair Tablets ... 1317
- Theolair-SR Tablets ... 1319
- TheoX Extended-Release Tablets ... 841
- Uniphyl 400 mg Tablets ... 1823

Theophylline Calcium Salicylate (Reduced theophylline clearance). Products include:
- Quadrinal Tablets ... 1183

Theophylline Sodium Glycinate (Reduced theophylline clearance). Products include:
- Asbron G ... 1997

Thyroxine (Lower-than-expected T3 concentration may result).
- No products indexed under this heading.

Verapamil Hydrochloride (Intravenous use of beta blocker and verapamil has resulted in serious adverse reactions in patients with severe cardiomyopathy, CHF or recent MI). Products include:
- Calan SR Caplets ... 2157
- Calan Tablets ... 2155
- Isoptin Injectable ... 1177
- Isoptin Oral Tablets ... 1179
- Isoptin SR Sustained Release Tablets ... 1181
- Verelan Capsules ... 1243
- Verelan Capsules ... 2535

INDERIDE TABLETS

(Propranolol Hydrochloride, Hydrochlorothiazide) ... 2463

May interact with antihypertensives, para-aminobenzoic acid based local anesthetics, catecholamine depleting drugs, cardiac glycosides, corticosteroids, calcium channel blockers, ganglionic blocking agents, insulin, non-steroidal anti-inflammatory agents, barbiturates, narcotic analgesics, xanthine bronchodilators, and certain other agents. Compounds in these categories include:

Acebutolol Hydrochloride (Potentiated or additive action). Products include:
- Sectral Capsules ... 2520

ACTH (Hypokalemia).
- No products indexed under this heading.

Alcohol (Slows the rate of absorption of propranolol).

Alfentanil Hydrochloride (Aggravates orthostatic hypotension). Products include:
- Alfenta Injection ... 1131

Aluminum Hydroxide (Greatly reduces intestinal absorption of propranolol). Products include:
- Cama Arthritis Pain Reliever ... ◘ 685
- Gaviscon Extra Strength Relief Formula Liquid Antacid ... ◘ 594
- Gaviscon Extra Strength Relief Formula Antacid Tablets ... ◘ 594
- Gaviscon Liquid Antacid ... ◘ 594
- Gelusil Liquid & Tablets ... ◘ 639
- Extra Strength Maalox Plus Suspension ... 1850
- Maalox TC Suspension ... 1851
- Maalox Plus Tablets ... ◘ 655
- Extra Strength Maalox Plus Tablets ... 1850
- Nephrox Suspension ... ◘ 563
- WinGel Liquid & Tablets ... ◘ 761

Aluminum Hydroxide Gel (Greatly reduces intestinal absorption of propranolol). Products include:
- ALternaGEL Liquid ... 1154
- Aludrox Oral Suspension ... 2428
- Amphojel Suspension ... 2429
- Amphojel Suspension without Flavor ... 2429
- Mylanta Liquid ... 1155
- Mylanta Double Strength Liquid ... 1155

Aluminum Hydroxide Gel, Dried (Greatly reduces intestinal absorption of propranolol). Products include:
- Alu-Tab/Alu-Cap ... 1309
- Amphojel Tablets ... 2429
- Ascriptin A/D Caplets ... 1850
- Regular Strength Ascriptin Tablets ... 1850
- Gaviscon Antacid Tablets ... ◘ 593
- Gaviscon-2 Antacid Tablets ... ◘ 594
- Mylanta Tablets ... 1155
- Mylanta Double Strength Tablets ... 1155

Aminophylline (Reduced theophylline clearance). Products include:
- Amesec ... ◘ 682
- Aminophyllin Tablets ... 2153

Antipyrine (Reduced clearance of antipyrine). Products include:
- Auralgan Otic Solution ... 2437

Aprobarbital (Aggravates orthostatic hypotension). Products include:
- Alurate Elixir ... 1883

Atenolol (Potentiated or additive action). Products include:
- Tenoretic Tablets ... 1105
- Tenormin Tablets and I.V. Injection ... 1107

Benazepril Hydrochloride (Potentiated or additive action). Products include:
- Lotensin Tablets ... 872

Bendroflumethiazide (Potentiated or additive action). Products include:
- Corzide Tablets ... 702
- Naturetin Tablets ... 1789
- Rauzide Tablets ... 1804

Bepridil Hydrochloride (Both agents may depress myocardial contractility or AV conduction resulting in increased adverse reactions). Products include:
- Vascor (200, 300 and 400 mg) Tablets ... 1383

Betamethasone Acetate (Hypokalemia). Products include:
- Celestone Soluspan Suspension ... 2081

Betamethasone Sodium Phosphate (Hypokalemia). Products include:
- Celestone Soluspan Suspension ... 2081

Betaxolol Hydrochloride (Potentiated or additive action). Products include:
- Betoptic Sterile Ophthalmic Solution ... 569
- Betoptic S Sterile Ophthalmic Suspension ... 570
- Kerlone Tablets ... 2172

Buprenorphine (Aggravates orthostatic hypotension).
- No products indexed under this heading.

Butabarbital (Aggravates orthostatic hypotension). Products include:
- Pyridium Plus ... 1764

Butalbital (Aggravates orthostatic hypotension). Products include:
- Esgic-Plus Tablets 1002
- Esgic Tablets & Capsules 1001
- Fioricet Tablets 2006
- Fiorinal Capsules 2007
- Fiorinal with Codeine Capsules 2008
- Fiorinal Tablets 2007
- Phrenilin 838
- Sedapap Tablets 50 mg/650 mg .. 1360

Captopril (Potentiated or additive action). Products include:
- Capoten 2255
- Capozide 2258

Carteolol Hydrochloride (Potentiated or additive action). Products include:
- Cartrol Tablets 507

Chlorothiazide (Potentiated or additive action). Products include:
- Aldoclor Tablets 1413
- Diupres Tablets 1461
- Diuril Oral 1464

Chlorothiazide Sodium (Potentiated or additive action). Products include:
- Diuril Sodium Intravenous 1463

Chlorpromazine (Increased plasma levels of both drugs). Products include:
- Thorazine 2234

Chlorthalidone (Potentiated or additive action). Products include:
- Combipres Tablets 678
- Tenoretic Tablets 1105
- Thalitone Tablets 687

Cimetidine (Decreases hepatic metabolism of propranolol resulting in increased blood levels). Products include:
- Tagamet Tablets 2228

Cimetidine Hydrochloride (Decreases hepatic metabolism of propranolol resulting in increased blood levels). Products include:
- Tagamet 2228

Clonidine (Potentiated or additive action). Products include:
- Catapres-TTS 677

Clonidine Hydrochloride (Potentiated or additive action). Products include:
- Catapres Tablets 676
- Combipres Tablets 678

Codeine (Aggravates orthostatic hypotension). Products include:
- Calcidrine Syrup 506

Codeine Phosphate (Aggravates orthostatic hypotension). Products include:
- Actifed with Codeine Cough Syrup.. 752
- Cheracol Cough Syrup 1853
- Codimal PH Syrup 846
- Dimetane-DC Cough Syrup 1857
- Empirin with Codeine Phosphate Nos. 2, 3 & 4 764
- Fiorinal with Codeine Capsules 2008
- Isoclor Expectorant 982
- Naldecon CX Adult Liquid .... ▣ 521
- Novahistine DH 1342
- Novahistine Expectorant 1343
- Nucofed Capsules 2219
- Nucofed Expectorant 2219
- Nucofed Pediatric Expectorant 2220
- Nucofed Syrup 2219
- Phenaphen with Codeine Capsules 1865
- Phenaphen-650 with Codeine Tablets 1866
- Phenergan with Codeine 2497
- Phenergan VC with Codeine 2501
- Robitussin A-C Syrup 1875
- Robitussin-DAC Syrup 1875
- Ryna .... ▣ 741
- Soma Compound w/Codeine Tablets 2390
- Triaminic Expectorant w/Codeine .. 1996
- Tussi-Organidin Liquid 2391
- Tylenol with Codeine 1381

Codeine Polistirex (Aggravates orthostatic hypotension).
- No products indexed under this heading.

Cortisone Acetate (Hypokalemia). Products include:
- Cortone Acetate Sterile Suspension 1437
- Cortone Acetate Tablets 1439

Deserpidine (May produce an excessive hypotension with bradycardia and orthostatic effects). Products include:
- Enduronyl 518
- Harmonyl Tablets 528
- Oreticyl 545

Deslanoside (Hypokalemia can sensitize or exaggerate the response of the heart to digitalis toxicity).
- No products indexed under this heading.

Dexamethasone (Hypokalemia). Products include:
- AK-Trol Ointment & Suspension .... ◉ 207
- Decadron Elixir 1445
- Decadron Tablets 1447
- Decaspray Topical Aerosol 1459
- Dexacidin .... ◉ 272
- Maxidex Sterile Ophthalmic Suspension .... ◉ 223
- Maxitrol Ophthalmic Ointment/Suspension .... ◉ 223
- TobraDex Ophthalmic Suspension and Ointment .... ◉ 228

Dexamethasone Acetate (Hypokalemia). Products include:
- Dalalone D.P. Injectable 999
- Decadron-LA Sterile Suspension 1457

Dexamethasone Sodium Phosphate (Hypokalemia). Products include:
- AK-Dex .... ◉ 203
- Decadron Phosphate Respihaler 1454
- Decadron Phosphate Sterile Ophthalmic Ointment 1453
- Decadron Phosphate Sterile Ophthalmic Solution 1453
- Decadron Phosphate Topical Cream 1455
- Decadron Phosphate Turbinaire 1456
- Maxidex Sterile Ophthalmic Ointment .... ◉ 222
- NeoDecadron Sterile Ophthalmic Ointment 1517
- NeoDecadron Sterile Ophthalmic Solution 1518
- NeoDecadron Topical Cream 1518

Dezocine (Aggravates orthostatic hypotension).

Diazoxide (Potentiated or additive action). Products include:
- Hyperstat I.V. Injection 2095
- Proglycem 649

Diclofenac Sodium (Blunting of the antihypertensive effect). Products include:
- Voltaren Ophthalmic Sterile Ophthalmic Solution .... ◉ 268
- Voltaren Tablets 1042

Digitoxin (Hypokalemia can sensitize or exaggerate the response of the heart to digitalis toxicity). Products include:
- Crystodigin Tablets 1253

Digoxin (Hypokalemia can sensitize or exaggerate the response of the heart to digitalis toxicity). Products include:
- Lanoxicaps 772
- Lanoxin Elixir Pediatric 775
- Lanoxin Injection 778
- Lanoxin Injection Pediatric 781
- Lanoxin Tablets 783

Diltiazem Hydrochloride (Both agents may depress myocardial contractility or AV conduction resulting in increased adverse reactions). Products include:
- Cardizem Tablets-30 mg, 60 mg, 90 mg and 120 mg 1329
- Cardizem SR Capsules-60 mg, 90 mg and 120 mg 1327

Doxazosin Mesylate (Potentiated or additive action). Products include:
- Cardura Tablets 1941

Dyphylline (Reduced theophylline clearance). Products include:
- Dilor 2079
- Dilor-G Tablets & Liquid 2079
- Lufyllin Elixir 2384
- Lufyllin & Lufyllin-400 Tablets 2384
- Lufyllin-GG Elixir & Tablets 2385

Enalapril Maleate (Potentiated or additive action). Products include:
- Vaseretic Tablets 1559
- Vasotec Tablets 1564

Enalaprilat (Potentiated or additive action). Products include:
- Vasotec I.V. 1562

Esmolol Hydrochloride (Potentiated or additive action). Products include:
- Brevibloc Injection 942

Etodolac (Blunting of the antihypertensive effect). Products include:
- Lodine Capsules 2468

Felodipine (Potentiated or additive action). Products include:
- Plendil Extended-Release Tablets 1526

Fenoprofen Calcium (Blunting of the antihypertensive effect). Products include:
- Nalfon Pulvules & Tablets 919

Fentanyl (Aggravates orthostatic hypotension). Products include:
- Duragesic Transdermal System 1133

Fentanyl Citrate (Aggravates orthostatic hypotension). Products include:
- Innovar Injection 1141
- Sublimaze Injection 1146

Flurbiprofen (Blunting of the antihypertensive effect). Products include:
- Ansaid Tablets 2319

Fosinopril Sodium (Potentiated or additive action). Products include:
- Monopril Tablets 1406

Furosemide (Potentiated or additive action). Products include:
- Lasix 1093

Guanabenz Acetate (Potentiated or additive action). Products include:
- Wytensin Tablets 2542

Guanethidine Monosulfate (Potentiation). Products include:
- Esimil Tablets 864
- Ismelin Tablets 869

Haloperidol (Concomitant use may result in hypotension and coronary arrest). Products include:
- Haldol Injection, Tablets and Concentrate 1373

Haloperidol Decanoate (Concomitant use may result in hypotension and coronary arrest). Products include:
- Haldol Decanoate 1375

Hydralazine Hydrochloride (Potentiated or additive action). Products include:
- Apresazide Capsules 854
- Apresoline Hydrochloride Parenteral (Ampuls) 856
- Apresoline Hydrochloride Tablets .. 855
- Apresoline-Esidrix Tablets 857
- Ser-Ap-Es Tablets 881
- Serpasil-Apresoline Tablets 884

Hydrocodone Bitartrate (Aggravates orthostatic hypotension). Products include:
- Anexsia 5/500 Tablets 2196
- Anexsia 7.5/650 Tablets 2197
- Azdōne Tablets 844
- Codiclear DH Syrup 845
- Codimal DH Syrup 846
- Damason-P 1356
- Hycodan Syrup, Tablets 927
- Hycomine Compound Tablets 929
- Hycomine Syrup 927
- Hycotuss Expectorant Syrup 930
- Hydrocet Capsules 835
- Lortab ASA Tablets 2414
- Lortab 2412
- Ru-Tuss with Hydrocodone 694
- Triaminic Expectorant DH 1995
- Vicodin Tablets 1187
- Vicodin ES Tablets 1189
- Zydone Capsules 941

Hydrocodone Polistirex (Aggravates orthostatic hypotension). Products include:
- Tussionex Extended-Release Suspension 988

Hydrocortisone (Hypokalemia). Products include:
- AK-Spore H.C. .... ◉ 206
- Bactine Hydrocortisone Anti-Itch Cream .... ▣ 625
- CaldeCORT Anti-Itch Hydrocortisone Spray .... ▣ 560
- Carmol HC Cream 1% 2296
- Cortaid Spray .... ▣ 735
- Cortenema 2244
- Cortisporin Ointment 758
- Cortisporin Ophthalmic Ointment Sterile 758
- Cortisporin Ophthalmic Suspension Sterile 759
- Cortisporin Otic Solution Sterile 760
- Cortisporin Otic Suspension Sterile 760
- Cortizone-5 Creme & Ointment .... ▣ 732
- Dermolate Anti-Itch Cream .... ▣ 697
- Eldecort Cream 1.0% 1113
- Eldecort Cream 1.0% and 2.5% 1113
- Fungoid HC Creme 1770
- Hydrocortone Tablets 1482
- Hytone 909
- LazerSporin-C Solution 1770
- Massengill Medicated Soft Cloth Towelettes 2192
- Nutracort Cream & Lotion 1684
- PediOtic Suspension Sterile 797
- Synacort Creams 1%, 2.5% 2296
- Vanoxide-HC Acne Lotion 911
- Vioform-Hydrocortisone Cream and Mild Cream 889
- Vioform-Hydrocortisone Ointment .. 889
- VōSoL HC Otic Solution 2392
- Vytone Cream 1% 911

Hydrocortisone Acetate (Hypokalemia). Products include:
- Analpram-HC Rectal Cream 1% and 2.5% 970
- Anusol-HC Cream 1690
- Anusol-HC Suppositories 1691
- Caldecort .... ▣ 560
- Carmol HC Cream 1% 2296
- Chloromycetin Hydrocortisone Ophthalmic 1694
- Coly-Mycin S Otic w/Neomycin & Hydrocortisone 1708
- Cortaid .... ▣ 735
- Cortef Feminine Itch Cream .... ▣ 735
- Corticaine .... ▣ 682
- Cortifoam 1827
- Cortisporin Cream 757
- Epifoam 1828
- Gynecort 5 Creme .... ▣ 556
- Hydrocortone Acetate Sterile Suspension 1479
- Lanacort 5 Creme and Ointment .. ▣ 557
- Mantadil Cream 789
- Ophthocort .... ◉ 301
- Orabase HCA Oral Paste 890
- Pramosone Cream, Lotion & Ointment 971
- ProctoCream-HC 1834
- Proctofoam-HC 1835

Hydrocortisone Sodium Phosphate (Hypokalemia). Products include:
- Hydrocortone Phosphate Injection, Sterile 1481

Hydrocortisone Sodium Succinate (Hypokalemia). Products include:
- Solu-Cortef Sterile Powder 2361

Hydroflumethiazide (Potentiated or additive action). Products include:
- Diucardin Tablets 2450
- Saluron 718
- Salutensin/Salutensin-Demi 719

Ibuprofen (Blunting of the antihypertensive effect). Products include:
- Advil Cold & Sinus Caplets (formerly CoAdvil) 2416
- Advil Ibuprofen Tablets and Caplets 2416
- Children's Advil Suspension 2426
- CoAdvil .... ▣ 748
- Dristan Sinus Caplets 2419

(▣ Described in PDR For Nonprescription Drugs) (◉ Described in PDR For Ophthalmology)

Haltran Tablets ⊞ 668
Ibuprofen ⊞ 631
Medipren ibuprofen Caplets and Tablets 1362
Midol 200 Cramp Relief Formula ⊞ 570
Motrin Tablets 2351
Motrin IB Caplets and Tablets ⊞ 736
Nuprin Ibuprofen/Analgesic Tablets & Caplets 752
PediaProfen Suspension 1363
Rufen Tablets 691
Trendar Ibuprofen Tablets ⊞ 756

Indapamide (Potentiated or additive action). Products include:
Lozol Tablets 1843

Indomethacin (Blunting of the antihypertensive effect). Products include:
Indocin 1487

Indomethacin Sodium Trihydrate (Blunting of the antihypertensive effect). Products include:
Indocin I.V. 1490

Insulin, Human (Insulin requirements may be altered).
No products indexed under this heading.

Insulin, Human Isophane Suspension (Insulin requirements may be altered). Products include:
Humulin N, 100 Units 1270

Insulin, Human NPH (Insulin requirements may be altered). Products include:
Insulatard NPH Human 1627
Novolin N 1627
Novolin N PenFill Cartridges 1628
Novolin N Prefilled 1628

Insulin, Human Regular (Insulin requirements may be altered). Products include:
Humulin BR, 100 Units 1268
Humulin R, 100 Units 1272
Novolin R 1627
Novolin R PenFill Cartridges 1628
Novolin R Prefilled 1629
Velosulin Human 1628

Insulin, Human, Zinc Suspension (Insulin requirements may be altered). Products include:
Humulin L, 100 Units 1268
Humulin U, 100 Units 1272
Novolin L 1627

Insulin, NPH (Insulin requirements may be altered). Products include:
NPH, 40 & 100 Units 1273
Beef NPH, 100 Units 1274
Pork NPH, 100 Units 1275
Insulatard NPH 1626
NPH Insulin 1626
NPH Purified Pork Isophane Insulin 1626

Insulin, Regular (Insulin requirements may be altered). Products include:
Regular, 40 & 100 Units 1273
Beef Regular, 100 Units 1275
Pork Regular, 100 Units 1275
Pork Regular (Concentrated), 500 Units 1276
Regular Insulin 1625
Regular Purified Pork Insulin 1626
Velosulin 1627

Insulin, Zinc Crystals (Insulin requirements may be altered). Products include:
NPH, 40 & 100 Units 1273

Insulin, Zinc Suspension (Insulin requirements may be altered). Products include:
Lente, 40 & 100 Units 1272
Protamine, Zinc, 40 & 100 Units 1273
Lente Iletin I 1272
Beef Lente, 100 Units 1274
Beef Protamine Zinc, 100 Units 1274
Pork Lente, 100 Units 1275
Pork, Protamine, Zinc, 100 Units 1275
Lente Insulin 1626
Lente Purified Pork Insulin 1626
Semilente Insulin 1625
Ultralente Insulin 1626

Isoproterenol Hydrochloride (Effects of propranolol reversed). Products include:
Isuprel Hydrochloride Injection 1:5000 2050
Isuprel Hydrochloride Mistometer 2051
Isuprel Hydrochloride Solution 1:200 & 1:100 2052
Norisodrine Aerotrol 540

Isoproterenol Sulfate (Effects of propranolol reversed).
No products indexed under this heading.

Isradipine (Potentiated or additive action). Products include:
DynaCirc Capsules 2004

Ketoprofen (Blunting of the antihypertensive effect). Products include:
Orudis Capsules 2488

Ketorolac Tromethamine (Blunting of the antihypertensive effect). Products include:
Toradol IM Injection 2302

Labetalol Hydrochloride (Potentiated or additive action). Products include:
Normodyne Injection 2108
Normodyne Tablets 2110
Normozide Tablets 2112
Trandate HCT Tablets 579
Trandate Injection 577
Trandate Tablets 579

Levorphanol Tartrate (Aggravates orthostatic hypotension). Products include:
Levo-Dromoran 1906

Lidocaine Hydrochloride (Reduced clearance of lidocaine). Products include:
Anestacon Solution 2394
Bactine Antiseptic/Anesthetic First Aid Spray ⊞ 624
Decadron Phosphate with Xylocaine Injection, Sterile 1451
Xylocaine Injections 637
Xylocaine Injections for Ventricular Arrhythmias 639
Xylocaine 2% Jelly 643
4% Xylocaine-MPF Sterile Solution 641
Xylocaine 2% Viscous Solution 646

Lisinopril (Potentiated or additive action). Products include:
Prinivil Tablets 1538
Prinzide Tablets 1540
Zestoretic 2274
Zestril Tablets 2277

Mecamylamine Hydrochloride (Potentiated or additive action). Products include:
Inversine Tablets 1492

Meclofenamate Sodium (Blunting of the antihypertensive effect). Products include:
Meclomen Capsules 1739

Mefenamic Acid (Blunting of the antihypertensive effect). Products include:
Ponstel 1758

Meperidine Hydrochloride (Aggravates orthostatic hypotension). Products include:
Demerol 2047
Mepergan Injection 2479

Mephobarbital (Aggravates orthostatic hypotension). Products include:
Mebaral Tablets 2061

Methadone Hydrochloride (Aggravates orthostatic hypotension). Products include:
Dolophine Hydrochloride Ampoules & Vials 1260
Dolophine Hydrochloride Tablets 1261
Methadone Hydrochloride Diskets 1284
Methadone Hydrochloride Oral Solution & Tablets 1987

Methyclothiazide (Potentiated or additive action). Products include:
Enduron Tablets 517
Enduronyl 518

Methyldopa (Potentiated or additive action). Products include:
Aldoclor Tablets 1413
Aldomet Oral 1415
Aldoril Tablets 1418

Methyldopate Hydrochloride (Potentiated or additive action). Products include:
Aldomet Ester HCl Injection 1417

Methylprednisolone Acetate (Hypokalemia). Products include:
Depo-Medrol Sterile Aqueous Suspension 2334

Methylprednisolone Sodium Succinate (Hypokalemia). Products include:
Solu-Medrol Sterile Powder 2363

Metolazone (Potentiated or additive action). Products include:
Diulo 2129
Mykrox ½ mg Tablets 984
Zaroxolyn Tablets 989

Metoprolol Tartrate (Potentiated or additive action). Products include:
Lopressor Ampuls 1032
Lopressor HCT Tablets 1034
Lopressor Tablets 1032

Metyrosine (Potentiated or additive action). Products include:
Demser Capsules 1460

Minoxidil (Potentiated or additive action). Products include:
Loniten Tablets 2346
Rogaine Topical Solution 2357

Morphine Sulfate (Aggravates orthostatic hypotension). Products include:
Astramorph/PF Injection, USP (Preservative-Free) 618
Duramorph 960
Infumorph 200 and Infumorph 500 Sterile Solutions 962
MS Contin Tablets 1814
MSIR 1817
Oramorph SR (Morphine Sulfate Sustained Release Tablets) 1988
Roxanol 1991

Nadolol (Potentiated or additive action). Products include:
Corgard Tablets 701
Corzide Tablets 702

Naproxen (Blunting of the antihypertensive effect). Products include:
Naprosyn 2297

Naproxen Sodium (Blunting of the antihypertensive effect). Products include:
Anaprox and Anaprox DS Tablets 2288

Nicardipine Hydrochloride (Both agents may depress myocardial contractility or AV conduction resulting in increased adverse reactions). Products include:
Cardene Capsules 2290

Nifedipine (Both agents may depress myocardial contractility or AV conduction resulting in increased adverse reactions). Products include:
Adalat Capsules (10 mg and 20 mg) 1587
Procardia Capsules 1781
Procardia XL Tablets 1783

Nimodipine (Both agents may depress myocardial contractility or AV conduction resulting in increased adverse reactions). Products include:
Nimotop Capsules 1607

Nitroglycerin (Potentiated or additive action). Products include:
Deponit NTG Transdermal Delivery System 2143
Minitran Transdermal Delivery System 1312
Nitro-Bid Ointment 1339
Nitro-Bid Capsules 1338
Nitrodisc 2176
Nitro-Dur (nitroglycerin) Transdermal Infusion System 1164
Nitrogard Tablets 1004
Nitrolingual Spray 1846
Nitrostat Tablets 1743
Transderm-Nitro Transdermal Therapeutic System 2283

Norepinephrine Bitartrate (Decreased arterial responsiveness to norepinephrine). Products include:
Levophed Bitartrate Injection 2054

Opium Alkaloids (Aggravates orthostatic hypotension). Products include:
B & O No. 15A & No. 16A Supprettes 2395
Pantopon Injectable 1911

Oxycodone Hydrochloride (Aggravates orthostatic hypotension). Products include:
Percocet Tablets 950
Percodan 951
Roxicodone Tablets, Oral Solution & Intensol (Oxycodone) 1992
Tylox Capsules 1382

Penbutolol Sulfate (Potentiated or additive action). Products include:
Levatol 1832

Pentobarbital Sodium (Aggravates orthostatic hypotension). Products include:
Nembutal Sodium Capsules 534
Nembutal Sodium Solution 536
Nembutal Sodium Suppositories 538

Phenobarbital (Accelerates propranolol clearance). Products include:
Arco-Lase Plus Tablets 607
Bellergal-S Tablets 1998
Bronkolixir ⊞ 761
Bronkotabs Tablets ⊞ 762
Donnatal 1858
Donnatal Extentabs 1859
Donnatal Tablets 1858
Donnazyme Tablets 1860
Kinesed Tablets 2272
Phenobarbital Elixir and Tablets 1293
Primatene Tablets-P Formula 2421
Quadrinal Tablets 1183
Tedral SA 1765

Phenoxybenzamine Hydrochloride (Potentiated or additive action). Products include:
Dibenzyline Capsules 2207

Phentolamine Mesylate (Potentiated or additive action). Products include:
Regitine 878

Phenylbutazone (Blunting of the antihypertensive effect). Products include:
Butazolidin Capsules & Tablets 1027

Phenytoin (Accelerates propranolol clearance). Products include:
Dilantin Infatabs 1710
Dilantin-30 Pediatric/Dilantin-125 Suspension 1713

Phenytoin Sodium (Accelerates propranolol clearance). Products include:
Dilantin Kapseals 1708
Dilantin Parenteral 1712
Dilantin with Phenobarbital Kapseals 1715

Pindolol (Potentiated or additive action). Products include:
Visken Tablets 2036

Piroxicam (Blunting of the antihypertensive effect). Products include:
Feldene Capsules 1777

Polythiazide (Potentiated or additive action). Products include:
Minizide Capsules 1779
Renese Tablets 1785
Renese-R Tablets 1786

Prazosin Hydrochloride (Potentiated or additive action). Products include:
Minipress Capsules 1778
Minizide Capsules 1779

Prednisolone Acetate (Hypokalemia). Products include:
AK-Cide Sterile Ophthalmic Ointment & Suspension ⊙ 202
Blephamide Liquifilm Sterile Ophthalmic Suspension 586

(⊞ Described in PDR For Nonprescription Drugs)

(⊙ Described in PDR For Ophthalmology)

Blephamide S.O.P. Sterile Ophthalmic Ointment 586
Cetapred Ointment .... ⊙ 220
⅛% Econopred & 1% Econopred Plus .... ⊙ 217
Isopto Cetapred Suspension .... ⊙ 220
Metimyd .... ⊙ 306
Poly-Pred Liquifilm .... ⊙ 250
Pred Forte .... ⊙ 252
Pred Mild .... ⊙ 254
Pred-G Liquifilm Sterile Ophthalmic Suspension .... ⊙ 252
Pred-G S.O.P. Sterile Ophthalmic Ointment .... ⊙ 253
Vasocidin Ointment .... ⊙ 275

Prednisolone Sodium Phosphate (Hypokalemia). Products include:
AK-Pred .... ⊙ 205
Hydeltrasol Injection, Sterile 1476
Inflamase .... ⊙ 274
Pediapred Oral Liquid 987
Vasocidin Ophthalmic Solution .... ⊙ 276

Prednisolone Tebutate (Hypokalemia). Products include:
Hydeltra-T.B.A. Sterile Suspension 1478

Prednisone (Hypokalemia). Products include:
Deltasone Tablets 2332

Propoxyphene Hydrochloride (Aggravates orthostatic hypotension). Products include:
Darvon 1256
Wygesic Tablets 2540

Propoxyphene Napsylate (Aggravates orthostatic hypotension). Products include:
Darvon-N/Darvocet-N 1254

Ramipril (Potentiated or additive action). Products include:
Altace Capsules 1086

Rauwolfia Serpentina (May produce an excessive hypotension with bradycardia and orthostatic effects). Products include:
Raudixin Tablets 1803
Rauzide Tablets 1804

Rescinnamine (May produce an excessive hypotension with bradycardia and orthostatic effects).
No products indexed under this heading.

Reserpine (May produce an excessive hypotension with bradycardia and orthostatic effects). Products include:
Diupres Tablets 1461
Hydromox R Tablets 1209
Hydropres Tablets 1485
Renese-R Tablets 1786
Salutensin/Salutensin-Demi 719
Ser-Ap-Es Tablets 881
Serpasil Tablets 883
Serpasil-Apresoline Tablets 884
Serpasil-Esidrix Tablets 886

Rifampin (Accelerates propranolol clearance). Products include:
Rifadin 1345
Rifamate Capsules 1347
Rimactane Capsules 879

Secobarbital Sodium (Aggravates orthostatic hypotension). Products include:
Seconal Sodium Pulvules 1296

Sodium Nitroprusside (Potentiated or additive action). Products include:
Nipride I.V. Infusion 1909

Sufentanil Citrate (Aggravates orthostatic hypotension). Products include:
Sufenta Injection 1147

Sulindac (Blunting of the antihypertensive effect). Products include:
Clinoril Tablets 1433

Terazosin Hydrochloride (Potentiated or additive action). Products include:
Hytrin Tablets 529

Theophylline (Reduced theophylline clearance). Products include:
Bronkaid Tablets .... ▣ 757
Bronkolixir .... ▣ 761
Bronkotabs Tablets .... ▣ 762
Constant-T Tablets 1029
Marax Tablets & DF Syrup 1954
Primatene Tablets 2421
Quibron Capsules 713
Quibron-T 714
Quibron-T/SR 716
Theolair Liquid 1317
Theo-Organidin Elixir 2391

Theophylline Anhydrous (Reduced theophylline clearance). Products include:
Aerolate 994
Primatene Tablets-M Formula .... ▣ 753
Primatene Tablets-Regular Formula 2421
Respbid Tablets 684
Slo-bid Gyrocaps 1847
T-PHYL (Uniphyl) 200 mg Tablets 1820
Tedral SA 1765
Theo-24 2179
Theo-Dur Sprinkle 1168
Theo-Dur Extended-Release Tablets 1166
Theolair Tablets 1317
Theolair-SR Tablets 1319
TheoX Extended-Release Tablets 841
Uniphyl 400 mg Tablets 1823

Theophylline Calcium Salicylate (Reduced theophylline clearance). Products include:
Quadrinal Tablets 1183

Theophylline Sodium Glycinate (Reduced theophylline clearance). Products include:
Asbron G 1997

Thiamylal Sodium (Aggravates orthostatic hypotension). Products include:
Surital Ampoules, Steri-Vials 1764

Thyroxine (Lower than expected T3 concentration).
No products indexed under this heading.

Thyroxine Sodium (Lower than expected T3 concentration).
No products indexed under this heading.

Timolol Maleate (Potentiated or additive action). Products include:
Blocadren Tablets 1429
Timolide Tablets 1547
Timoptic in Ocudose 1552
Timoptic Sterile Ophthalmic Solution 1550

Tolmetin Sodium (Blunting of the antihypertensive effect). Products include:
Tolectin (200, 400 and 600 mg) .. 1379

Triamcinolone (Hypokalemia).
No products indexed under this heading.

Triamcinolone Acetonide (Hypokalemia). Products include:
Aristocort A 1010
Azmacort Inhaler 1837
Kenalog Cream, Lotion & Ointment 2401
Kenalog-10 Injection 2402
Kenalog-40 Injection 2403
Kenalog in Orabase 604
Kenalog Spray 2401
Mycolog II Cream and Ointment 2407
Mytrex Cream & Ointment 2080
Nasacort Nasal Inhaler 1844

Triamcinolone Diacetate (Hypokalemia). Products include:
Aristocort Suspension 1008

Triamcinolone Hexacetonide (Hypokalemia). Products include:
Aristospan Suspension 1011

Trimethaphan Camsylate (Potentiated or additive action). Products include:
Arfonad Ampuls 1887

Tubocurarine Chloride (Increased responsiveness to tubocurarine).
No products indexed under this heading.

Verapamil Hydrochloride (Both agents may depress myocardial contractility or AV conduction resulting in increased adverse reactions). Products include:
Calan SR Caplets 2157
Calan Tablets 2155
Isoptin Injectable 1177
Isoptin Oral Tablets 1179
Isoptin SR Sustained Release Tablets 1181
Verelan Capsules 1243
Verelan Capsules 2535

INDERIDE LA LONG ACTING CAPSULES

(Propranolol Hydrochloride, Hydrochlorothiazide) 2465
May interact with antihypertensives, para-aminobenzoic acid based local anesthetics, catecholamine depleting drugs, cardiac glycosides, corticosteroids, insulin, ganglionic blocking agents, barbiturates, narcotic analgesics, and certain other agents. Compounds in these categories include:

Acebutolol Hydrochloride (Potentiated or additive action). Products include:
Sectral Capsules 2520

ACTH (Hypokalemia).
No products indexed under this heading.

Alcohol (May aggravate orthostatic hypotension).

Alfentanil Hydrochloride (May aggravate orthostatic hypotension). Products include:
Alfenta Injection 1131

Aprobarbital (May aggravate orthostatic hypotension). Products include:
Alurate Elixir 1883

Atenolol (Potentiated or additive action). Products include:
Tenoretic Tablets 1105
Tenormin Tablets and I.V. Injection 1107

Benazepril Hydrochloride (Potentiated or additive action). Products include:
Lotensin Tablets 872

Bendroflumethiazide (Potentiated or additive action). Products include:
Corzide Tablets 702
Naturetin Tablets 1789
Rauzide Tablets 1804

Betamethasone Acetate (Hypokalemia). Products include:
Celestone Soluspan Suspension 2081

Betamethasone Sodium Phosphate (Hypokalemia). Products include:
Celestone Soluspan Suspension 2081

Betaxolol Hydrochloride (Potentiated or additive action). Products include:
Betoptic Sterile Ophthalmic Solution 569
Betoptic S Sterile Ophthalmic Suspension 570
Kerlone Tablets 2172

Buprenorphine (May aggravate orthostatic hypotension).
No products indexed under this heading.

Butabarbital (May aggravate orthostatic hypotension). Products include:
Pyridium Plus 1764

Butalbital (May aggravate orthostatic hypotension). Products include:
Esgic-Plus Tablets 1002
Esgic Tablets & Capsules 1001
Fioricet Tablets 2006
Fiorinal Capsules 2007
Fiorinal with Codeine Capsules 2008
Fiorinal Tablets 2007
Phrenilin 838
Sedapap Tablets 50 mg/650 mg .. 1360

Captopril (Potentiated or additive action). Products include:
Capoten 2255
Capozide 2258

Carteolol Hydrochloride (Potentiated or additive action). Products include:
Cartrol Tablets 507

Chlorothiazide (Potentiated or additive action). Products include:
Aldoclor Tablets 1413
Diupres Tablets 1461
Diuril Oral 1464

Chlorothiazide Sodium (Potentiated or additive action). Products include:
Diuril Sodium Intravenous 1463

Chlorthalidone (Potentiated or additive action). Products include:
Combipres Tablets 678
Tenoretic Tablets 1105
Thalitone Tablets 687

Clonidine (Potentiated or additive action). Products include:
Catapres-TTS 677

Clonidine Hydrochloride (Potentiated or additive action). Products include:
Catapres Tablets 676
Combipres Tablets 678

Codeine (May aggravate orthostatic hypotension). Products include:
Calcidrine Syrup 506

Codeine Phosphate (May aggravate orthostatic hypotension). Products include:
Actifed with Codeine Cough Syrup.. 752
Cheracol Cough Syrup 1853
Codimal PH Syrup 846
Dimetane-DC Cough Syrup 1857
Empirin with Codeine Phosphate Nos. 2, 3 & 4 764
Fiorinal with Codeine Capsules 2008
Isoclor Expectorant 982
Naldecon CX Adult Liquid .... ▣ 521
Novahistine DH 1342
Novahistine Expectorant 1343
Nucofed Capsules 2219
Nucofed Expectorant 2219
Nucofed Pediatric Expectorant 2220
Nucofed Syrup 2219
Phenaphen with Codeine Capsules 1865
Phenaphen-650 with Codeine Tablets 1866
Phenergan with Codeine 2497
Phenergan VC with Codeine 2501
Robitussin A-C Syrup 1875
Robitussin-DAC Syrup 1875
Ryna .... ▣ 741
Soma Compound w/Codeine Tablets 2390
Triaminic Expectorant w/Codeine .. 1996
Tussi-Organidin Liquid 2391
Tylenol with Codeine 1381

Codeine Polistirex (May aggravate orthostatic hypotension).
No products indexed under this heading.

Cortisone Acetate (Hypokalemia). Products include:
Cortone Acetate Sterile Suspension 1437
Cortone Acetate Tablets 1439

Deserpidine (May produce an excessive hypotension with bradycardia and orthostatic effects). Products include:
Enduronyl 518
Harmonyl Tablets 528
Oreticyl 545

Deslanoside (Hypokalemia produced by thiazides can exaggerate cardiotoxicity of digitalis).
No products indexed under this heading.

Dexamethasone Acetate (Hypokalemia). Products include:
Dalalone D.P. Injectable 999
Decadron-LA Sterile Suspension 1457

Dexamethasone Sodium Phosphate (Hypokalemia). Products include:
AK-Dex ..... ⊙ 203
Decadron Phosphate Respihaler 1454
Decadron Phosphate Sterile Ophthalmic Ointment 1453
Decadron Phosphate Sterile Ophthalmic Solution 1453
Decadron Phosphate Topical Cream 1455
Decadron Phosphate Turbinaire 1456
Maxidex Sterile Ophthalmic Ointment ..... ⊙ 222
NeoDecadron Sterile Ophthalmic Ointment 1517
NeoDecadron Sterile Ophthalmic Solution 1518
NeoDecadron Topical Cream 1518

Dezocine (May aggravate orthostatic hypotension).

Diazoxide (Potentiated or additive action). Products include:
Hyperstat I.V. Injection 2095
Proglycem 649

Digitoxin (Hypokalemia produced by thiazides can exaggerate cardiotoxicity of digitalis). Products include:
Crystodigin Tablets 1253

Digoxin (Hypokalemia produced by thiazides can exaggerate cardiotoxicity of digitalis). Products include:
Lanoxicaps 772
Lanoxin Elixir Pediatric 775
Lanoxin Injection 778
Lanoxin Injection Pediatric 781
Lanoxin Tablets 783

Doxazosin Mesylate (Potentiated or additive action). Products include:
Cardura Tablets 1941

Enalapril Maleate (Potentiated or additive action). Products include:
Vaseretic Tablets 1559
Vasotec Tablets 1564

Enalaprilat (Potentiated or additive action). Products include:
Vasotec I.V. 1562

Esmolol Hydrochloride (Potentiated or additive action). Products include:
Brevibloc Injection 942

Felodipine (Potentiated or additive action). Products include:
Plendil Extended-Release Tablets 1526

Fentanyl (May aggravate orthostatic hypotension). Products include:
Duragesic Transdermal System 1133

Fentanyl Citrate (May aggravate orthostatic hypotension). Products include:
Innovar Injection 1141
Sublimaze Injection 1146

Fosinopril Sodium (Potentiated or additive action). Products include:
Monopril Tablets 1406

Furosemide (Potentiated or additive action). Products include:
Lasix 1093

Guanabenz Acetate (Potentiated or additive action). Products include:
Wytensin Tablets 2542

Guanethidine Monosulfate (Potentiated). Products include:
Esimil Tablets 864
Ismelin Tablets 869

Hydralazine Hydrochloride (Potentiated or additive action). Products include:
Apresazide Capsules 854
Apresoline Hydrochloride Parenteral (Ampuls) 856
Apresoline Hydrochloride Tablets 855
Apresoline-Esidrix Tablets 857
Ser-Ap-Es Tablets 881
Serpasil-Apresoline Tablets 884

Hydrocodone Bitartrate (May aggravate orthostatic hypotension). Products include:
Anexsia 5/500 Tablets 2196
Anexsia 7.5/650 Tablets 2197
Azdone Tablets 844
Codiclear DH Syrup 845
Codimal DH Syrup 846
Damason-P 1356
Hycodan Syrup, Tablets 927
Hycomine Compound Tablets 929
Hycomine Syrup 927
Hycotuss Expectorant Syrup 930
Hydrocet Capsules 835
Lortab ASA Tablets 2414
Lortab 2412
Ru-Tuss with Hydrocodone 694
Triaminic Expectorant DH 1995
Vicodin Tablets 1187
Vicodin ES Tablets 1189
Zydone Capsules 941

Hydrocodone Polistirex (May aggravate orthostatic hypotension). Products include:
Tussionex Extended-Release Suspension 988

Hydrocortisone (Hypokalemia). Products include:
AK-Spore H.C. ..... ⊙ 206
Bactine Hydrocortisone Anti-Itch Cream ..... ⊞ 625
CaldeCORT Anti-Itch Hydrocortisone Spray ..... ⊞ 560
Carmol HC Cream 1% 2296
Cortaid Spray ..... ⊞ 735
Cortenema 2244
Cortisporin Ointment 758
Cortisporin Ophthalmic Ointment Sterile 758
Cortisporin Ophthalmic Suspension Sterile 759
Cortisporin Otic Solution Sterile 760
Cortisporin Otic Suspension Sterile 760
Cortizone-5 Creme & Ointment ..... ⊞ 732
Dermolate Anti-Itch Cream ..... ⊞ 697
Eldecort Cream 1.0% 1113
Eldecort Cream 1.0% and 2.5% 1113
Fungoid HC Creme 1770
Hydrocortone Tablets 1482
Hytone 909
LazerSporin-C Solution 1770
Massengill Medicated Soft Cloth Towelettes 2192
Nutracort Cream & Lotion 1684
PediOtic Suspension Sterile 797
Synacort Creams 1%, 2.5% 2296
Vanoxide-HC Acne Lotion 911
Vioform-Hydrocortisone Cream and Mild Cream 889
Vioform-Hydrocortisone Ointment 889
VōSoL HC Otic Solution 2392
Vytone Cream 1% 911

Hydrocortisone Acetate (Hypokalemia). Products include:
Analpram-HC Rectal Cream 1% and 2.5% 970
Anusol-HC Cream 1690
Anusol-HC Suppositories 1691
Caldecort ..... ⊞ 560
Carmol HC Cream 1% 2296
Chloromycetin Hydrocortisone Ophthalmic 1694
Coly-Mycin S Otic w/Neomycin & Hydrocortisone 1708
Cortaid ..... ⊞ 735
Cortef Feminine Itch Cream ..... ⊞ 735
Corticaine ..... ⊞ 682
Cortifoam 1827
Cortisporin Cream 757
Epifoam 1828
Gynecort 5 Creme ..... ⊞ 556
Hydrocortone Acetate Sterile Suspension 1479
Lanacort 5 Creme and Ointment ..... ⊞ 557
Mantadil Cream 789
Ophthocort ..... ⊙ 301
Orabase HCA Oral Paste 890
Pramosone Cream, Lotion & Ointment 971
ProctoCream-HC 1834
Proctofoam-HC 1835

Hydrocortisone Sodium Phosphate (Hypokalemia). Products include:
Hydrocortone Phosphate Injection, Sterile 1481

Hydrocortisone Sodium Succinate (Hypokalemia). Products include:
Solu-Cortef Sterile Powder 2361

Hydroflumethiazide (Potentiated or additive action). Products include:
Diucardin Tablets 2450
Saluron 718
Salutensin/Salutensin-Demi 719

Indapamide (Potentiated or additive action). Products include:
Lozol Tablets 1843

Insulin, Human (Insulin requirements may be increased, decreased, or unchanged).
No products indexed under this heading.

Insulin, Human Isophane Suspension (Insulin requirements may be increased, decreased, or unchanged). Products include:
Humulin N, 100 Units 1270

Insulin, Human NPH (Insulin requirements may be increased, decreased, or unchanged). Products include:
Insulatard NPH Human 1627
Novolin N 1627
Novolin N PenFill Cartridges 1628
Novolin N Prefilled 1628

Insulin, Human Regular (Insulin requirements may be increased, decreased, or unchanged). Products include:
Humulin BR, 100 Units 1268
Humulin R, 100 Units 1272
Novolin R 1627
Novolin R PenFill Cartridges 1628
Novolin R Prefilled 1629
Velosulin Human 1628

Insulin, Human, Zinc Suspension (Insulin requirements may be increased, decreased, or unchanged). Products include:
Humulin L, 100 Units 1268
Humulin U, 100 Units 1272
Novolin L 1627

Insulin, NPH (Insulin requirements may be increased, decreased, or unchanged). Products include:
NPH, 40 & 100 Units 1273
Beef NPH, 100 Units 1274
Pork NPH, 100 Units 1275
Insulatard NPH 1626
NPH Insulin 1626
NPH Purified Pork Isophane Insulin 1626

Insulin, Regular (Insulin requirements may be increased, decreased, or unchanged). Products include:
Regular, 40 & 100 Units 1273
Beef Regular, 100 Units 1275
Pork Regular, 100 Units 1275
Pork Regular (Concentrated), 500 Units 1276
Regular Insulin 1625
Regular Purified Pork Insulin 1626
Velosulin 1627

Insulin, Zinc Crystals (Insulin requirements may be increased, decreased, or unchanged). Products include:
NPH, 40 & 100 Units 1273

Insulin, Zinc Suspension (Insulin requirements may be increased, decreased, or unchanged). Products include:
Lente, 40 & 100 Units 1272
Protamine, Zinc, 40 & 100 Units 1273
Lente Iletin I 1272
Beef Lente, 100 Units 1274
Beef Protamine Zinc, 100 Units 1274
Pork Lente, 100 Units 1275
Pork, Protamine, Zinc, 100 Units 1275
Lente Insulin 1626
Lente Purified Pork Insulin 1626
Semilente Insulin 1625
Ultralente Insulin 1626

Isradipine (Potentiated or additive action). Products include:
DynaCirc Capsules 2004

Labetalol Hydrochloride (Potentiated or additive action). Products include:
Normodyne Injection 2108
Normodyne Tablets 2110
Normozide Tablets 2112
Trandate HCT Tablets 579
Trandate Injection 577
Trandate Tablets 579

Levorphanol Tartrate (May aggravate orthostatic hypotension). Products include:
Levo-Dromoran 1906

Lisinopril (Potentiated or additive action). Products include:
Prinivil Tablets 1538
Prinzide Tablets 1540
Zestoretic 2274
Zestril Tablets 2277

Mecamylamine Hydrochloride (Potentiated or additive action). Products include:
Inversine Tablets 1492

Meperidine Hydrochloride (May aggravate orthostatic hypotension). Products include:
Demerol 2047
Mepergan Injection 2479

Mephobarbital (May aggravate orthostatic hypotension). Products include:
Mebaral Tablets 2061

Methadone Hydrochloride (May aggravate orthostatic hypotension). Products include:
Dolophine Hydrochloride Ampoules & Vials 1260
Dolophine Hydrochloride Tablets 1261
Methadone Hydrochloride Diskets 1284
Methadone Hydrochloride Oral Solution & Tablets 1987

Methyclothiazide (Potentiated or additive action). Products include:
Enduron Tablets 517
Enduronyl 518

Methyldopa (Potentiated or additive action). Products include:
Aldoclor Tablets 1413
Aldomet Oral 1415
Aldoril Tablets 1418

Methyldopate Hydrochloride (Potentiated or additive action). Products include:
Aldomet Ester HCl Injection 1417

Methylprednisolone Acetate (Hypokalemia). Products include:
Depo-Medrol Sterile Aqueous Suspension 2334

Methylprednisolone Sodium Succinate (Hypokalemia). Products include:
Solu-Medrol Sterile Powder 2363

Metolazone (Potentiated or additive action). Products include:
Diulo 2129
Mykrox ½ mg Tablets 984
Zaroxolyn Tablets 989

Metoprolol Tartrate (Potentiated or additive action). Products include:
Lopressor Ampuls 1032
Lopressor HCT Tablets 1034
Lopressor Tablets 1032

Metyrosine (Potentiated or additive action). Products include:
Demser Capsules 1460

Minoxidil (Potentiated or additive action). Products include:
Loniten Tablets 2346
Rogaine Topical Solution 2357

Morphine Sulfate (May aggravate orthostatic hypotension). Products include:

- Astramorph/PF Injection, USP (Preservative-Free) 618
- Duramorph 960
- Infumorph 200 and Infumorph 500 Sterile Solutions 962
- MS Contin Tablets 1814
- MSIR 1817
- Oramorph SR (Morphine Sulfate Sustained Release Tablets) 1988
- Roxanol 1991

Nadolol (Potentiated or additive action). Products include:

- Corgard Tablets 701
- Corzide Tablets 702

Nicardipine Hydrochloride (Potentiated or additive action). Products include:

- Cardene Capsules 2290

Nitroglycerin (Potentiated or additive action). Products include:

- Deponit NTG Transdermal Delivery System 2143
- Minitran Transdermal Delivery System 1312
- Nitro-Bid Ointment 1339
- Nitro-Bid Capsules 1338
- Nitrodisc 2176
- Nitro-Dur (nitroglycerin) Transdermal Infusion System 1164
- Nitrogard Tablets 1004
- Nitrolingual Spray 1846
- Nitrostat Tablets 1743
- Transderm-Nitro Transdermal Therapeutic System 2283

Norepinephrine Bitartrate (Decreased arterial responsiveness to norepinephrine). Products include:

- Levophed Bitartrate Injection 2054

Opium Alkaloids (May aggravate orthostatic hypotension). Products include:

- B & O No. 15A & No. 16A Supprettes 2395
- Pantopon Injectable 1911

Oxycodone Hydrochloride (May aggravate orthostatic hypotension). Products include:

- Percocet Tablets 950
- Percodan 951
- Roxicodone Tablets, Oral Solution & Intensol (Oxycodone) 1992
- Tylox Capsules 1382

Penbutolol Sulfate (Potentiated or additive action). Products include:

- Levatol 1832

Pentobarbital Sodium (May aggravate orthostatic hypotension). Products include:

- Nembutal Sodium Capsules 534
- Nembutal Sodium Solution 536
- Nembutal Sodium Suppositories 538

Phenobarbital (May aggravate orthostatic hypotension). Products include:

- Arco-Lase Plus Tablets 607
- Bellergal-S Tablets 1998
- Bronkolixir .... ▣ 761
- Bronkotabs Tablets .... ▣ 762
- Donnatal 1858
- Donnatal Extentabs 1859
- Donnatal Tablets 1858
- Donnazyme Tablets 1860
- Kinesed Tablets 2272
- Phenobarbital Elixir and Tablets 1293
- Primatene Tablets-P Formula 2421
- Quadrinal Tablets 1183
- Tedral SA 1765

Phenoxybenzamine Hydrochloride (Potentiated or additive action). Products include:

- Dibenzyline Capsules 2207

Phentolamine Mesylate (Potentiated or additive action). Products include:

- Regitine 878

Pindolol (Potentiated or additive action). Products include:

- Visken Tablets 2036

Polythiazide (Potentiated or additive action). Products include:

- Minizide Capsules 1779
- Renese Tablets 1785
- Renese-R Tablets 1786

Prazosin Hydrochloride (Potentiated). Products include:

- Minipress Capsules 1778
- Minizide Capsules 1779

Prednisolone Acetate (Hypokalemia). Products include:

- AK-Cide Sterile Ophthalmic Ointment & Suspension .... ⊙ 202
- Blephamide Liquifilm Sterile Ophthalmic Suspension 586
- Blephamide S.O.P. Sterile Ophthalmic Ointment 586
- Cetapred Ointment .... ⊙ 220
- ⅛ % Econopred & 1 % Econopred Plus .... ⊙ 217
- Isopto Cetapred Suspension .... ⊙ 220
- Metimyd .... ⊙ 306
- Poly-Pred Liquifilm .... ⊙ 250
- Pred Forte .... ⊙ 252
- Pred Mild .... ⊙ 254
- Pred-G Liquifilm Sterile Ophthalmic Suspension .... ⊙ 252
- Pred-G S.O.P. Sterile Ophthalmic Ointment .... ⊙ 253
- Vasocidin Ointment .... ⊙ 275

Prednisolone Sodium Phosphate (Hypokalemia). Products include:

- AK-Pred .... ⊙ 205
- Hydeltrasol Injection, Sterile 1476
- Inflamase .... ⊙ 274
- Pediapred Oral Liquid 987
- Vasocidin Ophthalmic Solution .... ⊙ 276

Prednisolone Tebutate (Hypokalemia). Products include:

- Hydeltra-T.B.A. Sterile Suspension 1478

Prednisone (Hypokalemia). Products include:

- Deltasone Tablets 2332

Propoxyphene Hydrochloride (May aggravate orthostatic hypotension). Products include:

- Darvon 1256
- Wygesic Tablets 2540

Propoxyphene Napsylate (May aggravate orthostatic hypotension). Products include:

- Darvon-N/Darvocet-N 1254

Ramipril (Potentiated or additive action). Products include:

- Altace Capsules 1086

Rauwolfia Serpentina (May produce an excessive hypotension with bradycardia and orthostatic effects). Products include:

- Raudixin Tablets 1803
- Rauzide Tablets 1804

Rescinnamine (May produce an excessive hypotension with bradycardia and orthostatic effects).

- No products indexed under this heading.

Reserpine (May produce an excessive hypotension with bradycardia and orthostatic effects). Products include:

- Diupres Tablets 1461
- Hydromox R Tablets 1209
- Hydropres Tablets 1485
- Renese-R Tablets 1786
- Salutensin/Salutensin-Demi 719
- Ser-Ap-Es Tablets 881
- Serpasil Tablets 883
- Serpasil-Apresoline Tablets 884
- Serpasil-Esidrix Tablets 886

Secobarbital Sodium (May aggravate orthostatic hypotension). Products include:

- Seconal Sodium Pulvules 1296

Sodium Nitroprusside (Potentiated or additive action). Products include:

- Nipride I.V. Infusion 1909

Sufentanil Citrate (May aggravate orthostatic hypotension). Products include:

- Sufenta Injection 1147

Terazosin Hydrochloride (Potentiated or additive action). Products include:

- Hytrin Tablets 529

Thiamylal Sodium (May aggravate orthostatic hypotension). Products include:

- Surital Ampoules, Steri-Vials 1764

Timolol Maleate (Potentiated or additive action). Products include:

- Blocadren Tablets 1429
- Timolide Tablets 1547
- Timoptic in Ocudose 1552
- Timoptic Sterile Ophthalmic Solution 1550

Triamcinolone (Hypokalemia).

- No products indexed under this heading.

Triamcinolone Acetonide (Hypokalemia). Products include:

- Aristocort A 1010
- Azmacort Inhaler 1837
- Kenalog Cream, Lotion & Ointment 2401
- Kenalog-10 Injection 2402
- Kenalog-40 Injection 2403
- Kenalog in Orabase 604
- Kenalog Spray 2401
- Mycolog II Cream and Ointment 2407
- Mytrex Cream & Ointment 2080
- Nasacort Nasal Inhaler 1844

Triamcinolone Diacetate (Hypokalemia). Products include:

- Aristocort Suspension 1008

Triamcinolone Hexacetonide (Hypokalemia). Products include:

- Aristospan Suspension 1011

Trimethaphan Camsylate (Potentiated). Products include:

- Arfonad Ampuls 1887

Tubocurarine Chloride (Increased responsiveness to tubocurarine).

- No products indexed under this heading.

INDOCIN CAPSULES

(Indomethacin) 1487

May interact with loop diuretics, oral anticoagulants, thiazides, potassium sparing diuretics, beta blockers, and certain other agents. Compounds in these categories include:

Acebutolol Hydrochloride (Blunting of antihypertensive effect of beta blockers). Products include:

- Sectral Capsules 2520

Amiloride Hydrochloride (Reduced diuretic, natriuretic, and antihypertensive effects and increased serum potassium levels). Products include:

- Midamor Tablets 1508
- Moduretic Tablets 1510

Aspirin (Decreases indomethacin blood levels). Products include:

- Alka-Seltzer Effervescent Antacid and Pain Reliever 1568
- Alka-Seltzer Extra Strength Effervescent Antacid and Pain Reliever 1570
- Alka-Seltzer (Flavored) Effervescent Antacid and Pain Reliever 1569
- Alka-Seltzer Plus Cold Medicine .... ▣ 623
- Alka-Seltzer Plus Night-Time Cold Medicine .... ▣ 623
- Alka Seltzer Plus Sinus Allergy Medicine .... ▣ 624
- Anacin Coated Analgesic Caplets 2417
- Anacin Coated Analgesic Tablets 2417
- Anacin Maximum Strength Analgesic Coated Tablets 2417
- Maximum Strength Arthritis Pain Formula By the Makers of Anacin Analgesic Tablets and Caplets 2418
- Arthritis Pain Formula by the Makers of Anacin Analgesic Tablets and Caplets .... ▣ 747
- Arthritis Strength BC Powder .... ▣ 516
- Ascriptin A/D Caplets 1850
- Regular Strength Ascriptin Tablets 1850
- Azdone Tablets 844
- BC Powder .... ▣ 517
- BC Cold Powder .... ▣ 517
- Children's Bayer Chewable Aspirin .... ▣ 564
- Genuine Bayer Aspirin Tablets & Caplets .... ▣ 564
- Maximum Bayer Aspirin Tablets & Caplets .... ▣ 566
- Bayer Plus Aspirin Tablets .... ▣ 567
- Therapy Bayer Aspirin Caplets .... ▣ 568
- 8 Hour Bayer Timed-Release Aspirin .... ▣ 566
- Arthritis Strength Bufferin Analgesic Caplets 744
- Extra Strength Bufferin Analgesic Tablets 745
- Bufferin Analgesic Tablets and Caplets 743
- Cama Arthritis Pain Reliever .... ▣ 685
- Damason-P 1356
- Easprin 1719
- Ecotrin Enteric Coated Aspirin Maximum Strength Tablets and Caplets 2189
- Ecotrin Enteric Coated Aspirin Regular Strength Tablets and Caplets 2189
- Empirin Aspirin .... ▣ 541
- Empirin with Codeine Phosphate Nos. 2, 3 & 4 764
- Equagesic Tablets 2451
- Excedrin Extra-Strength Analgesic Tablets & Caplets 749
- 4-Way Cold Tablets 750
- Fiorinal Capsules 2007
- Fiorinal with Codeine Capsules 2008
- Fiorinal Tablets 2007
- Lortab ASA Tablets 2414
- Momentum Muscular Backache Formula .... ▣ 751
- Norgesic 1314
- Norwich Extra-Strength Aspirin .... ▣ 546
- Norwich Regular Strength Aspirin ▣ 547
- P-A-C Analgesic Tablets .... ▣ 669
- Percodan 951
- Robaxisal Tablets 1872
- Sine-Off Sinus Medicine Tablets-Aspirin Formula .... ▣ 722
- Soma Compound w/Codeine Tablets 2390
- Soma Compound Tablets 2389
- St. Joseph Adult Chewable Aspirin (81 mg.) .... ▣ 703
- Synalgos-DC Capsules 2525
- Talwin Compound 2072
- Ursinus Inlay-Tabs .... ▣ 691
- Vanquish Analgesic Caplets .... ▣ 574
- Zorprin Tablets 698

Atenolol (Blunting of antihypertensive effect of beta blockers). Products include:

- Tenoretic Tablets 1105
- Tenormin Tablets and I.V. Injection 1107

Bendroflumethiazide (Reduced diuretic, natriuretic, and antihypertensive effects of thiazide diuretics). Products include:

- Corzide Tablets 702
- Naturetin Tablets 1789
- Rauzide Tablets 1804

Betaxolol Hydrochloride (Blunting of antihypertensive effect of beta blockers). Products include:

- Betoptic Sterile Ophthalmic Solution 569
- Betoptic S Sterile Ophthalmic Suspension 570
- Kerlone Tablets 2172

Bumetanide (Reduced diuretic, natriuretic, and antihypertensive effects of loop diuretics). Products include:

- Bumex 1895

Captopril (Reduced antihypertensive effect of captopril). Products include:

- Capoten 2255
- Capozide 2258

Carteolol Hydrochloride (Blunting of antihypertensive effect of beta blockers). Products include:

- Cartrol Tablets 507

(▣ Described in PDR For Nonprescription Drugs) (⊙ Described in PDR For Ophthalmology)

Chlorothiazide (Reduced diuretic, natriuretic, and antihypertensive effects of thiazide diuretics). Products include:
- Aldoclor Tablets 1413
- Diupres Tablets 1461
- Diuril Oral 1464

Chlorothiazide Sodium (Reduced diuretic, natriuretic, and antihypertensive effects of thiazide diuretics). Products include:
- Diuril Sodium Intravenous 1463

Cyclosporine (Increase in cyclosporine-induced toxicity). Products include:
- Sandimmune 2024

Dexamethasone (False-negative results in dexamethasone suppression test). Products include:
- AK-Trol Ointment & Suspension .... ⊙ 207
- Decadron Elixir 1445
- Decadron Tablets 1447
- Decaspray Topical Aerosol 1459
- Dexacidin .... ⊙ 272
- Maxidex Sterile Ophthalmic Suspension .... ⊙ 223
- Maxitrol Ophthalmic Ointment/Suspension .... ⊙ 223
- TobraDex Ophthalmic Suspension and Ointment .... ⊙ 228

Dexamethasone Acetate (False-negative results in dexamethasone suppression test). Products include:
- Dalalone D.P. Injectable 999
- Decadron-LA Sterile Suspension 1457

Dexamethasone Sodium Phosphate (False-negative results in dexamethasone suppression test). Products include:
- AK-Dex .... ⊙ 203
- Decadron Phosphate Respihaler 1454
- Decadron Phosphate Sterile Ophthalmic Ointment 1453
- Decadron Phosphate Sterile Ophthalmic Solution 1453
- Decadron Phosphate Topical Cream 1455
- Decadron Phosphate Turbinaire 1456
- Maxidex Sterile Ophthalmic Ointment .... ⊙ 222
- NeoDecadron Sterile Ophthalmic Ointment 1517
- NeoDecadron Sterile Ophthalmic Solution 1518
- NeoDecadron Topical Cream 1518

Dicumarol (Altered prothrombin time). Products include:
- Dicumarol Tablets 516

Diflunisal (Do not use concomitantly; fatal gastrointestinal hemorrhage). Products include:
- Dolobid Tablets 1465

Esmolol Hydrochloride (Blunting of antihypertensive effect of beta blockers). Products include:
- Brevibloc Injection 942

Ethacrynic Acid (Reduced diuretic, natriuretic, and antihypertensive effects of loop diuretics). Products include:
- Edecrin Tablets 1468

Furosemide (Reduced diuretic, natriuretic, and antihypertensive effects of loop diuretics). Products include:
- Lasix 1093

Hydrochlorothiazide (Reduced diuretic, natriuretic, and antihypertensive effects of thiazide diuretics). Products include:
- Aldactazide 2150
- Aldoril Tablets 1418
- Apresazide Capsules 854
- Apresoline-Esidrix Tablets 857
- Capozide 2258
- Dyazide Capsules 2208
- Esidrix Tablets 863
- Esimil Tablets 864
- HydroDIURIL Tablets 1484
- Hydropres Tablets 1485
- Inderide Tablets 2463
- Inderide LA Long Acting Capsules .. 2465
- Lopressor HCT Tablets 1034
- Maxzide 1215
- Moduretic Tablets 1510
- Normozide Tablets 2112
- Oretic Tablets 544
- Oreticyl 545
- Prinzide Tablets 1540
- Ser-Ap-Es Tablets 881
- Serpasil-Esidrix Tablets 886
- Timolide Tablets 1547
- Trandate HCT Tablets 579
- Vaseretic Tablets 1559
- Zestoretic 2274

Hydroflumethiazide (Reduced diuretic, natriuretic, and antihypertensive effects of thiazide diuretics). Products include:
- Diucardin Tablets 2450
- Saluron 718
- Salutensin/Salutensin-Demi 719

Labetalol Hydrochloride (Blunting of antihypertensive effect of beta blockers). Products include:
- Normodyne Injection 2108
- Normodyne Tablets 2110
- Normozide Tablets 2112
- Trandate HCT Tablets 579
- Trandate Injection 577
- Trandate Tablets 579

Lithium Carbonate (Elevated plasma lithium levels; toxicity). Products include:
- Eskalith 2214
- Lithane Tablets 1596
- Lithium Carbonate Capsules & Tablets 1984
- Lithobid Tablets 870

Lithium Citrate (Elevated plasma lithium levels; toxicity). Products include:
- Cibalith-S 870

Methotrexate Sodium (Potentiation of methotrexate toxicity). Products include:
- Methotrexate Tablets, Parenteral, LPF Parenteral 1217
- Rheumatrex Methotrexate Dose Pack 1234

Methyclothiazide (Reduced diuretic, natriuretic, and antihypertensive effects of thiazide diuretics). Products include:
- Enduron Tablets 517
- Enduronyl 518

Metoprolol Tartrate (Blunting of antihypertensive effect of beta blockers). Products include:
- Lopressor Ampuls 1032
- Lopressor HCT Tablets 1034
- Lopressor Tablets 1032

Nadolol (Blunting of antihypertensive effect of beta blockers). Products include:
- Corgard Tablets 701
- Corzide Tablets 702

Nephrotoxic Drugs (Overt renal decompensation).

Penbutolol Sulfate (Blunting of antihypertensive effect of beta blockers). Products include:
- Levatol 1832

Pindolol (Blunting of antihypertensive effect of beta blockers). Products include:
- Visken Tablets 2036

Polythiazide (Reduced diuretic, natriuretic, and antihypertensive effects of thiazide diuretics). Products include:
- Minizide Capsules 1779
- Renese Tablets 1785
- Renese-R Tablets 1786

Probenecid (Increased plasma levels of indomethacin). Products include:
- Benemid Tablets 1426
- ColBENEMID Tablets 1436
- Wycillin Injection and Probenecid Tablets 2539

Propranolol Hydrochloride (Blunting of antihypertensive effect of beta blockers). Products include:
- Inderal 2459
- Inderal LA Long Acting Capsules 2461
- Inderide Tablets 2463
- Inderide LA Long Acting Capsules .. 2465

Spironolactone (Reduced diuretic, natriuretic, and antihypertensive effects and increased serum potassium levels). Products include:
- Aldactazide 2150
- Aldactone 2152

Timolol Maleate (Blunting of antihypertensive effect of beta blockers). Products include:
- Blocadren Tablets 1429
- Timolide Tablets 1547
- Timoptic in Ocudose 1552
- Timoptic Sterile Ophthalmic Solution 1550

Triamterene (Potential for reversible acute renal failure and hyperkalemia). Products include:
- Dyazide Capsules 2208
- Dyrenium Capsules 2210
- Maxzide 1215

Warfarin Sodium (Altered prothrombin time). Products include:
- Coumadin Injection & Tablets 944
- Panwarfin Tablets 547

INDOCIN I.V.

(Indomethacin Sodium Trihydrate) 1490
May interact with cardiac glycosides and certain other agents. Compounds in these categories include:

Amikacin Sulfate (Serum levels of amikacin significantly elevated). Products include:
- Amikin Injectable 602

Deslanoside (Half-life of digitalis may be prolonged when given concomitantly).
- No products indexed under this heading.

Digitoxin (Half-life of digitalis may be prolonged when given concomitantly). Products include:
- Crystodigin Tablets 1253

Digoxin (Half-life of digitalis may be prolonged when given concomitantly). Products include:
- Lanoxicaps 772
- Lanoxin Elixir Pediatric 775
- Lanoxin Injection 778
- Lanoxin Injection Pediatric 781
- Lanoxin Tablets 783

Furosemide (Blunted natriuretic effect of furosemide). Products include:
- Lasix 1093

Gentamicin Sulfate (Serum levels of gentamicin significantly elevated). Products include:
- Garamycin Injectable 2093
- Garamycin Ophthalmic .... ⊙ 305
- Genoptic Liquifilm Sterile Ophthalmic Solution .... ⊙ 247
- Genoptic S.O.P. Sterile Ophthalmic Ointment .... ⊙ 247
- Gentacidin Ointment .... ⊙ 273
- Gentacidin Solution .... ⊙ 273
- Gentak Ointment & Solution .... ⊙ 208
- G-myticin Creme and Ointment 0.1% 1770
- Pred-G Liquifilm Sterile Ophthalmic Suspension .... ⊙ 252
- Pred-G S.O.P. Sterile Ophthalmic Ointment .... ⊙ 253

INDOCIN ORAL SUSPENSION

(Indomethacin) 1487
See **Indocin Capsules**

INDOCIN SR CAPSULES

(Indomethacin) 1487
See **Indocin Capsules**

INDOCIN SUPPOSITORIES

(Indomethacin) 1487
See **Indocin Capsules**

INFLAMASE FORTE 1%

(Prednisolone Sodium Phosphate) .. ⊙ 274
No interactions described in labeling.

INFLAMASE MILD ⅛%

(Prednisolone Sodium Phosphate) .. ⊙ 274
No interactions described in labeling.

INFUMORPH 200 AND INFUMORPH 500 STERILE SOLUTIONS

(Morphine Sulfate) 962
May interact with central nervous system depressants, antihistamines, neuromuscular blocking agents, and certain other agents. Compounds in these categories include:

Alcohol (Potentiates CNS depressant effects).

Alfentanil Hydrochloride (Potentiates CNS depressant effects). Products include:
- Alfenta Injection 1131

Alprazolam (Potentiates CNS depressant effects). Products include:
- Xanax Tablets 2367

Aprobarbital (Potentiates CNS depressant effects). Products include:
- Alurate Elixir 1883

Astemizole (Potentiates CNS depressant effects). Products include:
- Hismanal Tablets 1138

Azatadine Maleate (Potentiates CNS depressant effects). Products include:
- Optimine Tablets 2115
- Trinalin Repetabs Tablets 1170

Bromodiphenhydramine Hydrochloride (Potentiates CNS depressant effects).
- No products indexed under this heading.

Brompheniramine Maleate (Potentiates CNS depressant effects). Products include:
- Alka Seltzer Plus Sinus Allergy Medicine .... ▣ 624
- Atrohist Sprinkle Capsules 558
- Bromfed Capsules (Timed Release) 1615
- Bromfed Syrup .... ▣ 628
- Bromfed 1615
- Dimetane Decongestant .... ▣ 673
- Dimetane .... ▣ 672
- Dimetane-DC Cough Syrup 1857
- Dimetane-DX Cough Syrup 1858
- Dimetapp Elixir .... ▣ 673
- Dimetapp DM Elixir .... ▣ 674
- Dimetapp Extentabs .... ▣ 674
- Dimetapp Plus Caplets .... ▣ 675
- Dimetapp Tablets .... ▣ 675
- Drixoral Antihistamine/Nasal Decongestant Syrup .... ▣ 698

Buprenorphine (Potentiates CNS depressant effects).
- No products indexed under this heading.

Buspirone Hydrochloride (Potentiates CNS depressant effects). Products include:
- BuSpar 1401

Butabarbital (Potentiates CNS depressant effects). Products include:
- Pyridium Plus 1764

Butalbital (Potentiates CNS depressant effects). Products include:
- Esgic-Plus Tablets 1002
- Esgic Tablets & Capsules 1001
- Fioricet Tablets 2006
- Fiorinal Capsules 2007
- Fiorinal with Codeine Capsules 2008
- Fiorinal Tablets 2007
- Phrenilin 838
- Sedapap Tablets 50 mg/650 mg .. 1360

Chlordiazepoxide (Potentiates CNS depressant effects). Products include:
Libritabs Tablets 1930
Limbitrol 1933
Menrium Tablets 1934

Chlordiazepoxide Hydrochloride (Potentiates CNS depressant effects). Products include:
Librax Capsules 1929
Librium Capsules 1931
Librium Injectable 1932

Chlorpheniramine Maleate (Potentiates CNS depressant effects). Products include:
A.R.M. Allergy Relief Medicine Caplets ■ 615
Alka-Seltzer Plus Cold Medicine ■ 623
Allerest ■ 559
Ana-Kit Anaphylaxis Emergency Treatment Kit 1100
BC Cold Powder Multi-Symptom Formula ■ 517
Brexin L.A. Capsules 2078
Cerose-DM 2443
Cheracol Plus Head Cold/Cough Formula ■ 667
Chlor-Trimeton Allergy Syrup, Tablets & Long-Acting Repetabs Tablets ■ 693
Chlor-Trimeton Decongestant ■ 694
Comhist LA Capsules 1618
Allergy-Sinus Comtrex Multi-Symptom Allergy Sinus Formula Tablets & Caplets 746
Comtrex Multi-Symptom Cold Reliever Tablets/Caplets/Liqui-Gels/Liquid 745
Day-Night Comtrex 747
Contac Continuous Action Decongestant/Antihistamine Capsules ■ 710
Contac Maximum Strength Continuous Action Decongestant/Antihistamine Caplets ■ 709
Contac Severe Cold and Flu Formula Caplets ■ 711
Coricidin 'D' Decongestant Tablets ■ 695
Coricidin Demilets Tablets for Children ■ 696
Coricidin Tablets ■ 695
Deconamine 663
Demazin Nasal Decongestant/Antihistamine Repetabs Tablets & Syrup ■ 697
Dorcol Children's Liquid Cold Formula ■ 686
Dristan Decongestant/Antihistamine/ Analgesic Coated Caplets ■ 749
Dristan Cold Nasal Decongestant/Antihistamine/ Analgesic Coated Tablets 2419
Dristan Advanced Formula Decongestant/Antihistamine/Analgesic Tablets ■ 749
Extendryl 994
4-Way Cold Tablets 750
Fedahist Gyrocaps 2145
Fedahist Timecaps 2145
Hycomine Compound Tablets 929
Isoclor Timesule Capsules ■ 561
Kronofed-A 970
Medi-Flu Caplet, Liquid ■ 640
Naldecon Syrup, Tablets, Pediatric Drops and Pediatric Syrup 709
Nolamine Tablets 838
Novafed A Capsules 1342
Novahistine DH 1342
Novahistine Elixir ■ 596
Ornade Spansule Capsules 2221
Orthoxicol Cough Syrup ■ 668
PediaCare Allergy Relief Formula Liquid 1362
PediaCare Cough-Cold Formula Liquid 1362
PediaCare Night Rest Cough-Cold Formula Liquid 1362
PediaCare 6-12 Cough-Cold Formula Chewable Tablets 1362
Pyrroxate Capsules ■ 669
Quelidrine Syrup 556
Ru-Tuss II Capsules 693
Ru-Tuss Tablets 693
Ryna ■ 741
Sinarest Tablets & Extra Strength Tablets ■ 562
Sine-Off Maximum Strength Allergy/Sinus Formula Caplets ■ 721
Sine-Off Sinus Medicine Tablets-Aspirin Formula ■ 722
Singlet Tablets ■ 598
Sinulin 840
Sinutab Maximum Strength ■ 641
St. Joseph Nighttime Cold Medicine ■ 705
Sudafed Plus Liquid ■ 544
Sudafed Plus Tablets ■ 545
Teldrin Timed-Release Allergy Capsules, 12 mg 2192
TheraFlu Flu and Cold Medicine ■ 687
Triaminic Allergy Tablets ■ 688
Triaminic Chewables ■ 688
Triaminic Cold Tablets ■ 688
Triaminic Nite Light ■ 689
Triaminic Syrup ■ 689
Triaminic-12 Tablets ■ 690
Triaminicin Tablets ■ 690
Triaminicol Multi-Symptom Cold Tablets ■ 691
Triaminicol Multi-Symptom Relief ■ 691
Tylenol Allergy Sinus Medication Caplets and Gelcaps, Maximum Strength 1372
Children's Tylenol Cold Liquid Formula and Chewable Tablets 1368
Tylenol Cold & Flu Hot Medication, Packets 1369
Tylenol Cold Medication Caplets and Tablets 1370
Tylenol Cold Medication, Effervescent Tablets 1369
Vicks Children's NyQuil ■ 664
Vicks Formula 44 Cough Medicine ■ 661
Vicks Formula 44M Multi-Symptom Cough Medicine ■ 662
Vicks Pediatric Formula 44m Multi-Symptom Cough & Cold Medicine ■ 663

Chlorpheniramine Polistirex (Potentiates CNS depressant effects). Products include:
Tussionex Extended-Release Suspension 988

Chlorpheniramine Tannate (Potentiates CNS depressant effects). Products include:
Rynatan 2387
Rynatuss 2388

Chlorpromazine (Potentiates CNS depressant effects; increases the risk of respiratory depression). Products include:
Thorazine 2234

Chlorprothixene (Potentiates CNS depressant effects; increases the risk of respiratory depression). Products include:
Taractan Tablets 1920

Chlorprothixene Hydrochloride (Potentiates CNS depressant effects; increases the risk of respiratory depression). Products include:
Taractan 1920

Clemastine Fumarate (Potentiates CNS depressant effects). Products include:
Tavist Syrup 2033
Tavist Tablets 2035
Tavist-D Tablets 2035

Clorazepate Dipotassium (Potentiates CNS depressant effects). Products include:
Tranxene 556

Clozapine (Potentiates CNS depressant effects; increases the risk of respiratory depression). Products include:
Clozaril Tablets 2000

Codeine (Potentiates CNS depressant effects). Products include:
Calcidrine Syrup 506

Codeine Phosphate (Potentiates CNS depressant effects). Products include:
Actifed with Codeine Cough Syrup 752
Cheracol Cough Syrup 1853
Codimal PH Syrup 846
Dimetane-DC Cough Syrup 1857
Empirin with Codeine Phosphate Nos. 2, 3 & 4 764
Fiorinal with Codeine Capsules 2008
Isoclor Expectorant 982
Naldecon CX Adult Liquid ■ 521
Novahistine DH 1342
Novahistine Expectorant 1343
Nucofed Capsules 2219
Nucofed Expectorant 2219
Nucofed Pediatric Expectorant 2220
Nucofed Syrup 2219
Phenaphen with Codeine Capsules 1865
Phenaphen-650 with Codeine Tablets 1866
Phenergan with Codeine 2497
Phenergan VC with Codeine 2501
Robitussin A-C Syrup 1875
Robitussin-DAC Syrup 1875
Ryna ■ 741
Soma Compound w/Codeine Tablets 2390
Triaminic Expectorant w/Codeine 1996
Tussi-Organidin Liquid 2391
Tylenol with Codeine 1381

Codeine Polistirex (Potentiates CNS depressant effects).
No products indexed under this heading.

Cyproheptadine Hydrochloride (Potentiates CNS depressant effects). Products include:
Periactin 1525

Dexchlorpheniramine Maleate (Potentiates CNS depressant effects). Products include:
Polaramine 2116

Dezocine (Potentiates CNS depressant effects).

Diazepam (Potentiates CNS depressant effects). Products include:
Valium Injectable 1937
Valium Tablets 1939
Valrelease Capsules 1923

Diphenhydramine Citrate (Potentiates CNS depressant effects). Products include:
Alka-Seltzer Plus Night-Time Cold Medicine ■ 623
Bufferin AF Nite Time Analgesic/Sleeping Aid Caplets 744
Excedrin P.M. Analgesic/Sleeping Aid Tablets, Caplets and Liquid 749

Diphenhydramine Hydrochloride (Potentiates CNS depressant effects). Products include:
Benadryl Anti-Itch Cream ■ 635
Benadryl Capsules 1691
Benadryl Decongestant Elixir ■ 635
Benadryl Decongestant ■ 635
Benadryl Elixir ■ 636
Benadryl Kapseals 1691
Benadryl 25 Kapseals ■ 636
Benadryl Parenteral 1692
Benadryl Plus ■ 636
Benadryl Plus Nighttime ■ 637
Benadryl Spray, Maximum Strength ■ 637
Benadryl Spray, Regular Strength ■ 637
Benadryl Steri-Vials, Ampoules, and Steri-Dose Syringe 1692
Benadryl 25 Tablets ■ 636
Benylin Cough Syrup ■ 637
Benylin Decongestant ■ 638
Caladryl Cream, Lotion, Spray ■ 638
Miles Nervine Nighttime Sleep-Aid ■ 627
Nytol Tablets ■ 517
Sleep-ettes-D Tablets ■ 653
Sleep-eze 3 Tablets ■ 755
Sleepinal Night-time Sleep Aid Capsules ■ 734
Sominex Caplets and Tablets ■ 722
Sominex Liquid ■ 723
Sominex Pain Relief Formula ■ 723
Tylenol Cold Night Time Medication Liquid 1371
Tylenol PM, Extra Strength Caplets and Tablets 1368
Unisom Dual Relief Nighttime Sleep Aid/Analgesic 1774
Ziradryl Lotion ■ 643

Diphenylpyraline Hydrochloride (Potentiates CNS depressant effects).
No products indexed under this heading.

Droperidol (Potentiates CNS depressant effects). Products include:
Inapsine Injection 1140
Innovar Injection 1141

Enflurane (Potentiates CNS depressant effects). Products include:
Ethrane 599

Estazolam (Potentiates CNS depressant effects). Products include:
ProSom Tablets 554

Ethchlorvynol (Potentiates CNS depressant effects). Products include:
Placidyl Capsules 553

Ethinamate (Potentiates CNS depressant effects).
No products indexed under this heading.

Fentanyl (Potentiates CNS depressant effects). Products include:
Duragesic Transdermal System 1133

Fentanyl Citrate (Potentiates CNS depressant effects). Products include:
Innovar Injection 1141
Sublimaze Injection 1146

Fluphenazine Decanoate (Potentiates CNS depressant effects; increases the risk of respiratory depression). Products include:
Prolixin Decanoate 1795

Fluphenazine Enanthate (Potentiates CNS depressant effects; increases the risk of respiratory depression). Products include:
Prolixin Enanthate 1796

Fluphenazine Hydrochloride (Potentiates CNS depressant effects; increases the risk of respiratory depression). Products include:
Prolixin Elixir 1793
Prolixin Injection 1791
Prolixin Oral Concentrate 1792
Prolixin Tablets 1793

Flurazepam Hydrochloride (Potentiates CNS depressant effects). Products include:
Dalmane Capsules 1927

Glutethimide (Potentiates CNS depressant effects).
No products indexed under this heading.

Haloperidol (Potentiates CNS depressant effects; increases the risk of respiratory depression). Products include:
Haldol Injection, Tablets and Concentrate 1373

Haloperidol Decanoate (Potentiates CNS depressant effects; increases the risk of respiratory depression). Products include:
Haldol Decanoate 1375

Hydrocodone Bitartrate (Potentiates CNS depressant effects). Products include:
Anexsia 5/500 Tablets 2196
Anexsia 7.5/650 Tablets 2197
Azdone Tablets 844
Codiclear DH Syrup 845
Codimal DH Syrup 846
Damason-P 1356
Hycodan Syrup, Tablets 927
Hycomine Compound Tablets 929
Hycomine Syrup 927
Hycotuss Expectorant Syrup 930
Hydrocet Capsules 835
Lortab ASA Tablets 2414
Lortab 2412
Ru-Tuss with Hydrocodone 694
Triaminic Expectorant DH 1995
Vicodin Tablets 1187
Vicodin ES Tablets 1189
Zydone Capsules 941

Hydrocodone Polistirex (Potentiates CNS depressant effects). Products include:
Tussionex Extended-Release Suspension 988

Hydroxyzine Hydrochloride (Potentiates CNS depressant effects). Products include:
Atarax Tablets & Syrup 1941
Marax Tablets & DF Syrup 1954

Vistaril Intramuscular Solution 1970

Isoflurane (Potentiates CNS depressant effects). Products include:
- Forane 600

Ketamine Hydrochloride (Potentiates CNS depressant effects). Products include:
- Ketalar 1726

Levorphanol Tartrate (Potentiates CNS depressant effects). Products include:
- Levo-Dromoran 1906

Lithium Carbonate (Potentiates CNS depressant effects; increases the risk of respiratory depression). Products include:
- Eskalith 2214
- Lithane Tablets 1596
- Lithium Carbonate Capsules & Tablets 1984
- Lithobid Tablets 870

Lithium Citrate (Potentiates CNS depressant effects; increases the risk of respiratory depression). Products include:
- Cibalith-S 870

Lorazepam (Potentiates CNS depressant effects). Products include:
- Ativan Injection 2432
- Ativan Tablets 2434

Loxapine Hydrochloride (Potentiates CNS depressant effects; increases the risk of respiratory depression). Products include:
- Loxitane 1213

Loxapine Succinate (Potentiates CNS depressant effects; increases the risk of respiratory depression). Products include:
- Loxitane Capsules 1213

Meperidine Hydrochloride (Potentiates CNS depressant effects). Products include:
- Demerol 2047
- Mepergan Injection 2479

Mephobarbital (Potentiates CNS depressant effects). Products include:
- Mebaral Tablets 2061

Meprobamate (Potentiates CNS depressant effects). Products include:
- Deprol Tablets 2382
- Equagesic Tablets 2451
- Miltown Tablets 2386
- PMB 200 and PMB 400 2504

Mesoridazine (Potentiates CNS depressant effects). Products include:
- Serentil 686

Mesoridazine Besylate (Potentiates CNS depressant effects; increases the risk of respiratory depression).

Methadone Hydrochloride (Potentiates CNS depressant effects). Products include:
- Dolophine Hydrochloride Ampoules & Vials 1260
- Dolophine Hydrochloride Tablets 1261
- Methadone Hydrochloride Diskets 1284
- Methadone Hydrochloride Oral Solution & Tablets 1987

Methdilazine Hydrochloride (Potentiates CNS depressant effects). Products include:
- Tacaryl Syrup & Tablets 2409

Methohexital Sodium (Potentiates CNS depressant effects). Products include:
- Brevital Sodium Vials 1248

Methoxyflurane (Potentiates CNS depressant effects).
- No products indexed under this heading.

Midazolam Hydrochloride (Potentiates CNS depressant effects). Products include:
- Versed Injection 1924

Molindone Hydrochloride (Potentiates CNS depressant effects; increases the risk of respiratory depression). Products include:
- Moban Tablets & Concentrate 932

Opium Alkaloids (Potentiates CNS depressant effects). Products include:
- B & O No. 15A & No. 16A Supprettes 2395
- Pantopon Injectable 1911

Oxazepam (Potentiates CNS depressant effects). Products include:
- Serax Capsules 2522
- Serax Tablets 2522

Oxycodone Hydrochloride (Potentiates CNS depressant effects). Products include:
- Percocet Tablets 950
- Percodan 951
- Roxicodone Tablets, Oral Solution & Intensol (Oxycodone) 1992
- Tylox Capsules 1382

Pentobarbital Sodium (Potentiates CNS depressant effects). Products include:
- Nembutal Sodium Capsules 534
- Nembutal Sodium Solution 536
- Nembutal Sodium Suppositories 538

Perphenazine (Potentiates CNS depressant effects; increases the risk of respiratory depression). Products include:
- Etrafon 2087
- Triavil Tablets 1556
- Trilafon 2123

Phenobarbital (Potentiates CNS depressant effects). Products include:
- Arco-Lase Plus Tablets 607
- Bellergal-S Tablets 1998
- Bronkolixir .... ▣ 761
- Bronkotabs Tablets .... ▣ 762
- Donnatal 1858
- Donnatal Extentabs 1859
- Donnatal Tablets 1858
- Donnazyme Tablets 1860
- Kinesed Tablets 2272
- Phenobarbital Elixir and Tablets 1293
- Primatene Tablets-P Formula 2421
- Quadrinal Tablets 1183
- Tedral SA 1765

Pimozide (Potentiates CNS depressant effects; increases the risk of respiratory depression). Products include:
- Orap Tablets 1020

Prazepam (Potentiates CNS depressant effects). Products include:
- Centrax 1693

Prochlorperazine (Potentiates CNS depressant effects; increases the risk of respiratory depression). Products include:
- Compazine 2201

Promethazine Hydrochloride (Potentiates CNS depressant effects; increases the risk of respiratory depression). Products include:
- Mepergan Injection 2479
- Phenergan with Codeine 2497
- Phenergan with Dextromethorphan 2499
- Phenergan Injection 2493
- Phenergan Suppositories 2496
- Phenergan Syrup 2495
- Phenergan Tablets 2496
- Phenergan VC 2500
- Phenergan VC with Codeine 2501

Propofol (Potentiates CNS depressant effects). Products include:
- Diprivan Injection 2267

Propoxyphene Hydrochloride (Potentiates CNS depressant effects). Products include:
- Darvon 1256
- Wygesic Tablets 2540

Propoxyphene Napsylate (Potentiates CNS depressant effects). Products include:
- Darvon-N/Darvocet-N 1254

Pyrilamine Maleate (Potentiates CNS depressant effects). Products include:
- Codimal 846
- 4-Way Fast Acting Nasal Spray - Original Formula (regular & mentholated) & Metered Spray Pump (regular) 751
- Maximum Strength Midol Multi-Symptom Menstrual Formula .... ▣ 571
- Maximum Strength Midol PMS Premenstrual Syndrome Formula .... ▣ 570
- Regular Strength Midol Multi-Symptom Menstrual Formula .... ▣ 570
- Prefrin-A .... ⊙ 255
- Prēmsyn PMS Capsules & Caplets ▣ 547
- Primatene Tablets-M Formula 2421
- Robitussin Night Relief .... ▣ 677
- Ru-Tuss with Hydrocodone 694
- Triaminic Expectorant DH 1995
- Triaminic Oral Infant Drops 1996

Pyrilamine Tannate (Potentiates CNS depressant effects). Products include:
- Rynatan 2387

Quazepam (Potentiates CNS depressant effects). Products include:
- Doral Tablets 2383

Secobarbital Sodium (Potentiates CNS depressant effects). Products include:
- Seconal Sodium Pulvules 1296

Sufentanil Citrate (Potentiates CNS depressant effects). Products include:
- Sufenta Injection 1147

Temazepam (Potentiates CNS depressant effects). Products include:
- Restoril Capsules 2023

Terfenadine (Potentiates CNS depressant effects). Products include:
- Seldane Tablets 1349
- Seldane-D Extended-Release Tablets 1350

Thiamylal Sodium (Potentiates CNS depressant effects). Products include:
- Surital Ampoules, Steri-Vials 1764

Thioridazine Hydrochloride (Potentiates CNS depressant effects; increases the risk of respiratory depression). Products include:
- Mellaril 2011

Thiothixene (Potentiates CNS depressant effects; increases the risk of respiratory depression). Products include:
- Navane Capsules and Concentrate 1954
- Navane Intramuscular 1956

Triazolam (Potentiates CNS depressant effects). Products include:
- Halcion Tablets 2340

Trifluoperazine Hydrochloride (Potentiates CNS depressant effects; increases the risk of respiratory depression). Products include:
- Stelazine 2226

Trimeprazine Tartrate (Potentiates CNS depressant effects). Products include:
- Temaril Tablets, Syrup and Spansule Sustained Release Capsules 1085

Tripelennamine Hydrochloride (Potentiates CNS depressant effects). Products include:
- PBZ Tablets & Elixir 1037
- PBZ-SR Tablets 1037

Triprolidine Hydrochloride (Potentiates CNS depressant effects). Products include:
- Actidil .... ▣ 538
- Actifed Capsules .... ▣ 539
- Actifed Plus Caplets .... ▣ 539
- Actifed Plus Tablets .... ▣ 540
- Actifed with Codeine Cough Syrup .. 752
- Actifed Syrup .... ▣ 540
- Actifed Tablets .... ▣ 540
- Actifed 12-Hour Capsules .... ▣ 539

INNOVAR INJECTION

(Fentanyl Citrate, Droperidol) 1141

May interact with central nervous system depressants and certain other agents. Compounds in these categories include:

Alfentanil Hydrochloride (Additive or potentiating effects). Products include:
- Alfenta Injection 1131

Alprazolam (Additive or potentiating effects). Products include:
- Xanax Tablets 2367

Aprobarbital (Additive or potentiating effects). Products include:
- Alurate Elixir 1883

Buprenorphine (Additive or potentiating effects).
- No products indexed under this heading.

Buspirone Hydrochloride (Additive or potentiating effects). Products include:
- BuSpar 1401

Butabarbital (Additive or potentiating effects). Products include:
- Pyridium Plus 1764

Butalbital (Additive or potentiating effects). Products include:
- Esgic-Plus Tablets 1002
- Esgic Tablets & Capsules 1001
- Fioricet Tablets 2006
- Fiorinal Capsules 2007
- Fiorinal with Codeine Capsules 2008
- Fiorinal Tablets 2007
- Phrenilin 838
- Sedapap Tablets 50 mg/650 mg .. 1360

Chlordiazepoxide (Additive or potentiating effects). Products include:
- Libritabs Tablets 1930
- Limbitrol 1933
- Menrium Tablets 1934

Chlordiazepoxide Hydrochloride (Additive or potentiating effects). Products include:
- Librax Capsules 1929
- Librium Capsules 1931
- Librium Injectable 1932

Chlorpromazine (Additive or potentiating effects). Products include:
- Thorazine 2234

Chlorprothixene (Additive or potentiating effects). Products include:
- Taractan Tablets 1920

Chlorprothixene Hydrochloride (Additive or potentiating effects). Products include:
- Taractan 1920

Clorazepate Dipotassium (Additive or potentiating effects). Products include:
- Tranxene 556

Codeine (Additive or potentiating effects). Products include:
- Calcidrine Syrup 506

Codeine Phosphate (Additive or potentiating effects). Products include:
- Actifed with Codeine Cough Syrup .. 752
- Cheracol Cough Syrup 1853
- Codimal PH Syrup 846
- Dimetane-DC Cough Syrup 1857
- Empirin with Codeine Phosphate Nos. 2, 3 & 4 764
- Fiorinal with Codeine Capsules 2008
- Isoclor Expectorant 982
- Naldecon CX Adult Liquid .... ▣ 521
- Novahistine DH 1342
- Novahistine Expectorant 1343
- Nucofed Capsules 2219
- Nucofed Expectorant 2219
- Nucofed Pediatric Expectorant 2220
- Nucofed Syrup 2219

Phenaphen with Codeine Capsules 1865
Phenaphen-650 with Codeine Tablets 1866
Phenergan with Codeine 2497
Phenergan VC with Codeine 2501
Robitussin A-C Syrup 1875
Robitussin-DAC Syrup 1875
Ryna ▣ 741
Soma Compound w/Codeine Tablets 2390
Triaminic Expectorant w/Codeine .. 1996
Tussi-Organidin Liquid 2391
Tylenol with Codeine 1381

Codeine Polistirex (Additive or potentiating effects).
No products indexed under this heading.

Dezocine (Additive or potentiating effects).

Diazepam (Additive or potentiating effects). Products include:
Valium Injectable 1937
Valium Tablets 1939
Valrelease Capsules 1923

Enflurane (Additive or potentiating effects). Products include:
Ethrane 599

Epinephrine (Paradoxical decrease of blood pressure). Products include:
Ana-Kit Anaphylaxis Emergency Treatment Kit 1100
Bronkaid Mist ▣ 757
EpiPen 843
Marcaine Hydrochloride 0.5% with Epinephrine 1:200,000 (as bitartrate) 958
Marcaine Hydrochloride with Epinephrine 1:200,000 2055
Primatene Mist 2420
Sus-Phrine Injection 1006
Xylocaine with Epinephrine Injections 637

Estazolam (Additive or potentiating effects). Products include:
ProSom Tablets 554

Ethchlorvynol (Additive or potentiating effects). Products include:
Placidyl Capsules 553

Ethinamate (Additive or potentiating effects).
No products indexed under this heading.

Fentanyl (Additive or potentiating effects). Products include:
Duragesic Transdermal System 1133

Fluphenazine Decanoate (Additive or potentiating effects). Products include:
Prolixin Decanoate 1795

Fluphenazine Enanthate (Additive or potentiating effects). Products include:
Prolixin Enanthate 1796

Fluphenazine Hydrochloride (Additive or potentiating effects). Products include:
Prolixin Elixir 1793
Prolixin Injection 1791
Prolixin Oral Concentrate 1792
Prolixin Tablets 1793

Flurazepam Hydrochloride (Additive or potentiating effects). Products include:
Dalmane Capsules 1927

Glutethimide (Additive or potentiating effects).
No products indexed under this heading.

Haloperidol (Additive or potentiating effects). Products include:
Haldol Injection, Tablets and Concentrate 1373

Haloperidol Decanoate (Additive or potentiating effects). Products include:
Haldol Decanoate 1375

Hydrocodone Bitartrate (Additive or potentiating effects). Products include:
Anexsia 5/500 Tablets 2196
Anexsia 7.5/650 Tablets 2197
Azdone Tablets 844
Codiclear DH Syrup 845
Codimal DH Syrup 846
Damason-P 1356
Hycodan Syrup, Tablets 927
Hycomine Compound Tablets 929
Hycomine Syrup 927
Hycotuss Expectorant Syrup 930
Hydrocet Capsules 835
Lortab ASA Tablets 2414
Lortab 2412
Ru-Tuss with Hydrocodone 694
Triaminic Expectorant DH 1995
Vicodin Tablets 1187
Vicodin ES Tablets 1189
Zydone Capsules 941

Hydrocodone Polistirex (Additive or potentiating effects). Products include:
Tussionex Extended-Release Suspension 988

Hydroxyzine Hydrochloride (Additive or potentiating effects). Products include:
Atarax Tablets & Syrup 1941
Marax Tablets & DF Syrup 1954
Vistaril Intramuscular Solution 1970

Isoflurane (Additive or potentiating effects). Products include:
Forane 600

Ketamine Hydrochloride (Additive or potentiating effects). Products include:
Ketalar 1726

Levorphanol Tartrate (Additive or potentiating effects). Products include:
Levo-Dromoran 1906

Lorazepam (Additive or potentiating effects). Products include:
Ativan Injection 2432
Ativan Tablets 2434

Loxapine Hydrochloride (Additive or potentiating effects). Products include:
Loxitane 1213

Loxapine Succinate (Additive or potentiating effects). Products include:
Loxitane Capsules 1213

Meperidine Hydrochloride (Potentiation of CNS depressant effect). Products include:
Demerol 2047
Mepergan Injection 2479

Mephobarbital (Additive or potentiating effects). Products include:
Mebaral Tablets 2061

Meprobamate (Additive or potentiating effects). Products include:
Deprol Tablets 2382
Equagesic Tablets 2451
Miltown Tablets 2386
PMB 200 and PMB 400 2504

Mesoridazine (Additive or potentiating effects). Products include:
Serentil 686

Methadone Hydrochloride (Additive or potentiating effeccts). Products include:
Dolophine Hydrochloride Ampoules & Vials 1260
Dolophine Hydrochloride Tablets .. 1261
Methadone Hydrochloride Diskets .. 1284
Methadone Hydrochloride Oral Solution & Tablets 1987

Methohexital Sodium (Additive or potentiating effects). Products include:
Brevital Sodium Vials 1248

Methoxyflurane (Additive or potentiating effects).
No products indexed under this heading.

Midazolam Hydrochloride (Additive or potentiating effects). Products include:
Versed Injection 1924

Molindone Hydrochloride (Additive or potentiating effects). Products include:
Moban Tablets & Concentrate 932

Morphine Sulfate (Additive or potentiating effects). Products include:
Astramorph/PF Injection, USP (Preservative-Free) 618
Duramorph 960
Infumorph 200 and Infumorph 500 Sterile Solutions 962
MS Contin Tablets 1814
MSIR 1817
Oramorph SR (Morphine Sulfate Sustained Release Tablets) 1988
Roxanol 1991

Opium Alkaloids (Additive or potentiating effects). Products include:
B & O No. 15A & No. 16A Supprettes 2395
Pantopon Injectable 1911

Opium Preparations (Additive or potentiating effects).

Oxazepam (Additive or potentiating effects). Products include:
Serax Capsules 2522
Serax Tablets 2522

Oxycodone Hydrochloride (Additive or potentiating effects). Products include:
Percocet Tablets 950
Percodan 951
Roxicodone Tablets, Oral Solution & Intensol (Oxycodone) 1992
Tylox Capsules 1382

Pentobarbital Sodium (Additive or potentiating effects). Products include:
Nembutal Sodium Capsules 534
Nembutal Sodium Solution 536
Nembutal Sodium Suppositories 538

Perphenazine (Additive or potentiating effects). Products include:
Etrafon 2087
Triavil Tablets 1556
Trilafon 2123

Phenobarbital (Additive or potentiating effects). Products include:
Arco-Lase Plus Tablets 607
Bellergal-S Tablets 1998
Bronkolixir ▣ 761
Bronkotabs Tablets ▣ 762
Donnatal 1858
Donnatal Extentabs 1859
Donnatal Tablets 1858
Donnazyme Tablets 1860
Kinesed Tablets 2272
Phenobarbital Elixir and Tablets 1293
Primatene Tablets-P Formula 2421
Quadrinal Tablets 1183
Tedral SA 1765

Prazepam (Additive or potentiating effects). Products include:
Centrax 1693

Prochlorperazine (Additive or potentiating effects). Products include:
Compazine 2201

Promethazine Hydrochloride (Additive or potentiating effects). Products include:
Mepergan Injection 2479
Phenergan with Codeine 2497
Phenergan with Dextromethorphan 2499
Phenergan Injection 2493
Phenergan Suppositories 2496
Phenergan Syrup 2495
Phenergan Tablets 2496
Phenergan VC 2500
Phenergan VC with Codeine 2501

Propofol (Additive or potentiating effects). Products include:
Diprivan Injection 2267

Propoxyphene Hydrochloride (Additive or potentiating effects). Products include:
Darvon 1256
Wygesic Tablets 2540

Propoxyphene Napsylate (Additive or potentiating effects). Products include:
Darvon-N/Darvocet-N 1254

Quazepam (Additive or potentiating effects). Products include:
Doral Tablets 2383

Secobarbital Sodium (Additive or potentiating effects). Products include:
Seconal Sodium Pulvules 1296

Sufentanil Citrate (Additive or potentiating effects). Products include:
Sufenta Injection 1147

Temazepam (Additive or potentiating effects). Products include:
Restoril Capsules 2023

Thiamylal Sodium (Additive or potentiating effects). Products include:
Surital Ampoules, Steri-Vials 1764

Thioridazine Hydrochloride (Additive or potentiating effects). Products include:
Mellaril 2011

Thiothixene (Additive or potentiating effects). Products include:
Navane Capsules and Concentrate 1954
Navane Intramuscular 1956

Triazolam (Additive or potentiating effects). Products include:
Halcion Tablets 2340

Trifluoperazine Hydrochloride (Additive or potentiating effects). Products include:
Stelazine 2226

INOCOR LACTATE INJECTION
(Amrinone Lactate) 2048
May interact with:

Disopyramide Phosphate (Excessive hypotension; concurrent administration should be undertaken with caution). Products include:
Norpace 2177

INSTA-GLUCOSE
(Glucose) ▣ 575
No interactions described in labeling.

INSTAT COLLAGEN ABSORBABLE HEMOSTAT
(Collagen) 1151
No interactions described in labeling.

INSULATARD NPH
(Insulin, NPH) 1626
No interactions described in labeling.

INSULATARD NPH HUMAN
(Insulin, Human NPH) 1627
No interactions described in labeling.

INTAL CAPSULES
(Cromolyn Sodium) 978
May interact with:

Isoproterenol Hydrochloride (Concurrent use at extremely high doses of both drugs appears to have increased resorptions and malformations in animal studies). Products include:
Isuprel Hydrochloride Injection 1:5000 2050
Isuprel Hydrochloride Mistometer .. 2051
Isuprel Hydrochloride Solution 1:200 & 1:100 2052
Norisodrine Aerotrol 540

(▣ Described in PDR For Nonprescription Drugs) (⊙ Described in PDR For Ophthalmology)

INTAL INHALER
(Cromolyn Sodium) 979
May interact with:

Isoproterenol Hydrochloride (Increased incidence of both resorptions and malformations in animal studies). Products include:
Isuprel Hydrochloride Injection 1:5000 2050
Isuprel Hydrochloride Mistometer .. 2051
Isuprel Hydrochloride Solution 1:200 & 1:100 2052
Norisodrine Aerotrol 540

INTAL NEBULIZER SOLUTION
(Cromolyn Sodium) 980
May interact with:

Isoproterenol Hydrochloride (Extremely high doses of isoproterenol and cromolyn appear to have increased the incidence of both resorption and malformations in animal studies). Products include:
Isuprel Hydrochloride Injection 1:5000 2050
Isuprel Hydrochloride Mistometer .. 2051
Isuprel Hydrochloride Solution 1:200 & 1:100 2052
Norisodrine Aerotrol 540

INTERCEED (TC7) ABSORBABLE ADHESION BARRIER
(Oxidized Regenerated Cellulose) 969
No interactions described in labeling.

INTRON A
(Interferon alfa-2B, Recombinant) 2097
May interact with:

Bone Marrow Depressants, unspecified (Careful monitoring of the WBC count is indicated).
Zidovudine (Concomitant administration may result in a higher incidence of neutropenia). Products include:
Retrovir Capsules 802
Retrovir I.V. Infusion 805
Retrovir Syrup 802

INTROPIN INJECTION
(Dopamine Hydrochloride) 930
May interact with monoamine oxidase inhibitors, inhalant anesthetics, halogenated hydrocarbon anesthetics, and certain other agents. Compounds in these categories include:

Cyclopropane (Increases cardiac autonomic irritability).
Enflurane (Increases cardiac autonomic irritability). Products include:
Ethrane 599
Furazolidone (Increases effect of Intropin). Products include:
Furoxone 1855
Halothane (Increases cardiac autonomic irritability). Products include:
Fluothane 2453
Isocarboxazid (Increases effect of Intropin). Products include:
Marplan Tablets 1906
Isoflurane (Increases cardiac autonomic irritability). Products include:
Forane 600
Methoxyflurane (Increases cardiac autonomic irritability).
No products indexed under this heading.
Phenelzine Sulfate (Increases effect of Intropin). Products include:
Nardil 1742
Selegiline Hydrochloride (Increases effect of Intropin). Products include:
Eldepryl 2250
Tranylcypromine Sulfate (Increases effect of Intropin). Products include:
Parnate Tablets 2222

INVERSINE TABLETS
(Mecamylamine Hydrochloride)..........1492
May interact with sulfonamides, general anesthetics, antihypertensives, and certain other agents. Compounds in these categories include:

Acebutolol Hydrochloride (Potentiation of Inversine). Products include:
Sectral Capsules 2520
Alcohol (Potentiation of Inversine).
Antibiotics, unspecified (Patients receiving antibiotics generally should not be treated with ganglionic blockers).
Atenolol (Potentiation of Inversine). Products include:
Tenoretic Tablets 1105
Tenormin Tablets and I.V. Injection 1107
Benazepril Hydrochloride (Potentiation of Inversine). Products include:
Lotensin Tablets 872
Bendroflumethiazide (Potentiation of Inversine; patients receiving sulfonamides generally should not be treated with ganglion blockers). Products include:
Corzide Tablets 702
Naturetin Tablets 1789
Rauzide Tablets 1804
Betaxolol Hydrochloride (Potentiation of Inversine). Products include:
Betoptic Sterile Ophthalmic Solution 569
Betoptic S Sterile Ophthalmic Suspension 570
Kerlone Tablets 2172
Captopril (Potentiation of Inversine). Products include:
Capoten 2255
Capozide 2258
Carteolol Hydrochloride (Potentiation of Inversine). Products include:
Cartrol Tablets 507
Chlorothiazide (Potentiation of Inversine; patients receiving sulfonamides generally should not be treated with ganglion blockers). Products include:
Aldoclor Tablets 1413
Diupres Tablets 1461
Diuril Oral 1464
Chlorothiazide Sodium (Potentiation of Inversine; patients receiving sulfonamides generally should not be treated with ganglion blockers). Products include:
Diuril Sodium Intravenous 1463
Chlorpropamide (Patients receiving sulfonamides generally should not be treated with ganglionic blockers). Products include:
Diabinese Tablets 1775
Chlorthalidone (Potentiation of Inversine). Products include:
Combipres Tablets 678
Tenoretic Tablets 1105
Thalitone Tablets 687
Clonidine (Potentiation of Inversine). Products include:
Catapres-TTS 677
Clonidine Hydrochloride (Potentiation of Inversine). Products include:
Catapres Tablets 676
Combipres Tablets 678
Deserpidine (Potentiation of Inversine). Products include:
Enduronyl 518
Harmonyl Tablets 528
Oreticyl 545
Diazoxide (Potentiation of Inversine). Products include:
Hyperstat I.V. Injection 2095
Proglycem 649
Doxazosin Mesylate (Potentiation of Inversine). Products include:
Cardura Tablets 1941
Enalapril Maleate (Potentiation of Inversine). Products include:
Vaseretic Tablets 1559
Vasotec Tablets 1564
Enalaprilat (Potentiation of Inversine). Products include:
Vasotec I.V. 1562
Enflurane (Potentiation of Inversine). Products include:
Ethrane 599
Esmolol Hydrochloride (Potentiation of Inversine). Products include:
Brevibloc Injection 942
Felodipine (Potentiation of Inversine). Products include:
Plendil Extended-Release Tablets 1526
Fosinopril Sodium (Potentiation of Inversine). Products include:
Monopril Tablets 1406
Furosemide (Potentiation of Inversine). Products include:
Lasix 1093
Glipizide (Patients receiving sulfonamides generally should not be treated with ganglionic blockers). Products include:
Glucotrol 1952
Glyburide (Patients receiving sulfonamides generally should not be treated with ganglionic blockers). Products include:
DiaBeta 1091
Micronase Tablets 2350
Guanabenz Acetate (Potentiation of Inversine). Products include:
Wytensin Tablets 2542
Guanethidine Monosulfate (Potentiation of Inversine). Products include:
Esimil Tablets 864
Ismelin Tablets 869
Hydralazine Hydrochloride (Potentiation of Inversine). Products include:
Apresazide Capsules 854
Apresoline Hydrochloride Parenteral (Ampuls) 856
Apresoline Hydrochloride Tablets .. 855
Apresoline-Esidrix Tablets 857
Ser-Ap-Es Tablets 881
Serpasil-Apresoline Tablets 884
Hydrochlorothiazide (Potentiation of Inversine; patients receiving sulfonamides generally should not receive ganglion blockers). Products include:
Aldactazide 2150
Aldoril Tablets 1418
Apresazide Capsules 854
Apresoline-Esidrix Tablets 857
Capozide 2258
Dyazide Capsules 2208
Esidrix Tablets 863
Esimil Tablets 864
HydroDIURIL Tablets 1484
Hydropres Tablets 1485
Inderide Tablets 2463
Inderide LA Long Acting Capsules .. 2465
Lopressor HCT Tablets 1034
Maxzide 1215
Moduretic Tablets 1510
Normozide Tablets 2112
Oretic Tablets 544
Oreticyl 545
Prinzide Tablets 1540
Ser-Ap-Es Tablets 881
Serpasil-Esidrix Tablets 886
Timolide Tablets 1547
Trandate HCT Tablets 579
Vaseretic Tablets 1559
Zestoretic 2274
Hydroflumethiazide (Potentiation of Inversine; patients receiving sulfonamides generally should not be treated with ganglion blockers). Products include:
Diucardin Tablets 2450
Saluron 718
Salutensin/Salutensin-Demi 719
Indapamide (Potentiation of Inversine). Products include:
Lozol Tablets 1843
Isoflurane (Potentiation of Inversine). Products include:
Forane 600
Isradipine (Potentiation of Inversine). Products include:
DynaCirc Capsules 2004
Labetalol Hydrochloride (Potentiation of Inversine). Products include:
Normodyne Injection 2108
Normodyne Tablets 2110
Normozide Tablets 2112
Trandate HCT Tablets 579
Trandate Injection 577
Trandate Tablets 579
Lisinopril (Potentiation of Inversine). Products include:
Prinivil Tablets 1538
Prinzide Tablets 1540
Zestoretic 2274
Zestril Tablets 2277
Methohexital Sodium (Potentiation of Inversine). Products include:
Brevital Sodium Vials 1248
Methoxyflurane (Potentiation of Inversine).
No products indexed under this heading.
Methyclothiazide (Potentiation of Inversine; patients receiving sulfonamides generally should not be treated with ganglion blockers). Products include:
Enduron Tablets 517
Enduronyl 518
Methyldopa (Potentiation of Inversine). Products include:
Aldoclor Tablets 1413
Aldomet Oral 1415
Aldoril Tablets 1418
Methyldopate Hydrochloride (Potentiation of Inversine). Products include:
Aldomet Ester HCl Injection 1417
Metolazone (Potentiation of Inversine). Products include:
Diulo 2129
Mykrox ½ mg Tablets 984
Zaroxolyn Tablets 989
Metoprolol Tartrate (Potentiation of Inversine). Products include:
Lopressor Ampuls 1032
Lopressor HCT Tablets 1034
Lopressor Tablets 1032
Metyrosine (Potentiation of Inversine). Products include:
Demser Capsules 1460
Minoxidil (Potentiation of Inversine). Products include:
Loniten Tablets 2346
Rogaine Topical Solution 2357
Nadolol (Potentiation of Inversine). Products include:
Corgard Tablets 701
Corzide Tablets 702
Nicardipine Hydrochloride (Potentiation of Inversine). Products include:
Cardene Capsules 2290
Nitroglycerin (Potentiation of Inversine). Products include:
Deponit NTG Transdermal Delivery System 2143
Minitran Transdermal Delivery System 1312
Nitro-Bid Ointment 1339
Nitro-Bid Capsules 1338
Nitrodisc 2176

Nitro-Dur (nitroglycerin) Transdermal Infusion System ... 1164
Nitrogard Tablets ... 1004
Nitrolingual Spray ... 1846
Nitrostat Tablets ... 1743
Transderm-Nitro Transdermal Therapeutic System ... 2283

Penbutolol Sulfate (Potentiation of Inversine). Products include:
Levatol ... 1832

Phenoxybenzamine Hydrochloride (Potentiation of Inversine). Products include:
Dibenzyline Capsules ... 2207

Phentolamine Mesylate (Potentiation of Inversine). Products include:
Regitine ... 878

Pindolol (Potentiation of Inversine). Products include:
Visken Tablets ... 2036

Polythiazide (Potentiation of Inversine; patients receiving sulfonamides generally should not be treated with ganglion blockers). Products include:
Minizide Capsules ... 1779
Renese Tablets ... 1785
Renese-R Tablets ... 1786

Prazosin Hydrochloride (Potentiation of Inversine). Products include:
Minipress Capsules ... 1778
Minizide Capsules ... 1779

Propofol (Potentiation of Inversine). Products include:
Diprivan Injection ... 2267

Propranolol Hydrochloride (Potentiation of Inversine). Products include:
Inderal ... 2459
Inderal LA Long Acting Capsules ... 2461
Inderide Tablets ... 2463
Inderide LA Long Acting Capsules .. 2465

Ramipril (Potentiation of Inversine). Products include:
Altace Capsules ... 1086

Rauwolfia Serpentina (Potentiation of Inversine). Products include:
Raudixin Tablets ... 1803
Rauzide Tablets ... 1804

Rescinnamine (Potentiation of Inversine).
No products indexed under this heading.

Reserpine (Potentiation of Inversine). Products include:
Diupres Tablets ... 1461
Hydromox R Tablets ... 1209
Hydropres Tablets ... 1485
Renese-R Tablets ... 1786
Salutensin/Salutensin-Demi ... 719
Ser-Ap-Es Tablets ... 881
Serpasil Tablets ... 883
Serpasil-Apresoline Tablets ... 884
Serpasil-Esidrix Tablets ... 886

Sodium Nitroprusside (Potentiation of Inversine). Products include:
Nipride I.V. Infusion ... 1909

Sulfamethizole (Patients receiving sulfonamides generally should not be treated with ganglionic blockers). Products include:
Thiosulfil Forte Tablets ... 2526
Urobiotic-250 Capsules ... 1968

Sulfamethoxazole (Patients receiving sulfonamides generally should not be treated with ganglionic blockers). Products include:
Azo Gantanol Tablets ... 1887
Bactrim DS Tablets ... 1891
Bactrim I.V. Infusion ... 1889
Bactrim ... 1891
Gantanol ... 1899
Septra ... 813
Septra I.V. Infusion ... 808
Septra I.V. Infusion ADD-Vantage Vials ... 810
Septra ... 813

Sulfasalazine (Patients receiving sulfonamides generally should not be treated with ganglionic blockers). Products include:
Azulfidine Tablets, EN-tabs, Oral Suspension ... 1157

Sulfinpyrazone (Patients receiving sulfonamides generally should not be treated with ganglionic blockers). Products include:
Anturane ... 853

Sulfisoxazole (Patients receiving sulfonamides generally should not be treated with ganglionic blockers). Products include:
Azo Gantrisin Tablets ... 1888
Gantrisin Tablets ... 1901
Pediazole ... 1973

Sulfisoxazole Diolamine (Patients receiving sulfonamides generally should not be treated with ganglionic blockers). Products include:
Gantrisin Ophthalmic Ointment/Solution ... 1900

Terazosin Hydrochloride (Potentiation of Inversine). Products include:
Hytrin Tablets ... 529

Timolol Maleate (Potentiation of Inversine). Products include:
Blocadren Tablets ... 1429
Timolide Tablets ... 1547
Timoptic in Ocudose ... 1552
Timoptic Sterile Ophthalmic Solution ... 1550

Tolazamide (Patients receiving sulfonamides generally should not be treated with ganglionic blockers). Products include:
Tolinase Tablets ... 2365

Tolbutamide (Patients receiving sulfonamides generally should not be treated with ganglionic blockers). Products include:
Orinase Tablets ... 2354

Trimethaphan Camsylate (Potentiation of Inversine). Products include:
Arfonad Ampuls ... 1887

IONAMIN CAPSULES
(Phentermine Resin) ... 981
May interact with monoamine oxidase inhibitors, insulin, and certain other agents. Compounds in these categories include:

Alcohol (Possibility of adverse interactions).

Furazolidone (Hypertensive crisis may result; concurrent use is contraindicated). Products include:
Furoxone ... 1855

Guanethidine Monosulfate (Decreased hypotensive effect of guanethidine). Products include:
Esimil Tablets ... 864
Ismelin Tablets ... 869

Insulin, Human (Insulin requirement may be altered in diabetics).
No products indexed under this heading.

Insulin, Human Isophane Suspension (Insulin requirement may be altered in diabetics). Products include:
Humulin N, 100 Units ... 1270

Insulin, Human NPH (Insulin requirement may be altered in diabetics). Products include:
Insulatard NPH Human ... 1627
Novolin N ... 1627
Novolin N PenFill Cartridges ... 1628
Novolin N Prefilled ... 1628

Insulin, Human Regular (Insulin requirement may be altered in diabetics). Products include:
Humulin BR, 100 Units ... 1268
Humulin R, 100 Units ... 1272
Novolin R ... 1627
Novolin R PenFill Cartridges ... 1628
Novolin R Prefilled ... 1629
Velosulin Human ... 1628

Insulin, Human, Zinc Suspension (Insulin requirement may be altered in diabetics). Products include:
Humulin L, 100 Units ... 1268
Humulin U, 100 Units ... 1272
Novolin L ... 1627

Insulin, NPH (Insulin requirement may be altered in diabetics). Products include:
NPH, 40 & 100 Units ... 1273
Beef NPH, 100 Units ... 1274
Pork NPH, 100 Units ... 1275
Insulatard NPH ... 1626
NPH Insulin ... 1626
NPH Purified Pork Isophane Insulin ... 1626

Insulin, Regular (Insulin requirement may be altered in diabetics). Products include:
Regular, 40 & 100 Units ... 1273
Beef Regular, 100 Units ... 1275
Pork Regular, 100 Units ... 1275
Pork Regular (Concentrated), 500 Units ... 1276
Regular Insulin ... 1625
Regular Purified Pork Insulin ... 1626
Velosulin ... 1627

Insulin, Zinc Crystals (Insulin requirement may be altered in diabetics). Products include:
NPH, 40 & 100 Units ... 1273

Insulin, Zinc Suspension (Insulin requirement may be altered in diabetics). Products include:
Lente, 40 & 100 Units ... 1272
Protamine, Zinc, 40 & 100 Units ... 1273
Lente Iletin I ... 1272
Beef Lente, 100 Units ... 1274
Beef Protamine Zinc, 100 Units ... 1274
Pork Lente, 100 Units ... 1275
Pork, Protamine, Zinc, 100 Units ... 1275
Lente Insulin ... 1626
Lente Purified Pork Insulin ... 1626
Semilente Insulin ... 1625
Ultralente Insulin ... 1626

Isocarboxazid (Hypertensive crisis may result; concurrent use is contraindicated). Products include:
Marplan Tablets ... 1906

Phenelzine Sulfate (Hypertensive crisis may result; concurrent use is contraindicated). Products include:
Nardil ... 1742

Selegiline Hydrochloride (Hypertensive crisis may result; concurrent use is contraindicated). Products include:
Eldepryl ... 2250

Tranylcypromine Sulfate (Hypertensive crisis may result; concurrent use is contraindicated). Products include:
Parnate Tablets ... 2222

IONIL PLUS SHAMPOO
(Salicylic Acid) ... 1683
No interactions described in labeling.

IONIL SHAMPOO
(Salicylic Acid) ... 1683
No interactions described in labeling.

IONIL T PLUS SHAMPOO
(Tar Preparations) ... 1683
No interactions described in labeling.

IONIL T SHAMPOO
(Salicylic Acid, Tar Preparations) ... 1683
No interactions described in labeling.

IOPIDINE
(Apraclonidine Hydrochloride) ... ⊙ 232
May interact with monoamine oxidase inhibitors. Compounds in this category include:

Furazolidone (Concurrent therapy is contraindicated). Products include:
Furoxone ... 1855

Isocarboxazid (Concurrent therapy is contraindicated). Products include:
Marplan Tablets ... 1906

Phenelzine Sulfate (Concurrent therapy is contraindicated). Products include:
Nardil ... 1742

Selegiline Hydrochloride (Concurrent therapy is contraindicated). Products include:
Eldepryl ... 2250

Tranylcypromine Sulfate (Concurrent therapy is contraindicated). Products include:
Parnate Tablets ... 2222

IPECAC SYRUP, USP
(Ipecac) ... ▣ 633
No interactions described in labeling.

IPOL POLIOVIRUS VACCINE INACTIVATED
(Poliovirus Vaccine Inactivated, Trivalent Types 1,2,3) ... 894
No interactions described in labeling.

IROSPAN CAPSULES
(Ferrous Sulfate, Vitamin C) ... 972
No interactions described in labeling.

IROSPAN TABLETS
(Ferrous Sulfate) ... 972
No interactions described in labeling.

ISMELIN TABLETS
(Guanethidine Monosulfate) ... 869
May interact with monoamine oxidase inhibitors, tricyclic antidepressants, phenothiazines, estrogens, thiazides, oral contraceptives, cardiac glycosides, and certain other agents. Compounds in these categories include:

Alcohol (Aggravates orthostatic hypotensive effects).

Amitriptyline Hydrochloride (Reduces hypotensive effect). Products include:
Elavil ... 2269
Endep Tablets ... 1927
Etrafon ... 2087
Limbitrol ... 1933
Triavil Tablets ... 1556

Amoxapine (Reduces hypotensive effect). Products include:
Asendin Tablets ... 1196

Bendroflumethiazide (Enhances antihypertensive action of Ismelin). Products include:
Corzide Tablets ... 702
Naturetin Tablets ... 1789
Rauzide Tablets ... 1804

Chlorothiazide (Enhances antihypertensive action of Ismelin). Products include:
Aldoclor Tablets ... 1413
Diupres Tablets ... 1461
Diuril Oral ... 1464

Chlorothiazide Sodium (Enhances antihypertensive action of Ismelin). Products include:
Diuril Sodium Intravenous ... 1463

Chlorotrianisene (Reduces hypotensive effect). Products include:
TACE 12 and 25 mg ... 1353

Chlorpromazine (Reduces hypotensive effect). Products include:
Thorazine ... 2234

Clomipramine Hydrochloride (Reduces hypotensive effect). Products include:
Anafranil Capsules ... 650

Deserpidine (May result in excessive postural hypotension, bradycardia, and mental depression). Products include:
Enduronyl ... 518
Harmonyl Tablets ... 528
Oreticyl ... 545

Desipramine Hydrochloride (Reduces hypotensive effect). Products include:
Norpramin Tablets ... 1340

Deslanoside (Slow heart rate).
No products indexed under this heading.

Dienestrol (Reduces hypotensive effect). Products include:
Ortho Dienestrol Cream ... 1664

Diethylstilbestrol (Reduces hypotensive effect). Products include:
Diethylstilbestrol Tablets ... 1258

Digitoxin (Slow heart rate). Products include:
Crystodigin Tablets ... 1253

Digoxin (Slow heart rate). Products include:
Lanoxicaps ... 772
Lanoxin Elixir Pediatric ... 775
Lanoxin Injection ... 778
Lanoxin Injection Pediatric ... 781
Lanoxin Tablets ... 783

Doxepin Hydrochloride (Reduces hypotensive effect). Products include:
Sinequan ... 1960

Ephedrine Hydrochloride (Reduces hypotensive effect). Products include:
Amesec ... ▣ 682
Primatene Tablets-M Formula ... 2421
Primatene Tablets-P Formula ... 2421
Primatene Tablets-Regular Formula ... 2421
Quadrinal Tablets ... 1183
Quelidrine Syrup ... 556
Tedral SA ... 1765

Ephedrine Sulfate (Reduces hypotensive effect). Products include:
Bronkaid Tablets ... ▣ 757
Bronkolixir ... ▣ 761
Bronkotabs Tablets ... ▣ 762
Marax Tablets & DF Syrup ... 1954
Pazo Hemorrhoid Ointment & Suppositories ... 752
Vicks Vatronol Nose Drops ... ▣ 666

Ephedrine Tannate (Reduces hypotensive effect). Products include:
Rynatuss ... 2388

Estradiol (Reduces hypotensive effect). Products include:
Emcyt Capsules ... 1161
Estrace ... 1385
Estrace Vaginal Cream ... 1388
Estraderm Transdermal System ... 866

Estrogens, Conjugated (Reduces hypotensive effect). Products include:
Mediatric Capsules ... 2476
PMB 200 and PMB 400 ... 2504
Premarin Intravenous ... 2508
Premarin with Methyltestosterone ... 2515
Premarin Tablets ... 2510
Premarin Vaginal Cream ... 2512

Estrogens, Esterified (Reduces hypotensive effect). Products include:
Estratest ... 2245
Menrium Tablets ... 1934

Estropipate (Reduces hypotensive effect). Products include:
Ogen ... 540

Ethinyl Estradiol (Reduces hypotensive effect). Products include:
Brevicon ... 2304
Demulen ... 2161
Estinyl Tablets ... 2085
Jenest-28 Tablets ... 1636
Levlen/Tri-Levlen ... 665
Lo/Ovral Tablets ... 2471
Lo/Ovral-28 Tablets ... 2476
Loestrin ... 1728
Modicon ... 1667
Nordette-21 Tablets ... 2481
Nordette-28 Tablets ... 2483
Norethin ... 2133
Norinyl ... 2304
Norlestrin ... 1746
Ortho-Cyclen Tablets ... 1658
Ortho-Novum ... 1667
Ovcon ... 1391
Ovral Tablets ... 2490
Ovral-28 Tablets ... 2491
Levlen/Tri-Levlen ... 665
Tri-Norinyl ... 2304
Triphasil-21 Tablets ... 2527
Triphasil-28 Tablets ... 2532

Ethynodiol Diacetate (Reduces hypotensive effect). Products include:
Demulen ... 2161

Fluphenazine Decanoate (Reduces hypotensive effect). Products include:
Prolixin Decanoate ... 1795

Fluphenazine Enanthate (Reduces hypotensive effect). Products include:
Prolixin Enanthate ... 1796

Fluphenazine Hydrochloride (Reduces hypotensive effect). Products include:
Prolixin Elixir ... 1793
Prolixin Injection ... 1791
Prolixin Oral Concentrate ... 1792
Prolixin Tablets ... 1793

Furazolidone (Concurrent use contraindicated). Products include:
Furoxone ... 1855

Hydrochlorothiazide (Enhances antihypertensive action of Ismelin). Products include:
Aldactazide ... 2150
Aldoril Tablets ... 1418
Apresazide Capsules ... 854
Apresoline-Esidrix Tablets ... 857
Capozide ... 2258
Dyazide Capsules ... 2208
Esidrix Tablets ... 863
Esimil Tablets ... 864
HydroDIURIL Tablets ... 1484
Hydropres Tablets ... 1485
Inderide Tablets ... 2463
Inderide LA Long Acting Capsules ... 2465
Lopressor HCT Tablets ... 1034
Maxzide ... 1215
Moduretic Tablets ... 1510
Normozide Tablets ... 2112
Oretic Tablets ... 544
Oreticyl ... 545
Prinzide Tablets ... 1540
Ser-Ap-Es Tablets ... 881
Serpasil-Esidrix Tablets ... 886
Timolide Tablets ... 1547
Trandate HCT Tablets ... 579
Vaseretic Tablets ... 1559
Zestoretic ... 2274

Hydroflumethiazide (Enhances antihypertensive action of Ismelin). Products include:
Diucardin Tablets ... 2450
Saluron ... 718
Salutensin/Salutensin-Demi ... 719

Imipramine Hydrochloride (Reduces hypotensive effect). Products include:
Tofranil Ampuls ... 1038
Tofranil Tablets ... 1039

Imipramine Pamoate (Reduces hypotensive effect). Products include:
Tofranil-PM Capsules ... 1041

Isocarboxazid (Concurrent use contraindicated). Products include:
Marplan Tablets ... 1906

Levonorgestrel (Reduces hypotensive effect). Products include:
Levlen/Tri-Levlen ... 665
Nordette-21 Tablets ... 2481
Nordette-28 Tablets ... 2483
Norplant System ... 2484
Levlen/Tri-Levlen ... 665
Triphasil-21 Tablets ... 2527
Triphasil-28 Tablets ... 2532

Maprotiline Hydrochloride (Reduces hypotensive effect). Products include:
Ludiomil Tablets ... 874

Mesoridazine (Reduces hypotensive effect). Products include:
Serentil ... 686

Mestranol (Reduces hypotensive effect). Products include:
Enovid ... 2161
Norethin ... 2133
Norinyl ... 2304
Ortho-Novum ... 1667

Methyclothiazide (Reduces hypotensive effect). Products include:
Enduron Tablets ... 517
Enduronyl ... 518

Methylphenidate Hydrochloride (Reduces hypotensive effect). Products include:
Ritalin ... 880

Norethindrone (Reduces hypotensive effect). Products include:
Brevicon ... 2304
Jenest-28 Tablets ... 1636
Micronor Tablets ... 1667
Modicon ... 1667
Norethin ... 2133
Norinyl ... 2304
Norlutin ... 1755
Nor-Q D Tablets ... 2304
Ortho-Novum ... 1667
Ovcon ... 1391
Tri-Norinyl ... 2304

Norethynodrel (Reduces hypotensive effect). Products include:
Enovid ... 2161

Norgestimate (Reduces hypotensive effect). Products include:
Ortho-Cyclen Tablets ... 1658

Norgestrel (Reduces hypotensive effect). Products include:
Lo/Ovral Tablets ... 2471
Lo/Ovral-28 Tablets ... 2476
Ovral Tablets ... 2490
Ovral-28 Tablets ... 2491
Ovrette Tablets ... 2492

Nortriptyline Hydrochloride (Reduces hypotensive effect). Products include:
Pamelor ... 2019

Perphenazine (Reduces hypotensive effect). Products include:
Etrafon ... 2087
Triavil Tablets ... 1556
Trilafon ... 2123

Phenelzine Sulfate (Concurrent use contraindicated). Products include:
Nardil ... 1742

Polyestradiol Phosphate (Reduces hypotensive effect). Products include:
Estradurin ... 2452

Polythiazide (Enhances antihypertensive action of Ismelin). Products include:
Minizide Capsules ... 1779
Renese Tablets ... 1785
Renese-R Tablets ... 1786

Prochlorperazine (Reduces hypotensive effect). Products include:
Compazine ... 2201

Promethazine Hydrochloride (Reduces hypotensive effect). Products include:
Mepergan Injection ... 2479
Phenergan with Codeine ... 2497
Phenergan with Dextromethorphan ... 2499
Phenergan Injection ... 2493
Phenergan Suppositories ... 2496
Phenergan Syrup ... 2495
Phenergan Tablets ... 2496
Phenergan VC ... 2500
Phenergan VC with Codeine ... 2501

Protriptyline Hydrochloride (Reduces hypotensive effect). Products include:
Vivactil Tablets ... 1567

Quinestrol (Reduces hypotensive effect). Products include:
Estrovis ... 1721

Rauwolfia Serpentina (May result in excessive postural hypotension, bradycardia, and mental depression). Products include:
Raudixin Tablets ... 1803
Rauzide Tablets ... 1804

Rescinnamine (May result in excessive postural hypotension, bradycardia, and mental depression).
No products indexed under this heading.

Reserpine (May result in excessive postural hypotension, bradycardia, and mental depression). Products include:
Diupres Tablets ... 1461
Hydromox R Tablets ... 1209
Hydropres Tablets ... 1485
Renese-R Tablets ... 1786
Salutensin/Salutensin-Demi ... 719
Ser-Ap-Es Tablets ... 881
Serpasil Tablets ... 883
Serpasil-Apresoline Tablets ... 884
Serpasil-Esidrix Tablets ... 886

Selegiline Hydrochloride (Concurrent use contraindicated). Products include:
Eldepryl ... 2250

Thioridazine Hydrochloride (Reduces hypotensive effect). Products include:
Mellaril ... 2011

Tranylcypromine Sulfate (Concurrent use contraindicated). Products include:
Parnate Tablets ... 2222

Trifluoperazine Hydrochloride (Reduces hypotensive effect). Products include:
Stelazine ... 2226

Trimipramine Maleate (Reduces hypotensive effect). Products include:
Surmontil Capsules ... 2524

ISMOTIC
(Isosorbide) ... ◉ 233
No interactions described in labeling.

ISOCLOR EXPECTORANT
(Codeine Phosphate, Guaifenesin, Pseudoephedrine Hydrochloride) ... 982
No interactions described in labeling.

ISOCLOR TIMESULE CAPSULES
(Pseudoephedrine Hydrochloride, Chlorpheniramine Maleate) ... ▣ 561
May interact with antihypertensives, antidepressant drugs, and certain other agents. Compounds in these categories include:

Acebutolol Hydrochloride (Concurrent use not recommended). Products include:
Sectral Capsules ... 2520

Alcohol (May increase drowsiness effect).

Amitriptyline Hydrochloride (Concurrent use not recommended). Products include:
Elavil ... 2269
Endep Tablets ... 1927
Etrafon ... 2087
Limbitrol ... 1933
Triavil Tablets ... 1556

Amoxapine (Concurrent use not recommended). Products include:
Asendin Tablets ... 1196

Atenolol (Concurrent use not recommended). Products include:
Tenoretic Tablets ... 1105
Tenormin Tablets and I.V. Injection 1107

Benazepril Hydrochloride (Concurrent use not recommended). Products include:

Lotensin Tablets 872

Betaxolol Hydrochloride (Concurrent use not recommended). Products include:

Betoptic Sterile Ophthalmic Solution 569
Betoptic S Sterile Ophthalmic Suspension 570
Kerlone Tablets 2172

Bupropion Hydrochloride (Concurrent use not recommended). Products include:

Wellbutrin Tablets 821

Captopril (Concurrent use not recommended). Products include:

Capoten 2255
Capozide 2258

Carteolol Hydrochloride (Concurrent use not recommended). Products include:

Cartrol Tablets 507

Clonidine (Concurrent use not recommended). Products include:

Catapres-TTS 677

Clonidine Hydrochloride (Concurrent use not recommended). Products include:

Catapres Tablets 676
Combipres Tablets 678

Deserpidine (Concurrent use not recommended). Products include:

Enduronyl 518
Harmonyl Tablets 528
Oreticyl 545

Desipramine Hydrochloride (Concurrent use not recommended). Products include:

Norpramin Tablets 1340

Diazoxide (Concurrent use not recommended). Products include:

Hyperstat I.V. Injection 2095
Proglycem 649

Doxazosin Mesylate (Concurrent use not recommended). Products include:

Cardura Tablets 1941

Doxepin Hydrochloride (Concurrent use not recommended). Products include:

Sinequan 1960

Enalapril Maleate (Concurrent use not recommended). Products include:

Vaseretic Tablets 1559
Vasotec Tablets 1564

Enalaprilat (Concurrent use not recommended). Products include:

Vasotec I.V. 1562

Esmolol Hydrochloride (Concurrent use not recommended). Products include:

Brevibloc Injection 942

Felodipine (Concurrent use not recommended). Products include:

Plendil Extended-Release Tablets 1526

Fluoxetine Hydrochloride (Concurrent use not recommended). Products include:

Prozac Pulvules 920

Fosinopril Sodium (Concurrent use not recommended). Products include:

Monopril Tablets 1406

Guanabenz Acetate (Concurrent use not recommended). Products include:

Wytensin Tablets 2542

Guanethidine Monosulfate (Concurrent use not recommended). Products include:

Esimil Tablets 864
Ismelin Tablets 869

Hydralazine Hydrochloride (Concurrent use not recommended). Products include:

Apresazide Capsules 854
Apresoline Hydrochloride Parenteral (Ampuls) 856
Apresoline Hydrochloride Tablets 855
Apresoline-Esidrix Tablets 857
Ser-Ap-Es Tablets 881
Serpasil-Apresoline Tablets 884

Imipramine Hydrochloride (Concurrent use not recommended). Products include:

Tofranil Ampuls 1038
Tofranil Tablets 1039

Imipramine Pamoate (Concurrent use not recommended). Products include:

Tofranil-PM Capsules 1041

Isocarboxazid (Concurrent use not recommended). Products include:

Marplan Tablets 1906

Isradipine (Concurrent use not recommended). Products include:

DynaCirc Capsules 2004

Labetalol Hydrochloride (Concurrent use not recommended). Products include:

Normodyne Injection 2108
Normodyne Tablets 2110
Normozide Tablets 2112
Trandate HCT Tablets 579
Trandate Injection 577
Trandate Tablets 579

Lisinopril (Concurrent use not recommended). Products include:

Prinivil Tablets 1538
Prinzide Tablets 1540
Zestoretic 2274
Zestril Tablets 2277

Maprotiline Hydrochloride (Concurrent use not recommended). Products include:

Ludiomil Tablets 874

Mecamylamine Hydrochloride (Concurrent use not recommended). Products include:

Inversine Tablets 1492

Methyldopa (Concurrent use not recommended). Products include:

Aldoclor Tablets 1413
Aldomet Oral 1415
Aldoril Tablets 1418

Methyldopate Hydrochloride (Concurrent use not recommended). Products include:

Aldomet Ester HCl Injection 1417

Metoprolol Tartrate (Concurrent use not recommended). Products include:

Lopressor Ampuls 1032
Lopressor HCT Tablets 1034
Lopressor Tablets 1032

Metyrosine (Concurrent use not recommended). Products include:

Demser Capsules 1460

Minoxidil (Concurrent use not recommended). Products include:

Loniten Tablets 2346
Rogaine Topical Solution 2357

Nadolol (Concurrent use not recommended). Products include:

Corgard Tablets 701
Corzide Tablets 702

Nicardipine Hydrochloride (Concurrent use not recommended). Products include:

Cardene Capsules 2290

Nitroglycerin (Concurrent use not recommended). Products include:

Deponit NTG Transdermal Delivery System 2143
Minitran Transdermal Delivery System 1312
Nitro-Bid Ointment 1339
Nitro-Bid Capsules 1338
Nitrodisc 2176
Nitro-Dur (nitroglycerin) Transdermal Infusion System 1164
Nitrogard Tablets 1004
Nitrolingual Spray 1846
Nitrostat Tablets 1743
Transderm-Nitro Transdermal Therapeutic System 2283

Nortriptyline Hydrochloride (Concurrent use not recommended). Products include:

Pamelor 2019

Penbutolol Sulfate (Concurrent use not recommended). Products include:

Levatol 1832

Phenelzine Sulfate (Concurrent use not recommended). Products include:

Nardil 1742

Phenoxybenzamine Hydrochloride (Concurrent use not recommended). Products include:

Dibenzyline Capsules 2207

Phentolamine Mesylate (Concurrent use not recommended). Products include:

Regitine 878

Pindolol (Concurrent use not recommended). Products include:

Visken Tablets 2036

Prazosin Hydrochloride (Concurrent use not recommended). Products include:

Minipress Capsules 1778
Minizide Capsules 1779

Propranolol Hydrochloride (Concurrent use not recommended). Products include:

Inderal 2459
Inderal LA Long Acting Capsules 2461
Inderide Tablets 2463
Inderide LA Long Acting Capsules 2465

Protriptyline Hydrochloride (Concurrent use not recommended). Products include:

Vivactil Tablets 1567

Ramipril (Concurrent use not recommended). Products include:

Altace Capsules 1086

Rauwolfia Serpentina (Concurrent use not recommended). Products include:

Raudixin Tablets 1803
Rauzide Tablets 1804

Rescinnamine (Concurrent use not recommended).

No products indexed under this heading.

Reserpine (Concurrent use not recommended). Products include:

Diupres Tablets 1461
Hydromox R Tablets 1209
Hydropres Tablets 1485
Renese-R Tablets 1786
Salutensin/Salutensin-Demi 719
Ser-Ap-Es Tablets 881
Serpasil Tablets 883
Serpasil-Apresoline Tablets 884
Serpasil-Esidrix Tablets 886

Sodium Nitroprusside (Concurrent use not recommended). Products include:

Nipride I.V. Infusion 1909

Terazosin Hydrochloride (Concurrent use not recommended). Products include:

Hytrin Tablets 529

Timolol Maleate (Concurrent use not recommended). Products include:

Blocadren Tablets 1429
Timolide Tablets 1547
Timoptic in Ocudose 1552
Timoptic Sterile Ophthalmic Solution 1550

Tranylcypromine Sulfate (Concurrent use not recommended). Products include:

Parnate Tablets 2222

Trazodone Hydrochloride (Concurrent use not recommended). Products include:

Desyrel and Desyrel Dividose 1404

Trimethaphan Camsylate (Concurrent use not recommended). Products include:

Arfonad Ampuls 1887

Trimipramine Maleate (Concurrent use not recommended). Products include:

Surmontil Capsules 2524

ISOCOM CAPSULES
(Acetaminophen, Isometheptene Mucate, Dichloralphenazone) 1629
May interact with monoamine oxidase inhibitors. Compounds in this category include:

Furazolidone (Concurrent therapy is contraindicated). Products include:

Furoxone 1855

Isocarboxazid (Concurrent therapy is contraindicated). Products include:

Marplan Tablets 1906

Phenelzine Sulfate (Concurrent therapy is contraindicated). Products include:

Nardil 1742

Selegiline Hydrochloride (Concurrent therapy is contraindicated). Products include:

Eldepryl 2250

Tranylcypromine Sulfate (Concurrent therapy is contraindicated). Products include:

Parnate Tablets 2222

ISOPTIN AMPULES
(Verapamil Hydrochloride) 1177
May interact with beta blockers, alpha adrenergic blockers, inhalant anesthetics, nondepolarizing neuromuscular blocking agents, cardiac glycosides, lithium preparations, highly protein bound drugs (selected), and certain other agents. Compounds in these categories include:

Acebutolol Hydrochloride (Concomitant intravenous beta blocker therapy results in serious toxicity in patients with CHF, recent MI or severe cardiomyopathy). Products include:

Sectral Capsules 2520

Amiodarone Hydrochloride (Administer with caution to patients receiving other highly protein bound drugs). Products include:

Cordarone Tablets 2446

Amitriptyline Hydrochloride (Administer with caution to patients receiving other highly protein bound drugs). Products include:

Elavil 2269
Endep Tablets 1927
Etrafon 2087
Limbitrol 1933
Triavil Tablets 1556

Atenolol (Concomitant intravenous beta blocker therapy results in serious toxicity in patients with CHF, recent MI or severe cardiomyopathy). Products include:

Tenoretic Tablets 1105
Tenormin Tablets and I.V. Injection 1107

Atracurium Besylate (Verapamil may potentiate the activity of neuromuscular blocking agents). Products include:

Tracrium Injection 817

Betaxolol Hydrochloride (Concomitant intravenous beta blocker therapy results in serious toxicity in patients with CHF, recent MI or severe cardiomyopathy). Products include:

Betoptic Sterile Ophthalmic Solution 569

Betoptic S Sterile Ophthalmic Suspension 570
Kerlone Tablets 2172

Carbamazepine (Increased carbamazepine concentrations resulting in increased side effects of carbamazepine). Products include:
Tegretol Chewable Tablets 654
Tegretol Suspension 656
Tegretol Tablets 654

Carteolol Hydrochloride (Concomitant intravenous beta blocker therapy results in serious toxicity in patients with CHF, recent MI or severe cardiomyopathy). Products include:
Cartrol Tablets 507

Cefonicid Sodium (Administer with caution to patients receiving other highly protein bound drugs). Products include:
Monocid Injection 2217

Chlordiazepoxide (Administer with caution to patients receiving other highly protein bound drugs). Products include:
Libritabs Tablets 1930
Limbitrol 1933
Menrium Tablets 1934

Chlordiazepoxide Hydrochloride (Administer with caution to patients receiving other highly protein bound drugs). Products include:
Librax Capsules 1929
Librium Capsules 1931
Librium Injectable 1932

Chlorpromazine (Administer with caution to patients receiving other highly protein bound drugs). Products include:
Thorazine 2234

Cimetidine (Variable results on verapamil clearance). Products include:
Tagamet Tablets 2228

Cimetidine Hydrochloride (Variable results on verapamil clearance). Products include:
Tagamet 2228

Clomipramine Hydrochloride (Administer with caution to patients receiving other highly protein bound drugs). Products include:
Anafranil Capsules 650

Clozapine (Administer with caution to patients receiving other highly protein bound drugs). Products include:
Clozaril Tablets 2000

Cyclosporine (Increased serum levels of cyclosporin). Products include:
Sandimmune 2024

Dantrolene Sodium (Concomitant use of both drugs by intravenous route may result in cardiovascular collapse). Products include:
Dantrium Capsules 1619
Dantrium Intravenous 1620

Deslanoside (Both drugs slow AV conduction resulting in possible AV block or excessive bradycardia).
No products indexed under this heading.

Diazepam (Administer with caution to patients receiving other highly protein bound drugs). Products include:
Valium Injectable 1937
Valium Tablets 1939
Valrelease Capsules 1923

Diclofenac Sodium (Administer with caution to patients receiving other highly protein bound drugs). Products include:
Voltaren Ophthalmic Sterile Ophthalmic Solution .... ⊙ 268
Voltaren Tablets 1042

Digitoxin (Both drugs slow AV conduction resulting in possible AV block or excessive bradycardia). Products include:
Crystodigin Tablets 1253

Digoxin (Both drugs slow AV conduction resulting in possible AV block or excessive bradycardia). Products include:
Lanoxicaps 772
Lanoxin Elixir Pediatric 775
Lanoxin Injection 778
Lanoxin Injection Pediatric 781
Lanoxin Tablets 783

Dipyridamole (Administer with caution to patients receiving other highly protein bound drugs). Products include:
Persantine Tablets 683

Disopyramide Phosphate (Do not administer within 48 hours before or 24 hours after verapamil). Products include:
Norpace 2177

Doxazosin Mesylate (Exaggerated hypotensive response). Products include:
Cardura Tablets 1941

Enflurane (Excessive cardiovascular depression). Products include:
Ethrane 599

Esmolol Hydrochloride (Concomitant intravenous beta blocker therapy results in serious toxicity in patients with CHF, recent MI or severe cardiomyopathy). Products include:
Brevibloc Injection 942

Fenoprofen Calcium (Administer with caution to patients receiving other highly protein bound drugs). Products include:
Nalfon Pulvules & Tablets 919

Flecainide Acetate (Additive effects on myocardial contractility, AV conduction, and repolarization). Products include:
Tambocor Tablets 1315

Flurazepam Hydrochloride (Administer with caution to patients receiving other highly protein bound drugs). Products include:
Dalmane Capsules 1927

Flurbiprofen (Administer with caution to patients receiving other highly protein bound drugs). Products include:
Ansaid Tablets 2319

Glipizide (Administer with caution to patients receiving other highly protein bound drugs). Products include:
Glucotrol 1952

Halothane (Excessive cardiovascular depression). Products include:
Fluothane 2453

Ibuprofen (Administer with caution to patients receiving other highly protein bound drugs). Products include:
Advil Cold & Sinus Caplets (formerly CoAdvil) 2416
Advil Ibuprofen Tablets and Caplets 2416
Children's Advil Suspension 2426
CoAdvil .... ⊞ 748
Dristan Sinus Caplets 2419
Haltran Tablets .... ⊞ 668
Ibuprofen .... ⊞ 631
Medipren ibuprofen Caplets and Tablets 1362
Midol 200 Cramp Relief Formula .. ⊞ 570
Motrin Tablets 2351
Motrin IB Caplets and Tablets .... ⊞ 736
Nuprin Ibuprofen/Analgesic Tablets & Caplets 752
PediaProfen Suspension 1363
Rufen Tablets 691
Trendar Ibuprofen Tablets .... ⊞ 756

Imipramine Hydrochloride (Administer with caution to patients receiving other highly protein bound drugs). Products include:
Tofranil Ampuls 1038
Tofranil Tablets 1039

Imipramine Pamoate (Administer with caution to patients receiving other highly protein bound drugs). Products include:
Tofranil-PM Capsules 1041

Indomethacin (Administer with caution to patients receiving other highly protein bound drugs). Products include:
Indocin 1487

Indomethacin Sodium Trihydrate (Administer with caution to patients receiving other highly protein bound drugs). Products include:
Indocin I.V. 1490

Isoflurane (Excessive cardiovascular depression). Products include:
Forane 600

Ketoprofen (Administer with caution to patients receiving other highly protein bound drugs). Products include:
Orudis Capsules 2488

Ketorolac Tromethamine (Administer with caution to patients receiving other highly protein bound drugs). Products include:
Toradol IM Injection 2302

Labetalol Hydrochloride (Concomitant intravenous beta blocker therapy results in serious toxicity in patients with CHF, recent MI or severe cardiomyopathy). Products include:
Normodyne Injection 2108
Normodyne Tablets 2110
Normozide Tablets 2112
Trandate HCT Tablets 579
Trandate Injection 577
Trandate Tablets 579

Lithium Carbonate (Increased sensitivity to effects of lithium). Products include:
Eskalith 2214
Lithane Tablets 1596
Lithium Carbonate Capsules & Tablets 1984
Lithobid Tablets 870

Lithium Citrate (Increased sensitivity to effects of lithium). Products include:
Cibalith-S 870

Meclofenamate Sodium (Administer with caution to patients receiving other highly protein bound drugs). Products include:
Meclomen Capsules 1739

Mefenamic Acid (Administer with caution to patients receiving other highly protein bound drugs). Products include:
Ponstel 1758

Methoxyflurane (Excessive cardiovascular depression).
No products indexed under this heading.

Metocurine Iodide (Verapamil may potentiate the activity of neuromuscular blocking agents). Products include:
Metubine Iodide Vials 1285

Metoprolol Tartrate (Concomitant intravenous beta blocker therapy results in serious toxicity in patients with CHF, recent MI or severe cardiomyopathy). Products include:
Lopressor Ampuls 1032
Lopressor HCT Tablets 1034
Lopressor Tablets 1032

Midazolam Hydrochloride (Administer with caution to patients receiving other highly protein bound drugs). Products include:
Versed Injection 1924

Nadolol (Concomitant intravenous beta blocker therapy results in serious toxicity in patients with CHF, recent MI or severe cardiomyopathy). Products include:
Corgard Tablets 701
Corzide Tablets 702

Naproxen (Administer with caution to patients receiving other highly protein bound drugs). Products include:
Naprosyn 2297

Naproxen Sodium (Administer with caution to patients receiving other highly protein bound drugs). Products include:
Anaprox and Anaprox DS Tablets 2288

Nortriptyline Hydrochloride (Administer with caution to patients receiving other highly protein bound drugs). Products include:
Pamelor 2019

Oxazepam (Administer with caution to patients receiving other highly protein bound drugs). Products include:
Serax Capsules 2522
Serax Tablets 2522

Pancuronium Bromide Injection (Verapamil may potentiate the activity of neuromuscular blocking agents).
No products indexed under this heading.

Penbutolol Sulfate (Concomitant intravenous beta blocker therapy results in serious toxicity in patients with CHF, recent MI or severe cardiomyopathy). Products include:
Levatol 1832

Phenobarbital (Increases verapamil serum levels). Products include:
Arco-Lase Plus Tablets 607
Bellergal-S Tablets 1998
Bronkolixir .... ⊞ 761
Bronkotabs Tablets .... ⊞ 762
Donnatal 1858
Donnatal Extentabs 1859
Donnatal Tablets 1858
Donnazyme Tablets 1860
Kinesed Tablets 2272
Phenobarbital Elixir and Tablets 1293
Primatene Tablets-P Formula 2421
Quadrinal Tablets 1183
Tedral SA 1765

Phenylbutazone (Administer with caution to patients receiving other highly protein bound drugs). Products include:
Butazolidin Capsules & Tablets 1027

Pindolol (Concomitant intravenous beta blocker therapy results in serious toxicity in patients with CHF, recent MI or severe cardiomyopathy). Products include:
Visken Tablets 2036

Piroxicam (Administer with caution to patients receiving other highly protein bound drugs). Products include:
Feldene Capsules 1777

Prazosin Hydrochloride (Exaggerated hypotensive response). Products include:
Minipress Capsules 1778
Minizide Capsules 1779

Propranolol Hydrochloride (Administer with caution to patients receiving other highly protein bound drugs; concomitant intravenous beta blocker therapy results in serious toxicity in patients with CHF, recent MI or severe cardiomyopathy). Products include:
- Inderal 2459
- Inderal LA Long Acting Capsules 2461
- Inderide Tablets 2463
- Inderide LA Long Acting Capsules .. 2465

Quinidine Gluconate (Exaggerated hypotensive response). Products include:
- Quinaglute Dura-Tabs Tablets 663

Quinidine Polygalacturonate (Exaggerated hypotensive response). Products include:
- Cardioquin Tablets 1812

Quinidine Sulfate (Exggerated hypotensive response). Products include:
- Quinidex Extentabs 1868

Rifampin (Markedly reduces oral verapamil bioavailability). Products include:
- Rifadin 1345
- Rifamate Capsules 1347
- Rimactane Capsules 879

Sulindac (Administer with caution to patients receiving other highly protein bound drugs). Products include:
- Clinoril Tablets 1433

Temazepam (Administer with caution to patients receiving other highly protein bound drugs). Products include:
- Restoril Capsules 2023

Terazosin Hydrochloride (Exaggerated hypotensive response). Products include:
- Hytrin Tablets 529

Timolol Maleate (Concomitant intravenous beta blocker therapy results in serious toxicity in patients with CHF, recent MI or severe cardiomyopathy). Products include:
- Blocadren Tablets 1429
- Timolide Tablets 1547
- Timoptic in Ocudose 1552
- Timoptic Sterile Ophthalmic Solution 1550

Tolbutamide (Administer with caution to patients receiving other highly protein bound drugs). Products include:
- Orinase Tablets 2354

Tolmetin Sodium (Administer with caution to patients receiving other highly protein bound drugs). Products include:
- Tolectin (200, 400 and 600 mg) .. 1379

Trimipramine Maleate (Administer with caution to patients receiving other highly protein bound drugs). Products include:
- Surmontil Capsules 2524

Vecuronium Bromide (Verapamil may potentiate the activity of neuromuscular blocking agents). Products include:
- Norcuron 1642

Warfarin Sodium (Administer with caution to patients receiving other highly protein bound drugs). Products include:
- Coumadin Injection & Tablets 944
- Panwarfin Tablets 547

ISOPTIN FOR INTRAVENOUS INJECTION

(Verapamil Hydrochloride) 1177
See **Isoptin Ampules**

ISOPTIN ORAL TABLETS

(Verapamil Hydrochloride) 1179
May interact with antihypertensives, beta blockers, diuretics, inhalant anesthetics, nondepolarizing neuromuscular blocking agents, vasodilators, cardiac glycosides, lithium preparations, and ACE inhibitors. Compounds in these categories include:

Acebutolol Hydrochloride (Additive negative effects on heart rate, AV conduction and/or cardiac contractility). Products include:
- Sectral Capsules 2520

Amiloride Hydrochloride (Additive effect on lowering blood pressure). Products include:
- Midamor Tablets 1508
- Moduretic Tablets 1510

Atenolol (Additive negative effects on heart rate, AV conduction and/or cardiac contractility). Products include:
- Tenoretic Tablets 1105
- Tenormin Tablets and I.V. Injection 1107

Atracurium Besylate (Potentiated). Products include:
- Tracrium Injection 817

Benazepril Hydrochloride (Additive effect on lowering blood pressure). Products include:
- Lotensin Tablets 872

Bendroflumethiazide (Additive effect on lowering blood pressure). Products include:
- Corzide Tablets 702
- Naturetin Tablets 1789
- Rauzide Tablets 1804

Betaxolol Hydrochloride (Additive effect on lowering blood pressure). Products include:
- Betoptic Sterile Ophthalmic Solution 569
- Betoptic S Sterile Ophthalmic Suspension 570
- Kerlone Tablets 2172

Bumetanide (Additive effect on lowering blood pressure). Products include:
- Bumex 1895

Captopril (Additive effect on lowering blood pressure). Products include:
- Capoten 2255
- Capozide 2258

Carbamazepine (Increased carbamazepine concentrations). Products include:
- Tegretol Chewable Tablets 654
- Tegretol Suspension 656
- Tegretol Tablets 654

Carteolol Hydrochloride (Additive negative effects on heart rate, AV conduction and/or cardiac contractility). Products include:
- Cartrol Tablets 507

Chlorothiazide (Additive effect on lowering blood pressure). Products include:
- Aldoclor Tablets 1413
- Diupres Tablets 1461
- Diuril Oral 1464

Chlorothiazide Sodium (Additive effect on lowering blood pressure). Products include:
- Diuril Sodium Intravenous 1463

Chlorthalidone (Adverse effects on cardiac function; additive effect on lowering blood pressure). Products include:
- Combipres Tablets 678
- Tenoretic Tablets 1105
- Thalitone Tablets 687

Cimetidine (Possible reduced verapamil clearance). Products include:
- Tagamet Tablets 2228

Cimetidine Hydrochloride (Possible reduced verapamil clearance). Products include:
- Tagamet 2228

Clonidine (Additive effect on lowering blood pressure). Products include:
- Catapres-TTS 677

Clonidine Hydrochloride (Additive effect on lowering blood pressure; adverse effects on cardiac function). Products include:
- Catapres Tablets 676
- Combipres Tablets 678

Cyclosporine (Increased serum levels of cyclosporin). Products include:
- Sandimmune 2024

Deserpidine (Additive effect on lowering blood pressure). Products include:
- Enduronyl 518
- Harmonyl Tablets 528
- Oreticyl 545

Deslanoside (Chronic verapamil treatment can increase serum digoxin levels and this can result in digitalis toxicity).
No products indexed under this heading.

Diazoxide (Additive negative effects on heart rate, AV conduction and/or cardiac contractility). Products include:
- Hyperstat I.V. Injection 2095
- Proglycem 649

Digitoxin (Chronic verapamil treatment can increase serum digoxin levels and this can result in digitalis toxicity). Products include:
- Crystodigin Tablets 1253

Digoxin (Chronic verapamil treatment can increase serum digoxin levels and this can result in digitalis toxicity). Products include:
- Lanoxicaps 772
- Lanoxin Elixir Pediatric 775
- Lanoxin Injection 778
- Lanoxin Injection Pediatric 781
- Lanoxin Tablets 783

Disopyramide Phosphate (Should not be administered within 48 hours before or 24 hours after verapamil administration). Products include:
- Norpace 2177

Doxazosin Mesylate (Additive effect on lowering blood pressure). Products include:
- Cardura Tablets 1941

Enalapril Maleate (Additive effect on lowering blood pressure). Products include:
- Vaseretic Tablets 1559
- Vasotec Tablets 1564

Enalaprilat (Additive effect on lowering blood pressure). Products include:
- Vasotec I.V. 1562

Enflurane (Potential for excessive cardiovascular depression). Products include:
- Ethrane 599

Esmolol Hydrochloride (Additive negative effects on heart rate, AV conduction and/or cardiac contractility). Products include:
- Brevibloc Injection 942

Ethacrynic Acid (Additive effect on lowering blood pressure). Products include:
- Edecrin Tablets 1468

Felodipine (Additive effect on lowering blood pressure). Products include:
- Plendil Extended-Release Tablets 1526

Flecainide Acetate (Additive effects on myocardial contractility, AV conduction, and repolarization; concomitant therapy may result in negative inotropic effect and prolongation of atrioventricular conduction). Products include:
- Tambocor Tablets 1315

Fosinopril Sodium (Additive effect on lowering blood pressure). Products include:
- Monopril Tablets 1406

Furosemide (Additive effect on lowering blood pressure). Products include:
- Lasix 1093

Guanabenz Acetate (Additive effect on lowering blood pressure). Products include:
- Wytensin Tablets 2542

Guanethidine Monosulfate (Additive effect on lowering blood pressure). Products include:
- Esimil Tablets 864
- Ismelin Tablets 869

Halothane (Potential for excessive cardiovascular depression). Products include:
- Fluothane 2453

Hydralazine Hydrochloride (Additive effect on lowering blood pressure; adverse effects on cardiac function). Products include:
- Apresazide Capsules 854
- Apresoline Hydrochloride Parenteral (Ampuls) 856
- Apresoline Hydrochloride Tablets .. 855
- Apresoline-Esidrix Tablets 857
- Ser-Ap-Es Tablets 881
- Serpasil-Apresoline Tablets 884

Hydrochlorothiazide (Additive effect on lowering blood pressure). Products include:
- Aldactazide 2150
- Aldoril Tablets 1418
- Apresazide Capsules 854
- Apresoline-Esidrix Tablets 857
- Capozide 2258
- Dyazide Capsules 2208
- Esidrix Tablets 863
- Esimil Tablets 864
- HydroDIURIL Tablets 1484
- Hydropres Tablets 1485
- Inderide Tablets 2463
- Inderide LA Long Acting Capsules .. 2465
- Lopressor HCT Tablets 1034
- Maxzide 1215
- Moduretic Tablets 1510
- Normozide Tablets 2112
- Oretic Tablets 544
- Oreticyl 545
- Prinzide Tablets 1540
- Ser-Ap-Es Tablets 881
- Serpasil-Esidrix Tablets 886
- Timolide Tablets 1547
- Trandate HCT Tablets 579
- Vaseretic Tablets 1559
- Zestoretic 2274

Hydroflumethiazide (Additive effect on lowering blood pressure). Products include:
- Diucardin Tablets 2450
- Saluron 718
- Salutensin/Salutensin-Demi 719

Indapamide (Additive effect on lowering blood pressure). Products include:
- Lozol Tablets 1843

Isoflurane (Potential for excessive cardiovascular depression). Products include:
- Forane 600

Isradipine (Additive effect on lowering blood pressure). Products include:
- DynaCirc Capsules 2004

Labetalol Hydrochloride (Additive negative effects on heart rate, AV conduction and/or cardiac contractility). Products include:
- Normodyne Injection 2108

Normodyne Tablets 2110
Normozide Tablets 2112
Trandate HCT Tablets 579
Trandate Injection 577
Trandate Tablets 579

Lisinopril (Additive effect on lowering blood pressure). Products include:
Prinivil Tablets 1538
Prinzide Tablets 1540
Zestoretic 2274
Zestril Tablets 2277

Lithium Carbonate (May result in lowering of serum lithium levels and increased sensitivity to the effects of lithium). Products include:
Eskalith 2214
Lithane Tablets 1596
Lithium Carbonate Capsules & Tablets 1984
Lithobid Tablets 870

Lithium Citrate (May result in lowering of serum lithium levels and increased sensitivity to the effects of lithium). Products include:
Cibalith-S 870

Mecamylamine Hydrochloride (Additive effect on lowering blood pressure). Products include:
Inversine Tablets 1492

Methoxyflurane (Potential for excessive cardiovascular depression).
No products indexed under this heading.

Methyclothiazide (Additive effect on lowering blood pressure). Products include:
Enduron Tablets 517
Enduronyl 518

Methyldopa (Additive effect on lowering blood pressure). Products include:
Aldoclor Tablets 1413
Aldomet Oral 1415
Aldoril Tablets 1418

Methyldopate Hydrochloride (Additive effect on lowering blood pressure). Products include:
Aldomet Ester HCl Injection 1417

Metocurine Iodide (Potentiated). Products include:
Metubine Iodide Vials 1285

Metolazone (Additive effect on lowering blood pressure). Products include:
Diulo 2129
Mykrox ½ mg Tablets 984
Zaroxolyn Tablets 989

Metoprolol Tartrate (Additive negative effects on heart rate, AV conduction and/or cardiac contractility). Products include:
Lopressor Ampuls 1032
Lopressor HCT Tablets 1034
Lopressor Tablets 1032

Metyrosine (Additive effect on lowering blood pressure). Products include:
Demser Capsules 1460

Minoxidil (Additive effect on lowering blood pressure). Products include:
Loniten Tablets 2346
Rogaine Topical Solution 2357

Nadolol (Additive negative effects on heart rate, AV conduction and/or cardiac contractility). Products include:
Corgard Tablets 701
Corzide Tablets 702

Nicardipine Hydrochloride (Additive negative effects on heart rate, AV conduction and/or cardiac contractility). Products include:
Cardene Capsules 2290

Nitroglycerin (Additive effect on lowering blood pressure). Products include:
Deponit NTG Transdermal Delivery System 2143
Minitran Transdermal Delivery System 1312
Nitro-Bid Ointment 1339
Nitro-Bid Capsules 1338
Nitrodisc 2176
Nitro-Dur (nitroglycerin) Transdermal Infusion System 1164
Nitrogard Tablets 1004
Nitrolingual Spray 1846
Nitrostat Tablets 1743
Transderm-Nitro Transdermal Therapeutic System 2283

Pancuronium Bromide Injection (Potentiated).
No products indexed under this heading.

Penbutolol Sulfate (Additive negative effects on heart rate, AV conduction and/or cardiac contractility). Products include:
Levatol 1832

Phenoxybenzamine Hydrochloride (Additive effect on lowering blood pressure). Products include:
Dibenzyline Capsules 2207

Phentolamine Mesylate (Additive effect on lowering blood pressure). Products include:
Regitine 878

Pindolol (Additive negative effects on heart rate, AV conduction and/or cardiac contractility). Products include:
Visken Tablets 2036

Polythiazide (Additive effect on lowering blood pressure). Products include:
Minizide Capsules 1779
Renese Tablets 1785
Renese-R Tablets 1786

Prazosin Hydrochloride (May result in a reduction in blood pressure that is excessive in some patients). Products include:
Minipress Capsules 1778
Minizide Capsules 1779

Propranolol Hydrochloride (Additive negative effects on heart rate, AV conduction and/or cardiac contractility). Products include:
Inderal 2459
Inderal LA Long Acting Capsules 2461
Inderide Tablets 2463
Inderide LA Long Acting Capsules 2465

Quinidine Gluconate (Hypotension in patients with hypertrophic cardiomyopathy; increased quinidine levels). Products include:
Quinaglute Dura-Tabs Tablets 663

Quinidine Polygalacturonate (Hypotension in patients with hypertrophic cardiomyopathy; increased quinidine levels). Products include:
Cardioquin Tablets 1812

Quinidine Sulfate (Hypotension in patients with hypertrophic cardiomyopathy; increased quinidine levels). Products include:
Quinidex Extentabs 1868

Ramipril (Additive effect on lowering blood pressure). Products include:
Altace Capsules 1086

Rauwolfia Serpentina (Additive effect on lowering blood pressure). Products include:
Raudixin Tablets 1803
Rauzide Tablets 1804

Rescinnamine (Additive effect on lowering blood pressure).
No products indexed under this heading.

Reserpine (Additive effect on lowering blood pressure). Products include:
Diupres Tablets 1461
Hydromox R Tablets 1209
Hydropres Tablets 1485
Renese-R Tablets 1786
Salutensin/Salutensin-Demi 719
Ser-Ap-Es Tablets 881
Serpasil Tablets 883
Serpasil-Apresoline Tablets 884
Serpasil-Esidrix Tablets 886

Rifampin (Reduced verapamil bioavailability). Products include:
Rifadin 1345
Rifamate Capsules 1347
Rimactane Capsules 879

Sodium Nitroprusside (Additive effect on lowering blood pressure). Products include:
Nipride I.V. Infusion 1909

Spironolactone (Additive effect on lowering blood pressure). Products include:
Aldactazide 2150
Aldactone 2152

Terazosin Hydrochloride (May result in a reduction in blood pressure that is excessive in some patients). Products include:
Hytrin Tablets 529

Timolol Maleate (Additive negative effects on heart rate, AV conduction and/or cardiac contractility). Products include:
Blocadren Tablets 1429
Timolide Tablets 1547
Timoptic in Ocudose 1552
Timoptic Sterile Ophthalmic Solution 1550

Triamterene (Additive effect on lowering blood pressure). Products include:
Dyazide Capsules 2208
Dyrenium Capsules 2210
Maxzide 1215

Trimethaphan Camsylate (Additive effect on lowering blood pressure). Products include:
Arfonad Ampuls 1887

Vecuronium Bromide (Verapamil prolongs recovery from the neuromuscular blockade produced by vecuronium). Products include:
Norcuron 1642

ISOPTIN SR SUSTAINED RELEASE TABLETS
(Verapamil Hydrochloride) 1181
May interact with antihypertensives, beta blockers, diuretics, inhalant anesthetics, nondepolarizing neuromuscular blocking agents, vasodilators, ACE inhibitors, lithium preparations, alpha adrenergic blockers, cardiac glycosides, and certain other agents. Compounds in these categories include:

Acebutolol Hydrochloride (Additive negative effects on heart rate, AV conduction and/or cardiac contractility). Products include:
Sectral Capsules 2520

Amiloride Hydrochloride (Additive effect on lowering blood pressure). Products include:
Midamor Tablets 1508
Moduretic Tablets 1510

Atenolol (Additive negative effects on heart rate, AV conduction and/or cardiac contractility; a decrease in atenolol clearance). Products include:
Tenoretic Tablets 1105
Tenormin Tablets and I.V. Injection 1107

Atracurium Besylate (Verapamil may potentiate the activity of neuromuscular blocking agents). Products include:
Tracrium Injection 817

Benazepril Hydrochloride (Additive effect on lowering blood pressure). Products include:
Lotensin Tablets 872

Bendroflumethiazide (Additive effect on lowering blood pressure). Products include:
Corzide Tablets 702
Naturetin Tablets 1789
Rauzide Tablets 1804

Betaxolol Hydrochloride (Additive effect on lowering blood pressure). Products include:
Betoptic Sterile Ophthalmic Solution 569
Betoptic S Sterile Ophthalmic Suspension 570
Kerlone Tablets 2172

Bumetanide (Additive effect on lowering blood pressure). Products include:
Bumex 1895

Captopril (Additive effect on lowering blood pressure). Products include:
Capoten 2255
Capozide 2258

Carbamazepine (Increased carbamazepine concentrations). Products include:
Tegretol Chewable Tablets 654
Tegretol Suspension 656
Tegretol Tablets 654

Carteolol Hydrochloride (Additive negative effects on heart rate, AV conduction and/or cardiac contractility). Products include:
Cartrol Tablets 507

Chlorothiazide (Additive effect on lowering blood pressure). Products include:
Aldoclor Tablets 1413
Diupres Tablets 1461
Diuril Oral 1464

Chlorothiazide Sodium (Additive effect on lowering blood pressure). Products include:
Diuril Sodium Intravenous 1463

Chlorthalidone (Adverse effects on cardiac function; additive effect on lowering blood pressure). Products include:
Combipres Tablets 678
Tenoretic Tablets 1105
Thalitone Tablets 687

Cimetidine (Possible reduced verapamil clearance). Products include:
Tagamet Tablets 2228

Cimetidine Hydrochloride (Possible reduced verapamil clearance). Products include:
Tagamet 2228

Clonidine (Additive effect on lowering blood pressure). Products include:
Catapres-TTS 677

Clonidine Hydrochloride (Additive effect on lowering blood pressure; adverse effects on cardiac function). Products include:
Catapres Tablets 676
Combipres Tablets 678

Cyclosporine (Increased serum levels of cyclosporin). Products include:
Sandimmune 2024

Deserpidine (Additive effect on lowering blood pressure). Products include:
Enduronyl 518
Harmonyl Tablets 528
Oreticyl 545

Deslanoside (Chronic verapamil treatment can increase serum digoxin levels and this can result in digitalis toxicity).
No products indexed under this heading.

Diazoxide (Additive negative effects on heart rate, AV conduction and/or cardiac contractility). Products include:
- Hyperstat I.V. Injection ... 2095
- Proglycem ... 649

Digitoxin (Chronic verapamil treatment can increase serum digoxin levels and this can result in digitalis toxicity). Products include:
- Crystodigin Tablets ... 1253

Digoxin (Chronic verapamil treatment can increase serum digoxin levels and this can result in digitalis toxicity). Products include:
- Lanoxicaps ... 772
- Lanoxin Elixir Pediatric ... 775
- Lanoxin Injection ... 778
- Lanoxin Injection Pediatric ... 781
- Lanoxin Tablets ... 783

Disopyramide Phosphate (Should not be administered within 48 hours before or 24 hours after verapamil administration). Products include:
- Norpace ... 2177

Doxazosin Mesylate (May result in a reduction in blood pressure that is excessive in some patients). Products include:
- Cardura Tablets ... 1941

Enalapril Maleate (Additive effect on lowering blood pressure). Products include:
- Vaseretic Tablets ... 1559
- Vasotec Tablets ... 1564

Enalaprilat (Additive effect on lowering blood pressure). Products include:
- Vasotec I.V. ... 1562

Enflurane (Potential for excessive cardiovascular depression). Products include:
- Ethrane ... 599

Esmolol Hydrochloride (Additive negative effects on heart rate, AV conduction and/or cardiac contractility). Products include:
- Brevibloc Injection ... 942

Ethacrynic Acid (Additive effect on lowering blood pressure). Products include:
- Edecrin Tablets ... 1468

Felodipine (Additive effect on lowering blood pressure). Products include:
- Plendil Extended-Release Tablets ... 1526

Flecainide Acetate (Additive effects on myocardial contractility, AV conduction, and repolarization). Products include:
- Tambocor Tablets ... 1315

Fosinopril Sodium (Additive effect on lowering blood pressure). Products include:
- Monopril Tablets ... 1406

Furosemide (Additive effect on lowering blood pressure). Products include:
- Lasix ... 1093

Guanabenz Acetate (Additive effect on lowering blood pressure). Products include:
- Wytensin Tablets ... 2542

Guanethidine Monosulfate (Additive effect on lowering blood pressure). Products include:
- Esimil Tablets ... 864
- Ismelin Tablets ... 869

Halothane (Potential for excessive cardiovascular depression). Products include:
- Fluothane ... 2453

Hydralazine Hydrochloride (Additive effect on lowering blood pressure; adverse effects on cardiac function). Products include:
- Apresazide Capsules ... 854
- Apresoline Hydrochloride Parenteral (Ampuls) ... 856
- Apresoline Hydrochloride Tablets ... 855
- Apresoline-Esidrix Tablets ... 857
- Ser-Ap-Es Tablets ... 881
- Serpasil-Apresoline Tablets ... 884

Hydrochlorothiazide (Additive effect on lowering blood pressure). Products include:
- Aldactazide ... 2150
- Aldoril Tablets ... 1418
- Apresazide Capsules ... 854
- Apresoline-Esidrix Tablets ... 857
- Capozide ... 2258
- Dyazide Capsules ... 2208
- Esidrix Tablets ... 863
- Esimil Tablets ... 864
- HydroDIURIL Tablets ... 1484
- Hydropres Tablets ... 1485
- Inderide Tablets ... 2463
- Inderide LA Long Acting Capsules ... 2465
- Lopressor HCT Tablets ... 1034
- Maxzide ... 1215
- Moduretic Tablets ... 1510
- Normozide Tablets ... 2112
- Oretic Tablets ... 544
- Oreticyl ... 545
- Prinzide Tablets ... 1540
- Ser-Ap-Es Tablets ... 881
- Serpasil-Esidrix Tablets ... 886
- Timolide Tablets ... 1547
- Trandate HCT Tablets ... 579
- Vaseretic Tablets ... 1559
- Zestoretic ... 2274

Hydroflumethiazide (Additive effect on lowering blood pressure). Products include:
- Diucardin Tablets ... 2450
- Saluron ... 718
- Salutensin/Salutensin-Demi ... 719

Indapamide (Additive effect on lowering blood pressure). Products include:
- Lozol Tablets ... 1843

Isoflurane (Potential for excessive cardiovascular depression). Products include:
- Forane ... 600

Isradipine (Additive effect on lowering blood pressure). Products include:
- DynaCirc Capsules ... 2004

Labetalol Hydrochloride (Additive negative effects on heart rate, AV conduction and/or cardiac contractility). Products include:
- Normodyne Injection ... 2108
- Normodyne Tablets ... 2110
- Normozide Tablets ... 2112
- Trandate HCT Tablets ... 579
- Trandate Injection ... 577
- Trandate Tablets ... 579

Lisinopril (Additive effect on lowering blood pressure). Products include:
- Prinivil Tablets ... 1538
- Prinzide Tablets ... 1540
- Zestoretic ... 2274
- Zestril Tablets ... 2277

Lithium Carbonate (May result in lowering of serum lithium levels and increased sensitivity to the effects of lithium). Products include:
- Eskalith ... 2214
- Lithane Tablets ... 1596
- Lithium Carbonate Capsules & Tablets ... 1984
- Lithobid Tablets ... 870

Lithium Citrate (May result in lowering of serum lithium levels and increased sensitivity to the effects of lithium). Products include:
- Cibalith-S ... 870

Mecamylamine Hydrochloride (Additive effect on lowering blood pressure). Products include:
- Inversine Tablets ... 1492

Methoxyflurane (Potential for excessive cardiovascular depression).
- No products indexed under this heading.

Methyclothiazide (Additive effect on lowering blood pressure). Products include:
- Enduron Tablets ... 517
- Enduronyl ... 518

Methyldopa (Additive effect on lowering blood pressure). Products include:
- Aldoclor Tablets ... 1413
- Aldomet Oral ... 1415
- Aldoril Tablets ... 1418

Methyldopate Hydrochloride (Additive effect on lowering blood pressure). Products include:
- Aldomet Ester HCl Injection ... 1417

Metocurine Iodide (Verapamil may potentiate the activity of neuromuscular blocking agents). Products include:
- Metubine Iodide Vials ... 1285

Metolazone (Additive effect on lowering blood pressure). Products include:
- Diulo ... 2129
- Mykrox ½ mg Tablets ... 984
- Zaroxolyn Tablets ... 989

Metoprolol Tartrate (Additive negative effects on heart rate, AV conduction and/or cardiac contractility; a decrease in metoprolol clearance). Products include:
- Lopressor Ampuls ... 1032
- Lopressor HCT Tablets ... 1034
- Lopressor Tablets ... 1032

Metyrosine (Additive effect on lowering blood pressure). Products include:
- Demser Capsules ... 1460

Minoxidil (Additive effect on lowering blood pressure). Products include:
- Loniten Tablets ... 2346
- Rogaine Topical Solution ... 2357

Nadolol (Additive negative effects on heart rate, AV conduction and/or cardiac contractility). Products include:
- Corgard Tablets ... 701
- Corzide Tablets ... 702

Nicardipine Hydrochloride (Additive effect on lowering blood pressure). Products include:
- Cardene Capsules ... 2290

Pancuronium Bromide Injection (Verapamil may potentiate the activity of neuromuscular blocking agents).
- No products indexed under this heading.

Penbutolol Sulfate (Additive negative effects on heart rate, AV conduction and/or cardiac contractility). Products include:
- Levatol ... 1832

Phenobarbital (Increases verapamil clearance). Products include:
- Arco-Lase Plus Tablets ... 607
- Bellergal-S Tablets ... 1998
- Bronkolixir ... ▣ 761
- Bronkotabs Tablets ... ▣ 762
- Donnatal ... 1858
- Donnatal Extentabs ... 1859
- Donnatal Tablets ... 1858
- Donnazyme Tablets ... 1860
- Kinesed Tablets ... 2272
- Phenobarbital Elixir and Tablets ... 1293
- Primatene Tablets-P Formula ... 2421
- Quadrinal Tablets ... 1183
- Tedral SA ... 1765

Phenoxybenzamine Hydrochloride (Additive effect on lowering blood pressure). Products include:
- Dibenzyline Capsules ... 2207

Phentolamine Mesylate (Additive effect on lowering blood pressure). Products include:
- Regitine ... 878

Pindolol (Additive negative effects on heart rate, AV conduction and/or cardiac contractility). Products include:
- Visken Tablets ... 2036

Polythiazide (Additive effect on lowering blood pressure). Products include:
- Minizide Capsules ... 1779
- Renese Tablets ... 1785
- Renese-R Tablets ... 1786

Prazosin Hydrochloride (May result in a reduction in blood pressure that is excessive in some patients). Products include:
- Minipress Capsules ... 1778
- Minizide Capsules ... 1779

Propranolol Hydrochloride (Additive negative effects on heart rate, AV conduction and/or cardiac contractility). Products include:
- Inderal ... 2459
- Inderal LA Long Acting Capsules ... 2461
- Inderide Tablets ... 2463
- Inderide LA Long Acting Capsules ... 2465

Quinidine Gluconate (Hypotension (in patients with hypertrophic cardiomyopathy); increased quinidine levels). Products include:
- Quinaglute Dura-Tabs Tablets ... 663

Quinidine Polygalacturonate (Hypotension (in patients with hypertrophic cardiomyopathy); increased quinidine levels). Products include:
- Cardioquin Tablets ... 1812

Quinidine Sulfate (Hypotension (in patients with hypertrophic cardiomyopathy); increased quinidine levels). Products include:
- Quinidex Extentabs ... 1868

Ramipril (Additive effect on lowering blood pressure). Products include:
- Altace Capsules ... 1086

Rauwolfia Serpentina (Additive effect on lowering blood pressure). Products include:
- Raudixin Tablets ... 1803
- Rauzide Tablets ... 1804

Rescinnamine (Additive effect on lowering blood pressure).
- No products indexed under this heading.

Reserpine (Additive effect on lowering blood pressure). Products include:
- Diupres Tablets ... 1461
- Hydromox R Tablets ... 1209
- Hydropres Tablets ... 1485
- Renese-R Tablets ... 1786
- Salutensin/Salutensin-Demi ... 719
- Ser-Ap-Es Tablets ... 881
- Serpasil Tablets ... 883
- Serpasil-Apresoline Tablets ... 884
- Serpasil-Esidrix Tablets ... 886

Rifampin (Reduced verapamil bioavailability). Products include:
- Rifadin ... 1345
- Rifamate Capsules ... 1347
- Rimactane Capsules ... 879

Sodium Nitroprusside (Additive effect on lowering blood pressure). Products include:
- Nipride I.V. Infusion ... 1909

Spironolactone (Additive effect on lowering blood pressure). Products include:
- Aldactazide ... 2150
- Aldactone ... 2152

Succinylcholine Chloride (Verapamil may potentiate the activity of neuromuscular blocking agents). Products include:
- Anectine ... 755

Terazosin Hydrochloride (May result in a reduction in blood pressure that is excessive in some patients). Products include:
- Hytrin Tablets ... 529

Timolol Maleate (Additive negative effects on heart rate, AV conduction and/or cardiac contractility). Products include:
- Blocadren Tablets 1429
- Timolide Tablets 1547
- Timoptic in Ocudose 1552
- Timoptic Sterile Ophthalmic Solution 1550

Triamterene (Additive effect on lowering blood pressure). Products include:
- Dyazide Capsules 2208
- Dyrenium Capsules 2210
- Maxzide 1215

Trimethaphan Camsylate (Additive effect on lowering blood pressure). Products include:
- Arfonad Ampuls 1887

Vecuronium Bromide (Verapamil prolongs recovery from the neuromuscular blockade; may potentiate the activity of neuromuscular blocking agents). Products include:
- Norcuron 1642

Food Interactions

Food, unspecified (Produces decreased bioavailability (AUC) but a narrower peak to trough ratio).

ISOPTO ATROPINE
(Atropine Sulfate) ..... ⊚ 218
No interactions described in labeling.

ISOPTO CARBACHOL
(Carbachol) ..... ⊚ 219
No interactions described in labeling.

ISOPTO CARPINE
(Pilocarpine Hydrochloride) ..... ⊚ 219
No interactions described in labeling.

ISOPTO CETAMIDE SOLUTION
(Sulfacetamide Sodium) ..... ⊚ 220
May interact with silver preparations. Compounds in this category include:

Silver Nitrate (Incompatible).

ISOPTO CETAPRED SUSPENSION
(Prednisolone Acetate, Sulfacetamide Sodium) ..... ⊚ 220
No interactions described in labeling.

ISOPTO HOMATROPINE
(Homatropine Hydrobromide) ..... ⊚ 221
No interactions described in labeling.

ISOPTO HYOSCINE
(Scopolamine Hydrobromide) ..... ⊚ 222
No interactions described in labeling.

ISORDIL SUBLINGUAL TABLETS 2.5 MG, 5 MG & 10 MG
(Isosorbide Dinitrate) 2467
May interact with calcium channel blockers and certain other agents. Compounds in these categories include:

Alcohol (May enhance any marked sensitivity to the hypotensive effects).

Bepridil Hydrochloride (Marked orthostatic hypotension). Products include:
- Vascor (200, 300 and 400 mg) Tablets 1383

Diltiazem Hydrochloride (Marked orthostatic hypotension). Products include:
- Cardizem Tablets-30 mg, 60 mg, 90 mg and 120 mg 1329
- Cardizem SR Capsules-60 mg, 90 mg and 120 mg 1327

Felodipine (Marked orthostatic hypotension). Products include:
- Plendil Extended-Release Tablets 1526

Isradipine (Marked orthostatic hypotension). Products include:
- DynaCirc Capsules 2004

Nicardipine Hydrochloride (Marked orthostatic hypotension). Products include:
- Cardene Capsules 2290

Nifedipine (Marked orthostatic hypotension). Products include:
- Adalat Capsules (10 mg and 20 mg) 1587
- Procardia Capsules 1781
- Procardia XL Tablets 1783

Nimodipine (Marked orthostatic hypotension). Products include:
- Nimotop Capsules 1607

Verapamil Hydrochloride (Marked orthostatic hypotension). Products include:
- Calan SR Caplets 2157
- Calan Tablets 2155
- Isoptin Injectable 1177
- Isoptin Oral Tablets 1179
- Isoptin SR Sustained Release Tablets 1181
- Verelan Capsules 1243
- Verelan Capsules 2535

ISORDIL TEMBIDS CAPSULES (40 MG)
(Isosorbide Dinitrate) 2467
See **Isordil Sublingual Tablets 2.5 mg, 5 mg & 10 mg**

ISORDIL TEMBIDS TABLETS (40 MG)
(Isosorbide Dinitrate) 2467
See **Isordil Sublingual Tablets 2.5 mg, 5 mg & 10 mg**

ISORDIL 5 TITRADOSE TABLETS, 5 MG
(Isosorbide Dinitrate) 2467
See **Isordil Sublingual Tablets 2.5 mg, 5 mg & 10 mg**

ISORDIL 10 TITRADOSE TABLETS, 10 MG
(Isosorbide Dinitrate) 2467
See **Isordil Sublingual Tablets 2.5 mg, 5 mg & 10 mg**

ISORDIL 20 TITRADOSE TABLETS, 20 MG
(Isosorbide Dinitrate) 2467
See **Isordil Sublingual Tablets 2.5 mg, 5 mg & 10 mg**

ISORDIL 30 TITRADOSE TABLETS, 30 MG
(Isosorbide Dinitrate) 2467
See **Isordil Sublingual Tablets 2.5 mg, 5 mg & 10 mg**

ISORDIL 40 TITRADOSE TABLETS, 40 MG
(Isosorbide Dinitrate) 2467
See **Isordil Sublingual Tablets 2.5 mg, 5 mg & 10 mg**

ISUPREL HYDROCHLORIDE INJECTION 1:5000
(Isoproterenol Hydrochloride) 2050
May interact with inhalant anesthetics and certain other agents. Compounds in these categories include:

Enflurane (Myocardium sensitized to sympathomimetic amines). Products include:
- Ethrane 599

Epinephrine Hydrochloride (May induce serious arrhythmias). Products include:
- Adrenalin Chloride Solution 1:100 & 1:1,000 1689
- Epifrin ..... ⊚ 244
- Glaucon ..... ⊚ 218

Halothane (Myocardium sensitized to sympathomimetic amines). Products include:
- Fluothane 2453

Isoflurane (Myocardium sensitized to sympathomimetic amines). Products include:
- Forane 600

Methoxyflurane (Myocardium sensitized to sympathomimetic amines).
No products indexed under this heading.

ISUPREL HYDROCHLORIDE MISTOMETER
(Isoproterenol Hydrochloride) 2051
May interact with:

Epinephrine Hydrochloride (May induce serious arrhythmias). Products include:
- Adrenalin Chloride Solution 1:100 & 1:1,000 1689
- Epifrin ..... ⊚ 244
- Glaucon ..... ⊚ 218

ISUPREL HYDROCHLORIDE SOLUTION 1:200 & 1:100
(Isoproterenol Hydrochloride) 2052
May interact with:

Epinephrine Hydrochloride (May induce serious arrhythmias). Products include:
- Adrenalin Chloride Solution 1:100 & 1:1,000 1689
- Epifrin ..... ⊚ 244
- Glaucon ..... ⊚ 218

ITCH-X GEL
(Pramoxine Hydrochloride, Benzyl Alcohol) ..... ▣ 507
No interactions described in labeling.

JENEST-28 TABLETS
(Norethindrone, Ethinyl Estradiol) 1636
May interact with barbiturates, tetracyclines, and certain other agents. Compounds in these categories include:

Ampicillin Sodium (Reduces efficacy and increases incidence of breakthrough bleeding and menstrual irregularities). Products include:
- Unasyn 1965

Aprobarbital (Reduces efficacy and increases incidence of breakthrough bleeding and menstrual irregularities). Products include:
- Alurate Elixir 1883

Butabarbital (Reduces efficacy and increases incidence of breakthrough bleeding and menstrual irregularities). Products include:
- Pyridium Plus 1764

Butalbital (Reduces efficacy and increases incidence of breakthrough bleeding and menstrual irregularities). Products include:
- Esgic-Plus Tablets 1002
- Esgic Tablets & Capsules 1001
- Fioricet Tablets 2006
- Fiorinal Capsules 2007
- Fiorinal with Codeine Capsules 2008
- Fiorinal Tablets 2007
- Phrenilin 838
- Sedapap Tablets 50 mg/650 mg 1360

Demeclocycline Hydrochloride (Reduces efficacy and increases incidence of breakthrough bleeding and menstrual irregularities). Products include:
- Declomycin Capsules, Tablets 1199

Doxycycline Calcium (Reduces efficacy and increases incidence of breakthrough bleeding and menstrual irregularities).
No products indexed under this heading.

Doxycycline Hyclate (Reduces efficacy and increases incidence of breakthrough bleeding and menstrual irregularities). Products include:
- Doryx Capsules 1717
- Vibramycin Hyclate Capsules 1787
- Vibramycin Hyclate Intravenous 1968
- Vibra-Tabs Film Coated Tablets 1787

Doxycycline Monohydrate (Reduces efficacy and increases incidence of breakthrough bleeding and menstrual irregularities). Products include:
- Monodox Capsules 1630
- Vibramycin Monohydrate for Oral Suspension 1787

Griseofulvin (Reduces efficacy and increases incidence of breakthrough bleeding and menstrual irregularities). Products include:
- Fulvicin P/G Tablets 2090
- Fulvicin P/G 165 & 330 Tablets 2091
- Fulvicin-U/F Tablets 2092
- Grifulvin V (griseofulvin microsize) Tablets/Suspension 1678
- Grisactin 2454
- Grisactin Ultra Tablets 2455
- Gris-PEG Tablets, 125 mg & 250 mg 1083

Mephobarbital (Reduces efficacy and increases incidence of breakthrough bleeding and menstrual irregularities). Products include:
- Mebaral Tablets 2061

Methacycline Hydrochloride (Reduces efficacy and increases incidence of breakthrough bleeding and menstrual irregularities).
No products indexed under this heading.

Minocycline Hydrochloride (Reduces efficacy and increases incidence of breakthrough bleeding and menstrual irregularities). Products include:
- Minocin Intravenous 1221
- Minocin Oral Suspension 1224
- Minocin Pellet-Filled Capsules 1222

Oxytetracycline Hydrochloride (Reduces efficacy and increases incidence of breakthrough bleeding and menstrual irregularities). Products include:
- Terra-Cortril Ophthalmic Suspension 1963
- Terramycin Capsules 1786
- Terramycin Intramuscular Solution 1964
- Terramycin with Polymyxin B Sulfate Ophthalmic Ointment 1965

Pentobarbital Sodium (Reduces efficacy and increases incidence of breakthrough bleeding and menstrual irregularities). Products include:
- Nembutal Sodium Capsules 534
- Nembutal Sodium Solution 536
- Nembutal Sodium Suppositories 538

Phenobarbital (Reduces efficacy and increases incidence of breakthrough bleeding and menstrual irregularities). Products include:
- Arco-Lase Plus Tablets 607
- Bellergal-S Tablets 1998
- Bronkolixir ..... ▣ 761
- Bronkotabs Tablets ..... ▣ 762
- Donnatal 1858
- Donnatal Extentabs 1859
- Donnatal Tablets 1858
- Donnazyme Tablets 1860
- Kinesed Tablets 2272
- Phenobarbital Elixir and Tablets 1293
- Primatene Tablets-P Formula 2421
- Quadrinal Tablets 1183
- Tedral SA 1765

Phenylbutazone (Reduces efficacy and increases incidence of breakthrough bleeding and menstrual irregularities). Products include:
Butazolidin Capsules & Tablets........ 1027
Phenytoin Sodium (Reduces efficacy and increases incidence of breakthrough bleeding and menstrual irregularities). Products include:
Dilantin Kapseals 1708
Dilantin Parenteral 1712
Dilantin with Phenobarbital Kapseals 1715
Rifampin (Reduces efficacy and increases incidence of breakthrough bleeding and menstrual irregularities). Products include:
Rifadin 1345
Rifamate Capsules 1347
Rimactane Capsules 879
Secobarbital Sodium (Reduces efficacy and increases incidence of breakthrough bleeding and menstrual irregularities). Products include:
Seconal Sodium Pulvules 1296
Tetracycline Hydrochloride (Reduces efficacy and increases incidence of breakthrough bleeding and menstrual irregularities). Products include:
Achromycin V Capsules 1193
Achromycin Ophthalmic Ointment 1% .... ⊙ 307
Achromycin Ophthalmic Suspension 1% .... ⊙ 308
Topicycline for Topical Solution 1856
Thiamylal Sodium (Reduces efficacy and increases incidence of breakthrough bleeding and menstrual irregularities). Products include:
Surital Ampoules, Steri-Vials.......... 1764

JEVITY ISOTONIC LIQUID NUTRITION WITH FIBER
(Nutritional Supplement) 1972
No interactions described in labeling.

JOHNSON'S MEDICATED DIAPER RASH OINTMENT
(Zinc Oxide) .... ⊞ 577
No interactions described in labeling.

K-DUR MICROBURST RELEASE SYSTEM (POTASSIUM CHLORIDE, USP) E.R. TABLETS
(Potassium Chloride)..........1163
May interact with potassium sparing diuretics and ACE inhibitors. Compounds in these categories include:

Amiloride Hydrochloride (Severe hyperkalemia). Products include:
Midamor Tablets 1508
Moduretic Tablets 1510
Benazepril Hydrochloride (Potential for increased potassium retention). Products include:
Lotensin Tablets.......... 872
Captopril (Potential for increased potassium retention). Products include:
Capoten 2255
Capozide 2258
Enalapril Maleate (Potential for increased potassium retention). Products include:
Vaseretic Tablets 1559
Vasotec Tablets 1564
Enalaprilat (Potential for increased potassium retention). Products include:
Vasotec I.V. 1562
Fosinopril Sodium (Potential for increased potassium retention). Products include:
Monopril Tablets 1406
Lisinopril (Potential for increased potassium retention). Products include:
Prinivil Tablets 1538
Prinzide Tablets 1540
Zestoretic 2274
Zestril Tablets 2277
Ramipril (Potential for increased potassium retention). Products include:
Altace Capsules 1086
Spironolactone (Severe hyperkalemia). Products include:
Aldactazide.......... 2150
Aldactone 2152
Triamterene (Severe hyperkalemia). Products include:
Dyazide Capsules.......... 2208
Dyrenium Capsules.......... 2210
Maxzide 1215

K-LOR POWDER PACKETS
(Potassium Chloride).......... 531
May interact with potassium sparing diuretics and ACE inhibitors. Compounds in these categories include:

Amiloride Hydrochloride (Potential for severe hyperkalemia). Products include:
Midamor Tablets 1508
Moduretic Tablets 1510
Benazepril Hydrochloride (Potential for hyperkalemia). Products include:
Lotensin Tablets.......... 872
Captopril (Potential for hyperkalemia). Products include:
Capoten 2255
Capozide 2258
Enalapril Maleate (Potential for hyperkalemia). Products include:
Vaseretic Tablets 1559
Vasotec Tablets 1564
Enalaprilat (Potential for hyperkalemia). Products include:
Vasotec I.V. 1562
Fosinopril Sodium (Potential for hyperkalemia). Products include:
Monopril Tablets 1406
Lisinopril (Potential for hyperkalemia). Products include:
Prinivil Tablets 1538
Prinzide Tablets 1540
Zestoretic 2274
Zestril Tablets 2277
Ramipril (Potential for hyperkalemia). Products include:
Altace Capsules 1086
Spironolactone (Potential for severe hyperkalemia). Products include:
Aldactazide.......... 2150
Aldactone 2152
Triamterene (Potential for severe hyperkalemia). Products include:
Dyazide Capsules.......... 2208
Dyrenium Capsules.......... 2210
Maxzide 1215

K-LYTE/CL 50 EFFERVESCENT TABLETS
(Potassium Preparations).......... 707
See **K-Lyte & K-Lyte DS Effervescent Tablets**

K-LYTE/CL EFFERVESCENT TABLETS
(Potassium Preparations).......... 707
See **K-Lyte & K-Lyte DS Effervescent Tablets**

K-LYTE & K-LYTE DS EFFERVESCENT TABLETS
(Potassium Preparations).......... 707
May interact with:

Amiloride Hydrochloride (Severe hyperkalemia). Products include:
Midamor Tablets 1508
Moduretic Tablets 1510
Spironolactone (Severe hyperkalemia). Products include:
Aldactazide.......... 2150
Aldactone 2152
Triamterene (Severe hyperkalemia). Products include:
Dyazide Capsules.......... 2208
Dyrenium Capsules.......... 2210
Maxzide 1215

K-NORM CAPSULES
(Potassium Chloride).......... 982
May interact with potassium sparing diuretics. Compounds in this category include:

Amiloride Hydrochloride (Concurrent administration can produce severe hyperkalemia). Products include:
Midamor Tablets 1508
Moduretic Tablets 1510
Spironolactone (Concurrent administration can produce severe hyperkalemia). Products include:
Aldactazide.......... 2150
Aldactone 2152
Triamterene (Concurrent administration can produce severe hyperkalemia). Products include:
Dyazide Capsules.......... 2208
Dyrenium Capsules.......... 2210
Maxzide 1215

K-PHOS M.F. TABLETS
(Potassium Acid Phosphate, Sodium Acid Phosphate).......... 659
May interact with antacids, catecholamine depleting drugs, potassium sparing diuretics, salicylates, potassium-depleting corticosteroids, corticosteroids, and certain other agents. Compounds in these categories include:

ACTH (Hypernatremia).
Aluminum Carbonate Gel (May bind the phosphate and prevent its absorption). Products include:
Basaljel.......... 2438
Aluminum Hydroxide (May bind the phosphate and prevent its absorption). Products include:
Cama Arthritis Pain Reliever.......... ⊞ 685
Gaviscon Extra Strength Relief Formula Liquid Antacid.......... ⊞ 594
Gaviscon Extra Strength Relief Formula Antacid Tablets.......... ⊞ 594
Gaviscon Liquid Antacid.......... ⊞ 594
Gelusil Liquid & Tablets .... ⊞ 639
Extra Strength Maalox Plus Suspension.......... 1850
Maalox TC Suspension 1851
Maalox Plus Tablets .... ⊞ 655
Extra Strength Maalox Plus Tablets 1850
Nephrox Suspension .... ⊞ 563
WinGel Liquid & Tablets.......... ⊞ 761
Aluminum Hydroxide Gel (May bind the phosphate and prevent its absorption). Products include:
ALternaGEL Liquid 1154
Aludrox Oral Suspension 2428
Amphojel Suspension 2429
Amphojel Suspension without Flavor 2429
Mylanta Liquid 1155
Mylanta Double Strength Liquid 1155
Aluminum Hydroxide Gel, Dried (May bind the phosphate and prevent its absorption). Products include:
Alu-Tab/Alu-Cap 1309
Amphojel Tablets.......... 2429
Ascriptin A/D Caplets 1850
Regular Strength Ascriptin Tablets 1850
Gaviscon Antacid Tablets.......... ⊞ 593
Gaviscon-2 Antacid Tablets .... ⊞ 594
Mylanta Tablets 1155
Mylanta Double Strength Tablets 1155
Amiloride Hydrochloride (Hyperkalemia; monitor potassium levels periodically). Products include:
Midamor Tablets 1508
Moduretic Tablets 1510
Aspirin (Increased plasma salicylate levels). Products include:
Alka-Seltzer Effervescent Antacid and Pain Reliever.......... 1568
Alka-Seltzer Extra Strength Effervescent Antacid and Pain Reliever 1570
Alka-Seltzer (Flavored) Effervescent Antacid and Pain Reliever 1569
Alka-Seltzer Plus Cold Medicine .... ⊞ 623
Alka-Seltzer Plus Night-Time Cold Medicine .... ⊞ 623
Alka Seltzer Plus Sinus Allergy Medicine .... ⊞ 624
Anacin Coated Analgesic Caplets 2417
Anacin Coated Analgesic Tablets 2417
Anacin Maximum Strength Analgesic Coated Tablets.......... 2417
Maximum Strength Arthritis Pain Formula By the Makers of Anacin Analgesic Tablets and Caplets.......... 2418
Arthritis Pain Formula by the Makers of Anacin Analgesic Tablets and Caplets .... ⊞ 747
Arthritis Strength BC Powder.......... ⊞ 516
Ascriptin A/D Caplets 1850
Regular Strength Ascriptin Tablets 1850
Azdōne Tablets.......... 844
BC Powder .... ⊞ 517
BC Cold Powder.......... ⊞ 517
Children's Bayer Chewable Aspirin.......... ⊞ 564
Genuine Bayer Aspirin Tablets & Caplets.......... ⊞ 564
Maximum Bayer Aspirin Tablets & Caplets .... ⊞ 566
Bayer Plus Aspirin Tablets.......... ⊞ 567
Therapy Bayer Aspirin Caplets .... ⊞ 568
8 Hour Bayer Timed-Release Aspirin .... ⊞ 566
Arthritis Strength Bufferin Analgesic Caplets 744
Extra Strength Bufferin Analgesic Tablets 745
Bufferin Analgesic Tablets and Caplets 743
Cama Arthritis Pain Reliever.......... ⊞ 685
Damason-P.......... 1356
Easprin.......... 1719
Ecotrin Enteric Coated Aspirin Maximum Strength Tablets and Caplets.......... 2189
Ecotrin Enteric Coated Aspirin Regular Strength Tablets and Caplets.......... 2189
Empirin Aspirin.......... ⊞ 541
Empirin with Codeine Phosphate Nos. 2, 3 & 4.......... 764
Equagesic Tablets 2451
Excedrin Extra-Strength Analgesic Tablets & Caplets 749
4-Way Cold Tablets.......... 750
Fiorinal Capsules 2007
Fiorinal with Codeine Capsules 2008
Fiorinal Tablets.......... 2007
Lortab ASA Tablets.......... 2414
Momentum Muscular Backache Formula .... ⊞ 751
Norgesic.......... 1314
Norwich Extra-Strength Aspirin.......... ⊞ 546
Norwich Regular Strength Aspirin ⊞ 547
P-A-C Analgesic Tablets .... ⊞ 669
Percodan.......... 951
Robaxisal Tablets.......... 1872
Sine-Off Sinus Medicine Tablets-Aspirin Formula .... ⊞ 722
Soma Compound w/Codeine Tablets.......... 2390
Soma Compound Tablets.......... 2389
St. Joseph Adult Chewable Aspirin (81 mg.).......... ⊞ 703
Synalgos-DC Capsules.......... 2525
Talwin Compound 2072
Ursinus Inlay-Tabs.......... ⊞ 691
Vanquish Analgesic Caplets .... ⊞ 574
Zorprin Tablets.......... 698
Betamethasone Acetate (Hypernatremia). Products include:
Celestone Soluspan Suspension 2081

Betamethasone Sodium Phosphate (Hypernatremia). Products include:
Celestone Soluspan Suspension 2081

Choline Magnesium Trisalicylate (Increased plasma salicylate levels). Products include:
Trilisate 1822

Cortisone Acetate (Hypernatremia). Products include:
Cortone Acetate Sterile Suspension 1437
Cortone Acetate Tablets 1439

Deserpidine (Hypernatremia). Products include:
Enduronyl 518
Harmonyl Tablets 528
Oreticyl 545

Desoxycorticosterone Acetate (Hypernatremia).

Dexamethasone (Hypernatremia). Products include:
AK-Trol Ointment & Suspension .... ⊙ 207
Decadron Elixir 1445
Decadron Tablets 1447
Decaspray Topical Aerosol 1459
Dexacidin .... ⊙ 272
Maxidex Sterile Ophthalmic Suspension .... ⊙ 223
Maxitrol Ophthalmic Ointment/Suspension .... ⊙ 223
TobraDex Ophthalmic Suspension and Ointment .... ⊙ 228

Dexamethasone Acetate (Hypernatremia). Products include:
Dalalone D.P. Injectable 999
Decadron-LA Sterile Suspension 1457

Dexamethasone Sodium Phosphate (Hypernatremia). Products include:
AK-Dex .... ⊙ 203
Decadron Phosphate Respihaler 1454
Decadron Phosphate Sterile Ophthalmic Ointment 1453
Decadron Phosphate Sterile Ophthalmic Solution 1453
Decadron Phosphate Topical Cream 1455
Decadron Phosphate Turbinaire 1456
Maxidex Sterile Ophthalmic Ointment .... ⊙ 222
NeoDecadron Sterile Ophthalmic Ointment 1517
NeoDecadron Sterile Ophthalmic Solution 1518
NeoDecadron Topical Cream 1518

Diazoxide (Hypernatremia). Products include:
Hyperstat I.V. Injection 2095
Proglycem 649

Diflunisal (Increased plasma salicylate levels). Products include:
Dolobid Tablets 1465

Dihydroxyaluminum Sodium Carbonate (May bind the phosphate and prevent its absorption). Products include:
Rolaids .... ▣ 743

Guanethidine Monosulfate (Hypernatremia). Products include:
Esimil Tablets 864
Ismelin Tablets 869

Hydralazine Hydrochloride (Hypernatremia). Products include:
Apresazide Capsules 854
Apresoline Hydrochloride Parenteral (Ampuls) 856
Apresoline Hydrochloride Tablets .. 855
Apresoline-Esidrix Tablets 857
Ser-Ap-Es Tablets 881
Serpasil-Apresoline Tablets 884

Hydrocortisone (Hypernatremia). Products include:
AK-Spore H.C. .... ⊙ 206
Bactine Hydrocortisone Anti-Itch Cream .... ▣ 625
CaldeCORT Anti-Itch Hydrocortisone Spray .... ▣ 560
Carmol HC Cream 1% 2296
Cortaid Spray .... ▣ 735
Cortenema 2244
Cortisporin Ointment 758
Cortisporin Ophthalmic Ointment Sterile 758
Cortisporin Ophthalmic Suspension Sterile 759
Cortisporin Otic Solution Sterile 760
Cortisporin Otic Suspension Sterile 760
Cortizone-5 Creme & Ointment ...... ▣ 732
Dermolate Anti-Itch Cream .... ▣ 697
Eldecort Cream 1.0% 1113
Eldecort Cream 1.0% and 2.5% 1113
Fungoid HC Creme 1770
Hydrocortone Tablets 1482
Hytone 909
LazerSporin-C Solution 1770
Massengill Medicated Soft Cloth Towelettes 2192
Nutracort Cream & Lotion 1684
PediOtic Suspension Sterile 797
Synacort Creams 1%, 2.5% 2296
Vanoxide-HC Acne Lotion 911
Vioform-Hydrocortisone Cream and Mild Cream 889
Vioform-Hydrocortisone Ointment .. 889
VōSoL HC Otic Solution 2392
Vytone Cream 1% 911

Hydrocortisone Acetate (Hypernatremia). Products include:
Analpram-HC Rectal Cream 1% and 2.5% 970
Anusol-HC Cream 1690
Anusol-HC Suppositories 1691
Caldecort .... ▣ 560
Carmol HC Cream 1% 2296
Chloromycetin Hydrocortisone Ophthalmic 1694
Coly-Mycin S Otic w/Neomycin & Hydrocortisone 1708
Cortaid .... ▣ 735
Cortef Feminine Itch Cream .... ▣ 735
Corticaine .... ▣ 682
Cortifoam 1827
Cortisporin Cream 757
Epifoam 1828
Gynecort 5 Creme .... ▣ 556
Hydrocortone Acetate Sterile Suspension 1479
Lanacort 5 Creme and Ointment .. ▣ 557
Mantadil Cream 789
Ophthocort .... ⊙ 301
Orabase HCA Oral Paste 890
Pramosone Cream, Lotion & Ointment 971
ProctoCream-HC 1834
Proctofoam-HC 1835

Hydrocortisone Sodium Phosphate (Hypernatremia). Products include:
Hydrocortone Phosphate Injection, Sterile 1481

Hydrocortisone Sodium Succinate (Hypernatremia). Products include:
Solu-Cortef Sterile Powder 2361

Magaldrate (May bind the phosphate and prevent its absorption). Products include:
Riopan Antacid Chew Tablets .... ▣ 754
Riopan Antacid Chew Tablets in Rollpacks .... ▣ 754
Riopan Antacid Suspension 2421
Riopan Antacid Swallow Tablets 2421
Riopan Plus Chew Tablets 2422
Riopan Plus Chew Tablets in Rollpack 2422
Riopan Plus 2 Chew Tablets, Mint Flavor, Cherry Flavor 2422
Riopan Plus Suspension 2422
Riopan Plus 2 Suspension, Mint Flavor, Cherry Flavor 2422

Magnesium Hydroxide (May bind the phosphate and prevent its absorption). Products include:
Aludrox Oral Suspension 2428
Ascriptin A/D Caplets 1850
Regular Strength Ascriptin Tablets 1850
Di-Gel Antacid/Anti-Gas .... ▣ 697
Gelusil Liquid & Tablets .... ▣ 639
Haley's M-O, Regular & Flavored ... ▣ 569
Extra Strength Maalox Plus Suspension 1850
Maalox TC Suspension 1851
Maalox Plus Tablets .... ▣ 655
Extra Strength Maalox Plus Tablets 1850
Mylanta Liquid 1155
Mylanta Tablets 1155
Mylanta Double Strength Liquid 1155
Mylanta Double Strength Tablets 1155
Concentrated Phillips' Milk of Magnesia .... ▣ 573
Phillips' Milk of Magnesia Liquid .... ▣ 572
Phillips' Milk of Magnesia Tablets ▣ 573
WinGel Liquid & Tablets .... ▣ 761

Magnesium Oxide (May bind the phosphate and prevent its absorption). Products include:
Bayer Plus Aspirin Tablets .... ▣ 567
Beelith Tablets 659
Bufferin Analgesic Tablets and Caplets .... ▣ 524
Cama Arthritis Pain Reliever .... ▣ 685
Mag-Ox 400 673
Uro-Mag 673

Magnesium Salicylate (Increased plasma salicylate levels; toxic levels). Products include:
Doan's - Extra-Strength Analgesic ▣ 549
Doan's - Regular Strength Analgesic .... ▣ 549
Mobigesic Analgesic Tablets .... ▣ 507

Methyldopa (Hypernatremia). Products include:
Aldoclor Tablets 1413
Aldomet Oral 1415
Aldoril Tablets 1418

Methyldopate Hydrochloride (Hypernatremia). Products include:
Aldomet Ester HCl Injection 1417

Methylprednisolone Acetate (Hypernatremia). Products include:
Depo-Medrol Sterile Aqueous Suspension 2334

Methylprednisolone Sodium Succinate (Hypernatremia). Products include:
Solu-Medrol Sterile Powder 2363

Potassium Bicarbonate (Hyperkalemia; monitor potassium levels periodically). Products include:
Alka-Seltzer Advanced Formula Antacid & Non-Aspirin Pain Reliever .... ▣ 620
Alka-Seltzer Effervescent Antacid ▣ 622
K-Lyte 707
Klorvess Effervescent Granules 2010
Klorvess Effervescent Tablets 2011

Potassium Chloride (Hyperkalemia; monitor potassium levels periodically). Products include:
Chlor-3 Condiment 994
K-Dur Microburst Release System (potassium chloride, USP) E.R. Tablets 1163
K-Lor Powder Packets 531
K-Lyte 707
K-Norm Capsules 982
K-Tab Filmtab 532
Kato Potassium Supplement 1114
Klor-Con 8/Klor-Con 10 Extended-release Tablets 2374
Klorvess Effervescent Granules 2010
Klorvess Effervescent Tablets 2011
Klorvess 10% Liquid 2010
Klotrix 708
Kolyum Liquid 983
Micro-K 1863
Micro-K LS Packets 1864
NuLYTELY 699
Oral Rehydration Salts, Citrate 1150
Rum-K Syrup 995
Slow-K Tablets 2281
Ten-K Controlled-Release Tablets 2282
Thermotabs .... ▣ 619

Potassium Citrate (Hyperkalemia; monitor potassium levels periodically). Products include:
Alka-Seltzer Effervescent Antacid .. 1570
K-Lyte 707
Polycitra Syrup 2424
Polycitra-K 2424
Polycitra-LC—Sugar-Free 2424
Ricelyte, Rice-Based Oral Electrolyte Maintenance Solution .... ▣ 613

Potassium Gluconate (Hyperkalemia; monitor potassium levels periodically). Products include:
Kolyum Liquid 983

Potassium Phosphate, Dibasic (Hyperkalemia; monitor potassium levels periodically). Products include:
Neutra-Phos 2423

Potassium Phosphate, Monobasic (Hyperkalemia; monitor potassium levels periodically). Products include:
K-Phos M.F. Tablets 659
K-Phos Neutral Tablets 660
Neutra-Phos 2423

Prednisolone Acetate (Hypernatremia). Products include:
AK-Cide Sterile Ophthalmic Ointment & Suspension .... ⊙ 202
Blephamide Liquifilm Sterile Ophthalmic Suspension 586
Blephamide S.O.P. Sterile Ophthalmic Ointment 586
Cetapred Ointment .... ⊙ 220
⅛% Econopred & 1% Econopred Plus .... ⊙ 217
Isopto Cetapred Suspension .... ⊙ 220
Metimyd .... ⊙ 306
Poly-Pred Liquifilm .... ⊙ 250
Pred Forte .... ⊙ 252
Pred Mild .... ⊙ 254
Pred-G Liquifilm Sterile Ophthalmic Suspension .... ⊙ 252
Pred-G S.O.P. Sterile Ophthalmic Ointment .... ⊙ 253
Vasocidin Ointment .... ⊙ 275

Prednisolone Sodium Phosphate (Hypernatremia). Products include:
AK-Pred .... ⊙ 205
Hydeltrasol Injection, Sterile 1476
Inflamase .... ⊙ 274
Pediapred Oral Liquid 987
Vasocidin Ophthalmic Solution ...... ⊙ 276

Prednisolone Tebutate (Hypernatremia). Products include:
Hydeltra-T.B.A. Sterile Suspension 1478

Prednisone (Hypernatremia). Products include:
Deltasone Tablets 2332

Rauwolfia Serpentina (Hypernatremia). Products include:
Raudixin Tablets 1803
Rauzide Tablets 1804

Rescinnamine (Hypernatremia).
No products indexed under this heading.

Reserpine (Hypernatremia). Products include:
Diupres Tablets 1461
Hydromox R Tablets 1209
Hydropres Tablets 1485
Renese-R Tablets 1786
Salutensin/Salutensin-Demi 719
Ser-Ap-Es Tablets 881
Serpasil Tablets 883
Serpasil-Apresoline Tablets 884
Serpasil-Esidrix Tablets 886

Salsalate (Increased plasma salicylate levels). Products include:
Disalcid 1310
Mono-Gesic Tablets 846
Salflex 839

Spironolactone (Hyperkalemia; monitor potassium levels periodically). Products include:
Aldactazide 2150
Aldactone 2152

Triamcinolone (Hypernatremia).
No products indexed under this heading.

Triamcinolone Acetonide (Hypernatremia). Products include:
Aristocort A 1010
Azmacort Inhaler 1837
Kenalog Cream, Lotion & Ointment 2401
Kenalog-10 Injection 2402
Kenalog-40 Injection 2403
Kenalog in Orabase 604
Kenalog Spray 2401
Mycolog II Cream and Ointment 2407
Mytrex Cream & Ointment 2080
Nasacort Nasal Inhaler 1844

Triamcinolone Diacetate (Hypernatremia). Products include:
Aristocort Suspension 1008

Triamcinolone Hexacetonide (Hypernatremia). Products include:
Aristospan Suspension 1011

Triamterene (Hyperkalemia; monitor potassium levels periodically). Products include:
- Dyazide Capsules ... 2208
- Dyrenium Capsules ... 2210
- Maxzide ... 1215

K-PHOS NEUTRAL TABLETS
(Potassium Phosphate, Monobasic, Sodium Phosphate) ... 660
May interact with antacids, catecholamine depleting drugs, calcium preparations, salicylates, potassium-depleting corticosteroids, corticosteroids, potassium sparing diuretics, and certain other agents. Compounds in these categories include:

ACTH (Hypernatremia).

Aluminum Carbonate Gel (May bind phosphate and prevent its absorption). Products include:
- Basaljel ... 2438

Aluminum Hydroxide (May bind phosphate and prevent its absorption). Products include:
- Cama Arthritis Pain Reliever ... ■ 685
- Gaviscon Extra Strength Relief Formula Liquid Antacid ... ■ 594
- Gaviscon Extra Strength Relief Formula Antacid Tablets ... ■ 594
- Gaviscon Liquid Antacid ... ■ 594
- Gelusil Liquid & Tablets ... ■ 639
- Extra Strength Maalox Plus Suspension ... 1850
- Maalox TC Suspension ... 1851
- Maalox Plus Tablets ... ■ 655
- Extra Strength Maalox Plus Tablets 1850
- Nephrox Suspension ... ■ 563
- WinGel Liquid & Tablets ... ■ 761

Aluminum Hydroxide Gel (May bind phosphate and prevent its absorption). Products include:
- ALternaGEL Liquid ... 1154
- Aludrox Oral Suspension ... 2428
- Amphojel Suspension ... 2429
- Amphojel Suspension without Flavor ... 2429
- Mylanta Liquid ... 1155
- Mylanta Double Strength Liquid ... 1155

Aluminum Hydroxide Gel, Dried (May bind phosphate and prevent its absorption). Products include:
- Alu-Tab/Alu-Cap ... 1309
- Amphojel Tablets ... 2429
- Ascriptin A/D Caplets ... 1850
- Regular Strength Ascriptin Tablets 1850
- Gaviscon Antacid Tablets ... ■ 593
- Gaviscon-2 Antacid Tablets ... ■ 594
- Mylanta Tablets ... 1155
- Mylanta Double Strength Tablets ... 1155

Amiloride Hydrochloride (Hyperkalemia; monitor potassium levels periodically). Products include:
- Midamor Tablets ... 1508
- Moduretic Tablets ... 1510

Betamethasone Acetate (Hypernatremia). Products include:
- Celestone Soluspan Suspension ... 2081

Betamethasone Sodium Phosphate (Hypernatremia). Products include:
- Celestone Soluspan Suspension ... 2081

Calcium Carbonate (May antagonize effects of phosphates in treatment of hypercalcemia). Products include:
- Alka-Mints Chewable Antacid ... ■ 620
- Alka-Seltzer Advanced Formula Antacid & Non-Aspirin Pain Reliever ... ■ 620
- Ascriptin A/D Caplets ... 1850
- Regular Strength Ascriptin Tablets 1850
- Balmex Baby Powder ... ■ 590
- Bayer Plus Aspirin Tablets ... ■ 567
- Biocal 500 mg Tablet Calcium Supplement ... ■ 625
- Bufferin Analgesic Tablets and Caplets ... ■ 524
- Caltrate 600 ... ■ 583
- Caltrate 600 + Iron ... ■ 583
- Caltrate 600 + Vitamin D ... ■ 584
- Caltrate, Jr. ... ■ 583
- Centrum, Jr. (Children's Chewable) + Extra Calcium ... ■ 585
- Di-Gel Antacid/Anti-Gas ... ■ 697
- Gerimed Tablets ... 972
- Marblen ... ■ 563
- Natalins Rx ... 1391
- Natalins Tablets ... 1391
- Nephro-Calci Tablets ... 1826
- Os-Cal 500 Chewable Tablets ... ■ 596
- Os-Cal 500 Tablets ... ■ 597
- Os-Cal 250+D Tablets ... ■ 597
- Os-Cal 500+D Tablets ... ■ 597
- Pramet FA ... 1974
- Pramilet FA ... 1974
- Rolaids (Calcium Rich/Sodium Free) ... ■ 744
- Extra Strength Rolaids ... ■ 744
- Thermotabs ... ■ 619
- Total Formula-2 (multivitamin/multimineral) ... 2377
- Tums Liquid Extra ... ■ 726
- Zenate Tablets ... 2250

Calcium Chloride (May antagonize effects of phosphates in treatment of hypercalcemia).
- No products indexed under this heading.

Calcium Citrate (May antagonize effects of phosphates in treatment of hypercalcemia). Products include:
- Citracal Liquitab ... 1613
- Total Formula-2 (multivitamin/multimineral) ... 2377

Calcium Glubionate (May antagonize effects of phosphates in treatment of hypercalcemia). Products include:
- Neo-Calglucon Syrup ... 2018

Cortisone Acetate (Hypernatremia). Products include:
- Cortone Acetate Sterile Suspension ... 1437
- Cortone Acetate Tablets ... 1439

Deserpidine (Hypernatremia). Products include:
- Enduronyl ... 518
- Harmonyl Tablets ... 528
- Oreticyl ... 545

Desoxycorticosterone Acetate (Hypernatremia).

Dexamethasone (Hypernatremia). Products include:
- AK-Trol Ointment & Suspension ... ◉ 207
- Decadron Elixir ... 1445
- Decadron Tablets ... 1447
- Decaspray Topical Aerosol ... 1459
- Dexacidin ... ◉ 272
- Maxidex Sterile Ophthalmic Suspension ... ◉ 223
- Maxitrol Ophthalmic Ointment/Suspension ... ◉ 223
- TobraDex Ophthalmic Suspension and Ointment ... ◉ 228

Dexamethasone Acetate (Hypernatremia). Products include:
- Dalalone D.P. Injectable ... 999
- Decadron-LA Sterile Suspension ... 1457

Dexamethasone Sodium Phosphate (Hypernatremia). Products include:
- AK-Dex ... ◉ 203
- Decadron Phosphate Respihaler ... 1454
- Decadron Phosphate Sterile Ophthalmic Ointment ... 1453
- Decadron Phosphate Sterile Ophthalmic Solution ... 1453
- Decadron Phosphate Topical Cream ... 1455
- Decadron Phosphate Turbinaire ... 1456
- Maxidex Sterile Ophthalmic Ointment ... ◉ 222
- NeoDecadron Sterile Ophthalmic Ointment ... 1517
- NeoDecadron Sterile Ophthalmic Solution ... 1518
- NeoDecadron Topical Cream ... 1518

Diazoxide (Hypernatremia). Products include:
- Hyperstat I.V. Injection ... 2095
- Proglycem ... 649

Dihydroxyaluminum Sodium Carbonate (May bind phosphate and prevent its absorption). Products include:
- Rolaids ... ■ 743

Guanethidine Monosulfate (Hypernatremia). Products include:
- Esimil Tablets ... 864
- Ismelin Tablets ... 869

Hydralazine Hydrochloride (Hypernatremia). Products include:
- Apresazide Capsules ... 854
- Apresoline Hydrochloride Parenteral (Ampuls) ... 856
- Apresoline Hydrochloride Tablets .. 855
- Apresoline-Esidrix Tablets ... 857
- Ser-Ap-Es Tablets ... 881
- Serpasil-Apresoline Tablets ... 884

Hydrocortisone (Hypernatremia). Products include:
- AK-Spore H.C. ... ◉ 206
- Bactine Hydrocortisone Anti-Itch Cream ... ■ 625
- CaldeCORT Anti-Itch Hydrocortisone Spray ... ■ 560
- Carmol HC Cream 1% ... 2296
- Cortaid Spray ... ■ 735
- Cortenema ... 2244
- Cortisporin Ointment ... 758
- Cortisporin Ophthalmic Ointment Sterile ... 758
- Cortisporin Ophthalmic Suspension Sterile ... 759
- Cortisporin Otic Solution Sterile ... 760
- Cortisporin Otic Suspension Sterile 760
- Cortizone-5 Creme & Ointment ... ■ 732
- Dermolate Anti-Itch Cream ... ■ 697
- Eldecort Cream 1.0% ... 1113
- Eldecort Cream 1.0% and 2.5% ... 1113
- Fungoid HC Creme ... 1770
- Hydrocortone Tablets ... 1482
- Hytone ... 909
- LazerSporin-C Solution ... 1770
- Massengill Medicated Soft Cloth Towelettes ... 2192
- Nutracort Cream & Lotion ... 1684
- PediOtic Suspension Sterile ... 797
- Synacort Creams 1%, 2.5% ... 2296
- Vanoxide-HC Acne Lotion ... 911
- Vioform-Hydrocortisone Cream and Mild Cream ... 889
- Vioform-Hydrocortisone Ointment .. 889
- VōSoL HC Otic Solution ... 2392
- Vytone Cream 1% ... 911

Hydrocortisone Acetate (Hypernatremia). Products include:
- Analpram-HC Rectal Cream 1% and 2.5% ... 970
- Anusol-HC Cream ... 1690
- Anusol-HC Suppositories ... 1691
- Caldecort ... ■ 560
- Carmol HC Cream 1% ... 2296
- Chloromycetin Hydrocortisone Ophthalmic ... 1694
- Coly-Mycin S Otic w/Neomycin & Hydrocortisone ... 1708
- Cortaid ... ■ 735
- Cortef Feminine Itch Cream ... ■ 735
- Corticaine ... ■ 682
- Cortifoam ... 1827
- Cortisporin Cream ... 757
- Epifoam ... 1828
- Gynecort 5 Creme ... ■ 556
- Hydrocortone Acetate Sterile Suspension ... 1479
- Lanacort 5 Creme and Ointment .. ■ 557
- Mantadil Cream ... 789
- Ophthocort ... ◉ 301
- Orabase HCA Oral Paste ... 890
- Pramosone Cream, Lotion & Ointment ... 971
- ProctoCream-HC ... 1834
- Proctofoam-HC ... 1835

Hydrocortisone Sodium Phosphate (Hypernatremia). Products include:
- Hydrocortone Phosphate Injection, Sterile ... 1481

Hydrocortisone Sodium Succinate (Hypernatremia). Products include:
- Solu-Cortef Sterile Powder ... 2361

Magaldrate (May bind phosphate and prevent its absorption). Products include:
- Riopan Antacid Chew Tablets ... ■ 754
- Riopan Antacid Chew Tablets in Rollpacks ... ■ 754
- Riopan Antacid Suspension ... 2421
- Riopan Antacid Swallow Tablets ... 2421
- Riopan Plus Chew Tablets ... 2422
- Riopan Plus Chew Tablets in Rollpack ... 2422
- Riopan Plus 2 Chew Tablets, Mint Flavor, Cherry Flavor ... 2422
- Riopan Plus Suspension ... 2422
- Riopan Plus 2 Suspension, Mint Flavor, Cherry Flavor ... 2422

Magnesium Hydroxide (May bind phosphate and prevent its absorption). Products include:
- Aludrox Oral Suspension ... 2428
- Ascriptin A/D Caplets ... 1850
- Regular Strength Ascriptin Tablets 1850
- Di-Gel Antacid/Anti-Gas ... ■ 697
- Gelusil Liquid & Tablets ... ■ 639
- Haley's M-O, Regular & Flavored .. ■ 569
- Extra Strength Maalox Plus Suspension ... 1850
- Maalox TC Suspension ... 1851
- Maalox Plus Tablets ... ■ 655
- Extra Strength Maalox Plus Tablets 1850
- Mylanta Liquid ... 1155
- Mylanta Tablets ... 1155
- Mylanta Double Strength Liquid ... 1155
- Mylanta Double Strength Tablets ... 1155
- Concentrated Phillips' Milk of Magnesia ... ■ 573
- Phillips' Milk of Magnesia Liquid ... ■ 572
- Phillips' Milk of Magnesia Tablets ■ 573
- WinGel Liquid & Tablets ... ■ 761

Magnesium Oxide (May bind phosphate and prevent its absorption). Products include:
- Bayer Plus Aspirin Tablets ... ■ 567
- Beelith Tablets ... 659
- Bufferin Analgesic Tablets and Caplets ... ■ 524
- Cama Arthritis Pain Reliever ... ■ 685
- Mag-Ox 400 ... 673
- Uro-Mag ... 673

Methyldopa (Hypernatremia). Products include:
- Aldoclor Tablets ... 1413
- Aldomet Oral ... 1415
- Aldoril Tablets ... 1418

Methyldopate Hydrochloride (Hypernatremia). Products include:
- Aldomet Ester HCl Injection ... 1417

Methylprednisolone Acetate (Hypernatremia). Products include:
- Depo-Medrol Sterile Aqueous Suspension ... 2334

Methylprednisolone Sodium Succinate (Hypernatremia). Products include:
- Solu-Medrol Sterile Powder ... 2363

Potassium Acid Phosphate (Hyperkalemia; monitor potassium levels periodically). Products include:
- K-Phos M.F. Tablets ... 659
- K-Phos Original Formula 'Sodium Free' Tablets ... 660
- K-Phos No. 2 Tablets ... 659

Potassium Bicarbonate (Hyperkalemia; monitor potassium levels periodically). Products include:
- Alka-Seltzer Advanced Formula Antacid & Non-Aspirin Pain Reliever ... ■ 620
- Alka-Seltzer Effervescent Antacid ■ 622
- K-Lyte ... 707
- Klorvess Effervescent Granules ... 2010
- Klorvess Effervescent Tablets ... 2011

Potassium Chloride (Hyperkalemia; monitor potassium levels periodically). Products include:
- Chlor-3 Condiment ... 994
- K-Dur Microburst Release System (potassium chloride, USP) E.R. Tablets ... 1163
- K-Lor Powder Packets ... 531
- K-Lyte ... 707
- K-Norm Capsules ... 982
- K-Tab Filmtab ... 532
- Kato Potassium Supplement ... 1114
- Klor-Con 8/Klor-Con 10 Extended-release Tablets ... 2374
- Klorvess Effervescent Granules ... 2010
- Klorvess Effervescent Tablets ... 2011
- Klorvess 10% Liquid ... 2010
- Klotrix ... 708

Kolyum Liquid ... 983
Micro-K ... 1863
Micro-K LS Packets ... 1864
NuLYTELY ... 699
Oral Rehydration Salts, Citrate ... 1150
Rum-K Syrup ... 995
Slow-K Tablets ... 2281
Ten-K Controlled-Release Tablets ... 2282
Thermotabs ... ▣ 619

Potassium Citrate (Hyperkalemia; monitor potassium levels periodically). Products include:

Alka-Seltzer Effervescent Antacid ... 1570
K-Lyte ... 707
Polycitra Syrup ... 2424
Polycitra-K ... 2424
Polycitra-LC—Sugar-Free ... 2424
Ricelyte, Rice-Based Oral Electrolyte Maintenance Solution ... ▣ 613

Potassium Gluconate (Hyperkalemia; monitor potassium levels periodically). Products include:

Kolyum Liquid ... 983

Potassium Phosphate, Dibasic (Hyperkalemia; monitor potassium levels periodically). Products include:

Neutra-Phos ... 2423

Prednisolone Acetate (Hypernatremia). Products include:

AK-Cide Sterile Ophthalmic Ointment & Suspension ... ⊙ 202
Blephamide Liquifilm Sterile Ophthalmic Suspension ... 586
Blephamide S.O.P. Sterile Ophthalmic Ointment ... 586
Cetapred Ointment ... ⊙ 220
⅛% Econopred & 1% Econopred Plus ... ⊙ 217
Isopto Cetapred Suspension ... ⊙ 220
Metimyd ... ⊙ 306
Poly-Pred Liquifilm ... ⊙ 250
Pred Forte ... ⊙ 252
Pred Mild ... ⊙ 254
Pred-G Liquifilm Sterile Ophthalmic Suspension ... ⊙ 252
Pred-G S.O.P. Sterile Ophthalmic Ointment ... ⊙ 253
Vasocidin Ointment ... ⊙ 275

Prednisolone Sodium Phosphate (Hypernatremia). Products include:

AK-Pred ... ⊙ 205
Hydeltrasol Injection, Sterile ... 1476
Inflamase ... ⊙ 274
Pediapred Oral Liquid ... 987
Vasocidin Ophthalmic Solution ... ⊙ 276

Prednisolone Tebutate (Hypernatremia). Products include:

Hydeltra-T.B.A. Sterile Suspension 1478

Prednisone (Hypernatremia). Products include:

Deltasone Tablets ... 2332

Rauwolfia Serpentina (Hypernatremia). Products include:

Raudixin Tablets ... 1803
Rauzide Tablets ... 1804

Rescinnamine (Hypernatremia).

No products indexed under this heading.

Reserpine (Hypernatremia). Products include:

Diupres Tablets ... 1461
Hydromox R Tablets ... 1209
Hydropres Tablets ... 1485
Renese-R Tablets ... 1786
Salutensin/Salutensin-Demi ... 719
Ser-Ap-Es Tablets ... 881
Serpasil Tablets ... 883
Serpasil-Apresoline Tablets ... 884
Serpasil-Esidrix Tablets ... 886

Spironolactone (Hyperkalemia; monitor potassium levels periodically). Products include:

Aldactazide ... 2150
Aldactone ... 2152

Triamcinolone (Hypernatremia).

No products indexed under this heading.

Triamcinolone Acetonide (Hypernatremia). Products include:

Aristocort A ... 1010
Azmacort Inhaler ... 1837
Kenalog Cream, Lotion & Ointment 2401
Kenalog-10 Injection ... 2402
Kenalog-40 Injection ... 2403
Kenalog in Orabase ... 604
Kenalog Spray ... 2401
Mycolog II Cream and Ointment ... 2407
Mytrex Cream & Ointment ... 2080
Nasacort Nasal Inhaler ... 1844

Triamcinolone Diacetate (Hypernatremia). Products include:

Aristocort Suspension ... 1008

Triamcinolone Hexacetonide (Hypernatremia). Products include:

Aristospan Suspension ... 1011

Triamterene (Hyperkalemia; monitor potassium levels periodically). Products include:

Dyazide Capsules ... 2208
Dyrenium Capsules ... 2210
Maxzide ... 1215

Trichlormethiazide (Hypernatremia).

No products indexed under this heading.

Vitamin D (May antagonize effects of phosphates in treatment of hypercalcemia). Products include:

Bugs Bunny Children's Chewable Vitamins (Sugar Free) ... ▣ 625
Bugs Bunny With Extra C Children's Chewable Vitamins (Sugar Free) ... ▣ 626
Bugs Bunny Plus Iron Children's Chewable Vitamins (Sugar Free) ▣ 625
Calderol Capsules ... 1635
Caltrate 600 + Iron & Vitamin D ... 1198
Caltrate 600 + Vitamin D ... 1197
Caltrate, Jr. Tablets ... 1198
Flintstones Children's Chewable Vitamins ... ▣ 625
Flintstones Children's Chewable Vitamins With Extra C ... ▣ 626
Flintstones Children's Chewable Vitamins Plus Iron ... ▣ 625
Natalins Rx ... 1391
Natalins Tablets ... 1391
One-A-Day Essential Vitamins ... ▣ 627
One-A-Day Maximum Formula Vitamins and Minerals ... ▣ 627
One-A-Day Plus Extra C Vitamins .. ▣ 627
Os-Cal 250+D Tablets ... ▣ 597
Os-Cal 500+D Tablets ... ▣ 597
Os-Cal Fortified Tablets ... ▣ 597
Os-Cal Plus Tablets ... ▣ 597
Posture-D 600 mg ... 2420
Stressgard Stress Formula Vitamins ... ▣ 628
Tri-Vi-Flor 1.0 mg Vitamins with Fluoride Chewable Tablets ... 1400
Tri-Vi-Flor Drops ... 1400
Tri-Vi-Sol Vitamin Drops ... ▣ 614
Tri-Vi-Sol Vitamin Drops with Iron ▣ 614
Vi-Daylin ADC Vitamins Drops ... 1980
Vi-Daylin ADC Vitamins + Iron Drops ... 1980
Vi-Daylin/F ADC Vitamins Drops With Fluoride ... 1981
Vi-Daylin/F ADC Vitamins + Iron Drops With Fluoride ... 1981
Within Women's Formula Multivitamin with Calcium, Extra Iron and Zinc ... ▣ 628
Zymacap Capsules ... ▣ 670

K-PHOS ORIGINAL FORMULA 'SODIUM FREE' TABLETS

(Potassium Acid Phosphate) ... 660

May interact with antacids, potassium sparing diuretics, salicylates, potassium-depleting corticosteroids, and certain other agents. Compounds in these categories include:

Aluminum Carbonate Gel (May bind phosphate and prevent its absorption). Products include:

Basaljel ... 2438

Aluminum Hydroxide (May bind phosphate and prevent its absorption). Products include:

Cama Arthritis Pain Reliever ... ▣ 685
Gaviscon Extra Strength Relief Formula Liquid Antacid ... ▣ 594
Gaviscon Extra Strength Relief Formula Antacid Tablets ... ▣ 594
Gaviscon Liquid Antacid ... ▣ 594
Gelusil Liquid & Tablets ... ▣ 639
Extra Strength Maalox Plus Suspension ... 1850
Maalox TC Suspension ... 1851
Maalox Plus Tablets ... ▣ 655
Extra Strength Maalox Plus Tablets 1850
Nephrox Suspension ... ▣ 563
WinGel Liquid & Tablets ... ▣ 761

Aluminum Hydroxide Gel (May bind phosphate and prevent its absorption). Products include:

ALternaGEL Liquid ... 1154
Aludrox Oral Suspension ... 2428
Amphojel Suspension ... 2429
Amphojel Suspension without Flavor ... 2429
Mylanta Liquid ... 1155
Mylanta Double Strength Liquid ... 1155

Aluminum Hydroxide Gel, Dried (May bind phosphate and prevent its absorption). Products include:

Alu-Tab/Alu-Cap ... 1309
Amphojel Tablets ... 2429
Ascriptin A/D Caplets ... 1850
Regular Strength Ascriptin Tablets 1850
Gaviscon Antacid Tablets ... ▣ 593
Gaviscon-2 Antacid Tablets ... ▣ 594
Mylanta Tablets ... 1155
Mylanta Double Strength Tablets ... 1155

Amiloride Hydrochloride (Hyperkalemia). Products include:

Midamor Tablets ... 1508
Moduretic Tablets ... 1510

Aspirin (Increased serum salicylate levels; possible toxicity). Products include:

Alka-Seltzer Effervescent Antacid and Pain Reliever ... 1568
Alka-Seltzer Extra Strength Effervescent Antacid and Pain Reliever ... 1570
Alka-Seltzer (Flavored) Effervescent Antacid and Pain Reliever ... 1569
Alka-Seltzer Plus Cold Medicine ... ▣ 623
Alka-Seltzer Plus Night-Time Cold Medicine ... ▣ 623
Alka Seltzer Plus Sinus Allergy Medicine ... ▣ 624
Anacin Coated Analgesic Caplets ... 2417
Anacin Coated Analgesic Tablets ... 2417
Anacin Maximum Strength Analgesic Coated Tablets ... 2417
Maximum Strength Arthritis Pain Formula By the Makers of Anacin Analgesic Tablets and Caplets ... 2418
Arthritis Pain Formula by the Makers of Anacin Analgesic Tablets and Caplets ... ▣ 747
Arthritis Strength BC Powder ... ▣ 516
Ascriptin A/D Caplets ... 1850
Regular Strength Ascriptin Tablets 1850
Azdone Tablets ... 844
BC Powder ... ▣ 517
BC Cold Powder ... ▣ 517
Children's Bayer Chewable Aspirin ... ▣ 564
Genuine Bayer Aspirin Tablets & Caplets ... ▣ 564
Maximum Bayer Aspirin Tablets & Caplets ... ▣ 566
Bayer Plus Aspirin Tablets ... ▣ 567
Therapy Bayer Aspirin Caplets ... ▣ 568
8 Hour Bayer Timed-Release Aspirin ... ▣ 566
Arthritis Strength Bufferin Analgesic Caplets ... 744
Extra Strength Bufferin Analgesic Tablets ... 745
Bufferin Analgesic Tablets and Caplets ... 743
Cama Arthritis Pain Reliever ... ▣ 685
Damason-P ... 1356
Easprin ... 1719
Ecotrin Enteric Coated Aspirin Maximum Strength Tablets and Caplets ... 2189
Ecotrin Enteric Coated Aspirin Regular Strength Tablets and Caplets ... 2189
Empirin Aspirin ... ▣ 541
Empirin with Codeine Phosphate Nos. 2, 3 & 4 ... 764
Equagesic Tablets ... 2451
Excedrin Extra-Strength Analgesic Tablets & Caplets ... 749
4-Way Cold Tablets ... 750
Fiorinal Capsules ... 2007
Fiorinal with Codeine Capsules ... 2008
Fiorinal Tablets ... 2007
Lortab ASA Tablets ... 2414
Momentum Muscular Backache Formula ... ▣ 751
Norgesic ... 1314
Norwich Extra-Strength Aspirin ... ▣ 546
Norwich Regular Strength Aspirin ▣ 547
P-A-C Analgesic Tablets ... ▣ 669
Percodan ... 951
Robaxisal Tablets ... 1872
Sine-Off Sinus Medicine Tablets-Aspirin Formula ... ▣ 722
Soma Compound w/Codeine Tablets ... 2390
Soma Compound Tablets ... 2389
St. Joseph Adult Chewable Aspirin (81 mg.) ... ▣ 703
Synalgos-DC Capsules ... 2525
Talwin Compound ... 2072
Ursinus Inlay-Tabs ... ▣ 691
Vanquish Analgesic Caplets ... ▣ 574
Zorprin Tablets ... 698

Choline Magnesium Trisalicylate (Increased serum salicylate levels; possible toxicity). Products include:

Trilisate ... 1822

Diflunisal (Increased serum salicylate levels; possible toxicity). Products include:

Dolobid Tablets ... 1465

Dihydroxyaluminum Sodium Carbonate (May bind phosphate and prevent its absorption). Products include:

Rolaids ... ▣ 743

Magaldrate (May bind phosphate and prevent its absorption). Products include:

Riopan Antacid Chew Tablets ... ▣ 754
Riopan Antacid Chew Tablets in Rollpacks ... ▣ 754
Riopan Antacid Suspension ... 2421
Riopan Antacid Swallow Tablets ... 2421
Riopan Plus Chew Tablets ... 2422
Riopan Plus Chew Tablets in Rollpack ... 2422
Riopan Plus 2 Chew Tablets, Mint Flavor, Cherry Flavor ... 2422
Riopan Plus Suspension ... 2422
Riopan Plus 2 Suspension, Mint Flavor, Cherry Flavor ... 2422

Magnesium Hydroxide (May bind phosphate and prevent its absorption). Products include:

Aludrox Oral Suspension ... 2428
Ascriptin A/D Caplets ... 1850
Regular Strength Ascriptin Tablets 1850
Di-Gel Antacid/Anti-Gas ... ▣ 697
Gelusil Liquid & Tablets ... ▣ 639
Haley's M-O, Regular & Flavored ... ▣ 569
Extra Strength Maalox Plus Suspension ... 1850
Maalox TC Suspension ... 1851
Maalox Plus Tablets ... ▣ 655
Extra Strength Maalox Plus Tablets 1850
Mylanta Liquid ... 1155
Mylanta Tablets ... 1155
Mylanta Double Strength Liquid ... 1155
Mylanta Double Strength Tablets ... 1155
Concentrated Phillips' Milk of Magnesia ... ▣ 573
Phillips' Milk of Magnesia Liquid ... ▣ 572
Phillips' Milk of Magnesia Tablets ▣ 573
WinGel Liquid & Tablets ... ▣ 761

Magnesium Oxide (May bind phosphate and prevent its absorption). Products include:

Bayer Plus Aspirin Tablets ... ▣ 567
Beelith Tablets ... 659
Bufferin Analgesic Tablets and Caplets ... ▣ 524
Cama Arthritis Pain Reliever ... ▣ 685
Mag-Ox 400 ... 673
Uro-Mag ... 673

Magnesium Salicylate (Increased serum salicylate levels; possible toxicity). Products include:

Doan's - Extra-Strength Analgesic ▣ 549
Doan's - Regular Strength Analgesic ... ▣ 549
Mobigesic Analgesic Tablets ... ▣ 507

Potassium Bicarbonate (Potential for hyperkalemia). Products include:
- Alka-Seltzer Advanced Formula Antacid & Non-Aspirin Pain Reliever ...... ■ 620
- Alka-Seltzer Effervescent Antacid ■ 622
- K-Lyte 707
- Klorvess Effervescent Granules...... 2010
- Klorvess Effervescent Tablets 2011

Potassium Chloride (Potential for hyperkalemia). Products include:
- Chlor-3 Condiment 994
- K-Dur Microburst Release System (potassium chloride, USP) E.R. Tablets 1163
- K-Lor Powder Packets 531
- K-Lyte 707
- K-Norm Capsules 982
- K-Tab Filmtab 532
- Kato Potassium Supplement...... 1114
- Klor-Con 8/Klor-Con 10 Extended-release Tablets 2374
- Klorvess Effervescent Granules...... 2010
- Klorvess Effervescent Tablets 2011
- Klorvess 10% Liquid 2010
- Klotrix 708
- Kolyum Liquid 983
- Micro-K...... 1863
- Micro-K LS Packets...... 1864
- NuLYTELY...... 699
- Oral Rehydration Salts, Citrate 1150
- Rum-K Syrup 995
- Slow-K Tablets 2281
- Ten-K Controlled-Release Tablets.... 2282
- Thermotabs ...... ■ 619

Potassium Citrate (Potential for hyperkalemia). Products include:
- Alka-Seltzer Effervescent Antacid .. 1570
- K-Lyte 707
- Polycitra Syrup 2424
- Polycitra-K 2424
- Polycitra-LC—Sugar-Free...... 2424
- Ricelyte, Rice-Based Oral Electrolyte Maintenance Solution ...... ■ 613

Potassium Gluconate (Potential for hyperkalemia). Products include:
- Kolyum Liquid 983

Potassium Phosphate, Dibasic (Potential for hyperkalemia). Products include:
- Neutra-Phos 2423

Potassium Phosphate, Monobasic (Potential for hyperkalemia). Products include:
- K-Phos M.F. Tablets 659
- K-Phos Neutral Tablets 660
- Neutra-Phos 2423

Salsalate (Increased serum salicylate levels; possible toxicity). Products include:
- Disalcid 1310
- Mono-Gesic Tablets 846
- Salflex...... 839

Spironolactone (Hyperkalemia). Products include:
- Aldactazide...... 2150
- Aldactone 2152

Triamterene (Hyperkalemia). Products include:
- Dyazide Capsules...... 2208
- Dyrenium Capsules...... 2210
- Maxzide 1215

K-PHOS NO. 2 TABLETS
(Potassium Phosphate, Monobasic, Sodium Phosphate) 659
See **K-Phos M.F. Tablets**

K-TAB FILMTAB
(Potassium Chloride)...... 532
May interact with potassium sparing diuretics and ACE inhibitors. Compounds in these categories include:

Amiloride Hydrochloride (Potential for severe hyperkalemia). Products include:
- Midamor Tablets 1508
- Moduretic Tablets 1510

Benazepril Hydrochloride (Concomitant therapy may result in hyperkalemia; close monitoring is advised). Products include:
- Lotensin Tablets...... 872

Captopril (Concomitant therapy may result in hyperkalemia; close monitoring is advised). Products include:
- Capoten 2255
- Capozide 2258

Enalapril Maleate (Concomitant therapy may result in hyperkalemia; close monitoring is advised). Products include:
- Vaseretic Tablets 1559
- Vasotec Tablets 1564

Enalaprilat (Concomitant therapy may result in hyperkalemia; close monitoring is advised). Products include:
- Vasotec I.V...... 1562

Fosinopril Sodium (Concomitant therapy may result in hyperkalemia; close monitoring is advised). Products include:
- Monopril Tablets 1406

Lisinopril (Concomitant therapy may result in hyperkalemia; close monitoring is advised). Products include:
- Prinivil Tablets 1538
- Prinzide Tablets 1540
- Zestoretic 2274
- Zestril Tablets 2277

Ramipril (Concomitant therapy may result in hyperkalemia; close monitoring is advised). Products include:
- Altace Capsules 1086

Spironolactone (Potential for severe hyperkalemia). Products include:
- Aldactazide...... 2150
- Aldactone 2152

Triamterene (Potential for severe hyperkalemia). Products include:
- Dyazide Capsules...... 2208
- Dyrenium Capsules...... 2210
- Maxzide 1215

KAOPECTATE CONCENTRATED ANTI-DIARRHEAL, PEPPERMINT FLAVOR
(Attapulgite)...... ■ 736
No interactions described in labeling.

KAOPECTATE CONCENTRATED ANTI-DIARRHEAL, REGULAR FLAVOR
(Attapulgite)...... ■ 736
No interactions described in labeling.

KAOPECTATE CHILDREN'S CHEWABLE TABLETS
(Attapulgite)...... ■ 736
No interactions described in labeling.

KAOPECTATE MAXIMUM STRENGTH CAPLETS
(Attapulgite)...... ■ 736
No interactions described in labeling.

KATO POTASSIUM SUPPLEMENT
(Potassium Chloride)......1114
May interact with potassium sparing diuretics. Compounds in this category include:

Amiloride Hydrochloride (Severe hyperkalemia). Products include:
- Midamor Tablets 1508
- Moduretic Tablets 1510

Spironolactone (Severe hyperkalemia). Products include:
- Aldactazide...... 2150
- Aldactone 2152

Triamterene (Severe hyperkalemia). Products include:
- Dyazide Capsules...... 2208
- Dyrenium Capsules...... 2210
- Maxzide 1215

KAYEXALATE
(Sodium Polystyrene Sulfonate) 2053
May interact with antacids, cardiac glycosides, and certain other agents. Compounds in these categories include:

Aluminum Carbonate Gel (May reduce potassium exchange capability). Products include:
- Basaljel...... 2438

Aluminum Hydroxide (May reduce potassium exchange capability; potential for intestinal obstruction). Products include:
- Cama Arthritis Pain Reliever...... ■ 685
- Gaviscon Extra Strength Relief Formula Liquid Antacid...... ■ 594
- Gaviscon Extra Strength Relief Formula Antacid Tablets...... ■ 594
- Gaviscon Liquid Antacid ...... ■ 594
- Gelusil Liquid & Tablets ...... ■ 639
- Extra Strength Maalox Plus Suspension...... 1850
- Maalox TC Suspension 1851
- Maalox Plus Tablets ...... ■ 655
- Extra Strength Maalox Plus Tablets 1850
- Nephrox Suspension ...... ■ 563
- WinGel Liquid & Tablets...... ■ 761

Aluminum Hydroxide Gel (May reduce potassium exchange capability; potential for intestinal obstruction). Products include:
- ALternaGEL Liquid 1154
- Aludrox Oral Suspension 2428
- Amphojel Suspension 2429
- Amphojel Suspension without Flavor 2429
- Mylanta Liquid 1155
- Mylanta Double Strength Liquid 1155

Aluminum Hydroxide Gel, Dried (May reduce potassium exchange capability; potential for intestinal obstruction). Products include:
- Alu-Tab/Alu-Cap 1309
- Amphojel Tablets...... 2429
- Ascriptin A/D Caplets 1850
- Regular Strength Ascriptin Tablets 1850
- Gaviscon Antacid Tablets...... ■ 593
- Gaviscon-2 Antacid Tablets ...... ■ 594
- Mylanta Tablets 1155
- Mylanta Double Strength Tablets 1155

Deslanoside (Cardiac toxicity of digitalis may be exaggerated).
- No products indexed under this heading.

Digitoxin (Cardiac toxicity of digitalis may be exaggerated). Products include:
- Crystodigin Tablets...... 1253

Digoxin (Cardiac toxicity of digitalis may be exaggerated). Products include:
- Lanoxicaps 772
- Lanoxin Elixir Pediatric 775
- Lanoxin Injection 778
- Lanoxin Injection Pediatric...... 781
- Lanoxin Tablets 783

Dihydroxyaluminum Sodium Carbonate (May reduce potassium exchange capability). Products include:
- Rolaids ...... ■ 743

Magaldrate (May reduce potassium exchange capability). Products include:
- Riopan Antacid Chew Tablets...... ■ 754
- Riopan Antacid Chew Tablets in Rollpacks...... ■ 754
- Riopan Antacid Suspension 2421
- Riopan Antacid Swallow Tablets 2421
- Riopan Plus Chew Tablets 2422
- Riopan Plus Chew Tablets in Rollpack...... 2422
- Riopan Plus 2 Chew Tablets, Mint Flavor, Cherry Flavor 2422
- Riopan Plus Suspension 2422
- Riopan Plus 2 Suspension, Mint Flavor, Cherry Flavor 2422

Magnesium Hydroxide (May reduce potassium exchange capability; potential for grand mal seizure). Products include:
- Aludrox Oral Suspension 2428
- Ascriptin A/D Caplets 1850
- Regular Strength Ascriptin Tablets 1850
- Di-Gel Antacid/Anti-Gas ...... ■ 697
- Gelusil Liquid & Tablets ...... ■ 639
- Haley's M-O, Regular & Flavored .. ■ 569
- Extra Strength Maalox Plus Suspension...... 1850
- Maalox TC Suspension 1851
- Maalox Plus Tablets ...... ■ 655
- Extra Strength Maalox Plus Tablets 1850
- Mylanta Liquid 1155
- Mylanta Tablets 1155
- Mylanta Double Strength Liquid 1155
- Mylanta Double Strength Tablets 1155
- Concentrated Phillips' Milk of Magnesia ...... ■ 573
- Phillips' Milk of Magnesia Liquid.... ■ 572
- Phillips' Milk of Magnesia Tablets ■ 573
- WinGel Liquid & Tablets ...... ■ 761

Magnesium Oxide (May reduce potassium exchange capability). Products include:
- Bayer Plus Aspirin Tablets...... ■ 567
- Beelith Tablets 659
- Bufferin Analgesic Tablets and Caplets ...... ■ 524
- Cama Arthritis Pain Reliever...... ■ 685
- Mag-Ox 400 673
- Uro-Mag...... 673

KEFLEX PULVULES, ORAL SUSPENSION & PEDIATRIC DROPS
(Cephalexin) 916
No interactions described in labeling.

KEFTAB TABLETS
(Cephalexin Hydrochloride) 917
No interactions described in labeling.

KEFUROX VIALS, FASPAK & ADD-VANTAGE
(Cefuroxime Sodium) 1277
May interact with aminoglycosides and diuretics. Compounds in these categories include:

Amikacin Sulfate (Nephrotoxicity). Products include:
- Amikin Injectable 602

Amiloride Hydrochloride (Possible adverse effects on renal function). Products include:
- Midamor Tablets 1508
- Moduretic Tablets 1510

Bendroflumethiazide (Possible adverse effects on renal function). Products include:
- Corzide Tablets 702
- Naturetin Tablets 1789
- Rauzide Tablets 1804

Bumetanide (Possible adverse effects on renal function). Products include:
- Bumex 1895

Chlorothiazide (Possible adverse effects on renal function). Products include:
- Aldoclor Tablets 1413
- Diupres Tablets 1461
- Diuril Oral 1464

Chlorothiazide Sodium (Possible adverse effects on renal function). Products include:
- Diuril Sodium Intravenous 1463

Chlorthalidone (Possible adverse effects on renal function). Products include:
- Combipres Tablets 678
- Tenoretic Tablets...... 1105
- Thalitone Tablets 687

(■ Described in PDR For Nonprescription Drugs) (◉ Described in PDR For Ophthalmology)

Ethacrynic Acid (Possible adverse effects on renal function). Products include:
- Edecrin Tablets 1468

Furosemide (Possible adverse effects on renal function). Products include:
- Lasix 1093

Gentamicin Sulfate (Nephrotoxicity). Products include:
- Garamycin Injectable 2093
- Garamycin Ophthalmic ..... ◉ 305
- Genoptic Liquifilm Sterile Ophthalmic Solution ..... ◉ 247
- Genoptic S.O.P. Sterile Ophthalmic Ointment ..... ◉ 247
- Gentacidin Ointment ..... ◉ 273
- Gentacidin Solution ..... ◉ 273
- Gentak Ointment & Solution ..... ◉ 208
- G-myticin Creme and Ointment 0.1% 1770
- Pred-G Liquifilm Sterile Ophthalmic Suspension ..... ◉ 252
- Pred-G S.O.P. Sterile Ophthalmic Ointment ..... ◉ 253

Hydrochlorothiazide (Possible adverse effects on renal function). Products include:
- Aldactazide 2150
- Aldoril Tablets 1418
- Apresazide Capsules 854
- Apresoline-Esidrix Tablets 857
- Capozide 2258
- Dyazide Capsules 2208
- Esidrix Tablets 863
- Esimil Tablets 864
- HydroDIURIL Tablets 1484
- Hydropres Tablets 1485
- Inderide Tablets 2463
- Inderide LA Long Acting Capsules 2465
- Lopressor HCT Tablets 1034
- Maxzide 1215
- Moduretic Tablets 1510
- Normozide Tablets 2112
- Oretic Tablets 544
- Oreticyl 545
- Prinzide Tablets 1540
- Ser-Ap-Es Tablets 881
- Serpasil-Esidrix Tablets 886
- Timolide Tablets 1547
- Trandate HCT Tablets 579
- Vaseretic Tablets 1559
- Zestoretic 2274

Hydroflumethiazide (Possible adverse effects on renal function). Products include:
- Diucardin Tablets 2450
- Saluron 718
- Salutensin/Salutensin-Demi 719

Indapamide (Possible adverse effects on renal function). Products include:
- Lozol Tablets 1843

Kanamycin Sulfate (Nephrotoxicity). Products include:
- Kantrex Injection 601
- Kantrex Pediatric Injection 601

Methyclothiazide (Possible adverse effects on renal function). Products include:
- Enduron Tablets 517
- Enduronyl 518

Metolazone (Possible adverse effects on renal function). Products include:
- Diulo 2129
- Mykrox ½ mg Tablets 984
- Zaroxolyn Tablets 989

Polythiazide (Possible adverse effects on renal function). Products include:
- Minizide Capsules 1779
- Renese Tablets 1785
- Renese-R Tablets 1786

Spironolactone (Possible adverse effects on renal function). Products include:
- Aldactazide 2150
- Aldactone 2152

Streptomycin Sulfate (Nephrotoxicity).
- No products indexed under this heading.

Tobramycin (Nephrotoxicity). Products include:
- TobraDex Ophthalmic Suspension and Ointment ..... ◉ 228
- Tobrex Ophthalmic Ointment and Solution 572

Tobramycin Sulfate (Nephrotoxicity). Products include:
- Nebcin Vials, Hyporets & ADD-Vantage 1286

Triamterene (Possible adverse effects on renal function). Products include:
- Dyazide Capsules 2208
- Dyrenium Capsules 2210
- Maxzide 1215

KEFZOL VIALS, FASPAK & ADD-VANTAGE
(Cefazolin Sodium) 1279
May interact with:

Probenecid (Increases and prolongs cephalosporin blood levels). Products include:
- Benemid Tablets 1426
- ColBENEMID Tablets 1436
- Wycillin Injection and Probenecid Tablets 2539

KEMADRIN TABLETS
(Procyclidine Hydrochloride) 771
No interactions described in labeling.

KENALOG CREAM, LOTION & OINTMENT
(Triamcinolone Acetonide) 2401
No interactions described in labeling.

KENALOG-10 INJECTION
(Triamcinolone Acetonide) 2402
May interact with:

Immunization (Neurological complications; lack of antibody response).

KENALOG-40 INJECTION
(Triamcinolone Acetonide) 2403
May interact with:

Immunization (Neurological complications; lack of antibody response).

KENALOG IN ORABASE
(Triamcinolone Acetonide) 604
No interactions described in labeling.

KENALOG SPRAY
(Triamcinolone Acetonide) 2401
No interactions described in labeling.

KERALYT GEL
(Salicylic Acid) 2405
May interact with corticosteroids, antigout agents, and certain other agents. Compounds in these categories include:

Allopurinol (Effect inhibited). Products include:
- Zyloprim Tablets 830

Betamethasone Acetate (Decreased plasma salicylate levels). Products include:
- Celestone Soluspan Suspension 2081

Betamethasone Sodium Phosphate (Decreased plasma salicylate levels). Products include:
- Celestone Soluspan Suspension 2081

Clobetasol Propionate (Decreased plasma salicylate levels). Products include:
- Temovate 1056

Cortisone Acetate (Decreased plasma salicylate levels). Products include:
- Cortone Acetate Sterile Suspension 1437
- Cortone Acetate Tablets 1439

Dexamethasone (Decreased plasma salicylate levels). Products include:
- AK-Trol Ointment & Suspension ..... ◉ 207
- Decadron Elixir 1445
- Decadron Tablets 1447
- Decaspray Topical Aerosol 1459
- Dexacidin ..... ◉ 272
- Maxidex Sterile Ophthalmic Suspension ..... ◉ 223
- Maxitrol Ophthalmic Ointment/Suspension ..... ◉ 223
- TobraDex Ophthalmic Suspension and Ointment ..... ◉ 228

Dexamethasone Acetate (Decreased plasma salicylate levels). Products include:
- Dalalone D.P. Injectable 999
- Decadron-LA Sterile Suspension 1457

Dexamethasone Sodium Phosphate (Decreased plasma salicylate levels). Products include:
- AK-Dex ..... ◉ 203
- Decadron Phosphate Respihaler 1454
- Decadron Phosphate Sterile Ophthalmic Ointment 1453
- Decadron Phosphate Sterile Ophthalmic Solution 1453
- Decadron Phosphate Topical Cream 1455
- Decadron Phosphate Turbinaire 1456
- Maxidex Sterile Ophthalmic Ointment ..... ◉ 222
- NeoDecadron Sterile Ophthalmic Ointment 1517
- NeoDecadron Sterile Ophthalmic Solution 1518
- NeoDecadron Topical Cream 1518

Heparin Calcium (Interference with hemostasis). Products include:
- Calciparine Injection 925

Heparin Sodium (Interference with hemostasis). Products include:
- Heparin Lock Flush Solution 2456
- Heparin Sodium Vials 1264
- Heparin Sodium Injection 2457
- Heparin Sodium Injection, USP, Sterile Solution 2342

Hydrocortisone (Decreased plasma salicylate levels). Products include:
- AK-Spore H.C. ..... ◉ 206
- Bactine Hydrocortisone Anti-Itch Cream ..... ▣ 625
- CaldeCORT Anti-Itch Hydrocortisone Spray ..... ▣ 560
- Carmol HC Cream 1% 2296
- Cortaid Spray ..... ▣ 735
- Cortenema 2244
- Cortisporin Ointment 758
- Cortisporin Ophthalmic Ointment Sterile 758
- Cortisporin Ophthalmic Suspension Sterile 759
- Cortisporin Otic Solution Sterile 760
- Cortisporin Otic Suspension Sterile 760
- Cortizone-5 Creme & Ointment ..... ▣ 732
- Dermolate Anti-Itch Cream ..... ▣ 697
- Eldecort Cream 1.0% 1113
- Eldecort Cream 1.0% and 2.5% 1113
- Fungoid HC Creme 1770
- Hydrocortone Tablets 1482
- Hytone 909
- LazerSporin-C Solution 1770
- Massengill Medicated Soft Cloth Towelettes 2192
- Nutracort Cream & Lotion 1684
- PediOtic Suspension Sterile 797
- Synacort Creams 1%, 2.5% 2296
- Vanoxide-HC Acne Lotion 911
- Vioform-Hydrocortisone Cream and Mild Cream 889
- Vioform-Hydrocortisone Ointment 889
- VōSoL HC Otic Solution 2392
- Vytone Cream 1% 911

Hydrocortisone Acetate (Decreased plasma salicylate levels). Products include:
- Analpram-HC Rectal Cream 1% and 2.5% 970
- Anusol-HC Cream 1690
- Anusol-HC Suppositories 1691
- Caldecort ..... ▣ 560
- Carmol HC Cream 1% 2296
- Chloromycetin Hydrocortisone Ophthalmic 1694
- Coly-Mycin S Otic w/Neomycin & Hydrocortisone 1708
- Cortaid ..... ▣ 735
- Cortef Feminine Itch Cream ..... ▣ 735
- Corticaine ..... ▣ 682
- Cortifoam 1827
- Cortisporin Cream 757
- Epifoam 1828
- Gynecort 5 Creme ..... ▣ 556
- Hydrocortone Acetate Sterile Suspension 1479
- Lanacort 5 Creme and Ointment ..... ▣ 557
- Mantadil Cream 789
- Ophthocort ..... ◉ 301
- Orabase HCA Oral Paste 890
- Pramosone Cream, Lotion & Ointment 971
- ProctoCream-HC 1834
- Proctofoam-HC 1835

Hydrocortisone Sodium Phosphate (Decreased plasma salicylate levels). Products include:
- Hydrocortone Phosphate Injection, Sterile 1481

Hydrocortisone Sodium Succinate (Decreased plasma salicylate levels). Products include:
- Solu-Cortef Sterile Powder 2361

Methotrexate Sodium (Methotrexate toxicity can result). Products include:
- Methotrexate Tablets, Parenteral, LPF Parenteral 1217
- Rheumatrex Methotrexate Dose Pack 1234

Methylprednisolone Acetate (Decreased plasma salicylate levels). Products include:
- Depo-Medrol Sterile Aqueous Suspension 2334

Methylprednisolone Sodium Succinate (Decreased plasma salicylate levels). Products include:
- Solu-Medrol Sterile Powder 2363

Phenylbutazone (Effect inhibited). Products include:
- Butazolidin Capsules & Tablets 1027

Prednisolone Acetate (Decreased plasma salicylate levels). Products include:
- AK-Cide Sterile Ophthalmic Ointment & Suspension ..... ◉ 202
- Blephamide Liquifilm Sterile Ophthalmic Suspension 586
- Blephamide S.O.P. Sterile Ophthalmic Ointment 586
- Cetapred Ointment ..... ◉ 220
- ⅛% Econopred & 1% Econopred Plus ..... ◉ 217
- Isopto Cetapred Suspension ..... ◉ 220
- Metimyd ..... ◉ 306
- Poly-Pred Liquifilm ..... ◉ 250
- Pred Forte ..... ◉ 252
- Pred Mild ..... ◉ 254
- Pred-G Liquifilm Sterile Ophthalmic Suspension ..... ◉ 252
- Pred-G S.O.P. Sterile Ophthalmic Ointment ..... ◉ 253
- Vasocidin Ointment ..... ◉ 275

Prednisolone Sodium Phosphate (Decreased plasma salicylate levels). Products include:
- AK-Pred ..... ◉ 205
- Hydeltrasol Injection, Sterile 1476
- Inflamase ..... ◉ 274
- Pediapred Oral Liquid 987
- Vasocidin Ophthalmic Solution ..... ◉ 276

Prednisolone Tebutate (Decreased plasma salicylate levels). Products include:
- Hydeltra-T.B.A. Sterile Suspension 1478

Prednisone (Decreased plasma salicylate levels). Products include:
- Deltasone Tablets 2332

Probenecid (Effect inhibited). Products include:
- Benemid Tablets 1426
- ColBENEMID Tablets 1436
- Wycillin Injection and Probenecid Tablets 2539

Pyrazinamide (Pyrazinamide-induced hyperuricemia inhibited).
- No products indexed under this heading.

Sulfinpyrazone (Effect inhibited). Products include:
- Anturane ... 853

Tolbutamide (Hypoglycemia potentiated). Products include:
- Orinase Tablets ... 2354

Triamcinolone (Decreased plasma salicylate levels).
- No products indexed under this heading.

Triamcinolone Acetonide (Decreased plasma salicylate levels). Products include:
- Aristocort A ... 1010
- Azmacort Inhaler ... 1837
- Kenalog Cream, Lotion & Ointment 2401
- Kenalog-10 Injection ... 2402
- Kenalog-40 Injection ... 2403
- Kenalog in Orabase ... 604
- Kenalog Spray ... 2401
- Mycolog II Cream and Ointment ... 2407
- Mytrex Cream & Ointment ... 2080
- Nasacort Nasal Inhaler ... 1844

Triamcinolone Diacetate (Decreased plasma salicylate levels). Products include:
- Aristocort Suspension ... 1008

Triamcinolone Hexacetonide (Decreased plasma salicylate levels). Products include:
- Aristospan Suspension ... 1011

KERI LOTION - FRESH HERBAL SCENT
(Mineral Oil) ... ▣ 535
No interactions described in labeling.

KERI LOTION - ORIGINAL FORMULA
(Mineral Oil) ... ▣ 535
No interactions described in labeling.

KERI LOTION - SILKY SMOOTH FORMULA
(Glycerin, Petrolatum) ... ▣ 535
No interactions described in labeling.

KERLONE TABLETS
(Betaxolol Hydrochloride) ... 2172
May interact with catecholamine depleting drugs, calcium channel blockers, and certain other agents. Compounds in these categories include:

Bepridil Hydrochloride (Potential for hypotension, AV conduction disturbances, and LVF in patients with impaired cardiac function). Products include:
- Vascor (200, 300 and 400 mg) Tablets ... 1383

Clonidine (Potential for withdrawal reactions). Products include:
- Catapres-TTS ... 677

Clonidine Hydrochloride (Potential for withdrawal). Products include:
- Catapres Tablets ... 676
- Combipres Tablets ... 678

Deserpidine (Additive effect resulting in marked bradycardia, vertigo, syncope or postural hypotension). Products include:
- Enduronyl ... 518
- Harmonyl Tablets ... 528
- Oreticyl ... 545

Diltiazem Hydrochloride (Potential for hypotension, AV conduction disturbances, and LVF in patients with impaired cardiac function). Products include:
- Cardizem Tablets-30 mg, 60 mg, 90 mg and 120 mg ... 1329
- Cardizem SR Capsules-60 mg, 90 mg and 120 mg ... 1327

Felodipine (Potential for hypotension, AV conduction disturbances, and LVF in patients with impaired cardiac function). Products include:
- Plendil Extended-Release Tablets ... 1526

Isradipine (Potential for hypotension, AV conduction disturbances, and LVF in patients with impaired cardiac function). Products include:
- DynaCirc Capsules ... 2004

Nicardipine Hydrochloride (Potential for hypotension, AV conduction disturbances, and LVF in patients with impaired cardiac function). Products include:
- Cardene Capsules ... 2290

Nifedipine (Potential for hypotension, AV conduction disturbances, and LVF in patients with impaired cardiac function). Products include:
- Adalat Capsules (10 mg and 20 mg) ... 1587
- Procardia Capsules ... 1781
- Procardia XL Tablets ... 1783

Nimodipine (Potential for hypotension, AV conduction disturbances, and LVF in patients with impaired cardiac function). Products include:
- Nimotop Capsules ... 1607

Rauwolfia Serpentina (Additive effect resulting in marked bradycardia, vertigo, syncope or postural hypotension). Products include:
- Raudixin Tablets ... 1803
- Rauzide Tablets ... 1804

Rescinnamine (Additive effect resulting in marked bradycardia, vertigo, syncope or postural hypotension).
- No products indexed under this heading.

Reserpine (Additive effect resulting in marked bradycardia, vertigo, syncope or postural hypotension). Products include:
- Diupres Tablets ... 1461
- Hydromox R Tablets ... 1209
- Hydropres Tablets ... 1485
- Renese-R Tablets ... 1786
- Salutensin/Salutensin-Demi ... 719
- Ser-Ap-Es Tablets ... 881
- Serpasil Tablets ... 883
- Serpasil-Apresoline Tablets ... 884
- Serpasil-Esidrix Tablets ... 886

Verapamil Hydrochloride (Potential for hypotension, AV conduction disturbances, and LVF in patients with impaired cardiac function). Products include:
- Calan SR Caplets ... 2157
- Calan Tablets ... 2155
- Isoptin Injectable ... 1177
- Isoptin Oral Tablets ... 1179
- Isoptin SR Sustained Release Tablets ... 1181
- Verelan Capsules ... 1243
- Verelan Capsules ... 2535

KETALAR
(Ketamine Hydrochloride) ... 1726
May interact with barbiturates, narcotic analgesics, and certain other agents. Compounds in these categories include:

Alcohol (Effect not specified).

Alfentanil Hydrochloride (Prolonged recovery time). Products include:
- Alfenta Injection ... 1131

Aprobarbital (Prolonged recovery time). Products include:
- Alurate Elixir ... 1883

Buprenorphine (Prolonged recovery time).
- No products indexed under this heading.

Butabarbital (Prolonged recovery time). Products include:
- Pyridium Plus ... 1764

Butalbital (Prolonged recovery time). Products include:
- Esgic-Plus Tablets ... 1002
- Esgic Tablets & Capsules ... 1001
- Fioricet Tablets ... 2006
- Fiorinal Capsules ... 2007
- Fiorinal with Codeine Capsules ... 2008
- Fiorinal Tablets ... 2007
- Phrenilin ... 838
- Sedapap Tablets 50 mg/650 mg ... 1360

Codeine (Prolonged recovery time). Products include:
- Calcidrine Syrup ... 506

Codeine Phosphate (Prolonged recovery time). Products include:
- Actifed with Codeine Cough Syrup ... 752
- Cheracol Cough Syrup ... 1853
- Codimal PH Syrup ... 846
- Dimetane-DC Cough Syrup ... 1857
- Empirin with Codeine Phosphate Nos. 2, 3 & 4 ... 764
- Fiorinal with Codeine Capsules ... 2008
- Isoclor Expectorant ... 982
- Naldecon CX Adult Liquid ... ▣ 521
- Novahistine DH ... 1342
- Novahistine Expectorant ... 1343
- Nucofed Capsules ... 2219
- Nucofed Expectorant ... 2219
- Nucofed Pediatric Expectorant ... 2220
- Nucofed Syrup ... 2219
- Phenaphen with Codeine Capsules 1865
- Phenaphen-650 with Codeine Tablets ... 1866
- Phenergan with Codeine ... 2497
- Phenergan VC with Codeine ... 2501
- Robitussin A-C Syrup ... 1875
- Robitussin-DAC Syrup ... 1875
- Ryna ... ▣ 741
- Soma Compound w/Codeine Tablets ... 2390
- Triaminic Expectorant w/Codeine ... 1996
- Tussi-Organidin Liquid ... 2391
- Tylenol with Codeine ... 1381

Codeine Polistirex (Prolonged recovery time).
- No products indexed under this heading.

Dezocine (Prolonged recovery time).

Fentanyl (Prolonged recovery time). Products include:
- Duragesic Transdermal System ... 1133

Fentanyl Citrate (Prolonged recovery time). Products include:
- Innovar Injection ... 1141
- Sublimaze Injection ... 1146

Hydrocodone Bitartrate (Prolonged recovery time). Products include:
- Anexsia 5/500 Tablets ... 2196
- Anexsia 7.5/650 Tablets ... 2197
- Azdone Tablets ... 844
- Codiclear DH Syrup ... 845
- Codimal DH Syrup ... 846
- Damason-P ... 1356
- Hycodan Syrup, Tablets ... 927
- Hycomine Compound Tablets ... 929
- Hycomine Syrup ... 927
- Hycotuss Expectorant Syrup ... 930
- Hydrocet Capsules ... 835
- Lortab ASA Tablets ... 2414
- Lortab ... 2412
- Ru-Tuss with Hydrocodone ... 694
- Triaminic Expectorant DH ... 1995
- Vicodin Tablets ... 1187
- Vicodin ES Tablets ... 1189
- Zydone Capsules ... 941

Hydrocodone Polistirex (Prolonged recovery time). Products include:
- Tussionex Extended-Release Suspension ... 988

Levorphanol Tartrate (Prolonged recovery time). Products include:
- Levo-Dromoran ... 1906

Meperidine Hydrochloride (Prolonged recovery time). Products include:
- Demerol ... 2047
- Mepergan Injection ... 2479

Mephobarbital (Prolonged recovery time). Products include:
- Mebaral Tablets ... 2061

Methadone Hydrochloride (Prolonged recovery time). Products include:
- Dolophine Hydrochloride Ampoules & Vials ... 1260
- Dolophine Hydrochloride Tablets ... 1261
- Methadone Hydrochloride Diskets ... 1284
- Methadone Hydrochloride Oral Solution & Tablets ... 1987

Morphine Sulfate (Prolonged recovery time). Products include:
- Astramorph/PF Injection, USP (Preservative-Free) ... 618
- Duramorph ... 960
- Infumorph 200 and Infumorph 500 Sterile Solutions ... 962
- MS Contin Tablets ... 1814
- MSIR ... 1817
- Oramorph SR (Morphine Sulfate Sustained Release Tablets) ... 1988
- Roxanol ... 1991

Opium Alkaloids (Prolonged recovery time). Products include:
- B & O No. 15A & No. 16A Supprettes ... 2395
- Pantopon Injectable ... 1911

Oxycodone Hydrochloride (Prolonged recovery time). Products include:
- Percocet Tablets ... 950
- Percodan ... 951
- Roxicodone Tablets, Oral Solution & Intensol (Oxycodone) ... 1992
- Tylox Capsules ... 1382

Pentobarbital Sodium (Prolonged recovery time). Products include:
- Nembutal Sodium Capsules ... 534
- Nembutal Sodium Solution ... 536
- Nembutal Sodium Suppositories ... 538

Phenobarbital (Prolonged recovery time). Products include:
- Arco-Lase Plus Tablets ... 607
- Bellergal-S Tablets ... 1998
- Bronkolixir ... ▣ 761
- Bronkotabs Tablets ... ▣ 762
- Donnatal ... 1858
- Donnatal Extentabs ... 1859
- Donnatal Tablets ... 1858
- Donnazyme Tablets ... 1860
- Kinesed Tablets ... 2272
- Phenobarbital Elixir and Tablets ... 1293
- Primatene Tablets-P Formula ... 2421
- Quadrinal Tablets ... 1183
- Tedral SA ... 1765

Propoxyphene Hydrochloride (Prolonged recovery time). Products include:
- Darvon ... 1256
- Wygesic Tablets ... 2540

Propoxyphene Napsylate (Prolonged recovery time). Products include:
- Darvon-N/Darvocet-N ... 1254

Secobarbital Sodium (Prolonged recovery time). Products include:
- Seconal Sodium Pulvules ... 1296

Sufentanil Citrate (Prolonged recovery time). Products include:
- Sufenta Injection ... 1147

Thiamylal Sodium (Prolonged recovery time). Products include:
- Surital Ampoules, Steri-Vials ... 1764

KINESED TABLETS
(Belladonna Alkaloids, Phenobarbital) ... 2272
May interact with oral anticoagulants. Compounds in this category include:

Dicumarol (Decreased anticoagulant effect). Products include:
- Dicumarol Tablets ... 516

Warfarin Sodium (Decreased anticoagulant effect). Products include:
- Coumadin Injection & Tablets ... 944
- Panwarfin Tablets ... 547

KLONOPIN TABLETS
(Clonazepam) 1902
May interact with narcotic analgesics, barbiturates, hypnotics and sedatives, tranquilizers, phenothiazines, monoamine oxidase inhibitors, tricyclic antidepressants, anticonvulsants, and certain other agents. Compounds in these categories include:

Alcohol (Potentiates CNS-depressant action).

Alfentanil Hydrochloride (Potentiates CNS-depressant action). Products include:
Alfenta Injection 1131

Alprazolam (Potentiates CNS-depressant action). Products include:
Xanax Tablets 2367

Amitriptyline Hydrochloride (Potentiates CNS-depressant action). Products include:
Elavil 2269
Endep Tablets 1927
Etrafon 2087
Limbitrol 1933
Triavil Tablets 1556

Amoxapine (Potentiates CNS-depressant action). Products include:
Asendin Tablets 1196

Aprobarbital (Potentiates CNS-depressant action). Products include:
Alurate Elixir 1883

Buprenorphine (Potentiates CNS-depressant action).
No products indexed under this heading.

Buspirone Hydrochloride (Potentiates CNS-depressant action). Products include:
BuSpar 1401

Butabarbital (Potentiates CNS-depressant action). Products include:
Pyridium Plus 1764

Butalbital (Potentiates CNS-depressant action). Products include:
Esgic-Plus Tablets 1002
Esgic Tablets & Capsules 1001
Fioricet Tablets 2006
Fiorinal Capsules 2007
Fiorinal with Codeine Capsules 2008
Fiorinal Tablets 2007
Phrenilin 838
Sedapap Tablets 50 mg/650 mg .. 1360

Carbamazepine (Potentiates CNS-depressant action). Products include:
Tegretol Chewable Tablets 654
Tegretol Suspension 656
Tegretol Tablets 654

Chlordiazepoxide (Potentiates CNS-depressant action). Products include:
Libritabs Tablets 1930
Limbitrol 1933
Menrium Tablets 1934

Chlordiazepoxide Hydrochloride (Potentiates CNS-depressant action). Products include:
Librax Capsules 1929
Librium Capsules 1931
Librium Injectable 1932

Chlorpromazine (Potentiates CNS-depressant action). Products include:
Thorazine 2234

Chlorprothixene (Potentiates CNS-depressant action). Products include:
Taractan Tablets 1920

Chlorprothixene Hydrochloride (Potentiates CNS-depressant action). Products include:
Taractan 1920

Clomipramine Hydrochloride (Potentiates CNS-depressant action). Products include:
Anafranil Capsules 650

Clorazepate Dipotassium (Potentiates CNS-depressant action). Products include:
Tranxene 556

Codeine (Potentiates CNS-depressant action). Products include:
Calcidrine Syrup 506

Codeine Phosphate (Potentiates CNS-depressant action). Products include:
Actifed with Codeine Cough Syrup.. 752
Cheracol Cough Syrup 1853
Codimal PH Syrup 846
Dimetane-DC Cough Syrup 1857
Empirin with Codeine Phosphate Nos. 2, 3 & 4 764
Fiorinal with Codeine Capsules 2008
Isoclor Expectorant 982
Naldecon CX Adult Liquid .... ▣ 521
Novahistine DH 1342
Novahistine Expectorant 1343
Nucofed Capsules 2219
Nucofed Expectorant 2219
Nucofed Pediatric Expectorant 2220
Nucofed Syrup 2219
Phenaphen with Codeine Capsules 1865
Phenaphen-650 with Codeine Tablets 1866
Phenergan with Codeine 2497
Phenergan VC with Codeine 2501
Robitussin A-C Syrup 1875
Robitussin-DAC Syrup 1875
Ryna .... ▣ 741
Soma Compound w/Codeine Tablets 2390
Triaminic Expectorant w/Codeine .. 1996
Tussi-Organidin Liquid 2391
Tylenol with Codeine 1381

Codeine Polistirex (Potentiates CNS-depressant action).
No products indexed under this heading.

Desipramine Hydrochloride (Potentiates CNS-depressant action). Products include:
Norpramin Tablets 1340

Dezocine (Potentiates CNS-depressant action).

Diazepam (Potentiates CNS-depressant action). Products include:
Valium Injectable 1937
Valium Tablets 1939
Valrelease Capsules 1923

Divalproex Sodium (Potentiates CNS-depressant action). Products include:
Depakote 512

Doxepin Hydrochloride (Potentiates CNS-depressant action). Products include:
Sinequan 1960

Droperidol (Potentiates CNS-depressant action). Products include:
Inapsine Injection 1140
Innovar Injection 1141

Estazolam (Potentiates CNS-depressant action). Products include:
ProSom Tablets 554

Ethchlorvynol (Potentiates CNS-depressant action). Products include:
Placidyl Capsules 553

Ethinamate (Potentiates CNS-depressant action).
No products indexed under this heading.

Ethosuximide (Potentiates CNS-depressant action). Products include:
Zarontin Capsules 1768
Zarontin Syrup 1769

Ethotoin (Potentiates CNS-depressant action). Products include:
Peganone Tablets 551

Fentanyl (Potentiates CNS-depressant action). Products include:
Duragesic Transdermal System 1133

Fentanyl Citrate (Potentiates CNS-depressant action). Products include:
Innovar Injection 1141
Sublimaze Injection 1146

Fluphenazine Decanoate (Potentiates CNS-depressant action). Products include:
Prolixin Decanoate 1795

Fluphenazine Enanthate (Potentiates CNS-depressant action). Products include:
Prolixin Enanthate 1796

Fluphenazine Hydrochloride (Potentiates CNS-depressant action). Products include:
Prolixin Elixir 1793
Prolixin Injection 1791
Prolixin Oral Concentrate 1792
Prolixin Tablets 1793

Flurazepam Hydrochloride (Potentiates CNS-depressant action). Products include:
Dalmane Capsules 1927

Furazolidone (Potentiates CNS-depressant action). Products include:
Furoxone 1855

Glutethimide (Potentiates CNS-depressant action).
No products indexed under this heading.

Haloperidol (Potentiates CNS-depressant action). Products include:
Haldol Injection, Tablets and Concentrate 1373

Haloperidol Decanoate (Potentiates CNS-depressant action). Products include:
Haldol Decanoate 1375

Hydrocodone Bitartrate (Potentiates CNS-depressant action). Products include:
Anexsia 5/500 Tablets 2196
Anexsia 7.5/650 Tablets 2197
Azdone Tablets 844
Codiclear DH Syrup 845
Codimal DH Syrup 846
Damason-P 1356
Hycodan Syrup, Tablets 927
Hycomine Compound Tablets 929
Hycomine Syrup 927
Hycotuss Expectorant Syrup 930
Hydrocet Capsules 835
Lortab ASA Tablets 2414
Lortab 2412
Ru-Tuss with Hydrocodone 694
Triaminic Expectorant DH 1995
Vicodin Tablets 1187
Vicodin ES Tablets 1189
Zydone Capsules 941

Hydrocodone Polistirex (Potentiates CNS-depressant action). Products include:
Tussionex Extended-Release Suspension 988

Hydroxyzine Hydrochloride (Potentiates CNS-depressant action). Products include:
Atarax Tablets & Syrup 1941
Marax Tablets & DF Syrup 1954
Vistaril Intramuscular Solution 1970

Imipramine Hydrochloride (Potentiates CNS-depressant action). Products include:
Tofranil Ampuls 1038
Tofranil Tablets 1039

Imipramine Pamoate (Potentiates CNS-depressant action). Products include:
Tofranil-PM Capsules 1041

Isocarboxazid (Potentiates CNS-depressant action). Products include:
Marplan Tablets 1906

Levorphanol Tartrate (Potentiates CNS-depressant action). Products include:
Levo-Dromoran 1906

Lorazepam (Potentiates CNS-depressant action). Products include:
Ativan Injection 2432
Ativan Tablets 2434

Loxapine Hydrochloride (Potentiates CNS-depressant action). Products include:
Loxitane 1213

Maprotiline Hydrochloride (Potentiates CNS-depressant action). Products include:
Ludiomil Tablets 874

Meperidine Hydrochloride (Potentiates CNS-depressant action). Products include:
Demerol 2047
Mepergan Injection 2479

Mephenytoin (Potentiates CNS-depressant action). Products include:
Mesantoin Tablets 2013

Mephobarbital (Potentiates CNS-depressant action). Products include:
Mebaral Tablets 2061

Meprobamate (Potentiates CNS-depressant action). Products include:
Deprol Tablets 2382
Equagesic Tablets 2451
Miltown Tablets 2386
PMB 200 and PMB 400 2504

Mesoridazine (Potentiates CNS-depressant action). Products include:
Serentil 686

Methadone Hydrochloride (Potentiates CNS-depressant action). Products include:
Dolophine Hydrochloride Ampoules & Vials 1260
Dolophine Hydrochloride Tablets 1261
Methadone Hydrochloride Diskets .. 1284
Methadone Hydrochloride Oral Solution & Tablets 1987

Methsuximide (Potentiates CNS-depressant action). Products include:
Celontin 1692

Midazolam Hydrochloride (Potentiates CNS-depressant action). Products include:
Versed Injection 1924

Molindone Hydrochloride (Potentiates CNS-depressant action). Products include:
Moban Tablets & Concentrate 932

Morphine Sulfate (Potentiates CNS-depressant action). Products include:
Astramorph/PF Injection, USP (Preservative-Free) 618
Duramorph 960
Infumorph 200 and Infumorph 500 Sterile Solutions 962
MS Contin Tablets 1814
MSIR 1817
Oramorph SR (Morphine Sulfate Sustained Release Tablets) 1988
Roxanol 1991

Nortriptyline Hydrochloride (Potentiates CNS-depressant action). Products include:
Pamelor 2019

Opium Alkaloids (Potentiates CNS-depressant action). Products include:
B & O No. 15A & No. 16A Supprettes 2395
Pantopon Injectable 1911

Oxazepam (Potentiates CNS-depressant action). Products include:
Serax Capsules 2522
Serax Tablets 2522

Oxycodone Hydrochloride (Potentiates CNS-depressant action). Products include:
Percocet Tablets 950
Percodan 951
Roxicodone Tablets, Oral Solution & Intensol (Oxycodone) 1992
Tylox Capsules 1382

Paramethadione (Potentiates CNS-depressant action). Products include:
Paradione Capsules 548

Pentobarbital Sodium (Potentiates CNS-depressant action). Products include:
Nembutal Sodium Capsules 534
Nembutal Sodium Solution 536
Nembutal Sodium Suppositories 538

Perphenazine (Potentiates CNS-depressant action). Products include:
Etrafon 2087
Triavil Tablets 1556
Trilafon 2123

Phenacemide (Potentiates CNS-depressant action). Products include:
Phenurone Tablets 552

Phenelzine Sulfate (Potentiates CNS-depressant action). Products include:
Nardil 1742

Phenobarbital (Potentiates CNS-depressant action). Products include:
Arco-Lase Plus Tablets 607
Bellergal-S Tablets 1998
Bronkolixir ..... ▣ 761
Bronkotabs Tablets ..... ▣ 762
Donnatal 1858
Donnatal Extentabs 1859
Donnatal Tablets 1858
Donnazyme Tablets 1860
Kinesed Tablets 2272
Phenobarbital Elixir and Tablets 1293
Primatene Tablets-P Formula 2421
Quadrinal Tablets 1183
Tedral SA 1765

Phenothiazine Derivatives (Potentiates CNS-depressant action).

Phensuximide (Potentiates CNS-depressant action). Products include:
Milontin Kapseals 1741

Phenytoin (Potentiates CNS-depressant action). Products include:
Dilantin Infatabs 1710
Dilantin-30 Pediatric/Dilantin-125 Suspension 1713

Phenytoin Sodium (Potentiates CNS-depressant action). Products include:
Dilantin Kapseals 1708
Dilantin Parenteral 1712
Dilantin with Phenobarbital Kapseals 1715

Prazepam (Potentiates CNS-depressant action). Products include:
Centrax 1693

Primidone (Potentiates CNS-depressant action). Products include:
Mysoline 2480

Prochlorperazine (Potentiates CNS-depressant action). Products include:
Compazine 2201

Promethazine Hydrochloride (Potentiates CNS-depressant action). Products include:
Mepergan Injection 2479
Phenergan with Codeine 2497
Phenergan with Dextromethorphan 2499
Phenergan Injection 2493
Phenergan Suppositories 2496
Phenergan Syrup 2495
Phenergan Tablets 2496
Phenergan VC 2500
Phenergan VC with Codeine 2501

Propofol (Potentiates CNS-depressant action). Products include:
Diprivan Injection 2267

Propoxyphene Hydrochloride (Potentiates CNS-depressant action). Products include:
Darvon 1256
Wygesic Tablets 2540

Propoxyphene Napsylate (Potentiates CNS-depressant action). Products include:
Darvon-N/Darvocet-N 1254

Protriptyline Hydrochloride (Potentiates CNS-depressant action). Products include:
Vivactil Tablets 1567

Quazepam (Potentiates CNS-depressant action). Products include:
Doral Tablets 2383

Secobarbital Sodium (Potentiates CNS-depressant action). Products include:
Seconal Sodium Pulvules 1296

Selegiline Hydrochloride (Potentiates CNS-depressant action). Products include:
Eldepryl 2250

Sufentanil Citrate (Potentiates CNS-depressant action). Products include:
Sufenta Injection 1147

Temazepam (Potentiates CNS-depressant action). Products include:
Restoril Capsules 2023

Thiamylal Sodium (Potentiates CNS-depressant action). Products include:
Surital Ampoules, Steri-Vials 1764

Thioridazine Hydrochloride (Potentiates CNS-depressant action). Products include:
Mellaril 2011

Thiothixene (Potentiates CNS-depressant action). Products include:
Navane Capsules and Concentrate 1954
Navane Intramuscular 1956

Tranylcypromine Sulfate (Potentiates CNS-depressant action). Products include:
Parnate Tablets 2222

Triazolam (Potentiates CNS-depressant action). Products include:
Halcion Tablets 2340

Trifluoperazine Hydrochloride (Potentiates CNS-depressant action). Products include:
Stelazine 2226

Trimethadione (Potentiates CNS-depressant action). Products include:
Tridione 557

Trimipramine Maleate (Potentiates CNS-depressant action). Products include:
Surmontil Capsules 2524

Valproic Acid (Potentiates CNS-depressant action). Products include:
Depakene Capsules & Syrup 511

KLOR-CON 8/KLOR-CON 10 EXTENDED-RELEASE TABLETS
(Potassium Chloride) 2374
May interact with potassium sparing diuretics and ACE inhibitors. Compounds in these categories include:

Amiloride Hydrochloride (Severe hyperkalemia). Products include:
Midamor Tablets 1508
Moduretic Tablets 1510

Benazepril Hydrochloride (Possible hyperkalemia). Products include:
Lotensin Tablets 872

Captopril (Possible hyperkalemia). Products include:
Capoten 2255
Capozide 2258

Enalapril Maleate (Possible hyperkalemia). Products include:
Vaseretic Tablets 1559
Vasotec Tablets 1564

Enalaprilat (Possible hyperkalemia). Products include:
Vasotec I.V. 1562

Fosinopril Sodium (Possible hyperkalemia). Products include:
Monopril Tablets 1406

Lisinopril (Possible hyperkalemia). Products include:
Prinivil Tablets 1538
Prinzide Tablets 1540
Zestoretic 2274
Zestril Tablets 2277

Ramipril (Possible hyperkalemia). Products include:
Altace Capsules 1086

Spironolactone (Severe hyperkalemia). Products include:
Aldactazide 2150
Aldactone 2152

Triamterene (Severe hyperkalemia). Products include:
Dyazide Capsules 2208
Dyrenium Capsules 2210
Maxzide 1215

KLORVESS EFFERVESCENT GRANULES
(Potassium Chloride, Potassium Bicarbonate) 2010
May interact with potassium sparing diuretics and aldosterone-inhibiting diuretic agents. Compounds in these categories include:

Amiloride Hydrochloride (Concurrent administration is contraindicated). Products include:
Midamor Tablets 1508
Moduretic Tablets 1510

Spironolactone (Concurrent administration is contraindicated). Products include:
Aldactazide 2150
Aldactone 2152

Triamterene (Concurrent administration is contraindicated). Products include:
Dyazide Capsules 2208
Dyrenium Capsules 2210
Maxzide 1215

KLORVESS EFFERVESCENT TABLETS
(Potassium Chloride, Potassium Bicarbonate) 2011
May interact with potassium sparing diuretics and aldosterone-inhibiting diuretic agents. Compounds in these categories include:

Amiloride Hydrochloride (Concurrent administration is contraindicated). Products include:
Midamor Tablets 1508
Moduretic Tablets 1510

Spironolactone (Concurrent administration is contraindicated). Products include:
Aldactazide 2150
Aldactone 2152

Triamterene (Concurrent administration is contraindicated). Products include:
Dyazide Capsules 2208
Dyrenium Capsules 2210
Maxzide 1215

KLORVESS 10% LIQUID
(Potassium Chloride, Potassium Bicarbonate) 2010
See **Klorvess Effervescent Granules**

KLOTRIX
(Potassium Chloride) 708
May interact with potassium sparing diuretics and ACE inhibitors. Compounds in these categories include:

Amiloride Hydrochloride (Severe hyperkalemia). Products include:
Midamor Tablets 1508
Moduretic Tablets 1510

Benazepril Hydrochloride (Potential for hyperkalemia). Products include:
Lotensin Tablets 872

Captopril (Potential for hyperkalemia). Products include:
Capoten 2255
Capozide 2258

Enalapril Maleate (Potential for hyperkalemia). Products include:
Vaseretic Tablets 1559
Vasotec Tablets 1564

Enalaprilat (Potential for hyperkalemia). Products include:
Vasotec I.V. 1562

Fosinopril Sodium (Potential for hyperkalemia). Products include:
Monopril Tablets 1406

Lisinopril (Potential for hyperkalemia). Products include:
Prinivil Tablets 1538
Prinzide Tablets 1540
Zestoretic 2274
Zestril Tablets 2277

Ramipril (Potential for hyperkalemia). Products include:
Altace Capsules 1086

Spironolactone (Severe hyperkalemia). Products include:
Aldactazide 2150
Aldactone 2152

Triamterene (Severe hyperkalemia). Products include:
Dyazide Capsules 2208
Dyrenium Capsules 2210
Maxzide 1215

KOĀTE-HP ANTIHEMOPHILIC FACTOR (HUMAN)
(Antihemophilic Factor (Human), VIII, AHF, AHG) 1581
No interactions described in labeling.

KOĀTE-HS ANTIHEMOPHILIC FACTOR (HUMAN)
(Antihemophilic Factor (Human), VIII, AHF, AHG) 1580
No interactions described in labeling.

KOLYUM LIQUID
(Potassium Gluconate, Potassium Chloride) 983
May interact with potassium sparing diuretics. Compounds in this category include:

Amiloride Hydrochloride (Potential for severe hyperkalemia). Products include:
Midamor Tablets 1508
Moduretic Tablets 1510

Spironolactone (Potential for severe hyperkalemia). Products include:
Aldactazide 2150
Aldactone 2152

Triamterene (Potential for severe hyperkalemia). Products include:
Dyazide Capsules 2208
Dyrenium Capsules 2210
Maxzide 1215

KONAKION INJECTION
(Phytonadione) 1903
May interact with oral anticoagulants. Compounds in this category include:

Dicumarol (Concomitant use is not recommended except for excessive hypoprothrombinemia). Products include:

- Dicumarol Tablets ... 516

Warfarin Sodium (Concomitant use is not recommended except for excessive hypoprothrombinemia). Products include:

- Coumadin Injection & Tablets ... 944
- Panwarfin Tablets ... 547

KONINE 80 FACTOR IX COMPLEX

(Factor IX Complex (Human)) ...1571
No interactions described in labeling.

KONINE -HT FACTOR IX COMPLEX

(Factor IX Complex) ...1583
No interactions described in labeling.

KORO-FLEX ARCING SPRING DIAPHRAGM

(Vaginal Diaphragm & Apparatus) 2142
May interact with:

Petrolatum-containing body lubricants (Weakens diaphragm rubber).

Petrolatum-containing vaginal lubricants (Weakens diaphragm rubber).

KOROMEX COIL SPRING DIAPHRAGM

(Vaginal Diaphragm & Apparatus) 2142
May interact with:

Petrolatum-containing body lubricants (Weakens diaphragm rubber).

Petrolatum-containing vaginal lubricants (Weakens diaphragm rubber).

KRONOFED-A KRONOCAPS

(Chlorpheniramine Maleate, Pseudoephedrine Hydrochloride) ... 970
No interactions described in labeling.

KRONOFED-A-JR. KRONOCAPS

(Pseudoephedrine Hydrochloride, Chlorpheniramine Maleate) ... 970
No interactions described in labeling.

KUTAPRESSIN INJECTION

(Liver Preparations) ...2146
No interactions described in labeling.

KUTRASE CAPSULES

(Enzymes, Digestive) ...2146
No interactions described in labeling.

KU-ZYME CAPSULES

(Enzymes, Digestive) ...2146
No interactions described in labeling.

KU-ZYME HP CAPSULES

(Pancreatic Preparations) ...2147
May interact with:

Ferrous Fumarate (Decreased serum response to oral iron). Products include:

- Bugs Bunny Plus Iron Children's Chewable Vitamins (Sugar Free) ▣ 625
- Caltrate 600 + Iron & Vitamin D ... 1198
- Centrum, Jr. (Children's Chewable) + Iron ... ▣ 586
- Chromagen Capsules ... 2078
- FemIron Multi-Vitamins and Iron ... ▣ 617
- Ferancee Chewable Tablets ... 1155
- Ferancee-HP Tablets ... 1155
- Ferro-Sequels ... 1203
- Flintstones Children's Chewable Vitamins Plus Iron ... ▣ 625
- Natalins Rx ... 1391
- Natalins Tablets ... 1391
- Nephro-Fer Tablets ... 1826
- One-A-Day Maximum Formula Vitamins and Minerals ... ▣ 627
- Poly-Vi-Flor with Iron ... 1399
- Poly-Vi-Sol Vitamins with Iron, Chewable Tablets and Circus Shapes Chewable ... ▣ 612
- Pramilet FA ... 1974
- Stressgard Stress Formula Vitamins ... ▣ 628
- Stresstabs + Iron, Advanced Formula ... ▣ 589
- Stuartinic Tablets ... 1157
- Theragran-M Tablets ... ▣ 727
- Trinsicon Capsules ... 2415
- Within Women's Formula Multivitamin with Calcium, Extra Iron and Zinc ... ▣ 628
- Zenate Tablets ... 2250

Ferrous Gluconate (Decreased serum response to oral iron). Products include:

- Fergon ... ▣ 758

Ferrous Sulfate (Decreased serum response to oral iron). Products include:

- Dayalets Plus Iron Filmtab ... ▣ 502
- Feosol Capsules ... 2191
- Feosol Elixir ... 2191
- Feosol Tablets ... 2191
- Fero-Folic-500 Filmtab ... 527
- Fero-Grad-500 Filmtab ... 528
- Fero-Gradumet Filmtab ... 528
- Iberet Tablets ... 531
- Iberet-500 Liquid ... 531
- Iberet-Folic-500 Filmtab ... 527
- Iberet-Liquid ... 531
- Irospan ... 972
- Mol-Iron ... ▣ 703
- Poly-Vi-Sol Vitamins with Iron, Drops ... ▣ 612
- Pramet FA ... 1974
- Slow Fe Tablets ... 852
- Tri-Vi-Sol Vitamin Drops with Iron ▣ 614

Iron Preparations (Decreased serum response to oral iron). Products include:

- Allbee C-800 Plus Iron Tablets ... ▣ 670
- Bugs Bunny Children's Chewable Vitamins + Minerals with Iron and Calcium (Sugar Free) ... ▣ 626
- Bugs Bunny Plus Iron Children's Chewable Vitamins (Sugar Free) ▣ 625
- FemIron Multi-Vitamins and Iron ... ▣ 617
- Ferancee Chewable Tablets ... 1155
- Ferancee-HP Tablets ... 1155
- Fergon ... ▣ 758
- Fero-Folic-500 Filmtab ... 527
- Fero-Grad-500 Filmtab ... 528
- Fero-Gradumet Filmtab ... 528
- Ferro-Sequels ... 1203
- Flintstones Children's Chewable Vitamins Plus Iron ... ▣ 625
- Flintstones Complete With Calcium, Iron & Minerals Children's Chewable Vitamins ... ▣ 626
- Geritol Extend Tablets and Caplets ... ▣ 717
- Geritol Liquid - High Potency Iron & Vitamin Tonic ... ▣ 717
- Iberet Tablets ... 531
- Iberet-500 Liquid ... 531
- Iberet-Folic-500 Filmtab ... 527
- Iberet-Liquid ... 531
- Incremin w/Iron Syrup ... ▣ 588
- Irospan ... 972
- Mol-Iron ... ▣ 703
- Niferex ... 847
- Niferex-150 Forte Capsules ... 847
- Niferex Forte Elixir ... 847
- Niferex ... 847
- Niferex-PN Tablets ... 847
- One-A-Day Maximum Formula Vitamins and Minerals ... ▣ 627
- Peritinic Tablets ... ▣ 589
- Poly-Vi-Flor with Iron ... 1399
- Poly-Vi-Flor with Iron Drops ... 1399
- Poly-Vi-Sol Vitamins with Iron, Chewable Tablets and Circus Shapes Chewable ... ▣ 612
- Poly-Vi-Sol Vitamins with Iron, Drops ... ▣ 612
- SMA Iron Fortified Infant Formula, Concentrated, Ready-to-Feed and Powder ... ▣ 767
- Slow Fe Tablets ... ▣ 552
- The Stuart Formula Tablets ... ▣ 581
- Stuartinic Tablets ... 1157
- Surbex-750 with Iron ... ▣ 503
- Tri-Vi-Flor 0.25 mg Vitamins with Iron and Fluoride Drops ... 1401
- Unicap Plus Iron Vitamin Formula Tablets ... ▣ 738
- Vi-Daylin ADC Vitamins + Iron Drops ... 1980
- Vi-Daylin Multivitamin + Iron Drops ... 1981
- Vi-Daylin/F ADC Vitamins + Iron Drops With Fluoride ... 1981
- Vi-Daylin/F Multivitamin + Iron Drops With Fluoride ... 1981
- Vi-Daylin Multivitamin + Iron Chewable Tablets ... 1982
- Vi-Daylin/F Multivitamin + Iron Chewable Tablets With Fluoride .. 1982
- Vi-Daylin Multivitamin + Iron Liquid ... 1983

KWELL CREAM

(Lindane) ...1830
May interact with:

Oils, unspecified (May enhance absorption).

KWELL LOTION

(Lindane) ...1831
May interact with:

Oils, unspecified (May enhance absorption).

KWELL SHAMPOO

(Lindane) ...1832
May interact with:

Oils, unspecified (May enhance absorption).

KYOLIC

(Garlic Extract) ... ▣ 739
No interactions described in labeling.

LACRIL LUBRICANT OPHTHALMIC SOLUTION

(Gelatin A, Hydroxypropyl Methylcellulose) ... ⊙ 248
No interactions described in labeling.

LACRI-LUBE NP LUBRICANT OPHTHALMIC OINTMENT

(Emollient) ... ⊙ 249
No interactions described in labeling.

LACRI-LUBE S.O.P. STERILE OPHTHALMIC OINTMENT

(Mineral Oil, Petrolatum, White) ... ⊙ 249
No interactions described in labeling.

LACRISERT STERILE OPHTHALMIC INSERT

(Hydroxypropyl Cellulose) ...1493
No interactions described in labeling.

LACTAID CAPLETS

(Lactase (beta-d-Galactosidase)) ...1191
No interactions described in labeling.

LACTAID DROPS

(Lactase (beta-d-Galactosidase)) ...1191
No interactions described in labeling.

LACTINOL-E CREME

(Lactic Acid, Vitamin E) ...1770
No interactions described in labeling.

LAMPRENE CAPSULES

(Clofazimine) ...1030
No interactions described in labeling.

LANABIOTIC OINTMENT

(Bacitracin, Neomycin Sulfate, Polymyxin B Sulfate, Lidocaine) ... ▣ 556
No interactions described in labeling.

LANACANE CREME

(Benzocaine) ... ▣ 556
No interactions described in labeling.

LANACANE SPRAY

(Benzocaine) ... ▣ 557
No interactions described in labeling.

LANACORT 5 CREME AND OINTMENT

(Hydrocortisone) ... ▣ 557
No interactions described in labeling.

LANOXICAPS

(Digoxin) ... 772
May interact with thiazides, corticosteroids, mineralocorticoids, thyroid preparations, diuretics, antacids, sympathomimetic aerosol bronchodilators, beta blockers , calcium channel blockers, and certain other agents. Compounds in these categories include:

Acebutolol Hydrochloride (Additive effects on AV node conduction). Products include:

- Sectral Capsules ... 2520

Albuterol (Increased risk of cardiac arrhythmias). Products include:

- Proventil Inhalation Aerosol ... 2117
- Ventolin Inhalation Aerosol and Refill ... 583

Albuterol Sulfate (Increased risk of cardiac arrhythmias). Products include:

- Proventil Repetabs Tablets ... 2120
- Proventil Solutions for Inhalation 0.5% and 0.083% ... 2118
- Proventil Syrup ... 2119
- Proventil Tablets ... 2120
- Ventolin ... 583

Aluminum Carbonate Gel (Interferes with intestinal digoxin absorption). Products include:

- Basaljel ... 2438

Aluminum Hydroxide (Interferes with intestinal digoxin absorption). Products include:

- Cama Arthritis Pain Reliever ... ▣ 685
- Gaviscon Extra Strength Relief Formula Liquid Antacid ... ▣ 594
- Gaviscon Extra Strength Relief Formula Antacid Tablets ... ▣ 594
- Gaviscon Liquid Antacid ... ▣ 594
- Gelusil Liquid & Tablets ... ▣ 639
- Extra Strength Maalox Plus Suspension ... 1850
- Maalox TC Suspension ... 1851
- Maalox Plus Tablets ... ▣ 655
- Extra Strength Maalox Plus Tablets 1850
- Nephrox Suspension ... ▣ 563
- WinGel Liquid & Tablets ... ▣ 761

Aluminum Hydroxide Gel (Interferes with intestinal digoxin absorption). Products include:

- ALternaGEL Liquid ... 1154
- Aludrox Oral Suspension ... 2428
- Amphojel Suspension ... 2429
- Amphojel Suspension without Flavor ... 2429
- Mylanta Liquid ... 1155
- Mylanta Double Strength Liquid ... 1155

Aluminum Hydroxide Gel, Dried (Interferes with intestinal digoxin absorption). Products include:

- Alu-Tab/Alu-Cap ... 1309
- Amphojel Tablets ... 2429
- Ascriptin A/D Caplets ... 1850
- Regular Strength Ascriptin Tablets 1850
- Gaviscon Antacid Tablets ... ▣ 593
- Gaviscon-2 Antacid Tablets ... ▣ 594
- Mylanta Tablets ... 1155
- Mylanta Double Strength Tablets ... 1155

Amiodarone Hydrochloride (Rise in serum digoxin concentration). Products include:

- Cordarone Tablets ... 2446

Atenolol (Additive effects on AV node conduction). Products include:

- Tenoretic Tablets ... 1105
- Tenormin Tablets and I.V. Injection 1107

(▣ Described in PDR For Nonprescription Drugs) (⊙ Described in PDR For Ophthalmology)

Bendroflumethiazide (Contributing factor to digitalis toxicity). Products include:
- Corzide Tablets 702
- Naturetin Tablets 1789
- Rauzide Tablets 1804

Bepridil Hydrochloride (Additive effects on AV node conduction). Products include:
- Vascor (200, 300 and 400 mg) Tablets 1383

Betamethasone Acetate (Contributing factor to digitalis toxicity). Products include:
- Celestone Soluspan Suspension 2081

Betamethasone Sodium Phosphate (Contributing factor to digitalis toxicity). Products include:
- Celestone Soluspan Suspension 2081

Betaxolol Hydrochloride (Additive effects on AV node conduction). Products include:
- Betoptic Sterile Ophthalmic Solution 569
- Betoptic S Sterile Ophthalmic Suspension 570
- Kerlone Tablets 2172

Calcium, intravenous (May produce serious arrhythmias in digitalized patients).

Carteolol Hydrochloride (Additive effects on Av node conduction). Products include:
- Cartrol Tablets 507

Chlorothiazide (Contributing factor to digitalis toxicity). Products include:
- Aldoclor Tablets 1413
- Diupres Tablets 1461
- Diuril Oral 1464

Chlorothiazide Sodium (Contributing factor to digitalis toxicity). Products include:
- Diuril Sodium Intravenous 1463

Cholestyramine (Interferes with intestinal digoxin absorption). Products include:
- Cholybar 1705
- Questran Light 711
- Questran Powder 710

Cortisone Acetate (Contributing factor to digitalis toxicity). Products include:
- Cortone Acetate Sterile Suspension 1437
- Cortone Acetate Tablets 1439

Desoxycorticosterone Acetate (Contributing factor to digitalis toxicity).

Dexamethasone (Contriburing factor to digitalis toxicity). Products include:
- AK-Trol Ointment & Suspension ⊙ 207
- Decadron Elixir 1445
- Decadron Tablets 1447
- Decaspray Topical Aerosol 1459
- Dexacidin ⊙ 272
- Maxidex Sterile Ophthalmic Suspension ⊙ 223
- Maxitrol Ophthalmic Ointment/Suspension ⊙ 223
- TobraDex Ophthalmic Suspension and Ointment ⊙ 228

Dexamethasone Acetate (Contributing factor to digitalis toxicity). Products include:
- Dalalone D.P. Injectable 999
- Decadron-LA Sterile Suspension 1457

Dexamethasone Sodium Phosphate (Contributing factor to digitalis toxicity). Products include:
- AK-Dex ⊙ 203
- Decadron Phosphate Respihaler 1454
- Decadron Phosphate Sterile Ophthalmic Ointment 1453
- Decadron Phosphate Sterile Ophthalmic Solution 1453
- Decadron Phosphate Topical Cream 1455
- Decadron Phosphate Turbinaire 1456
- Maxidex Sterile Ophthalmic Ointment ⊙ 222
- NeoDecadron Sterile Ophthalmic Ointment 1517
- NeoDecadron Sterile Ophthalmic Solution 1518
- NeoDecadron Topical Cream 1518

Dihydroxyaluminum Sodium Carbonate (Interferes with intestinal digoxin absorption). Products include:
- Rolaids ▣ 743

Diltiazem Hydrochloride (Additive effects on AV node conduction). Products include:
- Cardizem Tablets-30 mg, 60 mg, 90 mg and 120 mg 1329
- Cardizem SR Capsules-60 mg, 90 mg and 120 mg 1327

Diphenoxylate Hydrochloride (Increases digoxin absorption). Products include:
- Lomotil 2174

Dobutamine Hydrochloride (Increased risk of cardiac arrhythmias). Products include:
- Dobutrex Solution Vials 1259

Dopamine Hydrochloride (Increased risk of cardiac arrhythmias). Products include:
- Intropin Injection 930

Ephedrine Hydrochloride (Increased risk of cardiac arrhythmias). Products include:
- Amesec ▣ 682
- Primatene Tablets-M Formula 2421
- Primatene Tablets-P Formula 2421
- Primatene Tablets-Regular Formula 2421
- Quadrinal Tablets 1183
- Quelidrine Syrup 556
- Tedral SA 1765

Ephedrine Sulfate (Increased risk of cardiac arrhythmias). Products include:
- Bronkaid Tablets ▣ 757
- Bronkolixir ▣ 761
- Bronkotabs Tablets ▣ 762
- Marax Tablets & DF Syrup 1954
- Pazo Hemorrhoid Ointment & Suppositories 752
- Vicks Vatronol Nose Drops ▣ 666

Ephedrine Tannate (Increased risk of cardiac arrhythmias). Products include:
- Rynatuss 2388

Epinephrine (Increased risk of cardiac arrhythmias). Products include:
- Ana-Kit Anaphylaxis Emergency Treatment Kit 1100
- Bronkaid Mist ▣ 757
- EpiPen 843
- Marcaine Hydrochloride 0.5% with Epinephrine 1:200,000 (as bitartrate) 958
- Marcaine Hydrochloride with Epinephrine 1:200,000 2055
- Primatene Mist 2420
- Sus-Phrine Injection 1006
- Xylocaine with Epinephrine Injections 637

Epinephrine Bitartrate (Increased risk of cardiac arrhythmias). Products include:
- AsthmaHaler Mist Epinephrine Bitartrate Bronchodilator ▣ 616
- Bronkaid Mist Suspension ▣ 757
- Primatene Mist Suspension 2421

Epinephrine Hydrochloride (Increased risk of cardiac arrhythmias). Products include:
- Adrenalin Chloride Solution 1:100 & 1:1,000 1689
- Epifrin ⊙ 244
- Glaucon ⊙ 218

Esmolol Hydrochloride (Additive effects on AV node conduction). Products include:
- Brevibloc Injection 942

Felodipine (Additive effects on AV node conduction). Products include:
- Plendil Extended-Release Tablets 1526

Hydrochlorothiazide (Contributing factor to digitalis toxicity). Products include:
- Aldactazide 2150
- Aldoril Tablets 1418
- Apresazide Capsules 854
- Apresoline-Esidrix Tablets 857
- Capozide 2258
- Dyazide Capsules 2208
- Esidrix Tablets 863
- Esimil Tablets 864
- HydroDIURIL Tablets 1484
- Hydropres Tablets 1485
- Inderide Tablets 2463
- Inderide LA Long Acting Capsules 2465
- Lopressor HCT Tablets 1034
- Maxzide 1215
- Moduretic Tablets 1510
- Normozide Tablets 2112
- Oretic Tablets 544
- Oreticyl 545
- Prinzide Tablets 1540
- Ser-Ap-Es Tablets 881
- Serpasil-Esidrix Tablets 886
- Timolide Tablets 1547
- Trandate HCT Tablets 579
- Vaseretic Tablets 1559
- Zestoretic 2274

Hydrocortisone (Contributing factor to digitalis toxicity). Products include:
- AK-Spore H.C. ⊙ 206
- Bactine Hydrocortisone Anti-Itch Cream ▣ 625
- CaldeCORT Anti-Itch Hydrocortisone Spray ▣ 560
- Carmol HC Cream 1% 2296
- Cortaid Spray ▣ 735
- Cortenema 2244
- Cortisporin Ointment 758
- Cortisporin Ophthalmic Ointment Sterile 758
- Cortisporin Ophthalmic Suspension Sterile 759
- Cortisporin Otic Solution Sterile 760
- Cortisporin Otic Suspension Sterile 760
- Cortizone-5 Creme & Ointment ▣ 732
- Dermolate Anti-Itch Cream ▣ 697
- Eldecort Cream 1.0% 1113
- Eldecort Cream 1.0% and 2.5% 1113
- Fungoid HC Creme 1770
- Hydrocortone Tablets 1482
- Hytone 909
- LazerSporin-C Solution 1770
- Massengill Medicated Soft Cloth Towelettes 2192
- Nutracort Cream & Lotion 1684
- PediOtic Suspension Sterile 797
- Synacort Creams 1%, 2.5% 2296
- Vanoxide-HC Acne Lotion 911
- Vioform-Hydrocortisone Cream and Mild Cream 889
- Vioform-Hydrocortisone Ointment 889
- VōSoL HC Otic Solution 2392
- Vytone Cream 1% 911

Hydrocortisone Acetate (Contributing factor to digitalis toxicity). Products include:
- Analpram-HC Rectal Cream 1% and 2.5% 970
- Anusol-HC Cream 1690
- Anusol-HC Suppositories 1691
- Caldecort ▣ 560
- Carmol HC Cream 1% 2296
- Chloromycetin Hydrocortisone Ophthalmic 1694
- Coly-Mycin S Otic w/Neomycin & Hydrocortisone 1708
- Cortaid ▣ 735
- Cortef Feminine Itch Cream ▣ 735
- Corticaine ▣ 682
- Cortifoam 1827
- Cortisporin Cream 757
- Epifoam 1828
- Gynecort 5 Creme ▣ 556
- Hydrocortone Acetate Sterile Suspension 1479
- Lanacort 5 Creme and Ointment ▣ 557
- Mantadil Cream 789
- Ophthocort ⊙ 301
- Orabase HCA Oral Paste 890
- Pramosone Cream, Lotion & Ointment 971
- ProctoCream-HC 1834
- Proctofoam-HC 1835

Hydrocortisone Sodium Phosphate (Contributing factor to digitalis toxicity). Products include:
- Hydrocortone Phosphate Injection, Sterile 1481

Hydrocortisone Sodium Succinate (Contributing factor to digitalis toxicity). Products include:
- Solu-Cortef Sterile Powder 2361

Hydroflumethiazide (Contributing factor to digitalis toxicity). Products include:
- Diucardin Tablets 2450
- Saluron 718
- Salutensin/Salutensin-Demi 719

Isoproterenol Hydrochloride (Increased risk of cardiac arrhythmias). Products include:
- Isuprel Hydrochloride Injection 1:5000 2050
- Isuprel Hydrochloride Mistometer 2051
- Isuprel Hydrochloride Solution 1:200 & 1:100 2052
- Norisodrine Aerotrol 540

Isradipine (Additive effects on AV node conduction). Products include:
- DynaCirc Capsules 2004

Kaolin (Interferes with intestinal digoxin absorption). Products include:
- Donnagel ▣ 675
- Donnagel-PG 1858

Labetalol Hydrochloride (Additive effects on AV node conduction). Products include:
- Normodyne Injection 2108
- Normodyne Tablets 2110
- Normozide Tablets 2112
- Trandate HCT Tablets 579
- Trandate Injection 577
- Trandate Tablets 579

Liothyronine Sodium (Hypothyroid patients may require increased digoxin dose). Products include:
- Cytomel Tablets 2203

Magaldrate (Interferes with intestinal digoxin absorption). Products include:
- Riopan Antacid Chew Tablets ▣ 754
- Riopan Antacid Chew Tablets in Rollpacks ▣ 754
- Riopan Antacid Suspension 2421
- Riopan Antacid Swallow Tablets 2421
- Riopan Plus Chew Tablets 2422
- Riopan Plus Chew Tablets in Rollpack 2422
- Riopan Plus 2 Chew Tablets, Mint Flavor, Cherry Flavor 2422
- Riopan Plus Suspension 2422
- Riopan Plus 2 Suspension, Mint Flavor, Cherry Flavor 2422

Magnesium Hydroxide (Interferes with intestinal digoxin absorption). Products include:
- Aludrox Oral Suspension 2428
- Ascriptin A/D Caplets 1850
- Regular Strength Ascriptin Tablets 1850
- Di-Gel Antacid/Anti-Gas ▣ 697
- Gelusil Liquid & Tablets ▣ 639
- Haley's M-O, Regular & Flavored ▣ 569
- Extra Strength Maalox Plus Suspension 1850
- Maalox TC Suspension 1851
- Maalox Plus Tablets ▣ 655
- Extra Strength Maalox Plus Tablets 1850
- Mylanta Liquid 1155
- Mylanta Tablets 1155
- Mylanta Double Strength Liquid 1155
- Mylanta Double Strength Tablets 1155
- Concentrated Phillips' Milk of Magnesia ▣ 573
- Phillips' Milk of Magnesia Liquid ▣ 572
- Phillips' Milk of Magnesia Tablets ▣ 573
- WinGel Liquid & Tablets ▣ 761

Magnesium Oxide (Interferes with intestinal digoxin absorption). Products include:
- Bayer Plus Aspirin Tablets ▣ 567
- Beelith Tablets 659
- Bufferin Analgesic Tablets and Caplets ▣ 524
- Cama Arthritis Pain Reliever ▣ 685
- Mag-Ox 400 673
- Uro-Mag 673

Metaproterenol Sulfate (Increased risk of cardiac arrhythmias). Products include:
- Alupent ... 674
- Arm-a-Med Metaproterenol Sulfate Inhalation Solution, USP ... 617
- Metaprel Inhalation Aerosol Bronchodilator ... 2014
- Metaprel Inhalation Solution ... 2015
- Metaprel ... 2015
- Metaproterenol Sulfate Inhalation Solution, USP ... 912

Metaraminol Bitartrate (Increased risk of cardiac arrhythmias). Products include:
- Aramine Injection ... 1424

Methoxamine Hydrochloride (Increased risk of cardiac arrhythmias). Products include:
- Vasoxyl Injection ... 819

Methyclothiazide (Contributing factor to digitalis toxicity). Products include:
- Enduron Tablets ... 517
- Enduronyl ... 518

Methylprednisolone Acetate (Contributing factor to digitalis toxicity). Products include:
- Depo-Medrol Sterile Aqueous Suspension ... 2334

Methylprednisolone Sodium Succinate (Contributing factor to digitalis toxicity). Products include:
- Solu-Medrol Sterile Powder ... 2363

Metoprolol Tartrate (Additive effects on AV node conduction). Products include:
- Lopressor Ampuls ... 1032
- Lopressor HCT Tablets ... 1034
- Lopressor Tablets ... 1032

Nadolol (Additive effects on AV node conduction). Products include:
- Corgard Tablets ... 701
- Corzide Tablets ... 702

Neomycin, oral (Interferes with intestinal digoxin absorption).

Nephrotoxic Drugs (May impair the excretion of digoxin).

Nicardipine Hydrochloride (Additive effects on AV node conduction). Products include:
- Cardene Capsules ... 2290

Nifedipine (Additive effects on AV node conduction). Products include:
- Adalat Capsules (10 mg and 20 mg) ... 1587
- Procardia Capsules ... 1781
- Procardia XL Tablets ... 1783

Nimodipine (Additive effects on AV node conduction). Products include:
- Nimotop Capsules ... 1607

Norepinephrine Bitartrate (Increased risk of cardiac arrhythmias). Products include:
- Levophed Bitartrate Injection ... 2054

Pectin (Interferes with intestinal digoxin absorption). Products include:
- Donnagel ... ▣ 675
- Donnagel-PG ... 1858

Penbutolol Sulfate (Additive effects on AV node conduction). Products include:
- Levatol ... 1832

Phenylephrine Bitartrate (Increased risk of cardiac arrhythmias).
- No products indexed under this heading.

Phenylephrine Hydrochloride (Increased risk of cardiac arrhythmias). Products include:
- AK-Dilate Solution 2.5% and 10% ... ⊙ 203
- Atrohist Sprinkle Capsules ... 558
- Cerose-DM ... 2443
- Codimal ... 846
- Comhist LA Capsules ... 1618
- Congespirin For Children Aspirin Free Chewable Cold Tablets ... 748
- Cyclomydril ... ⊙ 216
- Deconsal Sprinkle Capsules ... 559
- Dimetane Decongestant ... ▣ 673
- Dristan Decongestant/Antihistamine/ Analgesic Coated Caplets ... ▣ 749
- Dristan Cold Nasal Decongestant/ Antihistamine/ Analgesic Coated Tablets ... 2419
- Dristan Advanced Formula Decongestant/Antihistamine/ Analgesic Tablets ... ▣ 749
- Dristan Nasal Spray, Menthol ... 2419
- Dristan Nasal Spray, Regular and Regular with Metered Pump ... 2419
- Entex Capsules ... 1623
- Entex Liquid ... 1623
- Sinus Excedrin Analgesic, Decongestant Tablets & Caplets ... 750
- Extendryl ... 994
- 4-Way Fast Acting Nasal Spray - Original Formula (regular & mentholated) & Metered Spray Pump (regular) ... 751
- Hycomine Compound Tablets ... 929
- Murocoll-2 Sterile Ophthalmic Solution ... ⊙ 261
- Mydfrin 2.5% ... ⊙ 224
- Naldecon Syrup, Tablets, Pediatric Drops and Pediatric Syrup ... 709
- Neo-Synephrine Hydrochloride 1% Carpuject ... 2063
- Neo-Synephrine Hydrochloride 1% Injection ... 2063
- Neo-Synephrine Hydrochloride (Ophthalmic) ... 2064
- Neo-Synephrine ... ▣ 759
- Nōstril Nasal Decongestant ... ▣ 520
- Novahistine Elixir ... ▣ 596
- Phenergan VC ... 2500
- Phenergan VC with Codeine ... 2501
- Prefrin Liquifilm Vasoconstrictor and Lubricant Eye Drops ... ⊙ 254
- Prefrin-A ... ⊙ 255
- Quelidrine Syrup ... 556
- Relief Vasoconstrictor and Lubricant Eye Drops ... ⊙ 256
- Robitussin Night Relief ... ▣ 677
- Ru-Tuss with Hydrocodone ... 694
- Ru-Tuss Tablets ... 693
- Vasosulf ... ⊙ 279
- Vicks Sinex ... ▣ 665
- Zincfrin ... ⊙ 230

Phenylephrine Tannate (Increased risk of cardiac arrhythmias). Products include:
- Rynatan ... 2387
- Rynatuss ... 2388

Phenylpropanolamine Hydrochloride (Increased risk of cardiac arrhythmias). Products include:
- A.R.M. Allergy Relief Medicine Caplets ... ▣ 615
- Acutrim ... ▣ 548
- Allerest ... ▣ 559
- BC Cold Powder ... ▣ 517
- Cheracol Plus Head Cold/Cough Formula ... ▣ 667
- Codimal Expectorant ... 846
- Comtrex Multi-Symptom Cold Reliever Tablets/Caplets/Liqui-Gels/Liquid ... 745
- Contac Continuous Action Decongestant/Antihistamine Capsules ▣ 710
- Contac Maximum Strength Continuous Action Decongestant/ Antihistamine Caplets ... ▣ 709
- Contac Severe Cold and Flu Formula Caplets ... ▣ 711
- Coricidin 'D' Decongestant Tablets ... ▣ 695
- Coricidin Demilets Tablets for Children ... ▣ 696
- Demazin Nasal Decongestant/ Antihistamine Repetabs Tablets & Syrup ... ▣ 697
- Dexatrim ... ▣ 733
- Dimetane-DC Cough Syrup ... 1857
- Dimetapp Elixir ... ▣ 673
- Dimetapp DM Elixir ... ▣ 674
- Dimetapp Extentabs ... ▣ 674
- Dimetapp Plus Caplets ... ▣ 675
- Dimetapp Tablets ... ▣ 675
- Entex Capsules ... 1623
- Entex LA Tablets ... 1623
- Entex Liquid ... 1623
- 4-Way Cold Tablets ... 750
- Hycomine Syrup ... 927
- Naldecon CX Adult Liquid ... ▣ 521
- Naldecon DX Adult Liquid ... ▣ 521
- Naldecon DX Children's Syrup ... ▣ 522
- Naldecon DX Pediatric Drops ... ▣ 522
- Naldecon EX Children's Syrup ... ▣ 522
- Naldecon EX Pediatric Drops ... ▣ 523
- Naldecon Syrup, Tablets, Pediatric Drops and Pediatric Syrup ... 709
- Nolamine Tablets ... 838
- Nolex LA Tablets ... 838
- Ornade Spansule Capsules ... 2221
- Orthoxicol Cough Syrup ... ▣ 668
- Propagest ... 839
- Pyrroxate Capsules ... ▣ 669
- Robitussin-CF ... ▣ 676
- Ru-Tuss II Capsules ... 693
- Ru-Tuss with Hydrocodone ... 694
- Ru-Tuss Tablets ... 693
- Sine-Off Sinus Medicine Tablets-Aspirin Formula ... ▣ 722
- Sinulin ... 840
- St. Joseph Cold Tablets for Children ... ▣ 704
- Tavist-D Tablets ... 2035
- Triaminic Allergy Tablets ... ▣ 688
- Triaminic Chewables ... ▣ 688
- Triaminic Cold Tablets ... ▣ 688
- Triaminic Expectorant ... ▣ 688
- Triaminic Expectorant w/Codeine .. 1996
- Triaminic Expectorant DH ... 1995
- Triaminic Oral Infant Drops ... 1996
- Triaminic Syrup ... ▣ 689
- Triaminic-12 Tablets ... ▣ 690
- Triaminic-DM Syrup ... ▣ 689
- Triaminicin Tablets ... ▣ 690
- Triaminicol Multi-Symptom Cold Tablets ... ▣ 691
- Triaminicol Multi-Symptom Relief ▣ 691
- Tuss-Ornade Liquid ... 2242
- Tuss-Ornade Spansule Capsules ... 2242
- Tylenol Cold Medication, Effervescent Tablets ... 1369

Pindolol (Additive effects on AV node conduction). Products include:
- Visken Tablets ... 2036

Pirbuterol Acetate (Increased risk of cardiac arrhythmias). Products include:
- Maxair Inhaler ... 1311

Polythiazide (Contributing factor to digitalis toxicity). Products include:
- Minizide Capsules ... 1779
- Renese Tablets ... 1785
- Renese-R Tablets ... 1786

Prednisolone Acetate (Contributing factor to digitalis toxicity). Products include:
- AK-Cide Sterile Ophthalmic Ointment & Suspension ... ⊙ 202
- Blephamide Liquifilm Sterile Ophthalmic Suspension ... 586
- Blephamide S.O.P. Sterile Ophthalmic Ointment ... 586
- Cetapred Ointment ... ⊙ 220
- ⅛% Econopred & 1% Econopred Plus ... ⊙ 217
- Isopto Cetapred Suspension ... ⊙ 220
- Metimyd ... ⊙ 306
- Poly-Pred Liquifilm ... ⊙ 250
- Pred Forte ... ⊙ 252
- Pred Mild ... ⊙ 254
- Pred-G Liquifilm Sterile Ophthalmic Suspension ... ⊙ 252
- Pred-G S.O.P. Sterile Ophthalmic Ointment ... ⊙ 253
- Vasocidin Ointment ... ⊙ 275

Prednisolone Sodium Phosphate (Contributing factor to digitalis toxicity). Products include:
- AK-Pred ... ⊙ 205
- Hydeltrasol Injection, Sterile ... 1476
- Inflamase ... ⊙ 274
- Pediapred Oral Liquid ... 987
- Vasocidin Ophthalmic Solution ... ⊙ 276

Prednisolone Tebutate (Contributing factor to digitalis toxicity). Products include:
- Hydeltra-T.B.A. Sterile Suspension 1478

Prednisone (Contributing factor to digitalis toxicity). Products include:
- Deltasone Tablets ... 2332

Propantheline Bromide (Increases digoxin absorption). Products include:
- Pro-Banthīne Tablets ... 2141

Propranolol Hydrochloride (Additive effects on AV node conduction). Products include:
- Inderal ... 2459
- Inderal LA Long Acting Capsules ... 2461
- Inderide Tablets ... 2463
- Inderide LA Long Acting Capsules .. 2465

Pseudoephedrine Hydrochloride (Increased risk of cardiac arrhythmias). Products include:
- Actifed Capsules ... ▣ 539
- Actifed Plus Caplets ... ▣ 539
- Actifed Plus Tablets ... ▣ 540
- Actifed with Codeine Cough Syrup.. 752
- Actifed Syrup ... ▣ 540
- Actifed Tablets ... ▣ 540
- Actifed 12-Hour Capsules ... ▣ 539
- Advil Cold & Sinus Caplets (formerly CoAdvil) ... 2416
- Allerest ... ▣ 559
- Anatuss LA Tablets ... 1359
- Benadryl Decongestant Elixir ... ▣ 635
- Benadryl Decongestant ... ▣ 635
- Benadryl Plus ... ▣ 636
- Benadryl Plus Nighttime ... ▣ 637
- Benylin Decongestant ... ▣ 638
- Brexin L.A. Capsules ... 2078
- Bromfed Capsules (Timed Release) ... 1615
- Bromfed Syrup ... ▣ 628
- Bromfed ... 1615
- CoAdvil ... ▣ 748
- Allergy-Sinus Comtrex Multi-Symptom Allergy Sinus Formula Tablets & Caplets ... 746
- Cough Formula Comtrex ... 746
- Comtrex Multi-Symptom Cold Reliever Tablets/Caplets/Liqui-Gels/Liquid ... 745
- Day-Night Comtrex ... 747
- Non-Drowsy Comtrex ... 747
- Congess ... 994
- Congestac Caplets ... ▣ 617
- Contac Jr. Children's Cold Medicine ... ▣ 712
- Contac Nighttime Cold Medicine ... ▣ 713
- Contac Sinus Caplets Maximum Strength Non-Drowsy Formula ... ▣ 710
- Contac Sinus Tablets Maximum Strength Non-Drowsy Formula ... ▣ 710
- Deconamine ... 663
- Deconsal II Tablets ... 559
- Dimacol Caplets ... ▣ 672
- Dimetane-DX Cough Syrup ... 1858
- Dorcol Children's Cough Syrup ... ▣ 685
- Dorcol Children's Decongestant Liquid ... ▣ 685
- Dorcol Children's Liquid Cold Formula ... ▣ 686
- Maximum Strength Dristan Decongestant/Analgesic Coated Caplets ... ▣ 750
- No Drowsiness Dristan Cold Nasal Decongestant/Analgesic Coated Caplets ... 2420
- Dristan Sinus Caplets ... 2419
- Sinus Excedrin Analgesic, Decongestant Tablets & Caplets ... ▣ 533
- Fedahist Gyrocaps ... 2145
- Fedahist Timecaps ... 2145
- Guaifed ... 1615
- Guaifed Syrup ... ▣ 629
- Isoclor Expectorant ... 982
- Isoclor Timesule Capsules ... ▣ 561
- Kronofed-A ... 970
- Medi-Flu Caplet, Liquid ... ▣ 640
- Novafed A Capsules ... 1342
- Novafed Capsules ... 1342
- Novahistine DH ... 1342
- Novahistine DMX ... ▣ 595
- Novahistine Expectorant ... 1343
- Nucofed Capsules ... 2219
- Nucofed Expectorant ... 2219
- Nucofed Pediatric Expectorant ... 2220
- Nucofed Syrup ... 2219
- Ornex Caplets ... ▣ 618
- PediaCare Allergy Relief Formula Liquid ... 1362
- PediaCare Cough-Cold Formula Liquid ... 1362
- PediaCare Infants' Oral Decongestant Drops ... 1362
- PediaCare Night Rest Cough-Cold Formula Liquid ... 1362
- PediaCare 6-12 Cough-Cold Formula Chewable Tablets ... 1362
- Robitussin-DAC Syrup ... 1875
- Robitussin-PE ... ▣ 677
- Rondec ... 1975

Rondec-DM 1976
Rondec-TR Tablet 1975
Ru-Tuss DE Tablets 694
Ryna ▣ 741
Seldane-D Extended-Release Tablets 1350
Sinarest ▣ 562
Sine-Aid Maximum Strength Sinus Headache Caplets 1365
Sine-Aid Maximum Strength Sinus Headache Tablets 1365
Sine-Off Maximum Strength Allergy/Sinus Formula Caplets ▣ 721
Sine-Off Maximum Strength No Drowsiness Formula Caplets ▣ 722
Singlet Tablets ▣ 598
Sinutab Maximum Strength ▣ 641
Sinutab Maximum Strength Without Drowsiness Tablets & Caplets ▣ 642
Sinutab Regular Strength Without Drowsiness Formula ▣ 641
St. Joseph Nighttime Cold Medicine ▣ 705
Sudafed Children's Liquid ▣ 543
Sudafed Cough Syrup ▣ 543
Sudafed Plus Liquid ▣ 544
Sudafed Plus Tablets ▣ 545
Sudafed Sinus Caplets ▣ 545
Sudafed Sinus Tablets ▣ 545
Sudafed Tablets, 30 mg ▣ 544
Sudafed Tablets, Adult Strength, 60 mg ▣ 544
Sudafed 12 Hour Capsules ▣ 545
TheraFlu Flu and Cold Medicine ▣ 687
Triaminic Nite Light ▣ 689
Tylenol Allergy Sinus Medication Caplets and Gelcaps, Maximum Strength 1372
Children's Tylenol Cold Liquid Formula and Chewable Tablets 1368
Tylenol Cold & Flu Hot Medication, Packets 1369
Tylenol Cold & Flu No Drowsiness Hot Medication, Packets 1371
Tylenol Cold Medication Caplets and Tablets 1370
Tylenol Cold Medication No Drowsiness Formula Caplets 1370
Tylenol Cold Night Time Medication Liquid 1371
Tylenol Cough Medication Liquid with Decongestant, Maximum Strength 1372
Tylenol, Maximum Strength, Sinus Medication Gelcaps, Caplets and Tablets 1373
Ursinus Inlay-Tabs ▣ 691
Vicks Children's NyQuil ▣ 664
Vicks Daycare ▣ 660
Vicks Formula 44D Decongestant Cough Medicine ▣ 662
Vicks Formula 44M Multi-Symptom Cough Medicine ▣ 662
Vicks NyQuil Nighttime Colds Medicine-Original & Cherry Flavor ▣ 664
Vicks Pediatric Formula 44 Cough & Congestion Medicine ▣ 663
Vicks Pediatric Formula 44m Multi-Symptom Cough & Cold Medicine ▣ 663

Pseudoephedrine Sulfate (Increased risk of cardiac arrhythmias). Products include:
Afrin Tablets ▣ 693
Chlor-Trimeton Decongestant ▣ 694
Disophrol Chronotab Sustained-Action Tablets ▣ 698
Drixoral Antihistamine/Nasal Decongestant Syrup ▣ 698
Drixoral Non-Drowsy Formula ▣ 699
Drixoral Plus Extended-Release Tablets ▣ 699
Drixoral Sinus ▣ 700
Drixoral Sustained-Action Tablets ▣ 698
Sinutab Allergy Formula Sustained Action Tablets ▣ 640
Trinalin Repetabs Tablets 1170

Quinidine Gluconate (Causes rise in serum digoxin concentration). Products include:
Quinaglute Dura-Tabs Tablets 663

Quinidine Polygalacturonate (Causes rise in serum digoxin concentration). Products include:
Cardioquin Tablets 1812

Quinidine Sulfate (Causes rise in serum digoxin concentration). Products include:
Quinidex Extentabs 1868

Succinylcholine Chloride (May cause arrhythmias). Products include:
Anectine 755

Sulfasalazine (Interferes with intestinal digoxin absorption). Products include:
Azulfidine Tablets, EN-tabs, Oral Suspension 1157

Terbutaline Sulfate (Increased risk of cardiac arrhythmias). Products include:
Brethaire Inhaler 1024
Brethine Ampuls 1026
Brethine Tablets 1026
Bricanyl Injection 1324
Bricanyl Tablets 1325

Thyroid (Hypothyroid patients may require increased digoxin dose). Products include:
S-P-T "Liquid" Capsules 995

Thyroxine (Hypothyroid patients may require increased digoxin dose).
No products indexed under this heading.

Timolol Maleate (Additive effects on AV node conduction). Products include:
Blocadren Tablets 1429
Timolide Tablets 1547
Timoptic in Ocudose 1552
Timoptic Sterile Ophthalmic Solution 1550

Triamcinolone (Contributing factor to digitalis toxicity).
No products indexed under this heading.

Triamcinolone Acetonide (Contributing factor to digitalis toxicity). Products include:
Aristocort A 1010
Azmacort Inhaler 1837
Kenalog Cream, Lotion & Ointment 2401
Kenalog-10 Injection 2402
Kenalog-40 Injection 2403
Kenalog in Orabase 604
Kenalog Spray 2401
Mycolog II Cream and Ointment 2407
Mytrex Cream & Ointment 2080
Nasacort Nasal Inhaler 1844

Triamcinolone Diacetate (Contributing factor to digitalis toxicity). Products include:
Aristocort Suspension 1008

Triamcinolone Hexacetonide (Contributing factor to digitalis toxicity). Products include:
Aristospan Suspension 1011

Verapamil Hydrochloride (Causes rise in serum digoxin concentration; additive effects on AV node conduction). Products include:
Calan SR Caplets 2157
Calan Tablets 2155
Isoptin Injectable 1177
Isoptin Oral Tablets 1179
Isoptin SR Sustained Release Tablets 1181
Verelan Capsules 1243
Verelan Capsules 2535

Food Interactions

Meal, high in bran fiber (Reduces the amount of digoxin from an oral dose).

Meal, unspecified (The rate of absorption is slowed).

LANOXIN ELIXIR PEDIATRIC
(Digoxin) 775
May interact with potassium-depleting corticosteroids, potassium-depleting diuretics, antacids, sympathomimetic aerosol brochodilators, beta blockers, calcium channel blockers, thyroid preparations, mineralocorticoids, and certain other agents. Compounds in these categories include:

Acebutolol Hydrochloride (Additive effects on AV node conduction). Products include:
Sectral Capsules 2520

Albuterol (Increased risk of cardiac arrhythmias). Products include:
Proventil Inhalation Aerosol 2117
Ventolin Inhalation Aerosol and Refill 583

Albuterol Sulfate (Increased risk of cardiac arrhythmias). Products include:
Proventil Repetabs Tablets 2120
Proventil Solutions for Inhalation 0.5% and 0.083% 2118
Proventil Syrup 2119
Proventil Tablets 2120
Ventolin 583

Aluminum Carbonate Gel (Interferes with intestinal digoxin absorption). Products include:
Basaljel 2438

Aluminum Hydroxide (Interferes with intestinal digoxin absorption). Products include:
Cama Arthritis Pain Reliever ▣ 685
Gaviscon Extra Strength Relief Formula Liquid Antacid ▣ 594
Gaviscon Extra Strength Relief Formula Antacid Tablets ▣ 594
Gaviscon Liquid Antacid ▣ 594
Gelusil Liquid & Tablets ▣ 639
Extra Strength Maalox Plus Suspension 1850
Maalox TC Suspension 1851
Maalox Plus Tablets ▣ 655
Extra Strength Maalox Plus Tablets 1850
Nephrox Suspension ▣ 563
WinGel Liquid & Tablets ▣ 761

Aluminum Hydroxide Gel (Interferes with intestinal digoxin absorption). Products include:
ALternaGEL Liquid 1154
Aludrox Oral Suspension 2428
Amphojel Suspension 2429
Amphojel Suspension without Flavor 2429
Mylanta Liquid 1155
Mylanta Double Strength Liquid 1155

Aluminum Hydroxide Gel, Dried (Interferes with intestinal digoxin absorption). Products include:
Alu-Tab/Alu-Cap 1309
Amphojel Tablets 2429
Ascriptin A/D Caplets 1850
Regular Strength Ascriptin Tablets 1850
Gaviscon Antacid Tablets ▣ 593
Gaviscon-2 Antacid Tablets ▣ 594
Mylanta Tablets 1155
Mylanta Double Strength Tablets 1155

Amiodarone Hydrochloride (Causes rise in serum digoxin concentration). Products include:
Cordarone Tablets 2446

Antibiotics, unspecified (Increases digoxin absorption in patients who inactivate digoxin by bacterial metabolism).

Anticancer Drugs, unspecified (Interferes with intestinal digoxin absorption).

Atenolol (Additive effects on AV node conduction). Products include:
Tenoretic Tablets 1105
Tenormin Tablets and I.V. Injection 1107

Bendroflumethiazide (Major contributing factor to digitalis toxicity). Products include:
Corzide Tablets 702
Naturetin Tablets 1789
Rauzide Tablets 1804

Bepridil Hydrochloride (Additive effects on AV node conduction). Products include:
Vascor (200, 300 and 400 mg) Tablets 1383

Betamethasone Acetate (Major contributing factor to digitalis toxicity). Products include:
Celestone Soluspan Suspension 2081

Betamethasone Sodium Phosphate (Major contributing factor to digitalis toxicity). Products include:
Celestone Soluspan Suspension 2081

Betaxolol Hydrochloride (Additive effects on AV node conduction). Products include:
Betoptic Sterile Ophthalmic Solution 569
Betoptic S Sterile Ophthalmic Suspension 570
Kerlone Tablets 2172

Calcium, intravenous (May produce serious arrhythmias in digitalized patients).

Carteolol Hydrochloride (Additive effects on AV node conduction). Products include:
Cartrol Tablets 507

Chlorothiazide (Major contributing factor to digitalis toxicity). Products include:
Aldoclor Tablets 1413
Diupres Tablets 1461
Diuril Oral 1464

Chlorothiazide Sodium (Major contributing factor to digitalis toxicity). Products include:
Diuril Sodium Intravenous 1463

Cholestyramine (Interferes with intestinal digoxin absorption). Products include:
Cholybar 1705
Questran Light 711
Questran Powder 710

Cortisone Acetate (Major contributing factor to digitalis toxicity). Products include:
Cortone Acetate Sterile Suspension 1437
Cortone Acetate Tablets 1439

Dexamethasone (Major contributing factor to digitalis toxicity). Products include:
AK-Trol Ointment & Suspension ⊙ 207
Decadron Elixir 1445
Decadron Tablets 1447
Decaspray Topical Aerosol 1459
Dexacidin ⊙ 272
Maxidex Sterile Ophthalmic Suspension ⊙ 223
Maxitrol Ophthalmic Ointment/Suspension ⊙ 223
TobraDex Ophthalmic Suspension and Ointment ⊙ 228

Dexamethasone Acetate (Major contributing factor to digitalis toxicity). Products include:
Dalalone D.P. Injectable 999
Decadron-LA Sterile Suspension 1457

Dexamethasone Sodium Phosphate (Major contributing factor to digitalis toxicity). Products include:
AK-Dex ⊙ 203
Decadron Phosphate Respihaler 1454
Decadron Phosphate Sterile Ophthalmic Ointment 1453
Decadron Phosphate Sterile Ophthalmic Solution 1453
Decadron Phosphate Topical Cream 1455
Decadron Phosphate Turbinaire 1456
Maxidex Sterile Ophthalmic Ointment ⊙ 222
NeoDecadron Sterile Ophthalmic Ointment 1517
NeoDecadron Sterile Ophthalmic Solution 1518
NeoDecadron Topical Cream 1518

Dihydroxyaluminum Sodium Carbonate (Interferes with intestinal digoxin absorption). Products include:
Rolaids ▣ 743

Diltiazem Hydrochloride (Additive effects on AV node conduction). Products include:
- Cardizem Tablets-30 mg, 60 mg, 90 mg and 120 mg 1329
- Cardizem SR Capsules-60 mg, 90 mg and 120 mg 1327

Diphenoxylate Hydrochloride (Increases digoxin absorption). Products include:
- Lomotil 2174

Dobutamine Hydrochloride (Increased risk of cardiac arrhythmias). Products include:
- Dobutrex Solution Vials 1259

Dopamine Hydrochloride (Increased risk of cardiac arrhythmias). Products include:
- Intropin Injection 930

Ephedrine Hydrochloride (Increased risk of cardiac arrhythmias). Products include:
- Amesec ▣ 682
- Primatene Tablets-M Formula 2421
- Primatene Tablets-P Formula 2421
- Primatene Tablets-Regular Formula 2421
- Quadrinal Tablets 1183
- Quelidrine Syrup 556
- Tedral SA 1765

Ephedrine Sulfate (Increased risk of cardiac arrhythmias). Products include:
- Bronkaid Tablets ▣ 757
- Bronkolixir ▣ 761
- Bronkotabs Tablets ▣ 762
- Marax Tablets & DF Syrup 1954
- Pazo Hemorrhoid Ointment & Suppositories 752
- Vicks Vatronol Nose Drops ▣ 666

Ephedrine Tannate (Increased risk of cardiac arrhythmias). Products include:
- Rynatuss 2388

Epinephrine (Increased risk of cardiac arrhythmias). Products include:
- Ana-Kit Anaphylaxis Emergency Treatment Kit 1100
- Bronkaid Mist ▣ 757
- EpiPen 843
- Marcaine Hydrochloride 0.5% with Epinephrine 1:200,000 (as bitartrate) 958
- Marcaine Hydrochloride with Epinephrine 1:200,000 2055
- Primatene Mist 2420
- Sus-Phrine Injection 1006
- Xylocaine with Epinephrine Injections 637

Epinephrine Bitartrate (Increased risk of cardiac arrhythmias). Products include:
- AsthmaHaler Mist Epinephrine Bitartrate Bronchodilator ▣ 616
- Bronkaid Mist Suspension ▣ 757
- Primatene Mist Suspension 2421

Epinephrine Hydrochloride (Increased risk of cardiac arrhythmias). Products include:
- Adrenalin Chloride Solution 1:100 & 1:1,000 1689
- Epifrin ⊙ 244
- Glaucon ⊙ 218

Esmolol Hydrochloride (Additive effects on AV node conduction). Products include:
- Brevibloc Injection 942

Felodipine (Additive effects on AV node conduction). Products include:
- Plendil Extended-Release Tablets 1526

Hydrochlorothiazide (Major contributing factor to digitalis toxicity). Products include:
- Aldactazide 2150
- Aldoril Tablets 1418
- Apresazide Capsules 854
- Apresoline-Esidrix Tablets 857
- Capozide 2258
- Dyazide Capsules 2208
- Esidrix Tablets 863
- Esimil Tablets 864
- HydroDIURIL Tablets 1484
- Hydropres Tablets 1485
- Inderide Tablets 2463
- Inderide LA Long Acting Capsules 2465
- Lopressor HCT Tablets 1034
- Maxzide 1215
- Moduretic Tablets 1510
- Normozide Tablets 2112
- Oretic Tablets 544
- Oreticyl 545
- Prinzide Tablets 1540
- Ser-Ap-Es Tablets 881
- Serpasil-Esidrix Tablets 886
- Timolide Tablets 1547
- Trandate HCT Tablets 579
- Vaseretic Tablets 1559
- Zestoretic 2274

Hydrocortisone (Major contributing factor to digitalis toxicity). Products include:
- AK-Spore H.C. ⊙ 206
- Bactine Hydrocortisone Anti-Itch Cream ▣ 625
- CaldeCORT Anti-Itch Hydrocortisone Spray ▣ 560
- Carmol HC Cream 1% 2296
- Cortaid Spray ▣ 735
- Cortenema 2244
- Cortisporin Ointment 758
- Cortisporin Ophthalmic Ointment Sterile 758
- Cortisporin Ophthalmic Suspension Sterile 759
- Cortisporin Otic Solution Sterile 760
- Cortisporin Otic Suspension Sterile 760
- Cortizone-5 Creme & Ointment ▣ 732
- Dermolate Anti-Itch Cream ▣ 697
- Eldecort Cream 1.0% 1113
- Eldecort Cream 1.0% and 2.5% 1113
- Fungoid HC Creme 1770
- Hydrocortone Tablets 1482
- Hytone 909
- LazerSporin-C Solution 1770
- Massengill Medicated Soft Cloth Towelettes 2192
- Nutracort Cream & Lotion 1684
- PediOtic Suspension Sterile 797
- Synacort Creams 1%, 2.5% 2296
- Vanoxide-HC Acne Lotion 911
- Vioform-Hydrocortisone Cream and Mild Cream 889
- Vioform-Hydrocortisone Ointment 889
- VōSoL HC Otic Solution 2392
- Vytone Cream 1% 911

Hydrocortisone Acetate (Major contributing factor to digitalis toxicity). Products include:
- Analpram-HC Rectal Cream 1% and 2.5% 970
- Anusol-HC Cream 1690
- Anusol-HC Suppositories 1691
- Caldecort ▣ 560
- Carmol HC Cream 1% 2296
- Chloromycetin Hydrocortisone Ophthalmic 1694
- Coly-Mycin S Otic w/Neomycin & Hydrocortisone 1708
- Cortaid ▣ 735
- Cortef Feminine Itch Cream ▣ 735
- Corticaine ▣ 682
- Cortifoam 1827
- Cortisporin Cream 757
- Epifoam 1828
- Gynecort 5 Creme ▣ 556
- Hydrocortone Acetate Sterile Suspension 1479
- Lanacort 5 Creme and Ointment ▣ 557
- Mantadil Cream 789
- Ophthocort ⊙ 301
- Orabase HCA Oral Paste 890
- Pramosone Cream, Lotion & Ointment 971
- ProctoCream-HC 1834
- Proctofoam-HC 1835

Hydrocortisone Sodium Phosphate (Major contributing factor to digitalis toxicity). Products include:
- Hydrocortone Phosphate Injection, Sterile 1481

Hydrocortisone Sodium Succinate (Major contributing factor to digitalis toxicity). Products include:
- Solu-Cortef Sterile Powder 2361

Hydroflumethiazide (Major contributing factor to digitalis toxicity). Products include:
- Diucardin Tablets 2450
- Saluron 718
- Salutensin/Salutensin-Demi 719

Isoproterenol Hydrochloride (Increased risk of cardiac arrhythmias). Products include:
- Isuprel Hydrochloride Injection 1:5000 2050
- Isuprel Hydrochloride Mistometer 2051
- Isuprel Hydrochloride Solution 1:200 & 1:100 2052
- Norisodrine Aerotrol 540

Isradipine (Additive effects on AV node conduction). Products include:
- DynaCirc Capsules 2004

Labetalol Hydrochloride (Additive effects on AV node conduction). Products include:
- Normodyne Injection 2108
- Normodyne Tablets 2110
- Normozide Tablets 2112
- Trandate HCT Tablets 579
- Trandate Injection 577
- Trandate Tablets 579

Levothyroxine Sodium (Hypothyroid patients may require increased digoxin dose). Products include:
- Levothroid Tablets 1003
- Levoxine Tablets 904
- Synthroid 695

Liothyronine Sodium (Hypothyroid patients may require increased digoxin dose). Products include:
- Cytomel Tablets 2203

Liotrix (Hypothyroid patients may require increased digoxin dose). Products include:
- Euthroid 1724

Magaldrate (Interferes with intestinal digoxin absorption). Products include:
- Riopan Antacid Chew Tablets ▣ 754
- Riopan Antacid Chew Tablets in Rollpacks ▣ 754
- Riopan Antacid Suspension 2421
- Riopan Antacid Swallow Tablets 2421
- Riopan Plus Chew Tablets 2422
- Riopan Plus Chew Tablets in Rollpack 2422
- Riopan Plus 2 Chew Tablets, Mint Flavor, Cherry Flavor 2422
- Riopan Plus Suspension 2422
- Riopan Plus 2 Suspension, Mint Flavor, Cherry Flavor 2422

Magnesium Hydroxide (Interferes with intestinal digoxin absorption). Products include:
- Aludrox Oral Suspension 2428
- Ascriptin A/D Caplets 1850
- Regular Strength Ascriptin Tablets 1850
- Di-Gel Antacid/Anti-Gas ▣ 697
- Gelusil Liquid & Tablets ▣ 639
- Haley's M-O, Regular & Flavored ▣ 569
- Extra Strength Maalox Plus Suspension 1850
- Maalox TC Suspension 1851
- Maalox Plus Tablets ▣ 655
- Extra Strength Maalox Plus Tablets 1850
- Mylanta Liquid 1155
- Mylanta Tablets 1155
- Mylanta Double Strength Liquid 1155
- Mylanta Double Strength Tablets 1155
- Concentrated Phillips' Milk of Magnesia ▣ 573
- Phillips' Milk of Magnesia Liquid ▣ 572
- Phillips' Milk of Magnesia Tablets ▣ 573
- WinGel Liquid & Tablets ▣ 761

Magnesium Oxide (Interferes with intestinal digoxin absorption). Products include:
- Bayer Plus Aspirin Tablets ▣ 567
- Beelith Tablets 659
- Bufferin Analgesic Tablets and Caplets ▣ 524
- Cama Arthritis Pain Reliever ▣ 685
- Mag-Ox 400 673
- Uro-Mag 673

Metaproterenol Sulfate (Increased risk of cardiac arrhythmias). Products include:
- Alupent 674
- Arm-a-Med Metaproterenol Sulfate Inhalation Solution, USP 617
- Metaprel Inhalation Aerosol Bronchodilator 2014
- Metaprel Inhalation Solution 2015
- Metaprel 2015
- Metaproterenol Sulfate Inhalation Solution, USP 912

Metaraminol Bitartrate (Increased risk of cardiac arrhythmias). Products include:
- Aramine Injection 1424

Methoxamine Hydrochloride (Increased risk of cardiac arrhythmias). Products include:
- Vasoxyl Injection 819

Methyclothiazide (Major contributing factor to digitalis toxicity). Products include:
- Enduron Tablets 517
- Enduronyl 518

Methylprednisolone Acetate (Major contributing factor to digitalis toxicity). Products include:
- Depo-Medrol Sterile Aqueous Suspension 2334

Methylprednisolone Sodium Succinate (Major contributing factor to digitalis toxicity). Products include:
- Solu-Medrol Sterile Powder 2363

Metoprolol Tartrate (Additive effects on AV node conduction). Products include:
- Lopressor Ampuls 1032
- Lopressor HCT Tablets 1034
- Lopressor Tablets 1032

Nadolol (Additive effects on AV node conduction). Products include:
- Corgard Tablets 701
- Corzide Tablets 702

Neomycin, oral (Interferes with intestinal digoxin absorption).

Nephrotoxic Drugs (May impair the excretion of digoxin).

Nicardipine Hydrochloride (Additive effects on AV node conduction). Products include:
- Cardene Capsules 2290

Nifedipine (Additive effects on AV node conduction). Products include:
- Adalat Capsules (10 mg and 20 mg) 1587
- Procardia Capsules 1781
- Procardia XL Tablets 1783

Nimodipine (Additive effects on AV node conduction). Products include:
- Nimotop Capsules 1607

Norepinephrine Bitartrate (Increased risk of cardiac arrhythmias). Products include:
- Levophed Bitartrate Injection 2054

Pectin (Low digoxin serum concentration; interferes with intestinal digoxin absorption). Products include:
- Donnagel ▣ 675
- Donnagel-PG 1858

Penbutolol Sulfate (Additive effects on AV node conduction). Products include:
- Levatol 1832

Phenylephrine Bitartrate (Increased risk of cardiac arrhythmias).
- No products indexed under this heading.

Phenylephrine Hydrochloride (Increased risk of cardiac arrhythmias). Products include:
- AK-Dilate Solution 2.5% and 10% ⊙ 203
- Atrohist Sprinkle Capsules 558
- Cerose-DM 2443
- Codimal 846
- Comhist LA Capsules 1618
- Congespirin For Children Aspirin Free Chewable Cold Tablets 748
- Cyclomydril ⊙ 216
- Deconsal Sprinkle Capsules 559
- Dimetane Decongestant ▣ 673
- Dristan Decongestant/Antihistamine/ Analgesic Coated Caplets ▣ 749

Dristan Cold Nasal Decongestant/ Antihistamine/ Analgesic Coated Tablets 2419
Dristan Advanced Formula Decongestant/Antihistamine/ Analgesic Tablets .... ▣ 749
Dristan Nasal Spray, Menthol 2419
Dristan Nasal Spray, Regular and Regular with Metered Pump 2419
Entex Capsules 1623
Entex Liquid 1623
Sinus Excedrin Analgesic, Decongestant Tablets & Caplets 750
Extendryl 994
4-Way Fast Acting Nasal Spray - Original Formula (regular & mentholated) & Metered Spray Pump (regular) 751
Hycomine Compound Tablets 929
Murocoll-2 Sterile Ophthalmic Solution .... ⊙ 261
Mydfrin 2.5% .... ⊙ 224
Naldecon Syrup, Tablets, Pediatric Drops and Pediatric Syrup 709
Neo-Synephrine Hydrochloride 1% Carpuject 2063
Neo-Synephrine Hydrochloride 1% Injection 2063
Neo-Synephrine Hydrochloride (Ophthalmic) 2064
Neo-Synephrine .... ▣ 759
Nōstril Nasal Decongestant .... ▣ 520
Novahistine Elixir .... ▣ 596
Phenergan VC 2500
Phenergan VC with Codeine 2501
Prefrin Liquifilm Vasoconstrictor and Lubricant Eye Drops .... ⊙ 254
Prefrin-A .... ⊙ 255
Quelidrine Syrup 556
Relief Vasoconstrictor and Lubricant Eye Drops .... ⊙ 256
Robitussin Night Relief .... ▣ 677
Ru-Tuss with Hydrocodone 694
Ru-Tuss Tablets 693
Vasosulf .... ⊙ 279
Vicks Sinex .... ▣ 665
Zincfrin .... ⊙ 230

Phenylephrine Tannate (Increased risk of cardiac arrhythmias). Products include:

Rynatan 2387
Rynatuss 2388

Phenylpropanolamine Hydrochloride (Increased risk of cardiac arrhythmias). Products include:

A.R.M. Allergy Relief Medicine Caplets .... ▣ 615
Acutrim .... ▣ 548
Allerest .... ▣ 559
BC Cold Powder .... ▣ 517
Cheracol Plus Head Cold/Cough Formula .... ▣ 667
Codimal Expectorant 846
Comtrex Multi-Symptom Cold Reliever Tablets/Caplets/Liqui-Gels/Liquid 745
Contac Continuous Action Decongestant/Antihistamine Capsules ▣ 710
Contac Maximum Strength Continuous Action Decongestant/ Antihistamine Caplets .... ▣ 709
Contac Severe Cold and Flu Formula Caplets .... ▣ 711
Coricidin 'D' Decongestant Tablets .... ▣ 695
Coricidin Demilets Tablets for Children .... ▣ 696
Demazin Nasal Decongestant/ Antihistamine Repetabs Tablets & Syrup .... ▣ 697
Dexatrim .... ▣ 733
Dimetane-DC Cough Syrup 1857
Dimetapp Elixir .... ▣ 673
Dimetapp DM Elixir .... ▣ 674
Dimetapp Extentabs .... ▣ 674
Dimetapp Plus Caplets .... ▣ 675
Dimetapp Tablets .... ▣ 675
Entex Capsules 1623
Entex LA Tablets 1623
Entex Liquid 1623
4-Way Cold Tablets 750
Hycomine Syrup 927
Naldecon CX Adult Liquid .... ▣ 521
Naldecon DX Adult Liquid .... ▣ 521
Naldecon DX Children's Syrup .... ▣ 522
Naldecon DX Pediatric Drops .... ▣ 522
Naldecon EX Children's Syrup .... ▣ 522
Naldecon EX Pediatric Drops .... ▣ 523
Naldecon Syrup, Tablets, Pediatric Drops and Pediatric Syrup 709
Nolamine Tablets 838
Nolex LA Tablets 838
Ornade Spansule Capsules 2221
Orthoxicol Cough Syrup .... ▣ 668
Propagest 839
Pyrroxate Capsules .... ▣ 669
Robitussin-CF .... ▣ 676
Ru-Tuss II Capsules 693
Ru-Tuss with Hydrocodone 694
Ru-Tuss Tablets 693
Sine-Off Sinus Medicine Tablets-Aspirin Formula .... ▣ 722
Sinulin 840
St. Joseph Cold Tablets for Children .... ▣ 704
Tavist-D Tablets 2035
Triaminic Allergy Tablets .... ▣ 688
Triaminic Chewables .... ▣ 688
Triaminic Cold Tablets .... ▣ 688
Triaminic Expectorant .... ▣ 688
Triaminic Expectorant w/Codeine .. 1996
Triaminic Expectorant DH 1995
Triaminic Oral Infant Drops 1996
Triaminic Syrup .... ▣ 689
Triaminic-12 Tablets .... ▣ 690
Triaminic-DM Syrup .... ▣ 689
Triaminicin Tablets .... ▣ 690
Triaminicol Multi-Symptom Cold Tablets .... ▣ 691
Triaminicol Multi-Symptom Relief ▣ 691
Tuss-Ornade Liquid 2242
Tuss-Ornade Spansule Capsules 2242
Tylenol Cold Medication, Effervescent Tablets 1369

Pindolol (Additive effects on AV node conduction). Products include:

Visken Tablets 2036

Pirbuterol Acetate (Increased risk of cardiac arrhythmias). Products include:

Maxair Inhaler 1311

Polythiazide (Major contributing factor to digitalis toxicity). Products include:

Minizide Capsules 1779
Renese Tablets 1785
Renese-R Tablets 1786

Prednisolone Acetate (Major contributing factor to digitalis toxicity). Products include:

AK-Cide Sterile Ophthalmic Ointment & Suspension .... ⊙ 202
Blephamide Liquifilm Sterile Ophthalmic Suspension 586
Blephamide S.O.P. Sterile Ophthalmic Ointment 586
Cetapred Ointment .... ⊙ 220
⅛% Econopred & 1% Econopred Plus .... ⊙ 217
Isopto Cetapred Suspension .... ⊙ 220
Metimyd .... ⊙ 306
Poly-Pred Liquifilm .... ⊙ 250
Pred Forte .... ⊙ 252
Pred Mild .... ⊙ 254
Pred-G Liquifilm Sterile Ophthalmic Suspension .... ⊙ 252
Pred-G S.O.P. Sterile Ophthalmic Ointment .... ⊙ 253
Vasocidin Ointment .... ⊙ 275

Prednisolone Sodium Phosphate (Major contributing factor to digitalis toxicity). Products include:

AK-Pred .... ⊙ 205
Hydeltrasol Injection, Sterile 1476
Inflamase .... ⊙ 274
Pediapred Oral Liquid 987
Vasocidin Ophthalmic Solution .... ⊙ 276

Prednisolone Tebutate (Major contributing factor to digitalis toxicity). Products include:

Hydeltra-T.B.A. Sterile Suspension 1478

Prednisone (Major contributing factor to digitalis toxicity). Products include:

Deltasone Tablets 2332

Propantheline Bromide (Increases digoxin absorption). Products include:

Pro-Banthīne Tablets 2141

Propranolol Hydrochloride (Additive effects on AV node conduction). Products include:

Inderal 2459
Inderal LA Long Acting Capsules 2461
Inderide Tablets 2463
Inderide LA Long Acting Capsules .. 2465

Pseudoephedrine Hydrochloride (Increased risk of cardiac arrhythmias). Products include:

Actifed Capsules .... ▣ 539
Actifed Plus Caplets .... ▣ 539
Actifed Plus Tablets .... ▣ 540
Actifed with Codeine Cough Syrup .. 752
Actifed Syrup .... ▣ 540
Actifed Tablets .... ▣ 540
Actifed 12-Hour Capsules .... ▣ 539
Advil Cold & Sinus Caplets (formerly CoAdvil) 2416
Allerest .... ▣ 559
Anatuss LA Tablets 1359
Benadryl Decongestant Elixir .... ▣ 635
Benadryl Decongestant .... ▣ 635
Benadryl Plus .... ▣ 636
Benadryl Plus Nighttime .... ▣ 637
Benylin Decongestant .... ▣ 638
Brexin L.A. Capsules 2078
Bromfed Capsules (Timed Release) 1615
Bromfed Syrup .... ▣ 628
Bromfed 1615
CoAdvil .... ▣ 748
Allergy-Sinus Comtrex Multi-Symptom Allergy Sinus Formula Tablets & Caplets 746
Cough Formula Comtrex 746
Comtrex Multi-Symptom Cold Reliever Tablets/Caplets/Liqui-Gels/Liquid 745
Day-Night Comtrex 747
Non-Drowsy Comtrex 747
Congess 994
Congestac Caplets .... ▣ 617
Contac Jr. Children's Cold Medicine .... ▣ 712
Contac Nighttime Cold Medicine .... ▣ 713
Contac Sinus Caplets Maximum Strength Non-Drowsy Formula .... ▣ 710
Contac Sinus Tablets Maximum Strength Non-Drowsy Formula .... ▣ 710
Deconamine 663
Deconsal II Tablets 559
Dimacol Caplets .... ▣ 672
Dimetane-DX Cough Syrup 1858
Dorcol Children's Cough Syrup .... ▣ 685
Dorcol Children's Decongestant Liquid .... ▣ 685
Dorcol Children's Liquid Cold Formula .... ▣ 686
Maximum Strength Dristan Decongestant/Analgesic Coated Caplets .... ▣ 750
No Drowsiness Dristan Cold Nasal Decongestant/Analgesic Coated Caplets 2420
Dristan Sinus Caplets 2419
Sinus Excedrin Analgesic, Decongestant Tablets & Caplets .... ▣ 533
Fedahist Gyrocaps 2145
Fedahist Timecaps 2145
Guaifed 1615
Guaifed Syrup .... ▣ 629
Isoclor Expectorant 982
Isoclor Timesule Capsules .... ▣ 561
Kronofed-A 970
Medi-Flu Caplet, Liquid .... ▣ 640
Novafed A Capsules 1342
Novafed Capsules 1342
Novahistine DH 1342
Novahistine DMX .... ▣ 595
Novahistine Expectorant 1343
Nucofed Capsules 2219
Nucofed Expectorant 2219
Nucofed Pediatric Expectorant 2220
Nucofed Syrup 2219
Ornex Caplets .... ▣ 618
PediaCare Allergy Relief Formula Liquid 1362
PediaCare Cough-Cold Formula Liquid 1362
PediaCare Infants' Oral Decongestant Drops 1362
PediaCare Night Rest Cough-Cold Formula Liquid 1362
PediaCare 6-12 Cough-Cold Formula Chewable Tablets 1362
Robitussin-DAC Syrup 1875
Robitussin-PE .... ▣ 677
Rondec 1975
Rondec-DM 1976
Rondec-TR Tablet 1975
Ru-Tuss DE Tablets 694
Ryna .... ▣ 741
Seldane-D Extended-Release Tablets 1350
Sinarest .... ▣ 562
Sine-Aid Maximum Strength Sinus Headache Caplets 1365
Sine-Aid Maximum Strength Sinus Headache Tablets 1365
Sine-Off Maximum Strength Allergy/Sinus Formula Caplets .... ▣ 721
Sine-Off Maximum Strength No Drowsiness Formula Caplets .... ▣ 722
Singlet Tablets .... ▣ 598
Sinutab Maximum Strength .... ▣ 641
Sinutab Maximum Strength Without Drowsiness Tablets & Caplets .... ▣ 642
Sinutab Regular Strength Without Drowsiness Formula .... ▣ 641
St. Joseph Nighttime Cold Medicine .... ▣ 705
Sudafed Children's Liquid .... ▣ 543
Sudafed Cough Syrup .... ▣ 543
Sudafed Plus Liquid .... ▣ 544
Sudafed Plus Tablets .... ▣ 545
Sudafed Sinus Caplets .... ▣ 545
Sudafed Sinus Tablets .... ▣ 545
Sudafed Tablets, 30 mg .... ▣ 544
Sudafed Tablets, Adult Strength, 60 mg .... ▣ 544
Sudafed 12 Hour Capsules .... ▣ 545
TheraFlu Flu and Cold Medicine .... ▣ 687
Triaminic Nite Light .... ▣ 689
Tylenol Allergy Sinus Medication Caplets and Gelcaps, Maximum Strength 1372
Children's Tylenol Cold Liquid Formula and Chewable Tablets 1368
Tylenol Cold & Flu Hot Medication, Packets 1369
Tylenol Cold & Flu No Drowsiness Hot Medication, Packets 1371
Tylenol Cold Medication Caplets and Tablets 1370
Tylenol Cold Medication No Drowsiness Formula Caplets 1370
Tylenol Cold Night Time Medication Liquid 1371
Tylenol Cough Medication Liquid with Decongestant, Maximum Strength 1372
Tylenol, Maximum Strength, Sinus Medication Gelcaps, Caplets and Tablets 1373
Ursinus Inlay-Tabs .... ▣ 691
Vicks Children's NyQuil .... ▣ 664
Vicks Daycare .... ▣ 660
Vicks Formula 44D Decongestant Cough Medicine .... ▣ 662
Vicks Formula 44M Multi-Symptom Cough Medicine .... ▣ 662
Vicks NyQuil Nighttime Colds Medicine-Original & Cherry Flavor .... ▣ 664
Vicks Pediatric Formula 44 Cough & Congestion Medicine .... ▣ 663
Vicks Pediatric Formula 44m Multi-Symptom Cough & Cold Medicine .... ▣ 663

Pseudoephedrine Sulfate (Increased risk of cardiac arrhythmias). Products include:

Afrin Tablets .... ▣ 693
Chlor-Trimeton Decongestant .... ▣ 694
Disophrol Chronotab Sustained-Action Tablets .... ▣ 698
Drixoral Antihistamine/Nasal Decongestant Syrup .... ▣ 698
Drixoral Non-Drowsy Formula .... ▣ 699
Drixoral Plus Extended-Release Tablets .... ▣ 699
Drixoral Sinus .... ▣ 700
Drixoral Sustained-Action Tablets ▣ 698
Sinutab Allergy Formula Sustained Action Tablets .... ▣ 640
Trinalin Repetabs Tablets 1170

Quinidine Gluconate (Causes rise in serum digoxin concentration). Products include:

Quinaglute Dura-Tabs Tablets 663

Quinidine Polygalacturonate (Causes rise in serum digoxin concentration). Products include:

Cardioquin Tablets 1812

Quinidine Sulfate (Causes rise in serum digoxin concentration). Products include:

Quinidex Extentabs 1868

(▣ Described in PDR For Nonprescription Drugs) (⊙ Described in PDR For Ophthalmology)

Sodium Bicarbonate (Interferes with intestinal digoxin absorption). Products include:
Alka-Seltzer Advanced Formula Antacid & Non-Aspirin Pain Reliever ... ▣ 620
Alka-Seltzer Effervescent Antacid ... ▣ 622
Alka-Seltzer Effervescent Antacid and Pain Reliever ... 1568
Alka-Seltzer Extra Strength Effervescent Antacid and Pain Reliever ... ▣ 623
Alka-Seltzer (Flavored) Effervescent Antacid and Pain Reliever ... ▣ 621
Arm & Hammer Pure Baking Soda ... ▣ 548
Ceo-Two Rectal Suppositories ... 671
Citrocarbonate Antacid ... ▣ 668
Massengill Liquid Concentrate ... 2191
NuLYTELY ... 699

Succinylcholine Chloride (May cause arrhythmias). Products include:
Anectine ... 755

Sulfasalazine (Low digoxin serum concentration; interferes with intestinal digoxin absorption). Products include:
Azulfidine Tablets, EN-tabs, Oral Suspension ... 1157

Terbutaline Sulfate (Increased risk of cardiac arrhythmias). Products include:
Brethaire Inhaler ... 1024
Brethine Ampuls ... 1026
Brethine Tablets ... 1026
Bricanyl Injection ... 1324
Bricanyl Tablets ... 1325

Thyroglobulin (Hypothyroid patients may require increased digoxin dose). Products include:
Proloid Tablets ... 1761

Thyroid (Hypothyroid patients may require increased digoxin dose). Products include:
S-P-T "Liquid" Capsules ... 995

Thyroxine (Hypothyroid patients may require increased digoxin dose).
No products indexed under this heading.

Thyroxine Sodium (Hypothyroid patients may require increased digoxin dose).
No products indexed under this heading.

Timolol Maleate (Additive effects on AV node conduction). Products include:
Blocadren Tablets ... 1429
Timolide Tablets ... 1547
Timoptic in Ocudose ... 1552
Timoptic Sterile Ophthalmic Solution ... 1550

Triamcinolone (Major contributing factor to digitalis toxicity).
No products indexed under this heading.

Triamcinolone Acetonide (Major contributing factor to digitalis toxicity). Products include:
Aristocort A ... 1010
Azmacort Inhaler ... 1837
Kenalog Cream, Lotion & Ointment ... 2401
Kenalog-10 Injection ... 2402
Kenalog-40 Injection ... 2403
Kenalog in Orabase ... 604
Kenalog Spray ... 2401
Mycolog II Cream and Ointment ... 2407
Mytrex Cream & Ointment ... 2080
Nasacort Nasal Inhaler ... 1844

Triamcinolone Diacetate (Major contributing factor to digitalis toxicity). Products include:
Aristocort Suspension ... 1008

Triamcinolone Hexacetonide (Major contributing factor to digitalis toxicity). Products include:
Aristospan Suspension ... 1011

Verapamil Hydrochloride (Additive effects on AV node conduction; causes rise in serum digoxin concentration). Products include:
Calan SR Caplets ... 2157
Calan Tablets ... 2155
Isoptin Injectable ... 1177
Isoptin Oral Tablets ... 1179
Isoptin SR Sustained Release Tablets ... 1181
Verelan Capsules ... 1243
Verelan Capsules ... 2535

LANOXIN INJECTION
(Digoxin) ... **778**
May interact with potassium-depleting corticosteroids, potassium-depleting diuretics, antacids, sympathomimetic aerosal brochodilators, beta blockers, calcium channel blockers, thyroid preparations, mineralocorticoids, and certain other agents. Compounds in these categories include:

Acebutolol Hydrochloride (Additive effects on AV node conduction). Products include:
Sectral Capsules ... 2520

Albuterol (Increased risk of cardiac arrhythmias). Products include:
Proventil Inhalation Aerosol ... 2117
Ventolin Inhalation Aerosol and Refill ... 583

Albuterol Sulfate (Increased risk of cardiac arrhythmias). Products include:
Proventil Repetabs Tablets ... 2120
Proventil Solutions for Inhalation 0.5% and 0.083% ... 2118
Proventil Syrup ... 2119
Proventil Tablets ... 2120
Ventolin ... 583

Aluminum Carbonate Gel (Interferes with intestinal digoxin absorption). Products include:
Basaljel ... 2438

Aluminum Hydroxide (Interferes with intestinal digoxin absorption). Products include:
Cama Arthritis Pain Reliever ... ▣ 685
Gaviscon Extra Strength Relief Formula Liquid Antacid ... ▣ 594
Gaviscon Extra Strength Relief Formula Antacid Tablets ... ▣ 594
Gaviscon Liquid Antacid ... ▣ 594
Gelusil Liquid & Tablets ... ▣ 639
Extra Strength Maalox Plus Suspension ... 1850
Maalox TC Suspension ... 1851
Maalox Plus Tablets ... ▣ 655
Extra Strength Maalox Plus Tablets 1850
Nephrox Suspension ... ▣ 563
WinGel Liquid & Tablets ... ▣ 761

Aluminum Hydroxide Gel (Interferes with intestinal digoxin absorption). Products include:
ALternaGEL Liquid ... 1154
Aludrox Oral Suspension ... 2428
Amphojel Suspension ... 2429
Amphojel Suspension without Flavor ... 2429
Mylanta Liquid ... 1155
Mylanta Double Strength Liquid ... 1155

Aluminum Hydroxide Gel, Dried (Interferes with intestinal digoxin absorption). Products include:
Alu-Tab/Alu-Cap ... 1309
Amphojel Tablets ... 2429
Ascriptin A/D Caplets ... 1850
Regular Strength Ascriptin Tablets 1850
Gaviscon Antacid Tablets ... ▣ 593
Gaviscon-2 Antacid Tablets ... ▣ 594
Mylanta Tablets ... 1155
Mylanta Double Strength Tablets ... 1155

Amiodarone Hydrochloride (Causes rise in serum digoxin concentration). Products include:
Cordarone Tablets ... 2446

Antibiotics, unspecified (Increases digoxin absorption in patients who inactivate digoxin by bacterial metabolism).

Anticancer Drugs, unspecified (Interferes with intestinal digoxin absorption).

Atenolol (Additive effects on AV node conduction). Products include:
Tenoretic Tablets ... 1105
Tenormin Tablets and I.V. Injection 1107

Bendroflumethiazide (Major contributing factor to digitalis toxicity). Products include:
Corzide Tablets ... 702
Naturetin Tablets ... 1789
Rauzide Tablets ... 1804

Bepridil Hydrochloride (Additive effects on AV node conduction). Products include:
Vascor (200, 300 and 400 mg) Tablets ... 1383

Betamethasone Acetate (Major contributing factor to digitalis toxicity). Products include:
Celestone Soluspan Suspension ... 2081

Betamethasone Sodium Phosphate (Major contributing factor to digitalis toxicity). Products include:
Celestone Soluspan Suspension ... 2081

Betaxolol Hydrochloride (Additive effects on AV node conduction). Products include:
Betoptic Sterile Ophthalmic Solution ... 569
Betoptic S Sterile Ophthalmic Suspension ... 570
Kerlone Tablets ... 2172

Calcium, intravenous (May produce serious arrhythmias in digitalized patients).

Carteolol Hydrochloride (Additive effects on AV node conduction). Products include:
Cartrol Tablets ... 507

Chlorothiazide (Major contributing factor to digitalis toxicity). Products include:
Aldoclor Tablets ... 1413
Diupres Tablets ... 1461
Diuril Oral ... 1464

Chlorothiazide Sodium (Major contributing factor to digitalis toxicity). Products include:
Diuril Sodium Intravenous ... 1463

Cholestyramine (Interferes with intestinal digoxin absorption). Products include:
Cholybar ... 1705
Questran Light ... 711
Questran Powder ... 710

Cortisone Acetate (Major contributing factor to digitalis toxicity). Products include:
Cortone Acetate Sterile Suspension ... 1437
Cortone Acetate Tablets ... 1439

Dexamethasone (Major contributing factor to digitalis toxicity). Products include:
AK-Trol Ointment & Suspension ... ◉ 207
Decadron Elixir ... 1445
Decadron Tablets ... 1447
Decaspray Topical Aerosol ... 1459
Dexacidin ... ◉ 272
Maxidex Sterile Ophthalmic Suspension ... ◉ 223
Maxitrol Ophthalmic Ointment/Suspension ... ◉ 223
TobraDex Ophthalmic Suspension and Ointment ... ◉ 228

Dexamethasone Acetate (Major contributing factor to digitalis toxicity). Products include:
Dalalone D.P. Injectable ... 999
Decadron-LA Sterile Suspension ... 1457

Dexamethasone Sodium Phosphate (Major contributing factor to digitalis toxicity). Products include:
AK-Dex ... ◉ 203
Decadron Phosphate Respihaler ... 1454
Decadron Phosphate Sterile Ophthalmic Ointment ... 1453
Decadron Phosphate Sterile Ophthalmic Solution ... 1453
Decadron Phosphate Topical Cream ... 1455
Decadron Phosphate Turbinaire ... 1456
Maxidex Sterile Ophthalmic Ointment ... ◉ 222
NeoDecadron Sterile Ophthalmic Ointment ... 1517
NeoDecadron Sterile Ophthalmic Solution ... 1518
NeoDecadron Topical Cream ... 1518

Dihydroxyaluminum Sodium Carbonate (Interferes with intestinal digoxin absorption). Products include:
Rolaids ... ▣ 743

Diltiazem Hydrochloride (Additive effects on AV node conduction). Products include:
Cardizem Tablets-30 mg, 60 mg, 90 mg and 120 mg ... 1329
Cardizem SR Capsules-60 mg, 90 mg and 120 mg ... 1327

Diphenoxylate Hydrochloride (Increases digoxin absorption). Products include:
Lomotil ... 2174

Dobutamine Hydrochloride (Increased risk of cardiac arrhythmias). Products include:
Dobutrex Solution Vials ... 1259

Dopamine Hydrochloride (Increased risk of cardiac arrhythmias). Products include:
Intropin Injection ... 930

Ephedrine Hydrochloride (Increased risk of cardiac arrhythmias). Products include:
Amesec ... ▣ 682
Primatene Tablets-M Formula ... 2421
Primatene Tablets-P Formula ... 2421
Primatene Tablets-Regular Formula ... 2421
Quadrinal Tablets ... 1183
Quelidrine Syrup ... 556
Tedral SA ... 1765

Ephedrine Sulfate (Increased risk of cardiac arrhythmias). Products include:
Bronkaid Tablets ... ▣ 757
Bronkolixir ... ▣ 761
Bronkotabs Tablets ... ▣ 762
Marax Tablets & DF Syrup ... 1954
Pazo Hemorrhoid Ointment & Suppositories ... 752
Vicks Vatronol Nose Drops ... ▣ 666

Ephedrine Tannate (Increased risk of cardiac arrhythmias). Products include:
Rynatuss ... 2388

Epinephrine (Increased risk of cardiac arrhythmias). Products include:
Ana-Kit Anaphylaxis Emergency Treatment Kit ... 1100
Bronkaid Mist ... ▣ 757
EpiPen ... 843
Marcaine Hydrochloride 0.5% with Epinephrine 1:200,000 (as bitartrate) ... 958
Marcaine Hydrochloride with Epinephrine 1:200,000 ... 2055
Primatene Mist ... 2420
Sus-Phrine Injection ... 1006
Xylocaine with Epinephrine Injections ... 637

Epinephrine Bitartrate (Increased risk of cardiac arrhythmias). Products include:
AsthmaHaler Mist Epinephrine Bitartrate Bronchodilator ... ▣ 616
Bronkaid Mist Suspension ... ▣ 757
Primatene Mist Suspension ... 2421

Epinephrine Hydrochloride (Increased risk of cardiac arrhythmias). Products include:
Adrenalin Chloride Solution 1:100 & 1:1,000 ... 1689
Epifrin ... ◉ 244
Glaucon ... ◉ 218

Esmolol Hydrochloride (Additive effects on AV node conduction). Products include:
Brevibloc Injection 942

Felodipine (Additive effects on AV node conduction). Products include:
Plendil Extended-Release Tablets 1526

Hydrochlorothiazide (Major contributing factor to digitalis toxicity). Products include:
Aldactazide 2150
Aldoril Tablets 1418
Apresazide Capsules 854
Apresoline-Esidrix Tablets 857
Capozide 2258
Dyazide Capsules 2208
Esidrix Tablets 863
Esimil Tablets 864
HydroDIURIL Tablets 1484
Hydropres Tablets 1485
Inderide Tablets 2463
Inderide LA Long Acting Capsules .. 2465
Lopressor HCT Tablets 1034
Maxzide 1215
Moduretic Tablets 1510
Normozide Tablets 2112
Oretic Tablets 544
Oreticyl 545
Prinzide Tablets 1540
Ser-Ap-Es Tablets 881
Serpasil-Esidrix Tablets 886
Timolide Tablets 1547
Trandate HCT Tablets 579
Vaseretic Tablets 1559
Zestoretic 2274

Hydrocortisone (Major contributing factor to digitalis toxicity). Products include:
AK-Spore H.C. .... ⊙ 206
Bactine Hydrocortisone Anti-Itch Cream .... ▣ 625
CaldeCORT Anti-Itch Hydrocortisone Spray .... ▣ 560
Carmol HC Cream 1% 2296
Cortaid Spray .... ▣ 735
Cortenema 2244
Cortisporin Ointment 758
Cortisporin Ophthalmic Ointment Sterile 758
Cortisporin Ophthalmic Suspension Sterile 759
Cortisporin Otic Solution Sterile 760
Cortisporin Otic Suspension Sterile 760
Cortizone-5 Creme & Ointment .... ▣ 732
Dermolate Anti-Itch Cream .... ▣ 697
Eldecort Cream 1.0% 1113
Eldecort Cream 1.0% and 2.5% 1113
Fungoid HC Creme 1770
Hydrocortone Tablets 1482
Hytone 909
LazerSporin-C Solution 1770
Massengill Medicated Soft Cloth Towelettes 2192
Nutracort Cream & Lotion 1684
PediOtic Suspension Sterile 797
Synacort Creams 1%, 2.5% 2296
Vanoxide-HC Acne Lotion 911
Vioform-Hydrocortisone Cream and Mild Cream 889
Vioform-Hydrocortisone Ointment .. 889
VōSoL HC Otic Solution 2392
Vytone Cream 1% 911

Hydrocortisone Acetate (Major contributing factor to digitalis toxicity). Products include:
Analpram-HC Rectal Cream 1% and 2.5% 970
Anusol-HC Cream 1690
Anusol-HC Suppositories 1691
Caldecort .... ▣ 560
Carmol HC Cream 1% 2296
Chloromycetin Hydrocortisone Ophthalmic 1694
Coly-Mycin S Otic w/Neomycin & Hydrocortisone 1708
Cortaid .... ▣ 735
Cortef Feminine Itch Cream .... ▣ 735
Corticaine .... ▣ 682
Cortifoam 1827
Cortisporin Cream 757
Epifoam 1828
Gynecort 5 Creme .... ▣ 556
Hydrocortone Acetate Sterile Suspension 1479
Lanacort 5 Creme and Ointment .. ▣ 557
Mantadil Cream 789
Ophthocort .... ⊙ 301
Orabase HCA Oral Paste 890
Pramosone Cream, Lotion & Ointment 971
ProctoCream-HC 1834
Proctofoam-HC 1835

Hydrocortisone Sodium Phosphate (Major contributing factor to digitalis toxicity). Products include:
Hydrocortone Phosphate Injection, Sterile 1481

Hydrocortisone Sodium Succinate (Major contributing factor to digitalis toxicity). Products include:
Solu-Cortef Sterile Powder 2361

Hydroflumethiazide (Major contributing factor to digitalis toxicity). Products include:
Diucardin Tablets 2450
Saluron 718
Salutensin/Salutensin-Demi 719

Isoproterenol Hydrochloride (Increased risk of cardiac arrhythmias). Products include:
Isuprel Hydrochloride Injection 1:5000 2050
Isuprel Hydrochloride Mistometer .. 2051
Isuprel Hydrochloride Solution 1:200 & 1:100 2052
Norisodrine Aerotrol 540

Isradipine (Additive effects on AV node conduction). Products include:
DynaCirc Capsules 2004

Labetalol Hydrochloride (Additive effects on AV node conduction). Products include:
Normodyne Injection 2108
Normodyne Tablets 2110
Normozide Tablets 2112
Trandate HCT Tablets 579
Trandate Injection 577
Trandate Tablets 579

Levothyroxine Sodium (Hypothyroid patients may require increased digoxin dose). Products include:
Levothroid Tablets 1003
Levoxine Tablets 904
Synthroid 695

Liothyronine Sodium (Hypothyroid patients may require increased digoxin dose). Products include:
Cytomel Tablets 2203

Liotrix (Hypothyroid patients may require increased digoxin dose). Products include:
Euthroid 1724

Magaldrate (Interferes with intestinal digoxin absorption). Products include:
Riopan Antacid Chew Tablets .... ▣ 754
Riopan Antacid Chew Tablets in Rollpacks .... ▣ 754
Riopan Antacid Suspension 2421
Riopan Antacid Swallow Tablets 2421
Riopan Plus Chew Tablets 2422
Riopan Plus Chew Tablets in Rollpack 2422
Riopan Plus 2 Chew Tablets, Mint Flavor, Cherry Flavor 2422
Riopan Plus Suspension 2422
Riopan Plus 2 Suspension, Mint Flavor, Cherry Flavor 2422

Magnesium Hydroxide (Interferes with intestinal digoxin absorption). Products include:
Aludrox Oral Suspension 2428
Ascriptin A/D Caplets 1850
Regular Strength Ascriptin Tablets 1850
Di-Gel Antacid/Anti-Gas .... ▣ 697
Gelusil Liquid & Tablets .... ▣ 639
Haley's M-O, Regular & Flavored .. ▣ 569
Extra Strength Maalox Plus Suspension 1850
Maalox TC Suspension 1851
Maalox Plus Tablets .... ▣ 655
Extra Strength Maalox Plus Tablets 1850
Mylanta Liquid 1155
Mylanta Tablets 1155
Mylanta Double Strength Liquid 1155
Mylanta Double Strength Tablets 1155
Concentrated Phillips' Milk of Magnesia .... ▣ 573
Phillips' Milk of Magnesia Liquid .... ▣ 572
Phillips' Milk of Magnesia Tablets ▣ 573
WinGel Liquid & Tablets .... ▣ 761

Magnesium Oxide (Interferes with intestinal digoxin absorption). Products include:
Bayer Plus Aspirin Tablets .... ▣ 567
Beelith Tablets 659
Bufferin Analgesic Tablets and Caplets .... ▣ 524
Cama Arthritis Pain Reliever .... ▣ 685
Mag-Ox 400 673
Uro-Mag 673

Metaproterenol Sulfate (Increased risk of cardiac arrhythmias). Products include:
Alupent 674
Arm-a-Med Metaproterenol Sulfate Inhalation Solution, USP 617
Metaprel Inhalation Aerosol Bronchodilator 2014
Metaprel Inhalation Solution 2015
Metaprel 2015
Metaproterenol Sulfate Inhalation Solution, USP 912

Metaraminol Bitartrate (Increased risk of cardiac arrhythmias). Products include:
Aramine Injection 1424

Methoxamine Hydrochloride (Increased risk of cardiac arrhythmias). Products include:
Vasoxyl Injection 819

Methyclothiazide (Major contributing factor to digitalis toxicity). Products include:
Enduron Tablets 517
Enduronyl 518

Methylprednisolone Acetate (Major contributing factor to digitalis toxicity). Products include:
Depo-Medrol Sterile Aqueous Suspension 2334

Methylprednisolone Sodium Succinate (Major contributing factor to digitalis toxicity). Products include:
Solu-Medrol Sterile Powder 2363

Metoprolol Tartrate (Additive effects on AV node conduction). Products include:
Lopressor Ampuls 1032
Lopressor HCT Tablets 1034
Lopressor Tablets 1032

Nadolol (Additive effects on AV node conduction). Products include:
Corgard Tablets 701
Corzide Tablets 702

Neomycin, oral (Interferes with intestinal digoxin absorption).

Nephrotoxic Drugs (May impair the excretion of digoxin).

Nicardipine Hydrochloride (Additive effects on AV node conduction). Products include:
Cardene Capsules 2290

Nifedipine (Additive effects on AV node conduction). Products include:
Adalat Capsules (10 mg and 20 mg) 1587
Procardia Capsules 1781
Procardia XL Tablets 1783

Nimodipine (Additive effects on AV node conduction). Products include:
Nimotop Capsules 1607

Norepinephrine Bitartrate (Increased risk of cardiac arrhythmias). Products include:
Levophed Bitartrate Injection 2054

Pectin (Low digoxin serum concentration; interferes with intestinal digoxin absorption). Products include:
Donnagel .... ▣ 675
Donnagel-PG 1858

Penbutolol Sulfate (Additive effects on AV node conduction). Products include:
Levatol 1832

Phenylephrine Bitartrate (Increased risk of cardiac arrhythmias).
No products indexed under this heading.

Phenylephrine Hydrochloride (Increased risk of cardiac arrhythmias). Products include:
AK-Dilate Solution 2.5% and 10% .... ⊙ 203
Atrohist Sprinkle Capsules 558
Cerose-DM 2443
Codimal 846
Comhist LA Capsules 1618
Congespirin For Children Aspirin Free Chewable Cold Tablets 748
Cyclomydril .... ⊙ 216
Deconsal Sprinkle Capsules 559
Dimetane Decongestant .... ▣ 673
Dristan Decongestant/Antihistamine/ Analgesic Coated Caplets .... ▣ 749
Dristan Cold Nasal Decongestant/ Antihistamine/ Analgesic Coated Tablets 2419
Dristan Advanced Formula Decongestant/Antihistamine/ Analgesic Tablets .... ▣ 749
Dristan Nasal Spray, Menthol 2419
Dristan Nasal Spray, Regular and Regular with Metered Pump 2419
Entex Capsules 1623
Entex Liquid 1623
Sinus Excedrin Analgesic, Decongestant Tablets & Caplets 750
Extendryl 994
4-Way Fast Acting Nasal Spray - Original Formula (regular & mentholated) & Metered Spray Pump (regular) 751
Hycomine Compound Tablets 929
Murocoll-2 Sterile Ophthalmic Solution .... ⊙ 261
Mydfrin 2.5% .... ⊙ 224
Naldecon Syrup, Tablets, Pediatric Drops and Pediatric Syrup 709
Neo-Synephrine Hydrochloride 1% Carpuject 2063
Neo-Synephrine Hydrochloride 1% Injection 2063
Neo-Synephrine Hydrochloride (Ophthalmic) 2064
Neo-Synephrine .... ▣ 759
Nōstril Nasal Decongestant .... ▣ 520
Novahistine Elixir .... ▣ 596
Phenergan VC 2500
Phenergan VC with Codeine 2501
Prefrin Liquifilm Vasoconstrictor and Lubricant Eye Drops .... ⊙ 254
Prefrin-A .... ⊙ 255
Quelidrine Syrup 556
Relief Vasoconstrictor and Lubricant Eye Drops .... ⊙ 256
Robitussin Night Relief .... ▣ 677
Ru-Tuss with Hydrocodone 694
Ru-Tuss Tablets 693
Vasosulf .... ⊙ 279
Vicks Sinex .... ▣ 665
Zincfrin .... ⊙ 230

Phenylephrine Tannate (Increased risk of cardiac arrhythmias). Products include:
Rynatan 2387
Rynatuss 2388

Phenylpropanolamine Hydrochloride (Increased risk of cardiac arrhythmias). Products include:
A.R.M. Allergy Relief Medicine Caplets .... ▣ 615
Acutrim .... ▣ 548
Allerest .... ▣ 559
BC Cold Powder .... ▣ 517
Cheracol Plus Head Cold/Cough Formula .... ▣ 667
Codimal Expectorant 846
Comtrex Multi-Symptom Cold Reliever Tablets/Caplets/Liqui-Gels/Liquid 745
Contac Continuous Action Decongestant/Antihistamine Capsules ▣ 710
Contac Maximum Strength Continuous Action Decongestant/ Antihistamine Caplets .... ▣ 709
Contac Severe Cold and Flu Formula Caplets .... ▣ 711
Coricidin 'D' Decongestant Tablets .... ▣ 695
Coricidin Demilets Tablets for Children .... ▣ 696

- Demazin Nasal Decongestant/ Antihistamine Repetabs Tablets & Syrup ... ND 697
- Dexatrim ... ND 733
- Dimetane-DC Cough Syrup ... 1857
- Dimetapp Elixir ... ND 673
- Dimetapp DM Elixir ... ND 674
- Dimetapp Extentabs ... ND 674
- Dimetapp Plus Caplets ... ND 675
- Dimetapp Tablets ... ND 675
- Entex Capsules ... 1623
- Entex LA Tablets ... 1623
- Entex Liquid ... 1623
- 4-Way Cold Tablets ... 750
- Hycomine Syrup ... 927
- Naldecon CX Adult Liquid ... ND 521
- Naldecon DX Adult Liquid ... ND 521
- Naldecon DX Children's Syrup ... ND 522
- Naldecon DX Pediatric Drops ... ND 522
- Naldecon EX Children's Syrup ... ND 522
- Naldecon EX Pediatric Drops ... ND 523
- Naldecon Syrup, Tablets, Pediatric Drops and Pediatric Syrup ... 709
- Nolamine Tablets ... 838
- Nolex LA Tablets ... 838
- Ornade Spansule Capsules ... 2221
- Orthoxicol Cough Syrup ... ND 668
- Propagest ... 839
- Pyrroxate Capsules ... ND 669
- Robitussin-CF ... ND 676
- Ru-Tuss II Capsules ... 693
- Ru-Tuss with Hydrocodone ... 694
- Ru-Tuss Tablets ... 693
- Sine-Off Sinus Medicine Tablets-Aspirin Formula ... ND 722
- Sinulin ... 840
- St. Joseph Cold Tablets for Children ... ND 704
- Tavist-D Tablets ... 2035
- Triaminic Allergy Tablets ... ND 688
- Triaminic Chewables ... ND 688
- Triaminic Cold Tablets ... ND 688
- Triaminic Expectorant ... ND 688
- Triaminic Expectorant w/Codeine .. 1996
- Triaminic Expectorant DH ... 1995
- Triaminic Oral Infant Drops ... 1996
- Triaminic Syrup ... ND 689
- Triaminic-12 Tablets ... ND 690
- Triaminic-DM Syrup ... ND 689
- Triaminicin Tablets ... ND 690
- Triaminicol Multi-Symptom Cold Tablets ... ND 691
- Triaminicol Multi-Symptom Relief ND 691
- Tuss-Ornade Liquid ... 2242
- Tuss-Ornade Spansule Capsules ... 2242
- Tylenol Cold Medication, Effervescent Tablets ... 1369

Pindolol (Additive effects on AV node conduction). Products include:
- Visken Tablets ... 2036

Pirbuterol Acetate (Increased risk of cardiac arrhythmias). Products include:
- Maxair Inhaler ... 1311

Polythiazide (Major contributing factor to digitalis toxicity). Products include:
- Minizide Capsules ... 1779
- Renese Tablets ... 1785
- Renese-R Tablets ... 1786

Prednisolone Acetate (Major contributing factor to digitalis toxicity). Products include:
- AK-Cide Sterile Ophthalmic Ointment & Suspension ... ⊙ 202
- Blephamide Liquifilm Sterile Ophthalmic Suspension ... 586
- Blephamide S.O.P. Sterile Ophthalmic Ointment ... 586
- Cetapred Ointment ... ⊙ 220
- ⅛% Econopred & 1% Econopred Plus ... ⊙ 217
- Isopto Cetapred Suspension ... ⊙ 220
- Metimyd ... ⊙ 306
- Poly-Pred Liquifilm ... ⊙ 250
- Pred Forte ... ⊙ 252
- Pred Mild ... ⊙ 254
- Pred-G Liquifilm Sterile Ophthalmic Suspension ... ⊙ 252
- Pred-G S.O.P. Sterile Ophthalmic Ointment ... ⊙ 253
- Vasocidin Ointment ... ⊙ 275

Prednisolone Sodium Phosphate (Major contributing factor to digitalis toxicity). Products include:
- AK-Pred ... ⊙ 205
- Hydeltrasol Injection, Sterile ... 1476
- Inflamase ... ⊙ 274
- Pediapred Oral Liquid ... 987
- Vasocidin Ophthalmic Solution ... ⊙ 276

Prednisolone Tebutate (Major contributing factor to digitalis toxicity). Products include:
- Hydeltra-T.B.A. Sterile Suspension 1478

Prednisone (Major contributing factor to digitalis toxicity). Products include:
- Deltasone Tablets ... 2332

Propantheline Bromide (Increases digoxin absorption). Products include:
- Pro-Banthīne Tablets ... 2141

Propranolol Hydrochloride (Additive effects on AV node conduction). Products include:
- Inderal ... 2459
- Inderal LA Long Acting Capsules ... 2461
- Inderide Tablets ... 2463
- Inderide LA Long Acting Capsules .. 2465

Pseudoephedrine Hydrochloride (Increased risk of cardiac arrhythmias). Products include:
- Actifed Capsules ... ND 539
- Actifed Plus Caplets ... ND 539
- Actifed Plus Tablets ... ND 540
- Actifed with Codeine Cough Syrup .. 752
- Actifed Syrup ... ND 540
- Actifed Tablets ... ND 540
- Actifed 12-Hour Capsules ... ND 539
- Advil Cold & Sinus Caplets (formerly CoAdvil) ... 2416
- Allerest ... ND 559
- Anatuss LA Tablets ... 1359
- Benadryl Decongestant Elixir ... ND 635
- Benadryl Decongestant ... ND 635
- Benadryl Plus ... ND 636
- Benadryl Plus Nighttime ... ND 637
- Benylin Decongestant ... ND 638
- Brexin L.A. Capsules ... 2078
- Bromfed Capsules (Timed Release) ... 1615
- Bromfed Syrup ... ND 628
- Bromfed ... 1615
- CoAdvil ... ND 748
- Allergy-Sinus Comtrex Multi-Symptom Allergy Sinus Formula Tablets & Caplets ... 746
- Cough Formula Comtrex ... 746
- Comtrex Multi-Symptom Cold Reliever Tablets/Caplets/Liqui-Gels/Liquid ... 745
- Day-Night Comtrex ... 747
- Non-Drowsy Comtrex ... 747
- Congess ... 994
- Congestac Caplets ... ND 617
- Contac Jr. Children's Cold Medicine ... ND 712
- Contac Nighttime Cold Medicine ... ND 713
- Contac Sinus Caplets Maximum Strength Non-Drowsy Formula ... ND 710
- Contac Sinus Tablets Maximum Strength Non-Drowsy Formula ... ND 710
- Deconamine ... 663
- Deconsal II Tablets ... 559
- Dimacol Caplets ... ND 672
- Dimetane-DX Cough Syrup ... 1858
- Dorcol Children's Cough Syrup ... ND 685
- Dorcol Children's Decongestant Liquid ... ND 685
- Dorcol Children's Liquid Cold Formula ... ND 686
- Maximum Strength Dristan Decongestant/Analgesic Coated Caplets ... ND 750
- No Drowsiness Dristan Cold Nasal Decongestant/Analgesic Coated Caplets ... 2420
- Dristan Sinus Caplets ... 2419
- Sinus Excedrin Analgesic, Decongestant Tablets & Caplets ... ND 533
- Fedahist Gyrocaps ... 2145
- Fedahist Timecaps ... 2145
- Guaifed ... 1615
- Guaifed Syrup ... ND 629
- Isoclor Expectorant ... 982
- Isoclor Timesule Capsules ... ND 561
- Kronofed-A ... 970
- Medi-Flu Caplet, Liquid ... ND 640
- Novafed A Capsules ... 1342
- Novafed Capsules ... 1342
- Novahistine DH ... 1342
- Novahistine DMX ... ND 595
- Novahistine Expectorant ... 1343
- Nucofed Capsules ... 2219
- Nucofed Expectorant ... 2219
- Nucofed Pediatric Expectorant ... 2220
- Nucofed Syrup ... 2219
- Ornex Caplets ... ND 618
- PediaCare Allergy Relief Formula Liquid ... 1362
- PediaCare Cough-Cold Formula Liquid ... 1362
- PediaCare Infants' Oral Decongestant Drops ... 1362
- PediaCare Night Rest Cough-Cold Formula Liquid ... 1362
- PediaCare 6-12 Cough-Cold Formula Chewable Tablets ... 1362
- Robitussin-DAC Syrup ... 1875
- Robitussin-PE ... ND 677
- Rondec ... 1975
- Rondec-DM ... 1976
- Rondec-TR Tablet ... 1975
- Ru-Tuss DE Tablets ... 694
- Ryna ... ND 741
- Seldane-D Extended-Release Tablets ... 1350
- Sinarest ... ND 562
- Sine-Aid Maximum Strength Sinus Headache Caplets ... 1365
- Sine-Aid Maximum Strength Sinus Headache Tablets ... 1365
- Sine-Off Maximum Strength Allergy/Sinus Formula Caplets ... ND 721
- Sine-Off Maximum Strength No Drowsiness Formula Caplets ... ND 722
- Singlet Tablets ... ND 598
- Sinutab Maximum Strength ... ND 641
- Sinutab Maximum Strength Without Drowsiness Tablets & Caplets ... ND 642
- Sinutab Regular Strength Without Drowsiness Formula ... ND 641
- St. Joseph Nighttime Cold Medicine ... ND 705
- Sudafed Children's Liquid ... ND 543
- Sudafed Cough Syrup ... ND 543
- Sudafed Plus Liquid ... ND 544
- Sudafed Plus Tablets ... ND 545
- Sudafed Sinus Caplets ... ND 545
- Sudafed Sinus Tablets ... ND 545
- Sudafed Tablets, 30 mg ... ND 544
- Sudafed Tablets, Adult Strength, 60 mg ... ND 544
- Sudafed 12 Hour Capsules ... ND 545
- TheraFlu Flu and Cold Medicine ... ND 687
- Triaminic Nite Light ... ND 689
- Tylenol Allergy Sinus Medication Caplets and Gelcaps, Maximum Strength ... 1372
- Children's Tylenol Cold Liquid Formula and Chewable Tablets ... 1368
- Tylenol Cold & Flu Hot Medication, Packets ... 1369
- Tylenol Cold & Flu No Drowsiness Hot Medication, Packets ... 1371
- Tylenol Cold Medication Caplets and Tablets ... 1370
- Tylenol Cold Medication No Drowsiness Formula Caplets ... 1370
- Tylenol Cold Night Time Medication Liquid ... 1371
- Tylenol Cough Medication Liquid with Decongestant, Maximum Strength ... 1372
- Tylenol, Maximum Strength, Sinus Medication Gelcaps, Caplets and Tablets ... 1373
- Ursinus Inlay-Tabs ... ND 691
- Vicks Children's NyQuil ... ND 664
- Vicks Daycare ... ND 660
- Vicks Formula 44D Decongestant Cough Medicine ... ND 662
- Vicks Formula 44M Multi-Symptom Cough Medicine ... ND 662
- Vicks NyQuil Nighttime Colds Medicine-Original & Cherry Flavor ... ND 664
- Vicks Pediatric Formula 44 Cough & Congestion Medicine ... ND 663
- Vicks Pediatric Formula 44m Multi-Symptom Cough & Cold Medicine ... ND 663

Pseudoephedrine Sulfate (Increased risk of cardiac arrhythmias). Products include:
- Afrin Tablets ... ND 693
- Chlor-Trimeton Decongestant ... ND 694
- Disophrol Chronotab Sustained-Action Tablets ... ND 698
- Drixoral Antihistamine/Nasal Decongestant Syrup ... ND 698
- Drixoral Non-Drowsy Formula ... ND 699
- Drixoral Plus Extended-Release Tablets ... ND 699
- Drixoral Sinus ... ND 700
- Drixoral Sustained-Action Tablets ND 698
- Sinutab Allergy Formula Sustained Action Tablets ... ND 640
- Trinalin Repetabs Tablets ... 1170

Quinidine Gluconate (Causes rise in serum digoxin concentration). Products include:
- Quinaglute Dura-Tabs Tablets ... 663

Quinidine Polygalacturonate (Causes rise in serum digoxin concentration). Products include:
- Cardioquin Tablets ... 1812

Quinidine Sulfate (Causes rise in serum digoxin concentration). Products include:
- Quinidex Extentabs ... 1868

Sodium Bicarbonate (Interferes with intestinal digoxin absorption). Products include:
- Alka-Seltzer Advanced Formula Antacid & Non-Aspirin Pain Reliever ... ND 620
- Alka-Seltzer Effervescent Antacid ND 622
- Alka-Seltzer Effervescent Antacid and Pain Reliever ... 1568
- Alka-Seltzer Extra Strength Effervescent Antacid and Pain Reliever ... ND 623
- Alka-Seltzer (Flavored) Effervescent Antacid and Pain Reliever .. ND 621
- Arm & Hammer Pure Baking Soda ... ND 548
- Ceo-Two Rectal Suppositories ... 671
- Citrocarbonate Antacid ... ND 668
- Massengill Liquid Concentrate ... 2191
- NuLYTELY ... 699

Succinylcholine Chloride (May cause arrhythmias). Products include:
- Anectine ... 755

Sulfasalazine (Low digoxin serum concentration; interferes with intestinal digoxin absorption). Products include:
- Azulfidine Tablets, EN-tabs, Oral Suspension ... 1157

Terbutaline Sulfate (Increased risk of cardiac arrhythmias). Products include:
- Brethaire Inhaler ... 1024
- Brethine Ampuls ... 1026
- Brethine Tablets ... 1026
- Bricanyl Injection ... 1324
- Bricanyl Tablets ... 1325

Thyroglobulin (Hypothyroid patients may require increased digoxin dose). Products include:
- Proloid Tablets ... 1761

Thyroid (Hypothyroid patients may require increased digoxin dose). Products include:
- S-P-T "Liquid" Capsules ... 995

Thyroxine (Hypothyroid patients may require increased digoxin dose).
- No products indexed under this heading.

Thyroxine Sodium (Hypothyroid patients may require increased digoxin dose).
- No products indexed under this heading.

Timolol Maleate (Additive effects on AV node conduction). Products include:
- Blocadren Tablets ... 1429
- Timolide Tablets ... 1547
- Timoptic in Ocudose ... 1552
- Timoptic Sterile Ophthalmic Solution ... 1550

Triamcinolone (Major contributing factor to digitalis toxicity).
- No products indexed under this heading.

Triamcinolone Acetonide (Major contributing factor to digitalis toxicity). Products include:
- Aristocort A ... 1010
- Azmacort Inhaler ... 1837
- Kenalog Cream, Lotion & Ointment 2401
- Kenalog-10 Injection ... 2402
- Kenalog-40 Injection ... 2403
- Kenalog in Orabase ... 604

Kenalog Spray ... 2401
Mycolog II Cream and Ointment ... 2407
Mytrex Cream & Ointment ... 2080
Nasacort Nasal Inhaler ... 1844

Triamcinolone Diacetate (Major contributing factor to digitalis toxicity). Products include:
Aristocort Suspension ... 1008

Triamcinolone Hexacetonide (Major contributing factor to digitalis toxicity). Products include:
Aristospan Suspension ... 1011

Verapamil Hydrochloride (Additive effects on AV node conduction; causes rise in serum digoxin concentration). Products include:
Calan SR Caplets ... 2157
Calan Tablets ... 2155
Isoptin Injectable ... 1177
Isoptin Oral Tablets ... 1179
Isoptin SR Sustained Release Tablets ... 1181
Verelan Capsules ... 1243
Verelan Capsules ... 2535

LANOXIN INJECTION PEDIATRIC

(Digoxin) ... 781
May interact with potassium-depleting corticosteroids, potassium-depleting diuretics, antacids, sympathomimetic aerosal brochodilators, beta blockers, calcium channel blockers, thyroid preparations, mineralocorticoids, and certain other agents. Compounds in these categories include:

Acebutolol Hydrochloride (Additive effects on AV node conduction). Products include:
Sectral Capsules ... 2520

Albuterol (Increased risk of cardiac arrhythmias). Products include:
Proventil Inhalation Aerosol ... 2117
Ventolin Inhalation Aerosol and Refill ... 583

Albuterol Sulfate (Increased risk of cardiac arrhythmias). Products include:
Proventil Repetabs Tablets ... 2120
Proventil Solutions for Inhalation 0.5% and 0.083% ... 2118
Proventil Syrup ... 2119
Proventil Tablets ... 2120
Ventolin ... 583

Aluminum Carbonate Gel (Interferes with intestinal digoxin absorption). Products include:
Basaljel ... 2438

Aluminum Hydroxide (Interferes with intestinal digoxin absorption). Products include:
Cama Arthritis Pain Reliever ... ■ 685
Gaviscon Extra Strength Relief Formula Liquid Antacid ... ■ 594
Gaviscon Extra Strength Relief Formula Antacid Tablets ... ■ 594
Gaviscon Liquid Antacid ... ■ 594
Gelusil Liquid & Tablets ... ■ 639
Extra Strength Maalox Plus Suspension ... 1850
Maalox TC Suspension ... 1851
Maalox Plus Tablets ... ■ 655
Extra Strength Maalox Plus Tablets 1850
Nephrox Suspension ... ■ 563
WinGel Liquid & Tablets ... ■ 761

Aluminum Hydroxide Gel (Interferes with intestinal digoxin absorption). Products include:
ALternaGEL Liquid ... 1154
Aludrox Oral Suspension ... 2428
Amphojel Suspension ... 2429
Amphojel Suspension without Flavor ... 2429
Mylanta Liquid ... 1155
Mylanta Double Strength Liquid ... 1155

Aluminum Hydroxide Gel, Dried (Interferes with intestinal digoxin absorption). Products include:
Alu-Tab/Alu-Cap ... 1309
Amphojel Tablets ... 2429
Ascriptin A/D Caplets ... 1850
Regular Strength Ascriptin Tablets 1850
Gaviscon Antacid Tablets ... ■ 593
Gaviscon-2 Antacid Tablets ... ■ 594
Mylanta Tablets ... 1155
Mylanta Double Strength Tablets ... 1155

Amiodarone Hydrochloride (Causes rise in serum digoxin concentration). Products include:
Cordarone Tablets ... 2446

Antibiotics, unspecified (Increases digoxin absorption in patients who inactivate digoxin by bacterial metabolism).

Anticancer Drugs, unspecified (Interferes with intestinal digoxin absorption).

Atenolol (Additive effects on AV node conduction). Products include:
Tenoretic Tablets ... 1105
Tenormin Tablets and I.V. Injection 1107

Bendroflumethiazide (Major contributing factor to digitalis toxicity). Products include:
Corzide Tablets ... 702
Naturetin Tablets ... 1789
Rauzide Tablets ... 1804

Bepridil Hydrochloride (Additive effects on AV node conduction). Products include:
Vascor (200, 300 and 400 mg) Tablets ... 1383

Betamethasone Acetate (Major contributing factor to digitalis toxicity). Products include:
Celestone Soluspan Suspension ... 2081

Betamethasone Sodium Phosphate (Major contributing factor to digitalis toxicity). Products include:
Celestone Soluspan Suspension ... 2081

Betaxolol Hydrochloride (Additive effects on AV node conduction). Products include:
Betoptic Sterile Ophthalmic Solution ... 569
Betoptic S Sterile Ophthalmic Suspension ... 570
Kerlone Tablets ... 2172

Calcium, intravenous (May produce serious arrhythmias in digitalized patients).

Carteolol Hydrochloride (Additive effects on AV node conduction). Products include:
Cartrol Tablets ... 507

Chlorothiazide (Major contributing factor to digitalis toxicity). Products include:
Aldoclor Tablets ... 1413
Diupres Tablets ... 1461
Diuril Oral ... 1464

Chlorothiazide Sodium (Major contributing factor to digitalis toxicity). Products include:
Diuril Sodium Intravenous ... 1463

Cholestyramine (Interferes with intestinal digoxin absorption). Products include:
Cholybar ... 1705
Questran Light ... 711
Questran Powder ... 710

Cortisone Acetate (Major contributing factor to digitalis toxicity). Products include:
Cortone Acetate Sterile Suspension ... 1437
Cortone Acetate Tablets ... 1439

Dexamethasone (Major contributing factor to digitalis toxicity). Products include:
AK-Trol Ointment & Suspension ... ⊙ 207
Decadron Elixir ... 1445
Decadron Tablets ... 1447
Decaspray Topical Aerosol ... 1459
Dexacidin ... ⊙ 272
Maxidex Sterile Ophthalmic Suspension ... ⊙ 223
Maxitrol Ophthalmic Ointment/Suspension ... ⊙ 223
TobraDex Ophthalmic Suspension and Ointment ... ⊙ 228

Dexamethasone Acetate (Major contributing factor to digitalis toxicity). Products include:
Dalalone D.P. Injectable ... 999
Decadron-LA Sterile Suspension ... 1457

Dexamethasone Sodium Phosphate (Major contributing factor to digitalis toxicity). Products include:
AK-Dex ... ⊙ 203
Decadron Phosphate Respihaler ... 1454
Decadron Phosphate Sterile Ophthalmic Ointment ... 1453
Decadron Phosphate Sterile Ophthalmic Solution ... 1453
Decadron Phosphate Topical Cream ... 1455
Decadron Phosphate Turbinaire ... 1456
Maxidex Sterile Ophthalmic Ointment ... ⊙ 222
NeoDecadron Sterile Ophthalmic Ointment ... 1517
NeoDecadron Sterile Ophthalmic Solution ... 1518
NeoDecadron Topical Cream ... 1518

Dihydroxyaluminum Sodium Carbonate (Interferes with intestinal digoxin absorption). Products include:
Rolaids ... ■ 743

Diltiazem Hydrochloride (Additive effects on AV node conduction). Products include:
Cardizem Tablets-30 mg, 60 mg, 90 mg and 120 mg ... 1329
Cardizem SR Capsules-60 mg, 90 mg and 120 mg ... 1327

Diphenoxylate Hydrochloride (Increases digoxin absorption). Products include:
Lomotil ... 2174

Dobutamine Hydrochloride (Increased risk of cardiac arrhythmias). Products include:
Dobutrex Solution Vials ... 1259

Dopamine Hydrochloride (Increased risk of cardiac arrhythmias). Products include:
Intropin Injection ... 930

Ephedrine Hydrochloride (Increased risk of cardiac arrhythmias). Products include:
Amesec ... ■ 682
Primatene Tablets-M Formula ... 2421
Primatene Tablets-P Formula ... 2421
Primatene Tablets-Regular Formula ... 2421
Quadrinal Tablets ... 1183
Quelidrine Syrup ... 556
Tedral SA ... 1765

Ephedrine Sulfate (Increased risk of cardiac arrhythmias). Products include:
Bronkaid Tablets ... ■ 757
Bronkolixir ... ■ 761
Bronkotabs Tablets ... ■ 762
Marax Tablets & DF Syrup ... 1954
Pazo Hemorrhoid Ointment & Suppositories ... 752
Vicks Vatronol Nose Drops ... ■ 666

Ephedrine Tannate (Increased risk of cardiac arrhythmias). Products include:
Rynatuss ... 2388

Epinephrine (Increased risk of cardiac arrhythmias). Products include:
Ana-Kit Anaphylaxis Emergency Treatment Kit ... 1100
Bronkaid Mist ... ■ 757
EpiPen ... 843
Marcaine Hydrochloride 0.5% with Epinephrine 1:200,000 (as bitartrate) ... 958
Marcaine Hydrochloride with Epinephrine 1:200,000 ... 2055
Primatene Mist ... 2420
Sus-Phrine Injection ... 1006
Xylocaine with Epinephrine Injections ... 637

Epinephrine Bitartrate (Increased risk of cardiac arrhythmias). Products include:
AsthmaHaler Mist Epinephrine Bitartrate Bronchodilator ... ■ 616
Bronkaid Mist Suspension ... ■ 757
Primatene Mist Suspension ... 2421

Epinephrine Hydrochloride (Increased risk of cardiac arrhythmias). Products include:
Adrenalin Chloride Solution 1:100 & 1:1,000 ... 1689
Epifrin ... ⊙ 244
Glaucon ... ⊙ 218

Esmolol Hydrochloride (Additive effects on AV node conduction). Products include:
Brevibloc Injection ... 942

Felodipine (Additive effects on AV node conduction). Products include:
Plendil Extended-Release Tablets ... 1526

Hydrochlorothiazide (Major contributing factor to digitalis toxicity). Products include:
Aldactazide ... 2150
Aldoril Tablets ... 1418
Apresazide Capsules ... 854
Apresoline-Esidrix Tablets ... 857
Capozide ... 2258
Dyazide Capsules ... 2208
Esidrix Tablets ... 863
Esimil Tablets ... 864
HydroDIURIL Tablets ... 1484
Hydropres Tablets ... 1485
Inderide Tablets ... 2463
Inderide LA Long Acting Capsules .. 2465
Lopressor HCT Tablets ... 1034
Maxzide ... 1215
Moduretic Tablets ... 1510
Normozide Tablets ... 2112
Oretic Tablets ... 544
Oreticyl ... 545
Prinzide Tablets ... 1540
Ser-Ap-Es Tablets ... 881
Serpasil-Esidrix Tablets ... 886
Timolide Tablets ... 1547
Trandate HCT Tablets ... 579
Vaseretic Tablets ... 1559
Zestoretic ... 2274

Hydrocortisone (Major contributing factor to digitalis toxicity). Products include:
AK-Spore H.C. ... ⊙ 206
Bactine Hydrocortisone Anti-Itch Cream ... ■ 625
CaldeCORT Anti-Itch Hydrocortisone Spray ... ■ 560
Carmol HC Cream 1% ... 2296
Cortaid Spray ... ■ 735
Cortenema ... 2244
Cortisporin Ointment ... 758
Cortisporin Ophthalmic Ointment Sterile ... 758
Cortisporin Ophthalmic Suspension Sterile ... 759
Cortisporin Otic Solution Sterile ... 760
Cortisporin Otic Suspension Sterile 760
Cortizone-5 Creme & Ointment ... ■ 732
Dermolate Anti-Itch Cream ... ■ 697
Eldecort Cream 1.0% ... 1113
Eldecort Cream 1.0% and 2.5% ... 1113
Fungoid HC Creme ... 1770
Hydrocortone Tablets ... 1482
Hytone ... 909
LazerSporin-C Solution ... 1770
Massengill Medicated Soft Cloth Towelettes ... 2192
Nutracort Cream & Lotion ... 1684
PediOtic Suspension Sterile ... 797
Synacort Creams 1%, 2.5% ... 2296
Vanoxide-HC Acne Lotion ... 911
Vioform-Hydrocortisone Cream and Mild Cream ... 889
Vioform-Hydrocortisone Ointment .. 889
VōSoL HC Otic Solution ... 2392
Vytone Cream 1% ... 911

Hydrocortisone Acetate (Major contributing factor to digitalis toxicity). Products include:
Analpram-HC Rectal Cream 1% and 2.5% ... 970
Anusol-HC Cream ... 1690
Anusol-HC Suppositories ... 1691
Caldecort ... ■ 560
Carmol HC Cream 1% ... 2296
Chloromycetin Hydrocortisone Ophthalmic ... 1694

Coly-Mycin S Otic w/Neomycin & Hydrocortisone 1708
Cortaid ▣ 735
Cortef Feminine Itch Cream ▣ 735
Corticaine ▣ 682
Cortifoam 1827
Cortisporin Cream 757
Epifoam 1828
Gynecort 5 Creme ▣ 556
Hydrocortone Acetate Sterile Suspension 1479
Lanacort 5 Creme and Ointment ▣ 557
Mantadil Cream 789
Ophthocort ⊙ 301
Orabase HCA Oral Paste 890
Pramosone Cream, Lotion & Ointment 971
ProctoCream-HC 1834
Proctofoam-HC 1835

Hydrocortisone Sodium Phosphate (Major contributing factor to digitalis toxicity). Products include:
Hydrocortone Phosphate Injection, Sterile 1481

Hydrocortisone Sodium Succinate (Major contributing factor to digitalis toxicity). Products include:
Solu-Cortef Sterile Powder 2361

Hydroflumethiazide (Major contributing factor to digitalis toxicity). Products include:
Diucardin Tablets 2450
Saluron 718
Salutensin/Salutensin-Demi 719

Isoproterenol Hydrochloride (Increased risk of cardiac arrhythmias). Products include:
Isuprel Hydrochloride Injection 1:5000 2050
Isuprel Hydrochloride Mistometer 2051
Isuprel Hydrochloride Solution 1:200 & 1:100 2052
Norisodrine Aerotrol 540

Isradipine (Additive effects on AV node conduction). Products include:
DynaCirc Capsules 2004

Labetalol Hydrochloride (Additive effects on AV node conduction). Products include:
Normodyne Injection 2108
Normodyne Tablets 2110
Normozide Tablets 2112
Trandate HCT Tablets 579
Trandate Injection 577
Trandate Tablets 579

Levothyroxine Sodium (Hypothyroid patients may require increased digoxin dose). Products include:
Levothroid Tablets 1003
Levoxine Tablets 904
Synthroid 695

Liothyronine Sodium (Hypothyroid patients may require increased digoxin dose). Products include:
Cytomel Tablets 2203

Liotrix (Hypothyroid patients may require increased digoxin dose). Products include:
Euthroid 1724

Magaldrate (Interferes with intestinal digoxin absorption). Products include:
Riopan Antacid Chew Tablets ▣ 754
Riopan Antacid Chew Tablets in Rollpacks ▣ 754
Riopan Antacid Suspension 2421
Riopan Antacid Swallow Tablets 2421
Riopan Plus Chew Tablets 2422
Riopan Plus Chew Tablets in Rollpack 2422
Riopan Plus 2 Chew Tablets, Mint Flavor, Cherry Flavor 2422
Riopan Plus Suspension 2422
Riopan Plus 2 Suspension, Mint Flavor, Cherry Flavor 2422

Magnesium Hydroxide (Interferes with intestinal digoxin absorption). Products include:
Aludrox Oral Suspension 2428
Ascriptin A/D Caplets 1850
Regular Strength Ascriptin Tablets 1850
Di-Gel Antacid/Anti-Gas ▣ 697
Gelusil Liquid & Tablets ▣ 639
Haley's M-O, Regular & Flavored ▣ 569
Extra Strength Maalox Plus Suspension 1850
Maalox TC Suspension 1851
Maalox Plus Tablets ▣ 655
Extra Strength Maalox Plus Tablets 1850
Mylanta Liquid 1155
Mylanta Tablets 1155
Mylanta Double Strength Liquid 1155
Mylanta Double Strength Tablets 1155
Concentrated Phillips' Milk of Magnesia ▣ 573
Phillips' Milk of Magnesia Liquid ▣ 572
Phillips' Milk of Magnesia Tablets ▣ 573
WinGel Liquid & Tablets ▣ 761

Magnesium Oxide (Interferes with intestinal digoxin absorption). Products include:
Bayer Plus Aspirin Tablets ▣ 567
Beelith Tablets 659
Bufferin Analgesic Tablets and Caplets ▣ 524
Cama Arthritis Pain Reliever ▣ 685
Mag-Ox 400 673
Uro-Mag 673

Metaproterenol Sulfate (Increased risk of cardiac arrhythmias). Products include:
Alupent 674
Arm-a-Med Metaproterenol Sulfate Inhalation Solution, USP 617
Metaprel Inhalation Aerosol Bronchodilator 2014
Metaprel Inhalation Solution 2015
Metaprel 2015
Metaproterenol Sulfate Inhalation Solution, USP 912

Metaraminol Bitartrate (Increased risk of cardiac arrhythmias). Products include:
Aramine Injection 1424

Methoxamine Hydrochloride (Increased risk of cardiac arrhythmias). Products include:
Vasoxyl Injection 819

Methyclothiazide (Major contributing factor to digitalis toxicity). Products include:
Enduron Tablets 517
Enduronyl 518

Methylprednisolone Acetate (Major contributing factor to digitalis toxicity). Products include:
Depo-Medrol Sterile Aqueous Suspension 2334

Methylprednisolone Sodium Succinate (Major contributing factor to digitalis toxicity). Products include:
Solu-Medrol Sterile Powder 2363

Metoprolol Tartrate (Additive effects on AV node conduction). Products include:
Lopressor Ampuls 1032
Lopressor HCT Tablets 1034
Lopressor Tablets 1032

Nadolol (Additive effects on AV node conduction). Products include:
Corgard Tablets 701
Corzide Tablets 702

Neomycin, oral (Interferes with intestinal digoxin absorption).

Nephrotoxic Drugs (May impair the excretion of digoxin).

Nicardipine Hydrochloride (Additive effects on AV node conduction). Products include:
Cardene Capsules 2290

Nifedipine (Additive effects on AV node conduction). Products include:
Adalat Capsules (10 mg and 20 mg) 1587
Procardia Capsules 1781
Procardia XL Tablets 1783

Nimodipine (Additive effects on AV node conduction). Products include:
Nimotop Capsules 1607

Norepinephrine Bitartrate (Increased risk of cardiac arrhythmias). Products include:
Levophed Bitartrate Injection 2054

Pectin (Low digoxin serum concentration; interferes with intestinal digoxin absorption). Products include:
Donnagel ▣ 675
Donnagel-PG 1858

Penbutolol Sulfate (Additive effects on AV node conduction). Products include:
Levatol 1832

Phenylephrine Bitartrate (Increased risk of cardiac arrhythmias).
No products indexed under this heading.

Phenylephrine Hydrochloride (Increased risk of cardiac arrhythmias). Products include:
AK-Dilate Solution 2.5% and 10% ⊙ 203
Atrohist Sprinkle Capsules 558
Cerose-DM 2443
Codimal 846
Comhist LA Capsules 1618
Congespirin For Children Aspirin Free Chewable Cold Tablets 748
Cyclomydril ⊙ 216
Deconsal Sprinkle Capsules 559
Dimetane Decongestant ▣ 673
Dristan Decongestant/Antihistamine/ Analgesic Coated Caplets ▣ 749
Dristan Cold Nasal Decongestant/ Antihistamine/ Analgesic Coated Tablets 2419
Dristan Advanced Formula Decongestant/Antihistamine/ Analgesic Tablets ▣ 749
Dristan Nasal Spray, Menthol 2419
Dristan Nasal Spray, Regular and Regular with Metered Pump 2419
Entex Capsules 1623
Entex Liquid 1623
Sinus Excedrin Analgesic, Decongestant Tablets & Caplets 750
Extendryl 994
4-Way Fast Acting Nasal Spray - Original Formula (regular & mentholated) & Metered Spray Pump (regular) 751
Hycomine Compound Tablets 929
Murocoll-2 Sterile Ophthalmic Solution ⊙ 261
Mydfrin 2.5% ⊙ 224
Naldecon Syrup, Tablets, Pediatric Drops and Pediatric Syrup 709
Neo-Synephrine Hydrochloride 1% Carpuject 2063
Neo-Synephrine Hydrochloride 1% Injection 2063
Neo-Synephrine Hydrochloride (Ophthalmic) 2064
Neo-Synephrine ▣ 759
Nōstril Nasal Decongestant ▣ 520
Novahistine Elixir ▣ 596
Phenergan VC 2500
Phenergan VC with Codeine 2501
Prefrin Liquifilm Vasoconstrictor and Lubricant Eye Drops ⊙ 254
Prefrin-A ⊙ 255
Quelidrine Syrup 556
Relief Vasoconstrictor and Lubricant Eye Drops ⊙ 256
Robitussin Night Relief ▣ 677
Ru-Tuss with Hydrocodone 694
Ru-Tuss Tablets 693
Vasosulf ⊙ 279
Vicks Sinex ▣ 665
Zincfrin ⊙ 230

Phenylephrine Tannate (Increased risk of cardiac arrhythmias). Products include:
Rynatan 2387
Rynatuss 2388

Phenylpropanolamine Hydrochloride (Increased risk of cardiac arrhythmias). Products include:
A.R.M. Allergy Relief Medicine Caplets ▣ 615
Acutrim ▣ 548
Allerest ▣ 559
BC Cold Powder ▣ 517
Cheracol Plus Head Cold/Cough Formula ▣ 667
Codimal Expectorant 846
Comtrex Multi-Symptom Cold Reliever Tablets/Caplets/Liqui-Gels/Liquid 745
Contac Continuous Action Decongestant/Antihistamine Capsules ▣ 710
Contac Maximum Strength Continuous Action Decongestant/ Antihistamine Caplets ▣ 709
Contac Severe Cold and Flu Formula Caplets ▣ 711
Coricidin 'D' Decongestant Tablets ▣ 695
Coricidin Demilets Tablets for Children ▣ 696
Demazin Nasal Decongestant/ Antihistamine Repetabs Tablets & Syrup ▣ 697
Dexatrim ▣ 733
Dimetane-DC Cough Syrup 1857
Dimetapp Elixir ▣ 673
Dimetapp DM Elixir ▣ 674
Dimetapp Extentabs ▣ 674
Dimetapp Plus Caplets ▣ 675
Dimetapp Tablets ▣ 675
Entex Capsules 1623
Entex LA Tablets 1623
Entex Liquid 1623
4-Way Cold Tablets 750
Hycomine Syrup 927
Naldecon CX Adult Liquid ▣ 521
Naldecon DX Adult Liquid ▣ 521
Naldecon DX Children's Syrup ▣ 522
Naldecon DX Pediatric Drops ▣ 522
Naldecon EX Children's Syrup ▣ 522
Naldecon EX Pediatric Drops ▣ 523
Naldecon Syrup, Tablets, Pediatric Drops and Pediatric Syrup 709
Nolamine Tablets 838
Nolex LA Tablets 838
Ornade Spansule Capsules 2221
Orthoxicol Cough Syrup ▣ 668
Propagest 839
Pyrroxate Capsules ▣ 669
Robitussin-CF ▣ 676
Ru-Tuss II Capsules 693
Ru-Tuss with Hydrocodone 694
Ru-Tuss Tablets 693
Sine-Off Sinus Medicine Tablets-Aspirin Formula ▣ 722
Sinulin 840
St. Joseph Cold Tablets for Children ▣ 704
Tavist-D Tablets 2035
Triaminic Allergy Tablets ▣ 688
Triaminic Chewables ▣ 688
Triaminic Cold Tablets ▣ 688
Triaminic Expectorant ▣ 688
Triaminic Expectorant w/Codeine 1996
Triaminic Expectorant DH 1995
Triaminic Oral Infant Drops 1996
Triaminic Syrup ▣ 689
Triaminic-12 Tablets ▣ 690
Triaminic-DM Syrup ▣ 689
Triaminicin Tablets ▣ 690
Triaminicol Multi-Symptom Cold Tablets ▣ 691
Triaminicol Multi-Symptom Relief ▣ 691
Tuss-Ornade Liquid 2242
Tuss-Ornade Spansule Capsules 2242
Tylenol Cold Medication, Effervescent Tablets 1369

Pindolol (Additive effects on AV node conduction). Products include:
Visken Tablets 2036

Pirbuterol Acetate (Increased risk of cardiac arrhythmias). Products include:
Maxair Inhaler 1311

Polythiazide (Major contributing factor to digitalis toxicity). Products include:
Minizide Capsules 1779
Renese Tablets 1785
Renese-R Tablets 1786

Prednisolone Acetate (Major contributing factor to digitalis toxicity). Products include:
AK-Cide Sterile Ophthalmic Ointment & Suspension ⊙ 202
Blephamide Liquifilm Sterile Ophthalmic Suspension 586
Blephamide S.O.P. Sterile Ophthalmic Ointment 586
Cetapred Ointment ⊙ 220
⅛% Econopred & 1% Econopred Plus ⊙ 217
Isopto Cetapred Suspension ⊙ 220
Metimyd ⊙ 306
Poly-Pred Liquifilm ⊙ 250
Pred Forte ⊙ 252
Pred Mild ⊙ 254

Pred-G Liquifilm Sterile Ophthalmic Suspension ⊙ 252
Pred-G S.O.P. Sterile Ophthalmic Ointment ⊙ 253
Vasocidin Ointment ⊙ 275

Prednisolone Sodium Phosphate (Major contributing factor to digitalis toxicity). Products include:
AK-Pred ⊙ 205
Hydeltrasol Injection, Sterile 1476
Inflamase ⊙ 274
Pediapred Oral Liquid 987
Vasocidin Ophthalmic Solution ⊙ 276

Prednisolone Tebutate (Major contributing factor to digitalis toxicity). Products include:
Hydeltra-T.B.A. Sterile Suspension 1478

Prednisone (Major contributing factor to digitalis toxicity). Products include:
Deltasone Tablets 2332

Propantheline Bromide (Increases digoxin absorption). Products include:
Pro-Banthīne Tablets 2141

Propranolol Hydrochloride (Additive effects on AV node conduction). Products include:
Inderal 2459
Inderal LA Long Acting Capsules 2461
Inderide Tablets 2463
Inderide LA Long Acting Capsules 2465

Pseudoephedrine Hydrochloride (Increased risk of cardiac arrhythmias). Products include:
Actifed Capsules ▣ 539
Actifed Plus Caplets ▣ 539
Actifed Plus Tablets ▣ 540
Actifed with Codeine Cough Syrup 752
Actifed Syrup ▣ 540
Actifed Tablets ▣ 540
Actifed 12-Hour Capsules ▣ 539
Advil Cold & Sinus Caplets (formerly CoAdvil) 2416
Allerest ▣ 559
Anatuss LA Tablets 1359
Benadryl Decongestant Elixir ▣ 635
Benadryl Decongestant ▣ 635
Benadryl Plus ▣ 636
Benadryl Plus Nighttime ▣ 637
Benylin Decongestant ▣ 638
Brexin L.A. Capsules 2078
Bromfed Capsules (Timed Release) 1615
Bromfed Syrup ▣ 628
Bromfed 1615
CoAdvil ▣ 748
Allergy-Sinus Comtrex Multi-Symptom Allergy Sinus Formula Tablets & Caplets 746
Cough Formula Comtrex 746
Comtrex Multi-Symptom Cold Reliever Tablets/Caplets/Liqui-Gels/Liquid 745
Day-Night Comtrex 747
Non-Drowsy Comtrex 747
Congess 994
Congestac Caplets ▣ 617
Contac Jr. Children's Cold Medicine ▣ 712
Contac Nighttime Cold Medicine ▣ 713
Contac Sinus Caplets Maximum Strength Non-Drowsy Formula ▣ 710
Contac Sinus Tablets Maximum Strength Non-Drowsy Formula ▣ 710
Deconamine 663
Deconsal II Tablets 559
Dimacol Caplets ▣ 672
Dimetane-DX Cough Syrup 1858
Dorcol Children's Cough Syrup ▣ 685
Dorcol Children's Decongestant Liquid ▣ 685
Dorcol Children's Liquid Cold Formula ▣ 686
Maximum Strength Dristan Decongestant/Analgesic Coated Caplets ▣ 750
No Drowsiness Dristan Cold Nasal Decongestant/Analgesic Coated Caplets 2420
Dristan Sinus Caplets 2419
Sinus Excedrin Analgesic, Decongestant Tablets & Caplets ▣ 533
Fedahist Gyrocaps 2145
Fedahist Timecaps 2145
Guaifed 1615
Guaifed Syrup ▣ 629
Isoclor Expectorant 982
Isoclor Timesule Capsules ▣ 561
Kronofed-A 970
Medi-Flu Caplet, Liquid ▣ 640
Novafed A Capsules 1342
Novafed Capsules 1342
Novahistine DH 1342
Novahistine DMX ▣ 595
Novahistine Expectorant 1343
Nucofed Capsules 2219
Nucofed Expectorant 2219
Nucofed Pediatric Expectorant 2220
Nucofed Syrup 2219
Ornex Caplets ▣ 618
PediaCare Allergy Relief Formula Liquid 1362
PediaCare Cough-Cold Formula Liquid 1362
PediaCare Infants' Oral Decongestant Drops 1362
PediaCare Night Rest Cough-Cold Formula Liquid 1362
PediaCare 6-12 Cough-Cold Formula Chewable Tablets 1362
Robitussin-DAC Syrup 1875
Robitussin-PE ▣ 677
Rondec 1975
Rondec-DM 1976
Rondec-TR Tablet 1975
Ru-Tuss DE Tablets 694
Ryna ▣ 741
Seldane-D Extended-Release Tablets 1350
Sinarest ▣ 562
Sine-Aid Maximum Strength Sinus Headache Caplets 1365
Sine-Aid Maximum Strength Sinus Headache Tablets 1365
Sine-Off Maximum Strength Allergy/Sinus Formula Caplets ▣ 721
Sine-Off Maximum Strength No Drowsiness Formula Caplets ▣ 722
Singlet Tablets ▣ 598
Sinutab Maximum Strength ▣ 641
Sinutab Maximum Strength Without Drowsiness Tablets & Caplets ▣ 642
Sinutab Regular Strength Without Drowsiness Formula ▣ 641
St. Joseph Nighttime Cold Medicine ▣ 705
Sudafed Children's Liquid ▣ 543
Sudafed Cough Syrup ▣ 543
Sudafed Plus Liquid ▣ 544
Sudafed Plus Tablets ▣ 545
Sudafed Sinus Caplets ▣ 545
Sudafed Sinus Tablets ▣ 545
Sudafed Tablets, 30 mg ▣ 544
Sudafed Tablets, Adult Strength, 60 mg ▣ 544
Sudafed 12 Hour Capsules ▣ 545
TheraFlu Flu and Cold Medicine ▣ 687
Triaminic Nite Light ▣ 689
Tylenol Allergy Sinus Medication Caplets and Gelcaps, Maximum Strength 1372
Children's Tylenol Cold Liquid Formula and Chewable Tablets 1368
Tylenol Cold & Flu Hot Medication, Packets 1369
Tylenol Cold & Flu No Drowsiness Hot Medication, Packets 1371
Tylenol Cold Medication Caplets and Tablets 1370
Tylenol Cold Medication No Drowsiness Formula Caplets 1370
Tylenol Cold Night Time Medication Liquid 1371
Tylenol Cough Medication Liquid with Decongestant, Maximum Strength 1372
Tylenol, Maximum Strength, Sinus Medication Gelcaps, Caplets and Tablets 1373
Ursinus Inlay-Tabs ▣ 691
Vicks Children's NyQuil ▣ 664
Vicks Daycare ▣ 660
Vicks Formula 44D Decongestant Cough Medicine ▣ 662
Vicks Formula 44M Multi-Symptom Cough Medicine ▣ 662
Vicks NyQuil Nighttime Colds Medicine-Original & Cherry Flavor ▣ 664
Vicks Pediatric Formula 44 Cough & Congestion Medicine ▣ 663
Vicks Pediatric Formula 44m Multi-Symptom Cough & Cold Medicine ▣ 663

Pseudoephedrine Sulfate (Increased risk of cardiac arrhythmias). Products include:
Afrin Tablets ▣ 693
Chlor-Trimeton Decongestant ▣ 694
Disophrol Chronotab Sustained-Action Tablets ▣ 698
Drixoral Antihistamine/Nasal Decongestant Syrup ▣ 698
Drixoral Non-Drowsy Formula ▣ 699
Drixoral Plus Extended-Release Tablets ▣ 699
Drixoral Sinus ▣ 700
Drixoral Sustained-Action Tablets ▣ 698
Sinutab Allergy Formula Sustained Action Tablets ▣ 640
Trinalin Repetabs Tablets 1170

Quinidine Gluconate (Causes rise in serum digoxin concentration). Products include:
Quinaglute Dura-Tabs Tablets 663

Quinidine Polygalacturonate (Causes rise in serum digoxin concentration). Products include:
Cardioquin Tablets 1812

Quinidine Sulfate (Causes rise in serum digoxin concentration). Products include:
Quinidex Extentabs 1868

Sodium Bicarbonate (Interferes with intestinal digoxin absorption). Products include:
Alka-Seltzer Advanced Formula Antacid & Non-Aspirin Pain Reliever ▣ 620
Alka-Seltzer Effervescent Antacid ▣ 622
Alka-Seltzer Effervescent Antacid and Pain Reliever 1568
Alka-Seltzer Extra Strength Effervescent Antacid and Pain Reliever ▣ 623
Alka-Seltzer (Flavored) Effervescent Antacid and Pain Reliever ▣ 621
Arm & Hammer Pure Baking Soda ▣ 548
Ceo-Two Rectal Suppositories 671
Citrocarbonate Antacid ▣ 668
Massengill Liquid Concentrate 2191
NuLYTELY 699

Succinylcholine Chloride (May cause arrhythmias). Products include:
Anectine 755

Sulfasalazine (Low digoxin serum concentration; interferes with intestinal digoxin absorption). Products include:
Azulfidine Tablets, EN-tabs, Oral Suspension 1157

Terbutaline Sulfate (Increased risk of cardiac arrhythmias). Products include:
Brethaire Inhaler 1024
Brethine Ampuls 1026
Brethine Tablets 1026
Bricanyl Injection 1324
Bricanyl Tablets 1325

Thyroglobulin (Hypothyroid patients may require increased digoxin dose). Products include:
Proloid Tablets 1761

Thyroid (Hypothyroid patients may require increased digoxin dose). Products include:
S-P-T "Liquid" Capsules 995

Thyroxine (Hypothyroid patients may require increased digoxin dose).
No products indexed under this heading.

Thyroxine Sodium (Hypothyroid patients may require increased digoxin dose).
No products indexed under this heading.

Timolol Maleate (Additive effects on AV node conduction). Products include:
Blocadren Tablets 1429
Timolide Tablets 1547
Timoptic in Ocudose 1552
Timoptic Sterile Ophthalmic Solution 1550

Triamcinolone (Major contributing factor to digitalis toxicity).
No products indexed under this heading.

Triamcinolone Acetonide (Major contributing factor to digitalis toxicity). Products include:
Aristocort A 1010
Azmacort Inhaler 1837
Kenalog Cream, Lotion & Ointment 2401
Kenalog-10 Injection 2402
Kenalog-40 Injection 2403
Kenalog in Orabase 604
Kenalog Spray 2401
Mycolog II Cream and Ointment 2407
Mytrex Cream & Ointment 2080
Nasacort Nasal Inhaler 1844

Triamcinolone Diacetate (Major contributing factor to digitalis toxicity). Products include:
Aristocort Suspension 1008

Triamcinolone Hexacetonide (Major contributing factor to digitalis toxicity). Products include:
Aristospan Suspension 1011

Verapamil Hydrochloride (Additive effects on AV node conduction; causes rise in serum digoxin concentration). Products include:
Calan SR Caplets 2157
Calan Tablets 2155
Isoptin Injectable 1177
Isoptin Oral Tablets 1179
Isoptin SR Sustained Release Tablets 1181
Verelan Capsules 1243
Verelan Capsules 2535

LANOXIN TABLETS
(Digoxin) 783
May interact with potassium-depleting corticosteroids, potassium-depleting diuretics, antacids, sympathomimetic aerosal brochodilators, beta blockers, calcium channel blockers, thyroid preparations, mineralocorticoids, and certain other agents. Compounds in these categories include:

Acebutolol Hydrochloride (Additive effects on AV node conduction). Products include:
Sectral Capsules 2520

Albuterol (Increased risk of cardiac arrhythmias). Products include:
Proventil Inhalation Aerosol 2117
Ventolin Inhalation Aerosol and Refill 583

Albuterol Sulfate (Increased risk of cardiac arrhythmias). Products include:
Proventil Repetabs Tablets 2120
Proventil Solutions for Inhalation 0.5% and 0.083% 2118
Proventil Syrup 2119
Proventil Tablets 2120
Ventolin 583

Aluminum Carbonate Gel (Interferes with intestinal digoxin absorption). Products include:
Basaljel 2438

Aluminum Hydroxide (Interferes with intestinal digoxin absorption). Products include:
Cama Arthritis Pain Reliever ▣ 685
Gaviscon Extra Strength Relief Formula Liquid Antacid ▣ 594
Gaviscon Extra Strength Relief Formula Antacid Tablets ▣ 594
Gaviscon Liquid Antacid ▣ 594
Gelusil Liquid & Tablets ▣ 639
Extra Strength Maalox Plus Suspension 1850
Maalox TC Suspension 1851
Maalox Plus Tablets ▣ 655
Extra Strength Maalox Plus Tablets 1850
Nephrox Suspension ▣ 563
WinGel Liquid & Tablets ▣ 761

Aluminum Hydroxide Gel (Interferes with intestinal digoxin absorption). Products include:
ALternaGEL Liquid 1154
Aludrox Oral Suspension 2428

Amphojel Suspension 2429
Amphojel Suspension without Flavor 2429
Mylanta Liquid 1155
Mylanta Double Strength Liquid 1155

Aluminum Hydroxide Gel, Dried (Interferes with intestinal digoxin absorption). Products include:
Alu-Tab/Alu-Cap 1309
Amphojel Tablets 2429
Ascriptin A/D Caplets 1850
Regular Strength Ascriptin Tablets 1850
Gaviscon Antacid Tablets ⊞ 593
Gaviscon-2 Antacid Tablets ⊞ 594
Mylanta Tablets 1155
Mylanta Double Strength Tablets 1155

Amiodarone Hydrochloride (Causes rise in serum digoxin concentration). Products include:
Cordarone Tablets 2446

Antibiotics, unspecified (Increases digoxin absorption in patients who inactivate digoxin by bacterial metabolism).

Anticancer Drugs, unspecified (Interferes with intestinal digoxin absorption).

Atenolol (Additive effects on AV node conduction). Products include:
Tenoretic Tablets 1105
Tenormin Tablets and I.V. Injection 1107

Bendroflumethiazide (Major contributing factor to digitalis toxicity). Products include:
Corzide Tablets 702
Naturetin Tablets 1789
Rauzide Tablets 1804

Bepridil Hydrochloride (Additive effects on AV node conduction). Products include:
Vascor (200, 300 and 400 mg) Tablets 1383

Betamethasone Acetate (Major contributing factor to digitalis toxicity). Products include:
Celestone Soluspan Suspension 2081

Betamethasone Sodium Phosphate (Major contributing factor to digitalis toxicity). Products include:
Celestone Soluspan Suspension 2081

Betaxolol Hydrochloride (Additive effects on AV node conduction). Products include:
Betoptic Sterile Ophthalmic Solution 569
Betoptic S Sterile Ophthalmic Suspension 570
Kerlone Tablets 2172

Calcium, intravenous (May produce serious arrhythmias in digitalized patients).

Carteolol Hydrochloride (Additive effects on AV node conduction). Products include:
Cartrol Tablets 507

Chlorothiazide (Major contributing factor to digitalis toxicity). Products include:
Aldoclor Tablets 1413
Diupres Tablets 1461
Diuril Oral 1464

Chlorothiazide Sodium (Major contributing factor to digitalis toxicity). Products include:
Diuril Sodium Intravenous 1463

Cholestyramine (Interferes with intestinal digoxin absorption). Products include:
Cholybar 1705
Questran Light 711
Questran Powder 710

Cortisone Acetate (Major contributing factor to digitalis toxicity). Products include:
Cortone Acetate Sterile Suspension 1437
Cortone Acetate Tablets 1439

Dexamethasone (Major contributing factor to digitalis toxicity). Products include:
AK-Trol Ointment & Suspension ◉ 207
Decadron Elixir 1445
Decadron Tablets 1447
Decaspray Topical Aerosol 1459
Dexacidin ◉ 272
Maxidex Sterile Ophthalmic Suspension ◉ 223
Maxitrol Ophthalmic Ointment/Suspension ◉ 223
TobraDex Ophthalmic Suspension and Ointment ◉ 228

Dexamethasone Acetate (Major contributing factor to digitalis toxicity). Products include:
Dalalone D.P. Injectable 999
Decadron-LA Sterile Suspension 1457

Dexamethasone Sodium Phosphate (Major contributing factor to digitalis toxicity). Products include:
AK-Dex ◉ 203
Decadron Phosphate Respihaler 1454
Decadron Phosphate Sterile Ophthalmic Ointment 1453
Decadron Phosphate Sterile Ophthalmic Solution 1453
Decadron Phosphate Topical Cream 1455
Decadron Phosphate Turbinaire 1456
Maxidex Sterile Ophthalmic Ointment ◉ 222
NeoDecadron Sterile Ophthalmic Ointment 1517
NeoDecadron Sterile Ophthalmic Solution 1518
NeoDecadron Topical Cream 1518

Dihydroxyaluminum Sodium Carbonate (Interfers with intestinal digoxin absorption). Products include:
Rolaids ⊞ 743

Diltiazem Hydrochloride (Additive effects on AV node conduction). Products include:
Cardizem Tablets-30 mg, 60 mg, 90 mg and 120 mg 1329
Cardizem SR Capsules-60 mg, 90 mg and 120 mg 1327

Diphenoxylate Hydrochloride (Increases digoxin absorption). Products include:
Lomotil 2174

Dobutamine Hydrochloride (Increased risk of cardiac arrhythmias). Products include:
Dobutrex Solution Vials 1259

Dopamine Hydrochloride (Increased risk of cardiac arrhythmias). Products include:
Intropin Injection 930

Ephedrine Hydrochloride (Increased risk of cardiac arrhythmias). Products include:
Amesec ⊞ 682
Primatene Tablets-M Formula 2421
Primatene Tablets-P Formula 2421
Primatene Tablets-Regular Formula 2421
Quadrinal Tablets 1183
Quelidrine Syrup 556
Tedral SA 1765

Ephedrine Sulfate (Increased risk of cardiac arrhythmias). Products include:
Bronkaid Tablets ⊞ 757
Bronkolixir ⊞ 761
Bronkotabs Tablets ⊞ 762
Marax Tablets & DF Syrup 1954
Pazo Hemorrhoid Ointment & Suppositories 752
Vicks Vatronol Nose Drops ⊞ 666

Ephedrine Tannate (Increased risk of cardiac arrhythmias). Products include:
Rynatuss 2388

Epinephrine (Increased risk of cardiac arrhythmias). Products include:
Ana-Kit Anaphylaxis Emergency Treatment Kit 1100
Bronkaid Mist ⊞ 757
EpiPen 843
Marcaine Hydrochloride 0.5% with Epinephrine 1:200,000 (as bitartrate) 958
Marcaine Hydrochloride with Epinephrine 1:200,000 2055
Primatene Mist 2420
Sus-Phrine Injection 1006
Xylocaine with Epinephrine Injections 637

Epinephrine Bitartrate (Increased risk of cardiac arrhythmias). Products include:
AsthmaHaler Mist Epinephrine Bitartrate Bronchodilator ⊞ 616
Bronkaid Mist Suspension ⊞ 757
Primatene Mist Suspension 2421

Epinephrine Hydrochloride (Increased risk of cardiac arrhythmias). Products include:
Adrenalin Chloride Solution 1:100 & 1:1,000 1689
Epifrin ◉ 244
Glaucon ◉ 218

Esmolol Hydrochloride (Additive effects on AV node conduction). Products include:
Brevibloc Injection 942

Felodipine (Additive effects on AV node conduction). Products include:
Plendil Extended-Release Tablets 1526

Hydrochlorothiazide (Major contributing factor to digitalis toxicity). Products include:
Aldactazide 2150
Aldoril Tablets 1418
Apresazide Capsules 854
Apresoline-Esidrix Tablets 857
Capozide 2258
Dyazide Capsules 2208
Esidrix Tablets 863
Esimil Tablets 864
HydroDIURIL Tablets 1484
Hydropres Tablets 1485
Inderide Tablets 2463
Inderide LA Long Acting Capsules 2465
Lopressor HCT Tablets 1034
Maxzide 1215
Moduretic Tablets 1510
Normozide Tablets 2112
Oretic Tablets 544
Oreticyl 545
Prinzide Tablets 1540
Ser-Ap-Es Tablets 881
Serpasil-Esidrix Tablets 886
Timolide Tablets 1547
Trandate HCT Tablets 579
Vaseretic Tablets 1559
Zestoretic 2274

Hydrocortisone (Major contributing factor to digitalis toxicity). Products include:
AK-Spore H.C. ◉ 206
Bactine Hydrocortisone Anti-Itch Cream ⊞ 625
CaldeCORT Anti-Itch Hydrocortisone Spray ⊞ 560
Carmol HC Cream 1% 2296
Cortaid Spray ⊞ 735
Cortenema 2244
Cortisporin Ointment 758
Cortisporin Ophthalmic Ointment Sterile 758
Cortisporin Ophthalmic Suspension Sterile 759
Cortisporin Otic Solution Sterile 760
Cortisporin Otic Suspension Sterile 760
Cortizone-5 Creme & Ointment ⊞ 732
Dermolate Anti-Itch Cream ⊞ 697
Eldecort Cream 1.0% 1113
Eldecort Cream 1.0% and 2.5% 1113
Fungoid HC Creme 1770
Hydrocortone Tablets 1482
Hytone 909
LazerSporin-C Solution 1770
Massengill Medicated Soft Cloth Towelettes 2192
Nutracort Cream & Lotion 1684
PediOtic Suspension Sterile 797
Synacort Creams 1%, 2.5% 2296
Vanoxide-HC Acne Lotion 911
Vioform-Hydrocortisone Cream and Mild Cream 889
Vioform-Hydrocortisone Ointment 889
VōSoL HC Otic Solution 2392
Vytone Cream 1% 911

Hydrocortisone Acetate (Major contributing factor to digitalis toxicity). Products include:
Analpram-HC Rectal Cream 1% and 2.5% 970
Anusol-HC Cream 1690
Anusol-HC Suppositories 1691
Caldecort ⊞ 560
Carmol HC Cream 1% 2296
Chloromycetin Hydrocortisone Ophthalmic 1694
Coly-Mycin S Otic w/Neomycin & Hydrocortisone 1708
Cortaid ⊞ 735
Cortef Feminine Itch Cream ⊞ 735
Corticaine ⊞ 682
Cortifoam 1827
Cortisporin Cream 757
Epifoam 1828
Gynecort 5 Creme ⊞ 556
Hydrocortone Acetate Sterile Suspension 1479
Lanacort 5 Creme and Ointment ⊞ 557
Mantadil Cream 789
Ophthocort ◉ 301
Orabase HCA Oral Paste 890
Pramosone Cream, Lotion & Ointment 971
ProctoCream-HC 1834
Proctofoam-HC 1835

Hydrocortisone Sodium Phosphate (Major contributing factor to digitalis toxicity). Products include:
Hydrocortone Phosphate Injection, Sterile 1481

Hydrocortisone Sodium Succinate (Major contributing factor to digitalis toxicity). Products include:
Solu-Cortef Sterile Powder 2361

Hydroflumethiazide (Major contributing factor to digitalis toxicity). Products include:
Diucardin Tablets 2450
Saluron 718
Salutensin/Salutensin-Demi 719

Isoproterenol Hydrochloride (Increased risk of cardiac arrhythmias). Products include:
Isuprel Hydrochloride Injection 1:5000 2050
Isuprel Hydrochloride Mistometer 2051
Isuprel Hydrochloride Solution 1:200 & 1:100 2052
Norisodrine Aerotrol 540

Isradipine (Additive effects on AV node conduction). Products include:
DynaCirc Capsules 2004

Kaolin (Low digoxin serum concentration; interferes with intestinal digoxin absorption). Products include:
Donnagel ⊞ 675
Donnagel-PG 1858

Labetalol Hydrochloride (Additive effects on AV node conduction). Products include:
Normodyne Injection 2108
Normodyne Tablets 2110
Normozide Tablets 2112
Trandate HCT Tablets 579
Trandate Injection 577
Trandate Tablets 579

Liothyronine Sodium (Hypothyroid patients may require increased digoxin dose). Products include:
Cytomel Tablets 2203

Magaldrate (Interferes with intestinal digoxin absorption). Products include:
Riopan Antacid Chew Tablets ⊞ 754
Riopan Antacid Chew Tablets in Rollpacks ⊞ 754
Riopan Antacid Suspension 2421
Riopan Antacid Swallow Tablets 2421
Riopan Plus Chew Tablets 2422
Riopan Plus Chew Tablets in Rollpack 2422
Riopan Plus 2 Chew Tablets, Mint Flavor, Cherry Flavor 2422
Riopan Plus Suspension 2422
Riopan Plus 2 Suspension, Mint Flavor, Cherry Flavor 2422

Magnesium Hydroxide (Interferes with intestinal digoxin absorption). Products include:
- Aludrox Oral Suspension ... 2428
- Ascriptin A/D Caplets ... 1850
- Regular Strength Ascriptin Tablets 1850
- Di-Gel Antacid/Anti-Gas ... ▣ 697
- Gelusil Liquid & Tablets ... ▣ 639
- Haley's M-O, Regular & Flavored .. ▣ 569
- Extra Strength Maalox Plus Suspension ... 1850
- Maalox TC Suspension ... 1851
- Maalox Plus Tablets ... ▣ 655
- Extra Strength Maalox Plus Tablets 1850
- Mylanta Liquid ... 1155
- Mylanta Tablets ... 1155
- Mylanta Double Strength Liquid ... 1155
- Mylanta Double Strength Tablets ... 1155
- Concentrated Phillips' Milk of Magnesia ... ▣ 573
- Phillips' Milk of Magnesia Liquid ... ▣ 572
- Phillips' Milk of Magnesia Tablets ▣ 573
- WinGel Liquid & Tablets ... ▣ 761

Magnesium Oxide (Interferes with intestinal digoxin absorption). Products include:
- Bayer Plus Aspirin Tablets ... ▣ 567
- Beelith Tablets ... 659
- Bufferin Analgesic Tablets and Caplets ... ▣ 524
- Cama Arthritis Pain Reliever ... ▣ 685
- Mag-Ox 400 ... 673
- Uro-Mag ... 673

Metaproterenol Sulfate (Increased risk of cardiac arrhythmias). Products include:
- Alupent ... 674
- Arm-a-Med Metaproterenol Sulfate Inhalation Solution, USP ... 617
- Metaprel Inhalation Aerosol Bronchodilator ... 2014
- Metaprel Inhalation Solution ... 2015
- Metaprel ... 2015
- Metaproterenol Sulfate Inhalation Solution, USP ... 912

Metaraminol Bitartrate (Increased risk of cardiac arrhythmias). Products include:
- Aramine Injection ... 1424

Methoxamine Hydrochloride (Increased risk of cardiac arrhythmias). Products include:
- Vasoxyl Injection ... 819

Methyclothiazide (Major contributing factor to digitalis toxicity). Products include:
- Enduron Tablets ... 517
- Enduronyl ... 518

Methylprednisolone Acetate (Major contributing factor to digitalis toxicity). Products include:
- Depo-Medrol Sterile Aqueous Suspension ... 2334

Methylprednisolone Sodium Succinate (Major contributing factor to digitalis toxicity). Products include:
- Solu-Medrol Sterile Powder ... 2363

Metoprolol Tartrate (Additive effects on AV node conduction). Products include:
- Lopressor Ampuls ... 1032
- Lopressor HCT Tablets ... 1034
- Lopressor Tablets ... 1032

Nadolol (Additive effects on AV node conduction). Products include:
- Corgard Tablets ... 701
- Corzide Tablets ... 702

Neomycin, oral (Interferes with intestinal digoxin absorption).

Nephrotoxic Drugs (May impair the excretion of digoxin).

Nicardipine Hydrochloride (Additive effects on AV node conduction). Products include:
- Cardene Capsules ... 2290

Nifedipine (Additive effects on AV node conduction). Products include:
- Adalat Capsules (10 mg and 20 mg) ... 1587
- Procardia Capsules ... 1781
- Procardia XL Tablets ... 1783

Nimodipine (Additive effects on AV node conduction). Products include:
- Nimotop Capsules ... 1607

Norepinephrine Bitartrate (Increase risk of cardiac arrhythmias). Products include:
- Levophed Bitartrate Injection ... 2054

Pectin (Low digoxin serum concentration; interferes with intestinal digoxin absorption). Products include:
- Donnagel ... ▣ 675
- Donnagel-PG ... 1858

Penbutolol Sulfate (Additive effects on AV node conduction). Products include:
- Levatol ... 1832

Phenylephrine Bitartrate (Increased risk of cardiac arrhythmias).
- No products indexed under this heading.

Phenylephrine Hydrochloride (Increased risk of cardiac arrhythmias). Products include:
- AK-Dilate Solution 2.5% and 10% ... ◉ 203
- Atrohist Sprinkle Capsules ... 558
- Cerose-DM ... 2443
- Codimal ... 846
- Comhist LA Capsules ... 1618
- Congespirin For Children Aspirin Free Chewable Cold Tablets ... 748
- Cyclomydril ... ◉ 216
- Deconsal Sprinkle Capsules ... 559
- Dimetane Decongestant ... ▣ 673
- Dristan Decongestant/Antihistamine/ Analgesic Coated Caplets ... ▣ 749
- Dristan Cold Nasal Decongestant/ Antihistamine/ Analgesic Coated Tablets ... 2419
- Dristan Advanced Formula Decongestant/Antihistamine/ Analgesic Tablets ... ▣ 749
- Dristan Nasal Spray, Menthol ... 2419
- Dristan Nasal Spray, Regular and Regular with Metered Pump ... 2419
- Entex Capsules ... 1623
- Entex Liquid ... 1623
- Sinus Excedrin Analgesic, Decongestant Tablets & Caplets ... 750
- Extendryl ... 994
- 4-Way Fast Acting Nasal Spray - Original Formula (regular & mentholated) & Metered Spray Pump (regular) ... 751
- Hycomine Compound Tablets ... 929
- Murocoll-2 Sterile Ophthalmic Solution ... ◉ 261
- Mydfrin 2.5% ... ◉ 224
- Naldecon Syrup, Tablets, Pediatric Drops and Pediatric Syrup ... 709
- Neo-Synephrine Hydrochloride 1% Carpuject ... 2063
- Neo-Synephrine Hydrochloride 1% Injection ... 2063
- Neo-Synephrine Hydrochloride (Ophthalmic) ... 2064
- Neo-Synephrine ... ▣ 759
- Nōstril Nasal Decongestant ... ▣ 520
- Novahistine Elixir ... ▣ 596
- Phenergan VC ... 2500
- Phenergan VC with Codeine ... 2501
- Prefrin Liquifilm Vasoconstrictor and Lubricant Eye Drops ... ◉ 254
- Prefrin-A ... ◉ 255
- Quelidrine Syrup ... 556
- Relief Vasoconstrictor and Lubricant Eye Drops ... ◉ 256
- Robitussin Night Relief ... ▣ 677
- Ru-Tuss with Hydrocodone ... 694
- Ru-Tuss Tablets ... 693
- Vasosulf ... ◉ 279
- Vicks Sinex ... ▣ 665
- Zincfrin ... ◉ 230

Phenylephrine Tannate (Increased risk of cardiac arrhythmias). Products include:
- Rynatan ... 2387
- Rynatuss ... 2388

Phenylpropanolamine Hydrochloride (Increased risk of cardiac arrhythmias). Products include:
- A.R.M. Allergy Relief Medicine Caplets ... ▣ 615
- Acutrim ... ▣ 548
- Allerest ... ▣ 559
- BC Cold Powder ... ▣ 517
- Cheracol Plus Head Cold/Cough Formula ... ▣ 667
- Codimal Expectorant ... 846
- Comtrex Multi-Symptom Cold Reliever Tablets/Caplets/Liqui-Gels/Liquid ... 745
- Contac Continuous Action Decongestant/Antihistamine Capsules ▣ 710
- Contac Maximum Strength Continuous Action Decongestant/ Antihistamine Caplets ... ▣ 709
- Contac Severe Cold and Flu Formula Caplets ... ▣ 711
- Coricidin 'D' Decongestant Tablets ... ▣ 695
- Coricidin Demilets Tablets for Children ... ▣ 696
- Demazin Nasal Decongestant/ Antihistamine Repetabs Tablets & Syrup ... ▣ 697
- Dexatrim ... ▣ 733
- Dimetane-DC Cough Syrup ... 1857
- Dimetapp Elixir ... ▣ 673
- Dimetapp DM Elixir ... ▣ 674
- Dimetapp Extentabs ... ▣ 674
- Dimetapp Plus Caplets ... ▣ 675
- Dimetapp Tablets ... ▣ 675
- Entex Capsules ... 1623
- Entex LA Tablets ... 1623
- Entex Liquid ... 1623
- 4-Way Cold Tablets ... 750
- Hycomine Syrup ... 927
- Naldecon CX Adult Liquid ... ▣ 521
- Naldecon DX Adult Liquid ... ▣ 521
- Naldecon DX Children's Syrup ... ▣ 522
- Naldecon DX Pediatric Drops ... ▣ 522
- Naldecon EX Children's Syrup ... ▣ 522
- Naldecon EX Pediatric Drops ... ▣ 523
- Naldecon Syrup, Tablets, Pediatric Drops and Pediatric Syrup ... 709
- Nolamine Tablets ... 838
- Nolex LA Tablets ... 838
- Ornade Spansule Capsules ... 2221
- Orthoxicol Cough Syrup ... ▣ 668
- Propagest ... 839
- Pyrroxate Capsules ... ▣ 669
- Robitussin-CF ... ▣ 676
- Ru-Tuss II Capsules ... 693
- Ru-Tuss with Hydrocodone ... 694
- Ru-Tuss Tablets ... 693
- Sine-Off Sinus Medicine Tablets-Aspirin Formula ... ▣ 722
- Sinulin ... 840
- St. Joseph Cold Tablets for Children ... ▣ 704
- Tavist-D Tablets ... 2035
- Triaminic Allergy Tablets ... ▣ 688
- Triaminic Chewables ... ▣ 688
- Triaminic Cold Tablets ... ▣ 688
- Triaminic Expectorant ... ▣ 688
- Triaminic Expectorant w/Codeine .. 1996
- Triaminic Expectorant DH ... 1995
- Triaminic Oral Infant Drops ... 1996
- Triaminic Syrup ... ▣ 689
- Triaminic-12 Tablets ... ▣ 690
- Triaminic-DM Syrup ... ▣ 689
- Triaminicin Tablets ... ▣ 690
- Triaminicol Multi-Symptom Cold Tablets ... ▣ 691
- Triaminicol Multi-Symptom Relief ▣ 691
- Tuss-Ornade Liquid ... 2242
- Tuss-Ornade Spansule Capsules ... 2242
- Tylenol Cold Medication, Effervescent Tablets ... 1369

Pindolol (Additive effects on AV node conduction). Products include:
- Visken Tablets ... 2036

Pirbuterol Acetate (Increased risk of cardiac arrhythmias). Products include:
- Maxair Inhaler ... 1311

Polythiazide (Major contributing factor to digitalis toxicity). Products include:
- Minizide Capsules ... 1779
- Renese Tablets ... 1785
- Renese-R Tablets ... 1786

Prednisolone Acetate (Major contributing factor to digitalis toxicity). Products include:
- AK-Cide Sterile Ophthalmic Ointment & Suspension ... ◉ 202
- Blephamide Liquifilm Sterile Ophthalmic Suspension ... 586
- Blephamide S.O.P. Sterile Ophthalmic Ointment ... 586
- Cetapred Ointment ... ◉ 220
- ⅛% Econopred & 1% Econopred Plus ... ◉ 217
- Isopto Cetapred Suspension ... ◉ 220
- Metimyd ... ◉ 306
- Poly-Pred Liquifilm ... ◉ 250
- Pred Forte ... ◉ 252
- Pred Mild ... ◉ 254
- Pred-G Liquifilm Sterile Ophthalmic Suspension ... ◉ 252
- Pred-G S.O.P. Sterile Ophthalmic Ointment ... ◉ 253
- Vasocidin Ointment ... ◉ 275

Prednisolone Sodium Phosphate (Major contributing factor to digitalis toxicity). Products include:
- AK-Pred ... ◉ 205
- Hydeltrasol Injection, Sterile ... 1476
- Inflamase ... ◉ 274
- Pediapred Oral Liquid ... 987
- Vasocidin Ophthalmic Solution ... ◉ 276

Prednisolone Tebutate (Major contributing factor to digitalis toxicity). Products include:
- Hydeltra-T.B.A. Sterile Suspension 1478

Prednisone (Major contributing factor to digitalis toxicity). Products include:
- Deltasone Tablets ... 2332

Propantheline Bromide (Increases digoxin absorption). Products include:
- Pro-Banthine Tablets ... 2141

Propranolol Hydrochloride (Additive effects on AV node conduction). Products include:
- Inderal ... 2459
- Inderal LA Long Acting Capsules ... 2461
- Inderide Tablets ... 2463
- Inderide LA Long Acting Capsules .. 2465

Pseudoephedrine Hydrochloride (Increased risk of cardiac arrhythmias). Products include:
- Actifed Capsules ... ▣ 539
- Actifed Plus Caplets ... ▣ 539
- Actifed Plus Tablets ... ▣ 540
- Actifed with Codeine Cough Syrup.. 752
- Actifed Syrup ... ▣ 540
- Actifed Tablets ... ▣ 540
- Actifed 12-Hour Capsules ... ▣ 539
- Advil Cold & Sinus Caplets (formerly CoAdvil) ... 2416
- Allerest ... ▣ 559
- Anatuss LA Tablets ... 1359
- Benadryl Decongestant Elixir ... ▣ 635
- Benadryl Decongestant ... ▣ 635
- Benadryl Plus ... ▣ 636
- Benadryl Plus Nighttime ... ▣ 637
- Benylin Decongestant ... ▣ 638
- Brexin L.A. Capsules ... 2078
- Bromfed Capsules (Timed Release) ... 1615
- Bromfed Syrup ... ▣ 628
- Bromfed ... 1615
- CoAdvil ... ▣ 748
- Allergy-Sinus Comtrex Multi-Symptom Allergy Sinus Formula Tablets & Caplets ... 746
- Cough Formula Comtrex ... 746
- Comtrex Multi-Symptom Cold Reliever Tablets/Caplets/Liqui-Gels/Liquid ... 745
- Day-Night Comtrex ... 747
- Non-Drowsy Comtrex ... 747
- Congess ... 994
- Congestac Caplets ... ▣ 617
- Contac Jr. Children's Cold Medicine ... ▣ 712
- Contac Nighttime Cold Medicine ... ▣ 713
- Contac Sinus Caplets Maximum Strength Non-Drowsy Formula ... ▣ 710
- Contac Sinus Tablets Maximum Strength Non-Drowsy Formula ... ▣ 710
- Deconamine ... 663
- Deconsal II Tablets ... 559
- Dimacol Caplets ... ▣ 672
- Dimetane-DX Cough Syrup ... 1858
- Dorcol Children's Cough Syrup ... ▣ 685
- Dorcol Children's Decongestant Liquid ... ▣ 685
- Dorcol Children's Liquid Cold Formula ... ▣ 686
- Maximum Strength Dristan Decongestant/Analgesic Coated Caplets ... ▣ 750

No Drowsiness Dristan Cold Nasal Decongestant/Analgesic Coated Caplets 2420
Dristan Sinus Caplets 2419
Sinus Excedrin Analgesic, Decongestant Tablets & Caplets .... ⊞ 533
Fedahist Gyrocaps 2145
Fedahist Timecaps 2145
Guaifed 1615
Guaifed Syrup .... ⊞ 629
Isoclor Expectorant 982
Isoclor Timesule Capsules .... ⊞ 561
Kronofed-A 970
Medi-Flu Caplet, Liquid .... ⊞ 640
Novafed A Capsules 1342
Novafed Capsules 1342
Novahistine DH 1342
Novahistine DMX .... ⊞ 595
Novahistine Expectorant 1343
Nucofed Capsules 2219
Nucofed Expectorant 2219
Nucofed Pediatric Expectorant 2220
Nucofed Syrup 2219
Ornex Caplets .... ⊞ 618
PediaCare Allergy Relief Formula Liquid 1362
PediaCare Cough-Cold Formula Liquid 1362
PediaCare Infants' Oral Decongestant Drops 1362
PediaCare Night Rest Cough-Cold Formula Liquid 1362
PediaCare 6-12 Cough-Cold Formula Chewable Tablets 1362
Robitussin-DAC Syrup 1875
Robitussin-PE .... ⊞ 677
Rondec 1975
Rondec-DM 1976
Rondec-TR Tablet 1975
Ru-Tuss DE Tablets 694
Ryna .... ⊞ 741
Seldane-D Extended-Release Tablets 1350
Sinarest .... ⊞ 562
Sine-Aid Maximum Strength Sinus Headache Caplets 1365
Sine-Aid Maximum Strength Sinus Headache Tablets 1365
Sine-Off Maximum Strength Allergy/Sinus Formula Caplets .... ⊞ 721
Sine-Off Maximum Strength No Drowsiness Formula Caplets .... ⊞ 722
Singlet Tablets .... ⊞ 598
Sinutab Maximum Strength .... ⊞ 641
Sinutab Maximum Strength Without Drowsiness Tablets & Caplets .... ⊞ 642
Sinutab Regular Strength Without Drowsiness Formula .... ⊞ 641
St. Joseph Nighttime Cold Medicine .... ⊞ 705
Sudafed Children's Liquid .... ⊞ 543
Sudafed Cough Syrup .... ⊞ 543
Sudafed Plus Liquid .... ⊞ 544
Sudafed Plus Tablets .... ⊞ 545
Sudafed Sinus Caplets .... ⊞ 545
Sudafed Sinus Tablets .... ⊞ 545
Sudafed Tablets, 30 mg .... ⊞ 544
Sudafed Tablets, Adult Strength, 60 mg .... ⊞ 544
Sudafed 12 Hour Capsules .... ⊞ 545
TheraFlu Flu and Cold Medicine .... ⊞ 687
Triaminic Nite Light .... ⊞ 689
Tylenol Allergy Sinus Medication Caplets and Gelcaps, Maximum Strength 1372
Children's Tylenol Cold Liquid Formula and Chewable Tablets 1368
Tylenol Cold & Flu Hot Medication, Packets 1369
Tylenol Cold & Flu No Drowsiness Hot Medication, Packets 1371
Tylenol Cold Medication Caplets and Tablets 1370
Tylenol Cold Medication No Drowsiness Formula Caplets 1370
Tylenol Cold Night Time Medication Liquid 1371
Tylenol Cough Medication Liquid with Decongestant, Maximum Strength 1372
Tylenol, Maximum Strength, Sinus Medication Gelcaps, Caplets and Tablets 1373
Ursinus Inlay-Tabs .... ⊞ 691
Vicks Children's NyQuil .... ⊞ 664
Vicks Daycare .... ⊞ 660
Vicks Formula 44D Decongestant Cough Medicine .... ⊞ 662
Vicks Formula 44M Multi-Symptom Cough Medicine .... ⊞ 662
Vicks NyQuil Nighttime Colds Medicine-Original & Cherry Flavor .... ⊞ 664
Vicks Pediatric Formula 44 Cough & Congestion Medicine .... ⊞ 663
Vicks Pediatric Formula 44m Multi-Symptom Cough & Cold Medicine .... ⊞ 663

Pseudoephedrine Sulfate (Increased risk of cardiac arrhythmias). Products include:
Afrin Tablets .... ⊞ 693
Chlor-Trimeton Decongestant .... ⊞ 694
Disophrol Chronotab Sustained-Action Tablets .... ⊞ 698
Drixoral Antihistamine/Nasal Decongestant Syrup .... ⊞ 698
Drixoral Non-Drowsy Formula .... ⊞ 699
Drixoral Plus Extended-Release Tablets .... ⊞ 699
Drixoral Sinus .... ⊞ 700
Drixoral Sustained-Action Tablets .... ⊞ 698
Sinutab Allergy Formula Sustained Action Tablets .... ⊞ 640
Trinalin Repetabs Tablets 1170

Quinidine Gluconate (Causes rise in serum digoxin concentration). Products include:
Quinaglute Dura-Tabs Tablets 663

Quinidine Polygalacturonate (Causes rise in serum digoxin concentration). Products include:
Cardioquin Tablets 1812

Quinidine Sulfate (Causes rise in serum digoxin concentration). Products include:
Quinidex Extentabs 1868

Succinylcholine Chloride (May cause arrhythmias). Products include:
Anectine 755

Sulfasalazine (Low serum digoxin; interferes with intestinal digoxin absorption). Products include:
Azulfidine Tablets, EN-tabs, Oral Suspension 1157

Terbutaline Sulfate (Increased risk of cardiac arrhythmias). Products include:
Brethaire Inhaler 1024
Brethine Ampuls 1026
Brethine Tablets 1026
Bricanyl Injection 1324
Bricanyl Tablets 1325

Thyroid (Hypothyroid patients may require increased digoxin dose). Products include:
S-P-T "Liquid" Capsules 995

Thyroxine (Hypothyroid patients may require increased digoxin dose).
No products indexed under this heading.

Timolol Maleate (Additive effects on AV node conduction). Products include:
Blocadren Tablets 1429
Timolide Tablets 1547
Timoptic in Ocudose 1552
Timoptic Sterile Ophthalmic Solution 1550

Triamcinolone (Major contributing factor to digitalis toxicity).
No products indexed under this heading.

Triamcinolone Acetonide (Major contributing factor to digitalis toxicity). Products include:
Aristocort A 1010
Azmacort Inhaler 1837
Kenalog Cream, Lotion & Ointment 2401
Kenalog-10 Injection 2402
Kenalog-40 Injection 2403
Kenalog in Orabase 604
Kenalog Spray 2401
Mycolog II Cream and Ointment 2407
Mytrex Cream & Ointment 2080
Nasacort Nasal Inhaler 1844

Triamcinolone Diacetate (Major contributing factor to digitalis toxicity). Products include:
Aristocort Suspension 1008

Triamcinolone Hexacetonide (Major contributing factor to digitalis toxicity). Products include:
Aristospan Suspension 1011

Verapamil Hydrochloride (Causes rise in serum digoxin concentration; additive effects on AV node conduction). Products include:
Calan SR Caplets 2157
Calan Tablets 2155
Isoptin Injectable 1177
Isoptin Oral Tablets 1179
Isoptin SR Sustained Release Tablets 1181
Verelan Capsules 1243
Verelan Capsules 2535

Food Interactions

Meal, high in bran fiber (The amount of digoxin from an oral dose may be reduced).

Meal, unspecified (Slows the rate of absorption).

LARIAM TABLETS
(Mefloquine Hydrochloride) 1904
May interact with beta blockers, anticonvulsants, and certain other agents. Compounds in these categories include:

Acebutolol Hydrochloride (May produce electrocardiographic abnormalities). Products include:
Sectral Capsules 2520

Atenolol (May produce electrocardiographic abnormalities). Products include:
Tenoretic Tablets 1105
Tenormin Tablets and I.V. Injection 1107

Betaxolol Hydrochloride (May produce electrocardiographic abnormalities). Products include:
Betoptic Sterile Ophthalmic Solution 569
Betoptic S Sterile Ophthalmic Suspension 570
Kerlone Tablets 2172

Carbamazepine (Potential for loss of seizure control and lower than expected serum levels). Products include:
Tegretol Chewable Tablets 654
Tegretol Suspension 656
Tegretol Tablets 654

Carteolol Hydrochloride (May produce electrocardiographic abnormalities). Products include:
Cartrol Tablets 507

Chloroquine Hydrochloride (Increased risk of convulsions). Products include:
Aralen Hydrochloride Injection 2038

Chloroquine Phosphate (Increased risk of convulsions). Products include:
Aralen Phosphate with Primaquine Phosphate Tablets 2040
Aralen Phosphate Tablets 2039

Divalproex Sodium (Potential for loss of seizure control and lower than expected serum levels). Products include:
Depakote 512

Esmolol Hydrochloride (May produce electrocardiographic abnormalities). Products include:
Brevibloc Injection 942

Ethosuximide (Potential for loss of seizure control and lower than expected serum levels). Products include:
Zarontin Capsules 1768
Zarontin Syrup 1769

Ethotoin (Potential for loss of seizure control and lower than expected serum levels). Products include:
Peganone Tablets 551

Labetalol Hydrochloride (May produce electrocardiographic abnormalities). Products include:
Normodyne Injection 2108
Normodyne Tablets 2110
Normozide Tablets 2112
Trandate HCT Tablets 579
Trandate Injection 577
Trandate Tablets 579

Mephenytoin (Potential for loss of seizure control and lower than expected serum levels). Products include:
Mesantoin Tablets 2013

Methsuximide (Potential for loss of seizure control and lower than expected serum levels). Products include:
Celontin 1692

Metoprolol Tartrate (May produce electrocardiographic abnormalities). Products include:
Lopressor Ampuls 1032
Lopressor HCT Tablets 1034
Lopressor Tablets 1032

Nadolol (May produce electrocardiographic abnormalities). Products include:
Corgard Tablets 701
Corzide Tablets 702

Paramethadione (Potential for loss of seizure control and lower than expected serum levels). Products include:
Paradione Capsules 548

Penbutolol Sulfate (May produce electrocardiographic abnormalities). Products include:
Levatol 1832

Phenacemide (Potential for loss of seizure control and lower than expected serum levels). Products include:
Phenurone Tablets 552

Phenobarbital (Potential for loss of seizure control and lower than expected serum levels). Products include:
Arco-Lase Plus Tablets 607
Bellergal-S Tablets 1998
Bronkolixir .... ⊞ 761
Bronkotabs Tablets .... ⊞ 762
Donnatal 1858
Donnatal Extentabs 1859
Donnatal Tablets 1858
Donnazyme Tablets 1860
Kinesed Tablets 2272
Phenobarbital Elixir and Tablets 1293
Primatene Tablets-P Formula 2421
Quadrinal Tablets 1183
Tedral SA 1765

Phensuximide (Potential for loss of seizure control and lower than expected serum levels). Products include:
Milontin Kapseals 1741

Phenytoin (Potential for loss of seizure control and lower than expected serum levels). Products include:
Dilantin Infatabs 1710
Dilantin-30 Pediatric/Dilantin-125 Suspension 1713

Phenytoin Sodium (Potential for loss of seizure control and lower than expected serum levels). Products include:
Dilantin Kapseals 1708
Dilantin Parenteral 1712
Dilantin with Phenobarbital Kapseals 1715

Pindolol (May produce electrocardiographic abnormalities). Products include:
Visken Tablets 2036

Primidone (Potential for loss of seizure control and lower than expected serum levels). Products include:
Mysoline 2480

Propranolol Hydrochloride (Potential for cardiopulmonary arrest; may produce electrocardiographic abnormalities). Products include:

- Inderal ... 2459
- Inderal LA Long Acting Capsules ... 2461
- Inderide Tablets ... 2463
- Inderide LA Long Acting Capsules .. 2465

Quinidine Gluconate (May produce electrocardiographic abnormalities or cardiac arrest). Products include:

- Quinaglute Dura-Tabs Tablets ... 663

Quinidine Polygalacturonate (May produce electrocardiographic abnormalities or cardiac arrest). Products include:

- Cardioquin Tablets ... 1812

Quinidine Sulfate (May produce electrocardiographic abnormalities or cardiac arrest). Products include:

- Quinidex Extentabs ... 1868

Quinine Sulfate (Increased risk of convulsions). Products include:

- Legatrin ... ◘ 556
- Quinamm Tablets ... 1344
- Q-vel Muscle Relaxant Pain Reliever ... ◘ 552

Timolol Maleate (May produce electrocardiographic abnormalities). Products include:

- Blocadren Tablets ... 1429
- Timolide Tablets ... 1547
- Timoptic in Ocudose ... 1552
- Timoptic Sterile Ophthalmic Solution ... 1550

Trimethadione (Potential for loss of seizure control and lower than expected serum levels). Products include:

- Tridione ... 557

Valproic Acid (Potential for loss of seizure control and lower than expected serum levels). Products include:

- Depakene Capsules & Syrup ... 511

LAROBEC TABLETS
(Vitamins with Minerals, Therapeutic) ... 1905
No interactions described in labeling.

LARODOPA TABLETS
(Levodopa) ... 1905
May interact with monoamine oxidase inhibitors and antihypertensives. Compounds in these categories include:

Acebutolol Hydrochloride (Postural hypotensive episodes have been reported). Products include:

- Sectral Capsules ... 2520

Atenolol (Postural hypotensive episodes have been reported). Products include:

- Tenoretic Tablets ... 1105
- Tenormin Tablets and I.V. Injection 1107

Benazepril Hydrochloride (Postural hypotensive episodes have been reported). Products include:

- Lotensin Tablets ... 872

Bendroflumethiazide (Postural hypotensive episodes have been reported). Products include:

- Corzide Tablets ... 702
- Naturetin Tablets ... 1789
- Rauzide Tablets ... 1804

Betaxolol Hydrochloride (Postural hypotensive episodes have been reported). Products include:

- Betoptic Sterile Ophthalmic Solution ... 569
- Betoptic S Sterile Ophthalmic Suspension ... 570
- Kerlone Tablets ... 2172

Captopril (Postural hypotensive episodes have been reported). Products include:

- Capoten ... 2255
- Capozide ... 2258

Carteolol Hydrochloride (Postural hypotensive episodes have been reported). Products include:

- Cartrol Tablets ... 507

Chlorothiazide (Postural hypotensive episodes have been reported). Products include:

- Aldoclor Tablets ... 1413
- Diupres Tablets ... 1461
- Diuril Oral ... 1464

Chlorothiazide Sodium (Postural hypotensive episodes have been reported). Products include:

- Diuril Sodium Intravenous ... 1463

Chlorthalidone (Postural hypotensive episodes have been reported). Products include:

- Combipres Tablets ... 678
- Tenoretic Tablets ... 1105
- Thalitone Tablets ... 687

Clonidine (Postural hypotensive episodes have been reported). Products include:

- Catapres-TTS ... 677

Clonidine Hydrochloride (Postural hypotensive episodes have been reported). Products include:

- Catapres Tablets ... 676
- Combipres Tablets ... 678

Deserpidine (Postural hypotensive episodes have been reported). Products include:

- Enduronyl ... 518
- Harmonyl Tablets ... 528
- Oreticyl ... 545

Diazoxide (Postural hypotensive episodes have been reported). Products include:

- Hyperstat I.V. Injection ... 2095
- Proglycem ... 649

Doxazosin Mesylate (Postural hypotensive episodes have been reported). Products include:

- Cardura Tablets ... 1941

Enalapril Maleate (Postural hypotensive episodes have been reported). Products include:

- Vaseretic Tablets ... 1559
- Vasotec Tablets ... 1564

Enalaprilat (Postural hypotensive episodes have been reported). Products include:

- Vasotec I.V. ... 1562

Esmolol Hydrochloride (Postural hypotensive episodes have been reported). Products include:

- Brevibloc Injection ... 942

Felodipine (Postural hypotensive episodes have been reported). Products include:

- Plendil Extended-Release Tablets ... 1526

Fosinopril Sodium (Postural hypotensive episodes have been reported). Products include:

- Monopril Tablets ... 1406

Furazolidone (Concurrent administration is contraindicated). Products include:

- Furoxone ... 1855

Furosemide (Postural hypotensive episodes have been reported). Products include:

- Lasix ... 1093

Guanabenz Acetate (Postural hypotensive episodes have been reported). Products include:

- Wytensin Tablets ... 2542

Guanethidine Monosulfate (Postural hypotensive episodes have been reported). Products include:

- Esimil Tablets ... 864
- Ismelin Tablets ... 869

Hydralazine Hydrochloride (Postural hypotensive episodes have been reported). Products include:

- Apresazide Capsules ... 854
- Apresoline Hydrochloride Parenteral (Ampuls) ... 856
- Apresoline Hydrochloride Tablets .. 855
- Apresoline-Esidrix Tablets ... 857
- Ser-Ap-Es Tablets ... 881
- Serpasil-Apresoline Tablets ... 884

Hydrochlorothiazide (Postural hypotensive episodes have been reported). Products include:

- Aldactazide ... 2150
- Aldoril Tablets ... 1418
- Apresazide Capsules ... 854
- Apresoline-Esidrix Tablets ... 857
- Capozide ... 2258
- Dyazide Capsules ... 2208
- Esidrix Tablets ... 863
- Esimil Tablets ... 864
- HydroDIURIL Tablets ... 1484
- Hydropres Tablets ... 1485
- Inderide Tablets ... 2463
- Inderide LA Long Acting Capsules .. 2465
- Lopressor HCT Tablets ... 1034
- Maxzide ... 1215
- Moduretic Tablets ... 1510
- Normozide Tablets ... 2112
- Oretic Tablets ... 544
- Oreticyl ... 545
- Prinzide Tablets ... 1540
- Ser-Ap-Es Tablets ... 881
- Serpasil-Esidrix Tablets ... 886
- Timolide Tablets ... 1547
- Trandate HCT Tablets ... 579
- Vaseretic Tablets ... 1559
- Zestoretic ... 2274

Hydroflumethiazide (Postural hypotensive episodes have been reported). Products include:

- Diucardin Tablets ... 2450
- Saluron ... 718
- Salutensin/Salutensin-Demi ... 719

Indapamide (Postural hypotensive episodes have been reported). Products include:

- Lozol Tablets ... 1843

Isocarboxazid (Concurrent administration is contraindicated). Products include:

- Marplan Tablets ... 1906

Isradipine (Postural hypotensive episodes have been reported). Products include:

- DynaCirc Capsules ... 2004

Labetalol Hydrochloride (Postural hypotensive episodes have been reported). Products include:

- Normodyne Injection ... 2108
- Normodyne Tablets ... 2110
- Normozide Tablets ... 2112
- Trandate HCT Tablets ... 579
- Trandate Injection ... 577
- Trandate Tablets ... 579

Lisinopril (Postural hypotensive episodes have been reported). Products include:

- Prinivil Tablets ... 1538
- Prinzide Tablets ... 1540
- Zestoretic ... 2274
- Zestril Tablets ... 2277

Mecamylamine Hydrochloride (Postural hypotensive episodes have been reported). Products include:

- Inversine Tablets ... 1492

Methyclothiazide (Postural hypotensive episodes have been reported). Products include:

- Enduron Tablets ... 517
- Enduronyl ... 518

Methyldopa (Postural hypotensive episodes have been reported). Products include:

- Aldoclor Tablets ... 1413
- Aldomet Oral ... 1415
- Aldoril Tablets ... 1418

Methyldopate Hydrochloride (Postural hypotensive episodes have been reported). Products include:

- Aldomet Ester HCl Injection ... 1417

Metolazone (Postural hypotensive episodes have been reported). Products include:

- Diulo ... 2129
- Mykrox ½ mg Tablets ... 984
- Zaroxolyn Tablets ... 989

Metoprolol Tartrate (Postural hypotensive episodes have been reported). Products include:

- Lopressor Ampuls ... 1032
- Lopressor HCT Tablets ... 1034
- Lopressor Tablets ... 1032

Metyrosine (Postural hypotensive episodes have been reported). Products include:

- Demser Capsules ... 1460

Minoxidil (Postural hypotensive episodes have been reported). Products include:

- Loniten Tablets ... 2346
- Rogaine Topical Solution ... 2357

Nadolol (Postural hypotensive episodes have been reported). Products include:

- Corgard Tablets ... 701
- Corzide Tablets ... 702

Nicardipine Hydrochloride (Postural hypotensive episodes have been reported). Products include:

- Cardene Capsules ... 2290

Nitroglycerin (Postural hypotensive episodes have been reported). Products include:

- Deponit NTG Transdermal Delivery System ... 2143
- Minitran Transdermal Delivery System ... 1312
- Nitro-Bid Ointment ... 1339
- Nitro-Bid Capsules ... 1338
- Nitrodisc ... 2176
- Nitro-Dur (nitroglycerin) Transdermal Infusion System ... 1164
- Nitrogard Tablets ... 1004
- Nitrolingual Spray ... 1846
- Nitrostat Tablets ... 1743
- Transderm-Nitro Transdermal Therapeutic System ... 2283

Penbutolol Sulfate (Postural hypotensive episodes have been reported). Products include:

- Levatol ... 1832

Phenelzine Sulfate (Concurrent administration is contraindicated). Products include:

- Nardil ... 1742

Phenoxybenzamine Hydrochloride (Postural hypotensive episodes have been reported). Products include:

- Dibenzyline Capsules ... 2207

Phentolamine Mesylate (Postural hypotensive episodes have been reported). Products include:

- Regitine ... 878

Pindolol (Postural hypotensive episodes have been reported). Products include:

- Visken Tablets ... 2036

Polythiazide (Postural hypotensive episodes have been reported). Products include:

- Minizide Capsules ... 1779
- Renese Tablets ... 1785
- Renese-R Tablets ... 1786

Prazosin Hydrochloride (Postural hypotensive episodes have been reported). Products include:

- Minipress Capsules ... 1778
- Minizide Capsules ... 1779

Propranolol Hydrochloride (Postural hypotensive episodes have been reported). Products include:

- Inderal ... 2459
- Inderal LA Long Acting Capsules ... 2461
- Inderide Tablets ... 2463
- Inderide LA Long Acting Capsules .. 2465

Ramipril (Postural hypotensive episodes have been reported). Products include:

- Altace Capsules ... 1086

Rauwolfia Serpentina (Postural hypotensive episodes have been reported). Products include:
Raudixin Tablets 1803
Rauzide Tablets 1804

Rescinnamine (Postural hypotensive episodes have been reported).
No products indexed under this heading.

Reserpine (Postural hypotensive episodes have been reported). Products include:
Diupres Tablets 1461
Hydromox R Tablets 1209
Hydropres Tablets 1485
Renese-R Tablets 1786
Salutensin/Salutensin-Demi 719
Ser-Ap-Es Tablets 881
Serpasil Tablets 883
Serpasil-Apresoline Tablets 884
Serpasil-Esidrix Tablets 886

Selegiline Hydrochloride (Concurrent administration is contraindicated). Products include:
Eldepryl 2250

Sodium Nitroprusside (Postural hypotensive episodes have been reported). Products include:
Nipride I.V. Infusion 1909

Terazosin Hydrochloride (Postural hypotensive episodes have been reported). Products include:
Hytrin Tablets 529

Timolol Maleate (Postural hypotensive episodes have been reported). Products include:
Blocadren Tablets 1429
Timolide Tablets 1547
Timoptic in Ocudose 1552
Timoptic Sterile Ophthalmic Solution 1550

Tranylcypromine Sulfate (Concurrent administration is contraindicated). Products include:
Parnate Tablets 2222

Trimethaphan Camsylate (Postural hypotensive episodes have been reported). Products include:
Arfonad Ampuls 1887

LASIX ORAL SOLUTION
(Furosemide) 1093
May interact with aminoglycosides, salicylates, lithium preparations, antihypertensives, ganglionic blocking agents, para-aminobenzoic acid based local anesthetics, and certain other agents. Compounds in these categories include:

Acebutolol Hydrochloride (Added therapeutic effect). Products include:
Sectral Capsules 2520

Amikacin Sulfate (Increased ototoxic potential). Products include:
Amikin Injectable 602

Aspirin (Salicylate toxicity at lower doses; reduced creatinine clearance in patients with chronic renal insufficiency). Products include:
Alka-Seltzer Effervescent Antacid and Pain Reliever 1568
Alka-Seltzer Extra Strength Effervescent Antacid and Pain Reliever 1570
Alka-Seltzer (Flavored) Effervescent Antacid and Pain Reliever 1569
Alka-Seltzer Plus Cold Medicine ▣ 623
Alka-Seltzer Plus Night-Time Cold Medicine ▣ 623
Alka Seltzer Plus Sinus Allergy Medicine ▣ 624
Anacin Coated Analgesic Caplets 2417
Anacin Coated Analgesic Tablets 2417
Anacin Maximum Strength Analgesic Coated Tablets 2417
Maximum Strength Arthritis Pain Formula By the Makers of Anacin Analgesic Tablets and Caplets 2418
Arthritis Pain Formula by the Makers of Anacin Analgesic Tablets and Caplets ▣ 747
Arthritis Strength BC Powder ▣ 516
Ascriptin A/D Caplets 1850
Regular Strength Ascriptin Tablets 1850
Azdone Tablets 844
BC Powder ▣ 517
BC Cold Powder ▣ 517
Children's Bayer Chewable Aspirin ▣ 564
Genuine Bayer Aspirin Tablets & Caplets ▣ 564
Maximum Bayer Aspirin Tablets & Caplets ▣ 566
Bayer Plus Aspirin Tablets ▣ 567
Therapy Bayer Aspirin Caplets ▣ 568
8 Hour Bayer Timed-Release Aspirin ▣ 566
Arthritis Strength Bufferin Analgesic Caplets 744
Extra Strength Bufferin Analgesic Tablets 745
Bufferin Analgesic Tablets and Caplets 743
Cama Arthritis Pain Reliever ▣ 685
Damason-P 1356
Easprin 1719
Ecotrin Enteric Coated Aspirin Maximum Strength Tablets and Caplets 2189
Ecotrin Enteric Coated Aspirin Regular Strength Tablets and Caplets 2189
Empirin Aspirin ▣ 541
Empirin with Codeine Phosphate Nos. 2, 3 & 4 764
Equagesic Tablets 2451
Excedrin Extra-Strength Analgesic Tablets & Caplets 749
4-Way Cold Tablets 750
Fiorinal Capsules 2007
Fiorinal with Codeine Capsules 2008
Fiorinal Tablets 2007
Lortab ASA Tablets 2414
Momentum Muscular Backache Formula ▣ 751
Norgesic 1314
Norwich Extra-Strength Aspirin ▣ 546
Norwich Regular Strength Aspirin ▣ 547
P-A-C Analgesic Tablets ▣ 669
Percodan 951
Robaxisal Tablets 1872
Sine-Off Sinus Medicine Tablets-Aspirin Formula ▣ 722
Soma Compound w/Codeine Tablets 2390
Soma Compound Tablets 2389
St. Joseph Adult Chewable Aspirin (81 mg.) ▣ 703
Synalgos-DC Capsules 2525
Talwin Compound 2072
Ursinus Inlay-Tabs ▣ 691
Vanquish Analgesic Caplets ▣ 574
Zorprin Tablets 698

Atenolol (Added therapeutic effect). Products include:
Tenoretic Tablets 1105
Tenormin Tablets and I.V. Injection 1107

Benazepril Hydrochloride (Added therapeutic effect). Products include:
Lotensin Tablets 872

Bendroflumethiazide (Added therapeutic effect). Products include:
Corzide Tablets 702
Naturetin Tablets 1789
Rauzide Tablets 1804

Betaxolol Hydrochloride (Added therapeutic effect). Products include:
Betoptic Sterile Ophthalmic Solution 569
Betoptic S Sterile Ophthalmic Suspension 570
Kerlone Tablets 2172

Captopril (Added therapeutic effect). Products include:
Capoten 2255
Capozide 2258

Carteolol Hydrochloride (Added therapeutic effect). Products include:
Cartrol Tablets 507

Chlorothiazide (Added therapeutic effect). Products include:
Aldoclor Tablets 1413
Diupres Tablets 1461
Diuril Oral 1464

Chlorothiazide Sodium (Added therapeutic effect). Products include:
Diuril Sodium Intravenous 1463

Chlorthalidone (Added therapeutic effect). Products include:
Combipres Tablets 678
Tenoretic Tablets 1105
Thalitone Tablets 687

Choline Magnesium Trisalicylate (Salicylate toxicity at lower doses). Products include:
Trilisate 1822

Clonidine (Added therapeutic effect). Products include:
Catapres-TTS 677

Clonidine Hydrochloride (Added therapeutic effect). Products include:
Catapres Tablets 676
Combipres Tablets 678

Deserpidine (Potentiated therapeutic effect). Products include:
Enduronyl 518
Harmonyl Tablets 528
Oreticyl 545

Diazoxide (Added therapeutic effect). Products include:
Hyperstat I.V. Injection 2095
Proglycem 649

Diflunisal (Salicylate toxicity at lower doses). Products include:
Dolobid Tablets 1465

Doxazosin Mesylate (Added therapeutic effect). Products include:
Cardura Tablets 1941

Enalapril Maleate (Added therapeutic effect). Products include:
Vaseretic Tablets 1559
Vasotec Tablets 1564

Enalaprilat (Added therapeutic effect). Products include:
Vasotec I.V. 1562

Esmolol Hydrochloride (Added therapeutic effect). Products include:
Brevibloc Injection 942

Ethacrynic Acid (Increased possibility of otoxicity). Products include:
Edecrin Tablets 1468

Felodipine (Added therapeutic effect). Products include:
Plendil Extended-Release Tablets 1526

Fosinopril Sodium (Added therapeutic effect). Products include:
Monopril Tablets 1406

Gentamicin Sulfate (Increased ototoxic potential). Products include:
Garamycin Injectable 2093
Garamycin Ophthalmic ⊙ 305
Genoptic Liquifilm Sterile Ophthalmic Solution ⊙ 247
Genoptic S.O.P. Sterile Ophthalmic Ointment ⊙ 247
Gentacidin Ointment ⊙ 273
Gentacidin Solution ⊙ 273
Gentak Ointment & Solution ⊙ 208
G-myticin Creme and Ointment 0.1% 1770
Pred-G Liquifilm Sterile Ophthalmic Suspension ⊙ 252
Pred-G S.O.P. Sterile Ophthalmic Ointment ⊙ 253

Guanabenz Acetate (Added therapeutic effect). Products include:
Wytensin Tablets 2542

Guanethidine Monosulfate (Potentiated therapeutic effect). Products include:
Esimil Tablets 864
Ismelin Tablets 869

Hydralazine Hydrochloride (Added therapeutic effect). Products include:
Apresazide Capsules 854
Apresoline Hydrochloride Parenteral (Ampuls) 856
Apresoline Hydrochloride Tablets 855
Apresoline-Esidrix Tablets 857
Ser-Ap-Es Tablets 881
Serpasil-Apresoline Tablets 884

Hydrochlorothiazide (Added therapeutic effect). Products include:
Aldactazide 2150
Aldoril Tablets 1418
Apresazide Capsules 854
Apresoline-Esidrix Tablets 857
Capozide 2258
Dyazide Capsules 2208
Esidrix Tablets 863
Esimil Tablets 864
HydroDIURIL Tablets 1484
Hydropres Tablets 1485
Inderide Tablets 2463
Inderide LA Long Acting Capsules 2465
Lopressor HCT Tablets 1034
Maxzide 1215
Moduretic Tablets 1510
Normozide Tablets 2112
Oretic Tablets 544
Oreticyl 545
Prinzide Tablets 1540
Ser-Ap-Es Tablets 881
Serpasil-Esidrix Tablets 886
Timolide Tablets 1547
Trandate HCT Tablets 579
Vaseretic Tablets 1559
Zestoretic 2274

Hydroflumethiazide (Added therapeutic effect). Products include:
Diucardin Tablets 2450
Saluron 718
Salutensin/Salutensin-Demi 719

Indapamide (Added therapeutic effect). Products include:
Lozol Tablets 1843

Indomethacin (Reduced natriuretic and antihypertensive effects of Lasix). Products include:
Indocin 1487

Indomethacin Sodium Trihydrate (Reduced natriuretic and antihypertensive effects of Lasix). Products include:
Indocin I.V. 1490

Isradipine (Added therapeutic effect). Products include:
DynaCirc Capsules 2004

Kanamycin Sulfate (Increased ototoxic potential). Products include:
Kantrex Injection 601
Kantrex Pediatric Injection 601

Labetalol Hydrochloride (Added therapeutic effect). Products include:
Normodyne Injection 2108
Normodyne Tablets 2110
Normozide Tablets 2112
Trandate HCT Tablets 579
Trandate Injection 577
Trandate Tablets 579

Lisinopril (Added therapeutic effect). Products include:
Prinivil Tablets 1538
Prinzide Tablets 1540
Zestoretic 2274
Zestril Tablets 2277

Lithium Carbonate (Reduced renal clearance of lithium; lithium toxicity). Products include:
Eskalith 2214
Lithane Tablets 1596
Lithium Carbonate Capsules & Tablets 1984
Lithobid Tablets 870

Lithium Citrate (Reduced renal clearance of lithium; lithium toxicity). Products include:
Cibalith-S 870

Magnesium Salicylate (Salicylate toxicity at lower doses). Products include:
Doan's - Extra-Strength Analgesic ▣ 549
Doan's - Regular Strength Analgesic ▣ 549
Mobigesic Analgesic Tablets ▣ 507

Mecamylamine Hydrochloride (Potentiated therapeutic effect). Products include:
Inversine Tablets 1492

Methyclothiazide (Added therapeutic effect). Products include:
Enduron Tablets 517
Enduronyl 518

Methyldopa (Added therapeutic effect). Products include:
Aldoclor Tablets 1413
Aldomet Oral 1415
Aldoril Tablets 1418

Methyldopate Hydrochloride (Added therapeutic effect). Products include:
- Aldomet Ester HCl Injection 1417

Metolazone (Added therapeutic effect). Products include:
- Diulo 2129
- Mykrox ½ mg Tablets 984
- Zaroxolyn Tablets 989

Metoprolol Tartrate (Added therapeutic effect). Products include:
- Lopressor Ampuls 1032
- Lopressor HCT Tablets 1034
- Lopressor Tablets 1032

Metyrosine (Added therapeutic effect). Products include:
- Demser Capsules 1460

Minoxidil (Added therapeutic effect). Products include:
- Loniten Tablets 2346
- Rogaine Topical Solution 2357

Nadolol (Added therapeutic effect). Products include:
- Corgard Tablets 701
- Corzide Tablets 702

Nicardipine Hydrochloride (Added therapeutic effect). Products include:
- Cardene Capsules 2290

Nitroglycerin (Added therapeutic effect). Products include:
- Deponit NTG Transdermal Delivery System 2143
- Minitran Transdermal Delivery System 1312
- Nitro-Bid Ointment 1339
- Nitro-Bid Capsules 1338
- Nitrodisc 2176
- Nitro-Dur (nitroglycerin) Transdermal Infusion System 1164
- Nitrogard Tablets 1004
- Nitrolingual Spray 1846
- Nitrostat Tablets 1743
- Transderm-Nitro Transdermal Therapeutic System 2283

Norepinephrine Bitartrate (Decreased arterial response to norepinephrine). Products include:
- Levophed Bitartrate Injection 2054

Penbutolol Sulfate (Added therapeutic effect). Products include:
- Levatol 1832

Phenoxybenzamine Hydrochloride (Added therapeutic effect). Products include:
- Dibenzyline Capsules 2207

Phentolamine Mesylate (Added therapeutic effect). Products include:
- Regitine 878

Pindolol (Added therapeutic effect). Products include:
- Visken Tablets 2036

Polythiazide (Added therapeutic effect). Products include:
- Minizide Capsules 1779
- Renese Tablets 1785
- Renese-R Tablets 1786

Prazosin Hydrochloride (Potentiated therapeutic effect). Products include:
- Minipress Capsules 1778
- Minizide Capsules 1779

Propranolol Hydrochloride (Added therapeutic effect). Products include:
- Inderal 2459
- Inderal LA Long Acting Capsules 2461
- Inderide Tablets 2463
- Inderide LA Long Acting Capsules 2465

Ramipril (Added therapeutic effect). Products include:
- Altace Capsules 1086

Rauwolfia Serpentina (Potentiated therapeutic effect). Products include:
- Raudixin Tablets 1803
- Rauzide Tablets 1804

Rescinnamine (Potentiated therapeutic effect).
- No products indexed under this heading.

Reserpine (Potentiated therapeutic effect). Products include:
- Diupres Tablets 1461
- Hydromox R Tablets 1209
- Hydropres Tablets 1485
- Renese-R Tablets 1786
- Salutensin/Salutensin-Demi 719
- Ser-Ap-Es Tablets 881
- Serpasil Tablets 883
- Serpasil-Apresoline Tablets 884
- Serpasil-Esidrix Tablets 886

Salsalate (Salicylate toxicity at lower doses). Products include:
- Disalcid 1310
- Mono-Gesic Tablets 846
- Salflex 839

Sodium Nitroprusside (Added therapeutic effect). Products include:
- Nipride I.V. Infusion 1909

Streptomycin Sulfate (Increased ototoxic potential).
- No products indexed under this heading.

Succinylcholine Chloride (Potentiated action of succinylcholine). Products include:
- Anectine 755

Terazosin Hydrochloride (Added therapeutic effect). Products include:
- Hytrin Tablets 529

Timolol Maleate (Added therapeutic effect). Products include:
- Blocadren Tablets 1429
- Timolide Tablets 1547
- Timoptic in Ocudose 1552
- Timoptic Sterile Ophthalmic Solution 1550

Tobramycin Sulfate (Increased ototoxic potential). Products include:
- Nebcin Vials, Hyporets & ADD-Vantage 1286

Trimethaphan Camsylate (Potentiated therapeutic effect). Products include:
- Arfonad Ampuls 1887

Tubocurarine Chloride (Antagonized skeletal muscle relaxing effect).
- No products indexed under this heading.

LASIX TABLETS AND INJECTION
(Furosemide) 1093
See **Lasix Oral Solution**

LAVOPTIK EYE WASH
(Isotonic Solution) [BD] 583
No interactions described in labeling.

LAZER CREME
(Vitamin A, Vitamin E) 1770
No interactions described in labeling.

LAZERFORMALYDE SOLUTION
(Formaldehyde) 1770
No interactions described in labeling.

LAZERSPORIN-C SOLUTION
(Hydrocortisone, Neomycin Sulfate, Polymyxin B Sulfate) 1770
No interactions described in labeling.

LEGATRIN
(Quinine Sulfate) [BD] 556
No interactions described in labeling.

LENTE INSULIN
(Insulin, Zinc Suspension) 1626
No interactions described in labeling.

LENTE PURIFIED PORK INSULIN
(Insulin, Regular) 1626
No interactions described in labeling.

LEUCOVORIN CALCIUM FOR INJECTION, WELLCOVORIN BRAND
(Leucovorin Calcium) 786
May interact with:

Fluorouracil (Concomitant administration results in enhanced toxicity of fluorouracil). Products include:
- Efudex 1880
- Fluoroplex Topical Solution & Cream 1% 1082
- Fluorouracil Injection 1897

Phenobarbital (May counteract antiepileptic effects and increases frequency of seizures). Products include:
- Arco-Lase Plus Tablets 607
- Bellergal-S Tablets 1998
- Bronkolixir [BD] 761
- Bronkotabs Tablets [BD] 762
- Donnatal 1858
- Donnatal Extentabs 1859
- Donnatal Tablets 1858
- Donnazyme Tablets 1860
- Kinesed Tablets 2272
- Phenobarbital Elixir and Tablets 1293
- Primatene Tablets-P Formula 2421
- Quadrinal Tablets 1183
- Tedral SA 1765

Phenytoin (May counteract antiepileptic effects and increases frequency of seizures). Products include:
- Dilantin Infatabs 1710
- Dilantin-30 Pediatric/Dilantin-125 Suspension 1713

Phenytoin Sodium (May counteract antiepileptic effects and increases frequency of seizures). Products include:
- Dilantin Kapseals 1708
- Dilantin Parenteral 1712
- Dilantin with Phenobarbital Kapseals 1715

Primidone (May counteract antiepileptic effects and increases frequency of seizures). Products include:
- Mysoline 2480

LEUCOVORIN CALCIUM INJECTION
(Leucovorin Calcium) 1210
May interact with:

Fluorouracil (Enhanced toxicity of fluorouracil). Products include:
- Efudex 1880
- Fluoroplex Topical Solution & Cream 1% 1082
- Fluorouracil Injection 1897

Methotrexate Sodium (High doses of leucovorin may reduce the efficacy of intrathecally administered methotrexate). Products include:
- Methotrexate Tablets, Parenteral, LPF Parenteral 1217
- Rheumatrex Methotrexate Dose Pack 1234

Phenobarbital (Antiepileptic effect counteracted by large amount of folic acid). Products include:
- Arco-Lase Plus Tablets 607
- Bellergal-S Tablets 1998
- Bronkolixir [BD] 761
- Bronkotabs Tablets [BD] 762
- Donnatal 1858
- Donnatal Extentabs 1859
- Donnatal Tablets 1858
- Donnazyme Tablets 1860
- Kinesed Tablets 2272
- Phenobarbital Elixir and Tablets 1293
- Primatene Tablets-P Formula 2421
- Quadrinal Tablets 1183
- Tedral SA 1765

Phenytoin (Antiepileptic effect counteracted by large amount of folic acid). Products include:
- Dilantin Infatabs 1710
- Dilantin-30 Pediatric/Dilantin-125 Suspension 1713

Phenytoin Sodium (Antiepileptic effect counteracted by large amount of folic acid). Products include:
- Dilantin Kapseals 1708
- Dilantin Parenteral 1712
- Dilantin with Phenobarbital Kapseals 1715

Primidone (Antiepileptic effect counteracted by large amount of folic acid). Products include:
- Mysoline 2480

LEUCOVORIN CALCIUM TABLETS, WELLCOVORIN BRAND
(Leucovorin Calcium) 787
May interact with:

Fluorouracil (Enhanced toxicity of fluorouracil). Products include:
- Efudex 1880
- Fluoroplex Topical Solution & Cream 1% 1082
- Fluorouracil Injection 1897

Phenobarbital (Increased frequency of seizures in children). Products include:
- Arco-Lase Plus Tablets 607
- Bellergal-S Tablets 1998
- Bronkolixir [BD] 761
- Bronkotabs Tablets [BD] 762
- Donnatal 1858
- Donnatal Extentabs 1859
- Donnatal Tablets 1858
- Donnazyme Tablets 1860
- Kinesed Tablets 2272
- Phenobarbital Elixir and Tablets 1293
- Primatene Tablets-P Formula 2421
- Quadrinal Tablets 1183
- Tedral SA 1765

Phenytoin (Increased frequency of seizures in children). Products include:
- Dilantin Infatabs 1710
- Dilantin-30 Pediatric/Dilantin-125 Suspension 1713

Phenytoin Sodium (Increased frequency of seizures in children). Products include:
- Dilantin Kapseals 1708
- Dilantin Parenteral 1712
- Dilantin with Phenobarbital Kapseals 1715

Primidone (Increased frequency of seizures in children). Products include:
- Mysoline 2480

LEUCOVORIN CALCIUM TABLETS
(Leucovorin Calcium) 1212
May interact with:

Fluorouracil (Enhanced toxicity of fluorouracil). Products include:
- Efudex 1880
- Fluoroplex Topical Solution & Cream 1% 1082
- Fluorouracil Injection 1897

Methotrexate Sodium (High doses of leucovorin may reduce the efficacy of intrathecally administered methotrexate). Products include:
- Methotrexate Tablets, Parenteral, LPF Parenteral 1217
- Rheumatrex Methotrexate Dose Pack 1234

Phenobarbital (Antiepileptic effect counteracted by large amount of folic acid). Products include:
- Arco-Lase Plus Tablets 607
- Bellergal-S Tablets 1998
- Bronkolixir [BD] 761
- Bronkotabs Tablets [BD] 762
- Donnatal 1858
- Donnatal Extentabs 1859

Donnatal Tablets 1858
Donnazyme Tablets 1860
Kinesed Tablets 2272
Phenobarbital Elixir and Tablets 1293
Primatene Tablets-P Formula 2421
Quadrinal Tablets 1183
Tedral SA 1765

Phenytoin (Antiepileptic effect counteracted by large amount of folic acid). Products include:
Dilantin Infatabs 1710
Dilantin-30 Pediatric/Dilantin-125 Suspension 1713

Phenytoin Sodium (Antiepileptic effect counteracted by large amount of folic acid). Products include:
Dilantin Kapseals 1708
Dilantin Parenteral 1712
Dilantin with Phenobarbital Kapseals 1715

Primidone (Antiepileptic effect counteracted by large amount of folic acid). Products include:
Mysoline 2480

LEUKERAN TABLETS

(Chlorambucil) 788
No interactions described in labeling.

LEUKINE FOR IV INFUSION

(Sargramostim) 1127
May interact with drugs with myeloproliferative effects and cytotoxic drugs. Compounds in these categories include:

Betamethasone Acetate (May potentiate the myeloproliferative effect). Products include:
Celestone Soluspan Suspension 2081

Betamethasone Sodium Phosphate (May potentiate the myeloproliferative effect). Products include:
Celestone Soluspan Suspension 2081

Bleomycin Sulfate (Coadministration within 24 hours preceding or following chemotherapy is not recommended because of potential sensitivity of rapidly dividing hematopoietic progenitor cells to cytotoxic therapy). Products include:
Blenoxane 724

Cortisone Acetate (May potentiate the myeloproliferative effect). Products include:
Cortone Acetate Sterile Suspension 1437
Cortone Acetate Tablets 1439

Daunorubicin Hydrochloride (Coadministration within 24 hours preceding or following chemotherapy is not recommended because of potential sensitivity of rapidly dividing hematopoietic progenitor cells to cytotoxic therapy). Products include:
Cerubidine 2443

Dexamethasone (May potentiate the myeloproliferative effect). Products include:
AK-Trol Ointment & Suspension .... ◉ 207
Decadron Elixir 1445
Decadron Tablets 1447
Decaspray Topical Aerosol 1459
Dexacidin .... ◉ 272
Maxidex Sterile Ophthalmic Suspension .... ◉ 223
Maxitrol Ophthalmic Ointment/Suspension .... ◉ 223
TobraDex Ophthalmic Suspension and Ointment .... ◉ 228

Dexamethasone Acetate (May potentiate the myeloproliferative effect). Products include:
Dalalone D.P. Injectable 999
Decadron-LA Sterile Suspension 1457

Dexamethasone Sodium Phosphate (May potentiate the myeloproliferative effect). Products include:
AK-Dex .... ◉ 203
Decadron Phosphate Respihaler 1454
Decadron Phosphate Sterile Ophthalmic Ointment 1453
Decadron Phosphate Sterile Ophthalmic Solution 1453
Decadron Phosphate Topical Cream 1455
Decadron Phosphate Turbinaire 1456
Maxidex Sterile Ophthalmic Ointment .... ◉ 222
NeoDecadron Sterile Ophthalmic Ointment 1517
NeoDecadron Sterile Ophthalmic Solution 1518
NeoDecadron Topical Cream 1518

Doxorubicin Hydrochloride (Coadministration within 24 hours preceding or following chemotherapy is not recommended because of potential sensitivity of rapidly dividing hematopoietic progenitor cells to cytotoxic therapy). Products include:
Adriamycin PFS 561
Adriamycin RDF 562
Doxorubicin Hydrochloride for Injection, USP 622
Doxorubicin Hydrochloride Injection, USP 848
Rubex 739

Fluorouracil (Coadministration within 24 hours preceding or following chemotherapy is not recommended because of potential sensitivity of rapidly dividing hematopoietic progenitor cells to cytotoxic therapy). Products include:
Efudex 1880
Fluoroplex Topical Solution & Cream 1% 1082
Fluorouracil Injection 1897

Hydrocortisone (May potentiate the myeloproliferative effect). Products include:
AK-Spore H.C. .... ◉ 206
Bactine Hydrocortisone Anti-Itch Cream .... ®D 625
CaldeCORT Anti-Itch Hydrocortisone Spray .... ®D 560
Carmol HC Cream 1% 2296
Cortaid Spray .... ®D 735
Cortenema 2244
Cortisporin Ointment 758
Cortisporin Ophthalmic Ointment Sterile 758
Cortisporin Ophthalmic Suspension Sterile 759
Cortisporin Otic Solution Sterile 760
Cortisporin Otic Suspension Sterile 760
Cortizone-5 Creme & Ointment .... ®D 732
Dermolate Anti-Itch Cream .... ®D 697
Eldecort Cream 1.0% 1113
Eldecort Cream 1.0% and 2.5% 1113
Fungoid HC Creme 1770
Hydrocortone Tablets 1482
Hytone 909
LazerSporin-C Solution 1770
Massengill Medicated Soft Cloth Towelettes 2192
Nutracort Cream & Lotion 1684
PediOtic Suspension Sterile 797
Synacort Creams 1%, 2.5% 2296
Vanoxide-HC Acne Lotion 911
Vioform-Hydrocortisone Cream and Mild Cream 889
Vioform-Hydrocortisone Ointment 889
VōSoL HC Otic Solution 2392
Vytone Cream 1% 911

Hydrocortisone Acetate (May potentiate the myeloproliferative effect). Products include:
Analpram-HC Rectal Cream 1% and 2.5% 970
Anusol-HC Cream 1690
Anusol-HC Suppositories 1691
Caldecort .... ®D 560
Carmol HC Cream 1% 2296
Chloromycetin Hydrocortisone Ophthalmic 1694
Coly-Mycin S Otic w/Neomycin & Hydrocortisone 1708
Cortaid .... ®D 735
Cortef Feminine Itch Cream .... ®D 735
Corticaine .... ®D 682
Cortifoam 1827
Cortisporin Cream 757
Epifoam 1828
Gynecort 5 Creme .... ®D 556
Hydrocortone Acetate Sterile Suspension 1479
Lanacort 5 Creme and Ointment .. ®D 557
Mantadil Cream 789
Ophthocort .... ◉ 301
Orabase HCA Oral Paste 890
Pramosone Cream, Lotion & Ointment 971
ProctoCream-HC 1834
Proctofoam-HC 1835

Hydrocortisone Sodium Phosphate (May potentiate the myeloproliferative effect). Products include:
Hydrocortone Phosphate Injection, Sterile 1481

Hydrocortisone Sodium Succinate (May potentiate the myeloproliferative effect). Products include:
Solu-Cortef Sterile Powder 2361

Hydroxyurea (Coadministration within 24 hours preceding or following chemotherapy is not recommended because of potential sensitivity of rapidly dividing hematopoietic progenitor cells to cytotoxic therapy). Products include:
Hydrea Capsules 728

Lithium Carbonate (May potentiate the myeloproliferative effect). Products include:
Eskalith 2214
Lithane Tablets 1596
Lithium Carbonate Capsules & Tablets 1984
Lithobid Tablets 870

Lithium Citrate (May potentiate the myeloproliferative effect). Products include:
Cibalith-S 870

Methotrexate Sodium (Coadministration within 24 hours preceding or following chemotherapy is not recommended because of potential sensitivity of rapidly dividing hematopoietic progenitor cells to cytotoxic therapy). Products include:
Methotrexate Tablets, Parenteral, LPF Parenteral 1217
Rheumatrex Methotrexate Dose Pack 1234

Methylprednisolone Acetate (May potentiate the myeloproliferative effect). Products include:
Depo-Medrol Sterile Aqueous Suspension 2334

Methylprednisolone Sodium Succinate (May potentiate the myeloproliferative effect). Products include:
Solu-Medrol Sterile Powder 2363

Mitotane (Coadministration within 24 hours preceding or following chemotherapy is not recommended because of potential sensitivity of rapidly dividing hematopoietic progenitor cells to cytotoxic therapy). Products include:
Lysodren 731

Mitoxantrone Hydrochloride (Coadministration within 24 hours preceding or following chemotherapy is not recommended because of potential sensitivity of rapidly dividing hematopoietic progenitor cells to cytotoxic therapy). Products include:
Novantrone for Injection Concentrate 1226

Prednisolone Acetate (May potentiate the myeloproliferative effect). Products include:
AK-Cide Sterile Ophthalmic Ointment & Suspension .... ◉ 202
Blephamide Liquifilm Sterile Ophthalmic Suspension 586
Blephamide S.O.P. Sterile Ophthalmic Ointment 586
Cetapred Ointment .... ◉ 220
⅛% Econopred & 1% Econopred Plus .... ◉ 217
Isopto Cetapred Suspension .... ◉ 220
Metimyd .... ◉ 306
Poly-Pred Liquifilm .... ◉ 250
Pred Forte .... ◉ 252
Pred Mild .... ◉ 254
Pred-G Liquifilm Sterile Ophthalmic Suspension .... ◉ 252
Pred-G S.O.P. Sterile Ophthalmic Ointment .... ◉ 253
Vasocidin Ointment .... ◉ 275

Prednisolone Sodium Phosphate (May potentiate the myeloproliferative effect). Products include:
AK-Pred .... ◉ 205
Hydeltrasol Injection, Sterile 1476
Inflamase .... ◉ 274
Pediapred Oral Liquid 987
Vasocidin Ophthalmic Solution .... ◉ 276

Prednisolone Tebutate (May potentiate the myeloproliferative effect). Products include:
Hydeltra-T.B.A. Sterile Suspension 1478

Prednisone (May potentiate the myeloproliferative effect). Products include:
Deltasone Tablets 2332

Procarbazine Hydrochloride (Coadministration within 24 hours preceding or following chemotherapy is not recommended because of potential sensitivity of rapidly dividing hematopoietic progenitor cells to cytotoxic therapy). Products include:
Matulane Capsules 1907

Tamoxifen Citrate (Coadministration within 24 hours preceding or following chemotherapy is not recommended because of potential sensitivity of rapidly dividing hematopoietic progenitor cells to cytotoxic therapy). Products include:
Nolvadex Tablets 1102

Triamcinolone (May potentiate the myeloproliferative effect).
No products indexed under this heading.

Triamcinolone Acetonide (May potentiate the myeloproliferative effect). Products include:
Aristocort A 1010
Azmacort Inhaler 1837
Kenalog Cream, Lotion & Ointment 2401
Kenalog-10 Injection 2402
Kenalog-40 Injection 2403
Kenalog in Orabase 604
Kenalog Spray 2401
Mycolog II Cream and Ointment 2407
Mytrex Cream & Ointment 2080
Nasacort Nasal Inhaler 1844

Triamcinolone Diacetate (May potentiate the myeloproliferative effect). Products include:
Aristocort Suspension 1008

Triamcinolone Hexacetonide (May potentiate the myeloproliferative effect). Products include:
Aristospan Suspension 1011

Vincristine Sulfate (Coadministration within 24 hours preceding or following chemotherapy is not recommended because of potential sensitivity of rapidly dividing hematopoietic progenitor cells to cytotoxic therapy). Products include:
Oncovin Solution Vials & Hyporets 1288

LEVATOL

(Penbutolol Sulfate) 1832
May interact with calcium channel blockers, catecholamine depleting drugs, insulin, and certain other agents. Compounds in these categories include:

Alcohol (Increased number of errors in the eye-hand psychomotor function test).

Bepridil Hydrochloride (Potential for synergistic hypotensive effects, bradycardia, and arrhythmias). Products include:
Vascor (200, 300 and 400 mg) Tablets ... 1383
Cyclopropane (Potential for excessive myocardial depression).
Deserpidine (Concurrent use is not recommended). Products include:
Enduronyl ... 518
Harmonyl Tablets ... 528
Oreticyl ... 545
Diltiazem Hydrochloride (Potential for synergistic hypotensive effects, bradycardia, and arrhythmias). Products include:
Cardizem Tablets-30 mg, 60 mg, 90 mg and 120 mg ... 1329
Cardizem SR Capsules-60 mg, 90 mg and 120 mg ... 1327
Ether (Potential for excessive myocardial depression).
Felodipine (Potential for synergistic hypotensive effects, bradycardia, and arrhythmias). Products include:
Plendil Extended-Release Tablets ... 1526
Insulin, Human (Beta-blockade reduces the release of insulin in response to hyperglycemia).
No products indexed under this heading.
Insulin, Human Isophane Suspension (Beta-blockade reduces the release of insulin in response to hyperglycemia). Products include:
Humulin N, 100 Units ... 1270
Insulin, Human NPH (Beta-blockade reduces the release of insulin in response to hyperglycemia). Products include:
Insulatard NPH Human ... 1627
Novolin N ... 1627
Novolin N PenFill Cartridges ... 1628
Novolin N Prefilled ... 1628
Insulin, Human Regular (Beta-blockade reduces the release of insulin in response to hyperglycemia). Products include:
Humulin BR, 100 Units ... 1268
Humulin R, 100 Units ... 1272
Novolin R ... 1627
Novolin R PenFill Cartridges ... 1628
Novolin R Prefilled ... 1629
Velosulin Human ... 1628
Insulin, Human, Zinc Suspension (Beta-blockade reduces the release of insulin in response to hyperglycemia). Products include:
Humulin L, 100 Units ... 1268
Humulin U, 100 Units ... 1272
Novolin L ... 1627
Insulin, NPH (Beta-blockade reduces the release of insulin in response to hyperglycemia). Products include:
NPH, 40 & 100 Units ... 1273
Beef NPH, 100 Units ... 1274
Pork NPH, 100 Units ... 1275
Insulatard NPH ... 1626
NPH Insulin ... 1626
NPH Purified Pork Isophane Insulin ... 1626
Insulin, Regular (Beta-blockade reduces the release of insulin in response to hyperglycemia). Products include:
Regular, 40 & 100 Units ... 1273
Beef Regular, 100 Units ... 1275
Pork Regular, 100 Units ... 1275
Pork Regular (Concentrated), 500 Units ... 1276
Regular Insulin ... 1625
Regular Purified Pork Insulin ... 1626
Velosulin ... 1627
Insulin, Zinc Crystals (Beta-blockade reduces the release of insulin in response to hyperglycemia). Products include:
NPH, 40 & 100 Units ... 1273
Insulin, Zinc Suspension (Beta-blockade reduces the release of insulin in response to hyperglycemia). Products include:
Lente, 40 & 100 Units ... 1272
Protamine, Zinc, 40 & 100 Units ... 1273
Lente Iletin I ... 1272
Beef Lente, 100 Units ... 1274
Beef Protamine Zinc, 100 Units ... 1274
Pork Lente, 100 Units ... 1275
Pork, Protamine, Zinc, 100 Units ... 1275
Lente Insulin ... 1626
Lente Purified Pork Insulin ... 1626
Semilente Insulin ... 1625
Ultralente Insulin ... 1626
Isradipine (Potential for synergistic hypotensive effects, bradycardia, and arrhythmias). Products include:
DynaCirc Capsules ... 2004
Lidocaine Hydrochloride (Increased volume of distribution of lidocaine). Products include:
Anestacon Solution ... 2394
Bactine Antiseptic/Anesthetic First Aid Spray ... ⊞ 624
Decadron Phosphate with Xylocaine Injection, Sterile ... 1451
Xylocaine Injections ... 637
Xylocaine Injections for Ventricular Arrhythmias ... 639
Xylocaine 2% Jelly ... 643
4% Xylocaine-MPF Sterile Solution ... 641
Xylocaine 2% Viscous Solution ... 646
Nicardipine Hydrochloride (Potential for synergistic hypotensive effects, bradycardia, and arrhythmias). Products include:
Cardene Capsules ... 2290
Nifedipine (Potential for synergistic hypotensive effects, bradycardia, and arrhythmias). Products include:
Adalat Capsules (10 mg and 20 mg) ... 1587
Procardia Capsules ... 1781
Procardia XL Tablets ... 1783
Nimodipine (Potential for synergistic hypotensive effects, bradycardia, and arrhythmias). Products include:
Nimotop Capsules ... 1607
Rauwolfia Serpentina (Concurrent use is not recommended). Products include:
Raudixin Tablets ... 1803
Rauzide Tablets ... 1804
Rescinnamine (Concurrent use is not recommended).
No products indexed under this heading.
Reserpine (Concurrent use is not recommended). Products include:
Diupres Tablets ... 1461
Hydromox R Tablets ... 1209
Hydropres Tablets ... 1485
Renese-R Tablets ... 1786
Salutensin/Salutensin-Demi ... 719
Ser-Ap-Es Tablets ... 881
Serpasil Tablets ... 883
Serpasil-Apresoline Tablets ... 884
Serpasil-Esidrix Tablets ... 886
Verapamil Hydrochloride (Potential for synergistic hypotensive effects, bradycardia, and arrhythmias). Products include:
Calan SR Caplets ... 2157
Calan Tablets ... 2155
Isoptin Injectable ... 1177
Isoptin Oral Tablets ... 1179
Isoptin SR Sustained Release Tablets ... 1181
Verelan Capsules ... 1243
Verelan Capsules ... 2535

LEVLEN 21 TABLETS
(Levonorgestrel, Ethinyl Estradiol) 665
May interact with barbiturates, tetracyclines, and certain other agents. Compounds in these categories include:
Ampicillin Sodium (Reduced efficacy; breakthrough bleeding). Products include:
Unasyn ... 1965
Aprobarbital (Reduced efficacy; breakthrough bleeding). Products include:
Alurate Elixir ... 1883
Butabarbital (Reduced efficacy; breakthrough bleeding). Products include:
Pyridium Plus ... 1764
Butalbital (Reduced efficacy; breakthrough bleeding). Products include:
Esgic-Plus Tablets ... 1002
Esgic Tablets & Capsules ... 1001
Fioricet Tablets ... 2006
Fiorinal Capsules ... 2007
Fiorinal with Codeine Capsules ... 2008
Fiorinal Tablets ... 2007
Phrenilin ... 838
Sedapap Tablets 50 mg/650 mg .. 1360
Demeclocycline Hydrochloride (Reduced efficacy; breakthrough bleeding). Products include:
Declomycin Capsules, Tablets ... 1199
Doxycycline Calcium (Reduced efficacy; breakthrough bleeding).
No products indexed under this heading.
Doxycycline Hyclate (Reduced efficacy; breakthrough bleeding). Products include:
Doryx Capsules ... 1717
Vibramycin Hyclate Capsules ... 1787
Vibramycin Hyclate Intravenous ... 1968
Vibra-Tabs Film Coated Tablets ... 1787
Doxycycline Monohydrate (Reduced efficacy; breakthrough bleeding). Products include:
Monodox Capsules ... 1630
Vibramycin Monohydrate for Oral Suspension ... 1787
Griseofulvin (Reduced efficacy; breakthrough bleeding). Products include:
Fulvicin P/G Tablets ... 2090
Fulvicin P/G 165 & 330 Tablets ... 2091
Fulvicin-U/F Tablets ... 2092
Grifulvin V (griseofulvin microsize) Tablets/Suspension ... 1678
Grisactin ... 2454
Grisactin Ultra Tablets ... 2455
Gris-PEG Tablets, 125 mg & 250 mg ... 1083
Mephobarbital (Reduced efficacy; breakthrough bleeding). Products include:
Mebaral Tablets ... 2061
Methacycline Hydrochloride (Reduced efficacy; breakthrough bleeding).
No products indexed under this heading.
Minocycline Hydrochloride (Reduced efficacy; breakthrough bleeding). Products include:
Minocin Intravenous ... 1221
Minocin Oral Suspension ... 1224
Minocin Pellet-Filled Capsules ... 1222
Oxytetracycline (Reduced efficacy; breakthrough bleeding). Products include:
Terramycin Intramuscular Solution 1964
Urobiotic-250 Capsules ... 1968
Oxytetracycline Hydrochloride (Reduced efficacy; breakthrough bleeding). Products include:
Terra-Cortril Ophthalmic Suspension ... 1963
Terramycin Capsules ... 1786
Terramycin Intramuscular Solution 1964
Terramycin with Polymyxin B Sulfate Ophthalmic Ointment ... 1965
Pentobarbital Sodium (Reduced efficacy; breakthrough bleeding). Products include:
Nembutal Sodium Capsules ... 534
Nembutal Sodium Solution ... 536
Nembutal Sodium Suppositories ... 538
Phenobarbital (Reduced efficacy; breakthrough bleeding). Products include:
Arco-Lase Plus Tablets ... 607
Bellergal-S Tablets ... 1998
Bronkolixir ... ⊞ 761
Bronkotabs Tablets ... ⊞ 762
Donnatal ... 1858
Donnatal Extentabs ... 1859
Donnatal Tablets ... 1858
Donnazyme Tablets ... 1860
Kinesed Tablets ... 2272
Phenobarbital Elixir and Tablets ... 1293
Primatene Tablets-P Formula ... 2421
Quadrinal Tablets ... 1183
Tedral SA ... 1765
Phenylbutazone (Reduced efficacy; breakthrough bleeding). Products include:
Butazolidin Capsules & Tablets ... 1027
Phenytoin Sodium (Reduced efficacy; breakthrough bleeding). Products include:
Dilantin Kapseals ... 1708
Dilantin Parenteral ... 1712
Dilantin with Phenobarbital Kapseals ... 1715
Rifampin (Reduced efficacy; breakthrough bleeding). Products include:
Rifadin ... 1345
Rifamate Capsules ... 1347
Rimactane Capsules ... 879
Secobarbital Sodium (Reduced efficacy; breakthrough bleeding). Products include:
Seconal Sodium Pulvules ... 1296
Tetracycline Hydrochloride (Reduced efficacy; breakthrough bleeding). Products include:
Achromycin V Capsules ... 1193
Achromycin Ophthalmic Ointment 1% ... ⊙ 307
Achromycin Ophthalmic Suspension 1% ... ⊙ 308
Topicycline for Topical Solution ... 1856
Thiamylal Sodium (Reduced efficacy; breakthrough bleeding). Products include:
Surital Ampoules, Steri-Vials ... 1764

LEVLEN 28 TABLETS
(Levonorgestrel, Ethinyl Estradiol) 665
See **Levlen 21 Tablets**

LEVO-DROMORAN INJECTABLE
(Levorphanol Tartrate) ... 1906
No interactions described in labeling.

LEVO-DROMORAN TABLETS
(Levorphanol Tartrate) ... 1906
No interactions described in labeling.

LEVOPHED BITARTRATE INJECTION
(Norepinephrine Bitartrate) ... 2054
May interact with monoamine oxidase inhibitors, tricyclic antidepressants, and certain other agents. Compounds in these categories include:
Amitriptyline Hydrochloride (Severe prolonged hypertension). Products include:
Elavil ... 2269
Endep Tablets ... 1927
Etrafon ... 2087
Limbitrol ... 1933
Triavil Tablets ... 1556
Amoxapine (Severe prolonged hypertension). Products include:
Asendin Tablets ... 1196
Clomipramine Hydrochloride (Severe prolonged hypertension). Products include:
Anafranil Capsules ... 650
Cyclopropane (Increases cardiac autonomic irritability).

Desipramine Hydrochloride (Severe prolonged hypertension). Products include:
Norpramin Tablets 1340
Doxepin Hydrochloride (Severe prolonged hypertension). Products include:
Sinequan 1960
Furazolidone (Severe prolonged hypertension). Products include:
Furoxone 1855
Halothane (Increases cardiac autonomic irritability). Products include:
Fluothane 2453
Imipramine Hydrochloride (Severe prolonged hypertension). Products include:
Tofranil Ampuls 1038
Tofranil Tablets 1039
Imipramine Pamoate (Severe prolonged hypertension). Products include:
Tofranil-PM Capsules 1041
Isocarboxazid (Severe prolonged hypertension). Products include:
Marplan Tablets 1906
Maprotiline Hydrochloride (Severe prolonged hypertension). Products include:
Ludiomil Tablets 874
Nortriptyline Hydrochloride (Severe prolonged hypertension). Products include:
Pamelor 2019
Phenelzine Sulfate (Severe prolonged hypertension). Products include:
Nardil 1742
Protriptyline Hydrochloride (Severe prolonged hypertension). Products include:
Vivactil Tablets 1567
Selegiline Hydrochloride (Severe prolonged hypertension). Products include:
Eldepryl 2250
Tranylcypromine Sulfate (Severe prolonged hypertension). Products include:
Parnate Tablets 2222
Trimipramine Maleate (Severe prolonged hypertension). Products include:
Surmontil Capsules 2524

LEVOTHROID TABLETS
(Levothyroxine Sodium) 1003
May interact with oral hypoglycemic agents, insulin, oral anticoagulants, and certain other agents. Compounds in these categories include:

Chlorpropamide (Dosage of hypoglycemic agent may need to be adjusted). Products include:
Diabinese Tablets 1775
Cholestyramine (Impairs the absorption of thyroid hormone). Products include:
Cholybar 1705
Questran Light 711
Questran Powder 710
Colestipol Hydrochloride (Impairs the absorption of thyroid hormone). Products include:
Colestid Granules 2328
Dicumarol (Anticoagulant effects may be potentiated; dosage adjustment should be made). Products include:
Dicumarol Tablets 516
Epinephrine Hydrochloride (Enhanced coronary insufficiency). Products include:
Adrenalin Chloride Solution 1:100 & 1:1,000 1689
Epifrin ◉ 244
Glaucon ◉ 218
Glipizide (Dosage of hypoglycemic agent may need to be adjusted). Products include:
Glucotrol 1952
Glyburide (Dosage of hypoglycemic agent may need to be adjusted). Products include:
DiaBeta 1091
Micronase Tablets 2350
Insulin, Human (Dosage of insulin may need to be adjusted).
No products indexed under this heading.
Insulin, Human Isophane Suspension (Dosage of insulin may need to be adjusted). Products include:
Humulin N, 100 Units 1270
Insulin, Human NPH (Dosage of insulin may need to be adjusted). Products include:
Insulatard NPH Human 1627
Novolin N 1627
Novolin N PenFill Cartridges 1628
Novolin N Prefilled 1628
Insulin, Human Regular (Dosage of insulin may need to be adjusted). Products include:
Humulin BR, 100 Units 1268
Humulin R, 100 Units 1272
Novolin R 1627
Novolin R PenFill Cartridges 1628
Novolin R Prefilled 1629
Velosulin Human 1628
Insulin, Human, Zinc Suspension (Dosage of insulin may need to be adjusted). Products include:
Humulin L, 100 Units 1268
Humulin U, 100 Units 1272
Novolin L 1627
Insulin, NPH (Dosage of insulin may need to be adjusted). Products include:
NPH, 40 & 100 Units 1273
Beef NPH, 100 Units 1274
Pork NPH, 100 Units 1275
Insulatard NPH 1626
NPH Insulin 1626
NPH Purified Pork Isophane Insulin 1626
Insulin, Regular (Dosage of insulin may need to be adjusted). Products include:
Regular, 40 & 100 Units 1273
Beef Regular, 100 Units 1275
Pork Regular, 100 Units 1275
Pork Regular (Concentrated), 500 Units 1276
Regular Insulin 1625
Regular Purified Pork Insulin 1626
Velosulin 1627
Insulin, Zinc Crystals (Dosage of insulin may need to be adjusted). Products include:
NPH, 40 & 100 Units 1273
Insulin, Zinc Suspension (Dosage of insulin may need to be adjusted). Products include:
Lente, 40 & 100 Units 1272
Protamine, Zinc, 40 & 100 Units 1273
Lente Iletin I 1272
Beef Lente, 100 Units 1274
Beef Protamine Zinc, 100 Units 1274
Pork Lente, 100 Units 1275
Pork, Protamine, Zinc, 100 Units 1275
Lente Insulin 1626
Lente Purified Pork Insulin 1626
Semilente Insulin 1625
Ultralente Insulin 1626
Tolazamide (Dosage of hypoglycemic agent may need to be adjusted). Products include:
Tolinase Tablets 2365
Tolbutamide (Dosage of hypoglycemic agent may need to be adjusted). Products include:
Orinase Tablets 2354
Warfarin Sodium (Anticoagulant effects may be potentiated; dosage adjustment should be made). Products include:
Coumadin Injection & Tablets 944
Panwarfin Tablets 547

LEVOXINE TABLETS
(Levothyroxine Sodium) 904
May interact with insulin, oral hypoglycemic agents, oral anticoagulants, estrogens, and certain other agents. Compounds in these categories include:

Chlorotrianisene (Possible need to increase thyroid dosage). Products include:
TACE 12 and 25 mg 1353
Chlorpropamide (May cause an increase in the required dosage of oral hypoglycemics). Products include:
Diabinese Tablets 1775
Cholestyramine (Impairs absorption; 4 to 5 hours should elapse between administration of cholestyramine and thyroid hormones). Products include:
Cholybar 1705
Questran Light 711
Questran Powder 710
Dicumarol (Close supervision is advised; possible reduction in anticoagulant dosage). Products include:
Dicumarol Tablets 516
Dienestrol (Possible need to increase thyroid dosage). Products include:
Ortho Dienestrol Cream 1664
Diethylstilbestrol (Possible need to increase thyroid dosage). Products include:
Diethylstilbestrol Tablets 1258
Estradiol (Possible need to increase thyroid dosage). Products include:
Emcyt Capsules 1161
Estrace 1385
Estrace Vaginal Cream 1388
Estraderm Transdermal System 866
Estrogens, Conjugated (Possible need to increase thyroid dosage). Products include:
Mediatric Capsules 2476
PMB 200 and PMB 400 2504
Premarin Intravenous 2508
Premarin with Methyltestosterone 2515
Premarin Tablets 2510
Premarin Vaginal Cream 2512
Estrogens, Esterified (Possible need to increase thyroid dosage). Products include:
Estratest 2245
Menrium Tablets 1934
Estropipate (Possible need to increase thyroid dosage). Products include:
Ogen 540
Ethinyl Estradiol (Possible need to increase thyroid dosage). Products include:
Brevicon 2304
Demulen 2161
Estinyl Tablets 2085
Jenest-28 Tablets 1636
Levlen/Tri-Levlen 665
Lo/Ovral Tablets 2471
Lo/Ovral-28 Tablets 2476
Loestrin 1728
Modicon 1667
Nordette-21 Tablets 2481
Nordette-28 Tablets 2483
Norethin 2133
Norinyl 2304
Norlestrin 1746
Ortho-Cyclen Tablets 1658
Ortho-Novum 1667
Ovcon 1391
Ovral Tablets 2490
Ovral-28 Tablets 2491
Levlen/Tri-Levlen 665
Tri-Norinyl 2304
Triphasil-21 Tablets 2527
Triphasil-28 Tablets 2532
Glipizide (May cause an increase in the required dosage of oral hypoglycemics). Products include:
Glucotrol 1952
Glyburide (May cause an increase in the required dosage of oral hypoglycemics). Products include:
DiaBeta 1091
Micronase Tablets 2350
Insulin, Human (May cause an increase in the required dosage of insulin).
No products indexed under this heading.
Insulin, Human Isophane Suspension (May cause an increase in the required dosage of insulin). Products include:
Humulin N, 100 Units 1270
Insulin, Human NPH (May cause an increase in the required dosage of insulin). Products include:
Insulatard NPH Human 1627
Novolin N 1627
Novolin N PenFill Cartridges 1628
Novolin N Prefilled 1628
Insulin, Human Regular (May cause an increase in the required dosage of insulin). Products include:
Humulin BR, 100 Units 1268
Humulin R, 100 Units 1272
Novolin R 1627
Novolin R PenFill Cartridges 1628
Novolin R Prefilled 1629
Velosulin Human 1628
Insulin, Human, Zinc Suspension (May cause an increase in the required dosage of insulin). Products include:
Humulin L, 100 Units 1268
Humulin U, 100 Units 1272
Novolin L 1627
Insulin, NPH (May cause an increase in the required dosage of insulin). Products include:
NPH, 40 & 100 Units 1273
Beef NPH, 100 Units 1274
Pork NPH, 100 Units 1275
Insulatard NPH 1626
NPH Insulin 1626
NPH Purified Pork Isophane Insulin 1626
Insulin, Regular (May cause an increase in the required dosage of insulin). Products include:
Regular, 40 & 100 Units 1273
Beef Regular, 100 Units 1275
Pork Regular, 100 Units 1275
Pork Regular (Concentrated), 500 Units 1276
Regular Insulin 1625
Regular Purified Pork Insulin 1626
Velosulin 1627
Insulin, Zinc Crystals (May cause an increase in the required dosage of insulin). Products include:
NPH, 40 & 100 Units 1273
Insulin, Zinc Suspension (May cause an increase in the required dosage of insulin). Products include:
Lente, 40 & 100 Units 1272
Protamine, Zinc, 40 & 100 Units 1273
Lente Iletin I 1272
Beef Lente, 100 Units 1274
Beef Protamine Zinc, 100 Units 1274
Pork Lente, 100 Units 1275
Pork, Protamine, Zinc, 100 Units 1275
Lente Insulin 1626
Lente Purified Pork Insulin 1626
Semilente Insulin 1625
Ultralente Insulin 1626
Polyestradiol Phosphate (Possible need to increase thyroid dosage). Products include:
Estradurin 2452
Quinestrol (Possible need to increase thyroid dosage). Products include:
Estrovis 1721

Tolazamide (May cause an increase in the required dosage of oral hypoglycemics). Products include:
Tolinase Tablets ... 2365
Tolbutamide (May cause an increase in the required dosage of oral hypoglycemics). Products include:
Orinase Tablets ... 2354
Warfarin Sodium (Close supervision is advised; possible reduction in anticoagulant dosage). Products include:
Coumadin Injection & Tablets ... 944
Panwarfin Tablets ... 547

LEVSIN DROPS
(Hyoscyamine Sulfate) ... 2147
May interact with antimuscarinic drugs, phenothiazines, monoamine oxidase inhibitors, tricyclic antidepressants, antihistamines, antacids, and certain other agents. Compounds in these categories include:

Aluminum Carbonate Gel (Interferes with absorption of Levsin). Products include:
Basaljel ... 2438
Aluminum Hydroxide (Interferes with absorption of Levsin). Products include:
Cama Arthritis Pain Reliever ... ⊞ 685
Gaviscon Extra Strength Relief Formula Liquid Antacid ... ⊞ 594
Gaviscon Extra Strength Relief Formula Antacid Tablets ... ⊞ 594
Gaviscon Liquid Antacid ... ⊞ 594
Gelusil Liquid & Tablets ... ⊞ 639
Extra Strength Maalox Plus Suspension ... 1850
Maalox TC Suspension ... 1851
Maalox Plus Tablets ... ⊞ 655
Extra Strength Maalox Plus Tablets 1850
Nephrox Suspension ... ⊞ 563
WinGel Liquid & Tablets ... ⊞ 761
Aluminum Hydroxide Gel (Interferes with absorption of Levsin). Products include:
ALternaGEL Liquid ... 1154
Aludrox Oral Suspension ... 2428
Amphojel Suspension ... 2429
Amphojel Suspension without Flavor ... 2429
Mylanta Liquid ... 1155
Mylanta Double Strength Liquid ... 1155
Aluminum Hydroxide Gel, Dried (Interferes with absorption of Levsin). Products include:
Alu-Tab/Alu-Cap ... 1309
Amphojel Tablets ... 2429
Ascriptin A/D Caplets ... 1850
Regular Strength Ascriptin Tablets 1850
Gaviscon Antacid Tablets ... ⊞ 593
Gaviscon-2 Antacid Tablets ... ⊞ 594
Mylanta Tablets ... 1155
Mylanta Double Strength Tablets ... 1155
Amantadine Hydrochloride (Additive adverse effects). Products include:
Symmetrel Capsules & Syrup ... 936
Amitriptyline Hydrochloride (Additive adverse effects). Products include:
Elavil ... 2269
Endep Tablets ... 1927
Etrafon ... 2087
Limbitrol ... 1933
Triavil Tablets ... 1556
Amoxapine (Additive adverse effects). Products include:
Asendin Tablets ... 1196
Astemizole (Additive adverse effects). Products include:
Hismanal Tablets ... 1138
Atropine Sulfate (Additive adverse effects). Products include:
Arco-Lase Plus Tablets ... 607
Atropine Sulfate Sterile Ophthalmic Solution and S.O.P. Sterile Ophthalmic Ointment ... ◉ 239
Donnagel ... ⊞ 675
Donnagel-PG ... 1858
Donnatal ... 1858
Donnatal Extentabs ... 1859
Donnatal Tablets ... 1858
Donnazyme Tablets ... 1860
Isopto Atropine ... ◉ 218
Lomotil ... 2174
Motofen Tablets ... 836
Ru-Tuss Tablets ... 693
Urised Tablets ... 2396
Azatadine Maleate (Additive adverse effects). Products include:
Optimine Tablets ... 2115
Trinalin Repetabs Tablets ... 1170
Belladonna Alkaloids (Additive adverse effects). Products include:
Bellergal-S Tablets ... 1998
Hyland's Bed Wetting Tablets ... ⊞ 728
Hyland's Teething Tablets ... ⊞ 728
Kinesed Tablets ... 2272
Bromodiphenhydramine Hydrochloride (Additive adverse effects).
No products indexed under this heading.
Brompheniramine Maleate (Additive adverse effects). Products include:
Alka Seltzer Plus Sinus Allergy Medicine ... ⊞ 624
Atrohist Sprinkle Capsules ... 558
Bromfed Capsules (Timed Release) ... 1615
Bromfed Syrup ... ⊞ 628
Bromfed ... 1615
Dimetane Decongestant ... ⊞ 673
Dimetane ... ⊞ 672
Dimetane-DC Cough Syrup ... 1857
Dimetane-DX Cough Syrup ... 1858
Dimetapp Elixir ... ⊞ 673
Dimetapp DM Elixir ... ⊞ 674
Dimetapp Extentabs ... ⊞ 674
Dimetapp Plus Caplets ... ⊞ 675
Dimetapp Tablets ... ⊞ 675
Drixoral Antihistamine/Nasal Decongestant Syrup ... ⊞ 698
Chlorpheniramine Maleate (Additive adverse effects). Products include:
A.R.M. Allergy Relief Medicine Caplets ... ⊞ 615
Alka-Seltzer Plus Cold Medicine ... ⊞ 623
Allerest ... ⊞ 559
Ana-Kit Anaphylaxis Emergency Treatment Kit ... 1100
BC Cold Powder Multi-Symptom Formula ... ⊞ 517
Brexin L.A. Capsules ... 2078
Cerose-DM ... 2443
Cheracol Plus Head Cold/Cough Formula ... ⊞ 667
Chlor-Trimeton Allergy Syrup, Tablets & Long-Acting Repetabs Tablets ... ⊞ 693
Chlor-Trimeton Decongestant ... ⊞ 694
Comhist LA Capsules ... 1618
Allergy-Sinus Comtrex Multi-Symptom Allergy Sinus Formula Tablets & Caplets ... 746
Comtrex Multi-Symptom Cold Reliever Tablets/Caplets/Liqui-Gels/Liquid ... 745
Day-Night Comtrex ... 747
Contac Continuous Action Decongestant/Antihistamine Capsules ⊞ 710
Contac Maximum Strength Continuous Action Decongestant/Antihistamine Caplets ... ⊞ 709
Contac Severe Cold and Flu Formula Caplets ... ⊞ 711
Coricidin 'D' Decongestant Tablets ... ⊞ 695
Coricidin Demilets Tablets for Children ... ⊞ 696
Coricidin Tablets ... ⊞ 695
Deconamine ... 663
Demazin Nasal Decongestant/Antihistamine Repetabs Tablets & Syrup ... ⊞ 697
Dorcol Children's Liquid Cold Formula ... ⊞ 686
Dristan Decongestant/Antihistamine/ Analgesic Coated Caplets ... ⊞ 749
Dristan Cold Nasal Decongestant/Antihistamine/ Analgesic Coated Tablets ... 2419
Dristan Advanced Formula Decongestant/Antihistamine/Analgesic Tablets ... ⊞ 749
Extendryl ... 994
4-Way Cold Tablets ... 750
Fedahist Gyrocaps ... 2145
Fedahist Timecaps ... 2145
Hycomine Compound Tablets ... 929
Isoclor Timesule Capsules ... ⊞ 561
Kronofed-A ... 970
Medi-Flu Caplet, Liquid ... ⊞ 640
Naldecon Syrup, Tablets, Pediatric Drops and Pediatric Syrup ... 709
Nolamine Tablets ... 838
Novafed A Capsules ... 1342
Novahistine DH ... 1342
Novahistine Elixir ... ⊞ 596
Ornade Spansule Capsules ... 2221
Orthoxicol Cough Syrup ... ⊞ 668
PediaCare Allergy Relief Formula Liquid ... 1362
PediaCare Cough-Cold Formula Liquid ... 1362
PediaCare Night Rest Cough-Cold Formula Liquid ... 1362
PediaCare 6-12 Cough-Cold Formula Chewable Tablets ... 1362
Pyrroxate Capsules ... ⊞ 669
Quelidrine Syrup ... 556
Ru-Tuss II Capsules ... 693
Ru-Tuss Tablets ... 693
Ryna ... ⊞ 741
Sinarest Tablets & Extra Strength Tablets ... ⊞ 562
Sine-Off Maximum Strength Allergy/Sinus Formula Caplets ... ⊞ 721
Sine-Off Sinus Medicine Tablets-Aspirin Formula ... ⊞ 722
Singlet Tablets ... ⊞ 598
Sinulin ... 840
Sinutab Maximum Strength ... ⊞ 641
St. Joseph Nighttime Cold Medicine ... ⊞ 705
Sudafed Plus Liquid ... ⊞ 544
Sudafed Plus Tablets ... ⊞ 545
Teldrin Timed-Release Allergy Capsules, 12 mg ... 2192
TheraFlu Flu and Cold Medicine ... ⊞ 687
Triaminic Allergy Tablets ... ⊞ 688
Triaminic Chewables ... ⊞ 688
Triaminic Cold Tablets ... ⊞ 688
Triaminic Nite Light ... ⊞ 689
Triaminic Syrup ... ⊞ 689
Triaminic-12 Tablets ... ⊞ 690
Triaminicin Tablets ... ⊞ 690
Triaminicol Multi-Symptom Cold Tablets ... ⊞ 691
Triaminicol Multi-Symptom Relief ⊞ 691
Tylenol Allergy Sinus Medication Caplets and Gelcaps, Maximum Strength ... 1372
Children's Tylenol Cold Liquid Formula and Chewable Tablets ... 1368
Tylenol Cold & Flu Hot Medication, Packets ... 1369
Tylenol Cold Medication Caplets and Tablets ... 1370
Tylenol Cold Medication, Effervescent Tablets ... 1369
Vicks Children's NyQuil ... ⊞ 664
Vicks Formula 44 Cough Medicine ... ⊞ 661
Vicks Formula 44M Multi-Symptom Cough Medicine ... ⊞ 662
Vicks Pediatric Formula 44m Multi-Symptom Cough & Cold Medicine ... ⊞ 663
Chlorpheniramine Polistirex (Additive adverse effects). Products include:
Tussionex Extended-Release Suspension ... 988
Chlorpheniramine Tannate (Additive adverse effects). Products include:
Rynatan ... 2387
Rynatuss ... 2388
Chlorpromazine (Additive adverse effects). Products include:
Thorazine ... 2234
Clemastine Fumarate (Additive adverse effects). Products include:
Tavist Syrup ... 2033
Tavist Tablets ... 2035
Tavist-D Tablets ... 2035
Clidinium Bromide (Additive adverse effects). Products include:
Librax Capsules ... 1929
Quarzan Capsules ... 1937
Clomipramine Hydrochloride (Additive adverse effects). Products include:
Anafranil Capsules ... 650
Cyproheptadine Hydrochloride (Additive adverse effects). Products include:
Periactin ... 1525
Desipramine Hydrochloride (Additive adverse effects). Products include:
Norpramin Tablets ... 1340
Dexchlorpheniramine Maleate (Additive adverse effects). Products include:
Polaramine ... 2116
Dicyclomine Hydrochloride (Additive adverse effects). Products include:
Bentyl ... 1322
Dihydroxyaluminum Sodium Carbonate (Interferes with absorption of Levsin). Products include:
Rolaids ... ⊞ 743
Diphenhydramine Citrate (Additive adverse effects). Products include:
Alka-Seltzer Plus Night-Time Cold Medicine ... ⊞ 623
Bufferin AF Nite Time Analgesic/Sleeping Aid Caplets ... 744
Excedrin P.M. Analgesic/Sleeping Aid Tablets, Caplets and Liquid ... 749
Diphenhydramine Hydrochloride (Additive adverse effects). Products include:
Benadryl Anti-Itch Cream ... ⊞ 635
Benadryl Capsules ... 1691
Benadryl Decongestant Elixir ... ⊞ 635
Benadryl Decongestant ... ⊞ 635
Benadryl Elixir ... ⊞ 636
Benadryl Kapseals ... 1691
Benadryl 25 Kapseals ... ⊞ 636
Benadryl Parenteral ... 1692
Benadryl Plus ... ⊞ 636
Benadryl Plus Nighttime ... ⊞ 637
Benadryl Spray, Maximum Strength ... ⊞ 637
Benadryl Spray, Regular Strength ⊞ 637
Benadryl Steri-Vials, Ampoules, and Steri-Dose Syringe ... 1692
Benadryl 25 Tablets ... ⊞ 636
Benylin Cough Syrup ... ⊞ 637
Benylin Decongestant ... ⊞ 638
Caladryl Cream, Lotion, Spray ... ⊞ 638
Miles Nervine Nighttime Sleep-Aid ⊞ 627
Nytol Tablets ... ⊞ 517
Sleep-ettes-D Tablets ... ⊞ 653
Sleep-eze 3 Tablets ... ⊞ 755
Sleepinal Night-time Sleep Aid Capsules ... ⊞ 734
Sominex Caplets and Tablets ... ⊞ 722
Sominex Liquid ... ⊞ 723
Sominex Pain Relief Formula ... ⊞ 723
Tylenol Cold Night Time Medication Liquid ... 1371
Tylenol PM, Extra Strength Caplets and Tablets ... 1368
Unisom Dual Relief Nighttime Sleep Aid/Analgesic ... 1774
Ziradryl Lotion ... ⊞ 643
Diphenylpyraline Hydrochloride (Additive adverse effects).
No products indexed under this heading.
Doxepin Hydrochloride (Additive adverse effects). Products include:
Sinequan ... 1960
Fluphenazine Decanoate (Additive adverse effects). Products include:
Prolixin Decanoate ... 1795
Fluphenazine Enanthate (Additive adverse effects). Products include:
Prolixin Enanthate ... 1796
Fluphenazine Hydrochloride (Additive adverse effects). Products include:
Prolixin Elixir ... 1793
Prolixin Injection ... 1791
Prolixin Oral Concentrate ... 1792
Prolixin Tablets ... 1793

(⊞ Described in PDR For Nonprescription Drugs) (◉ Described in PDR For Ophthalmology)

Furazolidone (Additive adverse effects). Products include:
- Furoxone 1855

Glycopyrrolate (Additive adverse effects). Products include:
- Robinul Forte Tablets 1873
- Robinul Injectable 1873
- Robinul Tablets 1873

Haloperidol (Additive adverse effects). Products include:
- Haldol Injection, Tablets and Concentrate 1373

Haloperidol Decanoate (Additive adverse effects). Products include:
- Haldol Decanoate 1375

Hyoscyamine (Additive adverse effects). Products include:
- Cystospaz Tablets 2395
- Urised Tablets 2396

Imipramine Hydrochloride (Additive adverse effects). Products include:
- Tofranil Ampuls 1038
- Tofranil Tablets 1039

Imipramine Pamoate (Additive adverse effects). Products include:
- Tofranil-PM Capsules 1041

Ipratropium Bromide (Additive adverse effects). Products include:
- Atrovent Inhalation Aerosol 675

Isocarboxazid (Additive adverse effects). Products include:
- Marplan Tablets 1906

Magaldrate (Interferes with absorption of Levsin). Products include:
- Riopan Antacid Chew Tablets .... ⊞ 754
- Riopan Antacid Chew Tablets in Rollpacks .... ⊞ 754
- Riopan Antacid Suspension 2421
- Riopan Antacid Swallow Tablets 2421
- Riopan Plus Chew Tablets 2422
- Riopan Plus Chew Tablets in Rollpack 2422
- Riopan Plus 2 Chew Tablets, Mint Flavor, Cherry Flavor 2422
- Riopan Plus Suspension 2422
- Riopan Plus 2 Suspension, Mint Flavor, Cherry Flavor 2422

Magnesium Hydroxide (Interferes with absorption of Levsin). Products include:
- Aludrox Oral Suspension 2428
- Ascriptin A/D Caplets 1850
- Regular Strength Ascriptin Tablets 1850
- Di-Gel Antacid/Anti-Gas .... ⊞ 697
- Gelusil Liquid & Tablets .... ⊞ 639
- Haley's M-O, Regular & Flavored .... ⊞ 569
- Extra Strength Maalox Plus Suspension 1850
- Maalox TC Suspension 1851
- Maalox Plus Tablets .... ⊞ 655
- Extra Strength Maalox Plus Tablets 1850
- Mylanta Liquid 1155
- Mylanta Tablets 1155
- Mylanta Double Strength Liquid 1155
- Mylanta Double Strength Tablets 1155
- Concentrated Phillips' Milk of Magnesia .... ⊞ 573
- Phillips' Milk of Magnesia Liquid .... ⊞ 572
- Phillips' Milk of Magnesia Tablets .... ⊞ 573
- WinGel Liquid & Tablets .... ⊞ 761

Magnesium Oxide (Interferes with absorption of Levsin). Products include:
- Bayer Plus Aspirin Tablets .... ⊞ 567
- Beelith Tablets 659
- Bufferin Analgesic Tablets and Caplets .... ⊞ 524
- Cama Arthritis Pain Reliever .... ⊞ 685
- Mag-Ox 400 673
- Uro-Mag 673

Maprotiline Hydrochloride (Additive adverse effects). Products include:
- Ludiomil Tablets 874

Mepenzolate Bromide (Additive adverse effects). Products include:
- Cantil Tablets 1326

Mesoridazine (Additive adverse effects). Products include:
- Serentil 686

Methdilazine Hydrochloride (Additive adverse effects). Products include:
- Tacaryl Syrup & Tablets 2409

Nortriptyline Hydrochloride (Additive adverse effects). Products include:
- Pamelor 2019

Perphenazine (Additive adverse effects). Products include:
- Etrafon 2087
- Triavil Tablets 1556
- Trilafon 2123

Phenelzine Sulfate (Additive adverse effects). Products include:
- Nardil 1742

Prochlorperazine (Additive adverse effect). Products include:
- Compazine 2201

Promethazine Hydrochloride (Additive adverse effects). Products include:
- Mepergan Injection 2479
- Phenergan with Codeine 2497
- Phenergan with Dextromethorphan 2499
- Phenergan Injection 2493
- Phenergan Suppositories 2496
- Phenergan Syrup 2495
- Phenergan Tablets 2496
- Phenergan VC 2500
- Phenergan VC with Codeine 2501

Propantheline Bromide (Additive adverse effects). Products include:
- Pro-Banthīne Tablets 2141

Protriptyline Hydrochloride (Additive adverse effects). Products include:
- Vivactil Tablets 1567

Pyrilamine Maleate (Additive adverse effects). Products include:
- Codimal 846
- 4-Way Fast Acting Nasal Spray - Original Formula (regular & mentholated) & Metered Spray Pump (regular) 751
- Maximum Strength Midol Multi-Symptom Menstrual Formula .... ⊞ 571
- Maximum Strength Midol PMS Premenstrual Syndrome Formula .... ⊞ 570
- Regular Strength Midol Multi-Symptom Menstrual Formula .... ⊞ 570
- Prefrin-A .... ⊙ 255
- Prēmsyn PMS Capsules & Caplets .... ⊞ 547
- Primatene Tablets-M Formula 2421
- Robitussin Night Relief .... ⊞ 677
- Ru-Tuss with Hydrocodone 694
- Triaminic Expectorant DH 1995
- Triaminic Oral Infant Drops 1996

Pyrilamine Tannate (Additive adverse effects). Products include:
- Rynatan 2387

Scopolamine Hydrobromide (Additive adverse effects). Products include:
- Donnagel .... ⊞ 675
- Donnagel-PG 1858
- Donnatal 1858
- Donnatal Extentabs 1859
- Donnatal Tablets 1858
- Donnazyme Tablets 1860
- Isopto Hyoscine .... ⊙ 222
- Murocoll-2 Sterile Ophthalmic Solution .... ⊙ 261
- Ru-Tuss Tablets 693

Scopolamine Preparations (Additive adverse effects). Products include:
- Transderm Scōp Transdermal Therapeutic System 887

Selegiline Hydrochloride (Additive adverse effects). Products include:
- Eldepryl 2250

Terfenadine (Additive adverse effects). Products include:
- Seldane Tablets 1349
- Seldane-D Extended-Release Tablets 1350

Thioridazine Hydrochloride (Additive adverse effects). Products include:
- Mellaril 2011

Tranylcypromine Sulfate (Additive adverse effects). Products include:
- Parnate Tablets 2222

Tridihexethyl Chloride (Additive adverse effects).
- No products indexed under this heading.

Trifluoperazine Hydrochloride (Additive adverse effects). Products include:
- Stelazine 2226

Trimeprazine Tartrate (Additive adverse effects). Products include:
- Temaril Tablets, Syrup and Spansule Sustained Release Capsules 1085

Trimipramine Maleate (Additive adverse effects). Products include:
- Surmontil Capsules 2524

Tripelennamine Hydrochloride (Additive adverse effects). Products include:
- PBZ Tablets & Elixir 1037
- PBZ-SR Tablets 1037

Triprolidine Hydrochloride (Additive adverse effects). Products include:
- Actidil .... ⊞ 538
- Actifed Capsules .... ⊞ 539
- Actifed Plus Caplets .... ⊞ 539
- Actifed Plus Tablets .... ⊞ 540
- Actifed with Codeine Cough Syrup 752
- Actifed Syrup .... ⊞ 540
- Actifed Tablets .... ⊞ 540
- Actifed 12-Hour Capsules .... ⊞ 539

LEVSIN ELIXIR
(Hyoscyamine Sulfate) 2147
See **Levsin Drops**

LEVSIN INJECTION
(Hyoscyamine Sulfate) 2147
See **Levsin Drops**

LEVSIN TABLETS
(Hyoscyamine Sulfate) 2147
See **Levsin Drops**

LEVSIN/SL TABLETS
(Hyoscyamine Sulfate) 2147
See **Levsin Drops**

LEVSINEX TIMECAPS
(Hyoscyamine Sulfate) 2147
See **Levsin Drops**

LIBRAX CAPSULES
(Chlordiazepoxide Hydrochloride, Clidinium Bromide) 1929
May interact with monoamine oxidase inhibitors, phenothiazines, psychotropics, central nervous system depressants, and certain other agents. Compounds in these categories include:

Alcohol (Additive effects).

Alfentanil Hydrochloride (Additive effects). Products include:
- Alfenta Injection 1131

Alprazolam (Additive effects; concomitant use not recommended). Products include:
- Xanax Tablets 2367

Amitriptyline Hydrochloride (Additive effects; concomitant use not recommended). Products include:
- Elavil 2269
- Endep Tablets 1927
- Etrafon 2087
- Limbitrol 1933
- Triavil Tablets 1556

Amoxapine (Concomitant use not recommended). Products include:
- Asendin Tablets 1196

Aprobarbital (Additive effects). Products include:
- Alurate Elixir 1883

Buprenorphine (Additive effects).
- No products indexed under this heading.

Buspirone Hydrochloride (Additive effects; concomitant use not recommended). Products include:
- BuSpar 1401

Butabarbital (Additive effects). Products include:
- Pyridium Plus 1764

Butalbital (Additive effects). Products include:
- Esgic-Plus Tablets 1002
- Esgic Tablets & Capsules 1001
- Fioricet Tablets 2006
- Fiorinal Capsules 2007
- Fiorinal with Codeine Capsules 2008
- Fiorinal Tablets 2007
- Phrenilin 838
- Sedapap Tablets 50 mg/650 mg 1360

Chlordiazepoxide (Additive effects). Products include:
- Libritabs Tablets 1930
- Limbitrol 1933
- Menrium Tablets 1934

Chlorpromazine (Additive effects; concomitant use not recommended; potentiates Librax). Products include:
- Thorazine 2234

Chlorprothixene (Additive effects; concomitant use not recommended). Products include:
- Taractan Tablets 1920

Chlorprothixene Hydrochloride (Additive effects; concomitant use not recommended). Products include:
- Taractan 1920

Clorazepate Dipotassium (Additive effects; concomitant use not recommended). Products include:
- Tranxene 556

Codeine (Additive effects). Products include:
- Calcidrine Syrup 506

Codeine Phosphate (Additive effects). Products include:
- Actifed with Codeine Cough Syrup 752
- Cheracol Cough Syrup 1853
- Codimal PH Syrup 846
- Dimetane-DC Cough Syrup 1857
- Empirin with Codeine Phosphate Nos. 2, 3 & 4 764
- Fiorinal with Codeine Capsules 2008
- Isoclor Expectorant 982
- Naldecon CX Adult Liquid .... ⊞ 521
- Novahistine DH 1342
- Novahistine Expectorant 1343
- Nucofed Capsules 2219
- Nucofed Expectorant 2219
- Nucofed Pediatric Expectorant 2220
- Nucofed Syrup 2219
- Phenaphen with Codeine Capsules 1865
- Phenaphen-650 with Codeine Tablets 1866
- Phenergan with Codeine 2497
- Phenergan VC with Codeine 2501
- Robitussin A-C Syrup 1875
- Robitussin-DAC Syrup 1875
- Ryna .... ⊞ 741
- Soma Compound w/Codeine Tablets 2390
- Triaminic Expectorant w/Codeine 1996
- Tussi-Organidin Liquid 2391
- Tylenol with Codeine 1381

Codeine Polistirex (Additive effects).
- No products indexed under this heading.

Desipramine Hydrochloride (Concomitant use not recommended). Products include:
- Norpramin Tablets 1340

Dezocine (Additive effects).

Diazepam (Additive effects; concomitant use not recommended). Products include:
- Valium Injectable 1937

Valium Tablets 1939
Valrelease Capsules 1923

Doxepin Hydrochloride (Concomitant use not recommended). Products include:
Sinequan 1960

Droperidol (Additive effects; concomitant use not recommended). Products include:
Inapsine Injection 1140
Innovar Injection 1141

Enflurane (Additive effects). Products include:
Ethrane 599

Estazolam (Additive effects). Products include:
ProSom Tablets 554

Ethchlorvynol (Additive effects). Products include:
Placidyl Capsules 553

Ethinamate (Additive effects).
No products indexed under this heading.

Fentanyl (Additive effects). Products include:
Duragesic Transdermal System 1133

Fentanyl Citrate (Additive effects). Products include:
Innovar Injection 1141
Sublimaze Injection 1146

Fluphenazine Decanoate (Additive effects; concomitant use not recommended; potentiates Librax). Products include:
Prolixin Decanoate 1795

Fluphenazine Enanthate (Additive effects; concomitant use not recommended; potentiates Librax). Products include:
Prolixin Enanthate 1796

Fluphenazine Hydrochloride (Additive effects; concomitant use not recommended; potentiates Librax). Products include:
Prolixin Elixir 1793
Prolixin Injection 1791
Prolixin Oral Concentrate 1792
Prolixin Tablets 1793

Flurazepam Hydrochloride (Additive effects). Products include:
Dalmane Capsules 1927

Furazolidone (Potentiates Librax; concomitant use not recommended). Products include:
Furoxone 1855

Glutethimide (Additive effects).
No products indexed under this heading.

Haloperidol (Additive effects; concomitant use not recommended). Products include:
Haldol Injection, Tablets and Concentrate 1373

Haloperidol Decanoate (Additive effects; concomitant use not recommended). Products include:
Haldol Decanoate 1375

Hydrocodone Bitartrate (Additive effects). Products include:
Anexsia 5/500 Tablets 2196
Anexsia 7.5/650 Tablets 2197
Azdōne Tablets 844
Codiclear DH Syrup 845
Codimal DH Syrup 846
Damason-P 1356
Hycodan Syrup, Tablets 927
Hycomine Compound Tablets 929
Hycomine Syrup 927
Hycotuss Expectorant Syrup 930
Hydrocet Capsules 835
Lortab ASA Tablets 2414
Lortab 2412
Ru-Tuss with Hydrocodone 694
Triaminic Expectorant DH 1995
Vicodin Tablets 1187
Vicodin ES Tablets 1189
Zydone Capsules 941

Hydrocodone Polistirex (Additive effects). Products include:
Tussionex Extended-Release Suspension 988

Hydroxyzine Hydrochloride (Additive effects; concomitant use not recommended). Products include:
Atarax Tablets & Syrup 1941
Marax Tablets & DF Syrup 1954
Vistaril Intramuscular Solution 1970

Imipramine Hydrochloride (Concomitant use not recommended). Products include:
Tofranil Ampuls 1038
Tofranil Tablets 1039

Imipramine Pamoate (Concomitant use not recommended). Products include:
Tofranil-PM Capsules 1041

Isocarboxazid (Potentiates Librax; concomitant use not recommended). Products include:
Marplan Tablets 1906

Isoflurane (Additive effects). Products include:
Forane 600

Ketamine Hydrochloride (Additive effects). Products include:
Ketalar 1726

Levorphanol Tartrate (Additive effects). Products include:
Levo-Dromoran 1906

Lithium Carbonate (Concomitant use not recommended). Products include:
Eskalith 2214
Lithane Tablets 1596
Lithium Carbonate Capsules & Tablets 1984
Lithobid Tablets 870

Lithium Citrate (Concomitant use not recommended). Products include:
Cibalith-S 870

Lorazepam (Additive effects; concomitant use not recommended). Products include:
Ativan Injection 2432
Ativan Tablets 2434

Loxapine Hydrochloride (Additive effects; concomitant use not recommended). Products include:
Loxitane 1213

Loxapine Succinate (Additive effects). Products include:
Loxitane Capsules 1213

Maprotiline Hydrochloride (Concomitant use not recommended). Products include:
Ludiomil Tablets 874

Meperidine Hydrochloride (Additive effects). Products include:
Demerol 2047
Mepergan Injection 2479

Mephobarbital (Additive effects). Products include:
Mebaral Tablets 2061

Meprobamate (Additive effects; concomitant use not recommended). Products include:
Deprol Tablets 2382
Equagesic Tablets 2451
Miltown Tablets 2386
PMB 200 and PMB 400 2504

Mesoridazine (Additive effects; concomitant use not recommended; potentiates Librax). Products include:
Serentil 686

Methadone Hydrochloride (Additive effects). Products include:
Dolophine Hydrochloride Ampoules & Vials 1260
Dolophine Hydrochloride Tablets 1261
Methadone Hydrochloride Diskets 1284
Methadone Hydrochloride Oral Solution & Tablets 1987

Methohexital Sodium (Additive effects). Products include:
Brevital Sodium Vials 1248

Methoxyflurane (Additive effects).
No products indexed under this heading.

Midazolam Hydrochloride (Additive effects; concomitant use not recommended). Products include:
Versed Injection 1924

Molindone Hydrochloride (Additive effects; concomitant use not recommended). Products include:
Moban Tablets & Concentrate 932

Morphine Sulfate (Additive effects). Products include:
Astramorph/PF Injection, USP (Preservative-Free) 618
Duramorph 960
Infumorph 200 and Infumorph 500 Sterile Solutions 962
MS Contin Tablets 1814
MSIR 1817
Oramorph SR (Morphine Sulfate Sustained Release Tablets) 1988
Roxanol 1991

Nortriptyline Hydrochloride (Concomitant use not recommended). Products include:
Pamelor 2019

Opium Alkaloids (Additive effects). Products include:
B & O No. 15A & No. 16A Supprettes 2395
Pantopon Injectable 1911

Oxazepam (Additive effects; concomitant use not recommended). Products include:
Serax Capsules 2522
Serax Tablets 2522

Oxycodone Hydrochloride (Additive effects). Products include:
Percocet Tablets 950
Percodan 951
Roxicodone Tablets, Oral Solution & Intensol (Oxycodone) 1992
Tylox Capsules 1382

Pentobarbital Sodium (Additive effects). Products include:
Nembutal Sodium Capsules 534
Nembutal Sodium Solution 536
Nembutal Sodium Suppositories 538

Perphenazine (Additive effects; concomitant use not recommended; potentiates Librax). Products include:
Etrafon 2087
Triavil Tablets 1556
Trilafon 2123

Phenelzine Sulfate (Potentiates Librax; concomitant use not recommended). Products include:
Nardil 1742

Phenobarbital (Additive effects). Products include:
Arco-Lase Plus Tablets 607
Bellergal-S Tablets 1998
Bronkolixir ▣ 761
Bronkotabs Tablets ▣ 762
Donnatal 1858
Donnatal Extentabs 1859
Donnatal Tablets 1858
Donnazyme Tablets 1860
Kinesed Tablets 2272
Phenobarbital Elixir and Tablets 1293
Primatene Tablets-P Formula 2421
Quadrinal Tablets 1183
Tedral SA 1765

Prazepam (Additive effects; concomitant use not recommended). Products include:
Centrax 1693

Prochlorperazine (Additive effects; concomitant use not recommended). Products include:
Compazine 2201

Promethazine Hydrochloride (Additive effects; concomitant use not recommended; potentiates Librax). Products include:
Mepergan Injection 2479
Phenergan with Codeine 2497
Phenergan with Dextromethorphan 2499
Phenergan Injection 2493
Phenergan Suppositories 2496
Phenergan Syrup 2495
Phenergan Tablets 2496
Phenergan VC 2500
Phenergan VC with Codeine 2501

Propofol (Additive effects). Products include:
Diprivan Injection 2267

Propoxyphene Hydrochloride (Additive effects). Products include:
Darvon 1256
Wygesic Tablets 2540

Propoxyphene Napsylate (Additive effects). Products include:
Darvon-N/Darvocet-N 1254

Protriptyline Hydrochloride (Concomitant use not recommended). Products include:
Vivactil Tablets 1567

Quazepam (Additive effects). Products include:
Doral Tablets 2383

Secobarbital Sodium (Additive effects). Products include:
Seconal Sodium Pulvules 1296

Selegiline Hydrochloride (Potentiates Librax; concomitant use not recommended). Products include:
Eldepryl 2250

Sufentanil Citrate (Additive effects). Products include:
Sufenta Injection 1147

Temazepam (Additive effects). Products include:
Restoril Capsules 2023

Thiamylal Sodium (Additive effects). Products include:
Surital Ampoules, Steri-Vials 1764

Thioridazine Hydrochloride (Additive effects; concomitant use not recommended; potentiates Librax). Products include:
Mellaril 2011

Thiothixene (Additive effects; concomitant use not recommended). Products include:
Navane Capsules and Concentrate 1954
Navane Intramuscular 1956

Tranylcypromine Sulfate (Potentiates Librax; concomitant use not recommended). Products include:
Parnate Tablets 2222

Triazolam (Additive effects). Products include:
Halcion Tablets 2340

Trifluoperazine Hydrochloride (Additive effects; concomitant use not recommended; potentiates Librax). Products include:
Stelazine 2226

Trimipramine Maleate (Concomitant use not recommended). Products include:
Surmontil Capsules 2524

LIBRITABS TABLETS
(Chlordiazepoxide Hydrochloride) 1930
May interact with central nervous system depressants, monoamine oxidase inhibitors, phenothiazines, oral anticoagulants, and certain other agents. Compounds in these categories include:

Alcohol (Additive effect).

Alfentanil Hydrochloride (Additive effect). Products include:
Alfenta Injection 1131

Alprazolam (Additive effect). Products include:
Xanax Tablets 2367

Aprobarbital (Additive effect). Products include:
Alurate Elixir 1883

Buprenorphine (Additive effect).
No products indexed under this heading.

Buspirone Hydrochloride (Additive effect). Products include:
BuSpar ... 1401

Butabarbital (Additive effect). Products include:
Pyridium Plus ... 1764

Butalbital (Additive effect). Products include:
Esgic-Plus Tablets ... 1002
Esgic Tablets & Capsules ... 1001
Fioricet Tablets ... 2006
Fiorinal Capsules ... 2007
Fiorinal with Codeine Capsules ... 2008
Fiorinal Tablets ... 2007
Phrenilin ... 838
Sedapap Tablets 50 mg/650 mg .. 1360

Chlordiazepoxide (Additive effect). Products include:
Libritabs Tablets ... 1930
Limbitrol ... 1933
Menrium Tablets ... 1934

Chlorpromazine (Additive effect; potentiates Librium). Products include:
Thorazine ... 2234

Chlorprothixene (Additive effects). Products include:
Taractan Tablets ... 1920

Chlorprothixene Hydrochloride (Additive effect). Products include:
Taractan ... 1920

Clorazepate Dipotassium (Additive effect). Products include:
Tranxene ... 556

Codeine (Additive effect). Products include:
Calcidrine Syrup ... 506

Codeine Phosphate (Additive effect). Products include:
Actifed with Codeine Cough Syrup.. 752
Cheracol Cough Syrup ... 1853
Codimal PH Syrup ... 846
Dimetane-DC Cough Syrup ... 1857
Empirin with Codeine Phosphate Nos. 2, 3 & 4 ... 764
Fiorinal with Codeine Capsules ... 2008
Isoclor Expectorant ... 982
Naldecon CX Adult Liquid ... ▣ 521
Novahistine DH ... 1342
Novahistine Expectorant ... 1343
Nucofed Capsules ... 2219
Nucofed Expectorant ... 2219
Nucofed Pediatric Expectorant ... 2220
Nucofed Syrup ... 2219
Phenaphen with Codeine Capsules 1865
Phenaphen-650 with Codeine Tablets ... 1866
Phenergan with Codeine ... 2497
Phenergan VC with Codeine ... 2501
Robitussin A-C Syrup ... 1875
Robitussin-DAC Syrup ... 1875
Ryna ... ▣ 741
Soma Compound w/Codeine Tablets ... 2390
Triaminic Expectorant w/Codeine .. 1996
Tussi-Organidin Liquid ... 2391
Tylenol with Codeine ... 1381

Codeine Polistirex (Additive effect).
No products indexed under this heading.

Dezocine (Additive effect).

Diazepam (Additive effect). Products include:
Valium Injectable ... 1937
Valium Tablets ... 1939
Valrelease Capsules ... 1923

Dicumarol (Potential for variable effects on blood coagulation). Products include:
Dicumarol Tablets ... 516

Droperidol (Additive effect). Products include:
Inapsine Injection ... 1140
Innovar Injection ... 1141

Enflurane (Additive effect). Products include:
Ethrane ... 599

Estazolam (Additive effect). Products include:
ProSom Tablets ... 554

Ethchlorvynol (Additive effect). Products include:
Placidyl Capsules ... 553

Ethinamate (Additive effect).
No products indexed under this heading.

Fentanyl (Additive effect). Products include:
Duragesic Transdermal System ... 1133

Fentanyl Citrate (Additive effect). Products include:
Innovar Injection ... 1141
Sublimaze Injection ... 1146

Fluphenazine Decanoate (Additive effect; potentiates Librium). Products include:
Prolixin Decanoate ... 1795

Fluphenazine Enanthate (Additive effect; potentiates Librium). Products include:
Prolixin Enanthate ... 1796

Fluphenazine Hydrochloride (Additive effect; potentiates Librium). Products include:
Prolixin Elixir ... 1793
Prolixin Injection ... 1791
Prolixin Oral Concentrate ... 1792
Prolixin Tablets ... 1793

Flurazepam Hydrochloride (Additive effect). Products include:
Dalmane Capsules ... 1927

Furazolidone (Potentiates Librium). Products include:
Furoxone ... 1855

Glutethimide (Additive effect).
No products indexed under this heading.

Haloperidol (Additive effect). Products include:
Haldol Injection, Tablets and Concentrate ... 1373

Haloperidol Decanoate (Additive effect). Products include:
Haldol Decanoate ... 1375

Hydrocodone Bitartrate (Additive effect). Products include:
Anexsia 5/500 Tablets ... 2196
Anexsia 7.5/650 Tablets ... 2197
Azdone Tablets ... 844
Codiclear DH Syrup ... 845
Codimal DH Syrup ... 846
Damason-P ... 1356
Hycodan Syrup, Tablets ... 927
Hycomine Compound Tablets ... 929
Hycomine Syrup ... 927
Hycotuss Expectorant Syrup ... 930
Hydrocet Capsules ... 835
Lortab ASA Tablets ... 2414
Lortab ... 2412
Ru-Tuss with Hydrocodone ... 694
Triaminic Expectorant DH ... 1995
Vicodin Tablets ... 1187
Vicodin ES Tablets ... 1189
Zydone Capsules ... 941

Hydrocodone Polistirex (Additive effect). Products include:
Tussionex Extended-Release Suspension ... 988

Hydroxyzine Hydrochloride (Additive effect). Products include:
Atarax Tablets & Syrup ... 1941
Marax Tablets & DF Syrup ... 1954
Vistaril Intramuscular Solution ... 1970

Isocarboxazid (Potentiates Librium). Products include:
Marplan Tablets ... 1906

Isoflurane (Additive effect). Products include:
Forane ... 600

Ketamine Hydrochloride (Additive effect). Products include:
Ketalar ... 1726

Levorphanol Tartrate (Additive effect). Products include:
Levo-Dromoran ... 1906

Lorazepam (Additive effect). Products include:
Ativan Injection ... 2432
Ativan Tablets ... 2434

Loxapine Hydrochloride (Additive effect). Products include:
Loxitane ... 1213

Loxapine Succinate (Additive effect). Products include:
Loxitane Capsules ... 1213

Meperidine Hydrochloride (Additive effect). Products include:
Demerol ... 2047
Mepergan Injection ... 2479

Mephobarbital (Additive effect). Products include:
Mebaral Tablets ... 2061

Meprobamate (Additive effect). Products include:
Deprol Tablets ... 2382
Equagesic Tablets ... 2451
Miltown Tablets ... 2386
PMB 200 and PMB 400 ... 2504

Mesoridazine (Additive effect; potentiates Librium). Products include:
Serentil ... 686

Methadone Hydrochloride (Additive effect). Products include:
Dolophine Hydrochloride Ampoules & Vials ... 1260
Dolophine Hydrochloride Tablets ... 1261
Methadone Hydrochloride Diskets .. 1284
Methadone Hydrochloride Oral Solution & Tablets ... 1987

Methohexital Sodium (Additive effect). Products include:
Brevital Sodium Vials ... 1248

Methoxyflurane (Additive effect).
No products indexed under this heading.

Midazolam Hydrochloride (Additive effect). Products include:
Versed Injection ... 1924

Molindone Hydrochloride (Additive effect). Products include:
Moban Tablets & Concentrate ... 932

Morphine Sulfate (Additive effect). Products include:
Astramorph/PF Injection, USP (Preservative-Free) ... 618
Duramorph ... 960
Infumorph 200 and Infumorph 500 Sterile Solutions ... 962
MS Contin Tablets ... 1814
MSIR ... 1817
Oramorph SR (Morphine Sulfate Sustained Release Tablets) ... 1988
Roxanol ... 1991

Opium Alkaloids (Additive effect). Products include:
B & O No. 15A & No. 16A Supprettes ... 2395
Pantopon Injectable ... 1911

Oxazepam (Additive effect). Products include:
Serax Capsules ... 2522
Serax Tablets ... 2522

Oxycodone Hydrochloride (Additive effect). Products include:
Percocet Tablets ... 950
Percodan ... 951
Roxicodone Tablets, Oral Solution & Intensol (Oxycodone) ... 1992
Tylox Capsules ... 1382

Pentobarbital Sodium (Additive effect). Products include:
Nembutal Sodium Capsules ... 534
Nembutal Sodium Solution ... 536
Nembutal Sodium Suppositories ... 538

Perphenazine (Additive effect; potentiates Librium). Products include:
Etrafon ... 2087
Triavil Tablets ... 1556
Trilafon ... 2123

Phenelzine Sulfate (Potentiates Librium). Products include:
Nardil ... 1742

Phenobarbital (Additive effect). Products include:
Arco-Lase Plus Tablets ... 607
Bellergal-S Tablets ... 1998
Bronkolixir ... ▣ 761
Bronkotabs Tablets ... ▣ 762
Donnatal ... 1858
Donnatal Extentabs ... 1859
Donnatal Tablets ... 1858
Donnazyme Tablets ... 1860
Kinesed Tablets ... 2272
Phenobarbital Elixir and Tablets ... 1293
Primatene Tablets-P Formula ... 2421
Quadrinal Tablets ... 1183
Tedral SA ... 1765

Prazepam (Additive effect). Products include:
Centrax ... 1693

Prochlorperazine (Additive effect; potentiates Librium). Products include:
Compazine ... 2201

Promethazine Hydrochloride (Additive effect; potentiates Librium). Products include:
Mepergan Injection ... 2479
Phenergan with Codeine ... 2497
Phenergan with Dextromethorphan 2499
Phenergan Injection ... 2493
Phenergan Suppositories ... 2496
Phenergan Syrup ... 2495
Phenergan Tablets ... 2496
Phenergan VC ... 2500
Phenergan VC with Codeine ... 2501

Propofol (Additive effect). Products include:
Diprivan Injection ... 2267

Propoxyphene Hydrochloride (Additive effect). Products include:
Darvon ... 1256
Wygesic Tablets ... 2540

Propoxyphene Napsylate (Additive effect). Products include:
Darvon-N/Darvocet-N ... 1254

Quazepam (Additive effect). Products include:
Doral Tablets ... 2383

Secobarbital Sodium (Additive effect). Products include:
Seconal Sodium Pulvules ... 1296

Selegiline Hydrochloride (Potentiates Librium). Products include:
Eldepryl ... 2250

Sufentanil Citrate (Additive effect). Products include:
Sufenta Injection ... 1147

Temazepam (Additive effect). Products include:
Restoril Capsules ... 2023

Thiamylal Sodium (Additive effect). Products include:
Surital Ampoules, Steri-Vials ... 1764

Thioridazine Hydrochloride (Additive effect; potentiates Librium). Products include:
Mellaril ... 2011

Thiothixene (Additive effect). Products include:
Navane Capsules and Concentrate 1954
Navane Intramuscular ... 1956

Tranylcypromine Sulfate (Potentiates Librium). Products include:
Parnate Tablets ... 2222

Triazolam (Additive effect). Products include:
Halcion Tablets ... 2340

Trifluoperazine Hydrochloride (Additive effect; potentiates Librium). Products include:
Stelazine ... 2226

Warfarin Sodium (Potential for variable effects on blood coagulation). Products include:
Coumadin Injection & Tablets ... 944
Panwarfin Tablets ... 547

LIBRIUM CAPSULES (Chlordiazepoxide) ... 1931
May interact with monoamine oxidase inhibitors, phenothiazines, and

oral anticoagulants. Compounds in these categories include:

Chlorpromazine (Combination therapy requires careful monitoring from pharmacological point of view). Products include:
- Thorazine 2234

Dicumarol (Variable effects on blood coagulation). Products include:
- Dicumarol Tablets 516

Fluphenazine Decanoate (Combination therapy requires careful monitoring from pharmacological point of view). Products include:
- Prolixin Decanoate 1795

Fluphenazine Enanthate (Combination therapy requires careful monitoring from pharmacological point of view). Products include:
- Prolixin Enanthate 1796

Fluphenazine Hydrochloride (Combination therapy requires careful monitoring from pharmacological point of view). Products include:
- Prolixin Elixir 1793
- Prolixin Injection 1791
- Prolixin Oral Concentrate 1792
- Prolixin Tablets 1793

Furazolidone (Combination therapy requires careful monitoring from pharmacological point of view). Products include:
- Furoxone 1855

Isocarboxazid (Combination therapy requires careful monitoring from pharmacological point of view). Products include:
- Marplan Tablets 1906

Mesoridazine Besylate (Combination therapy requires careful monitoring from pharmacological point of view).

Perphenazine (Combination therapy requires careful monitoring from pharmacological point of view). Products include:
- Etrafon 2087
- Triavil Tablets 1556
- Trilafon 2123

Phenelzine Sulfate (Combination therapy requires careful monitoring from pharmacological point of view). Products include:
- Nardil 1742

Prochlorperazine (Combination therapy requires careful monitoring from pharmacological point of view). Products include:
- Compazine 2201

Promethazine Hydrochloride (Combination therapy requires careful monitoring from pharmacological point of view). Products include:
- Mepergan Injection 2479
- Phenergan with Codeine 2497
- Phenergan with Dextromethorphan 2499
- Phenergan Injection 2493
- Phenergan Suppositories 2496
- Phenergan Syrup 2495
- Phenergan Tablets 2496
- Phenergan VC 2500
- Phenergan VC with Codeine 2501

Selegiline Hydrochloride (Combination therapy requires careful monitoring from pharmacological point of view). Products include:
- Eldepryl 2250

Thioridazine Hydrochloride (Combination therapy requires careful monitoring from pharmacological point of view). Products include:
- Mellaril 2011

Tranylcypromine Sulfate (Combination therapy requires careful monitoring from pharmacological point of view). Products include:
- Parnate Tablets 2222

Trifluoperazine Hydrochloride (Combination therapy requires careful monitoring from pharmacological point of view). Products include:
- Stelazine 2226

Warfarin Sodium (Variable effects on blood coagulation). Products include:
- Coumadin Injection & Tablets 944
- Panwarfin Tablets 547

LIBRIUM INJECTABLE
(Chlordiazepoxide Hydrochloride) 1932
May interact with central nervous system depressants, monoamine oxidase inhibitors, phenothiazines, and certain other agents. Compounds in these categories include:

Alcohol (Additive effect).

Alfentanil Hydrochloride (Additive effect). Products include:
- Alfenta Injection 1131

Alprazolam (Additive effect). Products include:
- Xanax Tablets 2367

Aprobarbital (Additive effect). Products include:
- Alurate Elixir 1883

Buprenorphine (Additive effect).
No products indexed under this heading.

Buspirone Hydrochloride (Additive effect). Products include:
- BuSpar 1401

Butabarbital (Additive effect). Products include:
- Pyridium Plus 1764

Butalbital (Additive effect). Products include:
- Esgic-Plus Tablets 1002
- Esgic Tablets & Capsules 1001
- Fioricet Tablets 2006
- Fiorinal Capsules 2007
- Fiorinal with Codeine Capsules 2008
- Fiorinal Tablets 2007
- Phrenilin 838
- Sedapap Tablets 50 mg/650 mg 1360

Chlordiazepoxide (Additive effect). Products include:
- Libritabs Tablets 1930
- Limbitrol 1933
- Menrium Tablets 1934

Chlorpromazine (Additive effect; potentiates Librium). Products include:
- Thorazine 2234

Chlorprothixene (Additive effect). Products include:
- Taractan Tablets 1920

Chlorprothixene Hydrochloride (Additive effect). Products include:
- Taractan 1920

Clorazepate Dipotassium (Additive effect). Products include:
- Tranxene 556

Codeine (Additive effect). Products include:
- Calcidrine Syrup 506

Codeine Phosphate (Additive effect). Products include:
- Actifed with Codeine Cough Syrup 752
- Cheracol Cough Syrup 1853
- Codimal PH Syrup 846
- Dimetane-DC Cough Syrup 1857
- Empirin with Codeine Phosphate Nos. 2, 3 & 4 764
- Fiorinal with Codeine Capsules 2008
- Isoclor Expectorant 982
- Naldecon CX Adult Liquid ⊞ 521
- Novahistine DH 1342
- Novahistine Expectorant 1343
- Nucofed Capsules 2219
- Nucofed Expectorant 2219
- Nucofed Pediatric Expectorant 2220
- Nucofed Syrup 2219
- Phenaphen with Codeine Capsules 1865
- Phenaphen-650 with Codeine Tablets 1866
- Phenergan with Codeine 2497
- Phenergan VC with Codeine 2501
- Robitussin A-C Syrup 1875
- Robitussin-DAC Syrup 1875
- Ryna ⊞ 741
- Soma Compound w/Codeine Tablets 2390
- Triaminic Expectorant w/Codeine 1996
- Tussi-Organidin Liquid 2391
- Tylenol with Codeine 1381

Codeine Polistirex (Additive effect).
No products indexed under this heading.

Dezocine (Additive effect).

Diazepam (Additive effect). Products include:
- Valium Injectable 1937
- Valium Tablets 1939
- Valrelease Capsules 1923

Droperidol (Additive effect). Products include:
- Inapsine Injection 1140
- Innovar Injection 1141

Enflurane (Additive effect). Products include:
- Ethrane 599

Estazolam (Additive effect). Products include:
- ProSom Tablets 554

Ethchlorvynol (Additive effect). Products include:
- Placidyl Capsules 553

Ethinamate (Additive effect).
No products indexed under this heading.

Fentanyl (Additive effect). Products include:
- Duragesic Transdermal System 1133

Fentanyl Citrate (Additive effect). Products include:
- Innovar Injection 1141
- Sublimaze Injection 1146

Fluphenazine Decanoate (Additive effect; potentiates Librium). Products include:
- Prolixin Decanoate 1795

Fluphenazine Enanthate (Additive effect; potentiates Librium). Products include:
- Prolixin Enanthate 1796

Fluphenazine Hydrochloride (Additive effect; potentiates Librium). Products include:
- Prolixin Elixir 1793
- Prolixin Injection 1791
- Prolixin Oral Concentrate 1792
- Prolixin Tablets 1793

Flurazepam Hydrochloride (Additive effect). Products include:
- Dalmane Capsules 1927

Furazolidone (Potentiates Librium). Products include:
- Furoxone 1855

Glutethimide (Additive effect).
No products indexed under this heading.

Haloperidol (Additive effect). Products include:
- Haldol Injection, Tablets and Concentrate 1373

Haloperidol Decanoate (Additive effect). Products include:
- Haldol Decanoate 1375

Hydrocodone Bitartrate (Additive effect). Products include:
- Anexsia 5/500 Tablets 2196
- Anexsia 7.5/650 Tablets 2197
- Azdōne Tablets 844
- Codiclear DH Syrup 845
- Codimal DH Syrup 846
- Damason-P 1356
- Hycodan Syrup, Tablets 927
- Hycomine Compound Tablets 929
- Hycomine Syrup 927
- Hycotuss Expectorant Syrup 930
- Hydrocet Capsules 835
- Lortab ASA Tablets 2414
- Lortab 2412
- Ru-Tuss with Hydrocodone 694
- Triaminic Expectorant DH 1995
- Vicodin Tablets 1187
- Vicodin ES Tablets 1189
- Zydone Capsules 941

Hydrocodone Polistirex (Additive effect). Products include:
- Tussionex Extended-Release Suspension 988

Hydroxyzine Hydrochloride (Additive effect). Products include:
- Atarax Tablets & Syrup 1941
- Marax Tablets & DF Syrup 1954
- Vistaril Intramuscular Solution 1970

Isocarboxazid (Potentiates Librium). Products include:
- Marplan Tablets 1906

Isoflurane (Additive effect). Products include:
- Forane 600

Ketamine Hydrochloride (Additive effect). Products include:
- Ketalar 1726

Levorphanol Tartrate (Additive effect). Products include:
- Levo-Dromoran 1906

Lorazepam (Additive effect). Products include:
- Ativan Injection 2432
- Ativan Tablets 2434

Loxapine Hydrochloride (Additive effect). Products include:
- Loxitane 1213

Loxapine Succinate (Additive effect). Products include:
- Loxitane Capsules 1213

Meperidine Hydrochloride (Additive effect). Products include:
- Demerol 2047
- Mepergan Injection 2479

Mephobarbital (Additive effect). Products include:
- Mebaral Tablets 2061

Meprobamate (Additive effect). Products include:
- Deprol Tablets 2382
- Equagesic Tablets 2451
- Miltown Tablets 2386
- PMB 200 and PMB 400 2504

Mesoridazine (Additive effect; potentiates Librium). Products include:
- Serentil 686

Methadone Hydrochloride (Additive effect). Products include:
- Dolophine Hydrochloride Ampoules & Vials 1260
- Dolophine Hydrochloride Tablets 1261
- Methadone Hydrochloride Diskets 1284
- Methadone Hydrochloride Oral Solution & Tablets 1987

Methohexital Sodium (Additive effect). Products include:
- Brevital Sodium Vials 1248

Methoxyflurane (Additive effect).
No products indexed under this heading.

Midazolam Hydrochloride (Additive effect). Products include:
- Versed Injection 1924

Molindone Hydrochloride (Additive effect). Products include:
- Moban Tablets & Concentrate 932

Morphine Sulfate (Additive effect). Products include:
- Astramorph/PF Injection, USP (Preservative-Free) 618
- Duramorph 960
- Infumorph 200 and Infumorph 500 Sterile Solutions 962
- MS Contin Tablets 1814
- MSIR 1817
- Oramorph SR (Morphine Sulfate Sustained Release Tablets) 1988
- Roxanol 1991

Opium Alkaloids (Additive effect). Products include:
- B & O No. 15A & No. 16A Supprettes 2395
- Pantopon Injectable 1911

Oxazepam (Additive effect). Products include:
- Serax Capsules 2522
- Serax Tablets 2522

Oxycodone Hydrochloride (Additive effect). Products include:
- Percocet Tablets ... 950
- Percodan ... 951
- Roxicodone Tablets, Oral Solution & Intensol (Oxycodone) ... 1992
- Tylox Capsules ... 1382

Pentobarbital Sodium (Additive effect). Products include:
- Nembutal Sodium Capsules ... 534
- Nembutal Sodium Solution ... 536
- Nembutal Sodium Suppositories ... 538

Perphenazine (Additive effect; potentiates Librium). Products include:
- Etrafon ... 2087
- Triavil Tablets ... 1556
- Trilafon ... 2123

Phenelzine Sulfate (Potentiates Librium). Products include:
- Nardil ... 1742

Phenobarbital (Additive effect). Products include:
- Arco-Lase Plus Tablets ... 607
- Bellergal-S Tablets ... 1998
- Bronkolixir ... ⊞ 761
- Bronkotabs Tablets ... ⊞ 762
- Donnatal ... 1858
- Donnatal Extentabs ... 1859
- Donnatal Tablets ... 1858
- Donnazyme Tablets ... 1860
- Kinesed Tablets ... 2272
- Phenobarbital Elixir and Tablets ... 1293
- Primatene Tablets-P Formula ... 2421
- Quadrinal Tablets ... 1183
- Tedral SA ... 1765

Prazepam (Additive effect). Products include:
- Centrax ... 1693

Prochlorperazine (Additive effect; potentiates Librium). Products include:
- Compazine ... 2201

Promethazine Hydrochloride (Additive effect; potentiates Librium). Products include:
- Mepergan Injection ... 2479
- Phenergan with Codeine ... 2497
- Phenergan with Dextromethorphan 2499
- Phenergan Injection ... 2493
- Phenergan Suppositories ... 2496
- Phenergan Syrup ... 2495
- Phenergan Tablets ... 2496
- Phenergan VC ... 2500
- Phenergan VC with Codeine ... 2501

Propofol (Additive effect). Products include:
- Diprivan Injection ... 2267

Propoxyphene Hydrochloride (Additive effect). Products include:
- Darvon ... 1256
- Wygesic Tablets ... 2540

Propoxyphene Napsylate (Additive effect). Products include:
- Darvon-N/Darvocet-N ... 1254

Quazepam (Additive effect). Products include:
- Doral Tablets ... 2383

Secobarbital Sodium (Additive effect). Products include:
- Seconal Sodium Pulvules ... 1296

Selegiline Hydrochloride (Potentiates Librium). Products include:
- Eldepryl ... 2250

Sufentanil Citrate (Additive effect). Products include:
- Sufenta Injection ... 1147

Temazepam (Additive effect). Products include:
- Restoril Capsules ... 2023

Thiamylal Sodium (Additive effect). Products include:
- Surital Ampoules, Steri-Vials ... 1764

Thioridazine Hydrochloride (Additive effect; potentiates Librium). Products include:
- Mellaril ... 2011

Thiothixene (Additive effect). Products include:
- Navane Capsules and Concentrate 1954
- Navane Intramuscular ... 1956

Tranylcypromine Sulfate (Potentiates Librium). Products include:
- Parnate Tablets ... 2222

Triazolam (Additive effect). Products include:
- Halcion Tablets ... 2340

Trifluoperazine Hydrochloride (Additive effect). Products include:
- Stelazine ... 2226

LICE•ENZ FOAM
(Pyrethrins, Piperonyl Butoxide) ... ⊞ 558
No interactions described in labeling.

LIDEX CREAM 0.05%
(Fluocinonide) ... 2296
No interactions described in labeling.

LIDEX GEL 0.05%
(Fluocinonide) ... 2296
No interactions described in labeling.

LIDEX OINTMENT 0.05%
(Fluocinonide) ... 2296
No interactions described in labeling.

LIDEX TOPICAL SOLUTION 0.05%
(Fluocinonide) ... 2296
No interactions described in labeling.

LIDEX-E CREAM 0.05%
(Fluocinonide) ... 2296
No interactions described in labeling.

LIMBITROL DS TABLETS
(Chlordiazepoxide, Amitriptyline Hydrochloride) ... 1933
See **Limbitrol Tablets**

LIMBITROL TABLETS
(Chlordiazepoxide, Amitriptyline Hydrochloride) ... 1933
May interact with monoamine oxidase inhibitors, anticholinergics, central nervous system depressants, and certain other agents. Compounds in these categories include:

Alcohol (Additive effects).

Alfentanil Hydrochloride (Additive effects). Products include:
- Alfenta Injection ... 1131

Alprazolam (Additive effects). Products include:
- Xanax Tablets ... 2367

Aprobarbital (Additive effects). Products include:
- Alurate Elixir ... 1883

Atropine Sulfate (Severe constipation). Products include:
- Arco-Lase Plus Tablets ... 607
- Atropine Sulfate Sterile Ophthalmic Solution and S.O.P. Sterile Ophthalmic Ointment ... ◉ 239
- Donnagel ... ⊞ 675
- Donnagel-PG ... 1858
- Donnatal ... 1858
- Donnatal Extentabs ... 1859
- Donnatal Tablets ... 1858
- Donnazyme Tablets ... 1860
- Isopto Atropine ... ◉ 218
- Lomotil ... 2174
- Motofen Tablets ... 836
- Ru-Tuss Tablets ... 693
- Urised Tablets ... 2396

Belladonna Alkaloids (Severe constipation). Products include:
- Bellergal-S Tablets ... 1998
- Hyland's Bed Wetting Tablets ... ⊞ 728
- Hyland's Teething Tablets ... ⊞ 728
- Kinesed Tablets ... 2272

Benztropine Mesylate (Severe constipation). Products include:
- Cogentin ... 1435

Biperiden (Severe constipation). Products include:
- Akineton ... 1171

Buprenorphine (Additive effects).
No products indexed under this heading.

Buspirone Hydrochloride (Additive effects). Products include:
- BuSpar ... 1401

Butabarbital (Additive effects). Products include:
- Pyridium Plus ... 1764

Butalbital (Additive effects). Products include:
- Esgic-Plus Tablets ... 1002
- Esgic Tablets & Capsules ... 1001
- Fioricet Tablets ... 2006
- Fiorinal Capsules ... 2007
- Fiorinal with Codeine Capsules ... 2008
- Fiorinal Tablets ... 2007
- Phrenilin ... 838
- Sedapap Tablets 50 mg/650 mg .. 1360

Chlordiazepoxide Hydrochloride (Additive effects). Products include:
- Librax Capsules ... 1929
- Librium Capsules ... 1931
- Librium Injectable ... 1932

Chlorpromazine (Additive effects). Products include:
- Thorazine ... 2234

Chlorprothixene (Additive effects). Products include:
- Taractan Tablets ... 1920

Chlorprothixene Hydrochloride (Additive effects). Products include:
- Taractan ... 1920

Cimetidine (Reduces hepatic metabolism of tricyclic antidepressants). Products include:
- Tagamet Tablets ... 2228

Cimetidine Hydrochloride (Reduces hepatic metabolism of tricyclic antidepressants). Products include:
- Tagamet ... 2228

Clidinium Bromide (Severe constipation). Products include:
- Librax Capsules ... 1929
- Quarzan Capsules ... 1937

Clorazepate Dipotassium (Additive effects). Products include:
- Tranxene ... 556

Codeine (Additive effects). Products include:
- Calcidrine Syrup ... 506

Codeine Phosphate (Additive effects). Products include:
- Actifed with Codeine Cough Syrup.. 752
- Cheracol Cough Syrup ... 1853
- Codimal PH Syrup ... 846
- Dimetane-DC Cough Syrup ... 1857
- Empirin with Codeine Phosphate Nos. 2, 3 & 4 ... 764
- Fiorinal with Codeine Capsules ... 2008
- Isoclor Expectorant ... 982
- Naldecon CX Adult Liquid ... ⊞ 521
- Novahistine DH ... 1342
- Novahistine Expectorant ... 1343
- Nucofed Capsules ... 2219
- Nucofed Expectorant ... 2219
- Nucofed Pediatric Expectorant ... 2220
- Nucofed Syrup ... 2219
- Phenaphen with Codeine Capsules 1865
- Phenaphen-650 with Codeine Tablets ... 1866
- Phenergan with Codeine ... 2497
- Phenergan VC with Codeine ... 2501
- Robitussin A-C Syrup ... 1875
- Robitussin-DAC Syrup ... 1875
- Ryna ... ⊞ 741
- Soma Compound w/Codeine Tablets ... 2390
- Triaminic Expectorant w/Codeine .. 1996
- Tussi-Organidin Liquid ... 2391
- Tylenol with Codeine ... 1381

Codeine Polistirex (Additive effects).
No products indexed under this heading.

Dezocine (Additive effects).

Diazepam (Additive effects). Products include:
- Valium Injectable ... 1937
- Valium Tablets ... 1939
- Valrelease Capsules ... 1923

Dicyclomine Hydrochloride (Severe constipation). Products include:
- Bentyl ... 1322

Droperidol (Additive effects). Products include:
- Inapsine Injection ... 1140
- Innovar Injection ... 1141

Enflurane (Additive effects). Products include:
- Ethrane ... 599

Estazolam (Additive effects). Products include:
- ProSom Tablets ... 554

Ethchlorvynol (Additive effects). Products include:
- Placidyl Capsules ... 553

Ethinamate (Additive effects).
No products indexed under this heading.

Fentanyl (Additive effects). Products include:
- Duragesic Transdermal System ... 1133

Fentanyl Citrate (Additive effects). Products include:
- Innovar Injection ... 1141
- Sublimaze Injection ... 1146

Fluphenazine Decanoate (Additive effects). Products include:
- Prolixin Decanoate ... 1795

Fluphenazine Enanthate (Additive effects). Products include:
- Prolixin Enanthate ... 1796

Fluphenazine Hydrochloride (Additive effects). Products include:
- Prolixin Elixir ... 1793
- Prolixin Injection ... 1791
- Prolixin Oral Concentrate ... 1792
- Prolixin Tablets ... 1793

Flurazepam Hydrochloride (Additive effects). Products include:
- Dalmane Capsules ... 1927

Furazolidone (Hyperpyretic crisis). Products include:
- Furoxone ... 1855

Glutethimide (Additive effects).
No products indexed under this heading.

Glycopyrrolate (Severe constipation). Products include:
- Robinul Forte Tablets ... 1873
- Robinul Injectable ... 1873
- Robinul Tablets ... 1873

Guanethidine Monosulfate (Blocked antihypertensive action of guanethidine). Products include:
- Esimil Tablets ... 864
- Ismelin Tablets ... 869

Haloperidol (Additive effects). Products include:
- Haldol Injection, Tablets and Concentrate ... 1373

Haloperidol Decanoate (Additive effects). Products include:
- Haldol Decanoate ... 1375

Hydrocodone Bitartrate (Additive effects). Products include:
- Anexsia 5/500 Tablets ... 2196
- Anexsia 7.5/650 Tablets ... 2197
- Azdōne Tablets ... 844
- Codiclear DH Syrup ... 845
- Codimal DH Syrup ... 846
- Damason-P ... 1356
- Hycodan Syrup, Tablets ... 927
- Hycomine Compound Tablets ... 929
- Hycomine Syrup ... 927
- Hycotuss Expectorant Syrup ... 930
- Hydrocet Capsules ... 835
- Lortab ASA Tablets ... 2414
- Lortab ... 2412
- Ru-Tuss with Hydrocodone ... 694
- Triaminic Expectorant DH ... 1995
- Vicodin Tablets ... 1187
- Vicodin ES Tablets ... 1189
- Zydone Capsules ... 941

Hydrocodone Polistirex (Additive effects). Products include:
- Tussionex Extended-Release Suspension ... 988

Hydroxyzine Hydrochloride (Additive effects). Products include:
- Atarax Tablets & Syrup ... 1941
- Marax Tablets & DF Syrup ... 1954
- Vistaril Intramuscular Solution ... 1970

Hyoscyamine (Severe constipation). Products include:
- Cystospaz Tablets ... 2395
- Urised Tablets ... 2396

Hyoscyamine Sulfate (Severe constipation). Products include:
- Arco-Lase Plus Tablets ... 607
- Cystospaz-M Capsules ... 2395
- Donnagel ... ⊞ 675
- Donnagel-PG ... 1858
- Donnatal ... 1858
- Donnatal Extentabs ... 1859
- Donnatal Tablets ... 1858
- Donnazyme Tablets ... 1860
- Kutrase Capsules ... 2146
- Levsin/Levsinex ... 2147
- Ru-Tuss Tablets ... 693

Ipratropium Bromide (Severe constipation). Products include:
- Atrovent Inhalation Aerosol ... 675

Isocarboxazid (Hyperpyretic crisis). Products include:
- Marplan Tablets ... 1906

Isoflurane (Additive effects). Products include:
- Forane ... 600

Ketamine Hydrochloride (Additive effects). Products include:
- Ketalar ... 1726

Levorphanol Tartrate (Additive effects). Products include:
- Levo-Dromoran ... 1906

Lorazepam (Additive effects). Products include:
- Ativan Injection ... 2432
- Ativan Tablets ... 2434

Loxapine Hydrochloride (Additive effects). Products include:
- Loxitane ... 1213

Loxapine Succinate (Additive effects). Products include:
- Loxitane Capsules ... 1213

Mepenzolate Bromide (Severe constipation). Products include:
- Cantil Tablets ... 1326

Meperidine Hydrochloride (Additive effects). Products include:
- Demerol ... 2047
- Mepergan Injection ... 2479

Mephobarbital (Additive effects). Products include:
- Mebaral Tablets ... 2061

Meprobamate (Additive effects). Products include:
- Deprol Tablets ... 2382
- Equagesic Tablets ... 2451
- Miltown Tablets ... 2386
- PMB 200 and PMB 400 ... 2504

Mesoridazine (Additive effects). Products include:
- Serentil ... 686

Methadone Hydrochloride (Additive effects). Products include:
- Dolophine Hydrochloride Ampoules & Vials ... 1260
- Dolophine Hydrochloride Tablets ... 1261
- Methadone Hydrochloride Diskets .. 1284
- Methadone Hydrochloride Oral Solution & Tablets ... 1987

Methohexital Sodium (Additive effects). Products include:
- Brevital Sodium Vials ... 1248

Methoxyflurane (Additive effects). No products indexed under this heading.

Midazolam Hydrochloride (Additive effects). Products include:
- Versed Injection ... 1924

Molindone Hydrochloride (Additive effects). Products include:
- Moban Tablets & Concentrate ... 932

Morphine Sulfate (Additive effects). Products include:
- Astramorph/PF Injection, USP (Preservative-Free) ... 618
- Duramorph ... 960
- Infumorph 200 and Infumorph 500 Sterile Solutions ... 962
- MS Contin Tablets ... 1814
- MSIR ... 1817
- Oramorph SR (Morphine Sulfate Sustained Release Tablets) ... 1988
- Roxanol ... 1991

Opium Alkaloids (Additive effect). Products include:
- B & O No. 15A & No. 16A Supprettes ... 2395
- Pantopon Injectable ... 1911

Oxazepam (Additive effects). Products include:
- Serax Capsules ... 2522
- Serax Tablets ... 2522

Oxybutynin Chloride (Severe constipation). Products include:
- Ditropan ... 1332

Oxycodone Hydrochloride (Additive effects). Products include:
- Percocet Tablets ... 950
- Percodan ... 951
- Roxicodone Tablets, Oral Solution & Intensol (Oxycodone) ... 1992
- Tylox Capsules ... 1382

Pentobarbital Sodium (Additive effects). Products include:
- Nembutal Sodium Capsules ... 534
- Nembutal Sodium Solution ... 536
- Nembutal Sodium Suppositories ... 538

Perphenazine (Additive effects). Products include:
- Etrafon ... 2087
- Triavil Tablets ... 1556
- Trilafon ... 2123

Phenelzine Sulfate (Hyperpyretic crisis). Products include:
- Nardil ... 1742

Phenobarbital (Additive effects). Products include:
- Arco-Lase Plus Tablets ... 607
- Bellergal-S Tablets ... 1998
- Bronkolixir ... ⊞ 761
- Bronkotabs Tablets ... ⊞ 762
- Donnatal ... 1858
- Donnatal Extentabs ... 1859
- Donnatal Tablets ... 1858
- Donnazyme Tablets ... 1860
- Kinesed Tablets ... 2272
- Phenobarbital Elixir and Tablets ... 1293
- Primatene Tablets-P Formula ... 2421
- Quadrinal Tablets ... 1183
- Tedral SA ... 1765

Prazepam (Additive effects). Products include:
- Centrax ... 1693

Prochlorperazine (Additive effects). Products include:
- Compazine ... 2201

Procyclidine Hydrochloride (Severe constipation). Products include:
- Kemadrin Tablets ... 771

Promethazine Hydrochloride (Additive effects). Products include:
- Mepergan Injection ... 2479
- Phenergan with Codeine ... 2497
- Phenergan with Dextromethorphan ... 2499
- Phenergan Injection ... 2493
- Phenergan Suppositories ... 2496
- Phenergan Syrup ... 2495
- Phenergan Tablets ... 2496
- Phenergan VC ... 2500
- Phenergan VC with Codeine ... 2501

Propantheline Bromide (Severe constipation). Products include:
- Pro-Banthine Tablets ... 2141

Propofol (Additive effects). Products include:
- Diprivan Injection ... 2267

Propoxyphene Hydrochloride (Additive effects). Products include:
- Darvon ... 1256
- Wygesic Tablets ... 2540

Propoxyphene Napsylate (Additive effects). Products include:
- Darvon-N/Darvocet-N ... 1254

Quazepam (Additive effects). Products include:
- Doral Tablets ... 2383

Scopolamine Hydrobromide (Severe constipation). Products include:
- Donnagel ... ⊞ 675
- Donnagel-PG ... 1858
- Donnatal ... 1858
- Donnatal Extentabs ... 1859
- Donnatal Tablets ... 1858
- Donnazyme Tablets ... 1860
- Isopto Hyoscine ... ◉ 222
- Murocoll-2 Sterile Ophthalmic Solution ... ◉ 261
- Ru-Tuss Tablets ... 693

Scopolamine Preparations (Severe constipation). Products include:
- Transderm Scōp Transdermal Therapeutic System ... 887

Secobarbital Sodium (Additive effects). Products include:
- Seconal Sodium Pulvules ... 1296

Selegiline Hydrochloride (Hyperpyretic crisis). Products include:
- Eldepryl ... 2250

Sufentanil Citrate (Additive effects). Products include:
- Sufenta Injection ... 1147

Temazepam (Additive effects). Products include:
- Restoril Capsules ... 2023

Thiamylal Sodium (Additive effects). Products include:
- Surital Ampoules, Steri-Vials ... 1764

Thioridazine Hydrochloride (Additive effects). Products include:
- Mellaril ... 2011

Thiothixene (Additive effects). Products include:
- Navane Capsules and Concentrate 1954
- Navane Intramuscular ... 1956

Tranylcypromine Sulfate (Hyperpyretic crisis). Products include:
- Parnate Tablets ... 2222

Triazolam (Additive effects). Products include:
- Halcion Tablets ... 2340

Tridihexethyl Chloride (Severe constipation). No products indexed under this heading.

Trifluoperazine Hydrochloride (Additive effects). Products include:
- Stelazine ... 2226

Trihexyphenidyl Hydrochloride (Severe constipation). Products include:
- Artane ... 1195

LINCOCIN CAPSULES
(Lincomycin Hydrochloride Monohydrate) ... 2344
May interact with nondepolarizing neuromuscular blocking agents. Compounds in this category include:

Atracurium Besylate (Enhanced neuromuscular blocking activity). Products include:
- Tracrium Injection ... 817

Diphenoxylate Hydrochloride (May prolong and/or worsen colitis). Products include:
- Lomotil ... 2174

Metocurine Iodide (Enhanced neuromuscular blocking activity). Products include:
- Metubine Iodide Vials ... 1285

Pancuronium Bromide Injection (Enhanced neuromuscular blocking activity). No products indexed under this heading.

Paregoric (Worsened colitis). Products include:
- Donnagel-PG ... 1858

Vecuronium Bromide (Enhanced neuromuscular blocking activity). Products include:
- Norcuron ... 1642

LINCOCIN PEDIATRIC CAPSULES
(Lincomycin Hydrochloride Monohydrate) ... 2344
See **Lincocin Capsules**

LINCOCIN STERILE SOLUTION
(Lincomycin Hydrochloride Monohydrate) ... 2344
See **Lincocin Capsules**

LIORESAL TABLETS
(Baclofen) ... 1031
May interact with central nervous system depressants and certain other agents. Compounds in these categories include:

Alcohol (Additive depressant effect).

Alfentanil Hydrochloride (Additive depressant effect). Products include:
- Alfenta Injection ... 1131

Alprazolam (Additive depressant effect). Products include:
- Xanax Tablets ... 2367

Aprobarbital (Additive depressant effect). Products include:
- Alurate Elixir ... 1883

Buprenorphine (Additive depressant effect). No products indexed under this heading.

Buspirone Hydrochloride (Additive depressant effect). Products include:
- BuSpar ... 1401

Butabarbital (Additive depressant effect). Products include:
- Pyridium Plus ... 1764

Butalbital (Additive depressant effect). Products include:
- Esgic-Plus Tablets ... 1002
- Esgic Tablets & Capsules ... 1001
- Fioricet Tablets ... 2006
- Fiorinal Capsules ... 2007
- Fiorinal with Codeine Capsules ... 2008
- Fiorinal Tablets ... 2007
- Phrenilin ... 838
- Sedapap Tablets 50 mg/650 mg .. 1360

Chlordiazepoxide (Additive depressant effect). Products include:
- Libritabs Tablets ... 1930
- Limbitrol ... 1933
- Menrium Tablets ... 1934

Chlordiazepoxide Hydrochloride (Additive depressant effect). Products include:
- Librax Capsules ... 1929
- Librium Capsules ... 1931
- Librium Injectable ... 1932

Chlorpromazine (Additive depressant effect). Products include:
- Thorazine ... 2234

Chlorprothixene (Additive depressant effect). Products include:
- Taractan Tablets ... 1920

Chlorprothixene Hydrochloride (Additive depressant effect). Products include:
- Taractan ... 1920

Chlorprothixene Lactate (Additive depressant effect). Products include:
- Taractan Concentrate ... 1920

Clorazepate Dipotassium (Additive depressant effect). Products include:
- Tranxene ... 556

Codeine (Additive depressant effect). Products include:
- Calcidrine Syrup ... 506

Codeine Phosphate (Additive depressant effect). Products include:
- Actifed with Codeine Cough Syrup.. 752
- Cheracol Cough Syrup ... 1853
- Codimal PH Syrup ... 846
- Dimetane-DC Cough Syrup ... 1857
- Empirin with Codeine Phosphate Nos. 2, 3 & 4 ... 764
- Fiorinal with Codeine Capsules ... 2008
- Isoclor Expectorant ... 982
- Naldecon CX Adult Liquid ... ▣ 521
- Novahistine DH ... 1342
- Novahistine Expectorant ... 1343
- Nucofed Capsules ... 2219
- Nucofed Expectorant ... 2219
- Nucofed Pediatric Expectorant ... 2219
- Nucofed Syrup ... 2219
- Phenaphen with Codeine Capsules 1865
- Phenaphen-650 with Codeine Tablets ... 1866
- Phenergan with Codeine ... 2497
- Phenergan VC with Codeine ... 2501
- Robitussin A-C Syrup ... 1875
- Robitussin-DAC Syrup ... 1875
- Ryna ... ▣ 741
- Soma Compound w/Codeine Tablets ... 2390
- Triaminic Expectorant w/Codeine .. 1996
- Tussi-Organidin Liquid ... 2391
- Tylenol with Codeine ... 1381

Codeine Polistirex (Additive depressant effect).
- No products indexed under this heading.

Dezocine (Additive depressant effect).

Diazepam (Additive depressant effect). Products include:
- Valium Injectable ... 1937
- Valium Tablets ... 1939
- Valrelease Capsules ... 1923

Droperidol (Additive depressant effect). Products include:
- Inapsine Injection ... 1140
- Innovar Injection ... 1141

Enflurane (Additive depressant effect). Products include:
- Ethrane ... 599

Estazolam (Additive depressant effect). Products include:
- ProSom Tablets ... 554

Ethchlorvynol (Additive depressant effect). Products include:
- Placidyl Capsules ... 553

Ethinamate (Additive depressant effect).
- No products indexed under this heading.

Fentanyl (Additive depressant effect). Products include:
- Duragesic Transdermal System ... 1133

Fentanyl Citrate (Additive depressant effect). Products include:
- Innovar Injection ... 1141
- Sublimaze Injection ... 1146

Fluphenazine Decanoate (Additive depressant effect). Products include:
- Prolixin Decanoate ... 1795

Fluphenazine Enanthate (Additive depressant effect). Products include:
- Prolixin Enanthate ... 1796

Fluphenazine Hydrochloride (Additive depressant effect). Products include:
- Prolixin Elixir ... 1793
- Prolixin Injection ... 1791
- Prolixin Oral Concentrate ... 1792
- Prolixin Tablets ... 1793

Flurazepam Hydrochloride (Additive depressant effect). Products include:
- Dalmane Capsules ... 1927

Glutethimide (Additive depressant effect).
- No products indexed under this heading.

Haloperidol (Additive depressant effect). Products include:
- Haldol Injection, Tablets and Concentrate ... 1373

Haloperidol Decanoate (Additive depressant effect). Products include:
- Haldol Decanoate ... 1375

Hydrocodone Bitartrate (Additive depressant effect). Products include:
- Anexsia 5/500 Tablets ... 2196
- Anexsia 7.5/650 Tablets ... 2197
- Azdone Tablets ... 844
- Codiclear DH Syrup ... 845
- Codimal DH Syrup ... 846
- Damason-P ... 1356
- Hycodan Syrup, Tablets ... 927
- Hycomine Compound Tablets ... 929
- Hycomine Syrup ... 927
- Hycotuss Expectorant Syrup ... 930
- Hydrocet Capsules ... 835
- Lortab ASA Tablets ... 2414
- Lortab ... 2412
- Ru-Tuss with Hydrocodone ... 694
- Triaminic Expectorant DH ... 1995
- Vicodin Tablets ... 1187
- Vicodin ES Tablets ... 1189
- Zydone Capsules ... 941

Hydrocodone Polistirex (Additive depressant effect). Products include:
- Tussionex Extended-Release Suspension ... 988

Hydroxyzine Hydrochloride (Additive depressant effect). Products include:
- Atarax Tablets & Syrup ... 1941
- Marax Tablets & DF Syrup ... 1954
- Vistaril Intramuscular Solution ... 1970

Isoflurane (Additive depressant effect). Products include:
- Forane ... 600

Ketamine Hydrochloride (Additive depressant effect). Products include:
- Ketalar ... 1726

Levorphanol Tartrate (Additive depressant effect). Products include:
- Levo-Dromoran ... 1906

Lorazepam (Additive depressant effect). Products include:
- Ativan Injection ... 2432
- Ativan Tablets ... 2434

Loxapine Hydrochloride (Additive depressant effect). Products include:
- Loxitane ... 1213

Loxapine Succinate (Additive depressant effect). Products include:
- Loxitane Capsules ... 1213

Meperidine Hydrochloride (Additive depressant effect). Products include:
- Demerol ... 2047
- Mepergan Injection ... 2479

Mephobarbital (Additive depressant effect). Products include:
- Mebaral Tablets ... 2061

Meprobamate (Additive depressant effect). Products include:
- Deprol Tablets ... 2382
- Equagesic Tablets ... 2451
- Miltown Tablets ... 2386
- PMB 200 and PMB 400 ... 2504

Mesoridazine (Additive depressant effect). Products include:
- Serentil ... 686

Methadone Hydrochloride (Additive depressant effect). Products include:
- Dolophine Hydrochloride Ampoules & Vials ... 1260
- Dolophine Hydrochloride Tablets ... 1261
- Methadone Hydrochloride Diskets ... 1284
- Methadone Hydrochloride Oral Solution & Tablets ... 1987

Methohexital Sodium (Additive depressant effect). Products include:
- Brevital Sodium Vials ... 1248

Methoxyflurane (Additive depressant effect).
- No products indexed under this heading.

Midazolam Hydrochloride (Additive depressant effect). Products include:
- Versed Injection ... 1924

Molindone Hydrochloride (Additive depressant effect). Products include:
- Moban Tablets & Concentrate ... 932

Morphine Sulfate (Additive depressant effect). Products include:
- Astramorph/PF Injection, USP (Preservative-Free) ... 618
- Duramorph ... 960
- Infumorph 200 and Infumorph 500 Sterile Solutions ... 962
- MS Contin Tablets ... 1814
- MSIR ... 1817
- Oramorph SR (Morphine Sulfate Sustained Release Tablets) ... 1988
- Roxanol ... 1991

Opium Alkaloids (Additive depressant effect). Products include:
- B & O No. 15A & No. 16A Supprettes ... 2395
- Pantopon Injectable ... 1911

Oxazepam (Additive depressant effect). Products include:
- Serax Capsules ... 2522
- Serax Tablets ... 2522

Oxycodone Hydrochloride (Additive depressant effect). Products include:
- Percocet Tablets ... 950
- Percodan ... 951
- Roxicodone Tablets, Oral Solution & Intensol (Oxycodone) ... 1992
- Tylox Capsules ... 1382

Pentobarbital Sodium (Additive depressant effects). Products include:
- Nembutal Sodium Capsules ... 534
- Nembutal Sodium Solution ... 536
- Nembutal Sodium Suppositories ... 538

Perphenazine (Additive depressant effect). Products include:
- Etrafon ... 2087
- Triavil Tablets ... 1556
- Trilafon ... 2123

Phenobarbital (Additive depressant effect). Products include:
- Arco-Lase Plus Tablets ... 607
- Bellergal-S Tablets ... 1998
- Bronkolixir ... ▣ 761
- Bronkotabs Tablets ... ▣ 762
- Donnatal ... 1858
- Donnatal Extentabs ... 1859
- Donnatal Tablets ... 1858
- Donnazyme Tablets ... 1860
- Kinesed Tablets ... 2272
- Phenobarbital Elixir and Tablets ... 1293
- Primatene Tablets-P Formula ... 2421
- Quadrinal Tablets ... 1183
- Tedral SA ... 1765

Prazepam (Additive depressant effect). Products include:
- Centrax ... 1693

Prochlorperazine (Additive depressant effect). Products include:
- Compazine ... 2201

Promethazine Hydrochloride (Additive depressant effect). Products include:
- Mepergan Injection ... 2479
- Phenergan with Codeine ... 2497
- Phenergan with Dextromethorphan 2499
- Phenergan Injection ... 2493
- Phenergan Suppositories ... 2496
- Phenergan Syrup ... 2495
- Phenergan Tablets ... 2496
- Phenergan VC ... 2500
- Phenergan VC with Codeine ... 2501

Propofol (Additive depressant effect). Products include:
- Diprivan Injection ... 2267

Propoxyphene Hydrochloride (Additive depressant effect). Products include:
- Darvon ... 1256
- Wygesic Tablets ... 2540

Propoxyphene Napsylate (Additive depressant effect). Products include:
- Darvon-N/Darvocet-N ... 1254

Quazepam (Additive depressant effect). Products include:
- Doral Tablets ... 2383

Secobarbital Sodium (Additive depressant effect). Products include:
- Seconal Sodium Pulvules ... 1296

Sufentanil Citrate (Additive depressant effect). Products include:
- Sufenta Injection ... 1147

Temazepam (Additive depressant effect). Products include:
- Restoril Capsules ... 2023

Thiamylal Sodium (Additive depressant effect). Products include:
- Surital Ampoules, Steri-Vials ... 1764

Thioridazine Hydrochloride (Additive depressant effect). Products include:
- Mellaril ... 2011

Thiothixene (Additive depressant effect). Products include:
- Navane Capsules and Concentrate 1954
- Navane Intramuscular ... 1956

Triazolam (Additive depressant effect). Products include:
- Halcion Tablets ... 2340

Trifluoperazine Hydrochloride (Additive depressant effect). Products include:
- Stelazine ... 2226

LIPPES LOOP INTRAUTERINE DOUBLE-S
(Intrauterine device) ... 1654
No interactions described in labeling.

LIQUIFILM FORTE LUBRICANT OPHTHALMIC SOLUTION
(Polyvinyl Alcohol) ... ⊙ 249
No interactions described in labeling.

LIQUIFILM TEARS LUBRICANT OPHTHALMIC SOLUTION
(Polyvinyl Alcohol) ... ⊙ 249
No interactions described in labeling.

LIQUIPRIN CHILDREN'S ELIXIR
(Acetaminophen) ... ▣ 618
No interactions described in labeling.

LIQUIPRIN INFANTS' DROPS
(Acetaminophen) ... ▣ 618
No interactions described in labeling.

LISTERINE ANTISEPTIC
(Eucalyptol, Menthol, Methyl Salicylate) ... ▣ 742
No interactions described in labeling.

LISTERINE ANTISEPTIC LOZENGES REGULAR STRENGTH
(Hexylresorcinol) ... ▣ 743
No interactions described in labeling.

LISTERINE MAXIMUM STRENGTH ANTISEPTIC LOZENGES
(Hexylresorcinol) ... ▣ 743
No interactions described in labeling.

LISTERMINT WITH FLUORIDE
(Sodium Fluoride) ... ▣ 743
No interactions described in labeling.

(▣ Described in PDR For Nonprescription Drugs)

(⊙ Described in PDR For Ophthalmology)

Oreticyl 545
Prinzide Tablets 1540
Ser-Ap-Es Tablets 881
Serpasil-Esidrix Tablets 886
Timolide Tablets 1547
Trandate HCT Tablets 579
Vaseretic Tablets 1559
Zestoretic 2274

Hydroflumethiazide (Increased serum lithium levels; risk of lithium toxicity). Products include:
Diucardin Tablets 2450
Saluron 718
Salutensin/Salutensin-Demi 719

Ibuprofen (Increased serum lithium levels). Products include:
Advil Cold & Sinus Caplets (formerly CoAdvil) 2416
Advil Ibuprofen Tablets and Caplets 2416
Children's Advil Suspension 2426
CoAdvil ..... ▣ 748
Dristan Sinus Caplets 2419
Haltran Tablets ..... ▣ 668
Ibuprofen ..... ▣ 631
Medipren ibuprofen Caplets and Tablets 1362
Midol 200 Cramp Relief Formula .. ▣ 570
Motrin Tablets 2351
Motrin IB Caplets and Tablets ..... ▣ 736
Nuprin Ibuprofen/Analgesic Tablets & Caplets 752
PediaProfen Suspension 1363
Rufen Tablets 691
Trendar Ibuprofen Tablets ..... ▣ 756

Indapamide (Increased serum lithium levels; risk of lithium toxicity). Products include:
Lozol Tablets 1843

Indomethacin (Increased serum lithium levels). Products include:
Indocin 1487

Indomethacin Sodium Trihydrate (Increased serum lithium levels). Products include:
Indocin I.V. 1490

Ketoprofen (Increased serum lithium levels). Products include:
Orudis Capsules 2488

Ketorolac Tromethamine (Increased serum lithium levels). Products include:
Toradol IM Injection 2302

Meclofenamate Sodium (Increased serum lithium levels). Products include:
Meclomen Capsules 1739

Mefenamic Acid (Increased serum lithium levels). Products include:
Ponstel 1758

Methyclothiazide (Increased serum lithium levels; risk of lithium toxicity). Products include:
Enduron Tablets 517
Enduronyl 518

Metolazone (Increased serum lithium levels; risk of lithium toxicity). Products include:
Diulo 2129
Mykrox ½ mg Tablets 984
Zaroxolyn Tablets 989

Naproxen (Increased serum lithium levels). Products include:
Naprosyn 2297

Naproxen Sodium (Increased serum lithium levels). Products include:
Anaprox and Anaprox DS Tablets 2288

Phenylbutazone (Increased serum lithium levels). Products include:
Butazolidin Capsules & Tablets 1027

Piroxicam (Increased serum lithium levels). Products include:
Feldene Capsules 1777

Polythiazide (Increased serum lithium levels; risk of lithium toxicity). Products include:
Minizide Capsules 1779
Renese Tablets 1785
Renese-R Tablets 1786

Spironolactone (Increased serum lithium levels; risk of lithium toxicity). Products include:
Aldactazide 2150
Aldactone 2152

Sulindac (Increased serum lithium levels). Products include:
Clinoril Tablets 1433

Tolmetin Sodium (Increased serum lithium levels). Products include:
Tolectin (200, 400 and 600 mg) .. 1379

Triamterene (Increased serum lithium levels; risk of lithium toxicity). Products include:
Dyazide Capsules 2208
Dyrenium Capsules 2210
Maxzide 1215

LITHIUM CARBONATE CAPSULES & TABLETS
(Lithium Carbonate) 1984
May interact with neuromuscular blocking agents, nondepolarizing neuromuscular blocking agents, non-steroidal anti-inflammatory agents, diuretics, ACE inhibitors, and certain other agents. Compounds in these categories include:

Amiloride Hydrochloride (High risk of lithium toxicity). Products include:
Midamor Tablets 1508
Moduretic Tablets 1510

Atracurium Besylate (Prolonged effects of neuromuscular blockers). Products include:
Tracrium Injection 817

Benazepril Hydrochloride (Reduces lithium clearance and increases serum lithium levels resulting in risk of lithium toxicity). Products include:
Lotensin Tablets 872

Bendroflumethiazide (High risk of lithium toxicity). Products include:
Corzide Tablets 702
Naturetin Tablets 1789
Rauzide Tablets 1804

Bumetanide (High risk of lithium toxicity). Products include:
Bumex 1895

Captopril (Reduces lithium clearance and increases serum lithium levels resulting in risk of lithium toxicity). Products include:
Capoten 2255
Capozide 2258

Chlorothiazide (High risk of lithium toxicity). Products include:
Aldoclor Tablets 1413
Diupres Tablets 1461
Diuril Oral 1464

Chlorothiazide Sodium (High risk of lithium toxicity). Products include:
Diuril Sodium Intravenous 1463

Chlorpromazine (Neurological toxicity has occurred; encephalopathic syndrome followed by irreversible brain damage). Products include:
Thorazine 2234

Chlorprothixene (Neurological toxicity has occurred; encephalopathic syndrome followed by irreversible brain damage). Products include:
Taractan Tablets 1920

Chlorprothixene Hydrochloride (Neurological toxicity has occurred; encephalopathic syndrome followed by irreversible brain damage). Products include:
Taractan 1920

Chlorthalidone (High risk of lithium toxicity). Products include:
Combipres Tablets 678
Tenoretic Tablets 1105
Thalitone Tablets 687

Clozapine (Neurological toxicity has occurred; encephalopathic syndrome followed by irreversible brain damage). Products include:
Clozaril Tablets 2000

Diclofenac Sodium (Significant increase in steady state plasma lithium levels; possible lithium toxicity). Products include:
Voltaren Ophthalmic Sterile Ophthalmic Solution ..... ⊙ 268
Voltaren Tablets 1042

Enalapril Maleate (Reduces lithium clearance and increases serum lithium levels resulting in risk of lithium toxicity). Products include:
Vaseretic Tablets 1559
Vasotec Tablets 1564

Enalaprilat (Reduces lithium clearance and increases serum lithium levels resulting in risk of lithium toxicity). Products include:
Vasotec I.V. 1562

Ethacrynic Acid (High risk of lithium toxicity). Products include:
Edecrin Tablets 1468

Etodolac (Significant increase in steady state plasma lithium levels; possible lithium toxicity). Products include:
Lodine Capsules 2468

Fenoprofen Calcium (Significant increase in steady state plasma lithium levels; possible lithium toxicity). Products include:
Nalfon Pulvules & Tablets 919

Fluphenazine Decanoate (Neurological toxicity has occurred; encephalopathic syndrome followed by irreversible brain damage). Products include:
Prolixin Decanoate 1795

Fluphenazine Enanthate (Neurological toxicity has occurred; encephalopathic syndrome followed by irreversible brain damage). Products include:
Prolixin Enanthate 1796

Fluphenazine Hydrochloride (Neurological toxicity has occurred; encephalopathic syndrome followed by irreversible brain damage). Products include:
Prolixin Elixir 1793
Prolixin Injection 1791
Prolixin Oral Concentrate 1792
Prolixin Tablets 1793

Flurbiprofen (Significant increase in steady state plasma lithium levels; possible lithium toxicity). Products include:
Ansaid Tablets 2319

Fosinopril Sodium (Reduces lithium clearance and increases serum lithium levels resulting in risk of lithium toxicity). Products include:
Monopril Tablets 1406

Furosemide (High risk of lithium toxicity). Products include:
Lasix 1093

Haloperidol (Neurological toxicity has occurred; encephalopathic syndrome followed by irreversible brain damage). Products include:
Haldol Injection, Tablets and Concentrate 1373

Haloperidol Decanoate (Neurological toxicity has occurred; encephalopathic syndrome followed by irreversible brain damage). Products include:
Haldol Decanoate 1375

Hydrochlorothiazide (High risk of lithium toxicity). Products include:
Aldactazide 2150
Aldoril Tablets 1418

(▣ Described in PDR For Nonprescription Drugs)

(⊙ Described in PDR For Ophthalmology)

Apresazide Capsules 854
Apresoline-Esidrix Tablets 857
Capozide 2258
Dyazide Capsules 2208
Esidrix Tablets 863
Esimil Tablets 864
HydroDIURIL Tablets 1484
Hydropres Tablets 1485
Inderide Tablets 2463
Inderide LA Long Acting Capsules .. 2465
Lopressor HCT Tablets 1034
Maxzide 1215
Moduretic Tablets 1510
Normozide Tablets 2112
Oretic Tablets 544
Oreticyl 545
Prinzide Tablets 1540
Ser-Ap-Es Tablets 881
Serpasil-Esidrix Tablets 886
Timolide Tablets 1547
Trandate HCT Tablets 579
Vaseretic Tablets 1559
Zestoretic 2274

Hydroflumethiazide (High risk of lithium toxicity). Products include:
Diucardin Tablets 2450
Saluron 718
Salutensin/Salutensin-Demi 719

Ibuprofen (Significant increase in steady state plasma lithium levels; possible lithium toxicity). Products include:
Advil Cold & Sinus Caplets (formerly CoAdvil) 2416
Advil Ibuprofen Tablets and Caplets 2416
Children's Advil Suspension 2426
CoAdvil .... ◘ 748
Dristan Sinus Caplets 2419
Haltran Tablets .... ◘ 668
Ibuprofen .... ◘ 631
Medipren ibuprofen Caplets and Tablets 1362
Midol 200 Cramp Relief Formula .. ◘ 570
Motrin Tablets 2351
Motrin IB Caplets and Tablets .... ◘ 736
Nuprin Ibuprofen/Analgesic Tablets & Caplets 752
PediaProfen Suspension 1363
Rufen Tablets 691
Trendar Ibuprofen Tablets .... ◘ 756

Indapamide (High risk of lithium toxicity). Products include:
Lozol Tablets 1843

Indomethacin (Significant increase in steady state plasma lithium levels; possible lithium toxicity). Products include:
Indocin 1487

Indomethacin Sodium Trihydrate (Significant increase in steady state plasma lithium levels; possible lithium toxicity). Products include:
Indocin I.V. 1490

Ketoprofen (Significant increase in steady state plasma lithium levels; possible lithium toxicity). Products include:
Orudis Capsules 2488

Ketorolac Tromethamine (Significant increase in steady state plasma lithium levels; possible lithium toxicity). Products include:
Toradol IM Injection 2302

Lisinopril (Reduces lithium clearance and increases serum lithium levels resulting in risk of lithium toxicity). Products include:
Prinivil Tablets 1538
Prinzide Tablets 1540
Zestoretic 2274
Zestril Tablets 2277

Loxapine Hydrochloride (Neurological toxicity has occurred; encephalopathic syndrome followed by irreversible brain damage). Products include:
Loxitane 1213

Meclofenamate Sodium (Significant increase in steady state plasma lithium levels; possible lithium toxicity). Products include:
Meclomen Capsules 1739

Mefenamic Acid (Significant increase in steady state plasma lithium levels; possible lithium toxicity). Products include:
Ponstel 1758

Mesoridazine (Neurological toxicity has occurred; encephalopathic syndrome followed by irreversible brain damage). Products include:
Serentil 686

Methyclothiazide (High risk of lithium toxicity). Products include:
Enduron Tablets 517
Enduronyl 518

Metocurine Iodide (Prolonged effects of neuromuscular blockers). Products include:
Metubine Iodide Vials 1285

Metolazone (High risk of lithium toxicity). Products include:
Diulo 2129
Mykrox ½ mg Tablets 984
Zaroxolyn Tablets 989

Molindone Hydrochloride (Neurological toxicity has occurred; encephalopathic syndrome followed by irreversible brain damage). Products include:
Moban Tablets & Concentrate 932

Naproxen (Significant increase in steady state plasma lithium levels; possible lithium toxicity). Products include:
Naprosyn 2297

Naproxen Sodium (Significant increase in steady state plasma lithium levels; possible lithium toxicity). Products include:
Anaprox and Anaprox DS Tablets 2288

Pancuronium Bromide Injection (Prolonged effects of neuromuscular blockers).
No products indexed under this heading.

Perphenazine (Neurological toxicity has occurred; encephalopathic syndrome followed by irreversible brain damage). Products include:
Etrafon 2087
Triavil Tablets 1556
Trilafon 2123

Phenylbutazone (Significant increase in steady state plasma lithium levels; possible lithium toxicity). Products include:
Butazolidin Capsules & Tablets 1027

Pimozide (Neurological toxicity has occurred; encephalopathic syndrome followed by irreversible brain damage). Products include:
Orap Tablets 1020

Piroxicam (Significant increase in steady state plasma lithium levels; possible lithium toxicity). Products include:
Feldene Capsules 1777

Polythiazide (High risk of lithium toxicity). Products include:
Minizide Capsules 1779
Renese Tablets 1785
Renese-R Tablets 1786

Prochlorperazine (Neurological toxicity has occurred; encephalopathic syndrome followed by irreversible brain damage). Products include:
Compazine 2201

Promethazine Hydrochloride (Neurological toxicity has occurred; encephalopathic syndrome followed by irreversible brain damage). Products include:
Mepergan Injection 2479
Phenergan with Codeine 2497
Phenergan with Dextromethorphan 2499
Phenergan Injection 2493
Phenergan Suppositories 2496
Phenergan Syrup 2495
Phenergan Tablets 2496
Phenergan VC 2500
Phenergan VC with Codeine 2501

Ramipril (Reduces lithium clearance and increases serum lithium levels resulting in risk of lithium toxicity). Products include:
Altace Capsules 1086

Spironolactone (High risk of lithium toxicity). Products include:
Aldactazide 2150
Aldactone 2152

Sulindac (Significant increase in steady state plasma lithium levels; possible lithium toxicity). Products include:
Clinoril Tablets 1433

Thioridazine Hydrochloride (Neurological toxicity has occurred; encephalopathic syndrome followed by irreversible brain damage). Products include:
Mellaril 2011

Thiothixene (Neurological toxicity has occurred; encephalopathic syndrome followed by irreversible brain damage). Products include:
Navane Capsules and Concentrate 1954
Navane Intramuscular 1956

Tolmetin Sodium (Significant increase in steady state plasma lithium levels; possible lithium toxicity). Products include:
Tolectin (200, 400 and 600 mg) .. 1379

Triamterene (High risk of lithium toxicity). Products include:
Dyazide Capsules 2208
Dyrenium Capsules 2210
Maxzide 1215

Trifluoperazine Hydrochloride (Neurological toxicity has occurred; encephalopathic syndrome followed by irreversible brain damage). Products include:
Stelazine 2226

Vecuronium Bromide (Prolonged effects of neuromuscular blockers). Products include:
Norcuron 1642

LITHOBID TABLETS
(Lithium Carbonate) 870
See **Cibalith-S**

LODINE CAPSULES
(Etodolac) 2468
May interact with lithium preparations, diuretics, antacids, and certain other agents. Compounds in these categories include:

Aluminum Carbonate Gel (Coadministration decreases the peak concentration reached by about 15 to 20%). Products include:
Basaljel 2438

Aluminum Hydroxide (Coadministration decreases the peak concentration reached by about 15 to 20%). Products include:
Cama Arthritis Pain Reliever .... ◘ 685
Gaviscon Extra Strength Relief Formula Liquid Antacid .... ◘ 594
Gaviscon Extra Strength Relief Formula Antacid Tablets .... ◘ 594
Gaviscon Liquid Antacid .... ◘ 594
Gelusil Liquid & Tablets .... ◘ 639
Extra Strength Maalox Plus Suspension 1850
Maalox TC Suspension 1851
Maalox Plus Tablets .... ◘ 655
Extra Strength Maalox Plus Tablets 1850
Nephrox Suspension .... ◘ 563
WinGel Liquid & Tablets .... ◘ 761

Aluminum Hydroxide Gel (Coadministration decreases the peak concentration reached by about 15 to 20%). Products include:
ALternaGEL Liquid 1154
Aludrox Oral Suspension 2428
Amphojel Suspension 2429
Amphojel Suspension without Flavor 2429
Mylanta Liquid 1155
Mylanta Double Strength Liquid 1155

Aluminum Hydroxide Gel, Dried (Coadministration decreases the peak concentration reached by about 15 to 20%). Products include:
Alu-Tab/Alu-Cap 1309
Amphojel Tablets 2429
Ascriptin A/D Caplets 1850
Regular Strength Ascriptin Tablets 1850
Gaviscon Antacid Tablets .... ◘ 593
Gaviscon-2 Antacid Tablets .... ◘ 594
Mylanta Tablets 1155
Mylanta Double Strength Tablets 1155

Amiloride Hydrochloride (Caution is recommended if coadministered to patients with cardiac, renal or hepatic failure). Products include:
Midamor Tablets 1508
Moduretic Tablets 1510

Aspirin (Potential for increased adverse effects). Products include:
Alka-Seltzer Effervescent Antacid and Pain Reliever 1568
Alka-Seltzer Extra Strength Effervescent Antacid and Pain Reliever 1570
Alka-Seltzer (Flavored) Effervescent Antacid and Pain Reliever 1569
Alka-Seltzer Plus Cold Medicine .... ◘ 623
Alka-Seltzer Plus Night-Time Cold Medicine .... ◘ 623
Alka Seltzer Plus Sinus Allergy Medicine .... ◘ 624
Anacin Coated Analgesic Caplets 2417
Anacin Coated Analgesic Tablets 2417
Anacin Maximum Strength Analgesic Coated Tablets 2417
Maximum Strength Arthritis Pain Formula By the Makers of Anacin Analgesic Tablets and Caplets 2418
Arthritis Pain Formula by the Makers of Anacin Analgesic Tablets and Caplets .... ◘ 747
Arthritis Strength BC Powder .... ◘ 516
Ascriptin A/D Caplets 1850
Regular Strength Ascriptin Tablets 1850
Azdone Tablets 844
BC Powder .... ◘ 517
BC Cold Powder .... ◘ 517
Children's Bayer Chewable Aspirin .... ◘ 564
Genuine Bayer Aspirin Tablets & Caplets .... ◘ 564
Maximum Bayer Aspirin Tablets & Caplets .... ◘ 566
Bayer Plus Aspirin Tablets .... ◘ 567
Therapy Bayer Aspirin Caplets .... ◘ 568
8 Hour Bayer Timed-Release Aspirin .... ◘ 566
Arthritis Strength Bufferin Analgesic Caplets 744
Extra Strength Bufferin Analgesic Tablets 745
Bufferin Analgesic Tablets and Caplets 743
Cama Arthritis Pain Reliever .... ◘ 685
Damason-P 1356
Easprin 1719
Ecotrin Enteric Coated Aspirin Maximum Strength Tablets and Caplets 2189
Ecotrin Enteric Coated Aspirin Regular Strength Tablets and Caplets 2189
Empirin Aspirin .... ◘ 541
Empirin with Codeine Phosphate Nos. 2, 3 & 4 764
Equagesic Tablets 2451
Excedrin Extra-Strength Analgesic Tablets & Caplets 749
4-Way Cold Tablets 750
Fiorinal Capsules 2007
Fiorinal with Codeine Capsules 2008
Fiorinal Tablets 2007
Lortab ASA Tablets 2414
Momentum Muscular Backache Formula .... ◘ 751
Norgesic 1314
Norwich Extra-Strength Aspirin .... ◘ 546
Norwich Regular Strength Aspirin ◘ 547
P-A-C Analgesic Tablets .... ◘ 669
Percodan 951
Robaxisal Tablets 1872
Sine-Off Sinus Medicine Tablets-Aspirin Formula .... ◘ 722

Soma Compound w/Codeine Tablets 2390
Soma Compound Tablets 2389
St. Joseph Adult Chewable Aspirin (81 mg.) .... ▣ 703
Synalgos-DC Capsules 2525
Talwin Compound 2072
Ursinus Inlay-Tabs .... ▣ 691
Vanquish Analgesic Caplets .... ▣ 574
Zorprin Tablets 698

Bendroflumethiazide (Caution is recommended if coadministered to patients with cardiac, renal or hepatic failure). Products include:
Corzide Tablets 702
Naturetin Tablets 1789
Rauzide Tablets 1804

Bumetanide (Caution is recommended if coadministered to patients with cardiac, renal or hepatic failure). Products include:
Bumex 1895

Chlorothiazide (Caution is recommended if coadministered to patients with cardiac, renal or hepatic failure). Products include:
Aldoclor Tablets 1413
Diupres Tablets 1461
Diuril Oral 1464

Chlorothiazide Sodium (Caution is recommended if coadministered to patients with cardiac, renal or hepatic failure). Products include:
Diuril Sodium Intravenous 1463

Chlorthalidone (Caution is recommended if coadministered to patients with cardiac, renal or hepatic failure). Products include:
Combipres Tablets 678
Tenoretic Tablets 1105
Thalitone Tablets 687

Cyclosporine (Potential for elevated serum levels of cyclosporine and increased nephrotoxicity). Products include:
Sandimmune 2024

Digoxin (Potential for elevated serum levels of digoxin and increased toxicity). Products include:
Lanoxicaps 772
Lanoxin Elixir Pediatric 775
Lanoxin Injection 778
Lanoxin Injection Pediatric 781
Lanoxin Tablets 783

Dihydroxyaluminum Sodium Carbonate (Coadministration decreases the peak concentration reached by about 15 to 20%). Products include:
Rolaids .... ▣ 743

Ethacrynic Acid (Caution is recommended if coadministered to patients with cardiac, renal or hepatic failure). Products include:
Edecrin Tablets 1468

Furosemide (Caution is recommended if coadministered to patients with cardiac, renal or hepatic failure). Products include:
Lasix 1093

Hydrochlorothiazide (Caution is recommended if coadministered to patients with cardiac, renal or hepatic failure). Products include:
Aldactazide 2150
Aldoril Tablets 1418
Apresazide Capsules 854
Apresoline-Esidrix Tablets 857
Capozide 2258
Dyazide Capsules 2208
Esidrix Tablets 863
Esimil Tablets 864
HydroDIURIL Tablets 1484
Hydropres Tablets 1485
Inderide Tablets 2463
Inderide LA Long Acting Capsules .. 2465
Lopressor HCT Tablets 1034
Maxzide 1215
Moduretic Tablets 1510
Normozide Tablets 2112
Oretic Tablets 544
Oreticyl 545
Prinzide Tablets 1540
Ser-Ap-Es Tablets 881
Serpasil-Esidrix Tablets 886
Timolide Tablets 1547
Trandate HCT Tablets 579
Vaseretic Tablets 1559
Zestoretic 2274

Hydroflumethiazide (Caution is recommended if coadministered to patients with cardiac, renal or hepatic failure). Products include:
Diucardin Tablets 2450
Saluron 718
Salutensin/Salutensin-Demi 719

Indapamide (Caution is recommended if coadministered to patients with cardiac, renal or hepatic failure). Products include:
Lozol Tablets 1843

Lithium Carbonate (Potential for elevated serum levels of lithium and increased toxicity). Products include:
Eskalith 2214
Lithane Tablets 1596
Lithium Carbonate Capsules & Tablets 1984
Lithobid Tablets 870

Lithium Citrate (Potential for elevated serum levels of lithium and increased toxicity). Products include:
Cibalith-S 870

Magaldrate (Coadministration decreases the peak concentration reached by about 15 to 20%). Products include:
Riopan Antacid Chew Tablets .... ▣ 754
Riopan Antacid Chew Tablets in Rollpacks .... ▣ 754
Riopan Antacid Suspension 2421
Riopan Antacid Swallow Tablets 2421
Riopan Plus Chew Tablets 2422
Riopan Plus Chew Tablets in Rollpack 2422
Riopan Plus 2 Chew Tablets, Mint Flavor, Cherry Flavor 2422
Riopan Plus Suspension 2422
Riopan Plus 2 Suspension, Mint Flavor, Cherry Flavor 2422

Magnesium Hydroxide (Coadministration decreases the peak concentration reached by about 15 to 20%). Products include:
Aludrox Oral Suspension 2428
Ascriptin A/D Caplets 1850
Regular Strength Ascriptin Tablets 1850
Di-Gel Antacid/Anti-Gas .... ▣ 697
Gelusil Liquid & Tablets .... ▣ 639
Haley's M-O, Regular & Flavored .. ▣ 569
Extra Strength Maalox Plus Suspension 1850
Maalox TC Suspension 1851
Maalox Plus Tablets .... ▣ 655
Extra Strength Maalox Plus Tablets 1850
Mylanta Liquid 1155
Mylanta Tablets 1155
Mylanta Double Strength Liquid 1155
Mylanta Double Strength Tablets 1155
Concentrated Phillips' Milk of Magnesia .... ▣ 573
Phillips' Milk of Magnesia Liquid .... ▣ 572
Phillips' Milk of Magnesia Tablets ▣ 573
WinGel Liquid & Tablets .... ▣ 761

Magnesium Oxide (Coadministration decreases the peak concentration reached by about 15 to 20%). Products include:
Bayer Plus Aspirin Tablets .... ▣ 567
Beelith Tablets 659
Bufferin Analgesic Tablets and Caplets .... ▣ 524
Cama Arthritis Pain Reliever .... ▣ 685
Mag-Ox 400 673
Uro-Mag 673

Methotrexate Sodium (Potential for elevated serum levels of methotrexate and increased toxicity). Products include:
Methotrexate Tablets, Parenteral, LPF Parenteral 1217
Rheumatrex Methotrexate Dose Pack 1234

Methyclothiazide (Caution is recommended if coadministered to patients with cardiac, renal or hepatic failure). Products include:
Enduron Tablets 517
Enduronyl 518

Metolazone (Caution is recommended if coadministered to patients with cardiac, renal or hepatic failure). Products include:
Diulo 2129
Mykrox ½ mg Tablets 984
Zaroxolyn Tablets 989

Phenylbutazone (Increases (by about 80%) in the free fraction of etodolac in vitro studies). Products include:
Butazolidin Capsules & Tablets 1027

Polythiazide (Caution is recommended if coadministered to patients with cardiac, renal or hepatic failure). Products include:
Minizide Capsules 1779
Renese Tablets 1785
Renese-R Tablets 1786

Sodium Bicarbonate (Coadministration decreases the peak concentration reached by about 15 to 20%). Products include:
Alka-Seltzer Advanced Formula Antacid & Non-Aspirin Pain Reliever .... ▣ 620
Alka-Seltzer Effervescent Antacid ▣ 622
Alka-Seltzer Effervescent Antacid and Pain Reliever 1568
Alka-Seltzer Extra Strength Effervescent Antacid and Pain Reliever .... ▣ 623
Alka-Seltzer (Flavored) Effervescent Antacid and Pain Reliever .. ▣ 621
Arm & Hammer Pure Baking Soda .... ▣ 548
Ceo-Two Rectal Suppositories 671
Citrocarbonate Antacid .... ▣ 668
Massengill Liquid Concentrate 2191
NuLYTELY 699

Spironolactone (Caution is recommended if coadministered to patients with cardiac, renal or hepatic failure). Products include:
Aldactazide 2150
Aldactone 2152

Triamterene (Caution is recommended if coadministered to patients with cardiac, renal or hepatic failure). Products include:
Dyazide Capsules 2208
Dyrenium Capsules 2210
Maxzide 1215

Warfarin Sodium (Reduced protein binding of warfarin). Products include:
Coumadin Injection & Tablets 944
Panwarfin Tablets 547

Food Interactions

Food, unspecified (Reduces the peak concentration reached by approximately one-half and increases the time-to-peak concentration by 1.4 to 3.8 hours).

LO/OVRAL TABLETS

(Norgestrel, Ethinyl Estradiol) 2471
May interact with barbiturates and certain other agents. Compounds in these categories include:

Ampicillin Sodium (Reduced efficacy; increased incidence of breakthrough bleeding). Products include:
Unasyn 1965

Aprobarbital (Reduced efficacy; increased incidence of breakthrough bleeding). Products include:
Alurate Elixir 1883

Butabarbital (Reduced efficacy; increased incidence of breakthrough bleeding). Products include:
Pyridium Plus 1764

Butalbital (Reduced efficacy; increased incidence of breakthrough bleeding). Products include:
Esgic-Plus Tablets 1002
Esgic Tablets & Capsules 1001
Fioricet Tablets 2006
Fiorinal Capsules 2007
Fiorinal with Codeine Capsules 2008
Fiorinal Tablets 2007
Phrenilin 838
Sedapap Tablets 50 mg/650 mg .. 1360

Mephobarbital (Reduced efficacy; increased incidence of breakthrough bleeding). Products include:
Mebaral Tablets 2061

Oxytetracycline (Reduced efficacy; increased incidence of breakthrough bleeding). Products include:
Terramycin Intramuscular Solution 1964
Urobiotic-250 Capsules 1968

Oxytetracycline Hydrochloride (Reduced efficacy; increased incidence of breakthrough bleeding). Products include:
Terra-Cortril Ophthalmic Suspension 1963
Terramycin Capsules 1786
Terramycin Intramuscular Solution 1964
Terramycin with Polymyxin B Sulfate Ophthalmic Ointment 1965

Pentobarbital Sodium (Reduced efficacy; increased incidence of breakthrough bleeding). Products include:
Nembutal Sodium Capsules 534
Nembutal Sodium Solution 536
Nembutal Sodium Suppositories 538

Phenobarbital (Reduced efficacy; increased incidence of breakthrough bleeding). Products include:
Arco-Lase Plus Tablets 607
Bellergal-S Tablets 1998
Bronkolixir .... ▣ 761
Bronkotabs Tablets .... ▣ 762
Donnatal 1858
Donnatal Extentabs 1859
Donnatal Tablets 1858
Donnazyme Tablets 1860
Kinesed Tablets 2272
Phenobarbital Elixir and Tablets 1293
Primatene Tablets-P Formula 2421
Quadrinal Tablets 1183
Tedral SA 1765

Phenylbutazone (Reduced efficacy; increased incidence of breakthrough bleeding). Products include:
Butazolidin Capsules & Tablets 1027

Phenytoin Sodium (Reduced efficacy; increased incidence of breakthrough bleeding). Products include:
Dilantin Kapseals 1708
Dilantin Parenteral 1712
Dilantin with Phenobarbital Kapseals 1715

Rifampin (Reduced efficacy; increased incidence of breakthrough bleeding). Products include:
Rifadin 1345
Rifamate Capsules 1347
Rimactane Capsules 879

Secobarbital Sodium (Reduced efficacy; increased incidence of breakthrough bleeding). Products include:
Seconal Sodium Pulvules 1296

Tetracycline Hydrochloride (Reduced efficacy; increased incidence of breakthrough bleeding). Products include:
Achromycin V Capsules 1193
Achromycin Ophthalmic Ointment 1% .... ⊙ 307
Achromycin Ophthalmic Suspension 1% .... ⊙ 308
Topicycline for Topical Solution 1856

Thiamylal Sodium (Reduced efficacy; increased incidence of breakthrough bleeding). Products include:
Surital Ampoules, Steri-Vials 1764

LO/OVRAL-28 TABLETS
(Norgestrel, Ethinyl Estradiol) 2476
See **Lo/Ovral Tablets**

LOCOID CREAM, OINTMENT AND TOPICAL SOLUTION
(Hydrocortisone Butyrate) 970
No interactions described in labeling.

LOESTRIN [Fe] 1/20
(Norethindrone Acetate, Ethinyl Estradiol)..................................1728
See **Loestrin [21] 1/20**

LOESTRIN [Fe] 1.5/30
(Norethindrone Acetate, Ethinyl Estradiol)..................................1728
See **Loestrin [21] 1/20**

LOESTRIN [21] 1/20
(Norethindrone Acetate, Ethinyl Estradiol)..................................1728
May interact with barbiturates, tetracyclines, and certain other agents. Compounds in these categories include:

Ampicillin Sodium (Reduced efficacy of Loestrin; increased incidence of breakthrough bleeding). Products include:
Unasyn 1965

Aprobarbital (Reduced efficacy of Loestrin; increased incidence of breakthrough bleeding). Products include:
Alurate Elixir 1883

Butabarbital (Reduced efficacy of Loestrin; increased incidence of breakthrough bleeding). Products include:
Pyridium Plus 1764

Butalbital (Reduced efficacy of Loestrin; increased incidence of breakthrough bleeding). Products include:
Esgic-Plus Tablets 1002
Esgic Tablets & Capsules 1001
Fioricet Tablets 2006
Fiorinal Capsules 2007
Fiorinal with Codeine Capsules 2008
Fiorinal Tablets 2007
Phrenilin 838
Sedapap Tablets 50 mg/650 mg .. 1360

Griseofulvin (Reduced efficacy of Loestrin; increased incidence of breakthrough bleeding). Products include:
Fulvicin P/G Tablets 2090
Fulvicin P/G 165 & 330 Tablets 2091
Fulvicin-U/F Tablets 2092
Grifulvin V (griseofulvin microsize) Tablets/Suspension 1678
Grisactin 2454
Grisactin Ultra Tablets 2455
Gris-PEG Tablets, 125 mg & 250 mg 1083

Mephobarbital (Reduced efficacy of Loestrin; increased incidence of breakthrough bleeding). Products include:
Mebaral Tablets 2061

Oxytetracycline (Reduced efficacy of Loestrin; increased incidence of breakthrough bleeding). Products include:
Terramycin Intramuscular Solution 1964
Urobiotic-250 Capsules 1968

Oxytetracycline Hydrochloride (Reduced efficacy of Loestrin; increased incidence of breakthrough bleeding). Products include:
Terra-Cortril Ophthalmic Suspension 1963
Terramycin Capsules 1786
Terramycin Intramuscular Solution 1964
Terramycin with Polymyxin B Sulfate Ophthalmic Ointment 1965

Pentobarbital Sodium (Reduced efficacy of Loestrin; increased incidence of breakthrough bleeding). Products include:
Nembutal Sodium Capsules 534
Nembutal Sodium Solution 536
Nembutal Sodium Suppositories...... 538

Phenobarbital (Reduced efficacy of Loestrin; increased incidence of breakthrough bleeding). Products include:
Arco-Lase Plus Tablets 607
Bellergal-S Tablets 1998
Bronkolixir .... ⊡ 761
Bronkotabs Tablets .... ⊡ 762
Donnatal 1858
Donnatal Extentabs 1859
Donnatal Tablets 1858
Donnazyme Tablets 1860
Kinesed Tablets 2272
Phenobarbital Elixir and Tablets 1293
Primatene Tablets-P Formula 2421
Quadrinal Tablets 1183
Tedral SA 1765

Phenylbutazone (Reduced efficacy of Loestrin; increased incidence of breakthrough bleeding). Products include:
Butazolidin Capsules & Tablets 1027

Phenytoin Sodium (Reduced efficacy of Loestrin; increased incidence of breakthrough bleeding). Products include:
Dilantin Kapseals 1708
Dilantin Parenteral 1712
Dilantin with Phenobarbital Kapseals 1715

Rifampin (Reduced efficacy of Loestrin; increased incidence of breakthrough bleeding). Products include:
Rifadin 1345
Rifamate Capsules 1347
Rimactane Capsules 879

Secobarbital Sodium (Reduced efficacy of Loestrin; increased incidence of breakthrough bleeding). Products include:
Seconal Sodium Pulvules 1296

Tetracycline Hydrochloride (Reduced efficacy of Loestrin; increased incidence of breakthrough bleeding). Products include:
Achromycin V Capsules 1193
Achromycin Ophthalmic Ointment 1% .... ⊙ 307
Achromycin Ophthalmic Suspension 1% .... ⊙ 308
Topicycline for Topical Solution 1856

Thiamylal Sodium (Reduced efficacy of Loestrin; increased incidence of breakthrough bleeding). Products include:
Surital Ampoules, Steri-Vials............ 1764

LOESTRIN [21] 1.5/30
(Norethindrone Acetate, Ethinyl Estradiol)..................................1728
See **Loestrin [21] 1/20**

LOMOTIL LIQUID
(Diphenoxylate Hydrochloride, Atropine Sulfate) 2174
May interact with monoamine oxidase inhibitors, barbiturates, tranquilizers, and certain other agents. Compounds in these categories include:

Alcohol (Potentiation of alcohol).

Alprazolam (Potentiation of tranquilizers). Products include:
Xanax Tablets 2367

Aprobarbital (Potentiation of barbiturates). Products include:
Alurate Elixir 1883

Buspirone Hydrochloride (Potentiation of tranquilizers). Products include:
BuSpar 1401

Butabarbital (Potentiation of barbiturates). Products include:
Pyridium Plus 1764

Butalbital (Potentiation of barbiturates). Products include:
Esgic-Plus Tablets 1002
Esgic Tablets & Capsules 1001
Fioricet Tablets 2006
Fiorinal Capsules 2007
Fiorinal with Codeine Capsules 2008
Fiorinal Tablets 2007
Phrenilin 838
Sedapap Tablets 50 mg/650 mg .. 1360

Chlordiazepoxide (Potentiation of tranquilizers). Products include:
Libritabs Tablets 1930
Limbitrol 1933
Menrium Tablets 1934

Chlordiazepoxide Hydrochloride (Potentiation of tranquilizers). Products include:
Librax Capsules 1929
Librium Capsules 1931
Librium Injectable 1932

Chlorpromazine (Potentiation of tranquilizers). Products include:
Thorazine 2234

Chlorprothixene (Potentiation of tranquilizers). Products include:
Taractan Tablets 1920

Chlorprothixene Lactate (Potentiation of tranquilizers). Products include:
Taractan Concentrate 1920

Clorazepate Dipotassium (Potentiation of tranquilizers). Products include:
Tranxene 556

Diazepam (Potentiation of tranquilizers). Products include:
Valium Injectable 1937
Valium Tablets 1939
Valrelease Capsules 1923

Droperidol (Potentiation of tranquilizers). Products include:
Inapsine Injection 1140
Innovar Injection 1141

Fluphenazine Decanoate (Potentiation of tranquilizers). Products include:
Prolixin Decanoate 1795

Fluphenazine Enanthate (Potentiation of tranquilizers). Products include:
Prolixin Enanthate 1796

Fluphenazine Hydrochloride (Potentiation of tranquilizers). Products include:
Prolixin Elixir 1793
Prolixin Injection 1791
Prolixin Oral Concentrate 1792
Prolixin Tablets 1793

Furazolidone (Hypertensive crisis). Products include:
Furoxone 1855

Haloperidol (Potentiation of tranquilizers). Products include:
Haldol Injection, Tablets and Concentrate 1373

Haloperidol Decanoate (Potentiation of tranquilizers). Products include:
Haldol Decanoate 1375

Hydroxyzine Hydrochloride (Potentiation of tranquilizers). Products include:
Atarax Tablets & Syrup 1941
Marax Tablets & DF Syrup 1954
Vistaril Intramuscular Solution 1970

Isocarboxazid (Hypertensive crisis). Products include:
Marplan Tablets 1906

Lorazepam (Potentiation of tranquilizers). Products include:
Ativan Injection 2432
Ativan Tablets 2434

Loxapine Hydrochloride (Potentiation of tranquilizers). Products include:
Loxitane 1213

Mephobarbital (Potentiation of barbiturates). Products include:
Mebaral Tablets 2061

Meprobamate (Potentiation of tranquilizers). Products include:
Deprol Tablets 2382
Equagesic Tablets 2451
Miltown Tablets 2386
PMB 200 and PMB 400 2504

Mesoridazine (Potentiation of tranquilizers). Products include:
Serentil 686

Molindone Hydrochloride (Potentiation of tranquilizers). Products include:
Moban Tablets & Concentrate 932

Oxazepam (Potentiation of tranquilizers). Products include:
Serax Capsules 2522
Serax Tablets 2522

Pentobarbital Sodium (Potentiation of barbiturates). Products include:
Nembutal Sodium Capsules 534
Nembutal Sodium Solution 536
Nembutal Sodium Suppositories...... 538

Perphenazine (Potentiation of tranquilizers). Products include:
Etrafon 2087
Triavil Tablets 1556
Trilafon 2123

Phenelzine Sulfate (Hypertensive crisis). Products include:
Nardil 1742

Phenobarbital (Potentiation of barbiturates). Products include:
Arco-Lase Plus Tablets 607
Bellergal-S Tablets 1998
Bronkolixir .... ⊡ 761
Bronkotabs Tablets .... ⊡ 762
Donnatal 1858
Donnatal Extentabs 1859
Donnatal Tablets 1858
Donnazyme Tablets 1860
Kinesed Tablets 2272
Phenobarbital Elixir and Tablets 1293
Primatene Tablets-P Formula 2421
Quadrinal Tablets 1183
Tedral SA 1765

Prazepam (Potentiation of tranquilizers). Products include:
Centrax 1693

Prochlorperazine (Potentiation of tranquilizers). Products include:
Compazine 2201

Promethazine Hydrochloride (Potentiation of tranquilizers). Products include:
Mepergan Injection 2479
Phenergan with Codeine 2497
Phenergan with Dextromethorphan 2499
Phenergan Injection 2493
Phenergan Suppositories 2496
Phenergan Syrup 2495
Phenergan Tablets 2496
Phenergan VC 2500
Phenergan VC with Codeine 2501

Secobarbital Sodium (Potentiation of barbiturates). Products include:
Seconal Sodium Pulvules 1296

Selegiline Hydrochloride (Hypertensive crisis). Products include:
Eldepryl 2250

Thiamylal Sodium (Potentiation of barbiturates). Products include:
Surital Ampoules, Steri-Vials............ 1764

Thioridazine Hydrochloride (Potentiation of tranquilizers). Products include:
Mellaril 2011

Thiothixene (Potentiation of tranquilizers). Products include:
Navane Capsules and Concentrate 1954
Navane Intramuscular 1956

Tranylcypromine Sulfate (Hypertensive crisis). Products include:
Parnate Tablets 2222
Trifluoperazine Hydrochloride (Potentiation of tranquilizers). Products include:
Stelazine 2226

LOMOTIL TABLETS
(Diphenoxylate Hydrochloride, Atropine Sulfate) 2174
See **Lomotil Liquid**

LONITEN TABLETS
(Minoxidil) 2346
May interact with:

Guanethidine Monosulfate (Profound orthostatic effects). Products include:
Esimil Tablets 864
Ismelin Tablets 869

LOPID CAPSULES AND TABLETS
(Gemfibrozil) 1736
May interact with anticoagulants and certain other agents. Compounds in these categories include:

Dicumarol (May affect prothrombin time resulting in bleeding complication). Products include:
Dicumarol Tablets 516
Heparin Calcium (May affect prothrombin time resulting in bleeding complication). Products include:
Calciparine Injection 925
Heparin Sodium (May affect prothrombin time resulting in bleeding complication). Products include:
Heparin Lock Flush Solution 2456
Heparin Sodium Vials 1264
Heparin Sodium Injection 2457
Heparin Sodium Injection, USP, Sterile Solution 2342
Lovastatin (Rhabdomyolysis has occurred from concomitant therapy). Products include:
Mevacor Tablets 1505
Warfarin Sodium (May affect prothrombin time resulting in bleeding complication). Products include:
Coumadin Injection & Tablets 944
Panwarfin Tablets 547

LOPRESSOR AMPULS
(Metoprolol Tartrate) 1032
May interact with catecholamine depleting drugs and certain other agents. Compounds in these categories include:

Deserpidine (Potential for additive effect). Products include:
Enduronyl 518
Harmonyl Tablets 528
Oreticyl 545
Epinephrine Hydrochloride (Potential for unresponsiveness to epinephrine to treat allergic reactions in certain patients). Products include:
Adrenalin Chloride Solution 1:100 & 1:1,000 1689
Epifrin ..... ◉ 244
Glaucon ..... ◉ 218
Rauwolfia Serpentina (Potential for additive effect). Products include:
Raudixin Tablets 1803
Rauzide Tablets 1804
Rescinnamine (Potential for additive effect).
No products indexed under this heading.
Reserpine (Potential for additive effect). Products include:
Diupres Tablets 1461
Hydromox R Tablets 1209
Hydropres Tablets 1485
Renese-R Tablets 1786
Salutensin/Salutensin-Demi 719
Ser-Ap-Es Tablets 881
Serpasil Tablets 883
Serpasil-Apresoline Tablets 884
Serpasil-Esidrix Tablets 886

LOPRESSOR HCT TABLETS
(Metoprolol Tartrate, Hydrochlorothiazide) 1034
May interact with catecholamine depleting drugs, cardiac glycosides, corticosteroids, para-aminobenzoic acid based local anesthetics, ganglionic blocking agents, antihypertensives, non-steroidal anti-inflammatory agents, barbiturates, narcotic analgesics, and certain other agents. Compounds in these categories include:

Acebutolol Hydrochloride (Potentiation of antihypertensive action). Products include:
Sectral Capsules 2520
ACTH (Hypokalemia may develop during concomitant use).
No products indexed under this heading.
Alcohol (Orthostatic hypotension may be potentiated).
Alfentanil Hydrochloride (Orthostatic hypotension may be potentiated). Products include:
Alfenta Injection 1131
Aprobarbital (Orthostatic hypotension may be potentiated). Products include:
Alurate Elixir 1883
Atenolol (Potentiation of antihypertensive action). Products include:
Tenoretic Tablets 1105
Tenormin Tablets and I.V. Injection 1107
Benazepril Hydrochloride (Potentiation of antihypertensive action). Products include:
Lotensin Tablets 872
Bendroflumethiazide (Potentiation of antihypertensive action). Products include:
Corzide Tablets 702
Naturetin Tablets 1789
Rauzide Tablets 1804
Betamethasone Acetate (Hypokalemia may develop during concomitant use). Products include:
Celestone Soluspan Suspension 2081
Betamethasone Sodium Phosphate (Hypokalemia may develop during concomitant use). Products include:
Celestone Soluspan Suspension 2081
Betaxolol Hydrochloride (Potentiation of antihypertensive action). Products include:
Betoptic Sterile Ophthalmic Solution 569
Betoptic S Sterile Ophthalmic Suspension 570
Kerlone Tablets 2172
Buprenorphine (Orthostatic hypotension may be potentiated).
No products indexed under this heading.
Butabarbital (Orthostatic hypotension may be potentiated). Products include:
Pyridium Plus 1764
Butalbital (Orthostatic hypotension may be potentiated). Products include:
Esgic-Plus Tablets 1002
Esgic Tablets & Capsules 1001
Fioricet Tablets 2006
Fiorinal Capsules 2007
Fiorinal with Codeine Capsules 2008
Fiorinal Tablets 2007
Phrenilin 838
Sedapap Tablets 50 mg/650 mg .. 1360
Captopril (Potentiation of antihypertensive action). Products include:
Capoten 2255
Capozide 2258
Carteolol Hydrochloride (Potentiation of antihypertensive action). Products include:
Cartrol Tablets 507
Chlorothiazide (Potentiation of antihypertensive action). Products include:
Aldoclor Tablets 1413
Diupres Tablets 1461
Diuril Oral 1464
Chlorothiazide Sodium (Potentiation of antihypertensive action). Products include:
Diuril Sodium Intravenous 1463
Chlorthalidone (Potentiation of antihypertensive action). Products include:
Combipres Tablets 678
Tenoretic Tablets 1105
Thalitone Tablets 687
Clonidine (Potentiation of antihypertensive action). Products include:
Catapres-TTS 677
Clonidine Hydrochloride (Potentiation of antihypertensive action). Products include:
Catapres Tablets 676
Combipres Tablets 678
Codeine (Orthostatic hypotension may be potentiated). Products include:
Calcidrine Syrup 506
Codeine Phosphate (Orthostatic hypotension may be potentiated). Products include:
Actifed with Codeine Cough Syrup.. 752
Cheracol Cough Syrup 1853
Codimal PH Syrup 846
Dimetane-DC Cough Syrup 1857
Empirin with Codeine Phosphate Nos. 2, 3 & 4 764
Fiorinal with Codeine Capsules 2008
Isoclor Expectorant 982
Naldecon CX Adult Liquid ..... ▣ 521
Novahistine DH 1342
Novahistine Expectorant 1343
Nucofed Capsules 2219
Nucofed Expectorant 2219
Nucofed Pediatric Expectorant 2220
Nucofed Syrup 2219
Phenaphen with Codeine Capsules 1865
Phenaphen-650 with Codeine Tablets 1866
Phenergan with Codeine 2497
Phenergan VC with Codeine 2501
Robitussin A-C Syrup 1875
Robitussin-DAC Syrup 1875
Ryna ..... ▣ 741
Soma Compound w/Codeine Tablets 2390
Triaminic Expectorant w/Codeine .. 1996
Tussi-Organidin Liquid 2391
Tylenol with Codeine 1381
Codeine Polistirex (Orthostatic hypotension may be potentiated).
No products indexed under this heading.
Cortisone Acetate (Hypokalemia may develop during concomitant use). Products include:
Cortone Acetate Sterile Suspension 1437
Cortone Acetate Tablets 1439
Deserpidine (Potentiation of antihypertensive action; potential for additive effects). Products include:
Enduronyl 518
Harmonyl Tablets 528
Oreticyl 545
Deslanoside (Potential for toxic effects of deslanoside on heart).
No products indexed under this heading.
Dexamethasone (Hypokalemia may develop during concomitant use). Products include:
AK-Trol Ointment & Suspension ..... ◉ 207
Decadron Elixir 1445
Decadron Tablets 1447
Decaspray Topical Aerosol 1459
Dexacidin ..... ◉ 272
Maxidex Sterile Ophthalmic Suspension ..... ◉ 223
Maxitrol Ophthalmic Ointment/Suspension ..... ◉ 223
TobraDex Ophthalmic Suspension and Ointment ..... ◉ 228
Dexamethasone Acetate (Hypokalemia may develop during concomitant use). Products include:
Dalalone D.P. Injectable 999
Decadron-LA Sterile Suspension 1457
Dexamethasone Sodium Phosphate (Hypokalemia may develop during concomitant use). Products include:
AK-Dex ..... ◉ 203
Decadron Phosphate Respihaler 1454
Decadron Phosphate Sterile Ophthalmic Ointment 1453
Decadron Phosphate Sterile Ophthalmic Solution 1453
Decadron Phosphate Topical Cream 1455
Decadron Phosphate Turbinaire 1456
Maxidex Sterile Ophthalmic Ointment ..... ◉ 222
NeoDecadron Sterile Ophthalmic Ointment 1517
NeoDecadron Sterile Ophthalmic Solution 1518
NeoDecadron Topical Cream 1518
Dezocine (Orthostatic hypotension may be potentiated).
Diazoxide (Potentiation of antihypertensive action). Products include:
Hyperstat I.V. Injection 2095
Proglycem 649
Diclofenac Sodium (Reduces diuretic, natriuretic and antihypertensive effects of thiazides). Products include:
Voltaren Ophthalmic Sterile Ophthalmic Solution ..... ◉ 268
Voltaren Tablets 1042
Digitoxin (Potential for toxic effects of digitalis on heart). Products include:
Crystodigin Tablets 1253
Digoxin (Potential for toxic effects of digitalis on heart). Products include:
Lanoxicaps 772
Lanoxin Elixir Pediatric 775
Lanoxin Injection 778
Lanoxin Injection Pediatric 781
Lanoxin Tablets 783
Doxazosin Mesylate (Potentiation of antihypertensive action). Products include:
Cardura Tablets 1941
Enalapril Maleate (Potentiation of antihypertensive action). Products include:
Vaseretic Tablets 1559
Vasotec Tablets 1564
Enalaprilat (Potentiation of antihypertensive effects). Products include:
Vasotec I.V. 1562
Epinephrine Hydrochloride (Potential for unresponsiveness to epinephrine to treat allergic reactions in certain patients). Products include:
Adrenalin Chloride Solution 1:100 & 1:1,000 1689
Epifrin ..... ◉ 244
Glaucon ..... ◉ 218
Esmolol Hydrochloride (Potentiation of antihypertensive action). Products include:
Brevibloc Injection 942
Etodolac (Reduces diuretic, natriuretic and antihypertensive effects of thiazides). Products include:
Lodine Capsules 2468

Felodipine (Potentiation of antihypertensive action). Products include:
- Plendil Extended-Release Tablets 1526

Fenoprofen Calcium (Reduces diuretic, natriuretic and antihypertensive effects of thiazides). Products include:
- Nalfon Pulvules & Tablets 919

Fentanyl (Orthostatic hypotension may be potentiated). Products include:
- Duragesic Transdermal System 1133

Fentanyl Citrate (Orthostatic hypotension may be potentiated). Products include:
- Innovar Injection 1141
- Sublimaze Injection 1146

Flurbiprofen (Reduces diuretic, natriuretic and antihypertensive effects of thiazides). Products include:
- Ansaid Tablets 2319

Fosinopril Sodium (Potentiation of antihypertensive action). Products include:
- Monopril Tablets 1406

Furosemide (Potentiation of antihypertensive action). Products include:
- Lasix 1093

Guanabenz Acetate (Potentiation of antihypertensive action). Products include:
- Wytensin Tablets 2542

Guanethidine Monosulfate (Potentiation of antihypertensive action). Products include:
- Esimil Tablets 864
- Ismelin Tablets 869

Hydralazine Hydrochloride (Potentiation of antihypertensive action). Products include:
- Apresazide Capsules 854
- Apresoline Hydrochloride Parenteral (Ampuls) 856
- Apresoline Hydrochloride Tablets .. 855
- Apresoline-Esidrix Tablets 857
- Ser-Ap-Es Tablets 881
- Serpasil-Apresoline Tablets 884

Hydrocodone Bitartrate (Orthostatic hypotension may be potentiated). Products include:
- Anexsia 5/500 Tablets 2196
- Anexsia 7.5/650 Tablets 2197
- Azdone Tablets 844
- Codiclear DH Syrup 845
- Codimal DH Syrup 846
- Damason-P 1356
- Hycodan Syrup, Tablets 927
- Hycomine Compound Tablets 929
- Hycomine Syrup 927
- Hycotuss Expectorant Syrup 930
- Hydrocet Capsules 835
- Lortab ASA Tablets 2414
- Lortab 2412
- Ru-Tuss with Hydrocodone 694
- Triaminic Expectorant DH 1995
- Vicodin Tablets 1187
- Vicodin ES Tablets 1189
- Zydone Capsules 941

Hydrocodone Polistirex (Orthostatic hypotension may be potentiated). Products include:
- Tussionex Extended-Release Suspension 988

Hydrocortisone (Hypokalemia may develop during concomitant use). Products include:
- AK-Spore H.C. .... ⊙ 206
- Bactine Hydrocortisone Anti-Itch Cream .... ▣ 625
- CaldeCORT Anti-Itch Hydrocortisone Spray .... ▣ 560
- Carmol HC Cream 1% 2296
- Cortaid Spray .... ▣ 735
- Cortenema 2244
- Cortisporin Ointment 758
- Cortisporin Ophthalmic Ointment Sterile 758
- Cortisporin Ophthalmic Suspension Sterile 759
- Cortisporin Otic Solution Sterile 760
- Cortisporin Otic Suspension Sterile 760
- Cortizone-5 Creme & Ointment .... ▣ 732
- Dermolate Anti-Itch Cream .... ▣ 697
- Eldecort Cream 1.0% 1113
- Eldecort Cream 1.0% and 2.5% 1113
- Fungoid HC Creme 1770
- Hydrocortone Tablets 1482
- Hytone 909
- LazerSporin-C Solution 1770
- Massengill Medicated Soft Cloth Towelettes 2192
- Nutracort Cream & Lotion 1684
- PediOtic Suspension Sterile 797
- Synacort Creams 1%, 2.5% 2296
- Vanoxide-HC Acne Lotion 911
- Vioform-Hydrocortisone Cream and Mild Cream 889
- Vioform-Hydrocortisone Ointment .. 889
- VōSoL HC Otic Solution 2392
- Vytone Cream 1% 911

Hydrocortisone Acetate (Hypokalemia may develop during concomitant use). Products include:
- Analpram-HC Rectal Cream 1% and 2.5% 970
- Anusol-HC Cream 1690
- Anusol-HC Suppositories 1691
- Caldecort .... ▣ 560
- Carmol HC Cream 1% 2296
- Chloromycetin Hydrocortisone Ophthalmic 1694
- Coly-Mycin S Otic w/Neomycin & Hydrocortisone 1708
- Cortaid .... ▣ 735
- Cortef Feminine Itch Cream .... ▣ 735
- Corticaine .... ▣ 682
- Cortifoam 1827
- Cortisporin Cream 757
- Epifoam 1828
- Gynecort 5 Creme .... ▣ 556
- Hydrocortone Acetate Sterile Suspension 1479
- Lanacort 5 Creme and Ointment .. ▣ 557
- Mantadil Cream 789
- Ophthocort .... ⊙ 301
- Orabase HCA Oral Paste 890
- Pramosone Cream, Lotion & Ointment 971
- ProctoCream-HC 1834
- Proctofoam-HC 1835

Hydrocortisone Sodium Phosphate (Hypokalemia may develop during concomitant use). Products include:
- Hydrocortone Phosphate Injection, Sterile 1481

Hydrocortisone Sodium Succinate (Hypokalemia may develop during concomitant use). Products include:
- Solu-Cortef Sterile Powder 2361

Hydroflumethiazide (Potentiation of antihypertensive action). Products include:
- Diucardin Tablets 2450
- Saluron 718
- Salutensin/Salutensin-Demi 719

Ibuprofen (Reduces diuretic, natriuretic and antihypertensive effects of thiazides). Products include:
- Advil Cold & Sinus Caplets (formerly CoAdvil) 2416
- Advil Ibuprofen Tablets and Caplets 2416
- Children's Advil Suspension 2426
- CoAdvil .... ▣ 748
- Dristan Sinus Caplets 2419
- Haltran Tablets .... ▣ 668
- Ibuprofen .... ▣ 631
- Medipren ibuprofen Caplets and Tablets 1362
- Midol 200 Cramp Relief Formula .. ▣ 570
- Motrin Tablets 2351
- Motrin IB Caplets and Tablets .... ▣ 736
- Nuprin Ibuprofen/Analgesic Tablets & Caplets 752
- PediaProfen Suspension 1363
- Rufen Tablets 691
- Trendar Ibuprofen Tablets .... ▣ 756

Indapamide (Potentiation of antihypertensive action). Products include:
- Lozol Tablets 1843

Indomethacin (Reduces diuretic, natriuretic and antihypertensive effects of thiazides). Products include:
- Indocin 1487

Indomethacin Sodium Trihydrate (Reduces diuretic, natriuretic and antihypertensive effects of thiazides). Products include:
- Indocin I.V. 1490

Isradipine (Potentiation of antihypertensive action). Products include:
- DynaCirc Capsules 2004

Ketoprofen (Reduces diuretic, natriuretic and antihypertensive effects of thiazides). Products include:
- Orudis Capsules 2488

Ketorolac Tromethamine (Reduces diuretic, natriuretic and antihypertensive effects of thiazides). Products include:
- Toradol IM Injection 2302

Labetalol Hydrochloride (Potentiation of antihypertensive action). Products include:
- Normodyne Injection 2108
- Normodyne Tablets 2110
- Normozide Tablets 2112
- Trandate HCT Tablets 579
- Trandate Injection 577
- Trandate Tablets 579

Levorphanol Tartrate (Orthostatic hypotension may be potentiated). Products include:
- Levo-Dromoran 1906

Lisinopril (Potentiation of antihypertensive effects). Products include:
- Prinivil Tablets 1538
- Prinzide Tablets 1540
- Zestoretic 2274
- Zestril Tablets 2277

Lithium Carbonate (Lithium renal clearance is reduced, increasing risk of lithium toxicity). Products include:
- Eskalith 2214
- Lithane Tablets 1596
- Lithium Carbonate Capsules & Tablets 1984
- Lithobid Tablets 870

Lithium Citrate (Lithium renal clearance is reduced, increasing risk of lithium toxicity). Products include:
- Cibalith-S 870

Mecamylamine Hydrochloride (Potentiation of antihypertensive action). Products include:
- Inversine Tablets 1492

Meclofenamate Sodium (Reduces diuretic, natriuretic and antihypertensive effects of thiazides). Products include:
- Meclomen Capsules 1739

Mefenamic Acid (Reduces diuretic, natriuretic and antihypertensive effects of thiazides). Products include:
- Ponstel 1758

Meperidine Hydrochloride (Orthostatic hypotension may be potentiated). Products include:
- Demerol 2047
- Mepergan Injection 2479

Mephobarbital (Orthostatic hypotension may be potentiated). Products include:
- Mebaral Tablets 2061

Methadone Hydrochloride (Orthostatic hypotension may be potentiated). Products include:
- Dolophine Hydrochloride Ampoules & Vials 1260
- Dolophine Hydrochloride Tablets 1261
- Methadone Hydrochloride Diskets .. 1284
- Methadone Hydrochloride Oral Solution & Tablets 1987

Methyclothiazide (Potentiation of antihypertensive action). Products include:
- Enduron Tablets 517
- Enduronyl 518

Methyldopa (Potentiation of antihypertensive action; hemolytic anemia). Products include:
- Aldoclor Tablets 1413
- Aldomet Oral 1415
- Aldoril Tablets 1418

Methyldopate Hydrochloride (Potentiation of antihypertensive action; hemolytic anemia). Products include:
- Aldomet Ester HCl Injection 1417

Methylprednisolone Acetate (Hypokalemia may develop during concomitant use). Products include:
- Depo-Medrol Sterile Aqueous Suspension 2334

Methylprednisolone Sodium Succinate (Hypokalemia may develop during concomitant use). Products include:
- Solu-Medrol Sterile Powder 2363

Metolazone (Potentiation of antihypertensive action). Products include:
- Diulo 2129
- Mykrox ½ mg Tablets 984
- Zaroxolyn Tablets 989

Metyrosine (Potentiation of antihypertensive action). Products include:
- Demser Capsules 1460

Minoxidil (Potentiation of antihypertensive action). Products include:
- Loniten Tablets 2346
- Rogaine Topical Solution 2357

Morphine Sulfate (Orthostatic hypotension may be potentiated). Products include:
- Astramorph/PF Injection, USP (Preservative-Free) 618
- Duramorph 960
- Infumorph 200 and Infumorph 500 Sterile Solutions 962
- MS Contin Tablets 1814
- MSIR 1817
- Oramorph SR (Morphine Sulfate Sustained Release Tablets) 1988
- Roxanol 1991

Nadolol (Potentiation of antihypertensive action). Products include:
- Corgard Tablets 701
- Corzide Tablets 702

Naproxen (Reduces diuretic, natriuretic and antihypertensive effects of thiazides). Products include:
- Naprosyn 2297

Naproxen Sodium (Reduces diuretic, natriuretic and antihypertensive effects of thiazides). Products include:
- Anaprox and Anaprox DS Tablets 2288

Nicardipine Hydrochloride (Potentiation of antihypertensive action). Products include:
- Cardene Capsules 2290

Nitroglycerin (Potentiation of antihypertensive action). Products include:
- Deponit NTG Transdermal Delivery System 2143
- Minitran Transdermal Delivery System 1312
- Nitro-Bid Ointment 1339
- Nitro-Bid Capsules 1338
- Nitrodisc 2176
- Nitro-Dur (nitroglycerin) Transdermal Infusion System 1164
- Nitrogard Tablets 1004
- Nitrolingual Spray 1846
- Nitrostat Tablets 1743
- Transderm-Nitro Transdermal Therapeutic System 2283

(▣ Described in PDR For Nonprescription Drugs)

(⊙ Described in PDR For Ophthalmology)

Norepinephrine Bitartrate (Arterial responsiveness may be decreased, but not enough to preclude effectiveness of pressor agent). Products include:

Levophed Bitartrate Injection **2054**

Opium Alkaloids (Orthostatic hypotension may be potentiated). Products include:

B & O No. 15A & No. 16A Supprettes **2395**
Pantopon Injectable **1911**

Oxycodone Hydrochloride (Orthostatic hypotension may be potentiated). Products include:

Percocet Tablets **950**
Percodan **951**
Roxicodone Tablets, Oral Solution & Intensol (Oxycodone) **1992**
Tylox Capsules **1382**

Penbutolol Sulfate (Potentiation of antihypertensive action). Products include:

Levatol **1832**

Pentobarbital Sodium (Orthostatic hypotension may be potentiated). Products include:

Nembutal Sodium Capsules **534**
Nembutal Sodium Solution **536**
Nembutal Sodium Suppositories **538**

Phenobarbital (Orthostatic hypotension may be potentiated). Products include:

Arco-Lase Plus Tablets **607**
Bellergal-S Tablets **1998**
Bronkolixir .... ⊞ **761**
Bronkotabs Tablets .... ⊞ **762**
Donnatal **1858**
Donnatal Extentabs **1859**
Donnatal Tablets **1858**
Donnazyme Tablets **1860**
Kinesed Tablets **2272**
Phenobarbital Elixir and Tablets **1293**
Primatene Tablets-P Formula **2421**
Quadrinal Tablets **1183**
Tedral SA **1765**

Phenoxybenzamine Hydrochloride (Potentiation of antihypertensive action). Products include:

Dibenzyline Capsules **2207**

Phentolamine Mesylate (Potentiation of antihypertensive action). Products include:

Regitine **878**

Phenylbutazone (Reduces diuretic, natriuretic and antihypertensive effects of thiazides). Products include:

Butazolidin Capsules & Tablets **1027**

Pindolol (Potentiation of antihypertensive action). Products include:

Visken Tablets **2036**

Piroxicam (Reduces diuretic, natriuretic and antihypertensive effects of thiazides). Products include:

Feldene Capsules **1777**

Polythiazide (Potentiation of antihypertensive action). Products include:

Minizide Capsules **1779**
Renese Tablets **1785**
Renese-R Tablets **1786**

Prazosin Hydrochloride (Potentiation of antihypertensive action). Products include:

Minipress Capsules **1778**
Minizide Capsules **1779**

Prednisolone Acetate (Hypokalemia may develop during concomitant use). Products include:

AK-Cide Sterile Ophthalmic Ointment & Suspension .... ◉ **202**
Blephamide Liquifilm Sterile Ophthalmic Suspension **586**
Blephamide S.O.P. Sterile Ophthalmic Ointment **586**
Cetapred Ointment .... ◉ **220**
⅛% Econopred & 1% Econopred Plus .... ◉ **217**
Isopto Cetapred Suspension .... ◉ **220**
Metimyd .... ◉ **306**
Poly-Pred Liquifilm .... ◉ **250**
Pred Forte .... ◉ **252**
Pred Mild .... ◉ **254**
Pred-G Liquifilm Sterile Ophthalmic Suspension .... ◉ **252**
Pred-G S.O.P. Sterile Ophthalmic Ointment .... ◉ **253**
Vasocidin Ointment .... ◉ **275**

Prednisolone Sodium Phosphate (Hypokalemia may develop during concomitant use). Products include:

AK-Pred .... ◉ **205**
Hydeltrasol Injection, Sterile **1476**
Inflamase .... ◉ **274**
Pediapred Oral Liquid **987**
Vasocidin Ophthalmic Solution .... ◉ **276**

Prednisolone Tebutate (Hypokalemia may develop during concomitant use). Products include:

Hydeltra-T.B.A. Sterile Suspension **1478**

Prednisone (Hypokalemia may develop during concomitant use). Products include:

Deltasone Tablets **2332**

Propoxyphene Hydrochloride (Orthostatic hypotension may be potentiated). Products include:

Darvon **1256**
Wygesic Tablets **2540**

Propoxyphene Napsylate (Orthostatic hypotension may be potentiated). Products include:

Darvon-N/Darvocet-N **1254**

Propranolol Hydrochloride (Potentiation of antihypertensive action). Products include:

Inderal **2459**
Inderal LA Long Acting Capsules **2461**
Inderide Tablets **2463**
Inderide LA Long Acting Capsules **2465**

Ramipril (Potentiation of antihypertensive action). Products include:

Altace Capsules **1086**

Rauwolfia Serpentina (Potentiation of antihypertensive action; potential for additive effects). Products include:

Raudixin Tablets **1803**
Rauzide Tablets **1804**

Rescinnamine (Potentiation of antihypertensive action; potential for additive effects).

No products indexed under this heading.

Reserpine (Potentiation of antihypertensive action; potential for additive effects). Products include:

Diupres Tablets **1461**
Hydromox R Tablets **1209**
Hydropres Tablets **1485**
Renese-R Tablets **1786**
Salutensin/Salutensin-Demi **719**
Ser-Ap-Es Tablets **881**
Serpasil Tablets **883**
Serpasil-Apresoline Tablets **884**
Serpasil-Esidrix Tablets **886**

Secobarbital Sodium (Orthostatic hypotension may be potentiated). Products include:

Seconal Sodium Pulvules **1296**

Sodium Nitroprusside (Potentiation of antihypertensive action). Products include:

Nipride I.V. Infusion **1909**

Sufentanil Citrate (Orthostatic hypotension may be potentiated). Products include:

Sufenta Injection **1147**

Sulindac (Reduces diuretic, natriuretic and antihypertensive effects of thiazides). Products include:

Clinoril Tablets **1433**

Terazosin Hydrochloride (Potentiation of antihypertensive action). Products include:

Hytrin Tablets **529**

Thiamylal Sodium (Orthostatic hypotension may be potentiated). Products include:

Surital Ampoules, Steri-Vials **1764**

Timolol Maleate (Potentiation of antihypertensive action). Products include:

Blocadren Tablets **1429**
Timolide Tablets **1547**
Timoptic in Ocudose **1552**
Timoptic Sterile Ophthalmic Solution **1550**

Tolmetin Sodium (Reduces diuretic, natriuretic and antihypertensive effects of thiazides). Products include:

Tolectin (200, 400 and 600 mg) .. **1379**

Triamcinolone (Hypokalemia may develop during concomitant use).

No products indexed under this heading.

Triamcinolone Acetonide (Hypokalemia may develop during concomitant use). Products include:

Aristocort A **1010**
Azmacort Inhaler **1837**
Kenalog Cream, Lotion & Ointment **2401**
Kenalog-10 Injection **2402**
Kenalog-40 Injection **2403**
Kenalog in Orabase **604**
Kenalog Spray **2401**
Mycolog II Cream and Ointment **2407**
Mytrex Cream & Ointment **2080**
Nasacort Nasal Inhaler **1844**

Triamcinolone Diacetate (Hypokalemia may develop during concomitant use). Products include:

Aristocort Suspension **1008**

Triamcinolone Hexacetonide (Hypokalemia may develop during concomitant use). Products include:

Aristospan Suspension **1011**

Trimethaphan Camsylate (Potentiation of antihypertensive action). Products include:

Arfonad Ampuls **1887**

Tubocurarine Chloride (Increase responsiveness to tubocurarine).

No products indexed under this heading.

LOPRESSOR TABLETS
(Metoprolol Tartrate) 1032
See **Lopressor Ampuls**

LOPROX CREAM 1% AND LOTION 1%
(Ciclopirox Olamine) 1095
No interactions described in labeling.

LORELCO TABLETS
(Probucol) 1333
May interact with drugs that prolong the qt interval and certain other agents. Compounds in these categories include:

Amiodarone Hydrochloride (Increases the risk of serious arrhythmia). Products include:

Cordarone Tablets **2446**

Amitriptyline Hydrochloride (Increases the risk of serious arrhythmia). Products include:

Elavil **2269**
Endep Tablets **1927**
Etrafon **2087**
Limbitrol **1933**
Triavil Tablets **1556**

Amoxapine (Increases the risk of serious arrhythmia). Products include:

Asendin Tablets **1196**

Bretylium Tosylate (Increases the risk of serious arrhythmia). Products include:

Bretylol Injection **923**

Chlorpromazine (Increases the risk of serious arrhythmia). Products include:

Thorazine **2234**

Clofibrate (Pronounced lowering of HDL-cholesterol). Products include:

Atromid-S Capsules **2435**

Clomipramine Hydrochloride (Increases the risk of serious arrhythmia). Products include:

Anafranil Capsules **650**

Desipramine Hydrochloride (Increases the risk of serious arrhythmia). Products include:

Norpramin Tablets **1340**

Disopyramide Phosphate (Increases the risk of serious arrhythmia). Products include:

Norpace **2177**

Doxepin Hydrochloride (Increases the risk of serious arrhythmia). Products include:

Sinequan **1960**

Flecainide Acetate (Increases the risk of serious arrhythmia). Products include:

Tambocor Tablets **1315**

Fluphenazine Decanoate (Increases the risk of serious arrhythmia). Products include:

Prolixin Decanoate **1795**

Fluphenazine Enanthate (Increases the risk of serious arrhythmia). Products include:

Prolixin Enanthate **1796**

Fluphenazine Hydrochloride (Increases the risk of serious arrhythmia). Products include:

Prolixin Elixir **1793**
Prolixin Injection **1791**
Prolixin Oral Concentrate **1792**
Prolixin Tablets **1793**

Imipramine Hydrochloride (Increases the risk of serious arrhythmia). Products include:

Tofranil Ampuls **1038**
Tofranil Tablets **1039**

Imipramine Pamoate (Increases the risk of serious arrhythmia). Products include:

Tofranil-PM Capsules **1041**

Lidocaine Hydrochloride (Increases the risk of serious arrhythmia). Products include:

Anestacon Solution **2394**
Bactine Antiseptic/Anesthetic First Aid Spray .... ⊞ **624**
Decadron Phosphate with Xylocaine Injection, Sterile **1451**
Xylocaine Injections **637**
Xylocaine Injections for Ventricular Arrhythmias **639**
Xylocaine 2% Jelly **643**
4% Xylocaine-MPF Sterile Solution **641**
Xylocaine 2% Viscous Solution **646**

Maprotiline Hydrochloride (Increases the risk of serious arrhythmia). Products include:

Ludiomil Tablets **874**

Mesoridazine (Increases the risk of serious arrhythmia). Products include:

Serentil **686**

Mexiletine Hydrochloride (Increases the risk of serious arrhythmia). Products include:

Mexitil Capsules **680**

Nortriptyline Hydrochloride (Increases the risk of serious arrhythmia). Products include:

Pamelor **2019**

Perphenazine (Increases the risk of serious arrhythmia). Products include:

Etrafon **2087**
Triavil Tablets **1556**
Trilafon **2123**

(⊞ Described in PDR For Nonprescription Drugs) (◉ Described in PDR For Ophthalmology)

Procainamide Hydrochloride (Increases the risk of serious arrhythmia). Products include:

Procan SR Tablets ... 1760
Pronestyl Capsules and Tablets ... 1800
Pronestyl Injection ... 1798
Pronestyl-SR Tablets ... 1801

Prochlorperazine (Increases the risk of serious arrhythmia). Products include:

Compazine ... 2201

Promethazine Hydrochloride (Increases the risk of serious arrhythmia). Products include:

Mepergan Injection ... 2479
Phenergan with Codeine ... 2497
Phenergan with Dextromethorphan 2499
Phenergan Injection ... 2493
Phenergan Suppositories ... 2496
Phenergan Syrup ... 2495
Phenergan Tablets ... 2496
Phenergan VC ... 2500
Phenergan VC with Codeine ... 2501

Propafenone Hydrochloride (Increases the risk of serious arrhythmia). Products include:

Rythmol Tablets ... 1184

Protriptyline Hydrochloride (Increases the risk of serious arrhythmia). Products include:

Vivactil Tablets ... 1567

Quinidine Gluconate (Increases the risk of serious arrhythmia). Products include:

Quinaglute Dura-Tabs Tablets ... 663

Quinidine Polygalacturonate (Increases the risk of serious arrhythmia). Products include:

Cardioquin Tablets ... 1812

Quinidine Sulfate (Increases the risk of serious arrhythmia). Products include:

Quinidex Extentabs ... 1868

Thioridazine Hydrochloride (Increases the risk of serious arrhythmia). Products include:

Mellaril ... 2011

Tocainide Hydrochloride (Increases the risk of serious arrhythmia). Products include:

Tonocard Tablets ... 1554

Trifluoperazine Hydrochloride (Increases the risk of serious arrhythmia). Products include:

Stelazine ... 2226

Trimipramine Maleate (Increases the risk of serious arrhythmia). Products include:

Surmontil Capsules ... 2524

LORTAB ASA TABLETS

(Hydrocodone Bitartrate, Aspirin) ... 2414
May interact with narcotic analgesics, monoamine oxidase inhibitors, tranquilizers, central nervous system depressants, psychotropics, anticholinergics, tricyclic antidepressants, oral anticoagulants, oral hypoglycemic agents, insulin, non-steroidal anti-inflammatory agents, corticosteroids, and certain other agents. Compounds in these categories include:

Alcohol (Additive CNS depression).

Alfentanil Hydrochloride (Additive CNS depression; the dose of one or both agents should be reduced). Products include:

Alfenta Injection ... 1131

Alprazolam (Additive CNS depression; the dose of one or both agents should be reduced). Products include:

Xanax Tablets ... 2367

Amitriptyline Hydrochloride (Additive CNS depression; the dose of one or both agents should be reduced; increased effect of either hydrocodone or antidepressant). Products include:

Elavil ... 2269
Endep Tablets ... 1927
Etrafon ... 2087
Limbitrol ... 1933
Triavil Tablets ... 1556

Amoxapine (Additive CNS depression; the dose of one or both agents should be reduced; increased effect of either hydrocodone or antidepressant). Products include:

Asendin Tablets ... 1196

Aprobarbital (Additive CNS depression; the dose of one or both agents should be reduced). Products include:

Alurate Elixir ... 1883

Atropine Sulfate (May produce paralytic ileus). Products include:

Arco-Lase Plus Tablets ... 607
Atropine Sulfate Sterile Ophthalmic Solution and S.O.P. Sterile Ophthalmic Ointment ... ◉ 239
Donnagel ... ▣ 675
Donnagel-PG ... 1858
Donnatal ... 1858
Donnatal Extentabs ... 1859
Donnatal Tablets ... 1858
Donnazyme Tablets ... 1860
Isopto Atropine ... ◉ 218
Lomotil ... 2174
Motofen Tablets ... 836
Ru-Tuss Tablets ... 693
Urised Tablets ... 2396

Belladonna Alkaloids (May produce paralytic ileus). Products include:

Bellergal-S Tablets ... 1998
Hyland's Bed Wetting Tablets ... ▣ 728
Hyland's Teething Tablets ... ▣ 728
Kinesed Tablets ... 2272

Benztropine Mesylate (May produce paralytic ileus). Products include:

Cogentin ... 1435

Betamethasone Acetate (Potential for enhanced effect). Products include:

Celestone Soluspan Suspension ... 2081

Betamethasone Sodium Phosphate (Potential for enhanced effect). Products include:

Celestone Soluspan Suspension ... 2081

Biperiden (May produce paralytic ileus). Products include:

Akineton ... 1171

Buprenorphine (Additive CNS depression; the dose of one or both agents should be reduced).

No products indexed under this heading.

Buspirone Hydrochloride (Additive CNS depression; the dose of one or both agents should be reduced). Products include:

BuSpar ... 1401

Butabarbital (Additive CNS depression; the dose of one or both agents should be reduced). Products include:

Pyridium Plus ... 1764

Butalbital (Additive CNS depression; the dose of one or both agents should be reduced). Products include:

Esgic-Plus Tablets ... 1002
Esgic Tablets & Capsules ... 1001
Fioricet Tablets ... 2006
Fiorinal Capsules ... 2007
Fiorinal with Codeine Capsules ... 2008
Fiorinal Tablets ... 2007
Phrenilin ... 838
Sedapap Tablets 50 mg/650 mg .. 1360

Chlordiazepoxide (Additive CNS depression; the dose of one or both agents should be reduced). Products include:

Libritabs Tablets ... 1930
Limbitrol ... 1933
Menrium Tablets ... 1934

Chlordiazepoxide Hydrochloride (Additive CNS depression; the dose of one or both agents should be reduced). Products include:

Librax Capsules ... 1929
Librium Capsules ... 1931
Librium Injectable ... 1932

Chlorpromazine (Additive CNS depression; the dose of one or both agents should be reduced). Products include:

Thorazine ... 2234

Chlorpropamide (Aspirin may enhance the effects of oral hypoglycemic agents). Products include:

Diabinese Tablets ... 1775

Chlorprothixene (Additive CNS depression; the dose of one or both agents should be reduced). Products include:

Taractan Tablets ... 1920

Chlorprothixene Hydrochloride (Additive CNS depression; the dose of one or both agents should be reduced). Products include:

Taractan ... 1920

Clidinium Bromide (May produce paralytic ileus). Products include:

Librax Capsules ... 1929
Quarzan Capsules ... 1937

Clomipramine Hydrochloride (Additive CNS depression; the dose of one or both agents should be reduced; increased effect of either hydrocodone or antidepressant). Products include:

Anafranil Capsules ... 650

Clorazepate Dipotassium (Additive CNS depression; the dose of one or both agents should be reduced). Products include:

Tranxene ... 556

Codeine (Additive CNS depression; the dose of one or both agents should be reduced). Products include:

Calcidrine Syrup ... 506

Codeine Phosphate (Additive CNS depression; the dose of one or both agents should be reduced). Products include:

Actifed with Codeine Cough Syrup.. 752
Cheracol Cough Syrup ... 1853
Codimal PH Syrup ... 846
Dimetane-DC Cough Syrup ... 1857
Empirin with Codeine Phosphate Nos. 2, 3 & 4 ... 764
Fiorinal with Codeine Capsules ... 2008
Isoclor Expectorant ... 982
Naldecon CX Adult Liquid ... ▣ 521
Novahistine DH ... 1342
Novahistine Expectorant ... 1343
Nucofed Capsules ... 2219
Nucofed Expectorant ... 2219
Nucofed Pediatric Expectorant ... 2220
Nucofed Syrup ... 2219
Phenaphen with Codeine Capsules 1865
Phenaphen-650 with Codeine Tablets ... 1866
Phenergan with Codeine ... 2497
Phenergan VC with Codeine ... 2501
Robitussin A-C Syrup ... 1875
Robitussin-DAC Syrup ... 1875
Ryna ... ▣ 741
Soma Compound w/Codeine Tablets ... 2390
Triaminic Expectorant w/Codeine .. 1996
Tussi-Organidin Liquid ... 2391
Tylenol with Codeine ... 1381

Codeine Polistirex (Additive CNS depression; the dose of one or both agents should be reduced).

No products indexed under this heading.

Cortisone Acetate (Potential for enhanced effect). Products include:

Cortone Acetate Sterile Suspension ... 1437
Cortone Acetate Tablets ... 1439

Desipramine Hydrochloride (Additive CNS depression; the dose of one or both agents should be reduced; increased effect of either hydrocodone or antidepressant). Products include:

Norpramin Tablets ... 1340

Dexamethasone (Potential for enhanced effect). Products include:

AK-Trol Ointment & Suspension ... ◉ 207
Decadron Elixir ... 1445
Decadron Tablets ... 1447
Decaspray Topical Aerosol ... 1459
Dexacidin ... ◉ 272
Maxidex Sterile Ophthalmic Suspension ... ◉ 223
Maxitrol Ophthalmic Ointment/Suspension ... ◉ 223
TobraDex Ophthalmic Suspension and Ointment ... ◉ 228

Dexamethasone Acetate (Potential for enhanced effect). Products include:

Dalalone D.P. Injectable ... 999
Decadron-LA Sterile Suspension ... 1457

Dexamethasone Sodium Phosphate (Potential for enhanced effect). Products include:

AK-Dex ... ◉ 203
Decadron Phosphate Respihaler ... 1454
Decadron Phosphate Sterile Ophthalmic Ointment ... 1453
Decadron Phosphate Sterile Ophthalmic Solution ... 1453
Decadron Phosphate Topical Cream ... 1455
Decadron Phosphate Turbinaire ... 1456
Maxidex Sterile Ophthalmic Ointment ... ◉ 222
NeoDecadron Sterile Ophthalmic Ointment ... 1517
NeoDecadron Sterile Ophthalmic Solution ... 1518
NeoDecadron Topical Cream ... 1518

Dezocine (Additive CNS depression; the dose of one or both agents should be reduced).

Diazepam (Additive CNS depression; the dose of one or both agents should be reduced). Products include:

Valium Injectable ... 1937
Valium Tablets ... 1939
Valrelease Capsules ... 1923

Diclofenac Sodium (Potential for enhanced effect). Products include:

Voltaren Ophthalmic Sterile Ophthalmic Solution ... ◉ 268
Voltaren Tablets ... 1042

Dicumarol (Aspirin may enhance the effects of oral anticoagulant). Products include:

Dicumarol Tablets ... 516

Dicyclomine Hydrochloride (May produce paralytic ileus). Products include:

Bentyl ... 1322

Doxepin Hydrochloride (Additive CNS depression; the dose of one or both agents should be reduced; increased effect of either hydrocodone or antidepressant). Products include:

Sinequan ... 1960

Droperidol (Additive CNS depression; the dose of one or both agents should be reduced). Products include:

Inapsine Injection ... 1140
Innovar Injection ... 1141

Enflurane (Additive CNS depression; the dose of one or both agents should be reduced). Products include:

Ethrane ... 599

Estazolam (Additive CNS depression; the dose of one or both agents should be reduced). Products include:
ProSom Tablets 554

Ethchlorvynol (Additive CNS depression; the dose of one or both agents should be reduced). Products include:
Placidyl Capsules 553

Ethinamate (Additive CNS depression; the dose of one or both agents should be reduced).
No products indexed under this heading.

Etodolac (Potential for enhanced effect). Products include:
Lodine Capsules 2468

Fenoprofen Calcium (Potential for enhanced effect). Products include:
Nalfon Pulvules & Tablets 919

Fentanyl (Additive CNS depression; the dose of one or both agents should be reduced). Products include:
Duragesic Transdermal System 1133

Fentanyl Citrate (Additive CNS depression; the dose of one or both agents should be reduced). Products include:
Innovar Injection 1141
Sublimaze Injection 1146

Fluphenazine Decanoate (Additive CNS depression; the dose of one or both agents should be reduced). Products include:
Prolixin Decanoate 1795

Fluphenazine Enanthate (Additive CNS depression; the dose of one or both agents should be reduced). Products include:
Prolixin Enanthate 1796

Fluphenazine Hydrochloride (Additive CNS depression; the dose of one or both agents should be reduced). Products include:
Prolixin Elixir 1793
Prolixin Injection 1791
Prolixin Oral Concentrate 1792
Prolixin Tablets 1793

Flurazepam Hydrochloride (Additive CNS depression; the dose of one or both agents should be reduced). Products include:
Dalmane Capsules 1927

Flurbiprofen (Potential for enhanced effect). Products include:
Ansaid Tablets 2319

Furazolidone (Additive CNS depression; the dose of one or both agents should be reduced; increased effect of either hydrocodone or MAO inhibitor). Products include:
Furoxone 1855

Glipizide (Aspirin may enhance the effects of oral hypoglycemic agents). Products include:
Glucotrol 1952

Glutethimide (Additive CNS depression; the dose of one or both agents should be reduced).
No products indexed under this heading.

Glyburide (Aspirin may enhance the effects of oral hypoglycemic agents). Products include:
DiaBeta 1091
Micronase Tablets 2350

Glycopyrrolate (May produce paralytic ileus). Products include:
Robinul Forte Tablets 1873
Robinul Injectable 1873
Robinul Tablets 1873

Haloperidol (Additive CNS depression; the dose of one or both agents should be reduced). Products include:
Haldol Injection, Tablets and Concentrate 1373

Haloperidol Decanoate (Additive CNS depression; the dose of one or both agents should be reduced). Products include:
Haldol Decanoate 1375

Hydrocodone Polistirex (Additive CNS depression; the dose of one or both agents should be reduced). Products include:
Tussionex Extended-Release Suspension 988

Hydrocortisone (Potential for enhanced effect). Products include:
AK-Spore H.C. ◉ 206
Bactine Hydrocortisone Anti-Itch Cream ▣ 625
CaldeCORT Anti-Itch Hydrocortisone Spray ▣ 560
Carmol HC Cream 1% 2296
Cortaid Spray ▣ 735
Cortenema 2244
Cortisporin Ointment 758
Cortisporin Ophthalmic Ointment Sterile 758
Cortisporin Ophthalmic Suspension Sterile 759
Cortisporin Otic Solution Sterile 760
Cortisporin Otic Suspension Sterile 760
Cortizone-5 Creme & Ointment ▣ 732
Dermolate Anti-Itch Cream ▣ 697
Eldecort Cream 1.0% 1113
Eldecort Cream 1.0% and 2.5% 1113
Fungoid HC Creme 1770
Hydrocortone Tablets 1482
Hytone 909
LazerSporin-C Solution 1770
Massengill Medicated Soft Cloth Towelettes 2192
Nutracort Cream & Lotion 1684
PediOtic Suspension Sterile 797
Synacort Creams 1%, 2.5% 2296
Vanoxide-HC Acne Lotion 911
Vioform-Hydrocortisone Cream and Mild Cream 889
Vioform-Hydrocortisone Ointment 889
VōSoL HC Otic Solution 2392
Vytone Cream 1% 911

Hydrocortisone Acetate (Potential for enhanced effect). Products include:
Analpram-HC Rectal Cream 1% and 2.5% 970
Anusol-HC Cream 1690
Anusol-HC Suppositories 1691
Caldecort ▣ 560
Carmol HC Cream 1% 2296
Chloromycetin Hydrocortisone Ophthalmic 1694
Coly-Mycin S Otic w/Neomycin & Hydrocortisone 1708
Cortaid ▣ 735
Cortef Feminine Itch Cream ▣ 735
Corticaine ▣ 682
Cortifoam 1827
Cortisporin Cream 757
Epifoam 1828
Gynecort 5 Creme ▣ 556
Hydrocortone Acetate Sterile Suspension 1479
Lanacort 5 Creme and Ointment ▣ 557
Mantadil Cream 789
Ophthocort ◉ 301
Orabase HCA Oral Paste 890
Pramosone Cream, Lotion & Ointment 971
ProctoCream-HC 1834
Proctofoam-HC 1835

Hydrocortisone Sodium Phosphate (Potential for enhanced effect). Products include:
Hydrocortone Phosphate Injection, Sterile 1481

Hydrocortisone Sodium Succinate (Potential for enhanced effect). Products include:
Solu-Cortef Sterile Powder 2361

Hydroxyzine Hydrochloride (Additive CNS depression; the dose of one or both agents should be reduced). Products include:
Atarax Tablets & Syrup 1941
Marax Tablets & DF Syrup 1954
Vistaril Intramuscular Solution 1970

Hyoscyamine (May produce paralytic ileus). Products include:
Cystospaz Tablets 2395
Urised Tablets 2396

Hyoscyamine Sulfate (May produce paralytic ileus). Products include:
Arco-Lase Plus Tablets 607
Cystospaz-M Capsules 2395
Donnagel ▣ 675
Donnagel-PG 1858
Donnatal 1858
Donnatal Extentabs 1859
Donnatal Tablets 1858
Donnazyme Tablets 1860
Kutrase Capsules 2146
Levsin/Levsinex 2147
Ru-Tuss Tablets 693

Ibuprofen (Potential for enhanced effect). Products include:
Advil Cold & Sinus Caplets (formerly CoAdvil) 2416
Advil Ibuprofen Tablets and Caplets 2416
Children's Advil Suspension 2426
CoAdvil ▣ 748
Dristan Sinus Caplets 2419
Haltran Tablets ▣ 668
Ibuprofen ▣ 631
Medipren ibuprofen Caplets and Tablets 1362
Midol 200 Cramp Relief Formula ▣ 570
Motrin Tablets 2351
Motrin IB Caplets and Tablets ▣ 736
Nuprin Ibuprofen/Analgesic Tablets & Caplets 752
PediaProfen Suspension 1363
Rufen Tablets 691
Trendar Ibuprofen Tablets ▣ 756

Imipramine Hydrochloride (Additive CNS depression; the dose of one or both agents should be reduced; increased effect of either hydrocodone or antidepressant). Products include:
Tofranil Ampuls 1038
Tofranil Tablets 1039

Imipramine Pamoate (Additive CNS depression; the dose of one or both agents should be reduced; increased effect of either hydrocodone or antidepressant). Products include:
Tofranil-PM Capsules 1041

Indomethacin (Potential for enhanced effect). Products include:
Indocin 1487

Indomethacin Sodium Trihydrate (Potential for enhanced effect). Products include:
Indocin I.V. 1490

Insulin, Human (Aspirin may enhance the effects of insulin).
No products indexed under this heading.

Insulin, Human Isophane Suspension (Aspirin may enhance the effects of insulin). Products include:
Humulin N, 100 Units 1270

Insulin, Human NPH (Aspirin may enhance the effects of insulin). Products include:
Insulatard NPH Human 1627
Novolin N 1627
Novolin N PenFill Cartridges 1628
Novolin N Prefilled 1628

Insulin, Human Regular (Aspirin may enhance the effects of insulin). Products include:
Humulin BR, 100 Units 1268
Humulin R, 100 Units 1272
Novolin R 1627
Novolin R PenFill Cartridges 1628
Novolin R Prefilled 1629
Velosulin Human 1628

Insulin, Human, Zinc Suspension (Aspirin may enhance the effects of insulin). Products include:
Humulin L, 100 Units 1268
Humulin U, 100 Units 1272
Novolin L 1627

Insulin, NPH (Aspirin may enhance the effects of insulin). Products include:
NPH, 40 & 100 Units 1273
Beef NPH, 100 Units 1274
Pork NPH, 100 Units 1275
Insulatard NPH 1626
NPH Insulin 1626
NPH Purified Pork Isophane Insulin 1626

Insulin, Regular (Aspirin may enhance the effects of insulin). Products include:
Regular, 40 & 100 Units 1273
Beef Regular, 100 Units 1275
Pork Regular, 100 Units 1275
Pork Regular (Concentrated), 500 Units 1276
Regular Insulin 1625
Regular Purified Pork Insulin 1626
Velosulin 1627

Insulin, Zinc Crystals (Aspirin may enhance the effects of insulin). Products include:
NPH, 40 & 100 Units 1273

Insulin, Zinc Suspension (Aspirin may enhance the effects of insulin). Products include:
Lente, 40 & 100 Units 1272
Protamine, Zinc, 40 & 100 Units 1273
Lente Iletin I 1272
Beef Lente, 100 Units 1274
Beef Protamine Zinc, 100 Units 1274
Pork Lente, 100 Units 1275
Pork, Protamine, Zinc, 100 Units 1275
Lente Insulin 1626
Lente Purified Pork Insulin 1626
Semilente Insulin 1625
Ultralente Insulin 1626

Ipratropium Bromide (May produce paralytic ileus). Products include:
Atrovent Inhalation Aerosol 675

Isocarboxazid (Additive CNS depression; the dose of one or both agents should be reduced; increased effect of either hydrocodone or MAO inhibitor). Products include:
Marplan Tablets 1906

Isoflurane (Additive CNS depression; the dose of one or both agents should be reduced). Products include:
Forane 600

Ketamine Hydrochloride (Additive CNS depression; the dose of one or both agents should be reduced). Products include:
Ketalar 1726

Ketoprofen (Potential for enhanced effect). Products include:
Orudis Capsules 2488

Ketorolac Tromethamine (Potential for enhanced effect). Products include:
Toradol IM Injection 2302

Levorphanol Tartrate (Additive CNS depression; the dose of one or both agents should be reduced). Products include:
Levo-Dromoran 1906

Lithium Carbonate (Additive CNS depression; the dose of one or both agents should be reduced). Products include:
Eskalith 2214
Lithane Tablets 1596
Lithium Carbonate Capsules & Tablets 1984
Lithobid Tablets 870

Lithium Citrate (Additive CNS depression; the dose of one or both agents should be reduced). Products include:
Cibalith-S 870

Lorazepam (Additive CNS depression; the dose of one or both agents should be reduced). Products include:
- Ativan Injection 2432
- Ativan Tablets 2434

Loxapine Hydrochloride (Additive CNS depression; the dose of one or both agents should be reduced). Products include:
- Loxitane 1213

Loxapine Succinate (Additive CNS depression; the dose of one or both agents should be reduced). Products include:
- Loxitane Capsules 1213

Maprotiline Hydrochloride (Additive CNS depression; the dose of one or both agents should be reduced; increased effect of either hydrocodone or antidepressant). Products include:
- Ludiomil Tablets 874

Meclofenamate Sodium (Potential for enhanced effect). Products include:
- Meclomen Capsules 1739

Mefenamic Acid (Potential for enhanced effect). Products include:
- Ponstel 1758

Mepenzolate Bromide (May produce paralytic ileus). Products include:
- Cantil Tablets 1326

Meperidine Hydrochloride (Additive CNS depression; the dose of one or both agents should be reduced). Products include:
- Demerol 2047
- Mepergan Injection 2479

Mephobarbital (Additive CNS depression; the dose of one or both agents should be reduced). Products include:
- Mebaral Tablets 2061

Meprobamate (Additive CNS depression; the dose of one or both agents should be reduced). Products include:
- Deprol Tablets 2382
- Equagesic Tablets 2451
- Miltown Tablets 2386
- PMB 200 and PMB 400 2504

Mercaptopurine (Potential for enhanced effect and bone marrow toxicity). Products include:
- Purinethol Tablets 800

Mesoridazine (Additive CNS depression; the dose of one or both agents should be reduced). Products include:
- Serentil 686

Mesoridazine Besylate (Additive CNS depression; the dose of one or both agents should be reduced).

Methadone Hydrochloride (Additive CNS depression; the dose of one or both agents should be reduced). Products include:
- Dolophine Hydrochloride Ampoules & Vials 1260
- Dolophine Hydrochloride Tablets 1261
- Methadone Hydrochloride Diskets 1284
- Methadone Hydrochloride Oral Solution & Tablets 1987

Methohexital Sodium (Additive CNS depression; the dose of one or both agents should be reduced). Products include:
- Brevital Sodium Vials 1248

Methoxyflurane (Additive CNS depression; the dose of one or both agents should be reduced).
- No products indexed under this heading.

Methylprednisolone Acetate (Potential for enhanced effect). Products include:
- Depo-Medrol Sterile Aqueous Suspension 2334

Methylprednisolone Sodium Succinate (Potential for enhanced effect). Products include:
- Solu-Medrol Sterile Powder 2363

Midazolam Hydrochloride (Additive CNS depression; the dose of one or both agents should be reduced). Products include:
- Versed Injection 1924

Molindone Hydrochloride (Additive CNS depression; the dose of one or both agents should be reduced). Products include:
- Moban Tablets & Concentrate 932

Morphine Sulfate (Additive CNS depression; the dose of one or both agents should be reduced). Products include:
- Astramorph/PF Injection, USP (Preservative-Free) 618
- Duramorph 960
- Infumorph 200 and Infumorph 500 Sterile Solutions 962
- MS Contin Tablets 1814
- MSIR 1817
- Oramorph SR (Morphine Sulfate Sustained Release Tablets) 1988
- Roxanol 1991

Naproxen (Potential for enhanced effect). Products include:
- Naprosyn 2297

Naproxen Sodium (Potential for enhanced effect). Products include:
- Anaprox and Anaprox DS Tablets 2288

Nortriptyline Hydrochloride (Additive CNS depression; the dose of one or both agents should be reduced; increased effect of either hydrocodone or antidepressant). Products include:
- Pamelor 2019

Opium Alkaloids (Additive CNS depression; the dose of one or both agents should be reduced). Products include:
- B & O No. 15A & No. 16A Supprettes 2395
- Pantopon Injectable 1911

Oxazepam (Additive CNS depression; the dose of one or both agents should be reduced). Products include:
- Serax Capsules 2522
- Serax Tablets 2522

Oxybutynin Chloride (May produce paralytic ileus). Products include:
- Ditropan 1332

Oxycodone Hydrochloride (Additive CNS depression; the dose of one or both agents should be reduced). Products include:
- Percocet Tablets 950
- Percodan 951
- Roxicodone Tablets, Oral Solution & Intensol (Oxycodone) 1992
- Tylox Capsules 1382

Pentobarbital Sodium (Additive CNS depression; the dose of one or both agents should be reduced). Products include:
- Nembutal Sodium Capsules 534
- Nembutal Sodium Solution 536
- Nembutal Sodium Suppositories 538

Perphenazine (Additive CNS depression; the dose of one or both agents should be reduced). Products include:
- Etrafon 2087
- Triavil Tablets 1556
- Trilafon 2123

Phenelzine Sulfate (Additive CNS depression; the dose of one or both agents should be reduced; increased effect of either hydrocodone or MAO inhibitor). Products include:
- Nardil 1742

Phenobarbital (Additive CNS depression; the dose of one or both agents should be reduced). Products include:
- Arco-Lase Plus Tablets 607
- Bellergal-S Tablets 1998
- Bronkolixir .... ▣ 761
- Bronkotabs Tablets .... ▣ 762
- Donnatal 1858
- Donnatal Extentabs 1859
- Donnatal Tablets 1858
- Donnazyme Tablets 1860
- Kinesed Tablets 2272
- Phenobarbital Elixir and Tablets 1293
- Primatene Tablets-P Formula 2421
- Quadrinal Tablets 1183
- Tedral SA 1765

Phenylbutazone (Potential for enhanced effect). Products include:
- Butazolidin Capsules & Tablets 1027

Piroxicam (Potential for enhanced effect). Products include:
- Feldene Capsules 1777

Prazepam (Additive CNS depression; the dose of one or both agents should be reduced). Products include:
- Centrax 1693

Prednisolone Acetate (Potential for enhanced effect). Products include:
- AK-Cide Sterile Ophthalmic Ointment & Suspension .... ⊙ 202
- Blephamide Liquifilm Sterile Ophthalmic Suspension 586
- Blephamide S.O.P. Sterile Ophthalmic Ointment 586
- Cetapred Ointment .... ⊙ 220
- ⅛ % Econopred & 1 % Econopred Plus .... ⊙ 217
- Isopto Cetapred Suspension .... ⊙ 220
- Metimyd .... ⊙ 306
- Poly-Pred Liquifilm .... ⊙ 250
- Pred Forte .... ⊙ 252
- Pred Mild .... ⊙ 254
- Pred-G Liquifilm Sterile Ophthalmic Suspension .... ⊙ 252
- Pred-G S.O.P. Sterile Ophthalmic Ointment .... ⊙ 253
- Vasocidin Ointment .... ⊙ 275

Prednisolone Sodium Phosphate (Potential for enhanced effect). Products include:
- AK-Pred .... ⊙ 205
- Hydeltrasol Injection, Sterile 1476
- Inflamase .... ⊙ 274
- Pediapred Oral Liquid 987
- Vasocidin Ophthalmic Solution .... ⊙ 276

Prednisolone Tebutate (Potential for enhanced effect). Products include:
- Hydeltra-T.B.A. Sterile Suspension 1478

Prednisone (Potential for enhanced effect). Products include:
- Deltasone Tablets 2332

Probenecid (Aspirin may diminish the effects of uricosuric agent). Products include:
- Benemid Tablets 1426
- ColBENEMID Tablets 1436
- Wycillin Injection and Probenecid Tablets 2539

Prochlorperazine (Additive CNS depression; the dose of one or both agents should be reduced). Products include:
- Compazine 2201

Procyclidine Hydrochloride (May produce paralytic ileus). Products include:
- Kemadrin Tablets 771

Promethazine Hydrochloride (Additive CNS depression; the dose of one or both agents should be reduced). Products include:
- Mepergan Injection 2479
- Phenergan with Codeine 2497
- Phenergan with Dextromethorphan 2499
- Phenergan Injection 2493
- Phenergan Suppositories 2496
- Phenergan Syrup 2495
- Phenergan Tablets 2496
- Phenergan VC 2500
- Phenergan VC with Codeine 2501

Propantheline Bromide (May produce paralytic ileus). Products include:
- Pro-Banthīne Tablets 2141

Propofol (Additive CNS depression; the dose of one or both agents should be reduced). Products include:
- Diprivan Injection 2267

Propoxyphene Hydrochloride (Additive CNS depression; the dose of one or both agents should be reduced). Products include:
- Darvon 1256
- Wygesic Tablets 2540

Propoxyphene Napsylate (Additive CNS depression; the dose of one or both agents should be reduced). Products include:
- Darvon-N/Darvocet-N 1254

Protriptyline Hydrochloride (Additive CNS depression; the dose of one or both agents should be reduced; increased effect of either hydrocodone or antidepressant). Products include:
- Vivactil Tablets 1567

Quazepam (Additive CNS depression; the dose of one or both agents should be reduced). Products include:
- Doral Tablets 2383

Scopolamine Hydrobromide (May produce paralytic ileus). Products include:
- Donnagel .... ▣ 675
- Donnagel-PG 1858
- Donnatal 1858
- Donnatal Extentabs 1859
- Donnatal Tablets 1858
- Donnazyme Tablets 1860
- Isopto Hyoscine .... ⊙ 222
- Murocoll-2 Sterile Ophthalmic Solution .... ⊙ 261
- Ru-Tuss Tablets 693

Scopolamine Preparations (May produce paralytic ileus). Products include:
- Transderm Scōp Transdermal Therapeutic System 887

Secobarbital Sodium (Additive CNS depression; the dose of one or both agents should be reduced). Products include:
- Seconal Sodium Pulvules 1296

Selegiline Hydrochloride (Additive CNS depression; the dose of one or both agents should be reduced; increased effect of either hydrocodone or MAO inhibitor). Products include:
- Eldepryl 2250

Sufentanil Citrate (Additive CNS depression; the dose of one or both agents should be reduced). Products include:
- Sufenta Injection 1147

Sulfinpyrazone (Aspirin may diminish the effects of uricosuric agent). Products include:
- Anturane 853

Sulindac (Potential for enhanced effect). Products include:
- Clinoril Tablets 1433

Temazepam (Additive CNS depression; the dose of one or both agents should be reduced). Products include:
- Restoril Capsules 2023

Thiamylal Sodium (Additive CNS depression; the dose of one or both agents should be reduced). Products include:
- Surital Ampoules, Steri-Vials 1764

Thioridazine Hydrochloride (Additive CNS depression; the dose of one or both agents should be reduced). Products include:
- Mellaril 2011

Thiothixene (Additive CNS depression; the dose of one or both agents should be reduced). Products include:
- Navane Capsules and Concentrate 1954
- Navane Intramuscular 1956

Tolazamide (Aspirin may enhance the effects of oral hypoglycemic agents). Products include:
- Tolinase Tablets 2365

Tolbutamide (Aspirin may enhance the effects of oral hypoglycemic agents). Products include:
- Orinase Tablets 2354

Tolmetin Sodium (Potential for enhanced effect). Products include:
- Tolectin (200, 400 and 600 mg) .. 1379

Tranylcypromine Sulfate (Additive CNS depression; the dose of one or both agents should be reduced; increased effect of either hydrocodone or MAO inhibitor). Products include:
- Parnate Tablets 2222

Triamcinolone (Potential for enhanced effect).
- No products indexed under this heading.

Triamcinolone Acetonide (Potential for enhanced effect). Products include:
- Aristocort A 1010
- Azmacort Inhaler 1837
- Kenalog Cream, Lotion & Ointment 2401
- Kenalog-10 Injection 2402
- Kenalog-40 Injection 2403
- Kenalog in Orabase 604
- Kenalog Spray 2401
- Mycolog II Cream and Ointment 2407
- Mytrex Cream & Ointment 2080
- Nasacort Nasal Inhaler 1844

Triamcinolone Diacetate (Potential for enhanced effect). Products include:
- Aristocort Suspension 1008

Triamcinolone Hexacetonide (Potential for enhanced effect). Products include:
- Aristospan Suspension 1011

Triazolam (Additive CNS depression; the dose of one or both agents should be reduced). Products include:
- Halcion Tablets 2340

Tridihexethyl Chloride (May produce paralytic ileus).
- No products indexed under this heading.

Trifluoperazine Hydrochloride (Additive CNS depression; the dose of one or both agents should be reduced). Products include:
- Stelazine 2226

Trihexyphenidyl Hydrochloride (May produce paralytic ileus). Products include:
- Artane 1195

Trimipramine Maleate (Additive CNS depression; the dose of one or both agents should be reduced; increased effect of either hydrocodone or antidepressant). Products include:
- Surmontil Capsules 2524

Warfarin Sodium (Aspirin may enhance the effects of oral anticoagulant). Products include:
- Coumadin Injection & Tablets 944
- Panwarfin Tablets 547

LORTAB LIQUID
(Hydrocodone Bitartrate, Acetaminophen) 2412
May interact with central nervous system depressants, narcotic analgesics, psychotropics, tranquilizers, monoamine oxidase inhibitors, tricyclic antidepressants, anticholinergics, and certain other agents. Compounds in these categories include:

Alcohol (Additive CNS depression).

Alfentanil Hydrochloride (Additive CNS depression; the dose of one or both agents should be reduced). Products include:
- Alfenta Injection 1131

Alprazolam (Additive CNS depression; the dose of one or both agents should be reduced). Products include:
- Xanax Tablets 2367

Amitriptyline Hydrochloride (Increased effect of either hydrocodone or antidepressant; additive CNS depression; the dose of one or both agents should be reduced). Products include:
- Elavil 2269
- Endep Tablets 1927
- Etrafon 2087
- Limbitrol 1933
- Triavil Tablets 1556

Amoxapine (Increased effect of either hydrocodone or antidepressant; additive CNS depression; the dose of one or both agents should be reduced). Products include:
- Asendin Tablets 1196

Aprobarbital (Additive CNS depression; the dose of one or both agents should be reduced). Products include:
- Alurate Elixir 1883

Atropine Sulfate (May produce paralytic ileus). Products include:
- Arco-Lase Plus Tablets 607
- Atropine Sulfate Sterile Ophthalmic Solution and S.O.P. Sterile Ophthalmic Ointment .... ⊙ 239
- Donnagel .... ▣ 675
- Donnagel-PG 1858
- Donnatal 1858
- Donnatal Extentabs 1859
- Donnatal Tablets 1858
- Donnazyme Tablets 1860
- Isopto Atropine .... ⊙ 218
- Lomotil 2174
- Motofen Tablets 836
- Ru-Tuss Tablets 693
- Urised Tablets 2396

Belladonna Alkaloids (May produce paralytic ileus). Products include:
- Bellergal-S Tablets 1998
- Hyland's Bed Wetting Tablets .... ▣ 728
- Hyland's Teething Tablets .... ▣ 728
- Kinesed Tablets 2272

Benztropine Mesylate (May produce paralytic ileus). Products include:
- Cogentin 1435

Biperiden (May produce paralytic ileus). Products include:
- Akineton 1171

Buprenorphine (Additive CNS depression; the dose of one or both agents should be reduced).
- No products indexed under this heading.

Buspirone Hydrochloride (Additive CNS depression; the dose of one or both agents should be reduced). Products include:
- BuSpar 1401

Butabarbital (Additive CNS depression; the dose of one or both agents should be reduced). Products include:
- Pyridium Plus 1764

Butalbital (Additive CNS depression; the dose of one or both agents should be reduced). Products include:
- Esgic-Plus Tablets 1002
- Esgic Tablets & Capsules 1001
- Fioricet Tablets 2006
- Fiorinal Capsules 2007
- Fiorinal with Codeine Capsules 2008
- Fiorinal Tablets 2007
- Phrenilin 838
- Sedapap Tablets 50 mg/650 mg .. 1360

Chlordiazepoxide (Additive CNS depression; the dose of one or both agents should be reduced). Products include:
- Libritabs Tablets 1930
- Limbitrol 1933
- Menrium Tablets 1934

Chlordiazepoxide Hydrochloride (Additive CNS depression; the dose of one or both agents should be reduced). Products include:
- Librax Capsules 1929
- Librium Capsules 1931
- Librium Injectable 1932

Chlorpromazine (Additive CNS depression; the dose of one or both agents should be reduced). Products include:
- Thorazine 2234

Chlorprothixene (Additive CNS depression; the dose of one or both agents should be reduced). Products include:
- Taractan Tablets 1920

Chlorprothixene Hydrochloride (Additive CNS depression; the dose of one or both agents should be reduced). Products include:
- Taractan 1920

Clidinium Bromide (May produce paralytic ileus). Products include:
- Librax Capsules 1929
- Quarzan Capsules 1937

Clomipramine Hydrochloride (Increased effect of either hydrocodone or antidepressant; additive CNS depression; the dose of one or both agents should be reduced). Products include:
- Anafranil Capsules 650

Clorazepate Dipotassium (Additive CNS depression; the dose of one or both agents should be reduced). Products include:
- Tranxene 556

Codeine (Additive CNS depression; the dose of one or both agents should be reduced). Products include:
- Calcidrine Syrup 506

Codeine Phosphate (Additive CNS depression; the dose of one or both agents should be reduced). Products include:
- Actifed with Codeine Cough Syrup.. 752
- Cheracol Cough Syrup 1853
- Codimal PH Syrup 846
- Dimetane-DC Cough Syrup 1857
- Empirin with Codeine Phosphate Nos. 2, 3 & 4 764
- Fiorinal with Codeine Capsules 2008
- Isoclor Expectorant 982
- Naldecon CX Adult Liquid .... ▣ 521
- Novahistine DH 1342
- Novahistine Expectorant 1343
- Nucofed Capsules 2219
- Nucofed Expectorant 2219
- Nucofed Pediatric Expectorant 2220
- Nucofed Syrup 2219
- Phenaphen with Codeine Capsules 1865
- Phenaphen-650 with Codeine Tablets 1866
- Phenergan with Codeine 2497
- Phenergan VC with Codeine 2501
- Robitussin A-C Syrup 1875
- Robitussin-DAC Syrup 1875
- Ryna .... ▣ 741
- Soma Compound w/Codeine Tablets 2390
- Triaminic Expectorant w/Codeine .. 1996
- Tussi-Organidin Liquid 2391
- Tylenol with Codeine 1381

Codeine Polistirex (Additive CNS depression; the dose of one or both agents should be reduced).
- No products indexed under this heading.

Desipramine Hydrochloride (Increased effect of either hydrocodone or antidepressant; additive CNS depression; the dose of one or both agents should be reduced). Products include:
- Norpramin Tablets 1340

Dezocine (Additive CNS depression; the dose of one or both agents should be reduced).

Diazepam (Additive CNS depression; the dose of one or both agents should be reduced). Products include:
- Valium Injectable 1937
- Valium Tablets 1939
- Valrelease Capsules 1923

Dicyclomine Hydrochloride (May produce paralytic ileus). Products include:
- Bentyl 1322

Doxepin Hydrochloride (Increased effect of either hydrocodone or antidepressant; additive CNS depression; the dose of one or both agents should be reduced). Products include:
- Sinequan 1960

Droperidol (Additive CNS depression; the dose of one or both agents should be reduced). Products include:
- Inapsine Injection 1140
- Innovar Injection 1141

Enflurane (Additive CNS depression; the dose of one or both agents should be reduced). Products include:
- Ethrane 599

Estazolam (Additive CNS depression; the dose of one or both agents should be reduced). Products include:
- ProSom Tablets 554

Ethchlorvynol (Additive CNS depression; the dose of one or both agents should be reduced). Products include:
- Placidyl Capsules 553

Ethinamate (Additive CNS depression; the dose of one or both agents should be reduced).
- No products indexed under this heading.

Fentanyl (Additive CNS depression; the dose of one or both agents should be reduced). Products include:
- Duragesic Transdermal System 1133

Fentanyl Citrate (Additive CNS depression; the dose of one or both agents should be reduced). Products include:
- Innovar Injection 1141
- Sublimaze Injection 1146

Fluphenazine Decanoate (Additive CNS depression; the dose of one or both agents should be reduced). Products include:
- Prolixin Decanoate 1795

Fluphenazine Enanthate (Additive CNS depression; the dose of one or both agents should be reduced). Products include:
- Prolixin Enanthate 1796

Fluphenazine Hydrochloride (Additive CNS depression; the dose of one or both agents should be reduced). Products include:
- Prolixin Elixir 1793
- Prolixin Injection 1791

Prolixin Oral Concentrate 1792
Prolixin Tablets 1793

Flurazepam Hydrochloride (Additive CNS depression; the dose of one or both agents should be reduced). Products include:
Dalmane Capsules 1927

Furazolidone (Increased effect of either hydrocodone or MAO inhibitor; additive CNS depression; the dose of one or both agents should be reduced). Products include:
Furoxone 1855

Glutethimide (Additive CNS depression; the dose of one or both agents should be reduced).
No products indexed under this heading.

Glycopyrrolate (May produce paralytic ileus). Products include:
Robinul Forte Tablets 1873
Robinul Injectable 1873
Robinul Tablets 1873

Haloperidol (Additive CNS depression; the dose of one or both agents should be reduced). Products include:
Haldol Injection, Tablets and Concentrate 1373

Haloperidol Decanoate (Additive CNS depression; the dose of one or both agents should be reduced). Products include:
Haldol Decanoate 1375

Hydrocodone Polistirex (Additive CNS depression; the dose of one or both agents should be reduced). Products include:
Tussionex Extended-Release Suspension 988

Hydroxyzine Hydrochloride (Additive CNS depression; the dose of one or both agents should be reduced). Products include:
Atarax Tablets & Syrup 1941
Marax Tablets & DF Syrup 1954
Vistaril Intramuscular Solution 1970

Hyoscyamine (May produce paralytic ileus). Products include:
Cystospaz Tablets 2395
Urised Tablets 2396

Hyoscyamine Sulfate (May produce paralytic ileus). Products include:
Arco-Lase Plus Tablets 607
Cystospaz-M Capsules 2395
Donnagel .... ▣ 675
Donnagel-PG 1858
Donnatal 1858
Donnatal Extentabs 1859
Donnatal Tablets 1858
Donnazyme Tablets 1860
Kutrase Capsules 2146
Levsin/Levsinex 2147
Ru-Tuss Tablets 693

Imipramine Hydrochloride (Increased effect of either hydrocodone or antidepressant; additive CNS depression; the dose of one or both agents should be reduced). Products include:
Tofranil Ampuls 1038
Tofranil Tablets 1039

Imipramine Pamoate (Increased effect of either hydrocodone or antidepressant; additive CNS depression; the dose of one or both agents should be reduced). Products include:
Tofranil-PM Capsules 1041

Ipratropium Bromide (May produce paralytic ileus). Products include:
Atrovent Inhalation Aerosol 675

Isocarboxazid (Increased effect of either hydrocodone or MAO inhibitor; additive CNS depression; the dose of one or both agents should be reduced). Products include:
Marplan Tablets 1906

Isoflurane (Additive CNS depression; the dose of one or both agents should be reduced). Products include:
Forane 600

Ketamine Hydrochloride (Additive CNS depression; the dose of one or both agents should be reduced). Products include:
Ketalar 1726

Levorphanol Tartrate (Additive CNS depression; the dose of one or both agents should be reduced). Products include:
Levo-Dromoran 1906

Lithium Carbonate (Additive CNS depression; the dose of one or both agents should be reduced). Products include:
Eskalith 2214
Lithane Tablets 1596
Lithium Carbonate Capsules & Tablets 1984
Lithobid Tablets 870

Lithium Citrate (Additive CNS depression; the dose of one or both agents should be reduced). Products include:
Cibalith-S 870

Lorazepam (Additive CNS depression; the dose of one or both agents should be reduced). Products include:
Ativan Injection 2432
Ativan Tablets 2434

Loxapine Hydrochloride (Additive CNS depression; the dose of one or both agents should be reduced). Products include:
Loxitane 1213

Loxapine Succinate (Additive CNS depression; the dose of one or both agents should be reduced). Products include:
Loxitane Capsules 1213

Maprotiline Hydrochloride (Increased effect of either hydrocodone or antidepressant; additive CNS depression; the dose of one or both agents should be reduced). Products include:
Ludiomil Tablets 874

Mepenzolate Bromide (May produce paralytic ileus). Products include:
Cantil Tablets 1326

Meperidine Hydrochloride (Additive CNS depression; the dose of one or both agents should be reduced). Products include:
Demerol 2047
Mepergan Injection 2479

Mephobarbital (Additive CNS depression; the dose of one or both agents should be reduced). Products include:
Mebaral Tablets 2061

Meprobamate (Additive CNS depression; the dose of one or both agents should be reduced). Products include:
Deprol Tablets 2382
Equagesic Tablets 2451
Miltown Tablets 2386
PMB 200 and PMB 400 2504

Mesoridazine (Additive CNS depression; the dose of one or both agents should be reduced). Products include:
Serentil 686

Methadone Hydrochloride (Additive CNS depression; the dose of one or both agents should be reduced). Products include:
Dolophine Hydrochloride Ampoules & Vials 1260
Dolophine Hydrochloride Tablets 1261
Methadone Hydrochloride Diskets 1284
Methadone Hydrochloride Oral Solution & Tablets 1987

Methohexital Sodium (Additive CNS depression; the dose of one or both agents should be reduced). Products include:
Brevital Sodium Vials 1248

Methoxyflurane (Additive CNS depression; the dose of one or both agents should be reduced).
No products indexed under this heading.

Midazolam Hydrochloride (Additive CNS depression; the dose of one or both agents should be reduced). Products include:
Versed Injection 1924

Molindone Hydrochloride (Additive CNS depression; the dose of one or both agents should be reduced). Products include:
Moban Tablets & Concentrate 932

Morphine Sulfate (Additive CNS depression; the dose of one or both agents should be reduced). Products include:
Astramorph/PF Injection, USP (Preservative-Free) 618
Duramorph 960
Infumorph 200 and Infumorph 500 Sterile Solutions 962
MS Contin Tablets 1814
MSIR 1817
Oramorph SR (Morphine Sulfate Sustained Release Tablets) 1988
Roxanol 1991

Nortriptyline Hydrochloride (Increased effect of either hydrocodone or antidepressant; additive CNS depression; the dose of one or both agents should be reduced). Products include:
Pamelor 2019

Opium Alkaloids (Additive CNS depression; the dose of one or both agents should be reduced). Products include:
B & O No. 15A & No. 16A Supprettes 2395
Pantopon Injectable 1911

Oxazepam (Additive CNS depression; the dose of one or both agents should be reduced). Products include:
Serax Capsules 2522
Serax Tablets 2522

Oxybutynin Chloride (May produce paralytic ileus). Products include:
Ditropan 1332

Oxycodone Hydrochloride (Additive CNS depression; the dose of one or both agents should be reduced). Products include:
Percocet Tablets 950
Percodan 951
Roxicodone Tablets, Oral Solution & Intensol (Oxycodone) 1992
Tylox Capsules 1382

Pentobarbital Sodium (Additive CNS depression; the dose of one or both agents should be reduced). Products include:
Nembutal Sodium Capsules 534
Nembutal Sodium Solution 536
Nembutal Sodium Suppositories 538

Perphenazine (Additive CNS depression; the dose of one or both agents should be reduced). Products include:
Etrafon 2087
Triavil Tablets 1556
Trilafon 2123

Phenelzine Sulfate (Increased effect of either hydrocodone or MAO inhibitor; additive CNS depression; the dose of one or both agents should be reduced). Products include:
Nardil 1742

Phenobarbital (Additive CNS depression; the dose of one or both agents should be reduced). Products include:
Arco-Lase Plus Tablets 607
Bellergal-S Tablets 1998
Bronkolixir .... ▣ 761
Bronkotabs Tablets .... ▣ 762
Donnatal 1858
Donnatal Extentabs 1859
Donnatal Tablets 1858
Donnazyme Tablets 1860
Kinesed Tablets 2272
Phenobarbital Elixir and Tablets 1293
Primatene Tablets-P Formula 2421
Quadrinal Tablets 1183
Tedral SA 1765

Prazepam (Additive CNS depression; the dose of one or both agents should be reduced). Products include:
Centrax 1693

Prochlorperazine (Additive CNS depression; the dose of one or both agents should be reduced). Products include:
Compazine 2201

Procyclidine Hydrochloride (May produce paralytic ileus). Products include:
Kemadrin Tablets 771

Promethazine Hydrochloride (Additive CNS depression; the dose of one or both agents should be reduced). Products include:
Mepergan Injection 2479
Phenergan with Codeine 2497
Phenergan with Dextromethorphan 2499
Phenergan Injection 2493
Phenergan Suppositories 2496
Phenergan Syrup 2495
Phenergan Tablets 2496
Phenergan VC 2500
Phenergan VC with Codeine 2501

Propantheline Bromide (May produce paralytic ileus). Products include:
Pro-Banthīne Tablets 2141

Propofol (Additive CNS depression; the dose of one or both agents should be reduced). Products include:
Diprivan Injection 2267

Propoxyphene Hydrochloride (Additive CNS depression; the dose of one or both agents should be reduced). Products include:
Darvon 1256
Wygesic Tablets 2540

Propoxyphene Napsylate (Additive CNS depression; the dose of one or both agents should be reduced). Products include:
Darvon-N/Darvocet-N 1254

Protriptyline Hydrochloride (Increased effect of either hydrocodone or antidepressant; additive CNS depression; the dose of one or both agents should be reduced). Products include:
Vivactil Tablets 1567

Quazepam (Additive CNS depression; the dose of one or both agents should be reduced). Products include:
Doral Tablets 2383

Scopolamine Hydrobromide (May produce paralytic ileus). Products include:
Donnagel .... ▣ 675
Donnagel-PG 1858
Donnatal 1858
Donnatal Extentabs 1859
Donnatal Tablets 1858
Donnazyme Tablets 1860
Isopto Hyoscine .... ⊙ 222
Murocoll-2 Sterile Ophthalmic Solution .... ⊙ 261
Ru-Tuss Tablets 693

Scopolamine Preparations (May produce paralytic ileus). Products include:
- Transderm Scōp Transdermal Therapeutic System ... 887

Secobarbital Sodium (Additive CNS depression; the dose of one or both agents should be reduced). Products include:
- Seconal Sodium Pulvules ... 1296

Selegiline Hydrochloride (Increased effect of either hydrocodone or MAO inhibitor). Products include:
- Eldepryl ... 2250

Sufentanil Citrate (Additive CNS depression; the dose of one or both agents should be reduced). Products include:
- Sufenta Injection ... 1147

Temazepam (Additive CNS depression; the dose of one or both agents should be reduced). Products include:
- Restoril Capsules ... 2023

Thiamylal Sodium (Additive CNS depression; the dose of one or both agents should be reduced). Products include:
- Surital Ampoules, Steri-Vials ... 1764

Thioridazine Hydrochloride (Additive CNS depression; the dose of one or both agents should be reduced). Products include:
- Mellaril ... 2011

Thiothixene (Additive CNS depression; the dose of one or both agents should be reduced). Products include:
- Navane Capsules and Concentrate 1954
- Navane Intramuscular ... 1956

Tranylcypromine Sulfate (Increased effect of either hydrocodone or MAO inhibitor; additive CNS depression; the dose of one or both agents should be reduced). Products include:
- Parnate Tablets ... 2222

Triazolam (Additive CNS depression; the dose of one or both agents should be reduced). Products include:
- Halcion Tablets ... 2340

Tridihexethyl Chloride (May produce paralytic ileus).
- No products indexed under this heading.

Trifluoperazine Hydrochloride (Additive CNS depression; the dose of one or both agents should be reduced). Products include:
- Stelazine ... 2226

Trihexyphenidyl Hydrochloride (May produce paralytic ileus). Products include:
- Artane ... 1195

Trimipramine Maleate (Increased effect of either hydrocodone or antidepressant; additive CNS depression; the dose of one or both agents should be reduced). Products include:
- Surmontil Capsules ... 2524

LORTAB 2.5/500 TABLETS
(Hydrocodone Bitartrate, Acetaminophen) ... 2412

See **Lortab Liquid**

LORTAB 5/500 TABLETS
(Hydrocodone Bitartrate, Acetaminophen) ... 2412

See **Lortab Liquid**

LORTAB 7.5/500 TABLETS
(Hydrocodone Bitartrate, Acetaminophen) ... 2412

See **Lortab Liquid**

LOTENSIN TABLETS
(Benazepril Hydrochloride) ... 872

May interact with diuretics, potassium sparing diuretics, potassium-depleting corticosteroids, lithium preparations, and certain other agents. Compounds in these categories include:

Amiloride Hydrochloride (Potential for excessive reduction of blood pressure; potential for hyperkalemia). Products include:
- Midamor Tablets ... 1508
- Moduretic Tablets ... 1510

Bendroflumethiazide (Potential for excessive reduction of blood pressure). Products include:
- Corzide Tablets ... 702
- Naturetin Tablets ... 1789
- Rauzide Tablets ... 1804

Bumetanide (Potential for excessive reduction of blood pressure). Products include:
- Bumex ... 1895

Chlorothiazide (Potential for excessive reduction of blood pressure). Products include:
- Aldoclor Tablets ... 1413
- Diupres Tablets ... 1461
- Diuril Oral ... 1464

Chlorothiazide Sodium (Potential for excessive reduction of blood pressure). Products include:
- Diuril Sodium Intravenous ... 1463

Chlorthalidone (Potential for excessive reduction of blood pressure). Products include:
- Combipres Tablets ... 678
- Tenoretic Tablets ... 1105
- Thalitone Tablets ... 687

Ethacrynic Acid (Potential for excessive reduction of blood pressure). Products include:
- Edecrin Tablets ... 1468

Furosemide (Potential for excessive reduction of blood pressure). Products include:
- Lasix ... 1093

Hydrochlorothiazide (Potential for excessive reduction of blood pressure). Products include:
- Aldactazide ... 2150
- Aldoril Tablets ... 1418
- Apresazide Capsules ... 854
- Apresoline-Esidrix Tablets ... 857
- Capozide ... 2258
- Dyazide Capsules ... 2208
- Esidrix Tablets ... 863
- Esimil Tablets ... 864
- HydroDIURIL Tablets ... 1484
- Hydropres Tablets ... 1485
- Inderide Tablets ... 2463
- Inderide LA Long Acting Capsules .. 2465
- Lopressor HCT Tablets ... 1034
- Maxzide ... 1215
- Moduretic Tablets ... 1510
- Normozide Tablets ... 2112
- Oretic Tablets ... 544
- Oreticyl ... 545
- Prinzide Tablets ... 1540
- Ser-Ap-Es Tablets ... 881
- Serpasil-Esidrix Tablets ... 886
- Timolide Tablets ... 1547
- Trandate HCT Tablets ... 579
- Vaseretic Tablets ... 1559
- Zestoretic ... 2274

Hydroflumethiazide (Potential for excessive reduction of blood pressure). Products include:
- Diucardin Tablets ... 2450
- Saluron ... 718
- Salutensin/Salutensin-Demi ... 719

Indapamide (Potential for excessive reduction of blood pressure). Products include:
- Lozol Tablets ... 1843

Lithium Carbonate (Increased serum lithium levels and symptoms of lithium toxicity). Products include:
- Eskalith ... 2214
- Lithane Tablets ... 1596
- Lithium Carbonate Capsules & Tablets ... 1984
- Lithobid Tablets ... 870

Lithium Citrate (Increased serum lithium levels and symptoms of lithium toxicity). Products include:
- Cibalith-S ... 870

Methyclothiazide (Potential for excessive reduction of blood pressure). Products include:
- Enduron Tablets ... 517
- Enduronyl ... 518

Metolazone (Potential for excessive reduction of blood pressure). Products include:
- Diulo ... 2129
- Mykrox ½ mg Tablets ... 984
- Zaroxolyn Tablets ... 989

Polythiazide (Potential for excessive reduction of blood pressure). Products include:
- Minizide Capsules ... 1779
- Renese Tablets ... 1785
- Renese-R Tablets ... 1786

Potassium Acid Phosphate (Potential for hyperkalemia). Products include:
- K-Phos M.F. Tablets ... 659
- K-Phos Original Formula 'Sodium Free' Tablets ... 660
- K-Phos No. 2 Tablets ... 659

Potassium Bicarbonate (Potential for hyperkalemia). Products include:
- Alka-Seltzer Advanced Formula Antacid & Non-Aspirin Pain Reliever ... ▣ 620
- Alka-Seltzer Effervescent Antacid ▣ 622
- K-Lyte ... 707
- Klorvess Effervescent Granules ... 2010
- Klorvess Effervescent Tablets ... 2011

Potassium Chloride (Potential for hyperkalemia). Products include:
- Chlor-3 Condiment ... 994
- K-Dur Microburst Release System (potassium chloride, USP) E.R. Tablets ... 1163
- K-Lor Powder Packets ... 531
- K-Lyte ... 707
- K-Norm Capsules ... 982
- K-Tab Filmtab ... 532
- Kato Potassium Supplement ... 1114
- Klor-Con 8/Klor-Con 10 Extended-release Tablets ... 2374
- Klorvess Effervescent Granules ... 2010
- Klorvess Effervescent Tablets ... 2011
- Klorvess 10% Liquid ... 2010
- Klotrix ... 708
- Kolyum Liquid ... 983
- Micro-K ... 1863
- Micro-K LS Packets ... 1864
- NuLYTELY ... 699
- Oral Rehydration Salts, Citrate ... 1150
- Rum-K Syrup ... 995
- Slow-K Tablets ... 2281
- Ten-K Controlled-Release Tablets ... 2282
- Thermotabs ... ▣ 619

Potassium Citrate (Potential for hyperkalemia). Products include:
- Alka-Seltzer Effervescent Antacid . 1570
- K-Lyte ... 707
- Polycitra Syrup ... 2424
- Polycitra-K ... 2424
- Polycitra-LC—Sugar-Free ... 2424
- Ricelyte, Rice-Based Oral Electrolyte Maintenance Solution ... ▣ 613

Potassium Gluconate (Potential for hyperkalemia). Products include:
- Kolyum Liquid ... 983

Potassium Phosphate, Dibasic (Potential for hyperkalemia). Products include:
- Neutra-Phos ... 2423

Potassium Phosphate, Monobasic (Potential for hyperkalemia). Products include:
- K-Phos M.F. Tablets ... 659
- K-Phos Neutral Tablets ... 660
- Neutra-Phos ... 2423

Spironolactone (Potential for excessive reduction of blood pressure; potential for hyperkalemia). Products include:
- Aldactazide ... 2150
- Aldactone ... 2152

Triamterene (Potential for excessive reduction of blood pressure; potential for hyperkalemia). Products include:
- Dyazide Capsules ... 2208
- Dyrenium Capsules ... 2210
- Maxzide ... 1215

LOTRIMIN CREAM 1%
(Clotrimazole) ... 2102

No interactions described in labeling.

LOTRIMIN LOTION 1%
(Clotrimazole) ... 2102

No interactions described in labeling.

LOTRIMIN SOLUTION 1%
(Clotrimazole) ... 2102

No interactions described in labeling.

LOTRIMIN AF ANTIFUNGAL CREAM, LOTION AND SOLUTION
(Clotrimazole) ... ▣ 702

No interactions described in labeling.

LOTRISONE CREAM
(Clotrimazole, Betamethasone Dipropionate) ... 2103

No interactions described in labeling.

LOXITANE C ORAL CONCENTRATE
(Loxapine Hydrochloride) ... 1213

See **Loxitane Capsules**

LOXITANE CAPSULES
(Loxapine Succinate) ... 1213

May interact with anticholinergic-type anitparkinsonism drugs, barbiturates, narcotic analgesics, general anesthetics, and certain other agents. Compounds in these categories include:

Alfentanil Hydrochloride (Loxitane is contraindicated in severe narcotic-induced depressed state). Products include:
- Alfenta Injection ... 1131

Aprobarbital (Loxitane is contraindicated in severe barbiturate-induced depressed state). Products include:
- Alurate Elixir ... 1883

Benztropine Mesylate (Use Loxitane cautiously). Products include:
- Cogentin ... 1435

Biperiden (Use Loxitane cautiously). Products include:
- Akineton ... 1171

Buprenorphine (Loxitane is contraindicated in severe narcotic-induced depressed state).
- No products indexed under this heading.

Butabarbital (Loxitane is contraindicated in severe barbiturate-induced depressed state). Products include:
- Pyridium Plus ... 1764

Butalbital (Loxitane is contraindicated in severe barbiturate-induced depressed state). Products include:
- Esgic-Plus Tablets ... 1002
- Esgic Tablets & Capsules ... 1001
- Fioricet Tablets ... 2006
- Fiorinal Capsules ... 2007
- Fiorinal with Codeine Capsules ... 2008
- Fiorinal Tablets ... 2007
- Phrenilin ... 838
- Sedapap Tablets 50 mg/650 mg .. 1360

Codeine (Loxitane is contraindicated in severe narcotic-induced depressed state). Products include:
- Calcidrine Syrup 506

Codeine Phosphate (Loxitane is contraindicated in severe narcotic-induced depressed state). Products include:
- Actifed with Codeine Cough Syrup.. 752
- Cheracol Cough Syrup 1853
- Codimal PH Syrup 846
- Dimetane-DC Cough Syrup 1857
- Empirin with Codeine Phosphate Nos. 2, 3 & 4 764
- Fiorinal with Codeine Capsules 2008
- Isoclor Expectorant 982
- Naldecon CX Adult Liquid 521
- Novahistine DH 1342
- Novahistine Expectorant 1343
- Nucofed Capsules 2219
- Nucofed Expectorant 2219
- Nucofed Pediatric Expectorant 2220
- Nucofed Syrup 2219
- Phenaphen with Codeine Capsules 1865
- Phenaphen-650 with Codeine Tablets 1866
- Phenergan with Codeine 2497
- Phenergan VC with Codeine 2501
- Robitussin A-C Syrup 1875
- Robitussin-DAC Syrup 1875
- Ryna 741
- Soma Compound w/Codeine Tablets 2390
- Triaminic Expectorant w/Codeine .. 1996
- Tussi-Organidin Liquid 2391
- Tylenol with Codeine 1381

Codeine Polistirex (Loxitane is contraindicated in severe narcotic-induced depressed state).
- No products indexed under this heading.

Dezocine (Loxitane is contraindicated in severe narcotic-induced depressed state).

Diphenhydramine Hydrochloride (Use Loxitane cautiously). Products include:
- Benadryl Anti-Itch Cream 635
- Benadryl Capsules 1691
- Benadryl Decongestant Elixir 635
- Benadryl Decongestant 635
- Benadryl Elixir 636
- Benadryl Kapseals 1691
- Benadryl 25 Kapseals 636
- Benadryl Parenteral 1692
- Benadryl Plus 636
- Benadryl Plus Nighttime 637
- Benadryl Spray, Maximum Strength 637
- Benadryl Spray, Regular Strength 637
- Benadryl Steri-Vials, Ampoules, and Steri-Dose Syringe 1692
- Benadryl 25 Tablets 636
- Benylin Cough Syrup 637
- Benylin Decongestant 638
- Caladryl Cream, Lotion, Spray 638
- Miles Nervine Nighttime Sleep-Aid 627
- Nytol Tablets 517
- Sleep-ettes-D Tablets 653
- Sleep-eze 3 Tablets 755
- Sleepinal Night-time Sleep Aid Capsules 734
- Sominex Caplets and Tablets 722
- Sominex Liquid 723
- Sominex Pain Relief Formula 723
- Tylenol Cold Night Time Medication Liquid 1371
- Tylenol PM, Extra Strength Caplets and Tablets 1368
- Unisom Dual Relief Nighttime Sleep Aid/Analgesic 1774
- Ziradryl Lotion 643

Enflurane (Loxitane is contraindicated in severe anesthetic-induced depressed state). Products include:
- Ethrane 599

Epinephrine (Inhibition of vasopressor effect by Loxitane). Products include:
- Ana-Kit Anaphylaxis Emergency Treatment Kit 1100
- Bronkaid Mist 757
- EpiPen 843
- Marcaine Hydrochloride 0.5% with Epinephrine 1:200,000 (as bitartrate) 958
- Marcaine Hydrochloride with Epinephrine 1:200,000 2055
- Primatene Mist 2420
- Sus-Phrine Injection 1006
- Xylocaine with Epinephrine Injections 637

Fentanyl (Loxitane is contraindicated in severe narcotic-induced depressed state). Products include:
- Duragesic Transdermal System 1133

Fentanyl Citrate (Loxitane is contraindicated in severe narcotic-induced depressed state). Products include:
- Innovar Injection 1141
- Sublimaze Injection 1146

Hydrocodone Bitartrate (Loxitane is contraindicated in severe narcotic-induced depressed state). Products include:
- Anexsia 5/500 Tablets 2196
- Anexsia 7.5/650 Tablets 2197
- Azdone Tablets 844
- Codiclear DH Syrup 845
- Codimal DH Syrup 846
- Damason-P 1356
- Hycodan Syrup, Tablets 927
- Hycomine Compound Tablets 929
- Hycomine Syrup 927
- Hycotuss Expectorant Syrup 930
- Hydrocet Capsules 835
- Lortab ASA Tablets 2414
- Lortab 2412
- Ru-Tuss with Hydrocodone 694
- Triaminic Expectorant DH 1995
- Vicodin Tablets 1187
- Vicodin ES Tablets 1189
- Zydone Capsules 941

Hydrocodone Polistirex (Loxitane is contraindicated in severe narcotic-induced depressed state). Products include:
- Tussionex Extended-Release Suspension 988

Isoflurane (Loxitane is contraindicated in severe anesthetic-induced depressed state). Products include:
- Forane 600

Ketamine Hydrochloride (Loxitane is contraindicated in severe anesthetic-induced depressed state). Products include:
- Ketalar 1726

Levorphanol Tartrate (Loxitane is contraindicated in severe narcotic-induced depressed state). Products include:
- Levo-Dromoran 1906

Meperidine Hydrochloride (Loxitane is contraindicated in severe narcotic-induced depressed state). Products include:
- Demerol 2047
- Mepergan Injection 2479

Mephobarbital (Loxitane is contraindicated in severe barbiturate-induced depressed state). Products include:
- Mebaral Tablets 2061

Methadone Hydrochloride (Loxitane is contraindicated in severe narcotic-induced depressed state). Products include:
- Dolophine Hydrochloride Ampoules & Vials 1260
- Dolophine Hydrochloride Tablets 1261
- Methadone Hydrochloride Diskets .. 1284
- Methadone Hydrochloride Oral Solution & Tablets 1987

Methohexital Sodium (Loxitane is contraindicated in severe anesthetic-induced depressed state). Products include:
- Brevital Sodium Vials 1248

Methoxyflurane (Loxitane is contraindicated in severe anesthetic-induced depressed state).
- No products indexed under this heading.

Morphine Sulfate (Loxitane is contraindicated in severe narcotic-induced depressed state). Products include:
- Astramorph/PF Injection, USP (Preservative-Free) 618
- Duramorph 960
- Infumorph 200 and Infumorph 500 Sterile Solutions 962
- MS Contin Tablets 1814
- MSIR 1817
- Oramorph SR (Morphine Sulfate Sustained Release Tablets) 1988
- Roxanol 1991

Opium Alkaloids (Loxitane is contraindicated in severe narcotic-induced depressed state). Products include:
- B & O No. 15A & No. 16A Supprettes 2395
- Pantopon Injectable 1911

Oxycodone Hydrochloride (Loxitane is contraindicated in severe narcotic-induced depressed state). Products include:
- Percocet Tablets 950
- Percodan 951
- Roxicodone Tablets, Oral Solution & Intensol (Oxycodone) 1992
- Tylox Capsules 1382

Pentobarbital Sodium (Loxitane is contraindicated in severe barbiturate-induced depressed state). Products include:
- Nembutal Sodium Capsules 534
- Nembutal Sodium Solution 536
- Nembutal Sodium Suppositories 538

Phenobarbital (Loxitane is contraindicated in severe barbiturate-induced depressed state). Products include:
- Arco-Lase Plus Tablets 607
- Bellergal-S Tablets 1998
- Bronkolixir 761
- Bronkotabs Tablets 762
- Donnatal 1858
- Donnatal Extentabs 1859
- Donnatal Tablets 1858
- Donnazyme Tablets 1860
- Kinesed Tablets 2272
- Phenobarbital Elixir and Tablets 1293
- Primatene Tablets-P Formula 2421
- Quadrinal Tablets 1183
- Tedral SA 1765

Procyclidine Hydrochloride (Use Loxitane cautiously). Products include:
- Kemadrin Tablets 771

Propofol (Loxitane is contraindicated in severe anesthetic-induced depressed state). Products include:
- Diprivan Injection 2267

Propoxyphene Hydrochloride (Loxitane is contraindicated in severe narcotic-induced depressed state). Products include:
- Darvon 1256
- Wygesic Tablets 2540

Propoxyphene Napsylate (Loxitane is contraindicated in severe narcotic-induced depressed state). Products include:
- Darvon-N/Darvocet-N 1254

Secobarbital Sodium (Loxitane is contraindicated in severe barbiturate-induced depressed state). Products include:
- Seconal Sodium Pulvules 1296

Sufentanil Citrate (Loxitane is contraindicated in severe narcotic-induced depressed state). Products include:
- Sufenta Injection 1147

Thiamylal Sodium (Loxitane is contraindicated in severe barbiturate-induced depressed state). Products include:
- Surital Ampoules, Steri-Vials 1764

Tridihexethyl Chloride (Use Loxitane cautiously).
- No products indexed under this heading.

Trihexyphenidyl Hydrochloride (Use Loxitane cautiously). Products include:
- Artane 1195

LOXITANE IM
(Loxapine Hydrochloride) 1213
See **Loxitane Capsules**

LOZOL TABLETS
(Indapamide) 1843
May interact with antihypertensives, lithium preparations, corticosteroids, insulin, cardiac glycosides, and certain other agents. Compounds in these categories include:

Acebutolol Hydrochloride (Additive or potentiated antihypertensive action). Products include:
- Sectral Capsules 2520

ACTH (Hypokalemia).
- No products indexed under this heading.

Atenolol (Additive or potentiated antihypertensive action). Products include:
- Tenoretic Tablets 1105
- Tenormin Tablets and I.V. Injection 1107

Benazepril Hydrochloride (Additive or potentiated antihypertensive action). Products include:
- Lotensin Tablets 872

Bendroflumethiazide (Additive or potentiated antihypertensive action). Products include:
- Corzide Tablets 702
- Naturetin Tablets 1789
- Rauzide Tablets 1804

Betamethasone Acetate (Hypokalemia). Products include:
- Celestone Soluspan Suspension 2081

Betamethasone Sodium Phosphate (Hypokalemia). Products include:
- Celestone Soluspan Suspension 2081

Betaxolol Hydrochloride (Additive or potentiated antihypertensive action). Products include:
- Betoptic Sterile Ophthalmic Solution 569
- Betoptic S Sterile Ophthalmic Suspension 570
- Kerlone Tablets 2172

Captopril (Additive or potentiated antihypertensive action). Products include:
- Capoten 2255
- Capozide 2258

Carteolol Hydrochloride (Additive or potentiated antihypertensive action). Products include:
- Cartrol Tablets 507

Chlorothiazide (Additive or potentiated antihypertensive action). Products include:
- Aldoclor Tablets 1413
- Diupres Tablets 1461
- Diuril Oral 1464

Chlorothiazide Sodium (Additive or potentiated antihypertensive action). Products include:
- Diuril Sodium Intravenous 1463

Chlorthalidone (Possible additive or potentiated antihypertensive action). Products include:
- Combipres Tablets 678
- Tenoretic Tablets 1105
- Thalitone Tablets 687

Clonidine (Additive or potentiated antihypertensive action). Products include:
- Catapres-TTS 677

Clonidine Hydrochloride (Additive or potentiated antihypertensive action). Products include:
- Catapres Tablets ... 676
- Combipres Tablets ... 678

Cortisone Acetate (Hypokalemia). Products include:
- Cortone Acetate Sterile Suspension ... 1437
- Cortone Acetate Tablets ... 1439

Deserpidine (Additive or potentiated antihypertensive action). Products include:
- Enduronyl ... 518
- Harmonyl Tablets ... 528
- Oreticyl ... 545

Deslanoside (Hypokalemia can sensitize or exaggerate digitalis toxicity).
- No products indexed under this heading.

Dexamethasone (Hypokalemia). Products include:
- AK-Trol Ointment & Suspension ... ⊙ 207
- Decadron Elixir ... 1445
- Decadron Tablets ... 1447
- Decaspray Topical Aerosol ... 1459
- Dexacidin ... ⊙ 272
- Maxidex Sterile Ophthalmic Suspension ... ⊙ 223
- Maxitrol Ophthalmic Ointment/Suspension ... ⊙ 223
- TobraDex Ophthalmic Suspension and Ointment ... ⊙ 228

Dexamethasone Acetate (Hypokalemia). Products include:
- Dalalone D.P. Injectable ... 999
- Decadron-LA Sterile Suspension ... 1457

Dexamethasone Sodium Phosphate (Hypokalemia). Products include:
- AK-Dex ... ⊙ 203
- Decadron Phosphate Respihaler ... 1454
- Decadron Phosphate Sterile Ophthalmic Ointment ... 1453
- Decadron Phosphate Sterile Ophthalmic Solution ... 1453
- Decadron Phosphate Topical Cream ... 1455
- Decadron Phosphate Turbinaire ... 1456
- Maxidex Sterile Ophthalmic Ointment ... ⊙ 222
- NeoDecadron Sterile Ophthalmic Ointment ... 1517
- NeoDecadron Sterile Ophthalmic Solution ... 1518
- NeoDecadron Topical Cream ... 1518

Diazoxide (Additive or potentiated antihypertensive action). Products include:
- Hyperstat I.V. Injection ... 2095
- Proglycem ... 649

Digitoxin (Hypokalemia can sensitize or exaggerate digitalis toxicity). Products include:
- Crystodigin Tablets ... 1253

Digoxin (Hypokalemia can sensitize or exaggerate digitalis toxicity). Products include:
- Lanoxicaps ... 772
- Lanoxin Elixir Pediatric ... 775
- Lanoxin Injection ... 778
- Lanoxin Injection Pediatric ... 781
- Lanoxin Tablets ... 783

Doxazosin Mesylate (Additive or potentiated antihypertensive action). Products include:
- Cardura Tablets ... 1941

Enalapril Maleate (Additive or potentiated antihypertensive action). Products include:
- Vaseretic Tablets ... 1559
- Vasotec Tablets ... 1564

Enalaprilat (Additive or potentiated antihypertensive action). Products include:
- Vasotec I.V. ... 1562

Esmolol Hydrochloride (Additive or potentiated antihypertensive action). Products include:
- Brevibloc Injection ... 942

Felodipine (Additive or potentiated antihypertensive action). Products include:
- Plendil Extended-Release Tablets ... 1526

Fosinopril Sodium (Additive or potentiated antihypertensive action). Products include:
- Monopril Tablets ... 1406

Furosemide (Additive or potentiated antihypertensive action). Products include:
- Lasix ... 1093

Guanabenz Acetate (Additive or potentiated antihypertensive action). Products include:
- Wytensin Tablets ... 2542

Guanethidine Monosulfate (Additive or potentiated antihypertensive action). Products include:
- Esimil Tablets ... 864
- Ismelin Tablets ... 869

Hydralazine Hydrochloride (Possible additive or potentiated antihypertensive action). Products include:
- Apresazide Capsules ... 854
- Apresoline Hydrochloride Parenteral (Ampuls) ... 856
- Apresoline Hydrochloride Tablets ... 855
- Apresoline-Esidrix Tablets ... 857
- Ser-Ap-Es Tablets ... 881
- Serpasil-Apresoline Tablets ... 884

Hydrochlorothiazide (Additive or potentiated antihypertensive action). Products include:
- Aldactazide ... 2150
- Aldoril Tablets ... 1418
- Apresazide Capsules ... 854
- Apresoline-Esidrix Tablets ... 857
- Capozide ... 2258
- Dyazide Capsules ... 2208
- Esidrix Tablets ... 863
- Esimil Tablets ... 864
- HydroDIURIL Tablets ... 1484
- Hydropres Tablets ... 1485
- Inderide Tablets ... 2463
- Inderide LA Long Acting Capsules ... 2465
- Lopressor HCT Tablets ... 1034
- Maxzide ... 1215
- Moduretic Tablets ... 1510
- Normozide Tablets ... 2112
- Oretic Tablets ... 544
- Oreticyl ... 545
- Prinzide Tablets ... 1540
- Ser-Ap-Es Tablets ... 881
- Serpasil-Esidrix Tablets ... 886
- Timolide Tablets ... 1547
- Trandate HCT Tablets ... 579
- Vaseretic Tablets ... 1559
- Zestoretic ... 2274

Hydrocortisone (Hypokalemia). Products include:
- AK-Spore H.C. ... ⊙ 206
- Bactine Hydrocortisone Anti-Itch Cream ... ▣ 625
- CaldeCORT Anti-Itch Hydrocortisone Spray ... ▣ 560
- Carmol HC Cream 1% ... 2296
- Cortaid Spray ... ▣ 735
- Cortenema ... 2244
- Cortisporin Ointment ... 758
- Cortisporin Ophthalmic Ointment Sterile ... 758
- Cortisporin Ophthalmic Suspension Sterile ... 759
- Cortisporin Otic Solution Sterile ... 760
- Cortisporin Otic Suspension Sterile ... 760
- Cortizone-5 Creme & Ointment ... ▣ 732
- Dermolate Anti-Itch Cream ... ▣ 697
- Eldecort Cream 1.0% ... 1113
- Eldecort Cream 1.0% and 2.5% ... 1113
- Fungoid HC Creme ... 1770
- Hydrocortone Tablets ... 1482
- Hytone ... 909
- LazerSporin-C Solution ... 1770
- Massengill Medicated Soft Cloth Towelettes ... 2192
- Nutracort Cream & Lotion ... 1684
- PediOtic Suspension Sterile ... 797
- Synacort Creams 1%, 2.5% ... 2296
- Vanoxide-HC Acne Lotion ... 911
- Vioform-Hydrocortisone Cream and Mild Cream ... 889
- Vioform-Hydrocortisone Ointment ... 889
- VōSoL HC Otic Solution ... 2392
- Vytone Cream 1% ... 911

Hydrocortisone Acetate (Hypokalemia). Products include:
- Analpram-HC Rectal Cream 1% and 2.5% ... 970
- Anusol-HC Cream ... 1690
- Anusol-HC Suppositories ... 1691
- Caldecort ... ▣ 560
- Carmol HC Cream 1% ... 2296
- Chloromycetin Hydrocortisone Ophthalmic ... 1694
- Coly-Mycin S Otic w/Neomycin & Hydrocortisone ... 1708
- Cortaid ... ▣ 735
- Cortef Feminine Itch Cream ... ▣ 735
- Corticaine ... ▣ 682
- Cortifoam ... 1827
- Cortisporin Cream ... 757
- Epifoam ... 1828
- Gynecort 5 Creme ... ▣ 556
- Hydrocortone Acetate Sterile Suspension ... 1479
- Lanacort 5 Creme and Ointment ... ▣ 557
- Mantadil Cream ... 789
- Ophthocort ... ⊙ 301
- Orabase HCA Oral Paste ... 890
- Pramosone Cream, Lotion & Ointment ... 971
- ProctoCream-HC ... 1834
- Proctofoam-HC ... 1835

Hydrocortisone Sodium Phosphate (Hypokalemia). Products include:
- Hydrocortone Phosphate Injection, Sterile ... 1481

Hydrocortisone Sodium Succinate (Hypokalemia). Products include:
- Solu-Cortef Sterile Powder ... 2361

Hydroflumethiazide (Additive or potentiated antihypertensive action). Products include:
- Diucardin Tablets ... 2450
- Saluron ... 718
- Salutensin/Salutensin-Demi ... 719

Insulin, Human (Insulin requirements may be altered).
- No products indexed under this heading.

Insulin, Human Isophane Suspension (Insulin requirements may be altered). Products include:
- Humulin N, 100 Units ... 1270

Insulin, Human NPH (Insulin requirements may be altered). Products include:
- Insulatard NPH Human ... 1627
- Novolin N ... 1627
- Novolin N PenFill Cartridges ... 1628
- Novolin N Prefilled ... 1628

Insulin, Human Regular (Insulin requirements may be altered). Products include:
- Humulin BR, 100 Units ... 1268
- Humulin R, 100 Units ... 1272
- Novolin R ... 1627
- Novolin R PenFill Cartridges ... 1628
- Novolin R Prefilled ... 1629
- Velosulin Human ... 1628

Insulin, Human, Zinc Suspension (Insulin requirements may be altered). Products include:
- Humulin L, 100 Units ... 1268
- Humulin U, 100 Units ... 1272
- Novolin L ... 1627

Insulin, NPH (Insulin requirements may be altered). Products include:
- NPH, 40 & 100 Units ... 1273
- Beef NPH, 100 Units ... 1274
- Pork NPH, 100 Units ... 1275
- Insulatard NPH ... 1626
- NPH Insulin ... 1626
- NPH Purified Pork Isophane Insulin ... 1626

Insulin, Regular (Insulin requirements may be altered). Products include:
- Regular, 40 & 100 Units ... 1273
- Beef Regular, 100 Units ... 1275
- Pork Regular, 100 Units ... 1275
- Pork Regular (Concentrated), 500 Units ... 1276
- Regular Insulin ... 1625
- Regular Purified Pork Insulin ... 1626
- Velosulin ... 1627

Insulin, Zinc Crystals (Insulin requirements may be altered). Products include:
- NPH, 40 & 100 Units ... 1273

Insulin, Zinc Suspension (Insulin requirements may be altered). Products include:
- Lente, 40 & 100 Units ... 1272
- Protamine, Zinc, 40 & 100 Units ... 1273
- Lente Iletin I ... 1272
- Beef Lente, 100 Units ... 1274
- Beef Protamine Zinc, 100 Units ... 1274
- Pork Lente, 100 Units ... 1275
- Pork, Protamine, Zinc, 100 Units ... 1275
- Lente Insulin ... 1626
- Lente Purified Pork Insulin ... 1626
- Semilente Insulin ... 1625
- Ultralente Insulin ... 1626

Isradipine (Additive or potentiated antihypertensive action). Products include:
- DynaCirc Capsules ... 2004

Labetalol Hydrochloride (Additive or potentiated antihypertensive action). Products include:
- Normodyne Injection ... 2108
- Normodyne Tablets ... 2110
- Normozide Tablets ... 2112
- Trandate HCT Tablets ... 579
- Trandate Injection ... 577
- Trandate Tablets ... 579

Lisinopril (Additive or potentiated antihypertensive action). Products include:
- Prinivil Tablets ... 1538
- Prinzide Tablets ... 1540
- Zestoretic ... 2274
- Zestril Tablets ... 2277

Lithium Carbonate (Reduced renal clearance; high risk of lithium toxicity). Products include:
- Eskalith ... 2214
- Lithane Tablets ... 1596
- Lithium Carbonate Capsules & Tablets ... 1984
- Lithobid Tablets ... 870

Lithium Citrate (Reduced renal clearance; high risk of lithium toxicity). Products include:
- Cibalith-S ... 870

Mecamylamine Hydrochloride (Additive or potentiated antihypertensive action). Products include:
- Inversine Tablets ... 1492

Methyclothiazide (Additive or potentiated antihypertensive action). Products include:
- Enduron Tablets ... 517
- Enduronyl ... 518

Methyldopa (Additive or potentiated antihypertensive action). Products include:
- Aldoclor Tablets ... 1413
- Aldomet Oral ... 1415
- Aldoril Tablets ... 1418

Methyldopate Hydrochloride (Additive or potentiated antihypertensive action). Products include:
- Aldomet Ester HCl Injection ... 1417

Methylprednisolone Acetate (Hypokalemia). Products include:
- Depo-Medrol Sterile Aqueous Suspension ... 2334

Methylprednisolone Sodium Succinate (Hypokalemia). Products include:
- Solu-Medrol Sterile Powder ... 2363

Metolazone (Additive or potentiated antihypertensive action). Products include:
- Diulo ... 2129
- Mykrox ½ mg Tablets ... 984
- Zaroxolyn Tablets ... 989

Metoprolol Tartrate (Additive or potentiated antihypertensive action). Products include:
- Lopressor Ampuls ... 1032
- Lopressor HCT Tablets ... 1034
- Lopressor Tablets ... 1032

Metyrosine (Additive or potentiated antihypertensive action). Products include:
- Demser Capsules ... 1460

Minoxidil (Additive or potentiated antihypertensive action). Products include:
- Loniten Tablets ... 2346
- Rogaine Topical Solution ... 2357

Nadolol (Additive or potentiated antihypertensive action). Products include:
- Corgard Tablets ... 701
- Corzide Tablets ... 702

Nicardipine Hydrochloride (Additive or potentiated antihypertensive action). Products include:
- Cardene Capsules ... 2290

Nitroglycerin (Additive or potentiated antihypertensive action). Products include:
- Deponit NTG Transdermal Delivery System ... 2143
- Minitran Transdermal Delivery System ... 1312
- Nitro-Bid Ointment ... 1339
- Nitro-Bid Capsules ... 1338
- Nitrodisc ... 2176
- Nitro-Dur (nitroglycerin) Transdermal Infusion System ... 1164
- Nitrogard Tablets ... 1004
- Nitrolingual Spray ... 1846
- Nitrostat Tablets ... 1743
- Transderm-Nitro Transdermal Therapeutic System ... 2283

Norepinephrine Bitartrate (Decreased arterial responsiveness to norepinephrine). Products include:
- Levophed Bitartrate Injection ... 2054

Penbutolol Sulfate (Additive or potentiated antihypertensive action). Products include:
- Levatol ... 1832

Phenoxybenzamine Hydrochloride (Additive or potentiated antihypertensive action). Products include:
- Dibenzyline Capsules ... 2207

Phentolamine Mesylate (Additive or potentiated antihypertensive action). Products include:
- Regitine ... 878

Pindolol (Additive or potentiated antihypertensive action). Products include:
- Visken Tablets ... 2036

Polythiazide (Additive or potentiated antihypertensive action). Products include:
- Minizide Capsules ... 1779
- Renese Tablets ... 1785
- Renese-R Tablets ... 1786

Prazosin Hydrochloride (Additive or potentiated antihypertensive action). Products include:
- Minipress Capsules ... 1778
- Minizide Capsules ... 1779

Prednisolone Acetate (Hypokalemia). Products include:
- AK-Cide Sterile Ophthalmic Ointment & Suspension ... ◉ 202
- Blephamide Liquifilm Sterile Ophthalmic Suspension ... 586
- Blephamide S.O.P. Sterile Ophthalmic Ointment ... 586
- Cetapred Ointment ... ◉ 220
- ⅛% Econopred & 1% Econopred Plus ... ◉ 217
- Isopto Cetapred Suspension ... ◉ 220
- Metimyd ... ◉ 306
- Poly-Pred Liquifilm ... ◉ 250
- Pred Forte ... ◉ 252
- Pred Mild ... ◉ 254
- Pred-G Liquifilm Sterile Ophthalmic Suspension ... ◉ 252
- Pred-G S.O.P. Sterile Ophthalmic Ointment ... ◉ 253
- Vasocidin Ointment ... ◉ 275

Prednisolone Sodium Phosphate (Hypokalemia). Products include:
- AK-Pred ... ◉ 205
- Hydeltrasol Injection, Sterile ... 1476
- Inflamase ... ◉ 274
- Pediapred Oral Liquid ... 987
- Vasocidin Ophthalmic Solution ... ◉ 276

Prednisolone Tebutate (Hypokalemia). Products include:
- Hydeltra-T.B.A. Sterile Suspension 1478

Prednisone (Hypokalemia). Products include:
- Deltasone Tablets ... 2332

Propranolol Hydrochloride (Additive or potentiated antihypertensive action). Products include:
- Inderal ... 2459
- Inderal LA Long Acting Capsules ... 2461
- Inderide Tablets ... 2463
- Inderide LA Long Acting Capsules ... 2465

Ramipril (Additive or potentiated antihypertensive action). Products include:
- Altace Capsules ... 1086

Rauwolfia Serpentina (Additive or potentiated antihypertensive action). Products include:
- Raudixin Tablets ... 1803
- Rauzide Tablets ... 1804

Rescinnamine (Additive or potentiated antihypertensive action).
- No products indexed under this heading.

Reserpine (Additive or potentiated antihypertensive action). Products include:
- Diupres Tablets ... 1461
- Hydromox R Tablets ... 1209
- Hydropres Tablets ... 1485
- Renese-R Tablets ... 1786
- Salutensin/Salutensin-Demi ... 719
- Ser-Ap-Es Tablets ... 881
- Serpasil Tablets ... 883
- Serpasil-Apresoline Tablets ... 884
- Serpasil-Esidrix Tablets ... 886

Sodium Nitroprusside (Additive or potentiated antihypertensive action). Products include:
- Nipride I.V. Infusion ... 1909

Terazosin Hydrochloride (Additive or potentiated antihypertensive action). Products include:
- Hytrin Tablets ... 529

Timolol Maleate (Additive or potentiated antihypertensive action). Products include:
- Blocadren Tablets ... 1429
- Timolide Tablets ... 1547
- Timoptic in Ocudose ... 1552
- Timoptic Sterile Ophthalmic Solution ... 1550

Triamcinolone (Hypokalemia).
- No products indexed under this heading.

Triamcinolone Acetonide (Hypokalemia). Products include:
- Aristocort A ... 1010
- Azmacort Inhaler ... 1837
- Kenalog Cream, Lotion & Ointment 2401
- Kenalog-10 Injection ... 2402
- Kenalog-40 Injection ... 2403
- Kenalog in Orabase ... 604
- Kenalog Spray ... 2401
- Mycolog II Cream and Ointment ... 2407
- Mytrex Cream & Ointment ... 2080
- Nasacort Nasal Inhaler ... 1844

Triamcinolone Diacetate (Hypokalemia). Products include:
- Aristocort Suspension ... 1008

Triamcinolone Hexacetonide (Hypokalemia). Products include:
- Aristospan Suspension ... 1011

Trimethaphan Camsylate (Additive or potentiated antihypertensive action). Products include:
- Arfonad Ampuls ... 1887

LUBRASEPTIC JELLY
(Lubricant) ... 1073
No interactions described in labeling.

LUBRIDERM CREAM
(Emollient) ... ▣ 743
No interactions described in labeling.

LUBRIDERM LOTION
(Emollient) ... ▣ 743
No interactions described in labeling.

LUBRIDERM SKIN CONDITIONING OIL
(Emollient) ... ▣ 743
No interactions described in labeling.

LUDIOMIL TABLETS
(Maprotiline Hydrochloride) ... 874
May interact with monoamine oxidase inhibitors, benzodiazepines, phenothiazines, barbiturates, anticholinergics, sympathomimetic aerosol brochodilators, thyroid preparations, central nervous system depressants, and certain other agents. Compounds in these categories include:

Albuterol (Possible additive atropine-like effect). Products include:
- Proventil Inhalation Aerosol ... 2117
- Ventolin Inhalation Aerosol and Refill ... 583

Albuterol Sulfate (Possible additive atropine-like effect). Products include:
- Proventil Repetabs Tablets ... 2120
- Proventil Solutions for Inhalation 0.5% and 0.083% ... 2118
- Proventil Syrup ... 2119
- Proventil Tablets ... 2120
- Ventolin ... 583

Alcohol (Enhanced response to alcohol).

Alfentanil Hydrochloride (Enhanced response to CNS depressants). Products include:
- Alfenta Injection ... 1131

Alprazolam (Risk of seizures). Products include:
- Xanax Tablets ... 2367

Aprobarbital (Enhanced response to barbiturates). Products include:
- Alurate Elixir ... 1883

Atropine Sulfate (Possible additive atropine-like effect). Products include:
- Arco-Lase Plus Tablets ... 607
- Atropine Sulfate Sterile Ophthalmic Solution and S.O.P. Sterile Ophthalmic Ointment ... ◉ 239
- Donnagel ... ▣ 675
- Donnagel-PG ... 1858
- Donnatal ... 1858
- Donnatal Extentabs ... 1859
- Donnatal Tablets ... 1858
- Donnazyme Tablets ... 1860
- Isopto Atropine ... ◉ 218
- Lomotil ... 2174
- Motofen Tablets ... 836
- Ru-Tuss Tablets ... 693
- Urised Tablets ... 2396

Belladonna Alkaloids (Possible additive atropine-like effect). Products include:
- Bellergal-S Tablets ... 1998
- Hyland's Bed Wetting Tablets ... ▣ 728
- Hyland's Teething Tablets ... ▣ 728
- Kinesed Tablets ... 2272

Benztropine Mesylate (Possible additive atropine-like effect). Products include:
- Cogentin ... 1435

Biperiden (Possible additive atropine-like effect). Products include:
- Akineton ... 1171

Buprenorphine (Enhanced response to CNS depressants).
- No products indexed under this heading.

Buspirone Hydrochloride (Enhanced response to CNS depressants). Products include:
- BuSpar ... 1401

Butabarbital (Enhanced response to barbiturates). Products include:
- Pyridium Plus ... 1764

Butalbital (Enhanced response to barbiturates). Products include:
- Esgic-Plus Tablets ... 1002
- Esgic Tablets & Capsules ... 1001
- Fioricet Tablets ... 2006
- Fiorinal Capsules ... 2007
- Fiorinal with Codeine Capsules ... 2008
- Fiorinal Tablets ... 2007
- Phrenilin ... 838
- Sedapap Tablets 50 mg/650 mg ... 1360

Chlordiazepoxide (Risk of seizures; enhanced response to CNS depressants). Products include:
- Libritabs Tablets ... 1930
- Limbitrol ... 1933
- Menrium Tablets ... 1934

Chlordiazepoxide Hydrochloride (Risk of seizures). Products include:
- Librax Capsules ... 1929
- Librium Capsules ... 1931
- Librium Injectable ... 1932

Chlorpromazine (Risk of seizures; enhanced response to CNS depressants). Products include:
- Thorazine ... 2234

Chlorprothixene (Enhanced response to CNS depressants). Products include:
- Taractan Tablets ... 1920

Chlorprothixene Hydrochloride (Enhanced response to CNS depressants). Products include:
- Taractan ... 1920

Cimetidine (Increases plasma levels of Ludiomil). Products include:
- Tagamet Tablets ... 2228

Cimetidine Hydrochloride (Increases plasma levels of Ludiomil). Products include:
- Tagamet ... 2228

Clidinium Bromide (Possible additive atropine-like effect). Products include:
- Librax Capsules ... 1929
- Quarzan Capsules ... 1937

Clorazepate Dipotassium (Risk of seizures; enhanced response to CNS depressants). Products include:
- Tranxene ... 556

Codeine (Enhanced response to CNS depressants). Products include:
- Calcidrine Syrup ... 506

Codeine Phosphate (Enhanced response to CNS depressants). Products include:
- Actifed with Codeine Cough Syrup ... 752
- Cheracol Cough Syrup ... 1853
- Codimal PH Syrup ... 846
- Dimetane-DC Cough Syrup ... 1857
- Empirin with Codeine Phosphate Nos. 2, 3 & 4 ... 764
- Fiorinal with Codeine Capsules ... 2008
- Isoclor Expectorant ... 982
- Naldecon CX Adult Liquid ... ▣ 521
- Novahistine DH ... 1342
- Novahistine Expectorant ... 1343
- Nucofed Capsules ... 2219
- Nucofed Expectorant ... 2219
- Nucofed Pediatric Expectorant ... 2220
- Nucofed Syrup ... 2219
- Phenaphen with Codeine Capsules 1865
- Phenaphen-650 with Codeine Tablets ... 1866
- Phenergan with Codeine ... 2497
- Phenergan VC with Codeine ... 2501
- Robitussin A-C Syrup ... 1875
- Robitussin-DAC Syrup ... 1875
- Ryna ... ▣ 741
- Soma Compound w/Codeine Tablets ... 2390
- Triaminic Expectorant w/Codeine ... 1996
- Tussi-Organidin Liquid ... 2391
- Tylenol with Codeine ... 1381

Codeine Polistirex (Enhanced response to CNS depressants).
- No products indexed under this heading.

Dezocine (Enhanced response to CNS depressants).

Diazepam (Risk of seizures; enhanced response to CNS depressants). Products include:
- Valium Injectable 1937
- Valium Tablets 1939
- Valrelease Capsules 1923

Dicyclomine Hydrochloride (Possible additive atropine-like effect). Products include:
- Bentyl 1322

Dobutamine Hydrochloride (Possible additive atropine-like effect). Products include:
- Dobutrex Solution Vials 1259

Dopamine Hydrochloride (Possible additive atropine-like effect). Products include:
- Intropin Injection 930

Droperidol (Enhanced response to CNS depressants). Products include:
- Inapsine Injection 1140
- Innovar Injection 1141

Enflurane (Enhanced response to CNS depressants). Products include:
- Ethrane 599

Ephedrine Hydrochloride (Possible additive atropine-like effect). Products include:
- Amesec .... ▣ 682
- Primatene Tablets-M Formula 2421
- Primatene Tablets-P Formula 2421
- Primatene Tablets-Regular Formula 2421
- Quadrinal Tablets 1183
- Quelidrine Syrup 556
- Tedral SA 1765

Ephedrine Sulfate (Possible additive atropine-like effect). Products include:
- Bronkaid Tablets .... ▣ 757
- Bronkolixir .... ▣ 761
- Bronkotabs Tablets .... ▣ 762
- Marax Tablets & DF Syrup 1954
- Pazo Hemorrhoid Ointment & Suppositories 752
- Vicks Vatronol Nose Drops .... ▣ 666

Ephedrine Tannate (Possible additive atropine-like effect). Products include:
- Rynatuss 2388

Epinephrine (Possible additive atropine-like effect). Products include:
- Ana-Kit Anaphylaxis Emergency Treatment Kit 1100
- Bronkaid Mist .... ▣ 757
- EpiPen 843
- Marcaine Hydrochloride 0.5% with Epinephrine 1:200,000 (as bitartrate) 958
- Marcaine Hydrochloride with Epinephrine 1:200,000 2055
- Primatene Mist 2420
- Sus-Phrine Injection 1006
- Xylocaine with Epinephrine Injections 637

Epinephrine Bitartrate (Possible additive atropine-like effect). Products include:
- AsthmaHaler Mist Epinephrine Bitartrate Bronchodilator .... ▣ 616
- Bronkaid Mist Suspension .... ▣ 757
- Primatene Mist Suspension 2421

Epinephrine Hydrochloride (Possible additive atropine-like effect). Products include:
- Adrenalin Chloride Solution 1:100 & 1:1,000 1689
- Epifrin .... ◉ 244
- Glaucon .... ◉ 218

Estazolam (Risk of seizures). Products include:
- ProSom Tablets 554

Ethchlorvynol (Enhanced response to CNS depressants). Products include:
- Placidyl Capsules 553

Ethinamate (Enhanced response to CNS depressants).
- No products indexed under this heading.

Fentanyl (Enhanced response to CNS depressants). Products include:
- Duragesic Transdermal System 1133

Fentanyl Citrate (Enhanced response to CNS depressants). Products include:
- Innovar Injection 1141
- Sublimaze Injection 1146

Fluphenazine Decanoate (Risk of seizures; enhanced response to CNS depressants). Products include:
- Prolixin Decanoate 1795

Fluphenazine Enanthate (Risk of seizures; enhanced response to CNS depressants). Products include:
- Prolixin Enanthate 1796

Fluphenazine Hydrochloride (Risk of seizures; enhanced response to CNS depressants). Products include:
- Prolixin Elixir 1793
- Prolixin Injection 1791
- Prolixin Oral Concentrate 1792
- Prolixin Tablets 1793

Flurazepam Hydrochloride (Enhanced response to CNS depressants). Products include:
- Dalmane Capsules 1927

Furazolidone (Concurrent use contraindicated). Products include:
- Furoxone 1855

Glutethimide (Enhanced response to CNS depressants).
- No products indexed under this heading.

Glycopyrrolate (Possible additive atropine-like effect). Products include:
- Robinul Forte Tablets 1873
- Robinul Injectable 1873
- Robinul Tablets 1873

Guanethidine Monosulfate (Blocked pharmacologic effect). Products include:
- Esimil Tablets 864
- Ismelin Tablets 869

Haloperidol (Enhanced response to CNS depressants). Products include:
- Haldol Injection, Tablets and Concentrate 1373

Haloperidol Decanoate (Enhanced response to CNS depressants). Products include:
- Haldol Decanoate 1375

Hydrocodone Bitartrate (Enhanced response to CNS depressants). Products include:
- Anexsia 5/500 Tablets 2196
- Anexsia 7.5/650 Tablets 2197
- Azdone Tablets 844
- Codiclear DH Syrup 845
- Codimal DH Syrup 846
- Damason-P 1356
- Hycodan Syrup, Tablets 927
- Hycomine Compound Tablets 929
- Hycomine Syrup 927
- Hycotuss Expectorant Syrup 930
- Hydrocet Capsules 835
- Lortab ASA Tablets 2414
- Lortab 2412
- Ru-Tuss with Hydrocodone 694
- Triaminic Expectorant DH 1995
- Vicodin Tablets 1187
- Vicodin ES Tablets 1189
- Zydone Capsules 941

Hydrocodone Polistirex (Enhanced response to CNS depressants). Products include:
- Tussionex Extended-Release Suspension 988

Hydroxyzine Hydrochloride (Enhanced response to CNS depressants). Products include:
- Atarax Tablets & Syrup 1941
- Marax Tablets & DF Syrup 1954
- Vistaril Intramuscular Solution 1970

Hyoscyamine (Possible additive atropine-like effect). Products include:
- Cystospaz Tablets 2395
- Urised Tablets 2396

Hyoscyamine Sulfate (Possible additive atropine-like effect). Products include:
- Arco-Lase Plus Tablets 607
- Cystospaz-M Capsules 2395
- Donnagel .... ▣ 675
- Donnagel-PG 1858
- Donnatal 1858
- Donnatal Extentabs 1859
- Donnatal Tablets 1858
- Donnazyme Tablets 1860
- Kutrase Capsules 2146
- Levsin/Levsinex 2147
- Ru-Tuss Tablets 693

Ipratropium Bromide (Possible additive atropine-like effect). Products include:
- Atrovent Inhalation Aerosol 675

Isocarboxazid (Concurrent use contraindicated). Products include:
- Marplan Tablets 1906

Isoflurane (Enhanced response to CNS depressants). Products include:
- Forane 600

Isoproterenol Hydrochloride (Possible additive atropine-like effect). Products include:
- Isuprel Hydrochloride Injection 1:5000 2050
- Isuprel Hydrochloride Mistometer .. 2051
- Isuprel Hydrochloride Solution 1:200 & 1:100 2052
- Norisodrine Aerotrol 540

Ketamine Hydrochloride (Enhanced response to CNS depressants). Products include:
- Ketalar 1726

Levorphanol Tartrate (Enhanced response to CNS depressants). Products include:
- Levo-Dromoran 1906

Levothyroxine Sodium (Enhanced potential for cardiovascular toxicity of Ludiomil). Products include:
- Levothroid Tablets 1003
- Levoxine Tablets 904
- Synthroid 695

Liothyronine Sodium (Enhanced potential for cardiovascular toxicity of Ludiomil). Products include:
- Cytomel Tablets 2203

Lorazepam (Risk of seizures; enhanced response to CNS depressants). Products include:
- Ativan Injection 2432
- Ativan Tablets 2434

Loxapine Hydrochloride (Enhanced response to CNS depressants). Products include:
- Loxitane 1213

Loxapine Succinate (Enhanced response to CNS depressants). Products include:
- Loxitane Capsules 1213

Mepenzolate Bromide (Possible additive atropine-like effect). Products include:
- Cantil Tablets 1326

Meperidine Hydrochloride (Enhanced response to CNS depressants). Products include:
- Demerol 2047
- Mepergan Injection 2479

Mephobarbital (Enhanced response to barbiturates). Products include:
- Mebaral Tablets 2061

Meprobamate (Enhanced response to CNS depressants). Products include:
- Deprol Tablets 2382
- Equagesic Tablets 2451
- Miltown Tablets 2386
- PMB 200 and PMB 400 2504

Mesoridazine (Risk of seizures; enhanced response to CNS depressants). Products include:
- Serentil 686

Metaproterenol Sulfate (Possible additive atropine-like effect). Products include:
- Alupent 674
- Arm-a-Med Metaproterenol Sulfate Inhalation Solution, USP 617
- Metaprel Inhalation Aerosol Bronchodilator 2014
- Metaprel Inhalation Solution 2015
- Metaprel 2015
- Metaproterenol Sulfate Inhalation Solution, USP 912

Metaraminol Bitartrate (Possible additive atropine-like effect). Products include:
- Aramine Injection 1424

Methadone Hydrochloride (Enhanced response to CNS depressants). Products include:
- Dolophine Hydrochloride Ampoules & Vials 1260
- Dolophine Hydrochloride Tablets 1261
- Methadone Hydrochloride Diskets .. 1284
- Methadone Hydrochloride Oral Solution & Tablets 1987

Methohexital Sodium (Enhanced response to CNS depressants). Products include:
- Brevital Sodium Vials 1248

Methoxamine Hydrochloride (Possible additive atropine-like effect). Products include:
- Vasoxyl Injection 819

Methoxyflurane (Enhanced response to CNS depressants).
- No products indexed under this heading.

Midazolam Hydrochloride (Risk of seizures). Products include:
- Versed Injection 1924

Molindone Hydrochloride (Enhanced response to CNS depressants). Products include:
- Moban Tablets & Concentrate 932

Morphine Sulfate (Enhanced response to CNS depressants). Products include:
- Astramorph/PF Injection, USP (Preservative-Free) 618
- Duramorph 960
- Infumorph 200 and Infumorph 500 Sterile Solutions 962
- MS Contin Tablets 1814
- MSIR 1817
- Oramorph SR (Morphine Sulfate Sustained Release Tablets) 1988
- Roxanol 1991

Norepinephrine Bitartrate (Possible additive atropine-like effect). Products include:
- Levophed Bitartrate Injection 2054

Opium Alkaloids (Enhanced response to CNS depressants). Products include:
- B & O No. 15A & No. 16A Supprettes 2395
- Pantopon Injectable 1911

Oxazepam (Risk of seizures; enhanced response to CNS depressants). Products include:
- Serax Capsules 2522
- Serax Tablets 2522

Oxybutynin Chloride (Possible additive atropine-like effect). Products include:
- Ditropan 1332

Oxycodone Hydrochloride (Enhanced response to CNS depressants). Products include:
- Percocet Tablets 950
- Percodan 951
- Roxicodone Tablets, Oral Solution & Intensol (Oxycodone) 1992
- Tylox Capsules 1382

Pentobarbital Sodium (Enhanced response to barbiturates; enhanced response to CNS depressants). Products include:
- Nembutal Sodium Capsules 534
- Nembutal Sodium Solution 536
- Nembutal Sodium Suppositories 538

Perphenazine (Risk of seizures; enhanced response to CNS depressants). Products include:

Etrafon 2087
Triavil Tablets 1556
Trilafon 2123

Phenelzine Sulfate (Concurrent use contraindicated). Products include:

Nardil 1742

Phenobarbital (Enhanced response to barbiturates). Products include:

Arco-Lase Plus Tablets 607
Bellergal-S Tablets 1998
Bronkolixir ▣ 761
Bronkotabs Tablets ▣ 762
Donnatal 1858
Donnatal Extentabs 1859
Donnatal Tablets 1858
Donnazyme Tablets 1860
Kinesed Tablets 2272
Phenobarbital Elixir and Tablets 1293
Primatene Tablets-P Formula 2421
Quadrinal Tablets 1183
Tedral SA 1765

Phenylephrine Bitartrate (Possible additive atropine-like effect).

No products indexed under this heading.

Phenylephrine Hydrochloride (Possible additive atropine-like effect). Products include:

AK-Dilate Solution 2.5% and 10% ⊙ 203
Atrohist Sprinkle Capsules 558
Cerose-DM 2443
Codimal 846
Comhist LA Capsules 1618
Congespirin For Children Aspirin Free Chewable Cold Tablets 748
Cyclomydril ⊙ 216
Deconsal Sprinkle Capsules 559
Dimetane Decongestant ▣ 673
Dristan Decongestant/Antihistamine/ Analgesic Coated Caplets ▣ 749
Dristan Cold Nasal Decongestant/ Antihistamine/ Analgesic Coated Tablets 2419
Dristan Advanced Formula Decongestant/Antihistamine/ Analgesic Tablets ▣ 749
Dristan Nasal Spray, Menthol 2419
Dristan Nasal Spray, Regular and Regular with Metered Pump 2419
Entex Capsules 1623
Entex Liquid 1623
Sinus Excedrin Analgesic, Decongestant Tablets & Caplets 750
Extendryl 994
4-Way Fast Acting Nasal Spray - Original Formula (regular & mentholated) & Metered Spray Pump (regular) 751
Hycomine Compound Tablets 929
Murocoll-2 Sterile Ophthalmic Solution ⊙ 261
Mydfrin 2.5% ⊙ 224
Naldecon Syrup, Tablets, Pediatric Drops and Pediatric Syrup 709
Neo-Synephrine Hydrochloride 1% Carpuject 2063
Neo-Synephrine Hydrochloride 1% Injection 2063
Neo-Synephrine Hydrochloride (Ophthalmic) 2064
Neo-Synephrine ▣ 759
Nōstril Nasal Decongestant ▣ 520
Novahistine Elixir ▣ 596
Phenergan VC 2500
Phenergan VC with Codeine 2501
Prefrin Liquifilm Vasoconstrictor and Lubricant Eye Drops ⊙ 254
Prefrin-A ⊙ 255
Quelidrine Syrup 556
Relief Vasoconstrictor and Lubricant Eye Drops ⊙ 256
Robitussin Night Relief ▣ 677
Ru-Tuss with Hydrocodone 694
Ru-Tuss Tablets 693
Vasosulf ⊙ 279
Vicks Sinex ▣ 665
Zincfrin ⊙ 230

Phenylephrine Tannate (Possible additive atropine-like effect). Products include:

Rynatan 2387
Rynatuss 2388

Phenylpropanolamine Hydrochloride (Possible additive atropine-like effect). Products include:

A.R.M. Allergy Relief Medicine Caplets ▣ 615
Acutrim ▣ 548
Allerest ▣ 559
BC Cold Powder ▣ 517
Cheracol Plus Head Cold/Cough Formula ▣ 667
Codimal Expectorant 846
Comtrex Multi-Symptom Cold Reliever Tablets/Caplets/Liqui-Gels/Liquid 745
Contac Continuous Action Decongestant/Antihistamine Capsules ▣ 710
Contac Maximum Strength Continuous Action Decongestant/ Antihistamine Caplets ▣ 709
Contac Severe Cold and Flu Formula Caplets ▣ 711
Coricidin 'D' Decongestant Tablets ▣ 695
Coricidin Demilets Tablets for Children ▣ 696
Demazin Nasal Decongestant/ Antihistamine Repetabs Tablets & Syrup ▣ 697
Dexatrim ▣ 733
Dimetane-DC Cough Syrup 1857
Dimetapp Elixir ▣ 673
Dimetapp DM Elixir ▣ 674
Dimetapp Extentabs ▣ 674
Dimetapp Plus Caplets ▣ 675
Dimetapp Tablets ▣ 675
Entex Capsules 1623
Entex LA Tablets 1623
Entex Liquid 1623
4-Way Cold Tablets 750
Hycomine Syrup 927
Naldecon CX Adult Liquid ▣ 521
Naldecon DX Adult Liquid ▣ 521
Naldecon DX Children's Syrup ▣ 522
Naldecon DX Pediatric Drops ▣ 522
Naldecon EX Children's Syrup ▣ 522
Naldecon EX Pediatric Drops ▣ 523
Naldecon Syrup, Tablets, Pediatric Drops and Pediatric Syrup 709
Nolamine Tablets 838
Nolex LA Tablets 838
Ornade Spansule Capsules 2221
Orthoxicol Cough Syrup ▣ 668
Propagest 839
Pyrroxate Capsules ▣ 669
Robitussin-CF ▣ 676
Ru-Tuss II Capsules 693
Ru-Tuss with Hydrocodone 694
Ru-Tuss Tablets 693
Sine-Off Sinus Medicine Tablets-Aspirin Formula ▣ 722
Sinulin 840
St. Joseph Cold Tablets for Children ▣ 704
Tavist-D Tablets 2035
Triaminic Allergy Tablets ▣ 688
Triaminic Chewables ▣ 688
Triaminic Cold Tablets ▣ 688
Triaminic Expectorant ▣ 688
Triaminic Expectorant w/Codeine 1996
Triaminic Expectorant DH 1995
Triaminic Oral Infant Drops 1996
Triaminic Syrup ▣ 689
Triaminic-12 Tablets ▣ 690
Triaminic-DM Syrup ▣ 689
Triaminicin Tablets ▣ 690
Triaminicol Multi-Symptom Cold Tablets ▣ 691
Triaminicol Multi-Symptom Relief ▣ 691
Tuss-Ornade Liquid 2242
Tuss-Ornade Spansule Capsules 2242
Tylenol Cold Medication, Effervescent Tablets 1369

Pirbuterol Acetate (Possible additive atropine-like effect). Products include:

Maxair Inhaler 1311

Prazepam (Risk of seizures; enhanced response to CNS depressants). Products include:

Centrax 1693

Prochlorperazine (Risk of seizures; enhanced response to CNS depressants). Products include:

Compazine 2201

Procyclidine Hydrochloride (Possible additive atropine-like effect). Products include:

Kemadrin Tablets 771

Promethazine Hydrochloride (Risk of seizures; enhanced response to CNS depressants). Products include:

Mepergan Injection 2479
Phenergan with Codeine 2497
Phenergan with Dextromethorphan 2499
Phenergan Injection 2493
Phenergan Suppositories 2496
Phenergan Syrup 2495
Phenergan Tablets 2496
Phenergan VC 2500
Phenergan VC with Codeine 2501

Propantheline Bromide (Possible additive atropine-like effect). Products include:

Pro-Banthine Tablets 2141

Propofol (Enhanced response to CNS depressants). Products include:

Diprivan Injection 2267

Propoxyphene Hydrochloride (Enhanced response to CNS depressants). Products include:

Darvon 1256
Wygesic Tablets 2540

Propoxyphene Napsylate (Enhanced response to CNS depressants). Products include:

Darvon-N/Darvocet-N 1254

Pseudoephedrine Hydrochloride (Possible additive atropine-like effect). Products include:

Actifed Capsules ▣ 539
Actifed Plus Caplets ▣ 539
Actifed Plus Tablets ▣ 540
Actifed with Codeine Cough Syrup 752
Actifed Syrup ▣ 540
Actifed Tablets ▣ 540
Actifed 12-Hour Capsules ▣ 539
Advil Cold & Sinus Caplets (formerly CoAdvil) 2416
Allerest ▣ 559
Anatuss LA Tablets 1359
Benadryl Decongestant Elixir ▣ 635
Benadryl Decongestant ▣ 635
Benadryl Plus ▣ 636
Benadryl Plus Nighttime ▣ 637
Benylin Decongestant ▣ 638
Brexin L.A. Capsules 2078
Bromfed Capsules (Timed Release) 1615
Bromfed Syrup ▣ 628
Bromfed 1615
CoAdvil ▣ 748
Allergy-Sinus Comtrex Multi-Symptom Allergy Sinus Formula Tablets & Caplets 746
Cough Formula Comtrex 746
Comtrex Multi-Symptom Cold Reliever Tablets/Caplets/Liqui-Gels/Liquid 745
Day-Night Comtrex 747
Non-Drowsy Comtrex 747
Congess 994
Congestac Caplets ▣ 617
Contac Jr. Children's Cold Medicine ▣ 712
Contac Nighttime Cold Medicine ▣ 713
Contac Sinus Caplets Maximum Strength Non-Drowsy Formula ▣ 710
Contac Sinus Tablets Maximum Strength Non-Drowsy Formula ▣ 710
Deconamine 663
Deconsal II Tablets 559
Dimacol Caplets ▣ 672
Dimetane-DX Cough Syrup 1858
Dorcol Children's Cough Syrup ▣ 685
Dorcol Children's Decongestant Liquid ▣ 685
Dorcol Children's Liquid Cold Formula ▣ 686
Maximum Strength Dristan Decongestant/Analgesic Coated Caplets ▣ 750
No Drowsiness Dristan Cold Nasal Decongestant/Analgesic Coated Caplets 2420
Dristan Sinus Caplets 2419
Sinus Excedrin Analgesic, Decongestant Tablets & Caplets ▣ 533
Fedahist Gyrocaps 2145
Fedahist Timecaps 2145
Guaifed 1615
Guaifed Syrup ▣ 629
Isoclor Expectorant 982
Isoclor Timesule Capsules ▣ 561
Kronofed-A 970
Medi-Flu Caplet, Liquid ▣ 640
Novafed A Capsules 1342
Novafed Capsules 1342
Novahistine DH 1342
Novahistine DMX ▣ 595
Novahistine Expectorant 1343
Nucofed Capsules 2219
Nucofed Expectorant 2219
Nucofed Pediatric Expectorant 2220
Nucofed Syrup 2219
Ornex Caplets ▣ 618
PediaCare Allergy Relief Formula Liquid 1362
PediaCare Cough-Cold Formula Liquid 1362
PediaCare Infants' Oral Decongestant Drops 1362
PediaCare Night Rest Cough-Cold Formula Liquid 1362
PediaCare 6-12 Cough-Cold Formula Chewable Tablets 1362
Robitussin-DAC Syrup 1875
Robitussin-PE ▣ 677
Rondec 1975
Rondec-DM 1976
Rondec-TR Tablet 1975
Ru-Tuss DE Tablets 694
Ryna ▣ 741
Seldane-D Extended-Release Tablets 1350
Sinarest ▣ 562
Sine-Aid Maximum Strength Sinus Headache Caplets 1365
Sine-Aid Maximum Strength Sinus Headache Tablets 1365
Sine-Off Maximum Strength Allergy/Sinus Formula Caplets ▣ 721
Sine-Off Maximum Strength No Drowsiness Formula Caplets ▣ 722
Singlet Tablets ▣ 598
Sinutab Maximum Strength ▣ 641
Sinutab Maximum Strength Without Drowsiness Tablets & Caplets ▣ 642
Sinutab Regular Strength Without Drowsiness Formula ▣ 641
St. Joseph Nighttime Cold Medicine ▣ 705
Sudafed Children's Liquid ▣ 543
Sudafed Cough Syrup ▣ 543
Sudafed Plus Liquid ▣ 544
Sudafed Plus Tablets ▣ 545
Sudafed Sinus Caplets ▣ 545
Sudafed Sinus Tablets ▣ 545
Sudafed Tablets, 30 mg ▣ 544
Sudafed Tablets, Adult Strength, 60 mg ▣ 544
Sudafed 12 Hour Capsules ▣ 545
TheraFlu Flu and Cold Medicine ▣ 687
Triaminic Nite Light ▣ 689
Tylenol Allergy Sinus Medication Caplets and Gelcaps, Maximum Strength 1372
Children's Tylenol Cold Liquid Formula and Chewable Tablets 1368
Tylenol Cold & Flu Hot Medication, Packets 1369
Tylenol Cold & Flu No Drowsiness Hot Medication, Packets 1371
Tylenol Cold Medication Caplets and Tablets 1370
Tylenol Cold Medication No Drowsiness Formula Caplets 1370
Tylenol Cold Night Time Medication Liquid 1371
Tylenol Cough Medication Liquid with Decongestant, Maximum Strength 1372
Tylenol, Maximum Strength, Sinus Medication Gelcaps, Caplets and Tablets 1373
Ursinus Inlay-Tabs ▣ 691
Vicks Children's NyQuil ▣ 664
Vicks Daycare ▣ 660
Vicks Formula 44D Decongestant Cough Medicine ▣ 662
Vicks Formula 44M Multi-Symptom Cough Medicine ▣ 662
Vicks NyQuil Nighttime Colds Medicine-Original & Cherry Flavor ▣ 664

Vicks Pediatric Formula 44 Cough & Congestion Medicine ▣ 663
Vicks Pediatric Formula 44m Multi-Symptom Cough & Cold Medicine ▣ 663

Pseudoephedrine Sulfate (Possible additive atropine-like effect). Products include:
Afrin Tablets ▣ 693
Chlor-Trimeton Decongestant ▣ 694
Disophrol Chronotab Sustained-Action Tablets ▣ 698
Drixoral Antihistamine/Nasal Decongestant Syrup ▣ 698
Drixoral Non-Drowsy Formula ▣ 699
Drixoral Plus Extended-Release Tablets ▣ 699
Drixoral Sinus ▣ 700
Drixoral Sustained-Action Tablets ▣ 698
Sinutab Allergy Formula Sustained Action Tablets ▣ 640
Trinalin Repetabs Tablets 1170

Quazepam (Risk of seizures). Products include:
Doral Tablets 2383

Scopolamine Hydrobromide (Possible additive atropine-like effect). Products include:
Donnagel ▣ 675
Donnagel-PG 1858
Donnatal 1858
Donnatal Extentabs 1859
Donnatal Tablets 1858
Donnazyme Tablets 1860
Isopto Hyoscine ⊙ 222
Murocoll-2 Sterile Ophthalmic Solution ⊙ 261
Ru-Tuss Tablets 693

Scopolamine Preparations (Possible additive atropine-like effect). Products include:
Transderm Scōp Transdermal Therapeutic System 887

Secobarbital Sodium (Enhanced response to barbiturates). Products include:
Seconal Sodium Pulvules 1296

Selegiline Hydrochloride (Concurrent use contraindicated). Products include:
Eldepryl 2250

Sufentanil Citrate (Enhanced response to CNS depressants). Products include:
Sufenta Injection 1147

Temazepam (Enhanced response to CNS depressants). Products include:
Restoril Capsules 2023

Terbutaline Sulfate (Possible additive atropine-like effect). Products include:
Brethaire Inhaler 1024
Brethine Ampuls 1026
Brethine Tablets 1026
Bricanyl Injection 1324
Bricanyl Tablets 1325

Thiamylal Sodium (Enhanced response to barbiturates). Products include:
Surital Ampoules, Steri-Vials 1764

Thioridazine Hydrochloride (Risk of seizures; enhanced response to CNS depressants). Products include:
Mellaril 2011

Thiothixene (Risk of seizures; enhanced response to CNS depressants). Products include:
Navane Capsules and Concentrate 1954
Navane Intramuscular 1956

Thyroid (Enhanced potential for cardiovascular toxicity of Ludiomil). Products include:
S-P-T "Liquid" Capsules 995

Tranylcypromine Sulfate (Concurrent use contraindicated). Products include:
Parnate Tablets 2222

Triazolam (Enhanced response to CNS depressants). Products include:
Halcion Tablets 2340

Tridihexethyl Chloride (Possible additive atropine-like effect).
No products indexed under this heading.

Trifluoperazine Hydrochloride (Risk of seizures; enhanced response to CNS depressants). Products include:
Stelazine 2226

Trihexyphenidyl Hydrochloride (Possible additive atropine-like effect). Products include:
Artane 1195

LUFYLLIN ELIXIR
(Dyphylline) 2384
May interact with sympathomimetic bronchodilators and certain other agents. Compounds in these categories include:

Albuterol (Synergism). Products include:
Proventil Inhalation Aerosol 2117
Ventolin Inhalation Aerosol and Refill 583

Albuterol Sulfate (Synergism). Products include:
Proventil Repetabs Tablets 2120
Proventil Solutions for Inhalation 0.5% and 0.083% 2118
Proventil Syrup 2119
Proventil Tablets 2120
Ventolin 583

Bitolterol Mesylate (Synergism). Products include:
Tornalate 2074

Ephedrine Hydrochloride (Synergism). Products include:
Amesec ▣ 682
Primatene Tablets-M Formula 2421
Primatene Tablets-P Formula 2421
Primatene Tablets-Regular Formula 2421
Quadrinal Tablets 1183
Quelidrine Syrup 556
Tedral SA 1765

Ephedrine Sulfate (Synergism). Products include:
Bronkaid Tablets ▣ 757
Bronkolixir ▣ 761
Bronkotabs Tablets ▣ 762
Marax Tablets & DF Syrup 1954
Pazo Hemorrhoid Ointment & Suppositories 752
Vicks Vatronol Nose Drops ▣ 666

Ephedrine Tannate (Synergism). Products include:
Rynatuss 2388

Epinephrine (Synergism). Products include:
Ana-Kit Anaphylaxis Emergency Treatment Kit 1100
Bronkaid Mist ▣ 757
EpiPen 843
Marcaine Hydrochloride 0.5% with Epinephrine 1:200,000 (as bitartrate) 958
Marcaine Hydrochloride with Epinephrine 1:200,000 2055
Primatene Mist 2420
Sus-Phrine Injection 1006
Xylocaine with Epinephrine Injections 637

Epinephrine Hydrochloride (Synergism). Products include:
Adrenalin Chloride Solution 1:100 & 1:1,000 1689
Epifrin ⊙ 244
Glaucon ⊙ 218

Ethylnorepinephrine Hydrochloride (Synergism). Products include:
Bronkephrine Injection 2042

Isoetharine (Synergism). Products include:
Arm-a-Med Isoetharine Inhalation Solution, USP 616
Bronkometer Aerosol 2042
Bronkosol Solution 2042

Isoproterenol Hydrochloride (Synergism). Products include:
Isuprel Hydrochloride Injection 1:5000 2050
Isuprel Hydrochloride Mistometer 2051
Isuprel Hydrochloride Solution 1:200 & 1:100 2052
Norisodrine Aerotrol 540

Metaproterenol Sulfate (Synergism). Products include:
Alupent 674
Arm-a-Med Metaproterenol Sulfate Inhalation Solution, USP 617
Metaprel Inhalation Aerosol Bronchodilator 2014
Metaprel Inhalation Solution 2015
Metaprel 2015
Metaproterenol Sulfate Inhalation Solution, USP 912

Pirbuterol Acetate (Synergism). Products include:
Maxair Inhaler 1311

Probenecid (Increased plasma half-life of dyphylline). Products include:
Benemid Tablets 1426
ColBENEMID Tablets 1436
Wycillin Injection and Probenecid Tablets 2539

Terbutaline Sulfate (Synergism). Products include:
Brethaire Inhaler 1024
Brethine Ampuls 1026
Brethine Tablets 1026
Bricanyl Injection 1324
Bricanyl Tablets 1325

LUFYLLIN & LUFYLLIN-400 TABLETS
(Dyphylline) 2384
May interact with sympathomimetic bronchodilators and certain other agents. Compounds in these categories include:

Albuterol (Synergism). Products include:
Proventil Inhalation Aerosol 2117
Ventolin Inhalation Aerosol and Refill 583

Albuterol Sulfate (Synergism). Products include:
Proventil Repetabs Tablets 2120
Proventil Solutions for Inhalation 0.5% and 0.083% 2118
Proventil Syrup 2119
Proventil Tablets 2120
Ventolin 583

Bitolterol Mesylate (Synergism). Products include:
Tornalate 2074

Ephedrine Hydrochloride (Synergism). Products include:
Amesec ▣ 682
Primatene Tablets-M Formula 2421
Primatene Tablets-P Formula 2421
Primatene Tablets-Regular Formula 2421
Quadrinal Tablets 1183
Quelidrine Syrup 556
Tedral SA 1765

Ephedrine Sulfate (Synergism). Products include:
Bronkaid Tablets ▣ 757
Bronkolixir ▣ 761
Bronkotabs Tablets ▣ 762
Marax Tablets & DF Syrup 1954
Pazo Hemorrhoid Ointment & Suppositories 752
Vicks Vatronol Nose Drops ▣ 666

Ephedrine Tannate (Synergism). Products include:
Rynatuss 2388

Epinephrine (Synergism). Products include:
Ana-Kit Anaphylaxis Emergency Treatment Kit 1100
Bronkaid Mist ▣ 757
EpiPen 843
Marcaine Hydrochloride 0.5% with Epinephrine 1:200,000 (as bitartrate) 958
Marcaine Hydrochloride with Epinephrine 1:200,000 2055
Primatene Mist 2420
Sus-Phrine Injection 1006
Xylocaine with Epinephrine Injections 637

Epinephrine Bitartrate (Synergism). Products include:
AsthmaHaler Mist Epinephrine Bitartrate Bronchodilator ▣ 616
Bronkaid Mist Suspension ▣ 757
Primatene Mist Suspension 2421

Ethylnorepinephrine Hydrochloride (Synergism). Products include:
Bronkephrine Injection 2042

Isoetharine (Synergism). Products include:
Arm-a-Med Isoetharine Inhalation Solution, USP 616
Bronkometer Aerosol 2042
Bronkosol Solution 2042

Isoproterenol Hydrochloride (Synergism). Products include:
Isuprel Hydrochloride Injection 1:5000 2050
Isuprel Hydrochloride Mistometer 2051
Isuprel Hydrochloride Solution 1:200 & 1:100 2052
Norisodrine Aerotrol 540

Metaproterenol Sulfate (Synergism). Products include:
Alupent 674
Arm-a-Med Metaproterenol Sulfate Inhalation Solution, USP 617
Metaprel Inhalation Aerosol Bronchodilator 2014
Metaprel Inhalation Solution 2015
Metaprel 2015
Metaproterenol Sulfate Inhalation Solution, USP 912

Pirbuterol Acetate (Synergism). Products include:
Maxair Inhaler 1311

Probenecid (Increased plasma half-life of dyphylline). Products include:
Benemid Tablets 1426
ColBENEMID Tablets 1436
Wycillin Injection and Probenecid Tablets 2539

Terbutaline Sulfate (Synergism). Products include:
Brethaire Inhaler 1024
Brethine Ampuls 1026
Brethine Tablets 1026
Bricanyl Injection 1324
Bricanyl Tablets 1325

LUFYLLIN-GG ELIXIR & TABLETS
(Dyphylline, Guaifenesin) 2385
May interact with sympathomimetic bronchodilators and certain other agents. Compounds in these categories include:

Albuterol (Synergism). Products include:
Proventil Inhalation Aerosol 2117
Ventolin Inhalation Aerosol and Refill 583

Albuterol Sulfate (Synergism). Products include:
Proventil Repetabs Tablets 2120
Proventil Solutions for Inhalation 0.5% and 0.083% 2118
Proventil Syrup 2119
Proventil Tablets 2120
Ventolin 583

Ephedrine Hydrochloride (Synergism). Products include:
Amesec ▣ 682
Primatene Tablets-M Formula 2421
Primatene Tablets-P Formula 2421
Primatene Tablets-Regular Formula 2421
Quadrinal Tablets 1183
Quelidrine Syrup 556
Tedral SA 1765

Ephedrine Sulfate (Synergism). Products include:
Bronkaid Tablets ▣ 757
Bronkolixir ▣ 761
Bronkotabs Tablets ▣ 762
Marax Tablets & DF Syrup 1954

Pazo Hemorrhoid Ointment & Suppositories ... 752
Vicks Vatronol Nose Drops ... ⊞ 666

Ephedrine Tannate (Synergism). Products include:
Rynatuss ... 2388

Epinephrine (Synergism). Products include:
Ana-Kit Anaphylaxis Emergency Treatment Kit ... 1100
Bronkaid Mist ... ⊞ 757
EpiPen ... 843
Marcaine Hydrochloride 0.5% with Epinephrine 1:200,000 (as bitartrate) ... 958
Marcaine Hydrochloride with Epinephrine 1:200,000 ... 2055
Primatene Mist ... 2420
Sus-Phrine Injection ... 1006
Xylocaine with Epinephrine Injections ... 637

Epinephrine Hydrochloride (Synergism). Products include:
Adrenalin Chloride Solution 1:100 & 1:1,000 ... 1689
Epifrin ... ⊙ 244
Glaucon ... ⊙ 218

Ethylnorepinephrine Hydrochloride (Synergism). Products include:
Bronkephrine Injection ... 2042

Isoetharine (Synergism). Products include:
Arm-a-Med Isoetharine Inhalation Solution, USP ... 616
Bronkometer Aerosol ... 2042
Bronkosol Solution ... 2042

Isoproterenol Hydrochloride (Synergism). Products include:
Isuprel Hydrochloride Injection 1:5000 ... 2050
Isuprel Hydrochloride Mistometer .. 2051
Isuprel Hydrochloride Solution 1:200 & 1:100 ... 2052
Norisodrine Aerotrol ... 540

Metaproterenol Sulfate (Synergism). Products include:
Alupent ... 674
Arm-a-Med Metaproterenol Sulfate Inhalation Solution, USP ... 617
Metaprel Inhalation Aerosol Bronchodilator ... 2014
Metaprel Inhalation Solution ... 2015
Metaprel ... 2015
Metaproterenol Sulfate Inhalation Solution, USP ... 912

Pirbuterol Acetate (Synergism). Products include:
Maxair Inhaler ... 1311

Probenecid (Increased plasma half-life of dyphylline). Products include:
Benemid Tablets ... 1426
ColBENEMID Tablets ... 1436
Wycillin Injection and Probenecid Tablets ... 2539

Terbutaline Sulfate (Synergism). Products include:
Brethaire Inhaler ... 1024
Brethine Ampuls ... 1026
Brethine Tablets ... 1026
Bricanyl Injection ... 1324
Bricanyl Tablets ... 1325

LUPRON DEPOT 3.75 MG
(Leuprolide Acetate) ... 2312
No interactions described in labeling.

LUPRON DEPOT 7.5 MG
(Leuprolide Acetate) ... 2311
No interactions described in labeling.

LUPRON INJECTION
(Leuprolide Acetate) ... 2310
No interactions described in labeling.

LURIDE DROPS
(Sodium Fluoride) ... 889

Food Interactions

Dairy products (Incompatibility of fluoride with dairy foods results in the formation of poorly absorbed calcium fluoride).

LURIDE LOZI-TABS TABLETS
(Sodium Fluoride) ... 890

Food Interactions

Dairy products (Incompatibility of fluoride with dairy foods results in the formation of poorly absorbed calcium fluoride).

LURLINE PMS TABLETS
(Acetaminophen, Pamabrom) ... 972
No interactions described in labeling.

LUROSCRUB ANTIMICROBIAL SKIN CLEANSER
(Chlorhexidine Gluconate) ... 912
No interactions described in labeling.

LUTREPULSE FOR INJECTION
(Gonadorelin Acetate) ... 1655
May interact with ovulation stimulators. Compounds in this category include:

Chorionic Gonadotropin (Lutrepulse should not be used concomitantly with other ovulation stimulators). Products include:
A.P.L. ... 2431
Pregnyl ... 1644
Profasi (human chorionic gonadotropin, USP) ... 2186

Clomiphene Citrate (Lutrepulse should not be used concomitantly with other ovulation stimulators). Products include:
Serophene (clomiphene citrate tablets, USP) ... 2186

Menotropins (Lutrepulse should not be used concomitantly with other ovulation stimulators). Products include:
Pergonal (menotropins for injection, USP) ... 2184

Urofollitropin (Lutrepulse should not be used concomitantly with other ovulation stimulators). Products include:
Metrodin (urofollitropin for injection) ... 2182

LYSODREN
(Mitotane) ... 731
May interact with oral anticoagulants. Compounds in this category include:

Dicumarol (Accelerated metabolism of dicumarol). Products include:
Dicumarol Tablets ... 516

Warfarin Sodium (Accelerated metabolism of warfarin). Products include:
Coumadin Injection & Tablets ... 944
Panwarfin Tablets ... 547

MG 217 PSORIASIS OINTMENT AND LOTION
(Coal Tar, Sulfur, Salicylic Acid) ... ⊞ 734
No interactions described in labeling.

MG 217 PSORIASIS SHAMPOO AND CONDITIONER
(Coal Tar, Sulfur (Colloidal), Salicylic Acid) ... ⊞ 734
No interactions described in labeling.

MICRHOGAM $RH_O(D)$ IMMUNE GLOBULIN (HUMAN)
(Immune Globulin (Human)) ... 1650
No interactions described in labeling.

M-M-R II
(Measles, Mumps & Rubella Virus Vaccine Live) ... 1494
May interact with immunosuppressive agents. Compounds in this category include:

Azathioprine (Concurrent administration is containdicated). Products include:
Imuran ... 768

Cyclosporine (Concurrent administration is containdicated). Products include:
Sandimmune ... 2024

Immune Globulin (Human) (Concurrent administration is containdicated). Products include:
MICRhoGAM $Rh_0(D)$ Immune Globulin (Human) ... 1650
RhoGAM $Rh_0(D)$ Immune Globulin (Human) ... 1651

Immune Globulin Intravenous (Human) (Concurrent administration is containdicated). Products include:
Gamimune N Immune Globulin Intravenous (Human) ... 1572
Gammagard Immune Globulin, Intravenous (Human) ... 658
Iveegam ... 1129
Sandoglobulin I.V. ... 2027

Muromonab-CD3 (Concurrent administration is containdicated). Products include:
Orthoclone OKT3 Sterile Solution .. 1645

M-R-VAX II
(Measles & Rubella Virus Vaccine Live) ... 1496
May interact with immunosuppressive agents. Compounds in this category include:

Azathioprine (Concurrent administration is containdicated). Products include:
Imuran ... 768

Cyclosporine (Concurrent administration is containdicated). Products include:
Sandimmune ... 2024

Immune Globulin (Human) (Concurrent administration is containdicated). Products include:
MICRhoGAM $Rh_0(D)$ Immune Globulin (Human) ... 1650
RhoGAM $Rh_0(D)$ Immune Globulin (Human) ... 1651

Immune Globulin Intravenous (Human) (Concurrent administration is containdicated). Products include:
Gamimune N Immune Globulin Intravenous (Human) ... 1572
Gammagard Immune Globulin, Intravenous (Human) ... 658
Iveegam ... 1129
Sandoglobulin I.V. ... 2027

Muromonab-CD3 (Concurrent administration is containdicated). Products include:
Orthoclone OKT3 Sterile Solution .. 1645

MS CONTIN TABLETS
(Morphine Sulfate) ... 1814
May interact with phenothiazines, general anesthetics, hypnotics and sedatives, tranquilizers, muscle relaxants, central nervous system depressants, and certain other agents. Compounds in these categories include:

Alcohol (Severe hypotension; respiratory depression; profound sedation; coma).

Alfentanil Hydrochloride (Profound sedation; coma; severe hypotension; respiratory depression). Products include:
Alfenta Injection ... 1131

Alprazolam (Profound sedation; coma; severe hypotension; respiratory depression). Products include:
Xanax Tablets ... 2367

Aprobarbital (Profound sedation; coma; severe hypotension; respiratory depression). Products include:
Alurate Elixir ... 1883

Atracurium Besylate (Increased respiratory depression). Products include:
Tracrium Injection ... 817

Baclofen (Increased respiratory depression). Products include:
Lioresal Tablets ... 1031

Buprenorphine (Profound sedation; coma; severe hypotension; respiratory depression).
No products indexed under this heading.

Buspirone Hydrochloride (Profound sedation; coma; severe hypotension; respiratory depression). Products include:
BuSpar ... 1401

Butabarbital (Profound sedation; coma; severe hypotension; respiratory depression). Products include:
Pyridium Plus ... 1764

Butalbital (Profound sedation; coma; severe hypotension; respiratory depression). Products include:
Esgic-Plus Tablets ... 1002
Esgic Tablets & Capsules ... 1001
Fioricet Tablets ... 2006
Fiorinal Capsules ... 2007
Fiorinal with Codeine Capsules ... 2008
Fiorinal Tablets ... 2007
Phrenilin ... 838
Sedapap Tablets 50 mg/650 mg .. 1360

Carisoprodol (Increased respiratory depression). Products include:
Soma Compound w/Codeine Tablets ... 2390
Soma Compound Tablets ... 2389
Soma Tablets ... 2388

Chlordiazepoxide (Profound sedation; coma; severe hypotension; respiratory depression). Products include:
Libritabs Tablets ... 1930
Limbitrol ... 1933
Menrium Tablets ... 1934

Chlordiazepoxide Hydrochloride (Profound sedation; coma; severe hypotension; respiratory depression). Products include:
Librax Capsules ... 1929
Librium Capsules ... 1931
Librium Injectable ... 1932

Chlorpromazine (Profound sedation; coma; severe hypotension; respiratory depression). Products include:
Thorazine ... 2234

Chlorprothixene (Profound sedation; coma; severe hypotension; respiratory depression). Products include:
Taractan Tablets ... 1920

Chlorprothixene Hydrochloride (Profound sedation; coma; severe hypotension; respiratory depression). Products include:
Taractan ... 1920

Chlorzoxazone (Increased respiratory depression). Products include:
Paraflex Caplets ... 1378
Parafon Forte DSC Caplets ... 1379

Clorazepate Dipotassium (Profound sedation; coma; severe hypotension; respiratory depression). Products include:
Tranxene ... 556

Codeine (Profound sedation; coma; severe hypotension; respiratory depression). Products include:
Calcidrine Syrup ... 506

Codeine Phosphate (Profound sedation; coma; severe hypotension; respiratory depression). Products include:
- Actifed with Codeine Cough Syrup.. 752
- Cheracol Cough Syrup ... 1853
- Codimal PH Syrup ... 846
- Dimetane-DC Cough Syrup ... 1857
- Empirin with Codeine Phosphate Nos. 2, 3 & 4 ... 764
- Fiorinal with Codeine Capsules ... 2008
- Isoclor Expectorant ... 982
- Naldecon CX Adult Liquid ... ⊞ 521
- Novahistine DH ... 1342
- Novahistine Expectorant ... 1343
- Nucofed Capsules ... 2219
- Nucofed Expectorant ... 2219
- Nucofed Pediatric Expectorant ... 2220
- Nucofed Syrup ... 2219
- Phenaphen with Codeine Capsules 1865
- Phenaphen-650 with Codeine Tablets ... 1866
- Phenergan with Codeine ... 2497
- Phenergan VC with Codeine ... 2501
- Robitussin A-C Syrup ... 1875
- Robitussin-DAC Syrup ... 1875
- Ryna ... ⊞ 741
- Soma Compound w/Codeine Tablets ... 2390
- Triaminic Expectorant w/Codeine .. 1996
- Tussi-Organidin Liquid ... 2391
- Tylenol with Codeine ... 1381

Codeine Polistirex (Profound sedation; coma; severe hypotension; respiratory depression).
- No products indexed under this heading.

Cyclobenzaprine Hydrochloride (Increased respiratory depression hypotension; respiratory depression). Products include:
- Flexeril Tablets ... 1471

Dantrolene Sodium (Increased respiratory depression). Products include:
- Dantrium Capsules ... 1619
- Dantrium Intravenous ... 1620

Dezocine (Profound sedation; coma; severe hypotension; respiratory depression).

Diazepam (Profound sedation; coma; severe hypotension; respiratory depression). Products include:
- Valium Injectable ... 1937
- Valium Tablets ... 1939
- Valrelease Capsules ... 1923

Doxacurium Chloride (Increased respiratory depression). Products include:
- Nuromax Injection ... 794

Droperidol (Profound sedation; coma; severe hypotension; respiratory depression). Products include:
- Inapsine Injection ... 1140
- Innovar Injection ... 1141

Enflurane (Profound sedation; coma; severe hypotension; respiratory depression). Products include:
- Ethrane ... 599

Estazolam (Profound sedation; coma; severe hypotension; respiratory depression). Products include:
- ProSom Tablets ... 554

Ethchlorvynol (Profound sedation; coma; severe hypotension; respiratory depression). Products include:
- Placidyl Capsules ... 553

Ethinamate (Profound sedation; coma; severe hypotension; respiratory depression).
- No products indexed under this heading.

Fentanyl (Profound sedation; coma; severe hypotension; respiratory depression). Products include:
- Duragesic Transdermal System ... 1133

Fentanyl Citrate (Profound sedation; coma; severe hypotension; respiratory depression). Products include:
- Innovar Injection ... 1141
- Sublimaze Injection ... 1146

Fluphenazine Decanoate (Profound sedation; coma; severe hypotension; respiratory depression). Products include:
- Prolixin Decanoate ... 1795

Fluphenazine Enanthate (Profound sedation; coma; severe hypotension; respiratory depression). Products include:
- Prolixin Enanthate ... 1796

Fluphenazine Hydrochloride (Profound sedation; coma; severe hypotension; respiratory depression). Products include:
- Prolixin Elixir ... 1793
- Prolixin Injection ... 1791
- Prolixin Oral Concentrate ... 1792
- Prolixin Tablets ... 1793

Flurazepam Hydrochloride (Profound sedation; coma; severe hypotension; respiratory depression). Products include:
- Dalmane Capsules ... 1927

Glutethimide (Profound sedation; coma; severe hypotension; respiratory depression).
- No products indexed under this heading.

Haloperidol (Profound sedation; coma; severe hypotension; respiratory depression). Products include:
- Haldol Injection, Tablets and Concentrate ... 1373

Haloperidol Decanoate (Profound sedation; coma; severe hypotension; respiratory depression). Products include:
- Haldol Decanoate ... 1375

Hydrocodone Bitartrate (Profound sedation; coma; severe hypotension; respiratory depression). Products include:
- Anexsia 5/500 Tablets ... 2196
- Anexsia 7.5/650 Tablets ... 2197
- Azdone Tablets ... 844
- Codiclear DH Syrup ... 845
- Codimal DH Syrup ... 846
- Damason-P ... 1356
- Hycodan Syrup, Tablets ... 927
- Hycomine Compound Tablets ... 929
- Hycomine Syrup ... 927
- Hycotuss Expectorant Syrup ... 930
- Hydrocet Capsules ... 835
- Lortab ASA Tablets ... 2414
- Lortab ... 2412
- Ru-Tuss with Hydrocodone ... 694
- Triaminic Expectorant DH ... 1995
- Vicodin Tablets ... 1187
- Vicodin ES Tablets ... 1189
- Zydone Capsules ... 941

Hydrocodone Polistirex (Profound sedation; coma; severe hypotension; respiratory depression). Products include:
- Tussionex Extended-Release Suspension ... 988

Hydroxyzine Hydrochloride (Profound sedation; coma; severe hypotension; respiratory depression). Products include:
- Atarax Tablets & Syrup ... 1941
- Marax Tablets & DF Syrup ... 1954
- Vistaril Intramuscular Solution ... 1970

Isoflurane (Profound sedation; coma; severe hypotension; respiratory depression). Products include:
- Forane ... 600

Ketamine Hydrochloride (Profound sedation; coma; severe hypotension; respiratory depression). Products include:
- Ketalar ... 1726

Levorphanol Tartrate (Profound sedation; coma; severe hypotension; respiratory depression). Products include:
- Levo-Dromoran ... 1906

Lorazepam (Profound sedation; coma; severe hypotension; respiratory depression). Products include:
- Ativan Injection ... 2432
- Ativan Tablets ... 2434

Loxapine Hydrochloride (Profound sedation; coma; severe hypotension; respiratory depression). Products include:
- Loxitane ... 1213

Loxapine Succinate (Profound sedation; coma; severe hypotension; respiratory depression). Products include:
- Loxitane Capsules ... 1213

Meperidine Hydrochloride (Profound sedation; coma; severe hypotension; respiratory depression). Products include:
- Demerol ... 2047
- Mepergan Injection ... 2479

Mephobarbital (Profound sedation; coma; severe hypotension; respiratory depression). Products include:
- Mebaral Tablets ... 2061

Meprobamate (Profound sedation; coma; severe hypotension; respiratory depression). Products include:
- Deprol Tablets ... 2382
- Equagesic Tablets ... 2451
- Miltown Tablets ... 2386
- PMB 200 and PMB 400 ... 2504

Mesoridazine (Profound sedation; coma; severe hypotension; respiratory depression). Products include:
- Serentil ... 686

Metaxalone (Increased respiratory depression). Products include:
- Skelaxin ... 840

Methadone Hydrochloride (Profound sedation; coma; severe hypotension; respiratory depression). Products include:
- Dolophine Hydrochloride Ampoules & Vials ... 1260
- Dolophine Hydrochloride Tablets ... 1261
- Methadone Hydrochloride Diskets .. 1284
- Methadone Hydrochloride Oral Solution & Tablets ... 1987

Methocarbamol (Increased respiratory depression). Products include:
- Robaxin Injectable ... 1871
- Robaxin Tablets ... 1872
- Robaxisal Tablets ... 1872

Methohexital Sodium (Profound sedation; coma; severe hypotension; respiratory depression). Products include:
- Brevital Sodium Vials ... 1248

Methoxyflurane (Profound sedation; coma; severe hypotension; respiratory depression).
- No products indexed under this heading.

Metocurine Iodide (Profound sedation; coma; severe hypotension; respiratory depression). Products include:
- Metubine Iodide Vials ... 1285

Midazolam Hydrochloride (Profound sedation; coma; severe hypotension; respiratory depression). Products include:
- Versed Injection ... 1924

Molindone Hydrochloride (Profound sedation; coma; severe hypotension; respiratory depression). Products include:
- Moban Tablets & Concentrate ... 932

Opium Alkaloids (Profound sedation; coma; severe hypotension; respiratory depression). Products include:
- B & O No. 15A & No. 16A Supprettes ... 2395
- Pantopon Injectable ... 1911

Orphenadrine Citrate (Increased respiratory depression). Products include:
- Norflex ... 1314
- Norgesic ... 1314

Oxazepam (Profound sedation; coma; severe hypotension; respiratory depression). Products include:
- Serax Capsules ... 2522
- Serax Tablets ... 2522

Oxycodone Hydrochloride (Profound sedation; coma; severe hypotension; respiratory depression). Products include:
- Percocet Tablets ... 950
- Percodan ... 951
- Roxicodone Tablets, Oral Solution & Intensol (Oxycodone) ... 1992
- Tylox Capsules ... 1382

Pancuronium Bromide Injection (Increased respiratory depression).
- No products indexed under this heading.

Pentazocine Hydrochloride (Reduced analgesic effect; precipitation of withdrawal). Products include:
- Talacen ... 2070
- Talwin Compound ... 2072
- Talwin Nx ... 2073

Pentazocine Lactate (Reduced analgesic effect; precipitation of withdrawal). Products include:
- Talwin Injection ... 2071

Pentobarbital Sodium (Profound sedation; coma; severe hypotension; respiratory depression). Products include:
- Nembutal Sodium Capsules ... 534
- Nembutal Sodium Solution ... 536
- Nembutal Sodium Suppositories ... 538

Perphenazine (Profound sedation; coma; severe hypotension; respiratory depression). Products include:
- Etrafon ... 2087
- Triavil Tablets ... 1556
- Trilafon ... 2123

Phenobarbital (Profound sedation; coma; severe hypotension; respiratory depression). Products include:
- Arco-Lase Plus Tablets ... 607
- Bellergal-S Tablets ... 1998
- Bronkolixir ... ⊞ 761
- Bronkotabs Tablets ... ⊞ 762
- Donnatal ... 1858
- Donnatal Extentabs ... 1859
- Donnatal Tablets ... 1858
- Donnazyme Tablets ... 1860
- Kinesed Tablets ... 2272
- Phenobarbital Elixir and Tablets ... 1293
- Primatene Tablets-P Formula ... 2421
- Quadrinal Tablets ... 1183
- Tedral SA ... 1765

Prazepam (Profound sedation; coma; severe hypotension; respiratory depression). Products include:
- Centrax ... 1693

Prochlorperazine (Profound sedation; coma; severe hypotension; respiratory depression). Products include:
- Compazine ... 2201

Promethazine Hydrochloride (Profound sedation; coma; severe hypotension; respiratory depression). Products include:
- Mepergan Injection ... 2479
- Phenergan with Codeine ... 2497
- Phenergan with Dextromethorphan 2499
- Phenergan Injection ... 2493
- Phenergan Suppositories ... 2496
- Phenergan Syrup ... 2495
- Phenergan Tablets ... 2496
- Phenergan VC ... 2500
- Phenergan VC with Codeine ... 2501

Propofol (Profound sedation; coma; severe hypotension; respiratory depression). Products include:
- Diprivan Injection ... 2267

Propoxyphene Hydrochloride (Profound sedation; coma; severe hypotension; respiratory depression). Products include:

Darvon ... 1256
Wygesic Tablets ... 2540

Propoxyphene Napsylate (Profound sedation; coma; severe hypotension; respiratory depression). Products include:

Darvon-N/Darvocet-N ... 1254

Quazepam (Profound sedation; coma; severe hypotension; respiratory depression). Products include:

Doral Tablets ... 2383

Secobarbital Sodium (Profound sedation; coma; severe hypotension; respiratory depression). Products include:

Seconal Sodium Pulvules ... 1296

Succinylcholine Chloride (Increased respiratory depression). Products include:

Anectine ... 755

Sufentanil Citrate (Profound sedation; coma; severe hypotension; respiratory depression). Products include:

Sufenta Injection ... 1147

Temazepam (Profound sedation; coma; severe hypotension; respiratory depression). Products include:

Restoril Capsules ... 2023

Thiamylal Sodium (Profound sedation; coma; severe hypotension; respiratory depression). Products include:

Surital Ampoules, Steri-Vials ... 1764

Thioridazine Hydrochloride (Profound sedation; coma; severe hypotension; respiratory depression). Products include:

Mellaril ... 2011

Thiothixene (Profound sedation; coma; severe hypotension; respiratory depression). Products include:

Navane Capsules and Concentrate 1954
Navane Intramuscular ... 1956

Triazolam (Profound sedation; coma; severe hypotension; respiratory depression). Products include:

Halcion Tablets ... 2340

Trifluoperazine Hydrochloride (Profound sedation; coma; severe hypotension; respiratory depression). Products include:

Stelazine ... 2226

Vecuronium Bromide (Increased respiratory depression). Products include:

Norcuron ... 1642

MSIR ORAL SOLUTION
(Morphine Sulfate) ... 1817
May interact with hypnotics and sedatives, general anesthetics, phenothiazines, tranquilizers, muscle relaxants, central nervous system depressants, and certain other agents. Compounds in these categories include:

Alcohol (Profound sedation; respiratory depression; hypotension; coma).

Alfentanil Hydrochloride (Profound sedation; respiratory depression; hypotension; coma). Products include:

Alfenta Injection ... 1131

Alprazolam (Profound sedation; respiratory depression; hypotension; coma). Products include:

Xanax Tablets ... 2367

Aprobarbital (Profound sedation; respiratory depression; hypotension; coma). Products include:

Alurate Elixir ... 1883

Atracurium Besylate (Increased respiratory depression). Products include:

Tracrium Injection ... 817

Baclofen (Increased respiratory depression). Products include:

Lioresal Tablets ... 1031

Buprenorphine (Profound sedation; respiratory depression; hypotension; coma).

No products indexed under this heading.

Buspirone Hydrochloride (Profound sedation; respiratory depression; hypotension; coma). Products include:

BuSpar ... 1401

Butabarbital (Profound sedation; respiratory depression; hypotension; coma). Products include:

Pyridium Plus ... 1764

Butalbital (Profound sedation; respiratory depression; hypotension; coma). Products include:

Esgic-Plus Tablets ... 1002
Esgic Tablets & Capsules ... 1001
Fioricet Tablets ... 2006
Fiorinal Capsules ... 2007
Fiorinal with Codeine Capsules ... 2008
Fiorinal Tablets ... 2007
Phrenilin ... 838
Sedapap Tablets 50 mg/650 mg .. 1360

Carisoprodol (Profound sedation; respiratory depression; hypotension; coma). Products include:

Soma Compound w/Codeine Tablets ... 2390
Soma Compound Tablets ... 2389
Soma Tablets ... 2388

Chlordiazepoxide (Profound sedation; respiratory depression; hypotension; coma). Products include:

Libritabs Tablets ... 1930
Limbitrol ... 1933
Menrium Tablets ... 1934

Chlordiazepoxide Hydrochloride (Profound sedation; respiratory depression; hypotension; coma). Products include:

Librax Capsules ... 1929
Librium Capsules ... 1931
Librium Injectable ... 1932

Chlorpromazine (Profound sedation; respiratory depression; hypotension; coma). Products include:

Thorazine ... 2234

Chlorprothixene (Profound sedation; respiratory depression; hypotension; coma). Products include:

Taractan Tablets ... 1920

Chlorprothixene Hydrochloride (Profound sedation; respiratory depression; hypotension; coma). Products include:

Taractan ... 1920

Chlorzoxazone (Increased respiratory depression hypotension; coma). Products include:

Paraflex Caplets ... 1378
Parafon Forte DSC Caplets ... 1379

Clorazepate Dipotassium (Profound sedation; respiratory depression; hypotension; coma). Products include:

Tranxene ... 556

Codeine (Profound sedation; respiratory depression; hypotension; coma). Products include:

Calcidrine Syrup ... 506

Codeine Phosphate (Profound sedation; respiratory depression; hypotension; coma). Products include:

Actifed with Codeine Cough Syrup.. 752
Cheracol Cough Syrup ... 1853
Codimal PH Syrup ... 846
Dimetane-DC Cough Syrup ... 1857
Empirin with Codeine Phosphate Nos. 2, 3 & 4 ... 764
Fiorinal with Codeine Capsules ... 2008
Isoclor Expectorant ... 982
Naldecon CX Adult Liquid ... 521
Novahistine DH ... 1342
Novahistine Expectorant ... 1343
Nucofed Capsules ... 2219
Nucofed Expectorant ... 2219
Nucofed Pediatric Expectorant ... 2220
Nucofed Syrup ... 2219
Phenaphen with Codeine Capsules 1865
Phenaphen-650 with Codeine Tablets ... 1866
Phenergan with Codeine ... 2497
Phenergan VC with Codeine ... 2501
Robitussin A-C Syrup ... 1875
Robitussin-DAC Syrup ... 1875
Ryna ... 741
Soma Compound w/Codeine Tablets ... 2390
Triaminic Expectorant w/Codeine .. 1996
Tussi-Organidin Liquid ... 2391
Tylenol with Codeine ... 1381

Codeine Polistirex (Profound sedation; respiratory depression; hypotension; coma).

No products indexed under this heading.

Cyclobenzaprine Hydrochloride (Increased respiratory depression). Products include:

Flexeril Tablets ... 1471

Dantrolene Sodium (Increased respiratory depression). Products include:

Dantrium Capsules ... 1619
Dantrium Intravenous ... 1620

Dezocine (Profound sedation; respiratory depression; hypotension; coma).

Diazepam (Profound sedation; respiratory depression; hypotension; coma). Products include:

Valium Injectable ... 1937
Valium Tablets ... 1939
Valrelease Capsules ... 1923

DOXACURIUM CHLORIDE (Increased respiratory depression). Products include:

Nuromax Injection ... 794

Droperidol (Profound sedation; respiratory depression; hypotension; coma). Products include:

Inapsine Injection ... 1140
Innovar Injection ... 1141

Enflurane (Profound sedation; respiratory depression; hypotension; coma). Products include:

Ethrane ... 599

Estazolam (Profound sedation; respiratory depression; hypotension; coma). Products include:

ProSom Tablets ... 554

Ethchlorvynol (Profound sedation; respiratory depression; hypotension; coma). Products include:

Placidyl Capsules ... 553

Ethinamate (Profound sedation; respiratory depression; hypotension; coma).

No products indexed under this heading.

Fentanyl (Profound sedation; respiratory depression; hypotension; coma). Products include:

Duragesic Transdermal System ... 1133

Fentanyl Citrate (Profound sedation; respiratory depression; hypotension; coma). Products include:

Innovar Injection ... 1141
Sublimaze Injection ... 1146

Fluphenazine Decanoate (Profound sedation; respiratory depression; hypotension; coma). Products include:

Prolixin Decanoate ... 1795

Fluphenazine Enanthate (Profound sedation; respiratory depression; hypotension; coma). Products include:

Prolixin Enanthate ... 1796

Fluphenazine Hydrochloride (Profound sedation; respiratory depression; hypotension; coma). Products include:

Prolixin Elixir ... 1793
Prolixin Injection ... 1791
Prolixin Oral Concentrate ... 1792
Prolixin Tablets ... 1793

Flurazepam Hydrochloride (Profound sedation; respiratory depression; hypotension; coma). Products include:

Dalmane Capsules ... 1927

Glutethimide (Profound sedation; respiratory depression; hypotension; coma).

No products indexed under this heading.

Haloperidol (Profound sedation; respiratory depression; hypotension; coma). Products include:

Haldol Injection, Tablets and Concentrate ... 1373

Haloperidol Decanoate (Profound sedation; respiratory depression; hypotension; coma). Products include:

Haldol Decanoate ... 1375

Hydrocodone Bitartrate (Profound sedation; respiratory depression; hypotension; coma). Products include:

Anexsia 5/500 Tablets ... 2196
Anexsia 7.5/650 Tablets ... 2197
Azdone Tablets ... 844
Codiclear DH Syrup ... 845
Codimal DH Syrup ... 846
Damason-P ... 1356
Hycodan Syrup, Tablets ... 927
Hycomine Compound Tablets ... 929
Hycomine Syrup ... 927
Hycotuss Expectorant Syrup ... 930
Hydrocet Capsules ... 835
Lortab ASA Tablets ... 2414
Lortab ... 2412
Ru-Tuss with Hydrocodone ... 694
Triaminic Expectorant DH ... 1995
Vicodin Tablets ... 1187
Vicodin ES Tablets ... 1189
Zydone Capsules ... 941

Hydrocodone Polistirex (Profound sedation; respiratory depression; hypotension; coma). Products include:

Tussionex Extended-Release Suspension ... 988

Hydroxyzine Hydrochloride (Profound sedation; respiratory depression; hypotension; coma). Products include:

Atarax Tablets & Syrup ... 1941
Marax Tablets & DF Syrup ... 1954
Vistaril Intramuscular Solution ... 1970

Isoflurane (Profound sedation; respiratory depression; hypotension; coma). Products include:

Forane ... 600

Ketamine Hydrochloride (Profound sedation; respiratory depression; hypotension; coma). Products include:

Ketalar ... 1726

Levorphanol Tartrate (Profound sedation; respiratory depression; hypotension; coma). Products include:

Levo-Dromoran ... 1906

Lorazepam (Profound sedation; respiratory depression; hypotension; coma). Products include:

Ativan Injection ... 2432
Ativan Tablets ... 2434

Loxapine Hydrochloride (Profound sedation; respiratory depression; hypotension; coma). Products include:

Loxitane ... 1213

Loxapine Succinate (Profound sedation; respiratory depression; hypotension; coma). Products include:

- Loxitane Capsules ... 1213

Meperidine Hydrochloride (Profound sedation; respiratory depression; hypotension; coma). Products include:

- Demerol ... 2047
- Mepergan Injection ... 2479

Mephobarbital (Profound sedation; respiratory depression; hypotension; coma). Products include:

- Mebaral Tablets ... 2061

Meprobamate (Profound sedation; respiratory depression; hypotension; coma). Products include:

- Deprol Tablets ... 2382
- Equagesic Tablets ... 2451
- Miltown Tablets ... 2386
- PMB 200 and PMB 400 ... 2504

Mesoridazine (Profound sedation; respiratory depression; hypotension; coma). Products include:

- Serentil ... 686

Metaxalone (Increased respiratory depression). Products include:

- Skelaxin ... 840

Methadone Hydrochloride (Profound sedation; respiratory depression; hypotension; coma). Products include:

- Dolophine Hydrochloride Ampoules & Vials ... 1260
- Dolophine Hydrochloride Tablets ... 1261
- Methadone Hydrochloride Diskets ... 1284
- Methadone Hydrochloride Oral Solution & Tablets ... 1987

Methocarbamol (Increased respiratory depression). Products include:

- Robaxin Injectable ... 1871
- Robaxin Tablets ... 1872
- Robaxisal Tablets ... 1872

Methohexital Sodium (Profound sedation; respiratory depression; hypotension; coma). Products include:

- Brevital Sodium Vials ... 1248

Methoxyflurane (Profound sedation; respiratory depression; hypotension; coma).

- No products indexed under this heading.

Metocurine Iodide (Increased respiratory depression). Products include:

- Metubine Iodide Vials ... 1285

Midazolam Hydrochloride (Profound sedation; respiratory depression; hypotension; coma). Products include:

- Versed Injection ... 1924

Molindone Hydrochloride (Profound sedation; respiratory depression; hypotension; coma). Products include:

- Moban Tablets & Concentrate ... 932

Opium Alkaloids (Profound sedation; respiratory depression; hypotension; coma). Products include:

- B & O No. 15A & No. 16A Supprettes ... 2395
- Pantopon Injectable ... 1911

Orphenadrine Citrate (Increased respiratory depression). Products include:

- Norflex ... 1314
- Norgesic ... 1314

Oxazepam (Profound sedation; respiratory depression; hypotension; coma). Products include:

- Serax Capsules ... 2522
- Serax Tablets ... 2522

Oxycodone Hydrochloride (Profound sedation; respiratory depression; hypotension; coma). Products include:

- Percocet Tablets ... 950
- Percodan ... 951
- Roxicodone Tablets, Oral Solution & Intensol (Oxycodone) ... 1992
- Tylox Capsules ... 1382

Pancuronium Bromide Injection (Increased respiratory depression).

- No products indexed under this heading.

Pentazocine Hydrochloride (Reduced analgesic effect; precipitation of withdrawal). Products include:

- Talacen ... 2070
- Talwin Compound ... 2072
- Talwin Nx ... 2073

Pentazocine Lactate (Reduced analgesic effect; precipitation of withdrawal). Products include:

- Talwin Injection ... 2071

Pentobarbital Sodium (Profound sedation; respiratory depression; hypotension; coma). Products include:

- Nembutal Sodium Capsules ... 534
- Nembutal Sodium Solution ... 536
- Nembutal Sodium Suppositories ... 538

Perphenazine (Profound sedation; respiratory depression; hypotension; coma). Products include:

- Etrafon ... 2087
- Triavil Tablets ... 1556
- Trilafon ... 2123

Phenobarbital (Profound sedation; respiratory depression; hypotension; coma). Products include:

- Arco-Lase Plus Tablets ... 607
- Bellergal-S Tablets ... 1998
- Bronkolixir ... ⊞ 761
- Bronkotabs Tablets ... ⊞ 762
- Donnatal ... 1858
- Donnatal Extentabs ... 1859
- Donnatal Tablets ... 1858
- Donnazyme Tablets ... 1860
- Kinesed Tablets ... 2272
- Phenobarbital Elixir and Tablets ... 1293
- Primatene Tablets-P Formula ... 2421
- Quadrinal Tablets ... 1183
- Tedral SA ... 1765

Prazepam (Profound sedation; respiratory depression; hypotension; coma). Products include:

- Centrax ... 1693

Prochlorperazine (Profound sedation; coma; severe hypotension; respiratory depression). Products include:

- Compazine ... 2201

Promethazine Hydrochloride (Profound sedation; respiratory depression; hypotension; coma). Products include:

- Mepergan Injection ... 2479
- Phenergan with Codeine ... 2497
- Phenergan with Dextromethorphan 2499
- Phenergan Injection ... 2493
- Phenergan Suppositories ... 2496
- Phenergan Syrup ... 2495
- Phenergan Tablets ... 2496
- Phenergan VC ... 2500
- Phenergan VC with Codeine ... 2501

Propofol (Profound sedation; respiratory depression; hypotension; coma). Products include:

- Diprivan Injection ... 2267

Propoxyphene Hydrochloride (Profound sedation; respiratory depression; hypotension; coma). Products include:

- Darvon ... 1256
- Wygesic Tablets ... 2540

Propoxyphene Napsylate (Profound sedation; respiratory depression; hypotension; coma). Products include:

- Darvon-N/Darvocet-N ... 1254

Quazepam (Profound sedation; respiratory depression; hypotension; coma). Products include:

- Doral Tablets ... 2383

Secobarbital Sodium (Profound sedation; respiratory depression; hypotension; coma). Products include:

- Seconal Sodium Pulvules ... 1296

Succinylcholine Chloride (Increased respiratory depression). Products include:

- Anectine ... 755

Sufentanil Citrate (Profound sedation; respiratory depression; hypotension; coma). Products include:

- Sufenta Injection ... 1147

Temazepam (Profound sedation; respiratory depression; hypotension; coma). Products include:

- Restoril Capsules ... 2023

Thiamylal Sodium (Profound sedation; respiratory depression; hypotension; coma). Products include:

- Surital Ampoules, Steri-Vials ... 1764

Thioridazine Hydrochloride (Profound sedation; respiratory depression; hypotension; coma). Products include:

- Mellaril ... 2011

Thiothixene (Profound sedation; respiratory depression; hypotension; coma). Products include:

- Navane Capsules and Concentrate 1954
- Navane Intramuscular ... 1956

Triazolam (Profound sedation; respiratory depression; hypotension; coma). Products include:

- Halcion Tablets ... 2340

Trifluoperazine Hydrochloride (Profound sedation; respiratory depression; hypotension; coma). Products include:

- Stelazine ... 2226

Vecuronium Bromide (Increased respiratory depression). Products include:

- Norcuron ... 1642

MSIR ORAL SOLUTION CONCENTRATE
(Morphine Sulfate) ... 1817
See **MSIR Oral Solution**

MSIR TABLETS
(Morphine Sulfate) ... 1817
See **MSIR Oral Solution**

EXTRA STRENGTH MAALOX PLUS SUSPENSION
(Aluminum Hydroxide, Magnesium Hydroxide, Simethicone) ... 1850
May interact with tetracyclines. Compounds in this category include:

Demeclocycline Hydrochloride (Antacids may prevent proper absorption of oral tetracyclines). Products include:

- Declomycin Capsules, Tablets ... 1199

Doxycycline Calcium (Antacids may prevent proper absorption of oral tetracyclines).

- No products indexed under this heading.

Doxycycline Hyclate (Antacids may prevent proper absorption of oral tetracyclines). Products include:

- Doryx Capsules ... 1717
- Vibramycin Hyclate Capsules ... 1787
- Vibramycin Hyclate Intravenous ... 1968
- Vibra-Tabs Film Coated Tablets ... 1787

Doxycycline Monohydrate (Antacids may prevent proper absorption of oral tetracyclines). Products include:

- Monodox Capsules ... 1630
- Vibramycin Monohydrate for Oral Suspension ... 1787

Methacycline Hydrochloride (Antacids may prevent proper absorption of oral tetracyclines).

- No products indexed under this heading.

Minocycline Hydrochloride (Antacids may prevent proper absorption of oral tetracyclines). Products include:

- Minocin Intravenous ... 1221
- Minocin Oral Suspension ... 1224
- Minocin Pellet-Filled Capsules ... 1222

Oxytetracycline Hydrochloride (Antacids may prevent proper absorption of oral tetracyclines). Products include:

- Terra-Cortril Ophthalmic Suspension ... 1963
- Terramycin Capsules ... 1786
- Terramycin Intramuscular Solution 1964
- Terramycin with Polymyxin B Sulfate Ophthalmic Ointment ... 1965

Tetracycline Hydrochloride (Antacids may prevent proper absorption of oral tetracyclines). Products include:

- Achromycin V Capsules ... 1193
- Achromycin Ophthalmic Ointment 1% ... ◉ 307
- Achromycin Ophthalmic Suspension 1% ... ◉ 308
- Topicycline for Topical Solution ... 1856

MAALOX TC SUSPENSION
(Aluminum Hydroxide, Magnesium Hydroxide) ... 1851
May interact with tetracyclines. Compounds in this category include:

Demeclocycline Hydrochloride (Antacids may prevent proper absorption of oral tetracyclines). Products include:

- Declomycin Capsules, Tablets ... 1199

Doxycycline Calcium (Antacids may prevent proper absorption of oral tetracyclines).

- No products indexed under this heading.

Doxycycline Hyclate (Antacids may prevent proper absorption of oral tetracyclines). Products include:

- Doryx Capsules ... 1717
- Vibramycin Hyclate Capsules ... 1787
- Vibramycin Hyclate Intravenous ... 1968
- Vibra-Tabs Film Coated Tablets ... 1787

Doxycycline Monohydrate (Antacids may prevent proper absorption of oral tetracyclines). Products include:

- Monodox Capsules ... 1630
- Vibramycin Monohydrate for Oral Suspension ... 1787

Methacycline Hydrochloride (Antacids may prevent proper absorption of oral tetracyclines).

- No products indexed under this heading.

Minocycline Hydrochloride (Antacids may prevent proper absorption of oral tetracyclines). Products include:

- Minocin Intravenous ... 1221
- Minocin Oral Suspension ... 1224
- Minocin Pellet-Filled Capsules ... 1222

Oxytetracycline Hydrochloride (Antacids may prevent proper absorption of oral tetracyclines). Products include:

- Terra-Cortril Ophthalmic Suspension ... 1963
- Terramycin Capsules ... 1786
- Terramycin Intramuscular Solution 1964
- Terramycin with Polymyxin B Sulfate Ophthalmic Ointment ... 1965

Tetracycline Hydrochloride (Antacids may prevent proper absorption of oral tetracyclines). Products include:

- Achromycin V Capsules ... 1193
- Achromycin Ophthalmic Ointment 1% ... ◉ 307

Achromycin Ophthalmic Suspension 1% ◉ 308
Topicycline for Topical Solution 1856

EXTRA STRENGTH MAALOX PLUS TABLETS
(Aluminum Hydroxide Gel, Dried, Magnesium Hydroxide) 1850
See **Extra Strength Maalox Plus Suspension**

MACRODANTIN CAPSULES
(Nitrofurantoin) 1624
May interact with:

Magnesium Trisilicate (Rate and extent of Macrodantin absorption reduced). Products include:
Gaviscon Antacid Tablets ▣ 593
Gaviscon-2 Antacid Tablets ▣ 594
Probenecid (Possible toxicity and decreased efficacy of Macrodantin). Products include:
Benemid Tablets 1426
ColBENEMID Tablets 1436
Wycillin Injection and Probenecid Tablets 2539
Sulfinpyrazone (Possible toxicity and decreased efficacy of Macrodantin). Products include:
Anturane 853

Food Interactions
Food, unspecified (Increases bioavailability of Macrodantin).

MAGONATE LIQUID
(Magnesium Gluconate) 994
No interactions described in labeling.

MAGONATE TABLETS AND LIQUID
(Magnesium Gluconate) ▣ 563
No interactions described in labeling.

MAG-OX 400
(Magnesium Oxide) 673
No interactions described in labeling.

MALTSUPEX LIQUID, POWDER & TABLETS
(Malt Soup Extract) ▣ 740
No interactions described in labeling.

MANDELAMINE GRANULES
(Methenamine Mandelate) 1738
May interact with:

Sulfamethizole (Forms an insoluble precipitate in acid urine). Products include:
Thiosulfil Forte Tablets 2526
Urobiotic-250 Capsules 1968

Food Interactions
Food that raises urinary pH (Acidic urine is essential for antibacterial activity; restrict alkalinizing food).

MANDELAMINE SUSPENSION AND SUSPENSION FORTE
(Methenamine Mandelate) 1738
See **Mandelamine Granules**

MANDELAMINE TABLETS
(Methenamine Mandelate) 1738
See **Mandelamine Granules**

MANDOL VIALS, FASPAK & ADD-VANTAGE
(Cefamandole Nafate) 1281
May interact with aminoglycosides and certain other agents. Compounds in these categories include:

Alcohol (Nausea; vomiting; vasomotor instability with hypotension; peripheral vasodilatation).
Amikacin Sulfate (Nephrotoxicity). Products include:
Amikin Injectable 602
Gentamicin Sulfate (Nephrotoxicity). Products include:
Garamycin Injectable 2093
Garamycin Ophthalmic ◉ 305
Genoptic Liquifilm Sterile Ophthalmic Solution ◉ 247
Genoptic S.O.P. Sterile Ophthalmic Ointment ◉ 247
Gentacidin Ointment ◉ 273
Gentacidin Solution ◉ 273
Gentak Ointment & Solution ◉ 208
G-myticin Creme and Ointment 0.1% 1770
Pred-G Liquifilm Sterile Ophthalmic Suspension ◉ 252
Pred-G S.O.P. Sterile Ophthalmic Ointment ◉ 253
Kanamycin Sulfate (Nephrotoxicity). Products include:
Kantrex Injection 601
Kantrex Pediatric Injection 601
Probenecid (Slows tubular excretion and doubles the peak serum levels). Products include:
Benemid Tablets 1426
ColBENEMID Tablets 1436
Wycillin Injection and Probenecid Tablets 2539
Streptomycin Sulfate (Nephrotoxicity).
No products indexed under this heading.
Tobramycin Sulfate (Nephrotoxicity). Products include:
Nebcin Vials, Hyporets & ADD-Vantage 1286

MANTADIL CREAM
(Chlorcyclizine Hydrochloride) 789
No interactions described in labeling.

MARAX TABLETS & DF SYRUP
(Ephedrine Sulfate, Theophylline, Hydroxyzine Hydrochloride) 1954
May interact with central nervous system depressants and certain other agents. Compounds in these categories include:

Alcohol (Potentiated).
Alfentanil Hydrochloride (Potentiated). Products include:
Alfenta Injection 1131
Alprazolam (Potentiated). Products include:
Xanax Tablets 2367
Aprobarbital (Potentiated). Products include:
Alurate Elixir 1883
Buprenorphine (Potentiated).
No products indexed under this heading.
Buspirone Hydrochloride (Potentiated). Products include:
BuSpar 1401
Butabarbital (Potentiated). Products include:
Pyridium Plus 1764
Butalbital (Potentiated). Products include:
Esgic-Plus Tablets 1002
Esgic Tablets & Capsules 1001
Fioricet Tablets 2006
Fiorinal Capsules 2007
Fiorinal with Codeine Capsules 2008
Fiorinal Tablets 2007
Phrenilin 838
Sedapap Tablets 50 mg/650 mg 1360
Chlordiazepoxide (Potentiated). Products include:
Libritabs Tablets 1930
Limbitrol 1933
Menrium Tablets 1934
Chlordiazepoxide Hydrochloride (Potentiated). Products include:
Librax Capsules 1929
Librium Capsules 1931
Librium Injectable 1932
Chlorpromazine (Potentiated). Products include:
Thorazine 2234
Chlorprothixene (Potentiated). Products include:
Taractan Tablets 1920
Chlorprothixene Hydrochloride (Potentiated). Products include:
Taractan 1920
Chlorprothixene Lactate (Potentiated). Products include:
Taractan Concentrate 1920
Clorazepate Dipotassium (Potentiated). Products include:
Tranxene 556
Codeine (Potentiated). Products include:
Calcidrine Syrup 506
Codeine Phosphate (Potentiated). Products include:
Actifed with Codeine Cough Syrup 752
Cheracol Cough Syrup 1853
Codimal PH Syrup 846
Dimetane-DC Cough Syrup 1857
Empirin with Codeine Phosphate Nos. 2, 3 & 4 764
Fiorinal with Codeine Capsules 2008
Isoclor Expectorant 982
Naldecon CX Adult Liquid ▣ 521
Novahistine DH 1342
Novahistine Expectorant 1343
Nucofed Capsules 2219
Nucofed Expectorant 2219
Nucofed Pediatric Expectorant 2220
Nucofed Syrup 2219
Phenaphen with Codeine Capsules 1865
Phenaphen-650 with Codeine Tablets 1866
Phenergan with Codeine 2497
Phenergan VC with Codeine 2501
Robitussin A-C Syrup 1875
Robitussin-DAC Syrup 1875
Ryna ▣ 741
Soma Compound w/Codeine Tablets 2390
Triaminic Expectorant w/Codeine 1996
Tussi-Organidin Liquid 2391
Tylenol with Codeine 1381
Codeine Polistirex (Potentiated).
No products indexed under this heading.
Dezocine (Potentiated).
Diazepam (Potentiated). Products include:
Valium Injectable 1937
Valium Tablets 1939
Valrelease Capsules 1923
Droperidol (Potentiated). Products include:
Inapsine Injection 1140
Innovar Injection 1141
Enflurane (Potentiated). Products include:
Ethrane 599
Estazolam (Potentiated). Products include:
ProSom Tablets 554
Ethchlorvynol (Potentiated). Products include:
Placidyl Capsules 553
Ethinamate (Potentiated).
No products indexed under this heading.
Fentanyl (Potentiated). Products include:
Duragesic Transdermal System 1133
Fentanyl Citrate (Potentiated). Products include:
Innovar Injection 1141
Sublimaze Injection 1146
Fluphenazine Decanoate (Potentiated). Products include:
Prolixin Decanoate 1795
Fluphenazine Enanthate (Potentiated). Products include:
Prolixin Enanthate 1796
Fluphenazine Hydrochloride (Potentiated). Products include:
Prolixin Elixir 1793
Prolixin Injection 1791
Prolixin Oral Concentrate 1792
Prolixin Tablets 1793
Flurazepam Hydrochloride (Potentiated). Products include:
Dalmane Capsules 1927
Glutethimide (Potentiated).
No products indexed under this heading.
Haloperidol (Potentiated). Products include:
Haldol Injection, Tablets and Concentrate 1373
Haloperidol Decanoate (Potentiated). Products include:
Haldol Decanoate 1375
Hydrocodone Bitartrate (Potentiated). Products include:
Anexsia 5/500 Tablets 2196
Anexsia 7.5/650 Tablets 2197
Azdone Tablets 844
Codiclear DH Syrup 845
Codimal DH Syrup 846
Damason-P 1356
Hycodan Syrup, Tablets 927
Hycomine Compound Tablets 929
Hycomine Syrup 927
Hycotuss Expectorant Syrup 930
Hydrocet Capsules 835
Lortab ASA Tablets 2414
Lortab 2412
Ru-Tuss with Hydrocodone 694
Triaminic Expectorant DH 1995
Vicodin Tablets 1187
Vicodin ES Tablets 1189
Zydone Capsules 941
Hydrocodone Polistirex (Potentiated). Products include:
Tussionex Extended-Release Suspension 988
Isoflurane (Potentiated). Products include:
Forane 600
Ketamine Hydrochloride (Potentiated). Products include:
Ketalar 1726
Levorphanol Tartrate (Potentiated). Products include:
Levo-Dromoran 1906
Lorazepam (Potentiated). Products include:
Ativan Injection 2432
Ativan Tablets 2434
Loxapine Hydrochloride (Potentiated). Products include:
Loxitane 1213
Loxapine Succinate (Potentiated). Products include:
Loxitane Capsules 1213
Meperidine Hydrochloride (Potentiated). Products include:
Demerol 2047
Mepergan Injection 2479
Mephobarbital (Potentiated). Products include:
Mebaral Tablets 2061
Meprobamate (Potentiated). Products include:
Deprol Tablets 2382
Equagesic Tablets 2451
Miltown Tablets 2386
PMB 200 and PMB 400 2504
Mesoridazine (Potentiated). Products include:
Serentil 686
Methadone Hydrochloride (Potentiated). Products include:
Dolophine Hydrochloride Ampoules & Vials 1260
Dolophine Hydrochloride Tablets 1261
Methadone Hydrochloride Diskets 1284
Methadone Hydrochloride Oral Solution & Tablets 1987
Methohexital Sodium (Potentiated). Products include:
Brevital Sodium Vials 1248
Methoxyflurane (Potentiated).
No products indexed under this heading.

Midazolam Hydrochloride (Potentiated). Products include:
Versed Injection 1924

Molindone Hydrochloride (Potentiated). Products include:
Moban Tablets & Concentrate 932

Morphine Sulfate (Potentiated). Products include:
Astramorph/PF Injection, USP (Preservative-Free) 618
Duramorph 960
Infumorph 200 and Infumorph 500 Sterile Solutions 962
MS Contin Tablets 1814
MSIR 1817
Oramorph SR (Morphine Sulfate Sustained Release Tablets) 1988
Roxanol 1991

Opium Alkaloids (Potentiated). Products include:
B & O No. 15A & No. 16A Supprettes 2395
Pantopon Injectable 1911

Oxazepam (Potentiated). Products include:
Serax Capsules 2522
Serax Tablets 2522

Oxycodone Hydrochloride (Potentiated). Products include:
Percocet Tablets 950
Percodan 951
Roxicodone Tablets, Oral Solution & Intensol (Oxycodone) 1992
Tylox Capsules 1382

Pentobarbital Sodium (Potentiated). Products include:
Nembutal Sodium Capsules 534
Nembutal Sodium Solution 536
Nembutal Sodium Suppositories 538

Perphenazine (Potentiated). Products include:
Etrafon 2087
Triavil Tablets 1556
Trilafon 2123

Phenobarbital (Potentiated). Products include:
Arco-Lase Plus Tablets 607
Bellergal-S Tablets 1998
Bronkolixir .... ⊞ 761
Bronkotabs Tablets .... ⊞ 762
Donnatal 1858
Donnatal Extentabs 1859
Donnatal Tablets 1858
Donnazyme Tablets 1860
Kinesed Tablets 2272
Phenobarbital Elixir and Tablets 1293
Primatene Tablets-P Formula 2421
Quadrinal Tablets 1183
Tedral SA 1765

Prazepam (Potentiated). Products include:
Centrax 1693

Prochlorperazine (Potentiated). Products include:
Compazine 2201

Promethazine Hydrochloride (Potentiated). Products include:
Mepergan Injection 2479
Phenergan with Codeine 2497
Phenergan with Dextromethorphan 2499
Phenergan Injection 2493
Phenergan Suppositories 2496
Phenergan Syrup 2495
Phenergan Tablets 2496
Phenergan VC 2500
Phenergan VC with Codeine 2501

Propofol (Potentiated). Products include:
Diprivan Injection 2267

Propoxyphene Hydrochloride (Potentiated). Products include:
Darvon 1256
Wygesic Tablets 2540

Propoxyphene Napsylate (Potentiated). Products include:
Darvon-N/Darvocet-N 1254

Quazepam (Potentiated). Products include:
Doral Tablets 2383

Secobarbital Sodium (Potentiated). Products include:
Seconal Sodium Pulvules 1296

Sufentanil Citrate (Potentiated). Products include:
Sufenta Injection 1147

Temazepam (Potentiated). Products include:
Restoril Capsules 2023

Thiamylal Sodium (Potentiated). Products include:
Surital Ampoules, Steri-Vials 1764

Thioridazine Hydrochloride (Potentiated). Products include:
Mellaril 2011

Thiothixene (Potentiated). Products include:
Navane Capsules and Concentrate 1954
Navane Intramuscular 1956

Triazolam (Potentiated). Products include:
Halcion Tablets 2340

Trifluoperazine Hydrochloride (Potentiated). Products include:
Stelazine 2226

MARBLEN SUSPENSION PEACH/APRICOT

(Calcium Carbonate, Magnesium Carbonate) .... ⊞ 563
No interactions described in labeling.

MARBLEN SUSPENSION UNFLAVORED

(Calcium Carbonate, Magnesium Carbonate) .... ⊞ 563
No interactions described in labeling.

MARBLEN TABLETS

(Calcium Carbonate, Magnesium Carbonate) .... ⊞ 563
No interactions described in labeling.

MARCAINE HYDROCHLORIDE 0.5% WITH EPINEPHRINE 1:200,000 (AS BITARTRATE) (KODAK)

(Bupivacaine Hydrochloride, Epinephrine Bitartrate) 958
May interact with monoamine oxidase inhibitors, tricyclic antidepressants, ergot-type oxytocic drugs, and certain other agents. Compounds in these categories include:

Amitriptyline Hydrochloride (Produces severe, prolonged hypotension; concurrent use should be avoided). Products include:
Elavil 2269
Endep Tablets 1927
Etrafon 2087
Limbitrol 1933
Triavil Tablets 1556

Amoxapine (Produces severe, prolonged hypotension; concurrent use should be avoided). Products include:
Asendin Tablets 1196

Clomipramine Hydrochloride (Produces severe, prolonged hypotension; concurrent use should be avoided). Products include:
Anafranil Capsules 650

Desipramine Hydrochloride (Produces severe, prolonged hypotension; concurrent use should be avoided). Products include:
Norpramin Tablets 1340

Doxepin Hydrochloride (Produces severe, prolonged hypotension; concurrent use should be avoided). Products include:
Sinequan 1960

Furazolidone (Produces severe, prolonged hypotension; concurrent use should be avoided). Products include:
Furoxone 1855

Imipramine Hydrochloride (Produces severe, prolonged hypotension; concurrent use should be avoided). Products include:
Tofranil Ampuls 1038
Tofranil Tablets 1039

Imipramine Pamoate (Produces severe, prolonged hypotension; concurrent use should be avoided). Products include:
Tofranil-PM Capsules 1041

Isocarboxazid (Produces severe, prolonged hypotension; concurrent use should be avoided). Products include:
Marplan Tablets 1906

Maprotiline Hydrochloride (Produces severe, prolonged hypotension; concurrent use should be avoided). Products include:
Ludiomil Tablets 874

Methylergonovine Maleate (May cause severe, persistent hypertension or cerebrovascular accidents). Products include:
Methergine 2016

Nortriptyline Hydrochloride (Produces severe, prolonged hypotension; concurrent use should be avoided). Products include:
Pamelor 2019

Phenelzine Sulfate (Produces severe, prolonged hypotension; concurrent use should be avoided). Products include:
Nardil 1742

Protriptyline Hydrochloride (Produces severe, prolonged hypotension; concurrent use should be avoided). Products include:
Vivactil Tablets 1567

Selegiline Hydrochloride (Produces severe, prolonged hypotension; concurrent use should be avoided). Products include:
Eldepryl 2250

Tranylcypromine Sulfate (Produces severe, prolonged hypotension; concurrent use should be avoided). Products include:
Parnate Tablets 2222

Trimipramine Maleate (Produces severe, prolonged hypotension; concurrent use should be avoided). Products include:
Surmontil Capsules 2524

MARCAINE HYDROCHLORIDE WITH EPINEPHRINE 1:200,000 (SANOFI)

(Bupivacaine Hydrochloride, Epinephrine) 2055
May interact with monoamine oxidase inhibitors, tricyclic antidepressants, vasopressors, phenothiazines, butyrophenones, and certain other agents. Compounds in these categories include:

Amitriptyline Hydrochloride (Severe, persistent hypertension). Products include:
Elavil 2269
Endep Tablets 1927
Etrafon 2087
Limbitrol 1933
Triavil Tablets 1556

Amoxapine (Severe, persistent hypertension). Products include:
Asendin Tablets 1196

Chlorpromazine (May reduce or reverse the pressor effect of epinephrine). Products include:
Thorazine 2234

Clomipramine Hydrochloride (Severe, persistent hypertension). Products include:
Anafranil Capsules 650

Desipramine Hydrochloride (Severe, persistent hypertension). Products include:
Norpramin Tablets 1340

Dopamine Hydrochloride (Severe, persistent hypertension). Products include:
Intropin Injection 930

Doxepin Hydrochloride (Severe, persistent hypertension). Products include:
Sinequan 1960

Epinephrine Hydrochloride (Severe, persistent hypertension). Products include:
Adrenalin Chloride Solution 1:100 & 1:1,000 1689
Epifrin .... ⊙ 244
Glaucon .... ⊙ 218

Fluphenazine Decanoate (May reduce or reverse the pressor effect of epinephrine). Products include:
Prolixin Decanoate 1795

Fluphenazine Enanthate (May reduce or reverse the pressor effect of epinephrine). Products include:
Prolixin Enanthate 1796

Fluphenazine Hydrochloride (May reduce or reverse the pressor effect of epinephrine). Products include:
Prolixin Elixir 1793
Prolixin Injection 1791
Prolixin Oral Concentrate 1792
Prolixin Tablets 1793

Furazolidone (Severe, persistent hypertension). Products include:
Furoxone 1855

Haloperidol (May reduce or reverse the pressor effect of epinephrine). Products include:
Haldol Injection, Tablets and Concentrate 1373

Haloperidol Decanoate (May reduce or reverse the pressor effect of epinephrine). Products include:
Haldol Decanoate 1375

Imipramine Hydrochloride (Severe, persistent hypertension). Products include:
Tofranil Ampuls 1038
Tofranil Tablets 1039

Imipramine Pamoate (Severe, persistent hypertension). Products include:
Tofranil-PM Capsules 1041

Isocarboxazid (Severe, persistent hypertension). Products include:
Marplan Tablets 1906

Maprotiline Hydrochloride (Severe, persistent hypertension). Products include:
Ludiomil Tablets 874

Mesoridazine (May reduce or reverse the pressor effect of epinephrine). Products include:
Serentil 686

Metaraminol Bitartrate (Severe, persistent hypertension). Products include:
Aramine Injection 1424

Methoxamine Hydrochloride (Severe, persistent hypertension). Products include:
Vasoxyl Injection 819

Norepinephrine Bitartrate (Severe, persistent hypertension). Products include:
Levophed Bitartrate Injection 2054

Nortriptyline Hydrochloride (Severe, persistent hypertension). Products include:
Pamelor 2019

Oxytocin (Injection) (Severe, persistent hypertension). Products include:
Oxytocin Injection 2492

Pitocin Injection, Ampoules, Steri-Dose Syringes 1757

Oxytocin (Nasal Spray) (Severe, persistent hypertension).
No products indexed under this heading.

Perphenazine (May reduce or reverse the pressor effect of epinephrine). Products include:
Etrafon 2087
Triavil Tablets 1556
Trilafon 2123

Phenelzine Sulfate (Severe, persistent hypertension). Products include:
Nardil 1742

Phenylephrine Hydrochloride (Severe, persistent hypertension). Products include:
AK-Dilate Solution 2.5% and 10% .... ⊙ 203
Atrohist Sprinkle Capsules 558
Cerose-DM 2443
Codimal 846
Comhist LA Capsules 1618
Congespirin For Children Aspirin Free Chewable Cold Tablets 748
Cyclomydril .... ⊙ 216
Deconsal Sprinkle Capsules 559
Dimetane Decongestant .... ▣ 673
Dristan Decongestant/Antihistamine/ Analgesic Coated Caplets .... ▣ 749
Dristan Cold Nasal Decongestant/ Antihistamine/ Analgesic Coated Tablets 2419
Dristan Advanced Formula Decongestant/Antihistamine/ Analgesic Tablets .... ▣ 749
Dristan Nasal Spray, Menthol 2419
Dristan Nasal Spray, Regular and Regular with Metered Pump 2419
Entex Capsules 1623
Entex Liquid 1623
Sinus Excedrin Analgesic, Decongestant Tablets & Caplets 750
Extendryl 994
4-Way Fast Acting Nasal Spray - Original Formula (regular & mentholated) & Metered Spray Pump (regular) 751
Hycomine Compound Tablets 929
Murocoll-2 Sterile Ophthalmic Solution .... ⊙ 261
Mydfrin 2.5% .... ⊙ 224
Naldecon Syrup, Tablets, Pediatric Drops and Pediatric Syrup 709
Neo-Synephrine Hydrochloride 1% Carpuject 2063
Neo-Synephrine Hydrochloride 1% Injection 2063
Neo-Synephrine Hydrochloride (Ophthalmic) 2064
Neo-Synephrine .... ▣ 759
Nōstril Nasal Decongestant .... ▣ 520
Novahistine Elixir .... ▣ 596
Phenergan VC 2500
Phenergan VC with Codeine 2501
Prefrin Liquifilm Vasoconstrictor and Lubricant Eye Drops .... ⊙ 254
Prefrin-A .... ⊙ 255
Quelidrine Syrup 556
Relief Vasoconstrictor and Lubricant Eye Drops .... ⊙ 256
Robitussin Night Relief .... ▣ 677
Ru-Tuss with Hydrocodone 694
Ru-Tuss Tablets 693
Vasosulf .... ⊙ 279
Vicks Sinex .... ▣ 665
Zincfrin .... ⊙ 230

Prochlorperazine (May reduce or reverse the pressor effect of epinephrine). Products include:
Compazine 2201

Promethazine Hydrochloride (May reduce or reverse the pressor effect of epinephrine). Products include:
Mepergan Injection 2479
Phenergan with Codeine 2497
Phenergan with Dextromethorphan 2499
Phenergan Injection 2493
Phenergan Suppositories 2496
Phenergan Syrup 2495
Phenergan Tablets 2496
Phenergan VC 2500
Phenergan VC with Codeine 2501

Protriptyline Hydrochloride (Severe, persistent hypertension). Products include:
Vivactil Tablets 1567

Selegiline Hydrochloride (Severe, persistent hypertension). Products include:
Eldepryl 2250

Thioridazine Hydrochloride (May reduce or reverse the pressor effect of epinephrine). Products include:
Mellaril 2011

Tranylcypromine Sulfate (Severe, persistent hypertension). Products include:
Parnate Tablets 2222

Trifluoperazine Hydrochloride (May reduce or reverse the pressor effect of epinephrine). Products include:
Stelazine 2226

Trimipramine Maleate (Severe, persistent hypertension). Products include:
Surmontil Capsules 2524

MARCAINE HYDROCHLORIDE INJECTION

(Bupivacaine Hydrochloride) 2055
See **Marcaine Hydrochloride with Epinephrine 1:200,000**

MARCAINE SPINAL

(Bupivacaine Hydrochloride) 2058
May interact with monoamine oxidase inhibitors, tricyclic antidepressants, vasopressors, and certain other agents. Compounds in these categories include:

Amitriptyline Hydrochloride (Severe, persistent hypertension). Products include:
Elavil 2269
Endep Tablets 1927
Etrafon 2087
Limbitrol 1933
Triavil Tablets 1556

Amoxapine (Severe, persistent hypertension). Products include:
Asendin Tablets 1196

Clomipramine Hydrochloride (Severe, persistent hypertension). Products include:
Anafranil Capsules 650

Desipramine Hydrochloride (Severe, persistent hypertension). Products include:
Norpramin Tablets 1340

Dopamine Hydrochloride (Severe, persistent hypertension). Products include:
Intropin Injection 930

Doxepin Hydrochloride (Severe, persistent hypertension). Products include:
Sinequan 1960

Epinephrine Hydrochloride (Severe, persistent hypertension). Products include:
Adrenalin Chloride Solution 1:100 & 1:1,000 1689
Epifrin .... ⊙ 244
Glaucon .... ⊙ 218

Furazolidone (Severe, persistent hypertension). Products include:
Furoxone 1855

Imipramine Hydrochloride (Severe, persistent hypertension). Products include:
Tofranil Ampuls 1038
Tofranil Tablets 1039

Imipramine Pamoate (Severe, persistent hypertension). Products include:
Tofranil-PM Capsules 1041

Isocarboxazid (Severe, persistent hypertension). Products include:
Marplan Tablets 1906

Maprotiline Hydrochloride (Severe, persistent hypertension). Products include:
Ludiomil Tablets 874

Metaraminol Bitartrate (Severe, persistent hypertension). Products include:
Aramine Injection 1424

Methoxamine Hydrochloride (Severe, persistent hypertension). Products include:
Vasoxyl Injection 819

Norepinephrine Bitartrate (Severe, persistent hypertension). Products include:
Levophed Bitartrate Injection 2054

Nortriptyline Hydrochloride (Severe, persistent hypertension). Products include:
Pamelor 2019

Oxytocin (Injection) (Severe, persistent hypertension). Products include:
Oxytocin Injection 2492
Pitocin Injection, Ampoules, Steri-Dose Syringes 1757

Oxytocin (Nasal Spray) (Severe, persistent hypertension).
No products indexed under this heading.

Phenelzine Sulfate (Severe, persistent hypertension). Products include:
Nardil 1742

Phenylephrine Hydrochloride (Severe, persistent hypertension). Products include:
AK-Dilate Solution 2.5% and 10% .... ⊙ 203
Atrohist Sprinkle Capsules 558
Cerose-DM 2443
Codimal 846
Comhist LA Capsules 1618
Congespirin For Children Aspirin Free Chewable Cold Tablets 748
Cyclomydril .... ⊙ 216
Deconsal Sprinkle Capsules 559
Dimetane Decongestant .... ▣ 673
Dristan Decongestant/Antihistamine/ Analgesic Coated Caplets .... ▣ 749
Dristan Cold Nasal Decongestant/ Antihistamine/ Analgesic Coated Tablets 2419
Dristan Advanced Formula Decongestant/Antihistamine/ Analgesic Tablets .... ▣ 749
Dristan Nasal Spray, Menthol 2419
Dristan Nasal Spray, Regular and Regular with Metered Pump 2419
Entex Capsules 1623
Entex Liquid 1623
Sinus Excedrin Analgesic, Decongestant Tablets & Caplets 750
Extendryl 994
4-Way Fast Acting Nasal Spray - Original Formula (regular & mentholated) & Metered Spray Pump (regular) 751
Hycomine Compound Tablets 929
Murocoll-2 Sterile Ophthalmic Solution .... ⊙ 261
Mydfrin 2.5% .... ⊙ 224
Naldecon Syrup, Tablets, Pediatric Drops and Pediatric Syrup 709
Neo-Synephrine Hydrochloride 1% Carpuject 2063
Neo-Synephrine Hydrochloride 1% Injection 2063
Neo-Synephrine Hydrochloride (Ophthalmic) 2064
Neo-Synephrine .... ▣ 759
Nōstril Nasal Decongestant .... ▣ 520
Novahistine Elixir .... ▣ 596
Phenergan VC 2500
Phenergan VC with Codeine 2501
Prefrin Liquifilm Vasoconstrictor and Lubricant Eye Drops .... ⊙ 254
Prefrin-A .... ⊙ 255
Quelidrine Syrup 556
Relief Vasoconstrictor and Lubricant Eye Drops .... ⊙ 256
Robitussin Night Relief .... ▣ 677
Ru-Tuss with Hydrocodone 694
Ru-Tuss Tablets 693
Vasosulf .... ⊙ 279
Vicks Sinex .... ▣ 665
Zincfrin .... ⊙ 230

Protriptyline Hydrochloride (Severe, persistent hypertension). Products include:
Vivactil Tablets 1567

Selegiline Hydrochloride (Severe, persistent hypertension). Products include:
Eldepryl 2250

Tranylcypromine Sulfate (Severe, persistent hypertension). Products include:
Parnate Tablets 2222

Trimipramine Maleate (Severe, persistent hypertension). Products include:
Surmontil Capsules 2524

MAREZINE TABLETS

(Cyclizine Hydrochloride) .... ▣ 541
May interact with hypnotics and sedatives, tranquilizers, and certain other agents. Compounds in these categories include:

Alcohol (Increases drowsiness).

Alprazolam (Increases drowsiness). Products include:
Xanax Tablets 2367

Buspirone Hydrochloride (Increases drowsiness). Products include:
BuSpar 1401

Chlordiazepoxide (Increases drowsiness). Products include:
Libritabs Tablets 1930
Limbitrol 1933
Menrium Tablets 1934

Chlordiazepoxide Hydrochloride (Increases drowsiness). Products include:
Librax Capsules 1929
Librium Capsules 1931
Librium Injectable 1932

Chlorpromazine (Increases drowsiness). Products include:
Thorazine 2234

Chlorprothixene (Increases drowsiness). Products include:
Taractan Tablets 1920

Chlorprothixene Hydrochloride (Increases drowsiness). Products include:
Taractan 1920

Clorazepate Dipotassium (Increases drowsiness). Products include:
Tranxene 556

Diazepam (Increases drowsiness). Products include:
Valium Injectable 1937
Valium Tablets 1939
Valrelease Capsules 1923

Droperidol (Increases drowsiness). Products include:
Inapsine Injection 1140
Innovar Injection 1141

Estazolam (Increases drowsiness). Products include:
ProSom Tablets 554

Ethchlorvynol (Increases drowsiness). Products include:
Placidyl Capsules 553

Ethinamate (Increases drowsiness).
No products indexed under this heading.

Fluphenazine Decanoate (Increases drowsiness). Products include:
Prolixin Decanoate 1795

Fluphenazine Enanthate (Increases drowsiness). Products include:
Prolixin Enanthate ... 1796

Fluphenazine Hydrochloride (Increases drowsiness). Products include:
Prolixin Elixir ... 1793
Prolixin Injection ... 1791
Prolixin Oral Concentrate ... 1792
Prolixin Tablets ... 1793

Flurazepam Hydrochloride (Increases drowsiness). Products include:
Dalmane Capsules ... 1927

Glutethimide (Increases drowsiness).
No products indexed under this heading.

Haloperidol (Increases drowsiness). Products include:
Haldol Injection, Tablets and Concentrate ... 1373

Haloperidol Decanoate (Increases drowsiness). Products include:
Haldol Decanoate ... 1375

Hydroxyzine Hydrochloride (Increases drowsiness). Products include:
Atarax Tablets & Syrup ... 1941
Marax Tablets & DF Syrup ... 1954
Vistaril Intramuscular Solution ... 1970

Lorazepam (Increases drowsiness). Products include:
Ativan Injection ... 2432
Ativan Tablets ... 2434

Loxapine Hydrochloride (Increases drowsiness). Products include:
Loxitane ... 1213

Loxapine Succinate (Increases drowsiness). Products include:
Loxitane Capsules ... 1213

Meprobamate (Increases drowsiness). Products include:
Deprol Tablets ... 2382
Equagesic Tablets ... 2451
Miltown Tablets ... 2386
PMB 200 and PMB 400 ... 2504

Mesoridazine (Increases drowsiness). Products include:
Serentil ... 686

Midazolam Hydrochloride (Increases drowsiness). Products include:
Versed Injection ... 1924

Molindone Hydrochloride (Increases drowsiness). Products include:
Moban Tablets & Concentrate ... 932

Oxazepam (Increases drowsiness). Products include:
Serax Capsules ... 2522
Serax Tablets ... 2522

Perphenazine (Increases drowsiness). Products include:
Etrafon ... 2087
Triavil Tablets ... 1556
Trilafon ... 2123

Prazepam (Increases drowsiness). Products include:
Centrax ... 1693

Prochlorperazine (Increases drowsiness). Products include:
Compazine ... 2201

Promethazine Hydrochloride (Increases drowsiness). Products include:
Mepergan Injection ... 2479
Phenergan with Codeine ... 2497
Phenergan with Dextromethorphan 2499
Phenergan Injection ... 2493
Phenergan Suppositories ... 2496
Phenergan Syrup ... 2495
Phenergan Tablets ... 2496
Phenergan VC ... 2500
Phenergan VC with Codeine ... 2501

Propofol (Increases drowsiness). Products include:
Diprivan Injection ... 2267

Quazepam (Increases drowsiness). Products include:
Doral Tablets ... 2383

Secobarbital Sodium (Increases drowsiness). Products include:
Seconal Sodium Pulvules ... 1296

Temazepam (Increases drowsiness). Products include:
Restoril Capsules ... 2023

Thioridazine Hydrochloride (Increases drowsiness). Products include:
Mellaril ... 2011

Thiothixene (Increases drowsiness). Products include:
Navane Capsules and Concentrate 1954
Navane Intramuscular ... 1956

Triazolam (Increases drowsiness). Products include:
Halcion Tablets ... 2340

Trifluoperazine Hydrochloride (Increases drowsiness). Products include:
Stelazine ... 2226

MARINOL (DRONABINOL) CAPSULES
(Dronabinol) ... 1985
May interact with barbiturates, hypnotics and sedatives, and certain other agents. Compounds in these categories include:

Alcohol (Absorption of alcohol delayed; additive CNS depression; avoid combination).

Aprobarbital (Additive CNS depression). Products include:
Alurate Elixir ... 1883

Butabarbital (Additive CNS depression). Products include:
Pyridium Plus ... 1764

Butalbital (Additive CNS depression). Products include:
Esgic-Plus Tablets ... 1002
Esgic Tablets & Capsules ... 1001
Fioricet Tablets ... 2006
Fiorinal Capsules ... 2007
Fiorinal with Codeine Capsules ... 2008
Fiorinal Tablets ... 2007
Phrenilin ... 838
Sedapap Tablets 50 mg/650 mg .. 1360

Estazolam (Marinol should not be taken concurrently). Products include:
ProSom Tablets ... 554

Ethchlorvynol (Marinol should not be taken concurrently). Products include:
Placidyl Capsules ... 553

Ethinamate (Marinol should not be taken concurrently).
No products indexed under this heading.

Flurazepam Hydrochloride (Marinol should not be taken concurrently). Products include:
Dalmane Capsules ... 1927

Glutethimide (Marinol should not be taken concurrently).
No products indexed under this heading.

Lorazepam (Marinol should not be taken concurrently). Products include:
Ativan Injection ... 2432
Ativan Tablets ... 2434

Mephobarbital (Additive CNS depression). Products include:
Mebaral Tablets ... 2061

Midazolam Hydrochloride (Marinol should not be taken concurrently). Products include:
Versed Injection ... 1924

Pentobarbital Sodium (Additive CNS depression). Products include:
Nembutal Sodium Capsules ... 534
Nembutal Sodium Solution ... 536
Nembutal Sodium Suppositories ... 538

Phenobarbital (Additive CNS depression). Products include:
Arco-Lase Plus Tablets ... 607
Bellergal-S Tablets ... 1998
Bronkolixir ... ▣ 761
Bronkotabs Tablets ... ▣ 762
Donnatal ... 1858
Donnatal Extentabs ... 1859
Donnatal Tablets ... 1858
Donnazyme Tablets ... 1860
Kinesed Tablets ... 2272
Phenobarbital Elixir and Tablets ... 1293
Primatene Tablets-P Formula ... 2421
Quadrinal Tablets ... 1183
Tedral SA ... 1765

Propofol (Marinol should not be taken concurrently). Products include:
Diprivan Injection ... 2267

Quazepam (Marinol should not be taken concurrently). Products include:
Doral Tablets ... 2383

Secobarbital Sodium (Additive CNS depression). Products include:
Seconal Sodium Pulvules ... 1296

Temazepam (Marinol should not be taken concurrently). Products include:
Restoril Capsules ... 2023

Thiamylal Sodium (Additive CNS depression). Products include:
Surital Ampoules, Steri-Vials ... 1764

Triazolam (Marinol should not be taken concurrently). Products include:
Halcion Tablets ... 2340

MARLYN FORMULA 50 CAPSULES
(Amino Acid Preparations, Vitamin B_6) ... 1356
No interactions described in labeling.

MARLYN FORMULA 50 MEGA FORTE CAPSULES
(Nutritional Supplement) ... 1356
No interactions described in labeling.

MARPLAN TABLETS
(Isocarboxazid) ... 1906
May interact with psychotropics, barbiturates, dibenzazepines, sympathomimetic aerosal brochodilators, antihypertensives, narcotic analgesics, monoamine oxidase inhibitors, and certain other agents. Compounds in these categories include:

Acebutolol Hydrochloride (Hypotension may result). Products include:
Sectral Capsules ... 2520

Albuterol (Hypertensive crisis). Products include:
Proventil Inhalation Aerosol ... 2117
Ventolin Inhalation Aerosol and Refill ... 583

Albuterol Sulfate (Hypertensive crisis). Products include:
Proventil Repetabs Tablets ... 2120
Proventil Solutions for Inhalation 0.5% and 0.083% ... 2118
Proventil Syrup ... 2119
Proventil Tablets ... 2120
Ventolin ... 583

Alcohol (Concomitant use contraindicated).

Alfentanil Hydrochloride (Concomitant use contraindicated). Products include:
Alfenta Injection ... 1131

Alprazolam (Concomitant use is not recommended). Products include:
Xanax Tablets ... 2367

Amitriptyline Hydrochloride (Hypertensive crisis). Products include:
Elavil ... 2269
Endep Tablets ... 1927
Etrafon ... 2087
Limbitrol ... 1933
Triavil Tablets ... 1556

Amoxapine (Hypertensive crisis). Products include:
Asendin Tablets ... 1196

Aprobarbital (When given concomitantly, dosage should be reduced). Products include:
Alurate Elixir ... 1883

Atenolol (Hypotension may result). Products include:
Tenoretic Tablets ... 1105
Tenormin Tablets and I.V. Injection 1107

Benazepril Hydrochloride (Hypotension may result). Products include:
Lotensin Tablets ... 872

Bendroflumethiazide (Hypotension may result). Products include:
Corzide Tablets ... 702
Naturetin Tablets ... 1789
Rauzide Tablets ... 1804

Betaxolol Hydrochloride (Hypotension may result). Products include:
Betoptic Sterile Ophthalmic Solution ... 569
Betoptic S Sterile Ophthalmic Suspension ... 570
Kerlone Tablets ... 2172

Buprenorphine (Concomitant use contraindicated).
No products indexed under this heading.

Buspirone Hydrochloride (Concomitant use is not recommended). Products include:
BuSpar ... 1401

Butabarbital (When given concomitantly, dosage should be reduced). Products include:
Pyridium Plus ... 1764

Butalbital (When given concomitantly, dosage should be reduced). Products include:
Esgic-Plus Tablets ... 1002
Esgic Tablets & Capsules ... 1001
Fioricet Tablets ... 2006
Fiorinal Capsules ... 2007
Fiorinal with Codeine Capsules ... 2008
Fiorinal Tablets ... 2007
Phrenilin ... 838
Sedapap Tablets 50 mg/650 mg .. 1360

Caffeine (Excessive amounts may cause hypertensive crisis). Products include:
Anacin Coated Analgesic Caplets ... 2417
Anacin Coated Analgesic Tablets ... 2417
Anacin Maximum Strength Analgesic Coated Tablets ... 2417
Cafergot/Cafergot P-B ... 1999
Esgic-Plus Tablets ... 1002
Esgic Tablets & Capsules ... 1001
Aspirin Free Excedrin Analgesic Caplets ... 748
Excedrin Extra-Strength Analgesic Tablets & Caplets ... 749
Fioricet Tablets ... 2006
Fiorinal Capsules ... 2007
Fiorinal with Codeine Capsules ... 2008
Fiorinal Tablets ... 2007
No Doz Fast Acting Alertness Aid Tablets ... 751
No Doz Maximum Strength Caplets 751
Norgesic ... 1314
P-A-C Analgesic Tablets ... ▣ 669
Synalgos-DC Capsules ... 2525
Vanquish Analgesic Caplets ... ▣ 574
Vivarin Stimulant Tablets ... ▣ 726
Wigraine Tablets & Suppositories .. 1645

Caffeine-containing medications (Concurrent use with caffeine

in excessive amounts should be avoided).

Captopril (Hypotension may result). Products include:
- Capoten ... 2255
- Capozide ... 2258

Carbamazepine (Hypertensive crisis). Products include:
- Tegretol Chewable Tablets ... 654
- Tegretol Suspension ... 656
- Tegretol Tablets ... 654

Carteolol Hydrochloride (Hypotension may result). Products include:
- Cartrol Tablets ... 507

Chlordiazepoxide (Concomitant use is not recommended). Products include:
- Libritabs Tablets ... 1930
- Limbitrol ... 1933
- Menrium Tablets ... 1934

Chlordiazepoxide Hydrochloride (Concomitant use is not recommended). Products include:
- Librax Capsules ... 1929
- Librium Capsules ... 1931
- Librium Injectable ... 1932

Chlorothiazide (Hypotension may result). Products include:
- Aldoclor Tablets ... 1413
- Diupres Tablets ... 1461
- Diuril Oral ... 1464

Chlorothiazide Sodium (Hypotension may result). Products include:
- Diuril Sodium Intravenous ... 1463

Chlorpromazine (Concomitant use is not recommended). Products include:
- Thorazine ... 2234

Chlorprothixene (Concomitant use is not recommended). Products include:
- Taractan Tablets ... 1920

Chlorprothixene Hydrochloride (Concomitant use is not recommended). Products include:
- Taractan ... 1920

Chlorthalidone (Hypotension may result). Products include:
- Combipres Tablets ... 678
- Tenoretic Tablets ... 1105
- Thalitone Tablets ... 687

Clomipramine Hydrochloride (Hypertensive crisis). Products include:
- Anafranil Capsules ... 650

Clonidine (Hypotension may result). Products include:
- Catapres-TTS ... 677

Clonidine Hydrochloride (Hypotension may result). Products include:
- Catapres Tablets ... 676
- Combipres Tablets ... 678

Clorazepate Dipotassium (Concomitant use is not recommended). Products include:
- Tranxene ... 556

Clozapine (Hypertensive crisis). Products include:
- Clozaril Tablets ... 2000

Cocaine Hydrochloride (Concomitant use is not recommended). Products include:
- Cocaine Hydrochloride Topical Solution ... 620

Codeine (Concomitant use contraindicated). Products include:
- Calcidrine Syrup ... 506

Codeine Phosphate (Concomitant use contraindicated). Products include:
- Actifed with Codeine Cough Syrup.. 752
- Cheracol Cough Syrup ... 1853
- Codimal PH Syrup ... 846
- Dimetane-DC Cough Syrup ... 1857
- Empirin with Codeine Phosphate Nos. 2, 3 & 4 ... 764
- Fiorinal with Codeine Capsules ... 2008
- Isoclor Expectorant ... 982
- Naldecon CX Adult Liquid ... ■ 521
- Novahistine DH ... 1342
- Novahistine Expectorant ... 1343
- Nucofed Capsules ... 2219
- Nucofed Expectorant ... 2219
- Nucofed Pediatric Expectorant ... 2220
- Nucofed Syrup ... 2219
- Phenaphen with Codeine Capsules 1865
- Phenaphen-650 with Codeine Tablets ... 1866
- Phenergan with Codeine ... 2497
- Phenergan VC with Codeine ... 2501
- Robitussin A-C Syrup ... 1875
- Robitussin-DAC Syrup ... 1875
- Ryna ... ■ 741
- Soma Compound w/Codeine Tablets ... 2390
- Triaminic Expectorant w/Codeine .. 1996
- Tussi-Organidin Liquid ... 2391
- Tylenol with Codeine ... 1381

Codeine Polistirex (Concomitant use contraindicated).
- No products indexed under this heading.

Cyclobenzaprine Hydrochloride (Hypertensive crisis). Products include:
- Flexeril Tablets ... 1471

Deserpidine (Hypotension may result). Products include:
- Enduronyl ... 518
- Harmonyl Tablets ... 528
- Oreticyl ... 545

Desipramine Hydrochloride (Hypertensive crisis). Products include:
- Norpramin Tablets ... 1340

Dextroamphetamine (Hypertensive crisis). Products include:
- Biphetamine Capsules ... 973

Dextroamphetamine Saccharate (Hypertensive crisis).
- No products indexed under this heading.

Dextroamphetamine Sulfate (Hypertensive crisis). Products include:
- Dexedrine ... 2206

Dextromethorphan Hydrobromide (May cause brief episodes of psychosis or bizarre behavior). Products include:
- Benylin DM ... ■ 638
- Benylin Expectorant ... ■ 638
- Cerose-DM ... 2443
- Cheracol D Cough Formula ... ■ 667
- Cheracol Plus Head Cold/Cough Formula ... ■ 667
- Codimal DM Syrup ... 846
- Cough Formula Comtrex ... 746
- Comtrex Multi-Symptom Cold Reliever Tablets/Caplets/Liqui-Gels/Liquid ... 745
- Day-Night Comtrex ... 747
- Non-Drowsy Comtrex ... 747
- Contac Cough Formula ... ■ 711
- Contac Cough & Sore Throat Formula ... ■ 712
- Contac Jr. Children's Cold Medicine ... ■ 712
- Contac Nighttime Cold Medicine ... ■ 713
- Contac Severe Cold and Flu Formula Caplets ... ■ 711
- Dimacol Caplets ... ■ 672
- Dimetane-DX Cough Syrup ... 1858
- Dimetapp DM Elixir ... ■ 674
- Dorcol Children's Cough Syrup ... ■ 685
- Hold Cough Suppressant Lozenge ■ 617
- Humibid DM Tablets ... 560
- Medi-Flu Caplet, Liquid ... ■ 640
- Naldecon DX Adult Liquid ... ■ 521
- Naldecon DX Children's Syrup ... ■ 522
- Naldecon DX Pediatric Drops ... ■ 522
- Naldecon Senior DX Cough/Cold Liquid ... ■ 523
- Novahistine DMX ... ■ 595
- Orthoxicol Cough Syrup ... ■ 668
- PediaCare Cough-Cold Formula Liquid ... 1362
- PediaCare Night Rest Cough-Cold Formula Liquid ... 1362
- PediaCare 6-12 Cough-Cold Formula Chewable Tablets ... 1362
- Phenergan with Dextromethorphan 2499
- Quelidrine Syrup ... 556
- Robitussin Cough Calmers ... ■ 677
- Robitussin Night Relief ... ■ 677
- Robitussin Pediatric ... ■ 678
- Robitussin-CF ... ■ 676
- Robitussin-DM ... ■ 676
- Rondec-DM ... 1976
- St. Joseph Cough Suppressant for Children ... ■ 705
- St. Joseph Nighttime Cold Medicine ... ■ 705
- Sucrets Cough Control Formula ... ■ 724
- Sudafed Cough Syrup ... ■ 543
- Triaminic Nite Light ... ■ 689
- Triaminic-DM Syrup ... ■ 689
- Triaminicol Multi-Symptom Cold Tablets ... ■ 691
- Triaminicol Multi-Symptom Relief ■ 691
- Tussi-Organidin DM Liquid ... 2392
- Tylenol Cold & Flu Hot Medication, Packets ... 1369
- Tylenol Cold & Flu No Drowsiness Hot Medication, Packets ... 1371
- Tylenol Cold Medication Caplets and Tablets ... 1370
- Tylenol Cold Medication No Drowsiness Formula Caplets ... 1370
- Tylenol Cold Night Time Medication Liquid ... 1371
- Tylenol Cough Medication Liquid, Maximum Strength ... 1372
- Tylenol Cough Medication Liquid with Decongestant, Maximum Strength ... 1372
- Vicks Children's Cough Syrup ... ■ 660
- Vicks Children's NyQuil ... ■ 664
- Vicks Cough Silencers Cough Drops ... ■ 660
- Vicks Daycare ... ■ 660
- Vicks Formula 44 Cough Control Discs ... ■ 661
- Vicks Formula 44 Cough Medicine ... ■ 661
- Vicks Formula 44D Decongestant Cough Medicine ... ■ 662
- Vicks Formula 44M Multi-Symptom Cough Medicine ... ■ 662
- Vicks NyQuil Nighttime Colds Medicine-Original & Cherry Flavor ... ■ 664
- Vicks Pediatric Formula 44 Cough Medicine ... ■ 662
- Vicks Pediatric Formula 44 Cough & Congestion Medicine ... ■ 663
- Vicks Pediatric Formula 44m Multi-Symptom Cough & Cold Medicine ... ■ 663

Dextromethorphan Polistirex (May cause brief episodes of psychosis or bizarre behavior). Products include:
- Delsym Cough Formula ... ■ 560

Dezocine (Concomitant use contraindicated).

Diazepam (Concomitant use is not recommended). Products include:
- Valium Injectable ... 1937
- Valium Tablets ... 1939
- Valrelease Capsules ... 1923

Diazoxide (Hypotension may result). Products include:
- Hyperstat I.V. Injection ... 2095
- Proglycem ... 649

Dobutamine Hydrochloride (Hypertensive crisis). Products include:
- Dobutrex Solution Vials ... 1259

Dopamine Hydrochloride (Hypertensive crisis). Products include:
- Intropin Injection ... 930

Doxazosin Mesylate (Hypotension may result). Products include:
- Cardura Tablets ... 1941

Doxepin Hydrochloride (Hypertensive crisis). Products include:
- Sinequan ... 1960

Droperidol (Concomitant use is not recommended). Products include:
- Inapsine Injection ... 1140
- Innovar Injection ... 1141

Enalapril Maleate (Hypotension may result). Products include:
- Vaseretic Tablets ... 1559
- Vasotec Tablets ... 1564

Enalaprilat (Hypotension may result). Products include:
- Vasotec I.V. ... 1562

Ephedrine Hydrochloride (Hypertensive crisis). Products include:
- Amesec ... ■ 682
- Primatene Tablets-M Formula ... 2421
- Primatene Tablets-P Formula ... 2421
- Primatene Tablets-Regular Formula ... 2421
- Quadrinal Tablets ... 1183
- Quelidrine Syrup ... 556
- Tedral SA ... 1765

Ephedrine Sulfate (Hypertensive crisis). Products include:
- Bronkaid Tablets ... ■ 757
- Bronkolixir ... ■ 761
- Bronkotabs Tablets ... ■ 762
- Marax Tablets & DF Syrup ... 1954
- Pazo Hemorrhoid Ointment & Suppositories ... 752
- Vicks Vatronol Nose Drops ... ■ 666

Ephedrine Tannate (Hypertensive crisis). Products include:
- Rynatuss ... 2388

Epinephrine (Hypertensive crisis). Products include:
- Ana-Kit Anaphylaxis Emergency Treatment Kit ... 1100
- Bronkaid Mist ... ■ 757
- EpiPen ... 843
- Marcaine Hydrochloride 0.5% with Epinephrine 1:200,000 (as bitartrate) ... 958
- Marcaine Hydrochloride with Epinephrine 1:200,000 ... 2055
- Primatene Mist ... 2420
- Sus-Phrine Injection ... 1006
- Xylocaine with Epinephrine Injections ... 637

Epinephrine Bitartrate (Hypertensive crisis). Products include:
- AsthmaHaler Mist Epinephrine Bitartrate Bronchodilator ... ■ 616
- Bronkaid Mist Suspension ... ■ 757
- Primatene Mist Suspension ... 2421

Epinephrine Hydrochloride (Hypertensive crisis). Products include:
- Adrenalin Chloride Solution 1:100 & 1:1,000 ... 1689
- Epifrin ... ⊙ 244
- Glaucon ... ⊙ 218

Esmolol Hydrochloride (Hypotension may result). Products include:
- Brevibloc Injection ... 942

Felodipine (Hypotension may result). Products include:
- Plendil Extended-Release Tablets ... 1526

Fentanyl (Concomitant use contraindicated). Products include:
- Duragesic Transdermal System ... 1133

Fentanyl Citrate (Concomitant use contraindicated). Products include:
- Innovar Injection ... 1141
- Sublimaze Injection ... 1146

Fluoxetine Hydrochloride (Potential for hyperthermia, hypertension, rigidity, myoclonus, and mental changes; concurrent or successive administration is contraindicated). Products include:
- Prozac Pulvules ... 920

Fluphenazine Decanoate (Concomitant use is not recommended). Products include:
- Prolixin Decanoate ... 1795

Fluphenazine Enanthate (Concomitant use is not recommended). Products include:
- Prolixin Enanthate ... 1796

Fluphenazine Hydrochloride (Concomitant use is not recommended). Products include:
- Prolixin Elixir ... 1793
- Prolixin Injection ... 1791
- Prolixin Oral Concentrate ... 1792
- Prolixin Tablets ... 1793

Fosinopril Sodium (Hypotension may result). Products include:
Monopril Tablets 1406

Furazolidone (Concomitant use is not recommended). Products include:
Furoxone 1855

Furosemide (Hypotension may result). Products include:
Lasix 1093

Guanabenz Acetate (Hypotension may result). Products include:
Wytensin Tablets 2542

Guanethidine Monosulfate (Hypotension may result). Products include:
Esimil Tablets 864
Ismelin Tablets 869

Haloperidol (Concomitant use is not recommended). Products include:
Haldol Injection, Tablets and Concentrate 1373

Haloperidol Decanoate (Concomitant use is not recommended). Products include:
Haldol Decanoate 1375

Hydralazine Hydrochloride (Hypotension may result). Products include:
Apresazide Capsules 854
Apresoline Hydrochloride Parenteral (Ampuls) 856
Apresoline Hydrochloride Tablets 855
Apresoline-Esidrix Tablets 857
Ser-Ap-Es Tablets 881
Serpasil-Apresoline Tablets 884

Hydrochlorothiazide (Hypotension may result). Products include:
Aldactazide 2150
Aldoril Tablets 1418
Apresazide Capsules 854
Apresoline-Esidrix Tablets 857
Capozide 2258
Dyazide Capsules 2208
Esidrix Tablets 863
Esimil Tablets 864
HydroDIURIL Tablets 1484
Hydropres Tablets 1485
Inderide Tablets 2463
Inderide LA Long Acting Capsules 2465
Lopressor HCT Tablets 1034
Maxzide 1215
Moduretic Tablets 1510
Normozide Tablets 2112
Oretic Tablets 544
Oreticyl 545
Prinzide Tablets 1540
Ser-Ap-Es Tablets 881
Serpasil-Esidrix Tablets 886
Timolide Tablets 1547
Trandate HCT Tablets 579
Vaseretic Tablets 1559
Zestoretic 2274

Hydrocodone Bitartrate (Concomitant use contraindicated). Products include:
Anexsia 5/500 Tablets 2196
Anexsia 7.5/650 Tablets 2197
Azdone Tablets 844
Codiclear DH Syrup 845
Codimal DH Syrup 846
Damason-P 1356
Hycodan Syrup, Tablets 927
Hycomine Compound Tablets 929
Hycomine Syrup 927
Hycotuss Expectorant Syrup 930
Hydrocet Capsules 835
Lortab ASA Tablets 2414
Lortab 2412
Ru-Tuss with Hydrocodone 694
Triaminic Expectorant DH 1995
Vicodin Tablets 1187
Vicodin ES Tablets 1189
Zydone Capsules 941

Hydrocodone Polistirex (Concomitant use contraindicated). Products include:
Tussionex Extended-Release Suspension 988

Hydroflumethiazide (Hypotension may result). Products include:
Diucardin Tablets 2450
Saluron 718
Salutensin/Salutensin-Demi 719

Hydroxyzine Hydrochloride (Concomitant use is not recommended). Products include:
Atarax Tablets & Syrup 1941
Marax Tablets & DF Syrup 1954
Vistaril Intramuscular Solution 1970

Imipramine Hydrochloride (Hypertensive crisis). Products include:
Tofranil Ampuls 1038
Tofranil Tablets 1039

Imipramine Pamoate (Hypertensive crisis). Products include:
Tofranil-PM Capsules 1041

Indapamide (Hypotension may result). Products include:
Lozol Tablets 1843

Isoproterenol Hydrochloride (Hypertensive crisis). Products include:
Isuprel Hydrochloride Injection 1:5000 2050
Isuprel Hydrochloride Mistometer 2051
Isuprel Hydrochloride Solution 1:200 & 1:100 2052
Norisodrine Aerotrol 540

Isradipine (Hypotension may result). Products include:
DynaCirc Capsules 2004

Labetalol Hydrochloride (Hypotension may result). Products include:
Normodyne Injection 2108
Normodyne Tablets 2110
Normozide Tablets 2112
Trandate HCT Tablets 579
Trandate Injection 577
Trandate Tablets 579

Levodopa (Hypertensive crisis). Products include:
Larodopa Tablets 1905
Sinemet Tablets 952
Sinemet CR Tablets 953

Levorphanol Tartrate (Concomitant use contraindicated). Products include:
Levo-Dromoran 1906

Lisinopril (Hypotension may result). Products include:
Prinivil Tablets 1538
Prinzide Tablets 1540
Zestoretic 2274
Zestril Tablets 2277

Lithium Carbonate (Concomitant use is not recommended). Products include:
Eskalith 2214
Lithane Tablets 1596
Lithium Carbonate Capsules & Tablets 1984
Lithobid Tablets 870

Lithium Citrate (Concomitant use is not recommended). Products include:
Cibalith-S 870

Lorazepam (Concomitant use is not recommended). Products include:
Ativan Injection 2432
Ativan Tablets 2434

Loxapine Hydrochloride (Concomitant use is not recommended). Products include:
Loxitane 1213

Maprotiline Hydrochloride (Hypertensive crisis). Products include:
Ludiomil Tablets 874

Mecamylamine Hydrochloride (Hypotension may result). Products include:
Inversine Tablets 1492

Meperidine Hydrochloride (May cause circulatory collapse; concomitant use contraindicated). Products include:
Demerol 2047
Mepergan Injection 2479

Mephobarbital (When given concomitantly, dosage should be reduced). Products include:
Mebaral Tablets 2061

Meprobamate (Concomitant use is not recommended). Products include:
Deprol Tablets 2382
Equagesic Tablets 2451
Miltown Tablets 2386
PMB 200 and PMB 400 2504

Mesoridazine (Concomitant use is not recommended). Products include:
Serentil 686

Metaproterenol Sulfate (Hypertensive crisis). Products include:
Alupent 674
Arm-a-Med Metaproterenol Sulfate Inhalation Solution, USP 617
Metaprel Inhalation Aerosol Bronchodilator 2014
Metaprel Inhalation Solution 2015
Metaprel 2015
Metaproterenol Sulfate Inhalation Solution, USP 912

Metaraminol Bitartrate (Hypertensive crisis). Products include:
Aramine Injection 1424

Methadone Hydrochloride (Concomitant use contraindicated). Products include:
Dolophine Hydrochloride Ampoules & Vials 1260
Dolophine Hydrochloride Tablets 1261
Methadone Hydrochloride Diskets 1284
Methadone Hydrochloride Oral Solution & Tablets 1987

Methoxamine Hydrochloride (Hypertensive crisis). Products include:
Vasoxyl Injection 819

Methyclothiazide (Hypotension may result). Products include:
Enduron Tablets 517
Enduronyl 518

Methyldopa (Hypertensive crisis; hypotension may result). Products include:
Aldoclor Tablets 1413
Aldomet Oral 1415
Aldoril Tablets 1418

Methyldopate Hydrochloride (Hypertensive crisis; hypotension may result). Products include:
Aldomet Ester HCl Injection 1417

Metolazone (Hypotension may result). Products include:
Diulo 2129
Mykrox ½ mg Tablets 984
Zaroxolyn Tablets 989

Metoprolol Tartrate (Hypotension may result). Products include:
Lopressor Ampuls 1032
Lopressor HCT Tablets 1034
Lopressor Tablets 1032

Metyrosine (Hypotension may result). Products include:
Demser Capsules 1460

Midazolam Hydrochloride (Concomitant use is not recommended). Products include:
Versed Injection 1924

Minoxidil (Hypotension may result). Products include:
Loniten Tablets 2346
Rogaine Topical Solution 2357

Molindone Hydrochloride (Concomitant use is not recommended). Products include:
Moban Tablets & Concentrate 932

Morphine Sulfate (Concomitant use contraindicated). Products include:
Astramorph/PF Injection, USP (Preservative-Free) 618
Duramorph 960
Infumorph 200 and Infumorph 500 Sterile Solutions 962
MS Contin Tablets 1814
MSIR 1817
Oramorph SR (Morphine Sulfate Sustained Release Tablets) 1988
Roxanol 1991

Nadolol (Hypotension may result). Products include:
Corgard Tablets 701
Corzide Tablets 702

Nicardipine Hydrochloride (Hypotension may result). Products include:
Cardene Capsules 2290

Nitroglycerin (Hypotension may result). Products include:
Deponit NTG Transdermal Delivery System 2143
Minitran Transdermal Delivery System 1312
Nitro-Bid Ointment 1339
Nitro-Bid Capsules 1338
Nitrodisc 2176
Nitro-Dur (nitroglycerin) Transdermal Infusion System 1164
Nitrogard Tablets 1004
Nitrolingual Spray 1846
Nitrostat Tablets 1743
Transderm-Nitro Transdermal Therapeutic System 2283

Norepinephrine Bitartrate (Hypertensive crisis). Products include:
Levophed Bitartrate Injection 2054

Nortriptyline Hydrochloride (Hypertensive crisis). Products include:
Pamelor 2019

Opium Alkaloids (Concomitant use contraindicated). Products include:
B & O No. 15A & No. 16A Supprettes 2395
Pantopon Injectable 1911

Oxazepam (Concomitant use is not recommended). Products include:
Serax Capsules 2522
Serax Tablets 2522

Oxycodone Hydrochloride (Concomitant use contraindicated). Products include:
Percocet Tablets 950
Percodan 951
Roxicodone Tablets, Oral Solution & Intensol (Oxycodone) 1992
Tylox Capsules 1382

Penbutolol Sulfate (Hypotension may result). Products include:
Levatol 1832

Pentobarbital Sodium (When given concomitantly, dosage should be reduced). Products include:
Nembutal Sodium Capsules 534
Nembutal Sodium Solution 536
Nembutal Sodium Suppositories 538

Perphenazine (Concomitant use is not recommended). Products include:
Etrafon 2087
Triavil Tablets 1556
Trilafon 2123

Phenelzine Sulfate (Concomitant use is not recommended). Products include:
Nardil 1742

Phenobarbital (When given concomitantly, dosage should be reduced). Products include:
Arco-Lase Plus Tablets 607
Bellergal-S Tablets 1998
Bronkolixir ▣ 761
Bronkotabs Tablets ▣ 762
Donnatal 1858
Donnatal Extentabs 1859
Donnatal Tablets 1858
Donnazyme Tablets 1860
Kinesed Tablets 2272
Phenobarbital Elixir and Tablets 1293
Primatene Tablets-P Formula 2421
Quadrinal Tablets 1183
Tedral SA 1765

Phenoxybenzamine Hydrochloride (Hypotension may result). Products include:
Dibenzyline Capsules 2207

Phentolamine Mesylate (Hypotension may result). Products include:

- Regitine ... 878

Phenylephrine Bitartrate (Hypertensive crisis).

- No products indexed under this heading.

Phenylephrine Hydrochloride (Hypertensive crisis). Products include:

- AK-Dilate Solution 2.5% and 10% ... ⊙ 203
- Atrohist Sprinkle Capsules ... 558
- Cerose-DM ... 2443
- Codimal ... 846
- Comhist LA Capsules ... 1618
- Congespirin For Children Aspirin Free Chewable Cold Tablets ... 748
- Cyclomydril ... ⊙ 216
- Deconsal Sprinkle Capsules ... 559
- Dimetane Decongestant ... ■ 673
- Dristan Decongestant/Antihistamine/ Analgesic Coated Caplets ... ■ 749
- Dristan Cold Nasal Decongestant/ Antihistamine/ Analgesic Coated Tablets ... 2419
- Dristan Advanced Formula Decongestant/Antihistamine/ Analgesic Tablets ... ■ 749
- Dristan Nasal Spray, Menthol ... 2419
- Dristan Nasal Spray, Regular and Regular with Metered Pump ... 2419
- Entex Capsules ... 1623
- Entex Liquid ... 1623
- Sinus Excedrin Analgesic, Decongestant Tablets & Caplets ... 750
- Extendryl ... 994
- 4-Way Fast Acting Nasal Spray - Original Formula (regular & mentholated) & Metered Spray Pump (regular) ... 751
- Hycomine Compound Tablets ... 929
- Murocoll-2 Sterile Ophthalmic Solution ... ⊙ 261
- Mydfrin 2.5% ... ⊙ 224
- Naldecon Syrup, Tablets, Pediatric Drops and Pediatric Syrup ... 709
- Neo-Synephrine Hydrochloride 1% Carpuject ... 2063
- Neo-Synephrine Hydrochloride 1% Injection ... 2063
- Neo-Synephrine Hydrochloride (Ophthalmic) ... 2064
- Neo-Synephrine ... ■ 759
- Nōstril Nasal Decongestant ... ■ 520
- Novahistine Elixir ... ■ 596
- Phenergan VC ... 2500
- Phenergan VC with Codeine ... 2501
- Prefrin Liquifilm Vasoconstrictor and Lubricant Eye Drops ... ⊙ 254
- Prefrin-A ... ⊙ 255
- Quelidrine Syrup ... 556
- Relief Vasoconstrictor and Lubricant Eye Drops ... ⊙ 256
- Robitussin Night Relief ... ■ 677
- Ru-Tuss with Hydrocodone ... 694
- Ru-Tuss Tablets ... 693
- Vasosulf ... ⊙ 279
- Vicks Sinex ... ■ 665
- Zincfrin ... ⊙ 230

Phenylephrine Tannate (Hypertensive crisis). Products include:

- Rynatan ... 2387
- Rynatuss ... 2388

Phenylpropanolamine Hydrochloride (Hypertensive crisis). Products include:

- A.R.M. Allergy Relief Medicine Caplets ... ■ 615
- Acutrim ... ■ 548
- Allerest ... ■ 559
- BC Cold Powder ... ■ 517
- Cheracol Plus Head Cold/Cough Formula ... ■ 667
- Codimal Expectorant ... 846
- Comtrex Multi-Symptom Cold Reliever Tablets/Caplets/Liqui-Gels/Liquid ... 745
- Contac Continuous Action Decongestant/Antihistamine Capsules ■ 710
- Contac Maximum Strength Continuous Action Decongestant/ Antihistamine Caplets ... ■ 709
- Contac Severe Cold and Flu Formula Caplets ... ■ 711
- Coricidin 'D' Decongestant Tablets ... ■ 695
- Coricidin Demilets Tablets for Children ... ■ 696
- Demazin Nasal Decongestant/ Antihistamine Repetabs Tablets & Syrup ... ■ 697
- Dexatrim ... ■ 733
- Dimetane-DC Cough Syrup ... 1857
- Dimetapp Elixir ... ■ 673
- Dimetapp DM Elixir ... ■ 674
- Dimetapp Extentabs ... ■ 674
- Dimetapp Plus Caplets ... ■ 675
- Dimetapp Tablets ... ■ 675
- Entex Capsules ... 1623
- Entex LA Tablets ... 1623
- Entex Liquid ... 1623
- 4-Way Cold Tablets ... 750
- Hycomine Syrup ... 927
- Naldecon CX Adult Liquid ... ■ 521
- Naldecon DX Adult Liquid ... ■ 521
- Naldecon DX Children's Syrup ... ■ 522
- Naldecon DX Pediatric Drops ... ■ 522
- Naldecon EX Children's Syrup ... ■ 522
- Naldecon EX Pediatric Drops ... ■ 523
- Naldecon Syrup, Tablets, Pediatric Drops and Pediatric Syrup ... 709
- Nolamine Tablets ... 838
- Nolex LA Tablets ... 838
- Ornade Spansule Capsules ... 2221
- Orthoxicol Cough Syrup ... ■ 668
- Propagest ... 839
- Pyrroxate Capsules ... ■ 669
- Robitussin-CF ... ■ 676
- Ru-Tuss II Capsules ... 693
- Ru-Tuss with Hydrocodone ... 694
- Ru-Tuss Tablets ... 693
- Sine-Off Sinus Medicine Tablets-Aspirin Formula ... ■ 722
- Sinulin ... 840
- St. Joseph Cold Tablets for Children ... ■ 704
- Tavist-D Tablets ... 2035
- Triaminic Allergy Tablets ... ■ 688
- Triaminic Chewables ... ■ 688
- Triaminic Cold Tablets ... ■ 688
- Triaminic Expectorant ... ■ 688
- Triaminic Expectorant w/Codeine ... 1996
- Triaminic Expectorant DH ... 1995
- Triaminic Oral Infant Drops ... 1996
- Triaminic Syrup ... ■ 689
- Triaminic-12 Tablets ... ■ 690
- Triaminic-DM Syrup ... ■ 689
- Triaminicin Tablets ... ■ 690
- Triaminicol Multi-Symptom Cold Tablets ... ■ 691
- Triaminicol Multi-Symptom Relief ■ 691
- Tuss-Ornade Liquid ... 2242
- Tuss-Ornade Spansule Capsules ... 2242
- Tylenol Cold Medication, Effervescent Tablets ... 1369

Pindolol (Hypotension may result). Products include:

- Visken Tablets ... 2036

Pirbuterol Acetate (Hypertensive crisis). Products include:

- Maxair Inhaler ... 1311

Polythiazide (Hypotension may result). Products include:

- Minizide Capsules ... 1779
- Renese Tablets ... 1785
- Renese-R Tablets ... 1786

Prazepam (Concomitant use is not recommended). Products include:

- Centrax ... 1693

Prazosin Hydrochloride (Hypotension may result). Products include:

- Minipress Capsules ... 1778
- Minizide Capsules ... 1779

Prochlorperazine (Concomitant use is not recommended). Products include:

- Compazine ... 2201

Promethazine Hydrochloride (Concomitant use is not recommended). Products include:

- Mepergan Injection ... 2479
- Phenergan with Codeine ... 2497
- Phenergan with Dextromethorphan 2499
- Phenergan Injection ... 2493
- Phenergan Suppositories ... 2496
- Phenergan Syrup ... 2495
- Phenergan Tablets ... 2496
- Phenergan VC ... 2500
- Phenergan VC with Codeine ... 2501

Propoxyphene Hydrochloride (Concomitant use contraindicated). Products include:

- Darvon ... 1256
- Wygesic Tablets ... 2540

Propoxyphene Napsylate (Concomitant use contraindicated). Products include:

- Darvon-N/Darvocet-N ... 1254

Propranolol Hydrochloride (Hypotension may result). Products include:

- Inderal ... 2459
- Inderal LA Long Acting Capsules ... 2461
- Inderide Tablets ... 2463
- Inderide LA Long Acting Capsules .. 2465

Protriptyline Hydrochloride (Hypertensive crisis). Products include:

- Vivactil Tablets ... 1567

Pseudoephedrine Hydrochloride (Hypertensive crisis). Products include:

- Actifed Capsules ... ■ 539
- Actifed Plus Caplets ... ■ 539
- Actifed Plus Tablets ... ■ 540
- Actifed with Codeine Cough Syrup .. 752
- Actifed Syrup ... ■ 540
- Actifed Tablets ... ■ 540
- Actifed 12-Hour Capsules ... ■ 539
- Advil Cold & Sinus Caplets (formerly CoAdvil) ... 2416
- Allerest ... ■ 559
- Anatuss LA Tablets ... 1359
- Benadryl Decongestant Elixir ... ■ 635
- Benadryl Decongestant ... ■ 635
- Benadryl Plus ... ■ 636
- Benadryl Plus Nighttime ... ■ 637
- Benylin Decongestant ... ■ 638
- Brexin L.A. Capsules ... 2078
- Bromfed Capsules (Timed Release) ... 1615
- Bromfed Syrup ... ■ 628
- Bromfed ... 1615
- CoAdvil ... ■ 748
- Allergy-Sinus Comtrex Multi-Symptom Allergy Sinus Formula Tablets & Caplets ... 746
- Cough Formula Comtrex ... 746
- Comtrex Multi-Symptom Cold Reliever Tablets/Caplets/Liqui-Gels/Liquid ... 745
- Day-Night Comtrex ... 747
- Non-Drowsy Comtrex ... 747
- Congess ... 994
- Congestac Caplets ... ■ 617
- Contac Jr. Children's Cold Medicine ... ■ 712
- Contac Nighttime Cold Medicine ... ■ 713
- Contac Sinus Caplets Maximum Strength Non-Drowsy Formula ... ■ 710
- Contac Sinus Tablets Maximum Strength Non-Drowsy Formula ... ■ 710
- Deconamine ... 663
- Deconsal II Tablets ... 559
- Dimacol Caplets ... ■ 672
- Dimetane-DX Cough Syrup ... 1858
- Dorcol Children's Cough Syrup ... ■ 685
- Dorcol Children's Decongestant Liquid ... ■ 685
- Dorcol Children's Liquid Cold Formula ... ■ 686
- Maximum Strength Dristan Decongestant/Analgesic Coated Caplets ... ■ 750
- No Drowsiness Dristan Cold Nasal Decongestant/Analgesic Coated Caplets ... 2420
- Dristan Sinus Caplets ... 2419
- Sinus Excedrin Analgesic, Decongestant Tablets & Caplets ... ■ 533
- Fedahist Gyrocaps ... 2145
- Fedahist Timecaps ... 2145
- Guaifed ... 1615
- Guaifed Syrup ... ■ 629
- Isoclor Expectorant ... 982
- Isoclor Timesule Capsules ... ■ 561
- Kronofed-A ... 970
- Medi-Flu Caplet, Liquid ... ■ 640
- Novafed A Capsules ... 1342
- Novafed Capsules ... 1342
- Novahistine DH ... 1342
- Novahistine DMX ... ■ 595
- Novahistine Expectorant ... 1343
- Nucofed Capsules ... 2219
- Nucofed Expectorant ... 2219
- Nucofed Pediatric Expectorant ... 2220
- Nucofed Syrup ... 2219
- Ornex Caplets ... ■ 618
- PediaCare Allergy Relief Formula Liquid ... 1362
- PediaCare Cough-Cold Formula Liquid ... 1362
- PediaCare Infants' Oral Decongestant Drops ... 1362
- PediaCare Night Rest Cough-Cold Formula Liquid ... 1362
- PediaCare 6-12 Cough-Cold Formula Chewable Tablets ... 1362
- Robitussin-DAC Syrup ... 1875
- Robitussin-PE ... ■ 677
- Rondec ... 1975
- Rondec-DM ... 1976
- Rondec-TR Tablet ... 1975
- Ru-Tuss DE Tablets ... 694
- Ryna ... ■ 741
- Seldane-D Extended-Release Tablets ... 1350
- Sinarest ... ■ 562
- Sine-Aid Maximum Strength Sinus Headache Caplets ... 1365
- Sine-Aid Maximum Strength Sinus Headache Tablets ... 1365
- Sine-Off Maximum Strength Allergy/Sinus Formula Caplets ... ■ 721
- Sine-Off Maximum Strength No Drowsiness Formula Caplets ... ■ 722
- Singlet Tablets ... ■ 598
- Sinutab Maximum Strength ... ■ 641
- Sinutab Maximum Strength Without Drowsiness Tablets & Caplets ... ■ 642
- Sinutab Regular Strength Without Drowsiness Formula ... ■ 641
- St. Joseph Nighttime Cold Medicine ... ■ 705
- Sudafed Children's Liquid ... ■ 543
- Sudafed Cough Syrup ... ■ 543
- Sudafed Plus Liquid ... ■ 544
- Sudafed Plus Tablets ... ■ 545
- Sudafed Sinus Caplets ... ■ 545
- Sudafed Sinus Tablets ... ■ 545
- Sudafed Tablets, 30 mg ... ■ 544
- Sudafed Tablets, Adult Strength, 60 mg ... ■ 544
- Sudafed 12 Hour Capsules ... ■ 545
- TheraFlu Flu and Cold Medicine ... ■ 687
- Triaminic Nite Light ... ■ 689
- Tylenol Allergy Sinus Medication Caplets and Gelcaps, Maximum Strength ... 1372
- Children's Tylenol Cold Liquid Formula and Chewable Tablets ... 1368
- Tylenol Cold & Flu Hot Medication, Packets ... 1369
- Tylenol Cold & Flu No Drowsiness Hot Medication, Packets ... 1371
- Tylenol Cold Medication Caplets and Tablets ... 1370
- Tylenol Cold Medication No Drowsiness Formula Caplets ... 1370
- Tylenol Cold Night Time Medication Liquid ... 1371
- Tylenol Cough Medication Liquid with Decongestant, Maximum Strength ... 1372
- Tylenol, Maximum Strength, Sinus Medication Gelcaps, Caplets and Tablets ... 1373
- Ursinus Inlay-Tabs ... ■ 691
- Vicks Children's NyQuil ... ■ 664
- Vicks Daycare ... ■ 660
- Vicks Formula 44D Decongestant Cough Medicine ... ■ 662
- Vicks Formula 44M Multi-Symptom Cough Medicine ... ■ 662
- Vicks NyQuil Nighttime Colds Medicine-Original & Cherry Flavor ... ■ 664
- Vicks Pediatric Formula 44 Cough & Congestion Medicine ... ■ 663
- Vicks Pediatric Formula 44m Multi-Symptom Cough & Cold Medicine ... ■ 663

Pseudoephedrine Sulfate (Hypertensive crisis). Products include:

- Afrin Tablets ... ■ 693
- Chlor-Trimeton Decongestant ... ■ 694
- Disophrol Chronotab Sustained-Action Tablets ... ■ 698
- Drixoral Antihistamine/Nasal Decongestant Syrup ... ■ 698
- Drixoral Non-Drowsy Formula ... ■ 699
- Drixoral Plus Extended-Release Tablets ... ■ 699
- Drixoral Sinus ... ■ 700
- Drixoral Sustained-Action Tablets ■ 698

Sinutab Allergy Formula Sustained Action Tablets ▣ 640
Trinalin Repetabs Tablets 1170

Ramipril (Hypotension may result). Products include:
Altace Capsules 1086

Rauwolfia Serpentina (Hypotension may result). Products include:
Raudixin Tablets 1803
Rauzide Tablets 1804

Rescinnamine (Hypotension may result).
No products indexed under this heading.

Reserpine (Hypotension may result). Products include:
Diupres Tablets 1461
Hydromox R Tablets 1209
Hydropres Tablets 1485
Renese-R Tablets 1786
Salutensin/Salutensin-Demi 719
Ser-Ap-Es Tablets 881
Serpasil Tablets 883
Serpasil-Apresoline Tablets 884
Serpasil-Esidrix Tablets 886

Secobarbital Sodium (When given concomitantly, dosage should be reduced). Products include:
Seconal Sodium Pulvules 1296

Selegiline Hydrochloride (Concomitant use is not recommended). Products include:
Eldepryl 2250

Sodium Nitroprusside (Hypotension may result). Products include:
Nipride I.V. Infusion 1909

Sufentanil Citrate (Concomitant use contraindicated). Products include:
Sufenta Injection 1147

Terazosin Hydrochloride (Hypotension may result). Products include:
Hytrin Tablets 529

Terbutaline Sulfate (Hypertensive crisis). Products include:
Brethaire Inhaler 1024
Brethine Ampuls 1026
Brethine Tablets 1026
Bricanyl Injection 1324
Bricanyl Tablets 1325

Thiamylal Sodium (When given concomitantly, dosage should be reduced). Products include:
Surital Ampoules, Steri-Vials 1764

Thioridazine Hydrochloride (Concomitant use is not recommended). Products include:
Mellaril 2011

Thiothixene (Concomitant use is not recommended). Products include:
Navane Capsules and Concentrate 1954
Navane Intramuscular 1956

Timolol Maleate (Hypotension may result). Products include:
Blocadren Tablets 1429
Timolide Tablets 1547
Timoptic in Ocudose 1552
Timoptic Sterile Ophthalmic Solution 1550

Tranylcypromine Sulfate (Concomitant use is not recommended). Products include:
Parnate Tablets 2222

Trifluoperazine Hydrochloride (Concomitant use is not recommended). Products include:
Stelazine 2226

Trimethaphan Camsylate (Hypotension may result). Products include:
Arfonad Ampuls 1887

Trimipramine Maleate (Hypertensive crisis). Products include:
Surmontil Capsules 2524

Tyramine (Concomitant use contraindicated).

Food Interactions

Beans, broad (Hypertensive reactions).
Beer, alcohol-free (Hypertensive reactions).
Beer, reduced-alcohol (Hypertensive reactions).
Beer, unspecified (Hypertensive reactions).
Beverages, caffeine-containing (Hypertensive reactions).
Cheese, unspecified (Hypertensive reactions).
Food, caffeine containing (Hypertensive reactions).
Herring, pickled (Hypertensive reactions).
Liver, chicken (Hypertensive reactions).
Wine products (Hypertensive reactions).
Wine, unspecified (Hypertensive reactions).
Yeast extract (Hypertensive reactions).

MASSENGILL BABY POWDER SOFT CLOTH TOWELETTE AND UNSCENTED SOFT CLOTH TOWELETTE
(Cleanser) ▣ 717
No interactions described in labeling.

MASSENGILL DISPOSABLE DOUCHE
(Cleanser) 2191
No interactions described in labeling.

MASSENGILL FRAGRANCE-FREE SOFT CLOTH TOWELETTE
(Cleanser) 2192
No interactions described in labeling.

MASSENGILL LIQUID CONCENTRATE
(Cleanser) 2191
No interactions described in labeling.

MASSENGILL MEDICATED DISPOSABLE DOUCHE
(Povidone Iodine) 2192
No interactions described in labeling.

MASSENGILL MEDICATED LIQUID CONCENTRATE
(Povidone Iodine) 2192
No interactions described in labeling.

MASSENGILL MEDICATED SOFT CLOTH TOWELETTES
(Hydrocortisone) 2192
No interactions described in labeling.

MASSENGILL POWDER
(Povidone Iodine) 2191
No interactions described in labeling.

MATERNA TABLETS
(Vitamin Preparation With Folic Acid or its Derivatives) 1214
No interactions described in labeling.

MATULANE CAPSULES
(Procarbazine Hydrochloride) 1907
May interact with barbiturates, antihistamines, narcotic analgesics, phenothiazines, sympathomimetic aerosal brochodilators, tricyclic antidepressants, antihypertensives, and certain other agents. Compounds in these categories include:

Acebutolol Hydrochloride (Possible potentiation and increased CNS depression). Products include:
Sectral Capsules 2520

Albuterol (Avoided because of some maoi activity). Products include:
Proventil Inhalation Aerosol 2117
Ventolin Inhalation Aerosol and Refill 583

Albuterol Sulfate (Avoided). Products include:
Proventil Repetabs Tablets 2120
Proventil Solutions for Inhalation 0.5% and 0.083% 2118
Proventil Syrup 2119
Proventil Tablets 2120
Ventolin 583

Alcohol (May result in disulfiram-like reaction).

Alfentanil Hydrochloride (CNS depression). Products include:
Alfenta Injection 1131

Amitriptyline Hydrochloride (Avoid concurrent use). Products include:
Elavil 2269
Endep Tablets 1927
Etrafon 2087
Limbitrol 1933
Triavil Tablets 1556

Amoxapine (Avoid concurrent use). Products include:
Asendin Tablets 1196

Aprobarbital (CNS depression). Products include:
Alurate Elixir 1883

Astemizole (CNS depression). Products include:
Hismanal Tablets 1138

Atenolol (Possible potentiation and increased CNS depression). Products include:
Tenoretic Tablets 1105
Tenormin Tablets and I.V. Injection 1107

Azatadine Maleate (CNS depression). Products include:
Optimine Tablets 2115
Trinalin Repetabs Tablets 1170

Benazepril Hydrochloride (Possible potentiation and increased CNS depression). Products include:
Lotensin Tablets 872

Bendroflumethiazide (Possible potentiation and increased CNS depression). Products include:
Corzide Tablets 702
Naturetin Tablets 1789
Rauzide Tablets 1804

Betaxolol Hydrochloride (Possible potentiation and increased CNS depression). Products include:
Betoptic Sterile Ophthalmic Solution 569
Betoptic S Sterile Ophthalmic Suspension 570
Kerlone Tablets 2172

Bromodiphenhydramine Hydrochloride (CNS depression).
No products indexed under this heading.

Brompheniramine Maleate (CNS depression). Products include:
Alka Seltzer Plus Sinus Allergy Medicine ▣ 624
Atrohist Sprinkle Capsules 558
Bromfed Capsules (Timed Release) 1615
Bromfed Syrup ▣ 628
Bromfed 1615
Dimetane Decongestant ▣ 673
Dimetane ▣ 672
Dimetane-DC Cough Syrup 1857
Dimetane-DX Cough Syrup 1858
Dimetapp Elixir ▣ 673
Dimetapp DM Elixir ▣ 674
Dimetapp Extentabs ▣ 674
Dimetapp Plus Caplets ▣ 675
Dimetapp Tablets ▣ 675
Drixoral Antihistamine/Nasal Decongestant Syrup ▣ 698

Buprenorphine (CNS depression).
No products indexed under this heading.

Butabarbital (CNS depression). Products include:
Pyridium Plus 1764

Butalbital (CNS depression). Products include:
Esgic-Plus Tablets 1002
Esgic Tablets & Capsules 1001
Fioricet Tablets 2006
Fiorinal Capsules 2007
Fiorinal with Codeine Capsules 2008
Fiorinal Tablets 2007
Phrenilin 838
Sedapap Tablets 50 mg/650 mg 1360

Captopril (Possible potentiation and increased CNS depression). Products include:
Capoten 2255
Capozide 2258

Carteolol Hydrochloride (Possible potentiation and increased CNS depression). Products include:
Cartrol Tablets 507

Chlorothiazide (Possible potentiation and increased CNS depression). Products include:
Aldoclor Tablets 1413
Diupres Tablets 1461
Diuril Oral 1464

Chlorothiazide Sodium (Possible potentiation and increased CNS depression). Products include:
Diuril Sodium Intravenous 1463

Chlorpheniramine Maleate (CNS depression). Products include:
A.R.M. Allergy Relief Medicine Caplets ▣ 615
Alka-Seltzer Plus Cold Medicine ▣ 623
Allerest ▣ 559
Ana-Kit Anaphylaxis Emergency Treatment Kit 1100
BC Cold Powder Multi-Symptom Formula ▣ 517
Brexin L.A. Capsules 2078
Cerose-DM 2443
Cheracol Plus Head Cold/Cough Formula ▣ 667
Chlor-Trimeton Allergy Syrup, Tablets & Long-Acting Repetabs Tablets ▣ 693
Chlor-Trimeton Decongestant ▣ 694
Comhist LA Capsules 1618
Allergy-Sinus Comtrex Multi-Symptom Allergy Sinus Formula Tablets & Caplets 746
Comtrex Multi-Symptom Cold Reliever Tablets/Caplets/Liqui-Gels/Liquid 745
Day-Night Comtrex 747
Contac Continuous Action Decongestant/Antihistamine Capsules ▣ 710
Contac Maximum Strength Continuous Action Decongestant/Antihistamine Caplets ▣ 709
Contac Severe Cold and Flu Formula Caplets ▣ 711
Coricidin 'D' Decongestant Tablets ▣ 695
Coricidin Demilets Tablets for Children ▣ 696
Coricidin Tablets ▣ 695
Deconamine 663
Demazin Nasal Decongestant/Antihistamine Repetabs Tablets & Syrup ▣ 697
Dorcol Children's Liquid Cold Formula ▣ 686
Dristan Decongestant/Antihistamine/ Analgesic Coated Caplets ▣ 749
Dristan Cold Nasal Decongestant/ Antihistamine/ Analgesic Coated Tablets 2419
Dristan Advanced Formula Decongestant/Antihistamine/ Analgesic Tablets ▣ 749
Extendryl 994
4-Way Cold Tablets 750
Fedahist Gyrocaps 2145
Fedahist Timecaps 2145
Hycomine Compound Tablets 929
Isoclor Timesule Capsules ▣ 561
Kronofed-A 970

Medi-Flu Caplet, Liquid ▣ 640
Naldecon Syrup, Tablets, Pediatric Drops and Pediatric Syrup 709
Nolamine Tablets 838
Novafed A Capsules 1342
Novahistine DH 1342
Novahistine Elixir ▣ 596
Ornade Spansule Capsules 2221
Orthoxicol Cough Syrup ▣ 668
PediaCare Allergy Relief Formula Liquid 1362
PediaCare Cough-Cold Formula Liquid 1362
PediaCare Night Rest Cough-Cold Formula Liquid 1362
PediaCare 6-12 Cough-Cold Formula Chewable Tablets 1362
Pyrroxate Capsules ▣ 669
Quelidrine Syrup 556
Ru-Tuss II Capsules 693
Ru-Tuss Tablets 693
Ryna ▣ 741
Sinarest Tablets & Extra Strength Tablets ▣ 562
Sine-Off Maximum Strength Allergy/Sinus Formula Caplets ▣ 721
Sine-Off Sinus Medicine Tablets-Aspirin Formula ▣ 722
Singlet Tablets ▣ 598
Sinulin 840
Sinutab Maximum Strength ▣ 641
St. Joseph Nighttime Cold Medicine ▣ 705
Sudafed Plus Liquid ▣ 544
Sudafed Plus Tablets ▣ 545
Teldrin Timed-Release Allergy Capsules, 12 mg 2192
TheraFlu Flu and Cold Medicine ▣ 687
Triaminic Allergy Tablets ▣ 688
Triaminic Chewables ▣ 688
Triaminic Cold Tablets ▣ 688
Triaminic Nite Light ▣ 689
Triaminic Syrup ▣ 689
Triaminic-12 Tablets ▣ 690
Triaminicin Tablets ▣ 690
Triaminicol Multi-Symptom Cold Tablets ▣ 691
Triaminicol Multi-Symptom Relief ▣ 691
Tylenol Allergy Sinus Medication Caplets and Gelcaps, Maximum Strength 1372
Children's Tylenol Cold Liquid Formula and Chewable Tablets 1368
Tylenol Cold & Flu Hot Medication, Packets 1369
Tylenol Cold Medication Caplets and Tablets 1370
Tylenol Cold Medication, Effervescent Tablets 1369
Vicks Children's NyQuil ▣ 664
Vicks Formula 44 Cough Medicine ▣ 661
Vicks Formula 44M Multi-Symptom Cough Medicine ▣ 662
Vicks Pediatric Formula 44m Multi-Symptom Cough & Cold Medicine ▣ 663

Chlorpheniramine Polistirex (CNS depression). Products include:
Tussionex Extended-Release Suspension 988

Chlorpheniramine Tannate (CNS depression). Products include:
Rynatan 2387
Rynatuss 2388

Chlorpromazine (CNS depression). Products include:
Thorazine 2234

Chlorthalidone (Possible potentiation and increased CNS depression). Products include:
Combipres Tablets 678
Tenoretic Tablets 1105
Thalitone Tablets 687

Clemastine Fumarate (CNS depression). Products include:
Tavist Syrup 2033
Tavist Tablets 2035
Tavist-D Tablets 2035

Clomipramine Hydrochloride (Avoid concurrent use). Products include:
Anafranil Capsules 650

Clonidine (Possible potentiation and increased CNS depression). Products include:
Catapres-TTS 677

Clonidine Hydrochloride (Possible potentiation and increased CNS depression). Products include:
Catapres Tablets 676
Combipres Tablets 678

Codeine (CNS depression). Products include:
Calcidrine Syrup 506

Codeine Phosphate (CNS depression). Products include:
Actifed with Codeine Cough Syrup 752
Cheracol Cough Syrup 1853
Codimal PH Syrup 846
Dimetane-DC Cough Syrup 1857
Empirin with Codeine Phosphate Nos. 2, 3 & 4 764
Fiorinal with Codeine Capsules 2008
Isoclor Expectorant 982
Naldecon CX Adult Liquid ▣ 521
Novahistine DH 1342
Novahistine Expectorant 1343
Nucofed Capsules 2219
Nucofed Expectorant 2219
Nucofed Pediatric Expectorant 2220
Nucofed Syrup 2219
Phenaphen with Codeine Capsules 1865
Phenaphen-650 with Codeine Tablets 1866
Phenergan with Codeine 2497
Phenergan VC with Codeine 2501
Robitussin A-C Syrup 1875
Robitussin-DAC Syrup 1875
Ryna ▣ 741
Soma Compound w/Codeine Tablets 2390
Triaminic Expectorant w/Codeine 1996
Tussi-Organidin Liquid 2391
Tylenol with Codeine 1381

Codeine Polistirex (CNS depression).
No products indexed under this heading.

Cyproheptadine Hydrochloride (CNS depression). Products include:
Periactin 1525

Deserpidine (Possible potentiation and increased CNS depression). Products include:
Enduronyl 518
Harmonyl Tablets 528
Oreticyl 545

Desipramine Hydrochloride (Avoid concurrent use). Products include:
Norpramin Tablets 1340

Dexchlorpheniramine Maleate (CNS depression). Products include:
Polaramine 2116

Dezocine (CNS depression).

Diazoxide (Possible potentiation and increased CNS depression). Products include:
Hyperstat I.V. Injection 2095
Proglycem 649

Diphenhydramine Citrate (CNS depression). Products include:
Alka-Seltzer Plus Night-Time Cold Medicine ▣ 623
Bufferin AF Nite Time Analgesic/Sleeping Aid Caplets 744
Excedrin P.M. Analgesic/Sleeping Aid Tablets, Caplets and Liquid 749

Diphenhydramine Hydrochloride (CNS depression). Products include:
Benadryl Anti-Itch Cream ▣ 635
Benadryl Capsules 1691
Benadryl Decongestant Elixir ▣ 635
Benadryl Decongestant ▣ 635
Benadryl Elixir ▣ 636
Benadryl Kapseals 1691
Benadryl 25 Kapseals ▣ 636
Benadryl Parenteral 1692
Benadryl Plus ▣ 636
Benadryl Plus Nighttime ▣ 637
Benadryl Spray, Maximum Strength ▣ 637
Benadryl Spray, Regular Strength ▣ 637
Benadryl Steri-Vials, Ampoules, and Steri-Dose Syringe 1692
Benadryl 25 Tablets ▣ 636
Benylin Cough Syrup ▣ 637
Benylin Decongestant ▣ 638
Caladryl Cream, Lotion, Spray ▣ 638
Miles Nervine Nighttime Sleep-Aid ▣ 627
Nytol Tablets ▣ 517
Sleep-ettes-D Tablets ▣ 653
Sleep-eze 3 Tablets ▣ 755
Sleepinal Night-time Sleep Aid Capsules ▣ 734
Sominex Caplets and Tablets ▣ 722
Sominex Liquid ▣ 723
Sominex Pain Relief Formula ▣ 723
Tylenol Cold Night Time Medication Liquid 1371
Tylenol PM, Extra Strength Caplets and Tablets 1368
Unisom Dual Relief Nighttime Sleep Aid/Analgesic 1774
Ziradryl Lotion ▣ 643

Diphenylpyraline Hydrochloride (CNS depression).
No products indexed under this heading.

Dobutamine Hydrochloride (Avoid concurrent use). Products include:
Dobutrex Solution Vials 1259

Dopamine Hydrochloride (Avoid concurrent use). Products include:
Intropin Injection 930

Doxazosin Mesylate (Possible potentiation and increased CNS depression). Products include:
Cardura Tablets 1941

Doxepin Hydrochloride (Avoid concurrent use). Products include:
Sinequan 1960

Enalapril Maleate (Possible potentiation and increased CNS depression). Products include:
Vaseretic Tablets 1559
Vasotec Tablets 1564

Enalaprilat (Possible potentiation and increased CNS depression). Products include:
Vasotec I.V. 1562

Ephedrine Hydrochloride (Avoid concurrent use). Products include:
Amesec ▣ 682
Primatene Tablets-M Formula 2421
Primatene Tablets-P Formula 2421
Primatene Tablets-Regular Formula 2421
Quadrinal Tablets 1183
Quelidrine Syrup 556
Tedral SA 1765

Ephedrine Sulfate (Avoid concurrent use). Products include:
Bronkaid Tablets ▣ 757
Bronkolixir ▣ 761
Bronkotabs Tablets ▣ 762
Marax Tablets & DF Syrup 1954
Pazo Hemorrhoid Ointment & Suppositories 752
Vicks Vatronol Nose Drops ▣ 666

Ephedrine Tannate (Avoid concurrent use). Products include:
Rynatuss 2388

Epinephrine (Avoid concurrent use). Products include:
Ana-Kit Anaphylaxis Emergency Treatment Kit 1100
Bronkaid Mist ▣ 757
EpiPen 843
Marcaine Hydrochloride 0.5% with Epinephrine 1:200,000 (as bitartrate) 958
Marcaine Hydrochloride with Epinephrine 1:200,000 2055
Primatene Mist 2420
Sus-Phrine Injection 1006
Xylocaine with Epinephrine Injections 637

Epinephrine Bitartrate (Avoid concurrent use). Products include:
AsthmaHaler Mist Epinephrine Bitartrate Bronchodilator ▣ 616
Bronkaid Mist Suspension ▣ 757
Primatene Mist Suspension 2421

Epinephrine Hydrochloride (Avoid concurrent use). Products include:
Adrenalin Chloride Solution 1:100 & 1:1,000 1689
Epifrin ◉ 244
Glaucon ◉ 218

Esmolol Hydrochloride (Possible potentiation and increased CNS depression). Products include:
Brevibloc Injection 942

Felodipine (Possible potentiation and increased CNS depression). Products include:
Plendil Extended-Release Tablets 1526

Fentanyl (CNS depression). Products include:
Duragesic Transdermal System 1133

Fentanyl Citrate (CNS depression). Products include:
Innovar Injection 1141
Sublimaze Injection 1146

Fluphenazine Decanoate (CNS depression). Products include:
Prolixin Decanoate 1795

Fluphenazine Enanthate (CNS depression). Products include:
Prolixin Enanthate 1796

Fluphenazine Hydrochloride (CNS depression). Products include:
Prolixin Elixir 1793
Prolixin Injection 1791
Prolixin Oral Concentrate 1792
Prolixin Tablets 1793

Fosinopril Sodium (Possible potentiation and increased CNS depression). Products include:
Monopril Tablets 1406

Furosemide (Possible potentiation and increased CNS depression). Products include:
Lasix 1093

Guanabenz Acetate (Possible potentiation and increased CNS depression). Products include:
Wytensin Tablets 2542

Guanethidine Monosulfate (Possible potentiation and increased CNS depression). Products include:
Esimil Tablets 864
Ismelin Tablets 869

Hydralazine Hydrochloride (Possible potentiation and increased CNS depression). Products include:
Apresazide Capsules 854
Apresoline Hydrochloride Parenteral (Ampuls) 856
Apresoline Hydrochloride Tablets 855
Apresoline-Esidrix Tablets 857
Ser-Ap-Es Tablets 881
Serpasil-Apresoline Tablets 884

Hydrochlorothiazide (Possible potentiation and increased CNS depression). Products include:
Aldactazide 2150
Aldoril Tablets 1418
Apresazide Capsules 854
Apresoline-Esidrix Tablets 857
Capozide 2258
Dyazide Capsules 2208
Esidrix Tablets 863
Esimil Tablets 864
HydroDIURIL Tablets 1484
Hydropres Tablets 1485
Inderide Tablets 2463
Inderide LA Long Acting Capsules 2465
Lopressor HCT Tablets 1034
Maxzide 1215
Moduretic Tablets 1510
Normozide Tablets 2112
Oretic Tablets 544
Oreticyl 545
Prinzide Tablets 1540
Ser-Ap-Es Tablets 881
Serpasil-Esidrix Tablets 886
Timolide Tablets 1547
Trandate HCT Tablets 579
Vaseretic Tablets 1559
Zestoretic 2274

Hydrocodone Bitartrate (CNS depression). Products include:
Anexsia 5/500 Tablets 2196
Anexsia 7.5/650 Tablets 2197
Azdone Tablets 844
Codiclear DH Syrup 845
Codimal DH Syrup 846
Damason-P 1356
Hycodan Syrup, Tablets 927
Hycomine Compound Tablets 929
Hycomine Syrup 927

Hycotuss Expectorant Syrup 930
Hydrocet Capsules 835
Lortab ASA Tablets 2414
Lortab 2412
Ru-Tuss with Hydrocodone 694
Triaminic Expectorant DH 1995
Vicodin Tablets 1187
Vicodin ES Tablets 1189
Zydone Capsules 941

Hydrocodone Polistirex (CNS depression). Products include:
Tussionex Extended-Release Suspension 988

Hydroflumethiazide (Possible potentiation and increased CNS depression). Products include:
Diucardin Tablets 2450
Saluron 718
Salutensin/Salutensin-Demi 719

Imipramine Hydrochloride (Avoid concurrent use). Products include:
Tofranil Ampuls 1038
Tofranil Tablets 1039

Imipramine Pamoate (Avoid concurrent use). Products include:
Tofranil-PM Capsules 1041

Indapamide (Possible potentiation and increased CNS depression). Products include:
Lozol Tablets 1843

Isoproterenol Hydrochloride (Avoid concurrent use). Products include:
Isuprel Hydrochloride Injection 1:5000 2050
Isuprel Hydrochloride Mistometer .. 2051
Isuprel Hydrochloride Solution 1:200 & 1:100 2052
Norisodrine Aerotrol 540

Isradipine (Possible potentiation and increased CNS depression). Products include:
DynaCirc Capsules 2004

Labetalol Hydrochloride (Possible potentiation and increased CNS depression). Products include:
Normodyne Injection 2108
Normodyne Tablets 2110
Normozide Tablets 2112
Trandate HCT Tablets 579
Trandate Injection 577
Trandate Tablets 579

Levorphanol Tartrate (CNS depression). Products include:
Levo-Dromoran 1906

Lisinopril (Possible potentiation and increased CNS depression). Products include:
Prinivil Tablets 1538
Prinzide Tablets 1540
Zestoretic 2274
Zestril Tablets 2277

Maprotiline Hydrochloride (Avoid concurrent use). Products include:
Ludiomil Tablets 874

Mecamylamine Hydrochloride (Possible potentiation and increased CNS depression). Products include:
Inversine Tablets 1492

Meperidine Hydrochloride (CNS depression). Products include:
Demerol 2047
Mepergan Injection 2479

Mephobarbital (CNS depression). Products include:
Mebaral Tablets 2061

Mesoridazine (CNS depression). Products include:
Serentil 686

Metaproterenol Sulfate (Avoid concurrent use). Products include:
Alupent 674
Arm-a-Med Metaproterenol Sulfate Inhalation Solution, USP 617
Metaprel Inhalation Aerosol Bronchodilator 2014
Metaprel Inhalation Solution 2015
Metaprel 2015
Metaproterenol Sulfate Inhalation Solution, USP 912

Metaraminol Bitartrate (Avoid concurrent use). Products include:
Aramine Injection 1424

Methadone Hydrochloride (CNS depression). Products include:
Dolophine Hydrochloride Ampoules & Vials 1260
Dolophine Hydrochloride Tablets 1261
Methadone Hydrochloride Diskets .. 1284
Methadone Hydrochloride Oral Solution & Tablets 1987

Methdilazine Hydrochloride (CNS depression). Products include:
Tacaryl Syrup & Tablets 2409

Methoxamine Hydrochloride (Avoid concurrent use). Products include:
Vasoxyl Injection 819

Methyclothiazide (Possible potentiation and increased CNS depression). Products include:
Enduron Tablets 517
Enduronyl 518

Methyldopa (Possible potentiation and increased CNS depression). Products include:
Aldoclor Tablets 1413
Aldomet Oral 1415
Aldoril Tablets 1418

Methyldopate Hydrochloride (Possible potentiation and increased CNS depression). Products include:
Aldomet Ester HCl Injection 1417

Metolazone (Possible potentiation and increased CNS depression). Products include:
Diulo 2129
Mykrox ½ mg Tablets 984
Zaroxolyn Tablets 989

Metoprolol Tartrate (Possible potentiation and increased CNS depression). Products include:
Lopressor Ampuls 1032
Lopressor HCT Tablets 1034
Lopressor Tablets 1032

Metyrosine (Possible potentiation and increased CNS depression). Products include:
Demser Capsules 1460

Minoxidil (Possible potentiation and increased CNS depression). Products include:
Loniten Tablets 2346
Rogaine Topical Solution 2357

Morphine Sulfate (CNS depression). Products include:
Astramorph/PF Injection, USP (Preservative-Free) 618
Duramorph 960
Infumorph 200 and Infumorph 500 Sterile Solutions 962
MS Contin Tablets 1814
MSIR 1817
Oramorph SR (Morphine Sulfate Sustained Release Tablets) 1988
Roxanol 1991

Nadolol (Possible potentiation and increased CNS depression). Products include:
Corgard Tablets 701
Corzide Tablets 702

Nicardipine Hydrochloride (Possible potentiation and increased CNS depression). Products include:
Cardene Capsules 2290

Nitroglycerin (Possible potentiation and increased CNS depression). Products include:
Deponit NTG Transdermal Delivery System 2143
Minitran Transdermal Delivery System 1312
Nitro-Bid Ointment 1339
Nitro-Bid Capsules 1338
Nitrodisc 2176
Nitro-Dur (nitroglycerin) Transdermal Infusion System 1164
Nitrogard Tablets 1004
Nitrolingual Spray 1846
Nitrostat Tablets 1743
Transderm-Nitro Transdermal Therapeutic System 2283

Norepinephrine Bitartrate (Avoid concurrent use). Products include:
Levophed Bitartrate Injection 2054

Nortriptyline Hydrochloride (Avoid concurrent use). Products include:
Pamelor 2019

Opium Alkaloids (CNS depression). Products include:
B & O No. 15A & No. 16A Supprettes 2395
Pantopon Injectable 1911

Oxycodone Hydrochloride (CNS depression). Products include:
Percocet Tablets 950
Percodan 951
Roxicodone Tablets, Oral Solution & Intensol (Oxycodone) 1992
Tylox Capsules 1382

Penbutolol Sulfate (Possible potentiation and increased CNS depression). Products include:
Levatol 1832

Pentobarbital Sodium (CNS depression). Products include:
Nembutal Sodium Capsules 534
Nembutal Sodium Solution 536
Nembutal Sodium Suppositories 538

Perphenazine (CNS depression). Products include:
Etrafon 2087
Triavil Tablets 1556
Trilafon 2123

Phenobarbital (CNS depression). Products include:
Arco-Lase Plus Tablets 607
Bellergal-S Tablets 1998
Bronkolixir .... ▣ 761
Bronkotabs Tablets .... ▣ 762
Donnatal 1858
Donnatal Extentabs 1859
Donnatal Tablets 1858
Donnazyme Tablets 1860
Kinesed Tablets 2272
Phenobarbital Elixir and Tablets 1293
Primatene Tablets-P Formula 2421
Quadrinal Tablets 1183
Tedral SA 1765

Phenoxybenzamine Hydrochloride (Possible potentiation and increased CNS depression). Products include:
Dibenzyline Capsules 2207

Phentolamine Mesylate (Possible potentiation and increased CNS depression). Products include:
Regitine 878

Phenylephrine Bitartrate (Avoid concurrent use).
No products indexed under this heading.

Phenylephrine Hydrochloride (Avoid concurrent use). Products include:
AK-Dilate Solution 2.5% and 10% .... ⊙ 203
Atrohist Sprinkle Capsules 558
Cerose-DM 2443
Codimal 846
Comhist LA Capsules 1618
Congespirin For Children Aspirin Free Chewable Cold Tablets 748
Cyclomydril .... ⊙ 216
Deconsal Sprinkle Capsules 559
Dimetane Decongestant .... ▣ 673
Dristan Decongestant/Antihistamine/ Analgesic Coated Caplets .... ▣ 749
Dristan Cold Nasal Decongestant/ Antihistamine/ Analgesic Coated Tablets 2419
Dristan Advanced Formula Decongestant/Antihistamine/ Analgesic Tablets .... ▣ 749
Dristan Nasal Spray, Menthol 2419
Dristan Nasal Spray, Regular and Regular with Metered Pump 2419
Entex Capsules 1623
Entex Liquid 1623
Sinus Excedrin Analgesic, Decongestant Tablets & Caplets 750
Extendryl 994
4-Way Fast Acting Nasal Spray - Original Formula (regular & mentholated) & Metered Spray Pump (regular) 751
Hycomine Compound Tablets 929
Murocoll-2 Sterile Ophthalmic Solution .... ⊙ 261
Mydfrin 2.5% .... ⊙ 224
Naldecon Syrup, Tablets, Pediatric Drops and Pediatric Syrup 709
Neo-Synephrine Hydrochloride 1% Carpuject 2063
Neo-Synephrine Hydrochloride 1% Injection 2063
Neo-Synephrine Hydrochloride (Ophthalmic) 2064
Neo-Synephrine .... ▣ 759
Nōstril Nasal Decongestant .... ▣ 520
Novahistine Elixir .... ▣ 596
Phenergan VC 2500
Phenergan VC with Codeine 2501
Prefrin Liquifilm Vasoconstrictor and Lubricant Eye Drops .... ⊙ 254
Prefrin-A .... ⊙ 255
Quelidrine Syrup 556
Relief Vasoconstrictor and Lubricant Eye Drops .... ⊙ 256
Robitussin Night Relief .... ▣ 677
Ru-Tuss with Hydrocodone 694
Ru-Tuss Tablets 693
Vasosulf .... ⊙ 279
Vicks Sinex .... ▣ 665
Zincfrin .... ⊙ 230

Phenylephrine Tannate (Avoid concurrent use). Products include:
Rynatan 2387
Rynatuss 2388

Phenylpropanolamine Hydrochloride (Avoid concurrent use). Products include:
A.R.M. Allergy Relief Medicine Caplets .... ▣ 615
Acutrim .... ▣ 548
Allerest .... ▣ 559
BC Cold Powder .... ▣ 517
Cheracol Plus Head Cold/Cough Formula .... ▣ 667
Codimal Expectorant 846
Comtrex Multi-Symptom Cold Reliever Tablets/Caplets/Liqui-Gels/Liquid 745
Contac Continuous Action Decongestant/Antihistamine Capsules ▣ 710
Contac Maximum Strength Continuous Action Decongestant/ Antihistamine Caplets .... ▣ 709
Contac Severe Cold and Flu Formula Caplets .... ▣ 711
Coricidin 'D' Decongestant Tablets .... ▣ 695
Coricidin Demilets Tablets for Children .... ▣ 696
Demazin Nasal Decongestant/ Antihistamine Repetabs Tablets & Syrup .... ▣ 697
Dexatrim .... ▣ 733
Dimetane-DC Cough Syrup 1857
Dimetapp Elixir .... ▣ 673
Dimetapp DM Elixir .... ▣ 674
Dimetapp Extentabs .... ▣ 674
Dimetapp Plus Caplets .... ▣ 675
Dimetapp Tablets .... ▣ 675
Entex Capsules 1623
Entex LA Tablets 1623
Entex Liquid 1623
4-Way Cold Tablets 750
Hycomine Syrup 927
Naldecon CX Adult Liquid .... ▣ 521
Naldecon DX Adult Liquid .... ▣ 521
Naldecon DX Children's Syrup .... ▣ 522
Naldecon DX Pediatric Drops .... ▣ 522
Naldecon EX Children's Syrup .... ▣ 522
Naldecon EX Pediatric Drops .... ▣ 523
Naldecon Syrup, Tablets, Pediatric Drops and Pediatric Syrup 709
Nolamine Tablets 838
Nolex LA Tablets 838
Ornade Spansule Capsules 2221
Orthoxicol Cough Syrup .... ▣ 668
Propagest 839
Pyrroxate Capsules .... ▣ 669
Robitussin-CF .... ▣ 676
Ru-Tuss II Capsules 693
Ru-Tuss with Hydrocodone 694
Ru-Tuss Tablets 693
Sine-Off Sinus Medicine Tablets-Aspirin Formula .... ▣ 722
Sinulin 840
St. Joseph Cold Tablets for Children .... ▣ 704

- Tavist-D Tablets 2035
- Triaminic Allergy Tablets ▣ 688
- Triaminic Chewables ▣ 688
- Triaminic Cold Tablets ▣ 688
- Triaminic Expectorant ▣ 688
- Triaminic Expectorant w/Codeine 1996
- Triaminic Expectorant DH 1995
- Triaminic Oral Infant Drops 1996
- Triaminic Syrup ▣ 689
- Triaminic-12 Tablets ▣ 690
- Triaminic-DM Syrup ▣ 689
- Triaminicin Tablets ▣ 690
- Triaminicol Multi-Symptom Cold Tablets ▣ 691
- Triaminicol Multi-Symptom Relief ▣ 691
- Tuss-Ornade Liquid 2242
- Tuss-Ornade Spansule Capsules 2242
- Tylenol Cold Medication, Effervescent Tablets 1369

Pindolol (Possible potentiation and increased CNS depression). Products include:
- Visken Tablets 2036

Pirbuterol Acetate (Avoid concurrent use). Products include:
- Maxair Inhaler 1311

Polythiazide (Possible potentiation and increased CNS depression). Products include:
- Minizide Capsules 1779
- Renese Tablets 1785
- Renese-R Tablets 1786

Prazosin Hydrochloride (Possible potentiation and increased CNS depression). Products include:
- Minipress Capsules 1778
- Minizide Capsules 1779

Prochlorperazine (CNS depression). Products include:
- Compazine 2201

Promethazine Hydrochloride (CNS depression). Products include:
- Mepergan Injection 2479
- Phenergan with Codeine 2497
- Phenergan with Dextromethorphan 2499
- Phenergan Injection 2493
- Phenergan Suppositories 2496
- Phenergan Syrup 2495
- Phenergan Tablets 2496
- Phenergan VC 2500
- Phenergan VC with Codeine 2501

Propoxyphene Hydrochloride (CNS depression). Products include:
- Darvon 1256
- Wygesic Tablets 2540

Propoxyphene Napsylate (CNS depression). Products include:
- Darvon-N/Darvocet-N 1254

Propranolol Hydrochloride (Possible potentiation and increased CNS depression). Products include:
- Inderal 2459
- Inderal LA Long Acting Capsules 2461
- Inderide Tablets 2463
- Inderide LA Long Acting Capsules 2465

Protriptyline Hydrochloride (Avoid concurrent use). Products include:
- Vivactil Tablets 1567

Pseudoephedrine Hydrochloride (Avoid concurrent use). Products include:
- Actifed Capsules ▣ 539
- Actifed Plus Caplets ▣ 539
- Actifed Plus Tablets ▣ 540
- Actifed with Codeine Cough Syrup 752
- Actifed Syrup ▣ 540
- Actifed Tablets ▣ 540
- Actifed 12-Hour Capsules ▣ 539
- Advil Cold & Sinus Caplets (formerly CoAdvil) 2416
- Allerest ▣ 559
- Anatuss LA Tablets 1359
- Benadryl Decongestant Elixir ▣ 635
- Benadryl Decongestant ▣ 635
- Benadryl Plus ▣ 636
- Benadryl Plus Nighttime ▣ 637
- Benylin Decongestant ▣ 638
- Brexin L.A. Capsules 2078
- Bromfed Capsules (Timed Release) 1615
- Bromfed Syrup ▣ 628
- Bromfed 1615
- CoAdvil ▣ 748
- Allergy-Sinus Comtrex Multi-Symptom Allergy Sinus Formula Tablets & Caplets 746
- Cough Formula Comtrex 746
- Comtrex Multi-Symptom Cold Reliever Tablets/Caplets/Liqui-Gels/Liquid 745
- Day-Night Comtrex 747
- Non-Drowsy Comtrex 747
- Congess 994
- Congestac Caplets ▣ 617
- Contac Jr. Children's Cold Medicine ▣ 712
- Contac Nighttime Cold Medicine ▣ 713
- Contac Sinus Caplets Maximum Strength Non-Drowsy Formula ▣ 710
- Contac Sinus Tablets Maximum Strength Non-Drowsy Formula ▣ 710
- Deconamine 663
- Deconsal II Tablets 559
- Dimacol Caplets ▣ 672
- Dimetane-DX Cough Syrup 1858
- Dorcol Children's Cough Syrup ▣ 685
- Dorcol Children's Decongestant Liquid ▣ 685
- Dorcol Children's Liquid Cold Formula ▣ 686
- Maximum Strength Dristan Decongestant/Analgesic Coated Caplets ▣ 750
- No Drowsiness Dristan Cold Nasal Decongestant/Analgesic Coated Caplets 2420
- Dristan Sinus Caplets 2419
- Sinus Excedrin Analgesic, Decongestant Tablets & Caplets ▣ 533
- Fedahist Gyrocaps 2145
- Fedahist Timecaps 2145
- Guaifed 1615
- Guaifed Syrup ▣ 629
- Isoclor Expectorant 982
- Isoclor Timesule Capsules ▣ 561
- Kronofed-A 970
- Medi-Flu Caplet, Liquid ▣ 640
- Novafed A Capsules 1342
- Novafed Capsules 1342
- Novahistine DH 1342
- Novahistine DMX ▣ 595
- Novahistine Expectorant 1343
- Nucofed Capsules 2219
- Nucofed Expectorant 2219
- Nucofed Pediatric Expectorant 2220
- Nucofed Syrup 2219
- Ornex Caplets ▣ 618
- PediaCare Allergy Relief Formula Liquid 1362
- PediaCare Cough-Cold Formula Liquid 1362
- PediaCare Infants' Oral Decongestant Drops 1362
- PediaCare Night Rest Cough-Cold Formula Liquid 1362
- PediaCare 6-12 Cough-Cold Formula Chewable Tablets 1362
- Robitussin-DAC Syrup 1875
- Robitussin-PE ▣ 677
- Rondec 1975
- Rondec-DM 1976
- Rondec-TR Tablet 1975
- Ru-Tuss DE Tablets 694
- Ryna ▣ 741
- Seldane-D Extended-Release Tablets 1350
- Sinarest ▣ 562
- Sine-Aid Maximum Strength Sinus Headache Caplets 1365
- Sine-Aid Maximum Strength Sinus Headache Tablets 1365
- Sine-Off Maximum Strength Allergy/Sinus Formula Caplets ▣ 721
- Sine-Off Maximum Strength No Drowsiness Formula Caplets ▣ 722
- Singlet Tablets ▣ 598
- Sinutab Maximum Strength ▣ 641
- Sinutab Maximum Strength Without Drowsiness Tablets & Caplets ▣ 642
- Sinutab Regular Strength Without Drowsiness Formula ▣ 641
- St. Joseph Nighttime Cold Medicine ▣ 705
- Sudafed Children's Liquid ▣ 543
- Sudafed Cough Syrup ▣ 543
- Sudafed Plus Liquid ▣ 544
- Sudafed Plus Tablets ▣ 545
- Sudafed Sinus Caplets ▣ 545
- Sudafed Sinus Tablets ▣ 545
- Sudafed Tablets, 30 mg ▣ 544
- Sudafed Tablets, Adult Strength, 60 mg ▣ 544
- Sudafed 12 Hour Capsules ▣ 545
- TheraFlu Flu and Cold Medicine ▣ 687
- Triaminic Nite Light ▣ 689
- Tylenol Allergy Sinus Medication Caplets and Gelcaps, Maximum Strength 1372
- Children's Tylenol Cold Liquid Formula and Chewable Tablets 1368
- Tylenol Cold & Flu Hot Medication, Packets 1369
- Tylenol Cold & Flu No Drowsiness Hot Medication, Packets 1371
- Tylenol Cold Medication Caplets and Tablets 1370
- Tylenol Cold Medication No Drowsiness Formula Caplets 1370
- Tylenol Cold Night Time Medication Liquid 1371
- Tylenol Cough Medication Liquid with Decongestant, Maximum Strength 1372
- Tylenol, Maximum Strength, Sinus Medication Gelcaps, Caplets and Tablets 1373
- Ursinus Inlay-Tabs ▣ 691
- Vicks Children's NyQuil ▣ 664
- Vicks Daycare ▣ 660
- Vicks Formula 44D Decongestant Cough Medicine ▣ 662
- Vicks Formula 44M Multi-Symptom Cough Medicine ▣ 662
- Vicks NyQuil Nighttime Colds Medicine-Original & Cherry Flavor ▣ 664
- Vicks Pediatric Formula 44 Cough & Congestion Medicine ▣ 663
- Vicks Pediatric Formula 44m Multi-Symptom Cough & Cold Medicine ▣ 663

Pseudoephedrine Sulfate (Avoid concurrent use). Products include:
- Afrin Tablets ▣ 693
- Chlor-Trimeton Decongestant ▣ 694
- Disophrol Chronotab Sustained-Action Tablets ▣ 698
- Drixoral Antihistamine/Nasal Decongestant Syrup ▣ 698
- Drixoral Non-Drowsy Formula ▣ 699
- Drixoral Plus Extended-Release Tablets ▣ 699
- Drixoral Sinus ▣ 700
- Drixoral Sustained-Action Tablets ▣ 698
- Sinutab Allergy Formula Sustained Action Tablets ▣ 640
- Trinalin Repetabs Tablets 1170

Pyrilamine Maleate (CNS depression). Products include:
- Codimal 846
- 4-Way Fast Acting Nasal Spray - Original Formula (regular & mentholated) & Metered Spray Pump (regular) 751
- Maximum Strength Midol Multi-Symptom Menstrual Formula ▣ 571
- Maximum Strength Midol PMS Premenstrual Syndrome Formula ▣ 570
- Regular Strength Midol Multi-Symptom Menstrual Formula ▣ 570
- Prefrin-A ⊙ 255
- Prēmsyn PMS Capsules & Caplets ▣ 547
- Primatene Tablets-M Formula 2421
- Robitussin Night Relief ▣ 677
- Ru-Tuss with Hydrocodone 694
- Triaminic Expectorant DH 1995
- Triaminic Oral Infant Drops 1996

Pyrilamine Tannate (CNS depression). Products include:
- Rynatan 2387

Ramipril (Possible potentiation and increased CNS depression). Products include:
- Altace Capsules 1086

Rauwolfia Serpentina (Possible potentiation and increased CNS depression). Products include:
- Raudixin Tablets 1803
- Rauzide Tablets 1804

Rescinnamine (Possible potentiation and increased CNS depression).
- No products indexed under this heading.

Reserpine (Possible potentiation and increased CNS depression). Products include:
- Diupres Tablets 1461
- Hydromox R Tablets 1209
- Hydropres Tablets 1485
- Renese-R Tablets 1786
- Salutensin/Salutensin-Demi 719
- Ser-Ap-Es Tablets 881
- Serpasil Tablets 883
- Serpasil-Apresoline Tablets 884
- Serpasil-Esidrix Tablets 886

Secobarbital Sodium (CNS depression). Products include:
- Seconal Sodium Pulvules 1296

Sodium Nitroprusside (Possible potentiation and increased CNS depression). Products include:
- Nipride I.V. Infusion 1909

Sufentanil Citrate (CNS depression). Products include:
- Sufenta Injection 1147

Terazosin Hydrochloride (Possible potentiation and increased CNS depression). Products include:
- Hytrin Tablets 529

Terbutaline Sulfate (Avoid concurrent use). Products include:
- Brethaire Inhaler 1024
- Brethine Ampuls 1026
- Brethine Tablets 1026
- Bricanyl Injection 1324
- Bricanyl Tablets 1325

Terfenadine (CNS depression). Products include:
- Seldane Tablets 1349
- Seldane-D Extended-Release Tablets 1350

Thiamylal Sodium (CNS depression). Products include:
- Surital Ampoules, Steri-Vials 1764

Thioridazine Hydrochloride (CNS depression). Products include:
- Mellaril 2011

Timolol Maleate (Possible potentiation and increased CNS depression). Products include:
- Blocadren Tablets 1429
- Timolide Tablets 1547
- Timoptic in Ocudose 1552
- Timoptic Sterile Ophthalmic Solution 1550

Trifluoperazine Hydrochloride (CNS depression). Products include:
- Stelazine 2226

Trimeprazine Tartrate (CNS depression). Products include:
- Temaril Tablets, Syrup and Spansule Sustained Release Capsules 1085

Trimethaphan Camsylate (Possible potentiation and increased CNS depression). Products include:
- Arfonad Ampuls 1887

Trimipramine Maleate (Avoid concurrent use). Products include:
- Surmontil Capsules 2524

Tripelennamine Hydrochloride (CNS depression). Products include:
- PBZ Tablets & Elixir 1037
- PBZ-SR Tablets 1037

Triprolidine Hydrochloride (CNS depression). Products include:
- Actidil ▣ 538
- Actifed Capsules ▣ 539
- Actifed Plus Caplets ▣ 539
- Actifed Plus Tablets ▣ 540
- Actifed with Codeine Cough Syrup 752
- Actifed Syrup ▣ 540
- Actifed Tablets ▣ 540
- Actifed 12-Hour Capsules ▣ 539

Food Interactions

Bananas (Concurrent use should be avoided).

Cheese, aged (Concurrent use should be avoided).

Food with high concentration of tyramine (Concurrent use should be avoided).

Wine, unspecified (Concurrent use should be avoided).

Yogurt (Concurrent use should be avoided).

(▣ Described in PDR For Nonprescription Drugs) (⊙ Described in PDR For Ophthalmology)

MAXAIR INHALER
(Pirbuterol Acetate) 1311
May interact with monoamine oxidase inhibitors, tricyclic antidepressants, and sympathomimetic aerosal brochodilators. Compounds in these categories include:

Albuterol (Potential for additive effects). Products include:
Proventil Inhalation Aerosol 2117
Ventolin Inhalation Aerosol and Refill 583

Amitriptyline Hydrochloride (Action of pirbuterol on vascular system may be potentiated). Products include:
Elavil 2269
Endep Tablets 1927
Etrafon 2087
Limbitrol 1933
Triavil Tablets 1556

Amoxapine (Action of pirbuterol on vascular system may be potentiated). Products include:
Asendin Tablets 1196

Bitolterol Mesylate (Potential for additive effects). Products include:
Tornalate 2074

Clomipramine Hydrochloride (Action of pirbuterol on vascular system may be potentiated). Products include:
Anafranil Capsules 650

Desipramine Hydrochloride (Action of pirbuterol on vascular system may be potentiated). Products include:
Norpramin Tablets 1340

Doxepin Hydrochloride (Action of pirbuterol on vascular system may be potentiated). Products include:
Sinequan 1960

Furazolidone (Action of pirbuterol on vascular system may be potentiated). Products include:
Furoxone 1855

Imipramine Hydrochloride (Action of pirbuterol on vascular system may be potentiated). Products include:
Tofranil Ampuls 1038
Tofranil Tablets 1039

Imipramine Pamoate (Action of pirbuterol on vascular system may be potentiated). Products include:
Tofranil-PM Capsules 1041

Isocarboxazid (Action of pirbuterol on vascular system may be potentiated). Products include:
Marplan Tablets 1906

Isoetharine (Potential for additive effects). Products include:
Arm-a-Med Isoetharine Inhalation Solution, USP 616
Bronkometer Aerosol 2042
Bronkosol Solution 2042

Isoproterenol Hydrochloride (Potential for additive effects). Products include:
Isuprel Hydrochloride Injection 1:5000 2050
Isuprel Hydrochloride Mistometer .. 2051
Isuprel Hydrochloride Solution 1:200 & 1:100 2052
Norisodrine Aerotrol 540

Maprotiline Hydrochloride (Action of pirbuterol on vascular system may be potentiated). Products include:
Ludiomil Tablets 874

Metaproterenol Sulfate (Potential for additive effects). Products include:
Alupent 674
Arm-a-Med Metaproterenol Sulfate Inhalation Solution, USP 617
Metaprel Inhalation Aerosol Bronchodilator 2014
Metaprel Inhalation Solution 2015
Metaprel 2015
Metaproterenol Sulfate Inhalation Solution, USP 912

Nortriptyline Hydrochloride (Action of pirbuterol on vascular system may be potentiated). Products include:
Pamelor 2019

Phenelzine Sulfate (Action of pirbuterol on vascular system may be potentiated). Products include:
Nardil 1742

Protriptyline Hydrochloride (Action of pirbuterol on vascular system may be potentiated). Products include:
Vivactil Tablets 1567

Selegiline Hydrochloride (Action of pirbuterol on vascular system may be potentiated). Products include:
Eldepryl 2250

Terbutaline Sulfate (Potential for additive effects). Products include:
Brethaire Inhaler 1024
Brethine Ampuls 1026
Brethine Tablets 1026
Bricanyl Injection 1324
Bricanyl Tablets 1325

Tranylcypromine Sulfate (Action of pirbuterol on vascular system may be potentiated). Products include:
Parnate Tablets 2222

Trimipramine Maleate (Action of pirbuterol on vascular system may be potentiated). Products include:
Surmontil Capsules 2524

MAXAMAID XP BAR
(Dietary Supplement) 2150
No interactions described in labeling.

MAXIDEX STERILE OPHTHALMIC OINTMENT
(Dexamethasone Sodium Phosphate) .... ◉ 222
No interactions described in labeling.

MAXIDEX STERILE OPHTHALMIC SUSPENSION
(Dexamethasone) .... ◉ 223
No interactions described in labeling.

MAXITROL OPHTHALMIC OINTMENT/SUSPENSION
(Dexamethasone, Neomycin Sulfate, Polymyxin B Sulfate) .... ◉ 223
No interactions described in labeling.

MAXIVATE CREAM, LOTION & OINTMENT 0.05%
(Betamethasone Dipropionate) 2406
No interactions described in labeling.

MAXZIDE TABLETS
(Triamterene, Hydrochlorothiazide) .. 1215
May interact with lithium preparations, antihypertensives, non-steroidal anti-inflammatory agents, barbiturates, narcotic analgesics, ACE inhibitors, insulin, potassium sparing diuretics, cardiac glycosides, and certain other agents. Compounds in these categories include:

Acebutolol Hydrochloride (Potentiated). Products include:
Sectral Capsules 2520

Alcohol (May aggravate orthostatic hypotension).

Alfentanil Hydrochloride (May aggravate orthostatic hypotension). Products include:
Alfenta Injection 1131

Amiloride Hydrochloride (Contraindication). Products include:
Midamor Tablets 1508
Moduretic Tablets 1510

Aprobarbital (May aggravate orthostatic hypotension). Products include:
Alurate Elixir 1883

Atenolol (Potentiated). Products include:
Tenoretic Tablets 1105
Tenormin Tablets and I.V. Injection 1107

Benazepril Hydrochloride (Increased risk of hyperkalemia and antihypertensive effect potentiated). Products include:
Lotensin Tablets 872

Bendroflumethiazide (Potentiated). Products include:
Corzide Tablets 702
Naturetin Tablets 1789
Rauzide Tablets 1804

Betaxolol Hydrochloride (Increased risk of hyperkalemia and antihypertensive effect potentiated). Products include:
Betoptic Sterile Ophthalmic Solution 569
Betoptic S Sterile Ophthalmic Suspension 570
Kerlone Tablets 2172

Buprenorphine (May aggravate orthostatic hypotension).
No products indexed under this heading.

Butabarbital (May aggravate orthostatic hypotension). Products include:
Pyridium Plus 1764

Butalbital (May aggravate orthostatic hypotension). Products include:
Esgic-Plus Tablets 1002
Esgic Tablets & Capsules 1001
Fioricet Tablets 2006
Fiorinal Capsules 2007
Fiorinal with Codeine Capsules 2008
Fiorinal Tablets 2007
Phrenilin 838
Sedapap Tablets 50 mg/650 mg .. 1360

Captopril (Increased risk of hyperkalemia and antihypertensive effect potentiated). Products include:
Capoten 2255
Capozide 2258

Carteolol Hydrochloride (Potentiated). Products include:
Cartrol Tablets 507

Chlorothiazide (Potentiated). Products include:
Aldoclor Tablets 1413
Diupres Tablets 1461
Diuril Oral 1464

Chlorothiazide Sodium (Potentiated). Products include:
Diuril Sodium Intravenous 1463

Chlorthalidone (Potentiated). Products include:
Combipres Tablets 678
Tenoretic Tablets 1105
Thalitone Tablets 687

Clonidine (Potentiated). Products include:
Catapres-TTS 677

Clonidine Hydrochloride (Potentiated). Products include:
Catapres Tablets 676
Combipres Tablets 678

Codeine (May aggravate orthostatic hypotension). Products include:
Calcidrine Syrup 506

Codeine Phosphate (May aggravate orthostatic hypotension). Products include:
Actifed with Codeine Cough Syrup.. 752
Cheracol Cough Syrup 1853
Codimal PH Syrup 846
Dimetane-DC Cough Syrup 1857
Empirin with Codeine Phosphate Nos. 2, 3 & 4 764
Fiorinal with Codeine Capsules 2008
Isoclor Expectorant 982
Naldecon CX Adult Liquid .... ▣ 521
Novahistine DH 1342
Novahistine Expectorant 1343
Nucofed Capsules 2219
Nucofed Expectorant 2219
Nucofed Pediatric Expectorant 2220
Nucofed Syrup 2219
Phenaphen with Codeine Capsules 1865
Phenaphen-650 with Codeine Tablets 1866
Phenergan with Codeine 2497
Phenergan VC with Codeine 2501
Robitussin A-C Syrup 1875
Robitussin-DAC Syrup 1875
Ryna .... ▣ 741
Soma Compound w/Codeine Tablets 2390
Triaminic Expectorant w/Codeine .. 1996
Tussi-Organidin Liquid 2391
Tylenol with Codeine 1381

Codeine Polistirex (May aggravate orthostatic hypotension).
No products indexed under this heading.

Deserpidine (Potentiated). Products include:
Enduronyl 518
Harmonyl Tablets 528
Oreticyl 545

Deslanoside (Potential for digitalis toxicity due to hypokalemia).
No products indexed under this heading.

Dezocine (May aggravate orthostatic hypotension).

Diazoxide (Potentiated). Products include:
Hyperstat I.V. Injection 2095
Proglycem 649

Diclofenac Sodium (Potential for acute renal failure). Products include:
Voltaren Ophthalmic Sterile Ophthalmic Solution .... ◉ 268
Voltaren Tablets 1042

Digitoxin (Potential for digitalis toxicity due to hypokalemia). Products include:
Crystodigin Tablets 1253

Digoxin (Potential for digitalis toxicity due to hypokalemia). Products include:
Lanoxicaps 772
Lanoxin Elixir Pediatric 775
Lanoxin Injection 778
Lanoxin Injection Pediatric 781
Lanoxin Tablets 783

Doxazosin Mesylate (Increased risk of hyperkalemia and antihypertensive effect potentiated). Products include:
Cardura Tablets 1941

Enalapril Maleate (Increased risk of hyperkalemia and antihypertensive effect potentiated). Products include:
Vaseretic Tablets 1559
Vasotec Tablets 1564

Enalaprilat (Increased risk of hyperkalemia and antihypertensive effect potentiated). Products include:
Vasotec I.V. 1562

Esmolol Hydrochloride (Potentiated). Products include:
Brevibloc Injection 942

Etodolac (Potential for acute renal failure). Products include:
Lodine Capsules 2468

Felodipine (Increased risk of hyperkalemia and antihypertensive effect potentiated). Products include:
Plendil Extended-Release Tablets.... 1526

Fenoprofen Calcium (Potential for acute renal failure). Products include:
Nalfon Pulvules & Tablets 919

Fentanyl (May aggravate orthostatic hypotension). Products include:
- Duragesic Transdermal System 1133

Fentanyl Citrate (May aggravate orthostatic hypotension). Products include:
- Innovar Injection 1141
- Sublimaze Injection 1146

Flurbiprofen (Potential for acute renal failure). Products include:
- Ansaid Tablets 2319

Fosinopril Sodium (Increased risk of hyperkalemia and antihypertensive effect potentiated). Products include:
- Monopril Tablets 1406

Furosemide (Potentiated). Products include:
- Lasix 1093

Guanabenz Acetate (Potentiated). Products include:
- Wytensin Tablets 2542

Guanethidine Monosulfate (Potentiated). Products include:
- Esimil Tablets 864
- Ismelin Tablets 869

Hydralazine Hydrochloride (Potentiated). Products include:
- Apresazide Capsules 854
- Apresoline Hydrochloride Parenteral (Ampuls) 856
- Apresoline Hydrochloride Tablets .. 855
- Apresoline-Esidrix Tablets 857
- Ser-Ap-Es Tablets 881
- Serpasil-Apresoline Tablets 884

Hydrocodone Bitartrate (May aggravate orthostatic hypotension). Products include:
- Anexsia 5/500 Tablets 2196
- Anexsia 7.5/650 Tablets 2197
- Azdone Tablets 844
- Codiclear DH Syrup 845
- Codimal DH Syrup 846
- Damason-P 1356
- Hycodan Syrup, Tablets 927
- Hycomine Compound Tablets 929
- Hycomine Syrup 927
- Hycotuss Expectorant Syrup 930
- Hydrocet Capsules 835
- Lortab ASA Tablets 2414
- Lortab 2412
- Ru-Tuss with Hydrocodone 694
- Triaminic Expectorant DH 1995
- Vicodin Tablets 1187
- Vicodin ES Tablets 1189
- Zydone Capsules 941

Hydrocodone Polistirex (May aggravate orthostatic hypotension). Products include:
- Tussionex Extended-Release Suspension 988

Hydroflumethiazide (Potentiated). Products include:
- Diucardin Tablets 2450
- Saluron 718
- Salutensin/Salutensin-Demi 719

Ibuprofen (Potential for acute renal failure). Products include:
- Advil Cold & Sinus Caplets (formerly CoAdvil) 2416
- Advil Ibuprofen Tablets and Caplets 2416
- Children's Advil Suspension 2426
- CoAdvil .... ■ 748
- Dristan Sinus Caplets 2419
- Haltran Tablets .... ■ 668
- Ibuprofen .... ■ 631
- Medipren ibuprofen Caplets and Tablets 1362
- Midol 200 Cramp Relief Formula .. ■ 570
- Motrin Tablets 2351
- Motrin IB Caplets and Tablets .... ■ 736
- Nuprin Ibuprofen/Analgesic Tablets & Caplets 752
- PediaProfen Suspension 1363
- Rufen Tablets 691
- Trendar Ibuprofen Tablets .... ■ 756

Indapamide (Potentiated). Products include:
- Lozol Tablets 1843

Indomethacin (Potential for acute renal failure). Products include:
- Indocin 1487

Indomethacin Sodium Trihydrate (Potential for acute renal failure). Products include:
- Indocin I.V. 1490

Insulin, Human (Insulin requirements in diabetics may be altered).
- No products indexed under this heading.

Insulin, Human Isophane Suspension (Insulin requirements in diabetics may be altered). Products include:
- Humulin N, 100 Units 1270

Insulin, Human NPH (Insulin requirements in diabetics may be altered). Products include:
- Insulatard NPH Human 1627
- Novolin N 1627
- Novolin N PenFill Cartridges 1628
- Novolin N Prefilled 1628

Insulin, Human Regular (Insulin requirements in diabetics may be altered). Products include:
- Humulin BR, 100 Units 1268
- Humulin R, 100 Units 1272
- Novolin R 1627
- Novolin R PenFill Cartridges 1628
- Novolin R Prefilled 1629
- Velosulin Human 1628

Insulin, Human, Zinc Suspension (Insulin requirements in diabetics may be altered). Products include:
- Humulin L, 100 Units 1268
- Humulin U, 100 Units 1272
- Novolin L 1627

Insulin, NPH (Insulin requirements in diabetics may be altered). Products include:
- NPH, 40 & 100 Units 1273
- Beef NPH, 100 Units 1274
- Pork NPH, 100 Units 1275
- Insulatard NPH 1626
- NPH Insulin 1626
- NPH Purified Pork Isophane Insulin 1626

Insulin, Regular (Insulin requirements in diabetics may be altered). Products include:
- Regular, 40 & 100 Units 1273
- Beef Regular, 100 Units 1275
- Pork Regular, 100 Units 1275
- Pork Regular (Concentrated), 500 Units 1276
- Regular Insulin 1625
- Regular Purified Pork Insulin 1626
- Velosulin 1627

Insulin, Zinc Crystals (Insulin requirements in diabetics may be altered). Products include:
- NPH, 40 & 100 Units 1273

Insulin, Zinc Suspension (Insulin requirements in diabetics may be altered). Products include:
- Lente, 40 & 100 Units 1272
- Protamine, Zinc, 40 & 100 Units 1273
- Lente Iletin I 1272
- Beef Lente, 100 Units 1274
- Beef Protamine Zinc, 100 Units 1274
- Pork Lente, 100 Units 1275
- Pork, Protamine, Zinc, 100 Units 1275
- Lente Insulin 1626
- Lente Purified Pork Insulin 1626
- Semilente Insulin 1625
- Ultralente Insulin 1626

Isradipine (Increased risk of hyperkalemia and antihypertensive effect potentiated). Products include:
- DynaCirc Capsules 2004

Ketoprofen (Potential for acute renal failure). Products include:
- Orudis Capsules 2488

Ketorolac Tromethamine (Potential for acute renal failure). Products include:
- Toradol IM Injection 2302

Labetalol Hydrochloride (Potentiated). Products include:
- Normodyne Injection 2108
- Normodyne Tablets 2110
- Normozide Tablets 2112
- Trandate HCT Tablets 579
- Trandate Injection 577
- Trandate Tablets 579

Levorphanol Tartrate (May aggravate orthostatic hypotension). Products include:
- Levo-Dromoran 1906

Lisinopril (Increased risk of hyperkalemia and antihypertensive effect potentiated). Products include:
- Prinivil Tablets 1538
- Prinzide Tablets 1540
- Zestoretic 2274
- Zestril Tablets 2277

Lithium Carbonate (High risk of lithium toxicity). Products include:
- Eskalith 2214
- Lithane Tablets 1596
- Lithium Carbonate Capsules & Tablets 1984
- Lithobid Tablets 870

Lithium Citrate (High risk of lithium toxicity). Products include:
- Cibalith-S 870

Mecamylamine Hydrochloride (Potentiated). Products include:
- Inversine Tablets 1492

Meclofenamate Sodium (Potential for acute renal failure). Products include:
- Meclomen Capsules 1739

Mefenamic Acid (Potential for acute renal failure). Products include:
- Ponstel 1758

Meperidine Hydrochloride (May aggravate orthostatic hypotension). Products include:
- Demerol 2047
- Mepergan Injection 2479

Mephobarbital (May aggravate orthostatic hypotension). Products include:
- Mebaral Tablets 2061

Methadone Hydrochloride (May aggravate orthostatic hypotension). Products include:
- Dolophine Hydrochloride Ampoules & Vials 1260
- Dolophine Hydrochloride Tablets 1261
- Methadone Hydrochloride Diskets .. 1284
- Methadone Hydrochloride Oral Solution & Tablets 1987

Methyclothiazide (Potentiated). Products include:
- Enduron Tablets 517
- Enduronyl 518

Methyldopa (Potentiated). Products include:
- Aldoclor Tablets 1413
- Aldomet Oral 1415
- Aldoril Tablets 1418

Methyldopate Hydrochloride (Potentiated). Products include:
- Aldomet Ester HCl Injection 1417

Metolazone (Potentiated). Products include:
- Diulo 2129
- Mykrox ½ mg Tablets 984
- Zaroxolyn Tablets 989

Metoprolol Tartrate (Potentiated). Products include:
- Lopressor Ampuls 1032
- Lopressor HCT Tablets 1034
- Lopressor Tablets 1032

Metyrosine (Potentiated). Products include:
- Demser Capsules 1460

Minoxidil (Potentiated). Products include:
- Loniten Tablets 2346
- Rogaine Topical Solution 2357

Morphine Sulfate (May aggravate orthostatic hypotension). Products include:
- Astramorph/PF Injection, USP (Preservative-Free) 618
- Duramorph 960
- Infumorph 200 and Infumorph 500 Sterile Solutions 962
- MS Contin Tablets 1814
- MSIR 1817
- Oramorph SR (Morphine Sulfate Sustained Release Tablets) 1988
- Roxanol 1991

Nadolol (Potentiated). Products include:
- Corgard Tablets 701
- Corzide Tablets 702

Naproxen (Potential for acute renal failure). Products include:
- Naprosyn 2297

Naproxen Sodium (Potential for acute renal failure). Products include:
- Anaprox and Anaprox DS Tablets 2288

Nicardipine Hydrochloride (Potentiated). Products include:
- Cardene Capsules 2290

Nitroglycerin (Potentiated). Products include:
- Deponit NTG Transdermal Delivery System 2143
- Minitran Transdermal Delivery System 1312
- Nitro-Bid Ointment 1339
- Nitro-Bid Capsules 1338
- Nitrodisc 2176
- Nitro-Dur (nitroglycerin) Transdermal Infusion System 1164
- Nitrogard Tablets 1004
- Nitrolingual Spray 1846
- Nitrostat Tablets 1743
- Transderm-Nitro Transdermal Therapeutic System 2283

Norepinephrine Bitartrate (Decreased arterial responsiveness to norepinephrine). Products include:
- Levophed Bitartrate Injection 2054

Opium Alkaloids (May aggravate orthostatic hypotension). Products include:
- B & O No. 15A & No. 16A Supprettes 2395
- Pantopon Injectable 1911

Oxycodone Hydrochloride (May aggravate orthostatic hypotension). Products include:
- Percocet Tablets 950
- Percodan 951
- Roxicodone Tablets, Oral Solution & Intensol (Oxycodone) 1992
- Tylox Capsules 1382

Penbutolol Sulfate (Potentiated). Products include:
- Levatol 1832

Pentobarbital Sodium (May aggravate orthostatic hypotension). Products include:
- Nembutal Sodium Capsules 534
- Nembutal Sodium Solution 536
- Nembutal Sodium Suppositories 538

Phenobarbital (May aggravate orthostatic hypotension). Products include:
- Arco-Lase Plus Tablets 607
- Bellergal-S Tablets 1998
- Bronkolixir .... ■ 761
- Bronkotabs Tablets .... ■ 762
- Donnatal 1858
- Donnatal Extentabs 1859
- Donnatal Tablets 1858
- Donnazyme Tablets 1860
- Kinesed Tablets 2272
- Phenobarbital Elixir and Tablets 1293
- Primatene Tablets-P Formula 2421
- Quadrinal Tablets 1183
- Tedral SA 1765

Phenoxybenzamine Hydrochloride (Potentiated). Products include:
- Dibenzyline Capsules 2207

Phentolamine Mesylate (Potentiated). Products include:
- Regitine 878

Phenylbutazone (Potential for acute renal failure). Products include:
- Butazolidin Capsules & Tablets 1027

Pindolol (Potentiated). Products include:
- Visken Tablets 2036

Piroxicam (Potential for acute renal failure). Products include:
- Feldene Capsules 1777

Polythiazide (Potentiated). Products include:
- Minizide Capsules 1779
- Renese Tablets 1785
- Renese-R Tablets 1786

Potassium Acid Phosphate (Contraindication). Products include:
- K-Phos M.F. Tablets 659
- K-Phos Original Formula 'Sodium Free' Tablets 660
- K-Phos No. 2 Tablets 659

Potassium Bicarbonate (Contraindication). Products include:
- Alka-Seltzer Advanced Formula Antacid & Non-Aspirin Pain Reliever .... ND 620
- Alka-Seltzer Effervescent Antacid ND 622
- K-Lyte 707
- Klorvess Effervescent Granules 2010
- Klorvess Effervescent Tablets 2011

Potassium Chloride (Contraindication). Products include:
- Chlor-3 Condiment 994
- K-Dur Microburst Release System (potassium chloride, USP) E.R. Tablets 1163
- K-Lor Powder Packets 531
- K-Lyte 707
- K-Norm Capsules 982
- K-Tab Filmtab 532
- Kato Potassium Supplement 1114
- Klor-Con 8/Klor-Con 10 Extended-release Tablets 2374
- Klorvess Effervescent Granules 2010
- Klorvess Effervescent Tablets 2011
- Klorvess 10% Liquid 2010
- Klotrix 708
- Kolyum Liquid 983
- Micro-K 1863
- Micro-K LS Packets 1864
- NuLYTELY 699
- Oral Rehydration Salts, Citrate 1150
- Rum-K Syrup 995
- Slow-K Tablets 2281
- Ten-K Controlled-Release Tablets 2282
- Thermotabs .... ND 619

Potassium Citrate (Contraindication). Products include:
- Alka-Seltzer Effervescent Antacid .. 1570
- K-Lyte 707
- Polycitra Syrup 2424
- Polycitra-K 2424
- Polycitra-LC—Sugar-Free 2424
- Ricelyte, Rice-Based Oral Electrolyte Maintenance Solution .... ND 613

Potassium Gluconate (Contraindication). Products include:
- Kolyum Liquid 983

Potassium Phosphate, Dibasic (Contraindication). Products include:
- Neutra-Phos 2423

Potassium Phosphate, Monobasic (Contraindication). Products include:
- K-Phos M.F. Tablets 659
- K-Phos Neutral Tablets 660
- Neutra-Phos 2423

Prazosin Hydrochloride (Potentiated). Products include:
- Minipress Capsules 1778
- Minizide Capsules 1779

Propoxyphene Hydrochloride (May aggravate orthostatic hypotension). Products include:
- Darvon 1256
- Wygesic Tablets 2540

Propoxyphene Napsylate (May aggravate orthostatic hypotension). Products include:
- Darvon-N/Darvocet-N 1254

Propranolol Hydrochloride (Potentiated). Products include:
- Inderal 2459
- Inderal LA Long Acting Capsules 2461
- Inderide Tablets 2463
- Inderide LA Long Acting Capsules .. 2465

Ramipril (Increased risk of hyperkalemia and antihypertensive effect potentiated). Products include:
- Altace Capsules 1086

Rauwolfia Serpentina (Potentiated). Products include:
- Raudixin Tablets 1803
- Rauzide Tablets 1804

Rescinnamine (Potentiated).
- No products indexed under this heading.

Reserpine (Potentiated). Products include:
- Diupres Tablets 1461
- Hydromox R Tablets 1209
- Hydropres Tablets 1485
- Renese-R Tablets 1786
- Salutensin/Salutensin-Demi 719
- Ser-Ap-Es Tablets 881
- Serpasil Tablets 883
- Serpasil-Apresoline Tablets 884
- Serpasil-Esidrix Tablets 886

Secobarbital Sodium (May aggravate orthostatic hypotension). Products include:
- Seconal Sodium Pulvules 1296

Sodium Nitroprusside (Potentiated). Products include:
- Nipride I.V. Infusion 1909

Spironolactone (Contraindication). Products include:
- Aldactazide 2150
- Aldactone 2152

Sufentanil Citrate (May aggravate orthostatic hypotension). Products include:
- Sufenta Injection 1147

Sulindac (Potential for acute renal failure). Products include:
- Clinoril Tablets 1433

Terazosin Hydrochloride (Potentiated). Products include:
- Hytrin Tablets 529

Thiamylal Sodium (May aggravate orthostatic hypotension). Products include:
- Surital Ampoules, Steri-Vials 1764

Timolol Maleate (Potentiated). Products include:
- Blocadren Tablets 1429
- Timolide Tablets 1547
- Timoptic in Ocudose 1552
- Timoptic Sterile Ophthalmic Solution 1550

Tolmetin Sodium (Potential for acute renal failure). Products include:
- Tolectin (200, 400 and 600 mg) .. 1379

Trimethaphan Camsylate (Potentiated). Products include:
- Arfonad Ampuls 1887

Tubocurarine Chloride (Increased responsiveness to tubocurarine).
- No products indexed under this heading.

MAXZIDE-25 MG TABLETS

(Triamterene, Hydrochlorothiazide) .. 1215

See **Maxzide Tablets**

MAY-VITA ELIXIR

(Vitamins with Minerals) 1359

No interactions described in labeling.

MEBARAL TABLETS

(Mephobarbital) 2061

May interact with corticosteroids, monoamine oxidase inhibitors, central nervous system depressants, oral anticoagulants, oral contraceptives, and certain other agents. Compounds in these categories include:

Alfentanil Hydrochloride (Additive depressant effects). Products include:
- Alfenta Injection 1131

Alprazolam (Additive depressant effects). Products include:
- Xanax Tablets 2367

Aprobarbital (Additive depressant effects). Products include:
- Alurate Elixir 1883

Betamethasone Acetate (Enhanced metabolism of exogenous corticosteroids). Products include:
- Celestone Soluspan Suspension 2081

Betamethasone Sodium Phosphate (Enhanced metabolism of exogenous corticosteroids). Products include:
- Celestone Soluspan Suspension 2081

Buprenorphine (Additive depressant effects).
- No products indexed under this heading.

Buspirone Hydrochloride (Additive depressant effects). Products include:
- BuSpar 1401

Butabarbital (Additive depressant effects). Products include:
- Pyridium Plus 1764

Butalbital (Additive depressant effects). Products include:
- Esgic-Plus Tablets 1002
- Esgic Tablets & Capsules 1001
- Fioricet Tablets 2006
- Fiorinal Capsules 2007
- Fiorinal with Codeine Capsules 2008
- Fiorinal Tablets 2007
- Phrenilin 838
- Sedapap Tablets 50 mg/650 mg .. 1360

Chlordiazepoxide (Additive depressant effects). Products include:
- Libritabs Tablets 1930
- Limbitrol 1933
- Menrium Tablets 1934

Chlordiazepoxide Hydrochloride (Additive depressant effects). Products include:
- Librax Capsules 1929
- Librium Capsules 1931
- Librium Injectable 1932

Chlorpromazine (Additive depressant effects). Products include:
- Thorazine 2234

Chlorprothixene (Additive depressant effects). Products include:
- Taractan Tablets 1920

Chlorprothixene Hydrochloride (Additive depressant effects). Products include:
- Taractan 1920

Chlorprothixene Lactate (Additive depressant effects). Products include:
- Taractan Concentrate 1920

Clorazepate Dipotassium (Additive depressant effects). Products include:
- Tranxene 556

Codeine (Additive depressant effects). Products include:
- Calcidrine Syrup 506

Codeine Phosphate (Additive depressant effects). Products include:
- Actifed with Codeine Cough Syrup .. 752
- Cheracol Cough Syrup 1853
- Codimal PH Syrup 846
- Dimetane-DC Cough Syrup 1857
- Empirin with Codeine Phosphate Nos. 2, 3 & 4 764
- Fiorinal with Codeine Capsules 2008
- Isoclor Expectorant 982
- Naldecon CX Adult Liquid .... ND 521
- Novahistine DH 1342
- Novahistine Expectorant 1343
- Nucofed Capsules 2219
- Nucofed Expectorant 2219
- Nucofed Pediatric Expectorant 2220
- Nucofed Syrup 2219
- Phenaphen with Codeine Capsules 1865
- Phenaphen-650 with Codeine Tablets 1866
- Phenergan with Codeine 2497
- Phenergan VC with Codeine 2501
- Robitussin A-C Syrup 1875
- Robitussin-DAC Syrup 1875
- Ryna .... ND 741
- Soma Compound w/Codeine Tablets 2390
- Triaminic Expectorant w/Codeine .. 1996
- Tussi-Organidin Liquid 2391
- Tylenol with Codeine 1381

Codeine Polistirex (Additive depressant effects).
- No products indexed under this heading.

Cortisone Acetate (Enhanced metabolism of exogenous corticosteroids). Products include:
- Cortone Acetate Sterile Suspension 1437
- Cortone Acetate Tablets 1439

Dexamethasone (Enhanced metabolism of exogenous corticosteroids). Products include:
- AK-Trol Ointment & Suspension .... ⊙ 207
- Decadron Elixir 1445
- Decadron Tablets 1447
- Decaspray Topical Aerosol 1459
- Dexacidin .... ⊙ 272
- Maxidex Sterile Ophthalmic Suspension .... ⊙ 223
- Maxitrol Ophthalmic Ointment/Suspension .... ⊙ 223
- TobraDex Ophthalmic Suspension and Ointment .... ⊙ 228

Dexamethasone Acetate (Enhanced metabolism of exogenous corticosteroids). Products include:
- Dalalone D.P. Injectable 999
- Decadron-LA Sterile Suspension 1457

Dexamethasone Sodium Phosphate (Enhanced metabolism of exogenous corticosteroids). Products include:
- AK-Dex .... ⊙ 203
- Decadron Phosphate Respihaler 1454
- Decadron Phosphate Sterile Ophthalmic Ointment 1453
- Decadron Phosphate Sterile Ophthalmic Solution 1453
- Decadron Phosphate Topical Cream 1455
- Decadron Phosphate Turbinaire 1456
- Maxidex Sterile Ophthalmic Ointment .... ⊙ 222
- NeoDecadron Sterile Ophthalmic Ointment 1517
- NeoDecadron Sterile Ophthalmic Solution 1518
- NeoDecadron Topical Cream 1518

Dezocine (Additive depressant effects).

Diazepam (Additive depressant effects). Products include:
- Valium Injectable 1937
- Valium Tablets 1939
- Valrelease Capsules 1923

Dicumarol (Decreased anticoagulant response). Products include:
- Dicumarol Tablets 516

Doxycycline Calcium (Half-life of doxycycline shortened).
- No products indexed under this heading.

Doxycycline Hyclate (Half-life of doxycycline shortened). Products include:
- Doryx Capsules 1717
- Vibramycin Hyclate Capsules 1787
- Vibramycin Hyclate Intravenous 1968
- Vibra-Tabs Film Coated Tablets 1787

Doxycycline Monohydrate (Half-life of doxycycline shortened). Products include:
- Monodox Capsules 1630
- Vibramycin Monohydrate for Oral Suspension 1787

Droperidol (Additive depressant effects). Products include:
Inapsine Injection ... 1140
Innovar Injection ... 1141

Enflurane (Additive depressant effects). Products include:
Ethrane ... 599

Estazolam (Additive depressant effects). Products include:
ProSom Tablets ... 554

Estradiol (Decreased effect of estradiol). Products include:
Emcyt Capsules ... 1161
Estrace ... 1385
Estrace Vaginal Cream ... 1388
Estraderm Transdermal System ... 866

Estrone (Decreased effect of estrone). Products include:
Ogen ... 540

Ethchlorvynol (Additive depressant effects). Products include:
Placidyl Capsules ... 553

Ethinamate (Additive depressant effects).
No products indexed under this heading.

Ethinyl Estradiol (Decreased contraceptive effect). Products include:
Brevicon ... 2304
Demulen ... 2161
Estinyl Tablets ... 2085
Jenest-28 Tablets ... 1636
Levlen/Tri-Levlen ... 665
Lo/Ovral Tablets ... 2471
Lo/Ovral-28 Tablets ... 2476
Loestrin ... 1728
Modicon ... 1667
Nordette-21 Tablets ... 2481
Nordette-28 Tablets ... 2483
Norethin ... 2133
Norinyl ... 2304
Norlestrin ... 1746
Ortho-Cyclen Tablets ... 1658
Ortho-Novum ... 1667
Ovcon ... 1391
Ovral Tablets ... 2490
Ovral-28 Tablets ... 2491
Levlen/Tri-Levlen ... 665
Tri-Norinyl ... 2304
Triphasil-21 Tablets ... 2527
Triphasil-28 Tablets ... 2532

Ethynodiol Diacetate (Decreased contraceptive effect). Products include:
Demulen ... 2161

Fentanyl (Additive depressant effects). Products include:
Duragesic Transdermal System ... 1133

Fentanyl Citrate (Additive depressant effects). Products include:
Innovar Injection ... 1141
Sublimaze Injection ... 1146

Fluphenazine Decanoate (Additive depressant effects). Products include:
Prolixin Decanoate ... 1795

Fluphenazine Enanthate (Additive depressant effects). Products include:
Prolixin Enanthate ... 1796

Fluphenazine Hydrochloride (Additive depressant effects). Products include:
Prolixin Elixir ... 1793
Prolixin Injection ... 1791
Prolixin Oral Concentrate ... 1792
Prolixin Tablets ... 1793

Flurazepam Hydrochloride (Additive depressant effects). Products include:
Dalmane Capsules ... 1927

Furazolidone (Prolongs effects of barbiturates). Products include:
Furoxone ... 1855

Glutethimide (Additive depressant effects).
No products indexed under this heading.

Griseofulvin (Decreased blood levels of griseofulvin). Products include:
Fulvicin P/G Tablets ... 2090
Fulvicin P/G 165 & 330 Tablets ... 2091
Fulvicin-U/F Tablets ... 2092
Grifulvin V (griseofulvin microsize) Tablets/Suspension ... 1678
Grisactin ... 2454
Grisactin Ultra Tablets ... 2455
Gris-PEG Tablets, 125 mg & 250 mg ... 1083

Haloperidol (Additive depressant effects). Products include:
Haldol Injection, Tablets and Concentrate ... 1373

Haloperidol Decanoate (Additive depressant effects). Products include:
Haldol Decanoate ... 1375

Hydrocodone Bitartrate (Additive depressant effects). Products include:
Anexsia 5/500 Tablets ... 2196
Anexsia 7.5/650 Tablets ... 2197
Azdōne Tablets ... 844
Codiclear DH Syrup ... 845
Codimal DH Syrup ... 846
Damason-P ... 1356
Hycodan Syrup, Tablets ... 927
Hycomine Compound Tablets ... 929
Hycomine Syrup ... 927
Hycotuss Expectorant Syrup ... 930
Hydrocet Capsules ... 835
Lortab ASA Tablets ... 2414
Lortab ... 2412
Ru-Tuss with Hydrocodone ... 694
Triaminic Expectorant DH ... 1995
Vicodin Tablets ... 1187
Vicodin ES Tablets ... 1189
Zydone Capsules ... 941

Hydrocodone Polistirex (Additive depressant effects). Products include:
Tussionex Extended-Release Suspension ... 988

Hydrocortisone (Enhanced metabolism of exogenous corticosteroids). Products include:
AK-Spore H.C. ... ⊙ 206
Bactine Hydrocortisone Anti-Itch Cream ... ⊞ 625
CaldeCORT Anti-Itch Hydrocortisone Spray ... ⊞ 560
Carmol HC Cream 1% ... 2296
Cortaid Spray ... ⊞ 735
Cortenema ... 2244
Cortisporin Ointment ... 758
Cortisporin Ophthalmic Ointment Sterile ... 758
Cortisporin Ophthalmic Suspension Sterile ... 759
Cortisporin Otic Solution Sterile ... 760
Cortisporin Otic Suspension Sterile ... 760
Cortizone-5 Creme & Ointment ... ⊞ 732
Dermolate Anti-Itch Cream ... ⊞ 697
Eldecort Cream 1.0% ... 1113
Eldecort Cream 1.0% and 2.5% ... 1113
Fungoid HC Creme ... 1770
Hydrocortone Tablets ... 1482
Hytone ... 909
LazerSporin-C Solution ... 1770
Massengill Medicated Soft Cloth Towelettes ... 2192
Nutracort Cream & Lotion ... 1684
PediOtic Suspension Sterile ... 797
Synacort Creams 1%, 2.5% ... 2296
Vanoxide-HC Acne Lotion ... 911
Vioform-Hydrocortisone Cream and Mild Cream ... 889
Vioform-Hydrocortisone Ointment ... 889
VōSoL HC Otic Solution ... 2392
Vytone Cream 1% ... 911

Hydrocortisone Acetate (Enhanced metabolism of exogenous corticosteroids). Products include:
Analpram-HC Rectal Cream 1% and 2.5% ... 970
Anusol-HC Cream ... 1690
Anusol-HC Suppositories ... 1691
Caldecort ... ⊞ 560
Carmol HC Cream 1% ... 2296
Chloromycetin Hydrocortisone Ophthalmic ... 1694
Coly-Mycin S Otic w/Neomycin & Hydrocortisone ... 1708
Cortaid ... ⊞ 735
Cortef Feminine Itch Cream ... ⊞ 735
Corticaine ... ⊞ 682
Cortifoam ... 1827
Cortisporin Cream ... 757
Epifoam ... 1828
Gynecort 5 Creme ... ⊞ 556
Hydrocortone Acetate Sterile Suspension ... 1479
Lanacort 5 Creme and Ointment ... ⊞ 557
Mantadil Cream ... 789
Ophthocort ... ⊙ 301
Orabase HCA Oral Paste ... 890
Pramosone Cream, Lotion & Ointment ... 971
ProctoCream-HC ... 1834
Proctofoam-HC ... 1835

Hydrocortisone Sodium Phosphate (Enhanced metabolism of exogenous corticosteroids). Products include:
Hydrocortone Phosphate Injection, Sterile ... 1481

Hydrocortisone Sodium Succinate (Enhanced metabolism of exogenous corticosteroids). Products include:
Solu-Cortef Sterile Powder ... 2361

Hydroxyzine Hydrochloride (Additive depressant effects). Products include:
Atarax Tablets & Syrup ... 1941
Marax Tablets & DF Syrup ... 1954
Vistaril Intramuscular Solution ... 1970

Isocarboxazid (Prolongs effects of barbiturates). Products include:
Marplan Tablets ... 1906

Isoflurane (Additive depressant effects). Products include:
Forane ... 600

Ketamine Hydrochloride (Additive depressant effects). Products include:
Ketalar ... 1726

Levonorgestrel (Decreased contraceptive effect). Products include:
Levlen/Tri-Levlen ... 665
Nordette-21 Tablets ... 2481
Nordette-28 Tablets ... 2483
Norplant System ... 2484
Levlen/Tri-Levlen ... 665
Triphasil-21 Tablets ... 2527
Triphasil-28 Tablets ... 2532

Levorphanol Tartrate (Additive depressant effects). Products include:
Levo-Dromoran ... 1906

Lorazepam (Additive depressant effects). Products include:
Ativan Injection ... 2432
Ativan Tablets ... 2434

Loxapine Hydrochloride (Additive depressant effects). Products include:
Loxitane ... 1213

Loxapine Succinate (Additive depressant effects). Products include:
Loxitane Capsules ... 1213

Meperidine Hydrochloride (Additive depressant effects). Products include:
Demerol ... 2047
Mepergan Injection ... 2479

Meprobamate (Additive depressant effects). Products include:
Deprol Tablets ... 2382
Equagesic Tablets ... 2451
Miltown Tablets ... 2386
PMB 200 and PMB 400 ... 2504

Mesoridazine (Additive depressant effects). Products include:
Serentil ... 686

Mestranol (Decreased contraceptive effect). Products include:
Enovid ... 2161
Norethin ... 2133
Norinyl ... 2304
Ortho-Novum ... 1667

Methadone Hydrochloride (Additive depressant effects). Products include:
Dolophine Hydrochloride Ampoules & Vials ... 1260
Dolophine Hydrochloride Tablets ... 1261
Methadone Hydrochloride Diskets ... 1284
Methadone Hydrochloride Oral Solution & Tablets ... 1987

Methohexital Sodium (Additive depressant effects). Products include:
Brevital Sodium Vials ... 1248

Methoxyflurane (Additive depressant effects).
No products indexed under this heading.

Methylprednisolone Acetate (Enhanced metabolism of exogenous corticosteroids). Products include:
Depo-Medrol Sterile Aqueous Suspension ... 2334

Methylprednisolone Sodium Succinate (Enhanced metabolism of exogenous corticosteroids). Products include:
Solu-Medrol Sterile Powder ... 2363

Midazolam Hydrochloride (Additive depressant effects). Products include:
Versed Injection ... 1924

Molindone Hydrochloride (Additive depressant effects). Products include:
Moban Tablets & Concentrate ... 932

Morphine Sulfate (Additive depressant effects). Products include:
Astramorph/PF Injection, USP (Preservative-Free) ... 618
Duramorph ... 960
Infumorph 200 and Infumorph 500 Sterile Solutions ... 962
MS Contin Tablets ... 1814
MSIR ... 1817
Oramorph SR (Morphine Sulfate Sustained Release Tablets) ... 1988
Roxanol ... 1991

Norethindrone (Decreased contraceptive effect). Products include:
Brevicon ... 2304
Jenest-28 Tablets ... 1636
Micronor Tablets ... 1667
Modicon ... 1667
Norethin ... 2133
Norinyl ... 2304
Norlutin ... 1755
Nor-Q D Tablets ... 2304
Ortho-Novum ... 1667
Ovcon ... 1391
Tri-Norinyl ... 2304

Norethynodrel (Decreased contraceptive effect). Products include:
Enovid ... 2161

Norgestimate (Decreased contraceptive effect). Products include:
Ortho-Cyclen Tablets ... 1658

Norgestrel (Decreased contraceptive effect). Products include:
Lo/Ovral Tablets ... 2471
Lo/Ovral-28 Tablets ... 2476
Ovral Tablets ... 2490
Ovral-28 Tablets ... 2491
Ovrette Tablets ... 2492

Opium Alkaloids (Additive depressant effects). Products include:
B & O No. 15A & No. 16A Supprettes ... 2395
Pantopon Injectable ... 1911

Oxazepam (Additive depressant effects). Products include:
Serax Capsules ... 2522
Serax Tablets ... 2522

Oxycodone Hydrochloride (Additive depressant effects). Products include:
Percocet Tablets ... 950
Percodan ... 951
Roxicodone Tablets, Oral Solution & Intensol (Oxycodone) ... 1992
Tylox Capsules ... 1382

Pentobarbital Sodium (Additive depressant effects). Products include:
- Nembutal Sodium Capsules 534
- Nembutal Sodium Solution 536
- Nembutal Sodium Suppositories...... 538

Perphenazine (Additive depressant effects). Products include:
- Etrafon 2087
- Triavil Tablets 1556
- Trilafon.......... 2123

Phenelzine Sulfate (Prolongs effects of barbiturates). Products include:
- Nardil 1742

Phenobarbital (Additive depressant effects). Products include:
- Arco-Lase Plus Tablets 607
- Bellergal-S Tablets 1998
- Bronkolixir .... ▣ 761
- Bronkotabs Tablets.......... ▣ 762
- Donnatal 1858
- Donnatal Extentabs.......... 1859
- Donnatal Tablets 1858
- Donnazyme Tablets 1860
- Kinesed Tablets 2272
- Phenobarbital Elixir and Tablets...... 1293
- Primatene Tablets-P Formula.......... 2421
- Quadrinal Tablets 1183
- Tedral SA 1765

Phenytoin (Unpredictable effects). Products include:
- Dilantin Infatabs.......... 1710
- Dilantin-30 Pediatric/Dilantin-125 Suspension.......... 1713

Phenytoin Sodium (Unpredictable effects). Products include:
- Dilantin Kapseals 1708
- Dilantin Parenteral 1712
- Dilantin with Phenobarbital Kapseals 1715

Prazepam (Additive depressant effects). Products include:
- Centrax.......... 1693

Prednisolone Acetate (Enhanced metabolism of exogenous corticosteroids). Products include:
- AK-Cide Sterile Ophthalmic Ointment & Suspension.......... ⊙ 202
- Blephamide Liquifilm Sterile Ophthalmic Suspension.......... 586
- Blephamide S.O.P. Sterile Ophthalmic Ointment.......... 586
- Cetapred Ointment .... ⊙ 220
- ⅛ % Econopred & 1 % Econopred Plus .... ⊙ 217
- Isopto Cetapred Suspension .... ⊙ 220
- Metimyd.......... ⊙ 306
- Poly-Pred Liquifilm .... ⊙ 250
- Pred Forte.......... ⊙ 252
- Pred Mild.......... ⊙ 254
- Pred-G Liquifilm Sterile Ophthalmic Suspension .... ⊙ 252
- Pred-G S.O.P. Sterile Ophthalmic Ointment .... ⊙ 253
- Vasocidin Ointment .... ⊙ 275

Prednisolone Sodium Phosphate (Enhanced metabolism of exogenous corticosteroids). Products include:
- AK-Pred .... ⊙ 205
- Hydeltrasol Injection, Sterile.......... 1476
- Inflamase.......... ⊙ 274
- Pediapred Oral Liquid 987
- Vasocidin Ophthalmic Solution ...... ⊙ 276

Prednisolone Tebutate (Enhanced metabolism of exogenous corticosteroids). Products include:
- Hydeltra-T.B.A. Sterile Suspension 1478

Prednisone (Enhanced metabolism of exogenous corticosteroids). Products include:
- Deltasone Tablets 2332

Prochlorperazine (Additive depressant effects). Products include:
- Compazine 2201

Progesterone (Decreased effect of progesterone).
- No products indexed under this heading.

Promethazine Hydrochloride (Additive depressant effects). Products include:
- Mepergan Injection 2479
- Phenergan with Codeine.......... 2497
- Phenergan with Dextromethorphan 2499
- Phenergan Injection 2493
- Phenergan Suppositories 2496
- Phenergan Syrup 2495
- Phenergan Tablets 2496
- Phenergan VC 2500
- Phenergan VC with Codeine 2501

Propofol (Additive depressant effects). Products include:
- Diprivan Injection.......... 2267

Propoxyphene Hydrochloride (Additive depressant effects). Products include:
- Darvon 1256
- Wygesic Tablets 2540

Propoxyphene Napsylate (Additive depressant effects). Products include:
- Darvon-N/Darvocet-N 1254

Quazepam (Additive depressant effects). Products include:
- Doral Tablets 2383

Secobarbital Sodium (Additive depressant effects). Products include:
- Seconal Sodium Pulvules 1296

Selegiline Hydrochloride (Prolongs effects of barbiturates). Products include:
- Eldepryl 2250

Sodium Valproate (Barbiturate metabolism decreased).

Sufentanil Citrate (Additive depressant effects). Products include:
- Sufenta Injection 1147

Temazepam (Additive depressant effects). Products include:
- Restoril Capsules.......... 2023

Thiamylal Sodium (Additive depressant effects). Products include:
- Surital Ampoules, Steri-Vials.......... 1764

Thioridazine Hydrochloride (Additive depressant effects). Products include:
- Mellaril 2011

Thiothixene (Additive depressant effects). Products include:
- Navane Capsules and Concentrate 1954
- Navane Intramuscular 1956

Tranylcypromine Sulfate (Prolongs effects of barbiturates). Products include:
- Parnate Tablets 2222

Triamcinolone (Enhanced metabolism of exogenous corticosteroids).
- No products indexed under this heading.

Triamcinolone Acetonide (Enhanced metabolism of exogenous corticosteroids). Products include:
- Aristocort A 1010
- Azmacort Inhaler 1837
- Kenalog Cream, Lotion & Ointment 2401
- Kenalog-10 Injection 2402
- Kenalog-40 Injection 2403
- Kenalog in Orabase.......... 604
- Kenalog Spray.......... 2401
- Mycolog II Cream and Ointment 2407
- Mytrex Cream & Ointment.......... 2080
- Nasacort Nasal Inhaler 1844

Triamcinolone Diacetate (Enhanced metabolism of exogenous corticosteroids). Products include:
- Aristocort Suspension 1008

Triamcinolone Hexacetonide (Enhanced metabolism of exogenous corticosteroids). Products include:
- Aristospan Suspension 1011

Triazolam (Additive depressant effects). Products include:
- Halcion Tablets.......... 2340

Trifluoperazine Hydrochloride (Additive depressant effects). Products include:
- Stelazine 2226

Valproic Acid (Decreased barbiturate metabolism). Products include:
- Depakene Capsules & Syrup.......... 511

Warfarin Sodium (Decreased anticoagulant response). Products include:
- Coumadin Injection & Tablets 944
- Panwarfin Tablets 547

MECLAN (MECLOCYCLINE SULFOSALICYLATE) CREAM

(Meclocycline Sulfosalicylate) 1679
No interactions described in labeling.

MECLOMEN CAPSULES

(Meclofenamate Sodium) 1739
May interact with:

Aspirin (Concurrent administration may lower Meclomen plasma levels and greater fecal blood loss results). Products include:
- Alka-Seltzer Effervescent Antacid and Pain Reliever.......... 1568
- Alka-Seltzer Extra Strength Effervescent Antacid and Pain Reliever 1570
- Alka-Seltzer (Flavored) Effervescent Antacid and Pain Reliever 1569
- Alka-Seltzer Plus Cold Medicine .... ▣ 623
- Alka-Seltzer Plus Night-Time Cold Medicine .... ▣ 623
- Alka Seltzer Plus Sinus Allergy Medicine .... ▣ 624
- Anacin Coated Analgesic Caplets 2417
- Anacin Coated Analgesic Tablets 2417
- Anacin Maximum Strength Analgesic Coated Tablets.......... 2417
- Maximum Strength Arthritis Pain Formula By the Makers of Anacin Analgesic Tablets and Caplets...... 2418
- Arthritis Pain Formula by the Makers of Anacin Analgesic Tablets and Caplets .... ▣ 747
- Arthritis Strength BC Powder.......... ▣ 516
- Ascriptin A/D Caplets 1850
- Regular Strength Ascriptin Tablets 1850
- Azdōne Tablets.......... 844
- BC Powder .... ▣ 517
- BC Cold Powder .... ▣ 517
- Children's Bayer Chewable Aspirin.......... ▣ 564
- Genuine Bayer Aspirin Tablets & Caplets.......... ▣ 564
- Maximum Bayer Aspirin Tablets & Caplets.......... ▣ 566
- Bayer Plus Aspirin Tablets.......... ▣ 567
- Therapy Bayer Aspirin Caplets .... ▣ 568
- 8 Hour Bayer Timed-Release Aspirin .... ▣ 566
- Arthritis Strength Bufferin Analgesic Caplets 744
- Extra Strength Bufferin Analgesic Tablets 745
- Bufferin Analgesic Tablets and Caplets.......... 743
- Cama Arthritis Pain Reliever.......... ▣ 685
- Damason-P.......... 1356
- Easprin.......... 1719
- Ecotrin Enteric Coated Aspirin Maximum Strength Tablets and Caplets.......... 2189
- Ecotrin Enteric Coated Aspirin Regular Strength Tablets and Caplets.......... 2189
- Empirin Aspirin.......... ▣ 541
- Empirin with Codeine Phosphate Nos. 2, 3 & 4.......... 764
- Equagesic Tablets 2451
- Excedrin Extra-Strength Analgesic Tablets & Caplets 749
- 4-Way Cold Tablets.......... 750
- Fiorinal Capsules 2007
- Fiorinal with Codeine Capsules 2008
- Fiorinal Tablets 2007
- Lortab ASA Tablets.......... 2414
- Momentum Muscular Backache Formula .... ▣ 751
- Norgesic.......... 1314
- Norwich Extra-Strength Aspirin...... ▣ 546
- Norwich Regular Strength Aspirin ▣ 547
- P-A-C Analgesic Tablets .... ▣ 669
- Percodan.......... 951
- Robaxisal Tablets.......... 1872
- Sine-Off Sinus Medicine Tablets-Aspirin Formula .... ▣ 722
- Soma Compound w/Codeine Tablets 2390
- Soma Compound Tablets.......... 2389
- St. Joseph Adult Chewable Aspirin (81 mg.).......... ▣ 703
- Synalgos-DC Capsules 2525
- Talwin Compound 2072
- Ursinus Inlay-Tabs.......... ▣ 691
- Vanquish Analgesic Caplets .... ▣ 574
- Zorprin Tablets.......... 698

Aspirin, Enteric Coated (Concurrent administration may lower Meclomen plasma levels and greater fecal blood loss results). Products include:
- Therapy Bayer Aspirin Caplets ...... ▣ 568
- Ecotrin 2189

Warfarin Sodium (Enhanced effect of warfarin; the dosage of warfarin should be reduced). Products include:
- Coumadin Injection & Tablets 944
- Panwarfin Tablets 547

Food Interactions

Food, unspecified (Decreases in rate and the extent of absorption).

MEDIATRIC CAPSULES

(Estrogens, Conjugated, Methyltestosterone)....................2476
May interact with progestins. Compounds in this category include:

Medroxyprogesterone Acetate (Potential for adverse effect of carbohydrate metabolism). Products include:
- Amen.......... 833
- Cycrin Tablets.......... 2449
- Depo-Provera Sterile Aqueous Suspension.......... 2336
- Provera Tablets 2356

Megestrol Acetate (Potential for adverse effect of carbohydrate metabolism). Products include:
- Megace Tablets 732

Norgestimate (Potential for adverse effect of carbohydrate metabolism). Products include:
- Ortho-Cyclen Tablets 1658

MEDI-FLU CAPLET, LIQUID

(Acetaminophen, Chlorpheniramine Maleate, Dextromethorphan Hydrobromide, Pseudoephedrine Hydrochloride).................................. ▣ 640
May interact with hypnotics and sedatives, tranquilizers, antihypertensives, antidepressant drugs, and certain other agents. Compounds in these categories include:

Acebutolol Hydrochloride (Effect not specified). Products include:
- Sectral Capsules 2520

Alcohol (Increases drowsiness effect).

Alprazolam (Increases drowsiness effect). Products include:
- Xanax Tablets 2367

Amitriptyline Hydrochloride (Effect not specified). Products include:
- Elavil 2269
- Endep Tablets 1927
- Etrafon 2087
- Limbitrol 1933
- Triavil Tablets 1556

Amoxapine (Effect not specified). Products include:
- Asendin Tablets 1196

Atenolol (Effect not specified). Products include:
- Tenoretic Tablets.......... 1105
- Tenormin Tablets and I.V. Injection 1107

Benazepril Hydrochloride (Effect not specified). Products include:
Lotensin Tablets ... 872

Bendroflumethiazide (Effect not specified). Products include:
Corzide Tablets ... 702
Naturetin Tablets ... 1789
Rauzide Tablets ... 1804

Betaxolol Hydrochloride (Effect not specified). Products include:
Betoptic Sterile Ophthalmic Solution ... 569
Betoptic S Sterile Ophthalmic Suspension ... 570
Kerlone Tablets ... 2172

Bupropion Hydrochloride (Effect not specified). Products include:
Wellbutrin Tablets ... 821

Buspirone Hydrochloride (Increases drowsiness effect). Products include:
BuSpar ... 1401

Captopril (Effect not specified). Products include:
Capoten ... 2255
Capozide ... 2258

Carteolol Hydrochloride (Effect not specified). Products include:
Cartrol Tablets ... 507

Chlordiazepoxide (Increases drowsiness effect). Products include:
Libritabs Tablets ... 1930
Limbitrol ... 1933
Menrium Tablets ... 1934

Chlordiazepoxide Hydrochloride (Increases drowsiness effect). Products include:
Librax Capsules ... 1929
Librium Capsules ... 1931
Librium Injectable ... 1932

Chlorothiazide (Effect not specified). Products include:
Aldoclor Tablets ... 1413
Diupres Tablets ... 1461
Diuril Oral ... 1464

Chlorothiazide Sodium (Effect not specified). Products include:
Diuril Sodium Intravenous ... 1463

Chlorpromazine (Increases drowsiness effect). Products include:
Thorazine ... 2234

Chlorprothixene (Increases drowsiness effect). Products include:
Taractan Tablets ... 1920

Chlorprothixene Hydrochloride (Increases drowsiness effect). Products include:
Taractan ... 1920

Chlorthalidone (Effect not specified). Products include:
Combipres Tablets ... 678
Tenoretic Tablets ... 1105
Thalitone Tablets ... 687

Clonidine (Effect not specified). Products include:
Catapres-TTS ... 677

Clonidine Hydrochloride (Effect not specified). Products include:
Catapres Tablets ... 676
Combipres Tablets ... 678

Clorazepate Dipotassium (Increases drowsiness effect). Products include:
Tranxene ... 556

Deserpidine (Effect not specified). Products include:
Enduronyl ... 518
Harmonyl Tablets ... 528
Oreticyl ... 545

Desipramine Hydrochloride (Effect not specified). Products include:
Norpramin Tablets ... 1340

Diazepam (Increases drowsiness effect). Products include:
Valium Injectable ... 1937
Valium Tablets ... 1939
Valrelease Capsules ... 1923

Diazoxide (Effect not specified). Products include:
Hyperstat I.V. Injection ... 2095
Proglycem ... 649

Doxazosin Mesylate (Effect not specified). Products include:
Cardura Tablets ... 1941

Doxepin Hydrochloride (Effect not specified). Products include:
Sinequan ... 1960

Droperidol (Increases drowsiness effect). Products include:
Inapsine Injection ... 1140
Innovar Injection ... 1141

Enalapril Maleate (Effect not specified). Products include:
Vaseretic Tablets ... 1559
Vasotec Tablets ... 1564

Enalaprilat (Effect not specified). Products include:
Vasotec I.V. ... 1562

Esmolol Hydrochloride (Effect not specified). Products include:
Brevibloc Injection ... 942

Estazolam (Increases drowsiness effect). Products include:
ProSom Tablets ... 554

Ethchlorvynol (Increases drowsiness effect). Products include:
Placidyl Capsules ... 553

Ethinamate (Increases drowsiness effect).
No products indexed under this heading.

Felodipine (Effect not specified). Products include:
Plendil Extended-Release Tablets ... 1526

Fluoxetine Hydrochloride (Effect not specified). Products include:
Prozac Pulvules ... 920

Fluphenazine Decanoate (Increases drowsiness effect). Products include:
Prolixin Decanoate ... 1795

Fluphenazine Enanthate (Increases drowsiness effect). Products include:
Prolixin Enanthate ... 1796

Fluphenazine Hydrochloride (Increases drowsiness effect). Products include:
Prolixin Elixir ... 1793
Prolixin Injection ... 1791
Prolixin Oral Concentrate ... 1792
Prolixin Tablets ... 1793

Flurazepam Hydrochloride (Increases drowsiness effect). Products include:
Dalmane Capsules ... 1927

Fosinopril Sodium (Effect not specified). Products include:
Monopril Tablets ... 1406

Furosemide (Effect not specified). Products include:
Lasix ... 1093

Glutethimide (Increases drowsiness effect).
No products indexed under this heading.

Guanabenz Acetate (Effect not specified). Products include:
Wytensin Tablets ... 2542

Guanethidine Monosulfate (Effect not specified). Products include:
Esimil Tablets ... 864
Ismelin Tablets ... 869

Haloperidol (Increases drowsiness effect). Products include:
Haldol Injection, Tablets and Concentrate ... 1373

Haloperidol Decanoate (Increases drowsiness effect). Products include:
Haldol Decanoate ... 1375

Hydralazine Hydrochloride (Effect not specified). Products include:
Apresazide Capsules ... 854
Apresoline Hydrochloride Parenteral (Ampuls) ... 856
Apresoline Hydrochloride Tablets .. 855
Apresoline-Esidrix Tablets ... 857
Ser-Ap-Es Tablets ... 881
Serpasil-Apresoline Tablets ... 884

Hydrochlorothiazide (Effect not specified). Products include:
Aldactazide ... 2150
Aldoril Tablets ... 1418
Apresazide Capsules ... 854
Apresoline-Esidrix Tablets ... 857
Capozide ... 2258
Dyazide Capsules ... 2208
Esidrix Tablets ... 863
Esimil Tablets ... 864
HydroDIURIL Tablets ... 1484
Hydropres Tablets ... 1485
Inderide Tablets ... 2463
Inderide LA Long Acting Capsules .. 2465
Lopressor HCT Tablets ... 1034
Maxzide ... 1215
Moduretic Tablets ... 1510
Normozide Tablets ... 2112
Oretic Tablets ... 544
Oreticyl ... 545
Prinzide Tablets ... 1540
Ser-Ap-Es Tablets ... 881
Serpasil-Esidrix Tablets ... 886
Timolide Tablets ... 1547
Trandate HCT Tablets ... 579
Vaseretic Tablets ... 1559
Zestoretic ... 2274

Hydroflumethiazide (Effect not specified). Products include:
Diucardin Tablets ... 2450
Saluron ... 718
Salutensin/Salutensin-Demi ... 719

Hydroxyzine Hydrochloride (Increases drowsiness effect). Products include:
Atarax Tablets & Syrup ... 1941
Marax Tablets & DF Syrup ... 1954
Vistaril Intramuscular Solution ... 1970

Imipramine Hydrochloride (Effect not specified). Products include:
Tofranil Ampuls ... 1038
Tofranil Tablets ... 1039

Imipramine Pamoate (Effect not specified). Products include:
Tofranil-PM Capsules ... 1041

Indapamide (Effect not specified). Products include:
Lozol Tablets ... 1843

Isocarboxazid (Effect not specified). Products include:
Marplan Tablets ... 1906

Isradipine (Effect not specified). Products include:
DynaCirc Capsules ... 2004

Labetalol Hydrochloride (Effect not specified). Products include:
Normodyne Injection ... 2108
Normodyne Tablets ... 2110
Normozide Tablets ... 2112
Trandate HCT Tablets ... 579
Trandate Injection ... 577
Trandate Tablets ... 579

Lisinopril (Effect not specified). Products include:
Prinivil Tablets ... 1538
Prinzide Tablets ... 1540
Zestoretic ... 2274
Zestril Tablets ... 2277

Lorazepam (Increases drowsiness effect). Products include:
Ativan Injection ... 2432
Ativan Tablets ... 2434

Loxapine Hydrochloride (Increases drowsiness effect). Products include:
Loxitane ... 1213

Loxapine Succinate (Increases drowsiness effect). Products include:
Loxitane Capsules ... 1213

Maprotiline Hydrochloride (Effect not specified). Products include:
Ludiomil Tablets ... 874

Mecamylamine Hydrochloride (Effect not specified). Products include:
Inversine Tablets ... 1492

Meprobamate (Increases drowsiness effect). Products include:
Deprol Tablets ... 2382
Equagesic Tablets ... 2451
Miltown Tablets ... 2386
PMB 200 and PMB 400 ... 2504

Mesoridazine (Increases drowsiness effect). Products include:
Serentil ... 686

Methyclothiazide (Effect not specified). Products include:
Enduron Tablets ... 517
Enduronyl ... 518

Methyldopa (Effect not specified). Products include:
Aldoclor Tablets ... 1413
Aldomet Oral ... 1415
Aldoril Tablets ... 1418

Methyldopate Hydrochloride (Effect not specified). Products include:
Aldomet Ester HCl Injection ... 1417

Metolazone (Effect not specified). Products include:
Diulo ... 2129
Mykrox ½ mg Tablets ... 984
Zaroxolyn Tablets ... 989

Metoprolol Tartrate (Effect not specified). Products include:
Lopressor Ampuls ... 1032
Lopressor HCT Tablets ... 1034
Lopressor Tablets ... 1032

Metyrosine (Effect not specified). Products include:
Demser Capsules ... 1460

Midazolam Hydrochloride (Increases drowsiness effect). Products include:
Versed Injection ... 1924

Minoxidil (Effect not specified). Products include:
Loniten Tablets ... 2346
Rogaine Topical Solution ... 2357

Molindone Hydrochloride (Increases drowsiness effect). Products include:
Moban Tablets & Concentrate ... 932

Nadolol (Effect not specified). Products include:
Corgard Tablets ... 701
Corzide Tablets ... 702

Nicardipine Hydrochloride (Effect not specified). Products include:
Cardene Capsules ... 2290

Nitroglycerin (Effect not specified). Products include:
Deponit NTG Transdermal Delivery System ... 2143
Minitran Transdermal Delivery System ... 1312
Nitro-Bid Ointment ... 1339
Nitro-Bid Capsules ... 1338
Nitrodisc ... 2176
Nitro-Dur (nitroglycerin) Transdermal Infusion System ... 1164
Nitrogard Tablets ... 1004
Nitrolingual Spray ... 1846
Nitrostat Tablets ... 1743
Transderm-Nitro Transdermal Therapeutic System ... 2283

Nortriptyline Hydrochloride (Effect not specified). Products include:
Pamelor ... 2019

Oxazepam (Increases drowsiness effect). Products include:
Serax Capsules ... 2522
Serax Tablets ... 2522

Penbutolol Sulfate (Effect not specified). Products include:
Levatol ... 1832

Perphenazine (Increases drowsiness effect). Products include:
Etrafon ... 2087
Triavil Tablets ... 1556
Trilafon ... 2123

Phenelzine Sulfate (Effect not specified). Products include:
Nardil 1742

Phenoxybenzamine Hydrochloride (Effect not specified). Products include:
Dibenzyline Capsules 2207

Phentolamine Mesylate (Effect not specified). Products include:
Regitine 878

Pindolol (Effect not specified). Products include:
Visken Tablets 2036

Polythiazide (Effect not specified). Products include:
Minizide Capsules 1779
Renese Tablets 1785
Renese-R Tablets 1786

Prazepam (Increases drowsiness effect). Products include:
Centrax 1693

Prazosin Hydrochloride (Effect not specified). Products include:
Minipress Capsules 1778
Minizide Capsules 1779

Prochlorperazine (Increases drowsiness effect). Products include:
Compazine 2201

Promethazine Hydrochloride (Increases drowsiness effect). Products include:
Mepergan Injection 2479
Phenergan with Codeine 2497
Phenergan with Dextromethorphan 2499
Phenergan Injection 2493
Phenergan Suppositories 2496
Phenergan Syrup 2495
Phenergan Tablets 2496
Phenergan VC 2500
Phenergan VC with Codeine 2501

Propofol (Increases drowsiness effect). Products include:
Diprivan Injection 2267

Propranolol Hydrochloride (Effect not specified). Products include:
Inderal 2459
Inderal LA Long Acting Capsules 2461
Inderide Tablets 2463
Inderide LA Long Acting Capsules .. 2465

Protriptyline Hydrochloride (Effect not specified). Products include:
Vivactil Tablets 1567

Quazepam (Increases drowsiness effect). Products include:
Doral Tablets 2383

Ramipril (Effect not specified). Products include:
Altace Capsules 1086

Rauwolfia Serpentina (Effect not specified). Products include:
Raudixin Tablets 1803
Rauzide Tablets 1804

Rescinnamine (Effect not specified).
No products indexed under this heading.

Reserpine (Effect not specified). Products include:
Diupres Tablets 1461
Hydromox R Tablets 1209
Hydropres Tablets 1485
Renese-R Tablets 1786
Salutensin/Salutensin-Demi 719
Ser-Ap-Es Tablets 881
Serpasil Tablets 883
Serpasil-Apresoline Tablets 884
Serpasil-Esidrix Tablets 886

Secobarbital Sodium (Increases drowsiness effect). Products include:
Seconal Sodium Pulvules 1296

Sodium Nitroprusside (Effect not specified). Products include:
Nipride I.V. Infusion 1909

Temazepam (Increases drowsiness effect). Products include:
Restoril Capsules 2023

Terazosin Hydrochloride (Effect not specified). Products include:
Hytrin Tablets 529

Thioridazine Hydrochloride (Increases drowsiness effect). Products include:
Mellaril 2011

Thiothixene (Increases drowsiness effect). Products include:
Navane Capsules and Concentrate 1954
Navane Intramuscular 1956

Timolol Maleate (Effect not specified). Products include:
Blocadren Tablets 1429
Timolide Tablets 1547
Timoptic in Ocudose 1552
Timoptic Sterile Ophthalmic Solution 1550

Tranylcypromine Sulfate (Effect not specified). Products include:
Parnate Tablets 2222

Trazodone Hydrochloride (Effect not specified). Products include:
Desyrel and Desyrel Dividose 1404

Triazolam (Increases drowsiness effect). Products include:
Halcion Tablets 2340

Trifluoperazine Hydrochloride (Increases drowsiness effect). Products include:
Stelazine 2226

Trimethaphan Camsylate (Effect not specified). Products include:
Arfonad Ampuls 1887

Trimipramine Maleate (Effect not specified). Products include:
Surmontil Capsules 2524

MEDIHALER ERGOTAMINE AEROSOL

(Ergotamine Tartrate) 1312
No interactions described in labeling.

MEDIPREN IBUPROFEN CAPLETS AND TABLETS

(Ibuprofen) 1362
May interact with aspirin and acetaminophen containing products and certain other agents. Compounds in these categories include:

Acetaminophen (Concurrent use is not recommended). Products include:
Acetaminophen Uniserts Suppositories 2374
Actifed Plus Caplets .... ▣ 539
Actifed Plus Tablets .... ▣ 540
Alka-Seltzer Advanced Formula Antacid & Non-Aspirin Pain Reliever .... ▣ 620
Allerest .... ▣ 559
Aspirin Free Anacin Maximum Strength Acetaminophen Film Coated Caplets 2417
Aspirin Free Anacin Maximum Strength Acetaminophen Film Coated Tablets 2417
Anacin-3 Regular Strength Acetaminophen Film Coated Tablets ▣ 746
Anexsia 5/500 Tablets 2196
Anexsia 7.5/650 Tablets 2197
Benadryl Plus .... ▣ 636
Benadryl Plus Nighttime .... ▣ 637
Bufferin AF Nite Time Analgesic/Sleeping Aid Caplets 744
Allergy-Sinus Comtrex Multi-Symptom Allergy Sinus Formula Tablets & Caplets 746
Cough Formula Comtrex 746
Comtrex Multi-Symptom Cold Reliever Tablets/Caplets/Liqui-Gels/Liquid 745
Day-Night Comtrex 747
Non-Drowsy Comtrex 747
Congespirin For Children Aspirin Free Chewable Cold Tablets 748
Contac Cough & Sore Throat Formula .... ▣ 712
Contac Jr. Children's Cold Medicine .... ▣ 712
Contac Nighttime Cold Medicine .... ▣ 713
Contac Severe Cold and Flu Formula Caplets .... ▣ 711
Contac Sinus Caplets Maximum Strength Non-Drowsy Formula .... ▣ 710
Contac Sinus Tablets Maximum Strength Non-Drowsy Formula .... ▣ 710
Coricidin 'D' Decongestant Tablets .... ▣ 695
Coricidin Demilets Tablets for Children .... ▣ 696
Coricidin Tablets .... ▣ 695
Darvon-N/Darvocet-N 1254
Datril Extra-Strength Analgesic Tablets 748
Dimetapp Plus Caplets .... ▣ 675
Dorcol Children's Fever & Pain Reducer .... ▣ 686
Dristan Decongestant/Antihistamine/ Analgesic Coated Caplets .... ▣ 749
Dristan Cold Nasal Decongestant/ Antihistamine/ Analgesic Coated Tablets 2419
Dristan Advanced Formula Decongestant/Antihistamine/ Analgesic Tablets .... ▣ 749
Maximum Strength Dristan Decongestant/Analgesic Coated Caplets .... ▣ 750
No Drowsiness Dristan Cold Nasal Decongestant/Analgesic Coated Caplets 2420
Drixoral Plus Extended-Release Tablets .... ▣ 699
Drixoral Sinus .... ▣ 700
Esgic-Plus Tablets 1002
Esgic Tablets & Capsules 1001
Aspirin Free Excedrin Analgesic Caplets 748
Excedrin Extra-Strength Analgesic Tablets & Caplets 749
Excedrin P.M. Analgesic/Sleeping Aid Tablets, Caplets and Liquid 749
Sinus Excedrin Analgesic, Decongestant Tablets & Caplets 750
4-Way Cold Tablets 750
Feverall Sprinkle Caps 2374
Feverall Suppositories 2374
Fioricet Tablets 2006
Hycomine Compound Tablets 929
Hydrocet Capsules 835
Isocom Capsules 1629
Liquiprin .... ▣ 618
Lortab 2412
Lurline PMS Tablets 972
Medi-Flu Caplet, Liquid .... ▣ 640
Maximum Strength Midol Multi-Symptom Menstrual Formula .... ▣ 571
Maximum Strength Midol PMS Premenstrual Syndrome Formula .... ▣ 570
Regular Strength Midol Multi-Symptom Menstrual Formula .... ▣ 570
Midrin Capsules 836
Ornex Caplets .... ▣ 618
Children's Panadol Chewable Tablets, Liquid, Infants' Drops .... ▣ 571
Junior Strength Panadol .... ▣ 571
Maximum Strength Panadol Tablets and Caplets .... ▣ 572
Percocet Tablets 950
Percogesic Analgesic Tablets .... ▣ 660
Phenaphen with Codeine Capsules 1865
Phenaphen-650 with Codeine Tablets 1866
Phrenilin 838
Prēmsyn PMS Capsules & Caplets ▣ 547
Pyrroxate Capsules .... ▣ 669
Robitussin Night Relief .... ▣ 677
Sedapap Tablets 50 mg/650 mg .. 1360
Sinarest .... ▣ 562
Sine-Aid Maximum Strength Sinus Headache Caplets 1365
Sine-Aid Maximum Strength Sinus Headache Tablets 1365
Sine-Off Maximum Strength Allergy/Sinus Formula Caplets .... ▣ 721
Sine-Off Maximum Strength No Drowsiness Formula Caplets .... ▣ 722
Singlet Tablets .... ▣ 598
Sinulin 840
Sinutab Maximum Strength .... ▣ 641
Sinutab Maximum Strength Without Drowsiness Tablets & Caplets .... ▣ 642
Sinutab Regular Strength Without Drowsiness Formula .... ▣ 641
Sominex Pain Relief Formula .... ▣ 723
St. Joseph Aspirin-Free Fever Reducer for Children Chewable Tablets, Liquid & Infant Drops .... ▣ 704
St. Joseph Cold Tablets for Children .... ▣ 704
St. Joseph Nighttime Cold Medicine .... ▣ 705
Sudafed Sinus Caplets .... ▣ 545
Sudafed Sinus Tablets .... ▣ 545
Talacen 2070
Tempra, Acetaminophen .... ▣ 613
TheraFlu Flu and Cold Medicine .... ▣ 687
Triaminicin Tablets .... ▣ 690
Tylenol acetaminophen Children's Chewable Tablets & Elixir 1366
Tylenol Allergy Sinus Medication Caplets and Gelcaps, Maximum Strength 1372
Tylenol with Codeine 1381
Children's Tylenol Cold Liquid Formula and Chewable Tablets 1368
Tylenol Cold & Flu Hot Medication, Packets 1369
Tylenol Cold & Flu No Drowsiness Hot Medication, Packets 1371
Tylenol Cold Medication Caplets and Tablets 1370
Tylenol Cold Medication, Effervescent Tablets 1369
Tylenol Cold Medication No Drowsiness Formula Caplets 1370
Tylenol Cold Night Time Medication Liquid 1371
Tylenol Cough Medication Liquid, Maximum Strength 1372
Tylenol Cough Medication Liquid with Decongestant, Maximum Strength 1372
Tylenol, Extra Strength, acetaminophen Adult Liquid Pain Reliever .. 1367
Tylenol, Extra Strength, acetaminophen Gelcaps, Caplets, Tablets 1367
Tylenol, Infants' Drops 1366
Tylenol, Junior Strength, acetaminophen Coated Caplets, Grape and Fruit Chewable Tablets 1366
Tylenol, Maximum Strength, Sinus Medication Gelcaps, Caplets and Tablets 1373
Tylenol, Regular Strength, acetaminophen Tablets and Caplets 1367
Tylenol PM, Extra Strength Caplets and Tablets 1368
Tylox Capsules 1382
Unisom Dual Relief Nighttime Sleep Aid/Analgesic 1774
Vanquish Analgesic Caplets .... ▣ 574
Vicks Daycare .... ▣ 660
Vicks Formula 44M Multi-Symptom Cough Medicine .... ▣ 662
Vicks NyQuil Nighttime Colds Medicine-Original & Cherry Flavor .... ▣ 664
Vicodin Tablets 1187
Vicodin ES Tablets 1189
Wygesic Tablets 2540
Zydone Capsules 941

Aspirin (Concurrent use is not recommended). Products include:
Alka-Seltzer Effervescent Antacid and Pain Reliever 1568
Alka-Seltzer Extra Strength Effervescent Antacid and Pain Reliever 1570
Alka-Seltzer (Flavored) Effervescent Antacid and Pain Reliever 1569
Alka-Seltzer Plus Cold Medicine .... ▣ 623
Alka-Seltzer Plus Night-Time Cold Medicine .... ▣ 623
Alka Seltzer Plus Sinus Allergy Medicine .... ▣ 624
Anacin Coated Analgesic Caplets 2417
Anacin Coated Analgesic Tablets 2417
Anacin Maximum Strength Analgesic Coated Tablets 2417
Maximum Strength Arthritis Pain Formula By the Makers of Anacin Analgesic Tablets and Caplets 2418
Arthritis Pain Formula by the Makers of Anacin Analgesic Tablets and Caplets .... ▣ 747
Arthritis Strength BC Powder .... ▣ 516
Ascriptin A/D Caplets 1850
Regular Strength Ascriptin Tablets 1850
Azdone Tablets 844
BC Powder .... ▣ 517
BC Cold Powder .... ▣ 517
Children's Bayer Chewable Aspirin .... ▣ 564
Genuine Bayer Aspirin Tablets & Caplets .... ▣ 564
Maximum Bayer Aspirin Tablets & Caplets .... ▣ 566
Bayer Plus Aspirin Tablets .... ▣ 567

Therapy Bayer Aspirin Caplets ...... ▣ 568
8 Hour Bayer Timed-Release Aspirin ...... ▣ 566
Arthritis Strength Bufferin Analgesic Caplets 744
Extra Strength Bufferin Analgesic Tablets 745
Bufferin Analgesic Tablets and Caplets 743
Cama Arthritis Pain Reliever ...... ▣ 685
Damason-P 1356
Easprin 1719
Ecotrin Enteric Coated Aspirin Maximum Strength Tablets and Caplets 2189
Ecotrin Enteric Coated Aspirin Regular Strength Tablets and Caplets 2189
Empirin Aspirin ...... ▣ 541
Empirin with Codeine Phosphate Nos. 2, 3 & 4 764
Equagesic Tablets 2451
Excedrin Extra-Strength Analgesic Tablets & Caplets 749
4-Way Cold Tablets 750
Fiorinal Capsules 2007
Fiorinal with Codeine Capsules 2008
Fiorinal Tablets 2007
Lortab ASA Tablets 2414
Momentum Muscular Backache Formula ...... ▣ 751
Norgesic 1314
Norwich Extra-Strength Aspirin ...... ▣ 546
Norwich Regular Strength Aspirin ▣ 547
P-A-C Analgesic Tablets ...... ▣ 669
Percodan 951
Robaxisal Tablets 1872
Sine-Off Sinus Medicine Tablets-Aspirin Formula ...... ▣ 722
Soma Compound w/Codeine Tablets 2390
Soma Compound Tablets 2389
St. Joseph Adult Chewable Aspirin (81 mg.) ...... ▣ 703
Synalgos-DC Capsules 2525
Talwin Compound 2072
Ursinus Inlay-Tabs ...... ▣ 691
Vanquish Analgesic Caplets ...... ▣ 574
Zorprin Tablets 698

Prescription Drugs, unspecified (Effect not specified).

MEDROL DOSEPAK UNIT OF USE

(Methylprednisolone) 2348
May interact with:

Cyclosporine (Potential for convulsions). Products include:
Sandimmune 2024

Immunization (Possible hazard of neurological complications and a lack of antibody response).

Smallpox Vaccine (Possible hazard of neurological complications and a lack of antibody response).

MEDROL TABLETS

(Methylprednisolone) 2348
See **Medrol Dosepak Unit of Use**

MEFOXIN

(Cefoxitin Sodium) 1498
May interact with aminoglycosides and certain other agents. Compounds in these categories include:

Amikacin Sulfate (Increased nephrotoxicity). Products include:
Amikin Injectable 602

Gentamicin Sulfate (Increased nephrotoxicity). Products include:
Garamycin Injectable 2093
Garamycin Ophthalmic ...... ◉ 305
Genoptic Liquifilm Sterile Ophthalmic Solution ...... ◉ 247
Genoptic S.O.P. Sterile Ophthalmic Ointment ...... ◉ 247
Gentacidin Ointment ...... ◉ 273
Gentacidin Solution ...... ◉ 273
Gentak Ointment & Solution ...... ◉ 208
G-myticin Creme and Ointment 0.1% 1770
Pred-G Liquifilm Sterile Ophthalmic Suspension ...... ◉ 252
Pred-G S.O.P. Sterile Ophthalmic Ointment ...... ◉ 253

Kanamycin Sulfate (Increased nephrotoxicity). Products include:
Kantrex Injection 601
Kantrex Pediatric Injection 601

Probenecid (Higher serum levels of cefoxitin). Products include:
Benemid Tablets 1426
ColBENEMID Tablets 1436
Wycillin Injection and Probenecid Tablets 2539

Streptomycin Sulfate (Increased nephrotoxicity).
No products indexed under this heading.

Tobramycin Sulfate (Increased nephrotoxicity). Products include:
Nebcin Vials, Hyporets & ADD-Vantage 1286

MEFOXIN PREMIXED INTRAVENOUS SOLUTION

(Cefoxitin Sodium) 1500
May interact with aminoglycosides and certain other agents. Compounds in these categories include:

Amikacin Sulfate (Increased nephrotoxicity). Products include:
Amikin Injectable 602

Gentamicin Sulfate (Increased nephrotoxicity). Products include:
Garamycin Injectable 2093
Garamycin Ophthalmic ...... ◉ 305
Genoptic Liquifilm Sterile Ophthalmic Solution ...... ◉ 247
Genoptic S.O.P. Sterile Ophthalmic Ointment ...... ◉ 247
Gentacidin Ointment ...... ◉ 273
Gentacidin Solution ...... ◉ 273
Gentak Ointment & Solution ...... ◉ 208
G-myticin Creme and Ointment 0.1% 1770
Pred-G Liquifilm Sterile Ophthalmic Suspension ...... ◉ 252
Pred-G S.O.P. Sterile Ophthalmic Ointment ...... ◉ 253

Kanamycin Sulfate (Increased nephrotoxicity). Products include:
Kantrex Injection 601
Kantrex Pediatric Injection 601

Probenecid (Higher serum levels of cefoxitin). Products include:
Benemid Tablets 1426
ColBENEMID Tablets 1436
Wycillin Injection and Probenecid Tablets 2539

Streptomycin Sulfate (Increased nephrotoxicity).
No products indexed under this heading.

Tobramycin Sulfate (Increased nephrotoxicity). Products include:
Nebcin Vials, Hyporets & ADD-Vantage 1286

MEGA-B

(Vitamin B Complex) 607
No interactions described in labeling.

MEGACE TABLETS

(Megestrol Acetate) 732
No interactions described in labeling.

MELLARIL CONCENTRATE

(Thioridazine Hydrochloride) 2011
May interact with central nervous system depressants, general anesthetics, and certain other agents. Compounds in these categories include:

Alcohol (Potentiated).

Alfentanil Hydrochloride (Potentiated). Products include:
Alfenta Injection 1131

Alprazolam (Potentiated). Products include:
Xanax Tablets 2367

Aprobarbital (Potentiated). Products include:
Alurate Elixir 1883

Atropine Derivatives (Potentiated).

Atropine Nitrate, Methyl (Potentiated).
No products indexed under this heading.

Atropine Sulfate (Potentiated). Products include:
Arco-Lase Plus Tablets 607
Atropine Sulfate Sterile Ophthalmic Solution and S.O.P. Sterile Ophthalmic Ointment ...... ◉ 239
Donnagel ...... ▣ 675
Donnagel-PG 1858
Donnatal 1858
Donnatal Extentabs 1859
Donnatal Tablets 1858
Donnazyme Tablets 1860
Isopto Atropine ...... ◉ 218
Lomotil 2174
Motofen Tablets 836
Ru-Tuss Tablets 693
Urised Tablets 2396

Buprenorphine (Potentiated).
No products indexed under this heading.

Buspirone Hydrochloride (Potentiated). Products include:
BuSpar 1401

Butabarbital (Potentiated). Products include:
Pyridium Plus 1764

Butalbital (Potentiated). Products include:
Esgic-Plus Tablets 1002
Esgic Tablets & Capsules 1001
Fioricet Tablets 2006
Fiorinal Capsules 2007
Fiorinal with Codeine Capsules 2008
Fiorinal Tablets 2007
Phrenilin 838
Sedapap Tablets 50 mg/650 mg 1360

Chlordiazepoxide (Potentiated). Products include:
Libritabs Tablets 1930
Limbitrol 1933
Menrium Tablets 1934

Chlordiazepoxide Hydrochloride (Potentiated). Products include:
Librax Capsules 1929
Librium Capsules 1931
Librium Injectable 1932

Chlorpromazine (Potentiated). Products include:
Thorazine 2234

Chlorprothixene (Potentiated). Products include:
Taractan Tablets 1920

Chlorprothixene Hydrochloride (Potentiated). Products include:
Taractan 1920

Clorazepate Dipotassium (Potentiated). Products include:
Tranxene 556

Codeine (Potentiated). Products include:
Calcidrine Syrup 506

Codeine Phosphate (Potentiated). Products include:
Actifed with Codeine Cough Syrup 752
Cheracol Cough Syrup 1853
Codimal PH Syrup 846
Dimetane-DC Cough Syrup 1857
Empirin with Codeine Phosphate Nos. 2, 3 & 4 764
Fiorinal with Codeine Capsules 2008
Isoclor Expectorant 982
Naldecon CX Adult Liquid ...... ▣ 521
Novahistine DH 1342
Novahistine Expectorant 1343
Nucofed Capsules 2219
Nucofed Expectorant 2219
Nucofed Pediatric Expectorant 2220
Nucofed Syrup 2219
Phenaphen with Codeine Capsules 1865
Phenaphen-650 with Codeine Tablets 1866
Phenergan with Codeine 2497
Phenergan VC with Codeine 2501
Robitussin A-C Syrup 1875
Robitussin-DAC Syrup 1875
Ryna ...... ▣ 741
Soma Compound w/Codeine Tablets 2390
Triaminic Expectorant w/Codeine 1996
Tussi-Organidin Liquid 2391
Tylenol with Codeine 1381

Codeine Polistirex (Potentiated).
No products indexed under this heading.

Dezocine (Potentiated).

Diazepam (Potentiated). Products include:
Valium Injectable 1937
Valium Tablets 1939
Valrelease Capsules 1923

Droperidol (Potentiated). Products include:
Inapsine Injection 1140
Innovar Injection 1141

Enflurane (Potentiated). Products include:
Ethrane 599

Epinephrine Hydrochloride (Reversed epinephrine effect). Products include:
Adrenalin Chloride Solution 1:100 & 1:1,000 1689
Epifrin ...... ◉ 244
Glaucon ...... ◉ 218

Estazolam (Potentiated). Products include:
ProSom Tablets 554

Ethchlorvynol (Potentiated). Products include:
Placidyl Capsules 553

Ethinamate (Potentiated).
No products indexed under this heading.

Fentanyl (Potentiated). Products include:
Duragesic Transdermal System 1133

Fentanyl Citrate (Potentiated). Products include:
Innovar Injection 1141
Sublimaze Injection 1146

Fluphenazine Decanoate (Potentiated). Products include:
Prolixin Decanoate 1795

Fluphenazine Enanthate (Potentiated). Products include:
Prolixin Enanthate 1796

Fluphenazine Hydrochloride (Potentiated). Products include:
Prolixin Elixir 1793
Prolixin Injection 1791
Prolixin Oral Concentrate 1792
Prolixin Tablets 1793

Flurazepam Hydrochloride (Potentiated). Products include:
Dalmane Capsules 1927

Glutethimide (Potentiated).
No products indexed under this heading.

Haloperidol (Potentiated). Products include:
Haldol Injection, Tablets and Concentrate 1373

Haloperidol Decanoate (Potentiated). Products include:
Haldol Decanoate 1375

Hydrocodone Bitartrate (Potentiated). Products include:
Anexsia 5/500 Tablets 2196
Anexsia 7.5/650 Tablets 2197
Azdone Tablets 844
Codiclear DH Syrup 845
Codimal DH Syrup 846
Damason-P 1356
Hycodan Syrup, Tablets 927
Hycomine Compound Tablets 929
Hycomine Syrup 927
Hycotuss Expectorant Syrup 930
Hydrocet Capsules 835
Lortab ASA Tablets 2414
Lortab 2412
Ru-Tuss with Hydrocodone 694
Triaminic Expectorant DH 1995
Vicodin Tablets 1187
Vicodin ES Tablets 1189
Zydone Capsules 941

Hydrocodone Polistirex (Potentiated). Products include:
Tussionex Extended-Release Suspension 988

Hydroxyzine Hydrochloride (Potentiated). Products include:
Atarax Tablets & Syrup 1941
Marax Tablets & DF Syrup 1954
Vistaril Intramuscular Solution 1970

Isoflurane (Potentiated). Products include:
Forane 600

Ketamine Hydrochloride (Potentiated). Products include:
Ketalar 1726

Levorphanol Tartrate (Potentiated). Products include:
Levo-Dromoran 1906

Lorazepam (Potentiated). Products include:
Ativan Injection 2432
Ativan Tablets 2434

Loxapine Hydrochloride (Potentiated). Products include:
Loxitane 1213

Loxapine Succinate (Potentiated). Products include:
Loxitane Capsules 1213

Meperidine Hydrochloride (Potentiated). Products include:
Demerol 2047
Mepergan Injection 2479

Mephobarbital (Potentiated). Products include:
Mebaral Tablets 2061

Meprobamate (Potentiated). Products include:
Deprol Tablets 2382
Equagesic Tablets 2451
Miltown Tablets 2386
PMB 200 and PMB 400 2504

Mesoridazine (Potentiated). Products include:
Serentil 686

Methadone Hydrochloride (Potentiated). Products include:
Dolophine Hydrochloride Ampoules & Vials 1260
Dolophine Hydrochloride Tablets 1261
Methadone Hydrochloride Diskets 1284
Methadone Hydrochloride Oral Solution & Tablets 1987

Methohexital Sodium (Potentiated). Products include:
Brevital Sodium Vials 1248

Methoxyflurane (Potentiated).
No products indexed under this heading.

Midazolam Hydrochloride (Potentiated). Products include:
Versed Injection 1924

Molindone Hydrochloride (Potentiated). Products include:
Moban Tablets & Concentrate 932

Morphine Sulfate (Potentiated). Products include:
Astramorph/PF Injection, USP (Preservative-Free) 618
Duramorph 960
Infumorph 200 and Infumorph 500 Sterile Solutions 962
MS Contin Tablets 1814
MSIR 1817
Oramorph SR (Morphine Sulfate Sustained Release Tablets) 1988
Roxanol 1991

Opium Alkaloids (Potentiated). Products include:
B & O No. 15A & No. 16A Supprettes 2395
Pantopon Injectable 1911

Oxazepam (Potentiated). Products include:
Serax Capsules 2522
Serax Tablets 2522

Oxycodone Hydrochloride (Potentiated). Products include:
Percocet Tablets 950
Percodan 951
Roxicodone Tablets, Oral Solution & Intensol (Oxycodone) 1992
Tylox Capsules 1382

Pentobarbital Sodium (Potentiated). Products include:
Nembutal Sodium Capsules 534
Nembutal Sodium Solution 536
Nembutal Sodium Suppositories 538

Perphenazine (Potentiated). Products include:
Etrafon 2087
Triavil Tablets 1556
Trilafon 2123

Phenobarbital (Potentiated). Products include:
Arco-Lase Plus Tablets 607
Bellergal-S Tablets 1998
Bronkolixir ⊞ 761
Bronkotabs Tablets ⊞ 762
Donnatal 1858
Donnatal Extentabs 1859
Donnatal Tablets 1858
Donnazyme Tablets 1860
Kinesed Tablets 2272
Phenobarbital Elixir and Tablets 1293
Primatene Tablets-P Formula 2421
Quadrinal Tablets 1183
Tedral SA 1765

Pindolol (Concurrent administration of both drugs have resulted in higher serum levels of both). Products include:
Visken Tablets 2036

Prazepam (Potentiated). Products include:
Centrax 1693

Prochlorperazine (Potentiated). Products include:
Compazine 2201

Promethazine Hydrochloride (Potentiated). Products include:
Mepergan Injection 2479
Phenergan with Codeine 2497
Phenergan with Dextromethorphan 2499
Phenergan Injection 2493
Phenergan Suppositories 2496
Phenergan Syrup 2495
Phenergan Tablets 2496
Phenergan VC 2500
Phenergan VC with Codeine 2501

Propofol (Potentiated). Products include:
Diprivan Injection 2267

Propoxyphene Hydrochloride (Potentiated). Products include:
Darvon 1256
Wygesic Tablets 2540

Propoxyphene Napsylate (Potentiated). Products include:
Darvon-N/Darvocet-N 1254

Propranolol Hydrochloride (Concurrent administration produces increases in plasma levels of thioridazine). Products include:
Inderal 2459
Inderal LA Long Acting Capsules 2461
Inderide Tablets 2463
Inderide LA Long Acting Capsules 2465

Quazepam (Potentiated). Products include:
Doral Tablets 2383

Secobarbital Sodium (Potentiated). Products include:
Seconal Sodium Pulvules 1296

Sufentanil Citrate (Potentiated). Products include:
Sufenta Injection 1147

Temazepam (Potentiated). Products include:
Restoril Capsules 2023

Thiamylal Sodium (Potentiated). Products include:
Surital Ampoules, Steri-Vials 1764

Thiothixene (Potentiated). Products include:
Navane Capsules and Concentrate 1954
Navane Intramuscular 1956

Triazolam (Potentiated). Products include:
Halcion Tablets 2340

Trifluoperazine Hydrochloride (Potentiated). Products include:
Stelazine 2226

MELLARIL TABLETS
(Thioridazine Hydrochloride) 2011
See **Mellaril Concentrate**

MELLARIL-S SUSPENSION
(Thioridazine Hydrochloride) 2011
See **Mellaril Concentrate**

MENRIUM TABLETS
(Chlordiazepoxide, Estrogens, Conjugated) 1934
May interact with psychotropics, monoamine oxidase inhibitors, phenothiazines, and certain other agents. Compounds in these categories include:

Alcohol (Concomitant administration not recommended).

Alprazolam (Concomitant administration not recommended). Products include:
Xanax Tablets 2367

Amitriptyline Hydrochloride (Concomitant administration not recommended). Products include:
Elavil 2269
Endep Tablets 1927
Etrafon 2087
Limbitrol 1933
Triavil Tablets 1556

Amoxapine (Concomitant administration not recommended). Products include:
Asendin Tablets 1196

Buspirone Hydrochloride (Concomitant administration not recommended). Products include:
BuSpar 1401

Chlordiazepoxide Hydrochloride (Concomitant administration not recommended). Products include:
Librax Capsules 1929
Librium Capsules 1931
Librium Injectable 1932

Chlorpromazine (A potentiating compound; concomitant administration not recommended). Products include:
Thorazine 2234

Chlorprothixene (Concomitant administration not recommended). Products include:
Taractan Tablets 1920

Chlorprothixene Hydrochloride (Concomitant administration not recommended). Products include:
Taractan 1920

Clorazepate Dipotassium (Concomitant administration not recommended). Products include:
Tranxene 556

Desipramine Hydrochloride (Concomitant administration not recommended). Products include:
Norpramin Tablets 1340

Diazepam (Concomitant administration not recommended). Products include:
Valium Injectable 1937
Valium Tablets 1939
Valrelease Capsules 1923

Doxepin Hydrochloride (Concomitant administration not recommended). Products include:
Sinequan 1960

Droperidol (Concomitant administration not recommended). Products include:
Inapsine Injection 1140
Innovar Injection 1141

Fluphenazine Decanoate (A potentiating compound; concomitant administration not recommended). Products include:
Prolixin Decanoate 1795

Fluphenazine Enanthate (A potentiating compound; concomitant administration not recommended). Products include:
Prolixin Enanthate 1796

Fluphenazine Hydrochloride (A potentiating compound; concomitant administration not recommended). Products include:
Prolixin Elixir 1793
Prolixin Injection 1791
Prolixin Oral Concentrate 1792
Prolixin Tablets 1793

Furazolidone (A potentiating compound; concomitant administration not recommended). Products include:
Furoxone 1855

Haloperidol (Concomitant administration not recommended). Products include:
Haldol Injection, Tablets and Concentrate 1373

Haloperidol Decanoate (Concomitant administration not recommended). Products include:
Haldol Decanoate 1375

Hydroxyzine Hydrochloride (Concomitant administration not recommended). Products include:
Atarax Tablets & Syrup 1941
Marax Tablets & DF Syrup 1954
Vistaril Intramuscular Solution 1970

Imipramine Hydrochloride (Concomitant administration not recommended). Products include:
Tofranil Ampuls 1038
Tofranil Tablets 1039

Imipramine Pamoate (Concomitant administration not recommended). Products include:
Tofranil-PM Capsules 1041

Isocarboxazid (A potentiating compound; concomitant administration not recommended). Products include:
Marplan Tablets 1906

Lithium Carbonate (Concomitant administration not recommended). Products include:
Eskalith 2214
Lithane Tablets 1596
Lithium Carbonate Capsules & Tablets 1984
Lithobid Tablets 870

Lithium Citrate (Concomitant administration not recommended). Products include:
Cibalith-S 870

Lorazepam (Concomitant administration not recommended). Products include:
Ativan Injection 2432
Ativan Tablets 2434

Loxapine Hydrochloride (Concomitant administration not recommended). Products include:
Loxitane 1213

Loxapine Succinate (Concomitant administration not recommended). Products include:
Loxitane Capsules 1213

Maprotiline Hydrochloride (Concomitant administration not recommended). Products include:
Ludiomil Tablets 874

Meprobamate (Concomitant administration not recommended). Products include:
Deprol Tablets 2382
Equagesic Tablets 2451
Miltown Tablets 2386
PMB 200 and PMB 400 2504

Mesoridazine (A potentiating compound; concomitant administration not recommended). Products include:
- Serentil ... 686

Midazolam Hydrochloride (Concomitant administration not recommended). Products include:
- Versed Injection ... 1924

Molindone Hydrochloride (Concomitant administration not recommended). Products include:
- Moban Tablets & Concentrate ... 932

Nortriptyline Hydrochloride (Concomitant administration not recommended). Products include:
- Pamelor ... 2019

Oxazepam (Concomitant administration not recommended). Products include:
- Serax Capsules ... 2522
- Serax Tablets ... 2522

Perphenazine (A potentiating compound; concomitant administration not recommended). Products include:
- Etrafon ... 2087
- Triavil Tablets ... 1556
- Trilafon ... 2123

Phenelzine Sulfate (A potentiating compound; concomitant administration not recommended). Products include:
- Nardil ... 1742

Prazepam (Concomitant administration not recommended). Products include:
- Centrax ... 1693

Prochlorperazine (A potentiating compound;. concomitant administration not recommended). Products include:
- Compazine ... 2201

Promethazine Hydrochloride (A potentiating compound; concomitant administration not recommended). Products include:
- Mepergan Injection ... 2479
- Phenergan with Codeine ... 2497
- Phenergan with Dextromethorphan 2499
- Phenergan Injection ... 2493
- Phenergan Suppositories ... 2496
- Phenergan Syrup ... 2495
- Phenergan Tablets ... 2496
- Phenergan VC ... 2500
- Phenergan VC with Codeine ... 2501

Protriptyline Hydrochloride (Concomitant administration not recommended). Products include:
- Vivactil Tablets ... 1567

Selegiline Hydrochloride (A potentiating compound; concomitant administration not recommended). Products include:
- Eldepryl ... 2250

Thioridazine Hydrochloride (A potentiating compound; concomitant administration not recommended). Products include:
- Mellaril ... 2011

Thiothixene (Concomitant administration not recommended). Products include:
- Navane Capsules and Concentrate 1954
- Navane Intramuscular ... 1956

Tranylcypromine Sulfate (A potentiating compound; concomitant administration not recommended). Products include:
- Parnate Tablets ... 2222

Trifluoperazine Hydrochloride (A potentiating compound; concomitant administration not recommended). Products include:
- Stelazine ... 2226

Trimipramine Maleate (Concomitant administration not recommended). Products include:
- Surmontil Capsules ... 2524

MEPERGAN INJECTION
(Meperidine Hydrochloride, Promethazine Hydrochloride) ... 2479
May interact with narcotic analgesics, general anesthetics, phenothiazines, tranquilizers, hypnotics and sedatives, tricyclic antidepressants, barbiturates, central nervous system depressants, monoamine oxidase inhibitors, and certain other agents. Compounds in these categories include:

Alcohol (Respiratory depression, hypotension, profound sedation or coma).

Alfentanil Hydrochloride (Respiratory depression, hypotension, profound sedation or coma). Products include:
- Alfenta Injection ... 1131

Alprazolam (Respiratory depression, hypotension, profound sedation or coma). Products include:
- Xanax Tablets ... 2367

Amitriptyline Hydrochloride (Respiratory depression, hypotension, profound sedation or coma). Products include:
- Elavil ... 2269
- Endep Tablets ... 1927
- Etrafon ... 2087
- Limbitrol ... 1933
- Triavil Tablets ... 1556

Amoxapine (Respiratory depression, hypotension, profound sedation or coma). Products include:
- Asendin Tablets ... 1196

Aprobarbital (Respiratory depression, hypotension, profound sedation or coma). Products include:
- Alurate Elixir ... 1883

Buprenorphine (Respiratory depression, hypotension, profound sedation or coma).
- No products indexed under this heading.

Buspirone Hydrochloride (Respiratory depression, hypotension, profound sedation or coma). Products include:
- BuSpar ... 1401

Butabarbital (Respiratory depression, hypotension, profound sedation or coma). Products include:
- Pyridium Plus ... 1764

Butalbital (Respiratory depression, hypotension, profound sedation or coma). Products include:
- Esgic-Plus Tablets ... 1002
- Esgic Tablets & Capsules ... 1001
- Fioricet Tablets ... 2006
- Fiorinal Capsules ... 2007
- Fiorinal with Codeine Capsules ... 2008
- Fiorinal Tablets ... 2007
- Phrenilin ... 838
- Sedapap Tablets 50 mg/650 mg .. 1360

Chlordiazepoxide (Respiratory depression, hypotension, profound sedation or coma). Products include:
- Libritabs Tablets ... 1930
- Limbitrol ... 1933
- Menrium Tablets ... 1934

Chlordiazepoxide Hydrochloride (Respiratory depression, hypotension, profound sedation or coma). Products include:
- Librax Capsules ... 1929
- Librium Capsules ... 1931
- Librium Injectable ... 1932

Chlorpromazine (Respiratory depression, hypotension, profound sedation or coma). Products include:
- Thorazine ... 2234

Chlorprothixene (Respiratory depression, hypotension, profound sedation or coma). Products include:
- Taractan Tablets ... 1920

Chlorprothixene Hydrochloride (Respiratory depression, hypotension, profound sedation or coma). Products include:
- Taractan ... 1920

Clomipramine Hydrochloride (Respiratory depression, hypotension, profound sedation or coma). Products include:
- Anafranil Capsules ... 650

Clorazepate Dipotassium (Respiratory depression, hypotension, profound sedation or coma). Products include:
- Tranxene ... 556

Codeine (Respiratory depression, hypotension, profound sedation or coma). Products include:
- Calcidrine Syrup ... 506

Codeine Phosphate (Respiratory depression, hypotension, profound sedation or coma). Products include:
- Actifed with Codeine Cough Syrup.. 752
- Cheracol Cough Syrup ... 1853
- Codimal PH Syrup ... 846
- Dimetane-DC Cough Syrup ... 1857
- Empirin with Codeine Phosphate Nos. 2, 3 & 4 ... 764
- Fiorinal with Codeine Capsules ... 2008
- Isoclor Expectorant ... 982
- Naldecon CX Adult Liquid ... ▣ 521
- Novahistine DH ... 1342
- Novahistine Expectorant ... 1343
- Nucofed Capsules ... 2219
- Nucofed Expectorant ... 2219
- Nucofed Pediatric Expectorant ... 2220
- Nucofed Syrup ... 2219
- Phenaphen with Codeine Capsules 1865
- Phenaphen-650 with Codeine Tablets ... 1866
- Phenergan with Codeine ... 2497
- Phenergan VC with Codeine ... 2501
- Robitussin A-C Syrup ... 1875
- Robitussin-DAC Syrup ... 1875
- Ryna ... ▣ 741
- Soma Compound w/Codeine Tablets ... 2390
- Triaminic Expectorant w/Codeine .. 1996
- Tussi-Organidin Liquid ... 2391
- Tylenol with Codeine ... 1381

Codeine Polistirex (Respiratory depression, hypotension, profound sedation or coma).
- No products indexed under this heading.

Desipramine Hydrochloride (Respiratory depression, hypotension, profound sedation or coma). Products include:
- Norpramin Tablets ... 1340

Dezocine (Respiratory depression, hypotension, profound sedation or coma).

Diazepam (Respiratory depression, hypotension, profound sedation or coma). Products include:
- Valium Injectable ... 1937
- Valium Tablets ... 1939
- Valrelease Capsules ... 1923

Doxepin Hydrochloride (Respiratory depression, hypotension, profound sedation or coma). Products include:
- Sinequan ... 1960

Droperidol (Respiratory depression, hypotension, profound sedation or coma). Products include:
- Inapsine Injection ... 1140
- Innovar Injection ... 1141

Enflurane (Respiratory depression, hypotension, profound sedation or coma). Products include:
- Ethrane ... 599

Estazolam (Respiratory depression, hypotension, profound sedation or coma). Products include:
- ProSom Tablets ... 554

Ethchlorvynol (Respiratory depression, hypotension, profound sedation or coma). Products include:
- Placidyl Capsules ... 553

Ethinamate (Respiratory depression, hypotension, profound sedation or coma).
- No products indexed under this heading.

Fentanyl (Respiratory depression, hypotension, profound sedation or coma). Products include:
- Duragesic Transdermal System ... 1133

Fentanyl Citrate (Respiratory depression, hypotension, profound sedation or coma). Products include:
- Innovar Injection ... 1141
- Sublimaze Injection ... 1146

Fluphenazine Decanoate (Respiratory depression, hypotension, profound sedation or coma). Products include:
- Prolixin Decanoate ... 1795

Fluphenazine Enanthate (Respiratory depression, hypotension, profound sedation or coma). Products include:
- Prolixin Enanthate ... 1796

Fluphenazine Hydrochloride (Respiratory depression, hypotension, profound sedation or coma). Products include:
- Prolixin Elixir ... 1793
- Prolixin Injection ... 1791
- Prolixin Oral Concentrate ... 1792
- Prolixin Tablets ... 1793

Flurazepam Hydrochloride (Respiratory depression, hypotension, profound sedation or coma). Products include:
- Dalmane Capsules ... 1927

Furazolidone (Concurrent administration is contraindicated). Products include:
- Furoxone ... 1855

Glutethimide (Respiratory depression, hypotension, profound sedation or coma).
- No products indexed under this heading.

Haloperidol (Respiratory depression, hypotension, profound sedation or coma). Products include;
- Haldol Injection, Tablets and Concentrate ... 1373

Haloperidol Decanoate (Respiratory depression, hypotension, profound sedation or coma). Products include:
- Haldol Decanoate ... 1375

Hydrocodone Bitartrate (Respiratory depression, hypotension, profound sedation or coma). Products include:
- Anexsia 5/500 Tablets ... 2196
- Anexsia 7.5/650 Tablets ... 2197
- Azdone Tablets ... 844
- Codiclear DH Syrup ... 845
- Codimal DH Syrup ... 846
- Damason-P ... 1356
- Hycodan Syrup, Tablets ... 927
- Hycomine Compound Tablets ... 929
- Hycomine Syrup ... 927
- Hycotuss Expectorant Syrup ... 930
- Hydrocet Capsules ... 835
- Lortab ASA Tablets ... 2414
- Lortab ... 2412
- Ru-Tuss with Hydrocodone ... 694
- Triaminic Expectorant DH ... 1995
- Vicodin Tablets ... 1187
- Vicodin ES Tablets ... 1189
- Zydone Capsules ... 941

Hydrocodone Polistirex (Respiratory depression, hypotension, profound sedation or coma). Products include:
- Tussionex Extended-Release Suspension ... 988

Hydroxyzine Hydrochloride (Respiratory depression, hypotension, profound sedation or coma). Products include:
Atarax Tablets & Syrup ... 1941
Marax Tablets & DF Syrup ... 1954
Vistaril Intramuscular Solution ... 1970

Imipramine Hydrochloride (Respiratory depression, hypotension, profound sedation or coma). Products include:
Tofranil Ampuls ... 1038
Tofranil Tablets ... 1039

Imipramine Pamoate (Respiratory depression, hypotension, profound sedation or coma). Products include:
Tofranil-PM Capsules ... 1041

Isocarboxazid (Concurrent administration is contraindicated). Products include:
Marplan Tablets ... 1906

Isoflurane (Respiratory depression, hypotension, profound sedation or coma). Products include:
Forane ... 600

Ketamine Hydrochloride (Respiratory depression, hypotension, profound sedation or coma). Products include:
Ketalar ... 1726

Levorphanol Tartrate (Respiratory depression, hypotension, profound sedation or coma). Products include:
Levo-Dromoran ... 1906

Lorazepam (Respiratory depression, hypotension, profound sedation or coma). Products include:
Ativan Injection ... 2432
Ativan Tablets ... 2434

Loxapine Hydrochloride (Respiratory depression, hypotension, profound sedation or coma). Products include:
Loxitane ... 1213

Loxapine Succinate (Respiratory depression, hypotension, profound sedation or coma). Products include:
Loxitane Capsules ... 1213

Maprotiline Hydrochloride (Respiratory depression, hypotension, profound sedation or coma). Products include:
Ludiomil Tablets ... 874

Mephobarbital (Respiratory depression, hypotension, profound sedation or coma). Products include:
Mebaral Tablets ... 2061

Meprobamate (Respiratory depression, hypotension, profound sedation or coma). Products include:
Deprol Tablets ... 2382
Equagesic Tablets ... 2451
Miltown Tablets ... 2386
PMB 200 and PMB 400 ... 2504

Mesoridazine (Respiratory depression, hypotension, profound sedation or coma). Products include:
Serentil ... 686

Methadone Hydrochloride (Respiratory depression, hypotension, profound sedation or coma). Products include:
Dolophine Hydrochloride Ampoules & Vials ... 1260
Dolophine Hydrochloride Tablets ... 1261
Methadone Hydrochloride Diskets ... 1284
Methadone Hydrochloride Oral Solution & Tablets ... 1987

Methohexital Sodium (Respiratory depression, hypotension, profound sedation or coma). Products include:
Brevital Sodium Vials ... 1248

Methoxyflurane (Respiratory depression, hypotension, profound sedation or coma).
No products indexed under this heading.

Midazolam Hydrochloride (Respiratory depression, hypotension, profound sedation or coma). Products include:
Versed Injection ... 1924

Molindone Hydrochloride (Respiratory depression, hypotension, profound sedation or coma). Products include:
Moban Tablets & Concentrate ... 932

Morphine Sulfate (Respiratory depression, hypotension, profound sedation or coma). Products include:
Astramorph/PF Injection, USP (Preservative-Free) ... 618
Duramorph ... 960
Infumorph 200 and Infumorph 500 Sterile Solutions ... 962
MS Contin Tablets ... 1814
MSIR ... 1817
Oramorph SR (Morphine Sulfate Sustained Release Tablets) ... 1988
Roxanol ... 1991

Nortriptyline Hydrochloride (Respiratory depression, hypotension, profound sedation or coma). Products include:
Pamelor ... 2019

Opium Alkaloids (Respiratory depression, hypotension, profound sedation or coma). Products include:
B & O No. 15A & No. 16A Supprettes ... 2395
Pantopon Injectable ... 1911

Oxazepam (Respiratory depression, hypotension, profound sedation or coma). Products include:
Serax Capsules ... 2522
Serax Tablets ... 2522

Oxycodone Hydrochloride (Respiratory depression, hypotension, profound sedation or coma). Products include:
Percocet Tablets ... 950
Percodan ... 951
Roxicodone Tablets, Oral Solution & Intensol (Oxycodone) ... 1992
Tylox Capsules ... 1382

Pentobarbital Sodium (Respiratory depression, hypotension, profound sedation or coma). Products include:
Nembutal Sodium Capsules ... 534
Nembutal Sodium Solution ... 536
Nembutal Sodium Suppositories ... 538

Perphenazine (Respiratory depression, hypotension, profound sedation or coma). Products include:
Etrafon ... 2087
Triavil Tablets ... 1556
Trilafon ... 2123

Phenelzine Sulfate (Concurrent administration is contraindicated). Products include:
Nardil ... 1742

Phenobarbital (Respiratory depression, hypotension, profound sedation or coma). Products include:
Arco-Lase Plus Tablets ... 607
Bellergal-S Tablets ... 1998
Bronkolixir ... ▣ 761
Bronkotabs Tablets ... ▣ 762
Donnatal ... 1858
Donnatal Extentabs ... 1859
Donnatal Tablets ... 1858
Donnazyme Tablets ... 1860
Kinesed Tablets ... 2272
Phenobarbital Elixir and Tablets ... 1293
Primatene Tablets-P Formula ... 2421
Quadrinal Tablets ... 1183
Tedral SA ... 1765

Prazepam (Respiratory depression, hypotension, profound sedation or coma). Products include:
Centrax ... 1693

Prochlorperazine (Respiratory depression, hypotension, profound sedation or coma). Products include:
Compazine ... 2201

Propofol (Respiratory depression, hypotension, profound sedation or coma). Products include:
Diprivan Injection ... 2267

Propoxyphene Hydrochloride (Respiratory depression, hypotension, profound sedation or coma). Products include:
Darvon ... 1256
Wygesic Tablets ... 2540

Propoxyphene Napsylate (Respiratory depression, hypotension, profound sedation or coma). Products include:
Darvon-N/Darvocet-N ... 1254

Protriptyline Hydrochloride (Respiratory depression, hypotension, profound sedation or coma). Products include:
Vivactil Tablets ... 1567

Quazepam (Respiratory depression, hypotension, profound sedation or coma). Products include:
Doral Tablets ... 2383

Secobarbital Sodium (Respiratory depression, hypotension, profound sedation or coma). Products include:
Seconal Sodium Pulvules ... 1296

Selegiline Hydrochloride (Concurrent administration is contraindicated). Products include:
Eldepryl ... 2250

Sufentanil Citrate (Respiratory depression, hypotension, profound sedation or coma). Products include:
Sufenta Injection ... 1147

Temazepam (Respiratory depression, hypotension, profound sedation or coma). Products include:
Restoril Capsules ... 2023

Thiamylal Sodium (Respiratory depression, hypotension, profound sedation or coma). Products include:
Surital Ampoules, Steri-Vials ... 1764

Thioridazine Hydrochloride (Respiratory depression, hypotension, profound sedation or coma). Products include:
Mellaril ... 2011

Thiothixene (Respiratory depression, hypotension, profound sedation or coma). Products include:
Navane Capsules and Concentrate ... 1954
Navane Intramuscular ... 1956

Tranylcypromine Sulfate (Concurrent administration is contraindicated). Products include:
Parnate Tablets ... 2222

Triazolam (Respiratory depression, hypotension, profound sedation or coma). Products include:
Halcion Tablets ... 2340

Trifluoperazine Hydrochloride (Respiratory depression, hypotension, profound sedation or coma). Products include:
Stelazine ... 2226

Trimipramine Maleate (Respiratory depression, hypotension, profound sedation or coma). Products include:
Surmontil Capsules ... 2524

MEPHYTON TABLETS
(Phytonadione) ... 1503
No interactions described in labeling.

MERUVAX[II]
(Rubella Virus Vaccine Live) ... 1503
May interact with immunosuppressive agents. Compounds in this category include:

Azathioprine (Concurrent administration is contraindicated). Products include:
Imuran ... 768

Cyclosporine (Concurrent administration is contraindicated). Products include:
Sandimmune ... 2024

Immune Globulin (Human) (Concurrent administration is contraindicated). Products include:
MICRhoGAM Rh_0(D) Immune Globulin (Human) ... 1650
RhoGAM Rh_0(D) Immune Globulin (Human) ... 1651

Immune Globulin Intravenous (Human) (Concurrent administration is contraindicated). Products include:
Gamimune N Immune Globulin Intravenous (Human) ... 1572
Gammagard Immune Globulin, Intravenous (Human) ... 658
Iveegam ... 1129
Sandoglobulin I.V. ... 2027

Muromonab-CD3 (Concurrent administration is contraindicated). Products include:
Orthoclone OKT3 Sterile Solution ... 1645

MESANTOIN TABLETS
(Mephenytoin) ... 2013
May interact with central nervous system depressants and certain other agents. Compounds in these categories include:

Alcohol (Acute alcohol intoxication may increase the anticonvulsant effect; chronic alcohol abuse may decrease anticonvulsant effect).

Alfentanil Hydrochloride (Additive effects). Products include:
Alfenta Injection ... 1131

Alprazolam (Additive effects). Products include:
Xanax Tablets ... 2367

Aprobarbital (Additive effects). Products include:
Alurate Elixir ... 1883

Buprenorphine (Additive effects).
No products indexed under this heading.

Buspirone Hydrochloride (Additive effects). Products include:
BuSpar ... 1401

Butabarbital (Additive effects). Products include:
Pyridium Plus ... 1764

Butalbital (Additive effects). Products include:
Esgic-Plus Tablets ... 1002
Esgic Tablets & Capsules ... 1001
Fioricet Tablets ... 2006
Fiorinal Capsules ... 2007
Fiorinal with Codeine Capsules ... 2008
Fiorinal Tablets ... 2007
Phrenilin ... 838
Sedapap Tablets 50 mg/650 mg ... 1360

Chlordiazepoxide (Additive effects). Products include:
Libritabs Tablets ... 1930
Limbitrol ... 1933
Menrium Tablets ... 1934

Chlordiazepoxide Hydrochloride (Additive effects). Products include:
Librax Capsules ... 1929
Librium Capsules ... 1931
Librium Injectable ... 1932

Chlorpromazine (Additive effects). Products include:
Thorazine ... 2234

Chlorprothixene (Additive effects). Products include:
Taractan Tablets ... 1920

(▣ Described in PDR For Nonprescription Drugs)

(⊙ Described in PDR For Ophthalmology)

Chlorprothixene Hydrochloride (Additive effects). Products include:
Taractan 1920

Chlorprothixene Lactate (Additive effects). Products include:
Taractan Concentrate 1920

Clorazepate Dipotassium (Additive effects). Products include:
Tranxene 556

Codeine (Additive effects). Products include:
Calcidrine Syrup 506

Codeine Phosphate (Additive effects). Products include:
Actifed with Codeine Cough Syrup.. 752
Cheracol Cough Syrup 1853
Codimal PH Syrup 846
Dimetane-DC Cough Syrup 1857
Empirin with Codeine Phosphate Nos. 2, 3 & 4 764
Fiorinal with Codeine Capsules 2008
Isoclor Expectorant 982
Naldecon CX Adult Liquid .... ▣ 521
Novahistine DH 1342
Novahistine Expectorant 1343
Nucofed Capsules 2219
Nucofed Expectorant 2219
Nucofed Pediatric Expectorant 2220
Nucofed Syrup 2219
Phenaphen with Codeine Capsules 1865
Phenaphen-650 with Codeine Tablets 1866
Phenergan with Codeine 2497
Phenergan VC with Codeine 2501
Robitussin A-C Syrup 1875
Robitussin-DAC Syrup 1875
Ryna .... ▣ 741
Soma Compound w/Codeine Tablets 2390
Triaminic Expectorant w/Codeine .. 1996
Tussi-Organidin Liquid 2391
Tylenol with Codeine 1381

Codeine Polistirex (Additive effects).
No products indexed under this heading.

Dezocine (Additive effects).

Diazepam (Additive effects). Products include:
Valium Injectable 1937
Valium Tablets 1939
Valrelease Capsules 1923

Droperidol (Additive effects). Products include:
Inapsine Injection 1140
Innovar Injection 1141

Enflurane (Additive effects). Products include:
Ethrane 599

Estazolam (Additive effects). Products include:
ProSom Tablets 554

Ethchlorvynol (Additive effects). Products include:
Placidyl Capsules 553

Ethinamate (Additive effects).
No products indexed under this heading.

Fentanyl (Additive effects). Products include:
Duragesic Transdermal System 1133

Fentanyl Citrate (Additive effects). Products include:
Innovar Injection 1141
Sublimaze Injection 1146

Fluphenazine Decanoate (Additive effects). Products include:
Prolixin Decanoate 1795

Fluphenazine Enanthate (Additive effects). Products include:
Prolixin Enanthate 1796

Fluphenazine Hydrochloride (Additive effects). Products include:
Prolixin Elixir 1793
Prolixin Injection 1791
Prolixin Oral Concentrate 1792
Prolixin Tablets 1793

Flurazepam Hydrochloride (Additive effects). Products include:
Dalmane Capsules 1927

Glutethimide (Additive effects).
No products indexed under this heading.

Haloperidol (Additive effects). Products include:
Haldol Injection, Tablets and Concentrate 1373

Haloperidol Decanoate (Additive effects). Products include:
Haldol Decanoate 1375

Hydrocodone Bitartrate (Additive effects). Products include:
Anexsia 5/500 Tablets 2196
Anexsia 7.5/650 Tablets 2197
Azdone Tablets 844
Codiclear DH Syrup 845
Codimal DH Syrup 846
Damason-P 1356
Hycodan Syrup, Tablets 927
Hycomine Compound Tablets 929
Hycomine Syrup 927
Hycotuss Expectorant Syrup 930
Hydrocet Capsules 835
Lortab ASA Tablets 2414
Lortab 2412
Ru-Tuss with Hydrocodone 694
Triaminic Expectorant DH 1995
Vicodin Tablets 1187
Vicodin ES Tablets 1189
Zydone Capsules 941

Hydrocodone Polistirex (Additive effects). Products include:
Tussionex Extended-Release Suspension 988

Hydroxyzine Hydrochloride (Additive effects). Products include:
Atarax Tablets & Syrup 1941
Marax Tablets & DF Syrup 1954
Vistaril Intramuscular Solution 1970

Isoflurane (Additive effects). Products include:
Forane 600

Ketamine Hydrochloride (Additive effects). Products include:
Ketalar 1726

Levorphanol Tartrate (Additive effects). Products include:
Levo-Dromoran 1906

Lorazepam (Additive effects). Products include:
Ativan Injection 2432
Ativan Tablets 2434

Loxapine Hydrochloride (Additive effects). Products include:
Loxitane 1213

Loxapine Succinate (Additive effects). Products include:
Loxitane Capsules 1213

Meperidine Hydrochloride (Additive effects). Products include:
Demerol 2047
Mepergan Injection 2479

Mephobarbital (Additive effects). Products include:
Mebaral Tablets 2061

Meprobamate (Additive effects). Products include:
Deprol Tablets 2382
Equagesic Tablets 2451
Miltown Tablets 2386
PMB 200 and PMB 400 2504

Mesoridazine (Additive effects). Products include:
Serentil 686

Methadone Hydrochloride (Additive effects). Products include:
Dolophine Hydrochloride Ampoules & Vials 1260
Dolophine Hydrochloride Tablets ... 1261
Methadone Hydrochloride Diskets .. 1284
Methadone Hydrochloride Oral Solution & Tablets 1987

Methohexital Sodium (Additive effects). Products include:
Brevital Sodium Vials 1248

Methoxyflurane (Additive effects).
No products indexed under this heading.

Midazolam Hydrochloride (Additive effects). Products include:
Versed Injection 1924

Molindone Hydrochloride (Additive effects). Products include:
Moban Tablets & Concentrate 932

Morphine Sulfate (Additive effects). Products include:
Astramorph/PF Injection, USP (Preservative-Free) 618
Duramorph 960
Infumorph 200 and Infumorph 500 Sterile Solutions 962
MS Contin Tablets 1814
MSIR 1817
Oramorph SR (Morphine Sulfate Sustained Release Tablets) 1988
Roxanol 1991

Opium Alkaloids (Additive effects). Products include:
B & O No. 15A & No. 16A Supprettes 2395
Pantopon Injectable 1911

Oxazepam (Additive effects). Products include:
Serax Capsules 2522
Serax Tablets 2522

Oxycodone Hydrochloride (Additive effects). Products include:
Percocet Tablets 950
Percodan 951
Roxicodone Tablets, Oral Solution & Intensol (Oxycodone) 1992
Tylox Capsules 1382

Pentobarbital Sodium (Additive effects). Products include:
Nembutal Sodium Capsules 534
Nembutal Sodium Solution 536
Nembutal Sodium Suppositories 538

Perphenazine (Additive effects). Products include:
Etrafon 2087
Triavil Tablets 1556
Trilafon 2123

Phenobarbital (Additive effects). Products include:
Arco-Lase Plus Tablets 607
Bellergal-S Tablets 1998
Bronkolixir .... ▣ 761
Bronkotabs Tablets .... ▣ 762
Donnatal 1858
Donnatal Extentabs 1859
Donnatal Tablets 1858
Donnazyme Tablets 1860
Kinesed Tablets 2272
Phenobarbital Elixir and Tablets 1293
Primatene Tablets-P Formula 2421
Quadrinal Tablets 1183
Tedral SA 1765

Prazepam (Additive effects). Products include:
Centrax 1693

Prochlorperazine (Additive effects). Products include:
Compazine 2201

Promethazine Hydrochloride (Additive effects). Products include:
Mepergan Injection 2479
Phenergan with Codeine 2497
Phenergan with Dextromethorphan 2499
Phenergan Injection 2493
Phenergan Suppositories 2496
Phenergan Syrup 2495
Phenergan Tablets 2496
Phenergan VC 2500
Phenergan VC with Codeine 2501

Propofol (Additive effects). Products include:
Diprivan Injection 2267

Propoxyphene Hydrochloride (Additive effects). Products include:
Darvon 1256
Wygesic Tablets 2540

Propoxyphene Napsylate (Additive effects). Products include:
Darvon-N/Darvocet-N 1254

Quazepam (Additive effects). Products include:
Doral Tablets 2383

Secobarbital Sodium (Additive effects). Products include:
Seconal Sodium Pulvules 1296

Sufentanil Citrate (Additive effects). Products include:
Sufenta Injection 1147

Temazepam (Additive effects). Products include:
Restoril Capsules 2023

Thiamylal Sodium (Additive effects). Products include:
Surital Ampoules, Steri-Vials 1764

Thioridazine Hydrochloride (Additive effects). Products include:
Mellaril 2011

Thiothixene (Additive effects). Products include:
Navane Capsules and Concentrate 1954
Navane Intramuscular 1956

Triazolam (Additive effects). Products include:
Halcion Tablets 2340

Trifluoperazine Hydrochloride (Additive effects). Products include:
Stelazine 2226

MESNEX INJECTION
(Mesna) 733
No interactions described in labeling.

MESTINON INJECTABLE
(Pyridostigmine Bromide) 1115
No interactions described in labeling.

MESTINON SYRUP
(Pyridostigmine Bromide) 1116
No interactions described in labeling.

MESTINON TABLETS
(Pyridostigmine Bromide) 1116
No interactions described in labeling.

MESTINON TIMESPAN TABLETS
(Pyridostigmine Bromide) 1116
No interactions described in labeling.

METAMUCIL EFFERVESCENT SUGAR FREE, LEMON-LIME FLAVOR
(Psyllium Preparations) 1806
No interactions described in labeling.

METAMUCIL EFFERVESCENT SUGAR FREE, ORANGE FLAVOR
(Psyllium Preparations) 1806
No interactions described in labeling.

METAMUCIL POWDER, ORANGE FLAVOR
(Psyllium Preparations) 1806
No interactions described in labeling.

METAMUCIL POWDER, REGULAR FLAVOR
(Psyllium Preparations) 1806
No interactions described in labeling.

METAMUCIL POWDER, SUGAR FREE, ORANGE FLAVOR
(Psyllium Preparations) 1806
No interactions described in labeling.

METAMUCIL, SUNRISE SMOOTH, CITRUS
(Psyllium Preparations) 1806
No interactions described in labeling.

METAMUCIL, SUNRISE SMOOTH, CITRUS, SUGAR FREE
(Psyllium Preparations) 1806
No interactions described in labeling.

METAMUCIL, SUNRISE SMOOTH, ORANGE
(Psyllium Preparations) 1806
No interactions described in labeling.

METAMUCIL, SUNRISE SMOOTH, ORANGE, SUGAR FREE
(Psyllium Preparations) 1806
No interactions described in labeling.

METAMUCIL, WAFERS, APPLE CRISP
(Psyllium Preparations) 1806
No interactions described in labeling.

METAMUCIL, WAFERS, CINNAMON SPICE
(Psyllium Preparations) 1806
No interactions described in labeling.

METANDREN LINGUETS AND TABLETS
(Methyltestosterone) 875
May interact with oral anticoagulants, insulin, and certain other agents. Compounds in these categories include:

Dicumarol (Decreased anticoagulant requirements). Products include:
- Dicumarol Tablets 516

Insulin, Human (Decreased blood glucose levels and insulin requirements).
- No products indexed under this heading.

Insulin, Human Isophane Suspension (Decreased blood glucose levels and insulin requirements). Products include:
- Humulin N, 100 Units 1270

Insulin, Human NPH (Decreased blood glucose levels and insulin requirements). Products include:
- Insulatard NPH Human 1627
- Novolin N 1627
- Novolin N PenFill Cartridges 1628
- Novolin N Prefilled 1628

Insulin, Human Regular (Decreased blood glucose levels and insulin requirements). Products include:
- Humulin BR, 100 Units 1268
- Humulin R, 100 Units 1272
- Novolin R 1627
- Novolin R PenFill Cartridges 1628
- Novolin R Prefilled 1629
- Velosulin Human 1628

Insulin, Human, Zinc Suspension (Decreased blood glucose levels and insulin requirements). Products include:
- Humulin L, 100 Units 1268
- Humulin U, 100 Units 1272
- Novolin L 1627

Insulin, NPH (Decreased blood glucose levels and insulin requirements). Products include:
- NPH, 40 & 100 Units 1273
- Beef NPH, 100 Units 1274
- Pork NPH, 100 Units 1275
- Insulatard NPH 1626
- NPH Insulin 1626
- NPH Purified Pork Isophane Insulin 1626

Insulin, Regular (Decreased blood glucose levels and insulin requirements). Products include:
- Regular, 40 & 100 Units 1273
- Beef Regular, 100 Units 1275
- Pork Regular, 100 Units 1275
- Pork Regular (Concentrated), 500 Units 1276
- Regular Insulin 1625
- Regular Purified Pork Insulin 1626
- Velosulin 1627

Insulin, Zinc Crystals (Decreased blood glucose levels and insulin requirements). Products include:
- NPH, 40 & 100 Units 1273

Insulin, Zinc Suspension (Decreased blood glucose levels and insulin requirements). Products include:
- Lente, 40 & 100 Units 1272
- Protamine, Zinc, 40 & 100 Units 1273
- Lente Iletin I 1272
- Beef Lente, 100 Units 1274
- Beef Protamine Zinc, 100 Units 1274
- Pork Lente, 100 Units 1275
- Pork, Protamine, Zinc, 100 Units 1275
- Lente Insulin 1626
- Lente Purified Pork Insulin 1626
- Semilente Insulin 1625
- Ultralente Insulin 1626

Oxyphenbutazone (Elevated serum levels of oxyphenbutazone).

Warfarin Sodium (Decreased anticoagulant requirements). Products include:
- Coumadin Injection & Tablets 944
- Panwarfin Tablets 547

METAPREL INHALATION AEROSOL BRONCHODILATOR
(Metaproterenol Sulfate) 2014
May interact with monoamine oxidase inhibitors, tricyclic antidepressants, and sympathomimetic aerosal bronchodilators. Compounds in these categories include:

Albuterol (Possible additive effects). Products include:
- Proventil Inhalation Aerosol 2117
- Ventolin Inhalation Aerosol and Refill 583

Amitriptyline Hydrochloride (Action of beta adrenergic agonists on the vascular system may be potentiated). Products include:
- Elavil 2269
- Endep Tablets 1927
- Etrafon 2087
- Limbitrol 1933
- Triavil Tablets 1556

Amoxapine (Action of beta adrenergic agonists on the vascular system may be potentiated). Products include:
- Asendin Tablets 1196

Bitolterol Mesylate (Possible additive effects). Products include:
- Tornalate 2074

Clomipramine Hydrochloride (Action of beta adrenergic agonists on the vascular system may be potentiated). Products include:
- Anafranil Capsules 650

Desipramine Hydrochloride (Action of beta adrenergic agonists on the vascular system may be potentiated). Products include:
- Norpramin Tablets 1340

Doxepin Hydrochloride (Action of beta adrenergic agonists on the vascular system may be potentiated). Products include:
- Sinequan 1960

Furazolidone (Action of beta adrenergic agonists on the vascular system may be potentiated). Products include:
- Furoxone 1855

Imipramine Hydrochloride (Action of beta adrenergic agonists on the vascular system may be potentiated). Products include:
- Tofranil Ampuls 1038
- Tofranil Tablets 1039

Imipramine Pamoate (Action of beta adrenergic agonists on the vascular system may be potentiated). Products include:
- Tofranil-PM Capsules 1041

Isocarboxazid (Action of beta adrenergic agonists on the vascular system may be potentiated). Products include:
- Marplan Tablets 1906

Isoetharine (Possible additive effects). Products include:
- Arm-a-Med Isoetharine Inhalation Solution, USP 616
- Bronkometer Aerosol 2042
- Bronkosol Solution 2042

Isoproterenol Hydrochloride (Possible additive effects). Products include:
- Isuprel Hydrochloride Injection 1:5000 2050
- Isuprel Hydrochloride Mistometer .. 2051
- Isuprel Hydrochloride Solution 1:200 & 1:100 2052
- Norisodrine Aerotrol 540

Maprotiline Hydrochloride (Action of beta adrenergic agonists on the vascular system may be potentiated). Products include:
- Ludiomil Tablets 874

Nortriptyline Hydrochloride (Action of beta adrenergic agonists on the vascular system may be potentiated). Products include:
- Pamelor 2019

Phenelzine Sulfate (Action of beta adrenergic agonists on the vascular system may be potentiated). Products include:
- Nardil 1742

Pirbuterol Acetate (Possible additive effects). Products include:
- Maxair Inhaler 1311

Protriptyline Hydrochloride (Action of beta adrenergic agonists on the vascular system may be potentiated). Products include:
- Vivactil Tablets 1567

Selegiline Hydrochloride (Action of beta adrenergic agonists on the vascular system may be potentiated). Products include:
- Eldepryl 2250

Terbutaline Sulfate (Possible additive effects). Products include:
- Brethaire Inhaler 1024
- Brethine Ampuls 1026
- Brethine Tablets 1026
- Bricanyl Injection 1324
- Bricanyl Tablets 1325

Tranylcypromine Sulfate (Action of beta adrenergic agonists on the vascular system may be potentiated). Products include:
- Parnate Tablets 2222

Trimipramine Maleate (Action of beta adrenergic agonists on the vascular system may be potentiated). Products include:
- Surmontil Capsules 2524

METAPREL INHALATION SOLUTION
(Metaproterenol Sulfate) 2015
May interact with sympathomimetic aerosal bronchodilators. Compounds in this category include:

Albuterol (Exercise extreme caution). Products include:
- Proventil Inhalation Aerosol 2117
- Ventolin Inhalation Aerosol and Refill 583

Albuterol Sulfate (Exercise extreme caution). Products include:
- Proventil Repetabs Tablets 2120
- Proventil Solutions for Inhalation 0.5% and 0.083% 2118
- Proventil Syrup 2119
- Proventil Tablets 2120
- Ventolin 583

Dobutamine Hydrochloride (Exercise extreme caution). Products include:
- Dobutrex Solution Vials 1259

Dopamine Hydrochloride (Exercise extreme caution). Products include:
- Intropin Injection 930

Ephedrine Hydrochloride (Exercise extreme caution). Products include:
- Amesec .... ■ 682
- Primatene Tablets-M Formula 2421
- Primatene Tablets-P Formula 2421
- Primatene Tablets-Regular Formula 2421
- Quadrinal Tablets 1183
- Quelidrine Syrup 556
- Tedral SA 1765

Ephedrine Sulfate (Exercise extreme caution). Products include:
- Bronkaid Tablets .... ■ 757
- Bronkolixir .... ■ 761
- Bronkotabs Tablets .... ■ 762
- Marax Tablets & DF Syrup 1954
- Pazo Hemorrhoid Ointment & Suppositories 752
- Vicks Vatronol Nose Drops .... ■ 666

Ephedrine Tannate (Exercise extreme caution). Products include:
- Rynatuss 2388

Epinephrine (Exercise extreme caution). Products include:
- Ana-Kit Anaphylaxis Emergency Treatment Kit 1100
- Bronkaid Mist .... ■ 757
- EpiPen 843
- Marcaine Hydrochloride 0.5% with Epinephrine 1:200,000 (as bitartrate) 958
- Marcaine Hydrochloride with Epinephrine 1:200,000 2055
- Primatene Mist 2420
- Sus-Phrine Injection 1006
- Xylocaine with Epinephrine Injections 637

Epinephrine Bitartrate (Exercise extreme caution). Products include:
- AsthmaHaler Mist Epinephrine Bitartrate Bronchodilator .... ■ 616
- Bronkaid Mist Suspension .... ■ 757
- Primatene Mist Suspension 2421

Epinephrine Hydrochloride (Exercise extreme caution). Products include:
- Adrenalin Chloride Solution 1:100 & 1:1,000 1689
- Epifrin .... ⊙ 244
- Glaucon .... ⊙ 218

Isoproterenol Hydrochloride (Exercise extreme caution). Products include:
- Isuprel Hydrochloride Injection 1:5000 2050
- Isuprel Hydrochloride Mistometer .. 2051
- Isuprel Hydrochloride Solution 1:200 & 1:100 2052
- Norisodrine Aerotrol 540

Metaraminol Bitartrate (Exercise extreme caution). Products include:
- Aramine Injection 1424

Methoxamine Hydrochloride (Exercise extreme caution). Products include:
- Vasoxyl Injection 819

Norepinephrine Bitartrate (Exercise extreme caution). Products include:
- Levophed Bitartrate Injection 2054

Phenylephrine Bitartrate (Exercise extreme caution).
- No products indexed under this heading.

Phenylephrine Hydrochloride (Exercise extreme caution). Products include:
- AK-Dilate Solution 2.5% and 10% .... ⊙ 203
- Atrohist Sprinkle Capsules 558
- Cerose-DM 2443
- Codimal 846
- Comhist LA Capsules 1618
- Congespirin For Children Aspirin Free Chewable Cold Tablets 748
- Cyclomydril .... ⊙ 216
- Deconsal Sprinkle Capsules 559

Dimetane Decongestant ◘ 673
Dristan Decongestant/Antihistamine/ Analgesic Coated Caplets ◘ 749
Dristan Cold Nasal Decongestant/ Antihistamine/ Analgesic Coated Tablets 2419
Dristan Advanced Formula Decongestant/Antihistamine/ Analgesic Tablets ◘ 749
Dristan Nasal Spray, Menthol 2419
Dristan Nasal Spray, Regular and Regular with Metered Pump 2419
Entex Capsules 1623
Entex Liquid 1623
Sinus Excedrin Analgesic, Decongestant Tablets & Caplets 750
Extendryl 994
4-Way Fast Acting Nasal Spray - Original Formula (regular & mentholated) & Metered Spray Pump (regular) 751
Hycomine Compound Tablets 929
Murocoll-2 Sterile Ophthalmic Solution ⊙ 261
Mydfrin 2.5% ⊙ 224
Naldecon Syrup, Tablets, Pediatric Drops and Pediatric Syrup 709
Neo-Synephrine Hydrochloride 1% Carpuject 2063
Neo-Synephrine Hydrochloride 1% Injection 2063
Neo-Synephrine Hydrochloride (Ophthalmic) 2064
Neo-Synephrine ◘ 759
Nōstril Nasal Decongestant ◘ 520
Novahistine Elixir ◘ 596
Phenergan VC 2500
Phenergan VC with Codeine 2501
Prefrin Liquifilm Vasoconstrictor and Lubricant Eye Drops ⊙ 254
Prefrin-A ⊙ 255
Quelidrine Syrup 556
Relief Vasoconstrictor and Lubricant Eye Drops ⊙ 256
Robitussin Night Relief ◘ 677
Ru-Tuss with Hydrocodone 694
Ru-Tuss Tablets 693
Vasosulf ⊙ 279
Vicks Sinex ◘ 665
Zincfrin ⊙ 230

Phenylephrine Tannate (Exercise extreme caution). Products include:
Rynatan 2387
Rynatuss 2388

Phenylpropanolamine Hydrochloride (Exercise extreme caution). Products include:
A.R.M. Allergy Relief Medicine Caplets ◘ 615
Acutrim ◘ 548
Allerest ◘ 559
BC Cold Powder ◘ 517
Cheracol Plus Head Cold/Cough Formula ◘ 667
Codimal Expectorant 846
Comtrex Multi-Symptom Cold Reliever Tablets/Caplets/Liqui-Gels/Liquid 745
Contac Continuous Action Decongestant/Antihistamine Capsules ◘ 710
Contac Maximum Strength Continuous Action Decongestant/ Antihistamine Caplets ◘ 709
Contac Severe Cold and Flu Formula Caplets ◘ 711
Coricidin 'D' Decongestant Tablets ◘ 695
Coricidin Demilets Tablets for Children ◘ 696
Demazin Nasal Decongestant/ Antihistamine Repetabs Tablets & Syrup ◘ 697
Dexatrim ◘ 733
Dimetane-DC Cough Syrup 1857
Dimetapp Elixir ◘ 673
Dimetapp DM Elixir ◘ 674
Dimetapp Extentabs ◘ 674
Dimetapp Plus Caplets ◘ 675
Dimetapp Tablets ◘ 675
Entex Capsules 1623
Entex LA Tablets 1623
Entex Liquid 1623
4-Way Cold Tablets 750
Hycomine Syrup 927
Naldecon CX Adult Liquid ◘ 521
Naldecon DX Adult Liquid ◘ 521
Naldecon DX Children's Syrup ◘ 522
Naldecon DX Pediatric Drops ◘ 522
Naldecon EX Children's Syrup ◘ 522
Naldecon EX Pediatric Drops ◘ 523
Naldecon Syrup, Tablets, Pediatric Drops and Pediatric Syrup 709
Nolamine Tablets 838
Nolex LA Tablets 838
Ornade Spansule Capsules 2221
Orthoxicol Cough Syrup ◘ 668
Propagest 839
Pyrroxate Capsules ◘ 669
Robitussin-CF ◘ 676
Ru-Tuss II Capsules 693
Ru-Tuss with Hydrocodone 694
Ru-Tuss Tablets 693
Sine-Off Sinus Medicine Tablets-Aspirin Formula ◘ 722
Sinulin 840
St. Joseph Cold Tablets for Children ◘ 704
Tavist-D Tablets 2035
Triaminic Allergy Tablets ◘ 688
Triaminic Chewables ◘ 688
Triaminic Cold Tablets ◘ 688
Triaminic Expectorant ◘ 688
Triaminic Expectorant w/Codeine 1996
Triaminic Expectorant DH 1995
Triaminic Oral Infant Drops 1996
Triaminic Syrup ◘ 689
Triaminic-12 Tablets ◘ 690
Triaminic-DM Syrup ◘ 689
Triaminicin Tablets ◘ 690
Triaminicol Multi-Symptom Cold Tablets ◘ 691
Triaminicol Multi-Symptom Relief ◘ 691
Tuss-Ornade Liquid 2242
Tuss-Ornade Spansule Capsules 2242
Tylenol Cold Medication, Effervescent Tablets 1369

Pirbuterol Acetate (Exercise extreme caution). Products include:
Maxair Inhaler 1311

Pseudoephedrine Hydrochloride (Exercise extreme caution). Products include:
Actifed Capsules ◘ 539
Actifed Plus Caplets ◘ 539
Actifed Plus Tablets ◘ 540
Actifed with Codeine Cough Syrup 752
Actifed Syrup ◘ 540
Actifed Tablets ◘ 540
Actifed 12-Hour Capsules ◘ 539
Advil Cold & Sinus Caplets (formerly CoAdvil) 2416
Allerest ◘ 559
Anatuss LA Tablets 1359
Benadryl Decongestant Elixir ◘ 635
Benadryl Decongestant ◘ 635
Benadryl Plus ◘ 636
Benadryl Plus Nighttime ◘ 637
Benylin Decongestant ◘ 638
Brexin L.A. Capsules 2078
Bromfed Capsules (Timed Release) 1615
Bromfed Syrup ◘ 628
Bromfed 1615
CoAdvil ◘ 748
Allergy-Sinus Comtrex Multi-Symptom Allergy Sinus Formula Tablets & Caplets 746
Cough Formula Comtrex 746
Comtrex Multi-Symptom Cold Reliever Tablets/Caplets/Liqui-Gels/Liquid 745
Day-Night Comtrex 747
Non-Drowsy Comtrex 747
Congess 994
Congestac Caplets ◘ 617
Contac Jr. Children's Cold Medicine ◘ 712
Contac Nighttime Cold Medicine ◘ 713
Contac Sinus Caplets Maximum Strength Non-Drowsy Formula ◘ 710
Contac Sinus Tablets Maximum Strength Non-Drowsy Formula ◘ 710
Deconamine 663
Deconsal II Tablets 559
Dimacol Caplets ◘ 672
Dimetane-DX Cough Syrup 1858
Dorcol Children's Cough Syrup ◘ 685
Dorcol Children's Decongestant Liquid ◘ 685
Dorcol Children's Liquid Cold Formula ◘ 686
Maximum Strength Dristan Decongestant/Analgesic Coated Caplets ◘ 750
No Drowsiness Dristan Cold Nasal Decongestant/Analgesic Coated Caplets 2420
Dristan Sinus Caplets 2419
Sinus Excedrin Analgesic, Decongestant Tablets & Caplets ◘ 533
Fedahist Gyrocaps 2145
Fedahist Timecaps 2145
Guaifed 1615
Guaifed Syrup ◘ 629
Isoclor Expectorant 982
Isoclor Timesule Capsules ◘ 561
Kronofed-A 970
Medi-Flu Caplet, Liquid ◘ 640
Novafed A Capsules 1342
Novafed Capsules 1342
Novahistine DH 1342
Novahistine DMX ◘ 595
Novahistine Expectorant 1343
Nucofed Capsules 2219
Nucofed Expectorant 2219
Nucofed Pediatric Expectorant 2220
Nucofed Syrup 2219
Ornex Caplets ◘ 618
PediaCare Allergy Relief Formula Liquid 1362
PediaCare Cough-Cold Formula Liquid 1362
PediaCare Infants' Oral Decongestant Drops 1362
PediaCare Night Rest Cough-Cold Formula Liquid 1362
PediaCare 6-12 Cough-Cold Formula Chewable Tablets 1362
Robitussin-DAC Syrup 1875
Robitussin-PE ◘ 677
Rondec 1975
Rondec-DM 1976
Rondec-TR Tablet 1975
Ru-Tuss DE Tablets 694
Ryna ◘ 741
Seldane-D Extended-Release Tablets 1350
Sinarest ◘ 562
Sine-Aid Maximum Strength Sinus Headache Caplets 1365
Sine-Aid Maximum Strength Sinus Headache Tablets 1365
Sine-Off Maximum Strength Allergy/Sinus Formula Caplets ◘ 721
Sine-Off Maximum Strength No Drowsiness Formula Caplets ◘ 722
Singlet Tablets ◘ 598
Sinutab Maximum Strength ◘ 641
Sinutab Maximum Strength Without Drowsiness Tablets & Caplets ◘ 642
Sinutab Regular Strength Without Drowsiness Formula ◘ 641
St. Joseph Nighttime Cold Medicine ◘ 705
Sudafed Children's Liquid ◘ 543
Sudafed Cough Syrup ◘ 543
Sudafed Plus Liquid ◘ 544
Sudafed Plus Tablets ◘ 545
Sudafed Sinus Caplets ◘ 545
Sudafed Sinus Tablets ◘ 545
Sudafed Tablets, 30 mg ◘ 544
Sudafed Tablets, Adult Strength, 60 mg ◘ 544
Sudafed 12 Hour Capsules ◘ 545
TheraFlu Flu and Cold Medicine ◘ 687
Triaminic Nite Light ◘ 689
Tylenol Allergy Sinus Medication Caplets and Gelcaps, Maximum Strength 1372
Children's Tylenol Cold Liquid Formula and Chewable Tablets 1368
Tylenol Cold & Flu Hot Medication, Packets 1369
Tylenol Cold & Flu No Drowsiness Hot Medication, Packets 1371
Tylenol Cold Medication Caplets and Tablets 1370
Tylenol Cold Medication No Drowsiness Formula Caplets 1370
Tylenol Cold Night Time Medication Liquid 1371
Tylenol Cough Medication Liquid with Decongestant, Maximum Strength 1372
Tylenol, Maximum Strength, Sinus Medication Gelcaps, Caplets and Tablets 1373
Ursinus Inlay-Tabs ◘ 691
Vicks Children's NyQuil ◘ 664
Vicks Daycare ◘ 660
Vicks Formula 44D Decongestant Cough Medicine ◘ 662
Vicks Formula 44M Multi-Symptom Cough Medicine ◘ 662
Vicks NyQuil Nighttime Colds Medicine-Original & Cherry Flavor ◘ 664
Vicks Pediatric Formula 44 Cough & Congestion Medicine ◘ 663
Vicks Pediatric Formula 44m Multi-Symptom Cough & Cold Medicine ◘ 663

Pseudoephedrine Sulfate (Exercise extreme caution). Products include:
Afrin Tablets ◘ 693
Chlor-Trimeton Decongestant ◘ 694
Disophrol Chronotab Sustained-Action Tablets ◘ 698
Drixoral Antihistamine/Nasal Decongestant Syrup ◘ 698
Drixoral Non-Drowsy Formula ◘ 699
Drixoral Plus Extended-Release Tablets ◘ 699
Drixoral Sinus ◘ 700
Drixoral Sustained-Action Tablets ◘ 698
Sinutab Allergy Formula Sustained Action Tablets ◘ 640
Trinalin Repetabs Tablets 1170

Terbutaline Sulfate (Exercise extreme caution). Products include:
Brethaire Inhaler 1024
Brethine Ampuls 1026
Brethine Tablets 1026
Bricanyl Injection 1324
Bricanyl Tablets 1325

METAPREL SYRUP
(Metaproterenol Sulfate) 2015
See **Metaprel Tablets**

METAPREL TABLETS
(Metaproterenol Sulfate) 2015
May interact with sympathomimetic aerosal brochodilators. Compounds in this category include:

Albuterol (Exercise extreme caution). Products include:
Proventil Inhalation Aerosol 2117
Ventolin Inhalation Aerosol and Refill 583

Albuterol Sulfate (Exercise extreme caution). Products include:
Proventil Repetabs Tablets 2120
Proventil Solutions for Inhalation 0.5% and 0.083% 2118
Proventil Syrup 2119
Proventil Tablets 2120
Ventolin 583

Bitolterol Mesylate (Exercise extreme caution). Products include:
Tornalate 2074

Dobutamine Hydrochloride (Exercise extreme caution). Products include:
Dobutrex Solution Vials 1259

Dopamine Hydrochloride (Exercise extreme caution). Products include:
Intropin Injection 930

Ephedrine Hydrochloride (Exercise extreme caution). Products include:
Amesec ◘ 682
Primatene Tablets-M Formula 2421
Primatene Tablets-P Formula 2421
Primatene Tablets-Regular Formula 2421
Quadrinal Tablets 1183
Quelidrine Syrup 556
Tedral SA 1765

Ephedrine Sulfate (Exercise extreme caution). Products include:
Bronkaid Tablets ◘ 757
Bronkolixir ◘ 761
Bronkotabs Tablets ◘ 762
Marax Tablets & DF Syrup 1954
Pazo Hemorrhoid Ointment & Suppositories 752
Vicks Vatronol Nose Drops ◘ 666

Ephedrine Tannate (Exercise extreme caution). Products include:
Rynatuss 2388

Epinephrine (Exercise extreme caution). Products include:
Ana-Kit Anaphylaxis Emergency Treatment Kit 1100
Bronkaid Mist ◘ 757
EpiPen 843
Marcaine Hydrochloride 0.5% with Epinephrine 1:200,000 (as

bitartrate) 958
Marcaine Hydrochloride with Epinephrine 1:200,000 2055
Primatene Mist 2420
Sus-Phrine Injection 1006
Xylocaine with Epinephrine Injections 637

Epinephrine Bitartrate (Exercise extreme caution). Products include:
AsthmaHaler Mist Epinephrine Bitartrate Bronchodilator ▣ 616
Bronkaid Mist Suspension ▣ 757
Primatene Mist Suspension 2421

Epinephrine Hydrochloride (Exercise extreme caution). Products include:
Adrenalin Chloride Solution 1:100 & 1:1,000 1689
Epifrin ⊙ 244
Glaucon ⊙ 218

Ethylnorepinephrine Hydrochloride (Exercise extreme caution). Products include:
Bronkephrine Injection 2042

Isoetharine (Exercise extreme caution). Products include:
Arm-a-Med Isoetharine Inhalation Solution, USP 616
Bronkometer Aerosol 2042
Bronkosol Solution 2042

Isoproterenol Hydrochloride (Exercise extreme caution). Products include:
Isuprel Hydrochloride Injection 1:5000 2050
Isuprel Hydrochloride Mistometer 2051
Isuprel Hydrochloride Solution 1:200 & 1:100 2052
Norisodrine Aerotrol 540

Metaraminol Bitartrate (Exercise extreme caution). Products include:
Aramine Injection 1424

Methoxamine Hydrochloride (Exercise extreme caution). Products include:
Vasoxyl Injection 819

Norepinephrine Bitartrate (Exercise extreme caution). Products include:
Levophed Bitartrate Injection 2054

Phenylephrine Bitartrate (Exercise extreme caution).
No products indexed under this heading.

Phenylephrine Hydrochloride (Exercise extreme caution). Products include:
AK-Dilate Solution 2.5% and 10% ⊙ 203
Atrohist Sprinkle Capsules 558
Cerose-DM 2443
Codimal 846
Comhist LA Capsules 1618
Congespirin For Children Aspirin Free Chewable Cold Tablets 748
Cyclomydril ⊙ 216
Deconsal Sprinkle Capsules 559
Dimetane Decongestant ▣ 673
Dristan Decongestant/Antihistamine/ Analgesic Coated Caplets ▣ 749
Dristan Cold Nasal Decongestant/ Antihistamine/ Analgesic Coated Tablets 2419
Dristan Advanced Formula Decongestant/Antihistamine/ Analgesic Tablets ▣ 749
Dristan Nasal Spray, Menthol 2419
Dristan Nasal Spray, Regular and Regular with Metered Pump 2419
Entex Capsules 1623
Entex Liquid 1623
Sinus Excedrin Analgesic, Decongestant Tablets & Caplets 750
Extendryl 994
4-Way Fast Acting Nasal Spray - Original Formula (regular & mentholated) & Metered Spray Pump (regular) 751
Hycomine Compound Tablets 929
Murocoll-2 Sterile Ophthalmic Solution ⊙ 261
Mydfrin 2.5% ⊙ 224
Naldecon Syrup, Tablets, Pediatric Drops and Pediatric Syrup 709
Neo-Synephrine Hydrochloride 1% Carpuject 2063
Neo-Synephrine Hydrochloride 1% Injection 2063
Neo-Synephrine Hydrochloride (Ophthalmic) 2064
Neo-Synephrine ▣ 759
Nōstril Nasal Decongestant ▣ 520
Novahistine Elixir ▣ 596
Phenergan VC 2500
Phenergan VC with Codeine 2501
Prefrin Liquifilm Vasoconstrictor and Lubricant Eye Drops ⊙ 254
Prefrin-A ⊙ 255
Quelidrine Syrup 556
Relief Vasoconstrictor and Lubricant Eye Drops ⊙ 256
Robitussin Night Relief ▣ 677
Ru-Tuss with Hydrocodone 694
Ru-Tuss Tablets 693
Vasosulf ⊙ 279
Vicks Sinex ▣ 665
Zincfrin ⊙ 230

Phenylephrine Tannate (Exercise extreme caution). Products include:
Rynatan 2387
Rynatuss 2388

Phenylpropanolamine Hydrochloride (Exercise extreme caution). Products include:
A.R.M. Allergy Relief Medicine Caplets ▣ 615
Acutrim ▣ 548
Allerest ▣ 559
BC Cold Powder ▣ 517
Cheracol Plus Head Cold/Cough Formula ▣ 667
Codimal Expectorant 846
Comtrex Multi-Symptom Cold Reliever Tablets/Caplets/Liqui-Gels/Liquid 745
Contac Continuous Action Decongestant/Antihistamine Capsules ▣ 710
Contac Maximum Strength Continuous Action Decongestant/ Antihistamine Caplets ▣ 709
Contac Severe Cold and Flu Formula Caplets ▣ 711
Coricidin 'D' Decongestant Tablets ▣ 695
Coricidin Demilets Tablets for Children ▣ 696
Demazin Nasal Decongestant/ Antihistamine Repetabs Tablets & Syrup ▣ 697
Dexatrim ▣ 733
Dimetane-DC Cough Syrup 1857
Dimetapp Elixir ▣ 673
Dimetapp DM Elixir ▣ 674
Dimetapp Extentabs ▣ 674
Dimetapp Plus Caplets ▣ 675
Dimetapp Tablets ▣ 675
Entex Capsules 1623
Entex LA Tablets 1623
Entex Liquid 1623
4-Way Cold Tablets 750
Hycomine Syrup 927
Naldecon CX Adult Liquid ▣ 521
Naldecon DX Adult Liquid ▣ 521
Naldecon DX Children's Syrup ▣ 522
Naldecon DX Pediatric Drops ▣ 522
Naldecon EX Children's Syrup ▣ 522
Naldecon EX Pediatric Drops ▣ 523
Naldecon Syrup, Tablets, Pediatric Drops and Pediatric Syrup 709
Nolamine Tablets 838
Nolex LA Tablets 838
Ornade Spansule Capsules 2221
Orthoxicol Cough Syrup ▣ 668
Propagest 839
Pyrroxate Capsules ▣ 669
Robitussin-CF ▣ 676
Ru-Tuss II Capsules 693
Ru-Tuss with Hydrocodone 694
Ru-Tuss Tablets 693
Sine-Off Sinus Medicine Tablets-Aspirin Formula ▣ 722
Sinulin 840
St. Joseph Cold Tablets for Children ▣ 704
Tavist-D Tablets 2035
Triaminic Allergy Tablets ▣ 688
Triaminic Chewables ▣ 688
Triaminic Cold Tablets ▣ 688
Triaminic Expectorant ▣ 688
Triaminic Expectorant w/Codeine 1996
Triaminic Expectorant DH 1995
Triaminic Oral Infant Drops 1996
Triaminic Syrup ▣ 689
Triaminic-12 Tablets ▣ 690
Triaminic-DM Syrup ▣ 689
Triaminicin Tablets ▣ 690
Triaminicol Multi-Symptom Cold Tablets ▣ 691
Triaminicol Multi-Symptom Relief ▣ 691
Tuss-Ornade Liquid 2242
Tuss-Ornade Spansule Capsules 2242
Tylenol Cold Medication, Effervescent Tablets 1369

Pirbuterol Acetate (Exercise extreme caution). Products include:
Maxair Inhaler 1311

Pseudoephedrine Hydrochloride (Exercise extreme caution). Products include:
Actifed Capsules ▣ 539
Actifed Plus Caplets ▣ 539
Actifed Plus Tablets ▣ 540
Actifed with Codeine Cough Syrup 752
Actifed Syrup ▣ 540
Actifed Tablets ▣ 540
Actifed 12-Hour Capsules ▣ 539
Advil Cold & Sinus Caplets (formerly CoAdvil) 2416
Allerest ▣ 559
Anatuss LA Tablets 1359
Benadryl Decongestant Elixir ▣ 635
Benadryl Decongestant ▣ 635
Benadryl Plus ▣ 636
Benadryl Plus Nighttime ▣ 637
Benylin Decongestant ▣ 638
Brexin L.A. Capsules 2078
Bromfed Capsules (Timed Release) 1615
Bromfed Syrup ▣ 628
Bromfed 1615
CoAdvil ▣ 748
Allergy-Sinus Comtrex Multi-Symptom Allergy Sinus Formula Tablets & Caplets 746
Cough Formula Comtrex 746
Comtrex Multi-Symptom Cold Reliever Tablets/Caplets/Liqui-Gels/Liquid 745
Day-Night Comtrex 747
Non-Drowsy Comtrex 747
Congess 994
Congestac Caplets ▣ 617
Contac Jr. Children's Cold Medicine ▣ 712
Contac Nighttime Cold Medicine ▣ 713
Contac Sinus Caplets Maximum Strength Non-Drowsy Formula ▣ 710
Contac Sinus Tablets Maximum Strength Non-Drowsy Formula ▣ 710
Deconamine 663
Deconsal II Tablets 559
Dimacol Caplets ▣ 672
Dimetane-DX Cough Syrup 1858
Dorcol Children's Cough Syrup ▣ 685
Dorcol Children's Decongestant Liquid ▣ 685
Dorcol Children's Liquid Cold Formula ▣ 686
Maximum Strength Dristan Decongestant/Analgesic Coated Caplets ▣ 750
No Drowsiness Dristan Cold Nasal Decongestant/Analgesic Coated Caplets 2420
Dristan Sinus Caplets 2419
Sinus Excedrin Analgesic, Decongestant Tablets & Caplets ▣ 533
Fedahist Gyrocaps 2145
Fedahist Timecaps 2145
Guaifed 1615
Guaifed Syrup ▣ 629
Isoclor Expectorant 982
Isoclor Timesule Capsules ▣ 561
Kronofed-A 970
Medi-Flu Caplet, Liquid ▣ 640
Novafed A Capsules 1342
Novafed Capsules 1342
Novahistine DH 1342
Novahistine DMX ▣ 595
Novahistine Expectorant 1343
Nucofed Capsules 2219
Nucofed Expectorant 2219
Nucofed Pediatric Expectorant 2220
Nucofed Syrup 2219
Ornex Caplets ▣ 618
PediaCare Allergy Relief Formula Liquid 1362
PediaCare Cough-Cold Formula Liquid 1362
PediaCare Infants' Oral Decongestant Drops 1362
PediaCare Night Rest Cough-Cold Formula Liquid 1362
PediaCare 6-12 Cough-Cold Formula Chewable Tablets 1362
Robitussin-DAC Syrup 1875
Robitussin-PE ▣ 677
Rondec 1975
Rondec-DM 1976
Rondec-TR Tablet 1975
Ru-Tuss DE Tablets 694
Ryna ▣ 741
Seldane-D Extended-Release Tablets 1350
Sinarest ▣ 562
Sine-Aid Maximum Strength Sinus Headache Caplets 1365
Sine-Aid Maximum Strength Sinus Headache Tablets 1365
Sine-Off Maximum Strength Allergy/Sinus Formula Caplets ▣ 721
Sine-Off Maximum Strength No Drowsiness Formula Caplets ▣ 722
Singlet Tablets ▣ 598
Sinutab Maximum Strength ▣ 641
Sinutab Maximum Strength Without Drowsiness Tablets & Caplets ▣ 642
Sinutab Regular Strength Without Drowsiness Formula ▣ 641
St. Joseph Nighttime Cold Medicine ▣ 705
Sudafed Children's Liquid ▣ 543
Sudafed Cough Syrup ▣ 543
Sudafed Plus Liquid ▣ 544
Sudafed Plus Tablets ▣ 545
Sudafed Sinus Caplets ▣ 545
Sudafed Sinus Tablets ▣ 545
Sudafed Tablets, 30 mg ▣ 544
Sudafed Tablets, Adult Strength, 60 mg ▣ 544
Sudafed 12 Hour Capsules ▣ 545
TheraFlu Flu and Cold Medicine ▣ 687
Triaminic Nite Light ▣ 689
Tylenol Allergy Sinus Medication Caplets and Gelcaps, Maximum Strength 1372
Children's Tylenol Cold Liquid Formula and Chewable Tablets 1368
Tylenol Cold & Flu Hot Medication, Packets 1369
Tylenol Cold & Flu No Drowsiness Hot Medication, Packets 1371
Tylenol Cold Medication Caplets and Tablets 1370
Tylenol Cold Medication No Drowsiness Formula Caplets 1370
Tylenol Cold Night Time Medication Liquid 1371
Tylenol Cough Medication Liquid with Decongestant, Maximum Strength 1372
Tylenol, Maximum Strength, Sinus Medication Gelcaps, Caplets and Tablets 1373
Ursinus Inlay-Tabs ▣ 691
Vicks Children's NyQuil ▣ 664
Vicks Daycare ▣ 660
Vicks Formula 44D Decongestant Cough Medicine ▣ 662
Vicks Formula 44M Multi-Symptom Cough Medicine ▣ 662
Vicks NyQuil Nighttime Colds Medicine-Original & Cherry Flavor ▣ 664
Vicks Pediatric Formula 44 Cough & Congestion Medicine ▣ 663
Vicks Pediatric Formula 44m Multi-Symptom Cough & Cold Medicine ▣ 663

Pseudoephedrine Sulfate (Exercise extreme caution). Products include:
Afrin Tablets ▣ 693
Chlor-Trimeton Decongestant ▣ 694
Disophrol Chronotab Sustained-Action Tablets ▣ 698
Drixoral Antihistamine/Nasal Decongestant Syrup ▣ 698
Drixoral Non-Drowsy Formula ▣ 699
Drixoral Plus Extended-Release Tablets ▣ 699
Drixoral Sinus ▣ 700
Drixoral Sustained-Action Tablets ▣ 698
Sinutab Allergy Formula Sustained Action Tablets ▣ 640
Trinalin Repetabs Tablets 1170

Terbutaline Sulfate (Exercise extreme caution). Products include:
- Brethaire Inhaler ... 1024
- Brethine Ampuls ... 1026
- Brethine Tablets ... 1026
- Bricanyl Injection ... 1324
- Bricanyl Tablets ... 1325

METHADONE HYDROCHLORIDE DISKETS
(Methadone Hydrochloride) ... 1284
May interact with central nervous system depressants, tranquilizers, tricyclic antidepressants, monoamine oxidase inhibitors, and certain other agents. Compounds in these categories include:

Alcohol (Respiratory depression; hypotension; profound sedation; or coma).

Alfentanil Hydrochloride (Respiratory depression; hypotension; profound sedation; or coma). Products include:
- Alfenta Injection ... 1131

Alprazolam (Respiratory depression; hypotension; profound sedation; or coma). Products include:
- Xanax Tablets ... 2367

Amitriptyline Hydrochloride (Respiratory depression; hypotension; profound sedation; or coma). Products include:
- Elavil ... 2269
- Endep Tablets ... 1927
- Etrafon ... 2087
- Limbitrol ... 1933
- Triavil Tablets ... 1556

Amoxapine (Respiratory depression; hypotension; profound sedation; or coma). Products include:
- Asendin Tablets ... 1196

Aprobarbital (Respiratory depression; hypotension; profound sedation; or coma). Products include:
- Alurate Elixir ... 1883

Buprenorphine (Respiratory depression; hypotension; profound sedation; or coma).
- No products indexed under this heading.

Buspirone Hydrochloride (Respiratory depression; hypotension; profound sedation; or coma). Products include:
- BuSpar ... 1401

Butabarbital (Respiratory depression; hypotension; profound sedation; or coma). Products include:
- Pyridium Plus ... 1764

Butalbital (Respiratory depression; hypotension; profound sedation; or coma). Products include:
- Esgic-Plus Tablets ... 1002
- Esgic Tablets & Capsules ... 1001
- Fioricet Tablets ... 2006
- Fiorinal Capsules ... 2007
- Fiorinal with Codeine Capsules ... 2008
- Fiorinal Tablets ... 2007
- Phrenilin ... 838
- Sedapap Tablets 50 mg/650 mg .. 1360

Chlordiazepoxide (Respiratory depression; hypotension; profound sedation; or coma). Products include:
- Libritabs Tablets ... 1930
- Limbitrol ... 1933
- Menrium Tablets ... 1934

Chlordiazepoxide Hydrochloride (Respiratory depression; hypotension; profound sedation; or coma). Products include:
- Librax Capsules ... 1929
- Librium Capsules ... 1931
- Librium Injectable ... 1932

Chlorpromazine (Respiratory depression; hypotension; profound sedation; or coma). Products include:
- Thorazine ... 2234

Chlorprothixene (Respiratory depression; hypotension; profound sedation; or coma). Products include:
- Taractan Tablets ... 1920

Chlorprothixene Hydrochloride (Respiratory depression; hypotension; profound sedation; or coma). Products include:
- Taractan ... 1920

Clomipramine Hydrochloride (Respiratory depression; hypotension; profound sedation; or coma). Products include:
- Anafranil Capsules ... 650

Clorazepate Dipotassium (Respiratory depression; hypotension; profound sedation; or coma). Products include:
- Tranxene ... 556

Codeine (Respiratory depression; hypotension; profound sedation; or coma). Products include:
- Calcidrine Syrup ... 506

Codeine Phosphate (Respiratory depression; hypotension; profound sedation; or coma). Products include:
- Actifed with Codeine Cough Syrup.. 752
- Cheracol Cough Syrup ... 1853
- Codimal PH Syrup ... 846
- Dimetane-DC Cough Syrup ... 1857
- Empirin with Codeine Phosphate Nos. 2, 3 & 4 ... 764
- Fiorinal with Codeine Capsules ... 2008
- Isoclor Expectorant ... 982
- Naldecon CX Adult Liquid ... ◘ 521
- Novahistine DH ... 1342
- Novahistine Expectorant ... 1343
- Nucofed Capsules ... 2219
- Nucofed Expectorant ... 2219
- Nucofed Pediatric Expectorant ... 2220
- Nucofed Syrup ... 2219
- Phenaphen with Codeine Capsules 1865
- Phenaphen-650 with Codeine Tablets ... 1866
- Phenergan with Codeine ... 2497
- Phenergan VC with Codeine ... 2501
- Robitussin A-C Syrup ... 1875
- Robitussin-DAC Syrup ... 1875
- Ryna ... ◘ 741
- Soma Compound w/Codeine Tablets ... 2390
- Triaminic Expectorant w/Codeine .. 1996
- Tussi-Organidin Liquid ... 2391
- Tylenol with Codeine ... 1381

Codeine Polistirex (Respiratory depression; hypotension; profound sedation; or coma).
- No products indexed under this heading.

Desipramine Hydrochloride (Respiratory depression; hypotension; profound sedation; or coma). Products include:
- Norpramin Tablets ... 1340

Dezocine (Respiratory depression; hypotension; profound sedation; or coma).

Diazepam (Respiratory depression; hypotension; profound sedation; or coma). Products include:
- Valium Injectable ... 1937
- Valium Tablets ... 1939
- Valrelease Capsules ... 1923

Doxepin Hydrochloride (Respiratory depression; hypotension; profound sedation; or coma). Products include:
- Sinequan ... 1960

Droperidol (Respiratory depression; hypotension; profound sedation; or coma). Products include:
- Inapsine Injection ... 1140
- Innovar Injection ... 1141

Enflurane (Respiratory depression; hypotension; profound sedation; or coma). Products include:
- Ethrane ... 599

Estazolam (Respiratory depression; hypotension; profound sedation; or coma). Products include:
- ProSom Tablets ... 554

Ethchlorvynol (Respiratory depression; hypotension; profound sedation; or coma). Products include:
- Placidyl Capsules ... 553

Ethinamate (Respiratory depression; hypotension; profound sedation; or coma).
- No products indexed under this heading.

Fentanyl (Respiratory depression; hypotension; profound sedation; or coma). Products include:
- Duragesic Transdermal System ... 1133

Fentanyl Citrate (Respiratory depression; hypotension; profound sedation; or coma). Products include:
- Innovar Injection ... 1141
- Sublimaze Injection ... 1146

Fluphenazine Decanoate (Respiratory depression; hypotension; profound sedation; or coma). Products include:
- Prolixin Decanoate ... 1795

Fluphenazine Enanthate (Respiratory depression; hypotension; profound sedation; or coma). Products include:
- Prolixin Enanthate ... 1796

Fluphenazine Hydrochloride (Respiratory depression; hypotension; profound sedation; or coma). Products include:
- Prolixin Elixir ... 1793
- Prolixin Injection ... 1791
- Prolixin Oral Concentrate ... 1792
- Prolixin Tablets ... 1793

Flurazepam Hydrochloride (Respiratory depression; hypotension; profound sedation; or coma). Products include:
- Dalmane Capsules ... 1927

Furazolidone (Potential for meperidine-MAOI type interaction). Products include:
- Furoxone ... 1855

Glutethimide (Respiratory depression; hypotension; profound sedation; or coma).
- No products indexed under this heading.

Haloperidol (Respiratory depression; hypotension; profound sedation; or coma). Products include:
- Haldol Injection, Tablets and Concentrate ... 1373

Haloperidol Decanoate (Respiratory depression; hypotension; profound sedation; or coma). Products include:
- Haldol Decanoate ... 1375

Hydrocodone Bitartrate (Respiratory depression; hypotension; profound sedation; or coma). Products include:
- Anexsia 5/500 Tablets ... 2196
- Anexsia 7.5/650 Tablets ... 2197
- Azdone Tablets ... 844
- Codiclear DH Syrup ... 845
- Codimal DH Syrup ... 846
- Damason-P ... 1356
- Hycodan Syrup, Tablets ... 927
- Hycomine Compound Tablets ... 929
- Hycomine Syrup ... 927
- Hycotuss Expectorant Syrup ... 930
- Hydrocet Capsules ... 835
- Lortab ASA Tablets ... 2414
- Lortab ... 2412
- Ru-Tuss with Hydrocodone ... 694
- Triaminic Expectorant DH ... 1995
- Vicodin Tablets ... 1187
- Vicodin ES Tablets ... 1189
- Zydone Capsules ... 941

Hydrocodone Polistirex (Respiratory depression; hypotension; profound sedation; or coma). Products include:
- Tussionex Extended-Release Suspension ... 988

Hydroxyzine Hydrochloride (Respiratory depression; hypotension; profound sedation; or coma). Products include:
- Atarax Tablets & Syrup ... 1941
- Marax Tablets & DF Syrup ... 1954
- Vistaril Intramuscular Solution ... 1970

Imipramine Hydrochloride (Respiratory depression; hypotension; profound sedation; or coma). Products include:
- Tofranil Ampuls ... 1038
- Tofranil Tablets ... 1039

Imipramine Pamoate (Respiratory depression; hypotension; profound sedation; or coma). Products include:
- Tofranil-PM Capsules ... 1041

Isocarboxazid (Potential for meperidine-MAOI type interaction). Products include:
- Marplan Tablets ... 1906

Isoflurane (Respiratory depression; hypotension; profound sedation; or coma). Products include:
- Forane ... 600

Ketamine Hydrochloride (Respiratory depression; hypotension; profound sedation; or coma). Products include:
- Ketalar ... 1726

Levorphanol Tartrate (Respiratory depression; hypotension; profound sedation; or coma). Products include:
- Levo-Dromoran ... 1906

Lorazepam (Respiratory depression; hypotension; profound sedation; or coma). Products include:
- Ativan Injection ... 2432
- Ativan Tablets ... 2434

Loxapine Hydrochloride (Respiratory depression; hypotension; profound sedation; or coma). Products include:
- Loxitane ... 1213

Loxapine Succinate (Respiratory depression; hypotension; profound sedation; or coma). Products include:
- Loxitane Capsules ... 1213

Maprotiline Hydrochloride (Respiratory depression; hypotension; profound sedation; or coma). Products include:
- Ludiomil Tablets ... 874

Meperidine Hydrochloride (Respiratory depression; hypotension; profound sedation; or coma). Products include:
- Demerol ... 2047
- Mepergan Injection ... 2479

Mephobarbital (Respiratory depression; hypotension; profound sedation; or coma). Products include:
- Mebaral Tablets ... 2061

Meprobamate (Respiratory depression; hypotension; profound sedation; or coma). Products include:
- Deprol Tablets ... 2382
- Equagesic Tablets ... 2451
- Miltown Tablets ... 2386
- PMB 200 and PMB 400 ... 2504

Mesoridazine (Respiratory depression; hypotension; profound sedation; or coma). Products include:
- Serentil ... 686

(◘ Described in PDR For Nonprescription Drugs) (◉ Described in PDR For Ophthalmology)

Methohexital Sodium (Respiratory depression; hypotension; profound sedation; or coma). Products include:
Brevital Sodium Vials 1248

Methoxyflurane (Respiratory depression; hypotension; profound sedation; or coma).
No products indexed under this heading.

Midazolam Hydrochloride (Respiratory depression; hypotension; profound sedation; or coma). Products include:
Versed Injection 1924

Molindone Hydrochloride (Respiratory depression; hypotension; profound sedation; or coma). Products include:
Moban Tablets & Concentrate 932

Morphine Sulfate (Respiratory depression; hypotension; profound sedation; or coma). Products include:
Astramorph/PF Injection, USP (Preservative-Free) 618
Duramorph 960
Infumorph 200 and Infumorph 500 Sterile Solutions 962
MS Contin Tablets 1814
MSIR 1817
Oramorph SR (Morphine Sulfate Sustained Release Tablets) 1988
Roxanol 1991

Nortriptyline Hydrochloride (Respiratory depression; hypotension; profound sedation; or coma). Products include:
Pamelor 2019

Opium Alkaloids (Respiratory depression; hypotension; profound sedation; or coma). Products include:
B & O No. 15A & No. 16A Supprettes 2395
Pantopon Injectable 1911

Oxazepam (Respiratory depression; hypotension; profound sedation; or coma). Products include:
Serax Capsules 2522
Serax Tablets 2522

Oxycodone Hydrochloride (Respiratory depression; hypotension; profound sedation; or coma). Products include:
Percocet Tablets 950
Percodan 951
Roxicodone Tablets, Oral Solution & Intensol (Oxycodone) 1992
Tylox Capsules 1382

Pentazocine Hydrochloride (Withdrawal symptoms). Products include:
Talacen 2070
Talwin Compound 2072
Talwin Nx 2073

Pentazocine Lactate (Withdrawal symptoms). Products include:
Talwin Injection 2071

Pentobarbital Sodium (Respiratory depression; hypotension; profound sedation; or coma). Products include:
Nembutal Sodium Capsules 534
Nembutal Sodium Solution 536
Nembutal Sodium Suppositories 538

Perphenazine (Respiratory depression; hypotension; profound sedation; or coma). Products include:
Etrafon 2087
Triavil Tablets 1556
Trilafon 2123

Phenelzine Sulfate (Potential for meperidine-MAOI type interaction). Products include:
Nardil 1742

Phenobarbital (Respiratory depression; hypotension; profound sedation; or coma). Products include:
Arco-Lase Plus Tablets 607
Bellergal-S Tablets 1998
Bronkolixir .... ▣ 761
Bronkotabs Tablets .... ▣ 762
Donnatal 1858
Donnatal Extentabs 1859
Donnatal Tablets 1858
Donnazyme Tablets 1860
Kinesed Tablets 2272
Phenobarbital Elixir and Tablets 1293
Primatene Tablets-P Formula 2421
Quadrinal Tablets 1183
Tedral SA 1765

Phenoxybenzamine Hydrochloride (Respiratory depression; hypotension; profound sedation; or coma). Products include:
Dibenzyline Capsules 2207

Prazepam (Respiratory depression; hypotension; profound sedation; or coma). Products include:
Centrax 1693

Prochlorperazine (Respiratory depression; hypotension; profound sedation; or coma). Products include:
Compazine 2201

Promethazine Hydrochloride (Respiratory depression; hypotension; profound sedation; or coma). Products include:
Mepergan Injection 2479
Phenergan with Codeine 2497
Phenergan with Dextromethorphan 2499
Phenergan Injection 2493
Phenergan Suppositories 2496
Phenergan Syrup 2495
Phenergan Tablets 2496
Phenergan VC 2500
Phenergan VC with Codeine 2501

Propofol (Respiratory depression; hypotension; profound sedation; or coma). Products include:
Diprivan Injection 2267

Propoxyphene Hydrochloride (Respiratory depression; hypotension; profound sedation; or coma). Products include:
Darvon 1256
Wygesic Tablets 2540

Propoxyphene Napsylate (Respiratory depression; hypotension; profound sedation; or coma). Products include:
Darvon-N/Darvocet-N 1254

Protriptyline Hydrochloride (Respiratory depression; hypotension; profound sedation; or coma). Products include:
Vivactil Tablets 1567

Quazepam (Respiratory depression; hypotension; profound sedation; or coma). Products include:
Doral Tablets 2383

Rifampin (Reduces blood concentration of methadone to a degree sufficient to produce withdrawal symptoms). Products include:
Rifadin 1345
Rifamate Capsules 1347
Rimactane Capsules 879

Secobarbital Sodium (Respiratory depression; hypotension; profound sedation; or coma). Products include:
Seconal Sodium Pulvules 1296

Selegiline Hydrochloride (Potential for meperidine-MAOI type interaction). Products include:
Eldepryl 2250

Sufentanil Citrate (Respiratory depression; hypotension; profound sedation; or coma). Products include:
Sufenta Injection 1147

Temazepam (Respiratory depression; hypotension; profound sedation; or coma). Products include:
Restoril Capsules 2023

Thiamylal Sodium (Respiratory depression; hypotension; profound sedation; or coma). Products include:
Surital Ampoules, Steri-Vials 1764

Thioridazine Hydrochloride (Respiratory depression; hypotension; profound sedation; or coma). Products include:
Mellaril 2011

Thiothixene (Respiratory depression; hypotension; profound sedation; or coma). Products include:
Navane Capsules and Concentrate 1954
Navane Intramuscular 1956

Tranylcypromine Sulfate (Potential for meperidine-MAOI type interaction). Products include:
Parnate Tablets 2222

Triazolam (Respiratory depression; hypotension; profound sedation; or coma). Products include:
Halcion Tablets 2340

Trifluoperazine Hydrochloride (Respiratory depression; hypotension; profound sedation; or coma). Products include:
Stelazine 2226

Trimipramine Maleate (Respiratory depression; hypotension; profound sedation; or coma). Products include:
Surmontil Capsules 2524

METHADONE HYDROCHLORIDE ORAL SOLUTION & TABLETS
(Methadone Hydrochloride) 1987
May interact with tricyclic antidepressants, central nervous system depressants, monoamine oxidase inhibitors, and certain other agents. Compounds in these categories include:

Alcohol (Respiratory depression, hypotension, and profound sedation or coma may result).

Alfentanil Hydrochloride (Respiratory depression, hypotension, and profound sedation or coma may result). Products include:
Alfenta Injection 1131

Alprazolam (Respiratory depression, hypotension, and profound sedation or coma may result). Products include:
Xanax Tablets 2367

Amitriptyline Hydrochloride (Respiratory depression, hypotension, and profound sedation or coma may result). Products include:
Elavil 2269
Endep Tablets 1927
Etrafon 2087
Limbitrol 1933
Triavil Tablets 1556

Amoxapine (Respiratory depression, hypotension, and profound sedation or coma may result). Products include:
Asendin Tablets 1196

Aprobarbital (Respiratory depression, hypotension, and profound sedation or coma may result). Products include:
Alurate Elixir 1883

Buprenorphine (Respiratory depression, hypotension, and profound sedation or coma may result).
No products indexed under this heading.

Buspirone Hydrochloride (Respiratory depression, hypotension, and profound sedation or coma may result). Products include:
BuSpar 1401

Butabarbital (Respiratory depression, hypotension, and profound sedation or coma may result). Products include:
Pyridium Plus 1764

Butalbital (Respiratory depression, hypotension, and profound sedation or coma may result). Products include:
Esgic-Plus Tablets 1002
Esgic Tablets & Capsules 1001
Fioricet Tablets 2006
Fiorinal Capsules 2007
Fiorinal with Codeine Capsules 2008
Fiorinal Tablets 2007
Phrenilin 838
Sedapap Tablets 50 mg/650 mg .. 1360

Chlordiazepoxide (Respiratory depression, hypotension, and profound sedation or coma may result). Products include:
Libritabs Tablets 1930
Limbitrol 1933
Menrium Tablets 1934

Chlordiazepoxide Hydrochloride (Respiratory depression, hypotension, and profound sedation or coma may result). Products include:
Librax Capsules 1929
Librium Capsules 1931
Librium Injectable 1932

Chlorpromazine (Respiratory depression, hypotension, and profound sedation or coma may result). Products include:
Thorazine 2234

Chlorprothixene (Respiratory depression, hypotension, and profound sedation or coma may result). Products include:
Taractan Tablets 1920

Chlorprothixene Hydrochloride (Respiratory depression, hypotension, and profound sedation or coma may result). Products include:
Taractan 1920

Chlorprothixene Lactate (Respiratory depression, hypotension, and profound sedation or coma may result). Products include:
Taractan Concentrate 1920

Clomipramine Hydrochloride (Respiratory depression, hypotension, and profound sedation or coma may result). Products include:
Anafranil Capsules 650

Clorazepate Dipotassium (Respiratory depression, hypotension, and profound sedation or coma may result). Products include:
Tranxene 556

Codeine (Respiratory depression, hypotension, and profound sedation or coma may result). Products include:
Calcidrine Syrup 506

Codeine Phosphate (Respiratory depression, hypotension, and profound sedation or coma may result). Products include:
Actifed with Codeine Cough Syrup.. 752
Cheracol Cough Syrup 1853
Codimal PH Syrup 846
Dimetane-DC Cough Syrup 1857
Empirin with Codeine Phosphate Nos. 2, 3 & 4 764
Fiorinal with Codeine Capsules 2008
Isoclor Expectorant 982
Naldecon CX Adult Liquid .... ▣ 521
Novahistine DH 1342
Novahistine Expectorant 1343
Nucofed Capsules 2219
Nucofed Expectorant 2219
Nucofed Pediatric Expectorant 2220
Nucofed Syrup 2219
Phenaphen with Codeine Capsules 1865

Phenaphen-650 with Codeine Tablets ... 1866
Phenergan with Codeine ... 2497
Phenergan VC with Codeine ... 2501
Robitussin A-C Syrup ... 1875
Robitussin-DAC Syrup ... 1875
Ryna ... ▣ 741
Soma Compound w/Codeine Tablets ... 2390
Triaminic Expectorant w/Codeine ... 1996
Tussi-Organidin Liquid ... 2391
Tylenol with Codeine ... 1381

Codeine Polistirex (Respiratory depression, hypotension, and profound sedation or coma may result).
No products indexed under this heading.

Desipramine Hydrochloride (Respiratory depression, hypotension, and profound sedation or coma may result). Products include:
Norpramin Tablets ... 1340

Dezocine (Respiratory depression, hypotension, and profound sedation or coma may result).

Diazepam (Respiratory depression, hypotension, and profound sedation or coma may result). Products include:
Valium Injectable ... 1937
Valium Tablets ... 1939
Valrelease Capsules ... 1923

Doxepin Hydrochloride (Respiratory depression, hypotension, and profound sedation or coma may result). Products include:
Sinequan ... 1960

Droperidol (Respiratory depression, hypotension, and profound sedation or coma may result). Products include:
Inapsine Injection ... 1140
Innovar Injection ... 1141

Enflurane (Respiratory depression, hypotension, and profound sedation or coma may result). Products include:
Ethrane ... 599

Estazolam (Respiratory depression, hypotension, and profound sedation or coma may result). Products include:
ProSom Tablets ... 554

Ethchlorvynol (Respiratory depression, hypotension, and profound sedation or coma may result). Products include:
Placidyl Capsules ... 553

Ethinamate (Respiratory depression, hypotension, and profound sedation or coma may result).
No products indexed under this heading.

Fentanyl (Respiratory depression, hypotension, and profound sedation or coma may result). Products include:
Duragesic Transdermal System ... 1133

Fentanyl Citrate (Respiratory depression, hypotension, and profound sedation or coma may result). Products include:
Innovar Injection ... 1141
Sublimaze Injection ... 1146

Fluphenazine Decanoate (Respiratory depression, hypotension, and profound sedation or coma may result). Products include:
Prolixin Decanoate ... 1795

Fluphenazine Enanthate (Respiratory depression, hypotension, and profound sedation or coma may result). Products include:
Prolixin Enanthate ... 1796

Fluphenazine Hydrochloride (Respiratory depression, hypotension, and profound sedation or coma may result). Products include:
Prolixin Elixir ... 1793
Prolixin Injection ... 1791
Prolixin Oral Concentrate ... 1792
Prolixin Tablets ... 1793

Flurazepam Hydrochloride (Respiratory depression, hypotension, and profound sedation or coma may result). Products include:
Dalmane Capsules ... 1927

Furazolidone (Severe reactions not reported, but a sensitivity test is advised). Products include:
Furoxone ... 1855

Glutethimide (Respiratory depression, hypotension, and profound sedation or coma may result).
No products indexed under this heading.

Haloperidol (Respiratory depression, hypotension, and profound sedation or coma may result). Products include:
Haldol Injection, Tablets and Concentrate ... 1373

Haloperidol Decanoate (Respiratory depression, hypotension, and profound sedation or coma may result). Products include:
Haldol Decanoate ... 1375

Hydrocodone Bitartrate (Respiratory depression, hypotension, and profound sedation or coma may result). Products include:
Anexsia 5/500 Tablets ... 2196
Anexsia 7.5/650 Tablets ... 2197
Azdone Tablets ... 844
Codiclear DH Syrup ... 845
Codimal DH Syrup ... 846
Damason-P ... 1356
Hycodan Syrup, Tablets ... 927
Hycomine Compound Tablets ... 929
Hycomine Syrup ... 927
Hycotuss Expectorant Syrup ... 930
Hydrocet Capsules ... 835
Lortab ASA Tablets ... 2414
Lortab ... 2412
Ru-Tuss with Hydrocodone ... 694
Triaminic Expectorant DH ... 1995
Vicodin Tablets ... 1187
Vicodin ES Tablets ... 1189
Zydone Capsules ... 941

Hydrocodone Polistirex (Respiratory depression, hypotension, and profound sedation or coma may result). Products include:
Tussionex Extended-Release Suspension ... 988

Hydroxyzine Hydrochloride (Respiratory depression, hypotension, and profound sedation or coma may result). Products include:
Atarax Tablets & Syrup ... 1941
Marax Tablets & DF Syrup ... 1954
Vistaril Intramuscular Solution ... 1970

Imipramine Hydrochloride (Respiratory depression, hypotension, and profound sedation or coma may result). Products include:
Tofranil Ampuls ... 1038
Tofranil Tablets ... 1039

Imipramine Pamoate (Respiratory depression, hypotension, and profound sedation or coma may result). Products include:
Tofranil-PM Capsules ... 1041

Isocarboxazid (Severe reactions not reported, but a sensitivity test is advised). Products include:
Marplan Tablets ... 1906

Isoflurane (Respiratory depression, hypotension, and profound sedation or coma may result). Products include:
Forane ... 600

Ketamine Hydrochloride (Respiratory depression, hypotension, and profound sedation or coma may result). Products include:
Ketalar ... 1726

Levorphanol Tartrate (Respiratory depression, hypotension, and profound sedation or coma may result). Products include:
Levo-Dromoran ... 1906

Lorazepam (Respiratory depression, hypotension, and profound sedation or coma may result). Products include:
Ativan Injection ... 2432
Ativan Tablets ... 2434

Loxapine Hydrochloride (Respiratory depression, hypotension, and profound sedation or coma may result). Products include:
Loxitane ... 1213

Loxapine Succinate (Respiratory depression, hypotension, and profound sedation or coma may result). Products include:
Loxitane Capsules ... 1213

Maprotiline Hydrochloride (Respiratory depression, hypotension, and profound sedation or coma may result). Products include:
Ludiomil Tablets ... 874

Meperidine Hydrochloride (Respiratory depression, hypotension, and profound sedation or coma may result). Products include:
Demerol ... 2047
Mepergan Injection ... 2479

Mephobarbital (Respiratory depression, hypotension, and profound sedation or coma may result). Products include:
Mebaral Tablets ... 2061

Meprobamate (Respiratory depression, hypotension, and profound sedation or coma may result). Products include:
Deprol Tablets ... 2382
Equagesic Tablets ... 2451
Miltown Tablets ... 2386
PMB 200 and PMB 400 ... 2504

Mesoridazine (Respiratory depression, hypotension, and profound sedation or coma may result). Products include:
Serentil ... 686

Methohexital Sodium (Respiratory depression, hypotension, and profound sedation or coma may result). Products include:
Brevital Sodium Vials ... 1248

Methoxyflurane (Respiratory depression, hypotension, and profound sedation or coma may result).
No products indexed under this heading.

Methyldopate Hydrochloride (Respiratory depression, hypotension, and profound sedation or coma may result). Products include:
Aldomet Ester HCl Injection ... 1417

Midazolam Hydrochloride (Respiratory depression, hypotension, and profound sedation or coma may result). Products include:
Versed Injection ... 1924

Molindone Hydrochloride (Respiratory depression, hypotension, and profound sedation or coma may result). Products include:
Moban Tablets & Concentrate ... 932

Morphine Sulfate (Respiratory depression, hypotension, and profound sedation or coma may result). Products include:
Astramorph/PF Injection, USP (Preservative-Free) ... 618
Duramorph ... 960
Infumorph 200 and Infumorph 500 Sterile Solutions ... 962
MS Contin Tablets ... 1814
MSIR ... 1817
Oramorph SR (Morphine Sulfate Sustained Release Tablets) ... 1988
Roxanol ... 1991

Nortriptyline Hydrochloride (Respiratory depression, hypotension, and profound sedation or coma may result). Products include:
Pamelor ... 2019

Opium Alkaloids (Respiratory depression, hypotension, and profound sedation or coma may result). Products include:
B & O No. 15A & No. 16A Supprettes ... 2395
Pantopon Injectable ... 1911

Oxazepam (Respiratory depression, hypotension, and profound sedation or coma may result). Products include:
Serax Capsules ... 2522
Serax Tablets ... 2522

Oxycodone Hydrochloride (Respiratory depression, hypotension, and profound sedation or coma may result). Products include:
Percocet Tablets ... 950
Percodan ... 951
Roxicodone Tablets, Oral Solution & Intensol (Oxycodone) ... 1992
Tylox Capsules ... 1382

Pentazocine Hydrochloride (Possible withdrawal symptoms). Products include:
Talacen ... 2070
Talwin Compound ... 2072
Talwin Nx ... 2073

Pentazocine Lactate (Possible withdrawal symptoms). Products include:
Talwin Injection ... 2071

Pentobarbital Sodium (Respiratory depression, hypotension, and profound sedation or coma may result). Products include:
Nembutal Sodium Capsules ... 534
Nembutal Sodium Solution ... 536
Nembutal Sodium Suppositories ... 538

Perphenazine (Respiratory depression, hypotension, and profound sedation or coma may result). Products include:
Etrafon ... 2087
Triavil Tablets ... 1556
Trilafon ... 2123

Phenelzine Sulfate (Severe reactions not reported, but a sensitivity test is advised). Products include:
Nardil ... 1742

Phenobarbital (Respiratory depression, hypotension, and profound sedation or coma may result). Products include:
Arco-Lase Plus Tablets ... 607
Bellergal-S Tablets ... 1998
Bronkolixir ... ▣ 761
Bronkotabs Tablets ... ▣ 762
Donnatal ... 1858
Donnatal Extentabs ... 1859
Donnatal Tablets ... 1858
Donnazyme Tablets ... 1860
Kinesed Tablets ... 2272
Phenobarbital Elixir and Tablets ... 1293
Primatene Tablets-P Formula ... 2421
Quadrinal Tablets ... 1183
Tedral SA ... 1765

Prazepam (Respiratory depression, hypotension, and profound sedation or coma may result). Products include:
Centrax ... 1693

Prochlorperazine (Respiratory depression, hypotension, and profound sedation or coma may result). Products include:
Compazine ... 2201

Promethazine Hydrochloride (Respiratory depression, hypotension, and profound sedation or coma may result). Products include:
Mepergan Injection ... 2479
Phenergan with Codeine ... 2497
Phenergan with Dextromethorphan ... 2499
Phenergan Injection ... 2493
Phenergan Suppositories ... 2496

Phenergan Syrup 2495
Phenergan Tablets 2496
Phenergan VC 2500
Phenergan VC with Codeine 2501

Propofol (Respiratory depression, hypotension, and profound sedation or coma may result). Products include:
Diprivan Injection 2267

Propoxyphene Hydrochloride (Respiratory depression, hypotension, and profound sedation or coma may result). Products include:
Darvon 1256
Wygesic Tablets 2540

Propoxyphene Napsylate (Respiratory depression, hypotension, and profound sedation or coma may result). Products include:
Darvon-N/Darvocet-N 1254

Protriptyline Hydrochloride (Respiratory depression, hypotension, and profound sedation or coma may result). Products include:
Vivactil Tablets 1567

Quazepam (Respiratory depression, hypotension, and profound sedation or coma may result). Products include:
Doral Tablets 2383

Rifampin (Reduced blood concentration of methadone). Products include:
Rifadin 1345
Rifamate Capsules 1347
Rimactane Capsules 879

Secobarbital Sodium (Respiratory depression, hypotension, and profound sedation or coma may result). Products include:
Seconal Sodium Pulvules 1296

Selegiline Hydrochloride (Severe reactions not reported, but a sensitivity test is advised). Products include:
Eldepryl 2250

Sufentanil Citrate (Respiratory depression, hypotension, and profound sedation or coma may result). Products include:
Sufenta Injection 1147

Temazepam (Respiratory depression, hypotension, and profound sedation or coma may result). Products include:
Restoril Capsules 2023

Thiamylal Sodium (Respiratory depression, hypotension, and profound sedation or coma may result). Products include:
Surital Ampoules, Steri-Vials 1764

Thioridazine Hydrochloride (Respiratory depression, hypotension, and profound sedation or coma may result). Products include:
Mellaril 2011

Thiothixene (Respiratory depression, hypotension, and profound sedation or coma may result). Products include:
Navane Capsules and Concentrate 1954
Navane Intramuscular 1956

Tranylcypromine Sulfate (Severe reactions not reported, but a sensitivity test is advised). Products include:
Parnate Tablets 2222

Triazolam (Respiratory depression, hypotension, and profound sedation or coma may result). Products include:
Halcion Tablets 2340

Trifluoperazine Hydrochloride (Respiratory depression, hypotension, and profound sedation or coma may result). Products include:
Stelazine 2226

Trimipramine Maleate (Respiratory depression, hypotension, and profound sedation or coma may result). Products include:
Surmontil Capsules 2524

METHERGINE INJECTION

(Methylergonovine Maleate) 2016
May interact with vasopressors and certain other agents. Compounds in these categories include:

Dopamine Hydrochloride (Use cautiously). Products include:
Intropin Injection 930

Epinephrine Hydrochloride (Use cautiously). Products include:
Adrenalin Chloride Solution 1:100 & 1:1,000 1689
Epifrin .... ◉ 244
Glaucon .... ◉ 218

Ergoloid Mesylates (Use cautiously). Products include:
Hydergine 2010

Ergonovine Maleate (Use cautiously).

Metaraminol Bitartrate (Use cautiously). Products include:
Aramine Injection 1424

Methoxamine Hydrochloride (Use cautiously). Products include:
Vasoxyl Injection 819

Methysergide Maleate (Use cautiously). Products include:
Sansert Tablets 2031

Norepinephrine Bitartrate (Use cautiously). Products include:
Levophed Bitartrate Injection 2054

Phenylephrine Hydrochloride (Use cautiously). Products include:
AK-Dilate Solution 2.5% and 10% .... ◉ 203
Atrohist Sprinkle Capsules 558
Cerose-DM 2443
Codimal 846
Comhist LA Capsules 1618
Congespirin For Children Aspirin Free Chewable Cold Tablets 748
Cyclomydril .... ◉ 216
Deconsal Sprinkle Capsules 559
Dimetane Decongestant .... ▣ 673
Dristan Decongestant/Antihistamine/ Analgesic Coated Caplets .... ▣ 749
Dristan Cold Nasal Decongestant/ Antihistamine/ Analgesic Coated Tablets 2419
Dristan Advanced Formula Decongestant/Antihistamine/ Analgesic Tablets .... ▣ 749
Dristan Nasal Spray, Menthol 2419
Dristan Nasal Spray, Regular and Regular with Metered Pump 2419
Entex Capsules 1623
Entex Liquid 1623
Sinus Excedrin Analgesic, Decongestant Tablets & Caplets 750
Extendryl 994
4-Way Fast Acting Nasal Spray - Original Formula (regular & mentholated) & Metered Spray Pump (regular) 751
Hycomine Compound Tablets 929
Murocoll-2 Sterile Ophthalmic Solution .... ◉ 261
Mydfrin 2.5% .... ◉ 224
Naldecon Syrup, Tablets, Pediatric Drops and Pediatric Syrup 709
Neo-Synephrine Hydrochloride 1% Carpuject 2063
Neo-Synephrine Hydrochloride 1% Injection 2063
Neo-Synephrine Hydrochloride (Ophthalmic) 2064
Neo-Synephrine .... ▣ 759
Nōstril Nasal Decongestant .... ▣ 520
Novahistine Elixir .... ▣ 596
Phenergan VC 2500
Phenergan VC with Codeine 2501
Prefrin Liquifilm Vasoconstrictor and Lubricant Eye Drops .... ◉ 254
Prefrin-A .... ◉ 255
Quelidrine Syrup 556
Relief Vasoconstrictor and Lubricant Eye Drops .... ◉ 256
Robitussin Night Relief .... ▣ 677
Ru-Tuss with Hydrocodone 694
Ru-Tuss Tablets 693
Vasosulf .... ◉ 279
Vicks Sinex .... ▣ 665
Zincfrin .... ◉ 230

METHERGINE TABLETS

(Methylergonovine Maleate) 2016
See **Methergine Injection**

METHOTREXATE TABLETS, PARENTERAL, LPF PARENTERAL

(Methotrexate Sodium) 1217
May interact with salicylates, sulfonamides, tetracyclines, non-steroidal anti-inflammatory agents, cytotoxic drugs, and certain other agents. Compounds in these categories include:

Antibiotics, nonabsorbable broad spectrum, unspecified (Decreases intestinal absorption and interferes with enterohepatic circulation).

Aspirin (Increased toxicity). Products include:
Alka-Seltzer Effervescent Antacid and Pain Reliever 1568
Alka-Seltzer Extra Strength Effervescent Antacid and Pain Reliever 1570
Alka-Seltzer (Flavored) Effervescent Antacid and Pain Reliever 1569
Alka-Seltzer Plus Cold Medicine .... ▣ 623
Alka-Seltzer Plus Night-Time Cold Medicine .... ▣ 623
Alka Seltzer Plus Sinus Allergy Medicine .... ▣ 624
Anacin Coated Analgesic Caplets 2417
Anacin Coated Analgesic Tablets 2417
Anacin Maximum Strength Analgesic Coated Tablets 2417
Maximum Strength Arthritis Pain Formula By the Makers of Anacin Analgesic Tablets and Caplets 2418
Arthritis Pain Formula by the Makers of Anacin Analgesic Tablets and Caplets .... ▣ 747
Arthritis Strength BC Powder .... ▣ 516
Ascriptin A/D Caplets 1850
Regular Strength Ascriptin Tablets 1850
Azdōne Tablets 844
BC Powder .... ▣ 517
BC Cold Powder .... ▣ 517
Children's Bayer Chewable Aspirin .... ▣ 564
Genuine Bayer Aspirin Tablets & Caplets .... ▣ 564
Maximum Bayer Aspirin Tablets & Caplets .... ▣ 566
Bayer Plus Aspirin Tablets .... ▣ 567
Therapy Bayer Aspirin Caplets .... ▣ 568
8 Hour Bayer Timed-Release Aspirin .... ▣ 566
Arthritis Strength Bufferin Analgesic Caplets 744
Extra Strength Bufferin Analgesic Tablets 745
Bufferin Analgesic Tablets and Caplets 743
Cama Arthritis Pain Reliever .... ▣ 685
Damason-P 1356
Easprin 1719
Ecotrin Enteric Coated Aspirin Maximum Strength Tablets and Caplets 2189
Ecotrin Enteric Coated Aspirin Regular Strength Tablets and Caplets 2189
Empirin Aspirin .... ▣ 541
Empirin with Codeine Phosphate Nos. 2, 3 & 4 764
Equagesic Tablets 2451
Excedrin Extra-Strength Analgesic Tablets & Caplets 749
4-Way Cold Tablets 750
Fiorinal Capsules 2007
Fiorinal with Codeine Capsules 2008
Fiorinal Tablets 2007
Lortab ASA Tablets 2414
Momentum Muscular Backache Formula .... ▣ 751
Norgesic 1314
Norwich Extra-Strength Aspirin .... ▣ 546
Norwich Regular Strength Aspirin ▣ 547
P-A-C Analgesic Tablets .... ▣ 669
Percodan 951
Robaxisal Tablets 1872
Sine-Off Sinus Medicine Tablets-Aspirin Formula .... ▣ 722
Soma Compound w/Codeine Tablets 2390
Soma Compound Tablets 2389
St. Joseph Adult Chewable Aspirin (81 mg.) .... ▣ 703
Synalgos-DC Capsules 2525
Talwin Compound 2072
Ursinus Inlay-Tabs .... ▣ 691
Vanquish Analgesic Caplets .... ▣ 574
Zorprin Tablets 698

Auranofin (Combined use has not been studied and may increase the incidence of adverse effects). Products include:
Ridaura Capsules 2224

Aurothioglucose (Combined use has not been studied and may increase the incidence of adverse effects). Products include:
Solganal Suspension 2122

Bleomycin Sulfate (Combined use has not been studied and may increase the incidence of adverse effects). Products include:
Blenoxane 724

Chloramphenicol (Decreases intestinal absorption and interferes with enterohepatic circulation). Products include:
AK-Chlor Sterile Ophthalmic Ointment & Solution .... ◉ 201
Chloromycetin Cream, 1% 1694
Chloromycetin Hydrocortisone Ophthalmic 1694
Chloromycetin Kapseals 1695
Chloromycetin Ophthalmic Ointment, 1% 1696
Chloromycetin Ophthalmic Solution 1696
Chloromycetin Otic 1697
Chloroptic S.O.P. .... ◉ 243
Chloroptic Sterile Ophthalmic Solution .... ◉ 243
Ophthochlor Ophthalmic Solution ◉ 300
Ophthocort .... ◉ 301

Chloramphenicol Palmitate (Decreases intestinal absorption and interferes with enterohepatic circulation). Products include:
Chloromycetin Palmitate, Oral Suspension 1697

Chloramphenicol Sodium Succinate (Increased toxicity). Products include:
Chloromycetin Sodium Succinate 1698

Choline Magnesium Trisalicylate (Increased toxicity). Products include:
Trilisate 1822

Cisplatin (Caution should be exercised if high-dose of methotrexate is used concurrently in the treatment of osteosarcoma). Products include:
Platinol 737
Platinol-AQ Injection 738

Daunorubicin Hydrochloride (Combined use has not been studied and may increase the incidence of adverse effects). Products include:
Cerubidine 2443

Demeclocycline Hydrochloride (Decreases intestinal absorption and interferes with enterohepatic circulation). Products include:
Declomycin Capsules, Tablets 1199

Diclofenac Sodium (May elevate and prolong serum methotrexate levels; reduces the tubular secretion of methotrexate). Products include:
Voltaren Ophthalmic Sterile Ophthalmic Solution .... ◉ 268
Voltaren Tablets 1042

Diflunisal (Increased toxicity). Products include:
Dolobid Tablets 1465

Doxorubicin Hydrochloride (Combined use has not been studied and may increase the incidence of adverse effects). Products include:

- Adriamycin PFS ... 561
- Adriamycin RDF ... 562
- Doxorubicin Hydrochloride for Injection, USP ... 622
- Doxorubicin Hydrochloride Injection, USP ... 848
- Rubex ... 739

Doxycycline Calcium (Decreases intestinal absorption and interferes with enterohepatic circulation).

No products indexed under this heading.

Doxycycline Hyclate (Decreases intestinal absorption and interferes with enterohepatic circulation). Products include:

- Doryx Capsules ... 1717
- Vibramycin Hyclate Capsules ... 1787
- Vibramycin Hyclate Intravenous ... 1968
- Vibra-Tabs Film Coated Tablets ... 1787

Doxycycline Monohydrate (Decreases intestinal absorption and interferes with enterohepatic circulation). Products include:

- Monodox Capsules ... 1630
- Vibramycin Monohydrate for Oral Suspension ... 1787

Etodolac (May elevate and prolong serum methotrexate levels; reduces the tubular secretion of methotrexate). Products include:

- Lodine Capsules ... 2468

Fenoprofen Calcium (May elevate and prolong serum methotrexate levels; reduces the tubular secretion of methotrexate). Products include:

- Nalfon Pulvules & Tablets ... 919

Fluorouracil (Combined use has not been studied and may increase the incidence of adverse effects). Products include:

- Efudex ... 1880
- Fluoroplex Topical Solution & Cream 1% ... 1082
- Fluorouracil Injection ... 1897

Flurbiprofen (May elevate and prolong serum methotrexate levels; reduces the tubular secretion of methotrexate). Products include:

- Ansaid Tablets ... 2319

Folic Acid (May decrease response to methotrexate). Products include:

- Allbee C-800 Plus Iron Tablets ... ▣ 670
- Biotin Forte 3mg. & Extra Strength Biotin Forte 5mg. ... 2377
- Bugs Bunny Children's Chewable Vitamins (Sugar Free) ... ▣ 625
- Bugs Bunny With Extra C Children's Chewable Vitamins (Sugar Free) ... ▣ 626
- Bugs Bunny Plus Iron Children's Chewable Vitamins (Sugar Free) ▣ 625
- Cefol Filmtab ... 509
- Fero-Folic-500 Filmtab ... 527
- Flintstones Children's Chewable Vitamins ... ▣ 625
- Flintstones Children's Chewable Vitamins With Extra C ... ▣ 626
- Flintstones Children's Chewable Vitamins Plus Iron ... ▣ 625
- Iberet-Folic-500 Filmtab ... 527
- Materna Tablets ... 1214
- May-Vita Elixir ... 1359
- Mega-B ... 607
- Nephro-Vite Rx ... 1826
- Niferex-150 Forte Capsules ... 847
- One-A-Day Essential Vitamins ... ▣ 627
- One-A-Day Maximum Formula Vitamins and Minerals ... ▣ 627
- One-A-Day Plus Extra C Vitamins .. ▣ 627
- Pramet FA ... 1974
- Pramilet FA ... 1974
- Sigtab Tablets ... ▣ 669
- Stressgard Stress Formula Vitamins ... ▣ 628
- Stuart Prenatal Tablets ... ▣ 731
- The Stuart Formula Tablets ... ▣ 581
- Stuartnatal 1+1 Tablets ... 2273
- Theragran Stress Formula ... ▣ 727
- Trinsicon Capsules ... 2415
- Vicon Forte Capsules ... 2416
- Within Women's Formula Multivitamin with Calcium, Extra Iron and Zinc ... ▣ 628
- Zenate Tablets ... 2250
- Zymacap Capsules ... ▣ 670

Gold Sodium Thiomalate (Combined use has not been studied and may increase the incidence of adverse effects). Products include:

- Myochrysine Injection ... 1516

Hydroxychloroquine Sulfate (Combined use has not been studied and may increase the incidence of adverse effects). Products include:

- Plaquenil Sulfate Tablets ... 2067

Hydroxyurea (Combined use has not been studied and may increase the incidence of adverse effects). Products include:

- Hydrea Capsules ... 728

Ibuprofen (May elevate and prolong serum methotrexate levels; reduces the tubular secretion of methotrexate). Products include:

- Advil Cold & Sinus Caplets (formerly CoAdvil) ... 2416
- Advil Ibuprofen Tablets and Caplets ... 2416
- Children's Advil Suspension ... 2426
- CoAdvil ... ▣ 748
- Dristan Sinus Caplets ... 2419
- Haltran Tablets ... ▣ 668
- Ibuprofen ... ▣ 631
- Medipren ibuprofen Caplets and Tablets ... 1362
- Midol 200 Cramp Relief Formula .. ▣ 570
- Motrin Tablets ... 2351
- Motrin IB Caplets and Tablets ... ▣ 736
- Nuprin Ibuprofen/Analgesic Tablets & Caplets ... 752
- PediaProfen Suspension ... 1363
- Rufen Tablets ... 691
- Trendar Ibuprofen Tablets ... ▣ 756

Indomethacin (May elevate and prolong serum methotrexate levels; reduces the tubular secretion of methotrexate). Products include:

- Indocin ... 1487

Indomethacin Sodium Trihydrate (May elevate and prolong serum methotrexate levels; reduces the tubular secretion of methotrexate). Products include:

- Indocin I.V. ... 1490

Ketoprofen (May elevate and prolong serum methotrexate levels; reduces the tubular secretion of methotrexate). Products include:

- Orudis Capsules ... 2488

Ketorolac Tromethamine (May elevate and prolong serum methotrexate levels; reduces the tubular secretion of methotrexate). Products include:

- Toradol IM Injection ... 2302

Leucovorin Calcium (High doses may reduce the efficacy of intrathecally administered methotrexate). Products include:

- Leucovorin Calcium for Injection, Wellcovorin Brand ... 786
- Leucovorin Calcium Injection ... 1210
- Leucovorin Calcium Tablets, Wellcovorin Brand ... 787
- Leucovorin Calcium Tablets ... 1212

Magnesium Salicylate (Increased toxicity). Products include:

- Doan's - Extra-Strength Analgesic ▣ 549
- Doan's - Regular Strength Analgesic ... ▣ 549
- Mobigesic Analgesic Tablets ... ▣ 507

Meclofenamate Sodium (May elevate and prolong serum methotrexate levels; reduces the tubular secretion of methotrexate). Products include:

- Meclomen Capsules ... 1739

Mefenamic Acid (May elevate and prolong serum methotrexate levels; reduces the tubular secretion of methotrexate). Products include:

- Ponstel ... 1758

Methacycline Hydrochloride (Decreases intestinal absorption and interferes with enterohepatic circulation).

No products indexed under this heading.

Minocycline Hydrochloride (Decreases intestinal absorption and interferes with enterohepatic circulation). Products include:

- Minocin Intravenous ... 1221
- Minocin Oral Suspension ... 1224
- Minocin Pellet-Filled Capsules ... 1222

Mitotane (Combined use has not been studied and may increase the incidence of adverse effects). Products include:

- Lysodren ... 731

Mitoxantrone Hydrochloride (Combined use has not been studied and may increase the incidence of adverse effects). Products include:

- Novantrone for Injection Concentrate ... 1226

Naproxen (May elevate and prolong serum methotrexate levels; reduces the tubular secretion of methotrexate). Products include:

- Naprosyn ... 2297

Naproxen Sodium (May elevate and prolong serum methotrexate levels; reduces the tubular secretion of methotrexate). Products include:

- Anaprox and Anaprox DS Tablets ... 2288

Oxytetracycline (Decreases intestinal absorption and interferes with enterohepatic circulation). Products include:

- Terramycin Intramuscular Solution 1964
- Urobiotic-250 Capsules ... 1968

Oxytetracycline Hydrochloride (Decreases intestinal absorption and interferes with enterohepatic circulation). Products include:

- Terra-Cortril Ophthalmic Suspension ... 1963
- Terramycin Capsules ... 1786
- Terramycin Intramuscular Solution 1964
- Terramycin with Polymyxin B Sulfate Ophthalmic Ointment ... 1965

Penicillamine (Combined use has not been studied and may increase the incidence of adverse effects). Products include:

- Cuprimine Capsules ... 1442
- Depen Titratable Tablets ... 2379

Phenylbutazone (Increased toxicity; may elevate and prolong serum methotrexate levels; reduces the tubular secretion of methotrexate). Products include:

- Butazolidin Capsules & Tablets ... 1027

Phenytoin (Increased toxicity). Products include:

- Dilantin Infatabs ... 1710
- Dilantin-30 Pediatric/Dilantin-125 Suspension ... 1713

Phenytoin Sodium (Increased toxicity). Products include:

- Dilantin Kapseals ... 1708
- Dilantin Parenteral ... 1712
- Dilantin with Phenobarbital Kapseals ... 1715

Piroxicam (May elevate and prolong serum methotrexate levels; reduces the tubular secretion of methotrexate). Products include:

- Feldene Capsules ... 1777

Probenecid (Reduces renal tubular transport). Products include:

- Benemid Tablets ... 1426
- ColBENEMID Tablets ... 1436
- Wycillin Injection and Probenecid Tablets ... 2539

Procarbazine Hydrochloride (Combined use has not been studied and may increase the incidence of adverse effects). Products include:

- Matulane Capsules ... 1907

Salsalate (Increased toxicity). Products include:

- Disalcid ... 1310
- Mono-Gesic Tablets ... 846
- Salflex ... 839

Sulfamethizole (Increased toxicity). Products include:

- Thiosulfil Forte Tablets ... 2526
- Urobiotic-250 Capsules ... 1968

Sulfamethoxazole (Increased toxicity). Products include:

- Azo Gantanol Tablets ... 1887
- Bactrim DS Tablets ... 1891
- Bactrim I.V. Infusion ... 1889
- Bactrim ... 1891
- Gantanol ... 1899
- Septra ... 813
- Septra I.V. Infusion ... 808
- Septra I.V. Infusion ADD-Vantage Vials ... 810
- Septra ... 813

Sulfasalazine (Increased toxicity). Products include:

- Azulfidine Tablets, EN-tabs, Oral Suspension ... 1157

Sulfinpyrazone (Increased toxicity). Products include:

- Anturane ... 853

Sulfisoxazole (Increased toxicity). Products include:

- Azo Gantrisin Tablets ... 1888
- Gantrisin Tablets ... 1901
- Pediazole ... 1973

Sulfisoxazole Diolamine (Increased toxicity). Products include:

- Gantrisin Ophthalmic Ointment/Solution ... 1900

Sulindac (May elevate and prolong serum methotrexate levels; reduces the tubular secretion of methotrexate). Products include:

- Clinoril Tablets ... 1433

Tamoxifen Citrate (Combined use has not been studied and may increase the incidence of adverse effects). Products include:

- Nolvadex Tablets ... 1102

Tetracycline Hydrochloride (Decreases intestinal absorption and interferes with enterohepatic circulation). Products include:

- Achromycin V Capsules ... 1193
- Achromycin Ophthalmic Ointment 1% ... ⊙ 307
- Achromycin Ophthalmic Suspension 1% ... ⊙ 308
- Topicycline for Topical Solution ... 1856

Tolmetin Sodium (May elevate and prolong serum methotrexate levels; reduces the tubular secretion of methotrexate). Products include:

- Tolectin (200, 400 and 600 mg) .. 1379

Trimethoprim (May increase bone marrow suppression). Products include:

- Bactrim DS Tablets ... 1891
- Bactrim I.V. Infusion ... 1889
- Bactrim ... 1891
- Proloprim Tablets ... 799
- Septra ... 813
- Septra I.V. Infusion ... 808
- Septra I.V. Infusion ADD-Vantage Vials ... 810
- Septra ... 813
- Trimpex Tablets ... 1922

Vincristine Sulfate (Combined use has not been studied and may increase the incidence of adverse effects). Products include:

- Oncovin Solution Vials & Hyporets 1288

Food Interactions

Food, unspecified (Delays absorption and reduces peak concentration).

METIMYD OPHTHALMIC OINTMENT—STERILE
(Prednisolone Acetate, Sulfacetamide Sodium) .... ◉ 306
No interactions described in labeling.

METIMYD OPHTHALMIC SUSPENSION—STERILE
(Prednisolone Acetate, Sulfacetamide Sodium) .... ◉ 306
No interactions described in labeling.

METOPIRONE TABLETS
(Metyrapone) 876
May interact with corticosteroids, estrogens, and certain other agents. Compounds in these categories include:

Betamethasone Acetate (Concurrent administration may produce false results). Products include:
Celestone Soluspan Suspension 2081

Betamethasone Dipropionate (Concurrent administration may produce false results). Products include:
Alphatrex Cream, Ointment & Lotion 2076
Diprolene 2083
Lotrisone Cream 2103
Maxivate Cream, Lotion & Ointment 0.05% 2406
Psorion Cream 0.05% 1121

Betamethasone Sodium Phosphate (Concurrent administration may produce false results). Products include:
Celestone Soluspan Suspension 2081

Betamethasone Valerate (Concurrent administration may produce false results). Products include:
Betatrex Cream, Ointment & Lotion 2077

Chlorotrianisene (Subnormal response). Products include:
TACE 12 and 25 mg 1353

Clobetasol Propionate (Concurrent administration may produce false results). Products include:
Temovate 1056

Cortisone Acetate (Concurrent administration may produce false results). Products include:
Cortone Acetate Sterile Suspension 1437
Cortone Acetate Tablets 1439

Desoximetasone (Concurrent administration may produce false results). Products include:
Topicort 1098

Dexamethasone Acetate (Concurrent administration may produce false results). Products include:
Dalalone D.P. Injectable 999
Decadron-LA Sterile Suspension 1457

Dexamethasone Sodium Phosphate (Concurrent administration may produce false results). Products include:
AK-Dex .... ◉ 203
Decadron Phosphate Respihaler 1454
Decadron Phosphate Sterile Ophthalmic Ointment 1453
Decadron Phosphate Sterile Ophthalmic Solution 1453
Decadron Phosphate Topical Cream 1455
Decadron Phosphate Turbinaire 1456
Maxidex Sterile Ophthalmic Ointment .... ◉ 222
NeoDecadron Sterile Ophthalmic Ointment 1517
NeoDecadron Sterile Ophthalmic Solution 1518
NeoDecadron Topical Cream 1518

Dienestrol (Subnormal response). Products include:
Ortho Dienestrol Cream 1664

Diethylstilbestrol (Subnormal response). Products include:
Diethylstilbestrol Tablets 1258

Estradiol (Subnormal response). Products include:
Emcyt Capsules 1161
Estrace 1385
Estrace Vaginal Cream 1388
Estraderm Transdermal System 866

Estrogens, Conjugated (Subnormal response). Products include:
Mediatric Capsules 2476
PMB 200 and PMB 400 2504
Premarin Intravenous 2508
Premarin with Methyltestosterone .. 2515
Premarin Tablets 2510
Premarin Vaginal Cream 2512

Estrogens, Esterified (Subnormal response). Products include:
Estratest 2245
Menrium Tablets 1934

Estropipate (Subnormal response). Products include:
Ogen 540

Ethinyl Estradiol (Subnormal response). Products include:
Brevicon 2304
Demulen 2161
Estinyl Tablets 2085
Jenest-28 Tablets 1636
Levlen/Tri-Levlen 665
Lo/Ovral Tablets 2471
Lo/Ovral-28 Tablets 2476
Loestrin 1728
Modicon 1667
Nordette-21 Tablets 2481
Nordette-28 Tablets 2483
Norethin 2133
Norinyl 2304
Norlestrin 1746
Ortho-Cyclen Tablets 1658
Ortho-Novum 1667
Ovcon 1391
Ovral Tablets 2490
Ovral-28 Tablets 2491
Levlen/Tri-Levlen 665
Tri-Norinyl 2304
Triphasil-21 Tablets 2527
Triphasil-28 Tablets 2532

Flunisolide (Concurrent administration may produce false results). Products include:
AeroBid Inhaler System 995
Nasalide Nasal Solution 0.025% 2299

Hydrocortisone (Concurrent administration may produce false results). Products include:
AK-Spore H.C. .... ◉ 206
Bactine Hydrocortisone Anti-Itch Cream .... ▣ 625
CaldeCORT Anti-Itch Hydrocortisone Spray .... ▣ 560
Carmol HC Cream 1% 2296
Cortaid Spray .... ▣ 735
Cortenema 2244
Cortisporin Ointment 758
Cortisporin Ophthalmic Ointment Sterile 758
Cortisporin Ophthalmic Suspension Sterile 759
Cortisporin Otic Solution Sterile 760
Cortisporin Otic Suspension Sterile 760
Cortizone-5 Creme & Ointment .... ▣ 732
Dermolate Anti-Itch Cream .... ▣ 697
Eldecort Cream 1.0% 1113
Eldecort Cream 1.0% and 2.5% 1113
Fungoid HC Creme 1770
Hydrocortone Tablets 1482
Hytone 909
LazerSporin-C Solution 1770
Massengill Medicated Soft Cloth Towelettes 2192
Nutracort Cream & Lotion 1684
PediOtic Suspension Sterile 797
Synacort Creams 1%, 2.5% 2296
Vanoxide-HC Acne Lotion 911
Vioform-Hydrocortisone Cream and Mild Cream 889
Vioform-Hydrocortisone Ointment .. 889
VōSoL HC Otic Solution 2392
Vytone Cream 1% 911

Hydrocortisone Acetate (Concurrent administration may produce false results). Products include:
Analpram-HC Rectal Cream 1% and 2.5% 970
Anusol-HC Cream 1690
Anusol-HC Suppositories 1691
Caldecort .... ▣ 560
Carmol HC Cream 1% 2296
Chloromycetin Hydrocortisone Ophthalmic 1694
Coly-Mycin S Otic w/Neomycin & Hydrocortisone 1708
Cortaid .... ▣ 735
Cortef Feminine Itch Cream .... ▣ 735
Corticaine .... ▣ 682
Cortifoam 1827
Cortisporin Cream 757
Epifoam 1828
Gynecort 5 Creme .... ▣ 556
Hydrocortone Acetate Sterile Suspension 1479
Lanacort 5 Creme and Ointment .. ▣ 557
Mantadil Cream 789
Ophthocort .... ◉ 301
Orabase HCA Oral Paste 890
Pramosone Cream, Lotion & Ointment 971
ProctoCream-HC 1834
Proctofoam-HC 1835

Hydrocortisone Butyrate (Concurrent administration may produce false results). Products include:
Locoid Cream, Ointment and Topical Solution 970

Hydrocortisone Sodium Phosphate (Concurrent administration may produce false results). Products include:
Hydrocortone Phosphate Injection, Sterile 1481

Hydrocortisone Sodium Succinate (Concurrent administration may produce false results). Products include:
Solu-Cortef Sterile Powder 2361

Hydrocortisone Valerate (Concurrent administration may produce false results). Products include:
Westcort 2411

Methylprednisolone (Concurrent administration may produce false results). Products include:
Medrol 2348

Methylprednisolone Acetate (Concurrent administration may produce false results). Products include:
Depo-Medrol Sterile Aqueous Suspension 2334

Methylprednisolone Sodium Succinate (Concurrent administration may produce false results). Products include:
Solu-Medrol Sterile Powder 2363

Phenytoin (Accelerates metabolism of Metopirone). Products include:
Dilantin Infatabs 1710
Dilantin-30 Pediatric/Dilantin-125 Suspension 1713

Phenytoin Sodium (Accelerates metabolism of Metopirone). Products include:
Dilantin Kapseals 1708
Dilantin Parenteral 1712
Dilantin with Phenobarbital Kapseals 1715

Polyestradiol Phosphate (Subnormal response). Products include:
Estradurin 2452

Prednisolone Acetate (Concurrent administration may produce false results). Products include:
AK-Cide Sterile Ophthalmic Ointment & Suspension .... ◉ 202
Blephamide Liquifilm Sterile Ophthalmic Suspension 586
Blephamide S.O.P. Sterile Ophthalmic Ointment 586
Cetapred Ointment .... ◉ 220
⅛% Econopred & 1% Econopred Plus .... ◉ 217
Isopto Cetapred Suspension .... ◉ 220
Metimyd .... ◉ 306
Poly-Pred Liquifilm .... ◉ 250
Pred Forte .... ◉ 252
Pred Mild .... ◉ 254
Pred-G Liquifilm Sterile Ophthalmic Suspension .... ◉ 252
Pred-G S.O.P. Sterile Ophthalmic Ointment .... ◉ 253
Vasocidin Ointment .... ◉ 275

Prednisolone Sodium Phosphate (Concurrent administration may produce false results). Products include:
AK-Pred .... ◉ 205
Hydeltrasol Injection, Sterile 1476
Inflamase .... ◉ 274
Pediapred Oral Liquid 987
Vasocidin Ophthalmic Solution ...... ◉ 276

Prednisolone Tebutate (Concurrent administration may produce false results). Products include:
Hydeltra-T.B.A. Sterile Suspension 1478

Prednisone (Concurrent administration may produce false results). Products include:
Deltasone Tablets 2332

Quinestrol (Subnormal response). Products include:
Estrovis 1721

Triamcinolone (Concurrent administration may produce false results).
No products indexed under this heading.

Triamcinolone Acetonide (Concurrent administration may produce false results). Products include:
Aristocort A 1010
Azmacort Inhaler 1837
Kenalog Cream, Lotion & Ointment 2401
Kenalog-10 Injection 2402
Kenalog-40 Injection 2403
Kenalog in Orabase 604
Kenalog Spray 2401
Mycolog II Cream and Ointment 2407
Mytrex Cream & Ointment 2080
Nasacort Nasal Inhaler 1844

Triamcinolone Diacetate (Concurrent administration may produce false results). Products include:
Aristocort Suspension 1008

Triamcinolone Hexacetonide (Concurrent administration may produce false results). Products include:
Aristospan Suspension 1011

METRODIN (UROFOLLITROPIN FOR INJECTION)
(Urofollitropin) 2182
No interactions described in labeling.

METROGEL
(Metronidazole) 903
May interact with oral anticoagulants. Compounds in this category include:

Dicumarol (Potentiation of anticoagulant effect with oral metronidazole; less likely to occur with topical use). Products include:
Dicumarol Tablets 516

Warfarin Sodium (Potentiation of anticoagulant effect with oral metronidazole; less likely to occur with topical use). Products include:
Coumadin Injection & Tablets 944
Panwarfin Tablets 547

METUBINE IODIDE VIALS
(Metocurine Iodide) 1285
May interact with general anesthetics, muscle relaxants, tetracyclines, and certain other agents. Compounds in these categories include:

Atracurium Besylate (Synergistic or antagonistic effect). Products include:
Tracrium Injection 817

(▣ Described in PDR For Nonprescription Drugs) (◉ Described in PDR For Ophthalmology)

Bacitracin (Intensified or similar neuroblocking action). Products include:
- Baciguent Antibiotic Ointment ⊡ 735
- Bactine First Aid Antibiotic Ointment ⊡ 625
- Campho-Phenique Triple Antibiotic Ointment Plus Pain Reliever ⊡ 758
- Lanabiotic Ointment ⊡ 556
- Mycitracin ⊡ 737

Baclofen (Synergistic or antagonistic effect). Products include:
- Lioresal Tablets 1031

Carisoprodol (Synergistic or antagonistic effect). Products include:
- Soma Compound w/Codeine Tablets 2390
- Soma Compound Tablets 2389
- Soma Tablets 2388

Chlorzoxazone (Synergistic or antagonistic effect). Products include:
- Paraflex Caplets 1378
- Parafon Forte DSC Caplets 1379

Colistimethate Sodium (Intensified or similar neuroblocking action). Products include:
- Coly-Mycin M Parenteral 1706

Colistin Sulfate (Intensified or similar neuroblocking action). Products include:
- Coly-Mycin S For Oral Suspension 1708
- Coly-Mycin S Otic w/Neomycin & Hydrocortisone 1708

Cyclobenzaprine Hydrochloride (Synergistic or antagonistic effect). Products include:
- Flexeril Tablets 1471

Dantrolene Sodium (Synergistic or antagonistic effect). Products include:
- Dantrium Capsules 1619
- Dantrium Intravenous 1620

Demeclocycline Hydrochloride (Intensified or similar neuroblocking action). Products include:
- Declomycin Capsules, Tablets 1199

Diethyl Ether (Potentiation of neuromuscular blocking action of metubine iodide).

Doxacurium Chloride (Synergistic or antagonistic effect). Products include:
- Nuromax Injection 794

Doxycycline Calcium (Intensified or similar neuroblocking action).
- No products indexed under this heading.

Doxycycline Hyclate (Intensified or similar neuroblocking action). Products include:
- Doryx Capsules 1717
- Vibramycin Hyclate Capsules 1787
- Vibramycin Hyclate Intravenous 1968
- Vibra-Tabs Film Coated Tablets 1787

Doxycycline Monohydrate (Intensified or similar neuroblocking action). Products include:
- Monodox Capsules 1630
- Vibramycin Monohydrate for Oral Suspension 1787

Enflurane (Synergistic action). Products include:
- Ethrane 599

Gentamicin Sulfate (Intensified or similar neuroblocking action). Products include:
- Garamycin Injectable 2093
- Garamycin Ophthalmic ⊙ 305
- Genoptic Liquifilm Sterile Ophthalmic Solution ⊙ 247
- Genoptic S.O.P. Sterile Ophthalmic Ointment ⊙ 247
- Gentacidin Ointment ⊙ 273
- Gentacidin Solution ⊙ 273
- Gentak Ointment & Solution ⊙ 208
- G-myticin Creme and Ointment 0.1% 1770
- Pred-G Liquifilm Sterile Ophthalmic Suspension ⊙ 252
- Pred-G S.O.P. Sterile Ophthalmic Ointment ⊙ 253

Halothane (Potentiation of neuromuscular blocking action of metubine iodide). Products include:
- Fluothane 2453

Isoflurane (Potentiation of neuromuscular blocking action of metubine iodide; synergistic action). Products include:
- Forane 600

Kanamycin Sulfate (Intensified or similar neuroblocking action). Products include:
- Kantrex Injection 601
- Kantrex Pediatric Injection 601

Magnesium Sulfate (Potentiation of both depolarizing and nondepolarizing drugs). Products include:
- Eldertonic 1359
- Vicon Forte Capsules 2416
- Vicon Plus ⊡ 682
- Vicon-C ⊡ 682

Metaxalone (Synergistic or antagonistic effect). Products include:
- Skelaxin 840

Methacycline Hydrochloride (Intensified or similar neuroblocking action).
- No products indexed under this heading.

Methocarbamol (Synegistic or antagonistic effect). Products include:
- Robaxin Injectable 1871
- Robaxin Tablets 1872
- Robaxisal Tablets 1872

Methohexital Sodium (Potentiation of neuromuscular action of metubine iodide; synergistic action). Products include:
- Brevital Sodium Vials 1248

Methoxyflurane (Potentiation of neuromuscular action of metubine iodide; synergistic action).
- No products indexed under this heading.

Minocycline Hydrochloride (Intensified or similar neuroblocking action). Products include:
- Minocin Intravenous 1221
- Minocin Oral Suspension 1224
- Minocin Pellet-Filled Capsules 1222

Neomycin Sulfate (Intensified or similar neuroblocking action). Products include:
- AK-Spore H.C. ⊙ 206
- AK-Spore ⊙ 205
- AK-Trol Ointment & Suspension ⊙ 207
- Bactine First Aid Antibiotic Ointment ⊡ 625
- Campho-Phenique Triple Antibiotic Ointment Plus Pain Reliever ⊡ 758
- Coly-Mycin S Otic w/Neomycin & Hydrocortisone 1708
- Cortisporin Cream 757
- Cortisporin Ointment 758
- Cortisporin Ophthalmic Ointment Sterile 758
- Cortisporin Ophthalmic Suspension Sterile 759
- Cortisporin Otic Solution Sterile 760
- Cortisporin Otic Suspension Sterile 760
- Dexacidin ⊙ 272
- Lanabiotic Ointment ⊡ 556
- LazerSporin-C Solution 1770
- Maxitrol Ophthalmic Ointment/Suspension ⊙ 223
- Myciguent Antibiotic Ointment ⊡ 737
- Mycitracin ⊡ 737
- NeoDecadron Sterile Ophthalmic Ointment 1517
- NeoDecadron Sterile Ophthalmic Solution 1518
- NeoDecadron Topical Cream 1518
- Neosporin Cream 792
- Neosporin G.U. Irrigant Sterile 793
- Neosporin Ointment 793
- Maximum Strength Neosporin Ointment 793
- Neosporin Ophthalmic Ointment Sterile 793
- Neosporin Ophthalmic Solution Sterile 794
- Neo-Synalar Cream 2296
- PediOtic Suspension Sterile 797
- Poly-Pred Liquifilm ⊙ 250

Orphenadrine Citrate (Synergistic or antagonistic effect). Products include:
- Norflex 1314
- Norgesic 1314

Oxytetracycline (Intensified or similar neuroblocking action). Products include:
- Terramycin Intramuscular Solution 1964
- Urobiotic-250 Capsules 1968

Oxytetracycline Hydrochloride (Intensified or similar neuroblocking action). Products include:
- Terra-Cortril Ophthalmic Suspension 1963
- Terramycin Capsules 1786
- Terramycin Intramuscular Solution 1964
- Terramycin with Polymyxin B Sulfate Ophthalmic Ointment 1965

Pancuronium Bromide Injection (Synergistic or antagonistic effect).
- No products indexed under this heading.

Polymyxin B Sulfate (Intensified or similar neuroblocking action). Products include:
- AK-Poly-Bac Ointment ⊙ 205
- AK-Spore H.C. ⊙ 206
- AK-Spore ⊙ 205
- AK-Trol Ointment & Suspension ⊙ 207
- Aquaphor Antibiotic Formula 662
- Bactine First Aid Antibiotic Ointment ⊡ 625
- Campho-Phenique Triple Antibiotic Ointment Plus Pain Reliever ⊡ 758
- Cortisporin Cream 757
- Cortisporin Ointment 758
- Cortisporin Ophthalmic Ointment Sterile 758
- Cortisporin Ophthalmic Suspension Sterile 759
- Cortisporin Otic Solution Sterile 760
- Cortisporin Otic Suspension Sterile 760
- Dexacidin ⊙ 272
- Lanabiotic Ointment ⊡ 556
- LazerSporin-C Solution 1770
- Maxitrol Ophthalmic Ointment/Suspension ⊙ 223
- Mycitracin ⊡ 737
- Neosporin Cream 792
- Neosporin G.U. Irrigant Sterile 793
- Neosporin Ointment 793
- Maximum Strength Neosporin Ointment 793
- Neosporin Ophthalmic Ointment Sterile 793
- Neosporin Ophthalmic Solution Sterile 794
- Ophthocort ⊙ 301
- PediOtic Suspension Sterile 797
- Polymyxin B Sulfate, Aerosporin Brand Sterile Powder 798
- Poly-Pred Liquifilm ⊙ 250
- Polysporin Ointment ⊡ 543
- Polysporin Ophthalmic Ointment Sterile 798
- Polysporin Powder ⊡ 543
- Polysporin Spray ⊡ 543
- Polytrim Ophthalmic Solution Sterile 588
- Terramycin with Polymyxin B Sulfate Ophthalmic Ointment 1965

Propofol (Synergistic action). Products include:
- Diprivan Injection 2267

Quinidine Gluconate (Recurrent paralysis). Products include:
- Quinaglute Dura-Tabs Tablets 663

Quinidine Polygalacturonate (Recurrent paralysis). Products include:
- Cardioquin Tablets 1812

Quinidine Sulfate (Recurrent paralysis). Products include:
- Quinidex Extentabs 1868

Streptomycin Sulfate (Intensified or similar neuroblocking action).
- No products indexed under this heading.

Succinylcholine Chloride (Synergistic or antagonistic effect). Products include:
- Anectine 755

Tetracycline Hydrochloride (Intensified or similar neuroblocking action). Products include:
- Achromycin V Capsules 1193
- Achromycin Ophthalmic Ointment 1% ⊙ 307
- Achromycin Ophthalmic Suspension 1% ⊙ 308
- Topicycline for Topical Solution 1856

Vecuronium Bromide (Synergistic or antagonistic effect). Products include:
- Norcuron 1642

MEVACOR TABLETS

(Lovastatin) 1505

May interact with immunosuppressive agents, fibrates, oral anticoagulants, and certain other agents. Compounds in these categories include:

Alcohol (Increased potential for liver dysfunction).

Azathioprine (Potential for myopathy and/or markedly elevated CPK levels). Products include:
- Imuran 768

Clofibrate (Potential for myopathy and/or markedly elevated CPK levels). Products include:
- Atromid-S Capsules 2435

Cyclosporine (Potential for myopathy, markedly elevated CPK levels and/or acute renal failure from rhabdomyolysis). Products include:
- Sandimmune 2024

Dicumarol (Potential for clinically evident bleeding and/or increased prothrombin time). Products include:
- Dicumarol Tablets 516

Erythromycin (Concomitant therapy in seriously ill patients may result in rhabdomyolysis with or without renal impairment). Products include:
- A/T/S Topical Gel and Topical Solution 1089
- AK-Mycin Ointment ⊙ 204
- Benzamycin Topical Gel 907
- E-Mycin Tablets 688
- ETS-2% 1685
- ERYC 1720
- Erycette (erythromycin 2%) Topical Solution 1678
- Ery-Tab Tablets 521
- Erythromycin Base Filmtab 525
- Erythromycin Delayed-Release Capsules, USP 526
- Ilotycin Ophthalmic Ointment 915
- PCE Dispertab Tablets 549
- Pediazole 1973
- T-Stat 2.0% Topical Solution and Pads 2409
- Theramycin Z Topical Solution 2% 1410

Erythromycin Estolate (Concomitant therapy in seriously ill patients may result in rhabdomyolysis with or without renal impairment). Products include:
- Ilosone 913

Erythromycin Ethylsuccinate (Concomitant therapy in seriously ill patients may result in rhabdomyolysis with or without renal impairment). Products include:
- E.E.S. 522
- EryPed 519
- Pediazole 1973

Erythromycin Gluceptate (Concomitant therapy in seriously ill patients may result in rhabdomyolysis with or without renal impairment). Products include:
- Ilotycin Gluceptate, IV, Vials 915

Erythromycin Stearate (Concomitant therapy in seriously ill patients may result in rhabdomyolysis with or without renal impairment). Products include:
Erythrocin Stearate Filmtab ... 523

Gemfibrozil (Potential for myopathy, markedly elevated CPK levels and/or acute renal failure from rhabdomyolysis). Products include:
Lopid Capsules and Tablets ... 1736

Immune Globulin (Human) (Potential for myopathy and/or markedly elevated CPK levels). Products include:
MICRhoGAM Rh_0(D) Immune Globulin (Human) ... 1650
RhoGAM Rh_0(D) Immune Globulin (Human) ... 1651

Immune Globulin Intravenous (Human) (Potential for myopathy and/or markedly elevated CPK levels). Products include:
Gamimune N Immune Globulin Intravenous (Human) ... 1572
Gammagard Immune Globulin, Intravenous (Human) ... 658
Iveegam ... 1129
Sandoglobulin I.V. ... 2027

Levothyroxine Sodium (Concurrent therapy results in rare reports of thyroid function test abnormalities). Products include:
Levothroid Tablets ... 1003
Levoxine Tablets ... 904
Synthroid ... 695

Muromonab-CD3 (Potential for myopathy and/or markedly elevated CPK levels). Products include:
Orthoclone OKT3 Sterile Solution ... 1645

Nicotinic Acid (Potential for myopathy and/or markedly elevated CPK levels with lipid-lowering doses of nicotinic acid). Products include:
Niacor Tablets ... 2376
Nicobid ... 1846
Nicolar Tablets ... 1846
Nicotinex Elixir ... ▪ 563
Slo-Niacin Tablets ... 2376

Warfarin Sodium (Potential for clinically evident bleeding and/or increased prothrombin time). Products include:
Coumadin Injection & Tablets ... 944
Panwarfin Tablets ... 547

MEXITIL CAPSULES
(Mexiletine Hydrochloride) ... **680**
May interact with narcotic analgesics and certain other agents. Compounds in these categories include:

Alfentanil Hydrochloride (Narcotics slow the absorption of Mexitil). Products include:
Alfenta Injection ... 1131

Atropine Sulfate (Slows the absorption of Mexitil). Products include:
Arco-Lase Plus Tablets ... 607
Atropine Sulfate Sterile Ophthalmic Solution and S.O.P. Sterile Ophthalmic Ointment ... ⊙ 239
Donnagel ... ▪ 675
Donnagel-PG ... 1858
Donnatal ... 1858
Donnatal Extentabs ... 1859
Donnatal Tablets ... 1858
Donnazyme Tablets ... 1860
Isopto Atropine ... ⊙ 218
Lomotil ... 2174
Motofen Tablets ... 836
Ru-Tuss Tablets ... 693
Urised Tablets ... 2396

Buprenorphine (Narcotics slow the absorption of Mexitil).
No products indexed under this heading.

Caffeine-containing medications (Caffeine clearance decreased 50%).

Cimetidine (May alter Mexitil plasma levels). Products include:
Tagamet Tablets ... 2228

Cimetidine Hydrochloride (May alter Mexitil plasma levels). Products include:
Tagamet ... 2228

Codeine (Narcotics slow the absorption of Mexitil). Products include:
Calcidrine Syrup ... 506

Codeine Phosphate (Narcotics slow the absorption of Mexitil). Products include:
Actifed with Codeine Cough Syrup ... 752
Cheracol Cough Syrup ... 1853
Codimal PH Syrup ... 846
Dimetane-DC Cough Syrup ... 1857
Empirin with Codeine Phosphate Nos. 2, 3 & 4 ... 764
Fiorinal with Codeine Capsules ... 2008
Isoclor Expectorant ... 982
Naldecon CX Adult Liquid ... ▪ 521
Novahistine DH ... 1342
Novahistine Expectorant ... 1343
Nucofed Capsules ... 2219
Nucofed Expectorant ... 2219
Nucofed Pediatric Expectorant ... 2220
Nucofed Syrup ... 2219
Phenaphen with Codeine Capsules ... 1865
Phenaphen-650 with Codeine Tablets ... 1866
Phenergan with Codeine ... 2497
Phenergan VC with Codeine ... 2501
Robitussin A-C Syrup ... 1875
Robitussin-DAC Syrup ... 1875
Ryna ... ▪ 741
Soma Compound w/Codeine Tablets ... 2390
Triaminic Expectorant w/Codeine ... 1996
Tussi-Organidin Liquid ... 2391
Tylenol with Codeine ... 1381

Codeine Polistirex (Narcotics slow the absorption of Mexitil).
No products indexed under this heading.

Dezocine (Narcotics slow the absorption of Mexitil).

Digoxin (Lowered serum digoxin levels in presence of magnesium-aluminum hydroxide). Products include:
Lanoxicaps ... 772
Lanoxin Elixir Pediatric ... 775
Lanoxin Injection ... 778
Lanoxin Injection Pediatric ... 781
Lanoxin Tablets ... 783

Fentanyl (Narcotics slow the absorption of Mexitil). Products include:
Duragesic Transdermal System ... 1133

Fentanyl Citrate (Narcotics slow the absorption of Mexitil). Products include:
Innovar Injection ... 1141
Sublimaze Injection ... 1146

Hydrocodone Bitartrate (Narcotics slow the absorption of Mexitil). Products include:
Anexsia 5/500 Tablets ... 2196
Anexsia 7.5/650 Tablets ... 2197
Azdone Tablets ... 844
Codiclear DH Syrup ... 845
Codimal DH Syrup ... 846
Damason-P ... 1356
Hycodan Syrup, Tablets ... 927
Hycomine Compound Tablets ... 929
Hycomine Syrup ... 927
Hycotuss Expectorant Syrup ... 930
Hydrocet Capsules ... 835
Lortab ASA Tablets ... 2414
Lortab ... 2412
Ru-Tuss with Hydrocodone ... 694
Triaminic Expectorant DH ... 1995
Vicodin Tablets ... 1187
Vicodin ES Tablets ... 1189
Zydone Capsules ... 941

Hydrocodone Polistirex (Narcotics slow the absorption of Mexitil). Products include:
Tussionex Extended-Release Suspension ... 988

Levorphanol Tartrate (Narcotics slow the absorption of Mexitil). Products include:
Levo-Dromoran ... 1906

Magaldrate (Slows the absorption of Mexitil). Products include:
Riopan Antacid Chew Tablets ... ▪ 754
Riopan Antacid Chew Tablets in Rollpacks ... ▪ 754
Riopan Antacid Suspension ... 2421
Riopan Antacid Swallow Tablets ... 2421
Riopan Plus Chew Tablets ... 2422
Riopan Plus Chew Tablets in Rollpack ... 2422
Riopan Plus 2 Chew Tablets, Mint Flavor, Cherry Flavor ... 2422
Riopan Plus Suspension ... 2422
Riopan Plus 2 Suspension, Mint Flavor, Cherry Flavor ... 2422

Meperidine Hydrochloride (Narcotics slow the absorption of Mexitil). Products include:
Demerol ... 2047
Mepergan Injection ... 2479

Methadone Hydrochloride (Narcotics slow the absorption of Mexitil). Products include:
Dolophine Hydrochloride Ampoules & Vials ... 1260
Dolophine Hydrochloride Tablets ... 1261
Methadone Hydrochloride Diskets ... 1284
Methadone Hydrochloride Oral Solution & Tablets ... 1987

Metoclopramide Hydrochloride (Accelerates the absorption). Products include:
Reglan ... 1869

Morphine Sulfate (Narcotics slow the absorption of Mexitil). Products include:
Astramorph/PF Injection, USP (Preservative-Free) ... 618
Duramorph ... 960
Infumorph 200 and Infumorph 500 Sterile Solutions ... 962
MS Contin Tablets ... 1814
MSIR ... 1817
Oramorph SR (Morphine Sulfate Sustained Release Tablets) ... 1988
Roxanol ... 1991

Opium Alkaloids (Narcotics slow the absorption of Mexitil). Products include:
B & O No. 15A & No. 16A Supprettes ... 2395
Pantopon Injectable ... 1911

Oxycodone Hydrochloride (Narcotics slow the absorption of Mexitil). Products include:
Percocet Tablets ... 950
Percodan ... 951
Roxicodone Tablets, Oral Solution & Intensol (Oxycodone) ... 1992
Tylox Capsules ... 1382

Phenobarbital (Lowers Mexitil plasma levels). Products include:
Arco-Lase Plus Tablets ... 607
Bellergal-S Tablets ... 1998
Bronkolixir ... ▪ 761
Bronkotabs Tablets ... ▪ 762
Donnatal ... 1858
Donnatal Extentabs ... 1859
Donnatal Tablets ... 1858
Donnazyme Tablets ... 1860
Kinesed Tablets ... 2272
Phenobarbital Elixir and Tablets ... 1293
Primatene Tablets-P Formula ... 2421
Quadrinal Tablets ... 1183
Tedral SA ... 1765

Phenytoin (Lowers Mexitil plasma levels). Products include:
Dilantin Infatabs ... 1710
Dilantin-30 Pediatric/Dilantin-125 Suspension ... 1713

Phenytoin Sodium (Lowers Mexitil plasma levels). Products include:
Dilantin Kapseals ... 1708
Dilantin Parenteral ... 1712
Dilantin with Phenobarbital Kapseals ... 1715

Propoxyphene Hydrochloride (Narcotics slow the absorption of Mexitil). Products include:
Darvon ... 1256
Wygesic Tablets ... 2540

Propoxyphene Napsylate (Narcotics slow the absorption of Mexitil). Products include:
Darvon-N/Darvocet-N ... 1254

Rifampin (Lowers Mexitil plasma levels). Products include:
Rifadin ... 1345
Rifamate Capsules ... 1347
Rimactane Capsules ... 879

Sufentanil Citrate (Narcotics slow the absorption of Mexitil). Products include:
Sufenta Injection ... 1147

Theophylline (Potential for increased plasma theophylline levels). Products include:
Bronkaid Tablets ... ▪ 757
Bronkolixir ... ▪ 761
Bronkotabs Tablets ... ▪ 762
Constant-T Tablets ... 1029
Marax Tablets & DF Syrup ... 1954
Primatene Tablets ... 2421
Quibron Capsules ... 713
Quibron-T ... 714
Quibron-T/SR ... 716
Theolair Liquid ... 1317
Theo-Organidin Elixir ... 2391

Theophylline Anhydrous (Potential for increased plasma theophylline levels). Products include:
Aerolate ... 994
Primatene Tablets-M Formula ... ▪ 753
Primatene Tablets-Regular Formula ... 2421
Respbid Tablets ... 684
Slo-bid Gyrocaps ... 1847
T-PHYL (Uniphyl) 200 mg Tablets ... 1820
Tedral SA ... 1765
Theo-24 ... 2179
Theo-Dur Sprinkle ... 1168
Theo-Dur Extended-Release Tablets ... 1166
Theolair Tablets ... 1317
Theolair-SR Tablets ... 1319
TheoX Extended-Release Tablets ... 841
Uniphyl 400 mg Tablets ... 1823

Theophylline Calcium Salicylate (Potential for increased plasma theophylline levels). Products include:
Quadrinal Tablets ... 1183

Theophylline Sodium Glycinate (Potential for increased plasma theophylline levels). Products include:
Asbron G ... 1997

MEYENBERG EVAPORATED GOAT MILK - 12 FL. OZ.
(Goat Milk) ... ▪ **576**
No interactions described in labeling.

MEYENBERG POWDERED GOAT MILK - 4 OZ. & 14 OZ.
(Goat Milk) ... ▪ **576**
No interactions described in labeling.

MEZLIN
(Mezlocillin Sodium) ... **1597**
May interact with aminoglycosides and certain other agents. Compounds in these categories include:

Amikacin Sulfate (Physical incompatibility resulting in substantial inactivation of the aminoglycoside). Products include:
Amikin Injectable ... 602

Gentamicin Sulfate (Physical incompatibility resulting in substantial inactivation of the aminoglycoside). Products include:
Garamycin Injectable ... 2093
Garamycin Ophthalmic ... ⊙ 305
Genoptic Liquifilm Sterile Ophthalmic Solution ... ⊙ 247
Genoptic S.O.P. Sterile Ophthalmic Ointment ... ⊙ 247
Gentacidin Ointment ... ⊙ 273
Gentacidin Solution ... ⊙ 273

Gentak Ointment & Solution ◉ 208
G-myticin Creme and Ointment 0.1% 1770
Pred-G Liquifilm Sterile Ophthalmic Suspension ◉ 252
Pred-G S.O.P. Sterile Ophthalmic Ointment ◉ 253

Kanamycin Sulfate (Physical incompatibility resulting in substantial inactivation of the aminoglycoside). Products include:
Kantrex Injection 601
Kantrex Pediatric Injection 601

Probenecid (Increased serum concentrations and prolonged serum half-life of mezlocillin). Products include:
Benemid Tablets 1426
ColBENEMID Tablets 1436
Wycillin Injection and Probenecid Tablets 2539

Streptomycin Sulfate (Physical incompatibility resulting in substantial inactivation of the aminoglycoside).
No products indexed under this heading.

Tobramycin Sulfate (Physical incompatibility resulting in substantial inactivation of the aminoglycoside). Products include:
Nebcin Vials, Hyporets & ADD-Vantage 1286

MEZLIN PHARMACY BULK PACKAGE
(Mezlocillin Sodium) 1599
May interact with:

Probenecid (Prolongs serum half-life of antibiotic). Products include:
Benemid Tablets 1426
ColBENEMID Tablets 1436
Wycillin Injection and Probenecid Tablets 2539

MIACALCIN INJECTION
(Calcitonin, Synthetic) 2017
No interactions described in labeling.

MICATIN ANTIFUNGAL CREAM
(Miconazole Nitrate) ▣ 632
No interactions described in labeling.

MICATIN ANTIFUNGAL DEODORANT SPRAY POWDER
(Miconazole Nitrate) ▣ 632
No interactions described in labeling.

MICATIN ANTIFUNGAL POWDER
(Miconazole Nitrate) ▣ 632
No interactions described in labeling.

MICATIN ANTIFUNGAL SPRAY LIQUID
(Miconazole Nitrate) ▣ 632
No interactions described in labeling.

MICATIN ANTIFUNGAL SPRAY POWDER
(Miconazole Nitrate) ▣ 632
No interactions described in labeling.

MICATIN JOCK ITCH CREAM
(Miconazole Nitrate) ▣ 633
No interactions described in labeling.

MICATIN JOCK ITCH SPRAY POWDER
(Miconazole Nitrate) ▣ 633
No interactions described in labeling.

MICRO-GUARD CREAM, ANTISEPTIC, ANTIFUNGAL SKIN CREAM
(Chloroxylenol) 2286
No interactions described in labeling.

MICRO-GUARD POWDER, ANTIFUNGAL POWDER
(Chloroxylenol) 2286
No interactions described in labeling.

MICRO-K EXTENCAPS
(Potassium Chloride) 1863
May interact with potassium sparing diuretics and ACE inhibitors. Compounds in these categories include:

Amiloride Hydrochloride (Hyperkalemia). Products include:
Midamor Tablets 1508
Moduretic Tablets 1510

Benazepril Hydrochloride (Potential for hyperkalemia). Products include:
Lotensin Tablets 872

Captopril (Potential for hyperkalemia). Products include:
Capoten 2255
Capozide 2258

Enalapril Maleate (Potential for hyperkalemia). Products include:
Vaseretic Tablets 1559
Vasotec Tablets 1564

Enalaprilat (Potential for hyperkalemia). Products include:
Vasotec I.V. 1562

Fosinopril Sodium (Potential for hyperkalemia). Products include:
Monopril Tablets 1406

Lisinopril (Potential for hyperkalemia). Products include:
Prinivil Tablets 1538
Prinzide Tablets 1540
Zestoretic 2274
Zestril Tablets 2277

Ramipril (Potential for hyperkalemia). Products include:
Altace Capsules 1086

Spironolactone (Hyperkalemia). Products include:
Aldactazide 2150
Aldactone 2152

Triamterene (Hyperkalemia). Products include:
Dyazide Capsules 2208
Dyrenium Capsules 2210
Maxzide 1215

MICRO-K 10 EXTENCAPS
(Potassium Chloride) 1863
See **Micro-K Extencaps**

MICRO-K LS PACKETS
(Potassium Chloride) 1864
May interact with potassium sparing diuretics and ACE inhibitors. Compounds in these categories include:

Amiloride Hydrochloride (Simultaneous administration can produce severe hyperkalemia). Products include:
Midamor Tablets 1508
Moduretic Tablets 1510

Benazepril Hydrochloride (Potential for hyperkalemia). Products include:
Lotensin Tablets 872

Captopril (Potential for hyperkalemia). Products include:
Capoten 2255
Capozide 2258

Enalapril Maleate (Potential for hyperkalemia). Products include:
Vaseretic Tablets 1559
Vasotec Tablets 1564

Enalaprilat (Potential for hyperkalemia). Products include:
Vasotec I.V. 1562

Fosinopril Sodium (Potential for hyperkalemia). Products include:
Monopril Tablets 1406

Lisinopril (Potential for hyperkalemia). Products include:
Prinivil Tablets 1538
Prinzide Tablets 1540
Zestoretic 2274
Zestril Tablets 2277

Ramipril (Potential for hyperkalemia). Products include:
Altace Capsules 1086

Spironolactone (Simultaneous administration can produce severe hyperkalemia). Products include:
Aldactazide 2150
Aldactone 2152

Triamterene (Simultaneous administration can produce severe hyperkalemia). Products include:
Dyazide Capsules 2208
Dyrenium Capsules 2210
Maxzide 1215

MICRONASE TABLETS
(Glyburide) 2350
May interact with beta blockers, salicylates, non-steroidal anti-inflammatory agents, sulfonamides, oral anticoagulants, monoamine oxidase inhibitors, thiazides, potassium sparing diuretics, estrogens, phenothiazines, corticosteroids, oral contraceptives, sympathomimetic aerosal brochodilators, calcium channel blockers, diuretics, thyroid preparations, and certain other agents. Compounds in these categories include:

Acebutolol Hydrochloride (Hypoglycemic action potentiated). Products include:
Sectral Capsules 2520

Albuterol (Hyperglycemia). Products include:
Proventil Inhalation Aerosol 2117
Ventolin Inhalation Aerosol and Refill 583

Albuterol Sulfate (Hyperglycemia). Products include:
Proventil Repetabs Tablets 2120
Proventil Solutions for Inhalation 0.5% and 0.083% 2118
Proventil Syrup 2119
Proventil Tablets 2120
Ventolin 583

Amiloride Hydrochloride (Hyperglycemia). Products include:
Midamor Tablets 1508
Moduretic Tablets 1510

Aspirin (Hypoglycemic action potentiated). Products include:
Alka-Seltzer Effervescent Antacid and Pain Reliever 1568
Alka-Seltzer Extra Strength Effervescent Antacid and Pain Reliever 1570
Alka-Seltzer (Flavored) Effervescent Antacid and Pain Reliever 1569
Alka-Seltzer Plus Cold Medicine ▣ 623
Alka-Seltzer Plus Night-Time Cold Medicine ▣ 623
Alka Seltzer Plus Sinus Allergy Medicine ▣ 624
Anacin Coated Analgesic Caplets 2417
Anacin Coated Analgesic Tablets 2417
Anacin Maximum Strength Analgesic Coated Tablets 2417
Maximum Strength Arthritis Pain Formula By the Makers of Anacin Analgesic Tablets and Caplets 2418
Arthritis Pain Formula by the Makers of Anacin Analgesic Tablets and Caplets ▣ 747
Arthritis Strength BC Powder ▣ 516
Ascriptin A/D Caplets 1850
Regular Strength Ascriptin Tablets 1850
Azdōne Tablets 844
BC Powder ▣ 517
BC Cold Powder ▣ 517
Children's Bayer Chewable Aspirin ▣ 564
Genuine Bayer Aspirin Tablets & Caplets ▣ 564
Maximum Bayer Aspirin Tablets & Caplets ▣ 566
Bayer Plus Aspirin Tablets ▣ 567
Therapy Bayer Aspirin Caplets ▣ 568
8 Hour Bayer Timed-Release Aspirin ▣ 566
Arthritis Strength Bufferin Analgesic Caplets 744
Extra Strength Bufferin Analgesic Tablets 745
Bufferin Analgesic Tablets and Caplets 743
Cama Arthritis Pain Reliever ▣ 685
Damason-P 1356
Easprin 1719
Ecotrin Enteric Coated Aspirin Maximum Strength Tablets and Caplets 2189
Ecotrin Enteric Coated Aspirin Regular Strength Tablets and Caplets 2189
Empirin Aspirin ▣ 541
Empirin with Codeine Phosphate Nos. 2, 3 & 4 764
Equagesic Tablets 2451
Excedrin Extra-Strength Analgesic Tablets & Caplets 749
4-Way Cold Tablets 750
Fiorinal Capsules 2007
Fiorinal with Codeine Capsules 2008
Fiorinal Tablets 2007
Lortab ASA Tablets 2414
Momentum Muscular Backache Formula ▣ 751
Norgesic 1314
Norwich Extra-Strength Aspirin ▣ 546
Norwich Regular Strength Aspirin ▣ 547
P-A-C Analgesic Tablets ▣ 669
Percodan 951
Robaxisal Tablets 1872
Sine-Off Sinus Medicine Tablets-Aspirin Formula ▣ 722
Soma Compound w/Codeine Tablets 2390
Soma Compound Tablets 2389
St. Joseph Adult Chewable Aspirin (81 mg.) ▣ 703
Synalgos-DC Capsules 2525
Talwin Compound 2072
Ursinus Inlay-Tabs ▣ 691
Vanquish Analgesic Caplets ▣ 574
Zorprin Tablets 698

Atenolol (Hypoglycemic action potentiated). Products include:
Tenoretic Tablets 1105
Tenormin Tablets and I.V. Injection 1107

Bendroflumethiazide (Hypoglycemic action potentiated; hyperglycemia). Products include:
Corzide Tablets 702
Naturetin Tablets 1789
Rauzide Tablets 1804

Bepridil Hydrochloride (Hyperglycemia). Products include:
Vascor (200, 300 and 400 mg) Tablets 1383

Betamethasone Acetate (Hyperglycemia). Products include:
Celestone Soluspan Suspension 2081

Betamethasone Sodium Phosphate (Hyperglycemia). Products include:
Celestone Soluspan Suspension 2081

Betaxolol Hydrochloride (Hypoglycemic action potentiated). Products include:
Betoptic Sterile Ophthalmic Solution 569
Betoptic S Sterile Ophthalmic Suspension 570
Kerlone Tablets 2172

Bumetanide (Hyperglycemia). Products include:
Bumex 1895

Carteolol Hydrochloride (Hypoglycemic action potentiated). Products include:
Cartrol Tablets 507

Chloramphenicol (Hypoglycemic action potentiated). Products include:
AK-Chlor Sterile Ophthalmic Ointment & Solution ◉ 201
Chloromycetin Cream, 1% 1694
Chloromycetin Hydrocortisone Ophthalmic 1694

Chloromycetin Kapseals 1695
Chloromycetin Ophthalmic Ointment, 1% 1696
Chloromycetin Ophthalmic Solution 1696
Chloromycetin Otic 1697
Chloroptic S.O.P. ..... ⊙ 243
Chloroptic Sterile Ophthalmic Solution ..... ⊙ 243
Ophthochlor Ophthalmic Solution ⊙ 300
Ophthocort ..... ⊙ 301

Chloramphenicol Palmitate (Hypoglycemic action potentiated). Products include:
Chloromycetin Palmitate, Oral Suspension 1697

Chloramphenicol Sodium Succinate (Hypoglycemic action potentiated). Products include:
Chloromycetin Sodium Succinate 1698

Chlorothiazide (Hyperglycemia). Products include:
Aldoclor Tablets 1413
Diupres Tablets 1461
Diuril Oral 1464

Chlorothiazide Sodium (Hyperglycemia). Products include:
Diuril Sodium Intravenous 1463

Chlorotrianisene (Hyperglycemia). Products include:
TACE 12 and 25 mg 1353

Chlorpromazine (Hyperglycemia). Products include:
Thorazine 2234

Chlorthalidone (Hyperglycemia). Products include:
Combipres Tablets 678
Tenoretic Tablets 1105
Thalitone Tablets 687

Choline Magnesium Trisalicylate (Hypoglycemic action potentiated). Products include:
Trilisate 1822

Cortisone Acetate (Hyperglycemia). Products include:
Cortone Acetate Sterile Suspension 1437
Cortone Acetate Tablets 1439

Dexamethasone (Hyperglycemia). Products include:
AK-Trol Ointment & Suspension ..... ⊙ 207
Decadron Elixir 1445
Decadron Tablets 1447
Decaspray Topical Aerosol 1459
Dexacidin ..... ⊙ 272
Maxidex Sterile Ophthalmic Suspension ..... ⊙ 223
Maxitrol Ophthalmic Ointment/Suspension ..... ⊙ 223
TobraDex Ophthalmic Suspension and Ointment ..... ⊙ 228

Dexamethasone Acetate (Hyperglycemia). Products include:
Dalalone D.P. Injectable 999
Decadron-LA Sterile Suspension 1457

Dexamethasone Sodium Phosphate (Hyperglycemia). Products include:
AK-Dex ..... ⊙ 203
Decadron Phosphate Respihaler 1454
Decadron Phosphate Sterile Ophthalmic Ointment 1453
Decadron Phosphate Sterile Ophthalmic Solution 1453
Decadron Phosphate Topical Cream 1455
Decadron Phosphate Turbinaire 1456
Maxidex Sterile Ophthalmic Ointment ..... ⊙ 222
NeoDecadron Sterile Ophthalmic Ointment 1517
NeoDecadron Sterile Ophthalmic Solution 1518
NeoDecadron Topical Cream 1518

Diclofenac Sodium (Hyperglycemia). Products include:
Voltaren Ophthalmic Sterile Ophthalmic Solution ..... ⊙ 268
Voltaren Tablets 1042

Dicumarol (Hypoglycemic action potentiated). Products include:
Dicumarol Tablets 516

Dienestrol (Hyperglycemia). Products include:
Ortho Dienestrol Cream 1664

Diethylstilbestrol (Hyperglycemia). Products include:
Diethylstilbestrol Tablets 1258

Diflunisal (Hypoglycemic action potentiated). Products include:
Dolobid Tablets 1465

Diltiazem Hydrochloride (Hyperglycemia). Products include:
Cardizem Tablets-30 mg, 60 mg, 90 mg and 120 mg 1329
Cardizem SR Capsules-60 mg, 90 mg and 120 mg 1327

Dobutamine Hydrochloride (Hyperglycemia). Products include:
Dobutrex Solution Vials 1259

Dopamine Hydrochloride (Hyperglycemia). Products include:
Intropin Injection 930

Ephedrine Hydrochloride (Hyperglycemia). Products include:
Amesec ..... ▣ 682
Primatene Tablets-M Formula 2421
Primatene Tablets-P Formula 2421
Primatene Tablets-Regular Formula 2421
Quadrinal Tablets 1183
Quelidrine Syrup 556
Tedral SA 1765

Ephedrine Sulfate (Hyperglycemia). Products include:
Bronkaid Tablets ..... ▣ 757
Bronkolixir ..... ▣ 761
Bronkotabs Tablets ..... ▣ 762
Marax Tablets & DF Syrup 1954
Pazo Hemorrhoid Ointment & Suppositories 752
Vicks Vatronol Nose Drops ..... ▣ 666

Ephedrine Tannate (Hyperglycemia). Products include:
Rynatuss 2388

Epinephrine (Hyperglycemia). Products include:
Ana-Kit Anaphylaxis Emergency Treatment Kit 1100
Bronkaid Mist ..... ▣ 757
EpiPen 843
Marcaine Hydrochloride 0.5% with Epinephrine 1:200,000 (as bitartrate) 958
Marcaine Hydrochloride with Epinephrine 1:200,000 2055
Primatene Mist 2420
Sus-Phrine Injection 1006
Xylocaine with Epinephrine Injections 637

Epinephrine Bitartrate (Hyperglycemia). Products include:
AsthmaHaler Mist Epinephrine Bitartrate Bronchodilator ..... ▣ 616
Bronkaid Mist Suspension ..... ▣ 757
Primatene Mist Suspension 2421

Epinephrine Hydrochloride (Hyperglycemia). Products include:
Adrenalin Chloride Solution 1:100 & 1:1,000 1689
Epifrin ..... ⊙ 244
Glaucon ..... ⊙ 218

Esmolol Hydrochloride (Hypoglycemic action potentiated). Products include:
Brevibloc Injection 942

Estradiol (Hyperglycemia). Products include:
Emcyt Capsules 1161
Estrace 1385
Estrace Vaginal Cream 1388
Estraderm Transdermal System 866

Estrogens, Conjugated (Hyperglycemia). Products include:
Mediatric Capsules 2476
PMB 200 and PMB 400 2504
Premarin Intravenous 2508
Premarin with Methyltestosterone 2515
Premarin Tablets 2510
Premarin Vaginal Cream 2512

Estrogens, Esterified (Hyperglycemia). Products include:
Estratest 2245
Menrium Tablets 1934

Estropipate (Hyperglycemia). Products include:
Ogen 540

Ethacrynic Acid (Hyperglycemia). Products include:
Edecrin Tablets 1468

Ethinyl Estradiol (Hyperglycemia). Products include:
Brevicon 2304
Demulen 2161
Estinyl Tablets 2085
Jenest-28 Tablets 1636
Levlen/Tri-Levlen 665
Lo/Ovral Tablets 2471
Lo/Ovral-28 Tablets 2476
Loestrin 1728
Modicon 1667
Nordette-21 Tablets 2481
Nordette-28 Tablets 2483
Norethin 2133
Norinyl 2304
Norlestrin 1746
Ortho-Cyclen Tablets 1658
Ortho-Novum 1667
Ovcon 1391
Ovral Tablets 2490
Ovral-28 Tablets 2491
Levlen/Tri-Levlen 665
Tri-Norinyl 2304
Triphasil-21 Tablets 2527
Triphasil-28 Tablets 2532

Ethynodiol Diacetate (Hyperglycemia). Products include:
Demulen 2161

Etodolac (Hyperglycemia). Products include:
Lodine Capsules 2468

Felodipine (Hyperglycemia). Products include:
Plendil Extended-Release Tablets 1526

Fenoprofen Calcium (Hypoglycemic action potentiated). Products include:
Nalfon Pulvules & Tablets 919

Fluphenazine Decanoate (Hyperglycemia). Products include:
Prolixin Decanoate 1795

Fluphenazine Enanthate (Hyperglycemia). Products include:
Prolixin Enanthate 1796

Fluphenazine Hydrochloride (Hyperglycemia). Products include:
Prolixin Elixir 1793
Prolixin Injection 1791
Prolixin Oral Concentrate 1792
Prolixin Tablets 1793

Flurbiprofen (Hypoglycemic action potentiated). Products include:
Ansaid Tablets 2319

Furazolidone (Hyperglycemia). Products include:
Furoxone 1855

Furosemide (Hyperglycemia). Products include:
Lasix 1093

Hydrochlorothiazide (Hyperglycemia). Products include:
Aldactazide 2150
Aldoril Tablets 1418
Apresazide Capsules 854
Apresoline-Esidrix Tablets 857
Capozide 2258
Dyazide Capsules 2208
Esidrix Tablets 863
Esimil Tablets 864
HydroDIURIL Tablets 1484
Hydropres Tablets 1485
Inderide Tablets 2463
Inderide LA Long Acting Capsules 2465
Lopressor HCT Tablets 1034
Maxzide 1215
Moduretic Tablets 1510
Normozide Tablets 2112
Oretic Tablets 544
Oreticyl 545
Prinzide Tablets 1540
Ser-Ap-Es Tablets 881
Serpasil-Esidrix Tablets 886
Timolide Tablets 1547
Trandate HCT Tablets 579
Vaseretic Tablets 1559
Zestoretic 2274

Hydrocortisone (Hyperglycemia). Products include:
AK-Spore H.C. ..... ⊙ 206
Bactine Hydrocortisone Anti-Itch Cream ..... ▣ 625
CaldeCORT Anti-Itch Hydrocortisone Spray ..... ▣ 560
Carmol HC Cream 1% 2296
Cortaid Spray ..... ▣ 735
Cortenema 2244
Cortisporin Ointment 758
Cortisporin Ophthalmic Ointment Sterile 758
Cortisporin Ophthalmic Suspension Sterile 759
Cortisporin Otic Solution Sterile 760
Cortisporin Otic Suspension Sterile 760
Cortizone-5 Creme & Ointment ..... ▣ 732
Dermolate Anti-Itch Cream ..... ▣ 697
Eldecort Cream 1.0% 1113
Eldecort Cream 1.0% and 2.5% 1113
Fungoid HC Creme 1770
Hydrocortone Tablets 1482
Hytone 909
LazerSporin-C Solution 1770
Massengill Medicated Soft Cloth Towelettes 2192
Nutracort Cream & Lotion 1684
PediOtic Suspension Sterile 797
Synacort Creams 1%, 2.5% 2296
Vanoxide-HC Acne Lotion 911
Vioform-Hydrocortisone Cream and Mild Cream 889
Vioform-Hydrocortisone Ointment 889
VōSoL HC Otic Solution 2392
Vytone Cream 1% 911

Hydrocortisone Acetate (Hyperglycemia). Products include:
Analpram-HC Rectal Cream 1% and 2.5% 970
Anusol-HC Cream 1690
Anusol-HC Suppositories 1691
Caldecort ..... ▣ 560
Carmol HC Cream 1% 2296
Chloromycetin Hydrocortisone Ophthalmic 1694
Coly-Mycin S Otic w/Neomycin & Hydrocortisone 1708
Cortaid ..... ▣ 735
Cortef Feminine Itch Cream ..... ▣ 735
Corticaine ..... ▣ 682
Cortifoam 1827
Cortisporin Cream 757
Epifoam 1828
Gynecort 5 Creme ..... ▣ 556
Hydrocortone Acetate Sterile Suspension 1479
Lanacort 5 Creme and Ointment ..... ▣ 557
Mantadil Cream 789
Ophthocort ..... ⊙ 301
Orabase HCA Oral Paste 890
Pramosone Cream, Lotion & Ointment 971
ProctoCream-HC 1834
Proctofoam-HC 1835

Hydrocortisone Sodium Phosphate (Hyperglycemia). Products include:
Hydrocortone Phosphate Injection, Sterile 1481

Hydrocortisone Sodium Succinate (Hyperglycemia). Products include:
Solu-Cortef Sterile Powder 2361

Hydroflumethiazide (Hyperglycemia). Products include:
Diucardin Tablets 2450
Saluron 718
Salutensin/Salutensin-Demi 719

Ibuprofen (Hyperglycemia). Products include:
Advil Cold & Sinus Caplets (formerly CoAdvil) 2416
Advil Ibuprofen Tablets and Caplets 2416
Children's Advil Suspension 2426
CoAdvil ..... ▣ 748
Dristan Sinus Caplets 2419
Haltran Tablets ..... ▣ 668
Ibuprofen ..... ▣ 631
Medipren ibuprofen Caplets and Tablets 1362
Midol 200 Cramp Relief Formula ..... ▣ 570
Motrin Tablets 2351
Motrin IB Caplets and Tablets ..... ▣ 736
Nuprin Ibuprofen/Analgesic Tablets & Caplets 752
PediaProfen Suspension 1363

Rufen Tablets ... 691
Trendar Ibuprofen Tablets ... ▣ 756

Indapamide (Hyperglycemia). Products include:
Lozol Tablets ... 1843

Indomethacin (Hyperglycemia). Products include:
Indocin ... 1487

Indomethacin Sodium Trihydrate (Hyperglycemia). Products include:
Indocin I.V. ... 1490

Isocarboxazid (Hyperglycemia). Products include:
Marplan Tablets ... 1906

Isoniazid (Hyperglycemia). Products include:
INH Tablets ... 868
Rifamate Capsules ... 1347

Isoproterenol Hydrochloride (Hyperglycemia). Products include:
Isuprel Hydrochloride Injection 1:5000 ... 2050
Isuprel Hydrochloride Mistometer .. 2051
Isuprel Hydrochloride Solution 1:200 & 1:100 ... 2052
Norisodrine Aerotrol ... 540

Isradipine (Hyperglycemia). Products include:
DynaCirc Capsules ... 2004

Ketoprofen (Hypoglycemic action potentiated). Products include:
Orudis Capsules ... 2488

Ketorolac Tromethamine (Hyperglycemia). Products include:
Toradol IM Injection ... 2302

Labetalol Hydrochloride (Hypoglycemic action potentiated). Products include:
Normodyne Injection ... 2108
Normodyne Tablets ... 2110
Normozide Tablets ... 2112
Trandate HCT Tablets ... 579
Trandate Injection ... 577
Trandate Tablets ... 579

Levonorgestrel (Hyperglycemia). Products include:
Levlen/Tri-Levlen ... 665
Nordette-21 Tablets ... 2481
Nordette-28 Tablets ... 2483
Norplant System ... 2484
Levlen/Tri-Levlen ... 665
Triphasil-21 Tablets ... 2527
Triphasil-28 Tablets ... 2532

Levothyroxine Sodium (Hyperglycemia). Products include:
Levothroid Tablets ... 1003
Levoxine Tablets ... 904
Synthroid ... 695

Liothyronine Sodium (Hyperglycemia). Products include:
Cytomel Tablets ... 2203

Liotrix (Hyperglycemia). Products include:
Euthroid ... 1724

Magnesium Salicylate (Hypoglycemic action potentiated). Products include:
Doan's - Extra-Strength Analgesic ▣ 549
Doan's - Regular Strength Analgesic ... ▣ 549
Mobigesic Analgesic Tablets ... ▣ 507

Meclofenamate Sodium (Hypoglycemic action potentiated). Products include:
Meclomen Capsules ... 1739

Mefenamic Acid (Hypoglycemic action potentiated). Products include:
Ponstel ... 1758

Mesoridazine (Hyperglycemia). Products include:
Serentil ... 686

Mestranol (Hyperglycemia). Products include:
Enovid ... 2161
Norethin ... 2133
Norinyl ... 2304
Ortho-Novum ... 1667

Metaproterenol Sulfate (Hyperglycemia). Products include:
Alupent ... 674
Arm-a-Med Metaproterenol Sulfate Inhalation Solution, USP ... 617
Metaprel Inhalation Aerosol Bronchodilator ... 2014
Metaprel Inhalation Solution ... 2015
Metaprel ... 2015
Metaproterenol Sulfate Inhalation Solution, USP ... 912

Metaraminol Bitartrate (Hyperglycemia). Products include:
Aramine Injection ... 1424

Methoxamine Hydrochloride (Hyperglycemia). Products include:
Vasoxyl Injection ... 819

Methyclothiazide (Hyperglycemia). Products include:
Enduron Tablets ... 517
Enduronyl ... 518

Methylprednisolone (Hyperglycemia). Products include:
Medrol ... 2348

Methylprednisolone Acetate (Hyperglycemia). Products include:
Depo-Medrol Sterile Aqueous Suspension ... 2334

Methylprednisolone Sodium Succinate (Hyperglycemia). Products include:
Solu-Medrol Sterile Powder ... 2363

Metolazone (Hyperglycemia). Products include:
Diulo ... 2129
Mykrox ½ mg Tablets ... 984
Zaroxolyn Tablets ... 989

Metoprolol Tartrate (Hypoglycemic action potentiated). Products include:
Lopressor Ampuls ... 1032
Lopressor HCT Tablets ... 1034
Lopressor Tablets ... 1032

Miconazole (Severe hypoglycemia). Products include:
Monistat I.V. ... 1143

Miconazole Nitrate (Severe hypoglycemia). Products include:
Micatin ... ▣ 632
Micatin for Jock Itch ... ▣ 633
Monistat Dual-Pak ... 1657
Monistat 3 Vaginal Suppositories ... 1657
Monistat-Derm (miconazole nitrate) Cream ... 1679

Nadolol (Hypoglycemic action potentiated). Products include:
Corgard Tablets ... 701
Corzide Tablets ... 702

Naproxen (Hypoglycemic action potentiated). Products include:
Naprosyn ... 2297

Naproxen Sodium (Hypoglycemic action potentiated). Products include:
Anaprox and Anaprox DS Tablets ... 2288

Nicardipine Hydrochloride (Hyperglycemia). Products include:
Cardene Capsules ... 2290

Nicotinic Acid (Hyperglycemia). Products include:
Niacor Tablets ... 2376
Nicobid ... 1846
Nicolar Tablets ... 1846
Nicotinex Elixir ... ▣ 563
Slo-Niacin Tablets ... 2376

Nifedipine (Hyperglycemia). Products include:
Adalat Capsules (10 mg and 20 mg) ... 1587
Procardia Capsules ... 1781
Procardia XL Tablets ... 1783

Nimodipine (Hyperglycemia). Products include:
Nimotop Capsules ... 1607

Norepinephrine Bitartrate (Hyperglycemia). Products include:
Levophed Bitartrate Injection ... 2054

Norethindrone (Hyperglycemia). Products include:
Brevicon ... 2304
Jenest-28 Tablets ... 1636
Micronor Tablets ... 1667
Modicon ... 1667
Norethin ... 2133
Norinyl ... 2304
Norlutin ... 1755
Nor-Q D Tablets ... 2304
Ortho-Novum ... 1667
Ovcon ... 1391
Tri-Norinyl ... 2304

Norethynodrel (Hyperglycemia). Products include:
Enovid ... 2161

Norgestimate (Hyperglycemia). Products include:
Ortho-Cyclen Tablets ... 1658

Norgestrel (Hyperglycemia). Products include:
Lo/Ovral Tablets ... 2471
Lo/Ovral-28 Tablets ... 2476
Ovral Tablets ... 2490
Ovral-28 Tablets ... 2491
Ovrette Tablets ... 2492

Penbutolol Sulfate (Hypoglycemic action potentiated). Products include:
Levatol ... 1832

Perphenazine (Hyperglycemia). Products include:
Etrafon ... 2087
Triavil Tablets ... 1556
Trilafon ... 2123

Phenelzine Sulfate (Hypoglycemic action potentiated). Products include:
Nardil ... 1742

Phenylbutazone (Hypoglycemic action potentiated). Products include:
Butazolidin Capsules & Tablets ... 1027

Phenylephrine Bitartrate (Hyperglycemia).
No products indexed under this heading.

Phenylephrine Hydrochloride (Hyperglycemia). Products include:
AK-Dilate Solution 2.5% and 10% ... ⊙ 203
Atrohist Sprinkle Capsules ... 558
Cerose-DM ... 2443
Codimal ... 846
Comhist LA Capsules ... 1618
Congespirin For Children Aspirin Free Chewable Cold Tablets ... 748
Cyclomydril ... ⊙ 216
Deconsal Sprinkle Capsules ... 559
Dimetane Decongestant ... ▣ 673
Dristan Decongestant/Antihistamine/ Analgesic Coated Caplets ... ▣ 749
Dristan Cold Nasal Decongestant/ Antihistamine/ Analgesic Coated Tablets ... 2419
Dristan Advanced Formula Decongestant/Antihistamine/ Analgesic Tablets ... ▣ 749
Dristan Nasal Spray, Menthol ... 2419
Dristan Nasal Spray, Regular and Regular with Metered Pump ... 2419
Entex Capsules ... 1623
Entex Liquid ... 1623
Sinus Excedrin Analgesic, Decongestant Tablets & Caplets ... 750
Extendryl ... 994
4-Way Fast Acting Nasal Spray - Original Formula (regular & mentholated) & Metered Spray Pump (regular) ... 751
Hycomine Compound Tablets ... 929
Murocoll-2 Sterile Ophthalmic Solution ... ⊙ 261
Mydfrin 2.5% ... ⊙ 224
Naldecon Syrup, Tablets, Pediatric Drops and Pediatric Syrup ... 709
Neo-Synephrine Hydrochloride 1% Carpuject ... 2063
Neo-Synephrine Hydrochloride 1% Injection ... 2063
Neo-Synephrine Hydrochloride (Ophthalmic) ... 2064
Neo-Synephrine ... ▣ 759
Nōstril Nasal Decongestant ... ▣ 520
Novahistine Elixir ... ▣ 596
Phenergan VC ... 2500
Phenergan VC with Codeine ... 2501
Prefrin Liquifilm Vasoconstrictor and Lubricant Eye Drops ... ⊙ 254
Prefrin-A ... ⊙ 255
Quelidrine Syrup ... 556
Relief Vasoconstrictor and Lubricant Eye Drops ... ⊙ 256
Robitussin Night Relief ... ▣ 677
Ru-Tuss with Hydrocodone ... 694
Ru-Tuss Tablets ... 693
Vasosulf ... ⊙ 279
Vicks Sinex ... ▣ 665
Zincfrin ... ⊙ 230

Phenylephrine Tannate (Hyperglycemia). Products include:
Rynatan ... 2387
Rynatuss ... 2388

Phenylpropanolamine Hydrochloride (Hyperglycemia). Products include:
A.R.M. Allergy Relief Medicine Caplets ... ▣ 615
Acutrim ... ▣ 548
Allerest ... ▣ 559
BC Cold Powder ... ▣ 517
Cheracol Plus Head Cold/Cough Formula ... ▣ 667
Codimal Expectorant ... 846
Comtrex Multi-Symptom Cold Reliever Tablets/Caplets/Liqui-Gels/Liquid ... 745
Contac Continuous Action Decongestant/Antihistamine Capsules ▣ 710
Contac Maximum Strength Continuous Action Decongestant/ Antihistamine Caplets ... ▣ 709
Contac Severe Cold and Flu Formula Caplets ... ▣ 711
Coricidin 'D' Decongestant Tablets ... ▣ 695
Coricidin Demilets Tablets for Children ... ▣ 696
Demazin Nasal Decongestant/ Antihistamine Repetabs Tablets & Syrup ... ▣ 697
Dexatrim ... ▣ 733
Dimetane-DC Cough Syrup ... 1857
Dimetapp Elixir ... ▣ 673
Dimetapp DM Elixir ... ▣ 674
Dimetapp Extentabs ... ▣ 674
Dimetapp Plus Caplets ... ▣ 675
Dimetapp Tablets ... ▣ 675
Entex Capsules ... 1623
Entex LA Tablets ... 1623
Entex Liquid ... 1623
4-Way Cold Tablets ... 750
Hycomine Syrup ... 927
Naldecon CX Adult Liquid ... ▣ 521
Naldecon DX Adult Liquid ... ▣ 521
Naldecon DX Children's Syrup ... ▣ 522
Naldecon DX Pediatric Drops ... ▣ 522
Naldecon EX Children's Syrup ... ▣ 522
Naldecon EX Pediatric Drops ... ▣ 523
Naldecon Syrup, Tablets, Pediatric Drops and Pediatric Syrup ... 709
Nolamine Tablets ... 838
Nolex LA Tablets ... 838
Ornade Spansule Capsules ... 2221
Orthoxicol Cough Syrup ... ▣ 668
Propagest ... 839
Pyrroxate Capsules ... ▣ 669
Robitussin-CF ... ▣ 676
Ru-Tuss II Capsules ... 693
Ru-Tuss with Hydrocodone ... 694
Ru-Tuss Tablets ... 693
Sine-Off Sinus Medicine Tablets-Aspirin Formula ... ▣ 722
Sinulin ... 840
St. Joseph Cold Tablets for Children ... ▣ 704
Tavist-D Tablets ... 2035
Triaminic Allergy Tablets ... ▣ 688
Triaminic Chewables ... ▣ 688
Triaminic Cold Tablets ... ▣ 688
Triaminic Expectorant ... ▣ 688
Triaminic Expectorant w/Codeine .. 1996
Triaminic Expectorant DH ... 1995
Triaminic Oral Infant Drops ... 1996
Triaminic Syrup ... ▣ 689
Triaminic-12 Tablets ... ▣ 690
Triaminic-DM Syrup ... ▣ 689
Triaminicin Tablets ... ▣ 690
Triaminicol Multi-Symptom Cold Tablets ... ▣ 691
Triaminicol Multi-Symptom Relief ▣ 691
Tuss-Ornade Liquid ... 2242
Tuss-Ornade Spansule Capsules ... 2242
Tylenol Cold Medication, Effervescent Tablets ... 1369

Phenytoin (Hyperglycemia). Products include:
Dilantin Infatabs 1710
Dilantin-30 Pediatric/Dilantin-125 Suspension 1713

Phenytoin Sodium (Hyperglycemia). Products include:
Dilantin Kapseals 1708
Dilantin Parenteral 1712
Dilantin with Phenobarbital Kapseals 1715

Pindolol (Hypoglycemic action potentiated). Products include:
Visken Tablets 2036

Pirbuterol Acetate (Hyperglycemia). Products include:
Maxair Inhaler 1311

Piroxicam (Hypoglycemic action potentiated). Products include:
Feldene Capsules 1777

Polyestradiol Phosphate (Hyperglycemia). Products include:
Estradurin 2452

Polythiazide (Hyperglycemia). Products include:
Minizide Capsules 1779
Renese Tablets 1785
Renese-R Tablets 1786

Prednisolone Acetate (Hyperglycemia). Products include:
AK-Cide Sterile Ophthalmic Ointment & Suspension ⊙ 202
Blephamide Liquifilm Sterile Ophthalmic Suspension 586
Blephamide S.O.P. Sterile Ophthalmic Ointment 586
Cetapred Ointment ⊙ 220
⅛% Econopred & 1% Econopred Plus ⊙ 217
Isopto Cetapred Suspension ⊙ 220
Metimyd ⊙ 306
Poly-Pred Liquifilm ⊙ 250
Pred Forte ⊙ 252
Pred Mild ⊙ 254
Pred-G Liquifilm Sterile Ophthalmic Suspension ⊙ 252
Pred-G S.O.P. Sterile Ophthalmic Ointment ⊙ 253
Vasocidin Ointment ⊙ 275

Prednisolone Sodium Phosphate (Hyperglycemia). Products include:
AK-Pred ⊙ 205
Hydeltrasol Injection, Sterile 1476
Inflamase ⊙ 274
Pediapred Oral Liquid 987
Vasocidin Ophthalmic Solution ⊙ 276

Prednisolone Tebutate (Hyperglycemia). Products include:
Hydeltra-T.B.A. Sterile Suspension 1478

Prednisone (Hyperglycemia). Products include:
Deltasone Tablets 2332

Probenecid (Hypoglycemic action potentiated). Products include:
Benemid Tablets 1426
ColBENEMID Tablets 1436
Wycillin Injection and Probenecid Tablets 2539

Prochlorperazine (Hyperglycemia). Products include:
Compazine 2201

Promethazine Hydrochloride (Hyperglycemia). Products include:
Mepergan Injection 2479
Phenergan with Codeine 2497
Phenergan with Dextromethorphan 2499
Phenergan Injection 2493
Phenergan Suppositories 2496
Phenergan Syrup 2495
Phenergan Tablets 2496
Phenergan VC 2500
Phenergan VC with Codeine 2501

Propranolol Hydrochloride (Hypoglycemic action potentiated). Products include:
Inderal 2459
Inderal LA Long Acting Capsules 2461
Inderide Tablets 2463
Inderide LA Long Acting Capsules 2465

Pseudoephedrine Hydrochloride (Hyperglycemia). Products include:
Actifed Capsules ⊞ 539
Actifed Plus Caplets ⊞ 539
Actifed Plus Tablets ⊞ 540
Actifed with Codeine Cough Syrup 752
Actifed Syrup ⊞ 540
Actifed Tablets ⊞ 540
Actifed 12-Hour Capsules ⊞ 539
Advil Cold & Sinus Caplets (formerly CoAdvil) 2416
Allerest ⊞ 559
Anatuss LA Tablets 1359
Benadryl Decongestant Elixir ⊞ 635
Benadryl Decongestant ⊞ 635
Benadryl Plus ⊞ 636
Benadryl Plus Nighttime ⊞ 637
Benylin Decongestant ⊞ 638
Brexin L.A. Capsules 2078
Bromfed Capsules (Timed Release) 1615
Bromfed Syrup ⊞ 628
Bromfed 1615
CoAdvil ⊞ 748
Allergy-Sinus Comtrex Multi-Symptom Allergy Sinus Formula Tablets & Caplets 746
Cough Formula Comtrex 746
Comtrex Multi-Symptom Cold Reliever Tablets/Caplets/Liqui-Gels/Liquid 745
Day-Night Comtrex 747
Non-Drowsy Comtrex 747
Congess 994
Congestac Caplets ⊞ 617
Contac Jr. Children's Cold Medicine ⊞ 712
Contac Nighttime Cold Medicine ⊞ 713
Contac Sinus Caplets Maximum Strength Non-Drowsy Formula ⊞ 710
Contac Sinus Tablets Maximum Strength Non-Drowsy Formula ⊞ 710
Deconamine 663
Deconsal II Tablets 559
Dimacol Caplets ⊞ 672
Dimetane-DX Cough Syrup 1858
Dorcol Children's Cough Syrup ⊞ 685
Dorcol Children's Decongestant Liquid ⊞ 685
Dorcol Children's Liquid Cold Formula ⊞ 686
Maximum Strength Dristan Decongestant/Analgesic Coated Caplets ⊞ 750
No Drowsiness Dristan Cold Nasal Decongestant/Analgesic Coated Caplets 2420
Dristan Sinus Caplets 2419
Sinus Excedrin Analgesic, Decongestant Tablets & Caplets ⊞ 533
Fedahist Gyrocaps 2145
Fedahist Timecaps 2145
Guaifed 1615
Guaifed Syrup ⊞ 629
Isoclor Expectorant 982
Isoclor Timesule Capsules ⊞ 561
Kronofed-A 970
Medi-Flu Caplet, Liquid ⊞ 640
Novafed A Capsules 1342
Novafed Capsules 1342
Novahistine DH 1342
Novahistine DMX ⊞ 595
Novahistine Expectorant 1343
Nucofed Capsules 2219
Nucofed Expectorant 2219
Nucofed Pediatric Expectorant 2220
Nucofed Syrup 2219
Ornex Caplets ⊞ 618
PediaCare Allergy Relief Formula Liquid 1362
PediaCare Cough-Cold Formula Liquid 1362
PediaCare Infants' Oral Decongestant Drops 1362
PediaCare Night Rest Cough-Cold Formula Liquid 1362
PediaCare 6-12 Cough-Cold Formula Chewable Tablets 1362
Robitussin-DAC Syrup 1875
Robitussin-PE ⊞ 677
Rondec 1975
Rondec-DM 1976
Rondec-TR Tablet 1975
Ru-Tuss DE Tablets 694
Ryna ⊞ 741
Seldane-D Extended-Release Tablets 1350
Sinarest ⊞ 562
Sine-Aid Maximum Strength Sinus Headache Caplets 1365
Sine-Aid Maximum Strength Sinus Headache Tablets 1365
Sine-Off Maximum Strength Allergy/Sinus Formula Caplets ⊞ 721
Sine-Off Maximum Strength No Drowsiness Formula Caplets ⊞ 722
Singlet Tablets ⊞ 598
Sinutab Maximum Strength ⊞ 641
Sinutab Maximum Strength Without Drowsiness Tablets & Caplets ⊞ 642
Sinutab Regular Strength Without Drowsiness Formula ⊞ 641
St. Joseph Nighttime Cold Medicine ⊞ 705
Sudafed Children's Liquid ⊞ 543
Sudafed Cough Syrup ⊞ 543
Sudafed Plus Liquid ⊞ 544
Sudafed Plus Tablets ⊞ 545
Sudafed Sinus Caplets ⊞ 545
Sudafed Sinus Tablets ⊞ 545
Sudafed Tablets, 30 mg ⊞ 544
Sudafed Tablets, Adult Strength, 60 mg ⊞ 544
Sudafed 12 Hour Capsules ⊞ 545
TheraFlu Flu and Cold Medicine ⊞ 687
Triaminic Nite Light ⊞ 689
Tylenol Allergy Sinus Medication Caplets and Gelcaps, Maximum Strength 1372
Children's Tylenol Cold Liquid Formula and Chewable Tablets 1368
Tylenol Cold & Flu Hot Medication, Packets 1369
Tylenol Cold & Flu No Drowsiness Hot Medication, Packets 1371
Tylenol Cold Medication Caplets and Tablets 1370
Tylenol Cold Medication No Drowsiness Formula Caplets 1370
Tylenol Cold Night Time Medication Liquid 1371
Tylenol Cough Medication Liquid with Decongestant, Maximum Strength 1372
Tylenol, Maximum Strength, Sinus Medication Gelcaps, Caplets and Tablets 1373
Ursinus Inlay-Tabs ⊞ 691
Vicks Children's NyQuil ⊞ 664
Vicks Daycare ⊞ 660
Vicks Formula 44D Decongestant Cough Medicine ⊞ 662
Vicks Formula 44M Multi-Symptom Cough Medicine ⊞ 662
Vicks NyQuil Nighttime Colds Medicine-Original & Cherry Flavor ⊞ 664
Vicks Pediatric Formula 44 Cough & Congestion Medicine ⊞ 663
Vicks Pediatric Formula 44m Multi-Symptom Cough & Cold Medicine ⊞ 663

Pseudoephedrine Sulfate (Hyperglycemia). Products include:
Afrin Tablets ⊞ 693
Chlor-Trimeton Decongestant ⊞ 694
Disophrol Chronotab Sustained-Action Tablets ⊞ 698
Drixoral Antihistamine/Nasal Decongestant Syrup ⊞ 698
Drixoral Non-Drowsy Formula ⊞ 699
Drixoral Plus Extended-Release Tablets ⊞ 699
Drixoral Sinus ⊞ 700
Drixoral Sustained-Action Tablets ⊞ 698
Sinutab Allergy Formula Sustained Action Tablets ⊞ 640
Trinalin Repetabs Tablets 1170

Quinestrol (Hyperglycemia). Products include:
Estrovis 1721

Salsalate (Hypoglycemic action potentiated). Products include:
Disalcid 1310
Mono-Gesic Tablets 846
Salflex 839

Selegiline Hydrochloride (Hyperglycemia). Products include:
Eldepryl 2250

Spironolactone (Hyperglycemia). Products include:
Aldactazide 2150
Aldactone 2152

Sulfamethizole (Hypoglycemic action potentiated). Products include:
Thiosulfil Forte Tablets 2526
Urobiotic-250 Capsules 1968

Sulfamethoxazole (Hypoglycemic action potentiated). Products include:
Azo Gantanol Tablets 1887
Bactrim DS Tablets 1891
Bactrim I.V. Infusion 1889
Bactrim 1891
Gantanol 1899
Septra 813
Septra I.V. Infusion 808
Septra I.V. Infusion ADD-Vantage Vials 810
Septra 813

Sulfasalazine (Hypoglycemic action potentiated). Products include:
Azulfidine Tablets, EN-tabs, Oral Suspension 1157

Sulfinpyrazone (Hypoglycemic action potentiated). Products include:
Anturane 853

Sulfisoxazole (Hypoglycemic action potentiated). Products include:
Azo Gantrisin Tablets 1888
Gantrisin Tablets 1901
Pediazole 1973

Sulfisoxazole Diolamine (Hypoglycemic action potentiated). Products include:
Gantrisin Ophthalmic Ointment/Solution 1900

Sulindac (Hypoglycemic action potentiated). Products include:
Clinoril Tablets 1433

Terbutaline Sulfate (Hyperglycemia). Products include:
Brethaire Inhaler 1024
Brethine Ampuls 1026
Brethine Tablets 1026
Bricanyl Injection 1324
Bricanyl Tablets 1325

Thioridazine Hydrochloride (Hyperglycemia). Products include:
Mellaril 2011

Thyroglobulin (Hyperglycemia). Products include:
Proloid Tablets 1761

Thyroid (Hyperglycemia). Products include:
S-P-T "Liquid" Capsules 995

Timolol Maleate (Hypoglycemic action potentiated). Products include:
Blocadren Tablets 1429
Timolide Tablets 1547
Timoptic in Ocudose 1552
Timoptic Sterile Ophthalmic Solution 1550

Tolmetin Sodium (Hypoglycemic action potentiated). Products include:
Tolectin (200, 400 and 600 mg) 1379

Tranylcypromine Sulfate (Hypoglycemic action potentiated). Products include:
Parnate Tablets 2222

Triamcinolone (Hyperglycemia).
No products indexed under this heading.

Triamcinolone Acetonide (Hyperglycemia). Products include:
Aristocort A 1010
Azmacort Inhaler 1837
Kenalog Cream, Lotion & Ointment 2401
Kenalog-10 Injection 2402
Kenalog-40 Injection 2403
Kenalog in Orabase 604
Kenalog Spray 2401
Mycolog II Cream and Ointment 2407
Mytrex Cream & Ointment 2080
Nasacort Nasal Inhaler 1844

Triamcinolone Diacetate (Hyperglycemia). Products include:
Aristocort Suspension 1008

(⊞ Described in PDR For Nonprescription Drugs) (⊙ Described in PDR For Ophthalmology)

Triamcinolone Hexacetonide (Hyperglycemia). Products include:
Aristospan Suspension 1011
Triamterene (Hyperglycemia). Products include:
Dyazide Capsules........ 2208
Dyrenium Capsules........ 2210
Maxzide........ 1215
Trifluoperazine Hydrochloride (Hyperglycemia). Products include:
Stelazine........ 2226
Verapamil Hydrochloride (Hyperglycemia). Products include:
Calan SR Caplets........ 2157
Calan Tablets........ 2155
Isoptin Injectable........ 1177
Isoptin Oral Tablets........ 1179
Isoptin SR Sustained Release Tablets........ 1181
Verelan Capsules........ 1243
Verelan Capsules........ 2535
Warfarin Sodium (Hypoglycemic action potentiated). Products include:
Coumadin Injection & Tablets........ 944
Panwarfin Tablets........ 547

MICRONOR TABLETS
(Norethindrone)........1667
May interact with barbiturates, tetracyclines, and certain other agents. Compounds in these categories include:

Ampicillin Sodium (Possible reduced efficacy and increased incidence of breakthrough bleeding and menstrual irregularities). Products include:
Unasyn........ 1965
Aprobarbital (Reduced efficacy and increased incidence of breakthrough bleeding and menstrual irregularities). Products include:
Alurate Elixir........ 1883
Butabarbital (Reduced efficacy and increased incidence of breakthrough bleeding and menstrual irregularities). Products include:
Pyridium Plus........ 1764
Butalbital (Reduced efficacy and increased incidence of breakthrough bleeding and menstrual irregularities). Products include:
Esgic-Plus Tablets........ 1002
Esgic Tablets & Capsules........ 1001
Fioricet Tablets........ 2006
Fiorinal Capsules........ 2007
Fiorinal with Codeine Capsules........ 2008
Fiorinal Tablets........ 2007
Phrenilin........ 838
Sedapap Tablets 50 mg/650 mg.. 1360
Demeclocycline Hydrochloride (Possible reduced efficacy and increased incidence of breakthrough bleeding and menstrual irregularities). Products include:
Declomycin Capsules, Tablets........ 1199
Doxycycline Calcium (Possible reduced efficacy and increased incidence of breakthrough bleeding and menstrual irregularities).
No products indexed under this heading.
Doxycycline Hyclate (Possible reduced efficacy and increased incidence of breakthrough bleeding and menstrual irregularities). Products include:
Doryx Capsules........ 1717
Vibramycin Hyclate Capsules........ 1787
Vibramycin Hyclate Intravenous........ 1968
Vibra-Tabs Film Coated Tablets........ 1787
Doxycycline Monohydrate (Possible reduced efficacy and increased incidence of breakthrough bleeding and menstrual irregularities). Products include:
Monodox Capsules........ 1630
Vibramycin Monohydrate for Oral Suspension........ 1787
Griseofulvin (Possible reduced efficacy and increased incidence of breakthrough bleeding and menstrual irregularities). Products include:
Fulvicin P/G Tablets........ 2090
Fulvicin P/G 165 & 330 Tablets.... 2091
Fulvicin-U/F Tablets........ 2092
Grifulvin V (griseofulvin microsize) Tablets/Suspension........ 1678
Grisactin........ 2454
Grisactin Ultra Tablets........ 2455
Gris-PEG Tablets, 125 mg & 250 mg........ 1083
Mephobarbital (Reduced efficacy and increased incidence of breakthrough bleeding and menstrual irregularities). Products include:
Mebaral Tablets........ 2061
Methacycline Hydrochloride (Possible reduced efficacy and increased incidence of breakthrough bleeding and menstrual irregularities).
No products indexed under this heading.
Minocycline Hydrochloride (Possible reduced efficacy and increased incidence of breakthrough bleeding and menstrual irregularities). Products include:
Minocin Intravenous........ 1221
Minocin Oral Suspension........ 1224
Minocin Pellet-Filled Capsules........ 1222
Oxytetracycline (Possible reduced efficacy and increased incidence of breakthrough bleeding and menstrual irregularities). Products include:
Terramycin Intramuscular Solution 1964
Urobiotic-250 Capsules........ 1968
Oxytetracycline Hydrochloride (Possible reduced efficacy and increased incidence of breakthrough bleeding and menstrual irregularities). Products include:
Terra-Cortril Ophthalmic Suspension........ 1963
Terramycin Capsules........ 1786
Terramycin Intramuscular Solution 1964
Terramycin with Polymyxin B Sulfate Ophthalmic Ointment........ 1965
Pentobarbital Sodium (Reduced efficacy and increased incidence of breakthrough bleeding and menstrual irregularities). Products include:
Nembutal Sodium Capsules........ 534
Nembutal Sodium Solution........ 536
Nembutal Sodium Suppositories........ 538
Phenobarbital (Reduced efficacy and increased incidence of breakthrough bleeding and menstrual irregularities). Products include:
Arco-Lase Plus Tablets........ 607
Bellergal-S Tablets........ 1998
Bronkolixir........ ▣ 761
Bronkotabs Tablets........ ▣ 762
Donnatal........ 1858
Donnatal Extentabs........ 1859
Donnatal Tablets........ 1858
Donnazyme Tablets........ 1860
Kinesed Tablets........ 2272
Phenobarbital Elixir and Tablets........ 1293
Primatene Tablets-P Formula........ 2421
Quadrinal Tablets........ 1183
Tedral SA........ 1765
Phenylbutazone (Reduced efficacy and increased incidence of breakthrough bleeding and menstrual irregularities). Products include:
Butazolidin Capsules & Tablets........ 1027
Phenytoin (Reduced efficacy and increased incidence of breakthrough bleeding and menstrual irregularities). Products include:
Dilantin Infatabs........ 1710
Dilantin-30 Pediatric/Dilantin-125 Suspension........ 1713
Phenytoin Sodium (Reduced efficacy and increased incidence of breakthrough bleeding and menstrual irregularities). Products include:
Dilantin Kapseals........ 1708
Dilantin Parenteral........ 1712
Dilantin with Phenobarbital Kapseals........ 1715
Rifampin (Reduced contraceptive efficacy and increased incidence of breakthrough bleeding and menstrual irregularities). Products include:
Rifadin........ 1345
Rifamate Capsules........ 1347
Rimactane Capsules........ 879
Secobarbital Sodium (Reduced efficacy and increased incidence of breakthrough bleeding and menstrual irregularities). Products include:
Seconal Sodium Pulvules........ 1296
Tetracycline Hydrochloride (Possible reduced efficacy and increased incidence of breakthrough bleeding and menstrual irregularities). Products include:
Achromycin V Capsules........ 1193
Achromycin Ophthalmic Ointment 1%........ ◉ 307
Achromycin Ophthalmic Suspension 1%........ ◉ 308
Topicycline for Topical Solution........ 1856
Thiamylal Sodium (Reduced efficacy and increased incidence of breakthrough bleeding and menstrual irregularities). Products include:
Surital Ampoules, Steri-Vials........ 1764

MIDAMOR TABLETS
(Amiloride Hydrochloride)........1508
May interact with diuretics, potassium sparing diuretics, lithium preparations, non-steroidal anti-inflammatory agents, potassium-depleting corticosteroids, ACE inhibitors, and certain other agents. Compounds in these categories include:

Benazepril Hydrochloride (Increased risk of hyperkalemia). Products include:
Lotensin Tablets........ 872
Bendroflumethiazide (Hyponatremia; hypochloremia; increases in BUN levels). Products include:
Corzide Tablets........ 702
Naturetin Tablets........ 1789
Rauzide Tablets........ 1804
Bumetanide (Hyponatremia; hypochloremia; increases in BUN levels). Products include:
Bumex........ 1895
Captopril (Increased risk of hyperkalemia). Products include:
Capoten........ 2255
Capozide........ 2258
Chlorothiazide (Hyponatremia; hypochloremia; increases in BUN levels). Products include:
Aldoclor Tablets........ 1413
Diupres Tablets........ 1461
Diuril Oral........ 1464
Chlorothiazide Sodium (Hyponatremia; hypochloremia; increases in BUN levels). Products include:
Diuril Sodium Intravenous........ 1463
Chlorthalidone (Hyponatremia; hypochloremia; increases in BUN levels). Products include:
Combipres Tablets........ 678
Tenoretic Tablets........ 1105
Thalitone Tablets........ 687
Diclofenac Sodium (Reduced diuretic, natriuretic, and antihypertensive effects of Midamor). Products include:
Voltaren Ophthalmic Sterile Ophthalmic Solution........ ◉ 268
Voltaren Tablets........ 1042
Enalapril Maleate (Increased risk of hyperkalemia). Products include:
Vaseretic Tablets........ 1559
Vasotec Tablets........ 1564
Enalaprilat (Increased risk of hyperkalemia). Products include:
Vasotec I.V........ 1562
Ethacrynic Acid (Hyponatremia; hypochloremia; increases in BUN levels). Products include:
Edecrin Tablets........ 1468
Etodolac (Reduced diuretic, natriuretic, and antihypertensive effects of Midamor). Products include:
Lodine Capsules........ 2468
Fenoprofen Calcium (Reduced diuretic, natriuretic, and antihypertensive effects of Midamor). Products include:
Nalfon Pulvules & Tablets........ 919
Flurbiprofen (Reduced diuretic, natriuretic, and antihypertensive effects of Midamor). Products include:
Ansaid Tablets........ 2319
Fosinopril Sodium (Increased risk of hyperkalemia). Products include:
Monopril Tablets........ 1406
Furosemide (Hyponatremia; hypochloremia; increases in BUN levels). Products include:
Lasix........ 1093
Hydrochlorothiazide (Hyponatremia; hypochloremia; increases in BUN levels). Products include:
Aldactazide........ 2150
Aldoril Tablets........ 1418
Apresazide Capsules........ 854
Apresoline-Esidrix Tablets........ 857
Capozide........ 2258
Dyazide Capsules........ 2208
Esidrix Tablets........ 863
Esimil Tablets........ 864
HydroDIURIL Tablets........ 1484
Hydropres Tablets........ 1485
Inderide Tablets........ 2463
Inderide LA Long Acting Capsules.. 2465
Lopressor HCT Tablets........ 1034
Maxzide........ 1215
Moduretic Tablets........ 1510
Normozide Tablets........ 2112
Oretic Tablets........ 544
Oreticyl........ 545
Prinzide Tablets........ 1540
Ser-Ap-Es Tablets........ 881
Serpasil-Esidrix Tablets........ 886
Timolide Tablets........ 1547
Trandate HCT Tablets........ 579
Vaseretic Tablets........ 1559
Zestoretic........ 2274
Hydroflumethiazide (Hyponatremia; hypochloremia; increases in BUN levels). Products include:
Diucardin Tablets........ 2450
Saluron........ 718
Salutensin/Salutensin-Demi........ 719
Ibuprofen (Reduced diuretic, natriuretic, and antihypertensive effects of Midamor). Products include:
Advil Cold & Sinus Caplets (formerly CoAdvil)........ 2416
Advil Ibuprofen Tablets and Caplets........ 2416
Children's Advil Suspension........ 2426
CoAdvil........ ▣ 748
Dristan Sinus Caplets........ 2419
Haltran Tablets........ ▣ 668
Ibuprofen........ ▣ 631
Medipren ibuprofen Caplets and Tablets........ 1362
Midol 200 Cramp Relief Formula.. ▣ 570
Motrin Tablets........ 2351
Motrin IB Caplets and Tablets........ ▣ 736
Nuprin Ibuprofen/Analgesic Tablets & Caplets........ 752
PediaProfen Suspension........ 1363
Rufen Tablets........ 691
Trendar Ibuprofen Tablets........ ▣ 756
Indapamide (Hyponatremia; hypochloremia; increases in BUN levels). Products include:
Lozol Tablets........ 1843

Indomethacin (Reduced diuretic, natriuretic, and antihypertensive effects of Midamor; increased serum potassium levels of both drugs). Products include:

Indocin 1487

Indomethacin Sodium Trihydrate (Reduced diuretic, natriuretic, and antihypertensive effects of Midamor; increased serum potassium levels of both drugs). Products include:

Indocin I.V. 1490

Ketoprofen (Reduced diuretic, natriuretic, and antihypertensive effects of Midamor). Products include:

Orudis Capsules 2488

Ketorolac Tromethamine (Reduced diuretic, natriuretic, and antihypertensive effects of Midamor). Products include:

Toradol IM Injection 2302

Lisinopril (Increased risk of hyperkalemia). Products include:

Prinivil Tablets 1538
Prinzide Tablets 1540
Zestoretic 2274
Zestril Tablets 2277

Lithium Carbonate (High risk of lithium toxicity). Products include:

Eskalith 2214
Lithane Tablets 1596
Lithium Carbonate Capsules & Tablets 1984
Lithobid Tablets 870

Lithium Citrate (High risk of lithium toxicity). Products include:

Cibalith-S 870

Meclofenamate Sodium (Reduced diuretic, natriuretic, and antihypertensive effects of Midamor). Products include:

Meclomen Capsules 1739

Mefenamic Acid (Reduced diuretic, natriuretic, and antihypertensive effects of Midamor). Products include:

Ponstel 1758

Methyclothiazide (Hyponatremia; hypochloremia; increases in BUN levels). Products include:

Enduron Tablets 517
Enduronyl 518

Metolazone (Hyponatremia; hypochloremia; increases in BUN levels). Products include:

Diulo 2129
Mykrox ½ mg Tablets 984
Zaroxolyn Tablets 989

Naproxen (Reduced diuretic, natriuretic, and antihypertensive effects of Midamor). Products include:

Naprosyn 2297

Naproxen Sodium (Reduced diuretic, natriuretic, and antihypertensive effects of Midamor). Products include:

Anaprox and Anaprox DS Tablets 2288

Phenylbutazone (Reduced diuretic, natriuretic, and antihypertensive effects of Midamor). Products include:

Butazolidin Capsules & Tablets 1027

Piroxicam (Reduced diuretic, natriuretic, and antihypertensive effects of Midamor). Products include:

Feldene Capsules 1777

Polythiazide (Hyponatremia; hypochloremia; increases in BUN levels). Products include:

Minizide Capsules 1779
Renese Tablets 1785
Renese-R Tablets 1786

Potassium Acid Phosphate (Concomitant therapy is contraindicated). Products Include:

K-Phos M.F. Tablets 659
K-Phos Original Formula 'Sodium Free' Tablets 660
K-Phos No. 2 Tablets 659

Potassium Bicarbonate (Concomitant therapy is contraindicated). Products include:

Alka-Seltzer Advanced Formula Antacid & Non-Aspirin Pain Reliever ▣ 620
Alka-Seltzer Effervescent Antacid ▣ 622
K-Lyte 707
Klorvess Effervescent Granules 2010
Klorvess Effervescent Tablets 2011

Potassium Chloride (Concomitant therapy is contraindicated). Products include:

Chlor-3 Condiment 994
K-Dur Microburst Release System (potassium chloride, USP) E.R. Tablets 1163
K-Lor Powder Packets 531
K-Lyte 707
K-Norm Capsules 982
K-Tab Filmtab 532
Kato Potassium Supplement 1114
Klor-Con 8/Klor-Con 10 Extended-release Tablets 2374
Klorvess Effervescent Granules 2010
Klorvess Effervescent Tablets 2011
Klorvess 10% Liquid 2010
Klotrix 708
Kolyum Liquid 983
Micro-K 1863
Micro-K LS Packets 1864
NuLYTELY 699
Oral Rehydration Salts, Citrate 1150
Rum-K Syrup 995
Slow-K Tablets 2281
Ten-K Controlled-Release Tablets 2282
Thermotabs ▣ 619

Potassium Citrate (Concomitant therapy is contraindicated). Products include:

Alka-Seltzer Effervescent Antacid 1570
K-Lyte 707
Polycitra Syrup 2424
Polycitra-K 2424
Polycitra-LC—Sugar-Free 2424
Ricelyte, Rice-Based Oral Electrolyte Maintenance Solution ▣ 613

Potassium Gluconate (Concomitant therapy is contraindicated). Products include:

Kolyum Liquid 983

Potassium Phosphate, Dibasic (Concomitant therapy is contraindicated). Products include:

Neutra-Phos 2423

Potassium Phosphate, Monobasic (Concomitant therapy is contraindicated). Products include:

K-Phos M.F. Tablets 659
K-Phos Neutral Tablets 660
Neutra-Phos 2423

Ramipril (Increased risk of hyperkalemia). Products include:

Altace Capsules 1086

Spironolactone (Do not administer concomitantly; rapid increases in serum potassium; hyponatremia; hypochloremia; increases in BUN levels). Products include:

Aldactazide 2150
Aldactone 2152

Sulindac (Reduced diuretic, natriuretic, and antihypertensive effects of Midamor). Products include:

Clinoril Tablets 1433

Tolmetin Sodium (Reduced diuretic, natriuretic, and antihypertensive effects of Midamor). Products include:

Tolectin (200, 400 and 600 mg) 1379

Triamterene (Do not administer concomitantly; rapid increases in serum potassium; hyponatremia; hypochloremia; increases in BUN levels). Products include:

Dyazide Capsules 2208
Dyrenium Capsules 2210
Maxzide 1215

Food Interactions

Diet, potassium-rich (Potential for rapid increases in serum potassium levels).

MIDOL 200 CRAMP RELIEF FORMULA

(Ibuprofen) ▣ 570

May interact with aspirin and acetaminophen containing products and certain other agents. Compounds in these categories include:

Acetaminophen (Concomitant administration is recommended only under physician's direction). Products include:

Acetaminophen Uniserts Suppositories 2374
Actifed Plus Caplets ▣ 539
Actifed Plus Tablets ▣ 540
Alka-Seltzer Advanced Formula Antacid & Non-Aspirin Pain Reliever ▣ 620
Allerest ▣ 559
Aspirin Free Anacin Maximum Strength Acetaminophen Film Coated Caplets 2417
Aspirin Free Anacin Maximum Strength Acetaminophen Film Coated Tablets 2417
Anacin-3 Regular Strength Acetaminophen Film Coated Tablets ▣ 746
Anexsia 5/500 Tablets 2196
Anexsia 7.5/650 Tablets 2197
Benadryl Plus ▣ 636
Benadryl Plus Nighttime ▣ 637
Bufferin AF Nite Time Analgesic/Sleeping Aid Caplets 744
Allergy-Sinus Comtrex Multi-Symptom Allergy Sinus Formula Tablets & Caplets 746
Cough Formula Comtrex 746
Comtrex Multi-Symptom Cold Reliever Tablets/Caplets/Liqui-Gels/Liquid 745
Day-Night Comtrex 747
Non-Drowsy Comtrex 747
Congespirin For Children Aspirin Free Chewable Cold Tablets 748
Contac Cough & Sore Throat Formula ▣ 712
Contac Jr. Children's Cold Medicine ▣ 712
Contac Nighttime Cold Medicine ▣ 713
Contac Severe Cold and Flu Formula Caplets ▣ 711
Contac Sinus Caplets Maximum Strength Non-Drowsy Formula ▣ 710
Contac Sinus Tablets Maximum Strength Non-Drowsy Formula ▣ 710
Coricidin 'D' Decongestant Tablets ▣ 695
Coricidin Demilets Tablets for Children ▣ 696
Coricidin Tablets ▣ 695
Darvon-N/Darvocet-N 1254
Datril Extra-Strength Analgesic Tablets 748
Dimetapp Plus Caplets ▣ 675
Dorcol Children's Fever & Pain Reducer ▣ 686
Dristan Decongestant/Antihistamine/ Analgesic Coated Caplets ▣ 749
Dristan Cold Nasal Decongestant/ Antihistamine/ Analgesic Coated Tablets 2419
Dristan Advanced Formula Decongestant/Antihistamine/ Analgesic Tablets ▣ 749
Maximum Strength Dristan Decongestant/Analgesic Coated Caplets ▣ 750
No Drowsiness Dristan Cold Nasal Decongestant/Analgesic Coated Caplets 2420
Drixoral Plus Extended-Release Tablets ▣ 699
Drixoral Sinus ▣ 700
Esgic-Plus Tablets 1002
Esgic Tablets & Capsules 1001
Aspirin Free Excedrin Analgesic Caplets 748
Excedrin Extra-Strength Analgesic Tablets & Caplets 749
Excedrin P.M. Analgesic/Sleeping Aid Tablets, Caplets and Liquid 749
Sinus Excedrin Analgesic, Decongestant Tablets & Caplets 750
4-Way Cold Tablets 750
Feverall Sprinkle Caps 2374
Feverall Suppositories 2374
Fioricet Tablets 2006
Hycomine Compound Tablets 929
Hydrocet Capsules 835
Isocom Capsules 1629
Liquiprin ▣ 618
Lortab 2412
Lurline PMS Tablets 972
Medi-Flu Caplet, Liquid ▣ 640
Maximum Strength Midol Multi-Symptom Menstrual Formula ▣ 571
Maximum Strength Midol PMS Premenstrual Syndrome Formula ▣ 570
Regular Strength Midol Multi-Symptom Menstrual Formula ▣ 570
Midrin Capsules 836
Ornex Caplets ▣ 618
Children's Panadol Chewable Tablets, Liquid, Infants' Drops ▣ 571
Junior Strength Panadol ▣ 571
Maximum Strength Panadol Tablets and Caplets ▣ 572
Percocet Tablets 950
Percogesic Analgesic Tablets ▣ 660
Phenaphen with Codeine Capsules 1865
Phenaphen-650 with Codeine Tablets 1866
Phrenilin 838
Prēmsyn PMS Capsules & Caplets ▣ 547
Pyrroxate Capsules ▣ 669
Robitussin Night Relief ▣ 677
Sedapap Tablets 50 mg/650 mg 1360
Sinarest ▣ 562
Sine-Aid Maximum Strength Sinus Headache Caplets 1365
Sine-Aid Maximum Strength Sinus Headache Tablets 1365
Sine-Off Maximum Strength Allergy/Sinus Formula Caplets ▣ 721
Sine-Off Maximum Strength No Drowsiness Formula Caplets ▣ 722
Singlet Tablets ▣ 598
Sinulin 840
Sinutab Maximum Strength ▣ 641
Sinutab Maximum Strength Without Drowsiness Tablets & Caplets ▣ 642
Sinutab Regular Strength Without Drowsiness Formula ▣ 641
Sominex Pain Relief Formula ▣ 723
St. Joseph Aspirin-Free Fever Reducer for Children Chewable Tablets, Liquid & Infant Drops ▣ 704
St. Joseph Cold Tablets for Children ▣ 704
St. Joseph Nighttime Cold Medicine ▣ 705
Sudafed Sinus Caplets ▣ 545
Sudafed Sinus Tablets ▣ 545
Talacen 2070
Tempra, Acetaminophen ▣ 613
TheraFlu Flu and Cold Medicine ▣ 687
Triaminicin Tablets ▣ 690
Tylenol acetaminophen Children's Chewable Tablets & Elixir 1366
Tylenol Allergy Sinus Medication Caplets and Gelcaps, Maximum Strength 1372
Tylenol with Codeine 1381
Children's Tylenol Cold Liquid Formula and Chewable Tablets 1368
Tylenol Cold & Flu Hot Medication, Packets 1369
Tylenol Cold & Flu No Drowsiness Hot Medication, Packets 1371
Tylenol Cold Medication Caplets and Tablets 1370
Tylenol Cold Medication, Effervescent Tablets 1369
Tylenol Cold Medication No Drowsiness Formula Caplets 1370
Tylenol Cold Night Time Medication Liquid 1371
Tylenol Cough Medication Liquid, Maximum Strength 1372
Tylenol Cough Medication Liquid with Decongestant, Maximum Strength 1372
Tylenol, Extra Strength, acetaminophen Adult Liquid Pain Reliever 1367
Tylenol, Extra Strength, acetaminophen Gelcaps, Caplets, Tablets 1367
Tylenol, Infants' Drops 1366
Tylenol, Junior Strength, acetaminophen Coated Caplets, Grape and Fruit Chewable Tablets 1366

Tylenol, Maximum Strength, Sinus Medication Gelcaps, Caplets and Tablets 1373
Tylenol, Regular Strength, acetaminophen Tablets and Caplets 1367
Tylenol PM, Extra Strength Caplets and Tablets 1368
Tylox Capsules 1382
Unisom Dual Relief Nighttime Sleep Aid/Analgesic 1774
Vanquish Analgesic Caplets .... ▣ 574
Vicks Daycare .... ▣ 660
Vicks Formula 44M Multi-Symptom Cough Medicine .... ▣ 662
Vicks NyQuil Nighttime Colds Medicine-Original & Cherry Flavor .... ▣ 664
Vicodin Tablets 1187
Vicodin ES Tablets 1189
Wygesic Tablets 2540
Zydone Capsules 941

Aspirin (Concomitant administration is recommended only under physician's direction). Products include:

Alka-Seltzer Effervescent Antacid and Pain Reliever 1568
Alka-Seltzer Extra Strength Effervescent Antacid and Pain Reliever 1570
Alka-Seltzer (Flavored) Effervescent Antacid and Pain Reliever 1569
Alka-Seltzer Plus Cold Medicine .... ▣ 623
Alka-Seltzer Plus Night-Time Cold Medicine .... ▣ 623
Alka Seltzer Plus Sinus Allergy Medicine .... ▣ 624
Anacin Coated Analgesic Caplets 2417
Anacin Coated Analgesic Tablets 2417
Anacin Maximum Strength Analgesic Coated Tablets 2417
Maximum Strength Arthritis Pain Formula By the Makers of Anacin Analgesic Tablets and Caplets 2418
Arthritis Pain Formula by the Makers of Anacin Analgesic Tablets and Caplets .... ▣ 747
Arthritis Strength BC Powder .... ▣ 516
Ascriptin A/D Caplets 1850
Regular Strength Ascriptin Tablets 1850
Azdone Tablets 844
BC Powder .... ▣ 517
BC Cold Powder .... ▣ 517
Children's Bayer Chewable Aspirin .... ▣ 564
Genuine Bayer Aspirin Tablets & Caplets .... ▣ 564
Maximum Bayer Aspirin Tablets & Caplets .... ▣ 566
Bayer Plus Aspirin Tablets .... ▣ 567
Therapy Bayer Aspirin Caplets .... ▣ 568
8 Hour Bayer Timed-Release Aspirin .... ▣ 566
Arthritis Strength Bufferin Analgesic Caplets 744
Extra Strength Bufferin Analgesic Tablets 745
Bufferin Analgesic Tablets and Caplets 743
Cama Arthritis Pain Reliever .... ▣ 685
Damason-P 1356
Easprin 1719
Ecotrin Enteric Coated Aspirin Maximum Strength Tablets and Caplets 2189
Ecotrin Enteric Coated Aspirin Regular Strength Tablets and Caplets 2189
Empirin Aspirin .... ▣ 541
Empirin with Codeine Phosphate Nos. 2, 3 & 4 764
Equagesic Tablets 2451
Excedrin Extra-Strength Analgesic Tablets & Caplets 749
4-Way Cold Tablets 750
Fiorinal Capsules 2007
Fiorinal with Codeine Capsules 2008
Fiorinal Tablets 2007
Lortab ASA Tablets 2414
Momentum Muscular Backache Formula .... ▣ 751
Norgesic 1314
Norwich Extra-Strength Aspirin .... ▣ 546
Norwich Regular Strength Aspirin ▣ 547
P-A-C Analgesic Tablets .... ▣ 669
Percodan 951
Robaxisal Tablets 1872
Sine-Off Sinus Medicine Tablets-Aspirin Formula .... ▣ 722
Soma Compound w/Codeine Tablets 2390
Soma Compound Tablets 2389
St. Joseph Adult Chewable Aspirin (81 mg.) .... ▣ 703
Synalgos-DC Capsules 2525
Talwin Compound 2072
Ursinus Inlay-Tabs .... ▣ 691
Vanquish Analgesic Caplets .... ▣ 574
Zorprin Tablets 698

MAXIMUM STRENGTH MIDOL MULTI-SYMPTOM MENSTRUAL FORMULA
(Cinnamedrine Hydrochloride, Acetaminophen) .... ▣ 571
May interact with hypnotics and sedatives, tranquilizers, and certain other agents. Compounds in these categories include:

Alcohol (May increase drowsiness).
Alprazolam (May increase drowsiness). Products include:
Xanax Tablets 2367
Buspirone Hydrochloride (May increase drowsiness). Products include:
BuSpar 1401
Chlordiazepoxide (May increase drowsiness). Products include:
Libritabs Tablets 1930
Limbitrol 1933
Menrium Tablets 1934
Chlordiazepoxide Hydrochloride (May increase drowsiness). Products include:
Librax Capsules 1929
Librium Capsules 1931
Librium Injectable 1932
Chlorpromazine (May increase drowsiness). Products include:
Thorazine 2234
Chlorprothixene (May increase drowsiness). Products include:
Taractan Tablets 1920
Chlorprothixene Hydrochloride (May increase drowsiness). Products include:
Taractan 1920
Clorazepate Dipotassium (May increase drowsiness). Products include:
Tranxene 556
Diazepam (May increase drowsiness). Products include:
Valium Injectable 1937
Valium Tablets 1939
Valrelease Capsules 1923
Droperidol (May increase drowsiness). Products include:
Inapsine Injection 1140
Innovar Injection 1141
Estazolam (May increase drowsiness). Products include:
ProSom Tablets 554
Ethchlorvynol (May increase drowsiness). Products include:
Placidyl Capsules 553
Ethinamate (May increase drowsiness).
No products indexed under this heading.
Fluphenazine Decanoate (May increase drowsiness). Products include:
Prolixin Decanoate 1795
Fluphenazine Enanthate (May increase drowsiness). Products include:
Prolixin Enanthate 1796
Fluphenazine Hydrochloride (May increase drowsiness). Products include:
Prolixin Elixir 1793
Prolixin Injection 1791
Prolixin Oral Concentrate 1792
Prolixin Tablets 1793
Flurazepam Hydrochloride (May increase drowsiness). Products include:
Dalmane Capsules 1927
Glutethimide (May increase drowsiness).
No products indexed under this heading.
Haloperidol (May increase drowsiness). Products include:
Haldol Injection, Tablets and Concentrate 1373
Haloperidol Decanoate (May increase drowsiness). Products include:
Haldol Decanoate 1375
Hydroxyzine Hydrochloride (May increase drowsiness). Products include:
Atarax Tablets & Syrup 1941
Marax Tablets & DF Syrup 1954
Vistaril Intramuscular Solution 1970
Lorazepam (May increase drowsiness). Products include:
Ativan Injection 2432
Ativan Tablets 2434
Loxapine Hydrochloride (May increase drowsiness). Products include:
Loxitane 1213
Loxapine Succinate (May increase drowsiness). Products include:
Loxitane Capsules 1213
Meprobamate (May increase drowsiness). Products include:
Deprol Tablets 2382
Equagesic Tablets 2451
Miltown Tablets 2386
PMB 200 and PMB 400 2504
Mesoridazine Besylate (May increase drowsiness).
Midazolam Hydrochloride (May increase drowsiness). Products include:
Versed Injection 1924
Molindone Hydrochloride (May increase drowsiness). Products include:
Moban Tablets & Concentrate 932
Oxazepam (May increase drowsiness). Products include:
Serax Capsules 2522
Serax Tablets 2522
Perphenazine (May increase drowsiness). Products include:
Etrafon 2087
Triavil Tablets 1556
Trilafon 2123
Prazepam (May increase drowsiness). Products include:
Centrax 1693
Prochlorperazine (May increase drowsiness). Products include:
Compazine 2201
Promethazine Hydrochloride (May increase drowsiness). Products include:
Mepergan Injection 2479
Phenergan with Codeine 2497
Phenergan with Dextromethorphan 2499
Phenergan Injection 2493
Phenergan Suppositories 2496
Phenergan Syrup 2495
Phenergan Tablets 2496
Phenergan VC 2500
Phenergan VC with Codeine 2501
Propofol (May increase drowsiness). Products include:
Diprivan Injection 2267
Quazepam (May increase drowsiness). Products include:
Doral Tablets 2383
Secobarbital Sodium (May increase drowsiness). Products include:
Seconal Sodium Pulvules 1296
Temazepam (May increase drowsiness). Products include:
Restoril Capsules 2023
Thioridazine Hydrochloride (May increase drowsiness). Products include:
Mellaril 2011
Thiothixene (May increase drowsiness). Products include:
Navane Capsules and Concentrate 1954
Navane Intramuscular 1956
Triazolam (May increase drowsiness). Products include:
Halcion Tablets 2340
Trifluoperazine Hydrochloride (May increase drowsiness). Products include:
Stelazine 2226

MAXIMUM STRENGTH MIDOL PMS PREMENSTRUAL SYNDROME FORMULA
(Acetaminophen, Pamabrom, Pyrilamine Maleate) .... ▣ 570
May interact with hypnotics and sedatives, tranquilizers, and certain other agents. Compounds in these categories include:

Alcohol (May increase drowsiness).
Alprazolam (May increase drowsiness). Products include:
Xanax Tablets 2367
Buspirone Hydrochloride (May increase drowsiness). Products include:
BuSpar 1401
Chlordiazepoxide (May increase drowsiness). Products include:
Libritabs Tablets 1930
Limbitrol 1933
Menrium Tablets 1934
Chlordiazepoxide Hydrochloride (May increase drowsiness). Products include:
Librax Capsules 1929
Librium Capsules 1931
Librium Injectable 1932
Chlorpromazine (May increase drowsiness). Products include:
Thorazine 2234
Chlorprothixene (May increase drowsiness). Products include:
Taractan Tablets 1920
Chlorprothixene Hydrochloride (May increase drowsiness). Products include:
Taractan 1920
Clorazepate Dipotassium (May increase drowsiness). Products include:
Tranxene 556
Diazepam (May increase drowsiness). Products include:
Valium Injectable 1937
Valium Tablets 1939
Valrelease Capsules 1923
Droperidol (May increase drowsiness). Products include:
Inapsine Injection 1140
Innovar Injection 1141
Estazolam (May increase drowsiness). Products include:
ProSom Tablets 554
Ethchlorvynol (May increase drowsiness). Products include:
Placidyl Capsules 553
Ethinamate (May increase drowsiness).
No products indexed under this heading.
Fluphenazine Decanoate (May increase drowsiness). Products include:
Prolixin Decanoate 1795
Fluphenazine Enanthate (May increase drowsiness). Products include:
Prolixin Enanthate 1796

Fluphenazine Hydrochloride (May increase drowsiness). Products include:
- Prolixin Elixir ... 1793
- Prolixin Injection ... 1791
- Prolixin Oral Concentrate ... 1792
- Prolixin Tablets ... 1793

Flurazepam Hydrochloride (May increase drowsiness). Products include:
- Dalmane Capsules ... 1927

Glutethimide (May increase drowsiness).
- No products indexed under this heading.

Haloperidol (May increase drowsiness). Products include:
- Haldol Injection, Tablets and Concentrate ... 1373

Haloperidol Decanoate (May increase drowsiness). Products include:
- Haldol Decanoate ... 1375

Hydroxyzine Hydrochloride (May increase drowsiness). Products include:
- Atarax Tablets & Syrup ... 1941
- Marax Tablets & DF Syrup ... 1954
- Vistaril Intramuscular Solution ... 1970

Lorazepam (May increase drowsiness). Products include:
- Ativan Injection ... 2432
- Ativan Tablets ... 2434

Loxapine Hydrochloride (May increase drowsiness). Products include:
- Loxitane ... 1213

Loxapine Succinate (May increase drowsiness). Products include:
- Loxitane Capsules ... 1213

Meprobamate (May increase drowsiness). Products include:
- Deprol Tablets ... 2382
- Equagesic Tablets ... 2451
- Miltown Tablets ... 2386
- PMB 200 and PMB 400 ... 2504

Mesoridazine Besylate (May increase drowsiness).

Midazolam Hydrochloride (May increase drowsiness). Products include:
- Versed Injection ... 1924

Molindone Hydrochloride (May increase drowsiness). Products include:
- Moban Tablets & Concentrate ... 932

Oxazepam (May increase drowsiness). Products include:
- Serax Capsules ... 2522
- Serax Tablets ... 2522

Perphenazine (May increase drowsiness). Products include:
- Etrafon ... 2087
- Triavil Tablets ... 1556
- Trilafon ... 2123

Prazepam (May increase drowsiness). Products include:
- Centrax ... 1693

Prochlorperazine (May increase drowsiness). Products include:
- Compazine ... 2201

Promethazine Hydrochloride (May increase drowsiness). Products include:
- Mepergan Injection ... 2479
- Phenergan with Codeine ... 2497
- Phenergan with Dextromethorphan ... 2499
- Phenergan Injection ... 2493
- Phenergan Suppositories ... 2496
- Phenergan Syrup ... 2495
- Phenergan Tablets ... 2496
- Phenergan VC ... 2500
- Phenergan VC with Codeine ... 2501

Propofol (May increase drowsiness). Products include:
- Diprivan Injection ... 2267

Quazepam (May increase drowsiness). Products include:
- Doral Tablets ... 2383

Secobarbital Sodium (May increase drowsiness). Products include:
- Seconal Sodium Pulvules ... 1296

Temazepam (May increase drowsiness). Products include:
- Restoril Capsules ... 2023

Thioridazine Hydrochloride (May increase drowsiness). Products include:
- Mellaril ... 2011

Thiothixene (May increase drowsiness). Products include:
- Navane Capsules and Concentrate 1954
- Navane Intramuscular ... 1956

Triazolam (May increase drowsiness). Products include:
- Halcion Tablets ... 2340

Trifluoperazine Hydrochloride (May increase drowsiness). Products include:
- Stelazine ... 2226

REGULAR STRENGTH MIDOL MULTI-SYMPTOM MENSTRUAL FORMULA

(Cinnamedrine Hydrochloride, Acetaminophen) ... ▣ 570

May interact with hypnotics and sedatives, tranquilizers, and certain other agents. Compounds in these categories include:

Alcohol (May increase drowsiness).

Alprazolam (May increase drowsiness). Products include:
- Xanax Tablets ... 2367

Buspirone Hydrochloride (May increase drowsiness). Products include:
- BuSpar ... 1401

Chlordiazepoxide (May increase drowsiness). Products include:
- Libritabs Tablets ... 1930
- Limbitrol ... 1933
- Menrium Tablets ... 1934

Chlordiazepoxide Hydrochloride (May increase drowsiness). Products include:
- Librax Capsules ... 1929
- Librium Capsules ... 1931
- Librium Injectable ... 1932

Chlorpromazine (May increase drowsiness). Products include:
- Thorazine ... 2234

Chlorprothixene (May increase drowsiness). Products include:
- Taractan Tablets ... 1920

Chlorprothixene Hydrochloride (May increase drowsiness). Products include:
- Taractan ... 1920

Clorazepate Dipotassium (May increase drowsiness). Products include:
- Tranxene ... 556

Diazepam (May increase drowsiness). Products include:
- Valium Injectable ... 1937
- Valium Tablets ... 1939
- Valrelease Capsules ... 1923

Droperidol (May increase drowsiness). Products include:
- Inapsine Injection ... 1140
- Innovar Injection ... 1141

Estazolam (May increase drowsiness). Products include:
- ProSom Tablets ... 554

Ethchlorvynol (May increase drowsiness). Products include:
- Placidyl Capsules ... 553

Ethinamate (May increase drowsiness).
- No products indexed under this heading.

Fluphenazine Decanoate (May increase drowsiness). Products include:
- Prolixin Decanoate ... 1795

Fluphenazine Enanthate (May increase drowsiness). Products include:
- Prolixin Enanthate ... 1796

Fluphenazine Hydrochloride (May increase drowsiness). Products include:
- Prolixin Elixir ... 1793
- Prolixin Injection ... 1791
- Prolixin Oral Concentrate ... 1792
- Prolixin Tablets ... 1793

Flurazepam Hydrochloride (May increase drowsiness). Products include:
- Dalmane Capsules ... 1927

Glutethimide (May increase drowsiness).
- No products indexed under this heading.

Haloperidol (May increase drowsiness). Products include:
- Haldol Injection, Tablets and Concentrate ... 1373

Haloperidol Decanoate (May increase drowsiness). Products include:
- Haldol Decanoate ... 1375

Hydroxyzine Hydrochloride (May increase drowsiness). Products include:
- Atarax Tablets & Syrup ... 1941
- Marax Tablets & DF Syrup ... 1954
- Vistaril Intramuscular Solution ... 1970

Lorazepam (May increase drowsiness). Products include:
- Ativan Injection ... 2432
- Ativan Tablets ... 2434

Loxapine Hydrochloride (May increase drowsiness). Products include:
- Loxitane ... 1213

Loxapine Succinate (May increase drowsiness). Products include:
- Loxitane Capsules ... 1213

Meprobamate (May increase drowsiness). Products include:
- Deprol Tablets ... 2382
- Equagesic Tablets ... 2451
- Miltown Tablets ... 2386
- PMB 200 and PMB 400 ... 2504

Mesoridazine Besylate (May increase drowsiness).

Midazolam Hydrochloride (May increase drowsiness). Products include:
- Versed Injection ... 1924

Molindone Hydrochloride (May increase drowsiness). Products include:
- Moban Tablets & Concentrate ... 932

Oxazepam (May increase drowsiness). Products include:
- Serax Capsules ... 2522
- Serax Tablets ... 2522

Perphenazine (May increase drowsiness). Products include:
- Etrafon ... 2087
- Triavil Tablets ... 1556
- Trilafon ... 2123

Prazepam (May increase drowsiness). Products include:
- Centrax ... 1693

Prochlorperazine (May increase drowsiness). Products include:
- Compazine ... 2201

Promethazine Hydrochloride (May increase drowsiness). Products include:
- Mepergan Injection ... 2479
- Phenergan with Codeine ... 2497
- Phenergan with Dextromethorphan 2499
- Phenergan Injection ... 2493
- Phenergan Suppositories ... 2496
- Phenergan Syrup ... 2495
- Phenergan Tablets ... 2496
- Phenergan VC ... 2500
- Phenergan VC with Codeine ... 2501

Propofol (May increase drowsiness). Products include:
- Diprivan Injection ... 2267

Quazepam (May increase drowsiness). Products include:
- Doral Tablets ... 2383

Secobarbital Sodium (May increase drowsiness). Products include:
- Seconal Sodium Pulvules ... 1296

Temazepam (May increase drowsiness). Products include:
- Restoril Capsules ... 2023

Thioridazine Hydrochloride (May increase drowsiness). Products include:
- Mellaril ... 2011

Thiothixene (May increase drowsiness). Products include:
- Navane Capsules and Concentrate 1954
- Navane Intramuscular ... 1956

Triazolam (May increase drowsiness). Products include:
- Halcion Tablets ... 2340

Trifluoperazine Hydrochloride (May increase drowsiness). Products include:
- Stelazine ... 2226

MIDRIN CAPSULES

(Isometheptene Mucate, Dichloralphenazone, Acetaminophen) ... 836

May interact with monoamine oxidase inhibitors. Compounds in this category include:

Furazolidone (Concurrent therapy contraindicated). Products include:
- Furoxone ... 1855

Isocarboxazid (Concurrent therapy contraindicated). Products include:
- Marplan Tablets ... 1906

Phenelzine Sulfate (Concurrent therapy contraindicated). Products include:
- Nardil ... 1742

Selegiline Hydrochloride (Concurrent therapy contraindicated). Products include:
- Eldepryl ... 2250

Tranylcypromine Sulfate (Concurrent therapy contraindicated). Products include:
- Parnate Tablets ... 2222

MILES NERVINE NIGHTTIME SLEEP-AID

(Diphenhydramine Hydrochloride) .. ▣ 627

May interact with hypnotics and sedatives, tranquilizers, and certain other agents. Compounds in these categories include:

Alcohol (Concurrent use not recommended).

Alprazolam (Concurrent use not recommended). Products include:
- Xanax Tablets ... 2367

Buspirone Hydrochloride (Concurrent use not recommended). Products include:
- BuSpar ... 1401

Chlordiazepoxide (Concurrent use not recommended). Products include:
- Libritabs Tablets ... 1930
- Limbitrol ... 1933
- Menrium Tablets ... 1934

Chlordiazepoxide Hydrochloride (Concurrent use not recommended). Products include:
- Librax Capsules ... 1929
- Librium Capsules ... 1931
- Librium Injectable ... 1932

Chlorpromazine (Concurrent use not recommended). Products include:
Thorazine ... 2234
Chlorprothixene (Concurrent use not recommended). Products include:
Taractan Tablets ... 1920
Chlorprothixene Hydrochloride (Concurrent use not recommended). Products include:
Taractan ... 1920
Clorazepate Dipotassium (Concurrent use not recommended). Products include:
Tranxene ... 556
Diazepam (Concurrent use not recommended). Products include:
Valium Injectable ... 1937
Valium Tablets ... 1939
Valrelease Capsules ... 1923
Droperidol (Concurrent use not recommended). Products include:
Inapsine Injection ... 1140
Innovar Injection ... 1141
Estazolam (Concurrent use not recommended). Products include:
ProSom Tablets ... 554
Ethchlorvynol (Concurrent use not recommended). Products include:
Placidyl Capsules ... 553
Ethinamate (Concurrent use not recommended).
No products indexed under this heading.
Fluphenazine Decanoate (Concurrent use not recommended). Products include:
Prolixin Decanoate ... 1795
Fluphenazine Enanthate (Concurrent use not recommended). Products include:
Prolixin Enanthate ... 1796
Fluphenazine Hydrochloride (Concurrent use not recommended). Products include:
Prolixin Elixir ... 1793
Prolixin Injection ... 1791
Prolixin Oral Concentrate ... 1792
Prolixin Tablets ... 1793
Flurazepam Hydrochloride (Concurrent use not recommended). Products include:
Dalmane Capsules ... 1927
Glutethimide (Concurrent use not recommended).
No products indexed under this heading.
Haloperidol (Concurrent use not recommended). Products include:
Haldol Injection, Tablets and Concentrate ... 1373
Haloperidol Decanoate (Concurrent use not recommended). Products include:
Haldol Decanoate ... 1375
Hydroxyzine Hydrochloride (Concurrent use not recommended). Products include:
Atarax Tablets & Syrup ... 1941
Marax Tablets & DF Syrup ... 1954
Vistaril Intramuscular Solution ... 1970
Lorazepam (Concurrent use not recommended). Products include:
Ativan Injection ... 2432
Ativan Tablets ... 2434
Loxapine Hydrochloride (Concurrent use not recommended). Products include:
Loxitane ... 1213
Loxapine Succinate (Concurrent use not recommended). Products include:
Loxitane Capsules ... 1213
Meprobamate (Concurrent use not recommended). Products include:
Deprol Tablets ... 2382
Equagesic Tablets ... 2451
Miltown Tablets ... 2386
PMB 200 and PMB 400 ... 2504
Mesoridazine Besylate (Concurrent use not recommended).
Midazolam Hydrochloride (Concurrent use not recommended). Products include:
Versed Injection ... 1924
Molindone Hydrochloride (Concurrent use not recommended). Products include:
Moban Tablets & Concentrate ... 932
Oxazepam (Concurrent use not recommended). Products include:
Serax Capsules ... 2522
Serax Tablets ... 2522
Perphenazine (Concurrent use not recommended). Products include:
Etrafon ... 2087
Triavil Tablets ... 1556
Trilafon ... 2123
Prazepam (Concurrent use not recommended). Products include:
Centrax ... 1693
Prochlorperazine (Concurrent use not recommended). Products include:
Compazine ... 2201
Promethazine Hydrochloride (Concurrent use not recommended). Products include:
Mepergan Injection ... 2479
Phenergan with Codeine ... 2497
Phenergan with Dextromethorphan ... 2499
Phenergan Injection ... 2493
Phenergan Suppositories ... 2496
Phenergan Syrup ... 2495
Phenergan Tablets ... 2496
Phenergan VC ... 2500
Phenergan VC with Codeine ... 2501
Propofol (Concurrent use not recommended). Products include:
Diprivan Injection ... 2267
Quazepam (Concurrent use not recommended). Products include:
Doral Tablets ... 2383
Secobarbital Sodium (Concurrent use not recommended). Products include:
Seconal Sodium Pulvules ... 1296
Temazepam (Concurrent use not recommended). Products include:
Restoril Capsules ... 2023
Thioridazine Hydrochloride (Concurrent use not recommended). Products include:
Mellaril ... 2011
Thiothixene (Concurrent use not recommended). Products include:
Navane Capsules and Concentrate ... 1954
Navane Intramuscular ... 1956
Triazolam (Concurrent use not recommended). Products include:
Halcion Tablets ... 2340
Trifluoperazine Hydrochloride (Concurrent use not recommended). Products include:
Stelazine ... 2226

MILONTIN KAPSEALS
(Phensuximide) ... 1741
May interact with anticonvulsants. Compounds in this category include:

Carbamazepine (Effect not specified; periodic serum level determination may be necessary). Products include:
Tegretol Chewable Tablets ... 654
Tegretol Suspension ... 656
Tegretol Tablets ... 654
Divalproex Sodium (Effect not specified; periodic serum level determination may be necessary). Products include:
Depakote ... 512
Ethosuximide (Effect not specified; periodic serum level determination may be necessary). Products include:
Zarontin Capsules ... 1768
Zarontin Syrup ... 1769
Ethotoin (Effect not specified; periodic serum level determination may be necessary). Products include:
Peganone Tablets ... 551
Mephenytoin (Effect not specified; periodic serum level determination may be necessary). Products include:
Mesantoin Tablets ... 2013
Methsuximide (Effect not specified; periodic serum level determination may be necessary). Products include:
Celontin ... 1692
Paramethadione (Effect not specified; periodic serum level determination may be necessary). Products include:
Paradione Capsules ... 548
Phenacemide (Effect not specified; periodic serum level determination may be necessary). Products include:
Phenurone Tablets ... 552
Phenobarbital (Effect not specified; periodic serum level determination may be necessary). Products include:
Arco-Lase Plus Tablets ... 607
Bellergal-S Tablets ... 1998
Bronkolixir ... [ND] 761
Bronkotabs Tablets ... [ND] 762
Donnatal ... 1858
Donnatal Extentabs ... 1859
Donnatal Tablets ... 1858
Donnazyme Tablets ... 1860
Kinesed Tablets ... 2272
Phenobarbital Elixir and Tablets ... 1293
Primatene Tablets-P Formula ... 2421
Quadrinal Tablets ... 1183
Tedral SA ... 1765
Phenytoin (Effect not specified; periodic serum level determination may be necessary). Products include:
Dilantin Infatabs ... 1710
Dilantin-30 Pediatric/Dilantin-125 Suspension ... 1713
Phenytoin Sodium (Effect not specified; periodic serum level determination may be necessary). Products include:
Dilantin Kapseals ... 1708
Dilantin Parenteral ... 1712
Dilantin with Phenobarbital Kapseals ... 1715
Primidone (Effect not specified; periodic serum level determination may be necessary). Products include:
Mysoline ... 2480
Trimethadione (Effect not specified; periodic serum level determination may be necessary). Products include:
Tridione ... 557
Valproic Acid (Effect not specified; periodic serum level determination may be necessary). Products include:
Depakene Capsules & Syrup ... 511

MILTOWN TABLETS
(Meprobamate) ... 2386
May interact with central nervous system depressants, psychotropics, and certain other agents. Compounds in these categories include:

Alcohol (Additive effects).
Alfentanil Hydrochloride (Additive effects). Products include:
Alfenta Injection ... 1131
Alprazolam (Additive effects). Products include:
Xanax Tablets ... 2367
Amitriptyline Hydrochloride (Additive effects). Products include:
Elavil ... 2269
Endep Tablets ... 1927
Etrafon ... 2087
Limbitrol ... 1933
Triavil Tablets ... 1556
Amoxapine (Additive effects). Products include:
Asendin Tablets ... 1196
Aprobarbital (Additive effects). Products include:
Alurate Elixir ... 1883
Buprenorphine (Additive effects).
No products indexed under this heading.
Buspirone Hydrochloride (Additive effects). Products include:
BuSpar ... 1401
Butabarbital (Additive effects). Products include:
Pyridium Plus ... 1764
Butalbital (Additive effects). Products include:
Esgic-Plus Tablets ... 1002
Esgic Tablets & Capsules ... 1001
Fioricet Tablets ... 2006
Fiorinal Capsules ... 2007
Fiorinal with Codeine Capsules ... 2008
Fiorinal Tablets ... 2007
Phrenilin ... 838
Sedapap Tablets 50 mg/650 mg ... 1360
Chlordiazepoxide (Additive effects). Products include:
Libritabs Tablets ... 1930
Limbitrol ... 1933
Menrium Tablets ... 1934
Chlordiazepoxide Hydrochloride (Additive effects). Products include:
Librax Capsules ... 1929
Librium Capsules ... 1931
Librium Injectable ... 1932
Chlorpromazine (Additive effects). Products include:
Thorazine ... 2234
Chlorprothixene (Additive effects). Products include:
Taractan Tablets ... 1920
Chlorprothixene Hydrochloride (Additive effects). Products include:
Taractan ... 1920
Clorazepate Dipotassium (Additive effects). Products include:
Tranxene ... 556
Codeine (Additive effects). Products include:
Calcidrine Syrup ... 506
Codeine Phosphate (Additive effects). Products include:
Actifed with Codeine Cough Syrup ... 752
Cheracol Cough Syrup ... 1853
Codimal PH Syrup ... 846
Dimetane-DC Cough Syrup ... 1857
Empirin with Codeine Phosphate Nos. 2, 3 & 4 ... 764
Fiorinal with Codeine Capsules ... 2008
Isoclor Expectorant ... 982
Naldecon CX Adult Liquid ... [ND] 521
Novahistine DH ... 1342
Novahistine Expectorant ... 1343
Nucofed Capsules ... 2219
Nucofed Expectorant ... 2219
Nucofed Pediatric Expectorant ... 2220
Nucofed Syrup ... 2219
Phenaphen with Codeine Capsules ... 1865
Phenaphen-650 with Codeine Tablets ... 1866
Phenergan with Codeine ... 2497
Phenergan VC with Codeine ... 2501
Robitussin A-C Syrup ... 1875
Robitussin-DAC Syrup ... 1875
Ryna ... [ND] 741
Soma Compound w/Codeine Tablets ... 2390
Triaminic Expectorant w/Codeine ... 1996
Tussi-Organidin Liquid ... 2391
Tylenol with Codeine ... 1381

Codeine Polistirex (Additive effects).
No products indexed under this heading.

Desipramine Hydrochloride (Additive effects). Products include:
Norpramin Tablets 1340

Dezocine (Additive effects).

Diazepam (Additive effects). Products include:
Valium Injectable 1937
Valium Tablets 1939
Valrelease Capsules 1923

Doxepin Hydrochloride (Additive effects). Products include:
Sinequan 1960

Droperidol (Additive effects). Products include:
Inapsine Injection 1140
Innovar Injection 1141

Enflurane (Additive effects). Products include:
Ethrane 599

Estazolam (Additive effects). Products include:
ProSom Tablets 554

Ethchlorvynol (Additive effects). Products include:
Placidyl Capsules 553

Ethinamate (Additive effects).
No products indexed under this heading.

Fentanyl (Additive effects). Products include:
Duragesic Transdermal System 1133

Fentanyl Citrate (Additive effects). Products include:
Innovar Injection 1141
Sublimaze Injection 1146

Fluphenazine Decanoate (Additive effects). Products include:
Prolixin Decanoate 1795

Fluphenazine Enanthate (Additive effects). Products include:
Prolixin Enanthate 1796

Fluphenazine Hydrochloride (Additive effects). Products include:
Prolixin Elixir 1793
Prolixin Injection 1791
Prolixin Oral Concentrate 1792
Prolixin Tablets 1793

Flurazepam Hydrochloride (Additive effects). Products include:
Dalmane Capsules 1927

Glutethimide (Additive effects).
No products indexed under this heading.

Haloperidol (Additive effects). Products include:
Haldol Injection, Tablets and Concentrate 1373

Haloperidol Decanoate (Additive effects). Products include:
Haldol Decanoate 1375

Hydrocodone Bitartrate (Additive effects). Products include:
Anexsia 5/500 Tablets 2196
Anexsia 7.5/650 Tablets 2197
Azdone Tablets 844
Codiclear DH Syrup 845
Codimal DH Syrup 846
Damason-P 1356
Hycodan Syrup, Tablets 927
Hycomine Compound Tablets 929
Hycomine Syrup 927
Hycotuss Expectorant Syrup 930
Hydrocet Capsules 835
Lortab ASA Tablets 2414
Lortab 2412
Ru-Tuss with Hydrocodone 694
Triaminic Expectorant DH 1995
Vicodin Tablets 1187
Vicodin ES Tablets 1189
Zydone Capsules 941

Hydrocodone Polistirex (Additive effects). Products include:
Tussionex Extended-Release Suspension 988

Hydroxyzine Hydrochloride (Additive effects). Products include:
Atarax Tablets & Syrup 1941
Marax Tablets & DF Syrup 1954
Vistaril Intramuscular Solution 1970

Imipramine Hydrochloride (Additive effects). Products include:
Tofranil Ampuls 1038
Tofranil Tablets 1039

Imipramine Pamoate (Additive effects). Products include:
Tofranil-PM Capsules 1041

Isocarboxazid (Additive effects). Products include:
Marplan Tablets 1906

Isoflurane (Additive effects). Products include:
Forane 600

Ketamine Hydrochloride (Additive effects). Products include:
Ketalar 1726

Levorphanol Tartrate (Additive effects). Products include:
Levo-Dromoran 1906

Lithium Carbonate (Additive effects). Products include:
Eskalith 2214
Lithane Tablets 1596
Lithium Carbonate Capsules & Tablets 1984
Lithobid Tablets 870

Lithium Citrate (Additive effects). Products include:
Cibalith-S 870

Lorazepam (Additive effects). Products include:
Ativan Injection 2432
Ativan Tablets 2434

Loxapine Hydrochloride (Additive effects). Products include:
Loxitane 1213

Loxapine Succinate (Additive effects). Products include:
Loxitane Capsules 1213

Maprotiline Hydrochloride (Additive effects). Products include:
Ludiomil Tablets 874

Meperidine Hydrochloride (Additive effects). Products include:
Demerol 2047
Mepergan Injection 2479

Mephobarbital (Additive effects). Products include:
Mebaral Tablets 2061

Mesoridazine (Additive effects). Products include:
Serentil 686

Methadone Hydrochloride (Additive effects). Products include:
Dolophine Hydrochloride Ampoules & Vials 1260
Dolophine Hydrochloride Tablets 1261
Methadone Hydrochloride Diskets 1284
Methadone Hydrochloride Oral Solution & Tablets 1987

Methohexital Sodium (Additive effects). Products include:
Brevital Sodium Vials 1248

Methoxyflurane (Additive effects).
No products indexed under this heading.

Midazolam Hydrochloride (Additive effects). Products include:
Versed Injection 1924

Molindone Hydrochloride (Additive effects). Products include:
Moban Tablets & Concentrate 932

Morphine Sulfate (Additive effects). Products include:
Astramorph/PF Injection, USP (Preservative-Free) 618
Duramorph 960
Infumorph 200 and Infumorph 500 Sterile Solutions 962
MS Contin Tablets 1814
MSIR 1817
Oramorph SR (Morphine Sulfate Sustained Release Tablets) 1988
Roxanol 1991

Nortriptyline Hydrochloride (Additive effects). Products include:
Pamelor 2019

Opium Alkaloids (Additive effects). Products include:
B & O No. 15A & No. 16A Supprettes 2395
Pantopon Injectable 1911

Oxazepam (Additive effects). Products include:
Serax Capsules 2522
Serax Tablets 2522

Oxycodone Hydrochloride (Additive effects). Products include:
Percocet Tablets 950
Percodan 951
Roxicodone Tablets, Oral Solution & Intensol (Oxycodone) 1992
Tylox Capsules 1382

Pentobarbital Sodium (Additive effects). Products include:
Nembutal Sodium Capsules 534
Nembutal Sodium Solution 536
Nembutal Sodium Suppositories 538

Perphenazine (Additive effects). Products include:
Etrafon 2087
Triavil Tablets 1556
Trilafon 2123

Phenelzine Sulfate (Additive effects). Products include:
Nardil 1742

Phenobarbital (Additive effects). Products include:
Arco-Lase Plus Tablets 607
Bellergal-S Tablets 1998
Bronkolixir [OTC] 761
Bronkotabs Tablets [OTC] 762
Donnatal 1858
Donnatal Extentabs 1859
Donnatal Tablets 1858
Donnazyme Tablets 1860
Kinesed Tablets 2272
Phenobarbital Elixir and Tablets 1293
Primatene Tablets-P Formula 2421
Quadrinal Tablets 1183
Tedral SA 1765

Prazepam (Additive effects). Products include:
Centrax 1693

Prochlorperazine (Additive effects). Products include:
Compazine 2201

Promethazine Hydrochloride (Additive effects). Products include:
Mepergan Injection 2479
Phenergan with Codeine 2497
Phenergan with Dextromethorphan 2499
Phenergan Injection 2493
Phenergan Suppositories 2496
Phenergan Syrup 2495
Phenergan Tablets 2496
Phenergan VC 2500
Phenergan VC with Codeine 2501

Propofol (Additive effects). Products include:
Diprivan Injection 2267

Propoxyphene Hydrochloride (Additive effects). Products include:
Darvon 1256
Wygesic Tablets 2540

Propoxyphene Napsylate (Additive effects). Products include:
Darvon-N/Darvocet-N 1254

Protriptyline Hydrochloride (Additive effects). Products include:
Vivactil Tablets 1567

Quazepam (Additive effects). Products include:
Doral Tablets 2383

Secobarbital Sodium (Additive effects). Products include:
Seconal Sodium Pulvules 1296

Sufentanil Citrate (Additive effects). Products include:
Sufenta Injection 1147

Temazepam (Additive effects). Products include:
Restoril Capsules 2023

Thiamylal Sodium (Additive effects). Products include:
Surital Ampoules, Steri-Vials 1764

Thioridazine Hydrochloride (Additive effects). Products include:
Mellaril 2011

Thiothixene (Additive effects). Products include:
Navane Capsules and Concentrate 1954
Navane Intramuscular 1956

Tranylcypromine Sulfate (Additive effects). Products include:
Parnate Tablets 2222

Triazolam (Additive effects). Products include:
Halcion Tablets 2340

Trifluoperazine Hydrochloride (Additive effects). Products include:
Stelazine 2226

Trimipramine Maleate (Additive effects). Products include:
Surmontil Capsules 2524

MINI-GAMULIN RH, RH_0(D) IMMUNE GLOBULIN (HUMAN)
(Rh_0(D) Immune Globulin (Human)) 612
No interactions described in labeling.

MINIPRESS CAPSULES
(Prazosin Hydrochloride) 1778
May interact with beta blockers, diuretics, antihypertensives, and certain other agents. Compounds in these categories include:

Acebutolol Hydrochloride (Additive hypotensive effect; dosage retitration may be required). Products include:
Sectral Capsules 2520

Amiloride Hydrochloride (Additive hypotensive effect). Products include:
Midamor Tablets 1508
Moduretic Tablets 1510

Atenolol (Additive hypotensive effect; dosage retitration may be required). Products include:
Tenoretic Tablets 1105
Tenormin Tablets and I.V. Injection 1107

Benazepril Hydrochloride (Additive hypotensive effect; dosage retitration may be required). Products include:
Lotensin Tablets 872

Bendroflumethiazide (Additive hypotensive effect; dosage retitration may be required). Products include:
Corzide Tablets 702
Naturetin Tablets 1789
Rauzide Tablets 1804

Betaxolol Hydrochloride (Additive hypotensive effect; dosage retitration may be required). Products include:
Betoptic Sterile Ophthalmic Solution 569
Betoptic S Sterile Ophthalmic Suspension 570
Kerlone Tablets 2172

Bumetanide (Additive hypotensive effect). Products include:
Bumex 1895

Captopril (Additive hypotensive effect; dosage retitration may be required). Products include:
Capoten 2255
Capozide 2258

Carteolol Hydrochloride (Additive hypotensive effect; dosage retitration may be required). Products include:
Cartrol Tablets 507

Chlorothiazide (Additive hypotensive effect; dosage retitration may be required). Products include:
Aldoclor Tablets 1413

Diupres Tablets 1461
Diuril Oral 1464

Chlorothiazide Sodium (Additive hypotensive effect; dosage retitration may be required). Products include:
Diuril Sodium Intravenous 1463

Chlorthalidone (Additive hypotensive effect; dosage retitration may be required). Products include:
Combipres Tablets 678
Tenoretic Tablets 1105
Thalitone Tablets 687

Clonidine (Additive hypotensive effect; dosage retitration may be required). Products include:
Catapres-TTS 677

Clonidine Hydrochloride (Additive hypotensive effect; dosage retitration may be required). Products include:
Catapres Tablets 676
Combipres Tablets 678

Deserpidine (Additive hypotensive effect; dosage retitration may be required). Products include:
Enduronyl 518
Harmonyl Tablets 528
Oreticyl 545

Diazoxide (Additive hypotensive effect; dosage retitration may be required). Products include:
Hyperstat I.V. Injection 2095
Proglycem 649

Doxazosin Mesylate (Additive hypotensive effect; dosage retitration may be required). Products include:
Cardura Tablets 1941

Enalapril Maleate (Additive hypotensive effect; dosage retitration may be required). Products include:
Vaseretic Tablets 1559
Vasotec Tablets 1564

Enalaprilat (Additive hypotensive effect; dosage retitration may be required). Products include:
Vasotec I.V. 1562

Esmolol Hydrochloride (Additive hypotensive effect; dosage retitration may be required). Products include:
Brevibloc Injection 942

Ethacrynic Acid (Additive hypotensive effect). Products include:
Edecrin Tablets 1468

Felodipine (Additive hypotensive effect; dosage retitration may be required). Products include:
Plendil Extended-Release Tablets 1526

Fosinopril Sodium (Additive hypotensive effect; dosage retitration may be required). Products include:
Monopril Tablets 1406

Furosemide (Additive hypotensive effect; dosage retitration may be required). Products include:
Lasix 1093

Guanabenz Acetate (Additive hypotensive effect; dosage retitration may be required). Products include:
Wytensin Tablets 2542

Guanethidine Monosulfate (Additive hypotensive effect; dosage retitration may be required). Products include:
Esimil Tablets 864
Ismelin Tablets 869

Hydralazine Hydrochloride (Additive hypotensive effect; dosage retitration may be required). Products include:
Apresazide Capsules 854
Apresoline Hydrochloride Parenteral (Ampuls) 856
Apresoline Hydrochloride Tablets 855
Apresoline-Esidrix Tablets 857
Ser-Ap-Es Tablets 881
Serpasil-Apresoline Tablets 884

Hydrochlorothiazide (Additive hypotensive effect; dosage retitration may be required). Products include:
Aldactazide 2150
Aldoril Tablets 1418
Apresazide Capsules 854
Apresoline-Esidrix Tablets 857
Capozide 2258
Dyazide Capsules 2208
Esidrix Tablets 863
Esimil Tablets 864
HydroDIURIL Tablets 1484
Hydropres Tablets 1485
Inderide Tablets 2463
Inderide LA Long Acting Capsules 2465
Lopressor HCT Tablets 1034
Maxzide 1215
Moduretic Tablets 1510
Normozide Tablets 2112
Oretic Tablets 544
Oreticyl 545
Prinzide Tablets 1540
Ser-Ap-Es Tablets 881
Serpasil-Esidrix Tablets 886
Timolide Tablets 1547
Trandate HCT Tablets 579
Vaseretic Tablets 1559
Zestoretic 2274

Hydroflumethiazide (Additive hypotensive effect; dosage retitration may be required). Products include:
Diucardin Tablets 2450
Saluron 718
Salutensin/Salutensin-Demi 719

Indapamide (Additive hypotensive effect; dosage retitration may be required). Products include:
Lozol Tablets 1843

Isradipine (Additive hypotensive effect; dosage retitration may be required). Products include:
DynaCirc Capsules 2004

Labetalol Hydrochloride (Additive hypotensive effect; dosage retitration may be required). Products include:
Normodyne Injection 2108
Normodyne Tablets 2110
Normozide Tablets 2112
Trandate HCT Tablets 579
Trandate Injection 577
Trandate Tablets 579

Lisinopril (Additive hypotensive effect; dosage retitration may be required). Products include:
Prinivil Tablets 1538
Prinzide Tablets 1540
Zestoretic 2274
Zestril Tablets 2277

Mecamylamine Hydrochloride (Additive hypotensive effect; dosage retitration may be required). Products include:
Inversine Tablets 1492

Methyclothiazide (Additive hypotensive effect; dosage retitration may be required). Products include:
Enduron Tablets 517
Enduronyl 518

Methyldopa (Additive hypotensive effect; dosage retitration may be required). Products include:
Aldoclor Tablets 1413
Aldomet Oral 1415
Aldoril Tablets 1418

Methyldopate Hydrochloride (Additive hypotensive effect; dosage retitration may be required). Products include:
Aldomet Ester HCl Injection 1417

Metolazone (Additive hypotensive effect; dosage retitration may be required). Products include:
Diulo 2129
Mykrox ½ mg Tablets 984
Zaroxolyn Tablets 989

Metoprolol Tartrate (Additive hypotensive effect; dosage retitration may be required). Products include:
Lopressor Ampuls 1032
Lopressor HCT Tablets 1034
Lopressor Tablets 1032

Metyrosine (Additive hypotensive effect; dosage retitration may be required). Products include:
Demser Capsules 1460

Minoxidil (Additive hypotensive effect; dosage retitration may be required). Products include:
Loniten Tablets 2346
Rogaine Topical Solution 2357

Nadolol (Additive hypotensive effect; dosage retitration may be required). Products include:
Corgard Tablets 701
Corzide Tablets 702

Nicardipine Hydrochloride (Additive hypotensive effect; dosage retitration may be required). Products include:
Cardene Capsules 2290

Nitroglycerin (Additive hypotensive effect; dosage retitration may be required). Products include:
Deponit NTG Transdermal Delivery System 2143
Minitran Transdermal Delivery System 1312
Nitro-Bid Ointment 1339
Nitro-Bid Capsules 1338
Nitrodisc 2176
Nitro-Dur (nitroglycerin) Transdermal Infusion System 1164
Nitrogard Tablets 1004
Nitrolingual Spray 1846
Nitrostat Tablets 1743
Transderm-Nitro Transdermal Therapeutic System 2283

Penbutolol Sulfate (Additive hypotensive effect; dosage retitration may be required). Products include:
Levatol 1832

Phenoxybenzamine Hydrochloride (Additive hypotensive effect; dosage retitration may be required). Products include:
Dibenzyline Capsules 2207

Phentolamine Mesylate (Additive hypotensive effect; dosage retitration may be required). Products include:
Regitine 878

Pindolol (Additive hypotensive effect; dosage retitration may be required). Products include:
Visken Tablets 2036

Polythiazide (Additive hypotensive effect; dosage retitration may be required). Products include:
Minizide Capsules 1779
Renese Tablets 1785
Renese-R Tablets 1786

Propranolol Hydrochloride (Additive hypotensive effect; dosage retitration may be required). Products include:
Inderal 2459
Inderal LA Long Acting Capsules 2461
Inderide Tablets 2463
Inderide LA Long Acting Capsules 2465

Ramipril (Additive hypotensive effect; dosage retitration may be required). Products include:
Altace Capsules 1086

Rauwolfia Serpentina (Additive hypotensive effect; dosage retitration may be required). Products include:
Raudixin Tablets 1803
Rauzide Tablets 1804

Rescinnamine (Additive hypotensive effect; dosage retitration may be required).
No products indexed under this heading.

Reserpine (Additive hypotensive effect; dosage retitration may be required). Products include:
Diupres Tablets 1461
Hydromox R Tablets 1209
Hydropres Tablets 1485
Renese-R Tablets 1786
Salutensin/Salutensin-Demi 719
Ser-Ap-Es Tablets 881
Serpasil Tablets 883
Serpasil-Apresoline Tablets 884
Serpasil-Esidrix Tablets 886

Sodium Nitroprusside (Additive hypotensive effect; dosage retitration may be required). Products include:
Nipride I.V. Infusion 1909

Spironolactone (Additive hypotensive effect). Products include:
Aldactazide 2150
Aldactone 2152

Terazosin Hydrochloride (Additive hypotensive effect; dosage retitration may be required). Products include:
Hytrin Tablets 529

Timolol Maleate (Additive hypotensive effect; dosage retitration may be required). Products include:
Blocadren Tablets 1429
Timolide Tablets 1547
Timoptic in Ocudose 1552
Timoptic Sterile Ophthalmic Solution 1550

Triamterene (Additive hypotensive effect). Products include:
Dyazide Capsules 2208
Dyrenium Capsules 2210
Maxzide 1215

Trimethaphan Camsylate (Additive hypotensive effect; dosage retitration may be required). Products include:
Arfonad Ampuls 1887

MINITRAN TRANSDERMAL DELIVERY SYSTEM

(Nitroglycerin) 1312

May interact with calcium channel blockers, vasodilators, and certain other agents. Compounds in these categories include:

Alcohol (Additive vasodilating effects).

Bepridil Hydrochloride (Potential for marked symptomatic orthostatic hypotension; dose adjustment of either drug may be necessary). Products include:
Vascor (200, 300 and 400 mg) Tablets 1383

Diazoxide (Additive vasodilating effects). Products include:
Hyperstat I.V. Injection 2095
Proglycem 649

Diltiazem Hydrochloride (Potential for marked symptomatic orthostatic hypotension; dose adjustment of either drug may be necessary). Products include:
Cardizem Tablets-30 mg, 60 mg, 90 mg and 120 mg 1329
Cardizem SR Capsules-60 mg, 90 mg and 120 mg 1327

Felodipine (Potential for marked symptomatic orthostatic hypotension; dose adjustment of either drug may be necessary). Products include:
Plendil Extended-Release Tablets 1526

Hydralazine Hydrochloride (Additive vasodilating effects). Products include:
Apresazide Capsules 854

- Apresoline Hydrochloride Parenteral (Ampuls) 856
- Apresoline Hydrochloride Tablets 855
- Apresoline-Esidrix Tablets 857
- Ser-Ap-Es Tablets 881
- Serpasil-Apresoline Tablets 884

Isradipine (Potential for marked symptomatic orthostatic hypotension; dose adjustment of either drug may be necessary). Products include:
- DynaCirc Capsules 2004

Minoxidil (Additive vasodilating effects). Products include:
- Loniten Tablets 2346
- Rogaine Topical Solution 2357

Nicardipine Hydrochloride (Potential for marked symptomatic orthostatic hypotension; dose adjustment of either drug may be necessary). Products include:
- Cardene Capsules 2290

Nifedipine (Potential for marked symptomatic orthostatic hypotension; dose adjustment of either drug may be necessary). Products include:
- Adalat Capsules (10 mg and 20 mg) 1587
- Procardia Capsules 1781
- Procardia XL Tablets 1783

Nimodipine (Potential for marked symptomatic orthostatic hypotension; dose adjustment of either drug may be necessary). Products include:
- Nimotop Capsules 1607

Verapamil Hydrochloride (Potential for marked symptomatic orthostatic hypotension; dose adjustment of either drug may be necessary). Products include:
- Calan SR Caplets 2157
- Calan Tablets 2155
- Isoptin Injectable 1177
- Isoptin Oral Tablets 1179
- Isoptin SR Sustained Release Tablets 1181
- Verelan Capsules 1243
- Verelan Capsules 2535

MINIZIDE CAPSULES

(Prazosin Hydrochloride, Polythiazide) 1779

May interact with thiazides, ganglionic blocking agents, para-aminobenzoic acid based local anesthetics, insulin, barbiturates, narcotic analgesics, corticosteroids, cardiac glycosides, and certain other agents. Compounds in these categories include:

ACTH (Hypokalemia may be aggravated).

Alcohol (Orthostatic hypotension).

Alfentanil Hydrochloride (Orthostatic hypotension). Products include:
- Alfenta Injection 1131

Aprobarbital (Orthostatic hypotension). Products include:
- Alurate Elixir 1883

Bendroflumethiazide (Potentiation of antihypertensive action). Products include:
- Corzide Tablets 702
- Naturetin Tablets 1789
- Rauzide Tablets 1804

Betamethasone Acetate (Hypokalemia may be aggravated). Products include:
- Celestone Soluspan Suspension 2081

Betamethasone Sodium Phosphate (Hypokalemia may be aggravated). Products include:
- Celestone Soluspan Suspension 2081

Buprenorphine (Orthostatic hypotension).
- No products indexed under this heading.

Butabarbital (Orthostatic hypotension). Products include:
- Pyridium Plus 1764

Butalbital (Orthostatic hypotension). Products include:
- Esgic-Plus Tablets 1002
- Esgic Tablets & Capsules 1001
- Fioricet Tablets 2006
- Fiorinal Capsules 2007
- Fiorinal with Codeine Capsules 2008
- Fiorinal Tablets 2007
- Phrenilin 838
- Sedapap Tablets 50 mg/650 mg 1360

Chlorothiazide (Potentiation of antihypertensive action). Products include:
- Aldoclor Tablets 1413
- Diupres Tablets 1461
- Diuril Oral 1464

Chlorothiazide Sodium (Potentiation of antihypertensive action). Products include:
- Diuril Sodium Intravenous 1463

Codeine (Orthostatic hypotension). Products include:
- Calcidrine Syrup 506

Codeine Phosphate (Orthostatic hypotension). Products include:
- Actifed with Codeine Cough Syrup 752
- Cheracol Cough Syrup 1853
- Codimal PH Syrup 846
- Dimetane-DC Cough Syrup 1857
- Empirin with Codeine Phosphate Nos. 2, 3 & 4 764
- Fiorinal with Codeine Capsules 2008
- Isoclor Expectorant 982
- Naldecon CX Adult Liquid ⊞ 521
- Novahistine DH 1342
- Novahistine Expectorant 1343
- Nucofed Capsules 2219
- Nucofed Expectorant 2219
- Nucofed Pediatric Expectorant 2220
- Nucofed Syrup 2219
- Phenaphen with Codeine Capsules 1865
- Phenaphen-650 with Codeine Tablets 1866
- Phenergan with Codeine 2497
- Phenergan VC with Codeine 2501
- Robitussin A-C Syrup 1875
- Robitussin-DAC Syrup 1875
- Ryna ⊞ 741
- Soma Compound w/Codeine Tablets 2390
- Triaminic Expectorant w/Codeine 1996
- Tussi-Organidin Liquid 2391
- Tylenol with Codeine 1381

Codeine Polistirex (Orthostatic hypotension).
- No products indexed under this heading.

Cortisone Acetate (Hypokalemia may be aggravated). Products include:
- Cortone Acetate Sterile Suspension 1437
- Cortone Acetate Tablets 1439

Deserpidine (Potentiation of antihypertensive action of deserpidine). Products include:
- Enduronyl 518
- Harmonyl Tablets 528
- Oreticyl 545

Deslanoside (May exaggerate the metabolic effects of hypokalemia).
- No products indexed under this heading.

Dexamethasone (Hypokalemia may be aggravated). Products include:
- AK-Trol Ointment & Suspension ◉ 207
- Decadron Elixir 1445
- Decadron Tablets 1447
- Decaspray Topical Aerosol 1459
- Dexacidin ◉ 272
- Maxidex Sterile Ophthalmic Suspension ◉ 223
- Maxitrol Ophthalmic Ointment/Suspension ◉ 223
- TobraDex Ophthalmic Suspension and Ointment ◉ 228

Dexamethasone Acetate (Hypokalemia may be aggravated). Products include:
- Dalalone D.P. Injectable 999
- Decadron-LA Sterile Suspension 1457

Dexamethasone Sodium Phosphate (Hypokalemia may be aggravated). Products include:
- AK-Dex ◉ 203
- Decadron Phosphate Respihaler 1454
- Decadron Phosphate Sterile Ophthalmic Ointment 1453
- Decadron Phosphate Sterile Ophthalmic Solution 1453
- Decadron Phosphate Topical Cream 1455
- Decadron Phosphate Turbinaire 1456
- Maxidex Sterile Ophthalmic Ointment ◉ 222
- NeoDecadron Sterile Ophthalmic Ointment 1517
- NeoDecadron Sterile Ophthalmic Solution 1518
- NeoDecadron Topical Cream 1518

Dezocine (Orthostatic hypotension).

Digitoxin (May exaggerate the metabolic effects of hypokalemia). Products include:
- Crystodigin Tablets 1253

Digoxin (May exaggerate the metabolic effects of hypokalemia). Products include:
- Lanoxicaps 772
- Lanoxin Elixir Pediatric 775
- Lanoxin Injection 778
- Lanoxin Injection Pediatric 781
- Lanoxin Tablets 783

Fentanyl (Orthostatic hypotension). Products include:
- Duragesic Transdermal System 1133

Fentanyl Citrate (Orthostatic hypotension). Products include:
- Innovar Injection 1141
- Sublimaze Injection 1146

Guanethidine Monosulfate (Potentiation of antihypertensive action of guanethidine). Products include:
- Esimil Tablets 864
- Ismelin Tablets 869

Hydrochlorothiazide (Potentiation of antihypertensive action). Products include:
- Aldactazide 2150
- Aldoril Tablets 1418
- Apresazide Capsules 854
- Apresoline-Esidrix Tablets 857
- Capozide 2258
- Dyazide Capsules 2208
- Esidrix Tablets 863
- Esimil Tablets 864
- HydroDIURIL Tablets 1484
- Hydropres Tablets 1485
- Inderide Tablets 2463
- Inderide LA Long Acting Capsules 2465
- Lopressor HCT Tablets 1034
- Maxzide 1215
- Moduretic Tablets 1510
- Normozide Tablets 2112
- Oretic Tablets 544
- Oreticyl 545
- Prinzide Tablets 1540
- Ser-Ap-Es Tablets 881
- Serpasil-Esidrix Tablets 886
- Timolide Tablets 1547
- Trandate HCT Tablets 579
- Vaseretic Tablets 1559
- Zestoretic 2274

Hydrocodone Bitartrate (Orthostatic hypotension). Products include:
- Anexsia 5/500 Tablets 2196
- Anexsia 7.5/650 Tablets 2197
- Azdone Tablets 844
- Codiclear DH Syrup 845
- Codimal DH Syrup 846
- Damason-P 1356
- Hycodan Syrup, Tablets 927
- Hycomine Compound Tablets 929
- Hycomine Syrup 927
- Hycotuss Expectorant Syrup 930
- Hydrocet Capsules 835
- Lortab ASA Tablets 2414
- Lortab 2412
- Ru-Tuss with Hydrocodone 694
- Triaminic Expectorant DH 1995
- Vicodin Tablets 1187
- Vicodin ES Tablets 1189
- Zydone Capsules 941

Hydrocodone Polistirex (Orthostatic hypotension). Products include:
- Tussionex Extended-Release Suspension 988

Hydrocortisone (Hypokalemia may be aggravated). Products include:
- AK-Spore H.C. ◉ 206
- Bactine Hydrocortisone Anti-Itch Cream ⊞ 625
- CaldeCORT Anti-Itch Hydrocortisone Spray ⊞ 560
- Carmol HC Cream 1% 2296
- Cortaid Spray ⊞ 735
- Cortenema 2244
- Cortisporin Ointment 758
- Cortisporin Ophthalmic Ointment Sterile 758
- Cortisporin Ophthalmic Suspension Sterile 759
- Cortisporin Otic Solution Sterile 760
- Cortisporin Otic Suspension Sterile 760
- Cortizone-5 Creme & Ointment ⊞ 732
- Dermolate Anti-Itch Cream ⊞ 697
- Eldecort Cream 1.0% 1113
- Eldecort Cream 1.0% and 2.5% 1113
- Fungoid HC Creme 1770
- Hydrocortone Tablets 1482
- Hytone 909
- LazerSporin-C Solution 1770
- Massengill Medicated Soft Cloth Towelettes 2192
- Nutracort Cream & Lotion 1684
- PediOtic Suspension Sterile 797
- Synacort Creams 1%, 2.5% 2296
- Vanoxide-HC Acne Lotion 911
- Vioform-Hydrocortisone Cream and Mild Cream 889
- Vioform-Hydrocortisone Ointment 889
- VōSoL HC Otic Solution 2392
- Vytone Cream 1% 911

Hydrocortisone Acetate (Hypokalemia may be aggravated). Products include:
- Analpram-HC Rectal Cream 1% and 2.5% 970
- Anusol-HC Cream 1690
- Anusol-HC Suppositories 1691
- Caldecort ⊞ 560
- Carmol HC Cream 1% 2296
- Chloromycetin Hydrocortisone Ophthalmic 1694
- Coly-Mycin S Otic w/Neomycin & Hydrocortisone 1708
- Cortaid ⊞ 735
- Cortef Feminine Itch Cream ⊞ 735
- Corticaine ⊞ 682
- Cortifoam 1827
- Cortisporin Cream 757
- Epifoam 1828
- Gynecort 5 Creme ⊞ 556
- Hydrocortone Acetate Sterile Suspension 1479
- Lanacort 5 Creme and Ointment ⊞ 557
- Mantadil Cream 789
- Ophthocort ◉ 301
- Orabase HCA Oral Paste 890
- Pramosone Cream, Lotion & Ointment 971
- ProctoCream-HC 1834
- Proctofoam-HC 1835

Hydrocortisone Sodium Phosphate (Hypokalemia may be aggravated). Products include:
- Hydrocortone Phosphate Injection, Sterile 1481

Hydrocortisone Sodium Succinate (Hypokalemia may be aggravated). Products include:
- Solu-Cortef Sterile Powder 2361

Hydroflumethiazide (Potentiation of antihypertensive action). Products include:
- Diucardin Tablets 2450
- Saluron 718
- Salutensin/Salutensin-Demi 719

Insulin, Human (Altered insulin requirements).
- No products indexed under this heading.

Insulin, Human Isophane Suspension (Altered insulin requirements). Products include:
- Humulin N, 100 Units 1270

Insulin, Human NPH (Altered insulin requirements). Products include:
Insulatard NPH Human 1627
Novolin N 1627
Novolin N PenFill Cartridges 1628
Novolin N Prefilled 1628

Insulin, Human Regular (Altered insulin requirements). Products include:
Humulin BR, 100 Units 1268
Humulin R, 100 Units 1272
Novolin R 1627
Novolin R PenFill Cartridges 1628
Novolin R Prefilled 1629
Velosulin Human 1628

Insulin, Human, Zinc Suspension (Altered insulin requirements). Products include:
Humulin L, 100 Units 1268
Humulin U, 100 Units 1272
Novolin L 1627

Insulin, NPH (Altered insulin requirements). Products include:
NPH, 40 & 100 Units 1273
Beef NPH, 100 Units 1274
Pork NPH, 100 Units 1275
Insulatard NPH 1626
NPH Insulin 1626
NPH Purified Pork Isophane Insulin 1626

Insulin, Regular (Altered insulin requirements). Products include:
Regular, 40 & 100 Units 1273
Beef Regular, 100 Units 1275
Pork Regular, 100 Units 1275
Pork Regular (Concentrated), 500 Units 1276
Regular Insulin 1625
Regular Purified Pork Insulin 1626
Velosulin 1627

Insulin, Zinc Crystals (Altered insulin requirements). Products include:
NPH, 40 & 100 Units 1273

Insulin, Zinc Suspension (Altered insulin requirements). Products include:
Lente, 40 & 100 Units 1272
Protamine, Zinc, 40 & 100 Units 1273
Lente Iletin I 1272
Beef Lente, 100 Units 1274
Beef Protamine Zinc, 100 Units 1274
Pork Lente, 100 Units 1275
Pork, Protamine, Zinc, 100 Units 1275
Lente Insulin 1626
Lente Purified Pork Insulin 1626
Semilente Insulin 1625
Ultralente Insulin 1626

Levorphanol Tartrate (Orthostatic hypotension). Products include:
Levo-Dromoran 1906

Mecamylamine Hydrochloride (Potentiation of antihypertensive action of mecamylamine). Products include:
Inversine Tablets 1492

Meperidine Hydrochloride (Orthostatic hypotension). Products include:
Demerol 2047
Mepergan Injection 2479

Mephobarbital (Orthostatic hypotension). Products include:
Mebaral Tablets 2061

Methadone Hydrochloride (Orthostatic hypotension). Products include:
Dolophine Hydrochloride Ampoules & Vials 1260
Dolophine Hydrochloride Tablets 1261
Methadone Hydrochloride Diskets 1284
Methadone Hydrochloride Oral Solution & Tablets 1987

Methyclothiazide (Potentiation of antihypertensive action). Products include:
Enduron Tablets 517
Enduronyl 518

Methylprednisolone Acetate (Hypokalemia may be aggravated). Products include:
Depo-Medrol Sterile Aqueous Suspension 2334

Methylprednisolone Sodium Succinate (Hypokalemia may be aggravated). Products include:
Solu-Medrol Sterile Powder 2363

Morphine Sulfate (Orthostatic hypotension). Products include:
Astramorph/PF Injection, USP (Preservative-Free) 618
Duramorph 960
Infumorph 200 and Infumorph 500 Sterile Solutions 962
MS Contin Tablets 1814
MSIR 1817
Oramorph SR (Morphine Sulfate Sustained Release Tablets) 1988
Roxanol 1991

Norepinephrine Bitartrate (Decreased arterial responsiveness to norepinephrine). Products include:
Levophed Bitartrate Injection 2054

Opium Alkaloids (Orthostatic hypotension). Products include:
B & O No. 15A & No. 16A Supprettes 2395
Pantopon Injectable 1911

Oxycodone Hydrochloride (Orthostatic hypotension). Products include:
Percocet Tablets 950
Percodan 951
Roxicodone Tablets, Oral Solution & Intensol (Oxycodone) 1992
Tylox Capsules 1382

Pentobarbital Sodium (Orthostatic hypotension). Products include:
Nembutal Sodium Capsules 534
Nembutal Sodium Solution 536
Nembutal Sodium Suppositories 538

Phenobarbital (Orthostatic hypotension). Products include:
Arco-Lase Plus Tablets 607
Bellergal-S Tablets 1998
Bronkolixir ▣ 761
Bronkotabs Tablets ▣ 762
Donnatal 1858
Donnatal Extentabs 1859
Donnatal Tablets 1858
Donnazyme Tablets 1860
Kinesed Tablets 2272
Phenobarbital Elixir and Tablets 1293
Primatene Tablets-P Formula 2421
Quadrinal Tablets 1183
Tedral SA 1765

Prednisolone Acetate (Hypokalemia may be aggravated). Products include:
AK-Cide Sterile Ophthalmic Ointment & Suspension ◉ 202
Blephamide Liquifilm Sterile Ophthalmic Suspension 586
Blephamide S.O.P. Sterile Ophthalmic Ointment 586
Cetapred Ointment ◉ 220
⅛% Econopred & 1% Econopred Plus ◉ 217
Isopto Cetapred Suspension ◉ 220
Metimyd ◉ 306
Poly-Pred Liquifilm ◉ 250
Pred Forte ◉ 252
Pred Mild ◉ 254
Pred-G Liquifilm Sterile Ophthalmic Suspension ◉ 252
Pred-G S.O.P. Sterile Ophthalmic Ointment ◉ 253
Vasocidin Ointment ◉ 275

Prednisolone Sodium Phosphate (Hypokalemia may be aggravated). Products include:
AK-Pred ◉ 205
Hydeltrasol Injection, Sterile 1476
Inflamase ◉ 274
Pediapred Oral Liquid 987
Vasocidin Ophthalmic Solution ◉ 276

Prednisolone Tebutate (Hypokalemia may be aggravated). Products include:
Hydeltra-T.B.A. Sterile Suspension 1478

Prednisone (Hypokalemia may be aggravated). Products include:
Deltasone Tablets 2332

Propoxyphene Hydrochloride (Orthostatic hypotension). Products include:
Darvon 1256
Wygesic Tablets 2540

Propoxyphene Napsylate (Orthostatic hypotension). Products include:
Darvon-N/Darvocet-N 1254

Rauwolfia Serpentina (Potentiation of antihypertensive action of rauwolfia alkaloids). Products include:
Raudixin Tablets 1803
Rauzide Tablets 1804

Rescinnamine (Potentiation of antihypertensive action of rescinnamine).
No products indexed under this heading.

Reserpine (Potentiation of antihypertensive action of reserpine). Products include:
Diupres Tablets 1461
Hydromox R Tablets 1209
Hydropres Tablets 1485
Renese-R Tablets 1786
Salutensin/Salutensin-Demi 719
Ser-Ap-Es Tablets 881
Serpasil Tablets 883
Serpasil-Apresoline Tablets 884
Serpasil-Esidrix Tablets 886

Secobarbital Sodium (Orthostatic hypotension). Products include:
Seconal Sodium Pulvules 1296

Sufentanil Citrate (Orthostatic hypotension). Products include:
Sufenta Injection 1147

Terazosin Hydrochloride (Potentiation of antihypertensive action of guanadrel). Products include:
Hytrin Tablets 529

Thiamylal Sodium (Orthostatic hypotension). Products include:
Surital Ampoules, Steri-Vials 1764

Triamcinolone (Hypokalemia may be aggravated).
No products indexed under this heading.

Triamcinolone Acetonide (Hypokalemia may be aggravated). Products include:
Aristocort A 1010
Azmacort Inhaler 1837
Kenalog Cream, Lotion & Ointment 2401
Kenalog-10 Injection 2402
Kenalog-40 Injection 2403
Kenalog in Orabase 604
Kenalog Spray 2401
Mycolog II Cream and Ointment 2407
Mytrex Cream & Ointment 2080
Nasacort Nasal Inhaler 1844

Triamcinolone Diacetate (Hypokalemia may be aggravated). Products include:
Aristocort Suspension 1008

Triamcinolone Hexacetonide (Hypokalemia may be aggravated). Products include:
Aristospan Suspension 1011

Trimethaphan Camsylate (Potentiation of antihypertensive action of trimethaphan). Products include:
Arfonad Ampuls 1887

Tubocurarine Chloride (Increased responsiveness to tubocurarine).
No products indexed under this heading.

MINOCIN INTRAVENOUS

(Minocycline Hydrochloride) 1221
May interact with penicillins, anticoagulants, oral contraceptives, and certain other agents. Compounds in these categories include:

Amoxicillin (Interference with bactericidal action of penicillins). Products include:
Amoxil 2193
Augmentin Tablets, Powder for Oral Suspension, and Chewable Tablets 2198

Ampicillin Sodium (Interference with bactericidal action of penicillins). Products include:
Unasyn 1965

Azlocillin Sodium (Interference with bactericidal action of penicillins).
No products indexed under this heading.

Bacampicillin Hydrochloride (Interference with bactericidal action of penicillins). Products include:
Spectrobid Tablets & Powder for Oral Suspension 1961

Carbenicillin Disodium (Interference with bactericidal action of penicillins).

Carbenicillin Indanyl Sodium (Interference with bactericidal action of penicillins). Products include:
Geocillin Tablets 1951

Dicumarol (Depressed plasma prothrombin activity). Products include:
Dicumarol Tablets 516

Ethinyl Estradiol (Reduced efficacy and increased incidence of breakthrough bleeding). Products include:
Brevicon 2304
Demulen 2161
Estinyl Tablets 2085
Jenest-28 Tablets 1636
Levlen/Tri-Levlen 665
Lo/Ovral Tablets 2471
Lo/Ovral-28 Tablets 2476
Loestrin 1728
Modicon 1667
Nordette-21 Tablets 2481
Nordette-28 Tablets 2483
Norethin 2133
Norinyl 2304
Norlestrin 1746
Ortho-Cyclen Tablets 1658
Ortho-Novum 1667
Ovcon 1391
Ovral Tablets 2490
Ovral-28 Tablets 2491
Levlen/Tri-Levlen 665
Tri-Norinyl 2304
Triphasil-21 Tablets 2527
Triphasil-28 Tablets 2532

Ethynodiol Diacetate (Reduced efficacy and increased incidence of breakthrough bleeding). Products include:
Demulen 2161

Heparin Calcium (Depressed plasma prothrombin activity). Products include:
Calciparine Injection 925

Heparin Sodium (Depressed plasma prothrombin activity). Products include:
Heparin Lock Flush Solution 2456
Heparin Sodium Vials 1264
Heparin Sodium Injection 2457
Heparin Sodium Injection, USP, Sterile Solution 2342

Levonorgestrel (Reduced efficacy and increased incidence of breakthrough bleeding). Products include:
Levlen/Tri-Levlen 665
Nordette-21 Tablets 2481
Nordette-28 Tablets 2483
Norplant System 2484
Levlen/Tri-Levlen 665
Triphasil-21 Tablets 2527
Triphasil-28 Tablets 2532

Mestranol (Reduced efficacy and increased incidence of breakthrough bleeding). Products include:
Enovid 2161
Norethin 2133
Norinyl 2304
Ortho-Novum 1667

Mezlocillin Sodium (Interference with bactericidal action of penicillins). Products include:
Mezlin 1597
Mezlin Pharmacy Bulk Package 1599

Nafcillin Sodium (Interference with bactericidal action of penicillins). Products include:
Unipen 2533

Norethindrone (Reduced efficacy and increased incidence of breakthrough bleeding). Products include:
Brevicon 2304
Jenest-28 Tablets 1636
Micronor Tablets 1667
Modicon 1667
Norethin 2133
Norinyl 2304
Norlutin 1755
Nor-Q D Tablets 2304
Ortho-Novum 1667
Ovcon 1391
Tri-Norinyl 2304

Norethynodrel (Reduced efficacy and increased incidence of breakthrough bleeding). Products include:
Enovid 2161

Norgestimate (Reduced efficacy and increased incidence of breakthrough bleeding). Products include:
Ortho-Cyclen Tablets 1658

Norgestrel (Reduced efficacy and increased incidence of breakthrough bleeding). Products include:
Lo/Ovral Tablets 2471
Lo/Ovral-28 Tablets 2476
Ovral Tablets 2490
Ovral-28 Tablets 2491
Ovrette Tablets 2492

Penicillin G Potassium (Interference with bactericidal action of penicillins). Products include:
Pfizerpen for Injection 1957

Penicillin G Procaine (Interference with bactericidal action of penicillins). Products include:
Bicillin C-R Injection 2438
Bicillin C-R 900/300 Injection 2440
Pfizerpen-AS Aqueous Suspension 1959
Wycillin Injection 2537
Wycillin Injection and Probenecid Tablets 2539

Penicillin G, Benzathine (Interference with bactericidal action of penicillins). Products include:
Bicillin C-R Injection 2438
Bicillin C-R 900/300 Injection 2440
Bicillin L-A Injection 2442

Penicillin V Potassium (Interference with bactericidal action of penicillins).
No products indexed under this heading.

Ticarcillin Disodium (Interference with bactericidal action of penicillins). Products include:
Ticar for Injection 2236
Timentin for Injection 2239

Warfarin Sodium (Depressed plasma prothrombin activity). Products include:
Coumadin Injection & Tablets 944
Panwarfin Tablets 547

MINOCIN ORAL SUSPENSION
(Minocycline Hydrochloride) 1224
May interact with anticoagulants, oral contraceptives, penicillins, antacids containing aluminium, calcium and magnesium, and certain other agents. Compounds in these categories include:

Aluminum Carbonate Gel (Absorption of tetracyclines is impaired). Products include:
Basaljel 2438

Aluminum Hydroxide (Absorption of tetracyclines is impaired). Products include:
Cama Arthritis Pain Reliever .... BD 685
Gaviscon Extra Strength Relief Formula Liquid Antacid .... BD 594
Gaviscon Extra Strength Relief Formula Antacid Tablets .... BD 594
Gaviscon Liquid Antacid .... BD 594
Gelusil Liquid & Tablets .... BD 639
Extra Strength Maalox Plus Suspension 1850
Maalox TC Suspension 1851
Maalox Plus Tablets .... BD 655
Extra Strength Maalox Plus Tablets 1850
Nephrox Suspension .... BD 563
WinGel Liquid & Tablets .... BD 761

Aluminum Hydroxide Gel (Absorption of tetracyclines is impaired). Products include:
ALternaGEL Liquid 1154
Aludrox Oral Suspension 2428
Amphojel Suspension 2429
Amphojel Suspension without Flavor 2429
Mylanta Liquid 1155
Mylanta Double Strength Liquid 1155

Aluminum Hydroxide Gel, Dried (Absorption of tetracyclines is impaired). Products include:
Alu-Tab/Alu-Cap 1309
Amphojel Tablets 2429
Ascriptin A/D Caplets 1850
Regular Strength Ascriptin Tablets 1850
Gaviscon Antacid Tablets .... BD 593
Gaviscon-2 Antacid Tablets .... BD 594
Mylanta Tablets 1155
Mylanta Double Strength Tablets 1155

Amoxicillin (Interference with bactericidal action of penicillin). Products include:
Amoxil 2193
Augmentin Tablets, Powder for Oral Suspension, and Chewable Tablets 2198

Ampicillin Sodium (Interference with bactericidal action of penicillin). Products include:
Unasyn 1965

Azlocillin Sodium (Interference with bactericidal action of penicillin).
No products indexed under this heading.

Bacampicillin Hydrochloride (Interference with bactericidal action of penicillin). Products include:
Spectrobid Tablets & Powder for Oral Suspension 1961

Carbenicillin Disodium (Interference with bactericidal action of penicillin).

Carbenicillin Indanyl Sodium (Interference with bactericidal action of penicillin). Products include:
Geocillin Tablets 1951

Dicumarol (Depressed plasma prothrombin activity; may require downward adjustment of the anticoagulant dosage). Products include:
Dicumarol Tablets 516

Dihydroxyaluminum Sodium Carbonate (Absorption of tetracyclines is impaired). Products include:
Rolaids .... BD 743

Ethinyl Estradiol (Concurrent use may render oral contraceptives less effective; potential for breakthrough bleeding). Products include:
Brevicon 2304
Demulen 2161
Estinyl Tablets 2085
Jenest-28 Tablets 1636
Levlen/Tri-Levlen 665
Lo/Ovral Tablets 2471
Lo/Ovral-28 Tablets 2476
Loestrin 1728
Modicon 1667
Nordette-21 Tablets 2481
Nordette-28 Tablets 2483
Norethin 2133
Norinyl 2304
Norlestrin 1746
Ortho-Cyclen Tablets 1658
Ortho-Novum 1667
Ovcon 1391
Ovral Tablets 2490
Ovral-28 Tablets 2491
Levlen/Tri-Levlen 665
Tri-Norinyl 2304
Triphasil-21 Tablets 2527
Triphasil-28 Tablets 2532

Ethynodiol Diacetate (Concurrent use may render oral contraceptives less effective; potential for breakthrough bleeding). Products include:
Demulen 2161

Ferrous Fumarate (Absorption of tetracyclines is impaired). Products include:
Bugs Bunny Plus Iron Children's Chewable Vitamins (Sugar Free) BD 625
Caltrate 600 + Iron & Vitamin D 1198
Centrum, Jr. (Children's Chewable) + Iron .... BD 586
Chromagen Capsules 2078
Femlron Multi-Vitamins and Iron .... BD 617
Feramcee Chewable Tablets 1155
Ferancee-HP Tablets 1155
Ferro-Sequels 1203
Flintstones Children's Chewable Vitamins Plus Iron .... BD 625
Natalins Rx 1391
Natalins Tablets 1391
Nephro-Fer Tablets 1826
One-A-Day Maximum Formula Vitamins and Minerals .... BD 627
Poly-Vi-Flor with Iron 1399
Poly-Vi-Sol Vitamins with Iron, Chewable Tablets and Circus Shapes Chewable .... BD 612
Pramilet FA 1974
Stressgard Stress Formula Vitamins .... BD 628
Stresstabs + Iron, Advanced Formula .... BD 589
Stuartinic Tablets 1157
Theragran-M Tablets .... BD 727
Trinsicon Capsules 2415
Within Women's Formula Multivitamin with Calcium, Extra Iron and Zinc .... BD 628
Zenate Tablets 2250

Ferrous Gluconate (Absorption of tetracyclines is impaired). Products include:
Fergon .... BD 758

Ferrous Sulfate (Absorption of tetracyclines is impaired). Products include:
Dayalets Plus Iron Filmtab .... BD 502
Feosol Capsules 2191
Feosol Elixir 2191
Feosol Tablets 2191
Fero-Folic-500 Filmtab 527
Fero-Grad-500 Filmtab 528
Fero-Gradumet Filmtab 528
Iberet Tablets 531
Iberet-500 Liquid 531
Iberet-Folic-500 Filmtab 527
Iberet-Liquid 531
Irospan 972
Mol-Iron .... BD 703
Poly-Vi-Sol Vitamins with Iron, Drops .... BD 612
Pramet FA 1974
Slow Fe Tablets 852
Tri-Vi-Sol Vitamin Drops with Iron BD 614

Heparin Calcium (Depressed plasma prothrombin activity; may require downward adjustment of the anticoagulant dosage). Products include:
Calciparine Injection 925

Heparin Sodium (Depressed plasma prothrombin activity; may require downward adjustment of the anticoagulant dosage). Products include:
Heparin Lock Flush Solution 2456
Heparin Sodium Vials 1264
Heparin Sodium Injection 2457
Heparin Sodium Injection, USP, Sterile Solution 2342

Levonorgestrel (Concurrent use may render oral contraceptives less effective; potential for breakthrough bleeding). Products include:
Levlen/Tri-Levlen 665
Nordette-21 Tablets 2481
Nordette-28 Tablets 2483
Norplant System 2484
Levlen/Tri-Levlen 665
Triphasil-21 Tablets 2527
Triphasil-28 Tablets 2532

Magaldrate (Absorption of tetracyclines is impaired). Products include:
Riopan Antacid Chew Tablets .... BD 754
Riopan Antacid Chew Tablets in Rollpacks .... BD 754
Riopan Antacid Suspension 2421
Riopan Antacid Swallow Tablets 2421
Riopan Plus Chew Tablets 2422
Riopan Plus Chew Tablets in Rollpack 2422
Riopan Plus 2 Chew Tablets, Mint Flavor, Cherry Flavor 2422
Riopan Plus Suspension 2422
Riopan Plus 2 Suspension, Mint Flavor, Cherry Flavor 2422

Magnesium Hydroxide (Absorption of tetracyclines is impaired). Products include:
Aludrox Oral Suspension 2428
Ascriptin A/D Caplets 1850
Regular Strength Ascriptin Tablets 1850
Di-Gel Antacid/Anti-Gas .... BD 697
Gelusil Liquid & Tablets .... BD 639
Haley's M-O, Regular & Flavored .... BD 569
Extra Strength Maalox Plus Suspension 1850
Maalox TC Suspension 1851
Maalox Plus Tablets .... BD 655
Extra Strength Maalox Plus Tablets 1850
Mylanta Liquid 1155
Mylanta Tablets 1155
Mylanta Double Strength Liquid 1155
Mylanta Double Strength Tablets 1155
Concentrated Phillips' Milk of Magnesia .... BD 573
Phillips' Milk of Magnesia Liquid .... BD 572
Phillips' Milk of Magnesia Tablets BD 573
WinGel Liquid & Tablets .... BD 761

Magnesium Oxide (Absorption of tetracyclines is impaired). Products include:
Bayer Plus Aspirin Tablets .... BD 567
Beelith Tablets 659
Bufferin Analgesic Tablets and Caplets .... BD 524
Cama Arthritis Pain Reliever .... BD 685
Mag-Ox 400 673
Uro-Mag 673

Mestranol (Concurrent use may render oral contraceptives less effective; potential for breakthrough bleeding). Products include:
Enovid 2161
Norethin 2133
Norinyl 2304
Ortho-Novum 1667

Methoxyflurane (Potential for fatal renal toxicity).
No products indexed under this heading.

Mezlocillin Sodium (Interference with bactericidal action of penicillin). Products include:
Mezlin 1597
Mezlin Pharmacy Bulk Package 1599

Nafcillin Sodium (Interference with bactericidal action of penicillin). Products include:
Unipen 2533

Norethindrone (Concurrent use may render oral contraceptives less effective; potential for breakthrough bleeding). Products include:
Brevicon 2304
Jenest-28 Tablets 1636
Micronor Tablets 1667
Modicon 1667
Norethin 2133
Norinyl 2304
Norlutin 1755
Nor-Q D Tablets 2304

Ortho-Novum 1667
Ovcon 1391
Tri-Norinyl 2304

Norethynodrel (Concurrent use may render oral contraceptives less effective; potential for breakthrough bleeding). Products include:
Enovid 2161

Norgestimate (Concurrent use may render oral contraceptives less effective; potential for breakthrough bleeding). Products include:
Ortho-Cyclen Tablets 1658

Norgestrel (Concurrent use may render oral contraceptives less effective; potential for breakthrough bleeding). Products include:
Lo/Ovral Tablets 2471
Lo/Ovral-28 Tablets 2476
Ovral Tablets 2490
Ovral-28 Tablets 2491
Ovrette Tablets 2492

Penicillin G Potassium (Interference with bactericidal action of penicillin). Products include:
Pfizerpen for Injection 1957

Penicillin G Procaine (Interference with bactericidal action of penicillin). Products include:
Bicillin C-R Injection 2438
Bicillin C-R 900/300 Injection 2440
Pfizerpen-AS Aqueous Suspension 1959
Wycillin Injection 2537
Wycillin Injection and Probenecid Tablets 2539

Penicillin G Sodium (Interference with bactericidal action of penicillin).
No products indexed under this heading.

Penicillin V Potassium (Interference with bactericidal action of penicillin).
No products indexed under this heading.

Ticarcillin Disodium (Interference with bactericidal action of penicillin). Products include:
Ticar for Injection 2236
Timentin for Injection 2239

Warfarin Sodium (Depressed plasma prothrombin activity; may require downward adjustment of the anticoagulant dosage). Products include:
Coumadin Injection & Tablets 944
Panwarfin Tablets 547

MINOCIN PELLET-FILLED CAPSULES
(Minocycline Hydrochloride) 1222
May interact with anticoagulants, oral contraceptives, penicillins, antacids containing aluminium, calcium and magnesium, and certain other agents. Compounds in these categories include:

Aluminum Carbonate Gel (Absorption of tetracyclines is impaired). Products include:
Basaljel 2438

Aluminum Hydroxide (Absorption of tetracyclines is impaired). Products include:
Cama Arthritis Pain Reliever .... ◘ 685
Gaviscon Extra Strength Relief Formula Liquid Antacid .... ◘ 594
Gaviscon Extra Strength Relief Formula Antacid Tablets .... ◘ 594
Gaviscon Liquid Antacid .... ◘ 594
Gelusil Liquid & Tablets .... ◘ 639
Extra Strength Maalox Plus Suspension 1850
Maalox TC Suspension 1851
Maalox Plus Tablets .... ◘ 655
Extra Strength Maalox Plus Tablets 1850
Nephrox Suspension .... ◘ 563
WinGel Liquid & Tablets .... ◘ 761

Aluminum Hydroxide Gel (Absorption of tetracyclines is impaired). Products include:
ALternaGEL Liquid 1154
Aludrox Oral Suspension 2428
Amphojel Suspension 2429
Amphojel Suspension without Flavor 2429
Mylanta Liquid 1155
Mylanta Double Strength Liquid 1155

Aluminum Hydroxide Gel, Dried (Absorption of tetracyclines is impaired). Products include:
Alu-Tab/Alu-Cap 1309
Amphojel Tablets 2429
Ascriptin A/D Caplets 1850
Regular Strength Ascriptin Tablets 1850
Gaviscon Antacid Tablets .... ◘ 593
Gaviscon-2 Antacid Tablets .... ◘ 594
Mylanta Tablets 1155
Mylanta Double Strength Tablets 1155

Amoxicillin (Interference with bactericidal action of penicillin). Products include:
Amoxil 2193
Augmentin Tablets, Powder for Oral Suspension, and Chewable Tablets 2198

Ampicillin Sodium (Interference with bactericidal action of penicillin). Products include:
Unasyn 1965

Azlocillin Sodium (Interference with bactericidal action of penicillin).
No products indexed under this heading.

Bacampicillin Hydrochloride (Interference with bactericidal action of penicillin). Products include:
Spectrobid Tablets & Powder for Oral Suspension 1961

Carbenicillin Disodium (Interference with bactericidal action of penicillin).

Carbenicillin Indanyl Sodium (Interference with bactericidal action of penicillin). Products include:
Geocillin Tablets 1951

Dicumarol (Depressed plasma prothrombin activity; may require downward adjustment of the anticoagulant dosage). Products include:
Dicumarol Tablets 516

Dihydroxyaluminum Sodium Carbonate (Absorption of tetracyclines is impaired). Products include:
Rolaids .... ◘ 743

Ethinyl Estradiol (Concurrent use may render oral contraceptives less effective; potential for breakthrough bleeding). Products include:
Brevicon 2304
Demulen 2161
Estinyl Tablets 2085
Jenest-28 Tablets 1636
Levlen/Tri-Levlen 665
Lo/Ovral Tablets 2471
Lo/Ovral-28 Tablets 2476
Loestrin 1728
Modicon 1667
Nordette-21 Tablets 2481
Nordette-28 Tablets 2483
Norethin 2133
Norinyl 2304
Norlestrin 1746
Ortho-Cyclen Tablets 1658
Ortho-Novum 1667
Ovcon 1391
Ovral Tablets 2490
Ovral-28 Tablets 2491
Levlen/Tri-Levlen 665
Tri-Norinyl 2304
Triphasil-21 Tablets 2527
Triphasil-28 Tablets 2532

Ethynodiol Diacetate (Concurrent use may render oral contraceptives less effective; potential for breakthrough bleeding). Products include:
Demulen 2161

Ferrous Fumarate (Absorption of tetracyclines is impaired). Products include:
Bugs Bunny Plus Iron Children's Chewable Vitamins (Sugar Free) ◘ 625
Caltrate 600 + Iron & Vitamin D 1198
Centrum, Jr. (Children's Chewable) + Iron .... ◘ 586
Chromagen Capsules 2078
Femlron Multi-Vitamins and Iron .... ◘ 617
Ferancee Chewable Tablets 1155
Ferancee-HP Tablets 1155
Ferro-Sequels 1203
Flintstones Children's Chewable Vitamins Plus Iron .... ◘ 625
Natalins Rx 1391
Natalins Tablets 1391
Nephro-Fer Tablets 1826
One-A-Day Maximum Formula Vitamins and Minerals .... ◘ 627
Poly-Vi-Flor with Iron 1399
Poly-Vi-Sol Vitamins with Iron, Chewable Tablets and Circus Shapes Chewable .... ◘ 612
Pramilet FA 1974
Stressgard Stress Formula Vitamins .... ◘ 628
Stresstabs + Iron, Advanced Formula .... ◘ 589
Stuartinic Tablets 1157
Theragran-M Tablets .... ◘ 727
Trinsicon Capsules 2415
Within Women's Formula Multivitamin with Calcium, Extra Iron and Zinc .... ◘ 628
Zenate Tablets 2250

Ferrous Gluconate (Absorption of tetracyclines is impaired). Products include:
Fergon .... ◘ 758

Ferrous Sulfate (Absorption of tetracyclines is impaired). Products include:
Dayalets Plus Iron Filmtab .... ◘ 502
Feosol Capsules 2191
Feosol Elixir 2191
Feosol Tablets 2191
Fero-Folic-500 Filmtab 527
Fero-Grad-500 Filmtab 528
Fero-Gradumet Filmtab 528
Iberet Tablets 531
Iberet-500 Liquid 531
Iberet-Folic-500 Filmtab 527
Iberet-Liquid 531
Irospan 972
Mol-Iron .... ◘ 703
Poly-Vi-Sol Vitamins with Iron, Drops .... ◘ 612
Pramet FA 1974
Slow Fe Tablets 852
Tri-Vi-Sol Vitamin Drops with Iron ◘ 614

Heparin Calcium (Depressed plasma prothrombin activity; may require downward adjustment of the anticoagulant dosage). Products include:
Calciparine Injection 925

Heparin Sodium (Depressed plasma prothrombin activity; may require downward adjustment of the anticoagulant dosage). Products include:
Heparin Lock Flush Solution 2456
Heparin Sodium Vials 1264
Heparin Sodium Injection 2457
Heparin Sodium Injection, USP, Sterile Solution 2342

Levonorgestrel (Concurrent use may render oral contraceptives less effective; potential for breakthrough bleeding). Products include:
Levlen/Tri-Levlen 665
Nordette-21 Tablets 2481
Nordette-28 Tablets 2483
Norplant System 2484
Levlen/Tri-Levlen 665
Triphasil-21 Tablets 2527
Triphasil-28 Tablets 2532

Magaldrate (Absorption of tetracyclines is impaired). Products include:
Riopan Antacid Chew Tablets .... ◘ 754
Riopan Antacid Chew Tablets in Rollpacks .... ◘ 754
Riopan Antacid Suspension 2421
Riopan Antacid Swallow Tablets 2421
Riopan Plus Chew Tablets 2422
Riopan Plus Chew Tablets in Rollpack 2422
Riopan Plus 2 Chew Tablets, Mint Flavor, Cherry Flavor 2422
Riopan Plus Suspension 2422
Riopan Plus 2 Suspension, Mint Flavor, Cherry Flavor 2422

Magnesium Hydroxide (Absorption of tetracyclines is impaired). Products include:
Aludrox Oral Suspension 2428
Ascriptin A/D Caplets 1850
Regular Strength Ascriptin Tablets 1850
Di-Gel Antacid/Anti-Gas .... ◘ 697
Gelusil Liquid & Tablets .... ◘ 639
Haley's M-O, Regular & Flavored .... ◘ 569
Extra Strength Maalox Plus Suspension 1850
Maalox TC Suspension 1851
Maalox Plus Tablets .... ◘ 655
Extra Strength Maalox Plus Tablets 1850
Mylanta Liquid 1155
Mylanta Tablets 1155
Mylanta Double Strength Liquid 1155
Mylanta Double Strength Tablets 1155
Concentrated Phillips' Milk of Magnesia .... ◘ 573
Phillips' Milk of Magnesia Liquid .... ◘ 572
Phillips' Milk of Magnesia Tablets ◘ 573
WinGel Liquid & Tablets .... ◘ 761

Magnesium Oxide (Absorption of tetracyclines is impaired). Products include:
Bayer Plus Aspirin Tablets .... ◘ 567
Beelith Tablets 659
Bufferin Analgesic Tablets and Caplets .... ◘ 524
Cama Arthritis Pain Reliever .... ◘ 685
Mag-Ox 400 673
Uro-Mag 673

Mestranol (Concurrent use may render oral contraceptives less effective; potential for breakthrough bleeding). Products include:
Enovid 2161
Norethin 2133
Norinyl 2304
Ortho-Novum 1667

Methoxyflurane (Potential for fatal renal toxicity).
No products indexed under this heading.

Mezlocillin Sodium (Interference with bactericidal action of penicillin). Products include:
Mezlin 1597
Mezlin Pharmacy Bulk Package 1599

Nafcillin Sodium (Interference with bactericidal action of penicillin). Products include:
Unipen 2533

Norethindrone (Concurrent use may render oral contraceptives less effective; potential for breakthrough bleeding). Products include:
Brevicon 2304
Jenest-28 Tablets 1636
Micronor Tablets 1667
Modicon 1667
Norethin 2133
Norinyl 2304
Norlutin 1755
Nor-Q D Tablets 2304
Ortho-Novum 1667
Ovcon 1391
Tri-Norinyl 2304

Norethynodrel (Concurrent use may render oral contraceptives less effective; potential for breakthrough bleeding). Products include:
Enovid 2161

Norgestimate (Concurrent use may render oral contraceptives less effective; potential for breakthrough bleeding). Products include:
Ortho-Cyclen Tablets 1658

Norgestrel (Concurrent use may render oral contraceptives less effective; potential for breakthrough bleeding). Products include:
Lo/Ovral Tablets 2471
Lo/Ovral-28 Tablets 2476
Ovral Tablets 2490
Ovral-28 Tablets 2491
Ovrette Tablets 2492

Penicillin G Potassium (Interference with bactericidal action of penicillin). Products include:
Pfizerpen for Injection 1957

Penicillin G Procaine (Interference with bactericidal action of penicillin). Products include:
- Bicillin C-R Injection 2438
- Bicillin C-R 900/300 Injection 2440
- Pfizerpen-AS Aqueous Suspension 1959
- Wycillin Injection 2537
- Wycillin Injection and Probenecid Tablets 2539

Penicillin G Sodium (Interference with bactericidal action of penicillin).
No products indexed under this heading.

Penicillin V Potassium (Interference with bactericidal action of penicillin).
No products indexed under this heading.

Ticarcillin Disodium (Interference with bactericidal action of penicillin). Products include:
- Ticar for Injection 2236
- Timentin for Injection 2239

Warfarin Sodium (Depressed plasma prothrombin activity; may require downward adjustment of the anticoagulant dosage). Products include:
- Coumadin Injection & Tablets 944
- Panwarfin Tablets 547

Food Interactions

Dairy products (The peak plasma concentrations were slightly decreased (11.2%) and delayed by 1 hour).

Meal with dairy products (The peak plasma concentrations were slightly decreased (11.2%) and delayed by 1 hour).

MINTEZOL CHEWABLE TABLETS
(Thiabendazole) 1510
May interact with xanthine bronchodilators. Compounds in this category include:

Aminophylline (Xanthine toxicity). Products include:
- Amesec .... ▣ 682
- Aminophyllin Tablets 2153

Dyphylline (Xanthine toxicity). Products include:
- Dilor 2079
- Dilor-G Tablets & Liquid 2079
- Lufyllin Elixir 2384
- Lufyllin & Lufyllin-400 Tablets 2384
- Lufyllin-GG Elixir & Tablets 2385

Theophylline (Xanthine toxicity). Products include:
- Bronkaid Tablets .... ▣ 757
- Bronkolixir .... ▣ 761
- Bronkotabs Tablets .... ▣ 762
- Constant-T Tablets 1029
- Marax Tablets & DF Syrup 1954
- Primatene Tablets 2421
- Quibron Capsules 713
- Quibron-T 714
- Quibron-T/SR 716
- Theolair Liquid 1317
- Theo-Organidin Elixir 2391

Theophylline Anhydrous (Xanthine toxicity). Products include:
- Aerolate 994
- Primatene Tablets-M Formula .... ▣ 753
- Primatene Tablets-Regular Formula 2421
- Respbid Tablets 684
- Slo-bid Gyrocaps 1847
- T-PHYL (Uniphyl) 200 mg Tablets 1820
- Tedral SA 1765
- Theo-24 2179
- Theo-Dur Sprinkle 1168
- Theo-Dur Extended-Release Tablets 1166
- Theolair Tablets 1317
- Theolair-SR Tablets 1319
- TheoX Extended-Release Tablets 841
- Uniphyl 400 mg Tablets 1823

Theophylline Calcium Salicylate (Xanthine toxicity). Products include:
- Quadrinal Tablets 1183

Theophylline Sodium Glycinate (Xanthine toxicity). Products include:
- Asbron G 1997

Xanthine Preparations (Xanthine toxicity).

MINTEZOL SUSPENSION
(Thiabendazole) 1510
See **Mintezol Chewable Tablets**

MIOCHOL WITH IOCARE STERI-TAGS, MIOCHOL SYSTEM PAK AND MIOCHOL SYSTEM PAK PLUS
(Acetylcholine Chloride) .... ⊙ 274
May interact with topical nonsteroidal anti-inflammatory agents. Compounds in this category include:

Flurbiprofen Sodium (Renders acetylcholine chloride ineffective). Products include:
- Ocufen .... ⊙ 237

MIOSTAT
(Carbachol) .... ⊙ 233
No interactions described in labeling.

MITHRACIN
(Plicamycin) 1602
No interactions described in labeling.

MITROLAN CHEWABLE TABLETS
(Calcium Polycarbophil) 1878
May interact with tetracyclines. Compounds in this category include:

Demeclocycline Hydrochloride (Impaired tetracycline absorption). Products include:
- Declomycin Capsules, Tablets 1199

Doxycycline Calcium (Impaired tetracycline absorption).
No products indexed under this heading.

Doxycycline Hyclate (Impaired tetracycline absorption). Products include:
- Doryx Capsules 1717
- Vibramycin Hyclate Capsules 1787
- Vibramycin Hyclate Intravenous 1968
- Vibra-Tabs Film Coated Tablets 1787

Doxycycline Monohydrate (Impaired tetracycline absorption). Products include:
- Monodox Capsules 1630
- Vibramycin Monohydrate for Oral Suspension 1787

Methacycline Hydrochloride (Impaired tetracycline absorption).
No products indexed under this heading.

Minocycline Hydrochloride (Impaired tetracycline absorption). Products include:
- Minocin Intravenous 1221
- Minocin Oral Suspension 1224
- Minocin Pellet-Filled Capsules 1222

Oxytetracycline (Impaired tetracycline absorption). Products include:
- Terramycin Intramuscular Solution 1964
- Urobiotic-250 Capsules 1968

Oxytetracycline Hydrochloride (Impaired tetracycline absorption). Products include:
- Terra-Cortril Ophthalmic Suspension 1963
- Terramycin Capsules 1786
- Terramycin Intramuscular Solution 1964
- Terramycin with Polymyxin B Sulfate Ophthalmic Ointment 1965

Tetracycline Hydrochloride (Impaired tetracycline absorption). Products include:
- Achromycin V Capsules 1193
- Achromycin Ophthalmic Ointment 1% .... ⊙ 307
- Achromycin Ophthalmic Suspension 1% .... ⊙ 308
- Topicycline for Topical Solution 1856

MIXTARD 70/30
(Insulin, Regular) 1627
No interactions described in labeling.

MIXTARD HUMAN 70/30
(Insulin, Human) 1628
No interactions described in labeling.

MOBAN TABLETS & CONCENTRATE
(Molindone Hydrochloride) 932
May interact with tetracyclines and certain other agents. Compounds in these categories include:

Demeclocycline Hydrochloride (Moban Tablets contain calcium sulfate as an excipient which may interfere with absorption of oral tetracyclines). Products include:
- Declomycin Capsules, Tablets 1199

Doxycycline Calcium (Moban Tablets contain calcium sulfate as an excipient which may interfere with absorption of oral tetracyclines).
No products indexed under this heading.

Doxycycline Hyclate (Moban Tablets contain calcium sulfate as an excipient which may interfere with absorption of oral tetracyclines). Products include:
- Doryx Capsules 1717
- Vibramycin Hyclate Capsules 1787
- Vibramycin Hyclate Intravenous 1968
- Vibra-Tabs Film Coated Tablets 1787

Doxycycline Monohydrate (Moban Tablets contain calcium sulfate as an excipient which may interfere with absorption of oral tetracyclines). Products include:
- Monodox Capsules 1630
- Vibramycin Monohydrate for Oral Suspension 1787

Methacycline Hydrochloride (Moban Tablets contain calcium sulfate as an excipient which may interfere with absorption of oral tetracyclines).
No products indexed under this heading.

Minocycline Hydrochloride (Moban Tablets contain calcium sulfate as an excipient which may interfere with absorption of oral tetracyclines). Products include:
- Minocin Intravenous 1221
- Minocin Oral Suspension 1224
- Minocin Pellet-Filled Capsules 1222

Oxytetracycline Hydrochloride (Moban Tablets contain calcium sulfate as an excipient which may interfere with absorption of oral tetracyclines). Products include:
- Terra-Cortril Ophthalmic Suspension 1963
- Terramycin Capsules 1786
- Terramycin Intramuscular Solution 1964
- Terramycin with Polymyxin B Sulfate Ophthalmic Ointment 1965

Phenytoin Sodium (Calcium sulfate present in tablets may interfere with absorption of phenytoin sodium). Products include:
- Dilantin Kapseals 1708
- Dilantin Parenteral 1712
- Dilantin with Phenobarbital Kapseals 1715

Tetracycline Hydrochloride (Moban Tablets contain calcium sulfate as an excipient which may interfere with absorption of oral tetracyclines). Products include:
- Achromycin V Capsules 1193
- Achromycin Ophthalmic Ointment 1% .... ⊙ 307
- Achromycin Ophthalmic Suspension 1% .... ⊙ 308
- Topicycline for Topical Solution 1856

MOBIGESIC ANALGESIC TABLETS
(Magnesium Salicylate, Phenyltoloxamine Citrate) .... ▣ 507
No interactions described in labeling.

MOBISYL ANALGESIC CREME
(Trolamine Salicylate) .... ▣ 507
No interactions described in labeling.

MODANE PLUS TABLETS
(Phenolphthalein, Docusate Sodium) .... ▣ 504
May interact with:

Mineral Oil (Increased intestinal absorption of mineral oil). Products include:
- AKWA Tears Ointment .... ⊙ 208
- Agoral .... ▣ 634
- Aqua Care Cream .... ▣ 616
- Aqua Care Lotion .... ▣ 616
- Aquaphor Antibiotic Formula 662
- Aquaphor Healing Ointment, Original Formula 662
- Aquaphor Natural Healing Formula 662
- Complex 15 Hand & Body Moisturizing Cream .... ▣ 694
- Complex 15 Hand & Body Moisturizing Lotion .... ▣ 695
- Complex 15 Moisturizing Face Cream .... ▣ 695
- Duolube Eye Ointment .... ⊙ 258
- Duratears Naturale .... ⊙ 216
- Eucerin Dry Skin Care Lotion 662
- Eucerin Moisturizing Creme (Unscented) 662
- Eucerin Dry Skin Care Lotion (Fragrace-free) .... ▣ 514
- Fleet Mineral Oil Enema 992
- Fleet Relief 993
- Haley's M-O, Regular & Flavored .. ▣ 569
- Keri Lotion - Original Formula .... ▣ 535
- Lacri-Lube NP Lubricant Ophthalmic Ointment .... ⊙ 249
- Lacri-Lube S.O.P. Sterile Ophthalmic Ointment .... ⊙ 249
- Nephrox Suspension .... ▣ 563
- Nivea Bath Silk Bath Oil .... ▣ 514
- Nivea Bath Silk Bath & Shower Gel (Extra-Dry Skin) .... ▣ 514
- Nivea Moisturizing Creme .... ▣ 514
- Nivea Moisturizing Lotion (Original Formula) .... ▣ 514
- Nivea Moisturizing Oil .... ▣ 515
- Nivea Skin Oil .... ▣ 515
- Nivea Sun After Sun Lotion .... ▣ 515
- Nutraderm Cream & Lotion 1684
- pHisoDerm For Baby .... ▣ 761
- pHisoDerm Skin Cleanser and Conditioner - Regular and Oily .... ▣ 760
- Refresh P.M. Lubricant Ophthalmic Ointment .... ⊙ 256
- Replens .... ▣ 556
- Tears Renewed Ointment .... ⊙ 209
- Theraplex ClearLotion 1410

MODANE TABLETS
(Phenolphthalein) .... ▣ 503
No interactions described in labeling.

MODICON 21 TABLETS
(Norethindrone, Ethinyl Estradiol) 1667
See **Micronor Tablets**

MODICON 28 TABLETS
(Norethindrone, Ethinyl Estradiol) 1667
See **Micronor Tablets**

MODURETIC TABLETS
(Amiloride Hydrochloride, Hydrochlorothiazide) 1510
May interact with antihypertensives, lithium preparations, non-steroidal anti-inflammatory agents, insulin, cardiac glycosides, corticosteroids, potassium-depleting corticosteroids, ACE inhibitors, oral hypoglycemic agents, barbiturates, narcotic analgesics, and certain other agents.

Compounds in these categories include:

Acebutolol Hydrochloride (Potentiated or additive action). Products include:
- Sectral Capsules 2520

ACTH (Hypokalemia).
- No products indexed under this heading.

Alcohol (Potentiation of orthostatic hypotension).

Alfentanil Hydrochloride (Potentiation of orthostatic hypotension). Products include:
- Alfenta Injection 1131

Aprobarbital (Potentiation of orthostatic hypotension). Products include:
- Alurate Elixir 1883

Atenolol (Potentiated or additive action). Products include:
- Tenoretic Tablets 1105
- Tenormin Tablets and I.V. Injection 1107

Benazepril Hydrochloride (Potentiated or additive action; increased risk of hyperkalemia). Products include:
- Lotensin Tablets 872

Bendroflumethiazide (Potentiated or additive action). Products include:
- Corzide Tablets 702
- Naturetin Tablets 1789
- Rauzide Tablets 1804

Betamethasone Acetate (Hypokalemia). Products include:
- Celestone Soluspan Suspension 2081

Betamethasone Sodium Phosphate (Hypokalemia). Products include:
- Celestone Soluspan Suspension 2081

Betaxolol Hydrochloride (Potentiated or additive action; increased risk of hyperkalemia). Products include:
- Betoptic Sterile Ophthalmic Solution 569
- Betoptic S Sterile Ophthalmic Suspension 570
- Kerlone Tablets 2172

Buprenorphine (Potentiation of orthostatic hypotension).
- No products indexed under this heading.

Butabarbital (Potentiation of orthostatic hypotension). Products include:
- Pyridium Plus 1764

Butalbital (Potentiation of orthostatic hypotension). Products include:
- Esgic-Plus Tablets 1002
- Esgic Tablets & Capsules 1001
- Fioricet Tablets 2006
- Fiorinal Capsules 2007
- Fiorinal with Codeine Capsules 2008
- Fiorinal Tablets 2007
- Phrenilin 838
- Sedapap Tablets 50 mg/650 mg .. 1360

Captopril (Potentiated or additive action; increased risk of hyperkalemia). Products include:
- Capoten 2255
- Capozide 2258

Carteolol Hydrochloride (Potentiated or additive action). Products include:
- Cartrol Tablets 507

Chlorothiazide (Potentiated or additive action). Products include:
- Aldoclor Tablets 1413
- Diupres Tablets 1461
- Diuril Oral 1464

Chlorothiazide Sodium (Potentiated or additive action). Products include:
- Diuril Sodium Intravenous 1463

Chlorpropamide (Dosage adjustment of the antidiabetic drug may be required). Products include:
- Diabinese Tablets 1775

Chlorthalidone (Potentiated or additive effects). Products include:
- Combipres Tablets 678
- Tenoretic Tablets 1105
- Thalitone Tablets 687

Clonidine (Potentiated or additive action). Products include:
- Catapres-TTS 677

Clonidine Hydrochloride (Potentiated or additive action). Products include:
- Catapres Tablets 676
- Combipres Tablets 678

Codeine (Potentiation of orthostatic hypotension). Products include:
- Calcidrine Syrup 506

Codeine Phosphate (Potentiation of orthostatic hypotension). Products include:
- Actifed with Codeine Cough Syrup.. 752
- Cheracol Cough Syrup 1853
- Codimal PH Syrup 846
- Dimetane-DC Cough Syrup 1857
- Empirin with Codeine Phosphate Nos. 2, 3 & 4 764
- Fiorinal with Codeine Capsules 2008
- Isoclor Expectorant 982
- Naldecon CX Adult Liquid .... ⊞ 521
- Novahistine DH 1342
- Novahistine Expectorant 1343
- Nucofed Capsules 2219
- Nucofed Expectorant 2219
- Nucofed Pediatric Expectorant 2220
- Nucofed Syrup 2219
- Phenaphen with Codeine Capsules 1865
- Phenaphen-650 with Codeine Tablets 1866
- Phenergan with Codeine 2497
- Phenergan VC with Codeine 2501
- Robitussin A-C Syrup 1875
- Robitussin-DAC Syrup 1875
- Ryna .... ⊞ 741
- Soma Compound w/Codeine Tablets 2390
- Triaminic Expectorant w/Codeine .. 1996
- Tussi-Organidin Liquid 2391
- Tylenol with Codeine 1381

Codeine Polistirex (Potentiation of orthostatic hypotension).
- No products indexed under this heading.

Cortisone Acetate (Hypokalemia). Products include:
- Cortone Acetate Sterile Suspension 1437
- Cortone Acetate Tablets 1439

Deserpidine (Potentiated or additive action). Products include:
- Enduronyl 518
- Harmonyl Tablets 528
- Oreticyl 545

Deslanoside (Potential for exaggerated response of the heart to the toxic effects of digitalis).
- No products indexed under this heading.

Dexamethasone (Hypokalemia). Products include:
- AK-Trol Ointment & Suspension .... ⊙ 207
- Decadron Elixir 1445
- Decadron Tablets 1447
- Decaspray Topical Aerosol 1459
- Dexacidin .... ⊙ 272
- Maxidex Sterile Ophthalmic Suspension .... ⊙ 223
- Maxitrol Ophthalmic Ointment/Suspension .... ⊙ 223
- TobraDex Ophthalmic Suspension and Ointment .... ⊙ 228

Dexamethasone Acetate (Hypokalemia). Products include:
- Dalalone D.P. Injectable 999
- Decadron-LA Sterile Suspension 1457

Dexamethasone Sodium Phosphate (Hypokalemia). Products include:
- AK-Dex .... ⊙ 203
- Decadron Phosphate Respihaler 1454
- Decadron Phosphate Sterile Ophthalmic Ointment 1453
- Decadron Phosphate Sterile Ophthalmic Solution 1453
- Decadron Phosphate Topical Cream 1455
- Decadron Phosphate Turbinaire 1456
- Maxidex Sterile Ophthalmic Ointment .... ⊙ 222
- NeoDecadron Sterile Ophthalmic Ointment 1517
- NeoDecadron Sterile Ophthalmic Solution 1518
- NeoDecadron Topical Cream 1518

Dezocine (Potentiation of orthostatic hypotension).

Diazoxide (Potentiated or additive action). Products include:
- Hyperstat I.V. Injection 2095
- Proglycem 649

Diclofenac Sodium (Reduced diuretic, natriuretic, and antihypertensive effects of Moduretic). Products include:
- Voltaren Ophthalmic Sterile Ophthalmic Solution .... ⊙ 268
- Voltaren Tablets 1042

Digitoxin (Potential for exaggerated response of the heart to the toxic effects of digitalis). Products include:
- Crystodigin Tablets 1253

Digoxin (Potential for exaggerated response of the heart to the toxic effects of digitalis). Products include:
- Lanoxicaps 772
- Lanoxin Elixir Pediatric 775
- Lanoxin Injection 778
- Lanoxin Injection Pediatric 781
- Lanoxin Tablets 783

Doxazosin Mesylate (Potentiated or additive action; increased risk of hyperkalemia). Products include:
- Cardura Tablets 1941

Enalapril Maleate (Potentiated or additive action; increased risk of hyperkalemia). Products include:
- Vaseretic Tablets 1559
- Vasotec Tablets 1564

Enalaprilat (Potentiated or additive action; increased risk of hyperkalemia). Products include:
- Vasotec I.V. 1562

Etodolac (Reduced diuretic, natriuretic, and antihypertensive effects of Moduretic). Products include:
- Lodine Capsules 2468

Felodipine (Potentiated or additive action; increased risk of hyperkalemia). Products include:
- Plendil Extended-Release Tablets.... 1526

Fenoprofen Calcium (Reduced diuretic, natriuretic, and antihypertensive effects of Moduretic). Products include:
- Nalfon Pulvules & Tablets 919

Fentanyl (Potentiation of orthostatic hypotension). Products include:
- Duragesic Transdermal System........ 1133

Fentanyl Citrate (Potentiation of orthostatic hypotension). Products include:
- Innovar Injection 1141
- Sublimaze Injection 1146

Flurbiprofen (Reduced diuretic, natriuretic, and antihypertensive effects of Moduretic). Products include:
- Ansaid Tablets 2319

Fosinopril Sodium (Potentiated or additive action; increased risk of hyperkalemia). Products include:
- Monopril Tablets 1406

Furosemide (Potentiated or additive action). Products include:
- Lasix 1093

Glipizide (Dosage adjustment of the antidiabetic drug may be required). Products include:
- Glucotrol 1952

Glyburide (Dosage adjustment of the antidiabetic drug may be required). Products include:
- DiaBeta 1091
- Micronase Tablets 2350

Guanabenz Acetate (Potentiated or additive action). Products include:
- Wytensin Tablets 2542

Guanethidine Monosulfate (Potentiated or additive action). Products include:
- Esimil Tablets 864
- Ismelin Tablets 869

Hydralazine Hydrochloride (Potentiated or additive effects). Products include:
- Apresazide Capsules 854
- Apresoline Hydrochloride Parenteral (Ampuls) 856
- Apresoline Hydrochloride Tablets .. 855
- Apresoline-Esidrix Tablets 857
- Ser-Ap-Es Tablets 881
- Serpasil-Apresoline Tablets 884

Hydrocodone Bitartrate (Potentiation of orthostatic hypotension). Products include:
- Anexsia 5/500 Tablets 2196
- Anexsia 7.5/650 Tablets 2197
- Azdōne Tablets 844
- Codiclear DH Syrup 845
- Codimal DH Syrup 846
- Damason-P 1356
- Hycodan Syrup, Tablets 927
- Hycomine Compound Tablets 929
- Hycomine Syrup 927
- Hycotuss Expectorant Syrup 930
- Hydrocet Capsules 835
- Lortab ASA Tablets 2414
- Lortab 2412
- Ru-Tuss with Hydrocodone 694
- Triaminic Expectorant DH 1995
- Vicodin Tablets 1187
- Vicodin ES Tablets 1189
- Zydone Capsules 941

Hydrocodone Polistirex (Potentiation of orthostatic hypotension). Products include:
- Tussionex Extended-Release Suspension 988

Hydrocortisone (Hypokalemia). Products include:
- AK-Spore H.C. .... ⊙ 206
- Bactine Hydrocortisone Anti-Itch Cream .... ⊞ 625
- CaldeCORT Anti-Itch Hydrocortisone Spray .... ⊞ 560
- Carmol HC Cream 1% 2296
- Cortaid Spray .... ⊞ 735
- Cortenema 2244
- Cortisporin Ointment 758
- Cortisporin Ophthalmic Ointment Sterile 758
- Cortisporin Ophthalmic Suspension Sterile 759
- Cortisporin Otic Solution Sterile 760
- Cortisporin Otic Suspension Sterile 760
- Cortizone-5 Creme & Ointment .... ⊞ 732
- Dermolate Anti-Itch Cream .... ⊞ 697
- Eldecort Cream 1.0% 1113
- Eldecort Cream 1.0% and 2.5% 1113
- Fungoid HC Creme 1770
- Hydrocortone Tablets 1482
- Hytone 909
- LazerSporin-C Solution 1770
- Massengill Medicated Soft Cloth Towelettes 2192
- Nutracort Cream & Lotion 1684
- PediOtic Suspension Sterile 797
- Synacort Creams 1%, 2.5% 2296
- Vanoxide-HC Acne Lotion 911
- Vioform-Hydrocortisone Cream and Mild Cream 889
- Vioform-Hydrocortisone Ointment .. 889
- VōSoL HC Otic Solution 2392
- Vytone Cream 1% 911

Hydrocortisone Acetate (Hypokalemia). Products include:
- Analpram-HC Rectal Cream 1% and 2.5% 970
- Anusol-HC Cream 1690
- Anusol-HC Suppositories 1691
- Caldecort .... ⊞ 560

Carmol HC Cream 1% 2296
Chloromycetin Hydrocortisone Ophthalmic 1694
Coly-Mycin S Otic w/Neomycin & Hydrocortisone 1708
Cortaid .... ▣ 735
Cortef Feminine Itch Cream .... ▣ 735
Corticaine .... ▣ 682
Cortifoam 1827
Cortisporin Cream 757
Epifoam 1828
Gynecort 5 Creme .... ▣ 556
Hydrocortone Acetate Sterile Suspension 1479
Lanacort 5 Creme and Ointment .. ▣ 557
Mantadil Cream 789
Ophthocort .... ◉ 301
Orabase HCA Oral Paste 890
Pramosone Cream, Lotion & Ointment 971
ProctoCream-HC 1834
Proctofoam-HC 1835

Hydrocortisone Sodium Phosphate (Hypokalemia). Products include:
Hydrocortone Phosphate Injection, Sterile 1481

Hydrocortisone Sodium Succinate (Hypokalemia). Products include:
Solu-Cortef Sterile Powder 2361

Hydroflumethiazide (Potentiated or additive action). Products include:
Diucardin Tablets 2450
Saluron 718
Salutensin/Salutensin-Demi 719

Ibuprofen (Reduced diuretic, natriuretic, and antihypertensive effects of Moduretic). Products include:
Advil Cold & Sinus Caplets (formerly CoAdvil) 2416
Advil Ibuprofen Tablets and Caplets 2416
Children's Advil Suspension 2426
CoAdvil .... ▣ 748
Dristan Sinus Caplets 2419
Haltran Tablets .... ▣ 668
Ibuprofen .... ▣ 631
Medipren ibuprofen Caplets and Tablets 1362
Midol 200 Cramp Relief Formula .. ▣ 570
Motrin Tablets 2351
Motrin IB Caplets and Tablets .... ▣ 736
Nuprin Ibuprofen/Analgesic Tablets & Caplets 752
PediaProfen Suspension 1363
Rufen Tablets 691
Trendar Ibuprofen Tablets .... ▣ 756

Indapamide (Potentiated or additive action). Products include:
Lozol Tablets 1843

Indomethacin (Reduced diuretic, natriuretic, and antihypertensive effects of Moduretic; increased serum potassium levels of both drugs). Products include:
Indocin 1487

Indomethacin Sodium Trihydrate (Reduced diuretic, natriuretic, and antihypertensive effects of Moduretic; increased serum potassium levels of both drugs). Products include:
Indocin I.V. 1490

Insulin, Human (Altered insulin requirements).
No products indexed under this heading.

Insulin, Human Isophane Suspension (Altered insulin requirements). Products include:
Humulin N, 100 Units 1270

Insulin, Human NPH (Altered insulin requirements). Products include:
Insulatard NPH Human 1627
Novolin N 1627
Novolin N PenFill Cartridges 1628
Novolin N Prefilled 1628

Insulin, Human Regular (Altered insulin requirements). Products include:
Humulin BR, 100 Units 1268
Humulin R, 100 Units 1272
Novolin R 1627
Novolin R PenFill Cartridges 1628
Novolin R Prefilled 1629
Velosulin Human 1628

Insulin, Human, Zinc Suspension (Altered insulin requirements). Products include:
Humulin L, 100 Units 1268
Humulin U, 100 Units 1272
Novolin L 1627

Insulin, NPH (Altered insulin requirements). Products include:
NPH, 40 & 100 Units 1273
Beef NPH, 100 Units 1274
Pork NPH, 100 Units 1275
Insulatard NPH 1626
NPH Insulin 1626
NPH Purified Pork Isophane Insulin 1626

Insulin, Regular (Altered insulin requirements). Products include:
Regular, 40 & 100 Units 1273
Beef Regular, 100 Units 1275
Pork Regular, 100 Units 1275
Pork Regular (Concentrated), 500 Units 1276
Regular Insulin 1625
Regular Purified Pork Insulin 1626
Velosulin 1627

Insulin, Zinc Crystals (Altered insulin requirements). Products include:
NPH, 40 & 100 Units 1273

Insulin, Zinc Suspension (Altered insulin requirements). Products include:
Lente, 40 & 100 Units 1272
Protamine, Zinc, 40 & 100 Units 1273
Lente Iletin I 1272
Beef Lente, 100 Units 1274
Beef Protamine Zinc, 100 Units 1274
Pork Lente, 100 Units 1275
Pork, Protamine, Zinc, 100 Units 1275
Lente Insulin 1626
Lente Purified Pork Insulin 1626
Semilente Insulin 1625
Ultralente Insulin 1626

Isradipine (Potentiated or additive action; increased risk of hyperkalemia). Products include:
DynaCirc Capsules 2004

Ketoprofen (Reduced diuretic, natriuretic, and antihypertensive effects of Moduretic). Products include:
Orudis Capsules 2488

Ketorolac Tromethamine (Reduced diuretic, natriuretic, and antihypertensive effects of Moduretic). Products include:
Toradol IM Injection 2302

Labetalol Hydrochloride (Potentiated or additive action). Products include:
Normodyne Injection 2108
Normodyne Tablets 2110
Normozide Tablets 2112
Trandate HCT Tablets 579
Trandate Injection 577
Trandate Tablets 579

Levorphanol Tartrate (Potentiation of orthostatic hypotension). Products include:
Levo-Dromoran 1906

Lisinopril (Potentiated or additive action; increased risk of hyperkalemia). Products include:
Prinivil Tablets 1538
Prinzide Tablets 1540
Zestoretic 2274
Zestril Tablets 2277

Lithium Carbonate (High risk of lithium toxicity). Products include:
Eskalith 2214
Lithane Tablets 1596
Lithium Carbonate Capsules & Tablets 1984
Lithobid Tablets 870

Lithium Citrate (High risk of lithium toxicity). Products include:
Cibalith-S 870

Mecamylamine Hydrochloride (Potentiated or additive action). Products include:
Inversine Tablets 1492

Meclofenamate Sodium (Reduced diuretic, natriuretic, and antihypertensive effects of Modiuretic). Products include:
Meclomen Capsules 1739

Mefenamic Acid (Reduced diuretic, natriuretic, and antihypertensive effects of Modiuretic). Products include:
Ponstel 1758

Meperidine Hydrochloride (Potentiation of orthostatic hypotension). Products include:
Demerol 2047
Mepergan Injection 2479

Mephobarbital (Potentiation of orthostatic hypotension). Products include:
Mebaral Tablets 2061

Methadone Hydrochloride (Potentiation of orthostatic hypotension). Products include:
Dolophine Hydrochloride Ampoules & Vials 1260
Dolophine Hydrochloride Tablets 1261
Methadone Hydrochloride Diskets .. 1284
Methadone Hydrochloride Oral Solution & Tablets 1987

Methyclothiazide (Potentiated or additive action). Products include:
Enduron Tablets 517
Enduronyl 518

Methyldopa (Potentiated or additive action). Products include:
Aldoclor Tablets 1413
Aldomet Oral 1415
Aldoril Tablets 1418

Methyldopate Hydrochloride (Potentiated or additive action). Products include:
Aldomet Ester HCl Injection 1417

Methylprednisolone Acetate (Hypokalemia). Products include:
Depo-Medrol Sterile Aqueous Suspension 2334

Methylprednisolone Sodium Succinate (Hypokalemia). Products include:
Solu-Medrol Sterile Powder 2363

Metolazone (Potentiated or additive action). Products include:
Diulo 2129
Mykrox ½ mg Tablets 984
Zaroxolyn Tablets 989

Metoprolol Tartrate (Potentiated or additive action). Products include:
Lopressor Ampuls 1032
Lopressor HCT Tablets 1034
Lopressor Tablets 1032

Metyrosine (Potentiated or additive action). Products include:
Demser Capsules 1460

Minoxidil (Potentiated or additive action). Products include:
Loniten Tablets 2346
Rogaine Topical Solution 2357

Morphine Sulfate (Potentiation of orthostatic hypotension). Products include:
Astramorph/PF Injection, USP (Preservative-Free) 618
Duramorph 960
Infumorph 200 and Infumorph 500 Sterile Solutions 962
MS Contin Tablets 1814
MSIR 1817
Oramorph SR (Morphine Sulfate Sustained Release Tablets) 1988
Roxanol 1991

Nadolol (Potentiated or additive action). Products include:
Corgard Tablets 701
Corzide Tablets 702

Naproxen (Reduced diuretic, natriuretic, and antihypertensive effects of Moduretic). Products include:
Naprosyn 2297

Naproxen Sodium (Reduced diuretic, natriuretic, and antihypertensive effects of Moduretic). Products include:
Anaprox and Anaprox DS Tablets 2288

Nicardipine Hydrochloride (Potentiated or additive action). Products include:
Cardene Capsules 2290

Nitroglycerin (Potentiated or additive action). Products include:
Deponit NTG Transdermal Delivery System 2143
Minitran Transdermal Delivery System 1312
Nitro-Bid Ointment 1339
Nitro-Bid Capsules 1338
Nitrodisc 2176
Nitro-Dur (nitroglycerin) Transdermal Infusion System 1164
Nitrogard Tablets 1004
Nitrolingual Spray 1846
Nitrostat Tablets 1743
Transderm-Nitro Transdermal Therapeutic System 2283

Norepinephrine Bitartrate (Possible decreased response to pressor amines). Products include:
Levophed Bitartrate Injection 2054

Opium Alkaloids (Potentiation of orthostatic hypotension). Products include:
B & O No. 15A & No. 16A Supprettes 2395
Pantopon Injectable 1911

Oxycodone Hydrochloride (Potentiation of orthostatic hypotension). Products include:
Percocet Tablets 950
Percodan 951
Roxicodone Tablets, Oral Solution & Intensol (Oxycodone) 1992
Tylox Capsules 1382

Penbutolol Sulfate (Potentiated or additive action). Products include:
Levatol 1832

Pentobarbital Sodium (Potentiation of orthostatic hypotension). Products include:
Nembutal Sodium Capsules 534
Nembutal Sodium Solution 536
Nembutal Sodium Suppositories 538

Phenobarbital (Potentiation of orthostatic hypotension). Products include:
Arco-Lase Plus Tablets 607
Bellergal-S Tablets 1998
Bronkolixir .... ▣ 761
Bronkotabs Tablets .... ▣ 762
Donnatal 1858
Donnatal Extentabs 1859
Donnatal Tablets 1858
Donnazyme Tablets 1860
Kinesed Tablets 2272
Phenobarbital Elixir and Tablets 1293
Primatene Tablets-P Formula 2421
Quadrinal Tablets 1183
Tedral SA 1765

Phenoxybenzamine Hydrochloride (Potentiated or additive action). Products include:
Dibenzyline Capsules 2207

Phentolamine Mesylate (Potentiated or additive action). Products include:
Regitine 878

Phenylbutazone (Reduced diuretic, natriuretic, and antihypertensive effects of Moduretic). Products include:
Butazolidin Capsules & Tablets 1027

Pindolol (Potentiated or additive action). Products include:
Visken Tablets 2036

Piroxicam (Reduced diuretic, natriuretic, and antihypertensive effects of Moduretic). Products include:
- Feldene Capsules ... 1777

Polythiazide (Potentiated or additive action). Products include:
- Minizide Capsules ... 1779
- Renese Tablets ... 1785
- Renese-R Tablets ... 1786

Potassium Acid Phosphate (Potential for rapid increase in serum potassium levels). Products include:
- K-Phos M.F. Tablets ... 659
- K-Phos Original Formula 'Sodium Free' Tablets ... 660
- K-Phos No. 2 Tablets ... 659

Potassium Bicarbonate (Potential for rapid increase in serum potassium levels). Products include:
- Alka-Seltzer Advanced Formula Antacid & Non-Aspirin Pain Reliever ... ▣ 620
- Alka-Seltzer Effervescent Antacid ▣ 622
- K-Lyte ... 707
- Klorvess Effervescent Granules ... 2010
- Klorvess Effervescent Tablets ... 2011

Potassium Chloride (Potential for rapid increase in serum potassium levels). Products include:
- Chlor-3 Condiment ... 994
- K-Dur Microburst Release System (potassium chloride, USP) E.R. Tablets ... 1163
- K-Lor Powder Packets ... 531
- K-Lyte ... 707
- K-Norm Capsules ... 982
- K-Tab Filmtab ... 532
- Kato Potassium Supplement ... 1114
- Klor-Con 8/Klor-Con 10 Extended-release Tablets ... 2374
- Klorvess Effervescent Granules ... 2010
- Klorvess Effervescent Tablets ... 2011
- Klorvess 10% Liquid ... 2010
- Klotrix ... 708
- Kolyum Liquid ... 983
- Micro-K ... 1863
- Micro-K LS Packets ... 1864
- NuLYTELY ... 699
- Oral Rehydration Salts, Citrate ... 1150
- Rum-K Syrup ... 995
- Slow-K Tablets ... 2281
- Ten-K Controlled-Release Tablets ... 2282
- Thermotabs ... ▣ 619

Potassium Citrate (Potential for rapid increase in serum potassium levels). Products include:
- Alka-Seltzer Effervescent Antacid .. 1570
- K-Lyte ... 707
- Polycitra Syrup ... 2424
- Polycitra-K ... 2424
- Polycitra-LC—Sugar-Free ... 2424
- Ricelyte, Rice-Based Oral Electrolyte Maintenance Solution ... ▣ 613

Potassium Gluconate (Potential for rapid increase in serum potassium levels). Products include:
- Kolyum Liquid ... 983

Potassium Phosphate, Dibasic (Potential for rapid increase in serum potassium levels). Products include:
- Neutra-Phos ... 2423

Potassium Phosphate, Monobasic (Potential for rapid increase in serum potassium levels). Products include:
- K-Phos M.F. Tablets ... 659
- K-Phos Neutral Tablets ... 660
- Neutra-Phos ... 2423

Prazosin Hydrochloride (Potentiated or additive action). Products include:
- Minipress Capsules ... 1778
- Minizide Capsules ... 1779

Prednisolone Acetate (Hypokalemia). Products include:
- AK-Cide Sterile Ophthalmic Ointment & Suspension ... ⊙ 202
- Blephamide Liquifilm Sterile Ophthalmic Suspension ... 586
- Blephamide S.O.P. Sterile Ophthalmic Ointment ... 586
- Cetapred Ointment ... ⊙ 220
- ⅛% Econopred & 1% Econopred Plus ... ⊙ 217
- Isopto Cetapred Suspension ... ⊙ 220
- Metimyd ... ⊙ 306
- Poly-Pred Liquifilm ... ⊙ 250
- Pred Forte ... ⊙ 252
- Pred Mild ... ⊙ 254
- Pred-G Liquifilm Sterile Ophthalmic Suspension ... ⊙ 252
- Pred-G S.O.P. Sterile Ophthalmic Ointment ... ⊙ 253
- Vasocidin Ointment ... ⊙ 275

Prednisolone Sodium Phosphate (Hypokalemia). Products include:
- AK-Pred ... ⊙ 205
- Hydeltrasol Injection, Sterile ... 1476
- Inflamase ... ⊙ 274
- Pediapred Oral Liquid ... 987
- Vasocidin Ophthalmic Solution ... ⊙ 276

Prednisolone Tebutate (Hypokalemia). Products include:
- Hydeltra-T.B.A. Sterile Suspension 1478

Prednisone (Hypokalemia). Products include:
- Deltasone Tablets ... 2332

Propoxyphene Hydrochloride (Potentiation of orthostatic hypotension). Products include:
- Darvon ... 1256
- Wygesic Tablets ... 2540

Propoxyphene Napsylate (Potentiation of orthostatic hypotension). Products include:
- Darvon-N/Darvocet-N ... 1254

Propranolol Hydrochloride (Potentiated or additive action). Products include:
- Inderal ... 2459
- Inderal LA Long Acting Capsules ... 2461
- Inderide Tablets ... 2463
- Inderide LA Long Acting Capsules .. 2465

Ramipril (Potentiated or additive action; increased risk of hyperkalemia). Products include:
- Altace Capsules ... 1086

Rauwolfia Serpentina (Potentiated or additive action). Products include:
- Raudixin Tablets ... 1803
- Rauzide Tablets ... 1804

Rescinnamine (Potentiated or additive action).
- No products indexed under this heading.

Reserpine (Potentiated or additive action). Products include:
- Diupres Tablets ... 1461
- Hydromox R Tablets ... 1209
- Hydropres Tablets ... 1485
- Renese-R Tablets ... 1786
- Salutensin/Salutensin-Demi ... 719
- Ser-Ap-Es Tablets ... 881
- Serpasil Tablets ... 883
- Serpasil-Apresoline Tablets ... 884
- Serpasil-Esidrix Tablets ... 886

Secobarbital Sodium (Potentiation of orthostatic hypotension). Products include:
- Seconal Sodium Pulvules ... 1296

Sodium Nitroprusside (Potentiated or additive action). Products include:
- Nipride I.V. Infusion ... 1909

Spironolactone (Potential for rapid increase in serum potassium levels). Products include:
- Aldactazide ... 2150
- Aldactone ... 2152

Sufentanil Citrate (Potentiation of orthostatic hypotension). Products include:
- Sufenta Injection ... 1147

Sulindac (Reduced diuretic, natriuretic, and antihypertensive effects of Moduretic). Products include:
- Clinoril Tablets ... 1433

Terazosin Hydrochloride (Potentiated or additive action). Products include:
- Hytrin Tablets ... 529

Thiamylal Sodium (Potentiation of orthostatic hypotension). Products include:
- Surital Ampoules, Steri-Vials ... 1764

Timolol Maleate (Potentiated or additive action). Products include:
- Blocadren Tablets ... 1429
- Timolide Tablets ... 1547
- Timoptic in Ocudose ... 1552
- Timoptic Sterile Ophthalmic Solution ... 1550

Tolazamide (Dosage adjustment of the antidiabetic drug may be required). Products include:
- Tolinase Tablets ... 2365

Tolbutamide (Dosage adjustment of the antidiabetic drug may be required). Products include:
- Orinase Tablets ... 2354

Tolmetin Sodium (Reduced diuretic, natriuretic, and antihypertensive effects of Moduretic). Products include:
- Tolectin (200, 400 and 600 mg) .. 1379

Triamcinolone (Hypokalemia).
- No products indexed under this heading.

Triamcinolone Acetonide (Hypokalemia). Products include:
- Aristocort A ... 1010
- Azmacort Inhaler ... 1837
- Kenalog Cream, Lotion & Ointment 2401
- Kenalog-10 Injection ... 2402
- Kenalog-40 Injection ... 2403
- Kenalog in Orabase ... 604
- Kenalog Spray ... 2401
- Mycolog II Cream and Ointment ... 2407
- Mytrex Cream & Ointment ... 2080
- Nasacort Nasal Inhaler ... 1844

Triamcinolone Diacetate (Hypokalemia). Products include:
- Aristocort Suspension ... 1008

Triamcinolone Hexacetonide (Hypokalemia). Products include:
- Aristospan Suspension ... 1011

Triamterene (Potential for rapid increase in serum potassium levels). Products include:
- Dyazide Capsules ... 2208
- Dyrenium Capsules ... 2210
- Maxzide ... 1215

Trimethaphan Camsylate (Potentiated or additive action). Products include:
- Arfonad Ampuls ... 1887

Tubocurarine Chloride (Increased responsiveness to tubocurarine).
- No products indexed under this heading.

Food Interactions

Diet, potassium-rich (Potential for rapid increases in serum potassium levels).

MOISTURE DROPS
(Dextran 70, Glycerin, Hydroxypropyl Methylcellulose) ... ⊙ 258
No interactions described in labeling.

MOISTUREL CREAM
(Emollient) ... 2407
No interactions described in labeling.

MOISTUREL LOTION
(Emollient) ... 2407
No interactions described in labeling.

MOL-IRON TABLETS
(Ferrous Sulfate) ... ▣ 703
No interactions described in labeling.

MOL-IRON W/VITAMIN C TABLETS
(Ferrous Sulfate, Vitamin C) ... ▣ 703
No interactions described in labeling.

MOMENTUM MUSCULAR BACKACHE FORMULA
(Aspirin, Phenyltoloxamine Citrate) ▣ 751
No interactions described in labeling.

MONISTAT DUAL-PAK
(Miconazole) ... 1657
No interactions described in labeling.

MONISTAT I.V.
(Miconazole) ... 1143
May interact with oral hypoglycemic agents, anticoagulants, and certain other agents. Compounds in these categories include:

Carbamazepine (May alter metabolism of one or both drugs). Products include:
- Tegretol Chewable Tablets ... 654
- Tegretol Suspension ... 656
- Tegretol Tablets ... 654

Chlorpropamide (Severe hypoglycemia). Products include:
- Diabinese Tablets ... 1775

Cyclosporine (Potential for increased blood levels of cyclosporine). Products include:
- Sandimmune ... 2024

Dicumarol (Enhanced anticoagulant effect). Products include:
- Dicumarol Tablets ... 516

Glipizide (Severe hypoglycemia). Products include:
- Glucotrol ... 1952

Glyburide (Severe hypoglycemia). Products include:
- DiaBeta ... 1091
- Micronase Tablets ... 2350

Heparin Calcium (Enhanced anticoagulant effect). Products include:
- Calciparine Injection ... 925

Heparin Sodium (Enhanced anticoagulant effect). Products include:
- Heparin Lock Flush Solution ... 2456
- Heparin Sodium Vials ... 1264
- Heparin Sodium Injection ... 2457
- Heparin Sodium Injection, USP, Sterile Solution ... 2342

Phenytoin (May alter metabolism of one or both drugs). Products include:
- Dilantin Infatabs ... 1710
- Dilantin-30 Pediatric/Dilantin-125 Suspension ... 1713

Phenytoin Sodium (May alter metabolism of one or both drugs). Products include:
- Dilantin Kapseals ... 1708
- Dilantin Parenteral ... 1712
- Dilantin with Phenobarbital Kapseals ... 1715

Rifampin (May reduce blood levels of an imidazole derivative (miconazole)). Products include:
- Rifadin ... 1345
- Rifamate Capsules ... 1347
- Rimactane Capsules ... 879

Tolazamide (Severe hypoglycemia). Products include:
- Tolinase Tablets ... 2365

Tolbutamide (Severe hypoglycemia). Products include:
- Orinase Tablets ... 2354

Warfarin Sodium (Enhanced anticoagulant effect). Products include:
- Coumadin Injection & Tablets ... 944
- Panwarfin Tablets ... 547

MONISTAT 3 VAGINAL SUPPOSITORIES
(Miconazole) ... 1657
No interactions described in labeling.

MONISTAT-DERM (MICONAZOLE NITRATE) CREAM
(Miconazole Nitrate) ... 1679
No interactions described in labeling.

MONOCID INJECTION
(Cefonicid Sodium) 2217
May interact with aminoglycosides. Compounds in this category include:

Amikacin Sulfate (Concomitant administration may result in nephrotoxicity). Products include:
Amikin Injectable 602

Gentamicin Sulfate (Concomitant administration may result in nephrotoxicity). Products include:
Garamycin Injectable 2093
Garamycin Ophthalmic .... ◉ 305
Genoptic Liquifilm Sterile Ophthalmic Solution .... ◉ 247
Genoptic S.O.P. Sterile Ophthalmic Ointment .... ◉ 247
Gentacidin Ointment .... ◉ 273
Gentacidin Solution .... ◉ 273
Gentak Ointment & Solution .... ◉ 208
G-myticin Creme and Ointment 0.1% 1770
Pred-G Liquifilm Sterile Ophthalmic Suspension .... ◉ 252
Pred-G S.O.P. Sterile Ophthalmic Ointment .... ◉ 253

Kanamycin Sulfate (Concomitant administration may result in nephrotoxicity). Products include:
Kantrex Injection 601
Kantrex Pediatric Injection 601

Probenecid (Produces higher peak serum levels). Products include:
Benemid Tablets 1426
ColBENEMID Tablets 1436
Wycillin Injection and Probenecid Tablets 2539

Streptomycin Sulfate (Concomitant administration may result in nephrotoxicity).
No products indexed under this heading.

Tobramycin Sulfate (Concomitant administration may result in nephrotoxicity). Products include:
Nebcin Vials, Hyporets & ADD-Vantage 1286

MONOCLATE-P FACTOR VIII:C, PASTEURIZED, ANTIHEMOPHILIC FACTOR (HUMAN)
(Antihemophilic Factor (Human)) 612
No interactions described in labeling.

MONODOX CAPSULES
(Doxycycline Monohydrate) 1630
May interact with barbiturates, oral contraceptives, penicillins, antacids containing aluminium, calcium and magnesium, oral anticoagulants, and certain other agents. Compounds in these categories include:

Aluminum Carbonate Gel (Absorption of tetracyclines is impaired). Products include:
Basaljel 2438

Aluminum Hydroxide (Absorption of tetracyclines is impaired). Products include:
Cama Arthritis Pain Reliever .... ▣ 685
Gaviscon Extra Strength Relief Formula Liquid Antacid .... ▣ 594
Gaviscon Extra Strength Relief Formula Antacid Tablets .... ▣ 594
Gaviscon Liquid Antacid .... ▣ 594
Gelusil Liquid & Tablets .... ▣ 639
Extra Strength Maalox Plus Suspension 1850
Maalox TC Suspension 1851
Maalox Plus Tablets .... ▣ 655
Extra Strength Maalox Plus Tablets 1850
Nephrox Suspension .... ▣ 563
WinGel Liquid & Tablets .... ▣ 761

Aluminum Hydroxide Gel (Absorption of tetracyclines is impaired). Products include:
ALternaGEL Liquid 1154
Aludrox Oral Suspension 2428
Amphojel Suspension 2429
Amphojel Suspension without Flavor 2429
Mylanta Liquid 1155
Mylanta Double Strength Liquid 1155

Aluminum Hydroxide Gel, Dried (Absorption of tetracyclines is impaired). Products include:
Alu-Tab/Alu-Cap 1309
Amphojel Tablets 2429
Ascriptin A/D Caplets 1850
Regular Strength Ascriptin Tablets 1850
Gaviscon Antacid Tablets .... ▣ 593
Gaviscon-2 Antacid Tablets .... ▣ 594
Mylanta Tablets 1155
Mylanta Double Strength Tablets 1155

Amoxicillin (Interference with penicillins' bactericidal action). Products include:
Amoxil 2193
Augmentin Tablets, Powder for Oral Suspension, and Chewable Tablets 2198

Ampicillin Sodium (Interference with penicillins' bactericidal action). Products include:
Unasyn 1965

Aprobarbital (Decreases the half-life of doxycycline). Products include:
Alurate Elixir 1883

Azlocillin Sodium (Interference with penicillins' bactericidal action).
No products indexed under this heading.

Bacampicillin Hydrochloride (Interference with penicillins' bactericidal action). Products include:
Spectrobid Tablets & Powder for Oral Suspension 1961

Butabarbital (Decreases the half-life of doxycycline). Products include:
Pyridium Plus 1764

Butalbital (Decreases the half-life of doxycycline). Products include:
Esgic-Plus Tablets 1002
Esgic Tablets & Capsules 1001
Fioricet Tablets 2006
Fiorinal Capsules 2007
Fiorinal with Codeine Capsules 2008
Fiorinal Tablets 2007
Phrenilin 838
Sedapap Tablets 50 mg/650 mg .. 1360

Carbenicillin Disodium (Interference with penicillins' bactericidal action).

Carbenicillin Indanyl Sodium (Interference with penicillins' bactericidal action). Products include:
Geocillin Tablets 1951

Dicumarol (Depressed plasma prothrombin activity). Products include:
Dicumarol Tablets 516

Dihydroxyaluminum Sodium Carbonate (Absorption of tetracyclines is impaired). Products include:
Rolaids .... ▣ 743

Ethinyl Estradiol (Concurrent use may render oral contraceptives less effective). Products include:
Brevicon 2304
Demulen 2161
Estinyl Tablets 2085
Jenest-28 Tablets 1636
Levlen/Tri-Levlen 665
Lo/Ovral Tablets 2471
Lo/Ovral-28 Tablets 2476
Loestrin 1728
Modicon 1667
Nordette-21 Tablets 2481
Nordette-28 Tablets 2483
Norethin 2133
Norinyl 2304
Norlestrin 1746
Ortho-Cyclen Tablets 1658
Ortho-Novum 1667
Ovcon 1391
Ovral Tablets 2490
Ovral-28 Tablets 2491
Levlen/Tri-Levlen 665
Tri-Norinyl 2304
Triphasil-21 Tablets 2527
Triphasil-28 Tablets 2532

Ethynodiol Diacetate (Concurrent use may render oral contraceptives less effective). Products include:
Demulen 2161

Iron Preparations (Absorption of tetracyclines is impaired). Products include:
Allbee C-800 Plus Iron Tablets .... ▣ 670
Bugs Bunny Children's Chewable Vitamins + Minerals with Iron and Calcium (Sugar Free) .... ▣ 626
Bugs Bunny Plus Iron Children's Chewable Vitamins (Sugar Free) ▣ 625
FemIron Multi-Vitamins and Iron .... ▣ 617
Ferancee Chewable Tablets 1155
Ferancee-HP Tablets 1155
Fergon .... ▣ 758
Fero-Folic-500 Filmtab 527
Fero-Grad-500 Filmtab 528
Fero-Gradumet Filmtab 528
Ferro-Sequels 1203
Flintstones Children's Chewable Vitamins Plus Iron .... ▣ 625
Flintstones Complete With Calcium, Iron & Minerals Children's Chewable Vitamins .... ▣ 626
Geritol Extend Tablets and Caplets .... ▣ 717
Geritol Liquid - High Potency Iron & Vitamin Tonic .... ▣ 717
Iberet Tablets 531
Iberet-500 Liquid 531
Iberet-Folic-500 Filmtab 527
Iberet-Liquid 531
Incremin w/Iron Syrup .... ▣ 588
Irospan 972
Mol-Iron .... ▣ 703
Niferex 847
Niferex-150 Forte Capsules 847
Niferex Forte Elixir 847
Niferex 847
Niferex-PN Tablets 847
One-A-Day Maximum Formula Vitamins and Minerals .... ▣ 627
Peritinic Tablets .... ▣ 589
Poly-Vi-Flor with Iron 1399
Poly-Vi-Flor with Iron Drops 1399
Poly-Vi-Sol Vitamins with Iron, Chewable Tablets and Circus Shapes Chewable .... ▣ 612
Poly-Vi-Sol Vitamins with Iron, Drops .... ▣ 612
SMA Iron Fortified Infant Formula, Concentrated, Ready-to-Feed and Powder .... ▣ 767
Slow Fe Tablets .... ▣ 552
The Stuart Formula Tablets .... ▣ 581
Stuartinic Tablets 1157
Surbex-750 with Iron .... ▣ 503
Tri-Vi-Flor 0.25 mg Vitamins with Iron and Fluoride Drops 1401
Unicap Plus Iron Vitamin Formula Tablets .... ▣ 738
Vi-Daylin ADC Vitamins + Iron Drops 1980
Vi-Daylin Multivitamin + Iron Drops 1981
Vi-Daylin/F ADC Vitamins + Iron Drops With Fluoride 1981
Vi-Daylin/F Multivitamin + Iron Drops With Fluoride 1981
Vi-Daylin Multivitamin + Iron Chewable Tablets 1982
Vi-Daylin/F Multivitamin + Iron Chewable Tablets With Fluoride .. 1982
Vi-Daylin Multivitamin + Iron Liquid 1983

Levonorgestrel (Concurrent use may render oral contraceptives less effective). Products include:
Levlen/Tri-Levlen 665
Nordette-21 Tablets 2481
Nordette-28 Tablets 2483
Norplant System 2484
Levlen/Tri-Levlen 665
Triphasil-21 Tablets 2527
Triphasil-28 Tablets 2532

Magaldrate (Absorption of tetracyclines is impaired). Products include:
Riopan Antacid Chew Tablets .... ▣ 754
Riopan Antacid Chew Tablets in Rollpacks .... ▣ 754
Riopan Antacid Suspension 2421
Riopan Antacid Swallow Tablets 2421
Riopan Plus Chew Tablets 2422
Riopan Plus Chew Tablets in Rollpack 2422
Riopan Plus 2 Chew Tablets, Mint Flavor, Cherry Flavor 2422
Riopan Plus Suspension 2422
Riopan Plus 2 Suspension, Mint Flavor, Cherry Flavor 2422

Magnesium Hydroxide (Absorption of tetracyclines is impaired). Products include:
Aludrox Oral Suspension 2428
Ascriptin A/D Caplets 1850
Regular Strength Ascriptin Tablets 1850
Di-Gel Antacid/Anti-Gas .... ▣ 697
Gelusil Liquid & Tablets .... ▣ 639
Haley's M-O, Regular & Flavored .. ▣ 569
Extra Strength Maalox Plus Suspension 1850
Maalox TC Suspension 1851
Maalox Plus Tablets .... ▣ 655
Extra Strength Maalox Plus Tablets 1850
Mylanta Liquid 1155
Mylanta Tablets 1155
Mylanta Double Strength Liquid 1155
Mylanta Double Strength Tablets 1155
Concentrated Phillips' Milk of Magnesia .... ▣ 573
Phillips' Milk of Magnesia Liquid .... ▣ 572
Phillips' Milk of Magnesia Tablets ▣ 573
WinGel Liquid & Tablets .... ▣ 761

Magnesium Oxide (Absorption of tetracyclines is impaired). Products include:
Bayer Plus Aspirin Tablets .... ▣ 567
Beelith Tablets 659
Bufferin Analgesic Tablets and Caplets .... ▣ 524
Cama Arthritis Pain Reliever .... ▣ 685
Mag-Ox 400 673
Uro-Mag 673

Mephobarbital (Decreases the half-life of doxycycline). Products include:
Mebaral Tablets 2061

Mestranol (Concurrent use may render oral contraceptives less effective). Products include:
Enovid 2161
Norethin 2133
Norinyl 2304
Ortho-Novum 1667

Methoxyflurane (Potential for fatal renal toxicity).
No products indexed under this heading.

Mezlocillin Sodium (Interference with penicillins' bactericidal action). Products include:
Mezlin 1597
Mezlin Pharmacy Bulk Package 1599

Nafcillin Sodium (Interference with penicillins' bactericidal action). Products include:
Unipen 2533

Norethindrone (Concurrent use may render oral contraceptives less effective). Products include:
Brevicon 2304
Jenest-28 Tablets 1636
Micronor Tablets 1667
Modicon 1667
Norethin 2133
Norinyl 2304
Norlutin 1755
Nor-Q D Tablets 2304
Ortho-Novum 1667
Ovcon 1391
Tri-Norinyl 2304

Norethynodrel (Concurrent use may render oral contraceptives less effective). Products include:
Enovid 2161

Norgestimate (Concurrent use may render oral contraceptives less effective). Products include:
Ortho-Cyclen Tablets 1658

Norgestrel (Concurrent use may render oral contraceptives less effective). Products include:
Lo/Ovral Tablets 2471
Lo/Ovral-28 Tablets 2476
Ovral Tablets 2490
Ovral-28 Tablets 2491
Ovrette Tablets 2492

Penicillin G Potassium (Interference with penicillins' bactericidal action). Products include:
- Pfizerpen for Injection 1957

Penicillin G Procaine (Interference with penicillins' bactericidal action). Products include:
- Bicillin C-R Injection 2438
- Bicillin C-R 900/300 Injection 2440
- Pfizerpen-AS Aqueous Suspension 1959
- Wycillin Injection 2537
- Wycillin Injection and Probenecid Tablets 2539

Penicillin G Sodium (Interference with penicillins' bactericidal action).
- No products indexed under this heading.

Penicillin G, Benzathine (Interference with penicillins' bactericidal action). Products include:
- Bicillin C-R Injection 2438
- Bicillin C-R 900/300 Injection 2440
- Bicillin L-A Injection 2442

Penicillin (Repository) (Interference with penicillins' bactericidal action). Products include:
- Bicillin C-R Injection 2438
- Bicillin C-R 900/300 Injection 2440
- Bicillin L-A Injection 2442

Penicillin V Potassium (Interference with penicillins' bactericidal action).
- No products indexed under this heading.

Pentobarbital Sodium (Decreases the half-life of doxycycline). Products include:
- Nembutal Sodium Capsules 534
- Nembutal Sodium Solution 536
- Nembutal Sodium Suppositories 538

Phenobarbital (Decreases the half-life of doxycycline). Products include:
- Arco-Lase Plus Tablets 607
- Bellergal-S Tablets 1998
- Bronkolixir ■ 761
- Bronkotabs Tablets ■ 762
- Donnatal 1858
- Donnatal Extentabs 1859
- Donnatal Tablets 1858
- Donnazyme Tablets 1860
- Kinesed Tablets 2272
- Phenobarbital Elixir and Tablets 1293
- Primatene Tablets-P Formula 2421
- Quadrinal Tablets 1183
- Tedral SA 1765

Phenytoin (Decreases the half-life of doxycycline). Products include:
- Dilantin Infatabs 1710
- Dilantin-30 Pediatric/Dilantin-125 Suspension 1713

Phenytoin Sodium (Decreases the half-life of doxycycline). Products include:
- Dilantin Kapseals 1708
- Dilantin Parenteral 1712
- Dilantin with Phenobarbital Kapseals 1715

Secobarbital Sodium (Decreases the half-life of doxycycline). Products include:
- Seconal Sodium Pulvules 1296

Thiamylal Sodium (Decreases the half-life of doxycycline). Products include:
- Surital Ampoules, Steri-Vials 1764

Ticarcillin Disodium (Interference with penicillins' bactericidal action). Products include:
- Ticar for Injection 2236
- Timentin for Injection 2239

Warfarin Sodium (Depressed plasma prothrombin activity). Products include:
- Coumadin Injection & Tablets 944
- Panwarfin Tablets 547

MONO-GESIC TABLETS

(Salsalate, Salicylsalicylic Acid) 846
May interact with thyroid preparations, salicylates, antigout agents, anticoagulants, oral hypoglycemic agents, corticosteroids, and penicillins. Compounds in these categories include:

Allopurinol (Uricosuric action of gout drugs antagonized). Products include:
- Zyloprim Tablets 830

Amoxicillin (Competition for protein-binding sites). Products include:
- Amoxil 2193
- Augmentin Tablets, Powder for Oral Suspension, and Chewable Tablets 2198

Ampicillin Sodium (Competition for protein-binding sites). Products include:
- Unasyn 1965

Aspirin (Potential toxicity). Products include:
- Alka-Seltzer Effervescent Antacid and Pain Reliever 1568
- Alka-Seltzer Extra Strength Effervescent Antacid and Pain Reliever 1570
- Alka-Seltzer (Flavored) Effervescent Antacid and Pain Reliever 1569
- Alka-Seltzer Plus Cold Medicine ■ 623
- Alka-Seltzer Plus Night-Time Cold Medicine ■ 623
- Alka Seltzer Plus Sinus Allergy Medicine ■ 624
- Anacin Coated Analgesic Caplets 2417
- Anacin Coated Analgesic Tablets 2417
- Anacin Maximum Strength Analgesic Coated Tablets 2417
- Maximum Strength Arthritis Pain Formula By the Makers of Anacin Analgesic Tablets and Caplets 2418
- Arthritis Pain Formula by the Makers of Anacin Analgesic Tablets and Caplets ■ 747
- Arthritis Strength BC Powder ■ 516
- Ascriptin A/D Caplets 1850
- Regular Strength Ascriptin Tablets 1850
- Azdone Tablets 844
- BC Powder ■ 517
- BC Cold Powder ■ 517
- Children's Bayer Chewable Aspirin ■ 564
- Genuine Bayer Aspirin Tablets & Caplets ■ 564
- Maximum Bayer Aspirin Tablets & Caplets ■ 566
- Bayer Plus Aspirin Tablets ■ 567
- Therapy Bayer Aspirin Caplets ■ 568
- 8 Hour Bayer Timed-Release Aspirin ■ 566
- Arthritis Strength Bufferin Analgesic Caplets 744
- Extra Strength Bufferin Analgesic Tablets 745
- Bufferin Analgesic Tablets and Caplets 743
- Cama Arthritis Pain Reliever ■ 685
- Damason-P 1356
- Easprin 1719
- Ecotrin Enteric Coated Aspirin Maximum Strength Tablets and Caplets 2189
- Ecotrin Enteric Coated Aspirin Regular Strength Tablets and Caplets 2189
- Empirin Aspirin ■ 541
- Empirin with Codeine Phosphate Nos. 2, 3 & 4 764
- Equagesic Tablets 2451
- Excedrin Extra-Strength Analgesic Tablets & Caplets 749
- 4-Way Cold Tablets 750
- Fiorinal Capsules 2007
- Fiorinal with Codeine Capsules 2008
- Fiorinal Tablets 2007
- Lortab ASA Tablets 2414
- Momentum Muscular Backache Formula ■ 751
- Norgesic 1314
- Norwich Extra-Strength Aspirin ■ 546
- Norwich Regular Strength Aspirin ■ 547
- P-A-C Analgesic Tablets ■ 669
- Percodan 951
- Robaxisal Tablets 1872
- Sine-Off Sinus Medicine Tablets-Aspirin Formula ■ 722
- Soma Compound w/Codeine Tablets 2390
- Soma Compound Tablets 2389
- St. Joseph Adult Chewable Aspirin (81 mg.) ■ 703
- Synalgos-DC Capsules 2525
- Talwin Compound 2072
- Ursinus Inlay-Tabs ■ 691
- Vanquish Analgesic Caplets ■ 574
- Zorprin Tablets 698

Azlocillin Sodium (Competition for protein-binding sites).
- No products indexed under this heading.

Bacampicillin Hydrochloride (Competition for protein-binding sites). Products include:
- Spectrobid Tablets & Powder for Oral Suspension 1961

Betamethasone Acetate (Competition for protein-binding sites). Products include:
- Celestone Soluspan Suspension 2081

Betamethasone Sodium Phosphate (Competition for protein-binding sites). Products include:
- Celestone Soluspan Suspension 2081

Carbenicillin Disodium (Competition for protein-binding sites).

Carbenicillin Indanyl Sodium (Competition for protein-binding sites). Products include:
- Geocillin Tablets 1951

Chlorpropamide (Hypoglycemic effect enhanced). Products include:
- Diabinese Tablets 1775

Choline Magnesium Trisalicylate (Potential toxicity). Products include:
- Trilisate 1822

Cortisone Acetate (Competition for protein-binding sites). Products include:
- Cortone Acetate Sterile Suspension 1437
- Cortone Acetate Tablets 1439

Dexamethasone (Competition for protein-binding sites). Products include:
- AK-Trol Ointment & Suspension ⊙ 207
- Decadron Elixir 1445
- Decadron Tablets 1447
- Decaspray Topical Aerosol 1459
- Dexacidin ⊙ 272
- Maxidex Sterile Ophthalmic Suspension ⊙ 223
- Maxitrol Ophthalmic Ointment/Suspension ⊙ 223
- TobraDex Ophthalmic Suspension and Ointment ⊙ 228

Dexamethasone Acetate (Competition for protein-binding sites). Products include:
- Dalalone D.P. Injectable 999
- Decadron-LA Sterile Suspension 1457

Dexamethasone Sodium Phosphate (Competition for protein-binding sites). Products include:
- AK-Dex ⊙ 203
- Decadron Phosphate Respihaler 1454
- Decadron Phosphate Sterile Ophthalmic Ointment 1453
- Decadron Phosphate Sterile Ophthalmic Solution 1453
- Decadron Phosphate Topical Cream 1455
- Decadron Phosphate Turbinaire 1456
- Maxidex Sterile Ophthalmic Ointment ⊙ 222
- NeoDecadron Sterile Ophthalmic Ointment 1517
- NeoDecadron Sterile Ophthalmic Solution 1518
- NeoDecadron Topical Cream 1518

Dicumarol (Competition for protein binding predisposes to systemic bleeding). Products include:
- Dicumarol Tablets 516

Diflunisal (Potential toxicity). Products include:
- Dolobid Tablets 1465

Glipizide (Hypoglycemic effect enhanced). Products include:
- Glucotrol 1952

Glyburide (Hypoglycemic effect enhanced). Products include:
- DiaBeta 1091
- Micronase Tablets 2350

Heparin Calcium (Competition for protein binding predisposes to systemic bleeding). Products include:
- Calciparine Injection 925

Heparin Sodium (Competition for protein binding predisposes to systemic bleeding). Products include:
- Heparin Lock Flush Solution 2456
- Heparin Sodium Vials 1264
- Heparin Sodium Injection 2457
- Heparin Sodium Injection, USP, Sterile Solution 2342

Hydrocortisone (Competition for protein-binding sites). Products include:
- AK-Spore H.C. ⊙ 206
- Bactine Hydrocortisone Anti-Itch Cream ■ 625
- CaldeCORT Anti-Itch Hydrocortisone Spray ■ 560
- Carmol HC Cream 1% 2296
- Cortaid Spray ■ 735
- Cortenema 2244
- Cortisporin Ointment 758
- Cortisporin Ophthalmic Ointment Sterile 758
- Cortisporin Ophthalmic Suspension Sterile 759
- Cortisporin Otic Solution Sterile 760
- Cortisporin Otic Suspension Sterile 760
- Cortizone-5 Creme & Ointment ■ 732
- Dermolate Anti-Itch Cream ■ 697
- Eldecort Cream 1.0% 1113
- Eldecort Cream 1.0% and 2.5% 1113
- Fungoid HC Creme 1770
- Hydrocortone Tablets 1482
- Hytone 909
- LazerSporin-C Solution 1770
- Massengill Medicated Soft Cloth Towelettes 2192
- Nutracort Cream & Lotion 1684
- PediOtic Suspension Sterile 797
- Synacort Creams 1%, 2.5% 2296
- Vanoxide-HC Acne Lotion 911
- Vioform-Hydrocortisone Cream and Mild Cream 889
- Vioform-Hydrocortisone Ointment 889
- VōSoL HC Otic Solution 2392
- Vytone Cream 1% 911

Hydrocortisone Acetate (Competition for protein-binding sites). Products include:
- Analpram-HC Rectal Cream 1% and 2.5% 970
- Anusol-HC Cream 1690
- Anusol-HC Suppositories 1691
- Caldecort ■ 560
- Carmol HC Cream 1% 2296
- Chloromycetin Hydrocortisone Ophthalmic 1694
- Coly-Mycin S Otic w/Neomycin & Hydrocortisone 1708
- Cortaid ■ 735
- Cortef Feminine Itch Cream ■ 735
- Corticaine ■ 682
- Cortifoam 1827
- Cortisporin Cream 757
- Epifoam 1828
- Gynecort 5 Creme ■ 556
- Hydrocortone Acetate Sterile Suspension 1479
- Lanacort 5 Creme and Ointment ■ 557
- Mantadil Cream 789
- Ophthocort ⊙ 301
- Orabase HCA Oral Paste 890
- Pramosone Cream, Lotion & Ointment 971
- ProctoCream-HC 1834
- Proctofoam-HC 1835

Hydrocortisone Sodium Phosphate (Competition for protein-binding sites). Products include:
- Hydrocortone Phosphate Injection, Sterile 1481

Hydrocortisone Sodium Succinate (Competition for protein-binding sites). Products include:
- Solu-Cortef Sterile Powder 2361

Levothyroxine Sodium (Depressed plasma T4 value). Products include:
- Levothroid Tablets 1003

(■ Described in PDR For Nonprescription Drugs) (⊙ Described in PDR For Ophthalmology)

Levoxine Tablets 904
Synthroid 695

Liothyronine Sodium (Depressed plasma T4 value). Products include:
Cytomel Tablets 2203

Magnesium Salicylate (Potential toxicity). Products include:
Doan's - Extra-Strength Analgesic ⊞ 549
Doan's - Regular Strength Analgesic ⊞ 549
Mobigesic Analgesic Tablets ⊞ 507

Methotrexate Sodium (Competition for protein-binding sites). Products include:
Methotrexate Tablets, Parenteral, LPF Parenteral 1217
Rheumatrex Methotrexate Dose Pack 1234

Methylprednisolone Acetate (Competition for protein-binding sites). Products include:
Depo-Medrol Sterile Aqueous Suspension 2334

Methylprednisolone Sodium Succinate (Competition for protein-binding sites). Products include:
Solu-Medrol Sterile Powder 2363

Mezlocillin Sodium (Competition for protein-binding sites). Products include:
Mezlin 1597
Mezlin Pharmacy Bulk Package 1599

Nafcillin Sodium (Competition for protein-binding sites). Products include:
Unipen 2533

Naproxen (Competition for protein-binding sites). Products include:
Naprosyn 2297

Naproxen Sodium (Competition for protein-binding sites). Products include:
Anaprox and Anaprox DS Tablets 2288

Penicillin G Potassium (Competition for protein-binding sites). Products include:
Pfizerpen for Injection 1957

Penicillin G Procaine (Competition for protein-binding sites). Products include:
Bicillin C-R Injection 2438
Bicillin C-R 900/300 Injection 2440
Pfizerpen-AS Aqueous Suspension 1959
Wycillin Injection 2537
Wycillin Injection and Probenecid Tablets 2539

Penicillin G Sodium (Competition for protein-binding sites).
No products indexed under this heading.

Penicillin G, Benzathine (Competition for protein-binding sites). Products include:
Bicillin C-R Injection 2438
Bicillin C-R 900/300 Injection 2440
Bicillin L-A Injection 2442

Penicillin V Potassium (Competition for protein-binding sites).
No products indexed under this heading.

Phenytoin (Competition for protein-binding sites). Products include:
Dilantin Infatabs 1710
Dilantin-30 Pediatric/Dilantin-125 Suspension 1713

Phenytoin Sodium (Competition for protein-binding sites). Products include:
Dilantin Kapseals 1708
Dilantin Parenteral 1712
Dilantin with Phenobarbital Kapseals 1715

Prednisolone Acetate (Competition for protein-binding sites). Products include:
AK-Cide Sterile Ophthalmic Ointment & Suspension ◉ 202
Blephamide Liquifilm Sterile Ophthalmic Suspension 586
Blephamide S.O.P. Sterile Ophthalmic Ointment 586
Cetapred Ointment ◉ 220
⅛% Econopred & 1% Econopred Plus ◉ 217
Isopto Cetapred Suspension ◉ 220
Metimyd ◉ 306
Poly-Pred Liquifilm ◉ 250
Pred Forte ◉ 252
Pred Mild ◉ 254
Pred-G Liquifilm Sterile Ophthalmic Suspension ◉ 252
Pred-G S.O.P. Sterile Ophthalmic Ointment ◉ 253
Vasocidin Ointment ◉ 275

Prednisolone Sodium Phosphate (Competition for protein-binding sites). Products include:
AK-Pred ◉ 205
Hydeltrasol Injection, Sterile 1476
Inflamase ◉ 274
Pediapred Oral Liquid 987
Vasocidin Ophthalmic Solution ◉ 276

Prednisolone Tebutate (Competition for protein-binding sites). Products include:
Hydeltra-T.B.A. Sterile Suspension 1478

Prednisone (Competition for protein-binding sites). Products include:
Deltasone Tablets 2332

Probenecid (Uricosuric action of gout drugs antagonized). Products include:
Benemid Tablets 1426
ColBENEMID Tablets 1436
Wycillin Injection and Probenecid Tablets 2539

Sulfinpyrazone (Uricosuric action of gout drugs antagonized). Products include:
Anturane 853

Thyroxine (Depressed plasma T4 value; competition for protein-binding sites).
No products indexed under this heading.

Thyroxine Sodium (Depressed plasma T4 value).
No products indexed under this heading.

Ticarcillin Disodium (Competition for protein-binding sites). Products include:
Ticar for Injection 2236
Timentin for Injection 2239

Tolazamide (Hypoglycemic effect enhanced). Products include:
Tolinase Tablets 2365

Tolbutamide (Hypoglycemic effect enhanced). Products include:
Orinase Tablets 2354

Triamcinolone (Competition for protein-binding sites).
No products indexed under this heading.

Triamcinolone Acetonide (Competition for protein-binding sites). Products include:
Aristocort A 1010
Azmacort Inhaler 1837
Kenalog Cream, Lotion & Ointment 2401
Kenalog-10 Injection 2402
Kenalog-40 Injection 2403
Kenalog in Orabase 604
Kenalog Spray 2401
Mycolog II Cream and Ointment 2407
Mytrex Cream & Ointment 2080
Nasacort Nasal Inhaler 1844

Triamcinolone Diacetate (Competition for protein-binding sites). Products include:
Aristocort Suspension 1008

Triamcinolone Hexacetonide (Competition for protein-binding sites). Products include:
Aristospan Suspension 1011

l-Triiodothyronine (Competition for protein-binding sites).

Warfarin Sodium (Competition for protein binding predisposes to systemic bleeding). Products include:
Coumadin Injection & Tablets 944
Panwarfin Tablets 547

Food Interactions

Food that lowers urinary pH (Decreases urinary excretion and increases plasma levels).

Food that raises urinary pH (Increases renal clearance and urinary excretion of salicylic acid).

MONOPRIL TABLETS
(Fosinopril Sodium) 1406
May interact with diuretics, potassium sparing diuretics, potassium-depleting corticosteroids, lithium preparations, and certain other agents. Compounds in these categories include:

Aluminum Carbonate Gel (Antacids may impair absorption of fosinopril). Products include:
Basaljel 2438

Aluminum Hydroxide (Antacids may impair absorption of fosinopril). Products include:
Cama Arthritis Pain Reliever ⊞ 685
Gaviscon Extra Strength Relief Formula Liquid Antacid ⊞ 594
Gaviscon Extra Strength Relief Formula Antacid Tablets ⊞ 594
Gaviscon Liquid Antacid ⊞ 594
Gelusil Liquid & Tablets ⊞ 639
Extra Strength Maalox Plus Suspension 1850
Maalox TC Suspension 1851
Maalox Plus Tablets ⊞ 655
Extra Strength Maalox Plus Tablets 1850
Nephrox Suspension ⊞ 563
WinGel Liquid & Tablets ⊞ 761

Aluminum Hydroxide Gel (Antacids may impair absorption of fosinopril). Products include:
ALternaGEL Liquid 1154
Aludrox Oral Suspension 2428
Amphojel Suspension 2429
Amphojel Suspension without Flavor 2429
Mylanta Liquid 1155
Mylanta Double Strength Liquid 1155

Aluminum Hydroxide Gel, Dried (Antacids may impair absorption of fosinopril). Products include:
Alu-Tab/Alu-Cap 1309
Amphojel Tablets 2429
Ascriptin A/D Caplets 1850
Regular Strength Ascriptin Tablets 1850
Gaviscon Antacid Tablets ⊞ 593
Gaviscon-2 Antacid Tablets ⊞ 594
Mylanta Tablets 1155
Mylanta Double Strength Tablets 1155

Amiloride Hydrochloride (Potential for hyperkalemia; potential for excessive reduction in blood pressure after initiation of Monopril therapy). Products include:
Midamor Tablets 1508
Moduretic Tablets 1510

Bendroflumethiazide (Potential for excessive reduction in blood pressure after initiation of Monopril therapy). Products include:
Corzide Tablets 702
Naturetin Tablets 1789
Rauzide Tablets 1804

Bumetanide (Potential for excessive reduction in blood pressure after initiation of Monopril therapy). Products include:
Bumex 1895

Chlorothiazide (Potential for excessive reduction in blood pressure after initiation of Monopril therapy). Products include:
Aldoclor Tablets 1413
Diupres Tablets 1461
Diuril Oral 1464

Chlorothiazide Sodium (Potential for excessive reduction in blood pressure after initiation of Monopril therapy). Products include:
Diuril Sodium Intravenous 1463

Chlorthalidone (Potential for excessive reduction in blood pressure after initiation of Monopril therapy). Products include:
Combipres Tablets 678
Tenoretic Tablets 1105
Thalitone Tablets 687

Dihydroxyaluminum Sodium Carbonate (Antacids may impair absorption of fosinopril). Products include:
Rolaids ⊞ 743

Ethacrynic Acid (Potential for excessive reduction in blood pressure after initiation of Monopril therapy). Products include:
Edecrin Tablets 1468

Furosemide (Potential for excessive reduction in blood pressure after initiation of Monopril therapy). Products include:
Lasix 1093

Hydrochlorothiazide (Potential for excessive reduction in blood pressure after initiation of Monopril therapy). Products include:
Aldactazide 2150
Aldoril Tablets 1418
Apresazide Capsules 854
Apresoline-Esidrix Tablets 857
Capozide 2258
Dyazide Capsules 2208
Esidrix Tablets 863
Esimil Tablets 864
HydroDIURIL Tablets 1484
Hydropres Tablets 1485
Inderide Tablets 2463
Inderide LA Long Acting Capsules 2465
Lopressor HCT Tablets 1034
Maxzide 1215
Moduretic Tablets 1510
Normozide Tablets 2112
Oretic Tablets 544
Oreticyl 545
Prinzide Tablets 1540
Ser-Ap-Es Tablets 881
Serpasil-Esidrix Tablets 886
Timolide Tablets 1547
Trandate HCT Tablets 579
Vaseretic Tablets 1559
Zestoretic 2274

Hydroflumethiazide (Potential for excessive reduction in blood pressure after initiation of Monopril therapy). Products include:
Diucardin Tablets 2450
Saluron 718
Salutensin/Salutensin-Demi 719

Indapamide (Potential for excessive reduction in blood pressure after initiation of Monopril therapy). Products include:
Lozol Tablets 1843

Lithium Carbonate (Potential for increased lithium levels and symptoms of lithium toxicity). Products include:
Eskalith 2214
Lithane Tablets 1596
Lithium Carbonate Capsules & Tablets 1984
Lithobid Tablets 870

Lithium Citrate (Potential for increased lithium levels and symptoms of lithium toxicity). Products include:
Cibalith-S 870

Magaldrate (Antacids may impair absorption of fosinopril). Products include:
Riopan Antacid Chew Tablets ⊞ 754
Riopan Antacid Chew Tablets in Rollpacks ⊞ 754
Riopan Antacid Suspension 2421
Riopan Antacid Swallow Tablets 2421
Riopan Plus Chew Tablets 2422

Riopan Plus Chew Tablets in Rollpack ... 2422
Riopan Plus 2 Chew Tablets, Mint Flavor, Cherry Flavor ... 2422
Riopan Plus Suspension ... 2422
Riopan Plus 2 Suspension, Mint Flavor, Cherry Flavor ... 2422

Magnesium Hydroxide (Antacids may impair absorption of fosinopril). Products include:
Aludrox Oral Suspension ... 2428
Ascriptin A/D Caplets ... 1850
Regular Strength Ascriptin Tablets 1850
Di-Gel Antacid/Anti-Gas ... ⊞ 697
Gelusil Liquid & Tablets ... ⊞ 639
Haley's M-O, Regular & Flavored .. ⊞ 569
Extra Strength Maalox Plus Suspension ... 1850
Maalox TC Suspension ... 1851
Maalox Plus Tablets ... ⊞ 655
Extra Strength Maalox Plus Tablets 1850
Mylanta Liquid ... 1155
Mylanta Tablets ... 1155
Mylanta Double Strength Liquid ... 1155
Mylanta Double Strength Tablets ... 1155
Concentrated Phillips' Milk of Magnesia ... ⊞ 573
Phillips' Milk of Magnesia Liquid.... ⊞ 572
Phillips' Milk of Magnesia Tablets ⊞ 573
WinGel Liquid & Tablets ... ⊞ 761

Magnesium Oxide (Antacids may impair absorption of fosinopril). Products include:
Bayer Plus Aspirin Tablets ... ⊞ 567
Beelith Tablets ... 659
Bufferin Analgesic Tablets and Caplets ... ⊞ 524
Cama Arthritis Pain Reliever ... ⊞ 685
Mag-Ox 400 ... 673
Uro-Mag ... 673

Methyclothiazide (Potential for excessive reduction in blood pressure after initiation of Monopril therapy). Products include:
Enduron Tablets ... 517
Enduronyl ... 518

Metolazone (Potential for excessive reduction in blood pressure after initiation of Monopril therapy). Products include:
Diulo ... 2129
Mykrox ½ mg Tablets ... 984
Zaroxolyn Tablets ... 989

Polythiazide (Potential for excessive reduction in blood pressure after initiation of Monopril therapy). Products include:
Minizide Capsules ... 1779
Renese Tablets ... 1785
Renese-R Tablets ... 1786

Potassium Acid Phosphate (Potential for hyperkalemia). Products include:
K-Phos M.F. Tablets ... 659
K-Phos Original Formula 'Sodium Free' Tablets ... 660
K-Phos No. 2 Tablets ... 659

Potassium Bicarbonate (Potential for hyperkalemia). Products include:
Alka-Seltzer Advanced Formula Antacid & Non-Aspirin Pain Reliever ... ⊞ 620
Alka-Seltzer Effervescent Antacid ⊞ 622
K-Lyte ... 707
Klorvess Effervescent Granules ... 2010
Klorvess Effervescent Tablets ... 2011

Potassium Chloride (Potential for hyperkalemia). Products include:
Chlor-3 Condiment ... 994
K-Dur Microburst Release System (potassium chloride, USP) E.R. Tablets ... 1163
K-Lor Powder Packets ... 531
K-Lyte ... 707
K-Norm Capsules ... 982
K-Tab Filmtab ... 532
Kato Potassium Supplement ... 1114
Klor-Con 8/Klor-Con 10 Extended-release Tablets ... 2374
Klorvess Effervescent Granules ... 2010
Klorvess Effervescent Tablets ... 2011
Klorvess 10% Liquid ... 2010
Klotrix ... 708
Kolyum Liquid ... 983
Micro-K ... 1863
Micro-K LS Packets ... 1864
NuLYTELY ... 699
Oral Rehydration Salts, Citrate ... 1150
Rum-K Syrup ... 995
Slow-K Tablets ... 2281
Ten-K Controlled-Release Tablets.... 2282
Thermotabs ... ⊞ 619

Potassium Citrate (Potential for hyperkalemia). Products include:
Alka-Seltzer Effervescent Antacid .. 1570
K-Lyte ... 707
Polycitra Syrup ... 2424
Polycitra-K ... 2424
Polycitra-LC—Sugar-Free ... 2424
Ricelyte, Rice-Based Oral Electrolyte Maintenance Solution ... ⊞ 613

Potassium Gluconate (Potential for hyperkalemia). Products include:
Kolyum Liquid ... 983

Potassium Phosphate, Dibasic (Potential for hyperkalemia). Products include:
Neutra-Phos ... 2423

Potassium Phosphate, Monobasic (Potential for hyperkalemia). Products include:
K-Phos M.F. Tablets ... 659
K-Phos Neutral Tablets ... 660
Neutra-Phos ... 2423

Spironolactone (Potential for hyperkalemia; potential for excessive reduction in blood pressure after initiation of Monopril therapy). Products include:
Aldactazide ... 2150
Aldactone ... 2152

Triamterene (Potential for hyperkalemia; potential for excessive reduction in blood pressure after initiation of Monopril therapy). Products include:
Dyazide Capsules ... 2208
Dyrenium Capsules ... 2210
Maxzide ... 1215

Food Interactions

Food, unspecified (Rate of absorption may be slowed by the presence of food in the GI tract; the extent of absorption is not affected).

MOTOFEN TABLETS
(Atropine Sulfate, Difenoxin Hydrochloride) ... 836
May interact with monoamine oxidase inhibitors, barbiturates, tranquilizers, narcotic analgesics, and certain other agents. Compounds in these categories include:

Alcohol (Effects potentiated).

Alfentanil Hydrochloride (Effects potentiated). Products include:
Alfenta Injection ... 1131

Alprazolam (Effects potentiated). Products include:
Xanax Tablets ... 2367

Aprobarbital (Effects potentiated). Products include:
Alurate Elixir ... 1883

Buprenorphine (Effects potentiated).
No products indexed under this heading.

Buspirone Hydrochloride (Effects potentiated). Products include:
BuSpar ... 1401

Butabarbital (Effects potentiated). Products include:
Pyridium Plus ... 1764

Butalbital (Effects potentiated). Products include:
Esgic-Plus Tablets ... 1002
Esgic Tablets & Capsules ... 1001
Fioricet Tablets ... 2006
Fiorinal Capsules ... 2007
Fiorinal with Codeine Capsules ... 2008
Fiorinal Tablets ... 2007
Phrenilin ... 838
Sedapap Tablets 50 mg/650 mg .. 1360

Chlordiazepoxide (Effects potentiated). Products include:
Libritabs Tablets ... 1930
Limbitrol ... 1933
Menrium Tablets ... 1934

Chlordiazepoxide Hydrochloride (Effects potentiated). Products include:
Librax Capsules ... 1929
Librium Capsules ... 1931
Librium Injectable ... 1932

Chlorpromazine (Effects potentiated). Products include:
Thorazine ... 2234

Chlorprothixene (Effects potentiated). Products include:
Taractan Tablets ... 1920

Chlorprothixene Hydrochloride (Effects potentiated). Products include:
Taractan ... 1920

Clorazepate Dipotassium (Effects potentiated). Products include:
Tranxene ... 556

Codeine (Effects potentiated). Products include:
Calcidrine Syrup ... 506

Codeine Phosphate (Effects potentiated). Products include:
Actifed with Codeine Cough Syrup.. 752
Cheracol Cough Syrup ... 1853
Codimal PH Syrup ... 846
Dimetane-DC Cough Syrup ... 1857
Empirin with Codeine Phosphate Nos. 2, 3 & 4 ... 764
Fiorinal with Codeine Capsules ... 2008
Isoclor Expectorant ... 982
Naldecon CX Adult Liquid ... ⊞ 521
Novahistine DH ... 1342
Novahistine Expectorant ... 1343
Nucofed Capsules ... 2219
Nucofed Expectorant ... 2219
Nucofed Pediatric Expectorant ... 2220
Nucofed Syrup ... 2219
Phenaphen with Codeine Capsules 1865
Phenaphen-650 with Codeine Tablets ... 1866
Phenergan with Codeine ... 2497
Phenergan VC with Codeine ... 2501
Robitussin A-C Syrup ... 1875
Robitussin-DAC Syrup ... 1875
Ryna ... ⊞ 741
Soma Compound w/Codeine Tablets ... 2390
Triaminic Expectorant w/Codeine .. 1996
Tussi-Organidin Liquid ... 2391
Tylenol with Codeine ... 1381

Codeine Polistirex (Effects potentiated).
No products indexed under this heading.

Dezocine (Effects potentiated).

Diazepam (Effects potentiated). Products include:
Valium Injectable ... 1937
Valium Tablets ... 1939
Valrelease Capsules ... 1923

Droperidol (Effects potentiated). Products include:
Inapsine Injection ... 1140
Innovar Injection ... 1141

Fentanyl (Effects potentiated). Products include:
Duragesic Transdermal System ... 1133

Fentanyl Citrate (Effects potentiated). Products include:
Innovar Injection ... 1141
Sublimaze Injection ... 1146

Fluphenazine Decanoate (Effects potentiated). Products include:
Prolixin Decanoate ... 1795

Fluphenazine Enanthate (Effects potentiated). Products include:
Prolixin Enanthate ... 1796

Fluphenazine Hydrochloride (Effects potentiated). Products include:
Prolixin Elixir ... 1793
Prolixin Injection ... 1791
Prolixin Oral Concentrate ... 1792
Prolixin Tablets ... 1793

Furazolidone (Concurrent use may precipitate hypertensive crisis). Products include:
Furoxone ... 1855

Haloperidol (Effects potentiated). Products include:
Haldol Injection, Tablets and Concentrate ... 1373

Haloperidol Decanoate (Effects potentiated). Products include:
Haldol Decanoate ... 1375

Hydrocodone Bitartrate (Effects potentiated). Products include:
Anexsia 5/500 Tablets ... 2196
Anexsia 7.5/650 Tablets ... 2197
Azdone Tablets ... 844
Codiclear DH Syrup ... 845
Codimal DH Syrup ... 846
Damason-P ... 1356
Hycodan Syrup, Tablets ... 927
Hycomine Compound Tablets ... 929
Hycomine Syrup ... 927
Hycotuss Expectorant Syrup ... 930
Hydrocet Capsules ... 835
Lortab ASA Tablets ... 2414
Lortab ... 2412
Ru-Tuss with Hydrocodone ... 694
Triaminic Expectorant DH ... 1995
Vicodin Tablets ... 1187
Vicodin ES Tablets ... 1189
Zydone Capsules ... 941

Hydrocodone Polistirex (Effects potentiated). Products include:
Tussionex Extended-Release Suspension ... 988

Hydroxyzine Hydrochloride (Effects potentiated). Products include:
Atarax Tablets & Syrup ... 1941
Marax Tablets & DF Syrup ... 1954
Vistaril Intramuscular Solution ... 1970

Isocarboxazid (Concurrent use may precipitate hypertensive crisis). Products include:
Marplan Tablets ... 1906

Levorphanol Tartrate (Effects potentiated). Products include:
Levo-Dromoran ... 1906

Lorazepam (Effects potentiated). Products include:
Ativan Injection ... 2432
Ativan Tablets ... 2434

Loxapine Hydrochloride (Effects potentiated). Products include:
Loxitane ... 1213

Loxapine Succinate (Effects potentiated). Products include:
Loxitane Capsules ... 1213

Meperidine Hydrochloride (Effects potentiated). Products include:
Demerol ... 2047
Mepergan Injection ... 2479

Mephobarbital (Effects potentiated). Products include:
Mebaral Tablets ... 2061

Meprobamate (Effects potentiated). Products include:
Deprol Tablets ... 2382
Equagesic Tablets ... 2451
Miltown Tablets ... 2386
PMB 200 and PMB 400 ... 2504

Mesoridazine (Effects potentiated). Products include:
Serentil ... 686

Methadone Hydrochloride (Effects potentiated). Products include:
Dolophine Hydrochloride Ampoules & Vials ... 1260
Dolophine Hydrochloride Tablets 1261
Methadone Hydrochloride Diskets .. 1284
Methadone Hydrochloride Oral Solution & Tablets ... 1987

Molindone Hydrochloride (Effects potentiated). Products include:
Moban Tablets & Concentrate ... 932

Morphine Sulfate (Effects potentiated). Products include:
Astramorph/PF Injection, USP (Preservative-Free) ... 618
Duramorph ... 960

Infumorph 200 and Infumorph 500 Sterile Solutions ... 962
MS Contin Tablets ... 1814
MSIR ... 1817
Oramorph SR (Morphine Sulfate Sustained Release Tablets) ... 1988
Roxanol ... 1991

Opium Alkaloids (Effects potentiated). Products include:
B & O No. 15A & No. 16A Supprettes ... 2395
Pantopon Injectable ... 1911

Oxazepam (Effects potentiated). Products include:
Serax Capsules ... 2522
Serax Tablets ... 2522

Oxycodone Hydrochloride (Effects potentiated). Products include:
Percocet Tablets ... 950
Percodan ... 951
Roxicodone Tablets, Oral Solution & Intensol (Oxycodone) ... 1992
Tylox Capsules ... 1382

Pentobarbital Sodium (Effects potentiated). Products include:
Nembutal Sodium Capsules ... 534
Nembutal Sodium Solution ... 536
Nembutal Sodium Suppositories ... 538

Perphenazine (Effects potentiated). Products include:
Etrafon ... 2087
Triavil Tablets ... 1556
Trilafon ... 2123

Phenelzine Sulfate (Concurrent use may precipitate hypertensive crisis). Products include:
Nardil ... 1742

Phenobarbital (Effects potentiated). Products include:
Arco-Lase Plus Tablets ... 607
Bellergal-S Tablets ... 1998
Bronkolixir ... ⊞ 761
Bronkotabs Tablets ... ⊞ 762
Donnatal ... 1858
Donnatal Extentabs ... 1859
Donnatal Tablets ... 1858
Donnazyme Tablets ... 1860
Kinesed Tablets ... 2272
Phenobarbital Elixir and Tablets ... 1293
Primatene Tablets-P Formula ... 2421
Quadrinal Tablets ... 1183
Tedral SA ... 1765

Prazepam (Effects potentiated). Products include:
Centrax ... 1693

Prochlorperazine (Effects potentiated). Products include:
Compazine ... 2201

Promethazine Hydrochloride (Effects potentiated). Products include:
Mepergan Injection ... 2479
Phenergan with Codeine ... 2497
Phenergan with Dextromethorphan 2499
Phenergan Injection ... 2493
Phenergan Suppositories ... 2496
Phenergan Syrup ... 2495
Phenergan Tablets ... 2496
Phenergan VC ... 2500
Phenergan VC with Codeine ... 2501

Propoxyphene Hydrochloride (Effects potentiated). Products include:
Darvon ... 1256
Wygesic Tablets ... 2540

Propoxyphene Napsylate (Effects potentiated). Products include:
Darvon-N/Darvocet-N ... 1254

Secobarbital Sodium (Effects potentiated). Products include:
Seconal Sodium Pulvules ... 1296

Selegiline Hydrochloride (Concurrent use may precipitate hypertensive crisis). Products include:
Eldepryl ... 2250

Sufentanil Citrate (Effects potentiated). Products include:
Sufenta Injection ... 1147

Thiamylal Sodium (Effects potentiated). Products include:
Surital Ampoules, Steri-Vials ... 1764

Thioridazine Hydrochloride (Effects potentiated). Products include:
Mellaril ... 2011

Thiothixene (Effects potentiated). Products include:
Navane Capsules and Concentrate 1954
Navane Intramuscular ... 1956

Tranylcypromine Sulfate (Concurrent use may precipitate hypertensive crisis). Products include:
Parnate Tablets ... 2222

Trifluoperazine Hydrochloride (Effects potentiated). Products include:
Stelazine ... 2226

MOTRIN TABLETS

(Ibuprofen) ... 2351
May interact with oral anticoagulants, thiazides, and certain other agents. Compounds in these categories include:

Aspirin (Decreased anti-inflammatory activity). Products include:
Alka-Seltzer Effervescent Antacid and Pain Reliever ... 1568
Alka-Seltzer Extra Strength Effervescent Antacid and Pain Reliever ... 1570
Alka-Seltzer (Flavored) Effervescent Antacid and Pain Reliever ... 1569
Alka-Seltzer Plus Cold Medicine ... ⊞ 623
Alka-Seltzer Plus Night-Time Cold Medicine ... ⊞ 623
Alka Seltzer Plus Sinus Allergy Medicine ... ⊞ 624
Anacin Coated Analgesic Caplets ... 2417
Anacin Coated Analgesic Tablets ... 2417
Anacin Maximum Strength Analgesic Coated Tablets ... 2417
Maximum Strength Arthritis Pain Formula By the Makers of Anacin Analgesic Tablets and Caplets ... 2418
Arthritis Pain Formula by the Makers of Anacin Analgesic Tablets and Caplets ... ⊞ 747
Arthritis Strength BC Powder ... ⊞ 516
Ascriptin A/D Caplets ... 1850
Regular Strength Ascriptin Tablets 1850
Azdone Tablets ... 844
BC Powder ... ⊞ 517
BC Cold Powder ... ⊞ 517
Children's Bayer Chewable Aspirin ... ⊞ 564
Genuine Bayer Aspirin Tablets & Caplets ... ⊞ 564
Maximum Bayer Aspirin Tablets & Caplets ... ⊞ 566
Bayer Plus Aspirin Tablets ... ⊞ 567
Therapy Bayer Aspirin Caplets ... ⊞ 568
8 Hour Bayer Timed-Release Aspirin ... ⊞ 566
Arthritis Strength Bufferin Analgesic Caplets ... 744
Extra Strength Bufferin Analgesic Tablets ... 745
Bufferin Analgesic Tablets and Caplets ... 743
Cama Arthritis Pain Reliever ... ⊞ 685
Damason-P ... 1356
Easprin ... 1719
Ecotrin Enteric Coated Aspirin Maximum Strength Tablets and Caplets ... 2189
Ecotrin Enteric Coated Aspirin Regular Strength Tablets and Caplets ... 2189
Empirin Aspirin ... ⊞ 541
Empirin with Codeine Phosphate Nos. 2, 3 & 4 ... 764
Equagesic Tablets ... 2451
Excedrin Extra-Strength Analgesic Tablets & Caplets ... 749
4-Way Cold Tablets ... 750
Fiorinal Capsules ... 2007
Fiorinal with Codeine Capsules ... 2008
Fiorinal Tablets ... 2007
Lortab ASA Tablets ... 2414
Momentum Muscular Backache Formula ... ⊞ 751
Norgesic ... 1314
Norwich Extra-Strength Aspirin ... ⊞ 546
Norwich Regular Strength Aspirin ⊞ 547
P-A-C Analgesic Tablets ... ⊞ 669
Percodan ... 951
Robaxisal Tablets ... 1872
Sine-Off Sinus Medicine Tablets-Aspirin Formula ... ⊞ 722
Soma Compound w/Codeine Tablets ... 2390
Soma Compound Tablets ... 2389
St. Joseph Adult Chewable Aspirin (81 mg.) ... ⊞ 703
Synalgos-DC Capsules ... 2525
Talwin Compound ... 2072
Ursinus Inlay-Tabs ... ⊞ 691
Vanquish Analgesic Caplets ... ⊞ 574
Zorprin Tablets ... 698

Aspirin, Enteric Coated (Decreased anti-inflammatory activity). Products include:
Therapy Bayer Aspirin Caplets ... ⊞ 568
Ecotrin ... 2189

Bendroflumethiazide (Reduced natriuretic effects). Products include:
Corzide Tablets ... 702
Naturetin Tablets ... 1789
Rauzide Tablets ... 1804

Chlorothiazide (Reduced natriuretic effects). Products include:
Aldoclor Tablets ... 1413
Diupres Tablets ... 1461
Diuril Oral ... 1464

Chlorothiazide Sodium (Reduced natriuretic effects). Products include:
Diuril Sodium Intravenous ... 1463

Dicumarol (Concurrent administration may cause bleeding). Products include:
Dicumarol Tablets ... 516

Furosemide (Reduced natriuretic effects). Products include:
Lasix ... 1093

Hydrochlorothiazide (Reduced natriuretic effects). Products include:
Aldactazide ... 2150
Aldoril Tablets ... 1418
Apresazide Capsules ... 854
Apresoline-Esidrix Tablets ... 857
Capozide ... 2258
Dyazide Capsules ... 2208
Esidrix Tablets ... 863
Esimil Tablets ... 864
HydroDIURIL Tablets ... 1484
Hydropres Tablets ... 1485
Inderide Tablets ... 2463
Inderide LA Long Acting Capsules .. 2465
Lopressor HCT Tablets ... 1034
Maxzide ... 1215
Moduretic Tablets ... 1510
Normozide Tablets ... 2112
Oretic Tablets ... 544
Oreticyl ... 545
Prinzide Tablets ... 1540
Ser-Ap-Es Tablets ... 881
Serpasil-Esidrix Tablets ... 886
Timolide Tablets ... 1547
Trandate HCT Tablets ... 579
Vaseretic Tablets ... 1559
Zestoretic ... 2274

Hydroflumethiazide (Reduced natriuretic effects). Products include:
Diucardin Tablets ... 2450
Saluron ... 718
Salutensin/Salutensin-Demi ... 719

Lithium Carbonate (Possible elevation of lithium serum levels and reduction in renal lithium clearance). Products include:
Eskalith ... 2214
Lithane Tablets ... 1596
Lithium Carbonate Capsules & Tablets ... 1984
Lithobid Tablets ... 870

Lithium Citrate (Possible elevation of lithium serum levels and reduction in renal lithium clearance). Products include:
Cibalith-S ... 870

Methotrexate Sodium (Enhanced methotrexate toxicity). Products include:
Methotrexate Tablets, Parenteral, LPF Parenteral ... 1217
Rheumatrex Methotrexate Dose Pack ... 1234

Methyclothiazide (Reduced natriuretic effects). Products include:
Enduron Tablets ... 517
Enduronyl ... 518

Polythiazide (Reduced natriuretic effects). Products include:
Minizide Capsules ... 1779
Renese Tablets ... 1785
Renese-R Tablets ... 1786

Warfarin Sodium (Concurrent administration may cause bleeding). Products include:
Coumadin Injection & Tablets ... 944
Panwarfin Tablets ... 547

Food Interactions

Food, unspecified (A reduction in the rate of absorption but no appreciable decrease in the extent of absorption).

MOTRIN IB CAPLETS AND TABLETS

(Ibuprofen) ... ⊞ 736
May interact with aspirin and acetaminophen containing products. Compounds in this category include:

Acetaminophen (Effect not specified). Products include:
Acetaminophen Uniserts Suppositories ... 2374
Actifed Plus Caplets ... ⊞ 539
Actifed Plus Tablets ... ⊞ 540
Alka-Seltzer Advanced Formula Antacid & Non-Aspirin Pain Reliever ... ⊞ 620
Allerest ... ⊞ 559
Aspirin Free Anacin Maximum Strength Acetaminophen Film Coated Caplets ... 2417
Aspirin Free Anacin Maximum Strength Acetaminophen Film Coated Tablets ... 2417
Anacin-3 Regular Strength Acetaminophen Film Coated Tablets ⊞ 746
Anexsia 5/500 Tablets ... 2196
Anexsia 7.5/650 Tablets ... 2197
Benadryl Plus ... ⊞ 636
Benadryl Plus Nighttime ... ⊞ 637
Bufferin AF Nite Time Analgesic/Sleeping Aid Caplets ... 744
Allergy-Sinus Comtrex Multi-Symptom Allergy Sinus Formula Tablets & Caplets ... 746
Cough Formula Comtrex ... 746
Comtrex Multi-Symptom Cold Reliever Tablets/Caplets/Liqui-Gels/Liquid ... 745
Day-Night Comtrex ... 747
Non-Drowsy Comtrex ... 747
Congespirin For Children Aspirin Free Chewable Cold Tablets ... 748
Contac Cough & Sore Throat Formula ... ⊞ 712
Contac Jr. Children's Cold Medicine ... ⊞ 712
Contac Nighttime Cold Medicine ... ⊞ 713
Contac Severe Cold and Flu Formula Caplets ... ⊞ 711
Contac Sinus Caplets Maximum Strength Non-Drowsy Formula ... ⊞ 710
Contac Sinus Tablets Maximum Strength Non-Drowsy Formula ... ⊞ 710
Coricidin 'D' Decongestant Tablets ... ⊞ 695
Coricidin Demilets Tablets for Children ... ⊞ 696
Coricidin Tablets ... ⊞ 695
Darvon-N/Darvocet-N ... 1254
Datril Extra-Strength Analgesic Tablets ... 748
Dimetapp Plus Caplets ... ⊞ 675
Dorcol Children's Fever & Pain Reducer ... ⊞ 686
Dristan Decongestant/Antihistamine/ Analgesic Coated Caplets ... ⊞ 749
Dristan Cold Nasal Decongestant/ Antihistamine/ Analgesic Coated Tablets ... 2419
Dristan Advanced Formula Decongestant/Antihistamine/ Analgesic Tablets ... ⊞ 749
Maximum Strength Dristan Decongestant/Analgesic Coated Caplets ... ⊞ 750

No Drowsiness Dristan Cold Nasal Decongestant/Analgesic Coated Caplets 2420
Drixoral Plus Extended-Release Tablets ▣ 699
Drixoral Sinus ▣ 700
Esgic-Plus Tablets 1002
Esgic Tablets & Capsules 1001
Aspirin Free Excedrin Analgesic Caplets 748
Excedrin Extra-Strength Analgesic Tablets & Caplets 749
Excedrin P.M. Analgesic/Sleeping Aid Tablets, Caplets and Liquid 749
Sinus Excedrin Analgesic, Decongestant Tablets & Caplets 750
4-Way Cold Tablets 750
Feverall Sprinkle Caps 2374
Feverall Suppositories 2374
Fioricet Tablets 2006
Hycomine Compound Tablets 929
Hydrocet Capsules 835
Isocom Capsules 1629
Liquiprin ▣ 618
Lortab 2412
Lurline PMS Tablets 972
Medi-Flu Caplet, Liquid ▣ 640
Maximum Strength Midol Multi-Symptom Menstrual Formula ▣ 571
Maximum Strength Midol PMS Premenstrual Syndrome Formula ▣ 570
Regular Strength Midol Multi-Symptom Menstrual Formula ▣ 570
Midrin Capsules 836
Ornex Caplets ▣ 618
Children's Panadol Chewable Tablets, Liquid, Infants' Drops ▣ 571
Junior Strength Panadol ▣ 571
Maximum Strength Panadol Tablets and Caplets ▣ 572
Percocet Tablets 950
Percogesic Analgesic Tablets ▣ 660
Phenaphen with Codeine Capsules 1865
Phenaphen-650 with Codeine Tablets 1866
Phrenilin 838
Prēmsyn PMS Capsules & Caplets ▣ 547
Pyrroxate Capsules ▣ 669
Robitussin Night Relief ▣ 677
Sedapap Tablets 50 mg/650 mg 1360
Sinarest ▣ 562
Sine-Aid Maximum Strength Sinus Headache Caplets 1365
Sine-Aid Maximum Strength Sinus Headache Tablets 1365
Sine-Off Maximum Strength Allergy/Sinus Formula Caplets ▣ 721
Sine-Off Maximum Strength No Drowsiness Formula Caplets ▣ 722
Singlet Tablets ▣ 598
Sinulin 840
Sinutab Maximum Strength ▣ 641
Sinutab Maximum Strength Without Drowsiness Tablets & Caplets ▣ 642
Sinutab Regular Strength Without Drowsiness Formula ▣ 641
Sominex Pain Relief Formula ▣ 723
St. Joseph Aspirin-Free Fever Reducer for Children Chewable Tablets, Liquid & Infant Drops ▣ 704
St. Joseph Cold Tablets for Children ▣ 704
St. Joseph Nighttime Cold Medicine ▣ 705
Sudafed Sinus Caplets ▣ 545
Sudafed Sinus Tablets ▣ 545
Talacen 2070
Tempra, Acetaminophen ▣ 613
TheraFlu Flu and Cold Medicine ▣ 687
Triaminicin Tablets ▣ 690
Tylenol acetaminophen Children's Chewable Tablets & Elixir 1366
Tylenol Allergy Sinus Medication Caplets and Gelcaps, Maximum Strength 1372
Tylenol with Codeine 1381
Children's Tylenol Cold Liquid Formula and Chewable Tablets 1368
Tylenol Cold & Flu Hot Medication, Packets 1369
Tylenol Cold & Flu No Drowsiness Hot Medication, Packets 1371
Tylenol Cold Medication Caplets and Tablets 1370
Tylenol Cold Medication, Effervescent Tablets 1369
Tylenol Cold Medication No Drowsiness Formula Caplets 1370
Tylenol Cold Night Time Medication Liquid 1371
Tylenol Cough Medication Liquid, Maximum Strength 1372
Tylenol Cough Medication Liquid with Decongestant, Maximum Strength 1372
Tylenol, Extra Strength, acetaminophen Adult Liquid Pain Reliever 1367
Tylenol, Extra Strength, acetaminophen Gelcaps, Caplets, Tablets 1367
Tylenol, Infants' Drops 1366
Tylenol, Junior Strength, acetaminophen Coated Caplets, Grape and Fruit Chewable Tablets 1366
Tylenol, Maximum Strength, Sinus Medication Gelcaps, Caplets and Tablets 1373
Tylenol, Regular Strength, acetaminophen Tablets and Caplets 1367
Tylenol PM, Extra Strength Caplets and Tablets 1368
Tylox Capsules 1382
Unisom Dual Relief Nighttime Sleep Aid/Analgesic 1774
Vanquish Analgesic Caplets ▣ 574
Vicks Daycare ▣ 660
Vicks Formula 44M Multi-Symptom Cough Medicine ▣ 662
Vicks NyQuil Nighttime Colds Medicine-Original & Cherry Flavor ▣ 664
Vicodin Tablets 1187
Vicodin ES Tablets 1189
Wygesic Tablets 2540
Zydone Capsules 941

Aspirin (Effect not specified). Products include:
Alka-Seltzer Effervescent Antacid and Pain Reliever 1568
Alka-Seltzer Extra Strength Effervescent Antacid and Pain Reliever 1570
Alka-Seltzer (Flavored) Effervescent Antacid and Pain Reliever 1569
Alka-Seltzer Plus Cold Medicine ▣ 623
Alka-Seltzer Plus Night-Time Cold Medicine ▣ 623
Alka Seltzer Plus Sinus Allergy Medicine ▣ 624
Anacin Coated Analgesic Caplets 2417
Anacin Coated Analgesic Tablets 2417
Anacin Maximum Strength Analgesic Coated Tablets 2417
Maximum Strength Arthritis Pain Formula By the Makers of Anacin Analgesic Tablets and Caplets 2418
Arthritis Pain Formula by the Makers of Anacin Analgesic Tablets and Caplets ▣ 747
Arthritis Strength BC Powder ▣ 516
Ascriptin A/D Caplets 1850
Regular Strength Ascriptin Tablets 1850
Azdōne Tablets 844
BC Powder ▣ 517
BC Cold Powder ▣ 517
Children's Bayer Chewable Aspirin ▣ 564
Genuine Bayer Aspirin Tablets & Caplets ▣ 564
Maximum Bayer Aspirin Tablets & Caplets ▣ 566
Bayer Plus Aspirin Tablets ▣ 567
Therapy Bayer Aspirin Caplets ▣ 568
8 Hour Bayer Timed-Release Aspirin ▣ 566
Arthritis Strength Bufferin Analgesic Caplets 744
Extra Strength Bufferin Analgesic Tablets 745
Bufferin Analgesic Tablets and Caplets 743
Cama Arthritis Pain Reliever ▣ 685
Damason-P 1356
Easprin 1719
Ecotrin Enteric Coated Aspirin Maximum Strength Tablets and Caplets 2189
Ecotrin Enteric Coated Aspirin Regular Strength Tablets and Caplets 2189
Empirin Aspirin ▣ 541
Empirin with Codeine Phosphate Nos. 2, 3 & 4 764
Equagesic Tablets 2451
Excedrin Extra-Strength Analgesic Tablets & Caplets 749
4-Way Cold Tablets 750
Fiorinal Capsules 2007
Fiorinal with Codeine Capsules 2008
Fiorinal Tablets 2007
Lortab ASA Tablets 2414
Momentum Muscular Backache Formula ▣ 751
Norgesic 1314
Norwich Extra-Strength Aspirin ▣ 546
Norwich Regular Strength Aspirin ▣ 547
P-A-C Analgesic Tablets ▣ 669
Percodan 951
Robaxisal Tablets 1872
Sine-Off Sinus Medicine Tablets-Aspirin Formula ▣ 722
Soma Compound w/Codeine Tablets 2390
Soma Compound Tablets 2389
St. Joseph Adult Chewable Aspirin (81 mg.) ▣ 703
Synalgos-DC Capsules 2525
Talwin Compound 2072
Ursinus Inlay-Tabs ▣ 691
Vanquish Analgesic Caplets ▣ 574
Zorprin Tablets 698

MULVIDREN-F SOFTAB TABLETS
(Vitamins with Fluoride) 2273
No interactions described in labeling.

MUMPSVAX
(Mumps Virus Vaccine, Live) 1513
May interact with immunosuppressive agents. Compounds in this category include:

Azathioprine (Concurrent administration is containdicated). Products include:
Imuran 768

Cyclosporine (Concurrent administration is containdicated). Products include:
Sandimmune 2024

Immune Globulin (Human) (Concurrent administration is containdicated). Products include:
MICRhoGAM $Rh_0(D)$ Immune Globulin (Human) 1650
RhoGAM $Rh_0(D)$ Immune Globulin (Human) 1651

Immune Globulin Intravenous (Human) (Concurrent administration is containdicated). Products include:
Gamimune N Immune Globulin Intravenous (Human) 1572
Gammagard Immune Globulin, Intravenous (Human) 658
Iveegam 1129
Sandoglobulin I.V. 2027

Muromonab-CD3 (Concurrent administration is containdicated). Products include:
Orthoclone OKT3 Sterile Solution 1645

MURO 128 SODIUM CHLORIDE OPHTHALMIC OINTMENT
(Sodium Chloride) ◉ 260
No interactions described in labeling.

MURO 128 SOLUTION 2% AND 5%
(Sodium Chloride) ◉ 260
No interactions described in labeling.

MUROCOLL-2 STERILE OPHTHALMIC SOLUTION
(Phenylephrine Hydrobromide, Scopolamine Hydrobromide) ◉ 261
May interact with monoamine oxidase inhibitors. Compounds in this category include:

Furazolidone (Potential for hypertensive crisis). Products include:
Furoxone 1855

Isocarboxazid (Potential for hypertensive crisis). Products include:
Marplan Tablets 1906

Phenelzine Sulfate (Potential for hypertensive crisis). Products include:
Nardil 1742

Selegiline Hydrochloride (Potential for hypertensive crisis). Products include:
Eldepryl 2250

Tranylcypromine Sulfate (Potential for hypertensive crisis). Products include:
Parnate Tablets 2222

MUSTARGEN
(Mechlorethamine Hydrochloride) 1514
May interact with antineoplastics. Compounds in this category include:

Altretamine (Hematopoiesis may be further compromised in patients who have been previously treated with chemotherapeutic agents). Products include:
Hexalen Capsules 2316

Asparaginase (Hematopoiesis may be further compromised in patients who have been previously treated with chemotherapeutic agents). Products include:
Elspar 1470

Bleomycin Sulfate (Hematopoiesis may be further compromised in patients who have been previously treated with chemotherapeutic agents). Products include:
Blenoxane 724

Busulfan (Hematopoiesis may be further compromised in patients who have been previously treated with chemotherapeutic agents). Products include:
Myleran Tablets 790

Carboplatin (Hematopoiesis may be further compromised in patients who have been previously treated with chemotherapeutic agents). Products include:
Paraplatin for Injection 735

Carmustine (BCNU) (Hematopoiesis may be further compromised in patients who have been previously treated with chemotherapeutic agents). Products include:
BiCNU 723

Chlorambucil (Hematopoiesis may be further compromised in patients who have been previously treated with chemotherapeutic agents). Products include:
Leukeran Tablets 788

Cisplatin (Hematopoiesis may be further compromised in patients who have been previously treated with chemotherapeutic agents). Products include:
Platinol 737
Platinol-AQ Injection 738

Cyclophosphamide (Hematopoiesis may be further compromised in patients who have been previously treated with chemotherapeutic agents). Products include:
Cytoxan for Injection 726
Neosar for Injection 566

Dacarbazine (Hematopoiesis may be further compromised in patients who have been previously treated with chemotherapeutic agents). Products include:
DTIC-Dome 1595

Daunorubicin Hydrochloride (Hematopoiesis may be further compromised in patients who have been previously treated with chemotherapeutic agents). Products include:
Cerubidine 2443

Doxorubicin Hydrochloride (Hematopoiesis may be further compromised in patients who have been previously treated with chemotherapeutic agents). Products include:
Adriamycin PFS 561

Adriamycin RDF 562
Doxorubicin Hydrochloride for Injection, USP 622
Doxorubicin Hydrochloride Injection, USP 848
Rubex 739

Estramustine Phosphate Sodium (Hematopoiesis may be further compromised in patients who have been previously treated with chemotherapeutic agents). Products include:
Emcyt Capsules 1161

Etoposide (Hematopoiesis may be further compromised in patients who have been previously treated with chemotherapeutic agents). Products include:
VePesid Capsules and Injection 741

Floxuridine (Hematopoiesis may be further compromised in patients who have been previously treated with chemotherapeutic agents). Products include:
Sterile FUDR 1898

Fluorouracil (Hematopoiesis may be further compromised in patients who have been previously treated with chemotherapeutic agents). Products include:
Efudex 1880
Fluoroplex Topical Solution & Cream 1% 1082
Fluorouracil Injection 1897

Flutamide (Hematopoiesis may be further compromised in patients who have been previously treated with chemotherapeutic agents). Products include:
Eulexin Capsules 2089

Hydroxyurea (Hematopoiesis may be further compromised in patients who have been previously treated with chemotherapeutic agents). Products include:
Hydrea Capsules 728

Ifosfamide (Hematopoiesis may be further compromised in patients who have been previously treated with chemotherapeutic agents). Products include:
IFEX 729

Interferon alfa-2A, Recombinant (Hematopoiesis may be further compromised in patients who have been previously treated with chemotherapeutic agents). Products include:
Roferon-A Injection 1916

Interferon alfa-2B, Recombinant (Hematopoiesis may be further compromised in patients who have been previously treated with chemotherapeutic agents). Products include:
Intron A 2097

Levamisole Hydrochloride (Hematopoiesis may be further compromised in patients who have been previously treated with chemotherapeutic agents). Products include:
Ergamisol Tablets 1136

Lomustine (CCNU) (Hematopoiesis may be further compromised in patients who have been previously treated with chemotherapeutic agents). Products include:
CeeNU 725

Megestrol Acetate (Hematopoiesis may be further compromised in patients who have been previously treated with chemotherapeutic agents). Products include:
Megace Tablets 732

Melphalan (Hematopoiesis may be further compromised in patients who have been previously treated with chemotherapeutic agents). Products include:
Alkeran Tablets 754

Mercaptopurine (Hematopoiesis may be further compromised in patients who have been previously treated with chemotherapeutic agents). Products include:
Purinethol Tablets 800

Methotrexate Sodium (Hematopoiesis may be further compromised in patients who have been previously treated with chemotherapeutic agents). Products include:
Methotrexate Tablets, Parenteral, LPF Parenteral 1217
Rheumatrex Methotrexate Dose Pack 1234

Mitomycin (Mitomycin-C) (Hematopoiesis may be further compromised in patients who have been previously treated with chemotherapeutic agents). Products include:
Mutamycin 733

Mitotane (Hematopoiesis may be further compromised in patients who have been previously treated with chemotherapeutic agents). Products include:
Lysodren 731

Mitoxantrone Hydrochloride (Hematopoiesis may be further compromised in patients who have been previously treated with chemotherapeutic agents). Products include:
Novantrone for Injection Concentrate 1226

Procarbazine Hydrochloride (Hematopoiesis may be further compromised in patients who have been previously treated with chemotherapeutic agents). Products include:
Matulane Capsules 1907

Streptozocin (Hematopoiesis may be further compromised in patients who have been previously treated with chemotherapeutic agents). Products include:
Zanosar Sterile Powder 2371

Tamoxifen Citrate (Hematopoiesis may be further compromised in patients who have been previously treated with chemotherapeutic agents). Products include:
Nolvadex Tablets 1102

Thioguanine (Hematopoiesis may be further compromised in patients who have been previously treated with chemotherapeutic agents). Products include:
Thioguanine Tablets, Tabloid Brand 815

Thiotepa (Hematopoiesis may be further compromised in patients who have been previously treated with chemotherapeutic agents). Products include:
Thiotepa Parenteral 1240

Vincristine Sulfate (Hematopoiesis may be further compromised in patients who have been previously treated with chemotherapeutic agents). Products include:
Oncovin Solution Vials & Hyporets 1288

MUTAMYCIN
(Mitomycin (Mitomycin-C)) 733
May interact with antineoplastics, cytotoxic drugs, nitrogen-mustard-type alkylating agents, and certain other agents. Compounds in these categories include:

Altretamine (Adult respiratory distress syndrome). Products include:
Hexalen Capsules 2316

Asparaginase (Adult respiratory distress syndrome). Products include:
Elspar 1470

Bleomycin Sulfate (Hemolytic uremic syndrome; adult respiratory distress syndrome). Products include:
Blenoxane 724

Busulfan (Adult respiratory distress syndrome). Products include:
Myleran Tablets 790

Carboplatin (Adult respiratory distress syndrome). Products include:
Paraplatin for Injection 735

Carmustine (BCNU) (Adult respiratory distress syndrome). Products include:
BiCNU 723

Chlorambucil (Adult respiratory distress syndrome). Products include:
Leukeran Tablets 788

Cisplatin (Adult respiratory distress syndrome). Products include:
Platinol 737
Platinol-AQ Injection 738

Cyclophosphamide (Adult respiratory distress syndrome). Products include:
Cytoxan for Injection 726
Neosar for Injection 566

Dacarbazine (Hemolytic uremic syndrome; adult respiratory distress syndrome). Products include:
DTIC-Dome 1595

Daunorubicin Hydrochloride (Hemolytic uremic syndrome; adult respiratory distress syndrome). Products include:
Cerubidine 2443

Doxorubicin Hydrochloride (Hemolytic uremic syndrome; adult respiratory distress syndrome). Products include:
Adriamycin PFS 561
Adriamycin RDF 562
Doxorubicin Hydrochloride for Injection, USP 622
Doxorubicin Hydrochloride Injection, USP 848
Rubex 739

Estramustine Phosphate Sodium (Adult respiratory distress syndrome). Products include:
Emcyt Capsules 1161

Etoposide (Adult respiratory distress syndrome). Products include:
VePesid Capsules and Injection 741

Floxuridine (Adult respiratory distress syndrome). Products include:
Sterile FUDR 1898

Fluorouracil (Hemolytic uremic syndrome; adult respiratory distress syndrome). Products include:
Efudex 1880
Fluoroplex Topical Solution & Cream 1% 1082
Fluorouracil Injection 1897

Flutamide (Adult respiratory distress syndrome). Products include:
Eulexin Capsules 2089

Hydroxyurea (Hemolytic uremic syndrome; adult respiratory distress syndrome). Products include:
Hydrea Capsules 728

Ifosfamide (Adult respiratory distress syndrome). Products include:
IFEX 729

Interferon alfa-2A, Recombinant (Adult respiratory distress syndrome). Products include:
Roferon-A Injection 1916

Interferon alfa-2B, Recombinant (Adult respiratory distress syndrome). Products include:
Intron A 2097

Levamisole Hydrochloride (Adult respiratory distress syndrome). Products include:
Ergamisol Tablets 1136

Lomustine (CCNU) (Adult respiratory distress syndrome). Products include:
CeeNU 725

Mechlorethamine Hydrochloride (Adult respiratory distress syndrome). Products include:
Mustargen 1514

Megestrol Acetate (Adult respiratory distress syndrome). Products include:
Megace Tablets 732

Melphalan (Adult respiratory distress syndrome). Products include:
Alkeran Tablets 754

Mercaptopurine (Adult respiratory distress syndrome). Products include:
Purinethol Tablets 800

Methotrexate Sodium (Hemolytic uremic syndrome; adult respiratory distress syndrome). Products include:
Methotrexate Tablets, Parenteral, LPF Parenteral 1217
Rheumatrex Methotrexate Dose Pack 1234

Mitotane (Hemolytic uremic syndrome; adult respiratory distress syndrome). Products include:
Lysodren 731

Mitoxantrone Hydrochloride (Hemolytic uremic syndrome; adult respiratory distress syndrome). Products include:
Novantrone for Injection Concentrate 1226

Procarbazine Hydrochloride (Hemolytic uremic syndrome; adult respiratory distress syndrome). Products include:
Matulane Capsules 1907

Streptozocin (Adult respiratory distress syndrome). Products include:
Zanosar Sterile Powder 2371

Tamoxifen Citrate (Hemolytic uremic syndrome; adult respiratory distress syndrome). Products include:
Nolvadex Tablets 1102

Thioguanine (Adult respiratory distress syndrome). Products include:
Thioguanine Tablets, Tabloid Brand 815

Thiotepa (Adult respiratory distress syndrome). Products include:
Thiotepa Parenteral 1240

Vinblastine Sulfate (Acute shortness of breath; severe bronchospasm). Products include:
Velban Vials 1305

Vincristine Sulfate (Hemolytic uremic syndrome; adult respiratory distress syndrome). Products include:
Oncovin Solution Vials & Hyporets 1288

MYADEC
(Multivitamins with Minerals) .... ▣ 640
No interactions described in labeling.

MYAMBUTOL TABLETS
(Ethambutol Hydrochloride)................1225
No interactions described in labeling.

MYCELEX 1% CREAM AND TOPICAL SOLUTION 1%
(Clotrimazole)..1604
No interactions described in labeling.

MYCELEX OTC ANTIFUNGAL CREAM AND SOLUTION
(Clotrimazole)..1571
No interactions described in labeling.

MYCELEX TROCHES
(Clotrimazole)..1605
No interactions described in labeling.

MYCELEX-G 1% VAGINAL CREAM
(Clotrimazole)..1605
No interactions described in labeling.

MYCELEX-G 100 MG VAGINAL TABLETS
(Clotrimazole)..1606
No interactions described in labeling.

MYCELEX-G 500 MG VAGINAL TABLETS
(Clotrimazole)..1606
No interactions described in labeling.

MYCIGUENT ANTIBIOTIC OINTMENT
(Neomycin Sulfate)............................⊞ 737
No interactions described in labeling.

MYCITRACIN PLUS PAIN RELIEVER
(Bacitracin, Neomycin Sulfate, Lidocaine, Polymyxin B Sulfate) ......⊞ 737
No interactions described in labeling.

MYCITRACIN TRIPLE ANTIBIOTIC OINTMENT
(Bacitracin, Neomycin Sulfate, Polymyxin B Sulfate) ....⊞ 737
No interactions described in labeling.

MYCOLOG II CREAM AND OINTMENT
(Nystatin, Triamcinolone Acetonide)..2407
No interactions described in labeling.

MYCOSTATIN CREAM, OINTMENT, TOPICAL POWDER
(Nystatin) 2408
No interactions described in labeling.

MYCOSTATIN ORAL SUSPENSION
(Nystatin) 605
No interactions described in labeling.

MYCOSTATIN ORAL TABLETS
(Nystatin) 605
No interactions described in labeling.

MYCOSTATIN PASTILLES
(Nystatin) 734
No interactions described in labeling.

MYDFRIN 2.5%
(Phenylephrine Hydrochloride)........ ◉ 224
May interact with monoamine oxidase inhibitors, beta$_2$ agonists, tricyclic antidepressants, and certain other agents. Compounds in these categories include:

Acebutolol Hydrochloride (Increased likelihood of systemic side effects). Products include:
Sectral Capsules 2520

Amitriptyline Hydrochloride (May potentiate pressor response of phenylephrine). Products include:
Elavil 2269
Endep Tablets 1927
Etrafon 2087
Limbitrol 1933
Triavil Tablets 1556

Amoxapine (May potentiate pressor response of phenylephrine). Products include:
Asendin Tablets 1196

Atenolol (Increased likelihood of systemic side effects). Products include:
Tenoretic Tablets.............................. 1105
Tenormin Tablets and I.V. Injection 1107

Atropine Sulfate (May enhance pressor effects, and induce tachycardia—especially in infants). Products include:
Arco-Lase Plus Tablets 607
Atropine Sulfate Sterile Ophthalmic Solution and S.O.P. Sterile Ophthalmic Ointment.................... ◉ 239
Donnagel..⊞ 675
Donnagel-PG 1858
Donnatal 1858
Donnatal Extentabs.......................... 1859
Donnatal Tablets 1858
Donnazyme Tablets 1860
Isopto Atropine.............................. ◉ 218
Lomotil 2174
Motofen Tablets 836
Ru-Tuss Tablets 693
Urised Tablets................................ 2396

Betaxolol Hydrochloride (Increased likelihood of systemic side effects). Products include:
Betoptic Sterile Ophthalmic Solution.. 569
Betoptic S Sterile Ophthalmic Suspension.. 570
Kerlone Tablets................................ 2172

Clomipramine Hydrochloride (May potentiate pressor response of phenylephrine). Products include:
Anafranil Capsules 650

Desipramine Hydrochloride (May potentiate pressor response of phenylephrine). Products include:
Norpramin Tablets 1340

Doxepin Hydrochloride (May potentiate pressor response of phenylephrine). Products include:
Sinequan 1960

Esmolol Hydrochloride (Increased likelihood of systemic side effects). Products include:
Brevibloc Injection.......................... 942

Furazolidone (Exaggerated adrenergic effects may result with simultaneous usage or up to 21 days after MAOIs). Products include:
Furoxone 1855

Imipramine Hydrochloride (May potentiate pressor response of phenylephrine). Products include:
Tofranil Ampuls 1038
Tofranil Tablets 1039

Imipramine Pamoate (May potentiate pressor response of phenylephrine). Products include:
Tofranil-PM Capsules........................ 1041

Isocarboxazid (Exaggerated adrenergic effects may result with simultaneous usage or up to 21 days after MAOIs). Products include:
Marplan Tablets 1906

Labetalol Hydrochloride (Increased likelihood of systemic side effects). Products include:
Normodyne Injection 2108
Normodyne Tablets 2110
Normozide Tablets 2112
Trandate HCT Tablets........................ 579
Trandate Injection............................ 577
Trandate Tablets 579

Maprotiline Hydrochloride (May potentiate pressor response of phenylephrine). Products include:
Ludiomil Tablets.............................. 874

Metoprolol Tartrate (Increased likelihood of systemic side effects). Products include:
Lopressor Ampuls 1032
Lopressor HCT Tablets...................... 1034
Lopressor Tablets 1032

Nadolol (Increased likelihood of systemic side effects). Products include:
Corgard Tablets 701
Corzide Tablets 702

Nortriptyline Hydrochloride (May potentiate pressor response of phenylephrine). Products include:
Pamelor.. 2019

Phenelzine Sulfate (Exaggerated adrenergic effects may result with simultaneous usage or up to 21 days after MAOIs). Products include:
Nardil 1742

Pindolol (Increased likelihood of systemic side effects). Products include:
Visken Tablets................................ 2036

Propranolol Hydrochloride (Increased likelihood of systemic side effects). Products include:
Inderal 2459
Inderal LA Long Acting Capsules 2461
Inderide Tablets 2463
Inderide LA Long Acting Capsules .. 2465

Protriptyline Hydrochloride (May potentiate pressor response of phenylephrine). Products include:
Vivactil Tablets 1567

Selegiline Hydrochloride (Exaggerated adrenergic effects may result with simultaneous usage or up to 21 days after MAOIs). Products include:
Eldepryl 2250

Timolol Maleate (Increased likelihood of systemic side effects). Products include:
Blocadren Tablets 1429
Timolide Tablets.............................. 1547
Timoptic in Ocudose 1552
Timoptic Sterile Ophthalmic Solution.. 1550

Tranylcypromine Sulfate (Exaggerated adrenergic effects may result with simultaneous usage or up to 21 days after MAOIs). Products include:
Parnate Tablets 2222

Trimipramine Maleate (May potentiate pressor response of phenylephrine). Products include:
Surmontil Capsules.......................... 2524

MYDRIACYL
(Tropicamide) .... ◉ 225
No interactions described in labeling.

MYKROX ½ MG TABLETS
(Metolazone).. 984
May interact with lithium preparations, antihypertensives, insulin, barbiturates, narcotic analgesics, loop diuretics, cardiac glycosides, corticosteroids, salicylates, non-steroidal anti-inflammatory agents, oral hypoglycemic agents, and certain other agents. Compounds in these categories include:

Acebutolol Hydrochloride (Orthostatic hypotension may occur with concurrent therapy). Products include:
Sectral Capsules 2520

ACTH (Potential for increased hypokalemia).
No products indexed under this heading.

Alcohol (Potentiates orthostatic hypotensive effects).

Alfentanil Hydrochloride (Potentiates orthostatic hypotensive effects). Products include:
Alfenta Injection 1131

Aprobarbital (Potentiates orthostatic hypotensive effects). Products include:
Alurate Elixir 1883

Aspirin (Antihypertensive effects of Mykrox may be decreased). Products include:
Alka-Seltzer Effervescent Antacid and Pain Reliever 1568
Alka-Seltzer Extra Strength Effervescent Antacid and Pain Reliever 1570
Alka-Seltzer (Flavored) Effervescent Antacid and Pain Reliever 1569
Alka-Seltzer Plus Cold Medicine ....⊞ 623
Alka-Seltzer Plus Night-Time Cold Medicine ....⊞ 623
Alka Seltzer Plus Sinus Allergy Medicine ....⊞ 624
Anacin Coated Analgesic Caplets 2417
Anacin Coated Analgesic Tablets 2417
Anacin Maximum Strength Analgesic Coated Tablets........................ 2417
Maximum Strength Arthritis Pain Formula By the Makers of Anacin Analgesic Tablets and Caplets...... 2418
Arthritis Pain Formula by the Makers of Anacin Analgesic Tablets and Caplets ....⊞ 747
Arthritis Strength BC Powder..........⊞ 516
Ascriptin A/D Caplets 1850
Regular Strength Ascriptin Tablets 1850
Azdone Tablets................................ 844
BC Powder ....⊞ 517
BC Cold Powder ....⊞ 517
Children's Bayer Chewable Aspirin ....⊞ 564
Genuine Bayer Aspirin Tablets & Caplets ....⊞ 564
Maximum Bayer Aspirin Tablets & Caplets ....⊞ 566
Bayer Plus Aspirin Tablets..............⊞ 567
Therapy Bayer Aspirin Caplets ......⊞ 568
8 Hour Bayer Timed-Release Aspirin ....⊞ 566
Arthritis Strength Bufferin Analgesic Caplets 744
Extra Strength Bufferin Analgesic Tablets 745
Bufferin Analgesic Tablets and Caplets 743
Cama Arthritis Pain Reliever............⊞ 685
Damason-P...................................... 1356
Easprin.. 1719
Ecotrin Enteric Coated Aspirin Maximum Strength Tablets and Caplets 2189
Ecotrin Enteric Coated Aspirin Regular Strength Tablets and Caplets 2189
Empirin Aspirin................................⊞ 541
Empirin with Codeine Phosphate Nos. 2, 3 & 4.................................. 764
Equagesic Tablets 2451
Excedrin Extra-Strength Analgesic Tablets & Caplets 749
4-Way Cold Tablets.......................... 750
Fiorinal Capsules 2007
Fiorinal with Codeine Capsules 2008
Fiorinal Tablets 2007
Lortab ASA Tablets.......................... 2414
Momentum Muscular Backache Formula ....⊞ 751
Norgesic.. 1314
Norwich Extra-Strength Aspirin......⊞ 546
Norwich Regular Strength Aspirin ⊞ 547
P-A-C Analgesic Tablets ....⊞ 669
Percodan.. 951
Robaxisal Tablets............................ 1872
Sine-Off Sinus Medicine Tablets-Aspirin Formula ....⊞ 722
Soma Compound w/Codeine Tablets 2390
Soma Compound Tablets.................. 2389
St. Joseph Adult Chewable Aspirin (81 mg.)..................................⊞ 703
Synalgos-DC Capsules...................... 2525
Talwin Compound 2072
Ursinus Inlay-Tabs............................⊞ 691
Vanquish Analgesic Caplets ....⊞ 574
Zorprin Tablets................................ 698

Atenolol (Orthostatic hypotension may occur with concurrent therapy). Products include:
- Tenoretic Tablets ... 1105
- Tenormin Tablets and I.V. Injection 1107

Benazepril Hydrochloride (Orthostatic hypotension may occur with concurrent therapy). Products include:
- Lotensin Tablets ... 872

Bendroflumethiazide (Orthostatic hypotension may occur with concurrent therapy). Products include:
- Corzide Tablets ... 702
- Naturetin Tablets ... 1789
- Rauzide Tablets ... 1804

Betamethasone Acetate (Potential for increased hypokalemia). Products include:
- Celestone Soluspan Suspension ... 2081

Betamethasone Sodium Phosphate (Potential for increased hypokalemia). Products include:
- Celestone Soluspan Suspension ... 2081

Betaxolol Hydrochloride (Orthostatic hypotension may occur with concurrent therapy). Products include:
- Betoptic Sterile Ophthalmic Solution ... 569
- Betoptic S Sterile Ophthalmic Suspension ... 570
- Kerlone Tablets ... 2172

Bumetanide (Large or prolonged losses of fluids and electrolytes may result). Products include:
- Bumex ... 1895

Buprenorphine (Potentiates orthostatic hypotensive effects).
- No products indexed under this heading.

Butabarbital (Potentiates orthostatic hypotensive effects). Products include:
- Pyridium Plus ... 1764

Butalbital (Potentiates orthostatic hypotensive effects). Products include:
- Esgic-Plus Tablets ... 1002
- Esgic Tablets & Capsules ... 1001
- Fioricet Tablets ... 2006
- Fiorinal Capsules ... 2007
- Fiorinal with Codeine Capsules ... 2008
- Fiorinal Tablets ... 2007
- Phrenilin ... 838
- Sedapap Tablets 50 mg/650 mg .. 1360

Captopril (Orthostatic hypotension may occur with concurrent therapy). Products include:
- Capoten ... 2255
- Capozide ... 2258

Carteolol Hydrochloride (Orthostatic hypotension may occur with concurrent therapy). Products include:
- Cartrol Tablets ... 507

Chlorothiazide (Orthostatic hypotension may occur with concurrent therapy). Products include:
- Aldoclor Tablets ... 1413
- Diupres Tablets ... 1461
- Diuril Oral ... 1464

Chlorothiazide Sodium (Orthostatic hypotension may occur with concurrent therapy). Products include:
- Diuril Sodium Intravenous ... 1463

Chlorpropamide (Blood glucose concentrations may be raised by metolazone in diabetics). Products include:
- Diabinese Tablets ... 1775

Chlorthalidone (Orthostatic hypotension may occur with concurrent therapy). Products include:
- Combipres Tablets ... 678
- Tenoretic Tablets ... 1105
- Thalitone Tablets ... 687

Choline Magnesium Trisalicylate (Antihypertensive effects of Mykrox may be decreased). Products include:
- Trilisate ... 1822

Clonidine (Orthostatic hypotension may occur with concurrent therapy). Products include:
- Catapres-TTS ... 677

Clonidine Hydrochloride (Orthostatic hypotension may occur with concurrent therapy). Products include:
- Catapres Tablets ... 676
- Combipres Tablets ... 678

Codeine (Potentiates orthostatic hypotensive effects). Products include:
- Calcidrine Syrup ... 506

Codeine Phosphate (Potentiates orthostatic hypotensive effects). Products include:
- Actifed with Codeine Cough Syrup.. 752
- Cheracol Cough Syrup ... 1853
- Codimal PH Syrup ... 846
- Dimetane-DC Cough Syrup ... 1857
- Empirin with Codeine Phosphate Nos. 2, 3 & 4 ... 764
- Fiorinal with Codeine Capsules ... 2008
- Isoclor Expectorant ... 982
- Naldecon CX Adult Liquid ... ▣ 521
- Novahistine DH ... 1342
- Novahistine Expectorant ... 1343
- Nucofed Capsules ... 2219
- Nucofed Expectorant ... 2219
- Nucofed Pediatric Expectorant ... 2220
- Nucofed Syrup ... 2219
- Phenaphen with Codeine Capsules 1865
- Phenaphen-650 with Codeine Tablets ... 1866
- Phenergan with Codeine ... 2497
- Phenergan VC with Codeine ... 2501
- Robitussin A-C Syrup ... 1875
- Robitussin-DAC Syrup ... 1875
- Ryna ... ▣ 741
- Soma Compound w/Codeine Tablets ... 2390
- Triaminic Expectorant w/Codeine .. 1996
- Tussi-Organidin Liquid ... 2391
- Tylenol with Codeine ... 1381

Codeine Polistirex (Potentiates orthostatic hypotensive effects).
- No products indexed under this heading.

Cortisone Acetate (Potential for increased hypokalemia). Products include:
- Cortone Acetate Sterile Suspension ... 1437
- Cortone Acetate Tablets ... 1439

Deserpidine (Orthostatic hypotension may occur with concurrent therapy). Products include:
- Enduronyl ... 518
- Harmonyl Tablets ... 528
- Oreticyl ... 545

Deslanoside (Hypokalemia increases sensitivity of the myocardium to digitalis toxicity).
- No products indexed under this heading.

Dexamethasone (Potential for increased hypokalemia). Products include:
- AK-Trol Ointment & Suspension ... ◉ 207
- Decadron Elixir ... 1445
- Decadron Tablets ... 1447
- Decaspray Topical Aerosol ... 1459
- Dexacidin ... ◉ 272
- Maxidex Sterile Ophthalmic Suspension ... ◉ 223
- Maxitrol Ophthalmic Ointment/Suspension ... ◉ 223
- TobraDex Ophthalmic Suspension and Ointment ... ◉ 228

Dexamethasone Acetate (Potential for increased hypokalemia). Products include:
- Dalalone D.P. Injectable ... 999
- Decadron-LA Sterile Suspension ... 1457

Dexamethasone Sodium Phosphate (Potential for increased hypokalemia). Products include:
- AK-Dex ... ◉ 203
- Decadron Phosphate Respihaler ... 1454
- Decadron Phosphate Sterile Ophthalmic Ointment ... 1453
- Decadron Phosphate Sterile Ophthalmic Solution ... 1453
- Decadron Phosphate Topical Cream ... 1455
- Decadron Phosphate Turbinaire ... 1456
- Maxidex Sterile Ophthalmic Ointment ... ◉ 222
- NeoDecadron Sterile Ophthalmic Ointment ... 1517
- NeoDecadron Sterile Ophthalmic Solution ... 1518
- NeoDecadron Topical Cream ... 1518

Dezocine (Potentiates orthostatic hypotensive effects).

Diazoxide (Orthostatic hypotension may occur with concurrent therapy). Products include:
- Hyperstat I.V. Injection ... 2095
- Proglycem ... 649

Diclofenac Sodium (Antihypertensive effects of Mykrox may be decreased). Products include:
- Voltaren Ophthalmic Sterile Ophthalmic Solution ... ◉ 268
- Voltaren Tablets ... 1042

Diflunisal (Antihypertensive effects of Mykrox may be decreased). Products include:
- Dolobid Tablets ... 1465

Digitoxin (Hypokalemia increases sensitivity of the myocardium to digitalis toxicity). Products include:
- Crystodigin Tablets ... 1253

Digoxin (Hypokalemia increases sensitivity of the myocardium to digitalis toxicity). Products include:
- Lanoxicaps ... 772
- Lanoxin Elixir Pediatric ... 775
- Lanoxin Injection ... 778
- Lanoxin Injection Pediatric ... 781
- Lanoxin Tablets ... 783

Doxazosin Mesylate (Orthostatic hypotension may occur with concurrent therapy). Products include:
- Cardura Tablets ... 1941

Enalapril Maleate (Orthostatic hypotension may occur with concurrent therapy). Products include:
- Vaseretic Tablets ... 1559
- Vasotec Tablets ... 1564

Enalaprilat (Orthostatic hypotension may occur with concurrent therapy). Products include:
- Vasotec I.V. ... 1562

Esmolol Hydrochloride (Orthostatic hypotension may occur with concurrent therapy). Products include:
- Brevibloc Injection ... 942

Ethacrynic Acid (Large or prolonged losses of fluids and electrolytes may result). Products include:
- Edecrin Tablets ... 1468

Etodolac (Antihypertensive effects of Mykrox may be decreased). Products include:
- Lodine Capsules ... 2468

Felodipine (Orthostatic hypotension may occur with concurrent therapy). Products include:
- Plendil Extended-Release Tablets ... 1526

Fenoprofen Calcium (Antihypertensive effects of Mykrox may be decreased). Products include:
- Nalfon Pulvules & Tablets ... 919

Fentanyl (Potentiates orthostatic hypotensive effects). Products include:
- Duragesic Transdermal System ... 1133

Fentanyl Citrate (Potentiates orthostatic hypotensive effects). Products include:
- Innovar Injection ... 1141
- Sublimaze Injection ... 1146

Flurbiprofen (Antihypertensive effects of Mykrox may be decreased). Products include:
- Ansaid Tablets ... 2319

Fosinopril Sodium (Orthostatic hypotension may occur with concurrent therapy). Products include:
- Monopril Tablets ... 1406

Furosemide (Large or prolonged losses of fluids and electrolytes may result; orthostatic hypotension may occur with concurrent therapy). Products include:
- Lasix ... 1093

Glipizide (Blood glucose concentrations may be raised by metolazone in diabetics). Products include:
- Glucotrol ... 1952

Glyburide (Blood glucose concentrations may be raised by metolazone in diabetics). Products include:
- DiaBeta ... 1091
- Micronase Tablets ... 2350

Guanabenz Acetate (Orthostatic hypotension may occur with concurrent therapy). Products include:
- Wytensin Tablets ... 2542

Guanethidine Monosulfate (Orthostatic hypotension may occur with concurrent therapy). Products include:
- Esimil Tablets ... 864
- Ismelin Tablets ... 869

Hydralazine Hydrochloride (Orthostatic hypotension may occur with concurrent therapy). Products include:
- Apresazide Capsules ... 854
- Apresoline Hydrochloride Parenteral (Ampuls) ... 856
- Apresoline Hydrochloride Tablets .. 855
- Apresoline-Esidrix Tablets ... 857
- Ser-Ap-Es Tablets ... 881
- Serpasil-Apresoline Tablets ... 884

Hydrochlorothiazide (Orthostatic hypotension may occur with concurrent therapy). Products include:
- Aldactazide ... 2150
- Aldoril Tablets ... 1418
- Apresazide Capsules ... 854
- Apresoline-Esidrix Tablets ... 857
- Capozide ... 2258
- Dyazide Capsules ... 2208
- Esidrix Tablets ... 863
- Esimil Tablets ... 864
- HydroDIURIL Tablets ... 1484
- Hydropres Tablets ... 1485
- Inderide Tablets ... 2463
- Inderide LA Long Acting Capsules .. 2465
- Lopressor HCT Tablets ... 1034
- Maxzide ... 1215
- Moduretic Tablets ... 1510
- Normozide Tablets ... 2112
- Oretic Tablets ... 544
- Oreticyl ... 545
- Prinzide Tablets ... 1540
- Ser-Ap-Es Tablets ... 881
- Serpasil-Esidrix Tablets ... 886
- Timolide Tablets ... 1547
- Trandate HCT Tablets ... 579
- Vaseretic Tablets ... 1559
- Zestoretic ... 2274

Hydrocodone Bitartrate (Potentiates orthostatic hypotensive effects). Products include:
- Anexsia 5/500 Tablets ... 2196
- Anexsia 7.5/650 Tablets ... 2197
- Azdōne Tablets ... 844
- Codiclear DH Syrup ... 845
- Codimal DH Syrup ... 846
- Damason-P ... 1356
- Hycodan Syrup, Tablets ... 927
- Hycomine Compound Tablets ... 929
- Hycomine Syrup ... 927
- Hycotuss Expectorant Syrup ... 930
- Hydrocet Capsules ... 835
- Lortab ASA Tablets ... 2414
- Lortab ... 2412

(▣ Described in PDR For Nonprescription Drugs)

(◉ Described in PDR For Ophthalmology)

Ru-Tuss with Hydrocodone 694
Triaminic Expectorant DH 1995
Vicodin Tablets 1187
Vicodin ES Tablets 1189
Zydone Capsules 941

Hydrocodone Polistirex (Potentiates orthostatic hypotensive effects). Products include:
Tussionex Extended-Release Suspension 988

Hydrocortisone (Potential for increased hypokalemia). Products include:
AK-Spore H.C. .... ◉ 206
Bactine Hydrocortisone Anti-Itch Cream .... ■ 625
CaldeCORT Anti-Itch Hydrocortisone Spray .... ■ 560
Carmol HC Cream 1% 2296
Cortaid Spray .... ■ 735
Cortenema 2244
Cortisporin Ointment 758
Cortisporin Ophthalmic Ointment Sterile 758
Cortisporin Ophthalmic Suspension Sterile 759
Cortisporin Otic Solution Sterile 760
Cortisporin Otic Suspension Sterile 760
Cortizone-5 Creme & Ointment .... ■ 732
Dermolate Anti-Itch Cream .... ■ 697
Eldecort Cream 1.0% 1113
Eldecort Cream 1.0% and 2.5% 1113
Fungoid HC Creme 1770
Hydrocortone Tablets 1482
Hytone 909
LazerSporin-C Solution 1770
Massengill Medicated Soft Cloth Towelettes 2192
Nutracort Cream & Lotion 1684
PediOtic Suspension Sterile 797
Synacort Creams 1%, 2.5% 2296
Vanoxide-HC Acne Lotion 911
Vioform-Hydrocortisone Cream and Mild Cream 889
Vioform-Hydrocortisone Ointment 889
VōSoL HC Otic Solution 2392
Vytone Cream 1% 911

Hydrocortisone Acetate (Potential for increased hypokalemia). Products include:
Analpram-HC Rectal Cream 1% and 2.5% 970
Anusol-HC Cream 1690
Anusol-HC Suppositories 1691
Caldecort .... ■ 560
Carmol HC Cream 1% 2296
Chloromycetin Hydrocortisone Ophthalmic 1694
Coly-Mycin S Otic w/Neomycin & Hydrocortisone 1708
Cortaid .... ■ 735
Cortef Feminine Itch Cream .... ■ 735
Corticaine .... ■ 682
Cortifoam 1827
Cortisporin Cream 757
Epifoam 1828
Gynecort 5 Creme .... ■ 556
Hydrocortone Acetate Sterile Suspension 1479
Lanacort 5 Creme and Ointment .... ■ 557
Mantadil Cream 789
Ophthocort .... ◉ 301
Orabase HCA Oral Paste 890
Pramosone Cream, Lotion & Ointment 971
ProctoCream-HC 1834
Proctofoam-HC 1835

Hydrocortisone Sodium Phosphate (Potential for increased hypokalemia). Products include:
Hydrocortone Phosphate Injection, Sterile 1481

Hydrocortisone Sodium Succinate (Potential for increased hypokalemia). Products include:
Solu-Cortef Sterile Powder 2361

Hydroflumethiazide (Orthostatic hypotension may occur with concurrent therapy). Products include:
Diucardin Tablets 2450
Saluron 718
Salutensin/Salutensin-Demi 719

Ibuprofen (Antihypertensive effects of Mykrox may be decreased). Products include:
Advil Cold & Sinus Caplets (formerly CoAdvil) 2416
Advil Ibuprofen Tablets and Caplets 2416
Children's Advil Suspension 2426
CoAdvil .... ■ 748
Dristan Sinus Caplets 2419
Haltran Tablets .... ■ 668
Ibuprofen .... ■ 631
Medipren ibuprofen Caplets and Tablets 1362
Midol 200 Cramp Relief Formula .... ■ 570
Motrin Tablets 2351
Motrin IB Caplets and Tablets .... ■ 736
Nuprin Ibuprofen/Analgesic Tablets & Caplets 752
PediaProfen Suspension 1363
Rufen Tablets 691
Trendar Ibuprofen Tablets .... ■ 756

Indapamide (Orthostatic hypotension may occur with concurrent therapy). Products include:
Lozol Tablets 1843

Indomethacin (Antihypertensive effects of Mykrox may be decreased). Products include:
Indocin 1487

Indomethacin Sodium Trihydrate (Antihypertensive effects of Mykrox may be decreased). Products include:
Indocin I.V. 1490

Insulin, Human (Blood glucose concentrations may be raised by metolazone in diabetics).
No products indexed under this heading.

Insulin, Human Isophane Suspension (Blood glucose concentrations may be raised by metolazone in diabetics). Products include:
Humulin N, 100 Units 1270

Insulin, Human NPH (Blood glucose concentrations may be raised by metolazone in diabetics). Products include:
Insulatard NPH Human 1627
Novolin N 1627
Novolin N PenFill Cartridges 1628
Novolin N Prefilled 1628

Insulin, Human Regular (Blood glucose concentrations may be raised by metolazone in diabetics). Products include:
Humulin BR, 100 Units 1268
Humulin R, 100 Units 1272
Novolin R 1627
Novolin R PenFill Cartridges 1628
Novolin R Prefilled 1629
Velosulin Human 1628

Insulin, Human, Zinc Suspension (Blood glucose concentrations may be raised by metolazone in diabetics). Products include:
Humulin L, 100 Units 1268
Humulin U, 100 Units 1272
Novolin L 1627

Insulin, NPH (Blood glucose concentrations may be raised by metolazone in diabetics). Products include:
NPH, 40 & 100 Units 1273
Beef NPH, 100 Units 1274
Pork NPH, 100 Units 1275
Insulatard NPH 1626
NPH Insulin 1626
NPH Purified Pork Isophane Insulin 1626

Insulin, Regular (Blood glucose concentrations may be raised by metolazone in diabetics). Products include:
Regular, 40 & 100 Units 1273
Beef Regular, 100 Units 1275
Pork Regular, 100 Units 1275
Pork Regular (Concentrated), 500 Units 1276
Regular Insulin 1625
Regular Purified Pork Insulin 1626
Velosulin 1627

Insulin, Zinc Crystals (Blood glucose concentrations may be raised by metolazone in diabetics). Products include:
NPH, 40 & 100 Units 1273

Insulin, Zinc Suspension (Blood glucose concentrations may be raised by metolazone in diabetics). Products include:
Lente, 40 & 100 Units 1272
Protamine, Zinc, 40 & 100 Units 1273
Lente Iletin I 1272
Beef Lente, 100 Units 1274
Beef Protamine Zinc, 100 Units 1274
Pork Lente, 100 Units 1275
Pork, Protamine, Zinc, 100 Units 1275
Lente Insulin 1626
Lente Purified Pork Insulin 1626
Semilente Insulin 1625
Ultralente Insulin 1626

Isradipine (Orthostatic hypotension may occur with concurrent therapy). Products include:
DynaCirc Capsules 2004

Ketoprofen (Antihypertensive effects of Mykrox may be decreased). Products include:
Orudis Capsules 2488

Ketorolac Tromethamine (Antihypertensive effects of Mykrox may be decreased). Products include:
Toradol IM Injection 2302

Labetalol Hydrochloride (Orthostatic hypotension may occur with concurrent therapy). Products include:
Normodyne Injection 2108
Normodyne Tablets 2110
Normozide Tablets 2112
Trandate HCT Tablets 579
Trandate Injection 577
Trandate Tablets 579

Levorphanol Tartrate (Potentiates orthostatic hypotensive effects). Products include:
Levo-Dromoran 1906

Lisinopril (Orthostatic hypotension may occur with concurrent therapy). Products include:
Prinivil Tablets 1538
Prinzide Tablets 1540
Zestoretic 2274
Zestril Tablets 2277

Lithium Carbonate (Reduced renal clearance of lithium; high risk of lithium toxicity). Products include:
Eskalith 2214
Lithane Tablets 1596
Lithium Carbonate Capsules & Tablets 1984
Lithobid Tablets 870

Lithium Citrate (Reduced renal clearance of lithium; high risk of lithium toxicity). Products include:
Cibalith-S 870

Magnesium Salicylate (Antihypertensive effects of Mykrox may be decreased). Products include:
Doan's - Extra-Strength Analgesic .... ■ 549
Doan's - Regular Strength Analgesic .... ■ 549
Mobigesic Analgesic Tablets .... ■ 507

Mecamylamine Hydrochloride (Orthostatic hypotension may occur with concurrent therapy). Products include:
Inversine Tablets 1492

Meclofenamate Sodium (Antihypertensive effects of Mykrox may be decreased). Products include:
Meclomen Capsules 1739

Mefenamic Acid (Antihypertensive effects of Mykrox may be decreased). Products include:
Ponstel 1758

Meperidine Hydrochloride (Potentiates orthostatic hypotensive effects). Products include:
Demerol 2047
Mepergan Injection 2479

Mephobarbital (Potentiates orthostatic hypotensive effects). Products include:
Mebaral Tablets 2061

Methadone Hydrochloride (Potentiates orthostatic hypotensive effects). Products include:
Dolophine Hydrochloride Ampoules & Vials 1260
Dolophine Hydrochloride Tablets 1261
Methadone Hydrochloride Diskets 1284
Methadone Hydrochloride Oral Solution & Tablets 1987

Methenamine (Efficacy of methenamine may be decreased). Products include:
Urised Tablets 2396

Methenamine Hippurate (Efficacy of methenamine may be decreased). Products include:
Hiprex Tablets 1333
Urex Tablets 1321

Methenamine Mandelate (Efficacy of methenamine may be decreased). Products include:
Mandelamine 1738
Uroqid-Acid 661

Methyclothiazide (Orthostatic hypotension may occur with concurrent therapy). Products include:
Enduron Tablets 517
Enduronyl 518

Methyldopa (Orthostatic hypotension may occur with concurrent therapy). Products include:
Aldoclor Tablets 1413
Aldomet Oral 1415
Aldoril Tablets 1418

Methyldopate Hydrochloride (Orthostatic hypotension may occur with concurrent therapy). Products include:
Aldomet Ester HCl Injection 1417

Methylprednisolone Acetate (Potential for increased hypokalemia). Products include:
Depo-Medrol Sterile Aqueous Suspension 2334

Methylprednisolone Sodium Succinate (Potential for increased hypokalemia). Products include:
Solu-Medrol Sterile Powder 2363

Metoprolol Tartrate (Orthostatic hypotension may occur with concurrent therapy). Products include:
Lopressor Ampuls 1032
Lopressor HCT Tablets 1034
Lopressor Tablets 1032

Metyrosine (Orthostatic hypotension may occur with concurrent therapy). Products include:
Demser Capsules 1460

Minoxidil (Orthostatic hypotension may occur with concurrent therapy). Products include:
Loniten Tablets 2346
Rogaine Topical Solution 2357

Morphine Sulfate (Potentiates orthostatic hypotensive effects). Products include:
Astramorph/PF Injection, USP (Preservative-Free) 618
Duramorph 960
Infumorph 200 and Infumorph 500 Sterile Solutions 962
MS Contin Tablets 1814
MSIR 1817
Oramorph SR (Morphine Sulfate Sustained Release Tablets) 1988
Roxanol 1991

Nadolol (Orthostatic hypotension may occur with concurrent therapy). Products include:
Corgard Tablets 701
Corzide Tablets 702

Naproxen (Antihypertensive effects of Mykrox may be decreased). Products include:
Naprosyn 2297

Naproxen Sodium (Antihypertensive effects of Mykrox may be decreased). Products include:
- Anaprox and Anaprox DS Tablets.... 2288

Nicardipine Hydrochloride (Orthostatic hypotension may occur with concurrent therapy). Products include:
- Cardene Capsules 2290

Nitroglycerin (Orthostatic hypotension may occur with concurrent therapy). Products include:
- Deponit NTG Transdermal Delivery System 2143
- Minitran Transdermal Delivery System 1312
- Nitro-Bid Ointment 1339
- Nitro-Bid Capsules 1338
- Nitrodisc 2176
- Nitro-Dur (nitroglycerin) Transdermal Infusion System 1164
- Nitrogard Tablets 1004
- Nitrolingual Spray 1846
- Nitrostat Tablets 1743
- Transderm-Nitro Transdermal Therapeutic System 2283

Norepinephrine Bitartrate (Arterial responsiveness to norepinephrine may be decreased). Products include:
- Levophed Bitartrate Injection 2054

Opium Alkaloids (Potentiates orthostatic hypotensive effects). Products include:
- B & O No. 15A & No. 16A Supprettes 2395
- Pantopon Injectable 1911

Oxycodone Hydrochloride (Potentiates orthostatic hypotensive effects). Products include:
- Percocet Tablets 950
- Percodan 951
- Roxicodone Tablets, Oral Solution & Intensol (Oxycodone) 1992
- Tylox Capsules 1382

Penbutolol Sulfate (Orthostatic hypotension may occur with concurrent therapy). Products include:
- Levatol 1832

Pentobarbital Sodium (Potentiates orthostatic hypotensive effects). Products include:
- Nembutal Sodium Capsules 534
- Nembutal Sodium Solution 536
- Nembutal Sodium Suppositories 538

Phenobarbital (Potentiates orthostatic hypotensive effects). Products include:
- Arco-Lase Plus Tablets 607
- Bellergal-S Tablets 1998
- Bronkolixir .... ▣ 761
- Bronkotabs Tablets .... ▣ 762
- Donnatal 1858
- Donnatal Extentabs 1859
- Donnatal Tablets 1858
- Donnazyme Tablets 1860
- Kinesed Tablets 2272
- Phenobarbital Elixir and Tablets 1293
- Primatene Tablets-P Formula 2421
- Quadrinal Tablets 1183
- Tedral SA 1765

Phenoxybenzamine Hydrochloride (Orthostatic hypotension may occur with concurrent therapy). Products include:
- Dibenzyline Capsules 2207

Phentolamine Mesylate (Orthostatic hypotension may occur with concurrent therapy). Products include:
- Regitine 878

Phenylbutazone (Antihypertensive effects of Mykrox may be decreased). Products include:
- Butazolidin Capsules & Tablets 1027

Pindolol (Orthostatic hypotension may occur with concurrent therapy). Products include:
- Visken Tablets 2036

Piroxicam (Antihypertensive effects of Mykrox may be decreased). Products include:
- Feldene Capsules 1777

Polythiazide (Orthostatic hypotension may occur with concurrent therapy). Products include:
- Minizide Capsules 1779
- Renese Tablets 1785
- Renese-R Tablets 1786

Prazosin Hydrochloride (Orthostatic hypotension may occur with concurrent therapy). Products include:
- Minipress Capsules 1778
- Minizide Capsules 1779

Prednisolone Acetate (Potential for increased hypokalemia). Products include:
- AK-Cide Sterile Ophthalmic Ointment & Suspension .... ⊙ 202
- Blephamide Liquifilm Sterile Ophthalmic Suspension 586
- Blephamide S.O.P. Sterile Ophthalmic Ointment 586
- Cetapred Ointment .... ⊙ 220
- ⅛% Econopred & 1% Econopred Plus .... ⊙ 217
- Isopto Cetapred Suspension .... ⊙ 220
- Metimyd .... ⊙ 306
- Poly-Pred Liquifilm .... ⊙ 250
- Pred Forte .... ⊙ 252
- Pred Mild .... ⊙ 254
- Pred-G Liquifilm Sterile Ophthalmic Suspension .... ⊙ 252
- Pred-G S.O.P. Sterile Ophthalmic Ointment .... ⊙ 253
- Vasocidin Ointment .... ⊙ 275

Prednisolone Sodium Phosphate (Potential for increased hypokalemia). Products include:
- AK-Pred .... ⊙ 205
- Hydeltrasol Injection, Sterile 1476
- Inflamase .... ⊙ 274
- Pediapred Oral Liquid 987
- Vasocidin Ophthalmic Solution .... ⊙ 276

Prednisolone Tebutate (Potential for increased hypokalemia). Products include:
- Hydeltra-T.B.A. Sterile Suspension 1478

Prednisone (Potential for increased hypokalemia). Products include:
- Deltasone Tablets 2332

Propoxyphene Hydrochloride (Potentiates orthostatic hypotensive effects). Products include:
- Darvon 1256
- Wygesic Tablets 2540

Propoxyphene Napsylate (Potentiates orthostatic hypotensive effects). Products include:
- Darvon-N/Darvocet-N 1254

Propranolol Hydrochloride (Orthostatic hypotension may occur with concurrent therapy). Products include:
- Inderal 2459
- Inderal LA Long Acting Capsules 2461
- Inderide Tablets 2463
- Inderide LA Long Acting Capsules .. 2465

Ramipril (Orthostatic hypotension may occur with concurrent therapy). Products include:
- Altace Capsules 1086

Rauwolfia Serpentina (Orthostatic hypotension may occur with concurrent therapy). Products include:
- Raudixin Tablets 1803
- Rauzide Tablets 1804

Rescinnamine (Orthostatic hypotension may occur with concurrent therapy).
- No products indexed under this heading.

Reserpine (Orthostatic hypotension may occur with concurrent therapy). Products include:
- Diupres Tablets 1461
- Hydromox R Tablets 1209
- Hydropres Tablets 1485
- Renese-R Tablets 1786
- Salutensin/Salutensin-Demi 719
- Ser-Ap-Es Tablets 881
- Serpasil Tablets 883
- Serpasil-Apresoline Tablets 884
- Serpasil-Esidrix Tablets 886

Salsalate (Antihypertensive effects of Mykrox may be decreased). Products include:
- Disalcid 1310
- Mono-Gesic Tablets 846
- Salflex 839

Secobarbital Sodium (Potentiates orthostatic hypotensive effects). Products include:
- Seconal Sodium Pulvules 1296

Sodium Nitroprusside (Orthostatic hypotension may occur with concurrent therapy). Products include:
- Nipride I.V. Infusion 1909

Sufentanil Citrate (Potentiates orthostatic hypotensive effects). Products include:
- Sufenta Injection 1147

Sulindac (Antihypertensive effects of Mykrox may be decreased). Products include:
- Clinoril Tablets 1433

Terazosin Hydrochloride (Orthostatic hypotension may occur with concurrent therapy). Products include:
- Hytrin Tablets 529

Thiamylal Sodium (Potentiates orthostatic hypotensive effects). Products include:
- Surital Ampoules, Steri-Vials 1764

Timolol Maleate (Orthostatic hypotension may occur with concurrent therapy). Products include:
- Blocadren Tablets 1429
- Timolide Tablets 1547
- Timoptic in Ocudose 1552
- Timoptic Sterile Ophthalmic Solution 1550

Tolazamide (Blood glucose concentrations may be raised by metolazone in diabetics). Products include:
- Tolinase Tablets 2365

Tolbutamide (Blood glucose concentrations may be raised by metolazone in diabetics). Products include:
- Orinase Tablets 2354

Tolmetin Sodium (Antihypertensive effects of Mykrox may be decreased). Products include:
- Tolectin (200, 400 and 600 mg) .. 1379

Triamcinolone (Potential for increased hypokalemia).
- No products indexed under this heading.

Triamcinolone Acetonide (Potential for increased hypokalemia). Products include:
- Aristocort A 1010
- Azmacort Inhaler 1837
- Kenalog Cream, Lotion & Ointment 2401
- Kenalog-10 Injection 2402
- Kenalog-40 Injection 2403
- Kenalog in Orabase 604
- Kenalog Spray 2401
- Mycolog II Cream and Ointment 2407
- Mytrex Cream & Ointment 2080
- Nasacort Nasal Inhaler 1844

Triamcinolone Diacetate (Potential for increased hypokalemia). Products include:
- Aristocort Suspension 1008

Triamcinolone Hexacetonide (Potential for increased hypokalemia). Products include:
- Aristospan Suspension 1011

Trimethaphan Camsylate (Orthostatic hypotension may occur with concurrent therapy). Products include:
- Arfonad Ampuls 1887

Tubocurarine Chloride (Neuromuscular blocking effects of curariform drugs may be enhanced).
- No products indexed under this heading.

MYLANTA LIQUID
(Aluminum Hydroxide Gel, Dried, Magnesium Hydroxide, Simethicone) 1155
May interact with tetracyclines. Compounds in this category include:

Demeclocycline Hydrochloride (Not specified). Products include:
- Declomycin Capsules, Tablets 1199

Doxycycline Calcium (Not specified).
- No products indexed under this heading.

Doxycycline Hyclate (Not specified). Products include:
- Doryx Capsules 1717
- Vibramycin Hyclate Capsules 1787
- Vibramycin Hyclate Intravenous 1968
- Vibra-Tabs Film Coated Tablets 1787

Doxycycline Monohydrate (Not specified). Products include:
- Monodox Capsules 1630
- Vibramycin Monohydrate for Oral Suspension 1787

Methacycline Hydrochloride (Not specified).
- No products indexed under this heading.

Minocycline Hydrochloride (Not specified). Products include:
- Minocin Intravenous 1221
- Minocin Oral Suspension 1224
- Minocin Pellet-Filled Capsules 1222

Oxytetracycline (Not specified). Products include:
- Terramycin Intramuscular Solution 1964
- Urobiotic-250 Capsules 1968

Oxytetracycline Hydrochloride (Not specified). Products include:
- Terra-Cortril Ophthalmic Suspension 1963
- Terramycin Capsules 1786
- Terramycin Intramuscular Solution 1964
- Terramycin with Polymyxin B Sulfate Ophthalmic Ointment 1965

Tetracycline Hydrochloride (Not specified). Products include:
- Achromycin V Capsules 1193
- Achromycin Ophthalmic Ointment 1% .... ⊙ 307
- Achromycin Ophthalmic Suspension 1% .... ⊙ 308
- Topicycline for Topical Solution 1856

MYLANTA TABLETS
(Aluminum Hydroxide Gel, Dried, Magnesium Hydroxide, Simethicone) 1155
See **Mylanta Liquid**

MYLANTA DOUBLE STRENGTH LIQUID
(Aluminum Hydroxide Gel, Dried, Magnesium Hydroxide, Simethicone) 1155
May interact with tetracyclines. Compounds in this category include:

Demeclocycline Hydrochloride (Effects not specified). Products include:
- Declomycin Capsules, Tablets 1199

Doxycycline Calcium (Effects not specified).
- No products indexed under this heading.

Doxycycline Hyclate (Effects not specified). Products include:
- Doryx Capsules 1717
- Vibramycin Hyclate Capsules 1787
- Vibramycin Hyclate Intravenous 1968
- Vibra-Tabs Film Coated Tablets 1787

Doxycycline Monohydrate (Effects not specified). Products include:
- Monodox Capsules 1630
- Vibramycin Monohydrate for Oral Suspension 1787

Methacycline Hydrochloride (Effects not specified).
No products indexed under this heading.

Minocycline Hydrochloride (Effects not specified). Products include:
- Minocin Intravenous ... 1221
- Minocin Oral Suspension ... 1224
- Minocin Pellet-Filled Capsules ... 1222

Oxytetracycline (Effects not specified). Products include:
- Terramycin Intramuscular Solution 1964
- Urobiotic-250 Capsules ... 1968

Oxytetracycline Hydrochloride (Effects not specified). Products include:
- Terra-Cortril Ophthalmic Suspension ... 1963
- Terramycin Capsules ... 1786
- Terramycin Intramuscular Solution 1964
- Terramycin with Polymyxin B Sulfate Ophthalmic Ointment ... 1965

Tetracycline Hydrochloride (Effects not specified). Products include:
- Achromycin V Capsules ... 1193
- Achromycin Ophthalmic Ointment 1% ... ◉ 307
- Achromycin Ophthalmic Suspension 1% ... ◉ 308
- Topicycline for Topical Solution ... 1856

MYLANTA DOUBLE STRENGTH TABLETS
(Aluminum Hydroxide Gel, Dried, Magnesium Hydroxide, Simethicone) 1155
See **Mylanta Double Strength Liquid**

MYLANTA'S BRAND MYLICON GAS TABLETS
(Simethicone) ... 1156
No interactions described in labeling.

MAXIMUM STRENGTH MYLANTA'S BRAND MYLICON GAS TABLETS
(Simethicone) ... 1156
No interactions described in labeling.

MYLERAN TABLETS
(Busulfan) ... 790
May interact with bone marrow depressants, antineoplastics, and certain other agents. Compounds in these categories include:

Altretamine (Potential for rare life-threatening hepatic veno-occlusive disease). Products include:
- Hexalen Capsules ... 2316

Asparaginase (Potential for rare life-threatening hepatic veno-occlusive disease). Products include:
- Elspar ... 1470

Bleomycin Sulfate (Potential for rare life-threatening hepatic veno-occlusive disease). Products include:
- Blenoxane ... 724

Bone Marrow Depressants, unspecified (Additive myelosuppression).

Carboplatin (Potential for rare life-threatening hepatic veno-occlusive disease). Products include:
- Paraplatin for Injection ... 735

Carmustine (BCNU) (Potential for rare life-threatening hepatic veno-occlusive disease). Products include:
- BiCNU ... 723

Chlorambucil (Potential for rare life-threatening hepatic veno-occlusive disease). Products include:
- Leukeran Tablets ... 788

Cisplatin (Potential for rare life-threatening hepatic veno-occlusive disease). Products include:
- Platinol ... 737
- Platinol-AQ Injection ... 738

Cyclophosphamide (Potential for rare life-threatening hepatic veno-occlusive disease). Products include:
- Cytoxan for Injection ... 726
- Neosar for Injection ... 566

Dacarbazine (Potential for rare life-threatening hepatic veno-occlusive disease). Products include:
- DTIC-Dome ... 1595

Daunorubicin Hydrochloride (Potential for rare life-threatening hepatic veno-occlusive disease). Products include:
- Cerubidine ... 2443

Doxorubicin Hydrochloride (Potential for rare life-threatening hepatic veno-occlusive disease). Products include:
- Adriamycin PFS ... 561
- Adriamycin RDF ... 562
- Doxorubicin Hydrochloride for Injection, USP ... 622
- Doxorubicin Hydrochloride Injection, USP ... 848
- Rubex ... 739

Estramustine Phosphate Sodium (Potential for rare life-threatening hepatic veno-occlusive disease). Products include:
- Emcyt Capsules ... 1161

Etoposide (Potential for rare life-threatening hepatic veno-occlusive disease). Products include:
- VePesid Capsules and Injection ... 741

Floxuridine (Potential for rare life-threatening hepatic veno-occlusive disease). Products include:
- Sterile FUDR ... 1898

Fluorouracil (Potential for rare life-threatening hepatic veno-occlusive disease). Products include:
- Efudex ... 1880
- Fluoroplex Topical Solution & Cream 1% ... 1082
- Fluorouracil Injection ... 1897

Flutamide (Potential for rare life-threatening hepatic veno-occlusive disease). Products include:
- Eulexin Capsules ... 2089

Hydroxyurea (Potential for rare life-threatening hepatic veno-occlusive disease). Products include:
- Hydrea Capsules ... 728

Ifosfamide (Potential for rare life-threatening hepatic veno-occlusive disease). Products include:
- IFEX ... 729

Interferon alfa-2A, Recombinant (Potential for rare life-threatening hepatic veno-occlusive disease). Products include:
- Roferon-A Injection ... 1916

Interferon alfa-2B, Recombinant (Potential for rare life-threatening hepatic veno-occlusive disease). Products include:
- Intron A ... 2097

Levamisole Hydrochloride (Potential for rare life-threatening hepatic veno-occlusive disease). Products include:
- Ergamisol Tablets ... 1136

Lomustine (CCNU) (Potential for rare life-threatening hepatic veno-occlusive disease). Products include:
- CeeNU ... 725

Mechlorethamine Hydrochloride (Potential for rare life-threatening hepatic veno-occlusive disease). Products include:
- Mustargen ... 1514

Megestrol Acetate (Potential for rare life-threatening hepatic veno-occlusive disease). Products include:
- Megace Tablets ... 732

Melphalan (Potential for rare life-threatening hepatic veno-occlusive disease). Products include:
- Alkeran Tablets ... 754

Mercaptopurine (Potential for rare life-threatening hepatic veno-occlusive disease). Products include:
- Purinethol Tablets ... 800

Methotrexate Sodium (Potential for rare life-threatening hepatic veno-occlusive disease). Products include:
- Methotrexate Tablets, Parenteral, LPF Parenteral ... 1217
- Rheumatrex Methotrexate Dose Pack ... 1234

Mitomycin (Mitomycin-C) (Potential for rare life-threatening hepatic veno-occlusive disease). Products include:
- Mutamycin ... 733

Mitotane (Potential for rare life-threatening hepatic veno-occlusive disease). Products include:
- Lysodren ... 731

Mitoxantrone Hydrochloride (Potential for rare life-threatening hepatic veno-occlusive disease). Products include:
- Novantrone for Injection Concentrate ... 1226

Procarbazine Hydrochloride (Potential for rare life-threatening hepatic veno-occlusive disease). Products include:
- Matulane Capsules ... 1907

Streptozocin (Potential for rare life-threatening hepatic veno-occlusive disease). Products include:
- Zanosar Sterile Powder ... 2371

Tamoxifen Citrate (Potential for rare life-threatening hepatic veno-occlusive disease). Products include:
- Nolvadex Tablets ... 1102

Thioguanine (Potential for esophageal varices associated with abnormal liver function tests; potential for rare life-threatening hepatic veno-occlusive disease). Products include:
- Thioguanine Tablets, Tabloid Brand ... 815

Thiotepa (Potential for rare life-threatening hepatic veno-occlusive disease). Products include:
- Thiotepa Parenteral ... 1240

Vincristine Sulfate (Potential for rare life-threatening hepatic veno-occlusive disease). Products include:
- Oncovin Solution Vials & Hyporets 1288

MYLICON DROPS
(Simethicone) ... 1156
No interactions described in labeling.

MYLICON TABLETS
(Simethicone) ... 1156
No interactions described in labeling.

MYOCHRYSINE INJECTION
(Gold Sodium Thiomalate) ... 1516
May interact with cytotoxic drugs and certain other agents. Compounds in these categories include:

Bleomycin Sulfate (Safety of coadministration has NOT been established). Products include:
- Blenoxane ... 724

Daunorubicin Hydrochloride (Safety of coadministration has NOT been established). Products include:
- Cerubidine ... 2443

Doxorubicin Hydrochloride (Safety of coadministration has NOT been established). Products include:
- Adriamycin PFS ... 561
- Adriamycin RDF ... 562
- Doxorubicin Hydrochloride for Injection, USP ... 622
- Doxorubicin Hydrochloride Injection, USP ... 848
- Rubex ... 739

Fluorouracil (Safety of coadministration has NOT been established). Products include:
- Efudex ... 1880
- Fluoroplex Topical Solution & Cream 1% ... 1082
- Fluorouracil Injection ... 1897

Hydroxyurea (Safety of coadministration has NOT been established). Products include:
- Hydrea Capsules ... 728

Methotrexate Sodium (Safety of coadministration has NOT been established). Products include:
- Methotrexate Tablets, Parenteral, LPF Parenteral ... 1217
- Rheumatrex Methotrexate Dose Pack ... 1234

Mitotane (Safety of coadministration has NOT been established). Products include:
- Lysodren ... 731

Mitoxantrone Hydrochloride (Safety of coadministration has NOT been established). Products include:
- Novantrone for Injection Concentrate ... 1226

Penicillamine (Do not use concomitantly). Products include:
- Cuprimine Capsules ... 1442
- Depen Titratable Tablets ... 2379

Procarbazine Hydrochloride (Safety of coadministration has NOT been established). Products include:
- Matulane Capsules ... 1907

Tamoxifen Citrate (Safety of coadministration has NOT been established). Products include:
- Nolvadex Tablets ... 1102

Vincristine Sulfate (Safety of coadministration has NOT been established). Products include:
- Oncovin Solution Vials & Hyporets 1288

MYSOLINE SUSPENSION
(Primidone) ... 2480
No interactions described in labeling.

MYSOLINE TABLETS
(Primidone) ... 2480
No interactions described in labeling.

MYTREX CREAM & OINTMENT
(Nystatin, Triamcinolone Acetonide) .. 2080
No interactions described in labeling.

NP-27 CREAM, SOLUTION, SPRAY POWDER & POWDER ANTIFUNGAL
(Tolnaftate) ... ▣ 734
No interactions described in labeling.

NPH INSULIN
(Insulin, NPH) ... 1626
No interactions described in labeling.

NPH PURIFIED PORK ISOPHANE INSULIN
(Insulin, NPH) ... 1626
No interactions described in labeling.

NTZ LONG ACTING NASAL SPRAY & DROPS 0.05%
(Oxymetazoline Hydrochloride) ... ▣ 760
No interactions described in labeling.

NAFTIN CREAM 1%
(Naftifine Hydrochloride) ... 1084
No interactions described in labeling.

NAFTIN GEL 1%
(Naftifine Hydrochloride) ... 1084
No interactions described in labeling.

NAIL SCRUB
(Isopropyl Myristate) 1771
No interactions described in labeling.

NALDECON CX ADULT LIQUID
(Phenylpropanolamine Hydrochloride, Guaifenesin, Codeine Phosphate) 521
May interact with antidepressant drugs and antihypertensives. Compounds in these categories include:

Acebutolol Hydrochloride (Concurrent therapy is not recommended). Products include:
Sectral Capsules 2520

Amitriptyline Hydrochloride (Concurrent therapy is not recommended). Products include:
Elavil 2269
Endep Tablets 1927
Etrafon 2087
Limbitrol 1933
Triavil Tablets 1556

Amoxapine (Concurrent therapy is not recommended). Products include:
Asendin Tablets 1196

Atenolol (Concurrent therapy is not recommended). Products include:
Tenoretic Tablets 1105
Tenormin Tablets and I.V. Injection 1107

Benazepril Hydrochloride (Concurrent therapy is not recommended). Products include:
Lotensin Tablets 872

Bendroflumethiazide (Concurrent therapy is not recommended). Products include:
Corzide Tablets 702
Naturetin Tablets 1789
Rauzide Tablets 1804

Betaxolol Hydrochloride (Concurrent therapy is not recommended). Products include:
Betoptic Sterile Ophthalmic Solution 569
Betoptic S Sterile Ophthalmic Suspension 570
Kerlone Tablets 2172

Bupropion Hydrochloride (Concurrent therapy is not recommended). Products include:
Wellbutrin Tablets 821

Captopril (Concurrent therapy is not recommended). Products include:
Capoten 2255
Capozide 2258

Carteolol Hydrochloride (Concurrent therapy is not recommended). Products include:
Cartrol Tablets 507

Chlorothiazide (Concurrent therapy is not recommended). Products include:
Aldoclor Tablets 1413
Diupres Tablets 1461
Diuril Oral 1464

Chlorothiazide Sodium (Concurrent therapy is not recommended). Products include:
Diuril Sodium Intravenous 1463

Chlorthalidone (Concurrent therapy is not recommended). Products include:
Combipres Tablets 678
Tenoretic Tablets 1105
Thalitone Tablets 687

Clonidine (Concurrent therapy is not recommended). Products include:
Catapres-TTS 677

Clonidine Hydrochloride (Concurrent therapy is not recommended). Products include:
Catapres Tablets 676
Combipres Tablets 678

Deserpidine (Concurrent therapy is not recommended). Products include:
Enduronyl 518
Harmonyl Tablets 528
Oreticyl 545

Desipramine Hydrochloride (Concurrent therapy is not recommended). Products include:
Norpramin Tablets 1340

Diazoxide (Concurrent therapy is not recommended). Products include:
Hyperstat I.V. Injection 2095
Proglycem 649

Doxazosin Mesylate (Concurrent therapy is not recommended). Products include:
Cardura Tablets 1941

Doxepin Hydrochloride (Concurrent therapy is not recommended). Products include:
Sinequan 1960

Enalapril Maleate (Concurrent therapy is not recommended). Products include:
Vaseretic Tablets 1559
Vasotec Tablets 1564

Enalaprilat (Concurrent therapy is not recommended). Products include:
Vasotec I.V. 1562

Esmolol Hydrochloride (Concurrent therapy is not recommended). Products include:
Brevibloc Injection 942

Felodipine (Concurrent therapy is not recommended). Products include:
Plendil Extended-Release Tablets 1526

Fluoxetine Hydrochloride (Concurrent therapy is not recommended). Products include:
Prozac Pulvules 920

Fosinopril Sodium (Concurrent therapy is not recommended). Products include:
Monopril Tablets 1406

Furosemide (Concurrent therapy is not recommended). Products include:
Lasix 1093

Guanabenz Acetate (Concurrent therapy is not recommended). Products include:
Wytensin Tablets 2542

Guanethidine Monosulfate (Concurrent therapy is not recommended). Products include:
Esimil Tablets 864
Ismelin Tablets 869

Hydralazine Hydrochloride (Concurrent therapy is not recommended). Products include:
Apresazide Capsules 854
Apresoline Hydrochloride Parenteral (Ampuls) 856
Apresoline Hydrochloride Tablets 855
Apresoline-Esidrix Tablets 857
Ser-Ap-Es Tablets 881
Serpasil-Apresoline Tablets 884

Hydrochlorothiazide (Concurrent therapy is not recommended). Products include:
Aldactazide 2150
Aldoril Tablets 1418
Apresazide Capsules 854
Apresoline-Esidrix Tablets 857
Capozide 2258
Dyazide Capsules 2208
Esidrix Tablets 863
Esimil Tablets 864
HydroDIURIL Tablets 1484
Hydropres Tablets 1485
Inderide Tablets 2463
Inderide LA Long Acting Capsules 2465
Lopressor HCT Tablets 1034
Maxzide 1215
Moduretic Tablets 1510
Normozide Tablets 2112
Oretic Tablets 544
Oreticyl 545
Prinzide Tablets 1540
Ser-Ap-Es Tablets 881
Serpasil-Esidrix Tablets 886
Timolide Tablets 1547
Trandate HCT Tablets 579
Vaseretic Tablets 1559
Zestoretic 2274

Hydroflumethiazide (Concurrent therapy is not recommended). Products include:
Diucardin Tablets 2450
Saluron 718
Salutensin/Salutensin-Demi 719

Imipramine Hydrochloride (Concurrent therapy is not recommended). Products include:
Tofranil Ampuls 1038
Tofranil Tablets 1039

Imipramine Pamoate (Concurrent therapy is not recommended). Products include:
Tofranil-PM Capsules 1041

Indapamide (Concurrent therapy is not recommended). Products include:
Lozol Tablets 1843

Isocarboxazid (Concurrent therapy is not recommended). Products include:
Marplan Tablets 1906

Isradipine (Concurrent therapy is not recommended). Products include:
DynaCirc Capsules 2004

Labetalol Hydrochloride (Concurrent therapy is not recommended). Products include:
Normodyne Injection 2108
Normodyne Tablets 2110
Normozide Tablets 2112
Trandate HCT Tablets 579
Trandate Injection 577
Trandate Tablets 579

Lisinopril (Concurrent therapy is not recommended). Products include:
Prinivil Tablets 1538
Prinzide Tablets 1540
Zestoretic 2274
Zestril Tablets 2277

Maprotiline Hydrochloride (Concurrent therapy is not recommended). Products include:
Ludiomil Tablets 874

Mecamylamine Hydrochloride (Concurrent therapy is not recommended). Products include:
Inversine Tablets 1492

Methyclothiazide (Concurrent therapy is not recommended). Products include:
Enduron Tablets 517
Enduronyl 518

Methyldopa (Concurrent therapy is not recommended). Products include:
Aldoclor Tablets 1413
Aldomet Oral 1415
Aldoril Tablets 1418

Methyldopate Hydrochloride (Concurrent therapy is not recommended). Products include:
Aldomet Ester HCl Injection 1417

Metolazone (Concurrent therapy is not recommended). Products include:
Diulo 2129
Mykrox ½ mg Tablets 984
Zaroxolyn Tablets 989

Metoprolol Tartrate (Concurrent therapy is not recommended). Products include:
Lopressor Ampuls 1032
Lopressor HCT Tablets 1034
Lopressor Tablets 1032

Metyrosine (Concurrent therapy is not recommended). Products include:
Demser Capsules 1460

Minoxidil (Concurrent therapy is not recommended). Products include:
Loniten Tablets 2346
Rogaine Topical Solution 2357

Nadolol (Concurrent therapy is not recommended). Products include:
Corgard Tablets 701
Corzide Tablets 702

Nicardipine Hydrochloride (Concurrent therapy is not recommended). Products include:
Cardene Capsules 2290

Nitroglycerin (Concurrent therapy is not recommended). Products include:
Deponit NTG Transdermal Delivery System 2143
Minitran Transdermal Delivery System 1312
Nitro-Bid Ointment 1339
Nitro-Bid Capsules 1338
Nitrodisc 2176
Nitro-Dur (nitroglycerin) Transdermal Infusion System 1164
Nitrogard Tablets 1004
Nitrolingual Spray 1846
Nitrostat Tablets 1743
Transderm-Nitro Transdermal Therapeutic System 2283

Nortriptyline Hydrochloride (Concurrent therapy is not recommended). Products include:
Pamelor 2019

Penbutolol Sulfate (Concurrent therapy is not recommended). Products include:
Levatol 1832

Phenelzine Sulfate (Concurrent therapy is not recommended). Products include:
Nardil 1742

Phenoxybenzamine Hydrochloride (Concurrent therapy is not recommended). Products include:
Dibenzyline Capsules 2207

Phentolamine Mesylate (Concurrent therapy is not recommended). Products include:
Regitine 878

Pindolol (Concurrent therapy is not recommended). Products include:
Visken Tablets 2036

Polythiazide (Concurrent therapy is not recommended). Products include:
Minizide Capsules 1779
Renese Tablets 1785
Renese-R Tablets 1786

Prazosin Hydrochloride (Concurrent therapy is not recommended). Products include:
Minipress Capsules 1778
Minizide Capsules 1779

Propranolol Hydrochloride (Concurrent therapy is not recommended). Products include:
Inderal 2459
Inderal LA Long Acting Capsules 2461
Inderide Tablets 2463
Inderide LA Long Acting Capsules 2465

Protriptyline Hydrochloride (Concurrent therapy is not recommended). Products include:
Vivactil Tablets 1567

Ramipril (Concurrent therapy is not recommended). Products include:
Altace Capsules 1086

Rauwolfia Serpentina (Concurrent therapy is not recommended). Products include:
Raudixin Tablets 1803
Rauzide Tablets 1804

Rescinnamine (Concurrent therapy is not recommended).
No products indexed under this heading.

Reserpine (Concurrent therapy is not recommended). Products include:
Diupres Tablets 1461
Hydromox R Tablets 1209
Hydropres Tablets 1485
Renese-R Tablets 1786
Salutensin/Salutensin-Demi 719
Ser-Ap-Es Tablets 881
Serpasil Tablets 883
Serpasil-Apresoline Tablets 884
Serpasil-Esidrix Tablets 886
Sodium Nitroprusside (Concurrent therapy is not recommended). Products include:
Nipride I.V. Infusion 1909
Terazosin Hydrochloride (Concurrent therapy is not recommended). Products include:
Hytrin Tablets 529
Timolol Maleate (Concurrent therapy is not recommended). Products include:
Blocadren Tablets 1429
Timolide Tablets 1547
Timoptic in Ocudose 1552
Timoptic Sterile Ophthalmic Solution 1550
Tranylcypromine Sulfate (Concurrent therapy is not recommended). Products include:
Parnate Tablets 2222
Trazodone Hydrochloride (Concurrent therapy is not recommended). Products include:
Desyrel and Desyrel Dividose 1404
Trimethaphan Camsylate (Concurrent therapy is not recommended). Products include:
Arfonad Ampuls 1887
Trimipramine Maleate (Concurrent therapy is not recommended). Products include:
Surmontil Capsules 2524

NALDECON DX ADULT LIQUID
(Phenylpropanolamine Hydrochloride, Guaifenesin, Dextromethorphan Hydrobromide) ®◘ 521
May interact with antidepressant drugs and antihypertensives. Compounds in these categories include:

Acebutolol Hydrochloride (Concurrent therapy is not recommended). Products include:
Sectral Capsules 2520
Amitriptyline Hydrochloride (Concurrent therapy is not recommended). Products include:
Elavil 2269
Endep Tablets 1927
Etrafon 2087
Limbitrol 1933
Triavil Tablets 1556
Amoxapine (Concurrent therapy is not recommended). Products include:
Asendin Tablets 1196
Atenolol (Concurrent therapy is not recommended). Products include:
Tenoretic Tablets 1105
Tenormin Tablets and I.V. Injection 1107
Benazepril Hydrochloride (Concurrent therapy is not recommended). Products include:
Lotensin Tablets 872
Bendroflumethiazide (Concurrent therapy is not recommended). Products include:
Corzide Tablets 702
Naturetin Tablets 1789
Rauzide Tablets 1804
Betaxolol Hydrochloride (Concurrent therapy is not recommended). Products include:
Betoptic Sterile Ophthalmic Solution 569
Betoptic S Sterile Ophthalmic Suspension 570
Kerlone Tablets 2172
Bupropion Hydrochloride (Concurrent therapy is not recommended). Products include:
Wellbutrin Tablets 821
Captopril (Concurrent therapy is not recommended). Products include:
Capoten 2255
Capozide 2258
Carteolol Hydrochloride (Concurrent therapy is not recommended). Products include:
Cartrol Tablets 507
Chlorothiazide (Concurrent therapy is not recommended). Products include:
Aldoclor Tablets 1413
Diupres Tablets 1461
Diuril Oral 1464
Chlorothiazide Sodium (Concurrent therapy is not recommended). Products include:
Diuril Sodium Intravenous 1463
Chlorthalidone (Concurrent therapy is not recommended). Products include:
Combipres Tablets 678
Tenoretic Tablets 1105
Thalitone Tablets 687
Clonidine (Concurrent therapy is not recommended). Products include:
Catapres-TTS 677
Clonidine Hydrochloride (Concurrent therapy is not recommended). Products include:
Catapres Tablets 676
Combipres Tablets 678
Deserpidine (Concurrent therapy is not recommended). Products include:
Enduronyl 518
Harmonyl Tablets 528
Oreticyl 545
Desipramine Hydrochloride (Concurrent therapy is not recommended). Products include:
Norpramin Tablets 1340
Diazoxide (Concurrent therapy is not recommended). Products include:
Hyperstat I.V. Injection 2095
Proglycem 649
Doxazosin Mesylate (Concurrent therapy is not recommended). Products include:
Cardura Tablets 1941
Doxepin Hydrochloride (Concurrent therapy is not recommended). Products include:
Sinequan 1960
Enalapril Maleate (Concurrent therapy is not recommended). Products include:
Vaseretic Tablets 1559
Vasotec Tablets 1564
Enalaprilat (Concurrent therapy is not recommended). Products include:
Vasotec I.V. 1562
Esmolol Hydrochloride (Concurrent therapy is not recommended). Products include:
Brevibloc Injection 942
Felodipine (Concurrent therapy is not recommended). Products include:
Plendil Extended-Release Tablets 1526
Fluoxetine Hydrochloride (Concurrent therapy is not recommended). Products include:
Prozac Pulvules 920
Fosinopril Sodium (Concurrent therapy is not recommended). Products include:
Monopril Tablets 1406
Furosemide (Concurrent therapy is not recommended). Products include:
Lasix 1093
Guanabenz Acetate (Concurrent therapy is not recommended). Products include:
Wytensin Tablets 2542
Guanethidine Monosulfate (Concurrent therapy is not recommended). Products include:
Esimil Tablets 864
Ismelin Tablets 869
Hydralazine Hydrochloride (Concurrent therapy is not recommended). Products include:
Apresazide Capsules 854
Apresoline Hydrochloride Parenteral (Ampuls) 856
Apresoline Hydrochloride Tablets 855
Apresoline-Esidrix Tablets 857
Ser-Ap-Es Tablets 881
Serpasil-Apresoline Tablets 884
Hydrochlorothiazide (Concurrent therapy is not recommended). Products include:
Aldactazide 2150
Aldoril Tablets 1418
Apresazide Capsules 854
Apresoline-Esidrix Tablets 857
Capozide 2258
Dyazide Capsules 2208
Esidrix Tablets 863
Esimil Tablets 864
HydroDIURIL Tablets 1484
Hydropres Tablets 1485
Inderide Tablets 2463
Inderide LA Long Acting Capsules 2465
Lopressor HCT Tablets 1034
Maxzide 1215
Moduretic Tablets 1510
Normozide Tablets 2112
Oretic Tablets 544
Oreticyl 545
Prinzide Tablets 1540
Ser-Ap-Es Tablets 881
Serpasil-Esidrix Tablets 886
Timolide Tablets 1547
Trandate HCT Tablets 579
Vaseretic Tablets 1559
Zestoretic 2274
Hydroflumethiazide (Concurrent therapy is not recommended). Products include:
Diucardin Tablets 2450
Saluron 718
Salutensin/Salutensin-Demi 719
Imipramine Hydrochloride (Concurrent therapy is not recommended). Products include:
Tofranil Ampuls 1038
Tofranil Tablets 1039
Imipramine Pamoate (Concurrent therapy is not recommended). Products include:
Tofranil-PM Capsules 1041
Indapamide (Concurrent therapy is not recommended). Products include:
Lozol Tablets 1843
Isocarboxazid (Concurrent therapy is not recommended). Products include:
Marplan Tablets 1906
Isradipine (Concurrent therapy is not recommended). Products include:
DynaCirc Capsules 2004
Labetalol Hydrochloride (Concurrent therapy is not recommended). Products include:
Normodyne Injection 2108
Normodyne Tablets 2110
Normozide Tablets 2112
Trandate HCT Tablets 579
Trandate Injection 577
Trandate Tablets 579
Lisinopril (Concurrent therapy is not recommended). Products include:
Prinivil Tablets 1538
Prinzide Tablets 1540
Zestoretic 2274
Zestril Tablets 2277
Maprotiline Hydrochloride (Concurrent therapy is not recommended). Products include:
Ludiomil Tablets 874
Mecamylamine Hydrochloride (Concurrent therapy is not recommended). Products include:
Inversine Tablets 1492
Methyclothiazide (Concurrent therapy is not recommended). Products include:
Enduron Tablets 517
Enduronyl 518
Methyldopa (Concurrent therapy is not recommended). Products include:
Aldoclor Tablets 1413
Aldomet Oral 1415
Aldoril Tablets 1418
Methyldopate Hydrochloride (Concurrent therapy is not recommended). Products include:
Aldomet Ester HCl Injection 1417
Metolazone (Concurrent therapy is not recommended). Products include:
Diulo 2129
Mykrox ½ mg Tablets 984
Zaroxolyn Tablets 989
Metoprolol Tartrate (Concurrent therapy is not recommended). Products include:
Lopressor Ampuls 1032
Lopressor HCT Tablets 1034
Lopressor Tablets 1032
Metyrosine (Concurrent therapy is not recommended). Products include:
Demser Capsules 1460
Minoxidil (Concurrent therapy is not recommended). Products include:
Loniten Tablets 2346
Rogaine Topical Solution 2357
Nadolol (Concurrent therapy is not recommended). Products include:
Corgard Tablets 701
Corzide Tablets 702
Nicardipine Hydrochloride (Concurrent therapy is not recommended). Products include:
Cardene Capsules 2290
Nitroglycerin (Concurrent therapy is not recommended). Products include:
Deponit NTG Transdermal Delivery System 2143
Minitran Transdermal Delivery System 1312
Nitro-Bid Ointment 1339
Nitro-Bid Capsules 1338
Nitrodisc 2176
Nitro-Dur (nitroglycerin) Transdermal Infusion System 1164
Nitrogard Tablets 1004
Nitrolingual Spray 1846
Nitrostat Tablets 1743
Transderm-Nitro Transdermal Therapeutic System 2283
Nortriptyline Hydrochloride (Concurrent therapy is not recommended). Products include:
Pamelor 2019
Penbutolol Sulfate (Concurrent therapy is not recommended). Products include:
Levatol 1832
Phenelzine Sulfate (Concurrent therapy is not recommended). Products include:
Nardil 1742

Phenoxybenzamine Hydrochloride (Concurrent therapy is not recommended). Products include:
Dibenzyline Capsules 2207

Phentolamine Mesylate (Concurrent therapy is not recommended). Products include:
Regitine 878

Pindolol (Concurrent therapy is not recommended). Products include:
Visken Tablets 2036

Polythiazide (Concurrent therapy is not recommended). Products include:
Minizide Capsules 1779
Renese Tablets 1785
Renese-R Tablets 1786

Prazosin Hydrochloride (Concurrent therapy is not recommended). Products include:
Minipress Capsules 1778
Minizide Capsules 1779

Propranolol Hydrochloride (Concurrent therapy is not recommended). Products include:
Inderal 2459
Inderal LA Long Acting Capsules 2461
Inderide Tablets 2463
Inderide LA Long Acting Capsules 2465

Protriptyline Hydrochloride (Concurrent therapy is not recommended). Products include:
Vivactil Tablets 1567

Ramipril (Concurrent therapy is not recommended). Products include:
Altace Capsules 1086

Rauwolfia Serpentina (Concurrent therapy is not recommended). Products include:
Raudixin Tablets 1803
Rauzide Tablets 1804

Rescinnamine (Concurrent therapy is not recommended).
No products indexed under this heading.

Reserpine (Concurrent therapy is not recommended). Products include:
Diupres Tablets 1461
Hydromox R Tablets 1209
Hydropres Tablets 1485
Renese-R Tablets 1786
Salutensin/Salutensin-Demi 719
Ser-Ap-Es Tablets 881
Serpasil Tablets 883
Serpasil-Apresoline Tablets 884
Serpasil-Esidrix Tablets 886

Sodium Nitroprusside (Concurrent therapy is not recommended). Products include:
Nipride I.V. Infusion 1909

Terazosin Hydrochloride (Concurrent therapy is not recommended). Products include:
Hytrin Tablets 529

Timolol Maleate (Concurrent therapy is not recommended). Products include:
Blocadren Tablets 1429
Timolide Tablets 1547
Timoptic in Ocudose 1552
Timoptic Sterile Ophthalmic Solution 1550

Tranylcypromine Sulfate (Concurrent therapy is not recommended). Products include:
Parnate Tablets 2222

Trazodone Hydrochloride (Concurrent therapy is not recommended). Products include:
Desyrel and Desyrel Dividose 1404

Trimethaphan Camsylate (Concurrent therapy is not recommended). Products include:
Arfonad Ampuls 1887

Trimipramine Maleate (Concurrent therapy is not recommended). Products include:
Surmontil Capsules 2524

NALDECON DX CHILDREN'S SYRUP
(Phenylpropanolamine Hydrochloride, Guaifenesin, Dextromethorphan Hydrobromide) ▣ 522
May interact with antidepressant drugs and antihypertensives. Compounds in these categories include:

Acebutolol Hydrochloride (Concurrent therapy is not recommended). Products include:
Sectral Capsules 2520

Amitriptyline Hydrochloride (Concurrent therapy is not recommended). Products include:
Elavil 2269
Endep Tablets 1927
Etrafon 2087
Limbitrol 1933
Triavil Tablets 1556

Amoxapine (Concurrent therapy is not recommended). Products include:
Asendin Tablets 1196

Atenolol (Concurrent therapy is not recommended). Products include:
Tenoretic Tablets 1105
Tenormin Tablets and I.V. Injection 1107

Benazepril Hydrochloride (Concurrent therapy is not recommended). Products include:
Lotensin Tablets 872

Bendroflumethiazide (Concurrent therapy is not recommended). Products include:
Corzide Tablets 702
Naturetin Tablets 1789
Rauzide Tablets 1804

Betaxolol Hydrochloride (Concurrent therapy is not recommended). Products include:
Betoptic Sterile Ophthalmic Solution 569
Betoptic S Sterile Ophthalmic Suspension 570
Kerlone Tablets 2172

Bupropion Hydrochloride (Concurrent therapy is not recommended). Products include:
Wellbutrin Tablets 821

Captopril (Concurrent therapy is not recommended). Products include:
Capoten 2255
Capozide 2258

Carteolol Hydrochloride (Concurrent therapy is not recommended). Products include:
Cartrol Tablets 507

Chlorothiazide (Concurrent therapy is not recommended). Products include:
Aldoclor Tablets 1413
Diupres Tablets 1461
Diuril Oral 1464

Chlorothiazide Sodium (Concurrent therapy is not recommended). Products include:
Diuril Sodium Intravenous 1463

Chlorthalidone (Concurrent therapy is not recommended). Products include:
Combipres Tablets 678
Tenoretic Tablets 1105
Thalitone Tablets 687

Clonidine (Concurrent therapy is not recommended). Products include:
Catapres-TTS 677

Clonidine Hydrochloride (Concurrent therapy is not recommended). Products include:
Catapres Tablets 676
Combipres Tablets 678

Deserpidine (Concurrent therapy is not recommended). Products include:
Enduronyl 518
Harmonyl Tablets 528
Oreticyl 545

Desipramine Hydrochloride (Concurrent therapy is not recommended). Products include:
Norpramin Tablets 1340

Diazoxide (Concurrent therapy is not recommended). Products include:
Hyperstat I.V. Injection 2095
Proglycem 649

Doxazosin Mesylate (Concurrent therapy is not recommended). Products include:
Cardura Tablets 1941

Doxepin Hydrochloride (Concurrent therapy is not recommended). Products include:
Sinequan 1960

Enalapril Maleate (Concurrent therapy is not recommended). Products include:
Vaseretic Tablets 1559
Vasotec Tablets 1564

Enalaprilat (Concurrent therapy is not recommended). Products include:
Vasotec I.V. 1562

Esmolol Hydrochloride (Concurrent therapy is not recommended). Products include:
Brevibloc Injection 942

Felodipine (Concurrent therapy is not recommended). Products include:
Plendil Extended-Release Tablets 1526

Fluoxetine Hydrochloride (Concurrent therapy is not recommended). Products include:
Prozac Pulvules 920

Fosinopril Sodium (Concurrent therapy is not recommended). Products include:
Monopril Tablets 1406

Furosemide (Concurrent therapy is not recommended). Products include:
Lasix 1093

Guanabenz Acetate (Concurrent therapy is not recommended). Products include:
Wytensin Tablets 2542

Guanethidine Monosulfate (Concurrent therapy is not recommended). Products include:
Esimil Tablets 864
Ismelin Tablets 869

Hydralazine Hydrochloride (Concurrent therapy is not recommended). Products include:
Apresazide Capsules 854
Apresoline Hydrochloride Parenteral (Ampuls) 856
Apresoline Hydrochloride Tablets 855
Apresoline-Esidrix Tablets 857
Ser-Ap-Es Tablets 881
Serpasil-Apresoline Tablets 884

Hydrochlorothiazide (Concurrent therapy is not recommended). Products include:
Aldactazide 2150
Aldoril Tablets 1418
Apresazide Capsules 854
Apresoline-Esidrix Tablets 857
Capozide 2258
Dyazide Capsules 2208
Esidrix Tablets 863
Esimil Tablets 864
HydroDIURIL Tablets 1484
Hydropres Tablets 1485
Inderide Tablets 2463
Inderide LA Long Acting Capsules 2465
Lopressor HCT Tablets 1034
Maxzide 1215
Moduretic Tablets 1510
Normozide Tablets 2112
Oretic Tablets 544
Oreticyl 545
Prinzide Tablets 1540
Ser-Ap-Es Tablets 881
Serpasil-Esidrix Tablets 886
Timolide Tablets 1547
Trandate HCT Tablets 579
Vaseretic Tablets 1559
Zestoretic 2274

Hydroflumethiazide (Concurrent therapy is not recommended). Products include:
Diucardin Tablets 2450
Saluron 718
Salutensin/Salutensin-Demi 719

Imipramine Hydrochloride (Concurrent therapy is not recommended). Products include:
Tofranil Ampuls 1038
Tofranil Tablets 1039

Imipramine Pamoate (Concurrent therapy is not recommended). Products include:
Tofranil-PM Capsules 1041

Indapamide (Concurrent therapy is not recommended). Products include:
Lozol Tablets 1843

Isocarboxazid (Concurrent therapy is not recommended). Products include:
Marplan Tablets 1906

Isradipine (Concurrent therapy is not recommended). Products include:
DynaCirc Capsules 2004

Labetalol Hydrochloride (Concurrent therapy is not recommended). Products include:
Normodyne Injection 2108
Normodyne Tablets 2110
Normozide Tablets 2112
Trandate HCT Tablets 579
Trandate Injection 577
Trandate Tablets 579

Lisinopril (Concurrent therapy is not recommended). Products include:
Prinivil Tablets 1538
Prinzide Tablets 1540
Zestoretic 2274
Zestril Tablets 2277

Maprotiline Hydrochloride (Concurrent therapy is not recommended). Products include:
Ludiomil Tablets 874

Mecamylamine Hydrochloride (Concurrent therapy is not recommended). Products include:
Inversine Tablets 1492

Methyclothiazide (Concurrent therapy is not recommended). Products include:
Enduron Tablets 517
Enduronyl 518

Methyldopa (Concurrent therapy is not recommended). Products include:
Aldoclor Tablets 1413
Aldomet Oral 1415
Aldoril Tablets 1418

Methyldopate Hydrochloride (Concurrent therapy is not recommended). Products include:
Aldomet Ester HCl Injection 1417

Metolazone (Concurrent therapy is not recommended). Products include:
Diulo 2129
Mykrox ½ mg Tablets 984
Zaroxolyn Tablets 989

Metoprolol Tartrate (Concurrent therapy is not recommended). Products include:
Lopressor Ampuls 1032
Lopressor HCT Tablets 1034
Lopressor Tablets 1032

Metyrosine (Concurrent therapy is not recommended). Products include:
- Demser Capsules ... 1460

Minoxidil (Concurrent therapy is not recommended). Products include:
- Loniten Tablets ... 2346
- Rogaine Topical Solution ... 2357

Nadolol (Concurrent therapy is not recommended). Products include:
- Corgard Tablets ... 701
- Corzide Tablets ... 702

Nicardipine Hydrochloride (Concurrent therapy is not recommended). Products include:
- Cardene Capsules ... 2290

Nitroglycerin (Concurrent therapy is not recommended). Products include:
- Deponit NTG Transdermal Delivery System ... 2143
- Minitran Transdermal Delivery System ... 1312
- Nitro-Bid Ointment ... 1339
- Nitro-Bid Capsules ... 1338
- Nitrodisc ... 2176
- Nitro-Dur (nitroglycerin) Transdermal Infusion System ... 1164
- Nitrogard Tablets ... 1004
- Nitrolingual Spray ... 1846
- Nitrostat Tablets ... 1743
- Transderm-Nitro Transdermal Therapeutic System ... 2283

Nortriptyline Hydrochloride (Concurrent therapy is not recommended). Products include:
- Pamelor ... 2019

Penbutolol Sulfate (Concurrent therapy is not recommended). Products include:
- Levatol ... 1832

Phenelzine Sulfate (Concurrent therapy is not recommended). Products include:
- Nardil ... 1742

Phenoxybenzamine Hydrochloride (Concurrent therapy is not recommended). Products include:
- Dibenzyline Capsules ... 2207

Phentolamine Mesylate (Concurrent therapy is not recommended). Products include:
- Regitine ... 878

Pindolol (Concurrent therapy is not recommended). Products include:
- Visken Tablets ... 2036

Polythiazide (Concurrent therapy is not recommended). Products include:
- Minizide Capsules ... 1779
- Renese Tablets ... 1785
- Renese-R Tablets ... 1786

Prazosin Hydrochloride (Concurrent therapy is not recommended). Products include:
- Minipress Capsules ... 1778
- Minizide Capsules ... 1779

Propranolol Hydrochloride (Concurrent therapy is not recommended). Products include:
- Inderal ... 2459
- Inderal LA Long Acting Capsules ... 2461
- Inderide Tablets ... 2463
- Inderide LA Long Acting Capsules .. 2465

Protriptyline Hydrochloride (Concurrent therapy is not recommended). Products include:
- Vivactil Tablets ... 1567

Ramipril (Concurrent therapy is not recommended). Products include:
- Altace Capsules ... 1086

Rauwolfia Serpentina (Concurrent therapy is not recommended). Products include:
- Raudixin Tablets ... 1803
- Rauzide Tablets ... 1804

Rescinnamine (Concurrent therapy is not recommended).
- No products indexed under this heading.

Reserpine (Concurrent therapy is not recommended). Products include:
- Diupres Tablets ... 1461
- Hydromox R Tablets ... 1209
- Hydropres Tablets ... 1485
- Renese-R Tablets ... 1786
- Salutensin/Salutensin-Demi ... 719
- Ser-Ap-Es Tablets ... 881
- Serpasil Tablets ... 883
- Serpasil-Apresoline Tablets ... 884
- Serpasil-Esidrix Tablets ... 886

Sodium Nitroprusside (Concurrent therapy is not recommended). Products include:
- Nipride I.V. Infusion ... 1909

Terazosin Hydrochloride (Concurrent therapy is not recommended). Products include:
- Hytrin Tablets ... 529

Timolol Maleate (Concurrent therapy is not recommended). Products include:
- Blocadren Tablets ... 1429
- Timolide Tablets ... 1547
- Timoptic in Ocudose ... 1552
- Timoptic Sterile Ophthalmic Solution ... 1550

Tranylcypromine Sulfate (Concurrent therapy is not recommended). Products include:
- Parnate Tablets ... 2222

Trazodone Hydrochloride (Concurrent therapy is not recommended). Products include:
- Desyrel and Desyrel Dividose ... 1404

Trimethaphan Camsylate (Concurrent therapy is not recommended). Products include:
- Arfonad Ampuls ... 1887

Trimipramine Maleate (Concurrent therapy is not recommended). Products include:
- Surmontil Capsules ... 2524

NALDECON DX PEDIATRIC DROPS
(Phenylpropanolamine Hydrochloride, Guaifenesin, Dextromethorphan Hydrobromide) ▣ 522
May interact with antidepressant drugs and antihypertensives. Compounds in these categories include:

Acebutolol Hydrochloride (Concurrent therapy is not recommended). Products include:
- Sectral Capsules ... 2520

Amitriptyline Hydrochloride (Concurrent therapy is not recommended). Products include:
- Elavil ... 2269
- Endep Tablets ... 1927
- Etrafon ... 2087
- Limbitrol ... 1933
- Triavil Tablets ... 1556

Amoxapine (Concurrent therapy is not recommended). Products include:
- Asendin Tablets ... 1196

Atenolol (Concurrent therapy is not recommended). Products include:
- Tenoretic Tablets ... 1105
- Tenormin Tablets and I.V. Injection 1107

Benazepril Hydrochloride (Concurrent therapy is not recommended). Products include:
- Lotensin Tablets ... 872

Bendroflumethiazide (Concurrent therapy is not recommended). Products include:
- Corzide Tablets ... 702
- Naturetin Tablets ... 1789
- Rauzide Tablets ... 1804

Betaxolol Hydrochloride (Concurrent therapy is not recommended). Products include:
- Betoptic Sterile Ophthalmic Solution ... 569
- Betoptic S Sterile Ophthalmic Suspension ... 570
- Kerlone Tablets ... 2172

Bupropion Hydrochloride (Concurrent therapy is not recommended). Products include:
- Wellbutrin Tablets ... 821

Captopril (Concurrent therapy is not recommended). Products include:
- Capoten ... 2255
- Capozide ... 2258

Carteolol Hydrochloride (Concurrent therapy is not recommended). Products include:
- Cartrol Tablets ... 507

Chlorothiazide (Concurrent therapy is not recommended). Products include:
- Aldoclor Tablets ... 1413
- Diupres Tablets ... 1461
- Diuril Oral ... 1464

Chlorothiazide Sodium (Concurrent therapy is not recommended). Products include:
- Diuril Sodium Intravenous ... 1463

Chlorthalidone (Concurrent therapy is not recommended). Products include:
- Combipres Tablets ... 678
- Tenoretic Tablets ... 1105
- Thalitone Tablets ... 687

Clonidine (Concurrent therapy is not recommended). Products include:
- Catapres-TTS ... 677

Clonidine Hydrochloride (Concurrent therapy is not recommended). Products include:
- Catapres Tablets ... 676
- Combipres Tablets ... 678

Deserpidine (Concurrent therapy is not recommended). Products include:
- Enduronyl ... 518
- Harmonyl Tablets ... 528
- Oreticyl ... 545

Desipramine Hydrochloride (Concurrent therapy is not recommended). Products include:
- Norpramin Tablets ... 1340

Diazoxide (Concurrent therapy is not recommended). Products include:
- Hyperstat I.V. Injection ... 2095
- Proglycem ... 649

Doxazosin Mesylate (Concurrent therapy is not recommended). Products include:
- Cardura Tablets ... 1941

Doxepin Hydrochloride (Concurrent therapy is not recommended). Products include:
- Sinequan ... 1960

Enalapril Maleate (Concurrent therapy is not recommended). Products include:
- Vaseretic Tablets ... 1559
- Vasotec Tablets ... 1564

Enalaprilat (Concurrent therapy is not recommended). Products include:
- Vasotec I.V. ... 1562

Esmolol Hydrochloride (Concurrent therapy is not recommended). Products include:
- Brevibloc Injection ... 942

Felodipine (Concurrent therapy is not recommended). Products include:
- Plendil Extended-Release Tablets ... 1526

Fluoxetine Hydrochloride (Concurrent therapy is not recommended). Products include:
- Prozac Pulvules ... 920

Fosinopril Sodium (Concurrent therapy is not recommended). Products include:
- Monopril Tablets ... 1406

Furosemide (Concurrent therapy is not recommended). Products include:
- Lasix ... 1093

Guanabenz Acetate (Concurrent therapy is not recommended). Products include:
- Wytensin Tablets ... 2542

Guanethidine Monosulfate (Concurrent therapy is not recommended). Products include:
- Esimil Tablets ... 864
- Ismelin Tablets ... 869

Hydralazine Hydrochloride (Concurrent therapy is not recommended). Products include:
- Apresazide Capsules ... 854
- Apresoline Hydrochloride Parenteral (Ampuls) ... 856
- Apresoline Hydrochloride Tablets .. 855
- Apresoline-Esidrix Tablets ... 857
- Ser-Ap-Es Tablets ... 881
- Serpasil-Apresoline Tablets ... 884

Hydrochlorothiazide (Concurrent therapy is not recommended). Products include:
- Aldactazide ... 2150
- Aldoril Tablets ... 1418
- Apresazide Capsules ... 854
- Apresoline-Esidrix Tablets ... 857
- Capozide ... 2258
- Dyazide Capsules ... 2208
- Esidrix Tablets ... 863
- Esimil Tablets ... 864
- HydroDIURIL Tablets ... 1484
- Hydropres Tablets ... 1485
- Inderide Tablets ... 2463
- Inderide LA Long Acting Capsules .. 2465
- Lopressor HCT Tablets ... 1034
- Maxzide ... 1215
- Moduretic Tablets ... 1510
- Normozide Tablets ... 2112
- Oretic Tablets ... 544
- Oreticyl ... 545
- Prinzide Tablets ... 1540
- Ser-Ap-Es Tablets ... 881
- Serpasil-Esidrix Tablets ... 886
- Timolide Tablets ... 1547
- Trandate HCT Tablets ... 579
- Vaseretic Tablets ... 1559
- Zestoretic ... 2274

Hydroflumethiazide (Concurrent therapy is not recommended). Products include:
- Diucardin Tablets ... 2450
- Saluron ... 718
- Salutensin/Salutensin-Demi ... 719

Imipramine Hydrochloride (Concurrent therapy is not recommended). Products include:
- Tofranil Ampuls ... 1038
- Tofranil Tablets ... 1039

Imipramine Pamoate (Concurrent therapy is not recommended). Products include:
- Tofranil-PM Capsules ... 1041

Indapamide (Concurrent therapy is not recommended). Products include:
- Lozol Tablets ... 1843

Isocarboxazid (Concurrent therapy is not recommended). Products include:
- Marplan Tablets ... 1906

Isradipine (Concurrent therapy is not recommended). Products include:
- DynaCirc Capsules ... 2004

Labetalol Hydrochloride (Concurrent therapy is not recommended). Products include:
- Normodyne Injection ... 2108
- Normodyne Tablets ... 2110
- Normozide Tablets ... 2112

Trandate HCT Tablets ... 579
Trandate Injection ... 577
Trandate Tablets ... 579

Lisinopril (Concurrent therapy is not recommended). Products include:
Prinivil Tablets ... 1538
Prinzide Tablets ... 1540
Zestoretic ... 2274
Zestril Tablets ... 2277

Maprotiline Hydrochloride (Concurrent therapy is not recommended). Products include:
Ludiomil Tablets ... 874

Mecamylamine Hydrochloride (Concurrent therapy is not recommended). Products include:
Inversine Tablets ... 1492

Methyclothiazide (Concurrent therapy is not recommended). Products include:
Enduron Tablets ... 517
Enduronyl ... 518

Methyldopa (Concurrent therapy is not recommended). Products include:
Aldoclor Tablets ... 1413
Aldomet Oral ... 1415
Aldoril Tablets ... 1418

Methyldopate Hydrochloride (Concurrent therapy is not recommended). Products include:
Aldomet Ester HCl Injection ... 1417

Metolazone (Concurrent therapy is not recommended). Products include:
Diulo ... 2129
Mykrox ½ mg Tablets ... 984
Zaroxolyn Tablets ... 989

Metoprolol Tartrate (Concurrent therapy is not recommended). Products include:
Lopressor Ampuls ... 1032
Lopressor HCT Tablets ... 1034
Lopressor Tablets ... 1032

Metyrosine (Concurrent therapy is not recommended). Products include:
Demser Capsules ... 1460

Minoxidil (Concurrent therapy is not recommended). Products include:
Loniten Tablets ... 2346
Rogaine Topical Solution ... 2357

Nadolol (Concurrent therapy is not recommended). Products include:
Corgard Tablets ... 701
Corzide Tablets ... 702

Nicardipine Hydrochloride (Concurrent therapy is not recommended). Products include:
Cardene Capsules ... 2290

Nitroglycerin (Concurrent therapy is not recommended). Products include:
Deponit NTG Transdermal Delivery System ... 2143
Minitran Transdermal Delivery System ... 1312
Nitro-Bid Ointment ... 1339
Nitro-Bid Capsules ... 1338
Nitrodisc ... 2176
Nitro-Dur (nitroglycerin) Transdermal Infusion System ... 1164
Nitrogard Tablets ... 1004
Nitrolingual Spray ... 1846
Nitrostat Tablets ... 1743
Transderm-Nitro Transdermal Therapeutic System ... 2283

Nortriptyline Hydrochloride (Concurrent therapy is not recommended). Products include:
Pamelor ... 2019

Penbutolol Sulfate (Concurrent therapy is not recommended). Products include:
Levatol ... 1832

Phenelzine Sulfate (Concurrent therapy is not recommended). Products include:
Nardil ... 1742

Phenoxybenzamine Hydrochloride (Concurrent therapy is not recommended). Products include:
Dibenzyline Capsules ... 2207

Phentolamine Mesylate (Concurrent therapy is not recommended). Products include:
Regitine ... 878

Pindolol (Concurrent therapy is not recommended). Products include:
Visken Tablets ... 2036

Polythiazide (Concurrent therapy is not recommended). Products include:
Minizide Capsules ... 1779
Renese Tablets ... 1785
Renese-R Tablets ... 1786

Prazosin Hydrochloride (Concurrent therapy is not recommended). Products include:
Minipress Capsules ... 1778
Minizide Capsules ... 1779

Propranolol Hydrochloride (Concurrent therapy is not recommended). Products include:
Inderal ... 2459
Inderal LA Long Acting Capsules ... 2461
Inderide Tablets ... 2463
Inderide LA Long Acting Capsules ... 2465

Protriptyline Hydrochloride (Concurrent therapy is not recommended). Products include:
Vivactil Tablets ... 1567

Ramipril (Concurrent therapy is not recommended). Products include:
Altace Capsules ... 1086

Rauwolfia Serpentina (Concurrent therapy is not recommended). Products include:
Raudixin Tablets ... 1803
Rauzide Tablets ... 1804

Rescinnamine (Concurrent therapy is not recommended).
No products indexed under this heading.

Reserpine (Concurrent therapy is not recommended). Products include:
Diupres Tablets ... 1461
Hydromox R Tablets ... 1209
Hydropres Tablets ... 1485
Renese-R Tablets ... 1786
Salutensin/Salutensin-Demi ... 719
Ser-Ap-Es Tablets ... 881
Serpasil Tablets ... 883
Serpasil-Apresoline Tablets ... 884
Serpasil-Esidrix Tablets ... 886

Sodium Nitroprusside (Concurrent therapy is not recommended). Products include:
Nipride I.V. Infusion ... 1909

Terazosin Hydrochloride (Concurrent therapy is not recommended). Products include:
Hytrin Tablets ... 529

Timolol Maleate (Concurrent therapy is not recommended). Products include:
Blocadren Tablets ... 1429
Timolide Tablets ... 1547
Timoptic in Ocudose ... 1552
Timoptic Sterile Ophthalmic Solution ... 1550

Tranylcypromine Sulfate (Concurrent therapy is not recommended). Products include:
Parnate Tablets ... 2222

Trazodone Hydrochloride (Concurrent therapy is not recommended). Products include:
Desyrel and Desyrel Dividose ... 1404

Trimethaphan Camsylate (Concurrent therapy is not recommended). Products include:
Arfonad Ampuls ... 1887

Trimipramine Maleate (Concurrent therapy is not recommended). Products include:
Surmontil Capsules ... 2524

NALDECON EX CHILDREN'S SYRUP
(Phenylpropanolamine Hydrochloride, Guaifenesin) ... ◘ 522
May interact with antidepressant drugs and antihypertensives. Compounds in these categories include:

Acebutolol Hydrochloride (Concurrent therapy is not recommended). Products include:
Sectral Capsules ... 2520

Amitriptyline Hydrochloride (Concurrent therapy is not recommended). Products include:
Elavil ... 2269
Endep Tablets ... 1927
Etrafon ... 2087
Limbitrol ... 1933
Triavil Tablets ... 1556

Amoxapine (Concurrent therapy is not recommended). Products include:
Asendin Tablets ... 1196

Atenolol (Concurrent therapy is not recommended). Products include:
Tenoretic Tablets ... 1105
Tenormin Tablets and I.V. Injection ... 1107

Benazepril Hydrochloride (Concurrent therapy is not recommended). Products include:
Lotensin Tablets ... 872

Bendroflumethiazide (Concurrent therapy is not recommended). Products include:
Corzide Tablets ... 702
Naturetin Tablets ... 1789
Rauzide Tablets ... 1804

Betaxolol Hydrochloride (Concurrent therapy is not recommended). Products include:
Betoptic Sterile Ophthalmic Solution ... ◉ 569
Betoptic S Sterile Ophthalmic Suspension ... ◉ 570
Kerlone Tablets ... 2172

Bupropion Hydrochloride (Concurrent therapy is not recommended). Products include:
Wellbutrin Tablets ... 821

Captopril (Concurrent therapy is not recommended). Products include:
Capoten ... 2255
Capozide ... 2258

Carteolol Hydrochloride (Concurrent therapy is not recommended). Products include:
Cartrol Tablets ... 507

Chlorothiazide (Concurrent therapy is not recommended). Products include:
Aldoclor Tablets ... 1413
Diupres Tablets ... 1461
Diuril Oral ... 1464

Chlorothiazide Sodium (Concurrent therapy is not recommended). Products include:
Diuril Sodium Intravenous ... 1463

Chlorthalidone (Concurrent therapy is not recommended). Products include:
Combipres Tablets ... 678
Tenoretic Tablets ... 1105
Thalitone Tablets ... 687

Clonidine (Concurrent therapy is not recommended). Products include:
Catapres-TTS ... 677

Clonidine Hydrochloride (Concurrent therapy is not recommended). Products include:
Catapres Tablets ... 676
Combipres Tablets ... 678

Deserpidine (Concurrent therapy is not recommended). Products include:
Enduronyl ... 518
Harmonyl Tablets ... 528
Oreticyl ... 545

Desipramine Hydrochloride (Concurrent therapy is not recommended). Products include:
Norpramin Tablets ... 1340

Diazoxide (Concurrent therapy is not recommended). Products include:
Hyperstat I.V. Injection ... 2095
Proglycem ... 649

Doxepin Hydrochloride (Concurrent therapy is not recommended). Products include:
Sinequan ... 1960

Enalapril Maleate (Concurrent therapy is not recommended). Products include:
Vaseretic Tablets ... 1559
Vasotec Tablets ... 1564

Enalaprilat (Concurrent therapy is not recommended). Products include:
Vasotec I.V. ... 1562

Esmolol Hydrochloride (Concurrent therapy is not recommended). Products include:
Brevibloc Injection ... 942

Felodipine (Concurrent therapy is not recommended). Products include:
Plendil Extended-Release Tablets ... 1526

Fluoxetine Hydrochloride (Concurrent therapy is not recommended). Products include:
Prozac Pulvules ... 920

Fosinopril Sodium (Concurrent therapy is not recommended). Products include:
Monopril Tablets ... 1406

Furosemide (Concurrent therapy is not recommended). Products include:
Lasix ... 1093

Guanabenz Acetate (Concurrent therapy is not recommended). Products include:
Wytensin Tablets ... 2542

Guanethidine Monosulfate (Concurrent therapy is not recommended). Products include:
Esimil Tablets ... 864
Ismelin Tablets ... 869

Hydralazine Hydrochloride (Concurrent therapy is not recommended). Products include:
Apresazide Capsules ... 854
Apresoline Hydrochloride Parenteral (Ampuls) ... 856
Apresoline Hydrochloride Tablets ... 855
Apresoline-Esidrix Tablets ... 857
Ser-Ap-Es Tablets ... 881
Serpasil-Apresoline Tablets ... 884

Hydrochlorothiazide (Concurrent therapy is not recommended). Products include:
Aldactazide ... 2150
Aldoril Tablets ... 1418
Apresazide Capsules ... 854
Apresoline-Esidrix Tablets ... 857
Capozide ... 2258
Dyazide Capsules ... 2208
Esidrix Tablets ... 863
Esimil Tablets ... 864
HydroDIURIL Tablets ... 1484
Hydropres Tablets ... 1485
Inderide Tablets ... 2463
Inderide LA Long Acting Capsules ... 2465
Lopressor HCT Tablets ... 1034
Maxzide ... 1215
Moduretic Tablets ... 1510
Normozide Tablets ... 2112
Oretic Tablets ... 544
Oreticyl ... 545
Prinzide Tablets ... 1540
Ser-Ap-Es Tablets ... 881
Serpasil-Esidrix Tablets ... 886

Timolide Tablets.................... 1547
Trandate HCT Tablets.................... 579
Vaseretic Tablets.................... 1559
Zestoretic.................... 2274

Hydroflumethiazide (Concurrent therapy is not recommended). Products include:
Diucardin Tablets.................... 2450
Saluron.................... 718
Salutensin/Salutensin-Demi.................... 719

Imipramine Hydrochloride (Concurrent therapy is not recommended). Products include:
Tofranil Ampuls.................... 1038
Tofranil Tablets.................... 1039

Imipramine Pamoate (Concurrent therapy is not recommended). Products include:
Tofranil-PM Capsules.................... 1041

Indapamide (Concurrent therapy is not recommended). Products include:
Lozol Tablets.................... 1843

Isocarboxazid (Concurrent therapy is not recommended). Products include:
Marplan Tablets.................... 1906

Labetalol Hydrochloride (Concurrent therapy is not recommended). Products include:
Normodyne Injection.................... 2108
Normodyne Tablets.................... 2110
Normozide Tablets.................... 2112
Trandate HCT Tablets.................... 579
Trandate Injection.................... 577
Trandate Tablets.................... 579

Lisinopril (Concurrent therapy is not recommended). Products include:
Prinivil Tablets.................... 1538
Prinzide Tablets.................... 1540
Zestoretic.................... 2274
Zestril Tablets.................... 2277

Maprotiline Hydrochloride (Concurrent therapy is not recommended). Products include:
Ludiomil Tablets.................... 874

Mecamylamine Hydrochloride (Concurrent therapy is not recommended). Products include:
Inversine Tablets.................... 1492

Methyclothiazide (Concurrent therapy is not recommended). Products include:
Enduron Tablets.................... 517
Enduronyl.................... 518

Methyldopa (Concurrent therapy is not recommended). Products include:
Aldoclor Tablets.................... 1413
Aldomet Oral.................... 1415
Aldoril Tablets.................... 1418

Methyldopate Hydrochloride (Concurrent therapy is not recommended). Products include:
Aldomet Ester HCl Injection.................... 1417

Metolazone (Concurrent therapy is not recommended). Products include:
Diulo.................... 2129
Mykrox ½ mg Tablets.................... 984
Zaroxolyn Tablets.................... 989

Metoprolol Tartrate (Concurrent therapy is not recommended). Products include:
Lopressor Ampuls.................... 1032
Lopressor HCT Tablets.................... 1034
Lopressor Tablets.................... 1032

Metyrosine (Concurrent therapy is not recommended). Products include:
Demser Capsules.................... 1460

Minoxidil (Concurrent therapy is not recommended). Products include:
Loniten Tablets.................... 2346
Rogaine Topical Solution.................... 2357

Nadolol (Concurrent therapy is not recommended). Products include:
Corgard Tablets.................... 701
Corzide Tablets.................... 702

Nicardipine Hydrochloride (Concurrent therapy is not recommended). Products include:
Cardene Capsules.................... 2290

Nitroglycerin (Concurrent therapy is not recommended). Products include:
Deponit NTG Transdermal Delivery System.................... 2143
Minitran Transdermal Delivery System.................... 1312
Nitro-Bid Ointment.................... 1339
Nitro-Bid Capsules.................... 1338
Nitrodisc.................... 2176
Nitro-Dur (nitroglycerin) Transdermal Infusion System.................... 1164
Nitrogard Tablets.................... 1004
Nitrolingual Spray.................... 1846
Nitrostat Tablets.................... 1743
Transderm-Nitro Transdermal Therapeutic System.................... 2283

Nortriptyline Hydrochloride (Concurrent therapy is not recommended). Products include:
Pamelor.................... 2019

Penbutolol Sulfate (Concurrent therapy is not recommended). Products include:
Levatol.................... 1832

Phenelzine Sulfate (Concurrent therapy is not recommended). Products include:
Nardil.................... 1742

Phenoxybenzamine Hydrochloride (Concurrent therapy is not recommended). Products include:
Dibenzyline Capsules.................... 2207

Phentolamine Mesylate (Concurrent therapy is not recommended). Products include:
Regitine.................... 878

Pindolol (Concurrent therapy is not recommended). Products include:
Visken Tablets.................... 2036

Polythiazide (Concurrent therapy is not recommended). Products include:
Minizide Capsules.................... 1779
Renese Tablets.................... 1785
Renese-R Tablets.................... 1786

Prazosin Hydrochloride (Concurrent therapy is not recommended). Products include:
Minipress Capsules.................... 1778
Minizide Capsules.................... 1779

Propranolol Hydrochloride (Concurrent therapy is not recommended). Products include:
Inderal.................... 2459
Inderal LA Long Acting Capsules.................... 2461
Inderide Tablets.................... 2463
Inderide LA Long Acting Capsules.................... 2465

Protriptyline Hydrochloride (Concurrent therapy is not recommended). Products include:
Vivactil Tablets.................... 1567

Rauwolfia Serpentina (Concurrent therapy is not recommended). Products include:
Raudixin Tablets.................... 1803
Rauzide Tablets.................... 1804

Rescinnamine (Concurrent therapy is not recommended).
No products indexed under this heading.

Reserpine (Concurrent therapy is not recommended). Products include:
Diupres Tablets.................... 1461
Hydromox R Tablets.................... 1209
Hydropres Tablets.................... 1485
Renese-R Tablets.................... 1786
Salutensin/Salutensin-Demi.................... 719
Ser-Ap-Es Tablets.................... 881
Serpasil Tablets.................... 883
Serpasil-Apresoline Tablets.................... 884
Serpasil-Esidrix Tablets.................... 886

Sodium Nitroprusside (Concurrent therapy is not recommended). Products include:
Nipride I.V. Infusion.................... 1909

Terazosin Hydrochloride (Concurrent therapy is not recommended). Products include:
Hytrin Tablets.................... 529

Timolol Maleate (Concurrent therapy is not recommended). Products include:
Blocadren Tablets.................... 1429
Timolide Tablets.................... 1547
Timoptic in Ocudose.................... 1552
Timoptic Sterile Ophthalmic Solution.................... 1550

Tranylcypromine Sulfate (Concurrent therapy is not recommended). Products include:
Parnate Tablets.................... 2222

Trazodone Hydrochloride (Concurrent therapy is not recommended). Products include:
Desyrel and Desyrel Dividose.................... 1404

Trimethaphan Camsylate (Concurrent therapy is not recommended). Products include:
Arfonad Ampuls.................... 1887

Trimipramine Maleate (Concurrent therapy is not recommended). Products include:
Surmontil Capsules.................... 2524

NALDECON EX PEDIATRIC DROPS
(Phenylpropanolamine Hydrochloride, Guaifenesin).................... ▣ 523
May interact with antidepressant drugs and antihypertensives. Compounds in these categories include:

Acebutolol Hydrochloride (Concurrent therapy is not recommended). Products include:
Sectral Capsules.................... 2520

Amitriptyline Hydrochloride (Concurrent therapy is not recommended). Products include:
Elavil.................... 2269
Endep Tablets.................... 1927
Etrafon.................... 2087
Limbitrol.................... 1933
Triavil Tablets.................... 1556

Amoxapine (Concurrent therapy is not recommended). Products include:
Asendin Tablets.................... 1196

Atenolol (Concurrent therapy is not recommended). Products include:
Tenoretic Tablets.................... 1105
Tenormin Tablets and I.V. Injection.................... 1107

Benazepril Hydrochloride (Concurrent therapy is not recommended). Products include:
Lotensin Tablets.................... 872

Bendroflumethiazide (Concurrent therapy is not recommended). Products include:
Corzide Tablets.................... 702
Naturetin Tablets.................... 1789
Rauzide Tablets.................... 1804

Betaxolol Hydrochloride (Concurrent therapy is not recommended). Products include:
Betoptic Sterile Ophthalmic Solution.................... 569
Betoptic S Sterile Ophthalmic Suspension.................... 570
Kerlone Tablets.................... 2172

Bupropion Hydrochloride (Concurrent therapy is not recommended). Products include:
Wellbutrin Tablets.................... 821

Captopril (Concurrent therapy is not recommended). Products include:
Capoten.................... 2255
Capozide.................... 2258

Carteolol Hydrochloride (Concurrent therapy is not recommended). Products include:
Cartrol Tablets.................... 507

Chlorothiazide (Concurrent therapy is not recommended). Products include:
Aldoclor Tablets.................... 1413
Diupres Tablets.................... 1461
Diuril Oral.................... 1464

Chlorothiazide Sodium (Concurrent therapy is not recommended). Products include:
Diuril Sodium Intravenous.................... 1463

Chlorthalidone (Concurrent therapy is not recommended). Products include:
Combipres Tablets.................... 678
Tenoretic Tablets.................... 1105
Thalitone Tablets.................... 687

Clonidine (Concurrent therapy is not recommended). Products include:
Catapres-TTS.................... 677

Clonidine Hydrochloride (Concurrent therapy is not recommended). Products include:
Catapres Tablets.................... 676
Combipres Tablets.................... 678

Deserpidine (Concurrent therapy is not recommended). Products include:
Enduronyl.................... 518
Harmonyl Tablets.................... 528
Oreticyl.................... 545

Desipramine Hydrochloride (Concurrent therapy is not recommended). Products include:
Norpramin Tablets.................... 1340

Diazoxide (Concurrent therapy is not recommended). Products include:
Hyperstat I.V. Injection.................... 2095
Proglycem.................... 649

Doxazosin Mesylate (Concurrent therapy is not recommended). Products include:
Cardura Tablets.................... 1941

Doxepin Hydrochloride (Concurrent therapy is not recommended). Products include:
Sinequan.................... 1960

Enalapril Maleate (Concurrent therapy is not recommended). Products include:
Vaseretic Tablets.................... 1559
Vasotec Tablets.................... 1564

Enalaprilat (Concurrent therapy is not recommended). Products include:
Vasotec I.V..................... 1562

Esmolol Hydrochloride (Concurrent therapy is not recommended). Products include:
Brevibloc Injection.................... 942

Felodipine (Concurrent therapy is not recommended). Products include:
Plendil Extended-Release Tablets.................... 1526

Fluoxetine Hydrochloride (Concurrent therapy is not recommended). Products include:
Prozac Pulvules.................... 920

Fosinopril Sodium (Concurrent therapy is not recommended). Products include:
Monopril Tablets.................... 1406

Furosemide (Concurrent therapy is not recommended). Products include:
Lasix.................... 1093

Guanabenz Acetate (Concurrent therapy is not recommended). Products include:
Wytensin Tablets.................... 2542

Guanethidine Monosulfate (Concurrent therapy is not recommended). Products include:
Esimil Tablets ... 864
Ismelin Tablets ... 869

Hydralazine Hydrochloride (Concurrent therapy is not recommended). Products include:
Apresazide Capsules ... 854
Apresoline Hydrochloride Parenteral (Ampuls) ... 856
Apresoline Hydrochloride Tablets ... 855
Apresoline-Esidrix Tablets ... 857
Ser-Ap-Es Tablets ... 881
Serpasil-Apresoline Tablets ... 884

Hydrochlorothiazide (Concurrent therapy is not recommended). Products include:
Aldactazide ... 2150
Aldoril Tablets ... 1418
Apresazide Capsules ... 854
Apresoline-Esidrix Tablets ... 857
Capozide ... 2258
Dyazide Capsules ... 2208
Esidrix Tablets ... 863
Esimil Tablets ... 864
HydroDIURIL Tablets ... 1484
Hydropres Tablets ... 1485
Inderide Tablets ... 2463
Inderide LA Long Acting Capsules ... 2465
Lopressor HCT Tablets ... 1034
Maxzide ... 1215
Moduretic Tablets ... 1510
Normozide Tablets ... 2112
Oretic Tablets ... 544
Oreticyl ... 545
Prinzide Tablets ... 1540
Ser-Ap-Es Tablets ... 881
Serpasil-Esidrix Tablets ... 886
Timolide Tablets ... 1547
Trandate HCT Tablets ... 579
Vaseretic Tablets ... 1559
Zestoretic ... 2274

Hydroflumethiazide (Concurrent therapy is not recommended). Products include:
Diucardin Tablets ... 2450
Saluron ... 718
Salutensin/Salutensin-Demi ... 719

Imipramine Hydrochloride (Concurrent therapy is not recommended). Products include:
Tofranil Ampuls ... 1038
Tofranil Tablets ... 1039

Imipramine Pamoate (Concurrent therapy is not recommended). Products include:
Tofranil-PM Capsules ... 1041

Indapamide (Concurrent therapy is not recommended). Products include:
Lozol Tablets ... 1843

Isocarboxazid (Concurrent therapy is not recommended). Products include:
Marplan Tablets ... 1906

Isradipine (Concurrent therapy is not recommended). Products include:
DynaCirc Capsules ... 2004

Labetalol Hydrochloride (Concurrent therapy is not recommended). Products include:
Normodyne Injection ... 2108
Normodyne Tablets ... 2110
Normozide Tablets ... 2112
Trandate HCT Tablets ... 579
Trandate Injection ... 577
Trandate Tablets ... 579

Lisinopril (Concurrent therapy is not recommended). Products include:
Prinivil Tablets ... 1538
Prinzide Tablets ... 1540
Zestoretic ... 2274
Zestril Tablets ... 2277

Maprotiline Hydrochloride (Concurrent therapy is not recommended). Products include:
Ludiomil Tablets ... 874

Mecamylamine Hydrochloride (Concurrent therapy is not recommended). Products include:
Inversine Tablets ... 1492

Methyclothiazide (Concurrent therapy is not recommended). Products include:
Enduron Tablets ... 517
Enduronyl ... 518

Methyldopa (Concurrent therapy is not recommended). Products include:
Aldoclor Tablets ... 1413
Aldomet Oral ... 1415
Aldoril Tablets ... 1418

Methyldopate Hydrochloride (Concurrent therapy is not recommended). Products include:
Aldomet Ester HCl Injection ... 1417

Metolazone (Concurrent therapy is not recommended). Products include:
Diulo ... 2129
Mykrox ½ mg Tablets ... 984
Zaroxolyn Tablets ... 989

Metoprolol Tartrate (Concurrent therapy is not recommended). Products include:
Lopressor Ampuls ... 1032
Lopressor HCT Tablets ... 1034
Lopressor Tablets ... 1032

Metyrosine (Concurrent therapy is not recommended). Products include:
Demser Capsules ... 1460

Minoxidil (Concurrent therapy is not recommended). Products include:
Loniten Tablets ... 2346
Rogaine Topical Solution ... 2357

Nadolol (Concurrent therapy is not recommended). Products include:
Corgard Tablets ... 701
Corzide Tablets ... 702

Nicardipine Hydrochloride (Concurrent therapy is not recommended). Products include:
Cardene Capsules ... 2290

Nitroglycerin (Concurrent therapy is not recommended). Products include:
Deponit NTG Transdermal Delivery System ... 2143
Minitran Transdermal Delivery System ... 1312
Nitro-Bid Ointment ... 1339
Nitro-Bid Capsules ... 1338
Nitrodisc ... 2176
Nitro-Dur (nitroglycerin) Transdermal Infusion System ... 1164
Nitrogard Tablets ... 1004
Nitrolingual Spray ... 1846
Nitrostat Tablets ... 1743
Transderm-Nitro Transdermal Therapeutic System ... 2283

Nortriptyline Hydrochloride (Concurrent therapy is not recommended). Products include:
Pamelor ... 2019

Penbutolol Sulfate (Concurrent therapy is not recommended). Products include:
Levatol ... 1832

Phenelzine Sulfate (Concurrent therapy is not recommended). Products include:
Nardil ... 1742

Phenoxybenzamine Hydrochloride (Concurrent therapy is not recommended). Products include:
Dibenzyline Capsules ... 2207

Phentolamine Mesylate (Concurrent therapy is not recommended). Products include:
Regitine ... 878

Pindolol (Concurrent therapy is not recommended). Products include:
Visken Tablets ... 2036

Polythiazide (Concurrent therapy is not recommended). Products include:
Minizide Capsules ... 1779
Renese Tablets ... 1785
Renese-R Tablets ... 1786

Prazosin Hydrochloride (Concurrent therapy is not recommended). Products include:
Minipress Capsules ... 1778
Minizide Capsules ... 1779

Propranolol Hydrochloride (Concurrent therapy is not recommended). Products include:
Inderal ... 2459
Inderal LA Long Acting Capsules ... 2461
Inderide Tablets ... 2463
Inderide LA Long Acting Capsules ... 2465

Protriptyline Hydrochloride (Concurrent therapy is not recommended). Products include:
Vivactil Tablets ... 1567

Ramipril (Concurrent therapy is not recommended). Products include:
Altace Capsules ... 1086

Rauwolfia Serpentina (Concurrent therapy is not recommended). Products include:
Raudixin Tablets ... 1803
Rauzide Tablets ... 1804

Rescinnamine (Concurrent therapy is not recommended).
No products indexed under this heading.

Reserpine (Concurrent therapy is not recommended). Products include:
Diupres Tablets ... 1461
Hydromox R Tablets ... 1209
Hydropres Tablets ... 1485
Renese-R Tablets ... 1786
Salutensin/Salutensin-Demi ... 719
Ser-Ap-Es Tablets ... 881
Serpasil Tablets ... 883
Serpasil-Apresoline Tablets ... 884
Serpasil-Esidrix Tablets ... 886

Sodium Nitroprusside (Concurrent therapy is not recommended). Products include:
Nipride I.V. Infusion ... 1909

Terazosin Hydrochloride (Concurrent therapy is not recommended). Products include:
Hytrin Tablets ... 529

Timolol Maleate (Concurrent therapy is not recommended). Products include:
Blocadren Tablets ... 1429
Timolide Tablets ... 1547
Timoptic in Ocudose ... 1552
Timoptic Sterile Ophthalmic Solution ... 1550

Tranylcypromine Sulfate (Concurrent therapy is not recommended). Products include:
Parnate Tablets ... 2222

Trazodone Hydrochloride (Concurrent therapy is not recommended). Products include:
Desyrel and Desyrel Dividose ... 1404

Trimethaphan Camsylate (Concurrent therapy is not recommended). Products include:
Arfonad Ampuls ... 1887

Trimipramine Maleate (Concurrent therapy is not recommended). Products include:
Surmontil Capsules ... 2524

NALDECON SENIOR DX COUGH/COLD LIQUID
(Dextromethorphan Hydrobromide, Guaifenesin) ... ⊞ 523
No interactions described in labeling.

NALDECON SENIOR EX COUGH/COLD LIQUID
(Guaifenesin) ... ⊞ 523
No interactions described in labeling.

NALDECON SYRUP, TABLETS, PEDIATRIC DROPS AND PEDIATRIC SYRUP
(Phenylpropanolamine Hydrochloride, Phenylephrine Hydrochloride, Phenyltoloxamine Citrate, Chlorpheniramine Maleate) ... 709
May interact with monoamine oxidase inhibitors, beta blockers, veratrum alkaloids, tricyclic antidepressants, barbiturates, central nervous system depressants, and certain other agents. Compounds in these categories include:

Acebutolol Hydrochloride (Increased effect of sympathomimetics). Products include:
Sectral Capsules ... 2520

Alcohol (Additive effect).

Alfentanil Hydrochloride (Additive effect). Products include:
Alfenta Injection ... 1131

Alprazolam (Additive effect). Products include:
Xanax Tablets ... 2367

Amitriptyline Hydrochloride (Additive effect). Products include:
Elavil ... 2269
Endep Tablets ... 1927
Etrafon ... 2087
Limbitrol ... 1933
Triavil Tablets ... 1556

Amoxapine (Additive effect). Products include:
Asendin Tablets ... 1196

Aprobarbital (Additive effect). Products include:
Alurate Elixir ... 1883

Atenolol (Increased effect of sympathomimetics). Products include:
Tenoretic Tablets ... 1105
Tenormin Tablets and I.V. Injection 1107

Betaxolol Hydrochloride (Increased effect of sympathomimetics). Products include:
Betoptic Sterile Ophthalmic Solution ... 569
Betoptic S Sterile Ophthalmic Suspension ... 570
Kerlone Tablets ... 2172

Buprenorphine (Additive effect).
No products indexed under this heading.

Buspirone Hydrochloride (Additive effect). Products include:
BuSpar ... 1401

Butabarbital (Additive effect). Products include:
Pyridium Plus ... 1764

Butalbital (Additive effect). Products include:
Esgic-Plus Tablets ... 1002
Esgic Tablets & Capsules ... 1001
Fioricet Tablets ... 2006
Fiorinal Capsules ... 2007
Fiorinal with Codeine Capsules ... 2008
Fiorinal Tablets ... 2007
Phrenilin ... 838
Sedapap Tablets 50 mg/650 mg ... 1360

Carteolol Hydrochloride (Increased effect of sympathomimetics). Products include:
Cartrol Tablets ... 507

Chlordiazepoxide (Additive effect). Products include:
Libritabs Tablets ... 1930
Limbitrol ... 1933
Menrium Tablets ... 1934

Chlordiazepoxide Hydrochloride (Additive effect). Products include:
Librax Capsules ... 1929
Librium Capsules ... 1931

- Librium Injectable ... 1932

Chlorpromazine (Additive effect). Products include:
- Thorazine ... 2234

Chlorprothixene (Additive effect). Products include:
- Taractan Tablets ... 1920

Chlorprothixene Hydrochloride (Additive effect). Products include:
- Taractan ... 1920

Clomipramine Hydrochloride (Additive effect). Products include:
- Anafranil Capsules ... 650

Clorazepate Dipotassium (Additive effect). Products include:
- Tranxene ... 556

Codeine (Additive effect). Products include:
- Calcidrine Syrup ... 506

Codeine Phosphate (Additive effect). Products include:
- Actifed with Codeine Cough Syrup ... 752
- Cheracol Cough Syrup ... 1853
- Codimal PH Syrup ... 846
- Dimetane-DC Cough Syrup ... 1857
- Empirin with Codeine Phosphate Nos. 2, 3 & 4 ... 764
- Fiorinal with Codeine Capsules ... 2008
- Isoclor Expectorant ... 982
- Naldecon CX Adult Liquid ... ▣ 521
- Novahistine DH ... 1342
- Novahistine Expectorant ... 1343
- Nucofed Capsules ... 2219
- Nucofed Expectorant ... 2219
- Nucofed Pediatric Expectorant ... 2220
- Nucofed Syrup ... 2219
- Phenaphen with Codeine Capsules 1865
- Phenaphen-650 with Codeine Tablets ... 1866
- Phenergan with Codeine ... 2497
- Phenergan VC with Codeine ... 2501
- Robitussin A-C Syrup ... 1875
- Robitussin-DAC Syrup ... 1875
- Ryna ... ▣ 741
- Soma Compound w/Codeine Tablets ... 2390
- Triaminic Expectorant w/Codeine ... 1996
- Tussi-Organidin Liquid ... 2391
- Tylenol with Codeine ... 1381

Codeine Polistirex (Additive effect).
- No products indexed under this heading.

Cryptenamine Preparations (Reduced antihypertensive effects).

Desipramine Hydrochloride (Additive effect). Products include:
- Norpramin Tablets ... 1340

Dezocine (Additive effect).

Diazepam (Additive effect). Products include:
- Valium Injectable ... 1937
- Valium Tablets ... 1939
- Valrelease Capsules ... 1923

Doxepin Hydrochloride (Additive effect). Products include:
- Sinequan ... 1960

Droperidol (Additive effect). Products include:
- Inapsine Injection ... 1140
- Innovar Injection ... 1141

Enflurane (Additive effect). Products include:
- Ethrane ... 599

Esmolol Hydrochloride (Increased effect of sympathomimetics). Products include:
- Brevibloc Injection ... 942

Estazolam (Additive effect). Products include:
- ProSom Tablets ... 554

Ethchlorvynol (Additive effect). Products include:
- Placidyl Capsules ... 553

Ethinamate (Additive effect).
- No products indexed under this heading.

Fentanyl (Additive effect). Products include:
- Duragesic Transdermal System ... 1133

Fentanyl Citrate (Additive effect). Products include:
- Innovar Injection ... 1141
- Sublimaze Injection ... 1146

Fluphenazine Decanoate (Additive effect). Products include:
- Prolixin Decanoate ... 1795

Fluphenazine Enanthate (Additive effect). Products include:
- Prolixin Enanthate ... 1796

Fluphenazine Hydrochloride (Additive effect). Products include:
- Prolixin Elixir ... 1793
- Prolixin Injection ... 1791
- Prolixin Oral Concentrate ... 1792
- Prolixin Tablets ... 1793

Flurazepam Hydrochloride (Additive effect). Products include:
- Dalmane Capsules ... 1927

Furazolidone (Increased effect of sympathomimetics; concurrent use is contraindicated). Products include:
- Furoxone ... 1855

Glutethimide (Additive effect).
- No products indexed under this heading.

Haloperidol (Additive effect). Products include:
- Haldol Injection, Tablets and Concentrate ... 1373

Haloperidol Decanoate (Additive effect). Products include:
- Haldol Decanoate ... 1375

Hydrocodone Bitartrate (Additive effect). Products include:
- Anexsia 5/500 Tablets ... 2196
- Anexsia 7.5/650 Tablets ... 2197
- Azdone Tablets ... 844
- Codiclear DH Syrup ... 845
- Codimal DH Syrup ... 846
- Damason-P ... 1356
- Hycodan Syrup, Tablets ... 927
- Hycomine Compound Tablets ... 929
- Hycomine Syrup ... 927
- Hycotuss Expectorant Syrup ... 930
- Hydrocet Capsules ... 835
- Lortab ASA Tablets ... 2414
- Lortab ... 2412
- Ru-Tuss with Hydrocodone ... 694
- Triaminic Expectorant DH ... 1995
- Vicodin Tablets ... 1187
- Vicodin ES Tablets ... 1189
- Zydone Capsules ... 941

Hydrocodone Polistirex (Additive effect). Products include:
- Tussionex Extended-Release Suspension ... 988

Hydroxyzine Hydrochloride (Additive effect). Products include:
- Atarax Tablets & Syrup ... 1941
- Marax Tablets & DF Syrup ... 1954
- Vistaril Intramuscular Solution ... 1970

Imipramine Hydrochloride (Additive effect). Products include:
- Tofranil Ampuls ... 1038
- Tofranil Tablets ... 1039

Imipramine Pamoate (Additive effect). Products include:
- Tofranil-PM Capsules ... 1041

Isocarboxazid (Increased effect of sympathomimetics; concurrent use is contraindicated). Products include:
- Marplan Tablets ... 1906

Isoflurane (Additive effect). Products include:
- Forane ... 600

Ketamine Hydrochloride (Additive effect). Products include:
- Ketalar ... 1726

Labetalol Hydrochloride (Increased effect of sympathomimetics). Products include:
- Normodyne Injection ... 2108
- Normodyne Tablets ... 2110
- Normozide Tablets ... 2112
- Trandate HCT Tablets ... 579
- Trandate Injection ... 577
- Trandate Tablets ... 579

Levorphanol Tartrate (Additive effect). Products include:
- Levo-Dromoran ... 1906

Lorazepam (Additive effect). Products include:
- Ativan Injection ... 2432
- Ativan Tablets ... 2434

Loxapine Hydrochloride (Additive effect). Products include:
- Loxitane ... 1213

Loxapine Succinate (Additive effect). Products include:
- Loxitane Capsules ... 1213

Maprotiline Hydrochloride (Additive effect). Products include:
- Ludiomil Tablets ... 874

Mecamylamine Hydrochloride (Reduced antihypertensive effects). Products include:
- Inversine Tablets ... 1492

Meperidine Hydrochloride (Additive effect). Products include:
- Demerol ... 2047
- Mepergan Injection ... 2479

Mephobarbital (Additive effect). Products include:
- Mebaral Tablets ... 2061

Meprobamate (Additive effect). Products include:
- Deprol Tablets ... 2382
- Equagesic Tablets ... 2451
- Miltown Tablets ... 2386
- PMB 200 and PMB 400 ... 2504

Mesoridazine (Additive effect). Products include:
- Serentil ... 686

Methadone Hydrochloride (Additive effect). Products include:
- Dolophine Hydrochloride Ampoules & Vials ... 1260
- Dolophine Hydrochloride Tablets ... 1261
- Methadone Hydrochloride Diskets ... 1284
- Methadone Hydrochloride Oral Solution & Tablets ... 1987

Methohexital Sodium (Additive effect). Products include:
- Brevital Sodium Vials ... 1248

Methoxyflurane (Additive effect).
- No products indexed under this heading.

Methyldopa (Reduced antihypertensive effects). Products include:
- Aldoclor Tablets ... 1413
- Aldomet Oral ... 1415
- Aldoril Tablets ... 1418

Methyldopate Hydrochloride (Reduced antihypertensive effects). Products include:
- Aldomet Ester HCl Injection ... 1417

Metoprolol Tartrate (Increased effect of sympathomimetics). Products include:
- Lopressor Ampuls ... 1032
- Lopressor HCT Tablets ... 1034
- Lopressor Tablets ... 1032

Midazolam Hydrochloride (Additive effect). Products include:
- Versed Injection ... 1924

Molindone Hydrochloride (Additive effect). Products include:
- Moban Tablets & Concentrate ... 932

Morphine Sulfate (Additive effect). Products include:
- Astramorph/PF Injection, USP (Preservative-Free) ... 618
- Duramorph ... 960
- Infumorph 200 and Infumorph 500 Sterile Solutions ... 962
- MS Contin Tablets ... 1814
- MSIR ... 1817
- Oramorph SR (Morphine Sulfate Sustained Release Tablets) ... 1988
- Roxanol ... 1991

Nadolol (Increased effect of sympathomimetics). Products include:
- Corgard Tablets ... 701
- Corzide Tablets ... 702

Nortriptyline Hydrochloride (Additive effect). Products include:
- Pamelor ... 2019

Opium Alkaloids (Additive effect). Products include:
- B & O No. 15A & No. 16A Supprettes ... 2395
- Pantopon Injectable ... 1911

Oxazepam (Additive effect). Products include:
- Serax Capsules ... 2522
- Serax Tablets ... 2522

Oxycodone Hydrochloride (Additive effect). Products include:
- Percocet Tablets ... 950
- Percodan ... 951
- Roxicodone Tablets, Oral Solution & Intensol (Oxycodone) ... 1992
- Tylox Capsules ... 1382

Pargyline Hydrochloride (Increased effect of sympathomimetics).
- No products indexed under this heading.

Penbutolol Sulfate (Increased effect of sympathomimetics). Products include:
- Levatol ... 1832

Pentobarbital Sodium (Additive effect). Products include:
- Nembutal Sodium Capsules ... 534
- Nembutal Sodium Solution ... 536
- Nembutal Sodium Suppositories ... 538

Perphenazine (Additive effect). Products include:
- Etrafon ... 2087
- Triavil Tablets ... 1556
- Trilafon ... 2123

Phenelzine Sulfate (Increased effect of sympathomimetics; concurrent use is contraindicated). Products include:
- Nardil ... 1742

Phenobarbital (Additive effect). Products include:
- Arco-Lase Plus Tablets ... 607
- Bellergal-S Tablets ... 1998
- Bronkolixir ... ▣ 761
- Bronkotabs Tablets ... ▣ 762
- Donnatal ... 1858
- Donnatal Extentabs ... 1859
- Donnatal Tablets ... 1858
- Donnazyme Tablets ... 1860
- Kinesed Tablets ... 2272
- Phenobarbital Elixir and Tablets ... 1293
- Primatene Tablets-P Formula ... 2421
- Quadrinal Tablets ... 1183
- Tedral SA ... 1765

Pindolol (Increased effect of sympathomimetics). Products include:
- Visken Tablets ... 2036

Prazepam (Additive effect). Products include:
- Centrax ... 1693

Prochlorperazine (Additive effect). Products include:
- Compazine ... 2201

Promethazine Hydrochloride (Additive effect). Products include:
- Mepergan Injection ... 2479
- Phenergan with Codeine ... 2497
- Phenergan with Dextromethorphan 2499
- Phenergan Injection ... 2493
- Phenergan Suppositories ... 2496
- Phenergan Syrup ... 2495
- Phenergan Tablets ... 2496
- Phenergan VC ... 2500
- Phenergan VC with Codeine ... 2501

Propofol (Additive effect). Products include:
- Diprivan Injection ... 2267

Propoxyphene Hydrochloride (Additive effect). Products include:
- Darvon ... 1256
- Wygesic Tablets ... 2540

Propoxyphene Napsylate (Additive effect). Products include:
- Darvon-N/Darvocet-N ... 1254

Propranolol Hydrochloride (Increased effect of sympathomimetics). Products include:
- Inderal ... 2459
- Inderal LA Long Acting Capsules ... 2461
- Inderide Tablets ... 2463
- Inderide LA Long Acting Capsules ... 2465

(▣ Described in PDR For Nonprescription Drugs)

(⊙ Described in PDR For Ophthalmology)

Protriptyline Hydrochloride (Additve effect). Products include:
Vivactil Tablets ... 1567

Quazepam (Additive effect). Products include:
Doral Tablets ... 2383

Reserpine (Reduced antihypertensive effects). Products include:
Diupres Tablets ... 1461
Hydromox R Tablets ... 1209
Hydropres Tablets ... 1485
Renese-R Tablets ... 1786
Salutensin/Salutensin-Demi ... 719
Ser-Ap-Es Tablets ... 881
Serpasil Tablets ... 883
Serpasil-Apresoline Tablets ... 884
Serpasil-Esidrix Tablets ... 886

Secobarbital Sodium (Additive effect). Products include:
Seconal Sodium Pulvules ... 1296

Selegiline Hydrochloride (Increased effect of sympathomimetics; concurrent use is contraindicated). Products include:
Eldepryl ... 2250

Sufentanil Citrate (Additive effect). Products include:
Sufenta Injection ... 1147

Temazepam (Additive effect). Products include:
Restoril Capsules ... 2023

Thiamylal Sodium (Additive effect). Products include:
Surital Ampoules, Steri-Vials ... 1764

Thioridazine Hydrochloride (Additive effect). Products include:
Mellaril ... 2011

Thiothixene (Additive effect). Products include:
Navane Capsules and Concentrate 1954
Navane Intramuscular ... 1956

Timolol Maleate (Increased effect of sympathomimetics). Products include:
Blocadren Tablets ... 1429
Timolide Tablets ... 1547
Timoptic in Ocudose ... 1552
Timoptic Sterile Ophthalmic Solution ... 1550

Tranylcypromine Sulfate (Increased effect of sympathomimetics; concurrent use is contraindicated). Products include:
Parnate Tablets ... 2222

Triazolam (Additive effect). Products include:
Halcion Tablets ... 2340

Trifluoperazine Hydrochloride (Additive effect). Products include:
Stelazine ... 2226

Trimipramine Maleate (Additive effect). Products include:
Surmontil Capsules ... 2524

NALFON PULVULES & TABLETS
(Fenoprofen Calcium) ... 919
May interact with sulfonamides, oral hypoglycemic agents, oral anticoagulants, loop diuretics, hydantoin anticonvulsants, salicylates, and certain other agents. Compounds in these categories include:

Aspirin (Decreases half-life of fenoprofen). Products include:
Alka-Seltzer Effervescent Antacid and Pain Reliever ... 1568
Alka-Seltzer Extra Strength Effervescent Antacid and Pain Reliever ... 1570
Alka-Seltzer (Flavored) Effervescent Antacid and Pain Reliever ... 1569
Alka-Seltzer Plus Cold Medicine ... ◙ 623
Alka-Seltzer Plus Night-Time Cold Medicine ... ◙ 623
Alka Seltzer Plus Sinus Allergy Medicine ... ◙ 624
Anacin Coated Analgesic Caplets ... 2417
Anacin Coated Analgesic Tablets ... 2417
Anacin Maximum Strength Analgesic Coated Tablets ... 2417
Maximum Strength Arthritis Pain Formula By the Makers of Anacin Analgesic Tablets and Caplets ... 2418
Arthritis Pain Formula by the Makers of Anacin Analgesic Tablets and Caplets ... ◙ 747
Arthritis Strength BC Powder ... ◙ 516
Ascriptin A/D Caplets ... 1850
Regular Strength Ascriptin Tablets 1850
Azdone Tablets ... 844
BC Powder ... ◙ 517
BC Cold Powder ... ◙ 517
Children's Bayer Chewable Aspirin ... ◙ 564
Genuine Bayer Aspirin Tablets & Caplets ... ◙ 564
Maximum Bayer Aspirin Tablets & Caplets ... ◙ 566
Bayer Plus Aspirin Tablets ... ◙ 567
Therapy Bayer Aspirin Caplets ... ◙ 568
8 Hour Bayer Timed-Release Aspirin ... ◙ 566
Arthritis Strength Bufferin Analgesic Caplets ... 744
Extra Strength Bufferin Analgesic Tablets ... 745
Bufferin Analgesic Tablets and Caplets ... 743
Cama Arthritis Pain Reliever ... ◙ 685
Damason-P ... 1356
Easprin ... 1719
Ecotrin Enteric Coated Aspirin Maximum Strength Tablets and Caplets ... 2189
Ecotrin Enteric Coated Aspirin Regular Strength Tablets and Caplets ... 2189
Empirin Aspirin ... ◙ 541
Empirin with Codeine Phosphate Nos. 2, 3 & 4 ... 764
Equagesic Tablets ... 2451
Excedrin Extra-Strength Analgesic Tablets & Caplets ... 749
4-Way Cold Tablets ... 750
Fiorinal Capsules ... 2007
Fiorinal with Codeine Capsules ... 2008
Fiorinal Tablets ... 2007
Lortab ASA Tablets ... 2414
Momentum Muscular Backache Formula ... ◙ 751
Norgesic ... 1314
Norwich Extra-Strength Aspirin ... ◙ 546
Norwich Regular Strength Aspirin ◙ 547
P-A-C Analgesic Tablets ... ◙ 669
Percodan ... 951
Robaxisal Tablets ... 1872
Sine-Off Sinus Medicine Tablets-Aspirin Formula ... ◙ 722
Soma Compound w/Codeine Tablets ... 2390
Soma Compound Tablets ... 2389
St. Joseph Adult Chewable Aspirin (81 mg.) ... ◙ 703
Synalgos-DC Capsules ... 2525
Talwin Compound ... 2072
Ursinus Inlay-Tabs ... ◙ 691
Vanquish Analgesic Caplets ... ◙ 574
Zorprin Tablets ... 698

Bumetanide (Patients treated with Nalfon may be resistant to the effects of loop diuretics). Products include:
Bumex ... 1895

Chlorpropamide (Sulfonylurea toxicity). Products include:
Diabinese Tablets ... 1775

Choline Magnesium Trisalicylate (Decreases half-life of fenoprofen). Products include:
Trilisate ... 1822

Dicumarol (Prolonged prothrombin time). Products include:
Dicumarol Tablets ... 516

Diflunisal (Decreases half-life of fenoprofen). Products include:
Dolobid Tablets ... 1465

Ethacrynic Acid (Patients treated with Nalfon may be resistant to the effects of loop diuretics). Products include:
Edecrin Tablets ... 1468

Ethotoin (Potential for increased activity and toxicity of ethotoin). Products include:
Peganone Tablets ... 551

Furosemide (Patients treated with Nalfon may be resistant to the effects of loop diuretics). Products include:
Lasix ... 1093

Glipizide (Sulfonylurea toxicity). Products include:
Glucotrol ... 1952

Glyburide (Sulfonylurea toxicity). Products include:
DiaBeta ... 1091
Micronase Tablets ... 2350

Magnesium Salicylate (Decreases half-life of fenoprofen). Products include:
Doan's - Extra-Strength Analgesic ◙ 549
Doan's - Regular Strength Analgesic ... ◙ 549
Mobigesic Analgesic Tablets ... ◙ 507

Mephenytoin (Potential for increased activity and toxicity of mephenytoin). Products include:
Mesantoin Tablets ... 2013

Phenobarbital (Decreases plasma half-life of fenoprofen). Products include:
Arco-Lase Plus Tablets ... 607
Bellergal-S Tablets ... 1998
Bronkolixir ... ◙ 761
Bronkotabs Tablets ... ◙ 762
Donnatal ... 1858
Donnatal Extentabs ... 1859
Donnatal Tablets ... 1858
Donnazyme Tablets ... 1860
Kinesed Tablets ... 2272
Phenobarbital Elixir and Tablets ... 1293
Primatene Tablets-P Formula ... 2421
Quadrinal Tablets ... 1183
Tedral SA ... 1765

Phenytoin (Potential for increased activity and toxicity of phenytoin). Products include:
Dilantin Infatabs ... 1710
Dilantin-30 Pediatric/Dilantin-125 Suspension ... 1713

Phenytoin Sodium (Potential for increased activity and toxicity of phenytoin). Products include:
Dilantin Kapseals ... 1708
Dilantin Parenteral ... 1712
Dilantin with Phenobarbital Kapseals ... 1715

Salsalate (Decreases half-life of fenoprofen). Products include:
Disalcid ... 1310
Mono-Gesic Tablets ... 846
Salflex ... 839

Sulfamethizole (Sulfonamide toxicity). Products include:
Thiosulfil Forte Tablets ... 2526
Urobiotic-250 Capsules ... 1968

Sulfamethoxazole (Sulfonamide toxicity). Products include:
Azo Gantanol Tablets ... 1887
Bactrim DS Tablets ... 1891
Bactrim I.V. Infusion ... 1889
Bactrim ... 1891
Gantanol ... 1899
Septra ... 813
Septra I.V. Infusion ... 808
Septra I.V. Infusion ADD-Vantage Vials ... 810
Septra ... 813

Sulfasalazine (Sulfonamide toxicity). Products include:
Azulfidine Tablets, EN-tabs, Oral Suspension ... 1157

Sulfinpyrazone (Sulfonamide toxicity). Products include:
Anturane ... 853

Sulfisoxazole (Sulfonamide toxicity). Products include:
Azo Gantrisin Tablets ... 1888
Gantrisin Tablets ... 1901
Pediazole ... 1973

Sulfisoxazole Diolamine (Sulfonamide toxicity). Products include:
Gantrisin Ophthalmic Ointment/Solution ... 1900

Tolazamide (Sulfonylurea toxicity). Products include:
Tolinase Tablets ... 2365

Tolbutamide (Sulfonylurea toxicity). Products include:
Orinase Tablets ... 2354

Warfarin Sodium (Prolonged prothrombin time). Products include:
Coumadin Injection & Tablets ... 944
Panwarfin Tablets ... 547

Food Interactions

Dairy products (Peak blood levels are delayed and diminished).

Meal, unspecified (Peak blood levels are delayed and diminished).

NAPHCON
(Naphazoline Hydrochloride) ... ⊙ 226
No interactions described in labeling.

NAPHCON FORTE
(Naphazoline Hydrochloride) ... ⊙ 226
May interact with monoamine oxidase inhibitors, tricyclic antidepressants, and certain other agents. Compounds in these categories include:

Amitriptyline Hydrochloride (May potentiate the pressor effect of naphazoline). Products include:
Elavil ... 2269
Endep Tablets ... 1927
Etrafon ... 2087
Limbitrol ... 1933
Triavil Tablets ... 1556

Amoxapine (May potentiate the pressor effect of naphazoline). Products include:
Asendin Tablets ... 1196

Clomipramine Hydrochloride (May potentiate the pressor effect of naphazoline). Products include:
Anafranil Capsules ... 650

Desipramine Hydrochloride (May potentiate the pressor effect of naphazoline). Products include:
Norpramin Tablets ... 1340

Doxepin Hydrochloride (May potentiate the pressor effect of naphazoline). Products include:
Sinequan ... 1960

Furazolidone (Severe hypertensive crisis). Products include:
Furoxone ... 1855

Imipramine Hydrochloride (May potentiate the pressor effect of naphazoline). Products include:
Tofranil Ampuls ... 1038
Tofranil Tablets ... 1039

Imipramine Pamoate (May potentiate the pressor effect of naphazoline). Products include:
Tofranil-PM Capsules ... 1041

Isocarboxazid (Severe hypertensive crisis). Products include:
Marplan Tablets ... 1906

Maprotiline Hydrochloride (May potentiate the pressor effect of naphazoline). Products include:
Ludiomil Tablets ... 874

Nortriptyline Hydrochloride (May potentiate the pressor effect of naphazoline). Products include:
Pamelor ... 2019

Phenelzine Sulfate (Severe hypertensive crisis). Products include:
Nardil ... 1742

Protriptyline Hydrochloride (May potentiate the pressor effect of naphazoline). Products include:
Vivactil Tablets ... 1567

Selegiline Hydrochloride (Severe hypertensive crisis). Products include:
Eldepryl ... 2250

Tranylcypromine Sulfate (Severe hypertensive crisis). Products include:
Parnate Tablets ... 2222

Trimipramine Maleate (May potentiate the pressor effect of naphazoline). Products include:
Surmontil Capsules ... 2524

NAPHCON-A OPHTHALMIC SOLUTION

(Naphazoline Hydrochloride, Pheniramine Maleate) ... 571
May interact with monoamine oxidase inhibitors. Compounds in this category include:

Furazolidone (Severe hypertensive crisis). Products include:
Furoxone ... 1855

Isocarboxazid (Severe hypertensive crisis). Products include:
Marplan Tablets ... 1906

Phenelzine Sulfate (Severe hypertensive crisis). Products include:
Nardil ... 1742

Selegiline Hydrochloride (Severe hypertensive crisis). Products include:
Eldepryl ... 2250

Tranylcypromine Sulfate (Severe hypertensive crisis). Products include:
Parnate Tablets ... 2222

NAPROSYN SUSPENSION

(Naproxen) ... 2297
May interact with oral anticoagulants, sulfonamides, oral hypoglycemic agents, lithium preparations, beta blockers, hydantoin anticonvulsants, and certain other agents. Compounds in these categories include:

Acebutolol Hydrochloride (Reduced antihypertensive effect of beta blockers). Products include:
Sectral Capsules ... 2520

Atenolol (Reduced antihypertensive effect of beta blockers). Products include:
Tenoretic Tablets ... 1105
Tenormin Tablets and I.V. Injection 1107

Betaxolol Hydrochloride (Reduced antihypertensive effect of beta blockers). Products include:
Betoptic Sterile Ophthalmic Solution ... 569
Betoptic S Sterile Ophthalmic Suspension ... 570
Kerlone Tablets ... 2172

Carteolol Hydrochloride (Reduced antihypertensive effect of beta blockers). Products include:
Cartrol Tablets ... 507

Chlorpropamide (Sulfonylurea toxicity). Products include:
Diabinese Tablets ... 1775

Dicumarol (Prothrombin times may be affected). Products include:
Dicumarol Tablets ... 516

Esmolol Hydrochloride (Reduced antihypertensive effect of beta blockers). Products include:
Brevibloc Injection ... 942

Ethotoin (Hydantoin toxicity). Products include:
Peganone Tablets ... 551

Furosemide (Natriuretic effect of furosemide may be inhibited). Products include:
Lasix ... 1093

Glipizide (Sulfonylurea toxicity). Products include:
Glucotrol ... 1952

Glyburide (Sulfonylurea toxicity). Products include:
DiaBeta ... 1091
Micronase Tablets ... 2350

Labetalol Hydrochloride (Reduced antihypertensive effect of beta blockers). Products include:
Normodyne Injection ... 2108
Normodyne Tablets ... 2110
Normozide Tablets ... 2112
Trandate HCT Tablets ... 579
Trandate Injection ... 577
Trandate Tablets ... 579

Lithium Carbonate (Renal lithium clearance inhibited; increased plasma lithium levels). Products include:
Eskalith ... 2214
Lithane Tablets ... 1596
Lithium Carbonate Capsules & Tablets ... 1984
Lithobid Tablets ... 870

Lithium Citrate (Renal lithium clearance inhibited; increased plasma lithium levels). Products include:
Cibalith-S ... 870

Mephenytoin (Hydantoin toxicity). Products include:
Mesantoin Tablets ... 2013

Methotrexate Sodium (Methotrexate toxicity may be enhanced). Products include:
Methotrexate Tablets, Parenteral, LPF Parenteral ... 1217
Rheumatrex Methotrexate Dose Pack ... 1234

Metoprolol Tartrate (Reduced antihypertensive effect of beta blockers). Products include:
Lopressor Ampuls ... 1032
Lopressor HCT Tablets ... 1034
Lopressor Tablets ... 1032

Nadolol (Reduced antihypertensive effect of beta blockers). Products include:
Corgard Tablets ... 701
Corzide Tablets ... 702

Naproxen Sodium (Naproxen anion increased; should not be used concomitantly). Products include:
Anaprox and Anaprox DS Tablets ... 2288

Penbutolol Sulfate (Reduced antihypertensive effect of beta blockers). Products include:
Levatol ... 1832

Phenytoin (Hydantoin toxicity). Products include:
Dilantin Infatabs ... 1710
Dilantin-30 Pediatric/Dilantin-125 Suspension ... 1713

Phenytoin Sodium (Hydantoin toxicity). Products include:
Dilantin Kapseals ... 1708
Dilantin Parenteral ... 1712
Dilantin with Phenobarbital Kapseals ... 1715

Pindolol (Reduced antihypertensive effect of beta blockers). Products include:
Visken Tablets ... 2036

Probenecid (Increased naproxen anion). Products include:
Benemid Tablets ... 1426
ColBENEMID Tablets ... 1436
Wycillin Injection and Probenecid Tablets ... 2539

Propranolol Hydrochloride (Reduced antihypertensive effect of beta blockers). Products include:
Inderal ... 2459
Inderal LA Long Acting Capsules ... 2461
Inderide Tablets ... 2463
Inderide LA Long Acting Capsules ... 2465

Sulfamethizole (Sulfonamide toxicity). Products include:
Thiosulfil Forte Tablets ... 2526
Urobiotic-250 Capsules ... 1968

Sulfamethoxazole (Sulfonamide toxicity). Products include:
Azo Gantanol Tablets ... 1887
Bactrim DS Tablets ... 1891
Bactrim I.V. Infusion ... 1889
Bactrim ... 1891
Gantanol ... 1899
Septra ... 813
Septra I.V. Infusion ... 808
Septra I.V. Infusion ADD-Vantage Vials ... 810
Septra ... 813

Sulfasalazine (Sulfonamide toxicity). Products include:
Azulfidine Tablets, EN-tabs, Oral Suspension ... 1157

Sulfinpyrazone (Sulfonamide toxicity). Products include:
Anturane ... 853

Sulfisoxazole (Sulfonamide toxicity). Products include:
Azo Gantrisin Tablets ... 1888
Gantrisin Tablets ... 1901
Pediazole ... 1973

Sulfisoxazole Diolamine (Sulfonamide toxicity). Products include:
Gantrisin Ophthalmic Ointment/Solution ... 1900

Timolol Maleate (Reduced antihypertensive effect of beta blockers). Products include:
Blocadren Tablets ... 1429
Timolide Tablets ... 1547
Timoptic in Ocudose ... 1552
Timoptic Sterile Ophthalmic Solution ... 1550

Tolazamide (Sulfonylurea toxicity). Products include:
Tolinase Tablets ... 2365

Tolbutamide (Sulfonylurea toxicity). Products include:
Orinase Tablets ... 2354

Warfarin Sodium (Prothrombin times may be affected). Products include:
Coumadin Injection & Tablets ... 944
Panwarfin Tablets ... 547

NAPROSYN TABLETS

(Naproxen) ... 2297
See **Naprosyn Suspension**

NARCAN INJECTION

(Naloxone Hydrochloride) ... 933
No interactions described in labeling.

NARDIL

(Phenelzine Sulfate) ... 1742
May interact with monoamine oxidase inhibitors, antihypertensives, sympathomimetic aerosal bronchodilators, dibenzazepines, tricyclic antidepressants, phenylpropanolamine containing anorectics, alpha adrenergic stimulants, anorexiants, narcotic analgesics, and certain other agents. Compounds in these categories include:

Acebutolol Hydrochloride (Exaggerated hypotensive effects). Products include:
Sectral Capsules ... 2520

Albuterol (Hypertensive crises). Products include:
Proventil Inhalation Aerosol ... 2117
Ventolin Inhalation Aerosol and Refill ... 583

Albuterol Sulfate (Hypertensive crises). Products include:
Proventil Repetabs Tablets ... 2120
Proventil Solutions for Inhalation 0.5% and 0.083% ... 2118
Proventil Syrup ... 2119
Proventil Tablets ... 2120
Ventolin ... 583

Alcohol (Hypertensive crises).

Alfentanil Hydrochloride (Meperidine contraindication is extended to other narcotics). Products include:
Alfenta Injection ... 1131

Amitriptyline Hydrochloride (Concurrent or in rapid succession administration is contraindicated). Products include:
Elavil ... 2269
Endep Tablets ... 1927
Etrafon ... 2087
Limbitrol ... 1933
Triavil Tablets ... 1556

Amoxapine (Concurrent or in rapid succession administration is contraindicated). Products include:
Asendin Tablets ... 1196

Amphetamine Aspartate (Hypertensive crises).
No products indexed under this heading.

Amphetamine Resins (Concurrent administration is not recommended). Products include:
Biphetamine Capsules ... 973

Amphetamine Sulfate (Hypertensive crises).
No products indexed under this heading.

Atenolol (Exaggerated hypotensive effects). Products include:
Tenoretic Tablets ... 1105
Tenormin Tablets and I.V. Injection 1107

Benazepril Hydrochloride (Exaggerated hypotensive effects). Products include:
Lotensin Tablets ... 872

Bendroflumethiazide (Exaggerated hypotensive effects). Products include:
Corzide Tablets ... 702
Naturetin Tablets ... 1789
Rauzide Tablets ... 1804

Benzphetamine Hydrochloride (Concurrent administration is not recommended). Products include:
Didrex Tablets ... 2338

Betaxolol Hydrochloride (Exaggerated hypotensive effects). Products include:
Betoptic Sterile Ophthalmic Solution ... 569
Betoptic S Sterile Ophthalmic Suspension ... 570
Kerlone Tablets ... 2172

Buprenorphine (Meperidine contraindication is extended to other narcotics).
No products indexed under this heading.

Bupropion Hydrochloride (Concurrent and/or administration is contraindicated). Products include:
Wellbutrin Tablets ... 821

Buspirone Hydrochloride (Elevated blood pressure; concurrent therapy is contraindicated). Products include:
BuSpar ... 1401

Caffeine-containing medications (Concurrent use with excessive caffeine intake should be avoided).

Captopril (Exaggerated hypotensive effects). Products include:
Capoten ... 2255
Capozide ... 2258

Carbamazepine (Effect unspecified). Products include:
Tegretol Chewable Tablets ... 654
Tegretol Suspension ... 656
Tegretol Tablets ... 654

Carteolol Hydrochloride (Exaggerated hypotensive effects). Products include:
Cartrol Tablets ... 507

Chlorothiazide (Exaggerated hypotensive effects). Products include:
Aldoclor Tablets ... 1413
Diupres Tablets ... 1461
Diuril Oral ... 1464

Chlorothiazide Sodium (Exaggerated hypotensive effects). Products include:
Diuril Sodium Intravenous ... 1463

Chlorthalidone (Exaggerated hypotensive effects). Products include:
Combipres Tablets ... 678
Tenoretic Tablets ... 1105
Thalitone Tablets ... 687

Clomipramine Hydrochloride (Concurrent or in rapid succession administration is contraindicated). Products include:
- Anafranil Capsules 650

Clonidine (Exaggerated hypotensive effects). Products include:
- Catapres-TTS 677

Clonidine Hydrochloride (Exaggerated hypotensive effects). Products include:
- Catapres Tablets 676
- Combipres Tablets 678

Clozapine (Effect unspecified). Products include:
- Clozaril Tablets 2000

Cocaine Hydrochloride (Hypertensive crises). Products include:
- Cocaine Hydrochloride Topical Solution 620

Codeine (Meperidine contraindication is extended to other narcotics). Products include:
- Calcidrine Syrup 506

Codeine Phosphate (Meperidine contraindication is extended to other narcotics). Products include:
- Actifed with Codeine Cough Syrup 752
- Cheracol Cough Syrup 1853
- Codimal PH Syrup 846
- Dimetane-DC Cough Syrup 1857
- Empirin with Codeine Phosphate Nos. 2, 3 & 4 764
- Fiorinal with Codeine Capsules 2008
- Isoclor Expectorant 982
- Naldecon CX Adult Liquid ■ 521
- Novahistine DH 1342
- Novahistine Expectorant 1343
- Nucofed Capsules 2219
- Nucofed Expectorant 2219
- Nucofed Pediatric Expectorant 2220
- Nucofed Syrup 2219
- Phenaphen with Codeine Capsules 1865
- Phenaphen-650 with Codeine Tablets 1866
- Phenergan with Codeine 2497
- Phenergan VC with Codeine 2501
- Robitussin A-C Syrup 1875
- Robitussin-DAC Syrup 1875
- Ryna ■ 741
- Soma Compound w/Codeine Tablets 2390
- Triaminic Expectorant w/Codeine 1996
- Tussi-Organidin Liquid 2391
- Tylenol with Codeine 1381

Codeine Polistirex (Meperidine contraindication is extended to other narcotics).
- No products indexed under this heading.

Cyclobenzaprine Hydrochloride (Effect unspecified). Products include:
- Flexeril Tablets 1471

Deserpidine (Exaggerated hypotensive effects). Products include:
- Enduronyl 518
- Harmonyl Tablets 528
- Oreticyl 545

Desipramine Hydrochloride (Concurrent or in rapid succession administration is contraindicated). Products include:
- Norpramin Tablets 1340

Dextroamphetamine (Hypertensive crises). Products include:
- Biphetamine Capsules 973

Dextroamphetamine Sulfate (Hypertensive crises; concurrent administration is not recommended). Products include:
- Dexedrine 2206

Dextromethorphan Hydrobromide (Concurrent administration is not recommended). Products include:
- Benylin DM ■ 638
- Benylin Expectorant ■ 638
- Cerose-DM 2443
- Cheracol D Cough Formula ■ 667
- Cheracol Plus Head Cold/Cough Formula ■ 667
- Codimal DM Syrup 846
- Cough Formula Comtrex 746
- Comtrex Multi-Symptom Cold Reliever Tablets/Caplets/Liqui-Gels/Liquid 745
- Day-Night Comtrex 747
- Non-Drowsy Comtrex 747
- Contac Cough Formula ■ 711
- Contac Cough & Sore Throat Formula ■ 712
- Contac Jr. Children's Cold Medicine ■ 712
- Contac Nighttime Cold Medicine ■ 713
- Contac Severe Cold and Flu Formula Caplets ■ 711
- Dimacol Caplets ■ 672
- Dimetane-DX Cough Syrup 1858
- Dimetapp DM Elixir ■ 674
- Dorcol Children's Cough Syrup ■ 685
- Hold Cough Suppressant Lozenge ■ 617
- Humibid DM Tablets 560
- Medi-Flu Caplet, Liquid ■ 640
- Naldecon DX Adult Liquid ■ 521
- Naldecon DX Children's Syrup ■ 522
- Naldecon DX Pediatric Drops ■ 522
- Naldecon Senior DX Cough/Cold Liquid ■ 523
- Novahistine DMX ■ 595
- Orthoxicol Cough Syrup ■ 668
- PediaCare Cough-Cold Formula Liquid 1362
- PediaCare Night Rest Cough-Cold Formula Liquid 1362
- PediaCare 6-12 Cough-Cold Formula Chewable Tablets 1362
- Phenergan with Dextromethorphan 2499
- Quelidrine Syrup 556
- Robitussin Cough Calmers ■ 677
- Robitussin Night Relief ■ 677
- Robitussin Pediatric ■ 678
- Robitussin-CF ■ 676
- Robitussin-DM ■ 676
- Rondec-DM 1976
- St. Joseph Cough Suppressant for Children ■ 705
- St. Joseph Nighttime Cold Medicine ■ 705
- Sucrets Cough Control Formula ■ 724
- Sudafed Cough Syrup ■ 543
- Triaminic Nite Light ■ 689
- Triaminic-DM Syrup ■ 689
- Triaminicol Multi-Symptom Cold Tablets ■ 691
- Triaminicol Multi-Symptom Relief ■ 691
- Tussi-Organidin DM Liquid 2392
- Tylenol Cold & Flu Hot Medication, Packets 1369
- Tylenol Cold & Flu No Drowsiness Hot Medication, Packets 1371
- Tylenol Cold Medication Caplets and Tablets 1370
- Tylenol Cold Medication No Drowsiness Formula Caplets 1370
- Tylenol Cold Night Time Medication Liquid 1371
- Tylenol Cough Medication Liquid, Maximum Strength 1372
- Tylenol Cough Medication Liquid with Decongestant, Maximum Strength 1372
- Vicks Children's Cough Syrup ■ 660
- Vicks Children's NyQuil ■ 664
- Vicks Cough Silencers Cough Drops ■ 660
- Vicks Daycare ■ 660
- Vicks Formula 44 Cough Control Discs ■ 661
- Vicks Formula 44 Cough Medicine ■ 661
- Vicks Formula 44D Decongestant Cough Medicine ■ 662
- Vicks Formula 44M Multi-Symptom Cough Medicine ■ 662
- Vicks NyQuil Nighttime Colds Medicine-Original & Cherry Flavor ■ 664
- Vicks Pediatric Formula 44 Cough Medicine ■ 662
- Vicks Pediatric Formula 44 Cough & Congestion Medicine ■ 663
- Vicks Pediatric Formula 44m Multi-Symptom Cough & Cold Medicine ■ 663

Dextromethorphan Polistirex (Concurrent administration is not recommended). Products include:
- Delsym Cough Formula ■ 560

Dezocine (Meperidine contraindication is extended to other narcotics).

Diazoxide (Exaggerated hypotensive effects). Products include:
- Hyperstat I.V. Injection 2095
- Proglycem 649

Diethylpropion Hydrochloride (Concurrent administration is not recommended). Products include:
- Tenuate 1354

Dobutamine Hydrochloride (Hypertensive crises). Products include:
- Dobutrex Solution Vials 1259

Dopamine Hydrochloride (Hypertensive crises). Products include:
- Intropin Injection 930

Doxazosin Mesylate (Exaggerated hypotensive effects). Products include:
- Cardura Tablets 1941

Doxepin Hydrochloride (Concurrent or in rapid succession administration is contraindicated). Products include:
- Sinequan 1960

Enalapril Maleate (Exaggerated hypotensive effects). Products include:
- Vaseretic Tablets 1559
- Vasotec Tablets 1564

Enalaprilat (Exaggerated hypotensive effects). Products include:
- Vasotec I.V. 1562

Ephedrine Hydrochloride (Hypertensive crises). Products include:
- Amesec ■ 682
- Primatene Tablets-M Formula 2421
- Primatene Tablets-P Formula 2421
- Primatene Tablets-Regular Formula 2421
- Quadrinal Tablets 1183
- Quelidrine Syrup 556
- Tedral SA 1765

Ephedrine Sulfate (Hypertensive crises). Products include:
- Bronkaid Tablets ■ 757
- Bronkolixir ■ 761
- Bronkotabs Tablets ■ 762
- Marax Tablets & DF Syrup 1954
- Pazo Hemorrhoid Ointment & Suppositories 752
- Vicks Vatronol Nose Drops ■ 666

Ephedrine Tannate (Hypertensive crises). Products include:
- Rynatuss 2388

Epinephrine (Hypertensive crises). Products include:
- Ana-Kit Anaphylaxis Emergency Treatment Kit 1100
- Bronkaid Mist ■ 757
- EpiPen 843
- Marcaine Hydrochloride 0.5% with Epinephrine 1:200,000 (as bitartrate) 958
- Marcaine Hydrochloride with Epinephrine 1:200,000 2055
- Primatene Mist 2420
- Sus-Phrine Injection 1006
- Xylocaine with Epinephrine Injections 637

Epinephrine Bitartrate (Hypertensive crises). Products include:
- AsthmaHaler Mist Epinephrine Bitartrate Bronchodilator ■ 616
- Bronkaid Mist Suspension ■ 757
- Primatene Mist Suspension 2421

Epinephrine Hydrochloride (Hypertensive crises). Products include:
- Adrenalin Chloride Solution 1:100 & 1:1,000 1689
- Epifrin ⊙ 244
- Glaucon ⊙ 218

Esmolol Hydrochloride (Exaggerated hypotensive effects). Products include:
- Brevibloc Injection 942

Felodipine (Exaggerated hypotensive effects). Products include:
- Plendil Extended-Release Tablets 1526

Fenfluramine Hydrochloride (Concurrent administration is not recommended). Products include:
- Pondimin Tablets 1867

Fentanyl (Meperidine contraindication is extended to other narcotics). Products include:
- Duragesic Transdermal System 1133

Fentanyl Citrate (Meperidine contraindication is extended to other narcotics). Products include:
- Innovar Injection 1141
- Sublimaze Injection 1146

Fluoxetine Hydrochloride (Concurrent or in rapid succession administration is contraindicated; serious reactions including hyperthermia, rigidity, myoclonic movements and death have been reported). Products include:
- Prozac Pulvules 920

Fosinopril Sodium (Exaggerated hypotensive effects). Products include:
- Monopril Tablets 1406

Furazolidone (Concurrent or in rapid succession administration is contraindicated). Products include:
- Furoxone 1855

Furosemide (Exaggerated hypotensive effects). Products include:
- Lasix 1093

Guanabenz Acetate (Exaggerated hypotensive effects). Products include:
- Wytensin Tablets 2542

Guanethidine Monosulfate (Exaggerated hypotensive effects; contraindication). Products include:
- Esimil Tablets 864
- Ismelin Tablets 869

Hydralazine Hydrochloride (Exaggerated hypotensive effects). Products include:
- Apresazide Capsules 854
- Apresoline Hydrochloride Parenteral (Ampuls) 856
- Apresoline Hydrochloride Tablets 855
- Apresoline-Esidrix Tablets 857
- Ser-Ap-Es Tablets 881
- Serpasil-Apresoline Tablets 884

Hydrochlorothiazide (Exaggerated hypotensive effects). Products include:
- Aldactazide 2150
- Aldoril Tablets 1418
- Apresazide Capsules 854
- Apresoline-Esidrix Tablets 857
- Capozide 2258
- Dyazide Capsules 2208
- Esidrix Tablets 863
- Esimil Tablets 864
- HydroDIURIL Tablets 1484
- Hydropres Tablets 1485
- Inderide Tablets 2463
- Inderide LA Long Acting Capsules 2465
- Lopressor HCT Tablets 1034
- Maxzide 1215
- Moduretic Tablets 1510
- Normozide Tablets 2112
- Oretic Tablets 544
- Oreticyl 545
- Prinzide Tablets 1540
- Ser-Ap-Es Tablets 881
- Serpasil-Esidrix Tablets 886
- Timolide Tablets 1547
- Trandate HCT Tablets 579
- Vaseretic Tablets 1559
- Zestoretic 2274

Hydrocodone Bitartrate (Meperidine contraindication is extended to other narcotics). Products include:
- Anexsia 5/500 Tablets 2196
- Anexsia 7.5/650 Tablets 2197
- Azdone Tablets 844
- Codiclear DH Syrup 845
- Codimal DH Syrup 846
- Damason-P 1356
- Hycodan Syrup, Tablets 927
- Hycomine Compound Tablets 929
- Hycomine Syrup 927
- Hycotuss Expectorant Syrup 930
- Hydrocet Capsules 835

(■ Described in PDR For Nonprescription Drugs) (⊙ Described in PDR For Ophthalmology)

Lortab ASA Tablets 2414
Lortab 2412
Ru-Tuss with Hydrocodone 694
Triaminic Expectorant DH 1995
Vicodin Tablets 1187
Vicodin ES Tablets 1189
Zydone Capsules 941

Hydrocodone Polistirex (Meperidine contraindication is extended to other narcotics). Products include:
Tussionex Extended-Release Suspension 988

Hydroflumethiazide (Exaggerated hypotensive effects). Products include:
Diucardin Tablets 2450
Saluron 718
Salutensin/Salutensin-Demi 719

Imipramine Hydrochloride (Concurrent or in rapid succession administration is contraindicated). Products include:
Tofranil Ampuls 1038
Tofranil Tablets 1039

Imipramine Pamoate (Concurrent or in rapid succession administration is contraindicated). Products include:
Tofranil-PM Capsules 1041

Indapamide (Exaggerated hypotensive effects). Products include:
Lozol Tablets 1843

Isocarboxazid (Hypertensive crises; at least 10 days should elapse between discontinuation of Nardil and institution of another MAOI). Products include:
Marplan Tablets 1906

Isoproterenol Hydrochloride (Hypertensive crises). Products include:
Isuprel Hydrochloride Injection 1:5000 2050
Isuprel Hydrochloride Mistometer 2051
Isuprel Hydrochloride Solution 1:200 & 1:100 2052
Norisodrine Aerotrol 540

Isradipine (Exaggerated hypotensive effects). Products include:
DynaCirc Capsules 2004

Labetalol Hydrochloride (Exaggerated hypotensive effects). Products include:
Normodyne Injection 2108
Normodyne Tablets 2110
Normozide Tablets 2112
Trandate HCT Tablets 579
Trandate Injection 577
Trandate Tablets 579

Levodopa (Concurrent use should be avoided). Products include:
Larodopa Tablets 1905
Sinemet Tablets 952
Sinemet CR Tablets 953

Levorphanol Tartrate (Meperidine contraindication is extended to other narcotics). Products include:
Levo-Dromoran 1906

Lisinopril (Exaggerated hypotensive effects). Products include:
Prinivil Tablets 1538
Prinzide Tablets 1540
Zestoretic 2274
Zestril Tablets 2277

Maprotiline Hydrochloride (Concurrent or in rapid succession administration is contraindicated). Products include:
Ludiomil Tablets 874

Mazindol (Concurrent administration is not recommended). Products include:
Sanorex Tablets 2030

Mecamylamine Hydrochloride (Exaggerated hypotensive effects). Products include:
Inversine Tablets 1492

Meperidine Hydrochloride (Concurrent therapy is contraindicated; circulatory collapse, seizures, coma and death have been reported). Products include:
Demerol 2047
Mepergan Injection 2479

Metaproterenol Sulfate (Hypertensive crises). Products include:
Alupent 674
Arm-a-Med Metaproterenol Sulfate Inhalation Solution, USP 617
Metaprel Inhalation Aerosol Bronchodilator 2014
Metaprel Inhalation Solution 2015
Metaprel 2015
Metaproterenol Sulfate Inhalation Solution, USP 912

Metaraminol Bitartrate (Hypertensive crises). Products include:
Aramine Injection 1424

Methadone Hydrochloride (Meperidine contraindication is extended to other narcotics). Products include:
Dolophine Hydrochloride Ampoules & Vials 1260
Dolophine Hydrochloride Tablets 1261
Methadone Hydrochloride Diskets 1284
Methadone Hydrochloride Oral Solution & Tablets 1987

Methamphetamine Hydrochloride (Concurrent administration is not recommended). Products include:
Desoxyn Gradumet Tablets 514

Methoxamine Hydrochloride (Hypertensive crises). Products include:
Vasoxyl Injection 819

Methyclothiazide (Exaggerated hypotensive effects). Products include:
Enduron Tablets 517
Enduronyl 518

Methyldopa (Hypertensive crises). Products include:
Aldoclor Tablets 1413
Aldomet Oral 1415
Aldoril Tablets 1418

Methyldopate Hydrochloride (Hypertensive crises). Products include:
Aldomet Ester HCl Injection 1417

Methylphenidate Hydrochloride (Hypertensive crises). Products include:
Ritalin 880

Metolazone (Exaggerated hypotensive effects). Products include:
Diulo 2129
Mykrox ½ mg Tablets 984
Zaroxolyn Tablets 989

Metoprolol Tartrate (Exaggerated hypotensive effects). Products include:
Lopressor Ampuls 1032
Lopressor HCT Tablets 1034
Lopressor Tablets 1032

Metyrosine (Exaggerated hypotensive effects). Products include:
Demser Capsules 1460

Minoxidil (Exaggerated hypotensive effects). Products include:
Loniten Tablets 2346
Rogaine Topical Solution 2357

Morphine Sulfate (Meperidine contraindication is extended to other narcotics). Products include:
Astramorph/PF Injection, USP (Preservative-Free) 618
Duramorph 960
Infumorph 200 and Infumorph 500 Sterile Solutions 962
MS Contin Tablets 1814
MSIR 1817
Oramorph SR (Morphine Sulfate Sustained Release Tablets) 1988
Roxanol 1991

Nadolol (Exaggerated hypotensive effects). Products include:
Corgard Tablets 701
Corzide Tablets 702

Naphazoline Hydrochloride (Contraindicated). Products include:
AK-Con .... ⊙ 202
AK-Con-A .... ⊙ 203
Albalon Solution with Liquifilm .... ⊙ 238
Albalon-A Liquifilm .... ⊙ 238
Allergy Drops .... ⊙ 258
Clear Eyes ACR .... ⊙ 305
Clear Eyes Lubricating Eye Redness Reliever .... ⊙ 304
4-Way Fast Acting Nasal Spray - Original Formula (regular & mentholated) & Metered Spray Pump (regular) 751
Naphcon .... ⊙ 226
Naphcon Forte .... ⊙ 226
Naphcon-A Ophthalmic Solution 571
Opcon-A Ophthalmic Solution .... ⊙ 262
Privine Nasal Solution .... ▣ 552
Privine Nasal Solution 878
Privine Nasal Spray .... ▣ 552
Privine Nasal Spray 878
Vasocon-A .... ⊙ 278

Nicardipine Hydrochloride (Exaggerated hypotensive effects). Products include:
Cardene Capsules 2290

Nitroglycerin (Exaggerated hypotensive effects). Products include:
Deponit NTG Transdermal Delivery System 2143
Minitran Transdermal Delivery System 1312
Nitro-Bid Ointment 1339
Nitro-Bid Capsules 1338
Nitrodisc 2176
Nitro-Dur (nitroglycerin) Transdermal Infusion System 1164
Nitrogard Tablets 1004
Nitrolingual Spray 1846
Nitrostat Tablets 1743
Transderm-Nitro Transdermal Therapeutic System 2283

Norepinephrine Bitartrate (Hypertensive crises). Products include:
Levophed Bitartrate Injection 2054

Nortriptyline Hydrochloride (Hypertensive crises; concurrent or in rapid succession administration is contraindicated). Products include:
Pamelor 2019

Opium Alkaloids (Meperidine contraindication is extended to other narcotics). Products include:
B & O No. 15A & No. 16A Supprettes 2395
Pantopon Injectable 1911

Oxycodone Hydrochloride (Meperidine contraindication is extended to other narcotics). Products include:
Percocet Tablets 950
Percodan 951
Roxicodone Tablets, Oral Solution & Intensol (Oxycodone) 1992
Tylox Capsules 1382

Oxymetazoline Hydrochloride (Contraindicated). Products include:
Afrin .... ▣ 692
Cheracol Nasal Spray Pump .... ▣ 667
Dristan Long Lasting Menthol Nasal Spray 2419
Dristan Long Lasting Nasal Spray, Regular and Regular with Metered Dose Pump 2419
Duration Nasal Spray .... ▣ 700
Duration 12 Hour Nasal Spray Pump .... ▣ 700
4-Way Long Lasting Nasal Spray & Metered Spray Pump 751
NTZ Long Acting Nasal Spray & Drops 0.05% .... ▣ 760
Neo-Synephrine Maximum Strength 12 Hour Nasal Spray .... ▣ 759
Neo-Synephrine Maximum Strength 12 Hour Nasal Spray Pump .... ▣ 759
Nōstrilla Long Acting Nasal Decongestant .... ▣ 520
OcuClear Eye Drops .... ⊙ 306
Vicks Sinex Long Acting .... ▣ 665
Visine L.R. Eye Drops .... ▣ 647
Visine L.R. Eye Drope .... ⊙ 303

Penbutolol Sulfate (Exaggerated hypotensive effects). Products include:
Levatol 1832

Phendimetrazine Tartrate (Concurrent administration is not recommended). Products include:
Bontril Slow-Release 834
Plegine Tablets 2504
Prelu-2 Capsules 683

Phenmetrazine Hydrochloride (Concurrent administration is not recommended).
No products indexed under this heading.

Phenoxybenzamine Hydrochloride (Exaggerated hypotensive effects). Products include:
Dibenzyline Capsules 2207

Phentolamine Mesylate (Exaggerated hypotensive effects). Products include:
Regitine 878

d-Phenylalanine (Concurrent use should be avoided).

L-Phenylalanine (Concurrent use should be avoided).

Phenylephrine Bitartrate (Hypertensive crises).
No products indexed under this heading.

Phenylephrine Hydrochloride (Hypertensive crises; contraindicated). Products include:
AK-Dilate Solution 2.5% and 10% .... ⊙ 203
Atrohist Sprinkle Capsules 558
Cerose-DM 2443
Codimal 846
Comhist LA Capsules 1618
Congespirin For Children Aspirin Free Chewable Cold Tablets 748
Cyclomydril .... ⊙ 216
Deconsal Sprinkle Capsules 559
Dimetane Decongestant .... ▣ 673
Dristan Decongestant/Antihistamine/ Analgesic Coated Caplets .... ▣ 749
Dristan Cold Nasal Decongestant/ Antihistamine/ Analgesic Coated Tablets 2419
Dristan Advanced Formula Decongestant/Antihistamine/ Analgesic Tablets .... ▣ 749
Dristan Nasal Spray, Menthol 2419
Dristan Nasal Spray, Regular and Regular with Metered Pump 2419
Entex Capsules 1623
Entex Liquid 1623
Sinus Excedrin Analgesic, Decongestant Tablets & Caplets 750
Extendryl 994
4-Way Fast Acting Nasal Spray - Original Formula (regular & mentholated) & Metered Spray Pump (regular) 751
Hycomine Compound Tablets 929
Murocoll-2 Sterile Ophthalmic Solution .... ⊙ 261
Mydfrin 2.5% .... ⊙ 224
Naldecon Syrup, Tablets, Pediatric Drops and Pediatric Syrup 709
Neo-Synephrine Hydrochloride 1% Carpuject 2063
Neo-Synephrine Hydrochloride 1% Injection 2063
Neo-Synephrine Hydrochloride (Ophthalmic) 2064
Neo-Synephrine .... ▣ 759
Nōstril Nasal Decongestant .... ▣ 520
Novahistine Elixir .... ▣ 596
Phenergan VC 2500
Phenergan VC with Codeine 2501
Prefrin Liquifilm Vasoconstrictor and Lubricant Eye Drops .... ⊙ 254
Prefrin-A .... ⊙ 255
Quelidrine Syrup 556
Relief Vasoconstrictor and Lubricant Eye Drops .... ⊙ 256
Robitussin Night Relief .... ▣ 677
Ru-Tuss with Hydrocodone 694
Ru-Tuss Tablets 693
Vasosulf .... ⊙ 279
Vicks Sinex .... ▣ 665
Zincfrin .... ⊙ 230

Phenylephrine Tannate (Hypertensive crises). Products include:
- Rynatan 2387
- Rynatuss 2388

Phenylpropanolamine Containing Anorectics (Concurrent administration is not recommended).

Phenylpropanolamine Hydrochloride (Hypertensive crises; contraindicated). Products include:
- A.R.M. Allergy Relief Medicine Caplets .... ▣ 615
- Acutrim .... ▣ 548
- Allerest .... ▣ 559
- BC Cold Powder .... ▣ 517
- Cheracol Plus Head Cold/Cough Formula .... ▣ 667
- Codimal Expectorant 846
- Comtrex Multi-Symptom Cold Reliever Tablets/Caplets/Liqui-Gels/Liquid 745
- Contac Continuous Action Decongestant/Antihistamine Capsules ▣ 710
- Contac Maximum Strength Continuous Action Decongestant/Antihistamine Caplets .... ▣ 709
- Contac Severe Cold and Flu Formula Caplets .... ▣ 711
- Coricidin 'D' Decongestant Tablets .... ▣ 695
- Coricidin Demilets Tablets for Children .... ▣ 696
- Demazin Nasal Decongestant/Antihistamine Repetabs Tablets & Syrup .... ▣ 697
- Dexatrim .... ▣ 733
- Dimetane-DC Cough Syrup 1857
- Dimetapp Elixir .... ▣ 673
- Dimetapp DM Elixir .... ▣ 674
- Dimetapp Extentabs .... ▣ 674
- Dimetapp Plus Caplets .... ▣ 675
- Dimetapp Tablets .... ▣ 675
- Entex Capsules 1623
- Entex LA Tablets 1623
- Entex Liquid 1623
- 4-Way Cold Tablets 750
- Hycomine Syrup 927
- Naldecon CX Adult Liquid .... ▣ 521
- Naldecon DX Adult Liquid .... ▣ 521
- Naldecon DX Children's Syrup .... ▣ 522
- Naldecon DX Pediatric Drops .... ▣ 522
- Naldecon EX Children's Syrup .... ▣ 522
- Naldecon EX Pediatric Drops .... ▣ 523
- Naldecon Syrup, Tablets, Pediatric Drops and Pediatric Syrup 709
- Nolamine Tablets 838
- Nolex LA Tablets 838
- Ornade Spansule Capsules 2221
- Orthoxicol Cough Syrup .... ▣ 668
- Propagest 839
- Pyrroxate Capsules .... ▣ 669
- Robitussin-CF .... ▣ 676
- Ru-Tuss II Capsules 693
- Ru-Tuss with Hydrocodone 694
- Ru-Tuss Tablets 693
- Sine-Off Sinus Medicine Tablets-Aspirin Formula .... ▣ 722
- Sinulin 840
- St. Joseph Cold Tablets for Children .... ▣ 704
- Tavist-D Tablets 2035
- Triaminic Allergy Tablets .... ▣ 688
- Triaminic Chewables .... ▣ 688
- Triaminic Cold Tablets .... ▣ 688
- Triaminic Expectorant .... ▣ 688
- Triaminic Expectorant w/Codeine .. 1996
- Triaminic Expectorant DH 1995
- Triaminic Oral Infant Drops 1996
- Triaminic Syrup .... ▣ 689
- Triaminic-12 Tablets .... ▣ 690
- Triaminic-DM Syrup .... ▣ 689
- Triaminicin Tablets .... ▣ 690
- Triaminicol Multi-Symptom Cold Tablets .... ▣ 691
- Triaminicol Multi-Symptom Relief ▣ 691
- Tuss-Ornade Liquid 2242
- Tuss-Ornade Spansule Capsules 2242
- Tylenol Cold Medication, Effervescent Tablets 1369

Pindolol (Exaggerated hypotensive effects). Products include:
- Visken Tablets 2036

Pirbuterol Acetate (Hypertensive crises). Products include:
- Maxair Inhaler 1311

Polythiazide (Exaggerated hypotensive effects). Products include:
- Minizide Capsules 1779
- Renese Tablets 1785
- Renese-R Tablets 1786

Prazosin Hydrochloride (Exaggerated hypotensive effects). Products include:
- Minipress Capsules 1778
- Minizide Capsules 1779

Propoxyphene Hydrochloride (Meperidine contraindication is extended to other narcotics). Products include:
- Darvon 1256
- Wygesic Tablets 2540

Propoxyphene Napsylate (Meperidine contraindication is extended to other narcotics). Products include:
- Darvon-N/Darvocet-N 1254

Propranolol Hydrochloride (Exaggerated hypotensive effects). Products include:
- Inderal 2459
- Inderal LA Long Acting Capsules 2461
- Inderide Tablets 2463
- Inderide LA Long Acting Capsules .. 2465

Protriptyline Hydrochloride (Concurrent or in rapid succession administration is contraindicated). Products include:
- Vivactil Tablets 1567

Pseudoephedrine Hydrochloride (Hypertensive crises; contraindicated). Products include:
- Actifed Capsules .... ▣ 539
- Actifed Plus Caplets .... ▣ 539
- Actifed Plus Tablets .... ▣ 540
- Actifed with Codeine Cough Syrup.. 752
- Actifed Syrup .... ▣ 540
- Actifed Tablets .... ▣ 540
- Actifed 12-Hour Capsules .... ▣ 539
- Advil Cold & Sinus Caplets (formerly CoAdvil) 2416
- Allerest .... ▣ 559
- Anatuss LA Tablets 1359
- Benadryl Decongestant Elixir .... ▣ 635
- Benadryl Decongestant .... ▣ 635
- Benadryl Plus .... ▣ 636
- Benadryl Plus Nighttime .... ▣ 637
- Benylin Decongestant .... ▣ 638
- Brexin L.A. Capsules 2078
- Bromfed Capsules (Timed Release) 1615
- Bromfed Syrup .... ▣ 628
- Bromfed 1615
- CoAdvil .... ▣ 748
- Allergy-Sinus Comtrex Multi-Symptom Allergy Sinus Formula Tablets & Caplets 746
- Cough Formula Comtrex 746
- Comtrex Multi-Symptom Cold Reliever Tablets/Caplets/Liqui-Gels/Liquid 745
- Day-Night Comtrex 747
- Non-Drowsy Comtrex 747
- Congess 994
- Congestac Caplets .... ▣ 617
- Contac Jr. Children's Cold Medicine .... ▣ 712
- Contac Nighttime Cold Medicine.... ▣ 713
- Contac Sinus Caplets Maximum Strength Non-Drowsy Formula.... ▣ 710
- Contac Sinus Tablets Maximum Strength Non-Drowsy Formula.... ▣ 710
- Deconamine 663
- Deconsal II Tablets 559
- Dimacol Caplets .... ▣ 672
- Dimetane-DX Cough Syrup 1858
- Dorcol Children's Cough Syrup .... ▣ 685
- Dorcol Children's Decongestant Liquid .... ▣ 685
- Dorcol Children's Liquid Cold Formula .... ▣ 686
- Maximum Strength Dristan Decongestant/Analgesic Coated Caplets .... ▣ 750
- No Drowsiness Dristan Cold Nasal Decongestant/Analgesic Coated Caplets 2420
- Dristan Sinus Caplets 2419
- Sinus Excedrin Analgesic, Decongestant Tablets & Caplets .... ▣ 533
- Fedahist Gyrocaps 2145
- Fedahist Timecaps 2145
- Guaifed 1615
- Guaifed Syrup .... ▣ 629
- Isoclor Expectorant 982
- Isoclor Timesule Capsules .... ▣ 561
- Kronofed-A 970
- Medi-Flu Caplet, Liquid .... ▣ 640
- Novafed A Capsules 1342
- Novafed Capsules 1342
- Novahistine DH 1342
- Novahistine DMX .... ▣ 595
- Novahistine Expectorant 1343
- Nucofed Capsules 2219
- Nucofed Expectorant 2219
- Nucofed Pediatric Expectorant 2220
- Nucofed Syrup 2219
- Ornex Caplets .... ▣ 618
- PediaCare Allergy Relief Formula Liquid 1362
- PediaCare Cough-Cold Formula Liquid 1362
- PediaCare Infants' Oral Decongestant Drops 1362
- PediaCare Night Rest Cough-Cold Formula Liquid 1362
- PediaCare 6-12 Cough-Cold Formula Chewable Tablets 1362
- Robitussin-DAC Syrup 1875
- Robitussin-PE .... ▣ 677
- Rondec 1975
- Rondec-DM 1976
- Rondec-TR Tablet 1975
- Ru-Tuss DE Tablets 694
- Ryna .... ▣ 741
- Seldane-D Extended-Release Tablets 1350
- Sinarest .... ▣ 562
- Sine-Aid Maximum Strength Sinus Headache Caplets 1365
- Sine-Aid Maximum Strength Sinus Headache Tablets 1365
- Sine-Off Maximum Strength Allergy/Sinus Formula Caplets .... ▣ 721
- Sine-Off Maximum Strength No Drowsiness Formula Caplets .... ▣ 722
- Singlet Tablets .... ▣ 598
- Sinutab Maximum Strength .... ▣ 641
- Sinutab Maximum Strength Without Drowsiness Tablets & Caplets .... ▣ 642
- Sinutab Regular Strength Without Drowsiness Formula .... ▣ 641
- St. Joseph Nighttime Cold Medicine .... ▣ 705
- Sudafed Children's Liquid .... ▣ 543
- Sudafed Cough Syrup .... ▣ 543
- Sudafed Plus Liquid .... ▣ 544
- Sudafed Plus Tablets .... ▣ 545
- Sudafed Sinus Caplets .... ▣ 545
- Sudafed Sinus Tablets .... ▣ 545
- Sudafed Tablets, 30 mg .... ▣ 544
- Sudafed Tablets, Adult Strength, 60 mg .... ▣ 544
- Sudafed 12 Hour Capsules .... ▣ 545
- TheraFlu Flu and Cold Medicine .... ▣ 687
- Triaminic Nite Light .... ▣ 689
- Tylenol Allergy Sinus Medication Caplets and Gelcaps, Maximum Strength 1372
- Children's Tylenol Cold Liquid Formula and Chewable Tablets 1368
- Tylenol Cold & Flu Hot Medication, Packets 1369
- Tylenol Cold & Flu No Drowsiness Hot Medication, Packets 1371
- Tylenol Cold Medication Caplets and Tablets 1370
- Tylenol Cold Medication No Drowsiness Formula Caplets 1370
- Tylenol Cold Night Time Medication Liquid 1371
- Tylenol Cough Medication Liquid with Decongestant, Maximum Strength 1372
- Tylenol, Maximum Strength, Sinus Medication Gelcaps, Caplets and Tablets 1373
- Ursinus Inlay-Tabs .... ▣ 691
- Vicks Children's NyQuil .... ▣ 664
- Vicks Daycare .... ▣ 660
- Vicks Formula 44D Decongestant Cough Medicine .... ▣ 662
- Vicks Formula 44M Multi-Symptom Cough Medicine .... ▣ 662
- Vicks NyQuil Nighttime Colds Medicine-Original & Cherry Flavor .... ▣ 664
- Vicks Pediatric Formula 44 Cough & Congestion Medicine.... ▣ 663
- Vicks Pediatric Formula 44m Multi-Symptom Cough & Cold Medicine .... ▣ 663

Pseudoephedrine Sulfate (Hypertensive crises). Products include:
- Afrin Tablets .... ▣ 693
- Chlor-Trimeton Decongestant .... ▣ 694
- Disophrol Chronotab Sustained-Action Tablets .... ▣ 698
- Drixoral Antihistamine/Nasal Decongestant Syrup .... ▣ 698
- Drixoral Non-Drowsy Formula .... ▣ 699
- Drixoral Plus Extended-Release Tablets .... ▣ 699
- Drixoral Sinus .... ▣ 700
- Drixoral Sustained-Action Tablets ▣ 698
- Sinutab Allergy Formula Sustained Action Tablets .... ▣ 640
- Trinalin Repetabs Tablets 1170

Ramipril (Exaggerated hypotensive effects). Products include:
- Altace Capsules 1086

Rauwolfia Serpentina (Exaggerated hypotensive effects). Products include:
- Raudixin Tablets 1803
- Rauzide Tablets 1804

Rescinnamine (Exaggerated hypotensive effects).
- No products indexed under this heading.

Reserpine (Exaggerated hypotensive effects). Products include:
- Diupres Tablets 1461
- Hydromox R Tablets 1209
- Hydropres Tablets 1485
- Renese-R Tablets 1786
- Salutensin/Salutensin-Demi 719
- Ser-Ap-Es Tablets 881
- Serpasil Tablets 883
- Serpasil-Apresoline Tablets 884
- Serpasil-Esidrix Tablets 886

Selegiline Hydrochloride (Hypertensive crises; at least 10 days should elapse between discontinuation of Nardil and institution of another MAOI). Products include:
- Eldepryl 2250

Sodium Nitroprusside (Exaggerated hypotensive effects). Products include:
- Nipride I.V. Infusion 1909

Sufentanil Citrate (Meperidine contraindication is extended to other narcotics). Products include:
- Sufenta Injection 1147

Terazosin Hydrochloride (Exaggerated hypotensive effects). Products include:
- Hytrin Tablets 529

Terbutaline Sulfate (Hypertensive crises). Products include:
- Brethaire Inhaler 1024
- Brethine Ampuls 1026
- Brethine Tablets 1026
- Bricanyl Injection 1324
- Bricanyl Tablets 1325

Tetrahydrozoline Hydrochloride (Contraindicated). Products include:
- Collyrium Fresh 2445
- Murine Plus Lubricating Eye Redness Reliever .... ⊙ 305
- Visine A.C. Eye Drops .... ▣ 646
- Visine A.C. Eye Drops .... ⊙ 303
- Visine EXTRA Eye Drops .... ▣ 647
- Visine EXTRA Eye Drops .... ⊙ 303
- Visine Eye Drops .... ▣ 646
- Visine Eye Drops .... ⊙ 303

Timolol Maleate (Exaggerated hypotensive effects). Products include:
- Blocadren Tablets 1429
- Timolide Tablets 1547
- Timoptic in Ocudose 1552
- Timoptic Sterile Ophthalmic Solution 1550

Tranylcypromine Sulfate (At least 10 days should elapse between discontinuation of Nardil and institution of another MAOI). Products include:
- Parnate Tablets 2222

Trimethaphan Camsylate (Exaggerated hypotensive effects). Products include:
- Arfonad Ampuls 1887

(▣ Described in PDR For Nonprescription Drugs)

(⊙ Described in PDR For Ophthalmology)

Trimipramine Maleate (Concurrent or in rapid succession administration is contraindicated). Products include:
Surmontil Capsules 2524
L-Tryptophan (Concurrent use should be avoided). Products include:
Saave 1358
Tropamine 1358
Tyramine (Concurrent use should be avoided).
L-Tyrosine (Concurrent use should be avoided). Products include:
Tropamine 1358

Food Interactions

Beans, broad (Concurrent and/or sequential intake must be avoided).
Beans, Fava (Concurrent and/or sequential intake must be avoided).
Beer, alcohol-free (Concurrent and/or sequential intake must be avoided).
Beer, reduced-alcohol (Concurrent and/or sequential intake must be avoided).
Beer, unspecified (Concurrent and/or sequential intake must be avoided).
Beverages, caffeine-containing (Excessive caffeine intake should be avoided).
Bologna, Lebanon (Concurrent and/or sequential intake must be avoided).
Cheese, aged (Concurrent and/or sequential intake must be avoided).
Cheese, unspecified (Concurrent and/or sequential intake must be avoided).
Chocolate (Concurrent and/or sequential intake must be avoided).
Fish, smoked (Concurrent and/or sequential intake must be avoided).
Food with high concentration of dopamine (Concurrent and/or sequential intake must be avoided).
Food with high concentration of tyramine (Concurrent and/or sequential intake must be avoided).
Herring, pickled (Concurrent and/or sequential intake must be avoided).
Liver (Concurrent and/or sequential intake must be avoided).
Meat extracts (Concurrent and/or sequential intake must be avoided).
Meat, unspecified (Concurrent and/or sequential intake must be avoided).
Pepperoni (Concurrent and/or sequential intake must be avoided).
Salami, hard (Concurrent and/or sequential intake must be avoided).
Salami, Genoa (Concurrent and/or sequential intake must be avoided).
Sauerkraut (Concurrent and/or sequential intake must be avoided).
Sausage, dry (Concurrent and/or sequential intake must be avoided).
Wine products (Concurrent and/or sequential intake must be avoided).
Wine, unspecified (Concurrent and/or sequential intake must be avoided).
Yeast extract (Concurrent and/or sequential intake must be avoided).
Yeast, brewer's (Concurrent and/or sequential intake must be avoided).
Yogurt (Concurrent and/or sequential intake must be avoided).

NASACORT NASAL INHALER
(Triamcinolone Acetonide) 1844
No interactions described in labeling.

NāSAL MOISTURIZING NASAL SPRAY
(Sodium Chloride) .... ▣ 759
No interactions described in labeling.

NāSAL MOISTURIZING NOSE DROPS
(Sodium Chloride) .... ▣ 759
No interactions described in labeling.

NASALCROM NASAL SOLUTION
(Cromolyn Sodium) 986
No interactions described in labeling.

NASALIDE NASAL SOLUTION 0.025%
(Flunisolide) 2299
No interactions described in labeling.

NATABEC KAPSEALS
(Multivitamins with Minerals) .... ▣ 640
No interactions described in labeling.

NATACYN
(Natamycin) .... ◉ 227
No interactions described in labeling.

NATALINS RX
(Vitamin Preparation With Folic Acid or its Derivatives) 1391
No interactions described in labeling.

NATALINS TABLETS
(Vitamins with Minerals) 1391
No interactions described in labeling.

NATURE'S REMEDY NATURAL VEGETABLE LAXATIVE
(Cascara Sagrada) .... ▣ 719
No interactions described in labeling.

NATURETIN TABLETS
(Bendroflumethiazide) 1789
May interact with antihypertensives, ganglionic blocking agents, para-aminobenzoic acid based local anesthetics, corticosteroids, insulin, barbiturates, narcotic analgesics, oral hypoglycemic agents, lithium preparations, calcium preparations, monoamine oxidase inhibitors, cardiac glycosides, non-steroidal anti-inflammatory agents, oral anticoagulants, antigout agents, and certain other agents. Compounds in these categories include:

Acebutolol Hydrochloride (Antihypertensive effect potentiated). Products include:
Sectral Capsules 2520
ACTH (May intensify electrolyte imbalance, particularly hypokalemia).
No products indexed under this heading.
Alcohol (Potentiation of orthostatic hypotension).
Alfentanil Hydrochloride (Potentiation of orthostatic hypotension). Products include:
Alfenta Injection 1131
Allopurinol (Bendroflumethiazide raises blood uric acid levels). Products include:
Zyloprim Tablets 830
Amphotericin B (May intensify electrolyte imbalance, particularly hypokalemia). Products include:
Fungizone Cream, Lotion and Ointment 2261
Fungizone Intravenous 2262
Aprobarbital (Potentiation of orthostatic hypotension). Products include:
Alurate Elixir 1883
Atenolol (Antihypertensive effect potentiated). Products include:
Tenoretic Tablets 1105
Tenormin Tablets and I.V. Injection 1107
Benazepril Hydrochloride (Antihypertensive effect potentiated). Products include:
Lotensin Tablets 872
Betamethasone Acetate (May intensify electrolyte imbalance, particularly hypokalemia). Products include:
Celestone Soluspan Suspension 2081
Betamethasone Sodium Phosphate (May intensify electrolyte imbalance, particularly hypokalemia). Products include:
Celestone Soluspan Suspension 2081
Betaxolol Hydrochloride (Antihypertensive effect potentiated). Products include:
Betoptic Sterile Ophthalmic Solution 569
Betoptic S Sterile Ophthalmic Suspension 570
Kerlone Tablets 2172
Buprenorphine (Potentiation of orthostatic hypotension).
No products indexed under this heading.
Butabarbital (Potentiation of orthostatic hypotension). Products include:
Pyridium Plus 1764
Butalbital (Potentiation of orthostatic hypotension). Products include:
Esgic-Plus Tablets 1002
Esgic Tablets & Capsules 1001
Fioricet Tablets 2006
Fiorinal Capsules 2007
Fiorinal with Codeine Capsules 2008
Fiorinal Tablets 2007
Phrenilin 838
Sedapap Tablets 50 mg/650 mg .. 1360
Calcium Carbonate (Increased calcium levels due to decreased excretion). Products include:
Alka-Mints Chewable Antacid .... ▣ 620
Alka-Seltzer Advanced Formula Antacid & Non-Aspirin Pain Reliever .... ▣ 620
Ascriptin A/D Caplets 1850
Regular Strength Ascriptin Tablets 1850
Balmex Baby Powder .... ▣ 590
Bayer Plus Aspirin Tablets .... ▣ 567
Biocal 500 mg Tablet Calcium Supplement .... ▣ 625
Bufferin Analgesic Tablets and Caplets .... ▣ 524
Caltrate 600 .... ▣ 583
Caltrate 600 + Iron .... ▣ 583
Caltrate 600 + Vitamin D .... ▣ 584
Caltrate, Jr. .... ▣ 583
Centrum, Jr. (Children's Chewable) + Extra Calcium .... ▣ 585
Di-Gel Antacid/Anti-Gas .... ▣ 697
Gerimed Tablets 972
Marblen .... ▣ 563
Natalins Rx 1391
Natalins Tablets 1391
Nephro-Calci Tablets 1826
Os-Cal 500 Chewable Tablets .... ▣ 596
Os-Cal 500 Tablets .... ▣ 597
Os-Cal 250+D Tablets .... ▣ 597
Os-Cal 500+D Tablets .... ▣ 597
Pramet FA 1974
Pramilet FA 1974
Rolaids (Calcium Rich/Sodium Free) .... ▣ 744
Extra Strength Rolaids .... ▣ 744
Thermotabs .... ▣ 619
Total Formula-2 (multivitamin/multimineral) 2377
Tums Liquid Extra .... ▣ 726
Zenate Tablets 2250
Calcium Chloride (Increased calcium levels due to decreased excretion).
No products indexed under this heading.
Calcium Citrate (Increased calcium levels due to decreased excretion). Products include:
Citracal Liquitab 1613
Total Formula-2 (multivitamin/multimineral) 2377
Calcium Glubionate (Increased calcium levels due to decreased excretion). Products include:
Neo-Calglucon Syrup 2018
Captopril (Antihypertensive effect potentiated). Products include:
Capoten 2255
Capozide 2258
Carteolol Hydrochloride (Antihypertensive effect potentiated). Products include:
Cartrol Tablets 507
Chlorothiazide (Antihypertensive effect potentiated). Products include:
Aldoclor Tablets 1413
Diupres Tablets 1461
Diuril Oral 1464
Chlorothiazide Sodium (Antihypertensive effect potentiated). Products include:
Diuril Sodium Intravenous 1463
Chlorpropamide (Thiazide elevates blood glucose levels; dosage adjustment of antidiabetic agent may be required). Products include:
Diabinese Tablets 1775
Chlorthalidone (Antihypertensive effect potentiated). Products include:
Combipres Tablets 678
Tenoretic Tablets 1105
Thalitone Tablets 687
Cholestyramine (Decreases absorption of bendroflumethiazide). Products include:
Cholybar 1705
Questran Light 711
Questran Powder 710
Clonidine (Antihypertensive effect potentiated). Products include:
Catapres-TTS 677
Clonidine Hydrochloride (Antihypertensive effect potentiated). Products include:
Catapres Tablets 676
Combipres Tablets 678
Codeine (Potentiation of orthostatic hypotension). Products include:
Calcidrine Syrup 506
Codeine Phosphate (Potentiation of orthostatic hypotension). Products include:
Actifed with Codeine Cough Syrup.. 752
Cheracol Cough Syrup 1853
Codimal PH Syrup 846
Dimetane-DC Cough Syrup 1857
Empirin with Codeine Phosphate Nos. 2, 3 & 4 764
Fiorinal with Codeine Capsules 2008
Isoclor Expectorant 982
Naldecon CX Adult Liquid .... ▣ 521
Novahistine DH 1342
Novahistine Expectorant 1343
Nucofed Capsules 2219
Nucofed Expectorant 2219
Nucofed Pediatric Expectorant 2220
Nucofed Syrup 2219
Phenaphen with Codeine Capsules 1865
Phenaphen-650 with Codeine Tablets 1866
Phenergan with Codeine 2497
Phenergan VC with Codeine 2501
Robitussin A-C Syrup 1875
Robitussin-DAC Syrup 1875
Ryna .... ▣ 741
Soma Compound w/Codeine Tablets 2390
Triaminic Expectorant w/Codeine .. 1996
Tussi-Organidin Liquid 2391
Tylenol with Codeine 1381
Codeine Polistirex (Potentiation of orthostatic hypotension).
No products indexed under this heading.

Colestipol Hydrochloride (Decreases absorption of bendroflumethiazide). Products include:
Colestid Granules 2328

Cortisone Acetate (May intensify electrolyte imbalance, particularly hypokalemia). Products include:
Cortone Acetate Sterile Suspension 1437
Cortone Acetate Tablets 1439

Deserpidine (Antihypertensive effect potentiated). Products include:
Enduronyl 518
Harmonyl Tablets 528
Oreticyl 545

Deslanoside (Enhanced possibility of digitalis toxicity associated with hypokalemia).
No products indexed under this heading.

Dexamethasone (May intensify electrolyte imbalance, particularly hypokalemia). Products include:
AK-Trol Ointment & Suspension ⊙ 207
Decadron Elixir 1445
Decadron Tablets 1447
Decaspray Topical Aerosol 1459
Dexacidin ⊙ 272
Maxidex Sterile Ophthalmic Suspension ⊙ 223
Maxitrol Ophthalmic Ointment/Suspension ⊙ 223
TobraDex Ophthalmic Suspension and Ointment ⊙ 228

Dexamethasone Acetate (May intensify electrolyte imbalance, particularly hypokalemia). Products include:
Dalalone D.P. Injectable 999
Decadron-LA Sterile Suspension 1457

Dexamethasone Sodium Phosphate (May intensify electrolyte imbalance, particularly hypokalemia). Products include:
AK-Dex ⊙ 203
Decadron Phosphate Respihaler 1454
Decadron Phosphate Sterile Ophthalmic Ointment 1453
Decadron Phosphate Sterile Ophthalmic Solution 1453
Decadron Phosphate Topical Cream 1455
Decadron Phosphate Turbinaire 1456
Maxidex Sterile Ophthalmic Ointment ⊙ 222
NeoDecadron Sterile Ophthalmic Ointment 1517
NeoDecadron Sterile Ophthalmic Solution 1518
NeoDecadron Topical Cream 1518

Dezocine (Potentiation of orthostatic hypotension).

Diazoxide (Enhanced hyperglycemic, hyperuricemic, and antihypertensive effects). Products include:
Hyperstat I.V. Injection 2095
Proglycem 649

Diclofenac Sodium (Reduces diuretic, natriuretic, and antihypertensive effects). Products include:
Voltaren Ophthalmic Sterile Ophthalmic Solution ⊙ 268
Voltaren Tablets 1042

Dicumarol (Decreased anticoagulant effects). Products include:
Dicumarol Tablets 516

Digitoxin (Enhanced possibility of digitalis toxicity associated with hypokalemia). Products include:
Crystodigin Tablets 1253

Digoxin (Enhanced possibility of digitalis toxicity associated with hypokalemia). Products include:
Lanoxicaps 772
Lanoxin Elixir Pediatric 775
Lanoxin Injection 778
Lanoxin Injection Pediatric 781
Lanoxin Tablets 783

Doxazosin Mesylate (Antihypertensive effect potentiated). Products include:
Cardura Tablets 1941

Enalapril Maleate (Antihypertensive effect potentiated). Products include:
Vaseretic Tablets 1559
Vasotec Tablets 1564

Enalaprilat (Antihypertensive effect potentiated). Products include:
Vasotec I.V. 1562

Esmolol Hydrochloride (Antihypertensive effect potentiated). Products include:
Brevibloc Injection 942

Etodolac (Reduces diuretic, natriuretic, and antihypertensive effects). Products include:
Lodine Capsules 2468

Felodipine (Antihypertensive effect potentiated). Products include:
Plendil Extended-Release Tablets 1526

Fenoprofen Calcium (Reduces diuretic, natriuretic, and antihypertensive effects). Products include:
Nalfon Pulvules & Tablets 919

Fentanyl (Potentiation of orthostatic hypotension). Products include:
Duragesic Transdermal System 1133

Fentanyl Citrate (Potentiation of orthostatic hypotension). Products include:
Innovar Injection 1141
Sublimaze Injection 1146

Flurbiprofen (Reduces diuretic, natriuretic, and antihypertensive effects). Products include:
Ansaid Tablets 2319

Fosinopril Sodium (Antihypertensive effect potentiated). Products include:
Monopril Tablets 1406

Furazolidone (Hypotensive effects enhanced; dosage adjustment of one or both agents may be necessary). Products include:
Furoxone 1855

Furosemide (Antihypertensive effect potentiated). Products include:
Lasix 1093

Glipizide (Thiazide elevates blood glucose levels; dosage adjustment of antidiabetic agent may be required). Products include:
Glucotrol 1952

Glyburide (Thiazide elevates blood glucose levels; dosage adjustment of antidiabetic agent may be required). Products include:
DiaBeta 1091
Micronase Tablets 2350

Guanabenz Acetate (Antihypertensive effect potentiated). Products include:
Wytensin Tablets 2542

Guanethidine Monosulfate (Antihypertensive effect potentiated). Products include:
Esimil Tablets 864
Ismelin Tablets 869

Hydralazine Hydrochloride (Antihypertensive effect potentiated). Products include:
Apresazide Capsules 854
Apresoline Hydrochloride Parenteral (Ampuls) 856
Apresoline Hydrochloride Tablets 855
Apresoline-Esidrix Tablets 857
Ser-Ap-Es Tablets 881
Serpasil-Apresoline Tablets 884

Hydrochlorothiazide (Antihypertensive effect potentiated). Products include:
Aldactazide 2150
Aldoril Tablets 1418
Apresazide Capsules 854
Apresoline-Esidrix Tablets 857
Capozide 2258
Dyazide Capsules 2208
Esidrix Tablets 863
Esimil Tablets 864
HydroDIURIL Tablets 1484
Hydropres Tablets 1485
Inderide Tablets 2463
Inderide LA Long Acting Capsules 2465
Lopressor HCT Tablets 1034
Maxzide 1215
Moduretic Tablets 1510
Normozide Tablets 2112
Oretic Tablets 544
Oreticyl 545
Prinzide Tablets 1540
Ser-Ap-Es Tablets 881
Serpasil-Esidrix Tablets 886
Timolide Tablets 1547
Trandate HCT Tablets 579
Vaseretic Tablets 1559
Zestoretic 2274

Hydrocodone Bitartrate (Potentiation of orthostatic hypotension). Products include:
Anexsia 5/500 Tablets 2196
Anexsia 7.5/650 Tablets 2197
Azdone Tablets 844
Codiclear DH Syrup 845
Codimal DH Syrup 846
Damason-P 1356
Hycodan Syrup, Tablets 927
Hycomine Compound Tablets 929
Hycomine Syrup 927
Hycotuss Expectorant Syrup 930
Hydrocet Capsules 835
Lortab ASA Tablets 2414
Lortab 2412
Ru-Tuss with Hydrocodone 694
Triaminic Expectorant DH 1995
Vicodin Tablets 1187
Vicodin ES Tablets 1189
Zydone Capsules 941

Hydrocodone Polistirex (Potentiation of orthostatic hypotension). Products include:
Tussionex Extended-Release Suspension 988

Hydrocortisone (May intensify electrolyte imbalance, particularly hypokalemia). Products include:
AK-Spore H.C. ⊙ 206
Bactine Hydrocortisone Anti-Itch Cream ▣ 625
CaldeCORT Anti-Itch Hydrocortisone Spray ▣ 560
Carmol HC Cream 1% 2296
Cortaid Spray ▣ 735
Cortenema 2244
Cortisporin Ointment 758
Cortisporin Ophthalmic Ointment Sterile 758
Cortisporin Ophthalmic Suspension Sterile 759
Cortisporin Otic Solution Sterile 760
Cortisporin Otic Suspension Sterile 760
Cortizone-5 Creme & Ointment ▣ 732
Dermolate Anti-Itch Cream ▣ 697
Eldecort Cream 1.0% 1113
Eldecort Cream 1.0% and 2.5% 1113
Fungoid HC Creme 1770
Hydrocortone Tablets 1482
Hytone 909
LazerSporin-C Solution 1770
Massengill Medicated Soft Cloth Towelettes 2192
Nutracort Cream & Lotion 1684
PediOtic Suspension Sterile 797
Synacort Creams 1%, 2.5% 2296
Vanoxide-HC Acne Lotion 911
Vioform-Hydrocortisone Cream and Mild Cream 889
Vioform-Hydrocortisone Ointment 889
VōSoL HC Otic Solution 2392
Vytone Cream 1% 911

Hydrocortisone Acetate (May intensify electrolyte imbalance, particularly hypokalemia). Products include:
Analpram-HC Rectal Cream 1% and 2.5% 970
Anusol-HC Cream 1690
Anusol-HC Suppositories 1691
Caldecort ▣ 560
Carmol HC Cream 1% 2296
Chloromycetin Hydrocortisone Ophthalmic 1694
Coly-Mycin S Otic w/Neomycin & Hydrocortisone 1708
Cortaid ▣ 735
Cortef Feminine Itch Cream ▣ 735
Corticaine ▣ 682
Cortifoam 1827
Cortisporin Cream 757
Epifoam 1828
Gynecort 5 Creme ▣ 556
Hydrocortone Acetate Sterile Suspension 1479
Lanacort 5 Creme and Ointment ▣ 557
Mantadil Cream 789
Ophthocort ⊙ 301
Orabase HCA Oral Paste 890
Pramosone Cream, Lotion & Ointment 971
ProctoCream-HC 1834
Proctofoam-HC 1835

Hydrocortisone Sodium Phosphate (May intensify electrolyte imbalance, particularly hypokalemia). Products include:
Hydrocortone Phosphate Injection, Sterile 1481

Hydrocortisone Sodium Succinate (May intensify electrolyte imbalance, particularly hypokalemia). Products include:
Solu-Cortef Sterile Powder 2361

Hydroflumethiazide (Antihypertensive effect potentiated). Products include:
Diucardin Tablets 2450
Saluron 718
Salutensin/Salutensin-Demi 719

Ibuprofen (Reduces diuretic, natriuretic, and antihypertensive effects). Products include:
Advil Cold & Sinus Caplets (formerly CoAdvil) 2416
Advil Ibuprofen Tablets and Caplets 2416
Children's Advil Suspension 2426
CoAdvil ▣ 748
Dristan Sinus Caplets 2419
Haltran Tablets ▣ 668
Ibuprofen ▣ 631
Medipren ibuprofen Caplets and Tablets 1362
Midol 200 Cramp Relief Formula ▣ 570
Motrin Tablets 2351
Motrin IB Caplets and Tablets ▣ 736
Nuprin Ibuprofen/Analgesic Tablets & Caplets 752
PediaProfen Suspension 1363
Rufen Tablets 691
Trendar Ibuprofen Tablets ▣ 756

Indapamide (Antihypertensive effect potentiated). Products include:
Lozol Tablets 1843

Indomethacin (Reduces diuretic, natriuretic, and antihypertensive effects). Products include:
Indocin 1487

Indomethacin Sodium Trihydrate (Reduces diuretic, natriuretic, and antihypertensive effects). Products include:
Indocin I.V. 1490

Insulin, Human (Thiazide elevates blood glucose levels; dosage adjustment of antidiabetic agent may be required).
No products indexed under this heading.

Insulin, Human Isophane Suspension (Thiazide elevates blood glucose levels; dosage adjustment of antidiabetic agent may be required). Products include:
Humulin N, 100 Units 1270

Insulin, Human NPH (Thiazide elevates blood glucose levels; dosage adjustment of antidiabetic agent may be required). Products include:
Insulatard NPH Human 1627
Novolin N 1627
Novolin N PenFill Cartridges 1628
Novolin N Prefilled 1628

(▣ Described in PDR For Nonprescription Drugs) (⊙ Described in PDR For Ophthalmology)

Insulin, Human Regular (Thiazide elevates blood glucose levels; dosage adjustment of antidiabetic agent may be required). Products include:
Humulin BR, 100 Units ... 1268
Humulin R, 100 Units ... 1272
Novolin R ... 1627
Novolin R PenFill Cartridges ... 1628
Novolin R Prefilled ... 1629
Velosulin Human ... 1628

Insulin, Human, Zinc Suspension (Thiazide elevates blood glucose levels; dosage adjustment of antidiabetic agent may be required). Products include:
Humulin L, 100 Units ... 1268
Humulin U, 100 Units ... 1272
Novolin L ... 1627

Insulin, NPH (Thiazide elevates blood glucose levels; dosage adjustment of antidiabetic agent may be required). Products include:
NPH, 40 & 100 Units ... 1273
Beef NPH, 100 Units ... 1274
Pork NPH, 100 Units ... 1275
Insulatard NPH ... 1626
NPH Insulin ... 1626
NPH Purified Pork Isophane Insulin ... 1626

Insulin, Regular (Thiazide elevates blood glucose levels; dosage adjustment of antidiabetic agent may be required). Products include:
Regular, 40 & 100 Units ... 1273
Beef Regular, 100 Units ... 1275
Pork Regular, 100 Units ... 1275
Pork Regular (Concentrated), 500 Units ... 1276
Regular Insulin ... 1625
Regular Purified Pork Insulin ... 1626
Velosulin ... 1627

Insulin, Zinc Crystals (Thiazide elevates blood glucose levels; dosage adjustment of antidiabetic agent may be required). Products include:
NPH, 40 & 100 Units ... 1273

Insulin, Zinc Suspension (Thiazide elevates blood glucose levels; dosage adjustment of antidiabetic agent may be required). Products include:
Lente, 40 & 100 Units ... 1272
Protamine, Zinc, 40 & 100 Units ... 1273
Lente Iletin I ... 1272
Beef Lente, 100 Units ... 1274
Beef Protamine Zinc, 100 Units ... 1274
Pork Lente, 100 Units ... 1275
Pork, Protamine, Zinc, 100 Units ... 1275
Lente Insulin ... 1626
Lente Purified Pork Insulin ... 1626
Semilente Insulin ... 1625
Ultralente Insulin ... 1626

Isocarboxazid (Hypotensive effects enhanced; dosage adjustment of one or both agents may be necessary). Products include:
Marplan Tablets ... 1906

Isradipine (Antihypertensive effect potentiated). Products include:
DynaCirc Capsules ... 2004

Ketoprofen (Reduces diuretic, natriuretic, and antihypertensive effects). Products include:
Orudis Capsules ... 2488

Ketorolac Tromethamine (Reduces diuretic, natriuretic, and antihypertensive effects). Products include:
Toradol IM Injection ... 2302

Labetalol Hydrochloride (Antihypertensive effect potentiated). Products include:
Normodyne Injection ... 2108
Normodyne Tablets ... 2110
Normozide Tablets ... 2112
Trandate HCT Tablets ... 579
Trandate Injection ... 577
Trandate Tablets ... 579

Levorphanol Tartrate (Potentiation of orthostatic hypotension). Products include:
Levo-Dromoran ... 1906

Lisinopril (Antihypertensive effect potentiated). Products include:
Prinivil Tablets ... 1538
Prinzide Tablets ... 1540
Zestoretic ... 2274
Zestril Tablets ... 2277

Lithium Carbonate (Enhanced lithium toxicity due to reduced renal clearance; avoid concurrent use). Products include:
Eskalith ... 2214
Lithane Tablets ... 1596
Lithium Carbonate Capsules & Tablets ... 1984
Lithobid Tablets ... 870

Lithium Citrate (Enhanced lithium toxicity due to reduced renal clearance; avoid concurrent use). Products include:
Cibalith-S ... 870

Mecamylamine Hydrochloride (Antihypertensive effect potentiated). Products include:
Inversine Tablets ... 1492

Meclofenamate Sodium (Reduces diuretic, natriuretic, and antihypertensive effects). Products include:
Meclomen Capsules ... 1739

Mefenamic Acid (Reduces diuretic, natriuretic, and antihypertensive effects). Products include:
Ponstel ... 1758

Meperidine Hydrochloride (Potentiation of orthostatic hypotension). Products include:
Demerol ... 2047
Mepergan Injection ... 2479

Mephobarbital (Potentiation of orthostatic hypotension). Products include:
Mebaral Tablets ... 2061

Methadone Hydrochloride (Potentiation of orthostatic hypotension). Products include:
Dolophine Hydrochloride Ampoules & Vials ... 1260
Dolophine Hydrochloride Tablets ... 1261
Methadone Hydrochloride Diskets ... 1284
Methadone Hydrochloride Oral Solution & Tablets ... 1987

Methenamine (Possible decreased effectiveness due to alkalinization of urine). Products include:
Urised Tablets ... 2396

Methenamine Hippurate (Possible decreased effectiveness due to alkalinization of urine). Products include:
Hiprex Tablets ... 1333
Urex Tablets ... 1321

Methenamine Mandelate (Possible decreased effectiveness due to alkalinization of urine). Products include:
Mandelamine ... 1738
Uroqid-Acid ... 661

Methyclothiazide (Antihypertensive effect potentiated). Products include:
Enduron Tablets ... 517
Enduronyl ... 518

Methyldopa (Antihypertensive effect potentiated). Products include:
Aldoclor Tablets ... 1413
Aldomet Oral ... 1415
Aldoril Tablets ... 1418

Methyldopate Hydrochloride (Antihypertensive effect potentiated). Products include:
Aldomet Ester HCl Injection ... 1417

Methylprednisolone Acetate (May intensify electrolyte imbalance, particularly hypokalemia). Products include:
Depo-Medrol Sterile Aqueous Suspension ... 2334

Methylprednisolone Sodium Succinate (May intensify electrolyte imbalance, particularly hypokalemia). Products include:
Solu-Medrol Sterile Powder ... 2363

Metolazone (Antihypertensive effect potentiated). Products include:
Diulo ... 2129
Mykrox ½ mg Tablets ... 984
Zaroxolyn Tablets ... 989

Metoprolol Tartrate (Antihypertensive effect potentiated). Products include:
Lopressor Ampuls ... 1032
Lopressor HCT Tablets ... 1034
Lopressor Tablets ... 1032

Metyrosine (Antihypertensive effect potentiated). Products include:
Demser Capsules ... 1460

Minoxidil (Antihypertensive effect potentiated). Products include:
Loniten Tablets ... 2346
Rogaine Topical Solution ... 2357

Morphine Sulfate (Potentiation of orthostatic hypotension). Products include:
Astramorph/PF Injection, USP (Preservative-Free) ... 618
Duramorph ... 960
Infumorph 200 and Infumorph 500 Sterile Solutions ... 962
MS Contin Tablets ... 1814
MSIR ... 1817
Oramorph SR (Morphine Sulfate Sustained Release Tablets) ... 1988
Roxanol ... 1991

Nadolol (Antihypertensive effect potentiated). Products include:
Corgard Tablets ... 701
Corzide Tablets ... 702

Naproxen (Reduces diuretic, natriuretic, and antihypertensive effects). Products include:
Naprosyn ... 2297

Naproxen Sodium (Reduces diuretic, natriuretic, and antihypertensive effects). Products include:
Anaprox and Anaprox DS Tablets ... 2288

Nicardipine Hydrochloride (Antihypertensive effect potentiated). Products include:
Cardene Capsules ... 2290

Nitroglycerin (Antihypertensive effect potentiated). Products include:
Deponit NTG Transdermal Delivery System ... 2143
Minitran Transdermal Delivery System ... 1312
Nitro-Bid Ointment ... 1339
Nitro-Bid Capsules ... 1338
Nitrodisc ... 2176
Nitro-Dur (nitroglycerin) Transdermal Infusion System ... 1164
Nitrogard Tablets ... 1004
Nitrolingual Spray ... 1846
Nitrostat Tablets ... 1743
Transderm-Nitro Transdermal Therapeutic System ... 2283

Norepinephrine Bitartrate (Decreased arterial responsiveness). Products include:
Levophed Bitartrate Injection ... 2054

Opium Alkaloids (Potentiation of orthostatic hypotension). Products include:
B & O No. 15A & No. 16A Supprettes ... 2395
Pantopon Injectable ... 1911

Oxycodone Hydrochloride (Potentiation of orthostatic hypotension). Products include:
Percocet Tablets ... 950
Percodan ... 951
Roxicodone Tablets, Oral Solution & Intensol (Oxycodone) ... 1992
Tylox Capsules ... 1382

Penbutolol Sulfate (Antihypertensive effect potentiated). Products include:
Levatol ... 1832

Pentobarbital Sodium (Potentiation of orthostatic hypotension). Products include:
Nembutal Sodium Capsules ... 534
Nembutal Sodium Solution ... 536
Nembutal Sodium Suppositories ... 538

Phenelzine Sulfate (Hypotensive effects enhanced; dosage adjustment of one or both agents may be necessary). Products include:
Nardil ... 1742

Phenobarbital (Potentiation of orthostatic hypotension). Products include:
Arco-Lase Plus Tablets ... 607
Bellergal-S Tablets ... 1998
Bronkolixir ... ▣ 761
Bronkotabs Tablets ... ▣ 762
Donnatal ... 1858
Donnatal Extentabs ... 1859
Donnatal Tablets ... 1858
Donnazyme Tablets ... 1860
Kinesed Tablets ... 2272
Phenobarbital Elixir and Tablets ... 1293
Primatene Tablets-P Formula ... 2421
Quadrinal Tablets ... 1183
Tedral SA ... 1765

Phenoxybenzamine Hydrochloride (Antihypertensive effect potentiated). Products include:
Dibenzyline Capsules ... 2207

Phentolamine Mesylate (Antihypertensive effect potentiated). Products include:
Regitine ... 878

Phenylbutazone (Reduces diuretic, natriuretic, and antihypertensive effects). Products include:
Butazolidin Capsules & Tablets ... 1027

Pindolol (Antihypertensive effect potentiated). Products include:
Visken Tablets ... 2036

Piroxicam (Reduces diuretic, natriuretic, and antihypertensive effects). Products include:
Feldene Capsules ... 1777

Polythiazide (Antihypertensive effect potentiated). Products include:
Minizide Capsules ... 1779
Renese Tablets ... 1785
Renese-R Tablets ... 1786

Prazosin Hydrochloride (Antihypertensive effect potentiated). Products include:
Minipress Capsules ... 1778
Minizide Capsules ... 1779

Prednisolone Acetate (May intensify electrolyte imbalance, particularly hypokalemia). Products include:
AK-Cide Sterile Ophthalmic Ointment & Suspension ... ⊙ 202
Blephamide Liquifilm Sterile Ophthalmic Suspension ... 586
Blephamide S.O.P. Sterile Ophthalmic Ointment ... 586
Cetapred Ointment ... ⊙ 220
⅛% Econopred & 1% Econopred Plus ... ⊙ 217
Isopto Cetapred Suspension ... ⊙ 220
Metimyd ... ⊙ 306
Poly-Pred Liquifilm ... ⊙ 250
Pred Forte ... ⊙ 252
Pred Mild ... ⊙ 254
Pred-G Liquifilm Sterile Ophthalmic Suspension ... ⊙ 252
Pred-G S.O.P. Sterile Ophthalmic Ointment ... ⊙ 253
Vasocidin Ointment ... ⊙ 275

Prednisolone Sodium Phosphate (May intensify electrolyte imbalance, particularly hypokalemia). Products include:
AK-Pred ⊙ 205
Hydeltrasol Injection, Sterile 1476
Inflamase ⊙ 274
Pediapred Oral Liquid 987
Vasocidin Ophthalmic Solution ⊙ 276

Prednisolone Tebutate (May intensify electrolyte imbalance, particularly hypokalemia). Products include:
Hydeltra-T.B.A. Sterile Suspension 1478

Prednisone (May intensify electrolyte imbalance, particularly hypokalemia). Products include:
Deltasone Tablets 2332

Probenecid (Bendroflumethiazide raises blood uric acid levels). Products include:
Benemid Tablets 1426
ColBENEMID Tablets 1436
Wycillin Injection and Probenecid Tablets 2539

Propoxyphene Hydrochloride (Potentiation of orthostatic hypotension). Products include:
Darvon 1256
Wygesic Tablets 2540

Propoxyphene Napsylate (Potentiation of orthostatic hypotension). Products include:
Darvon-N/Darvocet-N 1254

Propranolol Hydrochloride (Antihypertensive effect potentiated). Products include:
Inderal 2459
Inderal LA Long Acting Capsules 2461
Inderide Tablets 2463
Inderide LA Long Acting Capsules 2465

Ramipril (Antihypertensive effect potentiated). Products include:
Altace Capsules 1086

Rauwolfia Serpentina (Antihypertensive effect potentiated). Products include:
Raudixin Tablets 1803
Rauzide Tablets 1804

Rescinnamine (Antihypertensive effect potentiated).
No products indexed under this heading.

Reserpine (Antihypertensive effect potentiated). Products include:
Diupres Tablets 1461
Hydromox R Tablets 1209
Hydropres Tablets 1485
Renese-R Tablets 1786
Salutensin/Salutensin-Demi 719
Ser-Ap-Es Tablets 881
Serpasil Tablets 883
Serpasil-Apresoline Tablets 884
Serpasil-Esidrix Tablets 886

Secobarbital Sodium (Potentiation of orthostatic hypotension). Products include:
Seconal Sodium Pulvules 1296

Selegiline Hydrochloride (Hypotensive effects enhanced; dosage adjustment of one or both agents may be necessary). Products include:
Eldepryl 2250

Sodium Nitroprusside (Antihypertensive effect potentiated). Products include:
Nipride I.V. Infusion 1909

Sufentanil Citrate (Potentiation of orthostatic hypotension). Products include:
Sufenta Injection 1147

Sulfinpyrazone (Bendroflumethiazide raises blood uric acid levels). Products include:
Anturane 853

Sulindac (Reduces diuretic, natriuretic, and antihypertensive effects). Products include:
Clinoril Tablets 1433

Terazosin Hydrochloride (Antihypertensive effect potentiated). Products include:
Hytrin Tablets 529

Thiamylal Sodium (Potentiation of orthostatic hypotension). Products include:
Surital Ampoules, Steri-Vials 1764

Timolol Maleate (Antihypertensive effect potentiated). Products include:
Blocadren Tablets 1429
Timolide Tablets 1547
Timoptic in Ocudose 1552
Timoptic Sterile Ophthalmic Solution 1550

Tolazamide (Thiazide elevates blood glucose levels; dosage adjustment of antidiabetic agent may be required). Products include:
Tolinase Tablets 2365

Tolbutamide (Thiazide elevates blood glucose levels; dosage adjustment of antidiabetic agent may be required). Products include:
Orinase Tablets 2354

Tolmetin Sodium (Reduces diuretic, natriuretic, and antihypertensive effects). Products include:
Tolectin (200, 400 and 600 mg) 1379

Tranylcypromine Sulfate (Hypotensive effects enhanced; dosage adjustment of one or both agents may be necessary). Products include:
Parnate Tablets 2222

Triamcinolone (May intensify electrolyte imbalance, particularly hypokalemia).
No products indexed under this heading.

Triamcinolone Acetonide (May intensify electrolyte imbalance, particularly hypokalemia). Products include:
Aristocort A 1010
Azmacort Inhaler 1837
Kenalog Cream, Lotion & Ointment 2401
Kenalog-10 Injection 2402
Kenalog-40 Injection 2403
Kenalog in Orabase 604
Kenalog Spray 2401
Mycolog II Cream and Ointment 2407
Mytrex Cream & Ointment 2080
Nasacort Nasal Inhaler 1844

Triamcinolone Diacetate (May intensify electrolyte imbalance, particularly hypokalemia). Products include:
Aristocort Suspension 1008

Triamcinolone Hexacetonide (May intensify electrolyte imbalance, particularly hypokalemia). Products include:
Aristospan Suspension 1011

Trimethaphan Camsylate (Antihypertensive effect potentiated). Products include:
Arfonad Ampuls 1887

Warfarin Sodium (Decreased anticoagulant effects). Products include:
Coumadin Injection & Tablets 944
Panwarfin Tablets 547

NAVANE CAPSULES AND CONCENTRATE
(Thiothixene) 1954
May interact with phenothiazines, barbiturates, central nervous system depressants, belladona products, and certain other agents. Compounds in these categories include:

Alfentanil Hydrochloride (Dosage adjustments required). Products include:
Alfenta Injection 1131

Alprazolam (Dosage adjustments required). Products include:
Xanax Tablets 2367

Aprobarbital (Potentiated). Products include:
Alurate Elixir 1883

Atropine Sulfate (Weak anticholinergic effect of Navane necessitates cautious use of atropine related drugs). Products include:
Arco-Lase Plus Tablets 607
Atropine Sulfate Sterile Ophthalmic Solution and S.O.P. Sterile Ophthalmic Ointment ⊙ 239
Donnagel ▣ 675
Donnagel-PG 1858
Donnatal 1858
Donnatal Extentabs 1859
Donnatal Tablets 1858
Donnazyme Tablets 1860
Isopto Atropine ⊙ 218
Lomotil 2174
Motofen Tablets 836
Ru-Tuss Tablets 693
Urised Tablets 2396

Belladonna Alkaloids (Weak anticholinergic effect of Navane necessitates cautious use of atropine related drugs). Products include:
Bellergal-S Tablets 1998
Hyland's Bed Wetting Tablets ▣ 728
Hyland's Teething Tablets ▣ 728
Kinesed Tablets 2272

Buprenorphine (Dosage adjustments required).
No products indexed under this heading.

Buspirone Hydrochloride (Dosage adjustments required). Products include:
BuSpar 1401

Butabarbital (Potentiated). Products include:
Pyridium Plus 1764

Butalbital (Potentiated). Products include:
Esgic-Plus Tablets 1002
Esgic Tablets & Capsules 1001
Fioricet Tablets 2006
Fiorinal Capsules 2007
Fiorinal with Codeine Capsules 2008
Fiorinal Tablets 2007
Phrenilin 838
Sedapap Tablets 50 mg/650 mg 1360

Chlordiazepoxide (Dosage adjustments required). Products include:
Libritabs Tablets 1930
Limbitrol 1933
Menrium Tablets 1934

Chlordiazepoxide Hydrochloride (Dosage adjustments required). Products include:
Librax Capsules 1929
Librium Capsules 1931
Librium Injectable 1932

Chlorpromazine (Likelihood of tardive dyskinesia). Products include:
Thorazine 2234

Chlorprothixene (Dosage adjustments required). Products include:
Taractan Tablets 1920

Chlorprothixene Hydrochloride (Dosage adjustments required). Products include:
Taractan 1920

Clorazepate Dipotassium (Dosage adjustments required). Products include:
Tranxene 556

Codeine (Dosage adjustments required). Products include:
Calcidrine Syrup 506

Codeine Phosphate (Dosage adjustments required). Products include:
Actifed with Codeine Cough Syrup 752
Cheracol Cough Syrup 1853
Codimal PH Syrup 846
Dimetane-DC Cough Syrup 1857
Empirin with Codeine Phosphate Nos. 2, 3 & 4 764
Fiorinal with Codeine Capsules 2008
Isoclor Expectorant 982
Naldecon CX Adult Liquid ▣ 521
Novahistine DH 1342
Novahistine Expectorant 1343
Nucofed Capsules 2219
Nucofed Expectorant 2219
Nucofed Pediatric Expectorant 2220
Nucofed Syrup 2219
Phenaphen with Codeine Capsules 1865
Phenaphen-650 with Codeine Tablets 1866
Phenergan with Codeine 2497
Phenergan VC with Codeine 2501
Robitussin A-C Syrup 1875
Robitussin-DAC Syrup 1875
Ryna ▣ 741
Soma Compound w/Codeine Tablets 2390
Triaminic Expectorant w/Codeine 1996
Tussi-Organidin Liquid 2391
Tylenol with Codeine 1381

Codeine Polistirex (Dosage adjustments required).
No products indexed under this heading.

Dezocine (Dosage adjustments required).

Diazepam (Dosage adjustments required). Products include:
Valium Injectable 1937
Valium Tablets 1939
Valrelease Capsules 1923

Droperidol (Dosage adjustments required). Products include:
Inapsine Injection 1140
Innovar Injection 1141

Enflurane (Dosage adjustments required). Products include:
Ethrane 599

Epinephrine Hydrochloride (Paradoxical hypotension may occur). Products include:
Adrenalin Chloride Solution 1:100 & 1:1,000 1689
Epifrin ⊙ 244
Glaucon ⊙ 218

Estazolam (Dosage adjustments required). Products include:
ProSom Tablets 554

Ethchlorvynol (Dosage adjustments required). Products include:
Placidyl Capsules 553

Ethinamate (Dosage adjustments required).
No products indexed under this heading.

Fentanyl (Dosage adjustments required). Products include:
Duragesic Transdermal System 1133

Fentanyl Citrate (Dosage adjustments required). Products include:
Innovar Injection 1141
Sublimaze Injection 1146

Fluphenazine Decanoate (Likelihood of tardive dyskinesia). Products include:
Prolixin Decanoate 1795

Fluphenazine Enanthate (Likelihood of tardive dyskinesia). Products include:
Prolixin Enanthate 1796

Fluphenazine Hydrochloride (Likelihood of tardive dyskinesia). Products include:
Prolixin Elixir 1793
Prolixin Injection 1791
Prolixin Oral Concentrate 1792
Prolixin Tablets 1793

Flurazepam Hydrochloride (Dosage adjustments required). Products include:
Dalmane Capsules 1927

Glutethimide (Dosage adjustments required).
No products indexed under this heading.

Haloperidol (Dosage adjustments required). Products include:
Haldol Injection, Tablets and Concentrate 1373

Haloperidol Decanoate (Dosage adjustments required). Products include:
Haldol Decanoate 1375

Hydrocodone Bitartrate (Dosage adjustments required). Products include:
Anexsia 5/500 Tablets 2196
Anexsia 7.5/650 Tablets 2197
Azdōne Tablets 844
Codiclear DH Syrup 845
Codimal DH Syrup 846
Damason-P 1356
Hycodan Syrup, Tablets 927
Hycomine Compound Tablets 929
Hycomine Syrup 927
Hycotuss Expectorant Syrup 930
Hydrocet Capsules 835
Lortab ASA Tablets 2414
Lortab 2412
Ru-Tuss with Hydrocodone 694
Triaminic Expectorant DH 1995
Vicodin Tablets 1187
Vicodin ES Tablets 1189
Zydone Capsules 941

Hydrocodone Polistirex (Dosage adjustments required). Products include:
Tussionex Extended-Release Suspension 988

Hydroxyzine Hydrochloride (Dosage adjustments required). Products include:
Atarax Tablets & Syrup 1941
Marax Tablets & DF Syrup 1954
Vistaril Intramuscular Solution 1970

Hyoscyamine (Weak anticholinergic effect of Navane necessitates cautious use of atropine related drugs). Products include:
Cystospaz Tablets 2395
Urised Tablets 2396

Hyoscyamine Sulfate (Weak anticholinergic effect of Navane necessitates cautious use of atropine related drugs). Products include:
Arco-Lase Plus Tablets 607
Cystospaz-M Capsules 2395
Donnagel ..... ■ 675
Donnagel-PG 1858
Donnatal 1858
Donnatal Extentabs 1859
Donnatal Tablets 1858
Donnazyme Tablets 1860
Kutrase Capsules 2146
Levsin/Levsinex 2147
Ru-Tuss Tablets 693

Isoflurane (Dosage adjustments required). Products include:
Forane 600

Ketamine Hydrochloride (Dosage adjustments required). Products include:
Ketalar 1726

Levorphanol Tartrate (Dosage adjustments required). Products include:
Levo-Dromoran 1906

Lorazepam (Dosage adjustments required). Products include:
Ativan Injection 2432
Ativan Tablets 2434

Loxapine Hydrochloride (Dosage adjustments required). Products include:
Loxitane 1213

Loxapine Succinate (Dosage adjustments required). Products include:
Loxitane Capsules 1213

Meperidine Hydrochloride (Dosage adjustments required). Products include:
Demerol 2047
Mepergan Injection 2479

Mephobarbital (Potentiating action of barbiturates). Products include:
Mebaral Tablets 2061

Meprobamate (Dosage adjustments required). Products include:
Deprol Tablets 2382
Equagesic Tablets 2451
Miltown Tablets 2386
PMB 200 and PMB 400 2504

Mesoridazine (Likelihood of tardive dyskinesia). Products include:
Serentil 686

Methadone Hydrochloride (Dosage adjustments required). Products include:
Dolophine Hydrochloride Ampoules & Vials 1260
Dolophine Hydrochloride Tablets 1261
Methadone Hydrochloride Diskets 1284
Methadone Hydrochloride Oral Solution & Tablets 1987

Methohexital Sodium (Dosage adjustments required). Products include:
Brevital Sodium Vials 1248

Methoxyflurane (Dosage adjustments required).
No products indexed under this heading.

Midazolam Hydrochloride (Dosage adjustments required). Products include:
Versed Injection 1924

Molindone Hydrochloride (Dosage adjustments required). Products include:
Moban Tablets & Concentrate 932

Morphine Sulfate (Dosage adjustments required). Products include:
Astramorph/PF Injection, USP (Preservative-Free) 618
Duramorph 960
Infumorph 200 and Infumorph 500 Sterile Solutions 962
MS Contin Tablets 1814
MSIR 1817
Oramorph SR (Morphine Sulfate Sustained Release Tablets) 1988
Roxanol 1991

Opium Alkaloids (Dosage adjustments required). Products include:
B & O No. 15A & No. 16A Supprettes 2395
Pantopon Injectable 1911

Oxazepam (Dosage adjustments required). Products include:
Serax Capsules 2522
Serax Tablets 2522

Oxycodone Hydrochloride (Dosage adjustments required). Products include:
Percocet Tablets 950
Percodan 951
Roxicodone Tablets, Oral Solution & Intensol (Oxycodone) 1992
Tylox Capsules 1382

Pentobarbital Sodium (Potentiated). Products include:
Nembutal Sodium Capsules 534
Nembutal Sodium Solution 536
Nembutal Sodium Suppositories 538

Perphenazine (Likelihood of tardive dyskinesia). Products include:
Etrafon 2087
Triavil Tablets 1556
Trilafon 2123

Phenobarbital (Potentiated). Products include:
Arco-Lase Plus Tablets 607
Bellergal-S Tablets 1998
Bronkolixir ..... ■ 761
Bronkotabs Tablets ..... ■ 762
Donnatal 1858
Donnatal Extentabs 1859
Donnatal Tablets 1858
Donnazyme Tablets 1860
Kinesed Tablets 2272
Phenobarbital Elixir and Tablets 1293
Primatene Tablets-P Formula 2421
Quadrinal Tablets 1183
Tedral SA 1765

Prazepam (Dosage adjustments required). Products include:
Centrax 1693

Prochlorperazine (Likelihood of tardive dyskinesia). Products include:
Compazine 2201

Promethazine Hydrochloride (Likelihood of tardive dyskinesia). Products include:
Mepergan Injection 2479
Phenergan with Codeine 2497
Phenergan with Dextromethorphan 2499
Phenergan Injection 2493
Phenergan Suppositories 2496
Phenergan Syrup 2495
Phenergan Tablets 2496
Phenergan VC 2500
Phenergan VC with Codeine 2501

Propofol (Dosage adjustments required). Products include:
Diprivan Injection 2267

Propoxyphene Hydrochloride (Dosage adjustments required). Products include:
Darvon 1256
Wygesic Tablets 2540

Propoxyphene Napsylate (Dosage adjustments required). Products include:
Darvon-N/Darvocet-N 1254

Quazepam (Dosage adjustments required). Products include:
Doral Tablets 2383

Scopolamine Hydrobromide (Weak anticholinergic effect of Navane necessitates cautious use of atropine related drugs). Products include:
Donnagel ..... ■ 675
Donnagel-PG 1858
Donnatal 1858
Donnatal Extentabs 1859
Donnatal Tablets 1858
Donnazyme Tablets 1860
Isopto Hyoscine ..... ◎ 222
Murocoll-2 Sterile Ophthalmic Solution ..... ◎ 261
Ru-Tuss Tablets 693

Scopolamine Preparations (Weak anticholinergic effect of Navane necessitates cautious use of atropine related drugs). Products include:
Transderm Scōp Transdermal Therapeutic System 887

Secobarbital Sodium (Potentiated). Products include:
Seconal Sodium Pulvules 1296

Sufentanil Citrate (Dosage adjustments required). Products include:
Sufenta Injection 1147

Temazepam (Dosage adjustments required). Products include:
Restoril Capsules 2023

Thiamylal Sodium (Potentiated). Products include:
Surital Ampoules, Steri-Vials 1764

Thioridazine Hydrochloride (Likelihood of tardive dyskinesia). Products include:
Mellaril 2011

Triazolam (Dosage adjustments required). Products include:
Halcion Tablets 2340

Trifluoperazine Hydrochloride (Likelihood of tardive dyskinesia). Products include:
Stelazine 2226

NAVANE INTRAMUSCULAR

(Thiothixene) 1956
May interact with phenothiazines, barbiturates, central nervous system depressants, belladona products, and certain other agents. Compounds in these categories include:

Alfentanil Hydrochloride (Dosage adjustments required). Products include:
Alfenta Injection 1131

Alprazolam (Dosage adjustments required). Products include:
Xanax Tablets 2367

Aprobarbital (Potentiated). Products include:
Alurate Elixir 1883

Atropine Sulfate (Use with caution). Products include:
Arco-Lase Plus Tablets 607
Atropine Sulfate Sterile Ophthalmic Solution and S.O.P. Sterile Ophthalmic Ointment ..... ◎ 239
Donnagel ..... ■ 675
Donnagel-PG 1858
Donnatal 1858
Donnatal Extentabs 1859
Donnatal Tablets 1858
Donnazyme Tablets 1860
Isopto Atropine ..... ◎ 218
Lomotil 2174
Motofen Tablets 836
Ru-Tuss Tablets 693
Urised Tablets 2396

Belladonna Alkaloids (Use with caution). Products include:
Bellergal-S Tablets 1998
Hyland's Bed Wetting Tablets ..... ■ 728
Hyland's Teething Tablets ..... ■ 728
Kinesed Tablets 2272

Buprenorphine (Dosage adjustments required).
No products indexed under this heading.

Buspirone Hydrochloride (Dosage adjustments required). Products include:
BuSpar 1401

Butabarbital (Potentiated). Products include:
Pyridium Plus 1764

Butalbital (Potentiated). Products include:
Esgic-Plus Tablets 1002
Esgic Tablets & Capsules 1001
Fioricet Tablets 2006
Fiorinal Capsules 2007
Fiorinal with Codeine Capsules 2008
Fiorinal Tablets 2007
Phrenilin 838
Sedapap Tablets 50 mg/650 mg 1360

Chlordiazepoxide (Dosage adjustments required). Products include:
Libritabs Tablets 1930
Limbitrol 1933
Menrium Tablets 1934

Chlordiazepoxide Hydrochloride (Dosage adjustments required). Products include:
Librax Capsules 1929
Librium Capsules 1931
Librium Injectable 1932

Chlorpromazine (Likelihood of tardive dyskinesia). Products include:
Thorazine 2234

Chlorprothixene (Dosage adjustments required). Products include:
Taractan Tablets 1920

Chlorprothixene Hydrochloride (Dosage adjustments required). Products include:
Taractan 1920

Clorazepate Dipotassium (Dosage adjustments required). Products include:
Tranxene 556

Codeine (Dosage adjustments required). Products include:
Calcidrine Syrup ... 506

Codeine Phosphate (Dosage adjustments required). Products include:
Actifed with Codeine Cough Syrup .. 752
Cheracol Cough Syrup ... 1853
Codimal PH Syrup ... 846
Dimetane-DC Cough Syrup ... 1857
Empirin with Codeine Phosphate Nos. 2, 3 & 4 ... 764
Fiorinal with Codeine Capsules ... 2008
Isoclor Expectorant ... 982
Naldecon CX Adult Liquid ... ⊡ 521
Novahistine DH ... 1342
Novahistine Expectorant ... 1343
Nucofed Capsules ... 2219
Nucofed Expectorant ... 2219
Nucofed Pediatric Expectorant ... 2220
Nucofed Syrup ... 2219
Phenaphen with Codeine Capsules 1865
Phenaphen-650 with Codeine Tablets ... 1866
Phenergan with Codeine ... 2497
Phenergan VC with Codeine ... 2501
Robitussin A-C Syrup ... 1875
Robitussin-DAC Syrup ... 1875
Ryna ... ⊡ 741
Soma Compound w/Codeine Tablets ... 2390
Triaminic Expectorant w/Codeine .. 1996
Tussi-Organidin Liquid ... 2391
Tylenol with Codeine ... 1381

Codeine Polistirex (Dosage adjustments required).
No products indexed under this heading.

Dezocine (Dosage adjustments required).

Diazepam (Dosage adjustments required). Products include:
Valium Injectable ... 1937
Valium Tablets ... 1939
Valrelease Capsules ... 1923

Droperidol (Dosage adjustments required). Products include:
Inapsine Injection ... 1140
Innovar Injection ... 1141

Enflurane (Dosage adjustments required). Products include:
Ethrane ... 599

Epinephrine Hydrochloride (Paradoxical hypotension may occur). Products include:
Adrenalin Chloride Solution 1:100 & 1:1,000 ... 1689
Epifrin ... ⊙ 244
Glaucon ... ⊙ 218

Estazolam (Dosage adjustments required). Products include:
ProSom Tablets ... 554

Ethchlorvynol (Dosage adjustments required). Products include:
Placidyl Capsules ... 553

Ethinamate (Dosage adjustments required).
No products indexed under this heading.

Fentanyl (Dosage adjustments required). Products include:
Duragesic Transdermal System ... 1133

Fentanyl Citrate (Dosage adjustments required). Products include:
Innovar Injection ... 1141
Sublimaze Injection ... 1146

Fluphenazine Decanoate (Likelihood of tardive dyskinesia). Products include:
Prolixin Decanoate ... 1795

Fluphenazine Enanthate (Likelihood of tardive dyskinesia). Products include:
Prolixin Enanthate ... 1796

Fluphenazine Hydrochloride (Likelihood of tardive dyskinesia). Products include:
Prolixin Elixir ... 1793
Prolixin Injection ... 1791
Prolixin Oral Concentrate ... 1792
Prolixin Tablets ... 1793

Flurazepam Hydrochloride (Dosage adjustments required). Products include:
Dalmane Capsules ... 1927

Glutethimide (Dosage adjustments required).
No products indexed under this heading.

Haloperidol (Dosage adjustments required). Products include:
Haldol Injection, Tablets and Concentrate ... 1373

Haloperidol Decanoate (Dosage adjustments required). Products include:
Haldol Decanoate ... 1375

Hydrocodone Bitartrate (Dosage adjustments required). Products include:
Anexsia 5/500 Tablets ... 2196
Anexsia 7.5/650 Tablets ... 2197
Azdone Tablets ... 844
Codiclear DH Syrup ... 845
Codimal DH Syrup ... 846
Damason-P ... 1356
Hycodan Syrup, Tablets ... 927
Hycomine Compound Tablets ... 929
Hycomine Syrup ... 927
Hycotuss Expectorant Syrup ... 930
Hydrocet Capsules ... 835
Lortab ASA Tablets ... 2414
Lortab ... 2412
Ru-Tuss with Hydrocodone ... 694
Triaminic Expectorant DH ... 1995
Vicodin Tablets ... 1187
Vicodin ES Tablets ... 1189
Zydone Capsules ... 941

Hydrocodone Polistirex (Dosage adjustments required). Products include:
Tussionex Extended-Release Suspension ... 988

Hydroxyzine Hydrochloride (Dosage adjustments required). Products include:
Atarax Tablets & Syrup ... 1941
Marax Tablets & DF Syrup ... 1954
Vistaril Intramuscular Solution ... 1970

Hyoscyamine (Use with caution). Products include:
Cystospaz Tablets ... 2395
Urised Tablets ... 2396

Hyoscyamine Sulfate (Use with caution). Products include:
Arco-Lase Plus Tablets ... 607
Cystospaz-M Capsules ... 2395
Donnagel ... ⊡ 675
Donnagel-PG ... 1858
Donnatal ... 1858
Donnatal Extentabs ... 1859
Donnatal Tablets ... 1858
Donnazyme Tablets ... 1860
Kutrase Capsules ... 2146
Levsin/Levsinex ... 2147
Ru-Tuss Tablets ... 693

Isoflurane (Dosage adjustments required). Products include:
Forane ... 600

Ketamine Hydrochloride (Dosage adjustments required). Products include:
Ketalar ... 1726

Levorphanol Tartrate (Dosage adjustments required). Products include:
Levo-Dromoran ... 1906

Lorazepam (Dosage adjustments required). Products include:
Ativan Injection ... 2432
Ativan Tablets ... 2434

Loxapine Hydrochloride (Dosage adjustments required). Products include:
Loxitane ... 1213

Loxapine Succinate (Dosage adjustments required). Products include:
Loxitane Capsules ... 1213

Meperidine Hydrochloride (Dosage adjustments required). Products include:
Demerol ... 2047
Mepergan Injection ... 2479

Mephobarbital (Potentiating action of barbiturates). Products include:
Mebaral Tablets ... 2061

Meprobamate (Dosage adjustments required). Products include:
Deprol Tablets ... 2382
Equagesic Tablets ... 2451
Miltown Tablets ... 2386
PMB 200 and PMB 400 ... 2504

Mesoridazine (Likelihood of tardive dyskinesia). Products include:
Serentil ... 686

Methadone Hydrochloride (Dosage adjustments required). Products include:
Dolophine Hydrochloride Ampoules & Vials ... 1260
Dolophine Hydrochloride Tablets ... 1261
Methadone Hydrochloride Diskets .. 1284
Methadone Hydrochloride Oral Solution & Tablets ... 1987

Methohexital Sodium (Dosage adjustments required). Products include:
Brevital Sodium Vials ... 1248

Methoxyflurane (Dosage adjustments required).
No products indexed under this heading.

Midazolam Hydrochloride (Dosage adjustments required). Products include:
Versed Injection ... 1924

Molindone Hydrochloride (Dosage adjustments required). Products include:
Moban Tablets & Concentrate ... 932

Morphine Sulfate (Dosage adjustments required). Products include:
Astramorph/PF Injection, USP (Preservative-Free) ... 618
Duramorph ... 960
Infumorph 200 and Infumorph 500 Sterile Solutions ... 962
MS Contin Tablets ... 1814
MSIR ... 1817
Oramorph SR (Morphine Sulfate Sustained Release Tablets) ... 1988
Roxanol ... 1991

Opium Alkaloids (Dosage adjustments required). Products include:
B & O No. 15A & No. 16A Supprettes ... 2395
Pantopon Injectable ... 1911

Oxazepam (Dosage adjustments required). Products include:
Serax Capsules ... 2522
Serax Tablets ... 2522

Oxycodone Hydrochloride (Dosage adjustments required). Products include:
Percocet Tablets ... 950
Percodan ... 951
Roxicodone Tablets, Oral Solution & Intensol (Oxycodone) ... 1992
Tylox Capsules ... 1382

Pentobarbital Sodium (Potentiated). Products include:
Nembutal Sodium Capsules ... 534
Nembutal Sodium Solution ... 536
Nembutal Sodium Suppositories ... 538

Perphenazine (Likelihood of tardive dyskinesia). Products include:
Etrafon ... 2087
Triavil Tablets ... 1556
Trilafon ... 2123

Phenobarbital (Potentiated). Products include:
Arco-Lase Plus Tablets ... 607
Bellergal-S Tablets ... 1998
Bronkolixir ... ⊡ 761
Bronkotabs Tablets ... ⊡ 762
Donnatal ... 1858
Donnatal Extentabs ... 1859
Donnatal Tablets ... 1858
Donnazyme Tablets ... 1860
Kinesed Tablets ... 2272
Phenobarbital Elixir and Tablets ... 1293
Primatene Tablets-P Formula ... 2421
Quadrinal Tablets ... 1183
Tedral SA ... 1765

Prazepam (Dosage adjustments required). Products include:
Centrax ... 1693

Prochlorperazine (Likelihood of tardive dyskinesia). Products include:
Compazine ... 2201

Promethazine Hydrochloride (Likelihood of tardive dyskinesia). Products include:
Mepergan Injection ... 2479
Phenergan with Codeine ... 2497
Phenergan with Dextromethorphan 2499
Phenergan Injection ... 2493
Phenergan Suppositories ... 2496
Phenergan Syrup ... 2495
Phenergan Tablets ... 2496
Phenergan VC ... 2500
Phenergan VC with Codeine ... 2501

Propofol (Dosage adjustments required). Products include:
Diprivan Injection ... 2267

Propoxyphene Hydrochloride (Dosage adjustments required). Products include:
Darvon ... 1256
Wygesic Tablets ... 2540

Propoxyphene Napsylate (Dosage adjustments required). Products include:
Darvon-N/Darvocet-N ... 1254

Quazepam (Dosage adjustments required). Products include:
Doral Tablets ... 2383

Scopolamine Hydrobromide (Use with caution). Products include:
Donnagel ... ⊡ 675
Donnagel-PG ... 1858
Donnatal ... 1858
Donnatal Extentabs ... 1859
Donnatal Tablets ... 1858
Donnazyme Tablets ... 1860
Isopto Hyoscine ... ⊙ 222
Murocoll-2 Sterile Ophthalmic Solution ... ⊙ 261
Ru-Tuss Tablets ... 693

Scopolamine Preparations (Use with caution). Products include:
Transderm Scōp Transdermal Therapeutic System ... 887

Secobarbital Sodium (Potentiated). Products include:
Seconal Sodium Pulvules ... 1296

Sufentanil Citrate (Dosage adjustments required). Products include:
Sufenta Injection ... 1147

Temazepam (Dosage adjustments required). Products include:
Restoril Capsules ... 2023

Thiamylal Sodium (Potentiated). Products include:
Surital Ampoules, Steri-Vials ... 1764

Thioridazine Hydrochloride (Likelihood of tardive dyskinesia). Products include:
Mellaril ... 2011

Triazolam (Dosage adjustments required). Products include:
Halcion Tablets ... 2340

Trifluoperazine Hydrochloride (Likelihood of tardive dyskinesia). Products include:
Stelazine ... 2226

NEBCIN VIALS, HYPORETS & ADD-VANTAGE
(Tobramycin Sulfate) ... 1286
May interact with aminoglycosides, cephalosporins, and certain other

agents. Compounds in these categories include:

Amikacin Sulfate (Avoid concurrent and sequential use). Products include:
- Amikin Injectable 602

Cefaclor (Increased incidence of nephrotoxicity). Products include:
- Ceclor Pulvules & Suspension 1251

Cefadroxil Monohydrate (Increased incidence of nephrotoxicity). Products include:
- Duricef 1405
- Ultracef Capsules, Tablets & Oral Suspension 722

Cefamandole Nafate (Increased incidence of nephrotoxicity). Products include:
- Mandol Vials, Faspak & ADD-Vantage 1281

Cefazolin Sodium (Increased incidence of nephrotoxicity). Products include:
- Ancef Injection 2194
- Kefzol Vials, Faspak & ADD-Vantage 1279

Cefixime (Increased incidence of nephrotoxicity). Products include:
- Suprax 1235

Cefmetazole Sodium (Increased incidence of nephrotoxicity). Products include:
- Zefazone Sterile Powder 2372

Cefonicid Sodium (Increased incidence of nephrotoxicity). Products include:
- Monocid Injection 2217

Cefoperazone Sodium (Increased incidence of nephrotoxicity). Products include:
- Cefobid Intravenous/Intramuscular 1943
- Cefobid Pharmacy Bulk Package - Not for Direct Infusion 1945

Ceforanide (Increased incidence of nephrotoxicity).
- No products indexed under this heading.

Cefotaxime Sodium (Increased incidence of nephrotoxicity). Products include:
- Claforan Sterile Injection 1089

Cefotetan (Increased incidence of nephrotoxicity). Products include:
- Cefotan 2265

Cefoxitin Sodium (Increased incidence of nephrotoxicity). Products include:
- Mefoxin 1498
- Mefoxin Premixed Intravenous Solution 1500

Ceftazidime (Increased incidence of nephrotoxicity). Products include:
- Ceptaz for Injection 1057
- Fortaz 1060
- Tazicef for Injection 2231
- Tazidime Vials, Faspak & ADD-Vantage 1299

Ceftizoxime Sodium (Increased incidence of nephrotoxicity). Products include:
- Cefizox Injection 1012

Ceftriaxone Sodium (Increased incidence of nephrotoxicity). Products include:
- Rocephin Injectable Vials, ADD-Vantage 1914

Cefuroxime Axetil (Increased incidence of nephrotoxicity). Products include:
- Ceftin Tablets 575

Cefuroxime Sodium (Increased incidence of nephrotoxicity). Products include:
- Kefurox Vials, Faspak & ADD-Vantage 1277
- Zinacef 1066

Cephalexin (Increased incidence of nephrotoxicity). Products include:
- Keflex Pulvules, Oral Suspension & Pediatric Drops 916

Cephaloridine (Avoid concurrent and sequential use).

Cephalothin Sodium (Increased incidence of nephrotoxicity).

Cephapirin Sodium (Increased incidence of nephrotoxicity).
- No products indexed under this heading.

Cephradine (Increased incidence of nephrotoxicity). Products include:
- Velosef Capsules and for Oral Suspension 606

Cisplatin (Avoid concurrent and sequential use). Products include:
- Platinol 737
- Platinol-AQ Injection 738

Colistin Sulfate (Avoid concurrent and sequential use). Products include:
- Coly-Mycin S For Oral Suspension .. 1708
- Coly-Mycin S Otic w/Neomycin & Hydrocortisone 1708

Decamethonium (Concurrent therapy in anesthetized patients may result in prolonged or secondary apnea).

Ethacrynic Acid (Do not use concurrently; ototoxicity). Products include:
- Edecrin Tablets 1468

Furosemide (Do not use concurrently; ototoxicity). Products include:
- Lasix 1093

Gentamicin Sulfate (Avoid concurrent and sequential use). Products include:
- Garamycin Injectable 2093
- Garamycin Ophthalmic .... ⊙ 305
- Genoptic Liquifilm Sterile Ophthalmic Solution .... ⊙ 247
- Genoptic S.O.P. Sterile Ophthalmic Ointment .... ⊙ 247
- Gentacidin Ointment .... ⊙ 273
- Gentacidin Solution .... ⊙ 273
- Gentak Ointment & Solution .... ⊙ 208
- G-myticin Creme and Ointment 0.1% 1770
- Pred-G Liquifilm Sterile Ophthalmic Suspension .... ⊙ 252
- Pred-G S.O.P. Sterile Ophthalmic Ointment .... ⊙ 253

Kanamycin Sulfate (Avoid concurrent and sequential use). Products include:
- Kantrex Injection 601
- Kantrex Pediatric Injection 601

Neomycin Sulfate (Avoid concurrent and sequential use). Products include:
- AK-Spore H.C. .... ⊙ 206
- AK-Spore .... ⊙ 205
- AK-Trol Ointment & Suspension .... ⊙ 207
- Bactine First Aid Antibiotic Ointment .... ▣ 625
- Campho-Phenique Triple Antibiotic Ointment Plus Pain Reliever ▣ 758
- Coly-Mycin S Otic w/Neomycin & Hydrocortisone 1708
- Cortisporin Cream 757
- Cortisporin Ointment 758
- Cortisporin Ophthalmic Ointment Sterile 758
- Cortisporin Ophthalmic Suspension Sterile 759
- Cortisporin Otic Solution Sterile 760
- Cortisporin Otic Suspension Sterile 760
- Dexacidin .... ⊙ 272
- Lanabiotic Ointment .... ▣ 556
- LazerSporin-C Solution 1770
- Maxitrol Ophthalmic Ointment/Suspension .... ⊙ 223
- Myciguent Antibiotic Ointment ...... ▣ 737
- Mycitracin .... ▣ 737
- NeoDecadron Sterile Ophthalmic Ointment 1517
- NeoDecadron Sterile Ophthalmic Solution 1518
- NeoDecadron Topical Cream 1518
- Neosporin Cream 792
- Neosporin G.U. Irrigant Sterile 793
- Neosporin Ointment 793
- Maximum Strength Neosporin Ointment 793
- Neosporin Ophthalmic Ointment Sterile 793
- Neosporin Ophthalmic Solution Sterile 794
- Neo-Synalar Cream 2296
- PediOtic Suspension Sterile 797
- Poly-Pred Liquifilm .... ⊙ 250

Paromomycin Sulfate (Avoid concurrent and sequential use). Products include:
- Humatin Capsules 1726

Polymyxin B Sulfate (Avoid concurrent and sequential use). Products include:
- AK-Poly-Bac Ointment .... ⊙ 205
- AK-Spore H.C. .... ⊙ 206
- AK-Spore .... ⊙ 205
- AK-Trol Ointment & Suspension .... ⊙ 207
- Aquaphor Antibiotic Formula 662
- Bactine First Aid Antibiotic Ointment .... ▣ 625
- Campho-Phenique Triple Antibiotic Ointment Plus Pain Reliever ▣ 758
- Cortisporin Cream 757
- Cortisporin Ointment 758
- Cortisporin Ophthalmic Ointment Sterile 758
- Cortisporin Ophthalmic Suspension Sterile 759
- Cortisporin Otic Solution Sterile 760
- Cortisporin Otic Suspension Sterile 760
- Dexacidin .... ⊙ 272
- Lanabiotic Ointment .... ▣ 556
- LazerSporin-C Solution 1770
- Maxitrol Ophthalmic Ointment/Suspension .... ⊙ 223
- Mycitracin .... ▣ 737
- Neosporin Cream 792
- Neosporin G.U. Irrigant Sterile 793
- Neosporin Ointment 793
- Maximum Strength Neosporin Ointment 793
- Neosporin Ophthalmic Ointment Sterile 793
- Neosporin Ophthalmic Solution Sterile 794
- Ophthocort .... ⊙ 301
- PediOtic Suspension Sterile 797
- Polymyxin B Sulfate, Aerosporin Brand Sterile Powder 798
- Poly-Pred Liquifilm .... ⊙ 250
- Polysporin Ointment .... ▣ 543
- Polysporin Ophthalmic Ointment Sterile 798
- Polysporin Powder .... ▣ 543
- Polysporin Spray .... ▣ 543
- Polytrim Ophthalmic Solution Sterile 588
- Terramycin with Polymyxin B Sulfate Ophthalmic Ointment 1965

Streptomycin Sulfate (Avoid concurrent and sequential use).
- No products indexed under this heading.

Succinylcholine Chloride (Concurrent therapy in anesthetized patients may result in prolonged or secondary apnea). Products include:
- Anectine 755

Tubocurarine Chloride (Concurrent therapy in anesthetized patients may result in prolonged or secondary apnea).
- No products indexed under this heading.

Vancomycin Hydrochloride (Avoid concurrent and sequential use). Products include:
- Vancocin HCl, Oral Solution & Pulvules 1304
- Vancocin HCl, Vials & ADD-Vantage 1302

Viomycin (Avoid concurrent and sequential use).

NEBUPENT FOR INHALATION SOLUTION
(Pentamidine Isethionate) 1017
No interactions described in labeling.

NEGGRAM CAPLETS
(Nalidixic Acid) 2062
May interact with oral anticoagulants and certain other agents. Compounds in these categories include:

Dicumarol (Enhanced effects of oral anticoagulants). Products include:
- Dicumarol Tablets 516

Nitrofurantoin (Interference with therapeutic action of nalidixic acid). Products include:
- Macrodantin Capsules 1624

Nitrofurantoin Macrocrystals (Interference with therapeutic action of nalidixic acid). Products include:
- Macrodantin Capsules 1624

Warfarin Sodium (Enhanced effect of oral anticoagulants). Products include:
- Coumadin Injection & Tablets 944
- Panwarfin Tablets 547

NEGGRAM SUSPENSION
(Nalidixic Acid) 2062
See **NegGram Caplets**

NEMBUTAL SODIUM CAPSULES
(Pentobarbital Sodium) 534
May interact with central nervous system depressants, oral anticoagulants, corticosteroids, monoamine oxidase inhibitors, estrogens, and certain other agents. Compounds in these categories include:

Alfentanil Hydrochloride (Additive CNS depressant effects). Products include:
- Alfenta Injection 1131

Alprazolam (Additive CNS depressant effects). Products include:
- Xanax Tablets 2367

Aprobarbital (Additive CNS depressant effects). Products include:
- Alurate Elixir 1883

Betamethasone Acetate (Barbiturates enhance metabolism). Products include:
- Celestone Soluspan Suspension 2081

Betamethasone Sodium Phosphate (Barbiturates enhance metabolism). Products include:
- Celestone Soluspan Suspension 2081

Buprenorphine (Additive CNS depressant effects).
- No products indexed under this heading.

Buspirone Hydrochloride (Additive CNS depressant effects). Products include:
- BuSpar 1401

Butabarbital (Additive CNS depressant effects). Products include:
- Pyridium Plus 1764

Butalbital (Additive CNS depressant effects). Products include:
- Esgic-Plus Tablets 1002
- Esgic Tablets & Capsules 1001
- Fioricet Tablets 2006
- Fiorinal Capsules 2007
- Fiorinal with Codeine Capsules 2008
- Fiorinal Tablets 2007
- Phrenilin 838
- Sedapap Tablets 50 mg/650 mg .. 1360

Chlordiazepoxide (Additive CNS depressant effects). Products include:
- Libritabs Tablets 1930
- Limbitrol 1933
- Menrium Tablets 1934

Chlordiazepoxide Hydrochloride (Additive CNS depressant effects). Products include:
- Librax Capsules 1929
- Librium Capsules 1931
- Librium Injectable 1932

(▣ Described in PDR For Nonprescription Drugs) (⊙ Described in PDR For Ophthalmology)

Chlorotrianisene (Decreased effects of estrogens). Products include:
TACE 12 and 25 mg ... 1353

Chlorpromazine (Additive CNS depressant effects). Products include:
Thorazine ... 2234

Chlorprothixene (Additive CNS depressant effects). Products include:
Taractan Tablets ... 1920

Chlorprothixene Hydrochloride (Additive CNS depressant effects). Products include:
Taractan ... 1920

Chlorprothixene Lactate (Additive CNS depressant effects). Products include:
Taractan Concentrate ... 1920

Clorazepate Dipotassium (Additive CNS depressant effects). Products include:
Tranxene ... 556

Codeine (Additive CNS depressant effects). Products include:
Calcidrine Syrup ... 506

Codeine Phosphate (Additive CNS depressant effects). Products include:
Actifed with Codeine Cough Syrup.. 752
Cheracol Cough Syrup ... 1853
Codimal PH Syrup ... 846
Dimetane-DC Cough Syrup ... 1857
Empirin with Codeine Phosphate Nos. 2, 3 & 4 ... 764
Fiorinal with Codeine Capsules ... 2008
Isoclor Expectorant ... 982
Naldecon CX Adult Liquid ... ▣ 521
Novahistine DH ... 1342
Novahistine Expectorant ... 1343
Nucofed Capsules ... 2219
Nucofed Expectorant ... 2219
Nucofed Pediatric Expectorant ... 2220
Nucofed Syrup ... 2219
Phenaphen with Codeine Capsules 1865
Phenaphen-650 with Codeine Tablets ... 1866
Phenergan with Codeine ... 2497
Phenergan VC with Codeine ... 2501
Robitussin A-C Syrup ... 1875
Robitussin-DAC Syrup ... 1875
Ryna ... ▣ 741
Soma Compound w/Codeine Tablets ... 2390
Triaminic Expectorant w/Codeine .. 1996
Tussi-Organidin Liquid ... 2391
Tylenol with Codeine ... 1381

Codeine Polistirex (Additive CNS depressant effects).
No products indexed under this heading.

Cortisone Acetate (Barbiturates enhance metabolism). Products include:
Cortone Acetate Sterile Suspension ... 1437
Cortone Acetate Tablets ... 1439

Dexamethasone (Barbiturates enchance metabolism). Products include:
AK-Trol Ointment & Suspension ... ⊙ 207
Decadron Elixir ... 1445
Decadron Tablets ... 1447
Decaspray Topical Aerosol ... 1459
Dexacidin ... ⊙ 272
Maxidex Sterile Ophthalmic Suspension ... ⊙ 223
Maxitrol Ophthalmic Ointment/Suspension ... ⊙ 223
TobraDex Ophthalmic Suspension and Ointment ... ⊙ 228

Dexamethasone Acetate (Barbiturates enhance metabolism). Products include:
Dalalone D.P. Injectable ... 999
Decadron-LA Sterile Suspension ... 1457

Dexamethasone Sodium Phosphate (Barbiturates enhance metabolism). Products include:
AK-Dex ... ⊙ 203
Decadron Phosphate Respihaler ... 1454
Decadron Phosphate Sterile Ophthalmic Ointment ... 1453
Decadron Phosphate Sterile Ophthalmic Solution ... 1453
Decadron Phosphate Topical Cream ... 1455
Decadron Phosphate Turbinaire ... 1456
Maxidex Sterile Ophthalmic Ointment ... ⊙ 222
NeoDecadron Sterile Ophthalmic Ointment ... 1517
NeoDecadron Sterile Ophthalmic Solution ... 1518
NeoDecadron Topical Cream ... 1518

Dezocine (Additive CNS depressant effects).

Diazepam (Additive CNS depressant effects). Products include:
Valium Injectable ... 1937
Valium Tablets ... 1939
Valrelease Capsules ... 1923

Dicumarol (Increased metabolism, decreased anticoagulant response). Products include:
Dicumarol Tablets ... 516

Dienestrol (Decreased effects of estrogens). Products include:
Ortho Dienestrol Cream ... 1664

Diethylstilbestrol (Decreased effects of estrogens). Products include:
Diethylstilbestrol Tablets ... 1258

Doxycycline Calcium (Barbiturates shortens half-life of doxycycline).
No products indexed under this heading.

Doxycycline Hyclate (Barbiturates shorten half-life of doxycycline). Products include:
Doryx Capsules ... 1717
Vibramycin Hyclate Capsules ... 1787
Vibramycin Hyclate Intravenous ... 1968
Vibra-Tabs Film Coated Tablets ... 1787

Doxycycline Monohydrate (Barbiturates shorten half-life of doxycycline). Products include:
Monodox Capsules ... 1630
Vibramycin Monohydrate for Oral Suspension ... 1787

Droperidol (Additive CNS depressant effects). Products include:
Inapsine Injection ... 1140
Innovar Injection ... 1141

Enflurane (Additive CNS depressant effects). Products include:
Ethrane ... 599

Estazolam (Additive CNS depressant effects). Products include:
ProSom Tablets ... 554

Estradiol (Decreased effects of estrogens). Products include:
Emcyt Capsules ... 1161
Estrace ... 1385
Estrace Vaginal Cream ... 1388
Estraderm Transdermal System ... 866

Estrogens, Conjugated (Decreased effects of estrogens). Products include:
Mediatric Capsules ... 2476
PMB 200 and PMB 400 ... 2504
Premarin Intravenous ... 2508
Premarin with Methyltestosterone .. 2515
Premarin Tablets ... 2510
Premarin Vaginal Cream ... 2512

Estrogens, Esterified (Decreased effects of estrogens). Products include:
Estratest ... 2245
Menrium Tablets ... 1934

Estropipate (Decreased effects of estrogens). Products include:
Ogen ... 540

Ethchlorvynol (Additive CNS depressant effects). Products include:
Placidyl Capsules ... 553

Ethinamate (Additive CNS depressant effects).
No products indexed under this heading.

Ethinyl Estradiol (Decreased effects on estrogens). Products include:
Brevicon ... 2304
Demulen ... 2161
Estinyl Tablets ... 2085
Jenest-28 Tablets ... 1636
Levlen/Tri-Levlen ... 665
Lo/Ovral Tablets ... 2471
Lo/Ovral-28 Tablets ... 2476
Loestrin ... 1728
Modicon ... 1667
Nordette-21 Tablets ... 2481
Nordette-28 Tablets ... 2483
Norethin ... 2133
Norinyl ... 2304
Norlestrin ... 1746
Ortho-Cyclen Tablets ... 1658
Ortho-Novum ... 1667
Ovcon ... 1391
Ovral Tablets ... 2490
Ovral-28 Tablets ... 2491
Levlen/Tri-Levlen ... 665
Tri-Norinyl ... 2304
Triphasil-21 Tablets ... 2527
Triphasil-28 Tablets ... 2532

Fentanyl (Additive CNS depressant effects). Products include:
Duragesic Transdermal System ... 1133

Fentanyl Citrate (Additive CNS depressant effects). Products include:
Innovar Injection ... 1141
Sublimaze Injection ... 1146

Fluphenazine Decanoate (Additive CNS depressant effects). Products include:
Prolixin Decanoate ... 1795

Fluphenazine Enanthate (Additive CNS depressant effects). Products include:
Prolixin Enanthate ... 1796

Fluphenazine Hydrochloride (Additive CNS depressant effects). Products include:
Prolixin Elixir ... 1793
Prolixin Injection ... 1791
Prolixin Oral Concentrate ... 1792
Prolixin Tablets ... 1793

Flurazepam Hydrochloride (Additive CNS depressant effects). Products include:
Dalmane Capsules ... 1927

Furazolidone (Prolongs effects of barbiturates). Products include:
Furoxone ... 1855

Glutethimide (Additive CNS depressant effects).
No products indexed under this heading.

Griseofulvin (Phenobarbital interferes with absorption). Products include:
Fulvicin P/G Tablets ... 2090
Fulvicin P/G 165 & 330 Tablets ... 2091
Fulvicin-U/F Tablets ... 2092
Grifulvin V (griseofulvin microsize) Tablets/Suspension ... 1678
Grisactin ... 2454
Grisactin Ultra Tablets ... 2455
Gris-PEG Tablets, 125 mg & 250 mg ... 1083

Haloperidol (Additive CNS depressant effects). Products include:
Haldol Injection, Tablets and Concentrate ... 1373

Haloperidol Decanoate (Additive CNS depressant effects). Products include:
Haldol Decanoate ... 1375

Hydrocodone Bitartrate (Additive CNS depressant effects). Products include:
Anexsia 5/500 Tablets ... 2196
Anexsia 7.5/650 Tablets ... 2197
Azdone Tablets ... 844
Codiclear DH Syrup ... 845
Codimal DH Syrup ... 846
Damason-P ... 1356
Hycodan Syrup, Tablets ... 927
Hycomine Compound Tablets ... 929
Hycomine Syrup ... 927
Hycotuss Expectorant Syrup ... 930
Hydrocet Capsules ... 835
Lortab ASA Tablets ... 2414
Lortab ... 2412
Ru-Tuss with Hydrocodone ... 694
Triaminic Expectorant DH ... 1995
Vicodin Tablets ... 1187
Vicodin ES Tablets ... 1189
Zydone Capsules ... 941

Hydrocodone Polistirex (Additive CNS depressant effects). Products include:
Tussionex Extended-Release Suspension ... 988

Hydrocortisone (Barbiturates enhance metabolism). Products include:
AK-Spore H.C. ... ⊙ 206
Bactine Hydrocortisone Anti-Itch Cream ... ▣ 625
CaldeCORT Anti-Itch Hydrocortisone Spray ... ▣ 560
Carmol HC Cream 1% ... 2296
Cortaid Spray ... ▣ 735
Cortenema ... 2244
Cortisporin Ointment ... 758
Cortisporin Ophthalmic Ointment Sterile ... 758
Cortisporin Ophthalmic Suspension Sterile ... 759
Cortisporin Otic Solution Sterile ... 760
Cortisporin Otic Suspension Sterile 760
Cortizone-5 Creme & Ointment ... ▣ 732
Dermolate Anti-Itch Cream ... ▣ 697
Eldecort Cream 1.0% ... 1113
Eldecort Cream 1.0% and 2.5% ... 1113
Fungoid HC Creme ... 1770
Hydrocortone Tablets ... 1482
Hytone ... 909
LazerSporin-C Solution ... 1770
Massengill Medicated Soft Cloth Towelettes ... 2192
Nutracort Cream & Lotion ... 1684
PediOtic Suspension Sterile ... 797
Synacort Creams 1%, 2.5% ... 2296
Vanoxide-HC Acne Lotion ... 911
Vioform-Hydrocortisone Cream and Mild Cream ... 889
Vioform-Hydrocortisone Ointment .. 889
VōSoL HC Otic Solution ... 2392
Vytone Cream 1% ... 911

Hydrocortisone Acetate (Barbiturates enhance metabolism). Products include:
Analpram-HC Rectal Cream 1% and 2.5% ... 970
Anusol-HC Cream ... 1690
Anusol-HC Suppositories ... 1691
Caldecort ... ▣ 560
Carmol HC Cream 1% ... 2296
Chloromycetin Hydrocortisone Ophthalmic ... 1694
Coly-Mycin S Otic w/Neomycin & Hydrocortisone ... 1708
Cortaid ... ▣ 735
Cortef Feminine Itch Cream ... ▣ 735
Corticaine ... ▣ 682
Cortifoam ... 1827
Cortisporin Cream ... 757
Epifoam ... 1828
Gynecort 5 Creme ... ▣ 556
Hydrocortone Acetate Sterile Suspension ... 1479
Lanacort 5 Creme and Ointment .. ▣ 557
Mantadil Cream ... 789
Ophthocort ... ⊙ 301
Orabase HCA Oral Paste ... 890
Pramosone Cream, Lotion & Ointment ... 971
ProctoCream-HC ... 1834
Proctofoam-HC ... 1835

Hydrocortisone Sodium Phosphate (Barbiturates enhance metabolism). Products include:
Hydrocortone Phosphate Injection, Sterile ... 1481

Hydrocortisone Sodium Succinate (Barbiturates enhance metabolism). Products include:
Solu-Cortef Sterile Powder ... 2361

Hydroxyzine Hydrochloride (Additive CNS depressant effects). Products include:
Atarax Tablets & Syrup ... 1941
Marax Tablets & DF Syrup ... 1954
Vistaril Intramuscular Solution ... 1970

Isocarboxazid (Prolongs effects of barbiturates). Products include:
Marplan Tablets 1906
Isoflurane (Additive CNS depressant effects). Products include:
Forane 600
Ketamine Hydrochloride (Additive CNS depressant effects). Products include:
Ketalar 1726
Levorphanol Tartrate (Additive CNS depressant effects). Products include:
Levo-Dromoran 1906
Lorazepam (Additive CNS depressant effects). Products include:
Ativan Injection 2432
Ativan Tablets 2434
Loxapine Hydrochloride (Additive CNS depressant effects). Products include:
Loxitane 1213
Loxapine Succinate (Additive CNS depressant effects). Products include:
Loxitane Capsules 1213
Meperidine Hydrochloride (Additive CNS depressant effects). Products include:
Demerol 2047
Mepergan Injection 2479
Mephobarbital (Additive CNS depressant effects). Products include:
Mebaral Tablets 2061
Meprobamate (Additive CNS depressant effects). Products include:
Deprol Tablets 2382
Equagesic Tablets 2451
Miltown Tablets 2386
PMB 200 and PMB 400 2504
Mesoridazine (Additive CNS depressant effects). Products include:
Serentil 686
Methadone Hydrochloride (Additive CNS depressant effects). Products include:
Dolophine Hydrochloride Ampoules & Vials 1260
Dolophine Hydrochloride Tablets 1261
Methadone Hydrochloride Diskets 1284
Methadone Hydrochloride Oral Solution & Tablets 1987
Methohexital Sodium (Additive CNS depressant effects). Products include:
Brevital Sodium Vials 1248
Methoxyflurane (Additive CNS depressant effects).
No products indexed under this heading.
Methylprednisolone Acetate (Barbiturates enhance metabolism). Products include:
Depo-Medrol Sterile Aqueous Suspension 2334
Methylprednisolone Sodium Succinate (Barbiturates enhance metabolism). Products include:
Solu-Medrol Sterile Powder 2363
Midazolam Hydrochloride (Additive CNS depressant effects). Products include:
Versed Injection 1924
Molindone Hydrochloride (Additive CNS depressant effects). Products include:
Moban Tablets & Concentrate 932
Morphine Sulfate (Additive CNS depressant effects). Products include:
Astramorph/PF Injection, USP (Preservative-Free) 618
Duramorph 960
Infumorph 200 and Infumorph 500 Sterile Solutions 962
MS Contin Tablets 1814
MSIR 1817
Oramorph SR (Morphine Sulfate Sustained Release Tablets) 1988
Roxanol 1991
Opium Alkaloids (Additive CNS depressant effects). Products include:
B & O No. 15A & No. 16A Supprettes 2395
Pantopon Injectable 1911
Oxazepam (Additive CNS depressant effects). Products include:
Serax Capsules 2522
Serax Tablets 2522
Oxycodone Hydrochloride (Additive CNS depressant effects). Products include:
Percocet Tablets 950
Percodan 951
Roxicodone Tablets, Oral Solution & Intensol (Oxycodone) 1992
Tylox Capsules 1382
Perphenazine (Additive CNS depressant effects). Products include:
Etrafon 2087
Triavil Tablets 1556
Trilafon 2123
Phenelzine Sulfate (Prolongs effects of barbiturates). Products include:
Nardil 1742
Phenobarbital (Additive CNS depressant effects). Products include:
Arco-Lase Plus Tablets 607
Bellergal-S Tablets 1998
Bronkolixir ..... ▣ 761
Bronkotabs Tablets ..... ▣ 762
Donnatal 1858
Donnatal Extentabs 1859
Donnatal Tablets 1858
Donnazyme Tablets 1860
Kinesed Tablets 2272
Phenobarbital Elixir and Tablets 1293
Primatene Tablets-P Formula 2421
Quadrinal Tablets 1183
Tedral SA 1765
Phenytoin (Variable effect on metabolism of phenytoin). Products include:
Dilantin Infatabs 1710
Dilantin-30 Pediatric/Dilantin-125 Suspension 1713
Phenytoin Sodium (Variable effect on metabolism of phenytoin). Products include:
Dilantin Kapseals 1708
Dilantin Parenteral 1712
Dilantin with Phenobarbital Kapseals 1715
Polyestradiol Phosphate (Decreased effects of estrogens). Products include:
Estradurin 2452
Prazepam (Additive CNS depressant effects). Products include:
Centrax 1693
Prednisolone Acetate (Barbiturates enhance metabolism). Products include:
AK-Cide Sterile Ophthalmic Ointment & Suspension ..... ◉ 202
Blephamide Liquifilm Sterile Ophthalmic Suspension 586
Blephamide S.O.P. Sterile Ophthalmic Ointment 586
Cetapred Ointment ..... ◉ 220
⅛% Econopred & 1% Econopred Plus ..... ◉ 217
Isopto Cetapred Suspension ..... ◉ 220
Metimyd ..... ◉ 306
Poly-Pred Liquifilm ..... ◉ 250
Pred Forte ..... ◉ 252
Pred Mild ..... ◉ 254
Pred-G Liquifilm Sterile Ophthalmic Suspension ..... ◉ 252
Pred-G S.O.P. Sterile Ophthalmic Ointment ..... ◉ 253
Vasocidin Ointment ..... ◉ 275
Prednisolone Sodium Phosphate (Barbiturates enhance metabolism). Products include:
AK-Pred ..... ◉ 205
Hydeltrasol Injection, Sterile 1476
Inflamase ..... ◉ 274
Pediapred Oral Liquid 987
Vasocidin Ophthalmic Solution ..... ◉ 276
Prednisolone Tebutate (Barbiturates enhance metabolism). Products include:
Hydeltra-T.B.A. Sterile Suspension 1478
Prednisone (Barbiturates enhance metabolism). Products include:
Deltasone Tablets 2332
Prochlorperazine (Additive CNS depressant effects). Products include:
Compazine 2201
Promethazine Hydrochloride (Additive CNS depressant effects). Products include:
Mepergan Injection 2479
Phenergan with Codeine 2497
Phenergan with Dextromethorphan 2499
Phenergan Injection 2493
Phenergan Suppositories 2496
Phenergan Syrup 2495
Phenergan Tablets 2496
Phenergan VC 2500
Phenergan VC with Codeine 2501
Propofol (Additive CNS depressant effects). Products include:
Diprivan Injection 2267
Propoxyphene Hydrochloride (Additive CNS depressant effects). Products include:
Darvon 1256
Wygesic Tablets 2540
Propoxyphene Napsylate (Additive CNS depressant effects). Products include:
Darvon-N/Darvocet-N 1254
Quazepam (Additive CNS depressant effects). Products include:
Doral Tablets 2383
Quinestrol (Decreased effects of estrogens). Products include:
Estrovis 1721
Secobarbital Sodium (Additive CNS depressant effects). Products include:
Seconal Sodium Pulvules 1296
Selegiline Hydrochloride (Prolongs effects of barbiturates). Products include:
Eldepryl 2250
Sufentanil Citrate (Additive CNS depressant effects). Products include:
Sufenta Injection 1147
Temazepam (Additive CNS depressant effects). Products include:
Restoril Capsules 2023
Thiamylal Sodium (Additive CNS depressant effects). Products include:
Surital Ampoules, Steri-Vials 1764
Thioridazine Hydrochloride (Additive CNS depressant effects). Products include:
Mellaril 2011
Thiothixene (Additive CNS depressant effects). Products include:
Navane Capsules and Concentrate 1954
Navane Intramuscular 1956
Tranylcypromine Sulfate (Prolongs effects of barbiturates). Products include:
Parnate Tablets 2222
Triamcinolone (Barbiturates enhance metabolism).
No products indexed under this heading.
Triamcinolone Acetonide (Barbiturates enhance metabolism). Products include:
Aristocort A 1010
Azmacort Inhaler 1837
Kenalog Cream, Lotion & Ointment 2401
Kenalog-10 Injection 2402
Kenalog-40 Injection 2403
Kenalog in Orabase 604
Kenalog Spray 2401
Mycolog II Cream and Ointment 2407
Mytrex Cream & Ointment 2080
Nasacort Nasal Inhaler 1844
Triamcinolone Diacetate (Barbiturates enhance metabolism). Products include:
Aristocort Suspension 1008
Triamcinolone Hexacetonide (Barbiturates enhance metabolism). Products include:
Aristospan Suspension 1011
Triazolam (Additive CNS depressant effects). Products include:
Halcion Tablets 2340
Trifluoperazine Hydrochloride (Additive CNS depressant effects). Products include:
Stelazine 2226
Valproic Acid (Decreases barbiturate metabolism). Products include:
Depakene Capsules & Syrup 511
Warfarin Sodium (Increased metabolism, decreased anticoagulant response). Products include:
Coumadin Injection & Tablets 944
Panwarfin Tablets 547

NEMBUTAL SODIUM SOLUTION
(Pentobarbital Sodium) 536
May interact with central nervous system depressants, oral anticoagulants, corticosteroids, monoamine oxidase inhibitors, estrogens, and certain other agents. Compounds in these categories include:

Alfentanil Hydrochloride (Additive CNS depressant effects). Products include:
Alfenta Injection 1131
Alprazolam (Additive CNS depressant effects). Products include:
Xanax Tablets 2367
Aprobarbital (Additive CNS depressant effects). Products include:
Alurate Elixir 1883
Betamethasone Acetate (Barbiturates enhance metabolism). Products include:
Celestone Soluspan Suspension 2081
Betamethasone Sodium Phosphate (Barbiturates enhance metabolism). Products include:
Celestone Soluspan Suspension 2081
Buprenorphine (Additive CNS depressant effects).
No products indexed under this heading.
Buspirone Hydrochloride (Additive CNS depressant effects). Products include:
BuSpar 1401
Butabarbital (Additive CNS depressant effects). Products include:
Pyridium Plus 1764
Butalbital (Additive CNS depressant effects). Products include:
Esgic-Plus Tablets 1002
Esgic Tablets & Capsules 1001
Fioricet Tablets 2006
Fiorinal Capsules 2007
Fiorinal with Codeine Capsules 2008
Fiorinal Tablets 2007
Phrenilin 838
Sedapap Tablets 50 mg/650 mg 1360
Chlordiazepoxide (Additive CNS depressant effects). Products include:
Libritabs Tablets 1930
Limbitrol 1933
Menrium Tablets 1934
Chlordiazepoxide Hydrochloride (Additive CNS depressant effects). Products include:
Librax Capsules 1929
Librium Capsules 1931
Librium Injectable 1932

Chlorotrianisene (Decreased effects of estrogens). Products include:
TACE 12 and 25 mg ... 1353
Chlorpromazine (Additive CNS depressant effects). Products include:
Thorazine ... 2234
Chlorprothixene (Additive CNS depressant effects). Products include:
Taractan Tablets ... 1920
Chlorprothixene Hydrochloride (Additive CNS depressant effects). Products include:
Taractan ... 1920
Chlorprothixene Lactate (Additive CNS depressant effects). Products include:
Taractan Concentrate ... 1920
Clorazepate Dipotassium (Additive CNS depressant effects). Products include:
Tranxene ... 556
Codeine (Additive CNS depressant effects). Products include:
Calcidrine Syrup ... 506
Codeine Phosphate (Additive CNS depressant effects). Products include:
Actifed with Codeine Cough Syrup.. 752
Cheracol Cough Syrup ... 1853
Codimal PH Syrup ... 846
Dimetane-DC Cough Syrup ... 1857
Empirin with Codeine Phosphate Nos. 2, 3 & 4 ... 764
Fiorinal with Codeine Capsules ... 2008
Isoclor Expectorant ... 982
Naldecon CX Adult Liquid ... ◙ 521
Novahistine DH ... 1342
Novahistine Expectorant ... 1343
Nucofed Capsules ... 2219
Nucofed Expectorant ... 2219
Nucofed Pediatric Expectorant ... 2220
Nucofed Syrup ... 2219
Phenaphen with Codeine Capsules 1865
Phenaphen-650 with Codeine Tablets ... 1866
Phenergan with Codeine ... 2497
Phenergan VC with Codeine ... 2501
Robitussin A-C Syrup ... 1875
Robitussin-DAC Syrup ... 1875
Ryna ... ◙ 741
Soma Compound w/Codeine Tablets ... 2390
Triaminic Expectorant w/Codeine .. 1996
Tussi-Organidin Liquid ... 2391
Tylenol with Codeine ... 1381
Codeine Polistirex (Additive CNS depressant effects).
No products indexed under this heading.
Cortisone Acetate (Barbiturates enhance metabolism). Products include:
Cortone Acetate Sterile Suspension ... 1437
Cortone Acetate Tablets ... 1439
Dexamethasone (Barbiturates enhance metabolism). Products include:
AK-Trol Ointment & Suspension ... ⊙ 207
Decadron Elixir ... 1445
Decadron Tablets ... 1447
Decaspray Topical Aerosol ... 1459
Dexacidin ... ⊙ 272
Maxidex Sterile Ophthalmic Suspension ... ⊙ 223
Maxitrol Ophthalmic Ointment/Suspension ... ⊙ 223
TobraDex Ophthalmic Suspension and Ointment ... ⊙ 228
Dexamethasone Acetate (Barbiturates enhance metabolism). Products include:
Dalalone D.P. Injectable ... 999
Decadron-LA Sterile Suspension ... 1457
Dexamethasone Sodium Phosphate (Barbiturates enhance metabolism). Products include:
AK-Dex ... ⊙ 203
Decadron Phosphate Respihaler ... 1454
Decadron Phosphate Sterile Ophthalmic Ointment ... 1453
Decadron Phosphate Sterile Ophthalmic Solution ... 1453
Decadron Phosphate Topical Cream ... 1455
Decadron Phosphate Turbinaire ... 1456
Maxidex Sterile Ophthalmic Ointment ... ⊙ 222
NeoDecadron Sterile Ophthalmic Ointment ... 1517
NeoDecadron Sterile Ophthalmic Solution ... 1518
NeoDecadron Topical Cream ... 1518
Dezocine (Additive CNS depressant effects).
Diazepam (Additive CNS depressant effects). Products include:
Valium Injectable ... 1937
Valium Tablets ... 1939
Valrelease Capsules ... 1923
Dicumarol (Increased metabolism, decreased anticoagulant response). Products include:
Dicumarol Tablets ... 516
Dienestrol (Decreased effects of estrogens). Products include:
Ortho Dienestrol Cream ... 1664
Diethylstilbestrol (Decreased effects of estrogens). Products include:
Diethylstilbestrol Tablets ... 1258
Doxepin Hydrochloride (Phenobarbital shortens half-life). Products include:
Sinequan ... 1960
Doxycycline Calcium (Barbiturates shorten half-life of doxycycline).
No products indexed under this heading.
Doxycycline Hyclate (Barbiturates shorten half-life of doxycycline). Products include:
Doryx Capsules ... 1717
Vibramycin Hyclate Capsules ... 1787
Vibramycin Hyclate Intravenous ... 1968
Vibra-Tabs Film Coated Tablets ... 1787
Doxycycline Monohydrate (Barbiturates shorten half-life of doxycycline). Products include:
Monodox Capsules ... 1630
Vibramycin Monohydrate for Oral Suspension ... 1787
Droperidol (Additive CNS depressant effects). Products include:
Inapsine Injection ... 1140
Innovar Injection ... 1141
Enflurane (Additive CNS depressant effects). Products include:
Ethrane ... 599
Estazolam (Additive CNS depressant effects). Products include:
ProSom Tablets ... 554
Estradiol (Decreased effects of estrogens). Products include:
Emcyt Capsules ... 1161
Estrace ... 1385
Estrace Vaginal Cream ... 1388
Estraderm Transdermal System ... 866
Estrogens, Conjugated (Decreased effects of estrogens). Products include:
Mediatric Capsules ... 2476
PMB 200 and PMB 400 ... 2504
Premarin Intravenous ... 2508
Premarin with Methyltestosterone .. 2515
Premarin Tablets ... 2510
Premarin Vaginal Cream ... 2512
Estrogens, Esterified (Decreased effects of estrogens). Products include:
Estratest ... 2245
Menrium Tablets ... 1934
Estropipate (Decreased effects of estrogens). Products include:
Ogen ... 540
Ethchlorvynol (Additive CNS depressant effects). Products include:
Placidyl Capsules ... 553
Ethinamate (Additive CNS depressant effects).
No products indexed under this heading.
Ethinyl Estradiol (Decreased effects of estrogens). Products include:
Brevicon ... 2304
Demulen ... 2161
Estinyl Tablets ... 2085
Jenest-28 Tablets ... 1636
Levlen/Tri-Levlen ... 665
Lo/Ovral Tablets ... 2471
Lo/Ovral-28 Tablets ... 2476
Loestrin ... 1728
Modicon ... 1667
Nordette-21 Tablets ... 2481
Nordette-28 Tablets ... 2483
Norethin ... 2133
Norinyl ... 2304
Norlestrin ... 1746
Ortho-Cyclen Tablets ... 1658
Ortho-Novum ... 1667
Ovcon ... 1391
Ovral Tablets ... 2490
Ovral-28 Tablets ... 2491
Levlen/Tri-Levlen ... 665
Tri-Norinyl ... 2304
Triphasil-21 Tablets ... 2527
Triphasil-28 Tablets ... 2532
Fentanyl (Additive CNS depressant effects). Products include:
Duragesic Transdermal System ... 1133
Fentanyl Citrate (Additive CNS depressant effects). Products include:
Innovar Injection ... 1141
Sublimaze Injection ... 1146
Fluphenazine Decanoate (Additive CNS depressant effects). Products include:
Prolixin Decanoate ... 1795
Fluphenazine Enanthate (Additive CNS depressant effects). Products include:
Prolixin Enanthate ... 1796
Fluphenazine Hydrochloride (Additive CNS depressant effects). Products include:
Prolixin Elixir ... 1793
Prolixin Injection ... 1791
Prolixin Oral Concentrate ... 1792
Prolixin Tablets ... 1793
Flurazepam Hydrochloride (Additive CNS depressant effects). Products include:
Dalmane Capsules ... 1927
Furazolidone (Prolongs effects of barbiturates). Products include:
Furoxone ... 1855
Glutethimide (Additive CNS depressant effects).
No products indexed under this heading.
Griseofulvin (Phenobarbital interferes with absorption). Products include:
Fulvicin P/G Tablets ... 2090
Fulvicin P/G 165 & 330 Tablets ... 2091
Fulvicin-U/F Tablets ... 2092
Grifulvin V (griseofulvin microsize) Tablets/Suspension ... 1678
Grisactin ... 2454
Grisactin Ultra Tablets ... 2455
Gris-PEG Tablets, 125 mg & 250 mg ... 1083
Haloperidol (Additive CNS depressant effects). Products include:
Haldol Injection, Tablets and Concentrate ... 1373
Haloperidol Decanoate (Additive CNS depressant effects). Products include:
Haldol Decanoate ... 1375
Hydrocodone Bitartrate (Additive CNS depressant effects). Products include:
Anexsia 5/500 Tablets ... 2196
Anexsia 7.5/650 Tablets ... 2197
Azdōne Tablets ... 844
Codiclear DH Syrup ... 845
Codimal DH Syrup ... 846
Damason-P ... 1356
Hycodan Syrup, Tablets ... 927
Hycomine Compound Tablets ... 929
Hycomine Syrup ... 927
Hycotuss Expectorant Syrup ... 930
Hydrocet Capsules ... 835
Lortab ASA Tablets ... 2414
Lortab ... 2412
Ru-Tuss with Hydrocodone ... 694
Triaminic Expectorant DH ... 1995
Vicodin Tablets ... 1187
Vicodin ES Tablets ... 1189
Zydone Capsules ... 941
Hydrocodone Polistirex (Additive CNS depressant effects). Products include:
Tussionex Extended-Release Suspension ... 988
Hydrocortisone (Barbiturates enhance metabolism). Products include:
AK-Spore H.C. ... ⊙ 206
Bactine Hydrocortisone Anti-Itch Cream ... ◙ 625
CaldeCORT Anti-Itch Hydrocortisone Spray ... ◙ 560
Carmol HC Cream 1% ... 2296
Cortaid Spray ... ◙ 735
Cortenema ... 2244
Cortisporin Ointment ... 758
Cortisporin Ophthalmic Ointment Sterile ... 758
Cortisporin Ophthalmic Suspension Sterile ... 759
Cortisporin Otic Solution Sterile ... 760
Cortisporin Otic Suspension Sterile 760
Cortizone-5 Creme & Ointment ... ◙ 732
Dermolate Anti-Itch Cream ... ◙ 697
Eldecort Cream 1.0% ... 1113
Eldecort Cream 1.0% and 2.5% ... 1113
Fungoid HC Creme ... 1770
Hydrocortone Tablets ... 1482
Hytone ... 909
LazerSporin-C Solution ... 1770
Massengill Medicated Soft Cloth Towelettes ... 2192
Nutracort Cream & Lotion ... 1684
PediOtic Suspension Sterile ... 797
Synacort Creams 1%, 2.5% ... 2296
Vanoxide-HC Acne Lotion ... 911
Vioform-Hydrocortisone Cream and Mild Cream ... 889
Vioform-Hydrocortisone Ointment.. 889
VōSoL HC Otic Solution ... 2392
Vytone Cream 1% ... 911
Hydrocortisone Acetate (Barbiturates enhance metabolism). Products include:
Analpram-HC Rectal Cream 1% and 2.5% ... 970
Anusol-HC Cream ... 1690
Anusol-HC Suppositories ... 1691
Caldecort ... ◙ 560
Carmol HC Cream 1% ... 2296
Chloromycetin Hydrocortisone Ophthalmic ... 1694
Coly-Mycin S Otic w/Neomycin & Hydrocortisone ... 1708
Cortaid ... ◙ 735
Cortef Feminine Itch Cream ... ◙ 735
Corticaine ... ◙ 682
Cortifoam ... 1827
Cortisporin Cream ... 757
Epifoam ... 1828
Gynecort 5 Creme ... ◙ 556
Hydrocortone Acetate Sterile Suspension ... 1479
Lanacort 5 Creme and Ointment .. ◙ 557
Mantadil Cream ... 789
Ophthocort ... ⊙ 301
Orabase HCA Oral Paste ... 890
Pramosone Cream, Lotion & Ointment ... 971
ProctoCream-HC ... 1834
Proctofoam-HC ... 1835
Hydrocortisone Sodium Phosphate (Barbiturates enhance metabolism). Products include:
Hydrocortone Phosphate Injection, Sterile ... 1481
Hydrocortisone Sodium Succinate (Barbiturates enhance metabolism). Products include:
Solu-Cortef Sterile Powder ... 2361

Hydroxyzine Hydrochloride (Additive CNS depressant effects). Products include:
Atarax Tablets & Syrup 1941
Marax Tablets & DF Syrup 1954
Vistaril Intramuscular Solution 1970

Isocarboxazid (Prolongs effects of barbiturates). Products include:
Marplan Tablets 1906

Isoflurane (Additive CNS depressant effects). Products include:
Forane 600

Ketamine Hydrochloride (Additive CNS depressant effects). Products include:
Ketalar 1726

Levorphanol Tartrate (Additive CNS depressant effects). Products include:
Levo-Dromoran 1906

Lorazepam (Additive CNS depressant effects). Products include:
Ativan Injection 2432
Ativan Tablets 2434

Loxapine Hydrochloride (Additive CNS depressant effects). Products include:
Loxitane 1213

Loxapine Succinate (Additive CNS depressant effects). Products include:
Loxitane Capsules 1213

Meperidine Hydrochloride (Additive CNS depressant effects). Products include:
Demerol 2047
Mepergan Injection 2479

Mephobarbital (Additive CNS depressant effects). Products include:
Mebaral Tablets 2061

Meprobamate (Additive CNS depressant effects). Products include:
Deprol Tablets 2382
Equagesic Tablets 2451
Miltown Tablets 2386
PMB 200 and PMB 400 2504

Mesoridazine (Additive CNS depressant effects). Products include:
Serentil 686

Methadone Hydrochloride (Additive CNS depressant effects). Products include:
Dolophine Hydrochloride Ampoules & Vials 1260
Dolophine Hydrochloride Tablets 1261
Methadone Hydrochloride Diskets 1284
Methadone Hydrochloride Oral Solution & Tablets 1987

Methohexital Sodium (Additive CNS depressant effects). Products include:
Brevital Sodium Vials 1248

Methoxyflurane (Additive CNS depressant effects).
No products indexed under this heading.

Methylprednisolone Acetate (Barbiturates enhance metabolism). Products include:
Depo-Medrol Sterile Aqueous Suspension 2334

Methylprednisolone Sodium Succinate (Barbiturates enhance metabolism). Products include:
Solu-Medrol Sterile Powder 2363

Midazolam Hydrochloride (Additive CNS depressant effects). Products include:
Versed Injection 1924

Molindone Hydrochloride (Additive CNS depressant effects). Products include:
Moban Tablets & Concentrate 932

Morphine Sulfate (Additive CNS depressant effects). Products include:
Astramorph/PF Injection, USP (Preservative-Free) 618
Duramorph 960
Infumorph 200 and Infumorph 500 Sterile Solutions 962
MS Contin Tablets 1814
MSIR 1817
Oramorph SR (Morphine Sulfate Sustained Release Tablets) 1988
Roxanol 1991

Opium Alkaloids (Additive CNS depressant effects). Products include:
B & O No. 15A & No. 16A Supprettes 2395
Pantopon Injectable 1911

Oxazepam (Additive CNS depressant effects). Products include:
Serax Capsules 2522
Serax Tablets 2522

Oxycodone Hydrochloride (Additive CNS depressant effects). Products include:
Percocet Tablets 950
Percodan 951
Roxicodone Tablets, Oral Solution & Intensol (Oxycodone) 1992
Tylox Capsules 1382

Perphenazine (Additive CNS depressant effects). Products include:
Etrafon 2087
Triavil Tablets 1556
Trilafon 2123

Phenelzine Sulfate (Prolongs effects of barbiturates). Products include:
Nardil 1742

Phenobarbital (Additive CNS depressant effects). Products include:
Arco-Lase Plus Tablets 607
Bellergal-S Tablets 1998
Bronkolixir .... ■D 761
Bronkotabs Tablets .... ■D 762
Donnatal 1858
Donnatal Extentabs 1859
Donnatal Tablets 1858
Donnazyme Tablets 1860
Kinesed Tablets 2272
Phenobarbital Elixir and Tablets 1293
Primatene Tablets-P Formula 2421
Quadrinal Tablets 1183
Tedral SA 1765

Phenytoin (Variable effect on metabolism of phenytoin). Products include:
Dilantin Infatabs 1710
Dilantin-30 Pediatric/Dilantin-125 Suspension 1713

Phenytoin Sodium (Variable effect on metabolism of phenytoin). Products include:
Dilantin Kapseals 1708
Dilantin Parenteral 1712
Dilantin with Phenobarbital Kapseals 1715

Polyestradiol Phosphate (Decreased effects of estrogens). Products include:
Estradurin 2452

Prazepam (Additive CNS depressant effects). Products include:
Centrax 1693

Prednisolone Acetate (Barbiturates enhance metabolism). Products include:
AK-Cide Sterile Ophthalmic Ointment & Suspension .... ◉ 202
Blephamide Liquifilm Sterile Ophthalmic Suspension 586
Blephamide S.O.P. Sterile Ophthalmic Ointment 586
Cetapred Ointment .... ◉ 220
⅛% Econopred & 1% Econopred Plus .... ◉ 217
Isopto Cetapred Suspension .... ◉ 220
Metimyd .... ◉ 306
Poly-Pred Liquifilm .... ◉ 250
Pred Forte .... ◉ 252
Pred Mild .... ◉ 254
Pred-G Liquifilm Sterile Ophthalmic Suspension .... ◉ 252
Pred-G S.O.P. Sterile Ophthalmic Ointment .... ◉ 253
Vasocidin Ointment .... ◉ 275

Prednisolone Sodium Phosphate (Barbiturates enhance metabolism). Products include:
AK-Pred .... ◉ 205
Hydeltrasol Injection, Sterile 1476
Inflamase .... ◉ 274
Pediapred Oral Liquid 987
Vasocidin Ophthalmic Solution .... ◉ 276

Prednisolone Tebutate (Barbiturates enhance metabolism). Products include:
Hydeltra-T.B.A. Sterile Suspension 1478

Prednisone (Barbiturates enhance metabolism). Products include:
Deltasone Tablets 2332

Prochlorperazine (Additive CNS depressant effects). Products include:
Compazine 2201

Promethazine Hydrochloride (Additive CNS depressant effects). Products include:
Mepergan Injection 2479
Phenergan with Codeine 2497
Phenergan with Dextromethorphan 2499
Phenergan Injection 2493
Phenergan Suppositories 2496
Phenergan Syrup 2495
Phenergan Tablets 2496
Phenergan VC 2500
Phenergan VC with Codeine 2501

Propofol (Additive CNS depressant effects). Products include:
Diprivan Injection 2267

Propoxyphene Hydrochloride (Additive CNS depressant effects). Products include:
Darvon 1256
Wygesic Tablets 2540

Propoxyphene Napsylate (Additive CNS depressant effects). Products include:
Darvon-N/Darvocet-N 1254

Quazepam (Additive CNS depressant effects). Products include:
Doral Tablets 2383

Quinestrol (Decreased effects of estrogens). Products include:
Estrovis 1721

Secobarbital Sodium (Additive CNS depressant effects). Products include:
Seconal Sodium Pulvules 1296

Selegiline Hydrochloride (Prolongs effects of barbiturates). Products include:
Eldepryl 2250

Sufentanil Citrate (Additive CNS depressant effects). Products include:
Sufenta Injection 1147

Temazepam (Additive CNS depressant effects). Products include:
Restoril Capsules 2023

Thiamylal Sodium (Additive CNS depressant effects). Products include:
Surital Ampoules, Steri-Vials 1764

Thioridazine Hydrochloride (Additive CNS depressant effects). Products include:
Mellaril 2011

Thiothixene (Additive CNS depressant effects). Products include:
Navane Capsules and Concentrate 1954
Navane Intramuscular 1956

Tranylcypromine Sulfate (Prolongs effects of barbiturates). Products include:
Parnate Tablets 2222

Triamcinolone (Barbiturates enhance metabolism).
No products indexed under this heading.

Triamcinolone Acetonide (Barbiturates enhance metabolism). Products include:
Aristocort A 1010
Azmacort Inhaler 1837
Kenalog Cream, Lotion & Ointment 2401
Kenalog-10 Injection 2402
Kenalog-40 Injection 2403
Kenalog in Orabase 604
Kenalog Spray 2401
Mycolog II Cream and Ointment 2407
Mytrex Cream & Ointment 2080
Nasacort Nasal Inhaler 1844

Triamcinolone Diacetate (Barbiturates enhance metabolism). Products include:
Aristocort Suspension 1008

Triamcinolone Hexacetonide (Barbiturates enhance metabolism). Products include:
Aristospan Suspension 1011

Triazolam (Additive CNS depressant effects). Products include:
Halcion Tablets 2340

Trifluoperazine Hydrochloride (Additive CNS depressant effects). Products include:
Stelazine 2226

Valproic Acid (Decreases barbiturate metabolism). Products include:
Depakene Capsules & Syrup 511

Warfarin Sodium (Decreased anticoagulant response). Products include:
Coumadin Injection & Tablets 944
Panwarfin Tablets 547

NEMBUTAL SODIUM SUPPOSITORIES

(Pentobarbital Sodium) 538
May interact with central nervous system depressants, oral anticoagulants, corticosteroids, monoamine oxidase inhibitors, estrogens, and certain other agents. Compounds in these categories include:

Alfentanil Hydrochloride (Additive CNS depressant effects). Products include:
Alfenta Injection 1131

Alprazolam (Additive CNS depressant effects). Products include:
Xanax Tablets 2367

Aprobarbital (Additive CNS depressant effects). Products include:
Alurate Elixir 1883

Betamethasone Acetate (Barbiturates enhance metabolism). Products include:
Celestone Soluspan Suspension 2081

Betamethasone Sodium Phosphate (Barbiturates enhance metabolism). Products include:
Celestone Soluspan Suspension 2081

Buprenorphine (Additive CNS depressant effects).
No products indexed under this heading.

Buspirone Hydrochloride (Additive CNS depressant effects). Products include:
BuSpar 1401

Butabarbital (Additive CNS depressant effects). Products include:
Pyridium Plus 1764

Butalbital (Additive CNS depressant effects). Products include:
Esgic-Plus Tablets 1002
Esgic Tablets & Capsules 1001
Fioricet Tablets 2006
Fiorinal Capsules 2007
Fiorinal with Codeine Capsules 2008
Fiorinal Tablets 2007
Phrenilin 838
Sedapap Tablets 50 mg/650 mg 1360

Chlordiazepoxide (Additive CNS depressant effects). Products include:
Libritabs Tablets 1930

Limbitrol 1933
Menrium Tablets 1934

Chlordiazepoxide Hydrochloride (Additive CNS depressant effects). Products include:
Librax Capsules 1929
Librium Capsules 1931
Librium Injectable 1932

Chlorotrianisene (Decreased effects of estrogens). Products include:
TACE 12 and 25 mg 1353

Chlorpromazine (Additive CNS depressant effects). Products include:
Thorazine 2234

Chlorprothixene (Additive CNS depressant effects). Products include:
Taractan Tablets 1920

Chlorprothixene Hydrochloride (Additive CNS depressant effects). Products include:
Taractan 1920

Chlorprothixene Lactate (Additive CNS depressant effects). Products include:
Taractan Concentrate 1920

Clorazepate Dipotassium (Additive CNS depressant effects). Products include:
Tranxene 556

Codeine (Additive CNS depressant effects). Products include:
Calcidrine Syrup 506

Codeine Phosphate (Additive CNS depressant effects). Products include:
Actifed with Codeine Cough Syrup.. 752
Cheracol Cough Syrup 1853
Codimal PH Syrup 846
Dimetane-DC Cough Syrup 1857
Empirin with Codeine Phosphate Nos. 2, 3 & 4 764
Fiorinal with Codeine Capsules 2008
Isoclor Expectorant 982
Naldecon CX Adult Liquid .... ■ 521
Novahistine DH 1342
Novahistine Expectorant 1343
Nucofed Capsules 2219
Nucofed Expectorant 2219
Nucofed Pediatric Expectorant 2220
Nucofed Syrup 2219
Phenaphen with Codeine Capsules 1865
Phenaphen-650 with Codeine Tablets 1866
Phenergan with Codeine 2497
Phenergan VC with Codeine 2501
Robitussin A-C Syrup 1875
Robitussin-DAC Syrup 1875
Ryna .... ■ 741
Soma Compound w/Codeine Tablets 2390
Triaminic Expectorant w/Codeine .. 1996
Tussi-Organidin Liquid 2391
Tylenol with Codeine 1381

Codeine Polistirex (Additive CNS depressant effects).
No products indexed under this heading.

Cortisone Acetate (Barbiturates enhance metabolism). Products include:
Cortone Acetate Sterile Suspension 1437
Cortone Acetate Tablets 1439

Dexamethasone (Barbiturates enhance metabolism). Products include:
AK-Trol Ointment & Suspension .... ⊙ 207
Decadron Elixir 1445
Decadron Tablets 1447
Decaspray Topical Aerosol 1459
Dexacidin .... ⊙ 272
Maxidex Sterile Ophthalmic Suspension .... ⊙ 223
Maxitrol Ophthalmic Ointment/Suspension .... ⊙ 223
TobraDex Ophthalmic Suspension and Ointment .... ⊙ 228

Dexamethasone Acetate (Barbiturates enhance metabolism). Products include:
Dalalone D.P. Injectable 999
Decadron-LA Sterile Suspension 1457

Dexamethasone Sodium Phosphate (Barbiturates enhance metabolism). Products include:
AK-Dex .... ⊙ 203
Decadron Phosphate Respihaler 1454
Decadron Phosphate Sterile Ophthalmic Ointment 1453
Decadron Phosphate Sterile Ophthalmic Solution 1453
Decadron Phosphate Topical Cream 1455
Decadron Phosphate Turbinaire 1456
Maxidex Sterile Ophthalmic Ointment .... ⊙ 222
NeoDecadron Sterile Ophthalmic Ointment 1517
NeoDecadron Sterile Ophthalmic Solution 1518
NeoDecadron Topical Cream 1518

Dezocine (Additive CNS depressant effects).

Diazepam (Additive CNS depressant effects). Products include:
Valium Injectable 1937
Valium Tablets 1939
Valrelease Capsules 1923

Dicumarol (Decreased anticoagulant response). Products include:
Dicumarol Tablets 516

Dienestrol (Decreased effects of estrogens). Products include:
Ortho Dienestrol Cream 1664

Diethylstilbestrol (Decreased effects of estrogens). Products include:
Diethylstilbestrol Tablets 1258

Doxepin Hydrochloride (Phenobarbital shortens half-life). Products include:
Sinequan 1960

Doxycycline Hyclate (Barbiturates shorten half-life of doxycycline). Products include:
Doryx Capsules 1717
Vibramycin Hyclate Capsules 1787
Vibramycin Hyclate Intravenous 1968
Vibra-Tabs Film Coated Tablets 1787

Doxycycline Monohydrate (Barbiturates shorten half-life of doxycycline). Products include:
Monodox Capsules 1630
Vibramycin Monohydrate for Oral Suspension 1787

Droperidol (Additive CNS depressant effects). Products include:
Inapsine Injection 1140
Innovar Injection 1141

Enflurane (Additive CNS depressant effects). Products include:
Ethrane 599

Estazolam (Additive CNS depressant effects). Products include:
ProSom Tablets 554

Estradiol (Decreased effects of estrogens). Products include:
Emcyt Capsules 1161
Estrace 1385
Estrace Vaginal Cream 1388
Estraderm Transdermal System 866

Estrogens, Conjugated (Decreased effects of estrogens). Products include:
Mediatric Capsules 2476
PMB 200 and PMB 400 2504
Premarin Intravenous 2508
Premarin with Methyltestosterone .. 2515
Premarin Tablets 2510
Premarin Vaginal Cream 2512

Estrogens, Esterified (Decreased effects of estrogens). Products include:
Estratest 2245
Menrium Tablets 1934

Estropipate (Decreased effects of estrogens). Products include:
Ogen 540

Ethchlorvynol (Additive CNS depressant effects). Products include:
Placidyl Capsules 553

Ethinamate (Additive CNS depressant effects).
No products indexed under this heading.

Ethinyl Estradiol (Decreased effects of estrogens). Products include:
Brevicon 2304
Demulen 2161
Estinyl Tablets 2085
Jenest-28 Tablets 1636
Levlen/Tri-Levlen 665
Lo/Ovral Tablets 2471
Lo/Ovral-28 Tablets 2476
Loestrin 1728
Modicon 1667
Nordette-21 Tablets 2481
Nordette-28 Tablets 2483
Norethin 2133
Norinyl 2304
Norlestrin 1746
Ortho-Cyclen Tablets 1658
Ortho-Novum 1667
Ovcon 1391
Ovral Tablets 2490
Ovral-28 Tablets 2491
Levlen/Tri-Levlen 665
Tri-Norinyl 2304
Triphasil-21 Tablets 2527
Triphasil-28 Tablets 2532

Fentanyl (Additive CNS depressant effects). Products include:
Duragesic Transdermal System 1133

Fentanyl Citrate (Additive CNS depressant effects). Products include:
Innovar Injection 1141
Sublimaze Injection 1146

Fluphenazine Decanoate (Additive CNS depressant effects). Products include:
Prolixin Decanoate 1795

Fluphenazine Enanthate (Additive CNS depressant effects). Products include:
Prolixin Enanthate 1796

Fluphenazine Hydrochloride (Additive CNS depressant effects). Products include:
Prolixin Elixir 1793
Prolixin Injection 1791
Prolixin Oral Concentrate 1792
Prolixin Tablets 1793

Flurazepam Hydrochloride (Additive CNS depressant effects). Products include:
Dalmane Capsules 1927

Furazolidone (Prolongs effects of barbiturates). Products include:
Furoxone 1855

Glutethimide (Additive CNS depressant effects).
No products indexed under this heading.

Haloperidol (Additive CNS depressant effects). Products include:
Haldol Injection, Tablets and Concentrate 1373

Haloperidol Decanoate (Additive CNS depressant effects). Products include:
Haldol Decanoate 1375

Hydrocodone Bitartrate (Additive CNS depressant effects). Products include:
Anexsia 5/500 Tablets 2196
Anexsia 7.5/650 Tablets 2197
Azdōne Tablets 844
Codiclear DH Syrup 845
Codimal DH Syrup 846
Damason-P 1356
Hycodan Syrup, Tablets 927
Hycomine Compound Tablets 929
Hycomine Syrup 927
Hycotuss Expectorant Syrup 930
Hydrocet Capsules 835
Lortab ASA Tablets 2414
Lortab 2412
Ru-Tuss with Hydrocodone 694
Triaminic Expectorant DH 1995
Vicodin Tablets 1187
Vicodin ES Tablets 1189
Zydone Capsules 941

Hydrocodone Polistirex (Additive CNS depressant effects). Products include:
Tussionex Extended-Release Suspension 988

Hydrocortisone (Barbiturates enhance metabolism). Products include:
AK-Spore H.C. .... ⊙ 206
Bactine Hydrocortisone Anti-Itch Cream .... ■ 625
CaldeCORT Anti-Itch Hydrocortisone Spray .... ■ 560
Carmol HC Cream 1% 2296
Cortaid Spray .... ■ 735
Cortenema 2244
Cortisporin Ointment 758
Cortisporin Ophthalmic Ointment Sterile 758
Cortisporin Ophthalmic Suspension Sterile 759
Cortisporin Otic Solution Sterile 760
Cortisporin Otic Suspension Sterile 760
Cortizone-5 Creme & Ointment .... ■ 732
Dermolate Anti-Itch Cream .... ■ 697
Eldecort Cream 1.0% 1113
Eldecort Cream 1.0% and 2.5% 1113
Fungoid HC Creme 1770
Hydrocortone Tablets 1482
Hytone 909
LazerSporin-C Solution 1770
Massengill Medicated Soft Cloth Towelettes 2192
Nutracort Cream & Lotion 1684
PediOtic Suspension Sterile 797
Synacort Creams 1%, 2.5% 2296
Vanoxide-HC Acne Lotion 911
Vioform-Hydrocortisone Cream and Mild Cream 889
Vioform-Hydrocortisone Ointment.. 889
VōSoL HC Otic Solution 2392
Vytone Cream 1% 911

Hydrocortisone Acetate (Barbiturates enhance metabolism). Products include:
Analpram-HC Rectal Cream 1% and 2.5% 970
Anusol-HC Cream 1690
Anusol-HC Suppositories 1691
Caldecort .... ■ 560
Carmol HC Cream 1% 2296
Chloromycetin Hydrocortisone Ophthalmic 1694
Coly-Mycin S Otic w/Neomycin & Hydrocortisone 1708
Cortaid .... ■ 735
Cortef Feminine Itch Cream .... ■ 735
Corticaine .... ■ 682
Cortifoam 1827
Cortisporin Cream 757
Epifoam 1828
Gynecort 5 Creme .... ■ 556
Hydrocortone Acetate Sterile Suspension 1479
Lanacort 5 Creme and Ointment .. ■ 557
Mantadil Cream 789
Ophthocort .... ⊙ 301
Orabase HCA Oral Paste 890
Pramosone Cream, Lotion & Ointment 971
ProctoCream-HC 1834
Proctofoam-HC 1835

Hydrocortisone Sodium Phosphate (Barbiturates enhance metabolism). Products include:
Hydrocortone Phosphate Injection, Sterile 1481

Hydrocortisone Sodium Succinate (Barbiturates enhance metabolism). Products include:
Solu-Cortef Sterile Powder 2361

Hydroxyzine Hydrochloride (Additive CNS depressant effects). Products include:
Atarax Tablets & Syrup 1941
Marax Tablets & DF Syrup 1954
Vistaril Intramuscular Solution 1970

Isocarboxazid (Prolongs effects of barbiturates). Products include:
Marplan Tablets 1906

Isoflurane (Additive CNS depressant effects). Products include:
Forane 600
Ketamine Hydrochloride (Additive CNS depressant effects). Products include:
Ketalar 1726
Levorphanol Tartrate (Additive CNS depressant effects). Products include:
Levo-Dromoran 1906
Lorazepam (Additive CNS depressant effects). Products include:
Ativan Injection 2432
Ativan Tablets 2434
Loxapine Hydrochloride (Additive CNS depressant effects). Products include:
Loxitane 1213
Loxapine Succinate (Additive CNS depressant effects). Products include:
Loxitane Capsules 1213
Meperidine Hydrochloride (Additive CNS depressant effects). Products include:
Demerol 2047
Mepergan Injection 2479
Mephobarbital (Additive CNS depressant effects). Products include:
Mebaral Tablets 2061
Meprobamate (Additive CNS depressant effects). Products include:
Deprol Tablets 2382
Equagesic Tablets 2451
Miltown Tablets 2386
PMB 200 and PMB 400 2504
Mesoridazine (Additive CNS depressant effects). Products include:
Serentil 686
Methadone Hydrochloride (Additive CNS depressant effects). Products include:
Dolophine Hydrochloride Ampoules & Vials 1260
Dolophine Hydrochloride Tablets 1261
Methadone Hydrochloride Diskets 1284
Methadone Hydrochloride Oral Solution & Tablets 1987
Methohexital Sodium (Additive CNS depressant effects). Products include:
Brevital Sodium Vials 1248
Methoxyflurane (Additive CNS depressant effects).
No products indexed under this heading.
Methylprednisolone Acetate (Barbiturates enhance metabolism). Products include:
Depo-Medrol Sterile Aqueous Suspension 2334
Methylprednisolone Sodium Succinate (Barbiturates enhance metabolism). Products include:
Solu-Medrol Sterile Powder 2363
Midazolam Hydrochloride (Additive CNS depressant effects). Products include:
Versed Injection 1924
Molindone Hydrochloride (Additive CNS depressant effects). Products include:
Moban Tablets & Concentrate 932
Morphine Sulfate (Additive CNS depressant effects). Products include:
Astramorph/PF Injection, USP (Preservative-Free) 618
Duramorph 960
Infumorph 200 and Infumorph 500 Sterile Solutions 962
MS Contin Tablets 1814
MSIR 1817
Oramorph SR (Morphine Sulfate Sustained Release Tablets) 1988
Roxanol 1991
Opium Alkaloids (Additive CNS depressant effects). Products include:
B & O No. 15A & No. 16A Supprettes 2395
Pantopon Injectable 1911
Oxazepam (Additive CNS depressant effects). Products include:
Serax Capsules 2522
Serax Tablets 2522
Oxycodone Hydrochloride (Additive CNS depressant effects). Products include:
Percocet Tablets 950
Percodan 951
Roxicodone Tablets, Oral Solution & Intensol (Oxycodone) 1992
Tylox Capsules 1382
Perphenazine (Additive CNS depressant effects). Products include:
Etrafon 2087
Triavil Tablets 1556
Trilafon 2123
Phenelzine Sulfate (Prolongs effects of barbiturates). Products include:
Nardil 1742
Phenobarbital (Additive CNS depressant effects). Products include:
Arco-Lase Plus Tablets 607
Bellergal-S Tablets 1998
Bronkolixir ..... ⊞ 761
Bronkotabs Tablets ..... ⊞ 762
Donnatal 1858
Donnatal Extentabs 1859
Donnatal Tablets 1858
Donnazyme Tablets 1860
Kinesed Tablets 2272
Phenobarbital Elixir and Tablets 1293
Primatene Tablets-P Formula 2421
Quadrinal Tablets 1183
Tedral SA 1765
Phenytoin (Variable effect on metabolism of phenytoin). Products include:
Dilantin Infatabs 1710
Dilantin-30 Pediatric/Dilantin-125 Suspension 1713
Phenytoin Sodium (Variable effect on metabolism of phenytoin). Products include:
Dilantin Kapseals 1708
Dilantin Parenteral 1712
Dilantin with Phenobarbital Kapseals 1715
Polyestradiol Phosphate (Decreased effects of estrogens). Products include:
Estradurin 2452
Prazepam (Additive CNS depressant effects). Products include:
Centrax 1693
Prednisolone Acetate (Barbiturates enhance metabolism). Products include:
AK-Cide Sterile Ophthalmic Ointment & Suspension ..... ⊙ 202
Blephamide Liquifilm Sterile Ophthalmic Suspension 586
Blephamide S.O.P. Sterile Ophthalmic Ointment 586
Cetapred Ointment ..... ⊙ 220
⅛% Econopred & 1% Econopred Plus ..... ⊙ 217
Isopto Cetapred Suspension ..... ⊙ 220
Metimyd ..... ⊙ 306
Poly-Pred Liquifilm ..... ⊙ 250
Pred Forte ..... ⊙ 252
Pred Mild ..... ⊙ 254
Pred-G Liquifilm Sterile Ophthalmic Suspension ..... ⊙ 252
Pred-G S.O.P. Sterile Ophthalmic Ointment ..... ⊙ 253
Vasocidin Ointment ..... ⊙ 275
Prednisolone Sodium Phosphate (Barbiturates enhance metabolism). Products include:
AK-Pred ..... ⊙ 205
Hydeltrasol Injection, Sterile 1476
Inflamase ..... ⊙ 274
Pediapred Oral Liquid 987
Vasocidin Ophthalmic Solution ..... ⊙ 276
Prednisolone Tebutate (Barbiturates enhance metabolism). Products include:
Hydeltra-T.B.A. Sterile Suspension 1478
Prednisone (Barbiturates enhance metabolism). Products include:
Deltasone Tablets 2332
Prochlorperazine (Additive CNS depressant effects). Products include:
Compazine 2201
Promethazine Hydrochloride (Additive CNS depressant effects). Products include:
Mepergan Injection 2479
Phenergan with Codeine 2497
Phenergan with Dextromethorphan 2499
Phenergan Injection 2493
Phenergan Suppositories 2496
Phenergan Syrup 2495
Phenergan Tablets 2496
Phenergan VC 2500
Phenergan VC with Codeine 2501
Propofol (Additive CNS depressant effects). Products include:
Diprivan Injection 2267
Propoxyphene Hydrochloride (Additive CNS depressant effects). Products include:
Darvon 1256
Wygesic Tablets 2540
Propoxyphene Napsylate (Additive CNS depressant effects). Products include:
Darvon-N/Darvocet-N 1254
Quazepam (Additive CNS depressant effects). Products include:
Doral Tablets 2383
Quinestrol (Decreased effects of estrogens). Products include:
Estrovis 1721
Secobarbital Sodium (Additive CNS depressant effects). Products include:
Seconal Sodium Pulvules 1296
Selegiline Hydrochloride (Prolongs effects of barbiturates). Products include:
Eldepryl 2250
Sufentanil Citrate (Additive CNS depressant effects). Products include:
Sufenta Injection 1147
Temazepam (Additive CNS depressant effects). Products include:
Restoril Capsules 2023
Thiamylal Sodium (Additive CNS depressant effects). Products include:
Surital Ampoules, Steri-Vials 1764
Thioridazine Hydrochloride (Additive CNS depressant effects). Products include:
Mellaril 2011
Thiothixene (Additive CNS depressant effects). Products include:
Navane Capsules and Concentrate 1954
Navane Intramuscular 1956
Tranylcypromine Sulfate (Prolongs effects of barbiturates). Products include:
Parnate Tablets 2222
Triamcinolone (Barbiturates enhance metabolism).
No products indexed under this heading.
Triamcinolone Acetonide (Barbiturates enhance metabolism). Products include:
Aristocort A 1010
Azmacort Inhaler 1837
Kenalog Cream, Lotion & Ointment 2401
Kenalog-10 Injection 2402
Kenalog-40 Injection 2403
Kenalog in Orabase 604
Kenalog Spray 2401
Mycolog II Cream and Ointment 2407
Mytrex Cream & Ointment 2080
Nasacort Nasal Inhaler 1844
Triamcinolone Diacetate (Barbiturates enhance metabolism). Products include:
Aristocort Suspension 1008
Triamcinolone Hexacetonide (Barbiturates enhance metabolism). Products include:
Aristospan Suspension 1011
Triazolam (Additive CNS depressant effects). Products include:
Halcion Tablets 2340
Trifluoperazine Hydrochloride (Additive CNS depressant effects). Products include:
Stelazine 2226
Valproic Acid (Decreases barbiturates metabolism). Products include:
Depakene Capsules & Syrup 511
Warfarin Sodium (Increased metabolism, decreased anticoagulant response). Products include:
Coumadin Injection & Tablets 944
Panwarfin Tablets 547

NEO-CALGLUCON SYRUP
(Calcium Glubionate) 2018
May interact with corticosteroids and certain other agents. Compounds in these categories include:
Betamethasone Acetate (Interference with calcium absorption). Products include:
Celestone Soluspan Suspension 2081
Betamethasone Sodium Phosphate (Interference with calcium absorption). Products include:
Celestone Soluspan Suspension 2081
Cortisone Acetate (Interference with calcium absorption). Products include:
Cortone Acetate Sterile Suspension 1437
Cortone Acetate Tablets 1439
Dexamethasone (Interference with calcium absorption). Products include:
AK-Trol Ointment & Suspension ..... ⊙ 207
Decadron Elixir 1445
Decadron Tablets 1447
Decaspray Topical Aerosol 1459
Dexacidin ..... ⊙ 272
Maxidex Sterile Ophthalmic Suspension ..... ⊙ 223
Maxitrol Ophthalmic Ointment/Suspension ..... ⊙ 223
TobraDex Ophthalmic Suspension and Ointment ..... ⊙ 228
Dexamethasone Acetate (Interference with calcium absorption). Products include:
Dalalone D.P. Injectable 999
Decadron-LA Sterile Suspension 1457
Dexamethasone Sodium Phosphate (Interference with calcium absorption). Products include:
AK-Dex ..... ⊙ 203
Decadron Phosphate Respihaler 1454
Decadron Phosphate Sterile Ophthalmic Ointment 1453
Decadron Phosphate Sterile Ophthalmic Solution 1453
Decadron Phosphate Topical Cream 1455
Decadron Phosphate Turbinaire 1456
Maxidex Sterile Ophthalmic Ointment ..... ⊙ 222
NeoDecadron Sterile Ophthalmic Ointment 1517
NeoDecadron Sterile Ophthalmic Solution 1518
NeoDecadron Topical Cream 1518
Hydrocortisone (Interference with calcium absorption). Products include:
AK-Spore H.C. ..... ⊙ 206
Bactine Hydrocortisone Anti-Itch Cream ..... ⊞ 625
CaldeCORT Anti-Itch Hydrocortisone Spray ..... ⊞ 560
Carmol HC Cream 1% 2296
Cortaid Spray ..... ⊞ 735

Cortenema ... 2244
Cortisporin Ointment ... 758
Cortisporin Ophthalmic Ointment Sterile ... 758
Cortisporin Ophthalmic Suspension Sterile ... 759
Cortisporin Otic Solution Sterile ... 760
Cortisporin Otic Suspension Sterile 760
Cortizone-5 Creme & Ointment ... ▣ 732
Dermolate Anti-Itch Cream ... ▣ 697
Eldecort Cream 1.0% ... 1113
Eldecort Cream 1.0% and 2.5% ... 1113
Fungoid HC Creme ... 1770
Hydrocortone Tablets ... 1482
Hytone ... 909
LazerSporin-C Solution ... 1770
Massengill Medicated Soft Cloth Towelettes ... 2192
Nutracort Cream & Lotion ... 1684
PediOtic Suspension Sterile ... 797
Synacort Creams 1%, 2.5% ... 2296
Vanoxide-HC Acne Lotion ... 911
Vioform-Hydrocortisone Cream and Mild Cream ... 889
Vioform-Hydrocortisone Ointment ... 889
VōSoL HC Otic Solution ... 2392
Vytone Cream 1% ... 911

Hydrocortisone Acetate (Interference with calcium absorption). Products include:
Analpram-HC Rectal Cream 1% and 2.5% ... 970
Anusol-HC Cream ... 1690
Anusol-HC Suppositories ... 1691
Caldecort ... ▣ 560
Carmol HC Cream 1% ... 2296
Chloromycetin Hydrocortisone Ophthalmic ... 1694
Coly-Mycin S Otic w/Neomycin & Hydrocortisone ... 1708
Cortaid ... ▣ 735
Cortef Feminine Itch Cream ... ▣ 735
Corticaine ... ▣ 682
Cortifoam ... 1827
Cortisporin Cream ... 757
Epifoam ... 1828
Gynecort 5 Creme ... ▣ 556
Hydrocortone Acetate Sterile Suspension ... 1479
Lanacort 5 Creme and Ointment ... ▣ 557
Mantadil Cream ... 789
Ophthocort ... ◉ 301
Orabase HCA Oral Paste ... 890
Pramosone Cream, Lotion & Ointment ... 971
ProctoCream-HC ... 1834
Proctofoam-HC ... 1835

Hydrocortisone Sodium Phosphate (Interference with calcium absorption). Products include:
Hydrocortone Phosphate Injection, Sterile ... 1481

Hydrocortisone Sodium Succinate (Interference with calcium absorption). Products include:
Solu-Cortef Sterile Powder ... 2361

Methylprednisolone (Interference with calcium absorption). Products include:
Medrol ... 2348

Methylprednisolone Acetate (Interference with calcium absorption). Products include:
Depo-Medrol Sterile Aqueous Suspension ... 2334

Methylprednisolone Sodium Succinate (Interference with calcium absorption). Products include:
Solu-Medrol Sterile Powder ... 2363

Phosphorus Preparations (Interference with calcium absorption). Products include:
K-Phos M.F. Tablets ... 659
K-Phos Neutral Tablets ... 660
Neutra-Phos ... 2423

Prednisolone Acetate (Interference with calcium absorption). Products include:
AK-Cide Sterile Ophthalmic Ointment & Suspension ... ◉ 202
Blephamide Liquifilm Sterile Ophthalmic Suspension ... 586
Blephamide S.O.P. Sterile Ophthalmic Ointment ... 586
Cetapred Ointment ... ◉ 220
⅛% Econopred & 1% Econopred Plus ... ◉ 217
Isopto Cetapred Suspension ... ◉ 220
Metimyd ... ◉ 306
Poly-Pred Liquifilm ... ◉ 250
Pred Forte ... ◉ 252
Pred Mild ... ◉ 254
Pred-G Liquifilm Sterile Ophthalmic Suspension ... ◉ 252
Pred-G S.O.P. Sterile Ophthalmic Ointment ... ◉ 253
Vasocidin Ointment ... ◉ 275

Prednisolone Sodium Phosphate (Interference with calcium absorption). Products include:
AK-Pred ... ◉ 205
Hydeltrasol Injection, Sterile ... 1476
Inflamase ... ◉ 274
Pediapred Oral Liquid ... 987
Vasocidin Ophthalmic Solution ... ◉ 276

Prednisolone Tebutate (Interference with calcium absorption). Products include:
Hydeltra-T.B.A. Sterile Suspension 1478

Prednisone (Interference with calcium absorption). Products include:
Deltasone Tablets ... 2332

Triamcinolone (Interference with calcium absorption).
No products indexed under this heading.

Triamcinolone Acetonide (Interference with calcium absorption). Products include:
Aristocort A ... 1010
Azmacort Inhaler ... 1837
Kenalog Cream, Lotion & Ointment 2401
Kenalog-10 Injection ... 2402
Kenalog-40 Injection ... 2403
Kenalog in Orabase ... 604
Kenalog Spray ... 2401
Mycolog II Cream and Ointment ... 2407
Mytrex Cream & Ointment ... 2080
Nasacort Nasal Inhaler ... 1844

Triamcinolone Diacetate (Interference with calcium absorption). Products include:
Aristocort Suspension ... 1008

Triamcinolone Hexacetonide (Interference with calcium absorption). Products include:
Aristospan Suspension ... 1011

Food Interactions

Bran, unspecified (Large quantities of phytic acid found in bran interfere with absorption of calcium).

Cereals, whole (Large quantities of phytic acid found in whole cereals interfere with absorption of calcium).

Dairy products (Phosphorus from milk and other dairy products interferes with the absorption of calcium).

Rhubarb (Large quantities of oxalic acid found in rhubarb interfere with absorption of calcium).

Spinach (Large quantities of oxalic acid found in spinach interfere with absorption of calcium).

NEODECADRON STERILE OPHTHALMIC OINTMENT
(Neomycin Sulfate, Dexamethasone Sodium Phosphate) ... 1517
No interactions described in labeling.

NEODECADRON STERILE OPHTHALMIC SOLUTION
(Neomycin Sulfate, Dexamethasone Sodium Phosphate) ... 1518
No interactions described in labeling.

NEODECADRON TOPICAL CREAM
(Neomycin Sulfate, Dexamethasone Sodium Phosphate) ... 1518
No interactions described in labeling.

NEOLOID EMULSIFIED CASTOR OIL
(Castor Oil) ... 1226
No interactions described in labeling.

NEOSAR FOR INJECTION
(Cyclophosphamide) ... 566
May interact with cytotoxic drugs, general anesthetics, and certain other agents. Compounds in these categories include:

Bleomycin Sulfate (Administer cyclophosphamide cautiously). Products include:
Blenoxane ... 724

Daunorubicin Hydrochloride (Administer cyclophosphamide cautiously). Products include:
Cerubidine ... 2443

Doxorubicin Hydrochloride (Doxorubicin-induced cardiotoxicity potentiated). Products include:
Adriamycin PFS ... 561
Adriamycin RDF ... 562
Doxorubicin Hydrochloride for Injection, USP ... 622
Doxorubicin Hydrochloride Injection, USP ... 848
Rubex ... 739

Enflurane (Effect not specified). Products include:
Ethrane ... 599

Fluorouracil (Administer cyclophosphamide cautiously). Products include:
Efudex ... 1880
Fluoroplex Topical Solution & Cream 1% ... 1082
Fluorouracil Injection ... 1897

Hydroxyurea (Administer cyclophosphamide cautiously). Products include:
Hydrea Capsules ... 728

Isoflurane (Effect not specified). Products include:
Forane ... 600

Ketamine Hydrochloride (Effect not specified). Products include:
Ketalar ... 1726

Methohexital Sodium (Effect not specified). Products include:
Brevital Sodium Vials ... 1248

Methotrexate Sodium (Administer cyclophosphamide cautiously). Products include:
Methotrexate Tablets, Parenteral, LPF Parenteral ... 1217
Rheumatrex Methotrexate Dose Pack ... 1234

Methoxyflurane (Effect not specified).
No products indexed under this heading.

Mitotane (Administer cyclophosphamide cautiously). Products include:
Lysodren ... 731

Mitoxantrone Hydrochloride (Administer cyclophosphamide cautiously). Products include:
Novantrone for Injection Concentrate ... 1226

Phenobarbital (The rate of metabolism and the leukopenic activity are increased by chronic administration of high doses of phenobarbital). Products include:
Arco-Lase Plus Tablets ... 607
Bellergal-S Tablets ... 1998
Bronkolixir ... ▣ 761
Bronkotabs Tablets ... ▣ 762
Donnatal ... 1858
Donnatal Extentabs ... 1859
Donnatal Tablets ... 1858
Donnazyme Tablets ... 1860
Kinesed Tablets ... 2272
Phenobarbital Elixir and Tablets ... 1293
Primatene Tablets-P Formula ... 2421
Quadrinal Tablets ... 1183
Tedral SA ... 1765

Procarbazine Hydrochloride (Administer cyclophosphamide cautiously). Products include:
Matulane Capsules ... 1907

Propofol (Effect not specified). Products include:
Diprivan Injection ... 2267

Succinylcholine Chloride (Potentiation of succinylcholine effects). Products include:
Anectine ... 755

Tamoxifen Citrate (Administer cyclophosphamide cautiously). Products include:
Nolvadex Tablets ... 1102

Vincristine Sulfate (Administer cyclophosphamide cautiously). Products include:
Oncovin Solution Vials & Hyporets 1288

NEOSPORIN CREAM
(Polymyxin B Sulfate, Neomycin Sulfate) ... 792
No interactions described in labeling.

NEOSPORIN G.U. IRRIGANT STERILE
(Neomycin Sulfate, Polymyxin B Sulfate) ... 793
No interactions described in labeling.

NEOSPORIN OINTMENT
(Polymyxin B Sulfate, Bacitracin, Neomycin Sulfate) ... 793
No interactions described in labeling.

MAXIMUM STRENGTH NEOSPORIN OINTMENT
(Polymyxin B Sulfate, Bacitracin, Neomycin Sulfate) ... 793
No interactions described in labeling.

NEOSPORIN OPHTHALMIC OINTMENT STERILE
(Polymyxin B Sulfate, Bacitracin Zinc, Neomycin Sulfate) ... 793
No interactions described in labeling.

NEOSPORIN OPHTHALMIC SOLUTION STERILE
(Polymyxin B Sulfate, Neomycin Sulfate, Gramicidin) ... 794
No interactions described in labeling.

NEO-SYNALAR CREAM
(Neomycin Sulfate, Fluocinolone Acetonide) ... 2296
No interactions described in labeling.

NEO-SYNEPHRINE MAXIMUM STRENGTH 12 HOUR NASAL SPRAY
(Oxymetazoline Hydrochloride) ... ▣ 759
No interactions described in labeling.

NEO-SYNEPHRINE MAXIMUM STRENGTH 12 HOUR NASAL SPRAY PUMP
(Oxymetazoline Hydrochloride) ... ▣ 759
No interactions described in labeling.

NEO-SYNEPHRINE HYDROCHLORIDE 1% CARPUJECT
(Phenylephrine Hydrochloride) ... 2063
May interact with monoamine oxidase inhibitors, tricyclic antidepressants, oxytocic drugs, and certain other agents. Compounds in these categories include:

Amitriptyline Hydrochloride (Pressor response potentiated). Products include:
Elavil ... 2269
Endep Tablets ... 1927
Etrafon ... 2087
Limbitrol ... 1933

Triavil Tablets 1556

Amoxapine (Pressor response potentiated). Products include:

Asendin Tablets 1196

Clomipramine Hydrochloride (Pressor response potentiated). Products include:

Anafranil Capsules 650

Desipramine Hydrochloride (Pressor response potentiated). Products include:

Norpramin Tablets 1340

Doxepin Hydrochloride (Pressor response potentiated). Products include:

Sinequan 1960

Ergonovine Maleate (Potentiates pressor effect).

Furazolidone (Potentiates effect of sympathomimetic pressor amines). Products include:

Furoxone 1855

Halothane (May cause serious cardiac arrhythmias). Products include:

Fluothane 2453

Imipramine Hydrochloride (Pressor response potentiated). Products include:

Tofranil Ampuls 1038
Tofranil Tablets 1039

Imipramine Pamoate (Pressor response potentiated). Products include:

Tofranil-PM Capsules 1041

Isocarboxazid (Potentiates effect of sympathomimetic pressor amines). Products include:

Marplan Tablets 1906

Methylergonovine Maleate (Potentiates pressor effect). Products include:

Methergine 2016

Nortriptyline Hydrochloride (Pressor response potentiated). Products include:

Pamelor 2019

Oxytocin (Injection) (Potentiates pressor effect). Products include:

Oxytocin Injection 2492
Pitocin Injection, Ampoules, Steri-Dose Syringes 1757

Phenelzine Sulfate (Potentiates effect of sympathomimetic pressor amines). Products include:

Nardil 1742

Protriptyline Hydrochloride (Pressor response potentiated). Products include:

Vivactil Tablets 1567

Selegiline Hydrochloride (Potentiates effect of sympathomimetic pressor amines). Products include:

Eldepryl 2250

Tranylcypromine Sulfate (Potentiates effect of sympathomimetic pressor amines). Products include:

Parnate Tablets 2222

Trimipramine Maleate (Pressor response potentiated). Products include:

Surmontil Capsules 2524

NEO-SYNEPHRINE HYDROCHLORIDE 1% INJECTION
(Phenylephrine Hydrochloride) 2063
See **Neo-Synephrine Hydrochloride 1% Carpuject**

NEO-SYNEPHRINE HYDROCHLORIDE (OPHTHALMIC)
(Phenylephrine Hydrochloride) 2064
May interact with beta blockers, monoamine oxidase inhibitors, tricyclic antidepressants, inhalant anesthetics, and certain other agents. Compounds in these categories include:

Acebutolol Hydrochloride (Acute hypertension; ruptured congenital cerebral aneurysm may occur). Products include:

Sectral Capsules 2520

Amitriptyline Hydrochloride (Pressor response potentiated). Products include:

Elavil 2269
Endep Tablets 1927
Etrafon 2087
Limbitrol 1933
Triavil Tablets 1556

Amoxapine (Pressor response potentiated). Products include:

Asendin Tablets 1196

Atenolol (Acute hypertension; ruptured congenital cerebral aneurysm may occur). Products include:

Tenoretic Tablets 1105
Tenormin Tablets and I.V. Injection 1107

Betaxolol Hydrochloride (Acute hypertension; ruptured congenital cerebral aneurysm may occur). Products include:

Betoptic Sterile Ophthalmic Solution 569
Betoptic S Sterile Ophthalmic Suspension 570
Kerlone Tablets 2172

Carteolol Hydrochloride (Acute hypertension; ruptured congenital cerebral aneurysm may occur). Products include:

Cartrol Tablets 507

Clomipramine Hydrochloride (Pressor response potentiated). Products include:

Anafranil Capsules 650

Desipramine Hydrochloride (Pressor response potentiated). Products include:

Norpramin Tablets 1340

Doxepin Hydrochloride (Pressor response potentiated). Products include:

Sinequan 1960

Enflurane (Neo-Synephrine may potentiate the cardiovascular depressant effects of potent inhalation anesthetic agents). Products include:

Ethrane 599

Esmolol Hydrochloride (Acute hypertension; ruptured congenital cerebral aneurysm may occur). Products include:

Brevibloc Injection 942

Furazolidone (Exaggerated adrenergic effects may occur). Products include:

Furoxone 1855

Guanethidine Monosulfate (Pressor response potentiated). Products include:

Esimil Tablets 864
Ismelin Tablets 869

Halothane (Neo-Synephrine may potentiate the cardiovascular depressant effects of potent inhalation anesthetic agents). Products include:

Fluothane 2453

Imipramine Hydrochloride (Pressor response potentiated). Products include:

Tofranil Ampuls 1038
Tofranil Tablets 1039

Imipramine Pamoate (Pressor response potentiated). Products include:

Tofranil-PM Capsules 1041

Isocarboxazid (Exaggerated adrenergic effects may occur). Products include:

Marplan Tablets 1906

Isoflurane (Neo-Synephrine may potentiate the cardiovascular depressant effects of potent inhalation anesthetic agents). Products include:

Forane 600

Labetalol Hydrochloride (Acute hypertension; ruptured congenital cerebral aneurysm may occur). Products include:

Normodyne Injection 2108
Normodyne Tablets 2110
Normozide Tablets 2112
Trandate HCT Tablets 579
Trandate Injection 577
Trandate Tablets 579

Maprotiline Hydrochloride (Pressor response potentiated). Products include:

Ludiomil Tablets 874

Methoxyflurane (Neo-Synephrine may potentiate the cardiovascular depressant effects of potent inhalation anesthetic agents).

No products indexed under this heading.

Methyldopa (Pressor response potentiated). Products include:

Aldoclor Tablets 1413
Aldomet Oral 1415
Aldoril Tablets 1418

Methyldopate Hydrochloride (Pressor response potentiated). Products include:

Aldomet Ester HCl Injection 1417

Metoprolol Tartrate (Acute hypertension; ruptured congenital cerebral aneurysm may occur). Products include:

Lopressor Ampuls 1032
Lopressor HCT Tablets 1034
Lopressor Tablets 1032

Nadolol (Acute hypertension; ruptured congenital cerebral aneurysm may occur). Products include:

Corgard Tablets 701
Corzide Tablets 702

Nortriptyline Hydrochloride (Pressor response potentiated). Products include:

Pamelor 2019

Penbutolol Sulfate (Acute hypertension; ruptured congenital cerebral aneurysm may occur). Products include:

Levatol 1832

Phenelzine Sulfate (Exaggerated adrenergic effects may occur). Products include:

Nardil 1742

Pindolol (Acute hypertension; ruptured congenital cerebral aneurysm may occur). Products include:

Visken Tablets 2036

Propranolol Hydrochloride (Acute hypertension; ruptured congenital cerebral aneurysm may occur). Products include:

Inderal 2459
Inderal LA Long Acting Capsules 2461
Inderide Tablets 2463
Inderide LA Long Acting Capsules .. 2465

Protriptyline Hydrochloride (Pressor response potentiated). Products include:

Vivactil Tablets 1567

Selegiline Hydrochloride (Exaggerated adrenergic effects may occur). Products include:

Eldepryl 2250

Timolol Maleate (Acute hypertension; ruptured congenital cerebral aneurysm may occur). Products include:

Blocadren Tablets 1429
Timolide Tablets 1547
Timoptic in Ocudose 1552
Timoptic Sterile Ophthalmic Solution 1550

Tranylcypromine Sulfate (Exaggerated adrenergic effects may occur). Products include:

Parnate Tablets 2222

Trimipramine Maleate (Pressor response potentiated). Products include:

Surmontil Capsules 2524

NEO-SYNEPHRINE JELLY
(Phenylephrine Hydrochloride) .... ▣ 759
No interactions described in labeling.

NEO-SYNEPHRINE NASAL SPRAY (MENTHOLATED)
(Phenylephrine Hydrochloride) .... ▣ 759
No interactions described in labeling.

NEO-SYNEPHRINE NASAL SPRAYS
(Phenylephrine Hydrochloride) .... ▣ 759
No interactions described in labeling.

NEO-SYNEPHRINE NOSE DROPS
(Phenylephrine Hydrochloride) .... ▣ 759
No interactions described in labeling.

NEPHRO-CALCI TABLETS
(Calcium Carbonate) 1826
No interactions described in labeling.

NEPHROCAPS
(Vitamins A & D) 994
No interactions described in labeling.

NEPHRO-FER TABLETS
(Ferrous Fumarate) 1826
No interactions described in labeling.

NEPHRO-VITE RX
(Vitamins, Multiple) 1826
No interactions described in labeling.

NEPHROX SUSPENSION
(Aluminum Hydroxide Gel, Mineral Oil) .... ▣ 563
No interactions described in labeling.

NEPRO SPECIALIZED LIQUID NUTRITION
(Nutritional Supplement) 1972
No interactions described in labeling.

NEPTAZANE TABLETS
(Methazolamide) .... ⊙ 311
May interact with corticosteroids. Compounds in this category include:

Betamethasone Acetate (Potential for hypokalemic state). Products include:

Celestone Soluspan Suspension 2081

Betamethasone Sodium Phosphate (Potential for hypokalemic state). Products include:

Celestone Soluspan Suspension 2081

Cortisone Acetate (Potential for hypokalemic state). Products include:

Cortone Acetate Sterile Suspension 1437
Cortone Acetate Tablets 1439

Dexamethasone (Potential for hypokalemic state). Products include:

AK-Trol Ointment & Suspension .... ⊙ 207
Decadron Elixir 1445
Decadron Tablets 1447
Decaspray Topical Aerosol 1459
Dexacidin .... ⊙ 272
Maxidex Sterile Ophthalmic Suspension .... ⊙ 223
Maxitrol Ophthalmic Ointment/Suspension .... ⊙ 223
TobraDex Ophthalmic Suspension and Ointment .... ⊙ 228

Dexamethasone Acetate (Potential for hypokalemic state). Products include:
Dalalone D.P. Injectable 999
Decadron-LA Sterile Suspension 1457
Dexamethasone Sodium Phosphate (Potential for hypokalemic state). Products include:
AK-Dex ⊙ 203
Decadron Phosphate Respihaler 1454
Decadron Phosphate Sterile Ophthalmic Ointment 1453
Decadron Phosphate Sterile Ophthalmic Solution 1453
Decadron Phosphate Topical Cream 1455
Decadron Phosphate Turbinaire 1456
Maxidex Sterile Ophthalmic Ointment ⊙ 222
NeoDecadron Sterile Ophthalmic Ointment 1517
NeoDecadron Sterile Ophthalmic Solution 1518
NeoDecadron Topical Cream 1518
Hydrocortisone (Potential for hypokalemic state). Products include:
AK-Spore H.C. ⊙ 206
Bactine Hydrocortisone Anti-Itch Cream ◘ 625
CaldeCORT Anti-Itch Hydrocortisone Spray ◘ 560
Carmol HC Cream 1% 2296
Cortaid Spray ◘ 735
Cortenema 2244
Cortisporin Ointment 758
Cortisporin Ophthalmic Ointment Sterile 758
Cortisporin Ophthalmic Suspension Sterile 759
Cortisporin Otic Solution Sterile 760
Cortisporin Otic Suspension Sterile 760
Cortizone-5 Creme & Ointment ◘ 732
Dermolate Anti-Itch Cream ◘ 697
Eldecort Cream 1.0% 1113
Eldecort Cream 1.0% and 2.5% 1113
Fungoid HC Creme 1770
Hydrocortone Tablets 1482
Hytone 909
LazerSporin-C Solution 1770
Massengill Medicated Soft Cloth Towelettes 2192
Nutracort Cream & Lotion 1684
PediOtic Suspension Sterile 797
Synacort Creams 1%, 2.5% 2296
Vanoxide-HC Acne Lotion 911
Vioform-Hydrocortisone Cream and Mild Cream 889
Vioform-Hydrocortisone Ointment 889
VōSoL HC Otic Solution 2392
Vytone Cream 1% 911
Hydrocortisone Acetate (Potential for hypokalemic state). Products include:
Analpram-HC Rectal Cream 1% and 2.5% 970
Anusol-HC Cream 1690
Anusol-HC Suppositories 1691
Caldecort ◘ 560
Carmol HC Cream 1% 2296
Chloromycetin Hydrocortisone Ophthalmic 1694
Coly-Mycin S Otic w/Neomycin & Hydrocortisone 1708
Cortaid ◘ 735
Cortef Feminine Itch Cream ◘ 735
Corticaine ◘ 682
Cortifoam 1827
Cortisporin Cream 757
Epifoam 1828
Gynecort 5 Creme ◘ 556
Hydrocortone Acetate Sterile Suspension 1479
Lanacort 5 Creme and Ointment ◘ 557
Mantadil Cream 789
Ophthocort ⊙ 301
Orabase HCA Oral Paste 890
Pramosone Cream, Lotion & Ointment 971
ProctoCream-HC 1834
Proctofoam-HC 1835
Hydrocortisone Sodium Phosphate (Potential for hypokalemic state). Products include:
Hydrocortone Phosphate Injection, Sterile 1481
Hydrocortisone Sodium Succinate (Potential for hypokalemic state). Products include:
Solu-Cortef Sterile Powder 2361
Methylprednisolone Acetate (Potential for hypokalemic state). Products include:
Depo-Medrol Sterile Aqueous Suspension 2334
Methylprednisolone Sodium Succinate (Potential for hypokalemic state). Products include:
Solu-Medrol Sterile Powder 2363
Prednisolone Acetate (Potential for hypokalemic state). Products include:
AK-Cide Sterile Ophthalmic Ointment & Suspension ⊙ 202
Blephamide Liquifilm Sterile Ophthalmic Suspension 586
Blephamide S.O.P. Sterile Ophthalmic Ointment 586
Cetapred Ointment ⊙ 220
⅛% Econopred & 1% Econopred Plus ⊙ 217
Isopto Cetapred Suspension ⊙ 220
Metimyd ⊙ 306
Poly-Pred Liquifilm ⊙ 250
Pred Forte ⊙ 252
Pred Mild ⊙ 254
Pred-G Liquifilm Sterile Ophthalmic Suspension ⊙ 252
Pred-G S.O.P. Sterile Ophthalmic Ointment ⊙ 253
Vasocidin Ointment ⊙ 275
Prednisolone Sodium Phosphate (Potential for hypokalemic state). Products include:
AK-Pred ⊙ 205
Hydeltrasol Injection, Sterile 1476
Inflamase ⊙ 274
Pediapred Oral Liquid 987
Vasocidin Ophthalmic Solution ⊙ 276
Prednisolone Tebutate (Potential for hypokalemic state). Products include:
Hydeltra-T.B.A. Sterile Suspension 1478
Prednisone (Potential for hypokalemic state). Products include:
Deltasone Tablets 2332
Triamcinolone (Potential for hypokalemic state).
No products indexed under this heading.
Triamcinolone Acetonide (Potential for hypokalemic state). Products include:
Aristocort A 1010
Azmacort Inhaler 1837
Kenalog Cream, Lotion & Ointment 2401
Kenalog-10 Injection 2402
Kenalog-40 Injection 2403
Kenalog in Orabase 604
Kenalog Spray 2401
Mycolog II Cream and Ointment 2407
Mytrex Cream & Ointment 2080
Nasacort Nasal Inhaler 1844
Triamcinolone Diacetate (Potential for hypokalemic state). Products include:
Aristocort Suspension 1008
Triamcinolone Hexacetonide (Potential for hypokalemic state). Products include:
Aristospan Suspension 1011

NESACAINE INJECTIONS (Chloroprocaine Hydrochloride) 629
May interact with (with epinephrine solutions only), monoamine oxidase inhibitors, phenothiazines, sulfonamides, tricyclic antidepressants, vasopressors, and certain other agents. Compounds in these categories include:
Amitriptyline Hydrochloride (Severe, prolonged hypotension or hypertension). Products include:
Elavil 2269
Endep Tablets 1927
Etrafon 2087
Limbitrol 1933
Triavil Tablets 1556
Amoxapine (Severe, prolonged hypotension or hypertension). Products include:
Asendin Tablets 1196
Chlorpromazine (Severe, prolonged hypotension or hypertension). Products include:
Thorazine 2234
Clomipramine Hydrochloride (Severe, prolonged hypotension or hypertension). Products include:
Anafranil Capsules 650
Desipramine Hydrochloride (Severe, prolonged hypotension or hypertension). Products include:
Norpramin Tablets 1340
Dopamine Hydrochloride (Severe, persistent hypertension or cerebrovascular accidents). Products include:
Intropin Injection 930
Doxepin Hydrochloride (Severe, prolonged hypotension or hypertension). Products include:
Sinequan 1960
Epinephrine Bitartrate (Severe, persistent hypertension or cerebrovascular accidents). Products include:
AsthmaHaler Mist Epinephrine Bitartrate Bronchodilator ◘ 616
Bronkaid Mist Suspension ◘ 757
Primatene Mist Suspension 2421
Epinephrine Hydrochloride (Severe, persistent hypertension or cerebrovascular accidents). Products include:
Adrenalin Chloride Solution 1:100 & 1:1,000 1689
Epifrin ⊙ 244
Glaucon ⊙ 218
Ergonovine Maleate (Severe, persistent hypertension or cerebrovascular accidents).
Fluphenazine Decanoate (Severe, prolonged hypotension or hypertension). Products include:
Prolixin Decanoate 1795
Fluphenazine Enanthate (Severe, prolonged hypotension or hypertension). Products include:
Prolixin Enanthate 1796
Fluphenazine Hydrochloride (Severe, prolonged hypotension or hypertension). Products include:
Prolixin Elixir 1793
Prolixin Injection 1791
Prolixin Oral Concentrate 1792
Prolixin Tablets 1793
Furazolidone (Severe, prolonged hypotension or hypertension). Products include:
Furoxone 1855
Imipramine Hydrochloride (Severe, prolonged hypotension or hypertension). Products include:
Tofranil Ampuls 1038
Tofranil Tablets 1039
Imipramine Pamoate (Severe, prolonged hypotension or hypertension). Products include:
Tofranil-PM Capsules 1041
Isocarboxazid (Severe, prolonged hypotension or hypertension). Products include:
Marplan Tablets 1906
Maprotiline Hydrochloride (Severe, prolonged hypotension or hypertension). Products include:
Ludiomil Tablets 874
Mesoridazine (Severe, prolonged hypotension or hypertension). Products include:
Serentil 686
Metaraminol Bitartrate (Severe, persistent hypertension or cerebrovascular accidents). Products include:
Aramine Injection 1424
Methoxamine Hydrochloride (Severe, persistent hypertension or cerebrovascular accidents). Products include:
Vasoxyl Injection 819
Methyclothiazide (Action of sulfonamides inhibited). Products include:
Enduron Tablets 517
Enduronyl 518
Methylergonovine Maleate (Severe persistent hypertension or cerebrovascular accidents). Products include:
Methergine 2016
Norepinephrine Bitartrate (Severe, persistent hypertension or cerebrovascular accidents). Products include:
Levophed Bitartrate Injection 2054
Nortriptyline Hydrochloride (Severe, prolonged hypotension or hypertension). Products include:
Pamelor 2019
Perphenazine (Severe, prolonged hypotension or hypertension). Products include:
Etrafon 2087
Triavil Tablets 1556
Trilafon 2123
Phenelzine Sulfate (Severe, prolonged hypotension or hypertension). Products include:
Nardil 1742
Phenylephrine Hydrochloride (Severe, persistent hypertension or cerebrovascular accidents). Products include:
AK-Dilate Solution 2.5% and 10% ⊙ 203
Atrohist Sprinkle Capsules 558
Cerose-DM 2443
Codimal 846
Comhist LA Capsules 1618
Congespirin For Children Aspirin Free Chewable Cold Tablets 748
Cyclomydril ⊙ 216
Deconsal Sprinkle Capsules 559
Dimetane Decongestant ◘ 673
Dristan Decongestant/Antihistamine/ Analgesic Coated Caplets ◘ 749
Dristan Cold Nasal Decongestant/ Antihistamine/ Analgesic Coated Tablets 2419
Dristan Advanced Formula Decongestant/Antihistamine/ Analgesic Tablets ◘ 749
Dristan Nasal Spray, Menthol 2419
Dristan Nasal Spray, Regular and Regular with Metered Pump 2419
Entex Capsules 1623
Entex Liquid 1623
Sinus Excedrin Analgesic, Decongestant Tablets & Caplets 750
Extendryl 994
4-Way Fast Acting Nasal Spray - Original Formula (regular & mentholated) & Metered Spray Pump (regular) 751
Hycomine Compound Tablets 929
Murocoll-2 Sterile Ophthalmic Solution ⊙ 261
Mydfrin 2.5% ⊙ 224
Naldecon Syrup, Tablets, Pediatric Drops and Pediatric Syrup 709
Neo-Synephrine Hydrochloride 1% Carpuject 2063
Neo-Synephrine Hydrochloride 1% Injection 2063
Neo-Synephrine Hydrochloride (Ophthalmic) 2064
Neo-Synephrine ◘ 759
Nōstril Nasal Decongestant ◘ 520
Novahistine Elixir ◘ 596
Phenergan VC 2500
Phenergan VC with Codeine 2501
Prefrin Liquifilm Vasoconstrictor and Lubricant Eye Drops ⊙ 254
Prefrin-A ⊙ 255

Quelidrine Syrup 556
Relief Vasoconstrictor and Lubricant Eye Drops ..... ◉ 256
Robitussin Night Relief ..... ▣ 677
Ru-Tuss with Hydrocodone 694
Ru-Tuss Tablets 693
Vasosulf ..... ◉ 279
Vicks Sinex ..... ▣ 665
Zincfrin ..... ◉ 230

Prochlorperazine (Severe, prolonged hypotension or hypertension). Products include:
Compazine 2201

Promethazine Hydrochloride (Severe, prolonged hypotension or hypertension). Products include:
Mepergan Injection 2479
Phenergan with Codeine 2497
Phenergan with Dextromethorphan 2499
Phenergan Injection 2493
Phenergan Suppositories 2496
Phenergan Syrup 2495
Phenergan Tablets 2496
Phenergan VC 2500
Phenergan VC with Codeine 2501

Protriptyline Hydrochloride (Severe, prolonged hypotension or hypertension). Products include:
Vivactil Tablets 1567

Selegiline Hydrochloride (Severe, prolonged hypotension or hypertension). Products include:
Eldepryl 2250

Sulfamethizole (Action of sulfonamides inhibited). Products include:
Thiosulfil Forte Tablets 2526
Urobiotic-250 Capsules 1968

Sulfamethoxazole (Action of sulfonamides inhibited). Products include:
Azo Gantanol Tablets 1887
Bactrim DS Tablets 1891
Bactrim I.V. Infusion 1889
Bactrim 1891
Gantanol 1899
Septra 813
Septra I.V. Infusion 808
Septra I.V. Infusion ADD-Vantage Vials 810
Septra 813

Sulfasalazine (Action of sulfonamides inhibited). Products include:
Azulfidine Tablets, EN-tabs, Oral Suspension 1157

Sulfinpyrazone (Action of sulfonamides inhibited). Products include:
Anturane 853

Sulfisoxazole (Action of sulfonamides inhibited). Products include:
Azo Gantrisin Tablets 1888
Gantrisin Tablets 1901
Pediazole 1973

Sulfisoxazole Diolamine (Action of sulfonamides inhibited). Products include:
Gantrisin Ophthalmic Ointment/Solution 1900

Thioridazine Hydrochloride (Severe, prolonged hypotension or hypertension). Products include:
Mellaril 2011

Tranylcypromine Sulfate (Severe, prolonged hypotension or hypertension). Products include:
Parnate Tablets 2222

Trifluoperazine Hydrochloride (Severe, prolonged hypotension or hypertension). Products include:
Stelazine 2226

Trimipramine Maleate (Severe, prolonged hypotension or hypertension). Products include:
Surmontil Capsules 2524

NESACAINE-MPF INJECTION
(Chloroprocaine Hydrochloride) 629
See **Nesacaine Injections**

NESTABS FA TABLETS
(Vitamins with Minerals) 972
No interactions described in labeling.

NETROMYCIN INJECTION 100 MG/ML
(Netilmicin Sulfate) 2104
May interact with nondepolarizing neuromuscular blocking agents, diuretics, cephalosporins, penicillins, and certain other agents. Compounds in these categories include:

Acyclovir (Neurotoxicity and/or nephrotoxicity). Products include:
Zovirax Capsules 824
Zovirax Ointment 5% 827
Zovirax 824

Acyclovir Sodium (Neurotoxicity and/or nephrotoxicity). Products include:
Zovirax Sterile Powder 828

Amikacin Sulfate (Neurotoxicity and/or nephrotoxicity). Products include:
Amikin Injectable 602

Amiloride Hydrochloride (Ototoxicity). Products include:
Midamor Tablets 1508
Moduretic Tablets 1510

Amoxicillin (Mutual inactivation). Products include:
Amoxil 2193
Augmentin Tablets, Powder for Oral Suspension, and Chewable Tablets 2198

Amphotericin B (Neurotoxicity and/or nephrotoxicity). Products include:
Fungizone Cream, Lotion and Ointment 2261
Fungizone Intravenous 2262

Ampicillin Sodium (Mutual inactivation). Products include:
Unasyn 1965

Atracurium Besylate (Potential for increased neuromuscular blockade and respiratory paralysis). Products include:
Tracrium Injection 817

Azlocillin Sodium (Mutual inactivation).
No products indexed under this heading.

Bacampicillin Hydrochloride (Mutual inactivation). Products include:
Spectrobid Tablets & Powder for Oral Suspension 1961

Bacitracin (Neurotoxicity and/or nephrotoxicity). Products include:
Baciguent Antibiotic Ointment ..... ▣ 735
Bactine First Aid Antibiotic Ointment ..... ▣ 625
Campho-Phenique Triple Antibiotic Ointment Plus Pain Reliever ▣ 758
Lanabiotic Ointment ..... ▣ 556
Mycitracin ..... ▣ 737

Bacitracin Zinc (Neurotoxicity and/or nephrotoxicity). Products include:
AK-Poly-Bac Ointment ..... ◉ 205
AK-Spore H.C. Ointment ..... ◉ 206
AK-Spore Ointment ..... ◉ 205
Aquaphor Antibiotic Formula 662
Cortisporin Ointment 758
Cortisporin Ophthalmic Ointment Sterile 758
Neosporin Ointment 793
Maximum Strength Neosporin Ointment 793
Neosporin Ophthalmic Ointment Sterile 793
Polysporin Ointment ..... ▣ 543
Polysporin Ophthalmic Ointment Sterile 798
Polysporin Powder ..... ▣ 543
Polysporin Spray ..... ▣ 543

Bendroflumethiazide (Ototoxicity). Products include:
Corzide Tablets 702
Naturetin Tablets 1789
Rauzide Tablets 1804

Bumetanide (Ototoxicity). Products include:
Bumex 1895

Carbenicillin Disodium (Mutual inactivation).

Carbenicillin Indanyl Sodium (Mutual inactivation). Products include:
Geocillin Tablets 1951

Cefaclor (Nephrotoxicity). Products include:
Ceclor Pulvules & Suspension 1251

Cefadroxil Monohydrate (Nephrotoxicity). Products include:
Duricef 1405
Ultracef Capsules, Tablets & Oral Suspension 722

Cefamandole Nafate (Nephrotoxicity). Products include:
Mandol Vials, Faspak & ADD-Vantage 1281

Cefazolin Sodium (Nephrotoxicity). Products include:
Ancef Injection 2194
Kefzol Vials, Faspak & ADD-Vantage 1279

Cefixime (Nephrotoxicity). Products include:
Suprax 1235

Cefmetazole Sodium (Nephrotoxicity). Products include:
Zefazone Sterile Powder 2372

Cefonicid Sodium (Nephrotoxicity). Products include:
Monocid Injection 2217

Cefoperazone Sodium (Nephrotoxicity). Products include:
Cefobid Intravenous/Intramuscular 1943
Cefobid Pharmacy Bulk Package - Not for Direct Infusion 1945

Ceforanide (Nephrotoxicity).
No products indexed under this heading.

Cefotaxime Sodium (Nephrotoxicity). Products include:
Claforan Sterile Injection 1089

Cefotetan (Nephrotoxicity). Products include:
Cefotan 2265

Cefoxitin Sodium (Nephrotoxicity). Products include:
Mefoxin 1498
Mefoxin Premixed Intravenous Solution 1500

Ceftazidime (Nephrotoxicity). Products include:
Ceptaz for Injection 1057
Fortaz 1060
Tazicef for Injection 2231
Tazidime Vials, Faspak & ADD-Vantage 1299

Ceftizoxime Sodium (Nephrotoxicity). Products include:
Cefizox Injection 1012

Ceftriaxone Sodium (Nephrotoxicity). Products include:
Rocephin Injectable Vials, ADD-Vantage 1914

Cefuroxime Axetil (Nephrotoxicity). Products include:
Ceftin Tablets 575

Cefuroxime Sodium (Nephrotoxicity). Products include:
Kefurox Vials, Faspak & ADD-Vantage 1277
Zinacef 1066

Cephalexin (Nephrotoxicity). Products include:
Keflex Pulvules, Oral Suspension & Pediatric Drops 916

Cephalothin Sodium (Nephrotoxicity).

Cephapirin Sodium (Nephrotoxicity).
No products indexed under this heading.

Cephradine (Nephrotoxicity). Products include:
Velosef Capsules and for Oral Suspension 606

Chlorothiazide (Ototoxicity). Products include:
Aldoclor Tablets 1413
Diupres Tablets 1461
Diuril Oral 1464

Chlorothiazide Sodium (Ototoxicity). Products include:
Diuril Sodium Intravenous 1463

Chlorthalidone (Ototoxicity). Products include:
Combipres Tablets 678
Tenoretic Tablets 1105
Thalitone Tablets 687

Cisplatin (Neurotoxicity and/or nephrotoxicity). Products include:
Platinol 737
Platinol-AQ Injection 738

Colistin Sulfate (Neurotoxicity and/or nephrotoxicity). Products include:
Coly-Mycin S For Oral Suspension .. 1708
Coly-Mycin S Otic w/Neomycin & Hydrocortisone 1708

Decamethonium (Potential for increased neuromuscular blockade and respiratory paralysis).

Ethacrynic Acid (Ototoxicity). Products include:
Edecrin Tablets 1468

Furosemide (Ototoxicity). Products include:
Lasix 1093

Gentamicin (Neurotoxicity and/or nephrotoxicity).
No products indexed under this heading.

Gentamicin Sulfate (Neurotoxicity and/or nephrotoxicity). Products include:
Garamycin Injectable 2093
Garamycin Ophthalmic ..... ◉ 305
Genoptic Liquifilm Sterile Ophthalmic Solution ..... ◉ 247
Genoptic S.O.P. Sterile Ophthalmic Ointment ..... ◉ 247
Gentacidin Ointment ..... ◉ 273
Gentacidin Solution ..... ◉ 273
Gentak Ointment & Solution ..... ◉ 208
G-myticin Creme and Ointment 0.1% 1770
Pred-G Liquifilm Sterile Ophthalmic Suspension ..... ◉ 252
Pred-G S.O.P. Sterile Ophthalmic Ointment ..... ◉ 253

Hydrochlorothiazide (Ototoxicity). Products include:
Aldactazide 2150
Aldoril Tablets 1418
Apresazide Capsules 854
Apresoline-Esidrix Tablets 857
Capozide 2258
Dyazide Capsules 2208
Esidrix Tablets 863
Esimil Tablets 864
HydroDIURIL Tablets 1484
Hydropres Tablets 1485
Inderide Tablets 2463
Inderide LA Long Acting Capsules .. 2465
Lopressor HCT Tablets 1034
Maxzide 1215
Moduretic Tablets 1510
Normozide Tablets 2112
Oretic Tablets 544
Oreticyl 545
Prinzide Tablets 1540
Ser-Ap-Es Tablets 881
Serpasil-Esidrix Tablets 886
Timolide Tablets 1547
Trandate HCT Tablets 579
Vaseretic Tablets 1559
Zestoretic 2274

Hydroflumethiazide (Ototoxicity). Products include:
Diucardin Tablets 2450
Saluron 718
Salutensin/Salutensin-Demi 719

Indapamide (Ototoxicity). Products include:
Lozol Tablets 1843

Kanamycin Sulfate (Neurotoxicity and/or nephrotoxicity). Products include:
- Kantrex Injection ... 601
- Kantrex Pediatric Injection ... 601

Methyclothiazide (Ototoxicity). Products include:
- Enduron Tablets ... 517
- Enduronyl ... 518

Metocurine Iodide (Potential for increased neuromuscular blockade and respiratory paralysis). Products include:
- Metubine Iodide Vials ... 1285

Metolazone (Ototoxicity). Products include:
- Diulo ... 2129
- Mykrox ½ mg Tablets ... 984
- Zaroxolyn Tablets ... 989

Mezlocillin Sodium (Mutual inactivation). Products include:
- Mezlin ... 1597
- Mezlin Pharmacy Bulk Package ... 1599

Nafcillin Sodium (Mutual inactivation). Products include:
- Unipen ... 2533

Neomycin Sulfate (Neurotoxicity and/or nephrotoxicity). Products include:
- AK-Spore H.C. ... ⊙ 206
- AK-Spore ... ⊙ 205
- AK-Trol Ointment & Suspension ... ⊙ 207
- Bactine First Aid Antibiotic Ointment ... ▣ 625
- Campho-Phenique Triple Antibiotic Ointment Plus Pain Reliever ▣ 758
- Coly-Mycin S Otic w/Neomycin & Hydrocortisone ... 1708
- Cortisporin Cream ... 757
- Cortisporin Ointment ... 758
- Cortisporin Ophthalmic Ointment Sterile ... 758
- Cortisporin Ophthalmic Suspension Sterile ... 759
- Cortisporin Otic Solution Sterile ... 760
- Cortisporin Otic Suspension Sterile 760
- Dexacidin ... ⊙ 272
- Lanabiotic Ointment ... ▣ 556
- LazerSporin-C Solution ... 1770
- Maxitrol Ophthalmic Ointment/Suspension ... ⊙ 223
- Myciguent Antibiotic Ointment ... ▣ 737
- Mycitracin ... ▣ 737
- NeoDecadron Sterile Ophthalmic Ointment ... 1517
- NeoDecadron Sterile Ophthalmic Solution ... 1518
- NeoDecadron Topical Cream ... 1518
- Neosporin Cream ... 792
- Neosporin G.U. Irrigant Sterile ... 793
- Neosporin Ointment ... 793
- Maximum Strength Neosporin Ointment ... 793
- Neosporin Ophthalmic Ointment Sterile ... 793
- Neosporin Ophthalmic Solution Sterile ... 794
- Neo-Synalar Cream ... 2296
- PediOtic Suspension Sterile ... 797
- Poly-Pred Liquifilm ... ⊙ 250

Pancuronium Bromide Injection (Potential for increased neuromuscular blockade and respiratory paralysis).
- No products indexed under this heading.

Paromomycin Sulfate (Neurotoxicity and/or nephrotoxicity). Products include:
- Humatin Capsules ... 1726

Penicillin G Potassium (Mutual inactivation). Products include:
- Pfizerpen for Injection ... 1957

Penicillin G Procaine (Mutual inactivation). Products include:
- Bicillin C-R Injection ... 2438
- Bicillin C-R 900/300 Injection ... 2440
- Pfizerpen-AS Aqueous Suspension 1959
- Wycillin Injection ... 2537
- Wycillin Injection and Probenecid Tablets ... 2539

Penicillin G Sodium (Mutual inactivation).
- No products indexed under this heading.

Penicillin G, Benzathine (Mutual inactivation). Products include:
- Bicillin C-R Injection ... 2438
- Bicillin C-R 900/300 Injection ... 2440
- Bicillin L-A Injection ... 2442

Penicillin (Repository) (Mutual inactivation). Products include:
- Bicillin C-R Injection ... 2438
- Bicillin C-R 900/300 Injection ... 2440
- Bicillin L-A Injection ... 2442

Penicillin V Potassium (Mutual inactivation).
- No products indexed under this heading.

Polymyxin B Sulfate (Neurotoxicity and/or nephrotoxicity). Products include:
- AK-Poly-Bac Ointment ... ⊙ 205
- AK-Spore H.C. ... ⊙ 206
- AK-Spore ... ⊙ 205
- AK-Trol Ointment & Suspension ... ⊙ 207
- Aquaphor Antibiotic Formula ... 662
- Bactine First Aid Antibiotic Ointment ... ▣ 625
- Campho-Phenique Triple Antibiotic Ointment Plus Pain Reliever ▣ 758
- Cortisporin Cream ... 757
- Cortisporin Ointment ... 758
- Cortisporin Ophthalmic Ointment Sterile ... 758
- Cortisporin Ophthalmic Suspension Sterile ... 759
- Cortisporin Otic Solution Sterile ... 760
- Cortisporin Otic Suspension Sterile 760
- Dexacidin ... ⊙ 272
- Lanabiotic Ointment ... ▣ 556
- LazerSporin-C Solution ... 1770
- Maxitrol Ophthalmic Ointment/Suspension ... ⊙ 223
- Mycitracin ... ▣ 737
- Neosporin Cream ... 792
- Neosporin G.U. Irrigant Sterile ... 793
- Neosporin Ointment ... 793
- Maximum Strength Neosporin Ointment ... 793
- Neosporin Ophthalmic Ointment Sterile ... 793
- Neosporin Ophthalmic Solution Sterile ... 794
- Ophthocort ... ⊙ 301
- PediOtic Suspension Sterile ... 797
- Polymyxin B Sulfate, Aerosporin Brand Sterile Powder ... 798
- Poly-Pred Liquifilm ... ⊙ 250
- Polysporin Ointment ... ▣ 543
- Polysporin Ophthalmic Ointment Sterile ... 798
- Polysporin Powder ... ▣ 543
- Polysporin Spray ... ▣ 543
- Polytrim Ophthalmic Solution Sterile ... 588
- Terramycin with Polymyxin B Sulfate Ophthalmic Ointment ... 1965

Polythiazide (Ototoxicity). Products include:
- Minizide Capsules ... 1779
- Renese Tablets ... 1785
- Renese-R Tablets ... 1786

Spironolactone (Ototoxicity). Products include:
- Aldactazide ... 2150
- Aldactone ... 2152

Streptomycin Sulfate (Neurotoxicity and/or nephrotoxicity).
- No products indexed under this heading.

Succinylcholine Chloride (Potential for increased neuromuscular blockade and respiratory paralysis). Products include:
- Anectine ... 755

Ticarcillin Disodium (Mutual inactivation). Products include:
- Ticar for Injection ... 2236
- Timentin for Injection ... 2239

Tobramycin (Toxicity). Products include:
- TobraDex Ophthalmic Suspension and Ointment ... ⊙ 228
- Tobrex Ophthalmic Ointment and Solution ... 572

Tobramycin Sulfate (Toxicity). Products include:
- Nebcin Vials, Hyporets & ADD-Vantage ... 1286

Triamterene (Ototoxicity). Products include:
- Dyazide Capsules ... 2208
- Dyrenium Capsules ... 2210
- Maxzide ... 1215

Vancomycin Hydrochloride (Toxicity). Products include:
- Vancocin HCl, Oral Solution & Pulvules ... 1304
- Vancocin HCl, Vials & ADD-Vantage ... 1302

Vecuronium Bromide (Potential for increased neuromuscular blockade and respiratory paralysis). Products include:
- Norcuron ... 1642

NEUPOGEN FOR INJECTION
(Filgrastim) ... 595
No interactions described in labeling.

NEUTRA-PHOS POWDER, PACKETS & CAPSULES
(Phosphorus Preparations) ... 2423
No interactions described in labeling.

NEUTRA-PHOS-K POWDER, PACKETS & CAPSULES
(Phosphorus Preparations) ... 2423
No interactions described in labeling.

NEUTROGENA CLEANSING WASH
(Cleanser) ... ▣ 630
No interactions described in labeling.

NEUTROGENA MELANEX TOPICAL SOLUTION
(Hydroquinone) ... 1618
May interact with:

Hydrogen Peroxide (Concurrent use may result in transient dark staining of skin areas so treated).

NEUTROGENA MOISTURE
(Octyl Methoxycinnamate) ... ▣ 630
No interactions described in labeling.

NEUTROGENA MOISTURE SPF 15 UNTINTED
(Octyl Methoxycinnamate, Benzophenone-3) ... ▣ 630
No interactions described in labeling.

NEUTROGENA MOISTURE SPF 15 WITH SHEER TINT
(Octyl Methoxycinnamate, Benzophenone-3) ... ▣ 630
No interactions described in labeling.

NEUTROGENA SUNBLOCK
(Octyl Methoxycinnamate, Benzophenone-3) ... ▣ 630
No interactions described in labeling.

NIACOR TABLETS
(Niacin) ... 2376
May interact with oral hypoglycemic agents and antihypertensives. Compounds in these categories include:

Acebutolol Hydrochloride (Additive vasodilating effect and potential for postural hypotension). Products include:
- Sectral Capsules ... 2520

Atenolol (Additive vasodilating effect and potential for postural hypotension). Products include:
- Tenoretic Tablets ... 1105
- Tenormin Tablets and I.V. Injection 1107

Benazepril Hydrochloride (Additive vasodilating effect and potential for postural hypotension). Products include:
- Lotensin Tablets ... 872

Betaxolol Hydrochloride (Additive vasodilating effect and potential for postural hypotension). Products include:
- Betoptic Sterile Ophthalmic Solution ... 569
- Betoptic S Sterile Ophthalmic Suspension ... 570
- Kerlone Tablets ... 2172

Captopril (Additive vasodilating effect and potential for postural hypotension). Products include:
- Capoten ... 2255
- Capozide ... 2258

Carteolol Hydrochloride (Additive vasodilating effect and potential for postural hypotension). Products include:
- Cartrol Tablets ... 507

Chlorpropamide (Decreased glucose tolerance; adjustment of hypoglycemic therapy may be necessary). Products include:
- Diabinese Tablets ... 1775

Clonidine (Additive vasodilating effect and potential for postural hypotension). Products include:
- Catapres-TTS ... 677

Clonidine Hydrochloride (Additive vasodilating effect and potential for postural hypotension). Products include:
- Catapres Tablets ... 676
- Combipres Tablets ... 678

Deserpidine (Additive vasodilating effect and potential for postural hypotension). Products include:
- Enduronyl ... 518
- Harmonyl Tablets ... 528
- Oreticyl ... 545

Diazoxide (Additive vasodilating effect and potential for postural hypotension). Products include:
- Hyperstat I.V. Injection ... 2095
- Proglycem ... 649

Doxazosin Mesylate (Additive vasodilating effect and potential for postural hypotension). Products include:
- Cardura Tablets ... 1941

Enalapril Maleate (Additive vasodilating effect and potential for postural hypotension). Products include:
- Vaseretic Tablets ... 1559
- Vasotec Tablets ... 1564

Enalaprilat (Additive vasodilating effect and potential for postural hypotension). Products include:
- Vasotec I.V. ... 1562

Esmolol Hydrochloride (Additive vasodilating effect and potential for postural hypotension). Products include:
- Brevibloc Injection ... 942

Felodipine (Additive vasodilating effect and potential for postural hypotension). Products include:
- Plendil Extended-Release Tablets ... 1526

Fosinopril Sodium (Additive vasodilating effect and potential for postural hypotension). Products include:
- Monopril Tablets ... 1406

Glipizide (Decreased glucose tolerance; adjustment of hypoglycemic therapy may be necessary). Products include:
- Glucotrol ... 1952

Glyburide (Decreased glucose tolerance; adjustment of hypoglycemic therapy may be necessary). Products include:
- DiaBeta ... 1091
- Micronase Tablets ... 2350

Guanabenz Acetate (Additive vasodilating effect and potential for postural hypotension). Products include:
- Wytensin Tablets 2542

Guanethidine Monosulfate (Additive vasodilating effect and potential for postural hypotension). Products include:
- Esimil Tablets 864
- Ismelin Tablets 869

Hydralazine Hydrochloride (Additive vasodilating effect and potential for postural hypotension). Products include:
- Apresazide Capsules 854
- Apresoline Hydrochloride Parenteral (Ampuls) 856
- Apresoline Hydrochloride Tablets .. 855
- Apresoline-Esidrix Tablets 857
- Ser-Ap-Es Tablets 881
- Serpasil-Apresoline Tablets 884

Isradipine (Additive vasodilating effect and potential for postural hypotension). Products include:
- DynaCirc Capsules 2004

Labetalol Hydrochloride (Additive vasodilating effect and potential for postural hypotension). Products include:
- Normodyne Injection 2108
- Normodyne Tablets 2110
- Normozide Tablets 2112
- Trandate HCT Tablets 579
- Trandate Injection 577
- Trandate Tablets 579

Lisinopril (Additive vasodilating effect and potential for postural hypotension). Products include:
- Prinivil Tablets 1538
- Prinzide Tablets 1540
- Zestoretic 2274
- Zestril Tablets 2277

Mecamylamine Hydrochloride (Additive vasodilating effect and potential for postural hypotension). Products include:
- Inversine Tablets 1492

Methyldopa (Additive vasodilating effect and potential for postural hypotension). Products include:
- Aldoclor Tablets 1413
- Aldomet Oral 1415
- Aldoril Tablets 1418

Methyldopate Hydrochloride (Additive vasodilating effect and potential for postural hypotension). Products include:
- Aldomet Ester HCl Injection 1417

Metoprolol Tartrate (Additive vasodilating effect and potential for postural hypotension). Products include:
- Lopressor Ampuls 1032
- Lopressor HCT Tablets 1034
- Lopressor Tablets 1032

Metyrosine (Additive vasodilating effect and potential for postural hypotension). Products include:
- Demser Capsules 1460

Minoxidil (Additive vasodilating effect and potential for postural hypotension). Products include:
- Loniten Tablets 2346
- Rogaine Topical Solution 2357

Nadolol (Additive vasodilating effect and potential for postural hypotension). Products include:
- Corgard Tablets 701
- Corzide Tablets 702

Nicardipine Hydrochloride (Additive vasodilating effect and potential for postural hypotension). Products include:
- Cardene Capsules 2290

Nitroglycerin (Additive vasodilating effect and potential for postural hypotension). Products include:
- Deponit NTG Transdermal Delivery System 2143
- Minitran Transdermal Delivery System 1312
- Nitro-Bid Ointment 1339
- Nitro-Bid Capsules 1338
- Nitrodisc 2176
- Nitro-Dur (nitroglycerin) Transdermal Infusion System 1164
- Nitrogard Tablets 1004
- Nitrolingual Spray 1846
- Nitrostat Tablets 1743
- Transderm-Nitro Transdermal Therapeutic System 2283

Penbutolol Sulfate (Additive vasodilating effect and potential for postural hypotension). Products include:
- Levatol 1832

Phenoxybenzamine Hydrochloride (Additive vasodilating effect and potential for postural hypotension). Products include:
- Dibenzyline Capsules 2207

Phentolamine Mesylate (Additive vasodilating effect and potential for postural hypotension). Products include:
- Regitine 878

Pindolol (Additive vasodilating effect and potential for postural hypotension). Products include:
- Visken Tablets 2036

Prazosin Hydrochloride (Additive vasodilating effect and potential for postural hypotension). Products include:
- Minipress Capsules 1778
- Minizide Capsules 1779

Propranolol Hydrochloride (Additive vasodilating effect and potential for postural hypotension). Products include:
- Inderal 2459
- Inderal LA Long Acting Capsules 2461
- Inderide Tablets 2463
- Inderide LA Long Acting Capsules .. 2465

Ramipril (Additive vasodilating effect and potential for postural hypotension). Products include:
- Altace Capsules 1086

Rauwolfia Serpentina (Additive vasodilating effect and potential for postural hypotension). Products include:
- Raudixin Tablets 1803
- Rauzide Tablets 1804

Rescinnamine (Additive vasodilating effect and potential for postural hypotension).
- No products indexed under this heading.

Reserpine (Additive vasodilating effect and potential for postural hypotension). Products include:
- Diupres Tablets 1461
- Hydromox R Tablets 1209
- Hydropres Tablets 1485
- Renese-R Tablets 1786
- Salutensin/Salutensin-Demi 719
- Ser-Ap-Es Tablets 881
- Serpasil Tablets 883
- Serpasil-Apresoline Tablets 884
- Serpasil-Esidrix Tablets 886

Sodium Nitroprusside (Additive vasodilating effect and potential for postural hypotension). Products include:
- Nipride I.V. Infusion 1909

Terazosin Hydrochloride (Additive vasodilating effect and potential for postural hypotension). Products include:
- Hytrin Tablets 529

Timolol Maleate (Additive vasodilating effect and potential for postural hypotension). Products include:
- Blocadren Tablets 1429
- Timolide Tablets 1547
- Timoptic in Ocudose 1552
- Timoptic Sterile Ophthalmic Solution 1550

Tolazamide (Decreased glucose tolerance; adjustment of hypoglycemic therapy may be necessary). Products include:
- Tolinase Tablets 2365

Tolbutamide (Decreased glucose tolerance; adjustment of hypoglycemic therapy may be necessary). Products include:
- Orinase Tablets 2354

Trimethaphan Camsylate (Additive vasodilating effect and potential for postural hypotension). Products include:
- Arfonad Ampuls 1887

N'ICE MEDICATED SUGARLESS SORE THROAT AND COUGH LOZENGES
(Menthol) .... ▣ 719
No interactions described in labeling.

N'ICE SORE THROAT SPRAY
(Menthol) .... ▣ 719
No interactions described in labeling.

N'ICE SUGARLESS VITAMIN C DROPS
(Vitamin C) .... ▣ 719
No interactions described in labeling.

NICLOCIDE CHEWABLE TABLETS
(Niclosamide) 1607
No interactions described in labeling.

NICOBID
(Niacin) 1846
May interact with:

Patients taking antihypertensive drugs should consult physician before taking Nicobid.

NICOLAR TABLETS
(Niacin) 1846
May interact with antihypertensives, insulin, and oral hypoglycemic agents. Compounds in these categories include:

Acebutolol Hydrochloride (Possible additive vasodilating effect; postural hypotension). Products include:
- Sectral Capsules 2520

Atenolol (Possible additive vasodilating effect; postural hypotension). Products include:
- Tenoretic Tablets 1105
- Tenormin Tablets and I.V. Injection 1107

Benazepril Hydrochloride (Possible additive vasodilating effect; postural hypotension). Products include:
- Lotensin Tablets 872

Bendroflumethiazide (Possible additive vasodilating effect; postural hypotension). Products include:
- Corzide Tablets 702
- Naturetin Tablets 1789
- Rauzide Tablets 1804

Betaxolol Hydrochloride (Possible additive vasodilating effect; postural hypotension). Products include:
- Betoptic Sterile Ophthalmic Solution 569
- Betoptic S Sterile Ophthalmic Suspension 570
- Kerlone Tablets 2172

Captopril (Possible additive vasodilating effect; postural hypotension). Products include:
- Capoten 2255
- Capozide 2258

Carteolol Hydrochloride (Possible additive vasodilating effect; postural hypotension). Products include:
- Cartrol Tablets 507

Chlorothiazide (Possible additive vasodilating effect; postural hypotension). Products include:
- Aldoclor Tablets 1413
- Diupres Tablets 1461
- Diuril Oral 1464

Chlorothiazide Sodium (Possible additive vasodilating effect; postural hypotension). Products include:
- Diuril Sodium Intravenous 1463

Chlorpropamide (Adjustment in diet and/or hypoglycemic therapy may be necessary). Products include:
- Diabinese Tablets 1775

Chlorthalidone (Possible additive vasodilating effect; postural hypotension). Products include:
- Combipres Tablets 678
- Tenoretic Tablets 1105
- Thalitone Tablets 687

Clonidine (Possible additive vasodilating effect; postural hypotension). Products include:
- Catapres-TTS 677

Clonidine Hydrochloride (Possible additive vasodilating effect; postural hypotension). Products include:
- Catapres Tablets 676
- Combipres Tablets 678

Deserpidine (Possible additive vasodilating effect; postural hypotension). Products include:
- Enduronyl 518
- Harmonyl Tablets 528
- Oreticyl 545

Diazoxide (Possible additive vasodilating effect; postural hypotension). Products include:
- Hyperstat I.V. Injection 2095
- Proglycem 649

Doxazosin Mesylate (Possible additive vasodilating effect; postural hypotension). Products include:
- Cardura Tablets 1941

Enalapril Maleate (Possible additive vasodilating effect; postural hypotension). Products include:
- Vaseretic Tablets 1559
- Vasotec Tablets 1564

Enalaprilat (Possible additive vasodilating effect; postural hypotension). Products include:
- Vasotec I.V. 1562

Esmolol Hydrochloride (Possible additive vasodilating effect; postural hypotension). Products include:
- Brevibloc Injection 942

Felodipine (Possible additive vasodilating effect; postural hypotension). Products include:
- Plendil Extended-Release Tablets 1526

Fosinopril Sodium (Possible additive vasodilating effect; postural hypotension). Products include:
- Monopril Tablets 1406

Furosemide (Possible additive vasodilating effect; postural hypotension). Products include:
- Lasix 1093

Glipizide (Adjustment in diet and/or hypoglycemic therapy may be necessary). Products include:
- Glucotrol 1952

Glyburide (Adjustment in diet and/or hypoglycemic therapy may be necessary). Products include:
- DiaBeta 1091
- Micronase Tablets 2350

Guanabenz Acetate (Possible additive vasodilating effect; postural hypotension). Products include:
- Wytensin Tablets 2542

Guanethidine Monosulfate (Possible additive vasodilating effect; postural hypotension). Products include:
Esimil Tablets 864
Ismelin Tablets 869

Hydralazine Hydrochloride (Possible additive vasodilating effect; postural hypotension). Products include:
Apresazide Capsules 854
Apresoline Hydrochloride Parenteral (Ampuls) 856
Apresoline Hydrochloride Tablets 855
Apresoline-Esidrix Tablets 857
Ser-Ap-Es Tablets 881
Serpasil-Apresoline Tablets 884

Hydrochlorothiazide (Possible additive vasodilating effect; postural hypotension). Products include:
Aldactazide 2150
Aldoril Tablets 1418
Apresazide Capsules 854
Apresoline-Esidrix Tablets 857
Capozide 2258
Dyazide Capsules 2208
Esidrix Tablets 863
Esimil Tablets 864
HydroDIURIL Tablets 1484
Hydropres Tablets 1485
Inderide Tablets 2463
Inderide LA Long Acting Capsules 2465
Lopressor HCT Tablets 1034
Maxzide 1215
Moduretic Tablets 1510
Normozide Tablets 2112
Oretic Tablets 544
Oreticyl 545
Prinzide Tablets 1540
Ser-Ap-Es Tablets 881
Serpasil-Esidrix Tablets 886
Timolide Tablets 1547
Trandate HCT Tablets 579
Vaseretic Tablets 1559
Zestoretic 2274

Hydroflumethiazide (Possible additive vasodilating effect; postural hypotension). Products include:
Diucardin Tablets 2450
Saluron 718
Salutensin/Salutensin-Demi 719

Indapamide (Possible additive vasodilating effect; postural hypotension). Products include:
Lozol Tablets 1843

Insulin, Human (Adjustment in diet and/or hypoglycemic therapy may be necessary).
No products indexed under this heading.

Insulin, Human Isophane Suspension (Adjustment in diet and/or hypoglycemic therapy may be necessary). Products include:
Humulin N, 100 Units 1270

Insulin, Human NPH (Adjustment in diet and/or hypoglycemic therapy may be necessary). Products include:
Insulatard NPH Human 1627
Novolin N 1627
Novolin N PenFill Cartridges 1628
Novolin N Prefilled 1628

Insulin, Human Regular (Adjustment in diet and/or hypoglycemic therapy may be necessary). Products include:
Humulin BR, 100 Units 1268
Humulin R, 100 Units 1272
Novolin R 1627
Novolin R PenFill Cartridges 1628
Novolin R Prefilled 1629
Velosulin Human 1628

Insulin, Human, Zinc Suspension (Adjustment in diet and/or hypoglycemic therapy may be necessary). Products include:
Humulin L, 100 Units 1268
Humulin U, 100 Units 1272
Novolin L 1627

Insulin, NPH (Adjustment in diet and/or hypoglycemic therapy may be necessary). Products include:
NPH, 40 & 100 Units 1273
Beef NPH, 100 Units 1274
Pork NPH, 100 Units 1275
Insulatard NPH 1626
NPH Insulin 1626
NPH Purified Pork Isophane Insulin 1626

Insulin, Regular (Adjustment in diet and/or hypoglycemic therapy may be necessary). Products include:
Regular, 40 & 100 Units 1273
Beef Regular, 100 Units 1275
Pork Regular, 100 Units 1275
Pork Regular (Concentrated), 500 Units 1276
Regular Insulin 1625
Regular Purified Pork Insulin 1626
Velosulin 1627

Insulin, Zinc Crystals (Adjustment in diet and/or hypoglycemic therapy may be necessary). Products include:
NPH, 40 & 100 Units 1273

Insulin, Zinc Suspension (Adjustment in diet and/or hypoglycemic therapy may be necessary). Products include:
Lente, 40 & 100 Units 1272
Protamine, Zinc, 40 & 100 Units 1273
Lente Iletin I 1272
Beef Lente, 100 Units 1274
Beef Protamine Zinc, 100 Units 1274
Pork Lente, 100 Units 1275
Pork, Protamine, Zinc, 100 Units 1275
Lente Insulin 1626
Lente Purified Pork Insulin 1626
Semilente Insulin 1625
Ultralente Insulin 1626

Isradipine (Possible additive vasodilating effect; postural hypotension). Products include:
DynaCirc Capsules 2004

Labetalol Hydrochloride (Possible additive vasodilating effect; postural hypotension). Products include:
Normodyne Injection 2108
Normodyne Tablets 2110
Normozide Tablets 2112
Trandate HCT Tablets 579
Trandate Injection 577
Trandate Tablets 579

Lisinopril (Possible additive vasodilating effect; postural hypotension). Products include:
Prinivil Tablets 1538
Prinzide Tablets 1540
Zestoretic 2274
Zestril Tablets 2277

Mecamylamine Hydrochloride (Possible additive vasodilating effect; postural hypotension). Products include:
Inversine Tablets 1492

Methyclothiazide (Possible additive vasodilating effect; postural hypotension). Products include:
Enduron Tablets 517
Enduronyl 518

Methyldopa (Possible additive vasodilating effect; postural hypotension). Products include:
Aldoclor Tablets 1413
Aldomet Oral 1415
Aldoril Tablets 1418

Methyldopate Hydrochloride (Possible additive vasodilating effect; postural hypotension). Products include:
Aldomet Ester HCl Injection 1417

Metolazone (Possible additive vasodilating effect; postural hypotension). Products include:
Diulo 2129
Mykrox ½ mg Tablets 984
Zaroxolyn Tablets 989

Metoprolol Tartrate (Possible additive vasodilating effect; postural hypotension). Products include:
Lopressor Ampuls 1032
Lopressor HCT Tablets 1034
Lopressor Tablets 1032

Metyrosine (Possible additive vasodilating effect; postural hypotension). Products include:
Demser Capsules 1460

Minoxidil (Possible additive vasodilating effect; postural hypotension). Products include:
Loniten Tablets 2346
Rogaine Topical Solution 2357

Nadolol (Possible additive vasodilating effect; postural hypotension). Products include:
Corgard Tablets 701
Corzide Tablets 702

Nicardipine Hydrochloride (Possible additive vasodilating effect; postural hypotension). Products include:
Cardene Capsules 2290

Nitroglycerin (Possible additive vasodilating effect; postural hypotension). Products include:
Deponit NTG Transdermal Delivery System 2143
Minitran Transdermal Delivery System 1312
Nitro-Bid Ointment 1339
Nitro-Bid Capsules 1338
Nitrodisc 2176
Nitro-Dur (nitroglycerin) Transdermal Infusion System 1164
Nitrogard Tablets 1004
Nitrolingual Spray 1846
Nitrostat Tablets 1743
Transderm-Nitro Transdermal Therapeutic System 2283

Penbutolol Sulfate (Possible additive vasodilating effect; postural hypotension). Products include:
Levatol 1832

Phenoxybenzamine Hydrochloride (Possible additive vasodilating effect; postural hypotension). Products include:
Dibenzyline Capsules 2207

Phentolamine Mesylate (Possible additive vasodilating effect; postural hypotension). Products include:
Regitine 878

Pindolol (Possible additive vasodilating effect; postural hypotension). Products include:
Visken Tablets 2036

Polythiazide (Possible additive vasodilating effect; postural hypotension). Products include:
Minizide Capsules 1779
Renese Tablets 1785
Renese-R Tablets 1786

Prazosin Hydrochloride (Possible additive vasodilating effect; postural hypotension). Products include:
Minipress Capsules 1778
Minizide Capsules 1779

Propranolol Hydrochloride (Possible additive vasodilating effect; postural hypotension). Products include:
Inderal 2459
Inderal LA Long Acting Capsules 2461
Inderide Tablets 2463
Inderide LA Long Acting Capsules 2465

Ramipril (Possible additive vasodilating effect; postural hypotension). Products include:
Altace Capsules 1086

Rauwolfia Serpentina (Possible additive vasodilating effect; postural hypotension). Products include:
Raudixin Tablets 1803
Rauzide Tablets 1804

Rescinnamine (Possible additive vasodilating effect; postural hypotension).
No products indexed under this heading.

Reserpine (Possible additive vasodilating effect; postural hypotension). Products include:
Diupres Tablets 1461
Hydromox R Tablets 1209
Hydropres Tablets 1485
Renese-R Tablets 1786
Salutensin/Salutensin-Demi 719
Ser-Ap-Es Tablets 881
Serpasil Tablets 883
Serpasil-Apresoline Tablets 884
Serpasil-Esidrix Tablets 886

Sodium Nitroprusside (Possible additive vasodilating effect; postural hypotension). Products include:
Nipride I.V. Infusion 1909

Terazosin Hydrochloride (Possible additive vasodilating effect; postural hypotension). Products include:
Hytrin Tablets 529

Timolol Maleate (Possible additive vasodilating effect; postural hypotension). Products include:
Blocadren Tablets 1429
Timolide Tablets 1547
Timoptic in Ocudose 1552
Timoptic Sterile Ophthalmic Solution 1550

Tolazamide (Adjustment in diet and/or hypoglycemic therapy may be necessary). Products include:
Tolinase Tablets 2365

Tolbutamide (Adjustment in diet and/or hypoglycemic therapy may be necessary). Products include:
Orinase Tablets 2354

Trimethaphan Camsylate (Possible additive vasodilating effect; postural hypotension). Products include:
Arfonad Ampuls 1887

NICORETTE
(Nicotine Polacrilex) 1335
May interact with:

Adrenergic agonists and blockers (Adjust therapy).

Aminophylline (Increased drug levels). Products include:
Amesec ▣ 682
Aminophyllin Tablets 2153

Caffeine (Increased drug levels). Products include:
Anacin Coated Analgesic Caplets 2417
Anacin Coated Analgesic Tablets 2417
Anacin Maximum Strength Analgesic Coated Tablets 2417
Cafergot/Cafergot P-B 1999
Esgic-Plus Tablets 1002
Esgic Tablets & Capsules 1001
Aspirin Free Excedrin Analgesic Caplets 748
Excedrin Extra-Strength Analgesic Tablets & Caplets 749
Fioricet Tablets 2006
Fiorinal Capsules 2007
Fiorinal with Codeine Capsules 2008
Fiorinal Tablets 2007
No Doz Fast Acting Alertness Aid Tablets 751
No Doz Maximum Strength Caplets 751
Norgesic 1314
P-A-C Analgesic Tablets ▣ 669
Synalgos-DC Capsules 2525
Vanquish Analgesic Caplets ▣ 574
Vivarin Stimulant Tablets ▣ 726
Wigraine Tablets & Suppositories 1645

Caffeine Anhydrous (Increased drug levels).
No products indexed under this heading.

Caffeine Citrate (Increased drug levels).
No products indexed under this heading.

Caffeine Sodium Benzoate (Increased drug levels).
No products indexed under this heading.

Dyphylline (Increased drug levels). Products include:
- Dilor 2079
- Dilor-G Tablets & Liquid 2079
- Lufyllin Elixir 2384
- Lufyllin & Lufyllin-400 Tablets 2384
- Lufyllin-GG Elixir & Tablets 2385

Furosemide (Increased diuretic effects). Products include:
- Lasix 1093

Glutethimide (Decreased absorption).
No products indexed under this heading.

Imipramine Hydrochloride (Increased drug levels). Products include:
- Tofranil Ampuls 1038
- Tofranil Tablets 1039

Imipramine Pamoate (Increased drug levels). Products include:
- Tofranil-PM Capsules 1041

Pentazocine Hydrochloride (Increased drug levels). Products include:
- Talacen 2070
- Talwin Compound 2072
- Talwin Nx 2073

Pentazocine Lactate (Increased drug levels). Products include:
- Talwin Injection 2071

Phenacetin (Increased drug levels).

Propoxyphene Hydrochloride (Decreased absorption). Products include:
- Darvon 1256
- Wygesic Tablets 2540

Propoxyphene Napsylate (Decreased absorption). Products include:
- Darvon-N/Darvocet-N 1254

Propranolol Hydrochloride (Decreased blood pressure). Products include:
- Inderal 2459
- Inderal LA Long Acting Capsules 2461
- Inderide Tablets 2463
- Inderide LA Long Acting Capsules 2465

Theophylline (Increased drug levels). Products include:
- Bronkaid Tablets .... ⊞ 757
- Bronkolixir .... ⊞ 761
- Bronkotabs Tablets .... ⊞ 762
- Constant-T Tablets 1029
- Marax Tablets & DF Syrup 1954
- Primatene Tablets 2421
- Quibron Capsules 713
- Quibron-T 714
- Quibron-T/SR 716
- Theolair Liquid 1317
- Theo-Organidin Elixir 2391

Theophylline Anhydrous (Increased drug levels). Products include:
- Aerolate 994
- Primatene Tablets-M Formula .... ⊞ 753
- Primatene Tablets-Regular Formula 2421
- Respbid Tablets 684
- Slo-bid Gyrocaps 1847
- T-PHYL (Uniphyl) 200 mg Tablets 1820
- Tedral SA 1765
- Theo-24 2179
- Theo-Dur Sprinkle 1168
- Theo-Dur Extended-Release Tablets 1166
- Theolair Tablets 1317
- Theolair-SR Tablets 1319
- TheoX Extended-Release Tablets 841
- Uniphyl 400 mg Tablets 1823

Theophylline Calcium Salicylate (Increased drug levels). Products include:
- Quadrinal Tablets 1183

Theophylline Sodium Glycinate (Increased drug levels). Products include:
- Asbron G 1997

NICOTINEX ELIXIR
(Niacin) .... ⊞ 563
No interactions described in labeling.

NIFEREX-150 CAPSULES
(Iron Polysaccharide Complex) 847
No interactions described in labeling.

NIFEREX ELIXIR
(Iron Polysaccharide Complex) 847
No interactions described in labeling.

NIFEREX-150 FORTE CAPSULES
(Iron Polysaccharide Complex, Folic Acid, Vitamin B_{12}) 847
No interactions described in labeling.

NIFEREX FORTE ELIXIR
(Iron Polysaccharide Complex, Folic Acid, Vitamin B_{12}) 847
No interactions described in labeling.

NIFEREX TABLETS
(Iron Polysaccharide Complex) 847
No interactions described in labeling.

NIFEREX W/VITAMIN C TABLETS
(Iron Polysaccharide Complex, Vitamin C) 847
No interactions described in labeling.

NIFEREX-PN TABLETS
(Iron Polysaccharide Complex) 847
No interactions described in labeling.

NIMOTOP CAPSULES
(Nimodipine) 1607
May interact with antihypertensives, calcium channel blockers, and certain other agents. Compounds in these categories include:

Acebutolol Hydrochloride (Concomitant administration results in intensified effect). Products include:
- Sectral Capsules 2520

Atenolol (Concomitant administration results in intensified effect). Products include:
- Tenoretic Tablets 1105
- Tenormin Tablets and I.V. Injection 1107

Benazepril Hydrochloride (Concomitant administration results in intensified effect). Products include:
- Lotensin Tablets 872

Bendroflumethiazide (Concomitant administration results in intensified effect). Products include:
- Corzide Tablets 702
- Naturetin Tablets 1789
- Rauzide Tablets 1804

Bepridil Hydrochloride (Enhanced action). Products include:
- Vascor (200, 300 and 400 mg) Tablets 1383

Betaxolol Hydrochloride (Concomitant administration results in intensified effect). Products include:
- Betoptic Sterile Ophthalmic Solution 569
- Betoptic S Sterile Ophthalmic Suspension 570
- Kerlone Tablets 2172

Captopril (Concomitant administration results in intensified effect). Products include:
- Capoten 2255
- Capozide 2258

Carteolol Hydrochloride (Concomitant administration results in intensified effect). Products include:
- Cartrol Tablets 507

Chlorothiazide (Concomitant administration results in intensified effect). Products include:
- Aldoclor Tablets 1413
- Diupres Tablets 1461
- Diuril Oral 1464

Chlorothiazide Sodium (Concomitant administration results in intensified effect). Products include:
- Diuril Sodium Intravenous 1463

Chlorthalidone (Concomitant administration results in intensified effect). Products include:
- Combipres Tablets 678
- Tenoretic Tablets 1105
- Thalitone Tablets 687

Cimetidine (May increase peak nimodipine plasma concentrations and AUC). Products include:
- Tagamet Tablets 2228

Cimetidine Hydrochloride (May increase peak nimodipine plasma concentrations and AUC). Products include:
- Tagamet 2228

Clonidine (Concomitant administration results in intensified effect). Products include:
- Catapres-TTS 677

Clonidine Hydrochloride (Concomitant administration results in intensified effect). Products include:
- Catapres Tablets 676
- Combipres Tablets 678

Deserpidine (Concomitant administration results in intensified effect). Products include:
- Enduronyl 518
- Harmonyl Tablets 528
- Oreticyl 545

Diazoxide (Concomitant administration results in intensified effect). Products include:
- Hyperstat I.V. Injection 2095
- Proglycem 649

Diltiazem Hydrochloride (Enhanced action). Products include:
- Cardizem Tablets-30 mg, 60 mg, 90 mg and 120 mg 1329
- Cardizem SR Capsules-60 mg, 90 mg and 120 mg 1327

Doxazosin Mesylate (Concomitant administration results in intensified effect). Products include:
- Cardura Tablets 1941

Enalapril Maleate (Concomitant administration results in intensified effect). Products include:
- Vaseretic Tablets 1559
- Vasotec Tablets 1564

Enalaprilat (Concomitant administration results in intensified effect). Products include:
- Vasotec I.V. 1562

Esmolol Hydrochloride (Concomitant administration results in intensified effect). Products include:
- Brevibloc Injection 942

Felodipine (Concomitant administration results in intensified effect). Products include:
- Plendil Extended-Release Tablets 1526

Fosinopril Sodium (Concomitant administration results in intensified effect). Products include:
- Monopril Tablets 1406

Furosemide (Concomitant administration results in intensified effect). Products include:
- Lasix 1093

Guanabenz Acetate (Concomitant administration results in intensified effect). Products include:
- Wytensin Tablets 2542

Guanethidine Monosulfate (Concomitant administration results in intensified effect). Products include:
- Esimil Tablets 864
- Ismelin Tablets 869

Hydralazine Hydrochloride (Concomitant administration results in intensified effect). Products include:
- Apresazide Capsules 854
- Apresoline Hydrochloride Parenteral (Ampuls) 856
- Apresoline Hydrochloride Tablets 855
- Apresoline-Esidrix Tablets 857
- Ser-Ap-Es Tablets 881
- Serpasil-Apresoline Tablets 884

Hydrochlorothiazide (Concomitant administration results in intensified effect). Products include:
- Aldactazide 2150
- Aldoril Tablets 1418
- Apresazide Capsules 854
- Apresoline-Esidrix Tablets 857
- Capozide 2258
- Dyazide Capsules 2208
- Esidrix Tablets 863
- Esimil Tablets 864
- HydroDIURIL Tablets 1484
- Hydropres Tablets 1485
- Inderide Tablets 2463
- Inderide LA Long Acting Capsules 2465
- Lopressor HCT Tablets 1034
- Maxzide 1215
- Moduretic Tablets 1510
- Normozide Tablets 2112
- Oretic Tablets 544
- Oreticyl 545
- Prinzide Tablets 1540
- Ser-Ap-Es Tablets 881
- Serpasil-Esidrix Tablets 886
- Timolide Tablets 1547
- Trandate HCT Tablets 579
- Vaseretic Tablets 1559
- Zestoretic 2274

Hydroflumethiazide (Concomitant administration results in intensified effect). Products include:
- Diucardin Tablets 2450
- Saluron 718
- Salutensin/Salutensin-Demi 719

Indapamide (Concomitant administration results in intensified effect). Products include:
- Lozol Tablets 1843

Isradipine (Concomitant administration results in intensified effect). Products include:
- DynaCirc Capsules 2004

Labetalol Hydrochloride (Concomitant administration results in intensified effect). Products include:
- Normodyne Injection 2108
- Normodyne Tablets 2110
- Normozide Tablets 2112
- Trandate HCT Tablets 579
- Trandate Injection 577
- Trandate Tablets 579

Lisinopril (Concomitant administration results in intensified effect). Products include:
- Prinivil Tablets 1538
- Prinzide Tablets 1540
- Zestoretic 2274
- Zestril Tablets 2277

Mecamylamine Hydrochloride (Concomitant administration results in intensified effect). Products include:
- Inversine Tablets 1492

Methyclothiazide (Concomitant administration results in intensified effect). Products include:
- Enduron Tablets 517
- Enduronyl 518

Methyldopa (Concomitant administration results in intensified effect). Products include:
- Aldoclor Tablets 1413
- Aldomet Oral 1415
- Aldoril Tablets 1418

Methyldopate Hydrochloride (Concomitant administration results in intensified effect). Products include:
- Aldomet Ester HCl Injection 1417

Metolazone (Concomitant administration results in intensified effect). Products include:
- Diulo 2129
- Mykrox ½ mg Tablets 984
- Zaroxolyn Tablets 989

Metoprolol Tartrate (Concomitant administration results in intensified effect). Products include:
- Lopressor Ampuls 1032
- Lopressor HCT Tablets 1034
- Lopressor Tablets 1032

Metyrosine (Concomitant administration results in intensified effect). Products include:
- Demser Capsules 1460

Minoxidil (Concomitant administration results in intensified effect). Products include:
- Loniten Tablets 2346
- Rogaine Topical Solution 2357

Nadolol (Concomitant administration results in intensified effect). Products include:
- Corgard Tablets 701
- Corzide Tablets 702

Nicardipine Hydrochloride (Enhanced action; concomitant administration results in intensified effect). Products include:
- Cardene Capsules 2290

Nifedipine (Enhanced action). Products include:
- Adalat Capsules (10 mg and 20 mg) 1587
- Procardia Capsules 1781
- Procardia XL Tablets 1783

Nitroglycerin (Concomitant administration results in intensified effect). Products include:
- Deponit NTG Transdermal Delivery System 2143
- Minitran Transdermal Delivery System 1312
- Nitro-Bid Ointment 1339
- Nitro-Bid Capsules 1338
- Nitrodisc 2176
- Nitro-Dur (nitroglycerin) Transdermal Infusion System 1164
- Nitrogard Tablets 1004
- Nitrolingual Spray 1846
- Nitrostat Tablets 1743
- Transderm-Nitro Transdermal Therapeutic System 2283

Penbutolol Sulfate (Concomitant administration results in intensified effect). Products include:
- Levatol 1832

Phenoxybenzamine Hydrochloride (Concomitant administration results in intensified effect). Products include:
- Dibenzyline Capsules 2207

Phentolamine Mesylate (Concomitant administration results in intensified effect). Products include:
- Regitine 878

Phenytoin (Potential for phenytoin toxicity). Products include:
- Dilantin Infatabs 1710
- Dilantin-30 Pediatric/Dilantin-125 Suspension 1713

Phenytoin Sodium (Potential for phenytoin toxicity). Products include:
- Dilantin Kapseals 1708
- Dilantin Parenteral 1712
- Dilantin with Phenobarbital Kapseals 1715

Pindolol (Concomitant administration results in intensified effect). Products include:
- Visken Tablets 2036

Polythiazide (Concomitant administration results in intensified effect). Products include:
- Minizide Capsules 1779
- Renese Tablets 1785
- Renese-R Tablets 1786

Prazosin Hydrochloride (Concomitant administration results in intensified effect). Products include:
- Minipress Capsules 1778
- Minizide Capsules 1779

Propranolol Hydrochloride (Concomitant administration results in intensified effect). Products include:
- Inderal 2459
- Inderal LA Long Acting Capsules 2461
- Inderide Tablets 2463
- Inderide LA Long Acting Capsules .. 2465

Ramipril (Concomitant administration results in intensified effect). Products include:
- Altace Capsules 1086

Rauwolfia Serpentina (Concomitant administration results in intensified effect). Products include:
- Raudixin Tablets 1803
- Rauzide Tablets 1804

Rescinnamine (Concomitant administration results in intensified effect).
- No products indexed under this heading.

Reserpine (Concomitant administration results in intensified effect). Products include:
- Diupres Tablets 1461
- Hydromox R Tablets 1209
- Hydropres Tablets 1485
- Renese-R Tablets 1786
- Salutensin/Salutensin-Demi 719
- Ser-Ap-Es Tablets 881
- Serpasil Tablets 883
- Serpasil-Apresoline Tablets 884
- Serpasil-Esidrix Tablets 886

Sodium Nitroprusside (Concomitant administration results in intensified effect). Products include:
- Nipride I.V. Infusion 1909

Terazosin Hydrochloride (Concomitant administration results in intensified effect). Products include:
- Hytrin Tablets 529

Timolol Maleate (Concomitant administration results in intensified effect). Products include:
- Blocadren Tablets 1429
- Timolide Tablets 1547
- Timoptic in Ocudose 1552
- Timoptic Sterile Ophthalmic Solution 1550

Trimethaphan Camsylate (Concomitant administration results in intensified effect). Products include:
- Arfonad Ampuls 1887

Verapamil Hydrochloride (Enhanced action). Products include:
- Calan SR Caplets 2157
- Calan Tablets 2155
- Isoptin Injectable 1177
- Isoptin Oral Tablets 1179
- Isoptin SR Sustained Release Tablets 1181
- Verelan Capsules 1243
- Verelan Capsules 2535

NIPRIDE I.V. INFUSION
(Sodium Nitroprusside)............ 1909
May interact with negative inotropic agents, ganglionic blocking agents, antihypertensives, inhalant anesthetics, and certain other agents. Compounds in these categories include:

Acebutolol Hydrochloride (Hypotensive effect is augmented). Products include:
- Sectral Capsules 2520

Atenolol (Hypotensive effect is augmented). Products include:
- Tenoretic Tablets 1105
- Tenormin Tablets and I.V. Injection 1107

Benazepril Hydrochloride (Hypotensive effect is augmented). Products include:
- Lotensin Tablets 872

Bendroflumethiazide (Hypotensive effect is augmented). Products include:
- Corzide Tablets 702
- Naturetin Tablets 1789
- Rauzide Tablets 1804

Betaxolol Hydrochloride (Hypotensive effect is augmented). Products include:
- Betoptic Sterile Ophthalmic Solution 569
- Betoptic S Sterile Ophthalmic Suspension 570
- Kerlone Tablets 2172

Captopril (Hypotensive effect is augmented). Products include:
- Capoten 2255
- Capozide 2258

Carteolol Hydrochloride (Hypotensive effect is augmented). Products include:
- Cartrol Tablets 507

Chlorothiazide (Hypotensive effect is augmented). Products include:
- Aldoclor Tablets 1413
- Diupres Tablets 1461
- Diuril Oral 1464

Chlorothiazide Sodium (Hypotensive effect is augmented). Products include:
- Diuril Sodium Intravenous 1463

Chlorthalidone (Hypotensive effect is augmented). Products include:
- Combipres Tablets 678
- Tenoretic Tablets 1105
- Thalitone Tablets 687

Clonidine (Hypotensive effect is augmented). Products include:
- Catapres-TTS 677

Clonidine Hydrochloride (Hypotensive effect is augmented). Products include:
- Catapres Tablets 676
- Combipres Tablets 678

Deserpidine (Hypotensive effect is augmented). Products include:
- Enduronyl 518
- Harmonyl Tablets 528
- Oreticyl 545

Diazoxide (Hypotensive effect is augmented). Products include:
- Hyperstat I.V. Injection 2095
- Proglycem 649

Doxazosin Mesylate (Hypotensive effect is augmented). Products include:
- Cardura Tablets 1941

Enalapril Maleate (Hypotensive effect is augmented). Products include:
- Vaseretic Tablets 1559
- Vasotec Tablets 1564

Enalaprilat (Hypotensive effect is augmented). Products include:
- Vasotec I.V. 1562

Enflurane (Hypotensive effect is augmented). Products include:
- Ethrane 599

Esmolol Hydrochloride (Hypotensive effect is augmented). Products include:
- Brevibloc Injection 942

Felodipine (Hypotensive effect is augmented). Products include:
- Plendil Extended-Release Tablets.... 1526

Fosinopril Sodium (Hypotensive effect is augmented). Products include:
- Monopril Tablets 1406

Furosemide (Hypotensive effect is augmented). Products include:
- Lasix 1093

Guanabenz Acetate (Hypotensive effect is augmented). Products include:
- Wytensin Tablets 2542

Guanethidine Monosulfate (Hypotensive effect is augmented). Products include:
- Esimil Tablets 864
- Ismelin Tablets 869

Halothane (Hypotensive effect is augmented). Products include:
- Fluothane 2453

Hydralazine Hydrochloride (Hypotensive effect is augmented). Products include:
- Apresazide Capsules 854
- Apresoline Hydrochloride Parenteral (Ampuls) 856
- Apresoline Hydrochloride Tablets .. 855
- Apresoline-Esidrix Tablets 857
- Ser-Ap-Es Tablets 881
- Serpasil-Apresoline Tablets 884

Hydrochlorothiazide (Hypotensive effect is augmented). Products include:
- Aldactazide 2150
- Aldoril Tablets 1418
- Apresazide Capsules 854
- Apresoline-Esidrix Tablets 857
- Capozide 2258
- Dyazide Capsules 2208
- Esidrix Tablets 863
- Esimil Tablets 864
- HydroDIURIL Tablets 1484
- Hydropres Tablets 1485
- Inderide Tablets 2463
- Inderide LA Long Acting Capsules .. 2465
- Lopressor HCT Tablets 1034
- Maxzide 1215
- Moduretic Tablets 1510
- Normozide Tablets 2112
- Oretic Tablets 544
- Oreticyl 545
- Prinzide Tablets 1540
- Ser-Ap-Es Tablets 881
- Serpasil-Esidrix Tablets 886
- Timolide Tablets 1547
- Trandate HCT Tablets 579
- Vaseretic Tablets 1559
- Zestoretic 2274

Hydroflumethiazide (Hypotensive effect is augmented). Products include:
- Diucardin Tablets 2450
- Saluron 718
- Salutensin/Salutensin-Demi 719

Indapamide (Hypotensive effect is augmented). Products include:
- Lozol Tablets 1843

Isoflurane (Hypotensive effect is augmented). Products include:
- Forane 600

Isradipine (Hypotensive effect is augmented). Products include:
- DynaCirc Capsules 2004

Labetalol Hydrochloride (Hypotensive effect is augmented). Products include:
- Normodyne Injection 2108
- Normodyne Tablets 2110
- Normozide Tablets 2112
- Trandate HCT Tablets 579
- Trandate Injection 577
- Trandate Tablets 579

Lisinopril (Hypotensive effect is augmented). Products include:
- Prinivil Tablets 1538
- Prinzide Tablets 1540
- Zestoretic 2274
- Zestril Tablets 2277

Mecamylamine Hydrochloride (Hypotensive effect is augmented). Products include:
- Inversine Tablets 1492

Methoxyflurane (Hypotensive effect is augmented).
- No products indexed under this heading.

Methyclothiazide (Hypotensive effect is augmented). Products include:
- Enduron Tablets ... 517
- Enduronyl ... 518

Methyldopa (Hypotensive effect is augmented). Products include:
- Aldoclor Tablets ... 1413
- Aldomet Oral ... 1415
- Aldoril Tablets ... 1418

Methyldopate Hydrochloride (Hypotensive effect is augmented). Products include:
- Aldomet Ester HCl Injection ... 1417

Metolazone (Hypotensive effect is augmented). Products include:
- Diulo ... 2129
- Mykrox ½ mg Tablets ... 984
- Zaroxolyn Tablets ... 989

Metoprolol Tartrate (Hypotensive effect is augmented). Products include:
- Lopressor Ampuls ... 1032
- Lopressor HCT Tablets ... 1034
- Lopressor Tablets ... 1032

Metyrosine (Hypotensive effect is augmented). Products include:
- Demser Capsules ... 1460

Minoxidil (Hypotensive effect is augmented). Products include:
- Loniten Tablets ... 2346
- Rogaine Topical Solution ... 2357

Nadolol (Hypotensive effect is augmented). Products include:
- Corgard Tablets ... 701
- Corzide Tablets ... 702

Nicardipine Hydrochloride (Hypotensive effect is augmented). Products include:
- Cardene Capsules ... 2290

Nitroglycerin (Hypotensive effect is augmented). Products include:
- Deponit NTG Transdermal Delivery System ... 2143
- Minitran Transdermal Delivery System ... 1312
- Nitro-Bid Ointment ... 1339
- Nitro-Bid Capsules ... 1338
- Nitrodisc ... 2176
- Nitro-Dur (nitroglycerin) Transdermal Infusion System ... 1164
- Nitrogard Tablets ... 1004
- Nitrolingual Spray ... 1846
- Nitrostat Tablets ... 1743
- Transderm-Nitro Transdermal Therapeutic System ... 2283

Penbutolol Sulfate (Hypotensive effect is augmented). Products include:
- Levatol ... 1832

Phenoxybenzamine Hydrochloride (Hypotensive effect is augmented). Products include:
- Dibenzyline Capsules ... 2207

Phentolamine Mesylate (Hypotensive effect is augmented). Products include:
- Regitine ... 878

Pindolol (Hypotensive effect is augmented). Products include:
- Visken Tablets ... 2036

Polythiazide (Hypotensive effect is augmented). Products include:
- Minizide Capsules ... 1779
- Renese Tablets ... 1785
- Renese-R Tablets ... 1786

Prazosin Hydrochloride (Hypotensive effect is augmented). Products include:
- Minipress Capsules ... 1778
- Minizide Capsules ... 1779

Propranolol Hydrochloride (Hypotensive effect is augmented). Products include:
- Inderal ... 2459
- Inderal LA Long Acting Capsules ... 2461
- Inderide Tablets ... 2463
- Inderide LA Long Acting Capsules ... 2465

Ramipril (Hypotensive effect is augmented). Products include:
- Altace Capsules ... 1086

Rauwolfia Serpentina (Hypotensive effect is augmented). Products include:
- Raudixin Tablets ... 1803
- Rauzide Tablets ... 1804

Rescinnamine (Hypotensive effect is augmented).
- No products indexed under this heading.

Reserpine (Hypotensive effect is augmented). Products include:
- Diupres Tablets ... 1461
- Hydromox R Tablets ... 1209
- Hydropres Tablets ... 1485
- Renese-R Tablets ... 1786
- Salutensin/Salutensin-Demi ... 719
- Ser-Ap-Es Tablets ... 881
- Serpasil Tablets ... 883
- Serpasil-Apresoline Tablets ... 884
- Serpasil-Esidrix Tablets ... 886

Terazosin Hydrochloride (Hypotensive effect is augmented). Products include:
- Hytrin Tablets ... 529

Timolol Maleate (Hypotensive effect is augmented). Products include:
- Blocadren Tablets ... 1429
- Timolide Tablets ... 1547
- Timoptic in Ocudose ... 1552
- Timoptic Sterile Ophthalmic Solution ... 1550

Trimethaphan Camsylate (Hypotensive effect is augmented). Products include:
- Arfonad Ampuls ... 1887

NITRO-BID IV
(Nitroglycerin) ... 1338
No interactions described in labeling.

NITRO-BID OINTMENT
(Nitroglycerin) ... 1339
May interact with calcium channel blockers and certain other agents. Compounds in these categories include:

Alcohol (May enhance sensitivity to the hypotensive effects of nitrates).

Bepridil Hydrochloride (May produce marked symptomatic orthostatic hypotension). Products include:
- Vascor (200, 300 and 400 mg) Tablets ... 1383

Diltiazem Hydrochloride (May produce marked symptomatic orthostatic hypotension). Products include:
- Cardizem Tablets-30 mg, 60 mg, 90 mg and 120 mg ... 1329
- Cardizem SR Capsules-60 mg, 90 mg and 120 mg ... 1327

Felodipine (May produce marked symptomatic orthostatic hypotension). Products include:
- Plendil Extended-Release Tablets ... 1526

Isradipine (May produce marked symptomatic orthostatic hypotension). Products include:
- DynaCirc Capsules ... 2004

Nicardipine Hydrochloride (May produce marked symptomatic orthostatic hypotension). Products include:
- Cardene Capsules ... 2290

Nifedipine (May produce marked symptomatic orthostatic hypotension). Products include:
- Adalat Capsules (10 mg and 20 mg) ... 1587
- Procardia Capsules ... 1781
- Procardia XL Tablets ... 1783

Nimodipine (May produce marked symptomatic orthostatic hypotension). Products include:
- Nimotop Capsules ... 1607

Verapamil Hydrochloride (May produce marked symptomatic orthostatic hypotension). Products include:
- Calan SR Caplets ... 2157
- Calan Tablets ... 2155
- Isoptin Injectable ... 1177
- Isoptin Oral Tablets ... 1179
- Isoptin SR Sustained Release Tablets ... 1181
- Verelan Capsules ... 1243
- Verelan Capsules ... 2535

NITRO-BID 2.5 PLATEAU CAPS
(Nitroglycerin) ... 1338
May interact with:

Alcohol (May enhance adverse effects).

NITRO-BID 6.5 PLATEAU CAPS
(Nitroglycerin) ... 1338
See **Nitro-Bid 2.5 Plateau Caps**

NITRO-BID 9 PLATEAU CAPS
(Nitroglycerin) ... 1338
See **Nitro-Bid 2.5 Plateau Caps**

NITRODISC
(Nitroglycerin) ... 2176
May interact with vasodilators and certain other agents. Compounds in these categories include:

Alcohol (Exhibits additive effects).

Diazoxide (Vasodilating effects may be additive). Products include:
- Hyperstat I.V. Injection ... 2095
- Proglycem ... 649

Hydralazine Hydrochloride (Vasodilating effects may be additive). Products include:
- Apresazide Capsules ... 854
- Apresoline Hydrochloride Parenteral (Ampuls) ... 856
- Apresoline Hydrochloride Tablets ... 855
- Apresoline-Esidrix Tablets ... 857
- Ser-Ap-Es Tablets ... 881
- Serpasil-Apresoline Tablets ... 884

Minoxidil (Vasodilating effects may be additive). Products include:
- Loniten Tablets ... 2346
- Rogaine Topical Solution ... 2357

NITRO-DUR (NITROGLYCERIN) TRANSDERMAL INFUSION SYSTEM
(Nitroglycerin) ... 1164
May interact with:

Alcohol (Enhances sensitivity to the hypotensive effects).

NITROGARD TABLETS
(Nitroglycerin) ... 1004
May interact with calcium channel blockers, vasodilators, and certain other agents. Compounds in these categories include:

Alcohol (Additive vasodilating effects).

Bepridil Hydrochloride (Potential for marked symptomatic hypotension). Products include:
- Vascor (200, 300 and 400 mg) Tablets ... 1383

Diazoxide (Additive vasodilating effects). Products include:
- Hyperstat I.V. Injection ... 2095
- Proglycem ... 649

Diltiazem Hydrochloride (Potential for marked symptomatic hypotension). Products include:
- Cardizem Tablets-30 mg, 60 mg, 90 mg and 120 mg ... 1329
- Cardizem SR Capsules-60 mg, 90 mg and 120 mg ... 1327

Felodipine (Potential for marked symptomatic hypotension). Products include:
- Plendil Extended-Release Tablets ... 1526

Hydralazine Hydrochloride (Additive vasodilating effects). Products include:
- Apresazide Capsules ... 854
- Apresoline Hydrochloride Parenteral (Ampuls) ... 856
- Apresoline Hydrochloride Tablets ... 855
- Apresoline-Esidrix Tablets ... 857
- Ser-Ap-Es Tablets ... 881
- Serpasil-Apresoline Tablets ... 884

Isradipine (Potential for marked symptomatic hypotension). Products include:
- DynaCirc Capsules ... 2004

Minoxidil (Additive vasodilating effects). Products include:
- Loniten Tablets ... 2346
- Rogaine Topical Solution ... 2357

Nicardipine Hydrochloride (Potential for marked symptomatic hypotension). Products include:
- Cardene Capsules ... 2290

Nifedipine (Potential for marked symptomatic hypotension). Products include:
- Adalat Capsules (10 mg and 20 mg) ... 1587
- Procardia Capsules ... 1781
- Procardia XL Tablets ... 1783

Nimodipine (Potential for marked symptomatic hypotension). Products include:
- Nimotop Capsules ... 1607

Verapamil Hydrochloride (Potential for marked symptomatic hypotension). Products include:
- Calan SR Caplets ... 2157
- Calan Tablets ... 2155
- Isoptin Injectable ... 1177
- Isoptin Oral Tablets ... 1179
- Isoptin SR Sustained Release Tablets ... 1181
- Verelan Capsules ... 1243
- Verelan Capsules ... 2535

NITROLINGUAL SPRAY
(Nitroglycerin) ... 1846
May interact with calcium channel blockers and certain other agents. Compounds in these categories include:

Alcohol (Enhanced sensitivity to hypotensive effects).

Bepridil Hydrochloride (Marked symptomatic orthostatic hypotension). Products include:
- Vascor (200, 300 and 400 mg) Tablets ... 1383

Diltiazem Hydrochloride (Marked symptomatic orthostatic hypotension). Products include:
- Cardizem Tablets-30 mg, 60 mg, 90 mg and 120 mg ... 1329
- Cardizem SR Capsules-60 mg, 90 mg and 120 mg ... 1327

Drugs Depending On Vascular Smooth Muscle (Decreased or increased effect).

Felodipine (Marked symptomatic orthostatic hypotension). Products include:
- Plendil Extended-Release Tablets ... 1526

Isradipine (Marked symptomatic orthostatic hypotension). Products include:
- DynaCirc Capsules ... 2004

Nicardipine Hydrochloride (Marked symptomatic orthostatic hypotension). Products include:
Cardene Capsules 2290

Nifedipine (Marked symptomatic orthostatic hypotension). Products include:
Adalat Capsules (10 mg and 20 mg) 1587
Procardia Capsules 1781
Procardia XL Tablets 1783

Nimodipine (Marked symptomatic orthostatic hypotension). Products include:
Nimotop Capsules 1607

Verapamil Hydrochloride (Marked symptomatic orthostatic hypotension). Products include:
Calan SR Caplets 2157
Calan Tablets 2155
Isoptin Injectable 1177
Isoptin Oral Tablets 1179
Isoptin SR Sustained Release Tablets 1181
Verelan Capsules 1243
Verelan Capsules 2535

NITROSTAT IV AMPOULES & VIALS
(Nitroglycerin) 1744
No interactions described in labeling.

NITROSTAT IV INFUSION KIT
(Nitroglycerin) 1744
No interactions described in labeling.

NITROSTAT TABLETS
(Nitroglycerin) 1743
May interact with antihypertensives, beta blockers, phenothiazines, and certain other agents. Compounds in these categories include:

Acebutolol Hydrochloride (Additive hypotensive effects). Products include:
Sectral Capsules 2520

Alcohol (Hypotension).

Atenolol (Additive hypotensive effects). Products include:
Tenoretic Tablets 1105
Tenormin Tablets and I.V. Injection 1107

Benazepril Hydrochloride (Additive hypotensive effects). Products include:
Lotensin Tablets 872

Bendroflumethiazide (Additive hypotensive effects). Products include:
Corzide Tablets 702
Naturetin Tablets 1789
Rauzide Tablets 1804

Betaxolol Hydrochloride (Additive hypotensive effects). Products include:
Betoptic Sterile Ophthalmic Solution 569
Betoptic S Sterile Ophthalmic Suspension 570
Kerlone Tablets 2172

Captopril (Additive hypotensive effects). Products include:
Capoten 2255
Capozide 2258

Carteolol Hydrochloride (Additive hypotensive effects). Products include:
Cartrol Tablets 507

Chlorothiazide (Additive hypotensive effects). Products include:
Aldoclor Tablets 1413
Diupres Tablets 1461
Diuril Oral 1464

Chlorothiazide Sodium (Additive hypotensive effects). Products include:
Diuril Sodium Intravenous 1463

Chlorpromazine (Additive hypotensive effects). Products include:
Thorazine 2234

Chlorthalidone (Additive hypotensive effects). Products include:
Combipres Tablets 678
Tenoretic Tablets 1105
Thalitone Tablets 687

Clonidine (Additive hypotensive effects). Products include:
Catapres-TTS 677

Clonidine Hydrochloride (Additive hypotensive effects). Products include:
Catapres Tablets 676
Combipres Tablets 678

Deserpidine (Additive hypotensive effects). Products include:
Enduronyl 518
Harmonyl Tablets 528
Oreticyl 545

Diazoxide (Additive hypotensive effects). Products include:
Hyperstat I.V. Injection 2095
Proglycem 649

Doxazosin Mesylate (Additive hypotensive effects). Products include:
Cardura Tablets 1941

Enalapril Maleate (Additive hypotensive effects). Products include:
Vaseretic Tablets 1559
Vasotec Tablets 1564

Enalaprilat (Additive hypotensive effects). Products include:
Vasotec I.V. 1562

Erythrityl Tetranitrate (Additive hypotensive effects). Products include:
Cardilate Oral/Sublingual Tablets .. 757

Esmolol Hydrochloride (Additive hypotensive effects). Products include:
Brevibloc Injection 942

Felodipine (Additive hypotensive effects). Products include:
Plendil Extended-Release Tablets 1526

Fluphenazine Decanoate (Additive hypotensive effects). Products include:
Prolixin Decanoate 1795

Fluphenazine Enanthate (Additive hypotensive effects). Products include:
Prolixin Enanthate 1796

Fluphenazine Hydrochloride (Additive hypotensive effects). Products include:
Prolixin Elixir 1793
Prolixin Injection 1791
Prolixin Oral Concentrate 1792
Prolixin Tablets 1793

Fosinopril Sodium (Additive hypotensive effects). Products include:
Monopril Tablets 1406

Furosemide (Additive hypotensive effects). Products include:
Lasix 1093

Guanabenz Acetate (Additive hypotensive effects). Products include:
Wytensin Tablets 2542

Guanethidine Monosulfate (Additive hypotensive effects). Products include:
Esimil Tablets 864
Ismelin Tablets 869

Hydralazine Hydrochloride (Additive hypotensive effects). Products include:
Apresazide Capsules 854
Apresoline Hydrochloride Parenteral (Ampuls) 856
Apresoline Hydrochloride Tablets .. 855
Apresoline-Esidrix Tablets 857
Ser-Ap-Es Tablets 881
Serpasil-Apresoline Tablets 884

Hydrochlorothiazide (Additive hypotensive effects). Products include:
Aldactazide 2150
Aldoril Tablets 1418
Apresazide Capsules 854
Apresoline-Esidrix Tablets 857
Capozide 2258
Dyazide Capsules 2208
Esidrix Tablets 863
Esimil Tablets 864
HydroDIURIL Tablets 1484
Hydropres Tablets 1485
Inderide Tablets 2463
Inderide LA Long Acting Capsules .. 2465
Lopressor HCT Tablets 1034
Maxzide 1215
Moduretic Tablets 1510
Normozide Tablets 2112
Oretic Tablets 544
Oreticyl 545
Prinzide Tablets 1540
Ser-Ap-Es Tablets 881
Serpasil-Esidrix Tablets 886
Timolide Tablets 1547
Trandate HCT Tablets 579
Vaseretic Tablets 1559
Zestoretic 2274

Hydroflumethiazide (Additive hypotensive effects). Products include:
Diucardin Tablets 2450
Saluron 718
Salutensin/Salutensin-Demi 719

Indapamide (Additive hypotensive effects). Products include:
Lozol Tablets 1843

Isosorbide Dinitrate (Additive hypotensive effects). Products include:
Dilatrate-SR 1827
Isordil 2467
Sorbitrate 1103

Isradipine (Additive hypotensive effects). Products include:
DynaCirc Capsules 2004

Labetalol Hydrochloride (Additive hypotensive effects). Products include:
Normodyne Injection 2108
Normodyne Tablets 2110
Normozide Tablets 2112
Trandate HCT Tablets 579
Trandate Injection 577
Trandate Tablets 579

Lisinopril (Additive hypotensive effects). Products include:
Prinivil Tablets 1538
Prinzide Tablets 1540
Zestoretic 2274
Zestril Tablets 2277

Mecamylamine Hydrochloride (Additive hypotensive effects). Products include:
Inversine Tablets 1492

Mesoridazine (Additive hypotensive effects). Products include:
Serentil 686

Methyclothiazide (Additive hypotensive effects). Products include:
Enduron Tablets 517
Enduronyl 518

Methyldopa (Additive hypotensive effects). Products include:
Aldoclor Tablets 1413
Aldomet Oral 1415
Aldoril Tablets 1418

Methyldopate Hydrochloride (Additive hypotensive effects). Products include:
Aldomet Ester HCl Injection 1417

Metolazone (Additive hypotensive effects). Products include:
Diulo 2129
Mykrox ½ mg Tablets 984
Zaroxolyn Tablets 989

Metoprolol Tartrate (Additive hypotensive effects). Products include:
Lopressor Ampuls 1032
Lopressor HCT Tablets 1034
Lopressor Tablets 1032

Metyrosine (Additive hypotensive effects). Products include:
Demser Capsules 1460

Minoxidil (Additive hypotensive effects). Products include:
Loniten Tablets 2346
Rogaine Topical Solution 2357

Nadolol (Additive hypotensive effects). Products include:
Corgard Tablets 701
Corzide Tablets 702

Nicardipine Hydrochloride (Additive hypotensive effects). Products include:
Cardene Capsules 2290

Penbutolol Sulfate (Additive hypotensive effects). Products include:
Levatol 1832

Pentaerythritol Tetranitrate (Additive hypotensive effects). Products include:
Peritrate 1756

Perphenazine (Additive hypotensive effects). Products include:
Etrafon 2087
Triavil Tablets 1556
Trilafon 2123

Phenoxybenzamine Hydrochloride (Additive hypotensive effects). Products include:
Dibenzyline Capsules 2207

Phentolamine Mesylate (Additive hypotensive effects). Products include:
Regitine 878

Pindolol (Additive hypotensive effects). Products include:
Visken Tablets 2036

Polythiazide (Additive hypotensive effects). Products include:
Minizide Capsules 1779
Renese Tablets 1785
Renese-R Tablets 1786

Prazosin Hydrochloride (Additive hypotensive effects). Products include:
Minipress Capsules 1778
Minizide Capsules 1779

Prochlorperazine (Additive hypotensive effects). Products include:
Compazine 2201

Promethazine Hydrochloride (Additive hypotensive effects). Products include:
Mepergan Injection 2479
Phenergan with Codeine 2497
Phenergan with Dextromethorphan 2499
Phenergan Injection 2493
Phenergan Suppositories 2496
Phenergan Syrup 2495
Phenergan Tablets 2496
Phenergan VC 2500
Phenergan VC with Codeine 2501

Propranolol Hydrochloride (Additive hypotensive effects). Products include:
Inderal 2459
Inderal LA Long Acting Capsules 2461
Inderide Tablets 2463
Inderide LA Long Acting Capsules .. 2465

Ramipril (Additive hypotensive effects). Products include:
Altace Capsules 1086

Rauwolfia Serpentina (Additive hypotensive effects). Products include:
Raudixin Tablets 1803
Rauzide Tablets 1804

Rescinnamine (Additive hypotensive effects).
No products indexed under this heading.

Reserpine (Additive hypotensive effects). Products include:
Diupres Tablets 1461
Hydromox R Tablets 1209
Hydropres Tablets 1485
Renese-R Tablets 1786
Salutensin/Salutensin-Demi 719

Ser-Ap-Es Tablets ... 881
Serpasil Tablets ... 883
Serpasil-Apresoline Tablets ... 884
Serpasil-Esidrix Tablets ... 886

Sodium Nitroprusside (Additive hypotensive effects). Products include:
Nipride I.V. Infusion ... 1909

Terazosin Hydrochloride (Additive hypotensive effects). Products include:
Hytrin Tablets ... 529

Thioridazine Hydrochloride (Additive hypotensive effects). Products include:
Mellaril ... 2011

Timolol Maleate (Additive hypotensive effects). Products include:
Blocadren Tablets ... 1429
Timolide Tablets ... 1547
Timoptic in Ocudose ... 1552
Timoptic Sterile Ophthalmic Solution ... 1550

Trifluoperazine Hydrochloride (Additive hypotensive effects). Products include:
Stelazine ... 2226

Trimethaphan Camsylate (Additive hypotensive effects). Products include:
Arfonad Ampuls ... 1887

NIVEA BATH SILK BATH OIL
(Moisturizing formula) ... ◘ 514
No interactions described in labeling.

NIVEA BATH SILK BATH & SHOWER GEL (EXTRA-DRY SKIN)
(Moisturizing formula) ... ◘ 514
No interactions described in labeling.

NIVEA BATH SILK BATH & SHOWER GEL (NORMAL-TO-DRY SKIN)
(Moisturizing formula) ... ◘ 514
No interactions described in labeling.

NIVEA MOISTURIZING CREME
(Moisturizing formula) ... ◘ 514
No interactions described in labeling.

NIVEA MOISTURIZING LOTION (EXTRA ENRICHED)
(Moisturizing formula) ... ◘ 514
No interactions described in labeling.

NIVEA MOISTURIZING LOTION (ORIGINAL FORMULA)
(Moisturizing formula) ... ◘ 514
No interactions described in labeling.

NIVEA MOISTURIZING OIL
(Moisturizing formula) ... ◘ 515
No interactions described in labeling.

NIVEA SKIN OIL
(Mineral Oil) ... ◘ 515
No interactions described in labeling.

NIVEA SUN AFTER SUN LOTION
(Moisturizing formula) ... ◘ 515
No interactions described in labeling.

NIVEA SUN SPF 15
(Octyl Methoxycinnamate, Oxybenzone, Padimate O (Octyl Dimethyl Paba)) ... ◘ 515
No interactions described in labeling.

NIVEA VISAGE FACIAL NOURISHING CREME
(Octyl Methoxycinnamate, Benzophenone-3) ... ◘ 515
No interactions described in labeling.

NIVEA VISAGE FACIAL NOURISHING LOTION
(Octyl Methoxycinnamate, Benzophenone-3) ... ◘ 515
No interactions described in labeling.

NIX CREME RINSE
(Permethrin) ... ◘ 542
No interactions described in labeling.

NIZORAL 2% CREAM
(Ketoconazole) ... 1143
No interactions described in labeling.

NIZORAL 2% SHAMPOO
(Ketoconazole) ... 1144
No interactions described in labeling.

NIZORAL TABLETS
(Ketoconazole) ... 1145
May interact with oral anticoagulants, oral hypoglycemic agents, and certain other agents. Compounds in these categories include:

ACTH (ACTH-induced corticosteroid serum levels decreased at high doses).

Chlorpropamide (Severe hypoglycemia). Products include:
Diabinese Tablets ... 1775

Cyclosporine (Increased blood levels of cyclosporine). Products include:
Sandimmune ... 2024

Dicumarol (Anticoagulant effect enhanced). Products include:
Dicumarol Tablets ... 516

Glipizide (Severe hypoglycemia). Products include:
Glucotrol ... 1952

Glyburide (Severe hypoglycemia). Products include:
DiaBeta ... 1091
Micronase Tablets ... 2350

Isoniazid (Affects ketoconazole concentrations adversely). Products include:
INH Tablets ... 868
Rifamate Capsules ... 1347

Phenytoin (May alter metabolism of one or both drugs). Products include:
Dilantin Infatabs ... 1710
Dilantin-30 Pediatric/Dilantin-125 Suspension ... 1713

Phenytoin Sodium (May alter metabolism of one or both drugs). Products include:
Dilantin Kapseals ... 1708
Dilantin Parenteral ... 1712
Dilantin with Phenobarbital Kapseals ... 1715

Rifampin (Reduces blood levels of ketoconazole). Products include:
Rifadin ... 1345
Rifamate Capsules ... 1347
Rimactane Capsules ... 879

Terfenadine (Increased plasma concentration of terfenadine resulting in prolonged QT interval). Products include:
Seldane Tablets ... 1349
Seldane-D Extended-Release Tablets ... 1350

Tolazamide (Severe hypoglycemia). Products include:
Tolinase Tablets ... 2365

Tolbutamide (Severe hypoglycemia). Products include:
Orinase Tablets ... 2354

Warfarin Sodium (Anticoagulant effect enhanced). Products include:
Coumadin Injection & Tablets ... 944
Panwarfin Tablets ... 547

NO DOZ FAST ACTING ALERTNESS AID TABLETS
(Caffeine) ... 751
May interact with:

Caffeine-containing medications (May cause sleeplessness, irritability, nervousness and rapid heart beat).

Food Interactions

Beverages, caffeine-containing (May cause sleeplessness, irritability, nervousness and rapid heart beat).

Food, caffeine containing (May cause sleeplessness, irritability, nervousness and rapid heart beat).

NO DOZ MAXIMUM STRENGTH CAPLETS
(Caffeine) ... 751
May interact with:

Caffeine-containing medications (May cause sleeplessness, irritability, nervousness and rapid heart beat).

Food Interactions

Beverages, caffeine-containing (May cause sleeplessness, irritability, nervousness and rapid heart beat).

Food, caffeine containing (May cause sleeplessness, irritability, nervousness and rapid heart beat).

NOLAHIST
(Phenindamine Tartrate) ... 837
May interact with:

Alcohol (Increased drowsiness).

NOLAMINE TABLETS
(Phenindamine Tartrate, Phenylpropanolamine Hydrochloride, Chlorpheniramine Maleate) ... 838
May interact with monoamine oxidase inhibitors. Compounds in this category include:

Furazolidone (Concurrent therapy contraindicated). Products include:
Furoxone ... 1855

Isocarboxazid (Concurrent therapy contraindicated). Products include:
Marplan Tablets ... 1906

Phenelzine Sulfate (Concurrent therapy contraindicated). Products include:
Nardil ... 1742

Selegiline Hydrochloride (Concurrent therapy contraindicated). Products include:
Eldepryl ... 2250

Tranylcypromine Sulfate (Concurrent therapy contraindicated). Products include:
Parnate Tablets ... 2222

NOLEX LA TABLETS
(Phenylpropanolamine Hydrochloride, Guaifenesin) ... 838
May interact with monoamine oxidase inhibitors and sympathomimetic aerosal brochodilators. Compounds in these categories include:

Albuterol (Concurrent use is not recommended). Products include:
Proventil Inhalation Aerosol ... 2117
Ventolin Inhalation Aerosol and Refill ... 583

Albuterol Sulfate (Concurrent use is not recommended). Products include:
Proventil Repetabs Tablets ... 2120
Proventil Solutions for Inhalation 0.5% and 0.083% ... 2118
Proventil Syrup ... 2119
Proventil Tablets ... 2120
Ventolin ... 583

Dobutamine Hydrochloride (Concurrent use is not recommended). Products include:
Dobutrex Solution Vials ... 1259

Dopamine Hydrochloride (Concurrent use is not recommended). Products include:
Intropin Injection ... 930

Ephedrine Hydrochloride (Concurrent use is not recommended). Products include:
Amesec ... ◘ 682
Primatene Tablets-M Formula ... 2421
Primatene Tablets-P Formula ... 2421
Primatene Tablets-Regular Formula ... 2421
Quadrinal Tablets ... 1183
Quelidrine Syrup ... 556
Tedral SA ... 1765

Ephedrine Sulfate (Concurrent use is not recommended). Products include:
Bronkaid Tablets ... ◘ 757
Bronkolixir ... ◘ 761
Bronkotabs Tablets ... ◘ 762
Marax Tablets & DF Syrup ... 1954
Pazo Hemorrhoid Ointment & Suppositories ... 752
Vicks Vatronol Nose Drops ... ◘ 666

Ephedrine Tannate (Concurrent use is not recommended). Products include:
Rynatuss ... 2388

Epinephrine (Concurrent use is not recommended). Products include:
Ana-Kit Anaphylaxis Emergency Treatment Kit ... 1100
Bronkaid Mist ... ◘ 757
EpiPen ... 843
Marcaine Hydrochloride 0.5% with Epinephrine 1:200,000 (as bitartrate) ... 958
Marcaine Hydrochloride with Epinephrine 1:200,000 ... 2055
Primatene Mist ... 2420
Sus-Phrine Injection ... 1006
Xylocaine with Epinephrine Injections ... 637

Epinephrine Bitartrate (Concurrent use is not recommended). Products include:
AsthmaHaler Mist Epinephrine Bitartrate Bronchodilator ... ◘ 616
Bronkaid Mist Suspension ... ◘ 757
Primatene Mist Suspension ... 2421

Epinephrine Hydrochloride (Concurrent use is not recommended). Products include:
Adrenalin Chloride Solution 1:100 & 1:1,000 ... 1689
Epifrin ... ◉ 244
Glaucon ... ◉ 218

Furazolidone (Concurrent use is contraindicated). Products include:
Furoxone ... 1855

Isocarboxazid (Concurrent use is contraindicated). Products include:
Marplan Tablets ... 1906

Isoproterenol Hydrochloride (Concurrent use is not recommended). Products include:
Isuprel Hydrochloride Injection 1:5000 ... 2050
Isuprel Hydrochloride Mistometer ... 2051
Isuprel Hydrochloride Solution 1:200 & 1:100 ... 2052
Norisodrine Aerotrol ... 540

Metaproterenol Sulfate (Concurrent use is not recommended). Products include:
Alupent ... 674
Arm-a-Med Metaproterenol Sulfate Inhalation Solution, USP ... 617

Metaprel Inhalation Aerosol Bronchodilator ... 2014
Metaprel Inhalation Solution ... 2015
Metaprel ... 2015
Metaproterenol Sulfate Inhalation Solution, USP ... 912

Metaraminol Bitartrate (Concurrent use is not recommended). Products include:
Aramine Injection ... 1424

Methoxamine Hydrochloride (Concurrent use is not recommended). Products include:
Vasoxyl Injection ... 819

Norepinephrine Bitartrate (Concurrent use is not recommended). Products include:
Levophed Bitartrate Injection ... 2054

Phenelzine Sulfate (Concurrent use is contraindicated). Products include:
Nardil ... 1742

Phenylephrine Bitartrate (Concurrent use is not recommended).
No products indexed under this heading.

Phenylephrine Hydrochloride (Concurrent use is not recommended). Products include:
AK-Dilate Solution 2.5% and 10% ... ⊙ 203
Atrohist Sprinkle Capsules ... 558
Cerose-DM ... 2443
Codimal ... 846
Comhist LA Capsules ... 1618
Congespirin For Children Aspirin Free Chewable Cold Tablets ... 748
Cyclomydril ... ⊙ 216
Deconsal Sprinkle Capsules ... 559
Dimetane Decongestant ... ⊞ 673
Dristan Decongestant/Antihistamine/ Analgesic Coated Caplets ... ⊞ 749
Dristan Cold Nasal Decongestant/ Antihistamine/ Analgesic Coated Tablets ... 2419
Dristan Advanced Formula Decongestant/Antihistamine/ Analgesic Tablets ... ⊞ 749
Dristan Nasal Spray, Menthol ... 2419
Dristan Nasal Spray, Regular and Regular with Metered Pump ... 2419
Entex Capsules ... 1623
Entex Liquid ... 1623
Sinus Excedrin Analgesic, Decongestant Tablets & Caplets ... 750
Extendryl ... 994
4-Way Fast Acting Nasal Spray - Original Formula (regular & mentholated) & Metered Spray Pump (regular) ... 751
Hycomine Compound Tablets ... 929
Murocoll-2 Sterile Ophthalmic Solution ... ⊙ 261
Mydfrin 2.5% ... ⊙ 224
Naldecon Syrup, Tablets, Pediatric Drops and Pediatric Syrup ... 709
Neo-Synephrine Hydrochloride 1% Carpuject ... 2063
Neo-Synephrine Hydrochloride 1% Injection ... 2063
Neo-Synephrine Hydrochloride (Ophthalmic) ... 2064
Neo-Synephrine ... ⊞ 759
Nōstril Nasal Decongestant ... ⊞ 520
Novahistine Elixir ... ⊞ 596
Phenergan VC ... 2500
Phenergan VC with Codeine ... 2501
Prefrin Liquifilm Vasoconstrictor and Lubricant Eye Drops ... ⊙ 254
Prefrin-A ... ⊙ 255
Quelidrine Syrup ... 556
Relief Vasoconstrictor and Lubricant Eye Drops ... ⊙ 256
Robitussin Night Relief ... ⊞ 677
Ru-Tuss with Hydrocodone ... 694
Ru-Tuss Tablets ... 693
Vasosulf ... ⊙ 279
Vicks Sinex ... ⊞ 665
Zincfrin ... ⊙ 230

Phenylephrine Tannate (Concurrent use is not recommended). Products include:
Rynatan ... 2387
Rynatuss ... 2388

Pirbuterol Acetate (Concurrent use is not recommended). Products include:
Maxair Inhaler ... 1311

Pseudoephedrine Hydrochloride (Concurrent use is not recommended). Products include:
Actifed Capsules ... ⊞ 539
Actifed Plus Caplets ... ⊞ 539
Actifed Plus Tablets ... ⊞ 540
Actifed with Codeine Cough Syrup ... 752
Actifed Syrup ... ⊞ 540
Actifed Tablets ... ⊞ 540
Actifed 12-Hour Capsules ... ⊞ 539
Advil Cold & Sinus Caplets (formerly CoAdvil) ... 2416
Allerest ... ⊞ 559
Anatuss LA Tablets ... 1359
Benadryl Decongestant Elixir ... ⊞ 635
Benadryl Decongestant ... ⊞ 635
Benadryl Plus ... ⊞ 636
Benadryl Plus Nighttime ... ⊞ 637
Benylin Decongestant ... ⊞ 638
Brexin L.A. Capsules ... 2078
Bromfed Capsules (Timed Release) ... 1615
Bromfed Syrup ... ⊞ 628
Bromfed ... 1615
CoAdvil ... ⊞ 748
Allergy-Sinus Comtrex Multi-Symptom Allergy Sinus Formula Tablets & Caplets ... 746
Cough Formula Comtrex ... 746
Comtrex Multi-Symptom Cold Reliever Tablets/Caplets/Liqui-Gels/Liquid ... 745
Day-Night Comtrex ... 747
Non-Drowsy Comtrex ... 747
Congess ... 994
Congestac Caplets ... ⊞ 617
Contac Jr. Children's Cold Medicine ... ⊞ 712
Contac Nighttime Cold Medicine ... ⊞ 713
Contac Sinus Caplets Maximum Strength Non-Drowsy Formula ... ⊞ 710
Contac Sinus Tablets Maximum Strength Non-Drowsy Formula ... ⊞ 710
Deconamine ... 663
Deconsal II Tablets ... 559
Dimacol Caplets ... ⊞ 672
Dimetane-DX Cough Syrup ... 1858
Dorcol Children's Cough Syrup ... ⊞ 685
Dorcol Children's Decongestant Liquid ... ⊞ 685
Dorcol Children's Liquid Cold Formula ... ⊞ 686
Maximum Strength Dristan Decongestant/Analgesic Coated Caplets ... ⊞ 750
No Drowsiness Dristan Cold Nasal Decongestant/Analgesic Coated Caplets ... 2420
Dristan Sinus Caplets ... 2419
Sinus Excedrin Analgesic, Decongestant Tablets & Caplets ... ⊞ 533
Fedahist Gyrocaps ... 2145
Fedahist Timecaps ... 2145
Guaifed ... 1615
Guaifed Syrup ... ⊞ 629
Isoclor Expectorant ... 982
Isoclor Timesule Capsules ... ⊞ 561
Kronofed-A ... 970
Medi-Flu Caplet, Liquid ... ⊞ 640
Novafed A Capsules ... 1342
Novafed Capsules ... 1342
Novahistine DH ... 1342
Novahistine DMX ... ⊞ 595
Novahistine Expectorant ... 1343
Nucofed Capsules ... 2219
Nucofed Expectorant ... 2219
Nucofed Pediatric Expectorant ... 2220
Nucofed Syrup ... 2219
Ornex Caplets ... ⊞ 618
PediaCare Allergy Relief Formula Liquid ... 1362
PediaCare Cough-Cold Formula Liquid ... 1362
PediaCare Infants' Oral Decongestant Drops ... 1362
PediaCare Night Rest Cough-Cold Formula Liquid ... 1362
PediaCare 6-12 Cough-Cold Formula Chewable Tablets ... 1362
Robitussin-DAC Syrup ... 1875
Robitussin-PE ... ⊞ 677
Rondec ... 1975
Rondec-DM ... 1976
Rondec-TR Tablet ... 1975
Ru-Tuss DE Tablets ... 694
Ryna ... ⊞ 741
Seldane-D Extended-Release Tablets ... 1350
Sinarest ... ⊞ 562
Sine-Aid Maximum Strength Sinus Headache Caplets ... 1365
Sine-Aid Maximum Strength Sinus Headache Tablets ... 1365
Sine-Off Maximum Strength Allergy/Sinus Formula Caplets ... ⊞ 721
Sine-Off Maximum Strength No Drowsiness Formula Caplets ... ⊞ 722
Singlet Tablets ... ⊞ 598
Sinutab Maximum Strength ... ⊞ 641
Sinutab Maximum Strength Without Drowsiness Tablets & Caplets ... ⊞ 642
Sinutab Regular Strength Without Drowsiness Formula ... ⊞ 641
St. Joseph Nighttime Cold Medicine ... ⊞ 705
Sudafed Children's Liquid ... ⊞ 543
Sudafed Cough Syrup ... ⊞ 543
Sudafed Plus Liquid ... ⊞ 544
Sudafed Plus Tablets ... ⊞ 545
Sudafed Sinus Caplets ... ⊞ 545
Sudafed Sinus Tablets ... ⊞ 545
Sudafed Tablets, 30 mg ... ⊞ 544
Sudafed Tablets, Adult Strength, 60 mg ... ⊞ 544
Sudafed 12 Hour Capsules ... ⊞ 545
TheraFlu Flu and Cold Medicine ... ⊞ 687
Triaminic Nite Light ... ⊞ 689
Tylenol Allergy Sinus Medication Caplets and Gelcaps, Maximum Strength ... 1372
Children's Tylenol Cold Liquid Formula and Chewable Tablets ... 1368
Tylenol Cold & Flu Hot Medication, Packets ... 1369
Tylenol Cold & Flu No Drowsiness Hot Medication, Packets ... 1371
Tylenol Cold Medication Caplets and Tablets ... 1370
Tylenol Cold Medication No Drowsiness Formula Caplets ... 1370
Tylenol Cold Night Time Medication Liquid ... 1371
Tylenol Cough Medication Liquid with Decongestant, Maximum Strength ... 1372
Tylenol, Maximum Strength, Sinus Medication Gelcaps, Caplets and Tablets ... 1373
Ursinus Inlay-Tabs ... ⊞ 691
Vicks Children's NyQuil ... ⊞ 664
Vicks Daycare ... ⊞ 660
Vicks Formula 44D Decongestant Cough Medicine ... ⊞ 662
Vicks Formula 44M Multi-Symptom Cough Medicine ... ⊞ 662
Vicks NyQuil Nighttime Colds Medicine-Original & Cherry Flavor ... ⊞ 664
Vicks Pediatric Formula 44 Cough & Congestion Medicine ... ⊞ 663
Vicks Pediatric Formula 44m Multi-Symptom Cough & Cold Medicine ... ⊞ 663

Pseudoephedrine Sulfate (Concurrent use is not recommended). Products include:
Afrin Tablets ... ⊞ 693
Chlor-Trimeton Decongestant ... ⊞ 694
Disophrol Chronotab Sustained-Action Tablets ... ⊞ 698
Drixoral Antihistamine/Nasal Decongestant Syrup ... ⊞ 698
Drixoral Non-Drowsy Formula ... ⊞ 699
Drixoral Plus Extended-Release Tablets ... ⊞ 699
Drixoral Sinus ... ⊞ 700
Drixoral Sustained-Action Tablets ... ⊞ 698
Sinutab Allergy Formula Sustained Action Tablets ... ⊞ 640
Trinalin Repetabs Tablets ... 1170

Selegiline Hydrochloride (Concurrent use is contraindicated). Products include:
Eldepryl ... 2250

Terbutaline Sulfate (Concurrent use is not recommended). Products include:
Brethaire Inhaler ... 1024
Brethine Ampuls ... 1026
Brethine Tablets ... 1026
Bricanyl Injection ... 1324
Bricanyl Tablets ... 1325

Tranylcypromine Sulfate (Concurrent use is contraindicated). Products include:
Parnate Tablets ... 2222

NOLVADEX TABLETS
(Tamoxifen Citrate) ... 1102
May interact with oral anticoagulants. Compounds in this category include:

Dicumarol (Increased anticoagulant effect; monitor patient's prothrombin time). Products include:
Dicumarol Tablets ... 516

Warfarin Sodium (Increased anticoagulant effect; monitor patient's prothrombin time). Products include:
Coumadin Injection & Tablets ... 944
Panwarfin Tablets ... 547

NORCURON
(Vecuronium Bromide) ... 1642
May interact with nondepolarizing neuromuscular blocking agents, inhalant anesthetics, aminoglycosides, tetracyclines, and certain other agents. Compounds in these categories include:

Amikacin Sulfate (Possible prolongation of neuromuscular blockade). Products include:
Amikin Injectable ... 602

Atracurium Besylate (Additive effect). Products include:
Tracrium Injection ... 817

Bacitracin (Possible prolongation of neuromuscular blockade). Products include:
Baciguent Antibiotic Ointment ... ⊞ 735
Bactine First Aid Antibiotic Ointment ... ⊞ 625
Campho-Phenique Triple Antibiotic Ointment Plus Pain Reliever ⊞ 758
Lanabiotic Ointment ... ⊞ 556
Mycitracin ... ⊞ 737

Colistimethate Sodium (Possible prolongation of neuromuscular blockade). Products include:
Coly-Mycin M Parenteral ... 1706

Colistin Sulfate (Possible prolongation of neuromuscular blockade). Products include:
Coly-Mycin S For Oral Suspension ... 1708
Coly-Mycin S Otic w/Neomycin & Hydrocortisone ... 1708

Demeclocycline Hydrochloride (Possible prolongation of neuromuscular blockade). Products include:
Declomycin Capsules, Tablets ... 1199

Doxycycline Calcium (Possible prolongation of neuromuscular blockade).
No products indexed under this heading.

Doxycycline Hyclate (Possible prolongation of neuromuscular blockade). Products include:
Doryx Capsules ... 1717
Vibramycin Hyclate Capsules ... 1787
Vibramycin Hyclate Intravenous ... 1968
Vibra-Tabs Film Coated Tablets ... 1787

Doxycycline Monohydrate (Possible prolongation of neuromuscular blockade). Products include:
Monodox Capsules ... 1630
Vibramycin Monohydrate for Oral Suspension ... 1787

Enflurane (Pronounced enhancement of neuromuscular blockade). Products include:
Ethrane ... 599

Gentamicin Sulfate (Possible prolongation of neuromuscular blockade). Products include:
Garamycin Injectable ... 2093
Garamycin Ophthalmic ... ⊙ 305
Genoptic Liquifilm Sterile Ophthalmic Solution ... ⊙ 247

Genoptic S.O.P. Sterile Ophthalmic Ointment ⊙ 247
Gentacidin Ointment ⊙ 273
Gentacidin Solution ⊙ 273
Gentak Ointment & Solution ⊙ 208
G-myticin Creme and Ointment 0.1% 1770
Pred-G Liquifilm Sterile Ophthalmic Suspension ⊙ 252
Pred-G S.O.P. Sterile Ophthalmic Ointment ⊙ 253

Halothane (Pronounced enhancement of neuromuscular blockade). Products include:
Fluothane 2453

Isoflurane (Pronounced enhancement of neuromuscular blockade). Products include:
Forane 600

Kanamycin Sulfate (Possible prolongation of neuromuscular blockade). Products include:
Kantrex Injection 601
Kantrex Pediatric Injection 601

Magnesium Sulfate Injection (May enhance the neuromuscular blockade).

Methacycline Hydrochloride (Possible prolongation of neuromuscular blockade).
No products indexed under this heading.

Methoxyflurane (Pronounced enhancement of neuromuscular blockade).
No products indexed under this heading.

Metocurine Iodide (Additive effect). Products include:
Metubine Iodide Vials 1285

Minocycline Hydrochloride (Possible prolongation of neuromuscular blockade). Products include:
Minocin Intravenous 1221
Minocin Oral Suspension 1224
Minocin Pellet-Filled Capsules 1222

Neomycin, oral (Possible prolongation of neuromuscular blockade).

Oxytetracycline (Possible prolongation of neuromuscular blockade). Products include:
Terramycin Intramuscular Solution 1964
Urobiotic-250 Capsules 1968

Oxytetracycline Hydrochloride (Possible prolongation of neuromuscular blockade). Products include:
Terra-Cortril Ophthalmic Suspension 1963
Terramycin Capsules 1786
Terramycin Intramuscular Solution 1964
Terramycin with Polymyxin B Sulfate Ophthalmic Ointment 1965

Pancuronium Bromide Injection (Additive effect).
No products indexed under this heading.

Polymyxin B Sulfate (Possible prolongation of neuromuscular blockade). Products include:
AK-Poly-Bac Ointment ⊙ 205
AK-Spore H.C. ⊙ 206
AK-Spore ⊙ 205
AK-Trol Ointment & Suspension ⊙ 207
Aquaphor Antibiotic Formula 662
Bactine First Aid Antibiotic Ointment ▣ 625
Campho-Phenique Triple Antibiotic Ointment Plus Pain Reliever ▣ 758
Cortisporin Cream 757
Cortisporin Ointment 758
Cortisporin Ophthalmic Ointment Sterile 758
Cortisporin Ophthalmic Suspension Sterile 759
Cortisporin Otic Solution Sterile 760
Cortisporin Otic Suspension Sterile 760
Dexacidin ⊙ 272
Lanabiotic Ointment ▣ 556
LazerSporin-C Solution 1770
Maxitrol Ophthalmic Ointment/Suspension ⊙ 223
Mycitracin ▣ 737
Neosporin Cream 792
Neosporin G.U. Irrigant Sterile 793
Neosporin Ointment 793
Maximum Strength Neosporin Ointment 793
Neosporin Ophthalmic Ointment Sterile 793
Neosporin Ophthalmic Solution Sterile 794
Ophthocort ⊙ 301
PediOtic Suspension Sterile 797
Polymyxin B Sulfate, Aerosporin Brand Sterile Powder 798
Poly-Pred Liquifilm ⊙ 250
Polysporin Ointment ▣ 543
Polysporin Ophthalmic Ointment Sterile 798
Polysporin Powder ▣ 543
Polysporin Spray ▣ 543
Polytrim Ophthalmic Solution Sterile 588
Terramycin with Polymyxin B Sulfate Ophthalmic Ointment 1965

Quinidine Gluconate (Possible recurrent paralysis). Products include:
Quinaglute Dura-Tabs Tablets 663

Quinidine Polygalacturonate (Possible recurrent paralysis). Products include:
Cardioquin Tablets 1812

Quinidine Sulfate (Possible recurrent paralysis). Products include:
Quinidex Extentabs 1868

Streptomycin Sulfate (Possible prolongation of neuromuscular blockade).
No products indexed under this heading.

Succinylcholine Chloride (Prior administration may enhance neuromuscular blocking effect and duration of action of Norcuron). Products include:
Anectine 755

Tetracycline Hydrochloride (Possible prolongation of neuromuscular blockade). Products include:
Achromycin V Capsules 1193
Achromycin Ophthalmic Ointment 1% ⊙ 307
Achromycin Ophthalmic Suspension 1% ⊙ 308
Topicycline for Topical Solution 1856

Tobramycin (Possible prolongation of neuromuscular blockade). Products include:
TobraDex Ophthalmic Suspension and Ointment ⊙ 228
Tobrex Ophthalmic Ointment and Solution 572

Tobramycin Sulfate (Possible prolongation of neuromuscular blockade). Products include:
Nebcin Vials, Hyporets & ADD-Vantage 1286

NORDETTE-21 TABLETS
(Levonorgestrel, Ethinyl Estradiol) 2481
May interact with barbiturates and certain other agents. Compounds in these categories include:

Ampicillin Sodium (Reduced efficacy; increased incidence of breakthrough bleeding). Products include:
Unasyn 1965

Aprobarbital (Reduced efficacy; increased incidence of breakthrough bleeding). Products include:
Alurate Elixir 1883

Butabarbital (Reduced efficacy; increased incidence of breakthrough bleeding). Products include:
Pyridium Plus 1764

Butalbital (Reduced efficacy; increased incidence of breakthrough bleeding). Products include:
Esgic-Plus Tablets 1002
Esgic Tablets & Capsules 1001
Fioricet Tablets 2006
Fiorinal Capsules 2007
Fiorinal with Codeine Capsules 2008
Fiorinal Tablets 2007
Phrenilin 838
Sedapap Tablets 50 mg/650 mg 1360

Mephobarbital (Reduced efficacy; increased incidence of breakthrough bleeding). Products include:
Mebaral Tablets 2061

Oxytetracycline (Reduced efficacy; increased incidence of breakthrough bleeding). Products include:
Terramycin Intramuscular Solution 1964
Urobiotic-250 Capsules 1968

Oxytetracycline Hydrochloride (Reduced efficacy; increased incidence of breakthrough bleeding). Products include:
Terra-Cortril Ophthalmic Suspension 1963
Terramycin Capsules 1786
Terramycin Intramuscular Solution 1964
Terramycin with Polymyxin B Sulfate Ophthalmic Ointment 1965

Pentobarbital Sodium (Reduced efficacy; increased incidence of breakthrough bleeding). Products include:
Nembutal Sodium Capsules 534
Nembutal Sodium Solution 536
Nembutal Sodium Suppositories 538

Phenobarbital (Reduced efficacy; increased incidence of breakthrough bleeding). Products include:
Arco-Lase Plus Tablets 607
Bellergal-S Tablets 1998
Bronkolixir ▣ 761
Bronkotabs Tablets ▣ 762
Donnatal 1858
Donnatal Extentabs 1859
Donnatal Tablets 1858
Donnazyme Tablets 1860
Kinesed Tablets 2272
Phenobarbital Elixir and Tablets 1293
Primatene Tablets-P Formula 2421
Quadrinal Tablets 1183
Tedral SA 1765

Phenylbutazone (Reduced efficacy; increased incidence of breakthrough bleeding). Products include:
Butazolidin Capsules & Tablets 1027

Phenytoin Sodium (Reduced efficacy; increased incidence of breakthrough bleeding). Products include:
Dilantin Kapseals 1708
Dilantin Parenteral 1712
Dilantin with Phenobarbital Kapseals 1715

Rifampin (Reduced efficacy; increased incidence of breakthrough bleeding). Products include:
Rifadin 1345
Rifamate Capsules 1347
Rimactane Capsules 879

Secobarbital Sodium (Reduced efficacy; increased incidence of breakthrough bleeding). Products include:
Seconal Sodium Pulvules 1296

Tetracycline Hydrochloride (Reduced efficacy; increased incidence of breakthrough bleeding). Products include:
Achromycin V Capsules 1193
Achromycin Ophthalmic Ointment 1% ⊙ 307
Achromycin Ophthalmic Suspension 1% ⊙ 308
Topicycline for Topical Solution 1856

Thiamylal Sodium (Reduced efficacy; increased incidence of breakthrough bleeding). Products include:
Surital Ampoules, Steri-Vials 1764

NORDETTE-28 TABLETS
(Levonorgestrel, Ethinyl Estradiol) 2483
See **Nordette-21 Tablets**

NORETHIN 1/35E-21
(Ethinyl Estradiol, Norethindrone) 2133
See **Demulen 1/35-21**

NORETHIN 1/35E-28
(Ethinyl Estradiol, Norethindrone) 2133
See **Demulen 1/35-21**

NORETHIN 1/50M-21
(Mestranol, Norethindrone) 2133
See **Demulen 1/35-21**

NORETHIN 1/50M-28
(Mestranol, Norethindrone) 2133
See **Demulen 1/35-21**

NORFLEX INJECTABLE
(Orphenadrine Citrate) 1314
No interactions described in labeling.

NORFLEX SUSTAINED-RELEASE TABLETS
(Orphenadrine Citrate) 1314
No interactions described in labeling.

NORGESIC FORTE TABLETS
(Orphenadrine Citrate, Aspirin) 1314
See **Norgesic Tablets**

NORGESIC TABLETS
(Orphenadrine Citrate, Aspirin) 1314
May interact with:

Propoxyphene Hydrochloride (Potential for confusion, anxiety and tremors). Products include:
Darvon 1256
Wygesic Tablets 2540

Propoxyphene Napsylate (Potential for confusion, anxiety and tremors). Products include:
Darvon-N/Darvocet-N 1254

NORINYL 1+35 21-DAY TABLETS
(Norethindrone, Mestranol) 2304
See **Brevicon 21-Day Tablets**

NORINYL 1+35 28-DAY TABLETS
(Norethindrone, Mestranol) 2304
See **Brevicon 21-Day Tablets**

NORINYL 1+50 21-DAY TABLETS
(Norethindrone, Mestranol) 2304
See **Brevicon 21-Day Tablets**

NORINYL 1+50 28-DAY TABLETS
(Norethindrone, Mestranol) 2304
See **Brevicon 21-Day Tablets**

NORISODRINE AEROTROL
(Isoproterenol Hydrochloride) 540
May interact with:

Epinephrine (Should not be used concurrently). Products include:
Ana-Kit Anaphylaxis Emergency Treatment Kit 1100
Bronkaid Mist ▣ 757
EpiPen 843
Marcaine Hydrochloride 0.5% with Epinephrine 1:200,000 (as bitartrate) 958
Marcaine Hydrochloride with Epinephrine 1:200,000 2055
Primatene Mist 2420
Sus-Phrine Injection 1006
Xylocaine with Epinephrine Injections 637

Epinephrine Bitartrate (Should not be used concurrently). Products include:
AsthmaHaler Mist Epinephrine Bitartrate Bronchodilator ▣ 616
Bronkaid Mist Suspension ▣ 757
Primatene Mist Suspension 2421

NORLESTRIN [Fe] 1/50
(Norethindrone Acetate, Ethinyl Estradiol) 1746
See **Norlestrin [21] 1/50**

NORLESTRIN [Fe] 2.5/50
(Norethindrone Acetate, Ethinyl Estradiol) 1746
See **Norlestrin [21] 1/50**

NORLESTRIN [21] 1/50
(Norethindrone Acetate, Ethinyl Estradiol) 1746
May interact with barbiturates, tetracyclines, and certain other agents. Compounds in these categories include:

Ampicillin Sodium (Reduced efficacy of Norlestrin; increased incidence of breakthrough bleeding). Products include:
- Unasyn 1965

Aprobarbital (Reduced efficacy of Norlestrin; increased incidence of breakthrough bleeding). Products include:
- Alurate Elixir 1883

Butabarbital (Reduced efficacy of Norlestrin; increased incidence of breakthrough bleeding). Products include:
- Pyridium Plus 1764

Butalbital (Reduced efficacy of Norlestrin; increased incidence of breakthrough bleeding). Products include:
- Esgic-Plus Tablets 1002
- Esgic Tablets & Capsules 1001
- Fioricet Tablets 2006
- Fiorinal Capsules 2007
- Fiorinal with Codeine Capsules 2008
- Fiorinal Tablets 2007
- Phrenilin 838
- Sedapap Tablets 50 mg/650 mg .. 1360

Demeclocycline Hydrochloride (Reduced efficacy of Norlestrin; increased incidence of breakthrough bleeding). Products include:
- Declomycin Capsules, Tablets 1199

Doxycycline Calcium (Reduced efficacy of Norlestrin; increased incidence of breakthrough bleeding).
No products indexed under this heading.

Doxycycline Hyclate (Reduced efficacy of Norlestrin; increased incidence of breakthrough bleeding). Products include:
- Doryx Capsules 1717
- Vibramycin Hyclate Capsules 1787
- Vibramycin Hyclate Intravenous 1968
- Vibra-Tabs Film Coated Tablets 1787

Doxycycline Monohydrate (Reduced efficacy of Norlestrin; increased incidence of breakthrough bleeding). Products include:
- Monodox Capsules 1630
- Vibramycin Monohydrate for Oral Suspension 1787

Griseofulvin (Reduced efficacy of Norlestrin; increased incidence of breakthrough bleeding). Products include:
- Fulvicin P/G Tablets 2090
- Fulvicin P/G 165 & 330 Tablets 2091
- Fulvicin-U/F Tablets 2092
- Grifulvin V (griseofulvin microsize) Tablets/Suspension 1678
- Grisactin 2454
- Grisactin Ultra Tablets 2455
- Gris-PEG Tablets, 125 mg & 250 mg 1083

Mephobarbital (Reduced efficacy of Norlestrin; increased incidence of breakthrough bleeding). Products include:
- Mebaral Tablets 2061

Methacycline Hydrochloride (Reduced efficacy of Norlestrin; increased incidence of breakthrough bleeding).
No products indexed under this heading.

Minocycline Hydrochloride (Reduced efficacy of Norlestrin; increased incidence of breakthrough bleeding). Products include:
- Minocin Intravenous 1221
- Minocin Oral Suspension 1224
- Minocin Pellet-Filled Capsules 1222

Oxytetracycline (Reduced efficacy of Norlestrin; increased incidence of breakthrough bleeding). Products include:
- Terramycin Intramuscular Solution 1964
- Urobiotic-250 Capsules 1968

Oxytetracycline Hydrochloride (Reduced efficacy of Norlestrin; increased incidence of breakthrough bleeding). Products include:
- Terra-Cortril Ophthalmic Suspension 1963
- Terramycin Capsules 1786
- Terramycin Intramuscular Solution 1964
- Terramycin with Polymyxin B Sulfate Ophthalmic Ointment 1965

Pentobarbital Sodium (Reduced efficacy of Norlestrin; increased incidence of breakthrough bleeding). Products include:
- Nembutal Sodium Capsules 534
- Nembutal Sodium Solution 536
- Nembutal Sodium Suppositories 538

Phenobarbital (Reduced efficacy of Norlestrin; increased incidence of breakthrough bleeding). Products include:
- Arco-Lase Plus Tablets 607
- Bellergal-S Tablets 1998
- Bronkolixir .... ▣ 761
- Bronkotabs Tablets .... ▣ 762
- Donnatal 1858
- Donnatal Extentabs 1859
- Donnatal Tablets 1858
- Donnazyme Tablets 1860
- Kinesed Tablets 2272
- Phenobarbital Elixir and Tablets 1293
- Primatene Tablets-P Formula 2421
- Quadrinal Tablets 1183
- Tedral SA 1765

Phenylbutazone (Reduced efficacy of Norlestrin; increased incidence of breakthrough bleeding). Products include:
- Butazolidin Capsules & Tablets 1027

Phenytoin (Reduced efficacy of Norlestrin; increased incidence of breakthrough bleeding). Products include:
- Dilantin Infatabs 1710
- Dilantin-30 Pediatric/Dilantin-125 Suspension 1713

Phenytoin Sodium (Reduced efficacy of Norlestrin; increased incidence of breakthrough bleeding). Products include:
- Dilantin Kapseals 1708
- Dilantin Parenteral 1712
- Dilantin with Phenobarbital Kapseals 1715

Rifampin (Reduced efficacy of Norlestrin; increased incidence of breakthrough bleeding). Products include:
- Rifadin 1345
- Rifamate Capsules 1347
- Rimactane Capsules 879

Secobarbital Sodium (Reduced efficacy of Norlestrin; increased incidence of breakthrough bleeding). Products include:
- Seconal Sodium Pulvules 1296

Tetracycline Hydrochloride (Reduced efficacy of Norlestrin; increased incidence of breakthrough bleeding). Products include:
- Achromycin V Capsules 1193
- Achromycin Ophthalmic Ointment 1% .... ◉ 307
- Achromycin Ophthalmic Suspension 1% .... ◉ 308
- Topicycline for Topical Solution 1856

Thiamylal Sodium (Reduced efficacy of Norlestrin; increased incidence of breakthrough bleeding). Products include:
- Surital Ampoules, Steri-Vials 1764

NORLESTRIN [21] 2.5/50
(Norethindrone Acetate, Ethinyl Estradiol) 1746
See **Norlestrin [21] 1/50**

NORLESTRIN [28] 1/50
(Norethindrone Acetate, Ethinyl Estradiol) 1746
See **Norlestrin [21] 1/50**

NORLUTATE
(Norethindrone Acetate) 1754
May interact with:

Rifampin (Reduced efficacy and increased incidence of breakthrough bleeding). Products include:
- Rifadin 1345
- Rifamate Capsules 1347
- Rimactane Capsules 879

NORLUTIN
(Norethindrone) 1755
May interact with progestins and certain other agents. Compounds in these categories include:

Medroxyprogesterone Acetate (Potential for adverse effects on carbohydrate and lipid metabolism). Products include:
- Amen 833
- Cycrin Tablets 2449
- Depo-Provera Sterile Aqueous Suspension 2336
- Provera Tablets 2356

Megestrol Acetate (Potential for adverse effects on carbohydrate and lipid metabolism). Products include:
- Megace Tablets 732

Norgestimate (Potential for adverse effects on carbohydrate and lipid metabolism). Products include:
- Ortho-Cyclen Tablets 1658

Rifampin (Reduced efficacy and increased incidence of breakthrough bleeding). Products include:
- Rifadin 1345
- Rifamate Capsules 1347
- Rimactane Capsules 879

NORMODYNE INJECTION
(Labetalol Hydrochloride) 2108
May interact with oral hypoglycemic agents, insulin, tricyclic antidepressants, sympathomimetic bronchodilators, and certain other agents. Compounds in these categories include:

Albuterol (Blunted bronchodilator effect). Products include:
- Proventil Inhalation Aerosol 2117
- Ventolin Inhalation Aerosol and Refill 583

Albuterol Sulfate (Blunted bronchodilator effect). Products include:
- Proventil Repetabs Tablets 2120
- Proventil Solutions for Inhalation 0.5% and 0.083% 2118
- Proventil Syrup 2119
- Proventil Tablets 2120
- Ventolin 583

Amitriptyline Hydrochloride (Potential for tremor). Products include:
- Elavil 2269
- Endep Tablets 1927
- Etrafon 2087
- Limbitrol 1933
- Triavil Tablets 1556

Amoxapine (Potential for tremor). Products include:
- Asendin Tablets 1196

Bitolterol Mesylate (Blunted bronchodilator effect). Products include:
- Tornalate 2074

Chlorpropamide (Altered dosage requirements). Products include:
- Diabinese Tablets 1775

Cimetidine (Increases bioavailability of labetalol). Products include:
- Tagamet Tablets 2228

Cimetidine Hydrochloride (Increases bioavailability of labetalol). Products include:
- Tagamet 2228

Clomipramine Hydrochloride (Potential for tremor). Products include:
- Anafranil Capsules 650

Desipramine Hydrochloride (Potential for tremor). Products include:
- Norpramin Tablets 1340

Doxepin Hydrochloride (Potential for tremor). Products include:
- Sinequan 1960

Ephedrine Hydrochloride (Blunted bronchodilator effect). Products include:
- Amesec .... ▣ 682
- Primatene Tablets-M Formula 2421
- Primatene Tablets-P Formula 2421
- Primatene Tablets-Regular Formula 2421
- Quadrinal Tablets 1183
- Quelidrine Syrup 556
- Tedral SA 1765

Ephedrine Sulfate (Blunted bronchodilator effect). Products include:
- Bronkaid Tablets .... ▣ 757
- Bronkolixir .... ▣ 761
- Bronkotabs Tablets .... ▣ 762
- Marax Tablets & DF Syrup 1954
- Pazo Hemorrhoid Ointment & Suppositories 752
- Vicks Vatronol Nose Drops .... ▣ 666

Ephedrine Tannate (Blunted bronchodilator effect). Products include:
- Rynatuss 2388

Epinephrine (Blunted bronchodilator effect). Products include:
- Ana-Kit Anaphylaxis Emergency Treatment Kit 1100
- Bronkaid Mist .... ▣ 757
- EpiPen 843
- Marcaine Hydrochloride 0.5% with Epinephrine 1:200,000 (as bitartrate) 958
- Marcaine Hydrochloride with Epinephrine 1:200,000 2055
- Primatene Mist 2420
- Sus-Phrine Injection 1006
- Xylocaine with Epinephrine Injections 637

Epinephrine Hydrochloride (Blunted bronchodilator effect). Products include:
- Adrenalin Chloride Solution 1:100 & 1:1,000 1689
- Epifrin .... ◉ 244
- Glaucon .... ◉ 218

Ethylnorepinephrine Hydrochloride (Blunted bronchodilator effect). Products include:
- Bronkephrine Injection 2042

Glipizide (Altered dosage requirements). Products include:
- Glucotrol 1952

Glyburide (Altered dosage requirements). Products include:
- DiaBeta 1091
- Micronase Tablets 2350

Halothane (Synergism; hypotension). Products include:
- Fluothane 2453

Imipramine Hydrochloride (Potential for tremor). Products include:
- Tofranil Ampuls 1038
- Tofranil Tablets 1039

Imipramine Pamoate (Potential for tremor). Products include:
- Tofranil-PM Capsules 1041

Insulin, Human (Altered dosage requirements).
- No products indexed under this heading.

Insulin, Human Isophane Suspension (Altered dosage requirements). Products include:
- Humulin N, 100 Units 1270

Insulin, Human NPH (Altered dosage requirements). Products include:
- Insulatard NPH Human 1627
- Novolin N 1627
- Novolin N PenFill Cartridges 1628
- Novolin N Prefilled 1628

Insulin, Human Regular (Altered dosage requirements). Products include:
- Humulin BR, 100 Units 1268
- Humulin R, 100 Units 1272
- Novolin R 1627
- Novolin R PenFill Cartridges 1628
- Novolin R Prefilled 1629
- Velosulin Human 1628

Insulin, Human, Zinc Suspension (Altered dosage requirements). Products include:
- Humulin L, 100 Units 1268
- Humulin U, 100 Units 1272
- Novolin L 1627

Insulin, NPH (Altered dosage requirements). Products include:
- NPH, 40 & 100 Units 1273
- Beef NPH, 100 Units 1274
- Pork NPH, 100 Units 1275
- Insulatard NPH 1626
- NPH Insulin 1626
- NPH Purified Pork Isophane Insulin 1626

Insulin, Regular (Altered dosage requirements). Products include:
- Regular, 40 & 100 Units 1273
- Beef Regular, 100 Units 1275
- Pork Regular, 100 Units 1275
- Pork Regular (Concentrated), 500 Units 1276
- Regular Insulin 1625
- Regular Purified Pork Insulin 1626
- Velosulin 1627

Insulin, Zinc Crystals (Altered dosage requirements). Products include:
- NPH, 40 & 100 Units 1273

Insulin, Zinc Suspension (Altered dosage requirements). Products include:
- Lente, 40 & 100 Units 1272
- Protamine, Zinc, 40 & 100 Units 1273
- Lente Iletin I 1272
- Beef Lente, 100 Units 1274
- Beef Protamine Zinc, 100 Units 1274
- Pork Lente, 100 Units 1275
- Pork, Protamine, Zinc, 100 Units 1275
- Lente Insulin 1626
- Lente Purified Pork Insulin 1626
- Semilente Insulin 1625
- Ultralente Insulin 1626

Isoetharine (Blunted bronchodilator effect). Products include:
- Arm-a-Med Isoetharine Inhalation Solution, USP 616
- Bronkometer Aerosol 2042
- Bronkosol Solution 2042

Isoproterenol Hydrochloride (Blunted bronchodilator effect). Products include:
- Isuprel Hydrochloride Injection 1:5000 2050
- Isuprel Hydrochloride Mistometer .. 2051
- Isuprel Hydrochloride Solution 1:200 & 1:100 2052
- Norisodrine Aerotrol 540

Maprotiline Hydrochloride (Potential for tremor). Products include:
- Ludiomil Tablets 874

Metaproterenol Sulfate (Blunted bronchodilator effect). Products include:
- Alupent 674
- Arm-a-Med Metaproterenol Sulfate Inhalation Solution, USP 617
- Metaprel Inhalation Aerosol Bronchodilator 2014
- Metaprel Inhalation Solution 2015
- Metaprel 2015
- Metaproterenol Sulfate Inhalation Solution, USP 912

Nitroglycerin (Reflex tachycardia produced by nitroglycerin blunted). Products include:
- Deponit NTG Transdermal Delivery System 2143
- Minitran Transdermal Delivery System 1312
- Nitro-Bid Ointment 1339
- Nitro-Bid Capsules 1338
- Nitrodisc 2176
- Nitro-Dur (nitroglycerin) Transdermal Infusion System 1164
- Nitrogard Tablets 1004
- Nitrolingual Spray 1846
- Nitrostat Tablets 1743
- Transderm-Nitro Transdermal Therapeutic System 2283

Nortriptyline Hydrochloride (Potential for tremor). Products include:
- Pamelor 2019

Pirbuterol Acetate (Blunted bronchodilator effect). Products include:
- Maxair Inhaler 1311

Protriptyline Hydrochloride (Potential for tremor). Products include:
- Vivactil Tablets 1567

Terbutaline Sulfate (Blunted bronchodilator effect). Products include:
- Brethaire Inhaler 1024
- Brethine Ampuls 1026
- Brethine Tablets 1026
- Bricanyl Injection 1324
- Bricanyl Tablets 1325

Tolazamide (Altered dosage requirements). Products include:
- Tolinase Tablets 2365

Tolbutamide (Altered dosage requirements). Products include:
- Orinase Tablets 2354

Trimipramine Maleate (Potential for tremor). Products include:
- Surmontil Capsules 2524

NORMODYNE TABLETS
(Labetalol Hydrochloride) 2110
May interact with oral hypoglycemic agents, tricyclic antidepressants, sympathomimetic bronchodilators, insulin, and certain other agents. Compounds in these categories include:

Albuterol (Blunted bronchodilator effects). Products include:
- Proventil Inhalation Aerosol 2117
- Ventolin Inhalation Aerosol and Refill 583

Albuterol Sulfate (Blunted bronchodilator effects). Products include:
- Proventil Repetabs Tablets 2120
- Proventil Solutions for Inhalation 0.5% and 0.083% 2118
- Proventil Syrup 2119
- Proventil Tablets 2120
- Ventolin 583

Amitriptyline Hydrochloride (Potential for tremor). Products include:
- Elavil 2269
- Endep Tablets 1927
- Etrafon 2087
- Limbitrol 1933
- Triavil Tablets 1556

Amoxapine (Potential for tremor). Products include:
- Asendin Tablets 1196

Bitolterol Mesylate (Blunted bronchodilator effects). Products include:
- Tornalate 2074

Chlorpropamide (Altered dosage requirements). Products include:
- Diabinese Tablets 1775

Cimetidine (Increases bioavailability of labetalol). Products include:
- Tagamet Tablets 2228

Cimetidine Hydrochloride (Increases bioavailability of labetalol). Products include:
- Tagamet 2228

Clomipramine Hydrochloride (Potential for tremor). Products include:
- Anafranil Capsules 650

Desipramine Hydrochloride (Potential for tremor). Products include:
- Norpramin Tablets 1340

Doxepin Hydrochloride (Potential for tremor). Products include:
- Sinequan 1960

Ephedrine Hydrochloride (Blunted bronchodilator effects). Products include:
- Amesec .... ◙ 682
- Primatene Tablets-M Formula 2421
- Primatene Tablets-P Formula 2421
- Primatene Tablets-Regular Formula 2421
- Quadrinal Tablets 1183
- Quelidrine Syrup 556
- Tedral SA 1765

Ephedrine Sulfate (Blunted bronchodilator effects). Products include:
- Bronkaid Tablets .... ◙ 757
- Bronkolixir .... ◙ 761
- Bronkotabs Tablets .... ◙ 762
- Marax Tablets & DF Syrup 1954
- Pazo Hemorrhoid Ointment & Suppositories 752
- Vicks Vatronol Nose Drops .... ◙ 666

Ephedrine Tannate (Blunted bronchodilator effects). Products include:
- Rynatuss 2388

Epinephrine (Blunted bronchodilator effects). Products include:
- Ana-Kit Anaphylaxis Emergency Treatment Kit 1100
- Bronkaid Mist .... ◙ 757
- EpiPen 843
- Marcaine Hydrochloride 0.5% with Epinephrine 1:200,000 (as bitartrate) 958
- Marcaine Hydrochloride with Epinephrine 1:200,000 2055
- Primatene Mist 2420
- Sus-Phrine Injection 1006
- Xylocaine with Epinephrine Injections 637

Epinephrine Hydrochloride (Blunted bronchodilator effects). Products include:
- Adrenalin Chloride Solution 1:100 & 1:1,000 1689
- Epifrin .... ⊙ 244
- Glaucon .... ⊙ 218

Ethylnorepinephrine Hydrochloride (Blunted bronchodilator effects). Products include:
- Bronkephrine Injection 2042

Glipizide (Altered dosage requirements). Products include:
- Glucotrol 1952

Glyburide (Altered dosage requirements). Products include:
- DiaBeta 1091
- Micronase Tablets 2350

Halothane (Synergism). Products include:
- Fluothane 2453

Imipramine Hydrochloride (Potential for tremor). Products include:
- Tofranil Ampuls 1038
- Tofranil Tablets 1039

Imipramine Pamoate (Potential for tremor). Products include:
- Tofranil-PM Capsules 1041

Insulin, Human (Altered dosage requirements).
- No products indexed under this heading.

Insulin, Human Isophane Suspension (Altered dosage requirements). Products include:
- Humulin N, 100 Units 1270

Insulin, Human NPH (Altered dosage requirements). Products include:
- Insulatard NPH Human 1627
- Novolin N 1627
- Novolin N PenFill Cartridges 1628
- Novolin N Prefilled 1628

Insulin, Human Regular (Altered dosage requirements). Products include:
- Humulin BR, 100 Units 1268
- Humulin R, 100 Units 1272
- Novolin R 1627
- Novolin R PenFill Cartridges 1628
- Novolin R Prefilled 1629
- Velosulin Human 1628

Insulin, Human, Zinc Suspension (Altered dosage requirements). Products include:
- Humulin L, 100 Units 1268
- Humulin U, 100 Units 1272
- Novolin L 1627

Insulin, NPH (Altered dosage requirements). Products include:
- NPH, 40 & 100 Units 1273
- Beef NPH, 100 Units 1274
- Pork NPH, 100 Units 1275
- Insulatard NPH 1626
- NPH Insulin 1626
- NPH Purified Pork Isophane Insulin 1626

Insulin, Regular (Altered dosage requirements). Products include:
- Regular, 40 & 100 Units 1273
- Beef Regular, 100 Units 1275
- Pork Regular, 100 Units 1275
- Pork Regular (Concentrated), 500 Units 1276
- Regular Insulin 1625
- Regular Purified Pork Insulin 1626
- Velosulin 1627

Insulin, Zinc Crystals (Altered dosage requirements). Products include:
- NPH, 40 & 100 Units 1273

Insulin, Zinc Suspension (Altered dosage requirements). Products include:
- Lente, 40 & 100 Units 1272
- Protamine, Zinc, 40 & 100 Units 1273
- Lente Iletin I 1272
- Beef Lente, 100 Units 1274
- Beef Protamine Zinc, 100 Units 1274
- Pork Lente, 100 Units 1275
- Pork, Protamine, Zinc, 100 Units 1275
- Lente Insulin 1626
- Lente Purified Pork Insulin 1626
- Semilente Insulin 1625
- Ultralente Insulin 1626

Isoetharine (Blunted bronchodilator effects). Products include:
- Arm-a-Med Isoetharine Inhalation Solution, USP 616
- Bronkometer Aerosol 2042
- Bronkosol Solution 2042

Isoproterenol Hydrochloride (Blunted bronchodilator effects). Products include:
- Isuprel Hydrochloride Injection 1:5000 2050
- Isuprel Hydrochloride Mistometer .. 2051
- Isuprel Hydrochloride Solution 1:200 & 1:100 2052
- Norisodrine Aerotrol 540

Maprotiline Hydrochloride (Potential for tremor). Products include:
- Ludiomil Tablets 874

Metaproterenol Sulfate (Blunted bronchodilator effects). Products include:
- Alupent 674
- Arm-a-Med Metaproterenol Sulfate Inhalation Solution, USP 617
- Metaprel Inhalation Aerosol Bronchodilator 2014

Metaprel Inhalation Solution 2015
Metaprel 2015
Metaproterenol Sulfate Inhalation Solution, USP 912

Nitroglycerin (Reflex tachycardia produced by nitroglycerin blunted). Products include:

Deponit NTG Transdermal Delivery System 2143
Minitran Transdermal Delivery System 1312
Nitro-Bid Ointment 1339
Nitro-Bid Capsules 1338
Nitrodisc 2176
Nitro-Dur (nitroglycerin) Transdermal Infusion System 1164
Nitrogard Tablets 1004
Nitrolingual Spray 1846
Nitrostat Tablets 1743
Transderm-Nitro Transdermal Therapeutic System 2283

Nortriptyline Hydrochloride (Potential for tremor). Products include:

Pamelor 2019

Pirbuterol Acetate (Blunted bronchodilator effects). Products include:

Maxair Inhaler 1311

Protriptyline Hydrochloride (Potential for tremor). Products include:

Vivactil Tablets 1567

Terbutaline Sulfate (Blunted bronchodilator effects). Products include:

Brethaire Inhaler 1024
Brethine Ampuls 1026
Brethine Tablets 1026
Bricanyl Injection 1324
Bricanyl Tablets 1325

Tolazamide (Altered dosage requirements). Products include:

Tolinase Tablets 2365

Tolbutamide (Altered dosage requirements). Products include:

Orinase Tablets 2354

Trimipramine Maleate (Potential for tremor). Products include:

Surmontil Capsules 2524

NORMOZIDE TABLETS

(Labetalol Hydrochloride, Hydrochlorothiazide) 2112

May interact with oral hypoglycemic agents, tricyclic antidepressants, sympathomimetic bronchodilators, insulin, non-steroidal anti-inflammatory agents, lithium preparations, para-aminobenzoic acid based local anesthetics, antihypertensives, and certain other agents. Compounds in these categories include:

Acebutolol Hydrochloride (Potentiation of antihypertensive effects). Products include:

Sectral Capsules 2520

Albuterol (Blunted bronchodilator effect). Products include:

Proventil Inhalation Aerosol 2117
Ventolin Inhalation Aerosol and Refill 583

Albuterol Sulfate (Blunted bronchodilator effect). Products include:

Proventil Repetabs Tablets 2120
Proventil Solutions for Inhalation 0.5% and 0.083% 2118
Proventil Syrup 2119
Proventil Tablets 2120
Ventolin 583

Amitriptyline Hydrochloride (Potential for tremor). Products include:

Elavil 2269
Endep Tablets 1927
Etrafon 2087
Limbitrol 1933
Triavil Tablets 1556

Amoxapine (Potential for tremor). Products include:

Asendin Tablets 1196

Atenolol (Potentiation of antihypertensive effects). Products include:

Tenoretic Tablets 1105
Tenormin Tablets and I.V. Injection 1107

Benazepril Hydrochloride (Potentiation of antihypertensive effects). Products include:

Lotensin Tablets 872

Bendroflumethiazide (Potentiation of antihypertensive effects). Products include:

Corzide Tablets 702
Naturetin Tablets 1789
Rauzide Tablets 1804

Betaxolol Hydrochloride (Potentiation of antihypertensive effects). Products include:

Betoptic Sterile Ophthalmic Solution 569
Betoptic S Sterile Ophthalmic Suspension 570
Kerlone Tablets 2172

Bitolterol Mesylate (Blunted bronchodilator effect). Products include:

Tornalate 2074

Captopril (Potentiation of antihypertensive effects). Products include:

Capoten 2255
Capozide 2258

Carteolol Hydrochloride (Potentiation of antihypertensive effects). Products include:

Cartrol Tablets 507

Chlorothiazide (Potentiation of antihypertensive effects). Products include:

Aldoclor Tablets 1413
Diupres Tablets 1461
Diuril Oral 1464

Chlorothiazide Sodium (Potentiation of antihypertensive effects). Products include:

Diuril Sodium Intravenous 1463

Chlorpropamide (Altered dosage requirements). Products include:

Diabinese Tablets 1775

Chlorthalidone (Potentiation of antihypertensive effects). Products include:

Combipres Tablets 678
Tenoretic Tablets 1105
Thalitone Tablets 687

Cimetidine (Increases bioavailability of labetalol). Products include:

Tagamet Tablets 2228

Cimetidine Hydrochloride (Increases bioavailability for labetalol). Products include:

Tagamet 2228

Clomipramine Hydrochloride (Potential for tremor). Products include:

Anafranil Capsules 650

Clonidine (Potentiation of antihypertensive effects). Products include:

Catapres-TTS 677

Clonidine Hydrochloride (Potentiation of antihypertensive effects). Products include:

Catapres Tablets 676
Combipres Tablets 678

Deserpidine (Potentiation of antihypertensive effects). Products include:

Enduronyl 518
Harmonyl Tablets 528
Oreticyl 545

Desipramine Hydrochloride (Potential for tremor). Products include:

Norpramin Tablets 1340

Diazoxide (Potentiation of antihypertensive effects). Products include:

Hyperstat I.V. Injection 2095
Proglycem 649

Diclofenac Sodium (Reduces diuretic, natriuretic and antihypertensive effects). Products include:

Voltaren Ophthalmic Sterile Ophthalmic Solution ◉ 268
Voltaren Tablets 1042

Doxazosin Mesylate (Potentiation of antihypertensive effects). Products include:

Cardura Tablets 1941

Doxepin Hydrochloride (Potential for tremor). Products include:

Sinequan 1960

Enalapril Maleate (Potentiation of antihypertensive effects). Products include:

Vaseretic Tablets 1559
Vasotec Tablets 1564

Enalaprilat (Potentiation of antihypertensive effects). Products include:

Vasotec I.V. 1562

Ephedrine Hydrochloride (Blunted bronchodilator effect). Products include:

Amesec ⊞ 682
Primatene Tablets-M Formula 2421
Primatene Tablets-P Formula 2421
Primatene Tablets-Regular Formula 2421
Quadrinal Tablets 1183
Quelidrine Syrup 556
Tedral SA 1765

Ephedrine Sulfate (Blunted bronchodilator effect). Products include:

Bronkaid Tablets ⊞ 757
Bronkolixir ⊞ 761
Bronkotabs Tablets ⊞ 762
Marax Tablets & DF Syrup 1954
Pazo Hemorrhoid Ointment & Suppositories 752
Vicks Vatronol Nose Drops ⊞ 666

Ephedrine Tannate (Blunted bronchodilator effect). Products include:

Rynatuss 2388

Epinephrine (Blunted bronchodilator effect). Products include:

Ana-Kit Anaphylaxis Emergency Treatment Kit 1100
Bronkaid Mist ⊞ 757
EpiPen 843
Marcaine Hydrochloride 0.5% with Epinephrine 1:200,000 (as bitartrate) 958
Marcaine Hydrochloride with Epinephrine 1:200,000 2055
Primatene Mist 2420
Sus-Phrine Injection 1006
Xylocaine with Epinephrine Injections 637

Epinephrine Bitartrate (Blunted bronchodilator effect). Products include:

AsthmaHaler Mist Epinephrine Bitartrate Bronchodilator ⊞ 616
Bronkaid Mist Suspension ⊞ 757
Primatene Mist Suspension 2421

Epinephrine Hydrochloride (Blunted bronchodilator effect). Products include:

Adrenalin Chloride Solution 1:100 & 1:1,000 1689
Epifrin ◉ 244
Glaucon ◉ 218

Esmolol Hydrochloride (Potentiation of antihypertensive effects). Products include:

Brevibloc Injection 942

Ethylnorepinephrine Hydrochloride (Blunted bronchodilator effect). Products include:

Bronkephrine Injection 2042

Etodolac (Reduces diuretic, natriuretic and antihypertensive effects). Products include:

Lodine Capsules 2468

Felodipine (Potentiation of antihypertensive effects). Products include:

Plendil Extended-Release Tablets 1526

Fenoprofen Calcium (Reduces diuretic, natriuretic, and antihypertensive effects). Products include:

Nalfon Pulvules & Tablets 919

Flurbiprofen (Reduces diuretic, natriuretic, and antihypertensive effects). Products include:

Ansaid Tablets 2319

Fosinopril Sodium (Potentiation of antihypertensive effects). Products include:

Monopril Tablets 1406

Furosemide (Potentiation of antihypertensive effects). Products include:

Lasix 1093

Glipizide (Altered dosage requirements). Products include:

Glucotrol 1952

Glyburide (Altered dosage requirements). Products include:

DiaBeta 1091
Micronase Tablets 2350

Guanabenz Acetate (Potentiation of antihypertensive effects). Products include:

Wytensin Tablets 2542

Guanethidine Monosulfate (Potentiation of antihypertensive effects). Products include:

Esimil Tablets 864
Ismelin Tablets 869

Halothane (Synergism). Products include:

Fluothane 2453

Hydralazine Hydrochloride (Potentiation of antihypertensive effects). Products include:

Apresazide Capsules 854
Apresoline Hydrochloride Parenteral (Ampuls) 856
Apresoline Hydrochloride Tablets 855
Apresoline-Esidrix Tablets 857
Ser-Ap-Es Tablets 881
Serpasil-Apresoline Tablets 884

Hydroflumethiazide (Potentiation of antihypertensive effects). Products include:

Diucardin Tablets 2450
Saluron 718
Salutensin/Salutensin-Demi 719

Ibuprofen (Reduces diuretic, natriuretic and antihypertensive effects). Products include:

Advil Cold & Sinus Caplets (formerly CoAdvil) 2416
Advil Ibuprofen Tablets and Caplets 2416
Children's Advil Suspension 2426
CoAdvil ⊞ 748
Dristan Sinus Caplets 2419
Haltran Tablets ⊞ 668
Ibuprofen ⊞ 631
Medipren ibuprofen Caplets and Tablets 1362
Midol 200 Cramp Relief Formula ⊞ 570
Motrin Tablets 2351
Motrin IB Caplets and Tablets ⊞ 736
Nuprin Ibuprofen/Analgesic Tablets & Caplets 752
PediaProfen Suspension 1363
Rufen Tablets 691
Trendar Ibuprofen Tablets ⊞ 756

Imipramine Hydrochloride (Potential for tremor). Products include:

Tofranil Ampuls 1038
Tofranil Tablets 1039

Imipramine Pamoate (Potential for tremor). Products include:

Tofranil-PM Capsules 1041

Indapamide (Potentiation of antihypertensive effects). Products include:

Lozol Tablets 1843

Indomethacin (Reduces diuretic, natriuretic and antihypertensive effects). Products include:

Indocin 1487

Indomethacin Sodium Trihydrate (Reduces diuretic, natriuretic and antihypertensive effects). Products include:
Indocin I.V. ... 1490

Insulin, Human (Altered insulin requirements).
No products indexed under this heading.

Insulin, Human Isophane Suspension (Altered insulin requirements). Products include:
Humulin N, 100 Units ... 1270

Insulin, Human NPH (Altered insulin requirements). Products include:
Insulatard NPH Human ... 1627
Novolin N ... 1627
Novolin N PenFill Cartridges ... 1628
Novolin N Prefilled ... 1628

Insulin, Human Regular (Altered insulin requirements). Products include:
Humulin BR, 100 Units ... 1268
Humulin R, 100 Units ... 1272
Novolin R ... 1627
Novolin R PenFill Cartridges ... 1628
Novolin R Prefilled ... 1629
Velosulin Human ... 1628

Insulin, Human, Zinc Suspension (Altered insulin requirements). Products include:
Humulin L, 100 Units ... 1268
Humulin U, 100 Units ... 1272
Novolin L ... 1627

Insulin, NPH (Altered insulin requirements). Products include:
NPH, 40 & 100 Units ... 1273
Beef NPH, 100 Units ... 1274
Pork NPH, 100 Units ... 1275
Insulatard NPH ... 1626
NPH Insulin ... 1626
NPH Purified Pork Isophane Insulin ... 1626

Insulin, Regular (Altered insulin requirements). Products include:
Regular, 40 & 100 Units ... 1273
Beef Regular, 100 Units ... 1275
Pork Regular, 100 Units ... 1275
Pork Regular (Concentrated), 500 Units ... 1276
Regular Insulin ... 1625
Regular Purified Pork Insulin ... 1626
Velosulin ... 1627

Insulin, Zinc Crystals (Altered insulin requirements). Products include:
NPH, 40 & 100 Units ... 1273

Insulin, Zinc Suspension (Altered insulin requirements). Products include:
Lente, 40 & 100 Units ... 1272
Protamine, Zinc, 40 & 100 Units ... 1273
Lente Iletin I ... 1272
Beef Lente, 100 Units ... 1274
Beef Protamine Zinc, 100 Units ... 1274
Pork Lente, 100 Units ... 1275
Pork, Protamine, Zinc, 100 Units ... 1275
Lente Insulin ... 1626
Lente Purified Pork Insulin ... 1626
Semilente Insulin ... 1625
Ultralente Insulin ... 1626

Isoetharine (Blunted bronchodilator effect). Products include:
Arm-a-Med Isoetharine Inhalation Solution, USP ... 616
Bronkometer Aerosol ... 2042
Bronkosol Solution ... 2042

Isoproterenol Hydrochloride (Blunted bronchodilator effect). Products include:
Isuprel Hydrochloride Injection 1:5000 ... 2050
Isuprel Hydrochloride Mistometer .. 2051
Isuprel Hydrochloride Solution 1:200 & 1:100 ... 2052
Norisodrine Aerotrol ... 540

Isradipine (Potentiation of antihypertensive effects). Products include:
DynaCirc Capsules ... 2004

Ketoprofen (Reduces diuretic, natriuretic and antihypertensive effects). Products include:
Orudis Capsules ... 2488

Ketorolac Tromethamine (Reduces diuretic, natriuretic and antihypertensive effects). Products include:
Toradol IM Injection ... 2302

Lisinopril (Potentiation of antihypertensive effects). Products include:
Prinivil Tablets ... 1538
Prinzide Tablets ... 1540
Zestoretic ... 2274
Zestril Tablets ... 2277

Lithium Carbonate (Reduced renal clearance of lithium). Products include:
Eskalith ... 2214
Lithane Tablets ... 1596
Lithium Carbonate Capsules & Tablets ... 1984
Lithobid Tablets ... 870

Lithium Citrate (Reduced renal clearance of lithium). Products include:
Cibalith-S ... 870

Maprotiline Hydrochloride (Potential for tremor). Products include:
Ludiomil Tablets ... 874

Mecamylamine Hydrochloride (Potentiation of antihypertensive effects). Products include:
Inversine Tablets ... 1492

Meclofenamate Sodium (Reduces diuretic, natriuretic and antihypertensive effects). Products include:
Meclomen Capsules ... 1739

Mefenamic Acid (Reduces diuretic, natriuretic and antihypertensive effects). Products include:
Ponstel ... 1758

Metaproterenol Sulfate (Blunted bronchodilator effect). Products include:
Alupent ... 674
Arm-a-Med Metaproterenol Sulfate Inhalation Solution, USP ... 617
Metaprel Inhalation Aerosol Bronchodilator ... 2014
Metaprel Inhalation Solution ... 2015
Metaprel ... 2015
Metaproterenol Sulfate Inhalation Solution, USP ... 912

Methyclothiazide (Potentiation of antihypertensive effects). Products include:
Enduron Tablets ... 517
Enduronyl ... 518

Methyldopa (Potentiation of antihypertensive effects). Products include:
Aldoclor Tablets ... 1413
Aldomet Oral ... 1415
Aldoril Tablets ... 1418

Methyldopate Hydrochloride (Potentiation of antihypertensive effects). Products include:
Aldomet Ester HCl Injection ... 1417

Metolazone (Potentiation of antihypertensive effects). Products include:
Diulo ... 2129
Mykrox ½ mg Tablets ... 984
Zaroxolyn Tablets ... 989

Metoprolol Tartrate (Potentiation of antihypertensive effects). Products include:
Lopressor Ampuls ... 1032
Lopressor HCT Tablets ... 1034
Lopressor Tablets ... 1032

Metyrosine (Potentiation of antihypertensive effects). Products include:
Demser Capsules ... 1460

Minoxidil (Potentiation of antihypertensive effects). Products include:
Loniten Tablets ... 2346
Rogaine Topical Solution ... 2357

Nadolol (Potentiation of antihypertensive effects). Products include:
Corgard Tablets ... 701
Corzide Tablets ... 702

Naproxen (Reduces diuretic, natriuretic and antihypertensive effects). Products include:
Naprosyn ... 2297

Naproxen Sodium (Reduces diuretic, natriuretic and antihypertensive effects). Products include:
Anaprox and Anaprox DS Tablets ... 2288

Nicardipine Hydrochloride (Potentiation of antihypertensive effects). Products include:
Cardene Capsules ... 2290

Nitroglycerin (Reflex tachycardia produced by nitroglycerin blunted). Products include:
Deponit NTG Transdermal Delivery System ... 2143
Minitran Transdermal Delivery System ... 1312
Nitro-Bid Ointment ... 1339
Nitro-Bid Capsules ... 1338
Nitrodisc ... 2176
Nitro-Dur (nitroglycerin) Transdermal Infusion System ... 1164
Nitrogard Tablets ... 1004
Nitrolingual Spray ... 1846
Nitrostat Tablets ... 1743
Transderm-Nitro Transdermal Therapeutic System ... 2283

Norepinephrine Bitartrate (Decreased arterial responsiveness to norepinephrine). Products include:
Levophed Bitartrate Injection ... 2054

Nortriptyline Hydrochloride (Potential for tremor). Products include:
Pamelor ... 2019

Penbutolol Sulfate (Potentiation of antihypertensive effects). Products include:
Levatol ... 1832

Phenoxybenzamine Hydrochloride (Potentiation of antihypertensive effects). Products include:
Dibenzyline Capsules ... 2207

Phentolamine Mesylate (Potentiation of antihypertensive effects). Products include:
Regitine ... 878

Phenylbutazone (Reduces diuretic, natriuretic and antihypertensive effects). Products include:
Butazolidin Capsules & Tablets ... 1027

Pindolol (Potentiation of antihypertensive effects). Products include:
Visken Tablets ... 2036

Pirbuterol Acetate (Blunted bronchodilator effect). Products include:
Maxair Inhaler ... 1311

Piroxicam (Reduces diuretic, natriuretic and antihypertensive effects). Products include:
Feldene Capsules ... 1777

Polythiazide (Potentiation of antihypertensive effects). Products include:
Minizide Capsules ... 1779
Renese Tablets ... 1785
Renese-R Tablets ... 1786

Prazosin Hydrochloride (Potentiation of antihypertensive effects). Products include:
Minipress Capsules ... 1778
Minizide Capsules ... 1779

Propranolol Hydrochloride (Potentiation of antihypertensive effects). Products include:
Inderal ... 2459
Inderal LA Long Acting Capsules ... 2461
Inderide Tablets ... 2463
Inderide LA Long Acting Capsules .. 2465

Protriptyline Hydrochloride (Potential for tremor). Products include:
Vivactil Tablets ... 1567

Ramipril (Potentiation of antihypertensive effects). Products include:
Altace Capsules ... 1086

Rauwolfia Serpentina (Potentiation of antihypertensive effects). Products include:
Raudixin Tablets ... 1803
Rauzide Tablets ... 1804

Rescinnamine (Potentiation of antihypertensive effects).
No products indexed under this heading.

Reserpine (Potentiation of antihypertensive effects). Products include:
Diupres Tablets ... 1461
Hydromox R Tablets ... 1209
Hydropres Tablets ... 1485
Renese-R Tablets ... 1786
Salutensin/Salutensin-Demi ... 719
Ser-Ap-Es Tablets ... 881
Serpasil Tablets ... 883
Serpasil-Apresoline Tablets ... 884
Serpasil-Esidrix Tablets ... 886

Sodium Nitroprusside (Potentiation of antihypertensive effects). Products include:
Nipride I.V. Infusion ... 1909

Sulindac (Reduces diuretic, natriuretic and antihypertensive effects). Products include:
Clinoril Tablets ... 1433

Terazosin Hydrochloride (Potentiation of antihypertensive effects). Products include:
Hytrin Tablets ... 529

Terbutaline Sulfate (Blunted bronchodilator effect). Products include:
Brethaire Inhaler ... 1024
Brethine Ampuls ... 1026
Brethine Tablets ... 1026
Bricanyl Injection ... 1324
Bricanyl Tablets ... 1325

Timolol Maleate (Potentiation of antihypertensive effects). Products include:
Blocadren Tablets ... 1429
Timolide Tablets ... 1547
Timoptic in Ocudose ... 1552
Timoptic Sterile Ophthalmic Solution ... 1550

Tolazamide (Altered dosage requirements). Products include:
Tolinase Tablets ... 2365

Tolbutamide (Altered dosage requirements). Products include:
Orinase Tablets ... 2354

Tolmetin Sodium (Reduces diuretic, natriuretic and antihypertensive effects). Products include:
Tolectin (200, 400 and 600 mg) .. 1379

Trimethaphan Camsylate (Potentiation of antihypertensive effects). Products include:
Arfonad Ampuls ... 1887

Trimipramine Maleate (Potential for tremor). Products include:
Surmontil Capsules ... 2524

Tubocurarine Chloride (Increased responsiveness to tubocurarine).
No products indexed under this heading.

NOROXIN TABLETS
(Norfloxacin) ... 1519
May interact with antacids, xanthine bronchodilators, oral anticoagulants,

and certain other agents. Compounds in these categories include:

Aluminum Carbonate Gel (Concomitant administration not recommended). Products include:
- Basaljel ... 2438

Aluminum Hydroxide (Concomitant administration not recommended). Products include:
- Cama Arthritis Pain Reliever ... ▣ 685
- Gaviscon Extra Strength Relief Formula Liquid Antacid ... ▣ 594
- Gaviscon Extra Strength Relief Formula Antacid Tablets ... ▣ 594
- Gaviscon Liquid Antacid ... ▣ 594
- Gelusil Liquid & Tablets ... ▣ 639
- Extra Strength Maalox Plus Suspension ... 1850
- Maalox TC Suspension ... 1851
- Maalox Plus Tablets ... ▣ 655
- Extra Strength Maalox Plus Tablets 1850
- Nephrox Suspension ... ▣ 563
- WinGel Liquid & Tablets ... ▣ 761

Aluminum Hydroxide Gel (Concomitant administration not recommended). Products include:
- ALternaGEL Liquid ... 1154
- Aludrox Oral Suspension ... 2428
- Amphojel Suspension ... 2429
- Amphojel Suspension without Flavor ... 2429
- Mylanta Liquid ... 1155
- Mylanta Double Strength Liquid ... 1155

Aluminum Hydroxide Gel, Dried (Concomitant administration not recommended). Products include:
- Alu-Tab/Alu-Cap ... 1309
- Amphojel Tablets ... 2429
- Ascriptin A/D Caplets ... 1850
- Regular Strength Ascriptin Tablets 1850
- Gaviscon Antacid Tablets ... ▣ 593
- Gaviscon-2 Antacid Tablets ... ▣ 594
- Mylanta Tablets ... 1155
- Mylanta Double Strength Tablets ... 1155

Aminophylline (Elevated theophylline plasma levels). Products include:
- Amesec ... ▣ 682
- Aminophyllin Tablets ... 2153

Caffeine (May interfere with the metabolism of caffeine). Products include:
- Anacin Coated Analgesic Caplets ... 2417
- Anacin Coated Analgesic Tablets ... 2417
- Anacin Maximum Strength Analgesic Coated Tablets ... 2417
- Cafergot/Cafergot P-B ... 1999
- Esgic-Plus Tablets ... 1002
- Esgic Tablets & Capsules ... 1001
- Aspirin Free Excedrin Analgesic Caplets ... 748
- Excedrin Extra-Strength Analgesic Tablets & Caplets ... 749
- Fioricet Tablets ... 2006
- Fiorinal Capsules ... 2007
- Fiorinal with Codeine Capsules ... 2008
- Fiorinal Tablets ... 2007
- No Doz Fast Acting Alertness Aid Tablets ... 751
- No Doz Maximum Strength Caplets 751
- Norgesic ... 1314
- P-A-C Analgesic Tablets ... ▣ 669
- Synalgos-DC Capsules ... 2525
- Vanquish Analgesic Caplets ... ▣ 574
- Vivarin Stimulant Tablets ... ▣ 726
- Wigraine Tablets & Suppositories ... 1645

Cyclosporine (Elevated serum levels of cyclosporine). Products include:
- Sandimmune ... 2024

Dicumarol (Potential for enhanced effects of oral anticoagulant). Products include:
- Dicumarol Tablets ... 516

Dihydroxyaluminum Sodium Carbonate (Concomitant administration not recommended). Products include:
- Rolaids ... ▣ 743

Dyphylline (Elevated theophylline plasma levels). Products include:
- Dilor ... 2079
- Dilor-G Tablets & Liquid ... 2079
- Lufyllin Elixir ... 2384
- Lufyllin & Lufyllin-400 Tablets ... 2384
- Lufyllin-GG Elixir & Tablets ... 2385

Iron Preparations (May result in lower serum and urine levels of norfloxacin). Products include:
- Allbee C-800 Plus Iron Tablets ... ▣ 670
- Bugs Bunny Children's Chewable Vitamins + Minerals with Iron and Calcium (Sugar Free) ... ▣ 626
- Bugs Bunny Plus Iron Children's Chewable Vitamins (Sugar Free) ▣ 625
- FemIron Multi-Vitamins and Iron ... ▣ 617
- Ferancee Chewable Tablets ... 1155
- Ferancee-HP Tablets ... 1155
- Fergon ... ▣ 758
- Fero-Folic-500 Filmtab ... 527
- Fero-Grad-500 Filmtab ... 528
- Fero-Gradumet Filmtab ... 528
- Ferro-Sequels ... 1203
- Flintstones Children's Chewable Vitamins Plus Iron ... ▣ 625
- Flintstones Complete With Calcium, Iron & Minerals Children's Chewable Vitamins ... ▣ 626
- Geritol Extend Tablets and Caplets ... ▣ 717
- Geritol Liquid - High Potency Iron & Vitamin Tonic ... ▣ 717
- Iberet Tablets ... 531
- Iberet-500 Liquid ... 531
- Iberet-Folic-500 Filmtab ... 527
- Iberet-Liquid ... 531
- Incremin w/Iron Syrup ... ▣ 588
- Irospan ... 972
- Mol-Iron ... ▣ 703
- Niferex ... 847
- Niferex-150 Forte Capsules ... 847
- Niferex Forte Elixir ... 847
- Niferex ... 847
- Niferex-PN Tablets ... 847
- One-A-Day Maximum Formula Vitamins and Minerals ... ▣ 627
- Peritinic Tablets ... ▣ 589
- Poly-Vi-Flor with Iron ... 1399
- Poly-Vi-Flor with Iron Drops ... 1399
- Poly-Vi-Sol Vitamins with Iron, Chewable Tablets and Circus Shapes Chewable ... ▣ 612
- Poly-Vi-Sol Vitamins with Iron, Drops ... ▣ 612
- SMA Iron Fortified Infant Formula, Concentrated, Ready-to-Feed and Powder ... ▣ 767
- Slow Fe Tablets ... ▣ 552
- The Stuart Formula Tablets ... ▣ 581
- Stuartinic Tablets ... 1157
- Surbex-750 with Iron ... ▣ 503
- Tri-Vi-Flor 0.25 mg Vitamins with Iron and Fluoride Drops ... 1401
- Unicap Plus Iron Vitamin Formula Tablets ... ▣ 738
- Vi-Daylin ADC Vitamins + Iron Drops ... 1980
- Vi-Daylin Multivitamin + Iron Drops ... 1981
- Vi-Daylin/F ADC Vitamins + Iron Drops With Fluoride ... 1981
- Vi-Daylin/F Multivitamin + Iron Drops With Fluoride ... 1981
- Vi-Daylin Multivitamin + Iron Chewable Tablets ... 1982
- Vi-Daylin/F Multivitamin + Iron Chewable Tablets With Fluoride .. 1982
- Vi-Daylin Multivitamin + Iron Liquid ... 1983

Magaldrate (Concomitant administration not recommended). Products include:
- Riopan Antacid Chew Tablets ... ▣ 754
- Riopan Antacid Chew Tablets in Rollpacks ... ▣ 754
- Riopan Antacid Suspension ... 2421
- Riopan Antacid Swallow Tablets ... 2421
- Riopan Plus Chew Tablets ... 2422
- Riopan Plus Chew Tablets in Rollpack ... 2422
- Riopan Plus 2 Chew Tablets, Mint Flavor, Cherry Flavor ... 2422
- Riopan Plus Suspension ... 2422
- Riopan Plus 2 Suspension, Mint Flavor, Cherry Flavor ... 2422

Magnesium Hydroxide (Concomitant administration not recommended). Products include:
- Aludrox Oral Suspension ... 2428
- Ascriptin A/D Caplets ... 1850
- Regular Strength Ascriptin Tablets 1850
- Di-Gel Antacid/Anti-Gas ... ▣ 697
- Gelusil Liquid & Tablets ... ▣ 639
- Haley's M-O, Regular & Flavored .. ▣ 569
- Extra Strength Maalox Plus Suspension ... 1850
- Maalox TC Suspension ... 1851
- Maalox Plus Tablets ... ▣ 655
- Extra Strength Maalox Plus Tablets 1850
- Mylanta Liquid ... 1155
- Mylanta Tablets ... 1155
- Mylanta Double Strength Liquid ... 1155
- Mylanta Double Strength Tablets ... 1155
- Concentrated Phillips' Milk of Magnesia ... ▣ 573
- Phillips' Milk of Magnesia Liquid ... ▣ 572
- Phillips' Milk of Magnesia Tablets ▣ 573
- WinGel Liquid & Tablets ... ▣ 761

Magnesium Oxide (Concomitant administration not recommended). Products include:
- Bayer Plus Aspirin Tablets ... ▣ 567
- Beelith Tablets ... 659
- Bufferin Analgesic Tablets and Caplets ... ▣ 524
- Cama Arthritis Pain Reliever ... ▣ 685
- Mag-Ox 400 ... 673
- Uro-Mag ... 673

Nitrofurantoin (Concomitant use not recommended; antagonizes antibacterial effect of norfloxacin in urinary tract). Products include:
- Macrodantin Capsules ... 1624

Probenecid (Diminished urinary excretion of norfloxacin). Products include:
- Benemid Tablets ... 1426
- ColBENEMID Tablets ... 1436
- Wycillin Injection and Probenecid Tablets ... 2539

Sucralfate (May interfere with absorption resulting in lower levels of norfloxacin). Products include:
- Carafate Tablets ... 1326

Theophylline (Elevated theophylline plasma levels). Products include:
- Bronkaid Tablets ... ▣ 757
- Bronkolixir ... ▣ 761
- Bronkotabs Tablets ... ▣ 762
- Constant-T Tablets ... 1029
- Marax Tablets & DF Syrup ... 1954
- Primatene Tablets ... 2421
- Quibron Capsules ... 713
- Quibron-T ... 714
- Quibron-T/SR ... 716
- Theolair Liquid ... 1317
- Theo-Organidin Elixir ... 2391

Theophylline Anhydrous (Elevated theophylline plasma levels). Products include:
- Aerolate ... 994
- Primatene Tablets-M Formula ... ▣ 753
- Primatene Tablets-Regular Formula ... 2421
- Respbid Tablets ... 684
- Slo-bid Gyrocaps ... 1847
- T-PHYL (Uniphyl) 200 mg Tablets 1820
- Tedral SA ... 1765
- Theo-24 ... 2179
- Theo-Dur Sprinkle ... 1168
- Theo-Dur Extended-Release Tablets ... 1166
- Theolair Tablets ... 1317
- Theolair-SR Tablets ... 1319
- TheoX Extended-Release Tablets ... 841
- Uniphyl 400 mg Tablets ... 1823

Theophylline Calcium Salicylate (Elevated theophylline plasma levels). Products include:
- Quadrinal Tablets ... 1183

Theophylline Sodium Glycinate (Elevated theophylline plasma levels). Products include:
- Asbron G ... 1997

Vitamins with Iron (May result in lower serum and urine levels of norfloxacin). Products include:
- Geritol Extend Tablets and Caplets ... ▣ 717
- Poly-Vi-Flor with Iron ... 1399
- Poly-Vi-Flor with Iron Drops ... 1399

Warfarin Sodium (Potential for enhanced effects of oral anticoagulant). Products include:
- Coumadin Injection & Tablets ... 944
- Panwarfin Tablets ... 547

Zinc Sulfate (May result in lower serum and urine levels of norfloxacin). Products include:
- Clear Eyes ACR ... ⊙ 305
- Eldertonic ... 1359
- Surbex-750 with Zinc ... ▣ 503
- Vicon Forte Capsules ... 2416
- Visine A.C. Eye Drops ... ▣ 646
- Visine A.C. Eye Drops ... ⊙ 303
- Zincfrin ... ⊙ 230

Food Interactions

Food, unspecified (The presence of food may decrease the absorption).

NORPACE CAPSULES

(Disopyramide Phosphate) ... 2177

May interact with antiarrhythmics, hepatic microsomal emzyme inducers, and certain other agents. Compounds in these categories include:

Acebutolol Hydrochloride (Excessive widening of QRS complex and prolongation of Q-T interval). Products include:
- Sectral Capsules ... 2520

Adenosine (Excessive widening of QRS complex and prolongation of Q-T interval). Products include:
- Adenocard Injection ... 1007

Amiodarone Hydrochloride (Excessive widening of QRS complex and prolongation of Q-T interval). Products include:
- Cordarone Tablets ... 2446

Bretylium Tosylate (Excessive widening of QRS complex and prolongation of Q-T interval). Products include:
- Bretylol Injection ... 923

Carbamazepine (Concurrent administration with hepatic enzyme inducers may lower plasma levels of disopyramide). Products include:
- Tegretol Chewable Tablets ... 654
- Tegretol Suspension ... 656
- Tegretol Tablets ... 654

Chlorpropamide (Concurrent administration with hepatic enzyme inducers may lower plasma levels of disopyramide). Products include:
- Diabinese Tablets ... 1775

Glipizide (Concurrent administration with hepatic enzyme inducers may lower plasma levels of disopyramide). Products include:
- Glucotrol ... 1952

Glyburide (Concurrent administration with hepatic enzyme inducers may lower plasma levels of disopyramide). Products include:
- DiaBeta ... 1091
- Micronase Tablets ... 2350

Lidocaine Hydrochloride (Excessive widening of QRS complex and prolongation of Q-T interval). Products include:
- Anestacon Solution ... 2394
- Bactine Antiseptic/Anesthetic First Aid Spray ... ▣ 624
- Decadron Phosphate with Xylocaine Injection, Sterile ... 1451
- Xylocaine Injections ... 637
- Xylocaine Injections for Ventricular Arrhythmias ... 639
- Xylocaine 2% Jelly ... 643
- 4% Xylocaine-MPF Sterile Solution 641
- Xylocaine 2% Viscous Solution ... 646

Mexiletine Hydrochloride (Excessive widening of QRS complex and prolongation of Q-T interval). Products include:
- Mexitil Capsules ... 680

Moricizine Hydrochloride (Excessive widening of QRS complex and prolongation of Q-T interval). Products include:
- Ethmozine Tablets ... 946

Phenobarbital (Concurrent administration with hepatic enzyme inducers may lower plasma levels of disopyramide). Products include:

Arco-Lase Plus Tablets ... 607
Bellergal-S Tablets ... 1998
Bronkolixir ... ◘ 761
Bronkotabs Tablets ... ◘ 762
Donnatal ... 1858
Donnatal Extentabs ... 1859
Donnatal Tablets ... 1858
Donnazyme Tablets ... 1860
Kinesed Tablets ... 2272
Phenobarbital Elixir and Tablets ... 1293
Primatene Tablets-P Formula ... 2421
Quadrinal Tablets ... 1183
Tedral SA ... 1765

Phenylbutazone (Concurrent administration with hepatic enzyme inducers may lower plasma levels of disopyramide). Products include:

Butazolidin Capsules & Tablets ... 1027

Phenytoin (Concurrent administration with hepatic enzyme inducers may lower plasma levels of disopyramide). Products include:

Dilantin Infatabs ... 1710
Dilantin-30 Pediatric/Dilantin-125 Suspension ... 1713

Phenytoin Sodium (Concurrent administration with hepatic enzyme inducers may lower plasma levels of disopyramide). Products include:

Dilantin Kapseals ... 1708
Dilantin Parenteral ... 1712
Dilantin with Phenobarbital Kapseals ... 1715

Procainamide Hydrochloride (Excessive widening of QRS complex and prolongation of Q-T interval). Products include:

Procan SR Tablets ... 1760
Pronestyl Capsules and Tablets ... 1800
Pronestyl Injection ... 1798
Pronestyl-SR Tablets ... 1801

Propafenone Hydrochloride (Excessive widening of QRS complex and prolongation of Q-T interval). Products include:

Rythmol Tablets ... 1184

Propranolol Hydrochloride (Excessive widening of QRS complex and prolongation of Q-T interval). Products include:

Inderal ... 2459
Inderal LA Long Acting Capsules ... 2461
Inderide Tablets ... 2463
Inderide LA Long Acting Capsules ... 2465

Quinidine Gluconate (Excessive widening of QRS complex and prolongation of Q-T interval). Products include:

Quinaglute Dura-Tabs Tablets ... 663

Quinidine Polygalacturonate (Excessive widening of QRS complex and prolongation of Q-T interval). Products include:

Cardioquin Tablets ... 1812

Quinidine Sulfate (Excessive widening of QRS complex and prolongation of Q-T interval). Products include:

Quinidex Extentabs ... 1868

Rifampin (Concurrent administration with hepatic enzyme inducers may lower plasma levels of disopyramide). Products include:

Rifadin ... 1345
Rifamate Capsules ... 1347
Rimactane Capsules ... 879

Tocainide Hydrochloride (Excessive widening of QRS complex and prolongation of Q-T interval). Products include:

Tonocard Tablets ... 1554

Tolazamide (Concurrent administration with hepatic enzyme inducers may lower plasma levels of disopyramide). Products include:

Tolinase Tablets ... 2365

Tolbutamide (Concurrent administration with hepatic enzyme inducers may lower plasma levels of disopyramide). Products include:

Orinase Tablets ... 2354

Verapamil Hydrochloride (Excessive widening of QRS complex and prolongation of Q-T interval). Products include:

Calan SR Caplets ... 2157
Calan Tablets ... 2155
Isoptin Injectable ... 1177
Isoptin Oral Tablets ... 1179
Isoptin SR Sustained Release Tablets ... 1181
Verelan Capsules ... 1243
Verelan Capsules ... 2535

NORPACE CR CAPSULES
(Disopyramide Phosphate) ... 2177
See **Norpace Capsules**

NORPLANT SYSTEM
(Levonorgestrel) ... 2484
May interact with:

Carbamazepine (Reduces efficacy (pregnancy)). Products include:

Tegretol Chewable Tablets ... 654
Tegretol Suspension ... 656
Tegretol Tablets ... 654

Phenytoin (Reduces efficacy (pregnancy)). Products include:

Dilantin Infatabs ... 1710
Dilantin-30 Pediatric/Dilantin-125 Suspension ... 1713

Phenytoin Sodium (Reduces efficacy (pregnancy)). Products include:

Dilantin Kapseals ... 1708
Dilantin Parenteral ... 1712
Dilantin with Phenobarbital Kapseals ... 1715

NORPRAMIN TABLETS
(Desipramine Hydrochloride) ... 1340
May interact with thyroid preparations, anticholinergics, sympathomimetic aerosal brochodilators, benzodiazepines, tranquilizers, monoamine oxidase inhibitors, tricyclic antidepressants, and certain other agents. Compounds in these categories include:

Albuterol (Close supervision and careful dosage adjustment required). Products include:

Proventil Inhalation Aerosol ... 2117
Ventolin Inhalation Aerosol and Refill ... 583

Albuterol Sulfate (Close supervision and careful dosage adjustment required). Products include:

Proventil Repetabs Tablets ... 2120
Proventil Solutions for Inhalation 0.5% and 0.083% ... 2118
Proventil Syrup ... 2119
Proventil Tablets ... 2120
Ventolin ... 583

Alcohol (Exaggerated response to alcohol; potentiation; increased danger of suicide or overdose).

Alprazolam (Additive sedative and anticholinergic effects). Products include:

Xanax Tablets ... 2367

Amitriptyline Hydrochloride (Concurrent administration may result in clinically significant increase in plasma levels of antidepressant). Products include:

Elavil ... 2269
Endep Tablets ... 1927
Etrafon ... 2087
Limbitrol ... 1933
Triavil Tablets ... 1556

Amoxapine (Concurrent administration may result in clinically significant increase in plasma levels of antidepressant). Products include:

Asendin Tablets ... 1196

Atropine Sulfate (Close supervision and careful dosage adjustment required). Products include:

Arco-Lase Plus Tablets ... 607
Atropine Sulfate Sterile Ophthalmic Solution and S.O.P. Sterile Ophthalmic Ointment ... ◉ 239
Donnagel ... ◘ 675
Donnagel-PG ... 1858
Donnatal ... 1858
Donnatal Extentabs ... 1859
Donnatal Tablets ... 1858
Donnazyme Tablets ... 1860
Isopto Atropine ... ◉ 218
Lomotil ... 2174
Motofen Tablets ... 836
Ru-Tuss Tablets ... 693
Urised Tablets ... 2396

Belladonna Alkaloids (Close supervision and careful dosage adjustment required). Products include:

Bellergal-S Tablets ... 1998
Hyland's Bed Wetting Tablets ... ◘ 728
Hyland's Teething Tablets ... ◘ 728
Kinesed Tablets ... 2272

Benztropine Mesylate (Close supervision and careful dosage adjustment required). Products include:

Cogentin ... 1435

Biperiden (Close supervision and careful dosage adjustment required). Products include:

Akineton ... 1171

Buspirone Hydrochloride (Additive sedative and anticholinergic effects). Products include:

BuSpar ... 1401

Chlordiazepoxide (Additive sedative and anticholinergic effects). Products include:

Libritabs Tablets ... 1930
Limbitrol ... 1933
Menrium Tablets ... 1934

Chlordiazepoxide Hydrochloride (Additive sedative and anticholinergic effects). Products include:

Librax Capsules ... 1929
Librium Capsules ... 1931
Librium Injectable ... 1932

Chlorpromazine (Additive sedative and anticholinergic effects). Products include:

Thorazine ... 2234

Chlorprothixene (Additive sedative and anticholinergic effects). Products include:

Taractan Tablets ... 1920

Chlorprothixene Hydrochloride (Additive sedative and anticholinergic effects). Products include:

Taractan ... 1920

Cimetidine (Significant increases in tricyclic antidepressant plasma levels). Products include:

Tagamet Tablets ... 2228

Cimetidine Hydrochloride (Significant increases in tricyclic antidepressant plasma levels). Products include:

Tagamet ... 2228

Clidinium Bromide (Close supervision and careful dosage adjustment required). Products include:

Librax Capsules ... 1929
Quarzan Capsules ... 1937

Clomipramine Hydrochloride (Concurrent administration may result in clinically significant increase in plasma levels of antidepressant). Products include:

Anafranil Capsules ... 650

Clorazepate Dipotassium (Additive sedative and anticholinergic effects). Products include:

Tranxene ... 556

Diazepam (Additive sedative and anticholinergic effects). Products include:

Valium Injectable ... 1937
Valium Tablets ... 1939
Valrelease Capsules ... 1923

Dicyclomine Hydrochloride (Close supervision and careful dosage adjustment required). Products include:

Bentyl ... 1322

Dobutamine Hydrochloride (Close supervision and careful dosage adjustment required). Products include:

Dobutrex Solution Vials ... 1259

Dopamine Hydrochloride (Close supervision and careful dosage adjustment required). Products include:

Intropin Injection ... 930

Doxepin Hydrochloride (Concurrent administration may result in clinically significant increase in plasma levels of antidepressant). Products include:

Sinequan ... 1960

Droperidol (Additive sedative and anticholinergic effects). Products include:

Inapsine Injection ... 1140
Innovar Injection ... 1141

Ephedrine Hydrochloride (Close supervision and careful dosage adjustment required). Products include:

Amesec ... ◘ 682
Primatene Tablets-M Formula ... 2421
Primatene Tablets-P Formula ... 2421
Primatene Tablets-Regular Formula ... 2421
Quadrinal Tablets ... 1183
Quelidrine Syrup ... 556
Tedral SA ... 1765

Ephedrine Sulfate (Close supervision and careful dosage adjustments required). Products include:

Bronkaid Tablets ... ◘ 757
Bronkolixir ... ◘ 761
Bronkotabs Tablets ... ◘ 762
Marax Tablets & DF Syrup ... 1954
Pazo Hemorrhoid Ointment & Suppositories ... 752
Vicks Vatronol Nose Drops ... ◘ 666

Ephedrine Tannate (Close supervision and careful dosage adjustment required). Products include:

Rynatuss ... 2388

Epinephrine (Close supervision and careful dosage adjustment required). Products include:

Ana-Kit Anaphylaxis Emergency Treatment Kit ... 1100
Bronkaid Mist ... ◘ 757
EpiPen ... 843
Marcaine Hydrochloride 0.5% with Epinephrine 1:200,000 (as bitartrate) ... 958
Marcaine Hydrochloride with Epinephrine 1:200,000 ... 2055
Primatene Mist ... 2420
Sus-Phrine Injection ... 1006
Xylocaine with Epinephrine Injections ... 637

Epinephrine Bitartrate (Close supervision and careful dosage adjustment required). Products include:

AsthmaHaler Mist Epinephrine Bitartrate Bronchodilator ... ◘ 616
Bronkaid Mist Suspension ... ◘ 757
Primatene Mist Suspension ... 2421

Epinephrine Hydrochloride (Close supervision and careful dosage adjustment required). Products include:

Adrenalin Chloride Solution 1:100 & 1:1,000 ... 1689
Epifrin ... ◉ 244
Glaucon ... ◉ 218

Estazolam (Additive sedative and anticholinergic effects). Products include:
ProSom Tablets ... 554

Fluoxetine Hydrochloride (Combination therapy may produce greater than twofold increases of previously stable plasma levels of tricyclic antidepressant). Products include:
Prozac Pulvules ... 920

Fluphenazine Decanoate (Additive sedative and anticholinergic effects). Products include:
Prolixin Decanoate ... 1795

Fluphenazine Enanthate (Additive sedative and anticholinergic effects). Products include:
Prolixin Enanthate ... 1796

Fluphenazine Hydrochloride (Additive sedative and anticholinergic effects). Products include:
Prolixin Elixir ... 1793
Prolixin Injection ... 1791
Prolixin Oral Concentrate ... 1792
Prolixin Tablets ... 1793

Furazolidone (Contraindication; hyperpyretic crises; severe convulsions; death). Products include:
Furoxone ... 1855

Glycopyrrolate (Close supervision and careful dosage adjustment required). Products include:
Robinul Forte Tablets ... 1873
Robinul Injectable ... 1873
Robinul Tablets ... 1873

Guanethidine Monosulfate (Antihypertensive effect blocked). Products include:
Esimil Tablets ... 864
Ismelin Tablets ... 869

Haloperidol (Additive sedative and anticholinergic effects). Products include:
Haldol Injection, Tablets and Concentrate ... 1373

Haloperidol Decanoate (Additive sedative and anticholinergic effects). Products include:
Haldol Decanoate ... 1375

Hydroxyzine Hydrochloride (Additive sedative and anticholinergic effects). Products include:
Atarax Tablets & Syrup ... 1941
Marax Tablets & DF Syrup ... 1954
Vistaril Intramuscular Solution ... 1970

Hyoscyamine (Close supervision and careful dosage adjustment required). Products include:
Cystospaz Tablets ... 2395
Urised Tablets ... 2396

Hyoscyamine Sulfate (Close supervision and careful dosage adjustment required). Products include:
Arco-Lase Plus Tablets ... 607
Cystospaz-M Capsules ... 2395
Donnagel ... ▣ 675
Donnagel-PG ... 1858
Donnatal ... 1858
Donnatal Extentabs ... 1859
Donnatal Tablets ... 1858
Donnazyme Tablets ... 1860
Kutrase Capsules ... 2146
Levsin/Levsinex ... 2147
Ru-Tuss Tablets ... 693

Imipramine Hydrochloride (Concurrent administration may result in clinically significant increase in plasma levels of antidepressant). Products include:
Tofranil Ampuls ... 1038
Tofranil Tablets ... 1039

Imipramine Pamoate (Concurrent administration may result in clinically significant increase in plasma levels of antidepressant). Products include:
Tofranil-PM Capsules ... 1041

Ipratropium Bromide (Close supervision and careful dosage adjustment required). Products include:
Atrovent Inhalation Aerosol ... 675

Isocarboxazid (Contraindication; hyperpyretic crises; severe convulsions; death). Products include:
Marplan Tablets ... 1906

Isoproterenol Hydrochloride (Close supervision and careful dosage adjustment required). Products include:
Isuprel Hydrochloride Injection 1:5000 ... 2050
Isuprel Hydrochloride Mistometer .. 2051
Isuprel Hydrochloride Solution 1:200 & 1:100 ... 2052
Norisodrine Aerotrol ... 540

Lorazepam (Additive sedative and anticholinergic effects). Products include:
Ativan Injection ... 2432
Ativan Tablets ... 2434

Loxapine Hydrochloride (Additive sedative and anticholinergic effects). Products include:
Loxitane ... 1213

Loxapine Succinate (Additive sedative and anticholinergic effects). Products include:
Loxitane Capsules ... 1213

Maprotiline Hydrochloride (Concurrent administration may result in clinically significant increase in plasma levels of antidepressant). Products include:
Ludiomil Tablets ... 874

Mepenzolate Bromide (Close supervision and careful dosage adjustment required). Products include:
Cantil Tablets ... 1326

Meprobamate (Additive sedative and anticholinergic effects). Products include:
Deprol Tablets ... 2382
Equagesic Tablets ... 2451
Miltown Tablets ... 2386
PMB 200 and PMB 400 ... 2504

Mesoridazine (Additive sedative and anticholinergic effects). Products include:
Serentil ... 686

Metaproterenol Sulfate (Close supervision and careful dosage adjustment required). Products include:
Alupent ... 674
Arm-a-Med Metaproterenol Sulfate Inhalation Solution, USP ... 617
Metaprel Inhalation Aerosol Bronchodilator ... 2014
Metaprel Inhalation Solution ... 2015
Metaprel ... 2015
Metaproterenol Sulfate Inhalation Solution, USP ... 912

Metaraminol Bitartrate (Close supervision and careful dosage adjustment required). Products include:
Aramine Injection ... 1424

Methoxamine Hydrochloride (Close supervision and careful dosage adjustment required). Products include:
Vasoxyl Injection ... 819

Midazolam Hydrochloride (Additive sedative and anticholinergic effects). Products include:
Versed Injection ... 1924

Molindone Hydrochloride (Additive sedative and anticholinergic effects). Products include:
Moban Tablets & Concentrate ... 932

Norepinephrine Bitartrate (Close supervision and careful dosage adjustment required). Products include:
Levophed Bitartrate Injection ... 2054

Nortriptyline Hydrochloride (Concurrent administration may result in clinically significant increase in plasma levels of antidepressant). Products include:
Pamelor ... 2019

Oxazepam (Additive sedative and anticholinergic effects). Products include:
Serax Capsules ... 2522
Serax Tablets ... 2522

Oxybutynin Chloride (Close supervision and careful dosage adjustment required). Products include:
Ditropan ... 1332

Perphenazine (Additive sedative and anticholinergic effects). Products include:
Etrafon ... 2087
Triavil Tablets ... 1556
Trilafon ... 2123

Phenelzine Sulfate (Contraindication; hyperpyretic crises; severe convulsions; death). Products include:
Nardil ... 1742

Phenylephrine Hydrochloride (Close supervision and careful dosage adjustment required). Products include:
AK-Dilate Solution 2.5% and 10% ... ⊙ 203
Atrohist Sprinkle Capsules ... 558
Cerose-DM ... 2443
Codimal ... 846
Comhist LA Capsules ... 1618
Congespirin For Children Aspirin Free Chewable Cold Tablets ... 748
Cyclomydril ... ⊙ 216
Deconsal Sprinkle Capsules ... 559
Dimetane Decongestant ... ▣ 673
Dristan Decongestant/Antihistamine/ Analgesic Coated Caplets ... ▣ 749
Dristan Cold Nasal Decongestant/ Antihistamine/ Analgesic Coated Tablets ... 2419
Dristan Advanced Formula Decongestant/Antihistamine/ Analgesic Tablets ... ▣ 749
Dristan Nasal Spray, Menthol ... 2419
Dristan Nasal Spray, Regular and Regular with Metered Pump ... 2419
Entex Capsules ... 1623
Entex Liquid ... 1623
Sinus Excedrin Analgesic, Decongestant Tablets & Caplets ... 750
Extendryl ... 994
4-Way Fast Acting Nasal Spray - Original Formula (regular & mentholated) & Metered Spray Pump (regular) ... 751
Hycomine Compound Tablets ... 929
Murocoll-2 Sterile Ophthalmic Solution ... ⊙ 261
Mydfrin 2.5% ... ⊙ 224
Naldecon Syrup, Tablets, Pediatric Drops and Pediatric Syrup ... 709
Neo-Synephrine Hydrochloride 1% Carpuject ... 2063
Neo-Synephrine Hydrochloride 1% Injection ... 2063
Neo-Synephrine Hydrochloride (Ophthalmic) ... 2064
Neo-Synephrine ... ▣ 759
Nōstril Nasal Decongestant ... ▣ 520
Novahistine Elixir ... ▣ 596
Phenergan VC ... 2500
Phenergan VC with Codeine ... 2501
Prefrin Liquifilm Vasoconstrictor and Lubricant Eye Drops ... ⊙ 254
Prefrin-A ... ⊙ 255
Quelidrine Syrup ... 556
Relief Vasoconstrictor and Lubricant Eye Drops ... ⊙ 256
Robitussin Night Relief ... ▣ 677
Ru-Tuss with Hydrocodone ... 694
Ru-Tuss Tablets ... 693
Vasosulf ... ⊙ 279
Vicks Sinex ... ▣ 665
Zincfrin ... ⊙ 230

Phenylephrine Tannate (Close supervision and careful dosage adjustment required). Products include:
Rynatan ... 2387
Rynatuss ... 2388

Phenylpropanolamine Hydrochloride (Close supervision and careful dosage adjustment required). Products include:
A.R.M. Allergy Relief Medicine Caplets ... ▣ 615
Acutrim ... ▣ 548
Allerest ... ▣ 559
BC Cold Powder ... ▣ 517
Cheracol Plus Head Cold/Cough Formula ... ▣ 667
Codimal Expectorant ... 846
Comtrex Multi-Symptom Cold Reliever Tablets/Caplets/Liqui-Gels/Liquid ... 745
Contac Continuous Action Decongestant/Antihistamine Capsules ▣ 710
Contac Maximum Strength Continuous Action Decongestant/ Antihistamine Caplets ... ▣ 709
Contac Severe Cold and Flu Formula Caplets ... ▣ 711
Coricidin 'D' Decongestant Tablets ... ▣ 695
Coricidin Demilets Tablets for Children ... ▣ 696
Demazin Nasal Decongestant/ Antihistamine Repetabs Tablets & Syrup ... ▣ 697
Dexatrim ... ▣ 733
Dimetane-DC Cough Syrup ... 1857
Dimetapp Elixir ... ▣ 673
Dimetapp DM Elixir ... ▣ 674
Dimetapp Extentabs ... ▣ 674
Dimetapp Plus Caplets ... ▣ 675
Dimetapp Tablets ... ▣ 675
Entex Capsules ... 1623
Entex LA Tablets ... 1623
Entex Liquid ... 1623
4-Way Cold Tablets ... 750
Hycomine Syrup ... 927
Naldecon CX Adult Liquid ... ▣ 521
Naldecon DX Adult Liquid ... ▣ 521
Naldecon DX Children's Syrup ... ▣ 522
Naldecon DX Pediatric Drops ... ▣ 522
Naldecon EX Children's Syrup ... ▣ 522
Naldecon EX Pediatric Drops ... ▣ 523
Naldecon Syrup, Tablets, Pediatric Drops and Pediatric Syrup ... 709
Nolamine Tablets ... 838
Nolex LA Tablets ... 838
Ornade Spansule Capsules ... 2221
Orthoxicol Cough Syrup ... ▣ 668
Propagest ... 839
Pyrroxate Capsules ... ▣ 669
Robitussin-CF ... ▣ 676
Ru-Tuss II Capsules ... 693
Ru-Tuss with Hydrocodone ... 694
Ru-Tuss Tablets ... 693
Sine-Off Sinus Medicine Tablets-Aspirin Formula ... ▣ 722
Sinulin ... 840
St. Joseph Cold Tablets for Children ... ▣ 704
Tavist-D Tablets ... 2035
Triaminic Allergy Tablets ... ▣ 688
Triaminic Chewables ... ▣ 688
Triaminic Cold Tablets ... ▣ 688
Triaminic Expectorant ... ▣ 688
Triaminic Expectorant w/Codeine .. 1996
Triaminic Expectorant DH ... 1995
Triaminic Oral Infant Drops ... 1996
Triaminic Syrup ... ▣ 689
Triaminic-12 Tablets ... ▣ 690
Triaminic-DM Syrup ... ▣ 689
Triaminicin Tablets ... ▣ 690
Triaminicol Multi-Symptom Cold Tablets ... ▣ 691
Triaminicol Multi-Symptom Relief ▣ 691
Tuss-Ornade Liquid ... 2242
Tuss-Ornade Spansule Capsules ... 2242
Tylenol Cold Medication, Effervescent Tablets ... 1369

Pirbuterol Acetate (Close supervision and careful dosage adjustment required). Products include:
Maxair Inhaler ... 1311

Prazepam (Additive sedative and anticholinergic effects). Products include:
Centrax ... 1693

Prochlorperazine (Additive sedative and anticholinergic effects). Products include:

Compazine ... 2201

Procyclidine Hydrochloride (Close supervision and careful dosage adjustment required). Products include:

Kemadrin Tablets ... 771

Promethazine Hydrochloride (Additive sedative and anticholinergic effects). Products include:

Mepergan Injection ... 2479
Phenergan with Codeine ... 2497
Phenergan with Dextromethorphan 2499
Phenergan Injection ... 2493
Phenergan Suppositories ... 2496
Phenergan Syrup ... 2495
Phenergan Tablets ... 2496
Phenergan VC ... 2500
Phenergan VC with Codeine ... 2501

Propantheline Bromide (Close supervision and careful dosage adjustment required). Products include:

Pro-Banthine Tablets ... 2141

Protriptyline Hydrochloride (Concurrent administration may result in clinically significant increase in plasma levels of antidepressant). Products include:

Vivactil Tablets ... 1567

Pseudoephedrine Hydrochloride (Close supervision and careful dosage adjustment required). Products include:

Actifed Capsules ... ◘ 539
Actifed Plus Caplets ... ◘ 539
Actifed Plus Tablets ... ◘ 540
Actifed with Codeine Cough Syrup.. 752
Actifed Syrup ... ◘ 540
Actifed Tablets ... ◘ 540
Actifed 12-Hour Capsules ... ◘ 539
Advil Cold & Sinus Caplets (formerly CoAdvil) ... 2416
Allerest ... ◘ 559
Anatuss LA Tablets ... 1359
Benadryl Decongestant Elixir ... ◘ 635
Benadryl Decongestant ... ◘ 635
Benadryl Plus ... ◘ 636
Benadryl Plus Nighttime ... ◘ 637
Benylin Decongestant ... ◘ 638
Brexin L.A. Capsules ... 2078
Bromfed Capsules (Timed Release) ... 1615
Bromfed Syrup ... ◘ 628
Bromfed ... 1615
CoAdvil ... ◘ 748
Allergy-Sinus Comtrex Multi-Symptom Allergy Sinus Formula Tablets & Caplets ... 746
Cough Formula Comtrex ... 746
Comtrex Multi-Symptom Cold Reliever Tablets/Caplets/Liqui-Gels/Liquid ... 745
Day-Night Comtrex ... 747
Non-Drowsy Comtrex ... 747
Congess ... 994
Congestac Caplets ... ◘ 617
Contac Jr. Children's Cold Medicine ... ◘ 712
Contac Nighttime Cold Medicine ... ◘ 713
Contac Sinus Caplets Maximum Strength Non-Drowsy Formula ... ◘ 710
Contac Sinus Tablets Maximum Strength Non-Drowsy Formula ... ◘ 710
Deconamine ... 663
Deconsal II Tablets ... 559
Dimacol Caplets ... ◘ 672
Dimetane-DX Cough Syrup ... 1858
Dorcol Children's Cough Syrup ... ◘ 685
Dorcol Children's Decongestant Liquid ... ◘ 685
Dorcol Children's Liquid Cold Formula ... ◘ 686
Maximum Strength Dristan Decongestant/Analgesic Coated Caplets ... ◘ 750
No Drowsiness Dristan Cold Nasal Decongestant/Analgesic Coated Caplets ... 2420
Dristan Sinus Caplets ... 2419
Sinus Excedrin Analgesic, Decongestant Tablets & Caplets ... ◘ 533
Fedahist Gyrocaps ... 2145
Fedahist Timecaps ... 2145
Guaifed ... 1615
Guaifed Syrup ... ◘ 629
Isoclor Expectorant ... 982
Isoclor Timesule Capsules ... ◘ 561
Kronofed-A ... 970
Medi-Flu Caplet, Liquid ... ◘ 640
Novafed A Capsules ... 1342
Novafed Capsules ... 1342
Novahistine DH ... 1342
Novahistine DMX ... ◘ 595
Novahistine Expectorant ... 1343
Nucofed Capsules ... 2219
Nucofed Expectorant ... 2219
Nucofed Pediatric Expectorant ... 2220
Nucofed Syrup ... 2219
Ornex Caplets ... ◘ 618
PediaCare Allergy Relief Formula Liquid ... 1362
PediaCare Cough-Cold Formula Liquid ... 1362
PediaCare Infants' Oral Decongestant Drops ... 1362
PediaCare Night Rest Cough-Cold Formula Liquid ... 1362
PediaCare 6-12 Cough-Cold Formula Chewable Tablets ... 1362
Robitussin-DAC Syrup ... 1875
Robitussin-PE ... ◘ 677
Rondec ... 1975
Rondec-DM ... 1976
Rondec-TR Tablet ... 1975
Ru-Tuss DE Tablets ... 694
Ryna ... ◘ 741
Seldane-D Extended-Release Tablets ... 1350
Sinarest ... ◘ 562
Sine-Aid Maximum Strength Sinus Headache Caplets ... 1365
Sine-Aid Maximum Strength Sinus Headache Tablets ... 1365
Sine-Off Maximum Strength Allergy/Sinus Formula Caplets ... ◘ 721
Sine-Off Maximum Strength No Drowsiness Formula Caplets ... ◘ 722
Singlet Tablets ... ◘ 598
Sinutab Maximum Strength ... ◘ 641
Sinutab Maximum Strength Without Drowsiness Tablets & Caplets ... ◘ 642
Sinutab Regular Strength Without Drowsiness Formula ... ◘ 641
St. Joseph Nighttime Cold Medicine ... ◘ 705
Sudafed Children's Liquid ... ◘ 543
Sudafed Cough Syrup ... ◘ 543
Sudafed Plus Liquid ... ◘ 544
Sudafed Plus Tablets ... ◘ 545
Sudafed Sinus Caplets ... ◘ 545
Sudafed Sinus Tablets ... ◘ 545
Sudafed Tablets, 30 mg ... ◘ 544
Sudafed Tablets, Adult Strength, 60 mg ... ◘ 544
Sudafed 12 Hour Capsules ... ◘ 545
TheraFlu Flu and Cold Medicine ... ◘ 687
Triaminic Nite Light ... ◘ 689
Tylenol Allergy Sinus Medication Caplets and Gelcaps, Maximum Strength ... 1372
Children's Tylenol Cold Liquid Formula and Chewable Tablets ... 1368
Tylenol Cold & Flu Hot Medication, Packets ... 1369
Tylenol Cold & Flu No Drowsiness Hot Medication, Packets ... 1371
Tylenol Cold Medication Caplets and Tablets ... 1370
Tylenol Cold Medication No Drowsiness Formula Caplets ... 1370
Tylenol Cold Night Time Medication Liquid ... 1371
Tylenol Cough Medication Liquid with Decongestant, Maximum Strength ... 1372
Tylenol, Maximum Strength, Sinus Medication Gelcaps, Caplets and Tablets ... 1373
Ursinus Inlay-Tabs ... ◘ 691
Vicks Children's NyQuil ... ◘ 664
Vicks Daycare ... ◘ 660
Vicks Formula 44D Decongestant Cough Medicine ... ◘ 662
Vicks Formula 44M Multi-Symptom Cough Medicine ... ◘ 662
Vicks NyQuil Nighttime Colds Medicine-Original & Cherry Flavor ... ◘ 664
Vicks Pediatric Formula 44 Cough & Congestion Medicine ... ◘ 663
Vicks Pediatric Formula 44m Multi-Symptom Cough & Cold Medicine ... ◘ 663

Pseudoephedrine Sulfate (Close supervision and careful dosage adjustment required). Products include:

Afrin Tablets ... ◘ 693
Chlor-Trimeton Decongestant ... ◘ 694
Disophrol Chronotab Sustained-Action Tablets ... ◘ 698
Drixoral Antihistamine/Nasal Decongestant Syrup ... ◘ 698
Drixoral Non-Drowsy Formula ... ◘ 699
Drixoral Plus Extended-Release Tablets ... ◘ 699
Drixoral Sinus ... ◘ 700
Drixoral Sustained-Action Tablets ◘ 698
Sinutab Allergy Formula Sustained Action Tablets ... ◘ 640
Trinalin Repetabs Tablets ... 1170

Quazepam (Additive sedative and anticholinergic effects). Products include:

Doral Tablets ... 2383

Scopolamine Hydrobromide (Close supervision and careful dosage adjustment required). Products include:

Donnagel ... ◘ 675
Donnagel-PG ... 1858
Donnatal ... 1858
Donnatal Extentabs ... 1859
Donnatal Tablets ... 1858
Donnazyme Tablets ... 1860
Isopto Hyoscine ... ⊙ 222
Murocoll-2 Sterile Ophthalmic Solution ... ⊙ 261
Ru-Tuss Tablets ... 693

Scopolamine Preparations (Close supervision and careful dosage adjustment required). Products include:

Transderm Scōp Transdermal Therapeutic System ... 887

Selegiline Hydrochloride (Contraindication; hyperpyretic crises; severe convulsions; death). Products include:

Eldepryl ... 2250

Terbutaline Sulfate (Close supervision and careful dosage adjustment required). Products include:

Brethaire Inhaler ... 1024
Brethine Ampuls ... 1026
Brethine Tablets ... 1026
Bricanyl Injection ... 1324
Bricanyl Tablets ... 1325

Thioridazine Hydrochloride (Additive sedative and anticholinergic effects). Products include:

Mellaril ... 2011

Thiothixene (Additive sedative and anticholinergic effects). Products include:

Navane Capsules and Concentrate 1954
Navane Intramuscular ... 1956

Thyroid (Cardiovascular toxicity, including arrhythmias). Products include:

S-P-T "Liquid" Capsules ... 995

Tranylcypromine Sulfate (Contraindication; hyperpyretic crises; severe convulsions; death). Products include:

Parnate Tablets ... 2222

Tridihexethyl Chloride (Close supervision and careful dosage adjustment required).

No products indexed under this heading.

Trifluoperazine Hydrochloride (Additive sedative and anticholinergic effects). Products include:

Stelazine ... 2226

Trihexyphenidyl Hydrochloride (Close supervision and careful dosage adjustments required). Products include:

Artane ... 1195

Trimipramine Maleate (Concurrent administration may result in clinically significant increase in plasma levels of antidepressant). Products include:

Surmontil Capsules ... 2524

NOR-Q D TABLETS

(Norethindrone) ... 2304

See **Brevicon 21-Day Tablets**

NORWICH EXTRA-STRENGTH ASPIRIN

(Aspirin) ... ◘ 546

May interact with oral anticoagulants, antigout agents, and certain other agents. Compounds in these categories include:

Allopurinol (Effect not specified). Products include:

Zyloprim Tablets ... 830

Antiarthritic Drugs, unspecified (Effect not specified).

Antidiabetic Drugs, unspecified (Effect not specified).

Dicumarol (Effect not specified). Products include:

Dicumarol Tablets ... 516

Probenecid (Effect not specified). Products include:

Benemid Tablets ... 1426
ColBENEMID Tablets ... 1436
Wycillin Injection and Probenecid Tablets ... 2539

Sulfinpyrazone (Effect not specified). Products include:

Anturane ... 853

Warfarin Sodium (Effect not specified). Products include:

Coumadin Injection & Tablets ... 944
Panwarfin Tablets ... 547

NORWICH REGULAR STRENGTH ASPIRIN

(Aspirin) ... ◘ 547

May interact with oral anticoagulants, antigout agents, and certain other agents. Compounds in these categories include:

Allopurinol (Effect not specified). Products include:

Zyloprim Tablets ... 830

Antiarthritic Drugs, unspecified (Effect not specified).

Antidiabetic Drugs, unspecified (Effect not specified).

Dicumarol (Effect not specified). Products include:

Dicumarol Tablets ... 516

Probenecid (Effect not specified). Products include:

Benemid Tablets ... 1426
ColBENEMID Tablets ... 1436
Wycillin Injection and Probenecid Tablets ... 2539

Sulfinpyrazone (Effect not specified). Products include:

Anturane ... 853

Warfarin Sodium (Effect not specified). Products include:

Coumadin Injection & Tablets ... 944
Panwarfin Tablets ... 547

NORZINE AMPULS

(Thiethylperazine Maleate) ... 1818

May interact with central nervous system depressants, general anesthetics, and certain other agents. Compounds in these categories include:

Alcohol (Potentiated effects).

Alfentanil Hydrochloride (Potentiated effects). Products include:

Alfenta Injection ... 1131

Alprazolam (Potentiated effects). Products include:
- Xanax Tablets ... 2367

Aprobarbital (Potentiated effects). Products include:
- Alurate Elixir ... 1883

Atropine Nitrate, Methyl (Potentiated effects).
- No products indexed under this heading.

Atropine Sulfate (Potentiated effects). Products include:
- Arco-Lase Plus Tablets ... 607
- Atropine Sulfate Sterile Ophthalmic Solution and S.O.P. Sterile Ophthalmic Ointment ... ⊙ 239
- Donnagel ... ▣ 675
- Donnagel-PG ... 1858
- Donnatal ... 1858
- Donnatal Extentabs ... 1859
- Donnatal Tablets ... 1858
- Donnazyme Tablets ... 1860
- Isopto Atropine ... ⊙ 218
- Lomotil ... 2174
- Motofen Tablets ... 836
- Ru-Tuss Tablets ... 693
- Urised Tablets ... 2396

Buprenorphine (Potentiated effects).
- No products indexed under this heading.

Buspirone Hydrochloride (Potentiated effects). Products include:
- BuSpar ... 1401

Butabarbital (Potentiated effects). Products include:
- Pyridium Plus ... 1764

Butalbital (Potentiated effects). Products include:
- Esgic-Plus Tablets ... 1002
- Esgic Tablets & Capsules ... 1001
- Fioricet Tablets ... 2006
- Fiorinal Capsules ... 2007
- Fiorinal with Codeine Capsules ... 2008
- Fiorinal Tablets ... 2007
- Phrenilin ... 838
- Sedapap Tablets 50 mg/650 mg ... 1360

Chlordiazepoxide (Potentiated effects). Products include:
- Libritabs Tablets ... 1930
- Limbitrol ... 1933
- Menrium Tablets ... 1934

Chlordiazepoxide Hydrochloride (Potentiated effects). Products include:
- Librax Capsules ... 1929
- Librium Capsules ... 1931
- Librium Injectable ... 1932

Chlorpromazine (Potentiated effects). Products include:
- Thorazine ... 2234

Chlorprothixene (Potentiated effects). Products include:
- Taractan Tablets ... 1920

Chlorprothixene Hydrochloride (Potentiated effects). Products include:
- Taractan ... 1920

Clorazepate Dipotassium (Potentiated effects). Products include:
- Tranxene ... 556

Codeine (Potentiated effects). Products include:
- Calcidrine Syrup ... 506

Codeine Phosphate (Potentiated effects). Products include:
- Actifed with Codeine Cough Syrup ... 752
- Cheracol Cough Syrup ... 1853
- Codimal PH Syrup ... 846
- Dimetane-DC Cough Syrup ... 1857
- Empirin with Codeine Phosphate Nos. 2, 3 & 4 ... 764
- Fiorinal with Codeine Capsules ... 2008
- Isoclor Expectorant ... 982
- Naldecon CX Adult Liquid ... ▣ 521
- Novahistine DH ... 1342
- Novahistine Expectorant ... 1343
- Nucofed Capsules ... 2219
- Nucofed Expectorant ... 2219
- Nucofed Pediatric Expectorant ... 2220
- Nucofed Syrup ... 2219
- Phenaphen with Codeine Capsules ... 1865
- Phenaphen-650 with Codeine Tablets ... 1866
- Phenergan with Codeine ... 2497
- Phenergan VC with Codeine ... 2501
- Robitussin A-C Syrup ... 1875
- Robitussin-DAC Syrup ... 1875
- Ryna ... ▣ 741
- Soma Compound w/Codeine Tablets ... 2390
- Triaminic Expectorant w/Codeine ... 1996
- Tussi-Organidin Liquid ... 2391
- Tylenol with Codeine ... 1381

Codeine Polistirex (Potentiated effects).
- No products indexed under this heading.

Dezocine (Potentiated effects).

Diazepam (Potentiated effects). Products include:
- Valium Injectable ... 1937
- Valium Tablets ... 1939
- Valrelease Capsules ... 1923

Droperidol (Potentiated effects). Products include:
- Inapsine Injection ... 1140
- Innovar Injection ... 1141

Enflurane (Potentiated effects). Products include:
- Ethrane ... 599

Epinephrine (May induce a reversed epinephrine effect on occasion). Products include:
- Ana-Kit Anaphylaxis Emergency Treatment Kit ... 1100
- Bronkaid Mist ... ▣ 757
- EpiPen ... 843
- Marcaine Hydrochloride 0.5% with Epinephrine 1:200,000 (as bitartrate) ... 958
- Marcaine Hydrochloride with Epinephrine 1:200,000 ... 2055
- Primatene Mist ... 2420
- Sus-Phrine Injection ... 1006
- Xylocaine with Epinephrine Injections ... 637

Epinephrine Bitartrate (May induce a reversed epinephrine effect on occasion). Products include:
- AsthmaHaler Mist Epinephrine Bitartrate Bronchodilator ... ▣ 616
- Bronkaid Mist Suspension ... ▣ 757
- Primatene Mist Suspension ... 2421

Epinephrine Hydrochloride (May induce a reversed epinephrine effect on occasion). Products include:
- Adrenalin Chloride Solution 1:100 & 1:1,000 ... 1689
- Epifrin ... ⊙ 244
- Glaucon ... ⊙ 218

Estazolam (Potentiated effects). Products include:
- ProSom Tablets ... 554

Ethchlorvynol (Potentiated effects). Products include:
- Placidyl Capsules ... 553

Ethinamate (Potentiated effects).
- No products indexed under this heading.

Fentanyl (Potentiated effects). Products include:
- Duragesic Transdermal System ... 1133

Fentanyl Citrate (Potentiated effects). Products include:
- Innovar Injection ... 1141
- Sublimaze Injection ... 1146

Fluphenazine Decanoate (Potentiated effects). Products include:
- Prolixin Decanoate ... 1795

Fluphenazine Enanthate (Potentiated effects). Products include:
- Prolixin Enanthate ... 1796

Fluphenazine Hydrochloride (Potentiated effects). Products include:
- Prolixin Elixir ... 1793
- Prolixin Injection ... 1791
- Prolixin Oral Concentrate ... 1792
- Prolixin Tablets ... 1793

Flurazepam Hydrochloride (Potentiated effects). Products include:
- Dalmane Capsules ... 1927

Glutethimide (Potentiated effects).
- No products indexed under this heading.

Haloperidol (Potentiated effects). Products include:
- Haldol Injection, Tablets and Concentrate ... 1373

Haloperidol Decanoate (Potentiated effects). Products include:
- Haldol Decanoate ... 1375

Hydrocodone Bitartrate (Potentiated effects). Products include:
- Anexsia 5/500 Tablets ... 2196
- Anexsia 7.5/650 Tablets ... 2197
- Azdone Tablets ... 844
- Codiclear DH Syrup ... 845
- Codimal DH Syrup ... 846
- Damason-P ... 1356
- Hycodan Syrup, Tablets ... 927
- Hycomine Compound Tablets ... 929
- Hycomine Syrup ... 927
- Hycotuss Expectorant Syrup ... 930
- Hydrocet Capsules ... 835
- Lortab ASA Tablets ... 2414
- Lortab ... 2412
- Ru-Tuss with Hydrocodone ... 694
- Triaminic Expectorant DH ... 1995
- Vicodin Tablets ... 1187
- Vicodin ES Tablets ... 1189
- Zydone Capsules ... 941

Hydrocodone Polistirex (Potentiated effects). Products include:
- Tussionex Extended-Release Suspension ... 988

Hydroxyzine Hydrochloride (Potentiated effects). Products include:
- Atarax Tablets & Syrup ... 1941
- Marax Tablets & DF Syrup ... 1954
- Vistaril Intramuscular Solution ... 1970

Isoflurane (Potentiated effects). Products include:
- Forane ... 600

Ketamine Hydrochloride (Potentiated effects). Products include:
- Ketalar ... 1726

Levorphanol Tartrate (Potentiated effects). Products include:
- Levo-Dromoran ... 1906

Lorazepam (Potentiated effects). Products include:
- Ativan Injection ... 2432
- Ativan Tablets ... 2434

Loxapine Hydrochloride (Potentiated effects). Products include:
- Loxitane ... 1213

Loxapine Succinate (Potentiated effects). Products include:
- Loxitane Capsules ... 1213

Meperidine Hydrochloride (Potentiated effects). Products include:
- Demerol ... 2047
- Mepergan Injection ... 2479

Mephobarbital (Potentiated effects). Products include:
- Mebaral Tablets ... 2061

Meprobamate (Potentiated effects). Products include:
- Deprol Tablets ... 2382
- Equagesic Tablets ... 2451
- Miltown Tablets ... 2386
- PMB 200 and PMB 400 ... 2504

Mesoridazine (Potentiated effects). Products include:
- Serentil ... 686

Methadone Hydrochloride (Potentiated effects). Products include:
- Dolophine Hydrochloride Ampoules & Vials ... 1260
- Dolophine Hydrochloride Tablets ... 1261
- Methadone Hydrochloride Diskets ... 1284
- Methadone Hydrochloride Oral Solution & Tablets ... 1987

Methohexital Sodium (Potentiated effects). Products include:
- Brevital Sodium Vials ... 1248

Methoxyflurane (Potentiated effects).
- No products indexed under this heading.

Midazolam Hydrochloride (Potentiated effects). Products include:
- Versed Injection ... 1924

Molindone Hydrochloride (Potentiated effects). Products include:
- Moban Tablets & Concentrate ... 932

Morphine Sulfate (Potentiated effects). Products include:
- Astramorph/PF Injection, USP (Preservative-Free) ... 618
- Duramorph ... 960
- Infumorph 200 and Infumorph 500 Sterile Solutions ... 962
- MS Contin Tablets ... 1814
- MSIR ... 1817
- Oramorph SR (Morphine Sulfate Sustained Release Tablets) ... 1988
- Roxanol ... 1991

Opium Alkaloids (Potentiated effects). Products include:
- B & O No. 15A & No. 16A Supprettes ... 2395
- Pantopon Injectable ... 1911

Oxazepam (Potentiated effects). Products include:
- Serax Capsules ... 2522
- Serax Tablets ... 2522

Oxycodone Hydrochloride (Potentiated effects). Products include:
- Percocet Tablets ... 950
- Percodan ... 951
- Roxicodone Tablets, Oral Solution & Intensol (Oxycodone) ... 1992
- Tylox Capsules ... 1382

Pentobarbital Sodium (Potentiated effects). Products include:
- Nembutal Sodium Capsules ... 534
- Nembutal Sodium Solution ... 536
- Nembutal Sodium Suppositories ... 538

Perphenazine (Potentiated effects). Products include:
- Etrafon ... 2087
- Triavil Tablets ... 1556
- Trilafon ... 2123

Phenobarbital (Potentiated effects). Products include:
- Arco-Lase Plus Tablets ... 607
- Bellergal-S Tablets ... 1998
- Bronkolixir ... ▣ 761
- Bronkotabs Tablets ... ▣ 762
- Donnatal ... 1858
- Donnatal Extentabs ... 1859
- Donnatal Tablets ... 1858
- Donnazyme Tablets ... 1860
- Kinesed Tablets ... 2272
- Phenobarbital Elixir and Tablets ... 1293
- Primatene Tablets-P Formula ... 2421
- Quadrinal Tablets ... 1183
- Tedral SA ... 1765

Prazepam (Potentiated effects). Products include:
- Centrax ... 1693

Prochlorperazine (Potentiated effects). Products include:
- Compazine ... 2201

Promethazine Hydrochloride (Potentiated effects). Products include:
- Mepergan Injection ... 2479
- Phenergan with Codeine ... 2497
- Phenergan with Dextromethorphan ... 2499
- Phenergan Injection ... 2493
- Phenergan Suppositories ... 2496
- Phenergan Syrup ... 2495
- Phenergan Tablets ... 2496
- Phenergan VC ... 2500
- Phenergan VC with Codeine ... 2501

Propofol (Potentiated effects). Products include:
- Diprivan Injection ... 2267

Propoxyphene Hydrochloride (Potentiated effects). Products include:
- Darvon ... 1256
- Wygesic Tablets ... 2540

Propoxyphene Napsylate (Potentiated effects). Products include:
- Darvon-N/Darvocet-N ... 1254

Quazepam (Potentiated effects). Products include:
- Doral Tablets ... 2383

Secobarbital Sodium (Potentiated effects). Products include:
- Seconal Sodium Pulvules 1296

Sufentanil Citrate (Potentiated effects). Products include:
- Sufenta Injection 1147

Temazepam (Potentiated effects). Products include:
- Restoril Capsules 2023

Thiamylal Sodium (Potentiated effects). Products include:
- Surital Ampoules, Steri-Vials 1764

Thioridazine Hydrochloride (Potentiated effects). Products include:
- Mellaril 2011

Thiothixene (Potentiated effects). Products include:
- Navane Capsules and Concentrate 1954
- Navane Intramuscular 1956

Triazolam (Potentiated effects). Products include:
- Halcion Tablets 2340

Trifluoperazine Hydrochloride (Potentiated effects). Products include:
- Stelazine 2226

NORZINE TABLETS AND SUPPOSITORIES
(Thiethylperazine Maleate) 1818
See **Norzine Ampuls**

NŌSTRIL NASAL DECONGESTANT
(Phenylephrine Hydrochloride) 520
No interactions described in labeling.

NŌSTRILLA LONG ACTING NASAL DECONGESTANT
(Oxymetazoline Hydrochloride) 520
No interactions described in labeling.

NOVAFED A CAPSULES
(Pseudoephedrine Hydrochloride, Chlorpheniramine Maleate) 1342
May interact with monoamine oxidase inhibitors, beta blockers , veratrum alkaloids, tricyclic antidepressants, central nervous system depressants, and certain other agents. Compounds in these categories include:

Acebutolol Hydrochloride (Increased effects of sympathomimetic). Products include:
- Sectral Capsules 2520

Alcohol (Additive effects).

Alfentanil Hydrochloride (Additive effects). Products include:
- Alfenta Injection 1131

Alprazolam (Additive effects). Products include:
- Xanax Tablets 2367

Amitriptyline Hydrochloride (Additive effects). Products include:
- Elavil 2269
- Endep Tablets 1927
- Etrafon 2087
- Limbitrol 1933
- Triavil Tablets 1556

Amoxapine (Additive effects). Products include:
- Asendin Tablets 1196

Aprobarbital (Additive effects). Products include:
- Alurate Elixir 1883

Atenolol (Increased effects of sympathomimetic). Products include:
- Tenoretic Tablets 1105
- Tenormin Tablets and I.V. Injection 1107

Betaxolol Hydrochloride (Increased effects of sympathomimetic). Products include:
- Betoptic Sterile Ophthalmic Solution 569
- Betoptic S Sterile Ophthalmic Suspension 570
- Kerlone Tablets 2172

Buprenorphine (Additive effects). No products indexed under this heading.

Buspirone Hydrochloride (Additive effects). Products include:
- BuSpar 1401

Butabarbital (Additive effects). Products include:
- Pyridium Plus 1764

Butalbital (Additive effects). Products include:
- Esgic-Plus Tablets 1002
- Esgic Tablets & Capsules 1001
- Fioricet Tablets 2006
- Fiorinal Capsules 2007
- Fiorinal with Codeine Capsules 2008
- Fiorinal Tablets 2007
- Phrenilin 838
- Sedapap Tablets 50 mg/650 mg .. 1360

Carteolol Hydrochloride (Increased effects of sympathomimetic). Products include:
- Cartrol Tablets 507

Chlordiazepoxide (Additive effects). Products include:
- Libritabs Tablets 1930
- Limbitrol 1933
- Menrium Tablets 1934

Chlordiazepoxide Hydrochloride (Additive effects). Products include:
- Librax Capsules 1929
- Librium Capsules 1931
- Librium Injectable 1932

Chlorpromazine (Additive effects). Products include:
- Thorazine 2234

Chlorprothixene (Additive effects). Products include:
- Taractan Tablets 1920

Chlorprothixene Hydrochloride (Additive effects). Products include:
- Taractan 1920

Chlorprothixene Lactate (Additive effects). Products include:
- Taractan Concentrate 1920

Clomipramine Hydrochloride (Additive effects). Products include:
- Anafranil Capsules 650

Clorazepate Dipotassium (Additive effects). Products include:
- Tranxene 556

Codeine (Additive effects). Products include:
- Calcidrine Syrup 506

Codeine Phosphate (Additive effects). Products include:
- Actifed with Codeine Cough Syrup .. 752
- Cheracol Cough Syrup 1853
- Codimal PH Syrup 846
- Dimetane-DC Cough Syrup 1857
- Empirin with Codeine Phosphate Nos. 2, 3 & 4 764
- Fiorinal with Codeine Capsules 2008
- Isoclor Expectorant 982
- Naldecon CX Adult Liquid 521
- Novahistine DH 1342
- Novahistine Expectorant 1343
- Nucofed Capsules 2219
- Nucofed Expectorant 2219
- Nucofed Pediatric Expectorant 2220
- Nucofed Syrup 2219
- Phenaphen with Codeine Capsules 1865
- Phenaphen-650 with Codeine Tablets 1866
- Phenergan with Codeine 2497
- Phenergan VC with Codeine 2501
- Robitussin A-C Syrup 1875
- Robitussin-DAC Syrup 1875
- Ryna 741
- Soma Compound w/Codeine Tablets 2390
- Triaminic Expectorant w/Codeine .. 1996
- Tussi-Organidin Liquid 2391
- Tylenol with Codeine 1381

Codeine Polistirex (Additive effects). No products indexed under this heading.

Cryptenamine Preparations (Reduced antihypertensive effects).

Desipramine Hydrochloride (Additive effects). Products include:
- Norpramin Tablets 1340

Dezocine (Additive effects).

Diazepam (Additive effects). Products include:
- Valium Injectable 1937
- Valium Tablets 1939
- Valrelease Capsules 1923

Doxepin Hydrochloride (Additive effects). Products include:
- Sinequan 1960

Droperidol (Additive effects). Products include:
- Inapsine Injection 1140
- Innovar Injection 1141

Enflurane (Additive effects). Products include:
- Ethrane 599

Esmolol Hydrochloride (Increased effects of sympathomimetic). Products include:
- Brevibloc Injection 942

Estazolam (Additive effects). Products include:
- ProSom Tablets 554

Ethchlorvynol (Additive effects). Products include:
- Placidyl Capsules 553

Ethinamate (Additive effects). No products indexed under this heading.

Fentanyl (Additive effects). Products include:
- Duragesic Transdermal System 1133

Fentanyl Citrate (Additive effects). Products include:
- Innovar Injection 1141
- Sublimaze Injection 1146

Fluphenazine Decanoate (Additive effects). Products include:
- Prolixin Decanoate 1795

Fluphenazine Enanthate (Additive effects). Products include:
- Prolixin Enanthate 1796

Fluphenazine Hydrochloride (Additive effects). Products include:
- Prolixin Elixir 1793
- Prolixin Injection 1791
- Prolixin Oral Concentrate 1792
- Prolixin Tablets 1793

Flurazepam Hydrochloride (Additive effects). Products include:
- Dalmane Capsules 1927

Furazolidone (Increased effects of sympathomimetic). Products include:
- Furoxone 1855

Glutethimide (Additive effects). No products indexed under this heading.

Haloperidol (Additive effects). Products include:
- Haldol Injection, Tablets and Concentrate 1373

Haloperidol Decanoate (Additive effects). Products include:
- Haldol Decanoate 1375

Hydrocodone Bitartrate (Additive effects). Products include:
- Anexsia 5/500 Tablets 2196
- Anexsia 7.5/650 Tablets 2197
- Azdone Tablets 844
- Codiclear DH Syrup 845
- Codimal DH Syrup 846
- Damason-P 1356
- Hycodan Syrup, Tablets 927
- Hycomine Compound Tablets 929
- Hycomine Syrup 927
- Hycotuss Expectorant Syrup 930
- Hydrocet Capsules 835
- Lortab ASA Tablets 2414
- Lortab 2412
- Ru-Tuss with Hydrocodone 694
- Triaminic Expectorant DH 1995
- Vicodin Tablets 1187
- Vicodin ES Tablets 1189
- Zydone Capsules 941

Hydrocodone Polistirex (Additive effects). Products include:
- Tussionex Extended-Release Suspension 988

Hydroxyzine Hydrochloride (Additive effects). Products include:
- Atarax Tablets & Syrup 1941
- Marax Tablets & DF Syrup 1954
- Vistaril Intramuscular Solution 1970

Imipramine Hydrochloride (Additive effects). Products include:
- Tofranil Ampuls 1038
- Tofranil Tablets 1039

Imipramine Pamoate (Additive effects). Products include:
- Tofranil-PM Capsules 1041

Isocarboxazid (Increased effects of sympathomimetic). Products include:
- Marplan Tablets 1906

Isoflurane (Additive effects). Products include:
- Forane 600

Ketamine Hydrochloride (Additive effects). Products include:
- Ketalar 1726

Labetalol Hydrochloride (Increased effects of sympathomimetic). Products include:
- Normodyne Injection 2108
- Normodyne Tablets 2110
- Normozide Tablets 2112
- Trandate HCT Tablets 579
- Trandate Injection 577
- Trandate Tablets 579

Levorphanol Tartrate (Additive effects). Products include:
- Levo-Dromoran 1906

Lorazepam (Additive effects). Products include:
- Ativan Injection 2432
- Ativan Tablets 2434

Loxapine Hydrochloride (Additive effects). Products include:
- Loxitane 1213

Loxapine Succinate (Additive effects). Products include:
- Loxitane Capsules 1213

Maprotiline Hydrochloride (Additive effects). Products include:
- Ludiomil Tablets 874

Mecamylamine Hydrochloride (Reduced antihypertensive effects). Products include:
- Inversine Tablets 1492

Meperidine Hydrochloride (Additive effects). Products include:
- Demerol 2047
- Mepergan Injection 2479

Mephobarbital (Additive effects). Products include:
- Mebaral Tablets 2061

Meprobamate (Additive effects). Products include:
- Deprol Tablets 2382
- Equagesic Tablets 2451
- Miltown Tablets 2386
- PMB 200 and PMB 400 2504

Mesoridazine (Additive effects). Products include:
- Serentil 686

Methadone Hydrochloride (Additive effects). Products include:
- Dolophine Hydrochloride Ampoules & Vials 1260
- Dolophine Hydrochloride Tablets 1261
- Methadone Hydrochloride Diskets .. 1284
- Methadone Hydrochloride Oral Solution & Tablets 1987

Methohexital Sodium (Additive effects). Products include:
- Brevital Sodium Vials 1248

Methoxyflurane (Additive effects). No products indexed under this heading.

Methyldopa (Reduced antihypertensive effects). Products include:
- Aldoclor Tablets 1413
- Aldomet Oral 1415

(Described in PDR For Nonprescription Drugs)

(⊙ Described in PDR For Ophthalmology)

Aldoril Tablets ... 1418

Metoprolol Tartrate (Increased effects of sympathomimetic). Products include:

Lopressor Ampuls ... 1032
Lopressor HCT Tablets ... 1034
Lopressor Tablets ... 1032

Midazolam Hydrochloride (Additive effects). Products include:

Versed Injection ... 1924

Molindone Hydrochloride (Additive effects). Products include:

Moban Tablets & Concentrate ... 932

Morphine Sulfate (Additive effects). Products include:

Astramorph/PF Injection, USP (Preservative-Free) ... 618
Duramorph ... 960
Infumorph 200 and Infumorph 500 Sterile Solutions ... 962
MS Contin Tablets ... 1814
MSIR ... 1817
Oramorph SR (Morphine Sulfate Sustained Release Tablets) ... 1988
Roxanol ... 1991

Nadolol (Increased effects of sympathomimetic). Products include:

Corgard Tablets ... 701
Corzide Tablets ... 702

Nortriptyline Hydrochloride (Additive effects). Products include:

Pamelor ... 2019

Opium Alkaloids (Additive effects). Products include:

B & O No. 15A & No. 16A Supprettes ... 2395
Pantopon Injectable ... 1911

Oxazepam (Additive effects). Products include:

Serax Capsules ... 2522
Serax Tablets ... 2522

Oxycodone Hydrochloride (Additive effects). Products include:

Percocet Tablets ... 950
Percodan ... 951
Roxicodone Tablets, Oral Solution & Intensol (Oxycodone) ... 1992
Tylox Capsules ... 1382

Penbutolol Sulfate (Increased effects of sympathomimetic). Products include:

Levatol ... 1832

Pentobarbital Sodium (Additive effect). Products include:

Nembutal Sodium Capsules ... 534
Nembutal Sodium Solution ... 536
Nembutal Sodium Suppositories ... 538

Perphenazine (Additive effects). Products include:

Etrafon ... 2087
Triavil Tablets ... 1556
Trilafon ... 2123

Phenelzine Sulfate (Increased effects of sympathomimetic). Products include:

Nardil ... 1742

Phenobarbital (Additive effects). Products include:

Arco-Lase Plus Tablets ... 607
Bellergal-S Tablets ... 1998
Bronkolixir ... 761
Bronkotabs Tablets ... 762
Donnatal ... 1858
Donnatal Extentabs ... 1859
Donnatal Tablets ... 1858
Donnazyme Tablets ... 1860
Kinesed Tablets ... 2272
Phenobarbital Elixir and Tablets ... 1293
Primatene Tablets-P Formula ... 2421
Quadrinal Tablets ... 1183
Tedral SA ... 1765

Pindolol (Increased effects of sympathomimetic). Products include:

Visken Tablets ... 2036

Prazepam (Additive effects). Products include:

Centrax ... 1693

Prochlorperazine (Additive effects). Products include:

Compazine ... 2201

Promethazine Hydrochloride (Additive effects). Products include:

Mepergan Injection ... 2479
Phenergan with Codeine ... 2497
Phenergan with Dextromethorphan ... 2499
Phenergan Injection ... 2493
Phenergan Suppositories ... 2496
Phenergan Syrup ... 2495
Phenergan Tablets ... 2496
Phenergan VC ... 2500
Phenergan VC with Codeine ... 2501

Propofol (Additive effects). Products include:

Diprivan Injection ... 2267

Propoxyphene Hydrochloride (Additive effects). Products include:

Darvon ... 1256
Wygesic Tablets ... 2540

Propoxyphene Napsylate (Additive effects). Products include:

Darvon-N/Darvocet-N ... 1254

Propranolol Hydrochloride (Increased effects of sympathomimetic). Products include:

Inderal ... 2459
Inderal LA Long Acting Capsules ... 2461
Inderide Tablets ... 2463
Inderide LA Long Acting Capsules ... 2465

Protriptyline Hydrochloride (Additive effects). Products include:

Vivactil Tablets ... 1567

Quazepam (Additive effects). Products include:

Doral Tablets ... 2383

Reserpine (Reduced antihypertensive effects). Products include:

Diupres Tablets ... 1461
Hydromox R Tablets ... 1209
Hydropres Tablets ... 1485
Renese-R Tablets ... 1786
Salutensin/Salutensin-Demi ... 719
Ser-Ap-Es Tablets ... 881
Serpasil Tablets ... 883
Serpasil-Apresoline Tablets ... 884
Serpasil-Esidrix Tablets ... 886

Secobarbital Sodium (Additive effects). Products include:

Seconal Sodium Pulvules ... 1296

Selegiline Hydrochloride (Increased effects of sympathomimetic). Products include:

Eldepryl ... 2250

Sufentanil Citrate (Additive effects). Products include:

Sufenta Injection ... 1147

Temazepam (Additive effects). Products include:

Restoril Capsules ... 2023

Thiamylal Sodium (Additive effects). Products include:

Surital Ampoules, Steri-Vials ... 1764

Thioridazine Hydrochloride (Additive effects). Products include:

Mellaril ... 2011

Thiothixene (Additive effects). Products include:

Navane Capsules and Concentrate ... 1954
Navane Intramuscular ... 1956

Timolol Maleate (Increased effects of sympathomimetic). Products include:

Blocadren Tablets ... 1429
Timolide Tablets ... 1547
Timoptic in Ocudose ... 1552
Timoptic Sterile Ophthalmic Solution ... 1550

Tranylcypromine Sulfate (Increased effects of sympathomimetic). Products include:

Parnate Tablets ... 2222

Triazolam (Additive effects). Products include:

Halcion Tablets ... 2340

Trifluoperazine Hydrochloride (Additive effects). Products include:

Stelazine ... 2226

Trimipramine Maleate (Additive effects). Products include:

Surmontil Capsules ... 2524

NOVAFED CAPSULES
(Pseudoephedrine Hydrochloride) ... 1342
May interact with monoamine oxidase inhibitors, beta blockers, veratrum alkaloids, and certain other agents. Compounds in these categories include:

Acebutolol Hydrochloride (Increased effects of pseudoephedrine). Products include:

Sectral Capsules ... 2520

Atenolol (Increased effects of pseudoephedrine). Products include:

Tenoretic Tablets ... 1105
Tenormin Tablets and I.V. Injection 1107

Betaxolol Hydrochloride (Increased effects of pseudoephedrine). Products include:

Betoptic Sterile Ophthalmic Solution ... 569
Betoptic S Sterile Ophthalmic Suspension ... 570
Kerlone Tablets ... 2172

Carteolol Hydrochloride (Increased effects of pseudoephedrine). Products include:

Cartrol Tablets ... 507

Cryptenamine Preparations (Reduced antihypertensive effects).

Deserpidine (Reduced antihypertensive effects). Products include:

Enduronyl ... 518
Harmonyl Tablets ... 528
Oreticyl ... 545

Esmolol Hydrochloride (Increased effects of pseudoephedrine). Products include:

Brevibloc Injection ... 942

Furazolidone (Increased effects of pseudoephedrine). Products include:

Furoxone ... 1855

Isocarboxazid (Increased effects of pseudoephedrine). Products include:

Marplan Tablets ... 1906

Labetalol Hydrochloride (Increased effects of pseudoephedrine). Products include:

Normodyne Injection ... 2108
Normodyne Tablets ... 2110
Normozide Tablets ... 2112
Trandate HCT Tablets ... 579
Trandate Injection ... 577
Trandate Tablets ... 579

Mecamylamine Hydrochloride (Reduced antihypertensive effects). Products include:

Inversine Tablets ... 1492

Methyldopa (Reduced antihypertensive effects). Products include:

Aldoclor Tablets ... 1413
Aldomet Oral ... 1415
Aldoril Tablets ... 1418

Metoprolol Tartrate (Increased effects of pseudoephedrine). Products include:

Lopressor Ampuls ... 1032
Lopressor HCT Tablets ... 1034
Lopressor Tablets ... 1032

Nadolol (Increased effects of pseudoephedrine). Products include:

Corgard Tablets ... 701
Corzide Tablets ... 702

Penbutolol Sulfate (Increased effects of pseudoephedrine). Products include:

Levatol ... 1832

Phenelzine Sulfate (Increased effects of pseudoephedrine). Products include:

Nardil ... 1742

Pindolol (Increased effects of pseudoephedrine). Products include:

Visken Tablets ... 2036

Propranolol Hydrochloride (Increased effects of pseudoephedrine). Products include:

Inderal ... 2459
Inderal LA Long Acting Capsules ... 2461
Inderide Tablets ... 2463
Inderide LA Long Acting Capsules ... 2465

Rauwolfia Serpentina (Reduced antihypertensive effects). Products include:

Raudixin Tablets ... 1803
Rauzide Tablets ... 1804

Rescinnamine (Reduced antihypertensive effects).

No products indexed under this heading.

Reserpine (Reduced antihypertensive effects). Products include:

Diupres Tablets ... 1461
Hydromox R Tablets ... 1209
Hydropres Tablets ... 1485
Renese-R Tablets ... 1786
Salutensin/Salutensin-Demi ... 719
Ser-Ap-Es Tablets ... 881
Serpasil Tablets ... 883
Serpasil-Apresoline Tablets ... 884
Serpasil-Esidrix Tablets ... 886

Selegiline Hydrochloride (Increased effects of pseudoephedrine). Products include:

Eldepryl ... 2250

Timolol Maleate (Increased effects of pseudoephedrine). Products include:

Blocadren Tablets ... 1429
Timolide Tablets ... 1547
Timoptic in Ocudose ... 1552
Timoptic Sterile Ophthalmic Solution ... 1550

Tranylcypromine Sulfate (Increased effects of pseudoephedrine). Products include:

Parnate Tablets ... 2222

NOVAHISTINE DH
(Codeine Phosphate, Pseudoephedrine Hydrochloride, Chlorpheniramine Maleate) ... 1342
May interact with tricyclic antidepressants, monoamine oxidase inhibitors, central nervous system depressants, beta blockers, veratrum alkaloids, and certain other agents. Compounds in these categories include:

Acebutolol Hydrochloride (Potentiates effects of pseudoephedrine). Products include:

Sectral Capsules ... 2520

Alcohol (Potentiated effects).

Alfentanil Hydrochloride (Potentiated effects). Products include:

Alfenta Injection ... 1131

Alprazolam (Potentiated effects). Products include:

Xanax Tablets ... 2367

Amitriptyline Hydrochloride (Potentiated effects). Products include:

Elavil ... 2269
Endep Tablets ... 1927
Etrafon ... 2087
Limbitrol ... 1933
Triavil Tablets ... 1556

Amoxapine (Potentiated effects). Products include:

Asendin Tablets ... 1196

Aprobarbital (Potentiated effects). Products include:

Alurate Elixir ... 1883

Atenolol (Potentiates effects of pseudoephedrine). Products include:

Tenoretic Tablets ... 1105
Tenormin Tablets and I.V. Injection 1107

Betaxolol Hydrochloride (Potentiates effects of pseudoephedrine). Products include:

Betoptic Sterile Ophthalmic Solution ... 569
Betoptic S Sterile Ophthalmic Suspension ... 570
Kerlone Tablets ... 2172

Buprenorphine (Potentiated effects).
No products indexed under this heading.

Buspirone Hydrochloride (Potentiated effects). Products include:
BuSpar ... 1401

Butabarbital (Potentiated effects). Products include:
Pyridium Plus ... 1764

Butalbital (Potentiated effects). Products include:
Esgic-Plus Tablets ... 1002
Esgic Tablets & Capsules ... 1001
Fioricet Tablets ... 2006
Fiorinal Capsules ... 2007
Fiorinal with Codeine Capsules ... 2008
Fiorinal Tablets ... 2007
Phrenilin ... 838
Sedapap Tablets 50 mg/650 mg .. 1360

Carteolol Hydrochloride (Potentiates effects of pseudoephedrine). Products include:
Cartrol Tablets ... 507

Chlordiazepoxide (Potentiated effects). Products include:
Libritabs Tablets ... 1930
Limbitrol ... 1933
Menrium Tablets ... 1934

Chlordiazepoxide Hydrochloride (Potentiated effects). Products include:
Librax Capsules ... 1929
Librium Capsules ... 1931
Librium Injectable ... 1932

Chlorpromazine (Potentiated effects). Products include:
Thorazine ... 2234

Chlorprothixene (Potentiated effects). Products include:
Taractan Tablets ... 1920

Chlorprothixene Hydrochloride (Potentiated effects). Products include:
Taractan ... 1920

Clomipramine Hydrochloride (Potentiated effects). Products include:
Anafranil Capsules ... 650

Clorazepate Dipotassium (Potentiated effects). Products include:
Tranxene ... 556

Codeine (Potentiated effects). Products include:
Calcidrine Syrup ... 506

Codeine Polistirex (Potentiated effects).
No products indexed under this heading.

Cryptenamine Preparations (Reduced antihypertensive effects).

Desipramine Hydrochloride (Potentiated effects). Products include:
Norpramin Tablets ... 1340

Dezocine (Potentiated effects).

Diazepam (Potentiated effects). Products include:
Valium Injectable ... 1937
Valium Tablets ... 1939
Valrelease Capsules ... 1923

Doxepin Hydrochloride (Potentiated effects). Products include:
Sinequan ... 1960

Droperidol (Potentiated effects). Products include:
Inapsine Injection ... 1140
Innovar Injection ... 1141

Enflurane (Potentiated effects). Products include:
Ethrane ... 599

Esmolol Hydrochloride (Potentiates effects of pseudoephedrine). Products include:
Brevibloc Injection ... 942

Estazolam (Potentiated effects). Products include:
ProSom Tablets ... 554

Ethchlorvynol (Potentiated effects). Products include:
Placidyl Capsules ... 553

Ethinamate (Potentiated effects).
No products indexed under this heading.

Fentanyl (Potentiated effects). Products include:
Duragesic Transdermal System ... 1133

Fentanyl Citrate (Potentiated effects). Products include:
Innovar Injection ... 1141
Sublimaze Injection ... 1146

Fluphenazine Decanoate (Potentiated effects). Products include:
Prolixin Decanoate ... 1795

Fluphenazine Enanthate (Potentiated effects). Products include:
Prolixin Enanthate ... 1796

Fluphenazine Hydrochloride (Potentiated effects). Products include:
Prolixin Elixir ... 1793
Prolixin Injection ... 1791
Prolixin Oral Concentrate ... 1792
Prolixin Tablets ... 1793

Flurazepam Hydrochloride (Potentiated effects). Products include:
Dalmane Capsules ... 1927

Furazolidone (Potentiated effects of MAO inhibitors; potentiated effects of pseudoephedrine). Products include:
Furoxone ... 1855

Glutethimide (Potentiated effects).
No products indexed under this heading.

Haloperidol (Potentiated effects). Products include:
Haldol Injection, Tablets and Concentrate ... 1373

Haloperidol Decanoate (Potentiated effects). Products include:
Haldol Decanoate ... 1375

Hydrocodone Bitartrate (Potentiated effects). Products include:
Anexsia 5/500 Tablets ... 2196
Anexsia 7.5/650 Tablets ... 2197
Azdōne Tablets ... 844
Codiclear DH Syrup ... 845
Codimal DH Syrup ... 846
Damason-P ... 1356
Hycodan Syrup, Tablets ... 927
Hycomine Compound Tablets ... 929
Hycomine Syrup ... 927
Hycotuss Expectorant Syrup ... 930
Hydrocet Capsules ... 835
Lortab ASA Tablets ... 2414
Lortab ... 2412
Ru-Tuss with Hydrocodone ... 694
Triaminic Expectorant DH ... 1995
Vicodin Tablets ... 1187
Vicodin ES Tablets ... 1189
Zydone Capsules ... 941

Hydrocodone Polistirex (Potentiated effects). Products include:
Tussionex Extended-Release Suspension ... 988

Hydroxyzine Hydrochloride (Potentiated effects). Products include:
Atarax Tablets & Syrup ... 1941
Marax Tablets & DF Syrup ... 1954
Vistaril Intramuscular Solution ... 1970

Imipramine Hydrochloride (Potentiated effects). Products include:
Tofranil Ampuls ... 1038
Tofranil Tablets ... 1039

Imipramine Pamoate (Potentiated effects). Products include:
Tofranil-PM Capsules ... 1041

Isocarboxazid (Potentiated effects of MAO inhibitors; potentiated effects of pseudoephedrine). Products include:
Marplan Tablets ... 1906

Isoflurane (Potentiated effects). Products include:
Forane ... 600

Ketamine Hydrochloride (Potentiated effects). Products include:
Ketalar ... 1726

Labetalol Hydrochloride (Potentiates effects of pseudoephedrine). Products include:
Normodyne Injection ... 2108
Normodyne Tablets ... 2110
Normozide Tablets ... 2112
Trandate HCT Tablets ... 579
Trandate Injection ... 577
Trandate Tablets ... 579

Levorphanol Tartrate (Potentiated effects). Products include:
Levo-Dromoran ... 1906

Lorazepam (Potentiated effects). Products include:
Ativan Injection ... 2432
Ativan Tablets ... 2434

Loxapine Hydrochloride (Potentiated effects). Products include:
Loxitane ... 1213

Loxapine Succinate (Potentiated effects). Products include:
Loxitane Capsules ... 1213

Maprotiline Hydrochloride (Potentiated effects). Products include:
Ludiomil Tablets ... 874

Mecamylamine Hydrochloride (Reduced antihypertensive effects). Products include:
Inversine Tablets ... 1492

Meperidine Hydrochloride (Potentiated effects). Products include:
Demerol ... 2047
Mepergan Injection ... 2479

Mephobarbital (Potentiated effects). Products include:
Mebaral Tablets ... 2061

Meprobamate (Potentiated effects). Products include:
Deprol Tablets ... 2382
Equagesic Tablets ... 2451
Miltown Tablets ... 2386
PMB 200 and PMB 400 ... 2504

Mesoridazine (Potentiated effects). Products include:
Serentil ... 686

Methadone Hydrochloride (Potentiated effects). Products include:
Dolophine Hydrochloride Ampoules & Vials ... 1260
Dolophine Hydrochloride Tablets ... 1261
Methadone Hydrochloride Diskets .. 1284
Methadone Hydrochloride Oral Solution & Tablets ... 1987

Methohexital Sodium (Potentiated effects). Products include:
Brevital Sodium Vials ... 1248

Methoxyflurane (Potentiated effects).
No products indexed under this heading.

Methyldopa (Reduced antihypertensive effects). Products include:
Aldoclor Tablets ... 1413
Aldomet Oral ... 1415
Aldoril Tablets ... 1418

Metoprolol Tartrate (Potentiated effects of pseudoephedrine). Products include:
Lopressor Ampuls ... 1032
Lopressor HCT Tablets ... 1034
Lopressor Tablets ... 1032

Midazolam Hydrochloride (Potentiated effects). Products include:
Versed Injection ... 1924

Molindone Hydrochloride (Potentiated effects). Products include:
Moban Tablets & Concentrate ... 932

Morphine Sulfate (Potentiated effects). Products include:
Astramorph/PF Injection, USP (Preservative-Free) ... 618
Duramorph ... 960
Infumorph 200 and Infumorph 500 Sterile Solutions ... 962
MS Contin Tablets ... 1814
MSIR ... 1817
Oramorph SR (Morphine Sulfate Sustained Release Tablets) ... 1988
Roxanol ... 1991

Nadolol (Potentiates effects of pseudoephedrine). Products include:
Corgard Tablets ... 701
Corzide Tablets ... 702

Nortriptyline Hydrochloride (Potentiated effects). Products include:
Pamelor ... 2019

Opium Alkaloids (Potentiated effects). Products include:
B & O No. 15A & No. 16A Supprettes ... 2395
Pantopon Injectable ... 1911

Oxazepam (Potentiated effects). Products include:
Serax Capsules ... 2522
Serax Tablets ... 2522

Oxycodone Hydrochloride (Potentiated effects). Products include:
Percocet Tablets ... 950
Percodan ... 951
Roxicodone Tablets, Oral Solution & Intensol (Oxycodone) ... 1992
Tylox Capsules ... 1382

Penbutolol Sulfate (Potentiates effects of pseudoephedrine). Products include:
Levatol ... 1832

Pentobarbital Sodium (Potentiated effects of MAO inhibitors; potentiated effects of pseudoephedrine). Products include:
Nembutal Sodium Capsules ... 534
Nembutal Sodium Solution ... 536
Nembutal Sodium Suppositories ... 538

Perphenazine (Potentiated effects). Products include:
Etrafon ... 2087
Triavil Tablets ... 1556
Trilafon ... 2123

Phenelzine Sulfate (Potentiated effects of MAO inhibitors; potentiated effects of pseudoephedrine). Products include:
Nardil ... 1742

Phenobarbital (Potentiated effects). Products include:
Arco-Lase Plus Tablets ... 607
Bellergal-S Tablets ... 1998
Bronkolixir ... ▣ 761
Bronkotabs Tablets ... ▣ 762
Donnatal ... 1858
Donnatal Extentabs ... 1859
Donnatal Tablets ... 1858
Donnazyme Tablets ... 1860
Kinesed Tablets ... 2272
Phenobarbital Elixir and Tablets ... 1293
Primatene Tablets-P Formula ... 2421
Quadrinal Tablets ... 1183
Tedral SA ... 1765

Pindolol (Potentiated effects of pseudoephedrine). Products include:
Visken Tablets ... 2036

Prazepam (Potentiated effects). Products include:
Centrax ... 1693

Prochlorperazine (Potentiated effects). Products include:
Compazine ... 2201

Promethazine Hydrochloride (Potentiated effects). Products include:
Mepergan Injection ... 2479
Phenergan with Codeine ... 2497
Phenergan with Dextromethorphan 2499
Phenergan Injection ... 2493
Phenergan Suppositories ... 2496
Phenergan Syrup ... 2495
Phenergan Tablets ... 2496
Phenergan VC ... 2500
Phenergan VC with Codeine ... 2501

Propofol (Potentiated effects). Products include:
Diprivan Injection ... 2267

Propoxyphene Hydrochloride (Potentiated effects). Products include:
Darvon ... 1256
Wygesic Tablets ... 2540

Propoxyphene Napsylate (Potentiated effects). Products include:
- Darvon-N/Darvocet-N 1254

Propranolol Hydrochloride (Potentiated effects of pseudoephedrine). Products include:
- Inderal 2459
- Inderal LA Long Acting Capsules 2461
- Inderide Tablets 2463
- Inderide LA Long Acting Capsules 2465

Protriptyline Hydrochloride (Potentiated effects). Products include:
- Vivactil Tablets 1567

Quazepam (Potentiated effects). Products include:
- Doral Tablets 2383

Reserpine (Reduced antihypertensive effects). Products include:
- Diupres Tablets 1461
- Hydromox R Tablets 1209
- Hydropres Tablets 1485
- Renese-R Tablets 1786
- Salutensin/Salutensin-Demi 719
- Ser-Ap-Es Tablets 881
- Serpasil Tablets 883
- Serpasil-Apresoline Tablets 884
- Serpasil-Esidrix Tablets 886

Secobarbital Sodium (Potentiated effects). Products include:
- Seconal Sodium Pulvules 1296

Selegiline Hydrochloride (Potentiated effects of MAO inhibitors; potentiated effects of pseudoephedrine). Products include:
- Eldepryl 2250

Sufentanil Citrate (Potentiated effects). Products include:
- Sufenta Injection 1147

Temazepam (Potentiated effects). Products include:
- Restoril Capsules 2023

Thiamylal Sodium (Potentiated effects). Products include:
- Surital Ampoules, Steri-Vials 1764

Thioridazine Hydrochloride (Potentiated effects). Products include:
- Mellaril 2011

Thiothixene (Potentiated effects). Products include:
- Navane Capsules and Concentrate 1954
- Navane Intramuscular 1956

Timolol Maleate (Potentiates effects of pseudoephedrine). Products include:
- Blocadren Tablets 1429
- Timolide Tablets 1547
- Timoptic in Ocudose 1552
- Timoptic Sterile Ophthalmic Solution 1550

Tranylcypromine Sulfate (Potentiated effects of MAO inhibitors; potentiated effects of pseudoephedrine). Products include:
- Parnate Tablets 2222

Triazolam (Potentiated effects). Products include:
- Halcion Tablets 2340

Trifluoperazine Hydrochloride (Potentiated effects). Products include:
- Stelazine 2226

Trimipramine Maleate (Potentiated effects). Products include:
- Surmontil Capsules 2524

NOVAHISTINE DMX
(Dextromethorphan Hydrobromide, Guaifenesin, Pseudoephedrine Hydrochloride) .... ⊞ 595
May interact with monoamine oxidase inhibitors, beta$_2$ agonists, antidepressant drugs, antihypertensives, and certain other agents. Compounds in these categories include:

Acebutolol Hydrochloride (Increases effects of pseudoephedrine). Products include:
- Sectral Capsules 2520

Amitriptyline Hydrochloride (Effect not specified). Products include:
- Elavil 2269
- Endep Tablets 1927
- Etrafon 2087
- Limbitrol 1933
- Triavil Tablets 1556

Amoxapine (Effect not specified). Products include:
- Asendin Tablets 1196

Atenolol (Increases effects of pseudoephedrine). Products include:
- Tenoretic Tablets 1105
- Tenormin Tablets and I.V. Injection 1107

Benazepril Hydrochloride (Reduced antihypertensive effects). Products include:
- Lotensin Tablets 872

Betaxolol Hydrochloride (Reduced antihypertensive effects). Products include:
- Betoptic Sterile Ophthalmic Solution 569
- Betoptic S Sterile Ophthalmic Suspension 570
- Kerlone Tablets 2172

Bupropion Hydrochloride (Effect not specified). Products include:
- Wellbutrin Tablets 821

Cryptenamine Preparations (Reduced antihypertensive effects).

Desipramine Hydrochloride (Effect not specified). Products include:
- Norpramin Tablets 1340

Doxazosin Mesylate (Reduced antihypertensive effects). Products include:
- Cardura Tablets 1941

Doxepin Hydrochloride (Effect not specified). Products include:
- Sinequan 1960

Esmolol Hydrochloride (Increases effects of pseudoephedrine). Products include:
- Brevibloc Injection 942

Felodipine (Reduced antihypertensive effects). Products include:
- Plendil Extended-Release Tablets 1526

Fluoxetine Hydrochloride (Effect not specified). Products include:
- Prozac Pulvules 920

Fosinopril Sodium (Reduced antihypertensive effects). Products include:
- Monopril Tablets 1406

Furazolidone (Increases effects of pseudoephedrine). Products include:
- Furoxone 1855

Imipramine Hydrochloride (Effect not specified). Products include:
- Tofranil Ampuls 1038
- Tofranil Tablets 1039

Imipramine Pamoate (Effect not specified). Products include:
- Tofranil-PM Capsules 1041

Isocarboxazid (Increases effects of pseudoephedrine). Products include:
- Marplan Tablets 1906

Isradipine (Reduced antihypertensive effects). Products include:
- DynaCirc Capsules 2004

Labetalol Hydrochloride (Increases effects of pseudoephedrine). Products include:
- Normodyne Injection 2108
- Normodyne Tablets 2110
- Normozide Tablets 2112
- Trandate HCT Tablets 579
- Trandate Injection 577
- Trandate Tablets 579

Maprotiline Hydrochloride (Effect not specified). Products include:
- Ludiomil Tablets 874

Mecamylamine Hydrochloride (Reduced antihypertensive effects). Products include:
- Inversine Tablets 1492

Methyldopa (Reduced antihypertensive effects). Products include:
- Aldoclor Tablets 1413
- Aldomet Oral 1415
- Aldoril Tablets 1418

Metoprolol Tartrate (Increases effects of pseudoephedrine). Products include:
- Lopressor Ampuls 1032
- Lopressor HCT Tablets 1034
- Lopressor Tablets 1032

Nadolol (Increases effects of pseudoephedrine). Products include:
- Corgard Tablets 701
- Corzide Tablets 702

Nortriptyline Hydrochloride (Effect not specified). Products include:
- Pamelor 2019

Penbutolol Sulfate (Increases effects of pseudoephedrine). Products include:
- Levatol 1832

Phenelzine Sulfate (Increases effects of pseudoephedrine). Products include:
- Nardil 1742

Pindolol (Increases effects of pseudoephedrine). Products include:
- Visken Tablets 2036

Propranolol Hydrochloride (Increases effects of pseudoephedrine). Products include:
- Inderal 2459
- Inderal LA Long Acting Capsules 2461
- Inderide Tablets 2463
- Inderide LA Long Acting Capsules 2465

Protriptyline Hydrochloride (Effect not specified). Products include:
- Vivactil Tablets 1567

Ramipril (Reduced antihypertensive effects). Products include:
- Altace Capsules 1086

Reserpine (Reduced antihypertensive effects). Products include:
- Diupres Tablets 1461
- Hydromox R Tablets 1209
- Hydropres Tablets 1485
- Renese-R Tablets 1786
- Salutensin/Salutensin-Demi 719
- Ser-Ap-Es Tablets 881
- Serpasil Tablets 883
- Serpasil-Apresoline Tablets 884
- Serpasil-Esidrix Tablets 886

Selegiline Hydrochloride (Increases effects of pseudoephedrine). Products include:
- Eldepryl 2250

Timolol Maleate (Increases effects of pseudoephedrine). Products include:
- Blocadren Tablets 1429
- Timolide Tablets 1547
- Timoptic in Ocudose 1552
- Timoptic Sterile Ophthalmic Solution 1550

Tranylcypromine Sulfate (Increases effects of pseudoephedrine). Products include:
- Parnate Tablets 2222

Trazodone Hydrochloride (Effect not specified). Products include:
- Desyrel and Desyrel Dividose 1404

Trimipramine Maleate (Effect not specified). Products include:
- Surmontil Capsules 2524

NOVAHISTINE ELIXIR
(Chlorpheniramine Maleate, Phenylephrine Hydrochloride) .... ⊞ 596
May interact with monoamine oxidase inhibitors, beta$_2$ agonists, tricyclic antidepressants, barbiturates, central nervous system depressants, veratrum alkaloids, and certain other agents. Compounds in these categories include:

Acebutolol Hydrochloride (Increases effects of sympathomimetics). Products include:
- Sectral Capsules 2520

Alfentanil Hydrochloride (Effects enhanced by antihistamines). Products include:
- Alfenta Injection 1131

Alprazolam (Effects enhanced by antihistamines). Products include:
- Xanax Tablets 2367

Amitriptyline Hydrochloride (Effects enhanced by antihistamines). Products include:
- Elavil 2269
- Endep Tablets 1927
- Etrafon 2087
- Limbitrol 1933
- Triavil Tablets 1556

Amoxapine (Effects enhanced by antihistamines). Products include:
- Asendin Tablets 1196

Aprobarbital (Effects enhanced by antihistamines). Products include:
- Alurate Elixir 1883

Atenolol (Increases effects of sympathomimetics). Products include:
- Tenoretic Tablets 1105
- Tenormin Tablets and I.V. Injection 1107

Betaxolol Hydrochloride (Increases effects of sympathomimetics). Products include:
- Betoptic Sterile Ophthalmic Solution 569
- Betoptic S Sterile Ophthalmic Suspension 570
- Kerlone Tablets 2172

Buprenorphine (Effects enhanced by antihistamines).
No products indexed under this heading.

Buspirone Hydrochloride (Effects enhanced by antihistamines). Products include:
- BuSpar 1401

Butabarbital (Effects enhanced by antihistamines). Products include:
- Pyridium Plus 1764

Butalbital (Effects enhanced by antihistamines). Products include:
- Esgic-Plus Tablets 1002
- Esgic Tablets & Capsules 1001
- Fioricet Tablets 2006
- Fiorinal Capsules 2007
- Fiorinal with Codeine Capsules 2008
- Fiorinal Tablets 2007
- Phrenilin 838
- Sedapap Tablets 50 mg/650 mg 1360

Chlordiazepoxide (Effects enhanced by antihistamines). Products include:
- Libritabs Tablets 1930
- Limbitrol 1933
- Menrium Tablets 1934

Chlordiazepoxide Hydrochloride (Effects enhanced by antihistamines). Products include:
- Librax Capsules 1929
- Librium Capsules 1931
- Librium Injectable 1932

Chlorpromazine (Effects enhanced by antihistamines). Products include:
- Thorazine 2234

Chlorprothixene (Effects enhanced by antihistamines). Products include:
- Taractan Tablets 1920

Chlorprothixene Hydrochloride (Effects enhanced by antihistamines). Products include:
- Taractan 1920

Clomipramine Hydrochloride (Effects enhanced by antihistamines). Products include:
- Anafranil Capsules ... 650

Clorazepate Dipotassium (Effects enhanced by antihistamines). Products include:
- Tranxene ... 556

Codeine (Effects enhanced by antihistamines). Products include:
- Calcidrine Syrup ... 506

Codeine Phosphate (Effects enhanced by antihistamines). Products include:
- Actifed with Codeine Cough Syrup.. 752
- Cheracol Cough Syrup ... 1853
- Codimal PH Syrup ... 846
- Dimetane-DC Cough Syrup ... 1857
- Empirin with Codeine Phosphate Nos. 2, 3 & 4 ... 764
- Fiorinal with Codeine Capsules ... 2008
- Isoclor Expectorant ... 982
- Naldecon CX Adult Liquid ... ⊞ 521
- Novahistine DH ... 1342
- Novahistine Expectorant ... 1343
- Nucofed Capsules ... 2219
- Nucofed Expectorant ... 2219
- Nucofed Pediatric Expectorant ... 2220
- Nucofed Syrup ... 2219
- Phenaphen with Codeine Capsules 1865
- Phenaphen-650 with Codeine Tablets ... 1866
- Phenergan with Codeine ... 2497
- Phenergan VC with Codeine ... 2501
- Robitussin A-C Syrup ... 1875
- Robitussin-DAC Syrup ... 1875
- Ryna ... ⊞ 741
- Soma Compound w/Codeine Tablets ... 2390
- Triaminic Expectorant w/Codeine .. 1996
- Tussi-Organidin Liquid ... 2391
- Tylenol with Codeine ... 1381

Codeine Polistirex (Effects enhanced by antihistamines).
- No products indexed under this heading.

Cryptenamine Preparations (Reduced antihypertensive effect).

Desipramine Hydrochloride (Effects enhanced by antihistamines). Products include:
- Norpramin Tablets ... 1340

Dezocine (Effects enhanced by antihistamines).

Diazepam (Effects enhanced by antihistamines). Products include:
- Valium Injectable ... 1937
- Valium Tablets ... 1939
- Valrelease Capsules ... 1923

Doxepin Hydrochloride (Effects enhanced by antihistamines). Products include:
- Sinequan ... 1960

Droperidol (Effects enhanced by antihistamines). Products include:
- Inapsine Injection ... 1140
- Innovar Injection ... 1141

Enflurane (Effects enhanced by antihistamines). Products include:
- Ethrane ... 599

Esmolol Hydrochloride (Increases effects of sympathomimetics). Products include:
- Brevibloc Injection ... 942

Estazolam (Effects enhanced by antihistamines). Products include:
- ProSom Tablets ... 554

Ethchlorvynol (Effects enhanced by antihistamines). Products include:
- Placidyl Capsules ... 553

Ethinamate (Effects enhanced by antihistamines).
- No products indexed under this heading.

Fentanyl (Effects enhanced by antihistamines). Products include:
- Duragesic Transdermal System ... 1133

Fentanyl Citrate (Effects enhanced by antihistamines). Products include:
- Innovar Injection ... 1141
- Sublimaze Injection ... 1146

Fluphenazine Decanoate (Effects enhanced by antihistamines). Products include:
- Prolixin Decanoate ... 1795

Fluphenazine Enanthate (Effects enhanced by antihistamines). Products include:
- Prolixin Enanthate ... 1796

Fluphenazine Hydrochloride (Effects enhanced by antihistamines). Products include:
- Prolixin Elixir ... 1793
- Prolixin Injection ... 1791
- Prolixin Oral Concentrate ... 1792
- Prolixin Tablets ... 1793

Flurazepam Hydrochloride (Effects enhanced by antihistamines). Products include:
- Dalmane Capsules ... 1927

Furazolidone (Increases effects of sympathomimetics). Products include:
- Furoxone ... 1855

Glutethimide (Effects enhanced by antihistamines).
- No products indexed under this heading.

Haloperidol (Effects enhanced by antihistamines). Products include:
- Haldol Injection, Tablets and Concentrate ... 1373

Haloperidol Decanoate (Effects enhanced by antihistamines). Products include:
- Haldol Decanoate ... 1375

Hydrocodone Bitartrate (Effects enhanced by antihistamines). Products include:
- Anexsia 5/500 Tablets ... 2196
- Anexsia 7.5/650 Tablets ... 2197
- Azdone Tablets ... 844
- Codiclear DH Syrup ... 845
- Codimal DH Syrup ... 846
- Damason-P ... 1356
- Hycodan Syrup, Tablets ... 927
- Hycomine Compound Tablets ... 929
- Hycomine Syrup ... 927
- Hycotuss Expectorant Syrup ... 930
- Hydrocet Capsules ... 835
- Lortab ASA Tablets ... 2414
- Lortab ... 2412
- Ru-Tuss with Hydrocodone ... 694
- Triaminic Expectorant DH ... 1995
- Vicodin Tablets ... 1187
- Vicodin ES Tablets ... 1189
- Zydone Capsules ... 941

Hydrocodone Polistirex (Effects enhanced by antihistamines). Products include:
- Tussionex Extended-Release Suspension ... 988

Hydroxyzine Hydrochloride (Effects enhanced by antihistamines). Products include:
- Atarax Tablets & Syrup ... 1941
- Marax Tablets & DF Syrup ... 1954
- Vistaril Intramuscular Solution ... 1970

Imipramine Hydrochloride (Effects enhanced by antihistamines). Products include:
- Tofranil Ampuls ... 1038
- Tofranil Tablets ... 1039

Imipramine Pamoate (Effects enhanced by antihistamines). Products include:
- Tofranil-PM Capsules ... 1041

Isocarboxazid (Increases effects of sympathomimetics). Products include:
- Marplan Tablets ... 1906

Isoflurane (Effects enhanced by antihistamines). Products include:
- Forane ... 600

Ketamine Hydrochloride (Effects enhanced by antihistamines). Products include:
- Ketalar ... 1726

Labetalol Hydrochloride (Increases effects of sympathomimetics). Products include:
- Normodyne Injection ... 2108
- Normodyne Tablets ... 2110
- Normozide Tablets ... 2112
- Trandate HCT Tablets ... 579
- Trandate Injection ... 577
- Trandate Tablets ... 579

Levorphanol Tartrate (Effects enhanced by antihistamines). Products include:
- Levo-Dromoran ... 1906

Lorazepam (Effects enhanced by antihistamines). Products include:
- Ativan Injection ... 2432
- Ativan Tablets ... 2434

Loxapine Hydrochloride (Effects enhanced by antihistamines). Products include:
- Loxitane ... 1213

Loxapine Succinate (Effects enhanced by antihistamines). Products include:
- Loxitane Capsules ... 1213

Maprotiline Hydrochloride (Effects enhanced by antihistamines). Products include:
- Ludiomil Tablets ... 874

Mecamylamine Hydrochloride (Reduced antihypertensive effect). Products include:
- Inversine Tablets ... 1492

Meperidine Hydrochloride (Effects enhanced by antihistamines). Products include:
- Demerol ... 2047
- Mepergan Injection ... 2479

Mephobarbital (Effects enhanced by antihistamines). Products include:
- Mebaral Tablets ... 2061

Meprobamate (Effects enhanced by antihistamines). Products include:
- Deprol Tablets ... 2382
- Equagesic Tablets ... 2451
- Miltown Tablets ... 2386
- PMB 200 and PMB 400 ... 2504

Mesoridazine (Effects enhanced by antihistamines). Products include:
- Serentil ... 686

Methadone Hydrochloride (Effects enhanced by antihistamines). Products include:
- Dolophine Hydrochloride Ampoules & Vials ... 1260
- Dolophine Hydrochloride Tablets 1261
- Methadone Hydrochloride Diskets .. 1284
- Methadone Hydrochloride Oral Solution & Tablets ... 1987

Methohexital Sodium (Effects enhanced by antihistamines). Products include:
- Brevital Sodium Vials ... 1248

Methoxyflurane (Effects enhanced by antihistamines).
- No products indexed under this heading.

Methyldopa (Reduced antihypertensive effect). Products include:
- Aldoclor Tablets ... 1413
- Aldomet Oral ... 1415
- Aldoril Tablets ... 1418

Metoprolol Tartrate (Increases effects of sympathomimetics). Products include:
- Lopressor Ampuls ... 1032
- Lopressor HCT Tablets ... 1034
- Lopressor Tablets ... 1032

Midazolam Hydrochloride (Effects enhanced by antihistamines). Products include:
- Versed Injection ... 1924

Molindone Hydrochloride (Effects enhanced by antihistamines). Products include:
- Moban Tablets & Concentrate ... 932

Morphine Sulfate (Effects enhanced by antihistamines). Products include:
- Astramorph/PF Injection, USP (Preservative-Free) ... 618
- Duramorph ... 960
- Infumorph 200 and Infumorph 500 Sterile Solutions ... 962
- MS Contin Tablets ... 1814
- MSIR ... 1817
- Oramorph SR (Morphine Sulfate Sustained Release Tablets) ... 1988
- Roxanol ... 1991

Nadolol (Increases effects of sympathomimetics). Products include:
- Corgard Tablets ... 701
- Corzide Tablets ... 702

Nortriptyline Hydrochloride (Effects enhanced by antihistamines). Products include:
- Pamelor ... 2019

Opium Alkaloids (Effects enhanced by antihistamines). Products include:
- B & O No. 15A & No. 16A Supprettes ... 2395
- Pantopon Injectable ... 1911

Oxazepam (Effects enhanced by antihistamines). Products include:
- Serax Capsules ... 2522
- Serax Tablets ... 2522

Oxycodone Hydrochloride (Effects enhanced by antihistamines). Products include:
- Percocet Tablets ... 950
- Percodan ... 951
- Roxicodone Tablets, Oral Solution & Intensol (Oxycodone) ... 1992
- Tylox Capsules ... 1382

Penbutolol Sulfate (Increases effects of sympathomimetics). Products include:
- Levatol ... 1832

Pentobarbital Sodium (Effects enhanced by antihistamines). Products include:
- Nembutal Sodium Capsules ... 534
- Nembutal Sodium Solution ... 536
- Nembutal Sodium Suppositories ... 538

Perphenazine (Effects enhanced by antihistamines). Products include:
- Etrafon ... 2087
- Triavil Tablets ... 1556
- Trilafon ... 2123

Phenelzine Sulfate (Increases effects of sympathomimetics). Products include:
- Nardil ... 1742

Phenobarbital (Effects enhanced by antihistamines). Products include:
- Arco-Lase Plus Tablets ... 607
- Bellergal-S Tablets ... 1998
- Bronkolixir ... ⊞ 761
- Bronkotabs Tablets ... ⊞ 762
- Donnatal ... 1858
- Donnatal Extentabs ... 1859
- Donnatal Tablets ... 1858
- Donnazyme Tablets ... 1860
- Kinesed Tablets ... 2272
- Phenobarbital Elixir and Tablets ... 1293
- Primatene Tablets-P Formula ... 2421
- Quadrinal Tablets ... 1183
- Tedral SA ... 1765

Pindolol (Increases effects of sympathomimetics). Products include:
- Visken Tablets ... 2036

Prazepam (Effects enhanced by antihistamines). Products include:
- Centrax ... 1693

Prochlorperazine (Effects enhanced by antihistamines). Products include:
- Compazine ... 2201

Promethazine Hydrochloride (Effects enhanced by antihistamines). Products include:
- Mepergan Injection ... 2479
- Phenergan with Codeine ... 2497
- Phenergan with Dextromethorphan 2499
- Phenergan Injection ... 2493
- Phenergan Suppositories ... 2496
- Phenergan Syrup ... 2495

Phenergan Tablets 2496
Phenergan VC 2500
Phenergan VC with Codeine 2501

Propofol (Effects enhanced by antihistamines). Products include:
Diprivan Injection 2267

Propoxyphene Hydrochloride (Effects enhanced by antihistamines). Products include:
Darvon 1256
Wygesic Tablets 2540

Propoxyphene Napsylate (Effects enhanced by antihistamines). Products include:
Darvon-N/Darvocet-N 1254

Propranolol Hydrochloride (Increases effects of sympathomimetics). Products include:
Inderal 2459
Inderal LA Long Acting Capsules ... 2461
Inderide Tablets 2463
Inderide LA Long Acting Capsules .. 2465

Protriptyline Hydrochloride (Effects enhanced by antihistamines). Products include:
Vivactil Tablets 1567

Quazepam (Effects enhanced by antihistamines). Products include:
Doral Tablets 2383

Reserpine (Reduced antihypertensive effect). Products include:
Diupres Tablets 1461
Hydromox R Tablets 1209
Hydropres Tablets 1485
Renese-R Tablets 1786
Salutensin/Salutensin-Demi 719
Ser-Ap-Es Tablets 881
Serpasil Tablets 883
Serpasil-Apresoline Tablets 884
Serpasil-Esidrix Tablets 886

Secobarbital Sodium (Effects enhanced by antihistamines). Products include:
Seconal Sodium Pulvules 1296

Selegiline Hydrochloride (Increases effects of sympathomimetics). Products include:
Eldepryl 2250

Sufentanil Citrate (Effects enhanced by antihistamines). Products include:
Sufenta Injection 1147

Temazepam (Effects enhanced by antihistamines). Products include:
Restoril Capsules 2023

Thiamylal Sodium (Effects enhanced by antihistamines). Products include:
Surital Ampoules, Steri-Vials 1764

Thioridazine Hydrochloride (Effects enhanced by antihistamines). Products include:
Mellaril 2011

Thiothixene (Effects enhanced by antihistamines). Products include:
Navane Capsules and Concentrate 1954
Navane Intramuscular 1956

Timolol Maleate (Increases effects of sympathomimetics). Products include:
Blocadren Tablets 1429
Timolide Tablets 1547
Timoptic in Ocudose 1552
Timoptic Sterile Ophthalmic Solution 1550

Tranylcypromine Sulfate (Increases effects of sympathomimetics). Products include:
Parnate Tablets 2222

Triazolam (Effects enhanced by antihistamines). Products include:
Halcion Tablets 2340

Trifluoperazine Hydrochloride (Effects enhanced by antihistamines). Products include:
Stelazine 2226

Trimipramine Maleate (Effects enhanced by antihistamines). Products include:
Surmontil Capsules 2524

NOVAHISTINE EXPECTORANT

(Codeine Phosphate, Pseudoephedrine Hydrochloride, Guaifenesin) 1343

May interact with tricyclic antidepressants, monoamine oxidase inhibitors, central nervous system depressants, beta blockers, veratrum alkaloids, and certain other agents. Compounds in these categories include:

Acebutolol Hydrochloride (Potentiates effects of pseudoephedrine). Products include:
Sectral Capsules 2520

Alcohol (Potentiated effects).

Alfentanil Hydrochloride (Potentiated effects). Products include:
Alfenta Injection 1131

Alprazolam (Potentiated effects). Products include:
Xanax Tablets 2367

Amitriptyline Hydrochloride (Potentiated effects). Products include:
Elavil 2269
Endep Tablets 1927
Etrafon 2087
Limbitrol 1933
Triavil Tablets 1556

Amoxapine (Potentiated effects). Products include:
Asendin Tablets 1196

Aprobarbital (Potentiated effects). Products include:
Alurate Elixir 1883

Atenolol (Potentiates effects of pseudoephedrine). Products include:
Tenoretic Tablets 1105
Tenormin Tablets and I.V. Injection 1107

Betaxolol Hydrochloride (Potentiates effects of pseudoephedrine). Products include:
Betoptic Sterile Ophthalmic Solution 569
Betoptic S Sterile Ophthalmic Suspension 570
Kerlone Tablets 2172

Buprenorphine (Potentiated effects).
No products indexed under this heading.

Buspirone Hydrochloride (Potentiated effects). Products include:
BuSpar 1401

Butabarbital (Potentiated effects). Products include:
Pyridium Plus 1764

Butalbital (Potentiated effects). Products include:
Esgic-Plus Tablets 1002
Esgic Tablets & Capsules 1001
Fioricet Tablets 2006
Fiorinal Capsules 2007
Fiorinal with Codeine Capsules 2008
Fiorinal Tablets 2007
Phrenilin 838
Sedapap Tablets 50 mg/650 mg .. 1360

Carteolol Hydrochloride (Potentiates effects of pseudoephedrine). Products include:
Cartrol Tablets 507

Chlordiazepoxide (Potentiated effects). Products include:
Libritabs Tablets 1930
Limbitrol 1933
Menrium Tablets 1934

Chlordiazepoxide Hydrochloride (Potentiated effects). Products include:
Librax Capsules 1929
Librium Capsules 1931
Librium Injectable 1932

Chlorpromazine (Potentiated effects). Products include:
Thorazine 2234

Chlorprothixene (Potentiated effects). Products include:
Taractan Tablets 1920

Chlorprothixene Hydrochloride (Potentiated effects). Products include:
Taractan 1920

Clomipramine Hydrochloride (Potentiated effects). Products include:
Anafranil Capsules 650

Clorazepate Dipotassium (Potentiated effects). Products include:
Tranxene 556

Codeine (Potentiated effects). Products include:
Calcidrine Syrup 506

Codeine Polistirex (Potentiated effects).
No products indexed under this heading.

Cryptenamine Preparations (Reduced antihypertensive effects).

Desipramine Hydrochloride (Potentiated effects). Products include:
Norpramin Tablets 1340

Dezocine (Potentiated effects).

Diazepam (Potentiated effects). Products include:
Valium Injectable 1937
Valium Tablets 1939
Valrelease Capsules 1923

Doxepin Hydrochloride (Potentiated effects). Products include:
Sinequan 1960

Droperidol (Potentiated effects). Products include:
Inapsine Injection 1140
Innovar Injection 1141

Enflurane (Potentiated effects). Products include:
Ethrane 599

Esmolol Hydrochloride (Potentiates effects of pseudoephedrine). Products include:
Brevibloc Injection 942

Estazolam (Potentiated effects). Products include:
ProSom Tablets 554

Ethchlorvynol (Potentiated effects). Products include:
Placidyl Capsules 553

Ethinamate (Potentiated effects).
No products indexed under this heading.

Fentanyl (Potentiated effects). Products include:
Duragesic Transdermal System 1133

Fentanyl Citrate (Potentiated effects). Products include:
Innovar Injection 1141
Sublimaze Injection 1146

Fluphenazine Decanoate (Potentiated effects). Products include:
Prolixin Decanoate 1795

Fluphenazine Enanthate (Potentiated effects). Products include:
Prolixin Enanthate 1796

Fluphenazine Hydrochloride (Potentiated effects). Products include:
Prolixin Elixir 1793
Prolixin Injection 1791
Prolixin Oral Concentrate 1792
Prolixin Tablets 1793

Flurazepam Hydrochloride (Potentiated effects). Products include:
Dalmane Capsules 1927

Furazolidone (Potentiated effects of MAO inhibitors; potentiated effects of pseudoephedrine). Products include:
Furoxone 1855

Glutethimide (Potentiated effects).
No products indexed under this heading.

Haloperidol (Potentiated effects). Products include:
Haldol Injection, Tablets and Concentrate 1373

Haloperidol Decanoate (Potentiated effects). Products include:
Haldol Decanoate 1375

Hydrocodone Bitartrate (Potentiated effects). Products include:
Anexsia 5/500 Tablets 2196
Anexsia 7.5/650 Tablets 2197
Azdone Tablets 844
Codiclear DH Syrup 845
Codimal DH Syrup 846
Damason-P 1356
Hycodan Syrup, Tablets 927
Hycomine Compound Tablets 929
Hycomine Syrup 927
Hycotuss Expectorant Syrup 930
Hydrocet Capsules 835
Lortab ASA Tablets 2414
Lortab 2412
Ru-Tuss with Hydrocodone 694
Triaminic Expectorant DH 1995
Vicodin Tablets 1187
Vicodin ES Tablets 1189
Zydone Capsules 941

Hydrocodone Polistirex (Potentiated effects). Products include:
Tussionex Extended-Release Suspension 988

Hydroxyzine Hydrochloride (Potentiated effects). Products include:
Atarax Tablets & Syrup 1941
Marax Tablets & DF Syrup 1954
Vistaril Intramuscular Solution 1970

Imipramine Hydrochloride (Potentiated effects). Products include:
Tofranil Ampuls 1038
Tofranil Tablets 1039

Imipramine Pamoate (Potentiated effects). Products include:
Tofranil-PM Capsules 1041

Isocarboxazid (Potentiated effects of MAO inhibitors; potentiated effects of pseudoephedrine). Products include:
Marplan Tablets 1906

Isoflurane (Potentiated effects). Products include:
Forane 600

Ketamine Hydrochloride (Potentiated effects). Products include:
Ketalar 1726

Labetalol Hydrochloride (Potentiates effects of pseudoephedrine). Products include:
Normodyne Injection 2108
Normodyne Tablets 2110
Normozide Tablets 2112
Trandate HCT Tablets 579
Trandate Injection 577
Trandate Tablets 579

Levorphanol Tartrate (Potentiated effects). Products include:
Levo-Dromoran 1906

Lorazepam (Potentiated effects). Products include:
Ativan Injection 2432
Ativan Tablets 2434

Loxapine Hydrochloride (Potentiated effects). Products include:
Loxitane 1213

Loxapine Succinate (Potentiated effects). Products include:
Loxitane Capsules 1213

Maprotiline Hydrochloride (Potentiated effects). Products include:
Ludiomil Tablets 874

Mecamylamine Hydrochloride (Reduced antihypertensive effects). Products include:
Inversine Tablets 1492

Meperidine Hydrochloride (Potentiated effects). Products include:
- Demerol ... 2047
- Mepergan Injection ... 2479

Mephobarbital (Potentiated effects). Products include:
- Mebaral Tablets ... 2061

Meprobamate (Potentiated effects). Products include:
- Deprol Tablets ... 2382
- Equagesic Tablets ... 2451
- Miltown Tablets ... 2386
- PMB 200 and PMB 400 ... 2504

Mesoridazine (Potentiated effects). Products include:
- Serentil ... 686

Methadone Hydrochloride (Potentiated effects). Products include:
- Dolophine Hydrochloride Ampoules & Vials ... 1260
- Dolophine Hydrochloride Tablets ... 1261
- Methadone Hydrochloride Diskets .. 1284
- Methadone Hydrochloride Oral Solution & Tablets ... 1987

Methohexital Sodium (Potentiated effects). Products include:
- Brevital Sodium Vials ... 1248

Methoxyflurane (Potentiated effects).
- No products indexed under this heading.

Methyldopa (Reduced antihypertensive effects). Products include:
- Aldoclor Tablets ... 1413
- Aldomet Oral ... 1415
- Aldoril Tablets ... 1418

Metoprolol Tartrate (Potentiates effects of pseudoephedrine). Products include:
- Lopressor Ampuls ... 1032
- Lopressor HCT Tablets ... 1034
- Lopressor Tablets ... 1032

Midazolam Hydrochloride (Potentiated effects). Products include:
- Versed Injection ... 1924

Molindone Hydrochloride (Potentiated effects). Products include:
- Moban Tablets & Concentrate ... 932

Morphine Sulfate (Potentiated effects). Products include:
- Astramorph/PF Injection, USP (Preservative-Free) ... 618
- Duramorph ... 960
- Infumorph 200 and Infumorph 500 Sterile Solutions ... 962
- MS Contin Tablets ... 1814
- MSIR ... 1817
- Oramorph SR (Morphine Sulfate Sustained Release Tablets) ... 1988
- Roxanol ... 1991

Nadolol (Potentiates effects of pseudoephedrine). Products include:
- Corgard Tablets ... 701
- Corzide Tablets ... 702

Nortriptyline Hydrochloride (Potentiated effects). Products include:
- Pamelor ... 2019

Opium Alkaloids (Potentiated effects). Products include:
- B & O No. 15A & No. 16A Supprettes ... 2395
- Pantopon Injectable ... 1911

Oxazepam (Potentiated effects). Products include:
- Serax Capsules ... 2522
- Serax Tablets ... 2522

Oxycodone Hydrochloride (Potentiated effects). Products include:
- Percocet Tablets ... 950
- Percodan ... 951
- Roxicodone Tablets, Oral Solution & Intensol (Oxycodone) ... 1992
- Tylox Capsules ... 1382

Penbutolol Sulfate (Potentiates effects of pseudoephedrine). Products include:
- Levatol ... 1832

Pentobarbital Sodium (Potentiated effects of MAO inhibitors; potentiated effects of pseudoephedrine). Products include:
- Nembutal Sodium Capsules ... 534
- Nembutal Sodium Solution ... 536
- Nembutal Sodium Suppositories ... 538

Perphenazine (Potentiated effects). Products include:
- Etrafon ... 2087
- Triavil Tablets ... 1556
- Trilafon ... 2123

Phenelzine Sulfate (Potentiated effects of MAO inhibitors; potentiated effects of pseudoephedrine). Products include:
- Nardil ... 1742

Phenobarbital (Potentiated effects). Products include:
- Arco-Lase Plus Tablets ... 607
- Bellergal-S Tablets ... 1998
- Bronkolixir ... (■) 761
- Bronkotabs Tablets ... (■) 762
- Donnatal ... 1858
- Donnatal Extentabs ... 1859
- Donnatal Tablets ... 1858
- Donnazyme Tablets ... 1860
- Kinesed Tablets ... 2272
- Phenobarbital Elixir and Tablets ... 1293
- Primatene Tablets-P Formula ... 2421
- Quadrinal Tablets ... 1183
- Tedral SA ... 1765

Pindolol (Potentiates effects of pseudoephedrine). Products include:
- Visken Tablets ... 2036

Prazepam (Potentiated effects). Products include:
- Centrax ... 1693

Prochlorperazine (Potentiated effects). Products include:
- Compazine ... 2201

Promethazine Hydrochloride (Potentiated effects). Products include:
- Mepergan Injection ... 2479
- Phenergan with Codeine ... 2497
- Phenergan with Dextromethorphan 2499
- Phenergan Injection ... 2493
- Phenergan Suppositories ... 2496
- Phenergan Syrup ... 2495
- Phenergan Tablets ... 2496
- Phenergan VC ... 2500
- Phenergan VC with Codeine ... 2501

Propofol (Potentiated effects). Products include:
- Diprivan Injection ... 2267

Propoxyphene Hydrochloride (Potentiated effects). Products include:
- Darvon ... 1256
- Wygesic Tablets ... 2540

Propoxyphene Napsylate (Potentiated effects). Products include:
- Darvon-N/Darvocet-N ... 1254

Propranolol Hydrochloride (Potentiates effects of pseudoephedrine). Products include:
- Inderal ... 2459
- Inderal LA Long Acting Capsules ... 2461
- Inderide Tablets ... 2463
- Inderide LA Long Acting Capsules .. 2465

Protriptyline Hydrochloride (Potentiated effects). Products include:
- Vivactil Tablets ... 1567

Quazepam (Potentiated effects). Products include:
- Doral Tablets ... 2383

Reserpine (Reduced antihypertensive effects). Products include:
- Diupres Tablets ... 1461
- Hydromox R Tablets ... 1209
- Hydropres Tablets ... 1485
- Renese-R Tablets ... 1786
- Salutensin/Salutensin-Demi ... 719
- Ser-Ap-Es Tablets ... 881
- Serpasil Tablets ... 883
- Serpasil-Apresoline Tablets ... 884
- Serpasil-Esidrix Tablets ... 886

Secobarbital Sodium (Potentiated effects). Products include:
- Seconal Sodium Pulvules ... 1296

Selegiline Hydrochloride (Potentiated effects of MAO inhibitors; potentiated effects of pseudoephedrine). Products include:
- Eldepryl ... 2250

Sufentanil Citrate (Potentiated effects). Products include:
- Sufenta Injection ... 1147

Temazepam (Potentiated effects). Products include:
- Restoril Capsules ... 2023

Thiamylal Sodium (Potentiated effects). Products include:
- Surital Ampoules, Steri-Vials ... 1764

Thioridazine Hydrochloride (Potentiated effects). Products include:
- Mellaril ... 2011

Thiothixene (Potentiated effects). Products include:
- Navane Capsules and Concentrate 1954
- Navane Intramuscular ... 1956

Timolol Maleate (Potentiates effects of pseudoephedrine). Products include:
- Blocadren Tablets ... 1429
- Timolide Tablets ... 1547
- Timoptic in Ocudose ... 1552
- Timoptic Sterile Ophthalmic Solution ... 1550

Tranylcypromine Sulfate (Potentiated effects of MAO inhibitors; potentiated effects of pseudoephedrine). Products include:
- Parnate Tablets ... 2222

Triazolam (Potentiated effects). Products include:
- Halcion Tablets ... 2340

Trifluoperazine Hydrochloride (Potentiated effects). Products include:
- Stelazine ... 2226

Trimipramine Maleate (Potentiated effects). Products include:
- Surmontil Capsules ... 2524

NOVANTRONE FOR INJECTION CONCENTRATE
(Mitoxantrone Hydrochloride) ... 1226
May interact with:

Daunorubicin Hydrochloride (Possible danger of cardiac effects). Products include:
- Cerubidine ... 2443

Doxorubicin Hydrochloride (Possible danger of cardiac effects). Products include:
- Adriamycin PFS ... 561
- Adriamycin RDF ... 562
- Doxorubicin Hydrochloride for Injection, USP ... 622
- Doxorubicin Hydrochloride Injection, USP ... 848
- Rubex ... 739

NOVOCAIN HYDROCHLORIDE FOR SPINAL ANESTHESIA
(Procaine Hydrochloride) ... 2065
May interact with sulfonamides. Compounds in this category include:

Sulfamethizole (Action of sulfonamides inhibited). Products include:
- Thiosulfil Forte Tablets ... 2526
- Urobiotic-250 Capsules ... 1968

Sulfamethoxazole (Action of sulfonamides inhibited). Products include:
- Azo Gantanol Tablets ... 1887
- Bactrim DS Tablets ... 1891
- Bactrim I.V. Infusion ... 1889
- Bactrim ... 1891
- Gantanol ... 1899
- Septra ... 813
- Septra I.V. Infusion ... 808
- Septra I.V. Infusion ADD-Vantage Vials ... 810
- Septra ... 813

Sulfasalazine (Action of sulfonamides inhibited). Products include:
- Azulfidine Tablets, EN-tabs, Oral Suspension ... 1157

Sulfinpyrazone (Action of sulfonamides inhibited). Products include:
- Anturane ... 853

Sulfisoxazole (Action of sulfonamides inhibited). Products include:
- Azo Gantrisin Tablets ... 1888
- Gantrisin Tablets ... 1901
- Pediazole ... 1973

Sulfisoxazole Diolamine (Action of sulfonamides inhibited). Products include:
- Gantrisin Ophthalmic Ointment/ Solution ... 1900

NOVOLIN L
(Insulin, Human, Zinc Suspension) ... 1627
No interactions described in labeling.

NOVOLIN N
(Insulin, Human Isophane Suspension) ... 1627
No interactions described in labeling.

NOVOLIN N PENFILL CARTRIDGES
(Insulin, Human NPH) ... 1628
No interactions described in labeling.

NOVOLIN N PREFILLED
(Insulin, Human Isophane Suspension) ... 1628
No interactions described in labeling.

NOVOLIN 70/30
(Insulin, Human NPH, Insulin, Human Regular) ... 1627
No interactions described in labeling.

NOVOLIN 70/30 PENFILL CARTRIDGES
(Insulin, Human NPH, Insulin, Human Regular) ... 1628
No interactions described in labeling.

NOVOLIN 70/30 PREFILLED
(Insulin, Human Regular and Human NPH Mixture) ... 1629
No interactions described in labeling.

NOVOLIN R
(Insulin, Human Regular) ... 1627
No interactions described in labeling.

NOVOLIN R PENFILL CARTRIDGES
(Insulin, Human Regular) ... 1628
No interactions described in labeling.

NOVOLIN R PREFILLED
(Insulin, Human Regular) ... 1629
No interactions described in labeling.

NUBAIN INJECTION
(Nalbuphine Hydrochloride) ... 934
May interact with narcotic analgesics, phenothiazines, hypnotics and sedatives, general anesthetics, tranquilizers, and certain other agents. Compounds in these categories include:

Alcohol (Additive effect).

Alfentanil Hydrochloride (Additive effect). Products include:
- Alfenta Injection ... 1131

Alprazolam (Additive effect). Products include:
- Xanax Tablets ... 2367

Buprenorphine (Additive effect).
- No products indexed under this heading.

Buspirone Hydrochloride (Additive effect). Products include:
BuSpar ... 1401

Chlordiazepoxide (Additive effect). Products include:
Libritabs Tablets ... 1930
Limbitrol ... 1933
Menrium Tablets ... 1934

Chlordiazepoxide Hydrochloride (Additive effect). Products include:
Librax Capsules ... 1929
Librium Capsules ... 1931
Librium Injectable ... 1932

Chlorpromazine (Additive effect). Products include:
Thorazine ... 2234

Clorazepate Dipotassium (Additive effect). Products include:
Tranxene ... 556

Codeine (Additive effect). Products include:
Calcidrine Syrup ... 506

Codeine Phosphate (Additive effect). Products include:
Actifed with Codeine Cough Syrup .. 752
Cheracol Cough Syrup ... 1853
Codimal PH Syrup ... 846
Dimetane-DC Cough Syrup ... 1857
Empirin with Codeine Phosphate Nos. 2, 3 & 4 ... 764
Fiorinal with Codeine Capsules ... 2008
Isoclor Expectorant ... 982
Naldecon CX Adult Liquid ... ▣ 521
Novahistine DH ... 1342
Novahistine Expectorant ... 1343
Nucofed Capsules ... 2219
Nucofed Expectorant ... 2219
Nucofed Pediatric Expectorant ... 2220
Nucofed Syrup ... 2219
Phenaphen with Codeine Capsules 1865
Phenaphen-650 with Codeine Tablets ... 1866
Phenergan with Codeine ... 2497
Phenergan VC with Codeine ... 2501
Robitussin A-C Syrup ... 1875
Robitussin-DAC Syrup ... 1875
Ryna ... ▣ 741
Soma Compound w/Codeine Tablets ... 2390
Triaminic Expectorant w/Codeine .. 1996
Tussi-Organidin Liquid ... 2391
Tylenol with Codeine ... 1381

Codeine Polistirex (Additive effect).
No products indexed under this heading.

Dezocine (Additive effect).

Diazepam (Additive effect). Products include:
Valium Injectable ... 1937
Valium Tablets ... 1939
Valrelease Capsules ... 1923

Droperidol (Additive effect). Products include:
Inapsine Injection ... 1140
Innovar Injection ... 1141

Enflurane (Additive effect). Products include:
Ethrane ... 599

Estazolam (Additive effect). Products include:
ProSom Tablets ... 554

Ethchlorvynol (Additive effect). Products include:
Placidyl Capsules ... 553

Ethinamate (Additive effect).
No products indexed under this heading.

Fentanyl (Additive effect). Products include:
Duragesic Transdermal System ... 1133

Fentanyl Citrate (Additive effect). Products include:
Innovar Injection ... 1141
Sublimaze Injection ... 1146

Fluphenazine Decanoate (Additive effect). Products include:
Prolixin Decanoate ... 1795

Fluphenazine Enanthate (Additive effect). Products include:
Prolixin Enanthate ... 1796

Fluphenazine Hydrochloride (Additive effect). Products include:
Prolixin Elixir ... 1793
Prolixin Injection ... 1791
Prolixin Oral Concentrate ... 1792
Prolixin Tablets ... 1793

Flurazepam Hydrochloride (Additive effect). Products include:
Dalmane Capsules ... 1927

Glutethimide (Additive effect).
No products indexed under this heading.

Haloperidol (Additive effect). Products include:
Haldol Injection, Tablets and Concentrate ... 1373

Haloperidol Decanoate (Additive effect). Products include:
Haldol Decanoate ... 1375

Hydrocodone Bitartrate (Additive effect). Products include:
Anexsia 5/500 Tablets ... 2196
Anexsia 7.5/650 Tablets ... 2197
Azdone Tablets ... 844
Codiclear DH Syrup ... 845
Codimal DH Syrup ... 846
Damason-P ... 1356
Hycodan Syrup, Tablets ... 927
Hycomine Compound Tablets ... 929
Hycomine Syrup ... 927
Hycotuss Expectorant Syrup ... 930
Hydrocet Capsules ... 835
Lortab ASA Tablets ... 2414
Lortab ... 2412
Ru-Tuss with Hydrocodone ... 694
Triaminic Expectorant DH ... 1995
Vicodin Tablets ... 1187
Vicodin ES Tablets ... 1189
Zydone Capsules ... 941

Hydrocodone Polistirex (Additive effect). Products include:
Tussionex Extended-Release Suspension ... 988

Hydroxyzine Hydrochloride (Additive effect). Products include:
Atarax Tablets & Syrup ... 1941
Marax Tablets & DF Syrup ... 1954
Vistaril Intramuscular Solution ... 1970

Isoflurane (Additive effect). Products include:
Forane ... 600

Levorphanol Tartrate (Additive effect). Products include:
Levo-Dromoran ... 1906

Lorazepam (Additive effect). Products include:
Ativan Injection ... 2432
Ativan Tablets ... 2434

Loxapine Hydrochloride (Additive effect). Products include:
Loxitane ... 1213

Meperidine Hydrochloride (Additive effect). Products include:
Demerol ... 2047
Mepergan Injection ... 2479

Meprobamate (Additive effect). Products include:
Deprol Tablets ... 2382
Equagesic Tablets ... 2451
Miltown Tablets ... 2386
PMB 200 and PMB 400 ... 2504

Mesoridazine (Additive effect). Products include:
Serentil ... 686

Methadone Hydrochloride (Additive effect). Products include:
Dolophine Hydrochloride Ampoules & Vials ... 1260
Dolophine Hydrochloride Tablets ... 1261
Methadone Hydrochloride Diskets .. 1284
Methadone Hydrochloride Oral Solution & Tablets ... 1987

Methohexital Sodium (Additive effect). Products include:
Brevital Sodium Vials ... 1248

Methoxyflurane (Additive effect).
No products indexed under this heading.

Midazolam Hydrochloride (Additive effect). Products include:
Versed Injection ... 1924

Molindone Hydrochloride (Additive effect). Products include:
Moban Tablets & Concentrate ... 932

Morphine Sulfate (Additive effect). Products include:
Astramorph/PF Injection, USP (Preservative-Free) ... 618
Duramorph ... 960
Infumorph 200 and Infumorph 500 Sterile Solutions ... 962
MS Contin Tablets ... 1814
MSIR ... 1817
Oramorph SR (Morphine Sulfate Sustained Release Tablets) ... 1988
Roxanol ... 1991

Opium Alkaloids (Additive effect). Products include:
B & O No. 15A & No. 16A Supprettes ... 2395
Pantopon Injectable ... 1911

Oxazepam (Additive effect). Products include:
Serax Capsules ... 2522
Serax Tablets ... 2522

Oxycodone Hydrochloride (Additive effect). Products include:
Percocet Tablets ... 950
Percodan ... 951
Roxicodone Tablets, Oral Solution & Intensol (Oxycodone) ... 1992
Tylox Capsules ... 1382

Perphenazine (Additive effect). Products include:
Etrafon ... 2087
Triavil Tablets ... 1556
Trilafon ... 2123

Prazepam (Additive effect). Products include:
Centrax ... 1693

Prochlorperazine (Additive effect). Products include:
Compazine ... 2201

Promethazine Hydrochloride (Additive effect). Products include:
Mepergan Injection ... 2479
Phenergan with Codeine ... 2497
Phenergan with Dextromethorphan 2499
Phenergan Injection ... 2493
Phenergan Suppositories ... 2496
Phenergan Syrup ... 2495
Phenergan Tablets ... 2496
Phenergan VC ... 2500
Phenergan VC with Codeine ... 2501

Propofol (Additive effect). Products include:
Diprivan Injection ... 2267

Propoxyphene Hydrochloride (Additive effect). Products include:
Darvon ... 1256
Wygesic Tablets ... 2540

Propoxyphene Napsylate (Additive effect). Products include:
Darvon-N/Darvocet-N ... 1254

Quazepam (Additive effect). Products include:
Doral Tablets ... 2383

Secobarbital Sodium (Additive effect). Products include:
Seconal Sodium Pulvules ... 1296

Sufentanil Citrate (Additive effect). Products include:
Sufenta Injection ... 1147

Temazepam (Additive effect). Products include:
Restoril Capsules ... 2023

Thioridazine Hydrochloride (Additive effect). Products include:
Mellaril ... 2011

Triazolam (Additive effect). Products include:
Halcion Tablets ... 2340

Trifluoperazine Hydrochloride (Additive effect). Products include:
Stelazine ... 2226

NUCOFED CAPSULES
(Codeine Phosphate, Pseudoephedrine Hydrochloride) 2219
May interact with beta blockers, veratrum alkaloids, sympathomimetic aerosal brochodilators, tricyclic antidepressants, central nervous system depressants, general anesthetics, anticholinergics, narcotic analgesics, and certain other agents. Compounds in these categories include:

Acebutolol Hydrochloride (Increased pressor effect of pseudoephedrine). Products include:
Sectral Capsules ... 2520

Albuterol (Increased effect of either agent; increased potential for side effects). Products include:
Proventil Inhalation Aerosol ... 2117
Ventolin Inhalation Aerosol and Refill ... 583

Albuterol Sulfate (Increased effect of either agent; increased potential for side effects). Products include:
Proventil Repetabs Tablets ... 2120
Proventil Solutions for Inhalation 0.5% and 0.083% ... 2118
Proventil Syrup ... 2119
Proventil Tablets ... 2120
Ventolin ... 583

Alcohol (Effect not specified).

Alfentanil Hydrochloride (Effect not specified). Products include:
Alfenta Injection ... 1131

Alprazolam (Effect not specified). Products include:
Xanax Tablets ... 2367

Amitriptyline Hydrochloride (May antagonize effects of pseudoephedrine; increased effect of antidepressants or the codeine component). Products include:
Elavil ... 2269
Endep Tablets ... 1927
Etrafon ... 2087
Limbitrol ... 1933
Triavil Tablets ... 1556

Amoxapine (May antagonize effects of pseudoephedrine; increased effect of antidepressants or the codeine component). Products include:
Asendin Tablets ... 1196

Aprobarbital (Effect not specified). Products include:
Alurate Elixir ... 1883

Atenolol (Increased pressor effect of pseudoephedrine). Products include:
Tenoretic Tablets ... 1105
Tenormin Tablets and I.V. Injection 1107

Atropine Sulfate (Paralytic ileus). Products include:
Arco-Lase Plus Tablets ... 607
Atropine Sulfate Sterile Ophthalmic Solution and S.O.P. Sterile Ophthalmic Ointment ... ⊙ 239
Donnagel ... ▣ 675
Donnagel-PG ... 1858
Donnatal ... 1858
Donnatal Extentabs ... 1859
Donnatal Tablets ... 1858
Donnazyme Tablets ... 1860
Isopto Atropine ... ⊙ 218
Lomotil ... 2174
Motofen Tablets ... 836
Ru-Tuss Tablets ... 693
Urised Tablets ... 2396

Belladonna Alkaloids (Paralytic ileus). Products include:
Bellergal-S Tablets ... 1998
Hyland's Bed Wetting Tablets ... ▣ 728
Hyland's Teething Tablets ... ▣ 728
Kinesed Tablets ... 2272

Benztropine Mesylate (Paralytic ileus). Products include:
Cogentin ... 1435

(▣ Described in PDR For Nonprescription Drugs)

(⊙ Described in PDR For Ophthalmology)

Betaxolol Hydrochloride (Increased pressor effect of pseudoephedrine). Products include:
- Betoptic Sterile Ophthalmic Solution ... 569
- Betoptic S Sterile Ophthalmic Suspension ... 570
- Kerlone Tablets ... 2172

Biperiden (Paralytic ileus). Products include:
- Akineton ... 1171

Buprenorphine (Effect not specified).
- No products indexed under this heading.

Buspirone Hydrochloride (Effect not specified). Products include:
- BuSpar ... 1401

Butabarbital (Effect not specified). Products include:
- Pyridium Plus ... 1764

Butalbital (Effect not specified). Products include:
- Esgic-Plus Tablets ... 1002
- Esgic Tablets & Capsules ... 1001
- Fioricet Tablets ... 2006
- Fiorinal Capsules ... 2007
- Fiorinal with Codeine Capsules ... 2008
- Fiorinal Tablets ... 2007
- Phrenilin ... 838
- Sedapap Tablets 50 mg/650 mg .. 1360

Carteolol Hydrochloride (Increased pressor effect of pseudoephedrine). Products include:
- Cartrol Tablets ... 507

Chlordiazepoxide (Effect not specified). Products include:
- Libritabs Tablets ... 1930
- Limbitrol ... 1933
- Menrium Tablets ... 1934

Chlordiazepoxide Hydrochloride (Effect not specified). Products include:
- Librax Capsules ... 1929
- Librium Capsules ... 1931
- Librium Injectable ... 1932

Chlorpromazine (Effect not specified). Products include:
- Thorazine ... 2234

Chlorprothixene (Effect not specified). Products include:
- Taractan Tablets ... 1920

Chlorprothixene Hydrochloride (Effect not specified). Products include:
- Taractan ... 1920

Clidinium Bromide (Paralytic ileus). Products include:
- Librax Capsules ... 1929
- Quarzan Capsules ... 1937

Clomipramine Hydrochloride (May antagonize effects of pseudoephedrine; increased effect of antidepressants or the codeine component). Products include:
- Anafranil Capsules ... 650

Clorazepate Dipotassium (Effect not specified). Products include:
- Tranxene ... 556

Codeine (Effect not specified). Products include:
- Calcidrine Syrup ... 506

Codeine Polistirex (Effect not specified).
- No products indexed under this heading.

Cryptenamine Preparations (Decreased hypotensive effects).

Desipramine Hydrochloride (May antagonize effects of pseudoephedrine; increased effect of antidepressants or the codeine component). Products include:
- Norpramin Tablets ... 1340

Deslanoside (Increased possibility of cardiac arrhythmias).
- No products indexed under this heading.

Dezocine (Effect not specified).

Diazepam (Effect not specified). Products include:
- Valium Injectable ... 1937
- Valium Tablets ... 1939
- Valrelease Capsules ... 1923

Dicyclomine Hydrochloride (Paralytic ileus). Products include:
- Bentyl ... 1322

Digitoxin (Increased possibility of cardiac arrhythmias). Products include:
- Crystodigin Tablets ... 1253

Digoxin (Increased possibility of cardiac arrhythmias). Products include:
- Lanoxicaps ... 772
- Lanoxin Elixir Pediatric ... 775
- Lanoxin Injection ... 778
- Lanoxin Injection Pediatric ... 781
- Lanoxin Tablets ... 783

Dobutamine Hydrochloride (Increased effect of either agent; increased potential for side effects). Products include:
- Dobutrex Solution Vials ... 1259

Dopamine Hydrochloride (Increased effect of either agent; increased potential for side effects). Products include:
- Intropin Injection ... 930

Doxepin Hydrochloride (May antagonize effects of pseudoephedrine; increased effect of antidepressants or the codeine component). Products include:
- Sinequan ... 1960

Droperidol (Effect not specified). Products include:
- Inapsine Injection ... 1140
- Innovar Injection ... 1141

Enflurane (Effect not specified). Products include:
- Ethrane ... 599

Ephedrine Hydrochloride (Increased effect of either agent; increased potential for side effects). Products include:
- Amesec ... ▣ 682
- Primatene Tablets-M Formula ... 2421
- Primatene Tablets-P Formula ... 2421
- Primatene Tablets-Regular Formula ... 2421
- Quadrinal Tablets ... 1183
- Quelidrine Syrup ... 556
- Tedral SA ... 1765

Ephedrine Sulfate (Increased effect of either agent; increased potential for side effects). Products include:
- Bronkaid Tablets ... ▣ 757
- Bronkolixir ... ▣ 761
- Bronkotabs Tablets ... ▣ 762
- Marax Tablets & DF Syrup ... 1954
- Pazo Hemorrhoid Ointment & Suppositories ... 752
- Vicks Vatronol Nose Drops ... ▣ 666

Ephedrine Tannate (Increased effect of either agent; increased potential for side effects). Products include:
- Rynatuss ... 2388

Epinephrine (Increased effect of either agent; increased potential for side effects). Products include:
- Ana-Kit Anaphylaxis Emergency Treatment Kit ... 1100
- Bronkaid Mist ... ▣ 757
- EpiPen ... 843
- Marcaine Hydrochloride 0.5% with Epinephrine 1:200,000 (as bitartrate) ... 958
- Marcaine Hydrochloride with Epinephrine 1:200,000 ... 2055
- Primatene Mist ... 2420
- Sus-Phrine Injection ... 1006
- Xylocaine with Epinephrine Injections ... 637

Epinephrine Bitartrate (Increased effect of either agent; increased potential for side effects). Products include:
- AsthmaHaler Mist Epinephrine Bitartrate Bronchodilator ... ▣ 616
- Bronkaid Mist Suspension ... ▣ 757
- Primatene Mist Suspension ... 2421

Epinephrine Hydrochloride (Increased effect of either agent; increased potential for side effects). Products include:
- Adrenalin Chloride Solution 1:100 & 1:1,000 ... 1689
- Epifrin ... ⊙ 244
- Glaucon ... ⊙ 218

Esmolol Hydrochloride (Increased pressor effect of pseudoephedrine). Products include:
- Brevibloc Injection ... 942

Estazolam (Effect not specified). Products include:
- ProSom Tablets ... 554

Ethchlorvynol (Effect not specified). Products include:
- Placidyl Capsules ... 553

Ethinamate (Effect not specified).
- No products indexed under this heading.

Ethopropazine Hydrochloride (Paralytic ileus).

Fentanyl (Effect not specified). Products include:
- Duragesic Transdermal System ... 1133

Fentanyl Citrate (Effect not specified). Products include:
- Innovar Injection ... 1141
- Sublimaze Injection ... 1146

Fluphenazine Decanoate (Effect not specified). Products include:
- Prolixin Decanoate ... 1795

Fluphenazine Enanthate (Effect not specified). Products include:
- Prolixin Enanthate ... 1796

Fluphenazine Hydrochloride (Effect not specified). Products include:
- Prolixin Elixir ... 1793
- Prolixin Injection ... 1791
- Prolixin Oral Concentrate ... 1792
- Prolixin Tablets ... 1793

Flurazepam Hydrochloride (Effect not specified). Products include:
- Dalmane Capsules ... 1927

Glutethimide (Effect not specified).
- No products indexed under this heading.

Glycopyrrolate (Paralytic ileus). Products include:
- Robinul Forte Tablets ... 1873
- Robinul Injectable ... 1873
- Robinul Tablets ... 1873

Haloperidol (Effect not specified). Products include:
- Haldol Injection, Tablets and Concentrate ... 1373

Haloperidol Decanoate (Effect not specified). Products include:
- Haldol Decanoate ... 1375

Hydrocodone Bitartrate (Effect not specified). Products include:
- Anexsia 5/500 Tablets ... 2196
- Anexsia 7.5/650 Tablets ... 2197
- Azdone Tablets ... 844
- Codiclear DH Syrup ... 845
- Codimal DH Syrup ... 846
- Damason-P ... 1356
- Hycodan Syrup, Tablets ... 927
- Hycomine Compound Tablets ... 929
- Hycomine Syrup ... 927
- Hycotuss Expectorant Syrup ... 930
- Hydrocet Capsules ... 835
- Lortab ASA Tablets ... 2414
- Lortab ... 2412
- Ru-Tuss with Hydrocodone ... 694
- Triaminic Expectorant DH ... 1995
- Vicodin Tablets ... 1187
- Vicodin ES Tablets ... 1189
- Zydone Capsules ... 941

Hydrocodone Polistirex (Effect not specified). Products include:
- Tussionex Extended-Release Suspension ... 988

Hydroxyzine Hydrochloride (Effect not specified). Products include:
- Atarax Tablets & Syrup ... 1941
- Marax Tablets & DF Syrup ... 1954
- Vistaril Intramuscular Solution ... 1970

Hyoscyamine (Paralytic ileus). Products include:
- Cystospaz Tablets ... 2395
- Urised Tablets ... 2396

Hyoscyamine Sulfate (Paralytic ileus). Products include:
- Arco-Lase Plus Tablets ... 607
- Cystospaz-M Capsules ... 2395
- Donnagel ... ▣ 675
- Donnagel-PG ... 1858
- Donnatal ... 1858
- Donnatal Extentabs ... 1859
- Donnatal Tablets ... 1858
- Donnazyme Tablets ... 1860
- Kutrase Capsules ... 2146
- Levsin/Levsinex ... 2147
- Ru-Tuss Tablets ... 693

Imipramine Hydrochloride (May antagonize effects of pseudoephedrine; increased effect of antidepressants or the codeine component). Products include:
- Tofranil Ampuls ... 1038
- Tofranil Tablets ... 1039

Imipramine Pamoate (May antagonize effects of pseudoephedrine; increased effect of antidepressants or the codeine component). Products include:
- Tofranil-PM Capsules ... 1041

Ipratropium Bromide (Paralytic ileus). Products include:
- Atrovent Inhalation Aerosol ... 675

Isocarboxazid (May potentiate pseudoephedrine's pressor effect; may result in a hypertensive crisis). Products include:
- Marplan Tablets ... 1906

Isoflurane (Effect not specified). Products include:
- Forane ... 600

Isoproterenol Hydrochloride (Increased effect of either agent; increased potential for side effects). Products include:
- Isuprel Hydrochloride Injection 1:5000 ... 2050
- Isuprel Hydrochloride Mistometer .. 2051
- Isuprel Hydrochloride Solution 1:200 & 1:100 ... 2052
- Norisodrine Aerotrol ... 540

Ketamine Hydrochloride (Effect not specified). Products include:
- Ketalar ... 1726

Labetalol Hydrochloride (Increased pressor effect of pseudoephedrine). Products include:
- Normodyne Injection ... 2108
- Normodyne Tablets ... 2110
- Normozide Tablets ... 2112
- Trandate HCT Tablets ... 579
- Trandate Injection ... 577
- Trandate Tablets ... 579

Levorphanol Tartrate (Effect not specified). Products include:
- Levo-Dromoran ... 1906

Lorazepam (Effect not specified). Products include:
- Ativan Injection ... 2432
- Ativan Tablets ... 2434

Loxapine Hydrochloride (Effect not specified). Products include:
- Loxitane ... 1213

Loxapine Succinate (Effect not specified). Products include:
- Loxitane Capsules ... 1213

Maprotiline Hydrochloride (May antagonize effects of pseudoephedrine; increased effect of antidepressants or the codeine component). Products include:
- Ludiomil Tablets ... 874

Mepenzolate Bromide (Paralytic ileus). Products include:
- Cantil Tablets ... 1326

Meperidine Hydrochloride (Effect not specified). Products include:
- Demerol ... 2047
- Mepergan Injection ... 2479

Mephobarbital (Effect not specified). Products include:
- Mebaral Tablets ... 2061

Meprobamate (Effect not specified). Products include:
- Deprol Tablets ... 2382
- Equagesic Tablets ... 2451
- Miltown Tablets ... 2386
- PMB 200 and PMB 400 ... 2504

Mesoridazine (Effect not specified). Products include:
- Serentil ... 686

Metaproterenol Sulfate (Increased effect of either agent; increased potential for side effects). Products include:
- Alupent ... 674
- Arm-a-Med Metaproterenol Sulfate Inhalation Solution, USP ... 617
- Metaprel Inhalation Aerosol Bronchodilator ... 2014
- Metaprel Inhalation Solution ... 2015
- Metaprel ... 2015
- Metaproterenol Sulfate Inhalation Solution, USP ... 912

Metaraminol Bitartrate (Increased effect of either agent; increased potential for side effects). Products include:
- Aramine Injection ... 1424

Methadone Hydrochloride (Effect not specified). Products include:
- Dolophine Hydrochloride Ampoules & Vials ... 1260
- Dolophine Hydrochloride Tablets ... 1261
- Methadone Hydrochloride Diskets ... 1284
- Methadone Hydrochloride Oral Solution & Tablets ... 1987

Methohexital Sodium (Effect not specified). Products include:
- Brevital Sodium Vials ... 1248

Methoxamine Hydrochloride (Increased effect of either agent; increased potential for side effects). Products include:
- Vasoxyl Injection ... 819

Methoxyflurane (Effect not specified).
- No products indexed under this heading.

Metoprolol Tartrate (Increased pressor effect of pseudoephedrine). Products include:
- Lopressor Ampuls ... 1032
- Lopressor HCT Tablets ... 1034
- Lopressor Tablets ... 1032

Midazolam Hydrochloride (Effect not specified). Products include:
- Versed Injection ... 1924

Molindone Hydrochloride (Effect not specified). Products include:
- Moban Tablets & Concentrate ... 932

Morphine Sulfate (Effect not specified). Products include:
- Astramorph/PF Injection, USP (Preservative-Free) ... 618
- Duramorph ... 960
- Infumorph 200 and Infumorph 500 Sterile Solutions ... 962
- MS Contin Tablets ... 1814
- MSIR ... 1817
- Oramorph SR (Morphine Sulfate Sustained Release Tablets) ... 1988
- Roxanol ... 1991

Nadolol (Increased pressor effect of pseudoephedrine). Products include:
- Corgard Tablets ... 701
- Corzide Tablets ... 702

Norepinephrine Bitartrate (Increased effect of either agent; increased potential for side effects). Products include:
- Levophed Bitartrate Injection ... 2054

Nortriptyline Hydrochloride (May antagonize effects of pseudoephedrine; increased effect of antidepressants or the codeine component). Products include:
- Pamelor ... 2019

Opium Alkaloids (Effect not specified). Products include:
- B & O No. 15A & No. 16A Supprettes ... 2395
- Pantopon Injectable ... 1911

Oxazepam (Effect not specified). Products include:
- Serax Capsules ... 2522
- Serax Tablets ... 2522

Oxybutynin Chloride (Paralytic ileus). Products include:
- Ditropan ... 1332

Oxycodone Hydrochloride (Effect not specified). Products include:
- Percocet Tablets ... 950
- Percodan ... 951
- Roxicodone Tablets, Oral Solution & Intensol (Oxycodone) ... 1992
- Tylox Capsules ... 1382

Pargyline Hydrochloride (May potentiate pseudoephedrine's pressor effect; may result in a hypertensive crisis).
- No products indexed under this heading.

Penbutolol Sulfate (Increased pressor effect of pseudoephedrine). Products include:
- Levatol ... 1832

Pentobarbital Sodium (Effect not specified). Products include:
- Nembutal Sodium Capsules ... 534
- Nembutal Sodium Solution ... 536
- Nembutal Sodium Suppositories ... 538

Perphenazine (Effect not specified). Products include:
- Etrafon ... 2087
- Triavil Tablets ... 1556
- Trilafon ... 2123

Phenelzine Sulfate (May potentiate pseudoephedrine's pressor effect; may result in a hypertensive crisis). Products include:
- Nardil ... 1742

Phenobarbital (Effect not specified). Products include:
- Arco-Lase Plus Tablets ... 607
- Bellergal-S Tablets ... 1998
- Bronkolixir ... [ND] 761
- Bronkotabs Tablets ... [ND] 762
- Donnatal ... 1858
- Donnatal Extentabs ... 1859
- Donnatal Tablets ... 1858
- Donnazyme Tablets ... 1860
- Kinesed Tablets ... 2272
- Phenobarbital Elixir and Tablets ... 1293
- Primatene Tablets-P Formula ... 2421
- Quadrinal Tablets ... 1183
- Tedral SA ... 1765

Phenylephrine Bitartrate (Increased effect of either agent; increased potential for side effects).
- No products indexed under this heading.

Phenylephrine Hydrochloride (Increased effect of either agent; increased potential for side effects). Products include:
- AK-Dilate Solution 2.5% and 10% ... ◉ 203
- Atrohist Sprinkle Capsules ... 558
- Cerose-DM ... 2443
- Codimal ... 846
- Comhist LA Capsules ... 1618
- Congespirin For Children Aspirin Free Chewable Cold Tablets ... 748
- Cyclomydril ... ◉ 216
- Deconsal Sprinkle Capsules ... 559
- Dimetane Decongestant ... [ND] 673
- Dristan Decongestant/Antihistamine/ Analgesic Coated Caplets ... [ND] 749
- Dristan Cold Nasal Decongestant/ Antihistamine/ Analgesic Coated Tablets ... 2419
- Dristan Advanced Formula Decongestant/Antihistamine/ Analgesic Tablets ... [ND] 749
- Dristan Nasal Spray, Menthol ... 2419
- Dristan Nasal Spray, Regular and Regular with Metered Pump ... 2419
- Entex Capsules ... 1623
- Entex Liquid ... 1623
- Sinus Excedrin Analgesic, Decongestant Tablets & Caplets ... 750
- Extendryl ... 994
- 4-Way Fast Acting Nasal Spray - Original Formula (regular & menth’olated) & Metered Spray Pump (regular) ... 751
- Hycomine Compound Tablets ... 929
- Murocoll-2 Sterile Ophthalmic Solution ... ◉ 261
- Mydfrin 2.5% ... ◉ 224
- Naldecon Syrup, Tablets, Pediatric Drops and Pediatric Syrup ... 709
- Neo-Synephrine Hydrochloride 1% Carpuject ... 2063
- Neo-Synephrine Hydrochloride 1% Injection ... 2063
- Neo-Synephrine Hydrochloride (Ophthalmic) ... 2064
- Neo-Synephrine ... [ND] 759
- Nōstril Nasal Decongestant ... [ND] 520
- Novahistine Elixir ... [ND] 596
- Phenergan VC ... 2500
- Phenergan VC with Codeine ... 2501
- Prefrin Liquifilm Vasoconstrictor and Lubricant Eye Drops ... ◉ 254
- Prefrin-A ... ◉ 255
- Quelidrine Syrup ... 556
- Relief Vasoconstrictor and Lubricant Eye Drops ... ◉ 256
- Robitussin Night Relief ... [ND] 677
- Ru-Tuss with Hydrocodone ... 694
- Ru-Tuss Tablets ... 693
- Vasosulf ... ◉ 279
- Vicks Sinex ... [ND] 665
- Zincfrin ... ◉ 230

Phenylephrine Tannate (Increased effect of either agent; increased potential for side effects). Products include:
- Rynatan ... 2387
- Rynatuss ... 2388

Phenylpropanolamine Hydrochloride (Increased effect of either agent; increased potential for side effects). Products include:
- A.R.M. Allergy Relief Medicine Caplets ... [ND] 615
- Acutrim ... [ND] 548
- Allerest ... [ND] 559
- BC Cold Powder ... [ND] 517
- Cheracol Plus Head Cold/Cough Formula ... [ND] 667
- Codimal Expectorant ... 846
- Comtrex Multi-Symptom Cold Reliever Tablets/Caplets/Liqui-Gels/Liquid ... 745
- Contac Continuous Action Decongestant/Antihistamine Capsules [ND] 710
- Contac Maximum Strength Continuous Action Decongestant/ Antihistamine Caplets ... [ND] 709
- Contac Severe Cold and Flu Formula Caplets ... [ND] 711
- Coricidin 'D' Decongestant Tablets ... [ND] 695
- Coricidin Demilets Tablets for Children ... [ND] 696
- Demazin Nasal Decongestant/ Antihistamine Repetabs Tablets & Syrup ... [ND] 697
- Dexatrim ... [ND] 733
- Dimetane-DC Cough Syrup ... 1857
- Dimetapp Elixir ... [ND] 673
- Dimetapp DM Elixir ... [ND] 674
- Dimetapp Extentabs ... [ND] 674
- Dimetapp Plus Caplets ... [ND] 675
- Dimetapp Tablets ... [ND] 675
- Entex Capsules ... 1623
- Entex LA Tablets ... 1623
- Entex Liquid ... 1623
- 4-Way Cold Tablets ... 750
- Hycomine Syrup ... 927
- Naldecon CX Adult Liquid ... [ND] 521
- Naldecon DX Adult Liquid ... [ND] 521
- Naldecon DX Children's Syrup ... [ND] 522
- Naldecon DX Pediatric Drops ... [ND] 522
- Naldecon EX Children's Syrup ... [ND] 522
- Naldecon EX Pediatric Drops ... [ND] 523
- Naldecon Syrup, Tablets, Pediatric Drops and Pediatric Syrup ... 709
- Nolamine Tablets ... 838
- Nolex LA Tablets ... 838
- Ornade Spansule Capsules ... 2221
- Orthoxicol Cough Syrup ... [ND] 668
- Propagest ... 839
- Pyrroxate Capsules ... [ND] 669
- Robitussin-CF ... [ND] 676
- Ru-Tuss II Capsules ... 693
- Ru-Tuss with Hydrocodone ... 694
- Ru-Tuss Tablets ... 693
- Sine-Off Sinus Medicine Tablets-Aspirin Formula ... [ND] 722
- Sinulin ... 840
- St. Joseph Cold Tablets for Children ... [ND] 704
- Tavist-D Tablets ... 2035
- Triaminic Allergy Tablets ... [ND] 688
- Triaminic Chewables ... [ND] 688
- Triaminic Cold Tablets ... [ND] 688
- Triaminic Expectorant ... [ND] 688
- Triaminic Expectorant w/Codeine ... 1996
- Triaminic Expectorant DH ... 1995
- Triaminic Oral Infant Drops ... 1996
- Triaminic Syrup ... [ND] 689
- Triaminic-12 Tablets ... [ND] 690
- Triaminic-DM Syrup ... [ND] 689
- Triaminicin Tablets ... [ND] 690
- Triaminicol Multi-Symptom Cold Tablets ... [ND] 691
- Triaminicol Multi-Symptom Relief [ND] 691
- Tuss-Ornade Liquid ... 2242
- Tuss-Ornade Spansule Capsules ... 2242
- Tylenol Cold Medication, Effervescent Tablets ... 1369

Pindolol (Increased pressor effect of pseudoephedrine side effects). Products include:
- Visken Tablets ... 2036

Pirbuterol Acetate (Increased effect of either agent; increased potential for side effects). Products include:
- Maxair Inhaler ... 1311

Potassium Iodide (Effect not specified). Products include:
- Hyland's C-Plus Cold Tablets ... [ND] 728
- Pima Syrup ... 994
- Quadrinal Tablets ... 1183

Prazepam (Effect not specified). Products include:
- Centrax ... 1693

Prochlorperazine (Effect not specified). Products include:
- Compazine ... 2201

Procyclidine Hydrochloride (Paralytic ileus). Products include:
- Kemadrin Tablets ... 771

Promethazine Hydrochloride (Effect not specified). Products include:
- Mepergan Injection ... 2479
- Phenergan with Codeine ... 2497
- Phenergan with Dextromethorphan 2499
- Phenergan Injection ... 2493
- Phenergan Suppositories ... 2496
- Phenergan Syrup ... 2495
- Phenergan Tablets ... 2496
- Phenergan VC ... 2500
- Phenergan VC with Codeine ... 2501

Propantheline Bromide (Paralytic ileus). Products include:
- Pro-Banthīne Tablets ... 2141

Propofol (Effect not specified). Products include:
- Diprivan Injection ... 2267

Propoxyphene Hydrochloride (Effect not specified). Products include:
- Darvon ... 1256
- Wygesic Tablets ... 2540

Propoxyphene Napsylate (Effect not specified). Products include:
- Darvon-N/Darvocet-N ... 1254

Propranolol Hydrochloride (Increased pressor effect of pseudoephedrine). Products include:
- Inderal ... 2459
- Inderal LA Long Acting Capsules ... 2461
- Inderide Tablets ... 2463
- Inderide LA Long Acting Capsules ... 2465

Protriptyline Hydrochloride (May antagonize effects of pseudoephedrine; increased effect of antidepressants or the codeine component). Products include:
- Vivactil Tablets ... 1567

Pseudoephedrine Sulfate (Increased effect of either agent; increased potential for side effects). Products include:
- Afrin Tablets ... ▣ 693
- Chlor-Trimeton Decongestant ... ▣ 694
- Disophrol Chronotab Sustained-Action Tablets ... ▣ 698
- Drixoral Antihistamine/Nasal Decongestant Syrup ... ▣ 698
- Drixoral Non-Drowsy Formula ... ▣ 699
- Drixoral Plus Extended-Release Tablets ... ▣ 699
- Drixoral Sinus ... ▣ 700
- Drixoral Sustained-Action Tablets ▣ 698
- Sinutab Allergy Formula Sustained Action Tablets ... ▣ 640
- Trinalin Repetabs Tablets ... 1170

Quazepam (Effect not specified). Products include:
- Doral Tablets ... 2383

Scopolamine Hydrobromide (Paralytic ileus). Products include:
- Donnagel ... ▣ 675
- Donnagel-PG ... 1858
- Donnatal ... 1858
- Donnatal Extentabs ... 1859
- Donnatal Tablets ... 1858
- Donnazyme Tablets ... 1860
- Isopto Hyoscine ... ◉ 222
- Murocoll-2 Sterile Ophthalmic Solution ... ◉ 261
- Ru-Tuss Tablets ... 693

Scopolamine Preparations (Paralytic ileus). Products include:
- Transderm Scōp Transdermal Therapeutic System ... 887

Secobarbital Sodium (Effect not specified). Products include:
- Seconal Sodium Pulvules ... 1296

Sufentanil Citrate (Effect not specified). Products include:
- Sufenta Injection ... 1147

Temazepam (Effect not specified). Products include:
- Restoril Capsules ... 2023

Terbutaline Sulfate (Increased effect of either agent; increased potential for side effects). Products include:
- Brethaire Inhaler ... 1024
- Brethine Ampuls ... 1026
- Brethine Tablets ... 1026
- Bricanyl Injection ... 1324
- Bricanyl Tablets ... 1325

Thiamylal Sodium (Effect not specified). Products include:
- Surital Ampoules, Steri-Vials ... 1764

Thioridazine Hydrochloride (Effect not specified). Products include:
- Mellaril ... 2011

Thiothixene (Effect not specified). Products include:
- Navane Capsules and Concentrate 1954
- Navane Intramuscular ... 1956

Timolol Maleate (Increased pressor effect of pseudoephedrine). Products include:
- Blocadren Tablets ... 1429
- Timolide Tablets ... 1547
- Timoptic in Ocudose ... 1552
- Timoptic Sterile Ophthalmic Solution ... 1550

Tranylcypromine Sulfate (May potentiate pseudoephedrine's pressor effect; may result in a hypertensive crisis). Products include:
- Parnate Tablets ... 2222

Triazolam (Effect not specified). Products include:
- Halcion Tablets ... 2340

Tridihexethyl Chloride (Paralytic ileus).
- No products indexed under this heading.

Trifluoperazine Hydrochloride (Effect not specified). Products include:
- Stelazine ... 2226

Trihexyphenidyl Hydrochloride (Paralytic ileus). Products include:
- Artane ... 1195

Trimipramine Maleate (May antagonize effects of pseudoephedrine; increased effect of antidepressants or the codeine component). Products include:
- Surmontil Capsules ... 2524

NUCOFED EXPECTORANT (Codeine Phosphate, Pseudoephedrine Hydrochloride, Guaifenesin) ... 2219

May interact with beta blockers, cardiac glycosides, veratrum alkaloids, monoamine oxidase inhibitors, sympathomimetic aerosal brochodilators, tricyclic antidepressants, central nervous system depressants, narcotic analgesics, general anesthetics, anticholinergics, and certain other agents. Compounds in these categories include:

Acebutolol Hydrochloride (Increased pressor effect of pseudoephedrine). Products include:
- Sectral Capsules ... 2520

Albuterol (Increased effect of either agent; increased potential for side effects). Products include:
- Proventil Inhalation Aerosol ... 2117
- Ventolin Inhalation Aerosol and Refill ... 583

Albuterol Sulfate (Increased effect of either agent; increased potential for side effects). Products include:
- Proventil Repetabs Tablets ... 2120
- Proventil Solutions for Inhalation 0.5% and 0.083% ... 2118
- Proventil Syrup ... 2119
- Proventil Tablets ... 2120
- Ventolin ... 583

Alcohol (Effect not specified).

Alfentanil Hydrochloride (Effect not specified). Products include:
- Alfenta Injection ... 1131

Alprazolam (Effect not specified). Products include:
- Xanax Tablets ... 2367

Amitriptyline Hydrochloride (May antagonize effects of pseudoephedrine; increased effects of antidepressants or the codeine component). Products include:
- Elavil ... 2269
- Endep Tablets ... 1927
- Etrafon ... 2087
- Limbitrol ... 1933
- Triavil Tablets ... 1556

Amoxapine (May antagonize effects of pseudoephedrine; increased effects of antidepressants or the codeine component). Products include:
- Asendin Tablets ... 1196

Aprobarbital (Effect not specified). Products include:
- Alurate Elixir ... 1883

Atenolol (Increased pressor effect of pseudoephedrine). Products include:
- Tenoretic Tablets ... 1105
- Tenormin Tablets and I.V. Injection 1107

Atropine Sulfate (Paralytic ileus). Products include:
- Arco-Lase Plus Tablets ... 607
- Atropine Sulfate Sterile Ophthalmic Solution and S.O.P. Sterile Ophthalmic Ointment ... ◉ 239
- Donnagel ... ▣ 675
- Donnagel-PG ... 1858
- Donnatal ... 1858
- Donnatal Extentabs ... 1859
- Donnatal Tablets ... 1858
- Donnazyme Tablets ... 1860
- Isopto Atropine ... ◉ 218
- Lomotil ... 2174
- Motofen Tablets ... 836
- Ru-Tuss Tablets ... 693
- Urised Tablets ... 2396

Belladonna Alkaloids (Paralytic ileus). Products include:
- Bellergal-S Tablets ... 1998
- Hyland's Bed Wetting Tablets ... ▣ 728
- Hyland's Teething Tablets ... ▣ 728
- Kinesed Tablets ... 2272

Benztropine Mesylate (Paralytic ileus). Products include:
- Cogentin ... 1435

Betaxolol Hydrochloride (Increased pressor effect of pseudoephedrine). Products include:
- Betoptic Sterile Ophthalmic Solution ... 569
- Betoptic S Sterile Ophthalmic Suspension ... 570
- Kerlone Tablets ... 2172

Biperiden (Paralytic ileus). Products include:
- Akineton ... 1171

Buprenorphine (Effect not specified).
- No products indexed under this heading.

Buspirone Hydrochloride (Effect not specified). Products include:
- BuSpar ... 1401

Butabarbital (Effect not specified). Products include:
- Pyridium Plus ... 1764

Butalbital (Effect not specified). Products include:
- Esgic-Plus Tablets ... 1002
- Esgic Tablets & Capsules ... 1001
- Fioricet Tablets ... 2006
- Fiorinal Capsules ... 2007
- Fiorinal with Codeine Capsules ... 2008
- Fiorinal Tablets ... 2007
- Phrenilin ... 838
- Sedapap Tablets 50 mg/650 mg .. 1360

Carteolol Hydrochloride (Increased pressor effect of pseudoephedrine). Products include:
- Cartrol Tablets ... 507

Chlordiazepoxide (Effect not specified). Products include:
- Libritabs Tablets ... 1930
- Limbitrol ... 1933
- Menrium Tablets ... 1934

Chlordiazepoxide Hydrochloride (Effect not specified). Products include:
- Librax Capsules ... 1929
- Librium Capsules ... 1931
- Librium Injectable ... 1932

Chlorpromazine (Effect not specified). Products include:
- Thorazine ... 2234

Chlorprothixene (Effect not specified). Products include:
- Taractan Tablets ... 1920

Chlorprothixene Hydrochloride (Effect not specified). Products include:
- Taractan ... 1920

Clidinium Bromide (Paralytic ileus). Products include:
- Librax Capsules ... 1929
- Quarzan Capsules ... 1937

Clomipramine Hydrochloride (May antagonize effects of pseudoephedrine; increased effects of antidepressants or the codeine component). Products include:
- Anafranil Capsules ... 650

Clorazepate Dipotassium (Effect not specified). Products include:
- Tranxene ... 556

Codeine (Effect not specified). Products include:
- Calcidrine Syrup ... 506

Codeine Polistirex (Effect not specified).
- No products indexed under this heading.

Cryptenamine Preparations (Decreased hypotensive effect).

Desipramine Hydrochloride (May antagonize effects of pseudoephedrine; increased effects of antidepressants or the codeine component). Products include:
- Norpramin Tablets ... 1340

Deslanoside (Increased possibility of cardiac arrhythmias).
- No products indexed under this heading.

Dezocine (Effect not specified).

Diazepam (Effect not specified). Products include:
- Valium Injectable ... 1937
- Valium Tablets ... 1939
- Valrelease Capsules ... 1923

Dicyclomine Hydrochloride (Paralytic ileus). Products include:
- Bentyl ... 1322

Digitoxin (Increased possibility of cardiac arrhythmias). Products include:
- Crystodigin Tablets ... 1253

Digoxin (Increased possibility of cardiac arrhythmias). Products include:
- Lanoxicaps ... 772
- Lanoxin Elixir Pediatric ... 775
- Lanoxin Injection ... 778
- Lanoxin Injection Pediatric ... 781
- Lanoxin Tablets ... 783

Dobutamine Hydrochloride (Increased effect of either agent; increased potential for side effects). Products include:
- Dobutrex Solution Vials ... 1259

Dopamine Hydrochloride (Increased effect of either agent; increased potential for side effects). Products include:
- Intropin Injection ... 930

Doxepin Hydrochloride (May antagonize effects of pseudoephedrine; increased effects of antidepressants or the codeine component). Products include:
- Sinequan ... 1960

Droperidol (Effect not specified). Products include:
- Inapsine Injection ... 1140
- Innovar Injection ... 1141

Enflurane (Effect not specified). Products include:
- Ethrane ... 599

Ephedrine Hydrochloride (Increased effect of either agent; increased potential for side effects). Products include:
- Amesec ... ▣ 682
- Primatene Tablets-M Formula ... 2421
- Primatene Tablets-P Formula ... 2421
- Primatene Tablets-Regular Formula ... 2421
- Quadrinal Tablets ... 1183
- Quelidrine Syrup ... 556
- Tedral SA ... 1765

Ephedrine Sulfate (Increased effect of either agent; increased potential for side effects). Products include:
- Bronkaid Tablets ... ▣ 757
- Bronkolixir ... ▣ 761
- Bronkotabs Tablets ... ▣ 762
- Marax Tablets & DF Syrup ... 1954
- Pazo Hemorrhoid Ointment & Suppositories ... 752
- Vicks Vatronol Nose Drops ... ▣ 666

Ephedrine Tannate (Increased effect of either agent; increased potential for side effects). Products include:
Rynatuss ... 2388

Epinephrine (Increased effect of either agent; increased potential for side effects). Products include:
Ana-Kit Anaphylaxis Emergency Treatment Kit ... 1100
Bronkaid Mist ... ⊞ 757
EpiPen ... 843
Marcaine Hydrochloride 0.5% with Epinephrine 1:200,000 (as bitartrate) ... 958
Marcaine Hydrochloride with Epinephrine 1:200,000 ... 2055
Primatene Mist ... 2420
Sus-Phrine Injection ... 1006
Xylocaine with Epinephrine Injections ... 637

Epinephrine Bitartrate (Increased effect of either agent; increased potential for side effects). Products include:
AsthmaHaler Mist Epinephrine Bitartrate Bronchodilator ... ⊞ 616
Bronkaid Mist Suspension ... ⊞ 757
Primatene Mist Suspension ... 2421

Epinephrine Hydrochloride (Increased effect of either agent; increased potential for side effects). Products include:
Adrenalin Chloride Solution 1:100 & 1:1,000 ... 1689
Epifrin ... ◉ 244
Glaucon ... ◉ 218

Esmolol Hydrochloride (Increased pressor effect of pseudoephedrine). Products include:
Brevibloc Injection ... 942

Estazolam (Effect not specified). Products include:
ProSom Tablets ... 554

Ethchlorvynol (Effect not specified). Products include:
Placidyl Capsules ... 553

Ethinamate (Effect not specified).
No products indexed under this heading.

Ethopropazine Hydrochloride (Paralytic ileus).

Fentanyl (Effect not specified). Products include:
Duragesic Transdermal System ... 1133

Fentanyl Citrate (Effect not specified). Products include:
Innovar Injection ... 1141
Sublimaze Injection ... 1146

Fluphenazine Decanoate (Effect not specified). Products include:
Prolixin Decanoate ... 1795

Fluphenazine Enanthate (Effect not specified). Products include:
Prolixin Enanthate ... 1796

Fluphenazine Hydrochloride (Effect not specified). Products include:
Prolixin Elixir ... 1793
Prolixin Injection ... 1791
Prolixin Oral Concentrate ... 1792
Prolixin Tablets ... 1793

Flurazepam Hydrochloride (Effect not specified). Products include:
Dalmane Capsules ... 1927

Furazolidone (May potentiate pseudoephedrine's pressor effect; may result in hypertensive crisis). Products include:
Furoxone ... 1855

Glutethimide (Effect not specified).
No products indexed under this heading.

Glycopyrrolate (Paralytic ileus). Products include:
Robinul Forte Tablets ... 1873
Robinul Injectable ... 1873
Robinul Tablets ... 1873

Haloperidol (Effect not specified). Products include:
Haldol Injection, Tablets and Concentrate ... 1373

Haloperidol Decanoate (Effect not specified). Products include:
Haldol Decanoate ... 1375

Hydrocodone Bitartrate (Effect not specified). Products include:
Anexsia 5/500 Tablets ... 2196
Anexsia 7.5/650 Tablets ... 2197
Azdone Tablets ... 844
Codiclear DH Syrup ... 845
Codimal DH Syrup ... 846
Damason-P ... 1356
Hycodan Syrup, Tablets ... 927
Hycomine Compound Tablets ... 929
Hycomine Syrup ... 927
Hycotuss Expectorant Syrup ... 930
Hydrocet Capsules ... 835
Lortab ASA Tablets ... 2414
Lortab ... 2412
Ru-Tuss with Hydrocodone ... 694
Triaminic Expectorant DH ... 1995
Vicodin Tablets ... 1187
Vicodin ES Tablets ... 1189
Zydone Capsules ... 941

Hydrocodone Polistirex (Effect not specified). Products include:
Tussionex Extended-Release Suspension ... 988

Hydroxyzine Hydrochloride (Effect not specified). Products include:
Atarax Tablets & Syrup ... 1941
Marax Tablets & DF Syrup ... 1954
Vistaril Intramuscular Solution ... 1970

Hyoscyamine (Paralytic ileus). Products include:
Cystospaz Tablets ... 2395
Urised Tablets ... 2396

Hyoscyamine Sulfate (Paralytic ileus). Products include:
Arco-Lase Plus Tablets ... 607
Cystospaz-M Capsules ... 2395
Donnagel ... ⊞ 675
Donnagel-PG ... 1858
Donnatal ... 1858
Donnatal Extentabs ... 1859
Donnatal Tablets ... 1858
Donnazyme Tablets ... 1860
Kutrase Capsules ... 2146
Levsin/Levsinex ... 2147
Ru-Tuss Tablets ... 693

Imipramine Hydrochloride (May antagonize effects of pseudoephedrine; increased effects of antidepressants or the codeine component). Products include:
Tofranil Ampuls ... 1038
Tofranil Tablets ... 1039

Imipramine Pamoate (May antagonize effects of pseudoephedrine; increased effects of antidepressants or the codeine component). Products include:
Tofranil-PM Capsules ... 1041

Ipratropium Bromide (Paralytic ileus). Products include:
Atrovent Inhalation Aerosol ... 675

Isocarboxazid (May potentiate pseudoephedrine's pressor effect; may result in hypertensive crisis). Products include:
Marplan Tablets ... 1906

Isoflurane (Effect not specified). Products include:
Forane ... 600

Isoproterenol Hydrochloride (Increased effect of either agent; increased potential for side effects). Products include:
Isuprel Hydrochloride Injection 1:5000 ... 2050
Isuprel Hydrochloride Mistometer .. 2051
Isuprel Hydrochloride Solution 1:200 & 1:100 ... 2052
Norisodrine Aerotrol ... 540

Ketamine Hydrochloride (Effect not specified). Products include:
Ketalar ... 1726

Labetalol Hydrochloride (Increased pressor effect of pseudoephedrine). Products include:
Normodyne Injection ... 2108
Normodyne Tablets ... 2110
Normozide Tablets ... 2112
Trandate HCT Tablets ... 579
Trandate Injection ... 577
Trandate Tablets ... 579

Levorphanol Tartrate (Effect not specified). Products include:
Levo-Dromoran ... 1906

Lorazepam (Effect not specified). Products include:
Ativan Injection ... 2432
Ativan Tablets ... 2434

Loxapine Hydrochloride (Effect not specified). Products include:
Loxitane ... 1213

Loxapine Succinate (Effect not specified). Products include:
Loxitane Capsules ... 1213

Maprotiline Hydrochloride (May antagonize effects of pseudoephedrine; increased effects of antidepressants or the codeine component). Products include:
Ludiomil Tablets ... 874

Mepenzolate Bromide (Paralytic ileus). Products include:
Cantil Tablets ... 1326

Meperidine Hydrochloride (Effect not specified). Products include:
Demerol ... 2047
Mepergan Injection ... 2479

Mephobarbital (Effect not specified). Products include:
Mebaral Tablets ... 2061

Meprobamate (Effect not specified). Products include:
Deprol Tablets ... 2382
Equagesic Tablets ... 2451
Miltown Tablets ... 2386
PMB 200 and PMB 400 ... 2504

Mesoridazine (Effect not specified). Products include:
Serentil ... 686

Metaproterenol Sulfate (Increased effect of either agent; increased potential for side effects). Products include:
Alupent ... 674
Arm-a-Med Metaproterenol Sulfate Inhalation Solution, USP ... 617
Metaprel Inhalation Aerosol Bronchodilator ... 2014
Metaprel Inhalation Solution ... 2015
Metaprel ... 2015
Metaproterenol Sulfate Inhalation Solution, USP ... 912

Metaraminol Bitartrate (Increased effect of either agent; increased potential for side effects). Products include:
Aramine Injection ... 1424

Methadone Hydrochloride (Effect not specified). Products include:
Dolophine Hydrochloride Ampoules & Vials ... 1260
Dolophine Hydrochloride Tablets 1261
Methadone Hydrochloride Diskets .. 1284
Methadone Hydrochloride Oral Solution & Tablets ... 1987

Methohexital Sodium (Effect not specified). Products include:
Brevital Sodium Vials ... 1248

Methoxamine Hydrochloride (Increased effect of either agent; increased potential for side effects). Products include:
Vasoxyl Injection ... 819

Methoxyflurane (Effect not specified).
No products indexed under this heading.

Metoprolol Tartrate (Increased pressor effect of pseudoephedrine). Products include:
Lopressor Ampuls ... 1032
Lopressor HCT Tablets ... 1034
Lopressor Tablets ... 1032

Midazolam Hydrochloride (Effect not specified). Products include:
Versed Injection ... 1924

Molindone Hydrochloride (Effect not specified). Products include:
Moban Tablets & Concentrate ... 932

Morphine Sulfate (Effect not specified). Products include:
Astramorph/PF Injection, USP (Preservative-Free) ... 618
Duramorph ... 960
Infumorph 200 and Infumorph 500 Sterile Solutions ... 962
MS Contin Tablets ... 1814
MSIR ... 1817
Oramorph SR (Morphine Sulfate Sustained Release Tablets) ... 1988
Roxanol ... 1991

Nadolol (Increased pressor effect of pseudoephedrine). Products include:
Corgard Tablets ... 701
Corzide Tablets ... 702

Norepinephrine Bitartrate (Increased effect of either agent; increased potential for side effects). Products include:
Levophed Bitartrate Injection ... 2054

Nortriptyline Hydrochloride (May antagonize effects of pseudoephedrine; increased effects of antidepressants or the codeine component). Products include:
Pamelor ... 2019

Opium Alkaloids (Effect not specified). Products include:
B & O No. 15A & No. 16A Supprettes ... 2395
Pantopon Injectable ... 1911

Oxazepam (Effect not specified). Products include:
Serax Capsules ... 2522
Serax Tablets ... 2522

Oxybutynin Chloride (Paralytic ileus). Products include:
Ditropan ... 1332

Oxycodone Hydrochloride (Effect not specified). Products include:
Percocet Tablets ... 950
Percodan ... 951
Roxicodone Tablets, Oral Solution & Intensol (Oxycodone) ... 1992
Tylox Capsules ... 1382

Penbutolol Sulfate (Increased pressor effect of pseudoephedrine). Products include:
Levatol ... 1832

Pentobarbital Sodium (Effect not specified). Products include:
Nembutal Sodium Capsules ... 534
Nembutal Sodium Solution ... 536
Nembutal Sodium Suppositories ... 538

Perphenazine (Effect not specified). Products include:
Etrafon ... 2087
Triavil Tablets ... 1556
Trilafon ... 2123

Phenelzine Sulfate (May potentiate pseudoephedrine's pressor effect; may result in hypertensive crisis). Products include:
Nardil ... 1742

Phenobarbital (Effect not specified). Products include:
Arco-Lase Plus Tablets ... 607
Bellergal-S Tablets ... 1998
Bronkolixir ... ⊞ 761
Bronkotabs Tablets ... ⊞ 762
Donnatal ... 1858
Donnatal Extentabs ... 1859
Donnatal Tablets ... 1858
Donnazyme Tablets ... 1860
Kinesed Tablets ... 2272
Phenobarbital Elixir and Tablets ... 1293
Primatene Tablets-P Formula ... 2421
Quadrinal Tablets ... 1183
Tedral SA ... 1765

Phenylephrine Bitartrate (Increased effect of either agent; increased potential for side effects).
No products indexed under this heading.

Phenylephrine Hydrochloride (Increased effect of either agent; increased potential for side effects). Products include:
AK-Dilate Solution 2.5% and 10% ⊙ 203
Atrohist Sprinkle Capsules 558
Cerose-DM 2443
Codimal 846
Comhist LA Capsules 1618
Congespirin For Children Aspirin Free Chewable Cold Tablets 748
Cyclomydril ⊙ 216
Deconsal Sprinkle Capsules 559
Dimetane Decongestant ▣ 673
Dristan Decongestant/Antihistamine/ Analgesic Coated Caplets ▣ 749
Dristan Cold Nasal Decongestant/ Antihistamine/ Analgesic Coated Tablets 2419
Dristan Advanced Formula Decongestant/Antihistamine/ Analgesic Tablets ▣ 749
Dristan Nasal Spray, Menthol 2419
Dristan Nasal Spray, Regular and Regular with Metered Pump 2419
Entex Capsules 1623
Entex Liquid 1623
Sinus Excedrin Analgesic, Decongestant Tablets & Caplets 750
Extendryl 994
4-Way Fast Acting Nasal Spray - Original Formula (regular & mentholated) & Metered Spray Pump (regular) 751
Hycomine Compound Tablets 929
Murocoll-2 Sterile Ophthalmic Solution ⊙ 261
Mydfrin 2.5% ⊙ 224
Naldecon Syrup, Tablets, Pediatric Drops and Pediatric Syrup 709
Neo-Synephrine Hydrochloride 1% Carpuject 2063
Neo-Synephrine Hydrochloride 1% Injection 2063
Neo-Synephrine Hydrochloride (Ophthalmic) 2064
Neo-Synephrine ▣ 759
Nōstril Nasal Decongestant ▣ 520
Novahistine Elixir ▣ 596
Phenergan VC 2500
Phenergan VC with Codeine 2501
Prefrin Liquifilm Vasoconstrictor and Lubricant Eye Drops ⊙ 254
Prefrin-A ⊙ 255
Quelidrine Syrup 556
Relief Vasoconstrictor and Lubricant Eye Drops ⊙ 256
Robitussin Night Relief ▣ 677
Ru-Tuss with Hydrocodone 694
Ru-Tuss Tablets 693
Vasosulf ⊙ 279
Vicks Sinex ▣ 665
Zincfrin ⊙ 230

Phenylephrine Tannate (Increased effect of either agent; increased potential for side effects). Products include:
Rynatan 2387
Rynatuss 2388

Phenylpropanolamine Hydrochloride (Increased effect of either agent; increased potential for side effects). Products include:
A.R.M. Allergy Relief Medicine Caplets ▣ 615
Acutrim ▣ 548
Allerest ▣ 559
BC Cold Powder ▣ 517
Cheracol Plus Head Cold/Cough Formula ▣ 667
Codimal Expectorant 846
Comtrex Multi-Symptom Cold Reliever Tablets/Caplets/Liqui-Gels/Liquid 745
Contac Continuous Action Decongestant/Antihistamine Capsules ▣ 710
Contac Maximum Strength Continuous Action Decongestant/ Antihistamine Caplets ▣ 709
Contac Severe Cold and Flu Formula Caplets ▣ 711
Coricidin 'D' Decongestant Tablets ▣ 695
Coricidin Demilets Tablets for Children ▣ 696
Demazin Nasal Decongestant/ Antihistamine Repetabs Tablets & Syrup ▣ 697
Dexatrim ▣ 733
Dimetane-DC Cough Syrup 1857
Dimetapp Elixir ▣ 673
Dimetapp DM Elixir ▣ 674
Dimetapp Extentabs ▣ 674
Dimetapp Plus Caplets ▣ 675
Dimetapp Tablets ▣ 675
Entex Capsules 1623
Entex LA Tablets 1623
Entex Liquid 1623
4-Way Cold Tablets 750
Hycomine Syrup 927
Naldecon CX Adult Liquid ▣ 521
Naldecon DX Adult Liquid ▣ 521
Naldecon DX Children's Syrup ▣ 522
Naldecon DX Pediatric Drops ▣ 522
Naldecon EX Children's Syrup ▣ 522
Naldecon EX Pediatric Drops ▣ 523
Naldecon Syrup, Tablets, Pediatric Drops and Pediatric Syrup 709
Nolamine Tablets 838
Nolex LA Tablets 838
Ornade Spansule Capsules 2221
Orthoxicol Cough Syrup ▣ 668
Propagest 839
Pyrroxate Capsules ▣ 669
Robitussin-CF ▣ 676
Ru-Tuss II Capsules 693
Ru-Tuss with Hydrocodone 694
Ru-Tuss Tablets 693
Sine-Off Sinus Medicine Tablets-Aspirin Formula ▣ 722
Sinulin 840
St. Joseph Cold Tablets for Children ▣ 704
Tavist-D Tablets 2035
Triaminic Allergy Tablets ▣ 688
Triaminic Chewables ▣ 688
Triaminic Cold Tablets ▣ 688
Triaminic Expectorant ▣ 688
Triaminic Expectorant w/Codeine 1996
Triaminic Expectorant DH 1995
Triaminic Oral Infant Drops 1996
Triaminic Syrup ▣ 689
Triaminic-12 Tablets ▣ 690
Triaminic-DM Syrup ▣ 689
Triaminicin Tablets ▣ 690
Triaminicol Multi-Symptom Cold Tablets ▣ 691
Triaminicol Multi-Symptom Relief ▣ 691
Tuss-Ornade Liquid 2242
Tuss-Ornade Spansule Capsules 2242
Tylenol Cold Medication, Effervescent Tablets 1369

Pindolol (Increased pressor effect of pseudoephedrine side effects). Products include:
Visken Tablets 2036

Pirbuterol Acetate (Increased effect of either agent; increased potential for side effects). Products include:
Maxair Inhaler 1311

Prazepam (Effect not specified). Products include:
Centrax 1693

Prochlorperazine (Effect not specified). Products include:
Compazine 2201

Procyclidine Hydrochloride (Paralytic ileus). Products include:
Kemadrin Tablets 771

Promethazine Hydrochloride (Effect not specified). Products include:
Mepergan Injection 2479
Phenergan with Codeine 2497
Phenergan with Dextromethorphan 2499
Phenergan Injection 2493
Phenergan Suppositories 2496
Phenergan Syrup 2495
Phenergan Tablets 2496
Phenergan VC 2500
Phenergan VC with Codeine 2501

Propantheline Bromide (Paralytic ileus). Products include:
Pro-Banthīne Tablets 2141

Propofol (Effect not specified). Products include:
Diprivan Injection 2267

Propoxyphene Hydrochloride (Effect not specified). Products include:
Darvon 1256
Wygesic Tablets 2540

Propoxyphene Napsylate (Effect not specified). Products include:
Darvon-N/Darvocet-N 1254

Propranolol Hydrochloride (Increased pressor effect of pseudoephedrine). Products include:
Inderal 2459
Inderal LA Long Acting Capsules 2461
Inderide Tablets 2463
Inderide LA Long Acting Capsules 2465

Protriptyline Hydrochloride (May antagonize effects of pseudoephedrine; increased effects of antidepressants or the codeine component). Products include:
Vivactil Tablets 1567

Pseudoephedrine Sulfate (Increased effect of either agent; increased potential for side effects). Products include:
Afrin Tablets ▣ 693
Chlor-Trimeton Decongestant ▣ 694
Disophrol Chronotab Sustained-Action Tablets ▣ 698
Drixoral Antihistamine/Nasal Decongestant Syrup ▣ 698
Drixoral Non-Drowsy Formula ▣ 699
Drixoral Plus Extended-Release Tablets ▣ 699
Drixoral Sinus ▣ 700
Drixoral Sustained-Action Tablets ▣ 698
Sinutab Allergy Formula Sustained Action Tablets ▣ 640
Trinalin Repetabs Tablets 1170

Quazepam (Effect not specified). Products include:
Doral Tablets 2383

Scopolamine Hydrobromide (Paralytic ileus). Products include:
Donnagel ▣ 675
Donnagel-PG 1858
Donnatal 1858
Donnatal Extentabs 1859
Donnatal Tablets 1858
Donnazyme Tablets 1860
Isopto Hyoscine ⊙ 222
Murocoll-2 Sterile Ophthalmic Solution ⊙ 261
Ru-Tuss Tablets 693

Scopolamine Preparations (Paralytic ileus). Products include:
Transderm Scōp Transdermal Therapeutic System 887

Secobarbital Sodium (Effect not specified). Products include:
Seconal Sodium Pulvules 1296

Selegiline Hydrochloride (May potentiate pseudoephedrine's pressor effect; may result in hypertensive crisis). Products include:
Eldepryl 2250

Sufentanil Citrate (Effect not specified). Products include:
Sufenta Injection 1147

Temazepam (Effect not specified). Products include:
Restoril Capsules 2023

Terbutaline Sulfate (Increased effect of either agent; increased potential for side effects). Products include:
Brethaire Inhaler 1024
Brethine Ampuls 1026
Brethine Tablets 1026
Bricanyl Injection 1324
Bricanyl Tablets 1325

Thiamylal Sodium (Effect not specified). Products include:
Surital Ampoules, Steri-Vials 1764

Thioridazine Hydrochloride (Effect not specified). Products include:
Mellaril 2011

Thiothixene (Effect not specified). Products include:
Navane Capsules and Concentrate 1954
Navane Intramuscular 1956

Timolol Maleate (Increased pressor effect of pseudoephedrine). Products include:
Blocadren Tablets 1429
Timolide Tablets 1547
Timoptic in Ocudose 1552
Timoptic Sterile Ophthalmic Solution 1550

Tranylcypromine Sulfate (May potentiate pseudoephedrine's pressor effect; may result in hypertensive crisis). Products include:
Parnate Tablets 2222

Triazolam (Effect not specified). Products include:
Halcion Tablets 2340

Tridihexethyl Chloride (Paralytic ileus).
No products indexed under this heading.

Trifluoperazine Hydrochloride (Effect not specified). Products include:
Stelazine 2226

Trihexyphenidyl Hydrochloride (Paralytic ileus). Products include:
Artane 1195

Trimipramine Maleate (May antagonize effects of pseudoephedrine; increased effects of antidepressants or the codeine component). Products include:
Surmontil Capsules 2524

NUCOFED PEDIATRIC EXPECTORANT

(Codeine Phosphate, Pseudoephedrine Hydrochloride, Guaifenesin) 2220

May interact with beta blockers, cardiac glycosides, monoamine oxidase inhibitors, sympathomimetic aerosal brochodilators, tricyclic antidepressants, central nervous system depressants, general anesthetics, anticholinergics, veratrum alkaloids, and certain other agents. Compounds in these categories include:

Acebutolol Hydrochloride (Increased pressor effect of pseudoephedrine). Products include:
Sectral Capsules 2520

Albuterol (Increased effect of either agent; increased potential for side effects). Products include:
Proventil Inhalation Aerosol 2117
Ventolin Inhalation Aerosol and Refill 583

Albuterol Sulfate (Increased effect of either agent; increased potential for side effects). Products include:
Proventil Repetabs Tablets 2120
Proventil Solutions for Inhalation 0.5% and 0.083% 2118
Proventil Syrup 2119
Proventil Tablets 2120
Ventolin 583

Alcohol (Effect not specified).

Alfentanil Hydrochloride (Effect not specified). Products include:
Alfenta Injection 1131

Alprazolam (Effect not specified). Products include:
Xanax Tablets 2367

Amitriptyline Hydrochloride (May antagonize effects of pseudoephedrine; increased effects of antidepressants or the codeine component). Products include:
Elavil 2269
Endep Tablets 1927
Etrafon 2087
Limbitrol 1933
Triavil Tablets 1556

Amoxapine (May antagonize effects of pseudoephedrine; increased effects of antidepressants or the codeine component). Products include:
- Asendin Tablets ... 1196

Aprobarbital (Effect not specified). Products include:
- Alurate Elixir ... 1883

Atenolol (Increased pressor effect of pseudoephedrine). Products include:
- Tenoretic Tablets ... 1105
- Tenormin Tablets and I.V. Injection 1107

Atropine Sulfate (Paralytic ileus). Products include:
- Arco-Lase Plus Tablets ... 607
- Atropine Sulfate Sterile Ophthalmic Solution and S.O.P. Sterile Ophthalmic Ointment ... ◉ 239
- Donnagel ... ⊞ 675
- Donnagel-PG ... 1858
- Donnatal ... 1858
- Donnatal Extentabs ... 1859
- Donnatal Tablets ... 1858
- Donnazyme Tablets ... 1860
- Isopto Atropine ... ◉ 218
- Lomotil ... 2174
- Motofen Tablets ... 836
- Ru-Tuss Tablets ... 693
- Urised Tablets ... 2396

Belladonna Alkaloids (Paralytic ileus). Products include:
- Bellergal-S Tablets ... 1998
- Hyland's Bed Wetting Tablets ... ⊞ 728
- Hyland's Teething Tablets ... ⊞ 728
- Kinesed Tablets ... 2272

Benztropine Mesylate (Paralytic ileus). Products include:
- Cogentin ... 1435

Betaxolol Hydrochloride (Increased pressor effect of pseudoephedrine). Products include:
- Betoptic Sterile Ophthalmic Solution ... 569
- Betoptic S Sterile Ophthalmic Suspension ... 570
- Kerlone Tablets ... 2172

Biperiden (Paralytic ileus). Products include:
- Akineton ... 1171

Buprenorphine (Effect not specified).
- No products indexed under this heading.

Buspirone Hydrochloride (Effect not specified). Products include:
- BuSpar ... 1401

Butabarbital (Effect not specified). Products include:
- Pyridium Plus ... 1764

Butalbital (Effect not specified). Products include:
- Esgic-Plus Tablets ... 1002
- Esgic Tablets & Capsules ... 1001
- Fioricet Tablets ... 2006
- Fiorinal Capsules ... 2007
- Fiorinal with Codeine Capsules ... 2008
- Fiorinal Tablets ... 2007
- Phrenilin ... 838
- Sedapap Tablets 50 mg/650 mg .. 1360

Carteolol Hydrochloride (Increased pressor effect of pseudoephedrine). Products include:
- Cartrol Tablets ... 507

Chlordiazepoxide (Effect not specified). Products include:
- Libritabs Tablets ... 1930
- Limbitrol ... 1933
- Menrium Tablets ... 1934

Chlordiazepoxide Hydrochloride (Effect not specified). Products include:
- Librax Capsules ... 1929
- Librium Capsules ... 1931
- Librium Injectable ... 1932

Chlorpromazine (Effect not specified). Products include:
- Thorazine ... 2234

Chlorprothixene (Effect not specified). Products include:
- Taractan Tablets ... 1920

Chlorprothixene Hydrochloride (Effect not specified). Products include:
- Taractan ... 1920

Clidinium Bromide (Paralytic ileus). Products include:
- Librax Capsules ... 1929
- Quarzan Capsules ... 1937

Clomipramine Hydrochloride (May antagonize effects of pseudoephedrine; increased effects of antidepressants or the codeine component). Products include:
- Anafranil Capsules ... 650

Clorazepate Dipotassium (Effect not specified). Products include:
- Tranxene ... 556

Codeine (Effect not specified). Products include:
- Calcidrine Syrup ... 506

Codeine Polistirex (Effect not specified).
- No products indexed under this heading.

Cryptenamine Preparations (Decreased hypotensive effect).

Desipramine Hydrochloride (May antagonize effects of pseudoephedrine; increased effects of antidepressants or the codeine component). Products include:
- Norpramin Tablets ... 1340

Deslanoside (Increased possibility of cardiac arrhythmias).
- No products indexed under this heading.

Dezocine (Effect not specified).

Diazepam (Effect not specified). Products include:
- Valium Injectable ... 1937
- Valium Tablets ... 1939
- Valrelease Capsules ... 1923

Dicyclomine Hydrochloride (Paralytic ileus). Products include:
- Bentyl ... 1322

Digitoxin (Increased possibility of cardiac arrhythmias). Products include:
- Crystodigin Tablets ... 1253

Digoxin (Increased possibility of cardiac arrhythmias). Products include:
- Lanoxicaps ... 772
- Lanoxin Elixir Pediatric ... 775
- Lanoxin Injection ... 778
- Lanoxin Injection Pediatric ... 781
- Lanoxin Tablets ... 783

Dobutamine Hydrochloride (Increased effect of either agent; increased potential for side effects). Products include:
- Dobutrex Solution Vials ... 1259

Dopamine Hydrochloride (Increased effect of either agent; increased potential for side effects). Products include:
- Intropin Injection ... 930

Doxepin Hydrochloride (May antagonize effects of pseudoephedrine; increased effects of antidepressants or the codeine component). Products include:
- Sinequan ... 1960

Droperidol (Effect not specified). Products include:
- Inapsine Injection ... 1140
- Innovar Injection ... 1141

Enflurane (Effect not specified). Products include:
- Ethrane ... 599

Ephedrine Hydrochloride (Increased effect of either agent; increased potential for side effects). Products include:
- Amesec ... ⊞ 682
- Primatene Tablets-M Formula ... 2421
- Primatene Tablets-P Formula ... 2421
- Primatene Tablets-Regular Formula ... 2421
- Quadrinal Tablets ... 1183
- Quelidrine Syrup ... 556
- Tedral SA ... 1765

Ephedrine Sulfate (Increased effect of either agent; increased potential for side effects). Products include:
- Bronkaid Tablets ... ⊞ 757
- Bronkolixir ... ⊞ 761
- Bronkotabs Tablets ... ⊞ 762
- Marax Tablets & DF Syrup ... 1954
- Pazo Hemorrhoid Ointment & Suppositories ... 752
- Vicks Vatronol Nose Drops ... ⊞ 666

Ephedrine Tannate (Increased effect of either agent; increased potential for side effects). Products include:
- Rynatuss ... 2388

Epinephrine (Increased effect of either agent; increased potential for side effects). Products include:
- Ana-Kit Anaphylaxis Emergency Treatment Kit ... 1100
- Bronkaid Mist ... ⊞ 757
- EpiPen ... 843
- Marcaine Hydrochloride 0.5% with Epinephrine 1:200,000 (as bitartrate) ... 958
- Marcaine Hydrochloride with Epinephrine 1:200,000 ... 2055
- Primatene Mist ... 2420
- Sus-Phrine Injection ... 1006
- Xylocaine with Epinephrine Injections ... 637

Epinephrine Bitartrate (Increased effect of either agent; increased potential for side effects). Products include:
- AsthmaHaler Mist Epinephrine Bitartrate Bronchodilator ... ⊞ 616
- Bronkaid Mist Suspension ... ⊞ 757
- Primatene Mist Suspension ... 2421

Epinephrine Hydrochloride (Increased effect of either agent; increased potential for side effects). Products include:
- Adrenalin Chloride Solution 1:100 & 1:1,000 ... 1689
- Epifrin ... ◉ 244
- Glaucon ... ◉ 218

Esmolol Hydrochloride (Increased pressor effect of pseudoephedrine). Products include:
- Brevibloc Injection ... 942

Estazolam (Effect not specified). Products include:
- ProSom Tablets ... 554

Ethchlorvynol (Effect not specified). Products include:
- Placidyl Capsules ... 553

Ethinamate (Effect not specified).
- No products indexed under this heading.

Ethopropazine Hydrochloride (Paralytic ileus).

Fentanyl (Effect not specified). Products include:
- Duragesic Transdermal System ... 1133

Fentanyl Citrate (Effect not specified). Products include:
- Innovar Injection ... 1141
- Sublimaze Injection ... 1146

Fluphenazine Decanoate (Effect not specified). Products include:
- Prolixin Decanoate ... 1795

Fluphenazine Enanthate (Effect not specified). Products include:
- Prolixin Enanthate ... 1796

Fluphenazine Hydrochloride (Effect not specified). Products include:
- Prolixin Elixir ... 1793
- Prolixin Injection ... 1791
- Prolixin Oral Concentrate ... 1792
- Prolixin Tablets ... 1793

Flurazepam Hydrochloride (Effect not specified). Products include:
- Dalmane Capsules ... 1927

Furazolidone (May potentiate pseudoephedrine's pressor effect; may result in hypertensive crisis). Products include:
- Furoxone ... 1855

Glutethimide (Effect not specified).
- No products indexed under this heading.

Glycopyrrolate (Paralytic ileus). Products include:
- Robinul Forte Tablets ... 1873
- Robinul Injectable ... 1873
- Robinul Tablets ... 1873

Haloperidol (Effect not specified). Products include:
- Haldol Injection, Tablets and Concentrate ... 1373

Haloperidol Decanoate (Effect not specified). Products include:
- Haldol Decanoate ... 1375

Hydrocodone Bitartrate (Effect not specified). Products include:
- Anexsia 5/500 Tablets ... 2196
- Anexsia 7.5/650 Tablets ... 2197
- Azdōne Tablets ... 844
- Codiclear DH Syrup ... 845
- Codimal DH Syrup ... 846
- Damason-P ... 1356
- Hycodan Syrup, Tablets ... 927
- Hycomine Compound Tablets ... 929
- Hycomine Syrup ... 927
- Hycotuss Expectorant Syrup ... 930
- Hydrocet Capsules ... 835
- Lortab ASA Tablets ... 2414
- Lortab ... 2412
- Ru-Tuss with Hydrocodone ... 694
- Triaminic Expectorant DH ... 1995
- Vicodin Tablets ... 1187
- Vicodin ES Tablets ... 1189
- Zydone Capsules ... 941

Hydrocodone Polistirex (Effect not specified). Products include:
- Tussionex Extended-Release Suspension ... 988

Hydroxyzine Hydrochloride (Effect not specified). Products include:
- Atarax Tablets & Syrup ... 1941
- Marax Tablets & DF Syrup ... 1954
- Vistaril Intramuscular Solution ... 1970

Hyoscyamine (Paralytic ileus). Products include:
- Cystospaz Tablets ... 2395
- Urised Tablets ... 2396

Hyoscyamine Sulfate (Paralytic ileus). Products include:
- Arco-Lase Plus Tablets ... 607
- Cystospaz-M Capsules ... 2395
- Donnagel ... ⊞ 675
- Donnagel-PG ... 1858
- Donnatal ... 1858
- Donnatal Extentabs ... 1859
- Donnatal Tablets ... 1858
- Donnazyme Tablets ... 1860
- Kutrase Capsules ... 2146
- Levsin/Levsinex ... 2147
- Ru-Tuss Tablets ... 693

Imipramine Hydrochloride (May antagonize effects of pseudoephedrine; increased effects of antidepressants or the codeine component). Products include:
- Tofranil Ampuls ... 1038
- Tofranil Tablets ... 1039

Imipramine Pamoate (May antagonize effects of pseudoephedrine; increased effects of antidepressants or the codeine component). Products include:
- Tofranil-PM Capsules ... 1041

Ipratropium Bromide (Paralytic ileus). Products include:
- Atrovent Inhalation Aerosol ... 675

Isocarboxazid (May potentiate pseudoephedrine's pressor effect; may result in hypertensive crisis). Products include:
- Marplan Tablets 1906

Isoflurane (Effect not specified). Products include:
- Forane 600

Isoproterenol Hydrochloride (Increased effect of either agent; increased potential for side effects). Products include:
- Isuprel Hydrochloride Injection 1:5000 2050
- Isuprel Hydrochloride Mistometer .. 2051
- Isuprel Hydrochloride Solution 1:200 & 1:100 2052
- Norisodrine Aerotrol 540

Ketamine Hydrochloride (Effect not specified). Products include:
- Ketalar 1726

Labetalol Hydrochloride (Increased pressor effect of pseudoephedrine). Products include:
- Normodyne Injection 2108
- Normodyne Tablets 2110
- Normozide Tablets 2112
- Trandate HCT Tablets 579
- Trandate Injection 577
- Trandate Tablets 579

Levorphanol Tartrate (Effect not specified). Products include:
- Levo-Dromoran 1906

Lorazepam (Effect not specified). Products include:
- Ativan Injection 2432
- Ativan Tablets 2434

Loxapine Hydrochloride (Effect not specified). Products include:
- Loxitane 1213

Loxapine Succinate (Effect not specified). Products include:
- Loxitane Capsules 1213

Maprotiline Hydrochloride (May antagonize effects of pseudoephedrine; increased effects of antidepressants or the codeine component). Products include:
- Ludiomil Tablets 874

Mepenzolate Bromide (Paralytic ileus). Products include:
- Cantil Tablets 1326

Meperidine Hydrochloride (Effect not specified). Products include:
- Demerol 2047
- Mepergan Injection 2479

Mephobarbital (Effect not specified). Products include:
- Mebaral Tablets 2061

Meprobamate (Effect not specified). Products include:
- Deprol Tablets 2382
- Equagesic Tablets 2451
- Miltown Tablets 2386
- PMB 200 and PMB 400 2504

Mesoridazine (Effect not specified). Products include:
- Serentil 686

Metaproterenol Sulfate (Increased effect of either agent; increased potential for side effects). Products include:
- Alupent 674
- Arm-a-Med Metaproterenol Sulfate Inhalation Solution, USP 617
- Metaprel Inhalation Aerosol Bronchodilator 2014
- Metaprel Inhalation Solution 2015
- Metaprel 2015
- Metaproterenol Sulfate Inhalation Solution, USP 912

Metaraminol Bitartrate (Increased effect of either agent; increased potential for side effects). Products include:
- Aramine Injection 1424

Methadone Hydrochloride (Effect not specified). Products include:
- Dolophine Hydrochloride Ampoules & Vials 1260
- Dolophine Hydrochloride Tablets 1261
- Methadone Hydrochloride Diskets .. 1284
- Methadone Hydrochloride Oral Solution & Tablets 1987

Methohexital Sodium (Effect not specified). Products include:
- Brevital Sodium Vials 1248

Methoxamine Hydrochloride (Increased effect of either agent; increased potential for side effects). Products include:
- Vasoxyl Injection 819

Methoxyflurane (Effect not specified).
- No products indexed under this heading.

Metoprolol Tartrate (Increased pressor effect of pseudoephedrine). Products include:
- Lopressor Ampuls 1032
- Lopressor HCT Tablets 1034
- Lopressor Tablets 1032

Midazolam Hydrochloride (Effect not specified). Products include:
- Versed Injection 1924

Molindone Hydrochloride (Effect not specified). Products include:
- Moban Tablets & Concentrate 932

Morphine Sulfate (Effect not specified). Products include:
- Astramorph/PF Injection, USP (Preservative-Free) 618
- Duramorph 960
- Infumorph 200 and Infumorph 500 Sterile Solutions 962
- MS Contin Tablets 1814
- MSIR 1817
- Oramorph SR (Morphine Sulfate Sustained Release Tablets) 1988
- Roxanol 1991

Nadolol (Increased pressor effect of pseudoephedrine). Products include:
- Corgard Tablets 701
- Corzide Tablets 702

Norepinephrine Bitartrate (Increased effect of either agent; increased potential for side effects). Products include:
- Levophed Bitartrate Injection 2054

Nortriptyline Hydrochloride (May antagonize effects of pseudoephedrine; increased effects of antidepressants or the codeine component). Products include:
- Pamelor 2019

Opium Alkaloids (Effect not specified). Products include:
- B & O No. 15A & No. 16A Supprettes 2395
- Pantopon Injectable 1911

Oxazepam (Effect not specified). Products include:
- Serax Capsules 2522
- Serax Tablets 2522

Oxybutynin Chloride (Paralytic ileus). Products include:
- Ditropan 1332

Oxycodone Hydrochloride (Effect not specified). Products include:
- Percocet Tablets 950
- Percodan 951
- Roxicodone Tablets, Oral Solution & Intensol (Oxycodone) 1992
- Tylox Capsules 1382

Penbutolol Sulfate (Increased pressor effect of pseudoephedrine). Products include:
- Levatol 1832

Pentobarbital Sodium (Effect not specified). Products include:
- Nembutal Sodium Capsules 534
- Nembutal Sodium Solution 536
- Nembutal Sodium Suppositories 538

Perphenazine (Effect not specified). Products include:
- Etrafon 2087
- Triavil Tablets 1556
- Trilafon 2123

Phenelzine Sulfate (May potentiate pseudoephedrine's pressor effect; may result in hypertensive crisis). Products include:
- Nardil 1742

Phenobarbital (Effect not specified). Products include:
- Arco-Lase Plus Tablets 607
- Bellergal-S Tablets 1998
- Bronkolixir .... ▣ 761
- Bronkotabs Tablets .... ▣ 762
- Donnatal 1858
- Donnatal Extentabs 1859
- Donnatal Tablets 1858
- Donnazyme Tablets 1860
- Kinesed Tablets 2272
- Phenobarbital Elixir and Tablets 1293
- Primatene Tablets-P Formula 2421
- Quadrinal Tablets 1183
- Tedral SA 1765

Phenylephrine Bitartrate (Increased effect of either agent; increased potential for side effects).
- No products indexed under this heading.

Phenylephrine Hydrochloride (Increased effect of either agent; increased potential for side effects). Products include:
- AK-Dilate Solution 2.5% and 10% .... ◉ 203
- Atrohist Sprinkle Capsules 558
- Cerose-DM 2443
- Codimal 846
- Comhist LA Capsules 1618
- Congespirin For Children Aspirin Free Chewable Cold Tablets 748
- Cyclomydril .... ◉ 216
- Deconsal Sprinkle Capsules 559
- Dimetane Decongestant .... ▣ 673
- Dristan Decongestant/Antihistamine/ Analgesic Coated Caplets .... ▣ 749
- Dristan Cold Nasal Decongestant/ Antihistamine/ Analgesic Coated Tablets 2419
- Dristan Advanced Formula Decongestant/Antihistamine/ Analgesic Tablets .... ▣ 749
- Dristan Nasal Spray, Menthol 2419
- Dristan Nasal Spray, Regular and Regular with Metered Pump 2419
- Entex Capsules 1623
- Entex Liquid 1623
- Sinus Excedrin Analgesic, Decongestant Tablets & Caplets 750
- Extendryl 994
- 4-Way Fast Acting Nasal Spray - Original Formula (regular & mentholated) & Metered Spray Pump (regular) 751
- Hycomine Compound Tablets 929
- Murocoll-2 Sterile Ophthalmic Solution .... ◉ 261
- Mydfrin 2.5% .... ◉ 224
- Naldecon Syrup, Tablets, Pediatric Drops and Pediatric Syrup 709
- Neo-Synephrine Hydrochloride 1% Carpuject 2063
- Neo-Synephrine Hydrochloride 1% Injection 2063
- Neo-Synephrine Hydrochloride (Ophthalmic) 2064
- Neo-Synephrine .... ▣ 759
- Nōstril Nasal Decongestant .... ▣ 520
- Novahistine Elixir .... ▣ 596
- Phenergan VC 2500
- Phenergan VC with Codeine 2501
- Prefrin Liquifilm Vasoconstrictor and Lubricant Eye Drops .... ◉ 254
- Prefrin-A .... ◉ 255
- Quelidrine Syrup 556
- Relief Vasoconstrictor and Lubricant Eye Drops .... ◉ 256
- Robitussin Night Relief .... ▣ 677
- Ru-Tuss with Hydrocodone 694
- Ru-Tuss Tablets 693
- Vasosulf .... ◉ 279
- Vicks Sinex .... ▣ 665
- Zincfrin .... ◉ 230

Phenylephrine Tannate (Increased effect of either agent; increased potential for side effects). Products include:
- Rynatan 2387
- Rynatuss 2388

Phenylpropanolamine Hydrochloride (Increased effect of either agent; increased potential for side effects). Products include:
- A.R.M. Allergy Relief Medicine Caplets .... ▣ 615
- Acutrim .... ▣ 548
- Allerest .... ▣ 559
- BC Cold Powder .... ▣ 517
- Cheracol Plus Head Cold/Cough Formula .... ▣ 667
- Codimal Expectorant 846
- Comtrex Multi-Symptom Cold Reliever Tablets/Caplets/Liqui-Gels/Liquid 745
- Contac Continuous Action Decongestant/Antihistamine Capsules ▣ 710
- Contac Maximum Strength Continuous Action Decongestant/ Antihistamine Caplets .... ▣ 709
- Contac Severe Cold and Flu Formula Caplets .... ▣ 711
- Coricidin 'D' Decongestant Tablets .... ▣ 695
- Coricidin Demilets Tablets for Children .... ▣ 696
- Demazin Nasal Decongestant/ Antihistamine Repetabs Tablets & Syrup .... ▣ 697
- Dexatrim .... ▣ 733
- Dimetane-DC Cough Syrup 1857
- Dimetapp Elixir .... ▣ 673
- Dimetapp DM Elixir .... ▣ 674
- Dimetapp Extentabs .... ▣ 674
- Dimetapp Plus Caplets .... ▣ 675
- Dimetapp Tablets .... ▣ 675
- Entex Capsules 1623
- Entex LA Tablets 1623
- Entex Liquid 1623
- 4-Way Cold Tablets 750
- Hycomine Syrup 927
- Naldecon CX Adult Liquid .... ▣ 521
- Naldecon DX Adult Liquid .... ▣ 521
- Naldecon DX Children's Syrup .... ▣ 522
- Naldecon DX Pediatric Drops .... ▣ 522
- Naldecon EX Children's Syrup .... ▣ 522
- Naldecon EX Pediatric Drops .... ▣ 523
- Naldecon Syrup, Tablets, Pediatric Drops and Pediatric Syrup 709
- Nolamine Tablets 838
- Nolex LA Tablets 838
- Ornade Spansule Capsules 2221
- Orthoxicol Cough Syrup .... ▣ 668
- Propagest 839
- Pyrroxate Capsules .... ▣ 669
- Robitussin-CF .... ▣ 676
- Ru-Tuss II Capsules 693
- Ru-Tuss with Hydrocodone 694
- Ru-Tuss Tablets 693
- Sine-Off Sinus Medicine Tablets-Aspirin Formula .... ▣ 722
- Sinulin 840
- St. Joseph Cold Tablets for Children .... ▣ 704
- Tavist-D Tablets 2035
- Triaminic Allergy Tablets .... ▣ 688
- Triaminic Chewables .... ▣ 688
- Triaminic Cold Tablets .... ▣ 688
- Triaminic Expectorant .... ▣ 688
- Triaminic Expectorant w/Codeine .. 1996
- Triaminic Expectorant DH 1995
- Triaminic Oral Infant Drops 1996
- Triaminic Syrup .... ▣ 689
- Triaminic-12 Tablets .... ▣ 690
- Triaminic-DM Syrup .... ▣ 689
- Triaminicin Tablets .... ▣ 690
- Triaminicol Multi-Symptom Cold Tablets .... ▣ 691
- Triaminicol Multi-Symptom Relief ▣ 691
- Tuss-Ornade Liquid 2242
- Tuss-Ornade Spansule Capsules 2242
- Tylenol Cold Medication, Effervescent Tablets 1369

Pindolol (Increased pressor effect of pseudoephedrine side effects). Products include:
- Visken Tablets 2036

Pirbuterol Acetate (Increased effect of either agent; increased potential for side effects). Products include:
- Maxair Inhaler 1311

Prazepam (Effect not specified). Products include:
- Centrax 1693

Prochlorperazine (Effect not specified). Products include:
- Compazine 2201

Procyclidine Hydrochloride (Paralytic ileus). Products include:
- Kemadrin Tablets ... 771

Promethazine Hydrochloride (Effect not specified). Products include:
- Mepergan Injection ... 2479
- Phenergan with Codeine ... 2497
- Phenergan with Dextromethorphan 2499
- Phenergan Injection ... 2493
- Phenergan Suppositories ... 2496
- Phenergan Syrup ... 2495
- Phenergan Tablets ... 2496
- Phenergan VC ... 2500
- Phenergan VC with Codeine ... 2501

Propantheline Bromide (Paralytic ileus). Products include:
- Pro-Banthīne Tablets ... 2141

Propofol (Effect not specified). Products include:
- Diprivan Injection ... 2267

Propoxyphene Hydrochloride (Effect not specified). Products include:
- Darvon ... 1256
- Wygesic Tablets ... 2540

Propoxyphene Napsylate (Effect not specified). Products include:
- Darvon-N/Darvocet-N ... 1254

Propranolol Hydrochloride (Increased pressor effect of pseudoephedrine). Products include:
- Inderal ... 2459
- Inderal LA Long Acting Capsules ... 2461
- Inderide Tablets ... 2463
- Inderide LA Long Acting Capsules ... 2465

Protriptyline Hydrochloride (May antagonize effects of pseudoephedrine; increased effects of antidepressants or the codeine component). Products include:
- Vivactil Tablets ... 1567

Pseudoephedrine Sulfate (Increased effect of either agent; increased potential for side effects). Products include:
- Afrin Tablets ... ▣ 693
- Chlor-Trimeton Decongestant ... ▣ 694
- Disophrol Chronotab Sustained-Action Tablets ... ▣ 698
- Drixoral Antihistamine/Nasal Decongestant Syrup ... ▣ 698
- Drixoral Non-Drowsy Formula ... ▣ 699
- Drixoral Plus Extended-Release Tablets ... ▣ 699
- Drixoral Sinus ... ▣ 700
- Drixoral Sustained-Action Tablets ▣ 698
- Sinutab Allergy Formula Sustained Action Tablets ... ▣ 640
- Trinalin Repetabs Tablets ... 1170

Quazepam (Effect not specified). Products include:
- Doral Tablets ... 2383

Scopolamine Hydrobromide (Paralytic ileus). Products include:
- Donnagel ... ▣ 675
- Donnagel-PG ... 1858
- Donnatal ... 1858
- Donnatal Extentabs ... 1859
- Donnatal Tablets ... 1858
- Donnazyme Tablets ... 1860
- Isopto Hyoscine ... ⊙ 222
- Murocoll-2 Sterile Ophthalmic Solution ... ⊙ 261
- Ru-Tuss Tablets ... 693

Scopolamine Preparations (Paralytic ileus). Products include:
- Transderm Scōp Transdermal Therapeutic System ... 887

Secobarbital Sodium (Effect not specified). Products include:
- Seconal Sodium Pulvules ... 1296

Selegiline Hydrochloride (May potentiate pseudoephedrine's pressor effect; may result in hypertensive crisis). Products include:
- Eldepryl ... 2250

Sufentanil Citrate (Effect not specified). Products include:
- Sufenta Injection ... 1147

Temazepam (Effect not specified). Products include:
- Restoril Capsules ... 2023

Terbutaline Sulfate (Increased effect of either agent; increased potential for side effects). Products include:
- Brethaire Inhaler ... 1024
- Brethine Ampuls ... 1026
- Brethine Tablets ... 1026
- Bricanyl Injection ... 1324
- Bricanyl Tablets ... 1325

Thiamylal Sodium (Effect not specified). Products include:
- Surital Ampoules, Steri-Vials ... 1764

Thioridazine Hydrochloride (Effect not specified). Products include:
- Mellaril ... 2011

Thiothixene (Effect not specified). Products include:
- Navane Capsules and Concentrate 1954
- Navane Intramuscular ... 1956

Timolol Maleate (Increased pressor effect of pseudoephedrine). Products include:
- Blocadren Tablets ... 1429
- Timolide Tablets ... 1547
- Timoptic in Ocudose ... 1552
- Timoptic Sterile Ophthalmic Solution ... 1550

Tranylcypromine Sulfate (May potentiate pseudoephedrine's pressor effect; may result in hypertensive crisis). Products include:
- Parnate Tablets ... 2222

Triazolam (Effect not specified). Products include:
- Halcion Tablets ... 2340

Tridihexethyl Chloride (Paralytic ileus).
- No products indexed under this heading.

Trifluoperazine Hydrochloride (Effect not specified). Products include:
- Stelazine ... 2226

Trihexyphenidyl Hydrochloride (Paralytic ileus). Products include:
- Artane ... 1195

Trimipramine Maleate (May antagonize effects of pseudoephedrine; increased effects of antidepressants or the codeine component). Products include:
- Surmontil Capsules ... 2524

NUCOFED SYRUP
(Codeine Phosphate, Pseudoephedrine Hydrochloride) ...2219
See **Nucofed Capsules**

NU-IRON 150 CAPS
(Iron Polysaccharide Complex) ...1359
No interactions described in labeling.

NU-IRON ELIXIR
(Iron Polysaccharide Complex) ...1359
No interactions described in labeling.

NULLO DEODORANT TABLETS
(Chlorophyllin Copper Complex) ... ▣ 547
No interactions described in labeling.

NULYTELY
(Polyethylene Glycol) ... 699
May interact with:

Oral Medications (Oral medications may not be absorbed if given within one hour).

Food Interactions

Food, unspecified (Solid food should not be given for at least two hours before the solution is given).

NUMORPHAN HYDROCHLORIDE INJECTION
(Oxymorphone Hydrochloride) ... 935
May interact with general anesthetics, hypnotics and sedatives, narcotic analgesics, phenothiazines, tranquilizers, and certain other agents. Compounds in these categories include:

Alcohol (Additive CNS depression).

Alfentanil Hydrochloride (Additive CNS depression). Products include:
- Alfenta Injection ... 1131

Alprazolam (Additive CNS depression). Products include:
- Xanax Tablets ... 2367

Buprenorphine (Additive CNS depression).
- No products indexed under this heading.

Buspirone Hydrochloride (Additive CNS depression). Products include:
- BuSpar ... 1401

Chlordiazepoxide (Additive CNS depression). Products include:
- Libritabs Tablets ... 1930
- Limbitrol ... 1933
- Menrium Tablets ... 1934

Chlordiazepoxide Hydrochloride (Additive CNS depression). Products include:
- Librax Capsules ... 1929
- Librium Capsules ... 1931
- Librium Injectable ... 1932

Chlorpromazine (Additive CNS depression). Products include:
- Thorazine ... 2234

Clorazepate Dipotassium (Additive CNS depression). Products include:
- Tranxene ... 556

Codeine (Additive CNS depression). Products include:
- Calcidrine Syrup ... 506

Codeine Phosphate (Additive CNS depression). Products include:
- Actifed with Codeine Cough Syrup.. 752
- Cheracol Cough Syrup ... 1853
- Codimal PH Syrup ... 846
- Dimetane-DC Cough Syrup ... 1857
- Empirin with Codeine Phosphate Nos. 2, 3 & 4 ... 764
- Fiorinal with Codeine Capsules ... 2008
- Isoclor Expectorant ... 982
- Naldecon CX Adult Liquid ... ▣ 521
- Novahistine DH ... 1342
- Novahistine Expectorant ... 1343
- Nucofed Capsules ... 2219
- Nucofed Expectorant ... 2219
- Nucofed Pediatric Expectorant ... 2220
- Nucofed Syrup ... 2219
- Phenaphen with Codeine Capsules 1865
- Phenaphen-650 with Codeine Tablets ... 1866
- Phenergan with Codeine ... 2497
- Phenergan VC with Codeine ... 2501
- Robitussin A-C Syrup ... 1875
- Robitussin-DAC Syrup ... 1875
- Ryna ... ▣ 741
- Soma Compound w/Codeine Tablets ... 2390
- Triaminic Expectorant w/Codeine .. 1996
- Tussi-Organidin Liquid ... 2391
- Tylenol with Codeine ... 1381

Codeine Polistirex (Additive CNS depression).
- No products indexed under this heading.

Dezocine (Additive CNS depression).

Diazepam (Additive CNS depression). Products include:
- Valium Injectable ... 1937
- Valium Tablets ... 1939
- Valrelease Capsules ... 1923

Droperidol (Additive CNS depression). Products include:
- Inapsine Injection ... 1140
- Innovar Injection ... 1141

Enflurane (Additive CNS depression). Products include:
- Ethrane ... 599

Estazolam (Additive CNS depression). Products include:
- ProSom Tablets ... 554

Ethchlorvynol (Additive CNS depression). Products include:
- Placidyl Capsules ... 553

Ethinamate (Additive CNS depression).
- No products indexed under this heading.

Fentanyl (Additive CNS depression). Products include:
- Duragesic Transdermal System ... 1133

Fentanyl Citrate (Additive CNS depression). Products include:
- Innovar Injection ... 1141
- Sublimaze Injection ... 1146

Fluphenazine Decanoate (Additive CNS depression). Products include:
- Prolixin Decanoate ... 1795

Fluphenazine Enanthate (Additive CNS depression). Products include:
- Prolixin Enanthate ... 1796

Fluphenazine Hydrochloride (Additive CNS depression). Products include:
- Prolixin Elixir ... 1793
- Prolixin Injection ... 1791
- Prolixin Oral Concentrate ... 1792
- Prolixin Tablets ... 1793

Flurazepam Hydrochloride (Additive CNS depression). Products include:
- Dalmane Capsules ... 1927

Glutethimide (Additive CNS depression).
- No products indexed under this heading.

Haloperidol (Additive CNS depression). Products include:
- Haldol Injection, Tablets and Concentrate ... 1373

Haloperidol Decanoate (Additive CNS depression). Products include:
- Haldol Decanoate ... 1375

Hydrocodone Bitartrate (Additive CNS depression). Products include:
- Anexsia 5/500 Tablets ... 2196
- Anexsia 7.5/650 Tablets ... 2197
- Azdone Tablets ... 844
- Codiclear DH Syrup ... 845
- Codimal DH Syrup ... 846
- Damason-P ... 1356
- Hycodan Syrup, Tablets ... 927
- Hycomine Compound Tablets ... 929
- Hycomine Syrup ... 927
- Hycotuss Expectorant Syrup ... 930
- Hydrocet Capsules ... 835
- Lortab ASA Tablets ... 2414
- Lortab ... 2412
- Ru-Tuss with Hydrocodone ... 694
- Triaminic Expectorant DH ... 1995
- Vicodin Tablets ... 1187
- Vicodin ES Tablets ... 1189
- Zydone Capsules ... 941

Hydrocodone Polistirex (Additive CNS depression). Products include:
- Tussionex Extended-Release Suspension ... 988

Hydroxyzine Hydrochloride (Additive CNS depression). Products include:
- Atarax Tablets & Syrup ... 1941
- Marax Tablets & DF Syrup ... 1954
- Vistaril Intramuscular Solution ... 1970

Isoflurane (Additive CNS depression). Products include:
- Forane ... 600

Levorphanol Tartrate (Additive CNS depression). Products include:
- Levo-Dromoran ... 1906

Morphine Sulfate (Additive CNS depression). Products include:
- Astramorph/PF Injection, USP (Preservative-Free) ... 618
- Duramorph ... 960
- Infumorph 200 and Infumorph 500 Sterile Solutions ... 962
- MS Contin Tablets ... 1814
- MSIR ... 1817
- Oramorph SR (Morphine Sulfate Sustained Release Tablets) ... 1988
- Roxanol ... 1991

Opium Alkaloids (Additive CNS depression). Products include:
- B & O No. 15A & No. 16A Supprettes ... 2395
- Pantopon Injectable ... 1911

Oxazepam (Additive CNS depression). Products include:
- Serax Capsules ... 2522
- Serax Tablets ... 2522

Oxycodone Hydrochloride (Additive CNS depression). Products include:
- Percocet Tablets ... 950
- Percodan ... 951
- Roxicodone Tablets, Oral Solution & Intensol (Oxycodone) ... 1992
- Tylox Capsules ... 1382

Perphenazine (Additive CNS depression). Products include:
- Etrafon ... 2087
- Triavil Tablets ... 1556
- Trilafon ... 2123

Prazepam (Additive CNS depression). Products include:
- Centrax ... 1693

Prochlorperazine (Additive CNS depression). Products include:
- Compazine ... 2201

Promethazine Hydrochloride (Additive CNS depression). Products include:
- Mepergan Injection ... 2479
- Phenergan with Codeine ... 2497
- Phenergan with Dextromethorphan ... 2499
- Phenergan Injection ... 2493
- Phenergan Suppositories ... 2496
- Phenergan Syrup ... 2495
- Phenergan Tablets ... 2496
- Phenergan VC ... 2500
- Phenergan VC with Codeine ... 2501

Propofol (Additive CNS depression). Products include:
- Diprivan Injection ... 2267

Propoxyphene Hydrochloride (Additive CNS depression). Products include:
- Darvon ... 1256
- Wygesic Tablets ... 2540

Propoxyphene Napsylate (Additive CNS depression). Products include:
- Darvon-N/Darvocet-N ... 1254

Quazepam (Additive CNS depression). Products include:
- Doral Tablets ... 2383

Secobarbital Sodium (Additive CNS depression). Products include:
- Seconal Sodium Pulvules ... 1296

Sufentanil Citrate (Additive CNS depression). Products include:
- Sufenta Injection ... 1147

Temazepam (Additive CNS depression). Products include:
- Restoril Capsules ... 2023

Thioridazine Hydrochloride (Additive CNS depression). Products include:
- Mellaril ... 2011

Triazolam (Additive CNS depression). Products include:
- Halcion Tablets ... 2340

Trifluoperazine Hydrochloride (Additive CNS depression). Products include:
- Stelazine ... 2226

NUPERCAINAL CREAM AND OINTMENT
(Dibucaine) ... 877
No interactions described in labeling.

NUPERCAINAL SUPPOSITORIES
(Zinc Oxide) ... 877
No interactions described in labeling.

NUPRIN IBUPROFEN/ANALGESIC TABLETS & CAPLETS
(Ibuprofen) ... 752
May interact with aspirin and acetaminophen containing products. Compounds in this category include:

Acetaminophen (Concomitant administration recommended only under a doctor's direction). Products include:
- Acetaminophen Uniserts Suppositories ... 2374
- Actifed Plus Caplets ... ⊞ 539
- Actifed Plus Tablets ... ⊞ 540
- Alka-Seltzer Advanced Formula Antacid & Non-Aspirin Pain Reliever ... ⊞ 620
- Allerest ... ⊞ 559
- Aspirin Free Anacin Maximum Strength Acetaminophen Film Coated Caplets ... 2417
- Aspirin Free Anacin Maximum Strength Acetaminophen Film Coated Tablets ... 2417
- Anacin-3 Regular Strength Acetaminophen Film Coated Tablets ⊞ 746
- Anexsia 5/500 Tablets ... 2196
- Anexsia 7.5/650 Tablets ... 2197
- Benadryl Plus ... ⊞ 636
- Benadryl Plus Nighttime ... ⊞ 637
- Bufferin AF Nite Time Analgesic/Sleeping Aid Caplets ... 744
- Allergy-Sinus Comtrex Multi-Symptom Allergy Sinus Formula Tablets & Caplets ... 746
- Cough Formula Comtrex ... 746
- Comtrex Multi-Symptom Cold Reliever Tablets/Caplets/Liqui-Gels/Liquid ... 745
- Day-Night Comtrex ... 747
- Non-Drowsy Comtrex ... 747
- Congespirin For Children Aspirin Free Chewable Cold Tablets ... 748
- Contac Cough & Sore Throat Formula ... ⊞ 712
- Contac Jr. Children's Cold Medicine ... ⊞ 712
- Contac Nighttime Cold Medicine ... ⊞ 713
- Contac Severe Cold and Flu Formula Caplets ... ⊞ 711
- Contac Sinus Caplets Maximum Strength Non-Drowsy Formula ... ⊞ 710
- Contac Sinus Tablets Maximum Strength Non-Drowsy Formula ... ⊞ 710
- Coricidin 'D' Decongestant Tablets ... ⊞ 695
- Coricidin Demilets Tablets for Children ... ⊞ 696
- Coricidin Tablets ... ⊞ 695
- Darvon-N/Darvocet-N ... 1254
- Datril Extra-Strength Analgesic Tablets ... 748
- Dimetapp Plus Caplets ... ⊞ 675
- Dorcol Children's Fever & Pain Reducer ... ⊞ 686
- Dristan Decongestant/Antihistamine/ Analgesic Coated Caplets ... ⊞ 749
- Dristan Cold Nasal Decongestant/ Antihistamine/ Analgesic Coated Tablets ... 2419
- Dristan Advanced Formula Decongestant/Antihistamine/ Analgesic Tablets ... ⊞ 749
- Maximum Strength Dristan Decongestant/Analgesic Coated Caplets ... ⊞ 750
- No Drowsiness Dristan Cold Nasal Decongestant/Analgesic Coated Caplets ... 2420
- Drixoral Plus Extended-Release Tablets ... ⊞ 699
- Drixoral Sinus ... ⊞ 700
- Esgic-Plus Tablets ... 1002
- Esgic Tablets & Capsules ... 1001
- Aspirin Free Excedrin Analgesic Caplets ... 748
- Excedrin Extra-Strength Analgesic Tablets & Caplets ... 749
- Excedrin P.M. Analgesic/Sleeping Aid Tablets, Caplets and Liquid ... 749
- Sinus Excedrin Analgesic, Decongestant Tablets & Caplets ... 750
- 4-Way Cold Tablets ... 750
- Feverall Sprinkle Caps ... 2374
- Feverall Suppositories ... 2374
- Fioricet Tablets ... 2006
- Hycomine Compound Tablets ... 929
- Hydrocet Capsules ... 835
- Isocom Capsules ... 1629
- Liquiprin ... ⊞ 618
- Lortab ... 2412
- Lurline PMS Tablets ... 972
- Medi-Flu Caplet, Liquid ... ⊞ 640
- Maximum Strength Midol Multi-Symptom Menstrual Formula ... ⊞ 571
- Maximum Strength Midol PMS Premenstrual Syndrome Formula ... ⊞ 570
- Regular Strength Midol Multi-Symptom Menstrual Formula ... ⊞ 570
- Midrin Capsules ... 836
- Ornex Caplets ... ⊞ 618
- Children's Panadol Chewable Tablets, Liquid, Infants' Drops ... ⊞ 571
- Junior Strength Panadol ... ⊞ 571
- Maximum Strength Panadol Tablets and Caplets ... ⊞ 572
- Percocet Tablets ... 950
- Percogesic Analgesic Tablets ... ⊞ 660
- Phenaphen with Codeine Capsules 1865
- Phenaphen-650 with Codeine Tablets ... 1866
- Phrenilin ... 838
- Prēmsyn PMS Capsules & Caplets ⊞ 547
- Pyrroxate Capsules ... ⊞ 669
- Robitussin Night Relief ... ⊞ 677
- Sedapap Tablets 50 mg/650 mg .. 1360
- Sinarest ... ⊞ 562
- Sine-Aid Maximum Strength Sinus Headache Caplets ... 1365
- Sine-Aid Maximum Strength Sinus Headache Tablets ... 1365
- Sine-Off Maximum Strength Allergy/Sinus Formula Caplets ... ⊞ 721
- Sine-Off Maximum Strength No Drowsiness Formula Caplets ... ⊞ 722
- Singlet Tablets ... ⊞ 598
- Sinulin ... 840
- Sinutab Maximum Strength ... ⊞ 641
- Sinutab Maximum Strength Without Drowsiness Tablets & Caplets ... ⊞ 642
- Sinutab Regular Strength Without Drowsiness Formula ... ⊞ 641
- Sominex Pain Relief Formula ... ⊞ 723
- St. Joseph Aspirin-Free Fever Reducer for Children Chewable Tablets, Liquid & Infant Drops ... ⊞ 704
- St. Joseph Cold Tablets for Children ... ⊞ 704
- St. Joseph Nighttime Cold Medicine ... ⊞ 705
- Sudafed Sinus Caplets ... ⊞ 545
- Sudafed Sinus Tablets ... ⊞ 545
- Talacen ... 2070
- Tempra, Acetaminophen ... ⊞ 613
- TheraFlu Flu and Cold Medicine ... ⊞ 687
- Triaminicin Tablets ... ⊞ 690
- Tylenol acetaminophen Children's Chewable Tablets & Elixir ... 1366
- Tylenol Allergy Sinus Medication Caplets and Gelcaps, Maximum Strength ... 1372
- Tylenol with Codeine ... 1381
- Children's Tylenol Cold Liquid Formula and Chewable Tablets ... 1368
- Tylenol Cold & Flu Hot Medication, Packets ... 1369
- Tylenol Cold & Flu No Drowsiness Hot Medication, Packets ... 1371
- Tylenol Cold Medication Caplets and Tablets ... 1370
- Tylenol Cold Medication, Effervescent Tablets ... 1369
- Tylenol Cold Medication No Drowsiness Formula Caplets ... 1370
- Tylenol Cold Night Time Medication Liquid ... 1371
- Tylenol Cough Medication Liquid, Maximum Strength ... 1372
- Tylenol Cough Medication Liquid with Decongestant, Maximum Strength ... 1372
- Tylenol, Extra Strength, acetaminophen Adult Liquid Pain Reliever .. 1367
- Tylenol, Extra Strength, acetaminophen Gelcaps, Caplets, Tablets ... 1367
- Tylenol, Infants' Drops ... 1366
- Tylenol, Junior Strength, acetaminophen Coated Caplets, Grape and Fruit Chewable Tablets ... 1366
- Tylenol, Maximum Strength, Sinus Medication Gelcaps, Caplets and Tablets ... 1373
- Tylenol, Regular Strength, acetaminophen Tablets and Caplets ... 1367
- Tylenol PM, Extra Strength Caplets and Tablets ... 1368
- Tylox Capsules ... 1382
- Unisom Dual Relief Nighttime Sleep Aid/Analgesic ... 1774
- Vanquish Analgesic Caplets ... ⊞ 574
- Vicks Daycare ... ⊞ 660
- Vicks Formula 44M Multi-Symptom Cough Medicine ... ⊞ 662
- Vicks NyQuil Nighttime Colds Medicine-Original & Cherry Flavor ... ⊞ 664
- Vicodin Tablets ... 1187
- Vicodin ES Tablets ... 1189
- Wygesic Tablets ... 2540
- Zydone Capsules ... 941

Aspirin (Concomitant administration recommended only under a doctor's direction). Products include:
- Alka-Seltzer Effervescent Antacid and Pain Reliever ... 1568
- Alka-Seltzer Extra Strength Effervescent Antacid and Pain Reliever ... 1570
- Alka-Seltzer (Flavored) Effervescent Antacid and Pain Reliever ... 1569
- Alka-Seltzer Plus Cold Medicine ... ⊞ 623
- Alka-Seltzer Plus Night-Time Cold Medicine ... ⊞ 623
- Alka Seltzer Plus Sinus Allergy Medicine ... ⊞ 624
- Anacin Coated Analgesic Caplets ... 2417
- Anacin Coated Analgesic Tablets ... 2417
- Anacin Maximum Strength Analgesic Coated Tablets ... 2417
- Maximum Strength Arthritis Pain Formula By the Makers of Anacin Analgesic Tablets and Caplets ... 2418
- Arthritis Pain Formula by the Makers of Anacin Analgesic Tablets and Caplets ... ⊞ 747
- Arthritis Strength BC Powder ... ⊞ 516
- Ascriptin A/D Caplets ... 1850
- Regular Strength Ascriptin Tablets 1850
- Azdōne Tablets ... 844
- BC Powder ... ⊞ 517
- BC Cold Powder ... ⊞ 517
- Children's Bayer Chewable Aspirin ... ⊞ 564
- Genuine Bayer Aspirin Tablets & Caplets ... ⊞ 564
- Maximum Bayer Aspirin Tablets & Caplets ... ⊞ 566
- Bayer Plus Aspirin Tablets ... ⊞ 567
- Therapy Bayer Aspirin Caplets ... ⊞ 568
- 8 Hour Bayer Timed-Release Aspirin ... ⊞ 566
- Arthritis Strength Bufferin Analgesic Caplets ... 744
- Extra Strength Bufferin Analgesic Tablets ... 745
- Bufferin Analgesic Tablets and Caplets ... 743
- Cama Arthritis Pain Reliever ... ⊞ 685
- Damason-P ... 1356
- Easprin ... 1719
- Ecotrin Enteric Coated Aspirin Maximum Strength Tablets and Caplets ... 2189
- Ecotrin Enteric Coated Aspirin Regular Strength Tablets and Caplets ... 2189
- Empirin Aspirin ... ⊞ 541
- Empirin with Codeine Phosphate Nos. 2, 3 & 4 ... 764
- Equagesic Tablets ... 2451
- Excedrin Extra-Strength Analgesic Tablets & Caplets ... 749
- 4-Way Cold Tablets ... 750
- Fiorinal Capsules ... 2007
- Fiorinal with Codeine Capsules ... 2008
- Fiorinal Tablets ... 2007
- Lortab ASA Tablets ... 2414
- Momentum Muscular Backache Formula ... ⊞ 751
- Norgesic ... 1314
- Norwich Extra-Strength Aspirin ... ⊞ 546
- Norwich Regular Strength Aspirin ⊞ 547
- P-A-C Analgesic Tablets ... ⊞ 669
- Percodan ... 951

Robaxisal Tablets........ 1872
Sine-Off Sinus Medicine Tablets-Aspirin Formula .... ▣ 722
Soma Compound w/Codeine Tablets 2390
Soma Compound Tablets........ 2389
St. Joseph Adult Chewable Aspirin (81 mg.) .... ▣ 703
Synalgos-DC Capsules........ 2525
Talwin Compound 2072
Ursinus Inlay-Tabs........ ▣ 691
Vanquish Analgesic Caplets .... ▣ 574
Zorprin Tablets........ 698

NUROMAX INJECTION
(Doxacurium Chloride)........ 794
May interact with inhalant anesthetics, aminoglycosides, tetracyclines, lithium preparations, local anesthetics, and certain other agents. Compounds in these categories include:

Amikacin Sulfate (Enhances the neuromuscular blocking action). Products include:
Amikin Injectable 602

Bacitracin (Enhances the neuromuscular blocking action). Products include:
Baciguent Antibiotic Ointment........ ▣ 735
Bactine First Aid Antibiotic Ointment .... ▣ 625
Campho-Phenique Triple Antibiotic Ointment Plus Pain Reliever ▣ 758
Lanabiotic Ointment........ ▣ 556
Mycitracin........ ▣ 737

Bupivacaine Hydrochloride (Enhances the neuromuscular blocking action). Products include:
Marcaine Hydrochloride 0.5% with Epinephrine 1:200,000 (as bitartrate) 958
Marcaine Hydrochloride with Epinephrine 1:200,000 2055
Marcaine Hydrochloride Injection.... 2055
Marcaine Spinal 2058
Sensorcaine 631
Sensorcaine-MPF Spinal 634

Carbamazepine (The time of onset of neuromuscular block is lengthened and the duration of block is shortened). Products include:
Tegretol Chewable Tablets 654
Tegretol Suspension........ 656
Tegretol Tablets 654

Chloroprocaine Hydrochloride (Enhances the neuromuscular blocking action). Products include:
Nescaine/Nescaine MPF........ 629

Clindamycin Hydrochloride (Enhances the neuromuscular blocking action). Products include:
Cleocin HCl Capsules........ 2322

Clindamycin Palmitate Hydrochloride (Enhances the neuromuscular blocking action). Products include:
Cleocin Pediatric Flavored Granules 2324

Clindamycin Phosphate (Enhances the neuromuscular blocking action). Products include:
Cleocin Phosphate Injection 2325
Cleocin T Topical 2327

Colistimethate Sodium (Enhances the neuromuscular blocking action). Products include:
Coly-Mycin M Parenteral........ 1706

Colistin Sulfate (Enhances the neuromuscular blocking action). Products include:
Coly-Mycin S For Oral Suspension.. 1708
Coly-Mycin S Otic w/Neomycin & Hydrocortisone........ 1708

Demeclocycline Hydrochloride (Enhances the neuromuscular blocking action). Products include:
Declomycin Capsules, Tablets 1199

Doxycycline Calcium (Enhances the neuromuscular blocking action).
No products indexed under this heading.

Doxycycline Hyclate (Enhances the neuromuscular blocking action). Products include:
Doryx Capsules........ 1717
Vibramycin Hyclate Capsules........ 1787
Vibramycin Hyclate Intravenous 1968
Vibra-Tabs Film Coated Tablets 1787

Doxycycline Monohydrate (Enhances the neuromuscular blocking action). Products include:
Monodox Capsules 1630
Vibramycin Monohydrate for Oral Suspension 1787

Enflurane (Decreases the ED$_{50}$ by 30% to 45%; prolongs the clinically effective duration of action by up to 25%). Products include:
Ethrane........ 599

Etidocaine Hydrochloride (Enhances the neuromuscular blocking action). Products include:
Duranest Injections........ 624

Gentamicin Sulfate (Enhances the neuromuscular blocking action). Products include:
Garamycin Injectable 2093
Garamycin Ophthalmic .... ⊙ 305
Genoptic Liquifilm Sterile Ophthalmic Solution .... ⊙ 247
Genoptic S.O.P. Sterile Ophthalmic Ointment........ ⊙ 247
Gentacidin Ointment .... ⊙ 273
Gentacidin Solution........ ⊙ 273
Gentak Ointment & Solution .... ⊙ 208
G-myticin Creme and Ointment 0.1% 1770
Pred-G Liquifilm Sterile Ophthalmic Suspension .... ⊙ 252
Pred-G S.O.P. Sterile Ophthalmic Ointment .... ⊙ 253

Halothane (Decreases the ED$_{50}$ by 30% to 45%; prolongs the clinically effective duration of action by up to 25%). Products include:
Fluothane 2453

Isoflurane (Decreases the ED$_{50}$ by 30% to 45%; prolongs the clinically effective duration of action by up to 25%). Products include:
Forane........ 600

Kanamycin Sulfate (Enhances the neuromuscular blocking action). Products include:
Kantrex Injection 601
Kantrex Pediatric Injection........ 601

Lidocaine Hydrochloride (Enhances the neuromuscular blocking action). Products include:
Anestacon Solution........ 2394
Bactine Antiseptic/Anesthetic First Aid Spray .... ▣ 624
Decadron Phosphate with Xylocaine Injection, Sterile 1451
Xylocaine Injections 637
Xylocaine Injections for Ventricular Arrhythmias........ 639
Xylocaine 2% Jelly 643
4% Xylocaine-MPF Sterile Solution 641
Xylocaine 2% Viscous Solution........ 646

Lincomycin Hydrochloride Monohydrate (Enhances the neuromuscular blocking action).
No products indexed under this heading.

Lithium Carbonate (Enhances the neuromuscular blocking action). Products include:
Eskalith 2214
Lithane Tablets 1596
Lithium Carbonate Capsules & Tablets 1984
Lithobid Tablets 870

Lithium Citrate (Enhances the neuromuscular blocking action). Products include:
Cibalith-S........ 870

Magnesium Salts (Enhances the neuromuscular blocking action).

Mepivacaine Hydrochloride Injection (Enhances the neuromuscular blocking action). Products include:
Carbocaine Hydrochloride 3% Injection 956
Carbocaine Hydrochloride Injection 2043
Carbocaine Hydrochloride 2% with Neo-Cobefrin 956

Methacycline Hydrochloride (Enhances the neuromuscular blocking action).
No products indexed under this heading.

Methoxyflurane (Decreases the ED$_{50}$ by 30% to 45%; prolongs the clinically effective duration of action by up to 25%).
No products indexed under this heading.

Minocycline Hydrochloride (Enhances the neuromuscular blocking action). Products include:
Minocin Intravenous........ 1221
Minocin Oral Suspension 1224
Minocin Pellet-Filled Capsules 1222

Oxytetracycline Hydrochloride (Enhances the neuromuscular blocking action). Products include:
Terra-Cortril Ophthalmic Suspension 1963
Terramycin Capsules 1786
Terramycin Intramuscular Solution 1964
Terramycin with Polymyxin B Sulfate Ophthalmic Ointment........ 1965

Phenytoin (The time of onset of neuromuscular block is lengthened and the duration of block is shortened). Products include:
Dilantin Infatabs........ 1710
Dilantin-30 Pediatric/Dilantin-125 Suspension 1713

Phenytoin Sodium (The time of onset of neuromuscular block is lengthened and the duration of block is shortened). Products include:
Dilantin Kapseals 1708
Dilantin Parenteral 1712
Dilantin with Phenobarbital Kapseals 1715

Polymyxin Preparations (Enhances the neuromuscular blocking action).

Procainamide Hydrochloride (Enhances the neuromuscular blocking action). Products include:
Procan SR Tablets........ 1760
Pronestyl Capsules and Tablets 1800
Pronestyl Injection........ 1798
Pronestyl-SR Tablets 1801

Procaine Hydrochloride (Enhances the neuromuscular blocking action). Products include:
Novocain Hydrochloride for Spinal Anesthesia 2065

Quinidine Gluconate (Enhances the neuromuscular blocking action). Products include:
Quinaglute Dura-Tabs Tablets 663

Quinidine Polygalacturonate (Enhances the neuromuscular blocking action). Products include:
Cardioquin Tablets 1812

Quinidine Sulfate (Enhances the neuromuscular blocking action). Products include:
Quinidex Extentabs........ 1868

Streptomycin Sulfate (Enhances the neuromuscular blocking action).
No products indexed under this heading.

Tetracaine Hydrochloride (Enhances the neuromuscular blocking action). Products include:
Cetacaine Topical Anesthetic 850
Pontocaine Hydrochloride for Spinal Anesthesia........ 2069

Tetracycline Hydrochloride (Enhances the neuromuscular blocking action). Products include:
Achromycin V Capsules 1193
Achromycin Ophthalmic Ointment 1% .... ⊙ 307
Achromycin Ophthalmic Suspension 1% .... ⊙ 308
Topicycline for Topical Solution 1856

Tobramycin (Enhances the neuromuscular blocking action). Products include:
TobraDex Ophthalmic Suspension and Ointment........ ⊙ 228
Tobrex Ophthalmic Ointment and Solution 572

Tobramycin Sulfate (Enhances the neuromuscular blocking action). Products include:
Nebcin Vials, Hyporets & ADD-Vantage 1286

NURSOY, SOY PROTEIN FORMULA FOR INFANTS, CONCENTRATED LIQUID, READY-TO-FEED, AND POWDER
(Protein Preparations)........ 2488
No interactions described in labeling.

NUTRACORT CREAM & LOTION
(Hydrocortisone) 1684
No interactions described in labeling.

NUTRADERM CREAM & LOTION
(Hydrocortisone) 1684
No interactions described in labeling.

NUTRADERM 30 LOTION
(Petrolatum) 1684
No interactions described in labeling.

NYSTATIN, USP FOR EXTEMPORANEOUS PREPARATION OF ORAL SUSPENSION
(Nystatin) 1685
No interactions described in labeling.

NYTOL TABLETS
(Diphenhydramine Hydrochloride).. ▣ 517
May interact with central nervous system depressants, hypnotics and sedatives, monoamine oxidase inhibitors, and certain other agents. Compounds in these categories include:

Alcohol (Heightens depressant effect).

Alfentanil Hydrochloride (Heightens depressant effect). Products include:
Alfenta Injection 1131

Alprazolam (Heightens depressant effect). Products include:
Xanax Tablets 2367

Aprobarbital (Heightens depressant effect). Products include:
Alurate Elixir 1883

Buprenorphine (Heightens depressant effect).
No products indexed under this heading.

Buspirone Hydrochloride (Heightens depressant effect). Products include:
BuSpar........ 1401

Butabarbital (Heightens depressant effect). Products include:
Pyridium Plus 1764

Butalbital (Heightens depressant effect). Products include:
Esgic-Plus Tablets 1002
Esgic Tablets & Capsules........ 1001
Fioricet Tablets........ 2006
Fiorinal Capsules 2007
Fiorinal with Codeine Capsules 2008

Fiorinal Tablets 2007
Phrenilin 838
Sedapap Tablets 50 mg/650 mg 1360

Chlordiazepoxide (Heightens depressant effect). Products include:
Libritabs Tablets 1930
Limbitrol 1933
Menrium Tablets 1934

Chlordiazepoxide Hydrochloride (Heightens depressant effect). Products include:
Librax Capsules 1929
Librium Capsules 1931
Librium Injectable 1932

Chlorpromazine (Heightens depressant effect). Products include:
Thorazine 2234

Chlorprothixene (Heightens depressant effect). Products include:
Taractan Tablets 1920

Chlorprothixene Hydrochloride (Heightens depressant effect). Products include:
Taractan 1920

Clorazepate Dipotassium (Heightens depressant effect). Products include:
Tranxene 556

Codeine (Heightens depressant effect). Products include:
Calcidrine Syrup 506

Codeine Phosphate (Heightens depressant effect). Products include:
Actifed with Codeine Cough Syrup 752
Cheracol Cough Syrup 1853
Codimal PH Syrup 846
Dimetane-DC Cough Syrup 1857
Empirin with Codeine Phosphate Nos. 2, 3 & 4 764
Fiorinal with Codeine Capsules 2008
Isoclor Expectorant 982
Naldecon CX Adult Liquid ◘ 521
Novahistine DH 1342
Novahistine Expectorant 1343
Nucofed Capsules 2219
Nucofed Expectorant 2219
Nucofed Pediatric Expectorant 2220
Nucofed Syrup 2219
Phenaphen with Codeine Capsules 1865
Phenaphen-650 with Codeine Tablets 1866
Phenergan with Codeine 2497
Phenergan VC with Codeine 2501
Robitussin A-C Syrup 1875
Robitussin-DAC Syrup 1875
Ryna ◘ 741
Soma Compound w/Codeine Tablets 2390
Triaminic Expectorant w/Codeine 1996
Tussi-Organidin Liquid 2391
Tylenol with Codeine 1381

Codeine Polistirex (Heightens depressant effect).
No products indexed under this heading.

Dezocine (Heightens depressant effect).

Diazepam (Heightens depressant effect). Products include:
Valium Injectable 1937
Valium Tablets 1939
Valrelease Capsules 1923

Droperidol (Heightens depressant effect). Products include:
Inapsine Injection 1140
Innovar Injection 1141

Enflurane (Heightens depressant effect). Products include:
Ethrane 599

Estazolam (Heightens depressant effect). Products include:
ProSom Tablets 554

Ethchlorvynol (Heightens depressant effect). Products include:
Placidyl Capsules 553

Ethinamate (Heightens depressant effect).
No products indexed under this heading.

Fentanyl (Heightens depressant effect). Products include:
Duragesic Transdermal System 1133

Fentanyl Citrate (Heightens depressant effect). Products include:
Innovar Injection 1141
Sublimaze Injection 1146

Fluphenazine Decanoate (Heightens depressant effect). Products include:
Prolixin Decanoate 1795

Fluphenazine Enanthate (Heightens depressant effect). Products include:
Prolixin Enanthate 1796

Fluphenazine Hydrochloride (Heightens depressant effect). Products include:
Prolixin Elixir 1793
Prolixin Injection 1791
Prolixin Oral Concentrate 1792
Prolixin Tablets 1793

Flurazepam Hydrochloride (Heightens depressant effect). Products include:
Dalmane Capsules 1927

Furazolidone (Prolongs and intensifies anticholinergic effects). Products include:
Furoxone 1855

Glutethimide (Heightens depressant effect).
No products indexed under this heading.

Haloperidol (Heightens depressant effect). Products include:
Haldol Injection, Tablets and Concentrate 1373

Haloperidol Decanoate (Heightens depressant effect). Products include:
Haldol Decanoate 1375

Hydrocodone Bitartrate (Heightens depressant effect). Products include:
Anexsia 5/500 Tablets 2196
Anexsia 7.5/650 Tablets 2197
Azdone Tablets 844
Codiclear DH Syrup 845
Codimal DH Syrup 846
Damason-P 1356
Hycodan Syrup, Tablets 927
Hycomine Compound Tablets 929
Hycomine Syrup 927
Hycotuss Expectorant Syrup 930
Hydrocet Capsules 835
Lortab ASA Tablets 2414
Lortab 2412
Ru-Tuss with Hydrocodone 694
Triaminic Expectorant DH 1995
Vicodin Tablets 1187
Vicodin ES Tablets 1189
Zydone Capsules 941

Hydrocodone Polistirex (Heightens depressant effect). Products include:
Tussionex Extended-Release Suspension 988

Hydroxyzine Hydrochloride (Heightens depressant effect). Products include:
Atarax Tablets & Syrup 1941
Marax Tablets & DF Syrup 1954
Vistaril Intramuscular Solution 1970

Isocarboxazid (Prolongs and intensifies anticholinergic effects). Products include:
Marplan Tablets 1906

Isoflurane (Heightens depressant effect). Products include:
Forane 600

Ketamine Hydrochloride (Heightens depressant effect). Products include:
Ketalar 1726

Levorphanol Tartrate (Heightens depressant effect). Products include:
Levo-Dromoran 1906

Lorazepam (Heightens depressant effect). Products include:
Ativan Injection 2432
Ativan Tablets 2434

Loxapine Hydrochloride (Heightens depressant effect). Products include:
Loxitane 1213

Loxapine Succinate (Heightens depressant effect). Products include:
Loxitane Capsules 1213

Meperidine Hydrochloride (Heightens depressant effect). Products include:
Demerol 2047
Mepergan Injection 2479

Mephobarbital (Heightens depressant effect). Products include:
Mebaral Tablets 2061

Meprobamate (Heightens depressant effect). Products include:
Deprol Tablets 2382
Equagesic Tablets 2451
Miltown Tablets 2386
PMB 200 and PMB 400 2504

Mesoridazine (Heightens depressant effect). Products include:
Serentil 686

Methadone Hydrochloride (Heightens depressant effect). Products include:
Dolophine Hydrochloride Ampoules & Vials 1260
Dolophine Hydrochloride Tablets 1261
Methadone Hydrochloride Diskets 1284
Methadone Hydrochloride Oral Solution & Tablets 1987

Methohexital Sodium (Heightens depressant effect). Products include:
Brevital Sodium Vials 1248

Methoxyflurane (Heightens depressant effect).
No products indexed under this heading.

Midazolam Hydrochloride (Heightens depressant effect). Products include:
Versed Injection 1924

Molindone Hydrochloride (Heightens depressant effect). Products include:
Moban Tablets & Concentrate 932

Morphine Sulfate (Heightens depressant effect). Products include:
Astramorph/PF Injection, USP (Preservative-Free) 618
Duramorph 960
Infumorph 200 and Infumorph 500 Sterile Solutions 962
MS Contin Tablets 1814
MSIR 1817
Oramorph SR (Morphine Sulfate Sustained Release Tablets) 1988
Roxanol 1991

Opium Alkaloids (Heightens depressant effect). Products include:
B & O No. 15A & No. 16A Supprettes 2395
Pantopon Injectable 1911

Oxazepam (Heightens depressant effect). Products include:
Serax Capsules 2522
Serax Tablets 2522

Oxycodone Hydrochloride (Heightens depressant effect). Products include:
Percocet Tablets 950
Percodan 951
Roxicodone Tablets, Oral Solution & Intensol (Oxycodone) 1992
Tylox Capsules 1382

Pentobarbital Sodium (Heightens depressant effect). Products include:
Nembutal Sodium Capsules 534
Nembutal Sodium Solution 536
Nembutal Sodium Suppositories 538

Perphenazine (Heightens depressant effect). Products include:
Etrafon 2087
Triavil Tablets 1556
Trilafon 2123

Phenelzine Sulfate (Prolongs and intensifies anticholinergic effects). Products include:
Nardil 1742

Phenobarbital (Heightens depressant effect). Products include:
Arco-Lase Plus Tablets 607
Bellergal-S Tablets 1998
Bronkolixir ◘ 761
Bronkotabs Tablets ◘ 762
Donnatal 1858
Donnatal Extentabs 1859
Donnatal Tablets 1858
Donnazyme Tablets 1860
Kinesed Tablets 2272
Phenobarbital Elixir and Tablets 1293
Primatene Tablets-P Formula 2421
Quadrinal Tablets 1183
Tedral SA 1765

Prazepam (Heightens depressant effect). Products include:
Centrax 1693

Prochlorperazine (Heightens depressant effect). Products include:
Compazine 2201

Promethazine Hydrochloride (Heightens depressant effect). Products include:
Mepergan Injection 2479
Phenergan with Codeine 2497
Phenergan with Dextromethorphan 2499
Phenergan Injection 2493
Phenergan Suppositories 2496
Phenergan Syrup 2495
Phenergan Tablets 2496
Phenergan VC 2500
Phenergan VC with Codeine 2501

Propofol (Heightens depressant effect). Products include:
Diprivan Injection 2267

Propoxyphene Hydrochloride (Heightens depressant effect). Products include:
Darvon 1256
Wygesic Tablets 2540

Propoxyphene Napsylate (Heightens depressant effect). Products include:
Darvon-N/Darvocet-N 1254

Quazepam (Heightens depressant effect). Products include:
Doral Tablets 2383

Secobarbital Sodium (Heightens depressant effect). Products include:
Seconal Sodium Pulvules 1296

Selegiline Hydrochloride (Prolongs and intensifies anticholinergic effects). Products include:
Eldepryl 2250

Sufentanil Citrate (Heightens depressant effect). Products include:
Sufenta Injection 1147

Temazepam (Heightens depressant effect). Products include:
Restoril Capsules 2023

Thiamylal Sodium (Heightens depressant effect). Products include:
Surital Ampoules, Steri-Vials 1764

Thioridazine Hydrochloride (Heightens depressant effect). Products include:
Mellaril 2011

Thiothixene (Heightens depressant effect). Products include:
Navane Capsules and Concentrate 1954
Navane Intramuscular 1956

Tranylcypromine Sulfate (Prolongs and intensifies anticholinergic effects). Products include:
Parnate Tablets 2222

Triazolam (Heightens depressant effect). Products include:
Halcion Tablets 2340

Trifluoperazine Hydrochloride (Heightens depressant effect). Products include:
Stelazine 2226

OCCLUSAL
(Salicylic Acid) 1045
No interactions described in labeling.

OCCLUSAL-HP
(Salicylic Acid) 1045
No interactions described in labeling.

OCCUCOAT
(Hydroxypropyl Methylcellulose) ◉ 312
No interactions described in labeling.

OCEAN NASAL MIST
(Sodium Chloride) ▣ 563
No interactions described in labeling.

OCUCLEAR EYE DROPS
(Oxymetazoline Hydrochloride) ◉ 306
No interactions described in labeling.

OCUFEN
(Flurbiprofen) ◉ 237
May interact with:

Acetylcholine Chloride (Ineffective when used in patients treated with Ocufen). Products include:
- Miochol with Iocare Steri-Tags, Miochol System Pak and Miochol System Pak Plus ◉ 274

Carbachol (Ineffective when used in patients treated with Ocufen). Products include:
- Isopto Carbachol ◉ 219
- MIOSTAT ◉ 233

OCULINUM FOR INJECTON
(Botulinum Toxin Type A) 587
No interactions described in labeling.

OCUSERT PILO-20 AND PILO-40 OCULAR THERAPEUTIC SYSTEMS
(Pilocarpine) ◉ 256
May interact with:

Epinephrine (Increased rate of absorption from the eye). Products include:
- Ana-Kit Anaphylaxis Emergency Treatment Kit 1100
- Bronkaid Mist ▣ 757
- EpiPen 843
- Marcaine Hydrochloride 0.5% with Epinephrine 1:200,000 (as bitartrate) 958
- Marcaine Hydrochloride with Epinephrine 1:200,000 2055
- Primatene Mist 2420
- Sus-Phrine Injection 1006
- Xylocaine with Epinephrine Injections 637

Epinephrine Bitartrate (Increased rate of absorption from the eye). Products include:
- AsthmaHaler Mist Epinephrine Bitartrate Bronchodilator ▣ 616
- Bronkaid Mist Suspension ▣ 757
- Primatene Mist Suspension 2421

ODOR-EATERS SPRAY POWDER
(Tolnaftate) ▣ 557
No interactions described in labeling.

OGEN TABLETS
(Estropipate) 540
May interact with insulin, hepatic microsomal emzyme inducers, and certain other agents. Compounds in these categories include:

Aprobarbital (Lowers estrogen levels). Products include:
- Alurate Elixir 1883

Butabarbital (Lowers estrogen levels). Products include:
- Pyridium Plus 1764

Carbamazepine (Lowers estrogen levels). Products include:
- Tegretol Chewable Tablets 654
- Tegretol Suspension 656
- Tegretol Tablets 654

Chlorpropamide (Lowers estrogen levels). Products include:
- Diabinese Tablets 1775

Glipizide (Lowers estrogen levels). Products include:
- Glucotrol 1952

Glyburide (Lowers estrogen levels). Products include:
- DiaBeta 1091
- Micronase Tablets 2350

Insulin, Human (Increased insulin requirements).
- No products indexed under this heading.

Insulin, Human Isophane Suspension (Increased insulin requirements). Products include:
- Humulin N, 100 Units 1270

Insulin, Human NPH (Increased insulin requirements). Products include:
- Insulatard NPH Human 1627
- Novolin N 1627
- Novolin N PenFill Cartridges 1628
- Novolin N Prefilled 1628

Insulin, Human Regular (Increased insulin requirements). Products include:
- Humulin BR, 100 Units 1268
- Humulin R, 100 Units 1272
- Novolin R 1627
- Novolin R PenFill Cartridges 1628
- Novolin R Prefilled 1629
- Velosulin Human 1628

Insulin, Human, Zinc Suspension (Increased insulin requirements). Products include:
- Humulin L, 100 Units 1268
- Humulin U, 100 Units 1272
- Novolin L 1627

Insulin, NPH (Increased insulin requirements). Products include:
- NPH, 40 & 100 Units 1273
- Beef NPH, 100 Units 1274
- Pork NPH, 100 Units 1275
- Insulatard NPH 1626
- NPH Insulin 1626
- NPH Purified Pork Isophane Insulin 1626

Insulin, Regular (Increased insulin requirements). Products include:
- Regular, 40 & 100 Units 1273
- Beef Regular, 100 Units 1275
- Pork Regular, 100 Units 1275
- Pork Regular (Concentrated), 500 Units 1276
- Regular Insulin 1625
- Regular Purified Pork Insulin 1626
- Velosulin 1627

Insulin, Zinc Crystals (Increased insulin requirements). Products include:
- NPH, 40 & 100 Units 1273

Insulin, Zinc Suspension (Increased insulin requirements). Products include:
- Lente, 40 & 100 Units 1272
- Protamine, Zinc, 40 & 100 Units 1273
- Lente Iletin I 1272
- Beef Lente, 100 Units 1274
- Beef Protamine Zinc, 100 Units 1274
- Pork Lente, 100 Units 1275
- Pork, Protamine, Zinc, 100 Units 1275
- Lente Insulin 1626
- Lente Purified Pork Insulin 1626
- Semilente Insulin 1625
- Ultralente Insulin 1626

Mephobarbital (Lowers estrogen levels). Products include:
- Mebaral Tablets 2061

Pentobarbital Sodium (Lowers estrogen levels). Products include:
- Nembutal Sodium Capsules 534
- Nembutal Sodium Solution 536
- Nembutal Sodium Suppositories 538

Phenobarbital (Lowers estrogen levels). Products include:
- Arco-Lase Plus Tablets 607
- Bellergal-S Tablets 1998
- Bronkolixir ▣ 761
- Bronkotabs Tablets ▣ 762
- Donnatal 1858
- Donnatal Extentabs 1859
- Donnatal Tablets 1858
- Donnazyme Tablets 1860
- Kinesed Tablets 2272
- Phenobarbital Elixir and Tablets 1293
- Primatene Tablets-P Formula 2421
- Quadrinal Tablets 1183
- Tedral SA 1765

Phenylbutazone (Lowers estrogen levels). Products include:
- Butazolidin Capsules & Tablets 1027

Phenytoin (Lowers estrogen levels). Products include:
- Dilantin Infatabs 1710
- Dilantin-30 Pediatric/Dilantin-125 Suspension 1713

Phenytoin Sodium (Lowers estrogen levels). Products include:
- Dilantin Kapseals 1708
- Dilantin Parenteral 1712
- Dilantin with Phenobarbital Kapseals 1715

Rifampin (Lowers estrogen levels). Products include:
- Rifadin 1345
- Rifamate Capsules 1347
- Rimactane Capsules 879

Thiamylal Sodium (Lowers estrogen levels). Products include:
- Surital Ampoules, Steri-Vials 1764

Tolazamide (Lowers estrogen levels). Products include:
- Tolinase Tablets 2365

Tolbutamide (Lowers estrogen levels). Products include:
- Orinase Tablets 2354

OGEN VAGINAL CREAM
(Estropipate) 540
See **Ogen Tablets**

OMNIPAQUE
(Iohexol) 2552
May interact with phenothiazines, monoamine oxidase inhibitors, tricyclic antidepressants, central nervous system stimulants, neuromuscular blocking agents, and certain other agents. Compounds in these categories include:

Amitriptyline Hydrochloride (Lowers seizure threshold). Products include:
- Elavil 2269
- Endep Tablets 1927
- Etrafon 2087
- Limbitrol 1933
- Triavil Tablets 1556

Amoxapine (Lowers seizure threshold). Products include:
- Asendin Tablets 1196

Amphetamine Resins (Lowers seizure threshold). Products include:
- Biphetamine Capsules 973

Chlorpromazine (Lowers seizure threshold). Products include:
- Thorazine 2234

Chlorprothixene (Lowers seizure threshold). Products include:
- Taractan Tablets 1920

Chlorprothixene Hydrochloride (Lowers seizure threshold). Products include:
- Taractan 1920

Clomipramine Hydrochloride (Lowers seizure threshold). Products include:
- Anafranil Capsules 650

Clozapine (Lowers seizure threshold). Products include:
- Clozaril Tablets 2000

Desipramine Hydrochloride (Lowers seizure threshold). Products include:
- Norpramin Tablets 1340

Dextroamphetamine Sulfate (Lowers seizure threshold). Products include:
- Dexedrine 2206

Doxepin Hydrochloride (Lowers seizure threshold). Products include:
- Sinequan 1960

Fluphenazine Decanoate (Lowers seizure threshold). Products include:
- Prolixin Decanoate 1795

Fluphenazine Enanthate (Lowers seizure threshold). Products include:
- Prolixin Enanthate 1796

Fluphenazine Hydrochloride (Lowers seizure threshold). Products include:
- Prolixin Elixir 1793
- Prolixin Injection 1791
- Prolixin Oral Concentrate 1792
- Prolixin Tablets 1793

Furazolidone (Lowers seizure threshold). Products include:
- Furoxone 1855

Haloperidol (Lowers seizure threshold). Products include:
- Haldol Injection, Tablets and Concentrate 1373

Haloperidol Decanoate (Lowers seizure threshold). Products include:
- Haldol Decanoate 1375

Imipramine Hydrochloride (Lowers seizure threshold). Products include:
- Tofranil Ampuls 1038
- Tofranil Tablets 1039

Imipramine Pamoate (Lowers seizure threshold). Products include:
- Tofranil-PM Capsules 1041

Isocarboxazid (Lowers seizure threshold). Products include:
- Marplan Tablets 1906

Lithium Carbonate (Lowers seizure threshold). Products include:
- Eskalith 2214
- Lithane Tablets 1596
- Lithium Carbonate Capsules & Tablets 1984
- Lithobid Tablets 870

Lithium Citrate (Lowers seizure threshold). Products include:
- Cibalith-S 870

Loxapine Hydrochloride (Lowers seizure threshold). Products include:
- Loxitane 1213

Maprotiline Hydrochloride (Lowers seizure threshold). Products include:
- Ludiomil Tablets 874

Mesoridazine (Lowers seizure threshold). Products include:
- Serentil 686

Methamphetamine Hydrochloride (Lowers seizure threshold). Products include:
- Desoxyn Gradumet Tablets 514

Methylphenidate Hydrochloride (Lowers seizure threshold). Products include:
- Ritalin 880

Molindone Hydrochloride (Lowers seizure threshold). Products include:
- Moban Tablets & Concentrate 932

Nortriptyline Hydrochloride (Lowers seizure threshold). Products include:
- Pamelor 2019

Pemoline (Lowers seizure threshold). Products include:
- Cylert Tablets 510

Perphenazine (Lowers seizure threshold). Products include:
- Etrafon 2087
- Triavil Tablets 1556
- Trilafon 2123

(▣ Described in PDR For Nonprescription Drugs) (◉ Described in PDR For Ophthalmology)

Phenelzine Sulfate (Lowers seizure threshold). Products include:
Nardil ... 1742
Pimozide (Lowers seizure threshold). Products include:
Orap Tablets ... 1020
Prochlorperazine (Lowers seizure threshold). Products include:
Compazine ... 2201
Promethazine Hydrochloride (Lowers seizure threshold). Products include:
Mepergan Injection ... 2479
Phenergan with Codeine ... 2497
Phenergan with Dextromethorphan 2499
Phenergan Injection ... 2493
Phenergan Suppositories ... 2496
Phenergan Syrup ... 2495
Phenergan Tablets ... 2496
Phenergan VC ... 2500
Phenergan VC with Codeine ... 2501
Protriptyline Hydrochloride (Lowers seizure threshold). Products include:
Vivactil Tablets ... 1567
Selegiline Hydrochloride (Lowers seizure threshold). Products include:
Eldepryl ... 2250
Thioridazine Hydrochloride (Lowers seizure threshold). Products include:
Mellaril ... 2011
Thiothixene (Lowers seizure threshold). Products include:
Navane Capsules and Concentrate 1954
Navane Intramuscular ... 1956
Tranylcypromine Sulfate (Lowers seizure threshold). Products include:
Parnate Tablets ... 2222
Trifluoperazine Hydrochloride (Lowers seizure threshold). Products include:
Stelazine ... 2226
Trimipramine Maleate (Lowers seizure threshold). Products include:
Surmontil Capsules ... 2524

ONCOVIN SOLUTION VIALS & HYPORETS
(Vincristine Sulfate) ... 1288
May interact with:
Mitomycin (Mitomycin-C) (Acute shortness of breath; severe bronchospasm). Products include:
Mutamycin ... 733
Neurotoxic Drugs (Potential for increased neurotoxicity).
Phenytoin (Increased seizure activity due to reduced phenytoin blood levels). Products include:
Dilantin Infatabs ... 1710
Dilantin-30 Pediatric/Dilantin-125 Suspension ... 1713
Phenytoin Sodium (Increased seizure activity due to reduced phenytoin blood levels). Products include:
Dilantin Kapseals ... 1708
Dilantin Parenteral ... 1712
Dilantin with Phenobarbital Kapseals ... 1715

ONE-A-DAY ESSENTIAL VITAMINS
(Multivitamins) ... ⊡ 627
No interactions described in labeling.

ONE-A-DAY MAXIMUM FORMULA VITAMINS AND MINERALS
(Multivitamins with Minerals) ... ⊡ 627
No interactions described in labeling.

ONE-A-DAY PLUS EXTRA C VITAMINS
(Multivitamins) ... ⊡ 627
No interactions described in labeling.

ONY-CLEAR NAIL SPRAY
(Triacetin) ... 1771
No interactions described in labeling.

ONYPLEX NAIL HARDENER/BITE DETERRENT
(TEVCO 50344) ... 1410
No interactions described in labeling.

OPCON-A OPHTHALMIC SOLUTION
(Naphazoline Hydrochloride, Pheniramine Maleate) ... ⊙ 262
May interact with monoamine oxidase inhibitors. Compounds in this category include:
Furazolidone (Potential for hypertensive crisis). Products include:
Furoxone ... 1855
Isocarboxazid (Potential for hypertensive crisis). Products include:
Marplan Tablets ... 1906
Phenelzine Sulfate (Potential for hypertensive crisis). Products include:
Nardil ... 1742
Selegiline Hydrochloride (Potential for hypertensive crisis). Products include:
Eldepryl ... 2250
Tranylcypromine Sulfate (Potential for hypertensive crisis). Products include:
Parnate Tablets ... 2222

OPHTHALGAN
(Glycerin) ... ⊙ 315
No interactions described in labeling.

OPHTHETIC
(Proparacaine Hydrochloride) ... ⊙ 249
No interactions described in labeling.

OPHTHOCHLOR OPHTHALMIC SOLUTION
(Chloramphenicol) ... ⊙ 300
No interactions described in labeling.

OPHTHOCORT
(Chloramphenicol, Polymyxin B Sulfate, Hydrocortisone Acetate) ... ⊙ 301
No interactions described in labeling.

OPTICROM 4%
(Cromolyn Sodium) ... 986
No interactions described in labeling.

OPTILETS-500 FILMTAB
(Multivitamins) ... ⊡ 502
No interactions described in labeling.

OPTILETS-M-500 FILMTAB
(Multivitamins with Minerals) ... ⊡ 502
No interactions described in labeling.

OPTIMINE TABLETS
(Azatadine Maleate) ... 2115
May interact with monoamine oxidase inhibitors, central nervous system depressants, hypnotics and sedatives, tranquilizers, oral anticoagulants, tricyclic antidepressants, and certain other agents. Compounds in these categories include:
Alcohol (Additive effects).
Alfentanil Hydrochloride (Additive effects). Products include:
Alfenta Injection ... 1131
Alprazolam (Additive effects). Products include:
Xanax Tablets ... 2367
Amitriptyline Hydrochloride (Additive effects). Products include:
Elavil ... 2269
Endep Tablets ... 1927
Etrafon ... 2087
Limbitrol ... 1933
Triavil Tablets ... 1556
Amoxapine (Additive effects). Products include:
Asendin Tablets ... 1196
Aprobarbital (Additive effects). Products include:
Alurate Elixir ... 1883
Buprenorphine (Additive effects).
No products indexed under this heading.
Buspirone Hydrochloride (Additive effects). Products include:
BuSpar ... 1401
Butabarbital (Additive effects). Products include:
Pyridium Plus ... 1764
Butalbital (Additive effects). Products include:
Esgic-Plus Tablets ... 1002
Esgic Tablets & Capsules ... 1001
Fioricet Tablets ... 2006
Fiorinal Capsules ... 2007
Fiorinal with Codeine Capsules ... 2008
Fiorinal Tablets ... 2007
Phrenilin ... 838
Sedapap Tablets 50 mg/650 mg .. 1360
Chlordiazepoxide (Additive effects). Products include:
Libritabs Tablets ... 1930
Limbitrol ... 1933
Menrium Tablets ... 1934
Chlordiazepoxide Hydrochloride (Additive effects). Products include:
Librax Capsules ... 1929
Librium Capsules ... 1931
Librium Injectable ... 1932
Chlorpromazine (Additive effects). Products include:
Thorazine ... 2234
Chlorprothixene (Additive effects). Products include:
Taractan Tablets ... 1920
Chlorprothixene Hydrochloride (Additive effects). Products include:
Taractan ... 1920
Chlorprothixene Lactate (Additive effects). Products include:
Taractan Concentrate ... 1920
Clomipramine Hydrochloride (Additive effects). Products include:
Anafranil Capsules ... 650
Clorazepate Dipotassium (Additive effects). Products include:
Tranxene ... 556
Codeine (Additive effects). Products include:
Calcidrine Syrup ... 506
Codeine Phosphate (Additive effects). Products include:
Actifed with Codeine Cough Syrup.. 752
Cheracol Cough Syrup ... 1853
Codimal PH Syrup ... 846
Dimetane-DC Cough Syrup ... 1857
Empirin with Codeine Phosphate Nos. 2, 3 & 4 ... 764
Fiorinal with Codeine Capsules ... 2008
Isoclor Expectorant ... 982
Naldecon CX Adult Liquid ... ⊡ 521
Novahistine DH ... 1342
Novahistine Expectorant ... 1343
Nucofed Capsules ... 2219
Nucofed Expectorant ... 2219
Nucofed Pediatric Expectorant ... 2220
Nucofed Syrup ... 2219
Phenaphen with Codeine Capsules 1865
Phenaphen-650 with Codeine Tablets ... 1866
Phenergan with Codeine ... 2497
Phenergan VC with Codeine ... 2501
Robitussin A-C Syrup ... 1875
Robitussin-DAC Syrup ... 1875
Ryna ... ⊡ 741
Soma Compound w/Codeine Tablets ... 2390
Triaminic Expectorant w/Codeine .. 1996
Tussi-Organidin Liquid ... 2391
Tylenol with Codeine ... 1381
Codeine Polistirex (Additive effects).
No products indexed under this heading.
Desipramine Hydrochloride (Additive effects). Products include:
Norpramin Tablets ... 1340
Dezocine (Additive effects).
Diazepam (Additive effects). Products include:
Valium Injectable ... 1937
Valium Tablets ... 1939
Valrelease Capsules ... 1923
Dicumarol (Diminished anticoagulant effects). Products include:
Dicumarol Tablets ... 516
Doxepin Hydrochloride (Additive effects). Products include:
Sinequan ... 1960
Droperidol (Additive effects). Products include:
Inapsine Injection ... 1140
Innovar Injection ... 1141
Enflurane (Additive effects). Products include:
Ethrane ... 599
Estazolam (Additive effects). Products include:
ProSom Tablets ... 554
Ethchlorvynol (Additive effects). Products include:
Placidyl Capsules ... 553
Ethinamate (Additive effects).
No products indexed under this heading.
Fentanyl (Additive effects). Products include:
Duragesic Transdermal System ... 1133
Fentanyl Citrate (Additive effects). Products include:
Innovar Injection ... 1141
Sublimaze Injection ... 1146
Fluphenazine Decanoate (Additive effects). Products include:
Prolixin Decanoate ... 1795
Fluphenazine Enanthate (Additive effects). Products include:
Prolixin Enanthate ... 1796
Fluphenazine Hydrochloride (Additive effects). Products include:
Prolixin Elixir ... 1793
Prolixin Injection ... 1791
Prolixin Oral Concentrate ... 1792
Prolixin Tablets ... 1793
Flurazepam Hydrochloride (Additive effects). Products include:
Dalmane Capsules ... 1927
Furazolidone (Prolonged anticholinergic effects of Optimine; concurrent administration is contraindicated). Products include:
Furoxone ... 1855
Glutethimide (Additive effects).
No products indexed under this heading.
Haloperidol (Additive effects). Products include:
Haldol Injection, Tablets and Concentrate ... 1373
Haloperidol Decanoate (Additive effects). Products include:
Haldol Decanoate ... 1375
Hydrocodone Bitartrate (Additive effects). Products include:
Anexsia 5/500 Tablets ... 2196
Anexsia 7.5/650 Tablets ... 2197
Azdone Tablets ... 844
Codiclear DH Syrup ... 845
Codimal DH Syrup ... 846
Damason-P ... 1356
Hycodan Syrup, Tablets ... 927
Hycomine Compound Tablets ... 929
Hycomine Syrup ... 927
Hycotuss Expectorant Syrup ... 930
Hydrocet Capsules ... 835
Lortab ASA Tablets ... 2414
Lortab ... 2412

Ru-Tuss with Hydrocodone 694
Triaminic Expectorant DH 1995
Vicodin Tablets 1187
Vicodin ES Tablets 1189
Zydone Capsules 941

Hydrocodone Polistirex (Additive effects). Products include:
Tussionex Extended-Release Suspension 988

Hydroxyzine Hydrochloride (Additive effects). Products include:
Atarax Tablets & Syrup 1941
Marax Tablets & DF Syrup 1954
Vistaril Intramuscular Solution 1970

Imipramine Hydrochloride (Additive effects). Products include:
Tofranil Ampuls 1038
Tofranil Tablets 1039

Imipramine Pamoate (Additive effects). Products include:
Tofranil-PM Capsules 1041

Isocarboxazid (Prolonged anticholinergic effects of Optimine; concurrent administration is contraindicated). Products include:
Marplan Tablets 1906

Isoflurane (Additive effects). Products include:
Forane 600

Ketamine Hydrochloride (Additive effects). Products include:
Ketalar 1726

Levorphanol Tartrate (Additive effects). Products include:
Levo-Dromoran 1906

Lorazepam (Additive effects). Products include:
Ativan Injection 2432
Ativan Tablets 2434

Loxapine Hydrochloride (Additive effects). Products include:
Loxitane 1213

Loxapine Succinate (Additive effects). Products include:
Loxitane Capsules 1213

Maprotiline Hydrochloride (Additive effects). Products include:
Ludiomil Tablets 874

Meperidine Hydrochloride (Additive effects). Products include:
Demerol 2047
Mepergan Injection 2479

Mephobarbital (Additive effects). Products include:
Mebaral Tablets 2061

Meprobamate (Additive effects). Products include:
Deprol Tablets 2382
Equagesic Tablets 2451
Miltown Tablets 2386
PMB 200 and PMB 400 2504

Mesoridazine (Additive effects). Products include:
Serentil 686

Methadone Hydrochloride (Additive effects). Products include:
Dolophine Hydrochloride Ampoules & Vials 1260
Dolophine Hydrochloride Tablets 1261
Methadone Hydrochloride Diskets 1284
Methadone Hydrochloride Oral Solution & Tablets 1987

Methohexital Sodium (Additive effects). Products include:
Brevital Sodium Vials 1248

Methoxyflurane (Additive effects).
No products indexed under this heading.

Midazolam Hydrochloride (Additive effects). Products include:
Versed Injection 1924

Molindone Hydrochloride (Additive effects). Products include:
Moban Tablets & Concentrate 932

Morphine Sulfate (Additive effects). Products include:
Astramorph/PF Injection, USP (Preservative-Free) 618
Duramorph 960
Infumorph 200 and Infumorph 500 Sterile Solutions 962
MS Contin Tablets 1814
MSIR 1817
Oramorph SR (Morphine Sulfate Sustained Release Tablets) 1988
Roxanol 1991

Nortriptyline Hydrochloride (Additive effects). Products include:
Pamelor 2019

Opium Alkaloids (Additive effects). Products include:
B & O No. 15A & No. 16A Supprettes 2395
Pantopon Injectable 1911

Oxazepam (Additive effects). Products include:
Serax Capsules 2522
Serax Tablets 2522

Oxycodone Hydrochloride (Additive effects). Products include:
Percocet Tablets 950
Percodan 951
Roxicodone Tablets, Oral Solution & Intensol (Oxycodone) 1992
Tylox Capsules 1382

Pentobarbital Sodium (Additive effects). Products include:
Nembutal Sodium Capsules 534
Nembutal Sodium Solution 536
Nembutal Sodium Suppositories 538

Perphenazine (Additive effects). Products include:
Etrafon 2087
Triavil Tablets 1556
Trilafon 2123

Phenelzine Sulfate (Prolonged anticholinergic effects of Optimine; concurrent administration is contraindicated). Products include:
Nardil 1742

Phenobarbital (Additive effects). Products include:
Arco-Lase Plus Tablets 607
Bellergal-S Tablets 1998
Bronkolixir ▣ 761
Bronkotabs Tablets ▣ 762
Donnatal 1858
Donnatal Extentabs 1859
Donnatal Tablets 1858
Donnazyme Tablets 1860
Kinesed Tablets 2272
Phenobarbital Elixir and Tablets 1293
Primatene Tablets-P Formula 2421
Quadrinal Tablets 1183
Tedral SA 1765

Prazepam (Additive effects). Products include:
Centrax 1693

Prochlorperazine (Additive effects). Products include:
Compazine 2201

Promethazine Hydrochloride (Additive effects). Products include:
Mepergan Injection 2479
Phenergan with Codeine 2497
Phenergan with Dextromethorphan 2499
Phenergan Injection 2493
Phenergan Suppositories 2496
Phenergan Syrup 2495
Phenergan Tablets 2496
Phenergan VC 2500
Phenergan VC with Codeine 2501

Propofol (Additive effects). Products include:
Diprivan Injection 2267

Propoxyphene Hydrochloride (Additive effects). Products include:
Darvon 1256
Wygesic Tablets 2540

Propoxyphene Napsylate (Additive effects). Products include:
Darvon-N/Darvocet-N 1254

Protriptyline Hydrochloride (Additive effects). Products include:
Vivactil Tablets 1567

Quazepam (Additive effects). Products include:
Doral Tablets 2383

Secobarbital Sodium (Additive effects). Products include:
Seconal Sodium Pulvules 1296

Selegiline Hydrochloride (Prolonged anticholinergic effects of Optimine; concurrent administration is contraindicated). Products include:
Eldepryl 2250

Sufentanil Citrate (Additive effects). Products include:
Sufenta Injection 1147

Temazepam (Additive effects). Products include:
Restoril Capsules 2023

Thiamylal Sodium (Additive effects). Products include:
Surital Ampoules, Steri-Vials 1764

Thioridazine Hydrochloride (Additive effects). Products include:
Mellaril 2011

Thiothixene (Additive effects). Products include:
Navane Capsules and Concentrate 1954
Navane Intramuscular 1956

Tranylcypromine Sulfate (Prolonged anticholinergic effects of Optimine; concurrent administration is contraindicated). Products include:
Parnate Tablets 2222

Triazolam (Additive effects). Products include:
Halcion Tablets 2340

Trifluoperazine Hydrochloride (Additive effects). Products include:
Stelazine 2226

Trimipramine Maleate (Additive effects). Products include:
Surmontil Capsules 2524

Warfarin Sodium (Diminished anticoagulant effects). Products include:
Coumadin Injection & Tablets 944
Panwarfin Tablets 547

OPTIPRANOLOL STERILE OPHTHALMIC SOLUTION
(Metipranolol Hydrochloride) ◉ 261
May interact with $beta_2$ agonists, catecholamine depleting drugs, adrenergic augmenting psychotropics, calcium channel blockers, cardiac glycosides, and certain other agents. Compounds in these categories include:

Acebutolol Hydrochloride (Potential for additive effects). Products include:
Sectral Capsules 2520

Atenolol (Potential for additive effects). Products include:
Tenoretic Tablets 1105
Tenormin Tablets and I.V. Injection 1107

Bepridil Hydrochloride (Possible precipitation of left ventricular failure and hypotension). Products include:
Vascor (200, 300 and 400 mg) Tablets 1383

Betaxolol Hydrochloride (Potential for additive effects). Products include:
Betoptic Sterile Ophthalmic Solution 569
Betoptic S Sterile Ophthalmic Suspension 570
Kerlone Tablets 2172

Carteolol Hydrochloride (Potential for additive effects). Products include:
Cartrol Tablets 507

Deserpidine (Possible additive effects and the production of hypotension and/or bradycardia). Products include:
Enduronyl 518
Harmonyl Tablets 528
Oreticyl 545

Deslanoside (The concomitant use of beta-adrenergic receptor blocking agents with digitalis and calcium channel antagonists may have additive effects, prolonging arterioventricular conduction time).
No products indexed under this heading.

Digitoxin (The concomitant use of beta-adrenergic receptor blocking agents with digitalis and calcium channel antagonists may have additive effects, prolonging arterioventricular conduction time). Products include:
Crystodigin Tablets 1253

Digoxin (The concomitant use of beta-adrenergic receptor blocking agents with digitalis and calcium channel antagonists may have additive effects, prolonging arterioventricular conduction time). Products include:
Lanoxicaps 772
Lanoxin Elixir Pediatric 775
Lanoxin Injection 778
Lanoxin Injection Pediatric 781
Lanoxin Tablets 783

Diltiazem Hydrochloride (Possible precipitation of left ventricular failure and hypotension). Products include:
Cardizem Tablets-30 mg, 60 mg, 90 mg and 120 mg 1329
Cardizem SR Capsules-60 mg, 90 mg and 120 mg 1327

Esmolol Hydrochloride (Potential for additive effects). Products include:
Brevibloc Injection 942

Felodipine (Possible precipitation of left ventricular failure and hypotension). Products include:
Plendil Extended-Release Tablets 1526

Isocarboxazid (Caution should be used in patients using concomitant adrenergic psychotropic drugs). Products include:
Marplan Tablets 1906

Isradipine (Possible precipitation of left ventricular failure and hypotension). Products include:
DynaCirc Capsules 2004

Labetalol Hydrochloride (Potential for additive effects). Products include:
Normodyne Injection 2108
Normodyne Tablets 2110
Normozide Tablets 2112
Trandate HCT Tablets 579
Trandate Injection 577
Trandate Tablets 579

Metoprolol Tartrate (Potential for additive effects). Products include:
Lopressor Ampuls 1032
Lopressor HCT Tablets 1034
Lopressor Tablets 1032

Nadolol (Potential for additive effects). Products include:
Corgard Tablets 701
Corzide Tablets 702

Nicardipine Hydrochloride (Possible precipitation of left ventricular failure and hypotension). Products include:
Cardene Capsules 2290

Nifedipine (Possible precipitation of left ventricular failure and hypotension). Products include:
Adalat Capsules (10 mg and 20 mg) 1587
Procardia Capsules 1781
Procardia XL Tablets 1783

Nimodipine (Possible precipitation of left ventricular failure and hypotension). Products include:
Nimotop Capsules 1607

Pargyline Hydrochloride (Caution should be used in patients using concomitant adrenergic psychotropic drugs).
No products indexed under this heading.

Penbutolol Sulfate (Potential for additive effects). Products include:
Levatol 1832

Phenelzine Sulfate (Caution should be used in patients using concomitant adrenergic psychotropic drugs). Products include:
Nardil 1742

Pindolol (Potential for additive effects). Products include:
Visken Tablets 2036

Propranolol Hydrochloride (Potential for additive effects). Products include:
Inderal 2459
Inderal LA Long Acting Capsules 2461
Inderide Tablets 2463
Inderide LA Long Acting Capsules 2465

Rauwolfia Serpentina (Possible additive effects and the production of hypotension and/or bradycardia). Products include:
Raudixin Tablets 1803
Rauzide Tablets 1804

Rescinnamine (Possible additive effects and the production of hypotension and/or bradycardia).
No products indexed under this heading.

Reserpine (Possible additive effects and the production of hypotension and/or bradycardia). Products include:
Diupres Tablets 1461
Hydromox R Tablets 1209
Hydropres Tablets 1485
Renese-R Tablets 1786
Salutensin/Salutensin-Demi 719
Ser-Ap-Es Tablets 881
Serpasil Tablets 883
Serpasil-Apresoline Tablets 884
Serpasil-Esidrix Tablets 886

Timolol Maleate (Potential for additive effects). Products include:
Blocadren Tablets 1429
Timolide Tablets 1547
Timoptic in Ocudose 1552
Timoptic Sterile Ophthalmic Solution 1550

Tranylcypromine Sulfate (Caution should be used in patients using concomitant adrenergic psychotropic drugs). Products include:
Parnate Tablets 2222

Verapamil Hydrochloride (Possible precipitation of left ventricular failure and hypotension). Products include:
Calan SR Caplets 2157
Calan Tablets 2155
Isoptin Injectable 1177
Isoptin Oral Tablets 1179
Isoptin SR Sustained Release Tablets 1181
Verelan Capsules 1243
Verelan Capsules 2535

ORABASE HCA ORAL PASTE
(Hydrocortisone Acetate) 890
No interactions described in labeling.

ORAL REHYDRATION SALTS, CITRATE
(Electrolyte Supplement) 1150
No interactions described in labeling.

ORAMORPH SR (MORPHINE SULFATE SUSTAINED RELEASE TABLETS)
(Morphine Sulfate) 1988
May interact with central nervous system depressants, hypnotics and sedatives, antihistamines, psychotropics, and certain other agents. Compounds in these categories include:

Alcohol (CNS depressant effects are potentiated).

Alfentanil Hydrochloride (CNS depressant effects are potentiated). Products include:
Alfenta Injection 1131

Alprazolam (CNS depressant effects are potentiated). Products include:
Xanax Tablets 2367

Amitriptyline Hydrochloride (CNS depressant effects are potentiated). Products include:
Elavil 2269
Endep Tablets 1927
Etrafon 2087
Limbitrol 1933
Triavil Tablets 1556

Amoxapine (CNS depressant effects are potentiated). Products include:
Asendin Tablets 1196

Aprobarbital (CNS depressant effects are potentiated). Products include:
Alurate Elixir 1883

Astemizole (CNS depressant effects are potentiated). Products include:
Hismanal Tablets 1138

Azatadine Maleate (CNS depressant effects are potentiated). Products include:
Optimine Tablets 2115
Trinalin Repetabs Tablets 1170

Bromodiphenhydramine Hydrochloride (CNS depressant effects are potentiated).
No products indexed under this heading.

Brompheniramine Maleate (CNS depressant effects are potentiated). Products include:
Alka Seltzer Plus Sinus Allergy Medicine ▣ 624
Atrohist Sprinkle Capsules 558
Bromfed Capsules (Timed Release) 1615
Bromfed Syrup ▣ 628
Bromfed 1615
Dimetane Decongestant ▣ 673
Dimetane ▣ 672
Dimetane-DC Cough Syrup 1857
Dimetane-DX Cough Syrup 1858
Dimetapp Elixir ▣ 673
Dimetapp DM Elixir ▣ 674
Dimetapp Extentabs ▣ 674
Dimetapp Plus Caplets ▣ 675
Dimetapp Tablets ▣ 675
Drixoral Antihistamine/Nasal Decongestant Syrup ▣ 698

Buprenorphine (CNS depressant effects are potentiated; may alter analgesic effect or may precipitate withdrawal symptoms).
No products indexed under this heading.

Buspirone Hydrochloride (CNS depressant effects are potentiated). Products include:
BuSpar 1401

Butabarbital (CNS depressant effects are potentiated). Products include:
Pyridium Plus 1764

Butalbital (CNS depressant effects are potentiated). Products include:
Esgic-Plus Tablets 1002
Esgic Tablets & Capsules 1001
Fioricet Tablets 2006
Fiorinal Capsules 2007
Fiorinal with Codeine Capsules 2008
Fiorinal Tablets 2007
Phrenilin 838
Sedapap Tablets 50 mg/650 mg 1360

Butorphanol Tartrate (May alter analgesic effect or may precipitate withdrawal symptoms). Products include:
Stadol 721

Chlordiazepoxide (CNS depressant effects are potentiated). Products include:
Libritabs Tablets 1930
Limbitrol 1933
Menrium Tablets 1934

Chlordiazepoxide Hydrochloride (CNS depressant effects are potentiated). Products include:
Librax Capsules 1929
Librium Capsules 1931
Librium Injectable 1932

Chlorpheniramine Maleate (CNS depressant effects are potentiated). Products include:
A.R.M. Allergy Relief Medicine Caplets ▣ 615
Alka-Seltzer Plus Cold Medicine ▣ 623
Allerest ▣ 559
Ana-Kit Anaphylaxis Emergency Treatment Kit 1100
BC Cold Powder Multi-Symptom Formula ▣ 517
Brexin L.A. Capsules 2078
Cerose-DM 2443
Cheracol Plus Head Cold/Cough Formula ▣ 667
Chlor-Trimeton Allergy Syrup, Tablets & Long-Acting Repetabs Tablets ▣ 693
Chlor-Trimeton Decongestant ▣ 694
Comhist LA Capsules 1618
Allergy-Sinus Comtrex Multi-Symptom Allergy Sinus Formula Tablets & Caplets 746
Comtrex Multi-Symptom Cold Reliever Tablets/Caplets/Liqui-Gels/Liquid 745
Day-Night Comtrex 747
Contac Continuous Action Decongestant/Antihistamine Capsules ▣ 710
Contac Maximum Strength Continuous Action Decongestant/Antihistamine Caplets ▣ 709
Contac Severe Cold and Flu Formula Caplets ▣ 711
Coricidin 'D' Decongestant Tablets ▣ 695
Coricidin Demilets Tablets for Children ▣ 696
Coricidin Tablets ▣ 695
Deconamine 663
Demazin Nasal Decongestant/Antihistamine Repetabs Tablets & Syrup ▣ 697
Dorcol Children's Liquid Cold Formula ▣ 686
Dristan Decongestant/Antihistamine/ Analgesic Coated Caplets ▣ 749
Dristan Cold Nasal Decongestant/Antihistamine/ Analgesic Coated Tablets 2419
Dristan Advanced Formula Decongestant/Antihistamine/ Analgesic Tablets ▣ 749
Extendryl 994
4-Way Cold Tablets 750
Fedahist Gyrocaps 2145
Fedahist Timecaps 2145
Hycomine Compound Tablets 929
Isoclor Timesule Capsules ▣ 561
Kronofed-A 970
Medi-Flu Caplet, Liquid ▣ 640
Naldecon Syrup, Tablets, Pediatric Drops and Pediatric Syrup 709
Nolamine Tablets 838
Novafed A Capsules 1342
Novahistine DH 1342
Novahistine Elixir ▣ 596
Ornade Spansule Capsules 2221
Orthoxicol Cough Syrup ▣ 668
PediaCare Allergy Relief Formula Liquid 1362
PediaCare Cough-Cold Formula Liquid 1362
PediaCare Night Rest Cough-Cold Formula Liquid 1362
PediaCare 6-12 Cough-Cold Formula Chewable Tablets 1362
Pyrroxate Capsules ▣ 669
Quelidrine Syrup 556
Ru-Tuss II Capsules 693
Ru-Tuss Tablets 693
Ryna ▣ 741
Sinarest Tablets & Extra Strength Tablets ▣ 562
Sine-Off Maximum Strength Allergy/Sinus Formula Caplets ▣ 721
Sine-Off Sinus Medicine Tablets-Aspirin Formula ▣ 722
Singlet Tablets ▣ 598
Sinulin 840
Sinutab Maximum Strength ▣ 641
St. Joseph Nighttime Cold Medicine ▣ 705
Sudafed Plus Liquid ▣ 544
Sudafed Plus Tablets ▣ 545
Teldrin Timed-Release Allergy Capsules, 12 mg 2192
TheraFlu Flu and Cold Medicine ▣ 687
Triaminic Allergy Tablets ▣ 688
Triaminic Chewables ▣ 688
Triaminic Cold Tablets ▣ 688
Triaminic Nite Light ▣ 689
Triaminic Syrup ▣ 689
Triaminic-12 Tablets ▣ 690
Triaminicin Tablets ▣ 690
Triaminicol Multi-Symptom Cold Tablets ▣ 691
Triaminicol Multi-Symptom Relief ▣ 691
Tylenol Allergy Sinus Medication Caplets and Gelcaps, Maximum Strength 1372
Children's Tylenol Cold Liquid Formula and Chewable Tablets 1368
Tylenol Cold & Flu Hot Medication, Packets 1369
Tylenol Cold Medication Caplets and Tablets 1370
Tylenol Cold Medication, Effervescent Tablets 1369
Vicks Children's NyQuil ▣ 664
Vicks Formula 44 Cough Medicine ▣ 661
Vicks Formula 44M Multi-Symptom Cough Medicine ▣ 662
Vicks Pediatric Formula 44m Multi-Symptom Cough & Cold Medicine ▣ 663

Chlorpheniramine Polistirex (CNS depressant effects are potentiated). Products include:
Tussionex Extended-Release Suspension 988

Chlorpheniramine Tannate (CNS depressant effects are potentiated). Products include:
Rynatan 2387
Rynatuss 2388

Chlorpromazine (CNS depressant effects are potentiated). Products include:
Thorazine 2234

Chlorprothixene (CNS depressant effects are potentiated). Products include:
Taractan Tablets 1920

Chlorprothixene Hydrochloride (CNS depressant effects are potentiated). Products include:
Taractan 1920

Clemastine Fumarate (CNS depressant effects are potentiated). Products include:
Tavist Syrup 2033
Tavist Tablets 2035
Tavist-D Tablets 2035

Clorazepate Dipotassium (CNS depressant effects are potentiated). Products include:
Tranxene 556

Codeine (CNS depressant effects are potentiated). Products include:
Calcidrine Syrup 506

Codeine Phosphate (CNS depressant effects are potentiated). Products include:
Actifed with Codeine Cough Syrup 752
Cheracol Cough Syrup 1853
Codimal PH Syrup 846
Dimetane-DC Cough Syrup 1857
Empirin with Codeine Phosphate Nos. 2, 3 & 4 764
Fiorinal with Codeine Capsules 2008
Isoclor Expectorant 982
Naldecon CX Adult Liquid ▣ 521
Novahistine DH 1342
Novahistine Expectorant 1343
Nucofed Capsules 2219

Nucofed Expectorant ... 2219
Nucofed Pediatric Expectorant ... 2220
Nucofed Syrup ... 2219
Phenaphen with Codeine Capsules 1865
Phenaphen-650 with Codeine Tablets ... 1866
Phenergan with Codeine ... 2497
Phenergan VC with Codeine ... 2501
Robitussin A-C Syrup ... 1875
Robitussin-DAC Syrup ... 1875
Ryna ... ■ 741
Soma Compound w/Codeine Tablets ... 2390
Triaminic Expectorant w/Codeine .. 1996
Tussi-Organidin Liquid ... 2391
Tylenol with Codeine ... 1381

Codeine Polistirex (CNS depressant effects are potentiated).
No products indexed under this heading.

Cyproheptadine Hydrochloride (CNS depressant effects are potentiated). Products include:
Periactin ... 1525

Desipramine Hydrochloride (CNS depressant effects are potentiated). Products include:
Norpramin Tablets ... 1340

Dexchlorpheniramine Maleate (CNS depressant effects are potentiated). Products include:
Polaramine ... 2116

Dezocine (CNS depressant effects are potentiated).

Diazepam (CNS depressant effects are potentiated). Products include:
Valium Injectable ... 1937
Valium Tablets ... 1939
Valrelease Capsules ... 1923

Diphenhydramine Citrate (CNS depressant effects are potentiated). Products include:
Alka-Seltzer Plus Night-Time Cold Medicine ... ■ 623
Bufferin AF Nite Time Analgesic/Sleeping Aid Caplets ... 744
Excedrin P.M. Analgesic/Sleeping Aid Tablets, Caplets and Liquid.... 749

Diphenhydramine Hydrochloride (CNS depressant effects are potentiated). Products include:
Benadryl Anti-Itch Cream ... ■ 635
Benadryl Capsules ... 1691
Benadryl Decongestant Elixir ... ■ 635
Benadryl Decongestant ... ■ 635
Benadryl Elixir ... ■ 636
Benadryl Kapseals ... 1691
Benadryl 25 Kapseals ... ■ 636
Benadryl Parenteral ... 1692
Benadryl Plus ... ■ 636
Benadryl Plus Nighttime ... ■ 637
Benadryl Spray, Maximum Strength ... ■ 637
Benadryl Spray, Regular Strength ■ 637
Benadryl Steri-Vials, Ampoules, and Steri-Dose Syringe ... 1692
Benadryl 25 Tablets ... ■ 636
Benylin Cough Syrup ... ■ 637
Benylin Decongestant ... ■ 638
Caladryl Cream, Lotion, Spray ... ■ 638
Miles Nervine Nighttime Sleep-Aid ■ 627
Nytol Tablets ... ■ 517
Sleep-ettes-D Tablets ... ■ 653
Sleep-eze 3 Tablets ... ■ 755
Sleepinal Night-time Sleep Aid Capsules ... ■ 734
Sominex Caplets and Tablets ... ■ 722
Sominex Liquid ... ■ 723
Sominex Pain Relief Formula ... ■ 723
Tylenol Cold Night Time Medication Liquid ... 1371
Tylenol PM, Extra Strength Caplets and Tablets ... 1368
Unisom Dual Relief Nighttime Sleep Aid/Analgesic ... 1774
Ziradryl Lotion ... ■ 643

Doxepin Hydrochloride (CNS depressant effects are potentiated). Products include:
Sinequan ... 1960

Droperidol (CNS depressant effects are potentiated). Products include:
Inapsine Injection ... 1140
Innovar Injection ... 1141

Enflurane (CNS depressant effects are potentiated). Products include:
Ethrane ... 599

Estazolam (CNS depressant effects are potentiated). Products include:
ProSom Tablets ... 554

Ethchlorvynol (CNS depressant effects are potentiated). Products include:
Placidyl Capsules ... 553

Ethinamate (CNS depressant effects are potentiated).
No products indexed under this heading.

Fentanyl (CNS depressant effects are potentiated). Products include:
Duragesic Transdermal System ... 1133

Fentanyl Citrate (CNS depressant effects are potentiated). Products include:
Innovar Injection ... 1141
Sublimaze Injection ... 1146

Fluphenazine Decanoate (CNS depressant effects are potentiated). Products include:
Prolixin Decanoate ... 1795

Fluphenazine Enanthate (CNS depressant effects are potentiated). Products include:
Prolixin Enanthate ... 1796

Fluphenazine Hydrochloride (CNS depressant effects are potentiated). Products include:
Prolixin Elixir ... 1793
Prolixin Injection ... 1791
Prolixin Oral Concentrate ... 1792
Prolixin Tablets ... 1793

Flurazepam Hydrochloride (CNS depressant effects are potentiated). Products include:
Dalmane Capsules ... 1927

Glutethimide (CNS depressant effects are potentiated).
No products indexed under this heading.

Haloperidol (CNS depressant effects are potentiated). Products include:
Haldol Injection, Tablets and Concentrate ... 1373

Haloperidol Decanoate (CNS depressant effects are potentiated). Products include:
Haldol Decanoate ... 1375

Hydrocodone Bitartrate (CNS depressant effects are potentiated). Products include:
Anexsia 5/500 Tablets ... 2196
Anexsia 7.5/650 Tablets ... 2197
Azdone Tablets ... 844
Codiclear DH Syrup ... 845
Codimal DH Syrup ... 846
Damason-P ... 1356
Hycodan Syrup, Tablets ... 927
Hycomine Compound Tablets ... 929
Hycomine Syrup ... 927
Hycotuss Expectorant Syrup ... 930
Hydrocet Capsules ... 835
Lortab ASA Tablets ... 2414
Lortab ... 2412
Ru-Tuss with Hydrocodone ... 694
Triaminic Expectorant DH ... 1995
Vicodin Tablets ... 1187
Vicodin ES Tablets ... 1189
Zydone Capsules ... 941

Hydrocodone Polistirex (CNS depressant effects are potentiated). Products include:
Tussionex Extended-Release Suspension ... 988

Hydroxyzine Hydrochloride (CNS depressant effects are potentiated). Products include:
Atarax Tablets & Syrup ... 1941
Marax Tablets & DF Syrup ... 1954
Vistaril Intramuscular Solution ... 1970

Imipramine Hydrochloride (CNS depressant effects are potentiated). Products include:
Tofranil Ampuls ... 1038
Tofranil Tablets ... 1039

Imipramine Pamoate (CNS depressant effects are potentiated). Products include:
Tofranil-PM Capsules ... 1041

Isocarboxazid (CNS depressant effects are potentiated). Products include:
Marplan Tablets ... 1906

Isoflurane (CNS depressant effects are potentiated). Products include:
Forane ... 600

Ketamine Hydrochloride (CNS depressant effects are potentiated). Products include:
Ketalar ... 1726

Levorphanol Tartrate (CNS depressant effects are potentiated). Products include:
Levo-Dromoran ... 1906

Lithium Carbonate (CNS depressant effects are potentiated). Products include:
Eskalith ... 2214
Lithane Tablets ... 1596
Lithium Carbonate Capsules & Tablets ... 1984
Lithobid Tablets ... 870

Lithium Citrate (CNS depressant effects are potentiated). Products include:
Cibalith-S ... 870

Lorazepam (CNS depressant effects are potentiated). Products include:
Ativan Injection ... 2432
Ativan Tablets ... 2434

Loxapine Hydrochloride (CNS depressant effects are potentiated). Products include:
Loxitane ... 1213

Loxapine Succinate (CNS depressant effects are potentiated). Products include:
Loxitane Capsules ... 1213

Maprotiline Hydrochloride (CNS depressant effects are potentiated). Products include:
Ludiomil Tablets ... 874

Meperidine Hydrochloride (CNS depressant effects are potentiated). Products include:
Demerol ... 2047
Mepergan Injection ... 2479

Mephobarbital (CNS depressant effects are potentiated). Products include:
Mebaral Tablets ... 2061

Meprobamate (CNS depressant effects are potentiated). Products include:
Deprol Tablets ... 2382
Equagesic Tablets ... 2451
Miltown Tablets ... 2386
PMB 200 and PMB 400 ... 2504

Mesoridazine (CNS depressant effects are potentiated). Products include:
Serentil ... 686

Mesoridazine Besylate (CNS depressant effects are potentiated).

Methadone Hydrochloride (CNS depressant effects are potentiated). Products include:
Dolophine Hydrochloride Ampoules & Vials ... 1260
Dolophine Hydrochloride Tablets 1261
Methadone Hydrochloride Diskets .. 1284
Methadone Hydrochloride Oral Solution & Tablets ... 1987

Methdilazine Hydrochloride (CNS depressant effects are potentiated). Products include:
Tacaryl Syrup & Tablets ... 2409

Methohexital Sodium (CNS depressant effects are potentiated). Products include:
Brevital Sodium Vials ... 1248

Methoxyflurane (CNS depressant effects are potentiated).
No products indexed under this heading.

Midazolam Hydrochloride (CNS depressant effects are potentiated). Products include:
Versed Injection ... 1924

Molindone Hydrochloride (CNS depressant effects are potentiated). Products include:
Moban Tablets & Concentrate ... 932

Nalbuphine Hydrochloride (May alter analgesic effect or may precipitate withdrawal symptoms). Products include:
Nubain Injection ... 934

Nortriptyline Hydrochloride (CNS depressant effects are potentiated). Products include:
Pamelor ... 2019

Opium Alkaloids (CNS depressant effects are potentiated). Products include:
B & O No. 15A & No. 16A Supprettes ... 2395
Pantopon Injectable ... 1911

Oxazepam (CNS depressant effects are potentiated). Products include:
Serax Capsules ... 2522
Serax Tablets ... 2522

Oxycodone Hydrochloride (CNS depressant effects are potentiated). Products include:
Percocet Tablets ... 950
Percodan ... 951
Roxicodone Tablets, Oral Solution & Intensol (Oxycodone) ... 1992
Tylox Capsules ... 1382

Pentazocine Hydrochloride (May alter analgesic effect or may precipitate withdrawal symptoms). Products include:
Talacen ... 2070
Talwin Compound ... 2072
Talwin Nx ... 2073

Pentazocine Lactate (May alter analgesic effect or may precipitate withdrawal symptoms). Products include:
Talwin Injection ... 2071

Pentobarbital Sodium (CNS depressant effects are potentiated). Products include:
Nembutal Sodium Capsules ... 534
Nembutal Sodium Solution ... 536
Nembutal Sodium Suppositories ... 538

Perphenazine (CNS depressant effects are potentiated). Products include:
Etrafon ... 2087
Triavil Tablets ... 1556
Trilafon ... 2123

Phenelzine Sulfate (CNS depressant effects are potentiated). Products include:
Nardil ... 1742

Phenobarbital (CNS depressant effects are potentiated). Products include:
Arco-Lase Plus Tablets ... 607
Bellergal-S Tablets ... 1998
Bronkolixir ... ■ 761
Bronkotabs Tablets ... ■ 762
Donnatal ... 1858
Donnatal Extentabs ... 1859
Donnatal Tablets ... 1858
Donnazyme Tablets ... 1860
Kinesed Tablets ... 2272
Phenobarbital Elixir and Tablets ... 1293
Primatene Tablets-P Formula ... 2421
Quadrinal Tablets ... 1183
Tedral SA ... 1765

Prazepam (CNS depressant effects are potentiated). Products include:
- Centrax ... 1693

Prochlorperazine (CNS depressant effects are potentiated). Products include:
- Compazine ... 2201

Promethazine Hydrochloride (CNS depressant effects are potentiated). Products include:
- Mepergan Injection ... 2479
- Phenergan with Codeine ... 2497
- Phenergan with Dextromethorphan 2499
- Phenergan Injection ... 2493
- Phenergan Suppositories ... 2496
- Phenergan Syrup ... 2495
- Phenergan Tablets ... 2496
- Phenergan VC ... 2500
- Phenergan VC with Codeine ... 2501

Propofol (CNS depressant effects are potentiated). Products include:
- Diprivan Injection ... 2267

Propoxyphene Hydrochloride (CNS depressant effects are potentiated). Products include:
- Darvon ... 1256
- Wygesic Tablets ... 2540

Propoxyphene Napsylate (CNS depressant effects are potentiated). Products include:
- Darvon-N/Darvocet-N ... 1254

Protriptyline Hydrochloride (CNS depressant effects are potentiated). Products include:
- Vivactil Tablets ... 1567

Pyrilamine Maleate (CNS depressant effects are potentiated). Products include:
- Codimal ... 846
- 4-Way Fast Acting Nasal Spray - Original Formula (regular & mentholated) & Metered Spray Pump (regular) ... 751
- Maximum Strength Midol Multi-Symptom Menstrual Formula ... ⊡ 571
- Maximum Strength Midol PMS Premenstrual Syndrome Formula ... ⊡ 570
- Regular Strength Midol Multi-Symptom Menstrual Formula ... ⊡ 570
- Prefrin-A ... ◉ 255
- Prēmsyn PMS Capsules & Caplets ⊡ 547
- Primatene Tablets-M Formula ... 2421
- Robitussin Night Relief ... ⊡ 677
- Ru-Tuss with Hydrocodone ... 694
- Triaminic Expectorant DH ... 1995
- Triaminic Oral Infant Drops ... 1996

Pyrilamine Tannate (CNS depressant effects are potentiated). Products include:
- Rynatan ... 2387

Quazepam (CNS depressant effects are potentiated). Products include:
- Doral Tablets ... 2383

Secobarbital Sodium (CNS depressant effects are potentiated). Products include:
- Seconal Sodium Pulvules ... 1296

Sufentanil Citrate (CNS depressant effects are potentiated). Products include:
- Sufenta Injection ... 1147

Temazepam (CNS depressant effects are potentiated). Products include:
- Restoril Capsules ... 2023

Terfenadine (CNS depressant effects are potentiated). Products include:
- Seldane Tablets ... 1349
- Seldane-D Extended-Release Tablets ... 1350

Thiamylal Sodium (CNS depressant effects are potentiated). Products include:
- Surital Ampoules, Steri-Vials ... 1764

Thioridazine Hydrochloride (CNS depressant effects are potentiated). Products include:
- Mellaril ... 2011

Thiothixene (CNS depressant effects are potentiated). Products include:
- Navane Capsules and Concentrate 1954
- Navane Intramuscular ... 1956

Tranylcypromine Sulfate (CNS depressant effects are potentiated). Products include:
- Parnate Tablets ... 2222

Triazolam (CNS depressant effects are potentiated). Products include:
- Halcion Tablets ... 2340

Trifluoperazine Hydrochloride (CNS depressant effects are potentiated). Products include:
- Stelazine ... 2226

Trimeprazine Tartrate (CNS depressant effects are potentiated). Products include:
- Temaril Tablets, Syrup and Spansule Sustained Release Capsules 1085

Trimipramine Maleate (CNS depressant effects are potentiated). Products include:
- Surmontil Capsules ... 2524

Tripelennamine Hydrochloride (CNS depressant effects are potentiated). Products include:
- PBZ Tablets & Elixir ... 1037
- PBZ-SR Tablets ... 1037

Tripelennamine Preparations (CNS depressant effects are potentiated).

Triprolidine Hydrochloride (CNS depressant effects are potentiated). Products include:
- Actidil ... ⊡ 538
- Actifed Capsules ... ⊡ 539
- Actifed Plus Caplets ... ⊡ 539
- Actifed Plus Tablets ... ⊡ 540
- Actifed with Codeine Cough Syrup .. 752
- Actifed Syrup ... ⊡ 540
- Actifed Tablets ... ⊡ 540
- Actifed 12-Hour Capsules ... ⊡ 539

ORAP TABLETS

(Pimozide) ... 1020

May interact with phenothiazines, tricyclic antidepressants, antiarrhythmics, benzodiazepines, hypnotics and sedatives, narcotic analgesics, tranquilizers, central nervous system depressants, and certain other agents. Compounds in these categories include:

Acebutolol Hydrochloride (Prolonged QT interval). Products include:
- Sectral Capsules ... 2520

Adenosine (Prolonged QT interval). Products include:
- Adenocard Injection ... 1007

Alcohol (Potentiated CNS depressant effect).

Alfentanil Hydrochloride (Potentiated CNS depressant effect). Products include:
- Alfenta Injection ... 1131

Alprazolam (Potentiated CNS depressant effect). Products include:
- Xanax Tablets ... 2367

Amiodarone Hydrochloride (Prolonged QT interval on ECG). Products include:
- Cordarone Tablets ... 2446

Amitriptyline Hydrochloride (Prolonged QT interval on ECG). Products include:
- Elavil ... 2269
- Endep Tablets ... 1927
- Etrafon ... 2087
- Limbitrol ... 1933
- Triavil Tablets ... 1556

Amoxapine (Prolonged QT interval on ECG). Products include:
- Asendin Tablets ... 1196

Aprobarbital (Potentiated CNS depressant effect). Products include:
- Alurate Elixir ... 1883

Bretylium Tosylate (Prolonged QT interval on ECG). Products include:
- Bretylol Injection ... 923

Buprenorphine (Potentiated CNS depressant effect).
- No products indexed under this heading.

Buspirone Hydrochloride (Potentiated CNS depressant effect). Products include:
- BuSpar ... 1401

Butabarbital (Potentiated CNS depressant effect). Products include:
- Pyridium Plus ... 1764

Butalbital (Potentiated CNS depressant effect). Products include:
- Esgic-Plus Tablets ... 1002
- Esgic Tablets & Capsules ... 1001
- Fioricet Tablets ... 2006
- Fiorinal Capsules ... 2007
- Fiorinal with Codeine Capsules ... 2008
- Fiorinal Tablets ... 2007
- Phrenilin ... 838
- Sedapap Tablets 50 mg/650 mg .. 1360

Chlordiazepoxide (Potentiated CNS depressant effect). Products include:
- Libritabs Tablets ... 1930
- Limbitrol ... 1933
- Menrium Tablets ... 1934

Chlordiazepoxide Hydrochloride (Potentiated CNS depressant effect). Products include:
- Librax Capsules ... 1929
- Librium Capsules ... 1931
- Librium Injectable ... 1932

Chlorpromazine (Prolonged QT interval on ECG; potentiated CNS depressant effect). Products include:
- Thorazine ... 2234

Chlorprothixene (Potentiated CNS depressant effect). Products include:
- Taractan Tablets ... 1920

Chlorprothixene Hydrochloride (Potentiated CNS depressant effect). Products include:
- Taractan ... 1920

Clomipramine Hydrochloride (Prolonged QT interval on ECG). Products include:
- Anafranil Capsules ... 650

Clorazepate Dipotassium (Potentiated CNS depressant effect). Products include:
- Tranxene ... 556

Codeine (Potentiated CNS depressant effect). Products include:
- Calcidrine Syrup ... 506

Codeine Phosphate (Potentiated CNS depressant effect). Products include:
- Actifed with Codeine Cough Syrup .. 752
- Cheracol Cough Syrup ... 1853
- Codimal PH Syrup ... 846
- Dimetane-DC Cough Syrup ... 1857
- Empirin with Codeine Phosphate Nos. 2, 3 & 4 ... 764
- Fiorinal with Codeine Capsules ... 2008
- Isoclor Expectorant ... 982
- Naldecon CX Adult Liquid ... ⊡ 521
- Novahistine DH ... 1342
- Novahistine Expectorant ... 1343
- Nucofed Capsules ... 2219
- Nucofed Expectorant ... 2219
- Nucofed Pediatric Expectorant ... 2220
- Nucofed Syrup ... 2219
- Phenaphen with Codeine Capsules 1865
- Phenaphen-650 with Codeine Tablets ... 1866
- Phenergan with Codeine ... 2497
- Phenergan VC with Codeine ... 2501
- Robitussin A-C Syrup ... 1875
- Robitussin-DAC Syrup ... 1875
- Ryna ... ⊡ 741
- Soma Compound w/Codeine Tablets ... 2390
- Triaminic Expectorant w/Codeine .. 1996
- Tussi-Organidin Liquid ... 2391
- Tylenol with Codeine ... 1381

Codeine Polistirex (Potentiated CNS depressant effect).
- No products indexed under this heading.

Desipramine Hydrochloride (Prolonged QT interval on ECG). Products include:
- Norpramin Tablets ... 1340

Dezocine (Potentiated CNS depressant effect).

Diazepam (Potentiated CNS depressant effect). Products include:
- Valium Injectable ... 1937
- Valium Tablets ... 1939
- Valrelease Capsules ... 1923

Disopyramide Phosphate (Prolonged QT interval on ECG). Products include:
- Norpace ... 2177

Doxepin Hydrochloride (Prolonged QT interval on ECG). Products include:
- Sinequan ... 1960

Droperidol (Potentiated CNS depressant effect). Products include:
- Inapsine Injection ... 1140
- Innovar Injection ... 1141

Enflurane (Potentiated CNS depressant effect). Products include:
- Ethrane ... 599

Estazolam (Potentiated CNS depressant effect). Products include:
- ProSom Tablets ... 554

Ethchlorvynol (Potentiated CNS depressant effect). Products include:
- Placidyl Capsules ... 553

Ethinamate (Potentiated CNS depressant effect).
- No products indexed under this heading.

Fentanyl (Potentiated CNS depressant effect). Products include:
- Duragesic Transdermal System ... 1133

Fentanyl Citrate (Potentiated CNS depressant effect). Products include:
- Innovar Injection ... 1141
- Sublimaze Injection ... 1146

Fluphenazine Decanoate (Prolonged QT interval on ECG; potentiated CNS depressant effect). Products include:
- Prolixin Decanoate ... 1795

Fluphenazine Enanthate (Prolonged QT interval on ECG; potentiated CNS depressant effect). Products include:
- Prolixin Enanthate ... 1796

Fluphenazine Hydrochloride (Prolonged QT interval on ECG; potentiated CNS depressant effect). Products include:
- Prolixin Elixir ... 1793
- Prolixin Injection ... 1791
- Prolixin Oral Concentrate ... 1792
- Prolixin Tablets ... 1793

Flurazepam Hydrochloride (Potentiated CNS depressant effect). Products include:
- Dalmane Capsules ... 1927

Glutethimide (Potentiated CNS depressant effect).
- No products indexed under this heading.

Haloperidol (Potentiated CNS depressant effect). Products include:
- Haldol Injection, Tablets and Concentrate ... 1373

Haloperidol Decanoate (Potentiated CNS depressant effect). Products include:
- Haldol Decanoate ... 1375

Hydrocodone Bitartrate (Potentiated CNS depressant effect). Products include:
- Anexsia 5/500 Tablets ... 2196
- Anexsia 7.5/650 Tablets ... 2197
- Azdōne Tablets ... 844
- Codiclear DH Syrup ... 845

Codimal DH Syrup ... 846
Damason-P ... 1356
Hycodan Syrup, Tablets ... 927
Hycomine Compound Tablets ... 929
Hycomine Syrup ... 927
Hycotuss Expectorant Syrup ... 930
Hydrocet Capsules ... 835
Lortab ASA Tablets ... 2414
Lortab ... 2412
Ru-Tuss with Hydrocodone ... 694
Triaminic Expectorant DH ... 1995
Vicodin Tablets ... 1187
Vicodin ES Tablets ... 1189
Zydone Capsules ... 941

Hydrocodone Polistirex (Potentiated CNS depressant effect). Products include:
Tussionex Extended-Release Suspension ... 988

Hydroxyzine Hydrochloride (Potentiated CNS depressant effect). Products include:
Atarax Tablets & Syrup ... 1941
Marax Tablets & DF Syrup ... 1954
Vistaril Intramuscular Solution ... 1970

Imipramine Hydrochloride (Prolonged QT interval on ECG). Products include:
Tofranil Ampuls ... 1038
Tofranil Tablets ... 1039

Imipramine Pamoate (Prolonged QT interval on ECG). Products include:
Tofranil-PM Capsules ... 1041

Isoflurane (Potentiated CNS depressant effect). Products include:
Forane ... 600

Ketamine Hydrochloride (Potentiated CNS depressant effect). Products include:
Ketalar ... 1726

Levorphanol Tartrate (Potentiated CNS depressant effect). Products include:
Levo-Dromoran ... 1906

Lidocaine Hydrochloride (Prolonged QT interval on ECG). Products include:
Anestacon Solution ... 2394
Bactine Antiseptic/Anesthetic First Aid Spray ▣ 624
Decadron Phosphate with Xylocaine Injection, Sterile ... 1451
Xylocaine Injections ... 637
Xylocaine Injections for Ventricular Arrhythmias ... 639
Xylocaine 2% Jelly ... 643
4% Xylocaine-MPF Sterile Solution ... 641
Xylocaine 2% Viscous Solution ... 646

Lorazepam (Potentiated CNS depressant effect). Products include:
Ativan Injection ... 2432
Ativan Tablets ... 2434

Loxapine Hydrochloride (Potentiated CNS depressant effect). Products include:
Loxitane ... 1213

Loxapine Succinate (Potentiated CNS depressant effect). Products include:
Loxitane Capsules ... 1213

Maprotiline Hydrochloride (Prolonged QT interval on ECG). Products include:
Ludiomil Tablets ... 874

Meperidine Hydrochloride (Potentiated CNS depressant effect). Products include:
Demerol ... 2047
Mepergan Injection ... 2479

Mephobarbital (Potentiated CNS depressant effect). Products include:
Mebaral Tablets ... 2061

Meprobamate (Potentiated CNS depressant effect). Products include:
Deprol Tablets ... 2382
Equagesic Tablets ... 2451
Miltown Tablets ... 2386
PMB 200 and PMB 400 ... 2504

Mesoridazine (Prolonged QT interval on ECG; potentiated CNS depressant effect). Products include:
Serentil ... 686

Methadone Hydrochloride (Potentiated CNS depressant effect). Products include:
Dolophine Hydrochloride Ampoules & Vials ... 1260
Dolophine Hydrochloride Tablets ... 1261
Methadone Hydrochloride Diskets ... 1284
Methadone Hydrochloride Oral Solution & Tablets ... 1987

Methohexital Sodium (Potentiated CNS depressant effect). Products include:
Brevital Sodium Vials ... 1248

Methoxyflurane (Potentiated CNS depressant effect).
No products indexed under this heading.

Mexiletine Hydrochloride (Prolonged QT interval on ECG). Products include:
Mexitil Capsules ... 680

Midazolam Hydrochloride (Potentiated CNS depressant effect). Products include:
Versed Injection ... 1924

Molindone Hydrochloride (Potentiated CNS depressant effect). Products include:
Moban Tablets & Concentrate ... 932

Moricizine Hydrochloride (Prolonged QT interval). Products include:
Ethmozine Tablets ... 946

Morphine Sulfate (Potentiated CNS depressant effect). Products include:
Astramorph/PF Injection, USP (Preservative-Free) ... 618
Duramorph ... 960
Infumorph 200 and Infumorph 500 Sterile Solutions ... 962
MS Contin Tablets ... 1814
MSIR ... 1817
Oramorph SR (Morphine Sulfate Sustained Release Tablets) ... 1988
Roxanol ... 1991

Nortriptyline Hydrochloride (Prolonged QT interval on ECG). Products include:
Pamelor ... 2019

Opium Alkaloids (Potentiated CNS depressant effect). Products include:
B & O No. 15A & No. 16A Supprettes ... 2395
Pantopon Injectable ... 1911

Oxazepam (Potentiated CNS depressant effect). Products include:
Serax Capsules ... 2522
Serax Tablets ... 2522

Oxycodone Hydrochloride (Potentiated CNS depressant effect). Products include:
Percocet Tablets ... 950
Percodan ... 951
Roxicodone Tablets, Oral Solution & Intensol (Oxycodone) ... 1992
Tylox Capsules ... 1382

Pentobarbital Sodium (Potentiated CNS depressant effect). Products include:
Nembutal Sodium Capsules ... 534
Nembutal Sodium Solution ... 536
Nembutal Sodium Suppositories ... 538

Perphenazine (Prolonged QT interval on ECG; potentiated CNS depressant effect). Products include:
Etrafon ... 2087
Triavil Tablets ... 1556
Trilafon ... 2123

Phenobarbital (Potentiated CNS depressant effect). Products include:
Arco-Lase Plus Tablets ... 607
Bellergal-S Tablets ... 1998
Bronkolixir ▣ 761
Bronkotabs Tablets ▣ 762
Donnatal ... 1858
Donnatal Extentabs ... 1859
Donnatal Tablets ... 1858
Donnazyme Tablets ... 1860
Kinesed Tablets ... 2272
Phenobarbital Elixir and Tablets ... 1293
Primatene Tablets-P Formula ... 2421
Quadrinal Tablets ... 1183
Tedral SA ... 1765

Prazepam (Potentiated CNS depressant effect). Products include:
Centrax ... 1693

Procainamide Hydrochloride (Prolonged QT interval on ECG). Products include:
Procan SR Tablets ... 1760
Pronestyl Capsules and Tablets ... 1800
Pronestyl Injection ... 1798
Pronestyl-SR Tablets ... 1801

Prochlorperazine (Prolonged QT interval on ECG; potentiated CNS depressant effect). Products include:
Compazine ... 2201

Promethazine Hydrochloride (Prolonged QT interval on ECG; potentiated CNS depressant effect). Products include:
Mepergan Injection ... 2479
Phenergan with Codeine ... 2497
Phenergan with Dextromethorphan 2499
Phenergan Injection ... 2493
Phenergan Suppositories ... 2496
Phenergan Syrup ... 2495
Phenergan Tablets ... 2496
Phenergan VC ... 2500
Phenergan VC with Codeine ... 2501

Propafenone Hydrochloride (Prolonged QT interval). Products include:
Rythmol Tablets ... 1184

Propofol (Potentiated CNS depressant effect). Products include:
Diprivan Injection ... 2267

Propoxyphene Hydrochloride (Potentiated CNS depressant effect). Products include:
Darvon ... 1256
Wygesic Tablets ... 2540

Propoxyphene Napsylate (Potentiated CNS depressant effect). Products include:
Darvon-N/Darvocet-N ... 1254

Propranolol Hydrochloride (Prolonged QT interval on ECG). Products include:
Inderal ... 2459
Inderal LA Long Acting Capsules ... 2461
Inderide Tablets ... 2463
Inderide LA Long Acting Capsules .. 2465

Protriptyline Hydrochloride (Prolonged QT interval on ECG). Products include:
Vivactil Tablets ... 1567

Quazepam (Potentiated CNS depressant effect). Products include:
Doral Tablets ... 2383

Quinidine Gluconate (Prolonged QT interval on ECG). Products include:
Quinaglute Dura-Tabs Tablets ... 663

Quinidine Polygalacturonate (Prolonged QT interval on ECG). Products include:
Cardioquin Tablets ... 1812

Quinidine Sulfate (Prolonged QT interval on ECG). Products include:
Quinidex Extentabs ... 1868

Secobarbital Sodium (Potentiated CNS depressant effect). Products include:
Seconal Sodium Pulvules ... 1296

Sufentanil Citrate (Potentiated CNS depressant effect). Products include:
Sufenta Injection ... 1147

Temazepam (Potentiated CNS depressant effect). Products include:
Restoril Capsules ... 2023

Thiamylal Sodium (Potentiated CNS depressant effect). Products include:
Surital Ampoules, Steri-Vials ... 1764

Thioridazine Hydrochloride (Prolonged QT Interval on ECG; potentiated CNS depressant effect). Products include:
Mellaril ... 2011

Thiothixene (Potentiated CNS depressant effect). Products include:
Navane Capsules and Concentrate 1954
Navane Intramuscular ... 1956

Tocainide Hydrochloride (Prolonged QT interval on ECG). Products include:
Tonocard Tablets ... 1554

Triazolam (Potentiated CNS depressant effect). Products include:
Halcion Tablets ... 2340

Trifluoperazine Hydrochloride (Prolonged QT interval on ECG; potentiated CNS depressant effect). Products include:
Stelazine ... 2226

Trimipramine Maleate (Prolonged QT interval on ECG). Products include:
Surmontil Capsules ... 2524

Verapamil Hydrochloride (Prolonged QT interval on ECG). Products include:
Calan SR Caplets ... 2157
Calan Tablets ... 2155
Isoptin Injectable ... 1177
Isoptin Oral Tablets ... 1179
Isoptin SR Sustained Release Tablets ... 1181
Verelan Capsules ... 1243
Verelan Capsules ... 2535

ORATECT GEL
(Benzocaine) ... 1309
No interactions described in labeling.

ORCOLON
(Polyacrylamide) ... ◉ 325
No interactions described in labeling.

ORETIC TABLETS
(Hydrochlorothiazide) ... 544
May interact with antihypertensives, ganglionic blocking agents, para-aminobenzoic acid based local anesthetics, corticosteroids, cardiac glycosides, insulin, barbiturates, narcotic analgesics, and certain other agents. Compounds in these categories include:

Acebutolol Hydrochloride (Additive or potentiative effects). Products include:
Sectral Capsules ... 2520

ACTH (Hypokalemia).
No products indexed under this heading.

Alcohol (May aggravate orthostatic hypotension).

Alfentanil Hydrochloride (May aggravate orthostatic hypotension). Products include:
Alfenta Injection ... 1131

Aprobarbital (May aggravate orthostatic hypotension). Products include:
Alurate Elixir ... 1883

Atenolol (Additive or potentiative effects). Products include:
Tenoretic Tablets ... 1105
Tenormin Tablets and I.V. Injection 1107

Benazepril Hydrochloride (Additive or potentiative effects). Products include:
Lotensin Tablets ... 872

Bendroflumethiazide (Additive or potentiative effects). Products include:
Corzide Tablets ... 702

(▣ Described in PDR For Nonprescription Drugs) (◉ Described in PDR For Ophthalmology)

Naturetin Tablets 1789
Rauzide Tablets 1804

Betamethasone Acetate (Hypokalemia). Products include:
Celestone Soluspan Suspension 2081

Betamethasone Sodium Phosphate (Hypokalemia). Products include:
Celestone Soluspan Suspension 2081

Betaxolol Hydrochloride (Additive or potentiative effects). Products include:
Betoptic Sterile Ophthalmic Solution 569
Betoptic S Sterile Ophthalmic Suspension 570
Kerlone Tablets 2172

Buprenorphine (May aggravate orthostatic hypotension).
No products indexed under this heading.

Butabarbital (May aggravate orthostatic hypotension). Products include:
Pyridium Plus 1764

Butalbital (May aggravate orthostatic hypotension). Products include:
Esgic-Plus Tablets 1002
Esgic Tablets & Capsules 1001
Fioricet Tablets 2006
Fiorinal Capsules 2007
Fiorinal with Codeine Capsules 2008
Fiorinal Tablets 2007
Phrenilin 838
Sedapap Tablets 50 mg/650 mg 1360

Captopril (Additive or potentiative effects). Products include:
Capoten 2255
Capozide 2258

Carteolol Hydrochloride (Additive or potentiative effects). Products include:
Cartrol Tablets 507

Chlorothiazide (Additive or potentiative effects). Products include:
Aldoclor Tablets 1413
Diupres Tablets 1461
Diuril Oral 1464

Chlorothiazide Sodium (Additive or potentiative effects). Products include:
Diuril Sodium Intravenous 1463

Chlorthalidone (Additive or potentiative effects). Products include:
Combipres Tablets 678
Tenoretic Tablets 1105
Thalitone Tablets 687

Clonidine (Additive or potentiative effects). Products include:
Catapres-TTS 677

Clonidine Hydrochloride (Additive or potentiative effects). Products include:
Catapres Tablets 676
Combipres Tablets 678

Codeine (May aggravate orthostatic hypotension). Products include:
Calcidrine Syrup 506

Codeine Phosphate (May aggravate orthostatic hypotension). Products include:
Actifed with Codeine Cough Syrup 752
Cheracol Cough Syrup 1853
Codimal PH Syrup 846
Dimetane-DC Cough Syrup 1857
Empirin with Codeine Phosphate Nos. 2, 3 & 4 764
Fiorinal with Codeine Capsules 2008
Isoclor Expectorant 982
Naldecon CX Adult Liquid ▣ 521
Novahistine DH 1342
Novahistine Expectorant 1343
Nucofed Capsules 2219
Nucofed Expectorant 2219
Nucofed Pediatric Expectorant 2220
Nucofed Syrup 2219
Phenaphen with Codeine Capsules 1865
Phenaphen-650 with Codeine Tablets 1866
Phenergan with Codeine 2497
Phenergan VC with Codeine 2501
Robitussin A-C Syrup 1875
Robitussin-DAC Syrup 1875
Ryna ▣ 741
Soma Compound w/Codeine Tablets 2390
Triaminic Expectorant w/Codeine 1996
Tussi-Organidin Liquid 2391
Tylenol with Codeine 1381

Codeine Polistirex (May aggravate orthostatic hypotension).
No products indexed under this heading.

Cortisone Acetate (Hypokalemia). Products include:
Cortone Acetate Sterile Suspension 1437
Cortone Acetate Tablets 1439

Deserpidine (Potentiation occurs). Products include:
Enduronyl 518
Harmonyl Tablets 528
Oreticyl 545

Deslanoside (Increased sensitization to effects).
No products indexed under this heading.

Dexamethasone (Hypokalemia). Products include:
AK-Trol Ointment & Suspension ◉ 207
Decadron Elixir 1445
Decadron Tablets 1447
Decaspray Topical Aerosol 1459
Dexacidin ◉ 272
Maxidex Sterile Ophthalmic Suspension ◉ 223
Maxitrol Ophthalmic Ointment/Suspension ◉ 223
TobraDex Ophthalmic Suspension and Ointment ◉ 228

Dexamethasone Acetate (Hypokalemia). Products include:
Dalalone D.P. Injectable 999
Decadron-LA Sterile Suspension 1457

Dexamethasone Sodium Phosphate (Hypokalemia). Products include:
AK-Dex ◉ 203
Decadron Phosphate Respihaler 1454
Decadron Phosphate Sterile Ophthalmic Ointment 1453
Decadron Phosphate Sterile Ophthalmic Solution 1453
Decadron Phosphate Topical Cream 1455
Decadron Phosphate Turbinaire 1456
Maxidex Sterile Ophthalmic Ointment ◉ 222
NeoDecadron Sterile Ophthalmic Ointment 1517
NeoDecadron Sterile Ophthalmic Solution 1518
NeoDecadron Topical Cream 1518

Dezocine (May aggravate orthostatic hypotension).

Diazoxide (Additive or potentiative effects). Products include:
Hyperstat I.V. Injection 2095
Proglycem 649

Digitoxin (Increased sensitization to effects). Products include:
Crystodigin Tablets 1253

Digoxin (Increased sensitization to effects). Products include:
Lanoxicaps 772
Lanoxin Elixir Pediatric 775
Lanoxin Injection 778
Lanoxin Injection Pediatric 781
Lanoxin Tablets 783

Doxazosin Mesylate (Additive or potentiative effects). Products include:
Cardura Tablets 1941

Enalapril Maleate (Additive or potentiative effects). Products include:
Vaseretic Tablets 1559
Vasotec Tablets 1564

Enalaprilat (Additive of potentiative effects). Products include:
Vasotec I.V. 1562

Esmolol Hydrochloride (Additive or potentiative effects). Products include:
Brevibloc Injection 942

Felodipine (Additive or potentiative effects). Products include:
Plendil Extended-Release Tablets 1526

Fentanyl (May aggravate orthostatic hypotension). Products include:
Duragesic Transdermal System 1133

Fentanyl Citrate (May aggravate orthostatic hypotension). Products include:
Innovar Injection 1141
Sublimaze Injection 1146

Fosinopril Sodium (Additive or potentiative effects). Products include:
Monopril Tablets 1406

Furosemide (Additive or potentiative effects). Products include:
Lasix 1093

Guanabenz Acetate (Additive or potentiative effects). Products include:
Wytensin Tablets 2542

Guanethidine Monosulfate (Potentiation occurs). Products include:
Esimil Tablets 864
Ismelin Tablets 869

Hydralazine Hydrochloride (Additive or potentiative effects). Products include:
Apresazide Capsules 854
Apresoline Hydrochloride Parenteral (Ampuls) 856
Apresoline Hydrochloride Tablets 855
Apresoline-Esidrix Tablets 857
Ser-Ap-Es Tablets 881
Serpasil-Apresoline Tablets 884

Hydrocodone Bitartrate (May aggravate orthostatic hypotension). Products include:
Anexsia 5/500 Tablets 2196
Anexsia 7.5/650 Tablets 2197
Azdone Tablets 844
Codiclear DH Syrup 845
Codimal DH Syrup 846
Damason-P 1356
Hycodan Syrup, Tablets 927
Hycomine Compound Tablets 929
Hycomine Syrup 927
Hycotuss Expectorant Syrup 930
Hydrocet Capsules 835
Lortab ASA Tablets 2414
Lortab 2412
Ru-Tuss with Hydrocodone 694
Triaminic Expectorant DH 1995
Vicodin Tablets 1187
Vicodin ES Tablets 1189
Zydone Capsules 941

Hydrocodone Polistirex (May aggravate orthostatic hypotension). Products include:
Tussionex Extended-Release Suspension 988

Hydrocortisone (Hypokalemia). Products include:
AK-Spore H.C. ◉ 206
Bactine Hydrocortisone Anti-Itch Cream ▣ 625
CaldeCORT Anti-Itch Hydrocortisone Spray ▣ 560
Carmol HC Cream 1% 2296
Cortaid Spray ▣ 735
Cortenema 2244
Cortisporin Ointment 758
Cortisporin Ophthalmic Ointment Sterile 758
Cortisporin Ophthalmic Suspension Sterile 759
Cortisporin Otic Solution Sterile 760
Cortisporin Otic Suspension Sterile 760
Cortizone-5 Creme & Ointment ▣ 732
Dermolate Anti-Itch Cream ▣ 697
Eldecort Cream 1.0% 1113
Eldecort Cream 1.0% and 2.5% 1113
Fungoid HC Creme 1770
Hydrocortone Tablets 1482
Hytone 909
LazerSporin-C Solution 1770
Massengill Medicated Soft Cloth Towelettes 2192
Nutracort Cream & Lotion 1684
PediOtic Suspension Sterile 797
Synacort Creams 1%, 2.5% 2296
Vanoxide-HC Acne Lotion 911
Vioform-Hydrocortisone Cream and Mild Cream 889
Vioform-Hydrocortisone Ointment 889
VōSoL HC Otic Solution 2392
Vytone Cream 1% 911

Hydrocortisone Acetate (Hypokalemia). Products include:
Analpram-HC Rectal Cream 1% and 2.5% 970
Anusol-HC Cream 1690
Anusol-HC Suppositories 1691
Caldecort ▣ 560
Carmol HC Cream 1% 2296
Chloromycetin Hydrocortisone Ophthalmic 1694
Coly-Mycin S Otic w/Neomycin & Hydrocortisone 1708
Cortaid ▣ 735
Cortef Feminine Itch Cream ▣ 735
Corticaine ▣ 682
Cortifoam 1827
Cortisporin Cream 757
Epifoam 1828
Gynecort 5 Creme ▣ 556
Hydrocortone Acetate Sterile Suspension 1479
Lanacort 5 Creme and Ointment ▣ 557
Mantadil Cream 789
Ophthocort ◉ 301
Orabase HCA Oral Paste 890
Pramosone Cream, Lotion & Ointment 971
ProctoCream-HC 1834
Proctofoam-HC 1835

Hydrocortisone Sodium Phosphate (Hypokalemia). Products include:
Hydrocortone Phosphate Injection, Sterile 1481

Hydrocortisone Sodium Succinate (Hypokalemia). Products include:
Solu-Cortef Sterile Powder 2361

Hydroflumethiazide (Additive or potentiative effects). Products include:
Diucardin Tablets 2450
Saluron 718
Salutensin/Salutensin-Demi 719

Indapamide (Additive or potentiative effects). Products include:
Lozol Tablets 1843

Insulin, Human (Increased or decreased insulin requirements).
No products indexed under this heading.

Insulin, Human Isophane Suspension (Increased or decreased insulin requirements). Products include:
Humulin N, 100 Units 1270

Insulin, Human NPH (Increased or decreased insulin requirements). Products include:
Insulatard NPH Human 1627
Novolin N 1627
Novolin N PenFill Cartridges 1628
Novolin N Prefilled 1628

Insulin, Human Regular (Increased or decreased insulin requirements). Products include:
Humulin BR, 100 Units 1268
Humulin R, 100 Units 1272
Novolin R 1627
Novolin R PenFill Cartridges 1628
Novolin R Prefilled 1629
Velosulin Human 1628

Insulin, Human, Zinc Suspension (Increased or decreased insulin requirements). Products include:
Humulin L, 100 Units 1268
Humulin U, 100 Units 1272
Novolin L 1627

Insulin, NPH (Increased or decreased insulin requirements). Products include:
NPH, 40 & 100 Units 1273
Beef NPH, 100 Units 1274
Pork NPH, 100 Units 1275
Insulatard NPH 1626

NPH Insulin ... 1626
NPH Purified Pork Isophane Insulin ... 1626

Insulin, Regular (Increased or decreased insulin requirements). Products include:
Regular, 40 & 100 Units ... 1273
Beef Regular, 100 Units ... 1275
Pork Regular, 100 Units ... 1275
Pork Regular (Concentrated), 500 Units ... 1276
Regular Insulin ... 1625
Regular Purified Pork Insulin ... 1626
Velosulin ... 1627

Insulin, Zinc Crystals (Increased or decreased insulin requirements). Products include:
NPH, 40 & 100 Units ... 1273

Insulin, Zinc Suspension (Increased or decreased insulin requirements). Products include:
Lente, 40 & 100 Units ... 1272
Protamine, Zinc, 40 & 100 Units ... 1273
Lente Iletin I ... 1272
Beef Lente, 100 Units ... 1274
Beef Protamine Zinc, 100 Units ... 1274
Pork Lente, 100 Units ... 1275
Pork, Protamine, Zinc, 100 Units ... 1275
Lente Insulin ... 1626
Lente Purified Pork Insulin ... 1626
Semilente Insulin ... 1625
Ultralente Insulin ... 1626

Isradipine (Additive or potentiative effects). Products include:
DynaCirc Capsules ... 2004

Labetalol Hydrochloride (Additive or potentiative effects). Products include:
Normodyne Injection ... 2108
Normodyne Tablets ... 2110
Normozide Tablets ... 2112
Trandate HCT Tablets ... 579
Trandate Injection ... 577
Trandate Tablets ... 579

Levorphanol Tartrate (May aggravate orthostatic hypotension). Products include:
Levo-Dromoran ... 1906

Lisinopril (Additive or potentiative effects). Products include:
Prinivil Tablets ... 1538
Prinzide Tablets ... 1540
Zestoretic ... 2274
Zestril Tablets ... 2277

Mecamylamine Hydrochloride (Potentiation occurs). Products include:
Inversine Tablets ... 1492

Meperidine Hydrochloride (May aggravate orthostatic hypotension). Products include:
Demerol ... 2047
Mepergan Injection ... 2479

Mephobarbital (May aggravate orthostatic hypotension). Products include:
Mebaral Tablets ... 2061

Methadone Hydrochloride (May aggravate orthostatic hypotension). Products include:
Dolophine Hydrochloride Ampoules & Vials ... 1260
Dolophine Hydrochloride Tablets ... 1261
Methadone Hydrochloride Diskets ... 1284
Methadone Hydrochloride Oral Solution & Tablets ... 1987

Methyclothiazide (Additive or potentiative effects). Products include:
Enduron Tablets ... 517
Enduronyl ... 518

Methyldopa (Additive or potentiative effects). Products include:
Aldoclor Tablets ... 1413
Aldomet Oral ... 1415
Aldoril Tablets ... 1418

Methyldopate Hydrochloride (Additive or potentiated effects). Products include:
Aldomet Ester HCl Injection ... 1417

Methylprednisolone Acetate (Hypokalemia). Products include:
Depo-Medrol Sterile Aqueous Suspension ... 2334

Methylprednisolone Sodium Succinate (Hypokalemia). Products include:
Solu-Medrol Sterile Powder ... 2363

Metolazone (Additive or potentiative effects). Products include:
Diulo ... 2129
Mykrox ½ mg Tablets ... 984
Zaroxolyn Tablets ... 989

Metoprolol Tartrate (Additive or potentiative effects). Products include:
Lopressor Ampuls ... 1032
Lopressor HCT Tablets ... 1034
Lopressor Tablets ... 1032

Metyrosine (Additive or potentiative effects). Products include:
Demser Capsules ... 1460

Minoxidil (Additive or potentiative effects). Products include:
Loniten Tablets ... 2346
Rogaine Topical Solution ... 2357

Morphine Sulfate (May aggravate orthostatic hypotension). Products include:
Astramorph/PF Injection, USP (Preservative-Free) ... 618
Duramorph ... 960
Infumorph 200 and Infumorph 500 Sterile Solutions ... 962
MS Contin Tablets ... 1814
MSIR ... 1817
Oramorph SR (Morphine Sulfate Sustained Release Tablets) ... 1988
Roxanol ... 1991

Nadolol (Additive or potentiative effects). Products include:
Corgard Tablets ... 701
Corzide Tablets ... 702

Nicardipine Hydrochloride (Additive or potentiative effects). Products include:
Cardene Capsules ... 2290

Nitroglycerin (Additive or potentiative effects). Products include:
Deponit NTG Transdermal Delivery System ... 2143
Minitran Transdermal Delivery System ... 1312
Nitro-Bid Ointment ... 1339
Nitro-Bid Capsules ... 1338
Nitrodisc ... 2176
Nitro-Dur (nitroglycerin) Transdermal Infusion System ... 1164
Nitrogard Tablets ... 1004
Nitrolingual Spray ... 1846
Nitrostat Tablets ... 1743
Transderm-Nitro Transdermal Therapeutic System ... 2283

Norepinephrine Bitartrate (Decreased arterial responsiveness). Products include:
Levophed Bitartrate Injection ... 2054

Opium Alkaloids (May aggravate orthostatic hypotension). Products include:
B & O No. 15A & No. 16A Supprettes ... 2395
Pantopon Injectable ... 1911

Oxycodone Hydrochloride (May aggravate orthostatic hypotension). Products include:
Percocet Tablets ... 950
Percodan ... 951
Roxicodone Tablets, Oral Solution & Intensol (Oxycodone) ... 1992
Tylox Capsules ... 1382

Pancuronium Bromide Injection (Decreased serum levels).
No products indexed under this heading.

Penbutolol Sulfate (Additive or potentiative effects). Products include:
Levatol ... 1832

Pentobarbital Sodium (May aggravate orthostatic hypotension). Products include:
Nembutal Sodium Capsules ... 534
Nembutal Sodium Solution ... 536
Nembutal Sodium Suppositories ... 538

Phenobarbital (May aggravate orthostatic hypotension). Products include:
Arco-Lase Plus Tablets ... 607
Bellergal-S Tablets ... 1998
Bronkolixir ... ▣ 761
Bronkotabs Tablets ... ▣ 762
Donnatal ... 1858
Donnatal Extentabs ... 1859
Donnatal Tablets ... 1858
Donnazyme Tablets ... 1860
Kinesed Tablets ... 2272
Phenobarbital Elixir and Tablets ... 1293
Primatene Tablets-P Formula ... 2421
Quadrinal Tablets ... 1183
Tedral SA ... 1765

Phenoxybenzamine Hydrochloride (Additive or potentiative effects). Products include:
Dibenzyline Capsules ... 2207

Phentolamine Mesylate (Additive or potentiative effects). Products include:
Regitine ... 878

Pindolol (Additive or potentiative effects). Products include:
Visken Tablets ... 2036

Polythiazide (Additive or potentiative effects). Products include:
Minizide Capsules ... 1779
Renese Tablets ... 1785
Renese-R Tablets ... 1786

Prazosin Hydrochloride (Potentiation occurs). Products include:
Minipress Capsules ... 1778
Minizide Capsules ... 1779

Prednisolone Acetate (Hypokalemia). Products include:
AK-Cide Sterile Ophthalmic Ointment & Suspension ... ⊙ 202
Blephamide Liquifilm Sterile Ophthalmic Suspension ... 586
Blephamide S.O.P. Sterile Ophthalmic Ointment ... 586
Cetapred Ointment ... ⊙ 220
⅛% Econopred & 1% Econopred Plus ... ⊙ 217
Isopto Cetapred Suspension ... ⊙ 220
Metimyd ... ⊙ 306
Poly-Pred Liquifilm ... ⊙ 250
Pred Forte ... ⊙ 252
Pred Mild ... ⊙ 254
Pred-G Liquifilm Sterile Ophthalmic Suspension ... ⊙ 252
Pred-G S.O.P. Sterile Ophthalmic Ointment ... ⊙ 253
Vasocidin Ointment ... ⊙ 275

Prednisolone Sodium Phosphate (Hypokalemia). Products include:
AK-Pred ... ⊙ 205
Hydeltrasol Injection, Sterile ... 1476
Inflamase ... ⊙ 274
Pediapred Oral Liquid ... 987
Vasocidin Ophthalmic Solution ... ⊙ 276

Prednisolone Tebutate (Hypokalemia). Products include:
Hydeltra-T.B.A. Sterile Suspension 1478

Prednisone (Hypokalemia). Products include:
Deltasone Tablets ... 2332

Propoxyphene Hydrochloride (May aggravate orthostatic hypotension). Products include:
Darvon ... 1256
Wygesic Tablets ... 2540

Propoxyphene Napsylate (May aggravate orthostatic hypotension). Products include:
Darvon-N/Darvocet-N ... 1254

Propranolol Hydrochloride (Additive or potentiative effects). Products include:
Inderal ... 2459
Inderal LA Long Acting Capsules ... 2461
Inderide Tablets ... 2463
Inderide LA Long Acting Capsules .. 2465

Ramipril (Additive or potentiative effects). Products include:
Altace Capsules ... 1086

Rauwolfia Serpentina (Potentiation occurs). Products include:
Raudixin Tablets ... 1803
Rauzide Tablets ... 1804

Rescinnamine (Potentiation occurs).
No products indexed under this heading.

Reserpine (Potentiation occurs). Products include:
Diupres Tablets ... 1461
Hydromox R Tablets ... 1209
Hydropres Tablets ... 1485
Renese-R Tablets ... 1786
Salutensin/Salutensin-Demi ... 719
Ser-Ap-Es Tablets ... 881
Serpasil Tablets ... 883
Serpasil-Apresoline Tablets ... 884
Serpasil-Esidrix Tablets ... 886

Secobarbital Sodium (May aggravate orthostatic hypotension). Products include:
Seconal Sodium Pulvules ... 1296

Sodium Nitroprusside (Additive or potentiative effects). Products include:
Nipride I.V. Infusion ... 1909

Sufentanil Citrate (May aggravate orthostatic hypotension). Products include:
Sufenta Injection ... 1147

Terazosin Hydrochloride (Additive or potentiative effects). Products include:
Hytrin Tablets ... 529

Thiamylal Sodium (May aggravate orthostatic hypotension). Products include:
Surital Ampoules, Steri-Vials ... 1764

Timolol Maleate (Additive or potentiative effects). Products include:
Blocadren Tablets ... 1429
Timolide Tablets ... 1547
Timoptic in Ocudose ... 1552
Timoptic Sterile Ophthalmic Solution ... 1550

Triamcinolone (Hypokalemia).
No products indexed under this heading.

Triamcinolone Acetonide (Hypokalemia). Products include:
Aristocort A ... 1010
Azmacort Inhaler ... 1837
Kenalog Cream, Lotion & Ointment 2401
Kenalog-10 Injection ... 2402
Kenalog-40 Injection ... 2403
Kenalog in Orabase ... 604
Kenalog Spray ... 2401
Mycolog II Cream and Ointment ... 2407
Mytrex Cream & Ointment ... 2080
Nasacort Nasal Inhaler ... 1844

Triamcinolone Diacetate (Hypokalemia). Products include:
Aristocort Suspension ... 1008

Triamcinolone Hexacetonide (Hypokalemia). Products include:
Aristospan Suspension ... 1011

Trimethaphan Camsylate (Potentiation occurs). Products include:
Arfonad Ampuls ... 1887

Tubocurarine Chloride (Increased responsiveness).
No products indexed under this heading.

ORETICYL FORTE TABLETS
(Hydrochlorothiazide, Deserpidine) .. 545
See **Oreticyl Tablets**

ORETICYL TABLETS
(Hydrochlorothiazide, Deserpidine) .. 545
May interact with antihypertensives, ganglionic blocking agents, para-aminobenzoic acid based local anesthetics, corticosteroids, cardiac glyco-

sides, insulin, barbiturates, narcotic analgesics, and certain other agents. Compounds in these categories include:

Acebutolol Hydrochloride (Additive or potentiative effects). Products include:
Sectral Capsules 2520

ACTH (Hypokalemia).
No products indexed under this heading.

Alcohol (May aggravate orthostatic hypotension).

Alfentanil Hydrochloride (May aggravate orthostatic hypotension). Products include:
Alfenta Injection 1131

Aprobarbital (May aggravate orthostatic hypotension). Products include:
Alurate Elixir 1883

Atenolol (Additive or potentiative effects). Products include:
Tenoretic Tablets 1105
Tenormin Tablets and I.V. Injection 1107

Benazepril Hydrochloride (Additive or potentiative effects). Products include:
Lotensin Tablets 872

Bendroflumethiazide (Additive or potentiative effects). Products include:
Corzide Tablets 702
Naturetin Tablets 1789
Rauzide Tablets 1804

Betamethasone Acetate (Hypokalemia). Products include:
Celestone Soluspan Suspension 2081

Betamethasone Sodium Phosphate (Hypokalemia). Products include:
Celestone Soluspan Suspension 2081

Betaxolol Hydrochloride (Additive or potentiative effects). Products include:
Betoptic Sterile Ophthalmic Solution 569
Betoptic S Sterile Ophthalmic Suspension 570
Kerlone Tablets 2172

Buprenorphine (May aggravate orthostatic hypotension).
No products indexed under this heading.

Butabarbital (May aggravate orthostatic hypotension). Products include:
Pyridium Plus 1764

Butalbital (May aggravate orthostatic hypotension). Products include:
Esgic-Plus Tablets 1002
Esgic Tablets & Capsules 1001
Fioricet Tablets 2006
Fiorinal Capsules 2007
Fiorinal with Codeine Capsules 2008
Fiorinal Tablets 2007
Phrenilin 838
Sedapap Tablets 50 mg/650 mg 1360

Captopril (Additive or potentiative effects). Products include:
Capoten 2255
Capozide 2258

Carteolol Hydrochloride (Additive or potentiative effects). Products include:
Cartrol Tablets 507

Chlorothiazide (Additive or potentiative effects). Products include:
Aldoclor Tablets 1413
Diupres Tablets 1461
Diuril Oral 1464

Chlorothiazide Sodium (Additive or potentiative effects). Products include:
Diuril Sodium Intravenous 1463

Chlorthalidone (Additive or potentiative effects). Products include:
Combipres Tablets 678
Tenoretic Tablets 1105
Thalitone Tablets 687

Clonidine (Additive or potentiative effects). Products include:
Catapres-TTS 677

Clonidine Hydrochloride (Additive or potentiative effects). Products include:
Catapres Tablets 676
Combipres Tablets 678

Codeine (May aggravate orthostatic hypotension). Products include:
Calcidrine Syrup 506

Codeine Phosphate (May aggravate orthostatic hypotension). Products include:
Actifed with Codeine Cough Syrup 752
Cheracol Cough Syrup 1853
Codimal PH Syrup 846
Dimetane-DC Cough Syrup 1857
Empirin with Codeine Phosphate Nos. 2, 3 & 4 764
Fiorinal with Codeine Capsules 2008
Isoclor Expectorant 982
Naldecon CX Adult Liquid ▣ 521
Novahistine DH 1342
Novahistine Expectorant 1343
Nucofed Capsules 2219
Nucofed Expectorant 2219
Nucofed Pediatric Expectorant 2220
Nucofed Syrup 2219
Phenaphen with Codeine Capsules 1865
Phenaphen-650 with Codeine Tablets 1866
Phenergan with Codeine 2497
Phenergan VC with Codeine 2501
Robitussin A-C Syrup 1875
Robitussin-DAC Syrup 1875
Ryna ▣ 741
Soma Compound w/Codeine Tablets 2390
Triaminic Expectorant w/Codeine 1996
Tussi-Organidin Liquid 2391
Tylenol with Codeine 1381

Codeine Polistirex (May aggravate orthostatic hypotension).
No products indexed under this heading.

Cortisone Acetate (Hypokalemia). Products include:
Cortone Acetate Sterile Suspension 1437
Cortone Acetate Tablets 1439

Deslanoside (Increased sensitization to effects).
No products indexed under this heading.

Dexamethasone (Hypokalemia). Products include:
AK-Trol Ointment & Suspension ⊙ 207
Decadron Elixir 1445
Decadron Tablets 1447
Decaspray Topical Aerosol 1459
Dexacidin ⊙ 272
Maxidex Sterile Ophthalmic Suspension ⊙ 223
Maxitrol Ophthalmic Ointment/Suspension ⊙ 223
TobraDex Ophthalmic Suspension and Ointment ⊙ 228

Dexamethasone Acetate (Hypokalemia). Products include:
Dalalone D.P. Injectable 999
Decadron-LA Sterile Suspension 1457

Dexamethasone Sodium Phosphate (Hypokalemia). Products include:
AK-Dex ⊙ 203
Decadron Phosphate Respihaler 1454
Decadron Phosphate Sterile Ophthalmic Ointment 1453
Decadron Phosphate Sterile Ophthalmic Solution 1453
Decadron Phosphate Topical Cream 1455
Decadron Phosphate Turbinaire 1456
Maxidex Sterile Ophthalmic Ointment ⊙ 222
NeoDecadron Sterile Ophthalmic Ointment 1517
NeoDecadron Sterile Ophthalmic Solution 1518
NeoDecadron Topical Cream 1518

Dezocine (May aggravate orthostatic hypotension).

Diazoxide (Additive or potentiative effects). Products include:
Hyperstat I.V. Injection 2095
Proglycem 649

Digitoxin (Increased sensitization to effects). Products include:
Crystodigin Tablets 1253

Digoxin (Increased sensitization to effects). Products include:
Lanoxicaps 772
Lanoxin Elixir Pediatric 775
Lanoxin Injection 778
Lanoxin Injection Pediatric 781
Lanoxin Tablets 783

Doxazosin Mesylate (Additive or potentiative effects). Products include:
Cardura Tablets 1941

Enalapril Maleate (Additive or potentiative effects). Products include:
Vaseretic Tablets 1559
Vasotec Tablets 1564

Enalaprilat (Additive or potentiative effects). Products include:
Vasotec I.V. 1562

Esmolol Hydrochloride (Additive or potentiative effects). Products include:
Brevibloc Injection 942

Felodipine (Additive or potentiative effects). Products include:
Plendil Extended-Release Tablets 1526

Fentanyl (May aggravate orthostatic hypotension). Products include:
Duragesic Transdermal System 1133

Fentanyl Citrate (May aggravate orthostatic hypotension). Products include:
Innovar Injection 1141
Sublimaze Injection 1146

Fosinopril Sodium (Additive or potentiative effects). Products include:
Monopril Tablets 1406

Furosemide (Additive or potentiative effects). Products include:
Lasix 1093

Guanabenz Acetate (Additive or potentiative effects). Products include:
Wytensin Tablets 2542

Guanethidine Monosulfate (Cardiac arrhythmias; additive or potentiative effects). Products include:
Esimil Tablets 864
Ismelin Tablets 869

Hydralazine Hydrochloride (Additive or potentiative effects). Products include:
Apresazide Capsules 854
Apresoline Hydrochloride Parenteral (Ampuls) 856
Apresoline Hydrochloride Tablets 855
Apresoline-Esidrix Tablets 857
Ser-Ap-Es Tablets 881
Serpasil-Apresoline Tablets 884

Hydrocodone Bitartrate (May aggravate orthostatic hypotension). Products include:
Anexsia 5/500 Tablets 2196
Anexsia 7.5/650 Tablets 2197
Azdone Tablets 844
Codiclear DH Syrup 845
Codimal DH Syrup 846
Damason-P 1356
Hycodan Syrup, Tablets 927
Hycomine Compound Tablets 929
Hycomine Syrup 927
Hycotuss Expectorant Syrup 930
Hydrocet Capsules 835
Lortab ASA Tablets 2414
Lortab 2412
Ru-Tuss with Hydrocodone 694
Triaminic Expectorant DH 1995
Vicodin Tablets 1187
Vicodin ES Tablets 1189
Zydone Capsules 941

Hydrocodone Polistirex (May aggravate orthostatic hypotension). Products include:
Tussionex Extended-Release Suspension 988

Hydrocortisone (Hypokalemia). Products include:
AK-Spore H.C. ⊙ 206
Bactine Hydrocortisone Anti-Itch Cream ▣ 625
CaldeCORT Anti-Itch Hydrocortisone Spray ▣ 560
Carmol HC Cream 1% 2296
Cortaid Spray ▣ 735
Cortenema 2244
Cortisporin Ointment 758
Cortisporin Ophthalmic Ointment Sterile 758
Cortisporin Ophthalmic Suspension Sterile 759
Cortisporin Otic Solution Sterile 760
Cortisporin Otic Suspension Sterile 760
Cortizone-5 Creme & Ointment ▣ 732
Dermolate Anti-Itch Cream ▣ 697
Eldecort Cream 1.0% 1113
Eldecort Cream 1.0% and 2.5% 1113
Fungoid HC Creme 1770
Hydrocortone Tablets 1482
Hytone 909
LazerSporin-C Solution 1770
Massengill Medicated Soft Cloth Towelettes 2192
Nutracort Cream & Lotion 1684
PediOtic Suspension Sterile 797
Synacort Creams 1%, 2.5% 2296
Vanoxide-HC Acne Lotion 911
Vioform-Hydrocortisone Cream and Mild Cream 889
Vioform-Hydrocortisone Ointment 889
VōSoL HC Otic Solution 2392
Vytone Cream 1% 911

Hydrocortisone Acetate (Hypokalemia). Products include:
Analpram-HC Rectal Cream 1% and 2.5% 970
Anusol-HC Cream 1690
Anusol-HC Suppositories 1691
Caldecort ▣ 560
Carmol HC Cream 1% 2296
Chloromycetin Hydrocortisone Ophthalmic 1694
Coly-Mycin S Otic w/Neomycin & Hydrocortisone 1708
Cortaid ▣ 735
Cortef Feminine Itch Cream ▣ 735
Corticaine ▣ 682
Cortifoam 1827
Cortisporin Cream 757
Epifoam 1828
Gynecort 5 Creme ▣ 556
Hydrocortone Acetate Sterile Suspension 1479
Lanacort 5 Creme and Ointment ▣ 557
Mantadil Cream 789
Ophthocort ⊙ 301
Orabase HCA Oral Paste 890
Pramosone Cream, Lotion & Ointment 971
ProctoCream-HC 1834
Proctofoam-HC 1835

Hydrocortisone Sodium Phosphate (Hypokalemia). Products include:
Hydrocortone Phosphate Injection, Sterile 1481

Hydrocortisone Sodium Succinate (Hypokalemia). Products include:
Solu-Cortef Sterile Powder 2361

Hydroflumethiazide (Additive or potentiative effects). Products include:
Diucardin Tablets 2450
Saluron 718
Salutensin/Salutensin-Demi 719

Indapamide (Additive or potentiative effects). Products include:
Lozol Tablets 1843

Insulin, Human (Increased or decreased insulin requirements).
No products indexed under this heading.

Insulin, Human Isophane Suspension (Increased or decreased insulin requirements). Products include:
Humulin N, 100 Units 1270

Insulin, Human NPH (Increased or decreased insulin requirements). Products include:
Insulatard NPH Human 1627
Novolin N 1627
Novolin N PenFill Cartridges 1628
Novolin N Prefilled 1628

Insulin, Human Regular (Increased or decreased insulin requirements). Products include:
Humulin BR, 100 Units 1268
Humulin R, 100 Units 1272
Novolin R 1627
Novolin R PenFill Cartridges 1628
Novolin R Prefilled 1629
Velosulin Human 1628

Insulin, Human, Zinc Suspension (Increased or decreased insulin requirements). Products include:
Humulin L, 100 Units 1268
Humulin U, 100 Units 1272
Novolin L 1627

Insulin, NPH (Increased or decreased insulin requirements). Products include:
NPH, 40 & 100 Units 1273
Beef NPH, 100 Units 1274
Pork NPH, 100 Units 1275
Insulatard NPH 1626
NPH Insulin 1626
NPH Purified Pork Isophane Insulin 1626

Insulin, Regular (Increased or decreased insulin requirements). Products include:
Regular, 40 & 100 Units 1273
Beef Regular, 100 Units 1275
Pork Regular, 100 Units 1275
Pork Regular (Concentrated), 500 Units 1276
Regular Insulin 1625
Regular Purified Pork Insulin 1626
Velosulin 1627

Insulin, Zinc Crystals (Increased or decreased insulin requirements). Products include:
NPH, 40 & 100 Units 1273

Insulin, Zinc Suspension (Increased or decreased insulin requirements). Products include:
Lente, 40 & 100 Units 1272
Protamine, Zinc, 40 & 100 Units 1273
Lente Iletin I 1272
Beef Lente, 100 Units 1274
Beef Protamine Zinc, 100 Units 1274
Pork Lente, 100 Units 1275
Pork, Protamine, Zinc, 100 Units 1275
Lente Insulin 1626
Lente Purified Pork Insulin 1626
Semilente Insulin 1625
Ultralente Insulin 1626

Isradipine (Additive or potentiative effects). Products include:
DynaCirc Capsules 2004

Labetalol Hydrochloride (Additive or potentiative effects). Products include:
Normodyne Injection 2108
Normodyne Tablets 2110
Normozide Tablets 2112
Trandate HCT Tablets 579
Trandate Injection 577
Trandate Tablets 579

Levorphanol Tartrate (May aggravate orthostatic hypotension). Products include:
Levo-Dromoran 1906

Lisinopril (Additive or potentiative effects). Products include:
Prinivil Tablets 1538
Prinzide Tablets 1540
Zestoretic 2274
Zestril Tablets 2277

Mecamylamine Hydrochloride (Potentiation occurs). Products include:
Inversine Tablets 1492

Meperidine Hydrochloride (May aggravate orthostatic hypotension). Products include:
Demerol 2047
Mepergan Injection 2479

Mephobarbital (May aggravate orthostatic hypotension). Products include:
Mebaral Tablets 2061

Methadone Hydrochloride (May aggravate orthostatic hypotension). Products include:
Dolophine Hydrochloride Ampoules & Vials 1260
Dolophine Hydrochloride Tablets 1261
Methadone Hydrochloride Diskets 1284
Methadone Hydrochloride Oral Solution & Tablets 1987

Methyclothiazide (Additive or potentiative effects). Products include:
Enduron Tablets 517
Enduronyl 518

Methyldopa (Additive or potentiative effects). Products include:
Aldoclor Tablets 1413
Aldomet Oral 1415
Aldoril Tablets 1418

Methyldopate Hydrochloride (Additive or potentiated effects). Products include:
Aldomet Ester HCl Injection 1417

Methylprednisolone Acetate (Hypokalemia). Products include:
Depo-Medrol Sterile Aqueous Suspension 2334

Methylprednisolone Sodium Succinate (Hypokalemia). Products include:
Solu-Medrol Sterile Powder 2363

Metolazone (Additive or potentiative effects). Products include:
Diulo 2129
Mykrox ½ mg Tablets 984
Zaroxolyn Tablets 989

Metoprolol Tartrate (Additive or potentiative effects). Products include:
Lopressor Ampuls 1032
Lopressor HCT Tablets 1034
Lopressor Tablets 1032

Metyrosine (Additive or potentiative effects). Products include:
Demser Capsules 1460

Minoxidil (Additive or potentiative effects). Products include:
Loniten Tablets 2346
Rogaine Topical Solution 2357

Morphine Sulfate (May aggravate orthostatic hypotension). Products include:
Astramorph/PF Injection, USP (Preservative-Free) 618
Duramorph 960
Infumorph 200 and Infumorph 500 Sterile Solutions 962
MS Contin Tablets 1814
MSIR 1817
Oramorph SR (Morphine Sulfate Sustained Release Tablets) 1988
Roxanol 1991

Nadolol (Additive or potentiative effects). Products include:
Corgard Tablets 701
Corzide Tablets 702

Nicardipine Hydrochloride (Additive or potentiative effects). Products include:
Cardene Capsules 2290

Nitroglycerin (Additive or potentiative effects). Products include:
Deponit NTG Transdermal Delivery System 2143
Minitran Transdermal Delivery System 1312
Nitro-Bid Ointment 1339
Nitro-Bid Capsules 1338
Nitrodisc 2176
Nitro-Dur (nitroglycerin) Transdermal Infusion System 1164
Nitrogard Tablets 1004
Nitrolingual Spray 1846
Nitrostat Tablets 1743
Transderm-Nitro Transdermal Therapeutic System 2283

Norepinephrine Bitartrate (Decreased arterial responsiveness). Products include:
Levophed Bitartrate Injection 2054

Opium Alkaloids (May aggravate orthostatic hypotension). Products include:
B & O No. 15A & No. 16A Supprettes 2395
Pantopon Injectable 1911

Oxycodone Hydrochloride (May aggravate orthostatic hypotension). Products include:
Percocet Tablets 950
Percodan 951
Roxicodone Tablets, Oral Solution & Intensol (Oxycodone) 1992
Tylox Capsules 1382

Pancuronium Bromide Injection (Decreased serum levels).
No products indexed under this heading.

Penbutolol Sulfate (Additive or potentiative effects). Products include:
Levatol 1832

Pentobarbital Sodium (May aggravate orthostatic hypotension). Products include:
Nembutal Sodium Capsules 534
Nembutal Sodium Solution 536
Nembutal Sodium Suppositories 538

Phenobarbital (May aggravate orthostatic hypotension). Products include:
Arco-Lase Plus Tablets 607
Bellergal-S Tablets 1998
Bronkolixir .... ▣ 761
Bronkotabs Tablets .... ▣ 762
Donnatal 1858
Donnatal Extentabs 1859
Donnatal Tablets 1858
Donnazyme Tablets 1860
Kinesed Tablets 2272
Phenobarbital Elixir and Tablets 1293
Primatene Tablets-P Formula 2421
Quadrinal Tablets 1183
Tedral SA 1765

Phenoxybenzamine Hydrochloride (Additive or potentiative effects). Products include:
Dibenzyline Capsules 2207

Phentolamine Mesylate (Additive or potentiative effects). Products include:
Regitine 878

Pindolol (Additive or potentiative effects). Products include:
Visken Tablets 2036

Polythiazide (Additive or potentiative effects). Products include:
Minizide Capsules 1779
Renese Tablets 1785
Renese-R Tablets 1786

Prazosin Hydrochloride (Potentiation occurs). Products include:
Minipress Capsules 1778
Minizide Capsules 1779

Prednisolone Acetate (Hypokalemia). Products include:
AK-Cide Sterile Ophthalmic Ointment & Suspension .... ◉ 202
Blephamide Liquifilm Sterile Ophthalmic Suspension 586
Blephamide S.O.P. Sterile Ophthalmic Ointment 586
Cetapred Ointment .... ◉ 220
⅛% Econopred & 1% Econopred Plus .... ◉ 217
Isopto Cetapred Suspension .... ◉ 220
Metimyd .... ◉ 306
Poly-Pred Liquifilm .... ◉ 250
Pred Forte .... ◉ 252
Pred Mild .... ◉ 254
Pred-G Liquifilm Sterile Ophthalmic Suspension .... ◉ 252
Pred-G S.O.P. Sterile Ophthalmic Ointment .... ◉ 253
Vasocidin Ointment .... ◉ 275

Prednisolone Sodium Phosphate (Hypokalemia). Products include:
AK-Pred .... ◉ 205
Hydeltrasol Injection, Sterile 1476
Inflamase .... ◉ 274
Pediapred Oral Liquid 987
Vasocidin Ophthalmic Solution .... ◉ 276

Prednisolone Tebutate (Hypokalemia). Products include:
Hydeltra-T.B.A. Sterile Suspension 1478

Prednisone (Hypokalemia). Products include:
Deltasone Tablets 2332

Propoxyphene Hydrochloride (May aggravate orthostatic hypotension). Products include:
Darvon 1256
Wygesic Tablets 2540

Propoxyphene Napsylate (May aggravate orthostatic hypotension). Products include:
Darvon-N/Darvocet-N 1254

Propranolol Hydrochloride (Additive or potentiative effects). Products include:
Inderal 2459
Inderal LA Long Acting Capsules 2461
Inderide Tablets 2463
Inderide LA Long Acting Capsules 2465

Ramipril (Additive or potentiative effects). Products include:
Altace Capsules 1086

Rauwolfia Serpentina (Potentiation occurs). Products include:
Raudixin Tablets 1803
Rauzide Tablets 1804

Rescinnamine (Potentiation occurs).
No products indexed under this heading.

Reserpine (Potentiation occurs). Products include:
Diupres Tablets 1461
Hydromox R Tablets 1209
Hydropres Tablets 1485
Renese-R Tablets 1786
Salutensin/Salutensin-Demi 719
Ser-Ap-Es Tablets 881
Serpasil Tablets 883
Serpasil-Apresoline Tablets 884
Serpasil-Esidrix Tablets 886

Secobarbital Sodium (May aggravate orthostatic hypotension). Products include:
Seconal Sodium Pulvules 1296

Sodium Nitroprusside (Additive or potentiative effects). Products include:
Nipride I.V. Infusion 1909

Sufentanil Citrate (May aggravate orthostatic hypotension). Products include:
Sufenta Injection 1147

Terazosin Hydrochloride (Additive or potentiative effects). Products include:
Hytrin Tablets 529

Thiamylal Sodium (May aggravate orthostatic hypotension). Products include:
Surital Ampoules, Steri-Vials 1764

Timolol Maleate (Additive or potentiative effects). Products include:
Blocadren Tablets 1429
Timolide Tablets 1547
Timoptic in Ocudose 1552
Timoptic Sterile Ophthalmic Solution 1550

Triamcinolone (Hypokalemia).
No products indexed under this heading.

Triamcinolone Acetonide (Hypokalemia). Products include:
Aristocort A 1010
Azmacort Inhaler 1837
Kenalog Cream, Lotion & Ointment 2401
Kenalog-10 Injection 2402
Kenalog-40 Injection 2403

Kenalog in Orabase ... 604
Kenalog Spray ... 2401
Mycolog II Cream and Ointment ... 2407
Mytrex Cream & Ointment ... 2080
Nasacort Nasal Inhaler ... 1844

Triamcinolone Diacetate (Hypokalemia). Products include:
Aristocort Suspension ... 1008

Triamcinolone Hexacetonide (Hypokalemia). Products include:
Aristospan Suspension ... 1011

Trimethaphan Camsylate (Potentiation occurs). Products include:
Arfonad Ampuls ... 1887

Tubocurarine Chloride (Increased responsiveness).
No products indexed under this heading.

OREXIN SOFTAB TABLETS
(Vitamin B Complex) ... 1157
No interactions described in labeling.

ORGANIDIN ELIXIR, SOLUTION & TABLETS
(Iodinated Glycerol) ... 2387
May interact with antithyroid agents and certain other agents. Compounds in these categories include:

Lithium Carbonate (Hypothyroid effect of lithium potentiated). Products include:
Eskalith ... 2214
Lithane Tablets ... 1596
Lithium Carbonate Capsules & Tablets ... 1984
Lithobid Tablets ... 870

Lithium Citrate (Hypothyroid effect of lithium potentiated). Products include:
Cibalith-S ... 870

Methimazole (Hypothyroid effect of antithyroid drugs potentiated). Products include:
Tapazole Tablets ... 1298

ORIMUNE POLIOVIRUS VACCINE LIVE ORAL TRIVALENT
(Poliovirus Vaccine, Live, Oral, Trivalent, Types 1,2,3 (Sabin)) ... 1228
May interact with antineoplastics and corticosteroids. Compounds in these categories include:

Altretamine (Contraindicated). Products include:
Hexalen Capsules ... 2316

Asparaginase (Contraindicated). Products include:
Elspar ... 1470

Betamethasone Acetate (Contraindicated). Products include:
Celestone Soluspan Suspension ... 2081

Betamethasone Sodium Phosphate (Contraindicated). Products include:
Celestone Soluspan Suspension ... 2081

Bleomycin Sulfate (Contraindicated). Products include:
Blenoxane ... 724

Busulfan (Contraindicated). Products include:
Myleran Tablets ... 790

Carboplatin (Contraindicated). Products include:
Paraplatin for Injection ... 735

Carmustine (BCNU) (Contraindicated). Products include:
BiCNU ... 723

Chlorambucil (Contraindicated). Products include:
Leukeran Tablets ... 788

Cisplatin (Contraindicated). Products include:
Platinol ... 737
Platinol-AQ Injection ... 738

Cortisone Acetate (Contraindicated). Products include:
Cortone Acetate Sterile Suspension ... 1437
Cortone Acetate Tablets ... 1439

Cyclophosphamide (Contraindicated). Products include:
Cytoxan for Injection ... 726
Neosar for Injection ... 566

Dacarbazine (Contraindicated). Products include:
DTIC-Dome ... 1595

Daunorubicin Hydrochloride (Contraindicated). Products include:
Cerubidine ... 2443

Dexamethasone (Contraindicated). Products include:
AK-Trol Ointment & Suspension ... ⊙ 207
Decadron Elixir ... 1445
Decadron Tablets ... 1447
Decaspray Topical Aerosol ... 1459
Dexacidin ... ⊙ 272
Maxidex Sterile Ophthalmic Suspension ... ⊙ 223
Maxitrol Ophthalmic Ointment/Suspension ... ⊙ 223
TobraDex Ophthalmic Suspension and Ointment ... ⊙ 228

Dexamethasone Acetate (Contraindicated). Products include:
Dalalone D.P. Injectable ... 999
Decadron-LA Sterile Suspension ... 1457

Dexamethasone Sodium Phosphate (Contraindicated). Products include:
AK-Dex ... ⊙ 203
Decadron Phosphate Respihaler ... 1454
Decadron Phosphate Sterile Ophthalmic Ointment ... 1453
Decadron Phosphate Sterile Ophthalmic Solution ... 1453
Decadron Phosphate Topical Cream ... 1455
Decadron Phosphate Turbinaire ... 1456
Maxidex Sterile Ophthalmic Ointment ... ⊙ 222
NeoDecadron Sterile Ophthalmic Ointment ... 1517
NeoDecadron Sterile Ophthalmic Solution ... 1518
NeoDecadron Topical Cream ... 1518

Doxorubicin Hydrochloride (Contraindicated). Products include:
Adriamycin PFS ... 561
Adriamycin RDF ... 562
Doxorubicin Hydrochloride for Injection, USP ... 622
Doxorubicin Hydrochloride Injection, USP ... 848
Rubex ... 739

Estramustine Phosphate Sodium (Contraindicated). Products include:
Emcyt Capsules ... 1161

Etoposide (Contraindicated). Products include:
VePesid Capsules and Injection ... 741

Floxuridine (Contraindicated). Products include:
Sterile FUDR ... 1898

Fluorouracil (Contraindicated). Products include:
Efudex ... 1880
Fluoroplex Topical Solution & Cream 1% ... 1082
Fluorouracil Injection ... 1897

Flutamide (Contraindicated). Products include:
Eulexin Capsules ... 2089

Hydrocortisone (Contraindicated). Products include:
AK-Spore H.C. ... ⊙ 206
Bactine Hydrocortisone Anti-Itch Cream ... ■ 625
CaldeCORT Anti-Itch Hydrocortisone Spray ... ■ 560
Carmol HC Cream 1% ... 2296
Cortaid Spray ... ■ 735
Cortenema ... 2244
Cortisporin Ointment ... 758
Cortisporin Ophthalmic Ointment Sterile ... 758
Cortisporin Ophthalmic Suspension Sterile ... 759
Cortisporin Otic Solution Sterile ... 760
Cortisporin Otic Suspension Sterile ... 760
Cortizone-5 Creme & Ointment ... ■ 732
Dermolate Anti-Itch Cream ... ■ 697
Eldecort Cream 1.0% ... 1113
Eldecort Cream 1.0% and 2.5% ... 1113
Fungoid HC Creme ... 1770
Hydrocortone Tablets ... 1482
Hytone ... 909
LazerSporin-C Solution ... 1770
Massengill Medicated Soft Cloth Towelettes ... 2192
Nutracort Cream & Lotion ... 1684
PediOtic Suspension Sterile ... 797
Synacort Creams 1%, 2.5% ... 2296
Vanoxide-HC Acne Lotion ... 911
Vioform-Hydrocortisone Cream and Mild Cream ... 889
Vioform-Hydrocortisone Ointment ... 889
VōSoL HC Otic Solution ... 2392
Vytone Cream 1% ... 911

Hydrocortisone Acetate (Contraindicated). Products include:
Analpram-HC Rectal Cream 1% and 2.5% ... 970
Anusol-HC Cream ... 1690
Anusol-HC Suppositories ... 1691
Caldecort ... ■ 560
Carmol HC Cream 1% ... 2296
Chloromycetin Hydrocortisone Ophthalmic ... 1694
Coly-Mycin S Otic w/Neomycin & Hydrocortisone ... 1708
Cortaid ... ■ 735
Cortef Feminine Itch Cream ... ■ 735
Corticaine ... ■ 682
Cortifoam ... 1827
Cortisporin Cream ... 757
Epifoam ... 1828
Gynecort 5 Creme ... ■ 556
Hydrocortone Acetate Sterile Suspension ... 1479
Lanacort 5 Creme and Ointment ... ■ 557
Mantadil Cream ... 789
Ophthocort ... ⊙ 301
Orabase HCA Oral Paste ... 890
Pramosone Cream, Lotion & Ointment ... 971
ProctoCream-HC ... 1834
Proctofoam-HC ... 1835

Hydrocortisone Sodium Phosphate (Contraindicated). Products include:
Hydrocortone Phosphate Injection, Sterile ... 1481

Hydrocortisone Sodium Succinate (Contraindicated). Products include:
Solu-Cortef Sterile Powder ... 2361

Hydroxyurea (Contraindicated). Products include:
Hydrea Capsules ... 728

Ifosfamide (Contraindicated). Products include:
IFEX ... 729

Interferon alfa-2A, Recombinant (Contraindicated). Products include:
Roferon-A Injection ... 1916

Interferon alfa-2B, Recombinant (Contraindicated). Products include:
Intron A ... 2097

Levamisole Hydrochloride (Contraindicated). Products include:
Ergamisol Tablets ... 1136

Lomustine (CCNU) (Contraindicated). Products include:
CeeNU ... 725

Mechlorethamine Hydrochloride (Contraindicated). Products include:
Mustargen ... 1514

Megestrol Acetate (Contraindicated). Products include:
Megace Tablets ... 732

Melphalan (Contraindicated). Products include:
Alkeran Tablets ... 754

Mercaptopurine (Contraindicated). Products include:
Purinethol Tablets ... 800

Methotrexate Sodium (Contraindicated). Products include:
Methotrexate Tablets, Parenteral, LPF Parenteral ... 1217
Rheumatrex Methotrexate Dose Pack ... 1234

Methylprednisolone Acetate (Contraindicated). Products include:
Depo-Medrol Sterile Aqueous Suspension ... 2334

Methylprednisolone Sodium Succinate (Contraindicated). Products include:
Solu-Medrol Sterile Powder ... 2363

Mitomycin (Mitomycin-C) (Contraindicated). Products include:
Mutamycin ... 733

Mitotane (Contraindicated). Products include:
Lysodren ... 731

Mitoxantrone Hydrochloride (Contraindicated). Products include:
Novantrone for Injection Concentrate ... 1226

Prednisolone Acetate (Contraindicated). Products include:
AK-Cide Sterile Ophthalmic Ointment & Suspension ... ⊙ 202
Blephamide Liquifilm Sterile Ophthalmic Suspension ... 586
Blephamide S.O.P. Sterile Ophthalmic Ointment ... 586
Cetapred Ointment ... ⊙ 220
⅛% Econopred & 1% Econopred Plus ... ⊙ 217
Isopto Cetapred Suspension ... ⊙ 220
Metimyd ... ⊙ 306
Poly-Pred Liquifilm ... ⊙ 250
Pred Forte ... ⊙ 252
Pred Mild ... ⊙ 254
Pred-G Liquifilm Sterile Ophthalmic Suspension ... ⊙ 252
Pred-G S.O.P. Sterile Ophthalmic Ointment ... ⊙ 253
Vasocidin Ointment ... ⊙ 275

Prednisolone Sodium Phosphate (Contraindicated). Products include:
AK-Pred ... ⊙ 205
Hydeltrasol Injection, Sterile ... 1476
Inflamase ... ⊙ 274
Pediapred Oral Liquid ... 987
Vasocidin Ophthalmic Solution ... ⊙ 276

Prednisolone Tebutate (Contraindicated). Products include:
Hydeltra-T.B.A. Sterile Suspension 1478

Prednisone (Contraindicated). Products include:
Deltasone Tablets ... 2332

Procarbazine Hydrochloride (Contraindicated). Products include:
Matulane Capsules ... 1907

Streptozocin (Contraindicated). Products include:
Zanosar Sterile Powder ... 2371

Tamoxifen Citrate (Contraindicated). Products include:
Nolvadex Tablets ... 1102

Thioguanine (Contraindicated). Products include:
Thioguanine Tablets, Tabloid Brand ... 815

Thiotepa (Contraindicated). Products include:
Thiotepa Parenteral ... 1240

Triamcinolone (Contraindicated).
No products indexed under this heading.

Triamcinolone Acetonide (Contraindicated). Products include:
Aristocort A ... 1010
Azmacort Inhaler ... 1837
Kenalog Cream, Lotion & Ointment 2401
Kenalog-10 Injection ... 2402
Kenalog-40 Injection ... 2403
Kenalog in Orabase ... 604
Kenalog Spray ... 2401
Mycolog II Cream and Ointment ... 2407

Mytrex Cream & Ointment 2080
Nasacort Nasal Inhaler 1844

Triamcinolone Diacetate (Contraindicated). Products include:
Aristocort Suspension 1008

Triamcinolone Hexacetonide (Contraindicated). Products include:
Aristospan Suspension 1011

Vincristine Sulfate (Contraindicated). Products include:
Oncovin Solution Vials & Hyporets 1288

ORINASE TABLETS
(Tolbutamide) 2354
May interact with non-steroidal anti-inflammatory agents, salicylates, sulfonamides, oral anticoagulants, beta blockers , monoamine oxidase inhibitors, thiazides, phenothiazines, corticosteroids, diuretics, thyroid preparations, estrogens, oral contraceptives, sympathomimetic aerosal brochodilators, calcium channel blockers, oral hypoglycemic agents, and certain other agents. Compounds in these categories include:

Acebutolol Hydrochloride (Hypoglycemic action potentiated). Products include:
Sectral Capsules 2520

Albuterol (Hyperglycemia; loss of control). Products include:
Proventil Inhalation Aerosol 2117
Ventolin Inhalation Aerosol and Refill 583

Albuterol Sulfate (Hyperglycemia; loss of control). Products include:
Proventil Repetabs Tablets 2120
Proventil Solutions for Inhalation 0.5% and 0.083% 2118
Proventil Syrup 2119
Proventil Tablets 2120
Ventolin 583

Amiloride Hydrochloride (Hyperglycemia; loss of control). Products include:
Midamor Tablets 1508
Moduretic Tablets 1510

Aspirin (Hypoglycemic action potentiated). Products include:
Alka-Seltzer Effervescent Antacid and Pain Reliever 1568
Alka-Seltzer Extra Strength Effervescent Antacid and Pain Reliever 1570
Alka-Seltzer (Flavored) Effervescent Antacid and Pain Reliever ... 1569
Alka-Seltzer Plus Cold Medicine .... ◘ 623
Alka-Seltzer Plus Night-Time Cold Medicine .... ◘ 623
Alka Seltzer Plus Sinus Allergy Medicine .... ◘ 624
Anacin Coated Analgesic Caplets 2417
Anacin Coated Analgesic Tablets 2417
Anacin Maximum Strength Analgesic Coated Tablets 2417
Maximum Strength Arthritis Pain Formula By the Makers of Anacin Analgesic Tablets and Caplets 2418
Arthritis Pain Formula by the Makers of Anacin Analgesic Tablets and Caplets .... ◘ 747
Arthritis Strength BC Powder .... ◘ 516
Ascriptin A/D Caplets 1850
Regular Strength Ascriptin Tablets 1850
Azdōne Tablets 844
BC Powder .... ◘ 517
BC Cold Powder .... ◘ 517
Children's Bayer Chewable Aspirin .... ◘ 564
Genuine Bayer Aspirin Tablets & Caplets .... ◘ 564
Maximum Bayer Aspirin Tablets & Caplets .... ◘ 566
Bayer Plus Aspirin Tablets .... ◘ 567
Therapy Bayer Aspirin Caplets ...... ◘ 568
8 Hour Bayer Timed-Release Aspirin .... ◘ 566
Arthritis Strength Bufferin Analgesic Caplets 744
Extra Strength Bufferin Analgesic Tablets 745
Bufferin Analgesic Tablets and Caplets 743
Cama Arthritis Pain Reliever .... ◘ 685
Damason-P 1356
Easprin 1719
Ecotrin Enteric Coated Aspirin Maximum Strength Tablets and Caplets 2189
Ecotrin Enteric Coated Aspirin Regular Strength Tablets and Caplets 2189
Empirin Aspirin .... ◘ 541
Empirin with Codeine Phosphate Nos. 2, 3 & 4 764
Equagesic Tablets 2451
Excedrin Extra-Strength Analgesic Tablets & Caplets 749
4-Way Cold Tablets 750
Fiorinal Capsules 2007
Fiorinal with Codeine Capsules 2008
Fiorinal Tablets 2007
Lortab ASA Tablets 2414
Momentum Muscular Backache Formula .... ◘ 751
Norgesic 1314
Norwich Extra-Strength Aspirin ...... ◘ 546
Norwich Regular Strength Aspirin ◘ 547
P-A-C Analgesic Tablets .... ◘ 669
Percodan 951
Robaxisal Tablets 1872
Sine-Off Sinus Medicine Tablets-Aspirin Formula .... ◘ 722
Soma Compound w/Codeine Tablets 2390
Soma Compound Tablets 2389
St. Joseph Adult Chewable Aspirin (81 mg.) .... ◘ 703
Synalgos-DC Capsules 2525
Talwin Compound 2072
Ursinus Inlay-Tabs .... ◘ 691
Vanquish Analgesic Caplets .... ◘ 574
Zorprin Tablets 698

Atenolol (Hypoglycemic action potentiated). Products include:
Tenoretic Tablets 1105
Tenormin Tablets and I.V. Injection 1107

Bendroflumethiazide (Hyperglycemia; loss of control). Products include:
Corzide Tablets 702
Naturetin Tablets 1789
Rauzide Tablets 1804

Bepridil Hydrochloride (Hyperglycemia; loss of control). Products include:
Vascor (200, 300 and 400 mg) Tablets 1383

Betamethasone Acetate (Hyperglycemia; loss of control). Products include:
Celestone Soluspan Suspension 2081

Betamethasone Sodium Phosphate (Hyperglycemia; loss of control). Products include:
Celestone Soluspan Suspension 2081

Betaxolol Hydrochloride (Hypoglycemic action potentiated). Products include:
Betoptic Sterile Ophthalmic Solution 569
Betoptic S Sterile Ophthalmic Suspension 570
Kerlone Tablets 2172

Bumetanide (Hyperglycemia; loss of control). Products include:
Bumex 1895

Carteolol Hydrochloride (Hypoglycemic action potentiated). Products include:
Cartrol Tablets 507

Chloramphenicol (Hypoglycemic action potentiated). Products include:
AK-Chlor Sterile Ophthalmic Ointment & Solution .... ⊙ 201
Chloromycetin Cream, 1% 1694
Chloromycetin Hydrocortisone Ophthalmic 1694
Chloromycetin Kapseals 1695
Chloromycetin Ophthalmic Ointment, 1% 1696
Chloromycetin Ophthalmic Solution 1696
Chloromycetin Otic 1697
Chloroptic S.O.P. .... ⊙ 243
Chloroptic Sterile Ophthalmic Solution .... ⊙ 243
Ophthochlor Ophthalmic Solution ⊙ 300
Ophthocort .... ⊙ 301

Chloramphenicol Palmitate (Hypoglycemic action potentiated). Products include:
Chloromycetin Palmitate, Oral Suspension 1697

Chloramphenicol Sodium Succinate (Hypoglycemic action potentiated). Products include:
Chloromycetin Sodium Succinate 1698

Chlorothiazide (Hyperglycemia; loss of control). Products include:
Aldoclor Tablets 1413
Diupres Tablets 1461
Diuril Oral 1464

Chlorothiazide Sodium (Hyperglycemia; loss of control). Products include:
Diuril Sodium Intravenous 1463

Chlorotrianisene (Hyperglycemia; loss of control). Products include:
TACE 12 and 25 mg 1353

Chlorpromazine (Hyperglycemia; loss of control). Products include:
Thorazine 2234

Chlorpropamide (Severe hypoglycemia). Products include:
Diabinese Tablets 1775

Chlorthalidone (Hyperglycemia; loss of control). Products include:
Combipres Tablets 678
Tenoretic Tablets 1105
Thalitone Tablets 687

Choline Magnesium Trisalicylate (Severe hypoglycemia). Products include:
Trilisate 1822

Cortisone Acetate (Hyperglycemia; loss of control). Products include:
Cortone Acetate Sterile Suspension 1437
Cortone Acetate Tablets 1439

Dexamethasone (Hyperglycemia; loss of control). Products include:
AK-Trol Ointment & Suspension .... ⊙ 207
Decadron Elixir 1445
Decadron Tablets 1447
Decaspray Topical Aerosol 1459
Dexacidin .... ⊙ 272
Maxidex Sterile Ophthalmic Suspension .... ⊙ 223
Maxitrol Ophthalmic Ointment/Suspension .... ⊙ 223
TobraDex Ophthalmic Suspension and Ointment .... ⊙ 228

Dexamethasone Acetate (Hyperglycemia; loss of control). Products include:
Dalalone D.P. Injectable 999
Decadron-LA Sterile Suspension 1457

Dexamethasone Sodium Phosphate (Hyperglycemia; loss of control). Products include:
AK-Dex .... ⊙ 203
Decadron Phosphate Respihaler 1454
Decadron Phosphate Sterile Ophthalmic Ointment 1453
Decadron Phosphate Sterile Ophthalmic Solution 1453
Decadron Phosphate Topical Cream 1455
Decadron Phosphate Turbinaire 1456
Maxidex Sterile Ophthalmic Ointment .... ⊙ 222
NeoDecadron Sterile Ophthalmic Ointment 1517
NeoDecadron Sterile Ophthalmic Solution 1518
NeoDecadron Topical Cream 1518

Diclofenac Sodium (Hypoglycemic action potentiated). Products include:
Voltaren Ophthalmic Sterile Ophthalmic Solution .... ⊙ 268
Voltaren Tablets 1042

Dicumarol (Hypoglycemic action potentiated). Products include:
Dicumarol Tablets 516

Dienestrol (Hyperglycemia; loss of control). Products include:
Ortho Dienestrol Cream 1664

Diethylstilbestrol (Hyperglycemia; loss of control). Products include:
Diethylstilbestrol Tablets 1258

Diflunisal (Hypoglycemic action potentiated). Products include:
Dolobid Tablets 1465

Diltiazem Hydrochloride (Hyperglycemia; loss of control). Products include:
Cardizem Tablets-30 mg, 60 mg, 90 mg and 120 mg 1329
Cardizem SR Capsules-60 mg, 90 mg and 120 mg 1327

Dobutamine Hydrochloride (Hyperglycemia; loss of control). Products include:
Dobutrex Solution Vials 1259

Dopamine Hydrochloride (Hyperglycemia; loss of control). Products include:
Intropin Injection 930

Ephedrine Hydrochloride (Hyperglycemia; loss of control). Products include:
Amesec .... ◘ 682
Primatene Tablets-M Formula 2421
Primatene Tablets-P Formula 2421
Primatene Tablets-Regular Formula 2421
Quadrinal Tablets 1183
Quelidrine Syrup 556
Tedral SA 1765

Ephedrine Sulfate (Hyperglycemia; loss of control). Products include:
Bronkaid Tablets .... ◘ 757
Bronkolixir .... ◘ 761
Bronkotabs Tablets .... ◘ 762
Marax Tablets & DF Syrup 1954
Pazo Hemorrhoid Ointment & Suppositories 752
Vicks Vatronol Nose Drops .... ◘ 666

Ephedrine Tannate (Hyperglycemia; loss of control). Products include:
Rynatuss 2388

Epinephrine (Hyperglycemia; loss of control). Products include:
Ana-Kit Anaphylaxis Emergency Treatment Kit 1100
Bronkaid Mist .... ◘ 757
EpiPen 843
Marcaine Hydrochloride 0.5% with Epinephrine 1:200,000 (as bitartrate) 958
Marcaine Hydrochloride with Epinephrine 1:200,000 2055
Primatene Mist 2420
Sus-Phrine Injection 1006
Xylocaine with Epinephrine Injections 637

Epinephrine Bitartrate (Hyperglycemia; loss of control). Products include:
AsthmaHaler Mist Epinephrine Bitartrate Bronchodilator .... ◘ 616
Bronkaid Mist Suspension .... ◘ 757
Primatene Mist Suspension 2421

Epinephrine Hydrochloride (Hyperglycemia; loss of control). Products include:
Adrenalin Chloride Solution 1:100 & 1:1,000 1689
Epifrin .... ⊙ 244
Glaucon .... ⊙ 218

Esmolol Hydrochloride (Hypoglycemic action potentiated). Products include:
Brevibloc Injection 942

Estradiol (Hyperglycemia; loss of control). Products include:
Emcyt Capsules 1161
Estrace 1385
Estrace Vaginal Cream 1388
Estraderm Transdermal System 866

Estrogens, Conjugated (Hyperglycemia; loss of control). Products include:
- Mediatric Capsules 2476
- PMB 200 and PMB 400 2504
- Premarin Intravenous 2508
- Premarin with Methyltestosterone .. 2515
- Premarin Tablets 2510
- Premarin Vaginal Cream 2512

Estrogens, Esterified (Hyperglycemia; loss of control). Products include:
- Estratest 2245
- Menrium Tablets 1934

Estropipate (Hyperglycemia; loss of control). Products include:
- Ogen 540

Ethacrynic Acid (Hyperglycemia; loss of control). Products include:
- Edecrin Tablets 1468

Ethinyl Estradiol (Hyperglycemia; loss of control). Products include:
- Brevicon 2304
- Demulen 2161
- Estinyl Tablets 2085
- Jenest-28 Tablets 1636
- Levlen/Tri-Levlen 665
- Lo/Ovral Tablets 2471
- Lo/Ovral-28 Tablets 2476
- Loestrin 1728
- Modicon 1667
- Nordette-21 Tablets 2481
- Nordette-28 Tablets 2483
- Norethin 2133
- Norinyl 2304
- Norlestrin 1746
- Ortho-Cyclen Tablets 1658
- Ortho-Novum 1667
- Ovcon 1391
- Ovral Tablets 2490
- Ovral-28 Tablets 2491
- Levlen/Tri-Levlen 665
- Tri-Norinyl 2304
- Triphasil-21 Tablets 2527
- Triphasil-28 Tablets 2532

Ethynodiol Diacetate (Hyperglycemia; loss of control). Products include:
- Demulen 2161

Etodolac (Hypoglycemic action potentiated). Products include:
- Lodine Capsules 2468

Felodipine (Hyperglycemia; loss of control). Products include:
- Plendil Extended-Release Tablets 1526

Fenoprofen Calcium (Hypoglycemic action potentiated). Products include:
- Nalfon Pulvules & Tablets 919

Fluphenazine Decanoate (Hyperglycemia; loss of control). Products include:
- Prolixin Decanoate 1795

Fluphenazine Enanthate (Hyperglycemia; loss of control). Products include:
- Prolixin Enanthate 1796

Fluphenazine Hydrochloride (Hyperglycemia; loss of control). Products include:
- Prolixin Elixir 1793
- Prolixin Injection 1791
- Prolixin Oral Concentrate 1792
- Prolixin Tablets 1793

Flurbiprofen (Hypoglycemic action potentiated). Products include:
- Ansaid Tablets 2319

Furazolidone (Hypoglycemic action potentiated). Products include:
- Furoxone 1855

Furosemide (Hyperglycemia; loss of control). Products include:
- Lasix 1093

Glipizide (Severe hypoglycemia). Products include:
- Glucotrol 1952

Glyburide (Severe hypoglycemia). Products include:
- DiaBeta 1091
- Micronase Tablets 2350

Hydrochlorothiazide (Hyperglycemia; loss of control). Products include:
- Aldactazide 2150
- Aldoril Tablets 1418
- Apresazide Capsules 854
- Apresoline-Esidrix Tablets 857
- Capozide 2258
- Dyazide Capsules 2208
- Esidrix Tablets 863
- Esimil Tablets 864
- HydroDIURIL Tablets 1484
- Hydropres Tablets 1485
- Inderide Tablets 2463
- Inderide LA Long Acting Capsules .. 2465
- Lopressor HCT Tablets 1034
- Maxzide 1215
- Moduretic Tablets 1510
- Normozide Tablets 2112
- Oretic Tablets 544
- Oreticyl 545
- Prinzide Tablets 1540
- Ser-Ap-Es Tablets 881
- Serpasil-Esidrix Tablets 886
- Timolide Tablets 1547
- Trandate HCT Tablets 579
- Vaseretic Tablets 1559
- Zestoretic 2274

Hydrocortisone (Hyperglycemia; loss of control). Products include:
- AK-Spore H.C. .... ⊙ 206
- Bactine Hydrocortisone Anti-Itch Cream .... ▣ 625
- CaldeCORT Anti-Itch Hydrocortisone Spray .... ▣ 560
- Carmol HC Cream 1% 2296
- Cortaid Spray .... ▣ 735
- Cortenema 2244
- Cortisporin Ointment 758
- Cortisporin Ophthalmic Ointment Sterile 758
- Cortisporin Ophthalmic Suspension Sterile 759
- Cortisporin Otic Solution Sterile 760
- Cortisporin Otic Suspension Sterile 760
- Cortizone-5 Creme & Ointment ..... ▣ 732
- Dermolate Anti-Itch Cream .... ▣ 697
- Eldecort Cream 1.0% 1113
- Eldecort Cream 1.0% and 2.5% 1113
- Fungoid HC Creme 1770
- Hydrocortone Tablets 1482
- Hytone 909
- LazerSporin-C Solution 1770
- Massengill Medicated Soft Cloth Towelettes 2192
- Nutracort Cream & Lotion 1684
- PediOtic Suspension Sterile 797
- Synacort Creams 1%, 2.5% 2296
- Vanoxide-HC Acne Lotion 911
- Vioform-Hydrocortisone Cream and Mild Cream 889
- Vioform-Hydrocortisone Ointment .. 889
- VōSoL HC Otic Solution 2392
- Vytone Cream 1% 911

Hydrocortisone Acetate (Hyperglycemia; loss of control). Products include:
- Analpram-HC Rectal Cream 1% and 2.5% 970
- Anusol-HC Cream 1690
- Anusol-HC Suppositories 1691
- Caldecort .... ▣ 560
- Carmol HC Cream 1% 2296
- Chloromycetin Hydrocortisone Ophthalmic 1694
- Coly-Mycin S Otic w/Neomycin & Hydrocortisone 1708
- Cortaid .... ▣ 735
- Cortef Feminine Itch Cream .... ▣ 735
- Corticaine .... ▣ 682
- Cortifoam 1827
- Cortisporin Cream 757
- Epifoam 1828
- Gynecort 5 Creme .... ▣ 556
- Hydrocortone Acetate Sterile Suspension 1479
- Lanacort 5 Creme and Ointment .. ▣ 557
- Mantadil Cream 789
- Ophthocort .... ⊙ 301
- Orabase HCA Oral Paste 890
- Pramosone Cream, Lotion & Ointment 971
- ProctoCream-HC 1834
- Proctofoam-HC 1835

Hydrocortisone Sodium Phosphate (Hyperglycemia; loss of control). Products include:
- Hydrocortone Phosphate Injection, Sterile 1481

Hydrocortisone Sodium Succinate (Hyperglycemia; loss of control). Products include:
- Solu-Cortef Sterile Powder 2361

Hydroflumethiazide (Hyperglycemia; loss of control). Products include:
- Diucardin Tablets 2450
- Saluron 718
- Salutensin/Salutensin-Demi 719

Ibuprofen (Hypoglycemic action potentiated). Products include:
- Advil Cold & Sinus Caplets (formerly CoAdvil) 2416
- Advil Ibuprofen Tablets and Caplets 2416
- Children's Advil Suspension 2426
- CoAdvil .... ▣ 748
- Dristan Sinus Caplets 2419
- Haltran Tablets .... ▣ 668
- Ibuprofen .... ▣ 631
- Medipren Ibuprofen Caplets and Tablets 1362
- Midol 200 Cramp Relief Formula .. ▣ 570
- Motrin Tablets 2351
- Motrin IB Caplets and Tablets .... ▣ 736
- Nuprin Ibuprofen/Analgesic Tablets & Caplets 752
- PediaProfen Suspension 1363
- Rufen Tablets 691
- Trendar Ibuprofen Tablets .... ▣ 756

Indapamide (Hyperglycemia; loss of control). Products include:
- Lozol Tablets 1843

Indomethacin (Hypoglycemic action potentiated). Products include:
- Indocin 1487

Indomethacin Sodium Trihydrate (Hypoglycemic action potentiated). Products include:
- Indocin I.V. 1490

Isocarboxazid (Hypoglycemic action potentiated). Products include:
- Marplan Tablets 1906

Isoniazid (Hyperglycemia; loss of control). Products include:
- INH Tablets 868
- Rifamate Capsules 1347

Isoproterenol Hydrochloride (Hyperglycemia; loss of control). Products include:
- Isuprel Hydrochloride Injection 1:5000 2050
- Isuprel Hydrochloride Mistometer .. 2051
- Isuprel Hydrochloride Solution 1:200 & 1:100 2052
- Norisodrine Aerotrol 540

Isradipine (Hyperglycemia; loss of control). Products include:
- DynaCirc Capsules 2004

Ketoprofen (Hypoglycemic action potentiated). Products include:
- Orudis Capsules 2488

Ketorolac Tromethamine (Hypoglycemic action potentiated). Products include:
- Toradol IM Injection 2302

Labetalol Hydrochloride (Hypoglycemic action potentiated). Products include:
- Normodyne Injection 2108
- Normodyne Tablets 2110
- Normozide Tablets 2112
- Trandate HCT Tablets 579
- Trandate Injection 577
- Trandate Tablets 579

Levonorgestrel (Hyperglycemia; loss of control). Products include:
- Levlen/Tri-Levlen 665
- Nordette-21 Tablets 2481
- Nordette-28 Tablets 2483
- Norplant System 2484
- Levlen/Tri-Levlen 665
- Triphasil-21 Tablets 2527
- Triphasil-28 Tablets 2532

Levothyroxine Sodium (Hyperglycemia; loss of control). Products include:
- Levothroid Tablets 1003
- Levoxine Tablets 904
- Synthroid 695

Liothyronine Sodium (Hyperglycemia; loss of control). Products include:
- Cytomel Tablets 2203

Liotrix (Hyperglycemia; loss of control). Products include:
- Euthroid 1724

Magnesium Salicylate (Hypoglycemic action potentiated). Products include:
- Doan's - Extra-Strength Analgesic ▣ 549
- Doan's - Regular Strength Analgesic .... ▣ 549
- Mobigesic Analgesic Tablets .... ▣ 507

Meclofenamate Sodium (Hypoglycemic action potentiated). Products include:
- Meclomen Capsules 1739

Mefenamic Acid (Hypoglycemic action potentiated). Products include:
- Ponstel 1758

Mesoridazine (Hyperglycemia; loss of control). Products include:
- Serentil 686

Mestranol (Hyperglycemia; loss of control). Products include:
- Enovid 2161
- Norethin 2133
- Norinyl 2304
- Ortho-Novum 1667

Metaproterenol Sulfate (Hyperglycemia; loss of control). Products include:
- Alupent 674
- Arm-a-Med Metaproterenol Sulfate Inhalation Solution, USP 617
- Metaprel Inhalation Aerosol Bronchodilator 2014
- Metaprel Inhalation Solution 2015
- Metaprel 2015
- Metaproterenol Sulfate Inhalation Solution, USP 912

Metaraminol Bitartrate (Hyperglycemia; loss of control). Products include:
- Aramine Injection 1424

Methoxamine Hydrochloride (Hyperglycemia; loss of control). Products include:
- Vasoxyl Injection 819

Methyclothiazide (Hyperglycemia; loss of control). Products include:
- Enduron Tablets 517
- Enduronyl 518

Methylprednisolone (Hyperglycemia; loss of control). Products include:
- Medrol 2348

Methylprednisolone Acetate (Hyperglycemia; loss of control). Products include:
- Depo-Medrol Sterile Aqueous Suspension 2334

Methylprednisolone Sodium Succinate (Hyperglycemia; loss of control). Products include:
- Solu-Medrol Sterile Powder 2363

Metoprolol Tartrate (Hypoglycemic action potentiated). Products include:
- Lopressor Ampuls 1032
- Lopressor HCT Tablets 1034
- Lopressor Tablets 1032

Miconazole (Hypoglycemia). Products include:
- Monistat I.V. 1143

Miconazole Nitrate (Hypoglycemia). Products include:
- Micatin .... ▣ 632
- Micatin for Jock Itch .... ▣ 633
- Monistat Dual-Pak 1657
- Monistat 3 Vaginal Suppositories 1657
- Monistat-Derm (miconazole nitrate) Cream 1679

Nadolol (Hypoglycemic action potentiated). Products include:
- Corgard Tablets 701

Corzide Tablets 702

Naproxen (Hypoglycemic action potentiated). Products include:

Naprosyn 2297

Naproxen Sodium (Hypoglycemic action potentiated). Products include:

Anaprox and Anaprox DS Tablets 2288

Nicardipine Hydrochloride (Hyperglycemia; loss of control). Products include:

Cardene Capsules 2290

Nicotinic Acid (Hyperglycemia; loss of control). Products include:

Niacor Tablets 2376
Nicobid 1846
Nicolar Tablets 1846
Nicotinex Elixir ■ 563
Slo-Niacin Tablets 2376

Nifedipine (Hyperglycemia; loss of control). Products include:

Adalat Capsules (10 mg and 20 mg) 1587
Procardia Capsules 1781
Procardia XL Tablets 1783

Nimodipine (Hyperglycemia; loss of control). Products include:

Nimotop Capsules 1607

Norepinephrine Bitartrate (Hyperglycemia; loss of control). Products include:

Levophed Bitartrate Injection 2054

Norethindrone (Hyperglycemia; loss of control). Products include:

Brevicon 2304
Jenest-28 Tablets 1636
Micronor Tablets 1667
Modicon 1667
Norethin 2133
Norinyl 2304
Norlutin 1755
Nor-Q D Tablets 2304
Ortho-Novum 1667
Ovcon 1391
Tri-Norinyl 2304

Norethynodrel (Hyperglycemia; loss of control). Products include:

Enovid 2161

Norgestimate (Hyperglycemia; loss of control). Products include:

Ortho-Cyclen Tablets 1658

Norgestrel (Hyperglycemia; loss of control). Products include:

Lo/Ovral Tablets 2471
Lo/Ovral-28 Tablets 2476
Ovral Tablets 2490
Ovral-28 Tablets 2491
Ovrette Tablets 2492

Penbutolol Sulfate (Hypoglycemic action potentiated). Products include:

Levatol 1832

Perphenazine (Hyperglycemia; loss of control). Products include:

Etrafon 2087
Triavil Tablets 1556
Trilafon 2123

Phenelzine Sulfate (Hypoglycemic action potentiated). Products include:

Nardil 1742

Phenylbutazone (Hypoglycemic action potentiated). Products include:

Butazolidin Capsules & Tablets 1027

Phenylephrine Bitartrate (Hyperglycemia; loss of control).

No products indexed under this heading.

Phenylephrine Hydrochloride (Hyperglycemia; loss of control). Products include:

AK-Dilate Solution 2.5% and 10% ⊙ 203
Atrohist Sprinkle Capsules 558
Cerose-DM 2443
Codimal 846
Comhist LA Capsules 1618
Congespirin For Children Aspirin Free Chewable Cold Tablets 748
Cyclomydril ⊙ 216
Deconsal Sprinkle Capsules 559
Dimetane Decongestant ■ 673
Dristan Decongestant/Antihistamine/ Analgesic Coated Caplets ■ 749
Dristan Cold Nasal Decongestant/ Antihistamine/ Analgesic Coated Tablets 2419
Dristan Advanced Formula Decongestant/Antihistamine/ Analgesic Tablets ■ 749
Dristan Nasal Spray, Menthol 2419
Dristan Nasal Spray, Regular and Regular with Metered Pump 2419
Entex Capsules 1623
Entex Liquid 1623
Sinus Excedrin Analgesic, Decongestant Tablets & Caplets 750
Extendryl 994
4-Way Fast Acting Nasal Spray - Original Formula (regular & mentholated) & Metered Spray Pump (regular) 751
Hycomine Compound Tablets 929
Murocoll-2 Sterile Ophthalmic Solution ⊙ 261
Mydfrin 2.5% ⊙ 224
Naldecon Syrup, Tablets, Pediatric Drops and Pediatric Syrup 709
Neo-Synephrine Hydrochloride 1% Carpuject 2063
Neo-Synephrine Hydrochloride 1% Injection 2063
Neo-Synephrine Hydrochloride (Ophthalmic) 2064
Neo-Synephrine ■ 759
Nōstril Nasal Decongestant ■ 520
Novahistine Elixir ■ 596
Phenergan VC 2500
Phenergan VC with Codeine 2501
Prefrin Liquifilm Vasoconstrictor and Lubricant Eye Drops ⊙ 254
Prefrin-A ⊙ 255
Quelidrine Syrup 556
Relief Vasoconstrictor and Lubricant Eye Drops ⊙ 256
Robitussin Night Relief ■ 677
Ru-Tuss with Hydrocodone 694
Ru-Tuss Tablets 693
Vasosulf ⊙ 279
Vicks Sinex ■ 665
Zincfrin ⊙ 230

Phenylephrine Tannate (Hyperglycemia; loss of control). Products include:

Rynatan 2387
Rynatuss 2388

Phenylpropanolamine Hydrochloride (Hyperglycemia; loss of control). Products include:

A.R.M. Allergy Relief Medicine Caplets ■ 615
Acutrim ■ 548
Allerest ■ 559
BC Cold Powder ■ 517
Cheracol Plus Head Cold/Cough Formula ■ 667
Codimal Expectorant 846
Comtrex Multi-Symptom Cold Reliever Tablets/Caplets/Liqui-Gels/Liquid 745
Contac Continuous Action Decongestant/Antihistamine Capsules ■ 710
Contac Maximum Strength Continuous Action Decongestant/ Antihistamine Caplets ■ 709
Contac Severe Cold and Flu Formula Caplets ■ 711
Coricidin 'D' Decongestant Tablets ■ 695
Coricidin Demilets Tablets for Children ■ 696
Demazin Nasal Decongestant/ Antihistamine Repetabs Tablets & Syrup ■ 697
Dexatrim ■ 733
Dimetane-DC Cough Syrup 1857
Dimetapp Elixir ■ 673
Dimetapp DM Elixir ■ 674
Dimetapp Extentabs ■ 674
Dimetapp Plus Caplets ■ 675
Dimetapp Tablets ■ 675
Entex Capsules 1623
Entex LA Tablets 1623
Entex Liquid 1623
4-Way Cold Tablets 750
Hycomine Syrup 927
Naldecon CX Adult Liquid ■ 521
Naldecon DX Adult Liquid ■ 521
Naldecon DX Children's Syrup ■ 522
Naldecon DX Pediatric Drops ■ 522
Naldecon EX Children's Syrup ■ 522
Naldecon EX Pediatric Drops ■ 523
Naldecon Syrup, Tablets, Pediatric Drops and Pediatric Syrup 709
Nolamine Tablets 838
Nolex LA Tablets 838
Ornade Spansule Capsules 2221
Orthoxicol Cough Syrup ■ 668
Propagest 839
Pyrroxate Capsules ■ 669
Robitussin-CF ■ 676
Ru-Tuss II Capsules 693
Ru-Tuss with Hydrocodone 694
Ru-Tuss Tablets 693
Sine-Off Sinus Medicine Tablets-Aspirin Formula ■ 722
Sinulin 840
St. Joseph Cold Tablets for Children ■ 704
Tavist-D Tablets 2035
Triaminic Allergy Tablets ■ 688
Triaminic Chewables ■ 688
Triaminic Cold Tablets ■ 688
Triaminic Expectorant ■ 688
Triaminic Expectorant w/Codeine 1996
Triaminic Expectorant DH 1995
Triaminic Oral Infant Drops 1996
Triaminic Syrup ■ 689
Triaminic-12 Tablets ■ 690
Triaminic-DM Syrup ■ 689
Triaminicin Tablets ■ 690
Triaminicol Multi-Symptom Cold Tablets ■ 691
Triaminicol Multi-Symptom Relief ■ 691
Tuss-Ornade Liquid 2242
Tuss-Ornade Spansule Capsules 2242
Tylenol Cold Medication, Effervescent Tablets 1369

Phenytoin (Hyperglycemia; loss of control). Products include:

Dilantin Infatabs 1710
Dilantin-30 Pediatric/Dilantin-125 Suspension 1713

Phenytoin Sodium (Hyperglycemia; loss of control). Products include:

Dilantin Kapseals 1708
Dilantin Parenteral 1712
Dilantin with Phenobarbital Kapseals 1715

Pindolol (Hypoglycemic action potentiated). Products include:

Visken Tablets 2036

Pirbuterol Acetate (Hyperglycemia; loss of control). Products include:

Maxair Inhaler 1311

Piroxicam (Hypoglycemic action potentiated). Products include:

Feldene Capsules 1777

Polyestradiol Phosphate (Hyperglycemia; loss of control). Products include:

Estradurin 2452

Polythiazide (Hyperglycemia; loss of control). Products include:

Minizide Capsules 1779
Renese Tablets 1785
Renese-R Tablets 1786

Prednisolone Acetate (Hyperglycemia; loss of control). Products include:

AK-Cide Sterile Ophthalmic Ointment & Suspension ⊙ 202
Blephamide Liquifilm Sterile Ophthalmic Suspension 586
Blephamide S.O.P. Sterile Ophthalmic Ointment 586
Cetapred Ointment ⊙ 220
⅛% Econopred & 1% Econopred Plus ⊙ 217
Isopto Cetapred Suspension ⊙ 220
Metimyd ⊙ 306
Poly-Pred Liquifilm ⊙ 250
Pred Forte ⊙ 252
Pred Mild ⊙ 254
Pred-G Liquifilm Sterile Ophthalmic Suspension ⊙ 252
Pred-G S.O.P. Sterile Ophthalmic Ointment ⊙ 253
Vasocidin Ointment ⊙ 275

Prednisolone Sodium Phosphate (Hyperglycemia; loss of control). Products include:

AK-Pred ⊙ 205
Hydeltrasol Injection, Sterile 1476
Inflamase ⊙ 274
Pediapred Oral Liquid 987
Vasocidin Ophthalmic Solution ⊙ 276

Prednisolone Tebutate (Hyperglycemia; loss of control). Products include:

Hydeltra-T.B.A. Sterile Suspension 1478

Prednisone (Hyperglycemia; loss of control). Products include:

Deltasone Tablets 2332

Probenecid (Hypoglycemic action potentiated). Products include:

Benemid Tablets 1426
ColBENEMID Tablets 1436
Wycillin Injection and Probenecid Tablets 2539

Prochlorperazine (Hyperglycemia; loss of control). Products include:

Compazine 2201

Promethazine Hydrochloride (Hyperglycemia; loss of control). Products include:

Mepergan Injection 2479
Phenergan with Codeine 2497
Phenergan with Dextromethorphan 2499
Phenergan Injection 2493
Phenergan Suppositories 2496
Phenergan Syrup 2495
Phenergan Tablets 2496
Phenergan VC 2500
Phenergan VC with Codeine 2501

Propranolol Hydrochloride (Hypoglycemic action potentiated). Products include:

Inderal 2459
Inderal LA Long Acting Capsules 2461
Inderide Tablets 2463
Inderide LA Long Acting Capsules 2465

Pseudoephedrine Hydrochloride (Hyperglycemia; loss of control). Products include:

Actifed Capsules ■ 539
Actifed Plus Caplets ■ 539
Actifed Plus Tablets ■ 540
Actifed with Codeine Cough Syrup 752
Actifed Syrup ■ 540
Actifed Tablets ■ 540
Actifed 12-Hour Capsules ■ 539
Advil Cold & Sinus Caplets (formerly CoAdvil) 2416
Allerest ■ 559
Anatuss LA Tablets 1359
Benadryl Decongestant Elixir ■ 635
Benadryl Decongestant ■ 635
Benadryl Plus ■ 636
Benadryl Plus Nighttime ■ 637
Benylin Decongestant ■ 638
Brexin L.A. Capsules 2078
Bromfed Capsules (Timed Release) 1615
Bromfed Syrup ■ 628
Bromfed 1615
CoAdvil ■ 748
Allergy-Sinus Comtrex Multi-Symptom Allergy Sinus Formula Tablets & Caplets 746
Cough Formula Comtrex 746
Comtrex Multi-Symptom Cold Reliever Tablets/Caplets/Liqui-Gels/Liquid 745
Day-Night Comtrex 747
Non-Drowsy Comtrex 747
Congess 994
Congestac Caplets ■ 617
Contac Jr. Children's Cold Medicine ■ 712
Contac Nighttime Cold Medicine ■ 713
Contac Sinus Caplets Maximum Strength Non-Drowsy Formula ■ 710
Contac Sinus Tablets Maximum Strength Non-Drowsy Formula ■ 710
Deconamine 663
Deconsal II Tablets 559
Dimacol Caplets ■ 672
Dimetane-DX Cough Syrup 1858
Dorcol Children's Cough Syrup ■ 685
Dorcol Children's Decongestant Liquid ■ 685
Dorcol Children's Liquid Cold Formula ■ 686
Maximum Strength Dristan Decongestant/Analgesic Coated Caplets ■ 750

(■ Described in PDR For Nonprescription Drugs) — (⊙ Described in PDR For Ophthalmology)

No Drowsiness Dristan Cold Nasal Decongestant/Analgesic Coated Caplets 2420
Dristan Sinus Caplets 2419
Sinus Excedrin Analgesic, Decongestant Tablets & Caplets ..... ▣ 533
Fedahist Gyrocaps 2145
Fedahist Timecaps 2145
Guaifed 1615
Guaifed Syrup ..... ▣ 629
Isoclor Expectorant 982
Isoclor Timesule Capsules ..... ▣ 561
Kronofed-A 970
Medi-Flu Caplet, Liquid ..... ▣ 640
Novafed A Capsules 1342
Novafed Capsules 1342
Novahistine DH 1342
Novahistine DMX ..... ▣ 595
Novahistine Expectorant 1343
Nucofed Capsules 2219
Nucofed Expectorant 2219
Nucofed Pediatric Expectorant 2220
Nucofed Syrup 2219
Ornex Caplets ..... ▣ 618
PediaCare Allergy Relief Formula Liquid 1362
PediaCare Cough-Cold Formula Liquid 1362
PediaCare Infants' Oral Decongestant Drops 1362
PediaCare Night Rest Cough-Cold Formula Liquid 1362
PediaCare 6-12 Cough-Cold Formula Chewable Tablets 1362
Robitussin-DAC Syrup 1875
Robitussin-PE ..... ▣ 677
Rondec 1975
Rondec-DM 1976
Rondec-TR Tablet 1975
Ru-Tuss DE Tablets 694
Ryna ..... ▣ 741
Seldane-D Extended-Release Tablets 1350
Sinarest ..... ▣ 562
Sine-Aid Maximum Strength Sinus Headache Caplets 1365
Sine-Aid Maximum Strength Sinus Headache Tablets 1365
Sine-Off Maximum Strength Allergy/Sinus Formula Caplets ..... ▣ 721
Sine-Off Maximum Strength No Drowsiness Formula Caplets ..... ▣ 722
Singlet Tablets ..... ▣ 598
Sinutab Maximum Strength ..... ▣ 641
Sinutab Maximum Strength Without Drowsiness Tablets & Caplets ..... ▣ 642
Sinutab Regular Strength Without Drowsiness Formula ..... ▣ 641
St. Joseph Nighttime Cold Medicine ..... ▣ 705
Sudafed Children's Liquid ..... ▣ 543
Sudafed Cough Syrup ..... ▣ 543
Sudafed Plus Liquid ..... ▣ 544
Sudafed Plus Tablets ..... ▣ 545
Sudafed Sinus Caplets ..... ▣ 545
Sudafed Sinus Tablets ..... ▣ 545
Sudafed Tablets, 30 mg ..... ▣ 544
Sudafed Tablets, Adult Strength, 60 mg ..... ▣ 544
Sudafed 12 Hour Capsules ..... ▣ 545
TheraFlu Flu and Cold Medicine ..... ▣ 687
Triaminic Nite Light ..... ▣ 689
Tylenol Allergy Sinus Medication Caplets and Gelcaps, Maximum Strength 1372
Children's Tylenol Cold Liquid Formula and Chewable Tablets 1368
Tylenol Cold & Flu Hot Medication, Packets 1369
Tylenol Cold & Flu No Drowsiness Hot Medication, Packets 1371
Tylenol Cold Medication Caplets and Tablets 1370
Tylenol Cold Medication No Drowsiness Formula Caplets 1370
Tylenol Cold Night Time Medication Liquid 1371
Tylenol Cough Medication Liquid with Decongestant, Maximum Strength 1372
Tylenol, Maximum Strength, Sinus Medication Gelcaps, Caplets and Tablets 1373
Ursinus Inlay-Tabs ..... ▣ 691
Vicks Children's NyQuil ..... ▣ 664
Vicks Daycare ..... ▣ 660
Vicks Formula 44D Decongestant Cough Medicine ..... ▣ 662
Vicks Formula 44M Multi-Symptom Cough Medicine ..... ▣ 662
Vicks NyQuil Nighttime Colds Medicine-Original & Cherry Flavor ..... ▣ 664
Vicks Pediatric Formula 44 Cough & Congestion Medicine ..... ▣ 663
Vicks Pediatric Formula 44m Multi-Symptom Cough & Cold Medicine ..... ▣ 663

Pseudoephedrine Sulfate (Hyperglycemia; loss of control). Products include:
Afrin Tablets ..... ▣ 693
Chlor-Trimeton Decongestant ..... ▣ 694
Disophrol Chronotab Sustained-Action Tablets ..... ▣ 698
Drixoral Antihistamine/Nasal Decongestant Syrup ..... ▣ 698
Drixoral Non-Drowsy Formula ..... ▣ 699
Drixoral Plus Extended-Release Tablets ..... ▣ 699
Drixoral Sinus ..... ▣ 700
Drixoral Sustained-Action Tablets ..... ▣ 698
Sinutab Allergy Formula Sustained Action Tablets ..... ▣ 640
Trinalin Repetabs Tablets 1170

Quinestrol (Hyperglycemia; loss of control). Products include:
Estrovis 1721

Salsalate (Hypoglycemic action potentiated). Products include:
Disalcid 1310
Mono-Gesic Tablets 846
Salflex 839

Selegiline Hydrochloride (Hypoglycemic action potentiated). Products include:
Eldepryl 2250

Spironolactone (Hyperglycemia; loss of control). Products include:
Aldactazide 2150
Aldactone 2152

Sulfamethizole (Hypoglycemic action potentiated). Products include:
Thiosulfil Forte Tablets 2526
Urobiotic-250 Capsules 1968

Sulfamethoxazole (Hypoglycemic action potentiated). Products include:
Azo Gantanol Tablets 1887
Bactrim DS Tablets 1891
Bactrim I.V. Infusion 1889
Bactrim 1891
Gantanol 1899
Septra 813
Septra I.V. Infusion 808
Septra I.V. Infusion ADD-Vantage Vials 810
Septra 813

Sulfasalazine (Hypoglycemic action potentiated). Products include:
Azulfidine Tablets, EN-tabs, Oral Suspension 1157

Sulfinpyrazone (Hypoglycemic action potentiated). Products include:
Anturane 853

Sulfisoxazole (Hypoglycemic action potentiated). Products include:
Azo Gantrisin Tablets 1888
Gantrisin Tablets 1901
Pediazole 1973

Sulfisoxazole Diolamine (Hypoglycemic action potentiated). Products include:
Gantrisin Ophthalmic Ointment/Solution 1900

Sulindac (Hypoglycemic action potentiated). Products include:
Clinoril Tablets 1433

Terbutaline Sulfate (Hyperglycemia; loss of control). Products include:
Brethaire Inhaler 1024
Brethine Ampuls 1026
Brethine Tablets 1026
Bricanyl Injection 1324
Bricanyl Tablets 1325

Thioridazine Hydrochloride (Hyperglycemia; loss of control). Products include:
Mellaril 2011

Thyroglobulin (Hyperglycemia; loss of control). Products include:
Proloid Tablets 1761

Thyroid (Hyperglycemia; loss of control). Products include:
S-P-T "Liquid" Capsules 995

Thyroxine (Hyperglycemia; loss of control).
No products indexed under this heading.

Thyroxine Sodium (Hyperglycemia; loss of control).
No products indexed under this heading.

Timolol Maleate (Hypoglycemic action potentiated). Products include:
Blocadren Tablets 1429
Timolide Tablets 1547
Timoptic in Ocudose 1552
Timoptic Sterile Ophthalmic Solution 1550

Tolazamide (Severe hypoglycemia). Products include:
Tolinase Tablets 2365

Tolmetin Sodium (Hypoglycemic action potentiated). Products include:
Tolectin (200, 400 and 600 mg) 1379

Tranylcypromine Sulfate (Hypoglycemic action potentiated). Products include:
Parnate Tablets 2222

Triamcinolone (Hyperglycemia; loss of control).
No products indexed under this heading.

Triamcinolone Acetonide (Hyperglycemia; loss of control). Products include:
Aristocort A 1010
Azmacort Inhaler 1837
Kenalog Cream, Lotion & Ointment 2401
Kenalog-10 Injection 2402
Kenalog-40 Injection 2403
Kenalog in Orabase 604
Kenalog Spray 2401
Mycolog II Cream and Ointment 2407
Mytrex Cream & Ointment 2080
Nasacort Nasal Inhaler 1844

Triamcinolone Diacetate (Hyperglycemia; loss of control). Products include:
Aristocort Suspension 1008

Triamcinolone Hexacetonide (Hyperglycemia; loss of control). Products include:
Aristospan Suspension 1011

Triamterene (Hyperglycemia; loss of control). Products include:
Dyazide Capsules 2208
Dyrenium Capsules 2210
Maxzide 1215

Trifluoperazine Hydrochloride (Hyperglycemia; loss of control). Products include:
Stelazine 2226

Verapamil Hydrochloride (Hyperglycemia; loss of control). Products include:
Calan SR Caplets 2157
Calan Tablets 2155
Isoptin Injectable 1177
Isoptin Oral Tablets 1179
Isoptin SR Sustained Release Tablets 1181
Verelan Capsules 1243
Verelan Capsules 2535

Warfarin Sodium (Hypoglycemic action potentiated). Products include:
Coumadin Injection & Tablets 944
Panwarfin Tablets 547

ORNADE SPANSULE CAPSULES
(Phenylpropanolamine Hydrochloride, Chlorpheniramine Maleate) 2221
May interact with central nervous system depressants, monoamine oxidase inhibitors, oral anticoagulants, ganglionic blocking agents, beta blockers, alpha adrenergic blockers, anticholinergics, corticosteroids, phenothiazines, and certain other agents. Compounds in these categories include:

Acebutolol Hydrochloride (Hypotensive action antagonized). Products include:
Sectral Capsules 2520

Alcohol (Potentiated).

Alfentanil Hydrochloride (Potentiated). Products include:
Alfenta Injection 1131

Alprazolam (Potentiated). Products include:
Xanax Tablets 2367

Amphetamine Resins (Additive effects). Products include:
Biphetamine Capsules 973

Aprobarbital (Potentiated). Products include:
Alurate Elixir 1883

Atenolol (Hypotensive action antagonized). Products include:
Tenoretic Tablets 1105
Tenormin Tablets and I.V. Injection 1107

Atropine Sulfate (Potentiation of CNS depressant and atropine-like effects). Products include:
Arco-Lase Plus Tablets 607
Atropine Sulfate Sterile Ophthalmic Solution and S.O.P. Sterile Ophthalmic Ointment ..... ⊙ 239
Donnagel ..... ▣ 675
Donnagel-PG 1858
Donnatal 1858
Donnatal Extentabs 1859
Donnatal Tablets 1858
Donnazyme Tablets 1860
Isopto Atropine ..... ⊙ 218
Lomotil 2174
Motofen Tablets 836
Ru-Tuss Tablets 693
Urised Tablets 2396

Belladonna Alkaloids (Potentiation of CNS depressant and atropine-like effects). Products include:
Bellergal-S Tablets 1998
Hyland's Bed Wetting Tablets ..... ▣ 728
Hyland's Teething Tablets ..... ▣ 728
Kinesed Tablets 2272

Benztropine Mesylate (Potentiation of CNS depressant and atropine-like effects). Products include:
Cogentin 1435

Betamethasone Acetate (Decreased effects of corticosteroids). Products include:
Celestone Soluspan Suspension 2081

Betamethasone Sodium Phosphate (Decreased effects of corticosteroids). Products include:
Celestone Soluspan Suspension 2081

Betaxolol Hydrochloride (Hypotensive action antagonized). Products include:
Betoptic Sterile Ophthalmic Solution 569
Betoptic S Sterile Ophthalmic Suspension 570
Kerlone Tablets 2172

Biperiden (Potentiation of CNS depressant and atropine-like effects). Products include:
Akineton 1171

Buprenorphine (Potentiated).
No products indexed under this heading.

Buspirone Hydrochloride (Potentiated). Products include:
BuSpar 1401

Butabarbital (Potentiated). Products include:
Pyridium Plus 1764

Butalbital (Potentiated). Products include:
Esgic-Plus Tablets ... 1002
Esgic Tablets & Capsules ... 1001
Fioricet Tablets ... 2006
Fiorinal Capsules ... 2007
Fiorinal with Codeine Capsules ... 2008
Fiorinal Tablets ... 2007
Phrenilin ... 838
Sedapap Tablets 50 mg/650 mg ... 1360

Carteolol Hydrochloride (Hypotensive action antagonized). Products include:
Cartrol Tablets ... 507

Chlordiazepoxide (Potentiated). Products include:
Libritabs Tablets ... 1930
Limbitrol ... 1933
Menrium Tablets ... 1934

Chlordiazepoxide Hydrochloride (Potentiated). Products include:
Librax Capsules ... 1929
Librium Capsules ... 1931
Librium Injectable ... 1932

Chlorpromazine (Additive CNS depressant effect; urinary retention; glaucoma;). Products include:
Thorazine ... 2234

Chlorprothixene (Potentiated). Products include:
Taractan Tablets ... 1920

Chlorprothixene Hydrochloride (Potentiated). Products include:
Taractan ... 1920

Clidinium Bromide (Potentiation of CNS depressant and atropine-like effects). Products include:
Librax Capsules ... 1929
Quarzan Capsules ... 1937

Clorazepate Dipotassium (Potentiated). Products include:
Tranxene ... 556

Codeine (Potentiated). Products include:
Calcidrine Syrup ... 506

Codeine Phosphate (Potentiated). Products include:
Actifed with Codeine Cough Syrup ... 752
Cheracol Cough Syrup ... 1853
Codimal PH Syrup ... 846
Dimetane-DC Cough Syrup ... 1857
Empirin with Codeine Phosphate Nos. 2, 3 & 4 ... 764
Fiorinal with Codeine Capsules ... 2008
Isoclor Expectorant ... 982
Naldecon CX Adult Liquid ... ▣ 521
Novahistine DH ... 1342
Novahistine Expectorant ... 1343
Nucofed Capsules ... 2219
Nucofed Expectorant ... 2219
Nucofed Pediatric Expectorant ... 2220
Nucofed Syrup ... 2219
Phenaphen with Codeine Capsules 1865
Phenaphen-650 with Codeine Tablets ... 1866
Phenergan with Codeine ... 2497
Phenergan VC with Codeine ... 2501
Robitussin A-C Syrup ... 1875
Robitussin-DAC Syrup ... 1875
Ryna ... ▣ 741
Soma Compound w/Codeine Tablets ... 2390
Triaminic Expectorant w/Codeine ... 1996
Tussi-Organidin Liquid ... 2391
Tylenol with Codeine ... 1381

Codeine Polistirex (Potentiated).
No products indexed under this heading.

Cortisone Acetate (Decreased effects of corticosteroids). Products include:
Cortone Acetate Sterile Suspension ... 1437
Cortone Acetate Tablets ... 1439

Dexamethasone (Decreased effects). Products include:
AK-Trol Ointment & Suspension ... ◉ 207
Decadron Elixir ... 1445
Decadron Tablets ... 1447
Decaspray Topical Aerosol ... 1459
Dexacidin ... ◉ 272
Maxidex Sterile Ophthalmic Suspension ... ◉ 223
Maxitrol Ophthalmic Ointment/Suspension ... ◉ 223
TobraDex Ophthalmic Suspension and Ointment ... ◉ 228

Dexamethasone Acetate (Decreased effects of corticosteroids). Products include:
Dalalone D.P. Injectable ... 999
Decadron-LA Sterile Suspension ... 1457

Dexamethasone Sodium Phosphate (Decreased effects of corticosteroids). Products include:
AK-Dex ... ◉ 203
Decadron Phosphate Respihaler ... 1454
Decadron Phosphate Sterile Ophthalmic Ointment ... 1453
Decadron Phosphate Sterile Ophthalmic Solution ... 1453
Decadron Phosphate Topical Cream ... 1455
Decadron Phosphate Turbinaire ... 1456
Maxidex Sterile Ophthalmic Ointment ... ◉ 222
NeoDecadron Sterile Ophthalmic Ointment ... 1517
NeoDecadron Sterile Ophthalmic Solution ... 1518
NeoDecadron Topical Cream ... 1518

Dextroamphetamine Sulfate (Additive effects). Products include:
Dexedrine ... 2206

Dezocine (Potentiated).

Diazepam (Potentiated). Products include:
Valium Injectable ... 1937
Valium Tablets ... 1939
Valrelease Capsules ... 1923

Dicumarol (Action of oral anticoagulants may be inhibited). Products include:
Dicumarol Tablets ... 516

Dicyclomine Hydrochloride (Potentiation of CNS depressant and atropine-like effects). Products include:
Bentyl ... 1322

Doxazosin Mesylate (Hypotensive action antagonized). Products include:
Cardura Tablets ... 1941

Droperidol (Potentiated). Products include:
Inapsine Injection ... 1140
Innovar Injection ... 1141

Enflurane (Potentiated). Products include:
Ethrane ... 599

Esmolol Hydrochloride (Hypotensive action antagonized). Products include:
Brevibloc Injection ... 942

Estazolam (Potentiated). Products include:
ProSom Tablets ... 554

Ethchlorvynol (Potentiated). Products include:
Placidyl Capsules ... 553

Ethinamate (Potentiated).
No products indexed under this heading.

Fentanyl (Potentiated). Products include:
Duragesic Transdermal System ... 1133

Fentanyl Citrate (Potentiated). Products include:
Innovar Injection ... 1141
Sublimaze Injection ... 1146

Fluphenazine Decanoate (Additive CNS depressant effect; urinary retention; glaucoma). Products include:
Prolixin Decanoate ... 1795

Fluphenazine Enanthate (Additive CNS depressant effect; urinary retention; glaucoma). Products include:
Prolixin Enanthate ... 1796

Fluphenazine Hydrochloride (Additive CNS depressant effect; urinary retention; glaucoma). Products include:
Prolixin Elixir ... 1793
Prolixin Injection ... 1791
Prolixin Oral Concentrate ... 1792
Prolixin Tablets ... 1793

Flurazepam Hydrochloride (Potentiated). Products include:
Dalmane Capsules ... 1927

Furazolidone (Contraindicated; prolongs and intensifies the anticholinergic effects and potentiates the pressor effects). Products include:
Furoxone ... 1855

Glutethimide (Potentiated).
No products indexed under this heading.

Glycopyrrolate (Potentiation of CNS depressant and atropine-like effects). Products include:
Robinul Forte Tablets ... 1873
Robinul Injectable ... 1873
Robinul Tablets ... 1873

Guanethidine Monosulfate (Hypotensive action antagonized). Products include:
Esimil Tablets ... 864
Ismelin Tablets ... 869

Haloperidol (Potentiated). Products include:
Haldol Injection, Tablets and Concentrate ... 1373

Haloperidol Decanoate (Potentiated). Products include:
Haldol Decanoate ... 1375

Hydrocodone Bitartrate (Potentiated). Products include:
Anexsia 5/500 Tablets ... 2196
Anexsia 7.5/650 Tablets ... 2197
Azdone Tablets ... 844
Codiclear DH Syrup ... 845
Codimal DH Syrup ... 846
Damason-P ... 1356
Hycodan Syrup, Tablets ... 927
Hycomine Compound Tablets ... 929
Hycomine Syrup ... 927
Hycotuss Expectorant Syrup ... 930
Hydrocet Capsules ... 835
Lortab ASA Tablets ... 2414
Lortab ... 2412
Ru-Tuss with Hydrocodone ... 694
Triaminic Expectorant DH ... 1995
Vicodin Tablets ... 1187
Vicodin ES Tablets ... 1189
Zydone Capsules ... 941

Hydrocodone Polistirex (Potentiated). Products include:
Tussionex Extended-Release Suspension ... 988

Hydrocortisone (Decreased effects of corticosteroids). Products include:
AK-Spore H.C. ... ◉ 206
Bactine Hydrocortisone Anti-Itch Cream ... ▣ 625
CaldeCORT Anti-Itch Hydrocortisone Spray ... ▣ 560
Carmol HC Cream 1% ... 2296
Cortaid Spray ... ▣ 735
Cortenema ... 2244
Cortisporin Ointment ... 758
Cortisporin Ophthalmic Ointment Sterile ... 758
Cortisporin Ophthalmic Suspension Sterile ... 759
Cortisporin Otic Solution Sterile ... 760
Cortisporin Otic Suspension Sterile 760
Cortizone-5 Creme & Ointment ... ▣ 732
Dermolate Anti-Itch Cream ... ▣ 697
Eldecort Cream 1.0% ... 1113
Eldecort Cream 1.0% and 2.5% ... 1113
Fungoid HC Creme ... 1770
Hydrocortone Tablets ... 1482
Hytone ... 909
LazerSporin-C Solution ... 1770
Massengill Medicated Soft Cloth Towelettes ... 2192
Nutracort Cream & Lotion ... 1684
PediOtic Suspension Sterile ... 797
Synacort Creams 1%, 2.5% ... 2296
Vanoxide-HC Acne Lotion ... 911
Vioform-Hydrocortisone Cream and Mild Cream ... 889
Vioform-Hydrocortisone Ointment ... 889
VōSoL HC Otic Solution ... 2392
Vytone Cream 1% ... 911

Hydrocortisone Acetate (Decreased effects of corticosteroids). Products include:
Analpram-HC Rectal Cream 1% and 2.5% ... 970
Anusol-HC Cream ... 1690
Anusol-HC Suppositories ... 1691
Caldecort ... ▣ 560
Carmol HC Cream 1% ... 2296
Chloromycetin Hydrocortisone Ophthalmic ... 1694
Coly-Mycin S Otic w/Neomycin & Hydrocortisone ... 1708
Cortaid ... ▣ 735
Cortef Feminine Itch Cream ... ▣ 735
Corticaine ... ▣ 682
Cortifoam ... 1827
Cortisporin Cream ... 757
Epifoam ... 1828
Gynecort 5 Creme ... ▣ 556
Hydrocortone Acetate Sterile Suspension ... 1479
Lanacort 5 Creme and Ointment ... ▣ 557
Mantadil Cream ... 789
Ophthocort ... ◉ 301
Orabase HCA Oral Paste ... 890
Pramosone Cream, Lotion & Ointment ... 971
ProctoCream-HC ... 1834
Proctofoam-HC ... 1835

Hydrocortisone Sodium Phosphate (Decreased effects of corticosteroids). Products include:
Hydrocortone Phosphate Injection, Sterile ... 1481

Hydrocortisone Sodium Succinate (Decreased effects of corticosteroids). Products include:
Solu-Cortef Sterile Powder ... 2361

Hydroxyzine Hydrochloride (Potentiated). Products include:
Atarax Tablets & Syrup ... 1941
Marax Tablets & DF Syrup ... 1954
Vistaril Intramuscular Solution ... 1970

Hyoscyamine (Potentiation of CNS depressant and atropine-like effects). Products include:
Cystospaz Tablets ... 2395
Urised Tablets ... 2396

Hyoscyamine Sulfate (Potentiation of CNS depressant and atropine-like effects). Products include:
Arco-Lase Plus Tablets ... 607
Cystospaz-M Capsules ... 2395
Donnagel ... ▣ 675
Donnagel-PG ... 1858
Donnatal ... 1858
Donnatal Extentabs ... 1859
Donnatal Tablets ... 1858
Donnazyme Tablets ... 1860
Kutrase Capsules ... 2146
Levsin/Levsinex ... 2147
Ru-Tuss Tablets ... 693

Imipramine Hydrochloride (Potentiation of CNS depressant and atropine-like effects). Products include:
Tofranil Ampuls ... 1038
Tofranil Tablets ... 1039

Imipramine Pamoate (Potentiation of CNS depressant and atropine-like effects). Products include:
Tofranil-PM Capsules ... 1041

Ipratropium Bromide (Potentiation of CNS depressant and atropine-like effects). Products include:
Atrovent Inhalation Aerosol ... 675

Isocarboxazid (Contraindicated; prolongs and intensifies the anticholinergic effects and potentiates the pressor effects). Products include:
Marplan Tablets ... 1906

Isoflurane (Potentiated). Products include:
Forane ... 600

Ketamine Hydrochloride (Potentiated). Products include:
Ketalar ... 1726

Labetalol Hydrochloride (Hypotensive action antagonized). Products include:
- Normodyne Injection 2108
- Normodyne Tablets 2110
- Normozide Tablets 2112
- Trandate HCT Tablets 579
- Trandate Injection 577
- Trandate Tablets 579

Levorphanol Tartrate (Potentiated). Products include:
- Levo-Dromoran 1906

Lorazepam (Potentiated). Products include:
- Ativan Injection 2432
- Ativan Tablets 2434

Loxapine Hydrochloride (Potentiated). Products include:
- Loxitane 1213

Loxapine Succinate (Potentiated). Products include:
- Loxitane Capsules 1213

Mecamylamine Hydrochloride (Potentiates reactions of sympathomimetics). Products include:
- Inversine Tablets 1492

Mepenzolate Bromide (Potentiation of CNS depressant and atropine-like effects). Products include:
- Cantil Tablets 1326

Meperidine Hydrochloride (Potentiated). Products include:
- Demerol 2047
- Mepergan Injection 2479

Mephobarbital (Potentiated). Products include:
- Mebaral Tablets 2061

Meprobamate (Potentiated). Products include:
- Deprol Tablets 2382
- Equagesic Tablets 2451
- Miltown Tablets 2386
- PMB 200 and PMB 400 2504

Mesoridazine (Additive CNS depressant effect; urinary retention; glaucoma). Products include:
- Serentil 686

Methadone Hydrochloride (Potentiated). Products include:
- Dolophine Hydrochloride Ampoules & Vials 1260
- Dolophine Hydrochloride Tablets 1261
- Methadone Hydrochloride Diskets 1284
- Methadone Hydrochloride Oral Solution & Tablets 1987

Methamphetamine Hydrochloride (Additive effects). Products include:
- Desoxyn Gradumet Tablets 514

Methohexital Sodium (Potentiated). Products include:
- Brevital Sodium Vials 1248

Methoxyflurane (Potentiated).
- No products indexed under this heading.

Methylprednisolone (Decreased effects of corticosteroids). Products include:
- Medrol 2348

Methylprednisolone Acetate (Decreased effects of corticosteroids). Products include:
- Depo-Medrol Sterile Aqueous Suspension 2334

Methylprednisolone Sodium Succinate (Decreased effects of corticosteroids). Products include:
- Solu-Medrol Sterile Powder 2363

Metoprolol Tartrate (Hypotensive action antagonized). Products include:
- Lopressor Ampuls 1032
- Lopressor HCT Tablets 1034
- Lopressor Tablets 1032

Midazolam Hydrochloride (Potentiated). Products include:
- Versed Injection 1924

Molindone Hydrochloride (Potentiated). Products include:
- Moban Tablets & Concentrate 932

Morphine Sulfate (Potentiated). Products include:
- Astramorph/PF Injection, USP (Preservative-Free) 618
- Duramorph 960
- Infumorph 200 and Infumorph 500 Sterile Solutions 962
- MS Contin Tablets 1814
- MSIR 1817
- Oramorph SR (Morphine Sulfate Sustained Release Tablets) 1988
- Roxanol 1991

Nadolol (Hypotensive action antagonized). Products include:
- Corgard Tablets 701
- Corzide Tablets 702

Norepinephrine Bitartrate (Cardiovascular effects potentiated). Products include:
- Levophed Bitartrate Injection 2054

Opium Alkaloids (Potentiated). Products include:
- B & O No. 15A & No. 16A Supprettes 2395
- Pantopon Injectable 1911

Oxazepam (Potentiated). Products include:
- Serax Capsules 2522
- Serax Tablets 2522

Oxybutynin Chloride (Potentiation of CNS depressant and atropine-like effects). Products include:
- Ditropan 1332

Oxycodone Hydrochloride (Potentiated). Products include:
- Percocet Tablets 950
- Percodan 951
- Roxicodone Tablets, Oral Solution & Intensol (Oxycodone) 1992
- Tylox Capsules 1382

Penbutolol Sulfate (Hypotensive action antagonized). Products include:
- Levatol 1832

Pentobarbital Sodium (Potentiated). Products include:
- Nembutal Sodium Capsules 534
- Nembutal Sodium Solution 536
- Nembutal Sodium Suppositories 538

Perphenazine (Additive CNS depressant effect; urinary retention; glaucoma). Products include:
- Etrafon 2087
- Triavil Tablets 1556
- Trilafon 2123

Phenelzine Sulfate (Contraindicated; prolongs and intensifies the anticholinergic effects and potentiates the pressor effects). Products include:
- Nardil 1742

Phenobarbital (Potentiated). Products include:
- Arco-Lase Plus Tablets 607
- Bellergal-S Tablets 1998
- Bronkolixir .... ▣ 761
- Bronkotabs Tablets .... ▣ 762
- Donnatal 1858
- Donnatal Extentabs 1859
- Donnatal Tablets 1858
- Donnazyme Tablets 1860
- Kinesed Tablets 2272
- Phenobarbital Elixir and Tablets 1293
- Primatene Tablets-P Formula 2421
- Quadrinal Tablets 1183
- Tedral SA 1765

Pindolol (Hypotensive action antagonized). Products include:
- Visken Tablets 2036

Prazepam (Potentiated). Products include:
- Centrax 1693

Prazosin Hydrochloride (Hypotensive action antagonized). Products include:
- Minipress Capsules 1778
- Minizide Capsules 1779

Prednisolone Acetate (Decreased effects of corticosteroids). Products include:
- AK-Cide Sterile Ophthalmic Ointment & Suspension .... ◉ 202
- Blephamide Liquifilm Sterile Ophthalmic Suspension 586
- Blephamide S.O.P. Sterile Ophthalmic Ointment 586
- Cetapred Ointment .... ◉ 220
- ⅛% Econopred & 1% Econopred Plus .... ◉ 217
- Isopto Cetapred Suspension .... ◉ 220
- Metimyd .... ◉ 306
- Poly-Pred Liquifilm .... ◉ 250
- Pred Forte .... ◉ 252
- Pred Mild .... ◉ 254
- Pred-G Liquifilm Sterile Ophthalmic Suspension .... ◉ 252
- Pred-G S.O.P. Sterile Ophthalmic Ointment .... ◉ 253
- Vasocidin Ointment .... ◉ 275

Prednisolone Sodium Phosphate (Decreased effects of corticosteroids). Products include:
- AK-Pred .... ◉ 205
- Hydeltrasol Injection, Sterile 1476
- Inflamase .... ◉ 274
- Pediapred Oral Liquid 987
- Vasocidin Ophthalmic Solution .... ◉ 276

Prednisolone Tebutate (Decreased effects of corticosteroids). Products include:
- Hydeltra-T.B.A. Sterile Suspension 1478

Prednisone (Decreased effects of corticosteroids). Products include:
- Deltasone Tablets 2332

Prochlorperazine (Additive CNS depressant effect; urinary retention; glaucoma;). Products include:
- Compazine 2201

Procyclidine Hydrochloride (Potentiation of CNS depressant and atropine-like effects). Products include:
- Kemadrin Tablets 771

Promethazine Hydrochloride (Additive CNS depressant effect; urinary retention; glaucoma). Products include:
- Mepergan Injection 2479
- Phenergan with Codeine 2497
- Phenergan with Dextromethorphan 2499
- Phenergan Injection 2493
- Phenergan Suppositories 2496
- Phenergan Syrup 2495
- Phenergan Tablets 2496
- Phenergan VC 2500
- Phenergan VC with Codeine 2501

Propantheline Bromide (Potentiation of CNS depressant and atropine-like effects). Products include:
- Pro-Banthine Tablets 2141

Propofol (Potentiated). Products include:
- Diprivan Injection 2267

Propoxyphene Hydrochloride (Potentiated). Products include:
- Darvon 1256
- Wygesic Tablets 2540

Propoxyphene Napsylate (Potentiated). Products include:
- Darvon-N/Darvocet-N 1254

Propranolol Hydrochloride (Hypotensive action antagonized). Products include:
- Inderal 2459
- Inderal LA Long Acting Capsules 2461
- Inderide Tablets 2463
- Inderide LA Long Acting Capsules 2465

Quazepam (Potentiated). Products include:
- Doral Tablets 2383

Scopolamine Hydrobromide (Potentiation of CNS depressant and atropine-like effects). Products include:
- Donnagel .... ▣ 675
- Donnagel-PG 1858
- Donnatal 1858
- Donnatal Extentabs 1859
- Donnatal Tablets 1858
- Donnazyme Tablets 1860
- Isopto Hyoscine .... ◉ 222
- Murocoll-2 Sterile Ophthalmic Solution .... ◉ 261
- Ru-Tuss Tablets 693

Scopolamine Preparations (Potentiation of CNS depressant and atropine-like effects). Products include:
- Transderm Scōp Transdermal Therapeutic System 887

Secobarbital Sodium (Potentiated). Products include:
- Seconal Sodium Pulvules 1296

Selegiline Hydrochloride (Contraindicated; prolongs and intensifies the anticholinergic effects and potentiates the pressor effects). Products include:
- Eldepryl 2250

Sufentanil Citrate (Potentiated). Products include:
- Sufenta Injection 1147

Temazepam (Potentiated). Products include:
- Restoril Capsules 2023

Terazosin Hydrochloride (Hypotensive action antagonized). Products include:
- Hytrin Tablets 529

Thiamylal Sodium (Potentiated). Products include:
- Surital Ampoules, Steri-Vials 1764

Thioridazine Hydrochloride (Additive CNS depressant effect; urinary retention; glaucoma). Products include:
- Mellaril 2011

Thiothixene (Additive effects). Products include:
- Navane Capsules and Concentrate 1954
- Navane Intramuscular 1956

Timolol Maleate (Hypotensive action antagonized). Products include:
- Blocadren Tablets 1429
- Timolide Tablets 1547
- Timoptic in Ocudose 1552
- Timoptic Sterile Ophthalmic Solution 1550

Tranylcypromine Sulfate (Contraindicated; prolongs and intensifies the anticholinergic effects and potentiates the pressor effects). Products include:
- Parnate Tablets 2222

Triamcinolone (Decreased effects of corticosteroids).
- No products indexed under this heading.

Triamcinolone Acetonide (Decreased effects of corticosteroids). Products include:
- Aristocort A 1010
- Azmacort Inhaler 1837
- Kenalog Cream, Lotion & Ointment 2401
- Kenalog-10 Injection 2402
- Kenalog-40 Injection 2403
- Kenalog in Orabase 604
- Kenalog Spray 2401
- Mycolog II Cream and Ointment 2407
- Mytrex Cream & Ointment 2080
- Nasacort Nasal Inhaler 1844

Triamcinolone Diacetate (Decreased effects of corticosteroids). Products include:
- Aristocort Suspension 1008

Triamcinolone Hexacetonide (Decreased effects of corticosteroids). Products include:
- Aristospan Suspension 1011

Triazolam (Potentiated). Products include:
- Halcion Tablets 2340

Tridihexethyl Chloride (Potentiation of CNS depressant and atropine-like effects).
- No products indexed under this heading.

Trifluoperazine Hydrochloride (Additive CNS depressant effect; urinary retention; glaucoma). Products include:
- Stelazine ... 2226

Trihexyphenidyl Hydrochloride (Potentiation of CNS depressant and atropine-like effects). Products include:
- Artane ... 1195

Trimethaphan Camsylate (Reactions potentiated). Products include:
- Arfonad Ampuls ... 1887

Warfarin Sodium (Action of oral anticoagulants may be inhibited; should not be taken together). Products include:
- Coumadin Injection & Tablets ... 944
- Panwarfin Tablets ... 547

ORNEX CAPLETS
(Acetaminophen, Pseudoephedrine Hydrochloride) ... ◘ 618
No interactions described in labeling.

ORTHO DIAPHRAGM KIT/ALL-FLEX ARCING SPRING
(Ortho Diaphragm) ... 1664
No interactions described in labeling.

ORTHO DIAPHRAGM KIT-COIL SPRING
(Ortho Diaphragm) ... 1664
No interactions described in labeling.

ORTHO DIENESTROL CREAM
(Dienestrol) ... 1664
No interactions described in labeling.

ORTHOCLONE OKT3 STERILE SOLUTION
(Muromonab-CD3) ... 1645
No interactions described in labeling.

ORTHO-CYCLEN TABLETS
(Norgestimate, Ethinyl Estradiol) ... 1658
May interact with tetracyclines, barbiturates, and certain other agents. Compounds in these categories include:

Ampicillin Sodium (Reduces efficacy and increases incidence of breakthrough bleeding and menstrual irregularities). Products include:
- Unasyn ... 1965

Aprobarbital (Reduces efficacy and increases incidence of breakthrough bleeding and menstrual irregularities). Products include:
- Alurate Elixir ... 1883

Butabarbital (Reduces efficacy and increases incidence of breakthrough bleeding and menstrual irregularities). Products include:
- Pyridium Plus ... 1764

Butalbital (Reduces efficacy and increases incidence of breakthrough bleeding and menstrual irregularities). Products include:
- Esgic-Plus Tablets ... 1002
- Esgic Tablets & Capsules ... 1001
- Fioricet Tablets ... 2006
- Fiorinal Capsules ... 2007
- Fiorinal with Codeine Capsules ... 2008
- Fiorinal Tablets ... 2007
- Phrenilin ... 838
- Sedapap Tablets 50 mg/650 mg ... 1360

Demeclocycline Hydrochloride (Reduces efficacy and increases incidence of breakthrough bleeding). Products include:
- Declomycin Capsules, Tablets ... 1199

Doxycycline Calcium (Reduces efficacy and increases incidence of breakthrough bleeding).
- No products indexed under this heading.

Doxycycline Hyclate (Reduces efficacy and increases incidence of breakthrough bleeding). Products include:
- Doryx Capsules ... 1717
- Vibramycin Hyclate Capsules ... 1787
- Vibramycin Hyclate Intravenous ... 1968
- Vibra-Tabs Film Coated Tablets ... 1787

Doxycycline Monohydrate (Reduces efficacy and increases incidence of breakthrough bleeding). Products include:
- Monodox Capsules ... 1630
- Vibramycin Monohydrate for Oral Suspension ... 1787

Griseofulvin (Reduces efficacy and increases incidence of breakthrough bleeding and menstrual irregularities). Products include:
- Fulvicin P/G Tablets ... 2090
- Fulvicin P/G 165 & 330 Tablets ... 2091
- Fulvicin-U/F Tablets ... 2092
- Grifulvin V (griseofulvin microsize) Tablets/Suspension ... 1678
- Grisactin ... 2454
- Grisactin Ultra Tablets ... 2455
- Gris-PEG Tablets, 125 mg & 250 mg ... 1083

Mephobarbital (Reduces efficacy and increases incidence of breakthrough bleeding and menstrual irregularities). Products include:
- Mebaral Tablets ... 2061

Methacycline Hydrochloride (Reduces efficacy and increases incidence of breakthrough bleeding).
- No products indexed under this heading.

Minocycline Hydrochloride (Reduces efficacy and increases incidence of breakthrough bleeding). Products include:
- Minocin Intravenous ... 1221
- Minocin Oral Suspension ... 1224
- Minocin Pellet-Filled Capsules ... 1222

Oxytetracycline Hydrochloride (Reduces efficacy and increases incidence of breakthrough bleeding). Products include:
- Terra-Cortril Ophthalmic Suspension ... 1963
- Terramycin Capsules ... 1786
- Terramycin Intramuscular Solution ... 1964
- Terramycin with Polymyxin B Sulfate Ophthalmic Ointment ... 1965

Pentobarbital Sodium (Reduces efficacy and increases incidence of breakthrough bleeding and menstrual irregularities). Products include:
- Nembutal Sodium Capsules ... 534
- Nembutal Sodium Solution ... 536
- Nembutal Sodium Suppositories ... 538

Phenobarbital (Reduces efficacy and increases incidence of breakthrough bleeding and menstrual irregularities). Products include:
- Arco-Lase Plus Tablets ... 607
- Bellergal-S Tablets ... 1998
- Bronkolixir ... ◘ 761
- Bronkotabs Tablets ... ◘ 762
- Donnatal ... 1858
- Donnatal Extentabs ... 1859
- Donnatal Tablets ... 1858
- Donnazyme Tablets ... 1860
- Kinesed Tablets ... 2272
- Phenobarbital Elixir and Tablets ... 1293
- Primatene Tablets-P Formula ... 2421
- Quadrinal Tablets ... 1183
- Tedral SA ... 1765

Phenylbutazone (Reduces efficacy and increases incidence of breakthrough bleeding and menstrual irregularities). Products include:
- Butazolidin Capsules & Tablets ... 1027

Phenytoin Sodium (Reduces efficacy and increases incidence of breakthrough bleeding and menstrual irregularities). Products include:
- Dilantin Kapseals ... 1708
- Dilantin Parenteral ... 1712
- Dilantin with Phenobarbital Kapseals ... 1715

Rifampin (Reduces efficacy and increases incidence of breakthrough bleeding and menstrual irregularities). Products include:
- Rifadin ... 1345
- Rifamate Capsules ... 1347
- Rimactane Capsules ... 879

Secobarbital Sodium (Reduces efficacy and increases incidence of breakthrough bleeding and menstrual irregularities). Products include:
- Seconal Sodium Pulvules ... 1296

Tetracycline Hydrochloride (Reduces efficacy and increases incidence of breakthrough bleeding). Products include:
- Achromycin V Capsules ... 1193
- Achromycin Ophthalmic Ointment 1% ... ⊙ 307
- Achromycin Ophthalmic Suspension 1% ... ⊙ 308
- Topicycline for Topical Solution ... 1856

Thiamylal Sodium (Reduces efficacy and increases incidence of breakthrough bleeding and menstrual irregularities). Products include:
- Surital Ampoules, Steri-Vials ... 1764

ORTHO-GYNOL CONTRACEPTIVE JELLY
(Octoxynol 9) ... ◘ 632
No interactions described in labeling.

ORTHO-NOVUM 1/35□21 TABLETS
(Norethindrone, Ethinyl Estradiol) ... 1667
See **Micronor Tablets**

ORTHO-NOVUM 1/35□28 TABLETS
(Norethindrone, Ethinyl Estradiol) ... 1667
See **Micronor Tablets**

ORTHO-NOVUM 1/50□21 TABLETS
(Norethindrone, Mestranol) ... 1667
See **Micronor Tablets**

ORTHO-NOVUM 1/50□28 TABLETS
(Norethindrone, Mestranol) ... 1667
See **Micronor Tablets**

ORTHO-NOVUM 7/7/7 □21 TABLETS
(Norethindrone, Ethinyl Estradiol) ... 1667
See **Micronor Tablets**

ORTHO-NOVUM 7/7/7 □28 TABLETS
(Norethindrone, Ethinyl Estradiol) ... 1667
See **Micronor Tablets**

ORTHO-NOVUM 10/11□21 TABLETS
(Norethindrone, Ethinyl Estradiol) ... 1667
See **Micronor Tablets**

ORTHO-NOVUM 10/11□28 TABLETS
(Norethindrone, Ethinyl Estradiol) ... 1667
See **Micronor Tablets**

ORTHO-WHITE DIAPHRAGM KIT-FLAT SPRING
(Ortho Diaphragm) ... 1664
No interactions described in labeling.

ORTHOXICOL COUGH SYRUP
(Phenylpropanolamine Hydrochloride, Chlorpheniramine Maleate, Dextromethorphan Hydrobromide) ... ◘ 668
May interact with monoamine oxidase inhibitors. Compounds in this category include:

Furazolidone (Effect not specified). Products include:
- Furoxone ... 1855

Isocarboxazid (Effect not specified). Products include:
- Marplan Tablets ... 1906

Phenelzine Sulfate (Effect not specified). Products include:
- Nardil ... 1742

Selegiline Hydrochloride (Effect not specified). Products include:
- Eldepryl ... 2250

Tranylcypromine Sulfate (Effect not specified). Products include:
- Parnate Tablets ... 2222

ORUDIS CAPSULES
(Ketoprofen) ... 2488
May interact with lithium preparations, diuretics, and certain other agents. Compounds in these categories include:

Amiloride Hydrochloride (Reduced urinary potassium and chloride excretion). Products include:
- Midamor Tablets ... 1508
- Moduretic Tablets ... 1510

Aspirin (Decreased protein-binding and increased plasma clearance of ketoprofen). Products include:
- Alka-Seltzer Effervescent Antacid and Pain Reliever ... 1568
- Alka-Seltzer Extra Strength Effervescent Antacid and Pain Reliever ... 1570
- Alka-Seltzer (Flavored) Effervescent Antacid and Pain Reliever ... 1569
- Alka-Seltzer Plus Cold Medicine ... ◘ 623
- Alka-Seltzer Plus Night-Time Cold Medicine ... ◘ 623
- Alka Seltzer Plus Sinus Allergy Medicine ... ◘ 624
- Anacin Coated Analgesic Caplets ... 2417
- Anacin Coated Analgesic Tablets ... 2417
- Anacin Maximum Strength Analgesic Coated Tablets ... 2417
- Maximum Strength Arthritis Pain Formula By the Makers of Anacin Analgesic Tablets and Caplets ... 2418
- Arthritis Pain Formula by the Makers of Anacin Analgesic Tablets and Caplets ... ◘ 747
- Arthritis Strength BC Powder ... ◘ 516
- Ascriptin A/D Caplets ... 1850
- Regular Strength Ascriptin Tablets ... 1850
- Azdōne Tablets ... 844
- BC Powder ... ◘ 517
- BC Cold Powder ... ◘ 517
- Children's Bayer Chewable Aspirin ... ◘ 564
- Genuine Bayer Aspirin Tablets & Caplets ... ◘ 564
- Maximum Bayer Aspirin Tablets & Caplets ... ◘ 566
- Bayer Plus Aspirin Tablets ... ◘ 567
- Therapy Bayer Aspirin Caplets ... ◘ 568
- 8 Hour Bayer Timed-Release Aspirin ... ◘ 566
- Arthritis Strength Bufferin Analgesic Caplets ... 744
- Extra Strength Bufferin Analgesic Tablets ... 745
- Bufferin Analgesic Tablets and Caplets ... 743
- Cama Arthritis Pain Reliever ... ◘ 685
- Damason-P ... 1356
- Easprin ... 1719
- Ecotrin Enteric Coated Aspirin Maximum Strength Tablets and Caplets ... 2189
- Ecotrin Enteric Coated Aspirin Regular Strength Tablets and Caplets ... 2189
- Empirin Aspirin ... ◘ 541

Empirin with Codeine Phosphate Nos. 2, 3 & 4 764
Equagesic Tablets 2451
Excedrin Extra-Strength Analgesic Tablets & Caplets 749
4-Way Cold Tablets 750
Fiorinal Capsules 2007
Fiorinal with Codeine Capsules 2008
Fiorinal Tablets 2007
Lortab ASA Tablets 2414
Momentum Muscular Backache Formula ..... ▣ 751
Norgesic 1314
Norwich Extra-Strength Aspirin ..... ▣ 546
Norwich Regular Strength Aspirin ▣ 547
P-A-C Analgesic Tablets ..... ▣ 669
Percodan 951
Robaxisal Tablets 1872
Sine-Off Sinus Medicine Tablets-Aspirin Formula ..... ▣ 722
Soma Compound w/Codeine Tablets 2390
Soma Compound Tablets 2389
St. Joseph Adult Chewable Aspirin (81 mg.) ..... ▣ 703
Synalgos-DC Capsules 2525
Talwin Compound 2072
Ursinus Inlay-Tabs ..... ▣ 691
Vanquish Analgesic Caplets ..... ▣ 574
Zorprin Tablets 698

Aspirin, Enteric Coated (Decreased protein-binding and increased plasma clearance of ketoprofen). Products include:
Therapy Bayer Aspirin Caplets ..... ▣ 568
Ecotrin 2189

Bendroflumethiazide (Reduced urinary potassium and chloride excretion). Products include:
Corzide Tablets 702
Naturetin Tablets 1789
Rauzide Tablets 1804

Bumetanide (Reduced urinary potassium and chloride excretion). Products include:
Bumex 1895

Chlorothiazide (Reduced urinary potassium and chloride excretion). Products include:
Aldoclor Tablets 1413
Diupres Tablets 1461
Diuril Oral 1464

Chlorothiazide Sodium (Reduced urinary potassium and chloride excretion). Products include:
Diuril Sodium Intravenous 1463

Chlorthalidone (Reduced urinary potassium and chloride excretion). Products include:
Combipres Tablets 678
Tenoretic Tablets 1105
Thalitone Tablets 687

Ethacrynic Acid (Reduced urinary potassium and chloride excretion). Products include:
Edecrin Tablets 1468

Furosemide (Reduced urinary potassium and chloride excretion). Products include:
Lasix 1093

Hydrochlorothiazide (Reduced urinary potassium and chloride excretion). Products include:
Aldactazide 2150
Aldoril Tablets 1418
Apresazide Capsules 854
Apresoline-Esidrix Tablets 857
Capozide 2258
Dyazide Capsules 2208
Esidrix Tablets 863
Esimil Tablets 864
HydroDIURIL Tablets 1484
Hydropres Tablets 1485
Inderide Tablets 2463
Inderide LA Long Acting Capsules .. 2465
Lopressor HCT Tablets 1034
Maxzide 1215
Moduretic Tablets 1510
Normozide Tablets 2112
Oretic Tablets 544
Oreticyl 545
Prinzide Tablets 1540
Ser-Ap-Es Tablets 881
Serpasil-Esidrix Tablets 886
Timolide Tablets 1547
Trandate HCT Tablets 579
Vaseretic Tablets 1559
Zestoretic 2274

Hydroflumethiazide (Reduced urinary potassium and chloride excretion). Products include:
Diucardin Tablets 2450
Saluron 718
Salutensin/Salutensin-Demi 719

Indapamide (Reduced urinary potassium and chloride excretion). Products include:
Lozol Tablets 1843

Lithium Carbonate (Increased steady-state plasma lithium levels). Products include:
Eskalith 2214
Lithane Tablets 1596
Lithium Carbonate Capsules & Tablets 1984
Lithobid Tablets 870

Lithium Citrate (Increased steady-state plasma lithium levels). Products include:
Cibalith-S 870

Methotrexate Sodium (Increased toxicity; avoid coadministration). Products include:
Methotrexate Tablets, Parenteral, LPF Parenteral 1217
Rheumatrex Methotrexate Dose Pack 1234

Methyclothiazide (Reduced urinary potassium and chloride excretion). Products include:
Enduron Tablets 517
Enduronyl 518

Metolazone (Reduced urinary potassium and chloride excretion). Products include:
Diulo 2129
Mykrox ½ mg Tablets 984
Zaroxolyn Tablets 989

Polythiazide (Reduced urinary potassium and chloride excretion). Products include:
Minizide Capsules 1779
Renese Tablets 1785
Renese-R Tablets 1786

Probenecid (Decreased protein-binding and increased plasma clearance of ketoprofen). Products include:
Benemid Tablets 1426
ColBENEMID Tablets 1436
Wycillin Injection and Probenecid Tablets 2539

Spironolactone (Reduced urinary potassium and chloride excretion). Products include:
Aldactazide 2150
Aldactone 2152

Triamterene (Reduced urinary potassium and chloride excretion). Products include:
Dyazide Capsules 2208
Dyrenium Capsules 2210
Maxzide 1215

Warfarin Sodium (Concurrent therapy requires close monitoring of patients on both drugs). Products include:
Coumadin Injection & Tablets 944
Panwarfin Tablets 547

Food Interactions

Food, unspecified (Slows rate of absorption resulting in delayed and reduced peak concentrations).

OS-CAL 500 CHEWABLE TABLETS
(Calcium Carbonate) ..... ▣ 596
No interactions described in labeling.

OS-CAL 250+D TABLETS
(Calcium (Oyster Shell), Vitamin D) ▣ 597
No interactions described in labeling.

OS-CAL FORTIFIED TABLETS
(Vitamins with Minerals, Calcium (Oyster Shell)) ..... ▣ 597
No interactions described in labeling.

OS-CAL PLUS TABLETS
(Vitamins with Minerals) ..... ▣ 597
No interactions described in labeling.

OSCILLOCOCCINUM
(Homeopathic Medications) ..... ▣ 520
No interactions described in labeling.

OSM_GLYN
(Glycerin) ..... ◉ 234
No interactions described in labeling.

OSMOLITE ISOTONIC LIQUID NUTRITION
(Nutritional Supplement) 1972
No interactions described in labeling.

OSMOLITE HN HIGH NITROGEN ISOTONIC LIQUID NUTRITION
(Nutritional Supplement) 1972
No interactions described in labeling.

OSTI-DERM LOTION
(Zinc Oxide, Magnesium Carbonate)..1771
No interactions described in labeling.

OTIC DOMEBORO SOLUTION
(Acetic Acid) 1609
No interactions described in labeling.

OTIC TRIDESILON SOLUTION 0.05%
(Desonide, Acetic Acid) 1612
No interactions described in labeling.

OTIX DROPS EAR WAX REMOVAL AID
(Carbamide Peroxide) ..... ▣ 548
No interactions described in labeling.

OTRIVIN NASAL SPRAY AND NASAL DROPS
(Xylometazoline Hydrochloride) 1036
No interactions described in labeling.

OTRIVIN PEDIATRIC NASAL DROPS
(Xylometazoline Hydrochloride) 1036
No interactions described in labeling.

OUTGRO SOLUTION
(Chlorobutanol, Tannic Acid) ..... ▣ 751
No interactions described in labeling.

OVCON 35
(Norethindrone, Ethinyl Estradiol) 1391
May interact with barbiturates and certain other agents. Compounds in these categories include:

Aprobarbital (Reduces efficacy; breakthrough bleeding). Products include:
Alurate Elixir 1883

Butabarbital (Reduces efficacy; breakthrough bleeding). Products include:
Pyridium Plus 1764

Butalbital (Reduces efficacy; breakthrough bleeding). Products include:
Esgic-Plus Tablets 1002
Esgic Tablets & Capsules 1001
Fioricet Tablets 2006
Fiorinal Capsules 2007
Fiorinal with Codeine Capsules 2008
Fiorinal Tablets 2007
Phrenilin 838
Sedapap Tablets 50 mg/650 mg .. 1360

Mephobarbital (Reduces efficacy; breakthrough bleeding). Products include:
Mebaral Tablets 2061

Oxytetracycline (Reduces efficacy; breakthrough bleeding). Products include:
Terramycin Intramuscular Solution 1964
Urobiotic-250 Capsules 1968

Oxytetracycline Hydrochloride (Reduces efficacy; breakthrough bleeding). Products include:
Terra-Cortril Ophthalmic Suspension 1963
Terramycin Capsules 1786
Terramycin Intramuscular Solution 1964
Terramycin with Polymyxin B Sulfate Ophthalmic Ointment 1965

Pentobarbital Sodium (Reduces efficacy; breakthrough bleeding). Products include:
Nembutal Sodium Capsules 534
Nembutal Sodium Solution 536
Nembutal Sodium Suppositories 538

Phenobarbital (Reduces efficacy; breakthrough bleeding). Products include:
Arco-Lase Plus Tablets 607
Bellergal-S Tablets 1998
Bronkolixir ..... ▣ 761
Bronkotabs Tablets ..... ▣ 762
Donnatal 1858
Donnatal Extentabs 1859
Donnatal Tablets 1858
Donnazyme Tablets 1860
Kinesed Tablets 2272
Phenobarbital Elixir and Tablets 1293
Primatene Tablets-P Formula 2421
Quadrinal Tablets 1183
Tedral SA 1765

Phenylbutazone (Reduces efficacy; breakthrough bleeding). Products include:
Butazolidin Capsules & Tablets 1027

Phenytoin (Reduces efficacy; breakthrough bleeding). Products include:
Dilantin Infatabs 1710
Dilantin-30 Pediatric/Dilantin-125 Suspension 1713

Phenytoin Sodium (Reduces efficacy; breakthrough bleeding). Products include:
Dilantin Kapseals 1708
Dilantin Parenteral 1712
Dilantin with Phenobarbital Kapseals 1715

Rifampin (Reduces efficacy; breakthrough bleeding). Products include:
Rifadin 1345
Rifamate Capsules 1347
Rimactane Capsules 879

Secobarbital Sodium (Reduces efficacy; breakthrough bleeding). Products include:
Seconal Sodium Pulvules 1296

Tetracycline Hydrochloride (Reduces efficacy; breakthrough bleeding). Products include:
Achromycin V Capsules 1193
Achromycin Ophthalmic Ointment 1% ..... ◉ 307
Achromycin Ophthalmic Suspension 1% ..... ◉ 308
Topicycline for Topical Solution 1856

Thiamylal Sodium (Reduces efficacy; breakthrough bleeding). Products include:
Surital Ampoules, Steri-Vials 1764

OVCON 50
(Norethindrone, Ethinyl Estradiol) 1391
See **Ovcon 35**

OVRAL TABLETS
(Norgestrel, Ethinyl Estradiol) 2490
See **Lo/Ovral Tablets**

OVRAL-28 TABLETS
(Norgestrel, Ethinyl Estradiol) 2491
See **Lo/Ovral Tablets**

OVRETTE TABLETS
(Norgestrel) 2492
See **Lo/Ovral Tablets**

OXIPOR VHC LOTION FOR PSORIASIS
(Benzocaine, Coal Tar, Salicylic Acid) ....▣ 751
No interactions described in labeling.

OXISTAT CREAM
(Oxiconazole Nitrate) 1055
No interactions described in labeling.

OXSORALEN LOTION 1%
(Methoxsalen) 1116
May interact with phenothiazines, sulfonamides, tetracyclines, thiazides, and certain other agents. Compounds in these categories include:

Anthralin (Possible photosensitivity effects). Products include:
- Anthra-Derm Ointment 1%, ½%, ¼%, 1/10% 907
- Drithocreme 590
- Dritho-Scalp 591

Bendroflumethiazide (Possible photosensitivity effects). Products include:
- Corzide Tablets 702
- Naturetin Tablets 1789
- Rauzide Tablets 1804

Chlorothiazide (Possible photosensitivity effects). Products include:
- Aldoclor Tablets 1413
- Diupres Tablets 1461
- Diuril Oral 1464

Chlorothiazide Sodium (Possible photosensitivity effects). Products include:
- Diuril Sodium Intravenous 1463

Chlorpromazine (Possible photosensitivity effects). Products include:
- Thorazine 2234

Coal Tar (Possible photosensitivity effects). Products include:
- DHS 1772
- Denorex Medicated Shampoo and Conditioner 2418
- Denorex Medicated Shampoo, Extra Strength 2418
- Denorex Medicated Shampoo, Extra Strength With Conditioners 2418
- Denorex Medicated Shampoo, Regular & Mountain Fresh Herbal Scent 2418
- Doctar Gel 2079
- Fototar Cream ....▣ 574
- Ionil T Plus Shampoo 1683
- Ionil T Shampoo 1683
- MG 217 ....▣ 734
- Oxipor VHC Lotion for Psoriasis ....▣ 751
- P & S Plus Tar Gel ....▣ 510
- Pentrax Tar Shampoo with Fractar 1045
- Sebutone and Sebutone Cream Antiseborrheic Tar Shampoos 2408
- Tegrin for Psoriasis Lotion, Cream & Soap ....▣ 518
- Tegrin Medicated Shampoo ....▣ 518
- Theraplex T Shampoo 1411
- X-Seb T Shampoo ....▣ 510
- X-Seb T Plus Conditioning Shampoo ....▣ 510
- Zetar Emulsion 911

Demeclocycline Hydrochloride (Possible photosensitivity effects). Products include:
- Declomycin Capsules, Tablets 1199

Doxycycline Calcium (Possible photosensitivity effects).
- No products indexed under this heading.

Doxycycline Hyclate (Possible photosensitivity effects). Products include:
- Doryx Capsules 1717
- Vibramycin Hyclate Capsules 1787
- Vibramycin Hyclate Intravenous 1968
- Vibra-Tabs Film Coated Tablets 1787

Doxycycline Monohydrate (Possible photosensitivity effects). Products include:
- Monodox Capsules 1630
- Vibramycin Monohydrate for Oral Suspension 1787

Fluphenazine Decanoate (Possible photosensitivity effects). Products include:
- Prolixin Decanoate 1795

Fluphenazine Enanthate (Possible photosensitivity effects). Products include:
- Prolixin Enanthate 1796

Fluphenazine Hydrochloride (Possible photosensitivity effects). Products include:
- Prolixin Elixir 1793
- Prolixin Injection 1791
- Prolixin Oral Concentrate 1792
- Prolixin Tablets 1793

Griseofulvin (Possible photosensitivity effects). Products include:
- Fulvicin P/G Tablets 2090
- Fulvicin P/G 165 & 330 Tablets 2091
- Fulvicin-U/F Tablets 2092
- Grifulvin V (griseofulvin microsize) Tablets/Suspension 1678
- Grisactin 2454
- Grisactin Ultra Tablets 2455
- Gris-PEG Tablets, 125 mg & 250 mg 1083

Hydrochlorothiazide (Possible photosensitivity effects). Products include:
- Aldactazide 2150
- Aldoril Tablets 1418
- Apresazide Capsules 854
- Apresoline-Esidrix Tablets 857
- Capozide 2258
- Dyazide Capsules 2208
- Esidrix Tablets 863
- Esimil Tablets 864
- HydroDIURIL Tablets 1484
- Hydropres Tablets 1485
- Inderide Tablets 2463
- Inderide LA Long Acting Capsules .. 2465
- Lopressor HCT Tablets 1034
- Maxzide 1215
- Moduretic Tablets 1510
- Normozide Tablets 2112
- Oretic Tablets 544
- Oreticyl 545
- Prinzide Tablets 1540
- Ser-Ap-Es Tablets 881
- Serpasil-Esidrix Tablets 886
- Timolide Tablets 1547
- Trandate HCT Tablets 579
- Vaseretic Tablets 1559
- Zestoretic 2274

Hydroflumethiazide (Possible photosensitivity effects). Products include:
- Diucardin Tablets 2450
- Saluron 718
- Salutensin/Salutensin-Demi 719

Mesoridazine (Possible photosensitivity effects). Products include:
- Serentil 686

Methacycline Hydrochloride (Possible photosensitivity effects).
- No products indexed under this heading.

Methyclothiazide (Possible photosensitivity effects). Products include:
- Enduron Tablets 517
- Enduronyl 518

Methylene Blue (Possible photosensitivity effects). Products include:
- Urised Tablets 2396

Minocycline Hydrochloride (Possible photosensitivity effects). Products include:
- Minocin Intravenous 1221
- Minocin Oral Suspension 1224
- Minocin Pellet-Filled Capsules 1222

Nalidixic Acid (Possible photosensitivity effects). Products include:
- NegGram 2062

Oxytetracycline (Possible photosensitivity effects). Products include:
- Terramycin Intramuscular Solution 1964
- Urobiotic-250 Capsules 1968

Oxytetracycline Hydrochloride (Possible photosensitivity effects). Products include:
- Terra-Cortril Ophthalmic Suspension 1963
- Terramycin Capsules 1786
- Terramycin Intramuscular Solution 1964
- Terramycin with Polymyxin B Sulfate Ophthalmic Ointment 1965

Perphenazine (Possible photosensitivity effects). Products include:
- Etrafon 2087
- Triavil Tablets 1556
- Trilafon 2123

Polythiazide (Possible photosensitivity effects). Products include:
- Minizide Capsules 1779
- Renese Tablets 1785
- Renese-R Tablets 1786

Prochlorperazine (Possible photosensitivity effects). Products include:
- Compazine 2201

Promethazine Hydrochloride (Possible photosensitivity effects). Products include:
- Mepergan Injection 2479
- Phenergan with Codeine 2497
- Phenergan with Dextromethorphan 2499
- Phenergan Injection 2493
- Phenergan Suppositories 2496
- Phenergan Syrup 2495
- Phenergan Tablets 2496
- Phenergan VC 2500
- Phenergan VC with Codeine 2501

Sulfamethizole (Possible photosensitivity effects). Products include:
- Thiosulfil Forte Tablets 2526
- Urobiotic-250 Capsules 1968

Sulfamethoxazole (Possible photosensitivity effects). Products include:
- Azo Gantanol Tablets 1887
- Bactrim DS Tablets 1891
- Bactrim I.V. Infusion 1889
- Bactrim 1891
- Gantanol 1899
- Septra 813
- Septra I.V. Infusion 808
- Septra I.V. Infusion ADD-Vantage Vials 810
- Septra 813

Sulfasalazine (Possible photosensitivity effects). Products include:
- Azulfidine Tablets, EN-tabs, Oral Suspension 1157

Sulfinpyrazone (Possible photosensitivity effects). Products include:
- Anturane 853

Sulfisoxazole (Possible photosensitivity effects). Products include:
- Azo Gantrisin Tablets 1888
- Gantrisin Tablets 1901
- Pediazole 1973

Sulfisoxazole Diolamine (Possible photosensitivity effects). Products include:
- Gantrisin Ophthalmic Ointment/ Solution 1900

Tetracycline Hydrochloride (Possible photosensitivity effects). Products include:
- Achromycin V Capsules 1193
- Achromycin Ophthalmic Ointment 1% ....⊙ 307
- Achromycin Ophthalmic Suspension 1% ....⊙ 308
- Topicycline for Topical Solution 1856

Thioridazine Hydrochloride (Possible photosensitivity effects). Products include:
- Mellaril 2011

Trifluoperazine Hydrochloride (Possible photosensitivity effects). Products include:
- Stelazine 2226

OXSORALEN-ULTRA CAPSULE
(Methoxsalen) 1117
May interact with phenothiazines, sulfonamides, tetracyclines, thiazides, and certain other agents. Compounds in these categories include:

Anthralin (Possible photosensitivity effects). Products include:
- Anthra-Derm Ointment 1%, ½%, ¼%, 1/10% 907
- Drithocreme 590
- Dritho-Scalp 591

Bendroflumethiazide (Possible photosensitivity effects). Products include:
- Corzide Tablets 702
- Naturetin Tablets 1789
- Rauzide Tablets 1804

Chlorothiazide (Possible photosensitivity effects). Products include:
- Aldoclor Tablets 1413
- Diupres Tablets 1461
- Diuril Oral 1464

Chlorothiazide Sodium (Possible photosensitivity effects). Products include:
- Diuril Sodium Intravenous 1463

Chlorpromazine (Possible photosensitivity effects). Products include:
- Thorazine 2234

Coal Tar (Possible photosensitivity effects). Products include:
- DHS 1772
- Denorex Medicated Shampoo and Conditioner 2418
- Denorex Medicated Shampoo, Extra Strength 2418
- Denorex Medicated Shampoo, Extra Strength With Conditioners 2418
- Denorex Medicated Shampoo, Regular & Mountain Fresh Herbal Scent 2418
- Doctar Gel 2079
- Fototar Cream ....▣ 574
- Ionil T Plus Shampoo 1683
- Ionil T Shampoo 1683
- MG 217 ....▣ 734
- Oxipor VHC Lotion for Psoriasis ....▣ 751
- P & S Plus Tar Gel ....▣ 510
- Pentrax Tar Shampoo with Fractar 1045
- Sebutone and Sebutone Cream Antiseborrheic Tar Shampoos 2408
- Tegrin for Psoriasis Lotion, Cream & Soap ....▣ 518
- Tegrin Medicated Shampoo ....▣ 518
- Theraplex T Shampoo 1411
- X-Seb T Shampoo ....▣ 510
- X-Seb T Plus Conditioning Shampoo ....▣ 510
- Zetar Emulsion 911

Demeclocycline Hydrochloride (Possible photosensitivity effects). Products include:
- Declomycin Capsules, Tablets 1199

Doxycycline Calcium (Possible photosensitivity effects).
- No products indexed under this heading.

Doxycycline Hyclate (Possible photosensitivity effects). Products include:
- Doryx Capsules 1717
- Vibramycin Hyclate Capsules 1787
- Vibramycin Hyclate Intravenous 1968
- Vibra-Tabs Film Coated Tablets 1787

Doxycycline Monohydrate (Possible photosensitivity effects). Products include:
- Monodox Capsules 1630
- Vibramycin Monohydrate for Oral Suspension 1787

Fluphenazine Decanoate (Possible photosensitivity effects). Products include:
- Prolixin Decanoate 1795

Fluphenazine Enanthate (Possible photosensitivity effects). Products include:
- Prolixin Enanthate 1796

Fluphenazine Hydrochloride (Possible photosensitivity effects). Products include:
- Prolixin Elixir 1793
- Prolixin Injection 1791

Prolixin Oral Concentrate 1792
Prolixin Tablets 1793

Griseofulvin (Possible photosensitivity effects). Products include:
Fulvicin P/G Tablets 2090
Fulvicin P/G 165 & 330 Tablets 2091
Fulvicin-U/F Tablets 2092
Grifulvin V (griseofulvin microsize) Tablets/Suspension 1678
Grisactin 2454
Grisactin Ultra Tablets 2455
Gris-PEG Tablets, 125 mg & 250 mg 1083

Hydrochlorothiazide (Possible photosensitivity effects). Products include:
Aldactazide 2150
Aldoril Tablets 1418
Apresazide Capsules 854
Apresoline-Esidrix Tablets 857
Capozide 2258
Dyazide Capsules 2208
Esidrix Tablets 863
Esimil Tablets 864
HydroDIURIL Tablets 1484
Hydropres Tablets 1485
Inderide Tablets 2463
Inderide LA Long Acting Capsules .. 2465
Lopressor HCT Tablets 1034
Maxzide 1215
Moduretic Tablets 1510
Normozide Tablets 2112
Oretic Tablets 544
Oreticyl 545
Prinzide Tablets 1540
Ser-Ap-Es Tablets 881
Serpasil-Esidrix Tablets 886
Timolide Tablets 1547
Trandate HCT Tablets 579
Vaseretic Tablets 1559
Zestoretic 2274

Hydroflumethiazide (Possible photosensitivity effects). Products include:
Diucardin Tablets 2450
Saluron 718
Salutensin/Salutensin-Demi 719

Mesoridazine (Possible photosensitivity effects). Products include:
Serentil 686

Methacycline Hydrochloride (Possible photosensitivity effects).
No products indexed under this heading.

Methyclothiazide (Possible photosensitivity effects). Products include:
Enduron Tablets 517
Enduronyl 518

Methylene Blue (Possible photosensitivity effects). Products include:
Urised Tablets 2396

Minocycline Hydrochloride (Possible photosensitivity effects). Products include:
Minocin Intravenous 1221
Minocin Oral Suspension 1224
Minocin Pellet-Filled Capsules 1222

Nalidixic Acid (Possible photosensitivity effects). Products include:
NegGram 2062

Oxytetracycline (Possible photosensitivity effects). Products include:
Terramycin Intramuscular Solution 1964
Urobiotic-250 Capsules 1968

Oxytetracycline Hydrochloride (Possible photosensitivity effects). Products include:
Terra-Cortril Ophthalmic Suspension 1963
Terramycin Capsules 1786
Terramycin Intramuscular Solution 1964
Terramycin with Polymyxin B Sulfate Ophthalmic Ointment 1965

Perphenazine (Possible photosensitivity effects). Products include:
Etrafon 2087
Triavil Tablets 1556
Trilafon 2123

Polythiazide (Possible photosensitivity effects). Products include:
Minizide Capsules 1779

Renese Tablets 1785
Renese-R Tablets 1786

Prochlorperazine (Possible photosensitivity effects). Products include:
Compazine 2201

Promethazine Hydrochloride (Possible photosensitivity effects). Products include:
Mepergan Injection 2479
Phenergan with Codeine 2497
Phenergan with Dextromethorphan 2499
Phenergan Injection 2493
Phenergan Suppositories 2496
Phenergan Syrup 2495
Phenergan Tablets 2496
Phenergan VC 2500
Phenergan VC with Codeine 2501

Sulfamethizole (Possible photosensitivity effects). Products include:
Thiosulfil Forte Tablets 2526
Urobiotic-250 Capsules 1968

Sulfamethoxazole (Possible photosensitivity effects). Products include:
Azo Gantanol Tablets 1887
Bactrim DS Tablets 1891
Bactrim I.V. Infusion 1889
Bactrim 1891
Gantanol 1899
Septra 813
Septra I.V. Infusion 808
Septra I.V. Infusion ADD-Vantage Vials 810
Septra 813

Sulfasalazine (Possible photosensitivity effects). Products include:
Azulfidine Tablets, EN-tabs, Oral Suspension 1157

Sulfinpyrazone (Possible photosensitivity effects). Products include:
Anturane 853

Sulfisoxazole (Possible photosensitivity effects). Products include:
Azo Gantrisin Tablets 1888
Gantrisin Tablets 1901
Pediazole 1973

Sulfisoxazole Diolamine (Possible photosensitivity effects). Products include:
Gantrisin Ophthalmic Ointment/Solution 1900

Tetracycline Hydrochloride (Possible photosensitivity effects). Products include:
Achromycin V Capsules 1193
Achromycin Ophthalmic Ointment 1% .... ◉ 307
Achromycin Ophthalmic Suspension 1% .... ◉ 308
Topicycline for Topical Solution 1856

Thioridazine Hydrochloride (Possible photosensitivity effects). Products include:
Mellaril 2011

Trifluoperazine Hydrochloride (Possible photosensitivity effects). Products include:
Stelazine 2226

OXY CLEAN LATHERING FACIAL SCRUB
(Cleanser) .... ▣ 720
No interactions described in labeling.

OXY CLEAN MEDICATED CLEANSER
(Alcohol, Salicylic Acid) .... ▣ 720
May interact with:

Topical Medications (Concurrent use of other topical acne medications may increase dryness or irritation).

OXY CLEAN MEDICATED PADS - REGULAR, SENSITIVE SKIN, AND MAXIMUM STRENGTH
(Alcohol, Salicylic Acid) .... ▣ 720
May interact with:

Topical Medications (Concurrent use of other topical acne medications may increase dryness or irritation).

OXY CLEAN MEDICATED SOAP
(Salicylic Acid) .... ▣ 720
See Oxy Clean Medicated Cleanser

OXY NIGHT WATCH NIGHTTIME ACNE MEDICATION-MAXIMUM STRENGTH AND SENSITIVE SKIN FORMULAS
(Salicylic Acid) .... ▣ 721
No interactions described in labeling.

OXY 10 DAILY FACE WASH ANTIBACTERIAL SKIN WASH
(Benzoyl Peroxide) .... ▣ 721
May interact with:

Topical Medications (Concurrent administration with other topical acne products may result in increased dryness or irritation).

OXY-5 AND OXY-10 TINTED AND VANISHING FORMULAS WITH SORBOXYL
(Benzoyl Peroxide) .... ▣ 719
May interact with:

Topical Medications (Concurrent use of other topical acne medications may increase dryness or irritation).

OXYTOCIN INJECTION
(Oxytocin (Injection)) 2492
May interact with vasopressors and certain other agents. Compounds in these categories include:

Cyclopropane (Hypotension; maternal sinus bradycardia with abnormal atrioventricular rhythms).

Dopamine Hydrochloride (Severe hypertension). Products include:
Intropin Injection 930

Epinephrine Hydrochloride (Severe hypertension). Products include:
Adrenalin Chloride Solution 1:100 & 1:1,000 1689
Epifrin .... ◉ 244
Glaucon .... ◉ 218

Metaraminol Bitartrate (Severe hypertension). Products include:
Aramine Injection 1424

Methoxamine Hydrochloride (Severe hypertension). Products include:
Vasoxyl Injection 819

Norepinephrine Bitartrate (Severe hypertension). Products include:
Levophed Bitartrate Injection 2054

P-A-C ANALGESIC TABLETS
(Aspirin, Caffeine Anhydrous) .... ▣ 669
May interact with oral anticoagulants, antigout agents, and certain other agents. Compounds in these categories include:

Allopurinol (Effect not specified). Products include:
Zyloprim Tablets 830

Antiarthritic Drugs, unspecified (Effect not specified).

Antidiabetic Drugs, unspecified (Effect not specified).

Dicumarol (Effect not specified). Products include:
Dicumarol Tablets 516

Probenecid (Effect not specified). Products include:
Benemid Tablets 1426
ColBENEMID Tablets 1436
Wycillin Injection and Probenecid Tablets 2539

Sulfinpyrazone (Effect not specified). Products include:
Anturane 853

Warfarin Sodium (Effect not specified). Products include:
Coumadin Injection & Tablets 944
Panwarfin Tablets 547

PBZ TABLETS & ELIXIR
(Tripelennamine Hydrochloride) 1037
May interact with central nervous system depressants and certain other agents. Compounds in these categories include:

Alcohol (CNS effects may be additive).

Alfentanil Hydrochloride (CNS effects may be additive). Products include:
Alfenta Injection 1131

Alprazolam (CNS effects may be additive). Products include:
Xanax Tablets 2367

Aprobarbital (CNS effects may be additive). Products include:
Alurate Elixir 1883

Buprenorphine (CNS effects may be additive).
No products indexed under this heading.

Buspirone Hydrochloride (CNS effects may be additive). Products include:
BuSpar 1401

Butabarbital (CNS effects may be additive). Products include:
Pyridium Plus 1764

Butalbital (CNS effects may be additive). Products include:
Esgic-Plus Tablets 1002
Esgic Tablets & Capsules 1001
Fioricet Tablets 2006
Fiorinal Capsules 2007
Fiorinal with Codeine Capsules 2008
Fiorinal Tablets 2007
Phrenilin 838
Sedapap Tablets 50 mg/650 mg .. 1360

Chlordiazepoxide (CNS effects may be additive). Products include:
Libritabs Tablets 1930
Limbitrol 1933
Menrium Tablets 1934

Chlordiazepoxide Hydrochloride (CNS effects may be additive). Products include:
Librax Capsules 1929
Librium Capsules 1931
Librium Injectable 1932

Chlorpromazine (CNS effects may be additive). Products include:
Thorazine 2234

Chlorprothixene (CNS effects may be additive). Products include:
Taractan Tablets 1920

Chlorprothixene Hydrochloride (CNS effects may be additive). Products include:
Taractan 1920

Chlorprothixene Lactate (CNS effects may be additive). Products include:
- Taractan Concentrate 1920

Clorazepate Dipotassium (CNS effects may be additive). Products include:
- Tranxene 556

Codeine (CNS effects may be additive). Products include:
- Calcidrine Syrup 506

Codeine Phosphate (CNS effects may be additive). Products include:
- Actifed with Codeine Cough Syrup.. 752
- Cheracol Cough Syrup 1853
- Codimal PH Syrup 846
- Dimetane-DC Cough Syrup 1857
- Empirin with Codeine Phosphate Nos. 2, 3 & 4 764
- Fiorinal with Codeine Capsules 2008
- Isoclor Expectorant 982
- Naldecon CX Adult Liquid .... ◙ 521
- Novahistine DH 1342
- Novahistine Expectorant 1343
- Nucofed Capsules 2219
- Nucofed Expectorant 2219
- Nucofed Pediatric Expectorant 2220
- Nucofed Syrup 2219
- Phenaphen with Codeine Capsules 1865
- Phenaphen-650 with Codeine Tablets 1866
- Phenergan with Codeine 2497
- Phenergan VC with Codeine 2501
- Robitussin A-C Syrup 1875
- Robitussin-DAC Syrup 1875
- [illegible]yna .... ◙ 741
- [illegible]ma Compound w/Codeine Tab[illegible]ts 2390
- [illegible]minic Expectorant w/Codeine .. 1996
- [illegible]Organidin Liquid 2391
- [illegible]with Codeine 1381

Code[illegible]olistirex (CNS effects may be additive).
- No products indexed under this heading.

Dezocine (CNS effects may be additive).

Diazepam (CNS effects may be additive). Products include:
- Valium Injectable 1937
- Valium Tablets 1939
- Valrelease Capsules 1923

Droperidol (CNS effects may be additive). Products include:
- Inapsine Injection 1140
- Innovar Injection 1141

Enflurane (CNS effects may be additive). Products include:
- Ethrane 599

Estazolam (CNS effects may be additive). Products include:
- ProSom Tablets 554

Ethchlorvynol (CNS effects may be additive). Products include:
- Placidyl Capsules 553

Ethinamate (CNS effects may be additive).
- No products indexed under this heading.

Fentanyl (CNS effects may be additive). Products include:
- Duragesic Transdermal System 1133

Fentanyl Citrate (CNS effects may be additive). Products include:
- Innovar Injection 1141
- Sublimaze Injection 1146

Fluphenazine Decanoate (CNS effects may be additive). Products include:
- Prolixin Decanoate 1795

Fluphenazine Enanthate (CNS effects may be additive). Products include:
- Prolixin Enanthate 1796

Fluphenazine Hydrochloride (CNS effects may be additive). Products include:
- Prolixin Elixir 1793
- Prolixin Injection 1791
- Prolixin Oral Concentrate 1792
- Prolixin Tablets 1793

Flurazepam Hydrochloride (CNS effects may be additive). Products include:
- Dalmane Capsules 1927

Glutethimide (CNS effects may be additive).
- No products indexed under this heading.

Haloperidol (CNS effects may be additive). Products include:
- Haldol Injection, Tablets and Concentrate 1373

Haloperidol Decanoate (CNS effects may be additive). Products include:
- Haldol Decanoate 1375

Hydrocodone Bitartrate (CNS effects may be additive). Products include:
- Anexsia 5/500 Tablets 2196
- Anexsia 7.5/650 Tablets 2197
- Azdone Tablets 844
- Codiclear DH Syrup 845
- Codimal DH Syrup 846
- Damason-P 1356
- Hycodan Syrup, Tablets 927
- Hycomine Compound Tablets 929
- Hycomine Syrup 927
- Hycotuss Expectorant Syrup 930
- Hydrocet Capsules 835
- Lortab ASA Tablets 2414
- Lortab 2412
- Ru-Tuss with Hydrocodone 694
- Triaminic Expectorant DH 1995
- Vicodin Tablets 1187
- Vicodin ES Tablets 1189
- Zydone Capsules 941

Hydrocodone Polistirex (CNS effects may be additive). Products include:
- Tussionex Extended-Release Suspension 988

Hydroxyzine Hydrochloride (CNS effects may be additive). Products include:
- Atarax Tablets & Syrup 1941
- Marax Tablets & DF Syrup 1954
- Vistaril Intramuscular Solution 1970

Isoflurane (CNS effects may be additive). Products include:
- Forane 600

Ketamine Hydrochloride (CNS effects may be additive). Products include:
- Ketalar 1726

Levorphanol Tartrate (CNS effects may be additive). Products include:
- Levo-Dromoran 1906

Lorazepam (CNS effects may be additive). Products include:
- Ativan Injection 2432
- Ativan Tablets 2434

Loxapine Hydrochloride (CNS effects may be additive). Products include:
- Loxitane 1213

Loxapine Succinate (CNS effects may be additive). Products include:
- Loxitane Capsules 1213

Meperidine Hydrochloride (CNS effects may be additive). Products include:
- Demerol 2047
- Mepergan Injection 2479

Mephobarbital (CNS effects may be additive). Products include:
- Mebaral Tablets 2061

Meprobamate (CNS effects may be additive). Products include:
- Deprol Tablets 2382
- Equagesic Tablets 2451
- Miltown Tablets 2386
- PMB 200 and PMB 400 2504

Mesoridazine (CNS effects may be additive). Products include:
- Serentil 686

Methadone Hydrochloride (CNS effects may be additive). Products include:
- Dolophine Hydrochloride Ampoules & Vials 1260
- Dolophine Hydrochloride Tablets 1261
- Methadone Hydrochloride Diskets .. 1284
- Methadone Hydrochloride Oral Solution & Tablets 1987

Methohexital Sodium (CNS effects may be additive). Products include:
- Brevital Sodium Vials 1248

Methoxyflurane (CNS effects may be additive).
- No products indexed under this heading.

Midazolam Hydrochloride (CNS effects may be additive). Products include:
- Versed Injection 1924

Molindone Hydrochloride (CNS effects may be additive). Products include:
- Moban Tablets & Concentrate 932

Morphine Sulfate (CNS effects may be additive). Products include:
- Astramorph/PF Injection, USP (Preservative-Free) 618
- Duramorph 960
- Infumorph 200 and Infumorph 500 Sterile Solutions 962
- MS Contin Tablets 1814
- MSIR 1817
- Oramorph SR (Morphine Sulfate Sustained Release Tablets) 1988
- Roxanol 1991

Opium Alkaloids (CNS effects may be additive). Products include:
- B & O No. 15A & No. 16A Supprettes 2395
- Pantopon Injectable 1911

Oxazepam (CNS effects may be additive). Products include:
- Serax Capsules 2522
- Serax Tablets 2522

Oxycodone Hydrochloride (CNS effects may be additive). Products include:
- Percocet Tablets 950
- Percodan 951
- Roxicodone Tablets, Oral Solution & Intensol (Oxycodone) 1992
- Tylox Capsules 1382

Pentobarbital Sodium (CNS effects may be additive). Products include:
- Nembutal Sodium Capsules 534
- Nembutal Sodium Solution 536
- Nembutal Sodium Suppositories 538

Perphenazine (CNS effects may be additive). Products include:
- Etrafon 2087
- Triavil Tablets 1556
- Trilafon 2123

Phenobarbital (CNS effects may be additive). Products include:
- Arco-Lase Plus Tablets 607
- Bellergal-S Tablets 1998
- Bronkolixir .... ◙ 761
- Bronkotabs Tablets .... ◙ 762
- Donnatal 1858
- Donnatal Extentabs 1859
- Donnatal Tablets 1858
- Donnazyme Tablets 1860
- Kinesed Tablets 2272
- Phenobarbital Elixir and Tablets 1293
- Primatene Tablets-P Formula 2421
- Quadrinal Tablets 1183
- Tedral SA 1765

Prazepam (CNS effects may be additive). Products include:
- Centrax 1693

Prochlorperazine (CNS effects may be additive). Products include:
- Compazine 2201

Promethazine Hydrochloride (CNS effects may be additive). Products include:
- Mepergan Injection 2479
- Phenergan with Codeine 2497
- Phenergan with Dextromethorphan 2499
- Phenergan Injection 2493
- Phenergan Suppositories 2496
- Phenergan Syrup 2495
- Phenergan Tablets 2496
- Phenergan VC 2500
- Phenergan VC with Codeine 2501

Propofol (CNS effects may be additive). Products include:
- Diprivan Injection 2267

Propoxyphene Hydrochloride (CNS effects may be additive). Products include:
- Darvon 1256
- Wygesic Tablets 2540

Propoxyphene Napsylate (CNS effects may be additive). Products include:
- Darvon-N/Darvocet-N 1254

Quazepam (CNS effects may be additive). Products include:
- Doral Tablets 2383

Secobarbital Sodium (CNS effects may be additive). Products include:
- Seconal Sodium Pulvules 1296

Sufentanil Citrate (CNS effects may be additive). Products include:
- Sufenta Injection 1147

Temazepam (CNS effects may be additive). Products include:
- Restoril Capsules 2023

Thiamylal Sodium (CNS effects may be additive). Products include:
- Surital Ampoules, Steri-Vials 1764

Thioridazine Hydrochloride (CNS effects may be additive). Products include:
- Mellaril 2011

Thiothixene (CNS effects may be additive). Products include:
- Navane Capsules and Concentrate 1954
- Navane Intramuscular 1956

Triazolam (CNS effects may be additive). Products include:
- Halcion Tablets 2340

Trifluoperazine Hydrochloride (CNS effects may be additive). Products include:
- Stelazine 2226

PBZ-SR TABLETS
(Tripelennamine Hydrochloride) 1037
May interact with central nervous system depressants, monoamine oxidase inhibitors, and certain other agents. Compounds in these categories include:

Alcohol (CNS effects may be additive).

Alfentanil Hydrochloride (CNS effects may be additive). Products include:
- Alfenta Injection 1131

Alprazolam (CNS effects may be additive). Products include:
- Xanax Tablets 2367

Aprobarbital (CNS effects may be additive). Products include:
- Alurate Elixir 1883

Buprenorphine (CNS effects may be additive).
- No products indexed under this heading.

Buspirone Hydrochloride (CNS effects may be additive). Products include:
- BuSpar 1401

Butabarbital (CNS effects may be additive). Products include:
- Pyridium Plus 1764

Butalbital (CNS effects may be additive). Products include:
- Esgic-Plus Tablets 1002
- Esgic Tablets & Capsules 1001
- Fioricet Tablets 2006
- Fiorinal Capsules 2007
- Fiorinal with Codeine Capsules 2008
- Fiorinal Tablets 2007

Phrenilin 838
Sedapap Tablets 50 mg/650 mg 1360

Chlordiazepoxide (CNS effects may be additive). Products include:
Libritabs Tablets 1930
Limbitrol 1933
Menrium Tablets 1934

Chlordiazepoxide Hydrochloride (CNS effects may be additive). Products include:
Librax Capsules 1929
Librium Capsules 1931
Librium Injectable 1932

Chlorpromazine (CNS effects may be additive). Products include:
Thorazine 2234

Chlorprothixene (CNS effects may be additive). Products include:
Taractan Tablets 1920

Chlorprothixene Hydrochloride (CNS effects may be additive). Products include:
Taractan 1920

Chlorprothixene Lactate (CNS effects may be additive). Products include:
Taractan Concentrate 1920

Clorazepate Dipotassium (CNS effects may be additive). Products include:
Tranxene 556

Codeine (CNS effects may be additive). Products include:
Calcidrine Syrup 506

Codeine Phosphate (CNS effects may be additive). Products include:
Actifed with Codeine Cough Syrup 752
Cheracol Cough Syrup 1853
Codimal PH Syrup 846
Dimetane-DC Cough Syrup 1857
Empirin with Codeine Phosphate Nos. 2, 3 & 4 764
Fiorinal with Codeine Capsules 2008
Isoclor Expectorant 982
Naldecon CX Adult Liquid ▣ 521
Novahistine DH 1342
Novahistine Expectorant 1343
Nucofed Capsules 2219
Nucofed Expectorant 2219
Nucofed Pediatric Expectorant 2220
Nucofed Syrup 2219
Phenaphen with Codeine Capsules 1865
Phenaphen-650 with Codeine Tablets 1866
Phenergan with Codeine 2497
Phenergan VC with Codeine 2501
Robitussin A-C Syrup 1875
Robitussin-DAC Syrup 1875
Ryna ▣ 741
Soma Compound w/Codeine Tablets 2390
Triaminic Expectorant w/Codeine 1996
Tussi-Organidin Liquid 2391
Tylenol with Codeine 1381

Codeine Polistirex (CNS effects may be additive).
No products indexed under this heading.

Dezocine (CNS effects may be additive).

Diazepam (CNS effects may be additive). Products include:
Valium Injectable 1937
Valium Tablets 1939
Valrelease Capsules 1923

Droperidol (CNS effects may be additive). Products include:
Inapsine Injection 1140
Innovar Injection 1141

Enflurane (CNS effects may be additive). Products include:
Ethrane 599

Estazolam (CNS effects may be additive). Products include:
ProSom Tablets 554

Ethchlorvynol (CNS effects may be additive). Products include:
Placidyl Capsules 553

Ethinamate (CNS effects may be additive).
No products indexed under this heading.

Fentanyl (CNS effects may be additive). Products include:
Duragesic Transdermal System 1133

Fentanyl Citrate (CNS effects may be additive). Products include:
Innovar Injection 1141
Sublimaze Injection 1146

Fluphenazine Decanoate (CNS effects may be additive). Products include:
Prolixin Decanoate 1795

Fluphenazine Enanthate (CNS effects may be additive). Products include:
Prolixin Enanthate 1796

Fluphenazine Hydrochloride (CNS effects may be additive). Products include:
Prolixin Elixir 1793
Prolixin Injection 1791
Prolixin Oral Concentrate 1792
Prolixin Tablets 1793

Flurazepam Hydrochloride (CNS effects may be additive). Products include:
Dalmane Capsules 1927

Furazolidone (Concurrent use contraindicated). Products include:
Furoxone 1855

Glutethimide (CNS effects may be additive).
No products indexed under this heading.

Haloperidol (CNS effects may be additive). Products include:
Haldol Injection, Tablets and Concentrate 1373

Haloperidol Decanoate (CNS effects may be additive). Products include:
Haldol Decanoate 1375

Hydrocodone Bitartrate (CNS effects may be additive). Products include:
Anexsia 5/500 Tablets 2196
Anexsia 7.5/650 Tablets 2197
Azdōne Tablets 844
Codiclear DH Syrup 845
Codimal DH Syrup 846
Damason-P 1356
Hycodan Syrup, Tablets 927
Hycomine Compound Tablets 929
Hycomine Syrup 927
Hycotuss Expectorant Syrup 930
Hydrocet Capsules 835
Lortab ASA Tablets 2414
Lortab 2412
Ru-Tuss with Hydrocodone 694
Triaminic Expectorant DH 1995
Vicodin Tablets 1187
Vicodin ES Tablets 1189
Zydone Capsules 941

Hydrocodone Polistirex (CNS effects may be additive). Products include:
Tussionex Extended-Release Suspension 988

Hydroxyzine Hydrochloride (CNS effects may be additive). Products include:
Atarax Tablets & Syrup 1941
Marax Tablets & DF Syrup 1954
Vistaril Intramuscular Solution 1970

Isocarboxazid (Concurrent use contraindicated). Products include:
Marplan Tablets 1906

Isoflurane (CNS effects may be additive). Products include:
Forane 600

Ketamine Hydrochloride (CNS effects may be additive). Products include:
Ketalar 1726

Levorphanol Tartrate (CNS effects may be additive). Products include:
Levo-Dromoran 1906

Lorazepam (CNS effects may be additive). Products include:
Ativan Injection 2432
Ativan Tablets 2434

Loxapine Hydrochloride (CNS effects may be additive). Products include:
Loxitane 1213

Loxapine Succinate (CNS effects may be additive). Products include:
Loxitane Capsules 1213

Meperidine Hydrochloride (CNS effects may be additive). Products include:
Demerol 2047
Mepergan Injection 2479

Mephobarbital (CNS effects may be additive). Products include:
Mebaral Tablets 2061

Meprobamate (CNS effects may be additive). Products include:
Deprol Tablets 2382
Equagesic Tablets 2451
Miltown Tablets 2386
PMB 200 and PMB 400 2504

Mesoridazine (CNS effects may be additive). Products include:
Serentil 686

Methadone Hydrochloride (CNS effects may be additive). Products include:
Dolophine Hydrochloride Ampoules & Vials 1260
Dolophine Hydrochloride Tablets 1261
Methadone Hydrochloride Diskets 1284
Methadone Hydrochloride Oral Solution & Tablets 1987

Methohexital Sodium (CNS effects may be additive). Products include:
Brevital Sodium Vials 1248

Methoxyflurane (CNS effects may be additive).
No products indexed under this heading.

Midazolam Hydrochloride (CNS effects may be additive). Products include:
Versed Injection 1924

Molindone Hydrochloride (CNS effects may be additive). Products include:
Moban Tablets & Concentrate 932

Morphine Sulfate (CNS effects may be additive). Products include:
Astramorph/PF Injection, USP (Preservative-Free) 618
Duramorph 960
Infumorph 200 and Infumorph 500 Sterile Solutions 962
MS Contin Tablets 1814
MSIR 1817
Oramorph SR (Morphine Sulfate Sustained Release Tablets) 1988
Roxanol 1991

Opium Alkaloids (CNS effects may be additive). Products include:
B & O No. 15A & No. 16A Supprettes 2395
Pantopon Injectable 1911

Oxazepam (CNS effects may be additive). Products include:
Serax Capsules 2522
Serax Tablets 2522

Oxycodone Hydrochloride (CNS effects may be additive). Products include:
Percocet Tablets 950
Percodan 951
Roxicodone Tablets, Oral Solution & Intensol (Oxycodone) 1992
Tylox Capsules 1382

Pentobarbital Sodium (CNS effects may be additive). Products include:
Nembutal Sodium Capsules 534
Nembutal Sodium Solution 536
Nembutal Sodium Suppositories 538

Perphenazine (CNS effects may be additive). Products include:
Etrafon 2087
Triavil Tablets 1556
Trilafon 2123

Phenelzine Sulfate (Concurrent use contraindicated). Products include:
Nardil 1742

Phenobarbital (CNS effects may be additive). Products include:
Arco-Lase Plus Tablets 607
Bellergal-S Tablets 1998
Bronkolixir ▣ 761
Bronkotabs Tablets ▣ 762
Donnatal 1858
Donnatal Extentabs 1859
Donnatal Tablets 1858
Donnazyme Tablets 1860
Kinesed Tablets 2272
Phenobarbital Elixir and Tablets 1293
Primatene Tablets-P Formula 2421
Quadrinal Tablets 1183
Tedral SA 1765

Prazepam (CNS effects may be additive). Products include:
Centrax 1693

Prochlorperazine (CNS effects may be additive). Products include:
Compazine 2201

Promethazine Hydrochloride (CNS effects may be additive). Products include:
Mepergan Injection 2479
Phenergan with Codeine 2497
Phenergan with Dextromethorphan 2499
Phenergan Injection 2493
Phenergan Suppositories 2496
Phenergan Syrup 2495
Phenergan Tablets 2496
Phenergan VC 2500
Phenergan VC with Codeine 2501

Propofol (CNS effects may be additive). Products include:
Diprivan Injection 2267

Propoxyphene Hydrochloride (CNS effects may be additive). Products include:
Darvon 1256
Wygesic Tablets 2540

Propoxyphene Napsylate (CNS effects may be additive). Products include:
Darvon-N/Darvocet-N 1254

Quazepam (CNS effects may be additive). Products include:
Doral Tablets 2383

Secobarbital Sodium (CNS effects may be additive). Products include:
Seconal Sodium Pulvules 1296

Selegiline Hydrochloride (Concurrent use contraindicated). Products include:
Eldepryl 2250

Sufentanil Citrate (CNS effects may be additive). Products include:
Sufenta Injection 1147

Temazepam (CNS effects may be additive). Products include:
Restoril Capsules 2023

Thiamylal Sodium (CNS effects may be additive). Products include:
Surital Ampoules, Steri-Vials 1764

Thioridazine Hydrochloride (CNS effects may be additive). Products include:
Mellaril 2011

Thiothixene (CNS effects may be additive). Products include:
Navane Capsules and Concentrate 1954
Navane Intramuscular 1956

Tranylcypromine Sulfate (Concurrent use contraindicated). Products include:
Parnate Tablets 2222

Triazolam (CNS effects may be additive). Products include:
- Halcion Tablets ... 2340

Trifluoperazine Hydrochloride (CNS effects may be additive). Products include:
- Stelazine ... 2226

PCE DISPERTAB TABLETS
(Erythromycin) ... 549

May interact with oral anticoagulants, xanthine bronchodilators, and certain other agents. Compounds in these categories include:

Aminophylline (Concomitant administration with high doses of theophylline may be associated with increased theophylline levels and potential toxicity). Products include:
- Amesec ... ◘ 682
- Aminophyllin Tablets ... 2153

Carbamazepine (Elevations in serum erythromycin and carbamazepine concentration). Products include:
- Tegretol Chewable Tablets ... 654
- Tegretol Suspension ... 656
- Tegretol Tablets ... 654

Cyclosporine (Elevations in serum erythromycin and cyclosporine concentration). Products include:
- Sandimmune ... 2024

Dicumarol (Increased anticoagulant effects). Products include:
- Dicumarol Tablets ... 516

Digoxin (Elevated digoxin serum levels). Products include:
- Lanoxicaps ... 772
- Lanoxin Elixir Pediatric ... 775
- Lanoxin Injection ... 778
- Lanoxin Injection Pediatric ... 781
- Lanoxin Tablets ... 783

Dihydroergotamine Mesylate (Potential for acute ergot toxicity characterized by severe peripheral vasospasm and dysesthesia). Products include:
- D.H.E. 45 Injection ... 2003

Dyphylline (Concomitant administration with high doses of theophylline may be associated with increased theophylline levels and potential toxicity). Products include:
- Dilor ... 2079
- Dilor-G Tablets & Liquid ... 2079
- Lufyllin Elixir ... 2384
- Lufyllin & Lufyllin-400 Tablets ... 2384
- Lufyllin-GG Elixir & Tablets ... 2385

Ergotamine Tartrate (Potential for acute ergot toxicity characterized by severe peripheral vasospasm and dysesthesia). Products include:
- Bellergal-S Tablets ... 1998
- Cafergot/Cafergot P-B ... 1999
- Ergostat ... 1719
- Medihaler Ergotamine Aerosol ... 1312
- Wigraine Tablets & Suppositories ... 1645

Hexobarbital (Elevations in serum erythromycin and hexobarbital concentration).

Lovastatin (Potential for rhabdomyolysis in seriously ill patients). Products include:
- Mevacor Tablets ... 1505

Phenytoin (Elevations in serum erythromycin and phenytoin concentration). Products include:
- Dilantin Infatabs ... 1710
- Dilantin-30 Pediatric/Dilantin-125 Suspension ... 1713

Phenytoin Sodium (Elevations in serum erythromycin and phenytoin concentration). Products include:
- Dilantin Kapseals ... 1708
- Dilantin Parenteral ... 1712
- Dilantin with Phenobarbital Kapseals ... 1715

Terfenadine (Potential for altered terfenadine metabolism). Products include:
- Seldane Tablets ... 1349
- Seldane-D Extended-Release Tablets ... 1350

Theophylline (Concomitant administration with high doses of theophylline may be associated with increased theophylline levels and potential toxicity). Products include:
- Bronkaid Tablets ... ◘ 757
- Bronkolixir ... ◘ 761
- Bronkotabs Tablets ... ◘ 762
- Constant-T Tablets ... 1029
- Marax Tablets & DF Syrup ... 1954
- Primatene Tablets ... 2421
- Quibron Capsules ... 713
- Quibron-T ... 714
- Quibron-T/SR ... 716
- Theolair Liquid ... 1317
- Theo-Organidin Elixir ... 2391

Theophylline Anhydrous (Concomitant administration with high doses of theophylline may be associated with increased theophylline levels and potential toxicity). Products include:
- Aerolate ... 994
- Primatene Tablets-M Formula ... ◘ 753
- Primatene Tablets-Regular Formula ... 2421
- Respbid Tablets ... 684
- Slo-bid Gyrocaps ... 1847
- T-PHYL (Uniphyl) 200 mg Tablets 1820
- Tedral SA ... 1765
- Theo-24 ... 2179
- Theo-Dur Sprinkle ... 1168
- Theo-Dur Extended-Release Tablets ... 1166
- Theolair Tablets ... 1317
- Theolair-SR Tablets ... 1319
- TheoX Extended-Release Tablets ... 841
- Uniphyl 400 mg Tablets ... 1823

Theophylline Calcium Salicylate (Concomitant administration with high doses of theophylline may be associated with increased theophylline levels and potential toxicity). Products include:
- Quadrinal Tablets ... 1183

Theophylline Sodium Glycinate (Concomitant administration with high doses of theophylline may be associated with increased theophylline levels and potential toxicity). Products include:
- Asbron G ... 1997

Triazolam (Decreased clearance of triazolam and increased the pharmacologic effect of triazolam). Products include:
- Halcion Tablets ... 2340

Warfarin Sodium (Increased anticoagulant effects). Products include:
- Coumadin Injection & Tablets ... 944
- Panwarfin Tablets ... 547

Food Interactions

Meal, unspecified (Optimal blood levels are obtained when PCE is given in the fasting state).

PHISODERM CLEANSING BAR
(Sodium Tallowate) ... ◘ 760

No interactions described in labeling.

PHISODERM FOR BABY
(Cleanser) ... ◘ 761

No interactions described in labeling.

PHISODERM SKIN CLEANSER AND CONDITIONER - REGULAR AND OILY
(Cleanser) ... ◘ 760

No interactions described in labeling.

PHISOHEX
(Hexachlorophene) ... 2066

No interactions described in labeling.

PHISOPUFF
(Cleanser) ... ◘ 761

No interactions described in labeling.

PMB 200 AND PMB 400
(Estrogens, Conjugated, Meprobamate) ... 2504

May interact with central nervous system depressants, psychotropics, narcotic analgesics, progestins, and certain other agents. Compounds in these categories include:

Alcohol (Additive effects).

Alfentanil Hydrochloride (Additive effects). Products include:
- Alfenta Injection ... 1131

Alprazolam (Additive effects). Products include:
- Xanax Tablets ... 2367

Amitriptyline Hydrochloride (Additive effects). Products include:
- Elavil ... 2269
- Endep Tablets ... 1927
- Etrafon ... 2087
- Limbitrol ... 1933
- Triavil Tablets ... 1556

Amoxapine (Additive effects). Products include:
- Asendin Tablets ... 1196

Aprobarbital (Additive effects). Products include:
- Alurate Elixir ... 1883

Buprenorphine (Additive effects).
- No products indexed under this heading.

Buspirone Hydrochloride (Additive effects). Products include:
- BuSpar ... 1401

Butabarbital (Additive effects). Products include:
- Pyridium Plus ... 1764

Butalbital (Additive effects). Products include:
- Esgic-Plus Tablets ... 1002
- Esgic Tablets & Capsules ... 1001
- Fioricet Tablets ... 2006
- Fiorinal Capsules ... 2007
- Fiorinal with Codeine Capsules ... 2008
- Fiorinal Tablets ... 2007
- Phrenilin ... 838
- Sedapap Tablets 50 mg/650 mg ... 1360

Chlordiazepoxide (Additive effects). Products include:
- Libritabs Tablets ... 1930
- Limbitrol ... 1933
- Menrium Tablets ... 1934

Chlordiazepoxide Hydrochloride (Additive effects). Products include:
- Librax Capsules ... 1929
- Librium Capsules ... 1931
- Librium Injectable ... 1932

Chlorpromazine (Additive effects). Products include:
- Thorazine ... 2234

Chlorprothixene (Additive effects). Products include:
- Taractan Tablets ... 1920

Chlorprothixene Hydrochloride (Additive effects). Products include:
- Taractan ... 1920

Clonidine (Additive effects). Products include:
- Catapres-TTS ... 677

Clonidine Hydrochloride (Additive effects). Products include:
- Catapres Tablets ... 676
- Combipres Tablets ... 678

Clorazepate Dipotassium (Additive effects). Products include:
- Tranxene ... 556

Codeine (Additive effects). Products include:
- Calcidrine Syrup ... 506

Codeine Phosphate (Additive effects). Products include:
- Actifed with Codeine Cough Syrup ... 752
- Cheracol Cough Syrup ... 1853
- Codimal PH Syrup ... 846
- Dimetane-DC Cough Syrup ... 1857
- Empirin with Codeine Phosphate Nos. 2, 3 & 4 ... 764
- Fiorinal with Codeine Capsules ... 2008
- Isoclor Expectorant ... 982
- Naldecon CX Adult Liquid ... ◘ 521
- Novahistine DH ... 1342
- Novahistine Expectorant ... 1343
- Nucofed Capsules ... 2219
- Nucofed Expectorant ... 2219
- Nucofed Pediatric Expectorant ... 2220
- Nucofed Syrup ... 2219
- Phenaphen with Codeine Capsules 1865
- Phenaphen-650 with Codeine Tablets ... 1866
- Phenergan with Codeine ... 2497
- Phenergan VC with Codeine ... 2501
- Robitussin A-C Syrup ... 1875
- Robitussin-DAC Syrup ... 1875
- Ryna ... ◘ 741
- Soma Compound w/Codeine Tablets ... 2390
- Triaminic Expectorant w/Codeine ... 1996
- Tussi-Organidin Liquid ... 2391
- Tylenol with Codeine ... 1381

Codeine Polistirex (Additive effects).
- No products indexed under this heading.

Desipramine Hydrochloride (Additive effects). Products include:
- Norpramin Tablets ... 1340

Dezocine (Additive effects).

Diazepam (Additive effects). Products include:
- Valium Injectable ... 1937
- Valium Tablets ... 1939
- Valrelease Capsules ... 1923

Doxepin Hydrochloride (Additive effects). Products include:
- Sinequan ... 1960

Droperidol (Additive effects). Products include:
- Inapsine Injection ... 1140
- Innovar Injection ... 1141

Enflurane (Additive effects). Products include:
- Ethrane ... 599

Estazolam (Additive effects). Products include:
- ProSom Tablets ... 554

Ethchlorvynol (Additive effects). Products include:
- Placidyl Capsules ... 553

Ethinamate (Additive effects).
- No products indexed under this heading.

Fentanyl (Additive effects). Products include:
- Duragesic Transdermal System ... 1133

Fentanyl Citrate (Additive effects). Products include:
- Innovar Injection ... 1141
- Sublimaze Injection ... 1146

Fluphenazine Decanoate (Additive effects). Products include:
- Prolixin Decanoate ... 1795

Fluphenazine Enanthate (Additive effects). Products include:
- Prolixin Enanthate ... 1796

Fluphenazine Hydrochloride (Additive effects). Products include:
- Prolixin Elixir ... 1793
- Prolixin Injection ... 1791
- Prolixin Oral Concentrate ... 1792
- Prolixin Tablets ... 1793

Flurazepam Hydrochloride (Additive effects). Products include:
- Dalmane Capsules ... 1927

Glutethimide (Additive effects).
- No products indexed under this heading.

Haloperidol (Additive effects). Products include:
- Haldol Injection, Tablets and Concentrate ... 1373

Haloperidol Decanoate (Additive effects). Products include:
- Haldol Decanoate ... 1375

Hydrocodone Bitartrate (Additive effects). Products include:
- Anexsia 5/500 Tablets ... 2196
- Anexsia 7.5/650 Tablets ... 2197
- Azdone Tablets ... 844
- Codiclear DH Syrup ... 845
- Codimal DH Syrup ... 846
- Damason-P ... 1356
- Hycodan Syrup, Tablets ... 927
- Hycomine Compound Tablets ... 929
- Hycomine Syrup ... 927
- Hycotuss Expectorant Syrup ... 930
- Hydrocet Capsules ... 835
- Lortab ASA Tablets ... 2414
- Lortab ... 2412
- Ru-Tuss with Hydrocodone ... 694
- Triaminic Expectorant DH ... 1995
- Vicodin Tablets ... 1187
- Vicodin ES Tablets ... 1189
- Zydone Capsules ... 941

Hydrocodone Polistirex (Additive effects). Products include:
- Tussionex Extended-Release Suspension ... 988

Hydroxyzine Hydrochloride (Additive effects). Products include:
- Atarax Tablets & Syrup ... 1941
- Marax Tablets & DF Syrup ... 1954
- Vistaril Intramuscular Solution ... 1970

Imipramine Hydrochloride (Additive effects). Products include:
- Tofranil Ampuls ... 1038
- Tofranil Tablets ... 1039

Imipramine Pamoate (Additive effects). Products include:
- Tofranil-PM Capsules ... 1041

Isocarboxazid (Additive effects). Products include:
- Marplan Tablets ... 1906

Isoflurane (Additive effects). Products include:
- Forane ... 600

Ketamine Hydrochloride (Additive effects). Products include:
- Ketalar ... 1726

Levorphanol Tartrate (Additive effects). Products include:
- Levo-Dromoran ... 1906

Lithium Carbonate (Additive effects). Products include:
- Eskalith ... 2214
- Lithane Tablets ... 1596
- Lithium Carbonate Capsules & Tablets ... 1984
- Lithobid Tablets ... 870

Lithium Citrate (Additive effects). Products include:
- Cibalith-S ... 870

Lorazepam (Additive effects). Products include:
- Ativan Injection ... 2432
- Ativan Tablets ... 2434

Loxapine Hydrochloride (Additive effects). Products include:
- Loxitane ... 1213

Loxapine Succinate (Additive effects). Products include:
- Loxitane Capsules ... 1213

Maprotiline Hydrochloride (Additive effects). Products include:
- Ludiomil Tablets ... 874

Medroxyprogesterone Acetate (Adverse effects on carbohydrate and lipid metabolism). Products include:
- Amen ... 833
- Cycrin Tablets ... 2449
- Depo-Provera Sterile Aqueous Suspension ... 2336
- Provera Tablets ... 2356

Megestrol Acetate (Adverse effects on carbohydrate and lipid metabolism). Products include:
- Megace Tablets ... 732

Meperidine Hydrochloride (Additive effects). Products include:
- Demerol ... 2047
- Mepergan Injection ... 2479

Mephobarbital (Additive effects). Products include:
- Mebaral Tablets ... 2061

Mesoridazine (Additive effects). Products include:
- Serentil ... 686

Methadone Hydrochloride (Additive effects). Products include:
- Dolophine Hydrochloride Ampoules & Vials ... 1260
- Dolophine Hydrochloride Tablets ... 1261
- Methadone Hydrochloride Diskets ... 1284
- Methadone Hydrochloride Oral Solution & Tablets ... 1987

Methohexital Sodium (Additive effects). Products include:
- Brevital Sodium Vials ... 1248

Methoxyflurane (Additive effects). Products include:
- No products indexed under this heading.

Midazolam Hydrochloride (Additive effects). Products include:
- Versed Injection ... 1924

Molindone Hydrochloride (Additive effects). Products include:
- Moban Tablets & Concentrate ... 932

Morphine Sulfate (Additive effects). Products include:
- Astramorph/PF Injection, USP (Preservative-Free) ... 618
- Duramorph ... 960
- Infumorph 200 and Infumorph 500 Sterile Solutions ... 962
- MS Contin Tablets ... 1814
- MSIR ... 1817
- Oramorph SR (Morphine Sulfate Sustained Release Tablets) ... 1988
- Roxanol ... 1991

Norgestimate (Adverse effects on carbohydrate and lipid metabolism). Products include:
- Ortho-Cyclen Tablets ... 1658

Nortriptyline Hydrochloride (Additive effects). Products include:
- Pamelor ... 2019

Opium Alkaloids (Additive effects). Products include:
- B & O No. 15A & No. 16A Supprettes ... 2395
- Pantopon Injectable ... 1911

Oxazepam (Additive effects). Products include:
- Serax Capsules ... 2522
- Serax Tablets ... 2522

Oxycodone Hydrochloride (Additive effects). Products include:
- Percocet Tablets ... 950
- Percodan ... 951
- Roxicodone Tablets, Oral Solution & Intensol (Oxycodone) ... 1992
- Tylox Capsules ... 1382

Pentobarbital Sodium (Additive effects). Products include:
- Nembutal Sodium Capsules ... 534
- Nembutal Sodium Solution ... 536
- Nembutal Sodium Suppositories ... 538

Perphenazine (Additive effects). Products include:
- Etrafon ... 2087
- Triavil Tablets ... 1556
- Trilafon ... 2123

Phenelzine Sulfate (Additive effects). Products include:
- Nardil ... 1742

Phenobarbital (Additive effects). Products include:
- Arco-Lase Plus Tablets ... 607
- Bellergal-S Tablets ... 1998
- Bronkolixir ... ▣ 761
- Bronkotabs Tablets ... ▣ 762
- Donnatal ... 1858
- Donnatal Extentabs ... 1859
- Donnatal Tablets ... 1858
- Donnazyme Tablets ... 1860
- Kinesed Tablets ... 2272
- Phenobarbital Elixir and Tablets ... 1293
- Primatene Tablets-P Formula ... 2421
- Quadrinal Tablets ... 1183
- Tedral SA ... 1765

Prazepam (Additive effects). Products include:
- Centrax ... 1693

Prochlorperazine (Additive effects). Products include:
- Compazine ... 2201

Promethazine Hydrochloride (Additive effects). Products include:
- Mepergan Injection ... 2479
- Phenergan with Codeine ... 2497
- Phenergan with Dextromethorphan ... 2499
- Phenergan Injection ... 2493
- Phenergan Suppositories ... 2496
- Phenergan Syrup ... 2495
- Phenergan Tablets ... 2496
- Phenergan VC ... 2500
- Phenergan VC with Codeine ... 2501

Propofol (Additive effects). Products include:
- Diprivan Injection ... 2267

Propoxyphene Hydrochloride (Additive effects). Products include:
- Darvon ... 1256
- Wygesic Tablets ... 2540

Propoxyphene Napsylate (Additive effects). Products include:
- Darvon-N/Darvocet-N ... 1254

Protriptyline Hydrochloride (Additive effects). Products include:
- Vivactil Tablets ... 1567

Quazepam (Additive effects). Products include:
- Doral Tablets ... 2383

Secobarbital Sodium (Additive effects). Products include:
- Seconal Sodium Pulvules ... 1296

Sufentanil Citrate (Additive effects). Products include:
- Sufenta Injection ... 1147

Temazepam (Additive effects). Products include:
- Restoril Capsules ... 2023

Thiamylal Sodium (Additive effects). Products include:
- Surital Ampoules, Steri-Vials ... 1764

Thioridazine Hydrochloride (Additive effects). Products include:
- Mellaril ... 2011

Thiothixene (Additive effects). Products include:
- Navane Capsules and Concentrate ... 1954
- Navane Intramuscular ... 1956

Tranylcypromine Sulfate (Additive effects). Products include:
- Parnate Tablets ... 2222

Triazolam (Additive effects). Products include:
- Halcion Tablets ... 2340

Trifluoperazine Hydrochloride (Additive effects). Products include:
- Stelazine ... 2226

Trimipramine Maleate (Additive effects). Products include:
- Surmontil Capsules ... 2524

PPD TINE TEST (Diagnostic aid) ... 2548
May interact with corticosteroids and immunosuppressive agents. Compounds in these categories include:

Azathioprine (Reactivity to the test may be suppressed). Products include:
- Imuran ... 768

Betamethasone Acetate (Reactivity to the test may be suppressed). Products include:
- Celestone Soluspan Suspension ... 2081

Betamethasone Sodium Phosphate (Reactivity to the test may be suppressed). Products include:
- Celestone Soluspan Suspension ... 2081

Cortisone Acetate (Reactivity to the test may be suppressed). Products include:
- Cortone Acetate Sterile Suspension ... 1437
- Cortone Acetate Tablets ... 1439

Cyclosporine (Reactivity to the test may be suppressed). Products include:
- Sandimmune ... 2024

Desoximetasone (Reactivity to the test may be suppressed). Products include:
- Topicort ... 1098

Dexamethasone Acetate (Reactivity to the test may be suppressed). Products include:
- Dalalone D.P. Injectable ... 999
- Decadron-LA Sterile Suspension ... 1457

Dexamethasone Sodium Phosphate (Reactivity to the test may be suppressed). Products include:
- AK-Dex ... ⊙ 203
- Decadron Phosphate Respihaler ... 1454
- Decadron Phosphate Sterile Ophthalmic Ointment ... 1453
- Decadron Phosphate Sterile Ophthalmic Solution ... 1453
- Decadron Phosphate Topical Cream ... 1455
- Decadron Phosphate Turbinaire ... 1456
- Maxidex Sterile Ophthalmic Ointment ... ⊙ 222
- NeoDecadron Sterile Ophthalmic Ointment ... 1517
- NeoDecadron Sterile Ophthalmic Solution ... 1518
- NeoDecadron Topical Cream ... 1518

Hydrocortisone (Reactivity to the test may be suppressed). Products include:
- AK-Spore H.C. ... ⊙ 206
- Bactine Hydrocortisone Anti-Itch Cream ... ▣ 625
- CaldeCORT Anti-Itch Hydrocortisone Spray ... ▣ 560
- Carmol HC Cream 1% ... 2296
- Cortaid Spray ... ▣ 735
- Cortenema ... 2244
- Cortisporin Ointment ... 758
- Cortisporin Ophthalmic Ointment Sterile ... 758
- Cortisporin Ophthalmic Suspension Sterile ... 759
- Cortisporin Otic Solution Sterile ... 760
- Cortisporin Otic Suspension Sterile ... 760
- Cortizone-5 Creme & Ointment ... ▣ 732
- Dermolate Anti-Itch Cream ... ▣ 697
- Eldecort Cream 1.0% ... 1113
- Eldecort Cream 1.0% and 2.5% ... 1113
- Fungoid HC Creme ... 1770
- Hydrocortone Tablets ... 1482
- Hytone ... 909
- LazerSporin-C Solution ... 1770
- Massengill Medicated Soft Cloth Towelettes ... 2192
- Nutracort Cream & Lotion ... 1684
- PediOtic Suspension Sterile ... 797
- Synacort Creams 1%, 2.5% ... 2296
- Vanoxide-HC Acne Lotion ... 911
- Vioform-Hydrocortisone Cream and Mild Cream ... 889
- Vioform-Hydrocortisone Ointment ... 889
- VōSoL HC Otic Solution ... 2392
- Vytone Cream 1% ... 911

Hydrocortisone Acetate (Reactivity to the test may be suppressed). Products include:
- Analpram-HC Rectal Cream 1% and 2.5% ... 970
- Anusol-HC Cream ... 1690
- Anusol-HC Suppositories ... 1691
- Caldecort ... ▣ 560
- Carmol HC Cream 1% ... 2296
- Chloromycetin Hydrocortisone Ophthalmic ... 1694
- Coly-Mycin S Otic w/Neomycin & Hydrocortisone ... 1708
- Cortaid ... ▣ 735
- Cortef Feminine Itch Cream ... ▣ 735
- Corticaine ... ▣ 682
- Cortifoam ... 1827
- Cortisporin Cream ... 757
- Epifoam ... 1828
- Gynecort 5 Creme ... ▣ 556
- Hydrocortone Acetate Sterile Suspension ... 1479
- Lanacort 5 Creme and Ointment ... ▣ 557
- Mantadil Cream ... 789
- Ophthocort ... ⊙ 301
- Orabase HCA Oral Paste ... 890
- Pramosone Cream, Lotion & Ointment ... 971

(▣ Described in PDR For Nonprescription Drugs)

(⊙ Described in PDR For Ophthalmology)

ProctoCream-HC 1834
Proctofoam-HC 1835

Hydrocortisone Sodium Phosphate (Reactivity to the test may be suppressed). Products include:
Hydrocortone Phosphate Injection, Sterile 1481

Hydrocortisone Sodium Succinate (Reactivity to the test may be suppressed). Products include:
Solu-Cortef Sterile Powder 2361

Immune Globulin (Human) (Reactivity to the test may be suppressed). Products include:
MICRhoGAM $Rh_o(D)$ Immune Globulin (Human) 1650
RhoGAM $Rh_o(D)$ Immune Globulin (Human) 1651

Immune Globulin Intravenous (Human) (Reactivity to the test may be suppressed). Products include:
Gamimune N Immune Globulin Intravenous (Human) 1572
Gammagard Immune Globulin, Intravenous (Human) 658
Iveegam 1129
Sandoglobulin I.V. 2027

Methylprednisolone Acetate (Reactivity to the test may be suppressed). Products include:
Depo-Medrol Sterile Aqueous Suspension 2334

Methylprednisolone Sodium Succinate (Reactivity to the test may be suppressed). Products include:
Solu-Medrol Sterile Powder 2363

Muromonab-CD3 (Reactivity to the test may be suppressed). Products include:
Orthoclone OKT3 Sterile Solution .. 1645

Prednisolone Acetate (Reactivity to the test may be suppressed). Products include:
AK-Cide Sterile Ophthalmic Ointment & Suspension .... ⊙ 202
Blephamide Liquifilm Sterile Ophthalmic Suspension 586
Blephamide S.O.P. Sterile Ophthalmic Ointment 586
Cetapred Ointment .... ⊙ 220
⅛% Econopred & 1% Econopred Plus .... ⊙ 217
Isopto Cetapred Suspension .... ⊙ 220
Metimyd .... ⊙ 306
Poly-Pred Liquifilm .... ⊙ 250
Pred Forte .... ⊙ 252
Pred Mild .... ⊙ 254
Pred-G Liquifilm Sterile Ophthalmic Suspension .... ⊙ 252
Pred-G S.O.P. Sterile Ophthalmic Ointment .... ⊙ 253
Vasocidin Ointment .... ⊙ 275

Prednisolone Sodium Phosphate (Reactivity to the test may be suppressed). Products include:
AK-Pred .... ⊙ 205
Hydeltrasol Injection, Sterile 1476
Inflamase .... ⊙ 274
Pediapred Oral Liquid 987
Vasocidin Ophthalmic Solution .... ⊙ 276

Prednisolone Tebutate (Reactivity to the test may be suppressed). Products include:
Hydeltra-T.B.A. Sterile Suspension 1478

Prednisone (Reactivity to the test may be suppressed). Products include:
Deltasone Tablets 2332

Triamcinolone (Reactivity to the test may be suppressed).
No products indexed under this heading.

Triamcinolone Acetonide (Reactivity to the test may be suppressed). Products include:
Aristocort A 1010
Azmacort Inhaler 1837
Kenalog Cream, Lotion & Ointment 2401
Kenalog-10 Injection 2402
Kenalog-40 Injection 2403
Kenalog in Orabase 604
Kenalog Spray 2401
Mycolog II Cream and Ointment 2407
Mytrex Cream & Ointment 2080
Nasacort Nasal Inhaler 1844

Triamcinolone Diacetate (Reactivity to the test may be suppressed). Products include:
Aristocort Suspension 1008

Triamcinolone Hexacetonide (Reactivity to the test may be suppressed). Products include:
Aristospan Suspension 1011

PRID SALVE
(Ichthammol) .... ▣ 740
No interactions described in labeling.

P & S LIQUID
(Mineral Oil) .... ▣ 509
No interactions described in labeling.

P & S PLUS TAR GEL
(Coal Tar, Ethyl Alcohol, Salicylic Acid) .... ▣ 510
No interactions described in labeling.

P & S SHAMPOO
(Salicylic Acid) .... ▣ 510
No interactions described in labeling.

PAMELOR CAPSULES
(Nortriptyline Hydrochloride) 2019
May interact with monoamine oxidase inhibitors, thyroid preparations, sympathomimetic aerosal bronchodilators, anticholinergics, and certain other agents. Compounds in these categories include:

Albuterol (Close supervision and dosage adjustment indicated). Products include:
Proventil Inhalation Aerosol 2117
Ventolin Inhalation Aerosol and Refill 583

Albuterol Sulfate (Close supervision and dosage adjustment indicated). Products include:
Proventil Repetabs Tablets 2120
Proventil Solutions for Inhalation 0.5% and 0.083% 2118
Proventil Syrup 2119
Proventil Tablets 2120
Ventolin 583

Alcohol (Response to alcohol may be exaggerated).

Atropine Sulfate (Close supervision and dosage adjustment indicated). Products include:
Arco-Lase Plus Tablets 607
Atropine Sulfate Sterile Ophthalmic Solution and S.O.P. Sterile Ophthalmic Ointment .... ⊙ 239
Donnagel .... ▣ 675
Donnagel-PG 1858
Donnatal 1858
Donnatal Extentabs 1859
Donnatal Tablets 1858
Donnazyme Tablets 1860
Isopto Atropine .... ⊙ 218
Lomotil 2174
Motofen Tablets 836
Ru-Tuss Tablets 693
Urised Tablets 2396

Belladonna Alkaloids (Close supervision and dosage adjustment indicated). Products include:
Bellergal-S Tablets 1998
Hyland's Bed Wetting Tablets .... ▣ 728
Hyland's Teething Tablets .... ▣ 728
Kinesed Tablets 2272

Benztropine Mesylate (Close supervision and dosage adjustment indicated). Products include:
Cogentin 1435

Biperiden (Close supervision and dosage adjustment indicated). Products include:
Akineton 1171

Chlorpropamide (A case of significant hypoglycemia has been reported in a type II diabetic patient maintained on chlorpropamide (250 mg/day), after the addition of nortriptyline (125 mg/day)). Products include:
Diabinese Tablets 1775

Cimetidine (Clinically significant increase in plasma concentrations of Pamelor). Products include:
Tagamet Tablets 2228

Cimetidine Hydrochloride (Clinically significant increase in plasma concentrations of Pamelor). Products include:
Tagamet 2228

Clidinium Bromide (Close supervision and dosage adjustment indicated). Products include:
Librax Capsules 1929
Quarzan Capsules 1937

Dicyclomine Hydrochloride (Close supervision and dosage adjustment indicated). Products include:
Bentyl 1322

Dobutamine Hydrochloride (Close supervision and dosage adjustment indicated). Products include:
Dobutrex Solution Vials 1259

Dopamine Hydrochloride (Close supervision and dosage adjustment indicated). Products include:
Intropin Injection 930

Ephedrine Hydrochloride (Close supervision and dosage adjustment indicated). Products include:
Amesec .... ▣ 682
Primatene Tablets-M Formula 2421
Primatene Tablets-P Formula 2421
Primatene Tablets-Regular Formula 2421
Quadrinal Tablets 1183
Quelidrine Syrup 556
Tedral SA 1765

Ephedrine Sulfate (Close supervision and dosage adjustment indicated). Products include:
Bronkaid Tablets .... ▣ 757
Bronkolixir .... ▣ 761
Bronkotabs Tablets .... ▣ 762
Marax Tablets & DF Syrup 1954
Pazo Hemorrhoid Ointment & Suppositories 752
Vicks Vatronol Nose Drops .... ▣ 666

Ephedrine Tannate (Close supervision and dosage adjustment indicated). Products include:
Rynatuss 2388

Epinephrine (Close supervision and dosage adjustment indicated). Products include:
Ana-Kit Anaphylaxis Emergency Treatment Kit 1100
Bronkaid Mist .... ▣ 757
EpiPen 843
Marcaine Hydrochloride 0.5% with Epinephrine 1:200,000 (as bitartrate) 958
Marcaine Hydrochloride with Epinephrine 1:200,000 2055
Primatene Mist 2420
Sus-Phrine Injection 1006
Xylocaine with Epinephrine Injections 637

Epinephrine Bitartrate (Close supervision and dosage adjustment indicated). Products include:
AsthmaHaler Mist Epinephrine Bitartrate Bronchodilator .... ▣ 616
Bronkaid Mist Suspension .... ▣ 757
Primatene Mist Suspension 2421

Epinephrine Hydrochloride (Close supervision and dosage adjustment indicated). Products include:
Adrenalin Chloride Solution 1:100 & 1:1,000 1689
Epifrin .... ⊙ 244
Glaucon .... ⊙ 218

Furazolidone (Concurrent administration can produce hyperpyretic crises, severe convulsions, and fatalities). Products include:
Furoxone 1855

Glycopyrrolate (Close supervision and dosage adjustment indicated). Products include:
Robinul Forte Tablets 1873
Robinul Injectable 1873
Robinul Tablets 1873

Guanethidine Monosulfate (Antihypertensive action of guanethidine blocked). Products include:
Esimil Tablets 864
Ismelin Tablets 869

Hyoscyamine (Close supervision and dosage adjustment indicated). Products include:
Cystospaz Tablets 2395
Urised Tablets 2396

Hyoscyamine Sulfate (Close supervision and dosage adjustment indicated). Products include:
Arco-Lase Plus Tablets 607
Cystospaz-M Capsules 2395
Donnagel .... ▣ 675
Donnagel-PG 1858
Donnatal 1858
Donnatal Extentabs 1859
Donnatal Tablets 1858
Donnazyme Tablets 1860
Kutrase Capsules 2146
Levsin/Levsinex 2147
Ru-Tuss Tablets 693

Ipratropium Bromide (Close supervision and dosage adjustment indicated). Products include:
Atrovent Inhalation Aerosol 675

Isocarboxazid (Concurrent administration can produce hyperpyretic crises, severe convulsions, and fatalities). Products include:
Marplan Tablets 1906

Isoproterenol Hydrochloride (Close supervision and dosage adjustment indicated). Products include:
Isuprel Hydrochloride Injection 1:5000 2050
Isuprel Hydrochloride Mistometer .. 2051
Isuprel Hydrochloride Solution 1:200 & 1:100 2052
Norisodrine Aerotrol 540

Levothyroxine Sodium (Cardiac arrhythmias). Products include:
Levothroid Tablets 1003
Levoxine Tablets 904
Synthroid 695

Liothyronine Sodium (Cardiac arrhythmias). Products include:
Cytomel Tablets 2203

Liotrix (Cardiac arrhythmias). Products include:
Euthroid 1724

Mepenzolate Bromide (Close supervision and dosage adjustment indicated). Products include:
Cantil Tablets 1326

Metaproterenol Sulfate (Close supervision and dosage adjustment indicated). Products include:
Alupent 674
Arm-a-Med Metaproterenol Sulfate Inhalation Solution, USP 617
Metaprel Inhalation Aerosol Bronchodilator 2014
Metaprel Inhalation Solution 2015
Metaprel 2015
Metaproterenol Sulfate Inhalation Solution, USP 912

Metaraminol Bitartrate (Close supervision and dosage adjustment indicated). Products include:
Aramine Injection 1424

Methoxamine Hydrochloride (Close supervision and dosage adjustment indicated). Products include:
Vasoxyl Injection 819

(▣ Described in PDR For Nonprescription Drugs) (⊙ Described in PDR For Ophthalmology)

Norepinephrine Bitartrate (Close supervision and dosage adjustment indicated). Products include:

Levophed Bitartrate Injection 2054

Oxybutynin Chloride (Close supervision and dosage adjustment indicated). Products include:

Ditropan 1332

Phenelzine Sulfate (Concurrent administration can produce hyperpyretic crises, severe convulsions, and fatalities). Products include:

Nardil 1742

Phenylephrine Bitartrate (Close supervision and dosage adjustment indicated).

No products indexed under this heading.

Phenylephrine Hydrochloride (Close supervision and dosage adjustment indicated). Products include:

AK-Dilate Solution 2.5% and 10% .... ⊙ 203
Atrohist Sprinkle Capsules 558
Cerose-DM 2443
Codimal 846
Comhist LA Capsules 1618
Congespirin For Children Aspirin Free Chewable Cold Tablets 748
Cyclomydril .... ⊙ 216
Deconsal Sprinkle Capsules 559
Dimetane Decongestant .... ▣ 673
Dristan Decongestant/Antihistamine/ Analgesic Coated Caplets .... ▣ 749
Dristan Cold Nasal Decongestant/ Antihistamine/ Analgesic Coated Tablets 2419
Dristan Advanced Formula Decongestant/Antihistamine/ Analgesic Tablets .... ▣ 749
Dristan Nasal Spray, Menthol 2419
Dristan Nasal Spray, Regular and Regular with Metered Pump 2419
Entex Capsules 1623
Entex Liquid 1623
Sinus Excedrin Analgesic, Decongestant Tablets & Caplets 750
Extendryl 994
4-Way Fast Acting Nasal Spray - Original Formula (regular & mentholated) & Metered Spray Pump (regular) 751
Hycomine Compound Tablets 929
Murocoll-2 Sterile Ophthalmic Solution .... ⊙ 261
Mydfrin 2.5% .... ⊙ 224
Naldecon Syrup, Tablets, Pediatric Drops and Pediatric Syrup 709
Neo-Synephrine Hydrochloride 1% Carpuject 2063
Neo-Synephrine Hydrochloride 1% Injection 2063
Neo-Synephrine Hydrochloride (Ophthalmic) 2064
Neo-Synephrine .... ▣ 759
Nōstril Nasal Decongestant .... ▣ 520
Novahistine Elixir .... ▣ 596
Phenergan VC 2500
Phenergan VC with Codeine 2501
Prefrin Liquifilm Vasoconstrictor and Lubricant Eye Drops .... ⊙ 254
Prefrin-A .... ⊙ 255
Quelidrine Syrup 556
Relief Vasoconstrictor and Lubricant Eye Drops .... ⊙ 256
Robitussin Night Relief .... ▣ 677
Ru-Tuss with Hydrocodone 694
Ru-Tuss Tablets 693
Vasosulf .... ⊙ 279
Vicks Sinex .... ▣ 665
Zincfrin .... ⊙ 230

Phenylephrine Tannate (Close supervision and dosage adjustment indicated). Products include:

Rynatan 2387
Rynatuss 2388

Phenylpropanolamine Hydrochloride (Close supervision and dosage adjustment indicated). Products include:

A.R.M. Allergy Relief Medicine Caplets .... ▣ 615
Acutrim .... ▣ 548
Allerest .... ▣ 559
BC Cold Powder .... ▣ 517
Cheracol Plus Head Cold/Cough Formula .... ▣ 667
Codimal Expectorant 846
Comtrex Multi-Symptom Cold Reliever Tablets/Caplets/Liqui-Gels/Liquid 745
Contac Continuous Action Decongestant/Antihistamine Capsules ▣ 710
Contac Maximum Strength Continuous Action Decongestant/ Antihistamine Caplets .... ▣ 709
Contac Severe Cold and Flu Formula Caplets .... ▣ 711
Coricidin 'D' Decongestant Tablets .... ▣ 695
Coricidin Demilets Tablets for Children .... ▣ 696
Demazin Nasal Decongestant/ Antihistamine Repetabs Tablets & Syrup .... ▣ 697
Dexatrim .... ▣ 733
Dimetane-DC Cough Syrup 1857
Dimetapp Elixir .... ▣ 673
Dimetapp DM Elixir .... ▣ 674
Dimetapp Extentabs .... ▣ 674
Dimetapp Plus Caplets .... ▣ 675
Dimetapp Tablets .... ▣ 675
Entex Capsules 1623
Entex LA Tablets 1623
Entex Liquid 1623
4-Way Cold Tablets 750
Hycomine Syrup 927
Naldecon CX Adult Liquid .... ▣ 521
Naldecon DX Adult Liquid .... ▣ 521
Naldecon DX Children's Syrup .... ▣ 522
Naldecon DX Pediatric Drops .... ▣ 522
Naldecon EX Children's Syrup .... ▣ 522
Naldecon EX Pediatric Drops .... ▣ 523
Naldecon Syrup, Tablets, Pediatric Drops and Pediatric Syrup 709
Nolamine Tablets 838
Nolex LA Tablets 838
Ornade Spansule Capsules 2221
Orthoxicol Cough Syrup .... ▣ 668
Propagest 839
Pyrroxate Capsules .... ▣ 669
Robitussin-CF .... ▣ 676
Ru-Tuss II Capsules 693
Ru-Tuss with Hydrocodone 694
Ru-Tuss Tablets 693
Sine-Off Sinus Medicine Tablets-Aspirin Formula .... ▣ 722
Sinulin 840
St. Joseph Cold Tablets for Children .... ▣ 704
Tavist-D Tablets 2035
Triaminic Allergy Tablets .... ▣ 688
Triaminic Chewables .... ▣ 688
Triaminic Cold Tablets .... ▣ 688
Triaminic Expectorant .... ▣ 688
Triaminic Expectorant w/Codeine .. 1996
Triaminic Expectorant DH 1995
Triaminic Oral Infant Drops 1996
Triaminic Syrup .... ▣ 689
Triaminic-12 Tablets .... ▣ 690
Triaminic-DM Syrup .... ▣ 689
Triaminicin Tablets .... ▣ 690
Triaminicol Multi-Symptom Cold Tablets .... ▣ 691
Triaminicol Multi-Symptom Relief ▣ 691
Tuss-Ornade Liquid 2242
Tuss-Ornade Spansule Capsules 2242
Tylenol Cold Medication, Effervescent Tablets 1369

Pirbuterol Acetate (Close supervision and dosage adjustment indicated). Products include:

Maxair Inhaler 1311

Procyclidine Hydrochloride (Close supervision and dosage adjustment indicated). Products include:

Kemadrin Tablets 771

Propantheline Bromide (Close supervision and dosage adjustment indicated). Products include:

Pro-Banthine Tablets 2141

Pseudoephedrine Hydrochloride (Close supervision and dosage adjustment indicated). Products include:

Actifed Capsules .... ▣ 539
Actifed Plus Caplets .... ▣ 539
Actifed Plus Tablets .... ▣ 540
Actifed with Codeine Cough Syrup.. 752
Actifed Syrup .... ▣ 540
Actifed Tablets .... ▣ 540
Actifed 12-Hour Capsules .... ▣ 539
Advil Cold & Sinus Caplets (formerly CoAdvil) 2416
Allerest .... ▣ 559
Anatuss LA Tablets 1359
Benadryl Decongestant Elixir .... ▣ 635
Benadryl Decongestant .... ▣ 635
Benadryl Plus .... ▣ 636
Benadryl Plus Nighttime .... ▣ 637
Benylin Decongestant .... ▣ 638
Brexin L.A. Capsules 2078
Bromfed Capsules (Timed Release) 1615
Bromfed Syrup .... ▣ 628
Bromfed 1615
CoAdvil .... ▣ 748
Allergy-Sinus Comtrex Multi-Symptom Allergy Sinus Formula Tablets & Caplets 746
Cough Formula Comtrex 746
Comtrex Multi-Symptom Cold Reliever Tablets/Caplets/Liqui-Gels/Liquid 745
Day-Night Comtrex 747
Non-Drowsy Comtrex 747
Congess 994
Congestac Caplets .... ▣ 617
Contac Jr. Children's Cold Medicine .... ▣ 712
Contac Nighttime Cold Medicine .... ▣ 713
Contac Sinus Caplets Maximum Strength Non-Drowsy Formula .... ▣ 710
Contac Sinus Tablets Maximum Strength Non-Drowsy Formula .... ▣ 710
Deconamine 663
Deconsal II Tablets 559
Dimacol Caplets .... ▣ 672
Dimetane-DX Cough Syrup 1858
Dorcol Children's Cough Syrup .... ▣ 685
Dorcol Children's Decongestant Liquid .... ▣ 685
Dorcol Children's Liquid Cold Formula .... ▣ 686
Maximum Strength Dristan Decongestant/Analgesic Coated Caplets .... ▣ 750
No Drowsiness Dristan Cold Nasal Decongestant/Analgesic Coated Caplets 2420
Dristan Sinus Caplets 2419
Sinus Excedrin Analgesic, Decongestant Tablets & Caplets .... ▣ 533
Fedahist Gyrocaps 2145
Fedahist Timecaps 2145
Guaifed 1615
Guaifed Syrup .... ▣ 629
Isoclor Expectorant 982
Isoclor Timesule Capsules .... ▣ 561
Kronofed-A 970
Medi-Flu Caplet, Liquid .... ▣ 640
Novafed A Capsules 1342
Novafed Capsules 1342
Novahistine DH 1342
Novahistine DMX .... ▣ 595
Novahistine Expectorant 1343
Nucofed Capsules 2219
Nucofed Expectorant 2219
Nucofed Pediatric Expectorant 2220
Nucofed Syrup 2219
Ornex Caplets .... ▣ 618
PediaCare Allergy Relief Formula Liquid 1362
PediaCare Cough-Cold Formula Liquid 1362
PediaCare Infants' Oral Decongestant Drops 1362
PediaCare Night Rest Cough-Cold Formula Liquid 1362
PediaCare 6-12 Cough-Cold Formula Chewable Tablets 1362
Robitussin-DAC Syrup 1875
Robitussin-PE .... ▣ 677
Rondec 1975
Rondec-DM 1976
Rondec-TR Tablet 1975
Ru-Tuss DE Tablets 694
Ryna .... ▣ 741
Seldane-D Extended-Release Tablets 1350
Sinarest .... ▣ 562
Sine-Aid Maximum Strength Sinus Headache Caplets 1365
Sine-Aid Maximum Strength Sinus Headache Tablets 1365
Sine-Off Maximum Strength Allergy/Sinus Formula Caplets .... ▣ 721
Sine-Off Maximum Strength No Drowsiness Formula Caplets .... ▣ 722
Singlet Tablets .... ▣ 598
Sinutab Maximum Strength .... ▣ 641
Sinutab Maximum Strength Without Drowsiness Tablets & Caplets .... ▣ 642
Sinutab Regular Strength Without Drowsiness Formula .... ▣ 641
St. Joseph Nighttime Cold Medicine .... ▣ 705
Sudafed Children's Liquid .... ▣ 543
Sudafed Cough Syrup .... ▣ 543
Sudafed Plus Liquid .... ▣ 544
Sudafed Plus Tablets .... ▣ 545
Sudafed Sinus Caplets .... ▣ 545
Sudafed Sinus Tablets .... ▣ 545
Sudafed Tablets, 30 mg .... ▣ 544
Sudafed Tablets, Adult Strength, 60 mg .... ▣ 544
Sudafed 12 Hour Capsules .... ▣ 545
TheraFlu Flu and Cold Medicine .... ▣ 687
Triaminic Nite Light .... ▣ 689
Tylenol Allergy Sinus Medication Caplets and Gelcaps, Maximum Strength 1372
Children's Tylenol Cold Liquid Formula and Chewable Tablets 1368
Tylenol Cold & Flu Hot Medication, Packets 1369
Tylenol Cold & Flu No Drowsiness Hot Medication, Packets 1371
Tylenol Cold Medication Caplets and Tablets 1370
Tylenol Cold Medication No Drowsiness Formula Caplets 1370
Tylenol Cold Night Time Medication Liquid 1371
Tylenol Cough Medication Liquid with Decongestant, Maximum Strength 1372
Tylenol, Maximum Strength, Sinus Medication Gelcaps, Caplets and Tablets 1373
Ursinus Inlay-Tabs .... ▣ 691
Vicks Children's NyQuil .... ▣ 664
Vicks Daycare .... ▣ 660
Vicks Formula 44D Decongestant Cough Medicine .... ▣ 662
Vicks Formula 44M Multi-Symptom Cough Medicine .... ▣ 662
Vicks NyQuil Nighttime Colds Medicine-Original & Cherry Flavor .... ▣ 664
Vicks Pediatric Formula 44 Cough & Congestion Medicine .... ▣ 663
Vicks Pediatric Formula 44m Multi-Symptom Cough & Cold Medicine .... ▣ 663

Pseudoephedrine Sulfate (Close supervision and dosage adjustment indicated). Products include:

Afrin Tablets .... ▣ 693
Chlor-Trimeton Decongestant .... ▣ 694
Disophrol Chronotab Sustained-Action Tablets .... ▣ 698
Drixoral Antihistamine/Nasal Decongestant Syrup .... ▣ 698
Drixoral Non-Drowsy Formula .... ▣ 699
Drixoral Plus Extended-Release Tablets .... ▣ 699
Drixoral Sinus .... ▣ 700
Drixoral Sustained-Action Tablets .... ▣ 698
Sinutab Allergy Formula Sustained Action Tablets .... ▣ 640
Trinalin Repetabs Tablets 1170

Quinidine Gluconate (Concomitant administration may result in longer plasma half-life, higher AUC and lower clearance of nortriptyline). Products include:

Quinaglute Dura-Tabs Tablets 663

Quinidine Polygalacturonate (Concomitant administration may result in longer plasma half-life, higher AUC and lower clearance of nortriptyline). Products include:

Cardioquin Tablets 1812

Quinidine Sulfate (Concomitant administration may result in longer plasma half-life, higher AUC and lower clearance of nortriptyline). Products include:

Quinidex Extentabs 1868

Reserpine (Stimulating effect). Products include:

Diupres Tablets 1461
Hydromox R Tablets 1209
Hydropres Tablets 1485
Renese-R Tablets 1786

Salutensin/Salutensin-Demi 719
Ser-Ap-Es Tablets 881
Serpasil Tablets 883
Serpasil-Apresoline Tablets 884
Serpasil-Esidrix Tablets 886

Scopolamine Hydrobromide (Close supervision and dosage adjustment indicated). Products include:
Donnagel ▣ 675
Donnagel-PG 1858
Donnatal 1858
Donnatal Extentabs 1859
Donnatal Tablets 1858
Donnazyme Tablets 1860
Isopto Hyoscine ⊙ 222
Murocoll-2 Sterile Ophthalmic Solution ⊙ 261
Ru-Tuss Tablets 693

Scopolamine Preparations (Close supervision and dosage adjustment indicated). Products include:
Transderm Scōp Transdermal Therapeutic System 887

Selegiline Hydrochloride (Concurrent administration can produce hyperpyretic crises, severe convulsions, and fatalities). Products include:
Eldepryl 2250

Terbutaline Sulfate (Close supervision and dosage adjustment indicated). Products include:
Brethaire Inhaler 1024
Brethine Ampuls 1026
Brethine Tablets 1026
Bricanyl Injection 1324
Bricanyl Tablets 1325

Thyroglobulin (Cardiac arrhythmias). Products include:
Proloid Tablets 1761

Thyroid (Cardiac arrhythmias). Products include:
S-P-T "Liquid" Capsules 995

Thyroxine (Cardiac arrhythmias).
No products indexed under this heading.

Tranylcypromine Sulfate (Concurrent administration can produce hyperpyretic crises, severe convulsions, and fatalities). Products include:
Parnate Tablets 2222

Tridihexethyl Chloride (Close supervision and dosage adjustment indicated).
No products indexed under this heading.

Trihexyphenidyl Hydrochloride (Close supervision and dosage adjustment indicated). Products include:
Artane 1195

PAMELOR SOLUTION
(Nortriptyline Hydrochloride) 2019
See **Pamelor Capsules**

CHILDREN'S PANADOL CHEWABLE TABLETS, LIQUID, INFANTS' DROPS
(Acetaminophen) ▣ 571
No interactions described in labeling.

JUNIOR STRENGTH PANADOL
(Acetaminophen) ▣ 571
No interactions described in labeling.

MAXIMUM STRENGTH PANADOL TABLETS AND CAPLETS
(Acetaminophen) ▣ 572
No interactions described in labeling.

PANAFIL OINTMENT
(Papain) 1995
No interactions described in labeling.

PANAFIL-WHITE OINTMENT
(Papain) 1995
No interactions described in labeling.

PANCREASE CAPSULES
(Pancrelipase) 1377
No interactions described in labeling.

PANCREASE MT CAPSULES
(Pancrelipase) 1378
No interactions described in labeling.

PANCREATIN 8X USP 900MG. (HIGH LIPASE)
(Pancreatic Preparations) 2377
No interactions described in labeling.

PANHEMATIN
(Hemin For Injection) 546
May interact with oral anticoagulants, estrogens, and barbiturates. Compounds in these categories include:

Aprobarbital (Increases delta-aminolevalinic acid synthetase). Products include:
Alurate Elixir 1883

Butabarbital (Increases delta-aminolevalinic acid synthetase). Products include:
Pyridium Plus 1764

Butalbital (Increases delta-aminolevalinic acid synthetase). Products include:
Esgic-Plus Tablets 1002
Esgic Tablets & Capsules 1001
Fioricet Tablets 2006
Fiorinal Capsules 2007
Fiorinal with Codeine Capsules 2008
Fiorinal Tablets 2007
Phrenilin 838
Sedapap Tablets 50 mg/650 mg 1360

Chlorotrianisene (Increases delta-aminolevalinic acid synthetase). Products include:
TACE 12 and 25 mg 1353

Dicumarol (Hypocoagulable state). Products include:
Dicumarol Tablets 516

Dienestrol (Increases delta-aminolevalinic acid synthetase). Products include:
Ortho Dienestrol Cream 1664

Diethylstilbestrol (Increases delta-aminolevalinic acid synthetase). Products include:
Diethylstilbestrol Tablets 1258

Estradiol (Increases delta-aminolevalinic acid synthetase). Products include:
Emcyt Capsules 1161
Estrace 1385
Estrace Vaginal Cream 1388
Estraderm Transdermal System 866

Estrogens, Conjugated (Increases delta-aminolevalinic acid synthetase). Products include:
Mediatric Capsules 2476
PMB 200 and PMB 400 2504
Premarin Intravenous 2508
Premarin with Methyltestosterone 2515
Premarin Tablets 2510
Premarin Vaginal Cream 2512

Estrogens, Esterified (Increases delta-aminolevalinic acid synthetase). Products include:
Estratest 2245
Menrium Tablets 1934

Estropipate (Increases delta-aminolevalinic acid synthetase). Products include:
Ogen 540

Ethinyl Estradiol (Increases delta-aminolevalinic acid synthetase). Products include:
Brevicon 2304
Demulen 2161
Estinyl Tablets 2085
Jenest-28 Tablets 1636
Levlen/Tri-Levlen 665
Lo/Ovral Tablets 2471
Lo/Ovral-28 Tablets 2476
Loestrin 1728
Modicon 1667
Nordette-21 Tablets 2481
Nordette-28 Tablets 2483
Norethin 2133
Norinyl 2304
Norlestrin 1746
Ortho-Cyclen Tablets 1658
Ortho-Novum 1667
Ovcon 1391
Ovral Tablets 2490
Ovral-28 Tablets 2491
Levlen/Tri-Levlen 665
Tri-Norinyl 2304
Triphasil-21 Tablets 2527
Triphasil-28 Tablets 2532

Mephobarbital (Increases delta-aminolevalinic acid synthetase). Products include:
Mebaral Tablets 2061

Pentobarbital Sodium (Increases delta-aminolevalinic acid synthetase). Products include:
Nembutal Sodium Capsules 534
Nembutal Sodium Solution 536
Nembutal Sodium Suppositories 538

Phenobarbital (Increases delta-aminolevalinic acid synthetase). Products include:
Arco-Lase Plus Tablets 607
Bellergal-S Tablets 1998
Bronkolixir ▣ 761
Bronkotabs Tablets ▣ 762
Donnatal 1858
Donnatal Extentabs 1859
Donnatal Tablets 1858
Donnazyme Tablets 1860
Kinesed Tablets 2272
Phenobarbital Elixir and Tablets 1293
Primatene Tablets-P Formula 2421
Quadrinal Tablets 1183
Tedral SA 1765

Polyestradiol Phosphate (Increases delta-aminolevalinic acid synthetase). Products include:
Estradurin 2452

Quinestrol (Increases delta-aminolevalinic acid synthetase). Products include:
Estrovis 1721

Secobarbital Sodium (Increases delta-aminolevalinic acid synthetase). Products include:
Seconal Sodium Pulvules 1296

Thiamylal Sodium (Increases delta-aminolevalinic acid synthetase). Products include:
Surital Ampoules, Steri-Vials 1764

Warfarin Sodium (Hypocoagulable state). Products include:
Coumadin Injection & Tablets 944
Panwarfin Tablets 547

PANTOPON INJECTABLE
(Opium Preparations) 1911
May interact with narcotic analgesics, general anesthetics, tranquilizers, hypnotics and sedatives, tricyclic antidepressants, monoamine oxidase inhibitors, central nervous system depressants, and certain other agents. Compounds in these categories include:

Alcohol (Respiratory depression and hypotension; profound sedation or coma).

Alfentanil Hydrochloride (Respiratory depression and hypotension; profound sedation or coma). Products include:
Alfenta Injection 1131

Alprazolam (Respiratory depression and hypotension; profound sedation or coma). Products include:
Xanax Tablets 2367

Amitriptyline Hydrochloride (Respiratory depression and hypotension; profound sedation or coma). Products include:
Elavil 2269
Endep Tablets 1927
Etrafon 2087
Limbitrol 1933
Triavil Tablets 1556

Amoxapine (Respiratory depression and hypotension; profound sedation or coma). Products include:
Asendin Tablets 1196

Aprobarbital (Respiratory depression and hypotension; profound sedation or coma). Products include:
Alurate Elixir 1883

Buprenorphine (Respiratory depression and hypotension; profound sedation or coma).
No products indexed under this heading.

Buspirone Hydrochloride (Respiratory depression and hypotension; profound sedation or coma). Products include:
BuSpar 1401

Butabarbital (Respiratory depression and hypotension; profound sedation or coma). Products include:
Pyridium Plus 1764

Butalbital (Respiratory depression and hypotension; profound sedation or coma). Products include:
Esgic-Plus Tablets 1002
Esgic Tablets & Capsules 1001
Fioricet Tablets 2006
Fiorinal Capsules 2007
Fiorinal with Codeine Capsules 2008
Fiorinal Tablets 2007
Phrenilin 838
Sedapap Tablets 50 mg/650 mg 1360

Chlordiazepoxide (Respiratory depression and hypotension; profound sedation or coma). Products include:
Libritabs Tablets 1930
Limbitrol 1933
Menrium Tablets 1934

Chlordiazepoxide Hydrochloride (Respiratory depression and hypotension; profound sedation or coma). Products include:
Librax Capsules 1929
Librium Capsules 1931
Librium Injectable 1932

Chlorpromazine (Respiratory depression and hypotension; profound sedation or coma). Products include:
Thorazine 2234

Chlorprothixene (Respiratory depression and hypotension; profound sedation or coma). Products include:
Taractan Tablets 1920

Chlorprothixene Hydrochloride (Respiratory depression and hypotension; profound sedation or coma). Products include:
Taractan 1920

Clomipramine Hydrochloride (Respiratory depression and hypotension; profound sedation or coma). Products include:
Anafranil Capsules 650

Clorazepate Dipotassium (Respiratory depression and hypotension; profound sedation or coma). Products include:
Tranxene 556

Codeine (Respiratory depression and hypotension; profound sedation or coma). Products include:
Calcidrine Syrup 506

Codeine Phosphate (Respiratory depression and hypotension; profound sedation or coma). Products include:
- Actifed with Codeine Cough Syrup.. 752
- Cheracol Cough Syrup 1853
- Codimal PH Syrup 846
- Dimetane-DC Cough Syrup 1857
- Empirin with Codeine Phosphate Nos. 2, 3 & 4 764
- Fiorinal with Codeine Capsules 2008
- Isoclor Expectorant 982
- Naldecon CX Adult Liquid ▣ 521
- Novahistine DH 1342
- Novahistine Expectorant 1343
- Nucofed Capsules 2219
- Nucofed Expectorant 2219
- Nucofed Pediatric Expectorant 2220
- Nucofed Syrup 2219
- Phenaphen with Codeine Capsules 1865
- Phenaphen-650 with Codeine Tablets 1866
- Phenergan with Codeine 2497
- Phenergan VC with Codeine 2501
- Robitussin A-C Syrup 1875
- Robitussin-DAC Syrup 1875
- Ryna ▣ 741
- Soma Compound w/Codeine Tablets 2390
- Triaminic Expectorant w/Codeine .. 1996
- Tussi-Organidin Liquid 2391
- Tylenol with Codeine 1381

Codeine Polistirex (Respiratory depression and hypotension; profound sedation or coma).
- No products indexed under this heading.

Desipramine Hydrochloride (Respiratory depression and hypotension; profound sedation or coma). Products include:
- Norpramin Tablets 1340

Dezocine (Respiratory depression and hypotension; profound sedation or coma).

Diazepam (Respiratory depression and hypotension; profound sedation or coma). Products include:
- Valium Injectable 1937
- Valium Tablets 1939
- Valrelease Capsules 1923

Doxepin Hydrochloride (Respiratory depression and hypotension; profound sedation or coma). Products include:
- Sinequan 1960

Droperidol (Respiratory depression and hypotension; profound sedation or coma). Products include:
- Inapsine Injection 1140
- Innovar Injection 1141

Enflurane (Respiratory depression and hypotension; profound sedation or coma). Products include:
- Ethrane 599

Estazolam (Respiratory depression and hypotension; profound sedation or coma). Products include:
- ProSom Tablets 554

Ethchlorvynol (Respiratory depression and hypotension; profound sedation or coma). Products include:
- Placidyl Capsules 553

Ethinamate (Respiratory depression and hypotension; profound sedation or coma).
- No products indexed under this heading.

Fentanyl (Respiratory depression and hypotension; profound sedation or coma). Products include:
- Duragesic Transdermal System 1133

Fentanyl Citrate (Respiratory depression and hypotension; profound sedation or coma). Products include:
- Innovar Injection 1141
- Sublimaze Injection 1146

Fluphenazine Decanoate (Respiratory depression and hypotension; profound sedation or coma). Products include:
- Prolixin Decanoate 1795

Fluphenazine Enanthate (Respiratory depression and hypotension; profound sedation or coma). Products include:
- Prolixin Enanthate 1796

Fluphenazine Hydrochloride (Respiratory depression and hypotension; profound sedation or coma). Products include:
- Prolixin Elixir 1793
- Prolixin Injection 1791
- Prolixin Oral Concentrate 1792
- Prolixin Tablets 1793

Flurazepam Hydrochloride (Respiratory depression and hypotension; profound sedation or coma). Products include:
- Dalmane Capsules 1927

Furazolidone (Respiratory depression and hypotension; profound sedation or coma). Products include:
- Furoxone 1855

Glutethimide (Respiratory depression and hypotension; profound sedation or coma).
- No products indexed under this heading.

Haloperidol (Respiratory depression and hypotension; profound sedation or coma). Products include:
- Haldol Injection, Tablets and Concentrate 1373

Haloperidol Decanoate (Respiratory depression and hypotension; profound sedation or coma). Products include:
- Haldol Decanoate 1375

Hydrocodone Bitartrate (Respiratory depression and hypotension; profound sedation or coma). Products include:
- Anexsia 5/500 Tablets 2196
- Anexsia 7.5/650 Tablets 2197
- Azdone Tablets 844
- Codiclear DH Syrup 845
- Codimal DH Syrup 846
- Damason-P 1356
- Hycodan Syrup, Tablets 927
- Hycomine Compound Tablets 929
- Hycomine Syrup 927
- Hycotuss Expectorant Syrup 930
- Hydrocet Capsules 835
- Lortab ASA Tablets 2414
- Lortab 2412
- Ru-Tuss with Hydrocodone 694
- Triaminic Expectorant DH 1995
- Vicodin Tablets 1187
- Vicodin ES Tablets 1189
- Zydone Capsules 941

Hydrocodone Polistirex (Respiratory depression and hypotension; profound sedation or coma). Products include:
- Tussionex Extended-Release Suspension 988

Hydroxyzine Hydrochloride (Respiratory depression and hypotension; profound sedation or coma). Products include:
- Atarax Tablets & Syrup 1941
- Marax Tablets & DF Syrup 1954
- Vistaril Intramuscular Solution 1970

Imipramine Hydrochloride (Respiratory depression and hypotension; profound sedation or coma). Products include:
- Tofranil Ampuls 1038
- Tofranil Tablets 1039

Imipramine Pamoate (Respiratory depression and hypotension; profound sedation or coma). Products include:
- Tofranil-PM Capsules 1041

Isocarboxazid (Respiratory depression and hypotension; profound sedation or coma). Products include:
- Marplan Tablets 1906

Isoflurane (Respiratory depression and hypotension; profound sedation or coma). Products include:
- Forane 600

Ketamine Hydrochloride (Respiratory depression and hypotension; profound sedation or coma). Products include:
- Ketalar 1726

Levorphanol Tartrate (Respiratory depression and hypotension; profound sedation or coma). Products include:
- Levo-Dromoran 1906

Lorazepam (Respiratory depression and hypotension; profound sedation or coma). Products include:
- Ativan Injection 2432
- Ativan Tablets 2434

Loxapine Hydrochloride (Respiratory depression and hypotension; profound sedation or coma). Products include:
- Loxitane 1213

Loxapine Succinate (Respiratory depression and hypotension; profound sedation or coma). Products include:
- Loxitane Capsules 1213

Maprotiline Hydrochloride (Respiratory depression and hypotension; profound sedation or coma). Products include:
- Ludiomil Tablets 874

Meperidine Hydrochloride (Respiratory depression and hypotension; profound sedation or coma). Products include:
- Demerol 2047
- Mepergan Injection 2479

Mephobarbital (Respiratory depression and hypotension; profound sedation or coma). Products include:
- Mebaral Tablets 2061

Meprobamate (Respiratory depression and hypotension; profound sedation or coma). Products include:
- Deprol Tablets 2382
- Equagesic Tablets 2451
- Miltown Tablets 2386
- PMB 200 and PMB 400 2504

Mesoridazine (Respiratory depression and hypotension; profound sedation or coma). Products include:
- Serentil 686

Methadone Hydrochloride (Respiratory depression and hypotension; profound sedation or coma). Products include:
- Dolophine Hydrochloride Ampoules & Vials 1260
- Dolophine Hydrochloride Tablets 1261
- Methadone Hydrochloride Diskets .. 1284
- Methadone Hydrochloride Oral Solution & Tablets 1987

Methohexital Sodium (Respiratory depression and hypotension; profound sedation or coma). Products include:
- Brevital Sodium Vials 1248

Methoxyflurane (Respiratory depression and hypotension; profound sedation or coma).
- No products indexed under this heading.

Midazolam Hydrochloride (Respiratory depression and hypotension; profound sedation or coma). Products include:
- Versed Injection 1924

Molindone Hydrochloride (Respiratory depression and hypotension; profound sedation or coma). Products include:
- Moban Tablets & Concentrate 932

Morphine Sulfate (Respiratory depression and hypotension; profound sedation or coma). Products include:
- Astramorph/PF Injection, USP (Preservative-Free) 618
- Duramorph 960
- Infumorph 200 and Infumorph 500 Sterile Solutions 962
- MS Contin Tablets 1814
- MSIR 1817
- Oramorph SR (Morphine Sulfate Sustained Release Tablets) 1988
- Roxanol 1991

Nortriptyline Hydrochloride (Respiratory depression and hypotension; profound sedation or coma). Products include:
- Pamelor 2019

Opium Alkaloids (Respiratory depression and hypotension; profound sedation or coma). Products include:
- B & O No. 15A & No. 16A Supprettes 2395
- Pantopon Injectable 1911

Oxazepam (Respiratory depression and hypotension; profound sedation or coma). Products include:
- Serax Capsules 2522
- Serax Tablets 2522

Oxycodone Hydrochloride (Respiratory depression and hypotension; profound sedation or coma). Products include:
- Percocet Tablets 950
- Percodan 951
- Roxicodone Tablets, Oral Solution & Intensol (Oxycodone) 1992
- Tylox Capsules 1382

Pentobarbital Sodium (Respiratory depression and hypotension; profound sedation or coma). Products include:
- Nembutal Sodium Capsules 534
- Nembutal Sodium Solution 536
- Nembutal Sodium Suppositories 538

Perphenazine (Respiratory depression and hypotension; profound sedation or coma). Products include:
- Etrafon 2087
- Triavil Tablets 1556
- Trilafon 2123

Phenelzine Sulfate (Respiratory depression and hypotension; profound sedation or coma). Products include:
- Nardil 1742

Phenobarbital (Respiratory depression and hypotension; profound sedation or coma). Products include:
- Arco-Lase Plus Tablets 607
- Bellergal-S Tablets 1998
- Bronkolixir ▣ 761
- Bronkotabs Tablets ▣ 762
- Donnatal 1858
- Donnatal Extentabs 1859
- Donnatal Tablets 1858
- Donnazyme Tablets 1860
- Kinesed Tablets 2272
- Phenobarbital Elixir and Tablets 1293
- Primatene Tablets-P Formula 2421
- Quadrinal Tablets 1183
- Tedral SA 1765

Prazepam (Respiratory depression and hypotension; profound sedation or coma). Products include:
- Centrax 1693

Prochlorperazine (Respiratory depression and hypotension; profound sedation or coma). Products include:
- Compazine 2201

Promethazine Hydrochloride (Respiratory depression and hypotension; profound sedation or coma). Products include:
- Mepergan Injection ... 2479
- Phenergan with Codeine ... 2497
- Phenergan with Dextromethorphan 2499
- Phenergan Injection ... 2493
- Phenergan Suppositories ... 2496
- Phenergan Syrup ... 2495
- Phenergan Tablets ... 2496
- Phenergan VC ... 2500
- Phenergan VC with Codeine ... 2501

Propofol (Respiratory depression and hypotension; profound sedation or coma). Products include:
- Diprivan Injection ... 2267

Propoxyphene Hydrochloride (Respiratory depression and hypotension; profound sedation or coma). Products include:
- Darvon ... 1256
- Wygesic Tablets ... 2540

Propoxyphene Napsylate (Respiratory depression and hypotension; profound sedation or coma). Products include:
- Darvon-N/Darvocet-N ... 1254

Protriptyline Hydrochloride (Respiratory depression and hypotension; profound sedation or coma). Products include:
- Vivactil Tablets ... 1567

Quazepam (Respiratory depression and hypotension; profound sedation or coma). Products include:
- Doral Tablets ... 2383

Secobarbital Sodium (Respiratory depression and hypotension; profound sedation or coma). Products include:
- Seconal Sodium Pulvules ... 1296

Selegiline Hydrochloride (Respiratory depression and hypotension; profound sedation or coma). Products include:
- Eldepryl ... 2250

Sufentanil Citrate (Respiratory depression and hypotension; profound sedation or coma). Products include:
- Sufenta Injection ... 1147

Temazepam (Respiratory depression and hypotension; profound sedation or coma). Products include:
- Restoril Capsules ... 2023

Thiamylal Sodium (Respiratory depression and hypotension; profound sedation or coma). Products include:
- Surital Ampoules, Steri-Vials ... 1764

Thioridazine Hydrochloride (Respiratory depression and hypotension; profound sedation or coma). Products include:
- Mellaril ... 2011

Thiothixene (Respiratory depression and hypotension; profound sedation or coma). Products include:
- Navane Capsules and Concentrate 1954
- Navane Intramuscular ... 1956

Tranylcypromine Sulfate (Respiratory depression and hypotension; profound sedation or coma). Products include:
- Parnate Tablets ... 2222

Triazolam (Respiratory depression and hypotension; profound sedation or coma). Products include:
- Halcion Tablets ... 2340

Trifluoperazine Hydrochloride (Respiratory depression and hypotension; profound sedation or coma). Products include:
- Stelazine ... 2226

Trimipramine Maleate (Respiratory depression and hypotension; profound sedation or coma). Products include:
- Surmontil Capsules ... 2524

PANWARFIN TABLETS (Warfarin Sodium) ... 547
May interact with narcotic analgesics, corticosteroids, diuretics, inhalant anesthetics, salicylates, antacids, antihistamines, barbiturates, oral contraceptives, oral hypoglycemic agents, anticonvulsants, androgens, and certain other agents. Compounds in these categories include:

ACTH (Decreased prothrombin time response).

Alcohol (Increased or decreased prothrombin time response).

Alfentanil Hydrochloride (Increased prothrombin time response). Products include:
- Alfenta Injection ... 1131

Allopurinol (Increased prothrombin time response). Products include:
- Zyloprim Tablets ... 830

Aluminum Carbonate Gel (Decreased prothrombin time response). Products include:
- Basaljel ... 2438

Aluminum Hydroxide (Decreased prothrombin time response). Products include:
- Cama Arthritis Pain Reliever ... ▣ 685
- Gaviscon Extra Strength Relief Formula Liquid Antacid ... ▣ 594
- Gaviscon Extra Strength Relief Formula Antacid Tablets ... ▣ 594
- Gaviscon Liquid Antacid ... ▣ 594
- Gelusil Liquid & Tablets ... ▣ 639
- Extra Strength Maalox Plus Suspension ... 1850
- Maalox TC Suspension ... 1851
- Maalox Plus Tablets ... ▣ 655
- Extra Strength Maalox Plus Tablets 1850
- Nephrox Suspension ... ▣ 563
- WinGel Liquid & Tablets ... ▣ 761

Aluminum Hydroxide Gel (Decreased prothrombin time response). Products include:
- ALternaGEL Liquid ... 1154
- Aludrox Oral Suspension ... 2428
- Amphojel Suspension ... 2429
- Amphojel Suspension without Flavor ... 2429
- Mylanta Liquid ... 1155
- Mylanta Double Strength Liquid ... 1155

Aluminum Hydroxide Gel, Dried (Decreased prothrombin time response). Products include:
- Alu-Tab/Alu-Cap ... 1309
- Amphojel Tablets ... 2429
- Ascriptin A/D Caplets ... 1850
- Regular Strength Ascriptin Tablets 1850
- Gaviscon Antacid Tablets ... ▣ 593
- Gaviscon-2 Antacid Tablets ... ▣ 594
- Mylanta Tablets ... 1155
- Mylanta Double Strength Tablets ... 1155

Amiloride Hydrochloride (Increased or decreased prothrombin time response). Products include:
- Midamor Tablets ... 1508
- Moduretic Tablets ... 1510

Aminosalicylic Acid (Increased prothrombin time response).

Amiodarone Hydrochloride (Increased prothrombin time response). Products include:
- Cordarone Tablets ... 2446

Antibiotics, unspecified (Increased prothrombin time response).

Aprobarbital (Decreased prothrombin time response). Products include:
- Alurate Elixir ... 1883

Aspirin (Increased prothrombin time response). Products include:
- Alka-Seltzer Effervescent Antacid and Pain Reliever ... 1568
- Alka-Seltzer Extra Strength Effervescent Antacid and Pain Reliever ... 1570
- Alka-Seltzer (Flavored) Effervescent Antacid and Pain Reliever ... 1569
- Alka-Seltzer Plus Cold Medicine ... ▣ 623
- Alka-Seltzer Plus Night-Time Cold Medicine ... ▣ 623
- Alka Seltzer Plus Sinus Allergy Medicine ... ▣ 624
- Anacin Coated Analgesic Caplets ... 2417
- Anacin Coated Analgesic Tablets ... 2417
- Anacin Maximum Strength Analgesic Coated Tablets ... 2417
- Maximum Strength Arthritis Pain Formula By the Makers of Anacin Analgesic Tablets and Caplets ... 2418
- Arthritis Pain Formula by the Makers of Anacin Analgesic Tablets and Caplets ... ▣ 747
- Arthritis Strength BC Powder ... ▣ 516
- Ascriptin A/D Caplets ... 1850
- Regular Strength Ascriptin Tablets 1850
- Azdone Tablets ... 844
- BC Powder ... ▣ 517
- BC Cold Powder ... ▣ 517
- Children's Bayer Chewable Aspirin ... ▣ 564
- Genuine Bayer Aspirin Tablets & Caplets ... ▣ 564
- Maximum Bayer Aspirin Tablets & Caplets ... ▣ 566
- Bayer Plus Aspirin Tablets ... ▣ 567
- Therapy Bayer Aspirin Caplets ... ▣ 568
- 8 Hour Bayer Timed-Release Aspirin ... ▣ 566
- Arthritis Strength Bufferin Analgesic Caplets ... 744
- Extra Strength Bufferin Analgesic Tablets ... 745
- Bufferin Analgesic Tablets and Caplets ... 743
- Cama Arthritis Pain Reliever ... ▣ 685
- Damason-P ... 1356
- Easprin ... 1719
- Ecotrin Enteric Coated Aspirin Maximum Strength Tablets and Caplets ... 2189
- Ecotrin Enteric Coated Aspirin Regular Strength Tablets and Caplets ... 2189
- Empirin Aspirin ... ▣ 541
- Empirin with Codeine Phosphate Nos. 2, 3 & 4 ... 764
- Equagesic Tablets ... 2451
- Excedrin Extra-Strength Analgesic Tablets & Caplets ... 749
- 4-Way Cold Tablets ... 750
- Fiorinal Capsules ... 2007
- Fiorinal with Codeine Capsules ... 2008
- Fiorinal Tablets ... 2007
- Lortab ASA Tablets ... 2414
- Momentum Muscular Backache Formula ... ▣ 751
- Norgesic ... 1314
- Norwich Extra-Strength Aspirin ... ▣ 546
- Norwich Regular Strength Aspirin ▣ 547
- P-A-C Analgesic Tablets ... ▣ 669
- Percodan ... 951
- Robaxisal Tablets ... 1872
- Sine-Off Sinus Medicine Tablets-Aspirin Formula ... ▣ 722
- Soma Compound w/Codeine Tablets ... 2390
- Soma Compound Tablets ... 2389
- St. Joseph Adult Chewable Aspirin (81 mg.) ... ▣ 703
- Synalgos-DC Capsules ... 2525
- Talwin Compound ... 2072
- Ursinus Inlay-Tabs ... ▣ 691
- Vanquish Analgesic Caplets ... ▣ 574
- Zorprin Tablets ... 698

Astemizole (Decreased prothrombin time response). Products include:
- Hismanal Tablets ... 1138

Azatadine Maleate (Decreased prothrombin time response). Products include:
- Optimine Tablets ... 2115
- Trinalin Repetabs Tablets ... 1170

Bendroflumethiazide (Increased or decreased prothrombin time response). Products include:
- Corzide Tablets ... 702
- Naturetin Tablets ... 1789
- Rauzide Tablets ... 1804

Betamethasone Acetate (Decreased prothrombin time response). Products include:
- Celestone Soluspan Suspension ... 2081

Betamethasone Sodium Phosphate (Decreased prothrombin time response). Products include:
- Celestone Soluspan Suspension ... 2081

Bromelains (Increased prothrombin time response). Products include:
- Bromase Capsules ... 672

Bromodiphenhydramine Hydrochloride (Decreased prothrombin time response).
- No products indexed under this heading.

Brompheniramine Maleate (Decreased prothrombin time response). Products include:
- Alka Seltzer Plus Sinus Allergy Medicine ... ▣ 624
- Atrohist Sprinkle Capsules ... 558
- Bromfed Capsules (Timed Release) ... 1615
- Bromfed Syrup ... ▣ 628
- Bromfed ... 1615
- Dimetane Decongestant ... ▣ 673
- Dimetane ... ▣ 672
- Dimetane-DC Cough Syrup ... 1857
- Dimetane-DX Cough Syrup ... 1858
- Dimetapp Elixir ... ▣ 673
- Dimetapp DM Elixir ... ▣ 674
- Dimetapp Extentabs ... ▣ 674
- Dimetapp Plus Caplets ... ▣ 675
- Dimetapp Tablets ... ▣ 675
- Drixoral Antihistamine/Nasal Decongestant Syrup ... ▣ 698

Bumetanide (Increased or decreased prothrombin time response). Products include:
- Bumex ... 1895

Buprenorphine (Increased prothrombin time response).
- No products indexed under this heading.

Butabarbital (Decreased prothrombin time response). Products include:
- Pyridium Plus ... 1764

Butalbital (Decreased prothrombin time response). Products include:
- Esgic-Plus Tablets ... 1002
- Esgic Tablets & Capsules ... 1001
- Fioricet Tablets ... 2006
- Fiorinal Capsules ... 2007
- Fiorinal with Codeine Capsules ... 2008
- Fiorinal Tablets ... 2007
- Phrenilin ... 838
- Sedapap Tablets 50 mg/650 mg .. 1360

Carbamazepine (Decreased prothrombin time response). Products include:
- Tegretol Chewable Tablets ... 654
- Tegretol Suspension ... 656
- Tegretol Tablets ... 654

Chloramphenicol (Increased prothrombin time response). Products include:
- AK-Chlor Sterile Ophthalmic Ointment & Solution ... ⊙ 201
- Chloromycetin Cream, 1% ... 1694
- Chloromycetin Hydrocortisone Ophthalmic ... 1694
- Chloromycetin Kapseals ... 1695
- Chloromycetin Ophthalmic Ointment, 1% ... 1696
- Chloromycetin Ophthalmic Solution ... 1696
- Chloromycetin Otic ... 1697
- Chloroptic S.O.P. ... ⊙ 243
- Chloroptic Sterile Ophthalmic Solution ... ⊙ 243
- Ophthochlor Ophthalmic Solution ⊙ 300
- Ophthocort ... ⊙ 301

Chloramphenicol Palmitate (Increased prothrombin time response). Products include:
- Chloromycetin Palmitate, Oral Suspension ... 1697

(▣ Described in PDR For Nonprescription Drugs) (⊙ Described in PDR For Ophthalmology)

Chloramphenicol Sodium Succinate (Increased prothrombin time response). Products include:
- Chloromycetin Sodium Succinate 1698

Chlordiazepoxide (Decreased prothrombin time response). Products include:
- Libritabs Tablets 1930
- Limbitrol 1933
- Menrium Tablets 1934

Chlordiazepoxide Hydrochloride (Decreased prothrombin time response). Products include:
- Librax Capsules 1929
- Librium Capsules 1931
- Librium Injectable 1932

Chlorothiazide (Increased or decreased prothrombin time response). Products include:
- Aldoclor Tablets 1413
- Diupres Tablets 1461
- Diuril Oral 1464

Chlorothiazide Sodium (Increased or decreased prothrombin time response). Products include:
- Diuril Sodium Intravenous 1463

Chlorpheniramine Maleate (Decreased prothrombin time response). Products include:
- A.R.M. Allergy Relief Medicine Caplets .... ■ 615
- Alka-Seltzer Plus Cold Medicine .... ■ 623
- Allerest .... ■ 559
- Ana-Kit Anaphylaxis Emergency Treatment Kit 1100
- BC Cold Powder Multi-Symptom Formula .... ■ 517
- Brexin L.A. Capsules 2078
- Cerose-DM 2443
- Cheracol Plus Head Cold/Cough Formula .... ■ 667
- Chlor-Trimeton Allergy Syrup, Tablets & Long-Acting Repetabs Tablets .... ■ 693
- Chlor-Trimeton Decongestant .... ■ 694
- Comhist LA Capsules 1618
- Allergy-Sinus Comtrex Multi-Symptom Allergy Sinus Formula Tablets & Caplets 746
- Comtrex Multi-Symptom Cold Reliever Tablets/Caplets/Liqui-Gels/Liquid 745
- Day-Night Comtrex 747
- Contac Continuous Action Decongestant/Antihistamine Capsules .... ■ 710
- Contac Maximum Strength Continuous Action Decongestant/Antihistamine Caplets .... ■ 709
- Contac Severe Cold and Flu Formula Caplets .... ■ 711
- Coricidin 'D' Decongestant Tablets .... ■ 695
- Coricidin Demilets Tablets for Children .... ■ 696
- Coricidin Tablets .... ■ 695
- Deconamine 663
- Demazin Nasal Decongestant/Antihistamine Repetabs Tablets & Syrup .... ■ 697
- Dorcol Children's Liquid Cold Formula .... ■ 686
- Dristan Decongestant/Antihistamine/ Analgesic Coated Caplets .... ■ 749
- Dristan Cold Nasal Decongestant/Antihistamine/ Analgesic Coated Tablets 2419
- Dristan Advanced Formula Decongestant/Antihistamine/Analgesic Tablets .... ■ 749
- Extendryl 994
- 4-Way Cold Tablets 750
- Fedahist Gyrocaps 2145
- Fedahist Timecaps 2145
- Hycomine Compound Tablets 929
- Isoclor Timesule Capsules .... ■ 561
- Kronofed-A 970
- Medi-Flu Caplet, Liquid .... ■ 640
- Naldecon Syrup, Tablets, Pediatric Drops and Pediatric Syrup 709
- Nolamine Tablets 838
- Novafed A Capsules 1342
- Novahistine DH 1342
- Novahistine Elixir .... ■ 596
- Ornade Spansule Capsules 2221
- Orthoxicol Cough Syrup .... ■ 668
- PediaCare Allergy Relief Formula Liquid 1362
- PediaCare Cough-Cold Formula Liquid 1362
- PediaCare Night Rest Cough-Cold Formula Liquid 1362
- PediaCare 6-12 Cough-Cold Formula Chewable Tablets 1362
- Pyrroxate Capsules .... ■ 669
- Quelidrine Syrup 556
- Ru-Tuss II Capsules 693
- Ru-Tuss Tablets 693
- Ryna .... ■ 741
- Sinarest Tablets & Extra Strength Tablets .... ■ 562
- Sine-Off Maximum Strength Allergy/Sinus Formula Caplets .... ■ 721
- Sine-Off Sinus Medicine Tablets-Aspirin Formula .... ■ 722
- Singlet Tablets .... ■ 598
- Sinulin 840
- Sinutab Maximum Strength .... ■ 641
- St. Joseph Nighttime Cold Medicine .... ■ 705
- Sudafed Plus Liquid .... ■ 544
- Sudafed Plus Tablets .... ■ 545
- Teldrin Timed-Release Allergy Capsules, 12 mg. 2192
- TheraFlu Flu and Cold Medicine .... ■ 687
- Triaminic Allergy Tablets .... ■ 688
- Triaminic Chewables .... ■ 688
- Triaminic Cold Tablets .... ■ 688
- Triaminic Nite Light .... ■ 689
- Triaminic Syrup .... ■ 689
- Triaminic-12 Tablets .... ■ 690
- Triaminicin Tablets .... ■ 690
- Triaminicol Multi-Symptom Cold Tablets .... ■ 691
- Triaminicol Multi-Symptom Relief .... ■ 691
- Tylenol Allergy Sinus Medication Caplets and Gelcaps, Maximum Strength 1372
- Children's Tylenol Cold Liquid Formula and Chewable Tablets 1368
- Tylenol Cold & Flu Hot Medication, Packets 1369
- Tylenol Cold Medication Caplets and Tablets 1370
- Tylenol Cold Medication, Effervescent Tablets 1369
- Vicks Children's NyQuil .... ■ 664
- Vicks Formula 44 Cough Medicine .... ■ 661
- Vicks Formula 44M Multi-Symptom Cough Medicine .... ■ 662
- Vicks Pediatric Formula 44m Multi-Symptom Cough & Cold Medicine .... ■ 663

Chlorpheniramine Polistirex (Decreased prothrombin time response). Products include:
- Tussionex Extended-Release Suspension 988

Chlorpheniramine Preparations (Decreased prothrombin time response).

Chlorpheniramine Tannate (Decreased prothrombin time response). Products include:
- Rynatan 2387
- Rynatuss 2388

Chlorpropamide (Increased prothrombin time response). Products include:
- Diabinese Tablets 1775

Chlorthalidone (Increased or decreased prothrombin time response). Products include:
- Combipres Tablets 678
- Tenoretic Tablets 1105
- Thalitone Tablets 687

Cholestyramine (Decreased prothrombin time response). Products include:
- Cholybar 1705
- Questran Light 711
- Questran Powder 710

Choline Magnesium Trisalicylate (Increased prothrombin time response). Products include:
- Trilisate 1822

Chymotrypsin (Increased prothrombin time response).
- No products indexed under this heading.

Cimetidine (Increased prothrombin time response). Products include:
- Tagamet Tablets 2228

Cimetidine Hydrochloride (Increased prothrombin time response). Products include:
- Tagamet 2228

Cinchophen (Increased prothrombin time response).

Clemastine Fumarate (Decreased prothrombin time response). Products include:
- Tavist Syrup 2033
- Tavist Tablets 2035
- Tavist-D Tablets 2035

Clofibrate (Increased prothrombin time response). Products include:
- Atromid-S Capsules 2435

Codeine (Increased prothrombin time response). Products include:
- Calcidrine Syrup 506

Codeine Phosphate (Increased prothrombin time response). Products include:
- Actifed with Codeine Cough Syrup .. 752
- Cheracol Cough Syrup 1853
- Codimal PH Syrup 846
- Dimetane-DC Cough Syrup 1857
- Empirin with Codeine Phosphate Nos. 2, 3 & 4 764
- Fiorinal with Codeine Capsules 2008
- Isoclor Expectorant 982
- Naldecon CX Adult Liquid .... ■ 521
- Novahistine DH 1342
- Novahistine Expectorant 1343
- Nucofed Capsules 2219
- Nucofed Expectorant 2219
- Nucofed Pediatric Expectorant 2220
- Nucofed Syrup 2219
- Phenaphen with Codeine Capsules 1865
- Phenaphen-650 with Codeine Tablets 1866
- Phenergan with Codeine 2497
- Phenergan VC with Codeine 2501
- Robitussin A-C Syrup 1875
- Robitussin-DAC Syrup 1875
- Ryna .... ■ 741
- Soma Compound w/Codeine Tablets 2390
- Triaminic Expectorant w/Codeine .. 1996
- Tussi-Organidin Liquid 2391
- Tylenol with Codeine 1381

Codeine Polistirex (Increased prothrombin time response).
- No products indexed under this heading.

Cortisone Acetate (Decreased prothrombin time response). Products include:
- Cortone Acetate Sterile Suspension 1437
- Cortone Acetate Tablets 1439

Cyproheptadine Hydrochloride (Decreased prothrombin time response). Products include:
- Periactin 1525

Dexamethasone (Decreased prothrombin time response). Products include:
- AK-Trol Ointment & Suspension .... ⊙ 207
- Decadron Elixir 1445
- Decadron Tablets 1447
- Decaspray Topical Aerosol 1459
- Dexacidin .... ⊙ 272
- Maxidex Sterile Ophthalmic Suspension .... ⊙ 223
- Maxitrol Ophthalmic Ointment/Suspension .... ⊙ 223
- TobraDex Ophthalmic Suspension and Ointment .... ⊙ 228

Dexamethasone Acetate (Decreased prothrombin time response). Products include:
- Dalalone D.P. Injectable 999
- Decadron-LA Sterile Suspension 1457

Dexamethasone Sodium Phosphate (Decreased prothrombin time response). Products include:
- AK-Dex .... ⊙ 203
- Decadron Phosphate Respihaler 1454
- Decadron Phosphate Sterile Ophthalmic Ointment 1453
- Decadron Phosphate Sterile Ophthalmic Solution 1453
- Decadron Phosphate Topical Cream 1455
- Decadron Phosphate Turbinaire 1456
- Maxidex Sterile Ophthalmic Ointment .... ⊙ 222
- NeoDecadron Sterile Ophthalmic Ointment 1517
- NeoDecadron Sterile Ophthalmic Solution 1518
- NeoDecadron Topical Cream 1518

Dexchlorpheniramine Maleate (Decreased prothrombin time response). Products include:
- Polaramine 2116

Dextran 40 (Increased prothrombin time response).
- No products indexed under this heading.

Dextran 70 (Increased prothrombin time response). Products include:
- Hyskon Hysteroscopy Fluid 1162
- Moisture Drops .... ⊙ 258
- Tears Naturale II 572

Dextrothyroxine Sodium (Increased prothrombin time response).
- No products indexed under this heading.

Dezocine (Increased prothrombin time response).

Diazoxide (Increased prothrombin time response). Products include:
- Hyperstat I.V. Injection 2095
- Proglycem 649

Diflunisal (Increased prothrombin time response). Products include:
- Dolobid Tablets 1465

Dihydroxyaluminum Sodium Carbonate (Decreased prothrombin time response). Products include:
- Rolaids .... ■ 743

Diphenhydramine Citrate (Decreased prothrombin time response). Products include:
- Alka-Seltzer Plus Night-Time Cold Medicine .... ■ 623
- Bufferin AF Nite Time Analgesic/Sleeping Aid Caplets 744
- Excedrin P.M. Analgesic/Sleeping Aid Tablets, Caplets and Liquid 749

Diphenhydramine Hydrochloride (Decreased prothrombin time response). Products include:
- Benadryl Anti-Itch Cream .... ■ 635
- Benadryl Capsules 1691
- Benadryl Decongestant Elixir .... ■ 635
- Benadryl Decongestant .... ■ 635
- Benadryl Elixir .... ■ 636
- Benadryl Kapseals 1691
- Benadryl 25 Kapseals .... ■ 636
- Benadryl Parenteral 1692
- Benadryl Plus .... ■ 636
- Benadryl Plus Nighttime .... ■ 637
- Benadryl Spray, Maximum Strength .... ■ 637
- Benadryl Spray, Regular Strength .... ■ 637
- Benadryl Steri-Vials, Ampoules, and Steri-Dose Syringe 1692
- Benadryl 25 Tablets .... ■ 636
- Benylin Cough Syrup .... ■ 637
- Benylin Decongestant .... ■ 638
- Caladryl Cream, Lotion, Spray .... ■ 638
- Miles Nervine Nighttime Sleep-Aid .... ■ 627
- Nytol Tablets .... ■ 517
- Sleep-ettes-D Tablets .... ■ 653
- Sleep-eze 3 Tablets .... ■ 755
- Sleepinal Night-time Sleep Aid Capsules .... ■ 734
- Sominex Caplets and Tablets .... ■ 722
- Sominex Liquid .... ■ 723
- Sominex Pain Relief Formula .... ■ 723
- Tylenol Cold Night Time Medication Liquid 1371
- Tylenol PM, Extra Strength Caplets and Tablets 1368
- Unisom Dual Relief Nighttime Sleep Aid/Analgesic 1774
- Ziradryl Lotion .... ■ 643

Diphenylpyraline Hydrochloride (Decreased prothrombin time response).
No products indexed under this heading.

Disulfiram (Increased prothrombin time response). Products include:
Antabuse Tablets ... 2429

Divalproex Sodium (Accumulation of anticonvulsants). Products include:
Depakote ... 512

Enflurane (Increased prothrombin time response). Products include:
Ethrane ... 599

Ethacrynic Acid (Increased or decreased prothrombin time response). Products include:
Edecrin Tablets ... 1468

Ethchlorvynol (Decreased prothrombin time response). Products include:
Placidyl Capsules ... 553

Ethinyl Estradiol (Decreased prothrombin time response). Products include:
Brevicon ... 2304
Demulen ... 2161
Estinyl Tablets ... 2085
Jenest-28 Tablets ... 1636
Levlen/Tri-Levlen ... 665
Lo/Ovral Tablets ... 2471
Lo/Ovral-28 Tablets ... 2476
Loestrin ... 1728
Modicon ... 1667
Nordette-21 Tablets ... 2481
Nordette-28 Tablets ... 2483
Norethin ... 2133
Norinyl ... 2304
Norlestrin ... 1746
Ortho-Cyclen Tablets ... 1658
Ortho-Novum ... 1667
Ovcon ... 1391
Ovral Tablets ... 2490
Ovral-28 Tablets ... 2491
Levlen/Tri-Levlen ... 665
Tri-Norinyl ... 2304
Triphasil-21 Tablets ... 2527
Triphasil-28 Tablets ... 2532

Ethosuximide (Accumulation of anticonvulsants). Products include:
Zarontin Capsules ... 1768
Zarontin Syrup ... 1769

Ethotoin (Accumulation of anticonvulsants). Products include:
Peganone Tablets ... 551

Ethynodiol Diacetate (Decreased prothrombin time response). Products include:
Demulen ... 2161

Fenoprofen Calcium (Increased prothrombin time response). Products include:
Nalfon Pulvules & Tablets ... 919

Fentanyl (Increased prothrombin time response). Products include:
Duragesic Transdermal System ... 1133

Fentanyl Citrate (Increased prothrombin time response). Products include:
Innovar Injection ... 1141
Sublimaze Injection ... 1146

Fluoxymesterone (Increased prothrombin time response). Products include:
Halotestin Tablets ... 2341

Furosemide (Increased or decreased prothrombin time response). Products include:
Lasix ... 1093

Glipizide (Accumulation of hypoglycemics). Products include:
Glucotrol ... 1952

Glucagon (Increased prothrombin time response). Products include:
Glucagon for Injection Vials and Emergency Kit ... 1263

Glutethimide (Decreased prothrombin time response).
No products indexed under this heading.

Glyburide (Accumulation of hypoglycemics). Products include:
DiaBeta ... 1091
Micronase Tablets ... 2350

Griseofulvin (Decreased prothrombin time response). Products include:
Fulvicin P/G Tablets ... 2090
Fulvicin P/G 165 & 330 Tablets ... 2091
Fulvicin-U/F Tablets ... 2092
Grifulvin V (griseofulvin microsize) Tablets/Suspension ... 1678
Grisactin ... 2454
Grisactin Ultra Tablets ... 2455
Gris-PEG Tablets, 125 mg & 250 mg ... 1083

Haloperidol (Decreased prothrombin time response). Products include:
Haldol Injection, Tablets and Concentrate ... 1373

Haloperidol Decanoate (Decreased prothrombin time response). Products include:
Haldol Decanoate ... 1375

Halothane (Increased prothrombin time response). Products include:
Fluothane ... 2453

Heparin Sodium (Affects prothrombin time). Products include:
Heparin Lock Flush Solution ... 2456
Heparin Sodium Vials ... 1264
Heparin Sodium Injection ... 2457
Heparin Sodium Injection, USP, Sterile Solution ... 2342

Hydrochlorothiazide (Increased or decreased prothrombin time response). Products include:
Aldactazide ... 2150
Aldoril Tablets ... 1418
Apresazide Capsules ... 854
Apresoline-Esidrix Tablets ... 857
Capozide ... 2258
Dyazide Capsules ... 2208
Esidrix Tablets ... 863
Esimil Tablets ... 864
HydroDIURIL Tablets ... 1484
Hydropres Tablets ... 1485
Inderide Tablets ... 2463
Inderide LA Long Acting Capsules ... 2465
Lopressor HCT Tablets ... 1034
Maxzide ... 1215
Moduretic Tablets ... 1510
Normozide Tablets ... 2112
Oretic Tablets ... 544
Oreticyl ... 545
Prinzide Tablets ... 1540
Ser-Ap-Es Tablets ... 881
Serpasil-Esidrix Tablets ... 886
Timolide Tablets ... 1547
Trandate HCT Tablets ... 579
Vaseretic Tablets ... 1559
Zestoretic ... 2274

Hydrocodone Bitartrate (Increased prothrombin time response). Products include:
Anexsia 5/500 Tablets ... 2196
Anexsia 7.5/650 Tablets ... 2197
Azdone Tablets ... 844
Codiclear DH Syrup ... 845
Codimal DH Syrup ... 846
Damason-P ... 1356
Hycodan Syrup, Tablets ... 927
Hycomine Compound Tablets ... 929
Hycomine Syrup ... 927
Hycotuss Expectorant Syrup ... 930
Hydrocet Capsules ... 835
Lortab ASA Tablets ... 2414
Lortab ... 2412
Ru-Tuss with Hydrocodone ... 694
Triaminic Expectorant DH ... 1995
Vicodin Tablets ... 1187
Vicodin ES Tablets ... 1189
Zydone Capsules ... 941

Hydrocodone Polistirex (Increased prothrombin time response). Products include:
Tussionex Extended-Release Suspension ... 988

Hydrocortisone (Decreased prothrombin time response). Products include:
AK-Spore H.C. ... ◉ 206
Bactine Hydrocortisone Anti-Itch Cream ... ▣ 625
CaldeCORT Anti-Itch Hydrocortisone Spray ... ▣ 560
Carmol HC Cream 1% ... 2296
Cortaid Spray ... ▣ 735
Cortenema ... 2244
Cortisporin Ointment ... 758
Cortisporin Ophthalmic Ointment Sterile ... 758
Cortisporin Ophthalmic Suspension Sterile ... 759
Cortisporin Otic Solution Sterile ... 760
Cortisporin Otic Suspension Sterile ... 760
Cortizone-5 Creme & Ointment ... ▣ 732
Dermolate Anti-Itch Cream ... ▣ 697
Eldecort Cream 1.0% ... 1113
Eldecort Cream 1.0% and 2.5% ... 1113
Fungoid HC Creme ... 1770
Hydrocortone Tablets ... 1482
Hytone ... 909
LazerSporin-C Solution ... 1770
Massengill Medicated Soft Cloth Towelettes ... 2192
Nutracort Cream & Lotion ... 1684
PediOtic Suspension Sterile ... 797
Synacort Creams 1%, 2.5% ... 2296
Vanoxide-HC Acne Lotion ... 911
Vioform-Hydrocortisone Cream and Mild Cream ... 889
Vioform-Hydrocortisone Ointment ... 889
VōSoL HC Otic Solution ... 2392
Vytone Cream 1% ... 911

Hydrocortisone Acetate (Decreased prothrombin time response). Products include:
Analpram-HC Rectal Cream 1% and 2.5% ... 970
Anusol-HC Cream ... 1690
Anusol-HC Suppositories ... 1691
Caldecort ... ▣ 560
Carmol HC Cream 1% ... 2296
Chloromycetin Hydrocortisone Ophthalmic ... 1694
Coly-Mycin S Otic w/Neomycin & Hydrocortisone ... 1708
Cortaid ... ▣ 735
Cortef Feminine Itch Cream ... ▣ 735
Corticaine ... ▣ 682
Cortifoam ... 1827
Cortisporin Cream ... 757
Epifoam ... 1828
Gynecort 5 Creme ... ▣ 556
Hydrocortone Acetate Sterile Suspension ... 1479
Lanacort 5 Creme and Ointment ... ▣ 557
Mantadil Cream ... 789
Ophthocort ... ◉ 301
Orabase HCA Oral Paste ... 890
Pramosone Cream, Lotion & Ointment ... 971
ProctoCream-HC ... 1834
Proctofoam-HC ... 1835

Hydrocortisone Sodium Phosphate (Decreased prothrombin time response). Products include:
Hydrocortone Phosphate Injection, Sterile ... 1481

Hydrocortisone Sodium Succinate (Decreased prothrombin time response). Products include:
Solu-Cortef Sterile Powder ... 2361

Hydroflumethiazide (Increased or decreased prothrombin time response). Products include:
Diucardin Tablets ... 2450
Saluron ... 718
Salutensin/Salutensin-Demi ... 719

Ibuprofen (Increased prothrombin time response). Products include:
Advil Cold & Sinus Caplets (formerly CoAdvil) ... 2416
Advil Ibuprofen Tablets and Caplets ... 2416
Children's Advil Suspension ... 2426
CoAdvil ... ▣ 748
Dristan Sinus Caplets ... 2419
Haltran Tablets ... ▣ 668
Ibuprofen ... ▣ 631
Medipren ibuprofen Caplets and Tablets ... 1362
Midol 200 Cramp Relief Formula ... ▣ 570
Motrin Tablets ... 2351
Motrin IB Caplets and Tablets ... ▣ 736
Nuprin Ibuprofen/Analgesic Tablets & Caplets ... 752
PediaProfen Suspension ... 1363
Rufen Tablets ... 691
Trendar Ibuprofen Tablets ... ▣ 756

Indapamide (Increased or decreased prothrombin time). Products include:
Lozol Tablets ... 1843

Indomethacin (Increased prothrombin time response). Products include:
Indocin ... 1487

Indomethacin Sodium Trihydrate (Increased prothrombin time response). Products include:
Indocin I.V. ... 1490

Influenza Virus Vaccine (Increased prothrombin time response). Products include:
Flu-Imune Influenza Virus Vaccine ... 1204

Isoflurane (Increased prothrombin time response). Products include:
Forane ... 600

Levonorgestrel (Decreased prothrombin time response). Products include:
Levlen/Tri-Levlen ... 665
Nordette-21 Tablets ... 2481
Nordette-28 Tablets ... 2483
Norplant System ... 2484
Levlen/Tri-Levlen ... 665
Triphasil-21 Tablets ... 2527
Triphasil-28 Tablets ... 2532

Levorphanol Tartrate (Increased prothrombin time response). Products include:
Levo-Dromoran ... 1906

Magaldrate (Decreased prothrombin time response). Products include:
Riopan Antacid Chew Tablets ... ▣ 754
Riopan Antacid Chew Tablets in Rollpacks ... ▣ 754
Riopan Antacid Suspension ... 2421
Riopan Antacid Swallow Tablets ... 2421
Riopan Plus Chew Tablets ... 2422
Riopan Plus Chew Tablets in Rollpack ... 2422
Riopan Plus 2 Chew Tablets, Mint Flavor, Cherry Flavor ... 2422
Riopan Plus Suspension ... 2422
Riopan Plus 2 Suspension, Mint Flavor, Cherry Flavor ... 2422

Magnesium Hydroxide (Decreased prothrombin time response). Products include:
Aludrox Oral Suspension ... 2428
Ascriptin A/D Caplets ... 1850
Regular Strength Ascriptin Tablets ... 1850
Di-Gel Antacid/Anti-Gas ... ▣ 697
Gelusil Liquid & Tablets ... ▣ 639
Haley's M-O, Regular & Flavored ... ▣ 569
Extra Strength Maalox Plus Suspension ... 1850
Maalox TC Suspension ... 1851
Maalox Plus Tablets ... ▣ 655
Extra Strength Maalox Plus Tablets ... 1850
Mylanta Liquid ... 1155
Mylanta Tablets ... 1155
Mylanta Double Strength Liquid ... 1155
Mylanta Double Strength Tablets ... 1155
Concentrated Phillips' Milk of Magnesia ... ▣ 573
Phillips' Milk of Magnesia Liquid ... ▣ 572
Phillips' Milk of Magnesia Tablets ... ▣ 573
WinGel Liquid & Tablets ... ▣ 761

Magnesium Oxide (Decreased prothrombin time response). Products include:
Bayer Plus Aspirin Tablets ... ▣ 567
Beelith Tablets ... 659
Bufferin Analgesic Tablets and Caplets ... ▣ 524
Cama Arthritis Pain Reliever ... ▣ 685
Mag-Ox 400 ... 673
Uro-Mag ... 673

Magnesium Salicylate (Increased prothrombin time response). Products include:
Doan's - Extra-Strength Analgesic ... ▣ 549
Doan's - Regular Strength Analgesic ... ▣ 549

(▣ Described in PDR For Nonprescription Drugs)

(◉ Described in PDR For Ophthalmology)

Mobigesic Analgesic Tablets ▣ 507

Mefenamic Acid (Increased prothrombin time response). Products include:
Ponstel 1758

Meperidine Hydrochloride (Increased prothrombin time response). Products include:
Demerol 2047
Mepergan Injection 2479

Mephenytoin (Accumulation of anticonvulsants). Products include:
Mesantoin Tablets 2013

Mephobarbital (Decreased prothrombin time response). Products include:
Mebaral Tablets 2061

Meprobamate (Decreased prothrombin time response). Products include:
Deprol Tablets 2382
Equagesic Tablets 2451
Miltown Tablets 2386
PMB 200 and PMB 400 2504

Mestranol (Decreased prothrombin time response). Products include:
Enovid 2161
Norethin 2133
Norinyl 2304
Ortho-Novum 1667

Methadone Hydrochloride (Increased prothrombin time response). Products include:
Dolophine Hydrochloride Ampoules & Vials 1260
Dolophine Hydrochloride Tablets 1261
Methadone Hydrochloride Diskets 1284
Methadone Hydrochloride Oral Solution & Tablets 1987

Methdilazine Hydrochloride (Decreased prothrombin time response). Products include:
Tacaryl Syrup & Tablets 2409

Methoxyflurane (Increased prothrombin time response).
No products indexed under this heading.

Methsuximide (Accumulation of anticonvulsants). Products include:
Celontin 1692

Methyclothiazide (Increased or decreased prothrombin time response). Products include:
Enduron Tablets 517
Enduronyl 518

Methyldopa (Increased prothrombin time response). Products include:
Aldoclor Tablets 1413
Aldomet Oral 1415
Aldoril Tablets 1418

Methyldopate Hydrochloride (Increased prothrombin time response). Products include:
Aldomet Ester HCl Injection 1417

Methylphenidate Hydrochloride (Increased prothrombin time response). Products include:
Ritalin 880

Methylprednisolone Acetate (Decreased prothrombin time response). Products include:
Depo-Medrol Sterile Aqueous Suspension 2334

Methylprednisolone Sodium Succinate (Decreased prothrombin time response). Products include:
Solu-Medrol Sterile Powder 2363

Methyltestosterone (Increased prothrombin time response). Products include:
Android 1111
Estratest 2245
Mediatric Capsules 2476
Metandren Linguets and Tablets 875
Premarin with Methyltestosterone 2515
Testred Capsules 1124

Methylthiouracil (Increased prothrombin time response).

Metolazone (Increased or decreased prothrombin time response). Products include:
Diulo 2129
Mykrox ½ mg Tablets 984
Zaroxolyn Tablets 989

Metronidazole (Increased prothrombin time response). Products include:
Flagyl I.V. RTU 2131
Flagyl Tablets 2170
MetroGel 903
Protostat Tablets 1674

Miconazole (Increased prothrombin time response). Products include:
Monistat I.V. 1143

Morphine Sulfate (Increased prothrombin time response). Products include:
Astramorph/PF Injection, USP (Preservative-Free) 618
Duramorph 960
Infumorph 200 and Infumorph 500 Sterile Solutions 962
MS Contin Tablets 1814
MSIR 1817
Oramorph SR (Morphine Sulfate Sustained Release Tablets) 1988
Roxanol 1991

Nalidixic Acid (Increased prothrombin time response). Products include:
NegGram 2062

Naproxen (Increased prothrombin time response). Products include:
Naprosyn 2297

Norethindrone (Decreased prothrombin time response). Products include:
Brevicon 2304
Jenest-28 Tablets 1636
Micronor Tablets 1667
Modicon 1667
Norethin 2133
Norinyl 2304
Norlutin 1755
Nor-Q D Tablets 2304
Ortho-Novum 1667
Ovcon 1391
Tri-Norinyl 2304

Norethynodrel (Decreased prothrombin time response). Products include:
Enovid 2161

Norgestimate (Decreased prothrombin time response). Products include:
Ortho-Cyclen Tablets 1658

Norgestrel (Decreased prothrombin time response). Products include:
Lo/Ovral Tablets 2471
Lo/Ovral-28 Tablets 2476
Ovral Tablets 2490
Ovral-28 Tablets 2491
Ovrette Tablets 2492

Nortriptyline Hydrochloride (Increased prothrombin time response). Products include:
Pamelor 2019

Opium Alkaloids (Increased prothrombin time response). Products include:
B & O No. 15A & No. 16A Supprettes 2395
Pantopon Injectable 1911

Oxandrolone (Increased prothrombin time response).
No products indexed under this heading.

Oxolinic Acid (Increased prothrombin time response).

Oxycodone Hydrochloride (Increased prothrombin time response). Products include:
Percocet Tablets 950
Percodan 951
Roxicodone Tablets, Oral Solution & Intensol (Oxycodone) 1992
Tylox Capsules 1382

Oxymetholone (Increased prothrombin time response). Products include:
Anadrol-50 Tablets 2287

Oxyphenbutazone (Increased prothrombin time response).

Paraldehyde (Decreased prothrombin time response).

Paramethadione (Accumulation of anticonvulsants). Products include:
Paradione Capsules 548

Pentobarbital Sodium (Decreased prothrombin time response). Products include:
Nembutal Sodium Capsules 534
Nembutal Sodium Solution 536
Nembutal Sodium Suppositories 538

Pentoxifylline (Increased prothrombin time response). Products include:
Trental 1099

Phenacemide (Accumulation of anticonvulsants). Products include:
Phenurone Tablets 552

Phenobarbital (Decreased prothrombin time response). Products include:
Arco-Lase Plus Tablets 607
Bellergal-S Tablets 1998
Bronkolixir ▣ 761
Bronkotabs Tablets ▣ 762
Donnatal 1858
Donnatal Extentabs 1859
Donnatal Tablets 1858
Donnazyme Tablets 1860
Kinesed Tablets 2272
Phenobarbital Elixir and Tablets 1293
Primatene Tablets-P Formula 2421
Quadrinal Tablets 1183
Tedral SA 1765

Phensuximide (Accumulation of anticonvulsants). Products include:
Milontin Kapseals 1741

Phenylbutazone (Increased prothrombin time response). Products include:
Butazolidin Capsules & Tablets 1027

Phenytoin (Accumulation of anticonvulsants). Products include:
Dilantin Infatabs 1710
Dilantin-30 Pediatric/Dilantin-125 Suspension 1713

Phenytoin Sodium (Accumulation of anticonvulsants). Products include:
Dilantin Kapseals 1708
Dilantin Parenteral 1712
Dilantin with Phenobarbital Kapseals 1715

Polythiazide (Increased or decreased prothrombin time). Products include:
Minizide Capsules 1779
Renese Tablets 1785
Renese-R Tablets 1786

Prednisolone Acetate (Decreased prothrombin time response). Products include:
AK-Cide Sterile Ophthalmic Ointment & Suspension ◎ 202
Blephamide Liquifilm Sterile Ophthalmic Suspension 586
Blephamide S.O.P. Sterile Ophthalmic Ointment 586
Cetapred Ointment ◎ 220
⅛% Econopred & 1% Econopred Plus ◎ 217
Isopto Cetapred Suspension ◎ 220
Metimyd ◎ 306
Poly-Pred Liquifilm ◎ 250
Pred Forte ◎ 252
Pred Mild ◎ 254
Pred-G Liquifilm Sterile Ophthalmic Suspension ◎ 252
Pred-G S.O.P. Sterile Ophthalmic Ointment ◎ 253
Vasocidin Ointment ◎ 275

Prednisolone Sodium Phosphate (Decreased prothrombin time response). Products include:
AK-Pred ◎ 205
Hydeltrasol Injection, Sterile 1476
Inflamase ◎ 274
Pediapred Oral Liquid 987
Vasocidin Ophthalmic Solution ◎ 276

Prednisolone Tebutate (Decreased prothrombin time response). Products include:
Hydeltra-T.B.A. Sterile Suspension 1478

Prednisone (Decreased prothrombin time response). Products include:
Deltasone Tablets 2332

Primidone (Accumulation of anticonvulsants). Products include:
Mysoline 2480

Promethazine Hydrochloride (Decreased prothrombin time response). Products include:
Mepergan Injection 2479
Phenergan with Codeine 2497
Phenergan with Dextromethorphan 2499
Phenergan Injection 2493
Phenergan Suppositories 2496
Phenergan Syrup 2495
Phenergan Tablets 2496
Phenergan VC 2500
Phenergan VC with Codeine 2501

Propoxyphene Hydrochloride (Increased prothrombin time response). Products include:
Darvon 1256
Wygesic Tablets 2540

Propoxyphene Napsylate (Increased prothrombin time response). Products include:
Darvon-N/Darvocet-N 1254

Propylthiouracil (Increased prothrombin time response).
No products indexed under this heading.

Pyrilamine Maleate (Decreased prothrombin time response). Products include:
Codimal 846
4-Way Fast Acting Nasal Spray - Original Formula (regular & mentholated) & Metered Spray Pump (regular) 751
Maximum Strength Midol Multi-Symptom Menstrual Formula ▣ 571
Maximum Strength Midol PMS Premenstrual Syndrome Formula ▣ 570
Regular Strength Midol Multi-Symptom Menstrual Formula ▣ 570
Prefrin-A ◎ 255
Prēmsyn PMS Capsules & Caplets ▣ 547
Primatene Tablets-M Formula 2421
Robitussin Night Relief ▣ 677
Ru-Tuss with Hydrocodone 694
Triaminic Expectorant DH 1995
Triaminic Oral Infant Drops 1996

Pyrilamine Tannate (Decreased prothrombin time response). Products include:
Rynatan 2387

Quinidine Gluconate (Increased prothrombin time response). Products include:
Quinaglute Dura-Tabs Tablets 663

Quinidine Polygalacturonate (Increased prothrombin time response). Products include:
Cardioquin Tablets 1812

Quinidine Sulfate (Increased prothrombin time response). Products include:
Quinidex Extentabs 1868

Quinine (Increased prothrombin time response).

Ranitidine Hydrochloride (Increased or decreased prothrombin time response). Products include:
Zantac Injection and Zantac Injection Premixed 1063
Zantac 1065

(▣ Described in PDR For Nonprescription Drugs)

(◎ Described in PDR For Ophthalmology)

Rifampin (Decreased prothrombin time response). Products include:

Rifadin ... 1345
Rifamate Capsules ... 1347
Rimactane Capsules ... 879

Salsalate (Increased prothrombin time response). Products include:

Disalcid ... 1310
Mono-Gesic Tablets ... 846
Salflex ... 839

Secobarbital Sodium (Decreased prothrombin time response). Products include:

Seconal Sodium Pulvules ... 1296

Sodium Bicarbonate (Decreased prothrombin time response). Products include:

Alka-Seltzer Advanced Formula Antacid & Non-Aspirin Pain Reliever ... ◘ 620
Alka-Seltzer Effervescent Antacid ◘ 622
Alka-Seltzer Effervescent Antacid and Pain Reliever ... 1568
Alka-Seltzer Extra Strength Effervescent Antacid and Pain Reliever ... ◘ 623
Alka-Seltzer (Flavored) Effervescent Antacid and Pain Reliever .. ◘ 621
Arm & Hammer Pure Baking Soda ... ◘ 548
Ceo-Two Rectal Suppositories ... 671
Citrocarbonate Antacid ... ◘ 668
Massengill Liquid Concentrate ... 2191
NuLYTELY ... 699

Spironolactone (Increased or decreased prothrombin time response). Products include:

Aldactazide ... 2150
Aldactone ... 2152

Stanozolol (Increased prothrombin time response). Products include:

Winstrol Tablets ... 2075

Sufentanil Citrate (Increased prothrombin time response). Products include:

Sufenta Injection ... 1147

Sulfinpyrazone (Increased prothrombin time response). Products include:

Anturane ... 853

Sulindac (Increased prothrombin time response). Products include:

Clinoril Tablets ... 1433

Terfenadine (Decreased prothrombin time response). Products include:

Seldane Tablets ... 1349
Seldane-D Extended-Release Tablets ... 1350

Thiamylal Sodium (Decreased prothrombin time response). Products include:

Surital Ampoules, Steri-Vials ... 1764

Thyroid (Increased prothrombin time response). Products include:

S-P-T "Liquid" Capsules ... 995

Tolazamide (Accumulation of anticonvulsants). Products include:

Tolinase Tablets ... 2365

Tolbutamide (Increased prothrombin time response). Products include:

Orinase Tablets ... 2354

Triamcinolone (Decreased prothrombin time response).

No products indexed under this heading.

Triamcinolone Acetonide (Decreased prothrombin time response). Products include:

Aristocort A ... 1010
Azmacort Inhaler ... 1837
Kenalog Cream, Lotion & Ointment 2401
Kenalog-10 Injection ... 2402
Kenalog-40 Injection ... 2403
Kenalog in Orabase ... 604
Kenalog Spray ... 2401
Mycolog II Cream and Ointment ... 2407
Mytrex Cream & Ointment ... 2080
Nasacort Nasal Inhaler ... 1844

Triamcinolone Diacetate (Decreased prothrombin time response). Products include:

Aristocort Suspension ... 1008

Triamcinolone Hexacetonide (Decreased prothrombin time response). Products include:

Aristospan Suspension ... 1011

Triamterene (Increased or decreased prothrombin time). Products include:

Dyazide Capsules ... 2208
Dyrenium Capsules ... 2210
Maxzide ... 1215

Trimeprazine Tartrate (Decreased prothrombin time response). Products include:

Temaril Tablets, Syrup and Spansule Sustained Release Capsules 1085

Trimethadione (Accumulation of anticonvulsants). Products include:

Tridione ... 557

Trimethoprim (Increased prothrombin time response). Products include:

Bactrim DS Tablets ... 1891
Bactrim I.V. Infusion ... 1889
Bactrim ... 1891
Proloprim Tablets ... 799
Septra ... 813
Septra I.V. Infusion ... 808
Septra I.V. Infusion ADD-Vantage Vials ... 810
Septra ... 813
Trimpex Tablets ... 1922

Tripelennamine Preparations (Decreased prothrombin time response).

Triprolidine Hydrochloride (Decreased prothrombin time response). Products include:

Actidil ... ◘ 538
Actifed Capsules ... ◘ 539
Actifed Plus Caplets ... ◘ 539
Actifed Plus Tablets ... ◘ 540
Actifed with Codeine Cough Syrup.. 752
Actifed Syrup ... ◘ 540
Actifed Tablets ... ◘ 540
Actifed 12-Hour Capsules ... ◘ 539

Valproic Acid (Accumulation of anticonvulsants). Products include:

Depakene Capsules & Syrup ... 511

Vitamin C (Decreased prothrombin time response). Products include:

Allbee with C Caplets ... ◘ 670
Allbee C-800 ... ◘ 670
Bromase Capsules ... 672
Bugs Bunny Children's Chewable Vitamins (Sugar Free) ... ◘ 625
Bugs Bunny With Extra C Children's Chewable Vitamins (Sugar Free) ... ◘ 626
Bugs Bunny Plus Iron Children's Chewable Vitamins (Sugar Free) ◘ 625
Cefol Filmtab ... 509
Centrum, Jr. (Children's Chewable) + Extra C ... ◘ 585
Cod Liver Oil Concentrate Tablets with Vitamin C ... ◘ 694
Ester-C Tablets ... ◘ 575
Ferancee Chewable Tablets ... 1155
Ferancee-HP Tablets ... 1155
Fero-Folic-500 Filmtab ... 527
Fero-Grad-500 Filmtab ... 528
Flintstones Children's Chewable Vitamins ... ◘ 625
Flintstones Children's Chewable Vitamins With Extra C ... ◘ 626
Flintstones Children's Chewable Vitamins Plus Iron ... ◘ 625
Halls Vitamin C Drops ... ◘ 742
Hyland's Vitamin C for Children ... ◘ 729
ICAPS Plus ... ⊙ 280
Mediatric Capsules ... 2476
Mol-Iron w/Vitamin C Tablets ... ◘ 703
Natalins Rx ... 1391
Natalins Tablets ... 1391
N'ICE Sugarless Vitamin C Drops.. ◘ 719
Niferex w/Vitamin C Tablets ... 847
Ocuvite Vitamin and Mineral Supplement ... ⊙ 312
One-A-Day Essential Vitamins ... ◘ 627
One-A-Day Maximum Formula Vitamins and Minerals ... ◘ 627
One-A-Day Plus Extra C Vitamins .. ◘ 627
Probec-T Tablets ... ◘ 581
Stressgard Stress Formula Vitamins ... ◘ 628
STUART PRENATAL Tablets ... ◘ 731
The Stuart Formula Tablets ... 1157
Stuartinic Tablets ... 1157
Sunkist Children's Chewable Multivitamins - Plus Extra C ... ◘ 553
Sunkist Vitamin C ... ◘ 553
Surbex with C ... ◘ 502
Trinsicon Capsules ... 2415
Tri-Vi-Flor 1.0 mg Vitamins with Fluoride Chewable Tablets ... 1400
Tri-Vi-Flor Drops ... 1400
Tri-Vi-Sol Vitamin Drops ... ◘ 614
Tri-Vi-Sol Vitamin Drops with Iron ◘ 614
Vicon Forte Capsules ... 2416
Vicon Plus ... ◘ 682
Vicon-C ... ◘ 682
Vi-Daylin ADC Vitamins Drops ... 1980
Vi-Daylin ADC Vitamins + Iron Drops ... 1980
Vi-Daylin/F ADC Vitamins Drops With Fluoride ... 1981
Vi-Daylin/F ADC Vitamins + Iron Drops With Fluoride ... 1981
Vi-Zac ... ◘ 682
Within Women's Formula Multivitamin with Calcium, Extra Iron and Zinc ... ◘ 628
Z-Bec Tablets ... ◘ 678

Food Interactions

Diet high in vitamin K (Decreased prothrombin time response).

PAPAVERINE HYDROCHLORIDE VIALS AND AMPOULES

(Papaverine Hydrochloride) ... 1290
No interactions described in labeling.

PAPLEX

(Salicylic Acid, Lactic Acid) ... 1410
No interactions described in labeling.

PAPLEX ULTRA

(Salicylic Acid) ... 1410
No interactions described in labeling.

PARADIONE CAPSULES

(Paramethadione) ... 548
May interact with:

Concurrent therapy with drugs known to cause toxic effects similar to those of the oxazolidinediones should be avoided or used with extreme caution ().

PARAFLEX CAPLETS

(Chlorzoxazone) ... 1378
May interact with central nervous system depressants and certain other agents. Compounds in these categories include:

Alcohol (May produce additive effect).

Alfentanil Hydrochloride (May produce additive effect). Products include:

Alfenta Injection ... 1131

Alprazolam (May produce additive effect). Products include:

Xanax Tablets ... 2367

Aprobarbital (May produce additive effect). Products include:

Alurate Elixir ... 1883

Buprenorphine (May produce additive effect).

No products indexed under this heading.

Buspirone Hydrochloride (May produce additive effect). Products include:

BuSpar ... 1401

Butabarbital (May produce additive effect). Products include:

Pyridium Plus ... 1764

Butalbital (May produce additive effect). Products include:

Esgic-Plus Tablets ... 1002
Esgic Tablets & Capsules ... 1001
Fioricet Tablets ... 2006
Fiorinal Capsules ... 2007
Fiorinal with Codeine Capsules ... 2008
Fiorinal Tablets ... 2007
Phrenilin ... 838
Sedapap Tablets 50 mg/650 mg .. 1360

Chlordiazepoxide (May produce additive effect). Products include:

Libritabs Tablets ... 1930
Limbitrol ... 1933
Menrium Tablets ... 1934

Chlordiazepoxide Hydrochloride (May produce additive effect). Products include:

Librax Capsules ... 1929
Librium Capsules ... 1931
Librium Injectable ... 1932

Chlorpromazine (May produce additive effect). Products include:

Thorazine ... 2234

Chlorprothixene (May produce additive effect). Products include:

Taractan Tablets ... 1920

Chlorprothixene Hydrochloride (May produce additive effect). Products include:

Taractan ... 1920

Chlorprothixene Lactate (May produce additive effect). Products include:

Taractan Concentrate ... 1920

Clorazepate Dipotassium (May produce additive effect). Products include:

Tranxene ... 556

Codeine (May produce additive effect). Products include:

Calcidrine Syrup ... 506

Codeine Phosphate (May produce additive effect). Products include:

Actifed with Codeine Cough Syrup.. 752
Cheracol Cough Syrup ... 1853
Codimal PH Syrup ... 846
Dimetane-DC Cough Syrup ... 1857
Empirin with Codeine Phosphate Nos. 2, 3 & 4 ... 764
Fiorinal with Codeine Capsules ... 2008
Isoclor Expectorant ... 982
Naldecon CX Adult Liquid ... ◘ 521
Novahistine DH ... 1342
Novahistine Expectorant ... 1343
Nucofed Capsules ... 2219
Nucofed Expectorant ... 2219
Nucofed Pediatric Expectorant ... 2220
Nucofed Syrup ... 2219
Phenaphen with Codeine Capsules 1865
Phenaphen-650 with Codeine Tablets ... 1866
Phenergan with Codeine ... 2497
Phenergan VC with Codeine ... 2501
Robitussin A-C Syrup ... 1875
Robitussin-DAC Syrup ... 1875
Ryna ... ◘ 741
Soma Compound w/Codeine Tablets ... 2390
Triaminic Expectorant w/Codeine .. 1996
Tussi-Organidin Liquid ... 2391
Tylenol with Codeine ... 1381

Codeine Polistirex (May produce additive effect).

No products indexed under this heading.

Dezocine (May produce additive effect).

Diazepam (May produce additive effect). Products include:

Valium Injectable ... 1937
Valium Tablets ... 1939
Valrelease Capsules ... 1923

Droperidol (May produce additive effect). Products include:

Inapsine Injection ... 1140
Innovar Injection ... 1141

Enflurane (May produce additive effect). Products include:

Ethrane ... 599

Estazolam (May produce additive effect). Products include:

ProSom Tablets ... 554

(◘ Described in PDR For Nonprescription Drugs)

(⊙ Described in PDR For Ophthalmology)

Ethchlorvynol (May produce additive effect). Products include:
- Placidyl Capsules ... 553

Ethinamate (May produce additive effect).
- No products indexed under this heading.

Fentanyl (May produce additive effect). Products include:
- Duragesic Transdermal System ... 1133

Fentanyl Citrate (May produce additive effect). Products include:
- Innovar Injection ... 1141
- Sublimaze Injection ... 1146

Fluphenazine Decanoate (May produce additive effect). Products include:
- Prolixin Decanoate ... 1795

Fluphenazine Enanthate (May produce additive effect). Products include:
- Prolixin Enanthate ... 1796

Fluphenazine Hydrochloride (May produce additive effect). Products include:
- Prolixin Elixir ... 1793
- Prolixin Injection ... 1791
- Prolixin Oral Concentrate ... 1792
- Prolixin Tablets ... 1793

Flurazepam Hydrochloride (May produce additive effect). Products include:
- Dalmane Capsules ... 1927

Glutethimide (May produce additive effect).
- No products indexed under this heading.

Haloperidol (May produce additive effect). Products include:
- Haldol Injection, Tablets and Concentrate ... 1373

Haloperidol Decanoate (May produce additive effect). Products include:
- Haldol Decanoate ... 1375

Hydrocodone Bitartrate (May produce additive effect). Products include:
- Anexsia 5/500 Tablets ... 2196
- Anexsia 7.5/650 Tablets ... 2197
- Azdone Tablets ... 844
- Codiclear DH Syrup ... 845
- Codimal DH Syrup ... 846
- Damason-P ... 1356
- Hycodan Syrup, Tablets ... 927
- Hycomine Compound Tablets ... 929
- Hycomine Syrup ... 927
- Hycotuss Expectorant Syrup ... 930
- Hydrocet Capsules ... 835
- Lortab ASA Tablets ... 2414
- Lortab ... 2412
- Ru-Tuss with Hydrocodone ... 694
- Triaminic Expectorant DH ... 1995
- Vicodin Tablets ... 1187
- Vicodin ES Tablets ... 1189
- Zydone Capsules ... 941

Hydrocodone Polistirex (May produce additive effect). Products include:
- Tussionex Extended-Release Suspension ... 988

Hydroxyzine Hydrochloride (May produce additive effect). Products include:
- Atarax Tablets & Syrup ... 1941
- Marax Tablets & DF Syrup ... 1954
- Vistaril Intramuscular Solution ... 1970

Isoflurane (May produce additive effect). Products include:
- Forane ... 600

Ketamine Hydrochloride (May produce additive effect). Products include:
- Ketalar ... 1726

Levorphanol Tartrate (May produce additive effect). Products include:
- Levo-Dromoran ... 1906

Lorazepam (May produce additive effect). Products include:
- Ativan Injection ... 2432
- Ativan Tablets ... 2434

Loxapine Hydrochloride (May produce additive effect). Products include:
- Loxitane ... 1213

Loxapine Succinate (May produce additive effect). Products include:
- Loxitane Capsules ... 1213

Meperidine Hydrochloride (May produce additive effect). Products include:
- Demerol ... 2047
- Mepergan Injection ... 2479

Mephobarbital (May produce additive effect). Products include:
- Mebaral Tablets ... 2061

Meprobamate (May produce additive effect). Products include:
- Deprol Tablets ... 2382
- Equagesic Tablets ... 2451
- Miltown Tablets ... 2386
- PMB 200 and PMB 400 ... 2504

Mesoridazine (May produce additive effect). Products include:
- Serentil ... 686

Methadone Hydrochloride (May produce additive effect). Products include:
- Dolophine Hydrochloride Ampoules & Vials ... 1260
- Dolophine Hydrochloride Tablets ... 1261
- Methadone Hydrochloride Diskets ... 1284
- Methadone Hydrochloride Oral Solution & Tablets ... 1987

Methohexital Sodium (May produce additive effect). Products include:
- Brevital Sodium Vials ... 1248

Methoxyflurane (May produce additive effect).
- No products indexed under this heading.

Midazolam Hydrochloride (May produce additive effect). Products include:
- Versed Injection ... 1924

Molindone Hydrochloride (May produce additive effect). Products include:
- Moban Tablets & Concentrate ... 932

Morphine Sulfate (May produce additive effect). Products include:
- Astramorph/PF Injection, USP (Preservative-Free) ... 618
- Duramorph ... 960
- Infumorph 200 and Infumorph 500 Sterile Solutions ... 962
- MS Contin Tablets ... 1814
- MSIR ... 1817
- Oramorph SR (Morphine Sulfate Sustained Release Tablets) ... 1988
- Roxanol ... 1991

Opium Alkaloids (May produce additive effect). Products include:
- B & O No. 15A & No. 16A Supprettes ... 2395
- Pantopon Injectable ... 1911

Oxazepam (May produce additive effect). Products include:
- Serax Capsules ... 2522
- Serax Tablets ... 2522

Oxycodone Hydrochloride (May produce additive effect). Products include:
- Percocet Tablets ... 950
- Percodan ... 951
- Roxicodone Tablets, Oral Solution & Intensol (Oxycodone) ... 1992
- Tylox Capsules ... 1382

Pentobarbital Sodium (May produce additive effect). Products include:
- Nembutal Sodium Capsules ... 534
- Nembutal Sodium Solution ... 536
- Nembutal Sodium Suppositories ... 538

Perphenazine (May produce additive effect). Products include:
- Etrafon ... 2087
- Triavil Tablets ... 1556
- Trilafon ... 2123

Phenobarbital (May produce additive effect). Products include:
- Arco-Lase Plus Tablets ... 607
- Bellergal-S Tablets ... 1998
- Bronkolixir ... ▣ 761
- Bronkotabs Tablets ... ▣ 762
- Donnatal ... 1858
- Donnatal Extentabs ... 1859
- Donnatal Tablets ... 1858
- Donnazyme Tablets ... 1860
- Kinesed Tablets ... 2272
- Phenobarbital Elixir and Tablets ... 1293
- Primatene Tablets-P Formula ... 2421
- Quadrinal Tablets ... 1183
- Tedral SA ... 1765

Prazepam (May produce additive effect). Products include:
- Centrax ... 1693

Prochlorperazine (May produce additive effect). Products include:
- Compazine ... 2201

Promethazine Hydrochloride (May produce additive effect). Products include:
- Mepergan Injection ... 2479
- Phenergan with Codeine ... 2497
- Phenergan with Dextromethorphan ... 2499
- Phenergan Injection ... 2493
- Phenergan Suppositories ... 2496
- Phenergan Syrup ... 2495
- Phenergan Tablets ... 2496
- Phenergan VC ... 2500
- Phenergan VC with Codeine ... 2501

Propofol (May produce additive effect). Products include:
- Diprivan Injection ... 2267

Propoxyphene Hydrochloride (May produce additive effect). Products include:
- Darvon ... 1256
- Wygesic Tablets ... 2540

Propoxyphene Napsylate (May produce additive effect). Products include:
- Darvon-N/Darvocet-N ... 1254

Quazepam (May produce additive effect). Products include:
- Doral Tablets ... 2383

Secobarbital Sodium (May produce additive effect). Products include:
- Seconal Sodium Pulvules ... 1296

Sufentanil Citrate (May produce additive effect). Products include:
- Sufenta Injection ... 1147

Temazepam (May produce additive effect). Products include:
- Restoril Capsules ... 2023

Thiamylal Sodium (May produce additive effect). Products include:
- Surital Ampoules, Steri-Vials ... 1764

Thioridazine Hydrochloride (May produce additive effect). Products include:
- Mellaril ... 2011

Thiothixene (May produce additive effect). Products include:
- Navane Capsules and Concentrate ... 1954
- Navane Intramuscular ... 1956

Triazolam (May produce additive effect). Products include:
- Halcion Tablets ... 2340

Trifluoperazine Hydrochloride (May produce additive effect). Products include:
- Stelazine ... 2226

PARAFON FORTE DSC CAPLETS
(Chlorzoxazone) ... 1379

May interact with central nervous system depressants and certain other agents. Compounds in these categories include:

Alcohol (May produce additive effect).

Alfentanil Hydrochloride (May produce additive effect). Products include:
- Alfenta Injection ... 1131

Alprazolam (May produce additive effect). Products include:
- Xanax Tablets ... 2367

Aprobarbital (May produce additive effect). Products include:
- Alurate Elixir ... 1883

Buprenorphine (May produce additive effect).
- No products indexed under this heading.

Buspirone Hydrochloride (May produce additive effect). Products include:
- BuSpar ... 1401

Butabarbital (May produce additive effect). Products include:
- Pyridium Plus ... 1764

Butalbital (May produce additive effect). Products include:
- Esgic-Plus Tablets ... 1002
- Esgic Tablets & Capsules ... 1001
- Fioricet Tablets ... 2006
- Fiorinal Capsules ... 2007
- Fiorinal with Codeine Capsules ... 2008
- Fiorinal Tablets ... 2007
- Phrenilin ... 838
- Sedapap Tablets 50 mg/650 mg ... 1360

Chlordiazepoxide (May produce additive effect). Products include:
- Libritabs Tablets ... 1930
- Limbitrol ... 1933
- Menrium Tablets ... 1934

Chlordiazepoxide Hydrochloride (May produce additive effect). Products include:
- Librax Capsules ... 1929
- Librium Capsules ... 1931
- Librium Injectable ... 1932

Chlorpromazine (May produce additive effect). Products include:
- Thorazine ... 2234

Chlorprothixene (May produce additive effect). Products include:
- Taractan Tablets ... 1920

Chlorprothixene Hydrochloride (May produce additive effect). Products include:
- Taractan ... 1920

Clorazepate Dipotassium (May produce additive effect). Products include:
- Tranxene ... 556

Codeine (May produce additive effect). Products include:
- Calcidrine Syrup ... 506

Codeine Phosphate (May produce additive effect). Products include:
- Actifed with Codeine Cough Syrup ... 752
- Cheracol Cough Syrup ... 1853
- Codimal PH Syrup ... 846
- Dimetane-DC Cough Syrup ... 1857
- Empirin with Codeine Phosphate Nos. 2, 3 & 4 ... 764
- Fiorinal with Codeine Capsules ... 2008
- Isoclor Expectorant ... 982
- Naldecon CX Adult Liquid ... ▣ 521
- Novahistine DH ... 1342
- Novahistine Expectorant ... 1343
- Nucofed Capsules ... 2219
- Nucofed Expectorant ... 2219
- Nucofed Pediatric Expectorant ... 2220
- Nucofed Syrup ... 2219
- Phenaphen with Codeine Capsules ... 1865
- Phenaphen-650 with Codeine Tablets ... 1866
- Phenergan with Codeine ... 2497
- Phenergan VC with Codeine ... 2501
- Robitussin A-C Syrup ... 1875
- Robitussin-DAC Syrup ... 1875
- Ryna ... ▣ 741
- Soma Compound w/Codeine Tablets ... 2390

Triaminic Expectorant w/Codeine .. 1996
Tussi-Organidin Liquid 2391
Tylenol with Codeine 1381

Codeine Polistirex (May produce additive effect).
No products indexed under this heading.

Dezocine (May produce additive effect).

Diazepam (May produce additive effect). Products include:
Valium Injectable 1937
Valium Tablets 1939
Valrelease Capsules 1923

Droperidol (May produce additive effect). Products include:
Inapsine Injection 1140
Innovar Injection 1141

Enflurane (May produce additive effect). Products include:
Ethrane 599

Estazolam (May produce additive effect). Products include:
ProSom Tablets 554

Ethchlorvynol (May produce additive effect). Products include:
Placidyl Capsules 553

Ethinamate (May produce additive effect).
No products indexed under this heading.

Fentanyl (May produce additive effect). Products include:
Duragesic Transdermal System 1133

Fentanyl Citrate (May produce additive effect). Products include:
Innovar Injection 1141
Sublimaze Injection 1146

Fluphenazine Decanoate (May produce additive effect). Products include:
Prolixin Decanoate 1795

Fluphenazine Enanthate (May produce additive effect). Products include:
Prolixin Enanthate 1796

Fluphenazine Hydrochloride (May produce additive effect). Products include:
Prolixin Elixir 1793
Prolixin Injection 1791
Prolixin Oral Concentrate 1792
Prolixin Tablets 1793

Flurazepam Hydrochloride (May produce additive effect). Products include:
Dalmane Capsules 1927

Glutethimide (May produce additive effect).
No products indexed under this heading.

Haloperidol (May produce additive effect). Products include:
Haldol Injection, Tablets and Concentrate 1373

Haloperidol Decanoate (May produce additive effect). Products include:
Haldol Decanoate 1375

Hydrocodone Bitartrate (May produce additive effect). Products include:
Anexsia 5/500 Tablets 2196
Anexsia 7.5/650 Tablets 2197
Azdone Tablets 844
Codiclear DH Syrup 845
Codimal DH Syrup 846
Damason-P 1356
Hycodan Syrup, Tablets 927
Hycomine Compound Tablets 929
Hycomine Syrup 927
Hycotuss Expectorant Syrup 930
Hydrocet Capsules 835
Lortab ASA Tablets 2414
Lortab 2412
Ru-Tuss with Hydrocodone 694
Triaminic Expectorant DH 1995
Vicodin Tablets 1187
Vicodin ES Tablets 1189
Zydone Capsules 941

Hydrocodone Polistirex (May produce additive effect). Products include:
Tussionex Extended-Release Suspension 988

Hydroxyzine Hydrochloride (May produce additive effect). Products include:
Atarax Tablets & Syrup 1941
Marax Tablets & DF Syrup 1954
Vistaril Intramuscular Solution 1970

Isoflurane (May produce additive effect). Products include:
Forane 600

Ketamine Hydrochloride (May produce additive effect). Products include:
Ketalar 1726

Levorphanol Tartrate (May produce additive effect). Products include:
Levo-Dromoran 1906

Lorazepam (May produce additive effect). Products include:
Ativan Injection 2432
Ativan Tablets 2434

Loxapine Hydrochloride (May produce additive effect). Products include:
Loxitane 1213

Loxapine Succinate (May produce additive effect). Products include:
Loxitane Capsules 1213

Meperidine Hydrochloride (May produce additive effect). Products include:
Demerol 2047
Mepergan Injection 2479

Mephobarbital (May produce additive effect). Products include:
Mebaral Tablets 2061

Meprobamate (May produce additive effect). Products include:
Deprol Tablets 2382
Equagesic Tablets 2451
Miltown Tablets 2386
PMB 200 and PMB 400 2504

Mesoridazine (May produce additive effect). Products include:
Serentil 686

Methadone Hydrochloride (May produce additive effect). Products include:
Dolophine Hydrochloride Ampoules & Vials 1260
Dolophine Hydrochloride Tablets 1261
Methadone Hydrochloride Diskets .. 1284
Methadone Hydrochloride Oral Solution & Tablets 1987

Methohexital Sodium (May produce additive effect). Products include:
Brevital Sodium Vials 1248

Methoxyflurane (May produce additive effect).
No products indexed under this heading.

Midazolam Hydrochloride (May produce additive effect). Products include:
Versed Injection 1924

Molindone Hydrochloride (May produce additive effect). Products include:
Moban Tablets & Concentrate 932

Morphine Sulfate (May produce additive effect). Products include:
Astramorph/PF Injection, USP (Preservative-Free) 618
Duramorph 960
Infumorph 200 and Infumorph 500 Sterile Solutions 962
MS Contin Tablets 1814
MSIR 1817
Oramorph SR (Morphine Sulfate Sustained Release Tablets) 1988
Roxanol 1991

Opium Alkaloids (May produce additive effect). Products include:
B & O No. 15A & No. 16A Supprettes 2395
Pantopon Injectable 1911

Oxazepam (May produce additive effect). Products include:
Serax Capsules 2522
Serax Tablets 2522

Oxycodone Hydrochloride (May produce additive effect). Products include:
Percocet Tablets 950
Percodan 951
Roxicodone Tablets, Oral Solution & Intensol (Oxycodone) 1992
Tylox Capsules 1382

Pentobarbital Sodium (May produce additive effect). Products include:
Nembutal Sodium Capsules 534
Nembutal Sodium Solution 536
Nembutal Sodium Suppositories 538

Perphenazine (May produce additive effect). Products include:
Etrafon 2087
Triavil Tablets 1556
Trilafon 2123

Phenobarbital (May produce additive effect). Products include:
Arco-Lase Plus Tablets 607
Bellergal-S Tablets 1998
Bronkolixir ...... ▣ 761
Bronkotabs Tablets ...... ▣ 762
Donnatal 1858
Donnatal Extentabs 1859
Donnatal Tablets 1858
Donnazyme Tablets 1860
Kinesed Tablets 2272
Phenobarbital Elixir and Tablets 1293
Primatene Tablets-P Formula 2421
Quadrinal Tablets 1183
Tedral SA 1765

Prazepam (May produce additive effect). Products include:
Centrax 1693

Prochlorperazine (May produce additive effect). Products include:
Compazine 2201

Promethazine Hydrochloride (May produce additive effect). Products include:
Mepergan Injection 2479
Phenergan with Codeine 2497
Phenergan with Dextromethorphan 2499
Phenergan Injection 2493
Phenergan Suppositories 2496
Phenergan Syrup 2495
Phenergan Tablets 2496
Phenergan VC 2500
Phenergan VC with Codeine 2501

Propofol (May produce additive effect). Products include:
Diprivan Injection 2267

Propoxyphene Hydrochloride (May produce additive effect). Products include:
Darvon 1256
Wygesic Tablets 2540

Propoxyphene Napsylate (May produce additive effect). Products include:
Darvon-N/Darvocet-N 1254

Quazepam (May produce additive effect). Products include:
Doral Tablets 2383

Secobarbital Sodium (May produce additive effect). Products include:
Seconal Sodium Pulvules 1296

Sufentanil Citrate (May produce additive effect). Products include:
Sufenta Injection 1147

Temazepam (May produce additive effect). Products include:
Restoril Capsules 2023

Thiamylal Sodium (May produce additive effect). Products include:
Surital Ampoules, Steri-Vials 1764

Thioridazine Hydrochloride (May produce additive effect). Products include:
Mellaril 2011

Thiothixene (May produce additive effect). Products include:
Navane Capsules and Concentrate 1954
Navane Intramuscular 1956

Triazolam (May produce additive effect). Products include:
Halcion Tablets 2340

Trifluoperazine Hydrochloride (May produce additive effect). Products include:
Stelazine 2226

PARAGARD T380A INTRAUTERINE COPPER CONTRACEPTIVE
(Intrauterine device) 411
May interact with anticoagulants and corticosteroids. Compounds in these categories include:

Betamethasone Acetate (Monitor carefully for infection following insertion). Products include:
Celestone Soluspan Suspension 2081

Betamethasone Sodium Phosphate (Monitor carefully for infection following insertion). Products include:
Celestone Soluspan Suspension 2081

Cortisone Acetate (Monitor carefully for infection following insertion). Products include:
Cortone Acetate Sterile Suspension 1437
Cortone Acetate Tablets 1439

Dexamethasone (Monitor carefully for infection following insertion). Products include:
AK-Trol Ointment & Suspension ...... ◉ 207
Decadron Elixir 1445
Decadron Tablets 1447
Decaspray Topical Aerosol 1459
Dexacidin ...... ◉ 272
Maxidex Sterile Ophthalmic Suspension ...... ◉ 223
Maxitrol Ophthalmic Ointment/Suspension ...... ◉ 223
TobraDex Ophthalmic Suspension and Ointment ...... ◉ 228

Dexamethasone Acetate (Monitor carefully for infection following insertion). Products include:
Dalalone D.P. Injectable 999
Decadron-LA Sterile Suspension 1457

Dexamethasone Sodium Phosphate (Monitor carefully for infection following insertion). Products include:
AK-Dex ...... ◉ 203
Decadron Phosphate Respihaler 1454
Decadron Phosphate Sterile Ophthalmic Ointment 1453
Decadron Phosphate Sterile Ophthalmic Solution 1453
Decadron Phosphate Topical Cream 1455
Decadron Phosphate Turbinaire 1456
Maxidex Sterile Ophthalmic Ointment ...... ◉ 222
NeoDecadron Sterile Ophthalmic Ointment 1517
NeoDecadron Sterile Ophthalmic Solution 1518
NeoDecadron Topical Cream 1518

Dicumarol (Greater risk of menorrhagia or hypermenorrhea). Products include:
Dicumarol Tablets 516

Heparin Calcium (Greater risk of menorrhagia or hypermenorrhea). Products include:
Calciparine Injection 925

Heparin Sodium (Greater risk of menorrhagia or hypermenorrhea). Products include:
Heparin Lock Flush Solution 2456
Heparin Sodium Vials 1264
Heparin Sodium Injection 2457

(▣ Described in PDR For Nonprescription Drugs)
(◉ Described in PDR For Ophthalmology)

Heparin Sodium Injection, USP, Sterile Solution ... 2342

Hydrocortisone (Monitor carefully for infection following insertion). Products include:

AK-Spore H.C. ... ◉ 206
Bactine Hydrocortisone Anti-Itch Cream ... ▣ 625
CaldeCORT Anti-Itch Hydrocortisone Spray ... ▣ 560
Carmol HC Cream 1% ... 2296
Cortaid Spray ... ▣ 735
Cortenema ... 2244
Cortisporin Ointment ... 758
Cortisporin Ophthalmic Ointment Sterile ... 758
Cortisporin Ophthalmic Suspension Sterile ... 759
Cortisporin Otic Solution Sterile ... 760
Cortisporin Otic Suspension Sterile 760
Cortizone-5 Creme & Ointment ... ▣ 732
Dermolate Anti-Itch Cream ... ▣ 697
Eldecort Cream 1.0% ... 1113
Eldecort Cream 1.0% and 2.5% ... 1113
Fungoid HC Creme ... 1770
Hydrocortone Tablets ... 1482
Hytone ... 909
LazerSporin-C Solution ... 1770
Massengill Medicated Soft Cloth Towelettes ... 2192
Nutracort Cream & Lotion ... 1684
PediOtic Suspension Sterile ... 797
Synacort Creams 1%, 2.5% ... 2296
Vanoxide-HC Acne Lotion ... 911
Vioform-Hydrocortisone Cream and Mild Cream ... 889
Vioform-Hydrocortisone Ointment .. 889
VōSoL HC Otic Solution ... 2392
Vytone Cream 1% ... 911

Hydrocortisone Acetate (Monitor carefully for infection following insertion). Products include:

Analpram-HC Rectal Cream 1% and 2.5% ... 970
Anusol-HC Cream ... 1690
Anusol-HC Suppositories ... 1691
Caldecort ... ▣ 560
Carmol HC Cream 1% ... 2296
Chloromycetin Hydrocortisone Ophthalmic ... 1694
Coly-Mycin S Otic w/Neomycin & Hydrocortisone ... 1708
Cortaid ... ▣ 735
Cortef Feminine Itch Cream ... ▣ 735
Corticaine ... ▣ 682
Cortifoam ... 1827
Cortisporin Cream ... 757
Epifoam ... 1828
Gynecort 5 Creme ... ▣ 556
Hydrocortone Acetate Sterile Suspension ... 1479
Lanacort 5 Creme and Ointment .. ▣ 557
Mantadil Cream ... 789
Ophthocort ... ◉ 301
Orabase HCA Oral Paste ... 890
Pramosone Cream, Lotion & Ointment ... 971
ProctoCream-HC ... 1834
Proctofoam-HC ... 1835

Hydrocortisone Sodium Phosphate (Monitor carefully for infection following insertion). Products include:

Hydrocortone Phosphate Injection, Sterile ... 1481

Hydrocortisone Sodium Succinate (Monitor carefully for infection following insertion). Products include:

Solu-Cortef Sterile Powder ... 2361

Methylprednisolone Acetate (Monitor carefully for infection following insertion). Products include:

Depo-Medrol Sterile Aqueous Suspension ... 2334

Methylprednisolone Sodium Succinate (Monitor carefully for infection following insertion). Products include:

Solu-Medrol Sterile Powder ... 2363

Prednisolone Acetate (Monitor carefully for infection following insertion). Products include:

AK-Cide Sterile Ophthalmic Ointment & Suspension ... ◉ 202
Blephamide Liquifilm Sterile Ophthalmic Suspension ... 586
Blephamide S.O.P. Sterile Ophthalmic Ointment ... 586
Cetapred Ointment ... ◉ 220
⅛% Econopred & 1% Econopred Plus ... ◉ 217
Isopto Cetapred Suspension ... ◉ 220
Metimyd ... ◉ 306
Poly-Pred Liquifilm ... ◉ 250
Pred Forte ... ◉ 252
Pred Mild ... ◉ 254
Pred-G Liquifilm Sterile Ophthalmic Suspension ... ◉ 252
Pred-G S.O.P. Sterile Ophthalmic Ointment ... ◉ 253
Vasocidin Ointment ... ◉ 275

Prednisolone Sodium Phosphate (Monitor carefully for infection following insertion). Products include:

AK-Pred ... ◉ 205
Hydeltrasol Injection, Sterile ... 1476
Inflamase ... ◉ 274
Pediapred Oral Liquid ... 987
Vasocidin Ophthalmic Solution ... ◉ 276

Prednisolone Tebutate (Monitor carefully for infection following insertion). Products include:

Hydeltra-T.B.A. Sterile Suspension 1478

Prednisone (Monitor carefully for infection following insertion). Products include:

Deltasone Tablets ... 2332

Triamcinolone (Monitor carefully for infection following insertion).

No products indexed under this heading.

Triamcinolone Acetonide (Monitor carefully for infection following insertion). Products include:

Aristocort A ... 1010
Azmacort Inhaler ... 1837
Kenalog Cream, Lotion & Ointment 2401
Kenalog-10 Injection ... 2402
Kenalog-40 Injection ... 2403
Kenalog in Orabase ... 604
Kenalog Spray ... 2401
Mycolog II Cream and Ointment ... 2407
Mytrex Cream & Ointment ... 2080
Nasacort Nasal Inhaler ... 1844

Triamcinolone Diacetate (Monitor carefully for infection following insertion). Products include:

Aristocort Suspension ... 1008

Triamcinolone Hexacetonide (Monitor carefully for infection following insertion). Products include:

Aristospan Suspension ... 1011

Warfarin Sodium (Greater risk of menorrhagia or hypermenorrhea). Products include:

Coumadin Injection & Tablets ... 944
Panwarfin Tablets ... 547

PARAPLATIN FOR INJECTION
(Carboplatin) ... 735
May interact with aminoglycosides and certain other agents. Compounds in these categories include:

Amikacin Sulfate (Concomitant treatment has resulted in increased renal and/or audiologic toxicity). Products include:

Amikin Injectable ... 602

Gentamicin Sulfate (Concomitant treatment has resulted in increased renal and/or audiologic toxicity). Products include:

Garamycin Injectable ... 2093
Garamycin Ophthalmic ... ◉ 305
Genoptic Liquifilm Sterile Ophthalmic Solution ... ◉ 247
Genoptic S.O.P. Sterile Ophthalmic Ointment ... ◉ 247
Gentacidin Ointment ... ◉ 273
Gentacidin Solution ... ◉ 273
Gentak Ointment & Solution ... ◉ 208
G-myticin Creme and Ointment 0.1% ... 1770
Pred-G Liquifilm Sterile Ophthalmic Suspension ... ◉ 252
Pred-G S.O.P. Sterile Ophthalmic Ointment ... ◉ 253

Kanamycin Sulfate (Concomitant treatment has resulted in increased renal and/or audiologic toxicity). Products include:

Kantrex Injection ... 601
Kantrex Pediatric Injection ... 601

Nephrotoxic Drugs (Renal effects may be potentiated).

Streptomycin Sulfate (Concomitant treatment has resulted in increased renal and/or audiologic toxicity).

No products indexed under this heading.

Tobramycin (Concomitant treatment has resulted in increased renal and/or audiologic toxicity). Products include:

TobraDex Ophthalmic Suspension and Ointment ... ◉ 228
Tobrex Ophthalmic Ointment and Solution ... 572

Tobramycin Sulfate (Concomitant treatment has resulted in increased renal and/or audiologic toxicity). Products include:

Nebcin Vials, Hyporets & ADD-Vantage ... 1286

PARLODEL CAPSULES
(Bromocriptine Mesylate) ... 2020
May interact with dopamine antagonists, butyrophenones, and certain other agents. Compounds in these categories include:

Chlorpromazine (Decrease in efficacy of Parlodel). Products include:

Thorazine ... 2234

Clozapine (Decrease in efficacy of Parlodel). Products include:

Clozaril Tablets ... 2000

Dihydroergotamine Mesylate (Concomitant use is not recommended). Products include:

D.H.E. 45 Injection ... 2003

Ergoloid Mesylates (Concomitant use is not recommended). Products include:

Hydergine ... 2010

Ergotamine Tartrate (Concomitant use is not recommended). Products include:

Bellergal-S Tablets ... 1998
Cafergot/Cafergot P-B ... 1999
Ergostat ... 1719
Medihaler Ergotamine Aerosol ... 1312
Wigraine Tablets & Suppositories .. 1645

Fluphenazine Decanoate (Decrease in efficacy of Parlodel). Products include:

Prolixin Decanoate ... 1795

Fluphenazine Enanthate (Decrease in efficacy of Parlodel). Products include:

Prolixin Enanthate ... 1796

Fluphenazine Hydrochloride (Decrease in efficacy of Parlodel). Products include:

Prolixin Elixir ... 1793
Prolixin Injection ... 1791
Prolixin Oral Concentrate ... 1792
Prolixin Tablets ... 1793

Haloperidol (Decrease in efficacy of Parlodel). Products include:

Haldol Injection, Tablets and Concentrate ... 1373

Haloperidol Decanoate (Decrease in efficacy of Parlodel). Products include:

Haldol Decanoate ... 1375

Mesoridazine (Decrease in efficacy of Parlodel). Products include:

Serentil ... 686

Methysergide Maleate (Concomitant use is not recommended). Products include:

Sansert Tablets ... 2031

Metoclopramide Hydrochloride (Decrease in efficacy of Parlodel). Products include:

Reglan ... 1869

Perphenazine (Decrease in efficacy of Parlodel). Products include:

Etrafon ... 2087
Triavil Tablets ... 1556
Trilafon ... 2123

Pimozide (Decrease in efficacy of Parlodel). Products include:

Orap Tablets ... 1020

Promethazine Hydrochloride (Decrease in efficacy of Parlodel). Products include:

Mepergan Injection ... 2479
Phenergan with Codeine ... 2497
Phenergan with Dextromethorphan 2499
Phenergan Injection ... 2493
Phenergan Suppositories ... 2496
Phenergan Syrup ... 2495
Phenergan Tablets ... 2496
Phenergan VC ... 2500
Phenergan VC with Codeine ... 2501

Thioridazine Hydrochloride (Decrease in efficacy of Parlodel). Products include:

Mellaril ... 2011

Trifluoperazine Hydrochloride (Decrease in efficacy of Parlodel). Products include:

Stelazine ... 2226

PARLODEL SNAPTABS
(Bromocriptine Mesylate) ... 2020
See **Parlodel Capsules**

PARNATE TABLETS
(Tranylcypromine Sulfate) ... 2222
May interact with monoamine oxidase inhibitors, dibenzazepines, tricyclic antidepressants, sympathomimetic aerosol brochodilators, antihypertensives, phenothiazines, insulin, oral hypoglycemic agents, narcotic analgesics, antihistamines, general anesthetics, anticholinergic-type antiparkinsonism drugs, central nervous system depressants, diuretics, hypnotics and sedatives, alpha adrenergic stimulants, phenylpropanolamine containing anorectics, anorexiants, and certain other agents. Compounds in these categories include:

Acebutolol Hydrochloride (Contraindicated; potentiated). Products include:

Sectral Capsules ... 2520

Albuterol (Contraindicated; hypertension, headache and related symptoms precipitated). Products include:

Proventil Inhalation Aerosol ... 2117
Ventolin Inhalation Aerosol and Refill ... 583

Albuterol Sulfate (Contraindicated; hypertension, headache and related symptoms precipitated). Products include:

Proventil Repetabs Tablets ... 2120
Proventil Solutions for Inhalation 0.5% and 0.083% ... 2118
Proventil Syrup ... 2119
Proventil Tablets ... 2120
Ventolin ... 583

Alcohol (Contraindicated; potentiated).

Alfentanil Hydrochloride (Contraindicated; potentiated). Products include:

Alfenta Injection ... 1131

Alprazolam (Contraindicated; potentiated). Products include:

Xanax Tablets ... 2367

Amitriptyline Hydrochloride (Contraindicated; hypertensive crises; severe convulsive seizures). Products include:
- Elavil ... 2269
- Endep Tablets ... 1927
- Etrafon ... 2087
- Limbitrol ... 1933
- Triavil Tablets ... 1556

Amoxapine (Contraindicated; hypertensive crises; severe convulsive seizures). Products include:
- Asendin Tablets ... 1196

Amphetamine Resins (Combined use contraindicated). Products include:
- Biphetamine Capsules ... 973

Aprobarbital (Contraindicated; potentiated). Products include:
- Alurate Elixir ... 1883

Astemizole (Contraindicated). Products include:
- Hismanal Tablets ... 1138

Atenolol (Contraindicated; potentiated). Products include:
- Tenoretic Tablets ... 1105
- Tenormin Tablets and I.V. Injection 1107

Azatadine Maleate (Contraindicated). Products include:
- Optimine Tablets ... 2115
- Trinalin Repetabs Tablets ... 1170

Benazepril Hydrochloride (Contraindicated; potentiated). Products include:
- Lotensin Tablets ... 872

Bendroflumethiazide (Contraindicated; potentiated). Products include:
- Corzide Tablets ... 702
- Naturetin Tablets ... 1789
- Rauzide Tablets ... 1804

Benzphetamine Hydrochloride (Combined use contraindicated). Products include:
- Didrex Tablets ... 2338

Benztropine Mesylate (Combined use contraindicated; severe reactions reported). Products include:
- Cogentin ... 1435

Betaxolol Hydrochloride (Contraindicated; potentiated). Products include:
- Betoptic Sterile Ophthalmic Solution ... 569
- Betoptic S Sterile Ophthalmic Suspension ... 570
- Kerlone Tablets ... 2172

Biperiden (Combined use contraindicated; severe reactions reported). Products include:
- Akineton ... 1171

Brompheniramine Maleate (Contraindicated). Products include:
- Alka Seltzer Plus Sinus Allergy Medicine ... ▣ 624
- Atrohist Sprinkle Capsules ... 558
- Bromfed Capsules (Timed Release) ... 1615
- Bromfed Syrup ... ▣ 628
- Bromfed ... 1615
- Dimetane Decongestant ... ▣ 673
- Dimetane ... ▣ 672
- Dimetane-DC Cough Syrup ... 1857
- Dimetane-DX Cough Syrup ... 1858
- Dimetapp Elixir ... ▣ 673
- Dimetapp DM Elixir ... ▣ 674
- Dimetapp Extentabs ... ▣ 674
- Dimetapp Plus Caplets ... ▣ 675
- Dimetapp Tablets ... ▣ 675
- Drixoral Antihistamine/Nasal Decongestant Syrup ... ▣ 698

Buprenorphine (Contraindicated; potentiated).
- No products indexed under this heading.

Buspirone Hydrochloride (Combined use contraindicated; several cases of elevated blood pressure have been reported). Products include:
- BuSpar ... 1401

Butabarbital (Contraindicated; potentiated). Products include:
- Pyridium Plus ... 1764

Butalbital (Contraindicated; potentiated). Products include:
- Esgic-Plus Tablets ... 1002
- Esgic Tablets & Capsules ... 1001
- Fioricet Tablets ... 2006
- Fiorinal Capsules ... 2007
- Fiorinal with Codeine Capsules ... 2008
- Fiorinal Tablets ... 2007
- Phrenilin ... 838
- Sedapap Tablets 50 mg/650 mg .. 1360

Caffeine (Excessive use contraindicated). Products include:
- Anacin Coated Analgesic Caplets ... 2417
- Anacin Coated Analgesic Tablets ... 2417
- Anacin Maximum Strength Analgesic Coated Tablets ... 2417
- Cafergot/Cafergot P-B ... 1999
- Esgic-Plus Tablets ... 1002
- Esgic Tablets & Capsules ... 1001
- Aspirin Free Excedrin Analgesic Caplets ... 748
- Excedrin Extra-Strength Analgesic Tablets & Caplets ... 749
- Fioricet Tablets ... 2006
- Fiorinal Capsules ... 2007
- Fiorinal with Codeine Capsules ... 2008
- Fiorinal Tablets ... 2007
- No Doz Fast Acting Alertness Aid Tablets ... 751
- No Doz Maximum Strength Caplets 751
- Norgesic ... 1314
- P-A-C Analgesic Tablets ... ▣ 669
- Synalgos-DC Capsules ... 2525
- Vanquish Analgesic Caplets ... ▣ 574
- Vivarin Stimulant Tablets ... ▣ 726
- Wigraine Tablets & Suppositories .. 1645

Captopril (Contraindicated; potentiated). Products include:
- Capoten ... 2255
- Capozide ... 2258

Carbamazepine (Contraindicated; hypertensive crises; severe convulsive seizures). Products include:
- Tegretol Chewable Tablets ... 654
- Tegretol Suspension ... 656
- Tegretol Tablets ... 654

Carteolol Hydrochloride (Contraindicated; potentiated). Products include:
- Cartrol Tablets ... 507

Chlordiazepoxide (Contraindicated; potentiated). Products include:
- Libritabs Tablets ... 1930
- Limbitrol ... 1933
- Menrium Tablets ... 1934

Chlordiazepoxide Hydrochloride (Contraindicated; potentiated). Products include:
- Librax Capsules ... 1929
- Librium Capsules ... 1931
- Librium Injectable ... 1932

Chlorothiazide (Contraindicated; potentiated). Products include:
- Aldoclor Tablets ... 1413
- Diupres Tablets ... 1461
- Diuril Oral ... 1464

Chlorothiazide Sodium (Contraindicated; potentiated). Products include:
- Diuril Sodium Intravenous ... 1463

Chlorpheniramine Maleate (Contraindicated). Products include:
- A.R.M. Allergy Relief Medicine Caplets ... ▣ 615
- Alka-Seltzer Plus Cold Medicine ... ▣ 623
- Allerest ... ▣ 559
- Ana-Kit Anaphylaxis Emergency Treatment Kit ... 1100
- BC Cold Powder Multi-Symptom Formula ... ▣ 517
- Brexin L.A. Capsules ... 2078
- Cerose-DM ... 2443
- Cheracol Plus Head Cold/Cough Formula ... ▣ 667
- Chlor-Trimeton Allergy Syrup, Tablets & Long-Acting Repetabs Tablets ... ▣ 693
- Chlor-Trimeton Decongestant ... ▣ 694
- Comhist LA Capsules ... 1618
- Allergy-Sinus Comtrex Multi-Symptom Allergy Sinus Formula Tablets & Caplets ... 746
- Comtrex Multi-Symptom Cold Reliever Tablets/Caplets/Liqui-Gels/Liquid ... 745
- Day-Night Comtrex ... 747
- Contac Continuous Action Decongestant/Antihistamine Capsules ▣ 710
- Contac Maximum Strength Continuous Action Decongestant/Antihistamine Caplets ... ▣ 709
- Contac Severe Cold and Flu Formula Caplets ... ▣ 711
- Coricidin 'D' Decongestant Tablets ... ▣ 695
- Coricidin Demilets Tablets for Children ... ▣ 696
- Coricidin Tablets ... ▣ 695
- Deconamine ... 663
- Demazin Nasal Decongestant/Antihistamine Repetabs Tablets & Syrup ... ▣ 697
- Dorcol Children's Liquid Cold Formula ... ▣ 686
- Dristan Decongestant/Antihistamine/ Analgesic Coated Caplets ... ▣ 749
- Dristan Cold Nasal Decongestant/Antihistamine/ Analgesic Coated Tablets ... 2419
- Dristan Advanced Formula Decongestant/Antihistamine/ Analgesic Tablets ... ▣ 749
- Extendryl ... 994
- 4-Way Cold Tablets ... 750
- Fedahist Gyrocaps ... 2145
- Fedahist Timecaps ... 2145
- Hycomine Compound Tablets ... 929
- Isoclor Timesule Capsules ... ▣ 561
- Kronofed-A ... 970
- Medi-Flu Caplet, Liquid ... ▣ 640
- Naldecon Syrup, Tablets, Pediatric Drops and Pediatric Syrup ... 709
- Nolamine Tablets ... 838
- Novafed A Capsules ... 1342
- Novahistine DH ... 1342
- Novahistine Elixir ... ▣ 596
- Ornade Spansule Capsules ... 2221
- Orthoxicol Cough Syrup ... ▣ 668
- PediaCare Allergy Relief Formula Liquid ... 1362
- PediaCare Cough-Cold Formula Liquid ... 1362
- PediaCare Night Rest Cough-Cold Formula Liquid ... 1362
- PediaCare 6-12 Cough-Cold Formula Chewable Tablets ... 1362
- Pyrroxate Capsules ... ▣ 669
- Quelidrine Syrup ... 556
- Ru-Tuss II Capsules ... 693
- Ru-Tuss Tablets ... 693
- Ryna ... ▣ 741
- Sinarest Tablets & Extra Strength Tablets ... ▣ 562
- Sine-Off Maximum Strength Allergy/Sinus Formula Caplets ... ▣ 721
- Sine-Off Sinus Medicine Tablets-Aspirin Formula ... ▣ 722
- Singlet Tablets ... ▣ 598
- Sinulin ... 840
- Sinutab Maximum Strength ... ▣ 641
- St. Joseph Nighttime Cold Medicine ... ▣ 705
- Sudafed Plus Liquid ... ▣ 544
- Sudafed Plus Tablets ... ▣ 545
- Teldrin Timed-Release Allergy Capsules, 12 mg ... 2192
- TheraFlu Flu and Cold Medicine ... ▣ 687
- Triaminic Allergy Tablets ... ▣ 688
- Triaminic Chewables ... ▣ 688
- Triaminic Cold Tablets ... ▣ 688
- Triaminic Nite Light ... ▣ 689
- Triaminic Syrup ... ▣ 689
- Triaminic-12 Tablets ... ▣ 690
- Triaminicin Tablets ... ▣ 690
- Triaminicol Multi-Symptom Cold Tablets ... ▣ 691
- Triaminicol Multi-Symptom Relief ▣ 691
- Tylenol Allergy Sinus Medication Caplets and Gelcaps, Maximum Strength ... 1372
- Children's Tylenol Cold Liquid Formula and Chewable Tablets ... 1368
- Tylenol Cold & Flu Hot Medication, Packets ... 1369
- Tylenol Cold Medication Caplets and Tablets ... 1370
- Tylenol Cold Medication, Effervescent Tablets ... 1369
- Vicks Children's NyQuil ... ▣ 664
- Vicks Formula 44 Cough Medicine ... ▣ 661
- Vicks Formula 44M Multi-Symptom Cough Medicine ... ▣ 662
- Vicks Pediatric Formula 44m Multi-Symptom Cough & Cold Medicine ... ▣ 663

Chlorpheniramine Polistirex (Contraindicated). Products include:
- Tussionex Extended-Release Suspension ... 988

Chlorpheniramine Tannate (Contraindicated). Products include:
- Rynatan ... 2387
- Rynatuss ... 2388

Chlorpromazine (Additive hypotensive effects). Products include:
- Thorazine ... 2234

Chlorpropamide (Hypoglycemic episodes). Products include:
- Diabinese Tablets ... 1775

Chlorprothixene (Contraindicated; potentiated). Products include:
- Taractan Tablets ... 1920

Chlorprothixene Hydrochloride (Contraindicated; potentiated). Products include:
- Taractan ... 1920

Chlorthalidone (Contraindicated; potentiated). Products include:
- Combipres Tablets ... 678
- Tenoretic Tablets ... 1105
- Thalitone Tablets ... 687

Clemastine Fumarate (Contraindicated). Products include:
- Tavist Syrup ... 2033
- Tavist Tablets ... 2035
- Tavist-D Tablets ... 2035

Clomipramine Hydrochloride (Contraindicated). Products include:
- Anafranil Capsules ... 650

Clonidine (Contraindicated; potentiated). Products include:
- Catapres-TTS ... 677

Clonidine Hydrochloride (Contraindicated; potentiated). Products include:
- Catapres Tablets ... 676
- Combipres Tablets ... 678

Clorazepate Dipotassium (Contraindicated; potentiated). Products include:
- Tranxene ... 556

Clozapine (Contraindicated; hypertensive crises; severe convulsive seizures). Products include:
- Clozaril Tablets ... 2000

Codeine (Contraindicated; potentiated). Products include:
- Calcidrine Syrup ... 506

Codeine Phosphate (Contraindicated; potentiated). Products include:
- Actifed with Codeine Cough Syrup .. 752
- Cheracol Cough Syrup ... 1853
- Codimal PH Syrup ... 846
- Dimetane-DC Cough Syrup ... 1857
- Empirin with Codeine Phosphate Nos. 2, 3 & 4 ... 764
- Fiorinal with Codeine Capsules ... 2008
- Isoclor Expectorant ... 982
- Naldecon CX Adult Liquid ... ▣ 521
- Novahistine DH ... 1342
- Novahistine Expectorant ... 1343
- Nucofed Capsules ... 2219
- Nucofed Expectorant ... 2219
- Nucofed Pediatric Expectorant ... 2220
- Nucofed Syrup ... 2219
- Phenaphen with Codeine Capsules 1865
- Phenaphen-650 with Codeine Tablets ... 1866
- Phenergan with Codeine ... 2497
- Phenergan VC with Codeine ... 2501
- Robitussin A-C Syrup ... 1875
- Robitussin-DAC Syrup ... 1875
- Ryna ... ▣ 741

(▣ Described in PDR For Nonprescription Drugs)

(⊙ Described in PDR For Ophthalmology)

Soma Compound w/Codeine Tablets 2390
Triaminic Expectorant w/Codeine .. 1996
Tussi-Organidin Liquid 2391
Tylenol with Codeine 1381

Codeine Polistirex (Contraindicated; potentiated).
No products indexed under this heading.

Cyclobenzaprine Hydrochloride (Contraindicated; hypertensive crises; severe convulsive seizures). Products include:
Flexeril Tablets 1471

Cyproheptadine Hydrochloride (Contraindicated). Products include:
Periactin 1525

Deserpidine (Contraindicated; potentiated). Products include:
Enduronyl 518
Harmonyl Tablets 528
Oreticyl 545

Desipramine Hydrochloride (Contraindicated; hypertensive crises; severe convulsive seizures). Products include:
Norpramin Tablets 1340

Dexchlorpheniramine Maleate (Contraindicated). Products include:
Polaramine 2116

Dextroamphetamine Sulfate (Combined use contraindicated). Products include:
Dexedrine 2206

Dextromethorphan Hydrobromide (May cause brief episodes of psychosis or bizarre behavior). Products include:
Benylin DM .... ▣ 638
Benylin Expectorant .... ▣ 638
Cerose-DM 2443
Cheracol D Cough Formula .... ▣ 667
Cheracol Plus Head Cold/Cough Formula .... ▣ 667
Codimal DM Syrup 846
Cough Formula Comtrex 746
Comtrex Multi-Symptom Cold Reliever Tablets/Caplets/Liqui-Gels/Liquid 745
Day-Night Comtrex 747
Non-Drowsy Comtrex 747
Contac Cough Formula .... ▣ 711
Contac Cough & Sore Throat Formula .... ▣ 712
Contac Jr. Children's Cold Medicine .... ▣ 712
Contac Nighttime Cold Medicine .... ▣ 713
Contac Severe Cold and Flu Formula Caplets .... ▣ 711
Dimacol Caplets .... ▣ 672
Dimetane-DX Cough Syrup 1858
Dimetapp DM Elixir .... ▣ 674
Dorcol Children's Cough Syrup .... ▣ 685
Hold Cough Suppressant Lozenge ▣ 617
Humibid DM Tablets 560
Medi-Flu Caplet, Liquid .... ▣ 640
Naldecon DX Adult Liquid .... ▣ 521
Naldecon DX Children's Syrup .... ▣ 522
Naldecon DX Pediatric Drops .... ▣ 522
Naldecon Senior DX Cough/Cold Liquid .... ▣ 523
Novahistine DMX .... ▣ 595
Orthoxicol Cough Syrup .... ▣ 668
PediaCare Cough-Cold Formula Liquid 1362
PediaCare Night Rest Cough-Cold Formula Liquid 1362
PediaCare 6-12 Cough-Cold Formula Chewable Tablets 1362
Phenergan with Dextromethorphan 2499
Quelidrine Syrup 556
Robitussin Cough Calmers .... ▣ 677
Robitussin Night Relief .... ▣ 677
Robitussin Pediatric .... ▣ 678
Robitussin-CF .... ▣ 676
Robitussin-DM .... ▣ 676
Rondec-DM 1976
St. Joseph Cough Suppressant for Children .... ▣ 705
St. Joseph Nighttime Cold Medicine .... ▣ 705
Sucrets Cough Control Formula .... ▣ 724
Sudafed Cough Syrup .... ▣ 543
Triaminic Nite Light .... ▣ 689
Triaminic-DM Syrup .... ▣ 689
Triaminicol Multi-Symptom Cold Tablets .... ▣ 691
Triaminicol Multi-Symptom Relief ▣ 691
Tussi-Organidin DM Liquid 2392
Tylenol Cold & Flu Hot Medication, Packets 1369
Tylenol Cold & Flu No Drowsiness Hot Medication, Packets 1371
Tylenol Cold Medication Caplets and Tablets 1370
Tylenol Cold Medication No Drowsiness Formula Caplets 1370
Tylenol Cold Night Time Medication Liquid 1371
Tylenol Cough Medication Liquid, Maximum Strength 1372
Tylenol Cough Medication Liquid with Decongestant, Maximum Strength 1372
Vicks Children's Cough Syrup .... ▣ 660
Vicks Children's NyQuil .... ▣ 664
Vicks Cough Silencers Cough Drops .... ▣ 660
Vicks Daycare .... ▣ 660
Vicks Formula 44 Cough Control Discs .... ▣ 661
Vicks Formula 44 Cough Medicine .... ▣ 661
Vicks Formula 44D Decongestant Cough Medicine .... ▣ 662
Vicks Formula 44M Multi-Symptom Cough Medicine .... ▣ 662
Vicks NyQuil Nighttime Colds Medicine-Original & Cherry Flavor .... ▣ 664
Vicks Pediatric Formula 44 Cough Medicine .... ▣ 662
Vicks Pediatric Formula 44 Cough & Congestion Medicine .... ▣ 663
Vicks Pediatric Formula 44m Multi-Symptom Cough & Cold Medicine .... ▣ 663

Dextromethorphan Polistirex (May cause brief episodes of psychosis or bizarre behavior). Products include:
Delsym Cough Formula .... ▣ 560

Dezocine (Contraindicated; potentiated).

Diazepam (Contraindicated; potentiated). Products include:
Valium Injectable 1937
Valium Tablets 1939
Valrelease Capsules 1923

Diazoxide (Contraindicated; potentiated). Products include:
Hyperstat I.V. Injection 2095
Proglycem 649

Diethylpropion Hydrochloride (Combined use contraindicated). Products include:
Tenuate 1354

Diphenhydramine Citrate (Contraindicated). Products include:
Alka-Seltzer Plus Night-Time Cold Medicine .... ▣ 623
Bufferin AF Nite Time Analgesic/Sleeping Aid Caplets 744
Excedrin P.M. Analgesic/Sleeping Aid Tablets, Caplets and Liquid 749

Diphenhydramine Hydrochloride (Contraindicated; combined use contraindicated; severe reactions reported). Products include:
Benadryl Anti-Itch Cream .... ▣ 635
Benadryl Capsules 1691
Benadryl Decongestant Elixir .... ▣ 635
Benadryl Decongestant .... ▣ 635
Benadryl Elixir .... ▣ 636
Benadryl Kapseals 1691
Benadryl 25 Kapseals .... ▣ 636
Benadryl Parenteral 1692
Benadryl Plus .... ▣ 636
Benadryl Plus Nighttime .... ▣ 637
Benadryl Spray, Maximum Strength .... ▣ 637
Benadryl Spray, Regular Strength ▣ 637
Benadryl Steri-Vials, Ampoules, and Steri-Dose Syringe 1692
Benadryl 25 Tablets .... ▣ 636
Benylin Cough Syrup .... ▣ 637
Benylin Decongestant .... ▣ 638
Caladryl Cream, Lotion, Spray .... ▣ 638
Miles Nervine Nighttime Sleep-Aid ▣ 627
Nytol Tablets .... ▣ 517
Sleep-ettes-D Tablets .... ▣ 653
Sleep-eze 3 Tablets .... ▣ 755
Sleepinal Night-time Sleep Aid Capsules .... ▣ 734
Sominex Caplets and Tablets .... ▣ 722
Sominex Liquid .... ▣ 723
Sominex Pain Relief Formula .... ▣ 723
Tylenol Cold Night Time Medication Liquid 1371
Tylenol PM, Extra Strength Caplets and Tablets 1368
Unisom Dual Relief Nighttime Sleep Aid/Analgesic 1774
Ziradryl Lotion .... ▣ 643

Diphenylpyraline Hydrochloride (Contraindicated).
No products indexed under this heading.

Disulfiram (Administer with caution). Products include:
Antabuse Tablets 2429

Dobutamine Hydrochloride (Contraindicated; hypertension, headache and related symptoms precipitated). Products include:
Dobutrex Solution Vials 1259

Dopamine Hydrochloride (Contraindicated; hypertension, headache and related symptoms precipitated). Products include:
Intropin Injection 930

Doxazosin Mesylate (Contraindicated; potentiated). Products include:
Cardura Tablets 1941

Doxepin Hydrochloride (Contraindicated; hypertensive crises; severe convulsive seizures). Products include:
Sinequan 1960

Droperidol (Contraindicated; potentiated). Products include:
Inapsine Injection 1140
Innovar Injection 1141

Enalapril Maleate (Contraindicated; potentiated). Products include:
Vaseretic Tablets 1559
Vasotec Tablets 1564

Enalaprilat (Contraindicated; potentiated). Products include:
Vasotec I.V. 1562

Enflurane (Contraindicated; potentiated). Products include:
Ethrane 599

Ephedrine Hydrochloride (Contraindicated; hypertension, headache and related symptoms precipitated). Products include:
Amesec .... ▣ 682
Primatene Tablets-M Formula 2421
Primatene Tablets-P Formula 2421
Primatene Tablets-Regular Formula 2421
Quadrinal Tablets 1183
Quelidrine Syrup 556
Tedral SA 1765

Ephedrine Sulfate (Contraindicated; hypertension, headache and related symptoms precipitated). Products include:
Bronkaid Tablets .... ▣ 757
Bronkolixir .... ▣ 761
Bronkotabs Tablets .... ▣ 762
Marax Tablets & DF Syrup 1954
Pazo Hemorrhoid Ointment & Suppositories 752
Vicks Vatronol Nose Drops .... ▣ 666

Ephedrine Tannate (Contraindicated; hypertension, headache and related symptoms precipitated). Products include:
Rynatuss 2388

Epinephrine (Contraindicated; hypertension, headache and related symptoms precipitated). Products include:
Ana-Kit Anaphylaxis Emergency Treatment Kit 1100
Bronkaid Mist .... ▣ 757
EpiPen 843
Marcaine Hydrochloride 0.5% with Epinephrine 1:200,000 (as bitartrate) 958
Marcaine Hydrochloride with Epinephrine 1:200,000 2055
Primatene Mist 2420
Sus-Phrine Injection 1006
Xylocaine with Epinephrine Injections 637

Epinephrine Bitartrate (Contraindicated; hypertension, headache and related symptoms precipitated). Products include:
AsthmaHaler Mist Epinephrine Bitartrate Bronchodilator .... ▣ 616
Bronkaid Mist Suspension .... ▣ 757
Primatene Mist Suspension 2421

Epinephrine Hydrochloride (Contraindicated; hypertension, headache and related symptoms precipitated). Products include:
Adrenalin Chloride Solution 1:100 & 1:1,000 1689
Epifrin .... ◉ 244
Glaucon .... ◉ 218

Esmolol Hydrochloride (Contraindicated; potentiated). Products include:
Brevibloc Injection 942

Estazolam (Contraindicated; potentiated). Products include:
ProSom Tablets 554

Ethchlorvynol (Contraindicated; potentiated). Products include:
Placidyl Capsules 553

Ethinamate (Contraindicated; potentiated).
No products indexed under this heading.

Felodipine (Contraindicated; potentiated). Products include:
Plendil Extended-Release Tablets 1526

Fenfluramine Hydrochloride (Combined use contraindicated). Products include:
Pondimin Tablets 1867

Fentanyl (Contraindicated; potentiated). Products include:
Duragesic Transdermal System 1133

Fentanyl Citrate (Contraindicated; potentiated). Products include:
Innovar Injection 1141
Sublimaze Injection 1146

Fluoxetine Hydrochloride (Concurrent administration contraindicated). Products include:
Prozac Pulvules 920

Fluphenazine Decanoate (Additive hypotensive effects; contraindicated; potentiated). Products include:
Prolixin Decanoate 1795

Fluphenazine Enanthate (Additive hypotensive effects; contraindicated; potentiated). Products include:
Prolixin Enanthate 1796

Fluphenazine Hydrochloride (Additive hypotensive effects; contraindicated; potentiated). Products include:
Prolixin Elixir 1793
Prolixin Injection 1791
Prolixin Oral Concentrate 1792
Prolixin Tablets 1793

Flurazepam Hydrochloride (Contraindicated; potentiated). Products include:
Dalmane Capsules 1927

Fosinopril Sodium (Contraindicated; potentiated). Products include:
Monopril Tablets 1406

Furazolidone (Contraindicated; hypertensive crises; severe convulsive seizures). Products include:
Furoxone 1855

Furosemide (Contraindicated; potentiated). Products include:
Lasix 1093

Glipizide (Hypoglycemic episodes). Products include:
Glucotrol 1952

Glutethimide (Contraindicated; potentiated).
No products indexed under this heading.

Glyburide (Hypoglycemic episodes). Products include:
DiaBeta 1091
Micronase Tablets 2350

Guanabenz Acetate (Contraindicated; potentiated). Products include:
Wytensin Tablets 2542

Guanethidine Monosulfate (Contraindicated; potentiated). Products include:
Esimil Tablets 864
Ismelin Tablets 869

Haloperidol (Contraindicated; potentiated). Products include:
Haldol Injection, Tablets and Concentrate 1373

Haloperidol Decanoate (Contraindicated; potentiated). Products include:
Haldol Decanoate 1375

Hydralazine Hydrochloride (Contraindicated; potentiated). Products include:
Apresazide Capsules 854
Apresoline Hydrochloride Parenteral (Ampuls) 856
Apresoline Hydrochloride Tablets 855
Apresoline-Esidrix Tablets 857
Ser-Ap-Es Tablets 881
Serpasil-Apresoline Tablets 884

Hydrochlorothiazide (Contraindicated; potentiated). Products include:
Aldactazide 2150
Aldoril Tablets 1418
Apresazide Capsules 854
Apresoline-Esidrix Tablets 857
Capozide 2258
Dyazide Capsules 2208
Esidrix Tablets 863
Esimil Tablets 864
HydroDIURIL Tablets 1484
Hydropres Tablets 1485
Inderide Tablets 2463
Inderide LA Long Acting Capsules 2465
Lopressor HCT Tablets 1034
Maxzide 1215
Moduretic Tablets 1510
Normozide Tablets 2112
Oretic Tablets 544
Oreticyl 545
Prinzide Tablets 1540
Ser-Ap-Es Tablets 881
Serpasil-Esidrix Tablets 886
Timolide Tablets 1547
Trandate HCT Tablets 579
Vaseretic Tablets 1559
Zestoretic 2274

Hydrocodone Bitartrate (Contraindicated; potentiated). Products include:
Anexsia 5/500 Tablets 2196
Anexsia 7.5/650 Tablets 2197
Azdone Tablets 844
Codiclear DH Syrup 845
Codimal DH Syrup 846
Damason-P 1356
Hycodan Syrup, Tablets 927
Hycomine Compound Tablets 929
Hycomine Syrup 927
Hycotuss Expectorant Syrup 930
Hydrocet Capsules 835
Lortab ASA Tablets 2414
Lortab 2412
Ru-Tuss with Hydrocodone 694
Triaminic Expectorant DH 1995
Vicodin Tablets 1187
Vicodin ES Tablets 1189
Zydone Capsules 941

Hydrocodone Polistirex (Contraindicated; potentiated). Products include:
Tussionex Extended-Release Suspension 988

Hydroflumethiazide (Contraindicated; potentiated). Products include:
Diucardin Tablets 2450
Saluron 718
Salutensin/Salutensin-Demi 719

Hydroxyzine Hydrochloride (Contraindicated; potentiated). Products include:
Atarax Tablets & Syrup 1941
Marax Tablets & DF Syrup 1954
Vistaril Intramuscular Solution 1970

Imipramine Hydrochloride (Contraindicated; hypertensive crises; severe convulsive seizures). Products include:
Tofranil Ampuls 1038
Tofranil Tablets 1039

Imipramine Pamoate (Contraindicated; hypertensive crises; severe convulsive seizures). Products include:
Tofranil-PM Capsules 1041

Indapamide (Contraindicated; potentiated). Products include:
Lozol Tablets 1843

Insulin, Human (Hypoglycemic episodes).
No products indexed under this heading.

Insulin, Human Isophane Suspension (Hypoglycemic episodes). Products include:
Humulin N, 100 Units 1270

Insulin, Human NPH (Hypoglycemic episodes). Products include:
Insulatard NPH Human 1627
Novolin N 1627
Novolin N PenFill Cartridges 1628
Novolin N Prefilled 1628

Insulin, Human Regular (Hypoglycemic episodes). Products include:
Humulin BR, 100 Units 1268
Humulin R, 100 Units 1272
Novolin R 1627
Novolin R PenFill Cartridges 1628
Novolin R Prefilled 1629
Velosulin Human 1628

Insulin, Human, Zinc Suspension (Hypoglycemic episodes). Products include:
Humulin L, 100 Units 1268
Humulin U, 100 Units 1272
Novolin L 1627

Insulin, NPH (Hypoglycemic episodes). Products include:
NPH, 40 & 100 Units 1273
Beef NPH, 100 Units 1274
Pork NPH, 100 Units 1275
Insulatard NPH 1626
NPH Insulin 1626
NPH Purified Pork Isophane Insulin 1626

Insulin, Regular (Hypoglycemic episodes). Products include:
Regular, 40 & 100 Units 1273
Beef Regular, 100 Units 1275
Pork Regular, 100 Units 1275
Pork Regular (Concentrated), 500 Units 1276
Regular Insulin 1625
Regular Purified Pork Insulin 1626
Velosulin 1627

Insulin, Zinc Crystals (Hypoglycemic episodes). Products include:
NPH, 40 & 100 Units 1273

Insulin, Zinc Suspension (Hypoglycemic episodes). Products include:
Lente, 40 & 100 Units 1272
Protamine, Zinc, 40 & 100 Units 1273
Lente Iletin I 1272
Beef Lente, 100 Units 1274
Beef Protamine Zinc, 100 Units 1274
Pork Lente, 100 Units 1275
Pork, Protamine, Zinc, 100 Units 1275
Lente Insulin 1626
Lente Purified Pork Insulin 1626
Semilente Insulin 1625
Ultralente Insulin 1626

Isocarboxazid (Contraindicated; hypertensive crises; severe convulsive seizures). Products include:
Marplan Tablets 1906

Isoflurane (Contraindicated; potentiated). Products include:
Forane 600

Isoproterenol Hydrochloride (Contraindicated; hypertension, headache and related symptoms precipitated). Products include:
Isuprel Hydrochloride Injection 1:5000 2050
Isuprel Hydrochloride Mistometer 2051
Isuprel Hydrochloride Solution 1:200 & 1:100 2052
Norisodrine Aerotrol 540

Isradipine (Contraindicated; potentiated). Products include:
DynaCirc Capsules 2004

Ketamine Hydrochloride (Contraindicated; potentiated). Products include:
Ketalar 1726

Labetalol Hydrochloride (Contraindicated; potentiated). Products include:
Normodyne Injection 2108
Normodyne Tablets 2110
Normozide Tablets 2112
Trandate HCT Tablets 579
Trandate Injection 577
Trandate Tablets 579

Levodopa (Contraindicated; hypertension, headache and related symptoms precipitated). Products include:
Larodopa Tablets 1905
Sinemet Tablets 952
Sinemet CR Tablets 953

Levorphanol Tartrate (Contraindicated; potentiated). Products include:
Levo-Dromoran 1906

Lisinopril (Contraindicated; potentiated). Products include:
Prinivil Tablets 1538
Prinzide Tablets 1540
Zestoretic 2274
Zestril Tablets 2277

Lorazepam (Contraindicated; potentiated). Products include:
Ativan Injection 2432
Ativan Tablets 2434

Loxapine Hydrochloride (Contraindicated; potentiated). Products include:
Loxitane 1213

Loxapine Succinate (Contraindicated; potentiated). Products include:
Loxitane Capsules 1213

Maprotiline Hydrochloride (Contraindicated; hypertensive crises; severe convulsive seizures). Products include:
Ludiomil Tablets 874

Mazindol (Combined use contraindicated). Products include:
Sanorex Tablets 2030

Mecamylamine Hydrochloride (Contraindicated; potentiated). Products include:
Inversine Tablets 1492

Meperidine Hydrochloride (Contraindicated; potentiated; serious reactions precipitated). Products include:
Demerol 2047
Mepergan Injection 2479

Mephobarbital (Contraindicated; potentiated). Products include:
Mebaral Tablets 2061

Meprobamate (Contraindicated; potentiated). Products include:
Deprol Tablets 2382
Equagesic Tablets 2451
Miltown Tablets 2386
PMB 200 and PMB 400 2504

Mesoridazine (Additive hypotensive effects). Products include:
Serentil 686

Metaproterenol Sulfate (Contraindicated; hypertension, headache and related symptoms precipitated). Products include:
Alupent 674
Arm-a-Med Metaproterenol Sulfate Inhalation Solution, USP 617
Metaprel Inhalation Aerosol Bronchodilator 2014
Metaprel Inhalation Solution 2015
Metaprel 2015
Metaproterenol Sulfate Inhalation Solution, USP 912

Metaraminol Bitartrate (Contraindicated; hypertension, headache and related symptoms precipitated). Products include:
Aramine Injection 1424

Methadone Hydrochloride (Contraindicated; potentiated). Products include:
Dolophine Hydrochloride Ampoules & Vials 1260
Dolophine Hydrochloride Tablets 1261
Methadone Hydrochloride Diskets 1284
Methadone Hydrochloride Oral Solution & Tablets 1987

Methamphetamine Hydrochloride (Combined use contraindicated). Products include:
Desoxyn Gradumet Tablets 514

Methdilazine Hydrochloride (Contraindicated). Products include:
Tacaryl Syrup & Tablets 2409

Methohexital Sodium (Contraindicated; potentiated). Products include:
Brevital Sodium Vials 1248

Methoxamine Hydrochloride (Contraindicated; hypertension, headache and related symptoms precipitated). Products include:
Vasoxyl Injection 819

Methoxyflurane (Contraindicated; potentiated).
No products indexed under this heading.

Methyclothiazide (Contraindicated; potentiated; hypertensive crises; severe convulsive seizures). Products include:
Enduron Tablets 517
Enduronyl 518

Methyldopa (Contraindicated; potentiated; hypertension headache and related symptoms precipitated). Products include:
Aldoclor Tablets 1413
Aldomet Oral 1415
Aldoril Tablets 1418

Methyldopate Hydrochloride (Contraindicated; potentiated; hypertension headache and related symptoms precipitated). Products include:
Aldomet Ester HCl Injection 1417

Metolazone (Contraindicated; potentiated). Products include:
Diulo 2129
Mykrox ½ mg Tablets 984
Zaroxolyn Tablets 989

Metoprolol Tartrate (Contraindicated; potentiated). Products include:
Lopressor Ampuls 1032
Lopressor HCT Tablets 1034
Lopressor Tablets 1032

Metyrosine (Contraindicated; potentiated). Products include:
Demser Capsules 1460

Midazolam Hydrochloride (Contraindicated; potentiated). Products include:
Versed Injection 1924

Minoxidil (Contraindicated; potentiated). Products include:
Loniten Tablets 2346
Rogaine Topical Solution 2357
Molindone Hydrochloride (Contraindicated; potentiated). Products include:
Moban Tablets & Concentrate 932
Morphine Sulfate (Contraindicated; potentiated). Products include:
Astramorph/PF Injection, USP (Preservative-Free) 618
Duramorph 960
Infumorph 200 and Infumorph 500 Sterile Solutions 962
MS Contin Tablets 1814
MSIR 1817
Oramorph SR (Morphine Sulfate Sustained Release Tablets) 1988
Roxanol 1991
Nadolol (Contraindicated; potentiated). Products include:
Corgard Tablets 701
Corzide Tablets 702
Naphazoline Hydrochloride (Combined use contraindicated). Products include:
AK-Con ◉ 202
AK-Con-A ◉ 203
Albalon Solution with Liquifilm ◉ 238
Albalon-A Liquifilm ◉ 238
Allergy Drops ◉ 258
Clear Eyes ACR ◉ 305
Clear Eyes Lubricating Eye Redness Reliever ◉ 304
4-Way Fast Acting Nasal Spray - Original Formula (regular & mentholated) & Metered Spray Pump (regular) 751
Naphcon ◉ 226
Naphcon Forte ◉ 226
Naphcon-A Ophthalmic Solution 571
Opcon-A Ophthalmic Solution ◉ 262
Privine Nasal Solution ▣ 552
Privine Nasal Solution 878
Privine Nasal Spray ▣ 552
Privine Nasal Spray 878
Vasocon-A ◉ 278
Nicardipine Hydrochloride (Contraindicated; potentiated). Products include:
Cardene Capsules 2290
Nitroglycerin (Contraindicated; potentiated). Products include:
Deponit NTG Transdermal Delivery System 2143
Minitran Transdermal Delivery System 1312
Nitro-Bid Ointment 1339
Nitro-Bid Capsules 1338
Nitrodisc 2176
Nitro-Dur (nitroglycerin) Transdermal Infusion System 1164
Nitrogard Tablets 1004
Nitrolingual Spray 1846
Nitrostat Tablets 1743
Transderm-Nitro Transdermal Therapeutic System 2283
Norepinephrine Bitartrate (Contraindicated; hypertension, headache and related symptoms precipitated). Products include:
Levophed Bitartrate Injection 2054
Nortriptyline Hydrochloride (Contraindicated; hypertensive crises; severe convulsive seizures). Products include:
Pamelor 2019
Opium Alkaloids (Contraindicated; potentiated). Products include:
B & O No. 15A & No. 16A Supprettes 2395
Pantopon Injectable 1911
Oxazepam (Contraindicated; potentiated). Products include:
Serax Capsules 2522
Serax Tablets 2522
Oxycodone Hydrochloride (Contraindicated; potentiated). Products include:
Percocet Tablets 950
Percodan 951
Roxicodone Tablets, Oral Solution & Intensol (Oxycodone) 1992
Tylox Capsules 1382
Oxymetazoline Hydrochloride (Combined use contraindicated). Products include:
Afrin ▣ 692
Cheracol Nasal Spray Pump ▣ 667
Dristan Long Lasting Menthol Nasal Spray 2419
Dristan Long Lasting Nasal Spray, Regular and Regular with Metered Dose Pump 2419
Duration Nasal Spray ▣ 700
Duration 12 Hour Nasal Spray Pump ▣ 700
4-Way Long Lasting Nasal Spray & Metered Spray Pump 751
NTZ Long Acting Nasal Spray & Drops 0.05% ▣ 760
Neo-Synephrine Maximum Strength 12 Hour Nasal Spray ▣ 759
Neo-Synephrine Maximum Strength 12 Hour Nasal Spray Pump ▣ 759
Nōstrilla Long Acting Nasal Decongestant ▣ 520
OcuClear Eye Drops ◉ 306
Vicks Sinex Long Acting ▣ 665
Visine L.R. Eye Drops ▣ 647
Visine L.R. Eye Drope ◉ 303
Penbutolol Sulfate (Contraindicated; potentiated). Products include:
Levatol 1832
Pentobarbital Sodium (Contraindicated; potentiated). Products include:
Nembutal Sodium Capsules 534
Nembutal Sodium Solution 536
Nembutal Sodium Suppositories 538
Perphenazine (Contraindicated; additive hypertensive effects; potentiated; hypertensive crises; severe convulsive seizures). Products include:
Etrafon 2087
Triavil Tablets 1556
Trilafon 2123
Phendimetrazine Tartrate (Combined use contraindicated). Products include:
Bontril Slow-Release 834
Plegine Tablets 2504
Prelu-2 Capsules 683
Phenelzine Sulfate (Contraindicated; hypertensive crises; severe convulsive seizures). Products include:
Nardil 1742
Phenmetrazine Hydrochloride (Combined use contraindicated).
No products indexed under this heading.
Phenobarbital (Contraindicated; potentiated). Products include:
Arco-Lase Plus Tablets 607
Bellergal-S Tablets 1998
Bronkolixir ▣ 761
Bronkotabs Tablets ▣ 762
Donnatal 1858
Donnatal Extentabs 1859
Donnatal Tablets 1858
Donnazyme Tablets 1860
Kinesed Tablets 2272
Phenobarbital Elixir and Tablets 1293
Primatene Tablets-P Formula 2421
Quadrinal Tablets 1183
Tedral SA 1765
Phenoxybenzamine Hydrochloride (Contraindicated; potentiated). Products include:
Dibenzyline Capsules 2207
Phentolamine Mesylate (Contraindicated; potentiated). Products include:
Regitine 878
Phenylephrine Bitartrate (Contraindicated; hypertension, headache and related symptoms precipitated).
No products indexed under this heading.
Phenylephrine Hydrochloride (Contraindicated; hypertension, headache and related symptoms precipitated; combined use contraindicated). Products include:
AK-Dilate Solution 2.5% and 10% ◉ 203
Atrohist Sprinkle Capsules 558
Cerose-DM 2443
Codimal 846
Comhist LA Capsules 1618
Congespirin For Children Aspirin Free Chewable Cold Tablets 748
Cyclomydril ◉ 216
Deconsal Sprinkle Capsules 559
Dimetane Decongestant ▣ 673
Dristan Decongestant/Antihistamine/ Analgesic Coated Caplets ▣ 749
Dristan Cold Nasal Decongestant/ Antihistamine/ Analgesic Coated Tablets 2419
Dristan Advanced Formula Decongestant/Antihistamine/ Analgesic Tablets ▣ 749
Dristan Nasal Spray, Menthol 2419
Dristan Nasal Spray, Regular and Regular with Metered Pump 2419
Entex Capsules 1623
Entex Liquid 1623
Sinus Excedrin Analgesic, Decongestant Tablets & Caplets 750
Extendryl 994
4-Way Fast Acting Nasal Spray - Original Formula (regular & mentholated) & Metered Spray Pump (regular) 751
Hycomine Compound Tablets 929
Murocoll-2 Sterile Ophthalmic Solution ◉ 261
Mydfrin 2.5% ◉ 224
Naldecon Syrup, Tablets, Pediatric Drops and Pediatric Syrup 709
Neo-Synephrine Hydrochloride 1% Carpuject 2063
Neo-Synephrine Hydrochloride 1% Injection 2063
Neo-Synephrine Hydrochloride (Ophthalmic) 2064
Neo-Synephrine ▣ 759
Nōstril Nasal Decongestant ▣ 520
Novahistine Elixir ▣ 596
Phenergan VC 2500
Phenergan VC with Codeine 2501
Prefrin Liquifilm Vasoconstrictor and Lubricant Eye Drops ◉ 254
Prefrin-A ◉ 255
Quelidrine Syrup 556
Relief Vasoconstrictor and Lubricant Eye Drops ◉ 256
Robitussin Night Relief ▣ 677
Ru-Tuss with Hydrocodone 694
Ru-Tuss Tablets 693
Vasosulf ◉ 279
Vicks Sinex ▣ 665
Zincfrin ◉ 230
Phenylephrine Tannate (Contraindicated; hypertension, headache and related symptoms precipitated). Products include:
Rynatan 2387
Rynatuss 2388
Phenylpropanolamine Containing Anorectics (Combined use contraindicated).
Phenylpropanolamine Hydrochloride (Contraindicated; hypertension, headache and related symptoms precipitated). Products include:
A.R.M. Allergy Relief Medicine Caplets ▣ 615
Acutrim ▣ 548
Allerest ▣ 559
BC Cold Powder ▣ 517
Cheracol Plus Head Cold/Cough Formula ▣ 667
Codimal Expectorant 846
Comtrex Multi-Symptom Cold Reliever Tablets/Caplets/Liqui-Gels/Liquid 745
Contac Continuous Action Decongestant/Antihistamine Capsules ▣ 710
Contac Maximum Strength Continuous Action Decongestant/ Antihistamine Caplets ▣ 709
Contac Severe Cold and Flu Formula Caplets ▣ 711
Coricidin 'D' Decongestant Tablets ▣ 695
Coricidin Demilets Tablets for Children ▣ 696
Demazin Nasal Decongestant/ Antihistamine Repetabs Tablets & Syrup ▣ 697
Dexatrim ▣ 733
Dimetane-DC Cough Syrup 1857
Dimetapp Elixir ▣ 673
Dimetapp DM Elixir ▣ 674
Dimetapp Extentabs ▣ 674
Dimetapp Plus Caplets ▣ 675
Dimetapp Tablets ▣ 675
Entex Capsules 1623
Entex LA Tablets 1623
Entex Liquid 1623
4-Way Cold Tablets 750
Hycomine Syrup 927
Naldecon CX Adult Liquid ▣ 521
Naldecon DX Adult Liquid ▣ 521
Naldecon DX Children's Syrup ▣ 522
Naldecon DX Pediatric Drops ▣ 522
Naldecon EX Children's Syrup ▣ 522
Naldecon EX Pediatric Drops ▣ 523
Naldecon Syrup, Tablets, Pediatric Drops and Pediatric Syrup 709
Nolamine Tablets 838
Nolex LA Tablets 838
Ornade Spansule Capsules 2221
Orthoxicol Cough Syrup ▣ 668
Propagest 839
Pyrroxate Capsules ▣ 669
Robitussin-CF ▣ 676
Ru-Tuss II Capsules 693
Ru-Tuss with Hydrocodone 694
Ru-Tuss Tablets 693
Sine-Off Sinus Medicine Tablets-Aspirin Formula ▣ 722
Sinulin 840
St. Joseph Cold Tablets for Children ▣ 704
Tavist-D Tablets 2035
Triaminic Allergy Tablets ▣ 688
Triaminic Chewables ▣ 688
Triaminic Cold Tablets ▣ 688
Triaminic Expectorant ▣ 688
Triaminic Expectorant w/Codeine 1996
Triaminic Expectorant DH 1995
Triaminic Oral Infant Drops 1996
Triaminic Syrup ▣ 689
Triaminic-12 Tablets ▣ 690
Triaminic-DM Syrup ▣ 689
Triaminicin Tablets ▣ 690
Triaminicol Multi-Symptom Cold Tablets ▣ 691
Triaminicol Multi-Symptom Relief ▣ 691
Tuss-Ornade Liquid 2242
Tuss-Ornade Spansule Capsules 2242
Tylenol Cold Medication, Effervescent Tablets 1369
Pindolol (Contraindicated; potentiated). Products include:
Visken Tablets 2036
Pirbuterol Acetate (Contraindicated; hypertension, headache and related symptoms precipitated). Products include:
Maxair Inhaler 1311
Polythiazide (Contraindicated; potentiated). Products include:
Minizide Capsules 1779
Renese Tablets 1785
Renese-R Tablets 1786
Prazepam (Contraindicated; potentiated). Products include:
Centrax 1693
Prazosin Hydrochloride (Contraindicated; potentiated). Products include:
Minipress Capsules 1778
Minizide Capsules 1779
Prochlorperazine (Additive hypotensive effects). Products include:
Compazine 2201
Procyclidine Hydrochloride (Combined use contraindicated; severe reactions reported). Products include:
Kemadrin Tablets 771
Promethazine Hydrochloride (Contraindicated; potentiated; additive hypotensive effects). Products include:
Mepergan Injection 2479
Phenergan with Codeine 2497

Phenergan with Dextromethorphan 2499
Phenergan Injection 2493
Phenergan Suppositories 2496
Phenergan Syrup 2495
Phenergan Tablets 2496
Phenergan VC 2500
Phenergan VC with Codeine 2501

Propofol (Contraindicated; potentiated). Products include:
Diprivan Injection 2267

Propoxyphene Hydrochloride (Contraindicated; potentiated). Products include:
Darvon 1256
Wygesic Tablets 2540

Propoxyphene Napsylate (Contraindicated; potentiated). Products include:
Darvon-N/Darvocet-N 1254

Propranolol Hydrochloride (Contraindicated; potentiated). Products include:
Inderal 2459
Inderal LA Long Acting Capsules 2461
Inderide Tablets 2463
Inderide LA Long Acting Capsules 2465

Protriptyline Hydrochloride (Contraindicated; hypertensive crises; severe convulsive seizures). Products include:
Vivactil Tablets 1567

Pseudoephedrine Hydrochloride (Contraindicated; hypertension, headache and related symptoms precipitated; combined use contraindicated). Products include:
Actifed Capsules ▣ 539
Actifed Plus Caplets ▣ 539
Actifed Plus Tablets ▣ 540
Actifed with Codeine Cough Syrup 752
Actifed Syrup ▣ 540
Actifed Tablets ▣ 540
Actifed 12-Hour Capsules ▣ 539
Advil Cold & Sinus Caplets (formerly CoAdvil) 2416
Allerest ▣ 559
Anatuss LA Tablets 1359
Benadryl Decongestant Elixir ▣ 635
Benadryl Decongestant ▣ 635
Benadryl Plus ▣ 636
Benadryl Plus Nighttime ▣ 637
Benylin Decongestant ▣ 638
Brexin L.A. Capsules 2078
Bromfed Capsules (Timed Release) 1615
Bromfed Syrup ▣ 628
Bromfed 1615
CoAdvil ▣ 748
Allergy-Sinus Comtrex Multi-Symptom Allergy Sinus Formula Tablets & Caplets 746
Cough Formula Comtrex 746
Comtrex Multi-Symptom Cold Reliever Tablets/Caplets/Liqui-Gels/Liquid 745
Day-Night Comtrex 747
Non-Drowsy Comtrex 747
Congess 994
Congestac Caplets ▣ 617
Contac Jr. Children's Cold Medicine ▣ 712
Contac Nighttime Cold Medicine ▣ 713
Contac Sinus Caplets Maximum Strength Non-Drowsy Formula ▣ 710
Contac Sinus Tablets Maximum Strength Non-Drowsy Formula ▣ 710
Deconamine 663
Deconsal II Tablets 559
Dimacol Caplets ▣ 672
Dimetane-DX Cough Syrup 1858
Dorcol Children's Cough Syrup ▣ 685
Dorcol Children's Decongestant Liquid ▣ 685
Dorcol Children's Liquid Cold Formula ▣ 686
Maximum Strength Dristan Decongestant/Analgesic Coated Caplets ▣ 750
No Drowsiness Dristan Cold Nasal Decongestant/Analgesic Coated Caplets 2420
Dristan Sinus Caplets 2419
Sinus Excedrin Analgesic, Decongestant Tablets & Caplets ▣ 533
Fedahist Gyrocaps 2145
Fedahist Timecaps 2145
Guaifed 1615
Guaifed Syrup ▣ 629
Isoclor Expectorant 982
Isoclor Timesule Capsules ▣ 561
Kronofed-A 970
Medi-Flu Caplet, Liquid ▣ 640
Novafed A Capsules 1342
Novafed Capsules 1342
Novahistine DH 1342
Novahistine DMX ▣ 595
Novahistine Expectorant 1343
Nucofed Capsules 2219
Nucofed Expectorant 2219
Nucofed Pediatric Expectorant 2220
Nucofed Syrup 2219
Ornex Caplets ▣ 618
PediaCare Allergy Relief Formula Liquid 1362
PediaCare Cough-Cold Formula Liquid 1362
PediaCare Infants' Oral Decongestant Drops 1362
PediaCare Night Rest Cough-Cold Formula Liquid 1362
PediaCare 6-12 Cough-Cold Formula Chewable Tablets 1362
Robitussin-DAC Syrup 1875
Robitussin-PE ▣ 677
Rondec 1975
Rondec-DM 1976
Rondec-TR Tablet 1975
Ru-Tuss DE Tablets 694
Ryna ▣ 741
Seldane-D Extended-Release Tablets 1350
Sinarest ▣ 562
Sine-Aid Maximum Strength Sinus Headache Caplets 1365
Sine-Aid Maximum Strength Sinus Headache Tablets 1365
Sine-Off Maximum Strength Allergy/Sinus Formula Caplets ▣ 721
Sine-Off Maximum Strength No Drowsiness Formula Caplets ▣ 722
Singlet Tablets ▣ 598
Sinutab Maximum Strength ▣ 641
Sinutab Maximum Strength Without Drowsiness Tablets & Caplets ▣ 642
Sinutab Regular Strength Without Drowsiness Formula ▣ 641
St. Joseph Nighttime Cold Medicine ▣ 705
Sudafed Children's Liquid ▣ 543
Sudafed Cough Syrup ▣ 543
Sudafed Plus Liquid ▣ 544
Sudafed Plus Tablets ▣ 545
Sudafed Sinus Caplets ▣ 545
Sudafed Sinus Tablets ▣ 545
Sudafed Tablets, 30 mg ▣ 544
Sudafed Tablets, Adult Strength, 60 mg ▣ 544
Sudafed 12 Hour Capsules ▣ 545
TheraFlu Flu and Cold Medicine ▣ 687
Triaminic Nite Light ▣ 689
Tylenol Allergy Sinus Medication Caplets and Gelcaps, Maximum Strength 1372
Children's Tylenol Cold Liquid Formula and Chewable Tablets 1368
Tylenol Cold & Flu Hot Medication, Packets 1369
Tylenol Cold & Flu No Drowsiness Hot Medication, Packets 1371
Tylenol Cold Medication Caplets and Tablets 1370
Tylenol Cold Medication No Drowsiness Formula Caplets 1370
Tylenol Cold Night Time Medication Liquid 1371
Tylenol Cough Medication Liquid with Decongestant, Maximum Strength 1372
Tylenol, Maximum Strength, Sinus Medication Gelcaps, Caplets and Tablets 1373
Ursinus Inlay-Tabs ▣ 691
Vicks Children's NyQuil ▣ 664
Vicks Daycare ▣ 660
Vicks Formula 44D Decongestant Cough Medicine ▣ 662
Vicks Formula 44M Multi-Symptom Cough Medicine ▣ 662
Vicks NyQuil Nighttime Colds Medicine-Original & Cherry Flavor ▣ 664
Vicks Pediatric Formula 44 Cough & Congestion Medicine ▣ 663
Vicks Pediatric Formula 44m Multi-Symptom Cough & Cold Medicine ▣ 663

Pseudoephedrine Sulfate (Contraindicated; hypertension, headache and related symptoms precipitated). Products include:
Afrin Tablets ▣ 693
Chlor-Trimeton Decongestant ▣ 694
Disophrol Chronotab Sustained-Action Tablets ▣ 698
Drixoral Antihistamine/Nasal Decongestant Syrup ▣ 698
Drixoral Non-Drowsy Formula ▣ 699
Drixoral Plus Extended-Release Tablets ▣ 699
Drixoral Sinus ▣ 700
Drixoral Sustained-Action Tablets ▣ 698
Sinutab Allergy Formula Sustained Action Tablets ▣ 640
Trinalin Repetabs Tablets 1170

Pyrilamine Maleate (Contraindicated). Products include:
Codimal 846
4-Way Fast Acting Nasal Spray - Original Formula (regular & mentholated) & Metered Spray Pump (regular) 751
Maximum Strength Midol Multi-Symptom Menstrual Formula ▣ 571
Maximum Strength Midol PMS Premenstrual Syndrome Formula ▣ 570
Regular Strength Midol Multi-Symptom Menstrual Formula ▣ 570
Prefrin-A ⊙ 255
Prēmsyn PMS Capsules & Caplets ▣ 547
Primatene Tablets-M Formula 2421
Robitussin Night Relief ▣ 677
Ru-Tuss with Hydrocodone 694
Triaminic Expectorant DH 1995
Triaminic Oral Infant Drops 1996

Pyrilamine Tannate (Contraindicated). Products include:
Rynatan 2387

Quazepam (Contraindicated; potentiated). Products include:
Doral Tablets 2383

Ramipril (Contraindicated; potentiated). Products include:
Altace Capsules 1086

Rauwolfia Serpentina (Contraindicated; potentiated). Products include:
Raudixin Tablets 1803
Rauzide Tablets 1804

Rescinnamine (Contraindicated; potentiated).
No products indexed under this heading.

Reserpine (Contraindicated; potentiated). Products include:
Diupres Tablets 1461
Hydromox R Tablets 1209
Hydropres Tablets 1485
Renese-R Tablets 1786
Salutensin/Salutensin-Demi 719
Ser-Ap-Es Tablets 881
Serpasil Tablets 883
Serpasil-Apresoline Tablets 884
Serpasil-Esidrix Tablets 886

Secobarbital Sodium (Contraindicated; potentiated). Products include:
Seconal Sodium Pulvules 1296

Selegiline Hydrochloride (Contraindicated; hypertensive crises; severe convulsive seizures). Products include:
Eldepryl 2250

Sodium Nitroprusside (Contraindicated; potentiated). Products include:
Nipride I.V. Infusion 1909

Sufentanil Citrate (Contraindicated; potentiated). Products include:
Sufenta Injection 1147

Temazepam (Contraindicated; potentiated). Products include:
Restoril Capsules 2023

Terazosin Hydrochloride (Contraindicated; potentiated). Products include:
Hytrin Tablets 529

Terbutaline Sulfate (Contraindicated; hypertension, headache and related symptoms precipitated). Products include:
Brethaire Inhaler 1024
Brethine Ampuls 1026
Brethine Tablets 1026
Bricanyl Injection 1324
Bricanyl Tablets 1325

Terfenadine (Contraindicated). Products include:
Seldane Tablets 1349
Seldane-D Extended-Release Tablets 1350

Tetrahydrozoline Hydrochloride (Combined use contraindicated). Products include:
Collyrium Fresh 2445
Murine Plus Lubricating Eye Redness Reliever ⊙ 305
Visine A.C. Eye Drops ▣ 646
Visine A.C. Eye Drops ⊙ 303
Visine EXTRA Eye Drops ▣ 647
Visine EXTRA Eye Drops ⊙ 303
Visine Eye Drops ▣ 646
Visine Eye Drops ⊙ 303

Thiamylal Sodium (Contraindicated; potentiated). Products include:
Surital Ampoules, Steri-Vials 1764

Thioridazine Hydrochloride (Additive hypotensive effects). Products include:
Mellaril 2011

Thiothixene (Contraindicated; potentiated). Products include:
Navane Capsules and Concentrate 1954
Navane Intramuscular 1956

Timolol Maleate (Contraindicated; potentiated). Products include:
Blocadren Tablets 1429
Timolide Tablets 1547
Timoptic in Ocudose 1552
Timoptic Sterile Ophthalmic Solution 1550

Tolazamide (Hypoglycemic episodes). Products include:
Tolinase Tablets 2365

Tolbutamide (Hypoglycemic episodes). Products include:
Orinase Tablets 2354

Triazolam (Contraindicated; potentiated). Products include:
Halcion Tablets 2340

Trifluoperazine Hydrochloride (Additive hypotensive effects). Products include:
Stelazine 2226

Trihexyphenidyl Hydrochloride (Combined use contraindicated; severe reactions reported). Products include:
Artane 1195

Trimeprazine Tartrate (Contraindicated). Products include:
Temaril Tablets, Syrup and Spansule Sustained Release Capsules 1085

Trimethaphan Camsylate (Contraindicated; potentiated). Products include:
Arfonad Ampuls 1887

Trimipramine Maleate (Contraindicated; hypertensive crises; severe convulsive seizures). Products include:
Surmontil Capsules 2524

Tripelennamine Hydrochloride (Contraindicated). Products include:
PBZ Tablets & Elixir 1037
PBZ-SR Tablets 1037

Triprolidine Hydrochloride (Contraindicated). Products include:
Actidil ▣ 538
Actifed Capsules ▣ 539
Actifed Plus Caplets ▣ 539
Actifed Plus Tablets ▣ 540
Actifed with Codeine Cough Syrup 752
Actifed Syrup ▣ 540
Actifed Tablets ▣ 540
Actifed 12-Hour Capsules ▣ 539

L-Tryptophan (Contraindicated; hypertension, headache and related symptoms precipitated). Products include:
Saave ... 1358
Tropamine ... 1358

Food Interactions

Anchovies (Potential for hypertensive crisis).
Avocados (Potential for hypertensive crisis).
Bananas (Potential for hypertensive crisis).
Beans, broad (Potential for hypertensive crisis).
Beans, Fava (Potential for hypertensive crisis).
Beer, alcohol-free (Potential for hypertensive crisis).
Beer, unspecified (Potential for hypertensive crisis).
Caviar (Potential for hypertensive crisis).
Cheese, aged (Potential for hypertensive crisis).
Cheese, strong, unpasteurized (Potential for hypertensive crisis).
Cheese, unspecified (Potential for hypertensive crisis).
Chocolate (Potential for hypertensive crisis).
Cream, sour (Potential for hypertensive crisis).
Figs, canned (Potential for hypertensive crisis).
Food with high concentration of tyramine (Potential for hypertensive crisis).
Herring, pickled (Potential for hypertensive crisis).
Liqueurs (Potential for hypertensive crisis).
Liver (Potential for hypertensive crisis).
Meat extracts (Potential for hypertensive crisis).
Meat prepared with tenderizers (Potential for hypertensive crisis).
Raisins (Potential for hypertensive crisis).
Sauerkraut (Potential for hypertensive crisis).
Sherry (Potential for hypertensive crisis).
Soy sauce (Potential for hypertensive crisis).
Wine, Chianti (Potential for hypertensive crisis).
Yeast extract (Potential for hypertensive crisis).
Yogurt (Potential for hypertensive crisis).

PAVABID CAPSULES
(Papaverine Hydrochloride) ... 1344
No interactions described in labeling.

PAVABID HP CAPSULETS
(Papaverine Hydrochloride) ... 1344
No interactions described in labeling.

PAZO HEMORRHOID OINTMENT & SUPPOSITORIES
(Ephedrine Sulfate, Zinc Oxide) ... 752
May interact with:

Antidepressant Medications, unspecified (Effects not specified).
Antihypertensive agents, unspecified (Effects not specified).

PEDIACARE ALLERGY RELIEF FORMULA LIQUID
(Pseudoephedrine Hydrochloride, Chlorpheniramine Maleate) ... 1362
May interact with antihypertensives and antidepressant drugs. Compounds in these categories include:

Acebutolol Hydrochloride (Effect not specified). Products include:
Sectral Capsules ... 2520
Amitriptyline Hydrochloride (Effect not specified). Products include:
Elavil ... 2269
Endep Tablets ... 1927
Etrafon ... 2087
Limbitrol ... 1933
Triavil Tablets ... 1556
Amoxapine (Effect not specified). Products include:
Asendin Tablets ... 1196
Atenolol (Effect not specified). Products include:
Tenoretic Tablets ... 1105
Tenormin Tablets and I.V. Injection 1107
Benazepril Hydrochloride (Effect not specified). Products include:
Lotensin Tablets ... 872
Betaxolol Hydrochloride (Effect not specified). Products include:
Betoptic Sterile Ophthalmic Solution ... 569
Betoptic S Sterile Ophthalmic Suspension ... 570
Kerlone Tablets ... 2172
Bupropion Hydrochloride (Effect not specified). Products include:
Wellbutrin Tablets ... 821
Captopril (Effect not specified). Products include:
Capoten ... 2255
Capozide ... 2258
Carteolol Hydrochloride (Effect not specified). Products include:
Cartrol Tablets ... 507
Clonidine (Effect not specified). Products include:
Catapres-TTS ... 677
Clonidine Hydrochloride (Effect not specified). Products include:
Catapres Tablets ... 676
Combipres Tablets ... 678
Deserpidine (Effect not specified). Products include:
Enduronyl ... 518
Harmonyl Tablets ... 528
Oreticyl ... 545
Desipramine Hydrochloride (Effect not specified). Products include:
Norpramin Tablets ... 1340
Diazoxide (Effect not specified). Products include:
Hyperstat I.V. Injection ... 2095
Proglycem ... 649
Doxazosin Mesylate (Effect not specified). Products include:
Cardura Tablets ... 1941
Doxepin Hydrochloride (Effect not specified). Products include:
Sinequan ... 1960
Enalapril Maleate (Effect not specified). Products include:
Vaseretic Tablets ... 1559
Vasotec Tablets ... 1564
Enalaprilat (Effect not specified). Products include:
Vasotec I.V. ... 1562
Esmolol Hydrochloride (Effect not specified). Products include:
Brevibloc Injection ... 942
Felodipine (Effect not specified). Products include:
Plendil Extended-Release Tablets ... 1526
Fluoxetine Hydrochloride (Effect not specified). Products include:
Prozac Pulvules ... 920
Fosinopril Sodium (Effect not specified). Products include:
Monopril Tablets ... 1406
Guanabenz Acetate (Effect not specified). Products include:
Wytensin Tablets ... 2542
Guanethidine Monosulfate (Effect not specified). Products include:
Esimil Tablets ... 864
Ismelin Tablets ... 869
Hydralazine Hydrochloride (Effect not specified). Products include:
Apresazide Capsules ... 854
Apresoline Hydrochloride Parenteral (Ampuls) ... 856
Apresoline Hydrochloride Tablets .. 855
Apresoline-Esidrix Tablets ... 857
Ser-Ap-Es Tablets ... 881
Serpasil-Apresoline Tablets ... 884
Imipramine Hydrochloride (Effect not specified). Products include:
Tofranil Ampuls ... 1038
Tofranil Tablets ... 1039
Imipramine Pamoate (Effect not specified). Products include:
Tofranil-PM Capsules ... 1041
Isocarboxazid (Effect not specified). Products include:
Marplan Tablets ... 1906
Isradipine (Effect not specified). Products include:
DynaCirc Capsules ... 2004
Labetalol Hydrochloride (Effect not specified). Products include:
Normodyne Injection ... 2108
Normodyne Tablets ... 2110
Normozide Tablets ... 2112
Trandate HCT Tablets ... 579
Trandate Injection ... 577
Trandate Tablets ... 579
Lisinopril (Effect not specified). Products include:
Prinivil Tablets ... 1538
Prinzide Tablets ... 1540
Zestoretic ... 2274
Zestril Tablets ... 2277
Maprotiline Hydrochloride (Effect not specified). Products include:
Ludiomil Tablets ... 874
Mecamylamine Hydrochloride (Effect not specified). Products include:
Inversine Tablets ... 1492
Methyldopa (Effect not specified). Products include:
Aldoclor Tablets ... 1413
Aldomet Oral ... 1415
Aldoril Tablets ... 1418
Methyldopate Hydrochloride (Effect not specified). Products include:
Aldomet Ester HCl Injection ... 1417
Metoprolol Tartrate (Effect not specified). Products include:
Lopressor Ampuls ... 1032
Lopressor HCT Tablets ... 1034
Lopressor Tablets ... 1032
Metyrosine (Effect not specified). Products include:
Demser Capsules ... 1460
Minoxidil (Effect not specified). Products include:
Loniten Tablets ... 2346
Rogaine Topical Solution ... 2357
Nadolol (Effect not specified). Products include:
Corgard Tablets ... 701
Corzide Tablets ... 702
Nicardipine Hydrochloride (Effect not specified). Products include:
Cardene Capsules ... 2290
Nitroglycerin (Effect not specified). Products include:
Deponit NTG Transdermal Delivery System ... 2143
Minitran Transdermal Delivery System ... 1312
Nitro-Bid Ointment ... 1339
Nitro-Bid Capsules ... 1338
Nitrodisc ... 2176
Nitro-Dur (nitroglycerin) Transdermal Infusion System ... 1164
Nitrogard Tablets ... 1004
Nitrolingual Spray ... 1846
Nitrostat Tablets ... 1743
Transderm-Nitro Transdermal Therapeutic System ... 2283
Nortriptyline Hydrochloride (Effect not specified). Products include:
Pamelor ... 2019
Penbutolol Sulfate (Effect not specified). Products include:
Levatol ... 1832
Phenelzine Sulfate (Effect not specified). Products include:
Nardil ... 1742
Phenoxybenzamine Hydrochloride (Effect not specified). Products include:
Dibenzyline Capsules ... 2207
Phentolamine Mesylate (Effect not specified). Products include:
Regitine ... 878
Pindolol (Effect not specified). Products include:
Visken Tablets ... 2036
Prazosin Hydrochloride (Effect not specified). Products include:
Minipress Capsules ... 1778
Minizide Capsules ... 1779
Propranolol Hydrochloride (Effect not specified). Products include:
Inderal ... 2459
Inderal LA Long Acting Capsules 2461
Inderide Tablets ... 2463
Inderide LA Long Acting Capsules .. 2465
Protriptyline Hydrochloride (Effect not specified). Products include:
Vivactil Tablets ... 1567
Ramipril (Effect not specified). Products include:
Altace Capsules ... 1086
Rauwolfia Serpentina (Effect not specified). Products include:
Raudixin Tablets ... 1803
Rauzide Tablets ... 1804
Rescinnamine (Effect not specified).
No products indexed under this heading.
Reserpine (Effect not specified). Products include:
Diupres Tablets ... 1461
Hydromox R Tablets ... 1209
Hydropres Tablets ... 1485
Renese-R Tablets ... 1786
Salutensin/Salutensin-Demi ... 719
Ser-Ap-Es Tablets ... 881
Serpasil Tablets ... 883
Serpasil-Apresoline Tablets ... 884
Serpasil-Esidrix Tablets ... 886
Sodium Nitroprusside (Effect not specified). Products include:
Nipride I.V. Infusion ... 1909
Terazosin Hydrochloride (Effect not specified). Products include:
Hytrin Tablets ... 529
Timolol Maleate (Effect not specified). Products include:
Blocadren Tablets ... 1429
Timolide Tablets ... 1547
Timoptic in Ocudose ... 1552
Timoptic Sterile Ophthalmic Solution ... 1550
Tranylcypromine Sulfate (Effect not specified). Products include:
Parnate Tablets ... 2222
Trazodone Hydrochloride (Effect not specified). Products include:
Desyrel and Desyrel Dividose ... 1404
Trimethaphan Camsylate (Effect not specified). Products include:
Arfonad Ampuls ... 1887
Trimipramine Maleate (Effect not specified). Products include:
Surmontil Capsules ... 2524

PEDIACARE COUGH-COLD FORMULA LIQUID
(Pseudoephedrine Hydrochloride, Chlorpheniramine Maleate, Dextromethorphan Hydrobromide)....1362
See **PediaCare Allergy Relief Formula Liquid**

PEDIACARE INFANTS' ORAL DECONGESTANT DROPS
(Pseudoephedrine Hydrochloride) 1362
See **PediaCare Allergy Relief Formula Liquid**

PEDIACARE NIGHT REST COUGH-COLD FORMULA LIQUID
(Chlorpheniramine Maleate, Dextromethorphan Hydrobromide, Pseudoephedrine Hydrochloride) 1362
See **PediaCare Allergy Relief Formula Liquid**

PEDIACARE 6-12 COUGH-COLD FORMULA CHEWABLE TABLETS
(Chlorpheniramine Maleate, Pseudoephedrine Hydrochloride, Dextromethorphan Hydrobromide)....1362
See **PediaCare Allergy Relief Formula Liquid**

PEDIAFLOR DROPS
(Sodium Fluoride) 1972
No interactions described in labeling.

PEDIALYTE ORAL ELECTROLYTE MAINTENANCE SOLUTION
(Electrolyte Supplement) 1972
No interactions described in labeling.

PEDIAPRED ORAL LIQUID
(Prednisolone Sodium Phosphate) 987
May interact with barbiturates. Compounds in this category include:

Aprobarbital (Increases dosage requirement of Pediapred). Products include:
- Alurate Elixir 1883

Butabarbital (Increases dosage requirement of Pediapred). Products include:
- Pyridium Plus 1764

Butalbital (Increases dosage requirement of Pediapred). Products include:
- Esgic-Plus Tablets 1002
- Esgic Tablets & Capsules 1001
- Fioricet Tablets 2006
- Fiorinal Capsules 2007
- Fiorinal with Codeine Capsules 2008
- Fiorinal Tablets 2007
- Phrenilin 838
- Sedapap Tablets 50 mg/650 mg .. 1360

Mephobarbital (Increases dosage requirement of Pediapred). Products include:
- Mebaral Tablets 2061

Pentobarbital Sodium (Increases dosage requirement of Pediapred). Products include:
- Nembutal Sodium Capsules 534
- Nembutal Sodium Solution 536
- Nembutal Sodium Suppositories.... 538

Phenobarbital (Increases dosage requirement of Pediapred). Products include:
- Arco-Lase Plus Tablets 607
- Bellergal-S Tablets 1998
- Bronkolixir .... ◼ 761
- Bronkotabs Tablets.... ◼ 762
- Donnatal 1858
- Donnatal Extentabs.... 1859
- Donnatal Tablets 1858
- Donnazyme Tablets 1860
- Kinesed Tablets 2272
- Phenobarbital Elixir and Tablets 1293
- Primatene Tablets-P Formula.... 2421
- Quadrinal Tablets 1183
- Tedral SA 1765

Secobarbital Sodium (Increases dosage requirement of Pediapred). Products include:
- Seconal Sodium Pulvules 1296

Thiamylal Sodium (Increases dosage requirement of Pediapred). Products include:
- Surital Ampoules, Steri-Vials.... 1764

PEDIAPROFEN SUSPENSION
(Ibuprofen) 1363
May interact with oral anticoagulants, thiazides, lithium preparations, and certain other agents. Compounds in these categories include:

Aspirin (Yields a net decrease in anti-inflammatory activity with lowered blood levels of the non-aspirin drug in animal studies). Products include:
- Alka-Seltzer Effervescent Antacid and Pain Reliever.... 1568
- Alka-Seltzer Extra Strength Effervescent Antacid and Pain Reliever 1570
- Alka-Seltzer (Flavored) Effervescent Antacid and Pain Reliever 1569
- Alka-Seltzer Plus Cold Medicine .... ◼ 623
- Alka-Seltzer Plus Night-Time Cold Medicine .... ◼ 623
- Alka Seltzer Plus Sinus Allergy Medicine .... ◼ 624
- Anacin Coated Analgesic Caplets 2417
- Anacin Coated Analgesic Tablets 2417
- Anacin Maximum Strength Analgesic Coated Tablets.... 2417
- Maximum Strength Arthritis Pain Formula By the Makers of Anacin Analgesic Tablets and Caplets 2418
- Arthritis Pain Formula by the Makers of Anacin Analgesic Tablets and Caplets .... ◼ 747
- Arthritis Strength BC Powder.... ◼ 516
- Ascriptin A/D Caplets 1850
- Regular Strength Ascriptin Tablets 1850
- Azdone Tablets.... 844
- BC Powder .... ◼ 517
- BC Cold Powder .... ◼ 517
- Children's Bayer Chewable Aspirin .... ◼ 564
- Genuine Bayer Aspirin Tablets & Caplets .... ◼ 564
- Maximum Bayer Aspirin Tablets & Caplets .... ◼ 566
- Bayer Plus Aspirin Tablets.... ◼ 567
- Therapy Bayer Aspirin Caplets .... ◼ 568
- 8 Hour Bayer Timed-Release Aspirin .... ◼ 566
- Arthritis Strength Bufferin Analgesic Caplets 744
- Extra Strength Bufferin Analgesic Tablets 745
- Bufferin Analgesic Tablets and Caplets 743
- Cama Arthritis Pain Reliever.... ◼ 685
- Damason-P.... 1356
- Easprin.... 1719
- Ecotrin Enteric Coated Aspirin Maximum Strength Tablets and Caplets 2189
- Ecotrin Enteric Coated Aspirin Regular Strength Tablets and Caplets 2189
- Empirin Aspirin.... ◼ 541
- Empirin with Codeine Phosphate Nos. 2, 3 & 4.... 764
- Equagesic Tablets 2451
- Excedrin Extra-Strength Analgesic Tablets & Caplets 749
- 4-Way Cold Tablets.... 750
- Fiorinal Capsules 2007
- Fiorinal with Codeine Capsules 2008
- Fiorinal Tablets.... 2007
- Lortab ASA Tablets.... 2414
- Momentum Muscular Backache Formula .... ◼ 751
- Norgesic.... 1314
- Norwich Extra-Strength Aspirin.... ◼ 546
- Norwich Regular Strength Aspirin ◼ 547
- P-A-C Analgesic Tablets .... ◼ 669
- Percodan.... 951
- Robaxisal Tablets.... 1872
- Sine-Off Sinus Medicine Tablets-Aspirin Formula .... ◼ 722
- Soma Compound w/Codeine Tablets 2390
- Soma Compound Tablets.... 2389
- St. Joseph Adult Chewable Aspirin (81 mg.) .... ◼ 703
- Synalgos-DC Capsules.... 2525
- Talwin Compound 2072
- Ursinus Inlay-Tabs.... ◼ 691
- Vanquish Analgesic Caplets .... ◼ 574
- Zorprin Tablets.... 698

Bendroflumethiazide (Reduced natriuretic effect). Products include:
- Corzide Tablets 702
- Naturetin Tablets.... 1789
- Rauzide Tablets 1804

Chlorothiazide (Reduced natriuretic effect). Products include:
- Aldoclor Tablets 1413
- Diupres Tablets 1461
- Diuril Oral 1464

Chlorothiazide Sodium (Reduced natriuretic effect). Products include:
- Diuril Sodium Intravenous 1463

Dicumarol (Potential for excessive bleeding). Products include:
- Dicumarol Tablets 516

Furosemide (Reduced natriuretic effect). Products include:
- Lasix 1093

Hydrochlorothiazide (Reduced natriuretic effect). Products include:
- Aldactazide.... 2150
- Aldoril Tablets.... 1418
- Apresazide Capsules 854
- Apresoline-Esidrix Tablets 857
- Capozide 2258
- Dyazide Capsules.... 2208
- Esidrix Tablets 863
- Esimil Tablets 864
- HydroDIURIL Tablets 1484
- Hydropres Tablets.... 1485
- Inderide Tablets.... 2463
- Inderide LA Long Acting Capsules .. 2465
- Lopressor HCT Tablets 1034
- Maxzide 1215
- Moduretic Tablets 1510
- Normozide Tablets 2112
- Oretic Tablets 544
- Oreticyl.... 545
- Prinzide Tablets 1540
- Ser-Ap-Es Tablets 881
- Serpasil-Esidrix Tablets.... 886
- Timolide Tablets.... 1547
- Trandate HCT Tablets 579
- Vaseretic Tablets 1559
- Zestoretic 2274

Hydroflumethiazide (Reduced natriuretic effect). Products include:
- Diucardin Tablets.... 2450
- Saluron.... 718
- Salutensin/Salutensin-Demi 719

Lithium Carbonate (Reduced renal lithium clearance and elevation of plasma lithium levels). Products include:
- Eskalith 2214
- Lithane Tablets 1596
- Lithium Carbonate Capsules & Tablets 1984
- Lithobid Tablets 870

Lithium Citrate (Reduced renal lithium clearance and elevation of plasma lithium levels). Products include:
- Cibalith-S.... 870

Methotrexate Sodium (Enhanced toxicity of methotrexate). Products include:
- Methotrexate Tablets, Parenteral, LPF Parenteral 1217
- Rheumatrex Methotrexate Dose Pack.... 1234

Methyclothiazide (Reduced natriuretic effect). Products include:
- Enduron Tablets.... 517
- Enduronyl 518

Polythiazide (Reduced natriuretic effect). Products include:
- Minizide Capsules 1779
- Renese Tablets 1785
- Renese-R Tablets.... 1786

Warfarin Sodium (Potential for excessive bleeding). Products include:
- Coumadin Injection & Tablets 944
- Panwarfin Tablets 547

Food Interactions

Food, unspecified (The peak levels are somewhat lower (up to 30%) and the time to reach peak levels is slightly prolonged (up to 30 min.) although the extent of absorption is unchanged).

PEDIASURE LIQUID NUTRITION FOR CHILDREN
(Nutritional Supplement) 1973
No interactions described in labeling.

PEDIAZOLE
(Erythromycin Ethylsuccinate, Acetyl Sulfisoxazole) 1973
May interact with xanthine bronchodilators. Compounds in this category include:

Aminophylline (Increased serum theophylline levels; potential theophylline toxicity). Products include:
- Amesec .... ◼ 682
- Aminophyllin Tablets 2153

Dyphylline (Increased serum theophylline levels; potential theophylline toxicity). Products include:
- Dilor.... 2079
- Dilor-G Tablets & Liquid.... 2079
- Lufyllin Elixir 2384
- Lufyllin & Lufyllin-400 Tablets 2384
- Lufyllin-GG Elixir & Tablets 2385

Theophylline (Increased serum theophylline levels; potential theophylline toxicity). Products include:
- Bronkaid Tablets .... ◼ 757
- Bronkolixir .... ◼ 761
- Bronkotabs Tablets.... ◼ 762
- Constant-T Tablets 1029
- Marax Tablets & DF Syrup.... 1954
- Primatene Tablets.... 2421
- Quibron Capsules 713
- Quibron-T 714
- Quibron-T/SR 716
- Theolair Liquid 1317
- Theo-Organidin Elixir 2391

Theophylline Anhydrous (Increased serum theophylline levels; potential theophylline toxicity). Products include:
- Aerolate 994
- Primatene Tablets-M Formula .... ◼ 753
- Primatene Tablets-Regular Formula 2421
- Respbid Tablets 684
- Slo-bid Gyrocaps 1847
- T-PHYL (Uniphyl) 200 mg Tablets 1820
- Tedral SA 1765
- Theo-24.... 2179
- Theo-Dur Sprinkle 1168
- Theo-Dur Extended-Release Tablets.... 1166
- Theolair Tablets 1317
- Theolair-SR Tablets.... 1319
- TheoX Extended-Release Tablets 841
- Uniphyl 400 mg Tablets.... 1823

Theophylline Calcium Salicylate (Increased serum theophylline levels; potential theophylline toxicity). Products include:
- Quadrinal Tablets 1183

Theophylline Sodium Glycinate (Increased serum theophylline levels; potential theophylline toxicity). Products include:
- Asbron G 1997

PEDI-BORO SOAK PAKS
(Aluminum Sulfate) 1771
No interactions described in labeling.

PEDI-DRI FOOT POWDER
(Aluminum Chlorhydroxide)....1771
No interactions described in labeling.

PEDIOTIC SUSPENSION STERILE
(Polymyxin B Sulfate, Neomycin Sulfate, Hydrocortisone) 797
No interactions described in labeling.

PEDI-PRO FOOT POWDER
(Aluminum Chlorhydroxide) 1771
No interactions described in labeling.

PEDVAXHIB
(Haemophilus B Conjugate Vaccine) 1521
May interact with immunosuppressive agents. Compounds in this category include:

Azathioprine (Expected immune response may not be observed). Products include:
Imuran 768

Cyclosporine (Expected immune response may not be observed). Products include:
Sandimmune 2024

Immune Globulin (Human) (Expected immune response may not be observed). Products include:
MICRhoGAM Rh$_0$(D) Immune Globulin (Human) 1650
RhoGAM Rh$_0$(D) Immune Globulin (Human) 1651

Immune Globulin Intravenous (Human) (Expected immune response may not be observed). Products include:
Gamimune N Immune Globulin Intravenous (Human) 1572
Gammagard Immune Globulin, Intravenous (Human) 658
Iveegam 1129
Sandoglobulin I.V. 2027

Muromonab-CD3 (Expected immune response may not be observed). Products include:
Orthoclone OKT3 Sterile Solution 1645

PEGANONE TABLETS
(Ethotoin) 551
May interact with oral anticoagulants and certain other agents. Compounds in these categories include:

Dicumarol (Possible interactions, not yet documented). Products include:
Dicumarol Tablets 516

Folic Acid (Interferes with folic acid metabolism). Products include:
Allbee C-800 Plus Iron Tablets ◆ 670
Biotin Forte 3mg. & Extra Strength Biotin Forte 5mg 2377
Bugs Bunny Children's Chewable Vitamins (Sugar Free) ◆ 625
Bugs Bunny With Extra C Children's Chewable Vitamins (Sugar Free) ◆ 626
Bugs Bunny Plus Iron Children's Chewable Vitamins (Sugar Free) ◆ 625
Cefol Filmtab 509
Fero-Folic-500 Filmtab 527
Flintstones Children's Chewable Vitamins ◆ 625
Flintstones Children's Chewable Vitamins With Extra C ◆ 626
Flintstones Children's Chewable Vitamins Plus Iron ◆ 625
Iberet-Folic-500 Filmtab 527
Materna Tablets 1214
May-Vita Elixir 1359
Mega-B 607
Nephro-Vite Rx 1826
Niferex-150 Forte Capsules 847
One-A-Day Essential Vitamins ◆ 627
One-A-Day Maximum Formula Vitamins and Minerals ◆ 627
One-A-Day Plus Extra C Vitamins ◆ 627
Pramet FA 1974
Pramilet FA 1974
Sigtab Tablets ◆ 669
Stressgard Stress Formula Vitamins ◆ 628
STUART PRENATAL Tablets ◆ 731
The Stuart Formula Tablets ◆ 581
Stuartnatal 1+1 Tablets 2273
Theragran Stress Formula ◆ 727
Trinsicon Capsules 2415
Vicon Forte Capsules 2416
Within Women's Formula Multivitamin with Calcium, Extra Iron and Zinc ◆ 628
Zenate Tablets 2250
Zymacap Capsules ◆ 670

Phenacemide (Paranoid symptoms). Products include:
Phenurone Tablets 552

Warfarin Sodium (Possible interactions, not yet documented). Products include:
Coumadin Injection & Tablets 944
Panwarfin Tablets 547

PEN•KERA CREME
(Emollient) ◆ 508
No interactions described in labeling.

PENTAM 300 INJECTION
(Pentamidine Isethionate) 1018
No interactions described in labeling.

PENTASPAN INJECTION
(Pentastarch) 949
No interactions described in labeling.

PENTRAX TAR SHAMPOO WITH FRACTAR
(Coal Tar) 1045
No interactions described in labeling.

PEPCID I.V.
(Famotidine) 1524
No interactions described in labeling.

PEPCID ORAL SUSPENSION
(Famotidine) 1524
May interact with antacids and certain other agents. Compounds in these categories include:

Aluminum Carbonate Gel (Bioavailability may be slightly decreased by antacids). Products include:
Basaljel 2438

Aluminum Hydroxide (Bioavailability may be slightly decreased by antacids). Products include:
Cama Arthritis Pain Reliever ◆ 685
Gaviscon Extra Strength Relief Formula Liquid Antacid ◆ 594
Gaviscon Extra Strength Relief Formula Antacid Tablets ◆ 594
Gaviscon Liquid Antacid ◆ 594
Gelusil Liquid & Tablets ◆ 639
Extra Strength Maalox Plus Suspension 1850
Maalox TC Suspension 1851
Maalox Plus Tablets ◆ 655
Extra Strength Maalox Plus Tablets 1850
Nephrox Suspension ◆ 563
WinGel Liquid & Tablets ◆ 761

Aluminum Hydroxide Gel (Bioavailability may be slightly decreased by antacids). Products include:
ALternaGEL Liquid 1154
Aludrox Oral Suspension 2428
Amphojel Suspension 2429
Amphojel Suspension without Flavor 2429
Mylanta Liquid 1155
Mylanta Double Strength Liquid 1155

Aluminum Hydroxide Gel, Dried (Bioavailability may be slightly decreased by antacids). Products include:
Alu-Tab/Alu-Cap 1309
Amphojel Tablets 2429
Ascriptin A/D Caplets 1850
Regular Strength Ascriptin Tablets 1850
Gaviscon Antacid Tablets ◆ 593
Gaviscon-2 Antacid Tablets ◆ 594
Mylanta Tablets 1155
Mylanta Double Strength Tablets 1155

Dihydroxyaluminum Sodium Carbonate (Bioavailability may be slightly decreased by antacids). Products include:
Rolaids ◆ 743

Magaldrate (Bioavailability may be slightly decreased by antacids). Products include:
Riopan Antacid Chew Tablets ◆ 754
Riopan Antacid Chew Tablets in Rollpacks ◆ 754
Riopan Antacid Suspension 2421
Riopan Antacid Swallow Tablets 2421
Riopan Plus Chew Tablets 2422
Riopan Plus Chew Tablets in Rollpack 2422
Riopan Plus 2 Chew Tablets, Mint Flavor, Cherry Flavor 2422
Riopan Plus Suspension 2422
Riopan Plus 2 Suspension, Mint Flavor, Cherry Flavor 2422

Magnesium Hydroxide (Bioavailability may be slightly decreased by antacids). Products include:
Aludrox Oral Suspension 2428
Ascriptin A/D Caplets 1850
Regular Strength Ascriptin Tablets 1850
Di-Gel Antacid/Anti-Gas ◆ 697
Gelusil Liquid & Tablets ◆ 639
Haley's M-O, Regular & Flavored ◆ 569
Extra Strength Maalox Plus Suspension 1850
Maalox TC Suspension 1851
Maalox Plus Tablets ◆ 655
Extra Strength Maalox Plus Tablets 1850
Mylanta Liquid 1155
Mylanta Tablets 1155
Mylanta Double Strength Liquid 1155
Mylanta Double Strength Tablets 1155
Concentrated Phillips' Milk of Magnesia ◆ 573
Phillips' Milk of Magnesia Liquid ◆ 572
Phillips' Milk of Magnesia Tablets ◆ 573
WinGel Liquid & Tablets ◆ 761

Magnesium Oxide (Bioavailability may be slightly decreased by antacids). Products include:
Bayer Plus Aspirin Tablets ◆ 567
Beelith Tablets 659
Bufferin Analgesic Tablets and Caplets ◆ 524
Cama Arthritis Pain Reliever ◆ 685
Mag-Ox 400 673
Uro-Mag 673

Sodium Bicarbonate (Bioavailability may be slightly decreased by antacids). Products include:
Alka-Seltzer Advanced Formula Antacid & Non-Aspirin Pain Reliever ◆ 620
Alka-Seltzer Effervescent Antacid ◆ 622
Alka-Seltzer Effervescent Antacid and Pain Reliever 1568
Alka-Seltzer Extra Strength Effervescent Antacid and Pain Reliever ◆ 623
Alka-Seltzer (Flavored) Effervescent Antacid and Pain Reliever ◆ 621
Arm & Hammer Pure Baking Soda ◆ 548
Ceo-Two Rectal Suppositories 671
Citrocarbonate Antacid ◆ 668
Massengill Liquid Concentrate 2191
NuLYTELY 699

Food Interactions

Food, unspecified (Bioavailability may be slightly increased by antacids).

PEPCID TABLETS
(Famotidine) 1524
See **Pepcid Oral Suspension**

PEPTAVLON
(Pentagastrin) 2563
No interactions described in labeling.

PEPTO-BISMOL LIQUID & TABLETS
(Bismuth Subsalicylate) 1807
May interact with oral anticoagulants, oral hypoglycemic agents, antigout agents, and certain other agents. Compounds in these categories include:

Allopurinol (Use cautiously). Products include:
Zyloprim Tablets 830

Chlorpropamide (Use cautiously). Products include:
Diabinese Tablets 1775

Dicumarol (Use cautiously). Products include:
Dicumarol Tablets 516

Glipizide (Use cautiously). Products include:
Glucotrol 1952

Glyburide (Use cautiously). Products include:
DiaBeta 1091
Micronase Tablets 2350

Probenecid (Use cautiously). Products include:
Benemid Tablets 1426
ColBENEMID Tablets 1436
Wycillin Injection and Probenecid Tablets 2539

Sulfinpyrazone (Use cautiously). Products include:
Anturane 853

Tolazamide (Use cautiously). Products include:
Tolinase Tablets 2365

Tolbutamide (Use cautiously). Products include:
Orinase Tablets 2354

Warfarin Sodium (Use cautiously). Products include:
Coumadin Injection & Tablets 944
Panwarfin Tablets 547

MAXIMUM STRENGTH PEPTO-BISMOL LIQUID
(Bismuth Subsalicylate) 1808
May interact with insulin, oral anticoagulants, antigout agents, and oral hypoglycemic agents. Compounds in these categories include:

Allopurinol (Use cautiously). Products include:
Zyloprim Tablets 830

Chlorpropamide (Use cautiously). Products include:
Diabinese Tablets 1775

Dicumarol (Use cautiously). Products include:
Dicumarol Tablets 516

Glipizide (Use cautiously). Products include:
Glucotrol 1952

Glyburide (Use cautiously). Products include:
DiaBeta 1091
Micronase Tablets 2350

Insulin, Human (Use cautiously).
No products indexed under this heading.

Insulin, Human Isophane Suspension (Use cautiously). Products include:
Humulin N, 100 Units 1270

Insulin, Human NPH (Use cautiously). Products include:
Insulatard NPH Human 1627
Novolin N 1627
Novolin N PenFill Cartridges 1628
Novolin N Prefilled 1628

Insulin, Human Regular (Use cautiously). Products include:
Humulin BR, 100 Units 1268
Humulin R, 100 Units 1272
Novolin R 1627
Novolin R PenFill Cartridges 1628
Novolin R Prefilled 1629
Velosulin Human 1628

Insulin, Human, Zinc Suspension (Use cautiously). Products include:
Humulin L, 100 Units 1268
Humulin U, 100 Units 1272

Novolin L 1627

Insulin, NPH (Use cautiously). Products include:

NPH, 40 & 100 Units 1273
Beef NPH, 100 Units 1274
Pork NPH, 100 Units 1275
Insulatard NPH 1626
NPH Insulin 1626
NPH Purified Pork Isophane Insulin 1626

Insulin, Regular (Use cautiously). Products include:

Regular, 40 & 100 Units 1273
Beef Regular, 100 Units 1275
Pork Regular, 100 Units 1275
Pork Regular (Concentrated), 500 Units 1276
Regular Insulin 1625
Regular Purified Pork Insulin 1626
Velosulin 1627

Insulin, Zinc Crystals (Use cautiously). Products include:

NPH, 40 & 100 Units 1273

Insulin, Zinc Suspension (Use cautiously). Products include:

Lente, 40 & 100 Units 1272
Protamine, Zinc, 40 & 100 Units 1273
Lente Iletin I 1272
Beef Lente, 100 Units 1274
Beef Protamine Zinc, 100 Units 1274
Pork Lente, 100 Units 1275
Pork, Protamine, Zinc, 100 Units 1275
Lente Insulin 1626
Lente Purified Pork Insulin 1626
Semilente Insulin 1625
Ultralente Insulin 1626

Probenecid (Use cautiously). Products include:

Benemid Tablets 1426
ColBENEMID Tablets 1436
Wycillin Injection and Probenecid Tablets 2539

Sulfinpyrazone (Use cautiously). Products include:

Anturane 853

Tolazamide (Use cautiously). Products include:

Tolinase Tablets 2365

Tolbutamide (Use cautiously). Products include:

Orinase Tablets 2354

Warfarin Sodium (Use cautiously). Products include:

Coumadin Injection & Tablets 944
Panwarfin Tablets 547

PERCOCET TABLETS
(Oxycodone Hydrochloride, Acetaminophen) 950

May interact with narcotic analgesics, general anesthetics, phenothiazines, tranquilizers, hypnotics and sedatives, central nervous system depressants, monoamine oxidase inhibitors, tricyclic antidepressants, anticholinergics, and certain other agents. Compounds in these categories include:

Alcohol (Additive CNS depression).

Alfentanil Hydrochloride (Additive CNS depression; dose of one or both agents should be reduced). Products include:

Alfenta Injection 1131

Alprazolam (Additive CNS depression). Products include:

Xanax Tablets 2367

Amitriptyline Hydrochloride (Increased effect of antidepressant). Products include:

Elavil 2269
Endep Tablets 1927
Etrafon 2087
Limbitrol 1933
Triavil Tablets 1556

Amoxapine (Increased effect of antidepressant). Products include:

Asendin Tablets 1196

Aprobarbital (Additive CNS depression; dose of one or both agents should be reduced). Products include:

Alurate Elixir 1883

Atropine Sulfate (May produce paralytic ileus). Products include:

Arco-Lase Plus Tablets 607
Atropine Sulfate Sterile Ophthalmic Solution and S.O.P. Sterile Ophthalmic Ointment ◉ 239
Donnagel ⊞ 675
Donnagel-PG 1858
Donnatal 1858
Donnatal Extentabs 1859
Donnatal Tablets 1858
Donnazyme Tablets 1860
Isopto Atropine ◉ 218
Lomotil 2174
Motofen Tablets 836
Ru-Tuss Tablets 693
Urised Tablets 2396

Belladonna Alkaloids (May produce paralytic ileus). Products include:

Bellergal-S Tablets 1998
Hyland's Bed Wetting Tablets ⊞ 728
Hyland's Teething Tablets ⊞ 728
Kinesed Tablets 2272

Benztropine Mesylate (May produce paralytic ileus). Products include:

Cogentin 1435

Biperiden (May produce paralytic ileus). Products include:

Akineton 1171

Buprenorphine (Additive CNS depression; dose of one or both agents should be reduced).

No products indexed under this heading.

Buspirone Hydrochloride (Additive CNS depression; dose of one or both agents should be reduced). Products include:

BuSpar 1401

Butabarbital (Additive CNS depression; dose of one or both agents should be reduced). Products include:

Pyridium Plus 1764

Butalbital (Additive CNS depression; dose of one or both agents should be reduced). Products include:

Esgic-Plus Tablets 1002
Esgic Tablets & Capsules 1001
Fioricet Tablets 2006
Fiorinal Capsules 2007
Fiorinal with Codeine Capsules 2008
Fiorinal Tablets 2007
Phrenilin 838
Sedapap Tablets 50 mg/650 mg 1360

Chlordiazepoxide (Additive CNS depression; dose of one or both agents should be reduced). Products include:

Libritabs Tablets 1930
Limbitrol 1933
Menrium Tablets 1934

Chlordiazepoxide Hydrochloride (Additive CNS depression; dose of one or both agents should be reduced). Products include:

Librax Capsules 1929
Librium Capsules 1931
Librium Injectable 1932

Chlorpromazine (Additive CNS depression; dose of one or both agents should be reduced). Products include:

Thorazine 2234

Chlorprothixene (Additive CNS depression; dose of one or both agents should be reduced). Products include:

Taractan Tablets 1920

Chlorprothixene Hydrochloride (Additive CNS depression; dose of one or both agents should be reduced). Products include:

Taractan 1920

Clomipramine Hydrochloride (Increased effect of antidepressant). Products include:

Anafranil Capsules 650

Clorazepate Dipotassium (Additive CNS depression; dose of one or both agents should be reduced). Products include:

Tranxene 556

Codeine (Additive CNS depression; dose of one or both agents should be reduced). Products include:

Calcidrine Syrup 506

Codeine Phosphate (Additive CNS depression; dose of one or both agents should be reduced). Products include:

Actifed with Codeine Cough Syrup 752
Cheracol Cough Syrup 1853
Codimal PH Syrup 846
Dimetane-DC Cough Syrup 1857
Empirin with Codeine Phosphate Nos. 2, 3 & 4 764
Fiorinal with Codeine Capsules 2008
Isoclor Expectorant 982
Naldecon CX Adult Liquid ⊞ 521
Novahistine DH 1342
Novahistine Expectorant 1343
Nucofed Capsules 2219
Nucofed Expectorant 2219
Nucofed Pediatric Expectorant 2220
Nucofed Syrup 2219
Phenaphen with Codeine Capsules 1865
Phenaphen-650 with Codeine Tablets 1866
Phenergan with Codeine 2497
Phenergan VC with Codeine 2501
Robitussin A-C Syrup 1875
Robitussin-DAC Syrup 1875
Ryna ⊞ 741
Soma Compound w/Codeine Tablets 2390
Triaminic Expectorant w/Codeine 1996
Tussi-Organidin Liquid 2391
Tylenol with Codeine 1381

Codeine Polistirex (Additive CNS depression; dose of one or both agents should be reduced).

No products indexed under this heading.

Desipramine Hydrochloride (Increased effect of antidepressant). Products include:

Norpramin Tablets 1340

Dezocine (Additive CNS depression; dose of one or both agents should be reduced).

Diazepam (Additive CNS depression; dose of one or both agents should be reduced). Products include:

Valium Injectable 1937
Valium Tablets 1939
Valrelease Capsules 1923

Dicyclomine Hydrochloride (May produce paralytic ileus). Products include:

Bentyl 1322

Doxepin Hydrochloride (Increased effect of antidepressant). Products include:

Sinequan 1960

Droperidol (Additive CNS depression; dose of one or both agents should be reduced). Products include:

Inapsine Injection 1140
Innovar Injection 1141

Enflurane (Additive CNS depression; dose of one or both agents should be reduced). Products include:

Ethrane 599

Estazolam (Additive CNS depression; dose of one or both agents should be reduced). Products include:

ProSom Tablets 554

Ethchlorvynol (Additive CNS depression; dose of one or both agents should be reduced). Products include:

Placidyl Capsules 553

Ethinamate (Additive CNS depression; dose of one or both agents should be reduced).

No products indexed under this heading.

Ethopropazine Hydrochloride (May produce paralytic ileus).

Fentanyl (Additive CNS depression; dose of one or both agents should be reduced). Products include:

Duragesic Transdermal System 1133

Fentanyl Citrate (Additive CNS depression; dose of one or both agents should be reduced). Products include:

Innovar Injection 1141
Sublimaze Injection 1146

Fluphenazine Decanoate (Additive CNS depression; dose of one or both agents should be reduced). Products include:

Prolixin Decanoate 1795

Fluphenazine Enanthate (Additive CNS depression; dose of one or both agents should be reduced). Products include:

Prolixin Enanthate 1796

Fluphenazine Hydrochloride (Additive CNS depression; dose of one or both agents should be reduced). Products include:

Prolixin Elixir 1793
Prolixin Injection 1791
Prolixin Oral Concentrate 1792
Prolixin Tablets 1793

Flurazepam Hydrochloride (Additive CNS depression; dose of one or both agents should be reduced). Products include:

Dalmane Capsules 1927

Furazolidone (Increased effect of either oxycodone or MAO inhibitor). Products include:

Furoxone 1855

Glutethimide (Additive CNS depression; dose of one or both agents should be reduced).

No products indexed under this heading.

Glycopyrrolate (May produce paralytic ileus). Products include:

Robinul Forte Tablets 1873
Robinul Injectable 1873
Robinul Tablets 1873

Haloperidol (Additive CNS depression; dose of one or both agents should be reduced). Products include:

Haldol Injection, Tablets and Concentrate 1373

Haloperidol Decanoate (Additive CNS depression; dose of one or both agents should be reduced). Products include:

Haldol Decanoate 1375

Hydrocodone Bitartrate (Additive CNS depression; dose of one or both agents should be reduced). Products include:

Anexsia 5/500 Tablets 2196
Anexsia 7.5/650 Tablets 2197
Azdōne Tablets 844
Codiclear DH Syrup 845
Codimal DH Syrup 846
Damason-P 1356
Hycodan Syrup, Tablets 927
Hycomine Compound Tablets 929
Hycomine Syrup 927
Hycotuss Expectorant Syrup 930

Hydrocet Capsules ... 835
Lortab ASA Tablets ... 2414
Lortab ... 2412
Ru-Tuss with Hydrocodone ... 694
Triaminic Expectorant DH ... 1995
Vicodin Tablets ... 1187
Vicodin ES Tablets ... 1189
Zydone Capsules ... 941

Hydrocodone Polistirex (Additive CNS depression; dose of one or both agents should be reduced). Products include:
Tussionex Extended-Release Suspension ... 988

Hydroxyzine Hydrochloride (Additive CNS depression; dose of one or both agents should be reduced). Products include:
Atarax Tablets & Syrup ... 1941
Marax Tablets & DF Syrup ... 1954
Vistaril Intramuscular Solution ... 1970

Hyoscyamine (May produce paralytic ileus). Products include:
Cystospaz Tablets ... 2395
Urised Tablets ... 2396

Hyoscyamine Sulfate (May produce paralytic ileus). Products include:
Arco-Lase Plus Tablets ... 607
Cystospaz-M Capsules ... 2395
Donnagel ... ▣ 675
Donnagel-PG ... 1858
Donnatal ... 1858
Donnatal Extentabs ... 1859
Donnatal Tablets ... 1858
Donnazyme Tablets ... 1860
Kutrase Capsules ... 2146
Levsin/Levsinex ... 2147
Ru-Tuss Tablets ... 693

Imipramine Hydrochloride (Increased effect of antidepressant). Products include:
Tofranil Ampuls ... 1038
Tofranil Tablets ... 1039

Imipramine Pamoate (Increased effect of antidepressant). Products include:
Tofranil-PM Capsules ... 1041

Ipratropium Bromide (May produce paralytic ileus). Products include:
Atrovent Inhalation Aerosol ... 675

Isocarboxazid (Increased effect of either oxycodone or MAO inhibitor). Products include:
Marplan Tablets ... 1906

Isoflurane (Additive CNS depression; dose of one or both agents should be reduced). Products include:
Forane ... 600

Ketamine Hydrochloride (Additive CNS depression; dose of one or both agents should be reduced). Products include:
Ketalar ... 1726

Levorphanol Tartrate (Additive CNS depression; dose of one or both agents should be reduced). Products include:
Levo-Dromoran ... 1906

Lorazepam (Additive CNS depression; dose of one or both agents should be reduced). Products include:
Ativan Injection ... 2432
Ativan Tablets ... 2434

Loxapine Hydrochloride (Additive CNS depression; dose of one or both agents should be reduced). Products include:
Loxitane ... 1213

Loxapine Succinate (Additive CNS depression; dose of one or both agents should be reduced). Products include:
Loxitane Capsules ... 1213

Maprotiline Hydrochloride (Increased effect of antidepressant). Products include:
Ludiomil Tablets ... 874

Mepenzolate Bromide (May produce paralytic ileus). Products include:
Cantil Tablets ... 1326

Meperidine Hydrochloride (Additive CNS depression; dose of one or both agents should be reduced). Products include:
Demerol ... 2047
Mepergan Injection ... 2479

Mephobarbital (Additive CNS depression; dose of one or both agents should be reduced). Products include:
Mebaral Tablets ... 2061

Meprobamate (Additive CNS depression; dose of one or both agents should be reduced). Products include:
Deprol Tablets ... 2382
Equagesic Tablets ... 2451
Miltown Tablets ... 2386
PMB 200 and PMB 400 ... 2504

Mesoridazine (Additive CNS depression; dose of one or both agents should be reduced). Products include:
Serentil ... 686

Methadone Hydrochloride (Additive CNS depression; dose of one or both agents should be reduced). Products include:
Dolophine Hydrochloride Ampoules & Vials ... 1260
Dolophine Hydrochloride Tablets ... 1261
Methadone Hydrochloride Diskets ... 1284
Methadone Hydrochloride Oral Solution & Tablets ... 1987

Methohexital Sodium (Additive CNS depression; dose of one or both agents should be reduced). Products include:
Brevital Sodium Vials ... 1248

Methoxyflurane (Additive CNS depression; dose of one or both agents should be reduced).
No products indexed under this heading.

Midazolam Hydrochloride (Additive CNS depression; dose of one or both agents should be reduced). Products include:
Versed Injection ... 1924

Molindone Hydrochloride (Additive CNS depression; dose of one or both agents should be reduced). Products include:
Moban Tablets & Concentrate ... 932

Morphine Sulfate (Additive CNS depression; dose of one or both agents should be reduced). Products include:
Astramorph/PF Injection, USP (Preservative-Free) ... 618
Duramorph ... 960
Infumorph 200 and Infumorph 500 Sterile Solutions ... 962
MS Contin Tablets ... 1814
MSIR ... 1817
Oramorph SR (Morphine Sulfate Sustained Release Tablets) ... 1988
Roxanol ... 1991

Nortriptyline Hydrochloride (Increased effect of antidepressant). Products include:
Pamelor ... 2019

Opium Alkaloids (Additive CNS depression; dose of one or both agents should be reduced). Products include:
B & O No. 15A & No. 16A Supprettes ... 2395
Pantopon Injectable ... 1911

Oxazepam (Additive CNS depression; dose of one or both agents should be reduced; increased effect of antidepressant). Products include:
Serax Capsules ... 2522
Serax Tablets ... 2522

Oxybutynin Chloride (May produce paralytic ileus). Products include:
Ditropan ... 1332

Oxyphenonium Bromide (May produce paralytic ileus).

Pentobarbital Sodium (Additive CNS depression; dose of one or both agents should be reduced). Products include:
Nembutal Sodium Capsules ... 534
Nembutal Sodium Solution ... 536
Nembutal Sodium Suppositories ... 538

Perphenazine (Additive CNS depression; dose of one or both agents should be reduced). Products include:
Etrafon ... 2087
Triavil Tablets ... 1556
Trilafon ... 2123

Phenelzine Sulfate (Increased effect of either oxycodone or MAO inhibitor). Products include:
Nardil ... 1742

Phenobarbital (Additive CNS depression; dose of one or both agents should be reduced). Products include:
Arco-Lase Plus Tablets ... 607
Bellergal-S Tablets ... 1998
Bronkolixir ... ▣ 761
Bronkotabs Tablets ... ▣ 762
Donnatal ... 1858
Donnatal Extentabs ... 1859
Donnatal Tablets ... 1858
Donnazyme Tablets ... 1860
Kinesed Tablets ... 2272
Phenobarbital Elixir and Tablets ... 1293
Primatene Tablets-P Formula ... 2421
Quadrinal Tablets ... 1183
Tedral SA ... 1765

Prazepam (Additive CNS depression; dose of one or both agents should be reduced). Products include:
Centrax ... 1693

Prochlorperazine (Additive CNS depression; dose of one or both agents should be reduced). Products include:
Compazine ... 2201

Procyclidine Hydrochloride (May produce paralytic ileus). Products include:
Kemadrin Tablets ... 771

Promethazine Hydrochloride (Additive CNS depression; dose of one or both agents should be reduced). Products include:
Mepergan Injection ... 2479
Phenergan with Codeine ... 2497
Phenergan with Dextromethorphan ... 2499
Phenergan Injection ... 2493
Phenergan Suppositories ... 2496
Phenergan Syrup ... 2495
Phenergan Tablets ... 2496
Phenergan VC ... 2500
Phenergan VC with Codeine ... 2501

Propantheline Bromide (May produce paralytic ileus). Products include:
Pro-Banthīne Tablets ... 2141

Propofol (Additive CNS depression; dose of one or both agents should be reduced). Products include:
Diprivan Injection ... 2267

Propoxyphene Hydrochloride (Additive CNS depression; dose of one or both agents should be reduced). Products include:
Darvon ... 1256
Wygesic Tablets ... 2540

Propoxyphene Napsylate (Additive CNS depression; dose of one or both agents should be reduced). Products include:
Darvon-N/Darvocet-N ... 1254

Protriptyline Hydrochloride (Increased effect of antidepressant). Products include:
Vivactil Tablets ... 1567

Quazepam (Additive CNS depression; dose of one or both agents should be reduced). Products include:
Doral Tablets ... 2383

Scopolamine Hydrobromide (May produce paralytic ileus). Products include:
Donnagel ... ▣ 675
Donnagel-PG ... 1858
Donnatal ... 1858
Donnatal Extentabs ... 1859
Donnatal Tablets ... 1858
Donnazyme Tablets ... 1860
Isopto Hyoscine ... ⊙ 222
Murocoll-2 Sterile Ophthalmic Solution ... ⊙ 261
Ru-Tuss Tablets ... 693

Secobarbital Sodium (Additive CNS depression; dose of one or both agents should be reduced). Products include:
Seconal Sodium Pulvules ... 1296

Selegiline Hydrochloride (Increased effect of either oxycodone or MAO inhibitor). Products include:
Eldepryl ... 2250

Sufentanil Citrate (Additive CNS depression; dose of one or both agents should be reduced). Products include:
Sufenta Injection ... 1147

Temazepam (Additive CNS depression; dose of one or both agents should be reduced). Products include:
Restoril Capsules ... 2023

Thiamylal Sodium (Additive CNS depression; dose of one or both agents should be reduced). Products include:
Surital Ampoules, Steri-Vials ... 1764

Thioridazine Hydrochloride (Additive CNS depression; dose of one or both agents should be reduced). Products include:
Mellaril ... 2011

Thiothixene (Additive CNS depression; dose of one or both agents should be reduced). Products include:
Navane Capsules and Concentrate 1954
Navane Intramuscular ... 1956

Tranylcypromine Sulfate (Increased effect of either oxycodone or MAO inhibitor). Products include:
Parnate Tablets ... 2222

Triazolam (Additive CNS depression; dose of one or both agents should be reduced). Products include:
Halcion Tablets ... 2340

Tridihexethyl Chloride (May produce paralytic ileus).
No products indexed under this heading.

Trifluoperazine Hydrochloride (Additive CNS depression; dose of one or both agents should be reduced). Products include:
Stelazine ... 2226

Trihexyphenidyl Hydrochloride (May produce paralytic ileus). Products include:
Artane ... 1195

Trimipramine Maleate (Increased effect of antidepressant). Products include:
Surmontil Capsules ... 2524

PERCODAN TABLETS
(Oxycodone Hydrochloride, Oxycodone Terephthalate, Aspirin).... 951
May interact with narcotic analgesics, general anesthetics, phenothiazines, tranquilizers, hypnotics and sedatives, anticoagulants, oral anticoagulants, and certain other agents. Compounds in these categories include:

Alcohol (Additive CNS depression).

Alfentanil Hydrochloride (Additive CNS depression). Products include:
- Alfenta Injection 1131

Alprazolam (Additive CNS depression). Products include:
- Xanax Tablets 2367

Buprenorphine (Additive CNS depression).
- No products indexed under this heading.

Buspirone Hydrochloride (Additive CNS depression). Products include:
- BuSpar 1401

Chlordiazepoxide (Additive CNS depression). Products include:
- Libritabs Tablets 1930
- Limbitrol 1933
- Menrium Tablets 1934

Chlordiazepoxide Hydrochloride (Additive CNS depression). Products include:
- Librax Capsules 1929
- Librium Capsules 1931
- Librium Injectable 1932

Chlorpromazine (Additive CNS depression). Products include:
- Thorazine 2234

Clorazepate Dipotassium (Additive CNS depression). Products include:
- Tranxene 556

Codeine (Additive CNS depression). Products include:
- Calcidrine Syrup 506

Codeine Phosphate (Additive CNS depression). Products include:
- Actifed with Codeine Cough Syrup .. 752
- Cheracol Cough Syrup 1853
- Codimal PH Syrup 846
- Dimetane-DC Cough Syrup 1857
- Empirin with Codeine Phosphate Nos. 2, 3 & 4 764
- Fiorinal with Codeine Capsules 2008
- Isoclor Expectorant 982
- Naldecon CX Adult Liquid .... ▣ 521
- Novahistine DH 1342
- Novahistine Expectorant 1343
- Nucofed Capsules 2219
- Nucofed Expectorant 2219
- Nucofed Pediatric Expectorant 2220
- Nucofed Syrup 2219
- Phenaphen with Codeine Capsules 1865
- Phenaphen-650 with Codeine Tablets 1866
- Phenergan with Codeine 2497
- Phenergan VC with Codeine 2501
- Robitussin A-C Syrup 1875
- Robitussin-DAC Syrup 1875
- Ryna .... ▣ 741
- Soma Compound w/Codeine Tablets 2390
- Triaminic Expectorant w/Codeine .. 1996
- Tussi-Organidin Liquid 2391
- Tylenol with Codeine 1381

Codeine Polistirex (Additive CNS depression).
- No products indexed under this heading.

Dezocine (Additive CNS depression).

Diazepam (Additive CNS depression). Products include:
- Valium Injectable 1937
- Valium Tablets 1939
- Valrelease Capsules 1923

Dicumarol (Enhanced effect of anticoagulant). Products include:
- Dicumarol Tablets 516

Droperidol (Additive CNS depression). Products include:
- Inapsine Injection 1140
- Innovar Injection 1141

Enflurane (Additive CNS depression). Products include:
- Ethrane 599

Estazolam (Additive CNS depression). Products include:
- ProSom Tablets 554

Ethchlorvynol (Additive CNS depression). Products include:
- Placidyl Capsules 553

Ethinamate (Additive CNS depression).
- No products indexed under this heading.

Fentanyl (Additive CNS depression). Products include:
- Duragesic Transdermal System 1133

Fentanyl Citrate (Additive CNS depression). Products include:
- Innovar Injection 1141
- Sublimaze Injection 1146

Fluphenazine Decanoate (Additive CNS depression). Products include:
- Prolixin Decanoate 1795

Fluphenazine Enanthate (Additive CNS depression). Products include:
- Prolixin Enanthate 1796

Fluphenazine Hydrochloride (Additive CNS depression). Products include:
- Prolixin Elixir 1793
- Prolixin Injection 1791
- Prolixin Oral Concentrate 1792
- Prolixin Tablets 1793

Flurazepam Hydrochloride (Additive CNS depression). Products include:
- Dalmane Capsules 1927

Glutethimide (Additive CNS depression).
- No products indexed under this heading.

Haloperidol (Additive CNS depression). Products include:
- Haldol Injection, Tablets and Concentrate 1373

Haloperidol Decanoate (Additive CNS depression). Products include:
- Haldol Decanoate 1375

Heparin Calcium (Enhanced effect of anticoagulant). Products include:
- Calciparine Injection 925

Heparin Sodium (Enhanced effect of anticoagulant). Products include:
- Heparin Lock Flush Solution 2456
- Heparin Sodium Vials 1264
- Heparin Sodium Injection 2457
- Heparin Sodium Injection, USP, Sterile Solution 2342

Hydrocodone Bitartrate (Additive CNS depression). Products include:
- Anexsia 5/500 Tablets 2196
- Anexsia 7.5/650 Tablets 2197
- Azdone Tablets 844
- Codiclear DH Syrup 845
- Codimal DH Syrup 846
- Damason-P 1356
- Hycodan Syrup, Tablets 927
- Hycomine Compound Tablets 929
- Hycomine Syrup 927
- Hycotuss Expectorant Syrup 930
- Hydrocet Capsules 835
- Lortab ASA Tablets 2414
- Lortab 2412
- Ru-Tuss with Hydrocodone 694
- Triaminic Expectorant DH 1995
- Vicodin Tablets 1187
- Vicodin ES Tablets 1189
- Zydone Capsules 941

Hydrocodone Polistirex (Additive CNS depression). Products include:
- Tussionex Extended-Release Suspension 988

Hydroxyzine Hydrochloride (Additive CNS depression). Products include:
- Atarax Tablets & Syrup 1941
- Marax Tablets & DF Syrup 1954
- Vistaril Intramuscular Solution 1970

Isoflurane (Additive CNS depression). Products include:
- Forane 600

Levorphanol Tartrate (Additive CNS depression). Products include:
- Levo-Dromoran 1906

Lorazepam (Additive CNS depression). Products include:
- Ativan Injection 2432
- Ativan Tablets 2434

Loxapine Hydrochloride (Additive CNS depression). Products include:
- Loxitane 1213

Meperidine Hydrochloride (Additive CNS depression). Products include:
- Demerol 2047
- Mepergan Injection 2479

Meprobamate (Additive CNS depression). Products include:
- Deprol Tablets 2382
- Equagesic Tablets 2451
- Miltown Tablets 2386
- PMB 200 and PMB 400 2504

Mesoridazine (Additive CNS depression). Products include:
- Serentil 686

Methadone Hydrochloride (Additive CNS depression). Products include:
- Dolophine Hydrochloride Ampoules & Vials 1260
- Dolophine Hydrochloride Tablets 1261
- Methadone Hydrochloride Diskets .. 1284
- Methadone Hydrochloride Oral Solution & Tablets 1987

Methohexital Sodium (Additive CNS depression). Products include:
- Brevital Sodium Vials 1248

Methoxyflurane (Additive CNS depression).
- No products indexed under this heading.

Midazolam Hydrochloride (Additive CNS depression). Products include:
- Versed Injection 1924

Molindone Hydrochloride (Additive CNS depression). Products include:
- Moban Tablets & Concentrate 932

Morphine Sulfate (Additive CNS depression). Products include:
- Astramorph/PF Injection, USP (Preservative-Free) 618
- Duramorph 960
- Infumorph 200 and Infumorph 500 Sterile Solutions 962
- MS Contin Tablets 1814
- MSIR 1817
- Oramorph SR (Morphine Sulfate Sustained Release Tablets) 1988
- Roxanol 1991

Opium Alkaloids (Additive CNS depression). Products include:
- B & O No. 15A & No. 16A Supprettes 2395
- Pantopon Injectable 1911

Oxazepam (Additive CNS depression). Products include:
- Serax Capsules 2522
- Serax Tablets 2522

Perphenazine (Additive CNS depression). Products include:
- Etrafon 2087
- Triavil Tablets 1556
- Trilafon 2123

Prazepam (Additive CNS depression). Products include:
- Centrax 1693

Probenecid (Aspirin may inhibit the uricosuric effects). Products include:
- Benemid Tablets 1426
- ColBENEMID Tablets 1436
- Wycillin Injection and Probenecid Tablets 2539

Prochlorperazine (Additive CNS depression). Products include:
- Compazine 2201

Promethazine Hydrochloride (Additive CNS depression). Products include:
- Mepergan Injection 2479
- Phenergan with Codeine 2497
- Phenergan with Dextromethorphan 2499
- Phenergan Injection 2493
- Phenergan Suppositories 2496
- Phenergan Syrup 2495
- Phenergan Tablets 2496
- Phenergan VC 2500
- Phenergan VC with Codeine 2501

Propofol (Additive CNS depression). Products include:
- Diprivan Injection 2267

Propoxyphene Hydrochloride (Additive CNS depression). Products include:
- Darvon 1256
- Wygesic Tablets 2540

Propoxyphene Napsylate (Additive CNS depression). Products include:
- Darvon-N/Darvocet-N 1254

Quazepam (Additive CNS depression). Products include:
- Doral Tablets 2383

Secobarbital Sodium (Additive CNS depression). Products include:
- Seconal Sodium Pulvules 1296

Sufentanil Citrate (Additive CNS depression). Products include:
- Sufenta Injection 1147

Sulfinpyrazone (Aspirin may inhibit the uricosuric effects). Products include:
- Anturane 853

Temazepam (Additive CNS depression). Products include:
- Restoril Capsules 2023

Thioridazine Hydrochloride (Additive CNS depression). Products include:
- Mellaril 2011

Triazolam (Additive CNS depression). Products include:
- Halcion Tablets 2340

Trifluoperazine Hydrochloride (Additive CNS depression). Products include:
- Stelazine 2226

Warfarin Sodium (Enhanced effect of anticoagulant). Products include:
- Coumadin Injection & Tablets 944
- Panwarfin Tablets 547

PERCODAN-DEMI TABLETS
(Oxycodone Hydrochloride, Oxycodone Terephthalate, Aspirin).... 951
See **Percodan Tablets**

PERDIEM FIBER GRANULES
(Psyllium Preparations) 1852
No interactions described in labeling.

PERDIEM GRANULES
(Psyllium Preparations, Senna) 1852
No interactions described in labeling.

PERGONAL (MENOTROPINS FOR INJECTION, USP)
(Menotropins) ... 2184
No interactions described in labeling.

PERIACTIN SYRUP
(Cyproheptadine Hydrochloride) ... 1525
May interact with central nervous system depressants and monoamine oxidase inhibitors. Compounds in these categories include:

Alcohol (Additive effects).

Alfentanil Hydrochloride (Additive effects). Products include:
- Alfenta Injection ... 1131

Alprazolam (Additive effects). Products include:
- Xanax Tablets ... 2367

Aprobarbital (Additive effects). Products include:
- Alurate Elixir ... 1883

Buprenorphine (Additive effects).
- No products indexed under this heading.

Buspirone Hydrochloride (Additive effects). Products include:
- BuSpar ... 1401

Butabarbital (Additive effects). Products include:
- Pyridium Plus ... 1764

Butalbital (Additive effects). Products include:
- Esgic-Plus Tablets ... 1002
- Esgic Tablets & Capsules ... 1001
- Fioricet Tablets ... 2006
- Fiorinal Capsules ... 2007
- Fiorinal with Codeine Capsules ... 2008
- Fiorinal Tablets ... 2007
- Phrenilin ... 838
- Sedapap Tablets 50 mg/650 mg .. 1360

Chlordiazepoxide (Additive effects). Products include:
- Libritabs Tablets ... 1930
- Limbitrol ... 1933
- Menrium Tablets ... 1934

Chlordiazepoxide Hydrochloride (Additive effects). Products include:
- Librax Capsules ... 1929
- Librium Capsules ... 1931
- Librium Injectable ... 1932

Chlorpromazine (Additive effects). Products include:
- Thorazine ... 2234

Chlorprothixene (Additive effects). Products include:
- Taractan Tablets ... 1920

Chlorprothixene Hydrochloride (Additive effects). Products include:
- Taractan ... 1920

Chlorprothixene Lactate (Additive effects). Products include:
- Taractan Concentrate ... 1920

Clorazepate Dipotassium (Additive effects). Products include:
- Tranxene ... 556

Codeine (Additive effects). Products include:
- Calcidrine Syrup ... 506

Codeine Phosphate (Additive effects). Products include:
- Actifed with Codeine Cough Syrup.. 752
- Cheracol Cough Syrup ... 1853
- Codimal PH Syrup ... 846
- Dimetane-DC Cough Syrup ... 1857
- Empirin with Codeine Phosphate Nos. 2, 3 & 4 ... 764
- Fiorinal with Codeine Capsules ... 2008
- Isoclor Expectorant ... 982
- Naldecon CX Adult Liquid ... ⊞ 521
- Novahistine DH ... 1342
- Novahistine Expectorant ... 1343
- Nucofed Capsules ... 2219
- Nucofed Expectorant ... 2219
- Nucofed Pediatric Expectorant ... 2220
- Nucofed Syrup ... 2219
- Phenaphen with Codeine Capsules 1865
- Phenaphen-650 with Codeine Tablets ... 1866
- Phenergan with Codeine ... 2497
- Phenergan VC with Codeine ... 2501
- Robitussin A-C Syrup ... 1875
- Robitussin-DAC Syrup ... 1875
- Ryna ... ⊞ 741
- Soma Compound w/Codeine Tablets ... 2390
- Triaminic Expectorant w/Codeine .. 1996
- Tussi-Organidin Liquid ... 2391
- Tylenol with Codeine ... 1381

Codeine Polistirex (Additive effects).
- No products indexed under this heading.

Dezocine (Additive effects).

Diazepam (Additive effects). Products include:
- Valium Injectable ... 1937
- Valium Tablets ... 1939
- Valrelease Capsules ... 1923

Droperidol (Additive effects). Products include:
- Inapsine Injection ... 1140
- Innovar Injection ... 1141

Enflurane (Additive effects). Products include:
- Ethrane ... 599

Estazolam (Additive effects). Products include:
- ProSom Tablets ... 554

Ethchlorvynol (Additive effects). Products include:
- Placidyl Capsules ... 553

Ethinamate (Additive effects).
- No products indexed under this heading.

Fentanyl (Additive effects). Products include:
- Duragesic Transdermal System ... 1133

Fentanyl Citrate (Additive effects). Products include:
- Innovar Injection ... 1141
- Sublimaze Injection ... 1146

Fluphenazine Decanoate (Additive effects). Products include:
- Prolixin Decanoate ... 1795

Fluphenazine Enanthate (Additive effects). Products include:
- Prolixin Enanthate ... 1796

Fluphenazine Hydrochloride (Additive effects). Products include:
- Prolixin Elixir ... 1793
- Prolixin Injection ... 1791
- Prolixin Oral Concentrate ... 1792
- Prolixin Tablets ... 1793

Flurazepam Hydrochloride (Additive effects). Products include:
- Dalmane Capsules ... 1927

Furazolidone (Contraindication; anticholinergic effects of antihistamines prolonged and intensified). Products include:
- Furoxone ... 1855

Glutethimide (Additive effects).
- No products indexed under this heading.

Haloperidol (Additive effects). Products include:
- Haldol Injection, Tablets and Concentrate ... 1373

Haloperidol Decanoate (Additive effects). Products include:
- Haldol Decanoate ... 1375

Hydrocodone Bitartrate (Additive effects). Products include:
- Anexsia 5/500 Tablets ... 2196
- Anexsia 7.5/650 Tablets ... 2197
- Azdone Tablets ... 844
- Codiclear DH Syrup ... 845
- Codimal DH Syrup ... 846
- Damason-P ... 1356
- Hycodan Syrup, Tablets ... 927
- Hycomine Compound Tablets ... 929
- Hycomine Syrup ... 927
- Hycotuss Expectorant Syrup ... 930
- Hydrocet Capsules ... 835
- Lortab ASA Tablets ... 2414
- Lortab ... 2412
- Ru-Tuss with Hydrocodone ... 694
- Triaminic Expectorant DH ... 1995
- Vicodin Tablets ... 1187
- Vicodin ES Tablets ... 1189
- Zydone Capsules ... 941

Hydrocodone Polistirex (Additive effects). Products include:
- Tussionex Extended-Release Suspension ... 988

Hydroxyzine Hydrochloride (Additive effects). Products include:
- Atarax Tablets & Syrup ... 1941
- Marax Tablets & DF Syrup ... 1954
- Vistaril Intramuscular Solution ... 1970

Isocarboxazid (Contraindication; anticholinergic effects of antihistamines prolonged and intensified). Products include:
- Marplan Tablets ... 1906

Isoflurane (Additive effects). Products include:
- Forane ... 600

Ketamine Hydrochloride (Additive effects). Products include:
- Ketalar ... 1726

Levorphanol Tartrate (Additive effects). Products include:
- Levo-Dromoran ... 1906

Lorazepam (Additive effects). Products include:
- Ativan Injection ... 2432
- Ativan Tablets ... 2434

Loxapine Hydrochloride (Additive effects). Products include:
- Loxitane ... 1213

Loxapine Succinate (Additive effects). Products include:
- Loxitane Capsules ... 1213

Meperidine Hydrochloride (Additive effects). Products include:
- Demerol ... 2047
- Mepergan Injection ... 2479

Mephobarbital (Additive effects). Products include:
- Mebaral Tablets ... 2061

Meprobamate (Additive effects). Products include:
- Deprol Tablets ... 2382
- Equagesic Tablets ... 2451
- Miltown Tablets ... 2386
- PMB 200 and PMB 400 ... 2504

Mesoridazine (Additive effects). Products include:
- Serentil ... 686

Methadone Hydrochloride (Additive effects). Products include:
- Dolophine Hydrochloride Ampoules & Vials ... 1260
- Dolophine Hydrochloride Tablets ... 1261
- Methadone Hydrochloride Diskets .. 1284
- Methadone Hydrochloride Oral Solution & Tablets ... 1987

Methohexital Sodium (Additive effects). Products include:
- Brevital Sodium Vials ... 1248

Methoxyflurane (Additive effects).
- No products indexed under this heading.

Midazolam Hydrochloride (Additive effects). Products include:
- Versed Injection ... 1924

Molindone Hydrochloride (Additive effects). Products include:
- Moban Tablets & Concentrate ... 932

Morphine Sulfate (Additive effects). Products include:
- Astramorph/PF Injection, USP (Preservative-Free) ... 618
- Duramorph ... 960
- Infumorph 200 and Infumorph 500 Sterile Solutions ... 962
- MS Contin Tablets ... 1814
- MSIR ... 1817
- Oramorph SR (Morphine Sulfate Sustained Release Tablets) ... 1988
- Roxanol ... 1991

Opium Alkaloids (Additive effects). Products include:
- B & O No. 15A & No. 16A Supprettes ... 2395
- Pantopon Injectable ... 1911

Oxazepam (Additive effects). Products include:
- Serax Capsules ... 2522
- Serax Tablets ... 2522

Oxycodone Hydrochloride (Additive effects). Products include:
- Percocet Tablets ... 950
- Percodan ... 951
- Roxicodone Tablets, Oral Solution & Intensol (Oxycodone) ... 1992
- Tylox Capsules ... 1382

Pentobarbital Sodium (Additive effects). Products include:
- Nembutal Sodium Capsules ... 534
- Nembutal Sodium Solution ... 536
- Nembutal Sodium Suppositories ... 538

Perphenazine (Additive effects). Products include:
- Etrafon ... 2087
- Triavil Tablets ... 1556
- Trilafon ... 2123

Phenelzine Sulfate (Contraindication; anticholinergic effects of antihistamines prolonged and intensified). Products include:
- Nardil ... 1742

Phenobarbital (Additive effects). Products include:
- Arco-Lase Plus Tablets ... 607
- Bellergal-S Tablets ... 1998
- Bronkolixir ... ⊞ 761
- Bronkotabs Tablets ... ⊞ 762
- Donnatal ... 1858
- Donnatal Extentabs ... 1859
- Donnatal Tablets ... 1858
- Donnazyme Tablets ... 1860
- Kinesed Tablets ... 2272
- Phenobarbital Elixir and Tablets ... 1293
- Primatene Tablets-P Formula ... 2421
- Quadrinal Tablets ... 1183
- Tedral SA ... 1765

Prazepam (Additive effects). Products include:
- Centrax ... 1693

Prochlorperazine (Additive effects). Products include:
- Compazine ... 2201

Promethazine Hydrochloride (Additive effects). Products include:
- Mepergan Injection ... 2479
- Phenergan with Codeine ... 2497
- Phenergan with Dextromethorphan 2499
- Phenergan Injection ... 2493
- Phenergan Suppositories ... 2496
- Phenergan Syrup ... 2495
- Phenergan Tablets ... 2496
- Phenergan VC ... 2500
- Phenergan VC with Codeine ... 2501

Propofol (Additive effects). Products include:
- Diprivan Injection ... 2267

Propoxyphene Hydrochloride (Additive effects). Products include:
- Darvon ... 1256
- Wygesic Tablets ... 2540

Propoxyphene Napsylate (Additive effects). Products include:
- Darvon-N/Darvocet-N ... 1254

Quazepam (Additive effects). Products include:
- Doral Tablets ... 2383

Secobarbital Sodium (Additive effects). Products include:
- Seconal Sodium Pulvules ... 1296

Selegiline Hydrochloride (Contraindication; anticholinergic effects of antihistamines prolonged and intensified). Products include:
- Eldepryl ... 2250

Sufentanil Citrate (Additive effects). Products include:
- Sufenta Injection ... 1147

Temazepam (Additive effects). Products include:
- Restoril Capsules ... 2023

Thiamylal Sodium (Additive effects). Products include:
- Surital Ampoules, Steri-Vials ... 1764

Thioridazine Hydrochloride (Additive effects). Products include:
- Mellaril 2011

Thiothixene (Additive effects). Products include:
- Navane Capsules and Concentrate 1954
- Navane Intramuscular 1956

Tranylcypromine Sulfate (Contraindication; anticholinergic effects of antihistamines prolonged and intensified). Products include:
- Parnate Tablets 2222

Triazolam (Additive effects). Products include:
- Halcion Tablets 2340

Trifluoperazine Hydrochloride (Additive effects). Products include:
- Stelazine 2226

PERIACTIN TABLETS
(Cyproheptadine Hydrochloride) 1525
See **Periactin Syrup**

PERI-COLACE
(Casanthranol, Docusate Sodium) 1409
No interactions described in labeling.

PERIDEX
(Chlorhexidine Gluconate) 1808
No interactions described in labeling.

PERITRATE SUSTAINED ACTION
(Pentaerythritol Tetranitrate) 1756
May interact with:

Alcohol (May enhance hypotensive effect of nitrates).

PERITRATE TABLETS
(Pentaerythritol Tetranitrate) 1756
See **Peritrate Sustained Action**

PERMAX TABLETS
(Pergolide Mesylate) 1291
May interact with dopamine antagonists, highly protein bound drugs (selected), and certain other agents. Compounds in these categories include:

Amiodarone Hydrochloride (Caution should be exercised if coadministered). Products include:
- Cordarone Tablets 2446

Amitriptyline Hydrochloride (Caution should be exercised if coadministered). Products include:
- Elavil 2269
- Endep Tablets 1927
- Etrafon 2087
- Limbitrol 1933
- Triavil Tablets 1556

Cefonicid Sodium (Caution should be exercised if coadministered). Products include:
- Monocid Injection 2217

Chlordiazepoxide (Caution should be exercised if coadministered). Products include:
- Libritabs Tablets 1930
- Limbitrol 1933
- Menrium Tablets 1934

Chlordiazepoxide Hydrochloride (Caution should be exercised if coadministered). Products include:
- Librax Capsules 1929
- Librium Capsules 1931
- Librium Injectable 1932

Chlorpromazine (May diminish the effectiveness of Permax; caution should be exercised if coadministered). Products include:
- Thorazine 2234

Clomipramine Hydrochloride (Caution should be exercised if coadministered). Products include:
- Anafranil Capsules 650

Clozapine (May diminish the effectiveness of Permax). Products include:
- Clozaril Tablets 2000

Cyclosporine (Caution should be exercised if coadministered). Products include:
- Sandimmune 2024

Diazepam (Caution should be exercised if coadministered). Products include:
- Valium Injectable 1937
- Valium Tablets 1939
- Valrelease Capsules 1923

Diclofenac Sodium (Caution should be exercised if coadministered). Products include:
- Voltaren Ophthalmic Sterile Ophthalmic Solution .... ⊙ 268
- Voltaren Tablets 1042

Dipyridamole (Caution should be exercised if coadministered). Products include:
- Persantine Tablets 683

Fenoprofen Calcium (Caution should be exercised if coadministered). Products include:
- Nalfon Pulvules & Tablets 919

Fluphenazine Decanoate (May diminish the effectiveness of Permax). Products include:
- Prolixin Decanoate 1795

Fluphenazine Enanthate (May diminish the effectiveness of Permax). Products include:
- Prolixin Enanthate 1796

Fluphenazine Hydrochloride (May diminish the effectiveness of Permax). Products include:
- Prolixin Elixir 1793
- Prolixin Injection 1791
- Prolixin Oral Concentrate 1792
- Prolixin Tablets 1793

Flurazepam Hydrochloride (Caution should be exercised if coadministered). Products include:
- Dalmane Capsules 1927

Flurbiprofen (Caution should be exercised if coadministered). Products include:
- Ansaid Tablets 2319

Glipizide (Caution should be exercised if coadministered). Products include:
- Glucotrol 1952

Haloperidol (May diminish the effectiveness of Permax). Products include:
- Haldol Injection, Tablets and Concentrate 1373

Haloperidol Decanoate (May diminish the effectiveness of Permax). Products include:
- Haldol Decanoate 1375

Ibuprofen (Caution should be exercised if coadministered). Products include:
- Advil Cold & Sinus Caplets (formerly CoAdvil) 2416
- Advil Ibuprofen Tablets and Caplets 2416
- Children's Advil Suspension 2426
- CoAdvil .... ▣ 748
- Dristan Sinus Caplets 2419
- Haltran Tablets .... ▣ 668
- Ibuprofen .... ▣ 631
- Medipren Ibuprofen Caplets and Tablets 1362
- Midol 200 Cramp Relief Formula .. ▣ 570
- Motrin Tablets 2351
- Motrin IB Caplets and Tablets .... ▣ 736
- Nuprin Ibuprofen/Analgesic Tablets & Caplets 752
- PediaProfen Suspension 1363
- Rufen Tablets 691
- Trendar Ibuprofen Tablets .... ▣ 756

Imipramine Hydrochloride (Caution should be exercised if coadministered). Products include:
- Tofranil Ampuls 1038
- Tofranil Tablets 1039

Imipramine Pamoate (Caution should be exercised if coadministered). Products include:
- Tofranil-PM Capsules 1041

Indomethacin (Caution should be exercised if coadministered). Products include:
- Indocin 1487

Indomethacin Sodium Trihydrate (Caution should be exercised if coadministered). Products include:
- Indocin I.V. 1490

Ketoprofen (Caution should be exercised if coadministered). Products include:
- Orudis Capsules 2488

Ketorolac Tromethamine (Caution should be exercised if coadministered). Products include:
- Toradol IM Injection 2302

Levodopa (Concomitant use may cause and/or exacerbate preexisting states of confusion and hallucination). Products include:
- Larodopa Tablets 1905
- Sinemet Tablets 952
- Sinemet CR Tablets 953

Meclofenamate Sodium (Caution should be exercised if coadministered). Products include:
- Meclomen Capsules 1739

Mefenamic Acid (Caution should be exercised if coadministered). Products include:
- Ponstel 1758

Mesoridazine Besylate (May diminish the effectiveness of Permax).

Metoclopramide Hydrochloride (May diminish the effectiveness of Permax). Products include:
- Reglan 1869

Midazolam Hydrochloride (Caution should be exercised if coadministered). Products include:
- Versed Injection 1924

Naproxen (Caution should be exercised if coadministered). Products include:
- Naprosyn 2297

Naproxen Sodium (Caution should be exercised if coadministered). Products include:
- Anaprox and Anaprox DS Tablets 2288

Nortriptyline Hydrochloride (Caution should be exercised if coadministered). Products include:
- Pamelor 2019

Oxazepam (Caution should be exercised if coadministered). Products include:
- Serax Capsules 2522
- Serax Tablets 2522

Perphenazine (May diminish the effectiveness of Permax). Products include:
- Etrafon 2087
- Triavil Tablets 1556
- Trilafon 2123

Phenylbutazone (Caution should be exercised if coadministered). Products include:
- Butazolidin Capsules & Tablets 1027

Pimozide (May diminish the effectiveness of Permax). Products include:
- Orap Tablets 1020

Piroxicam (Caution should be exercised if coadministered). Products include:
- Feldene Capsules 1777

Prochlorperazine (May diminish the effectiveness of Permax). Products include:
- Compazine 2201

Promethazine Hydrochloride (May diminish the effectiveness of Permax). Products include:
- Mepergan Injection 2479
- Phenergan with Codeine 2497
- Phenergan with Dextromethorphan 2499
- Phenergan Injection 2493
- Phenergan Suppositories 2496
- Phenergan Syrup 2495
- Phenergan Tablets 2496
- Phenergan VC 2500
- Phenergan VC with Codeine 2501

Propranolol Hydrochloride (Caution should be exercised if coadministered). Products include:
- Inderal 2459
- Inderal LA Long Acting Capsules 2461
- Inderide Tablets 2463
- Inderide LA Long Acting Capsules .. 2465

Sulindac (Caution should be exercised if coadministered). Products include:
- Clinoril Tablets 1433

Temazepam (Caution should be exercised if coadministered). Products include:
- Restoril Capsules 2023

Thioridazine Hydrochloride (May diminish the effectiveness of Permax). Products include:
- Mellaril 2011

Thiothixene (May diminish the effectiveness of Permax). Products include:
- Navane Capsules and Concentrate 1954
- Navane Intramuscular 1956

Tolbutamide (Caution should be exercised if coadministered). Products include:
- Orinase Tablets 2354

Tolmetin Sodium (Caution should be exercised if coadministered). Products include:
- Tolectin (200, 400 and 600 mg) .. 1379

Trifluoperazine Hydrochloride (May diminish the effectiveness of Permax). Products include:
- Stelazine 2226

Trimipramine Maleate (Caution should be exercised if coadministered). Products include:
- Surmontil Capsules 2524

Warfarin Sodium (Caution should be exercised if coadministered). Products include:
- Coumadin Injection & Tablets 944
- Panwarfin Tablets 547

PERSA-GEL (BENZOYL PEROXIDE)
(Benzoyl Peroxide) 1680
No interactions described in labeling.

PERSA-GEL W (BENZOYL PEROXIDE)
(Benzoyl Peroxide) 1680
No interactions described in labeling.

PERSANTINE TABLETS
(Dipyridamole) 683
No interactions described in labeling.

PFIZERPEN FOR INJECTION
(Penicillin G Potassium) 1957
May interact with tetracyclines and certain other agents. Compounds in these categories include:

Demeclocycline Hydrochloride (May diminish bactericidal effects of penicillins). Products include:
- Declomycin Capsules, Tablets 1199

Doxycycline Calcium (May diminish bactericidal effects of penicillins).
- No products indexed under this heading.

Doxycycline Hyclate (May diminish bactericidal effects of penicillins). Products include:
- Doryx Capsules ... 1717
- Vibramycin Hyclate Capsules ... 1787
- Vibramycin Hyclate Intravenous ... 1968
- Vibra-Tabs Film Coated Tablets ... 1787

Doxycycline Monohydrate (May diminish bactericidal effects of penicillins). Products include:
- Monodox Capsules ... 1630
- Vibramycin Monohydrate for Oral Suspension ... 1787

Erythromycin (May diminish bactericidal effects of penicillin). Products include:
- A/T/S Topical Gel and Topical Solution ... 1089
- AK-Mycin Ointment ... ⊙ 204
- Benzamycin Topical Gel ... 907
- E-Mycin Tablets ... 688
- ETS-2% ... 1685
- ERYC ... 1720
- Erycette (erythromycin 2%) Topical Solution ... 1678
- Ery-Tab Tablets ... 521
- Erythromycin Base Filmtab ... 525
- Erythromycin Delayed-Release Capsules, USP ... 526
- Ilotycin Ophthalmic Ointment ... 915
- PCE Dispertab Tablets ... 549
- Pediazole ... 1973
- T-Stat 2.0% Topical Solution and Pads ... 2409
- Theramycin Z Topical Solution 2% 1410

Erythromycin Estolate (May diminish bactericidal effects of penicillin). Products include:
- Ilosone ... 913

Erythromycin Ethylsuccinate (May diminish bactericidal effects of penicillin). Products include:
- E.E.S. ... 522
- EryPed ... 519
- Pediazole ... 1973

Erythromycin Gluceptate (May diminish bactericidal effects of penicillin). Products include:
- Ilotycin Gluceptate, IV, Vials ... 915

Erythromycin Stearate (May diminish bactericidal effects of penicillin). Products include:
- Erythrocin Stearate Filmtab ... 523

Methacycline Hydrochloride (May diminish bactericidal effects of penicillins).
- No products indexed under this heading.

Minocycline Hydrochloride (May diminish bactericidal effects of penicillins). Products include:
- Minocin Intravenous ... 1221
- Minocin Oral Suspension ... 1224
- Minocin Pellet-Filled Capsules ... 1222

Oxytetracycline Hydrochloride (May diminish bactericidal effects of penicillins). Products include:
- Terra-Cortril Ophthalmic Suspension ... 1963
- Terramycin Capsules ... 1786
- Terramycin Intramuscular Solution 1964
- Terramycin with Polymyxin B Sulfate Ophthalmic Ointment ... 1965

Probenecid (Penicillin blood levels may be prolonged). Products include:
- Benemid Tablets ... 1426
- ColBENEMID Tablets ... 1436
- Wycillin Injection and Probenecid Tablets ... 2539

Tetracycline Hydrochloride (May diminish bactericidal effects of penicillins). Products include:
- Achromycin V Capsules ... 1193
- Achromycin Ophthalmic Ointment 1% ... ⊙ 307
- Achromycin Ophthalmic Suspension 1% ... ⊙ 308
- Topicycline for Topical Solution ... 1856

PFIZERPEN-AS AQUEOUS SUSPENSION
(Penicillin G Procaine) ... 1959
May interact with tetracyclines and certain other agents. Compounds in these categories include:

Demeclocycline Hydrochloride (May diminish bactericidal effects of penicillin). Products include:
- Declomycin Capsules, Tablets ... 1199

Doxycycline Calcium (May diminish bactericidal effects of penicillin).
- No products indexed under this heading.

Doxycycline Hyclate (May diminish bactericidal effects of penicillin). Products include:
- Doryx Capsules ... 1717
- Vibramycin Hyclate Capsules ... 1787
- Vibramycin Hyclate Intravenous ... 1968
- Vibra-Tabs Film Coated Tablets ... 1787

Doxycycline Monohydrate (May diminish bactericidal effects of penicillin). Products include:
- Monodox Capsules ... 1630
- Vibramycin Monohydrate for Oral Suspension ... 1787

Erythromycin (May diminish bactericidal effects of penicillin). Products include:
- A/T/S Topical Gel and Topical Solution ... 1089
- AK-Mycin Ointment ... ⊙ 204
- Benzamycin Topical Gel ... 907
- E-Mycin Tablets ... 688
- ETS-2% ... 1685
- ERYC ... 1720
- Erycette (erythromycin 2%) Topical Solution ... 1678
- Ery-Tab Tablets ... 521
- Erythromycin Base Filmtab ... 525
- Erythromycin Delayed-Release Capsules, USP ... 526
- Ilotycin Ophthalmic Ointment ... 915
- PCE Dispertab Tablets ... 549
- Pediazole ... 1973
- T-Stat 2.0% Topical Solution and Pads ... 2409
- Theramycin Z Topical Solution 2% 1410

Erythromycin Estolate (May diminish bactericidal effects of penicillin). Products include:
- Ilosone ... 913

Erythromycin Ethylsuccinate (May diminish bactericidal effects of penicillin). Products include:
- E.E.S. ... 522
- EryPed ... 519
- Pediazole ... 1973

Erythromycin Gluceptate (May diminish bactericidal effects of penicillin). Products include:
- Ilotycin Gluceptate, IV, Vials ... 915

Erythromycin Stearate (May diminish bactericidal effects of penicillin). Products include:
- Erythrocin Stearate Filmtab ... 523

Methacycline Hydrochloride (May diminish bactericidal effects of penicillin).
- No products indexed under this heading.

Minocycline Hydrochloride (May diminish bactericidal effects of penicillin). Products include:
- Minocin Intravenous ... 1221
- Minocin Oral Suspension ... 1224
- Minocin Pellet-Filled Capsules ... 1222

Oxytetracycline Hydrochloride (May diminish bactericidal effects of penicillin). Products include:
- Terra-Cortril Ophthalmic Suspension ... 1963
- Terramycin Capsules ... 1786
- Terramycin Intramuscular Solution 1964
- Terramycin with Polymyxin B Sulfate Ophthalmic Ointment ... 1965

Probenecid (May prolong penicillin blood levels). Products include:
- Benemid Tablets ... 1426
- ColBENEMID Tablets ... 1436
- Wycillin Injection and Probenecid Tablets ... 2539

Tetracycline Hydrochloride (May diminish bactericidal effects of penicillin). Products include:
- Achromycin V Capsules ... 1193
- Achromycin Ophthalmic Ointment 1% ... ⊙ 307
- Achromycin Ophthalmic Suspension 1% ... ⊙ 308
- Topicycline for Topical Solution ... 1856

PHAZYME DROPS
(Simethicone) ... ▣ 651
No interactions described in labeling.

PHAZYME TABLETS
(Simethicone) ... ▣ 651
No interactions described in labeling.

PHAZYME-125 SOFTGELS MAXIMUM STRENGTH
(Simethicone) ... ▣ 651
No interactions described in labeling.

PHAZYME-95 TABLETS
(Simethicone) ... ▣ 651
No interactions described in labeling.

PHENAPHEN WITH CODEINE CAPSULES
(Codeine Phosphate, Acetaminophen) ... 1865
May interact with narcotic analgesics, phenothiazines, monoamine oxidase inhibitors, tricyclic antidepressants, anticholinergics, central nervous system depressants, neuromuscular blocking agents, and certain other agents. Compounds in these categories include:

Alcohol (Increased CNS depression).

Alfentanil Hydrochloride (Increased CNS depression). Products include:
- Alfenta Injection ... 1131

Alprazolam (Increased CNS depression). Products include:
- Xanax Tablets ... 2367

Amitriptyline Hydrochloride (Increased effect of antidepressant or codeine). Products include:
- Elavil ... 2269
- Endep Tablets ... 1927
- Etrafon ... 2087
- Limbitrol ... 1933
- Triavil Tablets ... 1556

Amoxapine (Increased effect of antidepressant or codeine). Products include:
- Asendin Tablets ... 1196

Aprobarbital (Increased CNS depression). Products include:
- Alurate Elixir ... 1883

Atropine Sulfate (May produce paralytic ileus). Products include:
- Arco-Lase Plus Tablets ... 607
- Atropine Sulfate Sterile Ophthalmic Solution and S.O.P. Sterile Ophthalmic Ointment ... ⊙ 239
- Donnagel ... ▣ 675
- Donnagel-PG ... 1858
- Donnatal ... 1858
- Donnatal Extentabs ... 1859
- Donnatal Tablets ... 1858
- Donnazyme Tablets ... 1860
- Isopto Atropine ... ⊙ 218
- Lomotil ... 2174
- Motofen Tablets ... 836
- Ru-Tuss Tablets ... 693
- Urised Tablets ... 2396

Belladonna Alkaloids (May produce paralytic ileus). Products include:
- Bellergal-S Tablets ... 1998
- Hyland's Bed Wetting Tablets ... ▣ 728
- Hyland's Teething Tablets ... ▣ 728
- Kinesed Tablets ... 2272

Benztropine Mesylate (May produce paralytic ileus). Products include:
- Cogentin ... 1435

Biperiden (May produce paralytic ileus). Products include:
- Akineton ... 1171

Buprenorphine (Increased CNS depression).
- No products indexed under this heading.

Buspirone Hydrochloride (Increased CNS depression). Products include:
- BuSpar ... 1401

Butabarbital (Increased CNS depression). Products include:
- Pyridium Plus ... 1764

Butalbital (Increased CNS depression). Products include:
- Esgic-Plus Tablets ... 1002
- Esgic Tablets & Capsules ... 1001
- Fioricet Tablets ... 2006
- Fiorinal Capsules ... 2007
- Fiorinal with Codeine Capsules ... 2008
- Fiorinal Tablets ... 2007
- Phrenilin ... 838
- Sedapap Tablets 50 mg/650 mg .. 1360

Chlordiazepoxide (Increased CNS depression). Products include:
- Libritabs Tablets ... 1930
- Limbitrol ... 1933
- Menrium Tablets ... 1934

Chlordiazepoxide Hydrochloride (Increased CNS depression). Products include:
- Librax Capsules ... 1929
- Librium Capsules ... 1931
- Librium Injectable ... 1932

Chlorpromazine (Increased CNS depression). Products include:
- Thorazine ... 2234

Chlorprothixene (Increased CNS depression). Products include:
- Taractan Tablets ... 1920

Chlorprothixene Hydrochloride (Increased CNS depression). Products include:
- Taractan ... 1920

Clidinium Bromide (May produce paralytic ileus). Products include:
- Librax Capsules ... 1929
- Quarzan Capsules ... 1937

Clomipramine Hydrochloride (Increased effect of antidepressant or codeine). Products include:
- Anafranil Capsules ... 650

Clorazepate Dipotassium (Increased CNS depression). Products include:
- Tranxene ... 556

Clozapine (Increased CNS depression). Products include:
- Clozaril Tablets ... 2000

Codeine (Increased CNS depression). Products include:
- Calcidrine Syrup ... 506

Codeine Polistirex (Increased CNS depression).
- No products indexed under this heading.

Desipramine Hydrochloride (Increased effect of antidepressant or codeine). Products include:
- Norpramin Tablets ... 1340

Dezocine (Increased CNS depression).

Diazepam (Increased CNS depression). Products include:
- Valium Injectable ... 1937
- Valium Tablets ... 1939
- Valrelease Capsules ... 1923

Dicyclomine Hydrochloride (May produce paralytic ileus). Products include:
- Bentyl ... 1322

Doxepin Hydrochloride (Increased effect of antidepressant or codeine). Products include:
- Sinequan 1960

Droperidol (Increased CNS depression). Products include:
- Inapsine Injection 1140
- Innovar Injection 1141

Enflurane (Increased CNS depression). Products include:
- Ethrane 599

Estazolam (Increased CNS depression). Products include:
- ProSom Tablets 554

Ethchlorvynol (Increased CNS depression). Products include:
- Placidyl Capsules 553

Ethinamate (Increased CNS depression).
- No products indexed under this heading.

Fentanyl (Increased CNS depression). Products include:
- Duragesic Transdermal System 1133

Fentanyl Citrate (Increased CNS depression). Products include:
- Innovar Injection 1141
- Sublimaze Injection 1146

Fluphenazine Decanoate (Increased CNS depression). Products include:
- Prolixin Decanoate 1795

Fluphenazine Enanthate (Increased CNS depression). Products include:
- Prolixin Enanthate 1796

Fluphenazine Hydrochloride (Increased CNS depression). Products include:
- Prolixin Elixir 1793
- Prolixin Injection 1791
- Prolixin Oral Concentrate 1792
- Prolixin Tablets 1793

Flurazepam Hydrochloride (Increased CNS depression). Products include:
- Dalmane Capsules 1927

Furazolidone (Increased effect of antidepressant or codeine). Products include:
- Furoxone 1855

Glutethimide (Increased CNS depression).
- No products indexed under this heading.

Glycopyrrolate (May produce paralytic ileus). Products include:
- Robinul Forte Tablets 1873
- Robinul Injectable 1873
- Robinul Tablets 1873

Haloperidol (Increased CNS depression). Products include:
- Haldol Injection, Tablets and Concentrate 1373

Haloperidol Decanoate (Increased CNS depression). Products include:
- Haldol Decanoate 1375

Hydrocodone Bitartrate (Increased CNS depression). Products include:
- Anexsia 5/500 Tablets 2196
- Anexsia 7.5/650 Tablets 2197
- Azdone Tablets 844
- Codiclear DH Syrup 845
- Codimal DH Syrup 846
- Damason-P 1356
- Hycodan Syrup, Tablets 927
- Hycomine Compound Tablets 929
- Hycomine Syrup 927
- Hycotuss Expectorant Syrup 930
- Hydrocet Capsules 835
- Lortab ASA Tablets 2414
- Lortab 2412
- Ru-Tuss with Hydrocodone 694
- Triaminic Expectorant DH 1995
- Vicodin Tablets 1187
- Vicodin ES Tablets 1189
- Zydone Capsules 941

Hydrocodone Polistirex (Increased CNS depression). Products include:
- Tussionex Extended-Release Suspension 988

Hydroxyzine Hydrochloride (Increased CNS depression). Products include:
- Atarax Tablets & Syrup 1941
- Marax Tablets & DF Syrup 1954
- Vistaril Intramuscular Solution 1970

Hyoscyamine (May produce paralytic ileus). Products include:
- Cystospaz Tablets 2395
- Urised Tablets 2396

Hyoscyamine Sulfate (May produce paralytic ileus). Products include:
- Arco-Lase Plus Tablets 607
- Cystospaz-M Capsules 2395
- Donnagel .... ▣ 675
- Donnagel-PG 1858
- Donnatal 1858
- Donnatal Extentabs 1859
- Donnatal Tablets 1858
- Donnazyme Tablets 1860
- Kutrase Capsules 2146
- Levsin/Levsinex 2147
- Ru-Tuss Tablets 693

Imipramine Hydrochloride (Increased effect of antidepressant or codeine). Products include:
- Tofranil Ampuls 1038
- Tofranil Tablets 1039

Imipramine Pamoate (Increased effect of antidepressant or codeine). Products include:
- Tofranil-PM Capsules 1041

Ipratropium Bromide (May produce paralytic ileus). Products include:
- Atrovent Inhalation Aerosol 675

Isocarboxazid (Increased effect of antidepressant or codeine). Products include:
- Marplan Tablets 1906

Isoflurane (Increased CNS depression). Products include:
- Forane 600

Ketamine Hydrochloride (Increased CNS depression). Products include:
- Ketalar 1726

Levorphanol Tartrate (Increased CNS depression). Products include:
- Levo-Dromoran 1906

Lithium Carbonate (Increased CNS depression). Products include:
- Eskalith 2214
- Lithane Tablets 1596
- Lithium Carbonate Capsules & Tablets 1984
- Lithobid Tablets 870

Lithium Citrate (Increased CNS depression). Products include:
- Cibalith-S 870

Lorazepam (Increased CNS depression). Products include:
- Ativan Injection 2432
- Ativan Tablets 2434

Loxapine Hydrochloride (Increased CNS depression). Products include:
- Loxitane 1213

Loxapine Succinate (Increased CNS depression). Products include:
- Loxitane Capsules 1213

Maprotiline Hydrochloride (Increased effect of antidepressant or codeine). Products include:
- Ludiomil Tablets 874

Mepenzolate Bromide (May produce paralytic ileus). Products include:
- Cantil Tablets 1326

Meperidine Hydrochloride (Increased CNS depression). Products include:
- Demerol 2047
- Mepergan Injection 2479

Mephobarbital (Increased CNS depression). Products include:
- Mebaral Tablets 2061

Meprobamate (Increased CNS depression). Products include:
- Deprol Tablets 2382
- Equagesic Tablets 2451
- Miltown Tablets 2386
- PMB 200 and PMB 400 2504

Mesoridazine (Increased CNS depression). Products include:
- Serentil 686

Methadone Hydrochloride (Increased CNS depression). Products include:
- Dolophine Hydrochloride Ampoules & Vials 1260
- Dolophine Hydrochloride Tablets 1261
- Methadone Hydrochloride Diskets 1284
- Methadone Hydrochloride Oral Solution & Tablets 1987

Methohexital Sodium (Increased CNS depression). Products include:
- Brevital Sodium Vials 1248

Methoxyflurane (Increased CNS depression).
- No products indexed under this heading.

Midazolam Hydrochloride (Increased CNS depression). Products include:
- Versed Injection 1924

Molindone Hydrochloride (Increased CNS depression). Products include:
- Moban Tablets & Concentrate 932

Morphine Sulfate (Increased CNS depression). Products include:
- Astramorph/PF Injection, USP (Preservative-Free) 618
- Duramorph 960
- Infumorph 200 and Infumorph 500 Sterile Solutions 962
- MS Contin Tablets 1814
- MSIR 1817
- Oramorph SR (Morphine Sulfate Sustained Release Tablets) 1988
- Roxanol 1991

Nortriptyline Hydrochloride (Increased effect of antidepressant or codeine). Products include:
- Pamelor 2019

Opium Alkaloids (Increased CNS depression). Products include:
- B & O No. 15A & No. 16A Supprettes 2395
- Pantopon Injectable 1911

Oxazepam (Increased CNS depression). Products include:
- Serax Capsules 2522
- Serax Tablets 2522

Oxybutynin Chloride (May produce paralytic ileus). Products include:
- Ditropan 1332

Oxycodone Hydrochloride (Increased CNS depression). Products include:
- Percocet Tablets 950
- Percodan 951
- Roxicodone Tablets, Oral Solution & Intensol (Oxycodone) 1992
- Tylox Capsules 1382

Pentobarbital Sodium (Increased CNS depression). Products include:
- Nembutal Sodium Capsules 534
- Nembutal Sodium Solution 536
- Nembutal Sodium Suppositories 538

Perphenazine (Increased CNS depression). Products include:
- Etrafon 2087
- Triavil Tablets 1556
- Trilafon 2123

Phenelzine Sulfate (Increased effect of antidepressant or codeine). Products include:
- Nardil 1742

Phenobarbital (Increased CNS depression). Products include:
- Arco-Lase Plus Tablets 607
- Bellergal-S Tablets 1998
- Bronkolixir .... ▣ 761
- Bronkotabs Tablets .... ▣ 762
- Donnatal 1858
- Donnatal Extentabs 1859
- Donnatal Tablets 1858
- Donnazyme Tablets 1860
- Kinesed Tablets 2272
- Phenobarbital Elixir and Tablets 1293
- Primatene Tablets-P Formula 2421
- Quadrinal Tablets 1183
- Tedral SA 1765

Pimozide (Increased CNS depression). Products include:
- Orap Tablets 1020

Prazepam (Increased CNS depression). Products include:
- Centrax 1693

Prochlorperazine (Increased CNS depression). Products include:
- Compazine 2201

Procyclidine Hydrochloride (May produce paralytic ileus). Products include:
- Kemadrin Tablets 771

Promethazine Hydrochloride (Increased CNS depression). Products include:
- Mepergan Injection 2479
- Phenergan with Codeine 2497
- Phenergan with Dextromethorphan 2499
- Phenergan Injection 2493
- Phenergan Suppositories 2496
- Phenergan Syrup 2495
- Phenergan Tablets 2496
- Phenergan VC 2500
- Phenergan VC with Codeine 2501

Propantheline Bromide (May produce paralytic ileus). Products include:
- Pro-Banthine Tablets 2141

Propofol (Increased CNS depression). Products include:
- Diprivan Injection 2267

Propoxyphene Hydrochloride (Increased CNS depression). Products include:
- Darvon 1256
- Wygesic Tablets 2540

Propoxyphene Napsylate (Increased CNS depression). Products include:
- Darvon-N/Darvocet-N 1254

Protriptyline Hydrochloride (Increased effect of antidepressant or codeine). Products include:
- Vivactil Tablets 1567

Quazepam (Increased CNS depression). Products include:
- Doral Tablets 2383

Scopolamine Hydrobromide (May produce paralytic ileus). Products include:
- Donnagel .... ▣ 675
- Donnagel-PG 1858
- Donnatal 1858
- Donnatal Extentabs 1859
- Donnatal Tablets 1858
- Donnazyme Tablets 1860
- Isopto Hyoscine .... ⊙ 222
- Murocoll-2 Sterile Ophthalmic Solution .... ⊙ 261
- Ru-Tuss Tablets 693

Scopolamine Preparations (May produce paralytic ileus). Products include:
- Transderm Scōp Transdermal Therapeutic System 887

Secobarbital Sodium (Increased CNS depression). Products include:
- Seconal Sodium Pulvules 1296

Selegiline Hydrochloride (Increased effect of antidepressant or codeine). Products include:
- Eldepryl 2250

Sodium Pentobarbital (Increased CNS depression). Products include:
- Nembutal Sodium Capsules 534

Nembutal Sodium Solution 536
Nembutal Sodium Suppositories...... 538

Sufentanil Citrate (Increased CNS depression). Products include:
Sufenta Injection 1147

Temazepam (Increased CNS depression). Products include:
Restoril Capsules 2023

Thiamylal Sodium (Increased CNS depression). Products include:
Surital Ampoules, Steri-Vials............ 1764

Thioridazine Hydrochloride (Increased CNS depression). Products include:
Mellaril 2011

Thiothixene (Increased CNS depression). Products include:
Navane Capsules and Concentrate 1954
Navane Intramuscular 1956

Tranylcypromine Sulfate (Increased effect of antidepressant or codeine). Products include:
Parnate Tablets 2222

Triazolam (Increased CNS depression). Products include:
Halcion Tablets.............................. 2340

Tridihexethyl Chloride (May produce paralytic ileus).
No products indexed under this heading.

Trifluoperazine Hydrochloride (Increased CNS depression). Products include:
Stelazine 2226

Trihexyphenidyl Hydrochloride (May produce paralytic ileus). Products include:
Artane... 1195

Trimipramine Maleate (Increased effect of antidepressant or codeine). Products include:
Surmontil Capsules.......................... 2524

PHENAPHEN-650 WITH CODEINE TABLETS

(Acetaminophen, Codeine Phosphate) 1866

May interact with central nervous system depressants, monoamine oxidase inhibitors, tricyclic antidepressants, anticholinergics, and certain other agents. Compounds in these categories include:

Alcohol (Additive CNS depression).

Alfentanil Hydrochloride (Additive CNS depression). Products include:
Alfenta Injection 1131

Alprazolam (Additive CNS depression). Products include:
Xanax Tablets 2367

Amitriptyline Hydrochloride (Increased effect of either drug). Products include:
Elavil 2269
Endep Tablets 1927
Etrafon 2087
Limbitrol 1933
Triavil Tablets 1556

Amoxapine (Increased effect of either drug). Products include:
Asendin Tablets 1196

Aprobarbital (Additive CNS depression). Products include:
Alurate Elixir 1883

Atropine Sulfate (Potential for paralytic ileus). Products include:
Arco-Lase Plus Tablets 607
Atropine Sulfate Sterile Ophthalmic Solution and S.O.P. Sterile Ophthalmic Ointment................. ◉ 239
Donnagel .... ▣ 675
Donnagel-PG 1858
Donnatal 1858
Donnatal Extentabs........................ 1859
Donnatal Tablets 1858
Donnazyme Tablets 1860
Isopto Atropine.............................. ◉ 218
Lomotil 2174

Motofen Tablets 836
Ru-Tuss Tablets 693
Urised Tablets............................... 2396

Belladonna Alkaloids (Potential for paralytic ileus). Products include:
Bellergal-S Tablets 1998
Hyland's Bed Wetting Tablets .... ▣ 728
Hyland's Teething Tablets .... ▣ 728
Kinesed Tablets 2272

Benztropine Mesylate (Potential for paralytic ileus). Products include:
Cogentin 1435

Biperiden (Potential for paralytic ileus). Products include:
Akineton 1171

Buprenorphine (Additive CNS depression).
No products indexed under this heading.

Buspirone Hydrochloride (Additive CNS depression). Products include:
BuSpar 1401

Butabarbital (Additive CNS depression). Products include:
Pyridium Plus 1764

Butalbital (Additive CNS depression). Products include:
Esgic-Plus Tablets 1002
Esgic Tablets & Capsules................ 1001
Fioricet Tablets.............................. 2006
Fiorinal Capsules 2007
Fiorinal with Codeine Capsules 2008
Fiorinal Tablets.............................. 2007
Phrenilin 838
Sedapap Tablets 50 mg/650 mg .. 1360

Chlordiazepoxide (Additive CNS depression). Products include:
Libritabs Tablets 1930
Limbitrol 1933
Menrium Tablets 1934

Chlordiazepoxide Hydrochloride (Additive CNS depression). Products include:
Librax Capsules 1929
Librium Capsules............................ 1931
Librium Injectable 1932

Chlorpromazine (Additive CNS depression). Products include:
Thorazine 2234

Chlorprothixene (Additive CNS depression). Products include:
Taractan Tablets 1920

Chlorprothixene Hydrochloride (Additive CNS depression). Products include:
Taractan 1920

Clidinium Bromide (Potential for paralytic ileus). Products include:
Librax Capsules 1929
Quarzan Capsules 1937

Clomipramine Hydrochloride (Increased effect of either drug). Products include:
Anafranil Capsules 650

Clorazepate Dipotassium (Additive CNS depression). Products include:
Tranxene 556

Codeine (Additive CNS depression). Products include:
Calcidrine Syrup............................. 506

Codeine Polistirex (Additive CNS depression).
No products indexed under this heading.

Desipramine Hydrochloride (Increased effect of either drug). Products include:
Norpramin Tablets 1340

Dezocine (Additive CNS depression).

Diazepam (Additive CNS depression). Products include:
Valium Injectable 1937
Valium Tablets 1939
Valrelease Capsules 1923

Dicyclomine Hydrochloride (Potential for paralytic ileus). Products include:
Bentyl 1322

Doxepin Hydrochloride (Increased effect of either drug). Products include:
Sinequan 1960

Droperidol (Additive CNS depression). Products include:
Inapsine Injection.......................... 1140
Innovar Injection............................ 1141

Enflurane (Additive CNS depression). Products include:
Ethrane.. 599

Estazolam (Additive CNS depression). Products include:
ProSom Tablets 554

Ethchlorvynol (Additive CNS depression). Products include:
Placidyl Capsules 553

Ethinamate (Additive CNS depression).
No products indexed under this heading.

Fentanyl (Additive CNS depression). Products include:
Duragesic Transdermal System........ 1133

Fentanyl Citrate (Additive CNS depression). Products include:
Innovar Injection............................ 1141
Sublimaze Injection........................ 1146

Fluphenazine Decanoate (Additive CNS depression). Products include:
Prolixin Decanoate 1795

Fluphenazine Enanthate (Additive CNS depression). Products include:
Prolixin Enanthate.......................... 1796

Fluphenazine Hydrochloride (Additive CNS depression). Products include:
Prolixin Elixir 1793
Prolixin Injection............................ 1791
Prolixin Oral Concentrate................ 1792
Prolixin Tablets.............................. 1793

Flurazepam Hydrochloride (Additive CNS depression). Products include:
Dalmane Capsules.......................... 1927

Furazolidone (Increased effect of either drug). Products include:
Furoxone 1855

Glutethimide (Additive CNS depression).
No products indexed under this heading.

Glycopyrrolate (Potential for paralytic ileus). Products include:
Robinul Forte Tablets..................... 1873
Robinul Injectable 1873
Robinul Tablets.............................. 1873

Haloperidol (Additive CNS depression). Products include:
Haldol Injection, Tablets and Concentrate 1373

Haloperidol Decanoate (Additive CNS depression). Products include:
Haldol Decanoate........................... 1375

Hydrocodone Bitartrate (Additive CNS depression). Products include:
Anexsia 5/500 Tablets.................... 2196
Anexsia 7.5/650 Tablets 2197
Azdōne Tablets.............................. 844
Codiclear DH Syrup 845
Codimal DH Syrup.......................... 846
Damason-P.................................... 1356
Hycodan Syrup, Tablets 927
Hycomine Compound Tablets 929
Hycomine Syrup............................. 927
Hycotuss Expectorant Syrup 930
Hydrocet Capsules 835
Lortab ASA Tablets........................ 2414
Lortab... 2412
Ru-Tuss with Hydrocodone 694
Triaminic Expectorant DH 1995
Vicodin Tablets.............................. 1187
Vicodin ES Tablets 1189

Zydone Capsules 941

Hydrocodone Polistirex (Additive CNS depression). Products include:
Tussionex Extended-Release Suspension.. 988

Hydroxyzine Hydrochloride (Additive CNS depression). Products include:
Atarax Tablets & Syrup.................. 1941
Marax Tablets & DF Syrup............. 1954
Vistaril Intramuscular Solution........ 1970

Hyoscyamine (Potential for paralytic ileus). Products include:
Cystospaz Tablets 2395
Urised Tablets............................... 2396

Hyoscyamine Sulfate (Potential for paralytic ileus). Products include:
Arco-Lase Plus Tablets 607
Cystospaz-M Capsules 2395
Donnagel .... ▣ 675
Donnagel-PG 1858
Donnatal 1858
Donnatal Extentabs........................ 1859
Donnatal Tablets 1858
Donnazyme Tablets 1860
Kutrase Capsules........................... 2146
Levsin/Levsinex 2147
Ru-Tuss Tablets 693

Imipramine Hydrochloride (Increased effect of either drug). Products include:
Tofranil Ampuls 1038
Tofranil Tablets 1039

Imipramine Pamoate (Increased effect of either drug). Products include:
Tofranil-PM Capsules..................... 1041

Ipratropium Bromide (Potential for paralytic ileus). Products include:
Atrovent Inhalation Aerosol............. 675

Isocarboxazid (Increased effect of either drug). Products include:
Marplan Tablets 1906

Isoflurane (Additive CNS depression). Products include:
Forane... 600

Ketamine Hydrochloride (Additive CNS depression). Products include:
Ketalar 1726

Levorphanol Tartrate (Additive CNS depression). Products include:
Levo-Dromoran............................... 1906

Lorazepam (Additive CNS depression). Products include:
Ativan Injection.............................. 2432
Ativan Tablets 2434

Loxapine Hydrochloride (Additive CNS depression). Products include:
Loxitane 1213

Loxapine Succinate (Additive CNS depression). Products include:
Loxitane Capsules 1213

Maprotiline Hydrochloride (Increased effect of either drug). Products include:
Ludiomil Tablets............................. 874

Mepenzolate Bromide (Potential for paralytic ileus). Products include:
Cantil Tablets 1326

Meperidine Hydrochloride (Additive CNS depression). Products include:
Demerol 2047
Mepergan Injection 2479

Mephobarbital (Additive CNS depression). Products include:
Mebaral Tablets 2061

Meprobamate (Additive CNS depression). Products include:
Deprol Tablets............................... 2382
Equagesic Tablets 2451
Miltown Tablets 2386
PMB 200 and PMB 400 2504

Mesoridazine (Additive CNS depression). Products include:
Serentil.. 686

Methadone Hydrochloride (Additive CNS depression). Products include:
- Dolophine Hydrochloride Ampoules & Vials 1260
- Dolophine Hydrochloride Tablets 1261
- Methadone Hydrochloride Diskets .. 1284
- Methadone Hydrochloride Oral Solution & Tablets 1987

Methohexital Sodium (Additive CNS depression). Products include:
- Brevital Sodium Vials 1248

Methoxyflurane (Additive CNS depression).
- No products indexed under this heading.

Midazolam Hydrochloride (Additive CNS depression). Products include:
- Versed Injection 1924

Molindone Hydrochloride (Additive CNS depression). Products include:
- Moban Tablets & Concentrate 932

Morphine Sulfate (Additive CNS depression). Products include:
- Astramorph/PF Injection, USP (Preservative-Free) 618
- Duramorph 960
- Infumorph 200 and Infumorph 500 Sterile Solutions 962
- MS Contin Tablets 1814
- MSIR 1817
- Oramorph SR (Morphine Sulfate Sustained Release Tablets) 1988
- Roxanol 1991

Nortriptyline Hydrochloride (Increased effect of either drug). Products include:
- Pamelor 2019

Opium Alkaloids (Additive CNS depression). Products include:
- B & O No. 15A & No. 16A Supprettes 2395
- Pantopon Injectable 1911

Oxazepam (Additive CNS depression). Products include:
- Serax Capsules 2522
- Serax Tablets 2522

Oxybutynin Chloride (Potential for paralytic ileus). Products include:
- Ditropan 1332

Oxycodone Hydrochloride (Additive CNS depression). Products include:
- Percocet Tablets 950
- Percodan 951
- Roxicodone Tablets, Oral Solution & Intensol (Oxycodone) 1992
- Tylox Capsules 1382

Pentobarbital Sodium (Additive CNS depression). Products include:
- Nembutal Sodium Capsules 534
- Nembutal Sodium Solution 536
- Nembutal Sodium Suppositories 538

Perphenazine (Additive CNS depression). Products include:
- Etrafon 2087
- Triavil Tablets 1556
- Trilafon 2123

Phenelzine Sulfate (Increased effect of either drug). Products include:
- Nardil 1742

Phenobarbital (Additive CNS depression). Products include:
- Arco-Lase Plus Tablets 607
- Bellergal-S Tablets 1998
- Bronkolixir .... ⊞ 761
- Bronkotabs Tablets .... ⊞ 762
- Donnatal 1858
- Donnatal Extentabs 1859
- Donnatal Tablets 1858
- Donnazyme Tablets 1860
- Kinesed Tablets 2272
- Phenobarbital Elixir and Tablets 1293
- Primatene Tablets-P Formula 2421
- Quadrinal Tablets 1183
- Tedral SA 1765

Prazepam (Additive CNS depression). Products include:
- Centrax 1693

Prochlorperazine (Additive CNS depression). Products include:
- Compazine 2201

Procyclidine Hydrochloride (Potential for paralytic ileus). Products include:
- Kemadrin Tablets 771

Promethazine Hydrochloride (Additive CNS depression). Products include:
- Mepergan Injection 2479
- Phenergan with Codeine 2497
- Phenergan with Dextromethorphan 2499
- Phenergan Injection 2493
- Phenergan Suppositories 2496
- Phenergan Syrup 2495
- Phenergan Tablets 2496
- Phenergan VC 2500
- Phenergan VC with Codeine 2501

Propantheline Bromide (Potential for paralytic ileus). Products include:
- Pro-Banthine Tablets 2141

Propofol (Additive CNS depression). Products include:
- Diprivan Injection 2267

Propoxyphene Hydrochloride (Additive CNS depression). Products include:
- Darvon 1256
- Wygesic Tablets 2540

Propoxyphene Napsylate (Additive CNS depression). Products include:
- Darvon-N/Darvocet-N 1254

Protriptyline Hydrochloride (Increased effect of either drug). Products include:
- Vivactil Tablets 1567

Quazepam (Additive CNS depression). Products include:
- Doral Tablets 2383

Scopolamine Hydrobromide (Potential for paralytic ileus). Products include:
- Donnagel .... ⊞ 675
- Donnagel-PG 1858
- Donnatal 1858
- Donnatal Extentabs 1859
- Donnatal Tablets 1858
- Donnazyme Tablets 1860
- Isopto Hyoscine .... ⊙ 222
- Murocoll-2 Sterile Ophthalmic Solution .... ⊙ 261
- Ru-Tuss Tablets 693

Scopolamine Preparations (Potential for paralytic ileus). Products include:
- Transderm Scōp Transdermal Therapeutic System 887

Secobarbital Sodium (Additive CNS depression). Products include:
- Seconal Sodium Pulvules 1296

Selegiline Hydrochloride (Increased effect of either drug). Products include:
- Eldepryl 2250

Sodium Pentobarbital (Additive CNS depression). Products include:
- Nembutal Sodium Capsules 534
- Nembutal Sodium Solution 536
- Nembutal Sodium Suppositories 538

Sufentanil Citrate (Additive CNS depression). Products include:
- Sufenta Injection 1147

Temazepam (Additive CNS depression). Products include:
- Restoril Capsules 2023

Thiamylal Sodium (Additive CNS depression). Products include:
- Surital Ampoules, Steri-Vials 1764

Thioridazine Hydrochloride (Additive CNS depression). Products include:
- Mellaril 2011

Thiothixene (Additive CNS depression). Products include:
- Navane Capsules and Concentrate 1954
- Navane Intramuscular 1956

Tranylcypromine Sulfate (Increased effect of either drug). Products include:
- Parnate Tablets 2222

Triazolam (Additive CNS depression). Products include:
- Halcion Tablets 2340

Tridihexethyl Chloride (Potential for paralytic ileus).
- No products indexed under this heading.

Trifluoperazine Hydrochloride (Additive CNS depression). Products include:
- Stelazine 2226

Trihexyphenidyl Hydrochloride (Potential for paralytic ileus). Products include:
- Artane 1195

Trimipramine Maleate (Increased effect of either drug). Products include:
- Surmontil Capsules 2524

PHENERGAN WITH CODEINE
(Codeine Phosphate, Promethazine Hydrochloride) 2497
May interact with narcotic analgesics, hypnotics and sedatives, tricyclic antidepressants, tranquilizers, monoamine oxidase inhibitors, and certain other agents. Compounds in these categories include:

Alcohol (Additive sedative effects).

Alfentanil Hydrochloride (Additive sedative effects). Products include:
- Alfenta Injection 1131

Alprazolam (Additive sedative effects). Products include:
- Xanax Tablets 2367

Amitriptyline Hydrochloride (Additive sedative effects). Products include:
- Elavil 2269
- Endep Tablets 1927
- Etrafon 2087
- Limbitrol 1933
- Triavil Tablets 1556

Amoxapine (Additive sedative effects). Products include:
- Asendin Tablets 1196

Buprenorphine (Additive sedative effects).
- No products indexed under this heading.

Buspirone Hydrochloride (Additive sedative effects). Products include:
- BuSpar 1401

Chlordiazepoxide (Additive sedative effects). Products include:
- Libritabs Tablets 1930
- Limbitrol 1933
- Menrium Tablets 1934

Chlordiazepoxide Hydrochloride (Additive sedative effects). Products include:
- Librax Capsules 1929
- Librium Capsules 1931
- Librium Injectable 1932

Chlorpromazine (Additive sedative effects). Products include:
- Thorazine 2234

Chlorprothixene (Additive sedative effects). Products include:
- Taractan Tablets 1920

Chlorprothixene Hydrochloride (Additive sedative effects). Products include:
- Taractan 1920

Clomipramine Hydrochloride (Additive sedative effects). Products include:
- Anafranil Capsules 650

Clorazepate Dipotassium (Additive sedative effects). Products include:
- Tranxene 556

Desipramine Hydrochloride (Additive sedative effects). Products include:
- Norpramin Tablets 1340

Dezocine (Additive sedative effects).

Diazepam (Additive sedative effects). Products include:
- Valium Injectable 1937
- Valium Tablets 1939
- Valrelease Capsules 1923

Doxepin Hydrochloride (Additive sedative effects). Products include:
- Sinequan 1960

Droperidol (Additive sedative effects). Products include:
- Inapsine Injection 1140
- Innovar Injection 1141

Estazolam (Additive sedative effects). Products include:
- ProSom Tablets 554

Ethchlorvynol (Additive sedative effects). Products include:
- Placidyl Capsules 553

Ethinamate (Additive sedative effects).
- No products indexed under this heading.

Fentanyl (Additive sedative effects). Products include:
- Duragesic Transdermal System 1133

Fentanyl Citrate (Additive sedative effects). Products include:
- Innovar Injection 1141
- Sublimaze Injection 1146

Fluphenazine Decanoate (Additive sedative effects). Products include:
- Prolixin Decanoate 1795

Fluphenazine Enanthate (Additive sedative effects). Products include:
- Prolixin Enanthate 1796

Fluphenazine Hydrochloride (Additive sedative effects). Products include:
- Prolixin Elixir 1793
- Prolixin Injection 1791
- Prolixin Oral Concentrate 1792
- Prolixin Tablets 1793

Flurazepam Hydrochloride (Additive sedative effects). Products include:
- Dalmane Capsules 1927

Furazolidone (Excessive narcotic effects). Products include:
- Furoxone 1855

Glutethimide (Additive sedative effects).
- No products indexed under this heading.

Haloperidol (Additive sedative effects). Products include:
- Haldol Injection, Tablets and Concentrate 1373

Haloperidol Decanoate (Additive sedative effects). Products include:
- Haldol Decanoate 1375

Hydrocodone Bitartrate (Additive sedative effects). Products include:
- Anexsia 5/500 Tablets 2196
- Anexsia 7.5/650 Tablets 2197
- Azdōne Tablets 844
- Codiclear DH Syrup 845
- Codimal DH Syrup 846
- Damason-P 1356
- Hycodan Syrup, Tablets 927
- Hycomine Compound Tablets 929
- Hycomine Syrup 927
- Hycotuss Expectorant Syrup 930
- Hydrocet Capsules 835
- Lortab ASA Tablets 2414
- Lortab 2412
- Ru-Tuss with Hydrocodone 694

Triaminic Expectorant DH ... 1995
Vicodin Tablets ... 1187
Vicodin ES Tablets ... 1189
Zydone Capsules ... 941

Hydrocodone Polistirex (Additive sedative effects). Products include:
Tussionex Extended-Release Suspension ... 988

Hydroxyzine Hydrochloride (Additive sedative effects). Products include:
Atarax Tablets & Syrup ... 1941
Marax Tablets & DF Syrup ... 1954
Vistaril Intramuscular Solution ... 1970

Imipramine Hydrochloride (Additive sedative effects). Products include:
Tofranil Ampuls ... 1038
Tofranil Tablets ... 1039

Imipramine Pamoate (Additive sedative effects). Products include:
Tofranil-PM Capsules ... 1041

Isocarboxazid (Excessive narcotic effects). Products include:
Marplan Tablets ... 1906

Levorphanol Tartrate (Additive sedative effects). Products include:
Levo-Dromoran ... 1906

Lorazepam (Additive sedative effects). Products include:
Ativan Injection ... 2432
Ativan Tablets ... 2434

Loxapine Hydrochloride (Additive sedative effects). Products include:
Loxitane ... 1213

Maprotiline Hydrochloride (Additive sedative effects). Products include:
Ludiomil Tablets ... 874

Meperidine Hydrochloride (Additive sedative effects). Products include:
Demerol ... 2047
Mepergan Injection ... 2479

Meprobamate (Additive sedative effects). Products include:
Deprol Tablets ... 2382
Equagesic Tablets ... 2451
Miltown Tablets ... 2386
PMB 200 and PMB 400 ... 2504

Mesoridazine (Additive sedative effects). Products include:
Serentil ... 686

Methadone Hydrochloride (Additive sedative effects). Products include:
Dolophine Hydrochloride Ampoules & Vials ... 1260
Dolophine Hydrochloride Tablets ... 1261
Methadone Hydrochloride Diskets ... 1284
Methadone Hydrochloride Oral Solution & Tablets ... 1987

Midazolam Hydrochloride (Additive sedative effects). Products include:
Versed Injection ... 1924

Molindone Hydrochloride (Additive sedative effects). Products include:
Moban Tablets & Concentrate ... 932

Morphine Sulfate (Additive sedative effects). Products include:
Astramorph/PF Injection, USP (Preservative-Free) ... 618
Duramorph ... 960
Infumorph 200 and Infumorph 500 Sterile Solutions ... 962
MS Contin Tablets ... 1814
MSIR ... 1817
Oramorph SR (Morphine Sulfate Sustained Release Tablets) ... 1988
Roxanol ... 1991

Nortriptyline Hydrochloride (Additive sedative effects). Products include:
Pamelor ... 2019

Opium Alkaloids (Additive sedative effects). Products include:
B & O No. 15A & No. 16A Supprettes ... 2395
Pantopon Injectable ... 1911

Oxazepam (Additive sedative effects). Products include:
Serax Capsules ... 2522
Serax Tablets ... 2522

Oxycodone Hydrochloride (Additive sedative effects). Products include:
Percocet Tablets ... 950
Percodan ... 951
Roxicodone Tablets, Oral Solution & Intensol (Oxycodone) ... 1992
Tylox Capsules ... 1382

Perphenazine (Additive sedative effects). Products include:
Etrafon ... 2087
Triavil Tablets ... 1556
Trilafon ... 2123

Phenelzine Sulfate (Excessive narcotic effects). Products include:
Nardil ... 1742

Prazepam (Additive sedative effects). Products include:
Centrax ... 1693

Prochlorperazine (Additive sedative effects). Products include:
Compazine ... 2201

Propofol (Additive sedative effects). Products include:
Diprivan Injection ... 2267

Propoxyphene Hydrochloride (Additive sedative effects). Products include:
Darvon ... 1256
Wygesic Tablets ... 2540

Propoxyphene Napsylate (Additive sedative effects). Products include:
Darvon-N/Darvocet-N ... 1254

Protriptyline Hydrochloride (Additive sedative effects). Products include:
Vivactil Tablets ... 1567

Quazepam (Additive sedative effects). Products include:
Doral Tablets ... 2383

Secobarbital Sodium (Additive sedative effects). Products include:
Seconal Sodium Pulvules ... 1296

Selegiline Hydrochloride (Excessive narcotic effects). Products include:
Eldepryl ... 2250

Sufentanil Citrate (Additive sedative effects). Products include:
Sufenta Injection ... 1147

Temazepam (Additive sedative effects). Products include:
Restoril Capsules ... 2023

Thioridazine Hydrochloride (Additive sedative effects). Products include:
Mellaril ... 2011

Thiothixene (Additive sedative effects). Products include:
Navane Capsules and Concentrate ... 1954
Navane Intramuscular ... 1956

Tranylcypromine Sulfate (Excessive narcotic effects). Products include:
Parnate Tablets ... 2222

Triazolam (Additive sedative effects). Products include:
Halcion Tablets ... 2340

Trifluoperazine Hydrochloride (Additive sedative effects). Products include:
Stelazine ... 2226

Trimipramine Maleate (Additive sedative effects). Products include:
Surmontil Capsules ... 2524

PHENERGAN WITH DEXTROMETHORPHAN
(Promethazine Hydrochloride, Dextromethorphan Hydrobromide) ... 2499
May interact with narcotic analgesics, hypnotics and sedatives, tricyclic antidepressants, tranquilizers, and certain other agents. Compounds in these categories include:

Alcohol (Additive sedative effects).

Alfentanil Hydrochloride (Additive sedative effects). Products include:
Alfenta Injection ... 1131

Alprazolam (Additive sedative effects). Products include:
Xanax Tablets ... 2367

Amitriptyline Hydrochloride (Additive sedative effects). Products include:
Elavil ... 2269
Endep Tablets ... 1927
Etrafon ... 2087
Limbitrol ... 1933
Triavil Tablets ... 1556

Amoxapine (Additive sedative effects). Products include:
Asendin Tablets ... 1196

Buprenorphine (Additive sedative effects).
No products indexed under this heading.

Buspirone Hydrochloride (Additive sedative effects). Products include:
BuSpar ... 1401

Chlordiazepoxide (Additive sedative effects). Products include:
Libritabs Tablets ... 1930
Limbitrol ... 1933
Menrium Tablets ... 1934

Chlordiazepoxide Hydrochloride (Additive sedative effects). Products include:
Librax Capsules ... 1929
Librium Capsules ... 1931
Librium Injectable ... 1932

Chlorpromazine (Additive sedative effects). Products include:
Thorazine ... 2234

Clomipramine Hydrochloride (Additive sedative effects). Products include:
Anafranil Capsules ... 650

Clorazepate Dipotassium (Additive sedative effects). Products include:
Tranxene ... 556

Codeine (Additive sedative effects). Products include:
Calcidrine Syrup ... 506

Codeine Phosphate (Additive sedative effects). Products include:
Actifed with Codeine Cough Syrup ... 752
Cheracol Cough Syrup ... 1853
Codimal PH Syrup ... 846
Dimetane-DC Cough Syrup ... 1857
Empirin with Codeine Phosphate Nos. 2, 3 & 4 ... 764
Fiorinal with Codeine Capsules ... 2008
Isoclor Expectorant ... 982
Naldecon CX Adult Liquid ... 521
Novahistine DH ... 1342
Novahistine Expectorant ... 1343
Nucofed Capsules ... 2219
Nucofed Expectorant ... 2219
Nucofed Pediatric Expectorant ... 2220
Nucofed Syrup ... 2219
Phenaphen with Codeine Capsules ... 1865
Phenaphen-650 with Codeine Tablets ... 1866
Phenergan with Codeine ... 2497
Phenergan VC with Codeine ... 2501
Robitussin A-C Syrup ... 1875
Robitussin-DAC Syrup ... 1875
Ryna ... 741
Soma Compound w/Codeine Tablets ... 2390
Triaminic Expectorant w/Codeine ... 1996
Tussi-Organidin Liquid ... 2391
Tylenol with Codeine ... 1381

Codeine Polistirex (Additive sedative effects).
No products indexed under this heading.

Desipramine Hydrochloride (Additive sedative effects). Products include:
Norpramin Tablets ... 1340

Dezocine (Additive sedative effects).

Diazepam (Additive sedative effects). Products include:
Valium Injectable ... 1937
Valium Tablets ... 1939
Valrelease Capsules ... 1923

Doxepin Hydrochloride (Additive sedative effects). Products include:
Sinequan ... 1960

Droperidol (Additive sedative effects). Products include:
Inapsine Injection ... 1140
Innovar Injection ... 1141

Estazolam (Additive sedative effects). Products include:
ProSom Tablets ... 554

Ethchlorvynol (Additive sedative effects). Products include:
Placidyl Capsules ... 553

Ethinamate (Additive sedative effects).
No products indexed under this heading.

Fentanyl (Additive sedative effects). Products include:
Duragesic Transdermal System ... 1133

Fentanyl Citrate (Additive sedative effects). Products include:
Innovar Injection ... 1141
Sublimaze Injection ... 1146

Fluphenazine Decanoate (Additive sedative effects). Products include:
Prolixin Decanoate ... 1795

Fluphenazine Enanthate (Additive sedative effects). Products include:
Prolixin Enanthate ... 1796

Fluphenazine Hydrochloride (Additive sedative effects). Products include:
Prolixin Elixir ... 1793
Prolixin Injection ... 1791
Prolixin Oral Concentrate ... 1792
Prolixin Tablets ... 1793

Flurazepam Hydrochloride (Additive sedative effects). Products include:
Dalmane Capsules ... 1927

Glutethimide (Additive sedative effects).
No products indexed under this heading.

Haloperidol (Additive sedative effects). Products include:
Haldol Injection, Tablets and Concentrate ... 1373

Haloperidol Decanoate (Additive sedative effects). Products include:
Haldol Decanoate ... 1375

Hydrocodone Bitartrate (Additive sedative effects). Products include:
Anexsia 5/500 Tablets ... 2196
Anexsia 7.5/650 Tablets ... 2197
Azdone Tablets ... 844
Codiclear DH Syrup ... 845
Codimal DH Syrup ... 846
Damason-P ... 1356
Hycodan Syrup, Tablets ... 927
Hycomine Compound Tablets ... 929
Hycomine Syrup ... 927
Hycotuss Expectorant Syrup ... 930
Hydrocet Capsules ... 835
Lortab ASA Tablets ... 2414
Lortab ... 2412
Ru-Tuss with Hydrocodone ... 694
Triaminic Expectorant DH ... 1995
Vicodin Tablets ... 1187
Vicodin ES Tablets ... 1189
Zydone Capsules ... 941

Hydrocodone Polistirex (Additive sedative effects). Products include:
Tussionex Extended-Release Suspension ... 988

Hydroxyzine Hydrochloride (Additive sedative effects). Products include:
Atarax Tablets & Syrup ... 1941
Marax Tablets & DF Syrup ... 1954
Vistaril Intramuscular Solution ... 1970

Imipramine Hydrochloride (Additive sedative effects). Products include:
Tofranil Ampuls ... 1038
Tofranil Tablets ... 1039

Imipramine Pamoate (Additive sedative effects). Products include:
Tofranil-PM Capsules ... 1041

Levorphanol Tartrate (Additive sedative effects). Products include:
Levo-Dromoran ... 1906

Lorazepam (Additive sedative effects). Products include:
Ativan Injection ... 2432
Ativan Tablets ... 2434

Loxapine Hydrochloride (Additive sedative effects). Products include:
Loxitane ... 1213

Maprotiline Hydrochloride (Additive sedative effects). Products include:
Ludiomil Tablets ... 874

Meperidine Hydrochloride (Additive sedative effects). Products include:
Demerol ... 2047
Mepergan Injection ... 2479

Meprobamate (Additive sedative effects). Products include:
Deprol Tablets ... 2382
Equagesic Tablets ... 2451
Miltown Tablets ... 2386
PMB 200 and PMB 400 ... 2504

Mesoridazine (Additive sedative effects). Products include:
Serentil ... 686

Methadone Hydrochloride (Additive sedative effects). Products include:
Dolophine Hydrochloride Ampoules & Vials ... 1260
Dolophine Hydrochloride Tablets ... 1261
Methadone Hydrochloride Diskets ... 1284
Methadone Hydrochloride Oral Solution & Tablets ... 1987

Midazolam Hydrochloride (Additive sedative effects). Products include:
Versed Injection ... 1924

Molindone Hydrochloride (Additive sedative effects). Products include:
Moban Tablets & Concentrate ... 932

Morphine Sulfate (Additive sedative effects). Products include:
Astramorph/PF Injection, USP (Preservative-Free) ... 618
Duramorph ... 960
Infumorph 200 and Infumorph 500 Sterile Solutions ... 962
MS Contin Tablets ... 1814
MSIR ... 1817
Oramorph SR (Morphine Sulfate Sustained Release Tablets) ... 1988
Roxanol ... 1991

Nortriptyline Hydrochloride (Additive sedative effects). Products include:
Pamelor ... 2019

Opium Alkaloids (Additive sedative effects). Products include:
B & O No. 15A & No. 16A Supprettes ... 2395
Pantopon Injectable ... 1911

Oxazepam (Additive sedative effects). Products include:
Serax Capsules ... 2522
Serax Tablets ... 2522

Oxycodone Hydrochloride (Additive sedative effects). Products include:
Percocet Tablets ... 950
Percodan ... 951
Roxicodone Tablets, Oral Solution & Intensol (Oxycodone) ... 1992
Tylox Capsules ... 1382

Perphenazine (Additive sedative effects). Products include:
Etrafon ... 2087
Triavil Tablets ... 1556
Trilafon ... 2123

Prazepam (Additive sedative effects). Products include:
Centrax ... 1693

Prochlorperazine (Additive sedative effects). Products include:
Compazine ... 2201

Propofol (Additive sedative effects). Products include:
Diprivan Injection ... 2267

Propoxyphene Hydrochloride (Additive sedative effects). Products include:
Darvon ... 1256
Wygesic Tablets ... 2540

Propoxyphene Napsylate (Additive sedative effects). Products include:
Darvon-N/Darvocet-N ... 1254

Protriptyline Hydrochloride (Additive sedative effects). Products include:
Vivactil Tablets ... 1567

Quazepam (Additive sedative effects). Products include:
Doral Tablets ... 2383

Secobarbital Sodium (Additive sedative effects). Products include:
Seconal Sodium Pulvules ... 1296

Sufentanil Citrate (Additive sedative effects). Products include:
Sufenta Injection ... 1147

Temazepam (Additive sedative effects). Products include:
Restoril Capsules ... 2023

Thioridazine Hydrochloride (Additive sedative effects). Products include:
Mellaril ... 2011

Thiothixene (Additive sedative effects). Products include:
Navane Capsules and Concentrate 1954
Navane Intramuscular ... 1956

Triazolam (Additive sedative effects). Products include:
Halcion Tablets ... 2340

Trifluoperazine Hydrochloride (Additive sedative effects). Products include:
Stelazine ... 2226

Trimipramine Maleate (Additive sedative effects). Products include:
Surmontil Capsules ... 2524

PHENERGAN INJECTION
(Promethazine Hydrochloride) ... 2493
May interact with narcotic analgesics, barbiturates, hypnotics and sedatives, general anesthetics, tranquilizers, central nervous system depressants, monoamine oxidase inhibitors, and certain other agents. Compounds in these categories include:

Alcohol (Additive sedative effects).

Alfentanil Hydrochloride (Additive sedative effects). Products include:
Alfenta Injection ... 1131

Alprazolam (Additive sedative effects). Products include:
Xanax Tablets ... 2367

Aprobarbital (Additive sedative effects). Products include:
Alurate Elixir ... 1883

Buprenorphine (Additive sedative effects).
No products indexed under this heading.

Buspirone Hydrochloride (Additive sedative effects). Products include:
BuSpar ... 1401

Butabarbital (Additive sedative effects). Products include:
Pyridium Plus ... 1764

Butalbital (Additive sedative effects). Products include:
Esgic-Plus Tablets ... 1002
Esgic Tablets & Capsules ... 1001
Fioricet Tablets ... 2006
Fiorinal Capsules ... 2007
Fiorinal with Codeine Capsules ... 2008
Fiorinal Tablets ... 2007
Phrenilin ... 838
Sedapap Tablets 50 mg/650 mg .. 1360

Chlordiazepoxide (Additive sedative effects). Products include:
Libritabs Tablets ... 1930
Limbitrol ... 1933
Menrium Tablets ... 1934

Chlordiazepoxide Hydrochloride (Additive sedative effects). Products include:
Librax Capsules ... 1929
Librium Capsules ... 1931
Librium Injectable ... 1932

Chlorpromazine (Additive sedative effects). Products include:
Thorazine ... 2234

Chlorprothixene (Additive sedative effects). Products include:
Taractan Tablets ... 1920

Chlorprothixene Hydrochloride (Additive sedative effects). Products include:
Taractan ... 1920

Clorazepate Dipotassium (Additive sedative effects). Products include:
Tranxene ... 556

Codeine (Additive sedative effects). Products include:
Calcidrine Syrup ... 506

Codeine Phosphate (Additive sedative effects). Products include:
Actifed with Codeine Cough Syrup.. 752
Cheracol Cough Syrup ... 1853
Codimal PH Syrup ... 846
Dimetane-DC Cough Syrup ... 1857
Empirin with Codeine Phosphate Nos. 2, 3 & 4 ... 764
Fiorinal with Codeine Capsules ... 2008
Isoclor Expectorant ... 982
Naldecon CX Adult Liquid ... ▣ 521
Novahistine DH ... 1342
Novahistine Expectorant ... 1343
Nucofed Capsules ... 2219
Nucofed Expectorant ... 2219
Nucofed Pediatric Expectorant ... 2220
Nucofed Syrup ... 2219
Phenaphen with Codeine Capsules 1865
Phenaphen-650 with Codeine Tablets ... 1866
Phenergan with Codeine ... 2497
Phenergan VC with Codeine ... 2501
Robitussin A-C Syrup ... 1875
Robitussin-DAC Syrup ... 1875
Ryna ... ▣ 741
Soma Compound w/Codeine Tablets ... 2390
Triaminic Expectorant w/Codeine .. 1996
Tussi-Organidin Liquid ... 2391
Tylenol with Codeine ... 1381

Codeine Polistirex (Additive sedative effects).
No products indexed under this heading.

Dezocine (Additive sedative effects).

Diazepam (Additive sedative effects). Products include:
Valium Injectable ... 1937
Valium Tablets ... 1939
Valrelease Capsules ... 1923

Droperidol (Additive sedative effects). Products include:
Inapsine Injection ... 1140
Innovar Injection ... 1141

Enflurane (Additive sedative effects). Products include:
Ethrane ... 599

Epinephrine Hydrochloride (Potential for reversal of the vasopressor effect). Products include:
Adrenalin Chloride Solution 1:100 & 1:1,000 ... 1689
Epifrin ... ⊙ 244
Glaucon ... ⊙ 218

Estazolam (Additive sedative effects). Products include:
ProSom Tablets ... 554

Ethchlorvynol (Additive sedative effects). Products include:
Placidyl Capsules ... 553

Ethinamate (Additive sedative effects).
No products indexed under this heading.

Fentanyl (Additive sedative effects). Products include:
Duragesic Transdermal System ... 1133

Fentanyl Citrate (Additive sedative effects). Products include:
Innovar Injection ... 1141
Sublimaze Injection ... 1146

Fluphenazine Decanoate (Additive sedative effects). Products include:
Prolixin Decanoate ... 1795

Fluphenazine Enanthate (Additive sedative effects). Products include:
Prolixin Enanthate ... 1796

Fluphenazine Hydrochloride (Additive sedative effects). Products include:
Prolixin Elixir ... 1793
Prolixin Injection ... 1791
Prolixin Oral Concentrate ... 1792
Prolixin Tablets ... 1793

Flurazepam Hydrochloride (Additive sedative effects). Products include:
Dalmane Capsules ... 1927

Furazolidone (Possibility of increased incidence of extrapyramidal effects). Products include:
Furoxone ... 1855

Glutethimide (Additive sedative effects).
No products indexed under this heading.

Haloperidol (Additive sedative effects). Products include:
Haldol Injection, Tablets and Concentrate ... 1373

Haloperidol Decanoate (Additive sedative effects). Products include:
Haldol Decanoate ... 1375

Hydrocodone Bitartrate (Additive sedative effects). Products include:
Anexsia 5/500 Tablets ... 2196
Anexsia 7.5/650 Tablets ... 2197
Azdone Tablets ... 844
Codiclear DH Syrup ... 845
Codimal DH Syrup ... 846
Damason-P ... 1356
Hycodan Syrup, Tablets ... 927
Hycomine Compound Tablets ... 929
Hycomine Syrup ... 927
Hycotuss Expectorant Syrup ... 930
Hydrocet Capsules ... 835
Lortab ASA Tablets ... 2414
Lortab ... 2412
Ru-Tuss with Hydrocodone ... 694
Triaminic Expectorant DH ... 1995
Vicodin Tablets ... 1187
Vicodin ES Tablets ... 1189
Zydone Capsules ... 941

Hydrocodone Polistirex (Additive sedative effects). Products include:
Tussionex Extended-Release Suspension ... 988
Hydroxyzine Hydrochloride (Additive sedative effects). Products include:
Atarax Tablets & Syrup ... 1941
Marax Tablets & DF Syrup ... 1954
Vistaril Intramuscular Solution ... 1970
Isocarboxazid (Possibility of increased incidence of extrapyramidal effects). Products include:
Marplan Tablets ... 1906
Isoflurane (Additive sedative effects). Products include:
Forane ... 600
Ketamine Hydrochloride (Additive sedative effects). Products include:
Ketalar ... 1726
Levorphanol Tartrate (Additive sedative effects). Products include:
Levo-Dromoran ... 1906
Lorazepam (Additive sedative effects). Products include:
Ativan Injection ... 2432
Ativan Tablets ... 2434
Loxapine Hydrochloride (Additive sedative effects). Products include:
Loxitane ... 1213
Loxapine Succinate (Additive sedative effects). Products include:
Loxitane Capsules ... 1213
Meperidine Hydrochloride (Additive sedative effects). Products include:
Demerol ... 2047
Mepergan Injection ... 2479
Mephobarbital (Additive sedative effects). Products include:
Mebaral Tablets ... 2061
Meprobamate (Additive sedative effects). Products include:
Deprol Tablets ... 2382
Equagesic Tablets ... 2451
Miltown Tablets ... 2386
PMB 200 and PMB 400 ... 2504
Mesoridazine (Additive sedative effects). Products include:
Serentil ... 686
Methadone Hydrochloride (Additive sedative effects). Products include:
Dolophine Hydrochloride Ampoules & Vials ... 1260
Dolophine Hydrochloride Tablets ... 1261
Methadone Hydrochloride Diskets ... 1284
Methadone Hydrochloride Oral Solution & Tablets ... 1987
Methohexital Sodium (Additive sedative effects). Products include:
Brevital Sodium Vials ... 1248
Methoxyflurane (Additive sedative effects).
No products indexed under this heading.
Midazolam Hydrochloride (Additive sedative effects). Products include:
Versed Injection ... 1924
Molindone Hydrochloride (Additive sedative effects). Products include:
Moban Tablets & Concentrate ... 932
Morphine Sulfate (Additive sedative effects). Products include:
Astramorph/PF Injection, USP (Preservative-Free) ... 618
Duramorph ... 960
Infumorph 200 and Infumorph 500 Sterile Solutions ... 962
MS Contin Tablets ... 1814
MSIR ... 1817
Oramorph SR (Morphine Sulfate Sustained Release Tablets) ... 1988
Roxanol ... 1991
Opium Alkaloids (Additive sedative effects). Products include:
B & O No. 15A & No. 16A Supprettes ... 2395
Pantopon Injectable ... 1911
Oxazepam (Additive sedative effects). Products include:
Serax Capsules ... 2522
Serax Tablets ... 2522
Oxycodone Hydrochloride (Additive sedative effects). Products include:
Percocet Tablets ... 950
Percodan ... 951
Roxicodone Tablets, Oral Solution & Intensol (Oxycodone) ... 1992
Tylox Capsules ... 1382
Pentobarbital Sodium (Additive sedative effects). Products include:
Nembutal Sodium Capsules ... 534
Nembutal Sodium Solution ... 536
Nembutal Sodium Suppositories ... 538
Perphenazine (Additive sedative effects). Products include:
Etrafon ... 2087
Triavil Tablets ... 1556
Trilafon ... 2123
Phenelzine Sulfate (Possibility of increased incidence of extrapyramidal effects). Products include:
Nardil ... 1742
Phenobarbital (Additive sedative effects). Products include:
Arco-Lase Plus Tablets ... 607
Bellergal-S Tablets ... 1998
Bronkolixir ... ▣ 761
Bronkotabs Tablets ... ▣ 762
Donnatal ... 1858
Donnatal Extentabs ... 1859
Donnatal Tablets ... 1858
Donnazyme Tablets ... 1860
Kinesed Tablets ... 2272
Phenobarbital Elixir and Tablets ... 1293
Primatene Tablets-P Formula ... 2421
Quadrinal Tablets ... 1183
Tedral SA ... 1765
Prazepam (Additive sedative effects). Products include:
Centrax ... 1693
Prochlorperazine (Additive sedative effects). Products include:
Compazine ... 2201
Propofol (Additive sedative effects). Products include:
Diprivan Injection ... 2267
Propoxyphene Hydrochloride (Additive sedative effects). Products include:
Darvon ... 1256
Wygesic Tablets ... 2540
Propoxyphene Napsylate (Additive sedative effects). Products include:
Darvon-N/Darvocet-N ... 1254
Quazepam (Additive sedative effects). Products include:
Doral Tablets ... 2383
Secobarbital Sodium (Additive sedative effects). Products include:
Seconal Sodium Pulvules ... 1296
Selegiline Hydrochloride (Possibility of increased incidence of extrapyramidal effects). Products include:
Eldepryl ... 2250
Sufentanil Citrate (Additive sedative effects). Products include:
Sufenta Injection ... 1147
Temazepam (Additive sedative effects). Products include:
Restoril Capsules ... 2023
Thiamylal Sodium (Additive sedative effects). Products include:
Surital Ampoules, Steri-Vials ... 1764
Thioridazine Hydrochloride (Additive sedative effects). Products include:
Mellaril ... 2011
Thiothixene (Additive sedative effects). Products include:
Navane Capsules and Concentrate ... 1954
Navane Intramuscular ... 1956
Tranylcypromine Sulfate (Possibility of increased incidence of extrapyramidal effects). Products include:
Parnate Tablets ... 2222
Triazolam (Additive sedative effects). Products include:
Halcion Tablets ... 2340
Trifluoperazine Hydrochloride (Additive sedative effects). Products include:
Stelazine ... 2226

PHENERGAN SUPPOSITORIES

(Promethazine Hydrochloride) ... 2496

May interact with narcotic analgesics, hypnotics and sedatives, tricyclic antidepressants, tranquilizers, central nervous system depressants, barbiturates, and certain other agents. Compounds in these categories include:

Alcohol (Additive sedative effects).
Alfentanil Hydrochloride (Additive sedative effects). Products include:
Alfenta Injection ... 1131
Alprazolam (Additive sedative effects). Products include:
Xanax Tablets ... 2367
Amitriptyline Hydrochloride (Additive sedative effects). Products include:
Elavil ... 2269
Endep Tablets ... 1927
Etrafon ... 2087
Limbitrol ... 1933
Triavil Tablets ... 1556
Amoxapine (Additive sedative effects). Products include:
Asendin Tablets ... 1196
Aprobarbital (Additive sedative effects; reduce the dose of barbiturate by one-half). Products include:
Alurate Elixir ... 1883
Buprenorphine (Additive sedative effects).
No products indexed under this heading.
Buspirone Hydrochloride (Additive sedative effects). Products include:
BuSpar ... 1401
Butabarbital (Additive sedative effects; reduce the dose of barbiturate by one-half). Products include:
Pyridium Plus ... 1764
Butalbital (Additive sedative effects; reduce the dose of barbiturate by one-half). Products include:
Esgic-Plus Tablets ... 1002
Esgic Tablets & Capsules ... 1001
Fioricet Tablets ... 2006
Fiorinal Capsules ... 2007
Fiorinal with Codeine Capsules ... 2008
Fiorinal Tablets ... 2007
Phrenilin ... 838
Sedapap Tablets 50 mg/650 mg ... 1360
Chlordiazepoxide (Additive sedative effects). Products include:
Libritabs Tablets ... 1930
Limbitrol ... 1933
Menrium Tablets ... 1934
Chlordiazepoxide Hydrochloride (Additive sedative effects). Products include:
Librax Capsules ... 1929
Librium Capsules ... 1931
Librium Injectable ... 1932
Chlorpromazine (Additive sedative effects). Products include:
Thorazine ... 2234
Chlorprothixene (Additive sedative effects). Products include:
Taractan Tablets ... 1920
Chlorprothixene Hydrochloride (Additive sedative effects). Products include:
Taractan ... 1920
Clomipramine Hydrochloride (Additive sedative effects). Products include:
Anafranil Capsules ... 650
Clorazepate Dipotassium (Additive sedative effects). Products include:
Tranxene ... 556
Codeine (Additive sedative effects). Products include:
Calcidrine Syrup ... 506
Codeine Phosphate (Additive sedative effects). Products include:
Actifed with Codeine Cough Syrup ... 752
Cheracol Cough Syrup ... 1853
Codimal PH Syrup ... 846
Dimetane-DC Cough Syrup ... 1857
Empirin with Codeine Phosphate Nos. 2, 3 & 4 ... 764
Fiorinal with Codeine Capsules ... 2008
Isoclor Expectorant ... 982
Naldecon CX Adult Liquid ... ▣ 521
Novahistine DH ... 1342
Novahistine Expectorant ... 1343
Nucofed Capsules ... 2219
Nucofed Expectorant ... 2219
Nucofed Pediatric Expectorant ... 2220
Nucofed Syrup ... 2219
Phenaphen with Codeine Capsules ... 1865
Phenaphen-650 with Codeine Tablets ... 1866
Phenergan with Codeine ... 2497
Phenergan VC with Codeine ... 2501
Robitussin A-C Syrup ... 1875
Robitussin-DAC Syrup ... 1875
Ryna ... ▣ 741
Soma Compound w/Codeine Tablets ... 2390
Triaminic Expectorant w/Codeine ... 1996
Tussi-Organidin Liquid ... 2391
Tylenol with Codeine ... 1381
Codeine Polistirex (Additive sedative effects).
No products indexed under this heading.
Desipramine Hydrochloride (Additive sedative effects). Products include:
Norpramin Tablets ... 1340
Dezocine (Additive sedative effects).
Diazepam (Additive sedative effects). Products include:
Valium Injectable ... 1937
Valium Tablets ... 1939
Valrelease Capsules ... 1923
Doxepin Hydrochloride (Additive sedative effects). Products include:
Sinequan ... 1960
Droperidol (Additive sedative effects). Products include:
Inapsine Injection ... 1140
Innovar Injection ... 1141
Enflurane (Additive sedative effects). Products include:
Ethrane ... 599
Epinephrine (Potential for reversal of the vasopressor effect). Products include:
Ana-Kit Anaphylaxis Emergency Treatment Kit ... 1100
Bronkaid Mist ... ▣ 757
EpiPen ... 843
Marcaine Hydrochloride 0.5% with Epinephrine 1:200,000 (as bitartrate) ... 958
Marcaine Hydrochloride with Epinephrine 1:200,000 ... 2055
Primatene Mist ... 2420
Sus-Phrine Injection ... 1006
Xylocaine with Epinephrine Injections ... 637
Estazolam (Additive sedative effects). Products include:
ProSom Tablets ... 554
Ethchlorvynol (Additive sedative effects). Products include:
Placidyl Capsules ... 553

Ethinamate (Additive sedative effects).
No products indexed under this heading.

Fentanyl (Additive sedative effects). Products include:
Duragesic Transdermal System........ 1133

Fentanyl Citrate (Additive sedative effects). Products include:
Innovar Injection........ 1141
Sublimaze Injection........ 1146

Fluphenazine Decanoate (Additive sedative effects). Products include:
Prolixin Decanoate........ 1795

Fluphenazine Enanthate (Additive sedative effects). Products include:
Prolixin Enanthate........ 1796

Fluphenazine Hydrochloride (Additive sedative effects). Products include:
Prolixin Elixir........ 1793
Prolixin Injection........ 1791
Prolixin Oral Concentrate........ 1792
Prolixin Tablets........ 1793

Flurazepam Hydrochloride (Additive sedative effects). Products include:
Dalmane Capsules........ 1927

Glutethimide (Additive sedative effects).
No products indexed under this heading.

Haloperidol (Additive sedative effects). Products include:
Haldol Injection, Tablets and Concentrate........ 1373

Haloperidol Decanoate (Additive sedative effects). Products include:
Haldol Decanoate........ 1375

Hydrocodone Bitartrate (Additive sedative effects). Products include:
Anexsia 5/500 Tablets........ 2196
Anexsia 7.5/650 Tablets........ 2197
Azdone Tablets........ 844
Codiclear DH Syrup........ 845
Codimal DH Syrup........ 846
Damason-P........ 1356
Hycodan Syrup, Tablets........ 927
Hycomine Compound Tablets........ 929
Hycomine Syrup........ 927
Hycotuss Expectorant Syrup........ 930
Hydrocet Capsules........ 835
Lortab ASA Tablets........ 2414
Lortab........ 2412
Ru-Tuss with Hydrocodone........ 694
Triaminic Expectorant DH........ 1995
Vicodin Tablets........ 1187
Vicodin ES Tablets........ 1189
Zydone Capsules........ 941

Hydrocodone Polistirex (Additive sedative effects). Products include:
Tussionex Extended-Release Suspension........ 988

Hydroxyzine Hydrochloride (Additive sedative effects). Products include:
Atarax Tablets & Syrup........ 1941
Marax Tablets & DF Syrup........ 1954
Vistaril Intramuscular Solution........ 1970

Imipramine Hydrochloride (Additive sedative effects). Products include:
Tofranil Ampuls........ 1038
Tofranil Tablets........ 1039

Imipramine Pamoate (Additive sedative effects). Products include:
Tofranil-PM Capsules........ 1041

Isoflurane (Additive sedative effects). Products include:
Forane........ 600

Ketamine Hydrochloride (Additive sedative effects). Products include:
Ketalar........ 1726

Levorphanol Tartrate (Additive sedative effects). Products include:
Levo-Dromoran........ 1906

Lorazepam (Additive sedative effects). Products include:
Ativan Injection........ 2432
Ativan Tablets........ 2434

Loxapine Hydrochloride (Additive sedative effects). Products include:
Loxitane........ 1213

Loxapine Succinate (Additive sedative effects). Products include:
Loxitane Capsules........ 1213

Maprotiline Hydrochloride (Additive sedative effects). Products include:
Ludiomil Tablets........ 874

Meperidine Hydrochloride (Additive sedative effects; reduce meperidine dose by one-fourth to one-half). Products include:
Demerol........ 2047
Mepergan Injection........ 2479

Mephobarbital (Additive sedative effects; reduce the dose of barbiturate by one-half). Products include:
Mebaral Tablets........ 2061

Meprobamate (Additive sedative effects). Products include:
Deprol Tablets........ 2382
Equagesic Tablets........ 2451
Miltown Tablets........ 2386
PMB 200 and PMB 400........ 2504

Mesoridazine (Additive sedative effects). Products include:
Serentil........ 686

Methadone Hydrochloride (Additive sedative effects). Products include:
Dolophine Hydrochloride Ampoules & Vials........ 1260
Dolophine Hydrochloride Tablets........ 1261
Methadone Hydrochloride Diskets........ 1284
Methadone Hydrochloride Oral Solution & Tablets........ 1987

Methohexital Sodium (Additive sedative effects). Products include:
Brevital Sodium Vials........ 1248

Methoxyflurane (Additive sedative effects).
No products indexed under this heading.

Midazolam Hydrochloride (Additive sedative effects). Products include:
Versed Injection........ 1924

Molindone Hydrochloride (Additive sedative effects). Products include:
Moban Tablets & Concentrate........ 932

Morphine Sulfate (Additive sedative effects; reduce the dose of morphine by one-fourth to one-half). Products include:
Astramorph/PF Injection, USP (Preservative-Free)........ 618
Duramorph........ 960
Infumorph 200 and Infumorph 500 Sterile Solutions........ 962
MS Contin Tablets........ 1814
MSIR........ 1817
Oramorph SR (Morphine Sulfate Sustained Release Tablets)........ 1988
Roxanol........ 1991

Nortriptyline Hydrochloride (Additive sedative effects). Products include:
Pamelor........ 2019

Opium Alkaloids (Additive sedative effects). Products include:
B & O No. 15A & No. 16A Supprettes........ 2395
Pantopon Injectable........ 1911

Oxazepam (Additive sedative effects). Products include:
Serax Capsules........ 2522
Serax Tablets........ 2522

Oxycodone Hydrochloride (Additive sedative effects). Products include:
Percocet Tablets........ 950
Percodan........ 951
Roxicodone Tablets, Oral Solution & Intensol (Oxycodone)........ 1992
Tylox Capsules........ 1382

Pentobarbital Sodium (Additive sedative effects; reduce the dose of barbiturate by one-half). Products include:
Nembutal Sodium Capsules........ 534
Nembutal Sodium Solution........ 536
Nembutal Sodium Suppositories........ 538

Perphenazine (Additive sedative effects). Products include:
Etrafon........ 2087
Triavil Tablets........ 1556
Trilafon........ 2123

Phenobarbital (Additive sedative effects; reduce the dose of barbiturate by one-half). Products include:
Arco-Lase Plus Tablets........ 607
Bellergal-S Tablets........ 1998
Bronkolixir........ ▣ 761
Bronkotabs Tablets........ ▣ 762
Donnatal........ 1858
Donnatal Extentabs........ 1859
Donnatal Tablets........ 1858
Donnazyme Tablets........ 1860
Kinesed Tablets........ 2272
Phenobarbital Elixir and Tablets........ 1293
Primatene Tablets-P Formula........ 2421
Quadrinal Tablets........ 1183
Tedral SA........ 1765

Prazepam (Additive sedative effects). Products include:
Centrax........ 1693

Prochlorperazine (Additive sedative effects). Products include:
Compazine........ 2201

Propofol (Additive sedative effects). Products include:
Diprivan Injection........ 2267

Propoxyphene Hydrochloride (Additive sedative effects). Products include:
Darvon........ 1256
Wygesic Tablets........ 2540

Propoxyphene Napsylate (Additive sedative effects). Products include:
Darvon-N/Darvocet-N........ 1254

Protriptyline Hydrochloride (Additive sedative effects). Products include:
Vivactil Tablets........ 1567

Quazepam (Additive sedative effects). Products include:
Doral Tablets........ 2383

Secobarbital Sodium (Additive sedative effects; reduce the dose of barbiturate by one-half). Products include:
Seconal Sodium Pulvules........ 1296

Sufentanil Citrate (Additive sedative effects). Products include:
Sufenta Injection........ 1147

Temazepam (Additive sedative effects). Products include:
Restoril Capsules........ 2023

Thiamylal Sodium (Additive sedative effects; reduce the dose of barbiturate by one-half). Products include:
Surital Ampoules, Steri-Vials........ 1764

Thioridazine Hydrochloride (Additive sedative effects). Products include:
Mellaril........ 2011

Thiothixene (Additive sedative effects). Products include:
Navane Capsules and Concentrate........ 1954
Navane Intramuscular........ 1956

Triazolam (Additive sedative effects). Products include:
Halcion Tablets........ 2340

Trifluoperazine Hydrochloride (Additive sedative effects). Products include:
Stelazine........ 2226

Trimipramine Maleate (Additive sedative effects). Products include:
Surmontil Capsules........ 2524

PHENERGAN SYRUP FORTIS
(Promethazine Hydrochloride)........ 2495
May interact with narcotic analgesics, hypnotics and sedatives, tricyclic antidepressants, tranquilizers, and certain other agents. Compounds in these categories include:

Alcohol (Additive sedative effects).

Alfentanil Hydrochloride (Additive sedative effects). Products include:
Alfenta Injection........ 1131

Alprazolam (Additive sedative effects). Products include:
Xanax Tablets........ 2367

Amitriptyline Hydrochloride (Additive sedative effects). Products include:
Elavil........ 2269
Endep Tablets........ 1927
Etrafon........ 2087
Limbitrol........ 1933
Triavil Tablets........ 1556

Amoxapine (Additive sedative effects). Products include:
Asendin Tablets........ 1196

Buprenorphine (Additive sedative effects).
No products indexed under this heading.

Buspirone Hydrochloride (Additive sedative effects). Products include:
BuSpar........ 1401

Chlordiazepoxide (Additive sedative effects). Products include:
Libritabs Tablets........ 1930
Limbitrol........ 1933
Menrium Tablets........ 1934

Chlordiazepoxide Hydrochloride (Additive sedative effects). Products include:
Librax Capsules........ 1929
Librium Capsules........ 1931
Librium Injectable........ 1932

Chlorpromazine (Additive sedative effects). Products include:
Thorazine........ 2234

Chlorprothixene (Additive sedative effects). Products include:
Taractan Tablets........ 1920

Chlorprothixene Hydrochloride (Additive sedative effects). Products include:
Taractan........ 1920

Clomipramine Hydrochloride (Additive sedative effects). Products include:
Anafranil Capsules........ 650

Clorazepate Dipotassium (Additive sedative effects). Products include:
Tranxene........ 556

Codeine (Additive sedative effects). Products include:
Calcidrine Syrup........ 506

Codeine Phosphate (Additive sedative effects). Products include:
Actifed with Codeine Cough Syrup........ 752
Cheracol Cough Syrup........ 1853
Codimal PH Syrup........ 846
Dimetane-DC Cough Syrup........ 1857
Empirin with Codeine Phosphate Nos. 2, 3 & 4........ 764
Fiorinal with Codeine Capsules........ 2008
Isoclor Expectorant........ 982
Naldecon CX Adult Liquid........ ▣ 521
Novahistine DH........ 1342
Novahistine Expectorant........ 1343
Nucofed Capsules........ 2219

Nucofed Expectorant 2219
Nucofed Pediatric Expectorant 2220
Nucofed Syrup 2219
Phenaphen with Codeine Capsules 1865
Phenaphen-650 with Codeine Tablets 1866
Phenergan with Codeine 2497
Phenergan VC with Codeine 2501
Robitussin A-C Syrup 1875
Robitussin-DAC Syrup 1875
Ryna ▣ 741
Soma Compound w/Codeine Tablets 2390
Triaminic Expectorant w/Codeine 1996
Tussi-Organidin Liquid 2391
Tylenol with Codeine 1381

Codeine Polistirex (Additive sedative effects).
No products indexed under this heading.

Desipramine Hydrochloride (Additive sedative effects). Products include:
Norpramin Tablets 1340

Dezocine (Additive sedative effects).

Diazepam (Additive sedative effects). Products include:
Valium Injectable 1937
Valium Tablets 1939
Valrelease Capsules 1923

Doxepin Hydrochloride (Additive sedative effects). Products include:
Sinequan 1960

Droperidol (Additive sedative effects). Products include:
Inapsine Injection 1140
Innovar Injection 1141

Estazolam (Additive sedative effects). Products include:
ProSom Tablets 554

Ethchlorvynol (Additive sedative effects). Products include:
Placidyl Capsules 553

Ethinamate (Additive sedative effects).
No products indexed under this heading.

Fentanyl (Additive sedative effects). Products include:
Duragesic Transdermal System 1133

Fentanyl Citrate (Additive sedative effects). Products include:
Innovar Injection 1141
Sublimaze Injection 1146

Fluphenazine Decanoate (Additive sedative effects). Products include:
Prolixin Decanoate 1795

Fluphenazine Enanthate (Additive sedative effects). Products include:
Prolixin Enanthate 1796

Fluphenazine Hydrochloride (Additive sedative effects). Products include:
Prolixin Elixir 1793
Prolixin Injection 1791
Prolixin Oral Concentrate 1792
Prolixin Tablets 1793

Flurazepam Hydrochloride (Additive sedative effects). Products include:
Dalmane Capsules 1927

Glutethimide (Additive sedative effects).
No products indexed under this heading.

Haloperidol (Additive sedative effects). Products include:
Haldol Injection, Tablets and Concentrate 1373

Haloperidol Decanoate (Additive sedative effects). Products include:
Haldol Decanoate 1375

Hydrocodone Bitartrate (Additive sedative effects). Products include:
Anexsia 5/500 Tablets 2196
Anexsia 7.5/650 Tablets 2197
Azdone Tablets 844
Codiclear DH Syrup 845
Codimal DH Syrup 846
Damason-P 1356
Hycodan Syrup, Tablets 927
Hycomine Compound Tablets 929
Hycomine Syrup 927
Hycotuss Expectorant Syrup 930
Hydrocet Capsules 835
Lortab ASA Tablets 2414
Lortab 2412
Ru-Tuss with Hydrocodone 694
Triaminic Expectorant DH 1995
Vicodin Tablets 1187
Vicodin ES Tablets 1189
Zydone Capsules 941

Hydrocodone Polistirex (Additive sedative effects). Products include:
Tussionex Extended-Release Suspension 988

Hydroxyzine Hydrochloride (Additive sedative effects). Products include:
Atarax Tablets & Syrup 1941
Marax Tablets & DF Syrup 1954
Vistaril Intramuscular Solution 1970

Imipramine Hydrochloride (Additive sedative effects). Products include:
Tofranil Ampuls 1038
Tofranil Tablets 1039

Imipramine Pamoate (Additive sedative effects). Products include:
Tofranil-PM Capsules 1041

Levorphanol Tartrate (Additive sedative effects). Products include:
Levo-Dromoran 1906

Lorazepam (Additive sedative effects). Products include:
Ativan Injection 2432
Ativan Tablets 2434

Loxapine Hydrochloride (Additive sedative effects). Products include:
Loxitane 1213

Loxapine Succinate (Additive sedative effects). Products include:
Loxitane Capsules 1213

Maprotiline Hydrochloride (Additive sedative effects). Products include:
Ludiomil Tablets 874

Meperidine Hydrochloride (Additive sedative effects). Products include:
Demerol 2047
Mepergan Injection 2479

Meprobamate (Additive sedative effects). Products include:
Deprol Tablets 2382
Equagesic Tablets 2451
Miltown Tablets 2386
PMB 200 and PMB 400 2504

Mesoridazine (Additive sedative effects). Products include:
Serentil 686

Methadone Hydrochloride (Additive sedative effects). Products include:
Dolophine Hydrochloride Ampoules & Vials 1260
Dolophine Hydrochloride Tablets 1261
Methadone Hydrochloride Diskets 1284
Methadone Hydrochloride Oral Solution & Tablets 1987

Midazolam Hydrochloride (Additive sedative effects). Products include:
Versed Injection 1924

Molindone Hydrochloride (Additive sedative effects). Products include:
Moban Tablets & Concentrate 932

Morphine Sulfate (Additive sedative effects). Products include:
Astramorph/PF Injection, USP (Preservative-Free) 618
Duramorph 960
Infumorph 200 and Infumorph 500 Sterile Solutions 962
MS Contin Tablets 1814
MSIR 1817
Oramorph SR (Morphine Sulfate Sustained Release Tablets) 1988
Roxanol 1991

Nortriptyline Hydrochloride (Additive sedative effects). Products include:
Pamelor 2019

Opium Alkaloids (Additive sedative effects). Products include:
B & O No. 15A & No. 16A Supprettes 2395
Pantopon Injectable 1911

Oxazepam (Additive sedative effects). Products include:
Serax Capsules 2522
Serax Tablets 2522

Oxycodone Hydrochloride (Additive sedative effects). Products include:
Percocet Tablets 950
Percodan 951
Roxicodone Tablets, Oral Solution & Intensol (Oxycodone) 1992
Tylox Capsules 1382

Perphenazine (Additive sedative effects). Products include:
Etrafon 2087
Triavil Tablets 1556
Trilafon 2123

Prazepam (Additive sedative effects). Products include:
Centrax 1693

Prochlorperazine (Additive sedative effects). Products include:
Compazine 2201

Propofol (Additive sedative effects). Products include:
Diprivan Injection 2267

Propoxyphene Hydrochloride (Additive sedative effects). Products include:
Darvon 1256
Wygesic Tablets 2540

Propoxyphene Napsylate (Additive sedative effects). Products include:
Darvon-N/Darvocet-N 1254

Protriptyline Hydrochloride (Additive sedative effects). Products include:
Vivactil Tablets 1567

Quazepam (Additive sedative effects). Products include:
Doral Tablets 2383

Secobarbital Sodium (Additive sedative effects). Products include:
Seconal Sodium Pulvules 1296

Sufentanil Citrate (Additive sedative effects). Products include:
Sufenta Injection 1147

Temazepam (Additive sedative effects). Products include:
Restoril Capsules 2023

Thioridazine Hydrochloride (Additive sedative effects). Products include:
Mellaril 2011

Thiothixene (Additive sedative effects). Products include:
Navane Capsules and Concentrate 1954
Navane Intramuscular 1956

Triazolam (Additive sedative effects). Products include:
Halcion Tablets 2340

Trifluoperazine Hydrochloride (Additive sedative effects). Products include:
Stelazine 2226

Trimipramine Maleate (Additive sedative effects). Products include:
Surmontil Capsules 2524

PHENERGAN SYRUP PLAIN
(Promethazine Hydrochloride) 2495
See **Phenergan Syrup Fortis**

PHENERGAN TABLETS
(Promethazine Hydrochloride) 2496
See **Phenergan Suppositories**

PHENERGAN VC
(Promethazine Hydrochloride, Phenylephrine Hydrochloride) 2500
May interact with narcotic analgesics, hypnotics and sedatives, tricyclic antidepressants, tranquilizers, monoamine oxidase inhibitors, sympathomimetic aerosol bronchodilators, sympathomimetic bronchodilators, beta blockers, alpha adrenergic blockers, and certain other agents. Compounds in these categories include:

Acebutolol Hydrochloride (Cardiostimulating effects blocked). Products include:
Sectral Capsules 2520

Albuterol (Tachycardia or arrhythmias may occur). Products include:
Proventil Inhalation Aerosol 2117
Ventolin Inhalation Aerosol and Refill 583

Albuterol Sulfate (Tachycardia or arrhythmias may occur). Products include:
Proventil Repetabs Tablets 2120
Proventil Solutions for Inhalation 0.5% and 0.083% 2118
Proventil Syrup 2119
Proventil Tablets 2120
Ventolin 583

Alcohol (Additive sedative effects).

Alfentanil Hydrochloride (Additive sedative effects). Products include:
Alfenta Injection 1131

Alprazolam (Additive sedative effects). Products include:
Xanax Tablets 2367

Amitriptyline Hydrochloride (Additive sedative effects; increased pressor response). Products include:
Elavil 2269
Endep Tablets 1927
Etrafon 2087
Limbitrol 1933
Triavil Tablets 1556

Amoxapine (Additive sedative effects; increased pressor response). Products include:
Asendin Tablets 1196

Amphetamine Aspartate (Synergistic adrenergic response).
No products indexed under this heading.

Amphetamine Resins (Synergistic adrenergic response). Products include:
Biphetamine Capsules 973

Amphetamine Sulfate (Synergistic adrenergic response).
No products indexed under this heading.

Atenolol (Cardiostimulating effects blocked). Products include:
Tenoretic Tablets 1105
Tenormin Tablets and I.V. Injection 1107

Atropine Sulfate (Enhanced pressor response; reflex bradycardia blocked). Products include:
Arco-Lase Plus Tablets 607
Atropine Sulfate Sterile Ophthalmic Solution and S.O.P. Sterile Ophthalmic Ointment ⊙ 239
Donnagel ▣ 675
Donnagel-PG 1858
Donnatal 1858
Donnatal Extentabs 1859
Donnatal Tablets 1858
Donnazyme Tablets 1860
Isopto Atropine ⊙ 218
Lomotil 2174
Motofen Tablets 836
Ru-Tuss Tablets 693
Urised Tablets 2396

Betaxolol Hydrochloride (Cardiostimulating effects blocked). Products include:
- Betoptic Sterile Ophthalmic Solution ... 569
- Betoptic S Sterile Ophthalmic Suspension ... 570
- Kerlone Tablets ... 2172

Bitolterol Mesylate (Tachycardia or arrhythmias may occur). Products include:
- Tornalate ... 2074

Buprenorphine (Additive sedative effects).
- No products indexed under this heading.

Buspirone Hydrochloride (Additive sedative effects). Products include:
- BuSpar ... 1401

Carteolol Hydrochloride (Cardiostimulating effects blocked). Products include:
- Cartrol Tablets ... 507

Chlordiazepoxide (Additive sedative effects). Products include:
- Libritabs Tablets ... 1930
- Limbitrol ... 1933
- Menrium Tablets ... 1934

Chlordiazepoxide Hydrochloride (Additive sedative effects). Products include:
- Librax Capsules ... 1929
- Librium Capsules ... 1931
- Librium Injectable ... 1932

Chlorpromazine (Additive sedative effects). Products include:
- Thorazine ... 2234

Chlorprothixene (Additive sedative effects). Products include:
- Taractan Tablets ... 1920

Chlorprothixene Hydrochloride (Additive sedative effects). Products include:
- Taractan ... 1920

Clomipramine Hydrochloride (Additive sedative effects; increased pressor response). Products include:
- Anafranil Capsules ... 650

Clorazepate Dipotassium (Additive sedative effects). Products include:
- Tranxene ... 556

Codeine (Additive sedative effects). Products include:
- Calcidrine Syrup ... 506

Codeine Phosphate (Additive sedative effects). Products include:
- Actifed with Codeine Cough Syrup.. 752
- Cheracol Cough Syrup ... 1853
- Codimal PH Syrup ... 846
- Dimetane-DC Cough Syrup ... 1857
- Empirin with Codeine Phosphate Nos. 2, 3 & 4 ... 764
- Fiorinal with Codeine Capsules ... 2008
- Isoclor Expectorant ... 982
- Naldecon CX Adult Liquid ... ⊞ 521
- Novahistine DH ... 1342
- Novahistine Expectorant ... 1343
- Nucofed Capsules ... 2219
- Nucofed Expectorant ... 2219
- Nucofed Pediatric Expectorant ... 2220
- Nucofed Syrup ... 2219
- Phenaphen with Codeine Capsules 1865
- Phenaphen-650 with Codeine Tablets ... 1866
- Phenergan with Codeine ... 2497
- Phenergan VC with Codeine ... 2501
- Robitussin A-C Syrup ... 1875
- Robitussin-DAC Syrup ... 1875
- Ryna ... ⊞ 741
- Soma Compound w/Codeine Tablets ... 2390
- Triaminic Expectorant w/Codeine .. 1996
- Tussi-Organidin Liquid ... 2391
- Tylenol with Codeine ... 1381

Codeine Polistirex (Additive sedative effects).
- No products indexed under this heading.

Desipramine Hydrochloride (Additive sedative effects; increased pressor response). Products include:
- Norpramin Tablets ... 1340

Dezocine (Additive sedative effects).

Diazepam (Additive sedative effects). Products include:
- Valium Injectable ... 1937
- Valium Tablets ... 1939
- Valrelease Capsules ... 1923

Dobutamine Hydrochloride (Tachycardia or arrhythmias may occur). Products include:
- Dobutrex Solution Vials ... 1259

Dopamine Hydrochloride (Tachycardia or arrhythmias may occur). Products include:
- Intropin Injection ... 930

Doxazosin Mesylate (Decreased pressor response). Products include:
- Cardura Tablets ... 1941

Doxepin Hydrochloride (Additive sedative effects; increased pressor response). Products include:
- Sinequan ... 1960

Droperidol (Additive sedative effects). Products include:
- Inapsine Injection ... 1140
- Innovar Injection ... 1141

Ephedrine Hydrochloride (Tachycardia or arrhythmias may occur). Products include:
- Amesec ... ⊞ 682
- Primatene Tablets-M Formula ... 2421
- Primatene Tablets-P Formula ... 2421
- Primatene Tablets-Regular Formula ... 2421
- Quadrinal Tablets ... 1183
- Quelidrine Syrup ... 556
- Tedral SA ... 1765

Ephedrine Sulfate (Tachycardia or arrhythmias may occur). Products include:
- Bronkaid Tablets ... ⊞ 757
- Bronkolixir ... ⊞ 761
- Bronkotabs Tablets ... ⊞ 762
- Marax Tablets & DF Syrup ... 1954
- Pazo Hemorrhoid Ointment & Suppositories ... 752
- Vicks Vatronol Nose Drops ... ⊞ 666

Ephedrine Tannate (Tachycardia or arrhythmias may occur). Products include:
- Rynatuss ... 2388

Epinephrine (Tachycardia or arrhythmias may occur). Products include:
- Ana-Kit Anaphylaxis Emergency Treatment Kit ... 1100
- Bronkaid Mist ... ⊞ 757
- EpiPen ... 843
- Marcaine Hydrochloride 0.5% with Epinephrine 1:200,000 (as bitartrate) ... 958
- Marcaine Hydrochloride with Epinephrine 1:200,000 ... 2055
- Primatene Mist ... 2420
- Sus-Phrine Injection ... 1006
- Xylocaine with Epinephrine Injections ... 637

Epinephrine Bitartrate (Tachycardia or arrhythmias may occur). Products include:
- AsthmaHaler Mist Epinephrine Bitartrate Bronchodilator ... ⊞ 616
- Bronkaid Mist Suspension ... ⊞ 757
- Primatene Mist Suspension ... 2421

Epinephrine Hydrochloride (Tachycardia or arrhythmias may occur). Products include:
- Adrenalin Chloride Solution 1:100 & 1:1,000 ... 1689
- Epifrin ... ⊙ 244
- Glaucon ... ⊙ 218

Ergot Alkaloids (Hydrogenated) (Excessive rise in blood pressure).

Ergotamine Tartrate (Excessive rise in blood pressure). Products include:
- Bellergal-S Tablets ... 1998
- Cafergot/Cafergot P-B ... 1999
- Ergostat ... 1719
- Medihaler Ergotamine Aerosol ... 1312
- Wigraine Tablets & Suppositories .. 1645

Esmolol Hydrochloride (Cardiostimulating effects blocked). Products include:
- Brevibloc Injection ... 942

Estazolam (Additive sedative effects). Products include:
- ProSom Tablets ... 554

Ethchlorvynol (Additive sedative effects). Products include:
- Placidyl Capsules ... 553

Ethinamate (Additive sedative effects).
- No products indexed under this heading.

Ethylnorepinephrine Hydrochloride (Tachycardia or arrhythmias may occur). Products include:
- Bronkephrine Injection ... 2042

Fentanyl (Additive sedative effects). Products include:
- Duragesic Transdermal System ... 1133

Fentanyl Citrate (Additive sedative effects). Products include:
- Innovar Injection ... 1141
- Sublimaze Injection ... 1146

Fluphenazine Decanoate (Additive sedative effects). Products include:
- Prolixin Decanoate ... 1795

Fluphenazine Enanthate (Additive sedative effects). Products include:
- Prolixin Enanthate ... 1796

Fluphenazine Hydrochloride (Additive sedative effects). Products include:
- Prolixin Elixir ... 1793
- Prolixin Injection ... 1791
- Prolixin Oral Concentrate ... 1792
- Prolixin Tablets ... 1793

Flurazepam Hydrochloride (Additive sedative effects). Products include:
- Dalmane Capsules ... 1927

Furazolidone (Acute hypertensive crisis; concurrent use is contraindicated). Products include:
- Furoxone ... 1855

Glutethimide (Additive sedative effects).
- No products indexed under this heading.

Haloperidol (Additive sedative effects). Products include:
- Haldol Injection, Tablets and Concentrate ... 1373

Haloperidol Decanoate (Additive sedative effects). Products include:
- Haldol Decanoate ... 1375

Hydrocodone Bitartrate (Additive sedative effects). Products include:
- Anexsia 5/500 Tablets ... 2196
- Anexsia 7.5/650 Tablets ... 2197
- Azdone Tablets ... 844
- Codiclear DH Syrup ... 845
- Codimal DH Syrup ... 846
- Damason-P ... 1356
- Hycodan Syrup, Tablets ... 927
- Hycomine Compound Tablets ... 929
- Hycomine Syrup ... 927
- Hycotuss Expectorant Syrup ... 930
- Hydrocet Capsules ... 835
- Lortab ASA Tablets ... 2414
- Lortab ... 2412
- Ru-Tuss with Hydrocodone ... 694
- Triaminic Expectorant DH ... 1995
- Vicodin Tablets ... 1187
- Vicodin ES Tablets ... 1189
- Zydone Capsules ... 941

Hydrocodone Polistirex (Additive sedative effects). Products include:
- Tussionex Extended-Release Suspension ... 988

Hydroxyzine Hydrochloride (Additive sedative effects). Products include:
- Atarax Tablets & Syrup ... 1941
- Marax Tablets & DF Syrup ... 1954
- Vistaril Intramuscular Solution ... 1970

Imipramine Hydrochloride (Additive sedative effects; increased pressor response). Products include:
- Tofranil Ampuls ... 1038
- Tofranil Tablets ... 1039

Imipramine Pamoate (Additive sedative effects; increased pressor response). Products include:
- Tofranil-PM Capsules ... 1041

Isocarboxazid (Acute hypertensive crisis; concurrent use is contraindicated). Products include:
- Marplan Tablets ... 1906

Isoetharine (Tachycardia or arrhythmias may occur). Products include:
- Arm-a-Med Isoetharine Inhalation Solution, USP ... 616
- Bronkometer Aerosol ... 2042
- Bronkosol Solution ... 2042

Isoproterenol Hydrochloride (Tachycardia or arrhythmias may occur). Products include:
- Isuprel Hydrochloride Injection 1:5000 ... 2050
- Isuprel Hydrochloride Mistometer .. 2051
- Isuprel Hydrochloride Solution 1:200 & 1:100 ... 2052
- Norisodrine Aerotrol ... 540

Labetalol Hydrochloride (Cardiostimulating effects blocked). Products include:
- Normodyne Injection ... 2108
- Normodyne Tablets ... 2110
- Normozide Tablets ... 2112
- Trandate HCT Tablets ... 579
- Trandate Injection ... 577
- Trandate Tablets ... 579

Levorphanol Tartrate (Additive sedative effects). Products include:
- Levo-Dromoran ... 1906

Lorazepam (Additive sedative effects). Products include:
- Ativan Injection ... 2432
- Ativan Tablets ... 2434

Loxapine Hydrochloride (Additive sedative effects). Products include:
- Loxitane ... 1213

Maprotiline Hydrochloride (Additive sedative effects; increased pressor response). Products include:
- Ludiomil Tablets ... 874

Meperidine Hydrochloride (Additive sedative effects). Products include:
- Demerol ... 2047
- Mepergan Injection ... 2479

Meprobamate (Additive sedative effects). Products include:
- Deprol Tablets ... 2382
- Equagesic Tablets ... 2451
- Miltown Tablets ... 2386
- PMB 200 and PMB 400 ... 2504

Mesoridazine (Additive sedative effects). Products include:
- Serentil ... 686

Metaproterenol Sulfate (Tachycardia or arrhythmias may occur). Products include:
- Alupent ... 674
- Arm-a-Med Metaproterenol Sulfate Inhalation Solution, USP ... 617
- Metaprel Inhalation Aerosol Bronchodilator ... 2014
- Metaprel Inhalation Solution ... 2015
- Metaprel ... 2015
- Metaproterenol Sulfate Inhalation Solution, USP ... 912

Metaraminol Bitartrate (Tachycardia or arrhythmias may occur). Products include:
Aramine Injection 1424

Methadone Hydrochloride (Additive sedative effects). Products include:
Dolophine Hydrochloride Ampoules & Vials 1260
Dolophine Hydrochloride Tablets 1261
Methadone Hydrochloride Diskets 1284
Methadone Hydrochloride Oral Solution & Tablets 1987

Methoxamine Hydrochloride (Tachycardia or arrhythmias may occur). Products include:
Vasoxyl Injection 819

Metoprolol Tartrate (Cardiostimulating effects blocked). Products include:
Lopressor Ampuls 1032
Lopressor HCT Tablets 1034
Lopressor Tablets 1032

Midazolam Hydrochloride (Additive sedative effects). Products include:
Versed Injection 1924

Molindone Hydrochloride (Additive sedative effects). Products include:
Moban Tablets & Concentrate 932

Morphine Sulfate (Additive sedative effects). Products include:
Astramorph/PF Injection, USP (Preservative-Free) 618
Duramorph 960
Infumorph 200 and Infumorph 500 Sterile Solutions 962
MS Contin Tablets 1814
MSIR 1817
Oramorph SR (Morphine Sulfate Sustained Release Tablets) 1988
Roxanol 1991

Nadolol (Cardiostimulating effects blocked). Products include:
Corgard Tablets 701
Corzide Tablets 702

Norepinephrine Bitartrate (Tachycardia or arrhythmias may occur). Products include:
Levophed Bitartrate Injection 2054

Nortriptyline Hydrochloride (Additive sedative effects; increased pressor response). Products include:
Pamelor 2019

Opium Alkaloids (Additive sedative effects). Products include:
B & O No. 15A & No. 16A Supprettes 2395
Pantopon Injectable 1911

Oxazepam (Additive sedative effects). Products include:
Serax Capsules 2522
Serax Tablets 2522

Oxycodone Hydrochloride (Additive sedative effects). Products include:
Percocet Tablets 950
Percodan 951
Roxicodone Tablets, Oral Solution & Intensol (Oxycodone) 1992
Tylox Capsules 1382

Penbutolol Sulfate (Cardiostimulating effects blocked). Products include:
Levatol 1832

Perphenazine (Additive sedative effects). Products include:
Etrafon 2087
Triavil Tablets 1556
Trilafon 2123

Phenelzine Sulfate (Acute hypertensive crisis; concurrent use is contraindicated). Products include:
Nardil 1742

Phentolamine Mesylate (Decreased pressor response). Products include:
Regitine 878

Phenylephrine Bitartrate (Tachycardia or arrhythmias may occur).
No products indexed under this heading.

Phenylephrine Tannate (Tachycardia or arrhythmias may occur). Products include:
Rynatan 2387
Rynatuss 2388

Phenylpropanolamine Hydrochloride (Tachycardia or arrhythmias may occur). Products include:
A.R.M. Allergy Relief Medicine Caplets ▣ 615
Acutrim ▣ 548
Allerest ▣ 559
BC Cold Powder ▣ 517
Cheracol Plus Head Cold/Cough Formula ▣ 667
Codimal Expectorant 846
Comtrex Multi-Symptom Cold Reliever Tablets/Caplets/Liqui-Gels/Liquid 745
Contac Continuous Action Decongestant/Antihistamine Capsules ▣ 710
Contac Maximum Strength Continuous Action Decongestant/Antihistamine Caplets ▣ 709
Contac Severe Cold and Flu Formula Caplets ▣ 711
Coricidin 'D' Decongestant Tablets ▣ 695
Coricidin Demilets Tablets for Children ▣ 696
Demazin Nasal Decongestant/Antihistamine Repetabs Tablets & Syrup ▣ 697
Dexatrim ▣ 733
Dimetane-DC Cough Syrup 1857
Dimetapp Elixir ▣ 673
Dimetapp DM Elixir ▣ 674
Dimetapp Extentabs ▣ 674
Dimetapp Plus Caplets ▣ 675
Dimetapp Tablets ▣ 675
Entex Capsules 1623
Entex LA Tablets 1623
Entex Liquid 1623
4-Way Cold Tablets 750
Hycomine Syrup 927
Naldecon CX Adult Liquid ▣ 521
Naldecon DX Adult Liquid ▣ 521
Naldecon DX Children's Syrup ▣ 522
Naldecon DX Pediatric Drops ▣ 522
Naldecon EX Children's Syrup ▣ 522
Naldecon EX Pediatric Drops ▣ 523
Naldecon Syrup, Tablets, Pediatric Drops and Pediatric Syrup 709
Nolamine Tablets 838
Nolex LA Tablets 838
Ornade Spansule Capsules 2221
Orthoxicol Cough Syrup ▣ 668
Propagest 839
Pyrroxate Capsules ▣ 669
Robitussin-CF ▣ 676
Ru-Tuss II Capsules 693
Ru-Tuss with Hydrocodone 694
Ru-Tuss Tablets 693
Sine-Off Sinus Medicine Tablets-Aspirin Formula ▣ 722
Sinulin 840
St. Joseph Cold Tablets for Children ▣ 704
Tavist-D Tablets 2035
Triaminic Allergy Tablets ▣ 688
Triaminic Chewables ▣ 688
Triaminic Cold Tablets ▣ 688
Triaminic Expectorant ▣ 688
Triaminic Expectorant w/Codeine 1996
Triaminic Expectorant DH 1995
Triaminic Oral Infant Drops 1996
Triaminic Syrup ▣ 689
Triaminic-12 Tablets ▣ 690
Triaminic-DM Syrup ▣ 689
Triaminicin Tablets ▣ 690
Triaminicol Multi-Symptom Cold Tablets ▣ 691
Triaminicol Multi-Symptom Relief ▣ 691
Tuss-Ornade Liquid 2242
Tuss-Ornade Spansule Capsules 2242
Tylenol Cold Medication, Effervescent Tablets 1369

Pindolol (Cardiostimulating effects blocked). Products include:
Visken Tablets 2036

Pirbuterol Acetate (Tachycardia or arrhythmias may occur). Products include:
Maxair Inhaler 1311

Prazepam (Additive sedative effects). Products include:
Centrax 1693

Prazosin Hydrochloride (Decreased pressor response). Products include:
Minipress Capsules 1778
Minizide Capsules 1779

Prochlorperazine (Additive sedative effects). Products include:
Compazine 2201

Propofol (Additive sedative effects). Products include:
Diprivan Injection 2267

Propoxyphene Hydrochloride (Additive sedative effects). Products include:
Darvon 1256
Wygesic Tablets 2540

Propoxyphene Napsylate (Additive sedative effects). Products include:
Darvon-N/Darvocet-N 1254

Propranolol Hydrochloride (Cardiostimulating effects blocked). Products include:
Inderal 2459
Inderal LA Long Acting Capsules 2461
Inderide Tablets 2463
Inderide LA Long Acting Capsules 2465

Protriptyline Hydrochloride (Additive sedative effects; increased pressor response). Products include:
Vivactil Tablets 1567

Pseudoephedrine Hydrochloride (Tachycardia or arrhythmias may occur). Products include:
Actifed Capsules ▣ 539
Actifed Plus Caplets ▣ 539
Actifed Plus Tablets ▣ 540
Actifed with Codeine Cough Syrup 752
Actifed Syrup ▣ 540
Actifed Tablets ▣ 540
Actifed 12-Hour Capsules ▣ 539
Advil Cold & Sinus Caplets (formerly CoAdvil) 2416
Allerest ▣ 559
Anatuss LA Tablets 1359
Benadryl Decongestant Elixir ▣ 635
Benadryl Decongestant ▣ 635
Benadryl Plus ▣ 636
Benadryl Plus Nighttime ▣ 637
Benylin Decongestant ▣ 638
Brexin L.A. Capsules 2078
Bromfed Capsules (Timed Release) 1615
Bromfed Syrup ▣ 628
Bromfed 1615
CoAdvil ▣ 748
Allergy-Sinus Comtrex Multi-Symptom Allergy Sinus Formula Tablets & Caplets 746
Cough Formula Comtrex 746
Comtrex Multi-Symptom Cold Reliever Tablets/Caplets/Liqui-Gels/Liquid 745
Day-Night Comtrex 747
Non-Drowsy Comtrex 747
Congess 994
Congestac Caplets ▣ 617
Contac Jr. Children's Cold Medicine ▣ 712
Contac Nighttime Cold Medicine ▣ 713
Contac Sinus Caplets Maximum Strength Non-Drowsy Formula ▣ 710
Contac Sinus Tablets Maximum Strength Non-Drowsy Formula ▣ 710
Deconamine 663
Deconsal II Tablets 559
Dimacol Caplets ▣ 672
Dimetane-DX Cough Syrup 1858
Dorcol Children's Cough Syrup ▣ 685
Dorcol Children's Decongestant Liquid ▣ 685
Dorcol Children's Liquid Cold Formula ▣ 686
Maximum Strength Dristan Decongestant/Analgesic Coated Caplets ▣ 750
No Drowsiness Dristan Cold Nasal Decongestant/Analgesic Coated Caplets 2420
Dristan Sinus Caplets 2419
Sinus Excedrin Analgesic, Decongestant Tablets & Caplets ▣ 533
Fedahist Gyrocaps 2145
Fedahist Timecaps 2145
Guaifed 1615
Guaifed Syrup ▣ 629
Isoclor Expectorant 982
Isoclor Timesule Capsules ▣ 561
Kronofed-A 970
Medi-Flu Caplet, Liquid ▣ 640
Novafed A Capsules 1342
Novafed Capsules 1342
Novahistine DH 1342
Novahistine DMX ▣ 595
Novahistine Expectorant 1343
Nucofed Capsules 2219
Nucofed Expectorant 2219
Nucofed Pediatric Expectorant 2220
Nucofed Syrup 2219
Ornex Caplets ▣ 618
PediaCare Allergy Relief Formula Liquid 1362
PediaCare Cough-Cold Formula Liquid 1362
PediaCare Infants' Oral Decongestant Drops 1362
PediaCare Night Rest Cough-Cold Formula Liquid 1362
PediaCare 6-12 Cough-Cold Formula Chewable Tablets 1362
Robitussin-DAC Syrup 1875
Robitussin-PE ▣ 677
Rondec 1975
Rondec-DM 1976
Rondec-TR Tablet 1975
Ru-Tuss DE Tablets 694
Ryna ▣ 741
Seldane-D Extended-Release Tablets 1350
Sinarest ▣ 562
Sine-Aid Maximum Strength Sinus Headache Caplets 1365
Sine-Aid Maximum Strength Sinus Headache Tablets 1365
Sine-Off Maximum Strength Allergy/Sinus Formula Caplets ▣ 721
Sine-Off Maximum Strength No Drowsiness Formula Caplets ▣ 722
Singlet Tablets ▣ 598
Sinutab Maximum Strength ▣ 641
Sinutab Maximum Strength Without Drowsiness Tablets & Caplets ▣ 642
Sinutab Regular Strength Without Drowsiness Formula ▣ 641
St. Joseph Nighttime Cold Medicine ▣ 705
Sudafed Children's Liquid ▣ 543
Sudafed Cough Syrup ▣ 543
Sudafed Plus Liquid ▣ 544
Sudafed Plus Tablets ▣ 545
Sudafed Sinus Caplets ▣ 545
Sudafed Sinus Tablets ▣ 545
Sudafed Tablets, 30 mg ▣ 544
Sudafed Tablets, Adult Strength, 60 mg ▣ 544
Sudafed 12 Hour Capsules ▣ 545
TheraFlu Flu and Cold Medicine ▣ 687
Triaminic Nite Light ▣ 689
Tylenol Allergy Sinus Medication Caplets and Gelcaps, Maximum Strength 1372
Children's Tylenol Cold Liquid Formula and Chewable Tablets 1368
Tylenol Cold & Flu Hot Medication, Packets 1369
Tylenol Cold & Flu No Drowsiness Hot Medication, Packets 1371
Tylenol Cold Medication Caplets and Tablets 1370
Tylenol Cold Medication No Drowsiness Formula Caplets 1370
Tylenol Cold Night Time Medication Liquid 1371
Tylenol Cough Medication Liquid with Decongestant, Maximum Strength 1372
Tylenol, Maximum Strength, Sinus Medication Gelcaps, Caplets and Tablets 1373
Ursinus Inlay-Tabs ▣ 691
Vicks Children's NyQuil ▣ 664
Vicks Daycare ▣ 660
Vicks Formula 44D Decongestant Cough Medicine ▣ 662
Vicks Formula 44M Multi-Symptom Cough Medicine ▣ 662
Vicks NyQuil Nighttime Colds Medicine-Original & Cherry Flavor ▣ 664
Vicks Pediatric Formula 44 Cough & Congestion Medicine ▣ 663

Vicks Pediatric Formula 44m Multi-Symptom Cough & Cold Medicine ⊞ 663

Pseudoephedrine Sulfate (Tachycardia or arrhythmias may occur). Products include:
Afrin Tablets ⊞ 693
Chlor-Trimeton Decongestant ⊞ 694
Disophrol Chronotab Sustained-Action Tablets ⊞ 698
Drixoral Antihistamine/Nasal Decongestant Syrup ⊞ 698
Drixoral Non-Drowsy Formula ⊞ 699
Drixoral Plus Extended-Release Tablets ⊞ 699
Drixoral Sinus ⊞ 700
Drixoral Sustained-Action Tablets ⊞ 698
Sinutab Allergy Formula Sustained Action Tablets ⊞ 640
Trinalin Repetabs Tablets 1170

Quazepam (Additive sedative effects). Products include:
Doral Tablets 2383

Secobarbital Sodium (Additive sedative effects). Products include:
Seconal Sodium Pulvules 1296

Selegiline Hydrochloride (Acute hypertensive crisis; concurrent use is contraindicated). Products include:
Eldepryl 2250

Sufentanil Citrate (Additive sedative effects). Products include:
Sufenta Injection 1147

Temazepam (Additive sedative effects). Products include:
Restoril Capsules 2023

Terazosin Hydrochloride (Decreased pressor response). Products include:
Hytrin Tablets 529

Terbutaline Sulfate (Tachycardia or arrhythmias may occur). Products include:
Brethaire Inhaler 1024
Brethine Ampuls 1026
Brethine Tablets 1026
Bricanyl Injection 1324
Bricanyl Tablets 1325

Thioridazine Hydrochloride (Additive sedative effects). Products include:
Mellaril 2011

Thiothixene (Additive sedative effects). Products include:
Navane Capsules and Concentrate 1954
Navane Intramuscular 1956

Timolol Maleate (Cardiostimulating effects blocked). Products include:
Blocadren Tablets 1429
Timolide Tablets 1547
Timoptic in Ocudose 1552
Timoptic Sterile Ophthalmic Solution 1550

Tranylcypromine Sulfate (Acute hypertensive crisis; concurrent use is contraindicated). Products include:
Parnate Tablets 2222

Triazolam (Additive sedative effects). Products include:
Halcion Tablets 2340

Trifluoperazine Hydrochloride (Additive sedative effects). Products include:
Stelazine 2226

Trimipramine Maleate (Additive sedative effects; increased pressor response). Products include:
Surmontil Capsules 2524

PHENERGAN VC WITH CODEINE
(Codeine Phosphate, Promethazine Hydrochloride, Phenylephrine Hydrochloride) 2501
May interact with narcotic analgesics, hypnotics and sedatives, tricyclic antidepressants, tranquilizers, monoamine oxidase inhibitors, sympathomimetic aerosol bronchodilators, sympathomimetic bronchodilators, beta blockers, alpha adrenergic blockers, and certain other agents. Compounds in these categories include:

Acebutolol Hydrochloride (Cardiostimulating effects blocked). Products include:
Sectral Capsules 2520

Albuterol (Tachycardia or arrhythmias may occur). Products include:
Proventil Inhalation Aerosol 2117
Ventolin Inhalation Aerosol and Refill 583

Albuterol Sulfate (Tachycardia or arrhythmias may occur). Products include:
Proventil Repetabs Tablets 2120
Proventil Solutions for Inhalation 0.5% and 0.083% 2118
Proventil Syrup 2119
Proventil Tablets 2120
Ventolin 583

Alcohol (Additive sedative effects).

Alfentanil Hydrochloride (Additive sedative effects). Products include:
Alfenta Injection 1131

Alprazolam (Additive sedative effects). Products include:
Xanax Tablets 2367

Amitriptyline Hydrochloride (Additive sedative effects; increased pressor response). Products include:
Elavil 2269
Endep Tablets 1927
Etrafon 2087
Limbitrol 1933
Triavil Tablets 1556

Amoxapine (Additive sedative effects; increased pressor response). Products include:
Asendin Tablets 1196

Atenolol (Cardiostimulating effects blocked). Products include:
Tenoretic Tablets 1105
Tenormin Tablets and I.V. Injection 1107

Atropine Sulfate (Enhanced pressor response; reflex bradycardia blocked). Products include:
Arco-Lase Plus Tablets 607
Atropine Sulfate Sterile Ophthalmic Solution and S.O.P. Sterile Ophthalmic Ointment ◉ 239
Donnagel ⊞ 675
Donnagel-PG 1858
Donnatal 1858
Donnatal Extentabs 1859
Donnatal Tablets 1858
Donnazyme Tablets 1860
Isopto Atropine ◉ 218
Lomotil 2174
Motofen Tablets 836
Ru-Tuss Tablets 693
Urised Tablets 2396

Betaxolol Hydrochloride (Cardiostimulating effects blocked). Products include:
Betoptic Sterile Ophthalmic Solution 569
Betoptic S Sterile Ophthalmic Suspension 570
Kerlone Tablets 2172

Bitolterol Mesylate (Tachycardia or arrhythmias may occur). Products include:
Tornalate 2074

Buprenorphine (Additive sedative effects).
No products indexed under this heading.

Buspirone Hydrochloride (Additive sedative effects). Products include:
BuSpar 1401

Carteolol Hydrochloride (Cardiostimulating effects blocked). Products include:
Cartrol Tablets 507

Chlordiazepoxide (Additive sedative effects). Products include:
Libritabs Tablets 1930
Limbitrol 1933
Menrium Tablets 1934

Chlordiazepoxide Hydrochloride (Additive sedative effects). Products include:
Librax Capsules 1929
Librium Capsules 1931
Librium Injectable 1932

Chlorpromazine (Additive sedative effects). Products include:
Thorazine 2234

Chlorprothixene (Additive sedative effects). Products include:
Taractan Tablets 1920

Chlorprothixene Hydrochloride (Additive sedative effects). Products include:
Taractan 1920

Clomipramine Hydrochloride (Additive sedative effects; increased pressor response). Products include:
Anafranil Capsules 650

Clorazepate Dipotassium (Additive sedative effects). Products include:
Tranxene 556

Desipramine Hydrochloride (Additive sedative effects; increased pressor response). Products include:
Norpramin Tablets 1340

Dezocine (Additive sedative effects).

Diazepam (Additive sedative effects). Products include:
Valium Injectable 1937
Valium Tablets 1939
Valrelease Capsules 1923

Dobutamine Hydrochloride (Tachycardia or arrhythmias may occur). Products include:
Dobutrex Solution Vials 1259

Dopamine Hydrochloride (Tachycardia or arrhythmias may occur). Products include:
Intropin Injection 930

Doxazosin Mesylate (Pressor response decreased). Products include:
Cardura Tablets 1941

Doxepin Hydrochloride (Additive sedative effects; increased pressor response). Products include:
Sinequan 1960

Droperidol (Additive sedative effects). Products include:
Inapsine Injection 1140
Innovar Injection 1141

Ephedrine Hydrochloride (Tachycardia or arrhythmias may occur). Products include:
Amesec ⊞ 682
Primatene Tablets-M Formula 2421
Primatene Tablets-P Formula 2421
Primatene Tablets-Regular Formula 2421
Quadrinal Tablets 1183
Quelidrine Syrup 556
Tedral SA 1765

Ephedrine Sulfate (Tachycardia or arrhythmias may occur). Products include:
Bronkaid Tablets ⊞ 757
Bronkolixir ⊞ 761
Bronkotabs Tablets ⊞ 762
Marax Tablets & DF Syrup 1954
Pazo Hemorrhoid Ointment & Suppositories 752
Vicks Vatronol Nose Drops ⊞ 666

Ephedrine Tannate (Tachycardia or arrhythmias may occur). Products include:
Rynatuss 2388

Epinephrine (Tachycardia or arrhythmias may occur). Products include:
Ana-Kit Anaphylaxis Emergency Treatment Kit 1100
Bronkaid Mist ⊞ 757
EpiPen 843
Marcaine Hydrochloride 0.5% with Epinephrine 1:200,000 (as bitartrate) 958
Marcaine Hydrochloride with Epinephrine 1:200,000 2055
Primatene Mist 2420
Sus-Phrine Injection 1006
Xylocaine with Epinephrine Injections 637

Epinephrine Bitartrate (Tachycardia or arrhythmias may occur). Products include:
AsthmaHaler Mist Epinephrine Bitartrate Bronchodilator ⊞ 616
Bronkaid Mist Suspension ⊞ 757
Primatene Mist Suspension 2421

Epinephrine Hydrochloride (Tachycardia or arrhythmias may occur). Products include:
Adrenalin Chloride Solution 1:100 & 1:1,000 1689
Epifrin ◉ 244
Glaucon ◉ 218

Ergotamine Tartrate (Excessive rise in blood pressure). Products include:
Bellergal-S Tablets 1998
Cafergot/Cafergot P-B 1999
Ergostat 1719
Medihaler Ergotamine Aerosol 1312
Wigraine Tablets & Suppositories 1645

Esmolol Hydrochloride (Cardiostimulating effects blocked). Products include:
Brevibloc Injection 942

Estazolam (Additive sedative effects). Products include:
ProSom Tablets 554

Ethchlorvynol (Additive sedative effects). Products include:
Placidyl Capsules 553

Ethinamate (Additive sedative effects).
No products indexed under this heading.

Ethylnorepinephrine Hydrochloride (Tachycardia or arrhythmias may occur). Products include:
Bronkephrine Injection 2042

Fentanyl (Additive sedative effects). Products include:
Duragesic Transdermal System 1133

Fentanyl Citrate (Additive sedative effects). Products include:
Innovar Injection 1141
Sublimaze Injection 1146

Fluphenazine Decanoate (Additive sedative effects). Products include:
Prolixin Decanoate 1795

Fluphenazine Enanthate (Additive sedative effects). Products include:
Prolixin Enanthate 1796

Fluphenazine Hydrochloride (Additive sedative effects). Products include:
Prolixin Elixir 1793
Prolixin Injection 1791
Prolixin Oral Concentrate 1792
Prolixin Tablets 1793

Flurazepam Hydrochloride (Additive sedative effects). Products include:
Dalmane Capsules 1927

Furazolidone (Acute hypertensive crisis; concurrent use is contraindicated). Products include:
Furoxone 1855

Glutethimide (Additive sedative effects).
No products indexed under this heading.

Haloperidol (Additive sedative effects). Products include:
- Haldol Injection, Tablets and Concentrate ... 1373

Haloperidol Decanoate (Additive sedative effects). Products include:
- Haldol Decanoate ... 1375

Hydrocodone Bitartrate (Additive sedative effects). Products include:
- Anexsia 5/500 Tablets ... 2196
- Anexsia 7.5/650 Tablets ... 2197
- Azdone Tablets ... 844
- Codiclear DH Syrup ... 845
- Codimal DH Syrup ... 846
- Damason-P ... 1356
- Hycodan Syrup, Tablets ... 927
- Hycomine Compound Tablets ... 929
- Hycomine Syrup ... 927
- Hycotuss Expectorant Syrup ... 930
- Hydrocet Capsules ... 835
- Lortab ASA Tablets ... 2414
- Lortab ... 2412
- Ru-Tuss with Hydrocodone ... 694
- Triaminic Expectorant DH ... 1995
- Vicodin Tablets ... 1187
- Vicodin ES Tablets ... 1189
- Zydone Capsules ... 941

Hydrocodone Polistirex (Additive sedative effects). Products include:
- Tussionex Extended-Release Suspension ... 988

Hydroxyzine Hydrochloride (Additive sedative effects). Products include:
- Atarax Tablets & Syrup ... 1941
- Marax Tablets & DF Syrup ... 1954
- Vistaril Intramuscular Solution ... 1970

Imipramine Hydrochloride (Additive sedative effects; increased pressor response). Products include:
- Tofranil Ampuls ... 1038
- Tofranil Tablets ... 1039

Imipramine Pamoate (Additive sedative effects; increased pressor response). Products include:
- Tofranil-PM Capsules ... 1041

Isocarboxazid (Acute hypertensive crisis; concurrent use is contraindicated). Products include:
- Marplan Tablets ... 1906

Isoetharine (Tachycardia or arrhythmias may occur). Products include:
- Arm-a-Med Isoetharine Inhalation Solution, USP ... 616
- Bronkometer Aerosol ... 2042
- Bronkosol Solution ... 2042

Isoproterenol Hydrochloride (Tachycardia or arrhythmias may occur). Products include:
- Isuprel Hydrochloride Injection 1:5000 ... 2050
- Isuprel Hydrochloride Mistometer ... 2051
- Isuprel Hydrochloride Solution 1:200 & 1:100 ... 2052
- Norisodrine Aerotrol ... 540

Labetalol Hydrochloride (Cardiostimulating effects blocked). Products include:
- Normodyne Injection ... 2108
- Normodyne Tablets ... 2110
- Normozide Tablets ... 2112
- Trandate HCT Tablets ... 579
- Trandate Injection ... 577
- Trandate Tablets ... 579

Levorphanol Tartrate (Additive sedative effects). Products include:
- Levo-Dromoran ... 1906

Lorazepam (Additive sedative effects). Products include:
- Ativan Injection ... 2432
- Ativan Tablets ... 2434

Loxapine Hydrochloride (Additive sedative effects). Products include:
- Loxitane ... 1213

Maprotiline Hydrochloride (Additive sedative effects; increased pressor response). Products include:
- Ludiomil Tablets ... 874

Meperidine Hydrochloride (Additive sedative effects). Products include:
- Demerol ... 2047
- Mepergan Injection ... 2479

Meprobamate (Additive sedative effects). Products include:
- Deprol Tablets ... 2382
- Equagesic Tablets ... 2451
- Miltown Tablets ... 2386
- PMB 200 and PMB 400 ... 2504

Mesoridazine (Additive sedative effects). Products include:
- Serentil ... 686

Metaproterenol Sulfate (Tachycardia or arrhythmias may occur). Products include:
- Alupent ... 674
- Arm-a-Med Metaproterenol Sulfate Inhalation Solution, USP ... 617
- Metaprel Inhalation Aerosol Bronchodilator ... 2014
- Metaprel Inhalation Solution ... 2015
- Metaprel ... 2015
- Metaproterenol Sulfate Inhalation Solution, USP ... 912

Metaraminol Bitartrate (Tachycardia or arrhythmias may occur). Products include:
- Aramine Injection ... 1424

Methadone Hydrochloride (Additive sedative effects). Products include:
- Dolophine Hydrochloride Ampoules & Vials ... 1260
- Dolophine Hydrochloride Tablets ... 1261
- Methadone Hydrochloride Diskets ... 1284
- Methadone Hydrochloride Oral Solution & Tablets ... 1987

Methoxamine Hydrochloride (Tachycardia or arrhythmias may occur). Products include:
- Vasoxyl Injection ... 819

Metoprolol Tartrate (Cardiostimulating effects blocked). Products include:
- Lopressor Ampuls ... 1032
- Lopressor HCT Tablets ... 1034
- Lopressor Tablets ... 1032

Midazolam Hydrochloride (Additive sedative effects). Products include:
- Versed Injection ... 1924

Molindone Hydrochloride (Additive sedative effects). Products include:
- Moban Tablets & Concentrate ... 932

Morphine Sulfate (Additive sedative effects). Products include:
- Astramorph/PF Injection, USP (Preservative-Free) ... 618
- Duramorph ... 960
- Infumorph 200 and Infumorph 500 Sterile Solutions ... 962
- MS Contin Tablets ... 1814
- MSIR ... 1817
- Oramorph SR (Morphine Sulfate Sustained Release Tablets) ... 1988
- Roxanol ... 1991

Nadolol (Cardiostimulating effects blocked). Products include:
- Corgard Tablets ... 701
- Corzide Tablets ... 702

Norepinephrine Bitartrate (Tachycardia or arrhythmias may occur). Products include:
- Levophed Bitartrate Injection ... 2054

Nortriptyline Hydrochloride (Additive sedative effects; increased pressor response). Products include:
- Pamelor ... 2019

Opium Alkaloids (Additive sedative effects). Products include:
- B & O No. 15A & No. 16A Supprettes ... 2395
- Pantopon Injectable ... 1911

Oxazepam (Additive sedative effects). Products include:
- Serax Capsules ... 2522
- Serax Tablets ... 2522

Oxycodone Hydrochloride (Additive sedative effects). Products include:
- Percocet Tablets ... 950
- Percodan ... 951
- Roxicodone Tablets, Oral Solution & Intensol (Oxycodone) ... 1992
- Tylox Capsules ... 1382

Penbutolol Sulfate (Cardiostimulating effects blocked). Products include:
- Levatol ... 1832

Perphenazine (Additive sedative effects). Products include:
- Etrafon ... 2087
- Triavil Tablets ... 1556
- Trilafon ... 2123

Phenelzine Sulfate (Acute hypertensive crisis; concurrent use is contraindicated). Products include:
- Nardil ... 1742

Phentolamine Mesylate (Decreased pressor response). Products include:
- Regitine ... 878

Phenylephrine Bitartrate (Tachycardia or arrhythmias may occur).
- No products indexed under this heading.

Phenylephrine Tannate (Tachycardia or arrhythmias may occur). Products include:
- Rynatan ... 2387
- Rynatuss ... 2388

Phenylpropanolamine Hydrochloride (Tachycardia or arrhythmias may occur). Products include:
- A.R.M. Allergy Relief Medicine Caplets ... ■ 615
- Acutrim ... ■ 548
- Allerest ... ■ 559
- BC Cold Powder ... ■ 517
- Cheracol Plus Head Cold/Cough Formula ... ■ 667
- Codimal Expectorant ... 846
- Comtrex Multi-Symptom Cold Reliever Tablets/Caplets/Liqui-Gels/Liquid ... 745
- Contac Continuous Action Decongestant/Antihistamine Capsules ■ 710
- Contac Maximum Strength Continuous Action Decongestant/Antihistamine Caplets ... ■ 709
- Contac Severe Cold and Flu Formula Caplets ... ■ 711
- Coricidin 'D' Decongestant Tablets ... ■ 695
- Coricidin Demilets Tablets for Children ... ■ 696
- Demazin Nasal Decongestant/Antihistamine Repetabs Tablets & Syrup ... ■ 697
- Dexatrim ... ■ 733
- Dimetane-DC Cough Syrup ... 1857
- Dimetapp Elixir ... ■ 673
- Dimetapp DM Elixir ... ■ 674
- Dimetapp Extentabs ... ■ 674
- Dimetapp Plus Caplets ... ■ 675
- Dimetapp Tablets ... ■ 675
- Entex Capsules ... 1623
- Entex LA Tablets ... 1623
- Entex Liquid ... 1623
- 4-Way Cold Tablets ... 750
- Hycomine Syrup ... 927
- Naldecon CX Adult Liquid ... ■ 521
- Naldecon DX Adult Liquid ... ■ 521
- Naldecon DX Children's Syrup ... ■ 522
- Naldecon DX Pediatric Drops ... ■ 522
- Naldecon EX Children's Syrup ... ■ 522
- Naldecon EX Pediatric Drops ... ■ 523
- Naldecon Syrup, Tablets, Pediatric Drops and Pediatric Syrup ... 709
- Nolamine Tablets ... 838
- Nolex LA Tablets ... 838
- Ornade Spansule Capsules ... 2221
- Orthoxicol Cough Syrup ... ■ 668
- Propagest ... 839
- Pyrroxate Capsules ... ■ 669
- Robitussin-CF ... ■ 676
- Ru-Tuss II Capsules ... 693
- Ru-Tuss with Hydrocodone ... 694
- Ru-Tuss Tablets ... 693
- Sine-Off Sinus Medicine Tablets-Aspirin Formula ... ■ 722
- Sinulin ... 840
- St. Joseph Cold Tablets for Children ... ■ 704
- Tavist-D Tablets ... 2035
- Triaminic Allergy Tablets ... ■ 688
- Triaminic Chewables ... ■ 688
- Triaminic Cold Tablets ... ■ 688
- Triaminic Expectorant ... ■ 688
- Triaminic Expectorant w/Codeine ... 1996
- Triaminic Expectorant DH ... 1995
- Triaminic Oral Infant Drops ... 1996
- Triaminic Syrup ... ■ 689
- Triaminic-12 Tablets ... ■ 690
- Triaminic-DM Syrup ... ■ 689
- Triaminicin Tablets ... ■ 690
- Triaminicol Multi-Symptom Cold Tablets ... ■ 691
- Triaminicol Multi-Symptom Relief ■ 691
- Tuss-Ornade Liquid ... 2242
- Tuss-Ornade Spansule Capsules ... 2242
- Tylenol Cold Medication, Effervescent Tablets ... 1369

Pindolol (Cardiostimulating effects blocked). Products include:
- Visken Tablets ... 2036

Pirbuterol Acetate (Tachycardia or arrhythmias may occur). Products include:
- Maxair Inhaler ... 1311

Prazepam (Additive sedative effects). Products include:
- Centrax ... 1693

Prazosin Hydrochloride (Pressor response decreased). Products include:
- Minipress Capsules ... 1778
- Minizide Capsules ... 1779

Prochlorperazine (Additive sedative effects). Products include:
- Compazine ... 2201

Propofol (Additive sedative effects). Products include:
- Diprivan Injection ... 2267

Propoxyphene Hydrochloride (Additive sedative effects). Products include:
- Darvon ... 1256
- Wygesic Tablets ... 2540

Propoxyphene Napsylate (Additive sedative effects). Products include:
- Darvon-N/Darvocet-N ... 1254

Propranolol Hydrochloride (Cardiostimulating effects blocked). Products include:
- Inderal ... 2459
- Inderal LA Long Acting Capsules ... 2461
- Inderide Tablets ... 2463
- Inderide LA Long Acting Capsules ... 2465

Protriptyline Hydrochloride (Additive sedative effects; increased pressor response). Products include:
- Vivactil Tablets ... 1567

Pseudoephedrine Hydrochloride (Tachycardia or arrhythmias may occur). Products include:
- Actifed Capsules ... ■ 539
- Actifed Plus Caplets ... ■ 539
- Actifed Plus Tablets ... ■ 540
- Actifed with Codeine Cough Syrup ... 752
- Actifed Syrup ... ■ 540
- Actifed Tablets ... ■ 540
- Actifed 12-Hour Capsules ... ■ 539
- Advil Cold & Sinus Caplets (formerly CoAdvil) ... 2416
- Allerest ... ■ 559
- Anatuss LA Tablets ... 1359
- Benadryl Decongestant Elixir ... ■ 635
- Benadryl Decongestant ... ■ 635
- Benadryl Plus ... ■ 636
- Benadryl Plus Nighttime ... ■ 637
- Benylin Decongestant ... ■ 638
- Brexin L.A. Capsules ... 2078
- Bromfed Capsules (Timed Release) ... 1615
- Bromfed Syrup ... ■ 628
- Bromfed ... 1615
- CoAdvil ... ■ 748
- Allergy-Sinus Comtrex Multi-Symptom Allergy Sinus Formula Tablets & Caplets ... 746
- Cough Formula Comtrex ... 746
- Comtrex Multi-Symptom Cold Reliever Tablets/Caplets/Liqui-Gels/Liquid ... 745
- Day-Night Comtrex ... 747

Non-Drowsy Comtrex 747
Congess 994
Congestac Caplets .... ▣ 617
Contac Jr. Children's Cold Medicine .... ▣ 712
Contac Nighttime Cold Medicine .... ▣ 713
Contac Sinus Caplets Maximum Strength Non-Drowsy Formula .... ▣ 710
Contac Sinus Tablets Maximum Strength Non-Drowsy Formula .... ▣ 710
Deconamine 663
Deconsal II Tablets 559
Dimacol Caplets .... ▣ 672
Dimetane-DX Cough Syrup 1858
Dorcol Children's Cough Syrup .... ▣ 685
Dorcol Children's Decongestant Liquid .... ▣ 685
Dorcol Children's Liquid Cold Formula .... ▣ 686
Maximum Strength Dristan Decongestant/Analgesic Coated Caplets .... ▣ 750
No Drowsiness Dristan Cold Nasal Decongestant/Analgesic Coated Caplets 2420
Dristan Sinus Caplets 2419
Sinus Excedrin Analgesic, Decongestant Tablets & Caplets .... ▣ 533
Fedahist Gyrocaps 2145
Fedahist Timecaps 2145
Guaifed 1615
Guaifed Syrup .... ▣ 629
Isoclor Expectorant 982
Isoclor Timesule Capsules .... ▣ 561
Kronofed-A 970
Medi-Flu Caplet, Liquid .... ▣ 640
Novafed A Capsules 1342
Novafed Capsules 1342
Novahistine DH 1342
Novahistine DMX .... ▣ 595
Novahistine Expectorant 1343
Nucofed Capsules 2219
Nucofed Expectorant 2219
Nucofed Pediatric Expectorant 2220
Nucofed Syrup 2219
Ornex Caplets .... ▣ 618
PediaCare Allergy Relief Formula Liquid 1362
PediaCare Cough-Cold Formula Liquid 1362
PediaCare Infants' Oral Decongestant Drops 1362
PediaCare Night Rest Cough-Cold Formula Liquid 1362
PediaCare 6-12 Cough-Cold Formula Chewable Tablets 1362
Robitussin-DAC Syrup 1875
Robitussin-PE .... ▣ 677
Rondec 1975
Rondec-DM 1976
Rondec-TR Tablet 1975
Ru-Tuss DE Tablets 694
Ryna .... ▣ 741
Seldane-D Extended-Release Tablets 1350
Sinarest .... ▣ 562
Sine-Aid Maximum Strength Sinus Headache Caplets 1365
Sine-Aid Maximum Strength Sinus Headache Tablets 1365
Sine-Off Maximum Strength Allergy/Sinus Formula Caplets .... ▣ 721
Sine-Off Maximum Strength No Drowsiness Formula Caplets .... ▣ 722
Singlet Tablets .... ▣ 598
Sinutab Maximum Strength .... ▣ 641
Sinutab Maximum Strength Without Drowsiness Tablets & Caplets .... ▣ 642
Sinutab Regular Strength Without Drowsiness Formula .... ▣ 641
St. Joseph Nighttime Cold Medicine .... ▣ 705
Sudafed Children's Liquid .... ▣ 543
Sudafed Cough Syrup .... ▣ 543
Sudafed Plus Liquid .... ▣ 544
Sudafed Plus Tablets .... ▣ 545
Sudafed Sinus Caplets .... ▣ 545
Sudafed Sinus Tablets .... ▣ 545
Sudafed Tablets, 30 mg .... ▣ 544
Sudafed Tablets, Adult Strength, 60 mg .... ▣ 544
Sudafed 12 Hour Capsules .... ▣ 545
TheraFlu Flu and Cold Medicine .... ▣ 687
Triaminic Nite Light .... ▣ 689
Tylenol Allergy Sinus Medication Caplets and Gelcaps, Maximum Strength 1372
Children's Tylenol Cold Liquid Formula and Chewable Tablets 1368
Tylenol Cold & Flu Hot Medication, Packets 1369
Tylenol Cold & Flu No Drowsiness Hot Medication, Packets 1371
Tylenol Cold Medication Caplets and Tablets 1370
Tylenol Cold Medication No Drowsiness Formula Caplets 1370
Tylenol Cold Night Time Medication Liquid 1371
Tylenol Cough Medication Liquid with Decongestant, Maximum Strength 1372
Tylenol, Maximum Strength, Sinus Medication Gelcaps, Caplets and Tablets 1373
Ursinus Inlay-Tabs .... ▣ 691
Vicks Children's NyQuil .... ▣ 664
Vicks Daycare .... ▣ 660
Vicks Formula 44D Decongestant Cough Medicine .... ▣ 662
Vicks Formula 44M Multi-Symptom Cough Medicine .... ▣ 662
Vicks NyQuil Nighttime Colds Medicine-Original & Cherry Flavor .... ▣ 664
Vicks Pediatric Formula 44 Cough & Congestion Medicine .... ▣ 663
Vicks Pediatric Formula 44m Multi-Symptom Cough & Cold Medicine .... ▣ 663

Pseudoephedrine Sulfate (Tachycardia or arrhythmias may occur). Products include:
Afrin Tablets .... ▣ 693
Chlor-Trimeton Decongestant .... ▣ 694
Disophrol Chronotab Sustained-Action Tablets .... ▣ 698
Drixoral Antihistamine/Nasal Decongestant Syrup .... ▣ 698
Drixoral Non-Drowsy Formula .... ▣ 699
Drixoral Plus Extended-Release Tablets .... ▣ 699
Drixoral Sinus .... ▣ 700
Drixoral Sustained-Action Tablets .... ▣ 698
Sinutab Allergy Formula Sustained Action Tablets .... ▣ 640
Trinalin Repetabs Tablets 1170

Quazepam (Additive sedative effects). Products include:
Doral Tablets 2383

Secobarbital Sodium (Additive sedative effects). Products include:
Seconal Sodium Pulvules 1296

Selegiline Hydrochloride (Acute hypertensive crisis; concurrent use is contraindicated). Products include:
Eldepryl 2250

Sufentanil Citrate (Additive sedative effects). Products include:
Sufenta Injection 1147

Temazepam (Additive sedative effects). Products include:
Restoril Capsules 2023

Terazosin Hydrochloride (Pressor response decreased). Products include:
Hytrin Tablets 529

Terbutaline Sulfate (Tachycardia or arrhythmias may occur). Products include:
Brethaire Inhaler 1024
Brethine Ampuls 1026
Brethine Tablets 1026
Bricanyl Injection 1324
Bricanyl Tablets 1325

Thioridazine Hydrochloride (Additive sedative effects). Products include:
Mellaril 2011

Thiothixene (Additive sedative effects). Products include:
Navane Capsules and Concentrate 1954
Navane Intramuscular 1956

Timolol Maleate (Cardiostimulating effects blocked). Products include:
Blocadren Tablets 1429
Timolide Tablets 1547
Timoptic in Ocudose 1552
Timoptic Sterile Ophthalmic Solution 1550

Tranylcypromine Sulfate (Acute hypertensive crisis; concurrent use is contraindicated). Products include:
Parnate Tablets 2222

Triazolam (Additive sedative effects). Products include:
Halcion Tablets 2340

Trifluoperazine Hydrochloride (Additive sedative effects). Products include:
Stelazine 2226

Trimipramine Maleate (Additive sedative effects; increased pressor response). Products include:
Surmontil Capsules 2524

PHENOBARBITAL ELIXIR AND TABLETS

(Phenobarbital) 1293

May interact with oral anticoagulants, corticosteroids, central nervous system depressants, antihistamines, tranquilizers, monoamine oxidase inhibitors, oral contraceptives, hypnotics and sedatives, and certain other agents. Compounds in these categories include:

Alcohol (Additive depressant effects).

Alfentanil Hydrochloride (Additive depressant effects). Products include:
Alfenta Injection 1131

Alprazolam (Additive depressant effects). Products include:
Xanax Tablets 2367

Aprobarbital (Additive depressant effects). Products include:
Alurate Elixir 1883

Astemizole (Additive depressant effects). Products include:
Hismanal Tablets 1138

Azatadine Maleate (Additive depressant effects). Products include:
Optimine Tablets 2115
Trinalin Repetabs Tablets 1170

Betamethasone Acetate (Enhanced metabolism of exogenous corticosteroids). Products include:
Celestone Soluspan Suspension 2081

Betamethasone Sodium Phosphate (Enhanced metabolism of exogenous corticosteroids). Products include:
Celestone Soluspan Suspension 2081

Bromodiphenhydramine Hydrochloride (Additive depressant effects).
No products indexed under this heading.

Brompheniramine Maleate (Additive depressant effects). Products include:
Alka Seltzer Plus Sinus Allergy Medicine .... ▣ 624
Atrohist Sprinkle Capsules 558
Bromfed Capsules (Timed Release) 1615
Bromfed Syrup .... ▣ 628
Bromfed 1615
Dimetane Decongestant .... ▣ 673
Dimetane .... ▣ 672
Dimetane-DC Cough Syrup 1857
Dimetane-DX Cough Syrup 1858
Dimetapp Elixir .... ▣ 673
Dimetapp DM Elixir .... ▣ 674
Dimetapp Extentabs .... ▣ 674
Dimetapp Plus Caplets .... ▣ 675
Dimetapp Tablets .... ▣ 675
Drixoral Antihistamine/Nasal Decongestant Syrup .... ▣ 698

Buprenorphine (Additive depressant effects).
No products indexed under this heading.

Buspirone Hydrochloride (Additive depressant effects). Products include:
BuSpar 1401

Butabarbital (Additive depressant effects). Products include:
Pyridium Plus 1764

Butalbital (Additive depressant effects). Products include:
Esgic-Plus Tablets 1002
Esgic Tablets & Capsules 1001
Fioricet Tablets 2006
Fiorinal Capsules 2007
Fiorinal with Codeine Capsules 2008
Fiorinal Tablets 2007
Phrenilin 838
Sedapap Tablets 50 mg/650 mg .. 1360

Chlordiazepoxide (Additive depressant effects). Products include:
Libritabs Tablets 1930
Limbitrol 1933
Menrium Tablets 1934

Chlordiazepoxide Hydrochloride (Additive depressant effects). Products include:
Librax Capsules 1929
Librium Capsules 1931
Librium Injectable 1932

Chlorpheniramine Maleate (Additive depressant effects). Products include:
A.R.M. Allergy Relief Medicine Caplets .... ▣ 615
Alka-Seltzer Plus Cold Medicine .... ▣ 623
Allerest .... ▣ 559
Ana-Kit Anaphylaxis Emergency Treatment Kit 1100
BC Cold Powder Multi-Symptom Formula .... ▣ 517
Brexin L.A. Capsules 2078
Cerose-DM 2443
Cheracol Plus Head Cold/Cough Formula .... ▣ 667
Chlor-Trimeton Allergy Syrup, Tablets & Long-Acting Repetabs Tablets .... ▣ 693
Chlor-Trimeton Decongestant .... ▣ 694
Comhist LA Capsules 1618
Allergy-Sinus Comtrex Multi-Symptom Allergy Sinus Formula Tablets & Caplets 746
Comtrex Multi-Symptom Cold Reliever Tablets/Caplets/Liqui-Gels/Liquid 745
Day-Night Comtrex 747
Contac Continuous Action Decongestant/Antihistamine Capsules ▣ 710
Contac Maximum Strength Continuous Action Decongestant/Antihistamine Caplets .... ▣ 709
Contac Severe Cold and Flu Formula Caplets .... ▣ 711
Coricidin 'D' Decongestant Tablets .... ▣ 695
Coricidin Demilets Tablets for Children .... ▣ 696
Coricidin Tablets .... ▣ 695
Deconamine 663
Demazin Nasal Decongestant/Antihistamine Repetabs Tablets & Syrup .... ▣ 697
Dorcol Children's Liquid Cold Formula .... ▣ 686
Dristan Decongestant/Antihistamine/Analgesic Coated Caplets .... ▣ 749
Dristan Cold Nasal Decongestant/Antihistamine/ Analgesic Coated Tablets 2419
Dristan Advanced Formula Decongestant/Antihistamine/Analgesic Tablets .... ▣ 749
Extendryl 994
4-Way Cold Tablets 750
Fedahist Gyrocaps 2145
Fedahist Timecaps 2145
Hycomine Compound Tablets 929
Isoclor Timesule Capsules .... ▣ 561
Kronofed-A 970
Medi-Flu Caplet, Liquid .... ▣ 640
Naldecon Syrup, Tablets, Pediatric Drops and Pediatric Syrup 709
Nolamine Tablets 838
Novafed A Capsules 1342
Novahistine DH 1342
Novahistine Elixir .... ▣ 596
Ornade Spansule Capsules 2221
Orthoxicol Cough Syrup .... ▣ 668

PediaCare Allergy Relief Formula Liquid 1362
PediaCare Cough-Cold Formula Liquid 1362
PediaCare Night Rest Cough-Cold Formula Liquid 1362
PediaCare 6-12 Cough-Cold Formula Chewable Tablets 1362
Pyrroxate Capsules .... ▣ 669
Quelidrine Syrup 556
Ru-Tuss II Capsules 693
Ru-Tuss Tablets 693
Ryna .... ▣ 741
Sinarest Tablets & Extra Strength Tablets .... ▣ 562
Sine-Off Maximum Strength Allergy/Sinus Formula Caplets .... ▣ 721
Sine-Off Sinus Medicine Tablets-Aspirin Formula .... ▣ 722
Singlet Tablets .... ▣ 598
Sinulin 840
Sinutab Maximum Strength .... ▣ 641
St. Joseph Nighttime Cold Medicine .... ▣ 705
Sudafed Plus Liquid .... ▣ 544
Sudafed Plus Tablets .... ▣ 545
Teldrin Timed-Release Allergy Capsules, 12 mg 2192
TheraFlu Flu and Cold Medicine .... ▣ 687
Triaminic Allergy Tablets .... ▣ 688
Triaminic Chewables .... ▣ 688
Triaminic Cold Tablets .... ▣ 688
Triaminic Nite Light .... ▣ 689
Triaminic Syrup .... ▣ 689
Triaminic-12 Tablets .... ▣ 690
Triaminicin Tablets .... ▣ 690
Triaminicol Multi-Symptom Cold Tablets .... ▣ 691
Triaminicol Multi-Symptom Relief .... ▣ 691
Tylenol Allergy Sinus Medication Caplets and Gelcaps, Maximum Strength 1372
Children's Tylenol Cold Liquid Formula and Chewable Tablets 1368
Tylenol Cold & Flu Hot Medication, Packets 1369
Tylenol Cold Medication Caplets and Tablets 1370
Tylenol Cold Medication, Effervescent Tablets 1369
Vicks Children's NyQuil .... ▣ 664
Vicks Formula 44 Cough Medicine .... ▣ 661
Vicks Formula 44M Multi-Symptom Cough Medicine .... ▣ 662
Vicks Pediatric Formula 44m Multi-Symptom Cough & Cold Medicine .... ▣ 663

Chlorpheniramine Polistirex (Additive depressant effects). Products include:
Tussionex Extended-Release Suspension 988

Chlorpheniramine Tannate (Additive depressant effects). Products include:
Rynatan 2387
Rynatuss 2388

Chlorpromazine (Additive depressant effects). Products include:
Thorazine 2234

Chlorprothixene (Additive depressant effects). Products include:
Taractan Tablets 1920

Chlorprothixene Hydrochloride (Additive depressant effects). Products include:
Taractan 1920

Clemastine Fumarate (Additive depressant effects). Products include:
Tavist Syrup 2033
Tavist Tablets 2035
Tavist-D Tablets 2035

Clorazepate Dipotassium (Additive depressant effects). Products include:
Tranxene 556

Codeine (Additive depressant effects). Products include:
Calcidrine Syrup 506

Codeine Phosphate (Additive depressant effects). Products include:
Actifed with Codeine Cough Syrup 752
Cheracol Cough Syrup 1853
Codimal PH Syrup 846
Dimetane-DC Cough Syrup 1857
Empirin with Codeine Phosphate Nos. 2, 3 & 4 764
Fiorinal with Codeine Capsules 2008
Isoclor Expectorant 982
Naldecon CX Adult Liquid .... ▣ 521
Novahistine DH 1342
Novahistine Expectorant 1343
Nucofed Capsules 2219
Nucofed Expectorant 2219
Nucofed Pediatric Expectorant 2220
Nucofed Syrup 2219
Phenaphen with Codeine Capsules 1865
Phenaphen-650 with Codeine Tablets 1866
Phenergan with Codeine 2497
Phenergan VC with Codeine 2501
Robitussin A-C Syrup 1875
Robitussin-DAC Syrup 1875
Ryna .... ▣ 741
Soma Compound w/Codeine Tablets 2390
Triaminic Expectorant w/Codeine 1996
Tussi-Organidin Liquid 2391
Tylenol with Codeine 1381

Codeine Polistirex (Additive depressant effects).
No products indexed under this heading.

Cortisone Acetate (Enhanced metabolism of exogenous corticosteroids). Products include:
Cortone Acetate Sterile Suspension 1437
Cortone Acetate Tablets 1439

Cyproheptadine Hydrochloride (Additive depressant effects). Products include:
Periactin 1525

Dexamethasone (Enhanced metabolism of exogenous corticosteroids). Products include:
AK-Trol Ointment & Suspension .... ◉ 207
Decadron Elixir 1445
Decadron Tablets 1447
Decaspray Topical Aerosol 1459
Dexacidin .... ◉ 272
Maxidex Sterile Ophthalmic Suspension .... ◉ 223
Maxitrol Ophthalmic Ointment/Suspension .... ◉ 223
TobraDex Ophthalmic Suspension and Ointment .... ◉ 228

Dexamethasone Acetate (Enhanced metabolism of exogenous corticosteroids). Products include:
Dalalone D.P. Injectable 999
Decadron-LA Sterile Suspension 1457

Dexamethasone Sodium Phosphate (Enhanced metabolism of exogenous corticosteroids). Products include:
AK-Dex .... ◉ 203
Decadron Phosphate Respihaler 1454
Decadron Phosphate Sterile Ophthalmic Ointment 1453
Decadron Phosphate Sterile Ophthalmic Solution 1453
Decadron Phosphate Topical Cream 1455
Decadron Phosphate Turbinaire 1456
Maxidex Sterile Ophthalmic Ointment .... ◉ 222
NeoDecadron Sterile Ophthalmic Ointment 1517
NeoDecadron Sterile Ophthalmic Solution 1518
NeoDecadron Topical Cream 1518

Dexchlorpheniramine Maleate (Additive depressant effects). Products include:
Polaramine 2116

Dezocine (Additive depressant effects).

Diazepam (Additive depressant effects). Products include:
Valium Injectable 1937
Valium Tablets 1939
Valrelease Capsules 1923

Dicumarol (Lowered plasma levels and decreased anticoagulant activity). Products include:
Dicumarol Tablets 516

Diphenhydramine Citrate (Additive depressant effects). Products include:
Alka-Seltzer Plus Night-Time Cold Medicine .... ▣ 623
Bufferin AF Nite Time Analgesic/Sleeping Aid Caplets 744
Excedrin P.M. Analgesic/Sleeping Aid Tablets, Caplets and Liquid 749

Diphenhydramine Hydrochloride (Additive depressant effects). Products include:
Benadryl Anti-Itch Cream .... ▣ 635
Benadryl Capsules 1691
Benadryl Decongestant Elixir .... ▣ 635
Benadryl Decongestant .... ▣ 635
Benadryl Elixir .... ▣ 636
Benadryl Kapseals 1691
Benadryl 25 Kapseals .... ▣ 636
Benadryl Parenteral 1692
Benadryl Plus .... ▣ 636
Benadryl Plus Nighttime .... ▣ 637
Benadryl Spray, Maximum Strength .... ▣ 637
Benadryl Spray, Regular Strength .... ▣ 637
Benadryl Steri-Vials, Ampoules, and Steri-Dose Syringe 1692
Benadryl 25 Tablets .... ▣ 636
Benylin Cough Syrup .... ▣ 637
Benylin Decongestant .... ▣ 638
Caladryl Cream, Lotion, Spray .... ▣ 638
Miles Nervine Nighttime Sleep-Aid .... ▣ 627
Nytol Tablets .... ▣ 517
Sleep-ettes-D Tablets .... ▣ 653
Sleep-eze 3 Tablets .... ▣ 755
Sleepinal Night-time Sleep Aid Capsules .... ▣ 734
Sominex Caplets and Tablets .... ▣ 722
Sominex Liquid .... ▣ 723
Sominex Pain Relief Formula .... ▣ 723
Tylenol Cold Night Time Medication Liquid 1371
Tylenol PM, Extra Strength Caplets and Tablets 1368
Unisom Dual Relief Nighttime Sleep Aid/Analgesic 1774
Ziradryl Lotion .... ▣ 643

Divalproex Sodium (Increases the phenobarbital serum levels). Products include:
Depakote 512

Doxycycline Calcium (Shortened half-life of doxycycline).
No products indexed under this heading.

Doxycycline Hyclate (Shortened half-life of doxycycline). Products include:
Doryx Capsules 1717
Vibramycin Hyclate Capsules 1787
Vibramycin Hyclate Intravenous 1968
Vibra-Tabs Film Coated Tablets 1787

Doxycycline Monohydrate (Shortened half-life of doxycycline). Products include:
Monodox Capsules 1630
Vibramycin Monohydrate for Oral Suspension 1787

Droperidol (Additive depressant effects). Products include:
Inapsine Injection 1140
Innovar Injection 1141

Enflurane (Additive depressant effects). Products include:
Ethrane 599

Estazolam (Additive depressant effects). Products include:
ProSom Tablets 554

Ethchlorvynol (Additive depressant effects). Products include:
Placidyl Capsules 553

Ethinamate (Additive depressant effects).
No products indexed under this heading.

Ethinyl Estradiol (Decreased estrogen effect). Products include:
Brevicon 2304
Demulen 2161
Estinyl Tablets 2085
Jenest-28 Tablets 1636
Levlen/Tri-Levlen 665
Lo/Ovral Tablets 2471
Lo/Ovral-28 Tablets 2476
Loestrin 1728
Modicon 1667
Nordette-21 Tablets 2481
Nordette-28 Tablets 2483
Norethin 2133
Norinyl 2304
Norlestrin 1746
Ortho-Cyclen Tablets 1658
Ortho-Novum 1667
Ovcon 1391
Ovral Tablets 2490
Ovral-28 Tablets 2491
Levlen/Tri-Levlen 665
Tri-Norinyl 2304
Triphasil-21 Tablets 2527
Triphasil-28 Tablets 2532

Ethynodiol Diacetate (Decreased estrogen effect). Products include:
Demulen 2161

Fentanyl (Additive depressant effects). Products include:
Duragesic Transdermal System 1133

Fentanyl Citrate (Additive depressant effects). Products include:
Innovar Injection 1141
Sublimaze Injection 1146

Fluphenazine Decanoate (Additive depressant effects). Products include:
Prolixin Decanoate 1795

Fluphenazine Enanthate (Additive depressant effects). Products include:
Prolixin Enanthate 1796

Fluphenazine Hydrochloride (Additive depressant effects). Products include:
Prolixin Elixir 1793
Prolixin Injection 1791
Prolixin Oral Concentrate 1792
Prolixin Tablets 1793

Flurazepam Hydrochloride (Additive depressant effects). Products include:
Dalmane Capsules 1927

Furazolidone (Prolongs the effects of barbiturates). Products include:
Furoxone 1855

Glutethimide (Additive depressant effects).
No products indexed under this heading.

Griseofulvin (Interference with griseofulvin absorption; decreased blood levels). Products include:
Fulvicin P/G Tablets 2090
Fulvicin P/G 165 & 330 Tablets 2091
Fulvicin-U/F Tablets 2092
Grifulvin V (griseofulvin microsize) Tablets/Suspension 1678
Grisactin 2454
Grisactin Ultra Tablets 2455
Gris-PEG Tablets, 125 mg & 250 mg 1083

Haloperidol (Additive depressant effects). Products include:
Haldol Injection, Tablets and Concentrate 1373

Haloperidol Decanoate (Additive depressant effects). Products include:
Haldol Decanoate 1375

Hydrocodone Bitartrate (Additive depressant effects). Products include:
Anexsia 5/500 Tablets 2196
Anexsia 7.5/650 Tablets 2197
Azdone Tablets 844
Codiclear DH Syrup 845
Codimal DH Syrup 846
Damason-P 1356
Hycodan Syrup, Tablets 927
Hycomine Compound Tablets 929
Hycomine Syrup 927
Hycotuss Expectorant Syrup 930
Hydrocet Capsules 835
Lortab ASA Tablets 2414
Lortab 2412
Ru-Tuss with Hydrocodone 694
Triaminic Expectorant DH 1995
Vicodin Tablets 1187
Vicodin ES Tablets 1189
Zydone Capsules 941

Hydrocodone Polistirex (Additive depressant effects). Products include:
- Tussionex Extended-Release Suspension ... 988

Hydrocortisone (Enhanced metabolism of exogenous corticosteroids). Products include:
- AK-Spore H.C. ... ◉ 206
- Bactine Hydrocortisone Anti-Itch Cream ... ⊡ 625
- CaldeCORT Anti-Itch Hydrocortisone Spray ... ⊡ 560
- Carmol HC Cream 1% ... 2296
- Cortaid Spray ... ⊡ 735
- Cortenema ... 2244
- Cortisporin Ointment ... 758
- Cortisporin Ophthalmic Ointment Sterile ... 758
- Cortisporin Ophthalmic Suspension Sterile ... 759
- Cortisporin Otic Solution Sterile ... 760
- Cortisporin Otic Suspension Sterile 760
- Cortizone-5 Creme & Ointment ... ⊡ 732
- Dermolate Anti-Itch Cream ... ⊡ 697
- Eldecort Cream 1.0% ... 1113
- Eldecort Cream 1.0% and 2.5% ... 1113
- Fungoid HC Creme ... 1770
- Hydrocortone Tablets ... 1482
- Hytone ... 909
- LazerSporin-C Solution ... 1770
- Massengill Medicated Soft Cloth Towelettes ... 2192
- Nutracort Cream & Lotion ... 1684
- PediOtic Suspension Sterile ... 797
- Synacort Creams 1%, 2.5% ... 2296
- Vanoxide-HC Acne Lotion ... 911
- Vioform-Hydrocortisone Cream and Mild Cream ... 889
- Vioform-Hydrocortisone Ointment ... 889
- VōSoL HC Otic Solution ... 2392
- Vytone Cream 1% ... 911

Hydrocortisone Acetate (Enhanced metabolism of exogenous corticosteroids). Products include:
- Analpram-HC Rectal Cream 1% and 2.5% ... 970
- Anusol-HC Cream ... 1690
- Anusol-HC Suppositories ... 1691
- Caldecort ... ⊡ 560
- Carmol HC Cream 1% ... 2296
- Chloromycetin Hydrocortisone Ophthalmic ... 1694
- Coly-Mycin S Otic w/Neomycin & Hydrocortisone ... 1708
- Cortaid ... ⊡ 735
- Cortef Feminine Itch Cream ... ⊡ 735
- Corticaine ... ⊡ 682
- Cortifoam ... 1827
- Cortisporin Cream ... 757
- Epifoam ... 1828
- Gynecort 5 Creme ... ⊡ 556
- Hydrocortone Acetate Sterile Suspension ... 1479
- Lanacort 5 Creme and Ointment ... ⊡ 557
- Mantadil Cream ... 789
- Ophthocort ... ◉ 301
- Orabase HCA Oral Paste ... 890
- Pramosone Cream, Lotion & Ointment ... 971
- ProctoCream-HC ... 1834
- Proctofoam-HC ... 1835

Hydrocortisone Sodium Phosphate (Enhanced metabolism of exogenous corticosteroids). Products include:
- Hydrocortone Phosphate Injection, Sterile ... 1481

Hydrocortisone Sodium Succinate (Enhanced metabolism of exogenous corticosteroids). Products include:
- Solu-Cortef Sterile Powder ... 2361

Hydroxyzine Hydrochloride (Additive depressant effects). Products include:
- Atarax Tablets & Syrup ... 1941
- Marax Tablets & DF Syrup ... 1954
- Vistaril Intramuscular Solution ... 1970

Isocarboxazid (Prolongs the effects of barbiturates). Products include:
- Marplan Tablets ... 1906

Isoflurane (Additive depressant effects). Products include:
- Forane ... 600

Ketamine Hydrochloride (Additive depressant effects). Products include:
- Ketalar ... 1726

Levonorgestrel (Decreased estrogen effect). Products include:
- Levlen/Tri-Levlen ... 665
- Nordette-21 Tablets ... 2481
- Nordette-28 Tablets ... 2483
- Norplant System ... 2484
- Levlen/Tri-Levlen ... 665
- Triphasil-21 Tablets ... 2527
- Triphasil-28 Tablets ... 2532

Levorphanol Tartrate (Additive depressant effects). Products include:
- Levo-Dromoran ... 1906

Lorazepam (Additive depressant effects). Products include:
- Ativan Injection ... 2432
- Ativan Tablets ... 2434

Loxapine Hydrochloride (Additive depressant effects). Products include:
- Loxitane ... 1213

Loxapine Succinate (Additive depressant effects). Products include:
- Loxitane Capsules ... 1213

Meperidine Hydrochloride (Additive depressant effects). Products include:
- Demerol ... 2047
- Mepergan Injection ... 2479

Mephobarbital (Additive depressant effects). Products include:
- Mebaral Tablets ... 2061

Meprobamate (Additive depressant effects). Products include:
- Deprol Tablets ... 2382
- Equagesic Tablets ... 2451
- Miltown Tablets ... 2386
- PMB 200 and PMB 400 ... 2504

Mesoridazine (Additive depressant effects). Products include:
- Serentil ... 686

Mesoridazine Besylate (Additive depressant effects).

Mestranol (Decreased estrogen effect). Products include:
- Enovid ... 2161
- Norethin ... 2133
- Norinyl ... 2304
- Ortho-Novum ... 1667

Methadone Hydrochloride (Additive depressant effects). Products include:
- Dolophine Hydrochloride Ampoules & Vials ... 1260
- Dolophine Hydrochloride Tablets ... 1261
- Methadone Hydrochloride Diskets ... 1284
- Methadone Hydrochloride Oral Solution & Tablets ... 1987

Methdilazine Hydrochloride (Additive depressant effects). Products include:
- Tacaryl Syrup & Tablets ... 2409

Methohexital Sodium (Additive depressant effects). Products include:
- Brevital Sodium Vials ... 1248

Methoxyflurane (Additive depressant effects).
- No products indexed under this heading.

Methylprednisolone Acetate (Enhanced metabolism of exogenous corticosteroids). Products include:
- Depo-Medrol Sterile Aqueous Suspension ... 2334

Methylprednisolone Sodium Succinate (Enhanced metabolism of exogenous corticosteroids). Products include:
- Solu-Medrol Sterile Powder ... 2363

Midazolam Hydrochloride (Additive depressant effects). Products include:
- Versed Injection ... 1924

Molindone Hydrochloride (Additive depressant effects). Products include:
- Moban Tablets & Concentrate ... 932

Morphine Sulfate (Additive depressant effects). Products include:
- Astramorph/PF Injection, USP (Preservative-Free) ... 618
- Duramorph ... 960
- Infumorph 200 and Infumorph 500 Sterile Solutions ... 962
- MS Contin Tablets ... 1814
- MSIR ... 1817
- Oramorph SR (Morphine Sulfate Sustained Release Tablets) ... 1988
- Roxanol ... 1991

Norethindrone (Decreased estrogen effect). Products include:
- Brevicon ... 2304
- Jenest-28 Tablets ... 1636
- Micronor Tablets ... 1667
- Modicon ... 1667
- Norethin ... 2133
- Norinyl ... 2304
- Norlutin ... 1755
- Nor-Q D Tablets ... 2304
- Ortho-Novum ... 1667
- Ovcon ... 1391
- Tri-Norinyl ... 2304

Norethynodrel (Decreased estrogen effect). Products include:
- Enovid ... 2161

Norgestimate (Decreased estrogen effect). Products include:
- Ortho-Cyclen Tablets ... 1658

Norgestrel (Decreased estrogen effect). Products include:
- Lo/Ovral Tablets ... 2471
- Lo/Ovral-28 Tablets ... 2476
- Ovral Tablets ... 2490
- Ovral-28 Tablets ... 2491
- Ovrette Tablets ... 2492

Opium Alkaloids (Additive depressant effects). Products include:
- B & O No. 15A & No. 16A Supprettes ... 2395
- Pantopon Injectable ... 1911

Oxazepam (Additive depressant effects). Products include:
- Serax Capsules ... 2522
- Serax Tablets ... 2522

Oxycodone Hydrochloride (Additive depressant effects). Products include:
- Percocet Tablets ... 950
- Percodan ... 951
- Roxicodone Tablets, Oral Solution & Intensol (Oxycodone) ... 1992
- Tylox Capsules ... 1382

Pentobarbital Sodium (Additive depressant effects). Products include:
- Nembutal Sodium Capsules ... 534
- Nembutal Sodium Solution ... 536
- Nembutal Sodium Suppositories ... 538

Perphenazine (Additive depressant effects). Products include:
- Etrafon ... 2087
- Triavil Tablets ... 1556
- Trilafon ... 2123

Phenelzine Sulfate (Prolongs the effects of barbiturates). Products include:
- Nardil ... 1742

Phenytoin (Variable effect on the metabolism of phenytoin). Products include:
- Dilantin Infatabs ... 1710
- Dilantin-30 Pediatric/Dilantin-125 Suspension ... 1713

Phenytoin Sodium (Variable effect on the metabolism of phenytoin). Products include:
- Dilantin Kapseals ... 1708
- Dilantin Parenteral ... 1712
- Dilantin with Phenobarbital Kapseals ... 1715

Prazepam (Additive depressant effects). Products include:
- Centrax ... 1693

Prednisolone Acetate (Enhanced metabolism of exogenous corticosteroids). Products include:
- AK-Cide Sterile Ophthalmic Ointment & Suspension ... ◉ 202
- Blephamide Liquifilm Sterile Ophthalmic Suspension ... 586
- Blephamide S.O.P. Sterile Ophthalmic Ointment ... 586
- Cetapred Ointment ... ◉ 220
- ⅛% Econopred & 1% Econopred Plus ... ◉ 217
- Isopto Cetapred Suspension ... ◉ 220
- Metimyd ... ◉ 306
- Poly-Pred Liquifilm ... ◉ 250
- Pred Forte ... ◉ 252
- Pred Mild ... ◉ 254
- Pred-G Liquifilm Sterile Ophthalmic Suspension ... ◉ 252
- Pred-G S.O.P. Sterile Ophthalmic Ointment ... ◉ 253
- Vasocidin Ointment ... ◉ 275

Prednisolone Sodium Phosphate (Enhanced metabolism of exogenous corticosteroids). Products include:
- AK-Pred ... ◉ 205
- Hydeltrasol Injection, Sterile ... 1476
- Inflamase ... ◉ 274
- Pediapred Oral Liquid ... 987
- Vasocidin Ophthalmic Solution ... ◉ 276

Prednisolone Tebutate (Enhanced metabolism of exogenous corticosteroids). Products include:
- Hydeltra-T.B.A. Sterile Suspension 1478

Prednisone (Enhanced metabolism of exogenous corticosteroids). Products include:
- Deltasone Tablets ... 2332

Prochlorperazine (Additive depressant effects). Products include:
- Compazine ... 2201

Promethazine Hydrochloride (Additive depressant effects). Products include:
- Mepergan Injection ... 2479
- Phenergan with Codeine ... 2497
- Phenergan with Dextromethorphan 2499
- Phenergan Injection ... 2493
- Phenergan Suppositories ... 2496
- Phenergan Syrup ... 2495
- Phenergan Tablets ... 2496
- Phenergan VC ... 2500
- Phenergan VC with Codeine ... 2501

Propofol (Additive depressant effects). Products include:
- Diprivan Injection ... 2267

Propoxyphene Hydrochloride (Additive depressant effects). Products include:
- Darvon ... 1256
- Wygesic Tablets ... 2540

Propoxyphene Napsylate (Additive depressant effects). Products include:
- Darvon-N/Darvocet-N ... 1254

Pyrilamine Maleate (Additive depressant effects). Products include:
- Codimal ... 846
- 4-Way Fast Acting Nasal Spray - Original Formula (regular & mentholated) & Metered Spray Pump (regular) ... 751
- Maximum Strength Midol Multi-Symptom Menstrual Formula ... ⊡ 571
- Maximum Strength Midol PMS Premenstrual Syndrome Formula ... ⊡ 570
- Regular Strength Midol Multi-Symptom Menstrual Formula ... ⊡ 570
- Prefrin-A ... ◉ 255
- Prēmsyn PMS Capsules & Caplets ⊡ 547
- Primatene Tablets-M Formula ... 2421
- Robitussin Night Relief ... ⊡ 677
- Ru-Tuss with Hydrocodone ... 694
- Triaminic Expectorant DH ... 1995
- Triaminic Oral Infant Drops ... 1996

Pyrilamine Tannate (Additive depressant effects). Products include:
- Rynatan ... 2387

Quazepam (Additive depressant effects). Products include:
- Doral Tablets 2383

Secobarbital Sodium (Additive depressant effects). Products include:
- Seconal Sodium Pulvules 1296

Selegiline Hydrochloride (Prolongs the effects of barbiturates). Products include:
- Eldepryl 2250

Sodium Valproate (Increases the phenobarbital serum levels).

Sufentanil Citrate (Additive depressant effects). Products include:
- Sufenta Injection 1147

Temazepam (Additive depressant effects). Products include:
- Restoril Capsules 2023

Terfenadine (Additive depressant effects). Products include:
- Seldane Tablets 1349
- Seldane-D Extended-Release Tablets 1350

Thiamylal Sodium (Additive depressant effects). Products include:
- Surital Ampoules, Steri-Vials 1764

Thioridazine Hydrochloride (Additive depressant effects). Products include:
- Mellaril 2011

Thiothixene (Additive depressant effects). Products include:
- Navane Capsules and Concentrate 1954
- Navane Intramuscular 1956

Tranylcypromine Sulfate (Prolongs the effects of barbiturates). Products include:
- Parnate Tablets 2222

Triamcinolone (Enhanced metabolism of exogenous corticosteroids).
- No products indexed under this heading.

Triamcinolone Acetonide (Enhanced metabolism of exogenous corticosteroids). Products include:
- Aristocort A 1010
- Azmacort Inhaler 1837
- Kenalog Cream, Lotion & Ointment 2401
- Kenalog-10 Injection 2402
- Kenalog-40 Injection 2403
- Kenalog in Orabase 604
- Kenalog Spray 2401
- Mycolog II Cream and Ointment 2407
- Mytrex Cream & Ointment 2080
- Nasacort Nasal Inhaler 1844

Triamcinolone Diacetate (Enhanced metabolism of exogenous corticosteroids). Products include:
- Aristocort Suspension 1008

Triamcinolone Hexacetonide (Enhanced metabolism of exogenous corticosteroids). Products include:
- Aristospan Suspension 1011

Triazolam (Additive depressant effects). Products include:
- Halcion Tablets 2340

Trifluoperazine Hydrochloride (Additive depressant effects). Products include:
- Stelazine 2226

Trimeprazine Tartrate (Additive depressant effects). Products include:
- Temaril Tablets, Syrup and Spansule Sustained Release Capsules 1085

Tripelennamine Hydrochloride (Additive depressant effects). Products include:
- PBZ Tablets & Elixir 1037
- PBZ-SR Tablets 1037

Triprolidine Hydrochloride (Additive depressant effects). Products include:
- Actidil .... ▣ 538
- Actifed Capsules .... ▣ 539
- Actifed Plus Caplets .... ▣ 539
- Actifed Plus Tablets .... ▣ 540
- Actifed with Codeine Cough Syrup.. 752
- Actifed Syrup .... ▣ 540
- Actifed Tablets .... ▣ 540
- Actifed 12-Hour Capsules .... ▣ 539

Valproic Acid (Increases the phenobarbital serum levels). Products include:
- Depakene Capsules & Syrup 511

Warfarin Sodium (Lowered plasma levels and decreased anticoagulant activity). Products include:
- Coumadin Injection & Tablets 944
- Panwarfin Tablets 547

PHENURONE TABLETS
(Phenacemide) 552
May interact with anticonvulsants and certain other agents. Compounds in these categories include:

Carbamazepine (Concurrent use requires extreme caution). Products include:
- Tegretol Chewable Tablets 654
- Tegretol Suspension 656
- Tegretol Tablets 654

Divalproex Sodium (Concurrent use requires extreme caution). Products include:
- Depakote 512

Ethosuximide (Concurrent use requires extreme caution). Products include:
- Zarontin Capsules 1768
- Zarontin Syrup 1769

Ethotoin (May result in paranoid symptoms). Products include:
- Peganone Tablets 551

Mephenytoin (Concurrent use requires extreme caution). Products include:
- Mesantoin Tablets 2013

Methsuximide (Concurrent use requires extreme caution). Products include:
- Celontin 1692

Paramethadione (Concurrent use requires extreme caution). Products include:
- Paradione Capsules 548

Phenobarbital (Concurrent use requires extreme caution). Products include:
- Arco-Lase Plus Tablets 607
- Bellergal-S Tablets 1998
- Bronkolixir .... ▣ 761
- Bronkotabs Tablets .... ▣ 762
- Donnatal 1858
- Donnatal Extentabs 1859
- Donnatal Tablets 1858
- Donnazyme Tablets 1860
- Kinesed Tablets 2272
- Phenobarbital Elixir and Tablets 1293
- Primatene Tablets-P Formula 2421
- Quadrinal Tablets 1183
- Tedral SA 1765

Phensuximide (Concurrent use requires extreme caution). Products include:
- Milontin Kapseals 1741

Phenytoin (Concurrent use requires extreme caution). Products include:
- Dilantin Infatabs 1710
- Dilantin-30 Pediatric/Dilantin-125 Suspension 1713

Phenytoin Sodium (Concurrent use requires extreme caution). Products include:
- Dilantin Kapseals 1708
- Dilantin Parenteral 1712
- Dilantin with Phenobarbital Kapseals 1715

Primidone (Concurrent use requires extreme caution). Products include:
- Mysoline 2480

Trimethadione (Concurrent use requires extreme caution). Products include:
- Tridione 557

Valproic Acid (Concurrent use requires extreme caution). Products include:
- Depakene Capsules & Syrup 511

PHILLIPS' LAXCAPS
(Docusate Sodium, Phenolphthalein) .... ▣ 572
No interactions described in labeling.

CONCENTRATED PHILLIPS' MILK OF MAGNESIA
(Magnesium Hydroxide) .... ▣ 573
May interact with:

Prescription Drugs, unspecified (Effect not specified).

PHILLIPS' MILK OF MAGNESIA LIQUID
(Magnesium Hydroxide) .... ▣ 572
May interact with:

Prescription Drugs, unspecified (Effect not specified).

PHILLIPS' MILK OF MAGNESIA TABLETS
(Magnesium Hydroxide) .... ▣ 573
No interactions described in labeling.

PHOSCHOL CONCENTRATE
(Phosphatidylcholine) 568
No interactions described in labeling.

PHOSCHOL 565 SOFTGELS
(Phosphatidylcholine) 568
No interactions described in labeling.

PHOSCHOL 900 SOFTGELS
(Phosphatidylcholine) 568
No interactions described in labeling.

PHOS-EX 167MG. & 250MG. (CALCIUM ACETATE)
(Calcium Acetate) 2377
No interactions described in labeling.

PHOSLO TABLETS
(Calcium Acetate) 700
May interact with cardiac glycosides, tetracyclines, and certain other agents. Compounds in these categories include:

Antacids, unspecified (Concurrent use should be avoided).

Demeclocycline Hydrochloride (Bioavailability of oral tetracyclines may be decreased). Products include:
- Declomycin Capsules, Tablets 1199

Deslanoside (Hypercalcemia may precipitate cardiac arrhythmia).
- No products indexed under this heading.

Digitoxin (Hypercalcemia may precipitate cardiac arrhythmia). Products include:
- Crystodigin Tablets 1253

Digoxin (Hypercalcemia may precipitate cardiac arrhythmia). Products include:
- Lanoxicaps 772
- Lanoxin Elixir Pediatric 775
- Lanoxin Injection 778
- Lanoxin Injection Pediatric 781
- Lanoxin Tablets 783

Doxycycline Calcium (Bioavailability of oral tetracyclines may be decreased).
- No products indexed under this heading.

Doxycycline Hyclate (Bioavailability of oral tetracyclines may be decreased). Products include:
- Doryx Capsules 1717
- Vibramycin Hyclate Capsules 1787
- Vibramycin Hyclate Intravenous 1968
- Vibra-Tabs Film Coated Tablets 1787

Doxycycline Monohydrate (Bioavailability of oral tetracyclines may be decreased). Products include:
- Monodox Capsules 1630
- Vibramycin Monohydrate for Oral Suspension 1787

Methacycline Hydrochloride (Bioavailability of oral tetracyclines may be decreased).
- No products indexed under this heading.

Minocycline Hydrochloride (Bioavailability of oral tetracyclines may be decreased). Products include:
- Minocin Intravenous 1221
- Minocin Oral Suspension 1224
- Minocin Pellet-Filled Capsules 1222

Oxytetracycline Hydrochloride (Bioavailability of oral tetracyclines may be decreased). Products include:
- Terra-Cortril Ophthalmic Suspension 1963
- Terramycin Capsules 1786
- Terramycin Intramuscular Solution 1964
- Terramycin with Polymyxin B Sulfate Ophthalmic Ointment 1965

Tetracycline Hydrochloride (Bioavailability of oral tetracyclines may be decreased). Products include:
- Achromycin V Capsules 1193
- Achromycin Ophthalmic Ointment 1% .... ⊙ 307
- Achromycin Ophthalmic Suspension 1% .... ⊙ 308
- Topicycline for Topical Solution 1856

PHOSPHOLINE IODIDE
(Echothiophate Iodide) .... ⊙ 315
May interact with:

Succinylcholine Chloride (Possible additive effects). Products include:
- Anectine 755

PHRENILIN FORTE CAPSULES
(Butalbital, Acetaminophen) 838
May interact with central nervous system depressants, hypnotics and sedatives, antihistamines, tranquilizers, oral anticoagulants, and certain other agents. Compounds in these categories include:

Alcohol (Additive depressant effect).

Alfentanil Hydrochloride (Additive depressant effect). Products include:
- Alfenta Injection 1131

Alprazolam (Additive depressant effect). Products include:
- Xanax Tablets 2367

Aprobarbital (Additive depressant effect). Products include:
- Alurate Elixir 1883

Astemizole (Additive depressant effect). Products include:
- Hismanal Tablets 1138

Azatadine Maleate (Additive depressant effect). Products include:
- Optimine Tablets 2115
- Trinalin Repetabs Tablets 1170

Bromodiphenhydramine Hydrochloride (Additive depressant effect).
- No products indexed under this heading.

Brompheniramine Maleate (Additive depressant effect). Products include:
- Alka Seltzer Plus Sinus Allergy Medicine ▣ 624
- Atrohist Sprinkle Capsules 558
- Bromfed Capsules (Timed Release) 1615
- Bromfed Syrup ▣ 628
- Bromfed 1615
- Dimetane Decongestant ▣ 673
- Dimetane ▣ 672
- Dimetane-DC Cough Syrup 1857
- Dimetane-DX Cough Syrup 1858
- Dimetapp Elixir ▣ 673
- Dimetapp DM Elixir ▣ 674
- Dimetapp Extentabs ▣ 674
- Dimetapp Plus Caplets ▣ 675
- Dimetapp Tablets ▣ 675
- Drixoral Antihistamine/Nasal Decongestant Syrup ▣ 698

Buprenorphine (Additive depressant effect).
- No products indexed under this heading.

Buspirone Hydrochloride (Additive depressant effect). Products include:
- BuSpar 1401

Butabarbital (Additive depressant effect). Products include:
- Pyridium Plus 1764

Chlordiazepoxide (Additive depressant effect). Products include:
- Libritabs Tablets 1930
- Limbitrol 1933
- Menrium Tablets 1934

Chlordiazepoxide Hydrochloride (Additive depressant effect). Products include:
- Librax Capsules 1929
- Librium Capsules 1931
- Librium Injectable 1932

Chlorpheniramine Maleate (Additive depressant effect). Products include:
- A.R.M. Allergy Relief Medicine Caplets ▣ 615
- Alka-Seltzer Plus Cold Medicine ▣ 623
- Allerest ▣ 559
- Ana-Kit Anaphylaxis Emergency Treatment Kit 1100
- BC Cold Powder Multi-Symptom Formula ▣ 517
- Brexin L.A. Capsules 2078
- Cerose-DM 2443
- Cheracol Plus Head Cold/Cough Formula ▣ 667
- Chlor-Trimeton Allergy Syrup, Tablets & Long-Acting Repetabs Tablets ▣ 693
- Chlor-Trimeton Decongestant ▣ 694
- Comhist LA Capsules 1618
- Allergy-Sinus Comtrex Multi-Symptom Allergy Sinus Formula Tablets & Caplets 746
- Comtrex Multi-Symptom Cold Reliever Tablets/Caplets/Liqui-Gels/Liquid 745
- Day-Night Comtrex 747
- Contac Continuous Action Decongestant/Antihistamine Capsules ▣ 710
- Contac Maximum Strength Continuous Action Decongestant/Antihistamine Caplets ▣ 709
- Contac Severe Cold and Flu Formula Caplets ▣ 711
- Coricidin 'D' Decongestant Tablets ▣ 695
- Coricidin Demilets Tablets for Children ▣ 696
- Coricidin Tablets ▣ 695
- Deconamine 663
- Demazin Nasal Decongestant/Antihistamine Repetabs Tablets & Syrup ▣ 697
- Dorcol Children's Liquid Cold Formula ▣ 686
- Dristan Decongestant/Antihistamine/Analgesic Coated Caplets ▣ 749
- Dristan Cold Nasal Decongestant/Antihistamine/Analgesic Coated Tablets 2419
- Dristan Advanced Formula Decongestant/Antihistamine/Analgesic Tablets ▣ 749
- Extendryl 994
- 4-Way Cold Tablets 750
- Fedahist Gyrocaps 2145
- Fedahist Timecaps 2145
- Hycomine Compound Tablets 929
- Isoclor Timesule Capsules ▣ 561
- Kronofed-A 970
- Medi-Flu Caplet, Liquid ▣ 640
- Naldecon Syrup, Tablets, Pediatric Drops and Pediatric Syrup 709
- Nolamine Tablets 838
- Novafed A Capsules 1342
- Novahistine DH 1342
- Novahistine Elixir ▣ 596
- Ornade Spansule Capsules 2221
- Orthoxicol Cough Syrup ▣ 668
- PediaCare Allergy Relief Formula Liquid 1362
- PediaCare Cough-Cold Formula Liquid 1362
- PediaCare Night Rest Cough-Cold Formula Liquid 1362
- PediaCare 6-12 Cough-Cold Formula Chewable Tablets 1362
- Pyrroxate Capsules ▣ 669
- Quelidrine Syrup 556
- Ru-Tuss II Capsules 693
- Ru-Tuss Tablets 693
- Ryna ▣ 741
- Sinarest Tablets & Extra Strength Tablets ▣ 562
- Sine-Off Maximum Strength Allergy/Sinus Formula Caplets ▣ 721
- Sine-Off Sinus Medicine Tablets-Aspirin Formula ▣ 722
- Singlet Tablets ▣ 598
- Sinulin 840
- Sinutab Maximum Strength ▣ 641
- St. Joseph Nighttime Cold Medicine ▣ 705
- Sudafed Plus Liquid ▣ 544
- Sudafed Plus Tablets ▣ 545
- Teldrin Timed-Release Allergy Capsules, 12 mg 2192
- TheraFlu Flu and Cold Medicine ▣ 687
- Triaminic Allergy Tablets ▣ 688
- Triaminic Chewables ▣ 688
- Triaminic Cold Tablets ▣ 688
- Triaminic Nite Light ▣ 689
- Triaminic Syrup ▣ 689
- Triaminic-12 Tablets ▣ 690
- Triaminicin Tablets ▣ 690
- Triaminicol Multi-Symptom Cold Tablets ▣ 691
- Triaminicol Multi-Symptom Relief ▣ 691
- Tylenol Allergy Sinus Medication Caplets and Gelcaps, Maximum Strength 1372
- Children's Tylenol Cold Liquid Formula and Chewable Tablets 1368
- Tylenol Cold & Flu Hot Medication, Packets 1369
- Tylenol Cold Medication Caplets and Tablets 1370
- Tylenol Cold Medication, Effervescent Tablets 1369
- Vicks Children's NyQuil ▣ 664
- Vicks Formula 44 Cough Medicine ▣ 661
- Vicks Formula 44M Multi-Symptom Cough Medicine ▣ 662
- Vicks Pediatric Formula 44m Multi-Symptom Cough & Cold Medicine ▣ 663

Chlorpheniramine Polistirex (Additive depressant effect). Products include:
- Tussionex Extended-Release Suspension 988

Chlorpheniramine Tannate (Additive depressant effect). Products include:
- Rynatan 2387
- Rynatuss 2388

Chlorpromazine (Additive depressant effect). Products include:
- Thorazine 2234

Chlorprothixene (Additive depressant effect). Products include:
- Taractan Tablets 1920

Chlorprothixene Hydrochloride (Additive depressant effect). Products include:
- Taractan 1920

Clemastine Fumarate (Additive depressant effect). Products include:
- Tavist Syrup 2033
- Tavist Tablets 2035
- Tavist-D Tablets 2035

Clomipramine Hydrochloride (Additive depressant effect). Products include:
- Anafranil Capsules 650

Clorazepate Dipotassium (Additive depressant effect). Products include:
- Tranxene 556

Codeine (Additive depressant effect). Products include:
- Calcidrine Syrup 506

Codeine Phosphate (Additive depressant effect). Products include:
- Actifed with Codeine Cough Syrup 752
- Cheracol Cough Syrup 1853
- Codimal PH Syrup 846
- Dimetane-DC Cough Syrup 1857
- Empirin with Codeine Phosphate Nos. 2, 3 & 4 764
- Fioricet with Codeine Capsules 2008
- Isoclor Expectorant 982
- Naldecon CX Adult Liquid ▣ 521
- Novahistine DH 1342
- Novahistine Expectorant 1343
- Nucofed Capsules 2219
- Nucofed Expectorant 2219
- Nucofed Pediatric Expectorant 2220
- Nucofed Syrup 2219
- Phenaphen with Codeine Capsules 1865
- Phenaphen-650 with Codeine Tablets 1866
- Phenergan with Codeine 2497
- Phenergan VC with Codeine 2501
- Robitussin A-C Syrup 1875
- Robitussin-DAC Syrup 1875
- Ryna ▣ 741
- Soma Compound w/Codeine Tablets 2390
- Triaminic Expectorant w/Codeine 1996
- Tussi-Organidin Liquid 2391
- Tylenol with Codeine 1381

Codeine Polistirex (Additive depressant effect).
- No products indexed under this heading.

Cyproheptadine Hydrochloride (Additive depressant effect). Products include:
- Periactin 1525

Dexchlorpheniramine Maleate (Additive depressant effect). Products include:
- Polaramine 2116

Dezocine (Additive depressant effect).

Diazepam (Additive depressant effect). Products include:
- Valium Injectable 1937
- Valium Tablets 1939
- Valrelease Capsules 1923

Dicumarol (Decreased anticoagulant effect). Products include:
- Dicumarol Tablets 516

Diphenhydramine Citrate (Additive depressant effect). Products include:
- Alka-Seltzer Plus Night-Time Cold Medicine ▣ 623
- Bufferin AF Nite Time Analgesic/Sleeping Aid Caplets 744
- Excedrin P.M. Analgesic/Sleeping Aid Tablets, Caplets and Liquid 749

Diphenhydramine Hydrochloride (Additive depressant effect). Products include:
- Benadryl Anti-Itch Cream ▣ 635
- Benadryl Capsules 1691
- Benadryl Decongestant Elixir ▣ 635
- Benadryl Decongestant ▣ 635
- Benadryl Elixir ▣ 636
- Benadryl Kapseals 1691
- Benadryl 25 Kapseals ▣ 636
- Benadryl Parenteral 1692
- Benadryl Plus ▣ 636
- Benadryl Plus Nighttime ▣ 637
- Benadryl Spray, Maximum Strength ▣ 637
- Benadryl Spray, Regular Strength ▣ 637
- Benadryl Steri-Vials, Ampoules, and Steri-Dose Syringe 1692
- Benadryl 25 Tablets ▣ 636
- Benylin Cough Syrup ▣ 637
- Benylin Decongestant ▣ 638
- Caladryl Cream, Lotion, Spray ▣ 638
- Miles Nervine Nighttime Sleep-Aid ▣ 627
- Nytol Tablets ▣ 517
- Sleep-ettes-D Tablets ▣ 653
- Sleep-eze 3 Tablets ▣ 755
- Sleepinal Night-time Sleep Aid Capsules ▣ 734
- Sominex Caplets and Tablets ▣ 722
- Sominex Liquid ▣ 723
- Sominex Pain Relief Formula ▣ 723
- Tylenol Cold Night Time Medication Liquid 1371
- Tylenol PM, Extra Strength Caplets and Tablets 1368
- Unisom Dual Relief Nighttime Sleep Aid/Analgesic 1774
- Ziradryl Lotion ▣ 643

Diphenylpyraline Hydrochloride (Additive depressant effect).
- No products indexed under this heading.

Droperidol (Additive depressant effect). Products include:
- Inapsine Injection 1140
- Innovar Injection 1141

Enflurane (Additive depressant effect). Products include:
- Ethrane 599

Estazolam (Additive depressant effect). Products include:
- ProSom Tablets 554

Ethchlorvynol (Additive depressant effect). Products include:
- Placidyl Capsules 553

Ethinamate (Additive depressant effect).
- No products indexed under this heading.

Fentanyl (Additive depressant effect). Products include:
- Duragesic Transdermal System 1133

Fentanyl Citrate (Additive depressant effect). Products include:
- Innovar Injection 1141
- Sublimaze Injection 1146

Fluphenazine Decanoate (Additive depressant effect). Products include:
- Prolixin Decanoate 1795

Fluphenazine Enanthate (Additive depressant effect). Products include:
- Prolixin Enanthate 1796

Fluphenazine Hydrochloride (Additive depressant effect). Products include:
- Prolixin Elixir 1793
- Prolixin Injection 1791
- Prolixin Oral Concentrate 1792
- Prolixin Tablets 1793

Flurazepam Hydrochloride (Additive depressant effect). Products include:
- Dalmane Capsules 1927

Glutethimide (Additive depressant effect).
- No products indexed under this heading.

Haloperidol (Additive depressant effect). Products include:
- Haldol Injection, Tablets and Concentrate 1373

Haloperidol Decanoate (Additive depressant effect). Products include:
- Haldol Decanoate 1375

Hydrocodone Bitartrate (Additive depressant effect). Products include:
- Anexsia 5/500 Tablets 2196
- Anexsia 7.5/650 Tablets 2197
- Azdone Tablets 844
- Codiclear DH Syrup 845
- Codimal DH Syrup 846
- Damason-P 1356
- Hycodan Syrup, Tablets 927
- Hycomine Compound Tablets 929
- Hycomine Syrup 927
- Hycotuss Expectorant Syrup 930
- Hydrocet Capsules 835
- Lortab ASA Tablets 2414
- Lortab 2412
- Ru-Tuss with Hydrocodone 694

Triaminic Expectorant DH 1995
Vicodin Tablets 1187
Vicodin ES Tablets 1189
Zydone Capsules 941

Hydrocodone Polistirex (Additive depressant effect). Products include:
Tussionex Extended-Release Suspension 988

Hydroxyzine Hydrochloride (Additive depressant effect). Products include:
Atarax Tablets & Syrup 1941
Marax Tablets & DF Syrup 1954
Vistaril Intramuscular Solution 1970

Isoflurane (Additive depressant effect). Products include:
Forane 600

Ketamine Hydrochloride (Additive depressant effect). Products include:
Ketalar 1726

Levorphanol Tartrate (Additive depressant effect). Products include:
Levo-Dromoran 1906

Lorazepam (Additive depressant effect). Products include:
Ativan Injection 2432
Ativan Tablets 2434

Loxapine Hydrochloride (Additive depressant effect). Products include:
Loxitane 1213

Loxapine Succinate (Additive depressant effect). Products include:
Loxitane Capsules 1213

Meperidine Hydrochloride (Additive depressant effect). Products include:
Demerol 2047
Mepergan Injection 2479

Mephobarbital (Additive depressant effect). Products include:
Mebaral Tablets 2061

Meprobamate (Additive depressant effect). Products include:
Deprol Tablets 2382
Equagesic Tablets 2451
Miltown Tablets 2386
PMB 200 and PMB 400 2504

Mesoridazine (Additive depressant effect). Products include:
Serentil 686

Methadone Hydrochloride (Additive depressant effect). Products include:
Dolophine Hydrochloride Ampoules & Vials 1260
Dolophine Hydrochloride Tablets 1261
Methadone Hydrochloride Diskets 1284
Methadone Hydrochloride Oral Solution & Tablets 1987

Methdilazine Hydrochloride (Additive depressant effect). Products include:
Tacaryl Syrup & Tablets 2409

Methohexital Sodium (Additive depressant effect). Products include:
Brevital Sodium Vials 1248

Methoxyflurane (Additive depressant effect).
No products indexed under this heading.

Midazolam Hydrochloride (Additive depressant effect). Products include:
Versed Injection 1924

Molindone Hydrochloride (Additive depressant effect). Products include:
Moban Tablets & Concentrate 932

Morphine Sulfate (Additive depressant effect). Products include:
Astramorph/PF Injection, USP (Preservative-Free) 618
Duramorph 960
Infumorph 200 and Infumorph 500 Sterile Solutions 962
MS Contin Tablets 1814
MSIR 1817
Oramorph SR (Morphine Sulfate Sustained Release Tablets) 1988
Roxanol 1991

Opium Alkaloids (Additive depressant effect). Products include:
B & O No. 15A & No. 16A Supprettes 2395
Pantopon Injectable 1911

Oxazepam (Additive depressant effect). Products include:
Serax Capsules 2522
Serax Tablets 2522

Oxycodone Hydrochloride (Additive depressant effect). Products include:
Percocet Tablets 950
Percodan 951
Roxicodone Tablets, Oral Solution & Intensol (Oxycodone) 1992
Tylox Capsules 1382

Pentobarbital Sodium (Additive depressant effect). Products include:
Nembutal Sodium Capsules 534
Nembutal Sodium Solution 536
Nembutal Sodium Suppositories 538

Perphenazine (Additive depressant effect). Products include:
Etrafon 2087
Triavil Tablets 1556
Trilafon 2123

Phenobarbital (Additive depressant effect). Products include:
Arco-Lase Plus Tablets 607
Bellergal-S Tablets 1998
Bronkolixir .... ▣ 761
Bronkotabs Tablets .... ▣ 762
Donnatal 1858
Donnatal Extentabs 1859
Donnatal Tablets 1858
Donnazyme Tablets 1860
Kinesed Tablets 2272
Phenobarbital Elixir and Tablets 1293
Primatene Tablets-P Formula 2421
Quadrinal Tablets 1183
Tedral SA 1765

Prazepam (Additive depressant effect). Products include:
Centrax 1693

Prochlorperazine (Additive depressant effect). Products include:
Compazine 2201

Promethazine Hydrochloride (Additive depressant effect). Products include:
Mepergan Injection 2479
Phenergan with Codeine 2497
Phenergan with Dextromethorphan 2499
Phenergan Injection 2493
Phenergan Suppositories 2496
Phenergan Syrup 2495
Phenergan Tablets 2496
Phenergan VC 2500
Phenergan VC with Codeine 2501

Propofol (Additive depressant effect). Products include:
Diprivan Injection 2267

Propoxyphene Hydrochloride (Additive depressant effect). Products include:
Darvon 1256
Wygesic Tablets 2540

Propoxyphene Napsylate (Additive depressant effect). Products include:
Darvon-N/Darvocet-N 1254

Pyrilamine Maleate (Additive depressant effect). Products include:
Codimal 846
4-Way Fast Acting Nasal Spray - Original Formula (regular & mentholated) & Metered Spray Pump (regular) 751
Maximum Strength Midol Multi-Symptom Menstrual Formula .... ▣ 571
Maximum Strength Midol PMS Premenstrual Syndrome Formula .... ▣ 570
Regular Strength Midol Multi-Symptom Menstrual Formula .... ▣ 570
Prefrin-A .... ⊙ 255
Prēmsyn PMS Capsules & Caplets ▣ 547
Primatene Tablets-M Formula 2421
Robitussin Night Relief .... ▣ 677
Ru-Tuss with Hydrocodone 694
Triaminic Expectorant DH 1995
Triaminic Oral Infant Drops 1996

Pyrilamine Tannate (Additive depressant effect). Products include:
Rynatan 2387

Quazepam (Additive depressant effect). Products include:
Doral Tablets 2383

Secobarbital Sodium (Additive depressant effect). Products include:
Seconal Sodium Pulvules 1296

Sufentanil Citrate (Additive depressant effect). Products include:
Sufenta Injection 1147

Temazepam (Additive depressant effect). Products include:
Restoril Capsules 2023

Terfenadine (Additive depressant effect). Products include:
Seldane Tablets 1349
Seldane-D Extended-Release Tablets 1350

Thiamylal Sodium (Additive depressant effect). Products include:
Surital Ampoules, Steri-Vials 1764

Thioridazine Hydrochloride (Additive depressant effect). Products include:
Mellaril 2011

Thiothixene (Additive depressant effect). Products include:
Navane Capsules and Concentrate 1954
Navane Intramuscular 1956

Triazolam (Additive depressant effect). Products include:
Halcion Tablets 2340

Trifluoperazine Hydrochloride (Additive depressant effect). Products include:
Stelazine 2226

Trimeprazine Tartrate (Additive depressant effect). Products include:
Temaril Tablets, Syrup and Spansule Sustained Release Capsules 1085

Tripelennamine Hydrochloride (Additive depressant effect). Products include:
PBZ Tablets & Elixir 1037
PBZ-SR Tablets 1037

Triprolidine Hydrochloride (Additive depressant effect). Products include:
Actidil .... ▣ 538
Actifed Capsules .... ▣ 539
Actifed Plus Caplets .... ▣ 539
Actifed Plus Tablets .... ▣ 540
Actifed with Codeine Cough Syrup 752
Actifed Syrup .... ▣ 540
Actifed Tablets .... ▣ 540
Actifed 12-Hour Capsules .... ▣ 539

Warfarin Sodium (Decreased anticoagulant effect). Products include:
Coumadin Injection & Tablets 944
Panwarfin Tablets 547

PHRENILIN TABLETS
(Butalbital, Acetaminophen) 838
See **Phrenilin Forte Capsules**

PILAGAN LIQUIFILM STERILE OPHTHALMIC SOLUTION
(Pilocarpine Nitrate) .... ⊙ 250
No interactions described in labeling.

PILAGAN LIQUIFILM STERILE OPHTHALMIC SOLUTION WITH C CAP COMPLIANCE CAP
(Pilocarpine Nitrate) .... ⊙ 250
No interactions described in labeling.

PILOCAR
(Pilocarpine Hydrochloride) .... ⊙ 275
No interactions described in labeling.

PILOCAR TWIN PACK
(Pilocarpine Hydrochloride) .... ⊙ 275
No interactions described in labeling.

PILOPINE HS GEL
(Pilocarpine Hydrochloride) .... ⊙ 227
No interactions described in labeling.

PILOSTAT STERILE OPHTHALMIC SOLUTION 0.5%, 1%, 2%, 3%, 4%, 5%, 6%
(Pilocarpine Hydrochloride) .... ⊙ 263
No interactions described in labeling.

PIMA SYRUP
(Potassium Iodide) 994
No interactions described in labeling.

PIPRACIL
(Piperacillin Sodium) 1230
May interact with aminoglycosides and certain other agents. Compounds in these categories include:

Amikacin Sulfate (Substantial inactivation of aminoglycosides *in vitro*). Products include:
Amikin Injectable 602

Gentamicin Sulfate (Substantial inactivation of aminoglycosides *in vitro*). Products include:
Garamycin Injectable 2093
Garamycin Ophthalmic .... ⊙ 305
Genoptic Liquifilm Sterile Ophthalmic Solution .... ⊙ 247
Genoptic S.O.P. Sterile Ophthalmic Ointment .... ⊙ 247
Gentacidin Ointment .... ⊙ 273
Gentacidin Solution .... ⊙ 273
Gentak Ointment & Solution .... ⊙ 208
G-myticin Creme and Ointment 0.1% 1770
Pred-G Liquifilm Sterile Ophthalmic Suspension .... ⊙ 252
Pred-G S.O.P. Sterile Ophthalmic Ointment .... ⊙ 253

Kanamycin Sulfate (Substantial inactivation of aminoglycosides *in vitro*). Products include:
Kantrex Injection 601
Kantrex Pediatric Injection 601

Probenecid (Increases peak serum level and area under the curve). Products include:
Benemid Tablets 1426
ColBENEMID Tablets 1436
Wycillin Injection and Probenecid Tablets 2539

Streptomycin Sulfate (Substantial inactivation of aminoglycosides *in vitro*).
No products indexed under this heading.

Tobramycin Sulfate (Substantial inactivation of aminoglycosides *in vitro*). Products include:
Nebcin Vials, Hyporets & ADD-Vantage 1286

PITOCIN INJECTION, AMPOULES, STERI-DOSE SYRINGES
(Oxytocin (Injection)) 1757
May interact with:

Bupivacaine Hydrochloride (Severe hypertension reported when vasoconstrictor was given prior to oxytocin). Products include:
Marcaine Hydrochloride 0.5% with Epinephrine 1:200,000 (as bitartrate) 958
Marcaine Hydrochloride with Epinephrine 1:200,000 2055
Marcaine Hydrochloride Injection 2055
Marcaine Spinal 2058
Sensorcaine 631
Sensorcaine-MPF Spinal 634

Chloroprocaine Hydrochloride (Severe hypertension reported when vasoconstrictor was given prior to oxytocin). Products include:
Nescaine/Nescaine MPF 629

Cyclopropane (May modify oxytocin's cardiovascular effects).

Etidocaine Hydrochloride (Severe hypertension reported when vasoconstrictor was given prior to oxytocin). Products include:
Duranest Injections 624

Mepivacaine Hydrochloride Injection (Severe hypertension reported when a vasoconstrictor was given prior to oxytocin). Products include:
Carbocaine Hydrochloride 3% Injection 956
Carbocaine Hydrochloride Injection 2043
Carbocaine Hydrochloride 2% with Neo-Cobefrin 956

PITRESSIN SYNTHETIC, AMPOULES
(Vasopressin) 1758
May interact with tricyclic antidepressants, lithium preparations, ganglionic blocking agents, and certain other agents. Compounds in these categories include:

Alcohol (Decreased antidiuretic effect of vasopressin).

Amitriptyline Hydrochloride (Potentiation of antidiuretic effect of vasopressin). Products include:
Elavil 2269
Endep Tablets 1927
Etrafon 2087
Limbitrol 1933
Triavil Tablets 1556

Amoxapine (Potentiation of antidiuretic effect of vasopressin). Products include:
Asendin Tablets 1196

Carbamazepine (Potentiation of antidiuretic effect of vasopressin). Products include:
Tegretol Chewable Tablets 654
Tegretol Suspension 656
Tegretol Tablets 654

Chlorpropamide (Potentiation of antidiuretic effect of vasopressin). Products include:
Diabinese Tablets 1775

Clofibrate (Potentiation of antidiuretic effect of vasopressin). Products include:
Atromid-S Capsules 2435

Clomipramine Hydrochloride (Potentiation of antidiuretic effect of vasopressin). Products include:
Anafranil Capsules 650

Demeclocycline Hydrochloride (Decreased antidiuretic effect of vasopressin). Products include:
Declomycin Capsules, Tablets 1199

Desipramine Hydrochloride (Potentiation of antidiuretic effect of vasopressin). Products include:
Norpramin Tablets 1340

Doxepin Hydrochloride (Potentiation of antidiuretic effect of vasopressin). Products include:
Sinequan 1960

Heparin Calcium (Decreased antidiuretic effect of vasopressin). Products include:
Calciparine Injection 925

Heparin Sodium (Decreased antidiuretic effect of vasopressin). Products include:
Heparin Lock Flush Solution 2456
Heparin Sodium Vials 1264
Heparin Sodium Injection 2457
Heparin Sodium Injection, USP, Sterile Solution 2342

Imipramine Hydrochloride (Potentiation of antidiuretic effect of vasopressin). Products include:
Tofranil Ampuls 1038
Tofranil Tablets 1039

Imipramine Pamoate (Potentiation of antidiuretic effect of vasopressin). Products include:
Tofranil-PM Capsules 1041

Lithium Carbonate (Decreased antidiuretic effect of vasopressin). Products include:
Eskalith 2214
Lithane Tablets 1596
Lithium Carbonate Capsules & Tablets 1984
Lithobid Tablets 870

Lithium Citrate (Decreased antidiuretic effect of vasopressin). Products include:
Cibalith-S 870

Maprotiline Hydrochloride (Potentiation of antidiuretic effect of vasopressin). Products include:
Ludiomil Tablets 874

Mecamylamine Hydrochloride (Increased sensitivity to the pressor effects of vasopressin). Products include:
Inversine Tablets 1492

Norepinephrine Bitartrate (Decreased antidiuretic effect of vasopressin). Products include:
Levophed Bitartrate Injection 2054

Nortriptyline Hydrochloride (Potentiation of antidiuretic effect of vasopressin). Products include:
Pamelor 2019

Protriptyline Hydrochloride (Potentiation of antidiuretic effect of vasopressin). Products include:
Vivactil Tablets 1567

Trimethaphan Camsylate (Increased sensitivity to the pressor effects of vasopressin). Products include:
Arfonad Ampuls 1887

Trimipramine Maleate (Potentiation of antidiuretic effect of vasopressin). Products include:
Surmontil Capsules 2524

PLACIDYL CAPSULES
(Ethchlorvynol) 553
May interact with central nervous system depressants, monoamine oxidase inhibitors, oral anticoagulants, and tricyclic antidepressants. Compounds in these categories include:

Alfentanil Hydrochloride (Exaggerated depressant effects). Products include:
Alfenta Injection 1131

Alprazolam (Exaggerated depressant effects). Products include:
Xanax Tablets 2367

Amitriptyline Hydrochloride (Transient delirium). Products include:
Elavil 2269
Endep Tablets 1927
Etrafon 2087
Limbitrol 1933
Triavil Tablets 1556

Amoxapine (Transient delirium). Products include:
Asendin Tablets 1196

Aprobarbital (Exaggerated depressant effects). Products include:
Alurate Elixir 1883

Buprenorphine (Exaggerated depressant effects).
No products indexed under this heading.

Buspirone Hydrochloride (Exaggerated depressant effects). Products include:
BuSpar 1401

Butabarbital (Exaggerated depressant effects). Products include:
Pyridium Plus 1764

Butalbital (Exaggerated depressant effects). Products include:
Esgic-Plus Tablets 1002
Esgic Tablets & Capsules 1001
Fioricet Tablets 2006
Fiorinal Capsules 2007
Fiorinal with Codeine Capsules 2008
Fiorinal Tablets 2007
Phrenilin 838
Sedapap Tablets 50 mg/650 mg .. 1360

Chlordiazepoxide (Exaggerated depressant effects). Products include:
Libritabs Tablets 1930
Limbitrol 1933
Menrium Tablets 1934

Chlordiazepoxide Hydrochloride (Exaggerated depressant effects). Products include:
Librax Capsules 1929
Librium Capsules 1931
Librium Injectable 1932

Chlorpromazine (Exaggerated depressant effects). Products include:
Thorazine 2234

Chlorprothixene (Exaggerated depressant effects). Products include:
Taractan Tablets 1920

Chlorprothixene Hydrochloride (Exaggerated depressant effects). Products include:
Taractan 1920

Clomipramine Hydrochloride (Transient delirium). Products include:
Anafranil Capsules 650

Clorazepate Dipotassium (Exaggerated depressant effects). Products include:
Tranxene 556

Codeine (Exaggerated depressant effects). Products include:
Calcidrine Syrup 506

Codeine Phosphate (Exaggerated depressant effects). Products include:
Actifed with Codeine Cough Syrup.. 752
Cheracol Cough Syrup 1853
Codimal PH Syrup 846
Dimetane-DC Cough Syrup 1857
Empirin with Codeine Phosphate Nos. 2, 3 & 4 764
Fiorinal with Codeine Capsules 2008
Isoclor Expectorant 982
Naldecon CX Adult Liquid ..... ⊞ 521
Novahistine DH 1342
Novahistine Expectorant 1343
Nucofed Capsules 2219
Nucofed Expectorant 2219
Nucofed Pediatric Expectorant 2220
Nucofed Syrup 2219
Phenaphen with Codeine Capsules 1865
Phenaphen-650 with Codeine Tablets 1866
Phenergan with Codeine 2497
Phenergan VC with Codeine 2501
Robitussin A-C Syrup 1875
Robitussin-DAC Syrup 1875
Ryna ..... ⊞ 741
Soma Compound w/Codeine Tablets 2390
Triaminic Expectorant w/Codeine .. 1996
Tussi-Organidin Liquid 2391
Tylenol with Codeine 1381

Codeine Polistirex (Exaggerated depressant effects).
No products indexed under this heading.

Desipramine Hydrochloride (Transient delirium). Products include:
Norpramin Tablets 1340

Dezocine (Exaggerated depressant effects).

Diazepam (Exaggerated depressant effects). Products include:
Valium Injectable 1937
Valium Tablets 1939
Valrelease Capsules 1923

Dicumarol (Decreased prothrombin time response). Products include:
Dicumarol Tablets 516

Doxepin Hydrochloride (Transient delirium). Products include:
Sinequan 1960

Droperidol (Exaggerated depressant effects). Products include:
Inapsine Injection 1140
Innovar Injection 1141

Enflurane (Exaggerated depressant effects). Products include:
Ethrane 599

Estazolam (Exaggerated depressant effects). Products include:
ProSom Tablets 554

Ethinamate (Exaggerated depressant effects).
No products indexed under this heading.

Fentanyl (Exaggerated depressant effects). Products include:
Duragesic Transdermal System 1133

Fentanyl Citrate (Exaggerated depressant effects). Products include:
Innovar Injection 1141
Sublimaze Injection 1146

Fluphenazine Decanoate (Exaggerated depressant effects). Products include:
Prolixin Decanoate 1795

Fluphenazine Enanthate (Exaggerated depressant effects). Products include:
Prolixin Enanthate 1796

Fluphenazine Hydrochloride (Exaggerated depressant effects). Products include:
Prolixin Elixir 1793
Prolixin Injection 1791
Prolixin Oral Concentrate 1792
Prolixin Tablets 1793

Flurazepam Hydrochloride (Exaggerated depressant effects). Products include:
Dalmane Capsules 1927

Furazolidone (Exaggerated depressant effects). Products include:
Furoxone 1855

Glutethimide (Exaggerated depressant effects).
No products indexed under this heading.

Haloperidol (Exaggerated depressant effects). Products include:
Haldol Injection, Tablets and Concentrate 1373

Haloperidol Decanoate (Exaggerated depressant effects). Products include:
Haldol Decanoate 1375

Hydrocodone Bitartrate (Exaggerated depressant effects). Products include:
Anexsia 5/500 Tablets 2196
Anexsia 7.5/650 Tablets 2197
Azdone Tablets 844
Codiclear DH Syrup 845
Codimal DH Syrup 846
Damason-P 1356
Hycodan Syrup, Tablets 927
Hycomine Compound Tablets 929
Hycomine Syrup 927
Hycotuss Expectorant Syrup 930
Hydrocet Capsules 835
Lortab ASA Tablets 2414
Lortab 2412
Ru-Tuss with Hydrocodone 694
Triaminic Expectorant DH 1995
Vicodin Tablets 1187
Vicodin ES Tablets 1189

Zydone Capsules ... 941

Hydrocodone Polistirex (Exaggerated depressant effects). Products include:

Tussionex Extended-Release Suspension ... 988

Hydroxyzine Hydrochloride (Exaggerated depressant effects). Products include:

Atarax Tablets & Syrup ... 1941
Marax Tablets & DF Syrup ... 1954
Vistaril Intramuscular Solution ... 1970

Imipramine Hydrochloride (Transient delirium). Products include:

Tofranil Ampuls ... 1038
Tofranil Tablets ... 1039

Imipramine Pamoate (Transient delirium). Products include:

Tofranil-PM Capsules ... 1041

Isocarboxazid (Exaggerated depressant effects). Products include:

Marplan Tablets ... 1906

Isoflurane (Exaggerated depressant effects). Products include:

Forane ... 600

Ketamine Hydrochloride (Exaggerated depressant effects). Products include:

Ketalar ... 1726

Levorphanol Tartrate (Exaggerated depressant effects). Products include:

Levo-Dromoran ... 1906

Lorazepam (Exaggerated depressant effects). Products include:

Ativan Injection ... 2432
Ativan Tablets ... 2434

Loxapine Hydrochloride (Exaggerated depressant effects). Products include:

Loxitane ... 1213

Loxapine Succinate (Exaggerated depressant effects). Products include:

Loxitane Capsules ... 1213

Maprotiline Hydrochloride (Transient delirium). Products include:

Ludiomil Tablets ... 874

Meperidine Hydrochloride (Exaggerated depressant effects). Products include:

Demerol ... 2047
Mepergan Injection ... 2479

Mephobarbital (Exaggerated depressant effects). Products include:

Mebaral Tablets ... 2061

Meprobamate (Exaggerated depressant effects). Products include:

Deprol Tablets ... 2382
Equagesic Tablets ... 2451
Miltown Tablets ... 2386
PMB 200 and PMB 400 ... 2504

Mesoridazine (Exaggerated depressant effects). Products include:

Serentil ... 686

Methadone Hydrochloride (Exaggerated depressant effects). Products include:

Dolophine Hydrochloride Ampoules & Vials ... 1260
Dolophine Hydrochloride Tablets ... 1261
Methadone Hydrochloride Diskets ... 1284
Methadone Hydrochloride Oral Solution & Tablets ... 1987

Methohexital Sodium (Exaggerated depressant effects). Products include:

Brevital Sodium Vials ... 1248

Methoxyflurane (Exaggerated depressant effects).

No products indexed under this heading.

Midazolam Hydrochloride (Exaggerated depressant effects). Products include:

Versed Injection ... 1924

Molindone Hydrochloride (Exaggerated depressant effects). Products include:

Moban Tablets & Concentrate ... 932

Morphine Sulfate (Exaggerated depressant effects). Products include:

Astramorph/PF Injection, USP (Preservative-Free) ... 618
Duramorph ... 960
Infumorph 200 and Infumorph 500 Sterile Solutions ... 962
MS Contin Tablets ... 1814
MSIR ... 1817
Oramorph SR (Morphine Sulfate Sustained Release Tablets) ... 1988
Roxanol ... 1991

Nortriptyline Hydrochloride (Transient delirium). Products include:

Pamelor ... 2019

Opium Alkaloids (Exaggerated depressant effects). Products include:

B & O No. 15A & No. 16A Supprettes ... 2395
Pantopon Injectable ... 1911

Oxazepam (Exaggerated depressant effects). Products include:

Serax Capsules ... 2522
Serax Tablets ... 2522

Oxycodone Hydrochloride (Exaggerated depressant effects). Products include:

Percocet Tablets ... 950
Percodan ... 951
Roxicodone Tablets, Oral Solution & Intensol (Oxycodone) ... 1992
Tylox Capsules ... 1382

Pentobarbital Sodium (Exaggerated depressant effects). Products include:

Nembutal Sodium Capsules ... 534
Nembutal Sodium Solution ... 536
Nembutal Sodium Suppositories ... 538

Perphenazine (Exaggerated depressant effects). Products include:

Etrafon ... 2087
Triavil Tablets ... 1556
Trilafon ... 2123

Phenelzine Sulfate (Exaggerated depressant effects). Products include:

Nardil ... 1742

Phenobarbital (Exaggerated depressant effects). Products include:

Arco-Lase Plus Tablets ... 607
Bellergal-S Tablets ... 1998
Bronkolixir ... ⊞ 761
Bronkotabs Tablets ... ⊞ 762
Donnatal ... 1858
Donnatal Extentabs ... 1859
Donnatal Tablets ... 1858
Donnazyme Tablets ... 1860
Kinesed Tablets ... 2272
Phenobarbital Elixir and Tablets ... 1293
Primatene Tablets-P Formula ... 2421
Quadrinal Tablets ... 1183
Tedral SA ... 1765

Prazepam (Exaggerated depressant effects). Products include:

Centrax ... 1693

Prochlorperazine (Exaggerated depressant effects). Products include:

Compazine ... 2201

Promethazine Hydrochloride (Exaggerated depressant effects). Products include:

Mepergan Injection ... 2479
Phenergan with Codeine ... 2497
Phenergan with Dextromethorphan ... 2499
Phenergan Injection ... 2493
Phenergan Suppositories ... 2496
Phenergan Syrup ... 2495
Phenergan Tablets ... 2496
Phenergan VC ... 2500
Phenergan VC with Codeine ... 2501

Propofol (Exaggerated depressant effects). Products include:

Diprivan Injection ... 2267

Propoxyphene Hydrochloride (Exaggerated depressant effects). Products include:

Darvon ... 1256
Wygesic Tablets ... 2540

Propoxyphene Napsylate (Exaggerated depressant effects). Products include:

Darvon-N/Darvocet-N ... 1254

Protriptyline Hydrochloride (Transient delirium). Products include:

Vivactil Tablets ... 1567

Quazepam (Exaggerated depressant effects). Products include:

Doral Tablets ... 2383

Secobarbital Sodium (Exaggerated depressant effects). Products include:

Seconal Sodium Pulvules ... 1296

Selegiline Hydrochloride (Exaggerated depressant effects). Products include:

Eldepryl ... 2250

Sufentanil Citrate (Exaggerated depressant effects). Products include:

Sufenta Injection ... 1147

Temazepam (Exaggerated depressant effects). Products include:

Restoril Capsules ... 2023

Thiamylal Sodium (Exaggerated depressant effects). Products include:

Surital Ampoules, Steri-Vials ... 1764

Thioridazine Hydrochloride (Exaggerated depressant effects). Products include:

Mellaril ... 2011

Thiothixene (Exaggerated depressant effects). Products include:

Navane Capsules and Concentrate 1954
Navane Intramuscular ... 1956

Tranylcypromine Sulfate (Exaggerated depressant effects). Products include:

Parnate Tablets ... 2222

Triazolam (Exaggerated depressant effects). Products include:

Halcion Tablets ... 2340

Trifluoperazine Hydrochloride (Exaggerated depressant effects). Products include:

Stelazine ... 2226

Trimipramine Maleate (Transient delirium). Products include:

Surmontil Capsules ... 2524

Warfarin Sodium (Decreased prothrombin time response). Products include:

Coumadin Injection & Tablets ... 944
Panwarfin Tablets ... 547

PLAGUE VACCINE
(Plague Vaccine) ... 1584
May interact with:

Cholera Vaccine (Concomitant administration accentuates side effects). Products include:

Cholera Vaccine ... 2445

Typhoid Vaccine (Concomitant administration accentuates side effects). Products include:

Typhoid Vaccine ... 2533

PLAQUENIL SULFATE TABLETS
(Hydroxychloroquine Sulfate) ... 2067
May interact with:

Hepatotoxic Drugs, unspecified (Use with caution).

PLASMA-PLEX PLASMA PROTEIN FRACTION (HUMAN)
(Plasma Protein Fraction (Human)) .. 613
No interactions described in labeling.

PLATINOL
(Cisplatin) ... 737
May interact with aminoglycosides and anticonvulsants. Compounds in these categories include:

Amikacin Sulfate (Potentiation of cumulative nephrotoxicity). Products include:

Amikin Injectable ... 602

Carbamazepine (Plasma levels of anticonvulsant agents may become subtherapeutic). Products include:

Tegretol Chewable Tablets ... 654
Tegretol Suspension ... 656
Tegretol Tablets ... 654

Divalproex Sodium (Plasma levels of anticonvulsant agents may become subtherapeutic). Products include:

Depakote ... 512

Ethosuximide (Plasma levels of anticonvulsant agents may become subtherapeutic). Products include:

Zarontin Capsules ... 1768
Zarontin Syrup ... 1769

Ethotoin (Plasma levels of anticonvulsant agents may become subtherapeutic). Products include:

Peganone Tablets ... 551

Gentamicin Sulfate (Potentiation of cumulative nephrotoxicity). Products include:

Garamycin Injectable ... 2093
Garamycin Ophthalmic ... ⊙ 305
Genoptic Liquifilm Sterile Ophthalmic Solution ... ⊙ 247
Genoptic S.O.P. Sterile Ophthalmic Ointment ... ⊙ 247
Gentacidin Ointment ... ⊙ 273
Gentacidin Solution ... ⊙ 273
Gentak Ointment & Solution ... ⊙ 208
G-myticin Creme and Ointment 0.1% ... 1770
Pred-G Liquifilm Sterile Ophthalmic Suspension ... ⊙ 252
Pred-G S.O.P. Sterile Ophthalmic Ointment ... ⊙ 253

Kanamycin Sulfate (Potentiation of cumulative nephrotoxicity). Products include:

Kantrex Injection ... 601
Kantrex Pediatric Injection ... 601

Mephenytoin (Plasma levels of anticonvulsant agents may become subtherapeutic). Products include:

Mesantoin Tablets ... 2013

Methsuximide (Plasma levels of anticonvulsant agents may become subtherapeutic). Products include:

Celontin ... 1692

Paramethadione (Plasma levels of anticonvulsant agents may become subtherapeutic). Products include:

Paradione Capsules ... 548

Phenacemide (Plasma levels of anticonvulsant agents may become subtherapeutic). Products include:

Phenurone Tablets ... 552

Phenobarbital (Plasma levels of anticonvulsant agents may become subtherapeutic). Products include:

Arco-Lase Plus Tablets ... 607
Bellergal-S Tablets ... 1998
Bronkolixir ... ⊞ 761
Bronkotabs Tablets ... ⊞ 762
Donnatal ... 1858
Donnatal Extentabs ... 1859
Donnatal Tablets ... 1858
Donnazyme Tablets ... 1860
Kinesed Tablets ... 2272
Phenobarbital Elixir and Tablets ... 1293
Primatene Tablets-P Formula ... 2421
Quadrinal Tablets ... 1183

Tedral SA 1765

Phensuximide (Plasma levels of anticonvulsant agents may become subtherapeutic). Products include:

Milontin Kapseals 1741

Phenytoin (Plasma levels of anticonvulsant agents may become subtherapeutic). Products include:

Dilantin Infatabs 1710
Dilantin-30 Pediatric/Dilantin-125 Suspension 1713

Phenytoin Sodium (Plasma levels of anticonvulsant agents may become subtherapeutic). Products include:

Dilantin Kapseals 1708
Dilantin Parenteral 1712
Dilantin with Phenobarbital Kapseals 1715

Primidone (Plasma levels of anticonvulsant agents may become subtherapeutic). Products include:

Mysoline 2480

Streptomycin Sulfate (Potentiation of cumulative nephrotoxicity).

No products indexed under this heading.

Tobramycin Sulfate (Potentiation of cumulative nephrotoxicity). Products include:

Nebcin Vials, Hyporets & ADD-Vantage 1286

Trimethadione (Plasma levels of anticonvulsant agents may become subtherapeutic). Products include:

Tridione 557

Valproic Acid (Plasma levels of anticonvulsant agents may become subtherapeutic). Products include:

Depakene Capsules & Syrup 511

PLATINOL-AQ INJECTION

(Cisplatin) 738

May interact with aminoglycosides and anticonvulsants. Compounds in these categories include:

Amikacin Sulfate (Concomitant administration potentiates nephrotoxicity). Products include:

Amikin Injectable 602

Carbamazepine (Plasma levels of anticonvulsant agents may become subtherapeutic). Products include:

Tegretol Chewable Tablets 654
Tegretol Suspension 656
Tegretol Tablets 654

Divalproex Sodium (Plasma levels of anticonvulsant agents may become subtherapeutic). Products include:

Depakote 512

Ethosuximide (Plasma levels of anticonvulsant agents may become subtherapeutic). Products include:

Zarontin Capsules 1768
Zarontin Syrup 1769

Ethotoin (Plasma levels of anticonvulsant agents may become subtherapeutic). Products include:

Peganone Tablets 551

Gentamicin Sulfate (Concomitant administration potentiates nephrotoxicity). Products include:

Garamycin Injectable 2093
Garamycin Ophthalmic ..... ⊙ 305
Genoptic Liquifilm Sterile Ophthalmic Solution ..... ⊙ 247
Genoptic S.O.P. Sterile Ophthalmic Ointment ..... ⊙ 247
Gentacidin Ointment ..... ⊙ 273
Gentacidin Solution ..... ⊙ 273
Gentak Ointment & Solution ..... ⊙ 208
G-myticin Creme and Ointment 0.1% 1770
Pred-G Liquifilm Sterile Ophthalmic Suspension ..... ⊙ 252
Pred-G S.O.P. Sterile Ophthalmic Ointment ..... ⊙ 253

Kanamycin Sulfate (Concomitant administration potentiates nephrotoxicity). Products include:

Kantrex Injection 601
Kantrex Pediatric Injection 601

Mephenytoin (Plasma levels of anticonvulsant agents may become subtherapeutic). Products include:

Mesantoin Tablets 2013

Methsuximide (Plasma levels of anticonvulsant agents may become subtherapeutic). Products include:

Celontin 1692

Paramethadione (Plasma levels of anticonvulsant agents may become subtherapeutic). Products include:

Paradione Capsules 548

Phenacemide (Plasma levels of anticonvulsant agents may become subtherapeutic). Products include:

Phenurone Tablets 552

Phenobarbital (Plasma levels of anticonvulsant agents may become subtherapeutic). Products include:

Arco-Lase Plus Tablets 607
Bellergal-S Tablets 1998
Bronkolixir ..... ▣ 761
Bronkotabs Tablets ..... ▣ 762
Donnatal 1858
Donnatal Extentabs 1859
Donnatal Tablets 1858
Donnazyme Tablets 1860
Kinesed Tablets 2272
Phenobarbital Elixir and Tablets 1293
Primatene Tablets-P Formula 2421
Quadrinal Tablets 1183
Tedral SA 1765

Phensuximide (Plasma levels of anticonvulsant agents may become subtherapeutic). Products include:

Milontin Kapseals 1741

Phenytoin (Plasma levels of anticonvulsant agents may become subtherapeutic). Products include:

Dilantin Infatabs 1710
Dilantin-30 Pediatric/Dilantin-125 Suspension 1713

Phenytoin Sodium (Plasma levels of anticonvulsant agents may become subtherapeutic). Products include:

Dilantin Kapseals 1708
Dilantin Parenteral 1712
Dilantin with Phenobarbital Kapseals 1715

Primidone (Plasma levels of anticonvulsant agents may become subtherapeutic). Products include:

Mysoline 2480

Streptomycin Sulfate (Concomitant administration potentiates nephrotoxicity).

No products indexed under this heading.

Tobramycin (Concomitant administration potentiates nephrotoxicity). Products include:

TobraDex Ophthalmic Suspension and Ointment ..... ⊙ 228
Tobrex Ophthalmic Ointment and Solution 572

Tobramycin Sulfate (Concomitant administration potentiates nephrotoxicity). Products include:

Nebcin Vials, Hyporets & ADD-Vantage 1286

Trimethadione (Plasma levels of anticonvulsant agents may become subtherapeutic). Products include:

Tridione 557

Valproic Acid (Plasma levels of anticonvulsant agents may become subtherapeutic). Products include:

Depakene Capsules & Syrup 511

PLEGINE TABLETS

(Phendimetrazine Tartrate) 2504

May interact with central nervous system stimulants, monoamine oxidase inhibitors, insulin, and certain other agents. Compounds in these categories include:

Amphetamine Resins (Contraindicated). Products include:

Biphetamine Capsules 973

Dextroamphetamine (Contraindicated). Products include:

Biphetamine Capsules 973

Dextroamphetamine Sulfate (Contraindicated). Products include:

Dexedrine 2206

Furazolidone (Hypertensive crisis; contraindicated). Products include:

Furoxone 1855

Guanethidine Monosulfate (Decreased hypotensive effect of guanethidine). Products include:

Esimil Tablets 864
Ismelin Tablets 869

Insulin, Human (Altered insulin requirements).

No products indexed under this heading.

Insulin, Human Isophane Suspension (Altered insulin requirements). Products include:

Humulin N, 100 Units 1270

Insulin, Human NPH (Altered insulin requirements). Products include:

Insulatard NPH Human 1627
Novolin N 1627
Novolin N PenFill Cartridges 1628
Novolin N Prefilled 1628

Insulin, Human Regular (Altered insulin requirements). Products include:

Humulin BR, 100 Units 1268
Humulin R, 100 Units 1272
Novolin R 1627
Novolin R PenFill Cartridges 1628
Novolin R Prefilled 1629
Velosulin Human 1628

Insulin, Human, Zinc Suspension (Altered insulin requirements). Products include:

Humulin L, 100 Units 1268
Humulin U, 100 Units 1272
Novolin L 1627

Insulin, NPH (Altered insulin requirements). Products include:

NPH, 40 & 100 Units 1273
Beef NPH, 100 Units 1274
Pork NPH, 100 Units 1275
Insulatard NPH 1626
NPH Insulin 1626
NPH Purified Pork Isophane Insulin 1626

Insulin, Regular (Altered insulin requirements). Products include:

Regular, 40 & 100 Units 1273
Beef Regular, 100 Units 1275
Pork Regular, 100 Units 1275
Pork Regular (Concentrated), 500 Units 1276
Regular Insulin 1625
Regular Purified Pork Insulin 1626
Velosulin 1627

Insulin, Zinc Crystals (Altered insulin requirements). Products include:

NPH, 40 & 100 Units 1273

Insulin, Zinc Suspension (Altered insulin requirements). Products include:

Lente, 40 & 100 Units 1272
Protamine, Zinc, 40 & 100 Units 1273
Lente Iletin I 1272
Beef Lente, 100 Units 1274
Beef Protamine Zinc, 100 Units 1274
Pork Lente, 100 Units 1275
Pork, Protamine, Zinc, 100 Units 1275
Lente Insulin 1626
Lente Purified Pork Insulin 1626
Semilente Insulin 1625
Ultralente Insulin 1626

Isocarboxazid (Hypertensive crisis; contraindicated). Products include:

Marplan Tablets 1906

Methamphetamine Hydrochloride (Contraindicated). Products include:

Desoxyn Gradumet Tablets 514

Methylphenidate Hydrochloride (Contraindicated). Products include:

Ritalin 880

Pemoline (Contraindicated). Products include:

Cylert Tablets 510

Phenelzine Sulfate (Hypertensive crisis; contraindicated). Products include:

Nardil 1742

Selegiline Hydrochloride (Hypertensive crisis; contraindicated). Products include:

Eldepryl 2250

Tranylcypromine Sulfate (Hypertensive crisis; contraindicated). Products include:

Parnate Tablets 2222

PLENDIL EXTENDED-RELEASE TABLETS

(Felodipine) 1526

May interact with:

Cimetidine (Increases AUC and C_{max} by 50%; low doses of Plendil should be used). Products include:

Tagamet Tablets 2228

Cimetidine Hydrochloride (Increases AUC and C_{max} by 50%; low doses of Plendil should be used). Products include:

Tagamet 2228

Digoxin (Increased peak plasma concentration of digoxin). Products include:

Lanoxicaps 772
Lanoxin Elixir Pediatric 775
Lanoxin Injection 778
Lanoxin Injection Pediatric 781
Lanoxin Tablets 783

Metoprolol Tartrate (Increased AUC and C_{max} of metoprolol approximately 31 and 38 percent respectively). Products include:

Lopressor Ampuls 1032
Lopressor HCT Tablets 1034
Lopressor Tablets 1032

Food Interactions

Grapefruit juice, doubly concentrated (Increases bioavailability more than two-fold).

PNEUMOVAX 23

(Pneumococcal Vaccine, Polyvalent) 1528

May interact with immunosuppressive agents. Compounds in this category include:

Azathioprine (Expected serum antibody response may not be obtained). Products include:

Imuran 768

Cyclosporine (Expected serum antibody response may not be obtained). Products include:

Sandimmune 2024

Immune Globulin (Human) (Expected serum antibody response may not be obtained). Products include:

MICRhoGAM Rh_0(D) Immune Globulin (Human) 1650
RhoGAM Rh_0(D) Immune Globulin (Human) 1651

Immune Globulin Intravenous (Human) (Expected serum antibody response may not be obtained). Products include:

Gamimune N Immune Globulin Intravenous (Human) 1572

Gammagard Immune Globulin, Intravenous (Human) 658
Iveegam 1129
Sandoglobulin I.V. 2027

Muromonab-CD3 (Expected serum antibody response may not be obtained). Products include:
Orthoclone OKT3 Sterile Solution .. 1645

PNU-IMUNE 23 PNEUMOCOCCAL VACCINE POLYVALENT
(Pneumococcal Vaccine, Polyvalent)..1233
May interact with immunosuppressive agents and antineoplastics. Compounds in these categories include:

Altretamine (Possible impaired serum antibody response to vaccine). Products include:
Hexalen Capsules 2316

Asparaginase (Possible impaired serum antibody response to vaccine). Products include:
Elspar 1470

Azathioprine (Reduction of antibody levels). Products include:
Imuran 768

Bleomycin Sulfate (Possible impaired serum antibody response to vaccine). Products include:
Blenoxane 724

Busulfan (Possible impaired serum antibody response to vaccine). Products include:
Myleran Tablets 790

Carboplatin (Possible impaired serum antibody response to vaccine). Products include:
Paraplatin for Injection 735

Carmustine (BCNU) (Possible impaired serum antibody response to vaccine). Products include:
BiCNU 723

Chlorambucil (Possible impaired serum antibody response to vaccine). Products include:
Leukeran Tablets 788

Cisplatin (Possible impaired serum antibody response to vaccine). Products include:
Platinol 737
Platinol-AQ Injection 738

Cyclophosphamide (Possible impaired serum antibody response to vaccine). Products include:
Cytoxan for Injection 726
Neosar for Injection 566

Cyclosporine (Reduction of antibody levels). Products include:
Sandimmune 2024

Dacarbazine (Possible impaired serum antibody response to vaccine). Products include:
DTIC-Dome 1595

Daunorubicin Hydrochloride (Possible impaired serum antibody response to vaccine). Products include:
Cerubidine 2443

Doxorubicin Hydrochloride (Possible impaired serum antibody response to vaccine). Products include:
Adriamycin PFS 561
Adriamycin RDF 562
Doxorubicin Hydrochloride for Injection, USP 622
Doxorubicin Hydrochloride Injection, USP 848
Rubex 739

Estramustine Phosphate Sodium (Possible impaired serum antibody response to vaccine). Products include:
Emcyt Capsules 1161

Etoposide (Possible impaired serum antibody response to vaccine). Products include:
VePesid Capsules and Injection 741

Floxuridine (Possible impaired serum antibody response to vaccine). Products include:
Sterile FUDR 1898

Fluorouracil (Possible impaired serum antibody response to vaccine). Products include:
Efudex 1880
Fluoroplex Topical Solution & Cream 1% 1082
Fluorouracil Injection 1897

Flutamide (Possible impaired serum antibody response to vaccine). Products include:
Eulexin Capsules 2089

Hydroxyurea (Possible impaired serum antibody response to vaccine). Products include:
Hydrea Capsules 728

Ifosfamide (Possible impaired serum antibody response to vaccine). Products include:
IFEX 729

Immune Globulin (Human) (Reduction of antibody levels). Products include:
MICRhoGAM Rh_0(D) Immune Globulin (Human) 1650
RhoGAM Rh_0(D) Immune Globulin (Human) 1651

Immune Globulin Intravenous (Human) (Reduction of antibody levels). Products include:
Gamimune N Immune Globulin Intravenous (Human) 1572
Gammagard Immune Globulin, Intravenous (Human) 658
Iveegam 1129
Sandoglobulin I.V. 2027

Interferon alfa-2A, Recombinant (Possible impaired serum antibody response to vaccine). Products include:
Roferon-A Injection 1916

Interferon alfa-2B, Recombinant (Possible impaired serum antibody response to vaccine). Products include:
Intron A 2097

Levamisole Hydrochloride (Possible impaired serum antibody response to vaccine). Products include:
Ergamisol Tablets 1136

Lomustine (CCNU) (Possible impaired serum antibody response to vaccine). Products include:
CeeNU 725

Mechlorethamine Hydrochloride (Possible impaired serum antibody response to vaccine). Products include:
Mustargen 1514

Megestrol Acetate (Possible impaired serum antibody response to vaccine). Products include:
Megace Tablets 732

Melphalan (Possible impaired serum antibody response to vaccine). Products include:
Alkeran Tablets 754

Mercaptopurine (Possible impaired serum antibody response to vaccine). Products include:
Purinethol Tablets 800

Methotrexate Sodium (Possible impaired serum antibody response to vaccine). Products include:
Methotrexate Tablets, Parenteral, LPF Parenteral 1217
Rheumatrex Methotrexate Dose Pack 1234

Mitomycin (Mitomycin-C) (Possible impaired serum antibody response to vaccine). Products include:
Mutamycin 733

Mitotane (Possible impaired serum antibody response to vaccine). Products include:
Lysodren 731

Mitoxantrone Hydrochloride (Possible impaired serum antibody response to vaccine). Products include:
Novantrone for Injection Concentrate 1226

Muromonab-CD3 (Reduction of antibody levels). Products include:
Orthoclone OKT3 Sterile Solution .. 1645

Procarbazine Hydrochloride (Possible impaired serum antibody response to vaccine). Products include:
Matulane Capsules 1907

Streptozocin (Possible impaired serum antibody response to vaccine). Products include:
Zanosar Sterile Powder 2371

Tamoxifen Citrate (Possible impaired serum antibody response to vaccine). Products include:
Nolvadex Tablets 1102

Thioguanine (Possible impaired serum antibody response to vaccine). Products include:
Thioguanine Tablets, Tabloid Brand 815

Thiotepa (Possible impaired serum antibody response to vaccine). Products include:
Thiotepa Parenteral 1240

Vincristine Sulfate (Possible impaired serum antibody response to vaccine). Products include:
Oncovin Solution Vials & Hyporets 1288

POLARAMINE REPETABS TABLETS
(Dexchlorpheniramine Maleate)..........2116
May interact with central nervous system depressants, hypnotics and sedatives, tranquilizers, monoamine oxidase inhibitors, oral anticoagulants, and certain other agents. Compounds in these categories include:

Alcohol (Additive effects).

Alfentanil Hydrochloride (Additive effects). Products include:
Alfenta Injection 1131

Alprazolam (Additive effects). Products include:
Xanax Tablets 2367

Aprobarbital (Additive effects). Products include:
Alurate Elixir 1883

Buprenorphine (Additive effects).
No products indexed under this heading.

Buspirone Hydrochloride (Additive effects). Products include:
BuSpar 1401

Butabarbital (Additive effects). Products include:
Pyridium Plus 1764

Butalbital (Additive effects). Products include:
Esgic-Plus Tablets 1002
Esgic Tablets & Capsules 1001
Fioricet Tablets 2006
Fiorinal Capsules 2007
Fiorinal with Codeine Capsules 2008
Fiorinal Tablets 2007
Phrenilin 838
Sedapap Tablets 50 mg/650 mg .. 1360

Chlordiazepoxide (Additive effects). Products include:
Libritabs Tablets 1930
Limbitrol 1933
Menrium Tablets 1934

Chlordiazepoxide Hydrochloride (Additive effects). Products include:
Librax Capsules 1929
Librium Capsules 1931
Librium Injectable 1932

Chlorpromazine (Additive effects). Products include:
Thorazine 2234

Chlorprothixene (Additive effects). Products include:
Taractan Tablets 1920

Chlorprothixene Hydrochloride (Additive effects). Products include:
Taractan 1920

Chlorprothixene Lactate (Additive effects). Products include:
Taractan Concentrate 1920

Clorazepate Dipotassium (Additive effects). Products include:
Tranxene 556

Codeine (Additive effects). Products include:
Calcidrine Syrup 506

Codeine Phosphate (Additive effects). Products include:
Actifed with Codeine Cough Syrup.. 752
Cheracol Cough Syrup 1853
Codimal PH Syrup 846
Dimetane-DC Cough Syrup 1857
Empirin with Codeine Phosphate Nos. 2, 3 & 4 764
Fiorinal with Codeine Capsules 2008
Isoclor Expectorant 982
Naldecon CX Adult Liquid .... ▣ 521
Novahistine DH 1342
Novahistine Expectorant 1343
Nucofed Capsules 2219
Nucofed Expectorant 2219
Nucofed Pediatric Expectorant 2220
Nucofed Syrup 2219
Phenaphen with Codeine Capsules 1865
Phenaphen-650 with Codeine Tablets 1866
Phenergan with Codeine 2497
Phenergan VC with Codeine 2501
Robitussin A-C Syrup 1875
Robitussin-DAC Syrup 1875
Ryna .... ▣ 741
Soma Compound w/Codeine Tablets 2390
Triaminic Expectorant w/Codeine .. 1996
Tussi-Organidin Liquid 2391
Tylenol with Codeine 1381

Codeine Polistirex (Additive effects).
No products indexed under this heading.

Dezocine (Additive effects).

Diazepam (Additive effects). Products include:
Valium Injectable 1937
Valium Tablets 1939
Valrelease Capsules 1923

Dicumarol (Inhibited anticoagulant action). Products include:
Dicumarol Tablets 516

Droperidol (Additive effects). Products include:
Inapsine Injection 1140
Innovar Injection 1141

Enflurane (Additive effects). Products include:
Ethrane 599

Estazolam (Additive effects). Products include:
ProSom Tablets 554

Ethchlorvynol (Additive effects). Products include:
Placidyl Capsules 553

Ethinamate (Additive effects).
No products indexed under this heading.

Fentanyl (Additive effects). Products include:
Duragesic Transdermal System 1133

Fentanyl Citrate (Additive effects). Products include:
Innovar Injection 1141
Sublimaze Injection 1146

Fluphenazine Decanoate (Additive effects). Products include:
Prolixin Decanoate 1795

Fluphenazine Enanthate (Additive effects). Products include:
Prolixin Enanthate 1796

Fluphenazine Hydrochloride (Additive effects). Products include:
Prolixin Elixir 1793
Prolixin Injection 1791
Prolixin Oral Concentrate 1792
Prolixin Tablets 1793

Flurazepam Hydrochloride (Additive effects). Products include:
Dalmane Capsules 1927

Furazolidone (Severe hypotension; concurrent therapy is contraindicated). Products include:
Furoxone 1855

Glutethimide (Additive effects).
No products indexed under this heading.

Haloperidol (Additive effects). Products include:
Haldol Injection, Tablets and Concentrate 1373

Haloperidol Decanoate (Additive effects). Products include:
Haldol Decanoate 1375

Hydrocodone Bitartrate (Additive effects). Products include:
Anexsia 5/500 Tablets 2196
Anexsia 7.5/650 Tablets 2197
Azdone Tablets 844
Codiclear DH Syrup 845
Codimal DH Syrup 846
Damason-P 1356
Hycodan Syrup, Tablets 927
Hycomine Compound Tablets 929
Hycomine Syrup 927
Hycotuss Expectorant Syrup 930
Hydrocet Capsules 835
Lortab ASA Tablets 2414
Lortab 2412
Ru-Tuss with Hydrocodone 694
Triaminic Expectorant DH 1995
Vicodin Tablets 1187
Vicodin ES Tablets 1189
Zydone Capsules 941

Hydrocodone Polistirex (Additive effects). Products include:
Tussionex Extended-Release Suspension 988

Hydroxyzine Hydrochloride (Additive effects). Products include:
Atarax Tablets & Syrup 1941
Marax Tablets & DF Syrup 1954
Vistaril Intramuscular Solution 1970

Isocarboxazid (Severe hypotension; concurrent therapy is contraindicated). Products include:
Marplan Tablets 1906

Isoflurane (Additive effects). Products include:
Forane 600

Ketamine Hydrochloride (Additive effects). Products include:
Ketalar 1726

Levorphanol Tartrate (Additive effects). Products include:
Levo-Dromoran 1906

Lorazepam (Additive effects). Products include:
Ativan Injection 2432
Ativan Tablets 2434

Loxapine Hydrochloride (Additive effects). Products include:
Loxitane 1213

Loxapine Succinate (Additive effects). Products include:
Loxitane Capsules 1213

Meperidine Hydrochloride (Additive effects). Products include:
Demerol 2047
Mepergan Injection 2479

Mephobarbital (Additive effects). Products include:
Mebaral Tablets 2061

Meprobamate (Additive effects). Products include:
Deprol Tablets 2382
Equagesic Tablets 2451
Miltown Tablets 2386
PMB 200 and PMB 400 2504

Mesoridazine (Additive effects). Products include:
Serentil 686

Methadone Hydrochloride (Additive effects). Products include:
Dolophine Hydrochloride Ampoules & Vials 1260
Dolophine Hydrochloride Tablets 1261
Methadone Hydrochloride Diskets 1284
Methadone Hydrochloride Oral Solution & Tablets 1987

Methohexital Sodium (Additive effects). Products include:
Brevital Sodium Vials 1248

Methoxyflurane (Additive effects).
No products indexed under this heading.

Midazolam Hydrochloride (Additive effects). Products include:
Versed Injection 1924

Molindone Hydrochloride (Additive effects). Products include:
Moban Tablets & Concentrate 932

Morphine Sulfate (Additive effects). Products include:
Astramorph/PF Injection, USP (Preservative-Free) 618
Duramorph 960
Infumorph 200 and Infumorph 500 Sterile Solutions 962
MS Contin Tablets 1814
MSIR 1817
Oramorph SR (Morphine Sulfate Sustained Release Tablets) 1988
Roxanol 1991

Opium Alkaloids (Additive effects). Products include:
B & O No. 15A & No. 16A Supprettes 2395
Pantopon Injectable 1911

Oxazepam (Additive effects). Products include:
Serax Capsules 2522
Serax Tablets 2522

Oxycodone Hydrochloride (Additive effects). Products include:
Percocet Tablets 950
Percodan 951
Roxicodone Tablets, Oral Solution & Intensol (Oxycodone) 1992
Tylox Capsules 1382

Pentobarbital Sodium (Additive effects). Products include:
Nembutal Sodium Capsules 534
Nembutal Sodium Solution 536
Nembutal Sodium Suppositories 538

Perphenazine (Additive effects). Products include:
Etrafon 2087
Triavil Tablets 1556
Trilafon 2123

Phenelzine Sulfate (Severe hypotension; concurrent therapy is contraindicated). Products include:
Nardil 1742

Phenobarbital (Additive effects). Products include:
Arco-Lase Plus Tablets 607
Bellergal-S Tablets 1998
Bronkolixir ◘ 761
Bronkotabs Tablets ◘ 762
Donnatal 1858
Donnatal Extentabs 1859
Donnatal Tablets 1858
Donnazyme Tablets 1860
Kinesed Tablets 2272
Phenobarbital Elixir and Tablets 1293
Primatene Tablets-P Formula 2421
Quadrinal Tablets 1183
Tedral SA 1765

Prazepam (Additive effects). Products include:
Centrax 1693

Prochlorperazine (Additive effects). Products include:
Compazine 2201

Promethazine Hydrochloride (Additive effects). Products include:
Mepergan Injection 2479
Phenergan with Codeine 2497
Phenergan with Dextromethorphan 2499
Phenergan Injection 2493
Phenergan Suppositories 2496
Phenergan Syrup 2495
Phenergan Tablets 2496
Phenergan VC 2500
Phenergan VC with Codeine 2501

Propofol (Additive effects). Products include:
Diprivan Injection 2267

Propoxyphene Hydrochloride (Additive effects). Products include:
Darvon 1256
Wygesic Tablets 2540

Propoxyphene Napsylate (Additive effects). Products include:
Darvon-N/Darvocet-N 1254

Quazepam (Additive effects). Products include:
Doral Tablets 2383

Secobarbital Sodium (Additive effects). Products include:
Seconal Sodium Pulvules 1296

Selegiline Hydrochloride (Severe hypotension; concurrent therapy is contraindicated). Products include:
Eldepryl 2250

Sufentanil Citrate (Additive effects). Products include:
Sufenta Injection 1147

Temazepam (Additive effects). Products include:
Restoril Capsules 2023

Thiamylal Sodium (Additive effects). Products include:
Surital Ampoules, Steri-Vials 1764

Thioridazine Hydrochloride (Additive effects). Products include:
Mellaril 2011

Thiothixene (Additive effects). Products include:
Navane Capsules and Concentrate 1954
Navane Intramuscular 1956

Tranylcypromine Sulfate (Severe hypotension; concurrent therapy is contraindicated). Products include:
Parnate Tablets 2222

Triazolam (Additive effects). Products include:
Halcion Tablets 2340

Trifluoperazine Hydrochloride (Additive effects). Products include:
Stelazine 2226

Warfarin Sodium (Inhibited anticoagulant action). Products include:
Coumadin Injection & Tablets 944
Panwarfin Tablets 547

POLARAMINE SYRUP
(Dexchlorpheniramine Maleate) 2116
See **Polaramine Repetabs Tablets**

POLARAMINE TABLETS
(Dexchlorpheniramine Maleate) 2116
See **Polaramine Repetabs Tablets**

POLYCITRA SYRUP
(Potassium Citrate, Sodium Citrate, Citric Acid) 2424
May interact with potassium-depleting corticosteroids, potassium sparing diuretics, cardiac glycosides, ACE inhibitors, and certain other agents. Compounds in these categories include:

Aluminum Carbonate Gel (Concurrent therapy in patients with renal insufficiency should be avoided). Products include:
Basaljel 2438

Aluminum Hydroxide (Concurrent therapy in patients with renal insufficiency should be avoided). Products include:
Cama Arthritis Pain Reliever ◘ 685
Gaviscon Extra Strength Relief Formula Liquid Antacid ◘ 594
Gaviscon Extra Strength Relief Formula Antacid Tablets ◘ 594
Gaviscon Liquid Antacid ◘ 594
Gelusil Liquid & Tablets ◘ 639
Extra Strength Maalox Plus Suspension 1850
Maalox TC Suspension 1851
Maalox Plus Tablets ◘ 655
Extra Strength Maalox Plus Tablets 1850
Nephrox Suspension ◘ 563
WinGel Liquid & Tablets ◘ 761

Aluminum Hydroxide Gel (Concurrent therapy in patients with renal insufficiency should be avoided). Products include:
ALternaGEL Liquid 1154
Aludrox Oral Suspension 2428
Amphojel Suspension 2429
Amphojel Suspension without Flavor 2429
Mylanta Liquid 1155
Mylanta Double Strength Liquid 1155

Aluminum Hydroxide Gel, Dried (Concurrent therapy in patients with renal insufficiency should be avoided). Products include:
Alu-Tab/Alu-Cap 1309
Amphojel Tablets 2429
Ascriptin A/D Caplets 1850
Regular Strength Ascriptin Tablets 1850
Gaviscon Antacid Tablets ◘ 593
Gaviscon-2 Antacid Tablets ◘ 594
Mylanta Tablets 1155
Mylanta Double Strength Tablets 1155

Amiloride Hydrochloride (Potential toxicity). Products include:
Midamor Tablets 1508
Moduretic Tablets 1510

Benazepril Hydrochloride (Potential toxicity). Products include:
Lotensin Tablets 872

Captopril (Potential toxicity). Products include:
Capoten 2255
Capozide 2258

Deslanoside (Potential toxicity).
No products indexed under this heading.

Digitoxin (Potential toxicity). Products include:
Crystodigin Tablets 1253

Digoxin (Potential toxicity). Products include:
Lanoxicaps 772
Lanoxin Elixir Pediatric 775
Lanoxin Injection 778
Lanoxin Injection Pediatric 781
Lanoxin Tablets 783

Enalapril Maleate (Potential toxicity). Products include:
Vaseretic Tablets 1559
Vasotec Tablets 1564

Enalaprilat (Potential toxicity). Products include:
Vasotec I.V. 1562

Fosinopril Sodium (Potential toxicity). Products include:
Monopril Tablets 1406

Lisinopril (Potential toxicity). Products include:
Prinivil Tablets 1538
Prinzide Tablets 1540
Zestoretic 2274
Zestril Tablets 2277

Potassium Acid Phosphate (Potential toxicity). Products include:
K-Phos M.F. Tablets 659
K-Phos Original Formula 'Sodium Free' Tablets 660
K-Phos No. 2 Tablets 659

Potassium Bicarbonate (Potential toxicity). Products include:
Alka-Seltzer Advanced Formula Antacid & Non-Aspirin Pain Reliever ◘ 620

Alka-Seltzer Effervescent Antacid ▣ 622
K-Lyte 707
Klorvess Effervescent Granules 2010
Klorvess Effervescent Tablets 2011

Potassium Chloride (Potential toxicity). Products include:
Chlor-3 Condiment 994
K-Dur Microburst Release System (potassium chloride, USP) E.R. Tablets 1163
K-Lor Powder Packets 531
K-Lyte 707
K-Norm Capsules 982
K-Tab Filmtab 532
Kato Potassium Supplement 1114
Klor-Con 8/Klor-Con 10 Extended-release Tablets 2374
Klorvess Effervescent Granules 2010
Klorvess Effervescent Tablets 2011
Klorvess 10% Liquid 2010
Klotrix 708
Kolyum Liquid 983
Micro-K 1863
Micro-K LS Packets 1864
NuLYTELY 699
Oral Rehydration Salts, Citrate 1150
Rum-K Syrup 995
Slow-K Tablets 2281
Ten-K Controlled-Release Tablets 2282
Thermotabs ▣ 619

Potassium Gluconate (Potential toxicity). Products include:
Kolyum Liquid 983

Potassium Phosphate, Dibasic (Potential toxicity). Products include:
Neutra-Phos 2423

Potassium Phosphate, Monobasic (Potential toxicity). Products include:
K-Phos M.F. Tablets 659
K-Phos Neutral Tablets 660
Neutra-Phos 2423

Ramipril (Potential toxicity). Products include:
Altace Capsules 1086

Spironolactone (Potential toxicity). Products include:
Aldactazide 2150
Aldactone 2152

Triamterene (Potential toxicity). Products include:
Dyazide Capsules 2208
Dyrenium Capsules 2210
Maxzide 1215

POLYCITRA-K CRYSTALS
(Potassium Citrate, Citric Acid) 2424
May interact with potassium-depleting corticosteroids, potassium sparing diuretics, ACE inhibitors, cardiac glycosides, and certain other agents. Compounds in these categories include:

Aluminum Carbonate Gel (Concurrent therapy in patients with renal insufficiency should be avoided). Products include:
Basaljel 2438

Aluminum Hydroxide (Concurrent therapy in patients with renal insufficiency should be avoided). Products include:
Cama Arthritis Pain Reliever ▣ 685
Gaviscon Extra Strength Relief Formula Liquid Antacid ▣ 594
Gaviscon Extra Strength Relief Formula Antacid Tablets ▣ 594
Gaviscon Liquid Antacid ▣ 594
Gelusil Liquid & Tablets ▣ 639
Extra Strength Maalox Plus Suspension 1850
Maalox TC Suspension 1851
Maalox Plus Tablets ▣ 655
Extra Strength Maalox Plus Tablets 1850
Nephrox Suspension ▣ 563
WinGel Liquid & Tablets ▣ 761

Aluminum Hydroxide Gel (Concurrent therapy in patients with renal insufficiency should be avoided). Products include:
ALternaGEL Liquid 1154
Aludrox Oral Suspension 2428
Amphojel Suspension 2429
Amphojel Suspension without Flavor 2429
Mylanta Liquid 1155
Mylanta Double Strength Liquid 1155

Aluminum Hydroxide Gel, Dried (Concurrent therapy in patients with renal insufficiency should be avoided). Products include:
Alu-Tab/Alu-Cap 1309
Amphojel Tablets 2429
Ascriptin A/D Caplets 1850
Regular Strength Ascriptin Tablets 1850
Gaviscon Antacid Tablets ▣ 593
Gaviscon-2 Antacid Tablets ▣ 594
Mylanta Tablets 1155
Mylanta Double Strength Tablets 1155

Amiloride Hydrochloride (Potential toxicity). Products include:
Midamor Tablets 1508
Moduretic Tablets 1510

Benazepril Hydrochloride (Potential toxicity). Products include:
Lotensin Tablets 872

Captopril (Potential toxicity). Products include:
Capoten 2255
Capozide 2258

Deslanoside (Potential toxicity).
No products indexed under this heading.

Digitoxin (Potential toxicity). Products include:
Crystodigin Tablets 1253

Digoxin (Potential toxicity). Products include:
Lanoxicaps 772
Lanoxin Elixir Pediatric 775
Lanoxin Injection 778
Lanoxin Injection Pediatric 781
Lanoxin Tablets 783

Enalapril Maleate (Potential toxicity). Products include:
Vaseretic Tablets 1559
Vasotec Tablets 1564

Enalaprilat (Potential toxicity). Products include:
Vasotec I.V. 1562

Fosinopril Sodium (Potential toxicity). Products include:
Monopril Tablets 1406

Lisinopril (Potential toxicity). Products include:
Prinivil Tablets 1538
Prinzide Tablets 1540
Zestoretic 2274
Zestril Tablets 2277

Potassium Acid Phosphate (Potential toxicity). Products include:
K-Phos M.F. Tablets 659
K-Phos Original Formula 'Sodium Free' Tablets 660
K-Phos No. 2 Tablets 659

Potassium Bicarbonate (Potential toxicity). Products include:
Alka-Seltzer Advanced Formula Antacid & Non-Aspirin Pain Reliever ▣ 620
Alka-Seltzer Effervescent Antacid ▣ 622
K-Lyte 707
Klorvess Effervescent Granules 2010
Klorvess Effervescent Tablets 2011

Potassium Chloride (Potential toxicity). Products include:
Chlor-3 Condiment 994
K-Dur Microburst Release System (potassium chloride, USP) E.R. Tablets 1163
K-Lor Powder Packets 531
K-Lyte 707
K-Norm Capsules 982
K-Tab Filmtab 532
Kato Potassium Supplement 1114
Klor-Con 8/Klor-Con 10 Extended-release Tablets 2374
Klorvess Effervescent Granules 2010
Klorvess Effervescent Tablets 2011
Klorvess 10% Liquid 2010
Klotrix 708
Kolyum Liquid 983
Micro-K 1863
Micro-K LS Packets 1864
NuLYTELY 699
Oral Rehydration Salts, Citrate 1150
Rum-K Syrup 995
Slow-K Tablets 2281
Ten-K Controlled-Release Tablets 2282
Thermotabs ▣ 619

Potassium Gluconate (Potential toxicity). Products include:
Kolyum Liquid 983

Potassium Phosphate, Dibasic (Potential toxicity). Products include:
Neutra-Phos 2423

Potassium Phosphate, Monobasic (Potential toxicity). Products include:
K-Phos M.F. Tablets 659
K-Phos Neutral Tablets 660
Neutra-Phos 2423

Ramipril (Potential toxicity). Products include:
Altace Capsules 1086

Spironolactone (Potential toxicity). Products include:
Aldactazide 2150
Aldactone 2152

Triamterene (Potential toxicity). Products include:
Dyazide Capsules 2208
Dyrenium Capsules 2210
Maxzide 1215

POLYCITRA-K ORAL SOLUTION
(Potassium Citrate, Citric Acid) 2424
See **Polycitra-K Crystals**

POLYCITRA-LC—SUGAR-FREE
(Potassium Citrate, Citric Acid, Sodium Citrate) 2424
See **Polycitra Syrup**

POLYCOSE GLUCOSE POLYMERS
(Glucose Polymers) 1974
No interactions described in labeling.

POLYMYXIN B SULFATE, AEROSPORIN BRAND STERILE POWDER
(Polymyxin B Sulfate) 798
May interact with aminoglycosides and certain other agents. Compounds in these categories include:

Amikacin Sulfate (Nephrotoxic/neurotoxic effects enhanced). Products include:
Amikin Injectable 602

Cephaloridine (Nephrotoxic/neurotoxic effects enhanced).

Colistin Sulfate (Nephrotoxic/neurotoxic effects enhanced). Products include:
Coly-Mycin S For Oral Suspension 1708
Coly-Mycin S Otic w/Neomycin & Hydrocortisone 1708

Decamethonium (Precipitation of respiratory depression).

Ether (Precipitation of respiratory depression).

Gallamine (Precipitation of respiratory depression).

Gentamicin Sulfate (Nephrotoxic/neurotoxic effects enhanced). Products include:
Garamycin Injectable 2093
Garamycin Ophthalmic ⊙ 305
Genoptic Liquifilm Sterile Ophthalmic Solution ⊙ 247
Genoptic S.O.P. Sterile Ophthalmic Ointment ⊙ 247
Gentacidin Ointment ⊙ 273
Gentacidin Solution ⊙ 273
Gentak Ointment & Solution ⊙ 208
G-myticin Creme and Ointment 0.1% 1770
Pred-G Liquifilm Sterile Ophthalmic Suspension ⊙ 252
Pred-G S.O.P. Sterile Ophthalmic Ointment ⊙ 253

Kanamycin Sulfate (Nephrotoxic/neurotoxic effects enhanced). Products include:
Kantrex Injection 601
Kantrex Pediatric Injection 601

Neomycin Sulfate (Nephrotoxic/neurotoxic effects enhanced). Products include:
AK-Spore H.C. ⊙ 206
AK-Spore ⊙ 205
AK-Trol Ointment & Suspension ⊙ 207
Bactine First Aid Antibiotic Ointment ▣ 625
Campho-Phenique Triple Antibiotic Ointment Plus Pain Reliever ▣ 758
Coly-Mycin S Otic w/Neomycin & Hydrocortisone 1708
Cortisporin Cream 757
Cortisporin Ointment 758
Cortisporin Ophthalmic Ointment Sterile 758
Cortisporin Ophthalmic Suspension Sterile 759
Cortisporin Otic Solution Sterile 760
Cortisporin Otic Suspension Sterile 760
Dexacidin ⊙ 272
Lanabiotic Ointment ▣ 556
LazerSporin-C Solution 1770
Maxitrol Ophthalmic Ointment/Suspension ⊙ 223
Myciguent Antibiotic Ointment ▣ 737
Mycitracin ▣ 737
NeoDecadron Sterile Ophthalmic Ointment 1517
NeoDecadron Sterile Ophthalmic Solution 1518
NeoDecadron Topical Cream 1518
Neosporin Cream 792
Neosporin G.U. Irrigant Sterile 793
Neosporin Ointment 793
Maximum Strength Neosporin Ointment 793
Neosporin Ophthalmic Ointment Sterile 793
Neosporin Ophthalmic Solution Sterile 794
Neo-Synalar Cream 2296
PediOtic Suspension Sterile 797
Poly-Pred Liquifilm ⊙ 250

Paromomycin Sulfate (Nephrotoxic/neurotoxic effects enhanced). Products include:
Humatin Capsules 1726

Sodium Citrate, Injection (Precipitation of respiratory depression).

Streptomycin Sulfate (Nephrotoxic/neurotoxic effects enhanced).
No products indexed under this heading.

Succinylcholine Chloride (Precipitation of respiratory depression). Products include:
Anectine 755

Tobramycin (Nephrotoxic/neurotoxic effects enhanced). Products include:
TobraDex Ophthalmic Suspension and Ointment ⊙ 228
Tobrex Ophthalmic Ointment and Solution 572

Tobramycin Sulfate (Nephrotoxic/neurotoxic effects enhanced). Products include:
Nebcin Vials, Hyporets & ADD-Vantage 1286

Tubocurarine Chloride (Precipitation of respiratory depression).
No products indexed under this heading.

Viomycin (Nephrotoxic/neurotoxic effects enhanced).

POLY-PRED LIQUIFILM
(Neomycin Sulfate, Polymyxin B Sulfate, Prednisolone Acetate) ⊙ 250
No interactions described in labeling.

POLYSPORIN OINTMENT
(Bacitracin Zinc, Polymyxin B Sulfate) ▣ 543
No interactions described in labeling.

(▣ Described in PDR For Nonprescription Drugs) (⊙ Described in PDR For Ophthalmology)

POLYSPORIN OPHTHALMIC OINTMENT STERILE
(Polymyxin B Sulfate, Bacitracin) 798
No interactions described in labeling.

POLYSPORIN POWDER
(Bacitracin Zinc, Polymyxin B Sulfate) .... ⊡ 543
No interactions described in labeling.

POLYSPORIN SPRAY
(Bacitracin Zinc, Polymyxin B Sulfate) .... ⊡ 543
No interactions described in labeling.

POLYTRIM OPHTHALMIC SOLUTION STERILE
(Polymyxin B Sulfate, Trimethoprim Sulfate) 588
No interactions described in labeling.

POLY-VI-FLOR 0.25 MG VITAMINS WITH FLUORIDE CHEWABLE TABLETS
(Vitamins with Fluoride) 1397
No interactions described in labeling.

POLY-VI-FLOR 0.5 MG VITAMINS WITH FLUORIDE CHEWABLE TABLETS
(Vitamins with Fluoride) 1397
No interactions described in labeling.

POLY-VI-FLOR 1.0 MG VITAMINS WITH FLUORIDE CHEWABLE TABLETS
(Vitamins with Fluoride) 1397
No interactions described in labeling.

POLY-VI-FLOR 0.25 MG VITAMINS WITH FLUORIDE DROPS
(Vitamins with Fluoride) 1398
No interactions described in labeling.

POLY-VI-FLOR 0.5 MG VITAMINS WITH FLUORIDE DROPS
(Vitamins with Fluoride) 1398
No interactions described in labeling.

POLY-VI-FLOR 0.25 MG VITAMINS WITH IRON AND FLUORIDE CHEWABLE TABLETS
(Vitamins with Fluoride, Ferrous Sulfate) 1399
No interactions described in labeling.

POLY-VI-FLOR 0.5 MG VITAMINS WITH IRON AND FLUORIDE CHEWABLE TABLETS
(Vitamins with Fluoride, Ferrous Sulfate) 1399
No interactions described in labeling.

POLY-VI-FLOR 1.0 MG VITAMINS WITH IRON AND FLUORIDE CHEWABLE TABLETS
(Vitamins with Fluoride, Ferrous Sulfate) 1399
No interactions described in labeling.

POLY-VI-FLOR 0.25 MG VITAMINS WITH IRON AND FLUORIDE DROPS
(Vitamins with Fluoride, Ferrous Sulfate) 1399
No interactions described in labeling.

POLY-VI-FLOR 0.5 MG VITAMINS WITH IRON AND FLUORIDE DROPS
(Vitamins with Fluoride, Ferrous Sulfate) 1399
No interactions described in labeling.

POLY-VI-SOL VITAMINS, CHEWABLE TABLETS AND DROPS (WITHOUT IRON)
(Vitamins, Multiple) .... ⊡ 612
No interactions described in labeling.

POLY-VI-SOL VITAMINS, CIRCUS SHAPES CHEWABLE (WITHOUT IRON)
(Vitamins, Multiple) .... ⊡ 612
No interactions described in labeling.

POLY-VI-SOL VITAMINS WITH IRON, CHEWABLE TABLETS AND CIRCUS SHAPES CHEWABLE
(Vitamins with Iron) .... ⊡ 612
No interactions described in labeling.

POLY-VI-SOL VITAMINS WITH IRON, DROPS
(Vitamins with Iron) .... ⊡ 612
No interactions described in labeling.

PONARIS NASAL MUCOSAL EMOLLIENT
(Oils, unspecified) 1131
No interactions described in labeling.

PONDIMIN TABLETS
(Fenfluramine Hydrochloride) 1867
May interact with central nervous system depressants, monoamine oxidase inhibitors, and certain other agents. Compounds in these categories include:

Alfentanil Hydrochloride (Possible additive effects of CNS depressants). Products include:
- Alfenta Injection 1131

Alprazolam (Possible additive effects of CNS depressants). Products include:
- Xanax Tablets 2367

Aprobarbital (Possible additive effects of CNS depressants). Products include:
- Alurate Elixir 1883

Buprenorphine (Possible additive effects of CNS depressants).
No products indexed under this heading.

Buspirone Hydrochloride (Possible additive effects of CNS depressants). Products include:
- BuSpar 1401

Butabarbital (Possible additive effects of CNS depressants). Products include:
- Pyridium Plus 1764

Butalbital (Possible additive effects of CNS depressants). Products include:
- Esgic-Plus Tablets 1002
- Esgic Tablets & Capsules 1001
- Fioricet Tablets 2006
- Fiorinal Capsules 2007
- Fiorinal with Codeine Capsules 2008
- Fiorinal Tablets 2007
- Phrenilin 838
- Sedapap Tablets 50 mg/650 mg .. 1360

Chlordiazepoxide (Possible additive effects of CNS depressants). Products include:
- Libritabs Tablets 1930
- Limbitrol 1933
- Menrium Tablets 1934

Chlordiazepoxide Hydrochloride (Possible additive effects of CNS depressants). Products include:
- Librax Capsules 1929
- Librium Capsules 1931
- Librium Injectable 1932

Chlorpromazine (Possible additive effects of CNS depressants). Products include:
- Thorazine 2234

Chlorprothixene (Possible additive effects of CNS depressants). Products include:
- Taractan Tablets 1920

Chlorprothixene Hydrochloride (Possible additive effects of CNS depressants). Products include:
- Taractan 1920

Clorazepate Dipotassium (Possible additive effects of CNS depressants). Products include:
- Tranxene 556

Codeine (Possible additive effects of CNS depressants). Products include:
- Calcidrine Syrup 506

Codeine Phosphate (Possible additive effects of CNS depressants). Products include:
- Actifed with Codeine Cough Syrup.. 752
- Cheracol Cough Syrup 1853
- Codimal PH Syrup 846
- Dimetane-DC Cough Syrup 1857
- Empirin with Codeine Phosphate Nos. 2, 3 & 4 764
- Fiorinal with Codeine Capsules 2008
- Isoclor Expectorant 982
- Naldecon CX Adult Liquid .... ⊡ 521
- Novahistine DH 1342
- Novahistine Expectorant 1343
- Nucofed Capsules 2219
- Nucofed Expectorant 2219
- Nucofed Pediatric Expectorant 2220
- Nucofed Syrup 2219
- Phenaphen with Codeine Capsules 1865
- Phenaphen-650 with Codeine Tablets 1866
- Phenergan with Codeine 2497
- Phenergan VC with Codeine 2501
- Robitussin A-C Syrup 1875
- Robitussin-DAC Syrup 1875
- Ryna .... ⊡ 741
- Soma Compound w/Codeine Tablets 2390
- Triaminic Expectorant w/Codeine .. 1996
- Tussi-Organidin Liquid 2391
- Tylenol with Codeine 1381

Codeine Polistirex (Possible additive effects of CNS depressants).
No products indexed under this heading.

Deserpidine (Increased effect of hypertensives). Products include:
- Enduronyl 518
- Harmonyl Tablets 528
- Oreticyl 545

Dezocine (Possible additive effects of CNS depressants).

Diazepam (Possible additive effects of CNS depressants). Products include:
- Valium Injectable 1937
- Valium Tablets 1939
- Valrelease Capsules 1923

Droperidol (Possible additive effects of CNS depressants). Products include:
- Inapsine Injection 1140
- Innovar Injection 1141

Enflurane (Possible additive effects of CNS depressants). Products include:
- Ethrane 599

Estazolam (Possible additive effects of CNS depressants). Products include:
- ProSom Tablets 554

Ethchlorvynol (Possible additive effects of CNS depressants). Products include:
- Placidyl Capsules 553

Ethinamate (Possible additive effects of CNS depressants).
No products indexed under this heading.

Fentanyl (Possible additive effects of CNS depressants). Products include:
- Duragesic Transdermal System 1133

Fentanyl Citrate (Possible additive effects of CNS depressants). Products include:
- Innovar Injection 1141
- Sublimaze Injection 1146

Fluphenazine Decanoate (Possible additive effects of CNS depressants). Products include:
- Prolixin Decanoate 1795

Fluphenazine Enanthate (Possible additive effects of CNS depressants). Products include:
- Prolixin Enanthate 1796

Fluphenazine Hydrochloride (Possible additive effects of CNS depressants). Products include:
- Prolixin Elixir 1793
- Prolixin Injection 1791
- Prolixin Oral Concentrate 1792
- Prolixin Tablets 1793

Flurazepam Hydrochloride (Possible additive effects of CNS depressants). Products include:
- Dalmane Capsules 1927

Furazolidone (Hypertensive crisis may result). Products include:
- Furoxone 1855

Glutethimide (Possible additive effects of CNS depressants).
No products indexed under this heading.

Guanadrel Sulfate (Increased effect of hypertensives). Products include:
- Hylorel Tablets 975

Guanethidine Monosulfate (Potential for slight increase in antihypertensive effect). Products include:
- Esimil Tablets 864
- Ismelin Tablets 869

Haloperidol (Possible additive effects of CNS depressants). Products include:
- Haldol Injection, Tablets and Concentrate 1373

Haloperidol Decanoate (Possible additive effects of CNS depressants). Products include:
- Haldol Decanoate 1375

Hydrocodone Bitartrate (Possible additive effects of CNS depressants). Products include:
- Anexsia 5/500 Tablets 2196
- Anexsia 7.5/650 Tablets 2197
- Azdone Tablets 844
- Codiclear DH Syrup 845
- Codimal DH Syrup 846
- Damason-P 1356
- Hycodan Syrup, Tablets 927
- Hycomine Compound Tablets 929
- Hycomine Syrup 927
- Hycotuss Expectorant Syrup 930
- Hydrocet Capsules 835
- Lortab ASA Tablets 2414
- Lortab 2412
- Ru-Tuss with Hydrocodone 694
- Triaminic Expectorant DH 1995
- Vicodin Tablets 1187
- Vicodin ES Tablets 1189
- Zydone Capsules 941

Hydrocodone Polistirex (Possible additive effects of CNS depressants). Products include:
- Tussionex Extended-Release Suspension 988

Hydroxyzine Hydrochloride (Possible additive effects of CNS depressants). Products include:
- Atarax Tablets & Syrup 1941
- Marax Tablets & DF Syrup 1954
- Vistaril Intramuscular Solution 1970

Isocarboxazid (Hypertensive crisis may result; concurrent or sequential use within 14 days is contraindicated). Products include:
- Marplan Tablets 1906

Isoflurane (Possible additive effects of CNS depressants). Products include:
- Forane 600

Ketamine Hydrochloride (Possible additive effects of CNS depressants). Products include:
- Ketalar 1726

Levorphanol Tartrate (Possible additive effects of CNS depressants). Products include:
- Levo-Dromoran 1906

Lorazepam (Possible additive effects of CNS depressants). Products include:
- Ativan Injection 2432
- Ativan Tablets 2434

Loxapine Hydrochloride (Possible additive effects of CNS depressants). Products include:
- Loxitane 1213

Loxapine Succinate (Possible additive effects of CNS depressants). Products include:
- Loxitane Capsules 1213

Meperidine Hydrochloride (Possible additive effects of CNS depressants). Products include:
- Demerol 2047
- Mepergan Injection 2479

Mephobarbital (Possible additive effects of CNS depressants). Products include:
- Mebaral Tablets 2061

Meprobamate (Possible additive effects of CNS depressants). Products include:
- Deprol Tablets 2382
- Equagesic Tablets 2451
- Miltown Tablets 2386
- PMB 200 and PMB 400 2504

Mesoridazine (Possible additive effects of CNS depressants). Products include:
- Serentil 686

Mesoridazine Besylate (Possible additive effects of CNS depressants).

Methadone Hydrochloride (Possible additive effects of CNS depressants). Products include:
- Dolophine Hydrochloride Ampoules & Vials 1260
- Dolophine Hydrochloride Tablets 1261
- Methadone Hydrochloride Diskets 1284
- Methadone Hydrochloride Oral Solution & Tablets 1987

Methohexital Sodium (Possible additive effects of CNS depressants). Products include:
- Brevital Sodium Vials 1248

Methoxyflurane (Possible additive effects of CNS depressants).
- No products indexed under this heading.

Methyldopa (Potential for slight increase in antihypertensive effect). Products include:
- Aldoclor Tablets 1413
- Aldomet Oral 1415
- Aldoril Tablets 1418

Methyldopate Hydrochloride (Potential for slight increase in antihypertensive effect). Products include:
- Aldomet Ester HCl Injection 1417

Midazolam Hydrochloride (Possible additive effects of CNS depressants). Products include:
- Versed Injection 1924

Molindone Hydrochloride (Possible additive effects of CNS depressants). Products include:
- Moban Tablets & Concentrate 932

Morphine Sulfate (Possible additive effects of CNS depressants). Products include:
- Astramorph/PF Injection, USP (Preservative-Free) 618
- Duramorph 960
- Infumorph 200 and Infumorph 500 Sterile Solutions 962
- MS Contin Tablets 1814
- MSIR 1817
- Oramorph SR (Morphine Sulfate Sustained Release Tablets) 1988
- Roxanol 1991

Opium Alkaloids (Possible additive effects of CNS depressants). Products include:
- B & O No. 15A & No. 16A Supprettes 2395
- Pantopon Injectable 1911

Oxazepam (Possible additive effects of CNS depressants). Products include:
- Serax Capsules 2522
- Serax Tablets 2522

Oxycodone Hydrochloride (Possible additive effects of CNS depressants). Products include:
- Percocet Tablets 950
- Percodan 951
- Roxicodone Tablets, Oral Solution & Intensol (Oxycodone) 1992
- Tylox Capsules 1382

Pentobarbital Sodium (Possible additive effects of CNS depressants). Products include:
- Nembutal Sodium Capsules 534
- Nembutal Sodium Solution 536
- Nembutal Sodium Suppositories 538

Perphenazine (Possible additive effects of CNS depressants). Products include:
- Etrafon 2087
- Triavil Tablets 1556
- Trilafon 2123

Phenelzine Sulfate (Hypertensive crisis may result; concurrent or sequential use within 14 days is contraindicated). Products include:
- Nardil 1742

Phenobarbital (Possible additive effects of CNS depressants). Products include:
- Arco-Lase Plus Tablets 607
- Bellergal-S Tablets 1998
- Bronkolixir .... ▣ 761
- Bronkotabs Tablets .... ▣ 762
- Donnatal 1858
- Donnatal Extentabs 1859
- Donnatal Tablets 1858
- Donnazyme Tablets 1860
- Kinesed Tablets 2272
- Phenobarbital Elixir and Tablets 1293
- Primatene Tablets-P Formula 2421
- Quadrinal Tablets 1183
- Tedral SA 1765

Prazepam (Possible additive effects of CNS depressants). Products include:
- Centrax 1693

Prochlorperazine (Possible additive effects of CNS depressants). Products include:
- Compazine 2201

Promethazine Hydrochloride (Possible additive effects of CNS depressants). Products include:
- Mepergan Injection 2479
- Phenergan with Codeine 2497
- Phenergan with Dextromethorphan 2499
- Phenergan Injection 2493
- Phenergan Suppositories 2496
- Phenergan Syrup 2495
- Phenergan Tablets 2496
- Phenergan VC 2500
- Phenergan VC with Codeine 2501

Propofol (Possible additive effects of CNS depressants). Products include:
- Diprivan Injection 2267

Propoxyphene Hydrochloride (Possible additive effects of CNS depressants). Products include:
- Darvon 1256
- Wygesic Tablets 2540

Propoxyphene Napsylate (Possible additive effects of CNS depressants). Products include:
- Darvon-N/Darvocet-N 1254

Quazepam (Possible additive effects of CNS depressants). Products include:
- Doral Tablets 2383

Rauwolfia Serpentina (Potential for slight increase in antihypertensive effect). Products include:
- Raudixin Tablets 1803
- Rauzide Tablets 1804

Rescinnamine (Potential for slight increase in antihypertensive effect).
- No products indexed under this heading.

Reserpine (Potential for slight increase in antihypertensive effect). Products include:
- Diupres Tablets 1461
- Hydromox R Tablets 1209
- Hydropres Tablets 1485
- Renese-R Tablets 1786
- Salutensin/Salutensin-Demi 719
- Ser-Ap-Es Tablets 881
- Serpasil Tablets 883
- Serpasil-Apresoline Tablets 884
- Serpasil-Esidrix Tablets 886

Secobarbital Sodium (Possible additive effects of CNS depressants). Products include:
- Seconal Sodium Pulvules 1296

Selegiline Hydrochloride (Hypertensive crisis may result; concurrent or sequential use within 14 days is contraindicated). Products include:
- Eldepryl 2250

Sufentanil Citrate (Possible additive effects of CNS depressants). Products include:
- Sufenta Injection 1147

Temazepam (Possible additive effects of CNS depressants). Products include:
- Restoril Capsules 2023

Thiamylal Sodium (Possible additive effects of CNS depressants). Products include:
- Surital Ampoules, Steri-Vials 1764

Thioridazine Hydrochloride (Possible additive effects of CNS depressants). Products include:
- Mellaril 2011

Thiothixene (Possible additive effects of CNS depressants). Products include:
- Navane Capsules and Concentrate 1954
- Navane Intramuscular 1956

Tranylcypromine Sulfate (Hypertensive crisis may result; concurrent or sequential use within 14 days is contraindicated). Products include:
- Parnate Tablets 2222

Triazolam (Possible additive effects of CNS depressants). Products include:
- Halcion Tablets 2340

Trifluoperazine Hydrochloride (Possible additive effects of CNS depressants). Products include:
- Stelazine 2226

PONSTEL
(Mefenamic Acid) 1758
May interact with oral anticoagulants. Compounds in this category include:

Dicumarol (Prolonged prothrombin time). Products include:
- Dicumarol Tablets 516

Warfarin Sodium (Prolonged prothrombin time). Products include:
- Coumadin Injection & Tablets 944
- Panwarfin Tablets 547

PONTOCAINE HYDROCHLORIDE FOR SPINAL ANESTHESIA
(Tetracaine Hydrochloride) 2069
May interact with sulfonamides. Compounds in this category include:

Sulfamethizole (Inhibited sulfonamide action). Products include:
- Thiosulfil Forte Tablets 2526
- Urobiotic-250 Capsules 1968

Sulfamethoxazole (Inhibited sulfonamide action). Products include:
- Azo Gantanol Tablets 1887
- Bactrim DS Tablets 1891
- Bactrim I.V. Infusion 1889
- Bactrim 1891
- Gantanol 1899
- Septra 813
- Septra I.V. Infusion 808
- Septra I.V. Infusion ADD-Vantage Vials 810
- Septra 813

Sulfasalazine (Inhibited sulfonamide action). Products include:
- Azulfidine Tablets, EN-tabs, Oral Suspension 1157

Sulfinpyrazone (Inhibited sulfonamide action). Products include:
- Anturane 853

Sulfisoxazole (Inhibited sulfonamide action). Products include:
- Azo Gantrisin Tablets 1888
- Gantrisin Tablets 1901
- Pediazole 1973

Sulfisoxazole Diolamine (Inhibited sulfonamide action). Products include:
- Gantrisin Ophthalmic Ointment/Solution 1900

POSTURE 600 MG
(Calcium Phosphate) 2420
No interactions described in labeling.

POSTURE-D 600 MG
(Calcium Phosphate, Vitamin D) 2420
No interactions described in labeling.

POTABA
(Aminobenzoate Potassium) 1071
May interact with sulfonamides. Compounds in this category include:

Bendroflumethiazide (Concurrent administration contraindicated). Products include:
- Corzide Tablets 702
- Naturetin Tablets 1789
- Rauzide Tablets 1804

Chlorothiazide (Concurrent administration contraindicated). Products include:
- Aldoclor Tablets 1413
- Diupres Tablets 1461
- Diuril Oral 1464

Chlorothiazide Sodium (Concurrent administration contraindicated). Products include:
- Diuril Sodium Intravenous 1463

Chlorpropamide (Concurrent administration contraindicated). Products include:
- Diabinese Tablets 1775

Glipizide (Concurrent administration contraindicated). Products include:
- Glucotrol 1952

Glyburide (Concurrent administration contraindicated). Products include:
DiaBeta 1091
Micronase Tablets 2350

Hydrochlorothiazide (Concurrent administration contraindicated). Products include:
Aldactazide 2150
Aldoril Tablets 1418
Apresazide Capsules 854
Apresoline-Esidrix Tablets 857
Capozide 2258
Dyazide Capsules 2208
Esidrix Tablets 863
Esimil Tablets 864
HydroDIURIL Tablets 1484
Hydropres Tablets 1485
Inderide Tablets 2463
Inderide LA Long Acting Capsules 2465
Lopressor HCT Tablets 1034
Maxzide 1215
Moduretic Tablets 1510
Normozide Tablets 2112
Oretic Tablets 544
Oreticyl 545
Prinzide Tablets 1540
Ser-Ap-Es Tablets 881
Serpasil-Esidrix Tablets 886
Timolide Tablets 1547
Trandate HCT Tablets 579
Vaseretic Tablets 1559
Zestoretic 2274

Hydroflumethiazide (Concurrent administration contraindicated). Products include:
Diucardin Tablets 2450
Saluron 718
Salutensin/Salutensin-Demi 719

Methyclothiazide (Concurrent administration contraindicated). Products include:
Enduron Tablets 517
Enduronyl 518

Polythiazide (Concurrent administration contraindicated). Products include:
Minizide Capsules 1779
Renese Tablets 1785
Renese-R Tablets 1786

Sulfamethizole (Concurrent administration contraindicated). Products include:
Thiosulfil Forte Tablets 2526
Urobiotic-250 Capsules 1968

Sulfamethoxazole (Concurrent administration contraindicated). Products include:
Azo Gantanol Tablets 1887
Bactrim DS Tablets 1891
Bactrim I.V. Infusion 1889
Bactrim 1891
Gantanol 1899
Septra 813
Septra I.V. Infusion 808
Septra I.V. Infusion ADD-Vantage Vials 810
Septra 813

Sulfasalazine (Concurrent administration contraindicated). Products include:
Azulfidine Tablets, EN-tabs, Oral Suspension 1157

Sulfinpyrazone (Concurrent administration contraindicated). Products include:
Anturane 853

Sulfisoxazole (Concurrent administration contraindicated). Products include:
Azo Gantrisin Tablets 1888
Gantrisin Tablets 1901
Pediazole 1973

Sulfisoxazole Diolamine (Concurrent administration contraindicated). Products include:
Gantrisin Ophthalmic Ointment/Solution 1900

Tolazamide (Concurrent administration contraindicated). Products include:
Tolinase Tablets 2365

Tolbutamide (Concurrent administration contraindicated). Products include:
Orinase Tablets 2354

PRAMEGEL
(Pramoxine Hydrochloride) 1045
No interactions described in labeling.

PRAMET FA
(Vitamins with Minerals) 1974
No interactions described in labeling.

PRAMILET FA
(Vitamins with Minerals) 1974
No interactions described in labeling.

PRAMOSONE CREAM, LOTION & OINTMENT
(Hydrocortisone Acetate, Pramoxine Hydrochloride) 971
No interactions described in labeling.

PRED FORTE
(Prednisolone Acetate) ◉ 252
No interactions described in labeling.

PRED MILD
(Prednisolone Acetate) ◉ 254
No interactions described in labeling.

PRED-G LIQUIFILM STERILE OPHTHALMIC SUSPENSION
(Gentamicin Sulfate, Prednisolone Acetate) ◉ 252
No interactions described in labeling.

PRED-G S.O.P. STERILE OPHTHALMIC OINTMENT
(Gentamicin Sulfate, Prednisolone Acetate) ◉ 253
No interactions described in labeling.

PREFRIN LIQUIFILM VASOCONSTRICTOR AND LUBRICANT EYE DROPS
(Phenylephrine Hydrochloride) ◉ 254
No interactions described in labeling.

PREFRIN-A
(Phenylephrine Hydrochloride, Pyrilamine Maleate) ◉ 255
No interactions described in labeling.

PREGNYL
(Chorionic Gonadotropin) 1644
No interactions described in labeling.

PRELU-2 CAPSULES
(Phendimetrazine Tartrate) 683
May interact with monoamine oxidase inhibitors, insulin, and certain other agents. Compounds in these categories include:

Furazolidone (Contraindicated; hypertensive crises may result). Products include:
Furoxone 1855

Guanethidine Monosulfate (Decreased hypotensive effect). Products include:
Esimil Tablets 864
Ismelin Tablets 869

Insulin, Human (Altered insulin requirements).
No products indexed under this heading.

Insulin, Human Isophane Suspension (Altered insulin requirements). Products include:
Humulin N, 100 Units 1270

Insulin, Human NPH (Altered insulin requirements). Products include:
Insulatard NPH Human 1627
Novolin N 1627
Novolin N PenFill Cartridges 1628
Novolin N Prefilled 1628

Insulin, Human Regular (Altered insulin requirements). Products include:
Humulin BR, 100 Units 1268
Humulin R, 100 Units 1272
Novolin R 1627
Novolin R PenFill Cartridges 1628
Novolin R Prefilled 1629
Velosulin Human 1628

Insulin, Human, Zinc Suspension (Altered insulin requirements). Products include:
Humulin L, 100 Units 1268
Humulin U, 100 Units 1272
Novolin L 1627

Insulin, NPH (Altered insulin requirements). Products include:
NPH, 40 & 100 Units 1273
Beef NPH, 100 Units 1274
Pork NPH, 100 Units 1275
Insulatard NPH 1626
NPH Insulin 1626
NPH Purified Pork Isophane Insulin 1626

Insulin, Regular (Altered insulin requirements). Products include:
Regular, 40 & 100 Units 1273
Beef Regular, 100 Units 1275
Pork Regular, 100 Units 1275
Pork Regular (Concentrated), 500 Units 1276
Regular Insulin 1625
Regular Purified Pork Insulin 1626
Velosulin 1627

Insulin, Zinc Crystals (Altered insulin requirements). Products include:
NPH, 40 & 100 Units 1273

Insulin, Zinc Suspension (Altered insulin requirements). Products include:
Lente, 40 & 100 Units 1272
Protamine, Zinc, 40 & 100 Units 1273
Lente Iletin I 1272
Beef Lente, 100 Units 1274
Beef Protamine Zinc, 100 Units 1274
Pork Lente, 100 Units 1275
Pork, Protamine, Zinc, 100 Units 1275
Lente Insulin 1626
Lente Purified Pork Insulin 1626
Semilente Insulin 1625
Ultralente Insulin 1626

Isocarboxazid (Contraindicated; hypertensive crises may result). Products include:
Marplan Tablets 1906

Phenelzine Sulfate (Contraindicated; hypertensive crises may result). Products include:
Nardil 1742

Selegiline Hydrochloride (Contraindicated; hypertensive crises may result). Products include:
Eldepryl 2250

Tranylcypromine Sulfate (Contraindicated; hypertensive crises may result). Products include:
Parnate Tablets 2222

PREMARIN INTRAVENOUS
(Estrogens, Conjugated) 2508
No interactions described in labeling.

PREMARIN WITH METHYLTESTOSTERONE
(Estrogens, Conjugated, Methyltestosterone) 2515
May interact with oral anticoagulants, insulin, progestins, and certain other agents. Compounds in these categories include:

Dicumarol (Decreased anticoagulant requirements). Products include:
Dicumarol Tablets 516

Insulin, Human (Decreased blood glucose and insulin requirements).
No products indexed under this heading.

Insulin, Human Isophane Suspension (Decreased blood glucose and insulin requirements). Products include:
Humulin N, 100 Units 1270

Insulin, Human NPH (Decreased blood glucose and insulin requirements). Products include:
Insulatard NPH Human 1627
Novolin N 1627
Novolin N PenFill Cartridges 1628
Novolin N Prefilled 1628

Insulin, Human Regular (Decreased blood glucose and insulin requirements). Products include:
Humulin BR, 100 Units 1268
Humulin R, 100 Units 1272
Novolin R 1627
Novolin R PenFill Cartridges 1628
Novolin R Prefilled 1629
Velosulin Human 1628

Insulin, Human, Zinc Suspension (Decreased blood glucose and insulin requirements). Products include:
Humulin L, 100 Units 1268
Humulin U, 100 Units 1272
Novolin L 1627

Insulin, NPH (Decreased blood glucose and insulin requirements). Products include:
NPH, 40 & 100 Units 1273
Beef NPH, 100 Units 1274
Pork NPH, 100 Units 1275
Insulatard NPH 1626
NPH Insulin 1626
NPH Purified Pork Isophane Insulin 1626

Insulin, Regular (Decreased blood glucose and insulin requirements). Products include:
Regular, 40 & 100 Units 1273
Beef Regular, 100 Units 1275
Pork Regular, 100 Units 1275
Pork Regular (Concentrated), 500 Units 1276
Regular Insulin 1625
Regular Purified Pork Insulin 1626
Velosulin 1627

Insulin, Zinc Crystals (Decreased blood glucose and insulin requirements). Products include:
NPH, 40 & 100 Units 1273

Insulin, Zinc Suspension (Decreased blood glucose and insulin requirements). Products include:
Lente, 40 & 100 Units 1272
Protamine, Zinc, 40 & 100 Units 1273
Lente Iletin I 1272
Beef Lente, 100 Units 1274
Beef Protamine Zinc, 100 Units 1274
Pork Lente, 100 Units 1275
Pork, Protamine, Zinc, 100 Units 1275
Lente Insulin 1626
Lente Purified Pork Insulin 1626
Semilente Insulin 1625
Ultralente Insulin 1626

Medroxyprogesterone Acetate (Adverse effects on carbohydrate and lipid metabolism). Products include:
Amen 833
Cycrin Tablets 2449
Depo-Provera Sterile Aqueous Suspension 2336
Provera Tablets 2356

Megestrol Acetate (Adverse effects on carbohydrate and lipid metabolism). Products include:
Megace Tablets 732

Norgestimate (Adverse effects on carbohydrate and lipid metabolism). Products include:
Ortho-Cyclen Tablets 1658

Oxyphenbutazone (Elevated serum levels of oxyphenbutazone).

Warfarin Sodium (Decreased anticoagulant requirements). Products include:
Coumadin Injection & Tablets 944
Panwarfin Tablets 547

PREMARIN TABLETS
(Estrogens, Conjugated) 2510
May interact with progestins. Compounds in this category include:

Medroxyprogesterone Acetate (Potential adverse effects on carbohydrate and lipid metabolism). Products include:
- Amen 833
- Cycrin Tablets 2449
- Depo-Provera Sterile Aqueous Suspension 2336
- Provera Tablets 2356

Megestrol Acetate (Potential adverse effects on carbohydrate and lipid metabolism). Products include:
- Megace Tablets 732

Norgestimate (Potential adverse effects on carbohydrate and lipid metabolism). Products include:
- Ortho-Cyclen Tablets 1658

PREMARIN VAGINAL CREAM
(Estrogens, Conjugated) 2512
May interact with progestins. Compounds in this category include:

Medroxyprogesterone Acetate (Potential adverse effects on carbohydrate and lipid metabolism). Products include:
- Amen 833
- Cycrin Tablets 2449
- Depo-Provera Sterile Aqueous Suspension 2336
- Provera Tablets 2356

Megestrol Acetate (Potential adverse effects on carbohydrate and lipid metabolism). Products include:
- Megace Tablets 732

Norgestimate (Potential adverse effects on carbohydrate and lipid metabolism). Products include:
- Ortho-Cyclen Tablets 1658

PREMSYN PMS CAPSULES & CAPLETS
(Acetaminophen, Pamabrom, Pyrilamine Maleate) .... ▣ 547
No interactions described in labeling.

PREPARATION H HEMORRHOIDAL CREAM
(Yeast Cell Derivative, Live) 2420
No interactions described in labeling.

PREPARATION H HEMORRHOIDAL OINTMENT
(Yeast Cell Derivative, Live) 2420
No interactions described in labeling.

PREPARATION H HEMORRHOIDAL SUPPOSITORIES
(Yeast Cell Derivative, Live) 2420
No interactions described in labeling.

PRE-PEN
(Benzylpenicilloyl-Polylysine) 2148
No interactions described in labeling.

PRESUN 15 FACIAL SUNSCREEN
(Octyl Dimethyl PABA, Oxybenzone) .... ▣ 537
No interactions described in labeling.

PRESUN FOR KIDS
(Octyl Methoxycinnamate)............... ▣ 537
No interactions described in labeling.

PRESUN 8, 15 AND 39 CREAMY SUNSCREENS
(Octyl Dimethyl PABA, Oxybenzone) .... ▣ 537
No interactions described in labeling.

PRESUN 15 AND 29 SENSITIVE SKIN SUNSCREEN
(Octyl Dimethyl PABA, Oxybenzone) .... ▣ 537
No interactions described in labeling.

PRESUN 23 SPRAY MIST
(Octyl Dimethyl PABA, Octyl Methoxycinnamate, Oxybenzone, Octyl Salicylate) .... ▣ 537
No interactions described in labeling.

PRILOSEC DELAYED-RELEASE CAPSULES
(Omeprazole) 1530
May interact with absorption of drugs where gastric ph is an important determinant in their bioavailability and certain other agents. Compounds in these categories include:

Bacampicillin Hydrochloride (Omeprazole may interfere with the gastric absorption). Products include:
- Spectrobid Tablets & Powder for Oral Suspension 1961

Cyclosporine (Potential of metabolism interaction via the cytochrome P-450 system). Products include:
- Sandimmune 2024

Diazepam (Prolonged elimination of diazepam). Products include:
- Valium Injectable 1937
- Valium Tablets 1939
- Valrelease Capsules 1923

Disulfiram (Potential of metabolism interaction via the cytochrome P-450 system). Products include:
- Antabuse Tablets 2429

Drugs which undergo biotransformation by cytochrome P-450 mixed function oxidase (Potential of metabolism interaction via the cytochrome P-450 system).

Ferrous Fumarate (Omeprazole may interfere with the gastric absorption). Products include:
- Bugs Bunny Plus Iron Children's Chewable Vitamins (Sugar Free) ▣ 625
- Caltrate 600 + Iron & Vitamin D 1198
- Centrum, Jr. (Children's Chewable) + Iron .... ▣ 586
- Chromagen Capsules 2078
- FemIron Multi-Vitamins and Iron .... ▣ 617
- Ferancee Chewable Tablets 1155
- Ferancee-HP Tablets 1155
- Ferro-Sequels 1203
- Flintstones Children's Chewable Vitamins Plus Iron .... ▣ 625
- Natalins Rx 1391
- Natalins Tablets 1391
- Nephro-Fer Tablets 1826
- One-A-Day Maximum Formula Vitamins and Minerals .... ▣ 627
- Poly-Vi-Flor with Iron 1399
- Poly-Vi-Sol Vitamins with Iron, Chewable Tablets and Circus Shapes Chewable .... ▣ 612
- Pramilet FA 1974
- Stressgard Stress Formula Vitamins .... ▣ 628
- Stresstabs + Iron, Advanced Formula .... ▣ 589
- Stuartinic Tablets 1157
- Theragran-M Tablets .... ▣ 727
- Trinsicon Capsules 2415
- Within Women's Formula Multivitamin with Calcium, Extra Iron and Zinc .... ▣ 628
- Zenate Tablets 2250

Ferrous Gluconate (Omeprazole may interfere with the gastric absorption). Products include:
- Fergon .... ▣ 758

Ferrous Sulfate (Omeprazole may interfere with the gastric absorption). Products include:
- Dayalets Plus Iron Filmtab .... ▣ 502
- Feosol Capsules 2191
- Feosol Elixir 2191
- Feosol Tablets 2191
- Fero-Folic-500 Filmtab 527
- Fero-Grad-500 Filmtab 528
- Fero-Gradumet Filmtab 528
- Iberet Tablets 531
- Iberet-500 Liquid 531
- Iberet-Folic-500 Filmtab 527
- Iberet-Liquid 531
- Irospan 972
- Mol-Iron .... ▣ 703
- Poly-Vi-Sol Vitamins with Iron, Drops .... ▣ 612
- Pramet FA 1974
- Slow Fe Tablets 852
- Tri-Vi-Sol Vitamin Drops with Iron ▣ 614

Ketoconazole (Omeprazole may interfere with the gastric absorption). Products include:
- Nizoral 2% Cream 1143
- Nizoral 2% Shampoo 1144
- Nizoral Tablets 1145

Phenytoin (Prolonged elimination of phenytoin). Products include:
- Dilantin Infatabs 1710
- Dilantin-30 Pediatric/Dilantin-125 Suspension 1713

Phenytoin Sodium (Prolonged elimination of phenytoin). Products include:
- Dilantin Kapseals 1708
- Dilantin Parenteral 1712
- Dilantin with Phenobarbital Kapseals 1715

Warfarin Sodium (Prolonged elimination of warfarin). Products include:
- Coumadin Injection & Tablets 944
- Panwarfin Tablets 547

PRIMATENE MIST
(Epinephrine) 2420
May interact with antihypertensives and antidepressant drugs. Compounds in these categories include:

Acebutolol Hydrochloride (Patients are advised to consult physician). Products include:
- Sectral Capsules 2520

Amitriptyline Hydrochloride (Patients are advised to consult physician). Products include:
- Elavil 2269
- Endep Tablets 1927
- Etrafon 2087
- Limbitrol 1933
- Triavil Tablets 1556

Amoxapine (Patients are advised to consult physician). Products include:
- Asendin Tablets 1196

Atenolol (Patients are advised to consult physician). Products include:
- Tenoretic Tablets 1105
- Tenormin Tablets and I.V. Injection 1107

Benazepril Hydrochloride (Patients are advised to consult physician). Products include:
- Lotensin Tablets 872

Betaxolol Hydrochloride (Patients are advised to consult physician). Products include:
- Betoptic Sterile Ophthalmic Solution 569
- Betoptic S Sterile Ophthalmic Suspension 570
- Kerlone Tablets 2172

Bupropion Hydrochloride (Patients are advised to consult physician). Products include:
- Wellbutrin Tablets 821

Captopril (Patients are advised to consult physician). Products include:
- Capoten 2255
- Capozide 2258

Carteolol Hydrochloride (Patients are advised to consult physician). Products include:
- Cartrol Tablets 507

Clonidine (Patients are advised to consult physician). Products include:
- Catapres-TTS 677

Clonidine Hydrochloride (Patients are advised to consult physician). Products include:
- Catapres Tablets 676
- Combipres Tablets 678

Deserpidine (Patients are advised to consult physician). Products include:
- Enduronyl 518
- Harmonyl Tablets 528
- Oreticyl 545

Desipramine Hydrochloride (Patients are advised to consult physician). Products include:
- Norpramin Tablets 1340

Diazoxide (Patients are advised to consult physician). Products include:
- Hyperstat I.V. Injection 2095
- Proglycem 649

Doxazosin Mesylate (Patients are advised to consult physician). Products include:
- Cardura Tablets 1941

Doxepin Hydrochloride (Patients are advised to consult physician). Products include:
- Sinequan 1960

Enalapril Maleate (Patients are advised to consult physician). Products include:
- Vaseretic Tablets 1559
- Vasotec Tablets 1564

Enalaprilat (Patients are advised to consult physician). Products include:
- Vasotec I.V. 1562

Esmolol Hydrochloride (Patients are advised to consult physician). Products include:
- Brevibloc Injection 942

Felodipine (Patients are advised to consult physician). Products include:
- Plendil Extended-Release Tablets 1526

Fluoxetine Hydrochloride (Patients are advised to consult physician). Products include:
- Prozac Pulvules 920

Fosinopril Sodium (Patients are advised to consult physician). Products include:
- Monopril Tablets 1406

Guanabenz Acetate (Patients are advised to consult physician). Products include:
- Wytensin Tablets 2542

Guanethidine Monosulfate (Patients are advised to consult physician). Products include:
- Esimil Tablets 864
- Ismelin Tablets 869

Hydralazine Hydrochloride (Patients are advised to consult physician). Products include:
- Apresazide Capsules 854
- Apresoline Hydrochloride Parenteral (Ampuls) 856
- Apresoline Hydrochloride Tablets 855
- Apresoline-Esidrix Tablets 857
- Ser-Ap-Es Tablets 881
- Serpasil-Apresoline Tablets 884

Imipramine Hydrochloride (Patients are advised to consult physician). Products include:
- Tofranil Ampuls 1038
- Tofranil Tablets 1039

Imipramine Pamoate (Patients are advised to consult physician). Products include:
- Tofranil-PM Capsules 1041

Isocarboxazid (Patients are advised to consult physician). Products include:
- Marplan Tablets 1906

Isradipine (Patients are advised to consult physician). Products include:
- DynaCirc Capsules 2004

Labetalol Hydrochloride (Patients are advised to consult physician). Products include:
- Normodyne Injection ... 2108
- Normodyne Tablets ... 2110
- Normozide Tablets ... 2112
- Trandate HCT Tablets ... 579
- Trandate Injection ... 577
- Trandate Tablets ... 579

Lisinopril (Patients are advised to consult physician). Products include:
- Prinivil Tablets ... 1538
- Prinzide Tablets ... 1540
- Zestoretic ... 2274
- Zestril Tablets ... 2277

Maprotiline Hydrochloride (Patients are advised to consult physician). Products include:
- Ludiomil Tablets ... 874

Mecamylamine Hydrochloride (Patients are advised to consult physician). Products include:
- Inversine Tablets ... 1492

Methyldopa (Patients are advised to consult physician). Products include:
- Aldoclor Tablets ... 1413
- Aldomet Oral ... 1415
- Aldoril Tablets ... 1418

Methyldopate Hydrochloride (Patients are advised to consult physician). Products include:
- Aldomet Ester HCl Injection ... 1417

Metoprolol Tartrate (Patients are advised to consult physician). Products include:
- Lopressor Ampuls ... 1032
- Lopressor HCT Tablets ... 1034
- Lopressor Tablets ... 1032

Metyrosine (Patients are advised to consult physician). Products include:
- Demser Capsules ... 1460

Minoxidil (Patients are advised to consult physician). Products include:
- Loniten Tablets ... 2346
- Rogaine Topical Solution ... 2357

Nadolol (Patients are advised to consult physician). Products include:
- Corgard Tablets ... 701
- Corzide Tablets ... 702

Nicardipine Hydrochloride (Patients are advised to consult physician). Products include:
- Cardene Capsules ... 2290

Nitroglycerin (Patients are advised to consult physician). Products include:
- Deponit NTG Transdermal Delivery System ... 2143
- Minitran Transdermal Delivery System ... 1312
- Nitro-Bid Ointment ... 1339
- Nitro-Bid Capsules ... 1338
- Nitrodisc ... 2176
- Nitro-Dur (nitroglycerin) Transdermal Infusion System ... 1164
- Nitrogard Tablets ... 1004
- Nitrolingual Spray ... 1846
- Nitrostat Tablets ... 1743
- Transderm-Nitro Transdermal Therapeutic System ... 2283

Nortriptyline Hydrochloride (Patients are advised to consult physician). Products include:
- Pamelor ... 2019

Penbutolol Sulfate (Patients are advised to consult physician). Products include:
- Levatol ... 1832

Phenelzine Sulfate (Patients are advised to consult physician). Products include:
- Nardil ... 1742

Phenoxybenzamine Hydrochloride (Patients are advised to consult physician). Products include:
- Dibenzyline Capsules ... 2207

Phentolamine Mesylate (Patients are advised to consult physician). Products include:
- Regitine ... 878

Pindolol (Patients are advised to consult physician). Products include:
- Visken Tablets ... 2036

Prazosin Hydrochloride (Patients are advised to consult physician). Products include:
- Minipress Capsules ... 1778
- Minizide Capsules ... 1779

Propranolol Hydrochloride (Patients are advised to consult physician). Products include:
- Inderal ... 2459
- Inderal LA Long Acting Capsules ... 2461
- Inderide Tablets ... 2463
- Inderide LA Long Acting Capsules ... 2465

Protriptyline Hydrochloride (Patients are advised to consult physician). Products include:
- Vivactil Tablets ... 1567

Ramipril (Patients are advised to consult physician). Products include:
- Altace Capsules ... 1086

Rauwolfia Serpentina (Patients are advised to consult physician). Products include:
- Raudixin Tablets ... 1803
- Rauzide Tablets ... 1804

Rescinnamine (Patients are advised to consult physician).
- No products indexed under this heading.

Reserpine (Patients are advised to consult physician). Products include:
- Diupres Tablets ... 1461
- Hydromox R Tablets ... 1209
- Hydropres Tablets ... 1485
- Renese-R Tablets ... 1786
- Salutensin/Salutensin-Demi ... 719
- Ser-Ap-Es Tablets ... 881
- Serpasil Tablets ... 883
- Serpasil-Apresoline Tablets ... 884
- Serpasil-Esidrix Tablets ... 886

Selegiline Hydrochloride (Patients are advised to consult a physician). Products include:
- Eldepryl ... 2250

Sodium Nitroprusside (Patients are advised to consult physician). Products include:
- Nipride I.V. Infusion ... 1909

Terazosin Hydrochloride (Patients are advised to consult physician). Products include:
- Hytrin Tablets ... 529

Timolol Maleate (Patients are advised to consult physician). Products include:
- Blocadren Tablets ... 1429
- Timolide Tablets ... 1547
- Timoptic in Ocudose ... 1552
- Timoptic Sterile Ophthalmic Solution ... 1550

Tranylcypromine Sulfate (Patients are advised to consult physician). Products include:
- Parnate Tablets ... 2222

Trazodone Hydrochloride (Patients are advised to consult physician). Products include:
- Desyrel and Desyrel Dividose ... 1404

Trimethaphan Camsylate (Patients are advised to consult physician). Products include:
- Arfonad Ampuls ... 1887

Trimipramine Maleate (Patients are advised to consult physician). Products include:
- Surmontil Capsules ... 2524

PRIMATENE MIST SUSPENSION
(Epinephrine Bitartrate) ... 2421
May interact with antihypertensives and antidepressant drugs. Compounds in these categories include:

Acebutolol Hydrochloride (Patients are advised to consult a physician). Products include:
- Sectral Capsules ... 2520

Atenolol (Patients are advised to consult a physician). Products include:
- Tenoretic Tablets ... 1105
- Tenormin Tablets and I.V. Injection 1107

Benazepril Hydrochloride (Patients are advised to consult a physician). Products include:
- Lotensin Tablets ... 872

Betaxolol Hydrochloride (Patients are advised to consult a physician). Products include:
- Betoptic Sterile Ophthalmic Solution ... 569
- Betoptic S Sterile Ophthalmic Suspension ... 570
- Kerlone Tablets ... 2172

Captopril (Patients are advised to consult a physician). Products include:
- Capoten ... 2255
- Capozide ... 2258

Carteolol Hydrochloride (Patients are advised to consult a physician). Products include:
- Cartrol Tablets ... 507

Clonidine (Patients are advised to consult a physician). Products include:
- Catapres-TTS ... 677

Clonidine Hydrochloride (Patients are advised to consult a physician). Products include:
- Catapres Tablets ... 676
- Combipres Tablets ... 678

Deserpidine (Patients are advised to consult a physician). Products include:
- Enduronyl ... 518
- Harmonyl Tablets ... 528
- Oreticyl ... 545

Diazoxide (Patients are advised to consult a physician). Products include:
- Hyperstat I.V. Injection ... 2095
- Proglycem ... 649

Doxazosin Mesylate (Patients are advised to consult a physician). Products include:
- Cardura Tablets ... 1941

Enalapril Maleate (Patients are advised to consult a physician). Products include:
- Vaseretic Tablets ... 1559
- Vasotec Tablets ... 1564

Enalaprilat (Patients are advised to consult a physician). Products include:
- Vasotec I.V. ... 1562

Esmolol Hydrochloride (Patients are advised to consult a physician). Products include:
- Brevibloc Injection ... 942

Felodipine (Patients are advised to consult a physician). Products include:
- Plendil Extended-Release Tablets ... 1526

Fosinopril Sodium (Patients are advised to consult a physician). Products include:
- Monopril Tablets ... 1406

Guanabenz Acetate (Patients are advised to consult a physician). Products include:
- Wytensin Tablets ... 2542

Guanethidine Monosulfate (Patients are advised to consult a physician). Products include:
- Esimil Tablets ... 864
- Ismelin Tablets ... 869

Hydralazine Hydrochloride (Patients are advised to consult a physician). Products include:
- Apresazide Capsules ... 854
- Apresoline Hydrochloride Parenteral (Ampuls) ... 856
- Apresoline Hydrochloride Tablets ... 855
- Apresoline-Esidrix Tablets ... 857
- Ser-Ap-Es Tablets ... 881
- Serpasil-Apresoline Tablets ... 884

Isocarboxazid (Patients are advised to consult a physician). Products include:
- Marplan Tablets ... 1906

Isradipine (Patients are advised to consult a physician). Products include:
- DynaCirc Capsules ... 2004

Labetalol Hydrochloride (Patients are advised to consult a physician). Products include:
- Normodyne Injection ... 2108
- Normodyne Tablets ... 2110
- Normozide Tablets ... 2112
- Trandate HCT Tablets ... 579
- Trandate Injection ... 577
- Trandate Tablets ... 579

Lisinopril (Patients are advised to consult a physician). Products include:
- Prinivil Tablets ... 1538
- Prinzide Tablets ... 1540
- Zestoretic ... 2274
- Zestril Tablets ... 2277

Mecamylamine Hydrochloride (Patients are advised to consult a physician). Products include:
- Inversine Tablets ... 1492

Methyclothiazide (Patients are advised to consult a physician). Products include:
- Enduron Tablets ... 517
- Enduronyl ... 518

Methyldopa (Patients are advised to consult a physician). Products include:
- Aldoclor Tablets ... 1413
- Aldomet Oral ... 1415
- Aldoril Tablets ... 1418

Methyldopate Hydrochloride (Patients are advised to consult a physician). Products include:
- Aldomet Ester HCl Injection ... 1417

Metoprolol Tartrate (Patients are advised to consult a physician). Products include:
- Lopressor Ampuls ... 1032
- Lopressor HCT Tablets ... 1034
- Lopressor Tablets ... 1032

Metyrosine (Patients are advised to consult a physician). Products include:
- Demser Capsules ... 1460

Minoxidil (Patients are advised to consult a physician). Products include:
- Loniten Tablets ... 2346
- Rogaine Topical Solution ... 2357

Nadolol (Patients are advised to consult a physician). Products include:
- Corgard Tablets ... 701
- Corzide Tablets ... 702

Nicardipine Hydrochloride (Patients are advised to consult a physician). Products include:
- Cardene Capsules ... 2290

Nitroglycerin (Patients are advised to consult a physician). Products include:
- Deponit NTG Transdermal Delivery System ... 2143
- Minitran Transdermal Delivery System ... 1312
- Nitro-Bid Ointment ... 1339
- Nitro-Bid Capsules ... 1338
- Nitrodisc ... 2176
- Nitro-Dur (nitroglycerin) Transdermal Infusion System ... 1164
- Nitrogard Tablets ... 1004
- Nitrolingual Spray ... 1846

Nitrostat Tablets 1743
Transderm-Nitro Transdermal Therapeutic System 2283

Penbutolol Sulfate (Patients are advised to consult a physician). Products include:
Levatol 1832

Phenelzine Sulfate (Patients are advised to consult a physician). Products include:
Nardil 1742

Phenoxybenzamine Hydrochloride (Patients are advised to consult a physician). Products include:
Dibenzyline Capsules 2207

Phentolamine Mesylate (Patients are advised to consult a physician). Products include:
Regitine 878

Pindolol (Patients are advised to consult a physician). Products include:
Visken Tablets 2036

Prazosin Hydrochloride (Patients are advised to consult a physician). Products include:
Minipress Capsules 1778
Minizide Capsules 1779

Propranolol Hydrochloride (Patients are advised to consult a physician). Products include:
Inderal 2459
Inderal LA Long Acting Capsules 2461
Inderide Tablets 2463
Inderide LA Long Acting Capsules 2465

Ramipril (Patients are advised to consult a physician). Products include:
Altace Capsules 1086

Rauwolfia Serpentina (Patients are advised to consult a physician). Products include:
Raudixin Tablets 1803
Rauzide Tablets 1804

Rescinnamine (Patients are advised to consult a physician).
No products indexed under this heading.

Reserpine (Patients are advised to consult a physician). Products include:
Diupres Tablets 1461
Hydromox R Tablets 1209
Hydropres Tablets 1485
Renese-R Tablets 1786
Salutensin/Salutensin-Demi 719
Ser-Ap-Es Tablets 881
Serpasil Tablets 883
Serpasil-Apresoline Tablets 884
Serpasil-Esidrix Tablets 886

Selegiline Hydrochloride (Patients are advised to consult a physician). Products include:
Eldepryl 2250

Sodium Nitroprusside (Patients are advised to consult a physician). Products include:
Nipride I.V. Infusion 1909

Terazosin Hydrochloride (Patients are advised to consult a physician). Products include:
Hytrin Tablets 529

Timolol Maleate (Patients are advised to consult a physician). Products include:
Blocadren Tablets 1429
Timolide Tablets 1547
Timoptic in Ocudose 1552
Timoptic Sterile Ophthalmic Solution 1550

Tranylcypromine Sulfate (Patients are advised to consult a physician). Products include:
Parnate Tablets 2222

Trimethaphan Camsylate (Patients are advised to consult a physician). Products include:
Arfonad Ampuls 1887

PRIMATENE TABLETS-M FORMULA
(Ephedrine Hydrochloride, Theophylline, Pyrilamine Maleate) 2421
No interactions described in labeling.

PRIMATENE TABLETS-P FORMULA
(Ephedrine Hydrochloride, Theophylline, Phenobarbital) 2421
No interactions described in labeling.

PRIMATENE TABLETS-REGULAR FORMULA
(Theophylline Anhydrous, Ephedrine Hydrochloride) 2421
No interactions described in labeling.

PRIMAXIN I.M.
(Imipenem-Cilastatin Sodium) 1532
May interact with:

Probenecid (Concomitant administration results in only minimal increase in plasma levels of imipenem). Products include:
Benemid Tablets 1426
ColBENEMID Tablets 1436
Wycillin Injection and Probenecid Tablets 2539

PRIMAXIN I.V.
(Imipenem-Cilastatin Sodium) 1535
May interact with:

Ganciclovir Sodium (Concomitant administration may result in generalized seizures). Products include:
Cytovene Sterile Powder 2292

Probenecid (Concomitant administration results in only minimal increase in plasma levels of imipenem). Products include:
Benemid Tablets 1426
ColBENEMID Tablets 1436
Wycillin Injection and Probenecid Tablets 2539

PRIMER UNNA BOOT
(Zinc Oxide) 1072
No interactions described in labeling.

PRINIVIL TABLETS
(Lisinopril) 1538
May interact with diuretics, potassium sparing diuretics, potassium-depleting corticosteroids, thiazides, lithium preparations, and certain other agents. Compounds in these categories include:

Amiloride Hydrochloride (Potential for significant hyperkalemia; possibility of excessive reduction in blood pressure). Products include:
Midamor Tablets 1508
Moduretic Tablets 1510

Bendroflumethiazide (Thiazide-induced potassium loss attenuated; possibility of excessive reduction in blood pressure). Products include:
Corzide Tablets 702
Naturetin Tablets 1789
Rauzide Tablets 1804

Bumetanide (Possibility of excessive reduction in blood pressure). Products include:
Bumex 1895

Chlorothiazide (Thiazide-induced potassium loss attenuated; possibility of excessive reduction in blood pressure). Products include:
Aldoclor Tablets 1413
Diupres Tablets 1461
Diuril Oral 1464

Chlorothiazide Sodium (Thiazide-induced potassium loss attenuated; possibility of excessive reduction in blood pressure). Products include:
Diuril Sodium Intravenous 1463

Chlorthalidone (Possibility of excessive reduction in blood pressure). Products include:
Combipres Tablets 678
Tenoretic Tablets 1105
Thalitone Tablets 687

Ethacrynic Acid (Possibility of excessive reduction in blood pressure). Products include:
Edecrin Tablets 1468

Furosemide (Possibility of excessive reduction in blood pressure). Products include:
Lasix 1093

Hydrochlorothiazide (Thiazide-induced potassium loss attenuated; possibility of excessive reduction in blood pressure). Products include:
Aldactazide 2150
Aldoril Tablets 1418
Apresazide Capsules 854
Apresoline-Esidrix Tablets 857
Capozide 2258
Dyazide Capsules 2208
Esidrix Tablets 863
Esimil Tablets 864
HydroDIURIL Tablets 1484
Hydropres Tablets 1485
Inderide Tablets 2463
Inderide LA Long Acting Capsules 2465
Lopressor HCT Tablets 1034
Maxzide 1215
Moduretic Tablets 1510
Normozide Tablets 2112
Oretic Tablets 544
Oreticyl 545
Prinzide Tablets 1540
Ser-Ap-Es Tablets 881
Serpasil-Esidrix Tablets 886
Timolide Tablets 1547
Trandate HCT Tablets 579
Vaseretic Tablets 1559
Zestoretic 2274

Hydroflumethiazide (Thiazide-induced potassium loss attenuated; possibility of excessive reduction in blood pressure). Products include:
Diucardin Tablets 2450
Saluron 718
Salutensin/Salutensin-Demi 719

Indapamide (Possibility of excessive reduction in blood pressure). Products include:
Lozol Tablets 1843

Indomethacin (Reduces antihypertensive effect). Products include:
Indocin 1487

Indomethacin Sodium Trihydrate (Reduces antihypertensive effect). Products include:
Indocin I.V. 1490

Lithium Carbonate (Potential for reversible lithium toxicity; frequent monitoring of lithium levels is recommended). Products include:
Eskalith 2214
Lithane Tablets 1596
Lithium Carbonate Capsules & Tablets 1984
Lithobid Tablets 870

Lithium Citrate (Potential for reversible lithium toxicity; frequent monitoring of lithium levels is recommended). Products include:
Cibalith-S 870

Methyclothiazide (Thiazide-induced potassium loss attenuated; possibility of excessive reduction in blood pressure). Products include:
Enduron Tablets 517
Enduronyl 518

Metolazone (Possibility of excessive reduction in blood pressure). Products include:
Diulo 2129
Mykrox ½ mg Tablets 984
Zaroxolyn Tablets 989

Polythiazide (Thiazide-induced potassium loss attenuated; possibility of excessive reduction in blood pressure). Products include:
Minizide Capsules 1779
Renese Tablets 1785
Renese-R Tablets 1786

Potassium Acid Phosphate (Potential for significant hyperkalemia). Products include:
K-Phos M.F. Tablets 659
K-Phos Original Formula 'Sodium Free' Tablets 660
K-Phos No. 2 Tablets 659

Potassium Bicarbonate (Potential for significant hyperkalemia). Products include:
Alka-Seltzer Advanced Formula Antacid & Non-Aspirin Pain Reliever ⊞ 620
Alka-Seltzer Effervescent Antacid ⊞ 622
K-Lyte 707
Klorvess Effervescent Granules 2010
Klorvess Effervescent Tablets 2011

Potassium Chloride (Potential for significant hyperkalemia). Products include:
Chlor-3 Condiment 994
K-Dur Microburst Release System (potassium chloride, USP) E.R. Tablets 1163
K-Lor Powder Packets 531
K-Lyte 707
K-Norm Capsules 982
K-Tab Filmtab 532
Kato Potassium Supplement 1114
Klor-Con 8/Klor-Con 10 Extended-release Tablets 2374
Klorvess Effervescent Granules 2010
Klorvess Effervescent Tablets 2011
Klorvess 10% Liquid 2010
Klotrix 708
Kolyum Liquid 983
Micro-K 1863
Micro-K LS Packets 1864
NuLYTELY 699
Oral Rehydration Salts, Citrate 1150
Rum-K Syrup 995
Slow-K Tablets 2281
Ten-K Controlled-Release Tablets 2282
Thermotabs ⊞ 619

Potassium Citrate (Potential for significant hyperkalemia). Products include:
Alka-Seltzer Effervescent Antacid 1570
K-Lyte 707
Polycitra Syrup 2424
Polycitra-K 2424
Polycitra-LC—Sugar-Free 2424
Ricelyte, Rice-Based Oral Electrolyte Maintenance Solution ⊞ 613

Potassium Gluconate (Potential for significant hyperkalemia). Products include:
Kolyum Liquid 983

Potassium Phosphate, Dibasic (Potential for significant hyperkalemia). Products include:
Neutra-Phos 2423

Potassium Phosphate, Monobasic (Potential for significant hyperkalemia). Products include:
K-Phos M.F. Tablets 659
K-Phos Neutral Tablets 660
Neutra-Phos 2423

Spironolactone (Potential for significant hyperkalemia; possibility of excessive reduction in blood pressure). Products include:
Aldactazide 2150
Aldactone 2152

Triamterene (Potential for significant hyperkalemia; possibility of excessive reduction in blood pressure). Products include:
Dyazide Capsules 2208
Dyrenium Capsules 2210
Maxzide 1215

PRINZIDE TABLETS
(Lisinopril, Hydrochlorothiazide) 1540
May interact with barbiturates, nar-

cotic analgesics, potassium sparing diuretics, potassium-depleting corticosteroids, antihypertensives, corticosteroids, lithium preparations, non-steroidal anti-inflammatory agents, diuretics, insulin, oral hypoglycemic agents, nondepolarizing neuromuscular blocking agents, and certain other agents. Compounds in these categories include:

Acebutolol Hydrochloride (Additive effect or potentiation). Products include:
- Sectral Capsules 2520

ACTH (Intensified electrolyte depletion, particularly hypokalemia).
- No products indexed under this heading.

Alcohol (Potentiates orthostatic hypotension).

Alfentanil Hydrochloride (Potentiates orthostatic hypotension). Products include:
- Alfenta Injection 1131

Amiloride Hydrochloride (Concomitant therapy may lead to hyperkalemia). Products include:
- Midamor Tablets 1508
- Moduretic Tablets 1510

Aprobarbital (Potentiates orthostatic hypotension). Products include:
- Alurate Elixir 1883

Atenolol (Additive effect or potentiation). Products include:
- Tenoretic Tablets 1105
- Tenormin Tablets and I.V. Injection 1107

Atracurium Besylate (Possible increased responsiveness to the muscle relaxant). Products include:
- Tracrium Injection 817

Benazepril Hydrochloride (Additive effect or potentiation). Products include:
- Lotensin Tablets 872

Bendroflumethiazide (Additive effect or potentiation). Products include:
- Corzide Tablets 702
- Naturetin Tablets 1789
- Rauzide Tablets 1804

Betamethasone Acetate (Intensified electrolyte depletion, particularly hypokalemia). Products include:
- Celestone Soluspan Suspension 2081

Betamethasone Sodium Phosphate (Intensified electrolyte depletion, particularly hypokalemia). Products include:
- Celestone Soluspan Suspension 2081

Betaxolol Hydrochloride (Additive effect or potentiation). Products include:
- Betoptic Sterile Ophthalmic Solution 569
- Betoptic S Sterile Ophthalmic Suspension 570
- Kerlone Tablets 2172

Buprenorphine (Potentiates orthostatic hypotension).
- No products indexed under this heading.

Butabarbital (Potentiates orthostatic hypotension). Products include:
- Pyridium Plus 1764

Butalbital (Potentiates orthostatic hypotension). Products include:
- Esgic-Plus Tablets 1002
- Esgic Tablets & Capsules 1001
- Fioricet Tablets 2006
- Fiorinal Capsules 2007
- Fiorinal with Codeine Capsules 2008
- Fiorinal Tablets 2007
- Phrenilin 838
- Sedapap Tablets 50 mg/650 mg .. 1360

Captopril (Additive effect or potentiation). Products include:
- Capoten 2255
- Capozide 2258

Carteolol Hydrochloride (Additive effect or potentiation). Products include:
- Cartrol Tablets 507

Chlorothiazide (Additive effect or potentiation). Products include:
- Aldoclor Tablets 1413
- Diupres Tablets 1461
- Diuril Oral 1464

Chlorothiazide Sodium (Additive effect or potentiation). Products include:
- Diuril Sodium Intravenous 1463

Chlorpropamide (Dosage adjustment of the antidiabetic drug may be required). Products include:
- Diabinese Tablets 1775

Chlorthalidone (Additive effect or potentiation). Products include:
- Combipres Tablets 678
- Tenoretic Tablets 1105
- Thalitone Tablets 687

Clonidine (Additive effect or potentiation). Products include:
- Catapres-TTS 677

Clonidine Hydrochloride (Additive effect or potentiation). Products include:
- Catapres Tablets 676
- Combipres Tablets 678

Codeine (Potentiates orthostatic hypotension). Products include:
- Calcidrine Syrup 506

Codeine Phosphate (Potentiates orthostatic hypotension). Products include:
- Actifed with Codeine Cough Syrup.. 752
- Cheracol Cough Syrup 1853
- Codimal PH Syrup 846
- Dimetane-DC Cough Syrup 1857
- Empirin with Codeine Phosphate Nos. 2, 3 & 4 764
- Fiorinal with Codeine Capsules 2008
- Isoclor Expectorant 982
- Naldecon CX Adult Liquid .... ▣ 521
- Novahistine DH 1342
- Novahistine Expectorant 1343
- Nucofed Capsules 2219
- Nucofed Expectorant 2219
- Nucofed Pediatric Expectorant 2220
- Nucofed Syrup 2219
- Phenaphen with Codeine Capsules 1865
- Phenaphen-650 with Codeine Tablets 1866
- Phenergan with Codeine 2497
- Phenergan VC with Codeine 2501
- Robitussin A-C Syrup 1875
- Robitussin-DAC Syrup 1875
- Ryna .... ▣ 741
- Soma Compound w/Codeine Tablets 2390
- Triaminic Expectorant w/Codeine .. 1996
- Tussi-Organidin Liquid 2391
- Tylenol with Codeine 1381

Codeine Polistirex (Potentiates orthostatic hypotension).
- No products indexed under this heading.

Cortisone Acetate (Intensified electrolyte depletion, particularly hypokalemia). Products include:
- Cortone Acetate Sterile Suspension 1437
- Cortone Acetate Tablets 1439

Deserpidine (Additive effect or potentiation). Products include:
- Enduronyl 518
- Harmonyl Tablets 528
- Oreticyl 545

Dexamethasone (Intensified electrolyte depletion, particularly hypokalemia). Products include:
- AK-Trol Ointment & Suspension .... ⊙ 207
- Decadron Elixir 1445
- Decadron Tablets 1447
- Decaspray Topical Aerosol 1459
- Dexacidin .... ⊙ 272
- Maxidex Sterile Ophthalmic Suspension .... ⊙ 223
- Maxitrol Ophthalmic Ointment/Suspension .... ⊙ 223
- TobraDex Ophthalmic Suspension and Ointment .... ⊙ 228

Dexamethasone Acetate (Intensified electrolyte depletion, particularly hypokalemia). Products include:
- Dalalone D.P. Injectable 999
- Decadron-LA Sterile Suspension 1457

Dexamethasone Sodium Phosphate (Intensified electrolyte depletion, particularly hypokalemia). Products include:
- AK-Dex .... ⊙ 203
- Decadron Phosphate Respihaler 1454
- Decadron Phosphate Sterile Ophthalmic Ointment 1453
- Decadron Phosphate Sterile Ophthalmic Solution 1453
- Decadron Phosphate Topical Cream 1455
- Decadron Phosphate Turbinaire 1456
- Maxidex Sterile Ophthalmic Ointment .... ⊙ 222
- NeoDecadron Sterile Ophthalmic Ointment 1517
- NeoDecadron Sterile Ophthalmic Solution 1518
- NeoDecadron Topical Cream 1518

Dezocine (Potentiates orthostatic hypotension).

Diazoxide (Additive effect or potentiation). Products include:
- Hyperstat I.V. Injection 2095
- Proglycem 649

Diclofenac Sodium (Reduces the diuretic, naturetic, and antihypertensive effects of thiazides). Products include:
- Voltaren Ophthalmic Sterile Ophthalmic Solution .... ⊙ 268
- Voltaren Tablets 1042

Doxazosin Mesylate (Additive effect or potentiation). Products include:
- Cardura Tablets 1941

Enalapril Maleate (Additive effect or potentiation). Products include:
- Vaseretic Tablets 1559
- Vasotec Tablets 1564

Enalaprilat (Additive effect or potentiation). Products include:
- Vasotec I.V. 1562

Esmolol Hydrochloride (Additive effect or potentiation). Products include:
- Brevibloc Injection 942

Etodolac (Reduces the diuretic, naturetic, and antihypertensive effects of thiazides). Products include:
- Lodine Capsules 2468

Felodipine (Additive effect or potentiation). Products include:
- Plendil Extended-Release Tablets.... 1526

Fenoprofen Calcium (Reduces the diuretic, naturetic, and antihypertensive effects of thiazides). Products include:
- Nalfon Pulvules & Tablets 919

Fentanyl (Potentiates orthostatic hypotension). Products include:
- Duragesic Transdermal System........ 1133

Fentanyl Citrate (Potentiates orthostatic hypotension). Products include:
- Innovar Injection 1141
- Sublimaze Injection 1146

Flurbiprofen (Reduces the diuretic, naturetic, and antihypertensive effects of thiazides). Products include:
- Ansaid Tablets 2319

Fosinopril Sodium (Additive effect or potentiation). Products include:
- Monopril Tablets 1406

Furosemide (Additive effect or potentiation). Products include:
- Lasix 1093

Glipizide (Dosage adjustment of the antidiabetic drug may be required). Products include:
- Glucotrol 1952

Glyburide (Dosage adjustment of the antidiabetic drug may be required). Products include:
- DiaBeta 1091
- Micronase Tablets 2350

Guanabenz Acetate (Additive effect or potentiation). Products include:
- Wytensin Tablets 2542

Guanethidine Monosulfate (Additive effect or potentiation). Products include:
- Esimil Tablets 864
- Ismelin Tablets 869

Hydralazine Hydrochloride (Additive effect or potentiation). Products include:
- Apresazide Capsules 854
- Apresoline Hydrochloride Parenteral (Ampuls) 856
- Apresoline Hydrochloride Tablets .. 855
- Apresoline-Esidrix Tablets 857
- Ser-Ap-Es Tablets 881
- Serpasil-Apresoline Tablets 884

Hydrocodone Bitartrate (Potentiates orthostatic hypotension). Products include:
- Anexsia 5/500 Tablets 2196
- Anexsia 7.5/650 Tablets 2197
- Azdone Tablets 844
- Codiclear DH Syrup 845
- Codimal DH Syrup 846
- Damason-P 1356
- Hycodan Syrup, Tablets 927
- Hycomine Compound Tablets 929
- Hycomine Syrup 927
- Hycotuss Expectorant Syrup 930
- Hydrocet Capsules 835
- Lortab ASA Tablets 2414
- Lortab 2412
- Ru-Tuss with Hydrocodone 694
- Triaminic Expectorant DH 1995
- Vicodin Tablets 1187
- Vicodin ES Tablets 1189
- Zydone Capsules 941

Hydrocodone Polistirex (Potentiates orthostatic hypotension). Products include:
- Tussionex Extended-Release Suspension 988

Hydrocortisone (Intensified electrolyte depletion, particularly hypokalemia). Products include:
- AK-Spore H.C. .... ⊙ 206
- Bactine Hydrocortisone Anti-Itch Cream .... ▣ 625
- CaldeCORT Anti-Itch Hydrocortisone Spray .... ▣ 560
- Carmol HC Cream 1% 2296
- Cortaid Spray .... ▣ 735
- Cortenema 2244
- Cortisporin Ointment 758
- Cortisporin Ophthalmic Ointment Sterile 758
- Cortisporin Ophthalmic Suspension Sterile 759
- Cortisporin Otic Solution Sterile 760
- Cortisporin Otic Suspension Sterile 760
- Cortizone-5 Creme & Ointment...... ▣ 732
- Dermolate Anti-Itch Cream .... ▣ 697
- Eldecort Cream 1.0% 1113
- Eldecort Cream 1.0% and 2.5% 1113
- Fungoid HC Creme 1770
- Hydrocortone Tablets 1482
- Hytone 909
- LazerSporin-C Solution 1770
- Massengill Medicated Soft Cloth Towelettes 2192
- Nutracort Cream & Lotion 1684
- PediOtic Suspension Sterile 797
- Synacort Creams 1%, 2.5% 2296
- Vanoxide-HC Acne Lotion 911
- Vioform-Hydrocortisone Cream and Mild Cream 889
- Vioform-Hydrocortisone Ointment.. 889
- VōSoL HC Otic Solution 2392
- Vytone Cream 1% 911

(▣ Described in PDR For Nonprescription Drugs)

(⊙ Described in PDR For Ophthalmology)

Hydrocortisone Acetate (Intensified electrolyte depletion, particularly hypokalemia). Products include:
Analpram-HC Rectal Cream 1% and 2.5% ... 970
Anusol-HC Cream ... 1690
Anusol-HC Suppositories ... 1691
Caldecort ... ▣ 560
Carmol HC Cream 1% ... 2296
Chloromycetin Hydrocortisone Ophthalmic ... 1694
Coly-Mycin S Otic w/Neomycin & Hydrocortisone ... 1708
Cortaid ... ▣ 735
Cortef Feminine Itch Cream ... ▣ 735
Corticaine ... ▣ 682
Cortifoam ... 1827
Cortisporin Cream ... 757
Epifoam ... 1828
Gynecort 5 Creme ... ▣ 556
Hydrocortone Acetate Sterile Suspension ... 1479
Lanacort 5 Creme and Ointment .. ▣ 557
Mantadil Cream ... 789
Ophthocort ... ◉ 301
Orabase HCA Oral Paste ... 890
Pramosone Cream, Lotion & Ointment ... 971
ProctoCream-HC ... 1834
Proctofoam-HC ... 1835

Hydrocortisone Sodium Phosphate (Intensified electrolyte depletion, particularly hypokalemia). Products include:
Hydrocortone Phosphate Injection, Sterile ... 1481

Hydrocortisone Sodium Succinate (Intensified electrolyte depletion, particularly hypokalemia). Products include:
Solu-Cortef Sterile Powder ... 2361

Hydroflumethiazide (Additive effect or potentiation). Products include:
Diucardin Tablets ... 2450
Saluron ... 718
Salutensin/Salutensin-Demi ... 719

Ibuprofen (Reduces the diuretic, naturetic, and antihypertensive effects of thiazides). Products include:
Advil Cold & Sinus Caplets (formerly CoAdvil) ... 2416
Advil Ibuprofen Tablets and Caplets ... 2416
Children's Advil Suspension ... 2426
CoAdvil ... ▣ 748
Dristan Sinus Caplets ... 2419
Haltran Tablets ... ▣ 668
Ibuprofen ... ▣ 631
Medipren ibuprofen Caplets and Tablets ... 1362
Midol 200 Cramp Relief Formula .. ▣ 570
Motrin Tablets ... 2351
Motrin IB Caplets and Tablets ... ▣ 736
Nuprin Ibuprofen/Analgesic Tablets & Caplets ... 752
PediaProfen Suspension ... 1363
Rufen Tablets ... 691
Trendar Ibuprofen Tablets ... ▣ 756

Indapamide (Additive effect or potentiation). Products include:
Lozol Tablets ... 1843

Indomethacin (Reduces lisinopril effects; reduces the diuretic, naturetic and antihypertensive effects of thiazides). Products include:
Indocin ... 1487

Indomethacin Sodium Trihydrate (Reduces the diuretic, naturetic, and antihypertensive effects of thiazides; reduces lisinopril effects). Products include:
Indocin I.V. ... 1490

Insulin, Human (Dosage adjustment of the antidiabetic drug may be required).
No products indexed under this heading.

Insulin, Human Isophane Suspension (Dosage adjustment of the antidiabetic drug may be required). Products include:
Humulin N, 100 Units ... 1270

Insulin, Human NPH (Dosage adjustment of the antidiabetic drug may be required). Products include:
Insulatard NPH Human ... 1627
Novolin N ... 1627
Novolin N PenFill Cartridges ... 1628
Novolin N Prefilled ... 1628

Insulin, Human Regular (Dosage adjustment of the antidiabetic drug may be required). Products include:
Humulin BR, 100 Units ... 1268
Humulin R, 100 Units ... 1272
Novolin R ... 1627
Novolin R PenFill Cartridges ... 1628
Novolin R Prefilled ... 1629
Velosulin Human ... 1628

Insulin, Human, Zinc Suspension (Dosage adjustment of the antidiabetic drug may be required). Products include:
Humulin L, 100 Units ... 1268
Humulin U, 100 Units ... 1272
Novolin L ... 1627

Insulin, NPH (Dosage adjustment of the antidiabetic drug may be required). Products include:
NPH, 40 & 100 Units ... 1273
Beef NPH, 100 Units ... 1274
Pork NPH, 100 Units ... 1275
Insulatard NPH ... 1626
NPH Insulin ... 1626
NPH Purified Pork Isophane Insulin ... 1626

Insulin, Regular (Dosage adjustment of the antidiabetic drug may be required). Products include:
Regular, 40 & 100 Units ... 1273
Beef Regular, 100 Units ... 1275
Pork Regular, 100 Units ... 1275
Pork Regular (Concentrated), 500 Units ... 1276
Regular Insulin ... 1625
Regular Purified Pork Insulin ... 1626
Velosulin ... 1627

Insulin, Zinc Crystals (Dosage adjustment of the antidiabetic drug may be required). Products include:
NPH, 40 & 100 Units ... 1273

Insulin, Zinc Suspension (Dosage adjustment of the antidiabetic drug may be required). Products include:
Lente, 40 & 100 Units ... 1272
Protamine, Zinc, 40 & 100 Units ... 1273
Lente Iletin I ... 1272
Beef Lente, 100 Units ... 1274
Beef Protamine Zinc, 100 Units ... 1274
Pork Lente, 100 Units ... 1275
Pork, Protamine, Zinc, 100 Units ... 1275
Lente Insulin ... 1626
Lente Purified Pork Insulin ... 1626
Semilente Insulin ... 1625
Ultralente Insulin ... 1626

Isradipine (Additive effect or potentiation). Products include:
DynaCirc Capsules ... 2004

Ketoprofen (Reduces the diuretic, naturetic, and antihypertensive effects of thiazides). Products include:
Orudis Capsules ... 2488

Ketorolac Tromethamine (Reduces the diuretic, naturetic, and antihypertensive effects of thiazides). Products include:
Toradol IM Injection ... 2302

Labetalol Hydrochloride (Additive effect or potentiation). Products include:
Normodyne Injection ... 2108
Normodyne Tablets ... 2110
Normozide Tablets ... 2112
Trandate HCT Tablets ... 579
Trandate Injection ... 577
Trandate Tablets ... 579

Levorphanol Tartrate (Potentiates orthostatic hypotension). Products include:
Levo-Dromoran ... 1906

Lithium Carbonate (Potential for lithium toxicity; monitor lithium levels frequently). Products include:
Eskalith ... 2214
Lithane Tablets ... 1596
Lithium Carbonate Capsules & Tablets ... 1984
Lithobid Tablets ... 870

Lithium Citrate (Potential for lithium toxicity; monitor lithium levels frequently). Products include:
Cibalith-S ... 870

Mecamylamine Hydrochloride (Additive effect or potentiation). Products include:
Inversine Tablets ... 1492

Meclofenamate Sodium (Reduces the diuretic, naturetic, and antihypertensive effects of thiazides). Products include:
Meclomen Capsules ... 1739

Mefenamic Acid (Reduces the diuretic, naturetic, and antihypertensive effects of thiazides). Products include:
Ponstel ... 1758

Meperidine Hydrochloride (Potentiates orthostatic hypotension). Products include:
Demerol ... 2047
Mepergan Injection ... 2479

Mephobarbital (Potentiates orthostatic hypotension). Products include:
Mebaral Tablets ... 2061

Methadone Hydrochloride (Potentiates orthostatic hypotension). Products include:
Dolophine Hydrochloride Ampoules & Vials ... 1260
Dolophine Hydrochloride Tablets ... 1261
Methadone Hydrochloride Diskets .. 1284
Methadone Hydrochloride Oral Solution & Tablets ... 1987

Methyclothiazide (Additive effect or potentiation). Products include:
Enduron Tablets ... 517
Enduronyl ... 518

Methyldopa (Additive effect or potentiation). Products include:
Aldoclor Tablets ... 1413
Aldomet Oral ... 1415
Aldoril Tablets ... 1418

Methyldopate Hydrochloride (Additive effect or potentiation). Products include:
Aldomet Ester HCl Injection ... 1417

Methylprednisolone Acetate (Intensified electrolyte depletion, particularly hypokalemia). Products include:
Depo-Medrol Sterile Aqueous Suspension ... 2334

Methylprednisolone Sodium Succinate (Intensified electrolyte depletion, particularly hypokalemia). Products include:
Solu-Medrol Sterile Powder ... 2363

Metocurine Iodide (Possible increased responsiveness to the muscle relaxant). Products include:
Metubine Iodide Vials ... 1285

Metolazone (Additive effect or potentiation). Products include:
Diulo ... 2129
Mykrox ½ mg Tablets ... 984
Zaroxolyn Tablets ... 989

Metoprolol Tartrate (Additive effect or potentiation). Products include:
Lopressor Ampuls ... 1032
Lopressor HCT Tablets ... 1034
Lopressor Tablets ... 1032

Metyrosine (Additive effect or potentiation). Products include:
Demser Capsules ... 1460

Minoxidil (Additive effect or potentiation). Products include:
Loniten Tablets ... 2346
Rogaine Topical Solution ... 2357

Morphine Sulfate (Potentiates orthostatic hypotension). Products include:
Astramorph/PF Injection, USP (Preservative-Free) ... 618
Duramorph ... 960
Infumorph 200 and Infumorph 500 Sterile Solutions ... 962
MS Contin Tablets ... 1814
MSIR ... 1817
Oramorph SR (Morphine Sulfate Sustained Release Tablets) ... 1988
Roxanol ... 1991

Nadolol (Additive effect or potentiation). Products include:
Corgard Tablets ... 701
Corzide Tablets ... 702

Naproxen (Reduces the diuretic, naturetic, and antihypertensive effects of thiazides). Products include:
Naprosyn ... 2297

Naproxen Sodium (Reduces the diuretic, naturetic, and antihypertensive effects of thiazides). Products include:
Anaprox and Anaprox DS Tablets ... 2288

Nicardipine Hydrochloride (Additive effect or potentiation). Products include:
Cardene Capsules ... 2290

Nitroglycerin (Additive effect or potentiation). Products include:
Deponit NTG Transdermal Delivery System ... 2143
Minitran Transdermal Delivery System ... 1312
Nitro-Bid Ointment ... 1339
Nitro-Bid Capsules ... 1338
Nitrodisc ... 2176
Nitro-Dur (nitroglycerin) Transdermal Infusion System ... 1164
Nitrogard Tablets ... 1004
Nitrolingual Spray ... 1846
Nitrostat Tablets ... 1743
Transderm-Nitro Transdermal Therapeutic System ... 2283

Norepinephrine Bitartrate (Possible decreased response to pressor amines). Products include:
Levophed Bitartrate Injection ... 2054

Opium Alkaloids (Potentiates orthostatic hypotension). Products include:
B & O No. 15A & No. 16A Supprettes ... 2395
Pantopon Injectable ... 1911

Oxycodone Hydrochloride (Potentiates orthostatic hypotension). Products include:
Percocet Tablets ... 950
Percodan ... 951
Roxicodone Tablets, Oral Solution & Intensol (Oxycodone) ... 1992
Tylox Capsules ... 1382

Pancuronium Bromide Injection (Possible increased responsiveness to the muscle relaxant).
No products indexed under this heading.

Penbutolol Sulfate (Additive effect or potentiation). Products include:
Levatol ... 1832

Pentobarbital Sodium (Potentiates orthostatic hypotension). Products include:
Nembutal Sodium Capsules ... 534
Nembutal Sodium Solution ... 536
Nembutal Sodium Suppositories ... 538

Phenobarbital (Potentiates orthostatic hypotension). Products include:
Arco-Lase Plus Tablets ... 607
Bellergal-S Tablets ... 1998
Bronkolixir ... ▣ 761
Bronkotabs Tablets ... ▣ 762
Donnatal ... 1858
Donnatal Extentabs ... 1859
Donnatal Tablets ... 1858
Donnazyme Tablets ... 1860
Kinesed Tablets ... 2272
Phenobarbital Elixir and Tablets ... 1293

Primatene Tablets-P Formula 2421
Quadrinal Tablets 1183
Tedral SA 1765

Phenoxybenzamine Hydrochloride (Additive effect or potentiation). Products include:
Dibenzyline Capsules 2207

Phentolamine Mesylate (Additive effect or potentiation). Products include:
Regitine 878

Phenylbutazone (Reduces the diuretic, naturetic, and antihypertensive effects of thiazides). Products include:
Butazolidin Capsules & Tablets 1027

Pindolol (Additive effect or potentiation). Products include:
Visken Tablets 2036

Piroxicam (Reduces the diuretic, naturetic, and antihypertensive effects of thiazides). Products include:
Feldene Capsules 1777

Polythiazide (Additive effect or potentiation). Products include:
Minizide Capsules 1779
Renese Tablets 1785
Renese-R Tablets 1786

Potassium Acid Phosphate (Concomitant therapy may lead to hyperkalemia). Products include:
K-Phos M.F. Tablets 659
K-Phos Original Formula 'Sodium Free' Tablets 660
K-Phos No. 2 Tablets 659

Potassium Bicarbonate (Concomitant therapy may lead to hyperkalemia). Products include:
Alka-Seltzer Advanced Formula Antacid & Non-Aspirin Pain Reliever ▣ 620
Alka-Seltzer Effervescent Antacid ▣ 622
K-Lyte 707
Klorvess Effervescent Granules 2010
Klorvess Effervescent Tablets 2011

Potassium Chloride (Concomitant therapy may lead to hyperkalemia). Products include:
Chlor-3 Condiment 994
K-Dur Microburst Release System (potassium chloride, USP) E.R. Tablets 1163
K-Lor Powder Packets 531
K-Lyte 707
K-Norm Capsules 982
K-Tab Filmtab 532
Kato Potassium Supplement 1114
Klor-Con 8/Klor-Con 10 Extended-release Tablets 2374
Klorvess Effervescent Granules 2010
Klorvess Effervescent Tablets 2011
Klorvess 10% Liquid 2010
Klotrix 708
Kolyum Liquid 983
Micro-K 1863
Micro-K LS Packets 1864
NuLYTELY 699
Oral Rehydration Salts, Citrate 1150
Rum-K Syrup 995
Slow-K Tablets 2281
Ten-K Controlled-Release Tablets 2282
Thermotabs ▣ 619

Potassium Citrate (Concomitant therapy may lead to hyperkalemia). Products include:
Alka-Seltzer Effervescent Antacid 1570
K-Lyte 707
Polycitra Syrup 2424
Polycitra-K 2424
Polycitra-LC—Sugar-Free 2424
Ricelyte, Rice-Based Oral Electrolyte Maintenance Solution ▣ 613

Potassium Gluconate (Concomitant therapy may lead to hyperkalemia). Products include:
Kolyum Liquid 983

Potassium Phosphate, Dibasic (Concomitant therapy may lead to hyperkalemia). Products include:
Neutra-Phos 2423

Potassium Phosphate, Monobasic (Concomitant therapy may lead to hyperkalemia). Products include:
K-Phos M.F. Tablets 659
K-Phos Neutral Tablets 660
Neutra-Phos 2423

Prazosin Hydrochloride (Additive effect or potentiation). Products include:
Minipress Capsules 1778
Minizide Capsules 1779

Prednisolone Acetate (Intensified electrolyte depletion, particularly hypokalemia). Products include:
AK-Cide Sterile Ophthalmic Ointment & Suspension ◉ 202
Blephamide Liquifilm Sterile Ophthalmic Suspension 586
Blephamide S.O.P. Sterile Ophthalmic Ointment 586
Cetapred Ointment ◉ 220
⅛% Econopred & 1% Econopred Plus ◉ 217
Isopto Cetapred Suspension ◉ 220
Metimyd ◉ 306
Poly-Pred Liquifilm ◉ 250
Pred Forte ◉ 252
Pred Mild ◉ 254
Pred-G Liquifilm Sterile Ophthalmic Suspension ◉ 252
Pred-G S.O.P. Sterile Ophthalmic Ointment ◉ 253
Vasocidin Ointment ◉ 275

Prednisolone Sodium Phosphate (Intensified electrolyte depletion, particularly hypokalemia). Products include:
AK-Pred ◉ 205
Hydeltrasol Injection, Sterile 1476
Inflamase ◉ 274
Pediapred Oral Liquid 987
Vasocidin Ophthalmic Solution ◉ 276

Prednisolone Tebutate (Intensified electrolyte depletion, particularly hypokalemia). Products include:
Hydeltra-T.B.A. Sterile Suspension 1478

Prednisone (Intensified electrolyte depletion, particularly hypokalemia). Products include:
Deltasone Tablets 2332

Propoxyphene Hydrochloride (Potentiates orthostatic hypotension). Products include:
Darvon 1256
Wygesic Tablets 2540

Propoxyphene Napsylate (Potentiates orthostatic hypotension). Products include:
Darvon-N/Darvocet-N 1254

Propranolol Hydrochloride (Additive effect or potentiation). Products include:
Inderal 2459
Inderal LA Long Acting Capsules 2461
Inderide Tablets 2463
Inderide LA Long Acting Capsules 2465

Ramipril (Additive effect or potentiation). Products include:
Altace Capsules 1086

Rauwolfia Serpentina (Additive effect or potentiation). Products include:
Raudixin Tablets 1803
Rauzide Tablets 1804

Rescinnamine (Additive effect or potentiation).
No products indexed under this heading.

Reserpine (Additive effect or potentiation). Products include:
Diupres Tablets 1461
Hydromox R Tablets 1209
Hydropres Tablets 1485
Renese-R Tablets 1786
Salutensin/Salutensin-Demi 719
Ser-Ap-Es Tablets 881
Serpasil Tablets 883
Serpasil-Apresoline Tablets 884
Serpasil-Esidrix Tablets 886

Secobarbital Sodium (Potentiates orthostatic hypotension). Products include:
Seconal Sodium Pulvules 1296

Sodium Nitroprusside (Additive effect or potentiation). Products include:
Nipride I.V. Infusion 1909

Spironolactone (Concomitant therapy may lead to hyperkalemia). Products include:
Aldactazide 2150
Aldactone 2152

Sufentanil Citrate (Potentiates orthostatic hypotension). Products include:
Sufenta Injection 1147

Sulindac (Reduces the diuretic, naturetic, and antihypertensive effects of thiazides). Products include:
Clinoril Tablets 1433

Terazosin Hydrochloride (Additive effect or potentiation). Products include:
Hytrin Tablets 529

Thiamylal Sodium (Potentiates orthostatic hypotension). Products include:
Surital Ampoules, Steri-Vials 1764

Timolol Maleate (Additive effect or potentiation). Products include:
Blocadren Tablets 1429
Timolide Tablets 1547
Timoptic in Ocudose 1552
Timoptic Sterile Ophthalmic Solution 1550

Tolazamide (Dosage adjustment of the antidiabetic drug may be required). Products include:
Tolinase Tablets 2365

Tolbutamide (Dosage adjustment of the antidiabetic drug may be required). Products include:
Orinase Tablets 2354

Tolmetin Sodium (Reduces the diuretic, naturetic, and antihypertensive effects of thiazides). Products include:
Tolectin (200, 400 and 600 mg) 1379

Triamcinolone (Intensified electrolyte depletion, particularly hypokalemia).
No products indexed under this heading.

Triamcinolone Acetonide (Intensified electrolyte depletion, particularly hypokalemia). Products include:
Aristocort A 1010
Azmacort Inhaler 1837
Kenalog Cream, Lotion & Ointment 2401
Kenalog-10 Injection 2402
Kenalog-40 Injection 2403
Kenalog in Orabase 604
Kenalog Spray 2401
Mycolog II Cream and Ointment 2407
Mytrex Cream & Ointment 2080
Nasacort Nasal Inhaler 1844

Triamcinolone Diacetate (Intensified electrolyte depletion, particularly hypokalemia). Products include:
Aristocort Suspension 1008

Triamcinolone Hexacetonide (Intensified electrolyte depletion, particularly hypokalemia). Products include:
Aristospan Suspension 1011

Triamterene (Concomitant therapy may lead to hyperkalemia). Products include:
Dyazide Capsules 2208
Dyrenium Capsules 2210
Maxzide 1215

Trimethaphan Camsylate (Additive effect or potentiation). Products include:
Arfonad Ampuls 1887

Vecuronium Bromide (Possible increased responsiveness to the muscle relaxant). Products include:
Norcuron 1642

PRISCOLINE HYDROCHLORIDE AMPULS
(Tolazoline Hydrochloride) 877
No interactions described in labeling.

PRIVINE NASAL SOLUTION
(Naphazoline Hydrochloride) 878
No interactions described in labeling.

PRIVINE NASAL SPRAY
(Naphazoline Hydrochloride) 878
No interactions described in labeling.

PRO-BANTHINE TABLETS
(Propantheline Bromide) 2141
May interact with antiarrhythmics, antihistamines, phenothiazines, tricyclic antidepressants, corticosteroids, anticholinergics, and certain other agents. Compounds in these categories include:

Acebutolol Hydrochloride (Excessive cholinergic blockade). Products include:
Sectral Capsules 2520

Adenosine (Excessive cholinergic blockade). Products include:
Adenocard Injection 1007

Amiodarone Hydrochloride (Excessive cholinergic blockade). Products include:
Cordarone Tablets 2446

Amitriptyline Hydrochloride (Excessive cholinergic blockade). Products include:
Elavil 2269
Endep Tablets 1927
Etrafon 2087
Limbitrol 1933
Triavil Tablets 1556

Amoxapine (Excessive cholinergic blockade). Products include:
Asendin Tablets 1196

Astemizole (Excessive cholinergic blockade). Products include:
Hismanal Tablets 1138

Atropine Sulfate (Excessive cholinergic blockade; increased intraocular pressure). Products include:
Arco-Lase Plus Tablets 607
Atropine Sulfate Sterile Ophthalmic Solution and S.O.P. Sterile Ophthalmic Ointment ◉ 239
Donnagel ▣ 675
Donnagel-PG 1858
Donnatal 1858
Donnatal Extentabs 1859
Donnatal Tablets 1858
Donnazyme Tablets 1860
Isopto Atropine ◉ 218
Lomotil 2174
Motofen Tablets 836
Ru-Tuss Tablets 693
Urised Tablets 2396

Azatadine Maleate (Excessive cholinergic blockade). Products include:
Optimine Tablets 2115
Trinalin Repetabs Tablets 1170

Belladonna Alkaloids (Excessive cholinergic blockade; increased intraocular pressure). Products include:
Bellergal-S Tablets 1998
Hyland's Bed Wetting Tablets ▣ 728
Hyland's Teething Tablets ▣ 728
Kinesed Tablets 2272

Benztropine Mesylate (Excessive cholinergic blockade; increased intraocular pressure). Products include:
Cogentin 1435

Betamethasone Acetate (Increased intraocular pressure). Products include:
Celestone Soluspan Suspension 2081

Betamethasone Sodium Phosphate (Increased intraocular pressure). Products include:
Celestone Soluspan Suspension 2081

Biperiden (Excessive cholinergic blockade; increased intraocular pressure). Products include:
Akineton 1171

Bretylium Tosylate (Excessive cholinergic blockade). Products include:
Bretylol Injection 923

Bromodiphenhydramine Hydrochloride (Excessive cholinergic blockade).
No products indexed under this heading.

Brompheniramine Maleate (Excessive cholinergic blockade). Products include:
Alka Seltzer Plus Sinus Allergy Medicine ..... ▣ 624
Atrohist Sprinkle Capsules 558
Bromfed Capsules (Timed Release) 1615
Bromfed Syrup ..... ▣ 628
Bromfed 1615
Dimetane Decongestant ..... ▣ 673
Dimetane ..... ▣ 672
Dimetane-DC Cough Syrup 1857
Dimetane-DX Cough Syrup 1858
Dimetapp Elixir ..... ▣ 673
Dimetapp DM Elixir ..... ▣ 674
Dimetapp Extentabs ..... ▣ 674
Dimetapp Plus Caplets ..... ▣ 675
Dimetapp Tablets ..... ▣ 675
Drixoral Antihistamine/Nasal Decongestant Syrup ..... ▣ 698

Chlorpheniramine Maleate (Excessive cholinergic blockade). Products include:
A.R.M. Allergy Relief Medicine Caplets ..... ▣ 615
Alka-Seltzer Plus Cold Medicine ..... ▣ 623
Allerest ..... ▣ 559
Ana-Kit Anaphylaxis Emergency Treatment Kit 1100
BC Cold Powder Multi-Symptom Formula ..... ▣ 517
Brexin L.A. Capsules 2078
Cerose-DM 2443
Cheracol Plus Head Cold/Cough Formula ..... ▣ 667
Chlor-Trimeton Allergy Syrup, Tablets & Long-Acting Repetabs Tablets ..... ▣ 693
Chlor-Trimeton Decongestant ..... ▣ 694
Comhist LA Capsules 1618
Allergy-Sinus Comtrex Multi-Symptom Allergy Sinus Formula Tablets & Caplets 746
Comtrex Multi-Symptom Cold Reliever Tablets/Caplets/Liqui-Gels/Liquid 745
Day-Night Comtrex 747
Contac Continuous Action Decongestant/Antihistamine Capsules ▣ 710
Contac Maximum Strength Continuous Action Decongestant/Antihistamine Caplets ..... ▣ 709
Contac Severe Cold and Flu Formula Caplets ..... ▣ 711
Coricidin 'D' Decongestant Tablets ..... ▣ 695
Coricidin Demilets Tablets for Children ..... ▣ 696
Coricidin Tablets ..... ▣ 695
Deconamine 663
Demazin Nasal Decongestant/Antihistamine Repetabs Tablets & Syrup ..... ▣ 697
Dorcol Children's Liquid Cold Formula ..... ▣ 686
Dristan Decongestant/Antihistamine/ Analgesic Coated Caplets ..... ▣ 749
Dristan Cold Nasal Decongestant/Antihistamine/ Analgesic Coated Tablets 2419
Dristan Advanced Formula Decongestant/Antihistamine/Analgesic Tablets ..... ▣ 749
Extendryl 994
4-Way Cold Tablets 750
Fedahist Gyrocaps 2145
Fedahist Timecaps 2145
Hycomine Compound Tablets 929
Isoclor Timesule Capsules ..... ▣ 561
Kronofed-A 970
Medi-Flu Caplet, Liquid ..... ▣ 640
Naldecon Syrup, Tablets, Pediatric Drops and Pediatric Syrup 709
Nolamine Tablets 838
Novafed A Capsules 1342
Novahistine DH 1342
Novahistine Elixir ..... ▣ 596
Ornade Spansule Capsules 2221
Orthoxicol Cough Syrup ..... ▣ 668
PediaCare Allergy Relief Formula Liquid 1362
PediaCare Cough-Cold Formula Liquid 1362
PediaCare Night Rest Cough-Cold Formula Liquid 1362
PediaCare 6-12 Cough-Cold Formula Chewable Tablets 1362
Pyrroxate Capsules ..... ▣ 669
Quelidrine Syrup 556
Ru-Tuss II Capsules 693
Ru-Tuss Tablets 693
Ryna ..... ▣ 741
Sinarest Tablets & Extra Strength Tablets ..... ▣ 562
Sine-Off Maximum Strength Allergy/Sinus Formula Caplets ..... ▣ 721
Sine-Off Sinus Medicine Tablets-Aspirin Formula ..... ▣ 722
Singlet Tablets ..... ▣ 598
Sinulin 840
Sinutab Maximum Strength ..... ▣ 641
St. Joseph Nighttime Cold Medicine ..... ▣ 705
Sudafed Plus Liquid ..... ▣ 544
Sudafed Plus Tablets ..... ▣ 545
Teldrin Timed-Release Allergy Capsules, 12 mg 2192
TheraFlu Flu and Cold Medicine ..... ▣ 687
Triaminic Allergy Tablets ..... ▣ 688
Triaminic Chewables ..... ▣ 688
Triaminic Cold Tablets ..... ▣ 688
Triaminic Nite Light ..... ▣ 689
Triaminic Syrup ..... ▣ 689
Triaminic-12 Tablets ..... ▣ 690
Triaminicin Tablets ..... ▣ 690
Triaminicol Multi-Symptom Cold Tablets ..... ▣ 691
Triaminicol Multi-Symptom Relief ▣ 691
Tylenol Allergy Sinus Medication Caplets and Gelcaps, Maximum Strength 1372
Children's Tylenol Cold Liquid Formula and Chewable Tablets 1368
Tylenol Cold & Flu Hot Medication, Packets 1369
Tylenol Cold Medication Caplets and Tablets 1370
Tylenol Cold Medication, Effervescent Tablets 1369
Vicks Children's NyQuil ..... ▣ 664
Vicks Formula 44 Cough Medicine ..... ▣ 661
Vicks Formula 44M Multi-Symptom Cough Medicine ..... ▣ 662
Vicks Pediatric Formula 44m Multi-Symptom Cough & Cold Medicine ..... ▣ 663

Chlorpheniramine Polistirex (Excessive cholinergic blockade). Products include:
Tussionex Extended-Release Suspension 988

Chlorpheniramine Tannate (Excessive cholinergic blockade). Products include:
Rynatan 2387
Rynatuss 2388

Chlorpromazine (Excessive cholinergic blockade; potentiated sedative effect). Products include:
Thorazine 2234

Clemastine Fumarate (Excessive cholinergic blockade). Products include:
Tavist Syrup 2033
Tavist Tablets 2035
Tavist-D Tablets 2035

Clidinium Bromide (Excessive cholinergic blockade; increased intraocular pressure). Products include:
Librax Capsules 1929
Quarzan Capsules 1937

Clomipramine Hydrochloride (Excessive cholinergic blockade). Products include:
Anafranil Capsules 650

Cortisone Acetate (Increased intraocular pressure). Products include:
Cortone Acetate Sterile Suspension 1437
Cortone Acetate Tablets 1439

Cyproheptadine Hydrochloride (Excessive cholinergic blockade). Products include:
Periactin 1525

Desipramine Hydrochloride (Excessive cholinergic blockade). Products include:
Norpramin Tablets 1340

Dexamethasone (Increased intraocular pressure). Products include:
AK-Trol Ointment & Suspension ..... ◉ 207
Decadron Elixir 1445
Decadron Tablets 1447
Decaspray Topical Aerosol 1459
Dexacidin ..... ◉ 272
Maxidex Sterile Ophthalmic Suspension ..... ◉ 223
Maxitrol Ophthalmic Ointment/Suspension ..... ◉ 223
TobraDex Ophthalmic Suspension and Ointment ..... ◉ 228

Dexamethasone Acetate (Increased intraocular pressure). Products include:
Dalalone D.P. Injectable 999
Decadron-LA Sterile Suspension 1457

Dexamethasone Sodium Phosphate (Increased intraocular pressure). Products include:
AK-Dex ..... ◉ 203
Decadron Phosphate Respihaler 1454
Decadron Phosphate Sterile Ophthalmic Ointment 1453
Decadron Phosphate Sterile Ophthalmic Solution 1453
Decadron Phosphate Topical Cream 1455
Decadron Phosphate Turbinaire 1456
Maxidex Sterile Ophthalmic Ointment ..... ◉ 222
NeoDecadron Sterile Ophthalmic Ointment 1517
NeoDecadron Sterile Ophthalmic Solution 1518
NeoDecadron Topical Cream 1518

Dexchlorpheniramine Maleate (Excessive cholinergic blockade). Products include:
Polaramine 2116

Dicyclomine Hydrochloride (Excessive cholinergic blockade; increased intraocular pressure). Products include:
Bentyl 1322

Digoxin (Increased serum digoxin levels in patients who are taking slow-dissolving tablets of digoxin). Products include:
Lanoxicaps 772
Lanoxin Elixir Pediatric 775
Lanoxin Injection 778
Lanoxin Injection Pediatric 781
Lanoxin Tablets 783

Diphenhydramine Citrate (Excessive cholinergic blockade). Products include:
Alka-Seltzer Plus Night-Time Cold Medicine ..... ▣ 623
Bufferin AF Nite Time Analgesic/Sleeping Aid Caplets 744
Excedrin P.M. Analgesic/Sleeping Aid Tablets, Caplets and Liquid 749

Diphenylpyraline Hydrochloride (Excessive cholinergic blockade).
No products indexed under this heading.

Disopyramide Phosphate (Excessive cholinergic blockade). Products include:
Norpace 2177

Doxepin Hydrochloride (Excessive cholinergic blockade). Products include:
Sinequan 1960

Fluphenazine Decanoate (Excessive cholinergic blockade; potentiated sedative effect). Products include:
Prolixin Decanoate 1795

Fluphenazine Enanthate (Excessive cholinergic blockade; potentiated sedative effect). Products include:
Prolixin Enanthate 1796

Fluphenazine Hydrochloride (Excessive cholinergic blockade; potentiated sedative effect). Products include:
Prolixin Elixir 1793
Prolixin Injection 1791
Prolixin Oral Concentrate 1792
Prolixin Tablets 1793

Glycopyrrolate (Excessive cholinergic blockade; increased intraocular pressure). Products include:
Robinul Forte Tablets 1873
Robinul Injectable 1873
Robinul Tablets 1873

Hydrocodone Bitartrate (Excessive cholinergic blockade). Products include:
Anexsia 5/500 Tablets 2196
Anexsia 7.5/650 Tablets 2197
Azdōne Tablets 844
Codiclear DH Syrup 845
Codimal DH Syrup 846
Damason-P 1356
Hycodan Syrup, Tablets 927
Hycomine Compound Tablets 929
Hycomine Syrup 927
Hycotuss Expectorant Syrup 930
Hydrocet Capsules 835
Lortab ASA Tablets 2414
Lortab 2412
Ru-Tuss with Hydrocodone 694
Triaminic Expectorant DH 1995
Vicodin Tablets 1187
Vicodin ES Tablets 1189
Zydone Capsules 941

Hydrocodone Polistirex (Excessive cholinergic blockade). Products include:
Tussionex Extended-Release Suspension 988

Hydrocortisone (Increased intraocular pressure). Products include:
AK-Spore H.C. ..... ◉ 206
Bactine Hydrocortisone Anti-Itch Cream ..... ▣ 625
CaldeCORT Anti-Itch Hydrocortisone Spray ..... ▣ 560
Carmol HC Cream 1% 2296
Cortaid Spray ..... ▣ 735
Cortenema 2244
Cortisporin Ointment 758
Cortisporin Ophthalmic Ointment Sterile 758
Cortisporin Ophthalmic Suspension Sterile 759
Cortisporin Otic Solution Sterile 760
Cortisporin Otic Suspension Sterile 760
Cortizone-5 Creme & Ointment ..... ▣ 732
Dermolate Anti-Itch Cream ..... ▣ 697
Eldecort Cream 1.0% 1113
Eldecort Cream 1.0% and 2.5% 1113
Fungoid HC Creme 1770
Hydrocortone Tablets 1482
Hytone 909
LazerSporin-C Solution 1770
Massengill Medicated Soft Cloth Towelettes 2192
Nutracort Cream & Lotion 1684
PediOtic Suspension Sterile 797
Synacort Creams 1%, 2.5% 2296
Vanoxide-HC Acne Lotion 911
Vioform-Hydrocortisone Cream and Mild Cream 889
Vioform-Hydrocortisone Ointment 889
VōSoL HC Otic Solution 2392
Vytone Cream 1% 911

Hydrocortisone Acetate (Increased intraocular pressure). Products include:
Analpram-HC Rectal Cream 1% and 2.5% 970

Anusol-HC Cream ... 1690
Anusol-HC Suppositories ... 1691
Caldecort ... ▣ 560
Carmol HC Cream 1% ... 2296
Chloromycetin Hydrocortisone Ophthalmic ... 1694
Coly-Mycin S Otic w/Neomycin & Hydrocortisone ... 1708
Cortaid ... ▣ 735
Cortef Feminine Itch Cream ... ▣ 735
Corticaine ... ▣ 682
Cortifoam ... 1827
Cortisporin Cream ... 757
Epifoam ... 1828
Gynecort 5 Creme ... ▣ 556
Hydrocortone Acetate Sterile Suspension ... 1479
Lanacort 5 Creme and Ointment .. ▣ 557
Mantadil Cream ... 789
Ophthocort ... ◉ 301
Orabase HCA Oral Paste ... 890
Pramosone Cream, Lotion & Ointment ... 971
ProctoCream-HC ... 1834
Proctofoam-HC ... 1835

Hydrocortisone Sodium Phosphate (Increased intraocular pressure). Products include:
Hydrocortone Phosphate Injection, Sterile ... 1481

Hydrocortisone Sodium Succinate (Increased intraocular pressure). Products include:
Solu-Cortef Sterile Powder ... 2361

Hyoscyamine (Excessive cholinergic blockade; increased intraocular pressure). Products include:
Cystospaz Tablets ... 2395
Urised Tablets ... 2396

Hyoscyamine Sulfate (Excessive cholinergic blockade; increased intraocular pressure). Products include:
Arco-Lase Plus Tablets ... 607
Cystospaz-M Capsules ... 2395
Donnagel ... ▣ 675
Donnagel-PG ... 1858
Donnatal ... 1858
Donnatal Extentabs ... 1859
Donnatal Tablets ... 1858
Donnazyme Tablets ... 1860
Kutrase Capsules ... 2146
Levsin/Levsinex ... 2147
Ru-Tuss Tablets ... 693

Imipramine Hydrochloride (Excessive cholinergic blockade). Products include:
Tofranil Ampuls ... 1038
Tofranil Tablets ... 1039

Imipramine Pamoate (Excessive cholinergic blockade). Products include:
Tofranil-PM Capsules ... 1041

Ipratropium Bromide (Excessive cholinergic blockade; increased intraocular pressure). Products include:
Atrovent Inhalation Aerosol ... 675

Lidocaine Hydrochloride (Excessive cholinergic blockade). Products include:
Anestacon Solution ... 2394
Bactine Antiseptic/Anesthetic First Aid Spray ... ▣ 624
Decadron Phosphate with Xylocaine Injection, Sterile ... 1451
Xylocaine Injections ... 637
Xylocaine Injections for Ventricular Arrhythmias ... 639
Xylocaine 2% Jelly ... 643
4% Xylocaine-MPF Sterile Solution ... 641
Xylocaine 2% Viscous Solution ... 646

Maprotiline Hydrochloride (Excessive cholinergic blockade). Products include:
Ludiomil Tablets ... 874

Mepenzolate Bromide (Excessive cholinergic blockade; increased intraocular pressure). Products include:
Cantil Tablets ... 1326

Meperidine Hydrochloride (Excessive cholinergic blockade). Products include:
Demerol ... 2047
Mepergan Injection ... 2479

Mesoridazine (Excessive cholinergic blockade; potentiated sedative effect). Products include:
Serentil ... 686

Methdilazine Hydrochloride (Excessive cholinergic blockade). Products include:
Tacaryl Syrup & Tablets ... 2409

Methylprednisolone Acetate (Increased intraocular pressure). Products include:
Depo-Medrol Sterile Aqueous Suspension ... 2334

Methylprednisolone Sodium Succinate (Increased intraocular pressure). Products include:
Solu-Medrol Sterile Powder ... 2363

Mexiletine Hydrochloride (Excessive cholinergic blockade). Products include:
Mexitil Capsules ... 680

Moricizine Hydrochloride (Excessive cholinergic blockade). Products include:
Ethmozine Tablets ... 946

Nortriptyline Hydrochloride (Excessive cholinergic blockade). Products include:
Pamelor ... 2019

Opium Alkaloids (Excessive cholinergic blockade). Products include:
B & O No. 15A & No. 16A Supprettes ... 2395
Pantopon Injectable ... 1911

Oxybutynin Chloride (Excessive cholinergic blockade; increased intraocular pressure). Products include:
Ditropan ... 1332

Oxycodone Hydrochloride (Excessive cholinergic blockade). Products include:
Percocet Tablets ... 950
Percodan ... 951
Roxicodone Tablets, Oral Solution & Intensol (Oxycodone) ... 1992
Tylox Capsules ... 1382

Perphenazine (Excessive cholinergic blockade; potentiated sedative effect). Products include:
Etrafon ... 2087
Triavil Tablets ... 1556
Trilafon ... 2123

Prednisolone Acetate (Increased intraocular pressure). Products include:
AK-Cide Sterile Ophthalmic Ointment & Suspension ... ◉ 202
Blephamide Liquifilm Sterile Ophthalmic Suspension ... 586
Blephamide S.O.P. Sterile Ophthalmic Ointment ... 586
Cetapred Ointment ... ◉ 220
⅛% Econopred & 1% Econopred Plus ... ◉ 217
Isopto Cetapred Suspension ... ◉ 220
Metimyd ... ◉ 306
Poly-Pred Liquifilm ... ◉ 250
Pred Forte ... ◉ 252
Pred Mild ... ◉ 254
Pred-G Liquifilm Sterile Ophthalmic Suspension ... ◉ 252
Pred-G S.O.P. Sterile Ophthalmic Ointment ... ◉ 253
Vasocidin Ointment ... ◉ 275

Prednisolone Sodium Phosphate (Increased intraocular pressure). Products include:
AK-Pred ... ◉ 205
Hydeltrasol Injection, Sterile ... 1476
Inflamase ... ◉ 274
Pediapred Oral Liquid ... 987
Vasocidin Ophthalmic Solution ... ◉ 276

Prednisolone Tebutate (Increased intraocular pressure). Products include:
Hydeltra-T.B.A. Sterile Suspension 1478

Prednisone (Increased intraocular pressure). Products include:
Deltasone Tablets ... 2332

Procainamide Hydrochloride (Excessive cholinergic blockade). Products include:
Procan SR Tablets ... 1760
Pronestyl Capsules and Tablets ... 1800
Pronestyl Injection ... 1798
Pronestyl-SR Tablets ... 1801

Prochlorperazine (Excessive cholinergic blockade; potentiated sedative effect). Products include:
Compazine ... 2201

Procyclidine Hydrochloride (Excessive cholinergic blockade; increased intraocular pressure). Products include:
Kemadrin Tablets ... 771

Promethazine Hydrochloride (Excessive cholinergic blockade; potentiated sedative effect). Products include:
Mepergan Injection ... 2479
Phenergan with Codeine ... 2497
Phenergan with Dextromethorphan 2499
Phenergan Injection ... 2493
Phenergan Suppositories ... 2496
Phenergan Syrup ... 2495
Phenergan Tablets ... 2496
Phenergan VC ... 2500
Phenergan VC with Codeine ... 2501

Propafenone Hydrochloride (Excessive cholinergic blockade). Products include:
Rythmol Tablets ... 1184

Propranolol Hydrochloride (Excessive cholinergic blockade). Products include:
Inderal ... 2459
Inderal LA Long Acting Capsules ... 2461
Inderide Tablets ... 2463
Inderide LA Long Acting Capsules .. 2465

Protriptyline Hydrochloride (Excessive cholinergic blockade). Products include:
Vivactil Tablets ... 1567

Pyrilamine Maleate (Excessive cholinergic blockade). Products include:
Codimal ... 846
4-Way Fast Acting Nasal Spray - Original Formula (regular & mentholated) & Metered Spray Pump (regular) ... 751
Maximum Strength Midol Multi-Symptom Menstrual Formula ... ▣ 571
Maximum Strength Midol PMS Premenstrual Syndrome Formula ... ▣ 570
Regular Strength Midol Multi-Symptom Menstrual Formula ... ▣ 570
Prefrin-A ... ◉ 255
Prēmsyn PMS Capsules & Caplets ▣ 547
Primatene Tablets-M Formula ... 2421
Robitussin Night Relief ... ▣ 677
Ru-Tuss with Hydrocodone ... 694
Triaminic Expectorant DH ... 1995
Triaminic Oral Infant Drops ... 1996

Pyrilamine Tannate (Excessive cholinergic blockade). Products include:
Rynatan ... 2387

Quinidine Gluconate (Excessive cholinergic blockade). Products include:
Quinaglute Dura-Tabs Tablets ... 663

Quinidine Polygalacturonate (Excessive cholinergic blockade). Products include:
Cardioquin Tablets ... 1812

Quinidine Sulfate (Excessive cholinergic blockade). Products include:
Quinidex Extentabs ... 1868

Scopolamine Hydrobromide (Excessive cholinergic blockade; increased intraocular pressure). Products include:
Donnagel ... ▣ 675
Donnagel-PG ... 1858
Donnatal ... 1858
Donnatal Extentabs ... 1859
Donnatal Tablets ... 1858
Donnazyme Tablets ... 1860
Isopto Hyoscine ... ◉ 222
Murocoll-2 Sterile Ophthalmic Solution ... ◉ 261
Ru-Tuss Tablets ... 693

Scopolamine Preparations (Excessive cholinergic blockade; increased intraocular pressure). Products include:
Transderm Scōp Transdermal Therapeutic System ... 887

Terfenadine (Excessive cholinergic blockade). Products include:
Seldane Tablets ... 1349
Seldane-D Extended-Release Tablets ... 1350

Thioridazine Hydrochloride (Excessive cholinergic blockade; potentiated sedative effect). Products include:
Mellaril ... 2011

Tocainide Hydrochloride (Excessive cholinergic blockade). Products include:
Tonocard Tablets ... 1554

Triamcinolone (Increased intraocular pressure).
No products indexed under this heading.

Triamcinolone Acetonide (Increased intraocular pressure). Products include:
Aristocort A ... 1010
Azmacort Inhaler ... 1837
Kenalog Cream, Lotion & Ointment 2401
Kenalog-10 Injection ... 2402
Kenalog-40 Injection ... 2403
Kenalog in Orabase ... 604
Kenalog Spray ... 2401
Mycolog II Cream and Ointment ... 2407
Mytrex Cream & Ointment ... 2080
Nasacort Nasal Inhaler ... 1844

Triamcinolone Diacetate (Increased intraocular pressure). Products include:
Aristocort Suspension ... 1008

Triamcinolone Hexacetonide (Increased intraocular pressure). Products include:
Aristospan Suspension ... 1011

Tridihexethyl Chloride (Excessive cholinergic blockade; increased intraocular pressure).
No products indexed under this heading.

Trifluoperazine Hydrochloride (Excessive cholinergic blockade; potentiated sedative effect). Products include:
Stelazine ... 2226

Trihexyphenidyl Hydrochloride (Excessive cholinergic blockade; increased intraocular pressure). Products include:
Artane ... 1195

Trimeprazine Tartrate (Excessive cholinergic blockade). Products include:
Temaril Tablets, Syrup and Spansule Sustained Release Capsules 1085

Trimipramine Maleate (Excessive cholinergic blockade). Products include:
Surmontil Capsules ... 2524

Tripelennamine Hydrochloride (Excessive cholinergic blockade). Products include:
PBZ Tablets & Elixir ... 1037
PBZ-SR Tablets ... 1037

Triprolidine Hydrochloride (Excessive cholinergic blockade). Products include:

Actidil ▣ 538
Actifed Capsules ▣ 539
Actifed Plus Caplets ▣ 539
Actifed Plus Tablets ▣ 540
Actifed with Codeine Cough Syrup.. 752
Actifed Syrup ▣ 540
Actifed Tablets ▣ 540
Actifed 12-Hour Capsules ▣ 539

Verapamil Hydrochloride (Excessive cholinergic blockade). Products include:

Calan SR Caplets 2157
Calan Tablets 2155
Isoptin Injectable 1177
Isoptin Oral Tablets 1179
Isoptin SR Sustained Release Tablets 1181
Verelan Capsules 1243
Verelan Capsules 2535

PROCAN SR TABLETS

(Procainamide Hydrochloride) 1760

May interact with antiarrhythmics, anticholinergics, type 1 antiarrhythmic drugs, cardiac glycosides, and certain other agents. Compounds in these categories include:

Acebutolol Hydrochloride (Additive cardiac effects). Products include:

Sectral Capsules 2520

Adenosine (Additive cardiac effects). Products include:

Adenocard Injection 1007

Amiodarone Hydrochloride (Additive cardiac effects). Products include:

Cordarone Tablets 2446

Atracurium Besylate (Potentiation of effects of skeletal muscle relaxants). Products include:

Tracrium Injection 817

Atropine Sulfate (Enhanced anticholinergic effects). Products include:

Arco-Lase Plus Tablets 607
Atropine Sulfate Sterile Ophthalmic Solution and S.O.P. Sterile Ophthalmic Ointment ⊙ 239
Donnagel ▣ 675
Donnagel-PG 1858
Donnatal 1858
Donnatal Extentabs 1859
Donnatal Tablets 1858
Donnazyme Tablets 1860
Isopto Atropine ⊙ 218
Lomotil 2174
Motofen Tablets 836
Ru-Tuss Tablets 693
Urised Tablets 2396

Belladonna Alkaloids (Enhanced anticholinergic effects). Products include:

Bellergal-S Tablets 1998
Hyland's Bed Wetting Tablets ▣ 728
Hyland's Teething Tablets ▣ 728
Kinesed Tablets 2272

Benztropine Mesylate (Enhanced anticholinergic effects). Products include:

Cogentin 1435

Biperiden (Enhanced anticholinergic effects). Products include:

Akineton 1171

Bretylium Tosylate (Additive cardiac effects; additive toxic effects). Products include:

Bretylol Injection 923

Clidinium Bromide (Enhanced anticholinergic effects). Products include:

Librax Capsules 1929
Quarzan Capsules 1937

Deslanoside (Additional depression of conduction and ventricular asystole or fibrillation may result in certain patients).

No products indexed under this heading.

Dicyclomine Hydrochloride (Enhanced anticholinergic effects). Products include:

Bentyl 1322

Digitoxin (Additional depression of conduction and ventricular asystole or fibrillation may result in certain patients). Products include:

Crystodigin Tablets 1253

Digoxin (Additional depression of conduction and ventricular asystole or fibrillation may result in certain patients). Products include:

Lanoxicaps 772
Lanoxin Elixir Pediatric 775
Lanoxin Injection 778
Lanoxin Injection Pediatric 781
Lanoxin Tablets 783

Disopyramide Phosphate (Enhanced prolongation of conduction or depression of contractility and hypotension). Products include:

Norpace 2177

Edrophonium Chloride (Antagonized effect). Products include:

Enlon Injection 598
Tensilon Injectable 1123

Glycopyrrolate (Enhanced anticholinergic effects). Products include:

Robinul Forte Tablets 1873
Robinul Injectable 1873
Robinul Tablets 1873

Hyoscyamine (Enhanced anticholinergic effects). Products include:

Cystospaz Tablets 2395
Urised Tablets 2396

Hyoscyamine Sulfate (Enhanced anticholinergic effects). Products include:

Arco-Lase Plus Tablets 607
Cystospaz-M Capsules 2395
Donnagel ▣ 675
Donnagel-PG 1858
Donnatal 1858
Donnatal Extentabs 1859
Donnatal Tablets 1858
Donnazyme Tablets 1860
Kutrase Capsules 2146
Levsin/Levsinex 2147
Ru-Tuss Tablets 693

Ipratropium Bromide (Enhanced anticholinergic effects). Products include:

Atrovent Inhalation Aerosol 675

Lidocaine Hydrochloride (Additive cardiac effects). Products include:

Anestacon Solution 2394
Bactine Antiseptic/Anesthetic First Aid Spray ▣ 624
Decadron Phosphate with Xylocaine Injection, Sterile 1451
Xylocaine Injections 637
Xylocaine Injections for Ventricular Arrhythmias 639
Xylocaine 2% Jelly 643
4% Xylocaine-MPF Sterile Solution 641
Xylocaine 2% Viscous Solution 646

Mepenzolate Bromide (Enhanced anticholinergic effects). Products include:

Cantil Tablets 1326

Metocurine Iodide (Potentiation of effects of skeletal muscle relaxants). Products include:

Metubine Iodide Vials 1285

Mexiletine Hydrochloride (Potential for agranulocytosis and additive cardiac effects). Products include:

Mexitil Capsules 680

Moricizine Hydrochloride (Additive cardiac effects). Products include:

Ethmozine Tablets 946

Oxybutynin Chloride (Enhanced anticholinergic effects). Products include:

Ditropan 1332

Pancuronium Bromide Injection (Potentiation of effects of skeletal muscle relaxants).

No products indexed under this heading.

Procyclidine Hydrochloride (Enhanced anticholinergic effects). Products include:

Kemadrin Tablets 771

Propafenone Hydrochloride (Additive cardiac effects). Products include:

Rythmol Tablets 1184

Propantheline Bromide (Enhanced anticholinergic effects). Products include:

Pro-Banthine Tablets 2141

Propranolol Hydrochloride (Additive cardiac effects). Products include:

Inderal 2459
Inderal LA Long Acting Capsules 2461
Inderide Tablets 2463
Inderide LA Long Acting Capsules 2465

Quinidine Gluconate (Enhanced prolongation of conduction or depression of contractility and hypotension). Products include:

Quinaglute Dura-Tabs Tablets 663

Quinidine Polygalacturonate (Enhanced prolongation of conduction or depression of contractility and hypotension). Products include:

Cardioquin Tablets 1812

Quinidine Sulfate (Enhanced prolongation of conduction or depression of contractility and hypotension). Products include:

Quinidex Extentabs 1868

Scopolamine Hydrobromide (Enhanced anticholinergic effects). Products include:

Donnagel ▣ 675
Donnagel-PG 1858
Donnatal 1858
Donnatal Extentabs 1859
Donnatal Tablets 1858
Donnazyme Tablets 1860
Isopto Hyoscine ⊙ 222
Murocoll-2 Sterile Ophthalmic Solution ⊙ 261
Ru-Tuss Tablets 693

Scopolamine Preparations (Enhanced anticholinergic effects). Products include:

Transderm Scōp Transdermal Therapeutic System 887

Succinylcholine Chloride (Procainamide reduces acetycholine release). Products include:

Anectine 755

Tocainide Hydrochloride (Additive cardiac effects). Products include:

Tonocard Tablets 1554

Trichlormethiazide (Potentiation of hypotensive effects of thiazide diuretics).

No products indexed under this heading.

Tridihexethyl Chloride (Enhanced anticholinergic effects).

No products indexed under this heading.

Trihexyphenidyl Hydrochloride (Enhanced anticholinergic effects). Products include:

Artane 1195

Trimethaphan Camsylate (Potentiation of hypotensive effects of antihypertensives). Products include:

Arfonad Ampuls 1887

Vecuronium Bromide (Potentiation of effects of skeletal muscle relaxants). Products include:

Norcuron 1642

Verapamil Hydrochloride (Additive cardiac effects). Products include:

Calan SR Caplets 2157
Calan Tablets 2155
Isoptin Injectable 1177
Isoptin Oral Tablets 1179
Isoptin SR Sustained Release Tablets 1181
Verelan Capsules 1243
Verelan Capsules 2535

PROCARDIA CAPSULES

(Nifedipine) 1781

May interact with beta blockers, oral anticoagulants, cardiac glycosides, and certain other agents. Compounds in these categories include:

Acebutolol Hydrochloride (Increased likelihood of congestive heart failure). Products include:

Sectral Capsules 2520

Atenolol (Increased likelihood of congestive heart failure). Products include:

Tenoretic Tablets 1105
Tenormin Tablets and I.V. Injection 1107

Betaxolol Hydrochloride (Increased likelihood of congestive heart failure). Products include:

Betoptic Sterile Ophthalmic Solution 569
Betoptic S Sterile Ophthalmic Suspension 570
Kerlone Tablets 2172

Carteolol Hydrochloride (Increased likelihood of congestive heart failure). Products include:

Cartrol Tablets 507

Cimetidine (Increases peak nifedipine plasma levels). Products include:

Tagamet Tablets 2228

Cimetidine Hydrochloride (Increases peak nifedipine plasma levels). Products include:

Tagamet 2228

Deslanoside (Increased digoxin levels).

No products indexed under this heading.

Dicumarol (Increased prothrombin time). Products include:

Dicumarol Tablets 516

Digitoxin (Increased digoxin levels). Products include:

Crystodigin Tablets 1253

Digoxin (Increased digoxin levels). Products include:

Lanoxicaps 772
Lanoxin Elixir Pediatric 775
Lanoxin Injection 778
Lanoxin Injection Pediatric 781
Lanoxin Tablets 783

Esmolol Hydrochloride (Increased likelihood of congestive heart failure). Products include:

Brevibloc Injection 942

Labetalol Hydrochloride (Increased likelihood of congestive heart failure). Products include:

Normodyne Injection 2108
Normodyne Tablets 2110
Normozide Tablets 2112
Trandate HCT Tablets 579
Trandate Injection 577
Trandate Tablets 579

(▣ Described in PDR For Nonprescription Drugs)

(⊙ Described in PDR For Ophthalmology)

Metoprolol Tartrate (Increased likelihood of congestive heart failure). Products include:
- Lopressor Ampuls 1032
- Lopressor HCT Tablets 1034
- Lopressor Tablets 1032

Nadolol (Increased likelihood of congestive heart failure). Products include:
- Corgard Tablets 701
- Corzide Tablets 702

Penbutolol Sulfate (Increased likelihood of congestive heart failure). Products include:
- Levatol 1832

Pindolol (Increased likelihood of congestive heart failure). Products include:
- Visken Tablets 2036

Propranolol Hydrochloride (Increased likelihood of congestive heart failure). Products include:
- Inderal 2459
- Inderal LA Long Acting Capsules 2461
- Inderide Tablets 2463
- Inderide LA Long Acting Capsules 2465

Timolol Maleate (Increased likelihood of congestive heart failure). Products include:
- Blocadren Tablets 1429
- Timolide Tablets 1547
- Timoptic in Ocudose 1552
- Timoptic Sterile Ophthalmic Solution 1550

Warfarin Sodium (Increased prothrombin time). Products include:
- Coumadin Injection & Tablets 944
- Panwarfin Tablets 547

PROCARDIA XL TABLETS
(Nifedipine) 1783

May interact with beta blockers, oral anticoagulants, diuretics, cardiac glycosides, and certain other agents. Compounds in these categories include:

Acebutolol Hydrochloride (Potential for congestive heart failure, severe hypotension, or exacerbation of angina). Products include:
- Sectral Capsules 2520

Amiloride Hydrochloride (Serum potassium slightly decreased). Products include:
- Midamor Tablets 1508
- Moduretic Tablets 1510

Atenolol (Potential for congestive heart failure, severe hypotension, or exacerbation of angina). Products include:
- Tenoretic Tablets 1105
- Tenormin Tablets and I.V. Injection 1107

Bendroflumethiazide (Serum potassium slightly decreased). Products include:
- Corzide Tablets 702
- Naturetin Tablets 1789
- Rauzide Tablets 1804

Betaxolol Hydrochloride (Potential for congestive heart failure, severe hypotension, or exacerbation of angina). Products include:
- Betoptic Sterile Ophthalmic Solution 569
- Betoptic S Sterile Ophthalmic Suspension 570
- Kerlone Tablets 2172

Bumetanide (Serum potassium slightly decreased). Products include:
- Bumex 1895

Carteolol Hydrochloride (Potential for congestive heart failure, severe hypotension, or exacerbation of angina). Products include:
- Cartrol Tablets 507

Chlorothiazide (Serum potassium slightly decreased). Products include:
- Aldoclor Tablets 1413
- Diupres Tablets 1461
- Diuril Oral 1464

Chlorothiazide Sodium (Serum potassium slightly decreased). Products include:
- Diuril Sodium Intravenous 1463

Chlorthalidone (Serum potassium slightly decreased). Products include:
- Combipres Tablets 678
- Tenoretic Tablets 1105
- Thalitone Tablets 687

Cimetidine (Significant increase peak nifedipine plasma levels and AUC). Products include:
- Tagamet Tablets 2228

Cimetidine Hydrochloride (Significant increase in peak nifedipine plasma levels and AUC). Products include:
- Tagamet 2228

Deslanoside (Potential for elevated digoxin levels).
- No products indexed under this heading.

Dicumarol (Rare reports of increased prothrombin time). Products include:
- Dicumarol Tablets 516

Digitoxin (Potential for elevated digoxin levels). Products include:
- Crystodigin Tablets 1253

Digoxin (Potential for elevated digoxin levels). Products include:
- Lanoxicaps 772
- Lanoxin Elixir Pediatric 775
- Lanoxin Injection 778
- Lanoxin Injection Pediatric 781
- Lanoxin Tablets 783

Esmolol Hydrochloride (Potential for congestive heart failure, severe hypotension, or exacerbation of angina). Products include:
- Brevibloc Injection 942

Ethacrynic Acid (Serum potassium slightly decreased). Products include:
- Edecrin Tablets 1468

Fentanyl Citrate (Severe hypotension and/or increased fluid volume requirements have been reported in patients receiving nifedipine together with a beta blocker undergoing high dose fentanyl anesthesia). Products include:
- Innovar Injection 1141
- Sublimaze Injection 1146

Furosemide (Serum potassium slightly decreased). Products include:
- Lasix 1093

Hydrochlorothiazide (Serum potassium slightly decreased). Products include:
- Aldactazide 2150
- Aldoril Tablets 1418
- Apresazide Capsules 854
- Apresoline-Esidrix Tablets 857
- Capozide 2258
- Dyazide Capsules 2208
- Esidrix Tablets 863
- Esimil Tablets 864
- HydroDIURIL Tablets 1484
- Hydropres Tablets 1485
- Inderide Tablets 2463
- Inderide LA Long Acting Capsules 2465
- Lopressor HCT Tablets 1034
- Maxzide 1215
- Moduretic Tablets 1510
- Normozide Tablets 2112
- Oretic Tablets 544
- Oreticyl 545
- Prinzide Tablets 1540
- Ser-Ap-Es Tablets 881
- Serpasil-Esidrix Tablets 886
- Timolide Tablets 1547
- Trandate HCT Tablets 579
- Vaseretic Tablets 1559
- Zestoretic 2274

Hydroflumethiazide (Serum potassium slightly decreased). Products include:
- Diucardin Tablets 2450
- Saluron 718
- Salutensin/Salutensin-Demi 719

Indapamide (Serum potassium slightly decreased). Products include:
- Lozol Tablets 1843

Labetalol Hydrochloride (Potential for congestive heart failure, severe hypotension, or exacerbation of angina). Products include:
- Normodyne Injection 2108
- Normodyne Tablets 2110
- Normozide Tablets 2112
- Trandate HCT Tablets 579
- Trandate Injection 577
- Trandate Tablets 579

Methyclothiazide (Serum potassium slightly decreased). Products include:
- Enduron Tablets 517
- Enduronyl 518

Metolazone (Serum potassium slightly decreased). Products include:
- Diulo 2129
- Mykrox ½ mg Tablets 984
- Zaroxolyn Tablets 989

Metoprolol Tartrate (Potential for congestive heart failure, severe hypotension, or exacerbation of angina). Products include:
- Lopressor Ampuls 1032
- Lopressor HCT Tablets 1034
- Lopressor Tablets 1032

Nadolol (Potential for congestive heart failure, severe hypotension, or exacerbation of angina). Products include:
- Corgard Tablets 701
- Corzide Tablets 702

Penbutolol Sulfate (Potential for congestive heart failure, severe hypotension, or exacerbation of angina). Products include:
- Levatol 1832

Pindolol (Potential for congestive heart failure, severe hypotension, or exacerbation of angina). Products include:
- Visken Tablets 2036

Polythiazide (Serum potassium slightly decreased). Products include:
- Minizide Capsules 1779
- Renese Tablets 1785
- Renese-R Tablets 1786

Propranolol Hydrochloride (Potential for congestive heart failure, severe hypotension, or exacerbation of angina). Products include:
- Inderal 2459
- Inderal LA Long Acting Capsules 2461
- Inderide Tablets 2463
- Inderide LA Long Acting Capsules 2465

Ranitidine Hydrochloride (Smaller non-significant increase in nifedipine plasma levels and AUC). Products include:
- Zantac Injection and Zantac Injection Premixed 1063
- Zantac 1065

Spironolactone (Serum potassium slightly decreased). Products include:
- Aldactazide 2150
- Aldactone 2152

Timolol Maleate (Potential for congestive heart failure, severe hypotension, or exacerbation of angina). Products include:
- Blocadren Tablets 1429
- Timolide Tablets 1547
- Timoptic in Ocudose 1552
- Timoptic Sterile Ophthalmic Solution 1550

Triamterene (Serum potassium slightly decreased). Products include:
- Dyazide Capsules 2208
- Dyrenium Capsules 2210
- Maxzide 1215

Warfarin Sodium (Rare reports of increased prothrombin time). Products include:
- Coumadin Injection & Tablets 944
- Panwarfin Tablets 547

Food Interactions

Food, unspecified (Presence of food slightly alters the early rate of drug absorption).

PRO-CEPTION
(Precoital douche) 1613

No interactions described in labeling.

PROCRIT FOR INJECTION
(Epoetin Alfa) 1647

No interactions described in labeling.

PROCTOCREAM-HC
(Hydrocortisone Acetate, Pramoxine Hydrochloride) 1834

No interactions described in labeling.

PROCTOFOAM/NON-STEROID
(Pramoxine Hydrochloride) .... ⊡ 651

No interactions described in labeling.

PROCTOFOAM-HC
(Hydrocortisone Acetate, Pramoxine Hydrochloride) 1835

No interactions described in labeling.

PROFASI (HUMAN CHORIONIC GONADOTROPIN, USP)
(Chorionic Gonadotropin) 2186

No interactions described in labeling.

PROFENAL STERILE OPHTHALMIC SOLUTION
(Suprofen) .... ⊙ 234

May interact with oral anticoagulants and certain other agents. Compounds in these categories include:

Dicumarol (Use with caution). Products include:
- Dicumarol Tablets 516

Warfarin Sodium (Use with caution). Products include:
- Coumadin Injection & Tablets 944
- Panwarfin Tablets 547

PROGAINE SHAMPOO
(TEA-Lauryl Sulfate) .... ⊡ 737

No interactions described in labeling.

PROGLYCEM CAPSULES
(Diazoxide) 649

May interact with oral anticoagulants, thiazides, diuretics, and certain other agents. Compounds in these categories include:

Amiloride Hydrochloride (Potentiates the hyperglycemic effects). Products include:
- Midamor Tablets 1508
- Moduretic Tablets 1510

Bendroflumethiazide (Potentiates the hyperglycemic effects). Products include:
- Corzide Tablets 702
- Naturetin Tablets 1789
- Rauzide Tablets 1804

Bumetanide (Potentiates the hyperglycemic effects). Products include:
- Bumex 1895

Chlorothiazide (Potentiates the hyperglycemic effects). Products include:

- Aldoclor Tablets **1413**
- Diupres Tablets **1461**
- Diuril Oral **1464**

Chlorothiazide Sodium (Potentiates the hyperglycemic effects). Products include:

- Diuril Sodium Intravenous **1463**

Chlorthalidone (Potentiates the hyperglycemic effects). Products include:

- Combipres Tablets **678**
- Tenoretic Tablets **1105**
- Thalitone Tablets **687**

Dicumarol (Increased blood levels of coumarin derivatives). Products include:

- Dicumarol Tablets **516**

Ethacrynic Acid (Potentiates the hyperglycemic effects). Products include:

- Edecrin Tablets **1468**

Furosemide (Potentiates the hyperglycemic effects). Products include:

- Lasix **1093**

Hydrochlorothiazide (Potentiates the hyperglycemic effects). Products include:

- Aldactazide **2150**
- Aldoril Tablets **1418**
- Apresazide Capsules **854**
- Apresoline-Esidrix Tablets **857**
- Capozide **2258**
- Dyazide Capsules **2208**
- Esidrix Tablets **863**
- Esimil Tablets **864**
- HydroDIURIL Tablets **1484**
- Hydropres Tablets **1485**
- Inderide Tablets **2463**
- Inderide LA Long Acting Capsules .. **2465**
- Lopressor HCT Tablets **1034**
- Maxzide **1215**
- Moduretic Tablets **1510**
- Normozide Tablets **2112**
- Oretic Tablets **544**
- Oreticyl **545**
- Prinzide Tablets **1540**
- Ser-Ap-Es Tablets **881**
- Serpasil-Esidrix Tablets **886**
- Timolide Tablets **1547**
- Trandate HCT Tablets **579**
- Vaseretic Tablets **1559**
- Zestoretic **2274**

Hydroflumethiazide (Potentiates the hyperglycemic effects). Products include:

- Diucardin Tablets **2450**
- Saluron **718**
- Salutensin/Salutensin-Demi **719**

Indapamide (Potentiates the hyperglycemic effects). Products include:

- Lozol Tablets **1843**

Methyclothiazide (Potentiates the hyperglycemic effects). Products include:

- Enduron Tablets **517**
- Enduronyl **518**

Metolazone (Potentiates the hyperglycemic effects). Products include:

- Diulo **2129**
- Mykrox ½ mg Tablets **984**
- Zaroxolyn Tablets **989**

Phenytoin (Concomitant administration may result in loss of seizure control). Products include:

- Dilantin Infatabs **1710**
- Dilantin-30 Pediatric/Dilantin-125 Suspension **1713**

Phenytoin Sodium (Concomitant administration may result in loss of seizure control). Products include:

- Dilantin Kapseals **1708**
- Dilantin Parenteral **1712**
- Dilantin with Phenobarbital Kapseals **1715**

Polythiazide (Potentiates the hyperglycemic effects). Products include:

- Minizide Capsules **1779**
- Renese Tablets **1785**
- Renese-R Tablets **1786**

Spironolactone (Potentiates the hyperglycemic effects). Products include:

- Aldactazide **2150**
- Aldactone **2152**

Triamterene (Potentiates the hyperglycemic effects). Products include:

- Dyazide Capsules **2208**
- Dyrenium Capsules **2210**
- Maxzide **1215**

Warfarin Sodium (Increased blood levels of coumarin derivatives). Products include:

- Coumadin Injection & Tablets **944**
- Panwarfin Tablets **547**

PROGLYCEM SUSPENSION

(Diazoxide) **649**

See **Proglycem Capsules**

PRO-HEPATONE CAPSULES

(Multivitamins, Amino Acid Preparations) **1356**

No interactions described in labeling.

PROHIBIT HAEMOPHILUS B CONJUGATE VACCINE (DIPHTHERIA TOXOID CONJUGATE)

(Diphtheria Toxoid, Conjugate) **896**

May interact with immunosuppressive agents. Compounds in this category include:

Azathioprine (Expected immune response may not be obtained). Products include:

- Imuran **768**

Cyclosporine (Expected immune response may not be obtained). Products include:

- Sandimmune **2024**

Immune Globulin (Human) (Expected immune response may not be obtained). Products include:

- MICRhoGAM $Rh_o(D)$ Immune Globulin (Human) **1650**
- RhoGAM $Rh_o(D)$ Immune Globulin (Human) **1651**

Immune Globulin Intravenous (Human) (Expected immune response may not be obtained). Products include:

- Gamimune N Immune Globulin Intravenous (Human) **1572**
- Gammagard Immune Globulin, Intravenous (Human) **658**
- Iveegam **1129**
- Sandoglobulin I.V. **2027**

Muromonab-CD3 (Expected immune response may not be obtained). Products include:

- Orthoclone OKT3 Sterile Solution .. **1645**

PROKINE FOR I.V. INFUSION

(Sargramostim) **1096**

May interact with drugs with myeloproliferative effects, cytotoxic drugs, and certain other agents. Compounds in these categories include:

Betamethasone Acetate (May potentiate the myeloproliferative effect). Products include:

- Celestone Soluspan Suspension **2081**

Betamethasone Sodium Phosphate (May potentiate the myeloproliferative effect). Products include:

- Celestone Soluspan Suspension **2081**

Bleomycin Sulfate (Coadministration within 24 hours preceding or following chemotherapy is not recommended because of potential sensitivity of rapidly dividing hematopoietic progenitor cells to cytotoxic therapy). Products include:

- Blenoxane **724**

Cortisone Acetate (May potentiate the myeloproliferative effect). Products include:

- Cortone Acetate Sterile Suspension **1437**
- Cortone Acetate Tablets **1439**

Daunorubicin Hydrochloride (Coadministration within 24 hours preceding or following chemotherapy is not recommended because of potential sensitivity of rapidly dividing hematopoietic progenitor cells to cytotoxic therapy). Products include:

- Cerubidine **2443**

Dexamethasone (May potentiate the myeloproliferative effect). Products include:

- AK-Trol Ointment & Suspension .... ⊙ **207**
- Decadron Elixir **1445**
- Decadron Tablets **1447**
- Decaspray Topical Aerosol **1459**
- Dexacidin .... ⊙ **272**
- Maxidex Sterile Ophthalmic Suspension .... ⊙ **223**
- Maxitrol Ophthalmic Ointment/Suspension .... ⊙ **223**
- TobraDex Ophthalmic Suspension and Ointment .... ⊙ **228**

Dexamethasone Acetate (May potentiate the myeloproliferative effect). Products include:

- Dalalone D.P. Injectable **999**
- Decadron-LA Sterile Suspension **1457**

Dexamethasone Sodium Phosphate (May potentiate the myeloproliferative effect). Products include:

- AK-Dex .... ⊙ **203**
- Decadron Phosphate Respihaler **1454**
- Decadron Phosphate Sterile Ophthalmic Ointment **1453**
- Decadron Phosphate Sterile Ophthalmic Solution **1453**
- Decadron Phosphate Topical Cream **1455**
- Decadron Phosphate Turbinaire **1456**
- Maxidex Sterile Ophthalmic Ointment .... ⊙ **222**
- NeoDecadron Sterile Ophthalmic Ointment **1517**
- NeoDecadron Sterile Ophthalmic Solution **1518**
- NeoDecadron Topical Cream **1518**

Doxorubicin Hydrochloride (Coadministration within 24 hours preceding or following chemotherapy is not recommended because of potential sensitivity of rapidly dividing hematopoietic progenitor cells to cytotoxic therapy). Products include:

- Adriamycin PFS **561**
- Adriamycin RDF **562**
- Doxorubicin Hydrochloride for Injection, USP **622**
- Doxorubicin Hydrochloride Injection, USP **848**
- Rubex **739**

Fluorouracil (Coadministration within 24 hours preceding or following chemotherapy is not recommended because of potential sensitivity of rapidly dividing hematopoietic progenitor cells to cytotoxic therapy). Products include:

- Efudex **1880**
- Fluoroplex Topical Solution & Cream 1% **1082**
- Fluorouracil Injection **1897**

Hydrocortisone (May potentiate the myeloproliferative effect). Products include:

- AK-Spore H.C. .... ⊙ **206**
- Bactine Hydrocortisone Anti-Itch Cream .... ■□ **625**
- CaldeCORT Anti-Itch Hydrocortisone Spray .... ■□ **560**
- Carmol HC Cream 1% **2296**
- Cortaid Spray .... ■□ **735**
- Cortenema **2244**
- Cortisporin Ointment **758**
- Cortisporin Ophthalmic Ointment Sterile **758**
- Cortisporin Ophthalmic Suspension Sterile **759**
- Cortisporin Otic Solution Sterile **760**
- Cortisporin Otic Suspension Sterile **760**
- Cortizone-5 Creme & Ointment .... ■□ **732**
- Dermolate Anti-Itch Cream .... ■□ **697**
- Eldecort Cream 1.0% **1113**
- Eldecort Cream 1.0% and 2.5% **1113**
- Fungoid HC Creme **1770**
- Hydrocortone Tablets **1482**
- Hytone **909**
- LazerSporin-C Solution **1770**
- Massengill Medicated Soft Cloth Towelettes **2192**
- Nutracort Cream & Lotion **1684**
- PediOtic Suspension Sterile **797**
- Synacort Creams 1%, 2.5% **2296**
- Vanoxide-HC Acne Lotion **911**
- Vioform-Hydrocortisone Cream and Mild Cream **889**
- Vioform-Hydrocortisone Ointment **889**
- VōSoL HC Otic Solution **2392**
- Vytone Cream 1% **911**

Hydrocortisone Acetate (May potentiate the myeloproliferative effect). Products include:

- Analpram-HC Rectal Cream 1% and 2.5% **970**
- Anusol-HC Cream **1690**
- Anusol-HC Suppositories **1691**
- Caldecort .... ■□ **560**
- Carmol HC Cream 1% **2296**
- Chloromycetin Hydrocortisone Ophthalmic **1694**
- Coly-Mycin S Otic w/Neomycin & Hydrocortisone **1708**
- Cortaid .... ■□ **735**
- Cortef Feminine Itch Cream .... ■□ **735**
- Corticaine .... ■□ **682**
- Cortifoam **1827**
- Cortisporin Cream **757**
- Epifoam **1828**
- Gynecort 5 Creme .... ■□ **556**
- Hydrocortone Acetate Sterile Suspension **1479**
- Lanacort 5 Creme and Ointment .... ■□ **557**
- Mantadil Cream **789**
- Ophthocort .... ⊙ **301**
- Orabase HCA Oral Paste **890**
- Pramosone Cream, Lotion & Ointment **971**
- ProctoCream-HC **1834**
- Proctofoam-HC **1835**

Hydrocortisone Sodium Phosphate (May potentiate the myeloproliferative effect). Products include:

- Hydrocortone Phosphate Injection, Sterile **1481**

Hydrocortisone Sodium Succinate (May potentiate the myeloproliferative effect). Products include:

- Solu-Cortef Sterile Powder **2361**

Hydroxyurea (Coadministration within 24 hours preceding or following chemotherapy is not recommended because of potential sensitivity of rapidly dividing hematopoietic progenitor cells to cytotoxic therapy). Products include:

- Hydrea Capsules **728**

Lithium Carbonate (May potentiate the myeloproliferative effect). Products include:

- Eskalith **2214**
- Lithane Tablets **1596**
- Lithium Carbonate Capsules & Tablets **1984**
- Lithobid Tablets **870**

Lithium Citrate (May potentiate the myeloproliferative effect). Products include:

- Cibalith-S **870**

Methotrexate Sodium (Coadministration within 24 hours preceding or following chemotherapy is not recommended because of potential sensitivity of rapidly dividing hematopoietic progenitor cells to cytotoxic therapy). Products include:
Methotrexate Tablets, Parenteral, LPF Parenteral 1217
Rheumatrex Methotrexate Dose Pack 1234

Methylprednisolone Acetate (May potentiate the myeloproliferative effect). Products include:
Depo-Medrol Sterile Aqueous Suspension 2334

Methylprednisolone Sodium Succinate (May potentiate the myeloproliferative effect). Products include:
Solu-Medrol Sterile Powder 2363

Mitotane (Coadministration within 24 hours preceding or following chemotherapy is not recommended because of potential sensitivity of rapidly dividing hematopoietic progenitor cells to cytotoxic therapy). Products include:
Lysodren 731

Mitoxantrone Hydrochloride (Coadministration within 24 hours preceding or following chemotherapy is not recommended because of potential sensitivity of rapidly dividing hematopoietic progenitor cells to cytotoxic therapy). Products include:
Novantrone for Injection Concentrate 1226

Prednisolone Sodium Phosphate (May potentiate the myeloproliferative effect). Products include:
AK-Pred .... ⊙ 205
Hydeltrasol Injection, Sterile 1476
Inflamase .... ⊙ 274
Pediapred Oral Liquid 987
Vasocidin Ophthalmic Solution .... ⊙ 276

Prednisolone Tebutate (May potentiate the myeloproliferative effect). Products include:
Hydeltra-T.B.A. Sterile Suspension 1478

Prednisone (May potentiate the myeloproliferative effect). Products include:
Deltasone Tablets 2332

Procarbazine Hydrochloride (Coadministration within 24 hours preceding or following chemotherapy is not recommended because of potential sensitivity of rapidly dividing hematopoietic progenitor cells to cytotoxic therapy). Products include:
Matulane Capsules 1907

Tamoxifen Citrate (Coadministration within 24 hours preceding or following chemotherapy is not recommended because of potential sensitivity of rapidly dividing hematopoietic progenitor cells to cytotoxic therapy). Products include:
Nolvadex Tablets 1102

Triamcinolone (May potentiate the myeloproliferative effect).
No products indexed under this heading.

Triamcinolone Acetonide (May potentiate the myeloproliferative effect). Products include:
Aristocort A 1010
Azmacort Inhaler 1837
Kenalog Cream, Lotion & Ointment 2401
Kenalog-10 Injection 2402
Kenalog-40 Injection 2403
Kenalog in Orabase 604
Kenalog Spray 2401
Mycolog II Cream and Ointment 2407
Mytrex Cream & Ointment 2080
Nasacort Nasal Inhaler 1844

Triamcinolone Diacetate (May potentiate the myeloproliferative effect). Products include:
Aristocort Suspension 1008

Triamcinolone Hexacetonide (May potentiate the myeloproliferative effect). Products include:
Aristospan Suspension 1011

Vincristine Sulfate (Coadministration within 24 hours preceding or following chemotherapy is not recommended because of potential sensitivity of rapidly dividing hematopoietic progenitor cells to cytotoxic therapy). Products include:
Oncovin Solution Vials & Hyporets 1288

PROLASTIN ALPHA$_1$-PROTEINASE INHIBITOR (HUMAN)

(Alpha$_1$-Proteinase Inhibitor (Human)) 1585
No interactions described in labeling.

PROLIXIN DECANOATE

(Fluphenazine Decanoate) 1795
May interact with hypnotics and sedatives, general anesthetics, central nervous system depressants, barbiturates, antihistamines, and certain other agents. Compounds in these categories include:

Alcohol (Potentiation of alcohol).

Alfentanil Hydrochloride (Potentiation of CNS depressants). Products include:
Alfenta Injection 1131

Alprazolam (Potentiation of CNS depressants). Products include:
Xanax Tablets 2367

Aprobarbital (Potentiation of CNS depressants). Products include:
Alurate Elixir 1883

Astemizole (Potentiation of antihistamines). Products include:
Hismanal Tablets 1138

Atropine Sulfate (Potentiation of atropine). Products include:
Arco-Lase Plus Tablets 607
Atropine Sulfate Sterile Ophthalmic Solution and S.O.P. Sterile Ophthalmic Ointment .... ⊙ 239
Donnagel .... ▣ 675
Donnagel-PG 1858
Donnatal 1858
Donnatal Extentabs 1859
Donnatal Tablets 1858
Donnazyme Tablets 1860
Isopto Atropine .... ⊙ 218
Lomotil 2174
Motofen Tablets 836
Ru-Tuss Tablets 693
Urised Tablets 2396

Azatadine Maleate (Potentiation of antihistamines). Products include:
Optimine Tablets 2115
Trinalin Repetabs Tablets 1170

Bromodiphenhydramine Hydrochloride (Potentiation of antihistamines).
No products indexed under this heading.

Brompheniramine Maleate (Potentiation of antihistamines). Products include:
Alka Seltzer Plus Sinus Allergy Medicine .... ▣ 624
Atrohist Sprinkle Capsules 558
Bromfed Capsules (Timed Release) 1615
Bromfed Syrup .... ▣ 628
Bromfed 1615
Dimetane Decongestant .... ▣ 673
Dimetane .... ▣ 672
Dimetane-DC Cough Syrup 1857
Dimetane-DX Cough Syrup 1858
Dimetapp Elixir .... ▣ 673
Dimetapp DM Elixir .... ▣ 674
Dimetapp Extentabs .... ▣ 674
Dimetapp Plus Caplets .... ▣ 675
Dimetapp Tablets .... ▣ 675
Drixoral Antihistamine/Nasal Decongestant Syrup .... ▣ 698

Buprenorphine (Potentiation of CNS depressants).
No products indexed under this heading.

Buspirone Hydrochloride (Potentiation of CNS depressants). Products include:
BuSpar 1401

Butabarbital (Potentiation of CNS depressants). Products include:
Pyridium Plus 1764

Butalbital (Potentiation of CNS depressants). Products include:
Esgic-Plus Tablets 1002
Esgic Tablets & Capsules 1001
Fioricet Tablets 2006
Fiorinal Capsules 2007
Fiorinal with Codeine Capsules 2008
Fiorinal Tablets 2007
Phrenilin 838
Sedapap Tablets 50 mg/650 mg .. 1360

Chlordiazepoxide (Potentiation of CNS depressants). Products include:
Libritabs Tablets 1930
Limbitrol 1933
Menrium Tablets 1934

Chlordiazepoxide Hydrochloride (Potentiation of CNS depressants). Products include:
Librax Capsules 1929
Librium Capsules 1931
Librium Injectable 1932

Chlorpheniramine Maleate (Potentiation of antihistamines). Products include:
A.R.M. Allergy Relief Medicine Caplets .... ▣ 615
Alka-Seltzer Plus Cold Medicine .... ▣ 623
Allerest .... ▣ 559
Ana-Kit Anaphylaxis Emergency Treatment Kit 1100
BC Cold Powder Multi-Symptom Formula .... ▣ 517
Brexin L.A. Capsules 2078
Cerose-DM 2443
Cheracol Plus Head Cold/Cough Formula .... ▣ 667
Chlor-Trimeton Allergy Syrup, Tablets & Long-Acting Repetabs Tablets .... ▣ 693
Chlor-Trimeton Decongestant .... ▣ 694
Comhist LA Capsules 1618
Allergy-Sinus Comtrex Multi-Symptom Allergy Sinus Formula Tablets & Caplets 746
Comtrex Multi-Symptom Cold Reliever Tablets/Caplets/Liqui-Gels/Liquid 745
Day-Night Comtrex 747
Contac Continuous Action Decongestant/Antihistamine Capsules ▣ 710
Contac Maximum Strength Continuous Action Decongestant/Antihistamine Caplets .... ▣ 709
Contac Severe Cold and Flu Formula Caplets .... ▣ 711
Coricidin 'D' Decongestant Tablets .... ▣ 695
Coricidin Demilets Tablets for Children .... ▣ 696
Coricidin Tablets .... ▣ 695
Deconamine 663
Demazin Nasal Decongestant/Antihistamine Repetabs Tablets & Syrup .... ▣ 697
Dorcol Children's Liquid Cold Formula .... ▣ 686
Dristan Decongestant/Antihistamine/ Analgesic Coated Caplets .... ▣ 749
Dristan Cold Nasal Decongestant/Antihistamine/ Analgesic Coated Tablets 2419
Dristan Advanced Formula Decongestant/Antihistamine/Analgesic Tablets .... ▣ 749
Extendryl 994
4-Way Cold Tablets 750
Fedahist Gyrocaps 2145
Fedahist Timecaps 2145
Hycomine Compound Tablets 929
Isoclor Timesule Capsules .... ▣ 561
Kronofed-A 970
Medi-Flu Caplet, Liquid .... ▣ 640
Naldecon Syrup, Tablets, Pediatric Drops and Pediatric Syrup 709
Nolamine Tablets 838
Novafed A Capsules 1342
Novahistine DH 1342
Novahistine Elixir .... ▣ 596
Ornade Spansule Capsules 2221
Orthoxicol Cough Syrup .... ▣ 668
PediaCare Allergy Relief Formula Liquid 1362
PediaCare Cough-Cold Formula Liquid 1362
PediaCare Night Rest Cough-Cold Formula Liquid 1362
PediaCare 6-12 Cough-Cold Formula Chewable Tablets 1362
Pyrroxate Capsules .... ▣ 669
Quelidrine Syrup 556
Ru-Tuss II Capsules 693
Ru-Tuss Tablets 693
Ryna .... ▣ 741
Sinarest Tablets & Extra Strength Tablets .... ▣ 562
Sine-Off Maximum Strength Allergy/Sinus Formula Caplets .... ▣ 721
Sine-Off Sinus Medicine Tablets-Aspirin Formula .... ▣ 722
Singlet Tablets .... ▣ 598
Sinulin 840
Sinutab Maximum Strength .... ▣ 641
St. Joseph Nighttime Cold Medicine .... ▣ 705
Sudafed Plus Liquid .... ▣ 544
Sudafed Plus Tablets .... ▣ 545
Teldrin Timed-Release Allergy Capsules, 12 mg 2192
TheraFlu Flu and Cold Medicine .... ▣ 687
Triaminic Allergy Tablets .... ▣ 688
Triaminic Chewables .... ▣ 688
Triaminic Cold Tablets .... ▣ 688
Triaminic Nite Light .... ▣ 689
Triaminic Syrup .... ▣ 689
Triaminic-12 Tablets .... ▣ 690
Triaminicin Tablets .... ▣ 690
Triaminicol Multi-Symptom Cold Tablets .... ▣ 691
Triaminicol Multi-Symptom Relief ▣ 691
Tylenol Allergy Sinus Medication Caplets and Gelcaps, Maximum Strength 1372
Children's Tylenol Cold Liquid Formula and Chewable Tablets 1368
Tylenol Cold & Flu Hot Medication, Packets 1369
Tylenol Cold Medication Caplets and Tablets 1370
Tylenol Cold Medication, Effervescent Tablets 1369
Vicks Children's NyQuil .... ▣ 664
Vicks Formula 44 Cough Medicine .... ▣ 661
Vicks Formula 44M Multi-Symptom Cough Medicine .... ▣ 662
Vicks Pediatric Formula 44m Multi-Symptom Cough & Cold Medicine .... ▣ 663

Chlorpheniramine Polistirex (Potentiation of antihistamines). Products include:
Tussionex Extended-Release Suspension 988

Chlorpheniramine Tannate (Potentiation of antihistamines). Products include:
Rynatan 2387
Rynatuss 2388

Chlorpromazine (Potentiation of CNS depressants). Products include:
Thorazine 2234

Chlorprothixene (Potentiation of CNS depressants). Products include:
Taractan Tablets 1920

Chlorprothixene Hydrochloride (Potentiation off CNS depressants). Products include:
Taractan 1920

Clemastine Fumarate (Potentiation of antihistamines). Products include:
Tavist Syrup 2033
Tavist Tablets 2035
Tavist-D Tablets 2035

Clorazepate Dipotassium (Potentiation of CNS depressants). Products include:
Tranxene 556

Codeine (Potentiation of CNS depressants). Products include:
- Calcidrine Syrup ... 506

Codeine Phosphate (Potentiation of CNS depressants). Products include:
- Actifed with Codeine Cough Syrup .. 752
- Cheracol Cough Syrup ... 1853
- Codimal PH Syrup ... 846
- Dimetane-DC Cough Syrup ... 1857
- Empirin with Codeine Phosphate Nos. 2, 3 & 4 ... 764
- Fiorinal with Codeine Capsules ... 2008
- Isoclor Expectorant ... 982
- Naldecon CX Adult Liquid ... ▣ 521
- Novahistine DH ... 1342
- Novahistine Expectorant ... 1343
- Nucofed Capsules ... 2219
- Nucofed Expectorant ... 2219
- Nucofed Pediatric Expectorant ... 2220
- Nucofed Syrup ... 2219
- Phenaphen with Codeine Capsules 1865
- Phenaphen-650 with Codeine Tablets ... 1866
- Phenergan with Codeine ... 2497
- Phenergan VC with Codeine ... 2501
- Robitussin A-C Syrup ... 1875
- Robitussin-DAC Syrup ... 1875
- Ryna ... ▣ 741
- Soma Compound w/Codeine Tablets ... 2390
- Triaminic Expectorant w/Codeine .. 1996
- Tussi-Organidin Liquid ... 2391
- Tylenol with Codeine ... 1381

Codeine Polistirex (Potentiation of CNS depressants).
- No products indexed under this heading.

Cyproheptadine Hydrochloride (Potentiation of antihistamines). Products include:
- Periactin ... 1525

Dexchlorpheniramine Maleate (Potentiation of antihistamines). Products include:
- Polaramine ... 2116

Dezocine (Potentiation of CNS depressants).

Diazepam (Potentiation of CNS depressants). Products include:
- Valium Injectable ... 1937
- Valium Tablets ... 1939
- Valrelease Capsules ... 1923

Diphenhydramine Citrate (Potentiation of antihistamines). Products include:
- Alka-Seltzer Plus Night-Time Cold Medicine ... ▣ 623
- Bufferin AF Nite Time Analgesic/Sleeping Aid Caplets ... 744
- Excedrin P.M. Analgesic/Sleeping Aid Tablets, Caplets and Liquid ... 749

Diphenhydramine Hydrochloride (Potentiation of antihistamines). Products include:
- Benadryl Anti-Itch Cream ... ▣ 635
- Benadryl Capsules ... 1691
- Benadryl Decongestant Elixir ... ▣ 635
- Benadryl Decongestant ... ▣ 635
- Benadryl Elixir ... ▣ 636
- Benadryl Kapseals ... 1691
- Benadryl 25 Kapseals ... ▣ 636
- Benadryl Parenteral ... 1692
- Benadryl Plus ... ▣ 636
- Benadryl Plus Nighttime ... ▣ 637
- Benadryl Spray, Maximum Strength ... ▣ 637
- Benadryl Spray, Regular Strength ▣ 637
- Benadryl Steri-Vials, Ampoules, and Steri-Dose Syringe ... 1692
- Benadryl 25 Tablets ... ▣ 636
- Benylin Cough Syrup ... ▣ 637
- Benylin Decongestant ... ▣ 638
- Caladryl Cream, Lotion, Spray ... ▣ 638
- Miles Nervine Nighttime Sleep-Aid ▣ 627
- Nytol Tablets ... ▣ 517
- Sleep-ettes-D Tablets ... ▣ 653
- Sleep-eze 3 Tablets ... ▣ 755
- Sleepinal Night-time Sleep Aid Capsules ... ▣ 734
- Sominex Caplets and Tablets ... ▣ 722
- Sominex Liquid ... ▣ 723
- Sominex Pain Relief Formula ... ▣ 723
- Tylenol Cold Night Time Medication Liquid ... 1371
- Tylenol PM, Extra Strength Caplets and Tablets ... 1368
- Unisom Dual Relief Nighttime Sleep Aid/Analgesic ... 1774
- Ziradryl Lotion ... ▣ 643

Diphenylpyraline Hydrochloride (Potentiation of antihistamines).
- No products indexed under this heading.

Droperidol (Potentiation of CNS depressants). Products include:
- Inapsine Injection ... 1140
- Innovar Injection ... 1141

Enflurane (Potentiation of CNS depressants). Products include:
- Ethrane ... 599

Epinephrine Hydrochloride (Action of epinephrine reversed). Products include:
- Adrenalin Chloride Solution 1:100 & 1:1,000 ... 1689
- Epifrin ... ⊙ 244
- Glaucon ... ⊙ 218

Estazolam (Potentiation of CNS depressants). Products include:
- ProSom Tablets ... 554

Ethchlorvynol (Potentiation of hypnotics). Products include:
- Placidyl Capsules ... 553

Ethinamate (Potentiation of hypnotics).
- No products indexed under this heading.

Fentanyl (Potentiation of CNS depressants). Products include:
- Duragesic Transdermal System ... 1133

Fentanyl Citrate (Potentiation of CNS depressants). Products include:
- Innovar Injection ... 1141
- Sublimaze Injection ... 1146

Fluphenazine Enanthate (Potentiation of CNS depressants). Products include:
- Prolixin Enanthate ... 1796

Fluphenazine Hydrochloride (Potentiation of CNS depressants). Products include:
- Prolixin Elixir ... 1793
- Prolixin Injection ... 1791
- Prolixin Oral Concentrate ... 1792
- Prolixin Tablets ... 1793

Flurazepam Hydrochloride (Potentiation of hypnotics). Products include:
- Dalmane Capsules ... 1927

Glutethimide (Potentiation of hypnotics).
- No products indexed under this heading.

Haloperidol (Potentiation of CNS depressants). Products include:
- Haldol Injection, Tablets and Concentrate ... 1373

Haloperidol Decanoate (Potentiation of CNS depressants). Products include:
- Haldol Decanoate ... 1375

Hydrocodone Bitartrate (Potentiation of CNS depressants). Products include:
- Anexsia 5/500 Tablets ... 2196
- Anexsia 7.5/650 Tablets ... 2197
- Azdone Tablets ... 844
- Codiclear DH Syrup ... 845
- Codimal DH Syrup ... 846
- Damason-P ... 1356
- Hycodan Syrup, Tablets ... 927
- Hycomine Compound Tablets ... 929
- Hycomine Syrup ... 927
- Hycotuss Expectorant Syrup ... 930
- Hydrocet Capsules ... 835
- Lortab ASA Tablets ... 2414
- Lortab ... 2412
- Ru-Tuss with Hydrocodone ... 694
- Triaminic Expectorant DH ... 1995
- Vicodin Tablets ... 1187
- Vicodin ES Tablets ... 1189
- Zydone Capsules ... 941

Hydrocodone Polistirex (Potentiation of CNS depressants). Products include:
- Tussionex Extended-Release Suspension ... 988

Hydroxyzine Hydrochloride (Potentiation of CNS depressants). Products include:
- Atarax Tablets & Syrup ... 1941
- Marax Tablets & DF Syrup ... 1954
- Vistaril Intramuscular Solution ... 1970

Isoflurane (Potentiation of CNS depressants). Products include:
- Forane ... 600

Ketamine Hydrochloride (Potentiation of CNS depressants). Products include:
- Ketalar ... 1726

Levorphanol Tartrate (Potentiation of CNS depressants). Products include:
- Levo-Dromoran ... 1906

Lorazepam (Potentiation of hypnotics). Products include:
- Ativan Injection ... 2432
- Ativan Tablets ... 2434

Loxapine Hydrochloride (Potentiation of hypnotics). Products include:
- Loxitane ... 1213

Loxapine Succinate (Potentiation of CNS depressants). Products include:
- Loxitane Capsules ... 1213

Meperidine Hydrochloride (Potentiation of CNS depressants). Products include:
- Demerol ... 2047
- Mepergan Injection ... 2479

Mephobarbital (Potentiation of CNS depressants). Products include:
- Mebaral Tablets ... 2061

Meprobamate (Potentiation of CNS depressants). Products include:
- Deprol Tablets ... 2382
- Equagesic Tablets ... 2451
- Miltown Tablets ... 2386
- PMB 200 and PMB 400 ... 2504

Mesoridazine (Potentiation of CNS depressants). Products include:
- Serentil ... 686

Methadone Hydrochloride (Potentiation of CNS depressants). Products include:
- Dolophine Hydrochloride Ampoules & Vials ... 1260
- Dolophine Hydrochloride Tablets 1261
- Methadone Hydrochloride Diskets .. 1284
- Methadone Hydrochloride Oral Solution & Tablets ... 1987

Methdilazine Hydrochloride (Potentiation of antihistamines). Products include:
- Tacaryl Syrup & Tablets ... 2409

Methohexital Sodium (Potentiation of CNS depressants). Products include:
- Brevital Sodium Vials ... 1248

Methoxyflurane (Potentiation of CNS depressants).
- No products indexed under this heading.

Midazolam Hydrochloride (Potentiation of hypnotics). Products include:
- Versed Injection ... 1924

Molindone Hydrochloride (Potentiation of CNS depressants). Products include:
- Moban Tablets & Concentrate ... 932

Morphine Sulfate (Potentiation of CNS depressants). Products include:
- Astramorph/PF Injection, USP (Preservative-Free) ... 618
- Duramorph ... 960
- Infumorph 200 and Infumorph 500 Sterile Solutions ... 962
- MS Contin Tablets ... 1814
- MSIR ... 1817
- Oramorph SR (Morphine Sulfate Sustained Release Tablets) ... 1988
- Roxanol ... 1991

Opium Alkaloids (Potentiation of CNS depressants). Products include:
- B & O No. 15A & No. 16A Supprettes ... 2395
- Pantopon Injectable ... 1911

Oxazepam (Potentiation of CNS depressants). Products include:
- Serax Capsules ... 2522
- Serax Tablets ... 2522

Oxycodone Hydrochloride (Potentiation of CNS depressants). Products include:
- Percocet Tablets ... 950
- Percodan ... 951
- Roxicodone Tablets, Oral Solution & Intensol (Oxycodone) ... 1992
- Tylox Capsules ... 1382

Pentobarbital Sodium (Potentiation of CNS depressants). Products include:
- Nembutal Sodium Capsules ... 534
- Nembutal Sodium Solution ... 536
- Nembutal Sodium Suppositories ... 538

Perphenazine (Potentiation of CNS depressants). Products include:
- Etrafon ... 2087
- Triavil Tablets ... 1556
- Trilafon ... 2123

Phenobarbital (Potentiation of CNS depressants). Products include:
- Arco-Lase Plus Tablets ... 607
- Bellergal-S Tablets ... 1998
- Bronkolixir ... ▣ 761
- Bronkotabs Tablets ... ▣ 762
- Donnatal ... 1858
- Donnatal Extentabs ... 1859
- Donnatal Tablets ... 1858
- Donnazyme Tablets ... 1860
- Kinesed Tablets ... 2272
- Phenobarbital Elixir and Tablets ... 1293
- Primatene Tablets-P Formula ... 2421
- Quadrinal Tablets ... 1183
- Tedral SA ... 1765

Prazepam (Potentiation of CNS depressants). Products include:
- Centrax ... 1693

Prochlorperazine (Potentiation of CNS depressants). Products include:
- Compazine ... 2201

Promethazine Hydrochloride (Potentiation of CNS depressants). Products include:
- Mepergan Injection ... 2479
- Phenergan with Codeine ... 2497
- Phenergan with Dextromethorphan 2499
- Phenergan Injection ... 2493
- Phenergan Suppositories ... 2496
- Phenergan Syrup ... 2495
- Phenergan Tablets ... 2496
- Phenergan VC ... 2500
- Phenergan VC with Codeine ... 2501

Propofol (Potentiation of CNS depressants). Products include:
- Diprivan Injection ... 2267

Propoxyphene Hydrochloride (Potentiation of CNS depressants). Products include:
- Darvon ... 1256
- Wygesic Tablets ... 2540

Propoxyphene Napsylate (Potentiation of CNS depressants). Products include:
- Darvon-N/Darvocet-N ... 1254

Pyrilamine Maleate (Potentiation of antihistamines). Products include:
- Codimal ... 846
- 4-Way Fast Acting Nasal Spray - Original Formula (regular & mentholated) & Metered Spray Pump (regular) ... 751
- Maximum Strength Midol Multi-Symptom Menstrual Formula ... ▣ 571
- Maximum Strength Midol PMS Premenstrual Syndrome Formula ... ▣ 570
- Regular Strength Midol Multi-Symptom Menstrual Formula ... ▣ 570
- Prefrin-A ... ⊙ 255
- Prēmsyn PMS Capsules & Caplets ▣ 547
- Primatene Tablets-M Formula ... 2421
- Robitussin Night Relief ... ▣ 677

Ru-Tuss with Hydrocodone 694
Triaminic Expectorant DH 1995
Triaminic Oral Infant Drops 1996

Pyrilamine Tannate (Potentiation of antihistamines). Products include:
Rynatan 2387

Quazepam (Potentiation of CNS depressants). Products include:
Doral Tablets 2383

Secobarbital Sodium (Potentiation of CNS depressants). Products include:
Seconal Sodium Pulvules 1296

Sufentanil Citrate (Potentiation of CNS depressants). Products include:
Sufenta Injection 1147

Temazepam (Potentiation of hypnotics). Products include:
Restoril Capsules 2023

Terfenadine (Potentiation of antihistamines). Products include:
Seldane Tablets 1349
Seldane-D Extended-Release Tablets 1350

Thiamylal Sodium (Potentiation of CNS depressants). Products include:
Surital Ampoules, Steri-Vials 1764

Thioridazine Hydrochloride (Potentiation of CNS depressants). Products include:
Mellaril 2011

Thiothixene (Potentiation of CNS depressants). Products include:
Navane Capsules and Concentrate 1954
Navane Intramuscular 1956

Triazolam (Potentiation of hypnotics). Products include:
Halcion Tablets 2340

Trifluoperazine Hydrochloride (Potentiation of CNS depressants). Products include:
Stelazine 2226

Trimeprazine Tartrate (Potentiation of antihistamines). Products include:
Temaril Tablets, Syrup and Spansule Sustained Release Capsules 1085

Tripelennamine Hydrochloride (Potentiation of antihistamines). Products include:
PBZ Tablets & Elixir 1037
PBZ-SR Tablets 1037

Triprolidine Hydrochloride (Potentiation of antihistamines). Products include:
Actidil ▣ 538
Actifed Capsules ▣ 539
Actifed Plus Caplets ▣ 539
Actifed Plus Tablets ▣ 540
Actifed with Codeine Cough Syrup 752
Actifed Syrup ▣ 540
Actifed Tablets ▣ 540
Actifed 12-Hour Capsules ▣ 539

PROLIXIN ELIXIR
(Fluphenazine Hydrochloride) 1793
May interact with hypnotics and sedatives, general anesthetics, central nervous system depressants, and certain other agents. Compounds in these categories include:

Alcohol (Potentiation of alcohol).

Alfentanil Hydrochloride (Potentiation of CNS depressants). Products include:
Alfenta Injection 1131

Alprazolam (Potentiation of CNS depressants). Products include:
Xanax Tablets 2367

Aprobarbital (Potentiation of CNS depressants). Products include:
Alurate Elixir 1883

Atropine Sulfate (Potentiation of atropine). Products include:
Arco-Lase Plus Tablets 607
Atropine Sulfate Sterile Ophthalmic Solution and S.O.P. Sterile Ophthalmic Ointment ⊙ 239
Donnagel ▣ 675
Donnagel-PG 1858
Donnatal 1858
Donnatal Extentabs 1859
Donnatal Tablets 1858
Donnazyme Tablets 1860
Isopto Atropine ⊙ 218
Lomotil 2174
Motofen Tablets 836
Ru-Tuss Tablets 693
Urised Tablets 2396

Azatadine Maleate (Potentiation of antihistamines). Products include:
Optimine Tablets 2115
Trinalin Repetabs Tablets 1170

Bromodiphenhydramine Hydrochloride (Potentiation of antihistamines).
No products indexed under this heading.

Brompheniramine Maleate (Potentiation of antihistamines). Products include:
Alka Seltzer Plus Sinus Allergy Medicine ▣ 624
Atrohist Sprinkle Capsules 558
Bromfed Capsules (Timed Release) 1615
Bromfed Syrup ▣ 628
Bromfed 1615
Dimetane Decongestant ▣ 673
Dimetane ▣ 672
Dimetane-DC Cough Syrup 1857
Dimetane-DX Cough Syrup 1858
Dimetapp Elixir ▣ 673
Dimetapp DM Elixir ▣ 674
Dimetapp Extentabs ▣ 674
Dimetapp Plus Caplets ▣ 675
Dimetapp Tablets ▣ 675
Drixoral Antihistamine/Nasal Decongestant Syrup ▣ 698

Buprenorphine (Potentiation of CNS depressants).
No products indexed under this heading.

Buspirone Hydrochloride (Potentiation of CNS depressants). Products include:
BuSpar 1401

Butabarbital (Potentiation of CNS depressants). Products include:
Pyridium Plus 1764

Butalbital (Potentiation of CNS depressants). Products include:
Esgic-Plus Tablets 1002
Esgic Tablets & Capsules 1001
Fioricet Tablets 2006
Fiorinal Capsules 2007
Fiorinal with Codeine Capsules 2008
Fiorinal Tablets 2007
Phrenilin 838
Sedapap Tablets 50 mg/650 mg 1360

Chlordiazepoxide (Potentiation of CNS depressants). Products include:
Libritabs Tablets 1930
Limbitrol 1933
Menrium Tablets 1934

Chlordiazepoxide Hydrochloride (Potentiation of CNS depressants). Products include:
Librax Capsules 1929
Librium Capsules 1931
Librium Injectable 1932

Chlorpheniramine Maleate (Potentiation of antihistamines). Products include:
A.R.M. Allergy Relief Medicine Caplets ▣ 615
Alka-Seltzer Plus Cold Medicine ▣ 623
Allerest ▣ 559
Ana-Kit Anaphylaxis Emergency Treatment Kit 1100
BC Cold Powder Multi-Symptom Formula ▣ 517
Brexin L.A. Capsules 2078
Cerose-DM 2443
Cheracol Plus Head Cold/Cough Formula ▣ 667
Chlor-Trimeton Allergy Syrup, Tablets & Long-Acting Repetabs Tablets ▣ 693
Chlor-Trimeton Decongestant ▣ 694
Comhist LA Capsules 1618
Allergy-Sinus Comtrex Multi-Symptom Allergy Sinus Formula Tablets & Caplets 746
Comtrex Multi-Symptom Cold Reliever Tablets/Caplets/Liqui-Gels/Liquid 745
Day-Night Comtrex 747
Contac Continuous Action Decongestant/Antihistamine Capsules ▣ 710
Contac Maximum Strength Continuous Action Decongestant/Antihistamine Caplets ▣ 709
Contac Severe Cold and Flu Formula Caplets ▣ 711
Coricidin 'D' Decongestant Tablets ▣ 695
Coricidin Demilets Tablets for Children ▣ 696
Coricidin Tablets ▣ 695
Deconamine 663
Demazin Nasal Decongestant/Antihistamine Repetabs Tablets & Syrup ▣ 697
Dorcol Children's Liquid Cold Formula ▣ 686
Dristan Decongestant/Antihistamine/ Analgesic Coated Caplets ▣ 749
Dristan Cold Nasal Decongestant/Antihistamine/ Analgesic Coated Tablets 2419
Dristan Advanced Formula Decongestant/Antihistamine/Analgesic Tablets ▣ 749
Extendryl 994
4-Way Cold Tablets 750
Fedahist Gyrocaps 2145
Fedahist Timecaps 2145
Hycomine Compound Tablets 929
Isoclor Timesule Capsules ▣ 561
Kronofed-A 970
Medi-Flu Caplet, Liquid ▣ 640
Naldecon Syrup, Tablets, Pediatric Drops and Pediatric Syrup 709
Nolamine Tablets 838
Novafed A Capsules 1342
Novahistine DH 1342
Novahistine Elixir ▣ 596
Ornade Spansule Capsules 2221
Orthoxicol Cough Syrup ▣ 668
PediaCare Allergy Relief Formula Liquid 1362
PediaCare Cough-Cold Formula Liquid 1362
PediaCare Night Rest Cough-Cold Formula Liquid 1362
PediaCare 6-12 Cough-Cold Formula Chewable Tablets 1362
Pyrroxate Capsules ▣ 669
Quelidrine Syrup 556
Ru-Tuss II Capsules 693
Ru-Tuss Tablets 693
Ryna ▣ 741
Sinarest Tablets & Extra Strength Tablets ▣ 562
Sine-Off Maximum Strength Allergy/Sinus Formula Caplets ▣ 721
Sine-Off Sinus Medicine Tablets-Aspirin Formula ▣ 722
Singlet Tablets ▣ 598
Sinulin 840
Sinutab Maximum Strength ▣ 641
St. Joseph Nighttime Cold Medicine ▣ 705
Sudafed Plus Liquid ▣ 544
Sudafed Plus Tablets ▣ 545
Teldrin Timed-Release Allergy Capsules, 12 mg 2192
TheraFlu Flu and Cold Medicine ▣ 687
Triaminic Allergy Tablets ▣ 688
Triaminic Chewables ▣ 688
Triaminic Cold Tablets ▣ 688
Triaminic Nite Light ▣ 689
Triaminic Syrup ▣ 689
Triaminic-12 Tablets ▣ 690
Triaminicin Tablets ▣ 690
Triaminicol Multi-Symptom Cold Tablets ▣ 691
Triaminicol Multi-Symptom Relief ▣ 691
Tylenol Allergy Sinus Medication Caplets and Gelcaps, Maximum Strength 1372
Children's Tylenol Cold Liquid Formula and Chewable Tablets 1368
Tylenol Cold & Flu Hot Medication, Packets 1369
Tylenol Cold Medication Caplets and Tablets 1370
Tylenol Cold Medication, Effervescent Tablets 1369
Vicks Children's NyQuil ▣ 664
Vicks Formula 44 Cough Medicine ▣ 661
Vicks Formula 44M Multi-Symptom Cough Medicine ▣ 662
Vicks Pediatric Formula 44m Multi-Symptom Cough & Cold Medicine ▣ 663

Chlorpheniramine Polistirex (Potentiation of antihistamines). Products include:
Tussionex Extended-Release Suspension 988

Chlorpheniramine Tannate (Potentiation of antihistamines). Products include:
Rynatan 2387
Rynatuss 2388

Chlorpromazine (Potentiation of CNS depressants). Products include:
Thorazine 2234

Chlorprothixene (Potentiation of CNS depressants). Products include:
Taractan Tablets 1920

Chlorprothixene Hydrochloride (Potentiation of CNS depressants). Products include:
Taractan 1920

Clemastine Fumarate (Potentiation of antihistamines). Products include:
Tavist Syrup 2033
Tavist Tablets 2035
Tavist-D Tablets 2035

Clorazepate Dipotassium (Potentiation of CNS depressants). Products include:
Tranxene 556

Codeine (Potentiation of CNS depressants). Products include:
Calcidrine Syrup 506

Codeine Phosphate (Potentiation of CNS depressants). Products include:
Actifed with Codeine Cough Syrup 752
Cheracol Cough Syrup 1853
Codimal PH Syrup 846
Dimetane-DC Cough Syrup 1857
Empirin with Codeine Phosphate Nos. 2, 3 & 4 764
Fiorinal with Codeine Capsules 2008
Isoclor Expectorant 982
Naldecon CX Adult Liquid ▣ 521
Novahistine DH 1342
Novahistine Expectorant 1343
Nucofed Capsules 2219
Nucofed Expectorant 2219
Nucofed Pediatric Expectorant 2220
Nucofed Syrup 2219
Phenaphen with Codeine Capsules 1865
Phenaphen-650 with Codeine Tablets 1866
Phenergan with Codeine 2497
Phenergan VC with Codeine 2501
Robitussin A-C Syrup 1875
Robitussin-DAC Syrup 1875
Ryna ▣ 741
Soma Compound w/Codeine Tablets 2390
Triaminic Expectorant w/Codeine 1996
Tussi-Organidin Liquid 2391
Tylenol with Codeine 1381

Codeine Polistirex (Potentiation of CNS depressants).
No products indexed under this heading.

Dezocine (Potentiation of CNS depressants).

Diazepam (Potentiation of CNS depressants). Products include:
Valium Injectable 1937
Valium Tablets 1939
Valrelease Capsules 1923

Diphenhydramine Citrate (Potentiation of antihistamines). Products include:
Alka-Seltzer Plus Night-Time Cold Medicine ▣ 623
Bufferin AF Nite Time Analgesic/Sleeping Aid Caplets 744
Excedrin P.M. Analgesic/Sleeping Aid Tablets, Caplets and Liquid 749

Diphenhydramine Hydrochloride (Potentiation of CNS depressants). Products include:
- Benadryl Anti-Itch Cream ◘ 635
- Benadryl Capsules 1691
- Benadryl Decongestant Elixir ◘ 635
- Benadryl Decongestant ◘ 635
- Benadryl Elixir ◘ 636
- Benadryl Kapseals 1691
- Benadryl 25 Kapseals ◘ 636
- Benadryl Parenteral 1692
- Benadryl Plus ◘ 636
- Benadryl Plus Nighttime ◘ 637
- Benadryl Spray, Maximum Strength ◘ 637
- Benadryl Spray, Regular Strength ◘ 637
- Benadryl Steri-Vials, Ampoules, and Steri-Dose Syringe 1692
- Benadryl 25 Tablets ◘ 636
- Benylin Cough Syrup ◘ 637
- Benylin Decongestant ◘ 638
- Caladryl Cream, Lotion, Spray ◘ 638
- Miles Nervine Nighttime Sleep-Aid ◘ 627
- Nytol Tablets ◘ 517
- Sleep-ettes-D Tablets ◘ 653
- Sleep-eze 3 Tablets ◘ 755
- Sleepinal Night-time Sleep Aid Capsules ◘ 734
- Sominex Caplets and Tablets ◘ 722
- Sominex Liquid ◘ 723
- Sominex Pain Relief Formula ◘ 723
- Tylenol Cold Night Time Medication Liquid 1371
- Tylenol PM, Extra Strength Caplets and Tablets 1368
- Unisom Dual Relief Nighttime Sleep Aid/Analgesic 1774
- Ziradryl Lotion ◘ 643

Diphenylpyraline Hydrochloride (Potentiation of antihistamines).
- No products indexed under this heading.

Droperidol (Potentiation of CNS depressants). Products include:
- Inapsine Injection 1140
- Innovar Injection 1141

Enflurane (Potentiation of CNS depressants). Products include:
- Ethrane 599

Epinephrine Hydrochloride (Action of epinephrine reversed). Products include:
- Adrenalin Chloride Solution 1:100 & 1:1,000 1689
- Epifrin ⊙ 244
- Glaucon ⊙ 218

Estazolam (Potentiation of CNS depressants). Products include:
- ProSom Tablets 554

Ethchlorvynol (Potentiation of hypnotics). Products include:
- Placidyl Capsules 553

Ethinamate (Potentiation of hypnotics).
- No products indexed under this heading.

Fentanyl (Potentiation of CNS depressants). Products include:
- Duragesic Transdermal System 1133

Fentanyl Citrate (Potentiation of CNS depressants). Products include:
- Innovar Injection 1141
- Sublimaze Injection 1146

Fluphenazine Decanoate (Potentiation of CNS depressants). Products include:
- Prolixin Decanoate 1795

Fluphenazine Enanthate (Potentiation of CNS depressants). Products include:
- Prolixin Enanthate 1796

Flurazepam Hydrochloride (Potentiation of hypnotics). Products include:
- Dalmane Capsules 1927

Glutethimide (Potentiation of hypnotics).
- No products indexed under this heading.

Haloperidol (Potentiation of CNS depressants). Products include:
- Haldol Injection, Tablets and Concentrate 1373

Haloperidol Decanoate (Potentiation of CNS depressants). Products include:
- Haldol Decanoate 1375

Hydrocodone Bitartrate (Potentiation of CNS depressants). Products include:
- Anexsia 5/500 Tablets 2196
- Anexsia 7.5/650 Tablets 2197
- Azdone Tablets 844
- Codiclear DH Syrup 845
- Codimal DH Syrup 846
- Damason-P 1356
- Hycodan Syrup, Tablets 927
- Hycomine Compound Tablets 929
- Hycomine Syrup 927
- Hycotuss Expectorant Syrup 930
- Hydrocet Capsules 835
- Lortab ASA Tablets 2414
- Lortab 2412
- Ru-Tuss with Hydrocodone 694
- Triaminic Expectorant DH 1995
- Vicodin Tablets 1187
- Vicodin ES Tablets 1189
- Zydone Capsules 941

Hydrocodone Polistirex (Potentiation of CNS depressants). Products include:
- Tussionex Extended-Release Suspension 988

Hydroxyzine Hydrochloride (Potentiation of CNS depressants). Products include:
- Atarax Tablets & Syrup 1941
- Marax Tablets & DF Syrup 1954
- Vistaril Intramuscular Solution 1970

Isoflurane (Potentiation of CNS depressants). Products include:
- Forane 600

Ketamine Hydrochloride (Potentiation of CNS depressants). Products include:
- Ketalar 1726

Levorphanol Tartrate (Potentiation of CNS depressants). Products include:
- Levo-Dromoran 1906

Lorazepam (Potentiation of hypnotics). Products include:
- Ativan Injection 2432
- Ativan Tablets 2434

Loxapine Hydrochloride (Potentiation of hypnotics). Products include:
- Loxitane 1213

Loxapine Succinate (Potentiation of CNS depressants). Products include:
- Loxitane Capsules 1213

Meperidine Hydrochloride (Potentiation of CNS depressants). Products include:
- Demerol 2047
- Mepergan Injection 2479

Mephobarbital (Potentiation of CNS depressants). Products include:
- Mebaral Tablets 2061

Meprobamate (Potentiation of CNS depressants). Products include:
- Deprol Tablets 2382
- Equagesic Tablets 2451
- Miltown Tablets 2386
- PMB 200 and PMB 400 2504

Mesoridazine (Potentiation of CNS depressants). Products include:
- Serentil 686

Methadone Hydrochloride (Potentiation of CNS depressants). Products include:
- Dolophine Hydrochloride Ampoules & Vials 1260
- Dolophine Hydrochloride Tablets 1261
- Methadone Hydrochloride Diskets 1284
- Methadone Hydrochloride Oral Solution & Tablets 1987

Methdilazine Hydrochloride (Potentiation of antihistamines). Products include:
- Tacaryl Syrup & Tablets 2409

Methohexital Sodium (Potentiation of CNS depressants). Products include:
- Brevital Sodium Vials 1248

Methoxyflurane (Potentiation of CNS depressants).
- No products indexed under this heading.

Midazolam Hydrochloride (Potentiation of hypnotics). Products include:
- Versed Injection 1924

Molindone Hydrochloride (Potentiation of CNS depressants). Products include:
- Moban Tablets & Concentrate 932

Morphine Sulfate (Potentiation of CNS depressants). Products include:
- Astramorph/PF Injection, USP (Preservative-Free) 618
- Duramorph 960
- Infumorph 200 and Infumorph 500 Sterile Solutions 962
- MS Contin Tablets 1814
- MSIR 1817
- Oramorph SR (Morphine Sulfate Sustained Release Tablets) 1988
- Roxanol 1991

Opium Alkaloids (Potentiation of CNS depressants). Products include:
- B & O No. 15A & No. 16A Supprettes 2395
- Pantopon Injectable 1911

Oxazepam (Potentiation of CNS depressants). Products include:
- Serax Capsules 2522
- Serax Tablets 2522

Oxycodone Hydrochloride (Potentiation of CNS depressants). Products include:
- Percocet Tablets 950
- Percodan 951
- Roxicodone Tablets, Oral Solution & Intensol (Oxycodone) 1992
- Tylox Capsules 1382

Pentobarbital Sodium (Potentiation of CNS depressants). Products include:
- Nembutal Sodium Capsules 534
- Nembutal Sodium Solution 536
- Nembutal Sodium Suppositories 538

Perphenazine (Potentiation of CNS depressants). Products include:
- Etrafon 2087
- Triavil Tablets 1556
- Trilafon 2123

Phenobarbital (Potentiation of CNS depressants). Products include:
- Arco-Lase Plus Tablets 607
- Bellergal-S Tablets 1998
- Bronkolixir ◘ 761
- Bronkotabs Tablets ◘ 762
- Donnatal 1858
- Donnatal Extentabs 1859
- Donnatal Tablets 1858
- Donnazyme Tablets 1860
- Kinesed Tablets 2272
- Phenobarbital Elixir and Tablets 1293
- Primatene Tablets-P Formula 2421
- Quadrinal Tablets 1183
- Tedral SA 1765

Prazepam (Potentiation of CNS depressants). Products include:
- Centrax 1693

Prochlorperazine (Potentiation of CNS depressants). Products include:
- Compazine 2201

Promethazine Hydrochloride (Potentiation of CNS depressants). Products include:
- Mepergan Injection 2479
- Phenergan with Codeine 2497
- Phenergan with Dextromethorphan 2499
- Phenergan Injection 2493
- Phenergan Suppositories 2496
- Phenergan Syrup 2495
- Phenergan Tablets 2496
- Phenergan VC 2500
- Phenergan VC with Codeine 2501

Propofol (Potentiation of CNS depressants). Products include:
- Diprivan Injection 2267

Propoxyphene Hydrochloride (Potentiation of CNS depressants). Products include:
- Darvon 1256
- Wygesic Tablets 2540

Propoxyphene Napsylate (Potentiation of CNS depressants). Products include:
- Darvon-N/Darvocet-N 1254

Pyrilamine Maleate (Potentiation of antihistamines). Products include:
- Codimal 846
- 4-Way Fast Acting Nasal Spray - Original Formula (regular & mentholated) & Metered Spray Pump (regular) 751
- Maximum Strength Midol Multi-Symptom Menstrual Formula ◘ 571
- Maximum Strength Midol PMS Premenstrual Syndrome Formula ◘ 570
- Regular Strength Midol Multi-Symptom Menstrual Formula ◘ 570
- Prefrin-A ⊙ 255
- Prēmsyn PMS Capsules & Caplets ◘ 547
- Primatene Tablets-M Formula 2421
- Robitussin Night Relief ◘ 677
- Ru-Tuss with Hydrocodone 694
- Triaminic Expectorant DH 1995
- Triaminic Oral Infant Drops 1996

Pyrilamine Tannate (Potentiation of antihistamines). Products include:
- Rynatan 2387

Quazepam (Potentiation of CNS depressants). Products include:
- Doral Tablets 2383

Secobarbital Sodium (Potentiation of CNS depressants). Products include:
- Seconal Sodium Pulvules 1296

Sufentanil Citrate (Potentiation of CNS depressants). Products include:
- Sufenta Injection 1147

Temazepam (Potentiation of hypnotics). Products include:
- Restoril Capsules 2023

Thiamylal Sodium (Potentiation of CNS depressants). Products include:
- Surital Ampoules, Steri-Vials 1764

Thioridazine Hydrochloride (Potentiation of CNS depressants). Products include:
- Mellaril 2011

Thiothixene (Potentiation of CNS depressants). Products include:
- Navane Capsules and Concentrate 1954
- Navane Intramuscular 1956

Triazolam (Potentiation of hypnotics). Products include:
- Halcion Tablets 2340

Trifluoperazine Hydrochloride (Potentiation of CNS depressants). Products include:
- Stelazine 2226

Tripelennamine Hydrochloride (Potentiation of antihistamines). Products include:
- PBZ Tablets & Elixir 1037
- PBZ-SR Tablets 1037

Triprolidine Hydrochloride (Potentiation of antihistamines). Products include:
- Actidil ◘ 538
- Actifed Capsules ◘ 539
- Actifed Plus Caplets ◘ 539
- Actifed Plus Tablets ◘ 540
- Actifed with Codeine Cough Syrup 752
- Actifed Syrup ◘ 540
- Actifed Tablets ◘ 540
- Actifed 12-Hour Capsules ◘ 539

PROLIXIN ENANTHATE (Fluphenazine Enanthate) 1796
May interact with hypnotics and sedatives, general anesthetics, central nervous system depressants,

barbiturates, antihistamines, and certain other agents. Compounds in these categories include:

Alcohol (Potentiation of alcohol).

Alfentanil Hydrochloride (Potentiation of CNS depressants). Products include:
- Alfenta Injection ... 1131

Alprazolam (Potentiation of CNS depressants). Products include:
- Xanax Tablets ... 2367

Aprobarbital (Potentiation of CNS depressants). Products include:
- Alurate Elixir ... 1883

Astemizole (Potentiation of antihistamines). Products include:
- Hismanal Tablets ... 1138

Atropine Sulfate (Potentiation of atropine). Products include:
- Arco-Lase Plus Tablets ... 607
- Atropine Sulfate Sterile Ophthalmic Solution and S.O.P. Sterile Ophthalmic Ointment ... ⊙ 239
- Donnagel ... ▣ 675
- Donnagel-PG ... 1858
- Donnatal ... 1858
- Donnatal Extentabs ... 1859
- Donnatal Tablets ... 1858
- Donnazyme Tablets ... 1860
- Isopto Atropine ... ⊙ 218
- Lomotil ... 2174
- Motofen Tablets ... 836
- Ru-Tuss Tablets ... 693
- Urised Tablets ... 2396

Azatadine Maleate (Potentiation of antihistamines). Products include:
- Optimine Tablets ... 2115
- Trinalin Repetabs Tablets ... 1170

Bromodiphenhydramine Hydrochloride (Potentiation of antihistamines).
- No products indexed under this heading.

Brompheniramine Maleate (Potentiation of antihistamines). Products include:
- Alka Seltzer Plus Sinus Allergy Medicine ... ▣ 624
- Atrohist Sprinkle Capsules ... 558
- Bromfed Capsules (Timed Release) ... 1615
- Bromfed Syrup ... ▣ 628
- Bromfed ... 1615
- Dimetane Decongestant ... ▣ 673
- Dimetane ... ▣ 672
- Dimetane-DC Cough Syrup ... 1857
- Dimetane-DX Cough Syrup ... 1858
- Dimetapp Elixir ... ▣ 673
- Dimetapp DM Elixir ... ▣ 674
- Dimetapp Extentabs ... ▣ 674
- Dimetapp Plus Caplets ... ▣ 675
- Dimetapp Tablets ... ▣ 675
- Drixoral Antihistamine/Nasal Decongestant Syrup ... ▣ 698

Buprenorphine (Potentiation of CNS depressants).
- No products indexed under this heading.

Buspirone Hydrochloride (Potentiation of CNS depressants). Products include:
- BuSpar ... 1401

Butabarbital (Potentiation of CNS depressants). Products include:
- Pyridium Plus ... 1764

Butalbital (Potentiation of CNS depressants). Products include:
- Esgic-Plus Tablets ... 1002
- Esgic Tablets & Capsules ... 1001
- Fioricet Tablets ... 2006
- Fiorinal Capsules ... 2007
- Fiorinal with Codeine Capsules ... 2008
- Fiorinal Tablets ... 2007
- Phrenilin ... 838
- Sedapap Tablets 50 mg/650 mg ... 1360

Chlordiazepoxide (Potentiation of CNS depressants). Products include:
- Libritabs Tablets ... 1930
- Limbitrol ... 1933
- Menrium Tablets ... 1934

Chlordiazepoxide Hydrochloride (Potentiation of CNS depressants). Products include:
- Librax Capsules ... 1929
- Librium Capsules ... 1931
- Librium Injectable ... 1932

Chlorpheniramine Maleate (Potentiation of antihistamines). Products include:
- A.R.M. Allergy Relief Medicine Caplets ... ▣ 615
- Alka-Seltzer Plus Cold Medicine ... ▣ 623
- Allerest ... ▣ 559
- Ana-Kit Anaphylaxis Emergency Treatment Kit ... 1100
- BC Cold Powder Multi-Symptom Formula ... ▣ 517
- Brexin L.A. Capsules ... 2078
- Cerose-DM ... 2443
- Cheracol Plus Head Cold/Cough Formula ... ▣ 667
- Chlor-Trimeton Allergy Syrup, Tablets & Long-Acting Repetabs Tablets ... ▣ 693
- Chlor-Trimeton Decongestant ... ▣ 694
- Comhist LA Capsules ... 1618
- Allergy-Sinus Comtrex Multi-Symptom Allergy Sinus Formula Tablets & Caplets ... 746
- Comtrex Multi-Symptom Cold Reliever Tablets/Caplets/Liqui-Gels/Liquid ... 745
- Day-Night Comtrex ... 747
- Contac Continuous Action Decongestant/Antihistamine Capsules ▣ 710
- Contac Maximum Strength Continuous Action Decongestant/Antihistamine Caplets ... ▣ 709
- Contac Severe Cold and Flu Formula Caplets ... ▣ 711
- Coricidin 'D' Decongestant Tablets ... ▣ 695
- Coricidin Demilets Tablets for Children ... ▣ 696
- Coricidin Tablets ... ▣ 695
- Deconamine ... 663
- Demazin Nasal Decongestant/Antihistamine Repetabs Tablets & Syrup ... ▣ 697
- Dorcol Children's Liquid Cold Formula ... ▣ 686
- Dristan Decongestant/Antihistamine/ Analgesic Coated Caplets ... ▣ 749
- Dristan Cold Nasal Decongestant/Antihistamine/ Analgesic Coated Tablets ... 2419
- Dristan Advanced Formula Decongestant/Antihistamine/Analgesic Tablets ... ▣ 749
- Extendryl ... 994
- 4-Way Cold Tablets ... 750
- Fedahist Gyrocaps ... 2145
- Fedahist Timecaps ... 2145
- Hycomine Compound Tablets ... 929
- Isoclor Timesule Capsules ... ▣ 561
- Kronofed-A ... 970
- Medi-Flu Caplet, Liquid ... ▣ 640
- Naldecon Syrup, Tablets, Pediatric Drops and Pediatric Syrup ... 709
- Nolamine Tablets ... 838
- Novafed A Capsules ... 1342
- Novahistine DH ... 1342
- Novahistine Elixir ... ▣ 596
- Ornade Spansule Capsules ... 2221
- Orthoxicol Cough Syrup ... ▣ 668
- PediaCare Allergy Relief Formula Liquid ... 1362
- PediaCare Cough-Cold Formula Liquid ... 1362
- PediaCare Night Rest Cough-Cold Formula Liquid ... 1362
- PediaCare 6-12 Cough-Cold Formula Chewable Tablets ... 1362
- Pyrroxate Capsules ... ▣ 669
- Quelidrine Syrup ... 556
- Ru-Tuss II Capsules ... 693
- Ru-Tuss Tablets ... 693
- Ryna ... ▣ 741
- Sinarest Tablets & Extra Strength Tablets ... ▣ 562
- Sine-Off Maximum Strength Allergy/Sinus Formula Caplets ... ▣ 721
- Sine-Off Sinus Medicine Tablets-Aspirin Formula ... ▣ 722
- Singlet Tablets ... ▣ 598
- Sinulin ... 840
- Sinutab Maximum Strength ... ▣ 641
- St. Joseph Nighttime Cold Medicine ... ▣ 705
- Sudafed Plus Liquid ... ▣ 544
- Sudafed Plus Tablets ... ▣ 545
- Teldrin Timed-Release Allergy Capsules, 12 mg ... 2192
- TheraFlu Flu and Cold Medicine ... ▣ 687
- Triaminic Allergy Tablets ... ▣ 688
- Triaminic Chewables ... ▣ 688
- Triaminic Cold Tablets ... ▣ 688
- Triaminic Nite Light ... ▣ 689
- Triaminic Syrup ... ▣ 689
- Triaminic-12 Tablets ... ▣ 690
- Triaminicin Tablets ... ▣ 690
- Triaminicol Multi-Symptom Cold Tablets ... ▣ 691
- Triaminicol Multi-Symptom Relief ▣ 691
- Tylenol Allergy Sinus Medication Caplets and Gelcaps, Maximum Strength ... 1372
- Children's Tylenol Cold Liquid Formula and Chewable Tablets ... 1368
- Tylenol Cold & Flu Hot Medication, Packets ... 1369
- Tylenol Cold Medication Caplets and Tablets ... 1370
- Tylenol Cold Medication, Effervescent Tablets ... 1369
- Vicks Children's NyQuil ... ▣ 664
- Vicks Formula 44 Cough Medicine ... ▣ 661
- Vicks Formula 44M Multi-Symptom Cough Medicine ... ▣ 662
- Vicks Pediatric Formula 44m Multi-Symptom Cough & Cold Medicine ... ▣ 663

Chlorpheniramine Polistirex (Potentiation of antihistamines). Products include:
- Tussionex Extended-Release Suspension ... 988

Chlorpheniramine Tannate (Potentiation of antihistamines). Products include:
- Rynatan ... 2387
- Rynatuss ... 2388

Chlorpromazine (Potentiation of CNS depressants). Products include:
- Thorazine ... 2234

Chlorprothixene (Potentiation of CNS depressants). Products include:
- Taractan Tablets ... 1920

Chlorprothixene Hydrochloride (Potentiation of CNS depressants). Products include:
- Taractan ... 1920

Clemastine Fumarate (Potentiation of antihistamines). Products include:
- Tavist Syrup ... 2033
- Tavist Tablets ... 2035
- Tavist-D Tablets ... 2035

Clorazepate Dipotassium (Potentiation of CNS depressants). Products include:
- Tranxene ... 556

Codeine (Potentiation of CNS depressants). Products include:
- Calcidrine Syrup ... 506

Codeine Phosphate (Potentiation of CNS depressants). Products include:
- Actifed with Codeine Cough Syrup ... 752
- Cheracol Cough Syrup ... 1853
- Codimal PH Syrup ... 846
- Dimetane-DC Cough Syrup ... 1857
- Empirin with Codeine Phosphate Nos. 2, 3 & 4 ... 764
- Fiorinal with Codeine Capsules ... 2008
- Isoclor Expectorant ... 982
- Naldecon CX Adult Liquid ... ▣ 521
- Novahistine DH ... 1342
- Novahistine Expectorant ... 1343
- Nucofed Capsules ... 2219
- Nucofed Expectorant ... 2219
- Nucofed Pediatric Expectorant ... 2220
- Nucofed Syrup ... 2219
- Phenaphen with Codeine Capsules 1865
- Phenaphen-650 with Codeine Tablets ... 1866
- Phenergan with Codeine ... 2497
- Phenergan VC with Codeine ... 2501
- Robitussin A-C Syrup ... 1875
- Robitussin-DAC Syrup ... 1875
- Ryna ... ▣ 741
- Soma Compound w/Codeine Tablets ... 2390
- Triaminic Expectorant w/Codeine ... 1996
- Tussi-Organidin Liquid ... 2391
- Tylenol with Codeine ... 1381

Codeine Polistirex (Potentiation of CNS depressants).
- No products indexed under this heading.

Cyproheptadine Hydrochloride (Potentiation of antihistamines). Products include:
- Periactin ... 1525

Dexchlorpheniramine Maleate (Potentiation of antihistamines). Products include:
- Polaramine ... 2116

Dezocine (Potentiation of CNS depressants).

Diazepam (Potentiation of CNS depressants). Products include:
- Valium Injectable ... 1937
- Valium Tablets ... 1939
- Valrelease Capsules ... 1923

Diphenhydramine Citrate (Potentiation of antihistamines). Products include:
- Alka-Seltzer Plus Night-Time Cold Medicine ... ▣ 623
- Bufferin AF Nite Time Analgesic/Sleeping Aid Caplets ... 744
- Excedrin P.M. Analgesic/Sleeping Aid Tablets, Caplets and Liquid ... 749

Diphenhydramine Hydrochloride (Potentiation of antihistamines). Products include:
- Benadryl Anti-Itch Cream ... ▣ 635
- Benadryl Capsules ... 1691
- Benadryl Decongestant Elixir ... ▣ 635
- Benadryl Decongestant ... ▣ 635
- Benadryl Elixir ... ▣ 636
- Benadryl Kapseals ... 1691
- Benadryl 25 Kapseals ... ▣ 636
- Benadryl Parenteral ... 1692
- Benadryl Plus ... ▣ 636
- Benadryl Plus Nighttime ... ▣ 637
- Benadryl Spray, Maximum Strength ... ▣ 637
- Benadryl Spray, Regular Strength ▣ 637
- Benadryl Steri-Vials, Ampoules, and Steri-Dose Syringe ... 1692
- Benadryl 25 Tablets ... ▣ 636
- Benylin Cough Syrup ... ▣ 637
- Benylin Decongestant ... ▣ 638
- Caladryl Cream, Lotion, Spray ... ▣ 638
- Miles Nervine Nighttime Sleep-Aid ▣ 627
- Nytol Tablets ... ▣ 517
- Sleep-ettes-D Tablets ... ▣ 653
- Sleep-eze 3 Tablets ... ▣ 755
- Sleepinal Night-time Sleep Aid Capsules ... ▣ 734
- Sominex Caplets and Tablets ... ▣ 722
- Sominex Liquid ... ▣ 723
- Sominex Pain Relief Formula ... ▣ 723
- Tylenol Cold Night Time Medication Liquid ... 1371
- Tylenol PM, Extra Strength Caplets and Tablets ... 1368
- Unisom Dual Relief Nighttime Sleep Aid/Analgesic ... 1774
- Ziradryl Lotion ... ▣ 643

Diphenylpyraline Hydrochloride (Potentiation of antihistamines).
- No products indexed under this heading.

Droperidol (Potentiation of CNS depressants). Products include:
- Inapsine Injection ... 1140
- Innovar Injection ... 1141

Enflurane (Potentiation of CNS depressants). Products include:
- Ethrane ... 599

Epinephrine Hydrochloride (Action of epinephrine reversed). Products include:
- Adrenalin Chloride Solution 1:100 & 1:1,000 ... 1689
- Epifrin ... ⊙ 244
- Glaucon ... ⊙ 218

Estazolam (Potentiation of CNS depressants). Products include:
- ProSom Tablets ... 554

Ethchlorvynol (Potentiation of hypnotics). Products include:
- Placidyl Capsules ... 553

Ethinamate (Potentiation of hypnotics).
No products indexed under this heading.

Fentanyl (Potentiation of CNS depressants). Products include:
Duragesic Transdermal System........ 1133

Fentanyl Citrate (Potentiation of CNS depressants). Products include:
Innovar Injection........ 1141
Sublimaze Injection........ 1146

Fluphenazine Decanoate (Potentiation of CNS depressants). Products include:
Prolixin Decanoate........ 1795

Fluphenazine Hydrochloride (Potentiation of CNS depressants). Products include:
Prolixin Elixir........ 1793
Prolixin Injection........ 1791
Prolixin Oral Concentrate........ 1792
Prolixin Tablets........ 1793

Flurazepam Hydrochloride (Potentiation of hypnotics). Products include:
Dalmane Capsules........ 1927

Glutethimide (Potentiation of hypnotics).
No products indexed under this heading.

Haloperidol (Potentiation of CNS depressants). Products include:
Haldol Injection, Tablets and Concentrate........ 1373

Haloperidol Decanoate (Potentiation of CNS depressants). Products include:
Haldol Decanoate........ 1375

Hydrocodone Bitartrate (Potentiation of CNS depressants). Products include:
Anexsia 5/500 Tablets........ 2196
Anexsia 7.5/650 Tablets........ 2197
Azdōne Tablets........ 844
Codiclear DH Syrup........ 845
Codimal DH Syrup........ 846
Damason-P........ 1356
Hycodan Syrup, Tablets........ 927
Hycomine Compound Tablets........ 929
Hycomine Syrup........ 927
Hycotuss Expectorant Syrup........ 930
Hydrocet Capsules........ 835
Lortab ASA Tablets........ 2414
Lortab........ 2412
Ru-Tuss with Hydrocodone........ 694
Triaminic Expectorant DH........ 1995
Vicodin Tablets........ 1187
Vicodin ES Tablets........ 1189
Zydone Capsules........ 941

Hydrocodone Polistirex (Potentiation of CNS depressants). Products include:
Tussionex Extended-Release Suspension........ 988

Hydroxyzine Hydrochloride (Potentiation of CNS depressants). Products include:
Atarax Tablets & Syrup........ 1941
Marax Tablets & DF Syrup........ 1954
Vistaril Intramuscular Solution........ 1970

Isoflurane (Potentiation of CNS depressants). Products include:
Forane........ 600

Ketamine Hydrochloride (Potentiation of CNS depressants). Products include:
Ketalar........ 1726

Levorphanol Tartrate (Potentiation of CNS depressants). Products include:
Levo-Dromoran........ 1906

Lorazepam (Potentiation of hypnotics). Products include:
Ativan Injection........ 2432
Ativan Tablets........ 2434

Loxapine Hydrochloride (Potentiation of hypnotics). Products include:
Loxitane........ 1213

Loxapine Succinate (Potentiation of CNS depressants). Products include:
Loxitane Capsules........ 1213

Meperidine Hydrochloride (Potentiation of CNS depressants). Products include:
Demerol........ 2047
Mepergan Injection........ 2479

Mephobarbital (Potentiation of CNS depressants). Products include:
Mebaral Tablets........ 2061

Meprobamate (Potentiation of CNS depressants). Products include:
Deprol Tablets........ 2382
Equagesic Tablets........ 2451
Miltown Tablets........ 2386
PMB 200 and PMB 400........ 2504

Mesoridazine (Potentiation of CNS depressants). Products include:
Serentil........ 686

Methadone Hydrochloride (Potentiation of CNS depressants). Products include:
Dolophine Hydrochloride Ampoules & Vials........ 1260
Dolophine Hydrochloride Tablets........ 1261
Methadone Hydrochloride Diskets........ 1284
Methadone Hydrochloride Oral Solution & Tablets........ 1987

Methdilazine Hydrochloride (Potentiation of antihistamines). Products include:
Tacaryl Syrup & Tablets........ 2409

Methohexital Sodium (Potentiation of CNS depressants). Products include:
Brevital Sodium Vials........ 1248

Methoxyflurane (Potentiation of CNS depressants).
No products indexed under this heading.

Midazolam Hydrochloride (Potentiation of hypnotics). Products include:
Versed Injection........ 1924

Molindone Hydrochloride (Potentiation of CNS depressants). Products include:
Moban Tablets & Concentrate........ 932

Morphine Sulfate (Potentiation of CNS depressants). Products include:
Astramorph/PF Injection, USP (Preservative-Free)........ 618
Duramorph........ 960
Infumorph 200 and Infumorph 500 Sterile Solutions........ 962
MS Contin Tablets........ 1814
MSIR........ 1817
Oramorph SR (Morphine Sulfate Sustained Release Tablets)........ 1988
Roxanol........ 1991

Opium Alkaloids (Potentiation of CNS depressants). Products include:
B & O No. 15A & No. 16A Supprettes........ 2395
Pantopon Injectable........ 1911

Oxazepam (Potentiation of CNS depressants). Products include:
Serax Capsules........ 2522
Serax Tablets........ 2522

Oxycodone Hydrochloride (Potentiation of CNS depressants). Products include:
Percocet Tablets........ 950
Percodan........ 951
Roxicodone Tablets, Oral Solution & Intensol (Oxycodone)........ 1992
Tylox Capsules........ 1382

Pentobarbital Sodium (Potentiation of CNS depressants). Products include:
Nembutal Sodium Capsules........ 534
Nembutal Sodium Solution........ 536
Nembutal Sodium Suppositories........ 538

Perphenazine (Potentiation of CNS depressants). Products include:
Etrafon........ 2087
Triavil Tablets........ 1556
Trilafon........ 2123

Phenobarbital (Potentiation of CNS depressants). Products include:
Arco-Lase Plus Tablets........ 607
Bellergal-S Tablets........ 1998
Bronkolixir........ ▣ 761
Bronkotabs Tablets........ ▣ 762
Donnatal........ 1858
Donnatal Extentabs........ 1859
Donnatal Tablets........ 1858
Donnazyme Tablets........ 1860
Kinesed Tablets........ 2272
Phenobarbital Elixir and Tablets........ 1293
Primatene Tablets-P Formula........ 2421
Quadrinal Tablets........ 1183
Tedral SA........ 1765

Prazepam (Potentiation of CNS depressants). Products include:
Centrax........ 1693

Prochlorperazine (Potentiation of CNS depressants). Products include:
Compazine........ 2201

Promethazine Hydrochloride (Potentiation of CNS depressants). Products include:
Mepergan Injection........ 2479
Phenergan with Codeine........ 2497
Phenergan with Dextromethorphan 2499
Phenergan Injection........ 2493
Phenergan Suppositories........ 2496
Phenergan Syrup........ 2495
Phenergan Tablets........ 2496
Phenergan VC........ 2500
Phenergan VC with Codeine........ 2501

Propofol (Potentiation of CNS depressants). Products include:
Diprivan Injection........ 2267

Propoxyphene Hydrochloride (Potentiation of CNS depressants). Products include:
Darvon........ 1256
Wygesic Tablets........ 2540

Propoxyphene Napsylate (Potentiation of CNS depressants). Products include:
Darvon-N/Darvocet-N........ 1254

Pyrilamine Maleate (Potentiation of antihistamines). Products include:
Codimal........ 846
4-Way Fast Acting Nasal Spray - Original Formula (regular & mentholated) & Metered Spray Pump (regular)........ 751
Maximum Strength Midol Multi-Symptom Menstrual Formula........ ▣ 571
Maximum Strength Midol PMS Premenstrual Syndrome Formula........ ▣ 570
Regular Strength Midol Multi-Symptom Menstrual Formula........ ▣ 570
Prefrin-A........ ⊙ 255
Prēmsyn PMS Capsules & Caplets ▣ 547
Primatene Tablets-M Formula........ 2421
Robitussin Night Relief........ ▣ 677
Ru-Tuss with Hydrocodone........ 694
Triaminic Expectorant DH........ 1995
Triaminic Oral Infant Drops........ 1996

Pyrilamine Tannate (Potentiation of antihistamines). Products include:
Rynatan........ 2387

Quazepam (Potentiation of CNS depressants). Products include:
Doral Tablets........ 2383

Secobarbital Sodium (Potentiation of CNS depressants). Products include:
Seconal Sodium Pulvules........ 1296

Sufentanil Citrate (Potentiation of CNS depressants). Products include:
Sufenta Injection........ 1147

Temazepam (Potentiation of hypnotics). Products include:
Restoril Capsules........ 2023

Terfenadine (Potentiation of antihistamines). Products include:
Seldane Tablets........ 1349
Seldane-D Extended-Release Tablets........ 1350

Thiamylal Sodium (Potentiation of CNS depressants). Products include:
Surital Ampoules, Steri-Vials........ 1764

Thioridazine Hydrochloride (Potentiation of CNS depressants). Products include:
Mellaril........ 2011

Thiothixene (Potentiation of CNS depressants). Products include:
Navane Capsules and Concentrate 1954
Navane Intramuscular........ 1956

Triazolam (Potentiation of hypnotics). Products include:
Halcion Tablets........ 2340

Trifluoperazine Hydrochloride (Potentiation of CNS depressants). Products include:
Stelazine........ 2226

Trimeprazine Tartrate (Potentiation of antihistamines). Products include:
Temaril Tablets, Syrup and Spansule Sustained Release Capsules 1085

Tripelennamine Hydrochloride (Potentiation of antihistamines). Products include:
PBZ Tablets & Elixir........ 1037
PBZ-SR Tablets........ 1037

Triprolidine Hydrochloride (Potentiation of antihistamines). Products include:
Actidil........ ▣ 538
Actifed Capsules........ ▣ 539
Actifed Plus Caplets........ ▣ 539
Actifed Plus Tablets........ ▣ 540
Actifed with Codeine Cough Syrup.. 752
Actifed Syrup........ ▣ 540
Actifed Tablets........ ▣ 540
Actifed 12-Hour Capsules........ ▣ 539

PROLIXIN INJECTION
(Fluphenazine Hydrochloride)........1791
May interact with central nervous system depressants, general anesthetics, and certain other agents. Compounds in these categories include:

Alcohol (Effects of alcohol potentiated).

Alfentanil Hydrochloride (Concurrent therapy may require reduced amounts of central nervous system depressants). Products include:
Alfenta Injection........ 1131

Alprazolam (Concurrent therapy may require reduced amounts of central nervous system depressants). Products include:
Xanax Tablets........ 2367

Aprobarbital (Concurrent therapy may require reduced amounts of central nervous system depressants). Products include:
Alurate Elixir........ 1883

Atropine Sulfate (Effects of atropine may be potentiated). Products include:
Arco-Lase Plus Tablets........ 607
Atropine Sulfate Sterile Ophthalmic Solution and S.O.P. Sterile Ophthalmic Ointment........ ⊙ 239
Donnagel........ ▣ 675
Donnagel-PG........ 1858
Donnatal........ 1858
Donnatal Extentabs........ 1859
Donnatal Tablets........ 1858
Donnazyme Tablets........ 1860
Isopto Atropine........ ⊙ 218
Lomotil........ 2174
Motofen Tablets........ 836
Ru-Tuss Tablets........ 693
Urised Tablets........ 2396

Belladonna Alkaloids (Effects of atropine may be potentiated). Products include:
Bellergal-S Tablets........ 1998
Hyland's Bed Wetting Tablets........ ▣ 728
Hyland's Teething Tablets........ ▣ 728
Kinesed Tablets........ 2272

Buprenorphine (Concurrent therapy may require reduced amounts of central nervous system depressants).
- No products indexed under this heading.

Buspirone Hydrochloride (Concurrent therapy may require reduced amounts of central nervous system depressants). Products include:
- BuSpar 1401

Butabarbital (Concurrent therapy may require reduced amounts of central nervous system depressants). Products include:
- Pyridium Plus 1764

Butalbital (Concurrent therapy may require reduced amounts of central nervous system depressants). Products include:
- Esgic-Plus Tablets 1002
- Esgic Tablets & Capsules 1001
- Fioricet Tablets 2006
- Fiorinal Capsules 2007
- Fiorinal with Codeine Capsules 2008
- Fiorinal Tablets 2007
- Phrenilin 838
- Sedapap Tablets 50 mg/650 mg .. 1360

Chlordiazepoxide (Concurrent therapy may require reduced amounts of central nervous system depressants). Products include:
- Libritabs Tablets 1930
- Limbitrol 1933
- Menrium Tablets 1934

Chlordiazepoxide Hydrochloride (Concurrent therapy may require reduced amounts of central nervous system depressants). Products include:
- Librax Capsules 1929
- Librium Capsules 1931
- Librium Injectable 1932

Chlorpromazine (Concurrent therapy may require reduced amounts of central nervous system depressants). Products include:
- Thorazine 2234

Chlorprothixene (Concurrent therapy may require reduced amounts of central nervous system depressants). Products include:
- Taractan Tablets 1920

Chlorprothixene Hydrochloride (Concurrent therapy may require reduced amounts of central nervous system depressants). Products include:
- Taractan 1920

Clorazepate Dipotassium (Concurrent therapy may require reduced amounts of central nervous system depressants). Products include:
- Tranxene 556

Codeine (Concurrent therapy may require reduced amounts of central nervous system depressants). Products include:
- Calcidrine Syrup 506

Codeine Phosphate (Concurrent therapy may require reduced amounts of central nervous system depressants). Products include:
- Actifed with Codeine Cough Syrup.. 752
- Cheracol Cough Syrup 1853
- Codimal PH Syrup 846
- Dimetane-DC Cough Syrup 1857
- Empirin with Codeine Phosphate Nos. 2, 3 & 4 764
- Fiorinal with Codeine Capsules 2008
- Isoclor Expectorant 982
- Naldecon CX Adult Liquid .... ⊞ 521
- Novahistine DH 1342
- Novahistine Expectorant 1343
- Nucofed Capsules 2219
- Nucofed Expectorant 2219
- Nucofed Pediatric Expectorant 2220
- Nucofed Syrup 2219
- Phenaphen with Codeine Capsules 1865
- Phenaphen-650 with Codeine Tablets 1866
- Phenergan with Codeine 2497
- Phenergan VC with Codeine 2501
- Robitussin A-C Syrup 1875
- Robitussin-DAC Syrup 1875
- Ryna .... ⊞ 741
- Soma Compound w/Codeine Tablets 2390
- Triaminic Expectorant w/Codeine .. 1996
- Tussi-Organidin Liquid 2391
- Tylenol with Codeine 1381

Codeine Polistirex (Concurrent therapy may require reduced amounts of central nervous system depressants).
- No products indexed under this heading.

Dezocine (Concurrent therapy may require reduced amounts of central nervous system depressants).

Diazepam (Concurrent therapy may require reduced amounts of central nervous system depressants). Products include:
- Valium Injectable 1937
- Valium Tablets 1939
- Valrelease Capsules 1923

Droperidol (Concurrent therapy may require reduced amounts of central nervous system depressants). Products include:
- Inapsine Injection 1140
- Innovar Injection 1141

Enflurane (Concurrent therapy may require reduced amounts of central nervous system depressants). Products include:
- Ethrane 599

Estazolam (Concurrent therapy may require reduced amounts of central nervous system depressants). Products include:
- ProSom Tablets 554

Ethchlorvynol (Concurrent therapy may require reduced amounts of central nervous system depressants). Products include:
- Placidyl Capsules 553

Ethinamate (Concurrent therapy may require reduced amounts of central nervous system depressants).
- No products indexed under this heading.

Fentanyl (Concurrent therapy may require reduced amounts of central nervous system depressants). Products include:
- Duragesic Transdermal System 1133

Fentanyl Citrate (Concurrent therapy may require reduced amounts of central nervous system depressants). Products include:
- Innovar Injection 1141
- Sublimaze Injection 1146

Fluphenazine Decanoate (Concurrent therapy may require reduced amounts of central nervous system depressants). Products include:
- Prolixin Decanoate 1795

Fluphenazine Enanthate (Concurrent therapy may require reduced amounts of central nervous system depressants). Products include:
- Prolixin Enanthate 1796

Flurazepam Hydrochloride (Concurrent therapy may require reduced amounts of central nervous system depressants). Products include:
- Dalmane Capsules 1927

Glutethimide (Concurrent therapy may require reduced amounts of central nervous system depressants).
- No products indexed under this heading.

Haloperidol (Concurrent therapy may require reduced amounts of central nervous system depressants). Products include:
- Haldol Injection, Tablets and Concentrate 1373

Haloperidol Decanoate (Concurrent therapy may require reduced amounts of central nervous system depressants). Products include:
- Haldol Decanoate 1375

Hydrocodone Bitartrate (Concurrent therapy may require reduced amounts of central nervous system depressants). Products include:
- Anexsia 5/500 Tablets 2196
- Anexsia 7.5/650 Tablets 2197
- Azdōne Tablets 844
- Codiclear DH Syrup 845
- Codimal DH Syrup 846
- Damason-P 1356
- Hycodan Syrup, Tablets 927
- Hycomine Compound Tablets 929
- Hycomine Syrup 927
- Hycotuss Expectorant Syrup 930
- Hydrocet Capsules 835
- Lortab ASA Tablets 2414
- Lortab 2412
- Ru-Tuss with Hydrocodone 694
- Triaminic Expectorant DH 1995
- Vicodin Tablets 1187
- Vicodin ES Tablets 1189
- Zydone Capsules 941

Hydrocodone Polistirex (Concurrent therapy may require reduced amounts of central nervous system depressants). Products include:
- Tussionex Extended-Release Suspension 988

Hydroxyzine Hydrochloride (Concurrent therapy may require reduced amounts of central nervous system depressants). Products include:
- Atarax Tablets & Syrup 1941
- Marax Tablets & DF Syrup 1954
- Vistaril Intramuscular Solution 1970

Isoflurane (Concurrent therapy may require reduced amounts of central nervous system depressants). Products include:
- Forane 600

Ketamine Hydrochloride (Concurrent therapy may require reduced amounts of central nervous system depressants). Products include:
- Ketalar 1726

Levorphanol Tartrate (Concurrent therapy may require reduced amounts of central nervous system depressants). Products include:
- Levo-Dromoran 1906

Lorazepam (Concurrent therapy may require reduced amounts of central nervous system depressants). Products include:
- Ativan Injection 2432
- Ativan Tablets 2434

Loxapine Hydrochloride (Concurrent therapy may require reduced amounts of central nervous system depressants). Products include:
- Loxitane 1213

Loxapine Succinate (Concurrent therapy may require reduced amounts of central nervous system depressants). Products include:
- Loxitane Capsules 1213

Meperidine Hydrochloride (Concurrent therapy may require reduced amounts of central nervous system depressants). Products include:
- Demerol 2047
- Mepergan Injection 2479

Mephobarbital (Concurrent therapy may require reduced amounts of central nervous system depressants). Products include:
- Mebaral Tablets 2061

Meprobamate (Concurrent therapy may require reduced amounts of central nervous system depressants). Products include:
- Deprol Tablets 2382
- Equagesic Tablets 2451
- Miltown Tablets 2386
- PMB 200 and PMB 400 2504

Mesoridazine (Concurrent therapy may require reduced amounts of central nervous system depressants). Products include:
- Serentil 686

Methadone Hydrochloride (Concurrent therapy may require reduced amounts of central nervous system depressants). Products include:
- Dolophine Hydrochloride Ampoules & Vials 1260
- Dolophine Hydrochloride Tablets 1261
- Methadone Hydrochloride Diskets .. 1284
- Methadone Hydrochloride Oral Solution & Tablets 1987

Methohexital Sodium (Concurrent therapy may require reduced amounts of central nervous system depressants). Products include:
- Brevital Sodium Vials 1248

Methoxyflurane (Concurrent therapy may require reduced amounts of central nervous system depressants).
- No products indexed under this heading.

Midazolam Hydrochloride (Concurrent therapy may require reduced amounts of central nervous system depressants). Products include:
- Versed Injection 1924

Molindone Hydrochloride (Concurrent therapy may require reduced amounts of central nervous system depressants). Products include:
- Moban Tablets & Concentrate 932

Morphine Sulfate (Concurrent therapy may require reduced amounts of central nervous system depressants). Products include:
- Astramorph/PF Injection, USP (Preservative-Free) 618
- Duramorph 960
- Infumorph 200 and Infumorph 500 Sterile Solutions 962
- MS Contin Tablets 1814
- MSIR 1817
- Oramorph SR (Morphine Sulfate Sustained Release Tablets) 1988
- Roxanol 1991

Opium Alkaloids (Concurrent therapy may require reduced amounts of central nervous system depressants). Products include:
- B & O No. 15A & No. 16A Supprettes 2395
- Pantopon Injectable 1911

Oxazepam (Concurrent therapy may require reduced amounts of central nervous system depressants). Products include:
- Serax Capsules 2522
- Serax Tablets 2522

Oxycodone Hydrochloride (Concurrent therapy may require reduced amounts of central nervous system depressants). Products include:
- Percocet Tablets 950
- Percodan 951
- Roxicodone Tablets, Oral Solution & Intensol (Oxycodone) 1992
- Tylox Capsules 1382

Pentobarbital Sodium (Concurrent therapy may require reduced amounts of central nervous system depressants). Products include:
- Nembutal Sodium Capsules 534
- Nembutal Sodium Solution 536
- Nembutal Sodium Suppositories 538

Perphenazine (Concurrent therapy may require reduced amounts of central nervous system depressants). Products include:
Etrafon ... 2087
Triavil Tablets ... 1556
Trilafon ... 2123
Phenobarbital (Concurrent therapy may require reduced amounts of central nervous system depressants). Products include:
Arco-Lase Plus Tablets ... 607
Bellergal-S Tablets ... 1998
Bronkolixir ... ▣ 761
Bronkotabs Tablets ... ▣ 762
Donnatal ... 1858
Donnatal Extentabs ... 1859
Donnatal Tablets ... 1858
Donnazyme Tablets ... 1860
Kinesed Tablets ... 2272
Phenobarbital Elixir and Tablets ... 1293
Primatene Tablets-P Formula ... 2421
Quadrinal Tablets ... 1183
Tedral SA ... 1765
Prazepam (Concurrent therapy may require reduced amounts of central nervous system depressants). Products include:
Centrax ... 1693
Prochlorperazine (Concurrent therapy may require reduced amounts of central nervous system depressants). Products include:
Compazine ... 2201
Promethazine Hydrochloride (Concurrent therapy may require reduced amounts of central nervous system depressants). Products include:
Mepergan Injection ... 2479
Phenergan with Codeine ... 2497
Phenergan with Dextromethorphan 2499
Phenergan Injection ... 2493
Phenergan Suppositories ... 2496
Phenergan Syrup ... 2495
Phenergan Tablets ... 2496
Phenergan VC ... 2500
Phenergan VC with Codeine ... 2501
Propofol (Concurrent therapy may require reduced amounts of central nervous system depressants). Products include:
Diprivan Injection ... 2267
Propoxyphene Hydrochloride (Concurrent therapy may require reduced amounts of central nervous system depressants). Products include:
Darvon ... 1256
Wygesic Tablets ... 2540
Propoxyphene Napsylate (Concurrent therapy may require reduced amounts of central nervous system depressants). Products include:
Darvon-N/Darvocet-N ... 1254
Quazepam (Concurrent therapy may require reduced amounts of central nervous system depressants). Products include:
Doral Tablets ... 2383
Secobarbital Sodium (Concurrent therapy may require reduced amounts of central nervous system depressants). Products include:
Seconal Sodium Pulvules ... 1296
Sufentanil Citrate (Concurrent therapy may require reduced amounts of central nervous system depressants). Products include:
Sufenta Injection ... 1147
Temazepam (Concurrent therapy may require reduced amounts of central nervous system depressants). Products include:
Restoril Capsules ... 2023
Thiamylal Sodium (Concurrent therapy may require reduced amounts of central nervous system depressants). Products include:
Surital Ampoules, Steri-Vials ... 1764
Thioridazine Hydrochloride (Concurrent therapy may require reduced amounts of central nervous system depressants). Products include:
Mellaril ... 2011
Thiothixene (Concurrent therapy may require reduced amounts of central nervous system depressants). Products include:
Navane Capsules and Concentrate 1954
Navane Intramuscular ... 1956
Triazolam (Concurrent therapy may require reduced amounts of central nervous system depressants). Products include:
Halcion Tablets ... 2340
Trifluoperazine Hydrochloride (Concurrent therapy may require reduced amounts of central nervous system depressants). Products include:
Stelazine ... 2226

PROLIXIN ORAL CONCENTRATE
(Fluphenazine Hydrochloride) ... 1792
May interact with central nervous system depressants, barbiturates, narcotic analgesics, antihistamines, and certain other agents. Compounds in these categories include:

Alcohol (Potentiation of central nervous system depressants may occur).
Alfentanil Hydrochloride (Potentiation of central nervous system depressants may occur). Products include:
Alfenta Injection ... 1131
Alprazolam (Potentiation of central nervous system depressants may occur). Products include:
Xanax Tablets ... 2367
Aprobarbital (Potentiation of central nervous system depressants may occur). Products include:
Alurate Elixir ... 1883
Astemizole (Potentiation of central nervous system depressants may occur). Products include:
Hismanal Tablets ... 1138
Atropine Sulfate (Potentiation of anticholinergic effects). Products include:
Arco-Lase Plus Tablets ... 607
Atropine Sulfate Sterile Ophthalmic Solution and S.O.P. Sterile Ophthalmic Ointment ... ◉ 239
Donnagel ... ▣ 675
Donnagel-PG ... 1858
Donnatal ... 1858
Donnatal Extentabs ... 1859
Donnatal Tablets ... 1858
Donnazyme Tablets ... 1860
Isopto Atropine ... ◉ 218
Lomotil ... 2174
Motofen Tablets ... 836
Ru-Tuss Tablets ... 693
Urised Tablets ... 2396
Azatadine Maleate (Potentiation of central nervous system depressants may occur). Products include:
Optimine Tablets ... 2115
Trinalin Repetabs Tablets ... 1170
Bromodiphenhydramine Hydrochloride (Potentiation of central nervous system depressants may occur).
No products indexed under this heading.
Brompheniramine Maleate (Potentiation of central nervous system depressants may occur). Products include:
Alka Seltzer Plus Sinus Allergy Medicine ... ▣ 624
Atrohist Sprinkle Capsules ... 558
Bromfed Capsules (Timed Release) ... 1615
Bromfed Syrup ... ▣ 628
Bromfed ... 1615
Dimetane Decongestant ... ▣ 673
Dimetane ... ▣ 672
Dimetane-DC Cough Syrup ... 1857
Dimetane-DX Cough Syrup ... 1858
Dimetapp Elixir ... ▣ 673
Dimetapp DM Elixir ... ▣ 674
Dimetapp Extentabs ... ▣ 674
Dimetapp Plus Caplets ... ▣ 675
Dimetapp Tablets ... ▣ 675
Drixoral Antihistamine/Nasal Decongestant Syrup ... ▣ 698
Buprenorphine (Potentiation of central nervous system depressants may occur).
No products indexed under this heading.
Buspirone Hydrochloride (Potentiation of central nervous system depressants may occur). Products include:
BuSpar ... 1401
Butabarbital (Potentiation of central nervous system depressants may occur). Products include:
Pyridium Plus ... 1764
Butalbital (Potentiation of central nervous system depressants may occur). Products include:
Esgic-Plus Tablets ... 1002
Esgic Tablets & Capsules ... 1001
Fioricet Tablets ... 2006
Fiorinal Capsules ... 2007
Fiorinal with Codeine Capsules ... 2008
Fiorinal Tablets ... 2007
Phrenilin ... 838
Sedapap Tablets 50 mg/650 mg .. 1360
Chlordiazepoxide (Potentiation of central nervous system depressants may occur). Products include:
Libritabs Tablets ... 1930
Limbitrol ... 1933
Menrium Tablets ... 1934
Chlordiazepoxide Hydrochloride (Potentiation of central nervous system depressants may occur). Products include:
Librax Capsules ... 1929
Librium Capsules ... 1931
Librium Injectable ... 1932
Chlorpheniramine Maleate (Potentiation of central nervous system depressants may occur). Products include:
A.R.M. Allergy Relief Medicine Caplets ... ▣ 615
Alka-Seltzer Plus Cold Medicine ... ▣ 623
Allerest ... ▣ 559
Ana-Kit Anaphylaxis Emergency Treatment Kit ... 1100
BC Cold Powder Multi-Symptom Formula ... ▣ 517
Brexin L.A. Capsules ... 2078
Cerose-DM ... 2443
Cheracol Plus Head Cold/Cough Formula ... ▣ 667
Chlor-Trimeton Allergy Syrup, Tablets & Long-Acting Repetabs Tablets ... ▣ 693
Chlor-Trimeton Decongestant ... ▣ 694
Comhist LA Capsules ... 1618
Allergy-Sinus Comtrex Multi-Symptom Allergy Sinus Formula Tablets & Caplets ... 746
Comtrex Multi-Symptom Cold Reliever Tablets/Caplets/Liqui-Gels/Liquid ... 745
Day-Night Comtrex ... 747
Contac Continuous Action Decongestant/Antihistamine Capsules ▣ 710
Contac Maximum Strength Continuous Action Decongestant/Antihistamine Caplets ... ▣ 709
Contac Severe Cold and Flu Formula Caplets ... ▣ 711
Coricidin 'D' Decongestant Tablets ... ▣ 695
Coricidin Demilets Tablets for Children ... ▣ 696
Coricidin Tablets ... ▣ 695
Deconamine ... 663
Demazin Nasal Decongestant/Antihistamine Repetabs Tablets & Syrup ... ▣ 697
Dorcol Children's Liquid Cold Formula ... ▣ 686
Dristan Decongestant/Antihistamine/ Analgesic Coated Caplets ... ▣ 749
Dristan Cold Nasal Decongestant/Antihistamine/ Analgesic Coated Tablets ... 2419
Dristan Advanced Formula Decongestant/Antihistamine/Analgesic Tablets ... ▣ 749
Extendryl ... 994
4-Way Cold Tablets ... 750
Fedahist Gyrocaps ... 2145
Fedahist Timecaps ... 2145
Hycomine Compound Tablets ... 929
Isoclor Timesule Capsules ... ▣ 561
Kronofed-A ... 970
Medi-Flu Caplet, Liquid ... ▣ 640
Naldecon Syrup, Tablets, Pediatric Drops and Pediatric Syrup ... 709
Nolamine Tablets ... 838
Novafed A Capsules ... 1342
Novahistine DH ... 1342
Novahistine Elixir ... ▣ 596
Ornade Spansule Capsules ... 2221
Orthoxicol Cough Syrup ... ▣ 668
PediaCare Allergy Relief Formula Liquid ... 1362
PediaCare Cough-Cold Formula Liquid ... 1362
PediaCare Night Rest Cough-Cold Formula Liquid ... 1362
PediaCare 6-12 Cough-Cold Formula Chewable Tablets ... 1362
Pyrroxate Capsules ... ▣ 669
Quelidrine Syrup ... 556
Ru-Tuss II Capsules ... 693
Ru-Tuss Tablets ... 693
Ryna ... ▣ 741
Sinarest Tablets & Extra Strength Tablets ... ▣ 562
Sine-Off Maximum Strength Allergy/Sinus Formula Caplets ... ▣ 721
Sine-Off Sinus Medicine Tablets-Aspirin Formula ... ▣ 722
Singlet Tablets ... ▣ 598
Sinulin ... 840
Sinutab Maximum Strength ... ▣ 641
St. Joseph Nighttime Cold Medicine ... ▣ 705
Sudafed Plus Liquid ... ▣ 544
Sudafed Plus Tablets ... ▣ 545
Teldrin Timed-Release Allergy Capsules, 12 mg ... 2192
TheraFlu Flu and Cold Medicine ... ▣ 687
Triaminic Allergy Tablets ... ▣ 688
Triaminic Chewables ... ▣ 688
Triaminic Cold Tablets ... ▣ 688
Triaminic Nite Light ... ▣ 689
Triaminic Syrup ... ▣ 689
Triaminic-12 Tablets ... ▣ 690
Triaminicin Tablets ... ▣ 690
Triaminicol Multi-Symptom Cold Tablets ... ▣ 691
Triaminicol Multi-Symptom Relief ▣ 691
Tylenol Allergy Sinus Medication Caplets and Gelcaps, Maximum Strength ... 1372
Children's Tylenol Cold Liquid Formula and Chewable Tablets ... 1368
Tylenol Cold & Flu Hot Medication, Packets ... 1369
Tylenol Cold Medication Caplets and Tablets ... 1370
Tylenol Cold Medication, Effervescent Tablets ... 1369
Vicks Children's NyQuil ... ▣ 664
Vicks Formula 44 Cough Medicine ... ▣ 661
Vicks Formula 44M Multi-Symptom Cough Medicine ... ▣ 662
Vicks Pediatric Formula 44m Multi-Symptom Cough & Cold Medicine ... ▣ 663
Chlorpheniramine Polistirex (Potentiation of central nervous system depressants may occur). Products include:
Tussionex Extended-Release Suspension ... 988
Chlorpheniramine Tannate (Potentiation of central nervous system depressants may occur). Products include:
Rynatan ... 2387
Rynatuss ... 2388

(▣ Described in PDR For Nonprescription Drugs) (◉ Described in PDR For Ophthalmology)

Chlorpromazine (Potentiation of central nervous system depressants may occur). Products include:
Thorazine ... 2234

Chlorprothixene (Potentiation of central nervous system depressants may occur). Products include:
Taractan Tablets ... 1920

Chlorprothixene Hydrochloride (Potentiation of central nervous system depressants may occur). Products include:
Taractan ... 1920

Clemastine Fumarate (Potentiation of central nervous system depressants may occur). Products include:
Tavist Syrup ... 2033
Tavist Tablets ... 2035
Tavist-D Tablets ... 2035

Clorazepate Dipotassium (Potentiation of central nervous system depressants may occur). Products include:
Tranxene ... 556

Codeine (Potentiation of central nervous system depressants may occur). Products include:
Calcidrine Syrup ... 506

Codeine Phosphate (Potentiation of central nervous system depressants may occur). Products include:
Actifed with Codeine Cough Syrup .. 752
Cheracol Cough Syrup ... 1853
Codimal PH Syrup ... 846
Dimetane-DC Cough Syrup ... 1857
Empirin with Codeine Phosphate Nos. 2, 3 & 4 ... 764
Fiorinal with Codeine Capsules ... 2008
Isoclor Expectorant ... 982
Naldecon CX Adult Liquid ... ◙ 521
Novahistine DH ... 1342
Novahistine Expectorant ... 1343
Nucofed Capsules ... 2219
Nucofed Expectorant ... 2219
Nucofed Pediatric Expectorant ... 2220
Nucofed Syrup ... 2219
Phenaphen with Codeine Capsules 1865
Phenaphen-650 with Codeine Tablets ... 1866
Phenergan with Codeine ... 2497
Phenergan VC with Codeine ... 2501
Robitussin A-C Syrup ... 1875
Robitussin-DAC Syrup ... 1875
Ryna ... ◙ 741
Soma Compound w/Codeine Tablets ... 2390
Triaminic Expectorant w/Codeine .. 1996
Tussi-Organidin Liquid ... 2391
Tylenol with Codeine ... 1381

Codeine Polistirex (Potentiation of central nervous system depressants may occur).
No products indexed under this heading.

Cyproheptadine Hydrochloride (Potentiation of central nervous system depressants may occur). Products include:
Periactin ... 1525

Dexchlorpheniramine Maleate (Potentiation of central nervous system depressants may occur). Products include:
Polaramine ... 2116

Dezocine (Potentiation of central nervous system depressants may occur).

Diazepam (Potentiation of central nervous system depressants may occur). Products include:
Valium Injectable ... 1937
Valium Tablets ... 1939
Valrelease Capsules ... 1923

Diphenhydramine Citrate (Potentiation of central nervous system depressants may occur). Products include:
Alka-Seltzer Plus Night-Time Cold Medicine ... ◙ 623
Bufferin AF Nite Time Analgesic/Sleeping Aid Caplets ... 744
Excedrin P.M. Analgesic/Sleeping Aid Tablets, Caplets and Liquid ... 749

Diphenhydramine Hydrochloride (Potentiation of central nervous system depressants may occur). Products include:
Benadryl Anti-Itch Cream ... ◙ 635
Benadryl Capsules ... 1691
Benadryl Decongestant Elixir ... ◙ 635
Benadryl Decongestant ... ◙ 635
Benadryl Elixir ... ◙ 636
Benadryl Kapseals ... 1691
Benadryl 25 Kapseals ... ◙ 636
Benadryl Parenteral ... 1692
Benadryl Plus ... ◙ 636
Benadryl Plus Nighttime ... ◙ 637
Benadryl Spray, Maximum Strength ... ◙ 637
Benadryl Spray, Regular Strength ◙ 637
Benadryl Steri-Vials, Ampoules, and Steri-Dose Syringe ... 1692
Benadryl 25 Tablets ... ◙ 636
Benylin Cough Syrup ... ◙ 637
Benylin Decongestant ... ◙ 638
Caladryl Cream, Lotion, Spray ... ◙ 638
Miles Nervine Nighttime Sleep-Aid ◙ 627
Nytol Tablets ... ◙ 517
Sleep-ettes-D Tablets ... ◙ 653
Sleep-eze 3 Tablets ... ◙ 755
Sleepinal Night-time Sleep Aid Capsules ... ◙ 734
Sominex Caplets and Tablets ... ◙ 722
Sominex Liquid ... ◙ 723
Sominex Pain Relief Formula ... ◙ 723
Tylenol Cold Night Time Medication Liquid ... 1371
Tylenol PM, Extra Strength Caplets and Tablets ... 1368
Unisom Dual Relief Nighttime Sleep Aid/Analgesic ... 1774
Ziradryl Lotion ... ◙ 643

Diphenylpyraline Hydrochloride (Potentiation of central nervous system depressants may occur).
No products indexed under this heading.

Droperidol (Potentiation of central nervous system depressants may occur). Products include:
Inapsine Injection ... 1140
Innovar Injection ... 1141

Enflurane (Potentiation of central nervous system depressants may occur). Products include:
Ethrane ... 599

Estazolam (Potentiation of central nervous system depressants may occur). Products include:
ProSom Tablets ... 554

Ethchlorvynol (Potentiation of central nervous system depressants may occur). Products include:
Placidyl Capsules ... 553

Ethinamate (Potentiation of central nervous system depressants may occur).
No products indexed under this heading.

Fentanyl (Potentiation of central nervous system depressants may occur). Products include:
Duragesic Transdermal System ... 1133

Fentanyl Citrate (Potentiation of central nervous system depressants may occur). Products include:
Innovar Injection ... 1141
Sublimaze Injection ... 1146

Fluphenazine Decanoate (Potentiation of central nervous system depressants may occur). Products include:
Prolixin Decanoate ... 1795

Fluphenazine Enanthate (Potentiation of central nervous system depressants may occur). Products include:
Prolixin Enanthate ... 1796

Flurazepam Hydrochloride (Potentiation of central nervous system depressants may occur). Products include:
Dalmane Capsules ... 1927

Glutethimide (Potentiation of central nervous system depressants may occur).
No products indexed under this heading.

Haloperidol (Potentiation of central nervous system depressants may occur). Products include:
Haldol Injection, Tablets and Concentrate ... 1373

Haloperidol Decanoate (Potentiation of central nervous system depressants may occur). Products include:
Haldol Decanoate ... 1375

Hydrocodone Bitartrate (Potentiation of central nervous system depressants may occur). Products include:
Anexsia 5/500 Tablets ... 2196
Anexsia 7.5/650 Tablets ... 2197
Azdone Tablets ... 844
Codiclear DH Syrup ... 845
Codimal DH Syrup ... 846
Damason-P ... 1356
Hycodan Syrup, Tablets ... 927
Hycomine Compound Tablets ... 929
Hycomine Syrup ... 927
Hycotuss Expectorant Syrup ... 930
Hydrocet Capsules ... 835
Lortab ASA Tablets ... 2414
Lortab ... 2412
Ru-Tuss with Hydrocodone ... 694
Triaminic Expectorant DH ... 1995
Vicodin Tablets ... 1187
Vicodin ES Tablets ... 1189
Zydone Capsules ... 941

Hydrocodone Polistirex (Potentiation of central nervous system depressants may occur). Products include:
Tussionex Extended-Release Suspension ... 988

Hydroxyzine Hydrochloride (Potentiation of central nervous system depressants may occur). Products include:
Atarax Tablets & Syrup ... 1941
Marax Tablets & DF Syrup ... 1954
Vistaril Intramuscular Solution ... 1970

Isoflurane (Potentiation of central nervous system depressants may occur). Products include:
Forane ... 600

Ketamine Hydrochloride (Potentiation of central nervous system depressants may occur). Products include:
Ketalar ... 1726

Levorphanol Tartrate (Potentiation of central nervous system depressants may occur). Products include:
Levo-Dromoran ... 1906

Lorazepam (Potentiation of central nervous system depressants may occur). Products include:
Ativan Injection ... 2432
Ativan Tablets ... 2434

Loxapine Hydrochloride (Potentiation of central nervous system depressants may occur). Products include:
Loxitane ... 1213

Loxapine Succinate (Potentiation of central nervous system depressants may occur). Products include:
Loxitane Capsules ... 1213

Meperidine Hydrochloride (Potentiation of central nervous system depressants may occur). Products include:
Demerol ... 2047
Mepergan Injection ... 2479

Mephobarbital (Potentiation of central nervous system depressants may occur). Products include:
Mebaral Tablets ... 2061

Meprobamate (Potentiation of central nervous system depressants may occur). Products include:
Deprol Tablets ... 2382
Equagesic Tablets ... 2451
Miltown Tablets ... 2386
PMB 200 and PMB 400 ... 2504

Mesoridazine (Potentiation of central nervous system depressants may occur). Products include:
Serentil ... 686

Methadone Hydrochloride (Potentiation of central nervous system depressants may occur). Products include:
Dolophine Hydrochloride Ampoules & Vials ... 1260
Dolophine Hydrochloride Tablets ... 1261
Methadone Hydrochloride Diskets .. 1284
Methadone Hydrochloride Oral Solution & Tablets ... 1987

Methdilazine Hydrochloride (Potentiation of central nervous system depressants may occur). Products include:
Tacaryl Syrup & Tablets ... 2409

Methohexital Sodium (Potentiation of central nervous system depressants may occur). Products include:
Brevital Sodium Vials ... 1248

Methoxyflurane (Potentiation of central nervous system depressants may occur).
No products indexed under this heading.

Midazolam Hydrochloride (Potentiation of central nervous system depressants may occur). Products include:
Versed Injection ... 1924

Molindone Hydrochloride (Potentiation of central nervous system depressants may occur). Products include:
Moban Tablets & Concentrate ... 932

Morphine Sulfate (Potentiation of central nervous system depressants may occur). Products include:
Astramorph/PF Injection, USP (Preservative-Free) ... 618
Duramorph ... 960
Infumorph 200 and Infumorph 500 Sterile Solutions ... 962
MS Contin Tablets ... 1814
MSIR ... 1817
Oramorph SR (Morphine Sulfate Sustained Release Tablets) ... 1988
Roxanol ... 1991

Opium Alkaloids (Potentiation of central nervous system depressants may occur). Products include:
B & O No. 15A & No. 16A Supprettes ... 2395
Pantopon Injectable ... 1911

Oxazepam (Potentiation of central nervous system depressants may occur). Products include:
Serax Capsules ... 2522
Serax Tablets ... 2522

Oxycodone Hydrochloride (Potentiation of central nervous system depressants may occur). Products include:
Percocet Tablets ... 950
Percodan ... 951
Roxicodone Tablets, Oral Solution & Intensol (Oxycodone) ... 1992
Tylox Capsules ... 1382

Pentobarbital Sodium (Potentiation of central nervous system depressants may occur). Products include:
Nembutal Sodium Capsules ... 534
Nembutal Sodium Solution ... 536
Nembutal Sodium Suppositories ... 538

Perphenazine (Potentiation of central nervous system depressants may occur). Products include:
Etrafon ... 2087
Triavil Tablets ... 1556

Trilafon 2123

Phenobarbital (Potentiation of central nervous system depressants may occur). Products include:
- Arco-Lase Plus Tablets 607
- Bellergal-S Tablets 1998
- Bronkolixir .... ▣ 761
- Bronkotabs Tablets .... ▣ 762
- Donnatal 1858
- Donnatal Extentabs 1859
- Donnatal Tablets 1858
- Donnazyme Tablets 1860
- Kinesed Tablets 2272
- Phenobarbital Elixir and Tablets 1293
- Primatene Tablets-P Formula 2421
- Quadrinal Tablets 1183
- Tedral SA 1765

Prazepam (Potentiation of central nervous system depressants may occur). Products include:
- Centrax 1693

Prochlorperazine (Potentiation of central nervous system depressants may occur). Products include:
- Compazine 2201

Promethazine Hydrochloride (Potentiation of central nervous system depressants may occur). Products include:
- Mepergan Injection 2479
- Phenergan with Codeine 2497
- Phenergan with Dextromethorphan 2499
- Phenergan Injection 2493
- Phenergan Suppositories 2496
- Phenergan Syrup 2495
- Phenergan Tablets 2496
- Phenergan VC 2500
- Phenergan VC with Codeine 2501

Propofol (Potentiation of central nervous system depressants may occur). Products include:
- Diprivan Injection 2267

Propoxyphene Hydrochloride (Potentiation of central nervous system depressants may occur). Products include:
- Darvon 1256
- Wygesic Tablets 2540

Propoxyphene Napsylate (Potentiation of central nervous system depressants may occur). Products include:
- Darvon-N/Darvocet-N 1254

Pyrilamine Maleate (Potentiation of central nervous system depressants may occur). Products include:
- Codimal 846
- 4-Way Fast Acting Nasal Spray - Original Formula (regular & mentholated) & Metered Spray Pump (regular) 751
- Maximum Strength Midol Multi-Symptom Menstrual Formula .... ▣ 571
- Maximum Strength Midol PMS Premenstrual Syndrome Formula .... ▣ 570
- Regular Strength Midol Multi-Symptom Menstrual Formula .... ▣ 570
- Prefrin-A .... ⊙ 255
- Prēmsyn PMS Capsules & Caplets ▣ 547
- Primatene Tablets-M Formula 2421
- Robitussin Night Relief .... ▣ 677
- Ru-Tuss with Hydrocodone 694
- Triaminic Expectorant DH 1995
- Triaminic Oral Infant Drops 1996

Pyrilamine Tannate (Potentiation of central nervous system depressants may occur). Products include:
- Rynatan 2387

Quazepam (Potentiation of central nervous system depressants may occur). Products include:
- Doral Tablets 2383

Secobarbital Sodium (Potentiation of central nervous system depressants may occur). Products include:
- Seconal Sodium Pulvules 1296

Sufentanil Citrate (Potentiation of central nervous system depressants may occur). Products include:
- Sufenta Injection 1147

Temazepam (Potentiation of central nervous system depressants may occur). Products include:
- Restoril Capsules 2023

Terfenadine (Potentiation of central nervous system depressants may occur). Products include:
- Seldane Tablets 1349
- Seldane-D Extended-Release Tablets 1350

Thiamylal Sodium (Potentiation of central nervous system depressants may occur). Products include:
- Surital Ampoules, Steri-Vials 1764

Thioridazine Hydrochloride (Potentiation of central nervous system depressants may occur). Products include:
- Mellaril 2011

Thiothixene (Potentiation of central nervous system depressants may occur). Products include:
- Navane Capsules and Concentrate 1954
- Navane Intramuscular 1956

Triazolam (Potentiation of central nervous system depressants may occur). Products include:
- Halcion Tablets 2340

Trifluoperazine Hydrochloride (Potentiation of central nervous system depressants may occur). Products include:
- Stelazine 2226

Trimeprazine Tartrate (Potentiation of central nervous system depressants may occur). Products include:
- Temaril Tablets, Syrup and Spansule Sustained Release Capsules 1085

Tripelennamine Hydrochloride (Potentiation of central nervous system depressants may occur). Products include:
- PBZ Tablets & Elixir 1037
- PBZ-SR Tablets 1037

Triprolidine Hydrochloride (Potentiation of central nervous system depressants may occur). Products include:
- Actidil .... ▣ 538
- Actifed Capsules .... ▣ 539
- Actifed Plus Caplets .... ▣ 539
- Actifed Plus Tablets .... ▣ 540
- Actifed with Codeine Cough Syrup.. 752
- Actifed Syrup .... ▣ 540
- Actifed Tablets .... ▣ 540
- Actifed 12-Hour Capsules .... ▣ 539

PROLIXIN TABLETS
(Fluphenazine Hydrochloride) 1793
See **Prolixin Elixir**

PROLOID TABLETS
(Thyroglobulin) 1761
May interact with oral anticoagulants, oral hypoglycemic agents, estrogens, oral contraceptives, insulin, and certain other agents. Compounds in these categories include:

Chlorotrianisene (Increased thyroid requirements). Products include:
- TACE 12 and 25 mg 1353

Chlorpropamide (Increased oral hypoglycemic requirements). Products include:
- Diabinese Tablets 1775

Cholestyramine (Impaired absorption of thyroid hormones). Products include:
- Cholybar 1705
- Questran Light 711
- Questran Powder 710

Dicumarol (Increases in clotting factor synthesis are impaired). Products include:
- Dicumarol Tablets 516

Dienestrol (Increased thyroid requirements). Products include:
- Ortho Dienestrol Cream 1664

Diethylstilbestrol (Increased thyroid requirements). Products include:
- Diethylstilbestrol Tablets 1258

Estradiol (Increased thyroid requirements). Products include:
- Emcyt Capsules 1161
- Estrace 1385
- Estrace Vaginal Cream 1388
- Estraderm Transdermal System 866

Estrogens, Conjugated (Increased thyroid requirements). Products include:
- Mediatric Capsules 2476
- PMB 200 and PMB 400 2504
- Premarin Intravenous 2508
- Premarin with Methyltestosterone .. 2515
- Premarin Tablets 2510
- Premarin Vaginal Cream 2512

Estrogens, Esterified (Increased thyroid requirements). Products include:
- Estratest 2245
- Menrium Tablets 1934

Estropipate (Increased thyroid requirements). Products include:
- Ogen 540

Ethinyl Estradiol (Increased thyroid requirements). Products include:
- Brevicon 2304
- Demulen 2161
- Estinyl Tablets 2085
- Jenest-28 Tablets 1636
- Levlen/Tri-Levlen 665
- Lo/Ovral Tablets 2471
- Lo/Ovral-28 Tablets 2476
- Loestrin 1728
- Modicon 1667
- Nordette-21 Tablets 2481
- Nordette-28 Tablets 2483
- Norethin 2133
- Norinyl 2304
- Norlestrin 1746
- Ortho-Cyclen Tablets 1658
- Ortho-Novum 1667
- Ovcon 1391
- Ovral Tablets 2490
- Ovral-28 Tablets 2491
- Levlen/Tri-Levlen 665
- Tri-Norinyl 2304
- Triphasil-21 Tablets 2527
- Triphasil-28 Tablets 2532

Ethynodiol Diacetate (Increased thyroid requirements). Products include:
- Demulen 2161

Glipizide (Increased oral hypoglycemic requirements). Products include:
- Glucotrol 1952

Glyburide (Increased oral hypoglycemic requirements). Products include:
- DiaBeta 1091
- Micronase Tablets 2350

Insulin, Human (Increased insulin requirements).
- No products indexed under this heading.

Insulin, Human Isophane Suspension (Increased insulin requirements). Products include:
- Humulin N, 100 Units 1270

Insulin, Human NPH (Increased insulin requirements). Products include:
- Insulatard NPH Human 1627
- Novolin N 1627
- Novolin N PenFill Cartridges 1628
- Novolin N Prefilled 1628

Insulin, Human Regular (Increased insulin requirements). Products include:
- Humulin BR, 100 Units 1268
- Humulin R, 100 Units 1272
- Novolin R 1627
- Novolin R PenFill Cartridges 1628
- Novolin R Prefilled 1629
- Velosulin Human 1628

Insulin, Human, Zinc Suspension (Increased insulin requirements). Products include:
- Humulin L, 100 Units 1268
- Humulin U, 100 Units 1272
- Novolin L 1627

Insulin, NPH (Increased insulin requirements). Products include:
- NPH, 40 & 100 Units 1273
- Beef NPH, 100 Units 1274
- Pork NPH, 100 Units 1275
- Insulatard NPH 1626
- NPH Insulin 1626
- NPH Purified Pork Isophane Insulin 1626

Insulin, Regular (Increased insulin requirements). Products include:
- Regular, 40 & 100 Units 1273
- Beef Regular, 100 Units 1275
- Pork Regular, 100 Units 1275
- Pork Regular (Concentrated), 500 Units 1276
- Regular Insulin 1625
- Regular Purified Pork Insulin 1626
- Velosulin 1627

Insulin, Zinc Crystals (Increased insulin requirements). Products include:
- NPH, 40 & 100 Units 1273

Insulin, Zinc Suspension (Increased insulin requirements). Products include:
- Lente, 40 & 100 Units 1272
- Protamine, Zinc, 40 & 100 Units.... 1273
- Lente Iletin I 1272
- Beef Lente, 100 Units 1274
- Beef Protamine Zinc, 100 Units 1274
- Pork Lente, 100 Units 1275
- Pork, Protamine, Zinc, 100 Units.... 1275
- Lente Insulin 1626
- Lente Purified Pork Insulin 1626
- Semilente Insulin 1625
- Ultralente Insulin 1626

Levonorgestrel (Increased thyroid requirements). Products include:
- Levlen/Tri-Levlen 665
- Nordette-21 Tablets 2481
- Nordette-28 Tablets 2483
- Norplant System 2484
- Levlen/Tri-Levlen 665
- Triphasil-21 Tablets 2527
- Triphasil-28 Tablets 2532

Mestranol (Increased thyroid requirements). Products include:
- Enovid 2161
- Norethin 2133
- Norinyl 2304
- Ortho-Novum 1667

Norethindrone (Increased thyroid requirements). Products include:
- Brevicon 2304
- Jenest-28 Tablets 1636
- Micronor Tablets 1667
- Modicon 1667
- Norethin 2133
- Norinyl 2304
- Norlutin 1755
- Nor-Q D Tablets 2304
- Ortho-Novum 1667
- Ovcon 1391
- Tri-Norinyl 2304

Norethynodrel (Increased thyroid requirements). Products include:
- Enovid 2161

Norgestimate (Increased thyroid requirements). Products include:
- Ortho-Cyclen Tablets 1658

Norgestrel (Increased thyroid requirements). Products include:
- Lo/Ovral Tablets 2471
- Lo/Ovral-28 Tablets 2476
- Ovral Tablets 2490
- Ovral-28 Tablets 2491
- Ovrette Tablets 2492

Polyestradiol Phosphate (Increased thyroid requirements). Products include:
- Estradurin 2452

Quinestrol (Increased thyroid requirements). Products include:
- Estrovis 1721

Tolazamide (Increased oral hypoglycemic requirements). Products include:
Tolinase Tablets ... 2365
Tolbutamide (Increased oral hypoglycemic requirements). Products include:
Orinase Tablets ... 2354
Warfarin Sodium (Increases in clotting factor synthesis are impaired). Products include:
Coumadin Injection & Tablets ... 944
Panwarfin Tablets ... 547

Food Interactions

Soybean formula, children's (May cause excessive fecal loss).

PROLOPRIM TABLETS
(Trimethoprim) ... 799
May interact with:

Phenytoin (Increased phenytoin half-life and decreased phenytoin metabolic clearance rate). Products include:
Dilantin Infatabs ... 1710
Dilantin-30 Pediatric/Dilantin-125 Suspension ... 1713
Phenytoin Sodium (Increased phenytoin half-life and decreased phenytoin metabolic clearance rate). Products include:
Dilantin Kapseals ... 1708
Dilantin Parenteral ... 1712
Dilantin with Phenobarbital Kapseals ... 1715

PROMISE TOOTHPASTE
(Potassium Nitrate) ... ■ 517
No interactions described in labeling.

PRONESTYL CAPSULES AND TABLETS
(Procainamide Hydrochloride) ... 1800
May interact with type 1 antiarrhythmic drugs, antiarrhythmics, anticholinergics, cardiac glycosides, and certain other agents. Compounds in these categories include:

Acebutolol Hydrochloride (Additive effect; hypotension). Products include:
Sectral Capsules ... 2520
Adenosine (Additive effect; hypotension). Products include:
Adenocard Injection ... 1007
Amiodarone Hydrochloride (Additive effect; hypotension). Products include:
Cordarone Tablets ... 2446
Atropine Sulfate (Additive antivagal effects on A-V nodal conduction). Products include:
Arco-Lase Plus Tablets ... 607
Atropine Sulfate Sterile Ophthalmic Solution and S.O.P. Sterile Ophthalmic Ointment ... ◉ 239
Donnagel ... ■ 675
Donnagel-PG ... 1858
Donnatal ... 1858
Donnatal Extentabs ... 1859
Donnatal Tablets ... 1858
Donnazyme Tablets ... 1860
Isopto Atropine ... ◉ 218
Lomotil ... 2174
Motofen Tablets ... 836
Ru-Tuss Tablets ... 693
Urised Tablets ... 2396
Belladonna Alkaloids (Additive antivagal effects on A-V nodal conduction). Products include:
Bellergal-S Tablets ... 1998
Hyland's Bed Wetting Tablets ... ■ 728
Hyland's Teething Tablets ... ■ 728
Kinesed Tablets ... 2272
Benztropine Mesylate (Additive antivagal effects on A-V nodal conduction). Products include:
Cogentin ... 1435
Biperiden (Additive antivagal effects on A-V nodal conduction). Products include:
Akineton ... 1171
Bretylium Tosylate (Additive effect; hypotension). Products include:
Bretylol Injection ... 923
Clidinium Bromide (Additive antivagal effects on A-V nodal conduction). Products include:
Librax Capsules ... 1929
Quarzan Capsules ... 1937
Deslanoside (Caution should be exercised in arrhythmias associated with digitalis intoxication).
No products indexed under this heading.
Dicyclomine Hydrochloride (Additive antivagal effects on A-V nodal conduction). Products include:
Bentyl ... 1322
Digitoxin (Caution should be exercised in arrhythmias associated with digitalis intoxication). Products include:
Crystodigin Tablets ... 1253
Digoxin (Caution should be exercised in arrhythmias associated with digitalis intoxication). Products include:
Lanoxicaps ... 772
Lanoxin Elixir Pediatric ... 775
Lanoxin Injection ... 778
Lanoxin Injection Pediatric ... 781
Lanoxin Tablets ... 783
Disopyramide Phosphate (Additive effect; may produce enhanced prolongation of conduction or depression of contractility and hypotension). Products include:
Norpace ... 2177
Glycopyrrolate (Additive antivagal effects on A-V nodal conduction). Products include:
Robinul Forte Tablets ... 1873
Robinul Injectable ... 1873
Robinul Tablets ... 1873
Hyoscyamine (Additive antivagal effects on A-V nodal conduction). Products include:
Cystospaz Tablets ... 2395
Urised Tablets ... 2396
Hyoscyamine Sulfate (Additive antivagal effects on A-V nodal conduction). Products include:
Arco-Lase Plus Tablets ... 607
Cystospaz-M Capsules ... 2395
Donnagel ... ■ 675
Donnagel-PG ... 1858
Donnatal ... 1858
Donnatal Extentabs ... 1859
Donnatal Tablets ... 1858
Donnazyme Tablets ... 1860
Kutrase Capsules ... 2146
Levsin/Levsinex ... 2147
Ru-Tuss Tablets ... 693
Ipratropium Bromide (Additive antivagal effects on A-V nodal conduction). Products include:
Atrovent Inhalation Aerosol ... 675
Lidocaine Hydrochloride (Additive effect; hypotension). Products include:
Anestacon Solution ... 2394
Bactine Antiseptic/Anesthetic First Aid Spray ... ■ 624
Decadron Phosphate with Xylocaine Injection, Sterile ... 1451
Xylocaine Injections ... 637
Xylocaine Injections for Ventricular Arrhythmias ... 639
Xylocaine 2% Jelly ... 643
4% Xylocaine-MPF Sterile Solution ... 641
Xylocaine 2% Viscous Solution ... 646
Mepenzolate Bromide (Additive antivagal effects on A-V nodal conduction). Products include:
Cantil Tablets ... 1326
Mexiletine Hydrochloride (Additive effect; hypotension). Products include:
Mexitil Capsules ... 680
Moricizine Hydrochloride (Additive effect; hypotension). Products include:
Ethmozine Tablets ... 946
Oxybutynin Chloride (Additive antivagal effects on A-V nodal conduction). Products include:
Ditropan ... 1332
Pancuronium Bromide Injection (Reduce neuromuscular blocker dosage).
No products indexed under this heading.
Procyclidine Hydrochloride (Additive antivagal effects on A-V nodal conduction). Products include:
Kemadrin Tablets ... 771
Propafenone Hydrochloride (Additive effect; hypotension). Products include:
Rythmol Tablets ... 1184
Propantheline Bromide (Additive antivagal effects on A-V nodal conduction). Products include:
Pro-Banthīne Tablets ... 2141
Propranolol Hydrochloride (Additive effect; hypotension). Products include:
Inderal ... 2459
Inderal LA Long Acting Capsules ... 2461
Inderide Tablets ... 2463
Inderide LA Long Acting Capsules ... 2465
Quinidine Gluconate (Additive effect; may produce enhanced prolongation of conduction or depression of contractility and hypotension). Products include:
Quinaglute Dura-Tabs Tablets ... 663
Quinidine Polygalacturonate (Additive effect; may produce enhanced prolongation of conduction or depression of contractility and hypotension). Products include:
Cardioquin Tablets ... 1812
Quinidine Sulfate (Additive effect; may produce enhanced prolongation of conduction or depression of contractility and hypotension). Products include:
Quinidex Extentabs ... 1868
Scopolamine Hydrobromide (Additive antivagal effects on A-V nodal conduction). Products include:
Donnagel ... ■ 675
Donnagel-PG ... 1858
Donnatal ... 1858
Donnatal Extentabs ... 1859
Donnatal Tablets ... 1858
Donnazyme Tablets ... 1860
Isopto Hyoscine ... ◉ 222
Murocoll-2 Sterile Ophthalmic Solution ... ◉ 261
Ru-Tuss Tablets ... 693
Scopolamine Preparations (Additive antivagal effects on A-V nodal conduction). Products include:
Transderm Scōp Transdermal Therapeutic System ... 887
Succinylcholine Chloride (Reduced acetylcholine release; reduced dosage of succinylcholine may be required). Products include:
Anectine ... 755
Tocainide Hydrochloride (Additive effect; hypotension). Products include:
Tonocard Tablets ... 1554
Tridihexethyl Chloride (Additive antivagal effects on A-V nodal conduction).
No products indexed under this heading.
Trihexyphenidyl Hydrochloride (Additive antivagal effects on A-V nodal conduction). Products include:
Artane ... 1195
Verapamil Hydrochloride (Additive effect; hypotension). Products include:
Calan SR Caplets ... 2157
Calan Tablets ... 2155
Isoptin Injectable ... 1177
Isoptin Oral Tablets ... 1179
Isoptin SR Sustained Release Tablets ... 1181
Verelan Capsules ... 1243
Verelan Capsules ... 2535

PRONESTYL INJECTION
(Procainamide Hydrochloride) ... 1798
May interact with type 1 antiarrhythmic drugs, antiarrhythmics, anticholinergics, and certain other agents. Compounds in these categories include:

Acebutolol Hydrochloride (Additive effects on the heart may occur with PA administration). Products include:
Sectral Capsules ... 2520
Adenosine (Additive effects on the heart may occur with PA administration). Products include:
Adenocard Injection ... 1007
Amiodarone Hydrochloride (Additive effects on the heart may occur with PA administration). Products include:
Cordarone Tablets ... 2446
Atropine Sulfate (Possible additive antivagal effects on A-V nodal conduction). Products include:
Arco-Lase Plus Tablets ... 607
Atropine Sulfate Sterile Ophthalmic Solution and S.O.P. Sterile Ophthalmic Ointment ... ◉ 239
Donnagel ... ■ 675
Donnagel-PG ... 1858
Donnatal ... 1858
Donnatal Extentabs ... 1859
Donnatal Tablets ... 1858
Donnazyme Tablets ... 1860
Isopto Atropine ... ◉ 218
Lomotil ... 2174
Motofen Tablets ... 836
Ru-Tuss Tablets ... 693
Urised Tablets ... 2396
Belladonna Alkaloids (Possible additive antivagal effects on A-V nodal conduction). Products include:
Bellergal-S Tablets ... 1998
Hyland's Bed Wetting Tablets ... ■ 728
Hyland's Teething Tablets ... ■ 728
Kinesed Tablets ... 2272
Benztropine Mesylate (Possible additive antivagal effects on A-V nodal conduction). Products include:
Cogentin ... 1435
Biperiden (Possible additive antivagal effects on A-V nodal conduction). Products include:
Akineton ... 1171
Bretylium Tosylate (Additive effects on the heart may occur with PA administration). Products include:
Bretylol Injection ... 923
Clidinium Bromide (Possible additive antivagal effects on A-V nodal conduction). Products include:
Librax Capsules ... 1929
Quarzan Capsules ... 1937
Dicyclomine Hydrochloride (Possible additive antivagal effects on A-V nodal conduction). Products include:
Bentyl ... 1322

Disopyramide Phosphate (Additive effects on the heart may occur with PA administration; may produce enhanced prolongation of conduction or depression of contractility and hypotension). Products include:

- Norpace 2177

Glycopyrrolate (Possible additive antivagal effects on A-V nodal conduction). Products include:

- Robinul Forte Tablets 1873
- Robinul Injectable 1873
- Robinul Tablets 1873

Hyoscyamine (Possible additive antivagal effects on A-V nodal conduction). Products include:

- Cystospaz Tablets 2395
- Urised Tablets 2396

Hyoscyamine Sulfate (Possible additive antivagal effects on A-V nodal conduction). Products include:

- Arco-Lase Plus Tablets 607
- Cystospaz-M Capsules 2395
- Donnagel .... ⊞ 675
- Donnagel-PG 1858
- Donnatal 1858
- Donnatal Extentabs 1859
- Donnatal Tablets 1858
- Donnazyme Tablets 1860
- Kutrase Capsules 2146
- Levsin/Levsinex 2147
- Ru-Tuss Tablets 693

Ipratropium Bromide (Possible additive antivagal effects on A-V nodal conduction). Products include:

- Atrovent Inhalation Aerosol 675

Lidocaine Hydrochloride (Additive effects on the heart may occur with PA administration). Products include:

- Anestacon Solution 2394
- Bactine Antiseptic/Anesthetic First Aid Spray .... ⊞ 624
- Decadron Phosphate with Xylocaine Injection, Sterile 1451
- Xylocaine Injections 637
- Xylocaine Injections for Ventricular Arrhythmias 639
- Xylocaine 2% Jelly 643
- 4% Xylocaine-MPF Sterile Solution 641
- Xylocaine 2% Viscous Solution 646

Mepenzolate Bromide (Possible additive antivagal effects on A-V nodal conduction). Products include:

- Cantil Tablets 1326

Mexiletine Hydrochloride (Additive effects on the heart may occur with PA administration). Products include:

- Mexitil Capsules 680

Moricizine Hydrochloride (Additive effects on the heart may occur with PA administration). Products include:

- Ethmozine Tablets 946

Oxybutynin Chloride (Possible additive antivagal effects on A-V nodal conduction). Products include:

- Ditropan 1332

Procyclidine Hydrochloride (Possible additive antivagal effects on A-V nodal conduction). Products include:

- Kemadrin Tablets 771

Propafenone Hydrochloride (Additive effects on the heart may occur with PA administration). Products include:

- Rythmol Tablets 1184

Propantheline Bromide (Possible additive antivagal effects on A-V nodal conduction). Products include:

- Pro-Banthīne Tablets 2141

Propranolol Hydrochloride (Additive effects on the heart may occur with PA administration). Products include:

- Inderal 2459
- Inderal LA Long Acting Capsules 2461
- Inderide Tablets 2463
- Inderide LA Long Acting Capsules 2465

Quinidine Gluconate (Additive effects on the heart may occur with PA administration; may produce enhanced prolongation of conduction or depression of contractility and hypotension). Products include:

- Quinaglute Dura-Tabs Tablets 663

Quinidine Polygalacturonate (Additive effects on the heart may occur with PA administration; may produce enhanced prolongation of conduction or depression of contractility and hypotension). Products include:

- Cardioquin Tablets 1812

Quinidine Sulfate (Additive effects on the heart may occur with PA administration; may produce enhanced prolongation of conduction or depression of contractility and hypotension). Products include:

- Quinidex Extentabs 1868

Scopolamine Hydrobromide (Possible additive antivagal effects on A-V nodal conduction). Products include:

- Donnagel .... ⊞ 675
- Donnagel-PG 1858
- Donnatal 1858
- Donnatal Extentabs 1859
- Donnatal Tablets 1858
- Donnazyme Tablets 1860
- Isopto Hyoscine .... ◉ 222
- Murocoll-2 Sterile Ophthalmic Solution .... ◉ 261
- Ru-Tuss Tablets 693

Scopolamine Preparations (Possible additive antivagal effects on A-V nodal conduction). Products include:

- Transderm Scōp Transdermal Therapeutic System 887

Succinylcholine Chloride (Concomitant administration may require reduced dose of neuromuscular blocking agent). Products include:

- Anectine 755

Tocainide Hydrochloride (Additive effects on the heart may occur with PA administration). Products include:

- Tonocard Tablets 1554

Tridihexethyl Chloride (Possible additive antivagal effects on A-V nodal conduction).

- No products indexed under this heading.

Trihexyphenidyl Hydrochloride (Possible additive antivagal effects on A-V nodal conduction). Products include:

- Artane 1195

Verapamil Hydrochloride (Additive effects on the heart may occur with PA administration). Products include:

- Calan SR Caplets 2157
- Calan Tablets 2155
- Isoptin Injectable 1177
- Isoptin Oral Tablets 1179
- Isoptin SR Sustained Release Tablets 1181
- Verelan Capsules 1243
- Verelan Capsules 2535

PRONESTYL-SR TABLETS
(Procainamide Hydrochloride) 1801
May interact with cardiac glycosides, antiarrhythmics, anticholinergics, and certain other agents. Compounds in these categories include:

Acebutolol Hydrochloride (May produce enhanced prolongation of conduction or depression of contractility and hypotension). Products include:

- Sectral Capsules 2520

Adenosine (May produce enhanced prolongation of conduction or depression of contractility and hypotension). Products include:

- Adenocard Injection 1007

Amiodarone Hydrochloride (May produce enhanced prolongation of conduction or depression of contractility and hypotension). Products include:

- Cordarone Tablets 2446

Atropine Sulfate (Additive antivagal effects on A-V nodal conduction). Products include:

- Arco-Lase Plus Tablets 607
- Atropine Sulfate Sterile Ophthalmic Solution and S.O.P. Sterile Ophthalmic Ointment .... ◉ 239
- Donnagel .... ⊞ 675
- Donnagel-PG 1858
- Donnatal 1858
- Donnatal Extentabs 1859
- Donnatal Tablets 1858
- Donnazyme Tablets 1860
- Isopto Atropine .... ◉ 218
- Lomotil 2174
- Motofen Tablets 836
- Ru-Tuss Tablets 693
- Urised Tablets 2396

Belladonna Alkaloids (Additive antivagal effects on A-V nodal conduction). Products include:

- Bellergal-S Tablets 1998
- Hyland's Bed Wetting Tablets .... ⊞ 728
- Hyland's Teething Tablets .... ⊞ 728
- Kinesed Tablets 2272

Benztropine Mesylate (Additive antivagal effects on A-V nodal conduction). Products include:

- Cogentin 1435

Biperiden (Additive antivagal effects on A-V nodal conduction). Products include:

- Akineton 1171

Bretylium Tosylate (May produce enhanced prolongation of conduction or depression of contractility and hypotension). Products include:

- Bretylol Injection 923

Clidinium Bromide (Additive antivagal effects on A-V nodal conduction). Products include:

- Librax Capsules 1929
- Quarzan Capsules 1937

Deslanoside (Caution should be exercised in arrhythmias associated with digitalis intoxication).

- No products indexed under this heading.

Dicyclomine Hydrochloride (Additive antivagal effects on A-V nodal conduction). Products include:

- Bentyl 1322

Digitoxin (Caution should be exercised in arrhythmias associated with digitalis intoxication). Products include:

- Crystodigin Tablets 1253

Digoxin (Caution should be exercised in arrhythmias associated with digitalis intoxication). Products include:

- Lanoxicaps 772
- Lanoxin Elixir Pediatric 775
- Lanoxin Injection 778
- Lanoxin Injection Pediatric 781
- Lanoxin Tablets 783

Disopyramide Phosphate (May produce enhanced prolongation of conduction or depression of contractility and hypotension). Products include:

- Norpace 2177

Ethopropazine Hydrochloride (Additive antivagal effects on A-V nodal conduction).

Glycopyrrolate (Additive antivagal effects on A-V nodal conduction). Products include:

- Robinul Forte Tablets 1873
- Robinul Injectable 1873
- Robinul Tablets 1873

Hyoscyamine (Additive antivagal effects on A-V nodal conduction). Products include:

- Cystospaz Tablets 2395
- Urised Tablets 2396

Hyoscyamine Sulfate (Additive antivagal effects on A-V nodal conduction). Products include:

- Arco-Lase Plus Tablets 607
- Cystospaz-M Capsules 2395
- Donnagel .... ⊞ 675
- Donnagel-PG 1858
- Donnatal 1858
- Donnatal Extentabs 1859
- Donnatal Tablets 1858
- Donnazyme Tablets 1860
- Kutrase Capsules 2146
- Levsin/Levsinex 2147
- Ru-Tuss Tablets 693

Ipratropium Bromide (Additive antivagal effects on A-V nodal conduction). Products include:

- Atrovent Inhalation Aerosol 675

Lidocaine Hydrochloride (May produce enhanced prolongation of conduction or depression of contractility and hypotension). Products include:

- Anestacon Solution 2394
- Bactine Antiseptic/Anesthetic First Aid Spray .... ⊞ 624
- Decadron Phosphate with Xylocaine Injection, Sterile 1451
- Xylocaine Injections 637
- Xylocaine Injections for Ventricular Arrhythmias 639
- Xylocaine 2% Jelly 643
- 4% Xylocaine-MPF Sterile Solution 641
- Xylocaine 2% Viscous Solution 646

Mepenzolate Bromide (Additive antivagal effects on A-V nodal conduction). Products include:

- Cantil Tablets 1326

Mexiletine Hydrochloride (May produce enhanced prolongation of conduction or depression of contractility and hypotension). Products include:

- Mexitil Capsules 680

Moricizine Hydrochloride (May produce enhanced prolongation of conduction or depression of contractility and hypotension). Products include:

- Ethmozine Tablets 946

Oxybutynin Chloride (Additive antivagal effects on A-V nodal conduction). Products include:

- Ditropan 1332

Oxyphenonium Bromide (Additive antivagal effects on A-V nodal conduction).

Procyclidine Hydrochloride (Additive antivagal effects on A-V nodal conduction). Products include:

- Kemadrin Tablets 771

Propafenone Hydrochloride (May produce enhanced prolongation of conduction or depression of contractility and hypotension). Products include:

- Rythmol Tablets 1184

Propantheline Bromide (Additive antivagal effects on A-V nodal conduction). Products include:

- Pro-Banthīne Tablets 2141

Propranolol Hydrochloride (May produce enhanced prolongation of conduction or depression of contractility and hypotension). Products include:

- Inderal 2459
- Inderal LA Long Acting Capsules 2461
- Inderide Tablets 2463
- Inderide LA Long Acting Capsules 2465

Quinidine Gluconate (May produce enhanced prolongation of conduction or depression of contractility and hypotension). Products include:
Quinaglute Dura-Tabs Tablets ... 663
Quinidine Polygalacturonate (May produce enhanced prolongation of conduction or depression of contractility and hypotension). Products include:
Cardioquin Tablets ... 1812
Quinidine Sulfate (May produce enhanced prolongation of conduction or depression of contractility and hypotension). Products include:
Quinidex Extentabs ... 1868
Scopolamine Hydrobromide (Additive antivagal effects on A-V nodal conduction). Products include:
Donnagel ... ■ 675
Donnagel-PG ... 1858
Donnatal ... 1858
Donnatal Extentabs ... 1859
Donnatal Tablets ... 1858
Donnazyme Tablets ... 1860
Isopto Hyoscine ... ⊙ 222
Murocoll-2 Sterile Ophthalmic Solution ... ⊙ 261
Ru-Tuss Tablets ... 693
Scopolamine Preparations (Additive antivagal effects on A-V nodal conduction). Products include:
Transderm Scōp Transdermal Therapeutic System ... 887
Succinylcholine Chloride (Reduced acetylcholine release). Products include:
Anectine ... 755
Tocainide Hydrochloride (May produce enhanced prolongation of conduction or depression of contractility and hypotension). Products include:
Tonocard Tablets ... 1554
Tridihexethyl Chloride (Additive antivagal effects on A-V nodal conduction).
No products indexed under this heading.
Trihexyphenidyl Hydrochloride (Additive antivagal effects on A-V nodal conduction). Products include:
Artane ... 1195
Verapamil Hydrochloride (May produce enhanced prolongation of conduction or depression of contractility and hypotension). Products include:
Calan SR Caplets ... 2157
Calan Tablets ... 2155
Isoptin Injectable ... 1177
Isoptin Oral Tablets ... 1179
Isoptin SR Sustained Release Tablets ... 1181
Verelan Capsules ... 1243
Verelan Capsules ... 2535

PROPAGEST
(Phenylpropanolamine Hydrochloride) ... 839
May interact with antihypertensives and antidepressant drugs. Compounds in these categories include:

Acebutolol Hydrochloride (Concurrent administration is not recommended). Products include:
Sectral Capsules ... 2520
Amitriptyline Hydrochloride (Concurrent administration is not recommended). Products include:
Elavil ... 2269
Endep Tablets ... 1927
Etrafon ... 2087
Limbitrol ... 1933
Triavil Tablets ... 1556
Amoxapine (Concurrent administration is not recommended). Products include:
Asendin Tablets ... 1196
Atenolol (Concurrent administration is not recommended). Products include:
Tenoretic Tablets ... 1105
Tenormin Tablets and I.V. Injection 1107
Benazepril Hydrochloride (Concurrent administration is not recommended). Products include:
Lotensin Tablets ... 872
Bendroflumethiazide (Concurrent administration is not recommended). Products include:
Corzide Tablets ... 702
Naturetin Tablets ... 1789
Rauzide Tablets ... 1804
Betaxolol Hydrochloride (Concurrent administration is not recommended). Products include:
Betoptic Sterile Ophthalmic Solution ... 569
Betoptic S Sterile Ophthalmic Suspension ... 570
Kerlone Tablets ... 2172
Bupropion Hydrochloride (Concurrent administration is not recommended). Products include:
Wellbutrin Tablets ... 821
Captopril (Concurrent administration is not recommended). Products include:
Capoten ... 2255
Capozide ... 2258
Carteolol Hydrochloride (Concurrent administration is not recommended). Products include:
Cartrol Tablets ... 507
Chlorothiazide (Concurrent administration is not recommended). Products include:
Aldoclor Tablets ... 1413
Diupres Tablets ... 1461
Diuril Oral ... 1464
Chlorothiazide Sodium (Concurrent administration is not recommended). Products include:
Diuril Sodium Intravenous ... 1463
Chlorthalidone (Concurrent administration is not recommended). Products include:
Combipres Tablets ... 678
Tenoretic Tablets ... 1105
Thalitone Tablets ... 687
Clonidine (Concurrent administration is not recommended). Products include:
Catapres-TTS ... 677
Clonidine Hydrochloride (Concurrent administration is not recommended). Products include:
Catapres Tablets ... 676
Combipres Tablets ... 678
Deserpidine (Concurrent administration is not recommended). Products include:
Enduronyl ... 518
Harmonyl Tablets ... 528
Oreticyl ... 545
Desipramine Hydrochloride (Concurrent administration is not recommended). Products include:
Norpramin Tablets ... 1340
Diazoxide (Concurrent administration is not recommended). Products include:
Hyperstat I.V. Injection ... 2095
Proglycem ... 649
Doxazosin Mesylate (Concurrent administration is not recommended). Products include:
Cardura Tablets ... 1941
Doxepin Hydrochloride (Concurrent administration is not recommended). Products include:
Sinequan ... 1960
Enalapril Maleate (Concurrent administration is not recommended). Products include:
Vaseretic Tablets ... 1559
Vasotec Tablets ... 1564
Enalaprilat (Concurrent administration is not recommended). Products include:
Vasotec I.V. ... 1562
Esmolol Hydrochloride (Concurrent administration is not recommended). Products include:
Brevibloc Injection ... 942
Felodipine (Concurrent administration is not recommended). Products include:
Plendil Extended-Release Tablets ... 1526
Fluoxetine Hydrochloride (Concurrent administration is not recommended). Products include:
Prozac Pulvules ... 920
Fosinopril Sodium (Concurrent administration is not recommended). Products include:
Monopril Tablets ... 1406
Furosemide (Concurrent administration is not recommended). Products include:
Lasix ... 1093
Guanabenz Acetate (Concurrent administration is not recommended). Products include:
Wytensin Tablets ... 2542
Guanethidine Monosulfate (Concurrent administration is not recommended). Products include:
Esimil Tablets ... 864
Ismelin Tablets ... 869
Hydralazine Hydrochloride (Concurrent administration is not recommended). Products include:
Apresazide Capsules ... 854
Apresoline Hydrochloride Parenteral (Ampuls) ... 856
Apresoline Hydrochloride Tablets ... 855
Apresoline-Esidrix Tablets ... 857
Ser-Ap-Es Tablets ... 881
Serpasil-Apresoline Tablets ... 884
Hydrochlorothiazide (Concurrent administration is not recommended). Products include:
Aldactazide ... 2150
Aldoril Tablets ... 1418
Apresazide Capsules ... 854
Apresoline-Esidrix Tablets ... 857
Capozide ... 2258
Dyazide Capsules ... 2208
Esidrix Tablets ... 863
Esimil Tablets ... 864
HydroDIURIL Tablets ... 1484
Hydropres Tablets ... 1485
Inderide Tablets ... 2463
Inderide LA Long Acting Capsules ... 2465
Lopressor HCT Tablets ... 1034
Maxzide ... 1215
Moduretic Tablets ... 1510
Normozide Tablets ... 2112
Oretic Tablets ... 544
Oreticyl ... 545
Prinzide Tablets ... 1540
Ser-Ap-Es Tablets ... 881
Serpasil-Esidrix Tablets ... 886
Timolide Tablets ... 1547
Trandate HCT Tablets ... 579
Vaseretic Tablets ... 1559
Zestoretic ... 2274
Hydroflumethiazide (Concurrent administration is not recommended). Products include:
Diucardin Tablets ... 2450
Saluron ... 718
Salutensin/Salutensin-Demi ... 719
Imipramine Hydrochloride (Concurrent administration is not recommended). Products include:
Tofranil Ampuls ... 1038
Tofranil Tablets ... 1039
Imipramine Pamoate (Concurrent administration is not recommended). Products include:
Tofranil-PM Capsules ... 1041
Indapamide (Concurrent administration is not recommended). Products include:
Lozol Tablets ... 1843
Isocarboxazid (Concurrent administration is not recommended). Products include:
Marplan Tablets ... 1906
Isradipine (Concurrent administration is not recommended). Products include:
DynaCirc Capsules ... 2004
Labetalol Hydrochloride (Concurrent administration is not recommended). Products include:
Normodyne Injection ... 2108
Normodyne Tablets ... 2110
Normozide Tablets ... 2112
Trandate HCT Tablets ... 579
Trandate Injection ... 577
Trandate Tablets ... 579
Lisinopril (Concurrent administration is not recommended). Products include:
Prinivil Tablets ... 1538
Prinzide Tablets ... 1540
Zestoretic ... 2274
Zestril Tablets ... 2277
Maprotiline Hydrochloride (Concurrent administration is not recommended). Products include:
Ludiomil Tablets ... 874
Mecamylamine Hydrochloride (Concurrent administration is not recommended). Products include:
Inversine Tablets ... 1492
Methyclothiazide (Concurrent administration is not recommended). Products include:
Enduron Tablets ... 517
Enduronyl ... 518
Methyldopa (Concurrent administration is not recommended). Products include:
Aldoclor Tablets ... 1413
Aldomet Oral ... 1415
Aldoril Tablets ... 1418
Methyldopate Hydrochloride (Concurrent administration is not recommended). Products include:
Aldomet Ester HCl Injection ... 1417
Metolazone (Concurrent administration is not recommended). Products include:
Diulo ... 2129
Mykrox ½ mg Tablets ... 984
Zaroxolyn Tablets ... 989
Metoprolol Tartrate (Concurrent administration is not recommended). Products include:
Lopressor Ampuls ... 1032
Lopressor HCT Tablets ... 1034
Lopressor Tablets ... 1032
Metyrosine (Concurrent administration is not recommended). Products include:
Demser Capsules ... 1460
Minoxidil (Concurrent administration is not recommended). Products include:
Loniten Tablets ... 2346
Rogaine Topical Solution ... 2357
Nadolol (Concurrent administration is not recommended). Products include:
Corgard Tablets ... 701
Corzide Tablets ... 702
Nicardipine Hydrochloride (Concurrent administration is not recommended). Products include:
Cardene Capsules ... 2290
Nitroglycerin (Concurrent administration is not recommended). Products include:
Deponit NTG Transdermal Delivery System ... 2143
Minitran Transdermal Delivery System ... 1312
Nitro-Bid Ointment ... 1339
Nitro-Bid Capsules ... 1338
Nitrodisc ... 2176
Nitro-Dur (nitroglycerin) Transdermal Infusion System ... 1164
Nitrogard Tablets ... 1004
Nitrolingual Spray ... 1846

Nitrostat Tablets 1743
Transderm-Nitro Transdermal Therapeutic System 2283

Nortriptyline Hydrochloride (Concurrent administration is not recommended). Products include:
Pamelor 2019

Penbutolol Sulfate (Concurrent administration is not recommended). Products include:
Levatol 1832

Phenelzine Sulfate (Concurrent administration is not recommended). Products include:
Nardil 1742

Phenoxybenzamine Hydrochloride (Concurrent administration is not recommended). Products include:
Dibenzyline Capsules 2207

Phentolamine Mesylate (Concurrent administration is not recommended). Products include:
Regitine 878

Pindolol (Concurrent administration is not recommended). Products include:
Visken Tablets 2036

Polythiazide (Concurrent administration is not recommended). Products include:
Minizide Capsules 1779
Renese Tablets 1785
Renese-R Tablets 1786

Prazosin Hydrochloride (Concurrent administration is not recommended). Products include:
Minipress Capsules 1778
Minizide Capsules 1779

Propranolol Hydrochloride (Concurrent administration is not recommended). Products include:
Inderal 2459
Inderal LA Long Acting Capsules 2461
Inderide Tablets 2463
Inderide LA Long Acting Capsules .. 2465

Protriptyline Hydrochloride (Concurrent administration is not recommended). Products include:
Vivactil Tablets 1567

Ramipril (Concurrent administration is not recommended). Products include:
Altace Capsules 1086

Rauwolfia Serpentina (Concurrent administration is not recommended). Products include:
Raudixin Tablets 1803
Rauzide Tablets 1804

Rescinnamine (Concurrent administration is not recommended).
No products indexed under this heading.

Reserpine (Concurrent administration is not recommended). Products include:
Diupres Tablets 1461
Hydromox R Tablets 1209
Hydropres Tablets 1485
Renese-R Tablets 1786
Salutensin/Salutensin-Demi 719
Ser-Ap-Es Tablets 881
Serpasil Tablets 883
Serpasil-Apresoline Tablets 884
Serpasil-Esidrix Tablets 886

Sodium Nitroprusside (Concurrent administration is not recommended). Products include:
Nipride I.V. Infusion 1909

Terazosin Hydrochloride (Concurrent administration is not recommended). Products include:
Hytrin Tablets 529

Timolol Maleate (Concurrent administration is not recommended). Products include:
Blocadren Tablets 1429
Timolide Tablets 1547
Timoptic in Ocudose 1552
Timoptic Sterile Ophthalmic Solution 1550

Tranylcypromine Sulfate (Concurrent administration is not recommended). Products include:
Parnate Tablets 2222

Trazodone Hydrochloride (Concurrent administration is not recommended). Products include:
Desyrel and Desyrel Dividose 1404

Trimethaphan Camsylate (Concurrent administration is not recommended). Products include:
Arfonad Ampuls 1887

Trimipramine Maleate (Concurrent administration is not recommended). Products include:
Surmontil Capsules 2524

PROPHYLLIN WET DRESSING POWDER AND OINTMENT
(Sodium Propionate, Chlorophyllin Copper Complex) 1995
No interactions described in labeling.

PROPINE WITH C CAP COMPLIANCE CAP
(Dipivefrin Hydrochloride) .... ⊛ 255
No interactions described in labeling.

PROSOM TABLETS
(Estazolam) 554
May interact with central nervous system depressants, anticonvulsants, antihistamines, barbiturates, monoamine oxidase inhibitors, narcotic analgesics, phenothiazines, and certain other agents. Compounds in these categories include:

Alcohol (Potentiates the action of benzodiazepines).

Alfentanil Hydrochloride (Potentiates the action of benzodiazepines). Products include:
Alfenta Injection 1131

Alprazolam (Potentiates the action of benzodiazepines). Products include:
Xanax Tablets 2367

Aprobarbital (Potentiates the action of benzodiazepines). Products include:
Alurate Elixir 1883

Astemizole (Potentiates the action of benzodiazepines). Products include:
Hismanal Tablets 1138

Azatadine Maleate (Potentiates the action of benzodiazepines). Products include:
Optimine Tablets 2115
Trinalin Repetabs Tablets 1170

Bromodiphenhydramine Hydrochloride (Potentiates the action of benzodiazepines).
No products indexed under this heading.

Brompheniramine Maleate (Potentiates the action of benzodiazepines). Products include:
Alka Seltzer Plus Sinus Allergy Medicine .... ▣ 624
Atrohist Sprinkle Capsules 558
Bromfed Capsules (Timed Release) 1615
Bromfed Syrup .... ▣ 628
Bromfed 1615
Dimetane Decongestant .... ▣ 673
Dimetane .... ▣ 672
Dimetane-DC Cough Syrup 1857
Dimetane-DX Cough Syrup 1858
Dimetapp Elixir .... ▣ 673
Dimetapp DM Elixir .... ▣ 674
Dimetapp Extentabs .... ▣ 674
Dimetapp Plus Caplets .... ▣ 675
Dimetapp Tablets .... ▣ 675
Drixoral Antihistamine/Nasal Decongestant Syrup .... ▣ 698

Buprenorphine (Potentiates the action of benzodiazepines).
No products indexed under this heading.

Buspirone Hydrochloride (Potentiates the action of benzodiazepines). Products include:
BuSpar 1401

Butabarbital (Potentiates the action of benzodiazepines). Products include:
Pyridium Plus 1764

Butalbital (Potentiates the action of benzodiazepines). Products include:
Esgic-Plus Tablets 1002
Esgic Tablets & Capsules 1001
Fioricet Tablets 2006
Fiorinal Capsules 2007
Fiorinal with Codeine Capsules 2008
Fiorinal Tablets 2007
Phrenilin 838
Sedapap Tablets 50 mg/650 mg .. 1360

Carbamazepine (Potentiates the action of benzodiazepines). Products include:
Tegretol Chewable Tablets 654
Tegretol Suspension 656
Tegretol Tablets 654

Chlordiazepoxide (Potentiates the action of benzodiazepines). Products include:
Libritabs Tablets 1930
Limbitrol 1933
Menrium Tablets 1934

Chlordiazepoxide Hydrochloride (Potentiates the action of benzodiazepines). Products include:
Librax Capsules 1929
Librium Capsules 1931
Librium Injectable 1932

Chlorpheniramine Maleate (Potentiates the action of benzodiazepines). Products include:
A.R.M. Allergy Relief Medicine Caplets .... ▣ 615
Alka-Seltzer Plus Cold Medicine .... ▣ 623
Allerest .... ▣ 559
Ana-Kit Anaphylaxis Emergency Treatment Kit 1100
BC Cold Powder Multi-Symptom Formula .... ▣ 517
Brexin L.A. Capsules 2078
Cerose-DM 2443
Cheracol Plus Head Cold/Cough Formula .... ▣ 667
Chlor-Trimeton Allergy Syrup, Tablets & Long-Acting Repetabs Tablets .... ▣ 693
Chlor-Trimeton Decongestant .... ▣ 694
Comhist LA Capsules 1618
Allergy-Sinus Comtrex Multi-Symptom Allergy Sinus Formula Tablets & Caplets 746
Comtrex Multi-Symptom Cold Reliever Tablets/Caplets/Liqui-Gels/Liquid 745
Day-Night Comtrex 747
Contac Continuous Action Decongestant/Antihistamine Capsules ▣ 710
Contac Maximum Strength Continuous Action Decongestant/Antihistamine Caplets .... ▣ 709
Contac Severe Cold and Flu Formula Caplets .... ▣ 711
Coricidin 'D' Decongestant Tablets .... ▣ 695
Coricidin Demilets Tablets for Children .... ▣ 696
Coricidin Tablets .... ▣ 695
Deconamine 663
Demazin Nasal Decongestant/Antihistamine Repetabs Tablets & Syrup .... ▣ 697
Dorcol Children's Liquid Cold Formula .... ▣ 686
Dristan Decongestant/Antihistamine/ Analgesic Coated Caplets .... ▣ 749
Dristan Cold Nasal Decongestant/Antihistamine/ Analgesic Coated Tablets 2419
Dristan Advanced Formula Decongestant/Antihistamine/ Analgesic Tablets .... ▣ 749
Extendryl 994
4-Way Cold Tablets 750
Fedahist Gyrocaps 2145
Fedahist Timecaps 2145
Hycomine Compound Tablets 929
Isoclor Timesule Capsules .... ▣ 561
Kronofed-A 970
Medi-Flu Caplet, Liquid .... ▣ 640
Naldecon Syrup, Tablets, Pediatric Drops and Pediatric Syrup 709
Nolamine Tablets 838
Novafed A Capsules 1342
Novahistine DH 1342
Novahistine Elixir .... ▣ 596
Ornade Spansule Capsules 2221
Orthoxicol Cough Syrup .... ▣ 668
PediaCare Allergy Relief Formula Liquid 1362
PediaCare Cough-Cold Formula Liquid 1362
PediaCare Night Rest Cough-Cold Formula Liquid 1362
PediaCare 6-12 Cough-Cold Formula Chewable Tablets 1362
Pyrroxate Capsules .... ▣ 669
Quelidrine Syrup 556
Ru-Tuss II Capsules 693
Ru-Tuss Tablets 693
Ryna .... ▣ 741
Sinarest Tablets & Extra Strength Tablets .... ▣ 562
Sine-Off Maximum Strength Allergy/Sinus Formula Caplets .... ▣ 721
Sine-Off Sinus Medicine Tablets-Aspirin Formula .... ▣ 722
Singlet Tablets .... ▣ 598
Sinulin 840
Sinutab Maximum Strength .... ▣ 641
St. Joseph Nighttime Cold Medicine .... ▣ 705
Sudafed Plus Liquid .... ▣ 544
Sudafed Plus Tablets .... ▣ 545
Teldrin Timed-Release Allergy Capsules, 12 mg 2192
TheraFlu Flu and Cold Medicine .... ▣ 687
Triaminic Allergy Tablets .... ▣ 688
Triaminic Chewables .... ▣ 688
Triaminic Cold Tablets .... ▣ 688
Triaminic Nite Light .... ▣ 689
Triaminic Syrup .... ▣ 689
Triaminic-12 Tablets .... ▣ 690
Triaminicin Tablets .... ▣ 690
Triaminicol Multi-Symptom Cold Tablets .... ▣ 691
Triaminicol Multi-Symptom Relief ▣ 691
Tylenol Allergy Sinus Medication Caplets and Gelcaps, Maximum Strength 1372
Children's Tylenol Cold Liquid Formula and Chewable Tablets 1368
Tylenol Cold & Flu Hot Medication, Packets 1369
Tylenol Cold Medication Caplets and Tablets 1370
Tylenol Cold Medication, Effervescent Tablets 1369
Vicks Children's NyQuil .... ▣ 664
Vicks Formula 44 Cough Medicine .... ▣ 661
Vicks Formula 44M Multi-Symptom Cough Medicine .... ▣ 662
Vicks Pediatric Formula 44m Multi-Symptom Cough & Cold Medicine .... ▣ 663

Chlorpheniramine Polistirex (Potentiates the action of benzodiazepines). Products include:
Tussionex Extended-Release Suspension 988

Chlorpheniramine Tannate (Potentiates the action of benzodiazepines). Products include:
Rynatan 2387
Rynatuss 2388

Chlorpromazine (Potentiates the action of benzodiazepines). Products include:
Thorazine 2234

Chlorprothixene (Potentiates the action of benzodiazepines). Products include:
Taractan Tablets 1920

Chlorprothixene Hydrochloride (Potentiates the action of benzodiazepines). Products include:
Taractan 1920

Clemastine Fumarate (Potentiates the action of benzodiazepines). Products include:
Tavist Syrup 2033
Tavist Tablets 2035
Tavist-D Tablets 2035

Clorazepate Dipotassium (Potentiates the action of benzodiazepines). Products include:
Tranxene 556

Codeine (Potentiates the action of benzodiazepines). Products include:
Calcidrine Syrup 506

Codeine Phosphate (Potentiates the action of benzodiazepines). Products include:
Actifed with Codeine Cough Syrup 752
Cheracol Cough Syrup 1853
Codimal PH Syrup 846
Dimetane-DC Cough Syrup 1857
Empirin with Codeine Phosphate Nos. 2, 3 & 4 764
Fiorinal with Codeine Capsules 2008
Isoclor Expectorant 982
Naldecon CX Adult Liquid ■ 521
Novahistine DH 1342
Novahistine Expectorant 1343
Nucofed Capsules 2219
Nucofed Expectorant 2219
Nucofed Pediatric Expectorant 2220
Nucofed Syrup 2219
Phenaphen with Codeine Capsules 1865
Phenaphen-650 with Codeine Tablets 1866
Phenergan with Codeine 2497
Phenergan VC with Codeine 2501
Robitussin A-C Syrup 1875
Robitussin-DAC Syrup 1875
Ryna ■ 741
Soma Compound w/Codeine Tablets 2390
Triaminic Expectorant w/Codeine 1996
Tussi-Organidin Liquid 2391
Tylenol with Codeine 1381

Codeine Polistirex (Potentiates the action of benzodiazepines).
No products indexed under this heading.

Cyproheptadine Hydrochloride (Potentiates the action of benzodiazepines). Products include:
Periactin 1525

Dexchlorpheniramine Maleate (Potentiates the action of benzodiazepines). Products include:
Polaramine 2116

Dezocine (Potentiates the action of benzodiazepines).

Diazepam (Potentiates the action of benzodiazepines). Products include:
Valium Injectable 1937
Valium Tablets 1939
Valrelease Capsules 1923

Diphenhydramine Citrate (Potentiates the action of benzodiazepines). Products include:
Alka-Seltzer Plus Night-Time Cold Medicine ■ 623
Bufferin AF Nite Time Analgesic/Sleeping Aid Caplets 744
Excedrin P.M. Analgesic/Sleeping Aid Tablets, Caplets and Liquid 749

Diphenhydramine Hydrochloride (Potentiates the action of benzodiazepines). Products include:
Benadryl Anti-Itch Cream ■ 635
Benadryl Capsules 1691
Benadryl Decongestant Elixir ■ 635
Benadryl Decongestant ■ 635
Benadryl Elixir ■ 636
Benadryl Kapseals 1691
Benadryl 25 Kapseals ■ 636
Benadryl Parenteral 1692
Benadryl Plus ■ 636
Benadryl Plus Nighttime ■ 637
Benadryl Spray, Maximum Strength ■ 637
Benadryl Spray, Regular Strength ■ 637
Benadryl Steri-Vials, Ampoules, and Steri-Dose Syringe 1692
Benadryl 25 Tablets ■ 636
Benylin Cough Syrup ■ 637
Benylin Decongestant ■ 638
Caladryl Cream, Lotion, Spray ■ 638
Miles Nervine Nighttime Sleep-Aid ■ 627
Nytol Tablets ■ 517
Sleep-ettes-D Tablets ■ 653
Sleep-eze 3 Tablets ■ 755
Sleepinal Night-time Sleep Aid Capsules ■ 734
Sominex Caplets and Tablets ■ 722
Sominex Liquid ■ 723
Sominex Pain Relief Formula ■ 723
Tylenol Cold Night Time Medication Liquid 1371
Tylenol PM, Extra Strength Caplets and Tablets 1368
Unisom Dual Relief Nighttime Sleep Aid/Analgesic 1774
Ziradryl Lotion ■ 643

Diphenylpyraline Hydrochloride (Potentiates the action of benzodiazepines).
No products indexed under this heading.

Divalproex Sodium (Potentiates the action of benzodiazepines). Products include:
Depakote 512

Droperidol (Potentiates the action of benzodiazepines). Products include:
Inapsine Injection 1140
Innovar Injection 1141

Enflurane (Potentiates the action of benzodiazepines). Products include:
Ethrane 599

Ethchlorvynol (Potentiates the action of benzodiazepines). Products include:
Placidyl Capsules 553

Ethinamate (Potentiates the action of benzodiazepines).
No products indexed under this heading.

Ethosuximide (Potentiates the action of benzodiazepines). Products include:
Zarontin Capsules 1768
Zarontin Syrup 1769

Ethotoin (Potentiates the action of benzodiazepines). Products include:
Peganone Tablets 551

Fentanyl (Potentiates the action of benzodiazepines). Products include:
Duragesic Transdermal System 1133

Fentanyl Citrate (Potentiates the action of benzodiazepines). Products include:
Innovar Injection 1141
Sublimaze Injection 1146

Fluphenazine Decanoate (Potentiates the action of benzodiazepines). Products include:
Prolixin Decanoate 1795

Fluphenazine Enanthate (Potentiates the action of benzodiazepines). Products include:
Prolixin Enanthate 1796

Fluphenazine Hydrochloride (Potentiates the action of benzodiazepines). Products include:
Prolixin Elixir 1793
Prolixin Injection 1791
Prolixin Oral Concentrate 1792
Prolixin Tablets 1793

Flurazepam Hydrochloride (Potentiates the action of benzodiazepines). Products include:
Dalmane Capsules 1927

Furazolidone (Potentiates the action of benzodiazepines). Products include:
Furoxone 1855

Glutethimide (Potentiates the action of benzodiazepines).
No products indexed under this heading.

Haloperidol (Potentiates the action of benzodiazepines). Products include:
Haldol Injection, Tablets and Concentrate 1373

Haloperidol Decanoate (Potentiates the action of benzodiazepines). Products include:
Haldol Decanoate 1375

Hydrocodone Bitartrate (Potentiates the action of benzodiazepines). Products include:
Anexsia 5/500 Tablets 2196
Anexsia 7.5/650 Tablets 2197
Azdone Tablets 844
Codiclear DH Syrup 845
Codimal DH Syrup 846
Damason-P 1356
Hycodan Syrup, Tablets 927
Hycomine Compound Tablets 929
Hycomine Syrup 927
Hycotuss Expectorant Syrup 930
Hydrocet Capsules 835
Lortab ASA Tablets 2414
Lortab 2412
Ru-Tuss with Hydrocodone 694
Triaminic Expectorant DH 1995
Vicodin Tablets 1187
Vicodin ES Tablets 1189
Zydone Capsules 941

Hydrocodone Polistirex (Potentiates the action of benzodiazepines). Products include:
Tussionex Extended-Release Suspension 988

Hydroxyzine Hydrochloride (Potentiates the action of benzodiazepines). Products include:
Atarax Tablets & Syrup 1941
Marax Tablets & DF Syrup 1954
Vistaril Intramuscular Solution 1970

Isocarboxazid (Potentiates the action of benzodiazepines). Products include:
Marplan Tablets 1906

Isoflurane (Potentiates the action of benzodiazepines). Products include:
Forane 600

Ketamine Hydrochloride (Potentiates the action of benzodiazepines). Products include:
Ketalar 1726

Levorphanol Tartrate (Potentiates the action of benzodiazepines). Products include:
Levo-Dromoran 1906

Lorazepam (Potentiates the action of benzodiazepines). Products include:
Ativan Injection 2432
Ativan Tablets 2434

Loxapine Hydrochloride (Potentiates the action of benzodiazepines). Products include:
Loxitane 1213

Loxapine Succinate (Potentiates the action of benzodiazepines). Products include:
Loxitane Capsules 1213

Meperidine Hydrochloride (Potentiates the action of benzodiazepines). Products include:
Demerol 2047
Mepergan Injection 2479

Mephenytoin (Potentiates the action of benzodiazepines). Products include:
Mesantoin Tablets 2013

Mephobarbital (Potentiates the action of benzodiazepines). Products include:
Mebaral Tablets 2061

Meprobamate (Potentiates the action of benzodiazepines). Products include:
Deprol Tablets 2382
Equagesic Tablets 2451
Miltown Tablets 2386
PMB 200 and PMB 400 2504

Mesoridazine (Potentiates the action of benzodiazepines). Products include:
Serentil 686

Mesoridazine Besylate (Potentiates the action of benzodiazepines).

Methadone Hydrochloride (Potentiates the action of benzodiazepines). Products include:
Dolophine Hydrochloride Ampoules & Vials 1260
Dolophine Hydrochloride Tablets 1261
Methadone Hydrochloride Diskets 1284
Methadone Hydrochloride Oral Solution & Tablets 1987

Methdilazine Hydrochloride (Potentiates the action of benzodiazepines). Products include:
Tacaryl Syrup & Tablets 2409

Methohexital Sodium (Potentiates the action of benzodiazepines). Products include:
Brevital Sodium Vials 1248

Methoxyflurane (Potentiates the action of benzodiazepines).
No products indexed under this heading.

Methsuximide (Potentiates the action of benzodiazepines). Products include:
Celontin 1692

Midazolam Hydrochloride (Potentiates the action of benzodiazepines). Products include:
Versed Injection 1924

Molindone Hydrochloride (Potentiates the action of benzodiazepines). Products include:
Moban Tablets & Concentrate 932

Morphine Sulfate (Potentiates the action of benzodiazepines). Products include:
Astramorph/PF Injection, USP (Preservative-Free) 618
Duramorph 960
Infumorph 200 and Infumorph 500 Sterile Solutions 962
MS Contin Tablets 1814
MSIR 1817
Oramorph SR (Morphine Sulfate Sustained Release Tablets) 1988
Roxanol 1991

Opium Alkaloids (Potentiates the action of benzodiazepines). Products include:
B & O No. 15A & No. 16A Supprettes 2395
Pantopon Injectable 1911

Oxazepam (Potentiates the action of benzodiazepines). Products include:
Serax Capsules 2522
Serax Tablets 2522

Oxycodone Hydrochloride (Potentiates the action of benzodiazepines). Products include:
Percocet Tablets 950
Percodan 951
Roxicodone Tablets, Oral Solution & Intensol (Oxycodone) 1992
Tylox Capsules 1382

Paramethadione (Potentiates the action of benzodiazepines). Products include:
Paradione Capsules 548

Pentobarbital Sodium (Potentiates the action of benzodiazepines). Products include:
Nembutal Sodium Capsules 534
Nembutal Sodium Solution 536
Nembutal Sodium Suppositories 538

Perphenazine (Potentiates the action of benzodiazepines). Products include:
Etrafon 2087
Triavil Tablets 1556
Trilafon 2123

Phenacemide (Potentiates the action of benzodiazepines). Products include:
- Phenurone Tablets ... 552

Phenelzine Sulfate (Potentiates the action of benzodiazepines). Products include:
- Nardil ... 1742

Phenobarbital (Potentiates the action of benzodiazepines). Products include:
- Arco-Lase Plus Tablets ... 607
- Bellergal-S Tablets ... 1998
- Bronkolixir ... ⊡ 761
- Bronkotabs Tablets ... ⊡ 762
- Donnatal ... 1858
- Donnatal Extentabs ... 1859
- Donnatal Tablets ... 1858
- Donnazyme Tablets ... 1860
- Kinesed Tablets ... 2272
- Phenobarbital Elixir and Tablets ... 1293
- Primatene Tablets-P Formula ... 2421
- Quadrinal Tablets ... 1183
- Tedral SA ... 1765

Phensuximide (Potentiates the action of benzodiazepines). Products include:
- Milontin Kapseals ... 1741

Phenytoin (Potentiates the action of benzodiazepines). Products include:
- Dilantin Infatabs ... 1710
- Dilantin-30 Pediatric/Dilantin-125 Suspension ... 1713

Phenytoin Sodium (Potentiates the action of benzodiazepines). Products include:
- Dilantin Kapseals ... 1708
- Dilantin Parenteral ... 1712
- Dilantin with Phenobarbital Kapseals ... 1715

Prazepam (Potentiates the action of benzodiazepines). Products include:
- Centrax ... 1693

Primidone (Potentiates the action of benzodiazepines). Products include:
- Mysoline ... 2480

Prochlorperazine (Potentiates the action of benzodiazepines). Products include:
- Compazine ... 2201

Promethazine Hydrochloride (Potentiates the action of benzodiazepines). Products include:
- Mepergan Injection ... 2479
- Phenergan with Codeine ... 2497
- Phenergan with Dextromethorphan 2499
- Phenergan Injection ... 2493
- Phenergan Suppositories ... 2496
- Phenergan Syrup ... 2495
- Phenergan Tablets ... 2496
- Phenergan VC ... 2500
- Phenergan VC with Codeine ... 2501

Propofol (Potentiates the action of benzodiazepines). Products include:
- Diprivan Injection ... 2267

Propoxyphene Hydrochloride (Potentiates the action of benzodiazepines). Products include:
- Darvon ... 1256
- Wygesic Tablets ... 2540

Propoxyphene Napsylate (Potentiates the action of benzodiazepines). Products include:
- Darvon-N/Darvocet-N ... 1254

Pyrilamine Maleate (Potentiates the action of benzodiazepines). Products include:
- Codimal ... 846
- 4-Way Fast Acting Nasal Spray - Original Formula (regular & mentholated) & Metered Spray Pump (regular) ... 751
- Maximum Strength Midol Multi-Symptom Menstrual Formula ... ⊡ 571
- Maximum Strength Midol PMS Premenstrual Syndrome Formula ... ⊡ 570
- Regular Strength Midol Multi-Symptom Menstrual Formula ... ⊡ 570
- Prefrin-A ... ⊙ 255
- Prēmsyn PMS Capsules & Caplets ⊡ 547
- Primatene Tablets-M Formula ... 2421
- Robitussin Night Relief ... ⊡ 677
- Ru-Tuss with Hydrocodone ... 694
- Triaminic Expectorant DH ... 1995
- Triaminic Oral Infant Drops ... 1996

Pyrilamine Tannate (Potentiates the action of benzodiazepines). Products include:
- Rynatan ... 2387

Quazepam (Potentiates the action of benzodiazepines). Products include:
- Doral Tablets ... 2383

Secobarbital Sodium (Potentiates the action of benzodiazepines). Products include:
- Seconal Sodium Pulvules ... 1296

Selegiline Hydrochloride (Potentiates the action of benzodiazepines). Products include:
- Eldepryl ... 2250

Sufentanil Citrate (Potentiates the action of benzodiazepines). Products include:
- Sufenta Injection ... 1147

Temazepam (Potentiates the action of benzodiazepines). Products include:
- Restoril Capsules ... 2023

Terfenadine (Potentiates the action of benzodiazepines). Products include:
- Seldane Tablets ... 1349
- Seldane-D Extended-Release Tablets ... 1350

Thiamylal Sodium (Potentiates the action of benzodiazepines). Products include:
- Surital Ampoules, Steri-Vials ... 1764

Thioridazine Hydrochloride (Potentiates the action of benzodiazepines). Products include:
- Mellaril ... 2011

Thiothixene (Potentiates the action of benzodiazepines). Products include:
- Navane Capsules and Concentrate 1954
- Navane Intramuscular ... 1956

Tranylcypromine Sulfate (Potentiates the action of benzodiazepines). Products include:
- Parnate Tablets ... 2222

Triazolam (Potentiates the action of benzodiazepines). Products include:
- Halcion Tablets ... 2340

Trifluoperazine Hydrochloride (Potentiates the action of benzodiazepines). Products include:
- Stelazine ... 2226

Trimeprazine Tartrate (Potentiates the action of benzodiazepines). Products include:
- Temaril Tablets, Syrup and Spansule Sustained Release Capsules 1085

Trimethadione (Potentiates the action of benzodiazepines). Products include:
- Tridione ... 557

Tripelennamine Hydrochloride (Potentiates the action of benzodiazepines). Products include:
- PBZ Tablets & Elixir ... 1037
- PBZ-SR Tablets ... 1037

Triprolidine Hydrochloride (Potentiates the action of benzodiazepines). Products include:
- Actidil ... ⊡ 538
- Actifed Capsules ... ⊡ 539
- Actifed Plus Caplets ... ⊡ 539
- Actifed Plus Tablets ... ⊡ 540
- Actifed with Codeine Cough Syrup.. 752
- Actifed Syrup ... ⊡ 540
- Actifed Tablets ... ⊡ 540
- Actifed 12-Hour Capsules ... ⊡ 539

Valproic Acid (Potentiates the action of benzodiazepines). Products include:
- Depakene Capsules & Syrup ... 511

PROSTIGMIN INJECTABLE
(Neostigmine Methylsulfate) ... 1120
May interact with antiarrhythmics, general anesthetics, and certain other agents. Compounds in these categories include:

Acebutolol Hydrochloride (Interferes with neuromuscular transmission). Products include:
- Sectral Capsules ... 2520

Adenosine (Interferes with neuromuscular transmission). Products include:
- Adenocard Injection ... 1007

Amiodarone Hydrochloride (Interferes with neuromuscular transmission). Products include:
- Cordarone Tablets ... 2446

Bretylium Tosylate (Interferes with neuromuscular transmission). Products include:
- Bretylol Injection ... 923

Decamethonium (Phase I block of depolarizing muscle relaxants may be prolonged).

Disopyramide Phosphate (Interferes with neuromuscular transmission). Products include:
- Norpace ... 2177

Enflurane (Caution should be exercised if used concurrently in myasthenia gravis). Products include:
- Ethrane ... 599

Isoflurane (Caution should be exercised if used concurrently in myasthenia gravis). Products include:
- Forane ... 600

Kanamycin Sulfate (May accentuate neuromuscular block). Products include:
- Kantrex Injection ... 601
- Kantrex Pediatric Injection ... 601

Ketamine Hydrochloride (Caution should be exercised if used concurrently in myasthenia gravis). Products include:
- Ketalar ... 1726

Lidocaine Hydrochloride (Interferes with neuromuscular transmission). Products include:
- Anestacon Solution ... 2394
- Bactine Antiseptic/Anesthetic First Aid Spray ... ⊡ 624
- Decadron Phosphate with Xylocaine Injection, Sterile ... 1451
- Xylocaine Injections ... 637
- Xylocaine Injections for Ventricular Arrhythmias ... 639
- Xylocaine 2% Jelly ... 643
- 4% Xylocaine-MPF Sterile Solution 641
- Xylocaine 2% Viscous Solution ... 646

Local Anesthetics (Prostigmin dosage increase may be required).

Methohexital Sodium (Caution should be exercised if used concurrently in myasthenia gravis). Products include:
- Brevital Sodium Vials ... 1248

Methoxyflurane (Caution should be exercised if used concurrently in myasthenia gravis).
- No products indexed under this heading.

Mexiletine Hydrochloride (Interferes with neuromuscular transmission). Products include:
- Mexitil Capsules ... 680

Moricizine Hydrochloride (Interferes with neuromuscular transmission). Products include:
- Ethmozine Tablets ... 946

Neomycin Sulfate (May accentuate neuromuscular block). Products include:
- AK-Spore H.C. ... ⊙ 206
- AK-Spore ... ⊙ 205
- AK-Trol Ointment & Suspension ... ⊙ 207
- Bactine First Aid Antibiotic Ointment ... ⊡ 625
- Campho-Phenique Triple Antibiotic Ointment Plus Pain Reliever ⊡ 758
- Coly-Mycin S Otic w/Neomycin & Hydrocortisone ... 1708
- Cortisporin Cream ... 757
- Cortisporin Ointment ... 758
- Cortisporin Ophthalmic Ointment Sterile ... 758
- Cortisporin Ophthalmic Suspension Sterile ... 759
- Cortisporin Otic Solution Sterile ... 760
- Cortisporin Otic Suspension Sterile 760
- Dexacidin ... ⊙ 272
- Lanabiotic Ointment ... ⊡ 556
- LazerSporin-C Solution ... 1770
- Maxitrol Ophthalmic Ointment/Suspension ... ⊙ 223
- Myciguent Antibiotic Ointment ... ⊡ 737
- Mycitracin ... ⊡ 737
- NeoDecadron Sterile Ophthalmic Ointment ... 1517
- NeoDecadron Sterile Ophthalmic Solution ... 1518
- NeoDecadron Topical Cream ... 1518
- Neosporin Cream ... 792
- Neosporin G.U. Irrigant Sterile ... 793
- Neosporin Ointment ... 793
- Maximum Strength Neosporin Ointment ... 793
- Neosporin Ophthalmic Ointment Sterile ... 793
- Neosporin Ophthalmic Solution Sterile ... 794
- Neo-Synalar Cream ... 2296
- PediOtic Suspension Sterile ... 797
- Poly-Pred Liquifilm ... ⊙ 250

Procainamide Hydrochloride (Interferes with neuromuscular transmission). Products include:
- Procan SR Tablets ... 1760
- Pronestyl Capsules and Tablets ... 1800
- Pronestyl Injection ... 1798
- Pronestyl-SR Tablets ... 1801

Propafenone Hydrochloride (Interferes with neuromuscular transmission). Products include:
- Rythmol Tablets ... 1184

Propofol (Caution should be exercised if used concurrently in myasthenia gravis). Products include:
- Diprivan Injection ... 2267

Propranolol Hydrochloride (Interferes with neuromuscular transmission). Products include:
- Inderal ... 2459
- Inderal LA Long Acting Capsules ... 2461
- Inderide Tablets ... 2463
- Inderide LA Long Acting Capsules .. 2465

Quinidine Gluconate (Interferes with neuromuscular transmission). Products include:
- Quinaglute Dura-Tabs Tablets ... 663

Quinidine Polygalacturonate (Interferes with neuromuscular transmission). Products include:
- Cardioquin Tablets ... 1812

Quinidine Sulfate (Interferes with neuromuscular transmission). Products include:
- Quinidex Extentabs ... 1868

Streptomycin Sulfate (May accentuate neuromuscular block).
- No products indexed under this heading.

Succinylcholine Chloride (Phase I block of depolarizing muscle relaxants may be prolonged). Products include:
- Anectine ... 755

Tocainide Hydrochloride (Interferes with neuromuscular transmission). Products include:
- Tonocard Tablets ... 1554

Verapamil Hydrochloride (Interferes with neuromuscular transmission). Products include:
Calan SR Caplets 2157
Calan Tablets 2155
Isoptin Injectable 1177
Isoptin Oral Tablets 1179
Isoptin SR Sustained Release Tablets 1181
Verelan Capsules 1243
Verelan Capsules 2535

PROSTIGMIN TABLETS
(Neostigmine Methylsulfate) 1121
May interact with anticholinergics, antiarrhythmics, and certain other agents. Compounds in these categories include:

Acebutolol Hydrochloride (Interferes with neuromuscular transmission). Products include:
Sectral Capsules 2520

Adenosine (Interferes with neuromuscular transmission). Products include:
Adenocard Injection 1007

Amiodarone Hydrochloride (Interferes with neuromuscular transmission). Products include:
Cordarone Tablets 2446

Atropine Sulfate (Decreased intestinal motility). Products include:
Arco-Lase Plus Tablets 607
Atropine Sulfate Sterile Ophthalmic Solution and S.O.P. Sterile Ophthalmic Ointment .... ◉ 239
Donnagel .... ■ 675
Donnagel-PG 1858
Donnatal 1858
Donnatal Extentabs 1859
Donnatal Tablets 1858
Donnazyme Tablets 1860
Isopto Atropine .... ◉ 218
Lomotil 2174
Motofen Tablets 836
Ru-Tuss Tablets 693
Urised Tablets 2396

Belladonna Alkaloids (Decreased intestinal motility). Products include:
Bellergal-S Tablets 1998
Hyland's Bed Wetting Tablets .... ■ 728
Hyland's Teething Tablets .... ■ 728
Kinesed Tablets 2272

Benztropine Mesylate (Decreased intestinal motility). Products include:
Cogentin 1435

Biperiden (Decreased intestinal motility). Products include:
Akineton 1171

Bretylium Tosylate (Interferes with neuromuscular transmission). Products include:
Bretylol Injection 923

Clidinium Bromide (Decreased intestinal motility). Products include:
Librax Capsules 1929
Quarzan Capsules 1937

Dicyclomine Hydrochloride (Decreased intestinal motility). Products include:
Bentyl 1322

Disopyramide Phosphate (Interferes with neuromuscular transmission). Products include:
Norpace 2177

Ethopropazine Hydrochloride (Decreased intestinal motility).

Glycopyrrolate (Decreased intestinal motility). Products include:
Robinul Forte Tablets 1873
Robinul Injectable 1873
Robinul Tablets 1873

Hyoscyamine (Decreased intestinal motility). Products include:
Cystospaz Tablets 2395
Urised Tablets 2396

Hyoscyamine Sulfate (Decreased intestinal motility). Products include:
Arco-Lase Plus Tablets 607
Cystospaz-M Capsules 2395
Donnagel .... ■ 675
Donnagel-PG 1858
Donnatal 1858
Donnatal Extentabs 1859
Donnatal Tablets 1858
Donnazyme Tablets 1860
Kutrase Capsules 2146
Levsin/Levsinex 2147
Ru-Tuss Tablets 693

Ipratropium Bromide (Decreased intestinal motility). Products include:
Atrovent Inhalation Aerosol 675

Kanamycin Sulfate (May accentuate neuromuscular block). Products include:
Kantrex Injection 601
Kantrex Pediatric Injection 601

Lidocaine Hydrochloride (Interferes with neuromuscular transmission). Products include:
Anestacon Solution 2394
Bactine Antiseptic/Anesthetic First Aid Spray .... ■ 624
Decadron Phosphate with Xylocaine Injection, Sterile 1451
Xylocaine Injections 637
Xylocaine Injections for Ventricular Arrhythmias 639
Xylocaine 2% Jelly 643
4% Xylocaine-MPF Sterile Solution 641
Xylocaine 2% Viscous Solution 646

Local Anesthetics (Prostigmin dosage increase may be required).

Mepenzolate Bromide (Decreased intestinal motility). Products include:
Cantil Tablets 1326

Mexiletine Hydrochloride (Interferes with neuromuscular transmission). Products include:
Mexitil Capsules 680

Moricizine Hydrochloride (Interferes with neuromuscular transmission). Products include:
Ethmozine Tablets 946

Oxybutynin Chloride (Decreased intestinal motility). Products include:
Ditropan 1332

Oxyphenonium Bromide (Decreased intestinal motility).

Procainamide Hydrochloride (Interferes with neuromuscular transmission). Products include:
Procan SR Tablets 1760
Pronestyl Capsules and Tablets 1800
Pronestyl Injection 1798
Pronestyl-SR Tablets 1801

Procyclidine Hydrochloride (Decreased intestinal motility). Products include:
Kemadrin Tablets 771

Propafenone Hydrochloride (Interferes with neuromuscular transmission). Products include:
Rythmol Tablets 1184

Propantheline Bromide (Decreased intestinal motility). Products include:
Pro-Banthine Tablets 2141

Propranolol Hydrochloride (Interferes with neuromuscular transmission). Products include:
Inderal 2459
Inderal LA Long Acting Capsules 2461
Inderide Tablets 2463
Inderide LA Long Acting Capsules 2465

Quinidine Gluconate (Interferes with neuromuscular transmission). Products include:
Quinaglute Dura-Tabs Tablets 663

Quinidine Polygalacturonate (Interferes with neuromuscular transmission). Products include:
Cardioquin Tablets 1812

Quinidine Sulfate (Interferes with neuromuscular transmission). Products include:
Quinidex Extentabs 1868

Scopolamine Hydrobromide (Decreased intestinal motility). Products include:
Donnagel .... ■ 675
Donnagel-PG 1858
Donnatal 1858
Donnatal Extentabs 1859
Donnatal Tablets 1858
Donnazyme Tablets 1860
Isopto Hyoscine .... ◉ 222
Murocoll-2 Sterile Ophthalmic Solution .... ◉ 261
Ru-Tuss Tablets 693

Scopolamine Preparations (Decreased intestinal motility). Products include:
Transderm Scōp Transdermal Therapeutic System 887

Streptomycin Sulfate (May accentuate neuromuscular block).
No products indexed under this heading.

Tocainide Hydrochloride (Interferes with neuromuscular transmission). Products include:
Tonocard Tablets 1554

Tridihexethyl Chloride (Decreased intestinal motility).
No products indexed under this heading.

Trihexyphenidyl Hydrochloride (Decreased intestinal motility). Products include:
Artane 1195

Verapamil Hydrochloride (Interferes with neuromuscular transmission). Products include:
Calan SR Caplets 2157
Calan Tablets 2155
Isoptin Injectable 1177
Isoptin Oral Tablets 1179
Isoptin SR Sustained Release Tablets 1181
Verelan Capsules 1243
Verelan Capsules 2535

PROSTIN VR PEDIATRIC STERILE SOLUTION
(Alprostadil) 2355
No interactions described in labeling.

PROTAMINE SULFATE AMPOULES & VIALS
(Protamine Sulfate) 1295
May interact with:

Antibiotics, unspecified (Incompatible with unspecified cephalosporins and penicillins in vitro).

PROTOPAM CHLORIDE FOR INJECTION
(Pralidoxime Chloride) 2518
May interact with barbiturates, xanthine bronchodilators, phenothiazines, and certain other agents. Compounds in these categories include:

Aminophylline (Concurrent use should be avoided in patients with organophosphate poisoning). Products include:
Amesec .... ■ 682
Aminophyllin Tablets 2153

Aprobarbital (Barbiturates are potentiated by the anticholinesterases, they should be used cautiously in the treatment of convulsions). Products include:
Alurate Elixir 1883

Atropine Nitrate, Methyl (Signs of atropinization may occur earlier than expected).
No products indexed under this heading.

Atropine Sulfate (Signs of atropinization may occur earlier than expected). Products include:
Arco-Lase Plus Tablets 607
Atropine Sulfate Sterile Ophthalmic Solution and S.O.P. Sterile Ophthalmic Ointment .... ◉ 239
Donnagel .... ■ 675
Donnagel-PG 1858
Donnatal 1858
Donnatal Extentabs 1859
Donnatal Tablets 1858
Donnazyme Tablets 1860
Isopto Atropine .... ◉ 218
Lomotil 2174
Motofen Tablets 836
Ru-Tuss Tablets 693
Urised Tablets 2396

Butabarbital (Barbiturates are potentiated by the anticholinesterases, they should be used cautiously in the treatment of convulsions). Products include:
Pyridium Plus 1764

Butalbital (Barbiturates are potentiated by the anticholinesterases, they should be used cautiously in the treatment of convulsions). Products include:
Esgic-Plus Tablets 1002
Esgic Tablets & Capsules 1001
Fioricet Tablets 2006
Fiorinal Capsules 2007
Fiorinal with Codeine Capsules 2008
Fiorinal Tablets 2007
Phrenilin 838
Sedapap Tablets 50 mg/650 mg 1360

Chlorpromazine (Concurrent use should be avoided in patients with organophosphate poisoning). Products include:
Thorazine 2234

Dyphylline (Concurrent use should be avoided in patients with organophosphate poisoning). Products include:
Dilor 2079
Dilor-G Tablets & Liquid 2079
Lufyllin Elixir 2384
Lufyllin & Lufyllin-400 Tablets 2384
Lufyllin-GG Elixir & Tablets 2385

Fluphenazine Decanoate (Concurrent use should be avoided in patients with organophosphate poisoning). Products include:
Prolixin Decanoate 1795

Fluphenazine Enanthate (Concurrent use should be avoided in patients with organophosphate poisoning). Products include:
Prolixin Enanthate 1796

Fluphenazine Hydrochloride (Concurrent use should be avoided in patients with organophosphate poisoning). Products include:
Prolixin Elixir 1793
Prolixin Injection 1791
Prolixin Oral Concentrate 1792
Prolixin Tablets 1793

Mephobarbital (Barbiturates are potentiated by the anticholinesterases, they should be used cautiously in the treatment of convulsions). Products include:
Mebaral Tablets 2061

Mesoridazine Besylate (Concurrent use should be avoided in patients with organophosphate poisoning).

Morphine Sulfate (Concurrent use should be avoided in patients with organophosphate poisoning). Products include:
Astramorph/PF Injection, USP (Preservative-Free) 618
Duramorph 960
Infumorph 200 and Infumorph 500 Sterile Solutions 962
MS Contin Tablets 1814
MSIR 1817
Oramorph SR (Morphine Sulfate Sustained Release Tablets) 1988
Roxanol 1991

Pentobarbital Sodium (Barbiturates are potentiated by the anticholinesterases, they should be used cautiously in the treatment of convulsions). Products include:

- Nembutal Sodium Capsules 534
- Nembutal Sodium Solution 536
- Nembutal Sodium Suppositories...... 538

Perphenazine (Concurrent use should be avoided in patients with organophosphate poisoning). Products include:

- Etrafon 2087
- Triavil Tablets 1556
- Trilafon............ 2123

Phenobarbital (Barbiturates are potentiated by the anticholinesterases, they should be used cautiously in the treatment of convulsions). Products include:

- Arco-Lase Plus Tablets 607
- Bellergal-S Tablets 1998
- Bronkolixir .... ▣ 761
- Bronkotabs Tablets............ ▣ 762
- Donnatal 1858
- Donnatal Extentabs............ 1859
- Donnatal Tablets 1858
- Donnazyme Tablets 1860
- Kinesed Tablets 2272
- Phenobarbital Elixir and Tablets 1293
- Primatene Tablets-P Formula............ 2421
- Quadrinal Tablets 1183
- Tedral SA 1765

Prochlorperazine (Concurrent use should be avoided in patients with organophosphate poisoning). Products include:

- Compazine 2201

Promethazine Hydrochloride (Concurrent use should be avoided in patients with organophosphate poisoning). Products include:

- Mepergan Injection 2479
- Phenergan with Codeine............ 2497
- Phenergan with Dextromethorphan 2499
- Phenergan Injection 2493
- Phenergan Suppositories 2496
- Phenergan Syrup 2495
- Phenergan Tablets 2496
- Phenergan VC 2500
- Phenergan VC with Codeine 2501

Reserpine (Concurrent use should be avoided in patients with organophosphate poisoning). Products include:

- Diupres Tablets 1461
- Hydromox R Tablets............ 1209
- Hydropres Tablets............ 1485
- Renese-R Tablets............ 1786
- Salutensin/Salutensin-Demi 719
- Ser-Ap-Es Tablets 881
- Serpasil Tablets 883
- Serpasil-Apresoline Tablets............ 884
- Serpasil-Esidrix Tablets............ 886

Secobarbital Sodium (Barbiturates are potentiated by the anticholinesterases, they should be used cautiously in the treatment of convulsions). Products include:

- Seconal Sodium Pulvules 1296

Succinylcholine Chloride (Concurrent use should be avoided in patients with organophosphate poisoning). Products include:

- Anectine............ 755

Theophylline (Concurrent use should be avoided in patients with organophosphate poisoning). Products include:

- Bronkaid Tablets .... ▣ 757
- Bronkolixir .... ▣ 761
- Bronkotabs Tablets............ ▣ 762
- Constant-T Tablets 1029
- Marax Tablets & DF Syrup............ 1954
- Primatene Tablets............ 2421
- Quibron Capsules 713
- Quibron-T 714
- Quibron-T/SR 716
- Theolair Liquid 1317
- Theo-Organidin Elixir 2391

Theophylline Anhydrous (Concurrent use should be avoided in patients with organophosphate poisoning). Products include:

- Aerolate 994
- Primatene Tablets-M Formula .... ▣ 753
- Primatene Tablets-Regular Formula 2421
- Respbid Tablets 684
- Slo-bid Gyrocaps 1847
- T-PHYL (Uniphyl) 200 mg Tablets 1820
- Tedral SA 1765
- Theo-24............ 2179
- Theo-Dur Sprinkle 1168
- Theo-Dur Extended-Release Tablets 1166
- Theolair Tablets 1317
- Theolair-SR Tablets............ 1319
- TheoX Extended-Release Tablets 841
- Uniphyl 400 mg Tablets............ 1823

Theophylline Calcium Salicylate (Concurrent use should be avoided in patients with organophosphate poisoning). Products include:

- Quadrinal Tablets 1183

Theophylline Sodium Glycinate (Concurrent use should be avoided in patients with organophosphate poisoning). Products include:

- Asbron G 1997

Thiamylal Sodium (Barbiturates are potentiated by the anticholinesterases, they should be used cautiously in the treatment of convulsions). Products include:

- Surital Ampoules, Steri-Vials............ 1764

Thioridazine Hydrochloride (Concurrent use should be avoided in patients with organophosphate poisoning). Products include:

- Mellaril 2011

Trifluoperazine Hydrochloride (Concurrent use should be avoided in patients with organophosphate poisoning). Products include:

- Stelazine 2226

PROTOSTAT TABLETS
(Metronidazole) 1674
May interact with oral anticoagulants and certain other agents. Compounds in these categories include:

Alcohol (Abdominal cramps, nausea, vomiting, headache, and flushing may occur; avoid concomitant use).

Cimetidine (Prolongs the half-life and decreases plasma clearance of metronidazole). Products include:

- Tagamet Tablets 2228

Cimetidine Hydrochloride (Prolongs the half-life and decreases plasma clearance of metronidazole). Products include:

- Tagamet............ 2228

Dicumarol (Potentiation of anticoagulant effect). Products include:

- Dicumarol Tablets 516

Phenobarbital (May accelerate the elimination of metronidazole reduced plasma levels). Products include:

- Arco-Lase Plus Tablets 607
- Bellergal-S Tablets 1998
- Bronkolixir .... ▣ 761
- Bronkotabs Tablets............ ▣ 762
- Donnatal 1858
- Donnatal Extentabs............ 1859
- Donnatal Tablets 1858
- Donnazyme Tablets 1860
- Kinesed Tablets 2272
- Phenobarbital Elixir and Tablets 1293
- Primatene Tablets-P Formula............ 2421
- Quadrinal Tablets 1183
- Tedral SA 1765

Phenytoin (May accelerate the elimination of metronidazole reduced plasma levels). Products include:

- Dilantin Infatabs 1710
- Dilantin-30 Pediatric/Dilantin-125 Suspension 1713

Phenytoin Sodium (May accelerate the elimination of metronidazole reduced plasma levels). Products include:

- Dilantin Kapseals 1708
- Dilantin Parenteral 1712
- Dilantin with Phenobarbital Kapseals 1715

Warfarin Sodium (Potentiation of anticoagulant effect). Products include:

- Coumadin Injection & Tablets 944
- Panwarfin Tablets 547

Food Interactions

Beverages, alcoholic (Alcoholic beverages should not be consumed during and for at least one day after therapy).

PROTROPIN
(Somatrem)............ 1049
May interact with glucocorticoids. Compounds in this category include:

Betamethasone Acetate (May inhibit growth-promoting effect of Protropin growth hormone). Products include:

- Celestone Soluspan Suspension 2081

Betamethasone Sodium Phosphate (May inhibit growth-promoting effect of Protropin growth hormone). Products include:

- Celestone Soluspan Suspension 2081

Cortisone Acetate (May inhibit growth-promoting effect of Protropin growth hormone). Products include:

- Cortone Acetate Sterile Suspension 1437
- Cortone Acetate Tablets............ 1439

Dexamethasone (May inhibit growth-promoting effect of Protropin growth hormone). Products include:

- AK-Trol Ointment & Suspension .... ⊙ 207
- Decadron Elixir 1445
- Decadron Tablets............ 1447
- Decaspray Topical Aerosol 1459
- Dexacidin............ ⊙ 272
- Maxidex Sterile Ophthalmic Suspension............ ⊙ 223
- Maxitrol Ophthalmic Ointment/Suspension............ ⊙ 223
- TobraDex Ophthalmic Suspension and Ointment............ ⊙ 228

Dexamethasone Acetate (May inhibit growth-promoting effect of Protropin growth hormone). Products include:

- Dalalone D.P. Injectable 999
- Decadron-LA Sterile Suspension...... 1457

Dexamethasone Sodium Phosphate (May inhibit growth-promoting effect of Protropin growth hormone). Products include:

- AK-Dex .... ⊙ 203
- Decadron Phosphate Respihaler...... 1454
- Decadron Phosphate Sterile Ophthalmic Ointment 1453
- Decadron Phosphate Sterile Ophthalmic Solution 1453
- Decadron Phosphate Topical Cream............ 1455
- Decadron Phosphate Turbinaire...... 1456
- Maxidex Sterile Ophthalmic Ointment .... ⊙ 222
- NeoDecadron Sterile Ophthalmic Ointment 1517
- NeoDecadron Sterile Ophthalmic Solution 1518
- NeoDecadron Topical Cream 1518

Hydrocortisone (May inhibit growth-promoting effect of Protropin growth hormone). Products include:

- AK-Spore H.C. .... ⊙ 206
- Bactine Hydrocortisone Anti-Itch Cream............ ▣ 625
- CaldeCORT Anti-Itch Hydrocortisone Spray .... ▣ 560
- Carmol HC Cream 1% 2296
- Cortaid Spray .... ▣ 735
- Cortenema 2244
- Cortisporin Ointment............ 758
- Cortisporin Ophthalmic Ointment Sterile 758
- Cortisporin Ophthalmic Suspension Sterile 759
- Cortisporin Otic Solution Sterile 760
- Cortisporin Otic Suspension Sterile 760
- Cortizone-5 Creme & Ointment...... ▣ 732
- Dermolate Anti-Itch Cream .... ▣ 697
- Eldecort Cream 1.0% 1113
- Eldecort Cream 1.0% and 2.5% 1113
- Fungoid HC Creme 1770
- Hydrocortone Tablets 1482
- Hytone 909
- LazerSporin-C Solution 1770
- Massengill Medicated Soft Cloth Towelettes............ 2192
- Nutracort Cream & Lotion 1684
- PediOtic Suspension Sterile 797
- Synacort Creams 1%, 2.5% 2296
- Vanoxide-HC Acne Lotion............ 911
- Vioform-Hydrocortisone Cream and Mild Cream 889
- Vioform-Hydrocortisone Ointment.. 889
- VōSoL HC Otic Solution............ 2392
- Vytone Cream 1%............ 911

Hydrocortisone Acetate (May inhibit growth-promoting effect of Protropin growth hormone). Products include:

- Analpram-HC Rectal Cream 1% and 2.5% 970
- Anusol-HC Cream 1690
- Anusol-HC Suppositories 1691
- Caldecort............ ▣ 560
- Carmol HC Cream 1% 2296
- Chloromycetin Hydrocortisone Ophthalmic............ 1694
- Coly-Mycin S Otic w/Neomycin & Hydrocortisone............ 1708
- Cortaid .... ▣ 735
- Cortef Feminine Itch Cream .... ▣ 735
- Corticaine .... ▣ 682
- Cortifoam 1827
- Cortisporin Cream............ 757
- Epifoam 1828
- Gynecort 5 Creme............ ▣ 556
- Hydrocortone Acetate Sterile Suspension............ 1479
- Lanacort 5 Creme and Ointment .. ▣ 557
- Mantadil Cream 789
- Ophthocort .... ⊙ 301
- Orabase HCA Oral Paste 890
- Pramosone Cream, Lotion & Ointment 971
- ProctoCream-HC 1834
- Proctofoam-HC............ 1835

Hydrocortisone Sodium Phosphate (May inhibit growth-promoting effect of Protropin growth hormone). Products include:

- Hydrocortone Phosphate Injection, Sterile 1481

Hydrocortisone Sodium Succinate (May inhibit growth-promoting effect of Protropin growth hormone). Products include:

- Solu-Cortef Sterile Powder............ 2361

Methylprednisolone Acetate (May inhibit growth-promoting effect of Protropin growth hormone). Products include:

- Depo-Medrol Sterile Aqueous Suspension............ 2334

Methylprednisolone Sodium Succinate (May inhibit growth-promoting effect of Protropin growth hormone). Products include:

- Solu-Medrol Sterile Powder............ 2363

Prednisolone Acetate (May inhibit growth-promoting effect of Protropin growth hormone). Products include:

- AK-Cide Sterile Ophthalmic Ointment & Suspension............ ⊙ 202
- Blephamide Liquifilm Sterile Ophthalmic Suspension............ 586
- Blephamide S.O.P. Sterile Ophthalmic Ointment............ 586
- Cetapred Ointment .... ⊙ 220
- ⅛% Econopred & 1% Econopred Plus .... ⊙ 217
- Isopto Cetapred Suspension............ ⊙ 220
- Metimyd............ ⊙ 306
- Poly-Pred Liquifilm .... ⊙ 250
- Pred Forte............ ⊙ 252

Pred Mild ◉ 254
Pred-G Liquifilm Sterile Ophthalmic Suspension ◉ 252
Pred-G S.O.P. Sterile Ophthalmic Ointment ◉ 253
Vasocidin Ointment ◉ 275

Prednisolone Sodium Phosphate (May inhibit growth-promoting effect of Protropin growth hormone). Products include:
AK-Pred ◉ 205
Hydeltrasol Injection, Sterile 1476
Inflamase ◉ 274
Pediapred Oral Liquid 987
Vasocidin Ophthalmic Solution ◉ 276

Prednisolone Tebutate (May inhibit growth-promoting effect of Protropin growth hormone). Products include:
Hydeltra-T.B.A. Sterile Suspension 1478

Prednisone (May inhibit growth-promoting effect of Protropin growth hormone). Products include:
Deltasone Tablets 2332

Triamcinolone (May inhibit growth-promoting effect of Protropin growth hormone).
No products indexed under this heading.

Triamcinolone Acetonide (May inhibit growth-promoting effect of Protropin growth hormone). Products include:
Aristocort A 1010
Azmacort Inhaler 1837
Kenalog Cream, Lotion & Ointment 2401
Kenalog-10 Injection 2402
Kenalog-40 Injection 2403
Kenalog in Orabase 604
Kenalog Spray 2401
Mycolog II Cream and Ointment 2407
Mytrex Cream & Ointment 2080
Nasacort Nasal Inhaler 1844

Triamcinolone Diacetate (May inhibit growth-promoting effect of Protropin growth hormone). Products include:
Aristocort Suspension 1008

Triamcinolone Hexacetonide (May inhibit growth-promoting effect of Protropin growth hormone). Products include:
Aristospan Suspension 1011

PROVENTIL INHALATION AEROSOL

(Albuterol) 2117

May interact with sympathomimetic aerosol bronchodilators, monoamine oxidase inhibitors, tricyclic antidepressants, and beta blockers. Compounds in these categories include:

Acebutolol Hydrochloride (Inhibited effects of both drugs). Products include:
Sectral Capsules 2520

Amitriptyline Hydrochloride (Potentiates albuterol's effects on the vascular system). Products include:
Elavil 2269
Endep Tablets 1927
Etrafon 2087
Limbitrol 1933
Triavil Tablets 1556

Amoxapine (Potentiates albuterol's effects on the vascular system). Products include:
Asendin Tablets 1196

Atenolol (Inhibited effects of both drugs). Products include:
Tenoretic Tablets 1105
Tenormin Tablets and I.V. Injection 1107

Betaxolol Hydrochloride (Inhibited effects of both drugs). Products include:
Betoptic Sterile Ophthalmic Solution 569
Betoptic S Sterile Ophthalmic Suspension 570
Kerlone Tablets 2172

Bitolterol Mesylate (Potentiates cardiovascular effects). Products include:
Tornalate 2074

Carteolol Hydrochloride (Inhibited effects of both drugs). Products include:
Cartrol Tablets 507

Clomipramine Hydrochloride (Potentiates albuterol's effects on the vascular system). Products include:
Anafranil Capsules 650

Desipramine Hydrochloride (Potentiates albuterol's effects on the vascular system). Products include:
Norpramin Tablets 1340

Doxepin Hydrochloride (Potentiates albuterol's effects on the vascular system). Products include:
Sinequan 1960

Furazolidone (Potentiates albuterol's effects on the vascular system). Products include:
Furoxone 1855

Imipramine Hydrochloride (Potentiates albuterol's effects on the vascular system). Products include:
Tofranil Ampuls 1038
Tofranil Tablets 1039

Imipramine Pamoate (Potentiates albuterol's effects on the vascular system). Products include:
Tofranil-PM Capsules 1041

Isocarboxazid (Potentiates albuterol's effects on the vascular system). Products include:
Marplan Tablets 1906

Isoetharine (Potentiates cardiovascular effects). Products include:
Arm-a-Med Isoetharine Inhalation Solution, USP 616
Bronkometer Aerosol 2042
Bronkosol Solution 2042

Isoproterenol Hydrochloride (Potentiates cardiovascular effects). Products include:
Isuprel Hydrochloride Injection 1:5000 2050
Isuprel Hydrochloride Mistometer 2051
Isuprel Hydrochloride Solution 1:200 & 1:100 2052
Norisodrine Aerotrol 540

Labetalol Hydrochloride (Inhibited effects of both drugs). Products include:
Normodyne Injection 2108
Normodyne Tablets 2110
Normozide Tablets 2112
Trandate HCT Tablets 579
Trandate Injection 577
Trandate Tablets 579

Maprotiline Hydrochloride (Potentiates albuterol's effects on the vascular system). Products include:
Ludiomil Tablets 874

Metaproterenol Sulfate (Potentiates cardiovascular effects). Products include:
Alupent 674
Arm-a-Med Metaproterenol Sulfate Inhalation Solution, USP 617
Metaprel Inhalation Aerosol Bronchodilator 2014
Metaprel Inhalation Solution 2015
Metaprel 2015
Metaproterenol Sulfate Inhalation Solution, USP 912

Metoprolol Tartrate (Inhibited effects of both drugs). Products include:
Lopressor Ampuls 1032
Lopressor HCT Tablets 1034
Lopressor Tablets 1032

Nadolol (Inhibited effects of both drugs). Products include:
Corgard Tablets 701
Corzide Tablets 702

Nortriptyline Hydrochloride (Potentiates albuterol's effects on the vascular system). Products include:
Pamelor 2019

Penbutolol Sulfate (Inhibited effects of both drugs). Products include:
Levatol 1832

Phenelzine Sulfate (Potentiates albuterol's effects on the vascular system). Products include:
Nardil 1742

Pindolol (Inhibited effects of both drugs). Products include:
Visken Tablets 2036

Pirbuterol Acetate (Potentiates cardiovascular effects). Products include:
Maxair Inhaler 1311

Propranolol Hydrochloride (Inhibited effects of both drugs). Products include:
Inderal 2459
Inderal LA Long Acting Capsules 2461
Inderide Tablets 2463
Inderide LA Long Acting Capsules 2465

Protriptyline Hydrochloride (Potentiates albuterol's effects on the vascular system). Products include:
Vivactil Tablets 1567

Selegiline Hydrochloride (Potentiates albuterol's effects on the vascular system). Products include:
Eldepryl 2250

Terbutaline Sulfate (Potentiates cardiovascular effects). Products include:
Brethaire Inhaler 1024
Brethine Ampuls 1026
Brethine Tablets 1026
Bricanyl Injection 1324
Bricanyl Tablets 1325

Timolol Maleate (Inhibited effects of both drugs). Products include:
Blocadren Tablets 1429
Timolide Tablets 1547
Timoptic in Ocudose 1552
Timoptic Sterile Ophthalmic Solution 1550

Tranylcypromine Sulfate (Potentiates albuterol's effects on the vascular system). Products include:
Parnate Tablets 2222

Trimipramine Maleate (Potentiates albuterol's effects on the vascular system). Products include:
Surmontil Capsules 2524

PROVENTIL REPETABS TABLETS

(Albuterol Sulfate) 2120

May interact with sympathomimetic bronchodilators, monoamine oxidase inhibitors, tricyclic antidepressants, beta blockers, and certain other agents. Compounds in these categories include:

Acebutolol Hydrochloride (Effect of both drugs inhibited). Products include:
Sectral Capsules 2520

Amitriptyline Hydrochloride (Potentiation of albuterol's action on vascular system). Products include:
Elavil 2269
Endep Tablets 1927
Etrafon 2087
Limbitrol 1933
Triavil Tablets 1556

Amoxapine (Potentiation of albuterol's action on vascular system). Products include:
Asendin Tablets 1196

Atenolol (Effect of both drugs inhibited). Products include:
Tenoretic Tablets 1105
Tenormin Tablets and I.V. Injection 1107

Betaxolol Hydrochloride (Effect of both drugs inhibited). Products include:
Betoptic Sterile Ophthalmic Solution 569
Betoptic S Sterile Ophthalmic Suspension 570
Kerlone Tablets 2172

Bitolterol Mesylate (Deleterious cardiovascular effects). Products include:
Tornalate 2074

Carteolol Hydrochloride (Effect of both drugs inhibited). Products include:
Cartrol Tablets 507

Clomipramine Hydrochloride (Potentiation of albuterol's action on vascular system). Products include:
Anafranil Capsules 650

Desipramine Hydrochloride (Potentiation of albuterol's action on vascular system). Products include:
Norpramin Tablets 1340

Doxepin Hydrochloride (Potentiation of albuterol's action on vascular system). Products include:
Sinequan 1960

Ephedrine Hydrochloride (Deleterious cardiovascular effects). Products include:
Amesec ▣ 682
Primatene Tablets-M Formula 2421
Primatene Tablets-P Formula 2421
Primatene Tablets-Regular Formula 2421
Quadrinal Tablets 1183
Quelidrine Syrup 556
Tedral SA 1765

Ephedrine Sulfate (Deleterious cardiovascular effects). Products include:
Bronkaid Tablets ▣ 757
Bronkolixir ▣ 761
Bronkotabs Tablets ▣ 762
Marax Tablets & DF Syrup 1954
Pazo Hemorrhoid Ointment & Suppositories 752
Vicks Vatronol Nose Drops ▣ 666

Ephedrine Tannate (Deleterious cardiovascular effects). Products include:
Rynatuss 2388

Epinephrine (Deleterious cardiovascular effects). Products include:
Ana-Kit Anaphylaxis Emergency Treatment Kit 1100
Bronkaid Mist ▣ 757
EpiPen 843
Marcaine Hydrochloride 0.5% with Epinephrine 1:200,000 (as bitartrate) 958
Marcaine Hydrochloride with Epinephrine 1:200,000 2055
Primatene Mist 2420
Sus-Phrine Injection 1006
Xylocaine with Epinephrine Injections 637

Epinephrine Bitartrate (Deleterious cardiovascular effects). Products include:
AsthmaHaler Mist Epinephrine Bitartrate Bronchodilator ▣ 616
Bronkaid Mist Suspension ▣ 757
Primatene Mist Suspension 2421

Epinephrine Hydrochloride (Deleterious cardiovascular effects). Products include:
Adrenalin Chloride Solution 1:100 & 1:1,000 1689
Epifrin ◉ 244
Glaucon ◉ 218

Esmolol Hydrochloride (Effect of both drugs inhibited). Products include:
Brevibloc Injection 942

Ethylnorepinephrine Hydrochloride (Deleterious cardiovascular effects). Products include:
Bronkephrine Injection 2042

Furazolidone (Potentiation of albuterol's action on vascular system). Products include:
- Furoxone 1855

Imipramine Hydrochloride (Potentiation of albuterol's action on vascular system). Products include:
- Tofranil Ampuls 1038
- Tofranil Tablets 1039

Imipramine Pamoate (Potentiation of albuterol's action on vascular system). Products include:
- Tofranil-PM Capsules 1041

Isocarboxazid (Potentiation of albuterol's action on vascular system). Products include:
- Marplan Tablets 1906

Isoetharine (Deleterious cardiovascular effects). Products include:
- Arm-a-Med Isoetharine Inhalation Solution, USP 616
- Bronkometer Aerosol 2042
- Bronkosol Solution 2042

Isoproterenol Hydrochloride (Deleterious cardiovascular effects). Products include:
- Isuprel Hydrochloride Injection 1:5000 2050
- Isuprel Hydrochloride Mistometer .. 2051
- Isuprel Hydrochloride Solution 1:200 & 1:100 2052
- Norisodrine Aerotrol 540

Labetalol Hydrochloride (Effect of both drugs inhibited). Products include:
- Normodyne Injection 2108
- Normodyne Tablets 2110
- Normozide Tablets 2112
- Trandate HCT Tablets 579
- Trandate Injection 577
- Trandate Tablets 579

Maprotiline Hydrochloride (Potentiation of albuterol's action on vascular system). Products include:
- Ludiomil Tablets 874

Metaproterenol Sulfate (Deleterious cardiovascular effects). Products include:
- Alupent 674
- Arm-a-Med Metaproterenol Sulfate Inhalation Solution, USP 617
- Metaprel Inhalation Aerosol Bronchodilator 2014
- Metaprel Inhalation Solution 2015
- Metaprel 2015
- Metaproterenol Sulfate Inhalation Solution, USP 912

Metoprolol Tartrate (Effect of both drugs inhibited). Products include:
- Lopressor Ampuls 1032
- Lopressor HCT Tablets 1034
- Lopressor Tablets 1032

Nadolol (Effect of both drugs inhibited). Products include:
- Corgard Tablets 701
- Corzide Tablets 702

Nortriptyline Hydrochloride (Potentiation of albuterol's action on vascular system). Products include:
- Pamelor 2019

Penbutolol Sulfate (Effect of both drugs inhibited). Products include:
- Levatol 1832

Phenelzine Sulfate (Potentiation of albuterol's action on vascular system). Products include:
- Nardil 1742

Pindolol (Effect of both drugs inhibited). Products include:
- Visken Tablets 2036

Pirbuterol Acetate (Deleterious cardiovascular effects). Products include:
- Maxair Inhaler 1311

Propranolol Hydrochloride (Effect of both drugs inhibited). Products include:
- Inderal 2459
- Inderal LA Long Acting Capsules 2461
- Inderide Tablets 2463
- Inderide LA Long Acting Capsules .. 2465

Protriptyline Hydrochloride (Potentiation of albuterol's action on vascular system). Products include:
- Vivactil Tablets 1567

Selegiline Hydrochloride (Potentiation of albuterol's action on vascular system). Products include:
- Eldepryl 2250

Terbutaline Sulfate (Deleterious cardiovascular effects). Products include:
- Brethaire Inhaler 1024
- Brethine Ampuls 1026
- Brethine Tablets 1026
- Bricanyl Injection 1324
- Bricanyl Tablets 1325

Timolol Maleate (Effect of both drugs inhibited). Products include:
- Blocadren Tablets 1429
- Timolide Tablets 1547
- Timoptic in Ocudose 1552
- Timoptic Sterile Ophthalmic Solution 1550

Tranylcypromine Sulfate (Potentiation of albuterol's action on vascular system). Products include:
- Parnate Tablets 2222

Trimipramine Maleate (Potentiation of albuterol's action on vascular system). Products include:
- Surmontil Capsules 2524

PROVENTIL SOLUTIONS FOR INHALATION 0.5% AND 0.083%

(Albuterol Sulfate) 2118

May interact with sympathomimetic aerosol bronchodilators, monoamine oxidase inhibitors, tricyclic antidepressants, and beta blockers. Compounds in these categories include:

Acebutolol Hydrochloride (Effects of both drugs inhibited). Products include:
- Sectral Capsules 2520

Amitriptyline Hydrochloride (Potentiation of albuterol's action on vascular system). Products include:
- Elavil 2269
- Endep Tablets 1927
- Etrafon 2087
- Limbitrol 1933
- Triavil Tablets 1556

Amoxapine (Potentiation of albuterol's action on vascular system). Products include:
- Asendin Tablets 1196

Atenolol (Effects of both drugs inhibited). Products include:
- Tenoretic Tablets 1105
- Tenormin Tablets and I.V. Injection 1107

Betaxolol Hydrochloride (Effects of both drugs inhibited). Products include:
- Betoptic Sterile Ophthalmic Solution 569
- Betoptic S Sterile Ophthalmic Suspension 570
- Kerlone Tablets 2172

Bitolterol Mesylate (Effect not specified). Products include:
- Tornalate 2074

Carteolol Hydrochloride (Effects of both drugs inhibited). Products include:
- Cartrol Tablets 507

Clomipramine Hydrochloride (Potentiation of albuterol's action on vascular system). Products include:
- Anafranil Capsules 650

Desipramine Hydrochloride (Potentiation of albuterol's action on vascular system). Products include:
- Norpramin Tablets 1340

Doxepin Hydrochloride (Potentiation of albuterol's action on vascular system). Products include:
- Sinequan 1960

Esmolol Hydrochloride (Effects of both drugs inhibited). Products include:
- Brevibloc Injection 942

Ethylnorepinephrine Hydrochloride (Effect not specified). Products include:
- Bronkephrine Injection 2042

Furazolidone (Potentiation of albuterol's action on vascular system). Products include:
- Furoxone 1855

Imipramine Hydrochloride (Potentiation of albuterol's action on vascular system). Products include:
- Tofranil Ampuls 1038
- Tofranil Tablets 1039

Imipramine Pamoate (Potentiation of albuterol's action on vascular system). Products include:
- Tofranil-PM Capsules 1041

Isocarboxazid (Potentiation of albuterol's action on vascular system). Products include:
- Marplan Tablets 1906

Isoetharine (Effect not specified). Products include:
- Arm-a-Med Isoetharine Inhalation Solution, USP 616
- Bronkometer Aerosol 2042
- Bronkosol Solution 2042

Isoproterenol Hydrochloride (Effect not specified). Products include:
- Isuprel Hydrochloride Injection 1:5000 2050
- Isuprel Hydrochloride Mistometer .. 2051
- Isuprel Hydrochloride Solution 1:200 & 1:100 2052
- Norisodrine Aerotrol 540

Labetalol Hydrochloride (Effects of both drugs inhibited). Products include:
- Normodyne Injection 2108
- Normodyne Tablets 2110
- Normozide Tablets 2112
- Trandate HCT Tablets 579
- Trandate Injection 577
- Trandate Tablets 579

Maprotiline Hydrochloride (Potentiation of albuterol's action on vascular system). Products include:
- Ludiomil Tablets 874

Metaproterenol Sulfate (Effect not specified). Products include:
- Alupent 674
- Arm-a-Med Metaproterenol Sulfate Inhalation Solution, USP 617
- Metaprel Inhalation Aerosol Bronchodilator 2014
- Metaprel Inhalation Solution 2015
- Metaprel 2015
- Metaproterenol Sulfate Inhalation Solution, USP 912

Metoprolol Tartrate (Effects of both drugs inhibited). Products include:
- Lopressor Ampuls 1032
- Lopressor HCT Tablets 1034
- Lopressor Tablets 1032

Nadolol (Effects of both drugs inhibited). Products include:
- Corgard Tablets 701
- Corzide Tablets 702

Nortriptyline Hydrochloride (Potentiation of albuterol's action on vascular system). Products include:
- Pamelor 2019

Penbutolol Sulfate (Effects of both drugs inhibited). Products include:
- Levatol 1832

Phenelzine Sulfate (Potentiation of albuterol's action on vascular system). Products include:
- Nardil 1742

Pindolol (Effects of both drugs inhibited). Products include:
- Visken Tablets 2036

Pirbuterol Acetate (Effect not specified). Products include:
- Maxair Inhaler 1311

Propranolol Hydrochloride (Effects of both drugs inhibited). Products include:
- Inderal 2459
- Inderal LA Long Acting Capsules 2461
- Inderide Tablets 2463
- Inderide LA Long Acting Capsules .. 2465

Protriptyline Hydrochloride (Potentiation of albuterol's action on vascular system). Products include:
- Vivactil Tablets 1567

Selegiline Hydrochloride (Potentiation of albuterol's action on vascular system). Products include:
- Eldepryl 2250

Terbutaline Sulfate (Effect not specified). Products include:
- Brethaire Inhaler 1024
- Brethine Ampuls 1026
- Brethine Tablets 1026
- Bricanyl Injection 1324
- Bricanyl Tablets 1325

Timolol Maleate (Effects of both drugs inhibited). Products include:
- Blocadren Tablets 1429
- Timolide Tablets 1547
- Timoptic in Ocudose 1552
- Timoptic Sterile Ophthalmic Solution 1550

Tranylcypromine Sulfate (Potentiation of albuterol's action on vascular system). Products include:
- Parnate Tablets 2222

Trimipramine Maleate (Potentiation of albuterol's action on vascular system). Products include:
- Surmontil Capsules 2524

PROVENTIL SYRUP

(Albuterol Sulfate) 2119

May interact with sympathomimetic bronchodilators, monoamine oxidase inhibitors, tricyclic antidepressants, and beta blockers. Compounds in these categories include:

Acebutolol Hydrochloride (Effects of both drugs inhibited). Products include:
- Sectral Capsules 2520

Amitriptyline Hydrochloride (Potentiation of albuterol's action on vascular system). Products include:
- Elavil 2269
- Endep Tablets 1927
- Etrafon 2087
- Limbitrol 1933
- Triavil Tablets 1556

Amoxapine (Potentiation of albuterol's action on vascular system). Products include:
- Asendin Tablets 1196

Atenolol (Effects of both drugs inhibited). Products include:
- Tenoretic Tablets 1105
- Tenormin Tablets and I.V. Injection 1107

Betaxolol Hydrochloride (Effects of both drugs inhibited). Products include:
- Betoptic Sterile Ophthalmic Solution 569
- Betoptic S Sterile Ophthalmic Suspension 570
- Kerlone Tablets 2172

Bitolterol Mesylate (Deleterious cardiovascular effects). Products include:
- Tornalate 2074

Carteolol Hydrochloride (Effects of both drugs inhibited). Products include:
- Cartrol Tablets 507

Clomipramine Hydrochloride (Potentiation of albuterol's action on vascular system). Products include:
Anafranil Capsules 650

Desipramine Hydrochloride (Potentiation of albuterol's action on vascular system). Products include:
Norpramin Tablets 1340

Doxepin Hydrochloride (Potentiation of albuterol's action on vascular system). Products include:
Sinequan 1960

Ephedrine Hydrochloride (Deleterious cardiovascular effects). Products include:
Amesec ◘ 682
Primatene Tablets-M Formula 2421
Primatene Tablets-P Formula 2421
Primatene Tablets-Regular Formula 2421
Quadrinal Tablets 1183
Quelidrine Syrup 556
Tedral SA 1765

Ephedrine Sulfate (Deleterious cardiovascular effects). Products include:
Bronkaid Tablets ◘ 757
Bronkolixir ◘ 761
Bronkotabs Tablets ◘ 762
Marax Tablets & DF Syrup 1954
Pazo Hemorrhoid Ointment & Suppositories 752
Vicks Vatronol Nose Drops ◘ 666

Ephedrine Tannate (Deleterious cardiovascular effects). Products include:
Rynatuss 2388

Epinephrine (Deleterious cardiovascular effects). Products include:
Ana-Kit Anaphylaxis Emergency Treatment Kit 1100
Bronkaid Mist ◘ 757
EpiPen 843
Marcaine Hydrochloride 0.5% with Epinephrine 1:200,000 (as bitartrate) 958
Marcaine Hydrochloride with Epinephrine 1:200,000 2055
Primatene Mist 2420
Sus-Phrine Injection 1006
Xylocaine with Epinephrine Injections 637

Epinephrine Bitartrate (Deleterious cardiovascular effects). Products include:
AsthmaHaler Mist Epinephrine Bitartrate Bronchodilator ◘ 616
Bronkaid Mist Suspension ◘ 757
Primatene Mist Suspension 2421

Epinephrine Hydrochloride (Deleterious cardiovascular effects). Products include:
Adrenalin Chloride Solution 1:100 & 1:1,000 1689
Epifrin ⊙ 244
Glaucon ⊙ 218

Esmolol Hydrochloride (Effects of both drugs inhibited). Products include:
Brevibloc Injection 942

Ethylnorepinephrine Hydrochloride (Deleterious cardiovascular effects). Products include:
Bronkephrine Injection 2042

Furazolidone (Potentiation of albuterol's action on vascular system). Products include:
Furoxone 1855

Imipramine Hydrochloride (Potentiation of albuterol's action on vascular system). Products include:
Tofranil Ampuls 1038
Tofranil Tablets 1039

Imipramine Pamoate (Potentiation of albuterol's action on vascular system). Products include:
Tofranil-PM Capsules 1041

Isocarboxazid (Potentiation of albuterol's action on vascular system). Products include:
Marplan Tablets 1906

Isoetharine (Deleterious cardiovascular effects). Products include:
Arm-a-Med Isoetharine Inhalation Solution, USP 616
Bronkometer Aerosol 2042
Bronkosol Solution 2042

Isoproterenol Hydrochloride (Deleterious cardiovascular effects). Products include:
Isuprel Hydrochloride Injection 1:5000 2050
Isuprel Hydrochloride Mistometer 2051
Isuprel Hydrochloride Solution 1:200 & 1:100 2052
Norisodrine Aerotrol 540

Labetalol Hydrochloride (Effects of both drugs inhibited). Products include:
Normodyne Injection 2108
Normodyne Tablets 2110
Normozide Tablets 2112
Trandate HCT Tablets 579
Trandate Injection 577
Trandate Tablets 579

Maprotiline Hydrochloride (Potentiation of albuterol's action on vascular system). Products include:
Ludiomil Tablets 874

Metaproterenol Sulfate (Deleterious cardiovascular effects). Products include:
Alupent 674
Arm-a-Med Metaproterenol Sulfate Inhalation Solution, USP 617
Metaprel Inhalation Aerosol Bronchodilator 2014
Metaprel Inhalation Solution 2015
Metaprel 2015
Metaproterenol Sulfate Inhalation Solution, USP 912

Metoprolol Tartrate (Effects of both drugs inhibited). Products include:
Lopressor Ampuls 1032
Lopressor HCT Tablets 1034
Lopressor Tablets 1032

Nadolol (Effects of both drugs inhibited). Products include:
Corgard Tablets 701
Corzide Tablets 702

Nortriptyline Hydrochloride (Potentiation of albuterol's action on vascular system). Products include:
Pamelor 2019

Penbutolol Sulfate (Effects of both drugs inhibited). Products include:
Levatol 1832

Phenelzine Sulfate (Potentiation of albuterol's action on vascular system). Products include:
Nardil 1742

Pindolol (Effects of both drugs inhibited). Products include:
Visken Tablets 2036

Pirbuterol Acetate (Deleterious cardiovascular effects). Products include:
Maxair Inhaler 1311

Propranolol Hydrochloride (Effects of both drugs inhibited). Products include:
Inderal 2459
Inderal LA Long Acting Capsules 2461
Inderide Tablets 2463
Inderide LA Long Acting Capsules 2465

Protriptyline Hydrochloride (Potentiation of albuterol's action on vascular system). Products include:
Vivactil Tablets 1567

Selegiline Hydrochloride (Potentiation of albuterol's action on vascular system). Products include:
Eldepryl 2250

Terbutaline Sulfate (Deleterious cardiovascular effects). Products include:
Brethaire Inhaler 1024
Brethine Ampuls 1026
Brethine Tablets 1026
Bricanyl Injection 1324
Bricanyl Tablets 1325

Timolol Maleate (Effects of both drugs inhibited). Products include:
Blocadren Tablets 1429
Timolide Tablets 1547
Timoptic in Ocudose 1552
Timoptic Sterile Ophthalmic Solution 1550

Tranylcypromine Sulfate (Potentiation of albuterol's action on vascular system). Products include:
Parnate Tablets 2222

Trimipramine Maleate (Potentiation of albuterol's action on vascular system). Products include:
Surmontil Capsules 2524

PROVENTIL TABLETS
(Albuterol Sulfate) 2120
See **Proventil Repetabs Tablets**

PROVERA TABLETS
(Medroxyprogesterone Acetate) 2356
May interact with:

Aminoglutethimide (Significantly depresses the bioavailability of Provera). Products include:
Cytadren Tablets 861

PROVOCHOLINE FOR INHALATION
(Metacholine Chloride) 1911
May interact with beta blockers. Compounds in this category include:

Acebutolol Hydrochloride (Response to methacholine can be exaggerated or prolonged). Products include:
Sectral Capsules 2520

Atenolol (Response to methacholine can be exaggerated or prolonged). Products include:
Tenoretic Tablets 1105
Tenormin Tablets and I.V. Injection 1107

Betaxolol Hydrochloride (Response to methacholine can be exaggerated or prolonged). Products include:
Betoptic Sterile Ophthalmic Solution 569
Betoptic S Sterile Ophthalmic Suspension 570
Kerlone Tablets 2172

Carteolol Hydrochloride (Response to methacholine can be exaggerated or prolonged). Products include:
Cartrol Tablets 507

Esmolol Hydrochloride (Response to methacholine can be exaggerated or prolonged). Products include:
Brevibloc Injection 942

Labetalol Hydrochloride (Response to methacholine can be exaggerated or prolonged). Products include:
Normodyne Injection 2108
Normodyne Tablets 2110
Normozide Tablets 2112
Trandate HCT Tablets 579
Trandate Injection 577
Trandate Tablets 579

Metoprolol Tartrate (Response to methacholine can be exaggerated or prolonged). Products include:
Lopressor Ampuls 1032
Lopressor HCT Tablets 1034
Lopressor Tablets 1032

Nadolol (Response to methacholine can be exaggerated or prolonged). Products include:
Corgard Tablets 701
Corzide Tablets 702

Penbutolol Sulfate (Response to methacholine can be exaggerated or prolonged). Products include:
Levatol 1832

Pindolol (Response to methacholine can be exaggerated or prolonged). Products include:
Visken Tablets 2036

Propranolol Hydrochloride (Response to methacholine can be exaggerated or prolonged). Products include:
Inderal 2459
Inderal LA Long Acting Capsules 2461
Inderide Tablets 2463
Inderide LA Long Acting Capsules 2465

Timolol Maleate (Response to methacholine can be exaggerated or prolonged). Products include:
Blocadren Tablets 1429
Timolide Tablets 1547
Timoptic in Ocudose 1552
Timoptic Sterile Ophthalmic Solution 1550

PROZAC PULVULES
(Fluoxetine Hydrochloride) 920
May interact with monoamine oxidase inhibitors, oral anticoagulants, antidepressant drugs, insulin, oral hypoglycemic agents, and certain other agents. Compounds in these categories include:

Amitriptyline Hydrochloride (Concomitant administration may result in greater increase in previously stable plasma levels of other antidepressants). Products include:
Elavil 2269
Endep Tablets 1927
Etrafon 2087
Limbitrol 1933
Triavil Tablets 1556

Amoxapine (Concomitant administration may result in greater increase in previously stable plasma levels of other antidepressants). Products include:
Asendin Tablets 1196

Bupropion Hydrochloride (Concomitant administration may result in greater increase in previously stable plasma levels of other antidepressants). Products include:
Wellbutrin Tablets 821

Chlorpropamide (Prozac may alter glycemic control; oral hypoglycemic dosage may need to be adjusted). Products include:
Diabinese Tablets 1775

Desipramine Hydrochloride (Concomitant administration may result in greater increase in previously stable plasma levels of other antidepressants). Products include:
Norpramin Tablets 1340

Diazepam (Half-life of concurrently administered diazepam may be prolonged). Products include:
Valium Injectable 1937
Valium Tablets 1939
Valrelease Capsules 1923

Dicumarol (Potential for adverse effects of either drug). Products include:
Dicumarol Tablets 516

Digitoxin (Potential for adverse effects of either drug). Products include:
Crystodigin Tablets 1253

Doxepin Hydrochloride (Concomitant administration may result in greater increase in previously stable plasma levels of other antidepressants). Products include:
Sinequan 1960

Furazolidone (Concomitant administration is contraindicated; at least five weeks should be allowed after stopping Prozac before starting a MAOI). Products include:
Furoxone 1855

Glipizide (Prozac may alter glycemic control; oral hypoglycemic dosage may need to be adjusted). Products include:
- Glucotrol 1952

Glyburide (Prozac may alter glycemic control; oral hypoglycemic dosage may need to be adjusted). Products include:
- DiaBeta 1091
- Micronase Tablets 2350

Imipramine Hydrochloride (Concomitant administration may result in greater increase in previously stable plasma levels of other antidepressants). Products include:
- Tofranil Ampuls 1038
- Tofranil Tablets 1039

Imipramine Pamoate (Concomitant administration may result in greater increase in previously stable plasma levels of other antidepressants). Products include:
- Tofranil-PM Capsules 1041

Insulin, Human (Prozac may alter glycemic control; insulin dosage may need to be adjusted).
- No products indexed under this heading.

Insulin, Human Isophane Suspension (Prozac may alter glycemic control; insulin dosage may need to be adjusted). Products include:
- Humulin N, 100 Units 1270

Insulin, Human NPH (Prozac may alter glycemic control; insulin dosage may need to be adjusted). Products include:
- Insulatard NPH Human 1627
- Novolin N 1627
- Novolin N PenFill Cartridges 1628
- Novolin N Prefilled 1628

Insulin, Human Regular (Prozac may alter glycemic control; insulin dosage may need to be adjusted). Products include:
- Humulin BR, 100 Units 1268
- Humulin R, 100 Units 1272
- Novolin R 1627
- Novolin R PenFill Cartridges 1628
- Novolin R Prefilled 1629
- Velosulin Human 1628

Insulin, Human, Zinc Suspension (Prozac may alter glycemic control; insulin dosage may need to be adjusted). Products include:
- Humulin L, 100 Units 1268
- Humulin U, 100 Units 1272
- Novolin L 1627

Insulin, NPH (Prozac may alter glycemic control; insulin dosage may need to be adjusted). Products include:
- NPH, 40 & 100 Units 1273
- Beef NPH, 100 Units 1274
- Pork NPH, 100 Units 1275
- Insulatard NPH 1626
- NPH Insulin 1626
- NPH Purified Pork Isophane Insulin 1626

Insulin, Regular (Prozac may alter glycemic control; insulin dosage may need to be adjusted). Products include:
- Regular, 40 & 100 Units 1273
- Beef Regular, 100 Units 1275
- Pork Regular, 100 Units 1275
- Pork Regular (Concentrated), 500 Units 1276
- Regular Insulin 1625
- Regular Purified Pork Insulin 1626
- Velosulin 1627

Insulin, Zinc Crystals (Prozac may alter glycemic control; insulin dosage may need to be adjusted). Products include:
- NPH, 40 & 100 Units 1273

Insulin, Zinc Suspension (Prozac may alter glycemic control; insulin dosage may need to be adjusted). Products include:
- Lente, 40 & 100 Units 1272
- Protamine, Zinc, 40 & 100 Units 1273
- Lente Iletin I 1272
- Beef Lente, 100 Units 1274
- Beef Protamine Zinc, 100 Units 1274
- Pork Lente, 100 Units 1275
- Pork, Protamine, Zinc, 100 Units 1275
- Lente Insulin 1626
- Lente Purified Pork Insulin 1626
- Semilente Insulin 1625
- Ultralente Insulin 1626

Isocarboxazid (Concomitant administration is contraindicated; at least five weeks should be allowed after stopping Prozac before starting a MAOI). Products include:
- Marplan Tablets 1906

Lithium Carbonate (Increased and decreased lithium levels; potential for lithium toxicity). Products include:
- Eskalith 2214
- Lithane Tablets 1596
- Lithium Carbonate Capsules & Tablets 1984
- Lithobid Tablets 870

Lithium Citrate (Increased and decreased lithium levels; potential for lithium toxicity). Products include:
- Cibalith-S 870

Maprotiline Hydrochloride (Concomitant administration may result in greater increase in previously stable plasma levels of other antidepressants). Products include:
- Ludiomil Tablets 874

Nortriptyline Hydrochloride (Concomitant administration may result in greater increase in previously stable plasma levels of other antidepressants). Products include:
- Pamelor 2019

Phenelzine Sulfate (Concomitant administration is contraindicated; at least five weeks should be allowed after stopping Prozac before starting a MAOI). Products include:
- Nardil 1742

Protriptyline Hydrochloride (Concomitant administration may result in greater increase in previously stable plasma levels of other antidepressants). Products include:
- Vivactil Tablets 1567

Selegiline Hydrochloride (Concomitant administration is contraindicated; at least five weeks should be allowed after stopping Prozac before starting a MAOI). Products include:
- Eldepryl 2250

Tolazamide (Prozac may alter glycemic control; oral hypoglycemic dosage may need to be adjusted). Products include:
- Tolinase Tablets 2365

Tolbutamide (Prozac may alter glycemic control; oral hypoglycemic dosage may need to be adjusted). Products include:
- Orinase Tablets 2354

Tranylcypromine Sulfate (Concomitant administration is contraindicated; at least five weeks should be allowed after stopping Prozac before starting a MAOI). Products include:
- Parnate Tablets 2222

Trazodone Hydrochloride (Concomitant administration may result in greater increase in previously stable plasma levels of other antidepressants). Products include:
- Desyrel and Desyrel Dividose 1404

Trimipramine Maleate (Concomitant administration may result in greater increase in previously stable plasma levels of other antidepressants). Products include:
- Surmontil Capsules 2524

L-Tryptophan (Potential for agitation, restlessness and gastrointestinal distress). Products include:
- Saave 1358
- Tropamine 1358

Warfarin Sodium (Potential for adverse effects of either drug). Products include:
- Coumadin Injection & Tablets 944
- Panwarfin Tablets 547

Food Interactions

Food, unspecified (May delay absorption of fluoxetine inconsequentially).

PSORCON OINTMENT 0.05%
(Diflorasone Diacetate) 909
No interactions described in labeling.

PSORION CREAM 0.05%
(Betamethasone Dipropionate) 1121
No interactions described in labeling.

PULMOCARE SPECIALIZED NUTRITION FOR PULMONARY PATIENTS
(Vitamins with Minerals) 1975
No interactions described in labeling.

PURGE CONCENTRATE
(Castor Oil) ..... ◘ 563
No interactions described in labeling.

PURI-CLENS, WOUND DEODORIZER AND CLEANSER
(Benzethonium Chloride) 2286
No interactions described in labeling.

PURINETHOL TABLETS
(Mercaptopurine) 800
May interact with:

Allopurinol (Delayed catabolism of mercaptopurine). Products include:
- Zyloprim Tablets 830

Doxorubicin Hydrochloride (Hepatotoxicity). Products include:
- Adriamycin PFS 561
- Adriamycin RDF 562
- Doxorubicin Hydrochloride for Injection, USP 622
- Doxorubicin Hydrochloride Injection, USP 848
- Rubex 739

Hepatotoxic Drugs, unspecified (Hepatotoxicity).

Sulfamethoxazole (Enhanced marrow suppression). Products include:
- Azo Gantanol Tablets 1887
- Bactrim DS Tablets 1891
- Bactrim I.V. Infusion 1889
- Bactrim 1891
- Gantanol 1899
- Septra 813
- Septra I.V. Infusion 808
- Septra I.V. Infusion ADD-Vantage Vials 810
- Septra 813

Thioguanine (Complete cross-resistance). Products include:
- Thioguanine Tablets, Tabloid Brand 815

Trimethoprim (Enhanced marrow suppression). Products include:
- Bactrim DS Tablets 1891
- Bactrim I.V. Infusion 1889
- Bactrim 1891
- Proloprim Tablets 799
- Septra 813
- Septra I.V. Infusion 808
- Septra I.V. Infusion ADD-Vantage Vials 810
- Septra 813
- Trimpex Tablets 1922

PURPOSE DUAL TREATMENT MOISTURIZER WITH SUNSCREEN (SPF 12)
(Octyl Methoxycinnamate, Oxybenzone) 1680
No interactions described in labeling.

PYRIDIUM
(Phenazopyridine Hydrochloride) 1763
No interactions described in labeling.

PYRIDIUM PLUS
(Phenazopyridine Hydrochloride, Hyoscyamine Hydrobromide, Butabarbital) 1764
No interactions described in labeling.

PYRROXATE CAPSULES
(Acetaminophen, Chlorpheniramine Maleate, Phenylpropanolamine Hydrochloride) ..... ◘ 669
May interact with monoamine oxidase inhibitors and certain other agents. Compounds in these categories include:

Alcohol (Concurrent use not recommended).

Furazolidone (Product labeling recommends physician's supervision for concurrent administration of these drugs). Products include:
- Furoxone 1855

Isocarboxazid (Product labeling recommends physician's supervision for concurrent administration of these drugs). Products include:
- Marplan Tablets 1906

Phenelzine Sulfate (Product labeling recommends physician's supervision for concurrent administration of these drugs). Products include:
- Nardil 1742

Selegiline Hydrochloride (Product labeling recommends physician's supervision for concurrent administration of these drugs). Products include:
- Eldepryl 2250

Tranylcypromine Sulfate (Product labeling recommends physician's supervision for concurrent administration of these drugs). Products include:
- Parnate Tablets 2222

QUADRINAL TABLETS
(Ephedrine, Phenobarbital) 1183
May interact with cardiac glycosides, general anesthetics, monoamine oxidase inhibitors, sympathomimetic aerosol bronchodilators, tricyclic antidepressants, central nervous system depressants, oral anticoagulants, corticosteroids, and certain other agents. Compounds in these categories include:

Albuterol (Increased effects). Products include:
- Proventil Inhalation Aerosol 2117
- Ventolin Inhalation Aerosol and Refill 583

Albuterol Sulfate (Increased effects). Products include:
- Proventil Repetabs Tablets 2120
- Proventil Solutions for Inhalation 0.5% and 0.083% 2118
- Proventil Syrup 2119
- Proventil Tablets 2120
- Ventolin 583

Alcohol (Increased effects).

Alfentanil Hydrochloride (Increased effects). Products include:
Alfenta Injection ... 1131
Alprazolam (Increased effects). Products include:
Xanax Tablets ... 2367
Amitriptyline Hydrochloride (Decreased effects; possible antagonized pressor effect of ephedrine). Products include:
Elavil ... 2269
Endep Tablets ... 1927
Etrafon ... 2087
Limbitrol ... 1933
Triavil Tablets ... 1556
Amoxapine (Decreased effects; possible antagonized pressor effect of ephedrine). Products include:
Asendin Tablets ... 1196
Aprobarbital (Increased effects). Products include:
Alurate Elixir ... 1883
Betamethasone Acetate (Decreased effects). Products include:
Celestone Soluspan Suspension ... 2081
Betamethasone Sodium Phosphate (Decreased effects). Products include:
Celestone Soluspan Suspension ... 2081
Buprenorphine (Increased effects).
No products indexed under this heading.
Buspirone Hydrochloride (Increased effects). Products include:
BuSpar ... 1401
Butabarbital (Increased effects). Products include:
Pyridium Plus ... 1764
Butalbital (Increased effects). Products include:
Esgic-Plus Tablets ... 1002
Esgic Tablets & Capsules ... 1001
Fioricet Tablets ... 2006
Fiorinal Capsules ... 2007
Fiorinal with Codeine Capsules ... 2008
Fiorinal Tablets ... 2007
Phrenilin ... 838
Sedapap Tablets 50 mg/650 mg .. 1360
Chlordiazepoxide (Fatty acid mobilization; increased effects). Products include:
Libritabs Tablets ... 1930
Limbitrol ... 1933
Menrium Tablets ... 1934
Chlordiazepoxide Hydrochloride (Fatty acid mobilization; increased effects). Products include:
Librax Capsules ... 1929
Librium Capsules ... 1931
Librium Injectable ... 1932
Chlorpromazine (Increased effects). Products include:
Thorazine ... 2234
Chlorprothixene (Increased effects). Products include:
Taractan Tablets ... 1920
Chlorprothixene Hydrochloride (Increased effects). Products include:
Taractan ... 1920
Cimetidine (Increased theophylline blood levels). Products include:
Tagamet Tablets ... 2228
Cimetidine Hydrochloride (Increased theophylline blood levels). Products include:
Tagamet ... 2228
Clindamycin Hydrochloride (Increased theophylline plasma levels). Products include:
Cleocin HCl Capsules ... 2322
Clindamycin Palmitate Hydrochloride (Increased theophylline plasma levels). Products include:
Cleocin Pediatric Flavored Granules ... 2324
Clindamycin Phosphate (Increased theophylline plasma levels). Products include:
Cleocin Phosphate Injection ... 2325
Cleocin T Topical ... 2327
Clomipramine Hydrochloride (Decreased effects; possible antagonized pressor effect of ephedrine). Products include:
Anafranil Capsules ... 650
Clorazepate Dipotassium (Increased effects). Products include:
Tranxene ... 556
Codeine (Increased effects). Products include:
Calcidrine Syrup ... 506
Codeine Phosphate (Increased effects). Products include:
Actifed with Codeine Cough Syrup.. 752
Cheracol Cough Syrup ... 1853
Codimal PH Syrup ... 846
Dimetane-DC Cough Syrup ... 1857
Empirin with Codeine Phosphate Nos. 2, 3 & 4 ... 764
Fiorinal with Codeine Capsules ... 2008
Isoclor Expectorant ... 982
Naldecon CX Adult Liquid ... ⊞ 521
Novahistine DH ... 1342
Novahistine Expectorant ... 1343
Nucofed Capsules ... 2219
Nucofed Expectorant ... 2219
Nucofed Pediatric Expectorant ... 2220
Nucofed Syrup ... 2219
Phenaphen with Codeine Capsules 1865
Phenaphen-650 with Codeine Tablets ... 1866
Phenergan with Codeine ... 2497
Phenergan VC with Codeine ... 2501
Robitussin A-C Syrup ... 1875
Robitussin-DAC Syrup ... 1875
Ryna ... ⊞ 741
Soma Compound w/Codeine Tablets ... 2390
Triaminic Expectorant w/Codeine .. 1996
Tussi-Organidin Liquid ... 2391
Tylenol with Codeine ... 1381
Codeine Polistirex (Increased effects).
No products indexed under this heading.
Cortisone Acetate (Decreased effects). Products include:
Cortone Acetate Sterile Suspension ... 1437
Cortone Acetate Tablets ... 1439
Desipramine Hydrochloride (Decreased effects; possible antagonized pressor effect of ephedrine). Products include:
Norpramin Tablets ... 1340
Deslanoside (Decreased effects; possible cardiac arrhythmias).
No products indexed under this heading.
Dexamethasone (Decreased effects). Products include:
AK-Trol Ointment & Suspension ... ⊙ 207
Decadron Elixir ... 1445
Decadron Tablets ... 1447
Decaspray Topical Aerosol ... 1459
Dexacidin ... ⊙ 272
Maxidex Sterile Ophthalmic Suspension ... ⊙ 223
Maxitrol Ophthalmic Ointment/Suspension ... ⊙ 223
TobraDex Ophthalmic Suspension and Ointment ... ⊙ 228
Dexamethasone Acetate (Decreased effects). Products include:
Dalalone D.P. Injectable ... 999
Decadron-LA Sterile Suspension ... 1457
Dexamethasone Sodium Phosphate (Decreased effects). Products include:
AK-Dex ... ⊙ 203
Decadron Phosphate Respihaler ... 1454
Decadron Phosphate Sterile Ophthalmic Ointment ... 1453
Decadron Phosphate Sterile Ophthalmic Solution ... 1453
Decadron Phosphate Topical Cream ... 1455
Decadron Phosphate Turbinaire ... 1456
Maxidex Sterile Ophthalmic Ointment ... ⊙ 222
NeoDecadron Sterile Ophthalmic Ointment ... 1517
NeoDecadron Sterile Ophthalmic Solution ... 1518
NeoDecadron Topical Cream ... 1518
Dezocine (Increased effects).
Diazepam (Increased effects). Products include:
Valium Injectable ... 1937
Valium Tablets ... 1939
Valrelease Capsules ... 1923
Dicumarol (Decreased anticoagulant effects). Products include:
Dicumarol Tablets ... 516
Digitoxin (Decreased effects; possible cardiac arrhythmias). Products include:
Crystodigin Tablets ... 1253
Digoxin (Decreased effects; possible cardiac arrhythmias). Products include:
Lanoxicaps ... 772
Lanoxin Elixir Pediatric ... 775
Lanoxin Injection ... 778
Lanoxin Injection Pediatric ... 781
Lanoxin Tablets ... 783
Dobutamine Hydrochloride (Increased effects). Products include:
Dobutrex Solution Vials ... 1259
Dopamine Hydrochloride (Increased effects). Products include:
Intropin Injection ... 930
Doxepin Hydrochloride (Decreased effects; possible antagonized pressor effect of ephedrine). Products include:
Sinequan ... 1960
Doxycycline Calcium (Decreased effects).
No products indexed under this heading.
Doxycycline Hyclate (Decreased effects). Products include:
Doryx Capsules ... 1717
Vibramycin Hyclate Capsules ... 1787
Vibramycin Hyclate Intravenous ... 1968
Vibra-Tabs Film Coated Tablets ... 1787
Doxycycline Monohydrate (Decreased effects). Products include:
Monodox Capsules ... 1630
Vibramycin Monohydrate for Oral Suspension ... 1787
Droperidol (Increased effects). Products include:
Inapsine Injection ... 1140
Innovar Injection ... 1141
Enflurane (Increased effects of medication; cardiac arrhythmias). Products include:
Ethrane ... 599
Epinephrine (Increased effects). Products include:
Ana-Kit Anaphylaxis Emergency Treatment Kit ... 1100
Bronkaid Mist ... ⊞ 757
EpiPen ... 843
Marcaine Hydrochloride 0.5% with Epinephrine 1:200,000 (as bitartrate) ... 958
Marcaine Hydrochloride with Epinephrine 1:200,000 ... 2055
Primatene Mist ... 2420
Sus-Phrine Injection ... 1006
Xylocaine with Epinephrine Injections ... 637
Epinephrine Bitartrate (Increased effects). Products include:
AsthmaHaler Mist Epinephrine Bitartrate Bronchodilator ... ⊞ 616
Bronkaid Mist Suspension ... ⊞ 757
Primatene Mist Suspension ... 2421
Epinephrine Hydrochloride (Increased effects). Products include:
Adrenalin Chloride Solution 1:100 & 1:1,000 ... 1689
Epifrin ... ⊙ 244
Glaucon ... ⊙ 218
Ergonovine Maleate (Hypertension).
Erythromycin (Increased theophylline plasma levels). Products include:
A/T/S Topical Gel and Topical Solution ... 1089
AK-Mycin Ointment ... ⊙ 204
Benzamycin Topical Gel ... 907
E-Mycin Tablets ... 688
ETS-2% ... 1685
ERYC ... 1720
Erycette (erythromycin 2%) Topical Solution ... 1678
Ery-Tab Tablets ... 521
Erythromycin Base Filmtab ... 525
Erythromycin Delayed-Release Capsules, USP ... 526
Ilotycin Ophthalmic Ointment ... 915
PCE Dispertab Tablets ... 549
Pediazole ... 1973
T-Stat 2.0% Topical Solution and Pads ... 2409
Theramycin Z Topical Solution 2% 1410
Erythromycin Estolate (Increased theophylline plasma levels). Products include:
Ilosone ... 913
Erythromycin Ethylsuccinate (Increased theophylline plasma levels). Products include:
E.E.S. ... 522
EryPed ... 519
Pediazole ... 1973
Erythromycin Gluceptate (Increased theophylline plasma levels). Products include:
Ilotycin Gluceptate, IV, Vials ... 915
Erythromycin Lactobionate (Increased theophylline plasma levels).
No products indexed under this heading.
Erythromycin Stearate (Increased theophylline plasma levels). Products include:
Erythrocin Stearate Filmtab ... 523
Estazolam (Increased effects). Products include:
ProSom Tablets ... 554
Ethchlorvynol (Increased effects). Products include:
Placidyl Capsules ... 553
Ethinamate (Increased effects).
No products indexed under this heading.
Fentanyl (Increased effects). Products include:
Duragesic Transdermal System ... 1133
Fentanyl Citrate (Increased effects). Products include:
Innovar Injection ... 1141
Sublimaze Injection ... 1146
Fluphenazine Decanoate (Increased effects). Products include:
Prolixin Decanoate ... 1795
Fluphenazine Enanthate (Increased effects). Products include:
Prolixin Enanthate ... 1796
Fluphenazine Hydrochloride (Increased effects). Products include:
Prolixin Elixir ... 1793
Prolixin Injection ... 1791
Prolixin Oral Concentrate ... 1792
Prolixin Tablets ... 1793
Flurazepam Hydrochloride (Increased effects). Products include:
Dalmane Capsules ... 1927
Furazolidone (Potentiated pressor effect of ephedrine). Products include:
Furoxone ... 1855
Furosemide (Increased diuresis). Products include:
Lasix ... 1093
Glutethimide (Increased effects).
No products indexed under this heading.

(⊞ Described in PDR For Nonprescription Drugs) (⊙ Described in PDR For Ophthalmology)

Griseofulvin (Decreased effects). Products include:
Fulvicin P/G Tablets 2090
Fulvicin P/G 165 & 330 Tablets 2091
Fulvicin-U/F Tablets 2092
Grifulvin V (griseofulvin microsize) Tablets/Suspension 1678
Grisactin 2454
Grisactin Ultra Tablets 2455
Gris-PEG Tablets, 125 mg & 250 mg 1083

Guanethidine Monosulfate (Decreased hypotensive effect). Products include:
Esimil Tablets 864
Ismelin Tablets 869

Haloperidol (Increased effects). Products include:
Haldol Injection, Tablets and Concentrate 1373

Haloperidol Decanoate (Increased effects). Products include:
Haldol Decanoate 1375

Hexamethonium (Decreased hexamethonium-induced chronotropic effect).

Hydrocodone Bitartrate (Increased effects). Products include:
Anexsia 5/500 Tablets 2196
Anexsia 7.5/650 Tablets 2197
Azdone Tablets 844
Codiclear DH Syrup 845
Codimal DH Syrup 846
Damason-P 1356
Hycodan Syrup, Tablets 927
Hycomine Compound Tablets 929
Hycomine Syrup 927
Hycotuss Expectorant Syrup 930
Hydrocet Capsules 835
Lortab ASA Tablets 2414
Lortab 2412
Ru-Tuss with Hydrocodone 694
Triaminic Expectorant DH 1995
Vicodin Tablets 1187
Vicodin ES Tablets 1189
Zydone Capsules 941

Hydrocodone Polistirex (Increased effects). Products include:
Tussionex Extended-Release Suspension 988

Hydrocortisone (Decreased effects). Products include:
AK-Spore H.C. .... ⊙ 206
Bactine Hydrocortisone Anti-Itch Cream .... ▣ 625
CaldeCORT Anti-Itch Hydrocortisone Spray .... ▣ 560
Carmol HC Cream 1% 2296
Cortaid Spray .... ▣ 735
Cortenema 2244
Cortisporin Ointment 758
Cortisporin Ophthalmic Ointment Sterile 758
Cortisporin Ophthalmic Suspension Sterile 759
Cortisporin Otic Solution Sterile 760
Cortisporin Otic Suspension Sterile 760
Cortizone-5 Creme & Ointment .... ▣ 732
Dermolate Anti-Itch Cream .... ▣ 697
Eldecort Cream 1.0% 1113
Eldecort Cream 1.0% and 2.5% 1113
Fungoid HC Creme 1770
Hydrocortone Tablets 1482
Hytone 909
LazerSporin-C Solution 1770
Massengill Medicated Soft Cloth Towelettes 2192
Nutracort Cream & Lotion 1684
PediOtic Suspension Sterile 797
Synacort Creams 1%, 2.5% 2296
Vanoxide-HC Acne Lotion 911
Vioform-Hydrocortisone Cream and Mild Cream 889
Vioform-Hydrocortisone Ointment 889
VōSoL HC Otic Solution 2392
Vytone Cream 1% 911

Hydrocortisone Acetate (Decreased effects). Products include:
Analpram-HC Rectal Cream 1% and 2.5% 970
Anusol-HC Cream 1690
Anusol-HC Suppositories 1691
Caldecort .... ▣ 560
Carmol HC Cream 1% 2296
Chloromycetin Hydrocortisone Ophthalmic 1694
Coly-Mycin S Otic w/Neomycin & Hydrocortisone 1708
Cortaid .... ▣ 735
Cortef Feminine Itch Cream .... ▣ 735
Corticaine .... ▣ 682
Cortifoam 1827
Cortisporin Cream 757
Epifoam 1828
Gynecort 5 Creme .... ▣ 556
Hydrocortone Acetate Sterile Suspension 1479
Lanacort 5 Creme and Ointment .. ▣ 557
Mantadil Cream 789
Ophthocort .... ⊙ 301
Orabase HCA Oral Paste 890
Pramosone Cream, Lotion & Ointment 971
ProctoCream-HC 1834
Proctofoam-HC 1835

Hydrocortisone Sodium Phosphate (Decreased effects). Products include:
Hydrocortone Phosphate Injection, Sterile 1481

Hydrocortisone Sodium Succinate (Decreased effects). Products include:
Solu-Cortef Sterile Powder 2361

Hydroxyzine Hydrochloride (Increased effects). Products include:
Atarax Tablets & Syrup 1941
Marax Tablets & DF Syrup 1954
Vistaril Intramuscular Solution 1970

Imipramine Hydrochloride (Decreased effects; possible antagonized pressor effect of ephedrine). Products include:
Tofranil Ampuls 1038
Tofranil Tablets 1039

Imipramine Pamoate (Decreased effects; possible antagonized pressor effect of ephedrine). Products include:
Tofranil-PM Capsules 1041

Isocarboxazid (Potentiated pressor effect of ephedrine). Products include:
Marplan Tablets 1906

Isoflurane (Increased effects of medication; cardiac arrhythmias). Products include:
Forane 600

Isoproterenol Hydrochloride (Increased effects). Products include:
Isuprel Hydrochloride Injection 1:5000 2050
Isuprel Hydrochloride Mistometer .. 2051
Isuprel Hydrochloride Solution 1:200 & 1:100 2052
Norisodrine Aerotrol 540

Ketamine Hydrochloride (Increased effects of medication; cardiac arrhythmias). Products include:
Ketalar 1726

Levorphanol Tartrate (Increased effects). Products include:
Levo-Dromoran 1906

Lincomycin Hydrochloride Monohydrate (Increased theophylline plasma levels).
No products indexed under this heading.

Lithium Carbonate (Increased excretion of lithium carbonate). Products include:
Eskalith 2214
Lithane Tablets 1596
Lithium Carbonate Capsules & Tablets 1984
Lithobid Tablets 870

Lorazepam (Increased effects). Products include:
Ativan Injection 2432
Ativan Tablets 2434

Loxapine Hydrochloride (Increased effects). Products include:
Loxitane 1213

Loxapine Succinate (Increased effects). Products include:
Loxitane Capsules 1213

Maprotiline Hydrochloride (Decreased effects; possible antagonized pressor effect of ephedrine). Products include:
Ludiomil Tablets 874

Meperidine Hydrochloride (Increased effects). Products include:
Demerol 2047
Mepergan Injection 2479

Mephobarbital (Increased effects). Products include:
Mebaral Tablets 2061

Meprobamate (Increased effects). Products include:
Deprol Tablets 2382
Equagesic Tablets 2451
Miltown Tablets 2386
PMB 200 and PMB 400 2504

Mesoridazine (Increased effects). Products include:
Serentil 686

Metaproterenol Sulfate (Increased effects). Products include:
Alupent 674
Arm-a-Med Metaproterenol Sulfate Inhalation Solution, USP 617
Metaprel Inhalation Aerosol Bronchodilator 2014
Metaprel Inhalation Solution 2015
Metaprel 2015
Metaproterenol Sulfate Inhalation Solution, USP 912

Metaraminol Bitartrate (Increased effects). Products include:
Aramine Injection 1424

Methadone Hydrochloride (Increased effects). Products include:
Dolophine Hydrochloride Ampoules & Vials 1260
Dolophine Hydrochloride Tablets 1261
Methadone Hydrochloride Diskets .. 1284
Methadone Hydrochloride Oral Solution & Tablets 1987

Methohexital Sodium (Increased effects of medication; cardiac arrhythmias). Products include:
Brevital Sodium Vials 1248

Methoxamine Hydrochloride (Increased effects). Products include:
Vasoxyl Injection 819

Methoxyflurane (Increased effects of medication; cardiac arrhythmias).
No products indexed under this heading.

Methylergonovine Maleate (Hypertension). Products include:
Methergine 2016

Methylprednisolone Acetate (Decreased effects). Products include:
Depo-Medrol Sterile Aqueous Suspension 2334

Methylprednisolone Sodium Succinate (Decreased effects). Products include:
Solu-Medrol Sterile Powder 2363

Midazolam Hydrochloride (Increased effects). Products include:
Versed Injection 1924

Molindone Hydrochloride (Increased effects). Products include:
Moban Tablets & Concentrate 932

Morphine Sulfate (Increased effects). Products include:
Astramorph/PF Injection, USP (Preservative-Free) 618
Duramorph 960
Infumorph 200 and Infumorph 500 Sterile Solutions 962
MS Contin Tablets 1814
MSIR 1817
Oramorph SR (Morphine Sulfate Sustained Release Tablets) 1988
Roxanol 1991

Norepinephrine Bitartrate (Increased effects). Products include:
Levophed Bitartrate Injection 2054

Nortriptyline Hydrochloride (Decreased effects; possible antagonized pressor effect of ephedrine). Products include:
Pamelor 2019

Opium Alkaloids (Increased effects). Products include:
B & O No. 15A & No. 16A Supprettes 2395
Pantopon Injectable 1911

Oxazepam (Increased effects). Products include:
Serax Capsules 2522
Serax Tablets 2522

Oxycodone Hydrochloride (Increased effects). Products include:
Percocet Tablets 950
Percodan 951
Roxicodone Tablets, Oral Solution & Intensol (Oxycodone) 1992
Tylox Capsules 1382

Oxytocin (Injection) (Hypertension). Products include:
Oxytocin Injection 2492
Pitocin Injection, Ampoules, Steri-Dose Syringes 1757

Oxytocin (Nasal Spray) (Hypertension).
No products indexed under this heading.

Pentobarbital Sodium (Increased effects). Products include:
Nembutal Sodium Capsules 534
Nembutal Sodium Solution 536
Nembutal Sodium Suppositories 538

Perphenazine (Increased effects). Products include:
Etrafon 2087
Triavil Tablets 1556
Trilafon 2123

Phenelzine Sulfate (Potentiated pressor effect of ephedrine). Products include:
Nardil 1742

Phenylephrine Bitartrate (Increased effects).
No products indexed under this heading.

Phenylephrine Hydrochloride (Increased effects). Products include:
AK-Dilate Solution 2.5% and 10% .... ⊙ 203
Atrohist Sprinkle Capsules 558
Cerose-DM 2443
Codimal 846
Comhist LA Capsules 1618
Congespirin For Children Aspirin Free Chewable Cold Tablets 748
Cyclomydril .... ⊙ 216
Deconsal Sprinkle Capsules 559
Dimetane Decongestant .... ▣ 673
Dristan Decongestant/Antihistamine/ Analgesic Coated Caplets .... ▣ 749
Dristan Cold Nasal Decongestant/ Antihistamine/ Analgesic Coated Tablets 2419
Dristan Advanced Formula Decongestant/Antihistamine/ Analgesic Tablets .... ▣ 749
Dristan Nasal Spray, Menthol 2419
Dristan Nasal Spray, Regular and Regular with Metered Pump 2419
Entex Capsules 1623
Entex Liquid 1623
Sinus Excedrin Analgesic, Decongestant Tablets & Caplets 750
Extendryl 994
4-Way Fast Acting Nasal Spray - Original Formula (regular & mentholated) & Metered Spray Pump (regular) 751
Hycomine Compound Tablets 929
Murocoll-2 Sterile Ophthalmic Solution .... ⊙ 261
Mydfrin 2.5% .... ⊙ 224
Naldecon Syrup, Tablets, Pediatric Drops and Pediatric Syrup 709
Neo-Synephrine Hydrochloride 1% Carpuject 2063

- Neo-Synephrine Hydrochloride 1% Injection ... 2063
- Neo-Synephrine Hydrochloride (Ophthalmic) ... 2064
- Neo-Synephrine ... ◘ 759
- Nōstril Nasal Decongestant ... ◘ 520
- Novahistine Elixir ... ◘ 596
- Phenergan VC ... 2500
- Phenergan VC with Codeine ... 2501
- Prefrin Liquifilm Vasoconstrictor and Lubricant Eye Drops ... ⊙ 254
- Prefrin-A ... ⊙ 255
- Quelidrine Syrup ... 556
- Relief Vasoconstrictor and Lubricant Eye Drops ... ⊙ 256
- Robitussin Night Relief ... ◘ 677
- Ru-Tuss with Hydrocodone ... 694
- Ru-Tuss Tablets ... 693
- Vasosulf ... ⊙ 279
- Vicks Sinex ... ◘ 665
- Zincfrin ... ⊙ 230

Phenylephrine Tannate (Increased effects). Products include:

- Rynatan ... 2387
- Rynatuss ... 2388

Phenylpropanolamine Hydrochloride (Increased effects). Products include:

- A.R.M. Allergy Relief Medicine Caplets ... ◘ 615
- Acutrim ... ◘ 548
- Allerest ... ◘ 559
- BC Cold Powder ... ◘ 517
- Cheracol Plus Head Cold/Cough Formula ... ◘ 667
- Codimal Expectorant ... 846
- Comtrex Multi-Symptom Cold Reliever Tablets/Caplets/Liqui-Gels/Liquid ... 745
- Contac Continuous Action Decongestant/Antihistamine Capsules ◘ 710
- Contac Maximum Strength Continuous Action Decongestant/Antihistamine Caplets ... ◘ 709
- Contac Severe Cold and Flu Formula Caplets ... ◘ 711
- Coricidin 'D' Decongestant Tablets ... ◘ 695
- Coricidin Demilets Tablets for Children ... ◘ 696
- Demazin Nasal Decongestant/Antihistamine Repetabs Tablets & Syrup ... ◘ 697
- Dexatrim ... ◘ 733
- Dimetane-DC Cough Syrup ... 1857
- Dimetapp Elixir ... ◘ 673
- Dimetapp DM Elixir ... ◘ 674
- Dimetapp Extentabs ... ◘ 674
- Dimetapp Plus Caplets ... ◘ 675
- Dimetapp Tablets ... ◘ 675
- Entex Capsules ... 1623
- Entex LA Tablets ... 1623
- Entex Liquid ... 1623
- 4-Way Cold Tablets ... 750
- Hycomine Syrup ... 927
- Naldecon CX Adult Liquid ... ◘ 521
- Naldecon DX Adult Liquid ... ◘ 521
- Naldecon DX Children's Syrup ... ◘ 522
- Naldecon DX Pediatric Drops ... ◘ 522
- Naldecon EX Children's Syrup ... ◘ 522
- Naldecon EX Pediatric Drops ... ◘ 523
- Naldecon Syrup, Tablets, Pediatric Drops and Pediatric Syrup ... 709
- Nolamine Tablets ... 838
- Nolex LA Tablets ... 838
- Ornade Spansule Capsules ... 2221
- Orthoxicol Cough Syrup ... ◘ 668
- Propagest ... 839
- Pyrroxate Capsules ... ◘ 669
- Robitussin-CF ... ◘ 676
- Ru-Tuss II Capsules ... 693
- Ru-Tuss with Hydrocodone ... 694
- Ru-Tuss Tablets ... 693
- Sine-Off Sinus Medicine Tablets-Aspirin Formula ... ◘ 722
- Sinulin ... 840
- St. Joseph Cold Tablets for Children ... ◘ 704
- Tavist-D Tablets ... 2035
- Triaminic Allergy Tablets ... ◘ 688
- Triaminic Chewables ... ◘ 688
- Triaminic Cold Tablets ... ◘ 688
- Triaminic Expectorant ... ◘ 688
- Triaminic Expectorant w/Codeine ... 1996
- Triaminic Expectorant DH ... 1995
- Triaminic Oral Infant Drops ... 1996
- Triaminic Syrup ... ◘ 689
- Triaminic-12 Tablets ... ◘ 690
- Triaminic-DM Syrup ... ◘ 689
- Triaminicin Tablets ... ◘ 690
- Triaminicol Multi-Symptom Cold Tablets ... ◘ 691
- Triaminicol Multi-Symptom Relief ◘ 691
- Tuss-Ornade Liquid ... 2242
- Tuss-Ornade Spansule Capsules ... 2242
- Tylenol Cold Medication, Effervescent Tablets ... 1369

Phenytoin (Decreased effects; decreased phenytoin levels). Products include:

- Dilantin Infatabs ... 1710
- Dilantin-30 Pediatric/Dilantin-125 Suspension ... 1713

Phenytoin Sodium (Decreased effects; decreased phenytoin levels). Products include:

- Dilantin Kapseals ... 1708
- Dilantin Parenteral ... 1712
- Dilantin with Phenobarbital Kapseals ... 1715

Pirbuterol Acetate (Increased effects). Products include:

- Maxair Inhaler ... 1311

Prazepam (Increased effects). Products include:

- Centrax ... 1693

Prednisolone Acetate (Decreased effects). Products include:

- AK-Cide Sterile Ophthalmic Ointment & Suspension ... ⊙ 202
- Blephamide Liquifilm Sterile Ophthalmic Suspension ... 586
- Blephamide S.O.P. Sterile Ophthalmic Ointment ... 586
- Cetapred Ointment ... ⊙ 220
- ⅛% Econopred & 1% Econopred Plus ... ⊙ 217
- Isopto Cetapred Suspension ... ⊙ 220
- Metimyd ... ⊙ 306
- Poly-Pred Liquifilm ... ⊙ 250
- Pred Forte ... ⊙ 252
- Pred Mild ... ⊙ 254
- Pred-G Liquifilm Sterile Ophthalmic Suspension ... ⊙ 252
- Pred-G S.O.P. Sterile Ophthalmic Ointment ... ⊙ 253
- Vasocidin Ointment ... ⊙ 275

Prednisolone Sodium Phosphate (Decreased effects). Products include:

- AK-Pred ... ⊙ 205
- Hydeltrasol Injection, Sterile ... 1476
- Inflamase ... ⊙ 274
- Pediapred Oral Liquid ... 987
- Vasocidin Ophthalmic Solution ... ⊙ 276

Prednisolone Tebutate (Decreased effects). Products include:

- Hydeltra-T.B.A. Sterile Suspension 1478

Prednisone (Decreased effects). Products include:

- Deltasone Tablets ... 2332

Prochlorperazine (Increased effects). Products include:

- Compazine ... 2201

Promethazine Hydrochloride (Increased effects). Products include:

- Mepergan Injection ... 2479
- Phenergan with Codeine ... 2497
- Phenergan with Dextromethorphan 2499
- Phenergan Injection ... 2493
- Phenergan Suppositories ... 2496
- Phenergan Syrup ... 2495
- Phenergan Tablets ... 2496
- Phenergan VC ... 2500
- Phenergan VC with Codeine ... 2501

Propofol (Increased effects). Products include:

- Diprivan Injection ... 2267

Propoxyphene Hydrochloride (Increased effects). Products include:

- Darvon ... 1256
- Wygesic Tablets ... 2540

Propoxyphene Napsylate (Increased effects). Products include:

- Darvon-N/Darvocet-N ... 1254

Propranolol Hydrochloride (Antagonism of propranolol effect). Products include:

- Inderal ... 2459
- Inderal LA Long Acting Capsules ... 2461
- Inderide Tablets ... 2463
- Inderide LA Long Acting Capsules .. 2465

Protriptyline Hydrochloride (Decreased effects; possible antagonized pressor effect of ephedrine). Products include:

- Vivactil Tablets ... 1567

Pseudoephedrine Hydrochloride (Increased effects). Products include:

- Actifed Capsules ... ◘ 539
- Actifed Plus Caplets ... ◘ 539
- Actifed Plus Tablets ... ◘ 540
- Actifed with Codeine Cough Syrup .. 752
- Actifed Syrup ... ◘ 540
- Actifed Tablets ... ◘ 540
- Actifed 12-Hour Capsules ... ◘ 539
- Advil Cold & Sinus Caplets (formerly CoAdvil) ... 2416
- Allerest ... ◘ 559
- Anatuss LA Tablets ... 1359
- Benadryl Decongestant Elixir ... ◘ 635
- Benadryl Decongestant ... ◘ 635
- Benadryl Plus ... ◘ 636
- Benadryl Plus Nighttime ... ◘ 637
- Benylin Decongestant ... ◘ 638
- Brexin L.A. Capsules ... 2078
- Bromfed Capsules (Timed Release) ... 1615
- Bromfed Syrup ... ◘ 628
- Bromfed ... 1615
- CoAdvil ... ◘ 748
- Allergy-Sinus Comtrex Multi-Symptom Allergy Sinus Formula Tablets & Caplets ... 746
- Cough Formula Comtrex ... 746
- Comtrex Multi-Symptom Cold Reliever Tablets/Caplets/Liqui-Gels/Liquid ... 745
- Day-Night Comtrex ... 747
- Non-Drowsy Comtrex ... 747
- Congess ... 994
- Congestac Caplets ... ◘ 617
- Contac Jr. Children's Cold Medicine ... ◘ 712
- Contac Nighttime Cold Medicine ... ◘ 713
- Contac Sinus Caplets Maximum Strength Non-Drowsy Formula ... ◘ 710
- Contac Sinus Tablets Maximum Strength Non-Drowsy Formula ... ◘ 710
- Deconamine ... 663
- Deconsal II Tablets ... 559
- Dimacol Caplets ... ◘ 672
- Dimetane-DX Cough Syrup ... 1858
- Dorcol Children's Cough Syrup ... ◘ 685
- Dorcol Children's Decongestant Liquid ... ◘ 685
- Dorcol Children's Liquid Cold Formula ... ◘ 686
- Maximum Strength Dristan Decongestant/Analgesic Coated Caplets ... ◘ 750
- No Drowsiness Dristan Cold Nasal Decongestant/Analgesic Coated Caplets ... 2420
- Dristan Sinus Caplets ... 2419
- Sinus Excedrin Analgesic, Decongestant Tablets & Caplets ... ◘ 533
- Fedahist Gyrocaps ... 2145
- Fedahist Timecaps ... 2145
- Guaifed ... 1615
- Guaifed Syrup ... ◘ 629
- Isoclor Expectorant ... 982
- Isoclor Timesule Capsules ... ◘ 561
- Kronofed-A ... 970
- Medi-Flu Caplet, Liquid ... ◘ 640
- Novafed A Capsules ... 1342
- Novafed Capsules ... 1342
- Novahistine DH ... 1342
- Novahistine DMX ... ◘ 595
- Novahistine Expectorant ... 1343
- Nucofed Capsules ... 2219
- Nucofed Expectorant ... 2219
- Nucofed Pediatric Expectorant ... 2220
- Nucofed Syrup ... 2219
- Ornex Caplets ... ◘ 618
- PediaCare Allergy Relief Formula Liquid ... 1362
- PediaCare Cough-Cold Formula Liquid ... 1362
- PediaCare Infants' Oral Decongestant Drops ... 1362
- PediaCare Night Rest Cough-Cold Formula Liquid ... 1362
- PediaCare 6-12 Cough-Cold Formula Chewable Tablets ... 1362
- Robitussin-DAC Syrup ... 1875
- Robitussin-PE ... ◘ 677
- Rondec ... 1975
- Rondec-DM ... 1976
- Rondec-TR Tablet ... 1975
- Ru-Tuss DE Tablets ... 694
- Ryna ... ◘ 741
- Seldane-D Extended-Release Tablets ... 1350
- Sinarest ... ◘ 562
- Sine-Aid Maximum Strength Sinus Headache Caplets ... 1365
- Sine-Aid Maximum Strength Sinus Headache Tablets ... 1365
- Sine-Off Maximum Strength Allergy/Sinus Formula Caplets ... ◘ 721
- Sine-Off Maximum Strength No Drowsiness Formula Caplets ... ◘ 722
- Singlet Tablets ... ◘ 598
- Sinutab Maximum Strength ... ◘ 641
- Sinutab Maximum Strength Without Drowsiness Tablets & Caplets ... ◘ 642
- Sinutab Regular Strength Without Drowsiness Formula ... ◘ 641
- St. Joseph Nighttime Cold Medicine ... ◘ 705
- Sudafed Children's Liquid ... ◘ 543
- Sudafed Cough Syrup ... ◘ 543
- Sudafed Plus Liquid ... ◘ 544
- Sudafed Plus Tablets ... ◘ 545
- Sudafed Sinus Caplets ... ◘ 545
- Sudafed Sinus Tablets ... ◘ 545
- Sudafed Tablets, 30 mg ... ◘ 544
- Sudafed Tablets, Adult Strength, 60 mg ... ◘ 544
- Sudafed 12 Hour Capsules ... ◘ 545
- TheraFlu Flu and Cold Medicine ... ◘ 687
- Triaminic Nite Light ... ◘ 689
- Tylenol Allergy Sinus Medication Caplets and Gelcaps, Maximum Strength ... 1372
- Children's Tylenol Cold Liquid Formula and Chewable Tablets ... 1368
- Tylenol Cold & Flu Hot Medication, Packets ... 1369
- Tylenol Cold & Flu No Drowsiness Hot Medication, Packets ... 1371
- Tylenol Cold Medication Caplets and Tablets ... 1370
- Tylenol Cold Medication No Drowsiness Formula Caplets ... 1370
- Tylenol Cold Night Time Medication Liquid ... 1371
- Tylenol Cough Medication Liquid with Decongestant, Maximum Strength ... 1372
- Tylenol, Maximum Strength, Sinus Medication Gelcaps, Caplets and Tablets ... 1373
- Ursinus Inlay-Tabs ... ◘ 691
- Vicks Children's NyQuil ... ◘ 664
- Vicks Daycare ... ◘ 660
- Vicks Formula 44D Decongestant Cough Medicine ... ◘ 662
- Vicks Formula 44M Multi-Symptom Cough Medicine ... ◘ 662
- Vicks NyQuil Nighttime Colds Medicine-Original & Cherry Flavor ... ◘ 664
- Vicks Pediatric Formula 44 Cough & Congestion Medicine ... ◘ 663
- Vicks Pediatric Formula 44m Multi-Symptom Cough & Cold Medicine ... ◘ 663

Pseudoephedrine Sulfate (Increased effects). Products include:

- Afrin Tablets ... ◘ 693
- Chlor-Trimeton Decongestant ... ◘ 694
- Disophrol Chronotab Sustained-Action Tablets ... ◘ 698
- Drixoral Antihistamine/Nasal Decongestant Syrup ... ◘ 698
- Drixoral Non-Drowsy Formula ... ◘ 699
- Drixoral Plus Extended-Release Tablets ... ◘ 699
- Drixoral Sinus ... ◘ 700
- Drixoral Sustained-Action Tablets ◘ 698
- Sinutab Allergy Formula Sustained Action Tablets ... ◘ 640
- Trinalin Repetabs Tablets ... 1170

Quazepam (Increased effects). Products include:

- Doral Tablets ... 2383

Reserpine (Tachycardia; decreased pressor effect of ephedrine). Products include:

(◘ Described in PDR For Nonprescription Drugs) (⊙ Described in PDR For Ophthalmology)

Diupres Tablets 1461
Hydromox R Tablets 1209
Hydropres Tablets 1485
Renese-R Tablets 1786
Salutensin/Salutensin-Demi 719
Ser-Ap-Es Tablets 881
Serpasil Tablets 883
Serpasil-Apresoline Tablets 884
Serpasil-Esidrix Tablets 886

Secobarbital Sodium (Increased effects). Products include:
Seconal Sodium Pulvules 1296

Selegiline Hydrochloride (Potentiated pressor effect of ephedrine). Products include:
Eldepryl 2250

Sufentanil Citrate (Increased effects). Products include:
Sufenta Injection 1147

Temazepam (Increased effects). Products include:
Restoril Capsules 2023

Terbutaline Sulfate (Increased effects). Products include:
Brethaire Inhaler 1024
Brethine Ampuls 1026
Brethine Tablets 1026
Bricanyl Injection 1324
Bricanyl Tablets 1325

Thiamylal Sodium (Increased effects). Products include:
Surital Ampoules, Steri-Vials 1764

Thioridazine Hydrochloride (Increased effects). Products include:
Mellaril 2011

Thiothixene (Increased effects). Products include:
Navane Capsules and Concentrate 1954
Navane Intramuscular 1956

Tranylcypromine Sulfate (Potentiated pressor effect of ephedrine). Products include:
Parnate Tablets 2222

Triamcinolone (Decreased effects).
No products indexed under this heading.

Triamcinolone Acetonide (Decreased effects). Products include:
Aristocort A 1010
Azmacort Inhaler 1837
Kenalog Cream, Lotion & Ointment 2401
Kenalog-10 Injection 2402
Kenalog-40 Injection 2403
Kenalog in Orabase 604
Kenalog Spray 2401
Mycolog II Cream and Ointment 2407
Mytrex Cream & Ointment 2080
Nasacort Nasal Inhaler 1844

Triamcinolone Diacetate (Decreased effects). Products include:
Aristocort Suspension 1008

Triamcinolone Hexacetonide (Decreased effects). Products include:
Aristospan Suspension 1011

Triazolam (Increased effects). Products include:
Halcion Tablets 2340

Trifluoperazine Hydrochloride (Increased effects). Products include:
Stelazine 2226

Trimipramine Maleate (Decreased effects; possible antagonized pressor effect of ephedrine). Products include:
Surmontil Capsules 2524

Troleandomycin (Increased theophylline plasma levels). Products include:
Tao Capsules 1963

Warfarin Sodium (Decreased anticoagulant effects). Products include:
Coumadin Injection & Tablets 944
Panwarfin Tablets 547

QUARZAN CAPSULES
(Clidinium Bromide) 1937
No interactions described in labeling.

QUELIDRINE SYRUP
(Dextromethorphan Hydrobromide, Chlorpheniramine Maleate, Ephedrine Hydrochloride, Phenylephrine Hydrochloride) 556
May interact with cardiac glycosides. Compounds in this category include:

Deslanoside (Use with caution).

Digitoxin (Use with caution). Products include:
Crystodigin Tablets 1253

Digoxin (Use with caution). Products include:
Lanoxicaps 772
Lanoxin Elixir Pediatric 775
Lanoxin Injection 778
Lanoxin Injection Pediatric 781
Lanoxin Tablets 783

QUESTRAN LIGHT
(Cholestyramine) 711
May interact with tetracyclines, thyroid preparations, cardiac glycosides, and certain other agents. Compounds in these categories include:

Chlorothiazide (Delayed or reduced absorption of concomitantly administered oral chlorothiazide (acidic)). Products include:
Aldoclor Tablets 1413
Diupres Tablets 1461
Diuril Oral 1464

Demeclocycline Hydrochloride (Delayed or reduced absorption of concomitantly administered oral tetracycline). Products include:
Declomycin Capsules, Tablets 1199

Deslanoside (Delayed or reduced absorption of concomitantly administered oral digitalis).
No products indexed under this heading.

Digitoxin (Delayed or reduced absorption of concomitantly administered oral digitalis). Products include:
Crystodigin Tablets 1253

Digoxin (Delayed or reduced absorption of concomitantly administered oral digitalis). Products include:
Lanoxicaps 772
Lanoxin Elixir Pediatric 775
Lanoxin Injection 778
Lanoxin Injection Pediatric 781
Lanoxin Tablets 783

Doxycycline Calcium (Delayed or reduced absorption of concomitantly administered oral tetracycline).
No products indexed under this heading.

Doxycycline Hyclate (Delayed or reduced absorption of concomitantly administered oral tetracycline). Products include:
Doryx Capsules 1717
Vibramycin Hyclate Capsules 1787
Vibramycin Hyclate Intravenous 1968
Vibra-Tabs Film Coated Tablets 1787

Doxycycline Monohydrate (Delayed or reduced absorption of concomitantly administered oral tetracycline). Products include:
Monodox Capsules 1630
Vibramycin Monohydrate for Oral Suspension 1787

Levothyroxine Sodium (Delayed or reduced absorption of concomitantly administered oral thyroid preparations). Products include:
Levothroid Tablets 1003
Levoxine Tablets 904
Synthroid 695

Liothyronine Sodium (Delayed or reduced absorption of concomitantly administered oral thyroid preparations). Products include:
Cytomel Tablets 2203

Liotrix (Delayed or reduced absorption of concomitantly administered oral thyroid preparations). Products include:
Euthroid 1724

Lovastatin (Cholesterol-lowering effects are additive). Products include:
Mevacor Tablets 1505

Methacycline Hydrochloride (Delayed or reduced absorption of concomitantly administered oral tetracycline).
No products indexed under this heading.

Minocycline Hydrochloride (Delayed or reduced absorption of concomitantly administered oral tetracycline). Products include:
Minocin Intravenous 1221
Minocin Oral Suspension 1224
Minocin Pellet-Filled Capsules 1222

Oxytetracycline Hydrochloride (Delayed or reduced absorption of concomitantly administered oral tetracycline). Products include:
Terra-Cortril Ophthalmic Suspension 1963
Terramycin Capsules 1786
Terramycin Intramuscular Solution 1964
Terramycin with Polymyxin B Sulfate Ophthalmic Ointment 1965

Penicillin G Potassium (Delayed or reduced absorption of concomitantly administered oral penicillin G). Products include:
Pfizerpen for Injection 1957

Phenobarbital (Delayed or reduced absorption of concomitantly administered oral phenobarbital). Products include:
Arco-Lase Plus Tablets 607
Bellergal-S Tablets 1998
Bronkolixir .... ◙ 761
Bronkotabs Tablets .... ◙ 762
Donnatal 1858
Donnatal Extentabs 1859
Donnatal Tablets 1858
Donnazyme Tablets 1860
Kinesed Tablets 2272
Phenobarbital Elixir and Tablets 1293
Primatene Tablets-P Formula 2421
Quadrinal Tablets 1183
Tedral SA 1765

Phenylbutazone (Delayed or reduced absorption of concomitantly administered oral phenylbutazone). Products include:
Butazolidin Capsules & Tablets 1027

Propranolol Hydrochloride (Delayed or reduced absorption of concomitantly administered oral propranolol (basic)). Products include:
Inderal 2459
Inderal LA Long Acting Capsules 2461
Inderide Tablets 2463
Inderide LA Long Acting Capsules .. 2465

Tetracycline Hydrochloride (Delayed or reduced absorption of concomitantly administered oral tetracycline). Products include:
Achromycin V Capsules 1193
Achromycin Ophthalmic Ointment 1% .... ⊙ 307
Achromycin Ophthalmic Suspension 1% .... ⊙ 308
Topicycline for Topical Solution 1856

Thyroglobulin (Delayed or reduced absorption of concomitantly administered oral thyroid preparations). Products include:
Proloid Tablets 1761

Thyroid (Delayed or reduced absorption of concomitantly administered oral thyroid preparations). Products include:
S-P-T "Liquid" Capsules 995

Vitamin A (Cholestyramine may interfere with oral absorption and digestion of fat soluble vitamin A). Products include:
Aquasol A Vitamin A Capsules, USP 615
Aquasol A Parenteral, USP 615
Bugs Bunny Children's Chewable Vitamins (Sugar Free) .... ◙ 625
Bugs Bunny With Extra C Children's Chewable Vitamins (Sugar Free) .... ◙ 626
Bugs Bunny/Flintstones .... ◙ 625
Flintstones Children's Chewable Vitamins With Extra C .... ◙ 626
Flintstones Children's Chewable Vitamins Plus Iron .... ◙ 625
Lazer Creme 1770
Myadec .... ◙ 640
Natalins Rx 1391
Natalins Tablets 1391
Ocuvite Vitamin and Mineral Supplement .... ⊙ 312
One-A-Day Essential Vitamins .... ◙ 627
One-A-Day Maximum Formula Vitamins and Minerals .... ◙ 627
One-A-Day Plus Extra C Vitamins .. ◙ 627
Stressgard Stress Formula Vitamins .... ◙ 628
Tri-Vi-Flor 1.0 mg Vitamins with Fluoride Chewable Tablets 1400
Tri-Vi-Flor Drops 1400
Tri-Vi-Sol Vitamin Drops .... ◙ 614
Tri-Vi-Sol Vitamin Drops with Iron ◙ 614
Vicon Forte Capsules 2416
Vicon Plus .... ◙ 682
Vi-Daylin ADC Vitamins Drops 1980
Vi-Daylin ADC Vitamins + Iron Drops 1980
Vi-Daylin/F ADC Vitamins Drops With Fluoride 1981
Vi-Daylin/F ADC Vitamins + Iron Drops With Fluoride 1981
Vi-Zac .... ◙ 682
Within Women's Formula Multivitamin with Calcium, Extra Iron and Zinc .... ◙ 628
Zymacap Capsules .... ◙ 670

Vitamin D (Cholestyramine may interfere with oral absorption and digestion of fat soluble vitamin D). Products include:
Bugs Bunny Children's Chewable Vitamins (Sugar Free) .... ◙ 625
Bugs Bunny With Extra C Children's Chewable Vitamins (Sugar Free) .... ◙ 626
Bugs Bunny Plus Iron Children's Chewable Vitamins (Sugar Free) ◙ 625
Calderol Capsules 1635
Caltrate 600 + Iron & Vitamin D 1198
Caltrate 600 + Vitamin D 1197
Caltrate, Jr. Tablets 1198
Flintstones Children's Chewable Vitamins .... ◙ 625
Flintstones Children's Chewable Vitamins With Extra C .... ◙ 626
Flintstones Children's Chewable Vitamins Plus Iron .... ◙ 625
Natalins Rx 1391
Natalins Tablets 1391
One-A-Day Essential Vitamins .... ◙ 627
One-A-Day Maximum Formula Vitamins and Minerals .... ◙ 627
One-A-Day Plus Extra C Vitamins .. ◙ 627
Os-Cal 250+D Tablets .... ◙ 597
Os-Cal 500+D Tablets .... ◙ 597
Os-Cal Fortified Tablets .... ◙ 597
Os-Cal Plus Tablets .... ◙ 597
Posture-D 600 mg 2420
Stressgard Stress Formula Vitamins .... ◙ 628
Tri-Vi-Flor 1.0 mg Vitamins with Fluoride Chewable Tablets 1400
Tri-Vi-Flor Drops 1400
Tri-Vi-Sol Vitamin Drops .... ◙ 614
Tri-Vi-Sol Vitamin Drops with Iron ◙ 614
Vi-Daylin ADC Vitamins Drops 1980
Vi-Daylin ADC Vitamins + Iron Drops 1980
Vi-Daylin/F ADC Vitamins Drops With Fluoride 1981
Vi-Daylin/F ADC Vitamins + Iron Drops With Fluoride 1981

Within Women's Formula Multivitamin with Calcium, Extra Iron and Zinc ▣ 628
Zymacap Capsules ▣ 670

Vitamin K (Cholestyramine may interfere with oral absorption and digestion of fat soluble vitamin K). Products include:
One-A-Day Maximum Formula Vitamins and Minerals ▣ 627
Synkayvite Injection 1919
Synkayvite Tablets 1920

Vitamin K₁ (Cholestyramine may interfere with oral absorption and digestion of fat soluble vitamin K). Products include:
AquaMEPHYTON Injection 1422
Konakion Injection 1903
Mephyton Tablets 1503

Warfarin Sodium (Delayed or reduced absorption of concomitantly administered oral warfarin). Products include:
Coumadin Injection & Tablets 944
Panwarfin Tablets 547

QUESTRAN POWDER
(Cholestyramine) 710
May interact with thyroid preparations, cardiac glycosides, tetracyclines, and certain other agents. Compounds in these categories include:

Chlorothiazide (Delayed or reduced absorption of concomitantly administered oral chlorothiazide (acidic)). Products include:
Aldoclor Tablets 1413
Diupres Tablets 1461
Diuril Oral 1464

Demeclocycline Hydrochloride (Delayed or reduced absorption of concomitantly administered oral tetracycline). Products include:
Declomycin Capsules, Tablets 1199

Deslanoside (Delayed or reduced absorption of concomitantly administered oral digitalis).
No products indexed under this heading.

Digitoxin (Delayed or reduced absorption of concomitantly administered oral digitalis). Products include:
Crystodigin Tablets 1253

Digoxin (Delayed or reduced absorption of concomitantly administered oral digitalis). Products include:
Lanoxicaps 772
Lanoxin Elixir Pediatric 775
Lanoxin Injection 778
Lanoxin Injection Pediatric 781
Lanoxin Tablets 783

Doxycycline Calcium (Delayed or reduced absorption of concomitantly administered oral tetracycline).
No products indexed under this heading.

Doxycycline Hyclate (Delayed or reduced absorption of concomitantly administered oral tetracycline). Products include:
Doryx Capsules 1717
Vibramycin Hyclate Capsules 1787
Vibramycin Hyclate Intravenous 1968
Vibra-Tabs Film Coated Tablets 1787

Doxycycline Monohydrate (Delayed or reduced absorption of concomitantly administered oral tetracycline). Products include:
Monodox Capsules 1630
Vibramycin Monohydrate for Oral Suspension 1787

Levothyroxine Sodium (Delayed or reduced absorption of concomitantly administered oral thyroid preparations). Products include:
Levothroid Tablets 1003
Levoxine Tablets 904
Synthroid 695

Liothyronine Sodium (Delayed or reduced absorption of concomitantly administered oral thyroid preparations). Products include:
Cytomel Tablets 2203

Liotrix (Delayed or reduced absorption of concomitantly administered oral thyroid preparations). Products include:
Euthroid 1724

Lovastatin (Cholesterol-lowering effects are additive). Products include:
Mevacor Tablets 1505

Methacycline Hydrochloride (Delayed or reduced absorption of concomitantly administered oral tetracycline).
No products indexed under this heading.

Minocycline Hydrochloride (Delayed or reduced absorption of concomitantly administered oral tetracycline). Products include:
Minocin Intravenous 1221
Minocin Oral Suspension 1224
Minocin Pellet-Filled Capsules 1222

Oxytetracycline Hydrochloride (Delayed or reduced absorption of concomitantly administered oral tetracycline). Products include:
Terra-Cortril Ophthalmic Suspension 1963
Terramycin Capsules 1786
Terramycin Intramuscular Solution 1964
Terramycin with Polymyxin B Sulfate Ophthalmic Ointment 1965

Penicillin G Potassium (Delayed or reduced absorption of concomitantly administered oral penicillin G). Products include:
Pfizerpen for Injection 1957

Phenobarbital (Delayed or reduced absorption of concomitantly administered oral phenobarbital). Products include:
Arco-Lase Plus Tablets 607
Bellergal-S Tablets 1998
Bronkolixir ▣ 761
Bronkotabs Tablets ▣ 762
Donnatal 1858
Donnatal Extentabs 1859
Donnatal Tablets 1858
Donnazyme Tablets 1860
Kinesed Tablets 2272
Phenobarbital Elixir and Tablets 1293
Primatene Tablets-P Formula 2421
Quadrinal Tablets 1183
Tedral SA 1765

Phenylbutazone (Delayed or reduced absorption of concomitantly administered oral phenylbutazone). Products include:
Butazolidin Capsules & Tablets 1027

Propranolol Hydrochloride (Delayed or reduced absorption of concomitantly administered oral propranolol (basic)). Products include:
Inderal 2459
Inderal LA Long Acting Capsules 2461
Inderide Tablets 2463
Inderide LA Long Acting Capsules 2465

Tetracycline Hydrochloride (Delayed or reduced absorption of concomitantly administered oral tetracycline). Products include:
Achromycin V Capsules 1193
Achromycin Ophthalmic Ointment 1% ⊙ 307
Achromycin Ophthalmic Suspension 1% ⊙ 308
Topicycline for Topical Solution 1856

Thyroglobulin (Delayed or reduced absorption of concomitantly administered oral thyroid preparations). Products include:
Proloid Tablets 1761

Thyroid (Delayed or reduced absorption of concomitantly administered oral thyroid preparations). Products include:
S-P-T "Liquid" Capsules 995

Vitamin A (Cholestyramine may interfere with oral absorption and digestion of fat soluble vitamin A). Products include:
Aquasol A Vitamin A Capsules, USP 615
Aquasol A Parenteral, USP 615
Bugs Bunny Children's Chewable Vitamins (Sugar Free) ▣ 625
Bugs Bunny With Extra C Children's Chewable Vitamins (Sugar Free) ▣ 626
Bugs Bunny/Flintstones ▣ 625
Flintstones Children's Chewable Vitamins With Extra C ▣ 626
Flintstones Children's Chewable Vitamins Plus Iron ▣ 625
Lazer Creme 1770
Myadec ▣ 640
Natalins Rx 1391
Natalins Tablets 1391
Ocuvite Vitamin and Mineral Supplement ⊙ 312
One-A-Day Essential Vitamins ▣ 627
One-A-Day Maximum Formula Vitamins and Minerals ▣ 627
One-A-Day Plus Extra C Vitamins ▣ 627
Stressgard Stress Formula Vitamins ▣ 628
Tri-Vi-Flor 1.0 mg Vitamins with Fluoride Chewable Tablets 1400
Tri-Vi-Flor Drops 1400
Tri-Vi-Sol Vitamin Drops ▣ 614
Tri-Vi-Sol Vitamin Drops with Iron ▣ 614
Vicon Forte Capsules 2416
Vicon Plus ▣ 682
Vi-Daylin ADC Vitamins Drops 1980
Vi-Daylin ADC Vitamins + Iron Drops 1980
Vi-Daylin/F ADC Vitamins Drops With Fluoride 1981
Vi-Daylin/F ADC Vitamins + Iron Drops With Fluoride 1981
Vi-Zac ▣ 682
Within Women's Formula Multivitamin with Calcium, Extra Iron and Zinc ▣ 628
Zymacap Capsules ▣ 670

Vitamin D (Cholestyramine may interfere with oral absorption and digestion of fat soluble vitamin D). Products include:
Bugs Bunny Children's Chewable Vitamins (Sugar Free) ▣ 625
Bugs Bunny With Extra C Children's Chewable Vitamins (Sugar Free) ▣ 626
Bugs Bunny Plus Iron Children's Chewable Vitamins (Sugar Free) ▣ 625
Calderol Capsules 1635
Caltrate 600 + Iron & Vitamin D 1198
Caltrate 600 + Vitamin D 1197
Caltrate, Jr. Tablets 1198
Flintstones Children's Chewable Vitamins ▣ 625
Flintstones Children's Chewable Vitamins With Extra C ▣ 626
Flintstones Children's Chewable Vitamins Plus Iron ▣ 625
Natalins Rx 1391
Natalins Tablets 1391
One-A-Day Essential Vitamins ▣ 627
One-A-Day Maximum Formula Vitamins and Minerals ▣ 627
One-A-Day Plus Extra C Vitamins ▣ 627
Os-Cal 250+D Tablets ▣ 597
Os-Cal 500+D Tablets ▣ 597
Os-Cal Fortified Tablets ▣ 597
Os-Cal Plus Tablets ▣ 597
Posture-D 600 mg 2420
Stressgard Stress Formula Vitamins ▣ 628
Tri-Vi-Flor 1.0 mg Vitamins with Fluoride Chewable Tablets 1400
Tri-Vi-Flor Drops 1400
Tri-Vi-Sol Vitamin Drops ▣ 614
Tri-Vi-Sol Vitamin Drops with Iron ▣ 614
Vi-Daylin ADC Vitamins Drops 1980
Vi-Daylin ADC Vitamins + Iron Drops 1980
Vi-Daylin/F ADC Vitamins Drops With Fluoride 1981
Vi-Daylin/F ADC Vitamins + Iron Drops With Fluoride 1981
Within Women's Formula Multivitamin with Calcium, Extra Iron and Zinc ▣ 628
Zymacap Capsules ▣ 670

Vitamin K (Cholestyramine may interfere with oral absorption and digestion of fat soluble vitamin K). Products include:
One-A-Day Maximum Formula Vitamins and Minerals ▣ 627
Synkayvite Injection 1919
Synkayvite Tablets 1920

Vitamin K₁ (Cholestyramine may interfere with oral absorption and digestion of fat soluble vitamin K). Products include:
AquaMEPHYTON Injection 1422
Konakion Injection 1903
Mephyton Tablets 1503

Warfarin Sodium (Delayed or reduced absorption of concomitantly administered oral warfarin). Products include:
Coumadin Injection & Tablets 944
Panwarfin Tablets 547

QUIBRON CAPSULES
(Theophylline, Guaifenesin) 713
May interact with sympathomimetic bronchodilators, macrolide antibiotics, oral contraceptives, and certain other agents. Compounds in these categories include:

Albuterol (Potential for toxic synergism). Products include:
Proventil Inhalation Aerosol 2117
Ventolin Inhalation Aerosol and Refill 583

Albuterol Sulfate (Potential for toxic synergism). Products include:
Proventil Repetabs Tablets 2120
Proventil Solutions for Inhalation 0.5% and 0.083% 2118
Proventil Syrup 2119
Proventil Tablets 2120
Ventolin 583

Allopurinol (Increases serum theophylline levels when high dose of allopurinol is used). Products include:
Zyloprim Tablets 830

Bitolterol Mesylate (Potential for toxic synergism). Products include:
Tornalate 2074

Cimetidine (Increases serum theophylline levels). Products include:
Tagamet Tablets 2228

Cimetidine Hydrochloride (Increases serum theophylline levels). Products include:
Tagamet 2228

Ciprofloxacin (Increases serum theophylline levels).
No products indexed under this heading.

Ciprofloxacin Hydrochloride (Increases serum theophylline levels). Products include:
Ciloxan Sterile Ophthalmic Solution ⊙ 214
Cipro I.V. 1592
Cipro Tablets 1589

Ephedrine Hydrochloride (Potential for toxic synergism). Products include:
Amesec ▣ 682
Primatene Tablets-M Formula 2421
Primatene Tablets-P Formula 2421
Primatene Tablets-Regular Formula 2421
Quadrinal Tablets 1183
Quelidrine Syrup 556
Tedral SA 1765

Ephedrine Sulfate (Potential for toxic synergism). Products include:
Bronkaid Tablets ▣ 757
Bronkolixir ▣ 761
Bronkotabs Tablets ▣ 762
Marax Tablets & DF Syrup 1954
Pazo Hemorrhoid Ointment & Suppositories 752

- Vicks Vatronol Nose Drops ▣ 666

Ephedrine Tannate (Potential for toxic synergism). Products include:

- Rynatuss 2388

Epinephrine (Potential for toxic synergism). Products include:

- Ana-Kit Anaphylaxis Emergency Treatment Kit 1100
- Bronkaid Mist ▣ 757
- EpiPen 843
- Marcaine Hydrochloride 0.5% with Epinephrine 1:200,000 (as bitartrate) 958
- Marcaine Hydrochloride with Epinephrine 1:200,000 2055
- Primatene Mist 2420
- Sus-Phrine Injection 1006
- Xylocaine with Epinephrine Injections 637

Epinephrine Hydrochloride (Potential for toxic synergism). Products include:

- Adrenalin Chloride Solution 1:100 & 1:1,000 1689
- Epifrin ⊙ 244
- Glaucon ⊙ 218

Erythromycin (Increases serum theophylline levels). Products include:

- A/T/S Topical Gel and Topical Solution 1089
- AK-Mycin Ointment ⊙ 204
- Benzamycin Topical Gel 907
- E-Mycin Tablets 688
- ETS-2% 1685
- ERYC 1720
- Erycette (erythromycin 2%) Topical Solution 1678
- Ery-Tab Tablets 521
- Erythromycin Base Filmtab 525
- Erythromycin Delayed-Release Capsules, USP 526
- Ilotycin Ophthalmic Ointment 915
- PCE Dispertab Tablets 549
- Pediazole 1973
- T-Stat 2.0% Topical Solution and Pads 2409
- Theramycin Z Topical Solution 2% 1410

Erythromycin Estolate (Increases serum theophylline levels). Products include:

- Ilosone 913

Erythromycin Ethylsuccinate (Increases serum theophylline levels). Products include:

- E.E.S. 522
- EryPed 519
- Pediazole 1973

Erythromycin Gluceptate (Increases serum theophylline levels). Products include:

- Ilotycin Gluceptate, IV, Vials 915

Erythromycin Stearate (Increases serum theophylline levels). Products include:

- Erythrocin Stearate Filmtab 523

Ethinyl Estradiol (Increases serum theophylline levels). Products include:

- Brevicon 2304
- Demulen 2161
- Estinyl Tablets 2085
- Jenest-28 Tablets 1636
- Levlen/Tri-Levlen 665
- Lo/Ovral Tablets 2471
- Lo/Ovral-28 Tablets 2476
- Loestrin 1728
- Modicon 1667
- Nordette-21 Tablets 2481
- Nordette-28 Tablets 2483
- Norethin 2133
- Norinyl 2304
- Norlestrin 1746
- Ortho-Cyclen Tablets 1658
- Ortho-Novum 1667
- Ovcon 1391
- Ovral Tablets 2490
- Ovral-28 Tablets 2491
- Levlen/Tri-Levlen 665
- Tri-Norinyl 2304
- Triphasil-21 Tablets 2527
- Triphasil-28 Tablets 2532

Ethylnorepinephrine Hydrochloride (Potential for toxic synergism). Products include:

- Bronkephrine Injection 2042

Ethynodiol Diacetate (Increases serum theophylline levels). Products include:

- Demulen 2161

Isoetharine (Potential for toxic synergism). Products include:

- Arm-a-Med Isoetharine Inhalation Solution, USP 616
- Bronkometer Aerosol 2042
- Bronkosol Solution 2042

Isoproterenol Hydrochloride (Potential for toxic synergism). Products include:

- Isuprel Hydrochloride Injection 1:5000 2050
- Isuprel Hydrochloride Mistometer 2051
- Isuprel Hydrochloride Solution 1:200 & 1:100 2052
- Norisodrine Aerotrol 540

Levonorgestrel (Increases serum theophylline levels). Products include:

- Levlen/Tri-Levlen 665
- Nordette-21 Tablets 2481
- Nordette-28 Tablets 2483
- Norplant System 2484
- Levlen/Tri-Levlen 665
- Triphasil-21 Tablets 2527
- Triphasil-28 Tablets 2532

Mestranol (Increases serum theophylline levels). Products include:

- Enovid 2161
- Norethin 2133
- Norinyl 2304
- Ortho-Novum 1667

Metaproterenol Sulfate (Potential for toxic synergism). Products include:

- Alupent 674
- Arm-a-Med Metaproterenol Sulfate Inhalation Solution, USP 617
- Metaprel Inhalation Aerosol Bronchodilator 2014
- Metaprel Inhalation Solution 2015
- Metaprel 2015
- Metaproterenol Sulfate Inhalation Solution, USP 912

Norethindrone (Increases serum theophylline levels). Products include:

- Brevicon 2304
- Jenest-28 Tablets 1636
- Micronor Tablets 1667
- Modicon 1667
- Norethin 2133
- Norinyl 2304
- Norlutin 1755
- Nor-Q D Tablets 2304
- Ortho-Novum 1667
- Ovcon 1391
- Tri-Norinyl 2304

Norethynodrel (Increases serum theophylline levels). Products include:

- Enovid 2161

Norgestimate (Increases serum theophylline levels). Products include:

- Ortho-Cyclen Tablets 1658

Norgestrel (Increases serum theophylline levels). Products include:

- Lo/Ovral Tablets 2471
- Lo/Ovral-28 Tablets 2476
- Ovral Tablets 2490
- Ovral-28 Tablets 2491
- Ovrette Tablets 2492

Phenytoin (Decreased theophylline and phenytoin serum levels). Products include:

- Dilantin Infatabs 1710
- Dilantin-30 Pediatric/Dilantin-125 Suspension 1713

Phenytoin Sodium (Decreased theophylline and phenytoin serum levels). Products include:

- Dilantin Kapseals 1708
- Dilantin Parenteral 1712
- Dilantin with Phenobarbital Kapseals 1715

Pirbuterol Acetate (Potential for toxic synergism). Products include:

- Maxair Inhaler 1311

Propranolol Hydrochloride (Increases serum theophylline levels). Products include:

- Inderal 2459
- Inderal LA Long Acting Capsules 2461
- Inderide Tablets 2463
- Inderide LA Long Acting Capsules 2465

Rifampin (Decreases serum theophylline levels). Products include:

- Rifadin 1345
- Rifamate Capsules 1347
- Rimactane Capsules 879

Terbutaline Sulfate (Potential for toxic synergism). Products include:

- Brethaire Inhaler 1024
- Brethine Ampuls 1026
- Brethine Tablets 1026
- Bricanyl Injection 1324
- Bricanyl Tablets 1325

Troleandomycin (Increases serum theophylline levels). Products include:

- Tao Capsules 1963

QUIBRON-T

(Theophylline Anhydrous) 714

May interact with xanthine bronchodilators, oral contraceptives, sympathomimetic bronchodilators, and certain other agents. Compounds in these categories include:

Albuterol (Toxic synergism may occur if administered concurrently). Products include:

- Proventil Inhalation Aerosol 2117
- Ventolin Inhalation Aerosol and Refill 583

Albuterol Sulfate (Toxic synergism may occur if administered concurrently). Products include:

- Proventil Repetabs Tablets 2120
- Proventil Solutions for Inhalation 0.5% and 0.083% 2118
- Proventil Syrup 2119
- Proventil Tablets 2120
- Ventolin 583

Allopurinol (Increases serum theophylline levels at high dose). Products include:

- Zyloprim Tablets 830

Aminophylline (Should not be administered concurrently). Products include:

- Amesec ▣ 682
- Aminophyllin Tablets 2153

Bitolterol Mesylate (Toxic synergism may occur if administered concurrently). Products include:

- Tornalate 2074

Cimetidine (Increased serum theophylline levels). Products include:

- Tagamet Tablets 2228

Cimetidine Hydrochloride (Increased serum theophylline levels). Products include:

- Tagamet 2228

Dyphylline (Should not be administered concurrently). Products include:

- Dilor 2079
- Dilor-G Tablets & Liquid 2079
- Lufyllin Elixir 2384
- Lufyllin & Lufyllin-400 Tablets 2384
- Lufyllin-GG Elixir & Tablets 2385

Ephedrine Hydrochloride (Toxic synergism may occur if administered concurrently). Products include:

- Amesec ▣ 682
- Primatene Tablets-M Formula 2421
- Primatene Tablets-P Formula 2421
- Primatene Tablets-Regular Formula 2421
- Quadrinal Tablets 1183
- Quelidrine Syrup 556
- Tedral SA 1765

Ephedrine Sulfate (Toxic synergism may occur if administered concurrently). Products include:

- Bronkaid Tablets ▣ 757
- Bronkolixir ▣ 761
- Bronkotabs Tablets ▣ 762
- Marax Tablets & DF Syrup 1954
- Pazo Hemorrhoid Ointment & Suppositories 752
- Vicks Vatronol Nose Drops ▣ 666

Ephedrine Tannate (Toxic synergism may occur if administered concurrently). Products include:

- Rynatuss 2388

Epinephrine (Toxic synergism may occur if administered concurrently). Products include:

- Ana-Kit Anaphylaxis Emergency Treatment Kit 1100
- Bronkaid Mist ▣ 757
- EpiPen 843
- Marcaine Hydrochloride 0.5% with Epinephrine 1:200,000 (as bitartrate) 958
- Marcaine Hydrochloride with Epinephrine 1:200,000 2055
- Primatene Mist 2420
- Sus-Phrine Injection 1006
- Xylocaine with Epinephrine Injections 637

Epinephrine Hydrochloride (Toxic synergism may occur if administered concurrently). Products include:

- Adrenalin Chloride Solution 1:100 & 1:1,000 1689
- Epifrin ⊙ 244
- Glaucon ⊙ 218

Erythromycin (Increased serum theophylline levels). Products include:

- A/T/S Topical Gel and Topical Solution 1089
- AK-Mycin Ointment ⊙ 204
- Benzamycin Topical Gel 907
- E-Mycin Tablets 688
- ETS-2% 1685
- ERYC 1720
- Erycette (erythromycin 2%) Topical Solution 1678
- Ery-Tab Tablets 521
- Erythromycin Base Filmtab 525
- Erythromycin Delayed-Release Capsules, USP 526
- Ilotycin Ophthalmic Ointment 915
- PCE Dispertab Tablets 549
- Pediazole 1973
- T-Stat 2.0% Topical Solution and Pads 2409
- Theramycin Z Topical Solution 2% 1410

Erythromycin Estolate (Increased serum theophylline levels). Products include:

- Ilosone 913

Erythromycin Gluceptate (Increased serum theophylline levels). Products include:

- Ilotycin Gluceptate, IV, Vials 915

Erythromycin Stearate (Increased serum theophylline levels). Products include:

- Erythrocin Stearate Filmtab 523

Ethinyl Estradiol (Increased serum theophylline levels). Products include:

- Brevicon 2304
- Demulen 2161
- Estinyl Tablets 2085
- Jenest-28 Tablets 1636
- Levlen/Tri-Levlen 665
- Lo/Ovral Tablets 2471
- Lo/Ovral-28 Tablets 2476
- Loestrin 1728
- Modicon 1667
- Nordette-21 Tablets 2481
- Nordette-28 Tablets 2483
- Norethin 2133
- Norinyl 2304
- Norlestrin 1746
- Ortho-Cyclen Tablets 1658
- Ortho-Novum 1667
- Ovcon 1391
- Ovral Tablets 2490
- Ovral-28 Tablets 2491
- Levlen/Tri-Levlen 665

Tri-Norinyl ... 2304
Triphasil-21 Tablets ... 2527
Triphasil-28 Tablets ... 2532

Ethylnorepinephrine Hydrochloride (Toxic synergism may occur if administered concurrently). Products include:
Bronkephrine Injection ... 2042

Ethynodiol Diacetate (Increased serum theophylline levels). Products include:
Demulen ... 2161

Isoetharine (Toxic synergism may occur if administered concurrently). Products include:
Arm-a-Med Isoetharine Inhalation Solution, USP ... 616
Bronkometer Aerosol ... 2042
Bronkosol Solution ... 2042

Isoproterenol Hydrochloride (Toxic synergism may occur if administered concurrently). Products include:
Isuprel Hydrochloride Injection 1:5000 ... 2050
Isuprel Hydrochloride Mistometer .. 2051
Isuprel Hydrochloride Solution 1:200 & 1:100 ... 2052
Norisodrine Aerotrol ... 540

Levonorgestrel (Increased serum theophylline levels). Products include:
Levlen/Tri-Levlen ... 665
Nordette-21 Tablets ... 2481
Nordette-28 Tablets ... 2483
Norplant System ... 2484
Levlen/Tri-Levlen ... 665
Triphasil-21 Tablets ... 2527
Triphasil-28 Tablets ... 2532

Lithium Carbonate (Increased renal excretion of lithium). Products include:
Eskalith ... 2214
Lithane Tablets ... 1596
Lithium Carbonate Capsules & Tablets ... 1984
Lithobid Tablets ... 870

Mestranol (Increased serum theophylline levels). Products include:
Enovid ... 2161
Norethin ... 2133
Norinyl ... 2304
Ortho-Novum ... 1667

Metaproterenol Sulfate (Toxic synergism may occur if administered concurrently). Products include:
Alupent ... 674
Arm-a-Med Metaproterenol Sulfate Inhalation Solution, USP ... 617
Metaprel Inhalation Aerosol Bronchodilator ... 2014
Metaprel Inhalation Solution ... 2015
Metaprel ... 2015
Metaproterenol Sulfate Inhalation Solution, USP ... 912

Norethindrone (Increased serum theophylline levels). Products include:
Brevicon ... 2304
Jenest-28 Tablets ... 1636
Micronor Tablets ... 1667
Modicon ... 1667
Norethin ... 2133
Norinyl ... 2304
Norlutin ... 1755
Nor-Q D Tablets ... 2304
Ortho-Novum ... 1667
Ovcon ... 1391
Tri-Norinyl ... 2304

Norethynodrel (Increased serum theophylline levels). Products include:
Enovid ... 2161

Norgestimate (Increased serum theophylline levels). Products include:
Ortho-Cyclen Tablets ... 1658

Norgestrel (Increased serum theophylline levels). Products include:
Lo/Ovral Tablets ... 2471
Lo/Ovral-28 Tablets ... 2476
Ovral Tablets ... 2490
Ovral-28 Tablets ... 2491
Ovrette Tablets ... 2492

Phenytoin (Decreased theophylline and phenytoin serum levels). Products include:
Dilantin Infatabs ... 1710
Dilantin-30 Pediatric/Dilantin-125 Suspension ... 1713

Phenytoin Sodium (Decreased theophylline and phenytoin serum levels). Products include:
Dilantin Kapseals ... 1708
Dilantin Parenteral ... 1712
Dilantin with Phenobarbital Kapseals ... 1715

Pirbuterol Acetate (Toxic synergism may occur if administered concurrently). Products include:
Maxair Inhaler ... 1311

Rifampin (Decresed serum theophylline levels). Products include:
Rifadin ... 1345
Rifamate Capsules ... 1347
Rimactane Capsules ... 879

Terbutaline Sulfate (Toxic synergism may occur if administered concurrently). Products include:
Brethaire Inhaler ... 1024
Brethine Ampuls ... 1026
Brethine Tablets ... 1026
Bricanyl Injection ... 1324
Bricanyl Tablets ... 1325

Theophylline (Should not be administered concurrently). Products include:
Bronkaid Tablets ... ▣ 757
Bronkolixir ... ▣ 761
Bronkotabs Tablets ... ▣ 762
Constant-T Tablets ... 1029
Marax Tablets & DF Syrup ... 1954
Primatene Tablets ... 2421
Quibron Capsules ... 713
Quibron-T ... 714
Quibron-T/SR ... 716
Theolair Liquid ... 1317
Theo-Organidin Elixir ... 2391

Theophylline Calcium Salicylate (Should not be administered concurrently). Products include:
Quadrinal Tablets ... 1183

Theophylline Sodium Glycinate (Should not be administered concurrently). Products include:
Asbron G ... 1997

Troleandomycin (Increased serum theophylline levels). Products include:
Tao Capsules ... 1963

QUIBRON-T/SR
(Theophylline Anhydrous) ... 716
May interact with macrolide antibiotics, sympathomimetic bronchodilators, and certain other agents. Compounds in these categories include:

Albuterol (Toxic synergism). Products include:
Proventil Inhalation Aerosol ... 2117
Ventolin Inhalation Aerosol and Refill ... 583

Albuterol Sulfate (Toxic synergism). Products include:
Proventil Repetabs Tablets ... 2120
Proventil Solutions for Inhalation 0.5% and 0.083% ... 2118
Proventil Syrup ... 2119
Proventil Tablets ... 2120
Ventolin ... 583

Aminophylline (Should not be administered concurrently). Products include:
Amesec ... ▣ 682
Aminophyllin Tablets ... 2153

Bitolterol Mesylate (Toxic synergism). Products include:
Tornalate ... 2074

Cimetidine (Increased serum theophylline levels). Products include:
Tagamet Tablets ... 2228

Cimetidine Hydrochloride (Increased serum theophylline levels). Products include:
Tagamet ... 2228

Dyphylline (Should not be administered concurrently). Products include:
Dilor ... 2079
Dilor-G Tablets & Liquid ... 2079
Lufyllin Elixir ... 2384
Lufyllin & Lufyllin-400 Tablets ... 2384
Lufyllin-GG Elixir & Tablets ... 2385

Ephedrine Hydrochloride (Toxic synergism). Products include:
Amesec ... ▣ 682
Primatene Tablets-M Formula ... 2421
Primatene Tablets-P Formula ... 2421
Primatene Tablets-Regular Formula ... 2421
Quadrinal Tablets ... 1183
Quelidrine Syrup ... 556
Tedral SA ... 1765

Ephedrine Sulfate (Toxic synergism). Products include:
Bronkaid Tablets ... ▣ 757
Bronkolixir ... ▣ 761
Bronkotabs Tablets ... ▣ 762
Marax Tablets & DF Syrup ... 1954
Pazo Hemorrhoid Ointment & Suppositories ... 752
Vicks Vatronol Nose Drops ... ▣ 666

Ephedrine Tannate (Toxic synergism). Products include:
Rynatuss ... 2388

Epinephrine (Toxic synergism). Products include:
Ana-Kit Anaphylaxis Emergency Treatment Kit ... 1100
Bronkaid Mist ... ▣ 757
EpiPen ... 843
Marcaine Hydrochloride 0.5% with Epinephrine 1:200,000 (as bitartrate) ... 958
Marcaine Hydrochloride with Epinephrine 1:200,000 ... 2055
Primatene Mist ... 2420
Sus-Phrine Injection ... 1006
Xylocaine with Epinephrine Injections ... 637

Epinephrine Hydrochloride (Toxic synergism). Products include:
Adrenalin Chloride Solution 1:100 & 1:1,000 ... 1689
Epifrin ... ⊙ 244
Glaucon ... ⊙ 218

Erythromycin (Increased serum theophylline levels). Products include:
A/T/S Topical Gel and Topical Solution ... 1089
AK-Mycin Ointment ... ⊙ 204
Benzamycin Topical Gel ... 907
E-Mycin Tablets ... 688
ETS-2% ... 1685
ERYC ... 1720
Erycette (erythromycin 2%) Topical Solution ... 1678
Ery-Tab Tablets ... 521
Erythromycin Base Filmtab ... 525
Erythromycin Delayed-Release Capsules, USP ... 526
Ilotycin Ophthalmic Ointment ... 915
PCE Dispertab Tablets ... 549
Pediazole ... 1973
T-Stat 2.0% Topical Solution and Pads ... 2409
Theramycin Z Topical Solution 2% 1410

Erythromycin Estolate (Increased serum theophylline levels). Products include:
Ilosone ... 913

Erythromycin Ethylsuccinate (Increased serum theophylline levels). Products include:
E.E.S. ... 522
EryPed ... 519
Pediazole ... 1973

Erythromycin Gluceptate (Increased serum theophylline levels). Products include:
Ilotycin Gluceptate, IV, Vials ... 915

Erythromycin Stearate (Increased serum theophylline levels). Products include:
Erythrocin Stearate Filmtab ... 523

Ethylnorepinephrine Hydrochloride (Toxic synergism). Products include:
Bronkephrine Injection ... 2042

Isoetharine (Toxic synergism). Products include:
Arm-a-Med Isoetharine Inhalation Solution, USP ... 616
Bronkometer Aerosol ... 2042
Bronkosol Solution ... 2042

Isoproterenol Hydrochloride (Toxic synergism). Products include:
Isuprel Hydrochloride Injection 1:5000 ... 2050
Isuprel Hydrochloride Mistometer .. 2051
Isuprel Hydrochloride Solution 1:200 & 1:100 ... 2052
Norisodrine Aerotrol ... 540

Lithium Carbonate (Increased renal excretion of lithium). Products include:
Eskalith ... 2214
Lithane Tablets ... 1596
Lithium Carbonate Capsules & Tablets ... 1984
Lithobid Tablets ... 870

Metaproterenol Sulfate (Toxic synergism). Products include:
Alupent ... 674
Arm-a-Med Metaproterenol Sulfate Inhalation Solution, USP ... 617
Metaprel Inhalation Aerosol Bronchodilator ... 2014
Metaprel Inhalation Solution ... 2015
Metaprel ... 2015
Metaproterenol Sulfate Inhalation Solution, USP ... 912

Pirbuterol Acetate (Toxic synergism). Products include:
Maxair Inhaler ... 1311

Propranolol Hydrochloride (Mutual antagonism of therapeutic effects). Products include:
Inderal ... 2459
Inderal LA Long Acting Capsules 2461
Inderide Tablets ... 2463
Inderide LA Long Acting Capsules .. 2465

Terbutaline Sulfate (Toxic synergism). Products include:
Brethaire Inhaler ... 1024
Brethine Ampuls ... 1026
Brethine Tablets ... 1026
Bricanyl Injection ... 1324
Bricanyl Tablets ... 1325

Troleandomycin (Increased serum theophylline levels). Products include:
Tao Capsules ... 1963

Food Interactions

Food, unspecified (May influence absorption).

QUINAGLUTE DURA-TABS TABLETS
(Quinidine Gluconate) ... 663
May interact with anticholinergics, cholinergic agents, carbonic anhydrase inhibitors, thiazides, oral anticoagulants, phenothiazines, and certain other agents. Compounds in these categories include:

Acetazolamide (Decreased excretion of quinidine). Products include:
Diamox Parenteral ... 1200
Diamox Parenteral ... ⊙ 308
Diamox Sequels (Sustained Release) ... 1201
Diamox Sequels (Sustained Release) ... ⊙ 310
Diamox Tablets ... 1200
Diamox Tablets ... ⊙ 308

Atropine Sulfate (Additive vagolytic effect). Products include:
Arco-Lase Plus Tablets ... 607
Atropine Sulfate Sterile Ophthalmic Solution and S.O.P. Sterile Ophthalmic Ointment ... ⊙ 239

(▣ Described in PDR For Nonprescription Drugs) (⊙ Described in PDR For Ophthalmology)

Donnagel ▣ 675
Donnagel-PG 1858
Donnatal 1858
Donnatal Extentabs 1859
Donnatal Tablets 1858
Donnazyme Tablets 1860
Isopto Atropine ◉ 218
Lomotil 2174
Motofen Tablets 836
Ru-Tuss Tablets 693
Urised Tablets 2396

Belladonna Alkaloids (Additive vagolytic effect). Products include:
Bellergal-S Tablets 1998
Hyland's Bed Wetting Tablets ▣ 728
Hyland's Teething Tablets ▣ 728
Kinesed Tablets 2272

Bendroflumethiazide (Decreased excretion of quinidine). Products include:
Corzide Tablets 702
Naturetin Tablets 1789
Rauzide Tablets 1804

Benztropine Mesylate (Additive vagolytic effect). Products include:
Cogentin 1435

Biperiden (Additive vagolytic effect). Products include:
Akineton 1171

Chlorothiazide (Decreased excretion of quinidine). Products include:
Aldoclor Tablets 1413
Diupres Tablets 1461
Diuril Oral 1464

Chlorothiazide Sodium (Decreased excretion of quinidine). Products include:
Diuril Sodium Intravenous 1463

Chlorpromazine (Additive cardiac depressive effects). Products include:
Thorazine 2234

Cimetidine (Potential for elevated quinidine plasma levels). Products include:
Tagamet Tablets 2228

Cimetidine Hydrochloride (Potential for elevated quinidine plasma levels). Products include:
Tagamet 2228

Clidinium Bromide (Additive vagolytic effect). Products include:
Librax Capsules 1929
Quarzan Capsules 1937

Decamethonium (Potentiation of neuromuscular blockade).

Dichlorphenamide (Decreased excretion of quinidine). Products include:
Daranide Tablets 1445

Dicumarol (Reduced clotting factor concentrations). Products include:
Dicumarol Tablets 516

Dicyclomine Hydrochloride (Additive vagolytic effect). Products include:
Bentyl 1322

Digitoxin (Increased digitoxin plasma concentrations). Products include:
Crystodigin Tablets 1253

Digoxin (Increased digoxin plasma concentrations). Products include:
Lanoxicaps 772
Lanoxin Elixir Pediatric 775
Lanoxin Injection 778
Lanoxin Injection Pediatric 781
Lanoxin Tablets 783

Edrophonium Chloride (Antagonism of cholinergic effects). Products include:
Enlon Injection 598
Tensilon Injectable 1123

Ethopropazine Hydrochloride (Additive vagolytic effect).

Fluphenazine Decanoate (Additive cardiac depressive effects). Products include:
Prolixin Decanoate 1795

Fluphenazine Enanthate (Additive cardiac depressive effects). Products include:
Prolixin Enanthate 1796

Fluphenazine Hydrochloride (Additive cardiac depressive effects). Products include:
Prolixin Elixir 1793
Prolixin Injection 1791
Prolixin Oral Concentrate 1792
Prolixin Tablets 1793

Glycopyrrolate (Additive vagolytic effect). Products include:
Robinul Forte Tablets 1873
Robinul Injectable 1873
Robinul Tablets 1873

Guanidine Hydrochloride (Antagonism of cholinergic effects).
No products indexed under this heading.

Hydrochlorothiazide (Decreased excretion of quinidine). Products include:
Aldactazide 2150
Aldoril Tablets 1418
Apresazide Capsules 854
Apresoline-Esidrix Tablets 857
Capozide 2258
Dyazide Capsules 2208
Esidrix Tablets 863
Esimil Tablets 864
HydroDIURIL Tablets 1484
Hydropres Tablets 1485
Inderide Tablets 2463
Inderide LA Long Acting Capsules 2465
Lopressor HCT Tablets 1034
Maxzide 1215
Moduretic Tablets 1510
Normozide Tablets 2112
Oretic Tablets 544
Oreticyl 545
Prinzide Tablets 1540
Ser-Ap-Es Tablets 881
Serpasil-Esidrix Tablets 886
Timolide Tablets 1547
Trandate HCT Tablets 579
Vaseretic Tablets 1559
Zestoretic 2274

Hydroflumethiazide (Decreased excretion of quinidine). Products include:
Diucardin Tablets 2450
Saluron 718
Salutensin/Salutensin-Demi 719

Hyoscyamine (Additive vagolytic effect). Products include:
Cystospaz Tablets 2395
Urised Tablets 2396

Hyoscyamine Sulfate (Additive vagolytic effect). Products include:
Arco-Lase Plus Tablets 607
Cystospaz-M Capsules 2395
Donnagel ▣ 675
Donnagel-PG 1858
Donnatal 1858
Donnatal Extentabs 1859
Donnatal Tablets 1858
Donnazyme Tablets 1860
Kutrase Capsules 2146
Levsin/Levsinex 2147
Ru-Tuss Tablets 693

Ipratropium Bromide (Additive vagolytic effect). Products include:
Atrovent Inhalation Aerosol 675

Mepenzolate Bromide (Additive vagolytic effect). Products include:
Cantil Tablets 1326

Mesoridazine (Additive cardiac depressive effects). Products include:
Serentil 686

Methazolamide (Decreased excretion of quinidine). Products include:
Neptazane Tablets ◉ 311

Methyclothiazide (Decreased excretion of quinidine). Products include:
Enduron Tablets 517
Enduronyl 518

Neostigmine Bromide (Antagonism of cholinergic effects). Products include:
Prostigmin Tablets 1121

Neostigmine Methylsulfate (Antagonism of cholinergic effects). Products include:
Prostigmin Injectable 1120

Oxybutynin Chloride (Additive vagolytic effect). Products include:
Ditropan 1332

Oxyphenonium Bromide (Additive vagolytic effect).

Perphenazine (Additive cardiac depressive effects). Products include:
Etrafon 2087
Triavil Tablets 1556
Trilafon 2123

Phenobarbital (Potential for reduced quinidine plasma levels). Products include:
Arco-Lase Plus Tablets 607
Bellergal-S Tablets 1998
Bronkolixir ▣ 761
Bronkotabs Tablets ▣ 762
Donnatal 1858
Donnatal Extentabs 1859
Donnatal Tablets 1858
Donnazyme Tablets 1860
Kinesed Tablets 2272
Phenobarbital Elixir and Tablets 1293
Primatene Tablets-P Formula 2421
Quadrinal Tablets 1183
Tedral SA 1765

Phenothiazine Derivatives (Additive cardiac depressive effects).

Phenytoin (Potential for reduced quinidine plasma levels). Products include:
Dilantin Infatabs 1710
Dilantin-30 Pediatric/Dilantin-125 Suspension 1713

Phenytoin Sodium (Potential for reduced quinidine plasma levels). Products include:
Dilantin Kapseals 1708
Dilantin Parenteral 1712
Dilantin with Phenobarbital Kapseals 1715

Polythiazide (Decreased excretion of quinidine). Products include:
Minizide Capsules 1779
Renese Tablets 1785
Renese-R Tablets 1786

Prochlorperazine (Additive cardiac depressive effects). Products include:
Compazine 2201

Procyclidine Hydrochloride (Additive vagolytic effect). Products include:
Kemadrin Tablets 771

Promethazine Hydrochloride (Additive cardiac depressive effects). Products include:
Mepergan Injection 2479
Phenergan with Codeine 2497
Phenergan with Dextromethorphan 2499
Phenergan Injection 2493
Phenergan Suppositories 2496
Phenergan Syrup 2495
Phenergan Tablets 2496
Phenergan VC 2500
Phenergan VC with Codeine 2501

Propantheline Bromide (Additive vagolytic effect). Products include:
Pro-Banthīne Tablets 2141

Pyridostigmine Bromide (Antagonism of cholinergic effects). Products include:
Mestinon Injectable 1115
Mestinon 1116

Reserpine (Additive cardiac depressive effects). Products include:
Diupres Tablets 1461
Hydromox R Tablets 1209
Hydropres Tablets 1485
Renese-R Tablets 1786
Salutensin/Salutensin-Demi 719
Ser-Ap-Es Tablets 881
Serpasil Tablets 883
Serpasil-Apresoline Tablets 884
Serpasil-Esidrix Tablets 886

Rifampin (Potential for reduced quinidine plasma levels). Products include:
Rifadin 1345
Rifamate Capsules 1347
Rimactane Capsules 879

Scopolamine Hydrobromide (Additive vagolytic effect). Products include:
Donnagel ▣ 675
Donnagel-PG 1858
Donnatal 1858
Donnatal Extentabs 1859
Donnatal Tablets 1858
Donnazyme Tablets 1860
Isopto Hyoscine ◉ 222
Murocoll-2 Sterile Ophthalmic Solution ◉ 261
Ru-Tuss Tablets 693

Scopolamine Preparations (Additive vagolytic effect). Products include:
Transderm Scōp Transdermal Therapeutic System 887

Sodium Bicarbonate (Decreased excretion of quinidine). Products include:
Alka-Seltzer Advanced Formula Antacid & Non-Aspirin Pain Reliever ▣ 620
Alka-Seltzer Effervescent Antacid ▣ 622
Alka-Seltzer Effervescent Antacid and Pain Reliever 1568
Alka-Seltzer Extra Strength Effervescent Antacid and Pain Reliever ▣ 623
Alka-Seltzer (Flavored) Effervescent Antacid and Pain Reliever ▣ 621
Arm & Hammer Pure Baking Soda ▣ 548
Ceo-Two Rectal Suppositories 671
Citrocarbonate Antacid ▣ 668
Massengill Liquid Concentrate 2191
NuLYTELY 699

Succinylcholine Chloride (Potentiaion of neuromuscular blockade). Products include:
Anectine 755

Thioridazine Hydrochloride (Additive cardiac depressive effects). Products include:
Mellaril 2011

Tridihexethyl Chloride (Additive vagolytic effect).
No products indexed under this heading.

Trifluoperazine Hydrochloride (Additive cardiac depressive effects). Products include:
Stelazine 2226

Trihexyphenidyl Hydrochloride (Additive vagolytic effect). Products include:
Artane 1195

Tubocurarine Chloride (Potentiation of neuromuscular blockade).
No products indexed under this heading.

Warfarin Sodium (Reduced clotting factor concentrations). Products include:
Coumadin Injection & Tablets 944
Panwarfin Tablets 547

QUINAMM TABLETS
(Quinine Sulfate) 1344
May interact with cardiac glycosides, oral anticoagulants, nondepolarizing neuromuscular blocking agents, urinary alkalizing agents, and certain other agents. Compounds in these categories include:

Acetazolamide (Quinine toxicity). Products include:
Diamox Parenteral 1200
Diamox Parenteral ◉ 308
Diamox Sequels (Sustained Release) 1201
Diamox Sequels (Sustained Release) ◉ 310
Diamox Tablets 1200
Diamox Tablets ◉ 308

Aluminum Carbonate Gel (Delayed or decreased absorption of quinine). Products include:
- Basaljel ... 2438

Aluminum Hydroxide (Delayed or decreased absorption of quinine). Products include:
- Cama Arthritis Pain Reliever ... ▣ 685
- Gaviscon Extra Strength Relief Formula Liquid Antacid ... ▣ 594
- Gaviscon Extra Strength Relief Formula Antacid Tablets ... ▣ 594
- Gaviscon Liquid Antacid ... ▣ 594
- Gelusil Liquid & Tablets ... ▣ 639
- Extra Strength Maalox Plus Suspension ... 1850
- Maalox TC Suspension ... 1851
- Maalox Plus Tablets ... ▣ 655
- Extra Strength Maalox Plus Tablets 1850
- Nephrox Suspension ... ▣ 563
- WinGel Liquid & Tablets ... ▣ 761

Aluminum Hydroxide Gel (Delayed or decreased absorption of quinine). Products include:
- ALternaGEL Liquid ... 1154
- Aludrox Oral Suspension ... 2428
- Amphojel Suspension ... 2429
- Amphojel Suspension without Flavor ... 2429
- Mylanta Liquid ... 1155
- Mylanta Double Strength Liquid ... 1155

Aluminum Hydroxide Gel, Dried (Delayed or decreased absorption of quinine). Products include:
- Alu-Tab/Alu-Cap ... 1309
- Amphojel Tablets ... 2429
- Ascriptin A/D Caplets ... 1850
- Regular Strength Ascriptin Tablets 1850
- Gaviscon Antacid Tablets ... ▣ 593
- Gaviscon-2 Antacid Tablets ... ▣ 594
- Mylanta Tablets ... 1155
- Mylanta Double Strength Tablets ... 1155

Atracurium Besylate (Potentiated; respiratory difficulties). Products include:
- Tracrium Injection ... 817

Deslanoside (Increased plasma levels of digoxin).
- No products indexed under this heading.

Dicumarol (Enhanced action of oral anticoagulants). Products include:
- Dicumarol Tablets ... 516

Digitoxin (Increased plasma levels of digoxin). Products include:
- Crystodigin Tablets ... 1253

Digoxin (Increased plasma levels of digoxin). Products include:
- Lanoxicaps ... 772
- Lanoxin Elixir Pediatric ... 775
- Lanoxin Injection ... 778
- Lanoxin Injection Pediatric ... 781
- Lanoxin Tablets ... 783

Metocurine Iodide (Potentiated; respiratory difficulties). Products include:
- Metubine Iodide Vials ... 1285

Pancuronium Bromide Injection (Potentiated; respiratory difficulties).
- No products indexed under this heading.

Potassium Citrate (Quinine toxicity). Products include:
- Alka-Seltzer Effervescent Antacid .. 1570
- K-Lyte ... 707
- Polycitra Syrup ... 2424
- Polycitra-K ... 2424
- Polycitra-LC—Sugar-Free ... 2424
- Ricelyte, Rice-Based Oral Electrolyte Maintenance Solution ... ▣ 613

Sodium Citrate (Quinine toxicity). Products include:
- Alka-Seltzer Effervescent Antacid .. 1570
- Alka-Seltzer Extra Strength Effervescent Antacid and Pain Reliever ... 1570
- Alka-Seltzer (Flavored) Effervescent Antacid and Pain Reliever ... 1569
- Bicitra—Sugar-Free ... 2423
- Citrocarbonate Antacid ... ▣ 668
- Polycitra ... 2424
- Ricelyte, Rice-Based Oral Electrolyte Maintenance Solution ... ▣ 613

Succinylcholine Chloride (Potentiated; respiratory difficulties). Products include:
- Anectine ... 755

Vecuronium Bromide (Potentiated; respiratory difficulties). Products include:
- Norcuron ... 1642

Warfarin Sodium (Enhanced action of oral anticoagulants). Products include:
- Coumadin Injection & Tablets ... 944
- Panwarfin Tablets ... 547

QUINIDEX EXTENTABS
(Quinidine Sulfate) ... 1868
May interact with anticholinergics, carbonic anhydrase inhibitors, thiazides, oral anticoagulants, nondepolarizing neuromuscular blocking agents, cholinergic agents, phenothiazines, and certain other agents. Compounds in these categories include:

Acetazolamide (Alkalinization of urine resulting in decreased excretion of quinidine). Products include:
- Diamox Parenteral ... 1200
- Diamox Parenteral ... ⊙ 308
- Diamox Sequels (Sustained Release) ... 1201
- Diamox Sequels (Sustained Release) ... ⊙ 310
- Diamox Tablets ... 1200
- Diamox Tablets ... ⊙ 308

Amiodarone Hydrochloride (Increased serum concentration of quinidine). Products include:
- Cordarone Tablets ... 2446

Atracurium Besylate (Potentiation of neuromuscular blockade). Products include:
- Tracrium Injection ... 817

Atropine Sulfate (Additive vagolytic effect). Products include:
- Arco-Lase Plus Tablets ... 607
- Atropine Sulfate Sterile Ophthalmic Solution and S.O.P. Sterile Ophthalmic Ointment ... ⊙ 239
- Donnagel ... ▣ 675
- Donnagel-PG ... 1858
- Donnatal ... 1858
- Donnatal Extentabs ... 1859
- Donnatal Tablets ... 1858
- Donnazyme Tablets ... 1860
- Isopto Atropine ... ⊙ 218
- Lomotil ... 2174
- Motofen Tablets ... 836
- Ru-Tuss Tablets ... 693
- Urised Tablets ... 2396

Belladonna Alkaloids (Additive vagolytic effect). Products include:
- Bellergal-S Tablets ... 1998
- Hyland's Bed Wetting Tablets ... ▣ 728
- Hyland's Teething Tablets ... ▣ 728
- Kinesed Tablets ... 2272

Bendroflumethiazide (Alkalinization of urine resulting in decreased excretion of quinidine). Products include:
- Corzide Tablets ... 702
- Naturetin Tablets ... 1789
- Rauzide Tablets ... 1804

Benztropine Mesylate (Additive vagolytic effect). Products include:
- Cogentin ... 1435

Biperiden (Additive vagolytic effect). Products include:
- Akineton ... 1171

Chlorothiazide (Alkalinization of urine resulting in decreased excretion of quinidine). Products include:
- Aldoclor Tablets ... 1413
- Diupres Tablets ... 1461
- Diuril Oral ... 1464

Chlorothiazide Sodium (Alkalinization of urine resulting in decreased excretion of quinidine). Products include:
- Diuril Sodium Intravenous ... 1463

Chlorpromazine (Additive cardiac depressive effects). Products include:
- Thorazine ... 2234

Cimetidine (Prolonged quinidine half-life; increase in serum quinidine level). Products include:
- Tagamet Tablets ... 2228

Cimetidine Hydrochloride (Prolonged quinidine half-life; increase in serum quinidine level). Products include:
- Tagamet ... 2228

Clidinium Bromide (Additive vagolytic effect). Products include:
- Librax Capsules ... 1929
- Quarzan Capsules ... 1937

Decamethonium (Potentiation of neuromuscular blockade).

Dichlorphenamide (Alkalinization of urine resulting in decreased excretion of quinidine). Products include:
- Daranide Tablets ... 1445

Dicumarol (Reduction of clotting factor concentrations). Products include:
- Dicumarol Tablets ... 516

Dicyclomine Hydrochloride (Additive vagolytic effect). Products include:
- Bentyl ... 1322

Digitoxin (Increased serum concentration of digitoxin). Products include:
- Crystodigin Tablets ... 1253

Digoxin (Increased serum concentration of digoxin). Products include:
- Lanoxicaps ... 772
- Lanoxin Elixir Pediatric ... 775
- Lanoxin Injection ... 778
- Lanoxin Injection Pediatric ... 781
- Lanoxin Tablets ... 783

Edrophonium Chloride (Antagonism of cholinergic effects). Products include:
- Enlon Injection ... 598
- Tensilon Injectable ... 1123

Ethopropazine Hydrochloride (Additive vagolytic effect).

Fluphenazine Decanoate (Additive cardiac depressive effects). Products include:
- Prolixin Decanoate ... 1795

Fluphenazine Enanthate (Additive cardiac depressive effects). Products include:
- Prolixin Enanthate ... 1796

Fluphenazine Hydrochloride (Additive cardiac depressive effects). Products include:
- Prolixin Elixir ... 1793
- Prolixin Injection ... 1791
- Prolixin Oral Concentrate ... 1792
- Prolixin Tablets ... 1793

Glycopyrrolate (Additive vagolytic effect). Products include:
- Robinul Forte Tablets ... 1873
- Robinul Injectable ... 1873
- Robinul Tablets ... 1873

Guanidine Hydrochloride (Antagonism of cholinergic effects).
- No products indexed under this heading.

Hydrochlorothiazide (Alkalinization of urine resulting in decreased excretion of quinidine). Products include:
- Aldactazide ... 2150
- Aldoril Tablets ... 1418
- Apresazide Capsules ... 854
- Apresoline-Esidrix Tablets ... 857
- Capozide ... 2258
- Dyazide Capsules ... 2208
- Esidrix Tablets ... 863
- Esimil Tablets ... 864
- HydroDIURIL Tablets ... 1484
- Hydropres Tablets ... 1485
- Inderide Tablets ... 2463
- Inderide LA Long Acting Capsules .. 2465
- Lopressor HCT Tablets ... 1034
- Maxzide ... 1215
- Moduretic Tablets ... 1510
- Normozide Tablets ... 2112
- Oretic Tablets ... 544
- Oreticyl ... 545
- Prinzide Tablets ... 1540
- Ser-Ap-Es Tablets ... 881
- Serpasil-Esidrix Tablets ... 886
- Timolide Tablets ... 1547
- Trandate HCT Tablets ... 579
- Vaseretic Tablets ... 1559
- Zestoretic ... 2274

Hydroflumethiazide (Alkalinization of urine resulting in decreased excretion of quinidine). Products include:
- Diucardin Tablets ... 2450
- Saluron ... 718
- Salutensin/Salutensin-Demi ... 719

Hyoscyamine (Additive vagolytic effect). Products include:
- Cystospaz Tablets ... 2395
- Urised Tablets ... 2396

Hyoscyamine Sulfate (Additive vagolytic effect). Products include:
- Arco-Lase Plus Tablets ... 607
- Cystospaz-M Capsules ... 2395
- Donnagel ... ▣ 675
- Donnagel-PG ... 1858
- Donnatal ... 1858
- Donnatal Extentabs ... 1859
- Donnatal Tablets ... 1858
- Donnazyme Tablets ... 1860
- Kutrase Capsules ... 2146
- Levsin/Levsinex ... 2147
- Ru-Tuss Tablets ... 693

Ipratropium Bromide (Additive vagolytic effect). Products include:
- Atrovent Inhalation Aerosol ... 675

Mepenzolate Bromide (Additive vagolytic effect). Products include:
- Cantil Tablets ... 1326

Mesoridazine (Additive cardiac depressive effects). Products include:
- Serentil ... 686

Methazolamide (Alkalinization of urine resulting in decreased excretion of quinidine). Products include:
- Neptazane Tablets ... ⊙ 311

Methyclothiazide (Alkalinization of urine resulting in decreased excretion of quinidine). Products include:
- Enduron Tablets ... 517
- Enduronyl ... 518

Metocurine Iodide (Potentiation of neuromuscular blockade). Products include:
- Metubine Iodide Vials ... 1285

Neostigmine Bromide (Antagonism of cholinergic effects). Products include:
- Prostigmin Tablets ... 1121

Neostigmine Methylsulfate (Antagonism of cholinergic effects). Products include:
- Prostigmin Injectable ... 1120

Nifedipine (Decreased serum concentrations of quinidine). Products include:
- Adalat Capsules (10 mg and 20 mg) ... 1587
- Procardia Capsules ... 1781
- Procardia XL Tablets ... 1783

Oxybutynin Chloride (Additive vagolytic effect). Products include:
- Ditropan ... 1332

Oxyphenonium Bromide (Additive vagolytic effect).

Pancuronium Bromide Injection (Potentiation of neuromuscular blockade).
- No products indexed under this heading.

Perphenazine (Additive cardiac depressive effects). Products include:
- Etrafon ... 2087
- Triavil Tablets ... 1556
- Trilafon ... 2123

Phenobarbital (Decreased plasma half-life of quinidine). Products include:
- Arco-Lase Plus Tablets ... 607
- Bellergal-S Tablets ... 1998
- Bronkolixir ... ▣ 761
- Bronkotabs Tablets ... ▣ 762
- Donnatal ... 1858
- Donnatal Extentabs ... 1859
- Donnatal Tablets ... 1858
- Donnazyme Tablets ... 1860
- Kinesed Tablets ... 2272
- Phenobarbital Elixir and Tablets ... 1293
- Primatene Tablets-P Formula ... 2421
- Quadrinal Tablets ... 1183
- Tedral SA ... 1765

Phenytoin (Decreased plasma half-life of quinidine). Products include:
- Dilantin Infatabs ... 1710
- Dilantin-30 Pediatric/Dilantin-125 Suspension ... 1713

Phenytoin Sodium (Decreased plasma half-life of quinidine). Products include:
- Dilantin Kapseals ... 1708
- Dilantin Parenteral ... 1712
- Dilantin with Phenobarbital Kapseals ... 1715

Polythiazide (Alkalinization of urine resulting in decreased excretion of quinidine). Products include:
- Minizide Capsules ... 1779
- Renese Tablets ... 1785
- Renese-R Tablets ... 1786

Prochlorperazine (Additive cardiac depressive effects). Products include:
- Compazine ... 2201

Procyclidine Hydrochloride (Additive vagolytic effect). Products include:
- Kemadrin Tablets ... 771

Promethazine Hydrochloride (Additive cardiac depressive effects). Products include:
- Mepergan Injection ... 2479
- Phenergan with Codeine ... 2497
- Phenergan with Dextromethorphan 2499
- Phenergan Injection ... 2493
- Phenergan Suppositories ... 2496
- Phenergan Syrup ... 2495
- Phenergan Tablets ... 2496
- Phenergan VC ... 2500
- Phenergan VC with Codeine ... 2501

Propantheline Bromide (Additive vagolytic effect). Products include:
- Pro-Banthine Tablets ... 2141

Pyridostigmine Bromide (Antagonism of cholinergic effects). Products include:
- Mestinon Injectable ... 1115
- Mestinon ... 1116

Ranitidine Hydrochloride (Premature ventricular contractions and/or bigeminy). Products include:
- Zantac Injection and Zantac Injection Premixed ... 1063
- Zantac ... 1065

Reserpine (Additive cardiac depressive effects). Products include:
- Diupres Tablets ... 1461
- Hydromox R Tablets ... 1209
- Hydropres Tablets ... 1485
- Renese-R Tablets ... 1786
- Salutensin/Salutensin-Demi ... 719
- Ser-Ap-Es Tablets ... 881
- Serpasil Tablets ... 883
- Serpasil-Apresoline Tablets ... 884
- Serpasil-Esidrix Tablets ... 886

Rifampin (Decreased plasma half-life of quinidine). Products include:
- Rifadin ... 1345
- Rifamate Capsules ... 1347
- Rimactane Capsules ... 879

Scopolamine Hydrobromide (Additive vagolytic effect). Products include:
- Donnagel ... ▣ 675
- Donnagel-PG ... 1858
- Donnatal ... 1858
- Donnatal Extentabs ... 1859
- Donnatal Tablets ... 1858
- Donnazyme Tablets ... 1860
- Isopto Hyoscine ... ◉ 222
- Murocoll-2 Sterile Ophthalmic Solution ... ◉ 261
- Ru-Tuss Tablets ... 693

Scopolamine Preparations (Additive vagolytic effect). Products include:
- Transderm Scōp Transdermal Therapeutic System ... 887

Sodium Bicarbonate (Alkalinization of urine resulting in decreased excretion of quinidine). Products include:
- Alka-Seltzer Advanced Formula Antacid & Non-Aspirin Pain Reliever ... ▣ 620
- Alka-Seltzer Effervescent Antacid ▣ 622
- Alka-Seltzer Effervescent Antacid and Pain Reliever ... 1568
- Alka-Seltzer Extra Strength Effervescent Antacid and Pain Reliever ... ▣ 623
- Alka-Seltzer (Flavored) Effervescent Antacid and Pain Reliever .. ▣ 621
- Arm & Hammer Pure Baking Soda ... ▣ 548
- Ceo-Two Rectal Suppositories ... 671
- Citrocarbonate Antacid ... ▣ 668
- Massengill Liquid Concentrate ... 2191
- NuLYTELY ... 699

Succinylcholine Chloride (Potentiation of neuromuscular blockade). Products include:
- Anectine ... 755

Tridihexethyl Chloride (Additive vagolytic effect).
- No products indexed under this heading.

Trifluoperazine Hydrochloride (Additive cardiac depressive effects). Products include:
- Stelazine ... 2226

Trihexyphenidyl Hydrochloride (Additive vagolytic effect). Products include:
- Artane ... 1195

Vecuronium Bromide (Potentiation of neuromuscular blockade). Products include:
- Norcuron ... 1642

Verapamil Hydrochloride (Increased quinidine half-life and increase in serum quinidine level; potential hypotensive reactions). Products include:
- Calan SR Caplets ... 2157
- Calan Tablets ... 2155
- Isoptin Injectable ... 1177
- Isoptin Oral Tablets ... 1179
- Isoptin SR Sustained Release Tablets ... 1181
- Verelan Capsules ... 1243
- Verelan Capsules ... 2535

Warfarin Sodium (Reduction of clotting factor concentrations). Products include:
- Coumadin Injection & Tablets ... 944
- Panwarfin Tablets ... 547

Q-VEL MUSCLE RELAXANT PAIN RELIEVER
(Quinine Sulfate) ... ▣ 552
No interactions described in labeling.

R&C SHAMPOO
(Pyrethrins) ... ▣ 652
No interactions described in labeling.

R&C SPRAY III
(Pyrethroids) ... ▣ 652
No interactions described in labeling.

RID LICE CONTROL SPRAY
(Pyrethroids) ... 1773
No interactions described in labeling.

RID LICE KILLING SHAMPOO
(Pyrethrins) ... 1774
No interactions described in labeling.

RAUDIXIN TABLETS
(Rauwolfia Serpentina) ... 1803
May interact with central nervous system depressants, antihypertensives, diuretics, cardiac glycosides, monoamine oxidase inhibitors, sympathomimetic aerosol bronchodilators, tricyclic antidepressants, catecholamine depleting drugs, and certain other agents. Compounds in these categories include:

Acebutolol Hydrochloride (Potentiation of antihypertensive effects). Products include:
- Sectral Capsules ... 2520

Alcohol (Increased CNS depressant effects; orthostatic hypotension).

Alfentanil Hydrochloride (Increased CNS depressant effects). Products include:
- Alfenta Injection ... 1131

Alprazolam (Increased CNS depressant effects). Products include:
- Xanax Tablets ... 2367

Amiloride Hydrochloride (Potentiation of antihypertensive effects). Products include:
- Midamor Tablets ... 1508
- Moduretic Tablets ... 1510

Amitriptyline Hydrochloride (Decreased antidepressant and antihypertensive effects). Products include:
- Elavil ... 2269
- Endep Tablets ... 1927
- Etrafon ... 2087
- Limbitrol ... 1933
- Triavil Tablets ... 1556

Amoxapine (Decreased antidepressant and antihypertensive effects). Products include:
- Asendin Tablets ... 1196

Aprobarbital (Increased CNS depressant effects). Products include:
- Alurate Elixir ... 1883

Atenolol (Potentiation of antihypertensive effects). Products include:
- Tenoretic Tablets ... 1105
- Tenormin Tablets and I.V. Injection 1107

Benazepril Hydrochloride (Potentiation of antihypertensive effects). Products include:
- Lotensin Tablets ... 872

Bendroflumethiazide (Potentiation of antihypertensive effects). Products include:
- Corzide Tablets ... 702
- Naturetin Tablets ... 1789
- Rauzide Tablets ... 1804

Betaxolol Hydrochloride (Potentiation of antihypertensive effects). Products include:
- Betoptic Sterile Ophthalmic Solution ... 569
- Betoptic S Sterile Ophthalmic Suspension ... 570
- Kerlone Tablets ... 2172

Bumetanide (Potentiation of antihypertensive effects). Products include:
- Bumex ... 1895

Buprenorphine (Increased CNS depressant effects).
- No products indexed under this heading.

Buspirone Hydrochloride (Increased CNS depressant effects). Products include:
- BuSpar ... 1401

Butabarbital (Increased CNS depressant effects). Products include:
- Pyridium Plus ... 1764

Butalbital (Increased CNS depressant effects). Products include:
- Esgic-Plus Tablets ... 1002
- Esgic Tablets & Capsules ... 1001
- Fioricet Tablets ... 2006
- Fiorinal Capsules ... 2007
- Fiorinal with Codeine Capsules ... 2008
- Fiorinal Tablets ... 2007
- Phrenilin ... 838
- Sedapap Tablets 50 mg/650 mg .. 1360

Captopril (Potentiation of antihypertensive effects). Products include:
- Capoten ... 2255
- Capozide ... 2258

Carteolol Hydrochloride (Potentiation of antihypertensive effects). Products include:
- Cartrol Tablets ... 507

Chlordiazepoxide (Increased CNS depressant effects). Products include:
- Libritabs Tablets ... 1930
- Limbitrol ... 1933
- Menrium Tablets ... 1934

Chlordiazepoxide Hydrochloride (Increased CNS depressant effects). Products include:
- Librax Capsules ... 1929
- Librium Capsules ... 1931
- Librium Injectable ... 1932

Chlorothiazide (Potentiation of antihypertensive effects). Products include:
- Aldoclor Tablets ... 1413
- Diupres Tablets ... 1461
- Diuril Oral ... 1464

Chlorothiazide Sodium (Potentiation of antihypertensive effects). Products include:
- Diuril Sodium Intravenous ... 1463

Chlorpromazine (Increased CNS depressant effects). Products include:
- Thorazine ... 2234

Chlorprothixene (Increased CNS depressant effects). Products include:
- Taractan Tablets ... 1920

Chlorprothixene Hydrochloride (Increased CNS depressant effects). Products include:
- Taractan ... 1920

Chlorthalidone (Potentiation of antihypertensive effects). Products include:
- Combipres Tablets ... 678
- Tenoretic Tablets ... 1105
- Thalitone Tablets ... 687

Clomipramine Hydrochloride (Decreased antidepressant and antihypertensive effects). Products include:
- Anafranil Capsules ... 650

Clonidine (Potentiation of antihypertensive effects). Products include:
- Catapres-TTS ... 677

Clonidine Hydrochloride (Potentiation of antihypertensive effects). Products include:
- Catapres Tablets ... 676
- Combipres Tablets ... 678

Clorazepate Dipotassium (Increased CNS depressant effects). Products include:
- Tranxene ... 556

Codeine (Increased CNS depressant effects). Products include:
- Calcidrine Syrup ... 506

Codeine Phosphate (Increased CNS depressant effects). Products include:
- Actifed with Codeine Cough Syrup.. 752
- Cheracol Cough Syrup ... 1853
- Codimal PH Syrup ... 846

Dimetane-DC Cough Syrup 1857
Empirin with Codeine Phosphate Nos. 2, 3 & 4 764
Fiorinal with Codeine Capsules 2008
Isoclor Expectorant 982
Naldecon CX Adult Liquid .... ⊞ 521
Novahistine DH 1342
Novahistine Expectorant 1343
Nucofed Capsules 2219
Nucofed Expectorant 2219
Nucofed Pediatric Expectorant 2220
Nucofed Syrup 2219
Phenaphen with Codeine Capsules 1865
Phenaphen-650 with Codeine Tablets 1866
Phenergan with Codeine 2497
Phenergan VC with Codeine 2501
Robitussin A-C Syrup 1875
Robitussin-DAC Syrup 1875
Ryna .... ⊞ 741
Soma Compound w/Codeine Tablets 2390
Triaminic Expectorant w/Codeine .. 1996
Tussi-Organidin Liquid 2391
Tylenol with Codeine 1381

Codeine Polistirex (Increased CNS depressant effects).
No products indexed under this heading.

Desipramine Hydrochloride (Decreased antidepressant and antihypertensive effects). Products include:
Norpramin Tablets 1340

Deslanoside (Cardiac arrhythmias).
No products indexed under this heading.

Dezocine (Increased CNS depressant effects).

Diazepam (Increased CNS depressant effects). Products include:
Valium Injectable 1937
Valium Tablets 1939
Valrelease Capsules 1923

Diazoxide (Potentiation of antihypertensive effects). Products include:
Hyperstat I.V. Injection 2095
Proglycem 649

Digitoxin (). Products include:
Crystodigin Tablets 1253

Digoxin (Cardiac arrhythmias). Products include:
Lanoxicaps 772
Lanoxin Elixir Pediatric 775
Lanoxin Injection 778
Lanoxin Injection Pediatric 781
Lanoxin Tablets 783

Dobutamine Hydrochloride (Prolonged effect of direct-acting sympathomimetic). Products include:
Dobutrex Solution Vials 1259

Dopamine Hydrochloride (Prolonged effect of direct-acting sympathomimetic). Products include:
Intropin Injection 930

Doxazosin Mesylate (Potentiation of antihypertensive effects). Products include:
Cardura Tablets 1941

Doxepin Hydrochloride (Decreased antidepressant and antihypertensive effects). Products include:
Sinequan 1960

Droperidol (Increased CNS depressant effects). Products include:
Inapsine Injection 1140
Innovar Injection 1141

Enalapril Maleate (Potentiation of antihypertensive effects). Products include:
Vaseretic Tablets 1559
Vasotec Tablets 1564

Enalaprilat (Potentiation of antihypertensive effects). Products include:
Vasotec I.V. 1562

Enflurane (Increased CNS depressant effects). Products include:
Ethrane 599

Ephedrine Hydrochloride (Sympathomimetic effect inhibited). Products include:
Amesec .... ⊞ 682
Primatene Tablets-M Formula 2421
Primatene Tablets-P Formula 2421
Primatene Tablets-Regular Formula 2421
Quadrinal Tablets 1183
Quelidrine Syrup 556
Tedral SA 1765

Ephedrine Sulfate (Sympathomimetic effect inhibited). Products include:
Bronkaid Tablets .... ⊞ 757
Bronkolixir .... ⊞ 761
Bronkotabs Tablets .... ⊞ 762
Marax Tablets & DF Syrup 1954
Pazo Hemorrhoid Ointment & Suppositories 752
Vicks Vatronol Nose Drops .... ⊞ 666

Ephedrine Tannate (Sympathomimetic effect inhibited). Products include:
Rynatuss 2388

Epinephrine (Prolonged effect of direct-acting sympathomimetic). Products include:
Ana-Kit Anaphylaxis Emergency Treatment Kit 1100
Bronkaid Mist .... ⊞ 757
EpiPen 843
Marcaine Hydrochloride 0.5% with Epinephrine 1:200,000 (as bitartrate) 958
Marcaine Hydrochloride with Epinephrine 1:200,000 2055
Primatene Mist 2420
Sus-Phrine Injection 1006
Xylocaine with Epinephrine Injections 637

Epinephrine Bitartrate (Prolonged effect of direct-acting sympathomimetic). Products include:
AsthmaHaler Mist Epinephrine Bitartrate Bronchodilator .... ⊞ 616
Bronkaid Mist Suspension .... ⊞ 757
Primatene Mist Suspension 2421

Epinephrine Hydrochloride (Prolonged effect of direct-acting sympathomimetic). Products include:
Adrenalin Chloride Solution 1:100 & 1:1,000 1689
Epifrin .... ⊙ 244
Glaucon .... ⊙ 218

Esmolol Hydrochloride (Potentiation of antihypertensive effects). Products include:
Brevibloc Injection 942

Estazolam (Increased CNS depressant effects). Products include:
ProSom Tablets 554

Ethacrynic Acid (Potentiation of antihypertensive effects). Products include:
Edecrin Tablets 1468

Ethchlorvynol (Increased CNS depressant effects). Products include:
Placidyl Capsules 553

Ethinamate (Increased CNS depressant effects).
No products indexed under this heading.

Felodipine (Potentiation of antihypertensive effects). Products include:
Plendil Extended-Release Tablets 1526

Fentanyl (Increased CNS depressant effects). Products include:
Duragesic Transdermal System 1133

Fentanyl Citrate (Increased CNS depressant effects). Products include:
Innovar Injection 1141
Sublimaze Injection 1146

Fluphenazine Decanoate (Increased CNS depressant effects). Products include:
Prolixin Decanoate 1795

Fluphenazine Enanthate (Increased CNS depressant effects). Products include:
Prolixin Enanthate 1796

Fluphenazine Hydrochloride (Increased CNS depressant effects). Products include:
Prolixin Elixir 1793
Prolixin Injection 1791
Prolixin Oral Concentrate 1792
Prolixin Tablets 1793

Flurazepam Hydrochloride (Increased CNS depressant effects). Products include:
Dalmane Capsules 1927

Fosinopril Sodium (Potentiation of antihypertensive effects). Products include:
Monopril Tablets 1406

Furazolidone (Excessive excitation; hypertension; sympathetic response). Products include:
Furoxone 1855

Furosemide (Potentiation of antihypertensive effects). Products include:
Lasix 1093

Glutethimide (Increased CNS depressant effects).
No products indexed under this heading.

Guanabenz Acetate (Potentiation of antihypertensive effects). Products include:
Wytensin Tablets 2542

Guanethidine Monosulfate (Potentiation of antihypertensive effects). Products include:
Esimil Tablets 864
Ismelin Tablets 869

Haloperidol (Increased CNS depressant effects). Products include:
Haldol Injection, Tablets and Concentrate 1373

Haloperidol Decanoate (Increased CNS depressant effects). Products include:
Haldol Decanoate 1375

Hydralazine Hydrochloride (Potentiation of antihypertensive effects). Products include:
Apresazide Capsules 854
Apresoline Hydrochloride Parenteral (Ampuls) 856
Apresoline Hydrochloride Tablets .. 855
Apresoline-Esidrix Tablets 857
Ser-Ap-Es Tablets 881
Serpasil-Apresoline Tablets 884

Hydrochlorothiazide (Potentiation of antihypertensive effects). Products include:
Aldactazide 2150
Aldoril Tablets 1418
Apresazide Capsules 854
Apresoline-Esidrix Tablets 857
Capozide 2258
Dyazide Capsules 2208
Esidrix Tablets 863
Esimil Tablets 864
HydroDIURIL Tablets 1484
Hydropres Tablets 1485
Inderide Tablets 2463
Inderide LA Long Acting Capsules .. 2465
Lopressor HCT Tablets 1034
Maxzide 1215
Moduretic Tablets 1510
Normozide Tablets 2112
Oretic Tablets 544
Oreticyl 545
Prinzide Tablets 1540
Ser-Ap-Es Tablets 881
Serpasil-Esidrix Tablets 886
Timolide Tablets 1547
Trandate HCT Tablets 579
Vaseretic Tablets 1559
Zestoretic 2274

Hydrocodone Bitartrate (Increased CNS depressant effects). Products include:
Anexsia 5/500 Tablets 2196
Anexsia 7.5/650 Tablets 2197
Azdone Tablets 844
Codiclear DH Syrup 845
Codimal DH Syrup 846
Damason-P 1356
Hycodan Syrup, Tablets 927
Hycomine Compound Tablets 929
Hycomine Syrup 927
Hycotuss Expectorant Syrup 930
Hydrocet Capsules 835
Lortab ASA Tablets 2414
Lortab 2412
Ru-Tuss with Hydrocodone 694
Triaminic Expectorant DH 1995
Vicodin Tablets 1187
Vicodin ES Tablets 1189
Zydone Capsules 941

Hydrocodone Polistirex (Increased CNS depressant effects). Products include:
Tussionex Extended-Release Suspension 988

Hydroflumethiazide (Potentiation of antihypertensive effects). Products include:
Diucardin Tablets 2450
Saluron 718
Salutensin/Salutensin-Demi 719

Hydroxyzine Hydrochloride (Increased CNS depressant effects). Products include:
Atarax Tablets & Syrup 1941
Marax Tablets & DF Syrup 1954
Vistaril Intramuscular Solution 1970

Imipramine Hydrochloride (Decreased antidepressant and antihypertensive effects). Products include:
Tofranil Ampuls 1038
Tofranil Tablets 1039

Imipramine Pamoate (Decreased antidepressant and antihypertensive effects). Products include:
Tofranil-PM Capsules 1041

Indapamide (Potentiation of antihypertensive effects). Products include:
Lozol Tablets 1843

Isocarboxazid (Excessive excitation; hypertension; sympathetic response). Products include:
Marplan Tablets 1906

Isoflurane (Increased CNS depressant effects). Products include:
Forane 600

Isoproterenol Hydrochloride (Prolonged effect of direct-acting sympathomimetic). Products include:
Isuprel Hydrochloride Injection 1:5000 2050
Isuprel Hydrochloride Mistometer .. 2051
Isuprel Hydrochloride Solution 1:200 & 1:100 2052
Norisodrine Aerotrol 540

Isradipine (Potentiation of antihypertensive effects). Products include:
DynaCirc Capsules 2004

Ketamine Hydrochloride (Increased CNS depressant effects). Products include:
Ketalar 1726

Labetalol Hydrochloride (Potentiation of antihypertensive effects). Products include:
Normodyne Injection 2108
Normodyne Tablets 2110
Normozide Tablets 2112
Trandate HCT Tablets 579
Trandate Injection 577
Trandate Tablets 579

Levodopa (Levodopa effects inhibited). Products include:
Larodopa Tablets 1905
Sinemet Tablets 952
Sinemet CR Tablets 953

Levorphanol Tartrate (Increased CNS depressant effects). Products include:
Levo-Dromoran 1906

Lisinopril (Potentiation of antihypertensive effects). Products include:
Prinivil Tablets 1538
Prinzide Tablets 1540
Zestoretic 2274
Zestril Tablets 2277

Lorazepam (Increased CNS depressant effects). Products include:
Ativan Injection 2432
Ativan Tablets 2434

Loxapine Hydrochloride (Increased CNS depressant effects). Products include:
Loxitane 1213

Loxapine Succinate (Increased CNS depressant effects). Products include:
Loxitane Capsules 1213

Maprotiline Hydrochloride (Decreased antidepressant and antihypertensive effects). Products include:
Ludiomil Tablets 874

Mecamylamine Hydrochloride (Potentiation of antihypertensive effects). Products include:
Inversine Tablets 1492

Meperidine Hydrochloride (Increased CNS depressant effects). Products include:
Demerol 2047
Mepergan Injection 2479

Mephobarbital (Increased CNS depressant effects). Products include:
Mebaral Tablets 2061

Meprobamate (Increased CNS depressant effects). Products include:
Deprol Tablets 2382
Equagesic Tablets 2451
Miltown Tablets 2386
PMB 200 and PMB 400 2504

Mesoridazine (Increased CNS depressant effects). Products include:
Serentil 686

Metaproterenol Sulfate (Sympathomimetic effect inhibited). Products include:
Alupent 674
Arm-a-Med Metaproterenol Sulfate Inhalation Solution, USP 617
Metaprel Inhalation Aerosol Bronchodilator 2014
Metaprel Inhalation Solution 2015
Metaprel 2015
Metaproterenol Sulfate Inhalation Solution, USP 912

Metaraminol Bitartrate (Sympathomimetic effect inhibited). Products include:
Aramine Injection 1424

Methadone Hydrochloride (Increased CNS depressant effects). Products include:
Dolophine Hydrochloride Ampoules & Vials 1260
Dolophine Hydrochloride Tablets 1261
Methadone Hydrochloride Diskets 1284
Methadone Hydrochloride Oral Solution & Tablets 1987

Methohexital Sodium (Increased CNS depressant effects). Products include:
Brevital Sodium Vials 1248

Methotrimeprazine (Increased orthostatic hypotension).
No products indexed under this heading.

Methoxamine Hydrochloride (Prolonged effect of direct-acting sympathomimetic). Products include:
Vasoxyl Injection 819

Methoxyflurane (Increased CNS depressant effects).
No products indexed under this heading.

Methyclothiazide (Potentiation of antihypertensive effects). Products include:
Enduron Tablets 517
Enduronyl 518

Methyldopa (Potentiation of antihypertensive effects). Products include:
Aldoclor Tablets 1413
Aldomet Oral 1415
Aldoril Tablets 1418

Methyldopate Hydrochloride (Potentiation of antihypertensive effects). Products include:
Aldomet Ester HCl Injection 1417

Metolazone (Potentiation of antihypertensive effects). Products include:
Diulo 2129
Mykrox ½ mg Tablets 984
Zaroxolyn Tablets 989

Metoprolol Tartrate (Potentiation of antihypertensive effects). Products include:
Lopressor Ampuls 1032
Lopressor HCT Tablets 1034
Lopressor Tablets 1032

Metyrosine (Potentiation of antihypertensive effects). Products include:
Demser Capsules 1460

Midazolam Hydrochloride (Increased CNS depressant effects). Products include:
Versed Injection 1924

Minoxidil (Potentiation of antihypertensive effects). Products include:
Loniten Tablets 2346
Rogaine Topical Solution 2357

Molindone Hydrochloride (Increased CNS depressant effects). Products include:
Moban Tablets & Concentrate 932

Morphine Sulfate (Increased CNS depressant effects). Products include:
Astramorph/PF Injection, USP (Preservative-Free) 618
Duramorph 960
Infumorph 200 and Infumorph 500 Sterile Solutions 962
MS Contin Tablets 1814
MSIR 1817
Oramorph SR (Morphine Sulfate Sustained Release Tablets) 1988
Roxanol 1991

Nadolol (Potentiation of antihypertensive effects). Products include:
Corgard Tablets 701
Corzide Tablets 702

Nicardipine Hydrochloride (Potentiation of antihypertensive effects). Products include:
Cardene Capsules 2290

Nitroglycerin (Potentiation of antihypertensive effects). Products include:
Deponit NTG Transdermal Delivery System 2143
Minitran Transdermal Delivery System 1312
Nitro-Bid Ointment 1339
Nitro-Bid Capsules 1338
Nitrodisc 2176
Nitro-Dur (nitroglycerin) Transdermal Infusion System 1164
Nitrogard Tablets 1004
Nitrolingual Spray 1846
Nitrostat Tablets 1743
Transderm-Nitro Transdermal Therapeutic System 2283

Norepinephrine Bitartrate (Prolonged effect of direct-acting sympathomimetic). Products include:
Levophed Bitartrate Injection 2054

Nortriptyline Hydrochloride (Decreased antidepressant and antihypertensive effects). Products include:
Pamelor 2019

Opium Alkaloids (Increased CNS depressant effects). Products include:
B & O No. 15A & No. 16A Supprettes 2395
Pantopon Injectable 1911

Oxazepam (Increased CNS depressant effects). Products include:
Serax Capsules 2522
Serax Tablets 2522

Oxycodone Hydrochloride (Increased CNS depressant effects). Products include:
Percocet Tablets 950
Percodan 951
Roxicodone Tablets, Oral Solution & Intensol (Oxycodone) 1992
Tylox Capsules 1382

Penbutolol Sulfate (Potentiation of antihypertensive effects). Products include:
Levatol 1832

Pentobarbital Sodium (Increased CNS depressant effects). Products include:
Nembutal Sodium Capsules 534
Nembutal Sodium Solution 536
Nembutal Sodium Suppositories 538

Perphenazine (Increased CNS depressant effects). Products include:
Etrafon 2087
Triavil Tablets 1556
Trilafon 2123

Phenelzine Sulfate (Excessive excitation; hypertension; sympathetic response). Products include:
Nardil 1742

Phenobarbital (Increased CNS depressant effects). Products include:
Arco-Lase Plus Tablets 607
Bellergal-S Tablets 1998
Bronkolixir .... ▣ 761
Bronkotabs Tablets .... ▣ 762
Donnatal 1858
Donnatal Extentabs 1859
Donnatal Tablets 1858
Donnazyme Tablets 1860
Kinesed Tablets 2272
Phenobarbital Elixir and Tablets 1293
Primatene Tablets-P Formula 2421
Quadrinal Tablets 1183
Tedral SA 1765

Phenoxybenzamine Hydrochloride (Potentiation of antihypertensive effects). Products include:
Dibenzyline Capsules 2207

Phentolamine Mesylate (Potentiation of antihypertensive effects). Products include:
Regitine 878

Phenylephrine Bitartrate (Sympathomimetic effect inhibited).
No products indexed under this heading.

Phenylephrine Hydrochloride (Sympathomimetic effect inhibited). Products include:
AK-Dilate Solution 2.5% and 10% .... ⊙ 203
Atrohist Sprinkle Capsules 558
Cerose-DM 2443
Codimal 846
Comhist LA Capsules 1618
Congespirin For Children Aspirin Free Chewable Cold Tablets 748
Cyclomydril .... ⊙ 216
Deconsal Sprinkle Capsules 559
Dimetane Decongestant .... ▣ 673
Dristan Decongestant/Antihistamine/Analgesic Coated Caplets .... ▣ 749
Dristan Cold Nasal Decongestant/Antihistamine/Analgesic Coated Tablets 2419
Dristan Advanced Formula Decongestant/Antihistamine/Analgesic Tablets .... ▣ 749
Dristan Nasal Spray, Menthol 2419
Dristan Nasal Spray, Regular and Regular with Metered Pump 2419
Entex Capsules 1623
Entex Liquid 1623
Sinus Excedrin Analgesic, Decongestant Tablets & Caplets 750
Extendryl 994
4-Way Fast Acting Nasal Spray - Original Formula (regular & mentholated) & Metered Spray Pump (regular) 751
Hycomine Compound Tablets 929
Murocoll-2 Sterile Ophthalmic Solution .... ⊙ 261
Mydfrin 2.5% .... ⊙ 224
Naldecon Syrup, Tablets, Pediatric Drops and Pediatric Syrup 709
Neo-Synephrine Hydrochloride 1% Carpuject 2063
Neo-Synephrine Hydrochloride 1% Injection 2063
Neo-Synephrine Hydrochloride (Ophthalmic) 2064
Neo-Synephrine .... ▣ 759
Nōstril Nasal Decongestant .... ▣ 520
Novahistine Elixir .... ▣ 596
Phenergan VC 2500
Phenergan VC with Codeine 2501
Prefrin Liquifilm Vasoconstrictor and Lubricant Eye Drops .... ⊙ 254
Prefrin-A .... ⊙ 255
Quelidrine Syrup 556
Relief Vasoconstrictor and Lubricant Eye Drops .... ⊙ 256
Robitussin Night Relief .... ▣ 677
Ru-Tuss with Hydrocodone 694
Ru-Tuss Tablets 693
Vasosulf .... ⊙ 279
Vicks Sinex .... ▣ 665
Zincfrin .... ⊙ 230

Phenylephrine Tannate (Sympathomimetic effect inhibited). Products include:
Rynatan 2387
Rynatuss 2388

Phenylpropanolamine Hydrochloride (Sympathomimetic effect inhibited). Products include:
A.R.M. Allergy Relief Medicine Caplets .... ▣ 615
Acutrim .... ▣ 548
Allerest .... ▣ 559
BC Cold Powder .... ▣ 517
Cheracol Plus Head Cold/Cough Formula .... ▣ 667
Codimal Expectorant 846
Comtrex Multi-Symptom Cold Reliever Tablets/Caplets/Liqui-Gels/Liquid 745
Contac Continuous Action Decongestant/Antihistamine Capsules ▣ 710
Contac Maximum Strength Continuous Action Decongestant/Antihistamine Caplets .... ▣ 709
Contac Severe Cold and Flu Formula Caplets .... ▣ 711
Coricidin 'D' Decongestant Tablets .... ▣ 695
Coricidin Demilets Tablets for Children .... ▣ 696
Demazin Nasal Decongestant/Antihistamine Repetabs Tablets & Syrup .... ▣ 697
Dexatrim .... ▣ 733
Dimetane-DC Cough Syrup 1857
Dimetapp Elixir .... ▣ 673
Dimetapp DM Elixir .... ▣ 674
Dimetapp Extentabs .... ▣ 674
Dimetapp Plus Caplets .... ▣ 675
Dimetapp Tablets .... ▣ 675
Entex Capsules 1623
Entex LA Tablets 1623
Entex Liquid 1623
4-Way Cold Tablets 750
Hycomine Syrup 927
Naldecon CX Adult Liquid .... ▣ 521
Naldecon DX Adult Liquid .... ▣ 521
Naldecon DX Children's Syrup .... ▣ 522
Naldecon DX Pediatric Drops .... ▣ 522
Naldecon EX Children's Syrup .... ▣ 522
Naldecon EX Pediatric Drops .... ▣ 523
Naldecon Syrup, Tablets, Pediatric Drops and Pediatric Syrup 709
Nolamine Tablets 838
Nolex LA Tablets 838
Ornade Spansule Capsules 2221

Orthoxicol Cough Syrup ■ 668
Propagest 839
Pyrroxate Capsules ■ 669
Robitussin-CF ■ 676
Ru-Tuss II Capsules 693
Ru-Tuss with Hydrocodone 694
Ru-Tuss Tablets 693
Sine-Off Sinus Medicine Tablets-Aspirin Formula ■ 722
Sinulin 840
St. Joseph Cold Tablets for Children ■ 704
Tavist-D Tablets 2035
Triaminic Allergy Tablets ■ 688
Triaminic Chewables ■ 688
Triaminic Cold Tablets ■ 688
Triaminic Expectorant ■ 688
Triaminic Expectorant w/Codeine 1996
Triaminic Expectorant DH 1995
Triaminic Oral Infant Drops 1996
Triaminic Syrup ■ 689
Triaminic-12 Tablets ■ 690
Triaminic-DM Syrup ■ 689
Triaminicin Tablets ■ 690
Triaminicol Multi-Symptom Cold Tablets ■ 691
Triaminicol Multi-Symptom Relief ■ 691
Tuss-Ornade Liquid 2242
Tuss-Ornade Spansule Capsules 2242
Tylenol Cold Medication, Effervescent Tablets 1369

Pindolol (Potentiation of antihypertensive effects). Products include:
Visken Tablets 2036

Pirbuterol Acetate (Sympathomimetic effect inhibited). Products include:
Maxair Inhaler 1311

Polythiazide (Potentiation of antihypertensive effects). Products include:
Minizide Capsules 1779
Renese Tablets 1785
Renese-R Tablets 1786

Prazepam (Increased CNS depressant effects). Products include:
Centrax 1693

Prazosin Hydrochloride (Potentiation of antihypertensive effects). Products include:
Minipress Capsules 1778
Minizide Capsules 1779

Prochlorperazine (Increased CNS depressant effects). Products include:
Compazine 2201

Promethazine Hydrochloride (Increased CNS depressant effects). Products include:
Mepergan Injection 2479
Phenergan with Codeine 2497
Phenergan with Dextromethorphan 2499
Phenergan Injection 2493
Phenergan Suppositories 2496
Phenergan Syrup 2495
Phenergan Tablets 2496
Phenergan VC 2500
Phenergan VC with Codeine 2501

Propofol (Increased CNS depressant effects). Products include:
Diprivan Injection 2267

Propoxyphene Hydrochloride (Increased CNS depressant effects). Products include:
Darvon 1256
Wygesic Tablets 2540

Propoxyphene Napsylate (Increased CNS depressant effects). Products include:
Darvon-N/Darvocet-N 1254

Propranolol Hydrochloride (Potentiation of antihypertensive effects). Products include:
Inderal 2459
Inderal LA Long Acting Capsules 2461
Inderide Tablets 2463
Inderide LA Long Acting Capsules 2465

Protriptyline Hydrochloride (Decreased antidepressant and antihypertensive effects). Products include:
Vivactil Tablets 1567

Pseudoephedrine Hydrochloride (Sympathomimetic effect inhibited). Products include:
Actifed Capsules ■ 539
Actifed Plus Caplets ■ 539
Actifed Plus Tablets ■ 540
Actifed with Codeine Cough Syrup 752
Actifed Syrup ■ 540
Actifed Tablets ■ 540
Actifed 12-Hour Capsules ■ 539
Advil Cold & Sinus Caplets (formerly CoAdvil) 2416
Allerest ■ 559
Anatuss LA Tablets 1359
Benadryl Decongestant Elixir ■ 635
Benadryl Decongestant ■ 635
Benadryl Plus ■ 636
Benadryl Plus Nighttime ■ 637
Benylin Decongestant ■ 638
Brexin L.A. Capsules 2078
Bromfed Capsules (Timed Release) 1615
Bromfed Syrup ■ 628
Bromfed 1615
CoAdvil ■ 748
Allergy-Sinus Comtrex Multi-Symptom Allergy Sinus Formula Tablets & Caplets 746
Cough Formula Comtrex 746
Comtrex Multi-Symptom Cold Reliever Tablets/Caplets/Liqui-Gels/Liquid 745
Day-Night Comtrex 747
Non-Drowsy Comtrex 747
Congess 994
Congestac Caplets ■ 617
Contac Jr. Children's Cold Medicine ■ 712
Contac Nighttime Cold Medicine ■ 713
Contac Sinus Caplets Maximum Strength Non-Drowsy Formula ■ 710
Contac Sinus Tablets Maximum Strength Non-Drowsy Formula ■ 710
Deconamine 663
Deconsal II Tablets 559
Dimacol Caplets ■ 672
Dimetane-DX Cough Syrup 1858
Dorcol Children's Cough Syrup ■ 685
Dorcol Children's Decongestant Liquid ■ 685
Dorcol Children's Liquid Cold Formula ■ 686
Maximum Strength Dristan Decongestant/Analgesic Coated Caplets ■ 750
No Drowsiness Dristan Cold Nasal Decongestant/Analgesic Coated Caplets 2420
Dristan Sinus Caplets 2419
Sinus Excedrin Analgesic, Decongestant Tablets & Caplets ■ 533
Fedahist Gyrocaps 2145
Fedahist Timecaps 2145
Guaifed 1615
Guaifed Syrup ■ 629
Isoclor Expectorant 982
Isoclor Timesule Capsules ■ 561
Kronofed-A 970
Medi-Flu Caplet, Liquid ■ 640
Novafed A Capsules 1342
Novafed Capsules 1342
Novahistine DH 1342
Novahistine DMX ■ 595
Novahistine Expectorant 1343
Nucofed Capsules 2219
Nucofed Expectorant 2219
Nucofed Pediatric Expectorant 2220
Nucofed Syrup 2219
Ornex Caplets ■ 618
PediaCare Allergy Relief Formula Liquid 1362
PediaCare Cough-Cold Formula Liquid 1362
PediaCare Infants' Oral Decongestant Drops 1362
PediaCare Night Rest Cough-Cold Formula Liquid 1362
PediaCare 6-12 Cough-Cold Formula Chewable Tablets 1362
Robitussin-DAC Syrup 1875
Robitussin-PE ■ 677
Rondec 1975
Rondec-DM 1976
Rondec-TR Tablet 1975
Ru-Tuss DE Tablets 694
Ryna ■ 741
Seldane-D Extended-Release Tablets 1350
Sinarest ■ 562
Sine-Aid Maximum Strength Sinus Headache Caplets 1365
Sine-Aid Maximum Strength Sinus Headache Tablets 1365
Sine-Off Maximum Strength Allergy/Sinus Formula Caplets ■ 721
Sine-Off Maximum Strength No Drowsiness Formula Caplets ■ 722
Singlet Tablets ■ 598
Sinutab Maximum Strength ■ 641
Sinutab Maximum Strength Without Drowsiness Tablets & Caplets ■ 642
Sinutab Regular Strength Without Drowsiness Formula ■ 641
St. Joseph Nighttime Cold Medicine ■ 705
Sudafed Children's Liquid ■ 543
Sudafed Cough Syrup ■ 543
Sudafed Plus Liquid ■ 544
Sudafed Plus Tablets ■ 545
Sudafed Sinus Caplets ■ 545
Sudafed Sinus Tablets ■ 545
Sudafed Tablets, 30 mg ■ 544
Sudafed Tablets, Adult Strength, 60 mg ■ 544
Sudafed 12 Hour Capsules ■ 545
TheraFlu Flu and Cold Medicine ■ 687
Triaminic Nite Light ■ 689
Tylenol Allergy Sinus Medication Caplets and Gelcaps, Maximum Strength 1372
Children's Tylenol Cold Liquid Formula and Chewable Tablets 1368
Tylenol Cold & Flu Hot Medication, Packets 1369
Tylenol Cold & Flu No Drowsiness Hot Medication, Packets 1371
Tylenol Cold Medication Caplets and Tablets 1370
Tylenol Cold Medication No Drowsiness Formula Caplets 1370
Tylenol Cold Night Time Medication Liquid 1371
Tylenol Cough Medication Liquid with Decongestant, Maximum Strength 1372
Tylenol, Maximum Strength, Sinus Medication Gelcaps, Caplets and Tablets 1373
Ursinus Inlay-Tabs ■ 691
Vicks Children's NyQuil ■ 664
Vicks Daycare ■ 660
Vicks Formula 44D Decongestant Cough Medicine ■ 662
Vicks Formula 44M Multi-Symptom Cough Medicine ■ 662
Vicks NyQuil Nighttime Colds Medicine-Original & Cherry Flavor ■ 664
Vicks Pediatric Formula 44 Cough & Congestion Medicine ■ 663
Vicks Pediatric Formula 44m Multi-Symptom Cough & Cold Medicine ■ 663

Pseudoephedrine Sulfate (Sympathomimetic effect inhibited). Products include:
Afrin Tablets ■ 693
Chlor-Trimeton Decongestant ■ 694
Disophrol Chronotab Sustained-Action Tablets ■ 698
Drixoral Antihistamine/Nasal Decongestant Syrup ■ 698
Drixoral Non-Drowsy Formula ■ 699
Drixoral Plus Extended-Release Tablets ■ 699
Drixoral Sinus ■ 700
Drixoral Sustained-Action Tablets ■ 698
Sinutab Allergy Formula Sustained Action Tablets ■ 640
Trinalin Repetabs Tablets 1170

Quazepam (Increased CNS depressant effects). Products include:
Doral Tablets 2383

Quinidine Gluconate (Cardiac arrhythmias). Products include:
Quinaglute Dura-Tabs Tablets 663

Quinidine Polygalacturonate (Cardiac arrhythmias). Products include:
Cardioquin Tablets 1812

Quinidine Sulfate (Cardiac arrhythmias). Products include:
Quinidex Extentabs 1868

Ramipril (Potentiation of antihypertensive effects). Products include:
Altace Capsules 1086

Rescinnamine (Potentiation of antihypertensive effects).
No products indexed under this heading.

Reserpine (Potentiation of antihypertensive effects). Products include:
Diupres Tablets 1461
Hydromox R Tablets 1209
Hydropres Tablets 1485
Renese-R Tablets 1786
Salutensin/Salutensin-Demi 719
Ser-Ap-Es Tablets 881
Serpasil Tablets 883
Serpasil-Apresoline Tablets 884
Serpasil-Esidrix Tablets 886

Secobarbital Sodium (Increased CNS depressant effects). Products include:
Seconal Sodium Pulvules 1296

Selegiline Hydrochloride (Excessive excitation; hypertension; sympathetic response). Products include:
Eldepryl 2250

Sodium Nitroprusside (Potentiation of antihypertensive effects). Products include:
Nipride I.V. Infusion 1909

Spironolactone (Potentiation of antihypertensive effects). Products include:
Aldactazide 2150
Aldactone 2152

Sufentanil Citrate (Increased CNS depressant effects). Products include:
Sufenta Injection 1147

Temazepam (Increased CNS depressant effects). Products include:
Restoril Capsules 2023

Terazosin Hydrochloride (Potentiation of antihypertensive effects). Products include:
Hytrin Tablets 529

Thiamylal Sodium (Increased CNS depressant effects). Products include:
Surital Ampoules, Steri-Vials 1764

Thioridazine Hydrochloride (Increased CNS depressant effects). Products include:
Mellaril 2011

Thiothixene (Increased CNS depressant effects). Products include:
Navane Capsules and Concentrate 1954
Navane Intramuscular 1956

Timolol Maleate (Potentiation of antihypertensive effects). Products include:
Blocadren Tablets 1429
Timolide Tablets 1547
Timoptic in Ocudose 1552
Timoptic Sterile Ophthalmic Solution 1550

Tranylcypromine Sulfate (Excessive excitation; hypertension; sympathetic response). Products include:
Parnate Tablets 2222

Triamterene (Potentiation of antihypertensive effects). Products include:
Dyazide Capsules 2208
Dyrenium Capsules 2210
Maxzide 1215

Triazolam (Increased CNS depressant effects). Products include:
Halcion Tablets 2340

Trifluoperazine Hydrochloride (Increased CNS depressant effects). Products include:
Stelazine 2226

Trimethaphan Camsylate (Potentiation of antihypertensive effects). Products include:
Arfonad Ampuls 1887

Trimipramine Maleate (Decreased antidepressant and antihypertensive effects). Products include:
- Surmontil Capsules 2524

RAUZIDE TABLETS
(Rauwolfia Serpentina, Bendroflumethiazide) 1804
May interact with central nervous system depressants, antihypertensives, diuretics, monoamine oxidase inhibitors, sympathomimetic aerosol bronchodilators, tricyclic antidepressants, lithium preparations, non-steroidal anti-inflammatory agents, barbiturates, narcotic analgesics, corticosteroids, oral anticoagulants, antigout agents, oral hypoglycemic agents, insulin, cardiac glycosides, nondepolarizing neuromuscular blocking agents, preanesthetic medications, general anesthetics, calcium preparations, and certain other agents. Compounds in these categories include:

Acebutolol Hydrochloride (Hyperglycemia; dosage adjustment may be required). Products include:
- Sectral Capsules 2520

ACTH (Electrolyte imbalance intensified; hypokalemia).
- No products indexed under this heading.

Alcohol (Increased CNS depressant effects; orthostatic hypotension potentiated).

Alfentanil Hydrochloride (Orthostatic hypotension aggravated; increased CNS depressant effects). Products include:
- Alfenta Injection 1131

Allopurinol (Blood uric acid level may be elevated). Products include:
- Zyloprim Tablets 830

Alprazolam (Increased CNS depressant effects). Products include:
- Xanax Tablets 2367

Amiloride Hydrochloride (Potentiation of antihypertensive effect). Products include:
- Midamor Tablets 1508
- Moduretic Tablets 1510

Amitriptyline Hydrochloride (Decreased antihypertensive and antidepressant effects). Products include:
- Elavil 2269
- Endep Tablets 1927
- Etrafon 2087
- Limbitrol 1933
- Triavil Tablets 1556

Amoxapine (Decreased antihypertensive and antidepressant effects). Products include:
- Asendin Tablets 1196

Amphotericin B (Electrolyte imbalance intensified; hypokalemia). Products include:
- Fungizone Cream, Lotion and Ointment 2261
- Fungizone Intravenous 2262

Aprobarbital (Orthostatic hypotension aggravated; increased CNS depressant effects). Products include:
- Alurate Elixir 1883

Atenolol (Potentiation of antihypertensive effect). Products include:
- Tenoretic Tablets 1105
- Tenormin Tablets and I.V. Injection 1107

Atracurium Besylate (Increased responsiveness to muscle relaxants). Products include:
- Tracrium Injection 817

Benazepril Hydrochloride (Potentiation of antihypertensive effect). Products include:
- Lotensin Tablets 872

Betamethasone Acetate (Electrolyte imbalance intensified; hypokalemia). Products include:
- Celestone Soluspan Suspension 2081

Betamethasone Sodium Phosphate (Electrolyte imbalance intensified; hypokalemia). Products include:
- Celestone Soluspan Suspension 2081

Betaxolol Hydrochloride (Potentiation of antihypertensive effect). Products include:
- Betoptic Sterile Ophthalmic Solution 569
- Betoptic S Sterile Ophthalmic Suspension 570
- Kerlone Tablets 2172

Bumetanide (Potentiation of antihypertensive effect). Products include:
- Bumex 1895

Buprenorphine (Orthostatic hypotension aggravated; increased CNS depressant effects).
- No products indexed under this heading.

Buspirone Hydrochloride (Increased CNS depressant effects). Products include:
- BuSpar 1401

Butabarbital (Orthostatic hypotension aggravated; increased CNS depressant effects). Products include:
- Pyridium Plus 1764

Butalbital (Orthostatic hypotension aggravated; increased CNS depressant effects). Products include:
- Esgic-Plus Tablets 1002
- Esgic Tablets & Capsules 1001
- Fioricet Tablets 2006
- Fiorinal Capsules 2007
- Fiorinal with Codeine Capsules 2008
- Fiorinal Tablets 2007
- Phrenilin 838
- Sedapap Tablets 50 mg/650 mg .. 1360

Calcium Carbonate (Potential for hypercalcemia due to decreased excretion). Products include:
- Alka-Mints Chewable Antacid .... ◘ 620
- Alka-Seltzer Advanced Formula Antacid & Non-Aspirin Pain Reliever .... ◘ 620
- Ascriptin A/D Caplets 1850
- Regular Strength Ascriptin Tablets 1850
- Balmex Baby Powder .... ◘ 590
- Bayer Plus Aspirin Tablets .... ◘ 567
- Biocal 500 mg Tablet Calcium Supplement .... ◘ 625
- Bufferin Analgesic Tablets and Caplets .... ◘ 524
- Caltrate 600 .... ◘ 583
- Caltrate 600 + Iron .... ◘ 583
- Caltrate 600 + Vitamin D .... ◘ 584
- Caltrate, Jr. .... ◘ 583
- Centrum, Jr. (Children's Chewable) + Extra Calcium .... ◘ 585
- Di-Gel Antacid/Anti-Gas .... ◘ 697
- Gerimed Tablets 972
- Marblen .... ◘ 563
- Natalins Rx 1391
- Natalins Tablets 1391
- Nephro-Calci Tablets 1826
- Os-Cal 500 Chewable Tablets .... ◘ 596
- Os-Cal 500 Tablets .... ◘ 597
- Os-Cal 250+D Tablets .... ◘ 597
- Os-Cal 500+D Tablets .... ◘ 597
- Pramet FA 1974
- Pramilet FA 1974
- Rolaids (Calcium Rich/Sodium Free) .... ◘ 744
- Extra Strength Rolaids .... ◘ 744
- Thermotabs .... ◘ 619
- Total Formula-2 (multivitamin/multimineral) 2377
- Tums Liquid Extra .... ◘ 726
- Zenate Tablets 2250

Calcium Chloride (Potential for hypercalcemia due to decreased excretion).
- No products indexed under this heading.

Calcium Citrate (Potential for hypercalcemia due to decreased excretion). Products include:
- Citracal Liquitab 1613
- Total Formula-2 (multivitamin/multimineral) 2377

Calcium Glubionate (Potential for hypercalcemia due to decreased excretion). Products include:
- Neo-Calglucon Syrup 2018

Captopril (Potentiation of antihypertensive effect). Products include:
- Capoten 2255
- Capozide 2258

Carteolol Hydrochloride (Hyperglycemia; dosage adjustment may be required). Products include:
- Cartrol Tablets 507

Chlordiazepoxide (Increased CNS depressant effects). Products include:
- Libritabs Tablets 1930
- Limbitrol 1933
- Menrium Tablets 1934

Chlordiazepoxide Hydrochloride (Increased CNS depressant effects). Products include:
- Librax Capsules 1929
- Librium Capsules 1931
- Librium Injectable 1932

Chlorothiazide (Potentiation of antihypertensive effect). Products include:
- Aldoclor Tablets 1413
- Diupres Tablets 1461
- Diuril Oral 1464

Chlorothiazide Sodium (Potentiation of antihypertensive effect). Products include:
- Diuril Sodium Intravenous 1463

Chlorpromazine (Increased CNS depressant effects). Products include:
- Thorazine 2234

Chlorpropamide (Hyperglycemia; dosage adjustment may be required). Products include:
- Diabinese Tablets 1775

Chlorprothixene (Increased CNS depressant effects). Products include:
- Taractan Tablets 1920

Chlorprothixene Hydrochloride (Increased CNS depressant effects). Products include:
- Taractan 1920

Chlorthalidone (Hyperglycemia; dosage adjustment may be required; potentiation of antihypertensive effects). Products include:
- Combipres Tablets 678
- Tenoretic Tablets 1105
- Thalitone Tablets 687

Cholestyramine (Delayed/decreased absorption of Rauzide). Products include:
- Cholybar 1705
- Questran Light 711
- Questran Powder 710

Clomipramine Hydrochloride (Decreased antihypertensive and antidepressant effects). Products include:
- Anafranil Capsules 650

Clonidine (Potentiation of antihypertensive effect). Products include:
- Catapres-TTS 677

Clonidine Hydrochloride (Potentiation of antihypertensive effect; hyperglycemia; dosage adjustment may be required). Products include:
- Catapres Tablets 676
- Combipres Tablets 678

Clorazepate Dipotassium (Increased CNS depressant effects). Products include:
- Tranxene 556

Codeine (Orthostatic hypotension aggravated; increased CNS depressant effects). Products include:
- Calcidrine Syrup 506

Codeine Phosphate (Orthostatic hypotension aggravated; increased CNS depressant effects). Products include:
- Actifed with Codeine Cough Syrup.. 752
- Cheracol Cough Syrup 1853
- Codimal PH Syrup 846
- Dimetane-DC Cough Syrup 1857
- Empirin with Codeine Phosphate Nos. 2, 3 & 4 764
- Fiorinal with Codeine Capsules 2008
- Isoclor Expectorant 982
- Naldecon CX Adult Liquid .... ◘ 521
- Novahistine DH 1342
- Novahistine Expectorant 1343
- Nucofed Capsules 2219
- Nucofed Expectorant 2219
- Nucofed Pediatric Expectorant 2220
- Nucofed Syrup 2219
- Phenaphen with Codeine Capsules 1865
- Phenaphen-650 with Codeine Tablets 1866
- Phenergan with Codeine 2497
- Phenergan VC with Codeine 2501
- Robitussin A-C Syrup 1875
- Robitussin-DAC Syrup 1875
- Ryna .... ◘ 741
- Soma Compound w/Codeine Tablets 2390
- Triaminic Expectorant w/Codeine .. 1996
- Tussi-Organidin Liquid 2391
- Tylenol with Codeine 1381

Codeine Polistirex (Orthostatic hypotension aggravated; increased CNS depressant effects).
- No products indexed under this heading.

Colestipol Hydrochloride (Delays or decreases absorption of Rauzide). Products include:
- Colestid Granules 2328

Cortisone Acetate (Electrolyte imbalance intensified; hypokalemia). Products include:
- Cortone Acetate Sterile Suspension 1437
- Cortone Acetate Tablets 1439

Deserpidine (Potentiation of antihypertensive effect). Products include:
- Enduronyl 518
- Harmonyl Tablets 528
- Oreticyl 545

Desipramine Hydrochloride (Decreased antihypertensive and antidepressant effects). Products include:
- Norpramin Tablets 1340

Deslanoside (Cardiac arrhythmias; hypokalemia; potential for digitalis toxicity associated with hypokalemia).
- No products indexed under this heading.

Dexamethasone (Electrolyte imbalance intensified; hypokalemia). Products include:
- AK-Trol Ointment & Suspension .... ⊙ 207
- Decadron Elixir 1445
- Decadron Tablets 1447
- Decaspray Topical Aerosol 1459
- Dexacidin .... ⊙ 272
- Maxidex Sterile Ophthalmic Suspension .... ⊙ 223
- Maxitrol Ophthalmic Ointment/Suspension .... ⊙ 223
- TobraDex Ophthalmic Suspension and Ointment .... ⊙ 228

Dexamethasone Acetate (Electrolyte imbalance intensified; hypokalemia). Products include:
- Dalalone D.P. Injectable 999
- Decadron-LA Sterile Suspension 1457

Dexamethasone Sodium Phosphate (Electrolyte imbalance intensified; hypokalemia). Products include:
- AK-Dex .... ⊙ 203
- Decadron Phosphate Respihaler 1454

(◘ Described in PDR For Nonprescription Drugs)

(⊙ Described in PDR For Ophthalmology)

Decadron Phosphate Sterile Ophthalmic Ointment ... 1453
Decadron Phosphate Sterile Ophthalmic Solution ... 1453
Decadron Phosphate Topical Cream ... 1455
Decadron Phosphate Turbinaire ... 1456
Maxidex Sterile Ophthalmic Ointment ... ◉ 222
NeoDecadron Sterile Ophthalmic Ointment ... 1517
NeoDecadron Sterile Ophthalmic Solution ... 1518
NeoDecadron Topical Cream ... 1518

Dezocine (Orthostatic hypotension aggravated; increased CNS depressant effects).

Diazepam (Increased CNS depressant effects). Products include:
Valium Injectable ... 1937
Valium Tablets ... 1939
Valrelease Capsules ... 1923

Diazoxide (Enhanced hyperglycemic, hyperuricemic, and antihypertensive effects). Products include:
Hyperstat I.V. Injection ... 2095
Proglycem ... 649

Diclofenac Sodium (Reduces the diuretic, natriuretic, and antihypertensive effect). Products include:
Voltaren Ophthalmic Sterile Ophthalmic Solution ... ◉ 268
Voltaren Tablets ... 1042

Dicumarol (Decreased anticoagulant effect). Products include:
Dicumarol Tablets ... 516

Digitoxin (Potential for digitalis toxicity associated with hypokalemia). Products include:
Crystodigin Tablets ... 1253

Digoxin (Potential for digitalis toxicity associated with hypokalemia). Products include:
Lanoxicaps ... 772
Lanoxin Elixir Pediatric ... 775
Lanoxin Injection ... 778
Lanoxin Injection Pediatric ... 781
Lanoxin Tablets ... 783

Dobutamine Hydrochloride (Effect of direct-acting sympathomimetics prolonged). Products include:
Dobutrex Solution Vials ... 1259

Dopamine Hydrochloride (Effect of direct-acting sympathomimetics prolonged). Products include:
Intropin Injection ... 930

Doxazosin Mesylate (Potentiation of antihypertensive effect). Products include:
Cardura Tablets ... 1941

Doxepin Hydrochloride (Decreased antihypertensive and antidepressant effects). Products include:
Sinequan ... 1960

Droperidol (Increased CNS depressant effects). Products include:
Inapsine Injection ... 1140
Innovar Injection ... 1141

Enalapril Maleate (Potentiation of antihypertensive effect). Products include:
Vaseretic Tablets ... 1559
Vasotec Tablets ... 1564

Enalaprilat (Potentiation of antihypertensive effect). Products include:
Vasotec I.V. ... 1562

Enflurane (Increased CNS depressant effects). Products include:
Ethrane ... 599

Ephedrine Hydrochloride (Effect of indirect-acting sympathomimetics inhibited). Products include:
Amesec ... ⊞ 682
Primatene Tablets-M Formula ... 2421
Primatene Tablets-P Formula ... 2421
Primatene Tablets-Regular Formula ... 2421
Quadrinal Tablets ... 1183
Quelidrine Syrup ... 556
Tedral SA ... 1765

Ephedrine Sulfate (Effect of indirect-acting sympathomimetics inhibited). Products include:
Bronkaid Tablets ... ⊞ 757
Bronkolixir ... ⊞ 761
Bronkotabs Tablets ... ⊞ 762
Marax Tablets & DF Syrup ... 1954
Pazo Hemorrhoid Ointment & Suppositories ... 752
Vicks Vatronol Nose Drops ... ⊞ 666

Ephedrine Tannate (Effect of indirect-acting sympathomimetics inhibited). Products include:
Rynatuss ... 2388

Epinephrine (Effect of direct-acting sympathomimetics prolonged). Products include:
Ana-Kit Anaphylaxis Emergency Treatment Kit ... 1100
Bronkaid Mist ... ⊞ 757
EpiPen ... 843
Marcaine Hydrochloride 0.5% with Epinephrine 1:200,000 (as bitartrate) ... 958
Marcaine Hydrochloride with Epinephrine 1:200,000 ... 2055
Primatene Mist ... 2420
Sus-Phrine Injection ... 1006
Xylocaine with Epinephrine Injections ... 637

Epinephrine Bitartrate (Effect of direct-acting sympathomimetics prolonged). Products include:
AsthmaHaler Mist Epinephrine Bitartrate Bronchodilator ... ⊞ 616
Bronkaid Mist Suspension ... ⊞ 757
Primatene Mist Suspension ... 2421

Epinephrine Hydrochloride (Effect of direct-acting sympathomimetics prolonged). Products include:
Adrenalin Chloride Solution 1:100 & 1:1,000 ... 1689
Epifrin ... ◉ 244
Glaucon ... ◉ 218

Esmolol Hydrochloride (Potentiation of antihypertensive effect). Products include:
Brevibloc Injection ... 942

Estazolam (Orthostatic hypotension aggravated; increased CNS depressant effects). Products include:
ProSom Tablets ... 554

Ethacrynic Acid (Potentiation of antihypertensive effect). Products include:
Edecrin Tablets ... 1468

Ethchlorvynol (Increased CNS depressant effects). Products include:
Placidyl Capsules ... 553

Ethinamate (Increased CNS depressant effects).
No products indexed under this heading.

Etodolac (Reduces the diuretic, natriuretic, and antihypertensive effect). Products include:
Lodine Capsules ... 2468

Felodipine (Potentiation of antihypertensive effect). Products include:
Plendil Extended-Release Tablets ... 1526

Fenoprofen Calcium (Reduces the diuretic, natriuretic, and antihypertensive effect). Products include:
Nalfon Pulvules & Tablets ... 919

Fentanyl (Orthostatic hypotension aggravated; increased CNS depressant effects). Products include:
Duragesic Transdermal System ... 1133

Fentanyl Citrate (Increased CNS depressant effects). Products include:
Innovar Injection ... 1141
Sublimaze Injection ... 1146

Fluphenazine Decanoate (Increased CNS depressant effects). Products include:
Prolixin Decanoate ... 1795

Fluphenazine Enanthate (Increased CNS depressant effects). Products include:
Prolixin Enanthate ... 1796

Fluphenazine Hydrochloride (Increased CNS depressant effects). Products include:
Prolixin Elixir ... 1793
Prolixin Injection ... 1791
Prolixin Oral Concentrate ... 1792
Prolixin Tablets ... 1793

Flurazepam Hydrochloride (Increased CNS depressant effects). Products include:
Dalmane Capsules ... 1927

Flurbiprofen (Reduces the diuretic, natriuretic, and antihypertensive effect). Products include:
Ansaid Tablets ... 2319

Fosinopril Sodium (Potentiation of antihypertensive effect). Products include:
Monopril Tablets ... 1406

Furazolidone (Excessive excitation, hypertension, sympathetic response; increased hypotensive effect). Products include:
Furoxone ... 1855

Furosemide (Potentiation of antihypertensive effect). Products include:
Lasix ... 1093

Glipizide (Hyperglycemia; dosage adjustment may be required). Products include:
Glucotrol ... 1952

Glutethimide (Increased CNS depressant effects).
No products indexed under this heading.

Glyburide (Hyperglycemia; dosage adjustment may be required). Products include:
DiaBeta ... 1091
Micronase Tablets ... 2350

Guanabenz Acetate (Potentiation of antihypertensive effect). Products include:
Wytensin Tablets ... 2542

Guanethidine Monosulfate (Potentiation of antihypertensive effect). Products include:
Esimil Tablets ... 864
Ismelin Tablets ... 869

Haloperidol (Increased CNS depressant effects). Products include:
Haldol Injection, Tablets and Concentrate ... 1373

Haloperidol Decanoate (Increased CNS depressant effects). Products include:
Haldol Decanoate ... 1375

Hydralazine Hydrochloride (Hyperglycemia; dosage adjustment may be required). Products include:
Apresazide Capsules ... 854
Apresoline Hydrochloride Parenteral (Ampuls) ... 856
Apresoline Hydrochloride Tablets ... 855
Apresoline-Esidrix Tablets ... 857
Ser-Ap-Es Tablets ... 881
Serpasil-Apresoline Tablets ... 884

Hydrochlorothiazide (Potentiation of antihypertensive effect). Products include:
Aldactazide ... 2150
Aldoril Tablets ... 1418
Apresazide Capsules ... 854
Apresoline-Esidrix Tablets ... 857
Capozide ... 2258
Dyazide Capsules ... 2208
Esidrix Tablets ... 863
Esimil Tablets ... 864
HydroDIURIL Tablets ... 1484
Hydropres Tablets ... 1485
Inderide Tablets ... 2463
Inderide LA Long Acting Capsules ... 2465
Lopressor HCT Tablets ... 1034
Maxzide ... 1215
Moduretic Tablets ... 1510
Normozide Tablets ... 2112
Oretic Tablets ... 544
Oreticyl ... 545
Prinzide Tablets ... 1540
Ser-Ap-Es Tablets ... 881
Serpasil-Esidrix Tablets ... 886
Timolide Tablets ... 1547
Trandate HCT Tablets ... 579
Vaseretic Tablets ... 1559
Zestoretic ... 2274

Hydrocodone Bitartrate (Increased CNS depressant effects). Products include:
Anexsia 5/500 Tablets ... 2196
Anexsia 7.5/650 Tablets ... 2197
Azdōne Tablets ... 844
Codiclear DH Syrup ... 845
Codimal DH Syrup ... 846
Damason-P ... 1356
Hycodan Syrup, Tablets ... 927
Hycomine Compound Tablets ... 929
Hycomine Syrup ... 927
Hycotuss Expectorant Syrup ... 930
Hydrocet Capsules ... 835
Lortab ASA Tablets ... 2414
Lortab ... 2412
Ru-Tuss with Hydrocodone ... 694
Triaminic Expectorant DH ... 1995
Vicodin Tablets ... 1187
Vicodin ES Tablets ... 1189
Zydone Capsules ... 941

Hydrocodone Polistirex (Increased CNS depressant effects). Products include:
Tussionex Extended-Release Suspension ... 988

Hydrocortisone (Electrolyte imbalance intensified; hypokalemia). Products include:
AK-Spore H.C. ... ◉ 206
Bactine Hydrocortisone Anti-Itch Cream ... ⊞ 625
CaldeCORT Anti-Itch Hydrocortisone Spray ... ⊞ 560
Carmol HC Cream 1% ... 2296
Cortaid Spray ... ⊞ 735
Cortenema ... 2244
Cortisporin Ointment ... 758
Cortisporin Ophthalmic Ointment Sterile ... 758
Cortisporin Ophthalmic Suspension Sterile ... 759
Cortisporin Otic Solution Sterile ... 760
Cortisporin Otic Suspension Sterile ... 760
Cortizone-5 Creme & Ointment ... ⊞ 732
Dermolate Anti-Itch Cream ... ⊞ 697
Eldecort Cream 1.0% ... 1113
Eldecort Cream 1.0% and 2.5% ... 1113
Fungoid HC Creme ... 1770
Hydrocortone Tablets ... 1482
Hytone ... 909
LazerSporin-C Solution ... 1770
Massengill Medicated Soft Cloth Towelettes ... 2192
Nutracort Cream & Lotion ... 1684
PediOtic Suspension Sterile ... 797
Synacort Creams 1%, 2.5% ... 2296
Vanoxide-HC Acne Lotion ... 911
Vioform-Hydrocortisone Cream and Mild Cream ... 889
Vioform-Hydrocortisone Ointment ... 889
VōSoL HC Otic Solution ... 2392
Vytone Cream 1% ... 911

Hydrocortisone Acetate (Electrolyte imbalance intensified; hypokalemia). Products include:
Analpram-HC Rectal Cream 1% and 2.5% ... 970
Anusol-HC Cream ... 1690
Anusol-HC Suppositories ... 1691
Caldecort ... ⊞ 560
Carmol HC Cream 1% ... 2296
Chloromycetin Hydrocortisone Ophthalmic ... 1694
Coly-Mycin S Otic w/Neomycin & Hydrocortisone ... 1708
Cortaid ... ⊞ 735
Cortef Feminine Itch Cream ... ⊞ 735
Corticaine ... ⊞ 682
Cortifoam ... 1827
Cortisporin Cream ... 757
Epifoam ... 1828
Gynecort 5 Creme ... ⊞ 556
Hydrocortone Acetate Sterile Suspension ... 1479
Lanacort 5 Creme and Ointment ... ⊞ 557
Mantadil Cream ... 789
Ophthocort ... ◉ 301
Orabase HCA Oral Paste ... 890

(⊞ Described in PDR For Nonprescription Drugs) (◉ Described in PDR For Ophthalmology)

Pramosone Cream, Lotion & Ointment 971
ProctoCream-HC 1834
Proctofoam-HC 1835

Hydrocortisone Sodium Phosphate (Electrolyte imbalance intensified; hypokalemia). Products include:
Hydrocortone Phosphate Injection, Sterile 1481

Hydrocortisone Sodium Succinate (Electrolyte imbalance intensified; hypokalemia). Products include:
Solu-Cortef Sterile Powder 2361

Hydroflumethiazide (Potentiation of antihypertensive effect). Products include:
Diucardin Tablets 2450
Saluron 718
Salutensin/Salutensin-Demi 719

Hydroxyzine Hydrochloride (Increased CNS depressant effects). Products include:
Atarax Tablets & Syrup 1941
Marax Tablets & DF Syrup 1954
Vistaril Intramuscular Solution 1970

Ibuprofen (Reduces the diuretic, natriuretic, and antihypertensive effect). Products include:
Advil Cold & Sinus Caplets (formerly CoAdvil) 2416
Advil Ibuprofen Tablets and Caplets 2416
Children's Advil Suspension 2426
CoAdvil .... ▣ 748
Dristan Sinus Caplets 2419
Haltran Tablets .... ▣ 668
Ibuprofen .... ▣ 631
Medipren ibuprofen Caplets and Tablets 1362
Midol 200 Cramp Relief Formula .. ▣ 570
Motrin Tablets 2351
Motrin IB Caplets and Tablets .... ▣ 736
Nuprin Ibuprofen/Analgesic Tablets & Caplets 752
PediaProfen Suspension 1363
Rufen Tablets 691
Trendar Ibuprofen Tablets .... ▣ 756

Imipramine Hydrochloride (Decreased antihypertensive and antidepressant effects). Products include:
Tofranil Ampuls 1038
Tofranil Tablets 1039

Imipramine Pamoate (Decreased antihypertensive and antidepressant effects). Products include:
Tofranil-PM Capsules 1041

Indapamide (Potentiation of antihypertensive effect). Products include:
Lozol Tablets 1843

Indomethacin (Reduces the diuretic, natriuretic, and antihypertensive effect). Products include:
Indocin 1487

Indomethacin Sodium Trihydrate (Reduces the diuretic, natriuretic, and antihypertensive effect). Products include:
Indocin I.V. 1490

Insulin, Human (Hyperglycemia; dosage adjustment).
No products indexed under this heading.

Insulin, Human Isophane Suspension (Hyperglycemia; dosage adjustment may be required). Products include:
Humulin N, 100 Units 1270

Insulin, Human NPH (Hyperglycemia; dosage adjustment may be required). Products include:
Insulatard NPH Human 1627
Novolin N 1627
Novolin N PenFill Cartridges 1628
Novolin N Prefilled 1628

Insulin, Human Regular (Hyperglycemia; dosage adjustment may be required). Products include:
Humulin BR, 100 Units 1268
Humulin R, 100 Units 1272
Novolin R 1627
Novolin R PenFill Cartridges 1628
Novolin R Prefilled 1629
Velosulin Human 1628

Insulin, Human, Zinc Suspension (Hyperglycemia; dosage adjustment may be required). Products include:
Humulin L, 100 Units 1268
Humulin U, 100 Units 1272
Novolin L 1627

Insulin, NPH (Hyperglycemia; dosage adjustment may be required). Products include:
NPH, 40 & 100 Units 1273
Beef NPH, 100 Units 1274
Pork NPH, 100 Units 1275
Insulatard NPH 1626
NPH Insulin 1626
NPH Purified Pork Isophane Insulin 1626

Insulin, Regular (Hyperglycemia; dosage adjustment may be required). Products include:
Regular, 40 & 100 Units 1273
Beef Regular, 100 Units 1275
Pork Regular, 100 Units 1275
Pork Regular (Concentrated), 500 Units 1276
Regular Insulin 1625
Regular Purified Pork Insulin 1626
Velosulin 1627

Insulin, Zinc Crystals (Hyperglycemia; dosage adjustment may be required). Products include:
NPH, 40 & 100 Units 1273

Insulin, Zinc Suspension (Hyperglycemia; dosage adjustment may be required). Products include:
Lente, 40 & 100 Units 1272
Protamine, Zinc, 40 & 100 Units 1273
Lente Iletin I 1272
Beef Lente, 100 Units 1274
Beef Protamine Zinc, 100 Units 1274
Pork Lente, 100 Units 1275
Pork, Protamine, Zinc, 100 Units 1275
Lente Insulin 1626
Lente Purified Pork Insulin 1626
Semilente Insulin 1625
Ultralente Insulin 1626

Isocarboxazid (Excessive excitation, hypertension, sympathetic response; increased hypotensive effect). Products include:
Marplan Tablets 1906

Isoflurane (Increased CNS depressant effects). Products include:
Forane 600

Isoproterenol Hydrochloride (Effect of direct-acting sympathomimetics prolonged). Products include:
Isuprel Hydrochloride Injection 1:5000 2050
Isuprel Hydrochloride Mistometer .. 2051
Isuprel Hydrochloride Solution 1:200 & 1:100 2052
Norisodrine Aerotrol 540

Isradipine (Potentiation of antihypertensive effect). Products include:
DynaCirc Capsules 2004

Ketamine Hydrochloride (Orthostatic hypotension aggravated; increased CNS depressant effects). Products include:
Ketalar 1726

Ketoprofen (Reduces the diuretic, natriuretic, and antihypertensive effect). Products include:
Orudis Capsules 2488

Ketorolac Tromethamine (Reduces the diuretic, natriuretic, and antihypertensive effect). Products include:
Toradol IM Injection 2302

Labetalol Hydrochloride (Potentiation of antihypertensive effect). Products include:
Normodyne Injection 2108
Normodyne Tablets 2110
Normozide Tablets 2112
Trandate HCT Tablets 579
Trandate Injection 577
Trandate Tablets 579

Levodopa (Effects inhibited). Products include:
Larodopa Tablets 1905
Sinemet Tablets 952
Sinemet CR Tablets 953

Levorphanol Tartrate (Increased CNS depressant effects). Products include:
Levo-Dromoran 1906

Lisinopril (Potentiation of antihypertensive effect). Products include:
Prinivil Tablets 1538
Prinzide Tablets 1540
Zestoretic 2274
Zestril Tablets 2277

Lithium Carbonate (Lithium toxicity). Products include:
Eskalith 2214
Lithane Tablets 1596
Lithium Carbonate Capsules & Tablets 1984
Lithobid Tablets 870

Lithium Citrate (Lithium toxicity). Products include:
Cibalith-S 870

Lorazepam (Increased CNS depressant effects). Products include:
Ativan Injection 2432
Ativan Tablets 2434

Loxapine Hydrochloride (Increased CNS depressant effects). Products include:
Loxitane 1213

Loxapine Succinate (Orthostatic hypotension aggravated; increased CNS depressant effects). Products include:
Loxitane Capsules 1213

Maprotiline Hydrochloride (Decreased antihypertensive and antidepressant effects). Products include:
Ludiomil Tablets 874

Mecamylamine Hydrochloride (Potentiation of antihypertensive effect). Products include:
Inversine Tablets 1492

Meclofenamate Sodium (Reduces the diuretic, natriuretic, and antihypertensive effect). Products include:
Meclomen Capsules 1739

Mefenamic Acid (Reduces the diuretic, natriuretic, and antihypertensive effect). Products include:
Ponstel 1758

Meperidine Hydrochloride (Orthostatic hypotension aggravated; increased CNS depressant effects). Products include:
Demerol 2047
Mepergan Injection 2479

Mephobarbital (Increased CNS depressant effects). Products include:
Mebaral Tablets 2061

Meprobamate (Increased CNS depressant effects). Products include:
Deprol Tablets 2382
Equagesic Tablets 2451
Miltown Tablets 2386
PMB 200 and PMB 400 2504

Mesoridazine (Increased CNS depressant effects). Products include:
Serentil 686

Metaraminol Bitartrate (Effect of indirect-acting sympathomimetics inhibited). Products include:
Aramine Injection 1424

Methadone Hydrochloride (Orthostatic hypotension aggravated; increased CNS depressant effects). Products include:
Dolophine Hydrochloride Ampoules & Vials 1260
Dolophine Hydrochloride Tablets .. 1261
Methadone Hydrochloride Diskets .. 1284
Methadone Hydrochloride Oral Solution & Tablets 1987

Methenamine (Decreased effectiveness of methenamine). Products include:
Urised Tablets 2396

Methenamine Hippurate (Decreased effectiveness of methenamine). Products include:
Hiprex Tablets 1333
Urex Tablets 1321

Methenamine Mandelate (Decreased effectiveness of methenamine). Products include:
Mandelamine 1738
Uroqid-Acid 661

Methohexital Sodium (Increased CNS depressant effects). Products include:
Brevital Sodium Vials 1248

Methoxamine Hydrochloride (Effect of direct-acting sympathomimetics prolonged). Products include:
Vasoxyl Injection 819

Methoxyflurane (Increased CNS depressant effects).
No products indexed under this heading.

Methyclothiazide (Potentiation of antihypertensive effect). Products include:
Enduron Tablets 517
Enduronyl 518

Methyldopa (Potentiation of antihypertensive effect). Products include:
Aldoclor Tablets 1413
Aldomet Oral 1415
Aldoril Tablets 1418

Methyldopate Hydrochloride (Potentiation of antihypertensive effect). Products include:
Aldomet Ester HCl Injection 1417

Methylprednisolone (Electrolyte imbalance intensified; hypokalemia). Products include:
Medrol 2348

Methylprednisolone Acetate (Electrolyte imbalance intensified; hypokalemia). Products include:
Depo-Medrol Sterile Aqueous Suspension 2334

Methylprednisolone Sodium Succinate (Electrolyte imbalance intensified; hypokalemia). Products include:
Solu-Medrol Sterile Powder 2363

Metocurine Iodide (Increased responsiveness to muscle relaxants). Products include:
Metubine Iodide Vials 1285

Metolazone (Potentiation of antihypertensive effect). Products include:
Diulo 2129
Mykrox ½ mg Tablets 984
Zaroxolyn Tablets 989

Metoprolol Tartrate (Potentiation of antihypertensive effect). Products include:
Lopressor Ampuls 1032
Lopressor HCT Tablets 1034
Lopressor Tablets 1032

Metyrosine (Potentiation of antihypertensive effect). Products include:
Demser Capsules 1460

Midazolam Hydrochloride (Increased CNS depressant effects). Products include:
Versed Injection 1924

Minoxidil (Potentiation of antihypertensive effect). Products include:
Loniten Tablets 2346
Rogaine Topical Solution 2357

Molindone Hydrochloride (Increased CNS depressant effects). Products include:
Moban Tablets & Concentrate 932

Morphine Sulfate (Orthostatic hypotension aggravated; increased CNS depressant effects). Products include:
Astramorph/PF Injection, USP (Preservative-Free) ... 618
Duramorph ... 960
Infumorph 200 and Infumorph 500 Sterile Solutions ... 962
MS Contin Tablets ... 1814
MSIR ... 1817
Oramorph SR (Morphine Sulfate Sustained Release Tablets) ... 1988
Roxanol ... 1991

Nadolol (Potentiation of antihypertensive effect). Products include:
Corgard Tablets ... 701
Corzide Tablets ... 702

Naproxen (Reduces the diuretic, natriuretic, and antihypertensive effect). Products include:
Naprosyn ... 2297

Naproxen Sodium (Reduces the diuretic, natriuretic, and antihypertensive effect). Products include:
Anaprox and Anaprox DS Tablets ... 2288

Nicardipine Hydrochloride (Hyperglycemia; dosage adjustment may be required). Products include:
Cardene Capsules ... 2290

Nitroglycerin (Potentiation of antihypertensive effect). Products include:
Deponit NTG Transdermal Delivery System ... 2143
Minitran Transdermal Delivery System ... 1312
Nitro-Bid Ointment ... 1339
Nitro-Bid Capsules ... 1338
Nitrodisc ... 2176
Nitro-Dur (nitroglycerin) Transdermal Infusion System ... 1164
Nitrogard Tablets ... 1004
Nitrolingual Spray ... 1846
Nitrostat Tablets ... 1743
Transderm-Nitro Transdermal Therapeutic System ... 2283

Norepinephrine Bitartrate (Effect of direct-acting sympathomimetics prolonged). Products include:
Levophed Bitartrate Injection ... 2054

Nortriptyline Hydrochloride (Decreased antihypertensive and antidepressant effects). Products include:
Pamelor ... 2019

Opium Alkaloids (Increased CNS depressant effects). Products include:
B & O No. 15A & No. 16A Supprettes ... 2395
Pantopon Injectable ... 1911

Oxazepam (Increased CNS depressant effects). Products include:
Serax Capsules ... 2522
Serax Tablets ... 2522

Oxycodone Hydrochloride (Orthostatic hypotension aggravated; increased CNS depressant effects). Products include:
Percocet Tablets ... 950
Percodan ... 951
Roxicodone Tablets, Oral Solution & Intensol (Oxycodone) ... 1992
Tylox Capsules ... 1382

Pancuronium Bromide Injection (Increased responsiveness to muscle relaxants).
No products indexed under this heading.

Penbutolol Sulfate (Hyperglycemia; dosage adjustment may be required). Products include:
Levatol ... 1832

Pentobarbital Sodium (Orthostatic hypotension aggravated; increased CNS depressant effects). Products include:
Nembutal Sodium Capsules ... 534
Nembutal Sodium Solution ... 536
Nembutal Sodium Suppositories ... 538

Perphenazine (Increased CNS depressant effects). Products include:
Etrafon ... 2087
Triavil Tablets ... 1556
Trilafon ... 2123

Phenelzine Sulfate (Excessive excitation, hypertension, sympathetic response; increased hypotensive effect). Products include:
Nardil ... 1742

Phenobarbital (Orthostatic hypotension aggravated; increased CNS depressant effects). Products include:
Arco-Lase Plus Tablets ... 607
Bellergal-S Tablets ... 1998
Bronkolixir ... ■ 761
Bronkotabs Tablets ... ■ 762
Donnatal ... 1858
Donnatal Extentabs ... 1859
Donnatal Tablets ... 1858
Donnazyme Tablets ... 1860
Kinesed Tablets ... 2272
Phenobarbital Elixir and Tablets ... 1293
Primatene Tablets-P Formula ... 2421
Quadrinal Tablets ... 1183
Tedral SA ... 1765

Phenoxybenzamine Hydrochloride (Potentiation of antihypertensive effect). Products include:
Dibenzyline Capsules ... 2207

Phentolamine Mesylate (Potentiation of antihypertensive effect). Products include:
Regitine ... 878

Phenylbutazone (Reduces the diuretic, natriuretic, and antihypertensive effect). Products include:
Butazolidin Capsules & Tablets ... 1027

Phenylephrine Bitartrate (Effect of indirect-acting sympathomimetics inhibited).
No products indexed under this heading.

Phenylephrine Hydrochloride (Effect of indirect-acting sympathomimetics inhibited). Products include:
AK-Dilate Solution 2.5% and 10% ... ◉ 203
Atrohist Sprinkle Capsules ... 558
Cerose-DM ... 2443
Codimal ... 846
Comhist LA Capsules ... 1618
Congespirin For Children Aspirin Free Chewable Cold Tablets ... 748
Cyclomydril ... ◉ 216
Deconsal Sprinkle Capsules ... 559
Dimetane Decongestant ... ■ 673
Dristan Decongestant/Antihistamine/ Analgesic Coated Caplets ... ■ 749
Dristan Cold Nasal Decongestant/ Antihistamine/ Analgesic Coated Tablets ... 2419
Dristan Advanced Formula Decongestant/Antihistamine/ Analgesic Tablets ... ■ 749
Dristan Nasal Spray, Menthol ... 2419
Dristan Nasal Spray, Regular and Regular with Metered Pump ... 2419
Entex Capsules ... 1623
Entex Liquid ... 1623
Sinus Excedrin Analgesic, Decongestant Tablets & Caplets ... 750
Extendryl ... 994
4-Way Fast Acting Nasal Spray - Original Formula (regular & mentholated) & Metered Spray Pump (regular) ... 751
Hycomine Compound Tablets ... 929
Murocoll-2 Sterile Ophthalmic Solution ... ◉ 261
Mydfrin 2.5% ... ◉ 224
Naldecon Syrup, Tablets, Pediatric Drops and Pediatric Syrup ... 709
Neo-Synephrine Hydrochloride 1% Carpuject ... 2063
Neo-Synephrine Hydrochloride 1% Injection ... 2063
Neo-Synephrine Hydrochloride (Ophthalmic) ... 2064
Neo-Synephrine ... ■ 759
Nōstril Nasal Decongestant ... ■ 520
Novahistine Elixir ... ■ 596
Phenergan VC ... 2500
Phenergan VC with Codeine ... 2501
Prefrin Liquifilm Vasoconstrictor and Lubricant Eye Drops ... ◉ 254
Prefrin-A ... ◉ 255
Quelidrine Syrup ... 556
Relief Vasoconstrictor and Lubricant Eye Drops ... ◉ 256
Robitussin Night Relief ... ■ 677
Ru-Tuss with Hydrocodone ... 694
Ru-Tuss Tablets ... 693
Vasosulf ... ◉ 279
Vicks Sinex ... ■ 665
Zincfrin ... ◉ 230

Phenylephrine Tannate (Effect of indirect-acting sympathomimetics inhibited). Products include:
Rynatan ... 2387
Rynatuss ... 2388

Phenylpropanolamine Hydrochloride (Effect of indirect-acting sympathomimetics inhibited). Products include:
A.R.M. Allergy Relief Medicine Caplets ... ■ 615
Acutrim ... ■ 548
Allerest ... ■ 559
BC Cold Powder ... ■ 517
Cheracol Plus Head Cold/Cough Formula ... ■ 667
Codimal Expectorant ... 846
Comtrex Multi-Symptom Cold Reliever Tablets/Caplets/Liqui-Gels/Liquid ... 745
Contac Continuous Action Decongestant/Antihistamine Capsules ■ 710
Contac Maximum Strength Continuous Action Decongestant/ Antihistamine Caplets ... ■ 709
Contac Severe Cold and Flu Formula Caplets ... ■ 711
Coricidin 'D' Decongestant Tablets ... ■ 695
Coricidin Demilets Tablets for Children ... ■ 696
Demazin Nasal Decongestant/ Antihistamine Repetabs Tablets & Syrup ... ■ 697
Dexatrim ... ■ 733
Dimetane-DC Cough Syrup ... 1857
Dimetapp Elixir ... ■ 673
Dimetapp DM Elixir ... ■ 674
Dimetapp Extentabs ... ■ 674
Dimetapp Plus Caplets ... ■ 675
Dimetapp Tablets ... ■ 675
Entex Capsules ... 1623
Entex LA Tablets ... 1623
Entex Liquid ... 1623
4-Way Cold Tablets ... 750
Hycomine Syrup ... 927
Naldecon CX Adult Liquid ... ■ 521
Naldecon DX Adult Liquid ... ■ 521
Naldecon DX Children's Syrup ... ■ 522
Naldecon DX Pediatric Drops ... ■ 522
Naldecon EX Children's Syrup ... ■ 522
Naldecon EX Pediatric Drops ... ■ 523
Naldecon Syrup, Tablets, Pediatric Drops and Pediatric Syrup ... 709
Nolamine Tablets ... 838
Nolex LA Tablets ... 838
Ornade Spansule Capsules ... 2221
Orthoxicol Cough Syrup ... ■ 668
Propagest ... 839
Pyrroxate Capsules ... ■ 669
Robitussin-CF ... ■ 676
Ru-Tuss II Capsules ... 693
Ru-Tuss with Hydrocodone ... 694
Ru-Tuss Tablets ... 693
Sine-Off Sinus Medicine Tablets-Aspirin Formula ... ■ 722
Sinulin ... 840
St. Joseph Cold Tablets for Children ... ■ 704
Tavist-D Tablets ... 2035
Triaminic Allergy Tablets ... ■ 688
Triaminic Chewables ... ■ 688
Triaminic Cold Tablets ... ■ 688
Triaminic Expectorant ... ■ 688
Triaminic Expectorant w/Codeine ... 1996
Triaminic Expectorant DH ... 1995
Triaminic Oral Infant Drops ... 1996
Triaminic Syrup ... ■ 689
Triaminic-12 Tablets ... ■ 690
Triaminic-DM Syrup ... ■ 689
Triaminicin Tablets ... ■ 690
Triaminicol Multi-Symptom Cold Tablets ... ■ 691
Triaminicol Multi-Symptom Relief ■ 691
Tuss-Ornade Liquid ... 2242
Tuss-Ornade Spansule Capsules ... 2242
Tylenol Cold Medication, Effervescent Tablets ... 1369

Pindolol (Potentiation of antihypertensive effect). Products include:
Visken Tablets ... 2036

Pirbuterol Acetate (Effect of indirect-acting sympathomimetics inhibited). Products include:
Maxair Inhaler ... 1311

Piroxicam (Reduces the diuretic, natriuretic, and antihypertensive effect). Products include:
Feldene Capsules ... 1777

Polythiazide (Potentiation of antihypertensive effect). Products include:
Minizide Capsules ... 1779
Renese Tablets ... 1785
Renese-R Tablets ... 1786

Prazepam (Increased CNS depressant effects). Products include:
Centrax ... 1693

Prazosin Hydrochloride (Potentiation of antihypertensive effect). Products include:
Minipress Capsules ... 1778
Minizide Capsules ... 1779

Prednisolone Acetate (Electrolyte imbalance intensified; hypokalemia). Products include:
AK-Cide Sterile Ophthalmic Ointment & Suspension ... ◉ 202
Blephamide Liquifilm Sterile Ophthalmic Suspension ... 586
Blephamide S.O.P. Sterile Ophthalmic Ointment ... 586
Cetapred Ointment ... ◉ 220
⅛% Econopred & 1% Econopred Plus ... ◉ 217
Isopto Cetapred Suspension ... ◉ 220
Metimyd ... ◉ 306
Poly-Pred Liquifilm ... ◉ 250
Pred Forte ... ◉ 252
Pred Mild ... ◉ 254
Pred-G Liquifilm Sterile Ophthalmic Suspension ... ◉ 252
Pred-G S.O.P. Sterile Ophthalmic Ointment ... ◉ 253
Vasocidin Ointment ... ◉ 275

Prednisolone Sodium Phosphate (Electrolyte imbalance intensified; hypokalemia). Products include:
AK-Pred ... ◉ 205
Hydeltrasol Injection, Sterile ... 1476
Inflamase ... ◉ 274
Pediapred Oral Liquid ... 987
Vasocidin Ophthalmic Solution ... ◉ 276

Prednisolone Tebutate (Electrolyte imbalance intensified; hypokalemia). Products include:
Hydeltra-T.B.A. Sterile Suspension 1478

Prednisone (Electrolyte imbalance intensified; hypokalemia). Products include:
Deltasone Tablets ... 2332

Pressor Amines (Decreased arterial responsiveness to pressors).

Probenecid (Dosage adjustments; increased dosage of probenecid). Products include:
Benemid Tablets ... 1426
ColBENEMID Tablets ... 1436
Wycillin Injection and Probenecid Tablets ... 2539

Prochlorperazine (Orthostatic hypotension aggravated; increased CNS depressant effects). Products include:
Compazine ... 2201

Promethazine Hydrochloride (Increased CNS depressant effects). Products include:
Mepergan Injection ... 2479
Phenergan with Codeine ... 2497
Phenergan with Dextromethorphan 2499
Phenergan Injection ... 2493
Phenergan Suppositories ... 2496
Phenergan Syrup ... 2495
Phenergan Tablets ... 2496
Phenergan VC ... 2500

Phenergan VC with Codeine 2501

Propofol (Orthostatic hypotension aggravated; increased CNS depressant effects). Products include:

Diprivan Injection 2267

Propoxyphene Hydrochloride (Orthostatic hypotension aggravated; increased CNS depressant effects). Products include:

Darvon 1256
Wygesic Tablets 2540

Propoxyphene Napsylate (Orthostatic hypotension aggravated; increased CNS depressant effects). Products include:

Darvon-N/Darvocet-N 1254

Propranolol Hydrochloride (Potentiation of antihypertensive effect). Products include:

Inderal 2459
Inderal LA Long Acting Capsules 2461
Inderide Tablets 2463
Inderide LA Long Acting Capsules .. 2465

Protriptyline Hydrochloride (Decreased antihypertensive and antidepressant effects). Products include:

Vivactil Tablets 1567

Pseudoephedrine Hydrochloride (Effect of indirect-acting sympathomimetics inhibited). Products include:

Actifed Capsules .... ▣ 539
Actifed Plus Caplets .... ▣ 539
Actifed Plus Tablets .... ▣ 540
Actifed with Codeine Cough Syrup.. 752
Actifed Syrup .... ▣ 540
Actifed Tablets .... ▣ 540
Actifed 12-Hour Capsules .... ▣ 539
Advil Cold & Sinus Caplets (formerly CoAdvil) 2416
Allerest .... ▣ 559
Anatuss LA Tablets 1359
Benadryl Decongestant Elixir .... ▣ 635
Benadryl Decongestant .... ▣ 635
Benadryl Plus .... ▣ 636
Benadryl Plus Nighttime .... ▣ 637
Benylin Decongestant .... ▣ 638
Brexin L.A. Capsules 2078
Bromfed Capsules (Timed Release) 1615
Bromfed Syrup .... ▣ 628
Bromfed 1615
CoAdvil .... ▣ 748
Allergy-Sinus Comtrex Multi-Symptom Allergy Sinus Formula Tablets & Caplets 746
Cough Formula Comtrex 746
Comtrex Multi-Symptom Cold Reliever Tablets/Caplets/Liqui-Gels/Liquid 745
Day-Night Comtrex 747
Non-Drowsy Comtrex 747
Congess 994
Congestac Caplets .... ▣ 617
Contac Jr. Children's Cold Medicine .... ▣ 712
Contac Nighttime Cold Medicine.... ▣ 713
Contac Sinus Caplets Maximum Strength Non-Drowsy Formula.... ▣ 710
Contac Sinus Tablets Maximum Strength Non-Drowsy Formula.... ▣ 710
Deconamine 663
Deconsal II Tablets 559
Dimacol Caplets .... ▣ 672
Dimetane-DX Cough Syrup 1858
Dorcol Children's Cough Syrup ...... ▣ 685
Dorcol Children's Decongestant Liquid .... ▣ 685
Dorcol Children's Liquid Cold Formula .... ▣ 686
Maximum Strength Dristan Decongestant/Analgesic Coated Caplets .... ▣ 750
No Drowsiness Dristan Cold Nasal Decongestant/Analgesic Coated Caplets 2420
Dristan Sinus Caplets 2419
Sinus Excedrin Analgesic, Decongestant Tablets & Caplets .... ▣ 533
Fedahist Gyrocaps 2145
Fedahist Timecaps 2145
Guaifed 1615
Guaifed Syrup .... ▣ 629
Isoclor Expectorant 982
Isoclor Timesule Capsules .... ▣ 561
Kronofed-A 970
Medi-Flu Caplet, Liquid .... ▣ 640
Novafed A Capsules 1342
Novafed Capsules 1342
Novahistine DH 1342
Novahistine DMX .... ▣ 595
Novahistine Expectorant 1343
Nucofed Capsules 2219
Nucofed Expectorant 2219
Nucofed Pediatric Expectorant 2220
Nucofed Syrup 2219
Ornex Caplets .... ▣ 618
PediaCare Allergy Relief Formula Liquid 1362
PediaCare Cough-Cold Formula Liquid 1362
PediaCare Infants' Oral Decongestant Drops 1362
PediaCare Night Rest Cough-Cold Formula Liquid 1362
PediaCare 6-12 Cough-Cold Formula Chewable Tablets 1362
Robitussin-DAC Syrup 1875
Robitussin-PE .... ▣ 677
Rondec 1975
Rondec-DM 1976
Rondec-TR Tablet 1975
Ru-Tuss DE Tablets 694
Ryna .... ▣ 741
Seldane-D Extended-Release Tablets 1350
Sinarest .... ▣ 562
Sine-Aid Maximum Strength Sinus Headache Caplets 1365
Sine-Aid Maximum Strength Sinus Headache Tablets 1365
Sine-Off Maximum Strength Allergy/Sinus Formula Caplets .... ▣ 721
Sine-Off Maximum Strength No Drowsiness Formula Caplets....... ▣ 722
Singlet Tablets .... ▣ 598
Sinutab Maximum Strength............. ▣ 641
Sinutab Maximum Strength Without Drowsiness Tablets & Caplets .... ▣ 642
Sinutab Regular Strength Without Drowsiness Formula .... ▣ 641
St. Joseph Nighttime Cold Medicine .... ▣ 705
Sudafed Children's Liquid .... ▣ 543
Sudafed Cough Syrup .... ▣ 543
Sudafed Plus Liquid .... ▣ 544
Sudafed Plus Tablets .... ▣ 545
Sudafed Sinus Caplets .... ▣ 545
Sudafed Sinus Tablets .... ▣ 545
Sudafed Tablets, 30 mg .... ▣ 544
Sudafed Tablets, Adult Strength, 60 mg .... ▣ 544
Sudafed 12 Hour Capsules .... ▣ 545
TheraFlu Flu and Cold Medicine .... ▣ 687
Triaminic Nite Light .... ▣ 689
Tylenol Allergy Sinus Medication Caplets and Gelcaps, Maximum Strength 1372
Children's Tylenol Cold Liquid Formula and Chewable Tablets 1368
Tylenol Cold & Flu Hot Medication, Packets 1369
Tylenol Cold & Flu No Drowsiness Hot Medication, Packets 1371
Tylenol Cold Medication Caplets and Tablets 1370
Tylenol Cold Medication No Drowsiness Formula Caplets 1370
Tylenol Cold Night Time Medication Liquid 1371
Tylenol Cough Medication Liquid with Decongestant, Maximum Strength 1372
Tylenol, Maximum Strength, Sinus Medication Gelcaps, Caplets and Tablets 1373
Ursinus Inlay-Tabs .... ▣ 691
Vicks Children's NyQuil .... ▣ 664
Vicks Daycare .... ▣ 660
Vicks Formula 44D Decongestant Cough Medicine .... ▣ 662
Vicks Formula 44M Multi-Symptom Cough Medicine .... ▣ 662
Vicks NyQuil Nighttime Colds Medicine-Original & Cherry Flavor .... ▣ 664
Vicks Pediatric Formula 44 Cough & Congestion Medicine .... ▣ 663
Vicks Pediatric Formula 44m Multi-Symptom Cough & Cold Medicine .... ▣ 663

Pseudoephedrine Sulfate (Effect of indirect-acting sympathomimetics inhibited). Products include:

Afrin Tablets .... ▣ 693
Chlor-Trimeton Decongestant .... ▣ 694
Disophrol Chronotab Sustained-Action Tablets .... ▣ 698
Drixoral Antihistamine/Nasal Decongestant Syrup .... ▣ 698
Drixoral Non-Drowsy Formula .... ▣ 699
Drixoral Plus Extended-Release Tablets .... ▣ 699
Drixoral Sinus .... ▣ 700
Drixoral Sustained-Action Tablets ▣ 698
Sinutab Allergy Formula Sustained Action Tablets .... ▣ 640
Trinalin Repetabs Tablets 1170

Quazepam (Orthostatic hypotension aggravated; increased CNS depressant effects). Products include:

Doral Tablets 2383

Quinidine Gluconate (Cardiac arrhythmias). Products include:

Quinaglute Dura-Tabs Tablets 663

Quinidine Polygalacturonate (Cardiac arrhythmias). Products include:

Cardioquin Tablets 1812

Quinidine Sulfate (Cardiac arrhythmias). Products include:

Quinidex Extentabs 1868

Ramipril (Potentiation of antihypertensive effect). Products include:

Altace Capsules 1086

Rescinnamine (Potentiation of antihypertensive effect).

No products indexed under this heading.

Reserpine (Potentiation of antihypertensive effect). Products include:

Diupres Tablets 1461
Hydromox R Tablets 1209
Hydropres Tablets 1485
Renese-R Tablets 1786
Salutensin/Salutensin-Demi 719
Ser-Ap-Es Tablets 881
Serpasil Tablets 883
Serpasil-Apresoline Tablets 884
Serpasil-Esidrix Tablets 886

Secobarbital Sodium (Orthostatic hypotension aggravated; increased CNS depressant effects). Products include:

Seconal Sodium Pulvules 1296

Selegiline Hydrochloride (Excessive excitation, hypertension, sympathetic response; increased hypotensive effect). Products include:

Eldepryl 2250

Sodium Nitroprusside (Potentiation of antihypertensive effect). Products include:

Nipride I.V. Infusion 1909

Spironolactone (Potentiation of antihypertensive effect). Products include:

Aldactazide 2150
Aldactone 2152

Sufentanil Citrate (Increased CNS depressant effects). Products include:

Sufenta Injection 1147

Sulfinpyrazone (Increased dosage of sulfinpyrazone may be required). Products include:

Anturane 853

Sulindac (Reduces the diuretic, natriuretic, and antihypertensive effect). Products include:

Clinoril Tablets 1433

Temazepam (Increased CNS depressant effects). Products include:

Restoril Capsules 2023

Terazosin Hydrochloride (Potentiation of antihypertensive effect). Products include:

Hytrin Tablets 529

Thiamylal Sodium (Increased CNS depressant effects). Products include:

Surital Ampoules, Steri-Vials............. 1764

Thioridazine Hydrochloride (Increased CNS depressant effects). Products include:

Mellaril 2011

Thiothixene (Increased CNS depressant effects). Products include:

Navane Capsules and Concentrate 1954
Navane Intramuscular 1956

Timolol Maleate (Potentiation of antihypertensive effect). Products include:

Blocadren Tablets 1429
Timolide Tablets 1547
Timoptic in Ocudose 1552
Timoptic Sterile Ophthalmic Solution 1550

Tolazamide (Hyperglycemia; dosage adjustment may be required). Products include:

Tolinase Tablets 2365

Tolbutamide (Hyperglycemia; dosage adjustment may be required). Products include:

Orinase Tablets 2354

Tolmetin Sodium (Reduces the diuretic, natriuretic, and antihypertensive effect). Products include:

Tolectin (200, 400 and 600 mg) .. 1379

Tranylcypromine Sulfate (Excessive excitation, hypertension, sympathetic response; increased hypotensive effect). Products include:

Parnate Tablets 2222

Triamcinolone (Electrolyte imbalance intensified; hypokalemia).

No products indexed under this heading.

Triamcinolone Acetonide (Electrolyte imbalance intensified; hypokalemia). Products include:

Aristocort A 1010
Azmacort Inhaler 1837
Kenalog Cream, Lotion & Ointment 2401
Kenalog-10 Injection 2402
Kenalog-40 Injection 2403
Kenalog in Orabase 604
Kenalog Spray 2401
Mycolog II Cream and Ointment 2407
Mytrex Cream & Ointment 2080
Nasacort Nasal Inhaler 1844

Triamcinolone Diacetate (Electrolyte imbalance intensified; hypokalemia). Products include:

Aristocort Suspension 1008

Triamcinolone Hexacetonide (Electrolyte imbalance intensified; hypokalemia). Products include:

Aristospan Suspension 1011

Triamterene (Potentiation of antihypertensive effect). Products include:

Dyazide Capsules 2208
Dyrenium Capsules 2210
Maxzide 1215

Triazolam (Increased CNS depressant effects). Products include:

Halcion Tablets 2340

Trifluoperazine Hydrochloride (Increased CNS depressant effects). Products include:

Stelazine 2226

Trimethaphan Camsylate (Potentiation of antihypertensive effect). Products include:

Arfonad Ampuls 1887

Trimipramine Maleate (Decreased antihypertensive and antidepressant effects). Products include:

Surmontil Capsules 2524

Vecuronium Bromide (Increased responsiveness to muscle relaxants). Products include:

Norcuron 1642

Warfarin Sodium (Decreased anticoagulant effect). Products include:

Coumadin Injection & Tablets 944
Panwarfin Tablets 547

RECOMBIVAX HB
(Hepatitis B Vaccine) 1544
No interactions described in labeling.

REESE'S PINWORM MEDICINE
(Pyrantel Pamoate) .... ◘ 653
No interactions described in labeling.

REFRESH LUBRICANT OPHTHALMIC SOLUTION
(Polyvinyl Alcohol, Povidone) .... ⊚ 256
No interactions described in labeling.

REFRESH P.M. LUBRICANT OPHTHALMIC OINTMENT
(Mineral Oil, Petrolatum, White) ...... ⊚ 256
No interactions described in labeling.

REGITINE
(Phentolamine Mesylate) 878

Withhold all medications, except those deemed essential, for at least 24 hours prior to Regitine blocking test for pheochromocytoma.

REGLAN INJECTABLE
(Metoclopramide Hydrochloride) 1869
May interact with anticholinergics, narcotic analgesics, central nervous system depressants, hypnotics and sedatives, tranquilizers, cardiac glycosides, insulin, monoamine oxidase inhibitors, and certain other agents. Compounds in these categories include:

Acetaminophen (Accelerated absorption from the small bowel). Products include:
- Acetaminophen Uniserts Suppositories 2374
- Actifed Plus Caplets .... ◘ 539
- Actifed Plus Tablets .... ◘ 540
- Alka-Seltzer Advanced Formula Antacid & Non-Aspirin Pain Reliever .... ◘ 620
- Allerest .... ◘ 559
- Aspirin Free Anacin Maximum Strength Acetaminophen Film Coated Caplets 2417
- Aspirin Free Anacin Maximum Strength Acetaminophen Film Coated Tablets 2417
- Anacin-3 Regular Strength Acetaminophen Film Coated Tablets ◘ 746
- Anexsia 5/500 Tablets 2196
- Anexsia 7.5/650 Tablets 2197
- Benadryl Plus .... ◘ 636
- Benadryl Plus Nighttime .... ◘ 637
- Bufferin AF Nite Time Analgesic/Sleeping Aid Caplets 744
- Allergy-Sinus Comtrex Multi-Symptom Allergy Sinus Formula Tablets & Caplets 746
- Cough Formula Comtrex 746
- Comtrex Multi-Symptom Cold Reliever Tablets/Caplets/Liqui-Gels/Liquid 745
- Day-Night Comtrex 747
- Non-Drowsy Comtrex 747
- Congespirin For Children Aspirin Free Chewable Cold Tablets 748
- Contac Cough & Sore Throat Formula .... ◘ 712
- Contac Jr. Children's Cold Medicine .... ◘ 712
- Contac Nighttime Cold Medicine .... ◘ 713
- Contac Severe Cold and Flu Formula Caplets .... ◘ 711
- Contac Sinus Caplets Maximum Strength Non-Drowsy Formula .... ◘ 710
- Contac Sinus Tablets Maximum Strength Non-Drowsy Formula .... ◘ 710
- Coricidin 'D' Decongestant Tablets .... ◘ 695
- Coricidin Demilets Tablets for Children .... ◘ 696
- Coricidin Tablets .... ◘ 695
- Darvon-N/Darvocet-N 1254
- Datril Extra-Strength Analgesic Tablets 748
- Dimetapp Plus Caplets .... ◘ 675
- Dorcol Children's Fever & Pain Reducer .... ◘ 686
- Dristan Decongestant/Antihistamine/Analgesic Coated Caplets .... ◘ 749
- Dristan Cold Nasal Decongestant/Antihistamine/Analgesic Coated Tablets 2419
- Dristan Advanced Formula Decongestant/Antihistamine/Analgesic Tablets .... ◘ 749
- Maximum Strength Dristan Decongestant/Analgesic Coated Caplets .... ◘ 750
- No Drowsiness Dristan Cold Nasal Decongestant/Analgesic Coated Caplets 2420
- Drixoral Plus Extended-Release Tablets .... ◘ 699
- Drixoral Sinus .... ◘ 700
- Esgic-Plus Tablets 1002
- Esgic Tablets & Capsules 1001
- Aspirin Free Excedrin Analgesic Caplets 748
- Excedrin Extra-Strength Analgesic Tablets & Caplets 749
- Excedrin P.M. Analgesic/Sleeping Aid Tablets, Caplets and Liquid 749
- Sinus Excedrin Analgesic, Decongestant Tablets & Caplets 750
- 4-Way Cold Tablets 750
- Feverall Sprinkle Caps 2374
- Feverall Suppositories 2374
- Fioricet Tablets 2006
- Hycomine Compound Tablets 929
- Hydrocet Capsules 835
- Isocom Capsules 1629
- Liquiprin .... ◘ 618
- Lortab 2412
- Lurline PMS Tablets 972
- Medi-Flu Caplet, Liquid .... ◘ 640
- Maximum Strength Midol Multi-Symptom Menstrual Formula .... ◘ 571
- Maximum Strength Midol PMS Premenstrual Syndrome Formula .... ◘ 570
- Regular Strength Midol Multi-Symptom Menstrual Formula .... ◘ 570
- Midrin Capsules 836
- Ornex Caplets .... ◘ 618
- Children's Panadol Chewable Tablets, Liquid, Infants' Drops .... ◘ 571
- Junior Strength Panadol .... ◘ 571
- Maximum Strength Panadol Tablets and Caplets .... ◘ 572
- Percocet Tablets 950
- Percogesic Analgesic Tablets .... ◘ 660
- Phenaphen with Codeine Capsules 1865
- Phenaphen-650 with Codeine Tablets 1866
- Phrenilin 838
- Prēmsyn PMS Capsules & Caplets ◘ 547
- Pyrroxate Capsules .... ◘ 669
- Robitussin Night Relief .... ◘ 677
- Sedapap Tablets 50 mg/650 mg .. 1360
- Sinarest .... ◘ 562
- Sine-Aid Maximum Strength Sinus Headache Caplets 1365
- Sine-Aid Maximum Strength Sinus Headache Tablets 1365
- Sine-Off Maximum Strength Allergy/Sinus Formula Caplets .... ◘ 721
- Sine-Off Maximum Strength No Drowsiness Formula Caplets .... ◘ 722
- Singlet Tablets .... ◘ 598
- Sinulin 840
- Sinutab Maximum Strength .... ◘ 641
- Sinutab Maximum Strength Without Drowsiness Tablets & Caplets .... ◘ 642
- Sinutab Regular Strength Without Drowsiness Formula .... ◘ 641
- Sominex Pain Relief Formula .... ◘ 723
- St. Joseph Aspirin-Free Fever Reducer for Children Chewable Tablets, Liquid & Infant Drops .... ◘ 704
- St. Joseph Cold Tablets for Children .... ◘ 704
- St. Joseph Nighttime Cold Medicine .... ◘ 705
- Sudafed Sinus Caplets .... ◘ 545
- Sudafed Sinus Tablets .... ◘ 545
- Talacen 2070
- Tempra, Acetaminophen .... ◘ 613
- TheraFlu Flu and Cold Medicine .... ◘ 687
- Triaminicin Tablets .... ◘ 690
- Tylenol acetaminophen Children's Chewable Tablets & Elixir 1366
- Tylenol Allergy Sinus Medication Caplets and Gelcaps, Maximum Strength 1372
- Tylenol with Codeine 1381
- Children's Tylenol Cold Liquid Formula and Chewable Tablets 1368
- Tylenol Cold & Flu Hot Medication, Packets 1369
- Tylenol Cold & Flu No Drowsiness Hot Medication, Packets 1371
- Tylenol Cold Medication Caplets and Tablets 1370
- Tylenol Cold Medication, Effervescent Tablets 1369
- Tylenol Cold Medication No Drowsiness Formula Caplets 1370
- Tylenol Cold Night Time Medication Liquid 1371
- Tylenol Cough Medication Liquid, Maximum Strength 1372
- Tylenol Cough Medication Liquid with Decongestant, Maximum Strength 1372
- Tylenol, Extra Strength, acetaminophen Adult Liquid Pain Reliever .. 1367
- Tylenol, Extra Strength, acetaminophen Gelcaps, Caplets, Tablets 1367
- Tylenol, Infants' Drops 1366
- Tylenol, Junior Strength, acetaminophen Coated Caplets, Grape and Fruit Chewable Tablets 1366
- Tylenol, Maximum Strength, Sinus Medication Gelcaps, Caplets and Tablets 1373
- Tylenol, Regular Strength, acetaminophen Tablets and Caplets 1367
- Tylenol PM, Extra Strength Caplets and Tablets 1368
- Tylox Capsules 1382
- Unisom Dual Relief Nighttime Sleep Aid/Analgesic 1774
- Vanquish Analgesic Caplets .... ◘ 574
- Vicks Daycare .... ◘ 660
- Vicks Formula 44M Multi-Symptom Cough Medicine .... ◘ 662
- Vicks NyQuil Nighttime Colds Medicine-Original & Cherry Flavor .... ◘ 664
- Vicodin Tablets 1187
- Vicodin ES Tablets 1189
- Wygesic Tablets 2540
- Zydone Capsules 941

Alcohol (Accelerated absorption from the small bowel; additive sedative effects).

Alfentanil Hydrochloride (Additive sedative effects; antagonizes gastrointestinal motility effects). Products include:
- Alfenta Injection 1131

Alprazolam (Additive sedative effects). Products include:
- Xanax Tablets 2367

Aprobarbital (Additive sedative effects). Products include:
- Alurate Elixir 1883

Atropine Sulfate (Antagonizes gastrointestinal motility effects). Products include:
- Arco-Lase Plus Tablets 607
- Atropine Sulfate Sterile Ophthalmic Solution and S.O.P. Sterile Ophthalmic Ointment .... ⊚ 239
- Donnagel .... ◘ 675
- Donnagel-PG 1858
- Donnatal 1858
- Donnatal Extentabs 1859
- Donnatal Tablets 1858
- Donnazyme Tablets 1860
- Isopto Atropine .... ⊚ 218
- Lomotil 2174
- Motofen Tablets 836
- Ru-Tuss Tablets 693
- Urised Tablets 2396

Belladonna Alkaloids (Antagonizes gastrointestinal motility effects). Products include:
- Bellergal-S Tablets 1998
- Hyland's Bed Wetting Tablets .... ◘ 728
- Hyland's Teething Tablets .... ◘ 728
- Kinesed Tablets 2272

Benztropine Mesylate (Antagonizes gastrointestinal motility effects). Products include:
- Cogentin 1435

Biperiden (Antagonizes gastrointestinal motility effects). Products include:
- Akineton 1171

Buprenorphine (Additive sedative effects; antagonizes gastrointestinal motility effects).
- No products indexed under this heading.

Buspirone Hydrochloride (Additive sedative effects). Products include:
- BuSpar 1401

Butabarbital (Additive sedative effects). Products include:
- Pyridium Plus 1764

Butalbital (Additive sedative effects). Products include:
- Esgic-Plus Tablets 1002
- Esgic Tablets & Capsules 1001
- Fioricet Tablets 2006
- Fiorinal Capsules 2007
- Fiorinal with Codeine Capsules 2008
- Fiorinal Tablets 2007
- Phrenilin 838
- Sedapap Tablets 50 mg/650 mg .. 1360

Chlordiazepoxide (Additive sedative effects). Products include:
- Libritabs Tablets 1930
- Limbitrol 1933
- Menrium Tablets 1934

Chlordiazepoxide Hydrochloride (Additive sedative effects). Products include:
- Librax Capsules 1929
- Librium Capsules 1931
- Librium Injectable 1932

Chlorpromazine (Additive sedative effects). Products include:
- Thorazine 2234

Chlorprothixene (Additive sedative effects). Products include:
- Taractan Tablets 1920

Chlorprothixene Hydrochloride (Additive sedative effects). Products include:
- Taractan 1920

Clidinium Bromide (Antagonizes gastrointestinal motility effects). Products include:
- Librax Capsules 1929
- Quarzan Capsules 1937

Clorazepate Dipotassium (Additive sedative effects). Products include:
- Tranxene 556

Codeine (Additive sedative effects; antagonizes gastrointestinal motility effects). Products include:
- Calcidrine Syrup 506

Codeine Phosphate (Additive sedative effects; antagonizes gastrointestinal motility effects). Products include:
- Actifed with Codeine Cough Syrup.. 752
- Cheracol Cough Syrup 1853
- Codimal PH Syrup 846
- Dimetane-DC Cough Syrup 1857
- Empirin with Codeine Phosphate Nos. 2, 3 & 4 764
- Fiorinal with Codeine Capsules 2008
- Isoclor Expectorant 982
- Naldecon CX Adult Liquid .... ◘ 521
- Novahistine DH 1342
- Novahistine Expectorant 1343
- Nucofed Capsules 2219
- Nucofed Expectorant 2219
- Nucofed Pediatric Expectorant 2220
- Nucofed Syrup 2219
- Phenaphen with Codeine Capsules 1865
- Phenaphen-650 with Codeine Tablets 1866
- Phenergan with Codeine 2497
- Phenergan VC with Codeine 2501
- Robitussin A-C Syrup 1875
- Robitussin-DAC Syrup 1875
- Ryna .... ◘ 741
- Soma Compound w/Codeine Tablets 2390
- Triaminic Expectorant w/Codeine .. 1996
- Tussi-Organidin Liquid 2391
- Tylenol with Codeine 1381

Codeine Polistirex (Additive sedative effects; antagonizes gastrointestinal motility effects).
No products indexed under this heading.

Deslanoside (Diminished absorption from the stomach).
No products indexed under this heading.

Dezocine (Additive sedative effects; antagonizes gastrointestinal motility effects).

Diazepam (Additive sedative effects). Products include:
Valium Injectable ... 1937
Valium Tablets ... 1939
Valrelease Capsules ... 1923

Dicyclomine Hydrochloride (Antagonizes gastrointestinal motility effects). Products include:
Bentyl ... 1322

Digitoxin (Diminished absorption from the stomach). Products include:
Crystodigin Tablets ... 1253

Digoxin (Diminished absorption from the stomach). Products include:
Lanoxicaps ... 772
Lanoxin Elixir Pediatric ... 775
Lanoxin Injection ... 778
Lanoxin Injection Pediatric ... 781
Lanoxin Tablets ... 783

Droperidol (Additive sedative effects). Products include:
Inapsine Injection ... 1140
Innovar Injection ... 1141

Enflurane (Additive sedative effects). Products include:
Ethrane ... 599

Estazolam (Additive sedative effects; antagonizes gastrointestinal motility effects). Products include:
ProSom Tablets ... 554

Ethchlorvynol (Additive sedative effects). Products include:
Placidyl Capsules ... 553

Ethinamate (Additive sedative effects).
No products indexed under this heading.

Fentanyl (Additive sedative effects; antagonizes gastrointestinal motility effects). Products include:
Duragesic Transdermal System ... 1133

Fentanyl Citrate (Additive sedative effects; antagonizes gastrointestinal motility effects). Products include:
Innovar Injection ... 1141
Sublimaze Injection ... 1146

Fluphenazine Decanoate (Additive sedative effects). Products include:
Prolixin Decanoate ... 1795

Fluphenazine Enanthate (Additive sedative effects). Products include:
Prolixin Enanthate ... 1796

Fluphenazine Hydrochloride (Additive sedative effects). Products include:
Prolixin Elixir ... 1793
Prolixin Injection ... 1791
Prolixin Oral Concentrate ... 1792
Prolixin Tablets ... 1793

Flurazepam Hydrochloride (Additive sedative effects). Products include:
Dalmane Capsules ... 1927

Furazolidone (Release of catecholamines). Products include:
Furoxone ... 1855

Glutethimide (Additive sedative effects).
No products indexed under this heading.

Glycopyrrolate (Antagonizes gastrointestinal motility effects). Products include:
Robinul Forte Tablets ... 1873
Robinul Injectable ... 1873
Robinul Tablets ... 1873

Haloperidol (Additive sedative effects). Products include:
Haldol Injection, Tablets and Concentrate ... 1373

Haloperidol Decanoate (Additive sedative effects). Products include:
Haldol Decanoate ... 1375

Hydrocodone Bitartrate (Additive sedative effects; antagonizes gastrointestinal motility effects). Products include:
Anexsia 5/500 Tablets ... 2196
Anexsia 7.5/650 Tablets ... 2197
Azdone Tablets ... 844
Codiclear DH Syrup ... 845
Codimal DH Syrup ... 846
Damason-P ... 1356
Hycodan Syrup, Tablets ... 927
Hycomine Compound Tablets ... 929
Hycomine Syrup ... 927
Hycotuss Expectorant Syrup ... 930
Hydrocet Capsules ... 835
Lortab ASA Tablets ... 2414
Lortab ... 2412
Ru-Tuss with Hydrocodone ... 694
Triaminic Expectorant DH ... 1995
Vicodin Tablets ... 1187
Vicodin ES Tablets ... 1189
Zydone Capsules ... 941

Hydrocodone Polistirex (Additive sedative effects; antagonizes gastrointestinal motility effects). Products include:
Tussionex Extended-Release Suspension ... 988

Hydroxyzine Hydrochloride (Additive sedative effects). Products include:
Atarax Tablets & Syrup ... 1941
Marax Tablets & DF Syrup ... 1954
Vistaril Intramuscular Solution ... 1970

Hyoscyamine (Antagonizes gastrointestinal motility effects). Products include:
Cystospaz Tablets ... 2395
Urised Tablets ... 2396

Hyoscyamine Sulfate (Antagonizes gastrointestinal motility effects). Products include:
Arco-Lase Plus Tablets ... 607
Cystospaz-M Capsules ... 2395
Donnagel ... 675
Donnagel-PG ... 1858
Donnatal ... 1858
Donnatal Extentabs ... 1859
Donnatal Tablets ... 1858
Donnazyme Tablets ... 1860
Kutrase Capsules ... 2146
Levsin/Levsinex ... 2147
Ru-Tuss Tablets ... 693

Insulin, Human (Potentiation of hypoglycemia).
No products indexed under this heading.

Insulin, Human Isophane Suspension (Potentiation of hypoglycemia). Products include:
Humulin N, 100 Units ... 1270

Insulin, Human NPH (Potentiation of hypoglycemia). Products include:
Insulatard NPH Human ... 1627
Novolin N ... 1627
Novolin N PenFill Cartridges ... 1628
Novolin N Prefilled ... 1628

Insulin, Human Regular (Potentiation of hypoglycemia). Products include:
Humulin BR, 100 Units ... 1268
Humulin R, 100 Units ... 1272
Novolin R ... 1627
Novolin R PenFill Cartridges ... 1628
Novolin R Prefilled ... 1629
Velosulin Human ... 1628

Insulin, Human, Zinc Suspension (Potentiation of hypoglycemia). Products include:
Humulin L, 100 Units ... 1268
Humulin U, 100 Units ... 1272
Novolin L ... 1627

Insulin, NPH (Potentiation of hypoglycemia). Products include:
NPH, 40 & 100 Units ... 1273
Beef NPH, 100 Units ... 1274
Pork NPH, 100 Units ... 1275
Insulatard NPH ... 1626
NPH Insulin ... 1626
NPH Purified Pork Isophane Insulin ... 1626

Insulin, Regular (Potentiation of hypoglycemia). Products include:
Regular, 40 & 100 Units ... 1273
Beef Regular, 100 Units ... 1275
Pork Regular, 100 Units ... 1275
Pork Regular (Concentrated), 500 Units ... 1276
Regular Insulin ... 1625
Regular Purified Pork Insulin ... 1626
Velosulin ... 1627

Insulin, Zinc Crystals (Potentiation of hypoglycemia). Products include:
NPH, 40 & 100 Units ... 1273

Insulin, Zinc Suspension (Potentiation of hypoglycemia). Products include:
Lente, 40 & 100 Units ... 1272
Protamine, Zinc, 40 & 100 Units ... 1273
Lente Iletin I ... 1272
Beef Lente, 100 Units ... 1274
Beef Protamine Zinc, 100 Units ... 1274
Pork Lente, 100 Units ... 1275
Pork, Protamine, Zinc, 100 Units ... 1275
Lente Insulin ... 1626
Lente Purified Pork Insulin ... 1626
Semilente Insulin ... 1625
Ultralente Insulin ... 1626

Ipratropium Bromide (Antagonizes gastrointestinal motility effects). Products include:
Atrovent Inhalation Aerosol ... 675

Isocarboxazid (Release of catecholamines). Products include:
Marplan Tablets ... 1906

Isoflurane (Additive sedative effects). Products include:
Forane ... 600

Ketamine Hydrochloride (Additive sedative effects; antagonizes gastrointestinal motility effects). Products include:
Ketalar ... 1726

Levodopa (Accelerated absorption from the small bowel). Products include:
Larodopa Tablets ... 1905
Sinemet Tablets ... 952
Sinemet CR Tablets ... 953

Levorphanol Tartrate (Additive sedative effects; antagonizes gastrointestinal motility effects). Products include:
Levo-Dromoran ... 1906

Lorazepam (Additive sedative effects). Products include:
Ativan Injection ... 2432
Ativan Tablets ... 2434

Loxapine Hydrochloride (Additive sedative effects). Products include:
Loxitane ... 1213

Loxapine Succinate (Additive sedative effects; antagonizes gastrointestinal motility effects). Products include:
Loxitane Capsules ... 1213

Mepenzolate Bromide (Antagonizes gastrointestinal motility effects). Products include:
Cantil Tablets ... 1326

Meperidine Hydrochloride (Additive sedative effects; antagonizes gastrointestinal motility effects). Products include:
Demerol ... 2047
Mepergan Injection ... 2479

Mephobarbital (Additive sedative effects). Products include:
Mebaral Tablets ... 2061

Meprobamate (Additive sedative effects). Products include:
Deprol Tablets ... 2382
Equagesic Tablets ... 2451
Miltown Tablets ... 2386
PMB 200 and PMB 400 ... 2504

Mesoridazine (Additive sedative effects). Products include:
Serentil ... 686

Methadone Hydrochloride (Additive sedative effects; antagonizes gastrointestinal motility effects). Products include:
Dolophine Hydrochloride Ampoules & Vials ... 1260
Dolophine Hydrochloride Tablets ... 1261
Methadone Hydrochloride Diskets ... 1284
Methadone Hydrochloride Oral Solution & Tablets ... 1987

Methohexital Sodium (Additive sedative effects). Products include:
Brevital Sodium Vials ... 1248

Methoxyflurane (Additive sedative effects).
No products indexed under this heading.

Midazolam Hydrochloride (Additive sedative effects). Products include:
Versed Injection ... 1924

Molindone Hydrochloride (Additive sedative effects). Products include:
Moban Tablets & Concentrate ... 932

Morphine Sulfate (Additive sedative effects; antagonizes gastrointestinal motility effects). Products include:
Astramorph/PF Injection, USP (Preservative-Free) ... 618
Duramorph ... 960
Infumorph 200 and Infumorph 500 Sterile Solutions ... 962
MS Contin Tablets ... 1814
MSIR ... 1817
Oramorph SR (Morphine Sulfate Sustained Release Tablets) ... 1988
Roxanol ... 1991

Opium Alkaloids (Additive sedative effects; antagonizes gastrointestinal motility effects). Products include:
B & O No. 15A & No. 16A Supprettes ... 2395
Pantopon Injectable ... 1911

Oxazepam (Additive sedative effects). Products include:
Serax Capsules ... 2522
Serax Tablets ... 2522

Oxybutynin Chloride (Antagonizes gastrointestinal motility effects). Products include:
Ditropan ... 1332

Oxycodone Hydrochloride (Additive sedative effects; antagonizes gastrointestinal motility effects). Products include:
Percocet Tablets ... 950
Percodan ... 951
Roxicodone Tablets, Oral Solution & Intensol (Oxycodone) ... 1992
Tylox Capsules ... 1382

Pentobarbital Sodium (Additive sedative effects). Products include:
Nembutal Sodium Capsules ... 534
Nembutal Sodium Solution ... 536
Nembutal Sodium Suppositories ... 538

Perphenazine (Additive sedative effects). Products include:
Etrafon ... 2087
Triavil Tablets ... 1556

Trilafon 2123

Phenelzine Sulfate (Release of catecholamines). Products include:
Nardil 1742

Phenobarbital (Additive sedative effects). Products include:
Arco-Lase Plus Tablets 607
Bellergal-S Tablets 1998
Bronkolixir .... ▣ 761
Bronkotabs Tablets .... ▣ 762
Donnatal 1858
Donnatal Extentabs 1859
Donnatal Tablets 1858
Donnazyme Tablets 1860
Kinesed Tablets 2272
Phenobarbital Elixir and Tablets 1293
Primatene Tablets-P Formula 2421
Quadrinal Tablets 1183
Tedral SA 1765

Prazepam (Additive sedative effects). Products include:
Centrax 1693

Prochlorperazine (Additive sedative effects). Products include:
Compazine 2201

Procyclidine Hydrochloride (Antagonizes gastrointestinal motility effects). Products include:
Kemadrin Tablets 771

Promethazine Hydrochloride (Additive sedative effects). Products include:
Mepergan Injection 2479
Phenergan with Codeine 2497
Phenergan with Dextromethorphan 2499
Phenergan Injection 2493
Phenergan Suppositories 2496
Phenergan Syrup 2495
Phenergan Tablets 2496
Phenergan VC 2500
Phenergan VC with Codeine 2501

Propantheline Bromide (Antagonizes gastrointestinal motility effects). Products include:
Pro-Banthīne Tablets 2141

Propofol (Additive sedative effects; antagonizes gastrointestinal motility effects). Products include:
Diprivan Injection 2267

Propoxyphene Hydrochloride (Additive sedative effects; antagonizes gastrointestinal motility effects). Products include:
Darvon 1256
Wygesic Tablets 2540

Propoxyphene Napsylate (Additive sedative effects; antagonizes gastrointestinal motility effects). Products include:
Darvon-N/Darvocet-N 1254

Quazepam (Additive sedative effects; antagonizes gastrointestinal motility effects). Products include:
Doral Tablets 2383

Scopolamine Hydrobromide (Antagonizes gastrointestinal motility effects). Products include:
Donnagel .... ▣ 675
Donnagel-PG 1858
Donnatal 1858
Donnatal Extentabs 1859
Donnatal Tablets 1858
Donnazyme Tablets 1860
Isopto Hyoscine .... ⊙ 222
Murocoll-2 Sterile Ophthalmic Solution .... ⊙ 261
Ru-Tuss Tablets 693

Scopolamine Preparations (Antagonizes gastrointestinal motility effects). Products include:
Transderm Scōp Transdermal Therapeutic System 887

Secobarbital Sodium (Additive sedative effects; antagonizes gastrointestinal motility effects). Products include:
Seconal Sodium Pulvules 1296

Selegiline Hydrochloride (Release of catecholamines). Products include:
Eldepryl 2250

Sufentanil Citrate (Additive sedative effects; antagonizes gastrointestinal motility effects). Products include:
Sufenta Injection 1147

Temazepam (Additive sedative effects). Products include:
Restoril Capsules 2023

Tetracycline Hydrochloride (Accelerated absorption from the small bowel). Products include:
Achromycin V Capsules 1193
Achromycin Ophthalmic Ointment 1% .... ⊙ 307
Achromycin Ophthalmic Suspension 1% .... ⊙ 308
Topicycline for Topical Solution 1856

Thiamylal Sodium (Additive sedative effects). Products include:
Surital Ampoules, Steri-Vials 1764

Thioridazine Hydrochloride (Additive sedative effects). Products include:
Mellaril 2011

Thiothixene (Additive sedative effects). Products include:
Navane Capsules and Concentrate 1954
Navane Intramuscular 1956

Tranylcypromine Sulfate (Release of catecholamines). Products include:
Parnate Tablets 2222

Triazolam (Additive sedative effects). Products include:
Halcion Tablets 2340

Tridihexethyl Chloride (Antagonizes gastrointestinal motility effects).
No products indexed under this heading.

Trifluoperazine Hydrochloride (Additive sedative effects). Products include:
Stelazine 2226

Trihexyphenidyl Hydrochloride (Antagonizes gastrointestinal motility effects). Products include:
Artane 1195

REGLAN SYRUP
(Metoclopramide Hydrochloride) 1869
See **Reglan Injectable**

REGLAN TABLETS
(Metoclopramide Hydrochloride) 1869
See **Reglan Injectable**

REGULAR INSULIN
(Insulin, Regular) 1625
No interactions described in labeling.

REGULAR PURIFIED PORK INSULIN
(Insulin, Regular) 1626
No interactions described in labeling.

REHYDRALYTE ORAL ELECTROLYTE REHYDRATION SOLUTION
(Electrolyte Supplement) 1975
No interactions described in labeling.

RELIEF VASOCONSTRICTOR AND LUBRICANT EYE DROPS
(Phenylephrine Hydrochloride) .... ⊙ 256
No interactions described in labeling.

RENESE TABLETS
(Polythiazide) 1785
May interact with antihypertensives, ganglionic blocking agents, para-aminobenzoic acid based local anesthetics, corticosteroids, insulin, barbiturates, narcotic analgesics, cardiac glycosides, and certain other agents. Compounds in these categories include:

Acebutolol Hydrochloride (Potentiation of antihypertensive effect). Products include:
Sectral Capsules 2520

ACTH (Hypokalemia).
No products indexed under this heading.

Alcohol (Orthostatic hypotension).

Alfentanil Hydrochloride (Orthostatic hypotension). Products include:
Alfenta Injection 1131

Aprobarbital (Orthostatic hypotension). Products include:
Alurate Elixir 1883

Atenolol (Potentiation of antihypertensive effect). Products include:
Tenoretic Tablets 1105
Tenormin Tablets and I.V. Injection 1107

Benazepril Hydrochloride (Potentiation of antihypertensive effect). Products include:
Lotensin Tablets 872

Bendroflumethiazide (Potentiation of antihypertensive effect). Products include:
Corzide Tablets 702
Naturetin Tablets 1789
Rauzide Tablets 1804

Betamethasone Acetate (Hypokalemia). Products include:
Celestone Soluspan Suspension 2081

Betamethasone Sodium Phosphate (Hypokalemia). Products include:
Celestone Soluspan Suspension 2081

Betaxolol Hydrochloride (Potentiation of antihypertensive effect). Products include:
Betoptic Sterile Ophthalmic Solution 569
Betoptic S Sterile Ophthalmic Suspension 570
Kerlone Tablets 2172

Buprenorphine (Orthostatic hypotension).
No products indexed under this heading.

Butabarbital (Orthostatic hypotension). Products include:
Pyridium Plus 1764

Butalbital (Orthostatic hypotension). Products include:
Esgic-Plus Tablets 1002
Esgic Tablets & Capsules 1001
Fioricet Tablets 2006
Fiorinal Capsules 2007
Fiorinal with Codeine Capsules 2008
Fiorinal Tablets 2007
Phrenilin 838
Sedapap Tablets 50 mg/650 mg .. 1360

Captopril (Potentiation of antihypertensive effect). Products include:
Capoten 2255
Capozide 2258

Carteolol Hydrochloride (Potentiation of antihypertensive effect). Products include:
Cartrol Tablets 507

Chlorothiazide (Potentiation of antihypertensive effect). Products include:
Aldoclor Tablets 1413
Diupres Tablets 1461
Diuril Oral 1464

Chlorothiazide Sodium (Potentiation of antihypertensive effect). Products include:
Diuril Sodium Intravenous 1463

Chlorthalidone (Potentiation of antihypertensive effect). Products include:
Combipres Tablets 678
Tenoretic Tablets 1105
Thalitone Tablets 687

Clonidine (Potentiation of antihypertensive effect). Products include:
Catapres-TTS 677

Clonidine Hydrochloride (Potentiation of antihypertensive effect). Products include:
Catapres Tablets 676
Combipres Tablets 678

Codeine (Orthostatic hypotension). Products include:
Calcidrine Syrup 506

Codeine Phosphate (Orthostatic hypotension). Products include:
Actifed with Codeine Cough Syrup .. 752
Cheracol Cough Syrup 1853
Codimal PH Syrup 846
Dimetane-DC Cough Syrup 1857
Empirin with Codeine Phosphate Nos. 2, 3 & 4 764
Fiorinal with Codeine Capsules 2008
Isoclor Expectorant 982
Naldecon CX Adult Liquid .... ▣ 521
Novahistine DH 1342
Novahistine Expectorant 1343
Nucofed Capsules 2219
Nucofed Expectorant 2219
Nucofed Pediatric Expectorant 2220
Nucofed Syrup 2219
Phenaphen with Codeine Capsules 1865
Phenaphen-650 with Codeine Tablets 1866
Phenergan with Codeine 2497
Phenergan VC with Codeine 2501
Robitussin A-C Syrup 1875
Robitussin-DAC Syrup 1875
Ryna .... ▣ 741
Soma Compound w/Codeine Tablets 2390
Triaminic Expectorant w/Codeine .. 1996
Tussi-Organidin Liquid 2391
Tylenol with Codeine 1381

Codeine Polistirex (Orthostatic hypotension).
No products indexed under this heading.

Cortisone Acetate (Hypokalemia). Products include:
Cortone Acetate Sterile Suspension 1437
Cortone Acetate Tablets 1439

Deserpidine (Potentiation of antihypertensive effect). Products include:
Enduronyl 518
Harmonyl Tablets 528
Oreticyl 545

Deslanoside (Exaggerated metabolic effects of hypokalemia).
No products indexed under this heading.

Dexamethasone (Hypokalemia). Products include:
AK-Trol Ointment & Suspension .... ⊙ 207
Decadron Elixir 1445
Decadron Tablets 1447
Decaspray Topical Aerosol 1459
Dexacidin .... ⊙ 272
Maxidex Sterile Ophthalmic Suspension .... ⊙ 223
Maxitrol Ophthalmic Ointment/Suspension .... ⊙ 223
TobraDex Ophthalmic Suspension and Ointment .... ⊙ 228

Dexamethasone Acetate (Hypokalemia). Products include:
Dalalone D.P. Injectable 999
Decadron-LA Sterile Suspension 1457

Dexamethasone Sodium Phosphate (Hypokalemia). Products include:
AK-Dex .... ⊙ 203
Decadron Phosphate Respihaler 1454
Decadron Phosphate Sterile Ophthalmic Ointment 1453
Decadron Phosphate Sterile Ophthalmic Solution 1453
Decadron Phosphate Topical Cream 1455
Decadron Phosphate Turbinaire 1456
Maxidex Sterile Ophthalmic Ointment .... ⊙ 222
NeoDecadron Sterile Ophthalmic Ointment 1517
NeoDecadron Sterile Ophthalmic Solution 1518

NeoDecadron Topical Cream 1518

Dezocine (Orthostatic hypotension).

Diazoxide (Potentiation of antihypertensive effect). Products include:
- Hyperstat I.V. Injection 2095
- Proglycem 649

Digitoxin (Exaggerated metabolic effects of hypokalemia). Products include:
- Crystodigin Tablets 1253

Digoxin (Exaggerated metabolic effects of hypokalemia). Products include:
- Lanoxicaps 772
- Lanoxin Elixir Pediatric 775
- Lanoxin Injection 778
- Lanoxin Injection Pediatric 781
- Lanoxin Tablets 783

Doxazosin Mesylate (Potentiation of antihypertensive effect). Products include:
- Cardura Tablets 1941

Enalapril Maleate (Potentiation of antihypertensive effect). Products include:
- Vaseretic Tablets 1559
- Vasotec Tablets 1564

Enalaprilat (Potentiation of antihypertensive effect). Products include:
- Vasotec I.V. 1562

Felodipine (Potentiation of antihypertensive effect). Products include:
- Plendil Extended-Release Tablets.... 1526

Fentanyl (Orthostatic hypotension). Products include:
- Duragesic Transdermal System........ 1133

Fentanyl Citrate (Orthostatic hypotension). Products include:
- Innovar Injection 1141
- Sublimaze Injection 1146

Fosinopril Sodium (Potentiation of antihypertensive effect). Products include:
- Monopril Tablets 1406

Furosemide (Potentiation of antihypertensive effect). Products include:
- Lasix 1093

Guanabenz Acetate (Potentiation of antihypertensive effect). Products include:
- Wytensin Tablets 2542

Guanethidine Monosulfate (Potentiation of antihypertensive effect). Products include:
- Esimil Tablets 864
- Ismelin Tablets 869

Hydralazine Hydrochloride (Potentiation of antihypertensive effect). Products include:
- Apresazide Capsules 854
- Apresoline Hydrochloride Parenteral (Ampuls) 856
- Apresoline Hydrochloride Tablets .. 855
- Apresoline-Esidrix Tablets 857
- Ser-Ap-Es Tablets 881
- Serpasil-Apresoline Tablets 884

Hydrochlorothiazide (Potentiation of antihypertensive effect). Products include:
- Aldactazide 2150
- Aldoril Tablets 1418
- Apresazide Capsules 854
- Apresoline-Esidrix Tablets 857
- Capozide 2258
- Dyazide Capsules 2208
- Esidrix Tablets 863
- Esimil Tablets 864
- HydroDIURIL Tablets 1484
- Hydropres Tablets 1485
- Inderide Tablets 2463
- Inderide LA Long Acting Capsules .. 2465
- Lopressor HCT Tablets 1034
- Maxzide 1215
- Moduretic Tablets 1510
- Normozide Tablets 2112
- Oretic Tablets 544
- Oreticyl 545
- Prinzide Tablets 1540
- Ser-Ap-Es Tablets 881
- Serpasil-Esidrix Tablets 886
- Timolide Tablets 1547
- Trandate HCT Tablets 579
- Vaseretic Tablets 1559
- Zestoretic 2274

Hydrocodone Bitartrate (Orthostatic hypotension). Products include:
- Anexsia 5/500 Tablets 2196
- Anexsia 7.5/650 Tablets 2197
- Azdone Tablets 844
- Codiclear DH Syrup 845
- Codimal DH Syrup 846
- Damason-P 1356
- Hycodan Syrup, Tablets 927
- Hycomine Compound Tablets 929
- Hycomine Syrup 927
- Hycotuss Expectorant Syrup 930
- Hydrocet Capsules 835
- Lortab ASA Tablets 2414
- Lortab 2412
- Ru-Tuss with Hydrocodone 694
- Triaminic Expectorant DH 1995
- Vicodin Tablets 1187
- Vicodin ES Tablets 1189
- Zydone Capsules 941

Hydrocodone Polistirex (Orthostatic hypotension). Products include:
- Tussionex Extended-Release Suspension 988

Hydrocortisone (Hypokalemia). Products include:
- AK-Spore H.C. .... ◉ 206
- Bactine Hydrocortisone Anti-Itch Cream .... ◘ 625
- CaldeCORT Anti-Itch Hydrocortisone Spray .... ◘ 560
- Carmol HC Cream 1% 2296
- Cortaid Spray .... ◘ 735
- Cortenema 2244
- Cortisporin Ointment 758
- Cortisporin Ophthalmic Ointment Sterile 758
- Cortisporin Ophthalmic Suspension Sterile 759
- Cortisporin Otic Solution Sterile 760
- Cortisporin Otic Suspension Sterile 760
- Cortizone-5 Creme & Ointment .... ◘ 732
- Dermolate Anti-Itch Cream .... ◘ 697
- Eldecort Cream 1.0% 1113
- Eldecort Cream 1.0% and 2.5% 1113
- Fungoid HC Creme 1770
- Hydrocortone Tablets 1482
- Hytone 909
- LazerSporin-C Solution 1770
- Massengill Medicated Soft Cloth Towelettes 2192
- Nutracort Cream & Lotion 1684
- PediOtic Suspension Sterile 797
- Synacort Creams 1%, 2.5% 2296
- Vanoxide-HC Acne Lotion 911
- Vioform-Hydrocortisone Cream and Mild Cream 889
- Vioform-Hydrocortisone Ointment.. 889
- VōSoL HC Otic Solution 2392
- Vytone Cream 1% 911

Hydrocortisone Acetate (Hypokalemia). Products include:
- Analpram-HC Rectal Cream 1% and 2.5% 970
- Anusol-HC Cream 1690
- Anusol-HC Suppositories 1691
- Caldecort .... ◘ 560
- Carmol HC Cream 1% 2296
- Chloromycetin Hydrocortisone Ophthalmic 1694
- Coly-Mycin S Otic w/Neomycin & Hydrocortisone 1708
- Cortaid .... ◘ 735
- Cortef Feminine Itch Cream .... ◘ 735
- Corticaine .... ◘ 682
- Cortifoam 1827
- Cortisporin Cream 757
- Epifoam 1828
- Gynecort 5 Creme .... ◘ 556
- Hydrocortone Acetate Sterile Suspension 1479
- Lanacort 5 Creme and Ointment .. ◘ 557
- Mantadil Cream 789
- Ophthocort .... ◉ 301
- Orabase HCA Oral Paste 890
- Pramosone Cream, Lotion & Ointment 971
- ProctoCream-HC 1834
- Proctofoam-HC 1835

Hydrocortisone Sodium Phosphate (Hypokalemia). Products include:
- Hydrocortone Phosphate Injection, Sterile 1481

Hydrocortisone Sodium Succinate (Hypokalemia). Products include:
- Solu-Cortef Sterile Powder 2361

Hydroflumethiazide (Potentiation of antihypertensive effect). Products include:
- Diucardin Tablets 2450
- Saluron 718
- Salutensin/Salutensin-Demi 719

Indapamide (Potentiation of antihypertensive effect). Products include:
- Lozol Tablets 1843

Insulin, Human (Altered insulin requirements).
- No products indexed under this heading.

Insulin, Human Isophane Suspension (Altered insulin requirements). Products include:
- Humulin N, 100 Units 1270

Insulin, Human NPH (Altered insulin requirements). Products include:
- Insulatard NPH Human 1627
- Novolin N 1627
- Novolin N PenFill Cartridges 1628
- Novolin N Prefilled 1628

Insulin, Human Regular (Altered insulin requirements). Products include:
- Humulin BR, 100 Units 1268
- Humulin R, 100 Units 1272
- Novolin R 1627
- Novolin R PenFill Cartridges 1628
- Novolin R Prefilled 1629
- Velosulin Human 1628

Insulin, Human, Zinc Suspension (Altered insulin requirements). Products include:
- Humulin L, 100 Units 1268
- Humulin U, 100 Units 1272
- Novolin L 1627

Insulin, NPH (Altered insulin requirements). Products include:
- NPH, 40 & 100 Units 1273
- Beef NPH, 100 Units 1274
- Pork NPH, 100 Units 1275
- Insulatard NPH 1626
- NPH Insulin 1626
- NPH Purified Pork Isophane Insulin 1626

Insulin, Regular (Altered insulin requirements). Products include:
- Regular, 40 & 100 Units 1273
- Beef Regular, 100 Units 1275
- Pork Regular, 100 Units 1275
- Pork Regular (Concentrated), 500 Units 1276
- Regular Insulin 1625
- Regular Purified Pork Insulin 1626
- Velosulin 1627

Insulin, Zinc Crystals (Altered insulin requirements). Products include:
- NPH, 40 & 100 Units 1273

Insulin, Zinc Suspension (Altered insulin requirements). Products include:
- Lente, 40 & 100 Units 1272
- Protamine, Zinc, 40 & 100 Units.... 1273
- Lente Iletin I 1272
- Beef Lente, 100 Units 1274
- Beef Protamine Zinc, 100 Units 1274
- Pork Lente, 100 Units 1275
- Pork, Protamine, Zinc, 100 Units.... 1275
- Lente Insulin 1626
- Lente Purified Pork Insulin 1626
- Semilente Insulin 1625
- Ultralente Insulin 1626

Isradipine (Potentiation of antihypertensive effect). Products include:
- DynaCirc Capsules 2004

Labetalol Hydrochloride (Potentiation of antihypertensive effect). Products include:
- Normodyne Injection 2108
- Normodyne Tablets 2110
- Normozide Tablets 2112
- Trandate HCT Tablets 579
- Trandate Injection 577
- Trandate Tablets 579

Levorphanol Tartrate (Orthostatic hypotension). Products include:
- Levo-Dromoran 1906

Lisinopril (Potentiation of antihypertensive effect). Products include:
- Prinivil Tablets 1538
- Prinzide Tablets 1540
- Zestoretic 2274
- Zestril Tablets 2277

Mecamylamine Hydrochloride (Potentiation of antihypertensive effect). Products include:
- Inversine Tablets 1492

Meperidine Hydrochloride (Orthostatic hypotension). Products include:
- Demerol 2047
- Mepergan Injection 2479

Mephobarbital (Orthostatic hypotension). Products include:
- Mebaral Tablets 2061

Methadone Hydrochloride (Orthostatic hypotension). Products include:
- Dolophine Hydrochloride Ampoules & Vials 1260
- Dolophine Hydrochloride Tablets 1261
- Methadone Hydrochloride Diskets .. 1284
- Methadone Hydrochloride Oral Solution & Tablets 1987

Methyclothiazide (Potentiation of antihypertensive effect). Products include:
- Enduron Tablets 517
- Enduronyl 518

Methyldopa (Potentiation of antihypertensive effect). Products include:
- Aldoclor Tablets 1413
- Aldomet Oral 1415
- Aldoril Tablets 1418

Methyldopate Hydrochloride (Potentiation of antihypertensive effect). Products include:
- Aldomet Ester HCl Injection 1417

Methylprednisolone (Hypokalemia). Products include:
- Medrol 2348

Methylprednisolone Acetate (Hypokalemia). Products include:
- Depo-Medrol Sterile Aqueous Suspension 2334

Methylprednisolone Sodium Succinate (Hypokalemia). Products include:
- Solu-Medrol Sterile Powder 2363

Metolazone (Potentiation of antihypertensive effect). Products include:
- Diulo 2129
- Mykrox ½ mg Tablets 984
- Zaroxolyn Tablets 989

Metoprolol Tartrate (Potentiation of antihypertensive effect). Products include:
- Lopressor Ampuls 1032
- Lopressor HCT Tablets 1034
- Lopressor Tablets 1032

Metyrosine (Potentiation of antihypertensive effect). Products include:
- Demser Capsules 1460

Minoxidil (Potentiation of antihypertensive effect). Products include:
- Loniten Tablets 2346
- Rogaine Topical Solution 2357

Morphine Sulfate (Orthostatic hypotension). Products include:
- Astramorph/PF Injection, USP (Preservative-Free) 618
- Duramorph 960

Infumorph 200 and Infumorph 500 Sterile Solutions ... 962
MS Contin Tablets ... 1814
MSIR ... 1817
Oramorph SR (Morphine Sulfate Sustained Release Tablets) ... 1988
Roxanol ... 1991

Nadolol (Potentiation of antihypertensive effect). Products include:
Corgard Tablets ... 701
Corzide Tablets ... 702

Nicardipine Hydrochloride (Potentiation of antihypertensive effect). Products include:
Cardene Capsules ... 2290

Nitroglycerin (Potentiation of antihypertensive effect). Products include:
Deponit NTG Transdermal Delivery System ... 2143
Minitran Transdermal Delivery System ... 1312
Nitro-Bid Ointment ... 1339
Nitro-Bid Capsules ... 1338
Nitrodisc ... 2176
Nitro-Dur (nitroglycerin) Transdermal Infusion System ... 1164
Nitrogard Tablets ... 1004
Nitrolingual Spray ... 1846
Nitrostat Tablets ... 1743
Transderm-Nitro Transdermal Therapeutic System ... 2283

Norepinephrine Bitartrate (Decreased arterial responsiveness to norepinephrine). Products include:
Levophed Bitartrate Injection ... 2054

Opium Alkaloids (Orthostatic hypotension). Products include:
B & O No. 15A & No. 16A Supprettes ... 2395
Pantopon Injectable ... 1911

Oxycodone Hydrochloride (Orthostatic hypotension). Products include:
Percocet Tablets ... 950
Percodan ... 951
Roxicodone Tablets, Oral Solution & Intensol (Oxycodone) ... 1992
Tylox Capsules ... 1382

Penbutolol Sulfate (Potentiation of antihypertensive effect). Products include:
Levatol ... 1832

Pentobarbital Sodium (Orthostatic hypotension). Products include:
Nembutal Sodium Capsules ... 534
Nembutal Sodium Solution ... 536
Nembutal Sodium Suppositories ... 538

Phenobarbital (Orthostatic hypotension). Products include:
Arco-Lase Plus Tablets ... 607
Bellergal-S Tablets ... 1998
Bronkolixir ... ▣ 761
Bronkotabs Tablets ... ▣ 762
Donnatal ... 1858
Donnatal Extentabs ... 1859
Donnatal Tablets ... 1858
Donnazyme Tablets ... 1860
Kinesed Tablets ... 2272
Phenobarbital Elixir and Tablets ... 1293
Primatene Tablets-P Formula ... 2421
Quadrinal Tablets ... 1183
Tedral SA ... 1765

Phenoxybenzamine Hydrochloride (Potentiation of antihypertensive effect). Products include:
Dibenzyline Capsules ... 2207

Phentolamine Mesylate (Potentiation of antihypertensive effect). Products include:
Regitine ... 878

Pindolol (Potentiation of antihypertensive effect). Products include:
Visken Tablets ... 2036

Prazosin Hydrochloride (Potentiation of antihypertensive effect). Products include:
Minipress Capsules ... 1778
Minizide Capsules ... 1779

Prednisolone Acetate (Hypokalemia). Products include:
AK-Cide Sterile Ophthalmic Ointment & Suspension ... ⊙ 202
Blephamide Liquifilm Sterile Ophthalmic Suspension ... 586
Blephamide S.O.P. Sterile Ophthalmic Ointment ... 586
Cetapred Ointment ... ⊙ 220
⅛% Econopred & 1% Econopred Plus ... ⊙ 217
Isopto Cetapred Suspension ... ⊙ 220
Metimyd ... ⊙ 306
Poly-Pred Liquifilm ... ⊙ 250
Pred Forte ... ⊙ 252
Pred Mild ... ⊙ 254
Pred-G Liquifilm Sterile Ophthalmic Suspension ... ⊙ 252
Pred-G S.O.P. Sterile Ophthalmic Ointment ... ⊙ 253
Vasocidin Ointment ... ⊙ 275

Prednisolone Sodium Phosphate (Hypokalemia). Products include:
AK-Pred ... ⊙ 205
Hydeltrasol Injection, Sterile ... 1476
Inflamase ... ⊙ 274
Pediapred Oral Liquid ... 987
Vasocidin Ophthalmic Solution ... ⊙ 276

Prednisolone Tebutate (Hypokalemia). Products include:
Hydeltra-T.B.A. Sterile Suspension 1478

Prednisone (Hypokalemia). Products include:
Deltasone Tablets ... 2332

Propoxyphene Hydrochloride (Orthostatic hypotension). Products include:
Darvon ... 1256
Wygesic Tablets ... 2540

Propoxyphene Napsylate (Orthostatic hypotension). Products include:
Darvon-N/Darvocet-N ... 1254

Propranolol Hydrochloride (Potentiation of antihypertensive effect). Products include:
Inderal ... 2459
Inderal LA Long Acting Capsules ... 2461
Inderide Tablets ... 2463
Inderide LA Long Acting Capsules ... 2465

Ramipril (Potentiation of antihypertensive effect). Products include:
Altace Capsules ... 1086

Rauwolfia Serpentina (Potentiation of antihypertensive effect). Products include:
Raudixin Tablets ... 1803
Rauzide Tablets ... 1804

Rescinnamine (Potentiation of antihypertensive effect).
No products indexed under this heading.

Secobarbital Sodium (Orthostatic hypotension). Products include:
Seconal Sodium Pulvules ... 1296

Sodium Nitroprusside (Potentiation of antihypertensive effect). Products include:
Nipride I.V. Infusion ... 1909

Sufentanil Citrate (Orthostatic hypotension). Products include:
Sufenta Injection ... 1147

Terazosin Hydrochloride (Potentiation of antihypertensive effect). Products include:
Hytrin Tablets ... 529

Thiamylal Sodium (Orthostatic hypotension). Products include:
Surital Ampoules, Steri-Vials ... 1764

Timolol Maleate (Potentiation of antihypertensive effect). Products include:
Blocadren Tablets ... 1429
Timolide Tablets ... 1547
Timoptic in Ocudose ... 1552
Timoptic Sterile Ophthalmic Solution ... 1550

Triamcinolone (Hypokalemia).
No products indexed under this heading.

Triamcinolone Acetonide (Hypokalemia). Products include:
Aristocort A ... 1010
Azmacort Inhaler ... 1837
Kenalog Cream, Lotion & Ointment 2401
Kenalog-10 Injection ... 2402
Kenalog-40 Injection ... 2403
Kenalog in Orabase ... 604
Kenalog Spray ... 2401
Mycolog II Cream and Ointment ... 2407
Mytrex Cream & Ointment ... 2080
Nasacort Nasal Inhaler ... 1844

Triamcinolone Diacetate (Hypokalemia). Products include:
Aristocort Suspension ... 1008

Triamcinolone Hexacetonide (Hypokalemia). Products include:
Aristospan Suspension ... 1011

Trimethaphan Camsylate (Potentiation of antihypertensive effect). Products include:
Arfonad Ampuls ... 1887

Tubocurarine Chloride (Increased response to tubocurarine).
No products indexed under this heading.

RENESE-R TABLETS
(Polythiazide, Reserpine) ... 1786
May interact with corticosteroids, antihypertensives, general anesthetics, cardiac glycosides, and certain other agents. Compounds in these categories include:

Acebutolol Hydrochloride (Altered dosage requirements). Products include:
Sectral Capsules ... 2520

Atenolol (Altered dosage requirements). Products include:
Tenoretic Tablets ... 1105
Tenormin Tablets and I.V. Injection 1107

Benazepril Hydrochloride (Altered dosage requirements). Products include:
Lotensin Tablets ... 872

Bendroflumethiazide (Altered dosage requirements). Products include:
Corzide Tablets ... 702
Naturetin Tablets ... 1789
Rauzide Tablets ... 1804

Betamethasone Acetate (Electrolyte imbalance). Products include:
Celestone Soluspan Suspension ... 2081

Betamethasone Sodium Phosphate (Electrolyte imbalance). Products include:
Celestone Soluspan Suspension ... 2081

Betaxolol Hydrochloride (Altered dosage requirements). Products include:
Betoptic Sterile Ophthalmic Solution ... 569
Betoptic S Sterile Ophthalmic Suspension ... 570
Kerlone Tablets ... 2172

Captopril (Altered dosage requirements). Products include:
Capoten ... 2255
Capozide ... 2258

Carteolol Hydrochloride (Altered dosage requirements). Products include:
Cartrol Tablets ... 507

Chlorothiazide (Altered dosage requirements). Products include:
Aldoclor Tablets ... 1413
Diupres Tablets ... 1461
Diuril Oral ... 1464

Chlorothiazide Sodium (Altered dosage requirements). Products include:
Diuril Sodium Intravenous ... 1463

Chlorthalidone (Altered dosage requirements). Products include:
Combipres Tablets ... 678
Tenoretic Tablets ... 1105
Thalitone Tablets ... 687

Clonidine (Altered dosage requirements). Products include:
Catapres-TTS ... 677

Clonidine Hydrochloride (Altered dosage requirements). Products include:
Catapres Tablets ... 676
Combipres Tablets ... 678

Cortisone Acetate (Electrolyte imbalance). Products include:
Cortone Acetate Sterile Suspension ... 1437
Cortone Acetate Tablets ... 1439

Deserpidine (Altered dosage requirements). Products include:
Enduronyl ... 518
Harmonyl Tablets ... 528
Oreticyl ... 545

Deslanoside (Arrhythmias).
No products indexed under this heading.

Dexamethasone (Electrolyte imbalance). Products include:
AK-Trol Ointment & Suspension ... ⊙ 207
Decadron Elixir ... 1445
Decadron Tablets ... 1447
Decaspray Topical Aerosol ... 1459
Dexacidin ... ⊙ 272
Maxidex Sterile Ophthalmic Suspension ... ⊙ 223
Maxitrol Ophthalmic Ointment/Suspension ... ⊙ 223
TobraDex Ophthalmic Suspension and Ointment ... ⊙ 228

Dexamethasone Acetate (Electrolyte imbalance). Products include:
Dalalone D.P. Injectable ... 999
Decadron-LA Sterile Suspension ... 1457

Dexamethasone Sodium Phosphate (Electrolyte imbalance). Products include:
AK-Dex ... ⊙ 203
Decadron Phosphate Respihaler ... 1454
Decadron Phosphate Sterile Ophthalmic Ointment ... 1453
Decadron Phosphate Sterile Ophthalmic Solution ... 1453
Decadron Phosphate Topical Cream ... 1455
Decadron Phosphate Turbinaire ... 1456
Maxidex Sterile Ophthalmic Ointment ... ⊙ 222
NeoDecadron Sterile Ophthalmic Ointment ... 1517
NeoDecadron Sterile Ophthalmic Solution ... 1518
NeoDecadron Topical Cream ... 1518

Diazoxide (Altered dosage requirements). Products include:
Hyperstat I.V. Injection ... 2095
Proglycem ... 649

Digitoxin (Arrhythmias). Products include:
Crystodigin Tablets ... 1253

Digoxin (Arrhythmias). Products include:
Lanoxicaps ... 772
Lanoxin Elixir Pediatric ... 775
Lanoxin Injection ... 778
Lanoxin Injection Pediatric ... 781
Lanoxin Tablets ... 783

Doxazosin Mesylate (Altered dosage requirements). Products include:
Cardura Tablets ... 1941

Enalapril Maleate (Altered dosage requirements). Products include:
Vaseretic Tablets ... 1559
Vasotec Tablets ... 1564

Enalaprilat (Altered dosage requirements). Products include:
Vasotec I.V. ... 1562

Enflurane (Potential for unexpected degree of hypotension and bradycardia). Products include:
Ethrane ... 599

Esmolol Hydrochloride (Altered dosage requirements). Products include:
- Brevibloc Injection 942

Felodipine (Altered dosage requirements). Products include:
- Plendil Extended-Release Tablets 1526

Fosinopril Sodium (Altered dosage requirements). Products include:
- Monopril Tablets 1406

Furosemide (Altered dosage requirements). Products include:
- Lasix 1093

Guanabenz Acetate (Altered dosage requirements). Products include:
- Wytensin Tablets 2542

Guanethidine Monosulfate (Altered dosage requirements). Products include:
- Esimil Tablets 864
- Ismelin Tablets 869

Hydralazine Hydrochloride (Altered dosage requirements). Products include:
- Apresazide Capsules 854
- Apresoline Hydrochloride Parenteral (Ampuls) 856
- Apresoline Hydrochloride Tablets 855
- Apresoline-Esidrix Tablets 857
- Ser-Ap-Es Tablets 881
- Serpasil-Apresoline Tablets 884

Hydrochlorothiazide (Altered dosage requirements). Products include:
- Aldactazide 2150
- Aldoril Tablets 1418
- Apresazide Capsules 854
- Apresoline-Esidrix Tablets 857
- Capozide 2258
- Dyazide Capsules 2208
- Esidrix Tablets 863
- Esimil Tablets 864
- HydroDIURIL Tablets 1484
- Hydropres Tablets 1485
- Inderide Tablets 2463
- Inderide LA Long Acting Capsules 2465
- Lopressor HCT Tablets 1034
- Maxzide 1215
- Moduretic Tablets 1510
- Normozide Tablets 2112
- Oretic Tablets 544
- Oreticyl 545
- Prinzide Tablets 1540
- Ser-Ap-Es Tablets 881
- Serpasil-Esidrix Tablets 886
- Timolide Tablets 1547
- Trandate HCT Tablets 579
- Vaseretic Tablets 1559
- Zestoretic 2274

Hydrocortisone (Electrolyte imbalance). Products include:
- AK-Spore H.C. ⊙ 206
- Bactine Hydrocortisone Anti-Itch Cream ⊞ 625
- CaldeCORT Anti-Itch Hydrocortisone Spray ⊞ 560
- Carmol HC Cream 1% 2296
- Cortaid Spray ⊞ 735
- Cortenema 2244
- Cortisporin Ointment 758
- Cortisporin Ophthalmic Ointment Sterile 758
- Cortisporin Ophthalmic Suspension Sterile 759
- Cortisporin Otic Solution Sterile 760
- Cortisporin Otic Suspension Sterile 760
- Cortizone-5 Creme & Ointment ⊞ 732
- Dermolate Anti-Itch Cream ⊞ 697
- Eldecort Cream 1.0% 1113
- Eldecort Cream 1.0% and 2.5% 1113
- Fungoid HC Creme 1770
- Hydrocortone Tablets 1482
- Hytone 909
- LazerSporin-C Solution 1770
- Massengill Medicated Soft Cloth Towelettes 2192
- Nutracort Cream & Lotion 1684
- PediOtic Suspension Sterile 797
- Synacort Creams 1%, 2.5% 2296
- Vanoxide-HC Acne Lotion 911
- Vioform-Hydrocortisone Cream and Mild Cream 889
- Vioform-Hydrocortisone Ointment 889
- VōSoL HC Otic Solution 2392
- Vytone Cream 1% 911

Hydrocortisone Acetate (Electrolyte imbalance). Products include:
- Analpram-HC Rectal Cream 1% and 2.5% 970
- Anusol-HC Cream 1690
- Anusol-HC Suppositories 1691
- Caldecort ⊞ 560
- Carmol HC Cream 1% 2296
- Chloromycetin Hydrocortisone Ophthalmic 1694
- Coly-Mycin S Otic w/Neomycin & Hydrocortisone 1708
- Cortaid ⊞ 735
- Cortef Feminine Itch Cream ⊞ 735
- Corticaine ⊞ 682
- Cortifoam 1827
- Cortisporin Cream 757
- Epifoam 1828
- Gynecort 5 Creme ⊞ 556
- Hydrocortone Acetate Sterile Suspension 1479
- Lanacort 5 Creme and Ointment ⊞ 557
- Mantadil Cream 789
- Ophthocort ⊙ 301
- Orabase HCA Oral Paste 890
- Pramosone Cream, Lotion & Ointment 971
- ProctoCream-HC 1834
- Proctofoam-HC 1835

Hydrocortisone Sodium Phosphate (Electrolyte imbalance). Products include:
- Hydrocortone Phosphate Injection, Sterile 1481

Hydrocortisone Sodium Succinate (Electrolyte imbalance). Products include:
- Solu-Cortef Sterile Powder 2361

Hydroflumethiazide (Altered dosage requirements). Products include:
- Diucardin Tablets 2450
- Saluron 718
- Salutensin/Salutensin-Demi 719

Indapamide (Altered dosage requirements). Products include:
- Lozol Tablets 1843

Isoflurane (Potential for unexpected degree of hypotension and bradycardia). Products include:
- Forane 600

Isradipine (Altered dosage requirements). Products include:
- DynaCirc Capsules 2004

Labetalol Hydrochloride (Altered dosage requirements). Products include:
- Normodyne Injection 2108
- Normodyne Tablets 2110
- Normozide Tablets 2112
- Trandate HCT Tablets 579
- Trandate Injection 577
- Trandate Tablets 579

Lisinopril (Altered dosage requirements). Products include:
- Prinivil Tablets 1538
- Prinzide Tablets 1540
- Zestoretic 2274
- Zestril Tablets 2277

Mecamylamine Hydrochloride (Altered dosage requirements). Products include:
- Inversine Tablets 1492

Methohexital Sodium (Potential for unexpected degree of hypotension and bradycardia). Products include:
- Brevital Sodium Vials 1248

Methoxyflurane (Potential for unexpected degree of hypotension and bradycardia).
- No products indexed under this heading.

Methyclothiazide (Altered dosage requirements). Products include:
- Enduron Tablets 517
- Enduronyl 518

Methyldopa (Altered dosage requirements). Products include:
- Aldoclor Tablets 1413
- Aldomet Oral 1415
- Aldoril Tablets 1418

Methyldopate Hydrochloride (Altered dosage requirements). Products include:
- Aldomet Ester HCl Injection 1417

Methylprednisolone (Electrolyte imbalance). Products include:
- Medrol 2348

Methylprednisolone Acetate (Electrolyte imbalance). Products include:
- Depo-Medrol Sterile Aqueous Suspension 2334

Methylprednisolone Sodium Succinate (Electrolyte imbalance). Products include:
- Solu-Medrol Sterile Powder 2363

Metolazone (Altered dosage requirements). Products include:
- Diulo 2129
- Mykrox ½ mg Tablets 984
- Zaroxolyn Tablets 989

Metoprolol Tartrate (Altered dosage requirements). Products include:
- Lopressor Ampuls 1032
- Lopressor HCT Tablets 1034
- Lopressor Tablets 1032

Metyrosine (Altered dosage requirements). Products include:
- Demser Capsules 1460

Minoxidil (Altered dosage requirements). Products include:
- Loniten Tablets 2346
- Rogaine Topical Solution 2357

Nadolol (Altered dosage requirements). Products include:
- Corgard Tablets 701
- Corzide Tablets 702

Nicardipine Hydrochloride (Altered dosage requirements). Products include:
- Cardene Capsules 2290

Nitroglycerin (Altered dosage requirements). Products include:
- Deponit NTG Transdermal Delivery System 2143
- Minitran Transdermal Delivery System 1312
- Nitro-Bid Ointment 1339
- Nitro-Bid Capsules 1338
- Nitrodisc 2176
- Nitro-Dur (nitroglycerin) Transdermal Infusion System 1164
- Nitrogard Tablets 1004
- Nitrolingual Spray 1846
- Nitrostat Tablets 1743
- Transderm-Nitro Transdermal Therapeutic System 2283

Norepinephrine Bitartrate (Decreased arterial responsiveness to norepinephrine). Products include:
- Levophed Bitartrate Injection 2054

Penbutolol Sulfate (Altered dosage requirements). Products include:
- Levatol 1832

Phenoxybenzamine Hydrochloride (Altered dosage requirements). Products include:
- Dibenzyline Capsules 2207

Phentolamine Mesylate (Altered dosage requirements). Products include:
- Regitine 878

Pindolol (Altered dosage requirements). Products include:
- Visken Tablets 2036

Prazosin Hydrochloride (Altered dosage requirements). Products include:
- Minipress Capsules 1778
- Minizide Capsules 1779

Prednisolone Acetate (Electrolyte imbalance). Products include:
- AK-Cide Sterile Ophthalmic Ointment & Suspension ⊙ 202
- Blephamide Liquifilm Sterile Ophthalmic Suspension 586
- Blephamide S.O.P. Sterile Ophthalmic Ointment 586
- Cetapred Ointment ⊙ 220
- ⅛% Econopred & 1% Econopred Plus ⊙ 217
- Isopto Cetapred Suspension ⊙ 220
- Metimyd ⊙ 306
- Poly-Pred Liquifilm ⊙ 250
- Pred Forte ⊙ 252
- Pred Mild ⊙ 254
- Pred-G Liquifilm Sterile Ophthalmic Suspension ⊙ 252
- Pred-G S.O.P. Sterile Ophthalmic Ointment ⊙ 253
- Vasocidin Ointment ⊙ 275

Prednisolone Sodium Phosphate (Electrolyte imbalance). Products include:
- AK-Pred ⊙ 205
- Hydeltrasol Injection, Sterile 1476
- Inflamase ⊙ 274
- Pediapred Oral Liquid 987
- Vasocidin Ophthalmic Solution ⊙ 276

Prednisolone Tebutate (Electrolyte imbalance). Products include:
- Hydeltra-T.B.A. Sterile Suspension 1478

Prednisone (Electrolyte imbalance). Products include:
- Deltasone Tablets 2332

Propofol (Potential for unexpected degree of hypotension and bradycardia). Products include:
- Diprivan Injection 2267

Propranolol Hydrochloride (Altered dosage requirements). Products include:
- Inderal 2459
- Inderal LA Long Acting Capsules 2461
- Inderide Tablets 2463
- Inderide LA Long Acting Capsules 2465

Quinidine Gluconate (Arrhythmias). Products include:
- Quinaglute Dura-Tabs Tablets 663

Quinidine Polygalacturonate (Arrhythmias). Products include:
- Cardioquin Tablets 1812

Quinidine Sulfate (Arrhythmias). Products include:
- Quinidex Extentabs 1868

Ramipril (Altered dosage requirements). Products include:
- Altace Capsules 1086

Rauwolfia Serpentina (Altered dosage requirements). Products include:
- Raudixin Tablets 1803
- Rauzide Tablets 1804

Rescinnamine (Altered dosage requirements).
- No products indexed under this heading.

Sodium Nitroprusside (Altered dosage requirements). Products include:
- Nipride I.V. Infusion 1909

Terazosin Hydrochloride (Altered dosage requirements). Products include:
- Hytrin Tablets 529

Timolol Maleate (Altered dosage requirements). Products include:
- Blocadren Tablets 1429
- Timolide Tablets 1547
- Timoptic in Ocudose 1552
- Timoptic Sterile Ophthalmic Solution 1550

Triamcinolone (Electrolyte imbalance).
- No products indexed under this heading.

Triamcinolone Acetonide (Electrolyte imbalance). Products include:
- Aristocort A 1010
- Azmacort Inhaler 1837
- Kenalog Cream, Lotion & Ointment 2401
- Kenalog-10 Injection 2402
- Kenalog-40 Injection 2403
- Kenalog in Orabase 604
- Kenalog Spray 2401
- Mycolog II Cream and Ointment 2407
- Mytrex Cream & Ointment 2080
- Nasacort Nasal Inhaler 1844

Triamcinolone Diacetate (Electrolyte imbalance). Products include:
- Aristocort Suspension 1008

Triamcinolone Hexacetonide (Electrolyte imbalance). Products include:
- Aristospan Suspension 1011

Trimethaphan Camsylate (Altered dosage requirements). Products include:
- Arfonad Ampuls 1887

Tubocurarine Chloride (Augmented paralyzing action).
- No products indexed under this heading.

REPLENS
(Lubricant) .... ▣ 556
No interactions described in labeling.

RESPBID TABLETS
(Theophylline) 684
May interact with sympathomimetic bronchodilators, oral contraceptives, macrolide antibiotics, and certain other agents. Compounds in these categories include:

Albuterol (Toxic synergism). Products include:
- Proventil Inhalation Aerosol 2117
- Ventolin Inhalation Aerosol and Refill 583

Albuterol Sulfate (Toxic synergism). Products include:
- Proventil Repetabs Tablets 2120
- Proventil Solutions for Inhalation 0.5% and 0.083% 2118
- Proventil Syrup 2119
- Proventil Tablets 2120
- Ventolin 583

Allopurinol (Increased serum theophylline levels). Products include:
- Zyloprim Tablets 830

Bitolterol Mesylate (Toxic synergism). Products include:
- Tornalate 2074

Cimetidine (Increased theophylline blood levels). Products include:
- Tagamet Tablets 2228

Ephedrine Hydrochloride (Toxic synergism). Products include:
- Amesec .... ▣ 682
- Primatene Tablets-M Formula 2421
- Primatene Tablets-P Formula 2421
- Primatene Tablets-Regular Formula 2421
- Quadrinal Tablets 1183
- Quelidrine Syrup 556
- Tedral SA 1765

Ephedrine Sulfate (Toxic synergism). Products include:
- Bronkaid Tablets .... ▣ 757
- Bronkolixir .... ▣ 761
- Bronkotabs Tablets .... ▣ 762
- Marax Tablets & DF Syrup 1954
- Pazo Hemorrhoid Ointment & Suppositories 752
- Vicks Vatronol Nose Drops .... ▣ 666

Ephedrine Tannate (Toxic synergism). Products include:
- Rynatuss 2388

Epinephrine (Toxic synergism). Products include:
- Ana-Kit Anaphylaxis Emergency Treatment Kit 1100
- Bronkaid Mist .... ▣ 757
- EpiPen 843
- Marcaine Hydrochloride 0.5% with Epinephrine 1:200,000 (as bitartrate) 958
- Marcaine Hydrochloride with Epinephrine 1:200,000 2055
- Primatene Mist 2420
- Sus-Phrine Injection 1006
- Xylocaine with Epinephrine Injections 637

Epinephrine Bitartrate (Toxic synergism). Products include:
- AsthmaHaler Mist Epinephrine Bitartrate Bronchodilator .... ▣ 616
- Bronkaid Mist Suspension .... ▣ 757
- Primatene Mist Suspension 2421

Epinephrine Hydrochloride (Toxic synergism). Products include:
- Adrenalin Chloride Solution 1:100 & 1:1,000 1689
- Epifrin .... ◉ 244
- Glaucon .... ◉ 218

Erythromycin (Increases theophylline blood levels). Products include:
- A/T/S Topical Gel and Topical Solution 1089
- AK-Mycin Ointment .... ◉ 204
- Benzamycin Topical Gel 907
- E-Mycin Tablets 688
- ETS-2% 1685
- ERYC 1720
- Erycette (erythromycin 2%) Topical Solution 1678
- Ery-Tab Tablets 521
- Erythromycin Base Filmtab 525
- Erythromycin Delayed-Release Capsules, USP 526
- Ilotycin Ophthalmic Ointment 915
- PCE Dispertab Tablets 549
- Pediazole 1973
- T-Stat 2.0% Topical Solution and Pads 2409
- Theramycin Z Topical Solution 2% 1410

Erythromycin Estolate (Increases theophylline blood levels). Products include:
- Ilosone 913

Erythromycin Ethylsuccinate (Increases theophylline blood levels). Products include:
- E.E.S. 522
- EryPed 519
- Pediazole 1973

Erythromycin Gluceptate (Increases theophylline blood levels). Products include:
- Ilotycin Gluceptate, IV, Vials 915

Erythromycin Stearate (Increases theophylline blood levels). Products include:
- Erythrocin Stearate Filmtab 523

Ethinyl Estradiol (Increased serum theophylline levels). Products include:
- Brevicon 2304
- Demulen 2161
- Estinyl Tablets 2085
- Jenest-28 Tablets 1636
- Levlen/Tri-Levlen 665
- Lo/Ovral Tablets 2471
- Lo/Ovral-28 Tablets 2476
- Loestrin 1728
- Modicon 1667
- Nordette-21 Tablets 2481
- Nordette-28 Tablets 2483
- Norethin 2133
- Norinyl 2304
- Norlestrin 1746
- Ortho-Cyclen Tablets 1658
- Ortho-Novum 1667
- Ovcon 1391
- Ovral Tablets 2490
- Ovral-28 Tablets 2491
- Levlen/Tri-Levlen 665
- Tri-Norinyl 2304
- Triphasil-21 Tablets 2527
- Triphasil-28 Tablets 2532

Ethylnorepinephrine Hydrochloride (Toxic synergism). Products include:
- Bronkephrine Injection 2042

Ethynodiol Diacetate (Increased serum theophylline levels). Products include:
- Demulen 2161

Isoetharine (Toxic synergism). Products include:
- Arm-a-Med Isoetharine Inhalation Solution, USP 616
- Bronkometer Aerosol 2042
- Bronkosol Solution 2042

Isoproterenol Hydrochloride (Toxic synergism). Products include:
- Isuprel Hydrochloride Injection 1:5000 2050
- Isuprel Hydrochloride Mistometer .. 2051
- Isuprel Hydrochloride Solution 1:200 & 1:100 2052
- Norisodrine Aerotrol 540

Levonorgestrel (Increased serum theophylline levels). Products include:
- Levlen/Tri-Levlen 665
- Nordette-21 Tablets 2481
- Nordette-28 Tablets 2483
- Norplant System 2484
- Levlen/Tri-Levlen 665
- Triphasil-21 Tablets 2527
- Triphasil-28 Tablets 2532

Lithium Carbonate (Increased excretion of lithium carbonate). Products include:
- Eskalith 2214
- Lithane Tablets 1596
- Lithium Carbonate Capsules & Tablets 1984
- Lithobid Tablets 870

Mestranol (Increased serum theophylline levels). Products include:
- Enovid 2161
- Norethin 2133
- Norinyl 2304
- Ortho-Novum 1667

Metaproterenol Sulfate (Toxic synergism). Products include:
- Alupent 674
- Arm-a-Med Metaproterenol Sulfate Inhalation Solution, USP 617
- Metaprel Inhalation Aerosol Bronchodilator 2014
- Metaprel Inhalation Solution 2015
- Metaprel 2015
- Metaproterenol Sulfate Inhalation Solution, USP 912

Norethindrone (Increased serum theophylline levels). Products include:
- Brevicon 2304
- Jenest-28 Tablets 1636
- Micronor Tablets 1667
- Modicon 1667
- Norethin 2133
- Norinyl 2304
- Norlutin 1755
- Nor-Q D Tablets 2304
- Ortho-Novum 1667
- Ovcon 1391
- Tri-Norinyl 2304

Norethynodrel (Increased serum theophylline levels). Products include:
- Enovid 2161

Norgestimate (Increased serum theophylline levels). Products include:
- Ortho-Cyclen Tablets 1658

Norgestrel (Increased serum theophylline levels). Products include:
- Lo/Ovral Tablets 2471
- Lo/Ovral-28 Tablets 2476
- Ovral Tablets 2490
- Ovral-28 Tablets 2491
- Ovrette Tablets 2492

Phenytoin (Decreased theophylline and phenytoin serum levels). Products include:
- Dilantin Infatabs 1710
- Dilantin-30 Pediatric/Dilantin-125 Suspension 1713

Phenytoin Sodium (Decreased theophylline and phenytoin serum levels). Products include:
- Dilantin Kapseals 1708
- Dilantin Parenteral 1712
- Dilantin with Phenobarbital Kapseals 1715

Pirbuterol Acetate (Toxic synergism). Products include:
- Maxair Inhaler 1311

Terbutaline Sulfate (Toxic synergism). Products include:
- Brethaire Inhaler 1024
- Brethine Ampuls 1026
- Brethine Tablets 1026
- Bricanyl Injection 1324
- Bricanyl Tablets 1325

Troleandomycin (Increases theophylline blood levels). Products include:
- Tao Capsules 1963

Food Interactions

Beverages, caffeine-containing (Avoid large quantities; increased side effects).

Chocolate (Eating large quantity of chocolate increases theophylline side effects).

Cola (Drinking large quantity of cola increases theophylline side effects).

Diet, high-lipid (Reduced plasma concentration levels; delay in time of peak plasma levels).

RESTORIL CAPSULES
(Temazepam) 2023
May interact with central nervous system depressants, hypnotics and sedatives, and certain other agents. Compounds in these categories include:

Alcohol (Additive effects).

Alfentanil Hydrochloride (Additive effects). Products include:
- Alfenta Injection 1131

Alprazolam (Additive effects). Products include:
- Xanax Tablets 2367

Aprobarbital (Additive effects). Products include:
- Alurate Elixir 1883

Buprenorphine (Additive effects).
- No products indexed under this heading.

Buspirone Hydrochloride (Additive effects). Products include:
- BuSpar 1401

Butabarbital (Additive effects). Products include:
- Pyridium Plus 1764

Butalbital (Additive effects). Products include:
- Esgic-Plus Tablets 1002
- Esgic Tablets & Capsules 1001
- Fioricet Tablets 2006
- Fiorinal Capsules 2007
- Fiorinal with Codeine Capsules 2008
- Fiorinal Tablets 2007
- Phrenilin 838
- Sedapap Tablets 50 mg/650 mg .. 1360

Chlordiazepoxide (Additive effects). Products include:
- Libritabs Tablets 1930
- Limbitrol 1933
- Menrium Tablets 1934

Chlordiazepoxide Hydrochloride (Additive effects). Products include:
- Librax Capsules 1929
- Librium Capsules 1931
- Librium Injectable 1932

Chlorpromazine (Additive effects). Products include:
- Thorazine 2234

Chlorprothixene (Additive effects). Products include:
- Taractan Tablets 1920

Chlorprothixene Hydrochloride (Additive effects). Products include:
- Taractan 1920

Clorazepate Dipotassium (Additive effects). Products include:
- Tranxene 556

Codeine (Additive effects). Products include:
- Calcidrine Syrup 506

Codeine Phosphate (Additive effects). Products include:
- Actifed with Codeine Cough Syrup.. 752
- Cheracol Cough Syrup 1853
- Codimal PH Syrup 846
- Dimetane-DC Cough Syrup 1857
- Empirin with Codeine Phosphate Nos. 2, 3 & 4 764
- Fiorinal with Codeine Capsules 2008
- Isoclor Expectorant 982
- Naldecon CX Adult Liquid .... ▣ 521
- Novahistine DH 1342
- Novahistine Expectorant 1343
- Nucofed Capsules 2219
- Nucofed Expectorant 2219

Nucofed Pediatric Expectorant 2220
Nucofed Syrup 2219
Phenaphen with Codeine Capsules 1865
Phenaphen-650 with Codeine Tablets 1866
Phenergan with Codeine 2497
Phenergan VC with Codeine 2501
Robitussin A-C Syrup 1875
Robitussin-DAC Syrup 1875
Ryna .... ▣ 741
Soma Compound w/Codeine Tablets 2390
Triaminic Expectorant w/Codeine .. 1996
Tussi-Organidin Liquid 2391
Tylenol with Codeine 1381

Codeine Polistirex (Additive effects).
No products indexed under this heading.

Dezocine (Additive effects).

Diazepam (Additive effects). Products include:
Valium Injectable 1937
Valium Tablets 1939
Valrelease Capsules 1923

Diphenhydramine Hydrochloride (Synergistic effect is possible). Products include:
Benadryl Anti-Itch Cream .... ▣ 635
Benadryl Capsules 1691
Benadryl Decongestant Elixir .... ▣ 635
Benadryl Decongestant .... ▣ 635
Benadryl Elixir .... ▣ 636
Benadryl Kapseals 1691
Benadryl 25 Kapseals .... ▣ 636
Benadryl Parenteral 1692
Benadryl Plus .... ▣ 636
Benadryl Plus Nighttime .... ▣ 637
Benadryl Spray, Maximum Strength .... ▣ 637
Benadryl Spray, Regular Strength ▣ 637
Benadryl Steri-Vials, Ampoules, and Steri-Dose Syringe 1692
Benadryl 25 Tablets .... ▣ 636
Benylin Cough Syrup .... ▣ 637
Benylin Decongestant .... ▣ 638
Caladryl Cream, Lotion, Spray .... ▣ 638
Miles Nervine Nighttime Sleep-Aid ▣ 627
Nytol Tablets .... ▣ 517
Sleep-ettes-D Tablets .... ▣ 653
Sleep-eze 3 Tablets .... ▣ 755
Sleepinal Night-time Sleep Aid Capsules .... ▣ 734
Sominex Caplets and Tablets .... ▣ 722
Sominex Liquid .... ▣ 723
Sominex Pain Relief Formula .... ▣ 723
Tylenol Cold Night Time Medication Liquid 1371
Tylenol PM, Extra Strength Caplets and Tablets 1368
Unisom Dual Relief Nighttime Sleep Aid/Analgesic 1774
Ziradryl Lotion .... ▣ 643

Droperidol (Additive effects). Products include:
Inapsine Injection 1140
Innovar Injection 1141

Enflurane (Additive effects). Products include:
Ethrane 599

Estazolam (Additive effects). Products include:
ProSom Tablets 554

Ethchlorvynol (Additive effects). Products include:
Placidyl Capsules 553

Ethinamate (Additive effects).
No products indexed under this heading.

Fentanyl (Additive effects). Products include:
Duragesic Transdermal System 1133

Fentanyl Citrate (Additive effects). Products include:
Innovar Injection 1141
Sublimaze Injection 1146

Fluphenazine Decanoate (Additive effects). Products include:
Prolixin Decanoate 1795

Fluphenazine Enanthate (Additive effects). Products include:
Prolixin Enanthate 1796

Fluphenazine Hydrochloride (Additive effects). Products include:
Prolixin Elixir 1793
Prolixin Injection 1791
Prolixin Oral Concentrate 1792
Prolixin Tablets 1793

Flurazepam Hydrochloride (Additive effects). Products include:
Dalmane Capsules 1927

Glutethimide (Additive effects).
No products indexed under this heading.

Haloperidol (Additive effects). Products include:
Haldol Injection, Tablets and Concentrate 1373

Haloperidol Decanoate (Additive effects). Products include:
Haldol Decanoate 1375

Hydrocodone Bitartrate (Additive effects). Products include:
Anexsia 5/500 Tablets 2196
Anexsia 7.5/650 Tablets 2197
Azdone Tablets 844
Codiclear DH Syrup 845
Codimal DH Syrup 846
Damason-P 1356
Hycodan Syrup, Tablets 927
Hycomine Compound Tablets 929
Hycomine Syrup 927
Hycotuss Expectorant Syrup 930
Hydrocet Capsules 835
Lortab ASA Tablets 2414
Lortab 2412
Ru-Tuss with Hydrocodone 694
Triaminic Expectorant DH 1995
Vicodin Tablets 1187
Vicodin ES Tablets 1189
Zydone Capsules 941

Hydrocodone Polistirex (Additive effects). Products include:
Tussionex Extended-Release Suspension 988

Hydroxyzine Hydrochloride (Additive effects). Products include:
Atarax Tablets & Syrup 1941
Marax Tablets & DF Syrup 1954
Vistaril Intramuscular Solution 1970

Isoflurane (Additive effects). Products include:
Forane 600

Ketamine Hydrochloride (Additive effects). Products include:
Ketalar 1726

Levorphanol Tartrate (Additive effects). Products include:
Levo-Dromoran 1906

Lorazepam (Additive effects). Products include:
Ativan Injection 2432
Ativan Tablets 2434

Loxapine Hydrochloride (Additive effects). Products include:
Loxitane 1213

Loxapine Succinate (Additive effects). Products include:
Loxitane Capsules 1213

Meperidine Hydrochloride (Additive effects). Products include:
Demerol 2047
Mepergan Injection 2479

Mephobarbital (Additive effects). Products include:
Mebaral Tablets 2061

Meprobamate (Additive effects). Products include:
Deprol Tablets 2382
Equagesic Tablets 2451
Miltown Tablets 2386
PMB 200 and PMB 400 2504

Mesoridazine (Additive effects). Products include:
Serentil 686

Methadone Hydrochloride (Additive effects). Products include:
Dolophine Hydrochloride Ampoules & Vials 1260
Dolophine Hydrochloride Tablets 1261
Methadone Hydrochloride Diskets .. 1284
Methadone Hydrochloride Oral Solution & Tablets 1987

Methohexital Sodium (Additive effects). Products include:
Brevital Sodium Vials 1248

Methoxyflurane (Additive effects).
No products indexed under this heading.

Midazolam Hydrochloride (Additive effects). Products include:
Versed Injection 1924

Molindone Hydrochloride (Additive effects). Products include:
Moban Tablets & Concentrate 932

Morphine Sulfate (Additive effects). Products include:
Astramorph/PF Injection, USP (Preservative-Free) 618
Duramorph 960
Infumorph 200 and Infumorph 500 Sterile Solutions 962
MS Contin Tablets 1814
MSIR 1817
Oramorph SR (Morphine Sulfate Sustained Release Tablets) 1988
Roxanol 1991

Opium Alkaloids (Additive effects). Products include:
B & O No. 15A & No. 16A Supprettes 2395
Pantopon Injectable 1911

Oxazepam (Additive effects). Products include:
Serax Capsules 2522
Serax Tablets 2522

Oxycodone Hydrochloride (Additive effects). Products include:
Percocet Tablets 950
Percodan 951
Roxicodone Tablets, Oral Solution & Intensol (Oxycodone) 1992
Tylox Capsules 1382

Pentobarbital Sodium (Additive effects). Products include:
Nembutal Sodium Capsules 534
Nembutal Sodium Solution 536
Nembutal Sodium Suppositories 538

Perphenazine (Additive effects). Products include:
Etrafon 2087
Triavil Tablets 1556
Trilafon 2123

Phenobarbital (Additive effects). Products include:
Arco-Lase Plus Tablets 607
Bellergal-S Tablets 1998
Bronkolixir .... ▣ 761
Bronkotabs Tablets .... ▣ 762
Donnatal 1858
Donnatal Extentabs 1859
Donnatal Tablets 1858
Donnazyme Tablets 1860
Kinesed Tablets 2272
Phenobarbital Elixir and Tablets 1293
Primatene Tablets-P Formula 2421
Quadrinal Tablets 1183
Tedral SA 1765

Prazepam (Additive effects). Products include:
Centrax 1693

Prochlorperazine (Additive effects). Products include:
Compazine 2201

Promethazine Hydrochloride (Additive effects). Products include:
Mepergan Injection 2479
Phenergan with Codeine 2497
Phenergan with Dextromethorphan 2499
Phenergan Injection 2493
Phenergan Suppositories 2496
Phenergan Syrup 2495
Phenergan Tablets 2496
Phenergan VC 2500
Phenergan VC with Codeine 2501

Propofol (Additive effects). Products include:
Diprivan Injection 2267

Propoxyphene Hydrochloride (Additive effects). Products include:
Darvon 1256
Wygesic Tablets 2540

Propoxyphene Napsylate (Additive effects). Products include:
Darvon-N/Darvocet-N 1254

Quazepam (Additive effects). Products include:
Doral Tablets 2383

Secobarbital Sodium (Additive effects). Products include:
Seconal Sodium Pulvules 1296

Sufentanil Citrate (Additive effects). Products include:
Sufenta Injection 1147

Thiamylal Sodium (Additive effects). Products include:
Surital Ampoules, Steri-Vials 1764

Thioridazine Hydrochloride (Additive effects). Products include:
Mellaril 2011

Thiothixene (Additive effects). Products include:
Navane Capsules and Concentrate 1954
Navane Intramuscular 1956

Triazolam (Additive effects). Products include:
Halcion Tablets 2340

Trifluoperazine Hydrochloride (Additive effects). Products include:
Stelazine 2226

RETIN-A (TRETINOIN) CREAM/GEL/LIQUID
(Tretinoin) 1680
May interact with:

Concomitant Topical Acne Therapy (Effect not specified).

Topical Medications (Effect not specified).

RETROVIR CAPSULES
(Zidovudine) 802
May interact with aspirin and acetaminophen containing products, cytotoxic drugs, experimental nucleoside analogues (selected) for AIDS and ARC, nephrotoxic drugs, and certain other agents. Compounds in these categories include:

Acetaminophen (May competitively inhibit glucuronidation; possible increased incidence of granulocytopenia). Products include:
Acetaminophen Uniserts Suppositories 2374
Actifed Plus Caplets .... ▣ 539
Actifed Plus Tablets .... ▣ 540
Alka-Seltzer Advanced Formula Antacid & Non-Aspirin Pain Reliever .... ▣ 620
Allerest .... ▣ 559
Aspirin Free Anacin Maximum Strength Acetaminophen Film Coated Caplets 2417
Aspirin Free Anacin Maximum Strength Acetaminophen Film Coated Tablets 2417
Anacin-3 Regular Strength Acetaminophen Film Coated Tablets ▣ 746
Anexsia 5/500 Tablets 2196
Anexsia 7.5/650 Tablets 2197
Benadryl Plus .... ▣ 636
Benadryl Plus Nighttime .... ▣ 637
Bufferin AF Nite Time Analgesic/Sleeping Aid Caplets 744
Allergy-Sinus Comtrex Multi-Symptom Allergy Sinus Formula Tablets & Caplets 746
Cough Formula Comtrex 746
Comtrex Multi-Symptom Cold Reliever Tablets/Caplets/Liqui-Gels/Liquid 745
Day-Night Comtrex 747
Non-Drowsy Comtrex 747
Congespirin For Children Aspirin Free Chewable Cold Tablets 748
Contac Cough & Sore Throat Formula .... ▣ 712
Contac Jr. Children's Cold Medicine .... ▣ 712
Contac Nighttime Cold Medicine .... ▣ 713
Contac Severe Cold and Flu Formula Caplets .... ▣ 711
Contac Sinus Caplets Maximum Strength Non-Drowsy Formula .... ▣ 710
Contac Sinus Tablets Maximum Strength Non-Drowsy Formula .... ▣ 710

Coricidin 'D' Decongestant Tablets ▣ 695
Coricidin Demilets Tablets for Children ▣ 696
Coricidin Tablets ▣ 695
Darvon-N/Darvocet-N 1254
Datril Extra-Strength Analgesic Tablets 748
Dimetapp Plus Caplets ▣ 675
Dorcol Children's Fever & Pain Reducer ▣ 686
Dristan Decongestant/Antihistamine/Analgesic Coated Caplets ▣ 749
Dristan Cold Nasal Decongestant/Antihistamine/Analgesic Coated Tablets 2419
Dristan Advanced Formula Decongestant/Antihistamine/Analgesic Tablets ▣ 749
Maximum Strength Dristan Decongestant/Analgesic Coated Caplets ▣ 750
No Drowsiness Dristan Cold Nasal Decongestant/Analgesic Coated Caplets 2420
Drixoral Plus Extended-Release Tablets ▣ 699
Drixoral Sinus ▣ 700
Esgic-Plus Tablets 1002
Esgic Tablets & Capsules 1001
Aspirin Free Excedrin Analgesic Caplets 748
Excedrin Extra-Strength Analgesic Tablets & Caplets 749
Excedrin P.M. Analgesic/Sleeping Aid Tablets, Caplets and Liquid 749
Sinus Excedrin Analgesic, Decongestant Tablets & Caplets 750
4-Way Cold Tablets 750
Feverall Sprinkle Caps 2374
Feverall Suppositories 2374
Fioricet Tablets 2006
Hycomine Compound Tablets 929
Hydrocet Capsules 835
Isocom Capsules 1629
Liquiprin ▣ 618
Lortab 2412
Lurline PMS Tablets 972
Medi-Flu Caplet, Liquid ▣ 640
Maximum Strength Midol Multi-Symptom Menstrual Formula ▣ 571
Maximum Strength Midol PMS Premenstrual Syndrome Formula ▣ 570
Regular Strength Midol Multi-Symptom Menstrual Formula ▣ 570
Midrin Capsules 836
Ornex Caplets ▣ 618
Children's Panadol Chewable Tablets, Liquid, Infants' Drops ▣ 571
Junior Strength Panadol ▣ 571
Maximum Strength Panadol Tablets and Caplets ▣ 572
Percocet Tablets 950
Percogesic Analgesic Tablets ▣ 660
Phenaphen with Codeine Capsules 1865
Phenaphen-650 with Codeine Tablets 1866
Phrenilin 838
Prēmsyn PMS Capsules & Caplets ▣ 547
Pyrroxate Capsules ▣ 669
Robitussin Night Relief ▣ 677
Sedapap Tablets 50 mg/650 mg 1360
Sinarest ▣ 562
Sine-Aid Maximum Strength Sinus Headache Caplets 1365
Sine-Aid Maximum Strength Sinus Headache Tablets 1365
Sine-Off Maximum Strength Allergy/Sinus Formula Caplets ▣ 721
Sine-Off Maximum Strength No Drowsiness Formula Caplets ▣ 722
Singlet Tablets ▣ 598
Sinulin 840
Sinutab Maximum Strength ▣ 641
Sinutab Maximum Strength Without Drowsiness Tablets & Caplets ▣ 642
Sinutab Regular Strength Without Drowsiness Formula ▣ 641
Sominex Pain Relief Formula ▣ 723
St. Joseph Aspirin-Free Fever Reducer for Children Chewable Tablets, Liquid & Infant Drops ▣ 704
St. Joseph Cold Tablets for Children ▣ 704
St. Joseph Nighttime Cold Medicine ▣ 705
Sudafed Sinus Caplets ▣ 545
Sudafed Sinus Tablets ▣ 545
Talacen 2070
Tempra, Acetaminophen ▣ 613
TheraFlu Flu and Cold Medicine ▣ 687
Triaminicin Tablets ▣ 690
Tylenol acetaminophen Children's Chewable Tablets & Elixir 1366
Tylenol Allergy Sinus Medication Caplets and Gelcaps, Maximum Strength 1372
Tylenol with Codeine 1381
Children's Tylenol Cold Liquid Formula and Chewable Tablets 1368
Tylenol Cold & Flu Hot Medication, Packets 1369
Tylenol Cold & Flu No Drowsiness Hot Medication, Packets 1371
Tylenol Cold Medication Caplets and Tablets 1370
Tylenol Cold Medication, Effervescent Tablets 1369
Tylenol Cold Medication No Drowsiness Formula Caplets 1370
Tylenol Cold Night Time Medication Liquid 1371
Tylenol Cough Medication Liquid, Maximum Strength 1372
Tylenol Cough Medication Liquid with Decongestant, Maximum Strength 1372
Tylenol, Extra Strength, acetaminophen Adult Liquid Pain Reliever 1367
Tylenol, Extra Strength, acetaminophen Gelcaps, Caplets, Tablets 1367
Tylenol, Infants' Drops 1366
Tylenol, Junior Strength, acetaminophen Coated Caplets, Grape and Fruit Chewable Tablets 1366
Tylenol, Maximum Strength, Sinus Medication Gelcaps, Caplets and Tablets 1373
Tylenol, Regular Strength, acetaminophen Tablets and Caplets 1367
Tylenol PM, Extra Strength Caplets and Tablets 1368
Tylox Capsules 1382
Unisom Dual Relief Nighttime Sleep Aid/Analgesic 1774
Vanquish Analgesic Caplets ▣ 574
Vicks Daycare ▣ 660
Vicks Formula 44M Multi-Symptom Cough Medicine ▣ 662
Vicks NyQuil Nighttime Colds Medicine-Original & Cherry Flavor ▣ 664
Vicodin Tablets 1187
Vicodin ES Tablets 1189
Wygesic Tablets 2540
Zydone Capsules 941

Acyclovir (Concomitant use may result in neurotoxicity (profound lethargy)). Products include:
Zovirax Capsules 824
Zovirax Ointment 5% 827
Zovirax 824

Acyclovir Sodium (Concomitant use may result in neurotoxicity (profound lethargy)). Products include:
Zovirax Sterile Powder 828

Amphotericin B (Increased risk of nephrotoxicity). Products include:
Fungizone Cream, Lotion and Ointment 2261
Fungizone Intravenous 2262

Aspirin (May competitively inhibit glucuronidation; possible increased incidence of granulocytopenia). Products include:
Alka-Seltzer Effervescent Antacid and Pain Reliever 1568
Alka-Seltzer Extra Strength Effervescent Antacid and Pain Reliever 1570
Alka-Seltzer (Flavored) Effervescent Antacid and Pain Reliever 1569
Alka-Seltzer Plus Cold Medicine ▣ 623
Alka-Seltzer Plus Night-Time Cold Medicine ▣ 623
Alka Seltzer Plus Sinus Allergy Medicine ▣ 624
Anacin Coated Analgesic Caplets 2417
Anacin Coated Analgesic Tablets 2417
Anacin Maximum Strength Analgesic Coated Tablets 2417
Maximum Strength Arthritis Pain Formula By the Makers of Anacin Analgesic Tablets and Caplets 2418
Arthritis Pain Formula by the Makers of Anacin Analgesic Tablets and Caplets ▣ 747
Arthritis Strength BC Powder ▣ 516
Ascriptin A/D Caplets 1850
Regular Strength Ascriptin Tablets 1850
Azdōne Tablets 844
BC Powder ▣ 517
BC Cold Powder ▣ 517
Children's Bayer Chewable Aspirin ▣ 564
Genuine Bayer Aspirin Tablets & Caplets ▣ 564
Maximum Bayer Aspirin Tablets & Caplets ▣ 566
Bayer Plus Aspirin Tablets ▣ 567
Therapy Bayer Aspirin Caplets ▣ 568
8 Hour Bayer Timed-Release Aspirin ▣ 566
Arthritis Strength Bufferin Analgesic Caplets 744
Extra Strength Bufferin Analgesic Tablets 745
Bufferin Analgesic Tablets and Caplets 743
Cama Arthritis Pain Reliever ▣ 685
Damason-P 1356
Easprin 1719
Ecotrin Enteric Coated Aspirin Maximum Strength Tablets and Caplets 2189
Ecotrin Enteric Coated Aspirin Regular Strength Tablets and Caplets 2189
Empirin Aspirin ▣ 541
Empirin with Codeine Phosphate Nos. 2, 3 & 4 764
Equagesic Tablets 2451
Excedrin Extra-Strength Analgesic Tablets & Caplets 749
4-Way Cold Tablets 750
Fiorinal Capsules 2007
Fiorinal with Codeine Capsules 2008
Fiorinal Tablets 2007
Lortab ASA Tablets 2414
Momentum Muscular Backache Formula ▣ 751
Norgesic 1314
Norwich Extra-Strength Aspirin ▣ 546
Norwich Regular Strength Aspirin ▣ 547
P-A-C Analgesic Tablets ▣ 669
Percodan 951
Robaxisal Tablets 1872
Sine-Off Sinus Medicine Tablets-Aspirin Formula ▣ 722
Soma Compound w/Codeine Tablets 2390
Soma Compound Tablets 2389
St. Joseph Adult Chewable Aspirin (81 mg.) ▣ 703
Synalgos-DC Capsules 2525
Talwin Compound 2072
Ursinus Inlay-Tabs ▣ 691
Vanquish Analgesic Caplets ▣ 574
Zorprin Tablets 698

Bleomycin Sulfate (Increased risk of toxicity). Products include:
Blenoxane 724

Dapsone (Increased risk of toxicity). Products include:
Dapsone USP 1130

Daunorubicin Hydrochloride (Increased risk of toxicity). Products include:
Cerubidine 2443

Doxorubicin Hydrochloride (Increased risk of toxicity). Products include:
Adriamycin PFS 561
Adriamycin RDF 562
Doxorubicin Hydrochloride for Injection, USP 622
Doxorubicin Hydrochloride Injection, USP 848
Rubex 739

Flucytosine (Increased risk of toxicity). Products include:
Ancobon Capsules 1886

Fluorouracil (Increased risk of toxicity). Products include:
Efudex 1880
Fluoroplex Topical Solution & Cream 1% 1082
Fluorouracil Injection 1897

Ganciclovir Sodium (May increase the potential for hematological toxicity). Products include:
Cytovene Sterile Powder 2292

Hydroxyurea (Increased risk of toxicity). Products include:
Hydrea Capsules 728

Indomethacin (Inhibits glucuronidation of Retrovir). Products include:
Indocin 1487

Indomethacin Sodium Trihydrate (Inhibits glucuronidation of Retrovir). Products include:
Indocin I.V. 1490

Interferon alfa-2A, Recombinant (Increased risk of toxicity). Products include:
Roferon-A Injection 1916

Interferon alfa-2B, Recombinant (Increased risk of toxicity). Products include:
Intron A 2097

Methotrexate Sodium (Increased risk of toxicity). Products include:
Methotrexate Tablets, Parenteral, LPF Parenteral 1217
Rheumatrex Methotrexate Dose Pack 1234

Mitotane (Increased risk of toxicity). Products include:
Lysodren 731

Mitoxantrone Hydrochloride (Increased risk of toxicity). Products include:
Novantrone for Injection Concentrate 1226

Nephrotoxic Drugs (Increased risk of toxicity).

Pentamidine Isethionate (Increased risk of toxicity). Products include:
NebuPent for Inhalation Solution 1017
Pentam 300 Injection 1018

Phenytoin (Possible alteration in the phenytoin plasma levels; low levels in some patients; high level documented in one case). Products include:
Dilantin Infatabs 1710
Dilantin-30 Pediatric/Dilantin-125 Suspension 1713

Phenytoin Sodium (Possible alteration in the phenytoin plasma levels; low levels in some patients; high level documented in one case). Products include:
Dilantin Kapseals 1708
Dilantin Parenteral 1712
Dilantin with Phenobarbital Kapseals 1715

Probenecid (Inhibits glucuronidation of Retrovir; may reduce renal excretion of Retrovir). Products include:
Benemid Tablets 1426
ColBENEMID Tablets 1436
Wycillin Injection and Probenecid Tablets 2539

Procarbazine Hydrochloride (Increased risk of toxicity). Products include:
Matulane Capsules 1907

Tamoxifen Citrate (Increased risk of toxicity). Products include:
Nolvadex Tablets 1102

Vinblastine Sulfate (Increased risk of toxicity). Products include:
Velban Vials 1305

Vincristine Sulfate (Increased risk of toxicity). Products include:
Oncovin Solution Vials & Hyporets 1288

RETROVIR I.V. INFUSION (Zidovudine) 805
May interact with nephrotoxic drugs, cytotoxic drugs, aspirin and acetaminophen containing products, experimental nucleoside analogues (selected) for AIDS and ARC, and certain

other agents. Compounds in these categories include:

Acetaminophen (May competitively inhibit glucuronidation; possible increased incidence of granulocytopenia). Products include:

Acetaminophen Uniserts Suppositories 2374
Actifed Plus Caplets ▣ 539
Actifed Plus Tablets ▣ 540
Alka-Seltzer Advanced Formula Antacid & Non-Aspirin Pain Reliever ▣ 620
Allerest ▣ 559
Aspirin Free Anacin Maximum Strength Acetaminophen Film Coated Caplets 2417
Aspirin Free Anacin Maximum Strength Acetaminophen Film Coated Tablets 2417
Anacin-3 Regular Strength Acetaminophen Film Coated Tablets ▣ 746
Anexsia 5/500 Tablets 2196
Anexsia 7.5/650 Tablets 2197
Benadryl Plus ▣ 636
Benadryl Plus Nighttime ▣ 637
Bufferin AF Nite Time Analgesic/Sleeping Aid Caplets 744
Allergy-Sinus Comtrex Multi-Symptom Allergy Sinus Formula Tablets & Caplets 746
Cough Formula Comtrex 746
Comtrex Multi-Symptom Cold Reliever Tablets/Caplets/Liqui-Gels/Liquid 745
Day-Night Comtrex 747
Non-Drowsy Comtrex 747
Congespirin For Children Aspirin Free Chewable Cold Tablets 748
Contac Cough & Sore Throat Formula ▣ 712
Contac Jr. Children's Cold Medicine ▣ 712
Contac Nighttime Cold Medicine ▣ 713
Contac Severe Cold and Flu Formula Caplets ▣ 711
Contac Sinus Caplets Maximum Strength Non-Drowsy Formula ▣ 710
Contac Sinus Tablets Maximum Strength Non-Drowsy Formula ▣ 710
Coricidin 'D' Decongestant Tablets ▣ 695
Coricidin Demilets Tablets for Children ▣ 696
Coricidin Tablets ▣ 695
Darvon-N/Darvocet-N 1254
Datril Extra-Strength Analgesic Tablets 748
Dimetapp Plus Caplets ▣ 675
Dorcol Children's Fever & Pain Reducer ▣ 686
Dristan Decongestant/Antihistamine/ Analgesic Coated Caplets ▣ 749
Dristan Cold Nasal Decongestant/ Antihistamine/ Analgesic Coated Tablets 2419
Dristan Advanced Formula Decongestant/Antihistamine/ Analgesic Tablets ▣ 749
Maximum Strength Dristan Decongestant/Analgesic Coated Caplets ▣ 750
No Drowsiness Dristan Cold Nasal Decongestant/Analgesic Coated Caplets 2420
Drixoral Plus Extended-Release Tablets ▣ 699
Drixoral Sinus ▣ 700
Esgic-Plus Tablets 1002
Esgic Tablets & Capsules 1001
Aspirin Free Excedrin Analgesic Caplets 748
Excedrin Extra-Strength Analgesic Tablets & Caplets 749
Excedrin P.M. Analgesic/Sleeping Aid Tablets, Caplets and Liquid 749
Sinus Excedrin Analgesic, Decongestant Tablets & Caplets 750
4-Way Cold Tablets 750
Feverall Sprinkle Caps 2374
Feverall Suppositories 2374
Fioricet Tablets 2006
Hycomine Compound Tablets 929
Hydrocet Capsules 835
Isocom Capsules 1629
Liquiprin ▣ 618
Lortab 2412
Lurline PMS Tablets 972
Medi-Flu Caplet, Liquid ▣ 640
Maximum Strength Midol Multi-Symptom Menstrual Formula ▣ 571
Maximum Strength Midol PMS Premenstrual Syndrome Formula ▣ 570
Regular Strength Midol Multi-Symptom Menstrual Formula ▣ 570
Midrin Capsules 836
Ornex Caplets ▣ 618
Children's Panadol Chewable Tablets, Liquid, Infants' Drops ▣ 571
Junior Strength Panadol ▣ 571
Maximum Strength Panadol Tablets and Caplets ▣ 572
Percocet Tablets 950
Percogesic Analgesic Tablets ▣ 660
Phenaphen with Codeine Capsules 1865
Phenaphen-650 with Codeine Tablets 1866
Phrenilin 838
Prēmsyn PMS Capsules & Caplets ▣ 547
Pyrroxate Capsules ▣ 669
Robitussin Night Relief ▣ 677
Sedapap Tablets 50 mg/650 mg 1360
Sinarest ▣ 562
Sine-Aid Maximum Strength Sinus Headache Caplets 1365
Sine-Aid Maximum Strength Sinus Headache Tablets 1365
Sine-Off Maximum Strength Allergy/Sinus Formula Caplets ▣ 721
Sine-Off Maximum Strength No Drowsiness Formula Caplets ▣ 722
Singlet Tablets ▣ 598
Sinulin 840
Sinutab Maximum Strength ▣ 641
Sinutab Maximum Strength Without Drowsiness Tablets & Caplets ▣ 642
Sinutab Regular Strength Without Drowsiness Formula ▣ 641
Sominex Pain Relief Formula ▣ 723
St. Joseph Aspirin-Free Fever Reducer for Children Chewable Tablets, Liquid & Infant Drops ▣ 704
St. Joseph Cold Tablets for Children ▣ 704
St. Joseph Nighttime Cold Medicine ▣ 705
Sudafed Sinus Caplets ▣ 545
Sudafed Sinus Tablets ▣ 545
Talacen 2070
Tempra, Acetaminophen ▣ 613
TheraFlu Flu and Cold Medicine ▣ 687
Triaminicin Tablets ▣ 690
Tylenol acetaminophen Children's Chewable Tablets & Elixir 1366
Tylenol Allergy Sinus Medication Caplets and Gelcaps, Maximum Strength 1372
Tylenol with Codeine 1381
Children's Tylenol Cold Liquid Formula and Chewable Tablets 1368
Tylenol Cold & Flu Hot Medication, Packets 1369
Tylenol Cold & Flu No Drowsiness Hot Medication, Packets 1371
Tylenol Cold Medication Caplets and Tablets 1370
Tylenol Cold Medication, Effervescent Tablets 1369
Tylenol Cold Medication No Drowsiness Formula Caplets 1370
Tylenol Cold Night Time Medication Liquid 1371
Tylenol Cough Medication Liquid, Maximum Strength 1372
Tylenol Cough Medication Liquid with Decongestant, Maximum Strength 1372
Tylenol, Extra Strength, acetaminophen Adult Liquid Pain Reliever 1367
Tylenol, Extra Strength, acetaminophen Gelcaps, Caplets, Tablets 1367
Tylenol, Infants' Drops 1366
Tylenol, Junior Strength, acetaminophen Coated Caplets, Grape and Fruit Chewable Tablets 1366
Tylenol, Maximum Strength, Sinus Medication Gelcaps, Caplets and Tablets 1373
Tylenol, Regular Strength, acetaminophen Tablets and Caplets 1367
Tylenol PM, Extra Strength Caplets and Tablets 1368
Tylox Capsules 1382
Unisom Dual Relief Nighttime Sleep Aid/Analgesic 1774
Vanquish Analgesic Caplets ▣ 574
Vicks Daycare ▣ 660
Vicks Formula 44M Multi-Symptom Cough Medicine ▣ 662
Vicks NyQuil Nighttime Colds Medicine-Original & Cherry Flavor ▣ 664
Vicodin Tablets 1187
Vicodin ES Tablets 1189
Wygesic Tablets 2540
Zydone Capsules 941

Acyclovir (One published report of neurotoxicity (profound lethargy) associated with concomitant use; may increase the potential for hematological toxicity). Products include:

Zovirax Capsules 824
Zovirax Ointment 5% 827
Zovirax 824

Acyclovir Sodium (One published report of neurotoxicity (profound lethargy) associated with concomitant use; may increase the potential for hematological toxicity). Products include:

Zovirax Sterile Powder 828

Amphotericin B (Increased risk of toxicity). Products include:

Fungizone Cream, Lotion and Ointment 2261
Fungizone Intravenous 2262

Aspirin (May competitively inhibit glucuronidation; possible increased incidence of granulocytopenia). Products include:

Alka-Seltzer Effervescent Antacid and Pain Reliever 1568
Alka-Seltzer Extra Strength Effervescent Antacid and Pain Reliever 1570
Alka-Seltzer (Flavored) Effervescent Antacid and Pain Reliever 1569
Alka-Seltzer Plus Cold Medicine ▣ 623
Alka-Seltzer Plus Night-Time Cold Medicine ▣ 623
Alka Seltzer Plus Sinus Allergy Medicine ▣ 624
Anacin Coated Analgesic Caplets 2417
Anacin Coated Analgesic Tablets 2417
Anacin Maximum Strength Analgesic Coated Tablets 2417
Maximum Strength Arthritis Pain Formula By the Makers of Anacin Analgesic Tablets and Caplets 2418
Arthritis Pain Formula by the Makers of Anacin Analgesic Tablets and Caplets ▣ 747
Arthritis Strength BC Powder ▣ 516
Ascriptin A/D Caplets 1850
Regular Strength Ascriptin Tablets 1850
Azdōne Tablets 844
BC Powder ▣ 517
BC Cold Powder ▣ 517
Children's Bayer Chewable Aspirin ▣ 564
Genuine Bayer Aspirin Tablets & Caplets ▣ 564
Maximum Bayer Aspirin Tablets & Caplets ▣ 566
Bayer Plus Aspirin Tablets ▣ 567
Therapy Bayer Aspirin Caplets ▣ 568
8 Hour Bayer Timed-Release Aspirin ▣ 566
Arthritis Strength Bufferin Analgesic Caplets 744
Extra Strength Bufferin Analgesic Tablets 745
Bufferin Analgesic Tablets and Caplets 743
Cama Arthritis Pain Reliever ▣ 685
Damason-P 1356
Easprin 1719
Ecotrin Enteric Coated Aspirin Maximum Strength Tablets and Caplets 2189
Ecotrin Enteric Coated Aspirin Regular Strength Tablets and Caplets 2189
Empirin Aspirin ▣ 541
Empirin with Codeine Phosphate Nos. 2, 3 & 4 764
Equagesic Tablets 2451
Excedrin Extra-Strength Analgesic Tablets & Caplets 749
4-Way Cold Tablets 750
Fiorinal Capsules 2007
Fiorinal with Codeine Capsules 2008
Fiorinal Tablets 2007
Lortab ASA Tablets 2414
Momentum Muscular Backache Formula ▣ 751
Norgesic 1314
Norwich Extra-Strength Aspirin ▣ 546
Norwich Regular Strength Aspirin ▣ 547
P-A-C Analgesic Tablets ▣ 669
Percodan 951
Robaxisal Tablets 1872
Sine-Off Sinus Medicine Tablets-Aspirin Formula ▣ 722
Soma Compound w/Codeine Tablets 2390
Soma Compound Tablets 2389
St. Joseph Adult Chewable Aspirin (81 mg.) ▣ 703
Synalgos-DC Capsules 2525
Talwin Compound 2072
Ursinus Inlay-Tabs ▣ 691
Vanquish Analgesic Caplets ▣ 574
Zorprin Tablets 698

Bleomycin Sulfate (Increased risk of toxicity). Products include:

Blenoxane 724

Dapsone (Increased risk of toxicity). Products include:

Dapsone USP 1130

Daunorubicin Hydrochloride (Increased risk of toxicity). Products include:

Cerubidine 2443

Doxorubicin Hydrochloride (Increased risk of toxicity). Products include:

Adriamycin PFS 561
Adriamycin RDF 562
Doxorubicin Hydrochloride for Injection, USP 622
Doxorubicin Hydrochloride Injection, USP 848
Rubex 739

Flucytosine (Increased risk of toxicity). Products include:

Ancobon Capsules 1886

Fluorouracil (Increased risk of toxicity). Products include:

Efudex 1880
Fluoroplex Topical Solution & Cream 1% 1082
Fluorouracil Injection 1897

Ganciclovir Sodium (May increase the potential for hematological toxicity). Products include:

Cytovene Sterile Powder 2292

Hydroxyurea (Increased risk of toxicity). Products include:

Hydrea Capsules 728

Indomethacin (May competitively inhibit glucuronidation). Products include:

Indocin 1487

Indomethacin Sodium Trihydrate (May competitively inhibit glucuronidation). Products include:

Indocin I.V. 1490

Interferon alfa-2A, Recombinant (Increased risk of toxicity). Products include:

Roferon-A Injection 1916

Interferon alfa-2B, Recombinant (Increased risk of toxicity). Products include:

Intron A 2097

Methotrexate Sodium (Increased risk of toxicity). Products include:

Methotrexate Tablets, Parenteral, LPF Parenteral 1217
Rheumatrex Methotrexate Dose Pack 1234

Mitotane (Increased risk of toxicity). Products include:

Lysodren 731

Mitoxantrone Hydrochloride (Increased risk of toxicity). Products include:

Novantrone for Injection Concentrate 1226

Nephrotoxic Drugs (Increased risk of toxicity).

Pentamidine Isethionate (Increased risk of toxicity). Products include:
- NebuPent for Inhalation Solution 1017
- Pentam 300 Injection 1018

Phenytoin (Low phenytoin levels reported in some patients; high level documented in one case). Products include:
- Dilantin Infatabs 1710
- Dilantin-30 Pediatric/Dilantin-125 Suspension 1713

Phenytoin Sodium (Low phenytoin levels reported in some patients; high level documented in one case). Products include:
- Dilantin Kapseals 1708
- Dilantin Parenteral 1712
- Dilantin with Phenobarbital Kapseals 1715

Probenecid (May inhibit glucuronidation and/or reduce renal excretion of zidovudine). Products include:
- Benemid Tablets 1426
- ColBENEMID Tablets 1436
- Wycillin Injection and Probenecid Tablets 2539

Procarbazine Hydrochloride (Increased risk of toxicity). Products include:
- Matulane Capsules 1907

Tamoxifen Citrate (Increased risk of toxicity). Products include:
- Nolvadex Tablets 1102

Vinblastine Sulfate (Increased risk of toxicity). Products include:
- Velban Vials 1305

Vincristine Sulfate (Increased risk of toxicity). Products include:
- Oncovin Solution Vials & Hyporets 1288

RETROVIR SYRUP
(Zidovudine) 802
See **Retrovir Capsules**

RĒV-EYES OPHTHALMIC EYEDROPS 0.5%
(Dapiprazole Hydrochloride) .... ⊙ 312
No interactions described in labeling.

RHEABAN MAXIMUM STRENGTH TABLETS
(Attapulgite, Activated) .... ▣ 644
No interactions described in labeling.

RHEUMATREX METHOTREXATE DOSE PACK
(Methotrexate Sodium) 1234
See **Methotrexate Tablets, Parenteral, LPF Parenteral**

RHOGAM RH_0(D) IMMUNE GLOBULIN (HUMAN)
(Immune Globulin (Human)) 1651
No interactions described in labeling.

RHULICREAM
(Benzocaine, Calamine) .... ▣ 684
No interactions described in labeling.

RHULIGEL
(Benzyl Alcohol, Camphor, Menthol) .... ▣ 684
No interactions described in labeling.

RHULISPRAY
(Benzocaine, Calamine, Camphor, Isopropyl Alcohol, Menthol) .... ▣ 684
No interactions described in labeling.

RICELYTE, RICE-BASED ORAL ELECTROLYTE MAINTENANCE SOLUTION
(Electrolyte Supplement) .... ▣ 613
No interactions described in labeling.

RIDAURA CAPSULES
(Auranofin) 2224
May interact with:

Phenytoin (Increased phenytoin blood levels). Products include:
- Dilantin Infatabs 1710
- Dilantin-30 Pediatric/Dilantin-125 Suspension 1713

Phenytoin Sodium (Increased phenytoin blood levels). Products include:
- Dilantin Kapseals 1708
- Dilantin Parenteral 1712
- Dilantin with Phenobarbital Kapseals 1715

RIFADIN CAPSULES
(Rifampin) 1345
May interact with oral anticoagulants, corticosteroids, cardiac glycosides, oral contraceptives, oral hypoglycemic agents, narcotic analgesics, barbiturates, beta blockers, anticonvulsants, xanthine bronchodilators, progestins, and certain other agents. Compounds in these categories include:

Acebutolol Hydrochloride (Diminished effects of concurrently administered beta blocker). Products include:
- Sectral Capsules 2520

Alfentanil Hydrochloride (Reduced activity of narcotics). Products include:
- Alfenta Injection 1131

Aminophylline (Diminished effects of concurrently administered theophylline). Products include:
- Amesec .... ▣ 682
- Aminophyllin Tablets 2153

Aprobarbital (Diminished effects of concurrently administered barbiturate). Products include:
- Alurate Elixir 1883

Atenolol (Diminished effects of concurrently administered beta blocker). Products include:
- Tenoretic Tablets 1105
- Tenormin Tablets and I.V. Injection 1107

Betamethasone Acetate (Reduced activity of corticosteroid). Products include:
- Celestone Soluspan Suspension 2081

Betamethasone Sodium Phosphate (Reduced activity of corticosteroid). Products include:
- Celestone Soluspan Suspension 2081

Betaxolol Hydrochloride (Diminished effects of concurrently administered beta blocker). Products include:
- Betoptic Sterile Ophthalmic Solution 569
- Betoptic S Sterile Ophthalmic Suspension 570
- Kerlone Tablets 2172

Buprenorphine (Reduced activity of narcotics).
No products indexed under this heading.

Butabarbital (Diminished effects of concurrently administered barbiturate). Products include:
- Pyridium Plus 1764

Butalbital (Diminished effects of concurrently administered barbiturate). Products include:
- Esgic-Plus Tablets 1002
- Esgic Tablets & Capsules 1001
- Fioricet Tablets 2006
- Fiorinal Capsules 2007
- Fiorinal with Codeine Capsules 2008
- Fiorinal Tablets 2007
- Phrenilin 838
- Sedapap Tablets 50 mg/650 mg .. 1360

Carbamazepine (Diminished effects of concurrently administered anticonvulsant). Products include:
- Tegretol Chewable Tablets 654
- Tegretol Suspension 656
- Tegretol Tablets 654

Carteolol Hydrochloride (Diminished effects of concurrently administered beta blocker). Products include:
- Cartrol Tablets 507

Chloramphenicol (Diminished effects of concurrently administered chloramphenicol). Products include:
- AK-Chlor Sterile Ophthalmic Ointment & Solution .... ⊙ 201
- Chloromycetin Cream, 1% 1694
- Chloromycetin Hydrocortisone Ophthalmic 1694
- Chloromycetin Kapseals 1695
- Chloromycetin Ophthalmic Ointment, 1% 1696
- Chloromycetin Ophthalmic Solution 1696
- Chloromycetin Otic 1697
- Chloroptic S.O.P. .... ⊙ 243
- Chloroptic Sterile Ophthalmic Solution .... ⊙ 243
- Ophthochlor Ophthalmic Solution ⊙ 300
- Ophthocort .... ⊙ 301

Chloramphenicol Palmitate (Diminished effects of concurrently administered chloramphenicol). Products include:
- Chloromycetin Palmitate, Oral Suspension 1697

Chloramphenicol Sodium Succinate (Diminished effects of concurrently administered chloramphenicol). Products include:
- Chloromycetin Sodium Succinate.... 1698

Chlorpropamide (Reduced activity of oral hypoglycemic agent). Products include:
- Diabinese Tablets 1775

Clofibrate (Diminished effects of concurrently administered clofibrate). Products include:
- Atromid-S Capsules 2435

Codeine (Reduced activity of narcotics). Products include:
- Calcidrine Syrup 506

Codeine Phosphate (Reduced activity of narcotics). Products include:
- Actifed with Codeine Cough Syrup.. 752
- Cheracol Cough Syrup 1853
- Codimal PH Syrup 846
- Dimetane-DC Cough Syrup 1857
- Empirin with Codeine Phosphate Nos. 2, 3 & 4 764
- Fiorinal with Codeine Capsules 2008
- Isoclor Expectorant 982
- Naldecon CX Adult Liquid .... ▣ 521
- Novahistine DH 1342
- Novahistine Expectorant 1343
- Nucofed Capsules 2219
- Nucofed Expectorant 2219
- Nucofed Pediatric Expectorant 2220
- Nucofed Syrup 2219
- Phenaphen with Codeine Capsules 1865
- Phenaphen-650 with Codeine Tablets 1866
- Phenergan with Codeine 2497
- Phenergan VC with Codeine 2501
- Robitussin A-C Syrup 1875
- Robitussin-DAC Syrup 1875
- Ryna .... ▣ 741
- Soma Compound w/Codeine Tablets 2390
- Triaminic Expectorant w/Codeine .. 1996
- Tussi-Organidin Liquid 2391
- Tylenol with Codeine 1381

Codeine Polistirex (Reduced activity of narcotics).
No products indexed under this heading.

Cortisone Acetate (Reduced activity of corticosteroid). Products include:
- Cortone Acetate Sterile Suspension 1437
- Cortone Acetate Tablets 1439

Cyclosporine (Reduced activity of cyclosporin). Products include:
- Sandimmune 2024

Dapsone (Reduced activity of dapsone). Products include:
- Dapsone USP 1130

Deslanoside (Reduced activity of cardiac glycoside).
No products indexed under this heading.

Dexamethasone (Reduced activity of corticosteroid). Products include:
- AK-Trol Ointment & Suspension .... ⊙ 207
- Decadron Elixir 1445
- Decadron Tablets 1447
- Decaspray Topical Aerosol 1459
- Dexacidin .... ⊙ 272
- Maxidex Sterile Ophthalmic Suspension .... ⊙ 223
- Maxitrol Ophthalmic Ointment/Suspension .... ⊙ 223
- TobraDex Ophthalmic Suspension and Ointment .... ⊙ 228

Dexamethasone Acetate (Reduced activity of corticosteroid). Products include:
- Dalalone D.P. Injectable 999
- Decadron-LA Sterile Suspension...... 1457

Dexamethasone Sodium Phosphate (Reduced activity of corticosteroid). Products include:
- AK-Dex .... ⊙ 203
- Decadron Phosphate Respihaler...... 1454
- Decadron Phosphate Sterile Ophthalmic Ointment 1453
- Decadron Phosphate Sterile Ophthalmic Solution 1453
- Decadron Phosphate Topical Cream 1455
- Decadron Phosphate Turbinaire 1456
- Maxidex Sterile Ophthalmic Ointment .... ⊙ 222
- NeoDecadron Sterile Ophthalmic Ointment 1517
- NeoDecadron Sterile Ophthalmic Solution 1518
- NeoDecadron Topical Cream 1518

Dezocine (Reduced activity of narcotics).

Diazepam (Diminished effects of concurrently administered diazepam). Products include:
- Valium Injectable 1937
- Valium Tablets 1939
- Valrelease Capsules 1923

Dicumarol (Reduced activity of anticoagulant). Products include:
- Dicumarol Tablets 516

Digitoxin (Reduced activity of cardiac glycoside). Products include:
- Crystodigin Tablets 1253

Digoxin (Reduced activity of cardiac glycoside). Products include:
- Lanoxicaps 772
- Lanoxin Elixir Pediatric 775
- Lanoxin Injection 778
- Lanoxin Injection Pediatric 781
- Lanoxin Tablets 783

Disopyramide Phosphate (Diminished effects of concurrently administered disopyramide). Products include:
- Norpace 2177

Divalproex Sodium (Diminished effects of concurrently administered anticonvulsant). Products include:
- Depakote 512

Dyphylline (Diminished effects of concurrently administered theophylline). Products include:
- Dilor 2079
- Dilor-G Tablets & Liquid 2079
- Lufyllin Elixir 2384
- Lufyllin & Lufyllin-400 Tablets 2384
- Lufyllin-GG Elixir & Tablets 2385

Esmolol Hydrochloride (Diminished effects of concurrently administered beta blocker). Products include:
- Brevibloc Injection 942

Ethinyl Estradiol (Reduced activity of oral contraceptives). Products include:
- Brevicon 2304
- Demulen 2161
- Estinyl Tablets 2085
- Jenest-28 Tablets 1636
- Levlen/Tri-Levlen 665
- Lo/Ovral Tablets 2471
- Lo/Ovral-28 Tablets 2476
- Loestrin 1728
- Modicon 1667
- Nordette-21 Tablets 2481
- Nordette-28 Tablets 2483
- Norethin 2133
- Norinyl 2304
- Norlestrin 1746
- Ortho-Cyclen Tablets 1658
- Ortho-Novum 1667
- Ovcon 1391
- Ovral Tablets 2490
- Ovral-28 Tablets 2491
- Levlen/Tri-Levlen 665
- Tri-Norinyl 2304
- Triphasil-21 Tablets 2527
- Triphasil-28 Tablets 2532

Ethosuximide (Diminished effects of concurrently administered anticonvulsant). Products include:
- Zarontin Capsules 1768
- Zarontin Syrup 1769

Ethotoin (Diminished effects of concurrently administered anticonvulsant). Products include:
- Peganone Tablets 551

Ethynodiol Diacetate (Reduced activity of oral contraceptives). Products include:
- Demulen 2161

Fentanyl (Reduced activity of narcotics). Products include:
- Duragesic Transdermal System 1133

Fentanyl Citrate (Reduced activity of narcotics). Products include:
- Innovar Injection 1141
- Sublimaze Injection 1146

Glipizide (Reduced activity of oral hypoglycemic agent). Products include:
- Glucotrol 1952

Glyburide (Reduced activity of oral hypoglycemic agent). Products include:
- DiaBeta 1091
- Micronase Tablets 2350

Halothane (Increased hepatotoxicity of both drugs). Products include:
- Fluothane 2453

Hydrocodone Bitartrate (Reduced activity of narcotics). Products include:
- Anexsia 5/500 Tablets 2196
- Anexsia 7.5/650 Tablets 2197
- Azdone Tablets 844
- Codiclear DH Syrup 845
- Codimal DH Syrup 846
- Damason-P 1356
- Hycodan Syrup, Tablets 927
- Hycomine Compound Tablets 929
- Hycomine Syrup 927
- Hycotuss Expectorant Syrup 930
- Hydrocet Capsules 835
- Lortab ASA Tablets 2414
- Lortab 2412
- Ru-Tuss with Hydrocodone 694
- Triaminic Expectorant DH 1995
- Vicodin Tablets 1187
- Vicodin ES Tablets 1189
- Zydone Capsules 941

Hydrocodone Polistirex (Reduced activity of narcotics). Products include:
- Tussionex Extended-Release Suspension 988

Hydrocortisone (Reduced activity of corticosteroid). Products include:
- AK-Spore H.C. .... ◉ 206
- Bactine Hydrocortisone Anti-Itch Cream .... ▣ 625
- CaldeCORT Anti-Itch Hydrocortisone Spray .... ▣ 560
- Carmol HC Cream 1% 2296
- Cortaid Spray .... ▣ 735
- Cortenema 2244
- Cortisporin Ointment 758
- Cortisporin Ophthalmic Ointment Sterile 758
- Cortisporin Ophthalmic Suspension Sterile 759
- Cortisporin Otic Solution Sterile 760
- Cortisporin Otic Suspension Sterile 760
- Cortizone-5 Creme & Ointment .... ▣ 732
- Dermolate Anti-Itch Cream .... ▣ 697
- Eldecort Cream 1.0% 1113
- Eldecort Cream 1.0% and 2.5% 1113
- Fungoid HC Creme 1770
- Hydrocortone Tablets 1482
- Hytone 909
- LazerSporin-C Solution 1770
- Massengill Medicated Soft Cloth Towelettes 2192
- Nutracort Cream & Lotion 1684
- PediOtic Suspension Sterile 797
- Synacort Creams 1%, 2.5% 2296
- Vanoxide-HC Acne Lotion 911
- Vioform-Hydrocortisone Cream and Mild Cream 889
- Vioform-Hydrocortisone Ointment 889
- VōSoL HC Otic Solution 2392
- Vytone Cream 1% 911

Hydrocortisone Acetate (Reduced activity of corticosteroid). Products include:
- Analpram-HC Rectal Cream 1% and 2.5% 970
- Anusol-HC Cream 1690
- Anusol-HC Suppositories 1691
- Caldecort .... ▣ 560
- Carmol HC Cream 1% 2296
- Chloromycetin Hydrocortisone Ophthalmic 1694
- Coly-Mycin S Otic w/Neomycin & Hydrocortisone 1708
- Cortaid .... ▣ 735
- Cortef Feminine Itch Cream .... ▣ 735
- Corticaine .... ▣ 682
- Cortifoam 1827
- Cortisporin Cream 757
- Epifoam 1828
- Gynecort 5 Creme .... ▣ 556
- Hydrocortone Acetate Sterile Suspension 1479
- Lanacort 5 Creme and Ointment .... ▣ 557
- Mantadil Cream 789
- Ophthocort .... ◉ 301
- Orabase HCA Oral Paste 890
- Pramosone Cream, Lotion & Ointment 971
- ProctoCream-HC 1834
- Proctofoam-HC 1835

Hydrocortisone Sodium Phosphate (Reduced activity of corticosteroid). Products include:
- Hydrocortone Phosphate Injection, Sterile 1481

Hydrocortisone Sodium Succinate (Reduced activity of corticosteroid). Products include:
- Solu-Cortef Sterile Powder 2361

Ketoconazole (Diminished serum concentrations of both drugs). Products include:
- Nizoral 2% Cream 1143
- Nizoral 2% Shampoo 1144
- Nizoral Tablets 1145

Labetalol Hydrochloride (Diminished effects of concurrently administered beta blocker). Products include:
- Normodyne Injection 2108
- Normodyne Tablets 2110
- Normozide Tablets 2112
- Trandate HCT Tablets 579
- Trandate Injection 577
- Trandate Tablets 579

Levonorgestrel (Reduced activity of oral contraceptives). Products include:
- Levlen/Tri-Levlen 665
- Nordette-21 Tablets 2481
- Nordette-28 Tablets 2483
- Norplant System 2484
- Levlen/Tri-Levlen 665
- Triphasil-21 Tablets 2527
- Triphasil-28 Tablets 2532

Levorphanol Tartrate (Reduced activity of narcotics). Products include:
- Levo-Dromoran 1906

Medroxyprogesterone Acetate (Diminished effects of concurrently administered progestin). Products include:
- Amen 833
- Cycrin Tablets 2449
- Depo-Provera Sterile Aqueous Suspension 2336
- Provera Tablets 2356

Megestrol Acetate (Diminished effects of concurrently administered progestin). Products include:
- Megace Tablets 732

Meperidine Hydrochloride (Reduced activity of narcotics). Products include:
- Demerol 2047
- Mepergan Injection 2479

Mephenytoin (Diminished effects of concurrently administered anticonvulsant). Products include:
- Mesantoin Tablets 2013

Mephobarbital (Diminished effects of concurrently administered barbiturate). Products include:
- Mebaral Tablets 2061

Mestranol (Reduced activity of oral contraceptives). Products include:
- Enovid 2161
- Norethin 2133
- Norinyl 2304
- Ortho-Novum 1667

Methadone Hydrochloride (Diminished effects of concurrently administered methadone; reduced activity of narcotics). Products include:
- Dolophine Hydrochloride Ampoules & Vials 1260
- Dolophine Hydrochloride Tablets 1261
- Methadone Hydrochloride Diskets 1284
- Methadone Hydrochloride Oral Solution & Tablets 1987

Methsuximide (Diminished effects of concurrently administered anticonvulsant). Products include:
- Celontin 1692

Methylprednisolone Acetate (Reduced activity of corticosteroid). Products include:
- Depo-Medrol Sterile Aqueous Suspension 2334

Methylprednisolone Sodium Succinate (Reduced activity of corticosteroid). Products include:
- Solu-Medrol Sterile Powder 2363

Metoprolol Tartrate (Diminished effects of concurrently administered beta blocker). Products include:
- Lopressor Ampuls 1032
- Lopressor HCT Tablets 1034
- Lopressor Tablets 1032

Mexiletine Hydrochloride (Diminished effects of concurrently administered mexiletine). Products include:
- Mexitil Capsules 680

Morphine Sulfate (Reduced activity of narcotics). Products include:
- Astramorph/PF Injection, USP (Preservative-Free) 618
- Duramorph 960
- Infumorph 200 and Infumorph 500 Sterile Solutions 962
- MS Contin Tablets 1814
- MSIR 1817
- Oramorph SR (Morphine Sulfate Sustained Release Tablets) 1988
- Roxanol 1991

Nadolol (Diminished effects of concurrently administered beta blocker). Products include:
- Corgard Tablets 701
- Corzide Tablets 702

Norethindrone (Reduced activity of oral contraceptives). Products include:
- Brevicon 2304
- Jenest-28 Tablets 1636
- Micronor Tablets 1667
- Modicon 1667
- Norethin 2133
- Norinyl 2304
- Norlutin 1755
- Nor-Q D Tablets 2304
- Ortho-Novum 1667
- Ovcon 1391
- Tri-Norinyl 2304

Norethynodrel (Reduced activity of oral contraceptives). Products include:
- Enovid 2161

Norgestimate (Reduced activity of oral contraceptives). Products include:
- Ortho-Cyclen Tablets 1658

Norgestrel (Reduced activity of oral contraceptives). Products include:
- Lo/Ovral Tablets 2471
- Lo/Ovral-28 Tablets 2476
- Ovral Tablets 2490
- Ovral-28 Tablets 2491
- Ovrette Tablets 2492

Opium Alkaloids (Reduced activity of narcotics). Products include:
- B & O No. 15A & No. 16A Supprettes 2395
- Pantopon Injectable 1911

Oxycodone Hydrochloride (Reduced activity of narcotics). Products include:
- Percocet Tablets 950
- Percodan 951
- Roxicodone Tablets, Oral Solution & Intensol (Oxycodone) 1992
- Tylox Capsules 1382

Para-Aminosalicylic Acid (Decreases serum rifampin levels).

Paramethadione (Diminished effects of concurrently administered anticonvulsant). Products include:
- Paradione Capsules 548

Penbutolol Sulfate (Diminished effects of concurrently administered beta blocker). Products include:
- Levatol 1832

Pentobarbital Sodium (Diminished effects of concurrently administered barbiturate). Products include:
- Nembutal Sodium Capsules 534
- Nembutal Sodium Solution 536
- Nembutal Sodium Suppositories 538

Phenacemide (Diminished effects of concurrently administered anticonvulsant). Products include:
- Phenurone Tablets 552

Phenobarbital (Diminished effects of concurrently administered barbiturate). Products include:
- Arco-Lase Plus Tablets 607
- Bellergal-S Tablets 1998
- Bronkolixir .... ▣ 761
- Bronkotabs Tablets .... ▣ 762
- Donnatal 1858
- Donnatal Extentabs 1859
- Donnatal Tablets 1858
- Donnazyme Tablets 1860
- Kinesed Tablets 2272
- Phenobarbital Elixir and Tablets 1293
- Primatene Tablets-P Formula 2421
- Quadrinal Tablets 1183
- Tedral SA 1765

Phensuximide (Diminished effects of concurrently administered anticonvulsant). Products include:
- Milontin Kapseals 1741

Phenytoin (Diminished effects of concurrently administered anticonvulsant). Products include:
- Dilantin Infatabs 1710
- Dilantin-30 Pediatric/Dilantin-125 Suspension 1713

Phenytoin Sodium (Diminished effects of concurrently administered anticonvulsant). Products include:
- Dilantin Kapseals 1708
- Dilantin Parenteral 1712
- Dilantin with Phenobarbital Kapseals 1715

Pindolol (Diminished effects of concurrently administered beta blocker). Products include:
- Visken Tablets ... 2036

Prednisolone Acetate (Reduced activity of corticosteroid). Products include:
- AK-Cide Sterile Ophthalmic Ointment & Suspension ... ◉ 202
- Blephamide Liquifilm Sterile Ophthalmic Suspension ... 586
- Blephamide S.O.P. Sterile Ophthalmic Ointment ... 586
- Cetapred Ointment ... ◉ 220
- ⅛% Econopred & 1% Econopred Plus ... ◉ 217
- Isopto Cetapred Suspension ... ◉ 220
- Metimyd ... ◉ 306
- Poly-Pred Liquifilm ... ◉ 250
- Pred Forte ... ◉ 252
- Pred Mild ... ◉ 254
- Pred-G Liquifilm Sterile Ophthalmic Suspension ... ◉ 252
- Pred-G S.O.P. Sterile Ophthalmic Ointment ... ◉ 253
- Vasocidin Ointment ... ◉ 275

Prednisolone Sodium Phosphate (Reduced activity of corticosteroid). Products include:
- AK-Pred ... ◉ 205
- Hydeltrasol Injection, Sterile ... 1476
- Inflamase ... ◉ 274
- Pediapred Oral Liquid ... 987
- Vasocidin Ophthalmic Solution ... ◉ 276

Prednisolone Tebutate (Reduced activity of corticosteroid). Products include:
- Hydeltra-T.B.A. Sterile Suspension 1478

Prednisone (Reduced activity of corticosteroid). Products include:
- Deltasone Tablets ... 2332

Primidone (Diminished effects of concurrently administered anticonvulsant). Products include:
- Mysoline ... 2480

Probenecid (Increases rifampin blood levels). Products include:
- Benemid Tablets ... 1426
- ColBENEMID Tablets ... 1436
- Wycillin Injection and Probenecid Tablets ... 2539

Propoxyphene Hydrochloride (Reduced activity of narcotics). Products include:
- Darvon ... 1256
- Wygesic Tablets ... 2540

Propoxyphene Napsylate (Reduced activity of narcotics). Products include:
- Darvon-N/Darvocet-N ... 1254

Propranolol Hydrochloride (Diminished effects of concurrently administered beta blocker). Products include:
- Inderal ... 2459
- Inderal LA Long Acting Capsules ... 2461
- Inderide Tablets ... 2463
- Inderide LA Long Acting Capsules .. 2465

Quinidine Gluconate (Reduced activity of quinidine). Products include:
- Quinaglute Dura-Tabs Tablets ... 663

Quinidine Polygalacturonate (Reduced activity of quinidine). Products include:
- Cardioquin Tablets ... 1812

Quinidine Sulfate (Reduced activity of quinidine). Products include:
- Quinidex Extentabs ... 1868

Secobarbital Sodium (Diminished effects of concurrently administered barbiturate). Products include:
- Seconal Sodium Pulvules ... 1296

Sufentanil Citrate (Reduced activity of narcotics). Products include:
- Sufenta Injection ... 1147

Theophylline (Diminished effects of concurrently administered theophylline). Products include:
- Bronkaid Tablets ... ▣ 757
- Bronkolixir ... ▣ 761
- Bronkotabs Tablets ... ▣ 762
- Constant-T Tablets ... 1029
- Marax Tablets & DF Syrup ... 1954
- Primatene Tablets ... 2421
- Quibron Capsules ... 713
- Quibron-T ... 714
- Quibron-T/SR ... 716
- Theolair Liquid ... 1317
- Theo-Organidin Elixir ... 2391

Theophylline Anhydrous (Diminished effects of concurrently administered theophylline). Products include:
- Aerolate ... 994
- Primatene Tablets-M Formula ... ▣ 753
- Primatene Tablets-Regular Formula ... 2421
- Respbid Tablets ... 684
- Slo-bid Gyrocaps ... 1847
- T-PHYL (Uniphyl) 200 mg Tablets 1820
- Tedral SA ... 1765
- Theo-24 ... 2179
- Theo-Dur Sprinkle ... 1168
- Theo-Dur Extended-Release Tablets ... 1166
- Theolair Tablets ... 1317
- Theolair-SR Tablets ... 1319
- TheoX Extended-Release Tablets ... 841
- Uniphyl 400 mg Tablets ... 1823

Theophylline Calcium Salicylate (Diminished effects of concurrently administered theophylline). Products include:
- Quadrinal Tablets ... 1183

Theophylline Sodium Glycinate (Diminished effects of concurrently administered theophylline). Products include:
- Asbron G ... 1997

Thiamylal Sodium (Diminished effects of concurrently administered barbiturate). Products include:
- Surital Ampoules, Steri-Vials ... 1764

Timolol Maleate (Diminished effects of concurrently administered beta blocker). Products include:
- Blocadren Tablets ... 1429
- Timolide Tablets ... 1547
- Timoptic in Ocudose ... 1552
- Timoptic Sterile Ophthalmic Solution ... 1550

Tolazamide (Reduced activity of oral hypoglycemic agent). Products include:
- Tolinase Tablets ... 2365

Tolbutamide (Reduced activity of oral hypoglycemic agent). Products include:
- Orinase Tablets ... 2354

Triamcinolone (Reduced activity of corticosteroid).
- No products indexed under this heading.

Triamcinolone Acetonide (Reduced activity of corticosteroid). Products include:
- Aristocort A ... 1010
- Azmacort Inhaler ... 1837
- Kenalog Cream, Lotion & Ointment 2401
- Kenalog-10 Injection ... 2402
- Kenalog-40 Injection ... 2403
- Kenalog in Orabase ... 604
- Kenalog Spray ... 2401
- Mycolog II Cream and Ointment ... 2407
- Mytrex Cream & Ointment ... 2080
- Nasacort Nasal Inhaler ... 1844

Triamcinolone Diacetate (Reduced activity of corticosteroid). Products include:
- Aristocort Suspension ... 1008

Triamcinolone Hexacetonide (Reduced activity of corticosteroid). Products include:
- Aristospan Suspension ... 1011

Trimethadione (Diminished effects of concurrently administered anticonvulsant). Products include:
- Tridione ... 557

Valproic Acid (Diminished effects of concurrently administered anticonvulsant). Products include:
- Depakene Capsules & Syrup ... 511

Verapamil Hydrochloride (Diminished effects of concurrently administered verapamil). Products include:
- Calan SR Caplets ... 2157
- Calan Tablets ... 2155
- Isoptin Injectable ... 1177
- Isoptin Oral Tablets ... 1179
- Isoptin SR Sustained Release Tablets ... 1181
- Verelan Capsules ... 1243
- Verelan Capsules ... 2535

Vitamin D (Effect not specified when used with rifampin-INH). Products include:
- Bugs Bunny Children's Chewable Vitamins (Sugar Free) ... ▣ 625
- Bugs Bunny With Extra C Children's Chewable Vitamins (Sugar Free) ... ▣ 626
- Bugs Bunny Plus Iron Children's Chewable Vitamins (Sugar Free) ▣ 625
- Calderol Capsules ... 1635
- Caltrate 600 + Iron & Vitamin D ... 1198
- Caltrate 600 + Vitamin D ... 1197
- Caltrate, Jr. Tablets ... 1198
- Flintstones Children's Chewable Vitamins ... ▣ 625
- Flintstones Children's Chewable Vitamins With Extra C ... ▣ 626
- Flintstones Children's Chewable Vitamins Plus Iron ... ▣ 625
- Natalins Rx ... 1391
- Natalins Tablets ... 1391
- One-A-Day Essential Vitamins ... ▣ 627
- One-A-Day Maximum Formula Vitamins and Minerals ... ▣ 627
- One-A-Day Plus Extra C Vitamins .. ▣ 627
- Os-Cal 250+D Tablets ... ▣ 597
- Os-Cal 500+D Tablets ... ▣ 597
- Os-Cal Fortified Tablets ... ▣ 597
- Os-Cal Plus Tablets ... ▣ 597
- Posture-D 600 mg ... 2420
- Stressgard Stress Formula Vitamins ... ▣ 628
- Tri-Vi-Flor 1.0 mg Vitamins with Fluoride Chewable Tablets ... 1400
- Tri-Vi-Flor Drops ... 1400
- Tri-Vi-Sol Vitamin Drops ... ▣ 614
- Tri-Vi-Sol Vitamin Drops with Iron ▣ 614
- Vi-Daylin ADC Vitamins Drops ... 1980
- Vi-Daylin ADC Vitamins + Iron Drops ... 1980
- Vi-Daylin/F ADC Vitamins Drops With Fluoride ... 1981
- Vi-Daylin/F ADC Vitamins + Iron Drops With Fluoride ... 1981
- Within Women's Formula Multivitamin with Calcium, Extra Iron and Zinc ... ▣ 628
- Zymacap Capsules ... ▣ 670

Warfarin Sodium (Reduced activity of anticoagulant). Products include:
- Coumadin Injection & Tablets ... 944
- Panwarfin Tablets ... 547

RIFADIN I.V.
(Rifampin) ... 1345

See **Rifadin Capsules**

RIFAMATE CAPSULES
(Rifampin, Isoniazid) ... 1347

May interact with oral anticoagulants, oral contraceptives, oral hypoglycemic agents, cardiac glycosides, and certain other agents. Compounds in these categories include:

Alcohol (Increased incidence of Isoniazid hepatitis).

Betamethasone (Pharmacologic activity decreased when rifampin is given in combination with other antituberculosis drugs).
- No products indexed under this heading.

Betamethasone Acetate (Pharmacologic activity decreased when rifampin is given with other antituberculosis drugs). Products include:
- Celestone Soluspan Suspension ... 2081

Betamethasone Sodium Phosphate (Pharmacologic activity decreased when rifampin is given with other antituberculosis drugs). Products include:
- Celestone Soluspan Suspension ... 2081

Chlorpropamide (Pharmacologic activity decreased when rifampin is given with other antituberculosis drugs). Products include:
- Diabinese Tablets ... 1775

Cortisone Acetate (Pharmacologic activity decreased when rifampin is given with other antituberculosis drugs). Products include:
- Cortone Acetate Sterile Suspension ... 1437
- Cortone Acetate Tablets ... 1439

Dapsone (Pharmacologic activity decreased when rifampin is given with other antituberculosis drugs). Products include:
- Dapsone USP ... 1130

Deslanoside (Pharmacologic activity decreased when rifampin is given with other antituberculosis drugs).
- No products indexed under this heading.

Dexamethasone (Pharmacologic activity decreased when rifampin is given with other antituberculosis drugs). Products include:
- AK-Trol Ointment & Suspension ... ◉ 207
- Decadron Elixir ... 1445
- Decadron Tablets ... 1447
- Decaspray Topical Aerosol ... 1459
- Dexacidin ... ◉ 272
- Maxidex Sterile Ophthalmic Suspension ... ◉ 223
- Maxitrol Ophthalmic Ointment/Suspension ... ◉ 223
- TobraDex Ophthalmic Suspension and Ointment ... ◉ 228

Dexamethasone Acetate (Pharmacologic activity decreased when rifampin is given with other antituberculosis drugs). Products include:
- Dalalone D.P. Injectable ... 999
- Decadron-LA Sterile Suspension ... 1457

Dexamethasone Phosphate (Pharmacologic activity decreased when rifampin is given with other antituberculosis drugs).
- No products indexed under this heading.

Dexamethasone Sodium Phosphate (Pharmacologic activity decreased when rifampin is given with other antituberculosis drugs). Products include:
- AK-Dex ... ◉ 203
- Decadron Phosphate Respihaler ... 1454
- Decadron Phosphate Sterile Ophthalmic Ointment ... 1453
- Decadron Phosphate Sterile Ophthalmic Solution ... 1453
- Decadron Phosphate Topical Cream ... 1455
- Decadron Phosphate Turbinaire ... 1456
- Maxidex Sterile Ophthalmic Ointment ... ◉ 222
- NeoDecadron Sterile Ophthalmic Ointment ... 1517
- NeoDecadron Sterile Ophthalmic Solution ... 1518
- NeoDecadron Topical Cream ... 1518

Dicumarol (Decreased anticoagulant dosage requirements). Products include:
- Dicumarol Tablets ... 516

Digitoxin (Pharmacologic activity decreased when rifampin is given with other antituberculosis drugs). Products include:
- Crystodigin Tablets 1253

Digoxin (Pharmacologic activity decreased when rifampin is given with other antituberculosis drugs). Products include:
- Lanoxicaps 772
- Lanoxin Elixir Pediatric 775
- Lanoxin Injection 778
- Lanoxin Injection Pediatric 781
- Lanoxin Tablets 783

Disopyramide Phosphate (Pharmacologic activity decreased when rifampin is given with other antituberculosis drugs). Products include:
- Norpace 2177

Ethambutol Hydrochloride (Potential for thrombocytopenia). Products include:
- Myambutol Tablets 1225

Ethinyl Estradiol (Reliability of oral contraceptive affected). Products include:
- Brevicon 2304
- Demulen 2161
- Estinyl Tablets 2085
- Jenest-28 Tablets 1636
- Levlen/Tri-Levlen 665
- Lo/Ovral Tablets 2471
- Lo/Ovral-28 Tablets 2476
- Loestrin 1728
- Modicon 1667
- Nordette-21 Tablets 2481
- Nordette-28 Tablets 2483
- Norethin 2133
- Norinyl 2304
- Norlestrin 1746
- Ortho-Cyclen Tablets 1658
- Ortho-Novum 1667
- Ovcon 1391
- Ovral Tablets 2490
- Ovral-28 Tablets 2491
- Levlen/Tri-Levlen 665
- Tri-Norinyl 2304
- Triphasil-21 Tablets 2527
- Triphasil-28 Tablets 2532

Ethynodiol Diacetate (Reliability of oral contraceptive affected). Products include:
- Demulen 2161

Glipizide (Pharmacologic activity decreased when rifampin is given with other antituberculosis drugs). Products include:
- Glucotrol 1952

Glyburide (Pharmacologic activity decreased when rifampin is given with other antituberculosis drugs). Products include:
- DiaBeta 1091
- Micronase Tablets 2350

Hepatotoxic Drugs, unspecified (Fatalities associated with jaundice).

Hydrocortisone (Pharmacologic activity decreased when rifampin is given with other antituberculosis drugs). Products include:
- AK-Spore H.C. ⊙ 206
- Bactine Hydrocortisone Anti-Itch Cream ⊞ 625
- CaldeCORT Anti-Itch Hydrocortisone Spray ⊞ 560
- Carmol HC Cream 1% 2296
- Cortaid Spray ⊞ 735
- Cortenema 2244
- Cortisporin Ointment 758
- Cortisporin Ophthalmic Ointment Sterile 758
- Cortisporin Ophthalmic Suspension Sterile 759
- Cortisporin Otic Solution Sterile 760
- Cortisporin Otic Suspension Sterile 760
- Cortizone-5 Creme & Ointment ⊞ 732
- Dermolate Anti-Itch Cream ⊞ 697
- Eldecort Cream 1.0% 1113
- Eldecort Cream 1.0% and 2.5% 1113
- Fungoid HC Creme 1770
- Hydrocortone Tablets 1482
- Hytone 909
- LazerSporin-C Solution 1770
- Massengill Medicated Soft Cloth Towelettes 2192
- Nutracort Cream & Lotion 1684
- PediOtic Suspension Sterile 797
- Synacort Creams 1%, 2.5% 2296
- Vanoxide-HC Acne Lotion 911
- Vioform-Hydrocortisone Cream and Mild Cream 889
- Vioform-Hydrocortisone Ointment 889
- VōSoL HC Otic Solution 2392
- Vytone Cream 1% 911

Hydrocortisone Acetate (Pharmacologic activity decreased when rifampin is given with other antituberculosis drugs). Products include:
- Analpram-HC Rectal Cream 1% and 2.5% 970
- Anusol-HC Cream 1690
- Anusol-HC Suppositories 1691
- Caldecort ⊞ 560
- Carmol HC Cream 1% 2296
- Chloromycetin Hydrocortisone Ophthalmic 1694
- Coly-Mycin S Otic w/Neomycin & Hydrocortisone 1708
- Cortaid ⊞ 735
- Cortef Feminine Itch Cream ⊞ 735
- Corticaine ⊞ 682
- Cortifoam 1827
- Cortisporin Cream 757
- Epifoam 1828
- Gynecort 5 Creme ⊞ 556
- Hydrocortone Acetate Sterile Suspension 1479
- Lanacort 5 Creme and Ointment ⊞ 557
- Mantadil Cream 789
- Ophthocort ⊙ 301
- Orabase HCA Oral Paste 890
- Pramosone Cream, Lotion & Ointment 971
- ProctoCream-HC 1834
- Proctofoam-HC 1835

Hydrocortisone Sodium Phosphate (Pharmacologic activity decreased when rifampin is given with other antituberculosis drugs). Products include:
- Hydrocortone Phosphate Injection, Sterile 1481

Hydrocortisone Sodium Succinate (Pharmacologic activity decreased when rifampin is given with other antituberculosis drugs). Products include:
- Solu-Cortef Sterile Powder 2361

Levonorgestrel (Reliability of oral contraceptive affected). Products include:
- Levlen/Tri-Levlen 665
- Nordette-21 Tablets 2481
- Nordette-28 Tablets 2483
- Norplant System 2484
- Levlen/Tri-Levlen 665
- Triphasil-21 Tablets 2527
- Triphasil-28 Tablets 2532

Mestranol (Reliability of oral contraceptive affected). Products include:
- Enovid 2161
- Norethin 2133
- Norinyl 2304
- Ortho-Novum 1667

Methadone Hydrochloride (Pharmacologic activity decreased when rifampin is given with other antituberculosis drugs). Products include:
- Dolophine Hydrochloride Ampoules & Vials 1260
- Dolophine Hydrochloride Tablets 1261
- Methadone Hydrochloride Diskets 1284
- Methadone Hydrochloride Oral Solution & Tablets 1987

Methylprednisolone Acetate (Pharmacologic activity decreased when rifampin is given with other antituberculosis drugs). Products include:
- Depo-Medrol Sterile Aqueous Suspension 2334

Methylprednisolone Sodium Succinate (Pharmacologic activity decreased when rifampin is given with other antituberculosis drugs). Products include:
- Solu-Medrol Sterile Powder 2363

Norethindrone (Reliability of oral contraceptive affected). Products include:
- Brevicon 2304
- Jenest-28 Tablets 1636
- Micronor Tablets 1667
- Modicon 1667
- Norethin 2133
- Norinyl 2304
- Norlutin 1755
- Nor-Q D Tablets 2304
- Ortho-Novum 1667
- Ovcon 1391
- Tri-Norinyl 2304

Norethynodrel (Reliability of oral contraceptive affected). Products include:
- Enovid 2161

Norgestimate (Reliability of oral contraceptive affected). Products include:
- Ortho-Cyclen Tablets 1658

Norgestrel (Reliability of oral contraceptive affected). Products include:
- Lo/Ovral Tablets 2471
- Lo/Ovral-28 Tablets 2476
- Ovral Tablets 2490
- Ovral-28 Tablets 2491
- Ovrette Tablets 2492

Phenytoin (Phenytoin intoxication). Products include:
- Dilantin Infatabs 1710
- Dilantin-30 Pediatric/Dilantin-125 Suspension 1713

Phenytoin Sodium (Phenytoin intoxication). Products include:
- Dilantin Kapseals 1708
- Dilantin Parenteral 1712
- Dilantin with Phenobarbital Kapseals 1715

Prednisolone (Pharmacologic activity decreased when rifampin is given with other antituberculosis drugs).
- No products indexed under this heading.

Prednisolone Acetate (Pharmacologic activity decreased when rifampin is given with other antituberculosis drugs). Products include:
- AK-Cide Sterile Ophthalmic Ointment & Suspension ⊙ 202
- Blephamide Liquifilm Sterile Ophthalmic Suspension 586
- Blephamide S.O.P. Sterile Ophthalmic Ointment 586
- Cetapred Ointment ⊙ 220
- ⅛% Econopred & 1% Econopred Plus ⊙ 217
- Isopto Cetapred Suspension ⊙ 220
- Metimyd ⊙ 306
- Poly-Pred Liquifilm ⊙ 250
- Pred Forte ⊙ 252
- Pred Mild ⊙ 254
- Pred-G Liquifilm Sterile Ophthalmic Suspension ⊙ 252
- Pred-G S.O.P. Sterile Ophthalmic Ointment ⊙ 253
- Vasocidin Ointment ⊙ 275

Prednisolone Sodium Phosphate (Pharmacologic activity decreased when rifampin is given with other antituberculosis drugs). Products include:
- AK-Pred ⊙ 205
- Hydeltrasol Injection, Sterile 1476
- Inflamase ⊙ 274
- Pediapred Oral Liquid 987
- Vasocidin Ophthalmic Solution ⊙ 276

Prednisolone Tebutate (Pharmacologic activity decreased when rifampin is given with other antituberculosis drugs). Products include:
- Hydeltra-T.B.A. Sterile Suspension 1478

Prednisone (Pharmacologic activity decreased when rifampin is given with other antituberculosis drugs). Products include:
- Deltasone Tablets 2332

Quinidine Gluconate (Pharmacologic activity decreased when rifampin is given with other antituberculosis drugs). Products include:
- Quinaglute Dura-Tabs Tablets 663

Quinidine Polygalacturonate (Pharmacologic activity decreased when rifampin is given with other antituberculosis drugs). Products include:
- Cardioquin Tablets 1812

Quinidine Sulfate (Pharmacologic activity decreased when rifampin is given with other antituberculosis drugs). Products include:
- Quinidex Extentabs 1868

Tolazamide (Pharmacologic activity decreased when rifampin is given with other antituberculosis drugs). Products include:
- Tolinase Tablets 2365

Tolbutamide (Pharmacologic activity decreased when rifampin is given with other antituberculosis drugs). Products include:
- Orinase Tablets 2354

Triamcinolone (Pharmacologic activity decreased when rifampin is given with other antituberculosis drugs).
- No products indexed under this heading.

Triamcinolone Acetonide (Pharmacologic activity decreased when rifampin is given with other antituberculosis drugs). Products include:
- Aristocort A 1010
- Azmacort Inhaler 1837
- Kenalog Cream, Lotion & Ointment 2401
- Kenalog-10 Injection 2402
- Kenalog-40 Injection 2403
- Kenalog in Orabase 604
- Kenalog Spray 2401
- Mycolog II Cream and Ointment 2407
- Mytrex Cream & Ointment 2080
- Nasacort Nasal Inhaler 1844

Triamcinolone Diacetate (Pharmacologic activity decreased when rifampin is given with other antituberculosis drugs). Products include:
- Aristocort Suspension 1008

Triamcinolone Hexacetonide (Pharmacologic activity decreased when rifampin is given with other antituberculosis drugs). Products include:
- Aristospan Suspension 1011

Warfarin Sodium (Increased anticoagulant dosage requirements). Products include:
- Coumadin Injection & Tablets 944
- Panwarfin Tablets 547

RIMACTANE CAPSULES
(Rifampin) 879
May interact with oral anticoagulants, oral contraceptives, oral hypoglycemic agents, corticosteroids, and cardiac glycosides. Compounds in these categories include:

Betamethasone Acetate (Diminished effects). Products include:
- Celestone Soluspan Suspension 2081

Betamethasone Sodium Phosphate (Diminished effects). Products include:
- Celestone Soluspan Suspension 2081

Chlorpropamide (Diminished effects). Products include:
- Diabinese Tablets 1775

(⊞ Described in PDR For Nonprescription Drugs) (⊙ Described in PDR For Ophthalmology)

Cortisone Acetate (Diminished effects). Products include:
Cortone Acetate Sterile Suspension ... 1437
Cortone Acetate Tablets ... 1439

Dapsone (Diminished effects). Products include:
Dapsone USP ... 1130

Deslanoside (Diminished effects).
No products indexed under this heading.

Dexamethasone (Diminished effects). Products include:
AK-Trol Ointment & Suspension ... ◉ 207
Decadron Elixir ... 1445
Decadron Tablets ... 1447
Decaspray Topical Aerosol ... 1459
Dexacidin ... ◉ 272
Maxidex Sterile Ophthalmic Suspension ... ◉ 223
Maxitrol Ophthalmic Ointment/Suspension ... ◉ 223
TobraDex Ophthalmic Suspension and Ointment ... ◉ 228

Dexamethasone Acetate (Diminished effects). Products include:
Dalalone D.P. Injectable ... 999
Decadron-LA Sterile Suspension ... 1457

Dexamethasone Sodium Phosphate (Diminished effects). Products include:
AK-Dex ... ◉ 203
Decadron Phosphate Respihaler ... 1454
Decadron Phosphate Sterile Ophthalmic Ointment ... 1453
Decadron Phosphate Sterile Ophthalmic Solution ... 1453
Decadron Phosphate Topical Cream ... 1455
Decadron Phosphate Turbinaire ... 1456
Maxidex Sterile Ophthalmic Ointment ... ◉ 222
NeoDecadron Sterile Ophthalmic Ointment ... 1517
NeoDecadron Sterile Ophthalmic Solution ... 1518
NeoDecadron Topical Cream ... 1518

Dicumarol (Increased requirements). Products include:
Dicumarol Tablets ... 516

Digitoxin (Diminished effects). Products include:
Crystodigin Tablets ... 1253

Digoxin (Diminished effects). Products include:
Lanoxicaps ... 772
Lanoxin Elixir Pediatric ... 775
Lanoxin Injection ... 778
Lanoxin Injection Pediatric ... 781
Lanoxin Tablets ... 783

Ethambutol Hydrochloride (Potential for thrombocytopenia). Products include:
Myambutol Tablets ... 1225

Ethinyl Estradiol (Reliability of oral contraceptive affected). Products include:
Brevicon ... 2304
Demulen ... 2161
Estinyl Tablets ... 2085
Jenest-28 Tablets ... 1636
Levlen/Tri-Levlen ... 665
Lo/Ovral Tablets ... 2471
Lo/Ovral-28 Tablets ... 2476
Loestrin ... 1728
Modicon ... 1667
Nordette-21 Tablets ... 2481
Nordette-28 Tablets ... 2483
Norethin ... 2133
Norinyl ... 2304
Norlestrin ... 1746
Ortho-Cyclen Tablets ... 1658
Ortho-Novum ... 1667
Ovcon ... 1391
Ovral Tablets ... 2490
Ovral-28 Tablets ... 2491
Levlen/Tri-Levlen ... 665
Tri-Norinyl ... 2304
Triphasil-21 Tablets ... 2527
Triphasil-28 Tablets ... 2532

Ethynodiol Diacetate (Reliability of oral contraceptive affected). Products include:
Demulen ... 2161

Glipizide (Diminished effects). Products include:
Glucotrol ... 1952

Glyburide (Diminished effects). Products include:
DiaBeta ... 1091
Micronase Tablets ... 2350

Hepatotoxic Drugs, unspecified (Increased risk of liver toxicity).

Hydrocortisone (Diminished effects). Products include:
AK-Spore H.C. ... ◉ 206
Bactine Hydrocortisone Anti-Itch Cream ... ▣ 625
CaldeCORT Anti-Itch Hydrocortisone Spray ... ▣ 560
Carmol HC Cream 1% ... 2296
Cortaid Spray ... ▣ 735
Cortenema ... 2244
Cortisporin Ointment ... 758
Cortisporin Ophthalmic Ointment Sterile ... 758
Cortisporin Ophthalmic Suspension Sterile ... 759
Cortisporin Otic Solution Sterile ... 760
Cortisporin Otic Suspension Sterile ... 760
Cortizone-5 Creme & Ointment ... ▣ 732
Dermolate Anti-Itch Cream ... ▣ 697
Eldecort Cream 1.0% ... 1113
Eldecort Cream 1.0% and 2.5% ... 1113
Fungoid HC Creme ... 1770
Hydrocortone Tablets ... 1482
Hytone ... 909
LazerSporin-C Solution ... 1770
Massengill Medicated Soft Cloth Towelettes ... 2192
Nutracort Cream & Lotion ... 1684
PediOtic Suspension Sterile ... 797
Synacort Creams 1%, 2.5% ... 2296
Vanoxide-HC Acne Lotion ... 911
Vioform-Hydrocortisone Cream and Mild Cream ... 889
Vioform-Hydrocortisone Ointment ... 889
VōSoL HC Otic Solution ... 2392
Vytone Cream 1% ... 911

Hydrocortisone Acetate (Diminished effects). Products include:
Analpram-HC Rectal Cream 1% and 2.5% ... 970
Anusol-HC Cream ... 1690
Anusol-HC Suppositories ... 1691
Caldecort ... ▣ 560
Carmol HC Cream 1% ... 2296
Chloromycetin Hydrocortisone Ophthalmic ... 1694
Coly-Mycin S Otic w/Neomycin & Hydrocortisone ... 1708
Cortaid ... ▣ 735
Cortef Feminine Itch Cream ... ▣ 735
Corticaine ... ▣ 682
Cortifoam ... 1827
Cortisporin Cream ... 757
Epifoam ... 1828
Gynecort 5 Creme ... ▣ 556
Hydrocortone Acetate Sterile Suspension ... 1479
Lanacort 5 Creme and Ointment ... ▣ 557
Mantadil Cream ... 789
Ophthocort ... ◉ 301
Orabase HCA Oral Paste ... 890
Pramosone Cream, Lotion & Ointment ... 971
ProctoCream-HC ... 1834
Proctofoam-HC ... 1835

Hydrocortisone Sodium Phosphate (Diminished effects). Products include:
Hydrocortone Phosphate Injection, Sterile ... 1481

Hydrocortisone Sodium Succinate (Diminished effects). Products include:
Solu-Cortef Sterile Powder ... 2361

Levonorgestrel (Reliability of oral contraceptive affected). Products include:
Levlen/Tri-Levlen ... 665
Nordette-21 Tablets ... 2481
Nordette-28 Tablets ... 2483
Norplant System ... 2484
Levlen/Tri-Levlen ... 665
Triphasil-21 Tablets ... 2527
Triphasil-28 Tablets ... 2532

Mestranol (Reliability of oral contraceptive affected). Products include:
Enovid ... 2161
Norethin ... 2133
Norinyl ... 2304
Ortho-Novum ... 1667

Methadone Hydrochloride (Diminished effects). Products include:
Dolophine Hydrochloride Ampoules & Vials ... 1260
Dolophine Hydrochloride Tablets ... 1261
Methadone Hydrochloride Diskets ... 1284
Methadone Hydrochloride Oral Solution & Tablets ... 1987

Methylprednisolone Acetate (Diminished effects). Products include:
Depo-Medrol Sterile Aqueous Suspension ... 2334

Methylprednisolone Sodium Succinate (Diminished effects). Products include:
Solu-Medrol Sterile Powder ... 2363

Norethindrone (Reliability of oral contraceptive affected). Products include:
Brevicon ... 2304
Jenest-28 Tablets ... 1636
Micronor Tablets ... 1667
Modicon ... 1667
Norethin ... 2133
Norinyl ... 2304
Norlutin ... 1755
Nor-Q D Tablets ... 2304
Ortho-Novum ... 1667
Ovcon ... 1391
Tri-Norinyl ... 2304

Norethynodrel (Reliability of oral contraceptive affected). Products include:
Enovid ... 2161

Norgestimate (Reliability of oral contraceptive affected). Products include:
Ortho-Cyclen Tablets ... 1658

Norgestrel (Reliability of oral contraceptive affected). Products include:
Lo/Ovral Tablets ... 2471
Lo/Ovral-28 Tablets ... 2476
Ovral Tablets ... 2490
Ovral-28 Tablets ... 2491
Ovrette Tablets ... 2492

Prednisolone Acetate (Diminished effects). Products include:
AK-Cide Sterile Ophthalmic Ointment & Suspension ... ◉ 202
Blephamide Liquifilm Sterile Ophthalmic Suspension ... 586
Blephamide S.O.P. Sterile Ophthalmic Ointment ... 586
Cetapred Ointment ... ◉ 220
⅛% Econopred & 1% Econopred Plus ... ◉ 217
Isopto Cetapred Suspension ... ◉ 220
Metimyd ... ◉ 306
Poly-Pred Liquifilm ... ◉ 250
Pred Forte ... ◉ 252
Pred Mild ... ◉ 254
Pred-G Liquifilm Sterile Ophthalmic Suspension ... ◉ 252
Pred-G S.O.P. Sterile Ophthalmic Ointment ... ◉ 253
Vasocidin Ointment ... ◉ 275

Prednisolone Sodium Phosphate (Diminished effects). Products include:
AK-Pred ... ◉ 205
Hydeltrasol Injection, Sterile ... 1476
Inflamase ... ◉ 274
Pediapred Oral Liquid ... 987
Vasocidin Ophthalmic Solution ... ◉ 276

Prednisolone Tebutate (Diminished effects). Products include:
Hydeltra-T.B.A. Sterile Suspension ... 1478

Prednisone (Diminished effects). Products include:
Deltasone Tablets ... 2332

Tolazamide (Diminished effects). Products include:
Tolinase Tablets ... 2365

Tolbutamide (Diminished effects). Products include:
Orinase Tablets ... 2354

Triamcinolone (Diminished effects).
No products indexed under this heading.

Triamcinolone Acetonide (Diminished effects). Products include:
Aristocort A ... 1010
Azmacort Inhaler ... 1837
Kenalog Cream, Lotion & Ointment ... 2401
Kenalog-10 Injection ... 2402
Kenalog-40 Injection ... 2403
Kenalog in Orabase ... 604
Kenalog Spray ... 2401
Mycolog II Cream and Ointment ... 2407
Mytrex Cream & Ointment ... 2080
Nasacort Nasal Inhaler ... 1844

Triamcinolone Diacetate (Diminished effects). Products include:
Aristocort Suspension ... 1008

Triamcinolone Hexacetonide (Diminished effects). Products include:
Aristospan Suspension ... 1011

Verapamil Hydrochloride (Reduced bioavailability and efficacy). Products include:
Calan SR Caplets ... 2157
Calan Tablets ... 2155
Isoptin Injectable ... 1177
Isoptin Oral Tablets ... 1179
Isoptin SR Sustained Release Tablets ... 1181
Verelan Capsules ... 1243
Verelan Capsules ... 2535

Warfarin Sodium (Increased requirements). Products include:
Coumadin Injection & Tablets ... 944
Panwarfin Tablets ... 547

RIMSO-50
(Dimethyl Sulfoxide) ... 1836
No interactions described in labeling.

RIOPAN ANTACID SUSPENSION
(Magaldrate) ... 2421
May interact with tetracyclines. Compounds in this category include:

Demeclocycline Hydrochloride (Concurrent use with any form of tetracycline should be avoided). Products include:
Declomycin Capsules, Tablets ... 1199

Doxycycline Calcium (Concurrent use with any form of tetracycline should be avoided).
No products indexed under this heading.

Doxycycline Hyclate (Concurrent use with any form of tetracycline should be avoided). Products include:
Doryx Capsules ... 1717
Vibramycin Hyclate Capsules ... 1787
Vibramycin Hyclate Intravenous ... 1968
Vibra-Tabs Film Coated Tablets ... 1787

Doxycycline Monohydrate (Concurrent use with any form of tetracycline should be avoided). Products include:
Monodox Capsules ... 1630
Vibramycin Monohydrate for Oral Suspension ... 1787

Methacycline Hydrochloride (Concurrent use with any form of tetracycline should be avoided).
No products indexed under this heading.

Minocycline Hydrochloride (Concurrent use with any form of tetracycline should be avoided). Products include:
Minocin Intravenous ... 1221
Minocin Oral Suspension ... 1224
Minocin Pellet-Filled Capsules ... 1222

(▣ Described in PDR For Nonprescription Drugs) (◉ Described in PDR For Ophthalmology)

Oxytetracycline Hydrochloride (Concurrent use with any form of tetracycline should be avoided). Products include:
Terra-Cortril Ophthalmic Suspension ... 1963
Terramycin Capsules ... 1786
Terramycin Intramuscular Solution 1964
Terramycin with Polymyxin B Sulfate Ophthalmic Ointment ... 1965
Tetracycline Hydrochloride (Concurrent use with any form of tetracycline should be avoided). Products include:
Achromycin V Capsules ... 1193
Achromycin Ophthalmic Ointment 1% ... ◉ 307
Achromycin Ophthalmic Suspension 1% ... ◉ 308
Topicycline for Topical Solution ... 1856

RIOPAN ANTACID SWALLOW TABLETS
(Magaldrate) ... 2421
See **Riopan Antacid Suspension**

RIOPAN PLUS CHEW TABLETS
(Magaldrate, Simethicone) ... 2422
May interact with:

Oxytetracycline (Effect not specified). Products include:
Terramycin Intramuscular Solution 1964
Urobiotic-250 Capsules ... 1968
Oxytetracycline Hydrochloride (Effect not specified). Products include:
Terra-Cortril Ophthalmic Suspension ... 1963
Terramycin Capsules ... 1786
Terramycin Intramuscular Solution 1964
Terramycin with Polymyxin B Sulfate Ophthalmic Ointment ... 1965
Tetracycline Hydrochloride (Effect not specified). Products include:
Achromycin V Capsules ... 1193
Achromycin Ophthalmic Ointment 1% ... ◉ 307
Achromycin Ophthalmic Suspension 1% ... ◉ 308
Topicycline for Topical Solution ... 1856

RIOPAN PLUS CHEW TABLETS IN ROLLPACK
(Magaldrate, Simethicone) ... 2422
See **Riopan Plus Chew Tablets**

RIOPAN PLUS 2 CHEW TABLETS, MINT FLAVOR, CHERRY FLAVOR
(Magaldrate, Simethicone) ... 2422
May interact with:

Oxytetracycline (Effect not specified). Products include:
Terramycin Intramuscular Solution 1964
Urobiotic-250 Capsules ... 1968
Oxytetracycline Hydrochloride (Effect not specified). Products include:
Terra-Cortril Ophthalmic Suspension ... 1963
Terramycin Capsules ... 1786
Terramycin Intramuscular Solution 1964
Terramycin with Polymyxin B Sulfate Ophthalmic Ointment ... 1965
Tetracycline Hydrochloride (Effect not specified). Products include:
Achromycin V Capsules ... 1193
Achromycin Ophthalmic Ointment 1% ... ◉ 307
Achromycin Ophthalmic Suspension 1% ... ◉ 308
Topicycline for Topical Solution ... 1856

RIOPAN PLUS SUSPENSION
(Magaldrate, Simethicone) ... 2422
See **Riopan Plus Chew Tablets**

RIOPAN PLUS 2 SUSPENSION, MINT FLAVOR, CHERRY FLAVOR
(Magaldrate, Simethicone) ... 2422
See **Riopan Plus Chew Tablets**

RITALIN TABLETS
(Methylphenidate Hydrochloride) ... 880
May interact with oral anticoagulants, vasopressors, monoamine oxidase inhibitors, tricyclic antidepressants, and certain other agents. Compounds in these categories include:

Amitriptyline Hydrochloride (Metabolism inhibited; downward dosage adjustment of antidepressant may be required). Products include:
Elavil ... 2269
Endep Tablets ... 1927
Etrafon ... 2087
Limbitrol ... 1933
Triavil Tablets ... 1556
Amoxapine (Metabolism inhibited; downward dosage adjustment of antidepressant may be required). Products include:
Asendin Tablets ... 1196
Clomipramine Hydrochloride (Metabolism inhibited; downward dosage adjustment of antidepressant may be required). Products include:
Anafranil Capsules ... 650
Desipramine Hydrochloride (Metabolism inhibited; downward dosage adjustment of antidepressant may be required). Products include:
Norpramin Tablets ... 1340
Dicumarol (Metabolism inhibited). Products include:
Dicumarol Tablets ... 516
Dopamine Hydrochloride (Concomitant use requires caution). Products include:
Intropin Injection ... 930
Doxepin Hydrochloride (Metabolism inhibited; downward dosage adjustment of antidepressant may be required). Products include:
Sinequan ... 1960
Epinephrine Hydrochloride (Concomitant use requires caution). Products include:
Adrenalin Chloride Solution 1:100 & 1:1,000 ... 1689
Epifrin ... ◉ 244
Glaucon ... ◉ 218
Furazolidone (Concomitant use requires caution). Products include:
Furoxone ... 1855
Guanethidine Monosulfate (Decreased hypotensive effect). Products include:
Esimil Tablets ... 864
Ismelin Tablets ... 869
Imipramine Hydrochloride (Metabolism inhibited; downward dosage adjustment of antidepressant may be required). Products include:
Tofranil Ampuls ... 1038
Tofranil Tablets ... 1039
Imipramine Pamoate (Metabolism inhibited; downward dosage adjustment of antidepressant may be required). Products include:
Tofranil-PM Capsules ... 1041
Isocarboxazid (Concomitant use requires caution). Products include:
Marplan Tablets ... 1906
Maprotiline Hydrochloride (Metabolism inhibited; downward dosage adjustment of antidepressant may be required). Products include:
Ludiomil Tablets ... 874
Metaraminol Bitartrate (Concomitant use requires caution). Products include:
Aramine Injection ... 1424
Methoxamine Hydrochloride (Concomitant use requires caution). Products include:
Vasoxyl Injection ... 819
Norepinephrine Bitartrate (Concomitant use requires caution). Products include:
Levophed Bitartrate Injection ... 2054
Nortriptyline Hydrochloride (Metabolism inhibited; downward dosage adjustment of antidepressant may be required). Products include:
Pamelor ... 2019
Phenelzine Sulfate (Concomitant use requires caution). Products include:
Nardil ... 1742
Phenylbutazone (Metabolism inhibited; downward dosage adjustment of phenylbutazone may be required). Products include:
Butazolidin Capsules & Tablets ... 1027
Phenylephrine Hydrochloride (Concomitant use requires caution). Products include:
AK-Dilate Solution 2.5% and 10% ... ◉ 203
Atrohist Sprinkle Capsules ... 558
Cerose-DM ... 2443
Codimal ... 846
Comhist LA Capsules ... 1618
Congespirin For Children Aspirin Free Chewable Cold Tablets ... 748
Cyclomydril ... ◉ 216
Deconsal Sprinkle Capsules ... 559
Dimetane Decongestant ... ▣ 673
Dristan Decongestant/Antihistamine/ Analgesic Coated Caplets ... ▣ 749
Dristan Cold Nasal Decongestant/ Antihistamine/ Analgesic Coated Tablets ... 2419
Dristan Advanced Formula Decongestant/Antihistamine/ Analgesic Tablets ... ▣ 749
Dristan Nasal Spray, Menthol ... 2419
Dristan Nasal Spray, Regular and Regular with Metered Pump ... 2419
Entex Capsules ... 1623
Entex Liquid ... 1623
Sinus Excedrin Analgesic, Decongestant Tablets & Caplets ... 750
Extendryl ... 994
4-Way Fast Acting Nasal Spray - Original Formula (regular & mentholated) & Metered Spray Pump (regular) ... 751
Hycomine Compound Tablets ... 929
Murocoll-2 Sterile Ophthalmic Solution ... ◉ 261
Mydfrin 2.5% ... ◉ 224
Naldecon Syrup, Tablets, Pediatric Drops and Pediatric Syrup ... 709
Neo-Synephrine Hydrochloride 1% Carpuject ... 2063
Neo-Synephrine Hydrochloride 1% Injection ... 2063
Neo-Synephrine Hydrochloride (Ophthalmic) ... 2064
Neo-Synephrine ... ▣ 759
Nōstril Nasal Decongestant ... ▣ 520
Novahistine Elixir ... ▣ 596
Phenergan VC ... 2500
Phenergan VC with Codeine ... 2501
Prefrin Liquifilm Vasoconstrictor and Lubricant Eye Drops ... ◉ 254
Prefrin-A ... ◉ 255
Quelidrine Syrup ... 556
Relief Vasoconstrictor and Lubricant Eye Drops ... ◉ 256
Robitussin Night Relief ... ▣ 677
Ru-Tuss with Hydrocodone ... 694
Ru-Tuss Tablets ... 693
Vasosulf ... ◉ 279
Vicks Sinex ... ▣ 665
Zincfrin ... ◉ 230
Phenytoin (Metabolism inhibited; downward dosage adjustment of anticonvulsant may be required). Products include:
Dilantin Infatabs ... 1710
Dilantin-30 Pediatric/Dilantin-125 Suspension ... 1713
Phenytoin Sodium (Metabolism inhibited; downward dosage adjustment of anticonvulsant may be required). Products include:
Dilantin Kapseals ... 1708
Dilantin Parenteral ... 1712
Dilantin with Phenobarbital Kapseals ... 1715
Primidone (Metabolism inhibited; downward dosage adjustment of anticonvulsant may be required). Products include:
Mysoline ... 2480
Protriptyline Hydrochloride (Metabolism inhibited; downward dosage adjustment of antidepressant may be required). Products include:
Vivactil Tablets ... 1567
Selegiline Hydrochloride (Concomitant use requires caution). Products include:
Eldepryl ... 2250
Tranylcypromine Sulfate (Concomitant use requires caution). Products include:
Parnate Tablets ... 2222
Trimipramine Maleate (Metabolism inhibited; downward dosage adjustment of antidepressant may be required). Products include:
Surmontil Capsules ... 2524
Warfarin Sodium (Metabolism inhibited). Products include:
Coumadin Injection & Tablets ... 944
Panwarfin Tablets ... 547

RITALIN-SR TABLETS
(Methylphenidate Hydrochloride) ... 880
See **Ritalin Tablets**

ROBAXIN INJECTABLE
(Methocarbamol) ... 1871
May interact with central nervous system depressants and certain other agents. Compounds in these categories include:

Alcohol (Increased depressant effect).
Alfentanil Hydrochloride (Increased CNS depressant effect). Products include:
Alfenta Injection ... 1131
Alprazolam (Increased CNS depressant effect). Products include:
Xanax Tablets ... 2367
Aprobarbital (Increased CNS depressant effect). Products include:
Alurate Elixir ... 1883
Buprenorphine (Increased CNS depressant effect).
No products indexed under this heading.
Buspirone Hydrochloride (Increased CNS depressant effect). Products include:
BuSpar ... 1401
Butabarbital (Increased CNS depressant effect). Products include:
Pyridium Plus ... 1764
Butalbital (Increased CNS depressant effect). Products include:
Esgic-Plus Tablets ... 1002
Esgic Tablets & Capsules ... 1001
Fioricet Tablets ... 2006
Fiorinal Capsules ... 2007
Fiorinal with Codeine Capsules ... 2008
Fiorinal Tablets ... 2007
Phrenilin ... 838
Sedapap Tablets 50 mg/650 mg ... 1360
Chlordiazepoxide (Increased CNS depressant effect). Products include:
Libritabs Tablets ... 1930
Limbitrol ... 1933
Menrium Tablets ... 1934
Chlordiazepoxide Hydrochloride (Increased CNS depressant effect). Products include:
Librax Capsules ... 1929

(▣ Described in PDR For Nonprescription Drugs) (◉ Described in PDR For Ophthalmology)

Librium Capsules 1931
Librium Injectable 1932

Chlorpromazine (Increased CNS depressant effect). Products include:
Thorazine 2234

Chlorprothixene (Increased CNS depressant effect). Products include:
Taractan Tablets 1920

Chlorprothixene Hydrochloride (Increased CNS depressant effect). Products include:
Taractan 1920

Chlorprothixene Lactate (Increased CNS depressant effect). Products include:
Taractan Concentrate 1920

Clorazepate Dipotassium (Increased CNS depressant effect). Products include:
Tranxene 556

Codeine (Increased CNS depressant effect). Products include:
Calcidrine Syrup 506

Codeine Phosphate (Increased CNS depressant effect). Products include:
Actifed with Codeine Cough Syrup.. 752
Cheracol Cough Syrup 1853
Codimal PH Syrup 846
Dimetane-DC Cough Syrup 1857
Empirin with Codeine Phosphate Nos. 2, 3 & 4 764
Fiorinal with Codeine Capsules 2008
Isoclor Expectorant 982
Naldecon CX Adult Liquid .... ■ 521
Novahistine DH 1342
Novahistine Expectorant 1343
Nucofed Capsules 2219
Nucofed Expectorant 2219
Nucofed Pediatric Expectorant 2220
Nucofed Syrup 2219
Phenaphen with Codeine Capsules 1865
Phenaphen-650 with Codeine Tablets 1866
Phenergan with Codeine 2497
Phenergan VC with Codeine 2501
Robitussin A-C Syrup 1875
Robitussin-DAC Syrup 1875
Ryna .... ■ 741
Soma Compound w/Codeine Tablets 2390
Triaminic Expectorant w/Codeine .. 1996
Tussi-Organidin Liquid 2391
Tylenol with Codeine 1381

Codeine Polistirex (Increased CNS depressant effect).
No products indexed under this heading.

Dezocine (Increased CNS depressant effect).

Diazepam (Increased CNS depressant effect). Products include:
Valium Injectable 1937
Valium Tablets 1939
Valrelease Capsules 1923

Droperidol (Increased CNS depressant effect). Products include:
Inapsine Injection 1140
Innovar Injection 1141

Enflurane (Increased CNS depressant effect). Products include:
Ethrane 599

Estazolam (Increased CNS depressant effect). Products include:
ProSom Tablets 554

Ethchlorvynol (Increased CNS depressant effect). Products include:
Placidyl Capsules 553

Ethinamate (Increased CNS depressant effect).
No products indexed under this heading.

Fentanyl (Increased CNS depressant effect). Products include:
Duragesic Transdermal System 1133

Fentanyl Citrate (Increased CNS depressant effect). Products include:
Innovar Injection 1141
Sublimaze Injection 1146

Fluphenazine Decanoate (Increased CNS depressant effect). Products include:
Prolixin Decanoate 1795

Fluphenazine Enanthate (Increased CNS depressant effect). Products include:
Prolixin Enanthate 1796

Fluphenazine Hydrochloride (Increased CNS depressant effect). Products include:
Prolixin Elixir 1793
Prolixin Injection 1791
Prolixin Oral Concentrate 1792
Prolixin Tablets 1793

Flurazepam Hydrochloride (Increased CNS depressant effect). Products include:
Dalmane Capsules 1927

Glutethimide (Increased CNS depressant effect).
No products indexed under this heading.

Haloperidol (Increased CNS depressant effect). Products include:
Haldol Injection, Tablets and Concentrate 1373

Haloperidol Decanoate (Increased CNS depressant effect). Products include:
Haldol Decanoate 1375

Hydrocodone Bitartrate (Increased CNS depressant effect). Products include:
Anexsia 5/500 Tablets 2196
Anexsia 7.5/650 Tablets 2197
Azdone Tablets 844
Codiclear DH Syrup 845
Codimal DH Syrup 846
Damason-P 1356
Hycodan Syrup, Tablets 927
Hycomine Compound Tablets 929
Hycomine Syrup 927
Hycotuss Expectorant Syrup 930
Hydrocet Capsules 835
Lortab ASA Tablets 2414
Lortab 2412
Ru-Tuss with Hydrocodone 694
Triaminic Expectorant DH 1995
Vicodin Tablets 1187
Vicodin ES Tablets 1189
Zydone Capsules 941

Hydrocodone Polistirex (Increased CNS depressant effect). Products include:
Tussionex Extended-Release Suspension 988

Hydroxyzine Hydrochloride (Increased CNS depressant effect). Products include:
Atarax Tablets & Syrup 1941
Marax Tablets & DF Syrup 1954
Vistaril Intramuscular Solution 1970

Isoflurane (Increased CNS depressant effect). Products include:
Forane 600

Ketamine Hydrochloride (Increased CNS depressant effect). Products include:
Ketalar 1726

Levorphanol Tartrate (Increased CNS depressant effect). Products include:
Levo-Dromoran 1906

Lorazepam (Increased CNS depressant effect). Products include:
Ativan Injection 2432
Ativan Tablets 2434

Loxapine Hydrochloride (Increased CNS depressant effect). Products include:
Loxitane 1213

Loxapine Succinate (Increased CNS depressant effect). Products include:
Loxitane Capsules 1213

Meperidine Hydrochloride (Increased CNS depressant effect). Products include:
Demerol 2047
Mepergan Injection 2479

Mephobarbital (Increased CNS depressant effect). Products include:
Mebaral Tablets 2061

Meprobamate (Increased CNS depressant effect). Products include:
Deprol Tablets 2382
Equagesic Tablets 2451
Miltown Tablets 2386
PMB 200 and PMB 400 2504

Mesoridazine (Increased CNS depressant effect). Products include:
Serentil 686

Methadone Hydrochloride (Increased CNS depressant effect). Products include:
Dolophine Hydrochloride Ampoules & Vials 1260
Dolophine Hydrochloride Tablets 1261
Methadone Hydrochloride Diskets .. 1284
Methadone Hydrochloride Oral Solution & Tablets 1987

Methohexital Sodium (Increased CNS depressant effect). Products include:
Brevital Sodium Vials 1248

Methoxyflurane (Increased CNS depressant effect).
No products indexed under this heading.

Midazolam Hydrochloride (Increased CNS depressant effect). Products include:
Versed Injection 1924

Molindone Hydrochloride (Increased CNS depressant effect). Products include:
Moban Tablets & Concentrate 932

Morphine Sulfate (Increased CNS depressant effect). Products include:
Astramorph/PF Injection, USP (Preservative-Free) 618
Duramorph 960
Infumorph 200 and Infumorph 500 Sterile Solutions 962
MS Contin Tablets 1814
MSIR 1817
Oramorph SR (Morphine Sulfate Sustained Release Tablets) 1988
Roxanol 1991

Opium Alkaloids (Increased CNS depressant effect). Products include:
B & O No. 15A & No. 16A Supprettes 2395
Pantopon Injectable 1911

Oxazepam (Increased CNS depressant effect). Products include:
Serax Capsules 2522
Serax Tablets 2522

Oxycodone Hydrochloride (Increased CNS depressant effect). Products include:
Percocet Tablets 950
Percodan 951
Roxicodone Tablets, Oral Solution & Intensol (Oxycodone) 1992
Tylox Capsules 1382

Pentobarbital Sodium (Increased additive effect). Products include:
Nembutal Sodium Capsules 534
Nembutal Sodium Solution 536
Nembutal Sodium Suppositories 538

Perphenazine (Increased CNS depressant effect). Products include:
Etrafon 2087
Triavil Tablets 1556
Trilafon 2123

Phenobarbital (Increased CNS depressant effect). Products include:
Arco-Lase Plus Tablets 607
Bellergal-S Tablets 1998
Bronkolixir .... ■ 761
Bronkotabs Tablets .... ■ 762
Donnatal 1858
Donnatal Extentabs 1859
Donnatal Tablets 1858
Donnazyme Tablets 1860
Kinesed Tablets 2272
Phenobarbital Elixir and Tablets 1293
Primatene Tablets-P Formula 2421
Quadrinal Tablets 1183
Tedral SA 1765

Prazepam (Increased CNS depressant effect). Products include:
Centrax 1693

Prochlorperazine (Increased CNS depressant effect). Products include:
Compazine 2201

Promethazine Hydrochloride (Increased CNS depressant effect). Products include:
Mepergan Injection 2479
Phenergan with Codeine 2497
Phenergan with Dextromethorphan 2499
Phenergan Injection 2493
Phenergan Suppositories 2496
Phenergan Syrup 2495
Phenergan Tablets 2496
Phenergan VC 2500
Phenergan VC with Codeine 2501

Propofol (Increased CNS depressant effect). Products include:
Diprivan Injection 2267

Propoxyphene Hydrochloride (Increased CNS depressant effect). Products include:
Darvon 1256
Wygesic Tablets 2540

Propoxyphene Napsylate (Increased CNS depressant effect). Products include:
Darvon-N/Darvocet-N 1254

Quazepam (Increased CNS depressant effect). Products include:
Doral Tablets 2383

Secobarbital Sodium (Increased CNS depressant effect). Products include:
Seconal Sodium Pulvules 1296

Sufentanil Citrate (Increased CNS depressant effect). Products include:
Sufenta Injection 1147

Temazepam (Increased CNS depressant effect). Products include:
Restoril Capsules 2023

Thiamylal Sodium (Increased CNS depressant effect). Products include:
Surital Ampoules, Steri-Vials 1764

Thioridazine Hydrochloride (Increased CNS depressant effect). Products include:
Mellaril 2011

Thiothixene (Increased CNS depressant effect). Products include:
Navane Capsules and Concentrate 1954
Navane Intramuscular 1956

Triazolam (Increased CNS depressant effect). Products include:
Halcion Tablets 2340

Trifluoperazine Hydrochloride (Increased CNS depressant effect). Products include:
Stelazine 2226

ROBAXIN TABLETS
(Methocarbamol) 1872
May interact with central nervous system depressants and certain other agents. Compounds in these categories include:

Alcohol (Increased CNS depressant effect).

Alfentanil Hydrochloride (Increased CNS depressant effect). Products include:
Alfenta Injection 1131

Alprazolam (Increased CNS depressant effect). Products include:
Xanax Tablets 2367

Aprobarbital (Increased CNS depressant effect). Products include:
Alurate Elixir 1883

Buprenorphine (Increased CNS depressant effect).
No products indexed under this heading.

Buspirone Hydrochloride (Increased CNS depressant effect). Products include:
- BuSpar ... 1401

Butabarbital (Increased CNS depressant effect). Products include:
- Pyridium Plus ... 1764

Butalbital (Increased CNS depressant effect). Products include:
- Esgic-Plus Tablets ... 1002
- Esgic Tablets & Capsules ... 1001
- Fioricet Tablets ... 2006
- Fiorinal Capsules ... 2007
- Fiorinal with Codeine Capsules ... 2008
- Fiorinal Tablets ... 2007
- Phrenilin ... 838
- Sedapap Tablets 50 mg/650 mg .. 1360

Chlordiazepoxide (Increased CNS depressant effect). Products include:
- Libritabs Tablets ... 1930
- Limbitrol ... 1933
- Menrium Tablets ... 1934

Chlordiazepoxide Hydrochloride (Increased CNS depressant effect). Products include:
- Librax Capsules ... 1929
- Librium Capsules ... 1931
- Librium Injectable ... 1932

Chlorpromazine (Increased CNS depressant effect). Products include:
- Thorazine ... 2234

Chlorprothixene (Increased CNS depressant effect). Products include:
- Taractan Tablets ... 1920

Chlorprothixene Hydrochloride (Increased CNS depressant effect). Products include:
- Taractan ... 1920

Chlorprothixene Lactate (Increased CNS depressant effect). Products include:
- Taractan Concentrate ... 1920

Clorazepate Dipotassium (Increased CNS depressant effect). Products include:
- Tranxene ... 556

Codeine (Increased CNS depressant effect). Products include:
- Calcidrine Syrup ... 506

Codeine Phosphate (Increased CNS depressant effect). Products include:
- Actifed with Codeine Cough Syrup.. 752
- Cheracol Cough Syrup ... 1853
- Codimal PH Syrup ... 846
- Dimetane-DC Cough Syrup ... 1857
- Empirin with Codeine Phosphate Nos. 2, 3 & 4 ... 764
- Fiorinal with Codeine Capsules ... 2008
- Isoclor Expectorant ... 982
- Naldecon CX Adult Liquid ... ◘ 521
- Novahistine DH ... 1342
- Novahistine Expectorant ... 1343
- Nucofed Capsules ... 2219
- Nucofed Expectorant ... 2219
- Nucofed Pediatric Expectorant ... 2220
- Nucofed Syrup ... 2219
- Phenaphen with Codeine Capsules 1865
- Phenaphen-650 with Codeine Tablets ... 1866
- Phenergan with Codeine ... 2497
- Phenergan VC with Codeine ... 2501
- Robitussin A-C Syrup ... 1875
- Robitussin-DAC Syrup ... 1875
- Ryna ... ◘ 741
- Soma Compound w/Codeine Tablets ... 2390
- Triaminic Expectorant w/Codeine .. 1996
- Tussi-Organidin Liquid ... 2391
- Tylenol with Codeine ... 1381

Codeine Polistirex (Increased CNS depressant effect).
- No products indexed under this heading.

Dezocine (Increased CNS depressant effect).

Diazepam (Increased CNS depressant effect). Products include:
- Valium Injectable ... 1937
- Valium Tablets ... 1939
- Valrelease Capsules ... 1923

Droperidol (Increased CNS depressant effect). Products include:
- Inapsine Injection ... 1140
- Innovar Injection ... 1141

Enflurane (Increased CNS depressant effect). Products include:
- Ethrane ... 599

Estazolam (Increased CNS depressant effect). Products include:
- ProSom Tablets ... 554

Ethchlorvynol (Increased CNS depressant effect). Products include:
- Placidyl Capsules ... 553

Ethinamate (Increased CNS depressant effect).
- No products indexed under this heading.

Fentanyl (Increased CNS depressant effect). Products include:
- Duragesic Transdermal System ... 1133

Fentanyl Citrate (Increased CNS depressant effect). Products include:
- Innovar Injection ... 1141
- Sublimaze Injection ... 1146

Fluphenazine Decanoate (Increased CNS depressant effect). Products include:
- Prolixin Decanoate ... 1795

Fluphenazine Enanthate (Increased CNS depressant effect). Products include:
- Prolixin Enanthate ... 1796

Fluphenazine Hydrochloride (Increased CNS depressant effect). Products include:
- Prolixin Elixir ... 1793
- Prolixin Injection ... 1791
- Prolixin Oral Concentrate ... 1792
- Prolixin Tablets ... 1793

Flurazepam Hydrochloride (Increased CNS depressant effect). Products include:
- Dalmane Capsules ... 1927

Glutethimide (Increased CNS depressant effect).
- No products indexed under this heading.

Haloperidol (Increased CNS depressant effect). Products include:
- Haldol Injection, Tablets and Concentrate ... 1373

Haloperidol Decanoate (Increased CNS depressant effect). Products include:
- Haldol Decanoate ... 1375

Hydrocodone Bitartrate (Increased CNS depressant effect). Products include:
- Anexsia 5/500 Tablets ... 2196
- Anexsia 7.5/650 Tablets ... 2197
- Azdone Tablets ... 844
- Codiclear DH Syrup ... 845
- Codimal DH Syrup ... 846
- Damason-P ... 1356
- Hycodan Syrup, Tablets ... 927
- Hycomine Compound Tablets ... 929
- Hycomine Syrup ... 927
- Hycotuss Expectorant Syrup ... 930
- Hydrocet Capsules ... 835
- Lortab ASA Tablets ... 2414
- Lortab ... 2412
- Ru-Tuss with Hydrocodone ... 694
- Triaminic Expectorant DH ... 1995
- Vicodin Tablets ... 1187
- Vicodin ES Tablets ... 1189
- Zydone Capsules ... 941

Hydrocodone Polistirex (Increased CNS depressant effect). Products include:
- Tussionex Extended-Release Suspension ... 988

Hydroxyzine Hydrochloride (Increased CNS depressant effect). Products include:
- Atarax Tablets & Syrup ... 1941
- Marax Tablets & DF Syrup ... 1954
- Vistaril Intramuscular Solution ... 1970

Isoflurane (Increased CNS depressant effect). Products include:
- Forane ... 600

Ketamine Hydrochloride (Increased CNS depressant effect). Products include:
- Ketalar ... 1726

Levorphanol Tartrate (Increased CNS depressant effect). Products include:
- Levo-Dromoran ... 1906

Lorazepam (Increased CNS depressant effect). Products include:
- Ativan Injection ... 2432
- Ativan Tablets ... 2434

Loxapine Hydrochloride (Increased CNS depressant effect). Products include:
- Loxitane ... 1213

Loxapine Succinate (Increased CNS depressant effect). Products include:
- Loxitane Capsules ... 1213

Meperidine Hydrochloride (Increased CNS depressant effect). Products include:
- Demerol ... 2047
- Mepergan Injection ... 2479

Mephobarbital (Increased CNS depressant effect). Products include:
- Mebaral Tablets ... 2061

Meprobamate (Increased CNS depressant effect). Products include:
- Deprol Tablets ... 2382
- Equagesic Tablets ... 2451
- Miltown Tablets ... 2386
- PMB 200 and PMB 400 ... 2504

Mesoridazine (Increased CNS depressant effect). Products include:
- Serentil ... 686

Methadone Hydrochloride (Increased CNS depressant effect). Products include:
- Dolophine Hydrochloride Ampoules & Vials ... 1260
- Dolophine Hydrochloride Tablets ... 1261
- Methadone Hydrochloride Diskets .. 1284
- Methadone Hydrochloride Oral Solution & Tablets ... 1987

Methohexital Sodium (Increased CNS depressant effect). Products include:
- Brevital Sodium Vials ... 1248

Methoxyflurane (Increased CNS depressant effect).
- No products indexed under this heading.

Midazolam Hydrochloride (Increased CNS depressant effect). Products include:
- Versed Injection ... 1924

Molindone Hydrochloride (Increased CNS depressant effect). Products include:
- Moban Tablets & Concentrate ... 932

Morphine Sulfate (Increased CNS depressant effect). Products include:
- Astramorph/PF Injection, USP (Preservative-Free) ... 618
- Duramorph ... 960
- Infumorph 200 and Infumorph 500 Sterile Solutions ... 962
- MS Contin Tablets ... 1814
- MSIR ... 1817
- Oramorph SR (Morphine Sulfate Sustained Release Tablets) ... 1988
- Roxanol ... 1991

Opium Alkaloids (Increased CNS depressant effect). Products include:
- B & O No. 15A & No. 16A Supprettes ... 2395
- Pantopon Injectable ... 1911

Oxazepam (Increased CNS depressant effect). Products include:
- Serax Capsules ... 2522
- Serax Tablets ... 2522

Oxycodone Hydrochloride (Increased CNS depressant effect). Products include:
- Percocet Tablets ... 950
- Percodan ... 951
- Roxicodone Tablets, Oral Solution & Intensol (Oxycodone) ... 1992

- Tylox Capsules ... 1382

Pentobarbital Sodium (Increased CNS depressant effect). Products include:
- Nembutal Sodium Capsules ... 534
- Nembutal Sodium Solution ... 536
- Nembutal Sodium Suppositories ... 538

Perphenazine (Increased CNS depressant effect). Products include:
- Etrafon ... 2087
- Triavil Tablets ... 1556
- Trilafon ... 2123

Phenobarbital (Increased CNS depressant effect). Products include:
- Arco-Lase Plus Tablets ... 607
- Bellergal-S Tablets ... 1998
- Bronkolixir ... ◘ 761
- Bronkotabs Tablets ... ◘ 762
- Donnatal ... 1858
- Donnatal Extentabs ... 1859
- Donnatal Tablets ... 1858
- Donnazyme Tablets ... 1860
- Kinesed Tablets ... 2272
- Phenobarbital Elixir and Tablets ... 1293
- Primatene Tablets-P Formula ... 2421
- Quadrinal Tablets ... 1183
- Tedral SA ... 1765

Prazepam (Increased CNS depressant effect). Products include:
- Centrax ... 1693

Prochlorperazine (Increased CNS depressant effect). Products include:
- Compazine ... 2201

Promethazine Hydrochloride (Increased CNS depressant effect). Products include:
- Mepergan Injection ... 2479
- Phenergan with Codeine ... 2497
- Phenergan with Dextromethorphan 2499
- Phenergan Injection ... 2493
- Phenergan Suppositories ... 2496
- Phenergan Syrup ... 2495
- Phenergan Tablets ... 2496
- Phenergan VC ... 2500
- Phenergan VC with Codeine ... 2501

Propofol (Increased CNS depressant effect). Products include:
- Diprivan Injection ... 2267

Propoxyphene Hydrochloride (Increased CNS depressant effect). Products include:
- Darvon ... 1256
- Wygesic Tablets ... 2540

Propoxyphene Napsylate (Increased CNS depressant effect). Products include:
- Darvon-N/Darvocet-N ... 1254

Quazepam (Increased CNS depressant effect). Products include:
- Doral Tablets ... 2383

Secobarbital Sodium (Increased CNS depressant effect). Products include:
- Seconal Sodium Pulvules ... 1296

Sufentanil Citrate (Increased CNS depressant effect). Products include:
- Sufenta Injection ... 1147

Temazepam (Increased CNS depressant effect). Products include:
- Restoril Capsules ... 2023

Thiamylal Sodium (Increased CNS depressant effect). Products include:
- Surital Ampoules, Steri-Vials ... 1764

Thioridazine Hydrochloride (Increased CNS depressant effect). Products include:
- Mellaril ... 2011

Thiothixene (Increased CNS depressant effect). Products include:
- Navane Capsules and Concentrate 1954
- Navane Intramuscular ... 1956

Triazolam (Increased CNS depressant effect). Products include:
- Halcion Tablets ... 2340

Trifluoperazine Hydrochloride (Increased CNS depressant effect). Products include:
- Stelazine ... 2226

ROBAXIN-750 TABLETS
(Methocarbamol) ... 1872
See **Robaxin Tablets**

ROBAXISAL TABLETS
(Methocarbamol, Aspirin) ... 1872
May interact with central nervous system depressants, anticoagulants, and certain other agents. Compounds in these categories include:

Alcohol (Increased depressant effect).

Alfentanil Hydrochloride (Increased depressant effect). Products include:
- Alfenta Injection ... 1131

Alprazolam (Increased depressant effect). Products include:
- Xanax Tablets ... 2367

Aprobarbital (Increased depressant effect). Products include:
- Alurate Elixir ... 1883

Buprenorphine (Increased depressant effect).
- No products indexed under this heading.

Buspirone Hydrochloride (Increased depressant effect). Products include:
- BuSpar ... 1401

Butabarbital (Increased depressant effect). Products include:
- Pyridium Plus ... 1764

Butalbital (Increased depressant effect). Products include:
- Esgic-Plus Tablets ... 1002
- Esgic Tablets & Capsules ... 1001
- Fioricet Tablets ... 2006
- Fiorinal Capsules ... 2007
- Fiorinal with Codeine Capsules ... 2008
- Fiorinal Tablets ... 2007
- Phrenilin ... 838
- Sedapap Tablets 50 mg/650 mg ... 1360

Chlordiazepoxide (Increased depressant effect). Products include:
- Libritabs Tablets ... 1930
- Limbitrol ... 1933
- Menrium Tablets ... 1934

Chlordiazepoxide Hydrochloride (Increased depressant effect). Products include:
- Librax Capsules ... 1929
- Librium Capsules ... 1931
- Librium Injectable ... 1932

Chlorpromazine (Increased depressant effect). Products include:
- Thorazine ... 2234

Chlorprothixene (Increased depressant effect). Products include:
- Taractan Tablets ... 1920

Chlorprothixene Hydrochloride (Increased depressant effect). Products include:
- Taractan ... 1920

Chlorprothixene Lactate (Increased depressant effect). Products include:
- Taractan Concentrate ... 1920

Clorazepate Dipotassium (Increased depressant effect). Products include:
- Tranxene ... 556

Codeine (Increased depressant effect). Products include:
- Calcidrine Syrup ... 506

Codeine Phosphate (Increased depressant effect). Products include:
- Actifed with Codeine Cough Syrup.. 752
- Cheracol Cough Syrup ... 1853
- Codimal PH Syrup ... 846
- Dimetane-DC Cough Syrup ... 1857
- Empirin with Codeine Phosphate Nos. 2, 3 & 4 ... 764
- Fiorinal with Codeine Capsules ... 2008
- Isoclor Expectorant ... 982
- Naldecon CX Adult Liquid ... ▣ 521
- Novahistine DH ... 1342
- Novahistine Expectorant ... 1343
- Nucofed Capsules ... 2219
- Nucofed Expectorant ... 2219
- Nucofed Pediatric Expectorant ... 2220
- Nucofed Syrup ... 2219
- Phenaphen with Codeine Capsules 1865
- Phenaphen-650 with Codeine Tablets ... 1866
- Phenergan with Codeine ... 2497
- Phenergan VC with Codeine ... 2501
- Robitussin A-C Syrup ... 1875
- Robitussin-DAC Syrup ... 1875
- Ryna ... ▣ 741
- Soma Compound w/Codeine Tablets ... 2390
- Triaminic Expectorant w/Codeine .. 1996
- Tussi-Organidin Liquid ... 2391
- Tylenol with Codeine ... 1381

Codeine Polistirex (Increased depressant effect).
- No products indexed under this heading.

Dezocine (Increased depressant effect).

Diazepam (Increased depressant effect). Products include:
- Valium Injectable ... 1937
- Valium Tablets ... 1939
- Valrelease Capsules ... 1923

Dicumarol (Increased anticoagulant effect). Products include:
- Dicumarol Tablets ... 516

Droperidol (Increased depressant effect). Products include:
- Inapsine Injection ... 1140
- Innovar Injection ... 1141

Enflurane (Increased depressant effect). Products include:
- Ethrane ... 599

Estazolam (Increased depressant effect). Products include:
- ProSom Tablets ... 554

Ethchlorvynol (Increased depressant effect). Products include:
- Placidyl Capsules ... 553

Ethinamate (Increased depressant effect).
- No products indexed under this heading.

Fentanyl (Increased depressant effect). Products include:
- Duragesic Transdermal System ... 1133

Fentanyl Citrate (Increased depressant effect). Products include:
- Innovar Injection ... 1141
- Sublimaze Injection ... 1146

Fluphenazine Decanoate (Increased depressant effect). Products include:
- Prolixin Decanoate ... 1795

Fluphenazine Enanthate (Increased depressant effect). Products include:
- Prolixin Enanthate ... 1796

Fluphenazine Hydrochloride (Increased depressant effect). Products include:
- Prolixin Elixir ... 1793
- Prolixin Injection ... 1791
- Prolixin Oral Concentrate ... 1792
- Prolixin Tablets ... 1793

Flurazepam Hydrochloride (Increased depressant effect). Products include:
- Dalmane Capsules ... 1927

Glutethimide (Increased depressant effect).
- No products indexed under this heading.

Haloperidol (Increased depressant effect). Products include:
- Haldol Injection, Tablets and Concentrate ... 1373

Haloperidol Decanoate (Increased depressant effect). Products include:
- Haldol Decanoate ... 1375

Heparin Calcium (Increased anticoagulant effect). Products include:
- Calciparine Injection ... 925

Heparin Sodium (Increased anticoagulant effect). Products include:
- Heparin Lock Flush Solution ... 2456
- Heparin Sodium Vials ... 1264
- Heparin Sodium Injection ... 2457
- Heparin Sodium Injection, USP, Sterile Solution ... 2342

Hydrocodone Bitartrate (Increased depressant effect). Products include:
- Anexsia 5/500 Tablets ... 2196
- Anexsia 7.5/650 Tablets ... 2197
- Azdone Tablets ... 844
- Codiclear DH Syrup ... 845
- Codimal DH Syrup ... 846
- Damason-P ... 1356
- Hycodan Syrup, Tablets ... 927
- Hycomine Compound Tablets ... 929
- Hycomine Syrup ... 927
- Hycotuss Expectorant Syrup ... 930
- Hydrocet Capsules ... 835
- Lortab ASA Tablets ... 2414
- Lortab ... 2412
- Ru-Tuss with Hydrocodone ... 694
- Triaminic Expectorant DH ... 1995
- Vicodin Tablets ... 1187
- Vicodin ES Tablets ... 1189
- Zydone Capsules ... 941

Hydrocodone Polistirex (Increased depressant effect). Products include:
- Tussionex Extended-Release Suspension ... 988

Hydroxyzine Hydrochloride (Increased depressant effect). Products include:
- Atarax Tablets & Syrup ... 1941
- Marax Tablets & DF Syrup ... 1954
- Vistaril Intramuscular Solution ... 1970

Isoflurane (Increased depressant effect). Products include:
- Forane ... 600

Ketamine Hydrochloride (Increased depressant effect). Products include:
- Ketalar ... 1726

Levorphanol Tartrate (Increased depressant effect). Products include:
- Levo-Dromoran ... 1906

Lorazepam (Increased depressant effect). Products include:
- Ativan Injection ... 2432
- Ativan Tablets ... 2434

Loxapine Hydrochloride (Increased depressant effect). Products include:
- Loxitane ... 1213

Loxapine Succinate (Increased depressant effect). Products include:
- Loxitane Capsules ... 1213

Meperidine Hydrochloride (Increased depressant effect). Products include:
- Demerol ... 2047
- Mepergan Injection ... 2479

Mephobarbital (Increased depressant effect). Products include:
- Mebaral Tablets ... 2061

Meprobamate (Increased depressant effect). Products include:
- Deprol Tablets ... 2382
- Equagesic Tablets ... 2451
- Miltown Tablets ... 2386
- PMB 200 and PMB 400 ... 2504

Mesoridazine (Increased depressant effect). Products include:
- Serentil ... 686

Methadone Hydrochloride (Increased depressant effect). Products include:
- Dolophine Hydrochloride Ampoules & Vials ... 1260
- Dolophine Hydrochloride Tablets ... 1261
- Methadone Hydrochloride Diskets .. 1284
- Methadone Hydrochloride Oral Solution & Tablets ... 1987

Methohexital Sodium (Increased depressant effect). Products include:
- Brevital Sodium Vials ... 1248

Methoxyflurane (Increased depressant effect).
- No products indexed under this heading.

Midazolam Hydrochloride (Increased depressant effect). Products include:
- Versed Injection ... 1924

Molindone Hydrochloride (Increased depressant effect). Products include:
- Moban Tablets & Concentrate ... 932

Morphine Sulfate (Increased depressant effect). Products include:
- Astramorph/PF Injection, USP (Preservative-Free) ... 618
- Duramorph ... 960
- Infumorph 200 and Infumorph 500 Sterile Solutions ... 962
- MS Contin Tablets ... 1814
- MSIR ... 1817
- Oramorph SR (Morphine Sulfate Sustained Release Tablets) ... 1988
- Roxanol ... 1991

Opium Alkaloids (Increased depressant effect). Products include:
- B & O No. 15A & No. 16A Supprettes ... 2395
- Pantopon Injectable ... 1911

Oxazepam (Increased depressant effect). Products include:
- Serax Capsules ... 2522
- Serax Tablets ... 2522

Oxycodone Hydrochloride (Increased depressant effect). Products include:
- Percocet Tablets ... 950
- Percodan ... 951
- Roxicodone Tablets, Oral Solution & Intensol (Oxycodone) ... 1992
- Tylox Capsules ... 1382

Pentobarbital Sodium (Increased depressant effect). Products include:
- Nembutal Sodium Capsules ... 534
- Nembutal Sodium Solution ... 536
- Nembutal Sodium Suppositories ... 538

Perphenazine (Increased depressant effect). Products include:
- Etrafon ... 2087
- Triavil Tablets ... 1556
- Trilafon ... 2123

Phenobarbital (Increased depressant effect). Products include:
- Arco-Lase Plus Tablets ... 607
- Bellergal-S Tablets ... 1998
- Bronkolixir ... ▣ 761
- Bronkotabs Tablets ... ▣ 762
- Donnatal ... 1858
- Donnatal Extentabs ... 1859
- Donnatal Tablets ... 1858
- Donnazyme Tablets ... 1860
- Kinesed Tablets ... 2272
- Phenobarbital Elixir and Tablets ... 1293
- Primatene Tablets-P Formula ... 2421
- Quadrinal Tablets ... 1183
- Tedral SA ... 1765

Prazepam (Increased depressant effect). Products include:
- Centrax ... 1693

Prochlorperazine (Increased depressant effect). Products include:
- Compazine ... 2201

Promethazine Hydrochloride (Increased depressant effect). Products include:
- Mepergan Injection ... 2479
- Phenergan with Codeine ... 2497
- Phenergan with Dextromethorphan 2499
- Phenergan Injection ... 2493
- Phenergan Suppositories ... 2496
- Phenergan Syrup ... 2495
- Phenergan Tablets ... 2496
- Phenergan VC ... 2500
- Phenergan VC with Codeine ... 2501

Propofol (Increased depressant effect). Products include:
- Diprivan Injection ... 2267

Propoxyphene Hydrochloride (Increased depressant effect). Products include:
- Darvon ... 1256
- Wygesic Tablets ... 2540

Propoxyphene Napsylate (Increased depressant effect). Products include:
Darvon-N/Darvocet-N 1254
Quazepam (Increased depressant effect). Products include:
Doral Tablets 2383
Secobarbital Sodium (Increased depressant effect). Products include:
Seconal Sodium Pulvules 1296
Sufentanil Citrate (Increased depressant effect). Products include:
Sufenta Injection 1147
Temazepam (Increased depressant effect). Products include:
Restoril Capsules 2023
Thiamylal Sodium (Increased depressant effect). Products include:
Surital Ampoules, Steri-Vials 1764
Thioridazine Hydrochloride (Increased depressant effect). Products include:
Mellaril 2011
Thiothixene (Increased depressant effect). Products include:
Navane Capsules and Concentrate 1954
Navane Intramuscular 1956
Triazolam (Increased depressant effect). Products include:
Halcion Tablets 2340
Trifluoperazine Hydrochloride (Increased depressant effect). Products include:
Stelazine 2226
Warfarin Sodium (Increased anticoagulant effect). Products include:
Coumadin Injection & Tablets 944
Panwarfin Tablets 547

ROBINUL FORTE TABLETS
(Glycopyrrolate) 1873
No interactions described in labeling.

ROBINUL INJECTABLE
(Glycopyrrolate) 1873
May interact with:

Cyclopropane (Potential ventricular arrhythmias).

ROBINUL TABLETS
(Glycopyrrolate) 1873
No interactions described in labeling.

ROBITUSSIN
(Guaifenesin) .... ▣ 676
No interactions described in labeling.

ROBITUSSIN A-C SYRUP
(Codeine, Guaifenesin) 1875
May interact with hypnotics and sedatives, tranquilizers, and monoamine oxidase inhibitors. Compounds in these categories include:

Alprazolam (Concurrent therapy may cause greater sedation). Products include:
Xanax Tablets 2367
Buspirone Hydrochloride (Concurrent therapy may cause greater sedation). Products include:
BuSpar 1401
Chlordiazepoxide (Concurrent therapy may cause greater sedation). Products include:
Libritabs Tablets 1930
Limbitrol 1933
Menrium Tablets 1934
Chlordiazepoxide Hydrochloride (Concurrent therapy may cause greater sedation). Products include:
Librax Capsules 1929
Librium Capsules 1931
Librium Injectable 1932
Chlorpromazine (Concurrent therapy may cause greater sedation). Products include:
Thorazine 2234
Chlorprothixene (Concurrent therapy may cause greater sedation). Products include:
Taractan Tablets 1920
Chlorprothixene Hydrochloride (Concurrent therapy may cause greater sedation). Products include:
Taractan 1920
Clorazepate Dipotassium (Concurrent therapy may cause greater sedation). Products include:
Tranxene 556
Diazepam (Concurrent therapy may cause greater sedation). Products include:
Valium Injectable 1937
Valium Tablets 1939
Valrelease Capsules 1923
Droperidol (Concurrent therapy may cause greater sedation). Products include:
Inapsine Injection 1140
Innovar Injection 1141
Estazolam (Concurrent therapy may cause greater sedation). Products include:
ProSom Tablets 554
Ethchlorvynol (Concurrent therapy may cause greater sedation). Products include:
Placidyl Capsules 553
Ethinamate (Concurrent therapy may cause greater sedation).
No products indexed under this heading.
Fluphenazine Decanoate (Concurrent therapy may cause greater sedation). Products include:
Prolixin Decanoate 1795
Fluphenazine Enanthate (Concurrent therapy may cause greater sedation). Products include:
Prolixin Enanthate 1796
Fluphenazine Hydrochloride (Concurrent therapy may cause greater sedation). Products include:
Prolixin Elixir 1793
Prolixin Injection 1791
Prolixin Oral Concentrate 1792
Prolixin Tablets 1793
Flurazepam Hydrochloride (Concurrent therapy may cause greater sedation). Products include:
Dalmane Capsules 1927
Furazolidone (Concurrent therapy may cause greater sedation). Products include:
Furoxone 1855
Glutethimide (Concurrent therapy may cause greater sedation).
No products indexed under this heading.
Haloperidol (Concurrent therapy may cause greater sedation). Products include:
Haldol Injection, Tablets and Concentrate 1373
Haloperidol Decanoate (Concurrent therapy may cause greater sedation). Products include:
Haldol Decanoate 1375
Hydroxyzine Hydrochloride (Concurrent therapy may cause greater sedation). Products include:
Atarax Tablets & Syrup 1941
Marax Tablets & DF Syrup 1954
Vistaril Intramuscular Solution 1970
Isocarboxazid (Concurrent therapy may cause greater sedation). Products include:
Marplan Tablets 1906
Lorazepam (Concurrent therapy may cause greater sedation). Products include:
Ativan Injection 2432
Ativan Tablets 2434
Loxapine Hydrochloride (Concurrent therapy may cause greater sedation). Products include:
Loxitane 1213
Loxapine Succinate (Concurrent therapy may cause greater sedation). Products include:
Loxitane Capsules 1213
Meprobamate (Concurrent therapy may cause greater sedation). Products include:
Deprol Tablets 2382
Equagesic Tablets 2451
Miltown Tablets 2386
PMB 200 and PMB 400 2504
Mesoridazine (Concurrent therapy may cause greater sedation). Products include:
Serentil 686
Midazolam Hydrochloride (Concurrent therapy may cause greater sedation). Products include:
Versed Injection 1924
Molindone Hydrochloride (Concurrent therapy may cause greater sedation). Products include:
Moban Tablets & Concentrate 932
Oxazepam (Concurrent therapy may cause greater sedation). Products include:
Serax Capsules 2522
Serax Tablets 2522
Perphenazine (Concurrent therapy may cause greater sedation). Products include:
Etrafon 2087
Triavil Tablets 1556
Trilafon 2123
Phenelzine Sulfate (Concurrent therapy may cause greater sedation). Products include:
Nardil 1742
Prazepam (Concurrent therapy may cause greater sedation). Products include:
Centrax 1693
Prochlorperazine (Concurrent therapy may cause greater sedation). Products include:
Compazine 2201
Promethazine Hydrochloride (Concurrent therapy may cause greater sedation). Products include:
Mepergan Injection 2479
Phenergan with Codeine 2497
Phenergan with Dextromethorphan 2499
Phenergan Injection 2493
Phenergan Suppositories 2496
Phenergan Syrup 2495
Phenergan Tablets 2496
Phenergan VC 2500
Phenergan VC with Codeine 2501
Propofol (Concurrent therapy may cause greater sedation). Products include:
Diprivan Injection 2267
Quazepam (Concurrent therapy may cause greater sedation). Products include:
Doral Tablets 2383
Secobarbital Sodium (Concurrent therapy may cause greater sedation). Products include:
Seconal Sodium Pulvules 1296
Selegiline Hydrochloride (Concurrent therapy may cause greater sedation). Products include:
Eldepryl 2250
Temazepam (Concurrent therapy may cause greater sedation). Products include:
Restoril Capsules 2023
Thioridazine Hydrochloride (Concurrent therapy may cause greater sedation). Products include:
Mellaril 2011
Thiothixene (Concurrent therapy may cause greater sedation). Products include:
Navane Capsules and Concentrate 1954
Navane Intramuscular 1956
Tranylcypromine Sulfate (Concurrent therapy may cause greater sedation). Products include:
Parnate Tablets 2222
Triazolam (Concurrent therapy may cause greater sedation). Products include:
Halcion Tablets 2340
Trifluoperazine Hydrochloride (Concurrent therapy may cause greater sedation). Products include:
Stelazine 2226

ROBITUSSIN COUGH CALMERS
(Dextromethorphan Hydrobromide) .... ▣ 677
May interact with monoamine oxidase inhibitors. Compounds in this category include:

Furazolidone (Concurrent use is contraindicated and may result in serious toxicity). Products include:
Furoxone 1855
Isocarboxazid (Concurrent use is contraindicated and may result in serious toxicity). Products include:
Marplan Tablets 1906
Phenelzine Sulfate (Concurrent use is contraindicated and may result in serious toxicity). Products include:
Nardil 1742
Selegiline Hydrochloride (Concurrent use is contraindicated and may result in serious toxicity). Products include:
Eldepryl 2250
Tranylcypromine Sulfate (Concurrent use is contraindicated and may result in serious toxicity). Products include:
Parnate Tablets 2222

ROBITUSSIN NIGHT RELIEF
(Acetaminophen, Dextromethorphan Hydrobromide, Phenylephrine Hydrochloride, Pyrilamine Maleate) .... ▣ 677
May interact with monoamine oxidase inhibitors, sympathomimetic aerosol bronchodilators, and certain other agents. Compounds in these categories include:

Albuterol (May produce additive effects and increased toxicity). Products include:
Proventil Inhalation Aerosol 2117
Ventolin Inhalation Aerosol and Refill 583
Albuterol Sulfate (May produce additive effects and increased toxicity). Products include:
Proventil Repetabs Tablets 2120
Proventil Solutions for Inhalation 0.5% and 0.083% 2118
Proventil Syrup 2119
Proventil Tablets 2120
Ventolin 583
Alcohol (Avoid concomitant use).
Antihypertensive agents, unspecified (Diminished antihypertensive effect).
Dobutamine Hydrochloride (May produce additive effects and increased toxicity). Products include:
Dobutrex Solution Vials 1259
Dopamine Hydrochloride (May produce additive effects and increased toxicity). Products include:
Intropin Injection 930

Ephedrine Hydrochloride (May produce additive effects and increased toxicity). Products include:

- Amesec ▣ 682
- Primatene Tablets-M Formula 2421
- Primatene Tablets-P Formula 2421
- Primatene Tablets-Regular Formula 2421
- Quadrinal Tablets 1183
- Quelidrine Syrup 556
- Tedral SA 1765

Ephedrine Sulfate (May produce additive effects and increased toxicity). Products include:

- Bronkaid Tablets ▣ 757
- Bronkolixir ▣ 761
- Bronkotabs Tablets ▣ 762
- Marax Tablets & DF Syrup 1954
- Pazo Hemorrhoid Ointment & Suppositories 752
- Vicks Vatronol Nose Drops ▣ 666

Ephedrine Tannate (May produce additive effects and increased toxicity). Products include:

- Rynatuss 2388

Epinephrine (May produce additive effects and increased toxicity). Products include:

- Ana-Kit Anaphylaxis Emergency Treatment Kit 1100
- Bronkaid Mist ▣ 757
- EpiPen 843
- Marcaine Hydrochloride 0.5% with Epinephrine 1:200,000 (as bitartrate) 958
- Marcaine Hydrochloride with Epinephrine 1:200,000 2055
- Primatene Mist 2420
- Sus-Phrine Injection 1006
- Xylocaine with Epinephrine Injections 637

Epinephrine Bitartrate (May produce additive effects and increased toxicity). Products include:

- AsthmaHaler Mist Epinephrine Bitartrate Bronchodilator ▣ 616
- Bronkaid Mist Suspension ▣ 757
- Primatene Mist Suspension 2421

Epinephrine Hydrochloride (May produce additive effects and increased toxicity). Products include:

- Adrenalin Chloride Solution 1:100 & 1:1,000 1689
- Epifrin ⊙ 244
- Glaucon ⊙ 218

Furazolidone (May produce hypertensive crisis; serious toxicity may result). Products include:

- Furoxone 1855

Isocarboxazid (May produce hypertensive crisis; serious toxicity may result). Products include:

- Marplan Tablets 1906

Metaproterenol Sulfate (May produce additive effects and increased toxicity). Products include:

- Alupent 674
- Arm-a-Med Metaproterenol Sulfate Inhalation Solution, USP 617
- Metaprel Inhalation Aerosol Bronchodilator 2014
- Metaprel Inhalation Solution 2015
- Metaprel 2015
- Metaproterenol Sulfate Inhalation Solution, USP 912

Metaraminol Bitartrate (May produce additive effects and increased toxicity). Products include:

- Aramine Injection 1424

Methoxamine Hydrochloride (May produce additive effects and increased toxicity). Products include:

- Vasoxyl Injection 819

Norepinephrine Bitartrate (May produce additive effects and increased toxicity). Products include:

- Levophed Bitartrate Injection 2054

Phenelzine Sulfate (May produce hypertensive crisis; serious toxicity may result). Products include:

- Nardil 1742

Phenylephrine Bitartrate (May produce additive effects and increased toxicity).

- No products indexed under this heading.

Phenylephrine Tannate (May produce additive effects and increased toxicity). Products include:

- Rynatan 2387
- Rynatuss 2388

Phenylpropanolamine Hydrochloride (May produce additive effects and increased toxicity). Products include:

- A.R.M. Allergy Relief Medicine Caplets ▣ 615
- Acutrim ▣ 548
- Allerest ▣ 559
- BC Cold Powder ▣ 517
- Cheracol Plus Head Cold/Cough Formula ▣ 667
- Codimal Expectorant 846
- Comtrex Multi-Symptom Cold Reliever Tablets/Caplets/Liqui-Gels/Liquid 745
- Contac Continuous Action Decongestant/Antihistamine Capsules ▣ 710
- Contac Maximum Strength Continuous Action Decongestant/Antihistamine Caplets ▣ 709
- Contac Severe Cold and Flu Formula Caplets ▣ 711
- Coricidin 'D' Decongestant Tablets ▣ 695
- Coricidin Demilets Tablets for Children ▣ 696
- Demazin Nasal Decongestant/Antihistamine Repetabs Tablets & Syrup ▣ 697
- Dexatrim ▣ 733
- Dimetane-DC Cough Syrup 1857
- Dimetapp Elixir ▣ 673
- Dimetapp DM Elixir ▣ 674
- Dimetapp Extentabs ▣ 674
- Dimetapp Plus Caplets ▣ 675
- Dimetapp Tablets ▣ 675
- Entex Capsules 1623
- Entex LA Tablets 1623
- Entex Liquid 1623
- 4-Way Cold Tablets 750
- Hycomine Syrup 927
- Naldecon CX Adult Liquid ▣ 521
- Naldecon DX Adult Liquid ▣ 521
- Naldecon DX Children's Syrup ▣ 522
- Naldecon DX Pediatric Drops ▣ 522
- Naldecon EX Children's Syrup ▣ 522
- Naldecon EX Pediatric Drops ▣ 523
- Naldecon Syrup, Tablets, Pediatric Drops and Pediatric Syrup 709
- Nolamine Tablets 838
- Nolex LA Tablets 838
- Ornade Spansule Capsules 2221
- Orthoxicol Cough Syrup ▣ 668
- Propagest 839
- Pyrroxate Capsules ▣ 669
- Robitussin-CF ▣ 676
- Ru-Tuss II Capsules 693
- Ru-Tuss with Hydrocodone 694
- Ru-Tuss Tablets 693
- Sine-Off Sinus Medicine Tablets-Aspirin Formula ▣ 722
- Sinulin 840
- St. Joseph Cold Tablets for Children ▣ 704
- Tavist-D Tablets 2035
- Triaminic Allergy Tablets ▣ 688
- Triaminic Chewables ▣ 688
- Triaminic Cold Tablets ▣ 688
- Triaminic Expectorant ▣ 688
- Triaminic Expectorant w/Codeine 1996
- Triaminic Expectorant DH 1995
- Triaminic Oral Infant Drops 1996
- Triaminic Syrup ▣ 689
- Triaminic-12 Tablets ▣ 690
- Triaminic-DM Syrup ▣ 689
- Triaminicin Tablets ▣ 690
- Triaminicol Multi-Symptom Cold Tablets ▣ 691
- Triaminicol Multi-Symptom Relief ▣ 691
- Tuss-Ornade Liquid 2242
- Tuss-Ornade Spansule Capsules 2242
- Tylenol Cold Medication, Effervescent Tablets 1369

Pirbuterol Acetate (May produce additive effects and increased toxicity). Products include:

- Maxair Inhaler 1311

Pseudoephedrine Hydrochloride (May produce additive effects and increased toxicity). Products include:

- Actifed Capsules ▣ 539
- Actifed Plus Caplets ▣ 539
- Actifed Plus Tablets ▣ 540
- Actifed with Codeine Cough Syrup 752
- Actifed Syrup ▣ 540
- Actifed Tablets ▣ 540
- Actifed 12-Hour Capsules ▣ 539
- Advil Cold & Sinus Caplets (formerly CoAdvil) 2416
- Allerest ▣ 559
- Anatuss LA Tablets 1359
- Benadryl Decongestant Elixir ▣ 635
- Benadryl Decongestant ▣ 635
- Benadryl Plus ▣ 636
- Benadryl Plus Nighttime ▣ 637
- Benylin Decongestant ▣ 638
- Brexin L.A. Capsules 2078
- Bromfed Capsules (Timed Release) 1615
- Bromfed Syrup ▣ 628
- Bromfed 1615
- CoAdvil ▣ 748
- Allergy-Sinus Comtrex Multi-Symptom Allergy Sinus Formula Tablets & Caplets 746
- Cough Formula Comtrex 746
- Comtrex Multi-Symptom Cold Reliever Tablets/Caplets/Liqui-Gels/Liquid 745
- Day-Night Comtrex 747
- Non-Drowsy Comtrex 747
- Congess 994
- Congestac Caplets ▣ 617
- Contac Jr. Children's Cold Medicine ▣ 712
- Contac Nighttime Cold Medicine ▣ 713
- Contac Sinus Caplets Maximum Strength Non-Drowsy Formula ▣ 710
- Contac Sinus Tablets Maximum Strength Non-Drowsy Formula ▣ 710
- Deconamine 663
- Deconsal II Tablets 559
- Dimacol Caplets ▣ 672
- Dimetane-DX Cough Syrup 1858
- Dorcol Children's Cough Syrup ▣ 685
- Dorcol Children's Decongestant Liquid ▣ 685
- Dorcol Children's Liquid Cold Formula ▣ 686
- Maximum Strength Dristan Decongestant/Analgesic Coated Caplets ▣ 750
- No Drowsiness Dristan Cold Nasal Decongestant/Analgesic Coated Caplets 2420
- Dristan Sinus Caplets 2419
- Sinus Excedrin Analgesic, Decongestant Tablets & Caplets ▣ 533
- Fedahist Gyrocaps 2145
- Fedahist Timecaps 2145
- Guaifed 1615
- Guaifed Syrup ▣ 629
- Isoclor Expectorant 982
- Isoclor Timesule Capsules ▣ 561
- Kronofed-A 970
- Medi-Flu Caplet, Liquid ▣ 640
- Novafed A Capsules 1342
- Novafed Capsules 1342
- Novahistine DH 1342
- Novahistine DMX ▣ 595
- Novahistine Expectorant 1343
- Nucofed Capsules 2219
- Nucofed Expectorant 2219
- Nucofed Pediatric Expectorant 2220
- Nucofed Syrup 2219
- Ornex Caplets ▣ 618
- PediaCare Allergy Relief Formula Liquid 1362
- PediaCare Cough-Cold Formula Liquid 1362
- PediaCare Infants' Oral Decongestant Drops 1362
- PediaCare Night Rest Cough-Cold Formula Liquid 1362
- PediaCare 6-12 Cough-Cold Formula Chewable Tablets 1362
- Robitussin-DAC Syrup 1875
- Robitussin-PE ▣ 677
- Rondec 1975
- Rondec-DM 1976
- Rondec-TR Tablet 1975
- Ru-Tuss DE Tablets 694
- Ryna ▣ 741
- Seldane-D Extended-Release Tablets 1350
- Sinarest ▣ 562
- Sine-Aid Maximum Strength Sinus Headache Caplets 1365
- Sine-Aid Maximum Strength Sinus Headache Tablets 1365
- Sine-Off Maximum Strength Allergy/Sinus Formula Caplets ▣ 721
- Sine-Off Maximum Strength No Drowsiness Formula Caplets ▣ 722
- Singlet Tablets ▣ 598
- Sinutab Maximum Strength ▣ 641
- Sinutab Maximum Strength Without Drowsiness Tablets & Caplets ▣ 642
- Sinutab Regular Strength Without Drowsiness Formula ▣ 641
- St. Joseph Nighttime Cold Medicine ▣ 705
- Sudafed Children's Liquid ▣ 543
- Sudafed Cough Syrup ▣ 543
- Sudafed Plus Liquid ▣ 544
- Sudafed Plus Tablets ▣ 545
- Sudafed Sinus Caplets ▣ 545
- Sudafed Sinus Tablets ▣ 545
- Sudafed Tablets, 30 mg ▣ 544
- Sudafed Tablets, Adult Strength, 60 mg ▣ 544
- Sudafed 12 Hour Capsules ▣ 545
- TheraFlu Flu and Cold Medicine ▣ 687
- Triaminic Nite Light ▣ 689
- Tylenol Allergy Sinus Medication Caplets and Gelcaps, Maximum Strength 1372
- Children's Tylenol Cold Liquid Formula and Chewable Tablets 1368
- Tylenol Cold & Flu Hot Medication, Packets 1369
- Tylenol Cold & Flu No Drowsiness Hot Medication, Packets 1371
- Tylenol Cold Medication Caplets and Tablets 1370
- Tylenol Cold Medication No Drowsiness Formula Caplets 1370
- Tylenol Cold Night Time Medication Liquid 1371
- Tylenol Cough Medication Liquid with Decongestant, Maximum Strength 1372
- Tylenol, Maximum Strength, Sinus Medication Gelcaps, Caplets and Tablets 1373
- Ursinus Inlay-Tabs ▣ 691
- Vicks Children's NyQuil ▣ 664
- Vicks Daycare ▣ 660
- Vicks Formula 44D Decongestant Cough Medicine ▣ 662
- Vicks Formula 44M Multi-Symptom Cough Medicine ▣ 662
- Vicks NyQuil Nighttime Colds Medicine-Original & Cherry Flavor ▣ 664
- Vicks Pediatric Formula 44 Cough & Congestion Medicine ▣ 663
- Vicks Pediatric Formula 44m Multi-Symptom Cough & Cold Medicine ▣ 663

Pseudoephedrine Sulfate (May produce additive effects and increased toxicity). Products include:

- Afrin Tablets ▣ 693
- Chlor-Trimeton Decongestant ▣ 694
- Disophrol Chronotab Sustained-Action Tablets ▣ 698
- Drixoral Antihistamine/Nasal Decongestant Syrup ▣ 698
- Drixoral Non-Drowsy Formula ▣ 699
- Drixoral Plus Extended-Release Tablets ▣ 699
- Drixoral Sinus ▣ 700
- Drixoral Sustained-Action Tablets ▣ 698
- Sinutab Allergy Formula Sustained Action Tablets ▣ 640
- Trinalin Repetabs Tablets 1170

Selegiline Hydrochloride (May produce hypertensive crisis; serious toxicity may result). Products include:

- Eldepryl 2250

Terbutaline Sulfate (May produce additive effects and increased toxicity). Products include:

- Brethaire Inhaler 1024
- Brethine Ampuls 1026
- Brethine Tablets 1026
- Bricanyl Injection 1324
- Bricanyl Tablets 1325

Tranylcypromine Sulfate (May produce hypertensive crisis; serious toxicity may result). Products include:

Parnate Tablets ... 2222

ROBITUSSIN PEDIATRIC
(Dextromethorphan Hydrobromide) ... ▣ 678
May interact with monoamine oxidase inhibitors. Compounds in this category include:

Furazolidone (Concurrent use is contraindicated and may result in serious toxicity). Products include:

Furoxone ... 1855

Isocarboxazid (Concurrent use is contraindicated and may result in serious toxicity). Products include:

Marplan Tablets ... 1906

Phenelzine Sulfate (Concurrent use is contraindicated and may result in serious toxicity). Products include:

Nardil ... 1742

Selegiline Hydrochloride (Concurrent use is contraindicated and may result in serious toxicity). Products include:

Eldepryl ... 2250

Tranylcypromine Sulfate (Concurrent use is contraindicated and may result in serious toxicity). Products include:

Parnate Tablets ... 2222

ROBITUSSIN-CF
(Dextromethorphan Hydrobromide, Guaifenesin, Phenylpropanolamine Hydrochloride) ... ▣ 676
May interact with monoamine oxidase inhibitors, sympathomimetic aerosol bronchodilators, and certain other agents. Compounds in these categories include:

Albuterol (May produce additive effects and increased toxicity). Products include:

Proventil Inhalation Aerosol ... 2117
Ventolin Inhalation Aerosol and Refill ... 583

Albuterol Sulfate (May produce additive effects and increased toxicity). Products include:

Proventil Repetabs Tablets ... 2120
Proventil Solutions for Inhalation 0.5% and 0.083% ... 2118
Proventil Syrup ... 2119
Proventil Tablets ... 2120
Ventolin ... 583

Antihypertensive agents, unspecified (Diminished antihypertensive effect).

Dobutamine Hydrochloride (May produce additive effects and increased toxicity). Products include:

Dobutrex Solution Vials ... 1259

Dopamine Hydrochloride (May produce additive effects and increased toxicity). Products include:

Intropin Injection ... 930

Ephedrine Hydrochloride (May produce additive effects and increased toxicity). Products include:

Amesec ... ▣ 682
Primatene Tablets-M Formula ... 2421
Primatene Tablets-P Formula ... 2421
Primatene Tablets-Regular Formula ... 2421
Quadrinal Tablets ... 1183
Quelidrine Syrup ... 556
Tedral SA ... 1765

Ephedrine Sulfate (May produce additive effects and increased toxicity). Products include:

Bronkaid Tablets ... ▣ 757
Bronkolixir ... ▣ 761
Bronkotabs Tablets ... ▣ 762
Marax Tablets & DF Syrup ... 1954
Pazo Hemorrhoid Ointment & Suppositories ... 752
Vicks Vatronol Nose Drops ... ▣ 666

Ephedrine Tannate (May produce additive effects and increased toxicity). Products include:

Rynatuss ... 2388

Epinephrine (May produce additive effects and increased toxicity). Products include:

Ana-Kit Anaphylaxis Emergency Treatment Kit ... 1100
Bronkaid Mist ... ▣ 757
EpiPen ... 843
Marcaine Hydrochloride 0.5% with Epinephrine 1:200,000 (as bitartrate) ... 958
Marcaine Hydrochloride with Epinephrine 1:200,000 ... 2055
Primatene Mist ... 2420
Sus-Phrine Injection ... 1006
Xylocaine with Epinephrine Injections ... 637

Epinephrine Bitartrate (May produce additive effects and increased toxicity). Products include:

AsthmaHaler Mist Epinephrine Bitartrate Bronchodilator ... ▣ 616
Bronkaid Mist Suspension ... ▣ 757
Primatene Mist Suspension ... 2421

Epinephrine Hydrochloride (May produce additive effects and increased toxicity). Products include:

Adrenalin Chloride Solution 1:100 & 1:1,000 ... 1689
Epifrin ... ◉ 244
Glaucon ... ◉ 218

Furazolidone (May produce a hypertensive crisis; concurrent use is contraindicated). Products include:

Furoxone ... 1855

Isocarboxazid (May produce a hypertensive crisis; concurrent use is contraindicated). Products include:

Marplan Tablets ... 1906

Metaproterenol Sulfate (May produce additive effects and increased toxicity). Products include:

Alupent ... 674
Arm-a-Med Metaproterenol Sulfate Inhalation Solution, USP ... 617
Metaprel Inhalation Aerosol Bronchodilator ... 2014
Metaprel Inhalation Solution ... 2015
Metaprel ... 2015
Metaproterenol Sulfate Inhalation Solution, USP ... 912

Metaraminol Bitartrate (May produce additive effects and increased toxicity). Products include:

Aramine Injection ... 1424

Methoxamine Hydrochloride (May produce additive effects and increased toxicity). Products include:

Vasoxyl Injection ... 819

Norepinephrine Bitartrate (May produce additive effects and increased toxicity). Products include:

Levophed Bitartrate Injection ... 2054

Phenelzine Sulfate (May produce a hypertensive crisis; concurrent use is contraindicated). Products include:

Nardil ... 1742

Phenylephrine Bitartrate (May produce additive effects and increased toxicity).

No products indexed under this heading.

Phenylephrine Hydrochloride (May produce additive effects and increased toxicity). Products include:

AK-Dilate Solution 2.5% and 10% ... ◉ 203
Atrohist Sprinkle Capsules ... 558
Cerose-DM ... 2443
Codimal ... 846
Comhist LA Capsules ... 1618
Congespirin For Children Aspirin Free Chewable Cold Tablets ... 748
Cyclomydril ... ◉ 216
Deconsal Sprinkle Capsules ... 559
Dimetane Decongestant ... ▣ 673
Dristan Decongestant/Antihistamine/ Analgesic Coated Caplets ... ▣ 749
Dristan Cold Nasal Decongestant/ Antihistamine/ Analgesic Coated Tablets ... 2419
Dristan Advanced Formula Decongestant/Antihistamine/ Analgesic Tablets ... ▣ 749
Dristan Nasal Spray, Menthol ... 2419
Dristan Nasal Spray, Regular and Regular with Metered Pump ... 2419
Entex Capsules ... 1623
Entex Liquid ... 1623
Sinus Excedrin Analgesic, Decongestant Tablets & Caplets ... 750
Extendryl ... 994
4-Way Fast Acting Nasal Spray - Original Formula (regular & mentholated) & Metered Spray Pump (regular) ... 751
Hycomine Compound Tablets ... 929
Murocoll-2 Sterile Ophthalmic Solution ... ◉ 261
Mydfrin 2.5% ... ◉ 224
Naldecon Syrup, Tablets, Pediatric Drops and Pediatric Syrup ... 709
Neo-Synephrine Hydrochloride 1% Carpuject ... 2063
Neo-Synephrine Hydrochloride 1% Injection ... 2063
Neo-Synephrine Hydrochloride (Ophthalmic) ... 2064
Neo-Synephrine ... ▣ 759
Nōstril Nasal Decongestant ... ▣ 520
Novahistine Elixir ... ▣ 596
Phenergan VC ... 2500
Phenergan VC with Codeine ... 2501
Prefrin Liquifilm Vasoconstrictor and Lubricant Eye Drops ... ◉ 254
Prefrin-A ... ◉ 255
Quelidrine Syrup ... 556
Relief Vasoconstrictor and Lubricant Eye Drops ... ◉ 256
Robitussin Night Relief ... ▣ 677
Ru-Tuss with Hydrocodone ... 694
Ru-Tuss Tablets ... 693
Vasosulf ... ◉ 279
Vicks Sinex ... ▣ 665
Zincfrin ... ◉ 230

Phenylephrine Tannate (May produce additive effects and increased toxicity). Products include:

Rynatan ... 2387
Rynatuss ... 2388

Pirbuterol Acetate (May produce additive effects and increased toxicity). Products include:

Maxair Inhaler ... 1311

Pseudoephedrine Hydrochloride (May produce additive effects and increased toxicity). Products include:

Actifed Capsules ... ▣ 539
Actifed Plus Caplets ... ▣ 539
Actifed Plus Tablets ... ▣ 540
Actifed with Codeine Cough Syrup ... 752
Actifed Syrup ... ▣ 540
Actifed Tablets ... ▣ 540
Actifed 12-Hour Capsules ... ▣ 539
Advil Cold & Sinus Caplets (formerly CoAdvil) ... 2416
Allerest ... ▣ 559
Anatuss LA Tablets ... 1359
Benadryl Decongestant Elixir ... ▣ 635
Benadryl Decongestant ... ▣ 635
Benadryl Plus ... ▣ 636
Benadryl Plus Nighttime ... ▣ 637
Benylin Decongestant ... ▣ 638
Brexin L.A. Capsules ... 2078
Bromfed Capsules (Timed Release) ... 1615
Bromfed Syrup ... ▣ 628
Bromfed ... 1615
CoAdvil ... ▣ 748
Allergy-Sinus Comtrex Multi-Symptom Allergy Sinus Formula Tablets & Caplets ... 746
Cough Formula Comtrex ... 746
Comtrex Multi-Symptom Cold Reliever Tablets/Caplets/Liqui-Gels/Liquid ... 745
Day-Night Comtrex ... 747
Non-Drowsy Comtrex ... 747
Congess ... 994
Congestac Caplets ... ▣ 617
Contac Jr. Children's Cold Medicine ... ▣ 712
Contac Nighttime Cold Medicine ... ▣ 713
Contac Sinus Caplets Maximum Strength Non-Drowsy Formula ... ▣ 710
Contac Sinus Tablets Maximum Strength Non-Drowsy Formula ... ▣ 710
Deconamine ... 663
Deconsal II Tablets ... 559
Dimacol Caplets ... ▣ 672
Dimetane-DX Cough Syrup ... 1858
Dorcol Children's Cough Syrup ... ▣ 685
Dorcol Children's Decongestant Liquid ... ▣ 685
Dorcol Children's Liquid Cold Formula ... ▣ 686
Maximum Strength Dristan Decongestant/Analgesic Coated Caplets ... ▣ 750
No Drowsiness Dristan Cold Nasal Decongestant/Analgesic Coated Caplets ... 2420
Dristan Sinus Caplets ... 2419
Sinus Excedrin Analgesic, Decongestant Tablets & Caplets ... ▣ 533
Fedahist Gyrocaps ... 2145
Fedahist Timecaps ... 2145
Guaifed ... 1615
Guaifed Syrup ... ▣ 629
Isoclor Expectorant ... 982
Isoclor Timesule Capsules ... ▣ 561
Kronofed-A ... 970
Medi-Flu Caplet, Liquid ... ▣ 640
Novafed A Capsules ... 1342
Novafed Capsules ... 1342
Novahistine DH ... 1342
Novahistine DMX ... ▣ 595
Novahistine Expectorant ... 1343
Nucofed Capsules ... 2219
Nucofed Expectorant ... 2219
Nucofed Pediatric Expectorant ... 2220
Nucofed Syrup ... 2219
Ornex Caplets ... ▣ 618
PediaCare Allergy Relief Formula Liquid ... 1362
PediaCare Cough-Cold Formula Liquid ... 1362
PediaCare Infants' Oral Decongestant Drops ... 1362
PediaCare Night Rest Cough-Cold Formula Liquid ... 1362
PediaCare 6-12 Cough-Cold Formula Chewable Tablets ... 1362
Robitussin-DAC Syrup ... 1875
Robitussin-PE ... ▣ 677
Rondec ... 1975
Rondec-DM ... 1976
Rondec-TR Tablet ... 1975
Ru-Tuss DE Tablets ... 694
Ryna ... ▣ 741
Seldane-D Extended-Release Tablets ... 1350
Sinarest ... ▣ 562
Sine-Aid Maximum Strength Sinus Headache Caplets ... 1365
Sine-Aid Maximum Strength Sinus Headache Tablets ... 1365
Sine-Off Maximum Strength Allergy/Sinus Formula Caplets ... ▣ 721
Sine-Off Maximum Strength No Drowsiness Formula Caplets ... ▣ 722
Singlet Tablets ... ▣ 598
Sinutab Maximum Strength ... ▣ 641
Sinutab Maximum Strength Without Drowsiness Tablets & Caplets ... ▣ 642
Sinutab Regular Strength Without Drowsiness Formula ... ▣ 641
St. Joseph Nighttime Cold Medicine ... ▣ 705
Sudafed Children's Liquid ... ▣ 543
Sudafed Cough Syrup ... ▣ 543
Sudafed Plus Liquid ... ▣ 544
Sudafed Plus Tablets ... ▣ 545
Sudafed Sinus Caplets ... ▣ 545
Sudafed Sinus Tablets ... ▣ 545
Sudafed Tablets, 30 mg ... ▣ 544
Sudafed Tablets, Adult Strength, 60 mg ... ▣ 544
Sudafed 12 Hour Capsules ... ▣ 545
TheraFlu Flu and Cold Medicine ... ▣ 687
Triaminic Nite Light ... ▣ 689
Tylenol Allergy Sinus Medication Caplets and Gelcaps, Maximum Strength ... 1372
Children's Tylenol Cold Liquid Formula and Chewable Tablets ... 1368
Tylenol Cold & Flu Hot Medication, Packets ... 1369
Tylenol Cold & Flu No Drowsiness Hot Medication, Packets ... 1371

Tylenol Cold Medication Caplets and Tablets ... 1370
Tylenol Cold Medication No Drowsiness Formula Caplets ... 1370
Tylenol Cold Night Time Medication Liquid ... 1371
Tylenol Cough Medication Liquid with Decongestant, Maximum Strength ... 1372
Tylenol, Maximum Strength, Sinus Medication Gelcaps, Caplets and Tablets ... 1373
Ursinus Inlay-Tabs ... ▣ 691
Vicks Children's NyQuil ... ▣ 664
Vicks Daycare ... ▣ 660
Vicks Formula 44D Decongestant Cough Medicine ... ▣ 662
Vicks Formula 44M Multi-Symptom Cough Medicine ... ▣ 662
Vicks NyQuil Nighttime Colds Medicine-Original & Cherry Flavor ... ▣ 664
Vicks Pediatric Formula 44 Cough & Congestion Medicine ... ▣ 663
Vicks Pediatric Formula 44m Multi-Symptom Cough & Cold Medicine ... ▣ 663

Pseudoephedrine Sulfate (May produce additive effects and increased toxicity). Products include:
Afrin Tablets ... ▣ 693
Chlor-Trimeton Decongestant ... ▣ 694
Disophrol Chronotab Sustained-Action Tablets ... ▣ 698
Drixoral Antihistamine/Nasal Decongestant Syrup ... ▣ 698
Drixoral Non-Drowsy Formula ... ▣ 699
Drixoral Plus Extended-Release Tablets ... ▣ 699
Drixoral Sinus ... ▣ 700
Drixoral Sustained-Action Tablets ▣ 698
Sinutab Allergy Formula Sustained Action Tablets ... ▣ 640
Trinalin Repetabs Tablets ... 1170

Selegiline Hydrochloride (May produce a hypertensive crisis; concurrent use is contraindicated). Products include:
Eldepryl ... 2250

Terbutaline Sulfate (May produce additive effects and increased toxicity). Products include:
Brethaire Inhaler ... 1024
Brethine Ampuls ... 1026
Brethine Tablets ... 1026
Bricanyl Injection ... 1324
Bricanyl Tablets ... 1325

Tranylcypromine Sulfate (May produce a hypertensive crisis; concurrent use is contraindicated). Products include:
Parnate Tablets ... 2222

ROBITUSSIN-DAC SYRUP
(Codeine Phosphate, Guaifenesin, Pseudoephedrine Hydrochloride) ... 1875
May interact with monoamine oxidase inhibitors. Compounds in this category include:

Furazolidone (Concurrent use is not recommended). Products include:
Furoxone ... 1855

Isocarboxazid (Concurrent use is not recommended). Products include:
Marplan Tablets ... 1906

Phenelzine Sulfate (Concurrent use is not recommended). Products include:
Nardil ... 1742

Selegiline Hydrochloride (Concurrent use is not recommended). Products include:
Eldepryl ... 2250

Tranylcypromine Sulfate (Concurrent use is not recommended). Products include:
Parnate Tablets ... 2222

ROBITUSSIN-DM
(Dextromethorphan Hydrobromide, Guaifenesin) ... ▣ 676
May interact with monoamine oxidase inhibitors. Compounds in this category include:

Furazolidone (Serious toxicity may develop). Products include:
Furoxone ... 1855

Isocarboxazid (Serious toxicity may develop). Products include:
Marplan Tablets ... 1906

Phenelzine Sulfate (Serious toxicity may develop). Products include:
Nardil ... 1742

Selegiline Hydrochloride (Serious toxicity may develop). Products include:
Eldepryl ... 2250

Tranylcypromine Sulfate (Serious toxicity may develop). Products include:
Parnate Tablets ... 2222

ROBITUSSIN-PE
(Guaifenesin, Pseudoephedrine Hydrochloride) ... ▣ 677
May interact with monoamine oxidase inhibitors, sympathomimetic aerosol bronchodilators, and certain other agents. Compounds in these categories include:

Albuterol (May produce additive effects and increased toxicity). Products include:
Proventil Inhalation Aerosol ... 2117
Ventolin Inhalation Aerosol and Refill ... 583

Albuterol Sulfate (May produce additive effects and increased toxicity). Products include:
Proventil Repetabs Tablets ... 2120
Proventil Solutions for Inhalation 0.5% and 0.083% ... 2118
Proventil Syrup ... 2119
Proventil Tablets ... 2120
Ventolin ... 583

Antihypertensive agents, unspecified (Diminished antihypertensive effect).

Dobutamine Hydrochloride (May produce additive effects and increased toxicity). Products include:
Dobutrex Solution Vials ... 1259

Dopamine Hydrochloride (May produce additive effects and increased toxicity). Products include:
Intropin Injection ... 930

Ephedrine Hydrochloride (May produce additive effects and increased toxicity). Products include:
Amesec ... ▣ 682
Primatene Tablets-M Formula ... 2421
Primatene Tablets-P Formula ... 2421
Primatene Tablets-Regular Formula ... 2421
Quadrinal Tablets ... 1183
Quelidrine Syrup ... 556
Tedral SA ... 1765

Ephedrine Sulfate (May produce additive effects and increased toxicity). Products include:
Bronkaid Tablets ... ▣ 757
Bronkolixir ... ▣ 761
Bronkotabs Tablets ... ▣ 762
Marax Tablets & DF Syrup ... 1954
Pazo Hemorrhoid Ointment & Suppositories ... 752
Vicks Vatronol Nose Drops ... ▣ 666

Ephedrine Tannate (May produce additive effects and increased toxicity). Products include:
Rynatuss ... 2388

Epinephrine (May produce additive effects and increased toxicity). Products include:
Ana-Kit Anaphylaxis Emergency Treatment Kit ... 1100
Bronkaid Mist ... ▣ 757
EpiPen ... 843
Marcaine Hydrochloride 0.5% with Epinephrine 1:200,000 (as bitartrate) ... 958
Marcaine Hydrochloride with Epinephrine 1:200,000 ... 2055
Primatene Mist ... 2420
Sus-Phrine Injection ... 1006
Xylocaine with Epinephrine Injections ... 637

Epinephrine Bitartrate (May produce additive effects and increased toxicity). Products include:
AsthmaHaler Mist Epinephrine Bitartrate Bronchodilator ... ▣ 616
Bronkaid Mist Suspension ... ▣ 757
Primatene Mist Suspension ... 2421

Epinephrine Hydrochloride (May produce additive effects and increased toxicity). Products include:
Adrenalin Chloride Solution 1:100 & 1:1,000 ... 1689
Epifrin ... ⊙ 244
Glaucon ... ⊙ 218

Furazolidone (May produce hypertensive crisis). Products include:
Furoxone ... 1855

Isocarboxazid (May produce hypertensive crisis). Products include:
Marplan Tablets ... 1906

Metaproterenol Sulfate (May produce additive effects and increased toxicity). Products include:
Alupent ... 674
Arm-a-Med Metaproterenol Sulfate Inhalation Solution, USP ... 617
Metaprel Inhalation Aerosol Bronchodilator ... 2014
Metaprel Inhalation Solution ... 2015
Metaprel ... 2015
Metaproterenol Sulfate Inhalation Solution, USP ... 912

Metaraminol Bitartrate (May produce additive effects and increased toxicity). Products include:
Aramine Injection ... 1424

Methoxamine Hydrochloride (May produce additive effects and increased toxicity). Products include:
Vasoxyl Injection ... 819

Norepinephrine Bitartrate (May produce additive effects and increased toxicity). Products include:
Levophed Bitartrate Injection ... 2054

Phenelzine Sulfate (May produce hypertensive crisis). Products include:
Nardil ... 1742

Phenylephrine Bitartrate (May produce additive effects and increased toxicity).
No products indexed under this heading.

Phenylephrine Hydrochloride (May produce additive effects and increased toxicity). Products include:
AK-Dilate Solution 2.5% and 10% ... ⊙ 203
Atrohist Sprinkle Capsules ... 558
Cerose-DM ... 2443
Codimal ... 846
Comhist LA Capsules ... 1618
Congespirin For Children Aspirin Free Chewable Cold Tablets ... 748
Cyclomydril ... ⊙ 216
Deconsal Sprinkle Capsules ... 559
Dimetane Decongestant ... ▣ 673
Dristan Decongestant/Antihistamine/ Analgesic Coated Caplets ... ▣ 749
Dristan Cold Nasal Decongestant/ Antihistamine/ Analgesic Coated Tablets ... 2419
Dristan Advanced Formula Decongestant/Antihistamine/ Analgesic Tablets ... ▣ 749
Dristan Nasal Spray, Menthol ... 2419
Dristan Nasal Spray, Regular and Regular with Metered Pump ... 2419
Entex Capsules ... 1623
Entex Liquid ... 1623
Sinus Excedrin Analgesic, Decongestant Tablets & Caplets ... 750
Extendryl ... 994
4-Way Fast Acting Nasal Spray - Original Formula (regular & mentholated) & Metered Spray Pump (regular) ... 751
Hycomine Compound Tablets ... 929
Murocoll-2 Sterile Ophthalmic Solution ... ⊙ 261
Mydfrin 2.5% ... ⊙ 224
Naldecon Syrup, Tablets, Pediatric Drops and Pediatric Syrup ... 709
Neo-Synephrine Hydrochloride 1% Carpuject ... 2063
Neo-Synephrine Hydrochloride 1% Injection ... 2063
Neo-Synephrine Hydrochloride (Ophthalmic) ... 2064
Neo-Synephrine ... ▣ 759
Nōstril Nasal Decongestant ... ▣ 520
Novahistine Elixir ... ▣ 596
Phenergan VC ... 2500
Phenergan VC with Codeine ... 2501
Prefrin Liquifilm Vasoconstrictor and Lubricant Eye Drops ... ⊙ 254
Prefrin-A ... ⊙ 255
Quelidrine Syrup ... 556
Relief Vasoconstrictor and Lubricant Eye Drops ... ⊙ 256
Robitussin Night Relief ... ▣ 677
Ru-Tuss with Hydrocodone ... 694
Ru-Tuss Tablets ... 693
Vasosulf ... ⊙ 279
Vicks Sinex ... ▣ 665
Zincfrin ... ⊙ 230

Phenylephrine Tannate (May produce additive effects and increased toxicity). Products include:
Rynatan ... 2387
Rynatuss ... 2388

Phenylpropanolamine Hydrochloride (May produce additive effects and increased toxicity). Products include:
A.R.M. Allergy Relief Medicine Caplets ... ▣ 615
Acutrim ... ▣ 548
Allerest ... ▣ 559
BC Cold Powder ... ▣ 517
Cheracol Plus Head Cold/Cough Formula ... ▣ 667
Codimal Expectorant ... 846
Comtrex Multi-Symptom Cold Reliever Tablets/Caplets/Liqui-Gels/Liquid ... 745
Contac Continuous Action Decongestant/Antihistamine Capsules ▣ 710
Contac Maximum Strength Continuous Action Decongestant/ Antihistamine Caplets ... ▣ 709
Contac Severe Cold and Flu Formula Caplets ... ▣ 711
Coricidin 'D' Decongestant Tablets ... ▣ 695
Coricidin Demilets Tablets for Children ... ▣ 696
Demazin Nasal Decongestant/ Antihistamine Repetabs Tablets & Syrup ... ▣ 697
Dexatrim ... ▣ 733
Dimetane-DC Cough Syrup ... 1857
Dimetapp Elixir ... ▣ 673
Dimetapp DM Elixir ... ▣ 674
Dimetapp Extentabs ... ▣ 674
Dimetapp Plus Caplets ... ▣ 675
Dimetapp Tablets ... ▣ 675
Entex Capsules ... 1623
Entex LA Tablets ... 1623
Entex Liquid ... 1623
4-Way Cold Tablets ... 750
Hycomine Syrup ... 927
Naldecon CX Adult Liquid ... ▣ 521
Naldecon DX Adult Liquid ... ▣ 521
Naldecon DX Children's Syrup ... ▣ 522
Naldecon DX Pediatric Drops ... ▣ 522
Naldecon EX Children's Syrup ... ▣ 522
Naldecon EX Pediatric Drops ... ▣ 523
Naldecon Syrup, Tablets, Pediatric Drops and Pediatric Syrup ... 709
Nolamine Tablets ... 838
Nolex LA Tablets ... 838
Ornade Spansule Capsules ... 2221
Orthoxicol Cough Syrup ... ▣ 668
Propagest ... 839
Pyrroxate Capsules ... ▣ 669
Robitussin-CF ... ▣ 676
Ru-Tuss II Capsules ... 693
Ru-Tuss with Hydrocodone ... 694
Ru-Tuss Tablets ... 693
Sine-Off Sinus Medicine Tablets-Aspirin Formula ... ▣ 722
Sinulin ... 840

St. Joseph Cold Tablets for Children ■ 704
Tavist-D Tablets 2035
Triaminic Allergy Tablets ■ 688
Triaminic Chewables ■ 688
Triaminic Cold Tablets ■ 688
Triaminic Expectorant ■ 688
Triaminic Expectorant w/Codeine 1996
Triaminic Expectorant DH 1995
Triaminic Oral Infant Drops 1996
Triaminic Syrup ■ 689
Triaminic-12 Tablets ■ 690
Triaminic-DM Syrup ■ 689
Triaminicin Tablets ■ 690
Triaminicol Multi-Symptom Cold Tablets ■ 691
Triaminicol Multi-Symptom Relief ■ 691
Tuss-Ornade Liquid 2242
Tuss-Ornade Spansule Capsules 2242
Tylenol Cold Medication, Effervescent Tablets 1369

Pirbuterol Acetate (May produce additive effects and increased toxicity). Products include:
Maxair Inhaler 1311

Pseudoephedrine Sulfate (May produce additive effects and increased toxicity). Products include:
Afrin Tablets ■ 693
Chlor-Trimeton Decongestant ■ 694
Disophrol Chronotab Sustained-Action Tablets ■ 698
Drixoral Antihistamine/Nasal Decongestant Syrup ■ 698
Drixoral Non-Drowsy Formula ■ 699
Drixoral Plus Extended-Release Tablets ■ 699
Drixoral Sinus ■ 700
Drixoral Sustained-Action Tablets ■ 698
Sinutab Allergy Formula Sustained Action Tablets ■ 640
Trinalin Repetabs Tablets 1170

Selegiline Hydrochloride (May produce hypertensive crisis). Products include:
Eldepryl 2250

Terbutaline Sulfate (May produce additive effects and increased toxicity). Products include:
Brethaire Inhaler 1024
Brethine Ampuls 1026
Brethine Tablets 1026
Bricanyl Injection 1324
Bricanyl Tablets 1325

Tranylcypromine Sulfate (May produce hypertensive crisis). Products include:
Parnate Tablets 2222

ROCALTROL CAPSULES
(Calcitriol) 1913
May interact with cardiac glycosides, magnesium-containing antacids, and certain other agents. Compounds in these categories include:

Cholestyramine (Reduced intestinal absorption of Rocaltrol). Products include:
Cholybar 1705
Questran Light 711
Questran Powder 710

Deslanoside (Increased risk of cardiac arrhythmias).
No products indexed under this heading.

Digitoxin (Increased risk of cardiac arrhythmias). Products include:
Crystodigin Tablets 1253

Digoxin (Increased risk of cardiac arrhythmias). Products include:
Lanoxicaps 772
Lanoxin Elixir Pediatric 775
Lanoxin Injection 778
Lanoxin Injection Pediatric 781
Lanoxin Tablets 783

Magaldrate (Potential for hypermagnesemia in patients on chronic renal dialysis). Products include:
Riopan Antacid Chew Tablets ■ 754
Riopan Antacid Chew Tablets in Rollpacks ■ 754
Riopan Antacid Suspension 2421
Riopan Antacid Swallow Tablets 2421
Riopan Plus Chew Tablets 2422
Riopan Plus Chew Tablets in Rollpack 2422
Riopan Plus 2 Chew Tablets, Mint Flavor, Cherry Flavor 2422
Riopan Plus Suspension 2422
Riopan Plus 2 Suspension, Mint Flavor, Cherry Flavor 2422

Magnesium Carbonate (Potential for hypermagnesemia in patients on chronic renal dialysis). Products include:
Bayer Plus Aspirin Tablets ■ 567
Gaviscon Extra Strength Relief Formula Liquid Antacid ■ 594
Gaviscon Extra Strength Relief Formula Antacid Tablets ■ 594
Gaviscon Liquid Antacid ■ 594
Marblen ■ 563
Osti-Derm Lotion 1771

Magnesium Hydroxide (Potential for hypermagnesemia in patients on chronic renal dialysis). Products include:
Aludrox Oral Suspension 2428
Ascriptin A/D Caplets 1850
Regular Strength Ascriptin Tablets 1850
Di-Gel Antacid/Anti-Gas ■ 697
Gelusil Liquid & Tablets ■ 639
Haley's M-O, Regular & Flavored ■ 569
Extra Strength Maalox Plus Suspension 1850
Maalox TC Suspension 1851
Maalox Plus Tablets ■ 655
Extra Strength Maalox Plus Tablets 1850
Mylanta Liquid 1155
Mylanta Tablets 1155
Mylanta Double Strength Liquid 1155
Mylanta Double Strength Tablets 1155
Concentrated Phillips' Milk of Magnesia ■ 573
Phillips' Milk of Magnesia Liquid ■ 572
Phillips' Milk of Magnesia Tablets ■ 573
WinGel Liquid & Tablets ■ 761

Magnesium Trisilicate (Potential for hypermagnesemia in patients on chronic renal dialysis). Products include:
Gaviscon Antacid Tablets ■ 593
Gaviscon-2 Antacid Tablets ■ 594

Vitamin D (Possible additive effect and hypercalcemia). Products include:
Bugs Bunny Children's Chewable Vitamins (Sugar Free) ■ 625
Bugs Bunny With Extra C Children's Chewable Vitamins (Sugar Free) ■ 626
Bugs Bunny Plus Iron Children's Chewable Vitamins (Sugar Free) ■ 625
Calderol Capsules 1635
Caltrate 600 + Iron & Vitamin D 1198
Caltrate 600 + Vitamin D 1197
Caltrate, Jr. Tablets 1198
Flintstones Children's Chewable Vitamins ■ 625
Flintstones Children's Chewable Vitamins With Extra C ■ 626
Flintstones Children's Chewable Vitamins Plus Iron ■ 625
Natalins Rx 1391
Natalins Tablets 1391
One-A-Day Essential Vitamins ■ 627
One-A-Day Maximum Formula Vitamins and Minerals ■ 627
One-A-Day Plus Extra C Vitamins ■ 627
Os-Cal 250+D Tablets ■ 597
Os-Cal 500+D Tablets ■ 597
Os-Cal Fortified Tablets ■ 597
Os-Cal Plus Tablets ■ 597
Posture-D 600 mg 2420
Stressgard Stress Formula Vitamins ■ 628
Tri-Vi-Flor 1.0 mg Vitamins with Fluoride Chewable Tablets 1400
Tri-Vi-Flor Drops 1400
Tri-Vi-Sol Vitamin Drops ■ 614
Tri-Vi-Sol Vitamin Drops with Iron ■ 614
Vi-Daylin ADC Vitamins Drops 1980
Vi-Daylin ADC Vitamins + Iron Drops 1980
Vi-Daylin/F ADC Vitamins Drops With Fluoride 1981
Vi-Daylin/F ADC Vitamins + Iron Drops With Fluoride 1981
Within Women's Formula Multivitamin with Calcium, Extra Iron and Zinc ■ 628
Zymacap Capsules ■ 670

ROCEPHIN INJECTABLE VIALS, ADD-VANTAGE
(Ceftriaxone Sodium) 1914
No interactions described in labeling.

ROFERON-A INJECTION
(Interferon alfa-2A, Recombinant) 1916
May interact with:

Aminophylline (Reduced clearance of theophylline). Products include:
Amesec ■ 682
Aminophyllin Tablets 2153

Bone Marrow Depressants, unspecified (Caution should be exercised when administered concomitantly with myelosuppressive agents).

Dyphylline (Reduced clearance of theophylline). Products include:
Dilor 2079
Dilor-G Tablets & Liquid 2079
Lufyllin Elixir 2384
Lufyllin & Lufyllin-400 Tablets 2384
Lufyllin-GG Elixir & Tablets 2385

Theophylline (Reduced clearance of theophylline). Products include:
Bronkaid Tablets ■ 757
Bronkolixir ■ 761
Bronkotabs Tablets ■ 762
Constant-T Tablets 1029
Marax Tablets & DF Syrup 1954
Primatene Tablets 2421
Quibron Capsules 713
Quibron-T 714
Quibron-T/SR 716
Theolair Liquid 1317
Theo-Organidin Elixir 2391

Theophylline Anhydrous (Reduced clearance of theophylline). Products include:
Aerolate 994
Primatene Tablets-M Formula ■ 753
Primatene Tablets-Regular Formula 2421
Respbid Tablets 684
Slo-bid Gyrocaps 1847
T-PHYL (Uniphyl) 200 mg Tablets 1820
Tedral SA 1765
Theo-24 2179
Theo-Dur Sprinkle 1168
Theo-Dur Extended-Release Tablets 1166
Theolair Tablets 1317
Theolair-SR Tablets 1319
TheoX Extended-Release Tablets 841
Uniphyl 400 mg Tablets 1823

Theophylline Calcium Salicylate (Reduced clearance of theophylline). Products include:
Quadrinal Tablets 1183

Theophylline Sodium Glycinate (Reduced clearance of theophylline). Products include:
Asbron G 1997

Zidovudine (Concomitant therapy may result in synergistic toxicity). Products include:
Retrovir Capsules 802
Retrovir I.V. Infusion 805
Retrovir Syrup 802

ROGAINE TOPICAL SOLUTION
(Minoxidil) 2357
May interact with:

Guanethidine Monosulfate (Theoretical possibility of potentiation of orthostatic hypotension). Products include:
Esimil Tablets 864
Ismelin Tablets 869

ROLAIDS
(Dihydroxyaluminum Sodium Carbonate) ■ 743
May interact with tetracyclines. Compounds in this category include:

Demeclocycline Hydrochloride (Concurrent oral administration is not recommended). Products include:
Declomycin Capsules, Tablets 1199

Doxycycline Calcium (Concurrent oral administration is not recommended).
No products indexed under this heading.

Doxycycline Hyclate (Concurrent oral administration is not recommended). Products include:
Doryx Capsules 1717
Vibramycin Hyclate Capsules 1787
Vibramycin Hyclate Intravenous 1968
Vibra-Tabs Film Coated Tablets 1787

Doxycycline Monohydrate (Concurrent oral administration is not recommended). Products include:
Monodox Capsules 1630
Vibramycin Monohydrate for Oral Suspension 1787

Methacycline Hydrochloride (Concurrent oral administration is not recommended).
No products indexed under this heading.

Minocycline Hydrochloride (Concurrent oral administration is not recommended). Products include:
Minocin Intravenous 1221
Minocin Oral Suspension 1224
Minocin Pellet-Filled Capsules 1222

Oxytetracycline Hydrochloride (Concurrent oral administration is not recommended). Products include:
Terra-Cortril Ophthalmic Suspension 1963
Terramycin Capsules 1786
Terramycin Intramuscular Solution 1964
Terramycin with Polymyxin B Sulfate Ophthalmic Ointment 1965

Tetracycline Hydrochloride (Concurrent oral administration is not recommended). Products include:
Achromycin V Capsules 1193
Achromycin Ophthalmic Ointment 1% ⊙ 307
Achromycin Ophthalmic Suspension 1% ⊙ 308
Topicycline for Topical Solution 1856

ROLAIDS (CALCIUM RICH/SODIUM FREE)
(Calcium Carbonate) ■ 744
No interactions described in labeling.

EXTRA STRENGTH ROLAIDS
(Calcium Carbonate) ■ 744
No interactions described in labeling.

RONDEC ORAL DROPS
(Carbinoxamine Maleate, Pseudoephedrine Hydrochloride) 1975
May interact with tricyclic antidepressants, central nervous system depressants, monoamine oxidase inhibitors, veratrum alkaloids, beta blockers, and certain other agents. Compounds in these categories include:

Acebutolol Hydrochloride (Effects of sympathomimetics increased). Products include:
Sectral Capsules 2520

Alcohol (Enhanced effects of alcohol).

Alfentanil Hydrochloride (Enhanced effects of CNS depressants). Products include:
Alfenta Injection 1131

Alprazolam (Enhanced effects of CNS depressants). Products include:
Xanax Tablets 2367

Amitriptyline Hydrochloride (Enhanced effects of tricyclic antidepressants). Products include:
Elavil 2269
Endep Tablets 1927
Etrafon 2087
Limbitrol 1933
Triavil Tablets 1556

Amoxapine (Enhanced effects of tricyclic antidepressants). Products include:
Asendin Tablets 1196

Aprobarbital (Enhanced effects of CNS depressants). Products include:
Alurate Elixir 1883

Atenolol (Effects of sympathomimetics increased). Products include:
Tenoretic Tablets 1105
Tenormin Tablets and I.V. Injection 1107

Betaxolol Hydrochloride (Effects of sympathomimetics increased). Products include:
Betoptic Sterile Ophthalmic Solution 569
Betoptic S Sterile Ophthalmic Suspension 570
Kerlone Tablets 2172

Buprenorphine (Enhanced effects of CNS depressants).
No products indexed under this heading.

Buspirone Hydrochloride (Enhanced effects of CNS depressants). Products include:
BuSpar 1401

Butabarbital (Enhanced effects of CNS depressants). Products include:
Pyridium Plus 1764

Butalbital (Enhanced effects of CNS depressants). Products include:
Esgic-Plus Tablets 1002
Esgic Tablets & Capsules 1001
Fioricet Tablets 2006
Fiorinal Capsules 2007
Fiorinal with Codeine Capsules 2008
Fiorinal Tablets 2007
Phrenilin 838
Sedapap Tablets 50 mg/650 mg .. 1360

Carteolol Hydrochloride (Effects of sympathomimetics increased). Products include:
Cartrol Tablets 507

Chlordiazepoxide (Enhanced effects of CNS depressants). Products include:
Libritabs Tablets 1930
Limbitrol 1933
Menrium Tablets 1934

Chlordiazepoxide Hydrochloride (Enhanced effects of CNS depressants). Products include:
Librax Capsules 1929
Librium Capsules 1931
Librium Injectable 1932

Chlorpromazine (Enhanced effects of CNS depressants). Products include:
Thorazine 2234

Chlorprothixene (Enhanced effects of CNS depressants). Products include:
Taractan Tablets 1920

Chlorprothixene Hydrochloride (Enhanced effects of CNS depressants). Products include:
Taractan 1920

Clomipramine Hydrochloride (Enhanced effects of tricyclic antidepressants). Products include:
Anafranil Capsules 650

Clorazepate Dipotassium (Enhanced effects of CNS depressants). Products include:
Tranxene 556

Codeine (Enhanced effects of CNS depressants). Products include:
Calcidrine Syrup 506

Codeine Phosphate (Enhanced effects of CNS depressants). Products include:
Actifed with Codeine Cough Syrup .. 752
Cheracol Cough Syrup 1853
Codimal PH Syrup 846
Dimetane-DC Cough Syrup 1857
Empirin with Codeine Phosphate Nos. 2, 3 & 4 764
Fiorinal with Codeine Capsules 2008
Isoclor Expectorant 982
Naldecon CX Adult Liquid .... ▣ 521
Novahistine DH 1342
Novahistine Expectorant 1343
Nucofed Capsules 2219
Nucofed Expectorant 2219
Nucofed Pediatric Expectorant 2220
Nucofed Syrup 2219
Phenaphen with Codeine Capsules 1865
Phenaphen-650 with Codeine Tablets 1866
Phenergan with Codeine 2497
Phenergan VC with Codeine 2501
Robitussin A-C Syrup 1875
Robitussin-DAC Syrup 1875
Ryna .... ▣ 741
Soma Compound w/Codeine Tablets 2390
Triaminic Expectorant w/Codeine .. 1996
Tussi-Organidin Liquid 2391
Tylenol with Codeine 1381

Codeine Polistirex (Enhanced effects of CNS depressants).
No products indexed under this heading.

Cryptenamine Preparations (Reduced antihypertensive effects).

Desipramine Hydrochloride (Enhanced effects of tricyclic antidepressants). Products include:
Norpramin Tablets 1340

Dezocine (Enhanced effects of CNS depressants).

Diazepam (Enhanced effects of CNS depressants). Products include:
Valium Injectable 1937
Valium Tablets 1939
Valrelease Capsules 1923

Doxepin Hydrochloride (Enhanced effects of tricyclic antidepressants). Products include:
Sinequan 1960

Droperidol (Enhanced effects of CNS depressants). Products include:
Inapsine Injection 1140
Innovar Injection 1141

Enflurane (Enhanced effects of CNS depressants). Products include:
Ethrane 599

Esmolol Hydrochloride (Effects of sympathomimetics increased). Products include:
Brevibloc Injection 942

Estazolam (Enhanced effects of CNS depressants). Products include:
ProSom Tablets 554

Ethchlorvynol (Enhanced effects of CNS depressants). Products include:
Placidyl Capsules 553

Ethinamate (Enhanced effects of CNS depressants).
No products indexed under this heading.

Fentanyl (Enhanced effects of CNS depressants). Products include:
Duragesic Transdermal System 1133

Fentanyl Citrate (Enhanced effects of CNS depressants). Products include:
Innovar Injection 1141
Sublimaze Injection 1146

Fluphenazine Decanoate (Enhanced effects of CNS depressants). Products include:
Prolixin Decanoate 1795

Fluphenazine Enanthate (Enhanced effects of CNS depressants). Products include:
Prolixin Enanthate 1796

Fluphenazine Hydrochloride (Enhanced effects of CNS depressants). Products include:
Prolixin Elixir 1793
Prolixin Injection 1791
Prolixin Oral Concentrate 1792
Prolixin Tablets 1793

Flurazepam Hydrochloride (Enhanced effects of CNS depressants). Products include:
Dalmane Capsules 1927

Furazolidone (Effects of sympathomimetics increased; anticholinergic effects of antihistamines prolonged and intensified). Products include:
Furoxone 1855

Glutethimide (Enhanced effects of CNS depressants).
No products indexed under this heading.

Haloperidol (Enhanced effects of CNS depressants). Products include:
Haldol Injection, Tablets and Concentrate 1373

Haloperidol Decanoate (Enhanced effects of CNS depressants). Products include:
Haldol Decanoate 1375

Hydrocodone Bitartrate (Enhanced effects of CNS depressants). Products include:
Anexsia 5/500 Tablets 2196
Anexsia 7.5/650 Tablets 2197
Azdōne Tablets 844
Codiclear DH Syrup 845
Codimal DH Syrup 846
Damason-P 1356
Hycodan Syrup, Tablets 927
Hycomine Compound Tablets 929
Hycomine Syrup 927
Hycotuss Expectorant Syrup 930
Hydrocet Capsules 835
Lortab ASA Tablets 2414
Lortab 2412
Ru-Tuss with Hydrocodone 694
Triaminic Expectorant DH 1995
Vicodin Tablets 1187
Vicodin ES Tablets 1189
Zydone Capsules 941

Hydrocodone Polistirex (Enhanced effects of CNS depressants). Products include:
Tussionex Extended-Release Suspension 988

Hydroxyzine Hydrochloride (Enhanced effects of CNS depressants). Products include:
Atarax Tablets & Syrup 1941
Marax Tablets & DF Syrup 1954
Vistaril Intramuscular Solution 1970

Imipramine Hydrochloride (Enhanced effects of tricyclic antidepressants). Products include:
Tofranil Ampuls 1038
Tofranil Tablets 1039

Imipramine Pamoate (Enhanced effects of tricyclic antidepressants). Products include:
Tofranil-PM Capsules 1041

Isocarboxazid (Effects of sympathomimetics increased; anticholinergic effects of antihistamines prolonged and intensified). Products include:
Marplan Tablets 1906

Isoflurane (Enhanced effects of CNS depressants). Products include:
Forane 600

Ketamine Hydrochloride (Enhanced effects of CNS depressants). Products include:
Ketalar 1726

Labetalol Hydrochloride (Effects of sympathomimetics increased). Products include:
Normodyne Injection 2108
Normodyne Tablets 2110
Normozide Tablets 2112
Trandate HCT Tablets 579
Trandate Injection 577
Trandate Tablets 579

Levorphanol Tartrate (Enhanced effects of CNS depressants). Products include:
Levo-Dromoran 1906

Lorazepam (Enhanced effects of CNS depressants). Products include:
Ativan Injection 2432
Ativan Tablets 2434

Loxapine Hydrochloride (Enhanced effects of CNS depressants). Products include:
Loxitane 1213

Loxapine Succinate (Enhanced effects of CNS depressants). Products include:
Loxitane Capsules 1213

Maprotiline Hydrochloride (Enhanced effects of tricyclic antidepressants). Products include:
Ludiomil Tablets 874

Mecamylamine Hydrochloride (Reduced antihypertensive effects). Products include:
Inversine Tablets 1492

Meperidine Hydrochloride (Enhanced effects of CNS depressants). Products include:
Demerol 2047
Mepergan Injection 2479

Mephobarbital (Enhanced effects of CNS depressants). Products include:
Mebaral Tablets 2061

Meprobamate (Enhanced effects of CNS depressants). Products include:
Deprol Tablets 2382
Equagesic Tablets 2451
Miltown Tablets 2386
PMB 200 and PMB 400 2504

Mesoridazine (Enhanced effects of CNS depressants). Products include:
Serentil 686

Methadone Hydrochloride (Enhanced effects of CNS depressants). Products include:
Dolophine Hydrochloride Ampoules & Vials 1260
Dolophine Hydrochloride Tablets 1261
Methadone Hydrochloride Diskets .. 1284
Methadone Hydrochloride Oral Solution & Tablets 1987

Methohexital Sodium (Enhanced effects of CNS depressants). Products include:
Brevital Sodium Vials 1248

Methoxyflurane (Enhanced effects of CNS depressants).
No products indexed under this heading.

Methyldopa (Reduced antihypertensive effects). Products include:
Aldoclor Tablets 1413
Aldomet Oral 1415
Aldoril Tablets 1418

Methyldopate Hydrochloride (Reduced antihypertensive effects). Products include:
Aldomet Ester HCl Injection 1417

Metoprolol Tartrate (Effects of sympathomimetics increased). Products include:
Lopressor Ampuls 1032
Lopressor HCT Tablets 1034
Lopressor Tablets 1032

Midazolam Hydrochloride (Enhanced effects of CNS depressants). Products include:
- Versed Injection ... 1924

Molindone Hydrochloride (Enhanced effects of CNS depressants). Products include:
- Moban Tablets & Concentrate ... 932

Morphine Sulfate (Enhanced effects of CNS depressants). Products include:
- Astramorph/PF Injection, USP (Preservative-Free) ... 618
- Duramorph ... 960
- Infumorph 200 and Infumorph 500 Sterile Solutions ... 962
- MS Contin Tablets ... 1814
- MSIR ... 1817
- Oramorph SR (Morphine Sulfate Sustained Release Tablets) ... 1988
- Roxanol ... 1991

Nadolol (Effects of sympathomimetics increased). Products include:
- Corgard Tablets ... 701
- Corzide Tablets ... 702

Nortriptyline Hydrochloride (Enhanced effects of tricyclic antidepressants). Products include:
- Pamelor ... 2019

Opium Alkaloids (Enhanced effects of CNS depressants). Products include:
- B & O No. 15A & No. 16A Supprettes ... 2395
- Pantopon Injectable ... 1911

Oxazepam (Enhanced effects of CNS depressants). Products include:
- Serax Capsules ... 2522
- Serax Tablets ... 2522

Oxycodone Hydrochloride (Enhanced effects of CNS depressants). Products include:
- Percocet Tablets ... 950
- Percodan ... 951
- Roxicodone Tablets, Oral Solution & Intensol (Oxycodone) ... 1992
- Tylox Capsules ... 1382

Penbutolol Sulfate (Effects of sympathomimetics increased). Products include:
- Levatol ... 1832

Pentobarbital Sodium (Enhanced effects of CNS depressants). Products include:
- Nembutal Sodium Capsules ... 534
- Nembutal Sodium Solution ... 536
- Nembutal Sodium Suppositories ... 538

Perphenazine (Enhanced effects of CNS depressants). Products include:
- Etrafon ... 2087
- Triavil Tablets ... 1556
- Trilafon ... 2123

Phenelzine Sulfate (Effects of sympathomimetics increased; anticholinergic effects of antihistamines prolonged and intensified). Products include:
- Nardil ... 1742

Phenobarbital (Enhanced effects of CNS depressants). Products include:
- Arco-Lase Plus Tablets ... 607
- Bellergal-S Tablets ... 1998
- Bronkolixir ... ⊡ 761
- Bronkotabs Tablets ... ⊡ 762
- Donnatal ... 1858
- Donnatal Extentabs ... 1859
- Donnatal Tablets ... 1858
- Donnazyme Tablets ... 1860
- Kinesed Tablets ... 2272
- Phenobarbital Elixir and Tablets ... 1293
- Primatene Tablets-P Formula ... 2421
- Quadrinal Tablets ... 1183
- Tedral SA ... 1765

Pindolol (Effects of sympathomimetics increased). Products include:
- Visken Tablets ... 2036

Prazepam (Enhanced effects of CNS depressants). Products include:
- Centrax ... 1693

Prochlorperazine (Enhanced effects of CNS depressants). Products include:
- Compazine ... 2201

Promethazine Hydrochloride (Enhanced effects of CNS depressants). Products include:
- Mepergan Injection ... 2479
- Phenergan with Codeine ... 2497
- Phenergan with Dextromethorphan 2499
- Phenergan Injection ... 2493
- Phenergan Suppositories ... 2496
- Phenergan Syrup ... 2495
- Phenergan Tablets ... 2496
- Phenergan VC ... 2500
- Phenergan VC with Codeine ... 2501

Propofol (Enhanced effects of CNS depressants). Products include:
- Diprivan Injection ... 2267

Propoxyphene Hydrochloride (Enhanced effects of CNS depressants). Products include:
- Darvon ... 1256
- Wygesic Tablets ... 2540

Propoxyphene Napsylate (Enhanced effects of CNS depressants). Products include:
- Darvon-N/Darvocet-N ... 1254

Propranolol Hydrochloride (Effects of sympathomimetics increased). Products include:
- Inderal ... 2459
- Inderal LA Long Acting Capsules ... 2461
- Inderide Tablets ... 2463
- Inderide LA Long Acting Capsules .. 2465

Protriptyline Hydrochloride (Enhanced effects of tricyclic antidepressants). Products include:
- Vivactil Tablets ... 1567

Quazepam (Enhanced effects of CNS depressants). Products include:
- Doral Tablets ... 2383

Reserpine (Reduced antihypertensive effects). Products include:
- Diupres Tablets ... 1461
- Hydromox R Tablets ... 1209
- Hydropres Tablets ... 1485
- Renese-R Tablets ... 1786
- Salutensin/Salutensin-Demi ... 719
- Ser-Ap-Es Tablets ... 881
- Serpasil Tablets ... 883
- Serpasil-Apresoline Tablets ... 884
- Serpasil-Esidrix Tablets ... 886

Secobarbital Sodium (Enhanced effects of CNS depressants). Products include:
- Seconal Sodium Pulvules ... 1296

Selegiline Hydrochloride (Effects of sympathomimetics increased; anticholinergic effects of antihistamines prolonged and intensified). Products include:
- Eldepryl ... 2250

Sufentanil Citrate (Enhanced effects of CNS depressants). Products include:
- Sufenta Injection ... 1147

Temazepam (Enhanced effects of CNS depressants). Products include:
- Restoril Capsules ... 2023

Thiamylal Sodium (Enhanced effects of CNS depressants). Products include:
- Surital Ampoules, Steri-Vials ... 1764

Thioridazine Hydrochloride (Enhanced effects of CNS depressants). Products include:
- Mellaril ... 2011

Thiothixene (Enhanced effects of CNS depressants). Products include:
- Navane Capsules and Concentrate 1954
- Navane Intramuscular ... 1956

Timolol Maleate (Effects of sympathomimetics increased). Products include:
- Blocadren Tablets ... 1429
- Timolide Tablets ... 1547
- Timoptic in Ocudose ... 1552
- Timoptic Sterile Ophthalmic Solution ... 1550

Tranylcypromine Sulfate (Effects of sympathomimetics increased; anticholinergic effects of antihistamines prolonged and intensified). Products include:
- Parnate Tablets ... 2222

Triazolam (Enhanced effects of CNS depressants). Products include:
- Halcion Tablets ... 2340

Trifluoperazine Hydrochloride (Enhanced effects of CNS depressants). Products include:
- Stelazine ... 2226

Trimipramine Maleate (Enhanced effects of tricyclic antidepressants). Products include:
- Surmontil Capsules ... 2524

RONDEC SYRUP
(Carbinoxamine Maleate, Pseudoephedrine Hydrochloride) 1975
See **Rondec Oral Drops**

RONDEC TABLET
(Carbinoxamine Maleate, Pseudoephedrine Hydrochloride) 1975
See **Rondec Oral Drops**

RONDEC-DM ORAL DROPS
(Carbinoxamine Maleate, Pseudoephedrine Hydrochloride, Dextromethorphan Hydrobromide)....1976
May interact with tricyclic antidepressants, central nervous system depressants, monoamine oxidase inhibitors, veratrum alkaloids, beta blockers, and certain other agents. Compounds in these categories include:

Acebutolol Hydrochloride (Effects of sympathomimetics increased). Products include:
- Sectral Capsules ... 2520

Alcohol (Enhanced effects of alcohol).

Alfentanil Hydrochloride (Enhanced effects of CNS depressants). Products include:
- Alfenta Injection ... 1131

Alprazolam (Enhanced effects of CNS depressants). Products include:
- Xanax Tablets ... 2367

Amitriptyline Hydrochloride (Enhanced effects of tricyclic antidepressants). Products include:
- Elavil ... 2269
- Endep Tablets ... 1927
- Etrafon ... 2087
- Limbitrol ... 1933
- Triavil Tablets ... 1556

Amoxapine (Enhanced effects of tricyclic antidepressants). Products include:
- Asendin Tablets ... 1196

Aprobarbital (Enhanced effects of CNS depressants). Products include:
- Alurate Elixir ... 1883

Atenolol (Effects of sympathomimetics increased). Products include:
- Tenoretic Tablets ... 1105
- Tenormin Tablets and I.V. Injection 1107

Betaxolol Hydrochloride (Effects of sympathomimetics increased). Products include:
- Betoptic Sterile Ophthalmic Solution ... 569
- Betoptic S Sterile Ophthalmic Suspension ... 570
- Kerlone Tablets ... 2172

Buprenorphine (Enhanced effects of CNS depressants).
- No products indexed under this heading.

Buspirone Hydrochloride (Enhanced effects of CNS depressants). Products include:
- BuSpar ... 1401

Butabarbital (Enhanced effects of CNS depressants). Products include:
- Pyridium Plus ... 1764

Butalbital (Enhanced effects of CNS depressants). Products include:
- Esgic-Plus Tablets ... 1002
- Esgic Tablets & Capsules ... 1001
- Fioricet Tablets ... 2006
- Fiorinal Capsules ... 2007
- Fiorinal with Codeine Capsules ... 2008
- Fiorinal Tablets ... 2007
- Phrenilin ... 838
- Sedapap Tablets 50 mg/650 mg .. 1360

Carteolol Hydrochloride (Effects of sympathomimetics increased). Products include:
- Cartrol Tablets ... 507

Chlordiazepoxide (Enhanced effects of CNS depressants). Products include:
- Libritabs Tablets ... 1930
- Limbitrol ... 1933
- Menrium Tablets ... 1934

Chlordiazepoxide Hydrochloride (Enhanced effects of CNS depressants). Products include:
- Librax Capsules ... 1929
- Librium Capsules ... 1931
- Librium Injectable ... 1932

Chlorpromazine (Enhanced effects of CNS depressants). Products include:
- Thorazine ... 2234

Chlorprothixene (Enhanced effects of CNS depressants). Products include:
- Taractan Tablets ... 1920

Chlorprothixene Hydrochloride (Enhanced effects of CNS depressants). Products include:
- Taractan ... 1920

Clomipramine Hydrochloride (Enhanced effects of tricyclic antidepressants). Products include:
- Anafranil Capsules ... 650

Clorazepate Dipotassium (Enhanced effects of CNS depressants). Products include:
- Tranxene ... 556

Codeine (Enhanced effects of CNS depressants). Products include:
- Calcidrine Syrup ... 506

Codeine Phosphate (Enhanced effects of CNS depressants). Products include:
- Actifed with Codeine Cough Syrup.. 752
- Cheracol Cough Syrup ... 1853
- Codimal PH Syrup ... 846
- Dimetane-DC Cough Syrup ... 1857
- Empirin with Codeine Phosphate Nos. 2, 3 & 4 ... 764
- Fiorinal with Codeine Capsules ... 2008
- Isoclor Expectorant ... 982
- Naldecon CX Adult Liquid ... ⊡ 521
- Novahistine DH ... 1342
- Novahistine Expectorant ... 1343
- Nucofed Capsules ... 2219
- Nucofed Expectorant ... 2219
- Nucofed Pediatric Expectorant ... 2220
- Nucofed Syrup ... 2219
- Phenaphen with Codeine Capsules 1865
- Phenaphen-650 with Codeine Tablets ... 1866
- Phenergan with Codeine ... 2497
- Phenergan VC with Codeine ... 2501
- Robitussin A-C Syrup ... 1875
- Robitussin-DAC Syrup ... 1875
- Ryna ... ⊡ 741
- Soma Compound w/Codeine Tablets ... 2390
- Triaminic Expectorant w/Codeine .. 1996
- Tussi-Organidin Liquid ... 2391
- Tylenol with Codeine ... 1381

Codeine Polistirex (Enhanced effects of CNS depressants).
- No products indexed under this heading.

Cryptenamine Preparations (Reduced antihypertensive effects).

Desipramine Hydrochloride (Enhanced effects of tricyclic antidepressants). Products include:

Norpramin Tablets 1340

Dezocine (Enhanced effects of CNS depressants).

Diazepam (Enhanced effects of CNS depressants). Products include:

Valium Injectable 1937
Valium Tablets 1939
Valrelease Capsules 1923

Doxepin Hydrochloride (Enhanced effects of tricyclic antidepressants). Products include:

Sinequan 1960

Droperidol (Enhanced effects of CNS depressants). Products include:

Inapsine Injection 1140
Innovar Injection 1141

Enflurane (Enhanced effects of CNS depressants). Products include:

Ethrane 599

Esmolol Hydrochloride (Effects of sympathomimetics increased). Products include:

Brevibloc Injection 942

Estazolam (Enhanced effects of CNS depressants). Products include:

ProSom Tablets 554

Ethchlorvynol (Enhanced effects of CNS depressants). Products include:

Placidyl Capsules 553

Ethinamate (Enhanced effects of CNS depressants).

No products indexed under this heading.

Fentanyl (Enhanced effects of CNS depressants). Products include:

Duragesic Transdermal System 1133

Fentanyl Citrate (Enhanced effects of CNS depressants). Products include:

Innovar Injection 1141
Sublimaze Injection 1146

Fluphenazine Decanoate (Enhanced effects of CNS depressants). Products include:

Prolixin Decanoate 1795

Fluphenazine Enanthate (Enhanced effects of CNS depressants). Products include:

Prolixin Enanthate 1796

Fluphenazine Hydrochloride (Enhanced effects of CNS depressants). Products include:

Prolixin Elixir 1793
Prolixin Injection 1791
Prolixin Oral Concentrate 1792
Prolixin Tablets 1793

Flurazepam Hydrochloride (Enhanced effects of CNS depressants). Products include:

Dalmane Capsules 1927

Furazolidone (Increased effects of sympathomimetics; anticholinergic effects of antihistamines prolonged and intensified). Products include:

Furoxone 1855

Glutethimide (Enhanced effects of CNS depressants).

No products indexed under this heading.

Haloperidol (Enhanced effects of CNS depressants). Products include:

Haldol Injection, Tablets and Concentrate 1373

Haloperidol Decanoate (Enhanced effects of CNS depressants). Products include:

Haldol Decanoate 1375

Hydrocodone Bitartrate (Enhanced effects of CNS depressants). Products include:

Anexsia 5/500 Tablets 2196
Anexsia 7.5/650 Tablets 2197
Azdone Tablets 844
Codiclear DH Syrup 845
Codimal DH Syrup 846
Damason-P 1356
Hycodan Syrup, Tablets 927
Hycomine Compound Tablets 929
Hycomine Syrup 927
Hycotuss Expectorant Syrup 930
Hydrocet Capsules 835
Lortab ASA Tablets 2414
Lortab 2412
Ru-Tuss with Hydrocodone 694
Triaminic Expectorant DH 1995
Vicodin Tablets 1187
Vicodin ES Tablets 1189
Zydone Capsules 941

Hydrocodone Polistirex (Enhanced effects of CNS depressants). Products include:

Tussionex Extended-Release Suspension 988

Hydroxyzine Hydrochloride (Enhanced effects of CNS depressants). Products include:

Atarax Tablets & Syrup 1941
Marax Tablets & DF Syrup 1954
Vistaril Intramuscular Solution 1970

Imipramine Hydrochloride (Enhanced effects of tricyclic antidepressants). Products include:

Tofranil Ampuls 1038
Tofranil Tablets 1039

Imipramine Pamoate (Enhanced effects of tricyclic antidepressants). Products include:

Tofranil-PM Capsules 1041

Isocarboxazid (Increased effects of sympathomimetics; anticholinergic effects of antihistamines prolonged and intensified). Products include:

Marplan Tablets 1906

Isoflurane (Enhanced effects of CNS depressants). Products include:

Forane 600

Ketamine Hydrochloride (Enhanced effects of CNS depressants). Products include:

Ketalar 1726

Labetalol Hydrochloride (Effects of sympathomimetics increased). Products include:

Normodyne Injection 2108
Normodyne Tablets 2110
Normozide Tablets 2112
Trandate HCT Tablets 579
Trandate Injection 577
Trandate Tablets 579

Levorphanol Tartrate (Enhanced effects of CNS depressants). Products include:

Levo-Dromoran 1906

Lorazepam (Enhanced effects of CNS depressants). Products include:

Ativan Injection 2432
Ativan Tablets 2434

Loxapine Hydrochloride (Enhanced effects of CNS depressants). Products include:

Loxitane 1213

Loxapine Succinate (Enhanced effects of CNS depressants). Products include:

Loxitane Capsules 1213

Maprotiline Hydrochloride (Enhanced effects of tricyclic antidepressants). Products include:

Ludiomil Tablets 874

Mecamylamine Hydrochloride (Reduced antihypertensive effects). Products include:

Inversine Tablets 1492

Meperidine Hydrochloride (Enhanced effects of CNS depressants). Products include:

Demerol 2047
Mepergan Injection 2479

Mephobarbital (Enhanced effects of CNS depressants). Products include:

Mebaral Tablets 2061

Meprobamate (Enhanced effects of CNS depressants). Products include:

Deprol Tablets 2382
Equagesic Tablets 2451
Miltown Tablets 2386
PMB 200 and PMB 400 2504

Mesoridazine (Enhanced effects of CNS depressants). Products include:

Serentil 686

Methadone Hydrochloride (Enhanced effects of CNS depressants). Products include:

Dolophine Hydrochloride Ampoules & Vials 1260
Dolophine Hydrochloride Tablets 1261
Methadone Hydrochloride Diskets 1284
Methadone Hydrochloride Oral Solution & Tablets 1987

Methohexital Sodium (Enhanced effects of CNS depressants). Products include:

Brevital Sodium Vials 1248

Methoxyflurane (Enhanced effects of CNS depressants).

No products indexed under this heading.

Methyldopa (Reduced antihypertensive effects). Products include:

Aldoclor Tablets 1413
Aldomet Oral 1415
Aldoril Tablets 1418

Methyldopate Hydrochloride (Reduced antihypertensive effects). Products include:

Aldomet Ester HCl Injection 1417

Metoprolol Tartrate (Effects of sympathomimetics increased). Products include:

Lopressor Ampuls 1032
Lopressor HCT Tablets 1034
Lopressor Tablets 1032

Midazolam Hydrochloride (Enhanced effects of CNS depressants). Products include:

Versed Injection 1924

Molindone Hydrochloride (Enhanced effects of CNS depressants). Products include:

Moban Tablets & Concentrate 932

Morphine Sulfate (Enhanced effects of CNS depressants). Products include:

Astramorph/PF Injection, USP (Preservative-Free) 618
Duramorph 960
Infumorph 200 and Infumorph 500 Sterile Solutions 962
MS Contin Tablets 1814
MSIR 1817
Oramorph SR (Morphine Sulfate Sustained Release Tablets) 1988
Roxanol 1991

Nadolol (Effects of sympathomimetics increased). Products include:

Corgard Tablets 701
Corzide Tablets 702

Nortriptyline Hydrochloride (Enhanced effects of tricyclic antidepressants). Products include:

Pamelor 2019

Opium Alkaloids (Enhanced effects of CNS depressants). Products include:

B & O No. 15A & No. 16A Supprettes 2395
Pantopon Injectable 1911

Oxazepam (Enhanced effects of CNS depressants). Products include:

Serax Capsules 2522
Serax Tablets 2522

Oxycodone Hydrochloride (Enhanced effects of CNS depressants). Products include:

Percocet Tablets 950
Percodan 951
Roxicodone Tablets, Oral Solution & Intensol (Oxycodone) 1992
Tylox Capsules 1382

Penbutolol Sulfate (Effects of sympathomimetics increased). Products include:

Levatol 1832

Pentobarbital Sodium (Enhanced effects of CNS depressants). Products include:

Nembutal Sodium Capsules 534
Nembutal Sodium Solution 536
Nembutal Sodium Suppositories 538

Perphenazine (Enhanced effects of CNS depressants). Products include:

Etrafon 2087
Triavil Tablets 1556
Trilafon 2123

Phenelzine Sulfate (Increased effects of sympathomimetics; anticholinergic effects of antihistamines prolonged and intensified). Products include:

Nardil 1742

Phenobarbital (Enhanced effects of CNS depressants). Products include:

Arco-Lase Plus Tablets 607
Bellergal-S Tablets 1998
Bronkolixir ⊞ 761
Bronkotabs Tablets ⊞ 762
Donnatal 1858
Donnatal Extentabs 1859
Donnatal Tablets 1858
Donnazyme Tablets 1860
Kinesed Tablets 2272
Phenobarbital Elixir and Tablets 1293
Primatene Tablets-P Formula 2421
Quadrinal Tablets 1183
Tedral SA 1765

Pindolol (Effects of sympathomimetics increased). Products include:

Visken Tablets 2036

Prazepam (Enhanced effects of CNS depressants). Products include:

Centrax 1693

Prochlorperazine (Enhanced effects of CNS depressants). Products include:

Compazine 2201

Promethazine Hydrochloride (Enhanced effects of CNS depressants). Products include:

Mepergan Injection 2479
Phenergan with Codeine 2497
Phenergan with Dextromethorphan 2499
Phenergan Injection 2493
Phenergan Suppositories 2496
Phenergan Syrup 2495
Phenergan Tablets 2496
Phenergan VC 2500
Phenergan VC with Codeine 2501

Propofol (Enhanced effects of CNS depressants). Products include:

Diprivan Injection 2267

Propoxyphene Hydrochloride (Enhanced effects of CNS depressants). Products include:

Darvon 1256
Wygesic Tablets 2540

Propoxyphene Napsylate (Enhanced effects of CNS depressants). Products include:

Darvon-N/Darvocet-N 1254

Propranolol Hydrochloride (Effects of sympathomimetics increased). Products include:

Inderal 2459
Inderal LA Long Acting Capsules 2461
Inderide Tablets 2463
Inderide LA Long Acting Capsules 2465

Protriptyline Hydrochloride (Enhanced effects of tricyclic antidepressants). Products include:

Vivactil Tablets 1567

Quazepam (Enhanced effects of CNS depressants). Products include:

Doral Tablets 2383

Reserpine (Reduced antihypertensive effects). Products include:

Diupres Tablets 1461
Hydromox R Tablets 1209
Hydropres Tablets 1485

Renese-R Tablets ... 1786
Salutensin/Salutensin-Demi ... 719
Ser-Ap-Es Tablets ... 881
Serpasil Tablets ... 883
Serpasil-Apresoline Tablets ... 884
Serpasil-Esidrix Tablets ... 886

Secobarbital Sodium (Enhanced effects of CNS depressants). Products include:
Seconal Sodium Pulvules ... 1296

Selegiline Hydrochloride (Increased effects of sympathomimetics; anticholinergic effects of antihistamines prolonged and intensified). Products include:
Eldepryl ... 2250

Sufentanil Citrate (Enhanced effects of CNS depressants). Products include:
Sufenta Injection ... 1147

Temazepam (Enhanced effects of CNS depressants). Products include:
Restoril Capsules ... 2023

Thiamylal Sodium (Enhanced effects of CNS depressants). Products include:
Surital Ampoules, Steri-Vials ... 1764

Thioridazine Hydrochloride (Enhanced effects of CNS depressants). Products include:
Mellaril ... 2011

Thiothixene (Enhanced effects of CNS depressants). Products include:
Navane Capsules and Concentrate 1954
Navane Intramuscular ... 1956

Timolol Maleate (Effects of sympathomimetics increased). Products include:
Blocadren Tablets ... 1429
Timolide Tablets ... 1547
Timoptic in Ocudose ... 1552
Timoptic Sterile Ophthalmic Solution ... 1550

Tranylcypromine Sulfate (Increased effects of sympathomimetics; anticholinergic effects of antihistamines prolonged and intensified). Products include:
Parnate Tablets ... 2222

Triazolam (Enhanced effects of CNS depressants). Products include:
Halcion Tablets ... 2340

Trifluoperazine Hydrochloride (Enhanced effects of CNS depressants). Products include:
Stelazine ... 2226

Trimipramine Maleate (Enhanced effects of tricyclic antidepressants). Products include:
Surmontil Capsules ... 2524

RONDEC-DM SYRUP
(Carbinoxamine Maleate, Pseudoephedrine Hydrochloride, Dextromethorphan Hydrobromide) ... 1976
See **Rondec-DM Oral Drops**

RONDEC-TR TABLET
(Carbinoxamine Maleate, Pseudoephedrine Hydrochloride) ... 1975
See **Rondec Oral Drops**

ROSE BENGAL 1%
(Rose Bengal) ... ⊙ 209
No interactions described in labeling.

ROWASA RECTAL SUPPOSITORIES
(Mesalamine) ... 2248
See **Rowasa Rectal Suspension Enema**

ROWASA RECTAL SUSPENSION ENEMA
(Mesalamine) ... 2248
May interact with:

Sulfasalazine (Patients on concurrent oral products which liberate mesalamine should be carefully monitored with urinalysis). Products include:
Azulfidine Tablets, EN-tabs, Oral Suspension ... 1157

ROXANOL (MORPHINE SULFATE CONCENTRATED ORAL SOLUTION)
(Morphine Sulfate) ... 1991
May interact with tricyclic antidepressants, central nervous system depressants, urinary alkalizing agents, monoamine oxidase inhibitors, antihistamines, beta blockers, anticoagulants, and certain other agents. Compounds in these categories include:

Acebutolol Hydrochloride (Depressant effects of morphine may be enhanced). Products include:
Sectral Capsules ... 2520

Alcohol (Respiratory depression, hypotension, and profound sedation or coma may result; depressant effects of morphine may be enhanced).

Alfentanil Hydrochloride (Respiratory depression, hypotension, and profound sedation or coma may result; depressant effects of morphine may be enhanced). Products include:
Alfenta Injection ... 1131

Alprazolam (Respiratory depression, hypotension, and profound sedation or coma may result; depressant effects of morphine may be enhanced). Products include:
Xanax Tablets ... 2367

Amitriptyline Hydrochloride (Respiratory depression, hypotension, and profound sedation or coma may result). Products include:
Elavil ... 2269
Endep Tablets ... 1927
Etrafon ... 2087
Limbitrol ... 1933
Triavil Tablets ... 1556

Amoxapine (Respiratory depression, hypotension, and profound sedation or coma may result). Products include:
Asendin Tablets ... 1196

Aprobarbital (Respiratory depression, hypotension, and profound sedation or coma may result; depressant effects of morphine may be enhanced). Products include:
Alurate Elixir ... 1883

Astemizole (Depressant effects of morphine may be enhanced). Products include:
Hismanal Tablets ... 1138

Atenolol (Depressant effects of morphine may be enhanced). Products include:
Tenoretic Tablets ... 1105
Tenormin Tablets and I.V. Injection 1107

Azatadine Maleate (Depressant effects of morphine may be enhanced). Products include:
Optimine Tablets ... 2115
Trinalin Repetabs Tablets ... 1170

Betaxolol Hydrochloride (Depressant effects of morphine may be enhanced). Products include:
Betoptic Sterile Ophthalmic Solution ... 569
Betoptic S Sterile Ophthalmic Suspension ... 570
Kerlone Tablets ... 2172

Bromodiphenhydramine Hydrochloride (Depressant effects of morphine may be enhanced).
No products indexed under this heading.

Brompheniramine Maleate (Depressant effects of morphine may be enhanced). Products include:
Alka Seltzer Plus Sinus Allergy Medicine ... ▣ 624
Atrohist Sprinkle Capsules ... 558
Bromfed Capsules (Timed Release) ... 1615
Bromfed Syrup ... ▣ 628
Bromfed ... 1615
Dimetane Decongestant ... ▣ 673
Dimetane ... ▣ 672
Dimetane-DC Cough Syrup ... 1857
Dimetane-DX Cough Syrup ... 1858
Dimetapp Elixir ... ▣ 673
Dimetapp DM Elixir ... ▣ 674
Dimetapp Extentabs ... ▣ 674
Dimetapp Plus Caplets ... ▣ 675
Dimetapp Tablets ... ▣ 675
Drixoral Antihistamine/Nasal Decongestant Syrup ... ▣ 698

Buprenorphine (Respiratory depression, hypotension, and profound sedation or coma may result; depressant effects of morphine may be enhanced).
No products indexed under this heading.

Buspirone Hydrochloride (Respiratory depression, hypotension, and profound sedation or coma may result; depressant effects of morphine may be enhanced). Products include:
BuSpar ... 1401

Butabarbital (Respiratory depression, hypotension, and profound sedation or coma may result; depressant effects of morphine may be enhanced). Products include:
Pyridium Plus ... 1764

Butalbital (Respiratory depression, hypotension, and profound sedation or coma may result; depressant effects of morphine may be enhanced). Products include:
Esgic-Plus Tablets ... 1002
Esgic Tablets & Capsules ... 1001
Fioricet Tablets ... 2006
Fiorinal Capsules ... 2007
Fiorinal with Codeine Capsules ... 2008
Fiorinal Tablets ... 2007
Phrenilin ... 838
Sedapap Tablets 50 mg/650 mg .. 1360

Carteolol Hydrochloride (Depressant effects of morphine may be enhanced). Products include:
Cartrol Tablets ... 507

Chloral Hydrate (Depressant effects of morphine may be enhanced).
No products indexed under this heading.

Chlordiazepoxide (Respiratory depression, hypotension, and profound sedation or coma may result; depressant effects of morphine may be enhanced). Products include:
Libritabs Tablets ... 1930
Limbitrol ... 1933
Menrium Tablets ... 1934

Chlordiazepoxide Hydrochloride (Respiratory depression, hypotension, and profound sedation or coma may result; depressant effects of morphine may be enhanced). Products include:
Librax Capsules ... 1929
Librium Capsules ... 1931
Librium Injectable ... 1932

Chlorpheniramine Maleate (Depressant effects of morphine may be enhanced). Products include:
A.R.M. Allergy Relief Medicine Caplets ... ▣ 615
Alka-Seltzer Plus Cold Medicine ... ▣ 623
Allerest ... ▣ 559
Ana-Kit Anaphylaxis Emergency Treatment Kit ... 1100
BC Cold Powder Multi-Symptom Formula ... ▣ 517
Brexin L.A. Capsules ... 2078
Cerose-DM ... 2443
Cheracol Plus Head Cold/Cough Formula ... ▣ 667
Chlor-Trimeton Allergy Syrup, Tablets & Long-Acting Repetabs Tablets ... ▣ 693
Chlor-Trimeton Decongestant ... ▣ 694
Comhist LA Capsules ... 1618
Allergy-Sinus Comtrex Multi-Symptom Allergy Sinus Formula Tablets & Caplets ... 746
Comtrex Multi-Symptom Cold Reliever Tablets/Caplets/Liqui-Gels/Liquid ... 745
Day-Night Comtrex ... 747
Contac Continuous Action Decongestant/Antihistamine Capsules ▣ 710
Contac Maximum Strength Continuous Action Decongestant/Antihistamine Caplets ... ▣ 709
Contac Severe Cold and Flu Formula Caplets ... ▣ 711
Coricidin 'D' Decongestant Tablets ... ▣ 695
Coricidin Demilets Tablets for Children ... ▣ 696
Coricidin Tablets ... ▣ 695
Deconamine ... 663
Demazin Nasal Decongestant/Antihistamine Repetabs Tablets & Syrup ... ▣ 697
Dorcol Children's Liquid Cold Formula ... ▣ 686
Dristan Decongestant/Antihistamine/Analgesic Coated Caplets ... ▣ 749
Dristan Cold Nasal Decongestant/Antihistamine/Analgesic Coated Tablets ... 2419
Dristan Advanced Formula Decongestant/Antihistamine/Analgesic Tablets ... ▣ 749
Extendryl ... 994
4-Way Cold Tablets ... 750
Fedahist Gyrocaps ... 2145
Fedahist Timecaps ... 2145
Hycomine Compound Tablets ... 929
Isoclor Timesule Capsules ... ▣ 561
Kronofed-A ... 970
Medi-Flu Caplet, Liquid ... ▣ 640
Naldecon Syrup, Tablets, Pediatric Drops and Pediatric Syrup ... 709
Nolamine Tablets ... 838
Novafed A Capsules ... 1342
Novahistine DH ... 1342
Novahistine Elixir ... ▣ 596
Ornade Spansule Capsules ... 2221
Orthoxicol Cough Syrup ... ▣ 668
PediaCare Allergy Relief Formula Liquid ... 1362
PediaCare Cough-Cold Formula Liquid ... 1362
PediaCare Night Rest Cough-Cold Formula Liquid ... 1362
PediaCare 6-12 Cough-Cold Formula Chewable Tablets ... 1362
Pyrroxate Capsules ... ▣ 669
Quelidrine Syrup ... 556
Ru-Tuss II Capsules ... 693
Ru-Tuss Tablets ... 693
Ryna ... ▣ 741
Sinarest Tablets & Extra Strength Tablets ... ▣ 562
Sine-Off Maximum Strength Allergy/Sinus Formula Caplets ... ▣ 721
Sine-Off Sinus Medicine Tablets-Aspirin Formula ... ▣ 722
Singlet Tablets ... ▣ 598
Sinulin ... 840
Sinutab Maximum Strength ... ▣ 641
St. Joseph Nighttime Cold Medicine ... ▣ 705
Sudafed Plus Liquid ... ▣ 544
Sudafed Plus Tablets ... ▣ 545
Teldrin Timed-Release Allergy Capsules, 12 mg ... 2192
TheraFlu Flu and Cold Medicine ... ▣ 687
Triaminic Allergy Tablets ... ▣ 688
Triaminic Chewables ... ▣ 688
Triaminic Cold Tablets ... ▣ 688
Triaminic Nite Light ... ▣ 689
Triaminic Syrup ... ▣ 689
Triaminic-12 Tablets ... ▣ 690
Triaminicin Tablets ... ▣ 690
Triaminicol Multi-Symptom Cold Tablets ... ▣ 691

Triaminicol Multi-Symptom Relief (ND) 691
Tylenol Allergy Sinus Medication Caplets and Gelcaps, Maximum Strength 1372
Children's Tylenol Cold Liquid Formula and Chewable Tablets 1368
Tylenol Cold & Flu Hot Medication, Packets 1369
Tylenol Cold Medication Caplets and Tablets 1370
Tylenol Cold Medication, Effervescent Tablets 1369
Vicks Children's NyQuil (ND) 664
Vicks Formula 44 Cough Medicine (ND) 661
Vicks Formula 44M Multi-Symptom Cough Medicine (ND) 662
Vicks Pediatric Formula 44m Multi-Symptom Cough & Cold Medicine (ND) 663

Chlorpheniramine Polistirex (Depressant effects of morphine may be enhanced). Products include:
Tussionex Extended-Release Suspension 988

Chlorpheniramine Tannate (Depressant effects of morphine may be enhanced). Products include:
Rynatan 2387
Rynatuss 2388

Chlorpromazine (Respiratory depression, hypotension, and profound sedation or coma may result; depressant effects of morphine may be enhanced; analgesic effect of morphine potentiated). Products include:
Thorazine 2234

Chlorprothixene (Respiratory depression, hypotension, and profound sedation or coma may result; depressant effects of morphine may be enhanced). Products include:
Taractan Tablets 1920

Chlorprothixene Hydrochloride (Respiratory depression, hypotension, and profound sedation or coma may result; depressant effects of morphine may be enhanced). Products include:
Taractan 1920

Clemastine Fumarate (Depressant effects of morphine may be enhanced). Products include:
Tavist Syrup 2033
Tavist Tablets 2035
Tavist-D Tablets 2035

Clomipramine Hydrochloride (Respiratory depression, hypotension, and profound sedation or coma may result). Products include:
Anafranil Capsules 650

Clorazepate Dipotassium (Respiratory depression, hypotension, and profound sedation or coma may result; depressant effects of morphine may be enhanced). Products include:
Tranxene 556

Codeine (Respiratory depression, hypotension, and profound sedation or coma may result; depressant effects of morphine may be enhanced). Products include:
Calcidrine Syrup 506

Codeine Phosphate (Respiratory depression, hypotension, and profound sedation or coma may result; depressant effects of morphine may be enhanced). Products include:
Actifed with Codeine Cough Syrup 752
Cheracol Cough Syrup 1853
Codimal PH Syrup 846
Dimetane-DC Cough Syrup 1857
Empirin with Codeine Phosphate Nos. 2, 3 & 4 764
Fiorinal with Codeine Capsules 2008
Isoclor Expectorant 982
Naldecon CX Adult Liquid (ND) 521
Novahistine DH 1342
Novahistine Expectorant 1343
Nucofed Capsules 2219
Nucofed Expectorant 2219
Nucofed Pediatric Expectorant 2220
Nucofed Syrup 2219
Phenaphen with Codeine Capsules 1865
Phenaphen-650 with Codeine Tablets 1866
Phenergan with Codeine 2497
Phenergan VC with Codeine 2501
Robitussin A-C Syrup 1875
Robitussin-DAC Syrup 1875
Ryna (ND) 741
Soma Compound w/Codeine Tablets 2390
Triaminic Expectorant w/Codeine 1996
Tussi-Organidin Liquid 2391
Tylenol with Codeine 1381

Codeine Polistirex (Respiratory depression, hypotension, and profound sedation or coma may result; depressant effects of morphine may be enhanced).
No products indexed under this heading.

Cyproheptadine Hydrochloride (Depressant effects of morphine may be enhanced). Products include:
Periactin 1525

Desipramine Hydrochloride (Respiratory depression, hypotension, and profound sedation or coma may result). Products include:
Norpramin Tablets 1340

Dexchlorpheniramine Maleate (Depressant effects of morphine may be enhanced). Products include:
Polaramine 2116

Dezocine (Respiratory depression, hypotension, and profound sedation or coma may result; depressant effects of morphine may be enhanced).

Diazepam (Respiratory depression, hypotension, and profound sedation or coma may result; depressant effects of morphine may be enhanced). Products include:
Valium Injectable 1937
Valium Tablets 1939
Valrelease Capsules 1923

Dicumarol (Anticoagulant activity may be increased). Products include:
Dicumarol Tablets 516

Diphenhydramine Citrate (Depressant effects of morphine may be enhanced). Products include:
Alka-Seltzer Plus Night-Time Cold Medicine (ND) 623
Bufferin AF Nite Time Analgesic/Sleeping Aid Caplets 744
Excedrin P.M. Analgesic/Sleeping Aid Tablets, Caplets and Liquid 749

Diphenhydramine Hydrochloride (Depressant effects of morphine may be enhanced). Products include:
Benadryl Anti-Itch Cream (ND) 635
Benadryl Capsules 1691
Benadryl Decongestant Elixir (ND) 635
Benadryl Decongestant (ND) 635
Benadryl Elixir (ND) 636
Benadryl Kapseals 1691
Benadryl 25 Kapseals (ND) 636
Benadryl Parenteral 1692
Benadryl Plus (ND) 636
Benadryl Plus Nighttime (ND) 637
Benadryl Spray, Maximum Strength (ND) 637
Benadryl Spray, Regular Strength (ND) 637
Benadryl Steri-Vials, Ampoules, and Steri-Dose Syringe 1692
Benadryl 25 Tablets (ND) 636
Benylin Cough Syrup (ND) 637
Benylin Decongestant (ND) 638
Caladryl Cream, Lotion, Spray (ND) 638
Miles Nervine Nighttime Sleep-Aid (ND) 627
Nytol Tablets (ND) 517
Sleep-ettes-D Tablets (ND) 653
Sleep-eze 3 Tablets (ND) 755
Sleepinal Night-time Sleep Aid Capsules (ND) 734
Sominex Caplets and Tablets (ND) 722
Sominex Liquid (ND) 723
Sominex Pain Relief Formula (ND) 723
Tylenol Cold Night Time Medication Liquid 1371
Tylenol PM, Extra Strength Caplets and Tablets 1368
Unisom Dual Relief Nighttime Sleep Aid/Analgesic 1774
Ziradryl Lotion (ND) 643

Diphenylpyraline Hydrochloride (Depressant effects of morphine may be enhanced).
No products indexed under this heading.

Doxepin Hydrochloride (Respiratory depression, hypotension, and profound sedation or coma may result). Products include:
Sinequan 1960

Droperidol (Respiratory depression, hypotension, and profound sedation or coma may result; depressant effects of morphine may be enhanced). Products include:
Inapsine Injection 1140
Innovar Injection 1141

Enflurane (Respiratory depression, hypotension, and profound sedation or coma may result; depressant effects of morphine may be enhanced). Products include:
Ethrane 599

Esmolol Hydrochloride (Depressant effects of morphine may be enhanced). Products include:
Brevibloc Injection 942

Estazolam (Respiratory depression, hypotension, and profound sedation or coma may result; depressant effects of morphine may be enhanced). Products include:
ProSom Tablets 554

Ethchlorvynol (Respiratory depression, hypotension, and profound sedation or coma may result; depressant effects of morphine may be enhanced). Products include:
Placidyl Capsules 553

Ethinamate (Respiratory depression, hypotension, and profound sedation or coma may result; depressant effects of morphine may be enhanced).
No products indexed under this heading.

Fentanyl (Respiratory depression, hypotension, and profound sedation or coma may result; depressant effects of morphine may be enhanced). Products include:
Duragesic Transdermal System 1133

Fentanyl Citrate (Respiratory depression, hypotension, and profound sedation or coma may result; depressant effects of morphine may be enhanced). Products include:
Innovar Injection 1141
Sublimaze Injection 1146

Fluphenazine Decanoate (Respiratory depression, hypotension, and profound sedation or coma may result; depressant effects of morphine may be enhanced). Products include:
Prolixin Decanoate 1795

Fluphenazine Enanthate (Respiratory depression, hypotension, and profound sedation or coma may result; depressant effects of morphine may be enhanced). Products include:
Prolixin Enanthate 1796

Fluphenazine Hydrochloride (Respiratory depression, hypotension, and profound sedation or coma may result; depressant effects of morphine may be enhanced). Products include:
Prolixin Elixir 1793
Prolixin Injection 1791
Prolixin Oral Concentrate 1792
Prolixin Tablets 1793

Flurazepam Hydrochloride (Respiratory depression, hypotension, and profound sedation or coma may result; depressant effects of morphine may be enhanced). Products include:
Dalmane Capsules 1927

Furazolidone (Depressant effects of morphine may be enhanced). Products include:
Furoxone 1855

Glutethimide (Respiratory depression, hypotension, and profound sedation or coma may result; depressant effects of morphine may be enhanced).
No products indexed under this heading.

Haloperidol (Respiratory depression, hypotension, and profound sedation or coma may result; depressant effects of morphine may be enhanced). Products include:
Haldol Injection, Tablets and Concentrate 1373

Haloperidol Decanoate (Respiratory depression, hypotension, and profound sedation or coma may result; depressant effects of morphine may be enhanced). Products include:
Haldol Decanoate 1375

Heparin Calcium (Anticoagulant activity may be increased). Products include:
Calciparine Injection 925

Heparin Sodium (Anticoagulant activity may be increased). Products include:
Heparin Lock Flush Solution 2456
Heparin Sodium Vials 1264
Heparin Sodium Injection 2457
Heparin Sodium Injection, USP, Sterile Solution 2342

Hydrocodone Bitartrate (Respiratory depression, hypotension, and profound sedation or coma may result; depressant effects of morphine may be enhanced). Products include:
Anexsia 5/500 Tablets 2196
Anexsia 7.5/650 Tablets 2197
Azdône Tablets 844
Codiclear DH Syrup 845
Codimal DH Syrup 846
Damason-P 1356
Hycodan Syrup, Tablets 927
Hycomine Compound Tablets 929
Hycomine Syrup 927
Hycotuss Expectorant Syrup 930
Hydrocet Capsules 835
Lortab ASA Tablets 2414
Lortab 2412
Ru-Tuss with Hydrocodone 694
Triaminic Expectorant DH 1995
Vicodin Tablets 1187
Vicodin ES Tablets 1189
Zydone Capsules 941

Hydrocodone Polistirex (Respiratory depression, hypotension, and profound sedation or coma may result; depressant effects of morphine may be enhanced). Products include:
Tussionex Extended-Release Suspension 988

Hydroxyzine Hydrochloride (Respiratory depression, hypotension, and profound sedation or coma may result; depressant effects of morphine may be enhanced). Products include:
Atarax Tablets & Syrup 1941
Marax Tablets & DF Syrup 1954
Vistaril Intramuscular Solution 1970

Imipramine Hydrochloride (Respiratory depression, hypotension, and profound sedation or coma may result). Products include:
Tofranil Ampuls 1038

Tofranil Tablets ... 1039

Imipramine Pamoate (Respiratory depression, hypotension, and profound sedation or coma may result). Products include:

Tofranil-PM Capsules ... 1041

Isocarboxazid (Depressant effects of morphine may be enhanced). Products include:

Marplan Tablets ... 1906

Isoflurane (Respiratory depression, hypotension, and profound sedation or coma may result; depressant effects of morphine may be enhanced). Products include:

Forane ... 600

Ketamine Hydrochloride (Respiratory depression, hypotension, and profound sedation or coma may result; depressant effects of morphine may be enhanced). Products include:

Ketalar ... 1726

Labetalol Hydrochloride (Depressant effects of morphine may be enhanced). Products include:

Normodyne Injection ... 2108
Normodyne Tablets ... 2110
Normozide Tablets ... 2112
Trandate HCT Tablets ... 579
Trandate Injection ... 577
Trandate Tablets ... 579

Levorphanol Tartrate (Respiratory depression, hypotension, and profound sedation or coma may result; depressant effects of morphine may be enhanced). Products include:

Levo-Dromoran ... 1906

Lorazepam (Respiratory depression, hypotension, and profound sedation or coma may result; depressant effects of morphine may be enhanced). Products include:

Ativan Injection ... 2432
Ativan Tablets ... 2434

Loxapine Hydrochloride (Respiratory depression, hypotension, and profound sedation or coma may result; depressant effects of morphine may be enhanced). Products include:

Loxitane ... 1213

Loxapine Succinate (Respiratory depression, hypotension, and profound sedation or coma may result; depressant effects of morphine may be enhanced). Products include:

Loxitane Capsules ... 1213

Maprotiline Hydrochloride (Respiratory depression, hypotension, and profound sedation or coma may result). Products include:

Ludiomil Tablets ... 874

Meperidine Hydrochloride (Respiratory depression, hypotension, and profound sedation or coma may result; depressant effects of morphine may be enhanced). Products include:

Demerol ... 2047
Mepergan Injection ... 2479

Mephobarbital (Respiratory depression, hypotension, and profound sedation or coma may result; depressant effects of morphine may be enhanced). Products include:

Mebaral Tablets ... 2061

Meprobamate (Respiratory depression, hypotension, and profound sedation or coma may result; depressant effects of morphine may be enhanced). Products include:

Deprol Tablets ... 2382
Equagesic Tablets ... 2451
Miltown Tablets ... 2386

PMB 200 and PMB 400 ... 2504

Mesoridazine (Respiratory depression, hypotension, and profound sedation or coma may result; depressant effects of morphine may be enhanced). Products include:

Serentil ... 686

Methadone Hydrochloride (Respiratory depression, hypotension, and profound sedation or coma may result; depressant effects of morphine may be enhanced). Products include:

Dolophine Hydrochloride Ampoules & Vials ... 1260
Dolophine Hydrochloride Tablets ... 1261
Methadone Hydrochloride Diskets ... 1284
Methadone Hydrochloride Oral Solution & Tablets ... 1987

Methdilazine Hydrochloride (Depressant effects of morphine may be enhanced). Products include:

Tacaryl Syrup & Tablets ... 2409

Methocarbamol (Analgesic effect of morphine potentiated). Products include:

Robaxin Injectable ... 1871
Robaxin Tablets ... 1872
Robaxisal Tablets ... 1872

Methohexital Sodium (Respiratory depression, hypotension, and profound sedation or coma may result; depressant effects of morphine may be enhanced). Products include:

Brevital Sodium Vials ... 1248

Methoxyflurane (Respiratory depression, hypotension, and profound sedation or coma may result; depressant effects of morphine may be enhanced).

No products indexed under this heading.

Metoprolol Tartrate (Depressant effects of morphine may be enhanced). Products include:

Lopressor Ampuls ... 1032
Lopressor HCT Tablets ... 1034
Lopressor Tablets ... 1032

Midazolam Hydrochloride (Respiratory depression, hypotension, and profound sedation or coma may result; depressant effects of morphine may be enhanced). Products include:

Versed Injection ... 1924

Molindone Hydrochloride (Respiratory depression, hypotension, and profound sedation or coma may result; depressant effects of morphine may be enhanced). Products include:

Moban Tablets & Concentrate ... 932

Nadolol (Depressant effects of morphine may be enhanced). Products include:

Corgard Tablets ... 701
Corzide Tablets ... 702

Nortriptyline Hydrochloride (Respiratory depression, hypotension, and profound sedation or coma may result). Products include:

Pamelor ... 2019

Opium Alkaloids (Respiratory depression hypotension, and profound sedation or coma may result; depressant effects of morphine may be enhanced). Products include:

B & O No. 15A & No. 16A Supprettes ... 2395
Pantopon Injectable ... 1911

Oxazepam (Respiratory depression, hypotension, and profound sedation or coma may result; depressant effects of morphine may be enhanced). Products include:

Serax Capsules ... 2522
Serax Tablets ... 2522

Oxycodone Hydrochloride (Respiratory depression, hypotension, and profound sedation or coma may result; depressant effects of morphine may be enhanced). Products include:

Percocet Tablets ... 950
Percodan ... 951
Roxicodone Tablets, Oral Solution & Intensol (Oxycodone) ... 1992
Tylox Capsules ... 1382

Penbutolol Sulfate (Depressant effects of morphine may be enhanced). Products include:

Levatol ... 1832

Pentobarbital Sodium (Respiratory depression, hypotension, and profound sedation or coma may result; depressant effects of morphine sulfate may be enhanced). Products include:

Nembutal Sodium Capsules ... 534
Nembutal Sodium Solution ... 536
Nembutal Sodium Suppositories ... 538

Perphenazine (Respiratory depression, hypotension, and profound sedation or coma may result; depressant effects of morphine may be enhanced). Products include:

Etrafon ... 2087
Triavil Tablets ... 1556
Trilafon ... 2123

Phenelzine Sulfate (Depressant effects of morphine may be enhanced). Products include:

Nardil ... 1742

Phenobarbital (Respiratory depression, hypotension, and profound sedation or coma may result; depressant effects of morphine may be enhanced). Products include:

Arco-Lase Plus Tablets ... 607
Bellergal-S Tablets ... 1998
Bronkolixir ... ▣ 761
Bronkotabs Tablets ... ▣ 762
Donnatal ... 1858
Donnatal Extentabs ... 1859
Donnatal Tablets ... 1858
Donnazyme Tablets ... 1860
Kinesed Tablets ... 2272
Phenobarbital Elixir and Tablets ... 1293
Primatene Tablets-P Formula ... 2421
Quadrinal Tablets ... 1183
Tedral SA ... 1765

Pindolol (Depressant effects of morphine may be enhanced). Products include:

Visken Tablets ... 2036

Potassium Acid Phosphate (Effects of morphine may be antagonized). Products include:

K-Phos M.F. Tablets ... 659
K-Phos Original Formula 'Sodium Free' Tablets ... 660
K-Phos No. 2 Tablets ... 659

Potassium Citrate (Effects of morphine may be potentiated). Products include:

Alka-Seltzer Effervescent Antacid ... 1570
K-Lyte ... 707
Polycitra Syrup ... 2424
Polycitra-K ... 2424
Polycitra-LC—Sugar-Free ... 2424
Ricelyte, Rice-Based Oral Electrolyte Maintenance Solution ... ▣ 613

Prazepam (Respiratory depression, hypotension, and profound sedation or coma may result; depressant effects of morphine may be enhanced). Products include:

Centrax ... 1693

Procarbazine Hydrochloride (Depressant effects of morphine may be enhanced). Products include:

Matulane Capsules ... 1907

Prochlorperazine (Respiratory depression, hypotension, and profound sedation or coma may result; depressant effects of morphine may be enhanced; analgesic effect of morphine potentiated). Products include:

Compazine ... 2201

Promethazine Hydrochloride (Respiratory depression, hypotension, and profound sedation or coma may result; depressant effects of morphine may be enhanced). Products include:

Mepergan Injection ... 2479
Phenergan with Codeine ... 2497
Phenergan with Dextromethorphan ... 2499
Phenergan Injection ... 2493
Phenergan Suppositories ... 2496
Phenergan Syrup ... 2495
Phenergan Tablets ... 2496
Phenergan VC ... 2500
Phenergan VC with Codeine ... 2501

Propofol (Respiratory depression, hypotension, and profound sedation or coma may result; depressant effects of morphine may be enhanced). Products include:

Diprivan Injection ... 2267

Propoxyphene Hydrochloride (Respiratory depression, hypotension, and profound sedation or coma may result; depressant effects of morphine may be enhanced). Products include:

Darvon ... 1256
Wygesic Tablets ... 2540

Propoxyphene Napsylate (Respiratory depression, hypotension, and profound sedation or coma may result; depressant effects of morphine may be enhanced). Products include:

Darvon-N/Darvocet-N ... 1254

Propranolol Hydrochloride (Depressant effects of morphine may be enhanced). Products include:

Inderal ... 2459
Inderal LA Long Acting Capsules ... 2461
Inderide Tablets ... 2463
Inderide LA Long Acting Capsules ... 2465

Protriptyline Hydrochloride (Respiratory depression, hypotension, and profound sedation or coma may result). Products include:

Vivactil Tablets ... 1567

Pyrilamine Maleate (Depressant effects of morphine may be enhanced). Products include:

Codimal ... 846
4-Way Fast Acting Nasal Spray - Original Formula (regular & mentholated) & Metered Spray Pump (regular) ... 751
Maximum Strength Midol Multi-Symptom Menstrual Formula ... ▣ 571
Maximum Strength Midol PMS Premenstrual Syndrome Formula ... ▣ 570
Regular Strength Midol Multi-Symptom Menstrual Formula ... ▣ 570
Prefrin-A ... ⊙ 255
Prēmsyn PMS Capsules & Caplets ▣ 547
Primatene Tablets-M Formula ... 2421
Robitussin Night Relief ... ▣ 677
Ru-Tuss with Hydrocodone ... 694
Triaminic Expectorant DH ... 1995
Triaminic Oral Infant Drops ... 1996

Pyrilamine Tannate (Depressant effects of morphine may be enhanced). Products include:

Rynatan ... 2387

Quazepam (Respiratory depression, hypotension, and profound sedation or coma may result; depressant effects of morphine may be enhanced). Products include:

Doral Tablets ... 2383

Secobarbital Sodium (Respiratory depression, hypotension, and profound sedation or coma may result; depressant effects of morphine may be enhanced). Products include:

Seconal Sodium Pulvules ... 1296

Selegiline Hydrochloride (Depressant effects of morphine may be enhanced). Products include:

Eldepryl ... 2250

Sodium Acid Phosphate (Effects of morphine may be antagonized). Products include:

K-Phos No. 2 Tablets ... 659
Uroqid-Acid ... 661

Sodium Citrate (Effects of morphine may be potentiated). Products include:

Alka-Seltzer Effervescent Antacid .. 1570
Alka-Seltzer Extra Strength Effervescent Antacid and Pain Reliever ... 1570
Alka-Seltzer (Flavored) Effervescent Antacid and Pain Reliever 1569
Bicitra—Sugar-Free ... 2423
Citrocarbonate Antacid ... ▣ 668
Polycitra ... 2424
Ricelyte, Rice-Based Oral Electrolyte Maintenance Solution ... ▣ 613

Sufentanil Citrate (Respiratory depression, hypotension, and profound sedation or coma may result; depressant effects of morphine may be enhanced). Products include:

Sufenta Injection ... 1147

Temazepam (Respiratory depression, hypotension, and profound sedation or coma may result; depressant effects of morphine may be enhanced). Products include:

Restoril Capsules ... 2023

Terfenadine (Depressant effects of morphine may be enhanced). Products include:

Seldane Tablets ... 1349
Seldane-D Extended-Release Tablets ... 1350

Thiamylal Sodium (Respiratory depression, hypotension, and profound sedation or coma may result; depressant effects of morphine may be enhanced). Products include:

Surital Ampoules, Steri-Vials ... 1764

Thioridazine Hydrochloride (Respiratory depression, hypotension, and profound sedation or coma may result; depressant effects of morphine may be enhanced). Products include:

Mellaril ... 2011

Thiothixene (Respiratory depression, hypotension, and profoundsedation or coma may result; depressant effects of morphine may be enhanced). Products include:

Navane Capsules and Concentrate 1954
Navane Intramuscular ... 1956

Timolol Maleate (Depressant effects of morphine may be enhanced). Products include:

Blocadren Tablets ... 1429
Timolide Tablets ... 1547
Timoptic in Ocudose ... 1552
Timoptic Sterile Ophthalmic Solution ... 1550

Tranylcypromine Sulfate (Depressant effects of morphine may be enhanced). Products include:

Parnate Tablets ... 2222

Triazolam (Respiratory depression, hypotension, and profound sedation or coma may result; depressant effects of morphine may be enhanced). Products include:

Halcion Tablets ... 2340

Trifluoperazine Hydrochloride (Respiratory depression, hypotension, and profound sedation or coma may result; depressant effects of morphine may be enhanced). Products include:

Stelazine ... 2226

Trimeprazine Tartrate (Depressant effects of morphine may be enhanced). Products include:

Temaril Tablets, Syrup and Spansule Sustained Release Capsules 1085

Trimipramine Maleate (Respiratory depression, hypotension, and profound sedation or coma may result). Products include:

Surmontil Capsules ... 2524

Tripelennamine Hydrochloride (Depressant effects of morphine may be enhanced). Products include:

PBZ Tablets & Elixir ... 1037
PBZ-SR Tablets ... 1037

Triprolidine Hydrochloride (Depressant effects of morphine may be enhanced). Products include:

Actidil ... ▣ 538
Actifed Capsules ... ▣ 539
Actifed Plus Caplets ... ▣ 539
Actifed Plus Tablets ... ▣ 540
Actifed with Codeine Cough Syrup.. 752
Actifed Syrup ... ▣ 540
Actifed Tablets ... ▣ 540
Actifed 12-Hour Capsules ... ▣ 539

Warfarin Sodium (Anticoagulant activity may be increased). Products include:

Coumadin Injection & Tablets ... 944
Panwarfin Tablets ... 547

ROXANOL 100 (MORPHINE SULFATE CONCENTRATED ORAL SOLUTION)
(Morphine Sulfate) ... 1991
See **Roxanol (Morphine Sulfate Concentrated Oral Solution)**

ROXANOL RESCUDOSE
(Morphine Sulfate) ... 1991
See **Roxanol (Morphine Sulfate Concentrated Oral Solution)**

ROXICODONE TABLETS, ORAL SOLUTION & INTENSOL (OXYCODONE)
(Oxycodone Hydrochloride) ... 1992
May interact with central nervous system depressants and certain other agents. Compounds in these categories include:

Alcohol (Possible additive CNS depression).

Alfentanil Hydrochloride (Possible additive CNS depression). Products include:

Alfenta Injection ... 1131

Alprazolam (Possible additive CNS depression). Products include:

Xanax Tablets ... 2367

Aprobarbital (Possible additive CNS depression). Products include:

Alurate Elixir ... 1883

Buprenorphine (Possible additive CNS depression).

No products indexed under this heading.

Buspirone Hydrochloride (Possible additive CNS depression). Products include:

BuSpar ... 1401

Butabarbital (Possible additive CNS depression). Products include:

Pyridium Plus ... 1764

Butalbital (Possible additive CNS depression). Products include:

Esgic-Plus Tablets ... 1002
Esgic Tablets & Capsules ... 1001
Fioricet Tablets ... 2006
Fiorinal Capsules ... 2007
Fiorinal with Codeine Capsules ... 2008
Fiorinal Tablets ... 2007
Phrenilin ... 838
Sedapap Tablets 50 mg/650 mg .. 1360

Chlordiazepoxide (Possible additive CNS depression). Products include:

Libritabs Tablets ... 1930
Limbitrol ... 1933
Menrium Tablets ... 1934

Chlordiazepoxide Hydrochloride (Possible additive CNS depression). Products include:

Librax Capsules ... 1929
Librium Capsules ... 1931
Librium Injectable ... 1932

Chlorpromazine (Possible additive CNS depression). Products include:

Thorazine ... 2234

Chlorprothixene (Possible additive CNS depression). Products include:

Taractan Tablets ... 1920

Chlorprothixene Hydrochloride (Possible additive CNS depression). Products include:

Taractan ... 1920

Chlorprothixene Lactate (Possible additive CNS depression). Products include:

Taractan Concentrate ... 1920

Clorazepate Dipotassium (Possible additive CNS depression). Products include:

Tranxene ... 556

Codeine (Possible additive CNS depression). Products include:

Calcidrine Syrup ... 506

Codeine Phosphate (Possible additive CNS depression). Products include:

Actifed with Codeine Cough Syrup.. 752
Cheracol Cough Syrup ... 1853
Codimal PH Syrup ... 846
Dimetane-DC Cough Syrup ... 1857
Empirin with Codeine Phosphate Nos. 2, 3 & 4 ... 764
Fiorinal with Codeine Capsules ... 2008
Isoclor Expectorant ... 982
Naldecon CX Adult Liquid ... ▣ 521
Novahistine DH ... 1342
Novahistine Expectorant ... 1343
Nucofed Capsules ... 2219
Nucofed Expectorant ... 2219
Nucofed Pediatric Expectorant ... 2220
Nucofed Syrup ... 2219
Phenaphen with Codeine Capsules 1865
Phenaphen-650 with Codeine Tablets ... 1866
Phenergan with Codeine ... 2497
Phenergan VC with Codeine ... 2501
Robitussin A-C Syrup ... 1875
Robitussin-DAC Syrup ... 1875
Ryna ... ▣ 741
Soma Compound w/Codeine Tablets ... 2390
Triaminic Expectorant w/Codeine .. 1996
Tussi-Organidin Liquid ... 2391
Tylenol with Codeine ... 1381

Codeine Polistirex (Possible additive CNS depression).

No products indexed under this heading.

Dezocine (Possible additive CNS depression).

Diazepam (Possible additive CNS depression). Products include:

Valium Injectable ... 1937
Valium Tablets ... 1939
Valrelease Capsules ... 1923

Droperidol (Possible additive CNS depression). Products include:

Inapsine Injection ... 1140
Innovar Injection ... 1141

Enflurane (Possible additive CNS depression). Products include:

Ethrane ... 599

Estazolam (Possible additive CNS depression). Products include:

ProSom Tablets ... 554

Ethchlorvynol (Possible additive CNS depression). Products include:

Placidyl Capsules ... 553

Ethinamate (Possible additive CNS depression).

No products indexed under this heading.

Fentanyl (Possible additive CNS depression). Products include:

Duragesic Transdermal System ... 1133

Fentanyl Citrate (Possible additive CNS depression). Products include:

Innovar Injection ... 1141
Sublimaze Injection ... 1146

Fluphenazine Decanoate (Possible additive CNS depression). Products include:

Prolixin Decanoate ... 1795

Fluphenazine Enanthate (Possible additive CNS depression). Products include:

Prolixin Enanthate ... 1796

Fluphenazine Hydrochloride (Possible additive CNS depression). Products include:

Prolixin Elixir ... 1793
Prolixin Injection ... 1791
Prolixin Oral Concentrate ... 1792
Prolixin Tablets ... 1793

Flurazepam Hydrochloride (Possible additive CNS depression). Products include:

Dalmane Capsules ... 1927

Glutethimide (Possible additive CNS depression).

No products indexed under this heading.

Haloperidol (Possible additive CNS depression). Products include:

Haldol Injection, Tablets and Concentrate ... 1373

Haloperidol Decanoate (Possible additive CNS depression). Products include:

Haldol Decanoate ... 1375

Hydrocodone Bitartrate (Possible additive CNS depression). Products include:

Anexsia 5/500 Tablets ... 2196
Anexsia 7.5/650 Tablets ... 2197
Azdone Tablets ... 844
Codiclear DH Syrup ... 845
Codimal DH Syrup ... 846
Damason-P ... 1356
Hycodan Syrup, Tablets ... 927
Hycomine Compound Tablets ... 929
Hycomine Syrup ... 927
Hycotuss Expectorant Syrup ... 930
Hydrocet Capsules ... 835
Lortab ASA Tablets ... 2414
Lortab ... 2412
Ru-Tuss with Hydrocodone ... 694
Triaminic Expectorant DH ... 1995
Vicodin Tablets ... 1187
Vicodin ES Tablets ... 1189
Zydone Capsules ... 941

Hydrocodone Polistirex (Possible additive CNS depression). Products include:

Tussionex Extended-Release Suspension ... 988

Hydroxyzine Hydrochloride (Possible additive CNS depression). Products include:

Atarax Tablets & Syrup ... 1941
Marax Tablets & DF Syrup ... 1954
Vistaril Intramuscular Solution ... 1970

Isoflurane (Possible additive CNS depression). Products include:

Forane ... 600

Ketamine Hydrochloride (Possible additive CNS depression). Products include:

Ketalar ... 1726

Levorphanol Tartrate (Possible additive CNS depression). Products include:

Levo-Dromoran ... 1906

Lorazepam (Possible additive CNS depression). Products include:
- Ativan Injection 2432
- Ativan Tablets 2434

Loxapine Hydrochloride (Possible additive CNS depression). Products include:
- Loxitane 1213

Loxapine Succinate (Possible additive CNS depression). Products include:
- Loxitane Capsules 1213

Meperidine Hydrochloride (Possible additive CNS depression). Products include:
- Demerol 2047
- Mepergan Injection 2479

Mephobarbital (Possible additive CNS depression). Products include:
- Mebaral Tablets 2061

Meprobamate (Possible additive CNS depression). Products include:
- Deprol Tablets 2382
- Equagesic Tablets 2451
- Miltown Tablets 2386
- PMB 200 and PMB 400 2504

Mesoridazine (Possible additive CNS depression). Products include:
- Serentil 686

Methadone Hydrochloride (Possible additive CNS depression). Products include:
- Dolophine Hydrochloride Ampoules & Vials 1260
- Dolophine Hydrochloride Tablets 1261
- Methadone Hydrochloride Diskets 1284
- Methadone Hydrochloride Oral Solution & Tablets 1987

Methohexital Sodium (Possible additive CNS depression). Products include:
- Brevital Sodium Vials 1248

Methoxyflurane (Possible additive CNS depression).
- No products indexed under this heading.

Midazolam Hydrochloride (Possible additive CNS depression). Products include:
- Versed Injection 1924

Molindone Hydrochloride (Possible additive CNS depression). Products include:
- Moban Tablets & Concentrate 932

Morphine Sulfate (Possible additive CNS depression). Products include:
- Astramorph/PF Injection, USP (Preservative-Free) 618
- Duramorph 960
- Infumorph 200 and Infumorph 500 Sterile Solutions 962
- MS Contin Tablets 1814
- MSIR 1817
- Oramorph SR (Morphine Sulfate Sustained Release Tablets) 1988
- Roxanol 1991

Opium Alkaloids (Possible additive CNS depression). Products include:
- B & O No. 15A & No. 16A Supprettes 2395
- Pantopon Injectable 1911

Oxazepam (Possible additive CNS depression). Products include:
- Serax Capsules 2522
- Serax Tablets 2522

Pentobarbital Sodium (Possible additive CNS depression). Products include:
- Nembutal Sodium Capsules 534
- Nembutal Sodium Solution 536
- Nembutal Sodium Suppositories 538

Perphenazine (Possible additive CNS depression). Products include:
- Etrafon 2087
- Triavil Tablets 1556
- Trilafon 2123

Phenobarbital (Possible additive CNS depression). Products include:
- Arco-Lase Plus Tablets 607
- Bellergal-S Tablets 1998
- Bronkolixir ▣ 761
- Bronkotabs Tablets ▣ 762
- Donnatal 1858
- Donnatal Extentabs 1859
- Donnatal Tablets 1858
- Donnazyme Tablets 1860
- Kinesed Tablets 2272
- Phenobarbital Elixir and Tablets 1293
- Primatene Tablets-P Formula 2421
- Quadrinal Tablets 1183
- Tedral SA 1765

Prazepam (Possible additive CNS depression). Products include:
- Centrax 1693

Prochlorperazine (Possible additive CNS depression). Products include:
- Compazine 2201

Promethazine Hydrochloride (Possible additive CNS depression). Products include:
- Mepergan Injection 2479
- Phenergan with Codeine 2497
- Phenergan with Dextromethorphan 2499
- Phenergan Injection 2493
- Phenergan Suppositories 2496
- Phenergan Syrup 2495
- Phenergan Tablets 2496
- Phenergan VC 2500
- Phenergan VC with Codeine 2501

Propofol (Possible additive CNS depression). Products include:
- Diprivan Injection 2267

Propoxyphene Hydrochloride (Possible additive CNS depression). Products include:
- Darvon 1256
- Wygesic Tablets 2540

Propoxyphene Napsylate (Possible additive CNS depression). Products include:
- Darvon-N/Darvocet-N 1254

Quazepam (Possible additive CNS depression). Products include:
- Doral Tablets 2383

Secobarbital Sodium (Possible additive CNS depression). Products include:
- Seconal Sodium Pulvules 1296

Sufentanil Citrate (Possible additive CNS depression). Products include:
- Sufenta Injection 1147

Temazepam (Possible additive CNS depression). Products include:
- Restoril Capsules 2023

Thiamylal Sodium (Possible additive CNS depression). Products include:
- Surital Ampoules, Steri-Vials 1764

Thioridazine Hydrochloride (Possible additive CNS depression). Products include:
- Mellaril 2011

Thiothixene (Possible additive CNS depression). Products include:
- Navane Capsules and Concentrate 1954
- Navane Intramuscular 1956

Triazolam (Possible additive CNS depression). Products include:
- Halcion Tablets 2340

Trifluoperazine Hydrochloride (Possible additive CNS depression). Products include:
- Stelazine 2226

ROYGEL 100 MG CAPSULES
(Vitamins, Supplement) ▣ 516
No interactions described in labeling.

ROYGEL ULTIMA CAPSULES
(Vitamins, Supplement) ▣ 516
No interactions described in labeling.

RUBEX
(Doxorubicin Hydrochloride) 739
May interact with antineoplastics and certain other agents. Compounds in these categories include:

Altretamine (Concomitant administration may potentiate toxicity). Products include:
- Hexalen Capsules 2316

Asparaginase (Concomitant administration may potentiate toxicity). Products include:
- Elspar 1470

Bleomycin Sulfate (Concomitant administration may potentiate toxicity). Products include:
- Blenoxane 724

Busulfan (Concomitant administration may potentiate toxicity). Products include:
- Myleran Tablets 790

Carboplatin (Concomitant administration may potentiate toxicity). Products include:
- Paraplatin for Injection 735

Carmustine (BCNU) (Concomitant administration may potentiate toxicity). Products include:
- BiCNU 723

Chlorambucil (Concomitant administration may potentiate toxicity). Products include:
- Leukeran Tablets 788

Cisplatin (Concomitant administration may potentiate toxicity). Products include:
- Platinol 737
- Platinol-AQ Injection 738

Cyclophosphamide (Concomitant administration may potentiate toxicity; exacerbation of cyclophosphamide induced hemorrhagic cystitis). Products include:
- Cytoxan for Injection 726
- Neosar for Injection 566

Dacarbazine (Concomitant administration may potentiate toxicity). Products include:
- DTIC-Dome 1595

Daunorubicin Hydrochloride (Concomitant administration may potentiate toxicity). Products include:
- Cerubidine 2443

Estramustine Phosphate Sodium (Concomitant administration may potentiate toxicity). Products include:
- Emcyt Capsules 1161

Etoposide (Concomitant administration may potentiate toxicity). Products include:
- VePesid Capsules and Injection 741

Floxuridine (Concomitant administration may potentiate toxicity). Products include:
- Sterile FUDR 1898

Fluorouracil (Concomitant administration may potentiate toxicity). Products include:
- Efudex 1880
- Fluoroplex Topical Solution & Cream 1% 1082
- Fluorouracil Injection 1897

Flutamide (Concomitant administration may potentiate toxicity). Products include:
- Eulexin Capsules 2089

Hydroxyurea (Concomitant administration may potentiate toxicity). Products include:
- Hydrea Capsules 728

Ifosfamide (Concomitant administration may potentiate toxicity). Products include:
- IFEX 729

Interferon alfa-2A, Recombinant (Concomitant administration may potentiate toxicity). Products include:
- Roferon-A Injection 1916

Interferon alfa-2B, Recombinant (Concomitant administration may potentiate toxicity). Products include:
- Intron A 2097

Levamisole Hydrochloride (Concomitant administration may potentiate toxicity). Products include:
- Ergamisol Tablets 1136

Lomustine (CCNU) (Concomitant administration may potentiate toxicity). Products include:
- CeeNU 725

Mechlorethamine Hydrochloride (Concomitant administration may potentiate toxicity). Products include:
- Mustargen 1514

Megestrol Acetate (Concomitant administration may potentiate toxicity). Products include:
- Megace Tablets 732

Melphalan (Concomitant administration may potentiate toxicity). Products include:
- Alkeran Tablets 754

Mercaptopurine (Concomitant administration enhances hepatotoxicity). Products include:
- Purinethol Tablets 800

Methotrexate Sodium (Concomitant administration may potentiate toxicity). Products include:
- Methotrexate Tablets, Parenteral, LPF Parenteral 1217
- Rheumatrex Methotrexate Dose Pack 1234

Mitomycin (Mitomycin-C) (Concomitant administration may potentiate toxicity). Products include:
- Mutamycin 733

Mitotane (Concomitant administration may potentiate toxicity). Products include:
- Lysodren 731

Mitoxantrone Hydrochloride (Concomitant administration may potentiate toxicity). Products include:
- Novantrone for Injection Concentrate 1226

Procarbazine Hydrochloride (Concomitant administration may potentiate toxicity). Products include:
- Matulane Capsules 1907

Streptozocin (Concomitant administration may potentiate toxicity). Products include:
- Zanosar Sterile Powder 2371

Tamoxifen Citrate (Concomitant administration may potentiate toxicity). Products include:
- Nolvadex Tablets 1102

Thioguanine (Concomitant administration may potentiate toxicity). Products include:
- Thioguanine Tablets, Tabloid Brand 815

Thiotepa (Concomitant administration may potentiate toxicity). Products include:
- Thiotepa Parenteral 1240

Vincristine Sulfate (Concomitant administration may potentiate toxicity). Products include:
- Oncovin Solution Vials & Hyporets 1288

RUFEN TABLETS
(Ibuprofen) 691
May interact with oral anticoagulants, thiazides, lithium preparations,

and certain other agents. Compounds in these categories include:

Aspirin (Lowered blood levels of non-aspirin drug; decreased anti-inflammatory activity). Products include:

- Alka-Seltzer Effervescent Antacid and Pain Reliever 1568
- Alka-Seltzer Extra Strength Effervescent Antacid and Pain Reliever 1570
- Alka-Seltzer (Flavored) Effervescent Antacid and Pain Reliever 1569
- Alka-Seltzer Plus Cold Medicine ▣ 623
- Alka-Seltzer Plus Night-Time Cold Medicine ▣ 623
- Alka Seltzer Plus Sinus Allergy Medicine ▣ 624
- Anacin Coated Analgesic Caplets 2417
- Anacin Coated Analgesic Tablets 2417
- Anacin Maximum Strength Analgesic Coated Tablets 2417
- Maximum Strength Arthritis Pain Formula By the Makers of Anacin Analgesic Tablets and Caplets 2418
- Arthritis Pain Formula by the Makers of Anacin Analgesic Tablets and Caplets ▣ 747
- Arthritis Strength BC Powder ▣ 516
- Ascriptin A/D Caplets 1850
- Regular Strength Ascriptin Tablets 1850
- Azdōne Tablets 844
- BC Powder ▣ 517
- BC Cold Powder ▣ 517
- Children's Bayer Chewable Aspirin ▣ 564
- Genuine Bayer Aspirin Tablets & Caplets ▣ 564
- Maximum Bayer Aspirin Tablets & Caplets ▣ 566
- Bayer Plus Aspirin Tablets ▣ 567
- Therapy Bayer Aspirin Caplets ▣ 568
- 8 Hour Bayer Timed-Release Aspirin ▣ 566
- Arthritis Strength Bufferin Analgesic Caplets 744
- Extra Strength Bufferin Analgesic Tablets 745
- Bufferin Analgesic Tablets and Caplets 743
- Cama Arthritis Pain Reliever ▣ 685
- Damason-P 1356
- Easprin 1719
- Ecotrin Enteric Coated Aspirin Maximum Strength Tablets and Caplets 2189
- Ecotrin Enteric Coated Aspirin Regular Strength Tablets and Caplets 2189
- Empirin Aspirin ▣ 541
- Empirin with Codeine Phosphate Nos. 2, 3 & 4 764
- Equagesic Tablets 2451
- Excedrin Extra-Strength Analgesic Tablets & Caplets 749
- 4-Way Cold Tablets 750
- Fiorinal Capsules 2007
- Fiorinal with Codeine Capsules 2008
- Fiorinal Tablets 2007
- Lortab ASA Tablets 2414
- Momentum Muscular Backache Formula ▣ 751
- Norgesic 1314
- Norwich Extra-Strength Aspirin ▣ 546
- Norwich Regular Strength Aspirin ▣ 547
- P-A-C Analgesic Tablets ▣ 669
- Percodan 951
- Robaxisal Tablets 1872
- Sine-Off Sinus Medicine Tablets-Aspirin Formula ▣ 722
- Soma Compound w/Codeine Tablets 2390
- Soma Compound Tablets 2389
- St. Joseph Adult Chewable Aspirin (81 mg.) ▣ 703
- Synalgos-DC Capsules 2525
- Talwin Compound 2072
- Ursinus Inlay-Tabs ▣ 691
- Vanquish Analgesic Caplets ▣ 574
- Zorprin Tablets 698

Aspirin, Enteric Coated (Lowered blood levels of non-aspirin drug; decreased anti-inflammatory activity). Products include:

- Therapy Bayer Aspirin Caplets ▣ 568
- Ecotrin 2189

Bendroflumethiazide (Reduced natriuretic effect). Products include:

- Corzide Tablets 702
- Naturetin Tablets 1789
- Rauzide Tablets 1804

Chlorothiazide (Reduced natriuretic effect). Products include:

- Aldoclor Tablets 1413
- Diupres Tablets 1461
- Diuril Oral 1464

Chlorothiazide Sodium (Reduced natriuretic effect). Products include:

- Diuril Sodium Intravenous 1463

Dicumarol (May affect prothrombin times or a variety of other clotting factors resulting in increased bleeding). Products include:

- Dicumarol Tablets 516

Furosemide (Reduced natriuretic effect). Products include:

- Lasix 1093

Hydrochlorothiazide (Reduced natriuretic effect). Products include:

- Aldactazide 2150
- Aldoril Tablets 1418
- Apresazide Capsules 854
- Apresoline-Esidrix Tablets 857
- Capozide 2258
- Dyazide Capsules 2208
- Esidrix Tablets 863
- Esimil Tablets 864
- HydroDIURIL Tablets 1484
- Hydropres Tablets 1485
- Inderide Tablets 2463
- Inderide LA Long Acting Capsules .. 2465
- Lopressor HCT Tablets 1034
- Maxzide 1215
- Moduretic Tablets 1510
- Normozide Tablets 2112
- Oretic Tablets 544
- Oreticyl 545
- Prinzide Tablets 1540
- Ser-Ap-Es Tablets 881
- Serpasil-Esidrix Tablets 886
- Timolide Tablets 1547
- Trandate HCT Tablets 579
- Vaseretic Tablets 1559
- Zestoretic 2274

Hydroflumethiazide (Reduced natriuretic effect). Products include:

- Diucardin Tablets 2450
- Saluron 718
- Salutensin/Salutensin-Demi 719

Lithium Carbonate (Elevation of plasma lithium levels and reduction of renal lithium clearance resulting in lithium toxicity). Products include:

- Eskalith 2214
- Lithane Tablets 1596
- Lithium Carbonate Capsules & Tablets 1984
- Lithobid Tablets 870

Lithium Citrate (Elevation of plasma lithium levels and reduction of renal lithium clearance resulting in lithium toxicity). Products include:

- Cibalith-S 870

Methotrexate Sodium (Potential for enhanced toxicity of methotrexate). Products include:

- Methotrexate Tablets, Parenteral, LPF Parenteral 1217
- Rheumatrex Methotrexate Dose Pack 1234

Methyclothiazide (Reduced natriuretic effect). Products include:

- Enduron Tablets 517
- Enduronyl 518

Polythiazide (Reduced natriuretic effect). Products include:

- Minizide Capsules 1779
- Renese Tablets 1785
- Renese-R Tablets 1786

Warfarin Sodium (May affect prothrombin times or a variety of other clotting factors resulting in increased bleeding). Products include:

- Coumadin Injection & Tablets 944
- Panwarfin Tablets 547

Food Interactions

Meal, unspecified (Reduces the rate of absorption but no appreciable decrease in the extent of absorption).

RUM-K SYRUP
(Potassium Chloride) 995
No interactions described in labeling.

RU-TUSS DE TABLETS
(Pseudoephedrine Hydrochloride, Guaifenesin) 694
May interact with monoamine oxidase inhibitors, beta blockers, veratrum alkaloids, catecholamine depleting drugs, and certain other agents. Compounds in these categories include:

Acebutolol Hydrochloride (Increases effects of sympathomimetics). Products include:

- Sectral Capsules 2520

Atenolol (Increases effects of sympathomimetics). Products include:

- Tenoretic Tablets 1105
- Tenormin Tablets and I.V. Injection 1107

Betaxolol Hydrochloride (Increases effects of sympathomimetics). Products include:

- Betoptic Sterile Ophthalmic Solution 569
- Betoptic S Sterile Ophthalmic Suspension 570
- Kerlone Tablets 2172

Carteolol Hydrochloride (Increases effects of sympathomimetics). Products include:

- Cartrol Tablets 507

Cryptenamine Preparations (Reduced antihypertensive effects).

Deserpidine (Reduced antihypertensive effects). Products include:

- Enduronyl 518
- Harmonyl Tablets 528
- Oreticyl 545

Esmolol Hydrochloride (Increases effects of sympathomimetics). Products include:

- Brevibloc Injection 942

Furazolidone (Increases effects of sympathomimetics; concurrent use is contraindicated). Products include:

- Furoxone 1855

Isocarboxazid (Increases effects of sympathomimetics; concurrent use is contraindicated). Products include:

- Marplan Tablets 1906

Labetalol Hydrochloride (Increases effects of sympathomimetics). Products include:

- Normodyne Injection 2108
- Normodyne Tablets 2110
- Normozide Tablets 2112
- Trandate HCT Tablets 579
- Trandate Injection 577
- Trandate Tablets 579

Mecamylamine Hydrochloride (Reduced antihypertensive effects). Products include:

- Inversine Tablets 1492

Methyldopa (Reduced antihypertensive effects). Products include:

- Aldoclor Tablets 1413
- Aldomet Oral 1415
- Aldoril Tablets 1418

Methyldopate Hydrochloride (Reduced antihypertensive effects). Products include:

- Aldomet Ester HCl Injection 1417

Metoprolol Tartrate (Increases effects of sympathomimetics). Products include:

- Lopressor Ampuls 1032
- Lopressor HCT Tablets 1034
- Lopressor Tablets 1032

Nadolol (Increases effects of sympathomimetics). Products include:

- Corgard Tablets 701
- Corzide Tablets 702

Penbutolol Sulfate (Increases effects of sympathomimetics). Products include:

- Levatol 1832

Phenelzine Sulfate (Increases effects of sympathomimetics; concurrent use is contraindicated). Products include:

- Nardil 1742

Pindolol (Increases effects of sympathomimetics). Products include:

- Visken Tablets 2036

Propranolol Hydrochloride (Increases effects of sympathomimetics). Products include:

- Inderal 2459
- Inderal LA Long Acting Capsules 2461
- Inderide Tablets 2463
- Inderide LA Long Acting Capsules .. 2465

Rauwolfia Serpentina (Reduced antihypertensive effects). Products include:

- Raudixin Tablets 1803
- Rauzide Tablets 1804

Rescinnamine (Reduced antihypertensive effects).

- No products indexed under this heading.

Reserpine (Reduced antihypertensive effects). Products include:

- Diupres Tablets 1461
- Hydromox R Tablets 1209
- Hydropres Tablets 1485
- Renese-R Tablets 1786
- Salutensin/Salutensin-Demi 719
- Ser-Ap-Es Tablets 881
- Serpasil Tablets 883
- Serpasil-Apresoline Tablets 884
- Serpasil-Esidrix Tablets 886

Selegiline Hydrochloride (Increases effects of sympathomimetics; concurrent use is contraindicated). Products include:

- Eldepryl 2250

Timolol Maleate (Increases effects of sympathomimetics). Products include:

- Blocadren Tablets 1429
- Timolide Tablets 1547
- Timoptic in Ocudose 1552
- Timoptic Sterile Ophthalmic Solution 1550

Tranylcypromine Sulfate (Increases effects of sympathomimetics; concurrent use is contraindicated). Products include:

- Parnate Tablets 2222

RU-TUSS II CAPSULES
(Phenylpropanolamine Hydrochloride, Chlorpheniramine Maleate) 693
May interact with monoamine oxidase inhibitors, central nervous system depressants, and certain other agents. Compounds in these categories include:

Alcohol (Additive effects).

Alfentanil Hydrochloride (Additive effects). Products include:

- Alfenta Injection 1131

Alprazolam (Additive effects). Products include:

- Xanax Tablets 2367

Aprobarbital (Additive effects). Products include:

- Alurate Elixir 1883

Buprenorphine (Additive effects).

- No products indexed under this heading.

Buspirone Hydrochloride (Additive effects). Products include:

- BuSpar 1401

Butabarbital (Additive effects). Products include:
Pyridium Plus 1764
Butalbital (Additive effects). Products include:
Esgic-Plus Tablets 1002
Esgic Tablets & Capsules 1001
Fioricet Tablets 2006
Fiorinal Capsules 2007
Fiorinal with Codeine Capsules 2008
Fiorinal Tablets 2007
Phrenilin 838
Sedapap Tablets 50 mg/650 mg 1360
Chlordiazepoxide (Additive effects). Products include:
Libritabs Tablets 1930
Limbitrol 1933
Menrium Tablets 1934
Chlordiazepoxide Hydrochloride (Additive effects). Products include:
Librax Capsules 1929
Librium Capsules 1931
Librium Injectable 1932
Chlorpromazine (Additive effects). Products include:
Thorazine 2234
Chlorprothixene (Additive effects). Products include:
Taractan Tablets 1920
Chlorprothixene Hydrochloride (Additive effects). Products include:
Taractan 1920
Clorazepate Dipotassium (Additive effects). Products include:
Tranxene 556
Codeine (Additive effects). Products include:
Calcidrine Syrup 506
Codeine Phosphate (Additive effects). Products include:
Actifed with Codeine Cough Syrup 752
Cheracol Cough Syrup 1853
Codimal PH Syrup 846
Dimetane-DC Cough Syrup 1857
Empirin with Codeine Phosphate Nos. 2, 3 & 4 764
Fiorinal with Codeine Capsules 2008
Isoclor Expectorant 982
Naldecon CX Adult Liquid 521
Novahistine DH 1342
Novahistine Expectorant 1343
Nucofed Capsules 2219
Nucofed Expectorant 2219
Nucofed Pediatric Expectorant 2220
Nucofed Syrup 2219
Phenaphen with Codeine Capsules 1865
Phenaphen-650 with Codeine Tablets 1866
Phenergan with Codeine 2497
Phenergan VC with Codeine 2501
Robitussin A-C Syrup 1875
Robitussin-DAC Syrup 1875
Ryna 741
Soma Compound w/Codeine Tablets 2390
Triaminic Expectorant w/Codeine 1996
Tussi-Organidin Liquid 2391
Tylenol with Codeine 1381
Codeine Polistirex (Additive effects).
No products indexed under this heading.
Dezocine (Additive effects).
Diazepam (Additive effects). Products include:
Valium Injectable 1937
Valium Tablets 1939
Valrelease Capsules 1923
Droperidol (Additive effects). Products include:
Inapsine Injection 1140
Innovar Injection 1141
Enflurane (Additive effects). Products include:
Ethrane 599
Estazolam (Additive effects). Products include:
ProSom Tablets 554
Ethchlorvynol (Additive effects). Products include:
Placidyl Capsules 553
Ethinamate (Additive effects).
No products indexed under this heading.
Fentanyl (Additive effects). Products include:
Duragesic Transdermal System 1133
Fentanyl Citrate (Additive effects). Products include:
Innovar Injection 1141
Sublimaze Injection 1146
Fluphenazine Decanoate (Additive effects). Products include:
Prolixin Decanoate 1795
Fluphenazine Enanthate (Additive effects). Products include:
Prolixin Enanthate 1796
Fluphenazine Hydrochloride (Additive effects). Products include:
Prolixin Elixir 1793
Prolixin Injection 1791
Prolixin Oral Concentrate 1792
Prolixin Tablets 1793
Flurazepam Hydrochloride (Additive effects). Products include:
Dalmane Capsules 1927
Furazolidone (Concomitant use contraindicated). Products include:
Furoxone 1855
Glutethimide (Additive effects).
No products indexed under this heading.
Haloperidol (Additive effects). Products include:
Haldol Injection, Tablets and Concentrate 1373
Haloperidol Decanoate (Additive effects). Products include:
Haldol Decanoate 1375
Hydrocodone Bitartrate (Additive effects). Products include:
Anexsia 5/500 Tablets 2196
Anexsia 7.5/650 Tablets 2197
Azdone Tablets 844
Codiclear DH Syrup 845
Codimal DH Syrup 846
Damason-P 1356
Hycodan Syrup, Tablets 927
Hycomine Compound Tablets 929
Hycomine Syrup 927
Hycotuss Expectorant Syrup 930
Hydrocet Capsules 835
Lortab ASA Tablets 2414
Lortab 2412
Ru-Tuss with Hydrocodone 694
Triaminic Expectorant DH 1995
Vicodin Tablets 1187
Vicodin ES Tablets 1189
Zydone Capsules 941
Hydrocodone Polistirex (Additive effects). Products include:
Tussionex Extended-Release Suspension 988
Hydroxyzine Hydrochloride (Additive effects). Products include:
Atarax Tablets & Syrup 1941
Marax Tablets & DF Syrup 1954
Vistaril Intramuscular Solution 1970
Isocarboxazid (Concomitant use contraindicated). Products include:
Marplan Tablets 1906
Isoflurane (Additive effects). Products include:
Forane 600
Ketamine Hydrochloride (Additive effects). Products include:
Ketalar 1726
Levorphanol Tartrate (Additive effects). Products include:
Levo-Dromoran 1906
Lorazepam (Additive effects). Products include:
Ativan Injection 2432
Ativan Tablets 2434
Loxapine Hydrochloride (Additive effects). Products include:
Loxitane 1213
Loxapine Succinate (Additive effects). Products include:
Loxitane Capsules 1213
Meperidine Hydrochloride (Additive effects). Products include:
Demerol 2047
Mepergan Injection 2479
Mephobarbital (Additive effects). Products include:
Mebaral Tablets 2061
Meprobamate (Additive effects). Products include:
Deprol Tablets 2382
Equagesic Tablets 2451
Miltown Tablets 2386
PMB 200 and PMB 400 2504
Mesoridazine (Additive effects). Products include:
Serentil 686
Methadone Hydrochloride (Additive effects). Products include:
Dolophine Hydrochloride Ampoules & Vials 1260
Dolophine Hydrochloride Tablets 1261
Methadone Hydrochloride Diskets 1284
Methadone Hydrochloride Oral Solution & Tablets 1987
Methohexital Sodium (Additive effects). Products include:
Brevital Sodium Vials 1248
Methoxyflurane (Additive effects).
No products indexed under this heading.
Midazolam Hydrochloride (Additive effects). Products include:
Versed Injection 1924
Molindone Hydrochloride (Additive effects). Products include:
Moban Tablets & Concentrate 932
Morphine Sulfate (Additive effects). Products include:
Astramorph/PF Injection, USP (Preservative-Free) 618
Duramorph 960
Infumorph 200 and Infumorph 500 Sterile Solutions 962
MS Contin Tablets 1814
MSIR 1817
Oramorph SR (Morphine Sulfate Sustained Release Tablets) 1988
Roxanol 1991
Opium Alkaloids (Additive effects). Products include:
B & O No. 15A & No. 16A Supprettes 2395
Pantopon Injectable 1911
Oxazepam (Additive effects). Products include:
Serax Capsules 2522
Serax Tablets 2522
Oxycodone Hydrochloride (Additive effects). Products include:
Percocet Tablets 950
Percodan 951
Roxicodone Tablets, Oral Solution & Intensol (Oxycodone) 1992
Tylox Capsules 1382
Pentobarbital Sodium (Additive effects). Products include:
Nembutal Sodium Capsules 534
Nembutal Sodium Solution 536
Nembutal Sodium Suppositories 538
Perphenazine (Additive effects). Products include:
Etrafon 2087
Triavil Tablets 1556
Trilafon 2123
Phenelzine Sulfate (Concomitant use contraindicated). Products include:
Nardil 1742
Phenobarbital (Additive effects). Products include:
Arco-Lase Plus Tablets 607
Bellergal-S Tablets 1998
Bronkolixir 761
Bronkotabs Tablets 762
Donnatal 1858
Donnatal Extentabs 1859
Donnatal Tablets 1858
Donnazyme Tablets 1860
Kinesed Tablets 2272
Phenobarbital Elixir and Tablets 1293
Primatene Tablets-P Formula 2421
Quadrinal Tablets 1183
Tedral SA 1765
Prazepam (Additive effects). Products include:
Centrax 1693
Prochlorperazine (Additive effects). Products include:
Compazine 2201
Promethazine Hydrochloride (Additive effects). Products include:
Mepergan Injection 2479
Phenergan with Codeine 2497
Phenergan with Dextromethorphan 2499
Phenergan Injection 2493
Phenergan Suppositories 2496
Phenergan Syrup 2495
Phenergan Tablets 2496
Phenergan VC 2500
Phenergan VC with Codeine 2501
Propofol (Additive effects). Products include:
Diprivan Injection 2267
Propoxyphene Hydrochloride (Additive effects). Products include:
Darvon 1256
Wygesic Tablets 2540
Propoxyphene Napsylate (Additive effects). Products include:
Darvon-N/Darvocet-N 1254
Quazepam (Additive effects). Products include:
Doral Tablets 2383
Secobarbital Sodium (Additive effects). Products include:
Seconal Sodium Pulvules 1296
Selegiline Hydrochloride (Concomitant use contraindicated). Products include:
Eldepryl 2250
Sufentanil Citrate (Additive effects). Products include:
Sufenta Injection 1147
Sulfabenzamide (Additive effects). Products include:
Sultrin 1675
Trysul Vaginal Cream 2081
Temazepam (Additive effects). Products include:
Restoril Capsules 2023
Thiamylal Sodium (Additive effects). Products include:
Surital Ampoules, Steri-Vials 1764
Thioridazine Hydrochloride (Additive effects). Products include:
Mellaril 2011
Thiothixene (Additive effects). Products include:
Navane Capsules and Concentrate 1954
Navane Intramuscular 1956
Tranylcypromine Sulfate (Concomitant use contraindicated). Products include:
Parnate Tablets 2222
Triazolam (Additive effects). Products include:
Halcion Tablets 2340
Trifluoperazine Hydrochloride (Additive effects). Products include:
Stelazine 2226

RU-TUSS WITH HYDROCODONE
(Hydrocodone Bitartrate, Phenylephrine Hydrochloride, Phenylpropanolamine Hydrochloride, Pheniramine Maleate, Pyrilamine Maleate) 694
May interact with monoamine oxidase inhibitors, hypnotics and sedatives, tranquilizers, and certain other agents. Compounds in these categories include:

Alcohol (Additive effects).
Alprazolam (Additive effects). Products include:
Xanax Tablets 2367
Buspirone Hydrochloride (Additive effects). Products include:
BuSpar 1401

Chlordiazepoxide (Additive effects). Products include:
Libritabs Tablets 1930
Limbitrol 1933
Menrium Tablets 1934

Chlordiazepoxide Hydrochloride (Additive effects). Products include:
Librax Capsules 1929
Librium Capsules 1931
Librium Injectable 1932

Chlorpromazine (Additive effects). Products include:
Thorazine 2234

Chlorprothixene (Additive effects). Products include:
Taractan Tablets 1920

Chlorprothixene Hydrochloride (Additive effects). Products include:
Taractan 1920

Clorazepate Dipotassium (Additive effects). Products include:
Tranxene 556

Diazepam (Additive effects). Products include:
Valium Injectable 1937
Valium Tablets 1939
Valrelease Capsules 1923

Droperidol (Additive effects). Products include:
Inapsine Injection 1140
Innovar Injection 1141

Estazolam (Additive effects). Products include:
ProSom Tablets 554

Ethchlorvynol (Additive effects). Products include:
Placidyl Capsules 553

Ethinamate (Additive effects).
No products indexed under this heading.

Fluphenazine Decanoate (Additive effects). Products include:
Prolixin Decanoate 1795

Fluphenazine Enanthate (Additive effects). Products include:
Prolixin Enanthate 1796

Fluphenazine Hydrochloride (Additive effects). Products include:
Prolixin Elixir 1793
Prolixin Injection 1791
Prolixin Oral Concentrate 1792
Prolixin Tablets 1793

Flurazepam Hydrochloride (Additive effects). Products include:
Dalmane Capsules 1927

Furazolidone (Concomitant use contraindicated). Products include:
Furoxone 1855

Glutethimide (Additive effects).
No products indexed under this heading.

Haloperidol (Additive effects). Products include:
Haldol Injection, Tablets and Concentrate 1373

Haloperidol Decanoate (Additive effects). Products include:
Haldol Decanoate 1375

Hydroxyzine Hydrochloride (Additive effects). Products include:
Atarax Tablets & Syrup 1941
Marax Tablets & DF Syrup 1954
Vistaril Intramuscular Solution 1970

Isocarboxazid (Concomitant use contraindicated). Products include:
Marplan Tablets 1906

Lorazepam (Additive effects). Products include:
Ativan Injection 2432
Ativan Tablets 2434

Loxapine Hydrochloride (Additive effects). Products include:
Loxitane 1213

Loxapine Succinate (Additive effects). Products include:
Loxitane Capsules 1213

Meprobamate (Additive effects). Products include:
Deprol Tablets 2382
Equagesic Tablets 2451
Miltown Tablets 2386
PMB 200 and PMB 400 2504

Mesoridazine (Additive effects). Products include:
Serentil 686

Midazolam Hydrochloride (Additive effects). Products include:
Versed Injection 1924

Molindone Hydrochloride (Additive effects). Products include:
Moban Tablets & Concentrate 932

Oxazepam (Additive effects). Products include:
Serax Capsules 2522
Serax Tablets 2522

Perphenazine (Additive effects). Products include:
Etrafon 2087
Triavil Tablets 1556
Trilafon 2123

Phenelzine Sulfate (Concomitant use contraindicated). Products include:
Nardil 1742

Prazepam (Additive effects). Products include:
Centrax 1693

Prochlorperazine (Additive effects). Products include:
Compazine 2201

Promethazine Hydrochloride (Additive effects). Products include:
Mepergan Injection 2479
Phenergan with Codeine 2497
Phenergan with Dextromethorphan 2499
Phenergan Injection 2493
Phenergan Suppositories 2496
Phenergan Syrup 2495
Phenergan Tablets 2496
Phenergan VC 2500
Phenergan VC with Codeine 2501

Propofol (Additive effects). Products include:
Diprivan Injection 2267

Quazepam (Additive effects). Products include:
Doral Tablets 2383

Secobarbital Sodium (Additive effects). Products include:
Seconal Sodium Pulvules 1296

Selegiline Hydrochloride (Concomitant use contraindicated). Products include:
Eldepryl 2250

Temazepam (Additive effects). Products include:
Restoril Capsules 2023

Thioridazine Hydrochloride (Additive effects). Products include:
Mellaril 2011

Thiothixene (Additive effects). Products include:
Navane Capsules and Concentrate 1954
Navane Intramuscular 1956

Tranylcypromine Sulfate (Concomitant use contraindicated). Products include:
Parnate Tablets 2222

Triazolam (Additive effects). Products include:
Halcion Tablets 2340

Trifluoperazine Hydrochloride (Additive effects). Products include:
Stelazine 2226

RU-TUSS TABLETS
(Phenylephrine Hydrochloride, Phenylpropanolamine Hydrochloride, Chlorpheniramine Maleate, Belladonna Alkaloids) 693
May interact with monoamine oxidase inhibitors, hypnotics and sedatives, tranquilizers, and certain other agents. Compounds in these categories include:

Alcohol (Additive effects).

Alprazolam (Additive effects). Products include:
Xanax Tablets 2367

Buspirone Hydrochloride (Additive effects). Products include:
BuSpar 1401

Chlordiazepoxide (Additive effects). Products include:
Libritabs Tablets 1930
Limbitrol 1933
Menrium Tablets 1934

Chlordiazepoxide Hydrochloride (Additive effects). Products include:
Librax Capsules 1929
Librium Capsules 1931
Librium Injectable 1932

Chlorpromazine (Additive effects). Products include:
Thorazine 2234

Clorazepate Dipotassium (Additive effects). Products include:
Tranxene 556

Diazepam (Additive effects). Products include:
Valium Injectable 1937
Valium Tablets 1939
Valrelease Capsules 1923

Droperidol (Additive effects). Products include:
Inapsine Injection 1140
Innovar Injection 1141

Estazolam (Additive effects). Products include:
ProSom Tablets 554

Ethchlorvynol (Additive effects). Products include:
Placidyl Capsules 553

Ethinamate (Additive effects).
No products indexed under this heading.

Fluphenazine Decanoate (Additive effects). Products include:
Prolixin Decanoate 1795

Fluphenazine Enanthate (Additive effects). Products include:
Prolixin Enanthate 1796

Fluphenazine Hydrochloride (Additive effects). Products include:
Prolixin Elixir 1793
Prolixin Injection 1791
Prolixin Oral Concentrate 1792
Prolixin Tablets 1793

Flurazepam Hydrochloride (Additive effects). Products include:
Dalmane Capsules 1927

Furazolidone (Concomitant use contraindicated). Products include:
Furoxone 1855

Glutethimide (Additive effects).
No products indexed under this heading.

Haloperidol (Additive effects). Products include:
Haldol Injection, Tablets and Concentrate 1373

Haloperidol Decanoate (Additive effects). Products include:
Haldol Decanoate 1375

Hydroxyzine Hydrochloride (Additive effects). Products include:
Atarax Tablets & Syrup 1941
Marax Tablets & DF Syrup 1954
Vistaril Intramuscular Solution 1970

Isocarboxazid (Concomitant use contraindicated). Products include:
Marplan Tablets 1906

Lorazepam (Additive effects). Products include:
Ativan Injection 2432
Ativan Tablets 2434

Loxapine Hydrochloride (Additive effects). Products include:
Loxitane 1213

Loxapine Succinate (Additive effects). Products include:
Loxitane Capsules 1213

Meprobamate (Additive effects). Products include:
Deprol Tablets 2382
Equagesic Tablets 2451
Miltown Tablets 2386
PMB 200 and PMB 400 2504

Mesoridazine (Additive effects). Products include:
Serentil 686

Midazolam Hydrochloride (Additive effects). Products include:
Versed Injection 1924

Molindone Hydrochloride (Additive effects). Products include:
Moban Tablets & Concentrate 932

Oxazepam (Additive effects). Products include:
Serax Capsules 2522
Serax Tablets 2522

Perphenazine (Additive effects). Products include:
Etrafon 2087
Triavil Tablets 1556
Trilafon 2123

Phenelzine Sulfate (Concomitant use contraindicated). Products include:
Nardil 1742

Prazepam (Additive effects). Products include:
Centrax 1693

Prochlorperazine (Additive effects). Products include:
Compazine 2201

Promethazine Hydrochloride (Additive effects). Products include:
Mepergan Injection 2479
Phenergan with Codeine 2497
Phenergan with Dextromethorphan 2499
Phenergan Injection 2493
Phenergan Suppositories 2496
Phenergan Syrup 2495
Phenergan Tablets 2496
Phenergan VC 2500
Phenergan VC with Codeine 2501

Propofol (Additive effects). Products include:
Diprivan Injection 2267

Quazepam (Additive effects). Products include:
Doral Tablets 2383

Secobarbital Sodium (Additive effects). Products include:
Seconal Sodium Pulvules 1296

Selegiline Hydrochloride (Concomitant use contraindicated). Products include:
Eldepryl 2250

Temazepam (Additive effects). Products include:
Restoril Capsules 2023

Thioridazine Hydrochloride (Additive effects). Products include:
Mellaril 2011

Tranylcypromine Sulfate (Concomitant use contraindicated). Products include:
Parnate Tablets 2222

Triazolam (Additive effects). Products include:
Halcion Tablets 2340

Trifluoperazine Hydrochloride (Additive effects). Products include:
Stelazine 2226

RYNA LIQUID
(Chlorpheniramine Maleate, Pseudoephedrine Hydrochloride) ▣ 741
May interact with antidepressant drugs, antihypertensives, and certain

other agents. Compounds in these categories include:

Acebutolol Hydrochloride (Concurrent use not recommended). Products include:
- Sectral Capsules ... 2520

Alcohol (Combined use may have an additive effect).

Amitriptyline Hydrochloride (Concurrent use not recommended). Products include:
- Elavil ... 2269
- Endep Tablets ... 1927
- Etrafon ... 2087
- Limbitrol ... 1933
- Triavil Tablets ... 1556

Amoxapine (Concurrent use not recommended). Products include:
- Asendin Tablets ... 1196

Atenolol (Concurrent use not recommended). Products include:
- Tenoretic Tablets ... 1105
- Tenormin Tablets and I.V. Injection 1107

Benazepril Hydrochloride (Concurrent use not recommended). Products include:
- Lotensin Tablets ... 872

Betaxolol Hydrochloride (Concurrent use not recommended). Products include:
- Betoptic Sterile Ophthalmic Solution ... 569
- Betoptic S Sterile Ophthalmic Suspension ... 570
- Kerlone Tablets ... 2172

Bupropion Hydrochloride (Concurrent use not recommended). Products include:
- Wellbutrin Tablets ... 821

Captopril (Concurrent use not recommended). Products include:
- Capoten ... 2255
- Capozide ... 2258

Carteolol Hydrochloride (Concurrent use not recommended). Products include:
- Cartrol Tablets ... 507

Clonidine (Concurrent use not recommended). Products include:
- Catapres-TTS ... 677

Clonidine Hydrochloride (Concurrent use not recommended). Products include:
- Catapres Tablets ... 676
- Combipres Tablets ... 678

Deserpidine (Concurrent use not recommended). Products include:
- Enduronyl ... 518
- Harmonyl Tablets ... 528
- Oreticyl ... 545

Desipramine Hydrochloride (Concurrent use not recommended). Products include:
- Norpramin Tablets ... 1340

Diazoxide (Concurrent use not recommended). Products include:
- Hyperstat I.V. Injection ... 2095
- Proglycem ... 649

Doxazosin Mesylate (Concurrent use not recommended). Products include:
- Cardura Tablets ... 1941

Doxepin Hydrochloride (Concurrent use not recommended). Products include:
- Sinequan ... 1960

Enalapril Maleate (Concurrent use not recommended). Products include:
- Vaseretic Tablets ... 1559
- Vasotec Tablets ... 1564

Enalaprilat (Concurrent use not recommended). Products include:
- Vasotec I.V. ... 1562

Esmolol Hydrochloride (Concurrent use not recommended). Products include:
- Brevibloc Injection ... 942

Felodipine (Concurrent use not recommended). Products include:
- Plendil Extended-Release Tablets ... 1526

Fluoxetine Hydrochloride (Concurrent use not recommended). Products include:
- Prozac Pulvules ... 920

Fosinopril Sodium (Concurrent use not recommended). Products include:
- Monopril Tablets ... 1406

Guanabenz Acetate (Concurrent use not recommended). Products include:
- Wytensin Tablets ... 2542

Guanethidine Monosulfate (Concurrent use not recommended). Products include:
- Esimil Tablets ... 864
- Ismelin Tablets ... 869

Hydralazine Hydrochloride (Concurrent use not recommended). Products include:
- Apresazide Capsules ... 854
- Apresoline Hydrochloride Parenteral (Ampuls) ... 856
- Apresoline Hydrochloride Tablets .. 855
- Apresoline-Esidrix Tablets ... 857
- Ser-Ap-Es Tablets ... 881
- Serpasil-Apresoline Tablets ... 884

Imipramine Hydrochloride (Concurrent use not recommended). Products include:
- Tofranil Ampuls ... 1038
- Tofranil Tablets ... 1039

Imipramine Pamoate (Concurrent use not recommended). Products include:
- Tofranil-PM Capsules ... 1041

Indapamide (Concurrent use not recommended). Products include:
- Lozol Tablets ... 1843

Isocarboxazid (Concurrent use not recommended). Products include:
- Marplan Tablets ... 1906

Isradipine (Concurrent use not recommended). Products include:
- DynaCirc Capsules ... 2004

Labetalol Hydrochloride (Concurrent use not recommended). Products include:
- Normodyne Injection ... 2108
- Normodyne Tablets ... 2110
- Normozide Tablets ... 2112
- Trandate HCT Tablets ... 579
- Trandate Injection ... 577
- Trandate Tablets ... 579

Lisinopril (Concurrent use not recommended). Products include:
- Prinivil Tablets ... 1538
- Prinzide Tablets ... 1540
- Zestoretic ... 2274
- Zestril Tablets ... 2277

Maprotiline Hydrochloride (Concurrent use not recommended). Products include:
- Ludiomil Tablets ... 874

Mecamylamine Hydrochloride (Concurrent use not recommended). Products include:
- Inversine Tablets ... 1492

Methyldopa (Concurrent use not recommended). Products include:
- Aldoclor Tablets ... 1413
- Aldomet Oral ... 1415
- Aldoril Tablets ... 1418

Methyldopate Hydrochloride (Concurrent use not recommended). Products include:
- Aldomet Ester HCl Injection ... 1417

Metoprolol Tartrate (Concurrent use not recommended). Products include:
- Lopressor Ampuls ... 1032
- Lopressor HCT Tablets ... 1034
- Lopressor Tablets ... 1032

Metyrosine (Concurrent use not recommended). Products include:
- Demser Capsules ... 1460

Minoxidil (Concurrent use not recommended). Products include:
- Loniten Tablets ... 2346
- Rogaine Topical Solution ... 2357

Nadolol (Concurrent use not recommended). Products include:
- Corgard Tablets ... 701
- Corzide Tablets ... 702

Nicardipine Hydrochloride (Concurrent use not recommended). Products include:
- Cardene Capsules ... 2290

Nitroglycerin (Concurrent use not recommended). Products include:
- Deponit NTG Transdermal Delivery System ... 2143
- Minitran Transdermal Delivery System ... 1312
- Nitro-Bid Ointment ... 1339
- Nitro-Bid Capsules ... 1338
- Nitrodisc ... 2176
- Nitro-Dur (nitroglycerin) Transdermal Infusion System ... 1164
- Nitrogard Tablets ... 1004
- Nitrolingual Spray ... 1846
- Nitrostat Tablets ... 1743
- Transderm-Nitro Transdermal Therapeutic System ... 2283

Nortriptyline Hydrochloride (Concurrent use not recommended). Products include:
- Pamelor ... 2019

Penbutolol Sulfate (Concurrent use not recommended). Products include:
- Levatol ... 1832

Phenelzine Sulfate (Concurrent use not recommended). Products include:
- Nardil ... 1742

Phenoxybenzamine Hydrochloride (Concurrent use not recommended). Products include:
- Dibenzyline Capsules ... 2207

Phentolamine Mesylate (Concurrent use not recommended). Products include:
- Regitine ... 878

Pindolol (Concurrent use not recommended). Products include:
- Visken Tablets ... 2036

Prazosin Hydrochloride (Concurrent use not recommended). Products include:
- Minipress Capsules ... 1778
- Minizide Capsules ... 1779

Propranolol Hydrochloride (Concurrent use not recommended). Products include:
- Inderal ... 2459
- Inderal LA Long Acting Capsules 2461
- Inderide Tablets ... 2463
- Inderide LA Long Acting Capsules .. 2465

Protriptyline Hydrochloride (Concurrent use not recommended). Products include:
- Vivactil Tablets ... 1567

Ramipril (Concurrent use not recommended). Products include:
- Altace Capsules ... 1086

Rauwolfia Serpentina (Concurrent use not recommended). Products include:
- Raudixin Tablets ... 1803
- Rauzide Tablets ... 1804

Rescinnamine (Concurrent use not recommended).
- No products indexed under this heading.

Reserpine (Concurrent use not recommended). Products include:
- Diupres Tablets ... 1461
- Hydromox R Tablets ... 1209
- Hydropres Tablets ... 1485
- Renese-R Tablets ... 1786
- Salutensin/Salutensin-Demi ... 719
- Ser-Ap-Es Tablets ... 881
- Serpasil Tablets ... 883
- Serpasil-Apresoline Tablets ... 884
- Serpasil-Esidrix Tablets ... 886

Sodium Nitroprusside (Concurrent use not recommended). Products include:
- Nipride I.V. Infusion ... 1909

Terazosin Hydrochloride (Concurrent use not recommended). Products include:
- Hytrin Tablets ... 529

Timolol Maleate (Concurrent use not recommended). Products include:
- Blocadren Tablets ... 1429
- Timolide Tablets ... 1547
- Timoptic in Ocudose ... 1552
- Timoptic Sterile Ophthalmic Solution ... 1550

Tranylcypromine Sulfate (Concurrent use not recommended). Products include:
- Parnate Tablets ... 2222

Trazodone Hydrochloride (Concurrent use not recommended). Products include:
- Desyrel and Desyrel Dividose ... 1404

Trimethaphan Camsylate (Concurrent use not recommended). Products include:
- Arfonad Ampuls ... 1887

Trimipramine Maleate (Concurrent use not recommended). Products include:
- Surmontil Capsules ... 2524

RYNA-C LIQUID
(Chlorpheniramine Maleate, Codeine Phosphate, Pseudoephedrine Hydrochloride) ... ▣ 741
May interact with antihypertensives, antidepressant drugs, central nervous system depressants, and certain other agents. Compounds in these categories include:

Acebutolol Hydrochloride (Concurrent use not recommended). Products include:
- Sectral Capsules ... 2520

Alcohol (Concurrent use should be avoided).

Alfentanil Hydrochloride (Effect not specified). Products include:
- Alfenta Injection ... 1131

Alprazolam (Effect not specified). Products include:
- Xanax Tablets ... 2367

Amitriptyline Hydrochloride (Concurrent use not recommended). Products include:
- Elavil ... 2269
- Endep Tablets ... 1927
- Etrafon ... 2087
- Limbitrol ... 1933
- Triavil Tablets ... 1556

Amoxapine (Concurrent use not recommended). Products include:
- Asendin Tablets ... 1196

Aprobarbital (Effect not specified). Products include:
- Alurate Elixir ... 1883

Atenolol (Concurrent use not recommended). Products include:
- Tenoretic Tablets ... 1105
- Tenormin Tablets and I.V. Injection 1107

Benazepril Hydrochloride (Concurrent use not recommended). Products include:
- Lotensin Tablets ... 872

Betaxolol Hydrochloride (Concurrent use not recommended). Products include:
- Betoptic Sterile Ophthalmic Solution ... 569
- Betoptic S Sterile Ophthalmic Suspension ... 570
- Kerlone Tablets ... 2172

Buprenorphine (Effect not specified).
- No products indexed under this heading.

Bupropion Hydrochloride (Concurrent use not recommended). Products include:
Wellbutrin Tablets ... 821
Buspirone Hydrochloride (Effect not specified). Products include:
BuSpar ... 1401
Butabarbital (Effect not specified). Products include:
Pyridium Plus ... 1764
Butalbital (Effect not specified). Products include:
Esgic-Plus Tablets ... 1002
Esgic Tablets & Capsules ... 1001
Fioricet Tablets ... 2006
Fiorinal Capsules ... 2007
Fiorinal with Codeine Capsules ... 2008
Fiorinal Tablets ... 2007
Phrenilin ... 838
Sedapap Tablets 50 mg/650 mg ... 1360
Captopril (Concurrent use not recommended). Products include:
Capoten ... 2255
Capozide ... 2258
Carteolol Hydrochloride (Concurrent use not recommended). Products include:
Cartrol Tablets ... 507
Chlordiazepoxide (Effect not specified). Products include:
Libritabs Tablets ... 1930
Limbitrol ... 1933
Menrium Tablets ... 1934
Chlordiazepoxide Hydrochloride (Effect not specified). Products include:
Librax Capsules ... 1929
Librium Capsules ... 1931
Librium Injectable ... 1932
Chlorpromazine (Effect not specified). Products include:
Thorazine ... 2234
Chlorprothixene (Effect not specified). Products include:
Taractan Tablets ... 1920
Chlorprothixene Hydrochloride (Effect not specified). Products include:
Taractan ... 1920
Clonidine (Concurrent use not recommended). Products include:
Catapres-TTS ... 677
Clonidine Hydrochloride (Concurrent use not recommended). Products include:
Catapres Tablets ... 676
Combipres Tablets ... 678
Clorazepate Dipotassium (Effect not specified). Products include:
Tranxene ... 556
Codeine (Effect not specified). Products include:
Calcidrine Syrup ... 506
Codeine Polistirex (Effect not specified).
No products indexed under this heading.
Deserpidine (Concurrent use not recommended). Products include:
Enduronyl ... 518
Harmonyl Tablets ... 528
Oreticyl ... 545
Desipramine Hydrochloride (Concurrent use not recommended). Products include:
Norpramin Tablets ... 1340
Dezocine (Effect not specified).
Diazepam (Effect not specified). Products include:
Valium Injectable ... 1937
Valium Tablets ... 1939
Valrelease Capsules ... 1923
Diazoxide (Concurrent use not recommended). Products include:
Hyperstat I.V. Injection ... 2095
Proglycem ... 649
Doxazosin Mesylate (Concurrent use not recommended). Products include:
Cardura Tablets ... 1941
Doxepin Hydrochloride (Concurrent use not recommended). Products include:
Sinequan ... 1960
Droperidol (Effect not specified). Products include:
Inapsine Injection ... 1140
Innovar Injection ... 1141
Enalapril Maleate (Concurrent use not recommended). Products include:
Vaseretic Tablets ... 1559
Vasotec Tablets ... 1564
Enalaprilat (Concurrent use not recommended). Products include:
Vasotec I.V. ... 1562
Enflurane (Effect not specified). Products include:
Ethrane ... 599
Esmolol Hydrochloride (Concurrent use not recommended). Products include:
Brevibloc Injection ... 942
Estazolam (Effect not specified). Products include:
ProSom Tablets ... 554
Ethchlorvynol (Effect not specified). Products include:
Placidyl Capsules ... 553
Ethinamate (Effect not specified).
No products indexed under this heading.
Felodipine (Concurrent use not recommended). Products include:
Plendil Extended-Release Tablets ... 1526
Fentanyl (Effect not specified). Products include:
Duragesic Transdermal System ... 1133
Fentanyl Citrate (Effect not specified). Products include:
Innovar Injection ... 1141
Sublimaze Injection ... 1146
Fluoxetine Hydrochloride (Concurrent use not recommended). Products include:
Prozac Pulvules ... 920
Fluphenazine Decanoate (Effect not specified). Products include:
Prolixin Decanoate ... 1795
Fluphenazine Enanthate (Effect not specified). Products include:
Prolixin Enanthate ... 1796
Fluphenazine Hydrochloride (Effect not specified). Products include:
Prolixin Elixir ... 1793
Prolixin Injection ... 1791
Prolixin Oral Concentrate ... 1792
Prolixin Tablets ... 1793
Flurazepam Hydrochloride (Effect not specified). Products include:
Dalmane Capsules ... 1927
Fosinopril Sodium (Concurrent use not recommended). Products include:
Monopril Tablets ... 1406
Glutethimide (Effect not specified).
No products indexed under this heading.
Guanabenz Acetate (Concurrent use not recommended). Products include:
Wytensin Tablets ... 2542
Guanethidine Monosulfate (Concurrent use not recommended). Products include:
Esimil Tablets ... 864
Ismelin Tablets ... 869
Haloperidol (Effect not specified). Products include:
Haldol Injection, Tablets and Concentrate ... 1373
Haloperidol Decanoate (Effect not specified). Products include:
Haldol Decanoate ... 1375
Hydralazine Hydrochloride (Concurrent use not recommended). Products include:
Apresazide Capsules ... 854
Apresoline Hydrochloride Parenteral (Ampuls) ... 856
Apresoline Hydrochloride Tablets ... 855
Apresoline-Esidrix Tablets ... 857
Ser-Ap-Es Tablets ... 881
Serpasil-Apresoline Tablets ... 884
Hydrocodone Bitartrate (Effect not specified). Products include:
Anexsia 5/500 Tablets ... 2196
Anexsia 7.5/650 Tablets ... 2197
Azdōne Tablets ... 844
Codiclear DH Syrup ... 845
Codimal DH Syrup ... 846
Damason-P ... 1356
Hycodan Syrup, Tablets ... 927
Hycomine Compound Tablets ... 929
Hycomine Syrup ... 927
Hycotuss Expectorant Syrup ... 930
Hydrocet Capsules ... 835
Lortab ASA Tablets ... 2414
Lortab ... 2412
Ru-Tuss with Hydrocodone ... 694
Triaminic Expectorant DH ... 1995
Vicodin Tablets ... 1187
Vicodin ES Tablets ... 1189
Zydone Capsules ... 941
Hydrocodone Polistirex (Effect not specified). Products include:
Tussionex Extended-Release Suspension ... 988
Hydroxyzine Hydrochloride (Effect not specified). Products include:
Atarax Tablets & Syrup ... 1941
Marax Tablets & DF Syrup ... 1954
Vistaril Intramuscular Solution ... 1970
Imipramine Hydrochloride (Concurrent use not recommended). Products include:
Tofranil Ampuls ... 1038
Tofranil Tablets ... 1039
Imipramine Pamoate (Concurrent use not recommended). Products include:
Tofranil-PM Capsules ... 1041
Indapamide (Concurrent use not recommended). Products include:
Lozol Tablets ... 1843
Isocarboxazid (Concurrent use not recommended). Products include:
Marplan Tablets ... 1906
Isoflurane (Effect not specified). Products include:
Forane ... 600
Isradipine (Concurrent use not recommended). Products include:
DynaCirc Capsules ... 2004
Ketamine Hydrochloride (Effect not specified). Products include:
Ketalar ... 1726
Labetalol Hydrochloride (Concurrent use not recommended). Products include:
Normodyne Injection ... 2108
Normodyne Tablets ... 2110
Normozide Tablets ... 2112
Trandate HCT Tablets ... 579
Trandate Injection ... 577
Trandate Tablets ... 579
Levorphanol Tartrate (Effect not specified). Products include:
Levo-Dromoran ... 1906
Lisinopril (Concurrent use not recommended). Products include:
Prinivil Tablets ... 1538
Prinzide Tablets ... 1540
Zestoretic ... 2274
Zestril Tablets ... 2277
Lorazepam (Effect not specified). Products include:
Ativan Injection ... 2432
Ativan Tablets ... 2434
Loxapine Hydrochloride (Effect not specified). Products include:
Loxitane ... 1213
Loxapine Succinate (Effect not specified). Products include:
Loxitane Capsules ... 1213
Maprotiline Hydrochloride (Concurrent use not recommended). Products include:
Ludiomil Tablets ... 874
Mecamylamine Hydrochloride (Concurrent use not recommended). Products include:
Inversine Tablets ... 1492
Meperidine Hydrochloride (Effect not specified). Products include:
Demerol ... 2047
Mepergan Injection ... 2479
Mephobarbital (Effect not specified). Products include:
Mebaral Tablets ... 2061
Meprobamate (Effect not specified). Products include:
Deprol Tablets ... 2382
Equagesic Tablets ... 2451
Miltown Tablets ... 2386
PMB 200 and PMB 400 ... 2504
Mesoridazine (Effect not specified). Products include:
Serentil ... 686
Methadone Hydrochloride (Effect not specified). Products include:
Dolophine Hydrochloride Ampoules & Vials ... 1260
Dolophine Hydrochloride Tablets ... 1261
Methadone Hydrochloride Diskets ... 1284
Methadone Hydrochloride Oral Solution & Tablets ... 1987
Methohexital Sodium (Effect not specified). Products include:
Brevital Sodium Vials ... 1248
Methoxyflurane (Effect not specified).
No products indexed under this heading.
Methyldopa (Concurrent use not recommended). Products include:
Aldoclor Tablets ... 1413
Aldomet Oral ... 1415
Aldoril Tablets ... 1418
Methyldopate Hydrochloride (Concurrent use not recommended). Products include:
Aldomet Ester HCl Injection ... 1417
Metoprolol Tartrate (Concurrent use not recommended). Products include:
Lopressor Ampuls ... 1032
Lopressor HCT Tablets ... 1034
Lopressor Tablets ... 1032
Metyrosine (Concurrent use not recommended). Products include:
Demser Capsules ... 1460
Midazolam Hydrochloride (Effect not specified). Products include:
Versed Injection ... 1924
Minoxidil (Concurrent use not recommended). Products include:
Loniten Tablets ... 2346
Rogaine Topical Solution ... 2357
Molindone Hydrochloride (Effect not specified). Products include:
Moban Tablets & Concentrate ... 932
Morphine Sulfate (Effect not specified). Products include:
Astramorph/PF Injection, USP (Preservative-Free) ... 618
Duramorph ... 960
Infumorph 200 and Infumorph 500 Sterile Solutions ... 962
MS Contin Tablets ... 1814
MSIR ... 1817
Oramorph SR (Morphine Sulfate Sustained Release Tablets) ... 1988
Roxanol ... 1991
Nadolol (Concurrent use not recommended). Products include:
Corgard Tablets ... 701
Corzide Tablets ... 702

Nicardipine Hydrochloride (Concurrent use not recommended). Products include:
- Cardene Capsules 2290

Nitroglycerin (Concurrent use not recommended). Products include:
- Deponit NTG Transdermal Delivery System 2143
- Minitran Transdermal Delivery System 1312
- Nitro-Bid Ointment 1339
- Nitro-Bid Capsules 1338
- Nitrodisc 2176
- Nitro-Dur (nitroglycerin) Transdermal Infusion System 1164
- Nitrogard Tablets 1004
- Nitrolingual Spray 1846
- Nitrostat Tablets 1743
- Transderm-Nitro Transdermal Therapeutic System 2283

Nortriptyline Hydrochloride (Concurrent use not recommended). Products include:
- Pamelor 2019

Opium Alkaloids (Effect not specified). Products include:
- B & O No. 15A & No. 16A Supprettes 2395
- Pantopon Injectable 1911

Oxazepam (Effect not specified). Products include:
- Serax Capsules 2522
- Serax Tablets 2522

Oxycodone Hydrochloride (Effect not specified). Products include:
- Percocet Tablets 950
- Percodan 951
- Roxicodone Tablets, Oral Solution & Intensol (Oxycodone) 1992
- Tylox Capsules 1382

Penbutolol Sulfate (Concurrent use not recommended). Products include:
- Levatol 1832

Pentobarbital Sodium (Effect not specified). Products include:
- Nembutal Sodium Capsules 534
- Nembutal Sodium Solution 536
- Nembutal Sodium Suppositories 538

Perphenazine (Effect not specified). Products include:
- Etrafon 2087
- Triavil Tablets 1556
- Trilafon 2123

Phenelzine Sulfate (Concurrent use not recommended). Products include:
- Nardil 1742

Phenobarbital (Effect not specified). Products include:
- Arco-Lase Plus Tablets 607
- Bellergal-S Tablets 1998
- Bronkolixir .... ◘ 761
- Bronkotabs Tablets .... ◘ 762
- Donnatal 1858
- Donnatal Extentabs 1859
- Donnatal Tablets 1858
- Donnazyme Tablets 1860
- Kinesed Tablets 2272
- Phenobarbital Elixir and Tablets 1293
- Primatene Tablets-P Formula 2421
- Quadrinal Tablets 1183
- Tedral SA 1765

Phenoxybenzamine Hydrochloride (Concurrent use not recommended). Products include:
- Dibenzyline Capsules 2207

Phentolamine Mesylate (Concurrent use not recommended). Products include:
- Regitine 878

Pindolol (Concurrent use not recommended). Products include:
- Visken Tablets 2036

Prazepam (Effect not specified). Products include:
- Centrax 1693

Prazosin Hydrochloride (Concurrent use not recommended). Products include:
- Minipress Capsules 1778
- Minizide Capsules 1779

Prochlorperazine (Effect not specified). Products include:
- Compazine 2201

Promethazine Hydrochloride (Effect not specified). Products include:
- Mepergan Injection 2479
- Phenergan with Codeine 2497
- Phenergan with Dextromethorphan 2499
- Phenergan Injection 2493
- Phenergan Suppositories 2496
- Phenergan Syrup 2495
- Phenergan Tablets 2496
- Phenergan VC 2500
- Phenergan VC with Codeine 2501

Propofol (Effect not specified). Products include:
- Diprivan Injection 2267

Propoxyphene Hydrochloride (Effect not specified). Products include:
- Darvon 1256
- Wygesic Tablets 2540

Propoxyphene Napsylate (Effect not specified). Products include:
- Darvon-N/Darvocet-N 1254

Propranolol Hydrochloride (Concurrent use not recommended). Products include:
- Inderal 2459
- Inderal LA Long Acting Capsules 2461
- Inderide Tablets 2463
- Inderide LA Long Acting Capsules 2465

Protriptyline Hydrochloride (Concurrent use not recommended). Products include:
- Vivactil Tablets 1567

Quazepam (Effect not specified). Products include:
- Doral Tablets 2383

Ramipril (Concurrent use not recommended). Products include:
- Altace Capsules 1086

Rauwolfia Serpentina (Concurrent use not recommended). Products include:
- Raudixin Tablets 1803
- Rauzide Tablets 1804

Rescinnamine (Concurrent use not recommended).
- No products indexed under this heading.

Reserpine (Concurrent use not recommended). Products include:
- Diupres Tablets 1461
- Hydromox R Tablets 1209
- Hydropres Tablets 1485
- Renese-R Tablets 1786
- Salutensin/Salutensin-Demi 719
- Ser-Ap-Es Tablets 881
- Serpasil Tablets 883
- Serpasil-Apresoline Tablets 884
- Serpasil-Esidrix Tablets 886

Secobarbital Sodium (Effect not specified). Products include:
- Seconal Sodium Pulvules 1296

Sodium Nitroprusside (Concurrent use not recommended). Products include:
- Nipride I.V. Infusion 1909

Sufentanil Citrate (Effect not specified). Products include:
- Sufenta Injection 1147

Temazepam (Effect not specified). Products include:
- Restoril Capsules 2023

Terazosin Hydrochloride (Concurrent use not recommended). Products include:
- Hytrin Tablets 529

Thiamylal Sodium (Effect not specified). Products include:
- Surital Ampoules, Steri-Vials 1764

Thioridazine Hydrochloride (Effect not specified). Products include:
- Mellaril 2011

Thiothixene (Effect not specified). Products include:
- Navane Capsules and Concentrate 1954
- Navane Intramuscular 1956

Timolol Maleate (Concurrent use not recommended). Products include:
- Blocadren Tablets 1429
- Timolide Tablets 1547
- Timoptic in Ocudose 1552
- Timoptic Sterile Ophthalmic Solution 1550

Tranylcypromine Sulfate (Concurrent use not recommended). Products include:
- Parnate Tablets 2222

Trazodone Hydrochloride (Concurrent use not recommended). Products include:
- Desyrel and Desyrel Dividose 1404

Triazolam (Effect not specified). Products include:
- Halcion Tablets 2340

Trifluoperazine Hydrochloride (Effect not specified). Products include:
- Stelazine 2226

Trimethaphan Camsylate (Concurrent use not recommended). Products include:
- Arfonad Ampuls 1887

Trimipramine Maleate (Concurrent use not recommended). Products include:
- Surmontil Capsules 2524

RYNA-CX LIQUID
(Codeine Phosphate, Guaifenesin, Pseudoephedrine Hydrochloride) .... ◘ 741
- See **Ryna-C Liquid**

RYNATAN TABLETS
(Chlorpheniramine Tannate, Pyrilamine Tannate) 2387
- See **Rynatan-S Pediatric Suspension**

RYNATAN-S PEDIATRIC SUSPENSION
(Phenylephrine Tannate, Chlorpheniramine Tannate, Pyrilamine Tannate) 2387

May interact with monoamine oxidase inhibitors, central nervous system depressants, and certain other agents. Compounds in these categories include:

Alcohol (Additive CNS effects).

Alfentanil Hydrochloride (Additive CNS effects). Products include:
- Alfenta Injection 1131

Alprazolam (Additive CNS effects). Products include:
- Xanax Tablets 2367

Aprobarbital (Additive CNS effects). Products include:
- Alurate Elixir 1883

Buprenorphine (Additive CNS effects).
- No products indexed under this heading.

Buspirone Hydrochloride (Additive CNS effects). Products include:
- BuSpar 1401

Butabarbital (Additive CNS effects). Products include:
- Pyridium Plus 1764

Butalbital (Additive CNS effects). Products include:
- Esgic-Plus Tablets 1002
- Esgic Tablets & Capsules 1001
- Fioricet Tablets 2006
- Fiorinal Capsules 2007
- Fiorinal with Codeine Capsules 2008
- Fiorinal Tablets 2007
- Phrenilin 838
- Sedapap Tablets 50 mg/650 mg 1360

Chlordiazepoxide (Additive CNS effects). Products include:
- Libritabs Tablets 1930
- Limbitrol 1933
- Menrium Tablets 1934

Chlordiazepoxide Hydrochloride (Additive CNS effects). Products include:
- Librax Capsules 1929
- Librium Capsules 1931
- Librium Injectable 1932

Chlorpromazine (Additive CNS effects). Products include:
- Thorazine 2234

Chlorprothixene (Additive CNS effects). Products include:
- Taractan Tablets 1920

Chlorprothixene Hydrochloride (Additive CNS effects). Products include:
- Taractan 1920

Clorazepate Dipotassium (Additive CNS effects). Products include:
- Tranxene 556

Codeine (Additive CNS effects). Products include:
- Calcidrine Syrup 506

Codeine Phosphate (Additive CNS effects). Products include:
- Actifed with Codeine Cough Syrup 752
- Cheracol Cough Syrup 1853
- Codimal PH Syrup 846
- Dimetane-DC Cough Syrup 1857
- Empirin with Codeine Phosphate Nos. 2, 3 & 4 764
- Fiorinal with Codeine Capsules 2008
- Isoclor Expectorant 982
- Naldecon CX Adult Liquid .... ◘ 521
- Novahistine DH 1342
- Novahistine Expectorant 1343
- Nucofed Capsules 2219
- Nucofed Expectorant 2219
- Nucofed Pediatric Expectorant 2220
- Nucofed Syrup 2219
- Phenaphen with Codeine Capsules 1865
- Phenaphen-650 with Codeine Tablets 1866
- Phenergan with Codeine 2497
- Phenergan VC with Codeine 2501
- Robitussin A-C Syrup 1875
- Robitussin-DAC Syrup 1875
- Ryna .... ◘ 741
- Soma Compound w/Codeine Tablets 2390
- Triaminic Expectorant w/Codeine 1996
- Tussi-Organidin Liquid 2391
- Tylenol with Codeine 1381

Codeine Polistirex (Additive CNS effects).
- No products indexed under this heading.

Dezocine (Additive CNS effects).

Diazepam (Additive CNS effects). Products include:
- Valium Injectable 1937
- Valium Tablets 1939
- Valrelease Capsules 1923

Droperidol (Additive CNS effects). Products include:
- Inapsine Injection 1140
- Innovar Injection 1141

Enflurane (Additive CNS effects). Products include:
- Ethrane 599

Estazolam (Additive CNS effects). Products include:
- ProSom Tablets 554

Ethchlorvynol (Additive CNS effects). Products include:
- Placidyl Capsules 553

Ethinamate (Additive CNS effects).
- No products indexed under this heading.

Fentanyl (Additive CNS effects). Products include:
- Duragesic Transdermal System 1133

Fentanyl Citrate (Additive CNS effects). Products include:
- Innovar Injection 1141
- Sublimaze Injection 1146

Fluphenazine Decanoate (Additive CNS effects). Products include:
- Prolixin Decanoate 1795

Fluphenazine Enanthate (Additive CNS effects). Products include:
- Prolixin Enanthate 1796

Fluphenazine Hydrochloride (Additive CNS effects). Products include:
- Prolixin Elixir ... 1793
- Prolixin Injection ... 1791
- Prolixin Oral Concentrate ... 1792
- Prolixin Tablets ... 1793

Flurazepam Hydrochloride (Additive CNS effects). Products include:
- Dalmane Capsules ... 1927

Furazolidone (Prolongs and intensifies anticholinergic effects of antihistamines and overall effects of sympathomimetics; use with caution or avoid concurrent use). Products include:
- Furoxone ... 1855

Glutethimide (Additive CNS effects).
- No products indexed under this heading.

Haloperidol (Additive CNS effects). Products include:
- Haldol Injection, Tablets and Concentrate ... 1373

Haloperidol Decanoate (Additive CNS effects). Products include:
- Haldol Decanoate ... 1375

Hydrocodone Bitartrate (Additive CNS effects). Products include:
- Anexsia 5/500 Tablets ... 2196
- Anexsia 7.5/650 Tablets ... 2197
- Azdōne Tablets ... 844
- Codiclear DH Syrup ... 845
- Codimal DH Syrup ... 846
- Damason-P ... 1356
- Hycodan Syrup, Tablets ... 927
- Hycomine Compound Tablets ... 929
- Hycomine Syrup ... 927
- Hycotuss Expectorant Syrup ... 930
- Hydrocet Capsules ... 835
- Lortab ASA Tablets ... 2414
- Lortab ... 2412
- Ru-Tuss with Hydrocodone ... 694
- Triaminic Expectorant DH ... 1995
- Vicodin Tablets ... 1187
- Vicodin ES Tablets ... 1189
- Zydone Capsules ... 941

Hydrocodone Polistirex (Additive CNS effects). Products include:
- Tussionex Extended-Release Suspension ... 988

Hydroxyzine Hydrochloride (Additive CNS effects). Products include:
- Atarax Tablets & Syrup ... 1941
- Marax Tablets & DF Syrup ... 1954
- Vistaril Intramuscular Solution ... 1970

Isocarboxazid (Prolongs and intensifies anticholinergic effects of antihistamines and overall effects of sympathomimetics; use with caution or avoid concurrent use). Products include:
- Marplan Tablets ... 1906

Isoflurane (Additive CNS effects). Products include:
- Forane ... 600

Ketamine Hydrochloride (Additive CNS effects). Products include:
- Ketalar ... 1726

Levorphanol Tartrate (Additive CNS effects). Products include:
- Levo-Dromoran ... 1906

Lorazepam (Additive CNS effects). Products include:
- Ativan Injection ... 2432
- Ativan Tablets ... 2434

Loxapine Hydrochloride (Additive CNS effects). Products include:
- Loxitane ... 1213

Loxapine Succinate (Additive CNS effects). Products include:
- Loxitane Capsules ... 1213

Meperidine Hydrochloride (Additive CNS effects). Products include:
- Demerol ... 2047
- Mepergan Injection ... 2479

Mephobarbital (Additive CNS effects). Products include:
- Mebaral Tablets ... 2061

Meprobamate (Additive CNS effects). Products include:
- Deprol Tablets ... 2382
- Equagesic Tablets ... 2451
- Miltown Tablets ... 2386
- PMB 200 and PMB 400 ... 2504

Mesoridazine (Additive CNS effects). Products include:
- Serentil ... 686

Methadone Hydrochloride (Additive CNS effects). Products include:
- Dolophine Hydrochloride Ampoules & Vials ... 1260
- Dolophine Hydrochloride Tablets ... 1261
- Methadone Hydrochloride Diskets ... 1284
- Methadone Hydrochloride Oral Solution & Tablets ... 1987

Methohexital Sodium (Additive CNS effects). Products include:
- Brevital Sodium Vials ... 1248

Methoxyflurane (Additive CNS effects).
- No products indexed under this heading.

Midazolam Hydrochloride (Additive CNS effects). Products include:
- Versed Injection ... 1924

Molindone Hydrochloride (Additive CNS effects). Products include:
- Moban Tablets & Concentrate ... 932

Morphine Sulfate (Additive CNS effects). Products include:
- Astramorph/PF Injection, USP (Preservative-Free) ... 618
- Duramorph ... 960
- Infumorph 200 and Infumorph 500 Sterile Solutions ... 962
- MS Contin Tablets ... 1814
- MSIR ... 1817
- Oramorph SR (Morphine Sulfate Sustained Release Tablets) ... 1988
- Roxanol ... 1991

Opium Alkaloids (Additive CNS effects). Products include:
- B & O No. 15A & No. 16A Supprettes ... 2395
- Pantopon Injectable ... 1911

Oxazepam (Additive CNS effects). Products include:
- Serax Capsules ... 2522
- Serax Tablets ... 2522

Oxycodone Hydrochloride (Additive CNS effects). Products include:
- Percocet Tablets ... 950
- Percodan ... 951
- Roxicodone Tablets, Oral Solution & Intensol (Oxycodone) ... 1992
- Tylox Capsules ... 1382

Pentobarbital Sodium (Additive CNS effects). Products include:
- Nembutal Sodium Capsules ... 534
- Nembutal Sodium Solution ... 536
- Nembutal Sodium Suppositories ... 538

Perphenazine (Additive CNS effects). Products include:
- Etrafon ... 2087
- Triavil Tablets ... 1556
- Trilafon ... 2123

Phenelzine Sulfate (Prolongs and intensifies anticholinergic effects of antihistamines and overall effects of sympathomimetics; use with caution or avoid concurrent use). Products include:
- Nardil ... 1742

Phenobarbital (Additive CNS effects). Products include:
- Arco-Lase Plus Tablets ... 607
- Bellergal-S Tablets ... 1998
- Bronkolixir ... ◙ 761
- Bronkotabs Tablets ... ◙ 762
- Donnatal ... 1858
- Donnatal Extentabs ... 1859
- Donnatal Tablets ... 1858
- Donnazyme Tablets ... 1860
- Kinesed Tablets ... 2272
- Phenobarbital Elixir and Tablets ... 1293
- Primatene Tablets-P Formula ... 2421
- Quadrinal Tablets ... 1183
- Tedral SA ... 1765

Prazepam (Additive CNS effects). Products include:
- Centrax ... 1693

Prochlorperazine (Additive CNS effects). Products include:
- Compazine ... 2201

Promethazine Hydrochloride (Additive CNS effects). Products include:
- Mepergan Injection ... 2479
- Phenergan with Codeine ... 2497
- Phenergan with Dextromethorphan ... 2499
- Phenergan Injection ... 2493
- Phenergan Suppositories ... 2496
- Phenergan Syrup ... 2495
- Phenergan Tablets ... 2496
- Phenergan VC ... 2500
- Phenergan VC with Codeine ... 2501

Propofol (Additive CNS effects). Products include:
- Diprivan Injection ... 2267

Propoxyphene Hydrochloride (Additive CNS effects). Products include:
- Darvon ... 1256
- Wygesic Tablets ... 2540

Propoxyphene Napsylate (Additive CNS effects). Products include:
- Darvon-N/Darvocet-N ... 1254

Quazepam (Additive CNS effects). Products include:
- Doral Tablets ... 2383

Secobarbital Sodium (Additive CNS effects). Products include:
- Seconal Sodium Pulvules ... 1296

Selegiline Hydrochloride (Prolongs and intensifies anticholinergic effects of antihistamines and overall effects of sympathomimetics; use with caution or avoid concurrent use). Products include:
- Eldepryl ... 2250

Sufentanil Citrate (Additive CNS effects). Products include:
- Sufenta Injection ... 1147

Temazepam (Additive CNS effects). Products include:
- Restoril Capsules ... 2023

Thiamylal Sodium (Additive CNS effects). Products include:
- Surital Ampoules, Steri-Vials ... 1764

Thioridazine Hydrochloride (Additive CNS effects). Products include:
- Mellaril ... 2011

Thiothixene (Additive CNS effects). Products include:
- Navane Capsules and Concentrate ... 1954
- Navane Intramuscular ... 1956

Tranylcypromine Sulfate (Prolongs and intensifies anticholinergic effects of antihistamines and overall effects of sympathomimetics; use with caution or avoid concurrent use). Products include:
- Parnate Tablets ... 2222

Triazolam (Additive CNS effects). Products include:
- Halcion Tablets ... 2340

Trifluoperazine Hydrochloride (Additive CNS effects). Products include:
- Stelazine ... 2226

RYNATUSS PEDIATRIC SUSPENSION (Carbetapentane Tannate, Chlorpheniramine Tannate, Ephedrine Tannate, Phenylephrine Tannate) ... 2388

May interact with monoamine oxidase inhibitors and central nervous system depressants. Compounds in these categories include:

Alcohol (Additive CNS effects).

Alfentanil Hydrochloride (Additive CNS effects). Products include:
- Alfenta Injection ... 1131

Alprazolam (Additive CNS effects). Products include:
- Xanax Tablets ... 2367

Aprobarbital (Additive CNS effects). Products include:
- Alurate Elixir ... 1883

Buprenorphine (Additive CNS effects).
- No products indexed under this heading.

Buspirone Hydrochloride (Additive CNS effects). Products include:
- BuSpar ... 1401

Butabarbital (Additive CNS effects). Products include:
- Pyridium Plus ... 1764

Butalbital (Additive CNS effects). Products include:
- Esgic-Plus Tablets ... 1002
- Esgic Tablets & Capsules ... 1001
- Fioricet Tablets ... 2006
- Fiorinal Capsules ... 2007
- Fiorinal with Codeine Capsules ... 2008
- Fiorinal Tablets ... 2007
- Phrenilin ... 838
- Sedapap Tablets 50 mg/650 mg ... 1360

Chlordiazepoxide (Additive CNS effects). Products include:
- Libritabs Tablets ... 1930
- Limbitrol ... 1933
- Menrium Tablets ... 1934

Chlordiazepoxide Hydrochloride (Additive CNS effects). Products include:
- Librax Capsules ... 1929
- Librium Capsules ... 1931
- Librium Injectable ... 1932

Chlorpromazine (Additive CNS effects). Products include:
- Thorazine ... 2234

Chlorprothixene (Additive CNS effects). Products include:
- Taractan Tablets ... 1920

Chlorprothixene Hydrochloride (Additive CNS effects). Products include:
- Taractan ... 1920

Clorazepate Dipotassium (Additive CNS effects). Products include:
- Tranxene ... 556

Codeine (Additive CNS effects). Products include:
- Calcidrine Syrup ... 506

Codeine Phosphate (Additive CNS effects). Products include:
- Actifed with Codeine Cough Syrup ... 752
- Cheracol Cough Syrup ... 1853
- Codimal PH Syrup ... 846
- Dimetane-DC Cough Syrup ... 1857
- Empirin with Codeine Phosphate Nos. 2, 3 & 4 ... 764
- Fiorinal with Codeine Capsules ... 2008
- Isoclor Expectorant ... 982
- Naldecon CX Adult Liquid ... ◙ 521
- Novahistine DH ... 1342
- Novahistine Expectorant ... 1343
- Nucofed Capsules ... 2219
- Nucofed Expectorant ... 2219
- Nucofed Pediatric Expectorant ... 2220
- Nucofed Syrup ... 2219
- Phenaphen with Codeine Capsules ... 1865
- Phenaphen-650 with Codeine Tablets ... 1866
- Phenergan with Codeine ... 2497
- Phenergan VC with Codeine ... 2501
- Robitussin A-C Syrup ... 1875
- Robitussin-DAC Syrup ... 1875
- Ryna ... ◙ 741
- Soma Compound w/Codeine Tablets ... 2390
- Triaminic Expectorant w/Codeine ... 1996
- Tussi-Organidin Liquid ... 2391
- Tylenol with Codeine ... 1381

Codeine Polistirex (Additive CNS effects).
No products indexed under this heading.

Dezocine (Additive CNS effects).

Diazepam (Additive CNS effects). Products include:
Valium Injectable ... 1937
Valium Tablets ... 1939
Valrelease Capsules ... 1923

Droperidol (Additive CNS effects). Products include:
Inapsine Injection ... 1140
Innovar Injection ... 1141

Enflurane (Additive CNS effects). Products include:
Ethrane ... 599

Estazolam (Additive CNS effects). Products include:
ProSom Tablets ... 554

Ethchlorvynol (Additive CNS effects). Products include:
Placidyl Capsules ... 553

Ethinamate (Additive CNS effects).
No products indexed under this heading.

Fentanyl (Additive CNS effects). Products include:
Duragesic Transdermal System ... 1133

Fentanyl Citrate (Additive CNS effects). Products include:
Innovar Injection ... 1141
Sublimaze Injection ... 1146

Fluphenazine Decanoate (Additive CNS effects). Products include:
Prolixin Decanoate ... 1795

Fluphenazine Enanthate (Additive CNS effects). Products include:
Prolixin Enanthate ... 1796

Fluphenazine Hydrochloride (Additive CNS effects). Products include:
Prolixin Elixir ... 1793
Prolixin Injection ... 1791
Prolixin Oral Concentrate ... 1792
Prolixin Tablets ... 1793

Flurazepam Hydrochloride (Additive CNS effects). Products include:
Dalmane Capsules ... 1927

Furazolidone (MAOIs may prolong and intensify anticholinergic effects of antihistamines and overall effects of sympathomimetics). Products include:
Furoxone ... 1855

Glutethimide (Additive CNS effects).
No products indexed under this heading.

Haloperidol (Additive CNS effects). Products include:
Haldol Injection, Tablets and Concentrate ... 1373

Haloperidol Decanoate (Additive CNS effects). Products include:
Haldol Decanoate ... 1375

Hydrocodone Bitartrate (Additive CNS effects). Products include:
Anexsia 5/500 Tablets ... 2196
Anexsia 7.5/650 Tablets ... 2197
Azdōne Tablets ... 844
Codiclear DH Syrup ... 845
Codimal DH Syrup ... 846
Damason-P ... 1356
Hycodan Syrup, Tablets ... 927
Hycomine Compound Tablets ... 929
Hycomine Syrup ... 927
Hycotuss Expectorant Syrup ... 930
Hydrocet Capsules ... 835
Lortab ASA Tablets ... 2414
Lortab ... 2412
Ru-Tuss with Hydrocodone ... 694
Triaminic Expectorant DH ... 1995
Vicodin Tablets ... 1187
Vicodin ES Tablets ... 1189
Zydone Capsules ... 941

Hydrocodone Polistirex (Additive CNS effects). Products include:
Tussionex Extended-Release Suspension ... 988

Hydroxyzine Hydrochloride (Additive CNS effects). Products include:
Atarax Tablets & Syrup ... 1941
Marax Tablets & DF Syrup ... 1954
Vistaril Intramuscular Solution ... 1970

Isocarboxazid (MAOIs may prolong and intensify anticholinergic effects of antihistamines and overall effects of sympathomimetics). Products include:
Marplan Tablets ... 1906

Isoflurane (Additive CNS effects). Products include:
Forane ... 600

Ketamine Hydrochloride (Additive CNS effects). Products include:
Ketalar ... 1726

Levorphanol Tartrate (Additive CNS effects). Products include:
Levo-Dromoran ... 1906

Lorazepam (Additive CNS effects). Products include:
Ativan Injection ... 2432
Ativan Tablets ... 2434

Loxapine Hydrochloride (Additive CNS effects). Products include:
Loxitane ... 1213

Loxapine Succinate (Additive CNS effects). Products include:
Loxitane Capsules ... 1213

Meperidine Hydrochloride (Additive CNS effects). Products include:
Demerol ... 2047
Mepergan Injection ... 2479

Mephobarbital (Additive CNS effects). Products include:
Mebaral Tablets ... 2061

Meprobamate (Additive CNS effects). Products include:
Deprol Tablets ... 2382
Equagesic Tablets ... 2451
Miltown Tablets ... 2386
PMB 200 and PMB 400 ... 2504

Mesoridazine (Additive CNS effects). Products include:
Serentil ... 686

Methadone Hydrochloride (Additive CNS effects). Products include:
Dolophine Hydrochloride Ampoules & Vials ... 1260
Dolophine Hydrochloride Tablets ... 1261
Methadone Hydrochloride Diskets ... 1284
Methadone Hydrochloride Oral Solution & Tablets ... 1987

Methohexital Sodium (Additive CNS effects). Products include:
Brevital Sodium Vials ... 1248

Methoxyflurane (Additive CNS effects).
No products indexed under this heading.

Midazolam Hydrochloride (Additive CNS effects). Products include:
Versed Injection ... 1924

Molindone Hydrochloride (Additive CNS effects). Products include:
Moban Tablets & Concentrate ... 932

Morphine Sulfate (Additive CNS effects). Products include:
Astramorph/PF Injection, USP (Preservative-Free) ... 618
Duramorph ... 960
Infumorph 200 and Infumorph 500 Sterile Solutions ... 962
MS Contin Tablets ... 1814
MSIR ... 1817
Oramorph SR (Morphine Sulfate Sustained Release Tablets) ... 1988
Roxanol ... 1991

Opium Alkaloids (Additive CNS effects). Products include:
B & O No. 15A & No. 16A Supprettes ... 2395
Pantopon Injectable ... 1911

Oxazepam (Additive CNS effects). Products include:
Serax Capsules ... 2522
Serax Tablets ... 2522

Oxycodone Hydrochloride (Additive CNS effects). Products include:
Percocet Tablets ... 950
Percodan ... 951
Roxicodone Tablets, Oral Solution & Intensol (Oxycodone) ... 1992
Tylox Capsules ... 1382

Pentobarbital Sodium (Additive CNS effects). Products include:
Nembutal Sodium Capsules ... 534
Nembutal Sodium Solution ... 536
Nembutal Sodium Suppositories ... 538

Perphenazine (Additive CNS effects). Products include:
Etrafon ... 2087
Triavil Tablets ... 1556
Trilafon ... 2123

Phenelzine Sulfate (MAOIs may prolong and intensify anticholinergic effects of antihistamines and overall effects of sympathomimetics). Products include:
Nardil ... 1742

Phenobarbital (Additive CNS effects). Products include:
Arco-Lase Plus Tablets ... 607
Bellergal-S Tablets ... 1998
Bronkolixir ... ▣ 761
Bronkotabs Tablets ... ▣ 762
Donnatal ... 1858
Donnatal Extentabs ... 1859
Donnatal Tablets ... 1858
Donnazyme Tablets ... 1860
Kinesed Tablets ... 2272
Phenobarbital Elixir and Tablets ... 1293
Primatene Tablets-P Formula ... 2421
Quadrinal Tablets ... 1183
Tedral SA ... 1765

Prazepam (Additive CNS effects). Products include:
Centrax ... 1693

Prochlorperazine (Additive CNS effects). Products include:
Compazine ... 2201

Promethazine Hydrochloride (Additive CNS effects). Products include:
Mepergan Injection ... 2479
Phenergan with Codeine ... 2497
Phenergan with Dextromethorphan ... 2499
Phenergan Injection ... 2493
Phenergan Suppositories ... 2496
Phenergan Syrup ... 2495
Phenergan Tablets ... 2496
Phenergan VC ... 2500
Phenergan VC with Codeine ... 2501

Propofol (Additive CNS effects). Products include:
Diprivan Injection ... 2267

Propoxyphene Hydrochloride (Additive CNS effects). Products include:
Darvon ... 1256
Wygesic Tablets ... 2540

Propoxyphene Napsylate (Additive CNS effects). Products include:
Darvon-N/Darvocet-N ... 1254

Quazepam (Additive CNS effects). Products include:
Doral Tablets ... 2383

Secobarbital Sodium (Additive CNS effects). Products include:
Seconal Sodium Pulvules ... 1296

Selegiline Hydrochloride (MAOIs may prolong and intensify anticholinergic effects of antihistamines and overall effects of sympathomimetics). Products include:
Eldepryl ... 2250

Sufentanil Citrate (Additive CNS effects). Products include:
Sufenta Injection ... 1147

Temazepam (Additive CNS effects). Products include:
Restoril Capsules ... 2023

Thiamylal Sodium (Additive CNS effects). Products include:
Surital Ampoules, Steri-Vials ... 1764

Thioridazine Hydrochloride (Additive CNS effects). Products include:
Mellaril ... 2011

Thiothixene (Additive CNS effects). Products include:
Navane Capsules and Concentrate 1954
Navane Intramuscular ... 1956

Tranylcypromine Sulfate (MAOIs may prolong and intensify anticholinergic effects of antihistamines and overall effects of sympathomimetics). Products include:
Parnate Tablets ... 2222

Triazolam (Additive CNS effects). Products include:
Halcion Tablets ... 2340

Trifluoperazine Hydrochloride (Additive CNS effects). Products include:
Stelazine ... 2226

RYNATUSS TABLETS
(Chlorpheniramine Tannate, Carbetapentane Tannate, Phenylephrine Tannate, Ephedrine Tannate) ... 2388
See **Rynatuss Pediatric Suspension**

RYTHMOL TABLETS
(Propafenone Hydrochloride) ... 1184
May interact with beta blockers, cardiac glycosides, local anesthetics, and certain other agents. Compounds in these categories include:

Acebutolol Hydrochloride (Potential for increased plasma concentration and elimination half-life of beta blockers; dosage reduction of beta-antagonist may be necessary). Products include:
Sectral Capsules ... 2520

Atenolol (Potential for increased plasma concentration and elimination half-life of beta blockers; dosage reduction of beta-antagonist may be necessary). Products include:
Tenoretic Tablets ... 1105
Tenormin Tablets and I.V. Injection 1107

Betaxolol Hydrochloride (Potential for increased plasma concentration and elimination half-life of beta blockers; dosage reduction of beta-antagonist may be necessary). Products include:
Betoptic Sterile Ophthalmic Solution ... 569
Betoptic S Sterile Ophthalmic Suspension ... 570
Kerlone Tablets ... 2172

Bupivacaine Hydrochloride (Concomitant use of local anesthetics may increase the risk of CNS side effects). Products include:
Marcaine Hydrochloride 0.5% with Epinephrine 1:200,000 (as bitartrate) ... 958
Marcaine Hydrochloride with Epinephrine 1:200,000 ... 2055
Marcaine Hydrochloride Injection ... 2055
Marcaine Spinal ... 2058
Sensorcaine ... 631
Sensorcaine-MPF Spinal ... 634

Carteolol Hydrochloride (Potential for increased plasma concentration and elimination half-life of beta blockers; dosage reduction of beta-antagonist may be necessary). Products include:
Cartrol Tablets ... 507

(▣ Described in PDR For Nonprescription Drugs) (◉ Described in PDR For Ophthalmology)

Chloroprocaine Hydrochloride (Concomitant use of local anesthetics may increase the risk of CNS side effects). Products include:
Nescaine/Nescaine MPF ... 629

Cimetidine (Increases steady-state plasma concentrations with no detectable changes in electrocardiographic parameters). Products include:
Tagamet Tablets ... 2228

Cimetidine Hydrochloride (Increases steady-state plasma concentrations with no detectable changes in electrocardiographic parameters). Products include:
Tagamet ... 2228

Deslanoside (Potential for elevated digoxin levels; dosage reduction of digitalis may be necessary).
No products indexed under this heading.

Digitoxin (Potential for elevated digoxin levels; dosage reduction of digitalis may be necessary). Products include:
Crystodigin Tablets ... 1253

Digoxin (Potential for elevated digoxin levels; dosage reduction of digitalis may be necessary). Products include:
Lanoxicaps ... 772
Lanoxin Elixir Pediatric ... 775
Lanoxin Injection ... 778
Lanoxin Injection Pediatric ... 781
Lanoxin Tablets ... 783

Esmolol Hydrochloride (Potential for increased plasma concentration and elimination half-life of beta blockers; dosage reduction of beta-antagonist may be necessary). Products include:
Brevibloc Injection ... 942

Etidocaine Hydrochloride (Concomitant use of local anesthetics may increase the risk of CNS side effects). Products include:
Duranest Injections ... 624

Labetalol Hydrochloride (Potential for increased plasma concentration and elimination half-life of beta blockers; dosage reduction of beta-antagonist may be necessary). Products include:
Normodyne Injection ... 2108
Normodyne Tablets ... 2110
Normozide Tablets ... 2112
Trandate HCT Tablets ... 579
Trandate Injection ... 577
Trandate Tablets ... 579

Lidocaine Hydrochloride (Concomitant use of local anesthetics may increase the risk of CNS side effects). Products include:
Anestacon Solution ... 2394
Bactine Antiseptic/Anesthetic First Aid Spray ... ⊞ 624
Decadron Phosphate with Xylocaine Injection, Sterile ... 1451
Xylocaine Injections ... 637
Xylocaine Injections for Ventricular Arrhythmias ... 639
Xylocaine 2% Jelly ... 643
4% Xylocaine-MPF Sterile Solution ... 641
Xylocaine 2% Viscous Solution ... 646

Mepivacaine Hydrochloride Injection (Concomitant use of local anesthetics may increase the risk of CNS side effects). Products include:
Carbocaine Hydrochloride 3% Injection ... 956
Carbocaine Hydrochloride Injection 2043
Carbocaine Hydrochloride 2% with Neo-Cobefrin ... 956

Metoprolol Tartrate (Potential for increased plasma concentration and elimination half-life of beta blockers; dosage reduction of beta-antagonist may be necessary). Products include:
Lopressor Ampuls ... 1032
Lopressor HCT Tablets ... 1034
Lopressor Tablets ... 1032

Nadolol (Potential for increased plasma concentration and elimination half-life of beta blockers; dosage reduction of beta-antagonist may be necessary). Products include:
Corgard Tablets ... 701
Corzide Tablets ... 702

Penbutolol Sulfate (Potential for increased plasma concentration and elimination half-life of beta blockers; dosage reduction of beta-antagonist may be necessary). Products include:
Levatol ... 1832

Pindolol (Potential for increased plasma concentration and elimination half-life of beta blockers; dosage reduction of beta-antagonist may be necessary). Products include:
Visken Tablets ... 2036

Procaine Hydrochloride (Concomitant use of local anesthetics may increase the risk of CNS side effects). Products include:
Novocain Hydrochloride for Spinal Anesthesia ... 2065

Propranolol Hydrochloride (Potential for increased plasma concentration and elimination half-life of beta blockers; dosage reduction of beta-antagonist may be necessary). Products include:
Inderal ... 2459
Inderal LA Long Acting Capsules ... 2461
Inderide Tablets ... 2463
Inderide LA Long Acting Capsules .. 2465

Quinidine Gluconate (Small doses of quinidine completely inhibit the hydroxylation metabolic pathway). Products include:
Quinaglute Dura-Tabs Tablets ... 663

Quinidine Polygalacturonate (Small doses of quinidine completely inhibit the hydroxylation metabolic pathway). Products include:
Cardioquin Tablets ... 1812

Quinidine Sulfate (Small doses of quinidine completely inhibit the hydroxylation metabolic pathway). Products include:
Quinidex Extentabs ... 1868

Tetracaine Hydrochloride (Concomitant use of local anesthetics may increase the risk of CNS side effects). Products include:
Cetacaine Topical Anesthetic ... 850
Pontocaine Hydrochloride for Spinal Anesthesia ... 2069

Timolol Maleate (Potential for increased plasma concentration and elimination half-life of beta blockers; dosage reduction of beta-antagonist may be necessary). Products include:
Blocadren Tablets ... 1429
Timolide Tablets ... 1547
Timoptic in Ocudose ... 1552
Timoptic Sterile Ophthalmic Solution ... 1550

Warfarin Sodium (Increase in mean steady-state plasma levels of warfarin resulting in increased prothrombin time). Products include:
Coumadin Injection & Tablets ... 944
Panwarfin Tablets ... 547

Food Interactions

Food, unspecified (Increased peak blood level and bioavailability in a single dose study).

SMA IRON FORTIFIED INFANT FORMULA, CONCENTRATED, READY-TO-FEED & POWDER
(Nutritional Supplement) ... 2523
No interactions described in labeling.

SMA LO-IRON INFANT FORMULA, CONCENTRATED, READY-TO-FEED & POWDER
(Nutritional Supplement) ... 2523
No interactions described in labeling.

S-P-T "LIQUID" CAPSULES
(Thyroid) ... 995
May interact with anorexiants. Compounds in this category include:

Amphetamine Resins (Potential for serious toxicity when S-P-T is used in larger dose with anorexiants). Products include:
Biphetamine Capsules ... 973

Benzphetamine Hydrochloride (Potential for serious toxicity when S-P-T is used in larger dose with anorexiants). Products include:
Didrex Tablets ... 2338

Dextroamphetamine Sulfate (Potential for serious toxicity when S-P-T is used in larger dose with anorexiants). Products include:
Dexedrine ... 2206

Diethylpropion Hydrochloride (Potential for serious toxicity when S-P-T is used in larger dose with anorexiants). Products include:
Tenuate ... 1354

Fenfluramine Hydrochloride (Potential for serious toxicity when S-P-T is used in larger dose with anorexiants). Products include:
Pondimin Tablets ... 1867

Mazindol (Potential for serious toxicity when S-P-T is used in larger dose with anorexiants). Products include:
Sanorex Tablets ... 2030

Methamphetamine Hydrochloride (Potential for serious toxicity when S-P-T is used in larger dose with anorexiants). Products include:
Desoxyn Gradumet Tablets ... 514

Phendimetrazine Tartrate (Potential for serious toxicity when S-P-T is used in larger dose with anorexiants). Products include:
Bontril Slow-Release ... 834
Plegine Tablets ... 2504
Prelu-2 Capsules ... 683

Phenmetrazine Hydrochloride (Potential for serious toxicity when S-P-T is used in larger dose with anorexiants).
No products indexed under this heading.

SSD CREAM
(Silver Sulfadiazine) ... 694
May interact with:

Cimetidine (Higher incidence of leukopenia). Products include:
Tagamet Tablets ... 2228

Cimetidine Hydrochloride (Higher incidence of leukopenia). Products include:
Tagamet ... 2228

SSD AF CREAM
(Silver Sulfadiazine) ... 694
See **SSD Cream**

SSD RP CREAM
(Silver Sulfadiazine) ... 690
May interact with:

Cimetidine (Higher incidence of leukopenia in patients treated concurrently with cimetidine). Products include:
Tagamet Tablets ... 2228

S.T.37 ANTISEPTIC SOLUTION
(Hexylresorcinol) ... ⊞ 618
No interactions described in labeling.

SAAVE
(Amino Acid Preparations) ... 1358
May interact with monoamine oxidase inhibitors. Compounds in this category include:

Furazolidone (Concurrent use is contraindicated). Products include:
Furoxone ... 1855

Isocarboxazid (Concurrent use is contraindicated). Products include:
Marplan Tablets ... 1906

Phenelzine Sulfate (Concurrent use is contraindicated). Products include:
Nardil ... 1742

Selegiline Hydrochloride (Concurrent use is contraindicated). Products include:
Eldepryl ... 2250

Tranylcypromine Sulfate (Concurrent use is contraindicated). Products include:
Parnate Tablets ... 2222

SAL-ACID PLASTERS
(Salicylic Acid) ... 1771
No interactions described in labeling.

SALAC
(Salicylic Acid) ... 1045
No interactions described in labeling.

SALACTIC FILM
(Salicylic Acid) ... 1771
No interactions described in labeling.

SALFLEX
(Salsalate) ... 839
May interact with antigout agents, salicylates, urinary alkalizing agents, oral anticoagulants, oral hypoglycemic agents, penicillins, corticosteroids, and certain other agents. Compounds in these categories include:

Allopurinol (Uricosuric action antagonized). Products include:
Zyloprim Tablets ... 830

Amoxicillin (Competition for protein binding site). Products include:
Amoxil ... 2193
Augmentin Tablets, Powder for Oral Suspension, and Chewable Tablets ... 2198

Ampicillin Sodium (Competition for protein binding site). Products include:
Unasyn ... 1965

Aspirin (Potential for additive effect and toxicity). Products include:
Alka-Seltzer Effervescent Antacid and Pain Reliever ... 1568
Alka-Seltzer Extra Strength Effervescent Antacid and Pain Reliever ... 1570
Alka-Seltzer (Flavored) Effervescent Antacid and Pain Reliever 1569
Alka-Seltzer Plus Cold Medicine .... ⊞ 623
Alka-Seltzer Plus Night-Time Cold Medicine ... ⊞ 623
Alka Seltzer Plus Sinus Allergy Medicine ... ⊞ 624
Anacin Coated Analgesic Caplets 2417
Anacin Coated Analgesic Tablets 2417
Anacin Maximum Strength Analgesic Coated Tablets ... 2417

Maximum Strength Arthritis Pain Formula By the Makers of Anacin Analgesic Tablets and Caplets 2418
Arthritis Pain Formula by the Makers of Anacin Analgesic Tablets and Caplets .... ▣ 747
Arthritis Strength BC Powder .... ▣ 516
Ascriptin A/D Caplets 1850
Regular Strength Ascriptin Tablets 1850
Azdōne Tablets 844
BC Powder .... ▣ 517
BC Cold Powder .... ▣ 517
Children's Bayer Chewable Aspirin .... ▣ 564
Genuine Bayer Aspirin Tablets & Caplets .... ▣ 564
Maximum Bayer Aspirin Tablets & Caplets .... ▣ 566
Bayer Plus Aspirin Tablets .... ▣ 567
Therapy Bayer Aspirin Caplets ...... ▣ 568
8 Hour Bayer Timed-Release Aspirin .... ▣ 566
Arthritis Strength Bufferin Analgesic Caplets 744
Extra Strength Bufferin Analgesic Tablets 745
Bufferin Analgesic Tablets and Caplets 743
Cama Arthritis Pain Reliever .... ▣ 685
Damason-P 1356
Easprin 1719
Ecotrin Enteric Coated Aspirin Maximum Strength Tablets and Caplets 2189
Ecotrin Enteric Coated Aspirin Regular Strength Tablets and Caplets 2189
Empirin Aspirin .... ▣ 541
Empirin with Codeine Phosphate Nos. 2, 3 & 4 764
Equagesic Tablets 2451
Excedrin Extra-Strength Analgesic Tablets & Caplets 749
4-Way Cold Tablets 750
Fiorinal Capsules 2007
Fiorinal with Codeine Capsules 2008
Fiorinal Tablets 2007
Lortab ASA Tablets 2414
Momentum Muscular Backache Formula .... ▣ 751
Norgesic 1314
Norwich Extra-Strength Aspirin ...... ▣ 546
Norwich Regular Strength Aspirin ▣ 547
P-A-C Analgesic Tablets .... ▣ 669
Percodan 951
Robaxisal Tablets 1872
Sine-Off Sinus Medicine Tablets-Aspirin Formula .... ▣ 722
Soma Compound w/Codeine Tablets 2390
Soma Compound Tablets 2389
St. Joseph Adult Chewable Aspirin (81 mg.) .... ▣ 703
Synalgos-DC Capsules 2525
Talwin Compound 2072
Ursinus Inlay-Tabs .... ▣ 691
Vanquish Analgesic Caplets .... ▣ 574
Zorprin Tablets 698

Azlocillin Sodium (Competition for protein binding site).
No products indexed under this heading.

Bacampicillin Hydrochloride (Competition for protein binding site). Products include:
Spectrobid Tablets & Powder for Oral Suspension 1961

Betamethasone Acetate (Competition for protein binding sites). Products include:
Celestone Soluspan Suspension 2081

Betamethasone Sodium Phosphate (Competition for protein binding sites). Products include:
Celestone Soluspan Suspension 2081

Carbenicillin Disodium (Competition for protein binding site).

Carbenicillin Indanyl Sodium (Competition for protein binding site). Products include:
Geocillin Tablets 1951

Chlorpropamide (Hypoglycemic effect may be enhanced). Products include:
Diabinese Tablets 1775

Choline Magnesium Trisalicylate (Potential for additive effect and toxicity). Products include:
Trilisate 1822

Cortisone Acetate (Competition for protein binding sites). Products include:
Cortone Acetate Sterile Suspension 1437
Cortone Acetate Tablets 1439

Dexamethasone (Competition for protein binding sites). Products include:
AK-Trol Ointment & Suspension .... ◉ 207
Decadron Elixir 1445
Decadron Tablets 1447
Decaspray Topical Aerosol 1459
Dexacidin .... ◉ 272
Maxidex Sterile Ophthalmic Suspension .... ◉ 223
Maxitrol Ophthalmic Ointment/Suspension .... ◉ 223
TobraDex Ophthalmic Suspension and Ointment .... ◉ 228

Dexamethasone Acetate (Competition for protein binding sites). Products include:
Dalalone D.P. Injectable 999
Decadron-LA Sterile Suspension 1457

Dexamethasone Sodium Phosphate (Competition for protein binding sites). Products include:
AK-Dex .... ◉ 203
Decadron Phosphate Respihaler 1454
Decadron Phosphate Sterile Ophthalmic Ointment 1453
Decadron Phosphate Sterile Ophthalmic Solution 1453
Decadron Phosphate Topical Cream 1455
Decadron Phosphate Turbinaire 1456
Maxidex Sterile Ophthalmic Ointment .... ◉ 222
NeoDecadron Sterile Ophthalmic Ointment 1517
NeoDecadron Sterile Ophthalmic Solution 1518
NeoDecadron Topical Cream 1518

Dicumarol (Increased potential for systemic bleeding). Products include:
Dicumarol Tablets 516

Diflunisal (Potential for additive effect and toxicity). Products include:
Dolobid Tablets 1465

Glipizide (Hypoglycemic effect may be enhanced). Products include:
Glucotrol 1952

Glyburide (Hypoglycemic effect may be enhanced). Products include:
DiaBeta 1091
Micronase Tablets 2350

Hydrocortisone (Competition for protein binding sites). Products include:
AK-Spore H.C. .... ◉ 206
Bactine Hydrocortisone Anti-Itch Cream .... ▣ 625
CaldeCORT Anti-Itch Hydrocortisone Spray .... ▣ 560
Carmol HC Cream 1% 2296
Cortaid Spray .... ▣ 735
Cortenema 2244
Cortisporin Ointment 758
Cortisporin Ophthalmic Ointment Sterile 758
Cortisporin Ophthalmic Suspension Sterile 759
Cortisporin Otic Solution Sterile 760
Cortisporin Otic Suspension Sterile 760
Cortizone-5 Creme & Ointment .... ▣ 732
Dermolate Anti-Itch Cream .... ▣ 697
Eldecort Cream 1.0% 1113
Eldecort Cream 1.0% and 2.5% 1113
Fungoid HC Creme 1770
Hydrocortone Tablets 1482
Hytone 909
LazerSporin-C Solution 1770
Massengill Medicated Soft Cloth Towelettes 2192
Nutracort Cream & Lotion 1684
PediOtic Suspension Sterile 797
Synacort Creams 1%, 2.5% 2296
Vanoxide-HC Acne Lotion 911
Vioform-Hydrocortisone Cream and Mild Cream 889
Vioform-Hydrocortisone Ointment .. 889
VōSoL HC Otic Solution 2392
Vytone Cream 1% 911

Hydrocortisone Acetate (Competition for protein binding sites). Products include:
Analpram-HC Rectal Cream 1% and 2.5% 970
Anusol-HC Cream 1690
Anusol-HC Suppositories 1691
Caldecort .... ▣ 560
Carmol HC Cream 1% 2296
Chloromycetin Hydrocortisone Ophthalmic 1694
Coly-Mycin S Otic w/Neomycin & Hydrocortisone 1708
Cortaid .... ▣ 735
Cortef Feminine Itch Cream .... ▣ 735
Corticaine .... ▣ 682
Cortifoam 1827
Cortisporin Cream 757
Epifoam 1828
Gynecort 5 Creme .... ▣ 556
Hydrocortone Acetate Sterile Suspension 1479
Lanacort 5 Creme and Ointment .. ▣ 557
Mantadil Cream 789
Ophthocort .... ◉ 301
Orabase HCA Oral Paste 890
Pramosone Cream, Lotion & Ointment 971
ProctoCream-HC 1834
Proctofoam-HC 1835

Hydrocortisone Sodium Phosphate (Competition for protein binding sites). Products include:
Hydrocortone Phosphate Injection, Sterile 1481

Hydrocortisone Sodium Succinate (Competition for protein binding sites). Products include:
Solu-Cortef Sterile Powder 2361

Magnesium Salicylate (Potential for additive effect and toxicity). Products include:
Doan's - Extra-Strength Analgesic ▣ 549
Doan's - Regular Strength Analgesic .... ▣ 549
Mobigesic Analgesic Tablets .... ▣ 507

Methotrexate Sodium (Competition for protein binding site). Products include:
Methotrexate Tablets, Parenteral, LPF Parenteral 1217
Rheumatrex Methotrexate Dose Pack 1234

Methylprednisolone Acetate (Competition for protein binding sites). Products include:
Depo-Medrol Sterile Aqueous Suspension 2334

Methylprednisolone Sodium Succinate (Competition for protein binding sites). Products include:
Solu-Medrol Sterile Powder 2363

Mezlocillin Sodium (Competition for protein binding site). Products include:
Mezlin 1597
Mezlin Pharmacy Bulk Package 1599

Nafcillin Sodium (Competition for protein binding site). Products include:
Unipen 2533

Naproxen (Competition for protein binding sites). Products include:
Naprosyn 2297

Naproxen Sodium (Competition for protein binding site). Products include:
Anaprox and Anaprox DS Tablets 2288

Penicillin G Potassium (Competition for protein binding site). Products include:
Pfizerpen for Injection 1957

Penicillin G Procaine (Competition for protein binding site). Products include:
Bicillin C-R Injection 2438
Bicillin C-R 900/300 Injection 2440
Pfizerpen-AS Aqueous Suspension 1959
Wycillin Injection 2537
Wycillin Injection and Probenecid Tablets 2539

Penicillin G Sodium (Competition for protein binding site).
No products indexed under this heading.

Penicillin G, Benzathine (Competition for protein binding site). Products include:
Bicillin C-R Injection 2438
Bicillin C-R 900/300 Injection 2440
Bicillin L-A Injection 2442

Penicillin V Potassium (Competition for protein binding site).
No products indexed under this heading.

Phenytoin (Competition for protein binding site). Products include:
Dilantin Infatabs 1710
Dilantin-30 Pediatric/Dilantin-125 Suspension 1713

Phenytoin Sodium (Competition for protein binding site). Products include:
Dilantin Kapseals 1708
Dilantin Parenteral 1712
Dilantin with Phenobarbital Kapseals 1715

Potassium Citrate (Lowers plasma levels of salicylic acid). Products include:
Alka-Seltzer Effervescent Antacid .. 1570
K-Lyte 707
Polycitra Syrup 2424
Polycitra-K 2424
Polycitra-LC—Sugar-Free 2424
Ricelyte, Rice-Based Oral Electrolyte Maintenance Solution .... ▣ 613

Prednisolone Acetate (Competition for protein binding sites). Products include:
AK-Cide Sterile Ophthalmic Ointment & Suspension .... ◉ 202
Blephamide Liquifilm Sterile Ophthalmic Suspension 586
Blephamide S.O.P. Sterile Ophthalmic Ointment 586
Cetapred Ointment .... ◉ 220
⅛% Econopred & 1% Econopred Plus .... ◉ 217
Isopto Cetapred Suspension .... ◉ 220
Metimyd .... ◉ 306
Poly-Pred Liquifilm .... ◉ 250
Pred Forte .... ◉ 252
Pred Mild .... ◉ 254
Pred-G Liquifilm Sterile Ophthalmic Suspension .... ◉ 252
Pred-G S.O.P. Sterile Ophthalmic Ointment .... ◉ 253
Vasocidin Ointment .... ◉ 275

Prednisolone Sodium Phosphate (Competition for protein binding sites). Products include:
AK-Pred .... ◉ 205
Hydeltrasol Injection, Sterile 1476
Inflamase .... ◉ 274
Pediapred Oral Liquid 987
Vasocidin Ophthalmic Solution ...... ◉ 276

Prednisolone Tebutate (Competition for protein binding sites). Products include:
Hydeltra-T.B.A. Sterile Suspension 1478

Prednisone (Competition for protein binding sites). Products include:
Deltasone Tablets 2332

Probenecid (Uricosuric action antagonized). Products include:
Benemid Tablets 1426
ColBENEMID Tablets 1436
Wycillin Injection and Probenecid Tablets 2539

Sodium Citrate (Lowers plasma levels of salicylic acid). Products include:
Alka-Seltzer Effervescent Antacid .. 1570
Alka-Seltzer Extra Strength Effervescent Antacid and Pain Reliever 1570
Alka-Seltzer (Flavored) Effervescent Antacid and Pain Reliever 1569
Bicitra—Sugar-Free 2423
Citrocarbonate Antacid .... ▣ 668

(▣ Described in PDR For Nonprescription Drugs) (◉ Described in PDR For Ophthalmology)

Polycitra 2424
Ricelyte, Rice-Based Oral Electrolyte Maintenance Solution .... ▣ 613

Sulfinpyrazone (Uricosuric action antagonized). Products include:
Anturane 853

Thyroxine Sodium (Competition for protein binding site).
No products indexed under this heading.

Ticarcillin Disodium (Competition for protein binding site). Products include:
Ticar for Injection 2236
Timentin for Injection 2239

Tolazamide (Hypoglycemic effect may be enhanced). Products include:
Tolinase Tablets 2365

Tolbutamide (Hypoglycemic effect may be enhanced). Products include:
Orinase Tablets 2354

Triamcinolone (Competition for protein binding sites).
No products indexed under this heading.

Triamcinolone Acetonide (Competition for protein binding sites). Products include:
Aristocort A 1010
Azmacort Inhaler 1837
Kenalog Cream, Lotion & Ointment 2401
Kenalog-10 Injection 2402
Kenalog-40 Injection 2403
Kenalog in Orabase 604
Kenalog Spray 2401
Mycolog II Cream and Ointment 2407
Mytrex Cream & Ointment 2080
Nasacort Nasal Inhaler 1844

Triamcinolone Diacetate (Competition for protein binding sites). Products include:
Aristocort Suspension 1008

Triamcinolone Hexacetonide (Competition for protein binding sites). Products include:
Aristospan Suspension 1011

l-Triiodothyronine (Competition for protein binding site).

Warfarin Sodium (Increased potential for systemic bleeding; competition for protein binding site). Products include:
Coumadin Injection & Tablets 944
Panwarfin Tablets 547

Food Interactions

Food, unspecified (Slows the absorption).

SALINEX NASAL MIST AND DROPS
(Sodium Chloride) .... ▣ 629
No interactions described in labeling.

SAL-PLANT GEL
(Salicylic Acid) 1771
No interactions described in labeling.

SALURON
(Hydroflumethiazide) 718
May interact with ganglionic blocking agents, para-aminobenzoic acid based local anesthetics, oral anticoagulants, antigout agents, antihypertensives, preanesthetic medications, general anesthetics, nondepolarizing neuromuscular blocking agents, corticosteroids, cardiac glycosides, oral hypoglycemic agents, lithium preparations, insulin, narcotic analgesics, barbiturates, non-steroidal anti-inflammatory agents, and certain other agents. Compounds in these categories include:

Acebutolol Hydrochloride (Potentiated). Products include:
Sectral Capsules 2520

ACTH (May intensify electrolyte imbalance, particularly hypokalemia).
No products indexed under this heading.

Alfentanil Hydrochloride (May aggravate orthostatic hypotension). Products include:
Alfenta Injection 1131

Allopurinol (Increased level of blood uric acid; dosage adjustment of allopurinol may be necessary). Products include:
Zyloprim Tablets 830

Amphotericin B (May intensify electrolyte imbalance, particularly hypokalemia). Products include:
Fungizone Cream, Lotion and Ointment 2261
Fungizone Intravenous 2262

Aprobarbital (May aggravate orthostatic hypotension). Products include:
Alurate Elixir 1883

Atenolol (Potentiated). Products include:
Tenoretic Tablets 1105
Tenormin Tablets and I.V. Injection 1107

Atracurium Besylate (Potentiated). Products include:
Tracrium Injection 817

Benazepril Hydrochloride (Potentiated). Products include:
Lotensin Tablets 872

Bendroflumethiazide (Potentiated). Products include:
Corzide Tablets 702
Naturetin Tablets 1789
Rauzide Tablets 1804

Betamethasone Acetate (May intensify electrolyte imbalance, particularly hypokalemia). Products include:
Celestone Soluspan Suspension 2081

Betamethasone Sodium Phosphate (May intensify electrolyte imbalance, particularly hypokalemia). Products include:
Celestone Soluspan Suspension 2081

Betaxolol Hydrochloride (Potentiated). Products include:
Betoptic Sterile Ophthalmic Solution 569
Betoptic S Sterile Ophthalmic Suspension 570
Kerlone Tablets 2172

Buprenorphine (May aggravate orthostatic hypotension).
No products indexed under this heading.

Butabarbital (May aggravate orthostatic hypotension). Products include:
Pyridium Plus 1764

Butalbital (May aggravate orthostatic hypotension). Products include:
Esgic-Plus Tablets 1002
Esgic Tablets & Capsules 1001
Fioricet Tablets 2006
Fiorinal Capsules 2007
Fiorinal with Codeine Capsules 2008
Fiorinal Tablets 2007
Phrenilin 838
Sedapap Tablets 50 mg/650 mg .. 1360

Captopril (Potentiated). Products include:
Capoten 2255
Capozide 2258

Carteolol Hydrochloride (Potentiated). Products include:
Cartrol Tablets 507

Chlorothiazide (Potentiated). Products include:
Aldoclor Tablets 1413
Diupres Tablets 1461
Diuril Oral 1464

Chlorothiazide Sodium (Potentiated). Products include:
Diuril Sodium Intravenous 1463

Chlorpropamide (Hypoglycemic dosage requirements may be affected). Products include:
Diabinese Tablets 1775

Chlorthalidone (Potentiated). Products include:
Combipres Tablets 678
Tenoretic Tablets 1105
Thalitone Tablets 687

Clobetasol Propionate (May intensify electrolyte imbalance, particularly hypokalemia). Products include:
Temovate 1056

Clonidine (Potentiated). Products include:
Catapres-TTS 677

Clonidine Hydrochloride (Potentiated). Products include:
Catapres Tablets 676
Combipres Tablets 678

Codeine (May aggravate orthostatic hypotension). Products include:
Calcidrine Syrup 506

Codeine Phosphate (May aggravate orthostatic hypotension). Products include:
Actifed with Codeine Cough Syrup .. 752
Cheracol Cough Syrup 1853
Codimal PH Syrup 846
Dimetane-DC Cough Syrup 1857
Empirin with Codeine Phosphate Nos. 2, 3 & 4 764
Fiorinal with Codeine Capsules 2008
Isoclor Expectorant 982
Naldecon CX Adult Liquid .... ▣ 521
Novahistine DH 1342
Novahistine Expectorant 1343
Nucofed Capsules 2219
Nucofed Expectorant 2219
Nucofed Pediatric Expectorant 2220
Nucofed Syrup 2219
Phenaphen with Codeine Capsules 1865
Phenaphen-650 with Codeine Tablets 1866
Phenergan with Codeine 2497
Phenergan VC with Codeine 2501
Robitussin A-C Syrup 1875
Robitussin-DAC Syrup 1875
Ryna .... ▣ 741
Soma Compound w/Codeine Tablets 2390
Triaminic Expectorant w/Codeine .. 1996
Tussi-Organidin Liquid 2391
Tylenol with Codeine 1381

Codeine Polistirex (May aggravate orthostatic hypotension).
No products indexed under this heading.

Colestipol Hydrochloride (May inhibit gastrointestinal absorption of thiazides). Products include:
Colestid Granules 2328

Cortisone Acetate (May intensify electrolyte imbalance, particularly hypokalemia). Products include:
Cortone Acetate Sterile Suspension 1437
Cortone Acetate Tablets 1439

Deserpidine (Potentiated). Products include:
Enduronyl 518
Harmonyl Tablets 528
Oreticyl 545

Deslanoside (Exaggerated metabolic effects of hypokalemia).
No products indexed under this heading.

Dexamethasone (May intensify electrolyte imbalance, particularly hypokalemia). Products include:
AK-Trol Ointment & Suspension .... ⊙ 207
Decadron Elixir 1445
Decadron Tablets 1447
Decaspray Topical Aerosol 1459
Dexacidin .... ⊙ 272
Maxidex Sterile Ophthalmic Suspension .... ⊙ 223
Maxitrol Ophthalmic Ointment/Suspension .... ⊙ 223
TobraDex Ophthalmic Suspension and Ointment .... ⊙ 228

Dexamethasone Acetate (May intensify electrolyte imbalance, particularly hypokalemia). Products include:
Dalalone D.P. Injectable 999
Decadron-LA Sterile Suspension 1457

Dexamethasone Sodium Phosphate (May intensify electrolyte imbalance, particularly hypokalemia). Products include:
AK-Dex .... ⊙ 203
Decadron Phosphate Respihaler 1454
Decadron Phosphate Sterile Ophthalmic Ointment 1453
Decadron Phosphate Sterile Ophthalmic Solution 1453
Decadron Phosphate Topical Cream 1455
Decadron Phosphate Turbinaire 1456
Maxidex Sterile Ophthalmic Ointment .... ⊙ 222
NeoDecadron Sterile Ophthalmic Ointment 1517
NeoDecadron Sterile Ophthalmic Solution 1518
NeoDecadron Topical Cream 1518

Dezocine (May aggravate orthostatic hypotension).

Diazepam (Potentiated). Products include:
Valium Injectable 1937
Valium Tablets 1939
Valrelease Capsules 1923

Diazoxide (Potentiated). Products include:
Hyperstat I.V. Injection 2095
Proglycem 649

Diclofenac Sodium (Concomitant administration can reduce effects of diuretics). Products include:
Voltaren Ophthalmic Sterile Ophthalmic Solution .... ⊙ 268
Voltaren Tablets 1042

Dicumarol (Decreased effects of dicumarol). Products include:
Dicumarol Tablets 516

Digitoxin (Exaggerated metabolic effects of hypokalemia). Products include:
Crystodigin Tablets 1253

Digoxin (Exaggerated metabolic effects of hypokalemia). Products include:
Lanoxicaps 772
Lanoxin Elixir Pediatric 775
Lanoxin Injection 778
Lanoxin Injection Pediatric 781
Lanoxin Tablets 783

Doxazosin Mesylate (Potentiated). Products include:
Cardura Tablets 1941

Droperidol (Potentiated). Products include:
Inapsine Injection 1140
Innovar Injection 1141

Enalapril Maleate (Potentiated). Products include:
Vaseretic Tablets 1559
Vasotec Tablets 1564

Enalaprilat (Potentiated). Products include:
Vasotec I.V. 1562

Enflurane (Potentiated). Products include:
Ethrane 599

Esmolol Hydrochloride (Potentiated). Products include:
Brevibloc Injection 942

Etodolac (Concomitant administration can reduce effects of diuretics). Products include:
Lodine Capsules 2468

Felodipine (Potentiated). Products include:
Plendil Extended-Release Tablets 1526

Fenoprofen Calcium (Concomitant administration can reduce effects of diuretics). Products include:
Nalfon Pulvules & Tablets ... 919

Fentanyl (May aggravate orthostatic hypotension). Products include:
Duragesic Transdermal System... 1133

Fentanyl Citrate (Potentiated). Products include:
Innovar Injection... 1141
Sublimaze Injection... 1146

Flunisolide (May intensify electrolyte imbalance, particularly hypokalemia). Products include:
AeroBid Inhaler System ... 995
Nasalide Nasal Solution 0.025% ... 2299

Flurbiprofen (Concomitant administration can reduce effects of diuretics). Products include:
Ansaid Tablets ... 2319

Fosinopril Sodium (Potentiated). Products include:
Monopril Tablets ... 1406

Furosemide (Potentiation of furosemide). Products include:
Lasix ... 1093

Glipizide (Hypoglycemic dosage requirements may be affected). Products include:
Glucotrol ... 1952

Glyburide (Hypoglycemic dosage requirements may be affected). Products include:
DiaBeta... 1091
Micronase Tablets... 2350

Guanabenz Acetate (Potentiated). Products include:
Wytensin Tablets ... 2542

Guanethidine Monosulfate (Potentiated). Products include:
Esimil Tablets ... 864
Ismelin Tablets ... 869

Hydralazine Hydrochloride (Potentiated). Products include:
Apresazide Capsules ... 854
Apresoline Hydrochloride Parenteral (Ampuls)... 856
Apresoline Hydrochloride Tablets .. 855
Apresoline-Esidrix Tablets ... 857
Ser-Ap-Es Tablets ... 881
Serpasil-Apresoline Tablets... 884

Hydrochlorothiazide (Potentiated). Products include:
Aldactazide... 2150
Aldoril Tablets... 1418
Apresazide Capsules ... 854
Apresoline-Esidrix Tablets ... 857
Capozide ... 2258
Dyazide Capsules... 2208
Esidrix Tablets ... 863
Esimil Tablets ... 864
HydroDIURIL Tablets ... 1484
Hydropres Tablets... 1485
Inderide Tablets ... 2463
Inderide LA Long Acting Capsules .. 2465
Lopressor HCT Tablets ... 1034
Maxzide ... 1215
Moduretic Tablets ... 1510
Normozide Tablets ... 2112
Oretic Tablets ... 544
Oreticyl... 545
Prinzide Tablets ... 1540
Ser-Ap-Es Tablets ... 881
Serpasil-Esidrix Tablets... 886
Timolide Tablets... 1547
Trandate HCT Tablets ... 579
Vaseretic Tablets ... 1559
Zestoretic ... 2274

Hydrocodone Bitartrate (May aggravate orthostatic hypotension). Products include:
Anexsia 5/500 Tablets... 2196
Anexsia 7.5/650 Tablets ... 2197
Azdone Tablets... 844
Codiclear DH Syrup ... 845
Codimal DH Syrup... 846
Damason-P ... 1356
Hycodan Syrup, Tablets ... 927
Hycomine Compound Tablets ... 929
Hycomine Syrup... 927
Hycotuss Expectorant Syrup ... 930
Hydrocet Capsules ... 835
Lortab ASA Tablets... 2414
Lortab... 2412
Ru-Tuss with Hydrocodone ... 694
Triaminic Expectorant DH ... 1995
Vicodin Tablets... 1187
Vicodin ES Tablets ... 1189
Zydone Capsules ... 941

Hydrocodone Polistirex (May aggravate orthostatic hypotension). Products include:
Tussionex Extended-Release Suspension... 988

Hydrocortisone (May intensify electrolyte imbalance, particularly hypokalemia). Products include:
AK-Spore H.C. ... ◉ 206
Bactine Hydrocortisone Anti-Itch Cream... ⊞ 625
CaldeCORT Anti-Itch Hydrocortisone Spray ... ⊞ 560
Carmol HC Cream 1% ... 2296
Cortaid Spray ... ⊞ 735
Cortenema ... 2244
Cortisporin Ointment... 758
Cortisporin Ophthalmic Ointment Sterile ... 758
Cortisporin Ophthalmic Suspension Sterile ... 759
Cortisporin Otic Solution Sterile ... 760
Cortisporin Otic Suspension Sterile ... 760
Cortizone-5 Creme & Ointment... ⊞ 732
Dermolate Anti-Itch Cream ... ⊞ 697
Eldecort Cream 1.0% ... 1113
Eldecort Cream 1.0% and 2.5% ... 1113
Fungoid HC Creme ... 1770
Hydrocortone Tablets ... 1482
Hytone ... 909
LazerSporin-C Solution ... 1770
Massengill Medicated Soft Cloth Towelettes... 2192
Nutracort Cream & Lotion ... 1684
PediOtic Suspension Sterile ... 797
Synacort Creams 1%, 2.5% ... 2296
Vanoxide-HC Acne Lotion... 911
Vioform-Hydrocortisone Cream and Mild Cream ... 889
Vioform-Hydrocortisone Ointment.. 889
VōSoL HC Otic Solution... 2392
Vytone Cream 1% ... 911

Hydrocortisone Acetate (May intensify electrolyte imbalance, particularly hypokalemia). Products include:
Analpram-HC Rectal Cream 1% and 2.5% ... 970
Anusol-HC Cream ... 1690
Anusol-HC Suppositories ... 1691
Caldecort... ⊞ 560
Carmol HC Cream 1% ... 2296
Chloromycetin Hydrocortisone Ophthalmic... 1694
Coly-Mycin S Otic w/Neomycin & Hydrocortisone... 1708
Cortaid ... ⊞ 735
Cortef Feminine Itch Cream ... ⊞ 735
Corticaine ... ⊞ 682
Cortifoam ... 1827
Cortisporin Cream... 757
Epifoam ... 1828
Gynecort 5 Creme... ⊞ 556
Hydrocortone Acetate Sterile Suspension... 1479
Lanacort 5 Creme and Ointment .. ⊞ 557
Mantadil Cream ... 789
Ophthocort... ◉ 301
Orabase HCA Oral Paste ... 890
Pramosone Cream, Lotion & Ointment ... 971
ProctoCream-HC ... 1834
Proctofoam-HC... 1835

Hydrocortisone Sodium Phosphate (May intensify electrolyte imbalance, particularly hypokalemia). Products include:
Hydrocortone Phosphate Injection, Sterile ... 1481

Hydrocortisone Sodium Succinate (May intensify electrolyte imbalance, particularly hypokalemia). Products include:
Solu-Cortef Sterile Powder... 2361

Hydroxyzine Hydrochloride (Potentiated). Products include:
Atarax Tablets & Syrup... 1941
Marax Tablets & DF Syrup... 1954
Vistaril Intramuscular Solution... 1970

Ibuprofen (Concomitant administration can reduce effects of diuretics). Products include:
Advil Cold & Sinus Caplets (formerly CoAdvil) ... 2416
Advil Ibuprofen Tablets and Caplets ... 2416
Children's Advil Suspension ... 2426
CoAdvil... ⊞ 748
Dristan Sinus Caplets... 2419
Haltran Tablets... ⊞ 668
Ibuprofen... ⊞ 631
Medipren ibuprofen Caplets and Tablets ... 1362
Midol 200 Cramp Relief Formula.. ⊞ 570
Motrin Tablets... 2351
Motrin IB Caplets and Tablets ... ⊞ 736
Nuprin Ibuprofen/Analgesic Tablets & Caplets ... 752
PediaProfen Suspension... 1363
Rufen Tablets ... 691
Trendar Ibuprofen Tablets... ⊞ 756

Indapamide (Potentiated). Products include:
Lozol Tablets ... 1843

Indomethacin (Concomitant administration can reduce effects of diuretics). Products include:
Indocin ... 1487

Indomethacin Sodium Trihydrate (Concomitant administration can reduce effects of diuretics). Products include:
Indocin I.V. ... 1490

Insulin, Human (Insulin requirements may be altered).
No products indexed under this heading.

Insulin, Human Isophane Suspension (Insulin requirements may be altered). Products include:
Humulin N, 100 Units ... 1270

Insulin, Human NPH (Insulin requirements may be altered). Products include:
Insulatard NPH Human... 1627
Novolin N... 1627
Novolin N PenFill Cartridges... 1628
Novolin N Prefilled ... 1628

Insulin, Human Regular (Insulin requirements may be altered). Products include:
Humulin BR, 100 Units ... 1268
Humulin R, 100 Units ... 1272
Novolin R... 1627
Novolin R PenFill Cartridges... 1628
Novolin R Prefilled... 1629
Velosulin Human ... 1628

Insulin, Human, Zinc Suspension (Insulin requirements may be altered). Products include:
Humulin L, 100 Units ... 1268
Humulin U, 100 Units... 1272
Novolin L ... 1627

Insulin, NPH (Insulin requirements may be altered). Products include:
NPH, 40 & 100 Units... 1273
Beef NPH, 100 Units... 1274
Pork NPH, 100 Units... 1275
Insulatard NPH ... 1626
NPH Insulin ... 1626
NPH Purified Pork Isophane Insulin ... 1626

Insulin, Regular (Insulin requirements may be altered). Products include:
Regular, 40 & 100 Units... 1273
Beef Regular, 100 Units... 1275
Pork Regular, 100 Units ... 1275
Pork Regular (Concentrated), 500 Units ... 1276
Regular Insulin ... 1625
Regular Purified Pork Insulin ... 1626
Velosulin ... 1627

Insulin, Zinc Crystals (Insulin requirements may be altered). Products include:
NPH, 40 & 100 Units ... 1273

Insulin, Zinc Suspension (Insulin requirements may be altered). Products include:
Lente, 40 & 100 Units ... 1272
Protamine, Zinc, 40 & 100 Units... 1273
Lente Iletin I ... 1272
Beef Lente, 100 Units... 1274
Beef Protamine Zinc, 100 Units ... 1274
Pork Lente, 100 Units... 1275
Pork, Protamine, Zinc, 100 Units... 1275
Lente Insulin... 1626
Lente Purified Pork Insulin ... 1626
Semilente Insulin ... 1625
Ultralente Insulin ... 1626

Isoflurane (Potentiated). Products include:
Forane... 600

Isradipine (Potentiated). Products include:
DynaCirc Capsules ... 2004

Ketoprofen (Concomitant administration can reduce effects of diuretics). Products include:
Orudis Capsules... 2488

Ketorolac Tromethamine (Concomitant administration can reduce effects of diuretics). Products include:
Toradol IM Injection ... 2302

Labetalol Hydrochloride (Potentiated). Products include:
Normodyne Injection ... 2108
Normodyne Tablets ... 2110
Normozide Tablets ... 2112
Trandate HCT Tablets... 579
Trandate Injection ... 577
Trandate Tablets ... 579

Levorphanol Tartrate (May aggravate orthostatic hypotension). Products include:
Levo-Dromoran... 1906

Lisinopril (Potentiated). Products include:
Prinivil Tablets ... 1538
Prinzide Tablets ... 1540
Zestoretic ... 2274
Zestril Tablets ... 2277

Lithium Carbonate (May provoke lithium toxicity). Products include:
Eskalith ... 2214
Lithane Tablets... 1596
Lithium Carbonate Capsules & Tablets ... 1984
Lithobid Tablets ... 870

Lithium Citrate (May provoke lithium toxicity). Products include:
Cibalith-S... 870

Lorazepam (Potentiated). Products include:
Ativan Injection... 2432
Ativan Tablets ... 2434

Mecamylamine Hydrochloride (Potentiated). Products include:
Inversine Tablets ... 1492

Meclofenamate Sodium (Concomitant administration can reduce effects of diuretics). Products include:
Meclomen Capsules ... 1739

Mefenamic Acid (Concomitant administration can reduce effects of diuretics). Products include:
Ponstel ... 1758

Meperidine Hydrochloride (Potentiated; may aggravate orthostatic hypotension). Products include:
Demerol ... 2047
Mepergan Injection ... 2479

Mephobarbital (May aggravate orthostatic hypotension). Products include:
Mebaral Tablets ... 2061

Methadone Hydrochloride (May aggravate orthostatic hypotension). Products include:
Dolophine Hydrochloride Ampoules & Vials ... 1260
Dolophine Hydrochloride Tablets ... 1261
Methadone Hydrochloride Diskets .. 1284
Methadone Hydrochloride Oral Solution & Tablets... 1987

Methenamine (Decreased effectiveness due to alkalinization of urine). Products include:
Urised Tablets ... 2396
Methenamine Hippurate (Decreased effectiveness due to alkalinization of urine). Products include:
Hiprex Tablets ... 1333
Urex Tablets ... 1321
Methenamine Mandelate (Decreased effectiveness due to alkalinization of urine). Products include:
Mandelamine ... 1738
Uroqid-Acid ... 661
Methohexital Sodium (Potentiated). Products include:
Brevital Sodium Vials ... 1248
Methoxyflurane (Potentiated).
No products indexed under this heading.
Methyclothiazide (Potentiated). Products include:
Enduron Tablets ... 517
Enduronyl ... 518
Methyldopa (Potentiated). Products include:
Aldoclor Tablets ... 1413
Aldomet Oral ... 1415
Aldoril Tablets ... 1418
Methyldopate Hydrochloride (Potentiated). Products include:
Aldomet Ester HCl Injection ... 1417
Methylprednisolone Acetate (May intensify electrolyte imbalance, particularly hypokalemia). Products include:
Depo-Medrol Sterile Aqueous Suspension ... 2334
Methylprednisolone Sodium Succinate (May intensify electrolyte imbalance, particularly hypokalemia). Products include:
Solu-Medrol Sterile Powder ... 2363
Metocurine Iodide (Potentiated). Products include:
Metubine Iodide Vials ... 1285
Metolazone (Potentiated). Products include:
Diulo ... 2129
Mykrox ½ mg Tablets ... 984
Zaroxolyn Tablets ... 989
Metoprolol Tartrate (Potentiated). Products include:
Lopressor Ampuls ... 1032
Lopressor HCT Tablets ... 1034
Lopressor Tablets ... 1032
Metyrosine (Potentiated). Products include:
Demser Capsules ... 1460
Minoxidil (Potentiated). Products include:
Loniten Tablets ... 2346
Rogaine Topical Solution ... 2357
Morphine Sulfate (Potentiated). Products include:
Astramorph/PF Injection, USP (Preservative-Free) ... 618
Duramorph ... 960
Infumorph 200 and Infumorph 500 Sterile Solutions ... 962
MS Contin Tablets ... 1814
MSIR ... 1817
Oramorph SR (Morphine Sulfate Sustained Release Tablets) ... 1988
Roxanol ... 1991
Nadolol (Potentiated). Products include:
Corgard Tablets ... 701
Corzide Tablets ... 702
Naproxen (Concomitant administration can reduce effects of diuretics). Products include:
Naprosyn ... 2297
Naproxen Sodium (Concomitant administration can reduce effects of diuretics). Products include:
Anaprox and Anaprox DS Tablets ... 2288
Nicardipine Hydrochloride (Potentiated). Products include:
Cardene Capsules ... 2290
Nitroglycerin (Potentiated). Products include:
Deponit NTG Transdermal Delivery System ... 2143
Minitran Transdermal Delivery System ... 1312
Nitro-Bid Ointment ... 1339
Nitro-Bid Capsules ... 1338
Nitrodisc ... 2176
Nitro-Dur (nitroglycerin) Transdermal Infusion System ... 1164
Nitrogard Tablets ... 1004
Nitrolingual Spray ... 1846
Nitrostat Tablets ... 1743
Transderm-Nitro Transdermal Therapeutic System ... 2283
Norepinephrine Bitartrate (Concomitant administration may decrease arterial responsiveness). Products include:
Levophed Bitartrate Injection ... 2054
Opium Alkaloids (May aggravate orthostatic hypotension). Products include:
B & O No. 15A & No. 16A Supprettes ... 2395
Pantopon Injectable ... 1911
Oxycodone Hydrochloride (May aggravate orthostatic hypotension). Products include:
Percocet Tablets ... 950
Percodan ... 951
Roxicodone Tablets, Oral Solution & Intensol (Oxycodone) ... 1992
Tylox Capsules ... 1382
Pancuronium Bromide Injection (Potentiated).
No products indexed under this heading.
Penbutolol Sulfate (Potentiated). Products include:
Levatol ... 1832
Pentobarbital Sodium (Potentiated). Products include:
Nembutal Sodium Capsules ... 534
Nembutal Sodium Solution ... 536
Nembutal Sodium Suppositories ... 538
Phenobarbital (May aggravate orthostatic hypotension). Products include:
Arco-Lase Plus Tablets ... 607
Bellergal-S Tablets ... 1998
Bronkolixir ... ▣ 761
Bronkotabs Tablets ... ▣ 762
Donnatal ... 1858
Donnatal Extentabs ... 1859
Donnatal Tablets ... 1858
Donnazyme Tablets ... 1860
Kinesed Tablets ... 2272
Phenobarbital Elixir and Tablets ... 1293
Primatene Tablets-P Formula ... 2421
Quadrinal Tablets ... 1183
Tedral SA ... 1765
Phenoxybenzamine Hydrochloride (Potentiated). Products include:
Dibenzyline Capsules ... 2207
Phentolamine Mesylate (Potentiated). Products include:
Regitine ... 878
Phenylbutazone (Concomitant administration can reduce effects of diuretics). Products include:
Butazolidin Capsules & Tablets ... 1027
Pindolol (Potentiated). Products include:
Visken Tablets ... 2036
Piroxicam (Concomitant administration can reduce effects of diuretics). Products include:
Feldene Capsules ... 1777
Polythiazide (Potentiated). Products include:
Minizide Capsules ... 1779
Renese Tablets ... 1785
Renese-R Tablets ... 1786
Prazosin Hydrochloride (Potentiated). Products include:
Minipress Capsules ... 1778
Minizide Capsules ... 1779
Prednisolone Acetate (May intensify electrolyte imbalance, particularly hypokalemia). Products include:
AK-Cide Sterile Ophthalmic Ointment & Suspension ... ◉ 202
Blephamide Liquifilm Sterile Ophthalmic Suspension ... 586
Blephamide S.O.P. Sterile Ophthalmic Ointment ... 586
Cetapred Ointment ... ◉ 220
⅛% Econopred & 1% Econopred Plus ... ◉ 217
Isopto Cetapred Suspension ... ◉ 220
Metimyd ... ◉ 306
Poly-Pred Liquifilm ... ◉ 250
Pred Forte ... ◉ 252
Pred Mild ... ◉ 254
Pred-G Liquifilm Sterile Ophthalmic Suspension ... ◉ 252
Pred-G S.O.P. Sterile Ophthalmic Ointment ... ◉ 253
Vasocidin Ointment ... ◉ 275
Prednisolone Sodium Phosphate (May intensify electrolyte imbalance, particularly hypokalemia). Products include:
AK-Pred ... ◉ 205
Hydeltrasol Injection, Sterile ... 1476
Inflamase ... ◉ 274
Pediapred Oral Liquid ... 987
Vasocidin Ophthalmic Solution ... ◉ 276
Prednisolone Tebutate (May intensify electrolyte imbalance, particularly hypokalemia). Products include:
Hydeltra-T.B.A. Sterile Suspension 1478
Prednisone (May intensify electrolyte imbalance, particularly hypokalemia). Products include:
Deltasone Tablets ... 2332
Probenecid (Increased level of blood uric acid; dosage adjustment of probenecid may be necessary). Products include:
Benemid Tablets ... 1426
ColBENEMID Tablets ... 1436
Wycillin Injection and Probenecid Tablets ... 2539
Promethazine Hydrochloride (Potentiated). Products include:
Mepergan Injection ... 2479
Phenergan with Codeine ... 2497
Phenergan with Dextromethorphan 2499
Phenergan Injection ... 2493
Phenergan Suppositories ... 2496
Phenergan Syrup ... 2495
Phenergan Tablets ... 2496
Phenergan VC ... 2500
Phenergan VC with Codeine ... 2501
Propofol (Potentiated). Products include:
Diprivan Injection ... 2267
Propoxyphene Hydrochloride (May aggravate orthostatic hypotension). Products include:
Darvon ... 1256
Wygesic Tablets ... 2540
Propoxyphene Napsylate (May aggravate orthostatic hypotension). Products include:
Darvon-N/Darvocet-N ... 1254
Propranolol Hydrochloride (Potentiated). Products include:
Inderal ... 2459
Inderal LA Long Acting Capsules ... 2461
Inderide Tablets ... 2463
Inderide LA Long Acting Capsules .. 2465
Ramipril (Potentiated). Products include:
Altace Capsules ... 1086
Rauwolfia Serpentina (Potentiated). Products include:
Raudixin Tablets ... 1803
Rauzide Tablets ... 1804
Rescinnamine (Potentiated).
No products indexed under this heading.
Reserpine (Potentiated). Products include:
Diupres Tablets ... 1461
Hydromox R Tablets ... 1209
Hydropres Tablets ... 1485
Renese-R Tablets ... 1786
Salutensin/Salutensin-Demi ... 719
Ser-Ap-Es Tablets ... 881
Serpasil Tablets ... 883
Serpasil-Apresoline Tablets ... 884
Serpasil-Esidrix Tablets ... 886
Secobarbital Sodium (May aggravate orthostatic hypotension). Products include:
Seconal Sodium Pulvules ... 1296
Sodium Nitroprusside (Potentiated). Products include:
Nipride I.V. Infusion ... 1909
Sufentanil Citrate (May aggravate orthostatic hypotension). Products include:
Sufenta Injection ... 1147
Sulfinpyrazone (Increased level of blood uric acid; dosage adjustment of sulfinpyrazone may be necessary). Products include:
Anturane ... 853
Sulindac (Concomitant administration can reduce effects of diuretics). Products include:
Clinoril Tablets ... 1433
Terazosin Hydrochloride (Potentiated). Products include:
Hytrin Tablets ... 529
Thiamylal Sodium (May aggravate orthostatic hypotension). Products include:
Surital Ampoules, Steri-Vials ... 1764
Ticarcillin Disodium (Potentiated). Products include:
Ticar for Injection ... 2236
Timentin for Injection ... 2239
Timolol Maleate (Potentiated). Products include:
Blocadren Tablets ... 1429
Timolide Tablets ... 1547
Timoptic in Ocudose ... 1552
Timoptic Sterile Ophthalmic Solution ... 1550
Tolazamide (Hypoglycemic dosage requirements may be affected). Products include:
Tolinase Tablets ... 2365
Tolbutamide (Hypoglycemia requirements may be affected). Products include:
Orinase Tablets ... 2354
Tolmetin Sodium (Concomitant administration can reduce effects of diuretics). Products include:
Tolectin (200, 400 and 600 mg) .. 1379
Triamcinolone (May intensify electrolyte imbalance, particularly hypokalemia).
No products indexed under this heading.
Triamcinolone Acetonide (May intensify electrolyte imbalance, particularly hypokalemia). Products include:
Aristocort A ... 1010
Azmacort Inhaler ... 1837
Kenalog Cream, Lotion & Ointment 2401
Kenalog-10 Injection ... 2402
Kenalog-40 Injection ... 2403
Kenalog in Orabase ... 604
Kenalog Spray ... 2401
Mycolog II Cream and Ointment ... 2407
Mytrex Cream & Ointment ... 2080
Nasacort Nasal Inhaler ... 1844
Triamcinolone Diacetate (May intensify electrolyte imbalance, particularly hypokalemia). Products include:
Aristocort Suspension ... 1008
Triamcinolone Hexacetonide (May intensify electrolyte imbalance, particularly hypokalemia). Products include:
Aristospan Suspension ... 1011
Trimethaphan Camsylate (Potentiated). Products include:
Arfonad Ampuls ... 1887

Tubocurarine Chloride (Concomitant administration may increase responsiveness).
No products indexed under this heading.

Vecuronium Bromide (Potentiated). Products include:
Norcuron ... 1642

Warfarin Sodium (Decreased effects of warfarin). Products include:
Coumadin Injection & Tablets ... 944
Panwarfin Tablets ... 547

SALUTENSIN/SALUTENSIN-DEMI

(Hydroflumethiazide, Reserpine) ... 719
May interact with central nervous system depressants, narcotic analgesics, antihypertensives, diuretics, beta blockers , non-steroidal anti-inflammatory agents, monoamine oxidase inhibitors, tricyclic antidepressants, preanesthetic medications, general anesthetics, nondepolarizing neuromuscular blocking agents, cardiac glycosides, oral hypoglycemic agents, insulin, lithium preparations, corticosteroids, and certain other agents. Compounds in these categories include:

Acebutolol Hydrochloride (Additive and possibly excessive blockage). Products include:
Sectral Capsules ... 2520

ACTH (May intensify electrolyte imbalance, particularly hypokalemia).
No products indexed under this heading.

Alcohol (Orthostatic hypotension; enhanced CNS depressant effect).

Alfentanil Hydrochloride (Orthostatic hypotension; enhanced CNS depressant effects). Products include:
Alfenta Injection ... 1131

Alprazolam (Enhanced CNS depressant effects). Products include:
Xanax Tablets ... 2367

Amiloride Hydrochloride (Potentiation of antihypertensive effects). Products include:
Midamor Tablets ... 1508
Moduretic Tablets ... 1510

Amitriptyline Hydrochloride (Decreased hypotensive effect of rauwolfia alkaloids; interference with antidepressant effects). Products include:
Elavil ... 2269
Endep Tablets ... 1927
Etrafon ... 2087
Limbitrol ... 1933
Triavil Tablets ... 1556

Amoxapine (Decreased hypotensive effect of rauwolfia alkaloids; interference with antidepressant effects). Products include:
Asendin Tablets ... 1196

Amphetamine Resins (Action of indirect acting sympathomimetics inhibited). Products include:
Biphetamine Capsules ... 973

Amphetamine Sulfate (Action of indirect acting sympathomimetics inhibited).
No products indexed under this heading.

Amphotericin B (May intensify electrolyte imbalance, particularly hypokalemia). Products include:
Fungizone Cream, Lotion and Ointment ... 2261
Fungizone Intravenous ... 2262

Aprobarbital (Orthostatic hypotension; enhanced CNS depressant effects). Products include:
Alurate Elixir ... 1883

Atenolol (Additive and possibly excessive blockage). Products include:
Tenoretic Tablets ... 1105
Tenormin Tablets and I.V. Injection 1107

Atracurium Besylate (Potentiation of atracurium; dosage adjustments may be necessary). Products include:
Tracrium Injection ... 817

Benazepril Hydrochloride (Potentiation of antihypertensive effects). Products include:
Lotensin Tablets ... 872

Bendroflumethiazide (Potentiation of antihypertensive effects). Products include:
Corzide Tablets ... 702
Naturetin Tablets ... 1789
Rauzide Tablets ... 1804

Betamethasone Acetate (May intensify electrolyte imbalance, particularly hypokalemia). Products include:
Celestone Soluspan Suspension ... 2081

Betamethasone Sodium Phosphate (May intensify electrolyte imbalance, particularly hypokalemia). Products include:
Celestone Soluspan Suspension ... 2081

Betaxolol Hydrochloride (Potentiation of antihypertensive effects). Products include:
Betoptic Sterile Ophthalmic Solution ... 569
Betoptic S Sterile Ophthalmic Suspension ... 570
Kerlone Tablets ... 2172

Bumetanide (Potentiation of antihypertensive effects). Products include:
Bumex ... 1895

Buprenorphine (Orthostatic hypotension; enhanced CNS depressant effects).
No products indexed under this heading.

Buspirone Hydrochloride (Enhanced CNS depressant effects). Products include:
BuSpar ... 1401

Butabarbital (Orthostatic hypotension; enhanced CNS depressant effects). Products include:
Pyridium Plus ... 1764

Butalbital (Orthostatic hypotension; enhanced CNS depressant effects). Products include:
Esgic-Plus Tablets ... 1002
Esgic Tablets & Capsules ... 1001
Fioricet Tablets ... 2006
Fiorinal Capsules ... 2007
Fiorinal with Codeine Capsules ... 2008
Fiorinal Tablets ... 2007
Phrenilin ... 838
Sedapap Tablets 50 mg/650 mg .. 1360

Captopril (Potentiation of antihypertensive effects). Products include:
Capoten ... 2255
Capozide ... 2258

Carteolol Hydrochloride (Additive and possibly excessive blockage). Products include:
Cartrol Tablets ... 507

Chlordiazepoxide (Enhanced CNS depressant effects). Products include:
Libritabs Tablets ... 1930
Limbitrol ... 1933
Menrium Tablets ... 1934

Chlordiazepoxide Hydrochloride (Enhanced CNS depressant effects). Products include:
Librax Capsules ... 1929
Librium Capsules ... 1931
Librium Injectable ... 1932

Chlorothiazide (Potentiation of antihypertensive effects). Products include:
Aldoclor Tablets ... 1413
Diupres Tablets ... 1461
Diuril Oral ... 1464

Chlorothiazide Sodium (Potentiation of antihypertensive effects). Products include:
Diuril Sodium Intravenous ... 1463

Chlorpromazine (Enhanced CNS depressant effects). Products include:
Thorazine ... 2234

Chlorpropamide (Elevated blood glucose levels; dosage of hypoglycemics and insulin requirements may be affected). Products include:
Diabinese Tablets ... 1775

Chlorprothixene (Orthostatic hypotension; enhanced CNS depressant effects). Products include:
Taractan Tablets ... 1920

Chlorprothixene Hydrochloride (Orthostatic hypotension; enhanced CNS depressant effects). Products include:
Taractan ... 1920

Chlorthalidone (Additive and possibly excessive blockage; potentiation of antihypertensive effects). Products include:
Combipres Tablets ... 678
Tenoretic Tablets ... 1105
Thalitone Tablets ... 687

Clomipramine Hydrochloride (Decreased hypotensive effect of rauwolfia alkaloids; interference with antidepressant effects). Products include:
Anafranil Capsules ... 650

Clonidine (Potentiation of antihypertensive effects). Products include:
Catapres-TTS ... 677

Clonidine Hydrochloride (Additive and possibly excessive blockage). Products include:
Catapres Tablets ... 676
Combipres Tablets ... 678

Clorazepate Dipotassium (Enhanced CNS depressant effects). Products include:
Tranxene ... 556

Codeine (Orthostatic hypotension; enhanced CNS depressant effects). Products include:
Calcidrine Syrup ... 506

Codeine Phosphate (Orthostatic hypotension; enhanced CNS depressant effects). Products include:
Actifed with Codeine Cough Syrup.. 752
Cheracol Cough Syrup ... 1853
Codimal PH Syrup ... 846
Dimetane-DC Cough Syrup ... 1857
Empirin with Codeine Phosphate Nos. 2, 3 & 4 ... 764
Fiorinal with Codeine Capsules ... 2008
Isoclor Expectorant ... 982
Naldecon CX Adult Liquid ... ◘ 521
Novahistine DH ... 1342
Novahistine Expectorant ... 1343
Nucofed Capsules ... 2219
Nucofed Expectorant ... 2219
Nucofed Pediatric Expectorant ... 2220
Nucofed Syrup ... 2219
Phenaphen with Codeine Capsules 1865
Phenaphen-650 with Codeine Tablets ... 1866
Phenergan with Codeine ... 2497
Phenergan VC with Codeine ... 2501
Robitussin A-C Syrup ... 1875
Robitussin-DAC Syrup ... 1875
Ryna ... ◘ 741
Soma Compound w/Codeine Tablets ... 2390
Triaminic Expectorant w/Codeine .. 1996
Tussi-Organidin Liquid ... 2391
Tylenol with Codeine ... 1381

Codeine Polistirex (Orthostatic hypotension; enhanced CNS depressant effects).
No products indexed under this heading.

Colestipol Hydrochloride (May inhibit gastrointestinal absorption of thiazide diuretics). Products include:
Colestid Granules ... 2328

Cortisone Acetate (May intensify electrolyte imbalance, particularly hypokalemia). Products include:
Cortone Acetate Sterile Suspension ... 1437
Cortone Acetate Tablets ... 1439

Deserpidine (Potentiation of antihypertensive effects). Products include:
Enduronyl ... 518
Harmonyl Tablets ... 528
Oreticyl ... 545

Desipramine Hydrochloride (Decreased hypotensive effect of rauwolfia alkaloids; interference with antidepressant effects). Products include:
Norpramin Tablets ... 1340

Deslanoside (Enhanced possibility of digitalis toxicity associated with hypokalemia).
No products indexed under this heading.

Dexamethasone (May intensify electrolyte imbalance, particularly hypokalemia). Products include:
AK-Trol Ointment & Suspension ... ⊙ 207
Decadron Elixir ... 1445
Decadron Tablets ... 1447
Decaspray Topical Aerosol ... 1459
Dexacidin ... ⊙ 272
Maxidex Sterile Ophthalmic Suspension ... ⊙ 223
Maxitrol Ophthalmic Ointment/ Suspension ... ⊙ 223
TobraDex Ophthalmic Suspension and Ointment ... ⊙ 228

Dexamethasone Acetate (May intensify electrolyte imbalance, particularly hypokalemia). Products include:
Dalalone D.P. Injectable ... 999
Decadron-LA Sterile Suspension ... 1457

Dexamethasone Sodium Phosphate (May intensify electrolyte imbalance, particularly hypokalemia). Products include:
AK-Dex ... ⊙ 203
Decadron Phosphate Respihaler ... 1454
Decadron Phosphate Sterile Ophthalmic Ointment ... 1453
Decadron Phosphate Sterile Ophthalmic Solution ... 1453
Decadron Phosphate Topical Cream ... 1455
Decadron Phosphate Turbinaire ... 1456
Maxidex Sterile Ophthalmic Ointment ... ⊙ 222
NeoDecadron Sterile Ophthalmic Ointment ... 1517
NeoDecadron Sterile Ophthalmic Solution ... 1518
NeoDecadron Topical Cream ... 1518

Dezocine (Orthostatic hypotension; enhanced CNS depressant effects).

Diazepam (Potentiation of diazepam; dosage adjustments may be necessary; enhanced CNS depressant effects). Products include:
Valium Injectable ... 1937
Valium Tablets ... 1939
Valrelease Capsules ... 1923

Diazoxide (Additive and possibly excessive blockage). Products include:
Hyperstat I.V. Injection ... 2095
Proglycem ... 649

Diclofenac Sodium (Reduces diuretic and antihypertensive effect of thiazides). Products include:
Voltaren Ophthalmic Sterile Ophthalmic Solution ... ⊙ 268
Voltaren Tablets ... 1042

Digitoxin (Enhanced possibility of digitalis toxicity associated with hypokalemia). Products include:
- Crystodigin Tablets ... 1253

Digoxin (Enhanced possibility of digitalis toxicity associated with hypokalemia). Products include:
- Lanoxicaps ... 772
- Lanoxin Elixir Pediatric ... 775
- Lanoxin Injection ... 778
- Lanoxin Injection Pediatric ... 781
- Lanoxin Tablets ... 783

Doxazosin Mesylate (Potentiation of antihypertensive effects). Products include:
- Cardura Tablets ... 1941

Doxepin Hydrochloride (Decreased hypotensive effect of rauwolfia alkaloids; interference with antidepressant effects). Products include:
- Sinequan ... 1960

Droperidol (Potentiation of droperidol; dosage adjustments may be necessary; enhanced CNS depressant effects). Products include:
- Inapsine Injection ... 1140
- Innovar Injection ... 1141

Enalapril Maleate (Potentiation of antihypertensive effects). Products include:
- Vaseretic Tablets ... 1559
- Vasotec Tablets ... 1564

Enalaprilat (Potentiation of antihypertensive effects). Products include:
- Vasotec I.V. ... 1562

Enflurane (Potentiation of enflurane; dosage adjustments may be necessary; enhanced CNS depressant effects). Products include:
- Ethrane ... 599

Ephedrine (Action of indirect-acting sympathomimetics inhibited).

Epinephrine (Prolonged action of direct-acting sympathomimetics). Products include:
- Ana-Kit Anaphylaxis Emergency Treatment Kit ... 1100
- Bronkaid Mist ... ■ 757
- EpiPen ... 843
- Marcaine Hydrochloride 0.5% with Epinephrine 1:200,000 (as bitartrate) ... 958
- Marcaine Hydrochloride with Epinephrine 1:200,000 ... 2055
- Primatene Mist ... 2420
- Sus-Phrine Injection ... 1006
- Xylocaine with Epinephrine Injections ... 637

Epinephrine Bitartrate (Prolonged action of direct-acting sympathomimetics). Products include:
- AsthmaHaler Mist Epinephrine Bitartrate Bronchodilator ... ■ 616
- Bronkaid Mist Suspension ... ■ 757
- Primatene Mist Suspension ... 2421

Esmolol Hydrochloride (Additive and possibly excessive blockage). Products include:
- Brevibloc Injection ... 942

Estazolam (Orthostatic hypotension; enhanced CNS depressant effects). Products include:
- ProSom Tablets ... 554

Ethacrynic Acid (Potentiation of antihypertensive effects). Products include:
- Edecrin Tablets ... 1468

Ethchlorvynol (Enhanced CNS depressant effects). Products include:
- Placidyl Capsules ... 553

Ethinamate (Enhanced CNS depressant effects).
- No products indexed under this heading.

Etodolac (Reduces diuretic and antihypertensive effect of thiazides). Products include:
- Lodine Capsules ... 2468

Felodipine (Potentiation of antihypertensive effects). Products include:
- Plendil Extended-Release Tablets ... 1526

Fenoprofen Calcium (Reduces diuretic and antihypertensive effect of thiazides). Products include:
- Nalfon Pulvules & Tablets ... 919

Fentanyl (Orthostatic hypotension; enhanced CNS depressant effects). Products include:
- Duragesic Transdermal System ... 1133

Fentanyl Citrate (Potentiation of fentanyl; dosage adjustments may be necessary). Products include:
- Innovar Injection ... 1141
- Sublimaze Injection ... 1146

Flunisolide (May intensify electrolyte imbalance, particularly hypokalemia). Products include:
- AeroBid Inhaler System ... 995
- Nasalide Nasal Solution 0.025% ... 2299

Fluphenazine Decanoate (Enhanced CNS depressant effects). Products include:
- Prolixin Decanoate ... 1795

Fluphenazine Enanthate (Enhanced CNS depressant effects). Products include:
- Prolixin Enanthate ... 1796

Fluphenazine Hydrochloride (Enhanced CNS depressant effects). Products include:
- Prolixin Elixir ... 1793
- Prolixin Injection ... 1791
- Prolixin Oral Concentrate ... 1792
- Prolixin Tablets ... 1793

Flurazepam Hydrochloride (Enhanced CNS depressant effects). Products include:
- Dalmane Capsules ... 1927

Flurbiprofen (Reduces diuretic and antihypertensive effect of thiazides). Products include:
- Ansaid Tablets ... 2319

Fosinopril Sodium (Potentiation of antihypertensive effects). Products include:
- Monopril Tablets ... 1406

Furazolidone (Hyperpyrexia reaching crisis levels; moderate to sudden and severe hypertension). Products include:
- Furoxone ... 1855

Furosemide (Potentiation of antihypertensive effects). Products include:
- Lasix ... 1093

Glipizide (Elevated blood glucose levels; dosage of hypoglycemics may be affected). Products include:
- Glucotrol ... 1952

Glutethimide (Enhanced CNS depressant effects).
- No products indexed under this heading.

Glyburide (Elevated blood glucose levels; dosage of hypoglycemics may be affected). Products include:
- DiaBeta ... 1091
- Micronase Tablets ... 2350

Guanabenz Acetate (Potentiation of antihypertensive effects). Products include:
- Wytensin Tablets ... 2542

Guanethidine Monosulfate (Potentiation of antihypertensive effects). Products include:
- Esimil Tablets ... 864
- Ismelin Tablets ... 869

Haloperidol (Enhanced CNS depressant effects). Products include:
- Haldol Injection, Tablets and Concentrate ... 1373

Haloperidol Decanoate (Enhanced CNS depressant effects). Products include:
- Haldol Decanoate ... 1375

Hydralazine Hydrochloride (Additive and possibly excessive blockage). Products include:
- Apresazide Capsules ... 854
- Apresoline Hydrochloride Parenteral (Ampuls) ... 856
- Apresoline Hydrochloride Tablets ... 855
- Apresoline-Esidrix Tablets ... 857
- Ser-Ap-Es Tablets ... 881
- Serpasil-Apresoline Tablets ... 884

Hydrochlorothiazide (Potentiation of antihypertensive effects). Products include:
- Aldactazide ... 2150
- Aldoril Tablets ... 1418
- Apresazide Capsules ... 854
- Apresoline-Esidrix Tablets ... 857
- Capozide ... 2258
- Dyazide Capsules ... 2208
- Esidrix Tablets ... 863
- Esimil Tablets ... 864
- HydroDIURIL Tablets ... 1484
- Hydropres Tablets ... 1485
- Inderide Tablets ... 2463
- Inderide LA Long Acting Capsules ... 2465
- Lopressor HCT Tablets ... 1034
- Maxzide ... 1215
- Moduretic Tablets ... 1510
- Normozide Tablets ... 2112
- Oretic Tablets ... 544
- Oreticyl ... 545
- Prinzide Tablets ... 1540
- Ser-Ap-Es Tablets ... 881
- Serpasil-Esidrix Tablets ... 886
- Timolide Tablets ... 1547
- Trandate HCT Tablets ... 579
- Vaseretic Tablets ... 1559
- Zestoretic ... 2274

Hydrocodone Bitartrate (Orthostatic hypotension; enhanced CNS depressant effects). Products include:
- Anexsia 5/500 Tablets ... 2196
- Anexsia 7.5/650 Tablets ... 2197
- Azdōne Tablets ... 844
- Codiclear DH Syrup ... 845
- Codimal DH Syrup ... 846
- Damason-P ... 1356
- Hycodan Syrup, Tablets ... 927
- Hycomine Compound Tablets ... 929
- Hycomine Syrup ... 927
- Hycotuss Expectorant Syrup ... 930
- Hydrocet Capsules ... 835
- Lortab ASA Tablets ... 2414
- Lortab ... 2412
- Ru-Tuss with Hydrocodone ... 694
- Triaminic Expectorant DH ... 1995
- Vicodin Tablets ... 1187
- Vicodin ES Tablets ... 1189
- Zydone Capsules ... 941

Hydrocodone Polistirex (Orthostatic hypotension; enhanced CNS depressant effects). Products include:
- Tussionex Extended-Release Suspension ... 988

Hydrocortisone (May intensify electrolyte imbalance, particularly hypokalemia). Products include:
- AK-Spore H.C. ... ⊙ 206
- Bactine Hydrocortisone Anti-Itch Cream ... ■ 625
- CaldeCORT Anti-Itch Hydrocortisone Spray ... ■ 560
- Carmol HC Cream 1% ... 2296
- Cortaid Spray ... ■ 735
- Cortenema ... 2244
- Cortisporin Ointment ... 758
- Cortisporin Ophthalmic Ointment Sterile ... 758
- Cortisporin Ophthalmic Suspension Sterile ... 759
- Cortisporin Otic Solution Sterile ... 760
- Cortisporin Otic Suspension Sterile ... 760
- Cortizone-5 Creme & Ointment ... ■ 732
- Dermolate Anti-Itch Cream ... ■ 697
- Eldecort Cream 1.0% ... 1113
- Eldecort Cream 1.0% and 2.5% ... 1113
- Fungoid HC Creme ... 1770
- Hydrocortone Tablets ... 1482
- Hytone ... 909
- LazerSporin-C Solution ... 1770
- Massengill Medicated Soft Cloth Towelettes ... 2192
- Nutracort Cream & Lotion ... 1684
- PediOtic Suspension Sterile ... 797
- Synacort Creams 1%, 2.5% ... 2296
- Vanoxide-HC Acne Lotion ... 911
- Vioform-Hydrocortisone Cream and Mild Cream ... 889
- Vioform-Hydrocortisone Ointment ... 889
- VōSoL HC Otic Solution ... 2392
- Vytone Cream 1% ... 911

Hydrocortisone Acetate (May intensify electrolyte imbalance, particularly hypokalemia). Products include:
- Analpram-HC Rectal Cream 1% and 2.5% ... 970
- Anusol-HC Cream ... 1690
- Anusol-HC Suppositories ... 1691
- Caldecort ... ■ 560
- Carmol HC Cream 1% ... 2296
- Chloromycetin Hydrocortisone Ophthalmic ... 1694
- Coly-Mycin S Otic w/Neomycin & Hydrocortisone ... 1708
- Cortaid ... ■ 735
- Cortef Feminine Itch Cream ... ■ 735
- Corticaine ... ■ 682
- Cortifoam ... 1827
- Cortisporin Cream ... 757
- Epifoam ... 1828
- Gynecort 5 Creme ... ■ 556
- Hydrocortone Acetate Sterile Suspension ... 1479
- Lanacort 5 Creme and Ointment ... ■ 557
- Mantadil Cream ... 789
- Ophthocort ... ⊙ 301
- Orabase HCA Oral Paste ... 890
- Pramosone Cream, Lotion & Ointment ... 971
- ProctoCream-HC ... 1834
- Proctofoam-HC ... 1835

Hydrocortisone Sodium Phosphate (May intensify electrolyte imbalance, particularly hypokalemia). Products include:
- Hydrocortone Phosphate Injection, Sterile ... 1481

Hydrocortisone Sodium Succinate (May intensify electrolyte imbalance, particularly hypokalemia). Products include:
- Solu-Cortef Sterile Powder ... 2361

Hydroxyzine Hydrochloride (Potentiation of hydroxyzine; dosage adjustments may be necessary; enhanced CNS depressant effects). Products include:
- Atarax Tablets & Syrup ... 1941
- Marax Tablets & DF Syrup ... 1954
- Vistaril Intramuscular Solution ... 1970

Ibuprofen (Reduces diuretic and antihypertensive effect of thiazides). Products include:
- Advil Cold & Sinus Caplets (formerly CoAdvil) ... 2416
- Advil Ibuprofen Tablets and Caplets ... 2416
- Children's Advil Suspension ... 2426
- CoAdvil ... ■ 748
- Dristan Sinus Caplets ... 2419
- Haltran Tablets ... ■ 668
- Ibuprofen ... ■ 631
- Medipren ibuprofen Caplets and Tablets ... 1362
- Midol 200 Cramp Relief Formula ... ■ 570
- Motrin Tablets ... 2351
- Motrin IB Caplets and Tablets ... ■ 736
- Nuprin Ibuprofen/Analgesic Tablets & Caplets ... 752
- PediaProfen Suspension ... 1363
- Rufen Tablets ... 691
- Trendar Ibuprofen Tablets ... ■ 756

Imipramine Hydrochloride (Decreased hypotensive effect of rauwolfia alkaloids; interference with antidepressant effects). Products include:
- Tofranil Ampuls ... 1038
- Tofranil Tablets ... 1039

(■ Described in PDR For Nonprescription Drugs) (⊙ Described in PDR For Ophthalmology)

Imipramine Pamoate (Decreased hypotensive effect of rauwolfia alkaloids; interference with antidepressant effects). Products include:
Tofranil-PM Capsules ... 1041

Indapamide (Potentiation of antihypertensive effects). Products include:
Lozol Tablets ... 1843

Indomethacin (Reduces diuretic and antihypertensive effect of thiazides). Products include:
Indocin ... 1487

Indomethacin Sodium Trihydrate (Reduces diuretic and antihypertensive effect of thiazides). Products include:
Indocin I.V. ... 1490

Insulin, Human (Insulin requirements may change).
No products indexed under this heading.

Insulin, Human Isophane Suspension (Insulin requirements may change). Products include:
Humulin N, 100 Units ... 1270

Insulin, Human NPH (Insulin requirements may change). Products include:
Insulatard NPH Human ... 1627
Novolin N ... 1627
Novolin N PenFill Cartridges ... 1628
Novolin N Prefilled ... 1628

Insulin, Human Regular (Insulin requirements may change). Products include:
Humulin BR, 100 Units ... 1268
Humulin R, 100 Units ... 1272
Novolin R ... 1627
Novolin R PenFill Cartridges ... 1628
Novolin R Prefilled ... 1629
Velosulin Human ... 1628

Insulin, Human, Zinc Suspension (Insulin requirements may change). Products include:
Humulin L, 100 Units ... 1268
Humulin U, 100 Units ... 1272
Novolin L ... 1627

Insulin, NPH (Insulin requirements may change). Products include:
NPH, 40 & 100 Units ... 1273
Beef NPH, 100 Units ... 1274
Pork NPH, 100 Units ... 1275
Insulatard NPH ... 1626
NPH Insulin ... 1626
NPH Purified Pork Isophane Insulin ... 1626

Insulin, Regular (Insulin requirements may change). Products include:
Regular, 40 & 100 Units ... 1273
Beef Regular, 100 Units ... 1275
Pork Regular, 100 Units ... 1275
Pork Regular (Concentrated), 500 Units ... 1276
Regular Insulin ... 1625
Regular Purified Pork Insulin ... 1626
Velosulin ... 1627

Insulin, Zinc Crystals (Insulin requirements may change). Products include:
NPH, 40 & 100 Units ... 1273

Insulin, Zinc Suspension (Insulin requirements may change). Products include:
Lente, 40 & 100 Units ... 1272
Protamine, Zinc, 40 & 100 Units ... 1273
Lente Iletin I ... 1272
Beef Lente, 100 Units ... 1274
Beef Protamine Zinc, 100 Units ... 1274
Pork Lente, 100 Units ... 1275
Pork, Protamine, Zinc, 100 Units ... 1275
Lente Insulin ... 1626
Lente Purified Pork Insulin ... 1626
Semilente Insulin ... 1625
Ultralente Insulin ... 1626

Isocarboxazid (Hyperpyrexia reaching crisis levels; moderate to sudden and severe hypertension). Products include:
Marplan Tablets ... 1906

Isoflurane (Potentiation of isoflurane; dosage adjustments may be necessary; enhanced CNS depressant effects). Products include:
Forane ... 600

Isoproterenol Hydrochloride (Prolonged action of direct-acting sympathomimetics). Products include:
Isuprel Hydrochloride Injection 1:5000 ... 2050
Isuprel Hydrochloride Mistometer .. 2051
Isuprel Hydrochloride Solution 1:200 & 1:100 ... 2052
Norisodrine Aerotrol ... 540

Isoproterenol Sulfate (Prolonged action of direct-acting sympathomimetics).
No products indexed under this heading.

Isradipine (Potentiation of antihypertensive effects). Products include:
DynaCirc Capsules ... 2004

Ketamine Hydrochloride (Orthostatic hypotension; enhanced CNS depressant effects). Products include:
Ketalar ... 1726

Ketoprofen (Reduces diuretic and antihypertensive effect of thiazides). Products include:
Orudis Capsules ... 2488

Ketorolac Tromethamine (Reduces diuretic and antihypertensive effect of thiazides). Products include:
Toradol IM Injection ... 2302

Labetalol Hydrochloride (Additive and possibly excessive blockage). Products include:
Normodyne Injection ... 2108
Normodyne Tablets ... 2110
Normozide Tablets ... 2112
Trandate HCT Tablets ... 579
Trandate Injection ... 577
Trandate Tablets ... 579

Levodopa (Concurrent use not recommended). Products include:
Larodopa Tablets ... 1905
Sinemet Tablets ... 952
Sinemet CR Tablets ... 953

Levorphanol Tartrate (Orthostatic hypotension; enhanced CNS depressant effects). Products include:
Levo-Dromoran ... 1906

Lisinopril (Potentiation of antihypertensive effects). Products include:
Prinivil Tablets ... 1538
Prinzide Tablets ... 1540
Zestoretic ... 2274
Zestril Tablets ... 2277

Lithium Carbonate (May provoke lithium toxicity). Products include:
Eskalith ... 2214
Lithane Tablets ... 1596
Lithium Carbonate Capsules & Tablets ... 1984
Lithobid Tablets ... 870

Lithium Citrate (May provoke lithium toxicity). Products include:
Cibalith-S ... 870

Lorazepam (Potentiation of lorazepam; dosage adjustments may be necessary; enhanced CNS depressant effects). Products include:
Ativan Injection ... 2432
Ativan Tablets ... 2434

Loxapine Hydrochloride (Enhanced CNS depressant effects). Products include:
Loxitane ... 1213

Loxapine Succinate (Orthostatic hypotension; enhanced CNS depressant effects). Products include:
Loxitane Capsules ... 1213

Maprotiline Hydrochloride (Decreased hypotensive effect of rauwolfia alkaloids; interference with antidepressant effects). Products include:
Ludiomil Tablets ... 874

Mecamylamine Hydrochloride (Potentiation of antihypertensive effects). Products include:
Inversine Tablets ... 1492

Meclofenamate Sodium (Reduces diuretic and antihypertensive effect of thiazides). Products include:
Meclomen Capsules ... 1739

Mefenamic Acid (Reduces diuretic and antihypertensive effect of thiazides). Products include:
Ponstel ... 1758

Meperidine Hydrochloride (Potentiation of meperidine; dosage adjustments may be necessary; enhanced CNS depressant effects). Products include:
Demerol ... 2047
Mepergan Injection ... 2479

Mephobarbital (Orthostatic hypertension; enhanced CNS depressant effects). Products include:
Mebaral Tablets ... 2061

Meprobamate (Enhanced CNS depressant effects). Products include:
Deprol Tablets ... 2382
Equagesic Tablets ... 2451
Miltown Tablets ... 2386
PMB 200 and PMB 400 ... 2504

Mesoridazine (Enhanced CNS depressant effects). Products include:
Serentil ... 686

Metaraminol Bitartrate (Prolonged action of direct-acting sympathomimetics). Products include:
Aramine Injection ... 1424

Methadone Hydrochloride (Orthostatic hypotension; enhanced CNS depressant effects). Products include:
Dolophine Hydrochloride Ampoules & Vials ... 1260
Dolophine Hydrochloride Tablets 1261
Methadone Hydrochloride Diskets .. 1284
Methadone Hydrochloride Oral Solution & Tablets ... 1987

Methamphetamine Hydrochloride (Action of indirect-acting sympathomimetics inhibited). Products include:
Desoxyn Gradumet Tablets ... 514

Methenamine (Effectiveness of methenamine may be decreased due to urinary alkalinization). Products include:
Urised Tablets ... 2396

Methohexital Sodium (Potentiation of methohexital; dosage adjustments may be necessary; enhanced CNS depressant effects). Products include:
Brevital Sodium Vials ... 1248

Methotrimeprazine (Additive hypotension).
No products indexed under this heading.

Methoxyflurane (Potentiation of methoxyflurane; dosage adjustments may be necessary; enhanced CNS depressant effects).
No products indexed under this heading.

Methyclothiazide (Potentiation of antihypertensive effects). Products include:
Enduron Tablets ... 517
Enduronyl ... 518

Methyldopa (Potentiation of antihypertensive effects). Products include:
Aldoclor Tablets ... 1413
Aldomet Oral ... 1415
Aldoril Tablets ... 1418

Methyldopate Hydrochloride (Potentiation of antihypertensive effects). Products include:
Aldomet Ester HCl Injection ... 1417

Methylphenidate Hydrochloride (Action of indirect-acting sympathomimetics inhibited). Products include:
Ritalin ... 880

Methylprednisolone Acetate (May intensify electrolyte imbalance, particularly hypokalemia). Products include:
Depo-Medrol Sterile Aqueous Suspension ... 2334

Methylprednisolone Sodium Succinate (May intensify electrolyte imbalance, particularly hypokalemia). Products include:
Solu-Medrol Sterile Powder ... 2363

Metocurine Iodide (Potentiation of metocurine; dosage adjustments may be necessary). Products include:
Metubine Iodide Vials ... 1285

Metolazone (Potentiation of antihypertensive effects). Products include:
Diulo ... 2129
Mykrox ½ mg Tablets ... 984
Zaroxolyn Tablets ... 989

Metoprolol Tartrate (Additive and possibly excessive blockage). Products include:
Lopressor Ampuls ... 1032
Lopressor HCT Tablets ... 1034
Lopressor Tablets ... 1032

Metyrosine (Potentiation of antihypertensive effects). Products include:
Demser Capsules ... 1460

Midazolam Hydrochloride (Orthostatic hypotension; enhanced CNS depressant effects). Products include:
Versed Injection ... 1924

Minoxidil (Potentiation of antihypertensive effects). Products include:
Loniten Tablets ... 2346
Rogaine Topical Solution ... 2357

Molindone Hydrochloride (Enhanced CNS depressant effects). Products include:
Moban Tablets & Concentrate ... 932

Morphine Sulfate (Potentiation of morphine; dosage adjustments may be necessary; enhanced CNS depressant effects). Products include:
Astramorph/PF Injection, USP (Preservative-Free) ... 618
Duramorph ... 960
Infumorph 200 and Infumorph 500 Sterile Solutions ... 962
MS Contin Tablets ... 1814
MSIR ... 1817
Oramorph SR (Morphine Sulfate Sustained Release Tablets) ... 1988
Roxanol ... 1991

Nadolol (Additive and possibly excessive blockage). Products include:
Corgard Tablets ... 701
Corzide Tablets ... 702

Naproxen (Reduces diuretic and antihypertensive effect of thiazides). Products include:
Naprosyn ... 2297

Naproxen Sodium (Reduces diuretic and antihypertensive effect of thiazides). Products include:
Anaprox and Anaprox DS Tablets ... 2288

Nicardipine Hydrochloride (Additive and possibly excessive blockage). Products include:
Cardene Capsules ... 2290

Nitroglycerin (Potentiation of antihypertensive effects). Products include:
Deponit NTG Transdermal Delivery System ... 2143
Minitran Transdermal Delivery System ... 1312
Nitro-Bid Ointment ... 1339
Nitro-Bid Capsules ... 1338
Nitrodisc ... 2176
Nitro-Dur (nitroglycerin) Transdermal Infusion System ... 1164
Nitrogard Tablets ... 1004
Nitrolingual Spray ... 1846
Nitrostat Tablets ... 1743
Transderm-Nitro Transdermal Therapeutic System ... 2283

Norepinephrine Bitartrate (Prolonged action of direct-acting sympathomimetics; decreased arterial responsiveness to norepinephrine). Products include:
Levophed Bitartrate Injection ... 2054

Nortriptyline Hydrochloride (Decreased hypotensive effect of rauwolfia alkaloids; interference with antidepressant effects). Products include:
Pamelor ... 2019

Opium Alkaloids (Orthostatic hypotension; enhanced CNS depressant effects). Products include:
B & O No. 15A & No. 16A Supprettes ... 2395
Pantopon Injectable ... 1911

Oxazepam (Enhanced CNS depressant effects). Products include:
Serax Capsules ... 2522
Serax Tablets ... 2522

Oxycodone Hydrochloride (Orthostatic hypotension; enhanced CNS depressant effects). Products include:
Percocet Tablets ... 950
Percodan ... 951
Roxicodone Tablets, Oral Solution & Intensol (Oxycodone) ... 1992
Tylox Capsules ... 1382

Pancuronium Bromide Injection (Potentiation of pancuronium; dosage adjustments may be necessary).
No products indexed under this heading.

Penbutolol Sulfate (Additive and possibly excessive blockage). Products include:
Levatol ... 1832

Pentobarbital Sodium (Orthostatic hypotension; potentiation of pentobarbital). Products include:
Nembutal Sodium Capsules ... 534
Nembutal Sodium Solution ... 536
Nembutal Sodium Suppositories ... 538

Perphenazine (Enhanced CNS depressant effects). Products include:
Etrafon ... 2087
Triavil Tablets ... 1556
Trilafon ... 2123

Phenelzine Sulfate (Hyperpyrexia reaching crisis levels; moderate to sudden and severe hypertension). Products include:
Nardil ... 1742

Phenobarbital (Orthostatic hypotension; enhanced CNS depressant effects). Products include:
Arco-Lase Plus Tablets ... 607
Bellergal-S Tablets ... 1998
Bronkolixir ... ▣ 761
Bronkotabs Tablets ... ▣ 762
Donnatal ... 1858
Donnatal Extentabs ... 1859
Donnatal Tablets ... 1858
Donnazyme Tablets ... 1860
Kinesed Tablets ... 2272
Phenobarbital Elixir and Tablets ... 1293
Primatene Tablets-P Formula ... 2421
Quadrinal Tablets ... 1183
Tedral SA ... 1765

Phenoxybenzamine Hydrochloride (Potentiation of antihypertensive effects). Products include:
Dibenzyline Capsules ... 2207

Phentolamine Mesylate (Potentiation of antihypertensive effects). Products include:
Regitine ... 878

Phenylbutazone (Reduces diuretic and antihypertensive effect of thiazides). Products include:
Butazolidin Capsules & Tablets ... 1027

Phenylephrine (Prolonged action of direct-acting sympathomimetics).

Phenylephrine Bitartrate (Prolonged action of direct-acting sympathomimetics).
No products indexed under this heading.

Phenylephrine Hydrochloride (Prolonged action of direct-acting sympathomimetics). Products include:
AK-Dilate Solution 2.5% and 10% ... ◉ 203
Atrohist Sprinkle Capsules ... 558
Cerose-DM ... 2443
Codimal ... 846
Comhist LA Capsules ... 1618
Congespirin For Children Aspirin Free Chewable Cold Tablets ... 748
Cyclomydril ... ◉ 216
Deconsal Sprinkle Capsules ... 559
Dimetane Decongestant ... ▣ 673
Dristan Decongestant/Antihistamine/ Analgesic Coated Caplets ... ▣ 749
Dristan Cold Nasal Decongestant/ Antihistamine/ Analgesic Coated Tablets ... 2419
Dristan Advanced Formula Decongestant/Antihistamine/ Analgesic Tablets ... ▣ 749
Dristan Nasal Spray, Menthol ... 2419
Dristan Nasal Spray, Regular and Regular with Metered Pump ... 2419
Entex Capsules ... 1623
Entex Liquid ... 1623
Sinus Excedrin Analgesic, Decongestant Tablets & Caplets ... 750
Extendryl ... 994
4-Way Fast Acting Nasal Spray - Original Formula (regular & mentholated) & Metered Spray Pump (regular) ... 751
Hycomine Compound Tablets ... 929
Murocoll-2 Sterile Ophthalmic Solution ... ◉ 261
Mydfrin 2.5% ... ◉ 224
Naldecon Syrup, Tablets, Pediatric Drops and Pediatric Syrup ... 709
Neo-Synephrine Hydrochloride 1% Carpuject ... 2063
Neo-Synephrine Hydrochloride 1% Injection ... 2063
Neo-Synephrine Hydrochloride (Ophthalmic) ... 2064
Neo-Synephrine ... ▣ 759
Nöstril Nasal Decongestant ... ▣ 520
Novahistine Elixir ... ▣ 596
Phenergan VC ... 2500
Phenergan VC with Codeine ... 2501
Prefrin Liquifilm Vasoconstrictor and Lubricant Eye Drops ... ◉ 254
Prefrin-A ... ◉ 255
Quelidrine Syrup ... 556
Relief Vasoconstrictor and Lubricant Eye Drops ... ◉ 256
Robitussin Night Relief ... ▣ 677
Ru-Tuss with Hydrocodone ... 694
Ru-Tuss Tablets ... 693
Vasosulf ... ◉ 279
Vicks Sinex ... ▣ 665
Zincfrin ... ◉ 230

Phenylephrine Tannate (Prolonged action of direct-acting sympathomimetics). Products include:
Rynatan ... 2387
Rynatuss ... 2388

Pindolol (Additive and possibly excessive blockage). Products include:
Visken Tablets ... 2036

Piroxicam (Reduces diuretic and antihypertensive effect of thiazides). Products include:
Feldene Capsules ... 1777

Polythiazide (Potentiation of antihypertensive effects). Products include:
Minizide Capsules ... 1779
Renese Tablets ... 1785
Renese-R Tablets ... 1786

Prazepam (Enhanced CNS depressant effects). Products include:
Centrax ... 1693

Prazosin Hydrochloride (Potentiation of antihypertensive effects). Products include:
Minipress Capsules ... 1778
Minizide Capsules ... 1779

Prednisolone Acetate (May intensify electrolyte imbalance, particularly hypokalemia). Products include:
AK-Cide Sterile Ophthalmic Ointment & Suspension ... ◉ 202
Blephamide Liquifilm Sterile Ophthalmic Suspension ... 586
Blephamide S.O.P. Sterile Ophthalmic Ointment ... 586
Cetapred Ointment ... ◉ 220
⅛% Econopred & 1% Econopred Plus ... ◉ 217
Isopto Cetapred Suspension ... ◉ 220
Metimyd ... ◉ 306
Poly-Pred Liquifilm ... ◉ 250
Pred Forte ... ◉ 252
Pred Mild ... ◉ 254
Pred-G Liquifilm Sterile Ophthalmic Suspension ... ◉ 252
Pred-G S.O.P. Sterile Ophthalmic Ointment ... ◉ 253
Vasocidin Ointment ... ◉ 275

Prednisolone Sodium Phosphate (May intensify electrolyte imbalance, particularly hypokalemia). Products include:
AK-Pred ... ◉ 205
Hydeltrasol Injection, Sterile ... 1476
Inflamase ... ◉ 274
Pediapred Oral Liquid ... 987
Vasocidin Ophthalmic Solution ... ◉ 276

Prednisolone Tebutate (May intensify electrolyte imbalance, particularly hypokalemia). Products include:
Hydeltra-T.B.A. Sterile Suspension 1478

Prednisone (May intensify electrolyte imbalance, particularly hypokalemia). Products include:
Deltasone Tablets ... 2332

Prochlorperazine (Enhanced CNS depressant effects). Products include:
Compazine ... 2201

Promethazine Hydrochloride (Potentiation of promethazine; dosage adjustments may be necessary; enhanced CNS depressant effects). Products include:
Mepergan Injection ... 2479
Phenergan with Codeine ... 2497
Phenergan with Dextromethorphan 2499
Phenergan Injection ... 2493
Phenergan Suppositories ... 2496
Phenergan Syrup ... 2495
Phenergan Tablets ... 2496
Phenergan VC ... 2500
Phenergan VC with Codeine ... 2501

Propofol (Orthostatic hypotension; enhanced CNS depressant effects). Products include:
Diprivan Injection ... 2267

Propoxyphene Hydrochloride (Orthostatic hypotension; enhanced CNS depressant effects). Products include:
Darvon ... 1256
Wygesic Tablets ... 2540

Propoxyphene Napsylate (Orthostatic hypotension; enhanced CNS depressant effects). Products include:
Darvon-N/Darvocet-N ... 1254

Propranolol Hydrochloride (Additive and possibly excessive blockage). Products include:
Inderal ... 2459
Inderal LA Long Acting Capsules ... 2461
Inderide Tablets ... 2463
Inderide LA Long Acting Capsules .. 2465

Protriptyline Hydrochloride (Decreased hypotensive effect of rauwolfia alkaloids interference with antidepressant effects). Products include:
Vivactil Tablets ... 1567

Pseudoephedrine Hydrochloride (Action of indirect-acting sympathomimetics inhibited). Products include:
Actifed Capsules ... ▣ 539
Actifed Plus Caplets ... ▣ 539
Actifed Plus Tablets ... ▣ 540
Actifed with Codeine Cough Syrup.. 752
Actifed Syrup ... ▣ 540
Actifed Tablets ... ▣ 540
Actifed 12-Hour Capsules ... ▣ 539
Advil Cold & Sinus Caplets (formerly CoAdvil) ... 2416
Allerest ... ▣ 559
Anatuss LA Tablets ... 1359
Benadryl Decongestant Elixir ... ▣ 635
Benadryl Decongestant ... ▣ 635
Benadryl Plus ... ▣ 636
Benadryl Plus Nighttime ... ▣ 637
Benylin Decongestant ... ▣ 638
Brexin L.A. Capsules ... 2078
Bromfed Capsules (Timed Release) ... 1615
Bromfed Syrup ... ▣ 628
Bromfed ... 1615
CoAdvil ... ▣ 748
Allergy-Sinus Comtrex Multi-Symptom Allergy Sinus Formula Tablets & Caplets ... 746
Cough Formula Comtrex ... 746
Comtrex Multi-Symptom Cold Reliever Tablets/Caplets/Liqui-Gels/Liquid ... 745
Day-Night Comtrex ... 747
Non-Drowsy Comtrex ... 747
Congess ... 994
Congestac Caplets ... ▣ 617
Contac Jr. Children's Cold Medicine ... ▣ 712
Contac Nighttime Cold Medicine ... ▣ 713
Contac Sinus Caplets Maximum Strength Non-Drowsy Formula ... ▣ 710
Contac Sinus Tablets Maximum Strength Non-Drowsy Formula ... ▣ 710
Deconamine ... 663
Deconsal II Tablets ... 559
Dimacol Caplets ... ▣ 672
Dimetane-DX Cough Syrup ... 1858
Dorcol Children's Cough Syrup ... ▣ 685
Dorcol Children's Decongestant Liquid ... ▣ 685
Dorcol Children's Liquid Cold Formula ... ▣ 686
Maximum Strength Dristan Decongestant/Analgesic Coated Caplets ... ▣ 750
No Drowsiness Dristan Cold Nasal Decongestant/Analgesic Coated Caplets ... 2420
Dristan Sinus Caplets ... 2419
Sinus Excedrin Analgesic, Decongestant Tablets & Caplets ... ▣ 533
Fedahist Gyrocaps ... 2145
Fedahist Timecaps ... 2145
Guaifed ... 1615
Guaifed Syrup ... ▣ 629
Isoclor Expectorant ... 982
Isoclor Timesule Capsules ... ▣ 561
Kronofed-A ... 970
Medi-Flu Caplet, Liquid ... ▣ 640
Novafed A Capsules ... 1342
Novafed Capsules ... 1342
Novahistine DH ... 1342
Novahistine DMX ... ▣ 595
Novahistine Expectorant ... 1343
Nucofed Capsules ... 2219
Nucofed Expectorant ... 2219
Nucofed Pediatric Expectorant ... 2220
Nucofed Syrup ... 2219

Ornex Caplets ▣ 618
PediaCare Allergy Relief Formula Liquid 1362
PediaCare Cough-Cold Formula Liquid 1362
PediaCare Infants' Oral Decongestant Drops 1362
PediaCare Night Rest Cough-Cold Formula Liquid 1362
PediaCare 6-12 Cough-Cold Formula Chewable Tablets 1362
Robitussin-DAC Syrup 1875
Robitussin-PE ▣ 677
Rondec 1975
Rondec-DM 1976
Rondec-TR Tablet 1975
Ru-Tuss DE Tablets 694
Ryna ▣ 741
Seldane-D Extended-Release Tablets 1350
Sinarest ▣ 562
Sine-Aid Maximum Strength Sinus Headache Caplets 1365
Sine-Aid Maximum Strength Sinus Headache Tablets 1365
Sine-Off Maximum Strength Allergy/Sinus Formula Caplets ▣ 721
Sine-Off Maximum Strength No Drowsiness Formula Caplets ▣ 722
Singlet Tablets ▣ 598
Sinutab Maximum Strength ▣ 641
Sinutab Maximum Strength Without Drowsiness Tablets & Caplets ▣ 642
Sinutab Regular Strength Without Drowsiness Formula ▣ 641
St. Joseph Nighttime Cold Medicine ▣ 705
Sudafed Children's Liquid ▣ 543
Sudafed Cough Syrup ▣ 543
Sudafed Plus Liquid ▣ 544
Sudafed Plus Tablets ▣ 545
Sudafed Sinus Caplets ▣ 545
Sudafed Sinus Tablets ▣ 545
Sudafed Tablets, 30 mg ▣ 544
Sudafed Tablets, Adult Strength, 60 mg ▣ 544
Sudafed 12 Hour Capsules ▣ 545
TheraFlu Flu and Cold Medicine ▣ 687
Triaminic Nite Light ▣ 689
Tylenol Allergy Sinus Medication Caplets and Gelcaps, Maximum Strength 1372
Children's Tylenol Cold Liquid Formula and Chewable Tablets 1368
Tylenol Cold & Flu Hot Medication, Packets 1369
Tylenol Cold & Flu No Drowsiness Hot Medication, Packets 1371
Tylenol Cold Medication Caplets and Tablets 1370
Tylenol Cold Medication No Drowsiness Formula Caplets 1370
Tylenol Cold Night Time Medication Liquid 1371
Tylenol Cough Medication Liquid with Decongestant, Maximum Strength 1372
Tylenol, Maximum Strength, Sinus Medication Gelcaps, Caplets and Tablets 1373
Ursinus Inlay-Tabs ▣ 691
Vicks Children's NyQuil ▣ 664
Vicks Daycare ▣ 660
Vicks Formula 44D Decongestant Cough Medicine ▣ 662
Vicks Formula 44M Multi-Symptom Cough Medicine ▣ 662
Vicks NyQuil Nighttime Colds Medicine-Original & Cherry Flavor ▣ 664
Vicks Pediatric Formula 44 Cough & Congestion Medicine ▣ 663
Vicks Pediatric Formula 44m Multi-Symptom Cough & Cold Medicine ▣ 663

Pseudoephedrine Sulfate (Action of indirect-acting sympathomimetics inhibited). Products include:
Afrin Tablets ▣ 693
Chlor-Trimeton Decongestant ▣ 694
Disophrol Chronotab Sustained-Action Tablets ▣ 698
Drixoral Antihistamine/Nasal Decongestant Syrup ▣ 698
Drixoral Non-Drowsy Formula ▣ 699
Drixoral Plus Extended-Release Tablets ▣ 699
Drixoral Sinus ▣ 700
Drixoral Sustained-Action Tablets ▣ 698
Sinutab Allergy Formula Sustained Action Tablets ▣ 640
Trinalin Repetabs Tablets 1170

Quazepam (Orthostatic hypotension; enhanced CNS depressant effects). Products include:
Doral Tablets 2383

Quinidine Gluconate (Cardiac arrhythmias). Products include:
Quinaglute Dura-Tabs Tablets 663

Quinidine Polygalacturonate (Cardiac arrhythmias). Products include:
Cardioquin Tablets 1812

Quinidine Sulfate (Cardiac arrhythmias). Products include:
Quinidex Extentabs 1868

Ramipril (Potentiation of antihypertensive effects). Products include:
Altace Capsules 1086

Rauwolfia Serpentina (Potentiation of antihypertensive effects). Products include:
Raudixin Tablets 1803
Rauzide Tablets 1804

Rescinnamine (Potentiation of antihypertensive effects).
No products indexed under this heading.

Secobarbital Sodium (Orthostatic hypotension; enhanced CNS depressant effects). Products include:
Seconal Sodium Pulvules 1296

Selegiline Hydrochloride (Hyperpyrexia reaching crisis levels; moderate to sudden and severe hypertension). Products include:
Eldepryl 2250

Sodium Nitroprusside (Potentiation of antihypertensive effects). Products include:
Nipride I.V. Infusion 1909

Spironolactone (Potentiation of antihypertensive effects). Products include:
Aldactazide 2150
Aldactone 2152

Sufentanil Citrate (Orthostatic hypotension; enhanced CNS depressant effects). Products include:
Sufenta Injection 1147

Sulindac (Reduces diuretic and antihypertensive effect of thiazides). Products include:
Clinoril Tablets 1433

Temazepam (Enhanced CNS depressant effects). Products include:
Restoril Capsules 2023

Terazosin Hydrochloride (Potentiation of antihypertensive effects). Products include:
Hytrin Tablets 529

Thiamylal Sodium (Orthostatic hypotension; enhanced CNS depressant effects). Products include:
Surital Ampoules, Steri-Vials 1764

Thioridazine Hydrochloride (Enhanced CNS depressant effects). Products include:
Mellaril 2011

Thiothixene (Enhanced CNS depressant effects). Products include:
Navane Capsules and Concentrate 1954
Navane Intramuscular 1956

Ticarcillin Disodium (Potentiation of antihypertensive effects). Products include:
Ticar for Injection 2236
Timentin for Injection 2239

Timolol Maleate (Additive and possibly excessive blockage). Products include:
Blocadren Tablets 1429
Timolide Tablets 1547
Timoptic in Ocudose 1552
Timoptic Sterile Ophthalmic Solution 1550

Tolazamide (Elevated blood glucose levels; dosage of hypoglycemic may be affected). Products include:
Tolinase Tablets 2365

Tolbutamide (Elevated blood glucose levels; dosage of hypoglycemic may be affected). Products include:
Orinase Tablets 2354

Tolmetin Sodium (Reduces diuretic and antihypertensive effect of thiazides). Products include:
Tolectin (200, 400 and 600 mg) 1379

Tranylcypromine Sulfate (Hyperpyrexia reaching crisis levels; moderate to sudden and severe hypertension). Products include:
Parnate Tablets 2222

Triamcinolone (May intensify electrolyte imbalance, particularly hypokalemia).
No products indexed under this heading.

Triamcinolone Acetonide (May intensify electrolyte imbalance, particularly hypokalemia). Products include:
Aristocort A 1010
Azmacort Inhaler 1837
Kenalog Cream, Lotion & Ointment 2401
Kenalog-10 Injection 2402
Kenalog-40 Injection 2403
Kenalog in Orabase 604
Kenalog Spray 2401
Mycolog II Cream and Ointment 2407
Mytrex Cream & Ointment 2080
Nasacort Nasal Inhaler 1844

Triamcinolone Diacetate (May intensify electrolyte imbalance, particularly hypokalemia). Products include:
Aristocort Suspension 1008

Triamcinolone Hexacetonide (May intensify electrolyte imbalance, particularly hypokalemia). Products include:
Aristospan Suspension 1011

Triamterene (Potentiation of antihypertensive effects). Products include:
Dyazide Capsules 2208
Dyrenium Capsules 2210
Maxzide 1215

Triazolam (Enhanced CNS depressant effects). Products include:
Halcion Tablets 2340

Trifluoperazine Hydrochloride (Enhanced CNS depressant effects). Products include:
Stelazine 2226

Trimethaphan Camsylate (Potentiation of antihypertensive effects). Products include:
Arfonad Ampuls 1887

Trimipramine Maleate (decreased hypotensive effect of rauwolfia alkaloids interference with antidepressant effects). Products include:
Surmontil Capsules 2524

Tyramine (Action of indirect-acting sympathomimetics inhibited).

Vecuronium Bromide (Potentiation of vecuronium; dosage adjustments may be necessary). Products include:
Norcuron 1642

SANDIMMUNE I.V. AMPULS FOR INFUSION
(Cyclosporine) 2024
May interact with immunosuppressive agents, potassium sparing diuretics, and certain other agents. Compounds in these categories include:

Amiloride Hydrochloride (Do not use with cyclosporine). Products include:
Midamor Tablets 1508
Moduretic Tablets 1510

Amphotericin B (Potential synergies of nephrotoxicity may occur). Products include:
Fungizone Cream, Lotion and Ointment 2261
Fungizone Intravenous 2262

Antibiotics, unspecified (Potential synergies of nephrotoxicity may occur).

Azapropazon (Potential nephrotoxic synergy).

Azathioprine (Increases susceptibility to infection). Products include:
Imuran 768

Bromocriptine Mesylate (Increases cyclosporine levels). Products include:
Parlodel 2020

Carbamazepine (Decreases cyclosporine plasma concentrations). Products include:
Tegretol Chewable Tablets 654
Tegretol Suspension 656
Tegretol Tablets 654

Cimetidine (Potential nephrotoxic synergy). Products include:
Tagamet Tablets 2228

Cimetidine Hydrochloride (Potential nephrotoxic synergy). Products include:
Tagamet 2228

Danazol (Increases cyclosporine plasma concentrations). Products include:
Danocrine Capsules 2046

Diclofenac Sodium (Potential nephrotoxic synergy). Products include:
Voltaren Ophthalmic Sterile Ophthalmic Solution ⊙ 268
Voltaren Tablets 1042

Digoxin (Reduced clearance of digoxin and potential for severe digitalis toxicity). Products include:
Lanoxicaps 772
Lanoxin Elixir Pediatric 775
Lanoxin Injection 778
Lanoxin Injection Pediatric 781
Lanoxin Tablets 783

Diltiazem Hydrochloride (Increases cyclosporine plasma concentrations). Products include:
Cardizem Tablets-30 mg, 60 mg, 90 mg and 120 mg 1329
Cardizem SR Capsules-60 mg, 90 mg and 120 mg 1327

Erythromycin (Increases cyclosporine plasma concentrations; dosage adjustments are essential). Products include:
A/T/S Topical Gel and Topical Solution 1089
AK-Mycin Ointment ⊙ 204
Benzamycin Topical Gel 907
E-Mycin Tablets 688
ETS-2% 1685
ERYC 1720
Erycette (erythromycin 2%) Topical Solution 1678
Ery-Tab Tablets 521
Erythromycin Base Filmtab 525
Erythromycin Delayed-Release Capsules, USP 526
Ilotycin Ophthalmic Ointment 915
PCE Dispertab Tablets 549
Pediazole 1973
T-Stat 2.0% Topical Solution and Pads 2409
Theramycin Z Topical Solution 2% 1410

Erythromycin Estolate (Increases cyclosporine plasma concentrations; dosage adjustments are essential). Products include:
- Ilosone 913

Erythromycin Ethylsuccinate (Increases cyclosporine plasma concentrations; dosage adjustments are essential). Products include:
- E.E.S. 522
- EryPed 519
- Pediazole 1973

Erythromycin Gluceptate (Increases cyclosporine plasma concentrations; dosage adjustments are essential). Products include:
- Ilotycin Gluceptate, IV, Vials 915

Erythromycin Lactobionate (Increases cyclosporine plasma concentrations; dosage adjustments are essential).
- No products indexed under this heading.

Erythromycin Stearate (Increases cyclosporine plasma concentrations; dosage adjustments are essential). Products include:
- Erythrocin Stearate Filmtab 523

Fluconazole (Increases cyclosporine levels). Products include:
- Diflucan Injection and Tablets 1948

Gentamicin Sulfate (Potential synergies of nephrotoxicity may occur). Products include:
- Garamycin Injectable 2093
- Garamyćin Ophthalmic .... ◉ 305
- Genoptic Liquifilm Sterile Ophthalmic Solution .... ◉ 247
- Genoptic S.O.P. Sterile Ophthalmic Ointment .... ◉ 247
- Gentacidin Ointment .... ◉ 273
- Gentacidin Solution .... ◉ 273
- Gentak Ointment & Solution .... ◉ 208
- G-myticin Creme and Ointment 0.1% 1770
- Pred-G Liquifilm Sterile Ophthalmic Suspension .... ◉ 252
- Pred-G S.O.P. Sterile Ophthalmic Ointment .... ◉ 253

Immune Globulin (Human) (Increases susceptibility to infection). Products include:
- MICRhoGAM Rh$_0$(D) Immune Globulin (Human) 1650
- RhoGAM Rh$_0$(D) Immune Globulin (Human) 1651

Immune Globulin Intravenous (Human) (Increases susceptibility to infection). Products include:
- Gamimune N Immune Globulin Intravenous (Human) 1572
- Gammagard Immune Globulin, Intravenous (Human) 658
- Iveegam 1129
- Sandoglobulin I.V. 2027

Itraconazole (Increases cyclosporine levels).

Ketoconazole (Increases cyclosporine plasma concentrations; dosage adjustments are essential). Products include:
- Nizoral 2% Cream 1143
- Nizoral 2% Shampoo 1144
- Nizoral Tablets 1145

Lovastatin (Concomitant administration associated with development of myositis). Products include:
- Mevacor Tablets 1505

Melphalan (Potential nephrotoxic synergy). Products include:
- Alkeran Tablets 754

Methylprednisolone (Increases cyclosporine plasma concentrations; dosage adjustments are essential). Products include:
- Medrol 2348

Methylprednisolone Acetate (Increases cyclosporine plasma concentrations; dosage adjustments are essential). Products include:
- Depo-Medrol Sterile Aqueous Suspension 2334

Methylprednisolone Sodium Succinate (Increases cyclosporine plasma concentrations; dosage adjustments are essential). Products include:
- Solu-Medrol Sterile Powder 2363

Metoclopramide Hydrochloride (Increases cyclosporine levels). Products include:
- Reglan 1869

Muromonab-CD3 (Increased susceptibility to infection and increased risk for development of lymphomas and malignancies). Products include:
- Orthoclone OKT3 Sterile Solution .. 1645

Nephrotoxic Drugs (Potential synergics of nephrotoxicity).

Nicardipine Hydrochloride (Increases cyclosporine plasma concentrations). Products include:
- Cardene Capsules 2290

Nifedipine (Potential for frequent gingival hyperplasia). Products include:
- Adalat Capsules (10 mg and 20 mg) 1587
- Procardia Capsules 1781
- Procardia XL Tablets 1783

Phenobarbital (Decreases cyclosporine plasma levels; dosage adjustments are essential). Products include:
- Arco-Lase Plus Tablets 607
- Bellergal-S Tablets 1998
- Bronkolixir .... ⊞ 761
- Bronkotabs Tablets .... ⊞ 762
- Donnatal 1858
- Donnatal Extentabs 1859
- Donnatal Tablets 1858
- Donnazyme Tablets 1860
- Kinesed Tablets 2272
- Phenobarbital Elixir and Tablets 1293
- Primatene Tablets-P Formula 2421
- Quadrinal Tablets 1183
- Tedral SA 1765

Phenytoin (Decreases cyclosporine plasma levels; dosage adjustments are essential). Products include:
- Dilantin Infatabs 1710
- Dilantin-30 Pediatric/Dilantin-125 Suspension 1713

Phenytoin Sodium (Decreases cyclosporine plasma levels; dosage adjustments are essential). Products include:
- Dilantin Kapseals 1708
- Dilantin Parenteral 1712
- Dilantin with Phenobarbital Kapseals 1715

Prednisolone (Reduced clearance of prednisolone).
- No products indexed under this heading.

Prednisolone Acetate (Reduced clearance of prednisolone). Products include:
- AK-Cide Sterile Ophthalmic Ointment & Suspension .... ◉ 202
- Blephamide Liquifilm Sterile Ophthalmic Suspension 586
- Blephamide S.O.P. Sterile Ophthalmic Ointment 586
- Cetapred Ointment .... ◉ 220
- ⅛% Econopred & 1% Econopred Plus .... ◉ 217
- Isopto Cetapred Suspension .... ◉ 220
- Metimyd .... ◉ 306
- Poly-Pred Liquifilm .... ◉ 250
- Pred Forte .... ◉ 252
- Pred Mild .... ◉ 254
- Pred-G Liquifilm Sterile Ophthalmic Suspension .... ◉ 252
- Pred-G S.O.P. Sterile Ophthalmic Ointment .... ◉ 253
- Vasocidin Ointment .... ◉ 275

Prednisolone Sodium Phosphate (Reduced clearance of prednisolone). Products include:
- AK-Pred .... ◉ 205
- Hydeltrasol Injection, Sterile 1476
- Inflamase .... ◉ 274
- Pediapred Oral Liquid 987
- Vasocidin Ophthalmic Solution .... ◉ 276

Prednisolone Tebutate (Reduced clearance of prednisolone). Products include:
- Hydeltra-T.B.A. Sterile Suspension 1478

Ranitidine Hydrochloride (Potential nephrotoxic synergy). Products include:
- Zantac Injection and Zantac Injection Premixed 1063
- Zantac 1065

Rifampin (Decreases cyclosporine plasma levels; dosage adjustments are essential). Products include:
- Rifadin 1345
- Rifamate Capsules 1347
- Rimactane Capsules 879

Spironolactone (Do not use with cyclosporine). Products include:
- Aldactazide 2150
- Aldactone 2152

Sulfamethoxazole (Decreases cyclosporine plasma levels; dosage adjustments are essential). Products include:
- Azo Gantanol Tablets 1887
- Bactrim DS Tablets 1891
- Bactrim I.V. Infusion 1889
- Bactrim 1891
- Gantanol 1899
- Septra 813
- Septra I.V. Infusion 808
- Septra I.V. Infusion ADD-Vantage Vials 810
- Septra 813

Tobramycin (Potential synergies of nephrotoxicity may occur). Products include:
- TobraDex Ophthalmic Suspension and Ointment .... ◉ 228
- Tobrex Ophthalmic Ointment and Solution 572

Tobramycin Sulfate (Potential synergies of nephrotoxicity may occur). Products include:
- Nebcin Vials, Hyporets & ADD-Vantage 1286

Triamterene (Do not use with cyclosporine). Products include:
- Dyazide Capsules 2208
- Dyrenium Capsules 2210
- Maxzide 1215

Trimethoprim (Decreases cyclosporine plasma levels; dosage adjustments are essential). Products include:
- Bactrim DS Tablets 1891
- Bactrim I.V. Infusion 1889
- Bactrim 1891
- Proloprim Tablets 799
- Septra 813
- Septra I.V. Infusion 808
- Septra I.V. Infusion ADD-Vantage Vials 810
- Septra 813
- Trimpex Tablets 1922

Vancomycin Hydrochloride (Potential nephrotoxic synergy). Products include:
- Vancocin HCl, Oral Solution & Pulvules 1304
- Vancocin HCl, Vials & ADD-Vantage 1302

Verapamil Hydrochloride (Increases cyclosporine levels). Products include:
- Calan SR Caplets 2157
- Calan Tablets 2155
- Isoptin Injectable 1177
- Isoptin Oral Tablets 1179
- Isoptin SR Sustained Release Tablets 1181
- Verelan Capsules 1243
- Verelan Capsules 2535

SANDIMMUNE ORAL SOLUTION
(Cyclosporine) 2024

See **Sandimmune I.V. Ampuls for Infusion**

SANDIMMUNE SOFT GELATIN CAPSULES
(Cyclosporine) 2024

See **Sandimmune I.V. Ampuls for Infusion**

SANDOGLOBULIN I.V.
(Immune Globulin (Human)) 2027

No interactions described in labeling.

SANDOSTATIN INJECTION
(Octreotide Acetate) 2029

May interact with oral hypoglycemic agents, insulin, beta blockers, and certain other agents. Compounds in these categories include:

Acebutolol Hydrochloride (Adjustment of the dosage of beta blockers may be required). Products include:
- Sectral Capsules 2520

Atenolol (Adjustment of the dosage of beta blockers may be required). Products include:
- Tenoretic Tablets 1105
- Tenormin Tablets and I.V. Injection 1107

Betaxolol Hydrochloride (Adjustment of the dosage of beta blockers may be required). Products include:
- Betoptic Sterile Ophthalmic Solution 569
- Betoptic S Sterile Ophthalmic Suspension 570
- Kerlone Tablets 2172

Carteolol Hydrochloride (Adjustment of the dosage of beta blockers may be required). Products include:
- Cartrol Tablets 507

Chlorpropamide (Adjustment of the dosage of hypoglycemic agents may be required). Products include:
- Diabinese Tablets 1775

Cyclosporine (A single case of transplant rejection episode in a patient immunosuppressed with cyclosporin has been reported). Products include:
- Sandimmune 2024

Diazoxide (Adjustment of the dosage of diazoxide may be required). Products include:
- Hyperstat I.V. Injection 2095
- Proglycem 649

Esmolol Hydrochloride (Adjustment of the dosage of beta blockers may be required). Products include:
- Brevibloc Injection 942

Glipizide (Adjustment of the dosage of hypoglycemic agents may be required). Products include:
- Glucotrol 1952

Glyburide (Adjustment of the dosage of hypoglycemic agents may be required). Products include:
- DiaBeta 1091
- Micronase Tablets 2350

Insulin, Human (Adjustment of the dosage of insulin may be required).
- No products indexed under this heading.

Insulin, Human Isophane Suspension (Adjustment of the dosage of insulin may be required). Products include:
- Humulin N, 100 Units 1270

Insulin, Human NPH (Adjustment of the dosage of insulin may be required). Products include:
- Insulatard NPH Human 1627

(⊞ Described in PDR For Nonprescription Drugs)

(◉ Described in PDR For Ophthalmology)

Novolin N 1627
Novolin N PenFill Cartridges 1628
Novolin N Prefilled 1628

Insulin, Human Regular (Adjustment of the dosage of insulin may be required). Products include:
Humulin BR, 100 Units 1268
Humulin R, 100 Units 1272
Novolin R 1627
Novolin R PenFill Cartridges 1628
Novolin R Prefilled 1629
Velosulin Human 1628

Insulin, Human, Zinc Suspension (Adjustment of the dosage of insulin may be required). Products include:
Humulin L, 100 Units 1268
Humulin U, 100 Units 1272
Novolin L 1627

Insulin, NPH (Adjustment of the dosage of insulin may be required). Products include:
NPH, 40 & 100 Units 1273
Beef NPH, 100 Units 1274
Pork NPH, 100 Units 1275
Insulatard NPH 1626
NPH Insulin 1626
NPH Purified Pork Isophane Insulin 1626

Insulin, Regular (Adjustment of the dosage of insulin may be required). Products include:
Regular, 40 & 100 Units 1273
Beef Regular, 100 Units 1275
Pork Regular, 100 Units 1275
Pork Regular (Concentrated), 500 Units 1276
Regular Insulin 1625
Regular Purified Pork Insulin 1626
Velosulin 1627

Insulin, Zinc Crystals (Adjustment of the dosage of insulin may be required). Products include:
NPH, 40 & 100 Units 1273

Insulin, Zinc Suspension (Adjustment of the dosage of insulin may be required). Products include:
Lente, 40 & 100 Units 1272
Protamine, Zinc, 40 & 100 Units 1273
Lente Iletin I 1272
Beef Lente, 100 Units 1274
Beef Protamine Zinc, 100 Units 1274
Pork Lente, 100 Units 1275
Pork, Protamine, Zinc, 100 Units 1275
Lente Insulin 1626
Lente Purified Pork Insulin 1626
Semilente Insulin 1625
Ultralente Insulin 1626

Labetalol Hydrochloride (Adjustment of the dosage of beta blockers may be required). Products include:
Normodyne Injection 2108
Normodyne Tablets 2110
Normozide Tablets 2112
Trandate HCT Tablets 579
Trandate Injection 577
Trandate Tablets 579

Metoprolol Tartrate (Adjustment of the dosage of beta blockers may be required). Products include:
Lopressor Ampuls 1032
Lopressor HCT Tablets 1034
Lopressor Tablets 1032

Nadolol (Adjustment of the dosage of beta blockers may be required). Products include:
Corgard Tablets 701
Corzide Tablets 702

Penbutolol Sulfate (Adjustment of the dosage of beta blockers may be required). Products include:
Levatol 1832

Pindolol (Adjustment of the dosage of beta blockers may be required). Products include:
Visken Tablets 2036

Propranolol Hydrochloride (Adjustment of the dosage of beta blockers may be required). Products include:
Inderal 2459
Inderal LA Long Acting Capsules 2461
Inderide Tablets 2463
Inderide LA Long Acting Capsules .. 2465

Timolol Maleate (Adjustment of the dosage of beta blockers may be required). Products include:
Blocadren Tablets 1429
Timolide Tablets 1547
Timoptic in Ocudose 1552
Timoptic Sterile Ophthalmic Solution 1550

Tolazamide (Adjustment of the dosage of hypoglycemic agents may be required). Products include:
Tolinase Tablets 2365

Tolbutamide (Adjustment of the dosage of hypoglycemic agents may be required). Products include:
Orinase Tablets 2354

SANOREX TABLETS
(Mazindol) 2030
May interact with monoamine oxidase inhibitors, insulin, vasopressors, and certain other agents. Compounds in these categories include:

Dopamine Hydrochloride (Potentiated pressor effects). Products include:
Intropin Injection 930

Epinephrine Hydrochloride (Potentiated pressor effects). Products include:
Adrenalin Chloride Solution 1:100 & 1:1,000 1689
Epifrin .... ◉ 244
Glaucon .... ◉ 218

Furazolidone (Concurrent use is contraindicated; potential for hypertensive crises). Products include:
Furoxone 1855

Guanethidine Monosulfate (Decreased hypotensive effect). Products include:
Esimil Tablets 864
Ismelin Tablets 869

Insulin, Human (Altered insulin requirements).
No products indexed under this heading.

Insulin, Human Isophane Suspension (Altered insulin requirements). Products include:
Humulin N, 100 Units 1270

Insulin, Human NPH (Altered insulin requirements). Products include:
Insulatard NPH Human 1627
Novolin N 1627
Novolin N PenFill Cartridges 1628
Novolin N Prefilled 1628

Insulin, Human Regular (Altered insulin requirements). Products include:
Humulin BR, 100 Units 1268
Humulin R, 100 Units 1272
Novolin R 1627
Novolin R PenFill Cartridges 1628
Novolin R Prefilled 1629
Velosulin Human 1628

Insulin, Human, Zinc Suspension (Altered insulin requirements). Products include:
Humulin L, 100 Units 1268
Humulin U, 100 Units 1272
Novolin L 1627

Insulin, NPH (Altered insulin requirements). Products include:
NPH, 40 & 100 Units 1273
Beef NPH, 100 Units 1274
Pork NPH, 100 Units 1275
Insulatard NPH 1626
NPH Insulin 1626
NPH Purified Pork Isophane Insulin 1626

Insulin, Regular (Altered insulin requirements). Products include:
Regular, 40 & 100 Units 1273
Beef Regular, 100 Units 1275
Pork Regular, 100 Units 1275
Pork Regular (Concentrated), 500 Units 1276
Regular Insulin 1625
Regular Purified Pork Insulin 1626
Velosulin 1627

Insulin, Zinc Crystals (Altered insulin requirements). Products include:
NPH, 40 & 100 Units 1273

Insulin, Zinc Suspension (Altered insulin requirements). Products include:
Lente, 40 & 100 Units 1272
Protamine, Zinc, 40 & 100 Units 1273
Lente Iletin I 1272
Beef Lente, 100 Units 1274
Beef Protamine Zinc, 100 Units 1274
Pork Lente, 100 Units 1275
Pork, Protamine, Zinc, 100 Units 1275
Lente Insulin 1626
Lente Purified Pork Insulin 1626
Semilente Insulin 1625
Ultralente Insulin 1626

Isocarboxazid (Concurrent use is contraindicated; potential for hypertensive crises). Products include:
Marplan Tablets 1906

Metaraminol Bitartrate (Potentiated pressor effects). Products include:
Aramine Injection 1424

Methoxamine Hydrochloride (Potentiated pressor effects). Products include:
Vasoxyl Injection 819

Norepinephrine Bitartrate (Potentiated pressor effects). Products include:
Levophed Bitartrate Injection 2054

Phenelzine Sulfate (Concurrent use is contraindicated; potential for hypertensive crises). Products include:
Nardil 1742

Phenylephrine Hydrochloride (Potentiated pressor effects). Products include:
AK-Dilate Solution 2.5% and 10% .... ◉ 203
Atrohist Sprinkle Capsules 558
Cerose-DM 2443
Codimal 846
Comhist LA Capsules 1618
Congespirin For Children Aspirin Free Chewable Cold Tablets 748
Cyclomydril .... ◉ 216
Deconsal Sprinkle Capsules 559
Dimetane Decongestant .... ▣ 673
Dristan Decongestant/Antihistamine/ Analgesic Coated Caplets .... ▣ 749
Dristan Cold Nasal Decongestant/ Antihistamine/ Analgesic Coated Tablets 2419
Dristan Advanced Formula Decongestant/Antihistamine/ Analgesic Tablets .... ▣ 749
Dristan Nasal Spray, Menthol 2419
Dristan Nasal Spray, Regular and Regular with Metered Pump 2419
Entex Capsules 1623
Entex Liquid 1623
Sinus Excedrin Analgesic, Decongestant Tablets & Caplets 750
Extendryl 994
4-Way Fast Acting Nasal Spray - Original Formula (regular & mentholated) & Metered Spray Pump (regular) 751
Hycomine Compound Tablets 929
Murocoll-2 Sterile Ophthalmic Solution .... ◉ 261
Mydfrin 2.5% .... ◉ 224
Naldecon Syrup, Tablets, Pediatric Drops and Pediatric Syrup 709
Neo-Synephrine Hydrochloride 1% Carpuject 2063
Neo-Synephrine Hydrochloride 1% Injection 2063
Neo-Synephrine Hydrochloride (Ophthalmic) 2064
Neo-Synephrine .... ▣ 759
Nōstril Nasal Decongestant .... ▣ 520
Novahistine Elixir .... ▣ 596
Phenergan VC 2500
Phenergan VC with Codeine 2501
Prefrin Liquifilm Vasoconstrictor and Lubricant Eye Drops .... ◉ 254
Prefrin-A .... ◉ 255
Quelidrine Syrup 556
Relief Vasoconstrictor and Lubricant Eye Drops .... ◉ 256
Robitussin Night Relief .... ▣ 677
Ru-Tuss with Hydrocodone 694
Ru-Tuss Tablets 693
Vasosulf .... ◉ 279
Vicks Sinex .... ▣ 665
Zincfrin .... ◉ 230

Selegiline Hydrochloride (Concurrent use is contraindicated; potential for hypertensive crises). Products include:
Eldepryl 2250

Tranylcypromine Sulfate (Concurrent use is contraindicated; potential for hypertensive crises). Products include:
Parnate Tablets 2222

SANSERT TABLETS
(Methysergide Maleate) 2031
No interactions described in labeling.

SARAPIN
(Sarracenia purpurea) 1086
No interactions described in labeling.

SCLEROMATE
(Morrhuate Sodium) 1685
No interactions described in labeling.

SEBULEX ANTISEBORRHEIC TREATMENT SHAMPOO
(Sulfur Preparations, Salicylic Acid) .. 2408
No interactions described in labeling.

SEBULEX SHAMPOO WITH CONDITIONERS
(Sulfur Preparations, Salicylic Acid) .. 2408
No interactions described in labeling.

SEBUTONE AND SEBUTONE CREAM ANTISEBORRHEIC TAR SHAMPOOS
(Sulfur Preparations, Salicylic Acid, Coal Tar) 2408
No interactions described in labeling.

SECONAL SODIUM PULVULES
(Secobarbital Sodium) 1296
May interact with central nervous system depressants, narcotic analgesics, tranquilizers, antihistamines, oral anticoagulants, corticosteroids, monoamine oxidase inhibitors, oral contraceptives, and certain other agents. Compounds in these categories include:

Alcohol (Concomitant use may produce additive CNS-depressant effects).

Alfentanil Hydrochloride (Concomitant use may produce additive CNS-depressant effects). Products include:
Alfenta Injection 1131

Alprazolam (Concomitant use may produce additive CNS-depressant effects). Products include:
Xanax Tablets 2367

Aprobarbital (Concomitant use may produce additive CNS-depressant effects). Products include:
Alurate Elixir 1883

Astemizole (Concomitant use may produce additive CNS-depressant effects). Products include:
Hismanal Tablets 1138

Azatadine Maleate (Concomitant use may produce additive CNS-depressant effects). Products include:
Optimine Tablets 2115

Trinalin Repetabs Tablets 1170

Betamethasone Acetate (Enhanced metabolism of exogenous corticosteroids). Products include:
Celestone Soluspan Suspension 2081

Betamethasone Sodium Phosphate (Enhanced metabolism of exogenous corticosteroids). Products include:
Celestone Soluspan Suspension 2081

Bromodiphenhydramine Hydrochloride (Concomitant use may produce additive CNS-depressant effects).
No products indexed under this heading.

Brompheniramine Maleate (Concomitant use may produce additive CNS-depressant effects). Products include:
Alka Seltzer Plus Sinus Allergy Medicine ▣ 624
Atrohist Sprinkle Capsules 558
Bromfed Capsules (Timed Release) 1615
Bromfed Syrup ▣ 628
Bromfed 1615
Dimetane Decongestant ▣ 673
Dimetane ▣ 672
Dimetane-DC Cough Syrup 1857
Dimetane-DX Cough Syrup 1858
Dimetapp Elixir ▣ 673
Dimetapp DM Elixir ▣ 674
Dimetapp Extentabs ▣ 674
Dimetapp Plus Caplets ▣ 675
Dimetapp Tablets ▣ 675
Drixoral Antihistamine/Nasal Decongestant Syrup ▣ 698

Buprenorphine (Concomitant use may produce additive CNS-depressant effects).
No products indexed under this heading.

Buspirone Hydrochloride (Concomitant use may produce additive CNS-depressant effects). Products include:
BuSpar 1401

Butabarbital (Concomitant use may produce additive CNS-depressant effects). Products include:
Pyridium Plus 1764

Butalbital (Concomitant use may produce additive CNS-depressant effects). Products include:
Esgic-Plus Tablets 1002
Esgic Tablets & Capsules 1001
Fioricet Tablets 2006
Fiorinal Capsules 2007
Fiorinal with Codeine Capsules 2008
Fiorinal Tablets 2007
Phrenilin 838
Sedapap Tablets 50 mg/650 mg 1360

Chlordiazepoxide (Concomitant use may produce additive CNS-depressant effects). Products include:
Libritabs Tablets 1930
Limbitrol 1933
Menrium Tablets 1934

Chlordiazepoxide Hydrochloride (Concomitant use may produce additive CNS-depressant effects). Products include:
Librax Capsules 1929
Librium Capsules 1931
Librium Injectable 1932

Chlorpheniramine Maleate (Concomitant use may produce additive CNS-depressant effects). Products include:
A.R.M. Allergy Relief Medicine Caplets ▣ 615
Alka-Seltzer Plus Cold Medicine ▣ 623
Allerest ▣ 559
Ana-Kit Anaphylaxis Emergency Treatment Kit 1100
BC Cold Powder Multi-Symptom Formula ▣ 517
Brexin L.A. Capsules 2078
Cerose-DM 2443
Cheracol Plus Head Cold/Cough Formula ▣ 667
Chlor-Trimeton Allergy Syrup, Tablets & Long-Acting Repetabs Tablets ▣ 693
Chlor-Trimeton Decongestant ▣ 694
Comhist LA Capsules 1618
Allergy-Sinus Comtrex Multi-Symptom Allergy Sinus Formula Tablets & Caplets 746
Comtrex Multi-Symptom Cold Reliever Tablets/Caplets/Liqui-Gels/Liquid 745
Day-Night Comtrex 747
Contac Continuous Action Decongestant/Antihistamine Capsules ▣ 710
Contac Maximum Strength Continuous Action Decongestant/Antihistamine Caplets ▣ 709
Contac Severe Cold and Flu Formula Caplets ▣ 711
Coricidin 'D' Decongestant Tablets ▣ 695
Coricidin Demilets Tablets for Children ▣ 696
Coricidin Tablets ▣ 695
Deconamine 663
Demazin Nasal Decongestant/Antihistamine Repetabs Tablets & Syrup ▣ 697
Dorcol Children's Liquid Cold Formula ▣ 686
Dristan Decongestant/Antihistamine/ Analgesic Coated Caplets ▣ 749
Dristan Cold Nasal Decongestant/ Antihistamine/ Analgesic Coated Tablets 2419
Dristan Advanced Formula Decongestant/Antihistamine/ Analgesic Tablets ▣ 749
Extendryl 994
4-Way Cold Tablets 750
Fedahist Gyrocaps 2145
Fedahist Timecaps 2145
Hycomine Compound Tablets 929
Isoclor Timesule Capsules ▣ 561
Kronofed-A 970
Medi-Flu Caplet, Liquid ▣ 640
Naldecon Syrup, Tablets, Pediatric Drops and Pediatric Syrup 709
Nolamine Tablets 838
Novafed A Capsules 1342
Novahistine DH 1342
Novahistine Elixir ▣ 596
Ornade Spansule Capsules 2221
Orthoxicol Cough Syrup ▣ 668
PediaCare Allergy Relief Formula Liquid 1362
PediaCare Cough-Cold Formula Liquid 1362
PediaCare Night Rest Cough-Cold Formula Liquid 1362
PediaCare 6-12 Cough-Cold Formula Chewable Tablets 1362
Pyrroxate Capsules ▣ 669
Quelidrine Syrup 556
Ru-Tuss II Capsules 693
Ru-Tuss Tablets 693
Ryna ▣ 741
Sinarest Tablets & Extra Strength Tablets ▣ 562
Sine-Off Maximum Strength Allergy/Sinus Formula Caplets ▣ 721
Sine-Off Sinus Medicine Tablets-Aspirin Formula ▣ 722
Singlet Tablets ▣ 598
Sinulin 840
Sinutab Maximum Strength ▣ 641
St. Joseph Nighttime Cold Medicine ▣ 705
Sudafed Plus Liquid ▣ 544
Sudafed Plus Tablets ▣ 545
Teldrin Timed-Release Allergy Capsules, 12 mg 2192
TheraFlu Flu and Cold Medicine ▣ 687
Triaminic Allergy Tablets ▣ 688
Triaminic Chewables ▣ 688
Triaminic Cold Tablets ▣ 688
Triaminic Nite Light ▣ 689
Triaminic Syrup ▣ 689
Triaminic-12 Tablets ▣ 690
Triaminicin Tablets ▣ 690
Triaminicol Multi-Symptom Cold Tablets ▣ 691
Triaminicol Multi-Symptom Relief ▣ 691
Tylenol Allergy Sinus Medication Caplets and Gelcaps, Maximum Strength 1372
Children's Tylenol Cold Liquid Formula and Chewable Tablets 1368
Tylenol Cold & Flu Hot Medication, Packets 1369
Tylenol Cold Medication Caplets and Tablets 1370
Tylenol Cold Medication, Effervescent Tablets 1369
Vicks Children's NyQuil ▣ 664
Vicks Formula 44 Cough Medicine ▣ 661
Vicks Formula 44M Multi-Symptom Cough Medicine ▣ 662
Vicks Pediatric Formula 44m Multi-Symptom Cough & Cold Medicine ▣ 663

Chlorpheniramine Polistirex (Concomitant use may produce additive CNS-depressant effects). Products include:
Tussionex Extended-Release Suspension 988

Chlorpheniramine Tannate (Concomitant use may produce additive CNS-depressant effects). Products include:
Rynatan 2387
Rynatuss 2388

Chlorpromazine (Concomitant use may produce additive CNS-depressant effects). Products include:
Thorazine 2234

Chlorprothixene (Concomitant use may produce additive CNS-depressant effects). Products include:
Taractan Tablets 1920

Chlorprothixene Hydrochloride (Concomitant use may produce additive CNS-depressant effects). Products include:
Taractan 1920

Clemastine Fumarate (Concomitant use may produce additive CNS-depressant effects). Products include:
Tavist Syrup 2033
Tavist Tablets 2035
Tavist-D Tablets 2035

Clorazepate Dipotassium (Concomitant use may produce additive CNS-depressant effects). Products include:
Tranxene 556

Codeine (Concomitant use may produce additive CNS-depressant effects). Products include:
Calcidrine Syrup 506

Codeine Phosphate (Concomitant use may produce additive CNS-depressant effects). Products include:
Actifed with Codeine Cough Syrup 752
Cheracol Cough Syrup 1853
Codimal PH Syrup 846
Dimetane-DC Cough Syrup 1857
Empirin with Codeine Phosphate Nos. 2, 3 & 4 764
Fiorinal with Codeine Capsules 2008
Isoclor Expectorant 982
Naldecon CX Adult Liquid ▣ 521
Novahistine DH 1342
Novahistine Expectorant 1343
Nucofed Capsules 2219
Nucofed Expectorant 2219
Nucofed Pediatric Expectorant 2220
Nucofed Syrup 2219
Phenaphen with Codeine Capsules 1865
Phenaphen-650 with Codeine Tablets 1866
Phenergan with Codeine 2497
Phenergan VC with Codeine 2501
Robitussin A-C Syrup 1875
Robitussin-DAC Syrup 1875
Ryna ▣ 741
Soma Compound w/Codeine Tablets 2390
Triaminic Expectorant w/Codeine 1996
Tussi-Organidin Liquid 2391
Tylenol with Codeine 1381

Codeine Polistirex (Concomitant use may produce additive CNS-depressant effects).
No products indexed under this heading.

Cortisone Acetate (Enhanced metabolism of exogenous corticosteroids). Products include:
Cortone Acetate Sterile Suspension 1437
Cortone Acetate Tablets 1439

Cyproheptadine Hydrochloride (Concomitant use may produce additive CNS-depressant effects). Products include:
Periactin 1525

Dexamethasone (Enhanced metabolism of exogenous corticosteroids). Products include:
AK-Trol Ointment & Suspension ⊙ 207
Decadron Elixir 1445
Decadron Tablets 1447
Decaspray Topical Aerosol 1459
Dexacidin ⊙ 272
Maxidex Sterile Ophthalmic Suspension ⊙ 223
Maxitrol Ophthalmic Ointment/ Suspension ⊙ 223
TobraDex Ophthalmic Suspension and Ointment ⊙ 228

Dexamethasone Acetate (Enhanced metabolism of exogenous corticosteroids). Products include:
Dalalone D.P. Injectable 999
Decadron-LA Sterile Suspension 1457

Dexamethasone Sodium Phosphate (Enhanced metabolism of exogenous corticosteroids). Products include:
AK-Dex ⊙ 203
Decadron Phosphate Respihaler 1454
Decadron Phosphate Sterile Ophthalmic Ointment 1453
Decadron Phosphate Sterile Ophthalmic Solution 1453
Decadron Phosphate Topical Cream 1455
Decadron Phosphate Turbinaire 1456
Maxidex Sterile Ophthalmic Ointment ⊙ 222
NeoDecadron Sterile Ophthalmic Ointment 1517
NeoDecadron Sterile Ophthalmic Solution 1518
NeoDecadron Topical Cream 1518

Dexchlorpheniramine Maleate (Concomitant use may produce additive CNS-depressant effects). Products include:
Polaramine 2116

Dezocine (Concomitant use may produce additive CNS-depressant effects).

Diazepam (Concomitant use may produce additive CNS-depressant effects). Products include:
Valium Injectable 1937
Valium Tablets 1939
Valrelease Capsules 1923

Dicumarol (Barbiturates can induce hepatic microsomal enzymes, resulting in increased or decreased anticoagulant response). Products include:
Dicumarol Tablets 516

Diphenhydramine Citrate (Concomitant use may produce additive CNS-depressant effects). Products include:
Alka-Seltzer Plus Night-Time Cold Medicine ▣ 623
Bufferin AF Nite Time Analgesic/ Sleeping Aid Caplets 744
Excedrin P.M. Analgesic/Sleeping Aid Tablets, Caplets and Liquid 749

Diphenhydramine Hydrochloride (Concomitant use may produce additive CNS-depressant effects). Products include:
Benadryl Anti-Itch Cream ▣ 635
Benadryl Capsules 1691
Benadryl Decongestant Elixir ▣ 635
Benadryl Decongestant ▣ 635
Benadryl Elixir ▣ 636
Benadryl Kapseals 1691
Benadryl 25 Kapseals ▣ 636
Benadryl Parenteral 1692
Benadryl Plus ▣ 636

Benadryl Plus Nighttime ▣ 637
Benadryl Spray, Maximum Strength ▣ 637
Benadryl Spray, Regular Strength ▣ 637
Benadryl Steri-Vials, Ampoules, and Steri-Dose Syringe 1692
Benadryl 25 Tablets ▣ 636
Benylin Cough Syrup ▣ 637
Benylin Decongestant ▣ 638
Caladryl Cream, Lotion, Spray ▣ 638
Miles Nervine Nighttime Sleep-Aid ▣ 627
Nytol Tablets ▣ 517
Sleep-ettes-D Tablets ▣ 653
Sleep-eze 3 Tablets ▣ 755
Sleepinal Night-time Sleep Aid Capsules ▣ 734
Sominex Caplets and Tablets ▣ 722
Sominex Liquid ▣ 723
Sominex Pain Relief Formula ▣ 723
Tylenol Cold Night Time Medication Liquid 1371
Tylenol PM, Extra Strength Caplets and Tablets 1368
Unisom Dual Relief Nighttime Sleep Aid/Analgesic 1774
Ziradryl Lotion ▣ 643

Divalproex Sodium (Increases blood levels of secobarbital sodium). Products include:
Depakote 512

Doxycycline Calcium (Half-life of doxycycline may be shortened).
No products indexed under this heading.

Doxycycline Hyclate (Half-life of doxycycline may be shortened). Products include:
Doryx Capsules 1717
Vibramycin Hyclate Capsules 1787
Vibramycin Hyclate Intravenous 1968
Vibra-Tabs Film Coated Tablets 1787

Doxycycline Monohydrate (Half-life of doxycycline may be shortened). Products include:
Monodox Capsules 1630
Vibramycin Monohydrate for Oral Suspension 1787

Droperidol (Concomitant use may produce additive CNS-depressant effects). Products include:
Inapsine Injection 1140
Innovar Injection 1141

Enflurane (Concomitant use may produce additive CNS-depressant effects). Products include:
Ethrane 599

Estazolam (Concomitant use may produce additive CNS-depressant effects). Products include:
ProSom Tablets 554

Ethchlorvynol (Concomitant use may produce additive CNS-depressant effects). Products include:
Placidyl Capsules 553

Ethinamate (Concomitant use may produce additive CNS-depressant effects).
No products indexed under this heading.

Ethinyl Estradiol (Decreased effect of estradiol by increasing its metabolism). Products include:
Brevicon 2304
Demulen 2161
Estinyl Tablets 2085
Jenest-28 Tablets 1636
Levlen/Tri-Levlen 665
Lo/Ovral Tablets 2471
Lo/Ovral-28 Tablets 2476
Loestrin 1728
Modicon 1667
Nordette-21 Tablets 2481
Nordette-28 Tablets 2483
Norethin 2133
Norinyl 2304
Norlestrin 1746
Ortho-Cyclen Tablets 1658
Ortho-Novum 1667
Ovcon 1391
Ovral Tablets 2490
Ovral-28 Tablets 2491
Levlen/Tri-Levlen 665
Tri-Norinyl 2304
Triphasil-21 Tablets 2527
Triphasil-28 Tablets 2532

Ethynodiol Diacetate (Decreased effect of estradiol by increasing its metabolism). Products include:
Demulen 2161

Fentanyl (Concomitant use may produce additive CNS-depressant effects). Products include:
Duragesic Transdermal System 1133

Fentanyl Citrate (Concomitant use may produce additive CNS-depressant effects). Products include:
Innovar Injection 1141
Sublimaze Injection 1146

Fluphenazine Decanoate (Concomitant use may produce additive CNS-depressant effects). Products include:
Prolixin Decanoate 1795

Fluphenazine Enanthate (Concomitant use may produce additive CNS-depressant effects). Products include:
Prolixin Enanthate 1796

Fluphenazine Hydrochloride (Concomitant use may produce additive CNS-depressant effects). Products include:
Prolixin Elixir 1793
Prolixin Injection 1791
Prolixin Oral Concentrate 1792
Prolixin Tablets 1793

Flurazepam Hydrochloride (Concomitant use may produce additive CNS-depressant effects). Products include:
Dalmane Capsules 1927

Furazolidone (Prolongs the effects of barbiturates). Products include:
Furoxone 1855

Glutethimide (Concomitant use may produce additive CNS-depressant effects).
No products indexed under this heading.

Griseofulvin (Interference with absorption of orally administered griseofulvin, thus decreasing its blood level). Products include:
Fulvicin P/G Tablets 2090
Fulvicin P/G 165 & 330 Tablets 2091
Fulvicin-U/F Tablets 2092
Grifulvin V (griseofulvin microsize) Tablets/Suspension 1678
Grisactin 2454
Grisactin Ultra Tablets 2455
Gris-PEG Tablets, 125 mg & 250 mg 1083

Haloperidol (Concomitant use may produce additive CNS-depressant effects). Products include:
Haldol Injection, Tablets and Concentrate 1373

Haloperidol Decanoate (Concomitant use may produce additive CNS-depressant effects). Products include:
Haldol Decanoate 1375

Hydrocodone Bitartrate (Concomitant use may produce additive CNS-depressant effects). Products include:
Anexsia 5/500 Tablets 2196
Anexsia 7.5/650 Tablets 2197
Azdone Tablets 844
Codiclear DH Syrup 845
Codimal DH Syrup 846
Damason-P 1356
Hycodan Syrup, Tablets 927
Hycomine Compound Tablets 929
Hycomine Syrup 927
Hycotuss Expectorant Syrup 930
Hydrocet Capsules 835
Lortab ASA Tablets 2414
Lortab 2412
Ru-Tuss with Hydrocodone 694
Triaminic Expectorant DH 1995
Vicodin Tablets 1187
Vicodin ES Tablets 1189
Zydone Capsules 941

Hydrocodone Polistirex (Concomitant use may produce additive CNS-depressant effects). Products include:
Tussionex Extended-Release Suspension 988

Hydrocortisone (Enhanced metabolism of exogenous corticosteroids). Products include:
AK-Spore H.C. ◉ 206
Bactine Hydrocortisone Anti-Itch Cream ▣ 625
CaldeCORT Anti-Itch Hydrocortisone Spray ▣ 560
Carmol HC Cream 1% 2296
Cortaid Spray ▣ 735
Cortenema 2244
Cortisporin Ointment 758
Cortisporin Ophthalmic Ointment Sterile 758
Cortisporin Ophthalmic Suspension Sterile 759
Cortisporin Otic Solution Sterile 760
Cortisporin Otic Suspension Sterile 760
Cortizone-5 Creme & Ointment ▣ 732
Dermolate Anti-Itch Cream ▣ 697
Eldecort Cream 1.0% 1113
Eldecort Cream 1.0% and 2.5% 1113
Fungoid HC Creme 1770
Hydrocortone Tablets 1482
Hytone 909
LazerSporin-C Solution 1770
Massengill Medicated Soft Cloth Towelettes 2192
Nutracort Cream & Lotion 1684
PediOtic Suspension Sterile 797
Synacort Creams 1%, 2.5% 2296
Vanoxide-HC Acne Lotion 911
Vioform-Hydrocortisone Cream and Mild Cream 889
Vioform-Hydrocortisone Ointment 889
VõSoL HC Otic Solution 2392
Vytone Cream 1% 911

Hydrocortisone Acetate (Enhanced metabolism of exogenous corticosteroids). Products include:
Analpram-HC Rectal Cream 1% and 2.5% 970
Anusol-HC Cream 1690
Anusol-HC Suppositories 1691
Caldecort ▣ 560
Carmol HC Cream 1% 2296
Chloromycetin Hydrocortisone Ophthalmic 1694
Coly-Mycin S Otic w/Neomycin & Hydrocortisone 1708
Cortaid ▣ 735
Cortef Feminine Itch Cream ▣ 735
Corticaine ▣ 682
Cortifoam 1827
Cortisporin Cream 757
Epifoam 1828
Gynecort 5 Creme ▣ 556
Hydrocortone Acetate Sterile Suspension 1479
Lanacort 5 Creme and Ointment ▣ 557
Mantadil Cream 789
Ophthocort ◉ 301
Orabase HCA Oral Paste 890
Pramosone Cream, Lotion & Ointment 971
ProctoCream-HC 1834
Proctofoam-HC 1835

Hydrocortisone Sodium Phosphate (Enhanced metabolism of exogenous corticosteroids). Products include:
Hydrocortone Phosphate Injection, Sterile 1481

Hydrocortisone Sodium Succinate (Enhanced metabolism of exogenous corticosteroids). Products include:
Solu-Cortef Sterile Powder 2361

Hydroxyzine Hydrochloride (Concomitant use may produce additive CNS-depressant effects). Products include:
Atarax Tablets & Syrup 1941
Marax Tablets & DF Syrup 1954
Vistaril Intramuscular Solution 1970

Isocarboxazid (Prolongs the effects of barbiturates). Products include:
Marplan Tablets 1906

Isoflurane (Concomitant use may produce additive CNS-depressant effects). Products include:
Forane 600

Ketamine Hydrochloride (Concomitant use may produce additive CNS-depressant effects). Products include:
Ketalar 1726

Levonorgestrel (Decreased effect of estradiol by increasing its metabolism). Products include:
Levlen/Tri-Levlen 665
Nordette-21 Tablets 2481
Nordette-28 Tablets 2483
Norplant System 2484
Levlen/Tri-Levlen 665
Triphasil-21 Tablets 2527
Triphasil-28 Tablets 2532

Levorphanol Tartrate (Concomitant use may produce additive CNS-depressant effects). Products include:
Levo-Dromoran 1906

Lorazepam (Concomitant use may produce additive CNS-depressant effects). Products include:
Ativan Injection 2432
Ativan Tablets 2434

Loxapine Hydrochloride (Concomitant use may produce additive CNS-depressant effects). Products include:
Loxitane 1213

Loxapine Succinate (Concomitant use may produce additive CNS-depressant effects). Products include:
Loxitane Capsules 1213

Meperidine Hydrochloride (Concomitant use may produce additive CNS-depressant effects). Products include:
Demerol 2047
Mepergan Injection 2479

Mephobarbital (Concomitant use may produce additive CNS-depressant effects). Products include:
Mebaral Tablets 2061

Meprobamate (Concomitant use may produce additive CNS-depressant effects). Products include:
Deprol Tablets 2382
Equagesic Tablets 2451
Miltown Tablets 2386
PMB 200 and PMB 400 2504

Mesoridazine (Concomitant use may produce additive CNS-depressant effects). Products include:
Serentil 686

Mestranol (Decreased effect of estradiol by increasing its metabolism). Products include:
Enovid 2161
Norethin 2133
Norinyl 2304
Ortho-Novum 1667

Methadone Hydrochloride (Concomitant use may produce additive CNS-depressant effects). Products include:
Dolophine Hydrochloride Ampoules & Vials 1260
Dolophine Hydrochloride Tablets 1261
Methadone Hydrochloride Diskets 1284
Methadone Hydrochloride Oral Solution & Tablets 1987

Methdilazine Hydrochloride (Concomitant use may produce additive CNS-depressant effects). Products include:
Tacaryl Syrup & Tablets 2409

Methohexital Sodium (Concomitant use may produce additive CNS-depressant effects). Products include:
Brevital Sodium Vials 1248

Methoxyflurane (Concomitant use may produce additive CNS-depressant effects).
No products indexed under this heading.

Methylprednisolone Acetate (Enhanced metabolism of exogenous corticosteroids). Products include:
Depo-Medrol Sterile Aqueous Suspension 2334

Methylprednisolone Sodium Succinate (Enhanced metabolism of exogenous corticosteroids). Products include:
Solu-Medrol Sterile Powder 2363

Midazolam Hydrochloride (Concomitant use may produce additive CNS-depressant effects). Products include:
Versed Injection 1924

Molindone Hydrochloride (Concomitant use may produce additive CNS-depressant effects). Products include:
Moban Tablets & Concentrate 932

Morphine Sulfate (Concomitant use may produce additive CNS-depressant effects). Products include:
Astramorph/PF Injection, USP (Preservative-Free) 618
Duramorph 960
Infumorph 200 and Infumorph 500 Sterile Solutions 962
MS Contin Tablets 1814
MSIR 1817
Oramorph SR (Morphine Sulfate Sustained Release Tablets) 1988
Roxanol 1991

Norethindrone (Decreased effect of estradiol by increasing its metabolism). Products include:
Brevicon 2304
Jenest-28 Tablets 1636
Micronor Tablets 1667
Modicon 1667
Norethin 2133
Norinyl 2304
Norlutin 1755
Nor-Q D Tablets 2304
Ortho-Novum 1667
Ovcon 1391
Tri-Norinyl 2304

Norethynodrel (Decreased effect of estradiol by increasing its metabolism). Products include:
Enovid 2161

Norgestimate (Decreased effect of estradiol by increasing its metabolism). Products include:
Ortho-Cyclen Tablets 1658

Norgestrel (Decreased effect of estradiol by increasing its metabolism). Products include:
Lo/Ovral Tablets 2471
Lo/Ovral-28 Tablets 2476
Ovral Tablets 2490
Ovral-28 Tablets 2491
Ovrette Tablets 2492

Opium Alkaloids (Concomitant use may produce additive CNS-depressant effects). Products include:
B & O No. 15A & No. 16A Supprettes 2395
Pantopon Injectable 1911

Oxazepam (Concomitant use may produce additive CNS-depressant effects). Products include:
Serax Capsules 2522
Serax Tablets 2522

Oxycodone Hydrochloride (Concomitant use may produce additive CNS-depressant effects). Products include:
Percocet Tablets 950
Percodan 951
Roxicodone Tablets, Oral Solution & Intensol (Oxycodone) 1992
Tylox Capsules 1382

Pentobarbital Sodium (Concomitant use may produce additive CNS-depressant effects). Products include:
Nembutal Sodium Capsules 534
Nembutal Sodium Solution 536
Nembutal Sodium Suppositories 538

Perphenazine (Concomitant use may produce additive CNS-depressant effects). Products include:
Etrafon 2087
Triavil Tablets 1556
Trilafon 2123

Phenelzine Sulfate (Prolongs the effects of barbiturates). Products include:
Nardil 1742

Phenobarbital (Concomitant use may produce additive CNS-depressant effects). Products include:
Arco-Lase Plus Tablets 607
Bellergal-S Tablets 1998
Bronkolixir .... ⊞ 761
Bronkotabs Tablets .... ⊞ 762
Donnatal 1858
Donnatal Extentabs 1859
Donnatal Tablets 1858
Donnazyme Tablets 1860
Kinesed Tablets 2272
Phenobarbital Elixir and Tablets 1293
Primatene Tablets-P Formula 2421
Quadrinal Tablets 1183
Tedral SA 1765

Phenytoin (Variable effect on the metabolism of phenytoin). Products include:
Dilantin Infatabs 1710
Dilantin-30 Pediatric/Dilantin-125 Suspension 1713

Phenytoin Sodium (Variable effect on the metabolism of phenytoin). Products include:
Dilantin Kapseals 1708
Dilantin Parenteral 1712
Dilantin with Phenobarbital Kapseals 1715

Prazepam (Concomitant use may produce additive CNS-depressant effects). Products include:
Centrax 1693

Prednisolone Acetate (Enhanced metabolism of exogenous corticosteroids). Products include:
AK-Cide Sterile Ophthalmic Ointment & Suspension .... ⊙ 202
Blephamide Liquifilm Sterile Ophthalmic Suspension 586
Blephamide S.O.P. Sterile Ophthalmic Ointment 586
Cetapred Ointment .... ⊙ 220
⅛% Econopred & 1% Econopred Plus .... ⊙ 217
Isopto Cetapred Suspension .... ⊙ 220
Metimyd .... ⊙ 306
Poly-Pred Liquifilm .... ⊙ 250
Pred Forte .... ⊙ 252
Pred Mild .... ⊙ 254
Pred-G Liquifilm Sterile Ophthalmic Suspension .... ⊙ 252
Pred-G S.O.P. Sterile Ophthalmic Ointment .... ⊙ 253
Vasocidin Ointment .... ⊙ 275

Prednisolone Sodium Phosphate (Enhanced metabolism of exogenous corticosteroids). Products include:
AK-Pred .... ⊙ 205
Hydeltrasol Injection, Sterile 1476
Inflamase .... ⊙ 274
Pediapred Oral Liquid 987
Vasocidin Ophthalmic Solution .... ⊙ 276

Prednisolone Tebutate (Enhanced metabolism of exogenous corticosteroids). Products include:
Hydeltra-T.B.A. Sterile Suspension 1478

Prednisone (Enhanced metabolism of exogenous corticosteroids). Products include:
Deltasone Tablets 2332

Prochlorperazine (Concomitant use may produce additive CNS-depressant effects). Products include:
Compazine 2201

Promethazine Hydrochloride (Concomitant use may produce additive CNS-depressant effects). Products include:
Mepergan Injection 2479
Phenergan with Codeine 2497
Phenergan with Dextromethorphan 2499
Phenergan Injection 2493
Phenergan Suppositories 2496
Phenergan Syrup 2495
Phenergan Tablets 2496
Phenergan VC 2500
Phenergan VC with Codeine 2501

Propofol (Concomitant use may produce additive CNS-depressant effects). Products include:
Diprivan Injection 2267

Propoxyphene Hydrochloride (Concomitant use may produce additive CNS-depressant effects). Products include:
Darvon 1256
Wygesic Tablets 2540

Propoxyphene Napsylate (Concomitant use may produce additive CNS-depressant effects). Products include:
Darvon-N/Darvocet-N 1254

Pyrilamine Maleate (Concomitant use may produce additive CNS-depressant effects). Products include:
Codimal 846
4-Way Fast Acting Nasal Spray - Original Formula (regular & mentholated) & Metered Spray Pump (regular) 751
Maximum Strength Midol Multi-Symptom Menstrual Formula .... ⊞ 571
Maximum Strength Midol PMS Premenstrual Syndrome Formula .... ⊞ 570
Regular Strength Midol Multi-Symptom Menstrual Formula .... ⊞ 570
Prefrin-A .... ⊙ 255
Prēmsyn PMS Capsules & Caplets ⊞ 547
Primatene Tablets-M Formula 2421
Robitussin Night Relief .... ⊞ 677
Ru-Tuss with Hydrocodone 694
Triaminic Expectorant DH 1995
Triaminic Oral Infant Drops 1996

Pyrilamine Tannate (Concomitant use may produce additive CNS-depressant effects). Products include:
Rynatan 2387

Quazepam (Concomitant use may produce additive CNS-depressant effects). Products include:
Doral Tablets 2383

Selegiline Hydrochloride (Prolongs the effects of barbiturates). Products include:
Eldepryl 2250

Sufentanil Citrate (Concomitant use may produce additive CNS-depressant effects). Products include:
Sufenta Injection 1147

Temazepam (Concomitant use may produce additive CNS-depressant effects). Products include:
Restoril Capsules 2023

Terfenadine (Concomitant use may produce additive CNS-depressant effects). Products include:
Seldane Tablets 1349
Seldane-D Extended-Release Tablets 1350

Thiamylal Sodium (Concomitant use may produce additive CNS-depressant effects). Products include:
Surital Ampoules, Steri-Vials 1764

Thioridazine Hydrochloride (Concomitant use may produce additive CNS-depressant effects). Products include:
Mellaril 2011

Thiothixene (Concomitant use may produce additive CNS-depressant effects). Products include:
Navane Capsules and Concentrate 1954
Navane Intramuscular 1956

Tranylcypromine Sulfate (Prolongs the effects of barbiturates). Products include:
Parnate Tablets 2222

Triamcinolone (Enhanced metabolism of exogenous corticosteroids).
No products indexed under this heading.

Triamcinolone Acetonide (Enhanced metabolism of exogenous corticosteroids). Products include:
Aristocort A 1010
Azmacort Inhaler 1837
Kenalog Cream, Lotion & Ointment 2401
Kenalog-10 Injection 2402
Kenalog-40 Injection 2403
Kenalog in Orabase 604
Kenalog Spray 2401
Mycolog II Cream and Ointment 2407
Mytrex Cream & Ointment 2080
Nasacort Nasal Inhaler 1844

Triamcinolone Diacetate (Enhanced metabolism of exogenous corticosteroids). Products include:
Aristocort Suspension 1008

Triamcinolone Hexacetonide (Enhanced metabolism of exogenous corticosteroids). Products include:
Aristospan Suspension 1011

Triazolam (Concomitant use may produce additive CNS-depressant effects). Products include:
Halcion Tablets 2340

Trifluoperazine Hydrochloride (Concomitant use may produce additive CNS-depressant effects). Products include:
Stelazine 2226

Trimeprazine Tartrate (Concomitant use may produce additive CNS-depressant effects). Products include:
Temaril Tablets, Syrup and Spansule Sustained Release Capsules 1085

Tripelennamine Hydrochloride (Concomitant use may produce additive CNS-depressant effects). Products include:
PBZ Tablets & Elixir 1037
PBZ-SR Tablets 1037

Triprolidine Hydrochloride (Concomitant use may produce additive CNS-depressant effects). Products include:
Actidil .... ⊞ 538
Actifed Capsules .... ⊞ 539
Actifed Plus Caplets .... ⊞ 539
Actifed Plus Tablets .... ⊞ 540
Actifed with Codeine Cough Syrup.. 752
Actifed Syrup .... ⊞ 540
Actifed Tablets .... ⊞ 540
Actifed 12-Hour Capsules .... ⊞ 539

Valproic Acid (Increases blood levels of secobarbital sodium). Products include:
Depakene Capsules & Syrup 511

Warfarin Sodium (Barbiturates can induce hepatic microsomal enzymes, resulting in increased or decreased anticoagulant response). Products include:
Coumadin Injection & Tablets 944
Panwarfin Tablets 547

SECRETIN-FERRING
(Secretin) 2547
No interactions described in labeling.

SECTRAL CAPSULES
(Acebutolol Hydrochloride) 2520
May interact with catecholamine depleting drugs, non-steroidal anti-inflammatory agents, alpha adrenergic stimulants, and insulin. Compounds in these categories include:

Deserpidine (Additive effect). Products include:
Enduronyl 518
Harmonyl Tablets 528

Oreticyl 545

Diclofenac Sodium (Blunting of the antihypertensive effect). Products include:
Voltaren Ophthalmic Sterile Ophthalmic Solution ⊙ 268
Voltaren Tablets 1042

Etodolac (Blunting of the antihypertensive effect). Products include:
Lodine Capsules 2468

Fenoprofen Calcium (Blunting of the antihypertensive effect). Products include:
Nalfon Pulvules & Tablets 919

Flurbiprofen (Blunting of the antihypertensive effect). Products include:
Ansaid Tablets 2319

Ibuprofen (Blunting of the antihypertensive effect). Products include:
Advil Cold & Sinus Caplets (formerly CoAdvil) 2416
Advil Ibuprofen Tablets and Caplets 2416
Children's Advil Suspension 2426
CoAdvil ▣ 748
Dristan Sinus Caplets 2419
Haltran Tablets ▣ 668
Ibuprofen ▣ 631
Medipren ibuprofen Caplets and Tablets 1362
Midol 200 Cramp Relief Formula ▣ 570
Motrin Tablets 2351
Motrin IB Caplets and Tablets ▣ 736
Nuprin Ibuprofen/Analgesic Tablets & Caplets 752
PediaProfen Suspension 1363
Rufen Tablets 691
Trendar Ibuprofen Tablets ▣ 756

Indomethacin (Blunting of the antihypertensive effect). Products include:
Indocin 1487

Indomethacin Sodium Trihydrate (Blunting of the antihypertensive effect). Products include:
Indocin I.V. 1490

Insulin, Human (Beta-blockers may potentiate insulin-induced hypoglycemia).
No products indexed under this heading.

Insulin, Human Isophane Suspension (Beta-blockers may potentiate insulin-induced hypoglycemia). Products include:
Humulin N, 100 Units 1270

Insulin, Human NPH (Beta-blockers may potentiate insulin-induced hypoglycemia). Products include:
Insulatard NPH Human 1627
Novolin N 1627
Novolin N PenFill Cartridges 1628
Novolin N Prefilled 1628

Insulin, Human Regular (Beta-blockers may potentiate insulin-induced hypoglycemia). Products include:
Humulin BR, 100 Units 1268
Humulin R, 100 Units 1272
Novolin R 1627
Novolin R PenFill Cartridges 1628
Novolin R Prefilled 1629
Velosulin Human 1628

Insulin, Human, Zinc Suspension (Beta-blockers may potentiate insulin-induced hypoglycemia). Products include:
Humulin L, 100 Units 1268
Humulin U, 100 Units 1272
Novolin L 1627

Insulin, NPH (Beta-blockers may potentiate insulin-induced hypoglycemia). Products include:
NPH, 40 & 100 Units 1273
Beef NPH, 100 Units 1274
Pork NPH, 100 Units 1275
Insulatard NPH 1626
NPH Insulin 1626
NPH Purified Pork Isophane Insulin 1626

Insulin, Regular (Beta-blockers may potentiate insulin-induced hypoglycemia). Products include:
Regular, 40 & 100 Units 1273
Beef Regular, 100 Units 1275
Pork Regular, 100 Units 1275
Pork Regular (Concentrated), 500 Units 1276
Regular Insulin 1625
Regular Purified Pork Insulin 1626
Velosulin 1627

Insulin, Zinc Crystals (Beta-blockers may potentiate insulin-induced hypoglycemia). Products include:
NPH, 40 & 100 Units 1273

Insulin, Zinc Suspension (Beta-blockers may potentiate insulin-induced hypoglycemia). Products include:
Lente, 40 & 100 Units 1272
Protamine, Zinc, 40 & 100 Units 1273
Lente Iletin I 1272
Beef Lente, 100 Units 1274
Beef Protamine Zinc, 100 Units 1274
Pork Lente, 100 Units 1275
Pork, Protamine, Zinc, 100 Units 1275
Lente Insulin 1626
Lente Purified Pork Insulin 1626
Semilente Insulin 1625
Ultralente Insulin 1626

Ketoprofen (Blunting of the antihypertensive effect). Products include:
Orudis Capsules 2488

Ketorolac Tromethamine (Blunting of the antihypertensive effect). Products include:
Toradol IM Injection 2302

Meclofenamate Sodium (Blunting of the antihypertensive effect). Products include:
Meclomen Capsules 1739

Mefenamic Acid (Blunting of the antihypertensive effect). Products include:
Ponstel 1758

Naphazoline Hydrochloride (Potential for exaggerated hypertensive response). Products include:
AK-Con ⊙ 202
AK-Con-A ⊙ 203
Albalon Solution with Liquifilm ⊙ 238
Albalon-A Liquifilm ⊙ 238
Allergy Drops ⊙ 258
Clear Eyes ACR ⊙ 305
Clear Eyes Lubricating Eye Redness Reliever ⊙ 304
4-Way Fast Acting Nasal Spray - Original Formula (regular & mentholated) & Metered Spray Pump (regular) 751
Naphcon ⊙ 226
Naphcon Forte ⊙ 226
Naphcon-A Ophthalmic Solution 571
Opcon-A Ophthalmic Solution ⊙ 262
Privine Nasal Solution ▣ 552
Privine Nasal Solution 878
Privine Nasal Spray ▣ 552
Privine Nasal Spray 878
Vasocon-A ⊙ 278

Naproxen (Blunting of the antihypertensive effect). Products include:
Naprosyn 2297

Naproxen Sodium (Blunting of the antihypertensive effect). Products include:
Anaprox and Anaprox DS Tablets 2288

Oxymetazoline Hydrochloride (Potential for exaggerated hypertensive response). Products include:
Afrin ▣ 692
Cheracol Nasal Spray Pump ▣ 667
Dristan Long Lasting Menthol Nasal Spray 2419
Dristan Long Lasting Nasal Spray, Regular and Regular with Metered Dose Pump 2419
Duration Nasal Spray ▣ 700
Duration 12 Hour Nasal Spray Pump ▣ 700
4-Way Long Lasting Nasal Spray & Metered Spray Pump 751
NTZ Long Acting Nasal Spray & Drops 0.05% ▣ 760
Neo-Synephrine Maximum Strength 12 Hour Nasal Spray ▣ 759
Neo-Synephrine Maximum Strength 12 Hour Nasal Spray Pump ▣ 759
Nöstrilla Long Acting Nasal Decongestant ▣ 520
OcuClear Eye Drops ⊙ 306
Vicks Sinex Long Acting ▣ 665
Visine L.R. Eye Drops ▣ 647
Visine L.R. Eye Drops ⊙ 303

Phenylbutazone (Blunting of the antihypertensive effect). Products include:
Butazolidin Capsules & Tablets 1027

Phenylephrine Hydrochloride (Potential for exaggerated hypertensive response). Products include:
AK-Dilate Solution 2.5% and 10% ⊙ 203
Atrohist Sprinkle Capsules 558
Cerose-DM 2443
Codimal 846
Comhist LA Capsules 1618
Congespirin For Children Aspirin Free Chewable Cold Tablets 748
Cyclomydril ⊙ 216
Deconsal Sprinkle Capsules 559
Dimetane Decongestant ▣ 673
Dristan Decongestant/Antihistamine/ Analgesic Coated Caplets ▣ 749
Dristan Cold Nasal Decongestant/ Antihistamine/ Analgesic Coated Tablets 2419
Dristan Advanced Formula Decongestant/Antihistamine/ Analgesic Tablets ▣ 749
Dristan Nasal Spray, Menthol 2419
Dristan Nasal Spray, Regular and Regular with Metered Pump 2419
Entex Capsules 1623
Entex Liquid 1623
Sinus Excedrin Analgesic, Decongestant Tablets & Caplets 750
Extendryl 994
4-Way Fast Acting Nasal Spray - Original Formula (regular & mentholated) & Metered Spray Pump (regular) 751
Hycomine Compound Tablets 929
Murocoll-2 Sterile Ophthalmic Solution ⊙ 261
Mydfrin 2.5% ⊙ 224
Naldecon Syrup, Tablets, Pediatric Drops and Pediatric Syrup 709
Neo-Synephrine Hydrochloride 1% Carpuject 2063
Neo-Synephrine Hydrochloride 1% Injection 2063
Neo-Synephrine Hydrochloride (Ophthalmic) 2064
Neo-Synephrine ▣ 759
Nöstril Nasal Decongestant ▣ 520
Novahistine Elixir ▣ 596
Phenergan VC 2500
Phenergan VC with Codeine 2501
Prefrin Liquifilm Vasoconstrictor and Lubricant Eye Drops ⊙ 254
Prefrin-A ⊙ 255
Quelidrine Syrup 556
Relief Vasoconstrictor and Lubricant Eye Drops ⊙ 256
Robitussin Night Relief ▣ 677
Ru-Tuss with Hydrocodone 694
Ru-Tuss Tablets 693
Vasosulf ⊙ 279
Vicks Sinex ▣ 665
Zincfrin ⊙ 230

Phenylpropanolamine Hydrochloride (Potential for exaggerated hypertensive response). Products include:
A.R.M. Allergy Relief Medicine Caplets ▣ 615
Acutrim ▣ 548
Allerest ▣ 559
BC Cold Powder ▣ 517
Cheracol Plus Head Cold/Cough Formula ▣ 667
Codimal Expectorant 846
Comtrex Multi-Symptom Cold Reliever Tablets/Caplets/Liqui-Gels/Liquid 745
Contac Continuous Action Decongestant/Antihistamine Capsules ▣ 710
Contac Maximum Strength Continuous Action Decongestant/ Antihistamine Caplets ▣ 709
Contac Severe Cold and Flu Formula Caplets ▣ 711
Coricidin 'D' Decongestant Tablets ▣ 695
Coricidin Demilets Tablets for Children ▣ 696
Demazin Nasal Decongestant/ Antihistamine Repetabs Tablets & Syrup ▣ 697
Dexatrim ▣ 733
Dimetane-DC Cough Syrup 1857
Dimetapp Elixir ▣ 673
Dimetapp DM Elixir ▣ 674
Dimetapp Extentabs ▣ 674
Dimetapp Plus Caplets ▣ 675
Dimetapp Tablets ▣ 675
Entex Capsules 1623
Entex LA Tablets 1623
Entex Liquid 1623
4-Way Cold Tablets 750
Hycomine Syrup 927
Naldecon CX Adult Liquid ▣ 521
Naldecon DX Adult Liquid ▣ 521
Naldecon DX Children's Syrup ▣ 522
Naldecon DX Pediatric Drops ▣ 522
Naldecon EX Children's Syrup ▣ 522
Naldecon EX Pediatric Drops ▣ 523
Naldecon Syrup, Tablets, Pediatric Drops and Pediatric Syrup 709
Nolamine Tablets 838
Nolex LA Tablets 838
Ornade Spansule Capsules 2221
Orthoxicol Cough Syrup ▣ 668
Propagest 839
Pyrroxate Capsules ▣ 669
Robitussin-CF ▣ 676
Ru-Tuss II Capsules 693
Ru-Tuss with Hydrocodone 694
Ru-Tuss Tablets 693
Sine-Off Sinus Medicine Tablets-Aspirin Formula ▣ 722
Sinulin 840
St. Joseph Cold Tablets for Children ▣ 704
Tavist-D Tablets 2035
Triaminic Allergy Tablets ▣ 688
Triaminic Chewables ▣ 688
Triaminic Cold Tablets ▣ 688
Triaminic Expectorant ▣ 688
Triaminic Expectorant w/Codeine 1996
Triaminic Expectorant DH 1995
Triaminic Oral Infant Drops 1996
Triaminic Syrup ▣ 689
Triaminic-12 Tablets ▣ 690
Triaminic-DM Syrup ▣ 689
Triaminicin Tablets ▣ 690
Triaminicol Multi-Symptom Cold Tablets ▣ 691
Triaminicol Multi-Symptom Relief ▣ 691
Tuss-Ornade Liquid 2242
Tuss-Ornade Spansule Capsules 2242
Tylenol Cold Medication, Effervescent Tablets 1369

Piroxicam (Blunting of the antihypertensive effect). Products include:
Feldene Capsules 1777

Pseudoephedrine Hydrochloride (Potential for exaggerated hypertensive response). Products include:
Actifed Capsules ▣ 539
Actifed Plus Caplets ▣ 539
Actifed Plus Tablets ▣ 540
Actifed with Codeine Cough Syrup 752
Actifed Syrup ▣ 540
Actifed Tablets ▣ 540
Actifed 12-Hour Capsules ▣ 539
Advil Cold & Sinus Caplets (formerly CoAdvil) 2416
Allerest ▣ 559
Anatuss LA Tablets 1359
Benadryl Decongestant Elixir ▣ 635
Benadryl Decongestant ▣ 635
Benadryl Plus ▣ 636
Benadryl Plus Nighttime ▣ 637
Benylin Decongestant ▣ 638
Brexin L.A. Capsules 2078
Bromfed Capsules (Timed Release) 1615
Bromfed Syrup ▣ 628
Bromfed 1615
CoAdvil ▣ 748
Allergy-Sinus Comtrex Multi-Symptom Allergy Sinus Formula Tablets & Caplets 746
Cough Formula Comtrex 746
Comtrex Multi-Symptom Cold Reliever Tablets/Caplets/Liqui-Gels/Liquid 745
Day-Night Comtrex 747

(▣ Described in PDR For Nonprescription Drugs)

(⊙ Described in PDR For Ophthalmology)

Non-Drowsy Comtrex 747
Congess 994
Congestac Caplets .... ▣ 617
Contac Jr. Children's Cold Medicine .... ▣ 712
Contac Nighttime Cold Medicine .... ▣ 713
Contac Sinus Caplets Maximum Strength Non-Drowsy Formula .... ▣ 710
Contac Sinus Tablets Maximum Strength Non-Drowsy Formula .... ▣ 710
Deconamine 663
Deconsal II Tablets 559
Dimacol Caplets .... ▣ 672
Dimetane-DX Cough Syrup 1858
Dorcol Children's Cough Syrup .... ▣ 685
Dorcol Children's Decongestant Liquid .... ▣ 685
Dorcol Children's Liquid Cold Formula .... ▣ 686
Maximum Strength Dristan Decongestant/Analgesic Coated Caplets .... ▣ 750
No Drowsiness Dristan Cold Nasal Decongestant/Analgesic Coated Caplets 2420
Dristan Sinus Caplets 2419
Sinus Excedrin Analgesic, Decongestant Tablets & Caplets .... ▣ 533
Fedahist Gyrocaps 2145
Fedahist Timecaps 2145
Guaifed 1615
Guaifed Syrup .... ▣ 629
Isoclor Expectorant 982
Isoclor Timesule Capsules .... ▣ 561
Kronofed-A 970
Medi-Flu Caplet, Liquid .... ▣ 640
Novafed A Capsules 1342
Novafed Capsules 1342
Novahistine DH 1342
Novahistine DMX .... ▣ 595
Novahistine Expectorant 1343
Nucofed Capsules 2219
Nucofed Expectorant 2219
Nucofed Pediatric Expectorant 2220
Nucofed Syrup 2219
Ornex Caplets .... ▣ 618
PediaCare Allergy Relief Formula Liquid 1362
PediaCare Cough-Cold Formula Liquid 1362
PediaCare Infants' Oral Decongestant Drops 1362
PediaCare Night Rest Cough-Cold Formula Liquid 1362
PediaCare 6-12 Cough-Cold Formula Chewable Tablets 1362
Robitussin-DAC Syrup 1875
Robitussin-PE .... ▣ 677
Rondec 1975
Rondec-DM 1976
Rondec-TR Tablet 1975
Ru-Tuss DE Tablets 694
Ryna .... ▣ 741
Seldane-D Extended-Release Tablets 1350
Sinarest .... ▣ 562
Sine-Aid Maximum Strength Sinus Headache Caplets 1365
Sine-Aid Maximum Strength Sinus Headache Tablets 1365
Sine-Off Maximum Strength Allergy/Sinus Formula Caplets .... ▣ 721
Sine-Off Maximum Strength No Drowsiness Formula Caplets .... ▣ 722
Singlet Tablets .... ▣ 598
Sinutab Maximum Strength .... ▣ 641
Sinutab Maximum Strength Without Drowsiness Tablets & Caplets .... ▣ 642
Sinutab Regular Strength Without Drowsiness Formula .... ▣ 641
St. Joseph Nighttime Cold Medicine .... ▣ 705
Sudafed Children's Liquid .... ▣ 543
Sudafed Cough Syrup .... ▣ 543
Sudafed Plus Liquid .... ▣ 544
Sudafed Plus Tablets .... ▣ 545
Sudafed Sinus Caplets .... ▣ 545
Sudafed Sinus Tablets .... ▣ 545
Sudafed Tablets, 30 mg .... ▣ 544
Sudafed Tablets, Adult Strength, 60 mg .... ▣ 544
Sudafed 12 Hour Capsules .... ▣ 545
TheraFlu Flu and Cold Medicine .... ▣ 687
Triaminic Nite Light .... ▣ 689
Tylenol Allergy Sinus Medication Caplets and Gelcaps, Maximum Strength 1372
Children's Tylenol Cold Liquid Formula and Chewable Tablets 1368
Tylenol Cold & Flu Hot Medication, Packets 1369
Tylenol Cold & Flu No Drowsiness Hot Medication, Packets 1371
Tylenol Cold Medication Caplets and Tablets 1370
Tylenol Cold Medication No Drowsiness Formula Caplets 1370
Tylenol Cold Night Time Medication Liquid 1371
Tylenol Cough Medication Liquid with Decongestant, Maximum Strength 1372
Tylenol, Maximum Strength, Sinus Medication Gelcaps, Caplets and Tablets 1373
Ursinus Inlay-Tabs .... ▣ 691
Vicks Children's NyQuil .... ▣ 664
Vicks Daycare .... ▣ 660
Vicks Formula 44D Decongestant Cough Medicine .... ▣ 662
Vicks Formula 44M Multi-Symptom Cough Medicine .... ▣ 662
Vicks NyQuil Nighttime Colds Medicine-Original & Cherry Flavor .... ▣ 664
Vicks Pediatric Formula 44 Cough & Congestion Medicine .... ▣ 663
Vicks Pediatric Formula 44m Multi-Symptom Cough & Cold Medicine .... ▣ 663

Rauwolfia Serpentina (Additive effect). Products include:
Raudixin Tablets 1803
Rauzide Tablets 1804

Rescinnamine (Additive effect).
No products indexed under this heading.

Reserpine (Additive effect). Products include:
Diupres Tablets 1461
Hydromox R Tablets 1209
Hydropres Tablets 1485
Renese-R Tablets 1786
Salutensin/Salutensin-Demi 719
Ser-Ap-Es Tablets 881
Serpasil Tablets 883
Serpasil-Apresoline Tablets 884
Serpasil-Esidrix Tablets 886

Sulindac (Blunting of the antihypertensive effect). Products include:
Clinoril Tablets 1433

Tetrahydrozoline Hydrochloride (Potential for exaggerated hypertensive response). Products include:
Collyrium Fresh 2445
Murine Plus Lubricating Eye Redness Reliever .... ⊙ 305
Visine A.C. Eye Drops .... ▣ 646
Visine A.C. Eye Drops .... ⊙ 303
Visine EXTRA Eye Drops .... ▣ 647
Visine EXTRA Eye Drops .... ⊙ 303
Visine Eye Drops .... ▣ 646
Visine Eye Drops .... ⊙ 303

Tolmetin Sodium (Blunting of the antihypertensive effect). Products include:
Tolectin (200, 400 and 600 mg) 1379

Food Interactions

Food, unspecified (Slightly decreases absorption and peak concentration).

SEDAPAP TABLETS 50 MG/650 MG

(Acetaminophen, Butalbital) 1360

May interact with central nervous system depressants, narcotic analgesics, tranquilizers, psychotropics, tricyclic antidepressants, oral anticoagulants, and certain other agents. Compounds in these categories include:

Alcohol (Additive CNS depression).

Alfentanil Hydrochloride (Additive CNS depression). Products include:
Alfenta Injection 1131

Alprazolam (Additive CNS depression). Products include:
Xanax Tablets 2367

Amitriptyline Hydrochloride (Additive CNS depression; decreased blood levels of the antidepressant). Products include:
Elavil 2269
Endep Tablets 1927
Etrafon 2087
Limbitrol 1933
Triavil Tablets 1556

Amoxapine (Additive CNS depression; decreased blood levels of the antidepressant). Products include:
Asendin Tablets 1196

Aprobarbital (Additive CNS depression). Products include:
Alurate Elixir 1883

Buprenorphine (Additive CNS depression).
No products indexed under this heading.

Buspirone Hydrochloride (Additive CNS depression). Products include:
BuSpar 1401

Butabarbital (Additive CNS depression). Products include:
Pyridium Plus 1764

Chlordiazepoxide (Additive CNS depression). Products include:
Libritabs Tablets 1930
Limbitrol 1933
Menrium Tablets 1934

Chlordiazepoxide Hydrochloride (Additive CNS depression). Products include:
Librax Capsules 1929
Librium Capsules 1931
Librium Injectable 1932

Chlorpromazine (Additive CNS depression). Products include:
Thorazine 2234

Chlorprothixene (Additive CNS depression). Products include:
Taractan Tablets 1920

Chlorprothixene Hydrochloride (Additive CNS depression). Products include:
Taractan 1920

Clomipramine Hydrochloride (Additive CNS depression; decreased blood levels of the antidepressant). Products include:
Anafranil Capsules 650

Clorazepate Dipotassium (Additive CNS depression). Products include:
Tranxene 556

Codeine (Additive CNS depression). Products include:
Calcidrine Syrup 506

Codeine Phosphate (Additive CNS depression). Products include:
Actifed with Codeine Cough Syrup 752
Cheracol Cough Syrup 1853
Codimal PH Syrup 846
Dimetane-DC Cough Syrup 1857
Empirin with Codeine Phosphate Nos. 2, 3 & 4 764
Fiorinal with Codeine Capsules 2008
Isoclor Expectorant 982
Naldecon CX Adult Liquid .... ▣ 521
Novahistine DH 1342
Novahistine Expectorant 1343
Nucofed Capsules 2219
Nucofed Expectorant 2219
Nucofed Pediatric Expectorant 2220
Nucofed Syrup 2219
Phenaphen with Codeine Capsules 1865
Phenaphen-650 with Codeine Tablets 1866
Phenergan with Codeine 2497
Phenergan VC with Codeine 2501
Robitussin A-C Syrup 1875
Robitussin-DAC Syrup 1875
Ryna .... ▣ 741
Soma Compound w/Codeine Tablets 2390
Triaminic Expectorant w/Codeine 1996
Tussi-Organidin Liquid 2391
Tylenol with Codeine 1381

Codeine Polistirex (Additive CNS depression).
No products indexed under this heading.

Desipramine Hydrochloride (Additive CNS depression; decreased blood levels of the antidepressant). Products include:
Norpramin Tablets 1340

Dezocine (Additive CNS depression).

Diazepam (Additive CNS depression). Products include:
Valium Injectable 1937
Valium Tablets 1939
Valrelease Capsules 1923

Dicumarol (Decreased effect of anticoagulant). Products include:
Dicumarol Tablets 516

Doxepin Hydrochloride (Additive CNS depression; decreased blood levels of the antidepressant). Products include:
Sinequan 1960

Droperidol (Additive CNS depression). Products include:
Inapsine Injection 1140
Innovar Injection 1141

Enflurane (Additive CNS depression). Products include:
Ethrane 599

Estazolam (Additive CNS depression). Products include:
ProSom Tablets 554

Ethchlorvynol (Additive CNS depression). Products include:
Placidyl Capsules 553

Ethinamate (Additive CNS depression).
No products indexed under this heading.

Fentanyl (Additive CNS depression). Products include:
Duragesic Transdermal System 1133

Fentanyl Citrate (Additive CNS depression). Products include:
Innovar Injection 1141
Sublimaze Injection 1146

Fluphenazine Decanoate (Additive CNS depression). Products include:
Prolixin Decanoate 1795

Fluphenazine Enanthate (Additive CNS depression). Products include:
Prolixin Enanthate 1796

Fluphenazine Hydrochloride (Additive CNS depression). Products include:
Prolixin Elixir 1793
Prolixin Injection 1791
Prolixin Oral Concentrate 1792
Prolixin Tablets 1793

Flurazepam Hydrochloride (Additive CNS depression). Products include:
Dalmane Capsules 1927

Glutethimide (Additive CNS depression).
No products indexed under this heading.

Haloperidol (Additive CNS depression). Products include:
Haldol Injection, Tablets and Concentrate 1373

Haloperidol Decanoate (Additive CNS depression). Products include:
Haldol Decanoate 1375

Hydrocodone Bitartrate (Additive CNS depression). Products include:
Anexsia 5/500 Tablets 2196
Anexsia 7.5/650 Tablets 2197
Azdōne Tablets 844
Codiclear DH Syrup 845
Codimal DH Syrup 846
Damason-P 1356
Hycodan Syrup, Tablets 927

Hycomine Compound Tablets 929
Hycomine Syrup 927
Hycotuss Expectorant Syrup 930
Hydrocet Capsules 835
Lortab ASA Tablets 2414
Lortab 2412
Ru-Tuss with Hydrocodone 694
Triaminic Expectorant DH 1995
Vicodin Tablets 1187
Vicodin ES Tablets 1189
Zydone Capsules 941

Hydrocodone Polistirex (Additive CNS depression). Products include:
Tussionex Extended-Release Suspension 988

Hydroxyzine Hydrochloride (Additive CNS depression). Products include:
Atarax Tablets & Syrup 1941
Marax Tablets & DF Syrup 1954
Vistaril Intramuscular Solution 1970

Imipramine Hydrochloride (Additive CNS depression; decreased blood levels of the antidepressant). Products include:
Tofranil Ampuls 1038
Tofranil Tablets 1039

Imipramine Pamoate (Additive CNS depression; decreased blood levels of the antidepressant). Products include:
Tofranil-PM Capsules 1041

Isocarboxazid (Additive CNS depression). Products include:
Marplan Tablets 1906

Isoflurane (Additive CNS depression). Products include:
Forane 600

Ketamine Hydrochloride (Additive CNS depression). Products include:
Ketalar 1726

Levorphanol Tartrate (Additive CNS depression). Products include:
Levo-Dromoran 1906

Lithium Carbonate (Additive CNS depression). Products include:
Eskalith 2214
Lithane Tablets 1596
Lithium Carbonate Capsules & Tablets 1984
Lithobid Tablets 870

Lithium Citrate (Additive CNS depression). Products include:
Cibalith-S 870

Lorazepam (Additive CNS depression). Products include:
Ativan Injection 2432
Ativan Tablets 2434

Loxapine Hydrochloride (Additive CNS depression). Products include:
Loxitane 1213

Loxapine Succinate (Additive CNS depression). Products include:
Loxitane Capsules 1213

Maprotiline Hydrochloride (Additive CNS depression; decreased blood levels of the antidepressant). Products include:
Ludiomil Tablets 874

Meperidine Hydrochloride (Additive CNS depression). Products include:
Demerol 2047
Mepergan Injection 2479

Mephobarbital (Additive CNS depression). Products include:
Mebaral Tablets 2061

Meprobamate (Additive CNS depression). Products include:
Deprol Tablets 2382
Equagesic Tablets 2451
Miltown Tablets 2386
PMB 200 and PMB 400 2504

Mesoridazine (Additive CNS depression). Products include:
Serentil 686

Methadone Hydrochloride (Additive CNS depression). Products include:
Dolophine Hydrochloride Ampoules & Vials 1260
Dolophine Hydrochloride Tablets 1261
Methadone Hydrochloride Diskets 1284
Methadone Hydrochloride Oral Solution & Tablets 1987

Methohexital Sodium (Additive CNS depression). Products include:
Brevital Sodium Vials 1248

Methoxyflurane (Additive CNS depression).
No products indexed under this heading.

Midazolam Hydrochloride (Additive CNS depression). Products include:
Versed Injection 1924

Molindone Hydrochloride (Additive CNS depression). Products include:
Moban Tablets & Concentrate 932

Morphine Sulfate (Additive CNS depression). Products include:
Astramorph/PF Injection, USP (Preservative-Free) 618
Duramorph 960
Infumorph 200 and Infumorph 500 Sterile Solutions 962
MS Contin Tablets 1814
MSIR 1817
Oramorph SR (Morphine Sulfate Sustained Release Tablets) 1988
Roxanol 1991

Nortriptyline Hydrochloride (Additive CNS depression; decreased blood levels of the antidepressant). Products include:
Pamelor 2019

Opium Alkaloids (Additive CNS depression). Products include:
B & O No. 15A & No. 16A Supprettes 2395
Pantopon Injectable 1911

Oxazepam (Additive CNS depression). Products include:
Serax Capsules 2522
Serax Tablets 2522

Oxycodone Hydrochloride (Additive CNS depression). Products include:
Percocet Tablets 950
Percodan 951
Roxicodone Tablets, Oral Solution & Intensol (Oxycodone) 1992
Tylox Capsules 1382

Pentobarbital Sodium (Additive CNS depression). Products include:
Nembutal Sodium Capsules 534
Nembutal Sodium Solution 536
Nembutal Sodium Suppositories 538

Perphenazine (Additive CNS depression). Products include:
Etrafon 2087
Triavil Tablets 1556
Trilafon 2123

Phenelzine Sulfate (Additive CNS depression). Products include:
Nardil 1742

Phenobarbital (Additive CNS depression). Products include:
Arco-Lase Plus Tablets 607
Bellergal-S Tablets 1998
Bronkolixir .... ▣ 761
Bronkotabs Tablets .... ▣ 762
Donnatal 1858
Donnatal Extentabs 1859
Donnatal Tablets 1858
Donnazyme Tablets 1860
Kinesed Tablets 2272
Phenobarbital Elixir and Tablets 1293
Primatene Tablets-P Formula 2421
Quadrinal Tablets 1183
Tedral SA 1765

Prazepam (Additive CNS depression). Products include:
Centrax 1693

Prochlorperazine (Additive CNS depression). Products include:
Compazine 2201

Promethazine Hydrochloride (Additive CNS depression). Products include:
Mepergan Injection 2479
Phenergan with Codeine 2497
Phenergan with Dextromethorphan 2499
Phenergan Injection 2493
Phenergan Suppositories 2496
Phenergan Syrup 2495
Phenergan Tablets 2496
Phenergan VC 2500
Phenergan VC with Codeine 2501

Propofol (Additive CNS depression). Products include:
Diprivan Injection 2267

Propoxyphene Hydrochloride (Additive CNS depression). Products include:
Darvon 1256
Wygesic Tablets 2540

Propoxyphene Napsylate (Additive CNS depression). Products include:
Darvon-N/Darvocet-N 1254

Protriptyline Hydrochloride (Additive CNS depression; decreased blood levels of the antidepressant). Products include:
Vivactil Tablets 1567

Quazepam (Additive CNS depression). Products include:
Doral Tablets 2383

Secobarbital Sodium (Additive CNS depression). Products include:
Seconal Sodium Pulvules 1296

Sufentanil Citrate (Additive CNS depression). Products include:
Sufenta Injection 1147

Temazepam (Additive CNS depression). Products include:
Restoril Capsules 2023

Thiamylal Sodium (Additive CNS depression). Products include:
Surital Ampoules, Steri-Vials 1764

Thioridazine Hydrochloride (Additive CNS depression). Products include:
Mellaril 2011

Thiothixene (Additive CNS depression). Products include:
Navane Capsules and Concentrate 1954
Navane Intramuscular 1956

Tranylcypromine Sulfate (Additive CNS depression). Products include:
Parnate Tablets 2222

Triazolam (Additive CNS depression). Products include:
Halcion Tablets 2340

Trifluoperazine Hydrochloride (Additive CNS depression). Products include:
Stelazine 2226

Trimipramine Maleate (Additive CNS depression; decreased blood levels of the antidepressant). Products include:
Surmontil Capsules 2524

Warfarin Sodium (Decreased effect of anticoagulant). Products include:
Coumadin Injection & Tablets 944
Panwarfin Tablets 547

SELDANE TABLETS
(Terfenadine) 1349
May interact with macrolide antibiotics and certain other agents. Compounds in these categories include:

Erythromycin (Significantly alters the metabolizing of terfenadine). Products include:
A/T/S Topical Gel and Topical Solution 1089
AK-Mycin Ointment .... ◉ 204
Benzamycin Topical Gel 907
E-Mycin Tablets 688
ETS-2% 1685
ERYC 1720
Erycette (erythromycin 2%) Topical Solution 1678
Ery-Tab Tablets 521
Erythromycin Base Filmtab 525
Erythromycin Delayed-Release Capsules, USP 526
Ilotycin Ophthalmic Ointment 915
PCE Dispertab Tablets 549
Pediazole 1973
T-Stat 2.0% Topical Solution and Pads 2409
Theramycin Z Topical Solution 2% 1410

Erythromycin Estolate (Significantly alters the metabolizing of terfenadine). Products include:
Ilosone 913

Erythromycin Ethylsuccinate (Significantly alters the metabolizing of terfenadine). Products include:
E.E.S. 522
EryPed 519
Pediazole 1973

Erythromycin Gluceptate (Significantly alters the metabolizing of terfenadine). Products include:
Ilotycin Gluceptate, IV, Vials 915

Erythromycin Stearate (Significantly alters the metabolizing of terfenadine). Products include:
Erythrocin Stearate Filmtab 523

Ketoconazole (Significantly alters the metabolizing of terfenadine). Products include:
Nizoral 2% Cream 1143
Nizoral 2% Shampoo 1144
Nizoral Tablets 1145

Troleandomycin (Significantly alters the metabolizing of terfenadine). Products include:
Tao Capsules 1963

SELDANE-D EXTENDED-RELEASE TABLETS
(Pseudoephedrine Hydrochloride, Terfenadine) 1350
May interact with monoamine oxidase inhibitors, macrolide antibiotics, beta blockers, and certain other agents. Compounds in these categories include:

Acebutolol Hydrochloride (Increases the effect of sympathomimetic amines). Products include:
Sectral Capsules 2520

Atenolol (Increases the effect of sympathomimetic amines). Products include:
Tenoretic Tablets 1105
Tenormin Tablets and I.V. Injection 1107

Betaxolol Hydrochloride (Increases the effect of sympathomimetic amines). Products include:
Betoptic Sterile Ophthalmic Solution 569
Betoptic S Sterile Ophthalmic Suspension 570
Kerlone Tablets 2172

Carteolol Hydrochloride (Increases the effect of sympathomimetic amines). Products include:
Cartrol Tablets 507

Deserpidine (Reduced antihypertensive effect). Products include:
Enduronyl 518
Harmonyl Tablets 528
Oreticyl 545

Erythromycin (Significantly alters the metabolism of terfenadine). Products include:
A/T/S Topical Gel and Topical Solution 1089
AK-Mycin Ointment .... ◉ 204
Benzamycin Topical Gel 907
E-Mycin Tablets 688
ETS-2% 1685
ERYC 1720
Erycette (erythromycin 2%) Topical Solution 1678
Ery-Tab Tablets 521
Erythromycin Base Filmtab 525

Erythromycin Delayed-Release Capsules, USP 526
Ilotycin Ophthalmic Ointment 915
PCE Dispertab Tablets 549
Pediazole 1973
T-Stat 2.0% Topical Solution and Pads 2409
Theramycin Z Topical Solution 2% 1410

Erythromycin Estolate (Significantly alters the metabolism of terfenadine). Products include:
Ilosone 913

Erythromycin Ethylsuccinate (Significantly alters the metabolism of terfenadine). Products include:
E.E.S. 522
EryPed 519
Pediazole 1973

Erythromycin Gluceptate (Significantly alters the metabolism of terfenadine). Products include:
Ilotycin Gluceptate, IV, Vials 915

Erythromycin Stearate (Significantly alters the metabolism of terfenadine). Products include:
Erythrocin Stearate Filmtab 523

Esmolol Hydrochloride (Increases the effect of sympathomimetic amines). Products include:
Brevibloc Injection 942

Furazolidone (Increases the effect of sympathomimetic amines; prolongs and intensifies effects of antihistamines; concurrent use is contraindicated). Products include:
Furoxone 1855

Isocarboxazid (Increases the effect of sympathomimetic amines; prolongs and intensifies effects of antihistamines; concurrent use is contraindicated). Products include:
Marplan Tablets 1906

Ketoconazole (Significantly alters the metabolism of terfenadine). Products include:
Nizoral 2% Cream 1143
Nizoral 2% Shampoo 1144
Nizoral Tablets 1145

Labetalol Hydrochloride (Increases the effect of sympathomimetic amines). Products include:
Normodyne Injection 2108
Normodyne Tablets 2110
Normozide Tablets 2112
Trandate HCT Tablets 579
Trandate Injection 577
Trandate Tablets 579

Mecamylamine Hydrochloride (Reduced antihypertensive effect). Products include:
Inversine Tablets 1492

Methyldopa (Reduced antihypertensive effect). Products include:
Aldoclor Tablets 1413
Aldomet Oral 1415
Aldoril Tablets 1418

Methyldopate Hydrochloride (Reduced antihypertensive effect). Products include:
Aldomet Ester HCl Injection 1417

Metoprolol Tartrate (Increases the effect of sympathomimetic amines). Products include:
Lopressor Ampuls 1032
Lopressor HCT Tablets 1034
Lopressor Tablets 1032

Nadolol (Increases the effect of sympathomimetic amines). Products include:
Corgard Tablets 701
Corzide Tablets 702

Penbutolol Sulfate (Increases the effect of sympathomimetic amines). Products include:
Levatol 1832

Phenelzine Sulfate (Increases the effect of sympathomimetic amines; prolongs and intensifies effects of antihistamines; concurrent use is contraindicated). Products include:
Nardil 1742

Pindolol (Increases the effect of sympathomimetic amines). Products include:
Visken Tablets 2036

Propranolol Hydrochloride (Increases the effect of sympathomimetic amines). Products include:
Inderal 2459
Inderal LA Long Acting Capsules 2461
Inderide Tablets 2463
Inderide LA Long Acting Capsules 2465

Rauwolfia Serpentina (Reduced antihypertensive effect). Products include:
Raudixin Tablets 1803
Rauzide Tablets 1804

Rescinnamine (Reduced antihypertensive effect).
No products indexed under this heading.

Reserpine (Reduced antihypertensive effect). Products include:
Diupres Tablets 1461
Hydromox R Tablets 1209
Hydropres Tablets 1485
Renese-R Tablets 1786
Salutensin/Salutensin-Demi 719
Ser-Ap-Es Tablets 881
Serpasil Tablets 883
Serpasil-Apresoline Tablets 884
Serpasil-Esidrix Tablets 886

Selegiline Hydrochloride (Increases the effect of sympathomimetic amines; prolongs and intensifies effects of antihistamines; concurrent use is contraindicated). Products include:
Eldepryl 2250

Timolol Maleate (Increases the effect of sympathomimetic amines). Products include:
Blocadren Tablets 1429
Timolide Tablets 1547
Timoptic in Ocudose 1552
Timoptic Sterile Ophthalmic Solution 1550

Tranylcypromine Sulfate (Increases the effect of sympathomimetic amines; prolongs and intensifies effects of antihistamines; concurrent use is contraindicated). Products include:
Parnate Tablets 2222

Troleandomycin (Significantly alters the metabolism of terfenadine). Products include:
Tao Capsules 1963

SELSUN BLUE DANDRUFF SHAMPOO
(Selenium Sulfide) 1978
No interactions described in labeling.

SELSUN RX 2.5% SELENIUM SULFIDE LOTION, USP
(Selenium Sulfide) 1977
No interactions described in labeling.

SEMICID VAGINAL CONTRACEPTIVE INSERTS
(Nonoxynol-9) 2422
No interactions described in labeling.

SEMILENTE INSULIN
(Insulin, Zinc Suspension) 1625
No interactions described in labeling.

SENNA X-PREP BOWEL EVACUANT LIQUID
(Senna Concentrates) 1073
No interactions described in labeling.

SENOKOT GRANULES
(Senna Concentrates) 1819
No interactions described in labeling.

SENOKOT SYRUP
(Senna Concentrates) 1819
No interactions described in labeling.

SENOKOT TABLETS
(Senna Concentrates) 1819
No interactions described in labeling.

SENOKOTXTRA TABLETS
(Senna Concentrates) 1819
No interactions described in labeling.

SENOKOT-S TABLETS
(Senna Concentrates, Docusate Sodium) 1820
No interactions described in labeling.

MINT GEL SENSODYNE
(Potassium Nitrate) ■ 518
No interactions described in labeling.

MINT SENSODYNE TOOTHPASTE
(Potassium Nitrate) ■ 518
No interactions described in labeling.

ORIGINAL SENSODYNE TOOTHPASTE
(Strontium Chloride Hexahydrate) ■ 518
No interactions described in labeling.

SENSORCAINE WITH EPINEPHRINE INJECTION
(Bupivacaine Hydrochloride, Epinephrine) 631
May interact with phenothiazines, butyrophenones, inhalant anesthetics, monoamine oxidase inhibitors, tricyclic antidepressants, vasopressors, ergot-type oxytocic drugs, and certain other agents. Compounds in these categories include:

Amitriptyline Hydrochloride (May produce severe and prolonged hypertension). Products include:
Elavil 2269
Endep Tablets 1927
Etrafon 2087
Limbitrol 1933
Triavil Tablets 1556

Amoxapine (May produce severe and prolonged hypertension). Products include:
Asendin Tablets 1196

Chlorpromazine (Reduces or reverses the pressor effect of epinephrine). Products include:
Thorazine 2234

Clomipramine Hydrochloride (May produce severe and prolonged hypertension). Products include:
Anafranil Capsules 650

Desipramine Hydrochloride (May produce severe and prolonged hypertension). Products include:
Norpramin Tablets 1340

Dopamine Hydrochloride (May produce severe and prolonged hypertension or cerebrovascular accidents). Products include:
Intropin Injection 930

Doxepin Hydrochloride (May produce severe and prolonged hypertension). Products include:
Sinequan 1960

Enflurane (Concurrent use may produce serious dose-related cardiac arrhythmias). Products include:
Ethrane 599

Epinephrine Hydrochloride (May produce severe and prolonged hypertension or cerebrovascular accidents). Products include:
Adrenalin Chloride Solution 1:100 & 1:1,000 1689
Epifrin ⊙ 244
Glaucon ⊙ 218

Fluphenazine Decanoate (Reduces or reverses the pressor effect of epinephrine). Products include:
Prolixin Decanoate 1795

Fluphenazine Enanthate (Reduces or reverses the pressor effect of epinephrine). Products include:
Prolixin Enanthate 1796

Fluphenazine Hydrochloride (Reduces or reverses the pressor effect of epinephrine). Products include:
Prolixin Elixir 1793
Prolixin Injection 1791
Prolixin Oral Concentrate 1792
Prolixin Tablets 1793

Furazolidone (May produce severe and prolonged hypertension). Products include:
Furoxone 1855

Haloperidol (Reduces or reverses the pressor effect of epinephrine). Products include:
Haldol Injection, Tablets and Concentrate 1373

Haloperidol Decanoate (Reduces or reverses the pressor effect of epinephrine). Products include:
Haldol Decanoate 1375

Halothane (Concurrent use may produce serious dose-related cardiac arrhythmias). Products include:
Fluothane 2453

Imipramine Hydrochloride (May produce severe and prolonged hypertension). Products include:
Tofranil Ampuls 1038
Tofranil Tablets 1039

Imipramine Pamoate (May produce severe and prolonged hypertension). Products include:
Tofranil-PM Capsules 1041

Isocarboxazid (May produce severe and prolonged hypertension). Products include:
Marplan Tablets 1906

Isoflurane (Concurrent use may produce serious dose-related cardiac arrhythmias). Products include:
Forane 600

Maprotiline Hydrochloride (May produce severe and prolonged hypertension). Products include:
Ludiomil Tablets 874

Mesoridazine (Reduces or reverses the pressor effect of epinephrine). Products include:
Serentil 686

Metaraminol Bitartrate (May produce severe and prolonged hypertension or cerebrovascular accidents). Products include:
Aramine Injection 1424

Methoxamine Hydrochloride (May produce severe and prolonged hypertension or cerebrovascular accidents). Products include:
Vasoxyl Injection 819

Methoxyflurane (Concurrent use may produce serious dose-related cardiac arrhythmias).
No products indexed under this heading.

Methylergonovine Maleate (May produce severe and prolonged hypertension or cerebrovascular accidents). Products include:
Methergine 2016

(■ Described in PDR For Nonprescription Drugs) (⊙ Described in PDR For Ophthalmology)

Norepinephrine Bitartrate (May produce severe and prolonged hypertension or cerebrovascular accidents). Products include:

Levophed Bitartrate Injection 2054

Nortriptyline Hydrochloride (May produce severe and prolonged hypertension). Products include:

Pamelor 2019

Perphenazine (Reduces or reverses the pressor effect of epinephrine). Products include:

Etrafon 2087
Triavil Tablets 1556
Trilafon 2123

Phenelzine Sulfate (May produce severe and prolonged hypertension). Products include:

Nardil 1742

Phenylephrine Hydrochloride (May produce severe and prolonged hypertension or cerebrovascular accidents). Products include:

AK-Dilate Solution 2.5% and 10% .... ⊙ 203
Atrohist Sprinkle Capsules 558
Cerose-DM 2443
Codimal 846
Comhist LA Capsules 1618
Congespirin For Children Aspirin Free Chewable Cold Tablets 748
Cyclomydril .... ⊙ 216
Deconsal Sprinkle Capsules 559
Dimetane Decongestant .... ▣ 673
Dristan Decongestant/Antihistamine/ Analgesic Coated Caplets .... ▣ 749
Dristan Cold Nasal Decongestant/ Antihistamine/ Analgesic Coated Tablets 2419
Dristan Advanced Formula Decongestant/Antihistamine/ Analgesic Tablets .... ▣ 749
Dristan Nasal Spray, Menthol 2419
Dristan Nasal Spray, Regular and Regular with Metered Pump 2419
Entex Capsules 1623
Entex Liquid 1623
Sinus Excedrin Analgesic, Decongestant Tablets & Caplets 750
Extendryl 994
4-Way Fast Acting Nasal Spray - Original Formula (regular & mentholated) & Metered Spray Pump (regular) 751
Hycomine Compound Tablets 929
Murocoll-2 Sterile Ophthalmic Solution .... ⊙ 261
Mydfrin 2.5% .... ⊙ 224
Naldecon Syrup, Tablets, Pediatric Drops and Pediatric Syrup 709
Neo-Synephrine Hydrochloride 1% Carpuject 2063
Neo-Synephrine Hydrochloride 1% Injection 2063
Neo-Synephrine Hydrochloride (Ophthalmic) 2064
Neo-Synephrine .... ▣ 759
Nöstril Nasal Decongestant .... ▣ 520
Novahistine Elixir .... ▣ 596
Phenergan VC 2500
Phenergan VC with Codeine 2501
Prefrin Liquifilm Vasoconstrictor and Lubricant Eye Drops .... ⊙ 254
Prefrin-A .... ⊙ 255
Quelidrine Syrup 556
Relief Vasoconstrictor and Lubricant Eye Drops .... ⊙ 256
Robitussin Night Relief .... ▣ 677
Ru-Tuss with Hydrocodone 694
Ru-Tuss Tablets 693
Vasosulf .... ⊙ 279
Vicks Sinex .... ▣ 665
Zincfrin .... ⊙ 230

Prochlorperazine (Reduces or reverses the pressor effect of epinephrine). Products include:

Compazine 2201

Promethazine Hydrochloride (Reduces or reverses the pressor effect of epinephrine). Products include:

Mepergan Injection 2479
Phenergan with Codeine 2497
Phenergan with Dextromethorphan 2499
Phenergan Injection 2493
Phenergan Suppositories 2496
Phenergan Syrup 2495
Phenergan Tablets 2496
Phenergan VC 2500
Phenergan VC with Codeine 2501

Protriptyline Hydrochloride (May produce severe and prolonged hypertension). Products include:

Vivactil Tablets 1567

Selegiline Hydrochloride (May produce severe and prolonged hypertension). Products include:

Eldepryl 2250

Thioridazine Hydrochloride (Reduces or reverses the pressor effect of epinephrine). Products include:

Mellaril 2011

Tranylcypromine Sulfate (May produce severe and prolonged hypertension). Products include:

Parnate Tablets 2222

Trifluoperazine Hydrochloride (Reduces or reverses the pressor effect of epinephrine). Products include:

Stelazine 2226

Trimipramine Maleate (May produce severe and prolonged hypertension). Products include:

Surmontil Capsules 2524

SENSORCAINE INJECTION
(Bupivacaine Hydrochloride) 631
See **Sensorcaine with Epinephrine Injection**

SENSORCAINE-MPF SPINAL
(Bupivacaine Hydrochloride) 634
See **Sensorcaine with Epinephrine Injection**

SEPTRA DS TABLETS
(Trimethoprim, Sulfamethoxazole) 813
May interact with thiazides, oral anticoagulants, and certain other agents. Compounds in these categories include:

Bendroflumethiazide (Potential for thrombocytopenia with purpura in elderly). Products include:

Corzide Tablets 702
Naturetin Tablets 1789
Rauzide Tablets 1804

Chlorothiazide (Potential for thrombocytopenia with purpura in elderly). Products include:

Aldoclor Tablets 1413
Diupres Tablets 1461
Diuril Oral 1464

Chlorothiazide Sodium (Potential for thrombocytopenia with purpura in elderly). Products include:

Diuril Sodium Intravenous 1463

Dicumarol (Septra prolongs prothrombin time in patients on anticoagulant). Products include:

Dicumarol Tablets 516

Hydrochlorothiazide (Potential for thrombocytopenia with purpura in elderly). Products include:

Aldactazide 2150
Aldoril Tablets 1418
Apresazide Capsules 854
Apresoline-Esidrix Tablets 857
Capozide 2258
Dyazide Capsules 2208
Esidrix Tablets 863
Esimil Tablets 864
HydroDIURIL Tablets 1484
Hydropres Tablets 1485
Inderide Tablets 2463
Inderide LA Long Acting Capsules .. 2465
Lopressor HCT Tablets 1034
Maxzide 1215
Moduretic Tablets 1510
Normozide Tablets 2112
Oretic Tablets 544
Oreticyl 545
Prinzide Tablets 1540
Ser-Ap-Es Tablets 881
Serpasil-Esidrix Tablets 886
Timolide Tablets 1547
Trandate HCT Tablets 579
Vaseretic Tablets 1559
Zestoretic 2274

Hydroflumethiazide (Potential for thrombocytopenia with purpura in elderly). Products include:

Diucardin Tablets 2450
Saluron 718
Salutensin/Salutensin-Demi 719

Methotrexate Sodium (Increased free methotrexate concentrations). Products include:

Methotrexate Tablets, Parenteral, LPF Parenteral 1217
Rheumatrex Methotrexate Dose Pack 1234

Methyclothiazide (Potential for thrombocytopenia with purpura in elderly). Products include:

Enduron Tablets 517
Enduronyl 518

Phenytoin (Decreased metabolism of phenytoin). Products include:

Dilantin Infatabs 1710
Dilantin-30 Pediatric/Dilantin-125 Suspension 1713

Phenytoin Sodium (Decreased metabolism of phenytoin). Products include:

Dilantin Kapseals 1708
Dilantin Parenteral 1712
Dilantin with Phenobarbital Kapseals 1715

Polythiazide (Potential for thrombocytopenia with purpura in elderly). Products include:

Minizide Capsules 1779
Renese Tablets 1785
Renese-R Tablets 1786

Warfarin Sodium (Prolongs prothrombin time). Products include:

Coumadin Injection & Tablets 944
Panwarfin Tablets 547

SEPTRA GRAPE SUSPENSION
(Trimethoprim, Sulfamethoxazole) 813
See **Septra DS Tablets**

SEPTRA I.V. INFUSION
(Trimethoprim, Sulfamethoxazole) 808
May interact with thiazides and certain other agents. Compounds in these categories include:

Bendroflumethiazide (Potential for thrombocytopenia with purpura in elderly). Products include:

Corzide Tablets 702
Naturetin Tablets 1789
Rauzide Tablets 1804

Chlorothiazide (Potential for thrombocytopenia with purpura in elderly patients). Products include:

Aldoclor Tablets 1413
Diupres Tablets 1461
Diuril Oral 1464

Chlorothiazide Sodium (Potential for thrombocytopenia with purpura in elderly). Products include:

Diuril Sodium Intravenous 1463

Hydrochlorothiazide (Potential for thrombocytopenia with purpura in elderly). Products include:

Aldactazide 2150
Aldoril Tablets 1418
Apresazide Capsules 854
Apresoline-Esidrix Tablets 857
Capozide 2258
Dyazide Capsules 2208
Esidrix Tablets 863
Esimil Tablets 864
HydroDIURIL Tablets 1484
Hydropres Tablets 1485
Inderide Tablets 2463
Inderide LA Long Acting Capsules .. 2465
Lopressor HCT Tablets 1034
Maxzide 1215
Moduretic Tablets 1510
Normozide Tablets 2112
Oretic Tablets 544
Oreticyl 545
Prinzide Tablets 1540
Ser-Ap-Es Tablets 881
Serpasil-Esidrix Tablets 886
Timolide Tablets 1547
Trandate HCT Tablets 579
Vaseretic Tablets 1559
Zestoretic 2274

Hydroflumethiazide (Potential for thrombocytopenia with purpura in elderly). Products include:

Diucardin Tablets 2450
Saluron 718
Salutensin/Salutensin-Demi 719

Methotrexate Sodium (Increased free methotrexate concentrations). Products include:

Methotrexate Tablets, Parenteral, LPF Parenteral 1217
Rheumatrex Methotrexate Dose Pack 1234

Methyclothiazide (Potential for thrombocytopenia with purpura in elderly). Products include:

Enduron Tablets 517
Enduronyl 518

Phenytoin (Decreased metabolism of phenytoin). Products include:

Dilantin Infatabs 1710
Dilantin-30 Pediatric/Dilantin-125 Suspension 1713

Phenytoin Sodium (Decreased metabolism of phenytoin). Products include:

Dilantin Kapseals 1708
Dilantin Parenteral 1712
Dilantin with Phenobarbital Kapseals 1715

Polythiazide (Potential for thrombocytopenia with purpura in elderly). Products include:

Minizide Capsules 1779
Renese Tablets 1785
Renese-R Tablets 1786

Warfarin Sodium (Prolonged prothrombin time). Products include:

Coumadin Injection & Tablets 944
Panwarfin Tablets 547

SEPTRA I.V. INFUSION ADD-VANTAGE VIALS
(Trimethoprim, Sulfamethoxazole) 810
May interact with thiazides and certain other agents. Compounds in these categories include:

Bendroflumethiazide (Potential for thrombocytopenia with purpura in elderly). Products include:

Corzide Tablets 702
Naturetin Tablets 1789
Rauzide Tablets 1804

Chlorothiazide (Potential for thrombocytopenia with purpura in elderly). Products include:

Aldoclor Tablets 1413
Diupres Tablets 1461
Diuril Oral 1464

Chlorothiazide Sodium (Potential for thrombocytopenia with purpura in elderly). Products include:

Diuril Sodium Intravenous 1463

Hydrochlorothiazide (Potential for thrombocytopenia with purpura in elderly). Products include:

Aldactazide 2150
Aldoril Tablets 1418
Apresazide Capsules 854
Apresoline-Esidrix Tablets 857
Capozide 2258
Dyazide Capsules 2208
Esidrix Tablets 863
Esimil Tablets 864
HydroDIURIL Tablets 1484
Hydropres Tablets 1485
Inderide Tablets 2463
Inderide LA Long Acting Capsules .. 2465
Lopressor HCT Tablets 1034
Maxzide 1215
Moduretic Tablets 1510
Normozide Tablets 2112
Oretic Tablets 544

Oreticyl ... 545
Prinzide Tablets ... 1540
Ser-Ap-Es Tablets ... 881
Serpasil-Esidrix Tablets ... 886
Timolide Tablets ... 1547
Trandate HCT Tablets ... 579
Vaseretic Tablets ... 1559
Zestoretic ... 2274

Hydroflumethiazide (Potential for thrombocytopenia with purpura in elderly). Products include:
Diucardin Tablets ... 2450
Saluron ... 718
Salutensin/Salutensin-Demi ... 719

Methotrexate Sodium (Increased free methotrexate concentrations). Products include:
Methotrexate Tablets, Parenteral, LPF Parenteral ... 1217
Rheumatrex Methotrexate Dose Pack ... 1234

Methyclothiazide (Potential for thrombocytopenia with purpura in elderly). Products include:
Enduron Tablets ... 517
Enduronyl ... 518

Phenytoin (Decreased metabolism of phenytoin). Products include:
Dilantin Infatabs ... 1710
Dilantin-30 Pediatric/Dilantin-125 Suspension ... 1713

Phenytoin Sodium (Decreased metabolism of phenytoin). Products include:
Dilantin Kapseals ... 1708
Dilantin Parenteral ... 1712
Dilantin with Phenobarbital Kapseals ... 1715

Polythiazide (Potential for thrombocytopenia with purpura in elderly). Products include:
Minizide Capsules ... 1779
Renese Tablets ... 1785
Renese-R Tablets ... 1786

Warfarin Sodium (Prolonged prothrombin time). Products include:
Coumadin Injection & Tablets ... 944
Panwarfin Tablets ... 547

SEPTRA SUSPENSION
(Trimethoprim, Sulfamethoxazole) ... 813
See **Septra DS Tablets**

SEPTRA TABLETS
(Trimethoprim, Sulfamethoxazole) ... 813
See **Septra DS Tablets**

SER-AP-ES TABLETS
(Hydralazine, Hydrochlorothiazide, Reserpine) ... 881
May interact with corticosteroids, lithium preparations, antihypertensives, monoamine oxidase inhibitors, insulin, cardiac glycosides, barbiturates, narcotic analgesics, non-steroidal anti-inflammatory agents, tricyclic antidepressants, direct-acting sympathomimetic amines, indirect-acting sympathomimetic amines, and certain other agents. Compounds in these categories include:

Acebutolol Hydrochloride (Additive or potentiated action). Products include:
Sectral Capsules ... 2520

ACTH (Hypokalemia).
No products indexed under this heading.

Alcohol (Orthostatic hypotension).

Alfentanil Hydrochloride (Orthostatic hypotension). Products include:
Alfenta Injection ... 1131

Amitriptyline Hydrochloride (Decreases the antihypertensive effect of reserpine). Products include:
Elavil ... 2269
Endep Tablets ... 1927
Etrafon ... 2087
Limbitrol ... 1933
Triavil Tablets ... 1556

Amoxapine (Decreases the antihypertensive effect of reserpine). Products include:
Asendin Tablets ... 1196

Amphetamine Resins (The action of indirect-acting sympathomimetic amines is inhibited). Products include:
Biphetamine Capsules ... 973

Aprobarbital (Orthostatic hypotension). Products include:
Alurate Elixir ... 1883

Atenolol (Additive or potentiated action). Products include:
Tenoretic Tablets ... 1105
Tenormin Tablets and I.V. Injection 1107

Benazepril Hydrochloride (Additive or potentiated action). Products include:
Lotensin Tablets ... 872

Bendroflumethiazide (Additive or potentiated action). Products include:
Corzide Tablets ... 702
Naturetin Tablets ... 1789
Rauzide Tablets ... 1804

Betamethasone Acetate (Hypokalemia). Products include:
Celestone Soluspan Suspension ... 2081

Betamethasone Sodium Phosphate (Hypokalemia). Products include:
Celestone Soluspan Suspension ... 2081

Betaxolol Hydrochloride (Additive or potentiated action). Products include:
Betoptic Sterile Ophthalmic Solution ... 569
Betoptic S Sterile Ophthalmic Suspension ... 570
Kerlone Tablets ... 2172

Buprenorphine (Orthostatic hypotension).
No products indexed under this heading.

Butabarbital (Orthostatic hypotension). Products include:
Pyridium Plus ... 1764

Butalbital (Orthostatic hypotension). Products include:
Esgic-Plus Tablets ... 1002
Esgic Tablets & Capsules ... 1001
Fioricet Tablets ... 2006
Fiorinal Capsules ... 2007
Fiorinal with Codeine Capsules ... 2008
Fiorinal Tablets ... 2007
Phrenilin ... 838
Sedapap Tablets 50 mg/650 mg .. 1360

Captopril (Additive or potentiated action). Products include:
Capoten ... 2255
Capozide ... 2258

Carteolol Hydrochloride (Additive or potentiated action). Products include:
Cartrol Tablets ... 507

Chlorothiazide (Additive or potentiated action). Products include:
Aldoclor Tablets ... 1413
Diupres Tablets ... 1461
Diuril Oral ... 1464

Chlorothiazide Sodium (Additive or potentiated action). Products include:
Diuril Sodium Intravenous ... 1463

Chlorthalidone (Additive or potentiated action). Products include:
Combipres Tablets ... 678
Tenoretic Tablets ... 1105
Thalitone Tablets ... 687

Clomipramine Hydrochloride (Decreases the antihypertensive effect of reserpine). Products include:
Anafranil Capsules ... 650

Clonidine (Additive or potentiated action). Products include:
Catapres-TTS ... 677

Clonidine Hydrochloride (Additive or potentiated action). Products include:
Catapres Tablets ... 676
Combipres Tablets ... 678

Codeine (Orthostatic hypotension). Products include:
Calcidrine Syrup ... 506

Codeine Phosphate (Orthostatic hypotension). Products include:
Actifed with Codeine Cough Syrup .. 752
Cheracol Cough Syrup ... 1853
Codimal PH Syrup ... 846
Dimetane-DC Cough Syrup ... 1857
Empirin with Codeine Phosphate Nos. 2, 3 & 4 ... 764
Fiorinal with Codeine Capsules ... 2008
Isoclor Expectorant ... 982
Naldecon CX Adult Liquid ... ⊞ 521
Novahistine DH ... 1342
Novahistine Expectorant ... 1343
Nucofed Capsules ... 2219
Nucofed Expectorant ... 2219
Nucofed Pediatric Expectorant ... 2220
Nucofed Syrup ... 2219
Phenaphen with Codeine Capsules 1865
Phenaphen-650 with Codeine Tablets ... 1866
Phenergan with Codeine ... 2497
Phenergan VC with Codeine ... 2501
Robitussin A-C Syrup ... 1875
Robitussin-DAC Syrup ... 1875
Ryna ... ⊞ 741
Soma Compound w/Codeine Tablets ... 2390
Triaminic Expectorant w/Codeine .. 1996
Tussi-Organidin Liquid ... 2391
Tylenol with Codeine ... 1381

Codeine Polistirex (Orthostatic hypotension).
No products indexed under this heading.

Cortisone Acetate (Hypokalemia). Products include:
Cortone Acetate Sterile Suspension ... 1437
Cortone Acetate Tablets ... 1439

Deserpidine (Additive or potentiated action). Products include:
Enduronyl ... 518
Harmonyl Tablets ... 528
Oreticyl ... 545

Desipramine Hydrochloride (Decreases the antihypertensive effect of reserpine). Products include:
Norpramin Tablets ... 1340

Deslanoside (Cardiac arrhythmia).
No products indexed under this heading.

Dexamethasone (Hypokalemia). Products include:
AK-Trol Ointment & Suspension ... ⊙ 207
Decadron Elixir ... 1445
Decadron Tablets ... 1447
Decaspray Topical Aerosol ... 1459
Dexacidin ... ⊙ 272
Maxidex Sterile Ophthalmic Suspension ... ⊙ 223
Maxitrol Ophthalmic Ointment/Suspension ... ⊙ 223
TobraDex Ophthalmic Suspension and Ointment ... ⊙ 228

Dexamethasone Acetate (Hypokalemia). Products include:
Dalalone D.P. Injectable ... 999
Decadron-LA Sterile Suspension ... 1457

Dexamethasone Sodium Phosphate (Hypokalemia). Products include:
AK-Dex ... ⊙ 203
Decadron Phosphate Respihaler ... 1454
Decadron Phosphate Sterile Ophthalmic Ointment ... 1453
Decadron Phosphate Sterile Ophthalmic Solution ... 1453
Decadron Phosphate Topical Cream ... 1455
Decadron Phosphate Turbinaire ... 1456
Maxidex Sterile Ophthalmic Ointment ... ⊙ 222
NeoDecadron Sterile Ophthalmic Ointment ... 1517
NeoDecadron Sterile Ophthalmic Solution ... 1518
NeoDecadron Topical Cream ... 1518

Dextroamphetamine Sulfate (The action of indirect-acting sympathomimetic amines is inhibited). Products include:
Dexedrine ... 2206

Dezocine (Orthostatic hypotension).

Diazoxide (Hypotension; additive or potentiated action). Products include:
Hyperstat I.V. Injection ... 2095
Proglycem ... 649

Diclofenac Sodium (May reduce the diuretic, natriuretic, and antihypertensive effects of thiazide diuretics). Products include:
Voltaren Ophthalmic Sterile Ophthalmic Solution ... ⊙ 268
Voltaren Tablets ... 1042

Digitoxin (Cardiac arrhythmia). Products include:
Crystodigin Tablets ... 1253

Digoxin (Cardiac arrhythmia). Products include:
Lanoxicaps ... 772
Lanoxin Elixir Pediatric ... 775
Lanoxin Injection ... 778
Lanoxin Injection Pediatric ... 781
Lanoxin Tablets ... 783

Doxazosin Mesylate (Additive or potentiated action). Products include:
Cardura Tablets ... 1941

Doxepin Hydrochloride (Decreases the antihypertensive effect of reserpine). Products include:
Sinequan ... 1960

Enalapril Maleate (Additive or potentiated action). Products include:
Vaseretic Tablets ... 1559
Vasotec Tablets ... 1564

Enalaprilat (Additive or potentiated action). Products include:
Vasotec I.V. ... 1562

Ephedrine Hydrochloride (The action of indirect-acting sympathomimetic amines is inhibited). Products include:
Amesec ... ⊞ 682
Primatene Tablets-M Formula ... 2421
Primatene Tablets-P Formula ... 2421
Primatene Tablets-Regular Formula ... 2421
Quadrinal Tablets ... 1183
Quelidrine Syrup ... 556
Tedral SA ... 1765

Ephedrine Sulfate (The action of indirect-acting sympathomimetic amines is inhibited). Products include:
Bronkaid Tablets ... ⊞ 757
Bronkolixir ... ⊞ 761
Bronkotabs Tablets ... ⊞ 762
Marax Tablets & DF Syrup ... 1954
Pazo Hemorrhoid Ointment & Suppositories ... 752
Vicks Vatronol Nose Drops ... ⊞ 666

Ephedrine Tannate (The action of indirect-acting sympathomimetic amines is inhibited). Products include:
Rynatuss ... 2388

Epinephrine Hydrochloride (The action of direct-acting sympathomimetic amines may be prolonged). Products include:
Adrenalin Chloride Solution 1:100 & 1:1,000 ... 1689
Epifrin ... ⊙ 244
Glaucon ... ⊙ 218

Esmolol Hydrochloride (Additive or potentiated action). Products include:
Brevibloc Injection ... 942

Etodolac (May reduce the diuretic, natriuretic, and antihypertensive effects of thiazide diuretics). Products include:
- Lodine Capsules 2468

Felodipine (Additive or potentiated action). Products include:
- Plendil Extended-Release Tablets 1526

Fenoprofen Calcium (May reduce the diuretic, natriuretic, and antihypertensive effects of thiazide diuretics). Products include:
- Nalfon Pulvules & Tablets 919

Fentanyl (Orthostatic hypotension). Products include:
- Duragesic Transdermal System 1133

Fentanyl Citrate (Orthostatic hypotension). Products include:
- Innovar Injection 1141
- Sublimaze Injection 1146

Flurbiprofen (May reduce the diuretic, natriuretic, and antihypertensive effects of thiazide diuretics). Products include:
- Ansaid Tablets 2319

Fosinopril Sodium (Additive or potentiated action). Products include:
- Monopril Tablets 1406

Furazolidone (Concurrent administration of MAOI should be avoided). Products include:
- Furoxone 1855

Furosemide (Additive or potentiated action). Products include:
- Lasix 1093

Guanabenz Acetate (Additive or potentiated action). Products include:
- Wytensin Tablets 2542

Guanethidine Monosulfate (Additive or potentiated action). Products include:
- Esimil Tablets 864
- Ismelin Tablets 869

Hydralazine Hydrochloride (Additive or potentiated action). Products include:
- Apresazide Capsules 854
- Apresoline Hydrochloride Parenteral (Ampuls) 856
- Apresoline Hydrochloride Tablets 855
- Apresoline-Esidrix Tablets 857
- Ser-Ap-Es Tablets 881
- Serpasil-Apresoline Tablets 884

Hydrocodone Bitartrate (Orthostatic hypotension). Products include:
- Anexsia 5/500 Tablets 2196
- Anexsia 7.5/650 Tablets 2197
- Azdōne Tablets 844
- Codiclear DH Syrup 845
- Codimal DH Syrup 846
- Damason-P 1356
- Hycodan Syrup, Tablets 927
- Hycomine Compound Tablets 929
- Hycomine Syrup 927
- Hycotuss Expectorant Syrup 930
- Hydrocet Capsules 835
- Lortab ASA Tablets 2414
- Lortab 2412
- Ru-Tuss with Hydrocodone 694
- Triaminic Expectorant DH 1995
- Vicodin Tablets 1187
- Vicodin ES Tablets 1189
- Zydone Capsules 941

Hydrocodone Polistirex (Orthostatic hypotension). Products include:
- Tussionex Extended-Release Suspension 988

Hydrocortisone (Hypokalemia). Products include:
- AK-Spore H.C. .... ⊙ 206
- Bactine Hydrocortisone Anti-Itch Cream .... ⊞ 625
- CaldeCORT Anti-Itch Hydrocortisone Spray .... ⊞ 560
- Carmol HC Cream 1% 2296
- Cortaid Spray .... ⊞ 735
- Cortenema 2244
- Cortisporin Ointment 758
- Cortisporin Ophthalmic Ointment Sterile 758
- Cortisporin Ophthalmic Suspension Sterile 759
- Cortisporin Otic Solution Sterile 760
- Cortisporin Otic Suspension Sterile 760
- Cortizone-5 Creme & Ointment .... ⊞ 732
- Dermolate Anti-Itch Cream .... ⊞ 697
- Eldecort Cream 1.0% 1113
- Eldecort Cream 1.0% and 2.5% 1113
- Fungoid HC Creme 1770
- Hydrocortone Tablets 1482
- Hytone 909
- LazerSporin-C Solution 1770
- Massengill Medicated Soft Cloth Towelettes 2192
- Nutracort Cream & Lotion 1684
- PediOtic Suspension Sterile 797
- Synacort Creams 1%, 2.5% 2296
- Vanoxide-HC Acne Lotion 911
- Vioform-Hydrocortisone Cream and Mild Cream 889
- Vioform-Hydrocortisone Ointment 889
- VōSoL HC Otic Solution 2392
- Vytone Cream 1% 911

Hydrocortisone Acetate (Hypokalemia). Products include:
- Analpram-HC Rectal Cream 1% and 2.5% 970
- Anusol-HC Cream 1690
- Anusol-HC Suppositories 1691
- Caldecort .... ⊞ 560
- Carmol HC Cream 1% 2296
- Chloromycetin Hydrocortisone Ophthalmic 1694
- Coly-Mycin S Otic w/Neomycin & Hydrocortisone 1708
- Cortaid .... ⊞ 735
- Cortef Feminine Itch Cream .... ⊞ 735
- Corticaine .... ⊞ 682
- Cortifoam 1827
- Cortisporin Cream 757
- Epifoam 1828
- Gynecort 5 Creme .... ⊞ 556
- Hydrocortone Acetate Sterile Suspension 1479
- Lanacort 5 Creme and Ointment .... ⊞ 557
- Mantadil Cream 789
- Ophthocort .... ⊙ 301
- Orabase HCA Oral Paste 890
- Pramosone Cream, Lotion & Ointment 971
- ProctoCream-HC 1834
- Proctofoam-HC 1835

Hydrocortisone Sodium Phosphate (Hypokalemia). Products include:
- Hydrocortone Phosphate Injection, Sterile 1481

Hydrocortisone Sodium Succinate (Hypokalemia). Products include:
- Solu-Cortef Sterile Powder 2361

Hydroflumethiazide (Additive or potentiated action). Products include:
- Diucardin Tablets 2450
- Saluron 718
- Salutensin/Salutensin-Demi 719

Ibuprofen (May reduce the diuretic, natriuretic, and antihypertensive effects of thiazide diuretics). Products include:
- Advil Cold & Sinus Caplets (formerly CoAdvil) 2416
- Advil Ibuprofen Tablets and Caplets 2416
- Children's Advil Suspension 2426
- CoAdvil .... ⊞ 748
- Dristan Sinus Caplets 2419
- Haltran Tablets .... ⊞ 668
- Ibuprofen .... ⊞ 631
- Medipren ibuprofen Caplets and Tablets 1362
- Midol 200 Cramp Relief Formula .... ⊞ 570
- Motrin Tablets 2351
- Motrin IB Caplets and Tablets .... ⊞ 736
- Nuprin Ibuprofen/Analgesic Tablets & Caplets 752
- PediaProfen Suspension 1363
- Rufen Tablets 691
- Trendar Ibuprofen Tablets .... ⊞ 756

Imipramine Hydrochloride (Decreases the antihypertensive effect of reserpine). Products include:
- Tofranil Ampuls 1038
- Tofranil Tablets 1039

Imipramine Pamoate (Decreases the antihypertensive effect of reserpine). Products include:
- Tofranil-PM Capsules 1041

Indapamide (Additive or potentiated action). Products include:
- Lozol Tablets 1843

Indomethacin (May reduce the diuretic, natriuretic, and antihypertensive effects of thiazide diuretics). Products include:
- Indocin 1487

Indomethacin Sodium Trihydrate (May reduce the diuretic, natriuretic, and antihypertensive effects of thiazide diuretics). Products include:
- Indocin I.V. 1490

Insulin, Human (Altered insulin requirements).
- No products indexed under this heading.

Insulin, Human Isophane Suspension (Altered insulin requirements). Products include:
- Humulin N, 100 Units 1270

Insulin, Human NPH (Altered insulin requirements). Products include:
- Insulatard NPH Human 1627
- Novolin N 1627
- Novolin N PenFill Cartridges 1628
- Novolin N Prefilled 1628

Insulin, Human Regular (Altered insulin requirements). Products include:
- Humulin BR, 100 Units 1268
- Humulin R, 100 Units 1272
- Novolin R 1627
- Novolin R PenFill Cartridges 1628
- Novolin R Prefilled 1629
- Velosulin Human 1628

Insulin, Human, Zinc Suspension (Altered insulin requirements). Products include:
- Humulin L, 100 Units 1268
- Humulin U, 100 Units 1272
- Novolin L 1627

Insulin, NPH (Altered insulin requirements). Products include:
- NPH, 40 & 100 Units 1273
- Beef NPH, 100 Units 1274
- Pork NPH, 100 Units 1275
- Insulatard NPH 1626
- NPH Insulin 1626
- NPH Purified Pork Isophane Insulin 1626

Insulin, Regular (Altered insulin requirements). Products include:
- Regular, 40 & 100 Units 1273
- Beef Regular, 100 Units 1275
- Pork Regular, 100 Units 1275
- Pork Regular (Concentrated), 500 Units 1276
- Regular Insulin 1625
- Regular Purified Pork Insulin 1626
- Velosulin 1627

Insulin, Zinc Crystals (Altered insulin requirements). Products include:
- NPH, 40 & 100 Units 1273

Insulin, Zinc Suspension (Altered insulin requirements). Products include:
- Lente, 40 & 100 Units 1272
- Protamine, Zinc, 40 & 100 Units 1273
- Lente Iletin I 1272
- Beef Lente, 100 Units 1274
- Beef Protamine Zinc, 100 Units 1274
- Pork Lente, 100 Units 1275
- Pork, Protamine, Zinc, 100 Units 1275
- Lente Insulin 1626
- Lente Purified Pork Insulin 1626
- Semilente Insulin 1625
- Ultralente Insulin 1626

Isocarboxazid (Concurrent administration of MAOI should be avoided). Products include:
- Marplan Tablets 1906

Isoproterenol Hydrochloride (The action of direct-acting sympathomimetic amines may be prolonged). Products include:
- Isuprel Hydrochloride Injection 1:5000 2050
- Isuprel Hydrochloride Mistometer 2051
- Isuprel Hydrochloride Solution 1:200 & 1:100 2052
- Norisodrine Aerotrol 540

Isradipine (Additive or potentiated action). Products include:
- DynaCirc Capsules 2004

Ketoprofen (May reduce the diuretic, natriuretic, and antihypertensive effects of thiazide diuretics). Products include:
- Orudis Capsules 2488

Ketorolac Tromethamine (May reduce the diuretic, natriuretic, and antihypertensive effects of thiazide diuretics). Products include:
- Toradol IM Injection 2302

Labetalol Hydrochloride (Additive or potentiated action). Products include:
- Normodyne Injection 2108
- Normodyne Tablets 2110
- Normozide Tablets 2112
- Trandate HCT Tablets 579
- Trandate Injection 577
- Trandate Tablets 579

Levorphanol Tartrate (Orthostatic hypotension). Products include:
- Levo-Dromoran 1906

Lisinopril (Additive or potentiated action). Products include:
- Prinivil Tablets 1538
- Prinzide Tablets 1540
- Zestoretic 2274
- Zestril Tablets 2277

Lithium Carbonate (Reduced renal clearance and increased risk of lithium toxicity). Products include:
- Eskalith 2214
- Lithane Tablets 1596
- Lithium Carbonate Capsules & Tablets 1984
- Lithobid Tablets 870

Lithium Citrate (Reduced renal clearance and increased risk of lithium toxicity). Products include:
- Cibalith-S 870

Maprotiline Hydrochloride (Decreases the antihypertensive effect of reserpine). Products include:
- Ludiomil Tablets 874

Mecamylamine Hydrochloride (Additive or potentiated action). Products include:
- Inversine Tablets 1492

Meclofenamate Sodium (May reduce the diuretic, natriuretic, and antihypertensive effects of thiazide diuretics). Products include:
- Meclomen Capsules 1739

Mefenamic Acid (May reduce the diuretic, natriuretic, and antihypertensive effects of thiazide diuretics). Products include:
- Ponstel 1758

Meperidine Hydrochloride (Orthostatic hypotension). Products include:
- Demerol 2047
- Mepergan Injection 2479

Mephobarbital (Orthostatic hypotension). Products include:
- Mebaral Tablets 2061

Metaraminol Bitartrate (The action of direct-acting sympathomimetic amines may be prolonged). Products include:
- Aramine Injection 1424

Methadone Hydrochloride (Orthostatic hypotension). Products include:
- Dolophine Hydrochloride Ampoules & Vials 1260
- Dolophine Hydrochloride Tablets 1261
- Methadone Hydrochloride Diskets 1284
- Methadone Hydrochloride Oral Solution & Tablets 1987

Methyclothiazide (Additive or potentiated action). Products include:
- Enduron Tablets 517
- Enduronyl 518

Methyldopa (Hemolytic anemia; additive or potentiated action). Products include:
- Aldoclor Tablets 1413
- Aldomet Oral 1415
- Aldoril Tablets 1418

Methyldopate Hydrochloride (Hemolytic anemia; additive or potentiated action). Products include:
- Aldomet Ester HCl Injection 1417

Methylprednisolone Acetate (Hypokalemia). Products include:
- Depo-Medrol Sterile Aqueous Suspension 2334

Methylprednisolone Sodium Succinate (Hypokalemia). Products include:
- Solu-Medrol Sterile Powder 2363

Metolazone (Additive or potentiated action). Products include:
- Diulo 2129
- Mykrox ½ mg Tablets 984
- Zaroxolyn Tablets 989

Metoprolol Tartrate (Additive or potentiated action). Products include:
- Lopressor Ampuls 1032
- Lopressor HCT Tablets 1034
- Lopressor Tablets 1032

Metyrosine (Additive or potentiated action). Products include:
- Demser Capsules 1460

Minoxidil (Additive or potentiated action). Products include:
- Loniten Tablets 2346
- Rogaine Topical Solution 2357

Morphine Sulfate (Orthostatic hypotension). Products include:
- Astramorph/PF Injection, USP (Preservative-Free) 618
- Duramorph 960
- Infumorph 200 and Infumorph 500 Sterile Solutions 962
- MS Contin Tablets 1814
- MSIR 1817
- Oramorph SR (Morphine Sulfate Sustained Release Tablets) 1988
- Roxanol 1991

Nadolol (Additive or potentiated action). Products include:
- Corgard Tablets 701
- Corzide Tablets 702

Naproxen (May reduce the diuretic, natriuretic, and antihypertensive effects of thiazide diuretics). Products include:
- Naprosyn 2297

Naproxen Sodium (May reduce the diuretic, natriuretic, and antihypertensive effects of thiazide diuretics). Products include:
- Anaprox and Anaprox DS Tablets 2288

Nicardipine Hydrochloride (Additive or potentiated action). Products include:
- Cardene Capsules 2290

Nitroglycerin (Additive or potentiated action). Products include:
- Deponit NTG Transdermal Delivery System 2143
- Minitran Transdermal Delivery System 1312
- Nitro-Bid Ointment 1339
- Nitro-Bid Capsules 1338
- Nitrodisc 2176
- Nitro-Dur (nitroglycerin) Transdermal Infusion System 1164
- Nitrogard Tablets 1004
- Nitrolingual Spray 1846
- Nitrostat Tablets 1743
- Transderm-Nitro Transdermal Therapeutic System 2283

Norepinephrine Bitartrate (Decreased arterial responsiveness to norepinephrine). Products include:
- Levophed Bitartrate Injection 2054

Norepinephrine Hydrochloride (The action of direct-acting sympathomimetic amines may be prolonged).

Nortriptyline Hydrochloride (Decreases the antihypertensive effect of reserpine). Products include:
- Pamelor 2019

Opium Alkaloids (Orthostatic hypotension). Products include:
- B & O No. 15A & No. 16A Supprettes 2395
- Pantopon Injectable 1911

Oxycodone Hydrochloride (Orthostatic hypotension). Products include:
- Percocet Tablets 950
- Percodan 951
- Roxicodone Tablets, Oral Solution & Intensol (Oxycodone) 1992
- Tylox Capsules 1382

Penbutolol Sulfate (Additive or potentiated action). Products include:
- Levatol 1832

Pentobarbital Sodium (Orthostatic hypotension). Products include:
- Nembutal Sodium Capsules 534
- Nembutal Sodium Solution 536
- Nembutal Sodium Suppositories 538

Phenelzine Sulfate (Concurrent administration of MAOI should be avoided). Products include:
- Nardil 1742

Phenobarbital (Orthostatic hypotension). Products include:
- Arco-Lase Plus Tablets 607
- Bellergal-S Tablets 1998
- Bronkolixir .... ▣ 761
- Bronkotabs Tablets .... ▣ 762
- Donnatal 1858
- Donnatal Extentabs 1859
- Donnatal Tablets 1858
- Donnazyme Tablets 1860
- Kinesed Tablets 2272
- Phenobarbital Elixir and Tablets 1293
- Primatene Tablets-P Formula 2421
- Quadrinal Tablets 1183
- Tedral SA 1765

Phenoxybenzamine Hydrochloride (Additive or potentiated action). Products include:
- Dibenzyline Capsules 2207

Phentolamine Mesylate (Additive or potentiated action). Products include:
- Regitine 878

Phenylbutazone (May reduce the diuretic, natriuretic, and antihypertensive effects of thiazide diuretics). Products include:
- Butazolidin Capsules & Tablets 1027

Phenylephrine Hydrochloride (The action of direct-acting sympathomimetic amines may be prolonged). Products include:
- AK-Dilate Solution 2.5% and 10% .... ⊙ 203
- Atrohist Sprinkle Capsules 558
- Cerose-DM 2443
- Codimal 846
- Comhist LA Capsules 1618
- Congespirin For Children Aspirin Free Chewable Cold Tablets 748
- Cyclomydril .... ⊙ 216
- Deconsal Sprinkle Capsules 559
- Dimetane Decongestant .... ▣ 673
- Dristan Decongestant/Antihistamine/ Analgesic Coated Caplets .... ▣ 749
- Dristan Cold Nasal Decongestant/ Antihistamine/ Analgesic Coated Tablets 2419
- Dristan Advanced Formula Decongestant/Antihistamine/ Analgesic Tablets .... ▣ 749
- Dristan Nasal Spray, Menthol 2419
- Dristan Nasal Spray, Regular and Regular with Metered Pump 2419
- Entex Capsules 1623
- Entex Liquid 1623
- Sinus Excedrin Analgesic, Decongestant Tablets & Caplets 750
- Extendryl 994
- 4-Way Fast Acting Nasal Spray - Original Formula (regular & mentholated) & Metered Spray Pump (regular) 751
- Hycomine Compound Tablets 929
- Murocoll-2 Sterile Ophthalmic Solution .... ⊙ 261
- Mydfrin 2.5% .... ⊙ 224
- Naldecon Syrup, Tablets, Pediatric Drops and Pediatric Syrup 709
- Neo-Synephrine Hydrochloride 1% Carpuject 2063
- Neo-Synephrine Hydrochloride 1% Injection 2063
- Neo-Synephrine Hydrochloride (Ophthalmic) 2064
- Neo-Synephrine .... ▣ 759
- Nōstril Nasal Decongestant .... ▣ 520
- Novahistine Elixir .... ▣ 596
- Phenergan VC 2500
- Phenergan VC with Codeine 2501
- Prefrin Liquifilm Vasoconstrictor and Lubricant Eye Drops .... ⊙ 254
- Prefrin-A .... ⊙ 255
- Quelidrine Syrup 556
- Relief Vasoconstrictor and Lubricant Eye Drops .... ⊙ 256
- Robitussin Night Relief .... ▣ 677
- Ru-Tuss with Hydrocodone 694
- Ru-Tuss Tablets 693
- Vasosulf .... ⊙ 279
- Vicks Sinex .... ▣ 665
- Zincfrin .... ⊙ 230

Phenylephrine Tannate (The action of direct-acting sympathomimetic amines may be prolonged). Products include:
- Rynatan 2387
- Rynatuss 2388

Pindolol (Additive or potentiated action). Products include:
- Visken Tablets 2036

Piroxicam (May reduce the diuretic, natriuretic, and antihypertensive effects of thiazide diuretics). Products include:
- Feldene Capsules 1777

Polythiazide (Additive or potentiated action). Products include:
- Minizide Capsules 1779
- Renese Tablets 1785
- Renese-R Tablets 1786

Prazosin Hydrochloride (Additive or potentiated action). Products include:
- Minipress Capsules 1778
- Minizide Capsules 1779

Prednisolone Acetate (Hypokalemia). Products include:
- AK-Cide Sterile Ophthalmic Ointment & Suspension .... ⊙ 202
- Blephamide Liquifilm Sterile Ophthalmic Suspension 586
- Blephamide S.O.P. Sterile Ophthalmic Ointment 586
- Cetapred Ointment .... ⊙ 220
- ⅛% Econopred & 1% Econopred Plus .... ⊙ 217
- Isopto Cetapred Suspension .... ⊙ 220
- Metimyd .... ⊙ 306
- Poly-Pred Liquifilm .... ⊙ 250
- Pred Forte .... ⊙ 252
- Pred Mild .... ⊙ 254
- Pred-G Liquifilm Sterile Ophthalmic Suspension .... ⊙ 252
- Pred-G S.O.P. Sterile Ophthalmic Ointment .... ⊙ 253
- Vasocidin Ointment .... ⊙ 275

Prednisolone Sodium Phosphate (Hypokalemia). Products include:
- AK-Pred .... ⊙ 205
- Hydeltrasol Injection, Sterile 1476
- Inflamase .... ⊙ 274
- Pediapred Oral Liquid 987
- Vasocidin Ophthalmic Solution .... ⊙ 276

Prednisolone Tebutate (Hypokalemia). Products include:
- Hydeltra-T.B.A. Sterile Suspension 1478

Prednisone (Hypokalemia). Products include:
- Deltasone Tablets 2332

Propoxyphene Hydrochloride (Orthostatic hypotension). Products include:
- Darvon 1256
- Wygesic Tablets 2540

Propoxyphene Napsylate (Orthostatic hypotension). Products include:
- Darvon-N/Darvocet-N 1254

Propranolol Hydrochloride (Additive or potentiated action). Products include:
- Inderal 2459
- Inderal LA Long Acting Capsules 2461
- Inderide Tablets 2463
- Inderide LA Long Acting Capsules 2465

Protriptyline Hydrochloride (Decreases the antihypertensive effect of reserpine). Products include:
- Vivactil Tablets 1567

Quinidine Gluconate (Potential for arrhythmias). Products include:
- Quinaglute Dura-Tabs Tablets 663

Quinidine Polygalacturonate (Potential for arrhythmias). Products include:
- Cardioquin Tablets 1812

Quinidine Sulfate (Potential for arrhythmias). Products include:
- Quinidex Extentabs 1868

Ramipril (Additive or potentiated action). Products include:
- Altace Capsules 1086

Rauwolfia Serpentina (Additive or potentiated action). Products include:
- Raudixin Tablets 1803
- Rauzide Tablets 1804

Rescinnamine (Additive or potentiated action).
- No products indexed under this heading.

Secobarbital Sodium (Orthostatic hypotension). Products include:
- Seconal Sodium Pulvules 1296

Selegiline Hydrochloride (Concurrent administration of MAOI should be avoided). Products include:
- Eldepryl 2250

Sodium Nitroprusside (Additive or potentiated action). Products include:
- Nipride I.V. Infusion 1909

Sufentanil Citrate (Orthostatic hypotension). Products include:
- Sufenta Injection 1147

Sulindac (May reduce the diuretic, natriuretic, and antihypertensive effects of thiazide diuretics). Products include:
- Clinoril Tablets 1433

Terazosin Hydrochloride (Additive or potentiated action). Products include:
- Hytrin Tablets 529

Thiamylal Sodium (Orthostatic hypotension). Products include:
- Surital Ampoules, Steri-Vials 1764

Timolol Maleate (Additive or potentiated action). Products include:
- Blocadren Tablets 1429
- Timolide Tablets 1547
- Timoptic in Ocudose 1552
- Timoptic Sterile Ophthalmic Solution 1550

Tolmetin Sodium (May reduce the diuretic, natriuretic, and antihypertensive effects of thiazide diuretics). Products include:
Tolectin (200, 400 and 600 mg) .. 1379
Tranylcypromine Sulfate (Concurrent administration of MAOI should be avoided). Products include:
Parnate Tablets 2222
Triamcinolone (Hypokalemia).
No products indexed under this heading.
Triamcinolone Acetonide (Hypokalemia). Products include:
Aristocort A 1010
Azmacort Inhaler 1837
Kenalog Cream, Lotion & Ointment 2401
Kenalog-10 Injection 2402
Kenalog-40 Injection 2403
Kenalog in Orabase 604
Kenalog Spray 2401
Mycolog II Cream and Ointment 2407
Mytrex Cream & Ointment 2080
Nasacort Nasal Inhaler 1844
Triamcinolone Diacetate (Hypokalemia). Products include:
Aristocort Suspension 1008
Triamcinolone Hexacetonide (Hypokalemia). Products include:
Aristospan Suspension 1011
Trimethaphan Camsylate (Additive or potentiated action). Products include:
Arfonad Ampuls 1887
Trimipramine Maleate (Decreases the antihypertensive effect of reserpine). Products include:
Surmontil Capsules 2524
Tubocurarine Chloride (Increased responsiveness to tubocurarine).
No products indexed under this heading.
Tyramine (The action of indirect-acting sympathomimetic amines is inhibited).

Food Interactions

Food, unspecified (Concomitant administration enhances gastrointestinal absorption of hydrochlorothiazide and results in higher plasma levels of hydralazine).

SERAX CAPSULES
(Oxazepam) 2522
May interact with central nervous system depressants and certain other agents. Compounds in these categories include:

Alcohol (Effects may be additive).
Alfentanil Hydrochloride (Effects may be additive). Products include:
Alfenta Injection 1131
Alprazolam (Effects may be additive). Products include:
Xanax Tablets 2367
Aprobarbital (Effects may be additive). Products include:
Alurate Elixir 1883
Buprenorphine (Effects may be additive).
No products indexed under this heading.
Buspirone Hydrochloride (Effects may be additive). Products include:
BuSpar 1401
Butabarbital (Effects may be additive). Products include:
Pyridium Plus 1764
Butalbital (Effects may be additive). Products include:
Esgic-Plus Tablets 1002
Esgic Tablets & Capsules 1001
Fioricet Tablets 2006
Fiorinal Capsules 2007
Fiorinal with Codeine Capsules 2008
Fiorinal Tablets 2007
Phrenilin 838
Sedapap Tablets 50 mg/650 mg .. 1360
Chlordiazepoxide (Effects may be additive). Products include:
Libritabs Tablets 1930
Limbitrol 1933
Menrium Tablets 1934
Chlordiazepoxide Hydrochloride (Effects may be additive). Products include:
Librax Capsules 1929
Librium Capsules 1931
Librium Injectable 1932
Chlorpromazine (Effects may be additive). Products include:
Thorazine 2234
Chlorprothixene (Effects may be additive). Products include:
Taractan Tablets 1920
Chlorprothixene Hydrochloride (Effects may be additive). Products include:
Taractan 1920
Clorazepate Dipotassium (Effects may be additive). Products include:
Tranxene 556
Codeine (Effects may be additive). Products include:
Calcidrine Syrup 506
Codeine Phosphate (Effects may be additive). Products include:
Actifed with Codeine Cough Syrup.. 752
Cheracol Cough Syrup 1853
Codimal PH Syrup 846
Dimetane-DC Cough Syrup 1857
Empirin with Codeine Phosphate Nos. 2, 3 & 4 764
Fiorinal with Codeine Capsules 2008
Isoclor Expectorant 982
Naldecon CX Adult Liquid .... ▣ 521
Novahistine DH 1342
Novahistine Expectorant 1343
Nucofed Capsules 2219
Nucofed Expectorant 2219
Nucofed Pediatric Expectorant 2220
Nucofed Syrup 2219
Phenaphen with Codeine Capsules 1865
Phenaphen-650 with Codeine Tablets 1866
Phenergan with Codeine 2497
Phenergan VC with Codeine 2501
Robitussin A-C Syrup 1875
Robitussin-DAC Syrup 1875
Ryna .... ▣ 741
Soma Compound w/Codeine Tablets 2390
Triaminic Expectorant w/Codeine .. 1996
Tussi-Organidin Liquid 2391
Tylenol with Codeine 1381
Codeine Polistirex (Effects may be additive).
No products indexed under this heading.
Dezocine (Effects may be additive).
Diazepam (Effects may be additive). Products include:
Valium Injectable 1937
Valium Tablets 1939
Valrelease Capsules 1923
Droperidol (Effects may be additive). Products include:
Inapsine Injection 1140
Innovar Injection 1141
Enflurane (Effects may be additive). Products include:
Ethrane 599
Estazolam (Effects may be additive). Products include:
ProSom Tablets 554
Ethchlorvynol (Effects may be additive). Products include:
Placidyl Capsules 553
Ethinamate (Effects may be additive).
No products indexed under this heading.
Fentanyl (Effects may be additive). Products include:
Duragesic Transdermal System 1133
Fentanyl Citrate (Effects may be additive). Products include:
Innovar Injection 1141
Sublimaze Injection 1146
Fluphenazine Decanoate (Effects may be additive). Products include:
Prolixin Decanoate 1795
Fluphenazine Enanthate (Effects may be additive). Products include:
Prolixin Enanthate 1796
Fluphenazine Hydrochloride (Effects may be additive). Products include:
Prolixin Elixir 1793
Prolixin Injection 1791
Prolixin Oral Concentrate 1792
Prolixin Tablets 1793
Flurazepam Hydrochloride (Effects may be additive). Products include:
Dalmane Capsules 1927
Glutethimide (Effects may be additive).
No products indexed under this heading.
Haloperidol (Effects may be additive). Products include:
Haldol Injection, Tablets and Concentrate 1373
Haloperidol Decanoate (Effects may be additive). Products include:
Haldol Decanoate 1375
Hydrocodone Bitartrate (Effects may be additive). Products include:
Anexsia 5/500 Tablets 2196
Anexsia 7.5/650 Tablets 2197
Azdone Tablets 844
Codiclear DH Syrup 845
Codimal DH Syrup 846
Damason-P 1356
Hycodan Syrup, Tablets 927
Hycomine Compound Tablets 929
Hycomine Syrup 927
Hycotuss Expectorant Syrup 930
Hydrocet Capsules 835
Lortab ASA Tablets 2414
Lortab 2412
Ru-Tuss with Hydrocodone 694
Triaminic Expectorant DH 1995
Vicodin Tablets 1187
Vicodin ES Tablets 1189
Zydone Capsules 941
Hydrocodone Polistirex (Effects may be additive). Products include:
Tussionex Extended-Release Suspension 988
Hydroxyzine Hydrochloride (Effects may be additive). Products include:
Atarax Tablets & Syrup 1941
Marax Tablets & DF Syrup 1954
Vistaril Intramuscular Solution 1970
Isoflurane (Effects may be additive). Products include:
Forane 600
Ketamine Hydrochloride (Effects may be additive). Products include:
Ketalar 1726
Levorphanol Tartrate (Effects may be additive). Products include:
Levo-Dromoran 1906
Lorazepam (Effects may be additive). Products include:
Ativan Injection 2432
Ativan Tablets 2434
Loxapine Hydrochloride (Effects may be additive). Products include:
Loxitane 1213
Loxapine Succinate (Effects may be additive). Products include:
Loxitane Capsules 1213
Meperidine Hydrochloride (Effects may be additive). Products include:
Demerol 2047
Mepergan Injection 2479
Mephobarbital (Effects may be additive). Products include:
Mebaral Tablets 2061
Meprobamate (Effects may be additive). Products include:
Deprol Tablets 2382
Equagesic Tablets 2451
Miltown Tablets 2386
PMB 200 and PMB 400 2504
Mesoridazine (Effects may be additive). Products include:
Serentil 686
Methadone Hydrochloride (Effects may be additive). Products include:
Dolophine Hydrochloride Ampoules & Vials 1260
Dolophine Hydrochloride Tablets 1261
Methadone Hydrochloride Diskets .. 1284
Methadone Hydrochloride Oral Solution & Tablets 1987
Methohexital Sodium (Effects may be additive). Products include:
Brevital Sodium Vials 1248
Methoxyflurane (Effects may be additive).
No products indexed under this heading.
Midazolam Hydrochloride (Effects may be additive). Products include:
Versed Injection 1924
Molindone Hydrochloride (Effects may be additive). Products include:
Moban Tablets & Concentrate 932
Morphine Sulfate (Effects may be additive). Products include:
Astramorph/PF Injection, USP (Preservative-Free) 618
Duramorph 960
Infumorph 200 and Infumorph 500 Sterile Solutions 962
MS Contin Tablets 1814
MSIR 1817
Oramorph SR (Morphine Sulfate Sustained Release Tablets) 1988
Roxanol 1991
Opium Alkaloids (Effects may be additive). Products include:
B & O No. 15A & No. 16A Supprettes 2395
Pantopon Injectable 1911
Oxycodone Hydrochloride (Effects may be additive). Products include:
Percocet Tablets 950
Percodan 951
Roxicodone Tablets, Oral Solution & Intensol (Oxycodone) 1992
Tylox Capsules 1382
Pentobarbital Sodium (Effects may be additive). Products include:
Nembutal Sodium Capsules 534
Nembutal Sodium Solution 536
Nembutal Sodium Suppositories 538
Perphenazine (Effects may be additive). Products include:
Etrafon 2087
Triavil Tablets 1556
Trilafon 2123
Phenobarbital (Effects may be additive). Products include:
Arco-Lase Plus Tablets 607
Bellergal-S Tablets 1998
Bronkolixir .... ▣ 761
Bronkotabs Tablets .... ▣ 762
Donnatal 1858
Donnatal Extentabs 1859
Donnatal Tablets 1858
Donnazyme Tablets 1860
Kinesed Tablets 2272
Phenobarbital Elixir and Tablets 1293
Primatene Tablets-P Formula 2421
Quadrinal Tablets 1183
Tedral SA 1765
Prazepam (Effects may be additive). Products include:
Centrax 1693

Prochlorperazine (Effects may be additive). Products include:
- Compazine ... 2201

Promethazine Hydrochloride (Effects may be additive). Products include:
- Mepergan Injection ... 2479
- Phenergan with Codeine ... 2497
- Phenergan with Dextromethorphan 2499
- Phenergan Injection ... 2493
- Phenergan Suppositories ... 2496
- Phenergan Syrup ... 2495
- Phenergan Tablets ... 2496
- Phenergan VC ... 2500
- Phenergan VC with Codeine ... 2501

Propofol (Effects may be additive). Products include:
- Diprivan Injection ... 2267

Propoxyphene Hydrochloride (Effects may be additive). Products include:
- Darvon ... 1256
- Wygesic Tablets ... 2540

Propoxyphene Napsylate (Effects may be additive). Products include:
- Darvon-N/Darvocet-N ... 1254

Quazepam (Effects may be additive). Products include:
- Doral Tablets ... 2383

Secobarbital Sodium (Effects may be additive). Products include:
- Seconal Sodium Pulvules ... 1296

Sufentanil Citrate (Effects may be additive). Products include:
- Sufenta Injection ... 1147

Temazepam (Effects may be additive). Products include:
- Restoril Capsules ... 2023

Thiamylal Sodium (Effects may be additive). Products include:
- Surital Ampoules, Steri-Vials ... 1764

Thioridazine Hydrochloride (Effects may be additive). Products include:
- Mellaril ... 2011

Thiothixene (Effects may be additive). Products include:
- Navane Capsules and Concentrate 1954
- Navane Intramuscular ... 1956

Triazolam (Effects may be additive). Products include:
- Halcion Tablets ... 2340

Trifluoperazine Hydrochloride (Effects may be additive). Products include:
- Stelazine ... 2226

SERAX TABLETS
(Oxazepam) ... 2522
See **Serax Capsules**

SERENTIL AMPULS
(Mesoridazine) ... 686
May interact with central nervous system depressants and certain other agents. Compounds in these categories include:

Alcohol (Potentiation).

Alfentanil Hydrochloride (Potentiation). Products include:
- Alfenta Injection ... 1131

Alprazolam (Potentiation). Products include:
- Xanax Tablets ... 2367

Aprobarbital (Potentiation). Products include:
- Alurate Elixir ... 1883

Atropine Nitrate, Methyl (Potentiation).
- No products indexed under this heading.

Atropine Sulfate (Potentiation). Products include:
- Arco-Lase Plus Tablets ... 607
- Atropine Sulfate Sterile Ophthalmic Solution and S.O.P. Sterile Ophthalmic Ointment ... ⊙ 239
- Donnagel ... ■ 675
- Donnagel-PG ... 1858
- Donnatal ... 1858
- Donnatal Extentabs ... 1859
- Donnatal Tablets ... 1858
- Donnazyme Tablets ... 1860
- Isopto Atropine ... ⊙ 218
- Lomotil ... 2174
- Motofen Tablets ... 836
- Ru-Tuss Tablets ... 693
- Urised Tablets ... 2396

Buprenorphine (Potentiation).
- No products indexed under this heading.

Buspirone Hydrochloride (Potentiation). Products include:
- BuSpar ... 1401

Butabarbital (Potentiation). Products include:
- Pyridium Plus ... 1764

Butalbital (Potentiation). Products include:
- Esgic-Plus Tablets ... 1002
- Esgic Tablets & Capsules ... 1001
- Fioricet Tablets ... 2006
- Fiorinal Capsules ... 2007
- Fiorinal with Codeine Capsules ... 2008
- Fiorinal Tablets ... 2007
- Phrenilin ... 838
- Sedapap Tablets 50 mg/650 mg .. 1360

Chlordiazepoxide (Potentiation). Products include:
- Libritabs Tablets ... 1930
- Limbitrol ... 1933
- Menrium Tablets ... 1934

Chlordiazepoxide Hydrochloride (Potentiation). Products include:
- Librax Capsules ... 1929
- Librium Capsules ... 1931
- Librium Injectable ... 1932

Chlorpromazine (Potentiation). Products include:
- Thorazine ... 2234

Chlorprothixene (Potentiation). Products include:
- Taractan Tablets ... 1920

Chlorprothixene Hydrochloride (Potentiation). Products include:
- Taractan ... 1920

Clorazepate Dipotassium (Potentiation). Products include:
- Tranxene ... 556

Codeine (Potentiation). Products include:
- Calcidrine Syrup ... 506

Codeine Phosphate (Potentiation). Products include:
- Actifed with Codeine Cough Syrup.. 752
- Cheracol Cough Syrup ... 1853
- Codimal PH Syrup ... 846
- Dimetane-DC Cough Syrup ... 1857
- Empirin with Codeine Phosphate Nos. 2, 3 & 4 ... 764
- Fiorinal with Codeine Capsules ... 2008
- Isoclor Expectorant ... 982
- Naldecon CX Adult Liquid ... ■ 521
- Novahistine DH ... 1342
- Novahistine Expectorant ... 1343
- Nucofed Capsules ... 2219
- Nucofed Expectorant ... 2219
- Nucofed Pediatric Expectorant ... 2220
- Nucofed Syrup ... 2219
- Phenaphen with Codeine Capsules 1865
- Phenaphen-650 with Codeine Tablets ... 1866
- Phenergan with Codeine ... 2497
- Phenergan VC with Codeine ... 2501
- Robitussin A-C Syrup ... 1875
- Robitussin-DAC Syrup ... 1875
- Ryna ... ■ 741
- Soma Compound w/Codeine Tablets ... 2390
- Triaminic Expectorant w/Codeine .. 1996
- Tussi-Organidin Liquid ... 2391
- Tylenol with Codeine ... 1381

Codeine Polistirex (Potentiation).
- No products indexed under this heading.

Dezocine (Potentiation).

Diazepam (Potentiation). Products include:
- Valium Injectable ... 1937
- Valium Tablets ... 1939
- Valrelease Capsules ... 1923

Droperidol (Potentiation). Products include:
- Inapsine Injection ... 1140
- Innovar Injection ... 1141

Enflurane (Potentiation). Products include:
- Ethrane ... 599

Estazolam (Potentiation). Products include:
- ProSom Tablets ... 554

Ethchlorvynol (Potentiation). Products include:
- Placidyl Capsules ... 553

Ethinamate (Potentiation).
- No products indexed under this heading.

Fentanyl (Potentiation). Products include:
- Duragesic Transdermal System ... 1133

Fentanyl Citrate (Potentiation). Products include:
- Innovar Injection ... 1141
- Sublimaze Injection ... 1146

Fluphenazine Decanoate (Potentiation). Products include:
- Prolixin Decanoate ... 1795

Fluphenazine Enanthate (Potentiation). Products include:
- Prolixin Enanthate ... 1796

Fluphenazine Hydrochloride (Potentiation). Products include:
- Prolixin Elixir ... 1793
- Prolixin Injection ... 1791
- Prolixin Oral Concentrate ... 1792
- Prolixin Tablets ... 1793

Flurazepam Hydrochloride (Potentiation). Products include:
- Dalmane Capsules ... 1927

Glutethimide (Potentiation).
- No products indexed under this heading.

Haloperidol (Potentiation). Products include:
- Haldol Injection, Tablets and Concentrate ... 1373

Haloperidol Decanoate (Potentiation). Products include:
- Haldol Decanoate ... 1375

Hydrocodone Bitartrate (Potentiation). Products include:
- Anexsia 5/500 Tablets ... 2196
- Anexsia 7.5/650 Tablets ... 2197
- Azdöne Tablets ... 844
- Codiclear DH Syrup ... 845
- Codimal DH Syrup ... 846
- Damason-P ... 1356
- Hycodan Syrup, Tablets ... 927
- Hycomine Compound Tablets ... 929
- Hycomine Syrup ... 927
- Hycotuss Expectorant Syrup ... 930
- Hydrocet Capsules ... 835
- Lortab ASA Tablets ... 2414
- Lortab ... 2412
- Ru-Tuss with Hydrocodone ... 694
- Triaminic Expectorant DH ... 1995
- Vicodin Tablets ... 1187
- Vicodin ES Tablets ... 1189
- Zydone Capsules ... 941

Hydrocodone Polistirex (Potentiation). Products include:
- Tussionex Extended-Release Suspension ... 988

Hydroxyzine Hydrochloride (Potentiation). Products include:
- Atarax Tablets & Syrup ... 1941
- Marax Tablets & DF Syrup ... 1954
- Vistaril Intramuscular Solution ... 1970

Isoflurane (Potentiation). Products include:
- Forane ... 600

Ketamine Hydrochloride (Potentiation). Products include:
- Ketalar ... 1726

Levorphanol Tartrate (Potentiation). Products include:
- Levo-Dromoran ... 1906

Lorazepam (Potentiation). Products include:
- Ativan Injection ... 2432
- Ativan Tablets ... 2434

Loxapine Hydrochloride (Potentiation). Products include:
- Loxitane ... 1213

Loxapine Succinate (Potentiation). Products include:
- Loxitane Capsules ... 1213

Meperidine Hydrochloride (Potentiation). Products include:
- Demerol ... 2047
- Mepergan Injection ... 2479

Mephobarbital (Potentiation). Products include:
- Mebaral Tablets ... 2061

Meprobamate (Potentiation). Products include:
- Deprol Tablets ... 2382
- Equagesic Tablets ... 2451
- Miltown Tablets ... 2386
- PMB 200 and PMB 400 ... 2504

Methadone Hydrochloride (Potentiation). Products include:
- Dolophine Hydrochloride Ampoules & Vials ... 1260
- Dolophine Hydrochloride Tablets 1261
- Methadone Hydrochloride Diskets .. 1284
- Methadone Hydrochloride Oral Solution & Tablets ... 1987

Methohexital Sodium (Potentiation). Products include:
- Brevital Sodium Vials ... 1248

Methoxyflurane (Potentiation).
- No products indexed under this heading.

Midazolam Hydrochloride (Potentiation). Products include:
- Versed Injection ... 1924

Molindone Hydrochloride (Potentiation). Products include:
- Moban Tablets & Concentrate ... 932

Morphine Sulfate (Potentiation). Products include:
- Astramorph/PF Injection, USP (Preservative-Free) ... 618
- Duramorph ... 960
- Infumorph 200 and Infumorph 500 Sterile Solutions ... 962
- MS Contin Tablets ... 1814
- MSIR ... 1817
- Oramorph SR (Morphine Sulfate Sustained Release Tablets) ... 1988
- Roxanol ... 1991

Opium Alkaloids (Potentiation). Products include:
- B & O No. 15A & No. 16A Supprettes ... 2395
- Pantopon Injectable ... 1911

Oxazepam (Potentiation). Products include:
- Serax Capsules ... 2522
- Serax Tablets ... 2522

Oxycodone Hydrochloride (Potentiation). Products include:
- Percocet Tablets ... 950
- Percodan ... 951
- Roxicodone Tablets, Oral Solution & Intensol (Oxycodone) ... 1992
- Tylox Capsules ... 1382

Pentobarbital Sodium (Potentiation). Products include:
- Nembutal Sodium Capsules ... 534
- Nembutal Sodium Solution ... 536
- Nembutal Sodium Suppositories ... 538

Perphenazine (Potentiation). Products include:
- Etrafon ... 2087
- Triavil Tablets ... 1556
- Trilafon ... 2123

Phenobarbital (Potentiation). Products include:
- Arco-Lase Plus Tablets ... 607
- Bellergal-S Tablets ... 1998
- Bronkolixir ... ■ 761
- Bronkotabs Tablets ... ■ 762
- Donnatal ... 1858
- Donnatal Extentabs ... 1859
- Donnatal Tablets ... 1858
- Donnazyme Tablets ... 1860

(■ Described in PDR For Nonprescription Drugs)

(⊙ Described in PDR For Ophthalmology)

- Kinesed Tablets ... 2272
- Phenobarbital Elixir and Tablets ... 1293
- Primatene Tablets-P Formula ... 2421
- Quadrinal Tablets ... 1183
- Tedral SA ... 1765

Prazepam (Potentiation). Products include:
- Centrax ... 1693

Prochlorperazine (Potentiation). Products include:
- Compazine ... 2201

Promethazine Hydrochloride (Potentiation). Products include:
- Mepergan Injection ... 2479
- Phenergan with Codeine ... 2497
- Phenergan with Dextromethorphan 2499
- Phenergan Injection ... 2493
- Phenergan Suppositories ... 2496
- Phenergan Syrup ... 2495
- Phenergan Tablets ... 2496
- Phenergan VC ... 2500
- Phenergan VC with Codeine ... 2501

Propofol (Potentiation). Products include:
- Diprivan Injection ... 2267

Propoxyphene Hydrochloride (Potentiation). Products include:
- Darvon ... 1256
- Wygesic Tablets ... 2540

Propoxyphene Napsylate (Potentiation). Products include:
- Darvon-N/Darvocet-N ... 1254

Quazepam (Potentiation). Products include:
- Doral Tablets ... 2383

Secobarbital Sodium (Potentiation). Products include:
- Seconal Sodium Pulvules ... 1296

Sufentanil Citrate (Potentiation). Products include:
- Sufenta Injection ... 1147

Temazepam (Potentiation). Products include:
- Restoril Capsules ... 2023

Thiamylal Sodium (Potentiation). Products include:
- Surital Ampoules, Steri-Vials ... 1764

Thioridazine Hydrochloride (Potentiation). Products include:
- Mellaril ... 2011

Thiothixene (Potentiation). Products include:
- Navane Capsules and Concentrate 1954
- Navane Intramuscular ... 1956

Triazolam (Potentiation). Products include:
- Halcion Tablets ... 2340

Trifluoperazine Hydrochloride (Potentiation). Products include:
- Stelazine ... 2226

SERENTIL CONCENTRATE
(Mesoridazine) ... 686

See **Serentil Ampuls**

SERENTIL TABLETS
(Mesoridazine) ... 686

See **Serentil Ampuls**

SEROMYCIN PULVULES
(Cycloserine) ... 1298

May interact with antituberculosis drugs and certain other agents. Compounds in these categories include:

Alcohol (Increases risk of epileptic episodes).

Ethambutol Hydrochloride (Concurrent use with other antituberculosis drugs may result in vitamin B_{12} and/or folic acid deficiency). Products include:
- Myambutol Tablets ... 1225

Ethionamide (Neurotoxic side effects potentiated). Products include:
- Trecator-SC Tablets ... 2527

Isoniazid (Concurrent use with other antituberculosis drugs may result in vitamin B_{12} and/or folic acid deficiency; increased incidence of CNS effects, such as dizziness or drowsiness; dosage adjustment may be necessary). Products include:
- INH Tablets ... 868
- Rifamate Capsules ... 1347

Rifampin (Concurrent use with other antituberculosis drugs may result in vitamin B_{12} and/or folic acid deficiency). Products include:
- Rifadin ... 1345
- Rifamate Capsules ... 1347
- Rimactane Capsules ... 879

SEROPHENE (CLOMIPHENE CITRATE TABLETS, USP)
(Clomiphene Citrate) ... 2186

No interactions described in labeling.

SERPASIL TABLETS
(Reserpine) ... 883

May interact with monoamine oxidase inhibitors, cardiac glycosides, antihypertensives, and certain other agents. Compounds in these categories include:

Acebutolol Hydrochloride (Concomitant use necessitates careful titration of dosage with each agent). Products include:
- Sectral Capsules ... 2520

Atenolol (Concomitant use necessitates careful titration of dosage with each agent). Products include:
- Tenoretic Tablets ... 1105
- Tenormin Tablets and I.V. Injection 1107

Benazepril Hydrochloride (Concomitant use necessitates careful titration of dosage with each agent). Products include:
- Lotensin Tablets ... 872

Bendroflumethiazide (Concomitant use necessitates careful titration of dosage with each agent). Products include:
- Corzide Tablets ... 702
- Naturetin Tablets ... 1789
- Rauzide Tablets ... 1804

Betaxolol Hydrochloride (Concomitant use necessitates careful titration of dosage with each agent). Products include:
- Betoptic Sterile Ophthalmic Solution ... 569
- Betoptic S Sterile Ophthalmic Suspension ... 570
- Kerlone Tablets ... 2172

Captopril (Concomitant use necessitates careful titration of dosage with each agent). Products include:
- Capoten ... 2255
- Capozide ... 2258

Carteolol Hydrochloride (Concomitant use necessitates careful titration of dosage with each agent). Products include:
- Cartrol Tablets ... 507

Chlorothiazide (Concomitant use necessitates careful titration of dosage with each agent). Products include:
- Aldoclor Tablets ... 1413
- Diupres Tablets ... 1461
- Diuril Oral ... 1464

Chlorothiazide Sodium (Concomitant use necessitates careful titration of dosage with each agent). Products include:
- Diuril Sodium Intravenous ... 1463

Chlorthalidone (Concomitant use necessitates careful titration of dosage with each agent). Products include:
- Combipres Tablets ... 678
- Tenoretic Tablets ... 1105
- Thalitone Tablets ... 687

Clonidine (Concomitant use necessitates careful titration of dosage with each agent). Products include:
- Catapres-TTS ... 677

Clonidine Hydrochloride (Concomitant use necessitates careful titration of dosage with each agent). Products include:
- Catapres Tablets ... 676
- Combipres Tablets ... 678

Deserpidine (Concomitant use necessitates careful titration of dosage with each agent). Products include:
- Enduronyl ... 518
- Harmonyl Tablets ... 528
- Oreticyl ... 545

Deslanoside (Cardiac arrhythmia).
- No products indexed under this heading.

Diazoxide (Concomitant use necessitates careful titration of dosage with each agent). Products include:
- Hyperstat I.V. Injection ... 2095
- Proglycem ... 649

Digitoxin (Cardiac arrhythmia). Products include:
- Crystodigin Tablets ... 1253

Digoxin (Cardiac arrhythmia). Products include:
- Lanoxicaps ... 772
- Lanoxin Elixir Pediatric ... 775
- Lanoxin Injection ... 778
- Lanoxin Injection Pediatric ... 781
- Lanoxin Tablets ... 783

Doxazosin Mesylate (Concomitant use necessitates careful titration of dosage with each agent). Products include:
- Cardura Tablets ... 1941

Enalapril Maleate (Concomitant use necessitates careful titration of dosage with each agent). Products include:
- Vaseretic Tablets ... 1559
- Vasotec Tablets ... 1564

Enalaprilat (Concomitant use necessitates careful titration of dosage with each agent). Products include:
- Vasotec I.V. ... 1562

Esmolol Hydrochloride (Concomitant use necessitates careful titration of dosage with each agent). Products include:
- Brevibloc Injection ... 942

Felodipine (Concomitant use necessitates careful titration of dosage with each agent). Products include:
- Plendil Extended-Release Tablets ... 1526

Fosinopril Sodium (Concomitant use necessitates careful titration of dosage with each agent). Products include:
- Monopril Tablets ... 1406

Furazolidone (Concurrent administration of MAOI should be avoided). Products include:
- Furoxone ... 1855

Furosemide (Concomitant use necessitates careful titration of dosage with each agent). Products include:
- Lasix ... 1093

Guanabenz Acetate (Concomitant use necessitates careful titration of dosage with each agent). Products include:
- Wytensin Tablets ... 2542

Guanethidine Monosulfate (Concomitant use necessitates careful titration of dosage with each agent). Products include:
- Esimil Tablets ... 864
- Ismelin Tablets ... 869

Hydralazine Hydrochloride (Concomitant use necessitates careful titration of dosage with each agent). Products include:
- Apresazide Capsules ... 854
- Apresoline Hydrochloride Parenteral (Ampuls) ... 856
- Apresoline Hydrochloride Tablets ... 855
- Apresoline-Esidrix Tablets ... 857
- Ser-Ap-Es Tablets ... 881
- Serpasil-Apresoline Tablets ... 884

Hydrochlorothiazide (Concomitant use necessitates careful titration of dosage with each agent). Products include:
- Aldactazide ... 2150
- Aldoril Tablets ... 1418
- Apresazide Capsules ... 854
- Apresoline-Esidrix Tablets ... 857
- Capozide ... 2258
- Dyazide Capsules ... 2208
- Esidrix Tablets ... 863
- Esimil Tablets ... 864
- HydroDIURIL Tablets ... 1484
- Hydropres Tablets ... 1485
- Inderide Tablets ... 2463
- Inderide LA Long Acting Capsules .. 2465
- Lopressor HCT Tablets ... 1034
- Maxzide ... 1215
- Moduretic Tablets ... 1510
- Normozide Tablets ... 2112
- Oretic Tablets ... 544
- Oreticyl ... 545
- Prinzide Tablets ... 1540
- Ser-Ap-Es Tablets ... 881
- Serpasil-Esidrix Tablets ... 886
- Timolide Tablets ... 1547
- Trandate HCT Tablets ... 579
- Vaseretic Tablets ... 1559
- Zestoretic ... 2274

Hydroflumethiazide (Concomitant use necessitates careful titration of dosage with each agent). Products include:
- Diucardin Tablets ... 2450
- Saluron ... 718
- Salutensin/Salutensin-Demi ... 719

Indapamide (Concomitant use necessitates careful titration of dosage with each agent). Products include:
- Lozol Tablets ... 1843

Isocarboxazid (Concurrent administration of MAOI should be avoided). Products include:
- Marplan Tablets ... 1906

Isradipine (Concomitant use necessitates careful titration of dosage with each agent). Products include:
- DynaCirc Capsules ... 2004

Labetalol Hydrochloride (Concomitant use necessitates careful titration of dosage with each agent). Products include:
- Normodyne Injection ... 2108
- Normodyne Tablets ... 2110
- Normozide Tablets ... 2112
- Trandate HCT Tablets ... 579
- Trandate Injection ... 577
- Trandate Tablets ... 579

Lisinopril (Concomitant use necessitates careful titration of dosage with each agent). Products include:
- Prinivil Tablets ... 1538
- Prinzide Tablets ... 1540
- Zestoretic ... 2274
- Zestril Tablets ... 2277

Mecamylamine Hydrochloride (Concomitant use necessitates careful titration of dosage with each agent). Products include:
- Inversine Tablets ... 1492

Methyclothiazide (Concomitant use necessitates careful titration of dosage with each agent). Products include:
- Enduron Tablets ... 517
- Enduronyl ... 518

Methyldopa (Concomitant use necessitates careful titration of dosage with each agent). Products include:
- Aldoclor Tablets ... 1413

Aldomet Oral 1415
Aldoril Tablets 1418

Methyldopate Hydrochloride (Concomitant use necessitates careful titration of dosage with each agent). Products include:
Aldomet Ester HCl Injection 1417

Metolazone (Concomitant use necessitates careful titration of dosage with each agent). Products include:
Diulo 2129
Mykrox ½ mg Tablets 984
Zaroxolyn Tablets 989

Metoprolol Tartrate (Concomitant use necessitates careful titration of dosage with each agent). Products include:
Lopressor Ampuls 1032
Lopressor HCT Tablets 1034
Lopressor Tablets 1032

Metyrosine (Concomitant use necessitates careful titration of dosage with each agent). Products include:
Demser Capsules 1460

Minoxidil (Concomitant use necessitates careful titration of dosage with each agent). Products include:
Loniten Tablets 2346
Rogaine Topical Solution 2357

Nadolol (Concomitant use necessitates careful titration of dosage with each agent). Products include:
Corgard Tablets 701
Corzide Tablets 702

Nicardipine Hydrochloride (Concomitant use necessitates careful titration of dosage with each agent). Products include:
Cardene Capsules 2290

Nitroglycerin (Concomitant use necessitates careful titration of dosage with each agent). Products include:
Deponit NTG Transdermal Delivery System 2143
Minitran Transdermal Delivery System 1312
Nitro-Bid Ointment 1339
Nitro-Bid Capsules 1338
Nitrodisc 2176
Nitro-Dur (nitroglycerin) Transdermal Infusion System 1164
Nitrogard Tablets 1004
Nitrolingual Spray 1846
Nitrostat Tablets 1743
Transderm-Nitro Transdermal Therapeutic System 2283

Penbutolol Sulfate (Concomitant use necessitates careful titration of dosage with each agent). Products include:
Levatol 1832

Phenelzine Sulfate (Concurrent administration of MAOI should be avoided). Products include:
Nardil 1742

Phenoxybenzamine Hydrochloride (Concomitant use necessitates careful titration of dosage with each agent). Products include:
Dibenzyline Capsules 2207

Phentolamine Mesylate (Concomitant use necessitates careful titration of dosage with each agent). Products include:
Regitine 878

Pindolol (Concomitant use necessitates careful titration of dosage with each agent). Products include:
Visken Tablets 2036

Polythiazide (Concomitant use necessitates careful titration of dosage with each agent). Products include:
Minizide Capsules 1779
Renese Tablets 1785
Renese-R Tablets 1786

Prazosin Hydrochloride (Concomitant use necessitates careful titration of dosage with each agent). Products include:
Minipress Capsules 1778
Minizide Capsules 1779

Propranolol Hydrochloride (Concomitant use necessitates careful titration of dosage with each agent). Products include:
Inderal 2459
Inderal LA Long Acting Capsules 2461
Inderide Tablets 2463
Inderide LA Long Acting Capsules 2465

Quinidine Gluconate (Cardiac arrhythmia). Products include:
Quinaglute Dura-Tabs Tablets 663

Quinidine Polygalacturonate (Cardiac arrhythmia). Products include:
Cardioquin Tablets 1812

Quinidine Sulfate (Cardiac arrhythmia). Products include:
Quinidex Extentabs 1868

Ramipril (Concomitant use necessitates careful titration of dosage with each agent). Products include:
Altace Capsules 1086

Rauwolfia Serpentina (Concomitant use necessitates careful titration of dosage with each agent). Products include:
Raudixin Tablets 1803
Rauzide Tablets 1804

Rescinnamine (Concomitant use necessitates careful titration of dosage with each agent).
No products indexed under this heading.

Selegiline Hydrochloride (Concurrent administration of MAOI should be avoided). Products include:
Eldepryl 2250

Sodium Nitroprusside (Concomitant use necessitates careful titration of dosage with each agent). Products include:
Nipride I.V. Infusion 1909

Terazosin Hydrochloride (Concomitant use necessitates careful titration of dosage with each agent). Products include:
Hytrin Tablets 529

Timolol Maleate (Concomitant use necessitates careful titration of dosage with each agent). Products include:
Blocadren Tablets 1429
Timolide Tablets 1547
Timoptic in Ocudose 1552
Timoptic Sterile Ophthalmic Solution 1550

Tranylcypromine Sulfate (Concurrent administration of MAOI should be avoided). Products include:
Parnate Tablets 2222

Trimethaphan Camsylate (Concomitant use necessitates careful titration of dosage with each agent). Products include:
Arfonad Ampuls 1887

SERPASIL-APRESOLINE TABLETS
(Reserpine, Hydralazine) 884
May interact with monoamine oxidase inhibitors, cardiac glycosides, tricyclic antidepressants, direct-acting sympathomimetic amines, indirect-acting sympathomimetic amines, and certain other agents. Compounds in these categories include:

Amitriptyline Hydrochloride (Decreases the antihypertensive effect of reserpine). Products include:
Elavil 2269
Endep Tablets 1927
Etrafon 2087
Limbitrol 1933
Triavil Tablets 1556

Amoxapine (Decreases the antihypertensive effect of reserpine). Products include:
Asendin Tablets 1196

Amphetamine Resins (The action of indirect sympathomimetic amines is inhibited). Products include:
Biphetamine Capsules 973

Clomipramine Hydrochloride (Decreases the antihypertensive effect of reserpine). Products include:
Anafranil Capsules 650

Desipramine Hydrochloride (Decreases the antihypertensive effect of reserpine). Products include:
Norpramin Tablets 1340

Deslanoside (Cardiac arrhythmia).
No products indexed under this heading.

Dextroamphetamine Sulfate (The action of indirect sympathomimetic amines is inhibited). Products include:
Dexedrine 2206

Diazoxide (Severe hypotension). Products include:
Hyperstat I.V. Injection 2095
Proglycem 649

Digitoxin (Cardiac arrhythmia). Products include:
Crystodigin Tablets 1253

Digoxin (Cardiac arrhythmia). Products include:
Lanoxicaps 772
Lanoxin Elixir Pediatric 775
Lanoxin Injection 778
Lanoxin Injection Pediatric 781
Lanoxin Tablets 783

Doxepin Hydrochloride (Decreases the antihypertensive effect of reserpine). Products include:
Sinequan 1960

Ephedrine Hydrochloride (The action of indirect sympathomimetic amines is inhibited). Products include:
Amesec .... ▣ 682
Primatene Tablets-M Formula 2421
Primatene Tablets-P Formula 2421
Primatene Tablets-Regular Formula 2421
Quadrinal Tablets 1183
Quelidrine Syrup 556
Tedral SA 1765

Ephedrine Sulfate (The action of indirect sympathomimetic amines is inhibited). Products include:
Bronkaid Tablets .... ▣ 757
Bronkolixir .... ▣ 761
Bronkotabs Tablets .... ▣ 762
Marax Tablets & DF Syrup 1954
Pazo Hemorrhoid Ointment & Suppositories 752
Vicks Vatronol Nose Drops .... ▣ 666

Ephedrine Tannate (The action of indirect sympathomimetic amines is inhibited). Products include:
Rynatuss 2388

Epinephrine (Pressor responses to epinephrine may be reduced). Products include:
Ana-Kit Anaphylaxis Emergency Treatment Kit 1100
Bronkaid Mist .... ▣ 757
EpiPen 843
Marcaine Hydrochloride 0.5% with Epinephrine 1:200,000 (as bitartrate) 958
Marcaine Hydrochloride with Epinephrine 1:200,000 2055
Primatene Mist 2420
Sus-Phrine Injection 1006
Xylocaine with Epinephrine Injections 637

Epinephrine Bitartrate (Pressor responses to epinephrine may be reduced). Products include:
AsthmaHaler Mist Epinephrine Bitartrate Bronchodilator .... ▣ 616
Bronkaid Mist Suspension .... ▣ 757
Primatene Mist Suspension 2421

Epinephrine Hydrochloride (The action of direct-acting sympathomimetic amines may be prolonged). Products include:
Adrenalin Chloride Solution 1:100 & 1:1,000 1689
Epifrin .... ⊙ 244
Glaucon .... ⊙ 218

Furazolidone (Concurrent administration of MAOI should be avoided). Products include:
Furoxone 1855

Imipramine Hydrochloride (Decreases the antihypertensive effect of reserpine). Products include:
Tofranil Ampuls 1038
Tofranil Tablets 1039

Imipramine Pamoate (Decreases the antihypertensive effect of reserpine). Products include:
Tofranil-PM Capsules 1041

Isocarboxazid (Concurrent administration of MAOI should be avoided). Products include:
Marplan Tablets 1906

Isoproterenol Hydrochloride (The action of direct-acting sympathomimetic amines may be prolonged). Products include:
Isuprel Hydrochloride Injection 1:5000 2050
Isuprel Hydrochloride Mistometer 2051
Isuprel Hydrochloride Solution 1:200 & 1:100 2052
Norisodrine Aerotrol 540

Maprotiline Hydrochloride (Decreases the antihypertensive effect of reserpine). Products include:
Ludiomil Tablets 874

Metaraminol Bitartrate (The action of direct-acting sympathomimetic amines may be prolonged). Products include:
Aramine Injection 1424

Norepinephrine Hydrochloride (The action of direct-acting sympathomimetic amines may be prolonged).

Nortriptyline Hydrochloride (Decreases the antihypertensive effect of reserpine). Products include:
Pamelor 2019

Phenelzine Sulfate (Concurrent administration of MAOI should be avoided). Products include:
Nardil 1742

Phenylephrine Hydrochloride (The action of direct-acting sympathomimetic amines may be prolonged). Products include:
AK-Dilate Solution 2.5% and 10% .... ⊙ 203
Atrohist Sprinkle Capsules 558
Cerose-DM 2443
Codimal 846
Comhist LA Capsules 1618
Congespirin For Children Aspirin Free Chewable Cold Tablets 748
Cyclomydril .... ⊙ 216
Deconsal Sprinkle Capsules 559
Dimetane Decongestant .... ▣ 673
Dristan Decongestant/Antihistamine/ Analgesic Coated Caplets .... ▣ 749

Dristan Cold Nasal Decongestant/ Antihistamine/ Analgesic Coated Tablets 2419
Dristan Advanced Formula Decongestant/Antihistamine/ Analgesic Tablets ..... ▣ 749
Dristan Nasal Spray, Menthol 2419
Dristan Nasal Spray, Regular and Regular with Metered Pump 2419
Entex Capsules 1623
Entex Liquid 1623
Sinus Excedrin Analgesic, Decongestant Tablets & Caplets 750
Extendryl 994
4-Way Fast Acting Nasal Spray - Original Formula (regular & mentholated) & Metered Spray Pump (regular) 751
Hycomine Compound Tablets 929
Murocoll-2 Sterile Ophthalmic Solution ..... ⊙ 261
Mydfrin 2.5% ..... ⊙ 224
Naldecon Syrup, Tablets, Pediatric Drops and Pediatric Syrup 709
Neo-Synephrine Hydrochloride 1% Carpuject 2063
Neo-Synephrine Hydrochloride 1% Injection 2063
Neo-Synephrine Hydrochloride (Ophthalmic) 2064
Neo-Synephrine ..... ▣ 759
Nōstril Nasal Decongestant ..... ▣ 520
Novahistine Elixir ..... ▣ 596
Phenergan VC 2500
Phenergan VC with Codeine 2501
Prefrin Liquifilm Vasoconstrictor and Lubricant Eye Drops ..... ⊙ 254
Prefrin-A ..... ⊙ 255
Quelidrine Syrup 556
Relief Vasoconstrictor and Lubricant Eye Drops ..... ⊙ 256
Robitussin Night Relief ..... ▣ 677
Ru-Tuss with Hydrocodone 694
Ru-Tuss Tablets 693
Vasosulf ..... ⊙ 279
Vicks Sinex ..... ▣ 665
Zincfrin ..... ⊙ 230

Phenylephrine Tannate (The action of direct-acting sympathomimetic amines may be prolonged). Products include:
Rynatan 2387
Rynatuss 2388

Protriptyline Hydrochloride (Decreases the antihypertensive effect of reserpine). Products include:
Vivactil Tablets 1567

Quinidine Gluconate (Cardiac arrhythmia). Products include:
Quinaglute Dura-Tabs Tablets 663

Quinidine Polygalacturonate (Cardiac arrhythmia). Products include:
Cardioquin Tablets 1812

Quinidine Sulfate (Cardiac arrhythmia). Products include:
Quinidex Extentabs 1868

Selegiline Hydrochloride (Concurrent administration of MAOI should be avoided). Products include:
Eldepryl 2250

Tranylcypromine Sulfate (Concurrent administration of MAOI should be avoided). Products include:
Parnate Tablets 2222

Trimipramine Maleate (Decreases the antihypertensive effect of reserpine). Products include:
Surmontil Capsules 2524

Tyramine (The action of indirect sympathomimetic amines is inhibited).

Food Interactions

Food, unspecified (Concomitant administration enhances gastrointestinal absorption of hydrochlorothiazide and results in higher plasma levels of hydralazine).

SERPASIL-ESIDRIX TABLETS

(Reserpine, Hydrochlorothiazide) 886

May interact with corticosteroids, antihypertensives, lithium preparations, monoamine oxidase inhibitors, cardiac glycosides, insulin, barbiturates, narcotic analgesics, non-steroidal anti-inflammatory agents, tricyclic antidepressants, direct-acting sympathomimetic amines, indirect-acting sympathomimetic amines, and certain other agents. Compounds in these categories include:

Acebutolol Hydrochloride (Additive or potentiated action). Products include:
Sectral Capsules 2520

ACTH (Hypokalemia).
No products indexed under this heading.

Alcohol (Orthostatic hypotension).

Alfentanil Hydrochloride (Orthostatic hypotension). Products include:
Alfenta Injection 1131

Amitriptyline Hydrochloride (Decreases the antihypertensive effect of reserpine). Products include:
Elavil 2269
Endep Tablets 1927
Etrafon 2087
Limbitrol 1933
Triavil Tablets 1556

Amoxapine (Decreases the antihypertensive effect of reserpine). Products include:
Asendin Tablets 1196

Amphetamine Resins (The action of indirect-acting sympathomimetic amines is inhibited). Products include:
Biphetamine Capsules 973

Aprobarbital (Orthostatic hypotension). Products include:
Alurate Elixir 1883

Atenolol (Additive or potentiated action). Products include:
Tenoretic Tablets 1105
Tenormin Tablets and I.V. Injection 1107

Benazepril Hydrochloride (Additive or potentiated action). Products include:
Lotensin Tablets 872

Bendroflumethiazide (Additive or potentiated action). Products include:
Corzide Tablets 702
Naturetin Tablets 1789
Rauzide Tablets 1804

Betamethasone Acetate (Hypokalemia). Products include:
Celestone Soluspan Suspension 2081

Betamethasone Sodium Phosphate (Hypokalemia). Products include:
Celestone Soluspan Suspension 2081

Betaxolol Hydrochloride (Additive or potentiated action). Products include:
Betoptic Sterile Ophthalmic Solution 569
Betoptic S Sterile Ophthalmic Suspension 570
Kerlone Tablets 2172

Buprenorphine (Orthostatic hypotension).
No products indexed under this heading.

Butabarbital (Orthostatic hypotension). Products include:
Pyridium Plus 1764

Butalbital (Orthostatic hypotension). Products include:
Esgic-Plus Tablets 1002
Esgic Tablets & Capsules 1001
Fioricet Tablets 2006
Fiorinal Capsules 2007
Fiorinal with Codeine Capsules 2008
Fiorinal Tablets 2007
Phrenilin 838
Sedapap Tablets 50 mg/650 mg 1360

Captopril (Additive or potentiated action). Products include:
Capoten 2255
Capozide 2258

Carteolol Hydrochloride (Additive or potentiated action). Products include:
Cartrol Tablets 507

Chlorothiazide (Additive or potentiated action). Products include:
Aldoclor Tablets 1413
Diupres Tablets 1461
Diuril Oral 1464

Chlorothiazide Sodium (Additive or potentiated action). Products include:
Diuril Sodium Intravenous 1463

Chlorthalidone (Additive or potentiated action). Products include:
Combipres Tablets 678
Tenoretic Tablets 1105
Thalitone Tablets 687

Clomipramine Hydrochloride (Decreases the antihypertensive effect of reserpine). Products include:
Anafranil Capsules 650

Clonidine (Additive or potentiated action). Products include:
Catapres-TTS 677

Clonidine Hydrochloride (Additive or potentiated action). Products include:
Catapres Tablets 676
Combipres Tablets 678

Codeine (Orthostatic hypotension). Products include:
Calcidrine Syrup 506

Codeine Phosphate (Orthostatic hypotension). Products include:
Actifed with Codeine Cough Syrup .. 752
Cheracol Cough Syrup 1853
Codimal PH Syrup 846
Dimetane-DC Cough Syrup 1857
Empirin with Codeine Phosphate Nos. 2, 3 & 4 764
Fiorinal with Codeine Capsules 2008
Isoclor Expectorant 982
Naldecon CX Adult Liquid ..... ▣ 521
Novahistine DH 1342
Novahistine Expectorant 1343
Nucofed Capsules 2219
Nucofed Expectorant 2219
Nucofed Pediatric Expectorant 2220
Nucofed Syrup 2219
Phenaphen with Codeine Capsules 1865
Phenaphen-650 with Codeine Tablets 1866
Phenergan with Codeine 2497
Phenergan VC with Codeine 2501
Robitussin A-C Syrup 1875
Robitussin-DAC Syrup 1875
Ryna ..... ▣ 741
Soma Compound w/Codeine Tablets 2390
Triaminic Expectorant w/Codeine .. 1996
Tussi-Organidin Liquid 2391
Tylenol with Codeine 1381

Codeine Polistirex (Orthostatic hypotension).
No products indexed under this heading.

Cortisone Acetate (Hypokalemia). Products include:
Cortone Acetate Sterile Suspension 1437
Cortone Acetate Tablets 1439

Deserpidine (Additive or potentiated action). Products include:
Enduronyl 518
Harmonyl Tablets 528
Oreticyl 545

Desipramine Hydrochloride (Decreases the antihypertensive effect of reserpine). Products include:
Norpramin Tablets 1340

Deslanoside (Cardiac arrhythmia).
No products indexed under this heading.

Dexamethasone (Hypokalemia). Products include:
AK-Trol Ointment & Suspension ..... ⊙ 207
Decadron Elixir 1445
Decadron Tablets 1447
Decaspray Topical Aerosol 1459
Dexacidin ..... ⊙ 272
Maxidex Sterile Ophthalmic Suspension ..... ⊙ 223
Maxitrol Ophthalmic Ointment/ Suspension ..... ⊙ 223
TobraDex Ophthalmic Suspension and Ointment ..... ⊙ 228

Dexamethasone Acetate (Hypokalemia). Products include:
Dalalone D.P. Injectable 999
Decadron-LA Sterile Suspension 1457

Dexamethasone Sodium Phosphate (Hypokalemia). Products include:
AK-Dex ..... ⊙ 203
Decadron Phosphate Respihaler 1454
Decadron Phosphate Sterile Ophthalmic Ointment 1453
Decadron Phosphate Sterile Ophthalmic Solution 1453
Decadron Phosphate Topical Cream 1455
Decadron Phosphate Turbinaire 1456
Maxidex Sterile Ophthalmic Ointment ..... ⊙ 222
NeoDecadron Sterile Ophthalmic Ointment 1517
NeoDecadron Sterile Ophthalmic Solution 1518
NeoDecadron Topical Cream 1518

Dextroamphetamine Sulfate (The action of indirect-acting sympathomimetic amines is inhibited). Products include:
Dexedrine 2206

Dezocine (Orthostatic hypotension).

Diazoxide (Additive or potentiated action). Products include:
Hyperstat I.V. Injection 2095
Proglycem 649

Diclofenac Sodium (May reduce the diuretic, natriuretic, and antihypertensive effects of thiazide diuretics). Products include:
Voltaren Ophthalmic Sterile Ophthalmic Solution ..... ⊙ 268
Voltaren Tablets 1042

Digitoxin (Cardiac arrhythmia). Products include:
Crystodigin Tablets 1253

Digoxin (Cardiac arrhythmia). Products include:
Lanoxicaps 772
Lanoxin Elixir Pediatric 775
Lanoxin Injection 778
Lanoxin Injection Pediatric 781
Lanoxin Tablets 783

Doxazosin Mesylate (Additive or potentiated action). Products include:
Cardura Tablets 1941

Doxepin Hydrochloride (Decreases the antihypertensive effect of reserpine). Products include:
Sinequan 1960

Enalapril Maleate (Additive or potentiated action). Products include:
Vaseretic Tablets 1559
Vasotec Tablets 1564

Enalaprilat (Additive or potentiated action). Products include:
Vasotec I.V. 1562

Ephedrine Hydrochloride (The action of indirect-acting sympathomimetic amines is inhibited). Products include:
Amesec ..... ▣ 682
Primatene Tablets-M Formula 2421
Primatene Tablets-P Formula 2421
Primatene Tablets-Regular Formula 2421

Quadrinal Tablets ... 1183
Quelidrine Syrup ... 556
Tedral SA ... 1765

Ephedrine Sulfate (The action of indirect-acting sympathomimetic amines is inhibited). Products include:
Bronkaid Tablets ... ▣ 757
Bronkolixir ... ▣ 761
Bronkotabs Tablets ... ▣ 762
Marax Tablets & DF Syrup ... 1954
Pazo Hemorrhoid Ointment & Suppositories ... 752
Vicks Vatronol Nose Drops ... ▣ 666

Ephedrine Tannate (The action of indirect-acting sympathomimetic amines is inhibited). Products include:
Rynatuss ... 2388

Epinephrine Hydrochloride (The action of direct-acting sympathomimetic amines may be prolonged). Products include:
Adrenalin Chloride Solution 1:100 & 1:1,000 ... 1689
Epifrin ... ⊙ 244
Glaucon ... ⊙ 218

Esmolol Hydrochloride (Additive or potentiated action). Products include:
Brevibloc Injection ... 942

Etodolac (May reduce the diuretic, natriuretic, and antihypertensive effects of thiazide diuretics). Products include:
Lodine Capsules ... 2468

Felodipine (Additive or potentiated action). Products include:
Plendil Extended-Release Tablets ... 1526

Fenoprofen Calcium (May reduce the diuretic, natriuretic, and antihypertensive effects of thiazide diuretics). Products include:
Nalfon Pulvules & Tablets ... 919

Fentanyl (Orthostatic hypotension). Products include:
Duragesic Transdermal System ... 1133

Fentanyl Citrate (Orthostatic hypotension). Products include:
Innovar Injection ... 1141
Sublimaze Injection ... 1146

Flurbiprofen (May reduce the diuretic, natriuretic, and antihypertensive effects of thiazide diuretics). Products include:
Ansaid Tablets ... 2319

Fosinopril Sodium (Additive or potentiated action). Products include:
Monopril Tablets ... 1406

Furazolidone (Concurrent administration of MAOI should be avoided). Products include:
Furoxone ... 1855

Furosemide (Additive or potentiated action). Products include:
Lasix ... 1093

Guanabenz Acetate (Additive or potentiated action). Products include:
Wytensin Tablets ... 2542

Guanethidine Monosulfate (Additive or potentiated action). Products include:
Esimil Tablets ... 864
Ismelin Tablets ... 869

Hydralazine Hydrochloride (Additive or potentiated action). Products include:
Apresazide Capsules ... 854
Apresoline Hydrochloride Parenteral (Ampuls) ... 856
Apresoline Hydrochloride Tablets ... 855
Apresoline-Esidrix Tablets ... 857
Ser-Ap-Es Tablets ... 881
Serpasil-Apresoline Tablets ... 884

Hydrocodone Bitartrate (Orthostatic hypotension). Products include:
Anexsia 5/500 Tablets ... 2196
Anexsia 7.5/650 Tablets ... 2197
Azdōne Tablets ... 844
Codiclear DH Syrup ... 845
Codimal DH Syrup ... 846
Damason-P ... 1356
Hycodan Syrup, Tablets ... 927
Hycomine Compound Tablets ... 929
Hycomine Syrup ... 927
Hycotuss Expectorant Syrup ... 930
Hydrocet Capsules ... 835
Lortab ASA Tablets ... 2414
Lortab ... 2412
Ru-Tuss with Hydrocodone ... 694
Triaminic Expectorant DH ... 1995
Vicodin Tablets ... 1187
Vicodin ES Tablets ... 1189
Zydone Capsules ... 941

Hydrocodone Polistirex (Orthostatic hypotension). Products include:
Tussionex Extended-Release Suspension ... 988

Hydrocortisone (Hypokalemia). Products include:
AK-Spore H.C. ... ⊙ 206
Bactine Hydrocortisone Anti-Itch Cream ... ▣ 625
CaldeCORT Anti-Itch Hydrocortisone Spray ... ▣ 560
Carmol HC Cream 1% ... 2296
Cortaid Spray ... ▣ 735
Cortenema ... 2244
Cortisporin Ointment ... 758
Cortisporin Ophthalmic Ointment Sterile ... 758
Cortisporin Ophthalmic Suspension Sterile ... 759
Cortisporin Otic Solution Sterile ... 760
Cortisporin Otic Suspension Sterile ... 760
Cortizone-5 Creme & Ointment ... ▣ 732
Dermolate Anti-Itch Cream ... ▣ 697
Eldecort Cream 1.0% ... 1113
Eldecort Cream 1.0% and 2.5% ... 1113
Fungoid HC Creme ... 1770
Hydrocortone Tablets ... 1482
Hytone ... 909
LazerSporin-C Solution ... 1770
Massengill Medicated Soft Cloth Towelettes ... 2192
Nutracort Cream & Lotion ... 1684
PediOtic Suspension Sterile ... 797
Synacort Creams 1%, 2.5% ... 2296
Vanoxide-HC Acne Lotion ... 911
Vioform-Hydrocortisone Cream and Mild Cream ... 889
Vioform-Hydrocortisone Ointment ... 889
VōSoL HC Otic Solution ... 2392
Vytone Cream 1% ... 911

Hydrocortisone Acetate (Hypokalemia). Products include:
Analpram-HC Rectal Cream 1% and 2.5% ... 970
Anusol-HC Cream ... 1690
Anusol-HC Suppositories ... 1691
Caldecort ... ▣ 560
Carmol HC Cream 1% ... 2296
Chloromycetin Hydrocortisone Ophthalmic ... 1694
Coly-Mycin S Otic w/Neomycin & Hydrocortisone ... 1708
Cortaid ... ▣ 735
Cortef Feminine Itch Cream ... ▣ 735
Corticaine ... ▣ 682
Cortifoam ... 1827
Cortisporin Cream ... 757
Epifoam ... 1828
Gynecort 5 Creme ... ▣ 556
Hydrocortone Acetate Sterile Suspension ... 1479
Lanacort 5 Creme and Ointment ... ▣ 557
Mantadil Cream ... 789
Ophthocort ... ⊙ 301
Orabase HCA Oral Paste ... 890
Pramosone Cream, Lotion & Ointment ... 971
ProctoCream-HC ... 1834
Proctofoam-HC ... 1835

Hydrocortisone Sodium Phosphate (Hypokalemia). Products include:
Hydrocortone Phosphate Injection, Sterile ... 1481

Hydrocortisone Sodium Succinate (Hypokalemia). Products include:
Solu-Cortef Sterile Powder ... 2361

Hydroflumethiazide (Additive or potentiated action). Products include:
Diucardin Tablets ... 2450
Saluron ... 718
Salutensin/Salutensin-Demi ... 719

Ibuprofen (May reduce the diuretic, natriuretic, and antihypertensive effects of thiazide diuretics). Products include:
Advil Cold & Sinus Caplets (formerly CoAdvil) ... 2416
Advil Ibuprofen Tablets and Caplets ... 2416
Children's Advil Suspension ... 2426
CoAdvil ... ▣ 748
Dristan Sinus Caplets ... 2419
Haltran Tablets ... ▣ 668
Ibuprofen ... ▣ 631
Medipren ibuprofen Caplets and Tablets ... 1362
Midol 200 Cramp Relief Formula ... ▣ 570
Motrin Tablets ... 2351
Motrin IB Caplets and Tablets ... ▣ 736
Nuprin Ibuprofen/Analgesic Tablets & Caplets ... 752
PediaProfen Suspension ... 1363
Rufen Tablets ... 691
Trendar Ibuprofen Tablets ... ▣ 756

Imipramine Hydrochloride (Decreases the antihypertensive effect of reserpine). Products include:
Tofranil Ampuls ... 1038
Tofranil Tablets ... 1039

Imipramine Pamoate (Decreases the antihypertensive effect of reserpine). Products include:
Tofranil-PM Capsules ... 1041

Indapamide (Additive or potentiated action). Products include:
Lozol Tablets ... 1843

Indomethacin (May reduce the diuretic, natriuretic, and antihypertensive effects of thiazide diuretics). Products include:
Indocin ... 1487

Indomethacin Sodium Trihydrate (May reduce the diuretic, natriuretic, and antihypertensive effects of thiazide diuretics). Products include:
Indocin I.V. ... 1490

Insulin, Human (In diabetic patients, insulin requirements may be increased, decreased or unchanged).
No products indexed under this heading.

Insulin, Human Isophane Suspension (In diabetic patients, insulin requirements may be increased, decreased or unchanged). Products include:
Humulin N, 100 Units ... 1270

Insulin, Human NPH (In diabetic patients, insulin requirements may be increased, decreased or unchanged). Products include:
Insulatard NPH Human ... 1627
Novolin N ... 1627
Novolin N PenFill Cartridges ... 1628
Novolin N Prefilled ... 1628

Insulin, Human Regular (In diabetic patients, insulin requirements may be increased, decreased or unchanged). Products include:
Humulin BR, 100 Units ... 1268
Humulin R, 100 Units ... 1272
Novolin R ... 1627
Novolin R PenFill Cartridges ... 1628
Novolin R Prefilled ... 1629
Velosulin Human ... 1628

Insulin, Human, Zinc Suspension (In diabetic patients, insulin requirements may be increased, decreased or unchanged). Products include:
Humulin L, 100 Units ... 1268
Humulin U, 100 Units ... 1272
Novolin L ... 1627

Insulin, NPH (In diabetic patients, insulin requirements may be increased, decreased or unchanged). Products include:
NPH, 40 & 100 Units ... 1273
Beef NPH, 100 Units ... 1274
Pork NPH, 100 Units ... 1275
Insulatard NPH ... 1626
NPH Insulin ... 1626
NPH Purified Pork Isophane Insulin ... 1626

Insulin, Regular (In diabetic patients, insulin requirements may be increased, decreased or unchanged). Products include:
Regular, 40 & 100 Units ... 1273
Beef Regular, 100 Units ... 1275
Pork Regular, 100 Units ... 1275
Pork Regular (Concentrated), 500 Units ... 1276
Regular Insulin ... 1625
Regular Purified Pork Insulin ... 1626
Velosulin ... 1627

Insulin, Zinc Crystals (In diabetic patients, insulin requirements may be increased, decreased or unchanged). Products include:
NPH, 40 & 100 Units ... 1273

Insulin, Zinc Suspension (In diabetic patients, insulin requirements may be increased, decreased or unchanged). Products include:
Lente, 40 & 100 Units ... 1272
Protamine, Zinc, 40 & 100 Units ... 1273
Lente Iletin I ... 1272
Beef Lente, 100 Units ... 1274
Beef Protamine Zinc, 100 Units ... 1274
Pork Lente, 100 Units ... 1275
Pork, Protamine, Zinc, 100 Units ... 1275
Lente Insulin ... 1626
Lente Purified Pork Insulin ... 1626
Semilente Insulin ... 1625
Ultralente Insulin ... 1626

Isocarboxazid (Concurrent administration of MAOI should be avoided). Products include:
Marplan Tablets ... 1906

Isoproterenol Hydrochloride (The action of direct-acting sympathomimetic amines may be prolonged). Products include:
Isuprel Hydrochloride Injection 1:5000 ... 2050
Isuprel Hydrochloride Mistometer ... 2051
Isuprel Hydrochloride Solution 1:200 & 1:100 ... 2052
Norisodrine Aerotrol ... 540

Isradipine (Additive or potentiated action). Products include:
DynaCirc Capsules ... 2004

Ketoprofen (May reduce the diuretic, natriuretic, and antihypertensive effects of thiazide diuretics). Products include:
Orudis Capsules ... 2488

Ketorolac Tromethamine (May reduce the diuretic, natriuretic, and antihypertensive effects of thiazide diuretics). Products include:
Toradol IM Injection ... 2302

Labetalol Hydrochloride (Additive or potentiated action). Products include:
Normodyne Injection ... 2108
Normodyne Tablets ... 2110
Normozide Tablets ... 2112
Trandate HCT Tablets ... 579
Trandate Injection ... 577
Trandate Tablets ... 579

Levorphanol Tartrate (Orthostatic hypotension). Products include:
Levo-Dromoran ... 1906

Lisinopril (Additive or potentiated action). Products include:
Prinivil Tablets ... 1538
Prinzide Tablets ... 1540
Zestoretic ... 2274
Zestril Tablets ... 2277

Lithium Carbonate (Reduced renal clearance and increased risk of lithium toxicity). Products include:
- Eskalith ... 2214
- Lithane Tablets ... 1596
- Lithium Carbonate Capsules & Tablets ... 1984
- Lithobid Tablets ... 870

Lithium Citrate (Reduced renal clearance and increased risk of lithium toxicity). Products include:
- Cibalith-S ... 870

Maprotiline Hydrochloride (Decreases the antihypertensive effect of reserpine). Products include:
- Ludiomil Tablets ... 874

Mecamylamine Hydrochloride (Additive or potentiated action). Products include:
- Inversine Tablets ... 1492

Meclofenamate Sodium (May reduce the diuretic, natriuretic, and antihypertensive effects of thiazide diuretics). Products include:
- Meclomen Capsules ... 1739

Mefenamic Acid (May reduce the diuretic, natriuretic, and antihypertensive effects of thiazide diuretics). Products include:
- Ponstel ... 1758

Meperidine Hydrochloride (Orthostatic hypotension). Products include:
- Demerol ... 2047
- Mepergan Injection ... 2479

Mephobarbital (Orthostatic hypotension). Products include:
- Mebaral Tablets ... 2061

Metaraminol Bitartrate (The action of direct-acting sympathomimetic amines may be prolonged). Products include:
- Aramine Injection ... 1424

Methadone Hydrochloride (Orthostatic hypotension). Products include:
- Dolophine Hydrochloride Ampoules & Vials ... 1260
- Dolophine Hydrochloride Tablets ... 1261
- Methadone Hydrochloride Diskets ... 1284
- Methadone Hydrochloride Oral Solution & Tablets ... 1987

Methyclothiazide (Additive or potentiated action). Products include:
- Enduron Tablets ... 517
- Enduronyl ... 518

Methyldopa (Hemolytic anemia; additive or potentiated action). Products include:
- Aldoclor Tablets ... 1413
- Aldomet Oral ... 1415
- Aldoril Tablets ... 1418

Methyldopate Hydrochloride (Additive or potentiated action). Products include:
- Aldomet Ester HCl Injection ... 1417

Methylprednisolone Acetate (Hypokalemia). Products include:
- Depo-Medrol Sterile Aqueous Suspension ... 2334

Methylprednisolone Sodium Succinate (Hypokalemia). Products include:
- Solu-Medrol Sterile Powder ... 2363

Metolazone (Additive or potentiated action). Products include:
- Diulo ... 2129
- Mykrox ½ mg Tablets ... 984
- Zaroxolyn Tablets ... 989

Metoprolol Tartrate (Additive or potentiated action). Products include:
- Lopressor Ampuls ... 1032
- Lopressor HCT Tablets ... 1034
- Lopressor Tablets ... 1032

Metyrosine (Additive or potentiated action). Products include:
- Demser Capsules ... 1460

Minoxidil (Additive or potentiated action). Products include:
- Loniten Tablets ... 2346
- Rogaine Topical Solution ... 2357

Morphine Sulfate (Orthostatic hypotension). Products include:
- Astramorph/PF Injection, USP (Preservative-Free) ... 618
- Duramorph ... 960
- Infumorph 200 and Infumorph 500 Sterile Solutions ... 962
- MS Contin Tablets ... 1814
- MSIR ... 1817
- Oramorph SR (Morphine Sulfate Sustained Release Tablets) ... 1988
- Roxanol ... 1991

Nadolol (Additive or potentiated action). Products include:
- Corgard Tablets ... 701
- Corzide Tablets ... 702

Naproxen (May reduce the diuretic, natriuretic, and antihypertensive effects of thiazide diuretics). Products include:
- Naprosyn ... 2297

Naproxen Sodium (May reduce the diuretic, natriuretic, and antihypertensive effects of thiazide diuretics). Products include:
- Anaprox and Anaprox DS Tablets ... 2288

Nicardipine Hydrochloride (Additive or potentiated action). Products include:
- Cardene Capsules ... 2290

Nitroglycerin (Additive or potentiated action). Products include:
- Deponit NTG Transdermal Delivery System ... 2143
- Minitran Transdermal Delivery System ... 1312
- Nitro-Bid Ointment ... 1339
- Nitro-Bid Capsules ... 1338
- Nitrodisc ... 2176
- Nitro-Dur (nitroglycerin) Transdermal Infusion System ... 1164
- Nitrogard Tablets ... 1004
- Nitrolingual Spray ... 1846
- Nitrostat Tablets ... 1743
- Transderm-Nitro Transdermal Therapeutic System ... 2283

Norepinephrine Bitartrate (Decreased arterial responsiveness to norepinephrine). Products include:
- Levophed Bitartrate Injection ... 2054

Norepinephrine Hydrochloride (The action of direct-acting sympathomimetic amines may be prolonged).

Nortriptyline Hydrochloride (Decreases the antihypertensive effect of reserpine). Products include:
- Pamelor ... 2019

Opium Alkaloids (Orthostatic hypotension). Products include:
- B & O No. 15A & No. 16A Supprettes ... 2395
- Pantopon Injectable ... 1911

Oxycodone Hydrochloride (Orthostatic hypotension). Products include:
- Percocet Tablets ... 950
- Percodan ... 951
- Roxicodone Tablets, Oral Solution & Intensol (Oxycodone) ... 1992
- Tylox Capsules ... 1382

Penbutolol Sulfate (Additive or potentiated action). Products include:
- Levatol ... 1832

Pentobarbital Sodium (Orthostatic hypotension). Products include:
- Nembutal Sodium Capsules ... 534
- Nembutal Sodium Solution ... 536
- Nembutal Sodium Suppositories ... 538

Phenelzine Sulfate (Concurrent administration of MAOI should be avoided). Products include:
- Nardil ... 1742

Phenobarbital (Orthostatic hypotension). Products include:
- Arco-Lase Plus Tablets ... 607
- Bellergal-S Tablets ... 1998
- Bronkolixir ... ▣ 761
- Bronkotabs Tablets ... ▣ 762
- Donnatal ... 1858
- Donnatal Extentabs ... 1859
- Donnatal Tablets ... 1858
- Donnazyme Tablets ... 1860
- Kinesed Tablets ... 2272
- Phenobarbital Elixir and Tablets ... 1293
- Primatene Tablets-P Formula ... 2421
- Quadrinal Tablets ... 1183
- Tedral SA ... 1765

Phenoxybenzamine Hydrochloride (Additive or potentiated action). Products include:
- Dibenzyline Capsules ... 2207

Phentolamine Mesylate (Additive or potentiated action). Products include:
- Regitine ... 878

Phenylbutazone (May reduce the diuretic, natriuretic, and antihypertensive effects of thiazide diuretics). Products include:
- Butazolidin Capsules & Tablets ... 1027

Phenylephrine Hydrochloride (The action of direct-acting sympathomimetic amines may be prolonged). Products include:
- AK-Dilate Solution 2.5% and 10% ... ⊙ 203
- Atrohist Sprinkle Capsules ... 558
- Cerose-DM ... 2443
- Codimal ... 846
- Comhist LA Capsules ... 1618
- Congespirin For Children Aspirin Free Chewable Cold Tablets ... 748
- Cyclomydril ... ⊙ 216
- Deconsal Sprinkle Capsules ... 559
- Dimetane Decongestant ... ▣ 673
- Dristan Decongestant/Antihistamine/ Analgesic Coated Caplets ... ▣ 749
- Dristan Cold Nasal Decongestant/ Antihistamine/ Analgesic Coated Tablets ... 2419
- Dristan Advanced Formula Decongestant/Antihistamine/ Analgesic Tablets ... ▣ 749
- Dristan Nasal Spray, Menthol ... 2419
- Dristan Nasal Spray, Regular and Regular with Metered Pump ... 2419
- Entex Capsules ... 1623
- Entex Liquid ... 1623
- Sinus Excedrin Analgesic, Decongestant Tablets & Caplets ... 750
- Extendryl ... 994
- 4-Way Fast Acting Nasal Spray - Original Formula (regular & mentholated) & Metered Spray Pump (regular) ... 751
- Hycomine Compound Tablets ... 929
- Murocoll-2 Sterile Ophthalmic Solution ... ⊙ 261
- Mydfrin 2.5% ... ⊙ 224
- Naldecon Syrup, Tablets, Pediatric Drops and Pediatric Syrup ... 709
- Neo-Synephrine Hydrochloride 1% Carpuject ... 2063
- Neo-Synephrine Hydrochloride 1% Injection ... 2063
- Neo-Synephrine Hydrochloride (Ophthalmic) ... 2064
- Neo-Synephrine ... ▣ 759
- Nōstril Nasal Decongestant ... ▣ 520
- Novahistine Elixir ... ▣ 596
- Phenergan VC ... 2500
- Phenergan VC with Codeine ... 2501
- Prefrin Liquifilm Vasoconstrictor and Lubricant Eye Drops ... ⊙ 254
- Prefrin-A ... ⊙ 255
- Quelidrine Syrup ... 556
- Relief Vasoconstrictor and Lubricant Eye Drops ... ⊙ 256
- Robitussin Night Relief ... ▣ 677
- Ru-Tuss with Hydrocodone ... 694
- Ru-Tuss Tablets ... 693
- Vasosulf ... ⊙ 279
- Vicks Sinex ... ▣ 665
- Zincfrin ... ⊙ 230

Phenylephrine Tannate (The action of direct-acting sympathomimetic amines may be prolonged). Products include:
- Rynatan ... 2387
- Rynatuss ... 2388

Pindolol (Additive or potentiated action). Products include:
- Visken Tablets ... 2036

Piroxicam (May reduce the diuretic, natriuretic, and antihypertensive effects of thiazide diuretics). Products include:
- Feldene Capsules ... 1777

Polythiazide (Additive or potentiated action). Products include:
- Minizide Capsules ... 1779
- Renese Tablets ... 1785
- Renese-R Tablets ... 1786

Prazosin Hydrochloride (Additive or potentiated action). Products include:
- Minipress Capsules ... 1778
- Minizide Capsules ... 1779

Prednisolone Acetate (Hypokalemia). Products include:
- AK-Cide Sterile Ophthalmic Ointment & Suspension ... ⊙ 202
- Blephamide Liquifilm Sterile Ophthalmic Suspension ... 586
- Blephamide S.O.P. Sterile Ophthalmic Ointment ... 586
- Cetapred Ointment ... ⊙ 220
- ⅛% Econopred & 1% Econopred Plus ... ⊙ 217
- Isopto Cetapred Suspension ... ⊙ 220
- Metimyd ... ⊙ 306
- Poly-Pred Liquifilm ... ⊙ 250
- Pred Forte ... ⊙ 252
- Pred Mild ... ⊙ 254
- Pred-G Liquifilm Sterile Ophthalmic Suspension ... ⊙ 252
- Pred-G S.O.P. Sterile Ophthalmic Ointment ... ⊙ 253
- Vasocidin Ointment ... ⊙ 275

Prednisolone Sodium Phosphate (Hypokalemia). Products include:
- AK-Pred ... ⊙ 205
- Hydeltrasol Injection, Sterile ... 1476
- Inflamase ... ⊙ 274
- Pediapred Oral Liquid ... 987
- Vasocidin Ophthalmic Solution ... ⊙ 276

Prednisolone Tebutate (Hypokalemia). Products include:
- Hydeltra-T.B.A. Sterile Suspension 1478

Prednisone (Hypokalemia). Products include:
- Deltasone Tablets ... 2332

Propoxyphene Hydrochloride (Orthostatic hypotension). Products include:
- Darvon ... 1256
- Wygesic Tablets ... 2540

Propoxyphene Napsylate (Orthostatic hypotension). Products include:
- Darvon-N/Darvocet-N ... 1254

Propranolol Hydrochloride (Additive or potentiated action). Products include:
- Inderal ... 2459
- Inderal LA Long Acting Capsules ... 2461
- Inderide Tablets ... 2463
- Inderide LA Long Acting Capsules ... 2465

Protriptyline Hydrochloride (Decreases the antihypertensive effect of reserpine). Products include:
- Vivactil Tablets ... 1567

Quinidine Gluconate (Potential for arrhythmias). Products include:
- Quinaglute Dura-Tabs Tablets ... 663

Quinidine Polygalacturonate (Potential for arrhythmias). Products include:
- Cardioquin Tablets ... 1812

Quinidine Sulfate (Potential for arrhythmias). Products include:
- Quinidex Extentabs ... 1868

Ramipril (Additive or potentiated action). Products include:
Altace Capsules ... 1086

Rauwolfia Serpentina (Additive or potentiated action). Products include:
Raudixin Tablets ... 1803
Rauzide Tablets ... 1804

Rescinnamine (Additive or potentiated action).
No products indexed under this heading.

Secobarbital Sodium (Orthostatic hypotension). Products include:
Seconal Sodium Pulvules ... 1296

Selegiline Hydrochloride (Concurrent administration of MAOI should be avoided). Products include:
Eldepryl ... 2250

Sodium Nitroprusside (Additive or potentiated action). Products include:
Nipride I.V. Infusion ... 1909

Sufentanil Citrate (Orthostatic hypotension). Products include:
Sufenta Injection ... 1147

Sulindac (May reduce the diuretic, natriuretic, and antihypertensive effects of thiazide diuretics). Products include:
Clinoril Tablets ... 1433

Terazosin Hydrochloride (Additive or potentiated action). Products include:
Hytrin Tablets ... 529

Thiamylal Sodium (Orthostatic hypotension). Products include:
Surital Ampoules, Steri-Vials ... 1764

Timolol Maleate (Additive or potentiated action). Products include:
Blocadren Tablets ... 1429
Timolide Tablets ... 1547
Timoptic in Ocudose ... 1552
Timoptic Sterile Ophthalmic Solution ... 1550

Tolmetin Sodium (May reduce the diuretic, natriuretic, and antihypertensive effects of thiazide diuretics). Products include:
Tolectin (200, 400 and 600 mg) ... 1379

Tranylcypromine Sulfate (Concurrent administration of MAOI should be avoided). Products include:
Parnate Tablets ... 2222

Triamcinolone (Hypokalemia).
No products indexed under this heading.

Triamcinolone Acetonide (Hypokalemia). Products include:
Aristocort A ... 1010
Azmacort Inhaler ... 1837
Kenalog Cream, Lotion & Ointment 2401
Kenalog-10 Injection ... 2402
Kenalog-40 Injection ... 2403
Kenalog in Orabase ... 604
Kenalog Spray ... 2401
Mycolog II Cream and Ointment ... 2407
Mytrex Cream & Ointment ... 2080
Nasacort Nasal Inhaler ... 1844

Triamcinolone Diacetate (Hypokalemia). Products include:
Aristocort Suspension ... 1008

Triamcinolone Hexacetonide (Hypokalemia). Products include:
Aristospan Suspension ... 1011

Trimethaphan Camsylate (Additive or potentiated action). Products include:
Arfonad Ampuls ... 1887

Trimipramine Maleate (Decreases the antihypertensive effect of reserpine). Products include:
Surmontil Capsules ... 2524

Tyramine (The action of indirect-acting sympathomimetic amines is inhibited).

Food Interactions

Food, unspecified (Enhances gastrointestinal absorption of hydrochlorothiazide).

SERUTAN TOASTED GRANULES
(Psyllium Preparations) ... ▣ 619
No interactions described in labeling.

SHADE OIL-FREE GEL SPF 15
(Ethylhexyl p-Methoxycinnamate, 2-Ethylhexyl Salicylate, Oxybenzone) ... ▣ 705
No interactions described in labeling.

SHADE OIL-FREE GEL SPF 25
(Ethylhexyl p-Methoxycinnamate, 2-Ethylhexyl Salicylate, Oxybenzone) ... ▣ 705
No interactions described in labeling.

SHADE SUNBLOCK LOTION SPF 15
(Ethylhexyl p-Methoxycinnamate, Oxybenzone) ... ▣ 705
No interactions described in labeling.

SHADE SUNBLOCK LOTION SPF 30
(Ethylhexyl p-Methoxycinnamate, Oxybenzone) ... ▣ 705
No interactions described in labeling.

SHADE SUNBLOCK LOTION SPF 45
(Ethylhexyl p-Methoxycinnamate, Oxybenzone) ... ▣ 705
No interactions described in labeling.

SHADE SUNBLOCK STICK SPF 30
(Ethylhexyl p-Methoxycinnamate, Homosalate) ... ▣ 705
No interactions described in labeling.

SIGTAB TABLETS
(Multivitamins) ... ▣ 669
No interactions described in labeling.

SILVADENE CREAM 1%
(Silver Sulfadiazine) ... 1352
No interactions described in labeling.

SINAREST NO DROWSINESS TABLETS
(Acetaminophen, Pseudoephedrine Hydrochloride) ... ▣ 562
See **Sinarest Tablets & Extra Strength Tablets**

SINAREST TABLETS & EXTRA STRENGTH TABLETS
(Acetaminophen, Chlorpheniramine Maleate, Pseudoephedrine Hydrochloride) ... ▣ 562
May interact with central nervous system depressants, antidepressant drugs, antihypertensives, and certain other agents. Compounds in these categories include:

Acebutolol Hydrochloride (Effect not specified). Products include:
Sectral Capsules ... 2520

Alcohol (Concurrent use produces additive effects).

Alfentanil Hydrochloride (Concurrent use produces additive effects). Products include:
Alfenta Injection ... 1131

Alprazolam (Concurrent use produces additive effects). Products include:
Xanax Tablets ... 2367

Amitriptyline Hydrochloride (Effect not specified). Products include:
Elavil ... 2269
Endep Tablets ... 1927
Etrafon ... 2087
Limbitrol ... 1933
Triavil Tablets ... 1556

Amoxapine (Effect not specified). Products include:
Asendin Tablets ... 1196

Aprobarbital (Concurrent use produces additive effects). Products include:
Alurate Elixir ... 1883

Atenolol (Effect not specified). Products include:
Tenoretic Tablets ... 1105
Tenormin Tablets and I.V. Injection 1107

Benazepril Hydrochloride (Effect not specified). Products include:
Lotensin Tablets ... 872

Bendroflumethiazide (Effect not specified). Products include:
Corzide Tablets ... 702
Naturetin Tablets ... 1789
Rauzide Tablets ... 1804

Betaxolol Hydrochloride (Effect not specified). Products include:
Betoptic Sterile Ophthalmic Solution ... 569
Betoptic S Sterile Ophthalmic Suspension ... 570
Kerlone Tablets ... 2172

Buprenorphine (Concurrent use produces additive effects).
No products indexed under this heading.

Bupropion Hydrochloride (Effect not specified). Products include:
Wellbutrin Tablets ... 821

Buspirone Hydrochloride (Concurrent use produces additive effects). Products include:
BuSpar ... 1401

Butabarbital (Concurrent use produces additive effects). Products include:
Pyridium Plus ... 1764

Butalbital (Concurrent use produces additive effects). Products include:
Esgic-Plus Tablets ... 1002
Esgic Tablets & Capsules ... 1001
Fioricet Tablets ... 2006
Fiorinal Capsules ... 2007
Fiorinal with Codeine Capsules ... 2008
Fiorinal Tablets ... 2007
Phrenilin ... 838
Sedapap Tablets 50 mg/650 mg .. 1360

Captopril (Effect not specified). Products include:
Capoten ... 2255
Capozide ... 2258

Carteolol Hydrochloride (Effect not specified). Products include:
Cartrol Tablets ... 507

Chlordiazepoxide (Concurrent use produces additive effects). Products include:
Libritabs Tablets ... 1930
Limbitrol ... 1933
Menrium Tablets ... 1934

Chlordiazepoxide Hydrochloride (Concurrent use produces additive effects). Products include:
Librax Capsules ... 1929
Librium Capsules ... 1931
Librium Injectable ... 1932

Chlorothiazide (Effect not specified). Products include:
Aldoclor Tablets ... 1413
Diupres Tablets ... 1461
Diuril Oral ... 1464

Chlorothiazide Sodium (Effect not specified). Products include:
Diuril Sodium Intravenous ... 1463

Chlorpromazine (Concurrent use produces additive effects). Products include:
Thorazine ... 2234

Chlorprothixene (Concurrent use produces additive effects). Products include:
Taractan Tablets ... 1920

Chlorprothixene Hydrochloride (Concurrent use produces additive effects). Products include:
Taractan ... 1920

Chlorthalidone (Effect not specified). Products include:
Combipres Tablets ... 678
Tenoretic Tablets ... 1105
Thalitone Tablets ... 687

Clonidine (Effect not specified). Products include:
Catapres-TTS ... 677

Clonidine Hydrochloride (Effect not specified). Products include:
Catapres Tablets ... 676
Combipres Tablets ... 678

Clorazepate Dipotassium (Concurrent use produces additive effects). Products include:
Tranxene ... 556

Codeine (Concurrent use produces additive effects). Products include:
Calcidrine Syrup ... 506

Codeine Phosphate (Concurrent use produces additive effects). Products include:
Actifed with Codeine Cough Syrup .. 752
Cheracol Cough Syrup ... 1853
Codimal PH Syrup ... 846
Dimetane-DC Cough Syrup ... 1857
Empirin with Codeine Phosphate Nos. 2, 3 & 4 ... 764
Fiorinal with Codeine Capsules ... 2008
Isoclor Expectorant ... 982
Naldecon CX Adult Liquid ... ▣ 521
Novahistine DH ... 1342
Novahistine Expectorant ... 1343
Nucofed Capsules ... 2219
Nucofed Expectorant ... 2219
Nucofed Pediatric Expectorant ... 2220
Nucofed Syrup ... 2219
Phenaphen with Codeine Capsules 1865
Phenaphen-650 with Codeine Tablets ... 1866
Phenergan with Codeine ... 2497
Phenergan VC with Codeine ... 2501
Robitussin A-C Syrup ... 1875
Robitussin-DAC Syrup ... 1875
Ryna ... ▣ 741
Soma Compound w/Codeine Tablets ... 2390
Triaminic Expectorant w/Codeine .. 1996
Tussi-Organidin Liquid ... 2391
Tylenol with Codeine ... 1381

Codeine Polistirex (Concurrent use produces additive effects).
No products indexed under this heading.

Deserpidine (Effect not specified). Products include:
Enduronyl ... 518
Harmonyl Tablets ... 528
Oreticyl ... 545

Desipramine Hydrochloride (Effect not specified). Products include:
Norpramin Tablets ... 1340

Dezocine (Concurrent use produces additive effects).

Diazepam (Concurrent use produces additive effects). Products include:
Valium Injectable ... 1937
Valium Tablets ... 1939
Valrelease Capsules ... 1923

Diazoxide (Effect not specified). Products include:
Hyperstat I.V. Injection ... 2095
Proglycem ... 649

Doxazosin Mesylate (Effect not specified). Products include:
Cardura Tablets ... 1941

Doxepin Hydrochloride (Effect not specified). Products include:
Sinequan ... 1960

Droperidol (Concurrent use produces additive effects). Products include:
Inapsine Injection ... 1140
Innovar Injection ... 1141

Enalapril Maleate (Effect not specified). Products include:
Vaseretic Tablets ... 1559
Vasotec Tablets ... 1564

Enalaprilat (Effect not specified). Products include:
Vasotec I.V. ... 1562

Enflurane (Concurrent use produces additive effects). Products include:
Ethrane ... 599

Esmolol Hydrochloride (Effect not specified). Products include:
Brevibloc Injection ... 942

Estazolam (Concurrent use produces additive effects). Products include:
ProSom Tablets ... 554

Ethchlorvynol (Concurrent use produces additive effects). Products include:
Placidyl Capsules ... 553

Ethinamate (Concurrent use produces additive effects).
No products indexed under this heading.

Felodipine (Effect not specified). Products include:
Plendil Extended-Release Tablets ... 1526

Fentanyl (Concurrent use produces additive effects). Products include:
Duragesic Transdermal System ... 1133

Fentanyl Citrate (Concurrent use produces additive effects). Products include:
Innovar Injection ... 1141
Sublimaze Injection ... 1146

Fluoxetine Hydrochloride (Effect not specified). Products include:
Prozac Pulvules ... 920

Fluphenazine Decanoate (Concurrent use produces additive effects). Products include:
Prolixin Decanoate ... 1795

Fluphenazine Enanthate (Concurrent use produces additive effects). Products include:
Prolixin Enanthate ... 1796

Fluphenazine Hydrochloride (Concurrent use produces additive effects). Products include:
Prolixin Elixir ... 1793
Prolixin Injection ... 1791
Prolixin Oral Concentrate ... 1792
Prolixin Tablets ... 1793

Flurazepam Hydrochloride (Concurrent use produces additive effects). Products include:
Dalmane Capsules ... 1927

Fosinopril Sodium (Effect not specified). Products include:
Monopril Tablets ... 1406

Furosemide (Effect not specified). Products include:
Lasix ... 1093

Glutethimide (Concurrent use produces additive effects).
No products indexed under this heading.

Guanabenz Acetate (Effect not specified). Products include:
Wytensin Tablets ... 2542

Guanethidine Monosulfate (Effect not specified). Products include:
Esimil Tablets ... 864
Ismelin Tablets ... 869

Haloperidol (Concurrent use produces additive effects). Products include:
Haldol Injection, Tablets and Concentrate ... 1373

Haloperidol Decanoate (Concurrent use produces additive effects). Products include:
Haldol Decanoate ... 1375

Hydralazine Hydrochloride (Effect not specified). Products include:
Apresazide Capsules ... 854
Apresoline Hydrochloride Parenteral (Ampuls) ... 856
Apresoline Hydrochloride Tablets .. 855
Apresoline-Esidrix Tablets ... 857
Ser-Ap-Es Tablets ... 881
Serpasil-Apresoline Tablets ... 884

Hydrochlorothiazide (Effect not specified). Products include:
Aldactazide ... 2150
Aldoril Tablets ... 1418
Apresazide Capsules ... 854
Apresoline-Esidrix Tablets ... 857
Capozide ... 2258
Dyazide Capsules ... 2208
Esidrix Tablets ... 863
Esimil Tablets ... 864
HydroDIURIL Tablets ... 1484
Hydropres Tablets ... 1485
Inderide Tablets ... 2463
Inderide LA Long Acting Capsules .. 2465
Lopressor HCT Tablets ... 1034
Maxzide ... 1215
Moduretic Tablets ... 1510
Normozide Tablets ... 2112
Oretic Tablets ... 544
Oreticyl ... 545
Prinzide Tablets ... 1540
Ser-Ap-Es Tablets ... 881
Serpasil-Esidrix Tablets ... 886
Timolide Tablets ... 1547
Trandate HCT Tablets ... 579
Vaseretic Tablets ... 1559
Zestoretic ... 2274

Hydrocodone Bitartrate (Concurrent use produces additive effects). Products include:
Anexsia 5/500 Tablets ... 2196
Anexsia 7.5/650 Tablets ... 2197
Azdōne Tablets ... 844
Codiclear DH Syrup ... 845
Codimal DH Syrup ... 846
Damason-P ... 1356
Hycodan Syrup, Tablets ... 927
Hycomine Compound Tablets ... 929
Hycomine Syrup ... 927
Hycotuss Expectorant Syrup ... 930
Hydrocet Capsules ... 835
Lortab ASA Tablets ... 2414
Lortab ... 2412
Ru-Tuss with Hydrocodone ... 694
Triaminic Expectorant DH ... 1995
Vicodin Tablets ... 1187
Vicodin ES Tablets ... 1189
Zydone Capsules ... 941

Hydrocodone Polistirex (Concurrent use produces additive effects). Products include:
Tussionex Extended-Release Suspension ... 988

Hydroflumethiazide (Effect not specified). Products include:
Diucardin Tablets ... 2450
Saluron ... 718
Salutensin/Salutensin-Demi ... 719

Hydroxyzine Hydrochloride (Concurrent use produces additive effects). Products include:
Atarax Tablets & Syrup ... 1941
Marax Tablets & DF Syrup ... 1954
Vistaril Intramuscular Solution ... 1970

Imipramine Hydrochloride (Effect not specified). Products include:
Tofranil Ampuls ... 1038
Tofranil Tablets ... 1039

Imipramine Pamoate (Effect not specified). Products include:
Tofranil-PM Capsules ... 1041

Indapamide (Effect not specified). Products include:
Lozol Tablets ... 1843

Isocarboxazid (Effect not specified). Products include:
Marplan Tablets ... 1906

Isoflurane (Concurrent use produces additive effects). Products include:
Forane ... 600

Isradipine (Effect not specified). Products include:
DynaCirc Capsules ... 2004

Ketamine Hydrochloride (Concurrent use produces additive effects). Products include:
Ketalar ... 1726

Labetalol Hydrochloride (Effect not specified). Products include:
Normodyne Injection ... 2108
Normodyne Tablets ... 2110
Normozide Tablets ... 2112
Trandate HCT Tablets ... 579
Trandate Injection ... 577
Trandate Tablets ... 579

Levorphanol Tartrate (Concurrent use produces additive effects). Products include:
Levo-Dromoran ... 1906

Lisinopril (Effect not specified). Products include:
Prinivil Tablets ... 1538
Prinzide Tablets ... 1540
Zestoretic ... 2274
Zestril Tablets ... 2277

Lorazepam (Concurrent use produces additive effects). Products include:
Ativan Injection ... 2432
Ativan Tablets ... 2434

Loxapine Hydrochloride (Concurrent use produces additive effects). Products include:
Loxitane ... 1213

Loxapine Succinate (Concurrent use produces additive effects). Products include:
Loxitane Capsules ... 1213

Maprotiline Hydrochloride (Effect not specified). Products include:
Ludiomil Tablets ... 874

Mecamylamine Hydrochloride (Effect not specified). Products include:
Inversine Tablets ... 1492

Meperidine Hydrochloride (Concurrent use produces additive effects). Products include:
Demerol ... 2047
Mepergan Injection ... 2479

Mephobarbital (Concurrent use produces additive effects). Products include:
Mebaral Tablets ... 2061

Meprobamate (Concurrent use produces additive effects). Products include:
Deprol Tablets ... 2382
Equagesic Tablets ... 2451
Miltown Tablets ... 2386
PMB 200 and PMB 400 ... 2504

Mesoridazine (Concurrent use produces additive effects). Products include:
Serentil ... 686

Methadone Hydrochloride (Concurrent use produces additive effects). Products include:
Dolophine Hydrochloride Ampoules & Vials ... 1260
Dolophine Hydrochloride Tablets ... 1261
Methadone Hydrochloride Diskets .. 1284
Methadone Hydrochloride Oral Solution & Tablets ... 1987

Methohexital Sodium (Concurrent use produces additive effects). Products include:
Brevital Sodium Vials ... 1248

Methoxyflurane (Concurrent use produces additive effects).
No products indexed under this heading.

Methyclothiazide (Effect not specified). Products include:
Enduron Tablets ... 517
Enduronyl ... 518

Methyldopa (Effect not specified). Products include:
Aldoclor Tablets ... 1413
Aldomet Oral ... 1415
Aldoril Tablets ... 1418

Methyldopate Hydrochloride (Effect not specified). Products include:
Aldomet Ester HCl Injection ... 1417

Metolazone (Effect not specified). Products include:
Diulo ... 2129
Mykrox ½ mg Tablets ... 984
Zaroxolyn Tablets ... 989

Metoprolol Tartrate (Effect not specified). Products include:
Lopressor Ampuls ... 1032
Lopressor HCT Tablets ... 1034
Lopressor Tablets ... 1032

Metyrosine (Effect not specified). Products include:
Demser Capsules ... 1460

Midazolam Hydrochloride (Concurrent use produces additive effects). Products include:
Versed Injection ... 1924

Minoxidil (Effect not specified). Products include:
Loniten Tablets ... 2346
Rogaine Topical Solution ... 2357

Molindone Hydrochloride (Concurrent use produces additive effects). Products include:
Moban Tablets & Concentrate ... 932

Morphine Sulfate (Concurrent use produces additive effects). Products include:
Astramorph/PF Injection, USP (Preservative-Free) ... 618
Duramorph ... 960
Infumorph 200 and Infumorph 500 Sterile Solutions ... 962
MS Contin Tablets ... 1814
MSIR ... 1817
Oramorph SR (Morphine Sulfate Sustained Release Tablets) ... 1988
Roxanol ... 1991

Nadolol (Effect not specified). Products include:
Corgard Tablets ... 701
Corzide Tablets ... 702

Nicardipine Hydrochloride (Effect not specified). Products include:
Cardene Capsules ... 2290

Nitroglycerin (Effect not specified). Products include:
Deponit NTG Transdermal Delivery System ... 2143
Minitran Transdermal Delivery System ... 1312
Nitro-Bid Ointment ... 1339
Nitro-Bid Capsules ... 1338
Nitrodisc ... 2176
Nitro-Dur (nitroglycerin) Transdermal Infusion System ... 1164
Nitrogard Tablets ... 1004
Nitrolingual Spray ... 1846
Nitrostat Tablets ... 1743
Transderm-Nitro Transdermal Therapeutic System ... 2283

Nortriptyline Hydrochloride (Effect not specified). Products include:
Pamelor ... 2019

Opium Alkaloids (Concurrent use produces additive effects). Products include:
B & O No. 15A & No. 16A Supprettes ... 2395
Pantopon Injectable ... 1911

Oxazepam (Concurrent use produces additive effects). Products include:
Serax Capsules ... 2522
Serax Tablets ... 2522

Oxycodone Hydrochloride (Concurrent use produces additive effects). Products include:
- Percocet Tablets ... 950
- Percodan ... 951
- Roxicodone Tablets, Oral Solution & Intensol (Oxycodone) ... 1992
- Tylox Capsules ... 1382

Penbutolol Sulfate (Effect not specified). Products include:
- Levatol ... 1832

Pentobarbital Sodium (Concurrent use produces additive effects). Products include:
- Nembutal Sodium Capsules ... 534
- Nembutal Sodium Solution ... 536
- Nembutal Sodium Suppositories ... 538

Perphenazine (Concurrent use produces additive effects). Products include:
- Etrafon ... 2087
- Triavil Tablets ... 1556
- Trilafon ... 2123

Phenelzine Sulfate (Effect not specified). Products include:
- Nardil ... 1742

Phenobarbital (Concurrent use produces additive effects). Products include:
- Arco-Lase Plus Tablets ... 607
- Bellergal-S Tablets ... 1998
- Bronkolixir ... ⊞ 761
- Bronkotabs Tablets ... ⊞ 762
- Donnatal ... 1858
- Donnatal Extentabs ... 1859
- Donnatal Tablets ... 1858
- Donnazyme Tablets ... 1860
- Kinesed Tablets ... 2272
- Phenobarbital Elixir and Tablets ... 1293
- Primatene Tablets-P Formula ... 2421
- Quadrinal Tablets ... 1183
- Tedral SA ... 1765

Phenoxybenzamine Hydrochloride (Effect not specified). Products include:
- Dibenzyline Capsules ... 2207

Phentolamine Mesylate (Effect not specified). Products include:
- Regitine ... 878

Pindolol (Effect not specified). Products include:
- Visken Tablets ... 2036

Polythiazide (Effect not specified). Products include:
- Minizide Capsules ... 1779
- Renese Tablets ... 1785
- Renese-R Tablets ... 1786

Prazepam (Concurrent use produces additive effects). Products include:
- Centrax ... 1693

Prazosin Hydrochloride (Effect not specified). Products include:
- Minipress Capsules ... 1778
- Minizide Capsules ... 1779

Prochlorperazine (Concurrent use produces additive effects). Products include:
- Compazine ... 2201

Promethazine Hydrochloride (Concurrent use produces additive effects). Products include:
- Mepergan Injection ... 2479
- Phenergan with Codeine ... 2497
- Phenergan with Dextromethorphan ... 2499
- Phenergan Injection ... 2493
- Phenergan Suppositories ... 2496
- Phenergan Syrup ... 2495
- Phenergan Tablets ... 2496
- Phenergan VC ... 2500
- Phenergan VC with Codeine ... 2501

Propofol (Concurrent use produces additive effects). Products include:
- Diprivan Injection ... 2267

Propoxyphene Hydrochloride (Concurrent use produces additive effects). Products include:
- Darvon ... 1256
- Wygesic Tablets ... 2540

Propoxyphene Napsylate (Concurrent use produces additive effects). Products include:
- Darvon-N/Darvocet-N ... 1254

Propranolol Hydrochloride (Effect not specified). Products include:
- Inderal ... 2459
- Inderal LA Long Acting Capsules ... 2461
- Inderide Tablets ... 2463
- Inderide LA Long Acting Capsules ... 2465

Protriptyline Hydrochloride (Effect not specified). Products include:
- Vivactil Tablets ... 1567

Quazepam (Concurrent use produces additive effects). Products include:
- Doral Tablets ... 2383

Ramipril (Effect not specified). Products include:
- Altace Capsules ... 1086

Rauwolfia Serpentina (Effect not specified). Products include:
- Raudixin Tablets ... 1803
- Rauzide Tablets ... 1804

Rescinnamine (Effect not specified).
- No products indexed under this heading.

Reserpine (Effect not specified). Products include:
- Diupres Tablets ... 1461
- Hydromox R Tablets ... 1209
- Hydropres Tablets ... 1485
- Renese-R Tablets ... 1786
- Salutensin/Salutensin-Demi ... 719
- Ser-Ap-Es Tablets ... 881
- Serpasil Tablets ... 883
- Serpasil-Apresoline Tablets ... 884
- Serpasil-Esidrix Tablets ... 886

Secobarbital Sodium (Concurrent use produces additive effects). Products include:
- Seconal Sodium Pulvules ... 1296

Sodium Nitroprusside (Effect not specified). Products include:
- Nipride I.V. Infusion ... 1909

Sufentanil Citrate (Concurrent use produces additive effects). Products include:
- Sufenta Injection ... 1147

Temazepam (Concurrent use produces additive effects). Products include:
- Restoril Capsules ... 2023

Terazosin Hydrochloride (Effect not specified). Products include:
- Hytrin Tablets ... 529

Thiamylal Sodium (Concurrent use produces additive effects). Products include:
- Surital Ampoules, Steri-Vials ... 1764

Thioridazine Hydrochloride (Concurrent use produces additive effects). Products include:
- Mellaril ... 2011

Thiothixene (Concurrent use produces additive effects). Products include:
- Navane Capsules and Concentrate ... 1954
- Navane Intramuscular ... 1956

Timolol Maleate (Effect not specified). Products include:
- Blocadren Tablets ... 1429
- Timolide Tablets ... 1547
- Timoptic in Ocudose ... 1552
- Timoptic Sterile Ophthalmic Solution ... 1550

Tranylcypromine Sulfate (Effect not specified). Products include:
- Parnate Tablets ... 2222

Trazodone Hydrochloride (Effect not specified). Products include:
- Desyrel and Desyrel Dividose ... 1404

Triazolam (Concurrent use produces additive effects). Products include:
- Halcion Tablets ... 2340

Trifluoperazine Hydrochloride (Concurrent use produces additive effects). Products include:
- Stelazine ... 2226

Trimethaphan Camsylate (Effect not specified). Products include:
- Arfonad Ampuls ... 1887

Trimipramine Maleate (Effect not specified). Products include:
- Surmontil Capsules ... 2524

SINE-AID MAXIMUM STRENGTH SINUS HEADACHE CAPLETS
(Acetaminophen, Pseudoephedrine Hydrochloride) ... 1365
May interact with antidepressant drugs and antihypertensives. Compounds in these categories include:

Acebutolol Hydrochloride (Effect not specified). Products include:
- Sectral Capsules ... 2520

Amitriptyline Hydrochloride (Effect not specified). Products include:
- Elavil ... 2269
- Endep Tablets ... 1927
- Etrafon ... 2087
- Limbitrol ... 1933
- Triavil Tablets ... 1556

Amoxapine (Effect not specified). Products include:
- Asendin Tablets ... 1196

Atenolol (Effect not specified). Products include:
- Tenoretic Tablets ... 1105
- Tenormin Tablets and I.V. Injection ... 1107

Benazepril Hydrochloride (Effect not specified). Products include:
- Lotensin Tablets ... 872

Betaxolol Hydrochloride (Effect not specified). Products include:
- Betoptic Sterile Ophthalmic Solution ... 569
- Betoptic S Sterile Ophthalmic Suspension ... 570
- Kerlone Tablets ... 2172

Bupropion Hydrochloride (Effect not specified). Products include:
- Wellbutrin Tablets ... 821

Captopril (Effect not specified). Products include:
- Capoten ... 2255
- Capozide ... 2258

Carteolol Hydrochloride (Effect not specified). Products include:
- Cartrol Tablets ... 507

Clonidine (Effect not specified). Products include:
- Catapres-TTS ... 677

Clonidine Hydrochloride (Effect not specified). Products include:
- Catapres Tablets ... 676
- Combipres Tablets ... 678

Deserpidine (Effect not specified). Products include:
- Enduronyl ... 518
- Harmonyl Tablets ... 528
- Oreticyl ... 545

Desipramine Hydrochloride (Effect not specified). Products include:
- Norpramin Tablets ... 1340

Diazoxide (Effect not specified). Products include:
- Hyperstat I.V. Injection ... 2095
- Proglycem ... 649

Doxazosin Mesylate (Effect not specified). Products include:
- Cardura Tablets ... 1941

Doxepin Hydrochloride (Effect not specified). Products include:
- Sinequan ... 1960

Enalapril Maleate (Effect not specified). Products include:
- Vaseretic Tablets ... 1559
- Vasotec Tablets ... 1564

Enalaprilat (Effect not specified). Products include:
- Vasotec I.V. ... 1562

Esmolol Hydrochloride (Effect not specified). Products include:
- Brevibloc Injection ... 942

Felodipine (Effect not specified). Products include:
- Plendil Extended-Release Tablets ... 1526

Fluoxetine Hydrochloride (Effect not specified). Products include:
- Prozac Pulvules ... 920

Fosinopril Sodium (Effect not specified). Products include:
- Monopril Tablets ... 1406

Guanabenz Acetate (Effect not specified). Products include:
- Wytensin Tablets ... 2542

Guanethidine Monosulfate (Effect not specified). Products include:
- Esimil Tablets ... 864
- Ismelin Tablets ... 869

Hydralazine Hydrochloride (Effect not specified). Products include:
- Apresazide Capsules ... 854
- Apresoline Hydrochloride Parenteral (Ampuls) ... 856
- Apresoline Hydrochloride Tablets ... 855
- Apresoline-Esidrix Tablets ... 857
- Ser-Ap-Es Tablets ... 881
- Serpasil-Apresoline Tablets ... 884

Imipramine Hydrochloride (Effect not specified). Products include:
- Tofranil Ampuls ... 1038
- Tofranil Tablets ... 1039

Imipramine Pamoate (Effect not specified). Products include:
- Tofranil-PM Capsules ... 1041

Isocarboxazid (Effect not specified). Products include:
- Marplan Tablets ... 1906

Isradipine (Effect not specified). Products include:
- DynaCirc Capsules ... 2004

Labetalol Hydrochloride (Effect not specified). Products include:
- Normodyne Injection ... 2108
- Normodyne Tablets ... 2110
- Normozide Tablets ... 2112
- Trandate HCT Tablets ... 579
- Trandate Injection ... 577
- Trandate Tablets ... 579

Lisinopril (Effect not specified). Products include:
- Prinivil Tablets ... 1538
- Prinzide Tablets ... 1540
- Zestoretic ... 2274
- Zestril Tablets ... 2277

Maprotiline Hydrochloride (Effect not specified). Products include:
- Ludiomil Tablets ... 874

Mecamylamine Hydrochloride (Effect not specified). Products include:
- Inversine Tablets ... 1492

Methyldopa (Effect not specified). Products include:
- Aldoclor Tablets ... 1413
- Aldomet Oral ... 1415
- Aldoril Tablets ... 1418

Methyldopate Hydrochloride (Effect not specified). Products include:
- Aldomet Ester HCl Injection ... 1417

Metoprolol Tartrate (Effect not specified). Products include:
- Lopressor Ampuls ... 1032
- Lopressor HCT Tablets ... 1034
- Lopressor Tablets ... 1032

Metyrosine (Effect not specified). Products include:
- Demser Capsules ... 1460

Minoxidil (Effect not specified). Products include:
- Loniten Tablets ... 2346
- Rogaine Topical Solution ... 2357

Nadolol (Effect not specified). Products include:
Corgard Tablets ... 701
Corzide Tablets ... 702

Nicardipine Hydrochloride (Effect not specified). Products include:
Cardene Capsules ... 2290

Nitroglycerin (Effect not specified). Products include:
Deponit NTG Transdermal Delivery System ... 2143
Minitran Transdermal Delivery System ... 1312
Nitro-Bid Ointment ... 1339
Nitro-Bid Capsules ... 1338
Nitrodisc ... 2176
Nitro-Dur (nitroglycerin) Transdermal Infusion System ... 1164
Nitrogard Tablets ... 1004
Nitrolingual Spray ... 1846
Nitrostat Tablets ... 1743
Transderm-Nitro Transdermal Therapeutic System ... 2283

Nortriptyline Hydrochloride (Effect not specified). Products include:
Pamelor ... 2019

Penbutolol Sulfate (Effect not specified). Products include:
Levatol ... 1832

Phenelzine Sulfate (Effect not specified). Products include:
Nardil ... 1742

Phenoxybenzamine Hydrochloride (Effect not specified). Products include:
Dibenzyline Capsules ... 2207

Phentolamine Mesylate (Effect not specified). Products include:
Regitine ... 878

Pindolol (Effect not specified). Products include:
Visken Tablets ... 2036

Prazosin Hydrochloride (Effect not specified). Products include:
Minipress Capsules ... 1778
Minizide Capsules ... 1779

Propranolol Hydrochloride (Effect not specified). Products include:
Inderal ... 2459
Inderal LA Long Acting Capsules ... 2461
Inderide Tablets ... 2463
Inderide LA Long Acting Capsules .. 2465

Protriptyline Hydrochloride (Effect not specified). Products include:
Vivactil Tablets ... 1567

Ramipril (Effect not specified). Products include:
Altace Capsules ... 1086

Rauwolfia Serpentina (Effect not specified). Products include:
Raudixin Tablets ... 1803
Rauzide Tablets ... 1804

Rescinnamine (Effect not specified).
No products indexed under this heading.

Reserpine (Effect not specified). Products include:
Diupres Tablets ... 1461
Hydromox R Tablets ... 1209
Hydropres Tablets ... 1485
Renese-R Tablets ... 1786
Salutensin/Salutensin-Demi ... 719
Ser-Ap-Es Tablets ... 881
Serpasil Tablets ... 883
Serpasil-Apresoline Tablets ... 884
Serpasil-Esidrix Tablets ... 886

Sodium Nitroprusside (Effect not specified). Products include:
Nipride I.V. Infusion ... 1909

Terazosin Hydrochloride (Effect not specified). Products include:
Hytrin Tablets ... 529

Timolol Maleate (Effect not specified). Products include:
Blocadren Tablets ... 1429
Timolide Tablets ... 1547
Timoptic in Ocudose ... 1552
Timoptic Sterile Ophthalmic Solution ... 1550

Tranylcypromine Sulfate (Effect not specified). Products include:
Parnate Tablets ... 2222

Trazodone Hydrochloride (Effect not specified). Products include:
Desyrel and Desyrel Dividose ... 1404

Trimethaphan Camsylate (Effect not specified). Products include:
Arfonad Ampuls ... 1887

Trimipramine Maleate (Effect not specified). Products include:
Surmontil Capsules ... 2524

SINE-AID MAXIMUM STRENGTH SINUS HEADACHE TABLETS
(Acetaminophen, Pseudoephedrine Hydrochloride) ... 1365

See **Sine-Aid Maximum Strength Sinus Headache Caplets**

SINEMET TABLETS
(Carbidopa, Levodopa) ... 952
May interact with monoamine oxidase inhibitors, antihypertensives, tricyclic antidepressants, phenothiazines, butyrophenones, and certain other agents. Compounds in these categories include:

Acebutolol Hydrochloride (Symptomatic postural hypotension). Products include:
Sectral Capsules ... 2520

Amitriptyline Hydrochloride (Hypertension; dyskinesia). Products include:
Elavil ... 2269
Endep Tablets ... 1927
Etrafon ... 2087
Limbitrol ... 1933
Triavil Tablets ... 1556

Amoxapine (Hypertension; dyskinesia). Products include:
Asendin Tablets ... 1196

Atenolol (Symptomatic postural hypotension). Products include:
Tenoretic Tablets ... 1105
Tenormin Tablets and I.V. Injection 1107

Benazepril Hydrochloride (Symptomatic postural hypotension). Products include:
Lotensin Tablets ... 872

Bendroflumethiazide (Symptomatic postural hypotension). Products include:
Corzide Tablets ... 702
Naturetin Tablets ... 1789
Rauzide Tablets ... 1804

Betaxolol Hydrochloride (Symptomatic postural hypotension). Products include:
Betoptic Sterile Ophthalmic Solution ... 569
Betoptic S Sterile Ophthalmic Suspension ... 570
Kerlone Tablets ... 2172

Captopril (Symptomatic postural hypotension). Products include:
Capoten ... 2255
Capozide ... 2258

Carteolol Hydrochloride (Symptomatic postural hypotension). Products include:
Cartrol Tablets ... 507

Chlorothiazide (Symptomatic postural hypotension). Products include:
Aldoclor Tablets ... 1413
Diupres Tablets ... 1461
Diuril Oral ... 1464

Chlorothiazide Sodium (Symptomatic postural hypotension). Products include:
Diuril Sodium Intravenous ... 1463

Chlorpromazine (Reduced therapeutic effects of levodopa). Products include:
Thorazine ... 2234

Chlorthalidone (Symptomatic postural hypotension). Products include:
Combipres Tablets ... 678
Tenoretic Tablets ... 1105
Thalitone Tablets ... 687

Clomipramine Hydrochloride (Hypertension; dyskinesia). Products include:
Anafranil Capsules ... 650

Clonidine (Symptomatic postural hypotension). Products include:
Catapres-TTS ... 677

Clonidine Hydrochloride (Symptomatic postural hypotension). Products include:
Catapres Tablets ... 676
Combipres Tablets ... 678

Deserpidine (Symptomatic postural hypotension). Products include:
Enduronyl ... 518
Harmonyl Tablets ... 528
Oreticyl ... 545

Desipramine Hydrochloride (Hypertension; dyskinesia). Products include:
Norpramin Tablets ... 1340

Diazoxide (Symptomatic postural hypotension). Products include:
Hyperstat I.V. Injection ... 2095
Proglycem ... 649

Doxazosin Mesylate (Symptomatic postural hypotension). Products include:
Cardura Tablets ... 1941

Doxepin Hydrochloride (Hypertension; dyskinesia). Products include:
Sinequan ... 1960

Enalapril Maleate (Symptomatic postural hypotension). Products include:
Vaseretic Tablets ... 1559
Vasotec Tablets ... 1564

Enalaprilat (Symptomatic postural hypotension). Products include:
Vasotec I.V. ... 1562

Esmolol Hydrochloride (Symptomatic postural hypotension). Products include:
Brevibloc Injection ... 942

Felodipine (Symptomatic postural hypotension). Products include:
Plendil Extended-Release Tablets ... 1526

Fluphenazine Decanoate (Reduced therapeutic effects of levodopa). Products include:
Prolixin Decanoate ... 1795

Fluphenazine Enanthate (Reduced therapeutic effects of levodopa). Products include:
Prolixin Enanthate ... 1796

Fluphenazine Hydrochloride (Reduced therapeutic effects of levodopa). Products include:
Prolixin Elixir ... 1793
Prolixin Injection ... 1791
Prolixin Oral Concentrate ... 1792
Prolixin Tablets ... 1793

Fosinopril Sodium (Symptomatic postural hypotension). Products include:
Monopril Tablets ... 1406

Furazolidone (Contraindication). Products include:
Furoxone ... 1855

Furosemide (Symptomatic postural hypotension). Products include:
Lasix ... 1093

Guanabenz Acetate (Symptomatic postural hypotension). Products include:
Wytensin Tablets ... 2542

Guanethidine Monosulfate (Symptomatic postural hypotension). Products include:
Esimil Tablets ... 864
Ismelin Tablets ... 869

Haloperidol (Reduced therapeutic effects of levodopa). Products include:
Haldol Injection, Tablets and Concentrate ... 1373

Haloperidol Decanoate (Reduced therapeutic effects of levodopa). Products include:
Haldol Decanoate ... 1375

Hydralazine Hydrochloride (Symptomatic postural hypotension). Products include:
Apresazide Capsules ... 854
Apresoline Hydrochloride Parenteral (Ampuls) ... 856
Apresoline Hydrochloride Tablets .. 855
Apresoline-Esidrix Tablets ... 857
Ser-Ap-Es Tablets ... 881
Serpasil-Apresoline Tablets ... 884

Hydrochlorothiazide (Symptomatic postural hypotension). Products include:
Aldactazide ... 2150
Aldoril Tablets ... 1418
Apresazide Capsules ... 854
Apresoline-Esidrix Tablets ... 857
Capozide ... 2258
Dyazide Capsules ... 2208
Esidrix Tablets ... 863
Esimil Tablets ... 864
HydroDIURIL Tablets ... 1484
Hydropres Tablets ... 1485
Inderide Tablets ... 2463
Inderide LA Long Acting Capsules .. 2465
Lopressor HCT Tablets ... 1034
Maxzide ... 1215
Moduretic Tablets ... 1510
Normozide Tablets ... 2112
Oretic Tablets ... 544
Oreticyl ... 545
Prinzide Tablets ... 1540
Ser-Ap-Es Tablets ... 881
Serpasil-Esidrix Tablets ... 886
Timolide Tablets ... 1547
Trandate HCT Tablets ... 579
Vaseretic Tablets ... 1559
Zestoretic ... 2274

Hydroflumethiazide (Symptomatic postural hypotension). Products include:
Diucardin Tablets ... 2450
Saluron ... 718
Salutensin/Salutensin-Demi ... 719

Imipramine Hydrochloride (Hypertension; dyskinesia). Products include:
Tofranil Ampuls ... 1038
Tofranil Tablets ... 1039

Imipramine Pamoate (Hypertension; dyskinesia). Products include:
Tofranil-PM Capsules ... 1041

Indapamide (Symptomatic postural hypotension). Products include:
Lozol Tablets ... 1843

Isocarboxazid (Contraindication). Products include:
Marplan Tablets ... 1906

Isradipine (Symptomatic postural hypotension). Products include:
DynaCirc Capsules ... 2004

Labetalol Hydrochloride (Symptomatic postural hypotension). Products include:
Normodyne Injection ... 2108
Normodyne Tablets ... 2110
Normozide Tablets ... 2112
Trandate HCT Tablets ... 579
Trandate Injection ... 577
Trandate Tablets ... 579

Lisinopril (Symptomatic postural hypotension). Products include:
Prinivil Tablets ... 1538
Prinzide Tablets ... 1540
Zestoretic ... 2274
Zestril Tablets ... 2277

Maprotiline Hydrochloride (Hypertension; dyskinesia). Products include:
- Ludiomil Tablets 874

Mecamylamine Hydrochloride (Symptomatic postural hypotension). Products include:
- Inversine Tablets 1492

Mesoridazine (Reduced therapeutic effects of levodopa). Products include:
- Serentil 686

Methyclothiazide (Symptomatic postural hypotension). Products include:
- Enduron Tablets 517
- Enduronyl 518

Methyldopa (Symptomatic postural hypotension). Products include:
- Aldoclor Tablets 1413
- Aldomet Oral 1415
- Aldoril Tablets 1418

Methyldopate Hydrochloride (Symptomatic postural hypotension). Products include:
- Aldomet Ester HCl Injection 1417

Metolazone (Symptomatic postural hypotension). Products include:
- Diulo 2129
- Mykrox ½ mg Tablets 984
- Zaroxolyn Tablets 989

Metoprolol Tartrate (Symptomatic postural hypotension). Products include:
- Lopressor Ampuls 1032
- Lopressor HCT Tablets 1034
- Lopressor Tablets 1032

Metyrosine (Symptomatic postural hypotension). Products include:
- Demser Capsules 1460

Minoxidil (Symptomatic postural hypotension). Products include:
- Loniten Tablets 2346
- Rogaine Topical Solution 2357

Nadolol (Symptomatic postural hypotension). Products include:
- Corgard Tablets 701
- Corzide Tablets 702

Nicardipine Hydrochloride (Symptomatic postural hypotension). Products include:
- Cardene Capsules 2290

Nitroglycerin (Symptomatic postural hypotension). Products include:
- Deponit NTG Transdermal Delivery System 2143
- Minitran Transdermal Delivery System 1312
- Nitro-Bid Ointment 1339
- Nitro-Bid Capsules 1338
- Nitrodisc 2176
- Nitro-Dur (nitroglycerin) Transdermal Infusion System 1164
- Nitrogard Tablets 1004
- Nitrolingual Spray 1846
- Nitrostat Tablets 1743
- Transderm-Nitro Transdermal Therapeutic System 2283

Nortriptyline Hydrochloride (Hypertension; dyskinesia). Products include:
- Pamelor 2019

Papaverine Hydrochloride (Beneficial effects of levodopa reversed in Parkinson's Disease). Products include:
- Papaverine Hydrochloride Vials and Ampoules 1290
- Pavabid Capsules 1344
- Pavabid HP Capsulets 1344

Penbutolol Sulfate (Symptomatic postural hypotension). Products include:
- Levatol 1832

Perphenazine (Reduced therapeutic effects of levodopa). Products include:
- Etrafon 2087
- Triavil Tablets 1556
- Trilafon 2123

Phenelzine Sulfate (Contraindication). Products include:
- Nardil 1742

Phenoxybenzamine Hydrochloride (Symptomatic postural hypotension). Products include:
- Dibenzyline Capsules 2207

Phentolamine Mesylate (Symptomatic postural hypotension). Products include:
- Regitine 878

Phenytoin (Beneficial effects of levodopa reversed in Parkinson's Disease). Products include:
- Dilantin Infatabs 1710
- Dilantin-30 Pediatric/Dilantin-125 Suspension 1713

Phenytoin Sodium (Beneficial effects of levodopa reversed in Parkinson's Disease). Products include:
- Dilantin Kapseals 1708
- Dilantin Parenteral 1712
- Dilantin with Phenobarbital Kapseals 1715

Pindolol (Symptomatic postural hypotension). Products include:
- Visken Tablets 2036

Polythiazide (Symptomatic postural hypotension). Products include:
- Minizide Capsules 1779
- Renese Tablets 1785
- Renese-R Tablets 1786

Prazosin Hydrochloride (Symptomatic postural hypotension). Products include:
- Minipress Capsules 1778
- Minizide Capsules 1779

Prochlorperazine (Reduced therapeutic effects of levodopa). Products include:
- Compazine 2201

Promethazine Hydrochloride (Reduced therapeutic effects of levodopa). Products include:
- Mepergan Injection 2479
- Phenergan with Codeine 2497
- Phenergan with Dextromethorphan 2499
- Phenergan Injection 2493
- Phenergan Suppositories 2496
- Phenergan Syrup 2495
- Phenergan Tablets 2496
- Phenergan VC 2500
- Phenergan VC with Codeine 2501

Propranolol Hydrochloride (Symptomatic postural hypotension). Products include:
- Inderal 2459
- Inderal LA Long Acting Capsules 2461
- Inderide Tablets 2463
- Inderide LA Long Acting Capsules 2465

Protriptyline Hydrochloride (Hypertension; dyskinesia). Products include:
- Vivactil Tablets 1567

Ramipril (Symptomatic postural hypotension). Products include:
- Altace Capsules 1086

Rauwolfia Serpentina (Symptomatic postural hypotension). Products include:
- Raudixin Tablets 1803
- Rauzide Tablets 1804

Rescinnamine (Symptomatic postural hypotension).
- No products indexed under this heading.

Reserpine (Symptomatic postural hypotension). Products include:
- Diupres Tablets 1461
- Hydromox R Tablets 1209
- Hydropres Tablets 1485
- Renese-R Tablets 1786
- Salutensin/Salutensin-Demi 719
- Ser-Ap-Es Tablets 881
- Serpasil Tablets 883
- Serpasil-Apresoline Tablets 884
- Serpasil-Esidrix Tablets 886

Sodium Nitroprusside (Symptomatic postural hypotension). Products include:
- Nipride I.V. Infusion 1909

Terazosin Hydrochloride (Symptomatic postural hypotension). Products include:
- Hytrin Tablets 529

Thioridazine Hydrochloride (Reduced therapeutic effects of levodopa). Products include:
- Mellaril 2011

Timolol Maleate (Symptomatic postural hypotension). Products include:
- Blocadren Tablets 1429
- Timolide Tablets 1547
- Timoptic in Ocudose 1552
- Timoptic Sterile Ophthalmic Solution 1550

Tranylcypromine Sulfate (Contraindication). Products include:
- Parnate Tablets 2222

Trifluoperazine Hydrochloride (Reduced therapeutic effects of levodopa). Products include:
- Stelazine 2226

Trimethaphan Camsylate (Symptomatic postural hypotension). Products include:
- Arfonad Ampuls 1887

Trimipramine Maleate (Hypertension; dyskinesia). Products include:
- Surmontil Capsules 2524

Food Interactions

Diet high in protein (Levodopa competes with certain amino acids, the absorption of levodopa may be impaired in some patients on a high protein diet).

SINEMET CR TABLETS

(Carbidopa, Levodopa) 953

May interact with antihypertensives, monoamine oxidase inhibitors, tricyclic antidepressants, phenothiazines, butyrophenones, and certain other agents. Compounds in these categories include:

Acebutolol Hydrochloride (Potential for postural hypertension). Products include:
- Sectral Capsules 2520

Amitriptyline Hydrochloride (Potential for hypertension and dyskinesia). Products include:
- Elavil 2269
- Endep Tablets 1927
- Etrafon 2087
- Limbitrol 1933
- Triavil Tablets 1556

Amoxapine (Potential for hypertension and dyskinesia). Products include:
- Asendin Tablets 1196

Atenolol (Potential for postural hypertension). Products include:
- Tenoretic Tablets 1105
- Tenormin Tablets and I.V. Injection 1107

Benazepril Hydrochloride (Potential for postural hypertension). Products include:
- Lotensin Tablets 872

Bendroflumethiazide (Potential for postural hypertension). Products include:
- Corzide Tablets 702
- Naturetin Tablets 1789
- Rauzide Tablets 1804

Betaxolol Hydrochloride (Potential for postural hypertension). Products include:
- Betoptic Sterile Ophthalmic Solution 569
- Betoptic S Sterile Ophthalmic Suspension 570
- Kerlone Tablets 2172

Captopril (Potential for postural hypertension). Products include:
- Capoten 2255
- Capozide 2258

Carteolol Hydrochloride (Potential for postural hypertension). Products include:
- Cartrol Tablets 507

Chlorothiazide (Potential for postural hypertension). Products include:
- Aldoclor Tablets 1413
- Diupres Tablets 1461
- Diuril Oral 1464

Chlorothiazide Sodium (Potential for postural hypertension). Products include:
- Diuril Sodium Intravenous 1463

Chlorpromazine (Reduces the therapeutic effects). Products include:
- Thorazine 2234

Chlorthalidone (Potential for postural hypertension). Products include:
- Combipres Tablets 678
- Tenoretic Tablets 1105
- Thalitone Tablets 687

Clomipramine Hydrochloride (Potential for hypertension and dyskinesia). Products include:
- Anafranil Capsules 650

Clonidine (Potential for postural hypertension). Products include:
- Catapres-TTS 677

Clonidine Hydrochloride (Potential for postural hypertension). Products include:
- Catapres Tablets 676
- Combipres Tablets 678

Deserpidine (Potential for postural hypertension). Products include:
- Enduronyl 518
- Harmonyl Tablets 528
- Oreticyl 545

Desipramine Hydrochloride (Potential for hypertension and dyskinesia). Products include:
- Norpramin Tablets 1340

Diazoxide (Potential for postural hypertension). Products include:
- Hyperstat I.V. Injection 2095
- Proglycem 649

Doxazosin Mesylate (Potential for postural hypertension). Products include:
- Cardura Tablets 1941

Doxepin Hydrochloride (Potential for hypertension and dyskinesia). Products include:
- Sinequan 1960

Enalapril Maleate (Potential for postural hypertension). Products include:
- Vaseretic Tablets 1559
- Vasotec Tablets 1564

Enalaprilat (Potential for postural hypertension). Products include:
- Vasotec I.V. 1562

Esmolol Hydrochloride (Potential for postural hypertension). Products include:
- Brevibloc Injection 942

Felodipine (Potential for postural hypertension). Products include:
- Plendil Extended-Release Tablets 1526

Fluphenazine Decanoate (Reduces the therapeutic effects). Products include:
- Prolixin Decanoate 1795

Fluphenazine Enanthate (Reduces the therapeutic effects). Products include:
- Prolixin Enanthate 1796

Fluphenazine Hydrochloride (Reduces the therapeutic effects). Products include:
- Prolixin Elixir 1793
- Prolixin Injection 1791
- Prolixin Oral Concentrate 1792
- Prolixin Tablets 1793

Fosinopril Sodium (Potential for postural hypertension). Products include:
Monopril Tablets ... 1406
Furazolidone (Concurrent administration is contraindicated). Products include:
Furoxone ... 1855
Furosemide (Potential for postural hypertension). Products include:
Lasix ... 1093
Guanabenz Acetate (Potential for postural hypertension). Products include:
Wytensin Tablets ... 2542
Guanethidine Monosulfate (Potential for postural hypertension). Products include:
Esimil Tablets ... 864
Ismelin Tablets ... 869
Haloperidol (Reduces the therapeutic effects). Products include:
Haldol Injection, Tablets and Concentrate ... 1373
Haloperidol Decanoate (Reduces the therapeutic effects). Products include:
Haldol Decanoate ... 1375
Hydralazine Hydrochloride (Potential for postural hypertension). Products include:
Apresazide Capsules ... 854
Apresoline Hydrochloride Parenteral (Ampuls) ... 856
Apresoline Hydrochloride Tablets .. 855
Apresoline-Esidrix Tablets ... 857
Ser-Ap-Es Tablets ... 881
Serpasil-Apresoline Tablets ... 884
Hydrochlorothiazide (Potential for postural hypertension). Products include:
Aldactazide ... 2150
Aldoril Tablets ... 1418
Apresazide Capsules ... 854
Apresoline-Esidrix Tablets ... 857
Capozide ... 2258
Dyazide Capsules ... 2208
Esidrix Tablets ... 863
Esimil Tablets ... 864
HydroDIURIL Tablets ... 1484
Hydropres Tablets ... 1485
Inderide Tablets ... 2463
Inderide LA Long Acting Capsules .. 2465
Lopressor HCT Tablets ... 1034
Maxzide ... 1215
Moduretic Tablets ... 1510
Normozide Tablets ... 2112
Oretic Tablets ... 544
Oreticyl ... 545
Prinzide Tablets ... 1540
Ser-Ap-Es Tablets ... 881
Serpasil-Esidrix Tablets ... 886
Timolide Tablets ... 1547
Trandate HCT Tablets ... 579
Vaseretic Tablets ... 1559
Zestoretic ... 2274
Hydroflumethiazide (Potential for postural hypertension). Products include:
Diucardin Tablets ... 2450
Saluron ... 718
Salutensin/Salutensin-Demi ... 719
Imipramine Hydrochloride (Potential for hypertension and dyskinesia). Products include:
Tofranil Ampuls ... 1038
Tofranil Tablets ... 1039
Imipramine Pamoate (Potential for hypertension and dyskinesia). Products include:
Tofranil-PM Capsules ... 1041
Indapamide (Potential for postural hypertension). Products include:
Lozol Tablets ... 1843
Isocarboxazid (Concurrent administration is contraindicated). Products include:
Marplan Tablets ... 1906
Isradipine (Potential for postural hypertension). Products include:
DynaCirc Capsules ... 2004
Labetalol Hydrochloride (Potential for postural hypertension). Products include:
Normodyne Injection ... 2108
Normodyne Tablets ... 2110
Normozide Tablets ... 2112
Trandate HCT Tablets ... 579
Trandate Injection ... 577
Trandate Tablets ... 579
Lisinopril (Potential for postural hypertension). Products include:
Prinivil Tablets ... 1538
Prinzide Tablets ... 1540
Zestoretic ... 2274
Zestril Tablets ... 2277
Maprotiline Hydrochloride (Potential for hypertension and dyskinesia). Products include:
Ludiomil Tablets ... 874
Mecamylamine Hydrochloride (Potential for postural hypertension). Products include:
Inversine Tablets ... 1492
Mesoridazine Besylate (Reduces the therapeutic effects).
Methyclothiazide (Potential for postural hypertension). Products include:
Enduron Tablets ... 517
Enduronyl ... 518
Methyldopa (Potential for postural hypertension). Products include:
Aldoclor Tablets ... 1413
Aldomet Oral ... 1415
Aldoril Tablets ... 1418
Methyldopate Hydrochloride (Potential for postural hypertension). Products include:
Aldomet Ester HCl Injection ... 1417
Metolazone (Potential for postural hypertension). Products include:
Diulo ... 2129
Mykrox ½ mg Tablets ... 984
Zaroxolyn Tablets ... 989
Metoprolol Tartrate (Potential for postural hypertension). Products include:
Lopressor Ampuls ... 1032
Lopressor HCT Tablets ... 1034
Lopressor Tablets ... 1032
Metyrosine (Potential for postural hypertension). Products include:
Demser Capsules ... 1460
Minoxidil (Potential for postural hypertension). Products include:
Loniten Tablets ... 2346
Rogaine Topical Solution ... 2357
Nadolol (Potential for postural hypertension). Products include:
Corgard Tablets ... 701
Corzide Tablets ... 702
Nicardipine Hydrochloride (Potential for postural hypertension). Products include:
Cardene Capsules ... 2290
Nitroglycerin (Potential for postural hypertension). Products include:
Deponit NTG Transdermal Delivery System ... 2143
Minitran Transdermal Delivery System ... 1312
Nitro-Bid Ointment ... 1339
Nitro-Bid Capsules ... 1338
Nitrodisc ... 2176
Nitro-Dur (nitroglycerin) Transdermal Infusion System ... 1164
Nitrogard Tablets ... 1004
Nitrolingual Spray ... 1846
Nitrostat Tablets ... 1743
Transderm-Nitro Transdermal Therapeutic System ... 2283
Nortriptyline Hydrochloride (Potential for hypertension and dyskinesia). Products include:
Pamelor ... 2019
Papaverine Hydrochloride (Reverses beneficial effects of levodopa). Products include:
Papaverine Hydrochloride Vials and Ampoules ... 1290
Pavabid Capsules ... 1344
Pavabid HP Capsules ... 1344
Penbutolol Sulfate (Potential for postural hypertension). Products include:
Levatol ... 1832
Perphenazine (Reduces the therapeutic effects). Products include:
Etrafon ... 2087
Triavil Tablets ... 1556
Trilafon ... 2123
Phenelzine Sulfate (Concurrent administration is contraindicated). Products include:
Nardil ... 1742
Phenoxybenzamine Hydrochloride (Potential for postural hypertension). Products include:
Dibenzyline Capsules ... 2207
Phentolamine Mesylate (Potential for postural hypertension). Products include:
Regitine ... 878
Phenytoin (Reverses beneficial effects of levodopa). Products include:
Dilantin Infatabs ... 1710
Dilantin-30 Pediatric/Dilantin-125 Suspension ... 1713
Phenytoin Sodium (Reverses beneficial effects of levodopa). Products include:
Dilantin Kapseals ... 1708
Dilantin Parenteral ... 1712
Dilantin with Phenobarbital Kapseals ... 1715
Pindolol (Potential for postural hypertension). Products include:
Visken Tablets ... 2036
Polythiazide (Potential for postural hypertension). Products include:
Minizide Capsules ... 1779
Renese Tablets ... 1785
Renese-R Tablets ... 1786
Prazosin Hydrochloride (Potential for postural hypertension). Products include:
Minipress Capsules ... 1778
Minizide Capsules ... 1779
Prochlorperazine (Reduces the therapeutic effects). Products include:
Compazine ... 2201
Promethazine Hydrochloride (Reduces the therapeutic effects). Products include:
Mepergan Injection ... 2479
Phenergan with Codeine ... 2497
Phenergan with Dextromethorphan 2499
Phenergan Injection ... 2493
Phenergan Suppositories ... 2496
Phenergan Syrup ... 2495
Phenergan Tablets ... 2496
Phenergan VC ... 2500
Phenergan VC with Codeine ... 2501
Propranolol Hydrochloride (Potential for postural hypertension). Products include:
Inderal ... 2459
Inderal LA Long Acting Capsules 2461
Inderide Tablets ... 2463
Inderide LA Long Acting Capsules .. 2465
Protriptyline Hydrochloride (Potential for hypertension and dyskinesia). Products include:
Vivactil Tablets ... 1567
Ramipril (Potential for postural hypertension). Products include:
Altace Capsules ... 1086
Rauwolfia Serpentina (Potential for postural hypertension). Products include:
Raudixin Tablets ... 1803
Rauzide Tablets ... 1804
Rescinnamine (Potential for postural hypertension).
No products indexed under this heading.
Reserpine (Potential for postural hypertension). Products include:
Diupres Tablets ... 1461
Hydromox R Tablets ... 1209
Hydropres Tablets ... 1485
Renese-R Tablets ... 1786
Salutensin/Salutensin-Demi ... 719
Ser-Ap-Es Tablets ... 881
Serpasil Tablets ... 883
Serpasil-Apresoline Tablets ... 884
Serpasil-Esidrix Tablets ... 886
Sodium Nitroprusside (Potential for postural hypertension). Products include:
Nipride I.V. Infusion ... 1909
Terazosin Hydrochloride (Potential for postural hypertension). Products include:
Hytrin Tablets ... 529
Thioridazine Hydrochloride (Reduces the therapeutic effects). Products include:
Mellaril ... 2011
Timolol Maleate (Potential for postural hypertension). Products include:
Blocadren Tablets ... 1429
Timolide Tablets ... 1547
Timoptic in Ocudose ... 1552
Timoptic Sterile Ophthalmic Solution ... 1550
Tranylcypromine Sulfate (Concurrent administration is contraindicated). Products include:
Parnate Tablets ... 2222
Trifluoperazine Hydrochloride (Reduces the therapeutic effects). Products include:
Stelazine ... 2226
Trimethaphan Camsylate (Potential for postural hypertension). Products include:
Arfonad Ampuls ... 1887
Trimipramine Maleate (Potential for hypertension and dyskinesia). Products include:
Surmontil Capsules ... 2524

Food Interactions

Food, unspecified (Increases the extent of availability and peak concentrations of levodopa).

SINE-OFF MAXIMUM STRENGTH ALLERGY/SINUS FORMULA CAPLETS
(Acetaminophen, Chlorpheniramine Maleate, Pseudoephedrine Hydrochloride) ... ▣ 721
May interact with hypnotics and sedatives, tranquilizers, and certain other agents. Compounds in these categories include:

Alcohol (Do not use concomitantly).
Alprazolam (Effect not specified). Products include:
Xanax Tablets ... 2367
Buspirone Hydrochloride (Effect not specified). Products include:
BuSpar ... 1401
Chlordiazepoxide (Effect not specified). Products include:
Libritabs Tablets ... 1930
Limbitrol ... 1933
Menrium Tablets ... 1934
Chlordiazepoxide Hydrochloride (Effect not specified). Products include:
Librax Capsules ... 1929
Librium Capsules ... 1931
Librium Injectable ... 1932
Chlorpromazine (Effect not specified). Products include:
Thorazine ... 2234
Chlorprothixene (Effect not specified). Products include:
Taractan Tablets ... 1920

Chlorprothixene Hydrochloride (Effect not specified). Products include:
Taractan ... 1920
Clorazepate Dipotassium (Effect not specified). Products include:
Tranxene ... 556
Diazepam (Effect not specified). Products include:
Valium Injectable ... 1937
Valium Tablets ... 1939
Valrelease Capsules ... 1923
Droperidol (Effect not specified). Products include:
Inapsine Injection ... 1140
Innovar Injection ... 1141
Estazolam (Effect not specified). Products include:
ProSom Tablets ... 554
Ethchlorvynol (Effect not specified). Products include:
Placidyl Capsules ... 553
Ethinamate (Effect not specified).
No products indexed under this heading.
Fluphenazine Decanoate (Effect not specified). Products include:
Prolixin Decanoate ... 1795
Fluphenazine Enanthate (Effect not specified). Products include:
Prolixin Enanthate ... 1796
Fluphenazine Hydrochloride (Effect not specified). Products include:
Prolixin Elixir ... 1793
Prolixin Injection ... 1791
Prolixin Oral Concentrate ... 1792
Prolixin Tablets ... 1793
Flurazepam Hydrochloride (Effect not specified). Products include:
Dalmane Capsules ... 1927
Glutethimide (Effect not specified).
No products indexed under this heading.
Haloperidol (Effect not specified). Products include:
Haldol Injection, Tablets and Concentrate ... 1373
Haloperidol Decanoate (Effect not specified). Products include:
Haldol Decanoate ... 1375
Hydroxyzine Hydrochloride (Effect not specified). Products include:
Atarax Tablets & Syrup ... 1941
Marax Tablets & DF Syrup ... 1954
Vistaril Intramuscular Solution ... 1970
Lorazepam (Effect not specified). Products include:
Ativan Injection ... 2432
Ativan Tablets ... 2434
Loxapine Hydrochloride (Effect not specified). Products include:
Loxitane ... 1213
Loxapine Succinate (Effect not specified). Products include:
Loxitane Capsules ... 1213
Meprobamate (Effect not specified). Products include:
Deprol Tablets ... 2382
Equagesic Tablets ... 2451
Miltown Tablets ... 2386
PMB 200 and PMB 400 ... 2504
Mesoridazine Besylate (Effect not specified).
Midazolam Hydrochloride (Effect not specified). Products include:
Versed Injection ... 1924
Molindone Hydrochloride (Effect not specified). Products include:
Moban Tablets & Concentrate ... 932
Oxazepam (Effect not specified). Products include:
Serax Capsules ... 2522
Serax Tablets ... 2522
Perphenazine (Effect not specified). Products include:
Etrafon ... 2087
Triavil Tablets ... 1556
Trilafon ... 2123
Prazepam (Effect not specified). Products include:
Centrax ... 1693
Prochlorperazine (Effect not specified). Products include:
Compazine ... 2201
Promethazine Hydrochloride (Effect not specified). Products include:
Mepergan Injection ... 2479
Phenergan with Codeine ... 2497
Phenergan with Dextromethorphan 2499
Phenergan Injection ... 2493
Phenergan Suppositories ... 2496
Phenergan Syrup ... 2495
Phenergan Tablets ... 2496
Phenergan VC ... 2500
Phenergan VC with Codeine ... 2501
Propofol (Effect not specified). Products include:
Diprivan Injection ... 2267
Quazepam (Effect not specified). Products include:
Doral Tablets ... 2383
Secobarbital Sodium (Effect not specified). Products include:
Seconal Sodium Pulvules ... 1296
Temazepam (Effect not specified). Products include:
Restoril Capsules ... 2023
Thioridazine Hydrochloride (Effect not specified). Products include:
Mellaril ... 2011
Thiothixene (Effect not specified). Products include:
Navane Capsules and Concentrate 1954
Navane Intramuscular ... 1956
Triazolam (Effect not specified). Products include:
Halcion Tablets ... 2340
Trifluoperazine Hydrochloride (Effect not specified). Products include:
Stelazine ... 2226

SINE-OFF MAXIMUM STRENGTH NO DROWSINESS FORMULA CAPLETS
(Acetaminophen, Pseudoephedrine Hydrochloride) ... ◘ 722
No interactions described in labeling.

SINE-OFF SINUS MEDICINE TABLETS-ASPIRIN FORMULA
(Aspirin, Chlorpheniramine Maleate, Phenylpropanolamine Hydrochloride) ... ◘ 722
May interact with phenylpropanolamine containing anorectics and certain other agents. Compounds in these categories include:

Alcohol (Do not use concomitantly).
Phenylpropanolamine Containing Anorectics (Effect not specified).

SINEQUAN CAPSULES
(Doxepin Hydrochloride) ... 1960
May interact with monoamine oxidase inhibitors and certain other agents. Compounds in these categories include:

Alcohol (Increases danger in Sinequan overdosage; response to alcohol may be potentiated).
Cimetidine (Increases serum concentrations of Sinequan). Products include:
Tagamet Tablets ... 2228
Cimetidine Hydrochloride (Increases serum concentrations of Sinequan). Products include:
Tagamet ... 2228
Furazolidone (Concurrent use is not recommended; potential for serious adverse effects). Products include:
Furoxone ... 1855
Guanethidine Monosulfate (Antihypertensive effect blocked by doxepin at dosage above 150 mg per day). Products include:
Esimil Tablets ... 864
Ismelin Tablets ... 869
Isocarboxazid (Concurrent use is not recommended; potential for serious adverse effects). Products include:
Marplan Tablets ... 1906
Phenelzine Sulfate (Concurrent use is not recommended; potential for serious adverse effects). Products include:
Nardil ... 1742
Selegiline Hydrochloride (Concurrent use is not recommended; potential for serious adverse effects). Products include:
Eldepryl ... 2250
Tolazamide (A case of severe hypoglycemia has been reported in a type II diabetic patient maintained on tolazamide (1 gm/day) 11 days after the addition of doxepin (75 mg/day)). Products include:
Tolinase Tablets ... 2365
Tranylcypromine Sulfate (Concurrent use is not recommended; potential for serious adverse effects). Products include:
Parnate Tablets ... 2222

SINEQUAN ORAL CONCENTRATE
(Doxepin Hydrochloride) ... 1960
See **Sinequan Capsules**

SINGLET TABLETS
(Acetaminophen, Chlorpheniramine Maleate, Pseudoephedrine Hydrochloride) ... ◘ 598
May interact with hypnotics and sedatives, tranquilizers, antihypertensives, antidepressant drugs, and certain other agents. Compounds in these categories include:

Acebutolol Hydrochloride (Effect not specified). Products include:
Sectral Capsules ... 2520
Alcohol (Increases drowsiness effect).
Alprazolam (Increases drowsiness effect). Products include:
Xanax Tablets ... 2367
Amitriptyline Hydrochloride (Effect not specified). Products include:
Elavil ... 2269
Endep Tablets ... 1927
Etrafon ... 2087
Limbitrol ... 1933
Triavil Tablets ... 1556
Amoxapine (Effect not specified). Products include:
Asendin Tablets ... 1196
Atenolol (Effect not specified). Products include:
Tenoretic Tablets ... 1105
Tenormin Tablets and I.V. Injection 1107
Benazepril Hydrochloride (Effect not specified). Products include:
Lotensin Tablets ... 872
Betaxolol Hydrochloride (Effect not specified). Products include:
Betoptic Sterile Ophthalmic Solution ... 569
Betoptic S Sterile Ophthalmic Suspension ... 570
Kerlone Tablets ... 2172
Bupropion Hydrochloride (Effect not specified). Products include:
Wellbutrin Tablets ... 821
Buspirone Hydrochloride (Increases drowsiness effect). Products include:
BuSpar ... 1401
Captopril (Effect not specified). Products include:
Capoten ... 2255
Capozide ... 2258
Carteolol Hydrochloride (Effect not specified). Products include:
Cartrol Tablets ... 507
Chlordiazepoxide (Increases drowsiness effect). Products include:
Libritabs Tablets ... 1930
Limbitrol ... 1933
Menrium Tablets ... 1934
Chlordiazepoxide Hydrochloride (Increases drowsiness effect). Products include:
Librax Capsules ... 1929
Librium Capsules ... 1931
Librium Injectable ... 1932
Chlorpromazine (Increases drowsiness effect). Products include:
Thorazine ... 2234
Chlorprothixene (Increases drowsiness effect). Products include:
Taractan Tablets ... 1920
Chlorprothixene Hydrochloride (Increases drowsiness effect). Products include:
Taractan ... 1920
Clonidine (Effect not specified). Products include:
Catapres-TTS ... 677
Clonidine Hydrochloride (Effect not specified). Products include:
Catapres Tablets ... 676
Combipres Tablets ... 678
Clorazepate Dipotassium (Increases drowsiness effect). Products include:
Tranxene ... 556
Deserpidine (Effect not specified). Products include:
Enduronyl ... 518
Harmonyl Tablets ... 528
Oreticyl ... 545
Desipramine Hydrochloride (Effect not specified). Products include:
Norpramin Tablets ... 1340
Diazepam (Increases drowsiness effect). Products include:
Valium Injectable ... 1937
Valium Tablets ... 1939
Valrelease Capsules ... 1923
Diazoxide (Effect not specified). Products include:
Hyperstat I.V. Injection ... 2095
Proglycem ... 649
Doxazosin Mesylate (Effect not specified). Products include:
Cardura Tablets ... 1941
Doxepin Hydrochloride (Effect not specified). Products include:
Sinequan ... 1960
Droperidol (Increases drowsiness effect). Products include:
Inapsine Injection ... 1140
Innovar Injection ... 1141
Enalapril Maleate (Effect not specified). Products include:
Vaseretic Tablets ... 1559
Vasotec Tablets ... 1564
Enalaprilat (Effect not specified). Products include:
Vasotec I.V. ... 1562

Esmolol Hydrochloride (Effect not specified). Products include:
Brevibloc Injection 942

Estazolam (Increases drowsiness effect). Products include:
ProSom Tablets 554

Ethchlorvynol (Increases drowsiness effect). Products include:
Placidyl Capsules 553

Ethinamate (Increases drowsiness effect).
No products indexed under this heading.

Felodipine (Effect not specified). Products include:
Plendil Extended-Release Tablets 1526

Fluoxetine Hydrochloride (Effect not specified). Products include:
Prozac Pulvules 920

Fluphenazine Decanoate (Increases drowsiness effect). Products include:
Prolixin Decanoate 1795

Fluphenazine Enanthate (Increases drowsiness effect). Products include:
Prolixin Enanthate 1796

Fluphenazine Hydrochloride (Increases drowsiness effect). Products include:
Prolixin Elixir 1793
Prolixin Injection 1791
Prolixin Oral Concentrate 1792
Prolixin Tablets 1793

Flurazepam Hydrochloride (Increases drowsiness effect). Products include:
Dalmane Capsules 1927

Fosinopril Sodium (Effect not specified). Products include:
Monopril Tablets 1406

Glutethimide (Increases drowsiness effect).
No products indexed under this heading.

Guanabenz Acetate (Effect not specified). Products include:
Wytensin Tablets 2542

Guanethidine Monosulfate (Effect not specified). Products include:
Esimil Tablets 864
Ismelin Tablets 869

Haloperidol (Increases drowsiness effect). Products include:
Haldol Injection, Tablets and Concentrate 1373

Haloperidol Decanoate (Increases drowsiness effect). Products include:
Haldol Decanoate 1375

Hydralazine Hydrochloride (Effect not specified). Products include:
Apresazide Capsules 854
Apresoline Hydrochloride Parenteral (Ampuls) 856
Apresoline Hydrochloride Tablets 855
Apresoline-Esidrix Tablets 857
Ser-Ap-Es Tablets 881
Serpasil-Apresoline Tablets 884

Hydroxyzine Hydrochloride (Increases drowsiness effect). Products include:
Atarax Tablets & Syrup 1941
Marax Tablets & DF Syrup 1954
Vistaril Intramuscular Solution 1970

Imipramine Hydrochloride (Effect not specified). Products include:
Tofranil Ampuls 1038
Tofranil Tablets 1039

Imipramine Pamoate (Effect not specified). Products include:
Tofranil-PM Capsules 1041

Isocarboxazid (Effect not specified). Products include:
Marplan Tablets 1906

Isradipine (Effect not specified). Products include:
DynaCirc Capsules 2004

Labetalol Hydrochloride (Effect not specified). Products include:
Normodyne Injection 2108
Normodyne Tablets 2110
Normozide Tablets 2112
Trandate HCT Tablets 579
Trandate Injection 577
Trandate Tablets 579

Lisinopril (Effect not specified). Products include:
Prinivil Tablets 1538
Prinzide Tablets 1540
Zestoretic 2274
Zestril Tablets 2277

Lorazepam (Increases drowsiness effect). Products include:
Ativan Injection 2432
Ativan Tablets 2434

Loxapine Hydrochloride (Increases drowsiness effect). Products include:
Loxitane 1213

Loxapine Succinate (Increases drowsiness effect). Products include:
Loxitane Capsules 1213

Maprotiline Hydrochloride (Effect not specified). Products include:
Ludiomil Tablets 874

Mecamylamine Hydrochloride (Effect not specified). Products include:
Inversine Tablets 1492

Meprobamate (Increases drowsiness effect). Products include:
Deprol Tablets 2382
Equagesic Tablets 2451
Miltown Tablets 2386
PMB 200 and PMB 400 2504

Mesoridazine (Increases drowsiness effect). Products include:
Serentil 686

Methyldopa (Effect not specified). Products include:
Aldoclor Tablets 1413
Aldomet Oral 1415
Aldoril Tablets 1418

Methyldopate Hydrochloride (Effect not specified). Products include:
Aldomet Ester HCl Injection 1417

Metolazone (Effect not specified). Products include:
Diulo 2129
Mykrox ½ mg Tablets 984
Zaroxolyn Tablets 989

Metoprolol Tartrate (Effect not specified). Products include:
Lopressor Ampuls 1032
Lopressor HCT Tablets 1034
Lopressor Tablets 1032

Metyrosine (Effect not specified). Products include:
Demser Capsules 1460

Midazolam Hydrochloride (Increases drowsiness effect). Products include:
Versed Injection 1924

Minoxidil (Effect not specified). Products include:
Loniten Tablets 2346
Rogaine Topical Solution 2357

Molindone Hydrochloride (Increases drowsiness effect). Products include:
Moban Tablets & Concentrate 932

Nadolol (Effect not specified). Products include:
Corgard Tablets 701
Corzide Tablets 702

Nicardipine Hydrochloride (Effect not specified). Products include:
Cardene Capsules 2290

Nitroglycerin (Effect not specified). Products include:
Deponit NTG Transdermal Delivery System 2143
Minitran Transdermal Delivery System 1312
Nitro-Bid Ointment 1339
Nitro-Bid Capsules 1338
Nitrodisc 2176
Nitro-Dur (nitroglycerin) Transdermal Infusion System 1164
Nitrogard Tablets 1004
Nitrolingual Spray 1846
Nitrostat Tablets 1743
Transderm-Nitro Transdermal Therapeutic System 2283

Nortriptyline Hydrochloride (Effect not specified). Products include:
Pamelor 2019

Oxazepam (Increases drowsiness effect). Products include:
Serax Capsules 2522
Serax Tablets 2522

Penbutolol Sulfate (Effect not specified). Products include:
Levatol 1832

Perphenazine (Increases drowsiness effect). Products include:
Etrafon 2087
Triavil Tablets 1556
Trilafon 2123

Phenelzine Sulfate (Effect not specified). Products include:
Nardil 1742

Phenoxybenzamine Hydrochloride (Effect not specified). Products include:
Dibenzyline Capsules 2207

Phentolamine Mesylate (Effect not specified). Products include:
Regitine 878

Pindolol (Effect not specified). Products include:
Visken Tablets 2036

Prazepam (Increases drowsiness effect). Products include:
Centrax 1693

Prazosin Hydrochloride (Effect not specified). Products include:
Minipress Capsules 1778
Minizide Capsules 1779

Prochlorperazine (Increases drowsiness effect). Products include:
Compazine 2201

Promethazine Hydrochloride (Increases drowsiness effect). Products include:
Mepergan Injection 2479
Phenergan with Codeine 2497
Phenergan with Dextromethorphan 2499
Phenergan Injection 2493
Phenergan Suppositories 2496
Phenergan Syrup 2495
Phenergan Tablets 2496
Phenergan VC 2500
Phenergan VC with Codeine 2501

Propofol (Increases drowsiness effect). Products include:
Diprivan Injection 2267

Propranolol Hydrochloride (Effect not specified). Products include:
Inderal 2459
Inderal LA Long Acting Capsules 2461
Inderide Tablets 2463
Inderide LA Long Acting Capsules 2465

Protriptyline Hydrochloride (Effect not specified). Products include:
Vivactil Tablets 1567

Quazepam (Increases drowsiness effect). Products include:
Doral Tablets 2383

Ramipril (Effect not specified). Products include:
Altace Capsules 1086

Rauwolfia Serpentina (Effect not specified). Products include:
Raudixin Tablets 1803
Rauzide Tablets 1804

Rescinnamine (Effect not specified).
No products indexed under this heading.

Reserpine (Effect not specified). Products include:
Diupres Tablets 1461
Hydromox R Tablets 1209
Hydropres Tablets 1485
Renese-R Tablets 1786
Salutensin/Salutensin-Demi 719
Ser-Ap-Es Tablets 881
Serpasil Tablets 883
Serpasil-Apresoline Tablets 884
Serpasil-Esidrix Tablets 886

Secobarbital Sodium (Increases drowsiness effect). Products include:
Seconal Sodium Pulvules 1296

Sodium Nitroprusside (Effect not specified). Products include:
Nipride I.V. Infusion 1909

Temazepam (Increases drowsiness effect). Products include:
Restoril Capsules 2023

Terazosin Hydrochloride (Effect not specified). Products include:
Hytrin Tablets 529

Thioridazine Hydrochloride (Increases drowsiness effect). Products include:
Mellaril 2011

Thiothixene (Increases drowsiness effect). Products include:
Navane Capsules and Concentrate 1954
Navane Intramuscular 1956

Timolol Maleate (Effect not specified). Products include:
Blocadren Tablets 1429
Timolide Tablets 1547
Timoptic in Ocudose 1552
Timoptic Sterile Ophthalmic Solution 1550

Tranylcypromine Sulfate (Effect not specified). Products include:
Parnate Tablets 2222

Trazodone Hydrochloride (Effect not specified). Products include:
Desyrel and Desyrel Dividose 1404

Triazolam (Increases drowsiness effect). Products include:
Halcion Tablets 2340

Trifluoperazine Hydrochloride (Increases drowsiness effect). Products include:
Stelazine 2226

Trimethaphan Camsylate (Effect not specified). Products include:
Arfonad Ampuls 1887

Trimipramine Maleate (Effect not specified). Products include:
Surmontil Capsules 2524

SINULIN
(Acetaminophen, Phenylpropanolamine Hydrochloride, Chlorpheniramine Maleate) 840
May interact with antihypertensives, antidepressant drugs, and certain other agents. Compounds in these categories include:

Acebutolol Hydrochloride (Effects not specified). Products include:
Sectral Capsules 2520

Alcohol (Increased drowsiness).

Amitriptyline Hydrochloride (Effects not specified). Products include:
Elavil 2269
Endep Tablets 1927
Etrafon 2087
Limbitrol 1933
Triavil Tablets 1556

Amoxapine (Effects not specified). Products include:
Asendin Tablets 1196

Atenolol (Effects not specified). Products include:
Tenoretic Tablets 1105

Tenormin Tablets and I.V. Injection 1107

Benazepril Hydrochloride (Effects not specified). Products include:
- Lotensin Tablets 872

Betaxolol Hydrochloride (Effects not specified). Products include:
- Betoptic Sterile Ophthalmic Solution 569
- Betoptic S Sterile Ophthalmic Suspension 570
- Kerlone Tablets 2172

Bupropion Hydrochloride (Effects not specified). Products include:
- Wellbutrin Tablets 821

Captopril (Effects not specified). Products include:
- Capoten 2255
- Capozide 2258

Carteolol Hydrochloride (Effects not specified). Products include:
- Cartrol Tablets 507

Clonidine (Effects not specified). Products include:
- Catapres-TTS 677

Clonidine Hydrochloride (Effects not specified). Products include:
- Catapres Tablets 676
- Combipres Tablets 678

Deserpidine (Effects not specified). Products include:
- Enduronyl 518
- Harmonyl Tablets 528
- Oreticyl 545

Desipramine Hydrochloride (Effects not specified). Products include:
- Norpramin Tablets 1340

Diazoxide (Effects not specified). Products include:
- Hyperstat I.V. Injection 2095
- Proglycem 649

Doxazosin Mesylate (Effects not specified). Products include:
- Cardura Tablets 1941

Doxepin Hydrochloride (Effects not specified). Products include:
- Sinequan 1960

Enalapril Maleate (Effects not specified). Products include:
- Vaseretic Tablets 1559
- Vasotec Tablets 1564

Enalaprilat (Effects not specified). Products include:
- Vasotec I.V. 1562

Esmolol Hydrochloride (Effects not specified). Products include:
- Brevibloc Injection 942

Felodipine (Effects not specified). Products include:
- Plendil Extended-Release Tablets 1526

Fluoxetine Hydrochloride (Effects not specified). Products include:
- Prozac Pulvules 920

Fosinopril Sodium (Effects not specified). Products include:
- Monopril Tablets 1406

Guanabenz Acetate (Effects not specified). Products include:
- Wytensin Tablets 2542

Guanethidine Monosulfate (Effects not specified). Products include:
- Esimil Tablets 864
- Ismelin Tablets 869

Hydralazine Hydrochloride (Effects not specified). Products include:
- Apresazide Capsules 854
- Apresoline Hydrochloride Parenteral (Ampuls) 856
- Apresoline Hydrochloride Tablets 855
- Apresoline-Esidrix Tablets 857
- Ser-Ap-Es Tablets 881
- Serpasil-Apresoline Tablets 884

Imipramine Hydrochloride (Effects not specified). Products include:
- Tofranil Ampuls 1038
- Tofranil Tablets 1039

Imipramine Pamoate (Effects not specified). Products include:
- Tofranil-PM Capsules 1041

Indapamide (Effects not specified). Products include:
- Lozol Tablets 1843

Isocarboxazid (Effects not specified). Products include:
- Marplan Tablets 1906

Isradipine (Effects not specified). Products include:
- DynaCirc Capsules 2004

Labetalol Hydrochloride (Effects not specified). Products include:
- Normodyne Injection 2108
- Normodyne Tablets 2110
- Normozide Tablets 2112
- Trandate HCT Tablets 579
- Trandate Injection 577
- Trandate Tablets 579

Lisinopril (Effects not specified). Products include:
- Prinivil Tablets 1538
- Prinzide Tablets 1540
- Zestoretic 2274
- Zestril Tablets 2277

Maprotiline Hydrochloride (Effects not specified). Products include:
- Ludiomil Tablets 874

Mecamylamine Hydrochloride (Effects not specified). Products include:
- Inversine Tablets 1492

Methyclothiazide (Effects not specified). Products include:
- Enduron Tablets 517
- Enduronyl 518

Methyldopa (Effects not specified). Products include:
- Aldoclor Tablets 1413
- Aldomet Oral 1415
- Aldoril Tablets 1418

Methyldopate Hydrochloride (Effects not specified). Products include:
- Aldomet Ester HCl Injection 1417

Metolazone (Effects not specified). Products include:
- Diulo 2129
- Mykrox ½ mg Tablets 984
- Zaroxolyn Tablets 989

Metoprolol Tartrate (Effects not specified). Products include:
- Lopressor Ampuls 1032
- Lopressor HCT Tablets 1034
- Lopressor Tablets 1032

Metyrosine (Effects not specified). Products include:
- Demser Capsules 1460

Minoxidil (Effects not specified). Products include:
- Loniten Tablets 2346
- Rogaine Topical Solution 2357

Nadolol (Effects not specified). Products include:
- Corgard Tablets 701
- Corzide Tablets 702

Nicardipine Hydrochloride (Effects not specified). Products include:
- Cardene Capsules 2290

Nitroglycerin (Effects not specified). Products include:
- Deponit NTG Transdermal Delivery System 2143
- Minitran Transdermal Delivery System 1312
- Nitro-Bid Ointment 1339
- Nitro-Bid Capsules 1338
- Nitrodisc 2176
- Nitro-Dur (nitroglycerin) Transdermal Infusion System 1164
- Nitrogard Tablets 1004
- Nitrolingual Spray 1846
- Nitrostat Tablets 1743
- Transderm-Nitro Transdermal Therapeutic System 2283

Nortriptyline Hydrochloride (Effects not specified). Products include:
- Pamelor 2019

Penbutolol Sulfate (Effects not specified). Products include:
- Levatol 1832

Phenelzine Sulfate (Effects not specified). Products include:
- Nardil 1742

Phenoxybenzamine Hydrochloride (Effects not specified). Products include:
- Dibenzyline Capsules 2207

Phentolamine Mesylate (Effects not specified). Products include:
- Regitine 878

Pindolol (Effects not specified). Products include:
- Visken Tablets 2036

Prazosin Hydrochloride (Effects not specified). Products include:
- Minipress Capsules 1778
- Minizide Capsules 1779

Propranolol Hydrochloride (Effects not specified). Products include:
- Inderal 2459
- Inderal LA Long Acting Capsules 2461
- Inderide Tablets 2463
- Inderide LA Long Acting Capsules 2465

Protriptyline Hydrochloride (Effects not specified). Products include:
- Vivactil Tablets 1567

Ramipril (Effects not specified). Products include:
- Altace Capsules 1086

Rauwolfia Serpentina (Effects not specified). Products include:
- Raudixin Tablets 1803
- Rauzide Tablets 1804

Rescinnamine (Effects not specified).
- No products indexed under this heading.

Reserpine (Effects not specified). Products include:
- Diupres Tablets 1461
- Hydromox R Tablets 1209
- Hydropres Tablets 1485
- Renese-R Tablets 1786
- Salutensin/Salutensin-Demi 719
- Ser-Ap-Es Tablets 881
- Serpasil Tablets 883
- Serpasil-Apresoline Tablets 884
- Serpasil-Esidrix Tablets 886

Sodium Nitroprusside (Effects not specified). Products include:
- Nipride I.V. Infusion 1909

Terazosin Hydrochloride (Effects not specified). Products include:
- Hytrin Tablets 529

Timolol Maleate (Effects not specified). Products include:
- Blocadren Tablets 1429
- Timolide Tablets 1547
- Timoptic in Ocudose 1552
- Timoptic Sterile Ophthalmic Solution 1550

Tranylcypromine Sulfate (Effects not specified). Products include:
- Parnate Tablets 2222

Trazodone Hydrochloride (Effects not specified). Products include:
- Desyrel and Desyrel Dividose 1404

Trimethaphan Camsylate (Effects not specified). Products include:
- Arfonad Ampuls 1887

Trimipramine Maleate (Effects not specified). Products include:
- Surmontil Capsules 2524

SINUTAB ALLERGY FORMULA SUSTAINED ACTION TABLETS
(Dexbrompheniramine Maleate, Pseudoephedrine Sulfate) .... ▣ 640
May interact with monoamine oxidase inhibitors and certain other agents. Compounds in these categories include:

Alcohol (May increase drowsiness effect).

Furazolidone (Effect not specified). Products include:
- Furoxone 1855

Isocarboxazid (Effect not specified). Products include:
- Marplan Tablets 1906

Phenelzine Sulfate (Effect not specified). Products include:
- Nardil 1742

Selegiline Hydrochloride (Effect not specified). Products include:
- Eldepryl 2250

Tranylcypromine Sulfate (Effect not specified). Products include:
- Parnate Tablets 2222

SINUTAB MAXIMUM STRENGTH CAPLETS
(Acetaminophen, Chlorpheniramine Maleate, Pseudoephedrine Hydrochloride) .... ▣ 641
May interact with antihypertensives, antidepressant drugs, and certain other agents. Compounds in these categories include:

Acebutolol Hydrochloride (Do not use concomitantly). Products include:
- Sectral Capsules 2520

Alcohol (Do not use concomitantly).

Amitriptyline Hydrochloride (Do not use concomitantly). Products include:
- Elavil 2269
- Endep Tablets 1927
- Etrafon 2087
- Limbitrol 1933
- Triavil Tablets 1556

Amoxapine (Do not use concomitantly). Products include:
- Asendin Tablets 1196

Atenolol (Do not use concomitantly). Products include:
- Tenoretic Tablets 1105
- Tenormin Tablets and I.V. Injection 1107

Benazepril Hydrochloride (Do not use concomitantly). Products include:
- Lotensin Tablets 872

Betaxolol Hydrochloride (Do not use concomitantly). Products include:
- Betoptic Sterile Ophthalmic Solution 569
- Betoptic S Sterile Ophthalmic Suspension 570
- Kerlone Tablets 2172

Bupropion Hydrochloride (Do not use concomitantly). Products include:
- Wellbutrin Tablets 821

Captopril (Do not use concomitantly). Products include:
- Capoten 2255
- Capozide 2258

Carteolol Hydrochloride (Do not use concomitantly). Products include:
- Cartrol Tablets 507

Clonidine (Do not use concomitantly). Products include:
- Catapres-TTS 677

Clonidine Hydrochloride (Do not use concomitantly). Products include:
- Catapres Tablets 676
- Combipres Tablets 678

Deserpidine (Do not use concomitantly). Products include:
- Enduronyl 518
- Harmonyl Tablets 528
- Oreticyl 545

Desipramine Hydrochloride (Do not use concomitantly). Products include:
- Norpramin Tablets 1340

Diazoxide (Do not use concomitantly). Products include:
- Hyperstat I.V. Injection 2095
- Proglycem 649

Doxazosin Mesylate (Do not use concomitantly). Products include:
- Cardura Tablets 1941

Doxepin Hydrochloride (Do not use concomitantly). Products include:
- Sinequan 1960

Enalapril Maleate (Do not use concomitantly). Products include:
- Vaseretic Tablets 1559
- Vasotec Tablets 1564

Enalaprilat (Do not use concomitantly). Products include:
- Vasotec I.V. 1562

Esmolol Hydrochloride (Do not use concomitantly). Products include:
- Brevibloc Injection 942

Felodipine (Do not use concomitantly). Products include:
- Plendil Extended-Release Tablets 1526

Fluoxetine Hydrochloride (Do not use concomitantly). Products include:
- Prozac Pulvules 920

Fosinopril Sodium (Do not use concomitantly). Products include:
- Monopril Tablets 1406

Furosemide (Do not use concomitantly). Products include:
- Lasix 1093

Guanabenz Acetate (Do not use concomitantly). Products include:
- Wytensin Tablets 2542

Guanethidine Monosulfate (Do not use concomitantly). Products include:
- Esimil Tablets 864
- Ismelin Tablets 869

Hydralazine Hydrochloride (Do not use concomitantly). Products include:
- Apresazide Capsules 854
- Apresoline Hydrochloride Parenteral (Ampuls) 856
- Apresoline Hydrochloride Tablets 855
- Apresoline-Esidrix Tablets 857
- Ser-Ap-Es Tablets 881
- Serpasil-Apresoline Tablets 884

Imipramine Hydrochloride (Do not use concomitantly). Products include:
- Tofranil Ampuls 1038
- Tofranil Tablets 1039

Imipramine Pamoate (Do not use concomitantly). Products include:
- Tofranil-PM Capsules 1041

Isocarboxazid (Do not use concomitantly). Products include:
- Marplan Tablets 1906

Isradipine (Do not use concomitantly). Products include:
- DynaCirc Capsules 2004

Labetalol Hydrochloride (Do not use concomitantly). Products include:
- Normodyne Injection 2108
- Normodyne Tablets 2110
- Normozide Tablets 2112
- Trandate HCT Tablets 579
- Trandate Injection 577
- Trandate Tablets 579

Lisinopril (Do not use concomitantly). Products include:
- Prinivil Tablets 1538
- Prinzide Tablets 1540
- Zestoretic 2274
- Zestril Tablets 2277

Maprotiline Hydrochloride (Do not use concomitantly). Products include:
- Ludiomil Tablets 874

Mecamylamine Hydrochloride (Do not use concomitantly). Products include:
- Inversine Tablets 1492

Methyldopa (Do not use concomitantly). Products include:
- Aldoclor Tablets 1413
- Aldomet Oral 1415
- Aldoril Tablets 1418

Methyldopate Hydrochloride (Do not use concomitantly). Products include:
- Aldomet Ester HCl Injection 1417

Metolazone (Do not use concomitantly). Products include:
- Diulo 2129
- Mykrox ½ mg Tablets 984
- Zaroxolyn Tablets 989

Metoprolol Tartrate (Do not use concomitantly). Products include:
- Lopressor Ampuls 1032
- Lopressor HCT Tablets 1034
- Lopressor Tablets 1032

Metyrosine (Do not use concomitantly). Products include:
- Demser Capsules 1460

Minoxidil (Do not use concomitantly). Products include:
- Loniten Tablets 2346
- Rogaine Topical Solution 2357

Nadolol (Do not use concomitantly). Products include:
- Corgard Tablets 701
- Corzide Tablets 702

Nicardipine Hydrochloride (Do not use concomitantly). Products include:
- Cardene Capsules 2290

Nitroglycerin (Do not use concomitantly). Products include:
- Deponit NTG Transdermal Delivery System 2143
- Minitran Transdermal Delivery System 1312
- Nitro-Bid Ointment 1339
- Nitro-Bid Capsules 1338
- Nitrodisc 2176
- Nitro-Dur (nitroglycerin) Transdermal Infusion System 1164
- Nitrogard Tablets 1004
- Nitrolingual Spray 1846
- Nitrostat Tablets 1743
- Transderm-Nitro Transdermal Therapeutic System 2283

Nortriptyline Hydrochloride (Do not use concomitantly). Products include:
- Pamelor 2019

Penbutolol Sulfate (Do not use concomitantly). Products include:
- Levatol 1832

Phenelzine Sulfate (Do not use concomitantly). Products include:
- Nardil 1742

Phenoxybenzamine Hydrochloride (Do not use concomitantly). Products include:
- Dibenzyline Capsules 2207

Phentolamine Mesylate (Do not use concomitantly). Products include:
- Regitine 878

Pindolol (Do not use concomitantly). Products include:
- Visken Tablets 2036

Prazosin Hydrochloride (Do not use concomitantly). Products include:
- Minipress Capsules 1778
- Minizide Capsules 1779

Propranolol Hydrochloride (Do not use concomitantly). Products include:
- Inderal 2459
- Inderal LA Long Acting Capsules 2461
- Inderide Tablets 2463
- Inderide LA Long Acting Capsules 2465

Protriptyline Hydrochloride (Do not use concomitantly). Products include:
- Vivactil Tablets 1567

Ramipril (Do not use concomitantly). Products include:
- Altace Capsules 1086

Rauwolfia Serpentina (Do not use concomitantly). Products include:
- Raudixin Tablets 1803
- Rauzide Tablets 1804

Rescinnamine (Do not use concomitantly).
- No products indexed under this heading.

Reserpine (Do not use concomitantly). Products include:
- Diupres Tablets 1461
- Hydromox R Tablets 1209
- Hydropres Tablets 1485
- Renese-R Tablets 1786
- Salutensin/Salutensin-Demi 719
- Ser-Ap-Es Tablets 881
- Serpasil Tablets 883
- Serpasil-Apresoline Tablets 884
- Serpasil-Esidrix Tablets 886

Sodium Nitroprusside (Do not use concomitantly). Products include:
- Nipride I.V. Infusion 1909

Terazosin Hydrochloride (Do not use concomitantly). Products include:
- Hytrin Tablets 529

Timolol Maleate (Do not use concomitantly). Products include:
- Blocadren Tablets 1429
- Timolide Tablets 1547
- Timoptic in Ocudose 1552
- Timoptic Sterile Ophthalmic Solution 1550

Tranylcypromine Sulfate (Do not use concomitantly). Products include:
- Parnate Tablets 2222

Trazodone Hydrochloride (Do not use concomitantly). Products include:
- Desyrel and Desyrel Dividose 1404

Trimethaphan Camsylate (Do not use concomitantly). Products include:
- Arfonad Ampuls 1887

Trimipramine Maleate (Do not use concomitantly). Products include:
- Surmontil Capsules 2524

SINUTAB MAXIMUM STRENGTH TABLETS
(Acetaminophen, Chlorpheniramine Maleate, Pseudoephedrine Hydrochloride) ..... ◘ 641
See **Sinutab Maximum Strength Caplets**

SINUTAB MAXIMUM STRENGTH WITHOUT DROWSINESS TABLETS & CAPLETS
(Acetaminophen, Pseudoephedrine Hydrochloride) ..... ◘ 642
May interact with antihypertensives and antidepressant drugs. Compounds in these categories include:

Acebutolol Hydrochloride (Concurrent use not recommended). Products include:
- Sectral Capsules 2520

Amitriptyline Hydrochloride (Concurrent use not recommended). Products include:
- Elavil 2269
- Endep Tablets 1927
- Etrafon 2087
- Limbitrol 1933
- Triavil Tablets 1556

Amoxapine (Concurrent use not recommended). Products include:
- Asendin Tablets 1196

Atenolol (Concurrent use not recommended). Products include:
- Tenoretic Tablets 1105
- Tenormin Tablets and I.V. Injection 1107

Benazepril Hydrochloride (Concurrent use not recommended). Products include:
- Lotensin Tablets 872

Betaxolol Hydrochloride (Concurrent use not recommended). Products include:
- Betoptic Sterile Ophthalmic Solution 569
- Betoptic S Sterile Ophthalmic Suspension 570
- Kerlone Tablets 2172

Bupropion Hydrochloride (Concurrent use not recommended). Products include:
- Wellbutrin Tablets 821

Captopril (Concurrent use not recommended). Products include:
- Capoten 2255
- Capozide 2258

Carteolol Hydrochloride (Concurrent use not recommended). Products include:
- Cartrol Tablets 507

Clonidine (Concurrent use not recommended). Products include:
- Catapres-TTS 677

Clonidine Hydrochloride (Concurrent use not recommended). Products include:
- Catapres Tablets 676
- Combipres Tablets 678

Deserpidine (Concurrent use not recommended). Products include:
- Enduronyl 518
- Harmonyl Tablets 528
- Oreticyl 545

Desipramine Hydrochloride (Concurrent use not recommended). Products include:
- Norpramin Tablets 1340

Diazoxide (Concurrent use not recommended). Products include:
- Hyperstat I.V. Injection 2095
- Proglycem 649

Doxazosin Mesylate (Concurrent use not recommended). Products include:
- Cardura Tablets 1941

Doxepin Hydrochloride (Concurrent use not recommended). Products include:
- Sinequan 1960

Enalapril Maleate (Concurrent use not recommended). Products include:
- Vaseretic Tablets 1559
- Vasotec Tablets 1564

Enalaprilat (Concurrent use not recommended). Products include:
- Vasotec I.V. 1562

Esmolol Hydrochloride (Concurrent use not recommended). Products include:
- Brevibloc Injection 942

Labetalol Hydrochloride (Concurrent use not recommended). Products include:
- Normodyne Injection ... 2108
- Normodyne Tablets ... 2110
- Normozide Tablets ... 2112
- Trandate HCT Tablets ... 579
- Trandate Injection ... 577
- Trandate Tablets ... 579

Lisinopril (Concurrent use not recommended). Products include:
- Prinivil Tablets ... 1538
- Prinzide Tablets ... 1540
- Zestoretic ... 2274
- Zestril Tablets ... 2277

Maprotiline Hydrochloride (Concurrent use not recommended). Products include:
- Ludiomil Tablets ... 874

Mecamylamine Hydrochloride (Concurrent use not recommended). Products include:
- Inversine Tablets ... 1492

Methyldopa (Concurrent use not recommended). Products include:
- Aldoclor Tablets ... 1413
- Aldomet Oral ... 1415
- Aldoril Tablets ... 1418

Methyldopate Hydrochloride (Concurrent use not recommended). Products include:
- Aldomet Ester HCl Injection ... 1417

Metoprolol Tartrate (Concurrent use not recommended). Products include:
- Lopressor Ampuls ... 1032
- Lopressor HCT Tablets ... 1034
- Lopressor Tablets ... 1032

Metyrosine (Concurrent use not recommended). Products include:
- Demser Capsules ... 1460

Minoxidil (Concurrent use not recommended). Products include:
- Loniten Tablets ... 2346
- Rogaine Topical Solution ... 2357

Nadolol (Concurrent use not recommended). Products include:
- Corgard Tablets ... 701
- Corzide Tablets ... 702

Nicardipine Hydrochloride (Concurrent use not recommended). Products include:
- Cardene Capsules ... 2290

Nitroglycerin (Concurrent use not recommended). Products include:
- Deponit NTG Transdermal Delivery System ... 2143
- Minitran Transdermal Delivery System ... 1312
- Nitro-Bid Ointment ... 1339
- Nitro-Bid Capsules ... 1338
- Nitrodisc ... 2176
- Nitro-Dur (nitroglycerin) Transdermal Infusion System ... 1164
- Nitrogard Tablets ... 1004
- Nitrolingual Spray ... 1846
- Nitrostat Tablets ... 1743
- Transderm-Nitro Transdermal Therapeutic System ... 2283

Nortriptyline Hydrochloride (Concurrent use not recommended). Products include:
- Pamelor ... 2019

Penbutolol Sulfate (Concurrent use not recommended). Products include:
- Levatol ... 1832

Phenelzine Sulfate (Concurrent use not recommended). Products include:
- Nardil ... 1742

Phenoxybenzamine Hydrochloride (Concurrent use not recommended). Products include:
- Dibenzyline Capsules ... 2207

Phentolamine Mesylate (Concurrent use not recommended). Products include:
- Regitine ... 878

Pindolol (Concurrent use not recommended). Products include:
- Visken Tablets ... 2036

Prazosin Hydrochloride (Concurrent use not recommended). Products include:
- Minipress Capsules ... 1778
- Minizide Capsules ... 1779

Propranolol Hydrochloride (Concurrent use not recommended). Products include:
- Inderal ... 2459
- Inderal LA Long Acting Capsules ... 2461
- Inderide Tablets ... 2463
- Inderide LA Long Acting Capsules .. 2465

Protriptyline Hydrochloride (Concurrent use not recommended). Products include:
- Vivactil Tablets ... 1567

Ramipril (Concurrent use not recommended). Products include:
- Altace Capsules ... 1086

Rauwolfia Serpentina (Concurrent use not recommended). Products include:
- Raudixin Tablets ... 1803
- Rauzide Tablets ... 1804

Rescinnamine (Concurrent use not recommended).
- No products indexed under this heading.

Reserpine (Concurrent use not recommended). Products include:
- Diupres Tablets ... 1461
- Hydromox R Tablets ... 1209
- Hydropres Tablets ... 1485
- Renese-R Tablets ... 1786
- Salutensin/Salutensin-Demi ... 719
- Ser-Ap-Es Tablets ... 881
- Serpasil Tablets ... 883
- Serpasil-Apresoline Tablets ... 884
- Serpasil-Esidrix Tablets ... 886

Sodium Nitroprusside (Concurrent use not recommended). Products include:
- Nipride I.V. Infusion ... 1909

Terazosin Hydrochloride (Concurrent use not recommended). Products include:
- Hytrin Tablets ... 529

Timolol Maleate (Concurrent use not recommended). Products include:
- Blocadren Tablets ... 1429
- Timolide Tablets ... 1547
- Timoptic in Ocudose ... 1552
- Timoptic Sterile Ophthalmic Solution ... 1550

Tranylcypromine Sulfate (Concurrent use not recommended). Products include:
- Parnate Tablets ... 2222

Trazodone Hydrochloride (Concurrent use not recommended). Products include:
- Desyrel and Desyrel Dividose ... 1404

Trimethaphan Camsylate (Concurrent use not recommended). Products include:
- Arfonad Ampuls ... 1887

Trimipramine Maleate (Concurrent use not recommended). Products include:
- Surmontil Capsules ... 2524

SKELAXIN

(Metaxalone) ... 840

No interactions described in labeling.

SLEEP-ETTES-D TABLETS

(Diphenhydramine Hydrochloride) .. ▣ 653

May interact with tranquilizers, hypnotics and sedatives, and certain other agents. Compounds in these categories include:

Alcohol (Effect not specified).

Alprazolam (Effect not specified). Products include:
- Xanax Tablets ... 2367

Buspirone Hydrochloride (Effect not specified). Products include:
- BuSpar ... 1401

Chlordiazepoxide (Effect not specified). Products include:
- Libritabs Tablets ... 1930
- Limbitrol ... 1933
- Menrium Tablets ... 1934

Chlordiazepoxide Hydrochloride (Effect not specified). Products include:
- Librax Capsules ... 1929
- Librium Capsules ... 1931
- Librium Injectable ... 1932

Chlorpromazine (Effect not specified). Products include:
- Thorazine ... 2234

Chlorprothixene (Effect not specified). Products include:
- Taractan Tablets ... 1920

Chlorprothixene Hydrochloride (Effect not specified). Products include:
- Taractan ... 1920

Clorazepate Dipotassium (Effect not specified). Products include:
- Tranxene ... 556

Diazepam (Effect not specified). Products include:
- Valium Injectable ... 1937
- Valium Tablets ... 1939
- Valrelease Capsules ... 1923

Droperidol (Effect not specified). Products include:
- Inapsine Injection ... 1140
- Innovar Injection ... 1141

Estazolam (Effect not specified). Products include:
- ProSom Tablets ... 554

Ethchlorvynol (Effect not specified). Products include:
- Placidyl Capsules ... 553

Ethinamate (Effect not specified).
- No products indexed under this heading.

Fluphenazine Decanoate (Effect not specified). Products include:
- Prolixin Decanoate ... 1795

Fluphenazine Enanthate (Effect not specified). Products include:
- Prolixin Enanthate ... 1796

Fluphenazine Hydrochloride (Effect not specified). Products include:
- Prolixin Elixir ... 1793
- Prolixin Injection ... 1791
- Prolixin Oral Concentrate ... 1792
- Prolixin Tablets ... 1793

Flurazepam Hydrochloride (Effect not specified). Products include:
- Dalmane Capsules ... 1927

Glutethimide (Effect not specified).
- No products indexed under this heading.

Haloperidol (Effect not specified). Products include:
- Haldol Injection, Tablets and Concentrate ... 1373

Haloperidol Decanoate (Effect not specified). Products include:
- Haldol Decanoate ... 1375

Hydroxyzine Hydrochloride (Effect not specified). Products include:
- Atarax Tablets & Syrup ... 1941
- Marax Tablets & DF Syrup ... 1954
- Vistaril Intramuscular Solution ... 1970

Lorazepam (Effect not specified). Products include:
- Ativan Injection ... 2432
- Ativan Tablets ... 2434

Loxapine Hydrochloride (Effect not specified). Products include:
- Loxitane ... 1213

Loxapine Succinate (Effect not specified). Products include:
- Loxitane Capsules ... 1213

Meprobamate (Effect not specified). Products include:
- Deprol Tablets ... 2382
- Equagesic Tablets ... 2451
- Miltown Tablets ... 2386
- PMB 200 and PMB 400 ... 2504

Mesoridazine Besylate (Effect not specified).

Midazolam Hydrochloride (Effect not specified). Products include:
- Versed Injection ... 1924

Molindone Hydrochloride (Effect not specified). Products include:
- Moban Tablets & Concentrate ... 932

Oxazepam (Effect not specified). Products include:
- Serax Capsules ... 2522
- Serax Tablets ... 2522

Perphenazine (Effect not specified). Products include:
- Etrafon ... 2087
- Triavil Tablets ... 1556
- Trilafon ... 2123

Prazepam (Effect not specified). Products include:
- Centrax ... 1693

Prochlorperazine (Effect not specified). Products include:
- Compazine ... 2201

Promethazine Hydrochloride (Effect not specified). Products include:
- Mepergan Injection ... 2479
- Phenergan with Codeine ... 2497
- Phenergan with Dextromethorphan 2499
- Phenergan Injection ... 2493
- Phenergan Suppositories ... 2496
- Phenergan Syrup ... 2495
- Phenergan Tablets ... 2496
- Phenergan VC ... 2500
- Phenergan VC with Codeine ... 2501

Propofol (Effect not specified). Products include:
- Diprivan Injection ... 2267

Quazepam (Effect not specified). Products include:
- Doral Tablets ... 2383

Secobarbital Sodium (Effect not specified). Products include:
- Seconal Sodium Pulvules ... 1296

Temazepam (Effect not specified). Products include:
- Restoril Capsules ... 2023

Thioridazine Hydrochloride (Effect not specified). Products include:
- Mellaril ... 2011

Thiothixene (Effect not specified). Products include:
- Navane Capsules and Concentrate 1954
- Navane Intramuscular ... 1956

Triazolam (Effect not specified). Products include:
- Halcion Tablets ... 2340

Trifluoperazine Hydrochloride (Effect not specified). Products include:
- Stelazine ... 2226

SLEEP-EZE 3 TABLETS

(Diphenhydramine Hydrochloride) .. ▣ 755

May interact with hypnotics and sedatives, tranquilizers, and certain other agents. Compounds in these categories include:

Alcohol (Effect not specified).

Alprazolam (Effect not specified). Products include:
- Xanax Tablets ... 2367

Buspirone Hydrochloride (Effect not specified). Products include:
- BuSpar ... 1401

Chlordiazepoxide (Effect not specified). Products include:
- Libritabs Tablets ... 1930
- Limbitrol ... 1933
- Menrium Tablets ... 1934

Chlordiazepoxide Hydrochloride (Effect not specified). Products include:
- Librax Capsules ... 1929
- Librium Capsules ... 1931
- Librium Injectable ... 1932

Chlorpromazine (Effect not specified). Products include:
- Thorazine ... 2234

Chlorprothixene (Effect not specified). Products include:
- Taractan Tablets ... 1920

Chlorprothixene Hydrochloride (Effect not specified). Products include:
- Taractan ... 1920

Clorazepate Dipotassium (Effect not specified). Products include:
- Tranxene ... 556

Diazepam (Effect not specified). Products include:
- Valium Injectable ... 1937
- Valium Tablets ... 1939
- Valrelease Capsules ... 1923

Droperidol (Effect not specified). Products include:
- Inapsine Injection ... 1140
- Innovar Injection ... 1141

Estazolam (Effect not specified). Products include:
- ProSom Tablets ... 554

Ethchlorvynol (Effect not specified). Products include:
- Placidyl Capsules ... 553

Ethinamate (Effect not specified).
- No products indexed under this heading.

Fluphenazine Decanoate (Effect not specified). Products include:
- Prolixin Decanoate ... 1795

Fluphenazine Enanthate (Effect not specified). Products include:
- Prolixin Enanthate ... 1796

Fluphenazine Hydrochloride (Effect not specified). Products include:
- Prolixin Elixir ... 1793
- Prolixin Injection ... 1791
- Prolixin Oral Concentrate ... 1792
- Prolixin Tablets ... 1793

Flurazepam Hydrochloride (Effect not specified). Products include:
- Dalmane Capsules ... 1927

Glutethimide (Effect not specified).
- No products indexed under this heading.

Haloperidol (Effect not specified). Products include:
- Haldol Injection, Tablets and Concentrate ... 1373

Haloperidol Decanoate (Effect not specified). Products include:
- Haldol Decanoate ... 1375

Hydroxyzine Hydrochloride (Effect not specified). Products include:
- Atarax Tablets & Syrup ... 1941
- Marax Tablets & DF Syrup ... 1954
- Vistaril Intramuscular Solution ... 1970

Lorazepam (Effect not specified). Products include:
- Ativan Injection ... 2432
- Ativan Tablets ... 2434

Loxapine Hydrochloride (Effect not specified). Products include:
- Loxitane ... 1213

Loxapine Succinate (Effect not specified). Products include:
- Loxitane Capsules ... 1213

Meprobamate (Effect not specified). Products include:
- Deprol Tablets ... 2382
- Equagesic Tablets ... 2451
- Miltown Tablets ... 2386
- PMB 200 and PMB 400 ... 2504

Mesoridazine Besylate (Effect not specified).

Midazolam Hydrochloride (Effect not specified). Products include:
- Versed Injection ... 1924

Molindone Hydrochloride (Effect not specified). Products include:
- Moban Tablets & Concentrate ... 932

Oxazepam (Effect not specified). Products include:
- Serax Capsules ... 2522
- Serax Tablets ... 2522

Perphenazine (Effect not specified). Products include:
- Etrafon ... 2087
- Triavil Tablets ... 1556
- Trilafon ... 2123

Prazepam (Effect not specified). Products include:
- Centrax ... 1693

Prochlorperazine (Effect not specified). Products include:
- Compazine ... 2201

Promethazine Hydrochloride (Effect not specified). Products include:
- Mepergan Injection ... 2479
- Phenergan with Codeine ... 2497
- Phenergan with Dextromethorphan 2499
- Phenergan Injection ... 2493
- Phenergan Suppositories ... 2496
- Phenergan Syrup ... 2495
- Phenergan Tablets ... 2496
- Phenergan VC ... 2500
- Phenergan VC with Codeine ... 2501

Propofol (Effect not specified). Products include:
- Diprivan Injection ... 2267

Quazepam (Effect not specified). Products include:
- Doral Tablets ... 2383

Secobarbital Sodium (Effect not specified). Products include:
- Seconal Sodium Pulvules ... 1296

Temazepam (Effect not specified). Products include:
- Restoril Capsules ... 2023

Thioridazine Hydrochloride (Effect not specified). Products include:
- Mellaril ... 2011

Thiothixene (Effect not specified). Products include:
- Navane Capsules and Concentrate 1954
- Navane Intramuscular ... 1956

Triazolam (Effect not specified). Products include:
- Halcion Tablets ... 2340

Trifluoperazine Hydrochloride (Effect not specified). Products include:
- Stelazine ... 2226

SLEEPINAL NIGHT-TIME SLEEP AID CAPSULES
(Diphenhydramine Hydrochloride) .. ▣ 734
May interact with hypnotics and sedatives, tranquilizers, and certain other agents. Compounds in these categories include:

Alcohol (Use with caution).

Alprazolam (Concomitant use is not recommended). Products include:
- Xanax Tablets ... 2367

Buspirone Hydrochloride (Concomitant use is not recommended). Products include:
- BuSpar ... 1401

Chlordiazepoxide (Concomitant use is not recommended). Products include:
- Libritabs Tablets ... 1930
- Limbitrol ... 1933
- Menrium Tablets ... 1934

Chlordiazepoxide Hydrochloride (Concomitant use is not recommended). Products include:
- Librax Capsules ... 1929
- Librium Capsules ... 1931
- Librium Injectable ... 1932

Chlorpromazine (Concomitant use is not recommended). Products include:
- Thorazine ... 2234

Chlorprothixene (Concomitant use is not recommended). Products include:
- Taractan Tablets ... 1920

Chlorprothixene Hydrochloride (Concomitant use is not recommended). Products include:
- Taractan ... 1920

Clorazepate Dipotassium (Concomitant use is not recommended). Products include:
- Tranxene ... 556

Diazepam (Concomitant use is not recommended). Products include:
- Valium Injectable ... 1937
- Valium Tablets ... 1939
- Valrelease Capsules ... 1923

Droperidol (Concomitant use is not recommended). Products include:
- Inapsine Injection ... 1140
- Innovar Injection ... 1141

Estazolam (Concomitant use is not recommended). Products include:
- ProSom Tablets ... 554

Ethchlorvynol (Concomitant use is not recommended). Products include:
- Placidyl Capsules ... 553

Ethinamate (Concomitant use is not recommended).
- No products indexed under this heading.

Fluphenazine Decanoate (Concomitant use is not recommended). Products include:
- Prolixin Decanoate ... 1795

Fluphenazine Enanthate (Concomitant use is not recommended). Products include:
- Prolixin Enanthate ... 1796

Fluphenazine Hydrochloride (Concomitant use is not recommended). Products include:
- Prolixin Elixir ... 1793
- Prolixin Injection ... 1791
- Prolixin Oral Concentrate ... 1792
- Prolixin Tablets ... 1793

Flurazepam Hydrochloride (Concomitant use is not recommended). Products include:
- Dalmane Capsules ... 1927

Glutethimide (Concomitant use is not recommended).
- No products indexed under this heading.

Haloperidol (Concomitant use is not recommended). Products include:
- Haldol Injection, Tablets and Concentrate ... 1373

Haloperidol Decanoate (Concomitant use is not recommended). Products include:
- Haldol Decanoate ... 1375

Hydroxyzine Hydrochloride (Concomitant use is not recommended). Products include:
- Atarax Tablets & Syrup ... 1941
- Marax Tablets & DF Syrup ... 1954
- Vistaril Intramuscular Solution ... 1970

Lorazepam (Concomitant use is not recommended). Products include:
- Ativan Injection ... 2432
- Ativan Tablets ... 2434

Loxapine Hydrochloride (Concomitant use is not recommended). Products include:
- Loxitane ... 1213

Loxapine Succinate (Concomitant use is not recommended). Products include:
- Loxitane Capsules ... 1213

Meprobamate (Concomitant use is not recommended). Products include:
- Deprol Tablets ... 2382
- Equagesic Tablets ... 2451
- Miltown Tablets ... 2386
- PMB 200 and PMB 400 ... 2504

Mesoridazine Besylate (Concomitant use is not recommended).

Midazolam Hydrochloride (Concomitant use is not recommended). Products include:
- Versed Injection ... 1924

Molindone Hydrochloride (Concomitant use is not recommended). Products include:
- Moban Tablets & Concentrate ... 932

Oxazepam (Concomitant use is not recommended). Products include:
- Serax Capsules ... 2522
- Serax Tablets ... 2522

Perphenazine (Concomitant use is not recommended). Products include:
- Etrafon ... 2087
- Triavil Tablets ... 1556
- Trilafon ... 2123

Prazepam (Concomitant use is not recommended). Products include:
- Centrax ... 1693

Prochlorperazine (Concomitant use is not recommended). Products include:
- Compazine ... 2201

Promethazine Hydrochloride (Concomitant use is not recommended). Products include:
- Mepergan Injection ... 2479
- Phenergan with Codeine ... 2497
- Phenergan with Dextromethorphan 2499
- Phenergan Injection ... 2493
- Phenergan Suppositories ... 2496
- Phenergan Syrup ... 2495
- Phenergan Tablets ... 2496
- Phenergan VC ... 2500
- Phenergan VC with Codeine ... 2501

Propofol (Concomitant use is not recommended). Products include:
- Diprivan Injection ... 2267

Quazepam (Concomitant use is not recommended). Products include:
- Doral Tablets ... 2383

Secobarbital Sodium (Concomitant use is not recommended). Products include:
- Seconal Sodium Pulvules ... 1296

Temazepam (Concomitant use is not recommended). Products include:
- Restoril Capsules ... 2023

Thioridazine Hydrochloride (Concomitant use is not recommended). Products include:
- Mellaril ... 2011

Thiothixene (Concomitant use is not recommended). Products include:
- Navane Capsules and Concentrate 1954
- Navane Intramuscular ... 1956

Triazolam (Concomitant use is not recommended). Products include:
- Halcion Tablets ... 2340

Trifluoperazine Hydrochloride (Concomitant use is not recommended). Products include:
- Stelazine ... 2226

SLO-BID GYROCAPS
(Theophylline Anhydrous) ... 1847
May interact with sympathomimetic bronchodilators, macrolide antibiotics, oral contraceptives, corticosteroids, thiazides, beta blockers, and

certain other agents. Compounds in these categories include:

Albuterol (Possible toxic synergism; xanthines can potentiate hypokalemia resulting from $beta_2$ agonist therapy). Products include:
Proventil Inhalation Aerosol ... 2117
Ventolin Inhalation Aerosol and Refill ... 583

Albuterol Sulfate (Possible toxic synergism; xanthines can potentiate hypokalemia resulting from $beta_2$ agonist therapy). Products include:
Proventil Repetabs Tablets ... 2120
Proventil Solutions for Inhalation 0.5% and 0.083% ... 2118
Proventil Syrup ... 2119
Proventil Tablets ... 2120
Ventolin ... 583

Allopurinol (Allopurinol in high doses increases serum theophylline levels). Products include:
Zyloprim Tablets ... 830

Bendroflumethiazide (Xanthines can potentiate hypokalemic effects). Products include:
Corzide Tablets ... 702
Naturetin Tablets ... 1789
Rauzide Tablets ... 1804

Betamethasone Acetate (Xanthines can potentiate hypokalemic effects). Products include:
Celestone Soluspan Suspension ... 2081

Betamethasone Sodium Phosphate (Xanthines can potentiate hypokalemic effects). Products include:
Celestone Soluspan Suspension ... 2081

Bitolterol Mesylate (Possible toxic synergism; xanthines can potentiate hypokalemia resulting from $beta_2$ agonist therapy). Products include:
Tornalate ... 2074

Chlorothiazide (Xanthines can potentiate hypokalemic effects). Products include:
Aldoclor Tablets ... 1413
Diupres Tablets ... 1461
Diuril Oral ... 1464

Chlorothiazide Sodium (Xanthines can potentiate hypokalemic effects). Products include:
Diuril Sodium Intravenous ... 1463

Cimetidine (Increased theophylline serum concentrations). Products include:
Tagamet Tablets ... 2228

Cimetidine Hydrochloride (Increased theophylline serum concentrations). Products include:
Tagamet ... 2228

Ciprofloxacin (Increased serum theophylline levels).
No products indexed under this heading.

Ciprofloxacin Hydrochloride (Increased serum theophylline levels). Products include:
Ciloxan Sterile Ophthalmic Solution ... ◉ 214
Cipro I.V. ... 1592
Cipro Tablets ... 1589

Cortisone Acetate (Xanthines can potentiate hypokalemic effects). Products include:
Cortone Acetate Sterile Suspension ... 1437
Cortone Acetate Tablets ... 1439

Dexamethasone (Xanthines can potentiate hypokalemic effects). Products include:
AK-Trol Ointment & Suspension ... ◉ 207
Decadron Elixir ... 1445
Decadron Tablets ... 1447
Decaspray Topical Aerosol ... 1459
Dexacidin ... ◉ 272
Maxidex Sterile Ophthalmic Suspension ... ◉ 223
Maxitrol Ophthalmic Ointment/Suspension ... ◉ 223
TobraDex Ophthalmic Suspension and Ointment ... ◉ 228

Dexamethasone Acetate (Xanthines can potentiate hypokalemic effects). Products include:
Dalalone D.P. Injectable ... 999
Decadron-LA Sterile Suspension ... 1457

Dexamethasone Sodium Phosphate (Xanthines can potentiate hypokalemic effects). Products include:
AK-Dex ... ◉ 203
Decadron Phosphate Respihaler ... 1454
Decadron Phosphate Sterile Ophthalmic Ointment ... 1453
Decadron Phosphate Sterile Ophthalmic Solution ... 1453
Decadron Phosphate Topical Cream ... 1455
Decadron Phosphate Turbinaire ... 1456
Maxidex Sterile Ophthalmic Ointment ... ◉ 222
NeoDecadron Sterile Ophthalmic Ointment ... 1517
NeoDecadron Sterile Ophthalmic Solution ... 1518
NeoDecadron Topical Cream ... 1518

Ephedrine Hydrochloride (Possible toxic synergism; xanthines can potentiate hypokalemia resulting from $beta_2$ agonist therapy). Products include:
Amesec ... ▣ 682
Primatene Tablets-M Formula ... 2421
Primatene Tablets-P Formula ... 2421
Primatene Tablets-Regular Formula ... 2421
Quadrinal Tablets ... 1183
Quelidrine Syrup ... 556
Tedral SA ... 1765

Ephedrine Sulfate (Possible toxic synergism; xanthines can potentiate hypokalemia resulting from $beta_2$ agonist therapy). Products include:
Bronkaid Tablets ... ▣ 757
Bronkolixir ... ▣ 761
Bronkotabs Tablets ... ▣ 762
Marax Tablets & DF Syrup ... 1954
Pazo Hemorrhoid Ointment & Suppositories ... 752
Vicks Vatronol Nose Drops ... ▣ 666

Ephedrine Tannate (Possible toxic synergism; xanthines can potentiate hypokalemia resulting from $beta_2$ agonist therapy). Products include:
Rynatuss ... 2388

Epinephrine (Possible toxic synergism; xanthines can potentiate hypokalemia resulting from $beta_2$ agonist therapy). Products include:
Ana-Kit Anaphylaxis Emergency Treatment Kit ... 1100
Bronkaid Mist ... ▣ 757
EpiPen ... 843
Marcaine Hydrochloride 0.5% with Epinephrine 1:200,000 (as bitartrate) ... 958
Marcaine Hydrochloride with Epinephrine 1:200,000 ... 2055
Primatene Mist ... 2420
Sus-Phrine Injection ... 1006
Xylocaine with Epinephrine Injections ... 637

Epinephrine Hydrochloride (Possible toxic synergism; xanthines can potentiate hypokalemia resulting from $beta_2$ agonist therapy). Products include:
Adrenalin Chloride Solution 1:100 & 1:1,000 ... 1689
Epifrin ... ◉ 244
Glaucon ... ◉ 218

Erythromycin (Increased theophylline serum concentrations). Products include:
A/T/S Topical Gel and Topical Solution ... 1089
AK-Mycin Ointment ... ◉ 204
Benzamycin Topical Gel ... 907
E-Mycin Tablets ... 688
ETS-2% ... 1685
ERYC ... 1720
Erycette (erythromycin 2%) Topical Solution ... 1678
Ery-Tab Tablets ... 521
Erythromycin Base Filmtab ... 525
Erythromycin Delayed-Release Capsules, USP ... 526
Ilotycin Ophthalmic Ointment ... 915
PCE Dispertab Tablets ... 549
Pediazole ... 1973
T-Stat 2.0% Topical Solution and Pads ... 2409
Theramycin Z Topical Solution 2% ... 1410

Erythromycin Estolate (Increased theophylline serum concentrations). Products include:
Ilosone ... 913

Erythromycin Ethylsuccinate (Increased theophylline serum concentrations). Products include:
E.E.S. ... 522
EryPed ... 519
Pediazole ... 1973

Erythromycin Gluceptate (Increased theophylline serum concentrations). Products include:
Ilotycin Gluceptate, IV, Vials ... 915

Erythromycin Stearate (Increased theophylline serum concentrations). Products include:
Erythrocin Stearate Filmtab ... 523

Ethinyl Estradiol (Increased serum theophylline levels). Products include:
Brevicon ... 2304
Demulen ... 2161
Estinyl Tablets ... 2085
Jenest-28 Tablets ... 1636
Levlen/Tri-Levlen ... 665
Lo/Ovral Tablets ... 2471
Lo/Ovral-28 Tablets ... 2476
Loestrin ... 1728
Modicon ... 1667
Nordette-21 Tablets ... 2481
Nordette-28 Tablets ... 2483
Norethin ... 2133
Norinyl ... 2304
Norlestrin ... 1746
Ortho-Cyclen Tablets ... 1658
Ortho-Novum ... 1667
Ovcon ... 1391
Ovral Tablets ... 2490
Ovral-28 Tablets ... 2491
Levlen/Tri-Levlen ... 665
Tri-Norinyl ... 2304
Triphasil-21 Tablets ... 2527
Triphasil-28 Tablets ... 2532

Ethylnorepinephrine Hydrochloride (Possible toxic synergism; xanthines can potentiate hypokalemia resulting from $beta_2$ agonist therapy). Products include:
Bronkephrine Injection ... 2042

Ethynodiol Diacetate (Increased serum theophylline levels). Products include:
Demulen ... 2161

Hydrochlorothiazide (Xanthines can potentiate hypokalemic effects). Products include:
Aldactazide ... 2150
Aldoril Tablets ... 1418
Apresazide Capsules ... 854
Apresoline-Esidrix Tablets ... 857
Capozide ... 2258
Dyazide Capsules ... 2208
Esidrix Tablets ... 863
Esimil Tablets ... 864
HydroDIURIL Tablets ... 1484
Hydropres Tablets ... 1485
Inderide Tablets ... 2463
Inderide LA Long Acting Capsules ... 2465
Lopressor HCT Tablets ... 1034
Maxzide ... 1215
Moduretic Tablets ... 1510
Normozide Tablets ... 2112
Oretic Tablets ... 544
Oreticyl ... 545
Prinzide Tablets ... 1540
Ser-Ap-Es Tablets ... 881
Serpasil-Esidrix Tablets ... 886
Timolide Tablets ... 1547
Trandate HCT Tablets ... 579
Vaseretic Tablets ... 1559
Zestoretic ... 2274

Hydrocortisone (Xanthines can potentiate hypokalemic effects). Products include:
AK-Spore H.C. ... ◉ 206
Bactine Hydrocortisone Anti-Itch Cream ... ▣ 625
CaldeCORT Anti-Itch Hydrocortisone Spray ... ▣ 560
Carmol HC Cream 1% ... 2296
Cortaid Spray ... ▣ 735
Cortenema ... 2244
Cortisporin Ointment ... 758
Cortisporin Ophthalmic Ointment Sterile ... 758
Cortisporin Ophthalmic Suspension Sterile ... 759
Cortisporin Otic Solution Sterile ... 760
Cortisporin Otic Suspension Sterile ... 760
Cortizone-5 Creme & Ointment ... ▣ 732
Dermolate Anti-Itch Cream ... ▣ 697
Eldecort Cream 1.0% ... 1113
Eldecort Cream 1.0% and 2.5% ... 1113
Fungoid HC Creme ... 1770
Hydrocortone Tablets ... 1482
Hytone ... 909
LazerSporin-C Solution ... 1770
Massengill Medicated Soft Cloth Towelettes ... 2192
Nutracort Cream & Lotion ... 1684
PediOtic Suspension Sterile ... 797
Synacort Creams 1%, 2.5% ... 2296
Vanoxide-HC Acne Lotion ... 911
Vioform-Hydrocortisone Cream and Mild Cream ... 889
Vioform-Hydrocortisone Ointment ... 889
VōSoL HC Otic Solution ... 2392
Vytone Cream 1% ... 911

Hydrocortisone Acetate (Xanthines can potentiate hypokalemic effects). Products include:
Analpram-HC Rectal Cream 1% and 2.5% ... 970
Anusol-HC Cream ... 1690
Anusol-HC Suppositories ... 1691
Caldecort ... ▣ 560
Carmol HC Cream 1% ... 2296
Chloromycetin Hydrocortisone Ophthalmic ... 1694
Coly-Mycin S Otic w/Neomycin & Hydrocortisone ... 1708
Cortaid ... ▣ 735
Cortef Feminine Itch Cream ... ▣ 735
Corticaine ... ▣ 682
Cortifoam ... 1827
Cortisporin Cream ... 757
Epifoam ... 1828
Gynecort 5 Creme ... ▣ 556
Hydrocortone Acetate Sterile Suspension ... 1479
Lanacort 5 Creme and Ointment ... ▣ 557
Mantadil Cream ... 789
Ophthocort ... ◉ 301
Orabase HCA Oral Paste ... 890
Pramosone Cream, Lotion & Ointment ... 971
ProctoCream-HC ... 1834
Proctofoam-HC ... 1835

Hydrocortisone Sodium Phosphate (Xanthines can potentiate hypokalemic effects). Products include:
Hydrocortone Phosphate Injection, Sterile ... 1481

Hydrocortisone Sodium Succinate (Xanthines can potentiate hypokalemic effects). Products include:
Solu-Cortef Sterile Powder ... 2361

Hydroflumethiazide (Xanthines can potentiate hypokalemic effects). Products include:
Diucardin Tablets ... 2450
Saluron ... 718
Salutensin/Salutensin-Demi ... 719

Influenza Virus Vaccine (Decreases theophylline clearance). Products include:
Flu-Imune Influenza Virus Vaccine ... 1204

Isoetharine (Possible toxic synergism; xanthines can potentiate hypokalemia resulting from $beta_2$ agonist therapy). Products include:
Arm-a-Med Isoetharine Inhalation Solution, USP ... 616
Bronkometer Aerosol ... 2042
Bronkosol Solution ... 2042

(▣ Described in PDR For Nonprescription Drugs)   (◉ Described in PDR For Ophthalmology)

Isoproterenol Hydrochloride (Possible toxic synergism; xanthines can potentiate hypokalemia resulting from $beta_2$ agonist therapy). Products include:
- Isuprel Hydrochloride Injection 1:5000 ... 2050
- Isuprel Hydrochloride Mistometer .. 2051
- Isuprel Hydrochloride Solution 1:200 & 1:100 ... 2052
- Norisodrine Aerotrol ... 540

Levonorgestrel (Increased serum theophylline levels). Products include:
- Levlen/Tri-Levlen ... 665
- Nordette-21 Tablets ... 2481
- Nordette-28 Tablets ... 2483
- Norplant System ... 2484
- Levlen/Tri-Levlen ... 665
- Triphasil-21 Tablets ... 2527
- Triphasil-28 Tablets ... 2532

Lithium Carbonate (Increased excretion of lithium carbonate). Products include:
- Eskalith ... 2214
- Lithane Tablets ... 1596
- Lithium Carbonate Capsules & Tablets ... 1984
- Lithobid Tablets ... 870

Mestranol (Increased serum theophylline levels). Products include:
- Enovid ... 2161
- Norethin ... 2133
- Norinyl ... 2304
- Ortho-Novum ... 1667

Metaproterenol Sulfate (Possible toxic synergism; xanthines can potentiate hypokalemia resulting from $beta_2$ agonist therapy). Products include:
- Alupent ... 674
- Arm-a-Med Metaproterenol Sulfate Inhalation Solution, USP ... 617
- Metaprel Inhalation Aerosol Bronchodilator ... 2014
- Metaprel Inhalation Solution ... 2015
- Metaprel ... 2015
- Metaproterenol Sulfate Inhalation Solution, USP ... 912

Methyclothiazide (Xanthines can potentiate hypokalemic effects). Products include:
- Enduron Tablets ... 517
- Enduronyl ... 518

Methylprednisolone Acetate (Xanthines can potentiate hypokalemic effects). Products include:
- Depo-Medrol Sterile Aqueous Suspension ... 2334

Methylprednisolone Sodium Succinate (Xanthines can potentiate hypokalemic effects). Products include:
- Solu-Medrol Sterile Powder ... 2363

Norethindrone (Increased serum theophylline levels). Products include:
- Brevicon ... 2304
- Jenest-28 Tablets ... 1636
- Micronor Tablets ... 1667
- Modicon ... 1667
- Norethin ... 2133
- Norinyl ... 2304
- Norlutin ... 1755
- Nor-Q D Tablets ... 2304
- Ortho-Novum ... 1667
- Ovcon ... 1391
- Tri-Norinyl ... 2304

Norethynodrel (Increased serum theophylline levels). Products include:
- Enovid ... 2161

Norgestimate (Increased serum theophylline levels). Products include:
- Ortho-Cyclen Tablets ... 1658

Norgestrel (Increased serum theophylline levels). Products include:
- Lo/Ovral Tablets ... 2471
- Lo/Ovral-28 Tablets ... 2476
- Ovral Tablets ... 2490
- Ovral-28 Tablets ... 2491
- Ovrette Tablets ... 2492

Phenytoin (Serum levels of both drugs decreased). Products include:
- Dilantin Infatabs ... 1710
- Dilantin-30 Pediatric/Dilantin-125 Suspension ... 1713

Phenytoin Sodium (Serum levels of both drugs decreased). Products include:
- Dilantin Kapseals ... 1708
- Dilantin Parenteral ... 1712
- Dilantin with Phenobarbital Kapseals ... 1715

Pirbuterol Acetate (Possible toxic synergism; xanthines can potentiate hypokalemia resulting from $beta_2$ agonist therapy). Products include:
- Maxair Inhaler ... 1311

Polythiazide (Xanthines can potentiate hypokalemic effects). Products include:
- Minizide Capsules ... 1779
- Renese Tablets ... 1785
- Renese-R Tablets ... 1786

Prednisolone Acetate (Xanthines can potentiate hypokalemic effects). Products include:
- AK-Cide Sterile Ophthalmic Ointment & Suspension ... ⊛ 202
- Blephamide Liquifilm Sterile Ophthalmic Suspension ... 586
- Blephamide S.O.P. Sterile Ophthalmic Ointment ... 586
- Cetapred Ointment ... ⊛ 220
- ⅛ % Econopred & 1 % Econopred Plus ... ⊛ 217
- Isopto Cetapred Suspension ... ⊛ 220
- Metimyd ... ⊛ 306
- Poly-Pred Liquifilm ... ⊛ 250
- Pred Forte ... ⊛ 252
- Pred Mild ... ⊛ 254
- Pred-G Liquifilm Sterile Ophthalmic Suspension ... ⊛ 252
- Pred-G S.O.P. Sterile Ophthalmic Ointment ... ⊛ 253
- Vasocidin Ointment ... ⊛ 275

Prednisolone Sodium Phosphate (Xanthines can potentiate hypokalemic effects). Products include:
- AK-Pred ... ⊛ 205
- Hydeltrasol Injection, Sterile ... 1476
- Inflamase ... ⊛ 274
- Pediapred Oral Liquid ... 987
- Vasocidin Ophthalmic Solution ... ⊛ 276

Prednisolone Tebutate (Xanthines can potentiate hypokalemic effects). Products include:
- Hydeltra-T.B.A. Sterile Suspension 1478

Prednisone (Xanthines can potentiate hypokalemic effects). Products include:
- Deltasone Tablets ... 2332

Propranolol Hydrochloride (Increased theophylline levels). Products include:
- Inderal ... 2459
- Inderal LA Long Acting Capsules 2461
- Inderide Tablets ... 2463
- Inderide LA Long Acting Capsules .. 2465

Rifampin (Decreased serum theophylline levels). Products include:
- Rifadin ... 1345
- Rifamate Capsules ... 1347
- Rimactane Capsules ... 879

Terbutaline Sulfate (Possible toxic synergism; xanthines can potentiate hypokalemia resulting from $beta_2$ agonist therapy). Products include:
- Brethaire Inhaler ... 1024
- Brethine Ampuls ... 1026
- Brethine Tablets ... 1026
- Bricanyl Injection ... 1324
- Bricanyl Tablets ... 1325

Triamcinolone (Xanthines can potentiate hypokalemic effects).
- No products indexed under this heading.

Triamcinolone Acetonide (Xanthines can potentiate hypokalemic effects). Products include:
- Aristocort A ... 1010
- Azmacort Inhaler ... 1837
- Kenalog Cream, Lotion & Ointment 2401
- Kenalog-10 Injection ... 2402
- Kenalog-40 Injection ... 2403
- Kenalog in Orabase ... 604
- Kenalog Spray ... 2401
- Mycolog II Cream and Ointment ... 2407
- Mytrex Cream & Ointment ... 2080
- Nasacort Nasal Inhaler ... 1844

Triamcinolone Diacetate (Xanthines can potentiate hypokalemic effects). Products include:
- Aristocort Suspension ... 1008

Triamcinolone Hexacetonide (Xanthines can potentiate hypokalemic effects). Products include:
- Aristospan Suspension ... 1011

Troleandomycin (Increased theophylline serum concentrations). Products include:
- Tao Capsules ... 1963

Food Interactions

Diet, high-lipid (Decreases in the rate of absorption, but with no significant difference in the extent of absorption).

SLO-NIACIN TABLETS
(Nicotinic Acid) ... 2376
No interactions described in labeling.

SLOW FE TABLETS
(Ferrous Sulfate) ... 852
May interact with tetracyclines. Compounds in this category include:

Demeclocycline Hydrochloride (Absorption of oral tetracycline impaired). Products include:
- Declomycin Capsules, Tablets ... 1199

Doxycycline Calcium (Absorption of oral tetracycline impaired).
- No products indexed under this heading.

Doxycycline Hyclate (Absorption of oral tetracycline impaired). Products include:
- Doryx Capsules ... 1717
- Vibramycin Hyclate Capsules ... 1787
- Vibramycin Hyclate Intravenous ... 1968
- Vibra-Tabs Film Coated Tablets ... 1787

Doxycycline Monohydrate (Absorption of oral tetracycline impaired). Products include:
- Monodox Capsules ... 1630
- Vibramycin Monohydrate for Oral Suspension ... 1787

Methacycline Hydrochloride (Absorption of oral tetracycline impaired).
- No products indexed under this heading.

Minocycline Hydrochloride (Absorption of oral tetracycline impaired). Products include:
- Minocin Intravenous ... 1221
- Minocin Oral Suspension ... 1224
- Minocin Pellet-Filled Capsules ... 1222

Oxytetracycline (Absorption of oral tetracycline impaired). Products include:
- Terramycin Intramuscular Solution 1964
- Urobiotic-250 Capsules ... 1968

Oxytetracycline Hydrochloride (Absorption of oral tetracycline impaired). Products include:
- Terra-Cortril Ophthalmic Suspension ... 1963
- Terramycin Capsules ... 1786
- Terramycin Intramuscular Solution 1964
- Terramycin with Polymyxin B Sulfate Ophthalmic Ointment ... 1965

Tetracycline Hydrochloride (Absorption of oral tetracycline impaired). Products include:
- Achromycin V Capsules ... 1193
- Achromycin Ophthalmic Ointment 1 % ... ⊛ 307
- Achromycin Ophthalmic Suspension 1 % ... ⊛ 308
- Topicycline for Topical Solution ... 1856

SLOW-K TABLETS
(Potassium Chloride) ... 2281
May interact with potassium sparing diuretics. Compounds in this category include:

Amiloride Hydrochloride (Hyperkalemia). Products include:
- Midamor Tablets ... 1508
- Moduretic Tablets ... 1510

Spironolactone (Hyperkalemia). Products include:
- Aldactazide ... 2150
- Aldactone ... 2152

Triamterene (Hyperkalemia). Products include:
- Dyazide Capsules ... 2208
- Dyrenium Capsules ... 2210
- Maxzide ... 1215

SNO STRIPS TEAR FLOW TEST STRIPS
(Diagnostic Agent) ... ⊛ 209
No interactions described in labeling.

SODIUM POLYSTYRENE SULFONATE SUSPENSION
(Sodium Polystyrene Sulfonate) ... 1993
May interact with cardiac glycosides, antacids containing aluminum, calcium and magnesium, and certain other agents. Compounds in these categories include:

Aluminum Carbonate Gel (Potential for systemic alkalosis). Products include:
- Basaljel ... 2438

Aluminum Hydroxide (Potential for systemic alkalosis). Products include:
- Cama Arthritis Pain Reliever ... ▣ 685
- Gaviscon Extra Strength Relief Formula Liquid Antacid ... ▣ 594
- Gaviscon Extra Strength Relief Formula Antacid Tablets ... ▣ 594
- Gaviscon Liquid Antacid ... ▣ 594
- Gelusil Liquid & Tablets ... ▣ 639
- Extra Strength Maalox Plus Suspension ... 1850
- Maalox TC Suspension ... 1851
- Maalox Plus Tablets ... ▣ 655
- Extra Strength Maalox Plus Tablets 1850
- Nephrox Suspension ... ▣ 563
- WinGel Liquid & Tablets ... ▣ 761

Aluminum Hydroxide Gel (Potential for systemic alkalosis). Products include:
- ALternaGEL Liquid ... 1154
- Aludrox Oral Suspension ... 2428
- Amphojel Suspension ... 2429
- Amphojel Suspension without Flavor ... 2429
- Mylanta Liquid ... 1155
- Mylanta Double Strength Liquid ... 1155

Aluminum Hydroxide Gel, Dried (Potential for systemic alkalosis). Products include:
- Alu-Tab/Alu-Cap ... 1309
- Amphojel Tablets ... 2429
- Ascriptin A/D Caplets ... 1850
- Regular Strength Ascriptin Tablets 1850
- Gaviscon Antacid Tablets ... ▣ 593
- Gaviscon-2 Antacid Tablets ... ▣ 594
- Mylanta Tablets ... 1155
- Mylanta Double Strength Tablets 1155

Deslanoside (Potential for digitalis toxicity exaggerated by hypokalemia).
- No products indexed under this heading.

Digitoxin (Potential for digitalis toxicity exaggerated by hypokalemia). Products include:
- Crystodigin Tablets ... 1253

Digoxin (Potential for digitalis toxicity exaggerated by hypokalemia). Products include:
- Lanoxicaps ... 772
- Lanoxin Elixir Pediatric ... 775
- Lanoxin Injection ... 778
- Lanoxin Injection Pediatric ... 781
- Lanoxin Tablets ... 783

(▣ Described in PDR For Nonprescription Drugs) (⊛ Described in PDR For Ophthalmology)

Dihydroxyaluminum Sodium Carbonate (Potential for systemic alkalosis). Products include:
- Rolaids ▣ 743

Magaldrate (Potential for systemic alkalosis). Products include:
- Riopan Antacid Chew Tablets ▣ 754
- Riopan Antacid Chew Tablets in Rollpacks ▣ 754
- Riopan Antacid Suspension 2421
- Riopan Antacid Swallow Tablets 2421
- Riopan Plus Chew Tablets 2422
- Riopan Plus Chew Tablets in Rollpack 2422
- Riopan Plus 2 Chew Tablets, Mint Flavor, Cherry Flavor 2422
- Riopan Plus Suspension 2422
- Riopan Plus 2 Suspension, Mint Flavor, Cherry Flavor 2422

Magnesium Hydroxide (Should not be administered concomitantly; potential for systemic alkalosis). Products include:
- Aludrox Oral Suspension 2428
- Ascriptin A/D Caplets 1850
- Regular Strength Ascriptin Tablets 1850
- Di-Gel Antacid/Anti-Gas ▣ 697
- Gelusil Liquid & Tablets ▣ 639
- Haley's M-O, Regular & Flavored ▣ 569
- Extra Strength Maalox Plus Suspension 1850
- Maalox TC Suspension 1851
- Maalox Plus Tablets ▣ 655
- Extra Strength Maalox Plus Tablets 1850
- Mylanta Liquid 1155
- Mylanta Tablets 1155
- Mylanta Double Strength Liquid 1155
- Mylanta Double Strength Tablets 1155
- Concentrated Phillips' Milk of Magnesia ▣ 573
- Phillips' Milk of Magnesia Liquid ▣ 572
- Phillips' Milk of Magnesia Tablets ▣ 573
- WinGel Liquid & Tablets ▣ 761

Magnesium Oxide (Potential for systemic alkalosis). Products include:
- Bayer Plus Aspirin Tablets ▣ 567
- Beelith Tablets 659
- Bufferin Analgesic Tablets and Caplets ▣ 524
- Cama Arthritis Pain Reliever ▣ 685
- Mag-Ox 400 673
- Uro-Mag 673

SODIUM SULAMYD OPHTHALMIC OINTMENT 10%-STERILE
(Sulfacetamide Sodium) 2122
No interactions described in labeling.

SODIUM SULAMYD OPHTHALMIC SOLUTION 10%-STERILE
(Sulfacetamide Sodium) 2122
No interactions described in labeling.

SODIUM SULAMYD OPHTHALMIC SOLUTION 30%-STERILE
(Sulfacetamide Sodium) 2122
No interactions described in labeling.

SOLAQUIN FORTE 4% CREAM
(Hydroquinone) 1122
No interactions described in labeling.

SOLAQUIN FORTE 4% GEL
(Hydroquinone) 1123
No interactions described in labeling.

SOLARCAINE
(Lidocaine, Benzocaine) ▣ 705
No interactions described in labeling.

SOLATENE CAPSULES
(Beta Carotene) 1881
May interact with:

Vitamin A (Patients should avoid supplementary Vitamin A intake). Products include:
- Aquasol A Vitamin A Capsules, USP 615
- Aquasol A Parenteral, USP 615
- Bugs Bunny Children's Chewable Vitamins (Sugar Free) ▣ 625
- Bugs Bunny With Extra C Children's Chewable Vitamins (Sugar Free) ▣ 626
- Bugs Bunny/Flintstones ▣ 625
- Flintstones Children's Chewable Vitamins With Extra C ▣ 626
- Flintstones Children's Chewable Vitamins Plus Iron ▣ 625
- Lazer Creme 1770
- Myadec ▣ 640
- Natalins Rx 1391
- Natalins Tablets 1391
- Ocuvite Vitamin and Mineral Supplement ⊙ 312
- One-A-Day Essential Vitamins ▣ 627
- One-A-Day Maximum Formula Vitamins and Minerals ▣ 627
- One-A-Day Plus Extra C Vitamins ▣ 627
- Stressgard Stress Formula Vitamins ▣ 628
- Tri-Vi-Flor 1.0 mg Vitamins with Fluoride Chewable Tablets 1400
- Tri-Vi-Flor Drops 1400
- Tri-Vi-Sol Vitamin Drops ▣ 614
- Tri-Vi-Sol Vitamin Drops with Iron ▣ 614
- Vicon Forte Capsules 2416
- Vicon Plus ▣ 682
- Vi-Daylin ADC Vitamins Drops 1980
- Vi-Daylin ADC Vitamins + Iron Drops 1980
- Vi-Daylin/F ADC Vitamins Drops With Fluoride 1981
- Vi-Daylin/F ADC Vitamins + Iron Drops With Fluoride 1981
- Vi-Zac ▣ 682
- Within Women's Formula Multivitamin with Calcium, Extra Iron and Zinc ▣ 628
- Zymacap Capsules ▣ 670

SOLBAR PF 15 CREAM (PABA FREE)
(Octyl Methoxycinnamate, Oxybenzone) 1772
No interactions described in labeling.

SOLBAR PF 15 LIQUID (PABA FREE)
(Octyl Methoxycinnamate, Oxybenzone) 1772
No interactions described in labeling.

SOLBAR PF ULTRA CREAM SPF 50 (PABA FREE)
(Oxybenzone) 1773
No interactions described in labeling.

SOLBAR PLUS 15 CREAM
(Oxybenzone, Dioxybenzone, Octyl Dimethyl PABA) 1772
No interactions described in labeling.

SOLGANAL SUSPENSION
(Aurothioglucose) 2122
May interact with antimalarials, immunosuppressive agents, and certain other agents. Compounds in these categories include:

Azathioprine (Safety of coadministration has not been established). Products include:
- Imuran 768

Chloroquine Hydrochloride (Concurrent use is contraindicated). Products include:
- Aralen Hydrochloride Injection 2038

Chloroquine Phosphate (Concurrent use is contraindicated). Products include:
- Aralen Phosphate with Primaquine Phosphate Tablets 2040
- Aralen Phosphate Tablets 2039

Cyclosporine (Safety of coadministration has not been established). Products include:
- Sandimmune 2024

Immune Globulin (Human) (Safety of coadministration has not been established). Products include:
- MICRhoGAM Rh_0(D) Immune Globulin (Human) 1650
- RhoGAM Rh_0(D) Immune Globulin (Human) 1651

Immune Globulin Intravenous (Human) (Safety of coadministration has not been established). Products include:
- Gamimune N Immune Globulin Intravenous (Human) 1572
- Gammagard Immune Globulin, Intravenous (Human) 658
- Iveegam 1129
- Sandoglobulin I.V. 2027

Mefloquine Hydrochloride (Concurrent use is contraindicated). Products include:
- Lariam Tablets 1904

Muromonab-CD3 (Safety of coadministration has not been established). Products include:
- Orthoclone OKT3 Sterile Solution 1645

Penicillamine (Concurrent use is contraindicated). Products include:
- Cuprimine Capsules 1442
- Depen Titratable Tablets 2379

Pyrimethamine (Concurrent use is contraindicated). Products include:
- Daraprim Tablets 761
- Fansidar Tablets 1896

SOLU-CORTEF STERILE POWDER
(Hydrocortisone Sodium Succinate) 2361
May interact with:

Immunization (Possible neurological complications; lack of antibody response).

Smallpox Vaccine (Possible neurological complications; lack of antibody response).

SOLU-MEDROL STERILE POWDER
(Methylprednisolone Sodium Succinate) 2363
May interact with:

Cyclosporine (Potential for convulsions). Products include:
- Sandimmune 2024

Immunization (Possible neurological complications; lack of antibody response).

Smallpox Vaccine (Possible neurological complications; lack of antibody response).

SOMA COMPOUND W/CODEINE TABLETS
(Carisoprodol, Aspirin, Codeine Phosphate) 2390
May interact with central nervous system depressants, psychotropics, oral anticoagulants, oral hypoglycemic agents, antacids, corticosteroids, and certain other agents. Compounds in these categories include:

Alcohol (Additive effects including gastrointestinal bleeding).

Alfentanil Hydrochloride (Additive effects). Products include:
- Alfenta Injection 1131

Alprazolam (Additive effects). Products include:
- Xanax Tablets 2367

Aluminum Carbonate Gel (May substantially decrease plasma salicylate concentration). Products include:
- Basaljel 2438

Aluminum Hydroxide (May substantially decrease plasma salicylate concentration). Products include:
- Cama Arthritis Pain Reliever ▣ 685
- Gaviscon Extra Strength Relief Formula Liquid Antacid ▣ 594
- Gaviscon Extra Strength Relief Formula Antacid Tablets ▣ 594
- Gaviscon Liquid Antacid ▣ 594
- Gelusil Liquid & Tablets ▣ 639
- Extra Strength Maalox Plus Suspension 1850
- Maalox TC Suspension 1851
- Maalox Plus Tablets ▣ 655
- Extra Strength Maalox Plus Tablets 1850
- Nephrox Suspension ▣ 563
- WinGel Liquid & Tablets ▣ 761

Aluminum Hydroxide Gel (May substantially decrease plasma salicylate concentration). Products include:
- ALternaGEL Liquid 1154
- Aludrox Oral Suspension 2428
- Amphojel Suspension 2429
- Amphojel Suspension without Flavor 2429
- Mylanta Liquid 1155
- Mylanta Double Strength Liquid 1155

Aluminum Hydroxide Gel, Dried (May substantially decrease plasma salicylate concentration). Products include:
- Alu-Tab/Alu-Cap 1309
- Amphojel Tablets 2429
- Ascriptin A/D Caplets 1850
- Regular Strength Ascriptin Tablets 1850
- Gaviscon Antacid Tablets ▣ 593
- Gaviscon-2 Antacid Tablets ▣ 594
- Mylanta Tablets 1155
- Mylanta Double Strength Tablets 1155

Amitriptyline Hydrochloride (Additive effects). Products include:
- Elavil 2269
- Endep Tablets 1927
- Etrafon 2087
- Limbitrol 1933
- Triavil Tablets 1556

Ammonium Chloride (Elevated plasma salicylate concentrations). Products include:
- Quelidrine Syrup 556

Amoxapine (Additive effects). Products include:
- Asendin Tablets 1196

Aprobarbital (Additive effects). Products include:
- Alurate Elixir 1883

Betamethasone Acetate (May decrease salicylate plasma levels). Products include:
- Celestone Soluspan Suspension 2081

Betamethasone Sodium Phosphate (May decrease salicylate plasma levels). Products include:
- Celestone Soluspan Suspension 2081

Buprenorphine (Additive effects).
- No products indexed under this heading.

Buspirone Hydrochloride (Additive effects). Products include:
- BuSpar 1401

Butabarbital (Additive effects). Products include:
- Pyridium Plus 1764

Butalbital (Additive effects). Products include:
- Esgic-Plus Tablets 1002
- Esgic Tablets & Capsules 1001
- Fioricet Tablets 2006
- Fiorinal Capsules 2007
- Fiorinal with Codeine Capsules 2008
- Fiorinal Tablets 2007
- Phrenilin 838
- Sedapap Tablets 50 mg/650 mg 1360

Chlordiazepoxide (Additive effects). Products include:
- Libritabs Tablets 1930

Limbitrol 1933
Menrium Tablets 1934

Chlordiazepoxide Hydrochloride (Additive effects). Products include:
Librax Capsules 1929
Librium Capsules 1931
Librium Injectable 1932

Chlorpromazine (Additive effects). Products include:
Thorazine 2234

Chlorpropamide (Possible enhancement of hypoglycemia). Products include:
Diabinese Tablets 1775

Chlorprothixene (Additive effects). Products include:
Taractan Tablets 1920

Chlorprothixene Hydrochloride (Additive effects). Products include:
Taractan 1920

Clorazepate Dipotassium (Additive effects). Products include:
Tranxene 556

Codeine (Additive effects). Products include:
Calcidrine Syrup 506

Codeine Polistirex (Additive effects).
No products indexed under this heading.

Cortisone Acetate (May decrease salicylate plasma levels). Products include:
Cortone Acetate Sterile Suspension 1437
Cortone Acetate Tablets 1439

Desipramine Hydrochloride (Additive effects). Products include:
Norpramin Tablets 1340

Dexamethasone (May decrease salicylate plasma levels). Products include:
AK-Trol Ointment & Suspension .... ◉ 207
Decadron Elixir 1445
Decadron Tablets 1447
Decaspray Topical Aerosol 1459
Dexacidin .... ◉ 272
Maxidex Sterile Ophthalmic Suspension .... ◉ 223
Maxitrol Ophthalmic Ointment/Suspension .... ◉ 223
TobraDex Ophthalmic Suspension and Ointment .... ◉ 228

Dexamethasone Acetate (May decrease salicylate plasma levels). Products include:
Dalalone D.P. Injectable 999
Decadron-LA Sterile Suspension 1457

Dexamethasone Sodium Phosphate (May decrease salicylate plasma levels). Products include:
AK-Dex .... ◉ 203
Decadron Phosphate Respihaler 1454
Decadron Phosphate Sterile Ophthalmic Ointment 1453
Decadron Phosphate Sterile Ophthalmic Solution 1453
Decadron Phosphate Topical Cream 1455
Decadron Phosphate Turbinaire 1456
Maxidex Sterile Ophthalmic Ointment .... ◉ 222
NeoDecadron Sterile Ophthalmic Ointment 1517
NeoDecadron Sterile Ophthalmic Solution 1518
NeoDecadron Topical Cream 1518

Dezocine (Additive effects).

Diazepam (Additive effects). Products include:
Valium Injectable 1937
Valium Tablets 1939
Valrelease Capsules 1923

Dicumarol (Enhanced potential for bleeding). Products include:
Dicumarol Tablets 516

Dihydroxyaluminum Sodium Carbonate (May substantially decrease plasma salicylate concentration). Products include:
Rolaids .... ▣ 743

Doxepin Hydrochloride (Additive effects). Products include:
Sinequan 1960

Droperidol (Additive effects). Products include:
Inapsine Injection 1140
Innovar Injection 1141

Enflurane (Additive effects). Products include:
Ethrane 599

Estazolam (Additive effects). Products include:
ProSom Tablets 554

Ethchlorvynol (Additive effects). Products include:
Placidyl Capsules 553

Ethinamate (Additive effects).
No products indexed under this heading.

Fentanyl (Additive effects). Products include:
Duragesic Transdermal System 1133

Fentanyl Citrate (Additive effects). Products include:
Innovar Injection 1141
Sublimaze Injection 1146

Fluphenazine Decanoate (Additive effects). Products include:
Prolixin Decanoate 1795

Fluphenazine Enanthate (Additive effects). Products include:
Prolixin Enanthate 1796

Fluphenazine Hydrochloride (Additive effects). Products include:
Prolixin Elixir 1793
Prolixin Injection 1791
Prolixin Oral Concentrate 1792
Prolixin Tablets 1793

Flurazepam Hydrochloride (Additive effects). Products include:
Dalmane Capsules 1927

Glipizide (Possible enhancement of hypoglycemia). Products include:
Glucotrol 1952

Glutethimide (Additive effects).
No products indexed under this heading.

Glyburide (Possible enhancement of hypoglycemia). Products include:
DiaBeta 1091
Micronase Tablets 2350

Haloperidol (Additive effects). Products include:
Haldol Injection, Tablets and Concentrate 1373

Haloperidol Decanoate (Additive effects). Products include:
Haldol Decanoate 1375

Hydrocodone Bitartrate (Additive effects). Products include:
Anexsia 5/500 Tablets 2196
Anexsia 7.5/650 Tablets 2197
Azdōne Tablets 844
Codiclear DH Syrup 845
Codimal DH Syrup 846
Damason-P 1356
Hycodan Syrup, Tablets 927
Hycomine Compound Tablets 929
Hycomine Syrup 927
Hycotuss Expectorant Syrup 930
Hydrocet Capsules 835
Lortab ASA Tablets 2414
Lortab 2412
Ru-Tuss with Hydrocodone 694
Triaminic Expectorant DH 1995
Vicodin Tablets 1187
Vicodin ES Tablets 1189
Zydone Capsules 941

Hydrocodone Polistirex (Additive effects). Products include:
Tussionex Extended-Release Suspension 988

Hydrocortisone (May decrease salicylate plasma levels). Products include:
AK-Spore H.C. .... ◉ 206
Bactine Hydrocortisone Anti-Itch Cream .... ▣ 625
CaldeCORT Anti-Itch Hydrocortisone Spray .... ▣ 560
Carmol HC Cream 1% 2296
Cortaid Spray .... ▣ 735
Cortenema 2244
Cortisporin Ointment 758
Cortisporin Ophthalmic Ointment Sterile 758
Cortisporin Ophthalmic Suspension Sterile 759
Cortisporin Otic Solution Sterile 760
Cortisporin Otic Suspension Sterile 760
Cortizone-5 Creme & Ointment .... ▣ 732
Dermolate Anti-Itch Cream .... ▣ 697
Eldecort Cream 1.0% 1113
Eldecort Cream 1.0% and 2.5% 1113
Fungoid HC Creme 1770
Hydrocortone Tablets 1482
Hytone 909
LazerSporin-C Solution 1770
Massengill Medicated Soft Cloth Towelettes 2192
Nutracort Cream & Lotion 1684
PediOtic Suspension Sterile 797
Synacort Creams 1%, 2.5% 2296
Vanoxide-HC Acne Lotion 911
Vioform-Hydrocortisone Cream and Mild Cream 889
Vioform-Hydrocortisone Ointment 889
VōSoL HC Otic Solution 2392
Vytone Cream 1% 911

Hydrocortisone Acetate (May decrease salicylate plasma levels). Products include:
Analpram-HC Rectal Cream 1% and 2.5% 970
Anusol-HC Cream 1690
Anusol-HC Suppositories 1691
Caldecort .... ▣ 560
Carmol HC Cream 1% 2296
Chloromycetin Hydrocortisone Ophthalmic 1694
Coly-Mycin S Otic w/Neomycin & Hydrocortisone 1708
Cortaid .... ▣ 735
Cortef Feminine Itch Cream .... ▣ 735
Corticaine .... ▣ 682
Cortifoam 1827
Cortisporin Cream 757
Epifoam 1828
Gynecort 5 Creme .... ▣ 556
Hydrocortone Acetate Sterile Suspension 1479
Lanacort 5 Creme and Ointment .... ▣ 557
Mantadil Cream 789
Ophthocort .... ◉ 301
Orabase HCA Oral Paste 890
Pramosone Cream, Lotion & Ointment 971
ProctoCream-HC 1834
Proctofoam-HC 1835

Hydrocortisone Sodium Phosphate (May decrease salicylate plasma levels). Products include:
Hydrocortone Phosphate Injection, Sterile 1481

Hydrocortisone Sodium Succinate (May decrease salicylate plasma levels). Products include:
Solu-Cortef Sterile Powder 2361

Hydroxyzine Hydrochloride (Additive effects). Products include:
Atarax Tablets & Syrup 1941
Marax Tablets & DF Syrup 1954
Vistaril Intramuscular Solution 1970

Imipramine Hydrochloride (Additive effects). Products include:
Tofranil Ampuls 1038
Tofranil Tablets 1039

Imipramine Pamoate (Additive effects). Products include:
Tofranil-PM Capsules 1041

Isocarboxazid (Additive effects). Products include:
Marplan Tablets 1906

Isoflurane (Additive effects). Products include:
Forane 600

Ketamine Hydrochloride (Additive effects). Products include:
Ketalar 1726

Levorphanol Tartrate (Additive effects). Products include:
Levo-Dromoran 1906

Lithium Carbonate (Additive effects). Products include:
Eskalith 2214
Lithane Tablets 1596
Lithium Carbonate Capsules & Tablets 1984
Lithobid Tablets 870

Lithium Citrate (Additive effects). Products include:
Cibalith-S 870

Lorazepam (Additive effects). Products include:
Ativan Injection 2432
Ativan Tablets 2434

Loxapine Hydrochloride (Additive effects). Products include:
Loxitane 1213

Loxapine Succinate (Additive effects). Products include:
Loxitane Capsules 1213

Magaldrate (May substantially decrease plasma salicylate concentration). Products include:
Riopan Antacid Chew Tablets .... ▣ 754
Riopan Antacid Chew Tablets in Rollpacks .... ▣ 754
Riopan Antacid Suspension 2421
Riopan Antacid Swallow Tablets 2421
Riopan Plus Chew Tablets 2422
Riopan Plus Chew Tablets in Rollpack 2422
Riopan Plus 2 Chew Tablets, Mint Flavor, Cherry Flavor 2422
Riopan Plus Suspension 2422
Riopan Plus 2 Suspension, Mint Flavor, Cherry Flavor 2422

Magnesium Hydroxide (May substantially decrease plasma salicylate concentration). Products include:
Aludrox Oral Suspension 2428
Ascriptin A/D Caplets 1850
Regular Strength Ascriptin Tablets 1850
Di-Gel Antacid/Anti-Gas .... ▣ 697
Gelusil Liquid & Tablets .... ▣ 639
Haley's M-O, Regular & Flavored .... ▣ 569
Extra Strength Maalox Plus Suspension 1850
Maalox TC Suspension 1851
Maalox Plus Tablets .... ▣ 655
Extra Strength Maalox Plus Tablets 1850
Mylanta Liquid 1155
Mylanta Tablets 1155
Mylanta Double Strength Liquid 1155
Mylanta Double Strength Tablets 1155
Concentrated Phillips' Milk of Magnesia .... ▣ 573
Phillips' Milk of Magnesia Liquid .... ▣ 572
Phillips' Milk of Magnesia Tablets .... ▣ 573
WinGel Liquid & Tablets .... ▣ 761

Magnesium Oxide (May substantially decrease plasma salicylate concentration). Products include:
Bayer Plus Aspirin Tablets .... ▣ 567
Beelith Tablets 659
Bufferin Analgesic Tablets and Caplets .... ▣ 524
Cama Arthritis Pain Reliever .... ▣ 685
Mag-Ox 400 673
Uro-Mag 673

Maprotiline Hydrochloride (Additive effects). Products include:
Ludiomil Tablets 874

Meperidine Hydrochloride (Additive effects). Products include:
Demerol 2047
Mepergan Injection 2479

Mephobarbital (Additive effects). Products include:
Mebaral Tablets 2061

Meprobamate (Additive effects). Products include:
Deprol Tablets 2382
Equagesic Tablets 2451
Miltown Tablets 2386
PMB 200 and PMB 400 2504

Mesoridazine (Additive effects). Products include:
Serentil 686
Methadone Hydrochloride (Additive effects). Products include:
Dolophine Hydrochloride Ampoules & Vials 1260
Dolophine Hydrochloride Tablets 1261
Methadone Hydrochloride Diskets .. 1284
Methadone Hydrochloride Oral Solution & Tablets 1987
Methohexital Sodium (Additive effects). Products include:
Brevital Sodium Vials 1248
Methotrexate Sodium (Toxic effects of methotrexate enhanced). Products include:
Methotrexate Tablets, Parenteral, LPF Parenteral 1217
Rheumatrex Methotrexate Dose Pack 1234
Methoxyflurane (Additive effects).
No products indexed under this heading.
Methylprednisolone Acetate (May decrease salicylate plasma levels). Products include:
Depo-Medrol Sterile Aqueous Suspension 2334
Methylprednisolone Sodium Succinate (May decrease salicylate plasma levels). Products include:
Solu-Medrol Sterile Powder 2363
Midazolam Hydrochloride (Additive effects). Products include:
Versed Injection 1924
Molindone Hydrochloride (Additive effects). Products include:
Moban Tablets & Concentrate 932
Morphine Sulfate (Additive effects). Products include:
Astramorph/PF Injection, USP (Preservative-Free) 618
Duramorph 960
Infumorph 200 and Infumorph 500 Sterile Solutions 962
MS Contin Tablets 1814
MSIR 1817
Oramorph SR (Morphine Sulfate Sustained Release Tablets) 1988
Roxanol 1991
Nortriptyline Hydrochloride (Additive effects). Products include:
Pamelor 2019
Opium Alkaloids (Additive effects). Products include:
B & O No. 15A & No. 16A Supprettes 2395
Pantopon Injectable 1911
Oxazepam (Additive effects). Products include:
Serax Capsules 2522
Serax Tablets 2522
Oxycodone Hydrochloride (Additive effects). Products include:
Percocet Tablets 950
Percodan 951
Roxicodone Tablets, Oral Solution & Intensol (Oxycodone) 1992
Tylox Capsules 1382
Pentobarbital Sodium (Additive effects). Products include:
Nembutal Sodium Capsules 534
Nembutal Sodium Solution 536
Nembutal Sodium Suppositories 538
Perphenazine (Additive effects). Products include:
Etrafon 2087
Triavil Tablets 1556
Trilafon 2123
Phenelzine Sulfate (Additive effects). Products include:
Nardil 1742
Phenobarbital (Additive effects). Products include:
Arco-Lase Plus Tablets 607
Bellergal-S Tablets 1998
Bronkolixir .... ▣ 761
Bronkotabs Tablets .... ▣ 762
Donnatal 1858
Donnatal Extentabs 1859
Donnatal Tablets 1858
Donnazyme Tablets 1860
Kinesed Tablets 2272
Phenobarbital Elixir and Tablets 1293
Primatene Tablets-P Formula 2421
Quadrinal Tablets 1183
Tedral SA 1765
Potassium Acid Phosphate (Elevated plasma salicylate concentrations). Products include:
K-Phos M.F. Tablets 659
K-Phos Original Formula 'Sodium Free' Tablets 660
K-Phos No. 2 Tablets 659
Prazepam (Additive effects). Products include:
Centrax 1693
Prednisolone Acetate (May decrease salicylate plasma levels). Products include:
AK-Cide Sterile Ophthalmic Ointment & Suspension .... ⊙ 202
Blephamide Liquifilm Sterile Ophthalmic Suspension 586
Blephamide S.O.P. Sterile Ophthalmic Ointment 586
Cetapred Ointment .... ⊙ 220
⅛% Econopred & 1% Econopred Plus .... ⊙ 217
Isopto Cetapred Suspension .... ⊙ 220
Metimyd .... ⊙ 306
Poly-Pred Liquifilm .... ⊙ 250
Pred Forte .... ⊙ 252
Pred Mild .... ⊙ 254
Pred-G Liquifilm Sterile Ophthalmic Suspension .... ⊙ 252
Pred-G S.O.P. Sterile Ophthalmic Ointment .... ⊙ 253
Vasocidin Ointment .... ⊙ 275
Prednisolone Sodium Phosphate (May decrease salicylate plasma levels). Products include:
AK-Pred .... ⊙ 205
Hydeltrasol Injection, Sterile 1476
Inflamase .... ⊙ 274
Pediapred Oral Liquid 987
Vasocidin Ophthalmic Solution .... ⊙ 276
Prednisolone Tebutate (May decrease salicylate plasma levels). Products include:
Hydeltra-T.B.A. Sterile Suspension 1478
Prednisone (May decrease salicylate plasma levels). Products include:
Deltasone Tablets 2332
Probenecid (Possible reduced renal excretion of salicylate). Products include:
Benemid Tablets 1426
ColBENEMID Tablets 1436
Wycillin Injection and Probenecid Tablets 2539
Prochlorperazine (Additive effects). Products include:
Compazine 2201
Promethazine Hydrochloride (Additive effects). Products include:
Mepergan Injection 2479
Phenergan with Codeine 2497
Phenergan with Dextromethorphan 2499
Phenergan Injection 2493
Phenergan Suppositories 2496
Phenergan Syrup 2495
Phenergan Tablets 2496
Phenergan VC 2500
Phenergan VC with Codeine 2501
Propofol (Additive effects). Products include:
Diprivan Injection 2267
Propoxyphene Hydrochloride (Additive effects). Products include:
Darvon 1256
Wygesic Tablets 2540
Propoxyphene Napsylate (Additive effects). Products include:
Darvon-N/Darvocet-N 1254
Protriptyline Hydrochloride (Additive effects). Products include:
Vivactil Tablets 1567
Quazepam (Additive effects). Products include:
Doral Tablets 2383
Secobarbital Sodium (Additive effects). Products include:
Seconal Sodium Pulvules 1296
Sodium Acid Phosphate (Elevated plasma salicylate concentrations). Products include:
K-Phos No. 2 Tablets 659
Uroqid-Acid 661
Sodium Bicarbonate (May substantially decrease plasma salicylate concentration). Products include:
Alka-Seltzer Advanced Formula Antacid & Non-Aspirin Pain Reliever .... ▣ 620
Alka-Seltzer Effervescent Antacid ▣ 622
Alka-Seltzer Effervescent Antacid and Pain Reliever 1568
Alka-Seltzer Extra Strength Effervescent Antacid and Pain Reliever .... ▣ 623
Alka-Seltzer (Flavored) Effervescent Antacid and Pain Reliever .. ▣ 621
Arm & Hammer Pure Baking Soda .... ▣ 548
Ceo-Two Rectal Suppositories 671
Citrocarbonate Antacid .... ▣ 668
Massengill Liquid Concentrate 2191
NuLYTELY 699
Sufentanil Citrate (Additive effects). Products include:
Sufenta Injection 1147
Sulfinpyrazone (Reduced uricosuric effect of both drugs; possible reduced renal excretion of salicylate). Products include:
Anturane 853
Temazepam (Additive effects). Products include:
Restoril Capsules 2023
Thiamylal Sodium (Additive effects). Products include:
Surital Ampoules, Steri-Vials 1764
Thioridazine Hydrochloride (Additive effects). Products include:
Mellaril 2011
Thiothixene (Additive effects). Products include:
Navane Capsules and Concentrate 1954
Navane Intramuscular 1956
Tolazamide (Possible enhancement of hypoglycemia). Products include:
Tolinase Tablets 2365
Tolbutamide (Possible enhancement of hypoglycemia). Products include:
Orinase Tablets 2354
Tranylcypromine Sulfate (Additive effects). Products include:
Parnate Tablets 2222
Triamcinolone (May decrease salicylate plasma levels).
No products indexed under this heading.
Triamcinolone Acetonide (May decrease salicylate plasma levels). Products include:
Aristocort A 1010
Azmacort Inhaler 1837
Kenalog Cream, Lotion & Ointment 2401
Kenalog-10 Injection 2402
Kenalog-40 Injection 2403
Kenalog in Orabase 604
Kenalog Spray 2401
Mycolog II Cream and Ointment 2407
Mytrex Cream & Ointment 2080
Nasacort Nasal Inhaler 1844
Triamcinolone Diacetate (May decrease salicylate plasma levels). Products include:
Aristocort Suspension 1008
Triamcinolone Hexacetonide (May decrease salicylate plasma levels). Products include:
Aristospan Suspension 1011
Triazolam (Additive effects). Products include:
Halcion Tablets 2340
Trifluoperazine Hydrochloride (Additive effects). Products include:
Stelazine 2226
Trimipramine Maleate (Additive effects). Products include:
Surmontil Capsules 2524
Warfarin Sodium (Enhanced potential for bleeding). Products include:
Coumadin Injection & Tablets 944
Panwarfin Tablets 547

SOMA COMPOUND TABLETS
(Carisoprodol, Aspirin) 2389
May interact with central nervous system depressants, psychotropics, oral anticoagulants, oral hypoglycemic agents, antacids, corticosteroids, and certain other agents. Compounds in these categories include:

Alcohol (Additive effects including gastrointestinal bleeding).
Alfentanil Hydrochloride (Additive effects). Products include:
Alfenta Injection 1131
Alprazolam (Additive effects). Products include:
Xanax Tablets 2367
Aluminum Carbonate Gel (May substantially decrease plasma salicylate concentration). Products include:
Basaljel 2438
Aluminum Hydroxide (May substantially decrease plasma salicylate concentration). Products include:
Cama Arthritis Pain Reliever .... ▣ 685
Gaviscon Extra Strength Relief Formula Liquid Antacid .... ▣ 594
Gaviscon Extra Strength Relief Formula Antacid Tablets .... ▣ 594
Gaviscon Liquid Antacid .... ▣ 594
Gelusil Liquid & Tablets .... ▣ 639
Extra Strength Maalox Plus Suspension 1850
Maalox TC Suspension 1851
Maalox Plus Tablets .... ▣ 655
Extra Strength Maalox Plus Tablets 1850
Nephrox Suspension .... ▣ 563
WinGel Liquid & Tablets .... ▣ 761
Aluminum Hydroxide Gel (May substantially decrease plasma salicylate concentration). Products include:
ALternaGEL Liquid 1154
Aludrox Oral Suspension 2428
Amphojel Suspension 2429
Amphojel Suspension without Flavor 2429
Mylanta Liquid 1155
Mylanta Double Strength Liquid 1155
Aluminum Hydroxide Gel, Dried (May substantially decrease plasma salicylate concentration). Products include:
Alu-Tab/Alu-Cap 1309
Amphojel Tablets 2429
Ascriptin A/D Caplets 1850
Regular Strength Ascriptin Tablets 1850
Gaviscon Antacid Tablets .... ▣ 593
Gaviscon-2 Antacid Tablets .... ▣ 594
Mylanta Tablets 1155
Mylanta Double Strength Tablets 1155
Amitriptyline Hydrochloride (Additive effects). Products include:
Elavil 2269
Endep Tablets 1927
Etrafon 2087
Limbitrol 1933
Triavil Tablets 1556
Ammonium Chloride (Elevated plasma salicylate concentrations). Products include:
Quelidrine Syrup 556
Amoxapine (Additive effects). Products include:
Asendin Tablets 1196
Aprobarbital (Additive effects). Products include:
Alurate Elixir 1883

Betamethasone Acetate (May decrease salicylate plasma levels). Products include:
- Celestone Soluspan Suspension 2081

Betamethasone Sodium Phosphate (May decrease salicylate plasma levels). Products include:
- Celestone Soluspan Suspension 2081

Buprenorphine (Additive effects).
- No products indexed under this heading.

Buspirone Hydrochloride (Additive effects). Products include:
- BuSpar 1401

Butabarbital (Additive effects). Products include:
- Pyridium Plus 1764

Butalbital (Additive effects). Products include:
- Esgic-Plus Tablets 1002
- Esgic Tablets & Capsules 1001
- Fioricet Tablets 2006
- Fiorinal Capsules 2007
- Fiorinal with Codeine Capsules 2008
- Fiorinal Tablets 2007
- Phrenilin 838
- Sedapap Tablets 50 mg/650 mg .. 1360

Chlordiazepoxide (Additive effects). Products include:
- Libritabs Tablets 1930
- Limbitrol 1933
- Menrium Tablets 1934

Chlordiazepoxide Hydrochloride (Additive effects). Products include:
- Librax Capsules 1929
- Librium Capsules 1931
- Librium Injectable 1932

Chlorpromazine (Additive effects). Products include:
- Thorazine 2234

Chlorpropamide (Possible enhancement of hypoglycemia). Products include:
- Diabinese Tablets 1775

Chlorprothixene (Additive effects). Products include:
- Taractan Tablets 1920

Chlorprothixene Hydrochloride (Additive effects). Products include:
- Taractan 1920

Clorazepate Dipotassium (Additive effects). Products include:
- Tranxene 556

Codeine (Additive effects). Products include:
- Calcidrine Syrup 506

Codeine Phosphate (Additive effects). Products include:
- Actifed with Codeine Cough Syrup.. 752
- Cheracol Cough Syrup 1853
- Codimal PH Syrup 846
- Dimetane-DC Cough Syrup 1857
- Empirin with Codeine Phosphate Nos. 2, 3 & 4 764
- Fiorinal with Codeine Capsules 2008
- Isoclor Expectorant 982
- Naldecon CX Adult Liquid ...... ▣ 521
- Novahistine DH 1342
- Novahistine Expectorant 1343
- Nucofed Capsules 2219
- Nucofed Expectorant 2219
- Nucofed Pediatric Expectorant 2220
- Nucofed Syrup 2219
- Phenaphen with Codeine Capsules 1865
- Phenaphen-650 with Codeine Tablets 1866
- Phenergan with Codeine 2497
- Phenergan VC with Codeine 2501
- Robitussin A-C Syrup 1875
- Robitussin-DAC Syrup 1875
- Ryna ...... ▣ 741
- Soma Compound w/Codeine Tablets 2390
- Triaminic Expectorant w/Codeine .. 1996
- Tussi-Organidin Liquid 2391
- Tylenol with Codeine 1381

Codeine Polistirex (Additive effect).
- No products indexed under this heading.

Cortisone Acetate (May decrease salicylate plasma levels). Products include:
- Cortone Acetate Sterile Suspension 1437
- Cortone Acetate Tablets 1439

Desipramine Hydrochloride (Additive effects). Products include:
- Norpramin Tablets 1340

Dexamethasone (May decrease salicylate plasma levels). Products include:
- AK-Trol Ointment & Suspension .... ◉ 207
- Decadron Elixir 1445
- Decadron Tablets 1447
- Decaspray Topical Aerosol 1459
- Dexacidin ...... ◉ 272
- Maxidex Sterile Ophthalmic Suspension ...... ◉ 223
- Maxitrol Ophthalmic Ointment/Suspension ...... ◉ 223
- TobraDex Ophthalmic Suspension and Ointment ...... ◉ 228

Dexamethasone Acetate (May decrease salicylate plasma levels). Products include:
- Dalalone D.P. Injectable 999
- Decadron-LA Sterile Suspension 1457

Dexamethasone Sodium Phosphate (May decrease salicylate plasma levels). Products include:
- AK-Dex ...... ◉ 203
- Decadron Phosphate Respihaler 1454
- Decadron Phosphate Sterile Ophthalmic Ointment 1453
- Decadron Phosphate Sterile Ophthalmic Solution 1453
- Decadron Phosphate Topical Cream 1455
- Decadron Phosphate Turbinaire 1456
- Maxidex Sterile Ophthalmic Ointment ...... ◉ 222
- NeoDecadron Sterile Ophthalmic Ointment 1517
- NeoDecadron Sterile Ophthalmic Solution 1518
- NeoDecadron Topical Cream 1518

Dezocine (Additive effects).

Diazepam (Additive effects). Products include:
- Valium Injectable 1937
- Valium Tablets 1939
- Valrelease Capsules 1923

Dicumarol (Enhanced potential for bleeding). Products include:
- Dicumarol Tablets 516

Dihydroxyaluminum Sodium Carbonate (May substantially decrease plasma salicylate concentration). Products include:
- Rolaids ...... ▣ 743

Doxepin Hydrochloride (Additive effects). Products include:
- Sinequan 1960

Droperidol (Additive effects). Products include:
- Inapsine Injection 1140
- Innovar Injection 1141

Enflurane (Additive effects). Products include:
- Ethrane 599

Estazolam (Additive effects). Products include:
- ProSom Tablets 554

Ethchlorvynol (Additive effects). Products include:
- Placidyl Capsules 553

Ethinamate (Additive effects).
- No products indexed under this heading.

Fentanyl (Additive effects). Products include:
- Duragesic Transdermal System 1133

Fentanyl Citrate (Additive effects). Products include:
- Innovar Injection 1141
- Sublimaze Injection 1146

Fluphenazine Decanoate (Additive effects). Products include:
- Prolixin Decanoate 1795

Fluphenazine Enanthate (Additive effects). Products include:
- Prolixin Enanthate 1796

Fluphenazine Hydrochloride (Additive effects). Products include:
- Prolixin Elixir 1793
- Prolixin Injection 1791
- Prolixin Oral Concentrate 1792
- Prolixin Tablets 1793

Flurazepam Hydrochloride (Additive effects). Products include:
- Dalmane Capsules 1927

Glipizide (Possible enhancement of hypoglycemia). Products include:
- Glucotrol 1952

Glutethimide (Additive effects).
- No products indexed under this heading.

Glyburide (Possible enhancement of hypoglycemia). Products include:
- DiaBeta 1091
- Micronase Tablets 2350

Haloperidol (Additive effects). Products include:
- Haldol Injection, Tablets and Concentrate 1373

Haloperidol Decanoate (Additive effects). Products include:
- Haldol Decanoate 1375

Hydrocodone Bitartrate (Additive effects). Products include:
- Anexsia 5/500 Tablets 2196
- Anexsia 7.5/650 Tablets 2197
- Azdöne Tablets 844
- Codiclear DH Syrup 845
- Codimal DH Syrup 846
- Damason-P 1356
- Hycodan Syrup, Tablets 927
- Hycomine Compound Tablets 929
- Hycomine Syrup 927
- Hycotuss Expectorant Syrup 930
- Hydrocet Capsules 835
- Lortab ASA Tablets 2414
- Lortab 2412
- Ru-Tuss with Hydrocodone 694
- Triaminic Expectorant DH 1995
- Vicodin Tablets 1187
- Vicodin ES Tablets 1189
- Zydone Capsules 941

Hydrocodone Polistirex (Additive effects). Products include:
- Tussionex Extended-Release Suspension 988

Hydrocortisone (May decrease salicylate plasma levels). Products include:
- AK-Spore H.C. ...... ◉ 206
- Bactine Hydrocortisone Anti-Itch Cream ...... ▣ 625
- CaldeCORT Anti-Itch Hydrocortisone Spray ...... ▣ 560
- Carmol HC Cream 1% 2296
- Cortaid Spray ...... ▣ 735
- Cortenema 2244
- Cortisporin Ointment 758
- Cortisporin Ophthalmic Ointment Sterile 758
- Cortisporin Ophthalmic Suspension Sterile 759
- Cortisporin Otic Solution Sterile 760
- Cortisporin Otic Suspension Sterile 760
- Cortizone-5 Creme & Ointment ...... ▣ 732
- Dermolate Anti-Itch Cream ...... ▣ 697
- Eldecort Cream 1.0% 1113
- Eldecort Cream 1.0% and 2.5% 1113
- Fungoid HC Creme 1770
- Hydrocortone Tablets 1482
- Hytone 909
- LazerSporin-C Solution 1770
- Massengill Medicated Soft Cloth Towelettes 2192
- Nutracort Cream & Lotion 1684
- PediOtic Suspension Sterile 797
- Synacort Creams 1%, 2.5% 2296
- Vanoxide-HC Acne Lotion 911
- Vioform-Hydrocortisone Cream and Mild Cream 889
- Vioform-Hydrocortisone Ointment.. 889
- VōSoL HC Otic Solution 2392
- Vytone Cream 1% 911

Hydrocortisone Acetate (May decrease salicylate plasma levels). Products include:
- Analpram-HC Rectal Cream 1% and 2.5% 970
- Anusol-HC Cream 1690
- Anusol-HC Suppositories 1691
- Caldecort ...... ▣ 560
- Carmol HC Cream 1% 2296
- Chloromycetin Hydrocortisone Ophthalmic 1694
- Coly-Mycin S Otic w/Neomycin & Hydrocortisone 1708
- Cortaid ...... ▣ 735
- Cortef Feminine Itch Cream ...... ▣ 735
- Corticaine ...... ▣ 682
- Cortifoam 1827
- Cortisporin Cream 757
- Epifoam 1828
- Gynecort 5 Creme ...... ▣ 556
- Hydrocortone Acetate Sterile Suspension 1479
- Lanacort 5 Creme and Ointment .. ▣ 557
- Mantadil Cream 789
- Ophthocort ...... ◉ 301
- Orabase HCA Oral Paste 890
- Pramosone Cream, Lotion & Ointment 971
- ProctoCream-HC 1834
- Proctofoam-HC 1835

Hydrocortisone Sodium Phosphate (May decrease salicylate plasma levels). Products include:
- Hydrocortone Phosphate Injection, Sterile 1481

Hydrocortisone Sodium Succinate (May decrease salicylate plasma levels). Products include:
- Solu-Cortef Sterile Powder 2361

Hydroxyzine Hydrochloride (Additive effects). Products include:
- Atarax Tablets & Syrup 1941
- Marax Tablets & DF Syrup 1954
- Vistaril Intramuscular Solution 1970

Imipramine Hydrochloride (Additive effects). Products include:
- Tofranil Ampuls 1038
- Tofranil Tablets 1039

Imipramine Pamoate (Additive effects). Products include:
- Tofranil-PM Capsules 1041

Isocarboxazid (Additive effects). Products include:
- Marplan Tablets 1906

Isoflurane (Additive effects). Products include:
- Forane 600

Ketamine Hydrochloride (Additive effects). Products include:
- Ketalar 1726

Levorphanol Tartrate (Additive effects). Products include:
- Levo-Dromoran 1906

Lithium Carbonate (Additive effects). Products include:
- Eskalith 2214
- Lithane Tablets 1596
- Lithium Carbonate Capsules & Tablets 1984
- Lithobid Tablets 870

Lithium Citrate (Additive effects). Products include:
- Cibalith-S 870

Lorazepam (Additive effects). Products include:
- Ativan Injection 2432
- Ativan Tablets 2434

Loxapine Hydrochloride (Additive effects). Products include:
- Loxitane 1213

Loxapine Succinate (Additive effects). Products include:
- Loxitane Capsules 1213

Magaldrate (May substantially decrease plasma salicylate concentration). Products include:
- Riopan Antacid Chew Tablets ...... ▣ 754
- Riopan Antacid Chew Tablets in Rollpacks ...... ▣ 754
- Riopan Antacid Suspension 2421
- Riopan Antacid Swallow Tablets 2421
- Riopan Plus Chew Tablets 2422
- Riopan Plus Chew Tablets in Rollpack 2422
- Riopan Plus 2 Chew Tablets, Mint Flavor, Cherry Flavor 2422
- Riopan Plus Suspension 2422

Riopan Plus 2 Suspension, Mint Flavor, Cherry Flavor 2422

Magnesium Hydroxide (May substantially decrease plasma salicylate concentration). Products include:
- Aludrox Oral Suspension 2428
- Ascriptin A/D Caplets 1850
- Regular Strength Ascriptin Tablets 1850
- Di-Gel Antacid/Anti-Gas .... ▣ 697
- Gelusil Liquid & Tablets .... ▣ 639
- Haley's M-O, Regular & Flavored .. ▣ 569
- Extra Strength Maalox Plus Suspension 1850
- Maalox TC Suspension 1851
- Maalox Plus Tablets .... ▣ 655
- Extra Strength Maalox Plus Tablets 1850
- Mylanta Liquid 1155
- Mylanta Tablets 1155
- Mylanta Double Strength Liquid 1155
- Mylanta Double Strength Tablets 1155
- Concentrated Phillips' Milk of Magnesia .... ▣ 573
- Phillips' Milk of Magnesia Liquid.... ▣ 572
- Phillips' Milk of Magnesia Tablets ▣ 573
- WinGel Liquid & Tablets .... ▣ 761

Magnesium Oxide (May substantially decrease plasma salicylate concentration). Products include:
- Bayer Plus Aspirin Tablets........ ▣ 567
- Beelith Tablets 659
- Bufferin Analgesic Tablets and Caplets .... ▣ 524
- Cama Arthritis Pain Reliever........ ▣ 685
- Mag-Ox 400 673
- Uro-Mag 673

Maprotiline Hydrochloride (Additive effects). Products include:
- Ludiomil Tablets 874

Meperidine Hydrochloride (Additive effects). Products include:
- Demerol 2047
- Mepergan Injection 2479

Mephobarbital (Additive effects). Products include:
- Mebaral Tablets 2061

Meprobamate (Additive effects). Products include:
- Deprol Tablets 2382
- Equagesic Tablets 2451
- Miltown Tablets 2386
- PMB 200 and PMB 400 2504

Mesoridazine (Additive effects). Products include:
- Serentil 686

Methadone Hydrochloride (Additive effects). Products include:
- Dolophine Hydrochloride Ampoules & Vials 1260
- Dolophine Hydrochloride Tablets 1261
- Methadone Hydrochloride Diskets .. 1284
- Methadone Hydrochloride Oral Solution & Tablets 1987

Methohexital Sodium (Additive effects). Products include:
- Brevital Sodium Vials 1248

Methotrexate Sodium (Toxic effects of metotrexate enhanced). Products include:
- Methotrexate Tablets, Parenteral, LPF Parenteral 1217
- Rheumatrex Methotrexate Dose Pack 1234

Methoxyflurane (Additive effects).
- No products indexed under this heading.

Methylprednisolone Acetate (May decrease salicylate plasma levels). Products include:
- Depo-Medrol Sterile Aqueous Suspension 2334

Methylprednisolone Sodium Succinate (May decrease salicylate plasma levels). Products include:
- Solu-Medrol Sterile Powder 2363

Midazolam Hydrochloride (Additive effects). Products include:
- Versed Injection 1924

Molindone Hydrochloride (Additive effects). Products include:
- Moban Tablets & Concentrate 932

Morphine Sulfate (Additive effects). Products include:
- Astramorph/PF Injection, USP (Preservative-Free) 618
- Duramorph 960
- Infumorph 200 and Infumorph 500 Sterile Solutions 962
- MS Contin Tablets 1814
- MSIR 1817
- Oramorph SR (Morphine Sulfate Sustained Release Tablets) 1988
- Roxanol 1991

Nortriptyline Hydrochloride (Additive effects). Products include:
- Pamelor 2019

Opium Alkaloids (Additive effects). Products include:
- B & O No. 15A & No. 16A Supprettes 2395
- Pantopon Injectable 1911

Oxazepam (Additive effects). Products include:
- Serax Capsules 2522
- Serax Tablets 2522

Oxycodone Hydrochloride (Additive effects). Products include:
- Percocet Tablets 950
- Percodan 951
- Roxicodone Tablets, Oral Solution & Intensol (Oxycodone) 1992
- Tylox Capsules 1382

Pentobarbital Sodium (Additive effects). Products include:
- Nembutal Sodium Capsules 534
- Nembutal Sodium Solution 536
- Nembutal Sodium Suppositories...... 538

Perphenazine (Additive effects). Products include:
- Etrafon 2087
- Triavil Tablets 1556
- Trilafon 2123

Phenelzine Sulfate (Additive effects). Products include:
- Nardil 1742

Phenobarbital (Additive effects). Products include:
- Arco-Lase Plus Tablets 607
- Bellergal-S Tablets 1998
- Bronkolixir .... ▣ 761
- Bronkotabs Tablets .... ▣ 762
- Donnatal 1858
- Donnatal Extentabs 1859
- Donnatal Tablets 1858
- Donnazyme Tablets 1860
- Kinesed Tablets 2272
- Phenobarbital Elixir and Tablets 1293
- Primatene Tablets-P Formula 2421
- Quadrinal Tablets 1183
- Tedral SA 1765

Potassium Acid Phosphate (Elevated plasma salicylate concentrations). Products include:
- K-Phos M.F. Tablets 659
- K-Phos Original Formula 'Sodium Free' Tablets 660
- K-Phos No. 2 Tablets 659

Prazepam (Additive effects). Products include:
- Centrax 1693

Prednisolone Acetate (May decrease salicylate plasma levels). Products include:
- AK-Cide Sterile Ophthalmic Ointment & Suspension .... ⊙ 202
- Blephamide Liquifilm Sterile Ophthalmic Suspension 586
- Blephamide S.O.P. Sterile Ophthalmic Ointment 586
- Cetapred Ointment .... ⊙ 220
- ⅛% Econopred & 1% Econopred Plus .... ⊙ 217
- Isopto Cetapred Suspension .... ⊙ 220
- Metimyd .... ⊙ 306
- Poly-Pred Liquifilm .... ⊙ 250
- Pred Forte .... ⊙ 252
- Pred Mild .... ⊙ 254
- Pred-G Liquifilm Sterile Ophthalmic Suspension .... ⊙ 252
- Pred-G S.O.P. Sterile Ophthalmic Ointment .... ⊙ 253
- Vasocidin Ointment .... ⊙ 275

Prednisolone Sodium Phosphate (May decrease salicylate plasma levels). Products include:
- AK-Pred .... ⊙ 205
- Hydeltrasol Injection, Sterile 1476
- Inflamase .... ⊙ 274
- Pediapred Oral Liquid 987
- Vasocidin Ophthalmic Solution ...... ⊙ 276

Prednisolone Tebutate (May decrease salicylate plasma levels). Products include:
- Hydeltra-T.B.A. Sterile Suspension 1478

Prednisone (May decrease salicylate plasma levels). Products include:
- Deltasone Tablets 2332

Probenecid (Reduced uricosuric effect of both drugs; possible reduced renal excretion of salicylate). Products include:
- Benemid Tablets 1426
- ColBENEMID Tablets 1436
- Wycillin Injection and Probenecid Tablets 2539

Prochlorperazine (Additive effects). Products include:
- Compazine 2201

Promethazine Hydrochloride (Additive effects). Products include:
- Mepergan Injection 2479
- Phenergan with Codeine 2497
- Phenergan with Dextromethorphan 2499
- Phenergan Injection 2493
- Phenergan Suppositories 2496
- Phenergan Syrup 2495
- Phenergan Tablets 2496
- Phenergan VC 2500
- Phenergan VC with Codeine 2501

Propofol (Additive effects). Products include:
- Diprivan Injection 2267

Propoxyphene Hydrochloride (Additive effects). Products include:
- Darvon 1256
- Wygesic Tablets 2540

Propoxyphene Napsylate (Additive effects). Products include:
- Darvon-N/Darvocet-N 1254

Protriptyline Hydrochloride (Additive effects). Products include:
- Vivactil Tablets 1567

Quazepam (Additive effects). Products include:
- Doral Tablets 2383

Secobarbital Sodium (Additive effects). Products include:
- Seconal Sodium Pulvules 1296

Sodium Acid Phosphate (Elevated plasma salicylate concentrations). Products include:
- K-Phos No. 2 Tablets 659
- Uroqid-Acid 661

Sodium Bicarbonate (May substantially decrease plasma salicylate concentration). Products include:
- Alka-Seltzer Advanced Formula Antacid & Non-Aspirin Pain Reliever .... ▣ 620
- Alka-Seltzer Effervescent Antacid ▣ 622
- Alka-Seltzer Effervescent Antacid and Pain Reliever 1568
- Alka-Seltzer Extra Strength Effervescent Antacid and Pain Reliever .... ▣ 623
- Alka-Seltzer (Flavored) Effervescent Antacid and Pain Reliever .. ▣ 621
- Arm & Hammer Pure Baking Soda .... ▣ 548
- Ceo-Two Rectal Suppositories 671
- Citrocarbonate Antacid .... ▣ 668
- Massengill Liquid Concentrate 2191
- NuLYTELY 699

Sufentanil Citrate (Additive effects). Products include:
- Sufenta Injection 1147

Sulfinpyrazone (Reduced uricosuric effect of both drugs; possible reduced renal excretion of salicylate). Products include:
- Anturane 853

Temazepam (Additive effects). Products include:
- Restoril Capsules 2023

Thiamylal Sodium (Additive effects). Products include:
- Surital Ampoules, Steri-Vials 1764

Thioridazine Hydrochloride (Additive effects). Products include:
- Mellaril 2011

Thiothixene (Additive effects). Products include:
- Navane Capsules and Concentrate 1954
- Navane Intramuscular 1956

Tolazamide (Possible enhancement of hypoglycemia). Products include:
- Tolinase Tablets 2365

Tolbutamide (Possible enhancement of hypoglycemia). Products include:
- Orinase Tablets 2354

Tranylcypromine Sulfate (Additive effects). Products include:
- Parnate Tablets 2222

Triamcinolone (May decrease salicylate plasma levels).
- No products indexed under this heading.

Triamcinolone Acetonide (May decrease salicylate plasma levels). Products include:
- Aristocort A 1010
- Azmacort Inhaler 1837
- Kenalog Cream, Lotion & Ointment 2401
- Kenalog-10 Injection 2402
- Kenalog-40 Injection 2403
- Kenalog in Orabase 604
- Kenalog Spray 2401
- Mycolog II Cream and Ointment 2407
- Mytrex Cream & Ointment 2080
- Nasacort Nasal Inhaler 1844

Triamcinolone Diacetate (May decrease salicylate plasma levels). Products include:
- Aristocort Suspension 1008

Triamcinolone Hexacetonide (May decrease salicylate plasma levels). Products include:
- Aristospan Suspension 1011

Triazolam (Additive effects). Products include:
- Halcion Tablets 2340

Trifluoperazine Hydrochloride (Additive effects). Products include:
- Stelazine 2226

Trimipramine Maleate (Additive effects). Products include:
- Surmontil Capsules 2524

Warfarin Sodium (Enhanced potential for bleeding). Products include:
- Coumadin Injection & Tablets 944
- Panwarfin Tablets 547

SOMA TABLETS
(Carisoprodol) 2388
May interact with central nervous system depressants and psychotropics. Compounds in these categories include:

Alcohol (Additive effects).

Alfentanil Hydrochloride (Additive effects). Products include:
- Alfenta Injection 1131

Alprazolam (Additive effects). Products include:
- Xanax Tablets 2367

Amitriptyline Hydrochloride (Additive effects). Products include:
- Elavil 2269
- Endep Tablets 1927
- Etrafon 2087
- Limbitrol 1933
- Triavil Tablets 1556

Amoxapine (Additive effects). Products include:
- Asendin Tablets 1196

Aprobarbital (Additive effects). Products include:
Alurate Elixir ... 1883

Buprenorphine (Additive effects).
No products indexed under this heading.

Buspirone Hydrochloride (Additive effects). Products include:
BuSpar ... 1401

Butabarbital (Additive effects). Products include:
Pyridium Plus ... 1764

Butalbital (Additive effects). Products include:
Esgic-Plus Tablets ... 1002
Esgic Tablets & Capsules ... 1001
Fioricet Tablets ... 2006
Fiorinal Capsules ... 2007
Fiorinal with Codeine Capsules ... 2008
Fiorinal Tablets ... 2007
Phrenilin ... 838
Sedapap Tablets 50 mg/650 mg .. 1360

Chlordiazepoxide (Additive effects). Products include:
Libritabs Tablets ... 1930
Limbitrol ... 1933
Menrium Tablets ... 1934

Chlordiazepoxide Hydrochloride (Additive effects). Products include:
Librax Capsules ... 1929
Librium Capsules ... 1931
Librium Injectable ... 1932

Chlorpromazine (Additive effects). Products include:
Thorazine ... 2234

Chlorprothixene (Additive effects). Products include:
Taractan Tablets ... 1920

Chlorprothixene Hydrochloride (Additive effects). Products include:
Taractan ... 1920

Clorazepate Dipotassium (Additive effects). Products include:
Tranxene ... 556

Codeine (Additive effects). Products include:
Calcidrine Syrup ... 506

Codeine Phosphate (Additive effects). Products include:
Actifed with Codeine Cough Syrup.. 752
Cheracol Cough Syrup ... 1853
Codimal PH Syrup ... 846
Dimetane-DC Cough Syrup ... 1857
Empirin with Codeine Phosphate Nos. 2, 3 & 4 ... 764
Fiorinal with Codeine Capsules ... 2008
Isoclor Expectorant ... 982
Naldecon CX Adult Liquid ... 521
Novahistine DH ... 1342
Novahistine Expectorant ... 1343
Nucofed Capsules ... 2219
Nucofed Expectorant ... 2219
Nucofed Pediatric Expectorant ... 2220
Nucofed Syrup ... 2219
Phenaphen with Codeine Capsules 1865
Phenaphen-650 with Codeine Tablets ... 1866
Phenergan with Codeine ... 2497
Phenergan VC with Codeine ... 2501
Robitussin A-C Syrup ... 1875
Robitussin-DAC Syrup ... 1875
Ryna ... 741
Soma Compound w/Codeine Tablets ... 2390
Triaminic Expectorant w/Codeine .. 1996
Tussi-Organidin Liquid ... 2391
Tylenol with Codeine ... 1381

Codeine Polistirex (Additive effects).
No products indexed under this heading.

Desipramine Hydrochloride (Additive effects). Products include:
Norpramin Tablets ... 1340

Dezocine (Additive effects).

Diazepam (Additive effects). Products include:
Valium Injectable ... 1937
Valium Tablets ... 1939
Valrelease Capsules ... 1923

Doxepin Hydrochloride (Additive effects). Products include:
Sinequan ... 1960

Droperidol (Additive effects). Products include:
Inapsine Injection ... 1140
Innovar Injection ... 1141

Enflurane (Additive effects). Products include:
Ethrane ... 599

Estazolam (Additive effects). Products include:
ProSom Tablets ... 554

Ethchlorvynol (Additive effects). Products include:
Placidyl Capsules ... 553

Ethinamate (Additive effects).
No products indexed under this heading.

Fentanyl (Additive effects). Products include:
Duragesic Transdermal System ... 1133

Fentanyl Citrate (Additive effects). Products include:
Innovar Injection ... 1141
Sublimaze Injection ... 1146

Fluphenazine Decanoate (Additive effects). Products include:
Prolixin Decanoate ... 1795

Fluphenazine Enanthate (Additive effects). Products include:
Prolixin Enanthate ... 1796

Fluphenazine Hydrochloride (Additive effects). Products include:
Prolixin Elixir ... 1793
Prolixin Injection ... 1791
Prolixin Oral Concentrate ... 1792
Prolixin Tablets ... 1793

Flurazepam Hydrochloride (Additive effects). Products include:
Dalmane Capsules ... 1927

Glutethimide (Additive effects).
No products indexed under this heading.

Haloperidol (Additive effects). Products include:
Haldol Injection, Tablets and Concentrate ... 1373

Haloperidol Decanoate (Additive effects). Products include:
Haldol Decanoate ... 1375

Hydrocodone Bitartrate (Additive effects). Products include:
Anexsia 5/500 Tablets ... 2196
Anexsia 7.5/650 Tablets ... 2197
Azdone Tablets ... 844
Codiclear DH Syrup ... 845
Codimal DH Syrup ... 846
Damason-P ... 1356
Hycodan Syrup, Tablets ... 927
Hycomine Compound Tablets ... 929
Hycomine Syrup ... 927
Hycotuss Expectorant Syrup ... 930
Hydrocet Capsules ... 835
Lortab ASA Tablets ... 2414
Lortab ... 2412
Ru-Tuss with Hydrocodone ... 694
Triaminic Expectorant DH ... 1995
Vicodin Tablets ... 1187
Vicodin ES Tablets ... 1189
Zydone Capsules ... 941

Hydrocodone Polistirex (Additive effects). Products include:
Tussionex Extended-Release Suspension ... 988

Hydroxyzine Hydrochloride (Additive effects). Products include:
Atarax Tablets & Syrup ... 1941
Marax Tablets & DF Syrup ... 1954
Vistaril Intramuscular Solution ... 1970

Imipramine Hydrochloride (Additive effects). Products include:
Tofranil Ampuls ... 1038
Tofranil Tablets ... 1039

Imipramine Pamoate (Additive effects). Products include:
Tofranil-PM Capsules ... 1041

Isocarboxazid (Additive effects). Products include:
Marplan Tablets ... 1906

Isoflurane (Additive effects). Products include:
Forane ... 600

Ketamine Hydrochloride (Additive effects). Products include:
Ketalar ... 1726

Levorphanol Tartrate (Additive effects). Products include:
Levo-Dromoran ... 1906

Lithium Carbonate (Additive effects). Products include:
Eskalith ... 2214
Lithane Tablets ... 1596
Lithium Carbonate Capsules & Tablets ... 1984
Lithobid Tablets ... 870

Lithium Citrate (Additive effects). Products include:
Cibalith-S ... 870

Lorazepam (Additive effects). Products include:
Ativan Injection ... 2432
Ativan Tablets ... 2434

Loxapine Hydrochloride (Additive effects). Products include:
Loxitane ... 1213

Loxapine Succinate (Additive effects). Products include:
Loxitane Capsules ... 1213

Maprotiline Hydrochloride (Additive effects). Products include:
Ludiomil Tablets ... 874

Meperidine Hydrochloride (Additive effects). Products include:
Demerol ... 2047
Mepergan Injection ... 2479

Mephobarbital (Additive effects). Products include:
Mebaral Tablets ... 2061

Meprobamate (Additive effects). Products include:
Deprol Tablets ... 2382
Equagesic Tablets ... 2451
Miltown Tablets ... 2386
PMB 200 and PMB 400 ... 2504

Mesoridazine (Additive effects). Products include:
Serentil ... 686

Methadone Hydrochloride (Additive effects). Products include:
Dolophine Hydrochloride Ampoules & Vials ... 1260
Dolophine Hydrochloride Tablets ... 1261
Methadone Hydrochloride Diskets .. 1284
Methadone Hydrochloride Oral Solution & Tablets ... 1987

Methohexital Sodium (Additive effects). Products include:
Brevital Sodium Vials ... 1248

Methoxyflurane (Additive effects).
No products indexed under this heading.

Midazolam Hydrochloride (Additive effects). Products include:
Versed Injection ... 1924

Molindone Hydrochloride (Additive effects). Products include:
Moban Tablets & Concentrate ... 932

Morphine Sulfate (Additive effects). Products include:
Astramorph/PF Injection, USP (Preservative-Free) ... 618
Duramorph ... 960
Infumorph 200 and Infumorph 500 Sterile Solutions ... 962
MS Contin Tablets ... 1814
MSIR ... 1817
Oramorph SR (Morphine Sulfate Sustained Release Tablets) ... 1988
Roxanol ... 1991

Nortriptyline Hydrochloride (Additive effects). Products include:
Pamelor ... 2019

Opium Alkaloids (Additive effects). Products include:
B & O No. 15A & No. 16A Supprettes ... 2395
Pantopon Injectable ... 1911

Oxazepam (Additive effects). Products include:
Serax Capsules ... 2522
Serax Tablets ... 2522

Oxycodone Hydrochloride (Additive effects). Products include:
Percocet Tablets ... 950
Percodan ... 951
Roxicodone Tablets, Oral Solution & Intensol (Oxycodone) ... 1992
Tylox Capsules ... 1382

Pentobarbital Sodium (Additive effects). Products include:
Nembutal Sodium Capsules ... 534
Nembutal Sodium Solution ... 536
Nembutal Sodium Suppositories ... 538

Perphenazine (Additive effects). Products include:
Etrafon ... 2087
Triavil Tablets ... 1556
Trilafon ... 2123

Phenelzine Sulfate (Additive effects). Products include:
Nardil ... 1742

Phenobarbital (Additive effects). Products include:
Arco-Lase Plus Tablets ... 607
Bellergal-S Tablets ... 1998
Bronkolixir ... 761
Bronkotabs Tablets ... 762
Donnatal ... 1858
Donnatal Extentabs ... 1859
Donnatal Tablets ... 1858
Donnazyme Tablets ... 1860
Kinesed Tablets ... 2272
Phenobarbital Elixir and Tablets ... 1293
Primatene Tablets-P Formula ... 2421
Quadrinal Tablets ... 1183
Tedral SA ... 1765

Prazepam (Additive effects). Products include:
Centrax ... 1693

Prochlorperazine (Additive effects). Products include:
Compazine ... 2201

Promethazine Hydrochloride (Additive effects). Products include:
Mepergan Injection ... 2479
Phenergan with Codeine ... 2497
Phenergan with Dextromethorphan 2499
Phenergan Injection ... 2493
Phenergan Suppositories ... 2496
Phenergan Syrup ... 2495
Phenergan Tablets ... 2496
Phenergan VC ... 2500
Phenergan VC with Codeine ... 2501

Propofol (Additive effects). Products include:
Diprivan Injection ... 2267

Propoxyphene Hydrochloride (Additive effects). Products include:
Darvon ... 1256
Wygesic Tablets ... 2540

Propoxyphene Napsylate (Additive effects). Products include:
Darvon-N/Darvocet-N ... 1254

Protriptyline Hydrochloride (Additive effects). Products include:
Vivactil Tablets ... 1567

Quazepam (Additive effects). Products include:
Doral Tablets ... 2383

Secobarbital Sodium (Additive effects). Products include:
Seconal Sodium Pulvules ... 1296

Sufentanil Citrate (Additive effects). Products include:
Sufenta Injection ... 1147

Temazepam (Additive effects). Products include:
Restoril Capsules ... 2023

Thiamylal Sodium (Additive effects). Products include:
Surital Ampoules, Steri-Vials ... 1764

Thioridazine Hydrochloride (Additive effects). Products include:
Mellaril ... 2011

Thiothixene (Additive effects). Products include:
Navane Capsules and Concentrate 1954
Navane Intramuscular ... 1956

Tranylcypromine Sulfate (Additive effects). Products include:
Parnate Tablets 2222
Triazolam (Additive effects). Products include:
Halcion Tablets 2340
Trifluoperazine Hydrochloride (Additive effects). Products include:
Stelazine 2226
Trimipramine Maleate (Additive effects). Products include:
Surmontil Capsules 2524

SOMINEX CAPLETS AND TABLETS
(Diphenhydramine Hydrochloride) .. ▣ 722
May interact with monoamine oxidase inhibitors, central nervous system depressants, hypnotics and sedatives, tranquilizers, and certain other agents. Compounds in these categories include:

Alcohol (CNS depressant effect heightened).
Alfentanil Hydrochloride (CNS depressant effect heightened). Products include:
Alfenta Injection 1131
Alprazolam (CNS depressant effect heightened). Products include:
Xanax Tablets 2367
Aprobarbital (CNS depressant effect heightened). Products include:
Alurate Elixir 1883
Buprenorphine (CNS depressant effect heightened).
No products indexed under this heading.
Buspirone Hydrochloride (CNS depressant effect heightened). Products include:
BuSpar 1401
Butabarbital (CNS depressant effect heightened). Products include:
Pyridium Plus 1764
Butalbital (CNS depressant effect heightened). Products include:
Esgic-Plus Tablets 1002
Esgic Tablets & Capsules 1001
Fioricet Tablets 2006
Fiorinal Capsules 2007
Fiorinal with Codeine Capsules 2008
Fiorinal Tablets 2007
Phrenilin 838
Sedapap Tablets 50 mg/650 mg .. 1360
Chlordiazepoxide (CNS depressant effect heightened). Products include:
Libritabs Tablets 1930
Limbitrol 1933
Menrium Tablets 1934
Chlordiazepoxide Hydrochloride (CNS depressant effect heightened). Products include:
Librax Capsules 1929
Librium Capsules 1931
Librium Injectable 1932
Chlorpromazine (CNS depressant effect heightened). Products include:
Thorazine 2234
Chlorprothixene (CNS depressant effect heightened). Products include:
Taractan Tablets 1920
Chlorprothixene Hydrochloride (CNS depressant effect heightened). Products include:
Taractan 1920
Clorazepate Dipotassium (CNS depressant effect heightened). Products include:
Tranxene 556
Codeine (CNS depressant effect heightened). Products include:
Calcidrine Syrup 506
Codeine Phosphate (CNS depressant effect heightened). Products include:
Actifed with Codeine Cough Syrup.. 752
Cheracol Cough Syrup 1853
Codimal PH Syrup 846
Dimetane-DC Cough Syrup 1857
Empirin with Codeine Phosphate Nos. 2, 3 & 4 764
Fiorinal with Codeine Capsules 2008
Isoclor Expectorant 982
Naldecon CX Adult Liquid .... ▣ 521
Novahistine DH 1342
Novahistine Expectorant 1343
Nucofed Capsules 2219
Nucofed Expectorant 2219
Nucofed Pediatric Expectorant 2220
Nucofed Syrup 2219
Phenaphen with Codeine Capsules 1865
Phenaphen-650 with Codeine Tablets 1866
Phenergan with Codeine 2497
Phenergan VC with Codeine 2501
Robitussin A-C Syrup 1875
Robitussin-DAC Syrup 1875
Ryna .... ▣ 741
Soma Compound w/Codeine Tablets 2390
Triaminic Expectorant w/Codeine .. 1996
Tussi-Organidin Liquid 2391
Tylenol with Codeine 1381
Codeine Polistirex (CNS depressant effect heightened).
No products indexed under this heading.
Dezocine (CNS depressant effect heightened).
Diazepam (CNS depressant effect heightened). Products include:
Valium Injectable 1937
Valium Tablets 1939
Valrelease Capsules 1923
Droperidol (CNS depressant effect heightened). Products include:
Inapsine Injection 1140
Innovar Injection 1141
Enflurane (CNS depressant effect heightened). Products include:
Ethrane 599
Estazolam (CNS depressant effect heightened). Products include:
ProSom Tablets 554
Ethchlorvynol (CNS depressant effect heightened). Products include:
Placidyl Capsules 553
Ethinamate (CNS depressant effect heightened).
No products indexed under this heading.
Fentanyl (CNS depressant effect heightened). Products include:
Duragesic Transdermal System 1133
Fentanyl Citrate (CNS depressant effect heightened). Products include:
Innovar Injection 1141
Sublimaze Injection 1146
Fluphenazine Decanoate (CNS depressant effect heightened). Products include:
Prolixin Decanoate 1795
Fluphenazine Enanthate (CNS depressant effect heightened). Products include:
Prolixin Enanthate 1796
Fluphenazine Hydrochloride (CNS depressant effect heightened). Products include:
Prolixin Elixir 1793
Prolixin Injection 1791
Prolixin Oral Concentrate 1792
Prolixin Tablets 1793
Flurazepam Hydrochloride (CNS depressant effect heightened). Products include:
Dalmane Capsules 1927
Furazolidone (Prolongs and intensifies anticholinergic effects). Products include:
Furoxone 1855
Glutethimide (CNS depressant effect heightened).
No products indexed under this heading.
Haloperidol (CNS depressant effect heightened). Products include:
Haldol Injection, Tablets and Concentrate 1373
Haloperidol Decanoate (CNS depressant effect heightened). Products include:
Haldol Decanoate 1375
Hydrocodone Bitartrate (CNS depressant effect heightened). Products include:
Anexsia 5/500 Tablets 2196
Anexsia 7.5/650 Tablets 2197
Azdone Tablets 844
Codiclear DH Syrup 845
Codimal DH Syrup 846
Damason-P 1356
Hycodan Syrup, Tablets 927
Hycomine Compound Tablets 929
Hycomine Syrup 927
Hycotuss Expectorant Syrup 930
Hydrocet Capsules 835
Lortab ASA Tablets 2414
Lortab 2412
Ru-Tuss with Hydrocodone 694
Triaminic Expectorant DH 1995
Vicodin Tablets 1187
Vicodin ES Tablets 1189
Zydone Capsules 941
Hydrocodone Polistirex (CNS depressant effect heightened). Products include:
Tussionex Extended-Release Suspension 988
Hydroxyzine Hydrochloride (CNS depressant effect heightened). Products include:
Atarax Tablets & Syrup 1941
Marax Tablets & DF Syrup 1954
Vistaril Intramuscular Solution 1970
Isocarboxazid (Prolongs and intensifies anticholinergic effects). Products include:
Marplan Tablets 1906
Isoflurane (CNS depressant effect heightened). Products include:
Forane 600
Ketamine Hydrochloride (CNS depressant effect heightened). Products include:
Ketalar 1726
Levorphanol Tartrate (CNS depressant effect heightened). Products include:
Levo-Dromoran 1906
Lorazepam (CNS depressant effect heightened). Products include:
Ativan Injection 2432
Ativan Tablets 2434
Loxapine Hydrochloride (CNS depressant effect heightened). Products include:
Loxitane 1213
Loxapine Succinate (CNS depressant effect heightened). Products include:
Loxitane Capsules 1213
Meperidine Hydrochloride (CNS depressant effect heightened). Products include:
Demerol 2047
Mepergan Injection 2479
Mephobarbital (CNS depressant effect heightened). Products include:
Mebaral Tablets 2061
Meprobamate (CNS depressant effect heightened). Products include:
Deprol Tablets 2382
Equagesic Tablets 2451
Miltown Tablets 2386
PMB 200 and PMB 400 2504
Mesoridazine (CNS depressant effect heightened). Products include:
Serentil 686
Methadone Hydrochloride (CNS depressant effect heightened). Products include:
Dolophine Hydrochloride Ampoules & Vials 1260
Dolophine Hydrochloride Tablets 1261
Methadone Hydrochloride Diskets .. 1284
Methadone Hydrochloride Oral Solution & Tablets 1987
Methohexital Sodium (CNS depressant effect heightened). Products include:
Brevital Sodium Vials 1248
Methoxyflurane (CNS depressant effect heightened).
No products indexed under this heading.
Midazolam Hydrochloride (CNS depressant effect heightened). Products include:
Versed Injection 1924
Molindone Hydrochloride (CNS depressant effect heightened). Products include:
Moban Tablets & Concentrate 932
Morphine Sulfate (CNS depressant effect heightened). Products include:
Astramorph/PF Injection, USP (Preservative-Free) 618
Duramorph 960
Infumorph 200 and Infumorph 500 Sterile Solutions 962
MS Contin Tablets 1814
MSIR 1817
Oramorph SR (Morphine Sulfate Sustained Release Tablets) 1988
Roxanol 1991
Opium Alkaloids (CNS depressant effect heightened). Products include:
B & O No. 15A & No. 16A Supprettes 2395
Pantopon Injectable 1911
Oxazepam (CNS depressant effect heightened). Products include:
Serax Capsules 2522
Serax Tablets 2522
Oxycodone Hydrochloride (CNS depressant effect heightened). Products include:
Percocet Tablets 950
Percodan 951
Roxicodone Tablets, Oral Solution & Intensol (Oxycodone) 1992
Tylox Capsules 1382
Pentobarbital Sodium (CNS depressant effect heightened). Products include:
Nembutal Sodium Capsules 534
Nembutal Sodium Solution 536
Nembutal Sodium Suppositories 538
Perphenazine (CNS depressant effect heightened). Products include:
Etrafon 2087
Triavil Tablets 1556
Trilafon 2123
Phenelzine Sulfate (Prolongs and intensifies anticholinergic effects). Products include:
Nardil 1742
Phenobarbital (CNS depressant effect heightened). Products include:
Arco-Lase Plus Tablets 607
Bellergal-S Tablets 1998
Bronkolixir .... ▣ 761
Bronkotabs Tablets .... ▣ 762
Donnatal 1858
Donnatal Extentabs 1859
Donnatal Tablets 1858
Donnazyme Tablets 1860
Kinesed Tablets 2272
Phenobarbital Elixir and Tablets 1293
Primatene Tablets-P Formula 2421
Quadrinal Tablets 1183
Tedral SA 1765
Prazepam (CNS depressant effect heightened). Products include:
Centrax 1693
Prochlorperazine (CNS depressant effect heightened). Products include:
Compazine 2201
Promethazine Hydrochloride (CNS depressant effect heightened). Products include:
Mepergan Injection 2479
Phenergan with Codeine 2497
Phenergan with Dextromethorphan 2499

Phenergan Injection 2493
Phenergan Suppositories 2496
Phenergan Syrup 2495
Phenergan Tablets 2496
Phenergan VC 2500
Phenergan VC with Codeine 2501

Propofol (CNS depressant effect heightened). Products include:
Diprivan Injection 2267

Propoxyphene Hydrochloride (CNS depressant effect heightened). Products include:
Darvon 1256
Wygesic Tablets 2540

Propoxyphene Napsylate (CNS depressant effect heightened). Products include:
Darvon-N/Darvocet-N 1254

Quazepam (CNS depressant effect heightened). Products include:
Doral Tablets 2383

Secobarbital Sodium (CNS depressant effect heightened). Products include:
Seconal Sodium Pulvules 1296

Selegiline Hydrochloride (Prolongs and intensifies anticholinergic effects). Products include:
Eldepryl 2250

Sufentanil Citrate (CNS depressant effect heightened). Products include:
Sufenta Injection 1147

Temazepam (CNS depressant effect heightened). Products include:
Restoril Capsules 2023

Thiamylal Sodium (CNS depressant effect heightened). Products include:
Surital Ampoules, Steri-Vials 1764

Thioridazine Hydrochloride (CNS depressant effect heightened). Products include:
Mellaril 2011

Thiothixene (CNS depressant effect heightened). Products include:
Navane Capsules and Concentrate 1954
Navane Intramuscular 1956

Tranylcypromine Sulfate (Prolongs and intensifies anticholinergic effects). Products include:
Parnate Tablets 2222

Triazolam (CNS depressant effect heightened). Products include:
Halcion Tablets 2340

Trifluoperazine Hydrochloride (CNS depressant effect heightened). Products include:
Stelazine 2226

SOMINEX LIQUID
(Diphenhydramine Hydrochloride) .. ▣ 723
May interact with monoamine oxidase inhibitors, central nervous system depressants, hypnotics and sedatives, tranquilizers, and certain other agents. Compounds in these categories include:

Alcohol (CNS depressant effect heightened).

Alfentanil Hydrochloride (CNS depressant effect heightened). Products include:
Alfenta Injection 1131

Alprazolam (CNS depressant effect heightened). Products include:
Xanax Tablets 2367

Aprobarbital (CNS depressant effect heightened). Products include:
Alurate Elixir 1883

Buprenorphine (CNS depressant effect heightened).
No products indexed under this heading.

Buspirone Hydrochloride (CNS depressant effect heightened). Products include:
BuSpar 1401

Butabarbital (CNS depressant effect heightened). Products include:
Pyridium Plus 1764

Butalbital (CNS depressant effect heightened). Products include:
Esgic-Plus Tablets 1002
Esgic Tablets & Capsules 1001
Fioricet Tablets 2006
Fiorinal Capsules 2007
Fiorinal with Codeine Capsules 2008
Fiorinal Tablets 2007
Phrenilin 838
Sedapap Tablets 50 mg/650 mg .. 1360

Chlordiazepoxide (CNS depressant effect heightened). Products include:
Libritabs Tablets 1930
Limbitrol 1933
Menrium Tablets 1934

Chlordiazepoxide Hydrochloride (CNS depressant effect heightened). Products include:
Librax Capsules 1929
Librium Capsules 1931
Librium Injectable 1932

Chlorpromazine (CNS depressant effect heightened). Products include:
Thorazine 2234

Chlorprothixene (CNS depressant effect heightened). Products include:
Taractan Tablets 1920

Chlorprothixene Hydrochloride (CNS depressant effect heightened). Products include:
Taractan 1920

Clorazepate Dipotassium (CNS depressant effect heightened). Products include:
Tranxene 556

Codeine (CNS depressant effect heightened). Products include:
Calcidrine Syrup 506

Codeine Phosphate (CNS depressant effect heightened). Products include:
Actifed with Codeine Cough Syrup.. 752
Cheracol Cough Syrup 1853
Codimal PH Syrup 846
Dimetane-DC Cough Syrup 1857
Empirin with Codeine Phosphate Nos. 2, 3 & 4 764
Fiorinal with Codeine Capsules 2008
Isoclor Expectorant 982
Naldecon CX Adult Liquid .... ▣ 521
Novahistine DH 1342
Novahistine Expectorant 1343
Nucofed Capsules 2219
Nucofed Expectorant 2219
Nucofed Pediatric Expectorant 2220
Nucofed Syrup 2219
Phenaphen with Codeine Capsules 1865
Phenaphen-650 with Codeine Tablets 1866
Phenergan with Codeine 2497
Phenergan VC with Codeine 2501
Robitussin A-C Syrup 1875
Robitussin-DAC Syrup 1875
Ryna .... ▣ 741
Soma Compound w/Codeine Tablets 2390
Triaminic Expectorant w/Codeine .. 1996
Tussi-Organidin Liquid 2391
Tylenol with Codeine 1381

Codeine Polistirex (CNS depressant effect heightened).
No products indexed under this heading.

Dezocine (CNS depressant effect heightened).

Diazepam (CNS depressant effect heightened). Products include:
Valium Injectable 1937
Valium Tablets 1939
Valrelease Capsules 1923

Droperidol (CNS depressant effect heightened). Products include:
Inapsine Injection 1140
Innovar Injection 1141

Enflurane (CNS depressant effect heightened). Products include:
Ethrane 599

Estazolam (CNS depressant effect heightened). Products include:
ProSom Tablets 554

Ethchlorvynol (CNS depressant effect heightened). Products include:
Placidyl Capsules 553

Ethinamate (CNS depressant effect heightened).
No products indexed under this heading.

Fentanyl (CNS depressant effect heightened). Products include:
Duragesic Transdermal System 1133

Fentanyl Citrate (CNS depressant effect heightened). Products include:
Innovar Injection 1141
Sublimaze Injection 1146

Fluphenazine Decanoate (CNS depressant effect heightened). Products include:
Prolixin Decanoate 1795

Fluphenazine Enanthate (CNS depressant effect heightened). Products include:
Prolixin Enanthate 1796

Fluphenazine Hydrochloride (CNS depressant effect heightened). Products include:
Prolixin Elixir 1793
Prolixin Injection 1791
Prolixin Oral Concentrate 1792
Prolixin Tablets 1793

Flurazepam Hydrochloride (CNS depressant effect heightened). Products include:
Dalmane Capsules 1927

Furazolidone (Prolongs and intensifies anticholinergic effects). Products include:
Furoxone 1855

Glutethimide (CNS depressant effect heightened).
No products indexed under this heading.

Haloperidol (CNS depressant effect heightened). Products include:
Haldol Injection, Tablets and Concentrate 1373

Haloperidol Decanoate (CNS depressant effect heightened). Products include:
Haldol Decanoate 1375

Hydrocodone Bitartrate (CNS depressant effect heightened). Products include:
Anexsia 5/500 Tablets 2196
Anexsia 7.5/650 Tablets 2197
Azdone Tablets 844
Codiclear DH Syrup 845
Codimal DH Syrup 846
Damason-P 1356
Hycodan Syrup, Tablets 927
Hycomine Compound Tablets 929
Hycomine Syrup 927
Hycotuss Expectorant Syrup 930
Hydrocet Capsules 835
Lortab ASA Tablets 2414
Lortab 2412
Ru-Tuss with Hydrocodone 694
Triaminic Expectorant DH 1995
Vicodin Tablets 1187
Vicodin ES Tablets 1189
Zydone Capsules 941

Hydrocodone Polistirex (CNS depressant effect heightened). Products include:
Tussionex Extended-Release Suspension 988

Hydroxyzine Hydrochloride (CNS depressant effect heightened). Products include:
Atarax Tablets & Syrup 1941
Marax Tablets & DF Syrup 1954
Vistaril Intramuscular Solution 1970

Isocarboxazid (Prolongs and intensifies anticholinergic effects). Products include:
Marplan Tablets 1906

Isoflurane (CNS depressant effect heightened). Products include:
Forane 600

Ketamine Hydrochloride (CNS depressant effect heightened). Products include:
Ketalar 1726

Levorphanol Tartrate (CNS depressant effect heightened). Products include:
Levo-Dromoran 1906

Lorazepam (CNS depressant effect heightened). Products include:
Ativan Injection 2432
Ativan Tablets 2434

Loxapine Hydrochloride (CNS depressant effect heightened). Products include:
Loxitane 1213

Loxapine Succinate (CNS depressant effect heightened). Products include:
Loxitane Capsules 1213

Meperidine Hydrochloride (CNS depressant effect heightened). Products include:
Demerol 2047
Mepergan Injection 2479

Mephobarbital (CNS depressant effect heightened). Products include:
Mebaral Tablets 2061

Meprobamate (CNS depressant effect heightened). Products include:
Deprol Tablets 2382
Equagesic Tablets 2451
Miltown Tablets 2386
PMB 200 and PMB 400 2504

Mesoridazine (CNS depressant effect heightened). Products include:
Serentil 686

Methadone Hydrochloride (CNS depressant effect heightened). Products include:
Dolophine Hydrochloride Ampoules & Vials 1260
Dolophine Hydrochloride Tablets 1261
Methadone Hydrochloride Diskets .. 1284
Methadone Hydrochloride Oral Solution & Tablets 1987

Methohexital Sodium (CNS depressant effect heightened). Products include:
Brevital Sodium Vials 1248

Methoxyflurane (CNS depressant effect heightened).
No products indexed under this heading.

Midazolam Hydrochloride (CNS depressant effect heightened). Products include:
Versed Injection 1924

Molindone Hydrochloride (CNS depressant effect heightened). Products include:
Moban Tablets & Concentrate 932

Morphine Sulfate (CNS depressant effect heightened). Products include:
Astramorph/PF Injection, USP (Preservative-Free) 618
Duramorph 960
Infumorph 200 and Infumorph 500 Sterile Solutions 962
MS Contin Tablets 1814
MSIR 1817
Oramorph SR (Morphine Sulfate Sustained Release Tablets) 1988
Roxanol 1991

Opium Alkaloids (CNS depressant effect heightened). Products include:
B & O No. 15A & No. 16A Supprettes 2395
Pantopon Injectable 1911

Oxazepam (CNS depressant effect heightened). Products include:
Serax Capsules 2522
Serax Tablets 2522

Oxycodone Hydrochloride (CNS depressant effect heightened). Products include:
- Percocet Tablets ... 950
- Percodan ... 951
- Roxicodone Tablets, Oral Solution & Intensol (Oxycodone) ... 1992
- Tylox Capsules ... 1382

Pentobarbital Sodium (CNS depressant effect heightened). Products include:
- Nembutal Sodium Capsules ... 534
- Nembutal Sodium Solution ... 536
- Nembutal Sodium Suppositories ... 538

Perphenazine (CNS depressant effect heightened). Products include:
- Etrafon ... 2087
- Triavil Tablets ... 1556
- Trilafon ... 2123

Phenelzine Sulfate (Prolongs and intensifies anticholinergic effects). Products include:
- Nardil ... 1742

Phenobarbital (CNS depressant effect heightened). Products include:
- Arco-Lase Plus Tablets ... 607
- Bellergal-S Tablets ... 1998
- Bronkolixir ... ⊞ 761
- Bronkotabs Tablets ... ⊞ 762
- Donnatal ... 1858
- Donnatal Extentabs ... 1859
- Donnatal Tablets ... 1858
- Donnazyme Tablets ... 1860
- Kinesed Tablets ... 2272
- Phenobarbital Elixir and Tablets ... 1293
- Primatene Tablets-P Formula ... 2421
- Quadrinal Tablets ... 1183
- Tedral SA ... 1765

Prazepam (CNS depressant effect heightened). Products include:
- Centrax ... 1693

Prochlorperazine (CNS depressant effect heightened). Products include:
- Compazine ... 2201

Promethazine Hydrochloride (CNS depressant effect heightened). Products include:
- Mepergan Injection ... 2479
- Phenergan with Codeine ... 2497
- Phenergan with Dextromethorphan 2499
- Phenergan Injection ... 2493
- Phenergan Suppositories ... 2496
- Phenergan Syrup ... 2495
- Phenergan Tablets ... 2496
- Phenergan VC ... 2500
- Phenergan VC with Codeine ... 2501

Propofol (CNS depressant effect heightened). Products include:
- Diprivan Injection ... 2267

Propoxyphene Hydrochloride (CNS depressant effect heightened). Products include:
- Darvon ... 1256
- Wygesic Tablets ... 2540

Propoxyphene Napsylate (CNS depressant effect heightened). Products include:
- Darvon-N/Darvocet-N ... 1254

Quazepam (CNS depressant effect heightened). Products include:
- Doral Tablets ... 2383

Secobarbital Sodium (CNS depressant effect heightened). Products include:
- Seconal Sodium Pulvules ... 1296

Selegiline Hydrochloride (Prolongs and intensifies anticholinergic effects). Products include:
- Eldepryl ... 2250

Sufentanil Citrate (CNS depressant effect heightened). Products include:
- Sufenta Injection ... 1147

Temazepam (CNS depressant effect heightened). Products include:
- Restoril Capsules ... 2023

Thiamylal Sodium (CNS depressant effect heightened). Products include:
- Surital Ampoules, Steri-Vials ... 1764

Thioridazine Hydrochloride (CNS depressant effect heightened). Products include:
- Mellaril ... 2011

Thiothixene (CNS depressant effect heightened). Products include:
- Navane Capsules and Concentrate 1954
- Navane Intramuscular ... 1956

Tranylcypromine Sulfate (Prolongs and intensifies anticholinergic effects). Products include:
- Parnate Tablets ... 2222

Triazolam (CNS depressant effect heightened). Products include:
- Halcion Tablets ... 2340

Trifluoperazine Hydrochloride (CNS depressant effect heightened). Products include:
- Stelazine ... 2226

SOMINEX PAIN RELIEF FORMULA
(Acetaminophen, Diphenhydramine Hydrochloride) ... ⊞ 723
May interact with monoamine oxidase inhibitors, central nervous system depressants, and certain other agents. Compounds in these categories include:

Alcohol (CNS depressant effect heightened).

Alfentanil Hydrochloride (CNS depressant effect heightened). Products include:
- Alfenta Injection ... 1131

Alprazolam (CNS depressant effect heightened). Products include:
- Xanax Tablets ... 2367

Aprobarbital (CNS depressant effect heightened). Products include:
- Alurate Elixir ... 1883

Buprenorphine (CNS depressant effect heightened).
- No products indexed under this heading.

Buspirone Hydrochloride (CNS depressant effect heightened). Products include:
- BuSpar ... 1401

Butabarbital (CNS depressant effect heightened). Products include:
- Pyridium Plus ... 1764

Butalbital (CNS depressant effect heightened). Products include:
- Esgic-Plus Tablets ... 1002
- Esgic Tablets & Capsules ... 1001
- Fioricet Tablets ... 2006
- Fiorinal Capsules ... 2007
- Fiorinal with Codeine Capsules ... 2008
- Fiorinal Tablets ... 2007
- Phrenilin ... 838
- Sedapap Tablets 50 mg/650 mg .. 1360

Chlordiazepoxide (CNS depressant effect heightened). Products include:
- Libritabs Tablets ... 1930
- Limbitrol ... 1933
- Menrium Tablets ... 1934

Chlordiazepoxide Hydrochloride (CNS depressant effect heightened). Products include:
- Librax Capsules ... 1929
- Librium Capsules ... 1931
- Librium Injectable ... 1932

Chlorpromazine (CNS depressant effect heightened). Products include:
- Thorazine ... 2234

Chlorprothixene (CNS depressant effect heightened). Products include:
- Taractan Tablets ... 1920

Chlorprothixene Hydrochloride (CNS depressant effect heightened). Products include:
- Taractan ... 1920

Clorazepate Dipotassium (CNS depressant effect heightened). Products include:
- Tranxene ... 556

Codeine (CNS depressant effect heightened). Products include:
- Calcidrine Syrup ... 506

Codeine Phosphate (CNS depressant effect heightened). Products include:
- Actifed with Codeine Cough Syrup.. 752
- Cheracol Cough Syrup ... 1853
- Codimal PH Syrup ... 846
- Dimetane-DC Cough Syrup ... 1857
- Empirin with Codeine Phosphate Nos. 2, 3 & 4 ... 764
- Fiorinal with Codeine Capsules ... 2008
- Isoclor Expectorant ... 982
- Naldecon CX Adult Liquid ... ⊞ 521
- Novahistine DH ... 1342
- Novahistine Expectorant ... 1343
- Nucofed Capsules ... 2219
- Nucofed Expectorant ... 2219
- Nucofed Pediatric Expectorant ... 2220
- Nucofed Syrup ... 2219
- Phenaphen with Codeine Capsules 1865
- Phenaphen-650 with Codeine Tablets ... 1866
- Phenergan with Codeine ... 2497
- Phenergan VC with Codeine ... 2501
- Robitussin A-C Syrup ... 1875
- Robitussin-DAC Syrup ... 1875
- Ryna ... ⊞ 741
- Soma Compound w/Codeine Tablets ... 2390
- Triaminic Expectorant w/Codeine .. 1996
- Tussi-Organidin Liquid ... 2391
- Tylenol with Codeine ... 1381

Codeine Polistirex (CNS depressant effect heightened).
- No products indexed under this heading.

Dezocine (CNS depressant effect heightened).

Diazepam (CNS depressant effect heightened). Products include:
- Valium Injectable ... 1937
- Valium Tablets ... 1939
- Valrelease Capsules ... 1923

Droperidol (CNS depressant effect heightened). Products include:
- Inapsine Injection ... 1140
- Innovar Injection ... 1141

Enflurane (CNS depressant effect heightened). Products include:
- Ethrane ... 599

Estazolam (CNS depressant effect heightened). Products include:
- ProSom Tablets ... 554

Ethchlorvynol (CNS depressant effect heightened). Products include:
- Placidyl Capsules ... 553

Ethinamate (CNS depressant effect heightened).
- No products indexed under this heading.

Fentanyl (CNS depressant effect heightened). Products include:
- Duragesic Transdermal System ... 1133

Fentanyl Citrate (CNS depressant effect heightened). Products include:
- Innovar Injection ... 1141
- Sublimaze Injection ... 1146

Fluphenazine Decanoate (CNS depressant effect heightened). Products include:
- Prolixin Decanoate ... 1795

Fluphenazine Enanthate (CNS depressant effect heightened). Products include:
- Prolixin Enanthate ... 1796

Fluphenazine Hydrochloride (CNS depressant effect heightened). Products include:
- Prolixin Elixir ... 1793
- Prolixin Injection ... 1791
- Prolixin Oral Concentrate ... 1792
- Prolixin Tablets ... 1793

Flurazepam Hydrochloride (CNS depressant effect heightened). Products include:
- Dalmane Capsules ... 1927

Furazolidone (Prolongs and intensifies anticholinergic effects). Products include:
- Furoxone ... 1855

Glutethimide (CNS depressant effect heightened).
- No products indexed under this heading.

Haloperidol (CNS depressant effect heightened). Products include:
- Haldol Injection, Tablets and Concentrate ... 1373

Haloperidol Decanoate (CNS depressant effect heightened). Products include:
- Haldol Decanoate ... 1375

Hydrocodone Bitartrate (CNS depressant effect heightened). Products include:
- Anexsia 5/500 Tablets ... 2196
- Anexsia 7.5/650 Tablets ... 2197
- Azdōne Tablets ... 844
- Codiclear DH Syrup ... 845
- Codimal DH Syrup ... 846
- Damason-P ... 1356
- Hycodan Syrup, Tablets ... 927
- Hycomine Compound Tablets ... 929
- Hycomine Syrup ... 927
- Hycotuss Expectorant Syrup ... 930
- Hydrocet Capsules ... 835
- Lortab ASA Tablets ... 2414
- Lortab ... 2412
- Ru-Tuss with Hydrocodone ... 694
- Triaminic Expectorant DH ... 1995
- Vicodin Tablets ... 1187
- Vicodin ES Tablets ... 1189
- Zydone Capsules ... 941

Hydrocodone Polistirex (CNS depressant effect heightened). Products include:
- Tussionex Extended-Release Suspension ... 988

Hydroxyzine Hydrochloride (CNS depressant effect heightened). Products include:
- Atarax Tablets & Syrup ... 1941
- Marax Tablets & DF Syrup ... 1954
- Vistaril Intramuscular Solution ... 1970

Isocarboxazid (Prolongs and intensifies anticholinergic effects). Products include:
- Marplan Tablets ... 1906

Isoflurane (CNS depressant effect heightened). Products include:
- Forane ... 600

Ketamine Hydrochloride (CNS depressant effect heightened). Products include:
- Ketalar ... 1726

Levorphanol Tartrate (CNS depressant effect heightened). Products include:
- Levo-Dromoran ... 1906

Lorazepam (CNS depressant effect heightened). Products include:
- Ativan Injection ... 2432
- Ativan Tablets ... 2434

Loxapine Hydrochloride (CNS depressant effect heightened). Products include:
- Loxitane ... 1213

Loxapine Succinate (CNS depressant effect heightened). Products include:
- Loxitane Capsules ... 1213

Meperidine Hydrochloride (CNS depressant effect heightened). Products include:
- Demerol ... 2047
- Mepergan Injection ... 2479

Mephobarbital (CNS depressant effect heightened). Products include:
- Mebaral Tablets ... 2061

Meprobamate (CNS depressant effect heightened). Products include:
- Deprol Tablets ... 2382

Equagesic Tablets 2451
Miltown Tablets 2386
PMB 200 and PMB 400 2504

Mesoridazine (CNS depressant effect heightened). Products include:
Serentil 686

Methadone Hydrochloride (CNS depressant effect heightened). Products include:
Dolophine Hydrochloride Ampoules & Vials 1260
Dolophine Hydrochloride Tablets 1261
Methadone Hydrochloride Diskets 1284
Methadone Hydrochloride Oral Solution & Tablets 1987

Methohexital Sodium (CNS depressant effect heightened). Products include:
Brevital Sodium Vials 1248

Methoxyflurane (CNS depressant effect heightened).
No products indexed under this heading.

Midazolam Hydrochloride (CNS depressant effect heightened). Products include:
Versed Injection 1924

Molindone Hydrochloride (CNS depressant effect heightened). Products include:
Moban Tablets & Concentrate 932

Morphine Sulfate (CNS depressant effect heightened). Products include:
Astramorph/PF Injection, USP (Preservative-Free) 618
Duramorph 960
Infumorph 200 and Infumorph 500 Sterile Solutions 962
MS Contin Tablets 1814
MSIR 1817
Oramorph SR (Morphine Sulfate Sustained Release Tablets) 1988
Roxanol 1991

Opium Alkaloids (CNS depressant effect heightened). Products include:
B & O No. 15A & No. 16A Supprettes 2395
Pantopon Injectable 1911

Oxazepam (CNS depressant effect heightened). Products include:
Serax Capsules 2522
Serax Tablets 2522

Oxycodone Hydrochloride (CNS depressant effect heightened). Products include:
Percocet Tablets 950
Percodan 951
Roxicodone Tablets, Oral Solution & Intensol (Oxycodone) 1992
Tylox Capsules 1382

Pentobarbital Sodium (CNS depressant effect heightened). Products include:
Nembutal Sodium Capsules 534
Nembutal Sodium Solution 536
Nembutal Sodium Suppositories 538

Perphenazine (CNS depressant effect heightened). Products include:
Etrafon 2087
Triavil Tablets 1556
Trilafon 2123

Phenelzine Sulfate (Prolongs and intensifies anticholinergic effects). Products include:
Nardil 1742

Phenobarbital (CNS depressant effect heightened). Products include:
Arco-Lase Plus Tablets 607
Bellergal-S Tablets 1998
Bronkolixir ▣ 761
Bronkotabs Tablets ▣ 762
Donnatal 1858
Donnatal Extentabs 1859
Donnatal Tablets 1858
Donnazyme Tablets 1860
Kinesed Tablets 2272
Phenobarbital Elixir and Tablets 1293
Primatene Tablets-P Formula 2421
Quadrinal Tablets 1183
Tedral SA 1765

Prazepam (CNS depressant effect heightened). Products include:
Centrax 1693

Prochlorperazine (CNS depressant effect heightened). Products include:
Compazine 2201

Promethazine Hydrochloride (CNS depressant effect heightened). Products include:
Mepergan Injection 2479
Phenergan with Codeine 2497
Phenergan with Dextromethorphan 2499
Phenergan Injection 2493
Phenergan Suppositories 2496
Phenergan Syrup 2495
Phenergan Tablets 2496
Phenergan VC 2500
Phenergan VC with Codeine 2501

Propofol (CNS depressant effect heightened). Products include:
Diprivan Injection 2267

Propoxyphene Hydrochloride (CNS depressant effect heightened). Products include:
Darvon 1256
Wygesic Tablets 2540

Propoxyphene Napsylate (CNS depressant effect heightened). Products include:
Darvon-N/Darvocet-N 1254

Quazepam (CNS depressant effect heightened). Products include:
Doral Tablets 2383

Secobarbital Sodium (CNS depressant effect heightened). Products include:
Seconal Sodium Pulvules 1296

Selegiline Hydrochloride (Prolongs and intensifies anticholinergic effects). Products include:
Eldepryl 2250

Sufentanil Citrate (CNS depressant effect heightened). Products include:
Sufenta Injection 1147

Temazepam (CNS depressant effect heightened). Products include:
Restoril Capsules 2023

Thiamylal Sodium (CNS depressant effect heightened). Products include:
Surital Ampoules, Steri-Vials 1764

Thioridazine Hydrochloride (CNS depressant effect heightened). Products include:
Mellaril 2011

Thiothixene (CNS depressant effect heightened). Products include:
Navane Capsules and Concentrate 1954
Navane Intramuscular 1956

Tranylcypromine Sulfate (Prolongs and intensifies anticholinergic effects). Products include:
Parnate Tablets 2222

Triazolam (CNS depressant effect heightened). Products include:
Halcion Tablets 2340

Trifluoperazine Hydrochloride (CNS depressant effect heightened). Products include:
Stelazine 2226

SOOTHE & CLEAN PERSONAL CLEANSING FOAM
(Glycerin, Witch Hazel) 1820
No interactions described in labeling.

SORBITRATE CHEWABLE TABLETS
(Isosorbide Dinitrate) 1103
May interact with calcium channel blockers and certain other agents. Compounds in these categories include:

Alcohol (Enhances sensitivity to hypotensive activity of nitrates).

Bepridil Hydrochloride (Symptomatic orthostatic hypotension). Products include:
Vascor (200, 300 and 400 mg) Tablets 1383

Diltiazem Hydrochloride (Symptomatic orthostatic hypotension). Products include:
Cardizem Tablets-30 mg, 60 mg, 90 mg and 120 mg 1329
Cardizem SR Capsules-60 mg, 90 mg and 120 mg 1327

Felodipine (Symptomatic orthostatic hypotension). Products include:
Plendil Extended-Release Tablets 1526

Isradipine (Symptomatic orthostatic hypotension). Products include:
DynaCirc Capsules 2004

Nicardipine Hydrochloride (Symptomatic orthostatic hypotension). Products include:
Cardene Capsules 2290

Nifedipine (Symptomatic orthostatic hypotension). Products include:
Adalat Capsules (10 mg and 20 mg) 1587
Procardia Capsules 1781
Procardia XL Tablets 1783

Nimodipine (Symptomatic orthostatic hypotension). Products include:
Nimotop Capsules 1607

Verapamil Hydrochloride (Symptomatic orthostatic hypotension). Products include:
Calan SR Caplets 2157
Calan Tablets 2155
Isoptin Injectable 1177
Isoptin Oral Tablets 1179
Isoptin SR Sustained Release Tablets 1181
Verelan Capsules 1243
Verelan Capsules 2535

SORBITRATE ORAL TABLETS
(Isosorbide Dinitrate) 1103
See **Sorbitrate Chewable Tablets**

SORBITRATE SUBLINGUAL TABLETS
(Isosorbide Dinitrate) 1103
See **Sorbitrate Chewable Tablets**

SORBITRATE SUSTAINED ACTION TABLETS
(Isosorbide Dinitrate) 1103
See **Sorbitrate Chewable Tablets**

SOTRADECOL (SODIUM TETRADECYL SULFATE INJECTION)
(Sodium Tetradecyl Sulfate) 964
May interact with oral contraceptives and certain other agents. Compounds in these categories include:

Ethinyl Estradiol (Use caution prior to initiating treatment with Sotradecol). Products include:
Brevicon 2304
Demulen 2161
Estinyl Tablets 2085
Jenest-28 Tablets 1636
Levlen/Tri-Levlen 665
Lo/Ovral Tablets 2471
Lo/Ovral-28 Tablets 2476
Loestrin 1728
Modicon 1667
Nordette-21 Tablets 2481
Nordette-28 Tablets 2483
Norethin 2133
Norinyl 2304
Norlestrin 1746
Ortho-Cyclen Tablets 1658
Ortho-Novum 1667
Ovcon 1391
Ovral Tablets 2490
Ovral-28 Tablets 2491
Levlen/Tri-Levlen 665
Tri-Norinyl 2304
Triphasil-21 Tablets 2527
Triphasil-28 Tablets 2532

Ethynodiol Diacetate (Use caution prior to initiating treatment with Sotradecol). Products include:
Demulen 2161

Heparin Calcium (*In Vitro* incompatibilities). Products include:
Calciparine Injection 925

Heparin Sodium (*In Vitro* incompatibilities). Products include:
Heparin Lock Flush Solution 2456
Heparin Sodium Vials 1264
Heparin Sodium Injection 2457
Heparin Sodium Injection, USP, Sterile Solution 2342

Levonorgestrel (Use caution prior to initiating treatment with Sotradecol). Products include:
Levlen/Tri-Levlen 665
Nordette-21 Tablets 2481
Nordette-28 Tablets 2483
Norplant System 2484
Levlen/Tri-Levlen 665
Triphasil-21 Tablets 2527
Triphasil-28 Tablets 2532

Mestranol (Use caution prior to initiating treatment with Sotradecol). Products include:
Enovid 2161
Norethin 2133
Norinyl 2304
Ortho-Novum 1667

Norethindrone (Use caution prior to initiating treatment with Sotradecol). Products include:
Brevicon 2304
Jenest-28 Tablets 1636
Micronor Tablets 1667
Modicon 1667
Norethin 2133
Norinyl 2304
Norlutin 1755
Nor-Q D Tablets 2304
Ortho-Novum 1667
Ovcon 1391
Tri-Norinyl 2304

Norethynodrel (Use caution prior to initiating treatment with Sotradecol). Products include:
Enovid 2161

Norgestimate (Use caution prior to initiating treatment with Sotradecol). Products include:
Ortho-Cyclen Tablets 1658

Norgestrel (Use caution prior to initiating treatment with Sotradecol). Products include:
Lo/Ovral Tablets 2471
Lo/Ovral-28 Tablets 2476
Ovral Tablets 2490
Ovral-28 Tablets 2491
Ovrette Tablets 2492

SPECTAZOLE (ECONAZOLE NITRATE) CREAM
(Econazole Nitrate) 1681
No interactions described in labeling.

SPECTROBID TABLETS & POWDER FOR ORAL SUSPENSION
(Bacampicillin Hydrochloride) 1961
May interact with antigout agents and certain other agents. Compounds in these categories include:

Allopurinol (Increased incidence of rashes). Products include:
Zyloprim Tablets 830

Disulfiram (Spectrobid should not be co-administered). Products include:
Antabuse Tablets 2429

Food Interactions

Food, unspecified (Spectrobid oral suspension absorption is affected by food).

ST. JOSEPH ADULT CHEWABLE ASPIRIN (81 MG.)
(Aspirin) ⊞ 703
No interactions described in labeling.

ST. JOSEPH ASPIRIN-FREE FEVER REDUCER FOR CHILDREN CHEWABLE TABLETS, LIQUID & INFANT DROPS
(Acetaminophen) ⊞ 704
No interactions described in labeling.

ST. JOSEPH NIGHTTIME COLD MEDICINE
(Chlorpheniramine Maleate, Pseudoephedrine Hydrochloride, Dextromethorphan Hydrobromide, Acetaminophen) ⊞ 705
No interactions described in labeling.

STADOL
(Butorphanol Tartrate) 721
May interact with narcotic analgesics and general anesthetics. Compounds in these categories include:

Alfentanil Hydrochloride (Difficulty in assessing addiction in patients who have recently received substantial amount of narcotic medication). Products include:
- Alfenta Injection 1131

Buprenorphine (Difficulty in assessing addiction in patients who have recently received substantial amount of narcotic medication).
- No products indexed under this heading.

Codeine (Difficulty in assessing addiction in patients who have recently received substantial amount of narcotic medication). Products include:
- Calcidrine Syrup 506

Codeine Phosphate (Difficulty in assessing addiction in patients who have recently received substantial amount of narcotic medication). Products include:
- Actifed with Codeine Cough Syrup.. 752
- Cheracol Cough Syrup 1853
- Codimal PH Syrup 846
- Dimetane-DC Cough Syrup 1857
- Empirin with Codeine Phosphate Nos. 2, 3 & 4 764
- Fiorinal with Codeine Capsules 2008
- Isoclor Expectorant 982
- Naldecon CX Adult Liquid ⊞ 521
- Novahistine DH 1342
- Novahistine Expectorant 1343
- Nucofed Capsules 2219
- Nucofed Expectorant 2219
- Nucofed Pediatric Expectorant 2220
- Nucofed Syrup 2219
- Phenaphen with Codeine Capsules 1865
- Phenaphen-650 with Codeine Tablets 1866
- Phenergan with Codeine 2497
- Phenergan VC with Codeine 2501
- Robitussin A-C Syrup 1875
- Robitussin-DAC Syrup 1875
- Ryna ⊞ 741
- Soma Compound w/Codeine Tablets 2390
- Triaminic Expectorant w/Codeine .. 1996
- Tussi-Organidin Liquid 2391
- Tylenol with Codeine 1381

Codeine Polistirex (Difficulty in assessing addiction in patients who have recently received substantial amount of narcotic medication).
- No products indexed under this heading.

Dezocine (Difficulty in assessing addiction in patients who have recently received substantial amount of narcotic medication).

Enflurane (Under-ventilation of apnea). Products include:
- Ethrane 599

Fentanyl (Difficulty in assessing addiction in patients who have recently received substantial amount of narcotic medication). Products include:
- Duragesic Transdermal System 1133

Fentanyl Citrate (Difficulty in assessing addiction in patients who have recently received substantial amount of narcotic medication). Products include:
- Innovar Injection 1141
- Sublimaze Injection 1146

Hydrocodone Bitartrate (Difficulty in assessing addiction in patients who have recently received substantial amount of narcotic medication). Products include:
- Anexsia 5/500 Tablets 2196
- Anexsia 7.5/650 Tablets 2197
- Azdone Tablets 844
- Codiclear DH Syrup 845
- Codimal DH Syrup 846
- Damason-P 1356
- Hycodan Syrup, Tablets 927
- Hycomine Compound Tablets 929
- Hycomine Syrup 927
- Hycotuss Expectorant Syrup 930
- Hydrocet Capsules 835
- Lortab ASA Tablets 2414
- Lortab 2412
- Ru-Tuss with Hydrocodone 694
- Triaminic Expectorant DH 1995
- Vicodin Tablets 1187
- Vicodin ES Tablets 1189
- Zydone Capsules 941

Hydrocodone Polistirex (Difficulty in assessing addiction in patients who have recently received substantial amount of narcotic medication). Products include:
- Tussionex Extended-Release Suspension 988

Isoflurane (Under-ventilation of apnea). Products include:
- Forane 600

Levorphanol Tartrate (Difficulty in assessing addiction in patients who have recently received substantial amount of narcotic medication). Products include:
- Levo-Dromoran 1906

Meperidine Hydrochloride (Difficulty in assessing addiction in patients who have recently received substantial amount of narcotic medication). Products include:
- Demerol 2047
- Mepergan Injection 2479

Methadone Hydrochloride (Difficulty in assessing addiction in patients who have recently received substantial amount of narcotic medication). Products include:
- Dolophine Hydrochloride Ampoules & Vials 1260
- Dolophine Hydrochloride Tablets 1261
- Methadone Hydrochloride Diskets .. 1284
- Methadone Hydrochloride Oral Solution & Tablets 1987

Methohexital Sodium (Under-ventilation of apnea). Products include:
- Brevital Sodium Vials 1248

Methoxyflurane (Under-ventilation of apnea).
- No products indexed under this heading.

Morphine Sulfate (Difficulty in assessing addiction in patients who have recently received substantial amount of narcotic medication). Products include:
- Astramorph/PF Injection, USP (Preservative-Free) 618
- Duramorph 960
- Infumorph 200 and Infumorph 500 Sterile Solutions 962
- MS Contin Tablets 1814
- MSIR 1817
- Oramorph SR (Morphine Sulfate Sustained Release Tablets) 1988
- Roxanol 1991

Opium Alkaloids (Difficulty in assessing addiction in patients who have recently received substantial amount of narcotic medication). Products include:
- B & O No. 15A & No. 16A Supprettes 2395
- Pantopon Injectable 1911

Oxycodone Hydrochloride (Difficulty in assessing addiction in patients who have recently received substantial amount of narcotic medication). Products include:
- Percocet Tablets 950
- Percodan 951
- Roxicodone Tablets, Oral Solution & Intensol (Oxycodone) 1992
- Tylox Capsules 1382

Propofol (Under-ventilation of apnea). Products include:
- Diprivan Injection 2267

Propoxyphene Hydrochloride (Difficulty in assessing addiction in patients who have recently received substantial amount of narcotic medication). Products include:
- Darvon 1256
- Wygesic Tablets 2540

Propoxyphene Napsylate (Difficulty in assessing addiction in patients who have recently received substantial amount of narcotic medication). Products include:
- Darvon-N/Darvocet-N 1254

Sufentanil Citrate (Difficulty in assessing addiction in patients who have recently received substantial amount of narcotic medication). Products include:
- Sufenta Injection 1147

STAPHAGE LYSATE (SPL)
(Staphylococcus Bacterial Antigen) .. 905
No interactions described in labeling.

STAR-OTIC EAR SOLUTION
(Acetic Acid, Boric Acid, Burow's Solution) ⊞ 729
No interactions described in labeling.

STELAZINE CONCENTRATE
(Trifluoperazine Hydrochloride) 2226
May interact with vasopressors, oral anticoagulants, thiazides, anticonvulsants, central nervous system depressants, and certain other agents. Compounds in these categories include:

Alcohol (Additive depressant effects).

Alfentanil Hydrochloride (Additive depressant effects). Products include:
- Alfenta Injection 1131

Alprazolam (Additive depressant effects). Products include:
- Xanax Tablets 2367

Aprobarbital (Additive depressant effects). Products include:
- Alurate Elixir 1883

Bendroflumethiazide (Orthostatic hypotension that occurs with phenothiazines may be accentuated). Products include:
- Corzide Tablets 702
- Naturetin Tablets 1789
- Rauzide Tablets 1804

Buprenorphine (Additive depressant effects).
- No products indexed under this heading.

Buspirone Hydrochloride (Additive depressant effects). Products include:
- BuSpar 1401

Butabarbital (Additive depressant effects). Products include:
- Pyridium Plus 1764

Butalbital (Additive depressant effects). Products include:
- Esgic-Plus Tablets 1002
- Esgic Tablets & Capsules 1001
- Fioricet Tablets 2006
- Fiorinal Capsules 2007
- Fiorinal with Codeine Capsules 2008
- Fiorinal Tablets 2007
- Phrenilin 838
- Sedapap Tablets 50 mg/650 mg .. 1360

Carbamazepine (Stelazine may lower convulsive thresholds; dosage adjustments of anticonvulsants may be necessary). Products include:
- Tegretol Chewable Tablets 654
- Tegretol Suspension 656
- Tegretol Tablets 654

Chlordiazepoxide (Additive depressant effects). Products include:
- Libritabs Tablets 1930
- Limbitrol 1933
- Menrium Tablets 1934

Chlordiazepoxide Hydrochloride (Additive depressant effects). Products include:
- Librax Capsules 1929
- Librium Capsules 1931
- Librium Injectable 1932

Chlorothiazide (Orthostatic hypotension that occurs with phenothiazines may be accentuated). Products include:
- Aldoclor Tablets 1413
- Diupres Tablets 1461
- Diuril Oral 1464

Chlorothiazide Sodium (Orthostatic hypotension that occurs with phenothiazines may be accentuated). Products include:
- Diuril Sodium Intravenous 1463

Chlorpromazine (Additive depressant effects). Products include:
- Thorazine 2234

Chlorprothixene (Additive depressant effects). Products include:
- Taractan Tablets 1920

Chlorprothixene Hydrochloride (Additive depressant effects). Products include:
- Taractan 1920

Clorazepate Dipotassium (Additive depressant effects). Products include:
- Tranxene 556

Codeine (Additive depressant effects). Products include:
- Calcidrine Syrup 506

Codeine Phosphate (Additive depressant effects). Products include:
- Actifed with Codeine Cough Syrup.. 752
- Cheracol Cough Syrup 1853
- Codimal PH Syrup 846
- Dimetane-DC Cough Syrup 1857
- Empirin with Codeine Phosphate Nos. 2, 3 & 4 764
- Fiorinal with Codeine Capsules 2008
- Isoclor Expectorant 982
- Naldecon CX Adult Liquid ⊞ 521
- Novahistine DH 1342
- Novahistine Expectorant 1343
- Nucofed Capsules 2219
- Nucofed Expectorant 2219

Nucofed Pediatric Expectorant 2220
Nucofed Syrup 2219
Phenaphen with Codeine Capsules 1865
Phenaphen-650 with Codeine Tablets 1866
Phenergan with Codeine 2497
Phenergan VC with Codeine 2501
Robitussin A-C Syrup 1875
Robitussin-DAC Syrup 1875
Ryna .... ▣ 741
Soma Compound w/Codeine Tablets 2390
Triaminic Expectorant w/Codeine .. 1996
Tussi-Organidin Liquid 2391
Tylenol with Codeine 1381

Codeine Polistirex (Additive depressant effects).
No products indexed under this heading.

Dezocine (Additive depressant effects).

Diazepam (Additive depressant effects). Products include:
Valium Injectable 1937
Valium Tablets 1939
Valrelease Capsules 1923

Dicumarol (Effect may be diminished). Products include:
Dicumarol Tablets 516

Divalproex Sodium (Stelazine may lower convulsive thresholds; dosage adjustments of anticonvulsants may be necessary). Products include:
Depakote 512

Dopamine Hydrochloride (May cause a paradoxical further lowering of blood pressure). Products include:
Intropin Injection 930

Droperidol (Additive depressant effects). Products include:
Inapsine Injection 1140
Innovar Injection 1141

Enflurane (Additive depressant effects). Products include:
Ethrane 599

Epinephrine Bitartrate (Reversed epinephrine effect; may cause a paradoxical further lowering of blood pressure). Products include:
AsthmaHaler Mist Epinephrine Bitartrate Bronchodilator .... ▣ 616
Bronkaid Mist Suspension .... ▣ 757
Primatene Mist Suspension 2421

Epinephrine Hydrochloride (Reversed epinephrine effect; may cause a paradoxical further lowering of blood pressure). Products include:
Adrenalin Chloride Solution 1:100 & 1:1,000 1689
Epifrin .... ⊙ 244
Glaucon .... ⊙ 218

Estazolam (Additive depressant effects). Products include:
ProSom Tablets 554

Ethchlorvynol (Additive depressant effects). Products include:
Placidyl Capsules 553

Ethinamate (Additive depressant effects).
No products indexed under this heading.

Ethosuximide (Stelazine may lower convulsive thresholds; dosage adjustments of anticonvulsants may be necessary). Products include:
Zarontin Capsules 1768
Zarontin Syrup 1769

Ethotoin (Stelazine may lower convulsive thresholds; dosage adjustments of anticonvulsants may be necessary). Products include:
Peganone Tablets 551

Fentanyl (Additive depressant effects). Products include:
Duragesic Transdermal System 1133

Fentanyl Citrate (Additive depressant effects). Products include:
Innovar Injection 1141
Sublimaze Injection 1146

Fluphenazine Decanoate (Additive depressant effects). Products include:
Prolixin Decanoate 1795

Fluphenazine Enanthate (Additive depressant effects). Products include:
Prolixin Enanthate 1796

Fluphenazine Hydrochloride (Additive depressant effects). Products include:
Prolixin Elixir 1793
Prolixin Injection 1791
Prolixin Oral Concentrate 1792
Prolixin Tablets 1793

Flurazepam Hydrochloride (Additive depressant effects). Products include:
Dalmane Capsules 1927

Glutethimide (Additive depressant effects).
No products indexed under this heading.

Guanethidine Monosulfate (Antihypertensive effects of guanethidine and related compounds may be counteracted when used concurrently). Products include:
Esimil Tablets 864
Ismelin Tablets 869

Haloperidol (Additive depressant effects). Products include:
Haldol Injection, Tablets and Concentrate 1373

Haloperidol Decanoate (Additive depressant effects). Products include:
Haldol Decanoate 1375

Hydrochlorothiazide (Orthostatic hypotension that occurs with Stelazine may be accentuated). Products include:
Aldactazide 2150
Aldoril Tablets 1418
Apresazide Capsules 854
Apresoline-Esidrix Tablets 857
Capozide 2258
Dyazide Capsules 2208
Esidrix Tablets 863
Esimil Tablets 864
HydroDIURIL Tablets 1484
Hydropres Tablets 1485
Inderide Tablets 2463
Inderide LA Long Acting Capsules .. 2465
Lopressor HCT Tablets 1034
Maxzide 1215
Moduretic Tablets 1510
Normozide Tablets 2112
Oretic Tablets 544
Oreticyl 545
Prinzide Tablets 1540
Ser-Ap-Es Tablets 881
Serpasil-Esidrix Tablets 886
Timolide Tablets 1547
Trandate HCT Tablets 579
Vaseretic Tablets 1559
Zestoretic 2274

Hydrocodone Bitartrate (Additive depressant effects). Products include:
Anexsia 5/500 Tablets 2196
Anexsia 7.5/650 Tablets 2197
Azdone Tablets 844
Codiclear DH Syrup 845
Codimal DH Syrup 846
Damason-P 1356
Hycodan Syrup, Tablets 927
Hycomine Compound Tablets 929
Hycomine Syrup 927
Hycotuss Expectorant Syrup 930
Hydrocet Capsules 835
Lortab ASA Tablets 2414
Lortab 2412
Ru-Tuss with Hydrocodone 694
Triaminic Expectorant DH 1995
Vicodin Tablets 1187
Vicodin ES Tablets 1189
Zydone Capsules 941

Hydrocodone Polistirex (Additive depressant effects). Products include:
Tussionex Extended-Release Suspension 988

Hydroflumethiazide (Orthostatic hypotension that occurs with Stelazine may be accentuated). Products include:
Diucardin Tablets 2450
Saluron 718
Salutensin/Salutensin-Demi 719

Hydroxyzine Hydrochloride (Additive depressant effects). Products include:
Atarax Tablets & Syrup 1941
Marax Tablets & DF Syrup 1954
Vistaril Intramuscular Solution 1970

Isoflurane (Additive depressant effects). Products include:
Forane 600

Ketamine Hydrochloride (Additive depressant effects). Products include:
Ketalar 1726

Levorphanol Tartrate (Additive depressant effects). Products include:
Levo-Dromoran 1906

Lorazepam (Additive depressant effects). Products include:
Ativan Injection 2432
Ativan Tablets 2434

Loxapine Hydrochloride (Additive depressant effects). Products include:
Loxitane 1213

Loxapine Succinate (Additive depressant effects). Products include:
Loxitane Capsules 1213

Meperidine Hydrochloride (Additive depressant effects). Products include:
Demerol 2047
Mepergan Injection 2479

Mephenytoin (Stelazine may lower convulsive thresholds; dosage adjustments of anticonvulsants may be necessary). Products include:
Mesantoin Tablets 2013

Mephobarbital (Additive depressant effects). Products include:
Mebaral Tablets 2061

Meprobamate (Additive depressant effects). Products include:
Deprol Tablets 2382
Equagesic Tablets 2451
Miltown Tablets 2386
PMB 200 and PMB 400 2504

Mesoridazine (Additive depressant effects). Products include:
Serentil 686

Metaraminol Bitartrate (May cause a paradoxical further lowering of blood pressure). Products include:
Aramine Injection 1424

Methadone Hydrochloride (Additive depressant effects). Products include:
Dolophine Hydrochloride Ampoules & Vials 1260
Dolophine Hydrochloride Tablets 1261
Methadone Hydrochloride Diskets .. 1284
Methadone Hydrochloride Oral Solution & Tablets 1987

Methohexital Sodium (Additive depressant effects). Products include:
Brevital Sodium Vials 1248

Methoxamine Hydrochloride (May cause a paradoxical further lowering of blood pressure). Products include:
Vasoxyl Injection 819

Methoxyflurane (Additive depressant effects).
No products indexed under this heading.

Methsuximide (Stelazine may lower convulsive thresholds; dosage adjustments of anticonvulsants may be necessary). Products include:
Celontin 1692

Methyclothiazide (Orthostatic hypotension that occurs with Stelazine may be accentuated). Products include:
Enduron Tablets 517
Enduronyl 518

Metrizamide (Stelazine may lower the seizure threshold; do not use concurrently).

Midazolam Hydrochloride (Additive depressant effects). Products include:
Versed Injection 1924

Molindone Hydrochloride (Additive depressant effects). Products include:
Moban Tablets & Concentrate 932

Morphine Sulfate (Additive depressant effects). Products include:
Astramorph/PF Injection, USP (Preservative-Free) 618
Duramorph 960
Infumorph 200 and Infumorph 500 Sterile Solutions 962
MS Contin Tablets 1814
MSIR 1817
Oramorph SR (Morphine Sulfate Sustained Release Tablets) 1988
Roxanol 1991

Norepinephrine Bitartrate (May cause a paradoxical further lowering of blood pressure). Products include:
Levophed Bitartrate Injection 2054

Opium Alkaloids (Additive depressant effects). Products include:
B & O No. 15A & No. 16A Supprettes 2395
Pantopon Injectable 1911

Oxazepam (Additive depressant effects). Products include:
Serax Capsules 2522
Serax Tablets 2522

Oxycodone Hydrochloride (Additive depressant effects). Products include:
Percocet Tablets 950
Percodan 951
Roxicodone Tablets, Oral Solution & Intensol (Oxycodone) 1992
Tylox Capsules 1382

Paramethadione (Stelazine may lower convulsive thresholds; dosage adjustments of anticonvulsants may be necessary). Products include:
Paradione Capsules 548

Pentobarbital Sodium (Additive depressant effects). Products include:
Nembutal Sodium Capsules 534
Nembutal Sodium Solution 536
Nembutal Sodium Suppositories 538

Perphenazine (Additive depressant effects). Products include:
Etrafon 2087
Triavil Tablets 1556
Trilafon 2123

Phenacemide (Stelazine may lower convulsive thresholds; dosage adjustments of anticonvulsants may be necessary). Products include:
Phenurone Tablets 552

Phenobarbital (Additive depressant effects). Products include:
Arco-Lase Plus Tablets 607
Bellergal-S Tablets 1998
Bronkolixir .... ▣ 761
Bronkotabs Tablets .... ▣ 762
Donnatal 1858
Donnatal Extentabs 1859
Donnatal Tablets 1858
Donnazyme Tablets 1860
Kinesed Tablets 2272
Phenobarbital Elixir and Tablets 1293
Primatene Tablets-P Formula 2421
Quadrinal Tablets 1183
Tedral SA 1765

(▣ Described in PDR For Nonprescription Drugs)

(⊙ Described in PDR For Ophthalmology)

Phensuximide (Phenothiazines may lower convulsive thresholds; dosage adjustments of anticonvulsants may be necessary). Products include:
- Milontin Kapseals 1741

Phenytoin (Phenytoin toxicity may be precipitated; Stelazine may lower convulsive thresholds; dosage adjustments of anticonvulsants may be necessary). Products include:
- Dilantin Infatabs 1710
- Dilantin-30 Pediatric/Dilantin-125 Suspension 1713

Phenytoin Sodium (Phenytoin toxicity may be precipitated; Stelazine may lower convulsive thresholds; dosage adjustments of anticonvulsants may be necessary). Products include:
- Dilantin Kapseals 1708
- Dilantin Parenteral 1712
- Dilantin with Phenobarbital Kapseals 1715

Polythiazide (Orthostatic hypotension that occurs with Stelazine may be accentuated). Products include:
- Minizide Capsules 1779
- Renese Tablets 1785
- Renese-R Tablets 1786

Prazepam (Additive depressant effects). Products include:
- Centrax 1693

Primidone (Stelazine may lower convulsive thresholds; dosage adjustments of anticonvulsants may be necessary). Products include:
- Mysoline 2480

Prochlorperazine (Additive depressant effects). Products include:
- Compazine 2201

Promethazine Hydrochloride (Additive depressant effects). Products include:
- Mepergan Injection 2479
- Phenergan with Codeine 2497
- Phenergan with Dextromethorphan 2499
- Phenergan Injection 2493
- Phenergan Suppositories 2496
- Phenergan Syrup 2495
- Phenergan Tablets 2496
- Phenergan VC 2500
- Phenergan VC with Codeine 2501

Propofol (Additive depressant effects). Products include:
- Diprivan Injection 2267

Propoxyphene Hydrochloride (Additive depressant effects). Products include:
- Darvon 1256
- Wygesic Tablets 2540

Propoxyphene Napsylate (Additive depressant effects). Products include:
- Darvon-N/Darvocet-N 1254

Propranolol Hydrochloride (Concomitant administration results in increased plasma levels of both drugs). Products include:
- Inderal 2459
- Inderal LA Long Acting Capsules 2461
- Inderide Tablets 2463
- Inderide LA Long Acting Capsules 2465

Quazepam (Additive depressant effects). Products include:
- Doral Tablets 2383

Secobarbital Sodium (Additive depressant effects). Products include:
- Seconal Sodium Pulvules 1296

Sufentanil Citrate (Additive depressant effects). Products include:
- Sufenta Injection 1147

Temazepam (Additive depressant effects). Products include:
- Restoril Capsules 2023

Thiamylal Sodium (Additive depressant effects). Products include:
- Surital Ampoules, Steri-Vials 1764

Thioridazine Hydrochloride (Additive depressant effects). Products include:
- Mellaril 2011

Thiothixene (Additive depressant effects). Products include:
- Navane Capsules and Concentrate 1954
- Navane Intramuscular 1956

Triazolam (Additive depressant effects). Products include:
- Halcion Tablets 2340

Trimethadione (Stelazine may lower convulsive thresholds; dosage adjustments of anticonvulsants may be necessary). Products include:
- Tridione 557

Valproic Acid (Stelazine may lower convulsive thresholds; dosage adjustments of anticonvulsants may be necessary). Products include:
- Depakene Capsules & Syrup 511

Warfarin Sodium (Effect may be diminished). Products include:
- Coumadin Injection & Tablets 944
- Panwarfin Tablets 547

STELAZINE INJECTION
(Trifluoperazine Hydrochloride) 2226
See **Stelazine Concentrate**

STELAZINE MULTI-DOSE VIALS
(Trifluoperazine Hydrochloride) 2226
See **Stelazine Concentrate**

STELAZINE TABLETS
(Trifluoperazine Hydrochloride) 2226
See **Stelazine Concentrate**

STILPHOSTROL TABLETS AND AMPULS
(Diethylstilbestrol Diphosphate) 1609
No interactions described in labeling.

STREPTASE FOR INFUSION
(Streptokinase) 635
May interact with anticoagulants and platelet inhibitors. Compounds in these categories include:

Aspirin (May cause bleeding complications). Products include:
- Alka-Seltzer Effervescent Antacid and Pain Reliever 1568
- Alka-Seltzer Extra Strength Effervescent Antacid and Pain Reliever 1570
- Alka-Seltzer (Flavored) Effervescent Antacid and Pain Reliever 1569
- Alka-Seltzer Plus Cold Medicine ▣ 623
- Alka-Seltzer Plus Night-Time Cold Medicine ▣ 623
- Alka Seltzer Plus Sinus Allergy Medicine ▣ 624
- Anacin Coated Analgesic Caplets 2417
- Anacin Coated Analgesic Tablets 2417
- Anacin Maximum Strength Analgesic Coated Tablets 2417
- Maximum Strength Arthritis Pain Formula By the Makers of Anacin Analgesic Tablets and Caplets 2418
- Arthritis Pain Formula by the Makers of Anacin Analgesic Tablets and Caplets ▣ 747
- Arthritis Strength BC Powder ▣ 516
- Ascriptin A/D Caplets 1850
- Regular Strength Ascriptin Tablets 1850
- Azdōne Tablets 844
- BC Powder ▣ 517
- BC Cold Powder ▣ 517
- Children's Bayer Chewable Aspirin ▣ 564
- Genuine Bayer Aspirin Tablets & Caplets ▣ 564
- Maximum Bayer Aspirin Tablets & Caplets ▣ 566
- Bayer Plus Aspirin Tablets ▣ 567
- Therapy Bayer Aspirin Caplets ▣ 568
- 8 Hour Bayer Timed-Release Aspirin ▣ 566
- Arthritis Strength Bufferin Analgesic Caplets 744
- Extra Strength Bufferin Analgesic Tablets 745
- Bufferin Analgesic Tablets and Caplets 743
- Cama Arthritis Pain Reliever ▣ 685
- Damason-P 1356
- Easprin 1719
- Ecotrin Enteric Coated Aspirin Maximum Strength Tablets and Caplets 2189
- Ecotrin Enteric Coated Aspirin Regular Strength Tablets and Caplets 2189
- Empirin Aspirin ▣ 541
- Empirin with Codeine Phosphate Nos. 2, 3 & 4 764
- Equagesic Tablets 2451
- Excedrin Extra-Strength Analgesic Tablets & Caplets 749
- 4-Way Cold Tablets 750
- Fiorinal Capsules 2007
- Fiorinal with Codeine Capsules 2008
- Fiorinal Tablets 2007
- Lortab ASA Tablets 2414
- Momentum Muscular Backache Formula ▣ 751
- Norgesic 1314
- Norwich Extra-Strength Aspirin ▣ 546
- Norwich Regular Strength Aspirin ▣ 547
- P-A-C Analgesic Tablets ▣ 669
- Percodan 951
- Robaxisal Tablets 1872
- Sine-Off Sinus Medicine Tablets-Aspirin Formula ▣ 722
- Soma Compound w/Codeine Tablets 2390
- Soma Compound Tablets 2389
- St. Joseph Adult Chewable Aspirin (81 mg.) ▣ 703
- Synalgos-DC Capsules 2525
- Talwin Compound 2072
- Ursinus Inlay-Tabs ▣ 691
- Vanquish Analgesic Caplets ▣ 574
- Zorprin Tablets 698

Azlocillin Sodium (May cause bleeding complications).
- No products indexed under this heading.

Carbenicillin Indanyl Sodium (May cause bleeding complications). Products include:
- Geocillin Tablets 1951

Choline Magnesium Trisalicylate (May cause bleeding complications). Products include:
- Trilisate 1822

Diclofenac Sodium (May cause bleeding complications). Products include:
- Voltaren Ophthalmic Sterile Ophthalmic Solution ⊙ 268
- Voltaren Tablets 1042

Dicumarol (May cause bleeding complications). Products include:
- Dicumarol Tablets 516

Diflunisal (May cause bleeding complications). Products include:
- Dolobid Tablets 1465

Dipyridamole (May cause bleeding complications). Products include:
- Persantine Tablets 683

Fenoprofen Calcium (May cause bleeding complications). Products include:
- Nalfon Pulvules & Tablets 919

Flurbiprofen (May cause bleeding complications). Products include:
- Ansaid Tablets 2319

Heparin Calcium (May cause bleeding complications). Products include:
- Calciparine Injection 925

Heparin Sodium (May cause bleeding complications). Products include:
- Heparin Lock Flush Solution 2456
- Heparin Sodium Vials 1264
- Heparin Sodium Injection 2457
- Heparin Sodium Injection, USP, Sterile Solution 2342

Ibuprofen (May cause bleeding complications). Products include:
- Advil Cold & Sinus Caplets (formerly CoAdvil) 2416
- Advil Ibuprofen Tablets and Caplets 2416
- Children's Advil Suspension 2426
- CoAdvil ▣ 748
- Dristan Sinus Caplets 2419
- Haltran Tablets ▣ 668
- Ibuprofen ▣ 631
- Medipren ibuprofen Caplets and Tablets 1362
- Midol 200 Cramp Relief Formula ▣ 570
- Motrin Tablets 2351
- Motrin IB Caplets and Tablets ▣ 736
- Nuprin Ibuprofen/Analgesic Tablets & Caplets 752
- PediaProfen Suspension 1363
- Rufen Tablets 691
- Trendar Ibuprofen Tablets ▣ 756

Indomethacin (May cause bleeding complications). Products include:
- Indocin 1487

Indomethacin Sodium Trihydrate (May cause bleeding complications). Products include:
- Indocin I.V. 1490

Ketoprofen (May cause bleeding complications). Products include:
- Orudis Capsules 2488

Magnesium Salicylate (May cause bleeding complications). Products include:
- Doan's - Extra-Strength Analgesic ▣ 549
- Doan's - Regular Strength Analgesic ▣ 549
- Mobigesic Analgesic Tablets ▣ 507

Meclofenamate Sodium (May cause bleeding complications). Products include:
- Meclomen Capsules 1739

Mefenamic Acid (May cause bleeding complications). Products include:
- Ponstel 1758

Mezlocillin Sodium (May cause bleeding complications). Products include:
- Mezlin 1597
- Mezlin Pharmacy Bulk Package 1599

Nafcillin Sodium (May cause bleeding complications). Products include:
- Unipen 2533

Naproxen (May cause bleeding complications). Products include:
- Naprosyn 2297

Naproxen Sodium (May cause bleeding complications). Products include:
- Anaprox and Anaprox DS Tablets 2288

Penicillin G Procaine (May cause bleeding complications). Products include:
- Bicillin C-R Injection 2438
- Bicillin C-R 900/300 Injection 2440
- Pfizerpen-AS Aqueous Suspension 1959
- Wycillin Injection 2537
- Wycillin Injection and Probenecid Tablets 2539

Penicillin G, Benzathine (May cause bleeding complications). Products include:
- Bicillin C-R Injection 2438
- Bicillin C-R 900/300 Injection 2440
- Bicillin L-A Injection 2442

Phenylbutazone (May cause bleeding complications). Products include:
- Butazolidin Capsules & Tablets 1027

Piroxicam (May cause bleeding complications). Products include:
- Feldene Capsules 1777

Salsalate (May cause bleeding complications). Products include:
- Disalcid 1310
- Mono-Gesic Tablets 846
- Salflex 839

Sulindac (May cause bleeding complications). Products include:
- Clinoril Tablets 1433

(▣ Described in PDR For Nonprescription Drugs) (⊙ Described in PDR For Ophthalmology)

Ticarcillin Disodium (May cause bleeding complications). Products include:
Ticar for Injection 2236
Timentin for Injection 2239

Tolmetin Sodium (May cause bleeding complications). Products include:
Tolectin (200, 400 and 600 mg) .. 1379

Warfarin Sodium (May cause bleeding complications). Products include:
Coumadin Injection & Tablets 944
Panwarfin Tablets 547

STRESSGARD STRESS FORMULA VITAMINS
(Multivitamins with Minerals) .... ▣ 628
No interactions described in labeling.

STRESSTABS
(Multivitamins) .... ▣ 589
No interactions described in labeling.

STRESSTABS + IRON, ADVANCED FORMULA
(Vitamins with Iron) .... ▣ 589
No interactions described in labeling.

STRESSTABS + ZINC
(Vitamins with Minerals) .... ▣ 589
No interactions described in labeling.

STRI-DEX DUAL TEXTURED MAXIMUM STRENGTH PADS
(Salicylic Acid) .... ▣ 573
May interact with:

Concomitant Topical Acne Therapy (May increase dryness or irritation of the skin).

STRI-DEX DUAL TEXTURED MAXIMUM STRENGTH BIG PADS
(Salicylic Acid) .... ▣ 573
See **Stri-Dex Dual Textured Maximum Strength Pads**

STRI-DEX DUAL TEXTURED REGULAR STRENGTH PADS
(Salicylic Acid) .... ▣ 573
See **Stri-Dex Dual Textured Maximum Strength Pads**

STRI-DEX DUAL TEXTURED REGULAR STRENGTH BIG PADS
(Salicylic Acid) .... ▣ 573
See **Stri-Dex Dual Textured Maximum Strength Pads**

STUART PRENATAL TABLETS
(Vitamins with Minerals) 2273
No interactions described in labeling.

THE STUART FORMULA TABLETS
(Vitamins with Minerals) 1157
No interactions described in labeling.

STUARTINIC TABLETS
(Vitamins with Minerals) 1157
No interactions described in labeling.

STUARTNATAL 1+1 TABLETS
(Vitamins with Minerals) 2273
No interactions described in labeling.

SUBLIMAZE INJECTION
(Fentanyl Citrate) 1146
May interact with central nervous system depressants and certain other agents. Compounds in these categories include:

Alfentanil Hydrochloride (Additive or potentiating effects). Products include:
Alfenta Injection 1131

Alprazolam (Additive or potentiating effects). Products include:
Xanax Tablets 2367

Aprobarbital (Additive or potentiating effects). Products include:
Alurate Elixir 1883

Buprenorphine (Additive or potentiating effects).
No products indexed under this heading.

Buspirone Hydrochloride (Additive or potentiating effects). Products include:
BuSpar 1401

Butabarbital (Additive or potentiating effects). Products include:
Pyridium Plus 1764

Butalbital (Additive or potentiating effects). Products include:
Esgic-Plus Tablets 1002
Esgic Tablets & Capsules 1001
Fioricet Tablets 2006
Fiorinal Capsules 2007
Fiorinal with Codeine Capsules 2008
Fiorinal Tablets 2007
Phrenilin 838
Sedapap Tablets 50 mg/650 mg .. 1360

Chlordiazepoxide (Additive or potentiating effects). Products include:
Libritabs Tablets 1930
Limbitrol 1933
Menrium Tablets 1934

Chlordiazepoxide Hydrochloride (Additive or potentiating effects). Products include:
Librax Capsules 1929
Librium Capsules 1931
Librium Injectable 1932

Chlorpromazine (Additive or potentiating effects). Products include:
Thorazine 2234

Chlorprothixene (Additive or potentiating effects). Products include:
Taractan Tablets 1920

Chlorprothixene Hydrochloride (Additive or potentiating effects). Products include:
Taractan 1920

Clorazepate Dipotassium (Additive or potentiating effects). Products include:
Tranxene 556

Codeine (Additive or potentiating effects). Products include:
Calcidrine Syrup 506

Codeine Phosphate (Additive or potentiating effects). Products include:
Actifed with Codeine Cough Syrup .. 752
Cheracol Cough Syrup 1853
Codimal PH Syrup 846
Dimetane-DC Cough Syrup 1857
Empirin with Codeine Phosphate Nos. 2, 3 & 4 764
Fiorinal with Codeine Capsules 2008
Isoclor Expectorant 982
Naldecon CX Adult Liquid .... ▣ 521
Novahistine DH 1342
Novahistine Expectorant 1343
Nucofed Capsules 2219
Nucofed Expectorant 2219
Nucofed Pediatric Expectorant 2220
Nucofed Syrup 2219
Phenaphen with Codeine Capsules 1865
Phenaphen-650 with Codeine Tablets 1866
Phenergan with Codeine 2497
Phenergan VC with Codeine 2501
Robitussin A-C Syrup 1875
Robitussin-DAC Syrup 1875
Ryna .... ▣ 741
Soma Compound w/Codeine Tablets 2390
Triaminic Expectorant w/Codeine .. 1996
Tussi-Organidin Liquid 2391
Tylenol with Codeine 1381

Codeine Polistirex (Additive or potentiating effects).
No products indexed under this heading.

Dezocine (Additive or potentiating effects).

Diazepam (Additive or potentiating effects; cardiovascular depression). Products include:
Valium Injectable 1937
Valium Tablets 1939
Valrelease Capsules 1923

Droperidol (Decreased pulmonary arterial pressure; additive or potentiating effects). Products include:
Inapsine Injection 1140
Innovar Injection 1141

Enflurane (Additive or potentiating effects). Products include:
Ethrane 599

Estazolam (Additive or potentiating effects). Products include:
ProSom Tablets 554

Ethchlorvynol (Additive or potentiating effects). Products include:
Placidyl Capsules 553

Ethinamate (Additive or potentiating effects).
No products indexed under this heading.

Fentanyl (Additive or potentiating effects). Products include:
Duragesic Transdermal System 1133

Fluphenazine Decanoate (Additive or potentiating effects). Products include:
Prolixin Decanoate 1795

Fluphenazine Enanthate (Additive or potentiating effects). Products include:
Prolixin Enanthate 1796

Fluphenazine Hydrochloride (Additive or potentiating effects). Products include:
Prolixin Elixir 1793
Prolixin Injection 1791
Prolixin Oral Concentrate 1792
Prolixin Tablets 1793

Flurazepam Hydrochloride (Additive or potentiating effects). Products include:
Dalmane Capsules 1927

Glutethimide (Additive or potentiating effects).
No products indexed under this heading.

Haloperidol (Additive or potentiating effects). Products include:
Haldol Injection, Tablets and Concentrate 1373

Haloperidol Decanoate (Additive or potentiating effects). Products include:
Haldol Decanoate 1375

Hydrocodone Bitartrate (Additive or potentiating effects). Products include:
Anexsia 5/500 Tablets 2196
Anexsia 7.5/650 Tablets 2197
Azdone Tablets 844
Codiclear DH Syrup 845
Codimal DH Syrup 846
Damason-P 1356
Hycodan Syrup, Tablets 927
Hycomine Compound Tablets 929
Hycomine Syrup 927
Hycotuss Expectorant Syrup 930
Hydrocet Capsules 835
Lortab ASA Tablets 2414
Lortab 2412
Ru-Tuss with Hydrocodone 694
Triaminic Expectorant DH 1995
Vicodin Tablets 1187
Vicodin ES Tablets 1189
Zydone Capsules 941

Hydrocodone Polistirex (Additive or potentiating effects). Products include:
Tussionex Extended-Release Suspension 988

Hydroxyzine Hydrochloride (Additive or potentiating effects). Products include:
Atarax Tablets & Syrup 1941
Marax Tablets & DF Syrup 1954
Vistaril Intramuscular Solution 1970

Isoflurane (Additive or potentiating effects). Products include:
Forane 600

Ketamine Hydrochloride (Additive or potentiating effects). Products include:
Ketalar 1726

Levorphanol Tartrate (Additive or potentiating effects). Products include:
Levo-Dromoran 1906

Lorazepam (Additive or potentiating effects). Products include:
Ativan Injection 2432
Ativan Tablets 2434

Loxapine Hydrochloride (Additive or potentiating effects). Products include:
Loxitane 1213

Loxapine Succinate (Additive or potentiating effects). Products include:
Loxitane Capsules 1213

Meperidine Hydrochloride (Additive or potentiating effects). Products include:
Demerol 2047
Mepergan Injection 2479

Mephobarbital (Additive or potentiating effects). Products include:
Mebaral Tablets 2061

Meprobamate (Additive or potentiating effects). Products include:
Deprol Tablets 2382
Equagesic Tablets 2451
Miltown Tablets 2386
PMB 200 and PMB 400 2504

Mesoridazine (Additive or potentiating effects). Products include:
Serentil 686

Methadone Hydrochloride (Additive or potentiating effects). Products include:
Dolophine Hydrochloride Ampoules & Vials 1260
Dolophine Hydrochloride Tablets 1261
Methadone Hydrochloride Diskets .. 1284
Methadone Hydrochloride Oral Solution & Tablets 1987

Methohexital Sodium (Additive or potentiating effects). Products include:
Brevital Sodium Vials 1248

Methoxyflurane (Additive or potentiating effects).
No products indexed under this heading.

Midazolam Hydrochloride (Additive of potentiating effects). Products include:
Versed Injection 1924

Molindone Hydrochloride (Additive or potentiating effects). Products include:
Moban Tablets & Concentrate 932

Morphine Sulfate (Additive or potentiating effects). Products include:
Astramorph/PF Injection, USP (Preservative-Free) 618
Duramorph 960
Infumorph 200 and Infumorph 500 Sterile Solutions 962
MS Contin Tablets 1814
MSIR 1817
Oramorph SR (Morphine Sulfate Sustained Release Tablets) 1988
Roxanol 1991

Nitrous Oxide (Cardiovascular depression).

Opium Alkaloids (Additive or potentiating effects). Products include:
- B & O No. 15A & No. 16A Supprettes ... 2395
- Pantopon Injectable ... 1911

Oxazepam (Additive or potentiating effects). Products include:
- Serax Capsules ... 2522
- Serax Tablets ... 2522

Oxycodone Hydrochloride (Additive or potentiating effects). Products include:
- Percocet Tablets ... 950
- Percodan ... 951
- Roxicodone Tablets, Oral Solution & Intensol (Oxycodone) ... 1992
- Tylox Capsules ... 1382

Pentobarbital Sodium (Additive or potentiating effects). Products include:
- Nembutal Sodium Capsules ... 534
- Nembutal Sodium Solution ... 536
- Nembutal Sodium Suppositories ... 538

Perphenazine (Additive or potentiating effects). Products include:
- Etrafon ... 2087
- Triavil Tablets ... 1556
- Trilafon ... 2123

Phenobarbital (Additive or potentiating effects). Products include:
- Arco-Lase Plus Tablets ... 607
- Bellergal-S Tablets ... 1998
- Bronkolixir ... ▣ 761
- Bronkotabs Tablets ... ▣ 762
- Donnatal ... 1858
- Donnatal Extentabs ... 1859
- Donnatal Tablets ... 1858
- Donnazyme Tablets ... 1860
- Kinesed Tablets ... 2272
- Phenobarbital Elixir and Tablets ... 1293
- Primatene Tablets-P Formula ... 2421
- Quadrinal Tablets ... 1183
- Tedral SA ... 1765

Prazepam (Additive or potentiating effects). Products include:
- Centrax ... 1693

Prochlorperazine (Additive or potentiating effects). Products include:
- Compazine ... 2201

Promethazine Hydrochloride (Additive or potentiating effects). Products include:
- Mepergan Injection ... 2479
- Phenergan with Codeine ... 2497
- Phenergan with Dextromethorphan 2499
- Phenergan Injection ... 2493
- Phenergan Suppositories ... 2496
- Phenergan Syrup ... 2495
- Phenergan Tablets ... 2496
- Phenergan VC ... 2500
- Phenergan VC with Codeine ... 2501

Propofol (Additive or potentiating effects). Products include:
- Diprivan Injection ... 2267

Propoxyphene Hydrochloride (Additive or potentiating effects). Products include:
- Darvon ... 1256
- Wygesic Tablets ... 2540

Propoxyphene Napsylate (Additive or potentiating effects). Products include:
- Darvon-N/Darvocet-N ... 1254

Quazepam (Additive or potentiating effects). Products include:
- Doral Tablets ... 2383

Secobarbital Sodium (Additive or potentiating effects). Products include:
- Seconal Sodium Pulvules ... 1296

Sufentanil Citrate (Additive or potentiating effects). Products include:
- Sufenta Injection ... 1147

Temazepam (Additive or potentiating effects). Products include:
- Restoril Capsules ... 2023

Thiamylal Sodium (Additive or potentiating effects). Products include:
- Surital Ampoules, Steri-Vials ... 1764

Thioridazine Hydrochloride (Additive or potentiating effects). Products include:
- Mellaril ... 2011

Thiothixene (Additive or potentiating effects). Products include:
- Navane Capsules and Concentrate 1954
- Navane Intramuscular ... 1956

Triazolam (Additive or potentiating effects). Products include:
- Halcion Tablets ... 2340

Trifluoperazine Hydrochloride (Additive or potentiating effects). Products include:
- Stelazine ... 2226

SUCCUS CINERARIA MARITIMA (SCM-WALKER)
(Senecio Cineraria Extracts) ... ◉ 313
No interactions described in labeling.

SUCRETS (ORIGINAL MINT AND MENTHOLATED MINT)
(Hexylresorcinol) ... ▣ 723
No interactions described in labeling.

SUCRETS CHILDREN'S CHERRY FLAVORED SORE THROAT LOZENGES
(Dyclonine Hydrochloride) ... ▣ 724
No interactions described in labeling.

SUCRETS COLD FORMULA
(Hexylresorcinol, Menthol) ... ▣ 724
No interactions described in labeling.

SUCRETS COUGH CONTROL FORMULA
(Dextromethorphan Hydrobromide) ... ▣ 724
No interactions described in labeling.

SUCRETS MAXIMUM STRENGTH WINTERGREEN AND SUCRETS WILD CHERRY (REGULAR STRENGTH) SORE THROAT LOZENGES
(Dyclonine Hydrochloride) ... ▣ 724
No interactions described in labeling.

SUCRETS MAXIMUM STRENGTH SPRAYS
(Dyclonine Hydrochloride) ... ▣ 725
No interactions described in labeling.

SUDAFED CHILDREN'S LIQUID
(Pseudoephedrine Hydrochloride) .. ▣ 543
May interact with antihypertensives and antidepressant drugs. Compounds in these categories include:

Acebutolol Hydrochloride (Concurrent use not recommended). Products include:
- Sectral Capsules ... 2520

Amitriptyline Hydrochloride (Concurrent use not recommended). Products include:
- Elavil ... 2269
- Endep Tablets ... 1927
- Etrafon ... 2087
- Limbitrol ... 1933
- Triavil Tablets ... 1556

Amoxapine (Concurrent use not recommended). Products include:
- Asendin Tablets ... 1196

Atenolol (Concurrent use not recommended). Products include:
- Tenoretic Tablets ... 1105
- Tenormin Tablets and I.V. Injection 1107

Benazepril Hydrochloride (Concurrent use not recommended). Products include:
- Lotensin Tablets ... 872

Betaxolol Hydrochloride (Concurrent use not recommended). Products include:
- Betoptic Sterile Ophthalmic Solution ... 569
- Betoptic S Sterile Ophthalmic Suspension ... 570
- Kerlone Tablets ... 2172

Bupropion Hydrochloride (Concurrent use not recommended). Products include:
- Wellbutrin Tablets ... 821

Captopril (Concurrent use not recommended). Products include:
- Capoten ... 2255
- Capozide ... 2258

Carteolol Hydrochloride (Concurrent use not recommended). Products include:
- Cartrol Tablets ... 507

Clonidine (Concurrent use not recommended). Products include:
- Catapres-TTS ... 677

Clonidine Hydrochloride (Concurrent use not recommended). Products include:
- Catapres Tablets ... 676
- Combipres Tablets ... 678

Deserpidine (Concurrent use not recommended). Products include:
- Enduronyl ... 518
- Harmonyl Tablets ... 528
- Oreticyl ... 545

Desipramine Hydrochloride (Concurrent use not recommended). Products include:
- Norpramin Tablets ... 1340

Diazoxide (Concurrent use not recommended). Products include:
- Hyperstat I.V. Injection ... 2095
- Proglycem ... 649

Doxazosin Mesylate (Concurrent use not recommended). Products include:
- Cardura Tablets ... 1941

Doxepin Hydrochloride (Concurrent use not recommended). Products include:
- Sinequan ... 1960

Enalapril Maleate (Concurrent use not recommended). Products include:
- Vaseretic Tablets ... 1559
- Vasotec Tablets ... 1564

Enalaprilat (Concurrent use not recommended). Products include:
- Vasotec I.V. ... 1562

Esmolol Hydrochloride (Concurrent use not recommended). Products include:
- Brevibloc Injection ... 942

Felodipine (Concurrent use not recommended). Products include:
- Plendil Extended-Release Tablets ... 1526

Fluoxetine Hydrochloride (Concurrent use not recommended). Products include:
- Prozac Pulvules ... 920

Fosinopril Sodium (Concurrent use not recommended). Products include:
- Monopril Tablets ... 1406

Guanabenz Acetate (Concurrent use not recommended). Products include:
- Wytensin Tablets ... 2542

Guanethidine Monosulfate (Concurrent use not recommended). Products include:
- Esimil Tablets ... 864
- Ismelin Tablets ... 869

Hydralazine Hydrochloride (Concurrent use not recommended). Products include:
- Apresazide Capsules ... 854
- Apresoline Hydrochloride Parenteral (Ampuls) ... 856
- Apresoline Hydrochloride Tablets .. 855
- Apresoline-Esidrix Tablets ... 857
- Ser-Ap-Es Tablets ... 881
- Serpasil-Apresoline Tablets ... 884

Imipramine Hydrochloride (Concurrent use not recommended). Products include:
- Tofranil Ampuls ... 1038
- Tofranil Tablets ... 1039

Imipramine Pamoate (Concurrent use not recommended). Products include:
- Tofranil-PM Capsules ... 1041

Indapamide (Concurrent use not recommended). Products include:
- Lozol Tablets ... 1843

Isocarboxazid (Concurrent use not recommended). Products include:
- Marplan Tablets ... 1906

Isradipine (Concurrent use not recommended). Products include:
- DynaCirc Capsules ... 2004

Labetalol Hydrochloride (Concurrent use not recommended). Products include:
- Normodyne Injection ... 2108
- Normodyne Tablets ... 2110
- Normozide Tablets ... 2112
- Trandate HCT Tablets ... 579
- Trandate Injection ... 577
- Trandate Tablets ... 579

Lisinopril (Concurrent use not recommended). Products include:
- Prinivil Tablets ... 1538
- Prinzide Tablets ... 1540
- Zestoretic ... 2274
- Zestril Tablets ... 2277

Maprotiline Hydrochloride (Concurrent use not recommended). Products include:
- Ludiomil Tablets ... 874

Mecamylamine Hydrochloride (Concurrent use not recommended). Products include:
- Inversine Tablets ... 1492

Methyldopa (Concurrent use not recommended). Products include:
- Aldoclor Tablets ... 1413
- Aldomet Oral ... 1415
- Aldoril Tablets ... 1418

Methyldopate Hydrochloride (Concurrent use not recommended). Products include:
- Aldomet Ester HCl Injection ... 1417

Metoprolol Tartrate (Concurrent use not recommended). Products include:
- Lopressor Ampuls ... 1032
- Lopressor HCT Tablets ... 1034
- Lopressor Tablets ... 1032

Metyrosine (Concurrent use not recommended). Products include:
- Demser Capsules ... 1460

Minoxidil (Concurrent use not recommended). Products include:
- Loniten Tablets ... 2346
- Rogaine Topical Solution ... 2357

Nadolol (Concurrent use not recommended). Products include:
- Corgard Tablets ... 701
- Corzide Tablets ... 702

Nicardipine Hydrochloride (Concurrent use not recommended). Products include:
- Cardene Capsules ... 2290

Nitroglycerin (Concurrent use not recommended). Products include:
- Deponit NTG Transdermal Delivery System ... 2143
- Minitran Transdermal Delivery System ... 1312
- Nitro-Bid Ointment ... 1339
- Nitro-Bid Capsules ... 1338
- Nitrodisc ... 2176

Nitro-Dur (nitroglycerin) Transdermal Infusion System 1164
Nitrogard Tablets................................ 1004
Nitrolingual Spray 1846
Nitrostat Tablets 1743
Transderm-Nitro Transdermal Therapeutic System 2283

Nortriptyline Hydrochloride (Concurrent use not recommended). Products include:
Pamelor 2019

Penbutolol Sulfate (Concurrent use not recommended). Products include:
Levatol 1832

Phenelzine Sulfate (Concurrent use not recommended). Products include:
Nardil 1742

Phenoxybenzamine Hydrochloride (Concurrent use not recommended). Products include:
Dibenzyline Capsules 2207

Phentolamine Mesylate (Concurrent use not recommended). Products include:
Regitine 878

Pindolol (Concurrent use not recommended). Products include:
Visken Tablets.. 2036

Prazosin Hydrochloride (Concurrent use not recommended). Products include:
Minipress Capsules.............................. 1778
Minizide Capsules................................ 1779

Propranolol Hydrochloride (Concurrent use not recommended). Products include:
Inderal 2459
Inderal LA Long Acting Capsules 2461
Inderide Tablets 2463
Inderide LA Long Acting Capsules .. 2465

Protriptyline Hydrochloride (Concurrent use not recommended). Products include:
Vivactil Tablets 1567

Ramipril (Concurrent use not recommended). Products include:
Altace Capsules 1086

Rauwolfia Serpentina (Concurrent use not recommended). Products include:
Raudixin Tablets.................................. 1803
Rauzide Tablets 1804

Rescinnamine (Concurrent use not recommended).
No products indexed under this heading.

Reserpine (Concurrent use not recommended). Products include:
Diupres Tablets 1461
Hydromox R Tablets............................ 1209
Hydropres Tablets................................ 1485
Renese-R Tablets................................ 1786
Salutensin/Salutensin-Demi 719
Ser-Ap-Es Tablets 881
Serpasil Tablets 883
Serpasil-Apresoline Tablets.............. 884
Serpasil-Esidrix Tablets...................... 886

Sodium Nitroprusside (Concurrent use not recommended). Products include:
Nipride I.V. Infusion 1909

Terazosin Hydrochloride (Concurrent use not recommended). Products include:
Hytrin Tablets 529

Timolol Maleate (Concurrent use not recommended). Products include:
Blocadren Tablets 1429
Timolide Tablets.................................. 1547
Timoptic in Ocudose 1552
Timoptic Sterile Ophthalmic Solution.. 1550

Tranylcypromine Sulfate (Concurrent use not recommended). Products include:
Parnate Tablets 2222

Trazodone Hydrochloride (Concurrent use not recommended). Products include:
Desyrel and Desyrel Dividose 1404

Trimethaphan Camsylate (Concurrent use not recommended). Products include:
Arfonad Ampuls 1887

Trimipramine Maleate (Concurrent use not recommended). Products include:
Surmontil Capsules.............................. 2524

SUDAFED COUGH SYRUP
(Dextromethorphan Hydrobromide, Guaifenesin, Pseudoephedrine Hydrochloride)................................▣ 543
May interact with monoamine oxidase inhibitors. Compounds in this category include:

Furazolidone (Concurrent administration is not recommended). Products include:
Furoxone 1855

Isocarboxazid (Concurrent administration is not recommended). Products include:
Marplan Tablets 1906

Phenelzine Sulfate (Concurrent administration is not recommended). Products include:
Nardil 1742

Selegiline Hydrochloride (Concurrent administration is not recommended). Products include:
Eldepryl 2250

Tranylcypromine Sulfate (Concurrent administration is not recommended). Products include:
Parnate Tablets 2222

SUDAFED PLUS LIQUID
(Chlorpheniramine Maleate, Pseudoephedrine Hydrochloride)....▣ 544
May interact with monoamine oxidase inhibitors and certain other agents. Compounds in these categories include:

Alcohol (Concurrent use not recommended).

Furazolidone (Concurrent administration is not recommended). Products include:
Furoxone 1855

Isocarboxazid (Concurrent administration is not recommended). Products include:
Marplan Tablets 1906

Phenelzine Sulfate (Concurrent administration is not recommended). Products include:
Nardil 1742

Selegiline Hydrochloride (Concurrent administration is not recommended). Products include:
Eldepryl 2250

Tranylcypromine Sulfate (Concurrent administration is not recommended). Products include:
Parnate Tablets 2222

SUDAFED PLUS TABLETS
(Chlorpheniramine Maleate, Pseudoephedrine Hydrochloride)....▣ 545
May interact with monoamine oxidase inhibitors and certain other agents. Compounds in these categories include:

Alcohol (Concurrent use not recommended).

Furazolidone (Concurrent administration is not recommended). Products include:
Furoxone 1855

Isocarboxazid (Concurrent administration is not recommended). Products include:
Marplan Tablets 1906

Phenelzine Sulfate (Concurrent administration is not recommended). Products include:
Nardil 1742

Selegiline Hydrochloride (Concurrent administration is not recommended). Products include:
Eldepryl 2250

Tranylcypromine Sulfate (Concurrent administration is not recommended). Products include:
Parnate Tablets 2222

SUDAFED SINUS CAPLETS
(Acetaminophen, Pseudoephedrine Hydrochloride)................................▣ 545
May interact with monoamine oxidase inhibitors. Compounds in this category include:

Furazolidone (Concurrent administration is not recommended). Products include:
Furoxone 1855

Isocarboxazid (Concurrent administration is not recommended). Products include:
Marplan Tablets 1906

Phenelzine Sulfate (Concurrent administration is not recommended). Products include:
Nardil 1742

Selegiline Hydrochloride (Concurrent administration is not recommended). Products include:
Eldepryl 2250

Tranylcypromine Sulfate (Concurrent administration is not recommended). Products include:
Parnate Tablets 2222

SUDAFED SINUS TABLETS
(Acetaminophen, Pseudoephedrine Hydrochloride)................................▣ 545
May interact with monoamine oxidase inhibitors. Compounds in this category include:

Furazolidone (Concurrent administration is not recommended). Products include:
Furoxone 1855

Isocarboxazid (Concurrent administration is not recommended). Products include:
Marplan Tablets 1906

Phenelzine Sulfate (Concurrent administration is not recommended). Products include:
Nardil 1742

Selegiline Hydrochloride (Concurrent administration is not recommended). Products include:
Eldepryl 2250

Tranylcypromine Sulfate (Concurrent administration is not recommended). Products include:
Parnate Tablets 2222

SUDAFED TABLETS, 30 MG
(Pseudoephedrine Hydrochloride) ..▣ 544
May interact with monoamine oxidase inhibitors. Compounds in this category include:

Furazolidone (Concurrent administration is not recommended). Products include:
Furoxone 1855

Isocarboxazid (Concurrent administration is not recommended). Products include:
Marplan Tablets 1906

Phenelzine Sulfate (Concurrent administration is not recommended). Products include:
Nardil 1742

Selegiline Hydrochloride (Concurrent administration is not recommended). Products include:
Eldepryl 2250

Tranylcypromine Sulfate (Concurrent administration is not recommended). Products include:
Parnate Tablets 2222

SUDAFED TABLETS, ADULT STRENGTH, 60 MG
(Pseudoephedrine Hydrochloride) ..▣ 544
May interact with monoamine oxidase inhibitors. Compounds in this category include:

Furazolidone (Concurrent administration is not recommended). Products include:
Furoxone 1855

Isocarboxazid (Concurrent administration is not recommended). Products include:
Marplan Tablets 1906

Phenelzine Sulfate (Concurrent administration is not recommended). Products include:
Nardil 1742

Selegiline Hydrochloride (Concurrent administration is not recommended). Products include:
Eldepryl 2250

Tranylcypromine Sulfate (Concurrent administration is not recommended). Products include:
Parnate Tablets 2222

SUDAFED 12 HOUR CAPSULES
(Pseudoephedrine Hydrochloride) ..▣ 545
May interact with monoamine oxidase inhibitors. Compounds in this category include:

Furazolidone (Concurrent administration is not recommended). Products include:
Furoxone 1855

Isocarboxazid (Concurrent administration is not recommended). Products include:
Marplan Tablets 1906

Phenelzine Sulfate (Concurrent administration is not recommended). Products include:
Nardil 1742

Selegiline Hydrochloride (Concurrent administration is not recommended). Products include:
Eldepryl 2250

Tranylcypromine Sulfate (Concurrent administration is not recommended). Products include:
Parnate Tablets 2222

SUFENTA INJECTION
(Sufentanil Citrate) 1147
May interact with central nervous system depressants, barbiturates, tranquilizers, narcotic analgesics, neuromuscular blocking agents, and certain other agents. Compounds in these categories include:

Alfentanil Hydrochloride (Enhanced magnitude and duration of CNS/cardiovascular effects; respiratory depression may be enhanced). Products include:
Alfenta Injection 1131

Alprazolam (Enhanced magnitude and duration of CNS/cardiovascular effects; respiratory depression may be enhanced). Products include:
Xanax Tablets 2367

Aprobarbital (Enhanced magnitude and duration of CNS/cardiovascular effects; respiratory depression may be enhanced). Products include:
- Alurate Elixir ... 1883

Atracurium Besylate (May produce bradycardia and hypotension; effect may be pronounced in the presence of calcium channel and/or beta-blockers). Products include:
- Tracrium Injection ... 817

Buprenorphine (Enhanced magnitude and duration of CNS/cardiovascular effects; respiratory depression may be enhanced).
- No products indexed under this heading.

Buspirone Hydrochloride (Enhanced magnitude and duration of CNS/cardiovascular effects; respiratory depression may be enhanced). Products include:
- BuSpar ... 1401

Butabarbital (Enhanced magnitude and duration of CNS/cardiovascular effects; respiratory depression may be enhanced). Products include:
- Pyridium Plus ... 1764

Butalbital (Enhanced magnitude and duration of CNS/cardiovascular effects; respiratory depression may be enhanced). Products include:
- Esgic-Plus Tablets ... 1002
- Esgic Tablets & Capsules ... 1001
- Fioricet Tablets ... 2006
- Fiorinal Capsules ... 2007
- Fiorinal with Codeine Capsules ... 2008
- Fiorinal Tablets ... 2007
- Phrenilin ... 838
- Sedapap Tablets 50 mg/650 mg .. 1360

Chlordiazepoxide (Enhanced magnitude and duration of CNS/cardiovascular effects; respiratory depression may be enhanced). Products include:
- Libritabs Tablets ... 1930
- Limbitrol ... 1933
- Menrium Tablets ... 1934

Chlordiazepoxide Hydrochloride (Enhanced magnitude and duration of CNS/cardiovascular effects; respiratory depression may be enhanced). Products include:
- Librax Capsules ... 1929
- Librium Capsules ... 1931
- Librium Injectable ... 1932

Chlorpromazine (Enhanced magnitude and duration of CNS/cardiovascular effects; respiratory depression may be enhanced). Products include:
- Thorazine ... 2234

Chlorprothixene (Enhanced magnitude and duration of CNS/cardiovascular effects; respiratory depression may be enhanced). Products include:
- Taractan Tablets ... 1920

Chlorprothixene Hydrochloride (Enhanced magnitude and duration of CNS/cardiovascular effects; respiratory depression may be enhanced). Products include:
- Taractan ... 1920

Clorazepate Dipotassium (Enhanced magnitude and duration of CNS/cardiovascular effects; respiratory depression may be enhanced). Products include:
- Tranxene ... 556

Codeine (Enhanced magnitude and duration of CNS/cardiovascular effects; respiratory depression may be enhanced). Products include:
- Calcidrine Syrup ... 506

Codeine Phosphate (Enhanced magnitude and duration of CNS/cardiovascular effects; respiratory depression may be enhanced). Products include:
- Actifed with Codeine Cough Syrup.. 752
- Cheracol Cough Syrup ... 1853
- Codimal PH Syrup ... 846
- Dimetane-DC Cough Syrup ... 1857
- Empirin with Codeine Phosphate Nos. 2, 3 & 4 ... 764
- Fiorinal with Codeine Capsules ... 2008
- Isoclor Expectorant ... 982
- Naldecon CX Adult Liquid ... 521
- Novahistine DH ... 1342
- Novahistine Expectorant ... 1343
- Nucofed Capsules ... 2219
- Nucofed Expectorant ... 2219
- Nucofed Pediatric Expectorant ... 2220
- Nucofed Syrup ... 2219
- Phenaphen with Codeine Capsules 1865
- Phenaphen-650 with Codeine Tablets ... 1866
- Phenergan with Codeine ... 2497
- Phenergan VC with Codeine ... 2501
- Robitussin A-C Syrup ... 1875
- Robitussin-DAC Syrup ... 1875
- Ryna ... 741
- Soma Compound w/Codeine Tablets ... 2390
- Triaminic Expectorant w/Codeine .. 1996
- Tussi-Organidin Liquid ... 2391
- Tylenol with Codeine ... 1381

Codeine Polistirex (Enhanced magnitude and duration of CNS/cardiovascular effects; respiratory depression may be enhanced).
- No products indexed under this heading.

Dezocine (Enhanced magnitude and duration of CNS/cardiovascular effects; respiratory depression may be enhanced).

Diazepam (Enhanced magnitude and duration of CNS/cardiovascular effects; respiratory depression may be enhanced). Products include:
- Valium Injectable ... 1937
- Valium Tablets ... 1939
- Valrelease Capsules ... 1923

DOXACURIUM CHLORIDE (May produce bradycardia and hypotension; effect may be pronounced in the presence of calcium channel and/or beta-blockers). Products include:
- Nuromax Injection ... 794

Droperidol (Enhanced magnitude and duration of CNS/cardiovascular effects; respiratory depression may be enhanced). Products include:
- Inapsine Injection ... 1140
- Innovar Injection ... 1141

Enflurane (Enhanced magnitude and duration of CNS/cardiovascular effects; respiratory depression may be enhanced). Products include:
- Ethrane ... 599

Estazolam (Enhanced magnitude and duration of CNS/cardiovascular effects; respiratory depression may be enhanced). Products include:
- ProSom Tablets ... 554

Ethchlorvynol (Enhanced magnitude and duration of CNS/cardiovascular effects; respiratory depression may be enhanced). Products include:
- Placidyl Capsules ... 553

Ethinamate (Enhanced magnitude and duration of CNS/cardiovascular effects; respiratory depression may be enhanced).
- No products indexed under this heading.

Fentanyl (Enhanced magnitude and duration of CNS/cardiovascular effects; respiratory depression may be enhanced). Products include:
- Duragesic Transdermal System ... 1133

Fentanyl Citrate (Enhanced magnitude and duration of CNS/cardiovascular effects; respiratory depression may be enhanced). Products include:
- Innovar Injection ... 1141
- Sublimaze Injection ... 1146

Fluphenazine Decanoate (Enhanced magnitude and duration of CNS/cardiovascular effects; respiratory depression may be enhanced). Products include:
- Prolixin Decanoate ... 1795

Fluphenazine Enanthate (Enhanced magnitude and duration of CNS/cardiovascular effects; respiratory depression may be enhanced). Products include:
- Prolixin Enanthate ... 1796

Fluphenazine Hydrochloride (Enhanced magnitude and duration of CNS/cardiovascular effects; respiratory depression may be enhanced). Products include:
- Prolixin Elixir ... 1793
- Prolixin Injection ... 1791
- Prolixin Oral Concentrate ... 1792
- Prolixin Tablets ... 1793

Flurazepam Hydrochloride (Enhanced magnitude and duration of CNS/cardiovascular effects; respiratory depression may be enhanced). Products include:
- Dalmane Capsules ... 1927

Glutethimide (Enhanced magnitude and duration of CNS/cardiovascular effects; respiratory depression may be enhanced).
- No products indexed under this heading.

Haloperidol (Enhanced magnitude and duration of CNS/cardiovascular effects; respiratory depression may be enhanced). Products include:
- Haldol Injection, Tablets and Concentrate ... 1373

Haloperidol Decanoate (Enhanced magnitude and duration of CNS/cardiovascular effects; respiratory depression may be enhanced). Products include:
- Haldol Decanoate ... 1375

Hydrocodone Bitartrate (Enhanced magnitude and duration of CNS/cardiovascular effects; respiratory depression may be enhanced). Products include:
- Anexsia 5/500 Tablets ... 2196
- Anexsia 7.5/650 Tablets ... 2197
- Azdōne Tablets ... 844
- Codiclear DH Syrup ... 845
- Codimal DH Syrup ... 846
- Damason-P ... 1356
- Hycodan Syrup, Tablets ... 927
- Hycomine Compound Tablets ... 929
- Hycomine Syrup ... 927
- Hycotuss Expectorant Syrup ... 930
- Hydrocet Capsules ... 835
- Lortab ASA Tablets ... 2414
- Lortab ... 2412
- Ru-Tuss with Hydrocodone ... 694
- Triaminic Expectorant DH ... 1995
- Vicodin Tablets ... 1187
- Vicodin ES Tablets ... 1189
- Zydone Capsules ... 941

Hydrocodone Polistirex (Enhanced magnitude and duration of CNS/cardiovascular effects; respiratory depression may be enhanced). Products include:
- Tussionex Extended-Release Suspension ... 988

Hydroxyzine Hydrochloride (Enhanced magnitude and duration of CNS/cardiovascular effects; respiratory depression may be enhanced). Products include:
- Atarax Tablets & Syrup ... 1941
- Marax Tablets & DF Syrup ... 1954
- Vistaril Intramuscular Solution ... 1970

Isoflurane (Enhanced magnitude and duration of CNS/cardiovascular effects; respiratory depression may be enhanced). Products include:
- Forane ... 600

Ketamine Hydrochloride (Enhanced magnitude and duration of CNS/cardiovascular effects; respiratory depression may be enhanced). Products include:
- Ketalar ... 1726

Levorphanol Tartrate (Enhanced magnitude and duration of CNS/cardiovascular effects; respiratory depression may be enhanced). Products include:
- Levo-Dromoran ... 1906

Lorazepam (Enhanced magnitude and duration of CNS/cardiovascular effects; respiratory depression may be enhanced). Products include:
- Ativan Injection ... 2432
- Ativan Tablets ... 2434

Loxapine Hydrochloride (Enhanced magnitude and duration of CNS/cardiovascular effects; respiratory depression may be enhanced). Products include:
- Loxitane ... 1213

Loxapine Succinate (Enhanced magnitude and duration of CNS/cardiovascular effects; respiratory depression may be enhanced). Products include:
- Loxitane Capsules ... 1213

Meperidine Hydrochloride (Enhanced magnitude and duration of CNS/cardiovascular effects; respiratory depression may be enhanced). Products include:
- Demerol ... 2047
- Mepergan Injection ... 2479

Mephobarbital (Enhanced magnitude and duration of CNS/cardiovascular effects; respiratory depression may be enhanced). Products include:
- Mebaral Tablets ... 2061

Meprobamate (Enhanced magnitude and duration of CNS/cardiovascular effects; respiratory depression may be enhanced). Products include:
- Deprol Tablets ... 2382
- Equagesic Tablets ... 2451
- Miltown Tablets ... 2386
- PMB 200 and PMB 400 ... 2504

Mesoridazine (Enhanced magnitude and duration of CNS/cardiovascular effects; respiratory depression may be enhanced). Products include:
- Serentil ... 686

Mesoridazine Besylate (Enhanced magnitude and duration of CNS/cardiovascular effects; respiratory depression may be enhanced).

Methadone Hydrochloride (Enhanced magnitude and duration of CNS/cardiovascular effects; respiratory depression may be enhanced). Products include:
- Dolophine Hydrochloride Ampoules & Vials ... 1260
- Dolophine Hydrochloride Tablets 1261
- Methadone Hydrochloride Diskets .. 1284
- Methadone Hydrochloride Oral Solution & Tablets ... 1987

Methohexital Sodium (Enhanced magnitude and duration of CNS/cardiovascular effects; respiratory depression may be enhanced). Products include:
- Brevital Sodium Vials ... 1248

Methoxyflurane (Enhanced magnitude and duration of CNS/cardiovascular effects; respiratory depression may be enhanced).
- No products indexed under this heading.

Metocurine Iodide (May produce bradycardia and hypotension; effect may be pronounced in the presence of calcium channel and/or beta-blockers). Products include:

- Metubine Iodide Vials 1285

Midazolam Hydrochloride (Enhanced magnitude and duration of CNS/cardiovascular effects; respiratory depression may be enhanced). Products include:

- Versed Injection 1924

Molindone Hydrochloride (Enhanced magnitude and duration of CNS/cardiovascular effects; respiratory depression may be enhanced). Products include:

- Moban Tablets & Concentrate 932

Morphine Sulfate (Enhanced magnitude and duration of CNS/cardiovascular effects; respiratory depression may be enhanced). Products include:

- Astramorph/PF Injection, USP (Preservative-Free) 618
- Duramorph 960
- Infumorph 200 and Infumorph 500 Sterile Solutions 962
- MS Contin Tablets 1814
- MSIR 1817
- Oramorph SR (Morphine Sulfate Sustained Release Tablets) 1988
- Roxanol 1991

Nitrous Oxide (Possible cardiovascular depression).

Opium Alkaloids (Additive or potentiating effects; respiratory depression may be enhanced). Products include:

- B & O No. 15A & No. 16A Supprettes 2395
- Pantopon Injectable 1911

Oxazepam (Enhanced magnitude and duration of CNS/cardiovascular effects; respiratory depression may be enhanced). Products include:

- Serax Capsules 2522
- Serax Tablets 2522

Oxycodone Hydrochloride (Enhanced magnitude and duration of CNS/cardiovascular effects; respiratory depression may be enhanced). Products include:

- Percocet Tablets 950
- Percodan 951
- Roxicodone Tablets, Oral Solution & Intensol (Oxycodone) 1992
- Tylox Capsules 1382

Pancuronium Bromide Injection (Elevated heart rate; may produce bradycardia and hypotension; effect may be pronounced in the presence of calcium channel and/or beta-blockers).

- No products indexed under this heading.

Pentobarbital Sodium (Enhanced magnitude and duration of CNS/cardiovascular effects; respiratory depression may be enhanced). Products include:

- Nembutal Sodium Capsules 534
- Nembutal Sodium Solution 536
- Nembutal Sodium Suppositories 538

Perphenazine (Enhanced magnitude and duration of CNS/cardiovascular effects; respiratory depression may be enhanced). Products include:

- Etrafon 2087
- Triavil Tablets 1556
- Trilafon 2123

Phenobarbital (Enhanced magnitude and duration of CNS/cardiovascular effects; respiratory depression may be enhanced). Products include:

- Arco-Lase Plus Tablets 607
- Bellergal-S Tablets 1998
- Bronkolixir .... ▣ 761
- Bronkotabs Tablets .... ▣ 762
- Donnatal 1858
- Donnatal Extentabs 1859
- Donnatal Tablets 1858
- Donnazyme Tablets 1860
- Kinesed Tablets 2272
- Phenobarbital Elixir and Tablets 1293
- Primatene Tablets-P Formula 2421
- Quadrinal Tablets 1183
- Tedral SA 1765

Prazepam (Enhanced magnitude and duration of CNS/cardiovascular effects; respiratory depression may be enhanced). Products include:

- Centrax 1693

Prochlorperazine (Enhanced magnitude and duration of CNS/cardiovascular effects; respiratory depression may be enhanced). Products include:

- Compazine 2201

Promethazine Hydrochloride (Enhanced magnitude and duration of CNS/cardiovascular effects; respiratory depression may be enhanced). Products include:

- Mepergan Injection 2479
- Phenergan with Codeine 2497
- Phenergan with Dextromethorphan 2499
- Phenergan Injection 2493
- Phenergan Suppositories 2496
- Phenergan Syrup 2495
- Phenergan Tablets 2496
- Phenergan VC 2500
- Phenergan VC with Codeine 2501

Propofol (Enhanced magnitude and duration of CNS/cardiovascular effects; respiratory depression may be enhanced). Products include:

- Diprivan Injection 2267

Propoxyphene Hydrochloride (Enhanced magnitude and duration of CNS/cardiovascular effects; respiratory depression may be enhanced). Products include:

- Darvon 1256
- Wygesic Tablets 2540

Propoxyphene Napsylate (Enhanced magnitude and duration of CNS/cardiovascular effects; respiratory depression may be enhanced). Products include:

- Darvon-N/Darvocet-N 1254

Quazepam (Enhanced magnitude and duration of CNS/cardiovascular effects; respiratory depression may be enhanced). Products include:

- Doral Tablets 2383

Secobarbital Sodium (Enhanced magnitude and duration of CNS/cardiovascular effects; respiratory depression may be enhanced). Products include:

- Seconal Sodium Pulvules 1296

Succinylcholine Chloride (May produce bradycardia and hypotension; effect may be pronounced in the presence of calcium channel and/or beta-blockers). Products include:

- Anectine 755

Temazepam (Enhanced magnitude and duration of CNS/cardiovascular effects; respiratory depression may be enhanced). Products include:

- Restoril Capsules 2023

Thiamylal Sodium (Enhanced magnitude and duration of CNS/cardiovascular effects; respiratory depression may be enhanced). Products include:

- Surital Ampoules, Steri-Vials 1764

Thioridazine Hydrochloride (Enhanced magnitude and duration of CNS/cardiovascular effects; respiratory depression may be enhanced). Products include:

- Mellaril 2011

Thiothixene (Enhanced magnitude and duration of CNS/cardiovascular effects; respiratory depression may be enhanced). Products include:

- Navane Capsules and Concentrate 1954
- Navane Intramuscular 1956

Triazolam (Enhanced magnitude and duration of CNS/cardiovascular effects; respiratory depression may be enhanced). Products include:

- Halcion Tablets 2340

Trifluoperazine Hydrochloride (Enhanced magnitude and duration of CNS/cardiovascular effects; respiratory depression may be enhanced). Products include:

- Stelazine 2226

Vecuronium Bromide (May produce bradycardia and hypotension; effect may be pronounced in the presence of calcium channel and/or beta-blockers). Products include:

- Norcuron 1642

SULFACET-R ACNE LOTION
(Sodium Sulfacetamide, Sulfur) 910
No interactions described in labeling.

SULTRIN TRIPLE SULFA CREAM
(Sulfathiazole, Sulfacetamide, Sulfabenzamide) 1675
No interactions described in labeling.

SULTRIN TRIPLE SULFA VAGINAL TABLETS
(Sulfathiazole, Sulfacetamide, Sulfabenzamide) 1675
No interactions described in labeling.

SUMMER'S EVE MEDICATED DOUCHE
(Povidone Iodine) 993
No interactions described in labeling.

SUNKIST CHILDREN'S CHEWABLE MULTIVITAMINS - COMPLETE
(Multivitamins with Minerals) .... ▣ 553
No interactions described in labeling.

SUNKIST CHILDREN'S CHEWABLE MULTIVITAMINS - PLUS EXTRA C
(Multivitamins, Vitamin C) .... ▣ 553
No interactions described in labeling.

SUNKIST CHILDREN'S CHEWABLE MULTIVITAMINS - PLUS IRON
(Vitamins with Iron) .... ▣ 553
No interactions described in labeling.

SUNKIST CHILDREN'S CHEWABLE MULTIVITAMINS - REGULAR
(Multivitamins) .... ▣ 553
No interactions described in labeling.

SUNKIST VITAMIN C - CHEWABLE
(Vitamin C) .... ▣ 553
No interactions described in labeling.

SUNKIST VITAMIN C - EASY TO SWALLOW
(Vitamin C) .... ▣ 553
No interactions described in labeling.

SUPLENA SPECIALIZED LIQUID NUTRITION
(Dietary Supplement) 1978
No interactions described in labeling.

SUPRAX POWDER FOR ORAL SUSPENSION
(Cefixime) 1235
No interactions described in labeling.

SUPRAX TABLETS
(Cefixime) 1235
No interactions described in labeling.

SURBEX
(Vitamin B Complex) .... ▣ 502
No interactions described in labeling.

SURBEX WITH C
(Vitamin B Complex With Vitamin C) .... ▣ 502
No interactions described in labeling.

SURBEX-750 WITH IRON
(Vitamin B Complex With Vitamin C, Ferrous Sulfate) .... ▣ 503
No interactions described in labeling.

SURBEX-750 WITH ZINC
(Multivitamins with Minerals, Zinc Sulfate) .... ▣ 503
No interactions described in labeling.

SURBEX-T
(Vitamin B Complex With Vitamin C) .... ▣ 502
No interactions described in labeling.

SURFAK CAPSULES
(Docusate Calcium) .... ▣ 737
No interactions described in labeling.

SURGICEL ABSORBABLE HEMOSTAT
(Oxidized Regenerated Cellulose) 1151
May interact with escharotic chemicals. Compounds in this category include:

Silver Nitrate (Absorption of Surgicel could be prevented in chemically cauterized areas, its use should not be preceded by application of escharotic chemicals).

SURGICEL NU-KNIT ABSORBABLE HEMOSTAT
(Oxidized Regenerated Cellulose) 1151
See **SURGICEL Absorbable Hemostat**

SURITAL AMPOULES, STERI-VIALS
(Thiamylal Sodium) 1764
No interactions described in labeling.

SURMONTIL CAPSULES
(Trimipramine Maleate) 2524
May interact with monoamine oxidase inhibitors, catecholamine depleting drugs, anticholinergics, and sympathomimetic aerosol bronchodilators. Compounds in these categories include:

Albuterol (Potentiated atropine-like effects). Products include:

- Proventil Inhalation Aerosol 2117
- Ventolin Inhalation Aerosol and Refill 583

Albuterol Sulfate (Potentiated atropine-like effects). Products include:

- Proventil Repetabs Tablets 2120
- Proventil Solutions for Inhalation 0.5% and 0.083% 2118
- Proventil Syrup 2119
- Proventil Tablets 2120
- Ventolin 583

Alcohol (Exaggerated effects).

Atropine Sulfate (Potentiated atropine-like effects). Products include:
- Arco-Lase Plus Tablets 607
- Atropine Sulfate Sterile Ophthalmic Solution and S.O.P. Sterile Ophthalmic Ointment .... ⊙ 239
- Donnagel .... ▣ 675
- Donnagel-PG 1858
- Donnatal 1858
- Donnatal Extentabs 1859
- Donnatal Tablets 1858
- Donnazyme Tablets 1860
- Isopto Atropine .... ⊙ 218
- Lomotil 2174
- Motofen Tablets 836
- Ru-Tuss Tablets 693
- Urised Tablets 2396

Belladonna Alkaloids (Potentiated atropine-like effects). Products include:
- Bellergal-S Tablets 1998
- Hyland's Bed Wetting Tablets .... ▣ 728
- Hyland's Teething Tablets .... ▣ 728
- Kinesed Tablets 2272

Benztropine Mesylate (Potentiated atropine-like effects). Products include:
- Cogentin 1435

Biperiden (Potentiated atropine-like effects). Products include:
- Akineton 1171

Cimetidine (Inhibits elimination of antidepressant). Products include:
- Tagamet Tablets 2228

Cimetidine Hydrochloride (Inhibits elimination of antidepressant). Products include:
- Tagamet 2228

Clidinium Bromide (Potentiated atropine-like effects). Products include:
- Librax Capsules 1929
- Quarzan Capsules 1937

Deserpidine (Potentiates effects). Products include:
- Enduronyl 518
- Harmonyl Tablets 528
- Oreticyl 545

Dicyclomine Hydrochloride (Potentiated atropine-like effects). Products include:
- Bentyl 1322

Dobutamine Hydrochloride (Potentiated atropine-like effects). Products include:
- Dobutrex Solution Vials 1259

Dopamine Hydrochloride (Potentiated atropine-like effects). Products include:
- Intropin Injection 930

Ephedrine Hydrochloride (Potentiated atropine-like effects). Products include:
- Amesec .... ▣ 682
- Primatene Tablets-M Formula 2421
- Primatene Tablets-P Formula 2421
- Primatene Tablets-Regular Formula 2421
- Quadrinal Tablets 1183
- Quelidrine Syrup 556
- Tedral SA 1765

Ephedrine Sulfate (Potentiated atropine-like effects). Products include:
- Bronkaid Tablets .... ▣ 757
- Bronkolixir .... ▣ 761
- Bronkotabs Tablets .... ▣ 762
- Marax Tablets & DF Syrup 1954
- Pazo Hemorrhoid Ointment & Suppositories 752
- Vicks Vatronol Nose Drops .... ▣ 666

Ephedrine Tannate (Potentiated atropine-like effects). Products include:
- Rynatuss 2388

Epinephrine (Potentiated atropine-like effects). Products include:
- Ana-Kit Anaphylaxis Emergency Treatment Kit 1100
- Bronkaid Mist .... ▣ 757
- EpiPen 843
- Marcaine Hydrochloride 0.5% with Epinephrine 1:200,000 (as bitartrate) 958
- Marcaine Hydrochloride with Epinephrine 1:200,000 2055
- Primatene Mist 2420
- Sus-Phrine Injection 1006
- Xylocaine with Epinephrine Injections 637

Epinephrine Bitartrate (Potentiated atropine-like effects). Products include:
- AsthmaHaler Mist Epinephrine Bitartrate Bronchodilator .... ▣ 616
- Bronkaid Mist Suspension .... ▣ 757
- Primatene Mist Suspension 2421

Epinephrine Hydrochloride (Potentiated atropine-like effects). Products include:
- Adrenalin Chloride Solution 1:100 & 1:1,000 1689
- Epifrin .... ⊙ 244
- Glaucon .... ⊙ 218

Ethopropazine Hydrochloride (Potentiated atropine-like effects).

Furazolidone (Severe hyperpyretic reactions, convulsions, deaths; concurrent use is contraindicated). Products include:
- Furoxone 1855

Glycopyrrolate (Potentiated atropine-like effects). Products include:
- Robinul Forte Tablets 1873
- Robinul Injectable 1873
- Robinul Tablets 1873

Hyoscyamine (Potentiated atropine-like effects). Products include:
- Cystospaz Tablets 2395
- Urised Tablets 2396

Hyoscyamine Sulfate (Potentiated atropine-like effects). Products include:
- Arco-Lase Plus Tablets 607
- Cystospaz-M Capsules 2395
- Donnagel .... ▣ 675
- Donnagel-PG 1858
- Donnatal 1858
- Donnatal Extentabs 1859
- Donnatal Tablets 1858
- Donnazyme Tablets 1860
- Kutrase Capsules 2146
- Levsin/Levsinex 2147
- Ru-Tuss Tablets 693

Ipratropium Bromide (Potentiated atropine-like effects). Products include:
- Atrovent Inhalation Aerosol 675

Isocarboxazid (Severe hyperpyretic reactions, convulsions, deaths; concurrent use is contraindicated). Products include:
- Marplan Tablets 1906

Isoproterenol Hydrochloride (Potentiated atropine-like effects). Products include:
- Isuprel Hydrochloride Injection 1:5000 2050
- Isuprel Hydrochloride Mistometer .. 2051
- Isuprel Hydrochloride Solution 1:200 & 1:100 2052
- Norisodrine Aerotrol 540

Mepenzolate Bromide (Potentiated atropine-like effects). Products include:
- Cantil Tablets 1326

Metaproterenol Sulfate (Potentiated atropine-like effects). Products include:
- Alupent 674
- Arm-a-Med Metaproterenol Sulfate Inhalation Solution, USP 617
- Metaprel Inhalation Aerosol Bronchodilator 2014
- Metaprel Inhalation Solution 2015
- Metaprel 2015
- Metaproterenol Sulfate Inhalation Solution, USP 912

Metaraminol Bitartrate (Potentiated atropine-like effects). Products include:
- Aramine Injection 1424

Methoxamine Hydrochloride (Potentiated atropine-like effects). Products include:
- Vasoxyl Injection 819

Norepinephrine Bitartrate (Potentiated atropine-like effects). Products include:
- Levophed Bitartrate Injection 2054

Oxybutynin Chloride (Potentiated atropine-like effects). Products include:
- Ditropan 1332

Oxyphenonium Bromide (Potentiated atropine-like effects).

Phenelzine Sulfate (Severe hyperpyretic reactions, convulsions, deaths; concurrent use is contraindicated). Products include:
- Nardil 1742

Phenylephrine Bitartrate (Potentiated atropine-like effects).
- No products indexed under this heading.

Phenylephrine Hydrochloride (Potentiated atropine-like effects). Products include:
- AK-Dilate Solution 2.5% and 10% .... ⊙ 203
- Atrohist Sprinkle Capsules 558
- Cerose-DM 2443
- Codimal 846
- Comhist LA Capsules 1618
- Congespirin For Children Aspirin Free Chewable Cold Tablets 748
- Cyclomydril .... ⊙ 216
- Deconsal Sprinkle Capsules 559
- Dimetane Decongestant .... ▣ 673
- Dristan Decongestant/Antihistamine/ Analgesic Coated Caplets .... ▣ 749
- Dristan Cold Nasal Decongestant/ Antihistamine/ Analgesic Coated Tablets 2419
- Dristan Advanced Formula Decongestant/Antihistamine/ Analgesic Tablets .... ▣ 749
- Dristan Nasal Spray, Menthol 2419
- Dristan Nasal Spray, Regular and Regular with Metered Pump 2419
- Entex Capsules 1623
- Entex Liquid 1623
- Sinus Excedrin Analgesic, Decongestant Tablets & Caplets 750
- Extendryl 994
- 4-Way Fast Acting Nasal Spray - Original Formula (regular & mentholated) & Metered Spray Pump (regular) 751
- Hycomine Compound Tablets 929
- Murocoll-2 Sterile Ophthalmic Solution .... ⊙ 261
- Mydfrin 2.5% .... ⊙ 224
- Naldecon Syrup, Tablets, Pediatric Drops and Pediatric Syrup 709
- Neo-Synephrine Hydrochloride 1% Carpuject 2063
- Neo-Synephrine Hydrochloride 1% Injection 2063
- Neo-Synephrine Hydrochloride (Ophthalmic) 2064
- Neo-Synephrine .... ▣ 759
- Nōstril Nasal Decongestant .... ▣ 520
- Novahistine Elixir .... ▣ 596
- Phenergan VC 2500
- Phenergan VC with Codeine 2501
- Prefrin Liquifilm Vasoconstrictor and Lubricant Eye Drops .... ⊙ 254
- Prefrin-A .... ⊙ 255
- Quelidrine Syrup 556
- Relief Vasoconstrictor and Lubricant Eye Drops .... ⊙ 256
- Robitussin Night Relief .... ▣ 677
- Ru-Tuss with Hydrocodone 694
- Ru-Tuss Tablets 693
- Vasosulf .... ⊙ 279
- Vicks Sinex .... ▣ 665
- Zincfrin .... ⊙ 230

Phenylephrine Tannate (Potentiated atropine-like effects). Products include:
- Rynatan 2387
- Rynatuss 2388

Phenylpropanolamine Hydrochloride (Potentiated atropine-like effects). Products include:
- A.R.M. Allergy Relief Medicine Caplets .... ▣ 615
- Acutrim .... ▣ 548
- Allerest .... ▣ 559
- BC Cold Powder .... ▣ 517
- Cheracol Plus Head Cold/Cough Formula .... ▣ 667
- Codimal Expectorant 846
- Comtrex Multi-Symptom Cold Reliever Tablets/Caplets/Liqui-Gels/Liquid 745
- Contac Continuous Action Decongestant/Antihistamine Capsules ▣ 710
- Contac Maximum Strength Continuous Action Decongestant/ Antihistamine Caplets .... ▣ 709
- Contac Severe Cold and Flu Formula Caplets .... ▣ 711
- Coricidin 'D' Decongestant Tablets .... ▣ 695
- Coricidin Demilets Tablets for Children .... ▣ 696
- Demazin Nasal Decongestant/ Antihistamine Repetabs Tablets & Syrup .... ▣ 697
- Dexatrim .... ▣ 733
- Dimetane-DC Cough Syrup 1857
- Dimetapp Elixir .... ▣ 673
- Dimetapp DM Elixir .... ▣ 674
- Dimetapp Extentabs .... ▣ 674
- Dimetapp Plus Caplets .... ▣ 675
- Dimetapp Tablets .... ▣ 675
- Entex Capsules 1623
- Entex LA Tablets 1623
- Entex Liquid 1623
- 4-Way Cold Tablets 750
- Hycomine Syrup 927
- Naldecon CX Adult Liquid .... ▣ 521
- Naldecon DX Adult Liquid .... ▣ 521
- Naldecon DX Children's Syrup .... ▣ 522
- Naldecon DX Pediatric Drops .... ▣ 522
- Naldecon EX Children's Syrup .... ▣ 522
- Naldecon EX Pediatric Drops .... ▣ 523
- Naldecon Syrup, Tablets, Pediatric Drops and Pediatric Syrup 709
- Nolamine Tablets 838
- Nolex LA Tablets 838
- Ornade Spansule Capsules 2221
- Orthoxicol Cough Syrup .... ▣ 668
- Propagest 839
- Pyrroxate Capsules .... ▣ 669
- Robitussin-CF .... ▣ 676
- Ru-Tuss II Capsules 693
- Ru-Tuss with Hydrocodone 694
- Ru-Tuss Tablets 693
- Sine-Off Sinus Medicine Tablets-Aspirin Formula .... ▣ 722
- Sinulin 840
- St. Joseph Cold Tablets for Children .... ▣ 704
- Tavist-D Tablets 2035
- Triaminic Allergy Tablets .... ▣ 688
- Triaminic Chewables .... ▣ 688
- Triaminic Cold Tablets .... ▣ 688
- Triaminic Expectorant .... ▣ 688
- Triaminic Expectorant w/Codeine .. 1996
- Triaminic Expectorant DH 1995
- Triaminic Oral Infant Drops 1996
- Triaminic Syrup .... ▣ 689
- Triaminic-12 Tablets .... ▣ 690
- Triaminic-DM Syrup .... ▣ 689
- Triaminicin Tablets .... ▣ 690
- Triaminicol Multi-Symptom Cold Tablets .... ▣ 691
- Triaminicol Multi-Symptom Relief ▣ 691
- Tuss-Ornade Liquid 2242
- Tuss-Ornade Spansule Capsules 2242
- Tylenol Cold Medication, Effervescent Tablets 1369

Pirbuterol Acetate (Potentiated atropine-like effects). Products include:
- Maxair Inhaler 1311

Procyclidine Hydrochloride (Potentiated atropine-like effects). Products include:
- Kemadrin Tablets 771

Propantheline Bromide (Potentiated atropine-like effects). Products include:
- Pro-Banthine Tablets 2141

Pseudoephedrine Hydrochloride (Potentiated atropine-like effects). Products include:
- Actifed Capsules .... ▣ 539

(▣ Described in PDR For Nonprescription Drugs)

(⊙ Described in PDR For Ophthalmology)

Actifed Plus Caplets ▣ 539
Actifed Plus Tablets ▣ 540
Actifed with Codeine Cough Syrup 752
Actifed Syrup ▣ 540
Actifed Tablets ▣ 540
Actifed 12-Hour Capsules ▣ 539
Advil Cold & Sinus Caplets (formerly CoAdvil) 2416
Allerest ▣ 559
Anatuss LA Tablets 1359
Benadryl Decongestant Elixir ▣ 635
Benadryl Decongestant ▣ 635
Benadryl Plus ▣ 636
Benadryl Plus Nighttime ▣ 637
Benylin Decongestant ▣ 638
Brexin L.A. Capsules 2078
Bromfed Capsules (Timed Release) 1615
Bromfed Syrup ▣ 628
Bromfed 1615
CoAdvil ▣ 748
Allergy-Sinus Comtrex Multi-Symptom Allergy Sinus Formula Tablets & Caplets 746
Cough Formula Comtrex 746
Comtrex Multi-Symptom Cold Reliever Tablets/Caplets/Liqui-Gels/Liquid 745
Day-Night Comtrex 747
Non-Drowsy Comtrex 747
Congess 994
Congestac Caplets ▣ 617
Contac Jr. Children's Cold Medicine ▣ 712
Contac Nighttime Cold Medicine ▣ 713
Contac Sinus Caplets Maximum Strength Non-Drowsy Formula ▣ 710
Contac Sinus Tablets Maximum Strength Non-Drowsy Formula ▣ 710
Deconamine 663
Deconsal II Tablets 559
Dimacol Caplets ▣ 672
Dimetane-DX Cough Syrup 1858
Dorcol Children's Cough Syrup ▣ 685
Dorcol Children's Decongestant Liquid ▣ 685
Dorcol Children's Liquid Cold Formula ▣ 686
Maximum Strength Dristan Decongestant/Analgesic Coated Caplets ▣ 750
No Drowsiness Dristan Cold Nasal Decongestant/Analgesic Coated Caplets 2420
Dristan Sinus Caplets 2419
Sinus Excedrin Analgesic, Decongestant Tablets & Caplets ▣ 533
Fedahist Gyrocaps 2145
Fedahist Timecaps 2145
Guaifed 1615
Guaifed Syrup ▣ 629
Isoclor Expectorant 982
Isoclor Timesule Capsules ▣ 561
Kronofed-A 970
Medi-Flu Caplet, Liquid ▣ 640
Novafed A Capsules 1342
Novafed Capsules 1342
Novahistine DH 1342
Novahistine DMX ▣ 595
Novahistine Expectorant 1343
Nucofed Capsules 2219
Nucofed Expectorant 2219
Nucofed Pediatric Expectorant 2220
Nucofed Syrup 2219
Ornex Caplets ▣ 618
PediaCare Allergy Relief Formula Liquid 1362
PediaCare Cough-Cold Formula Liquid 1362
PediaCare Infants' Oral Decongestant Drops 1362
PediaCare Night Rest Cough-Cold Formula Liquid 1362
PediaCare 6-12 Cough-Cold Formula Chewable Tablets 1362
Robitussin-DAC Syrup 1875
Robitussin-PE ▣ 677
Rondec 1975
Rondec-DM 1976
Rondec-TR Tablet 1975
Ru-Tuss DE Tablets 694
Ryna ▣ 741
Seldane-D Extended-Release Tablets 1350
Sinarest ▣ 562
Sine-Aid Maximum Strength Sinus Headache Caplets 1365
Sine-Aid Maximum Strength Sinus Headache Tablets 1365
Sine-Off Maximum Strength Allergy/Sinus Formula Caplets ▣ 721
Sine-Off Maximum Strength No Drowsiness Formula Caplets ▣ 722
Singlet Tablets ▣ 598
Sinutab Maximum Strength ▣ 641
Sinutab Maximum Strength Without Drowsiness Tablets & Caplets ▣ 642
Sinutab Regular Strength Without Drowsiness Formula ▣ 641
St. Joseph Nighttime Cold Medicine ▣ 705
Sudafed Children's Liquid ▣ 543
Sudafed Cough Syrup ▣ 543
Sudafed Plus Liquid ▣ 544
Sudafed Plus Tablets ▣ 545
Sudafed Sinus Caplets ▣ 545
Sudafed Sinus Tablets ▣ 545
Sudafed Tablets, 30 mg ▣ 544
Sudafed Tablets, Adult Strength, 60 mg ▣ 544
Sudafed 12 Hour Capsules ▣ 545
TheraFlu Flu and Cold Medicine ▣ 687
Triaminic Nite Light ▣ 689
Tylenol Allergy Sinus Medication Caplets and Gelcaps, Maximum Strength 1372
Children's Tylenol Cold Liquid Formula and Chewable Tablets 1368
Tylenol Cold & Flu Hot Medication, Packets 1369
Tylenol Cold & Flu No Drowsiness Hot Medication, Packets 1371
Tylenol Cold Medication Caplets and Tablets 1370
Tylenol Cold Medication No Drowsiness Formula Caplets 1370
Tylenol Cold Night Time Medication Liquid 1371
Tylenol Cough Medication Liquid with Decongestant, Maximum Strength 1372
Tylenol, Maximum Strength, Sinus Medication Gelcaps, Caplets and Tablets 1373
Ursinus Inlay-Tabs ▣ 691
Vicks Children's NyQuil ▣ 664
Vicks Daycare ▣ 660
Vicks Formula 44D Decongestant Cough Medicine ▣ 662
Vicks Formula 44M Multi-Symptom Cough Medicine ▣ 662
Vicks NyQuil Nighttime Colds Medicine-Original & Cherry Flavor ▣ 664
Vicks Pediatric Formula 44 Cough & Congestion Medicine ▣ 663
Vicks Pediatric Formula 44m Multi-Symptom Cough & Cold Medicine ▣ 663

Pseudoephedrine Sulfate (Potentiated atropine-like effects). Products include:

Afrin Tablets ▣ 693
Chlor-Trimeton Decongestant ▣ 694
Disophrol Chronotab Sustained-Action Tablets ▣ 698
Drixoral Antihistamine/Nasal Decongestant Syrup ▣ 698
Drixoral Non-Drowsy Formula ▣ 699
Drixoral Plus Extended-Release Tablets ▣ 699
Drixoral Sinus ▣ 700
Drixoral Sustained-Action Tablets ▣ 698
Sinutab Allergy Formula Sustained Action Tablets ▣ 640
Trinalin Repetabs Tablets 1170

Rauwolfia Serpentina (Potentiates effects). Products include:

Raudixin Tablets 1803
Rauzide Tablets 1804

Rescinnamine (Potentiates effects).

No products indexed under this heading.

Reserpine (Potentiates effects). Products include:

Diupres Tablets 1461
Hydromox R Tablets 1209
Hydropres Tablets 1485
Renese-R Tablets 1786
Salutensin/Salutensin-Demi 719
Ser-Ap-Es Tablets 881
Serpasil Tablets 883
Serpasil-Apresoline Tablets 884
Serpasil-Esidrix Tablets 886

Scopolamine Hydrobromide (Potentiated atropine-like effects). Products include:

Donnagel ▣ 675
Donnagel-PG 1858
Donnatal 1858
Donnatal Extentabs 1859
Donnatal Tablets 1858
Donnazyme Tablets 1860
Isopto Hyoscine ⊙ 222
Murocoll-2 Sterile Ophthalmic Solution ⊙ 261
Ru-Tuss Tablets 693

Scopolamine Preparations (Potentiated atropine-like effects). Products include:

Transderm Scōp Transdermal Therapeutic System 887

Selegiline Hydrochloride (Severe hyperpyretic reactions, convulsions, deaths; concurrent use is contraindicated). Products include:

Eldepryl 2250

Terbutaline Sulfate (Potentiated atropine-like effects). Products include:

Brethaire Inhaler 1024
Brethine Ampuls 1026
Brethine Tablets 1026
Bricanyl Injection 1324
Bricanyl Tablets 1325

Tranylcypromine Sulfate (Severe hyperpyretic reactions, convulsions, deaths; concurrent use is contraindicated). Products include:

Parnate Tablets 2222

Tridihexethyl Chloride (Potentiated atropine-like effects).

No products indexed under this heading.

Trihexyphenidyl Hydrochloride (Potentiated atropine-like effects). Products include:

Artane 1195

SURVANTA BERACTANT INTRATRACHEAL SUSPENSION

(Beractant) 1978
No interactions described in labeling.

SUS-PHRINE INJECTION

(Epinephrine) 1006
May interact with tricyclic antidepressants, cardiac glycosides, sympathomimetic aerosol bronchodilators, and certain other agents. Compounds in these categories include:

Albuterol (Combined effects on cardiovascular system may be deleterious). Products include:

Proventil Inhalation Aerosol 2117
Ventolin Inhalation Aerosol and Refill 583

Albuterol Sulfate (Combined effects on cardiovascular system may be deleterious). Products include:

Proventil Repetabs Tablets 2120
Proventil Solutions for Inhalation 0.5% and 0.083% 2118
Proventil Syrup 2119
Proventil Tablets 2120
Ventolin 583

Amitriptyline Hydrochloride (Epinephrine effects may be potentiated). Products include:

Elavil 2269
Endep Tablets 1927
Etrafon 2087
Limbitrol 1933
Triavil Tablets 1556

Amoxapine (Epinephrine effects may be potentiated). Products include:

Asendin Tablets 1196

Chlorpheniramine (Epinephrine effects may be potentiated).

Chlorpheniramine Maleate (Epinephrine effects may be potentiated). Products include:

A.R.M. Allergy Relief Medicine Caplets ▣ 615
Alka-Seltzer Plus Cold Medicine ▣ 623
Allerest ▣ 559
Ana-Kit Anaphylaxis Emergency Treatment Kit 1100
BC Cold Powder Multi-Symptom Formula ▣ 517
Brexin L.A. Capsules 2078
Cerose-DM 2443
Cheracol Plus Head Cold/Cough Formula ▣ 667
Chlor-Trimeton Allergy Syrup, Tablets & Long-Acting Repetabs Tablets ▣ 693
Chlor-Trimeton Decongestant ▣ 694
Comhist LA Capsules 1618
Allergy-Sinus Comtrex Multi-Symptom Allergy Sinus Formula Tablets & Caplets 746
Comtrex Multi-Symptom Cold Reliever Tablets/Caplets/Liqui-Gels/Liquid 745
Day-Night Comtrex 747
Contac Continuous Action Decongestant/Antihistamine Capsules ▣ 710
Contac Maximum Strength Continuous Action Decongestant/Antihistamine Caplets ▣ 709
Contac Severe Cold and Flu Formula Caplets ▣ 711
Coricidin 'D' Decongestant Tablets ▣ 695
Coricidin Demilets Tablets for Children ▣ 696
Coricidin Tablets ▣ 695
Deconamine 663
Demazin Nasal Decongestant/Antihistamine Repetabs Tablets & Syrup ▣ 697
Dorcol Children's Liquid Cold Formula ▣ 686
Dristan Decongestant/Antihistamine/ Analgesic Coated Caplets ▣ 749
Dristan Cold Nasal Decongestant/Antihistamine/ Analgesic Coated Tablets 2419
Dristan Advanced Formula Decongestant/Antihistamine/Analgesic Tablets ▣ 749
Extendryl 994
4-Way Cold Tablets 750
Fedahist Gyrocaps 2145
Fedahist Timecaps 2145
Hycomine Compound Tablets 929
Isoclor Timesule Capsules ▣ 561
Kronofed-A 970
Medi-Flu Caplet, Liquid ▣ 640
Naldecon Syrup, Tablets, Pediatric Drops and Pediatric Syrup 709
Nolamine Tablets 838
Novafed A Capsules 1342
Novahistine DH 1342
Novahistine Elixir ▣ 596
Ornade Spansule Capsules 2221
Orthoxicol Cough Syrup ▣ 668
PediaCare Allergy Relief Formula Liquid 1362
PediaCare Cough-Cold Formula Liquid 1362
PediaCare Night Rest Cough-Cold Formula Liquid 1362
PediaCare 6-12 Cough-Cold Formula Chewable Tablets 1362
Pyrroxate Capsules ▣ 669
Quelidrine Syrup 556
Ru-Tuss II Capsules 693
Ru-Tuss Tablets 693
Ryna ▣ 741
Sinarest Tablets & Extra Strength Tablets ▣ 562
Sine-Off Maximum Strength Allergy/Sinus Formula Caplets ▣ 721
Sine-Off Sinus Medicine Tablets-Aspirin Formula ▣ 722
Singlet Tablets ▣ 598
Sinulin 840
Sinutab Maximum Strength ▣ 641
St. Joseph Nighttime Cold Medicine ▣ 705
Sudafed Plus Liquid ▣ 544
Sudafed Plus Tablets ▣ 545
Teldrin Timed-Release Allergy Capsules, 12 mg 2192
TheraFlu Flu and Cold Medicine ▣ 687
Triaminic Allergy Tablets ▣ 688
Triaminic Chewables ▣ 688

Triaminic Cold Tablets ▣ 688
Triaminic Nite Light ▣ 689
Triaminic Syrup ▣ 689
Triaminic-12 Tablets ▣ 690
Triaminicin Tablets ▣ 690
Triaminicol Multi-Symptom Cold Tablets ▣ 691
Triaminicol Multi-Symptom Relief ▣ 691
Tylenol Allergy Sinus Medication Caplets and Gelcaps, Maximum Strength 1372
Children's Tylenol Cold Liquid Formula and Chewable Tablets 1368
Tylenol Cold & Flu Hot Medication, Packets 1369
Tylenol Cold Medication Caplets and Tablets 1370
Tylenol Cold Medication, Effervescent Tablets 1369
Vicks Children's NyQuil ▣ 664
Vicks Formula 44 Cough Medicine ▣ 661
Vicks Formula 44M Multi-Symptom Cough Medicine ▣ 662
Vicks Pediatric Formula 44m Multi-Symptom Cough & Cold Medicine ▣ 663

Chlorpheniramine Polistirex (Epinephrine effects may be potentiated). Products include:
Tussionex Extended-Release Suspension 988

Chlorpheniramine Preparations (Epinephrine effects may be potentiated).

Chlorpheniramine Tannate (Epinephrine effects may be potentiated). Products include:
Rynatan 2387
Rynatuss 2388

Clomipramine Hydrochloride (Epinephrine effects may be potentiated). Products include:
Anafranil Capsules 650

Desipramine Hydrochloride (Epinephrine effects may be potentiated). Products include:
Norpramin Tablets 1340

Deslanoside (Potential for arrhythmias).
No products indexed under this heading.

Digitoxin (Potential for arrhythmias). Products include:
Crystodigin Tablets 1253

Digoxin (Potential for arrhythmias). Products include:
Lanoxicaps 772
Lanoxin Elixir Pediatric 775
Lanoxin Injection 778
Lanoxin Injection Pediatric 781
Lanoxin Tablets 783

Diphenhydramine (Epinephrine effects may be potentiated).
No products indexed under this heading.

Diphenhydramine Citrate (Epinephrine effects may be potentiated). Products include:
Alka-Seltzer Plus Night-Time Cold Medicine ▣ 623
Bufferin AF Nite Time Analgesic/Sleeping Aid Caplets 744
Excedrin P.M. Analgesic/Sleeping Aid Tablets, Caplets and Liquid 749

Diphenhydramine Hydrochloride (Epinephrine effects may be potentiated). Products include:
Benadryl Anti-Itch Cream ▣ 635
Benadryl Capsules 1691
Benadryl Decongestant Elixir ▣ 635
Benadryl Decongestant ▣ 635
Benadryl Elixir ▣ 636
Benadryl Kapseals 1691
Benadryl 25 Kapseals ▣ 636
Benadryl Parenteral 1692
Benadryl Plus ▣ 636
Benadryl Plus Nighttime ▣ 637
Benadryl Spray, Maximum Strength ▣ 637
Benadryl Spray, Regular Strength ▣ 637
Benadryl Steri-Vials, Ampoules, and Steri-Dose Syringe 1692
Benadryl 25 Tablets ▣ 636
Benylin Cough Syrup ▣ 637
Benylin Decongestant ▣ 638
Caladryl Cream, Lotion, Spray ▣ 638
Miles Nervine Nighttime Sleep-Aid ▣ 627
Nytol Tablets ▣ 517
Sleep-ettes-D Tablets ▣ 653
Sleep-eze 3 Tablets ▣ 755
Sleepinal Night-time Sleep Aid Capsules ▣ 734
Sominex Caplets and Tablets ▣ 722
Sominex Liquid ▣ 723
Sominex Pain Relief Formula ▣ 723
Tylenol Cold Night Time Medication Liquid 1371
Tylenol PM, Extra Strength Caplets and Tablets 1368
Unisom Dual Relief Nighttime Sleep Aid/Analgesic 1774
Ziradryl Lotion ▣ 643

Dobutamine Hydrochloride (Combined effects on cardiovascular system may be deleterious). Products include:
Dobutrex Solution Vials 1259

Dopamine Hydrochloride (Combined effects on cardiovascular system may be deleterious). Products include:
Intropin Injection 930

Doxepin Hydrochloride (Epinephrine effects may be potentiated). Products include:
Sinequan 1960

Ephedrine Hydrochloride (Combined effects on cardiovascular system may be deleterious). Products include:
Amesec ▣ 682
Primatene Tablets-M Formula 2421
Primatene Tablets-P Formula 2421
Primatene Tablets-Regular Formula 2421
Quadrinal Tablets 1183
Quelidrine Syrup 556
Tedral SA 1765

Ephedrine Sulfate (Combined effects on cardiovascular system may be deleterious). Products include:
Bronkaid Tablets ▣ 757
Bronkolixir ▣ 761
Bronkotabs Tablets ▣ 762
Marax Tablets & DF Syrup 1954
Pazo Hemorrhoid Ointment & Suppositories 752
Vicks Vatronol Nose Drops ▣ 666

Ephedrine Tannate (Combined effects on cardiovascular system may be deleterious). Products include:
Rynatuss 2388

Epinephrine Bitartrate (Combined effects on cardiovascular system may be deleterious). Products include:
AsthmaHaler Mist Epinephrine Bitartrate Bronchodilator ▣ 616
Bronkaid Mist Suspension ▣ 757
Primatene Mist Suspension 2421

Epinephrine Hydrochloride (Combined effects on cardiovascular system may be deleterious). Products include:
Adrenalin Chloride Solution 1:100 & 1:1,000 1689
Epifrin ◉ 244
Glaucon ◉ 218

Imipramine Hydrochloride (Epinephrine effects may be potentiated). Products include:
Tofranil Ampuls 1038
Tofranil Tablets 1039

Imipramine Pamoate (Epinephrine effects may be potentiated). Products include:
Tofranil-PM Capsules 1041

Isoproterenol Hydrochloride (Combined effects on cardiovascular system may be deleterious). Products include:
Isuprel Hydrochloride Injection 1:5000 2050
Isuprel Hydrochloride Mistometer 2051
Isuprel Hydrochloride Solution 1:200 & 1:100 2052
Norisodrine Aerotrol 540

Maprotiline Hydrochloride (Epinephrine effects may be potentiated). Products include:
Ludiomil Tablets 874

Metaproterenol Sulfate (Combined effects on cardiovascular system may be deleterious). Products include:
Alupent 674
Arm-a-Med Metaproterenol Sulfate Inhalation Solution, USP 617
Metaprel Inhalation Aerosol Bronchodilator 2014
Metaprel Inhalation Solution 2015
Metaprel 2015
Metaproterenol Sulfate Inhalation Solution, USP 912

Metaraminol Bitartrate (Combined effects on cardiovascular system may be deleterious). Products include:
Aramine Injection 1424

Norepinephrine Bitartrate (Combined effects on cardiovascular system may be deleterious). Products include:
Levophed Bitartrate Injection 2054

Nortriptyline Hydrochloride (Epinephrine effects may be potentiated). Products include:
Pamelor 2019

Phenylephrine Bitartrate (Combined effects on cardiovascular system may be deleterious).
No products indexed under this heading.

Phenylephrine Hydrochloride (Combined effects on cardiovascular system may be deleterious). Products include:
AK-Dilate Solution 2.5% and 10% ◉ 203
Atrohist Sprinkle Capsules 558
Cerose-DM 2443
Codimal 846
Comhist LA Capsules 1618
Congespirin For Children Aspirin Free Chewable Cold Tablets 748
Cyclomydril ◉ 216
Deconsal Sprinkle Capsules 559
Dimetane Decongestant ▣ 673
Dristan Decongestant/Antihistamine/ Analgesic Coated Caplets ▣ 749
Dristan Cold Nasal Decongestant/ Antihistamine/ Analgesic Coated Tablets 2419
Dristan Advanced Formula Decongestant/Antihistamine/ Analgesic Tablets ▣ 749
Dristan Nasal Spray, Menthol 2419
Dristan Nasal Spray, Regular and Regular with Metered Pump 2419
Entex Capsules 1623
Entex Liquid 1623
Sinus Excedrin Analgesic, Decongestant Tablets & Caplets 750
Extendryl 994
4-Way Fast Acting Nasal Spray - Original Formula (regular & mentholated) & Metered Spray Pump (regular) 751
Hycomine Compound Tablets 929
Murocoll-2 Sterile Ophthalmic Solution ◉ 261
Mydfrin 2.5% ◉ 224
Naldecon Syrup, Tablets, Pediatric Drops and Pediatric Syrup 709
Neo-Synephrine Hydrochloride 1% Carpuject 2063
Neo-Synephrine Hydrochloride 1% Injection 2063
Neo-Synephrine Hydrochloride (Ophthalmic) 2064
Neo-Synephrine ▣ 759
Nōstril Nasal Decongestant ▣ 520
Novahistine Elixir ▣ 596
Phenergan VC 2500
Phenergan VC with Codeine 2501
Prefrin Liquifilm Vasoconstrictor and Lubricant Eye Drops ◉ 254
Prefrin-A ◉ 255
Quelidrine Syrup 556
Relief Vasoconstrictor and Lubricant Eye Drops ◉ 256
Robitussin Night Relief ▣ 677
Ru-Tuss with Hydrocodone 694
Ru-Tuss Tablets 693
Vasosulf ◉ 279
Vicks Sinex ▣ 665
Zincfrin ◉ 230

Phenylephrine Tannate (Combined effects on cardiovascular system may be deleterious). Products include:
Rynatan 2387
Rynatuss 2388

Phenylpropanolamine Hydrochloride (Combined effects on cardiovascular system may be deleterious). Products include:
A.R.M. Allergy Relief Medicine Caplets ▣ 615
Acutrim ▣ 548
Allerest ▣ 559
BC Cold Powder ▣ 517
Cheracol Plus Head Cold/Cough Formula ▣ 667
Codimal Expectorant 846
Comtrex Multi-Symptom Cold Reliever Tablets/Caplets/Liqui-Gels/Liquid 745
Contac Continuous Action Decongestant/Antihistamine Capsules ▣ 710
Contac Maximum Strength Continuous Action Decongestant/ Antihistamine Caplets ▣ 709
Contac Severe Cold and Flu Formula Caplets ▣ 711
Coricidin 'D' Decongestant Tablets ▣ 695
Coricidin Demilets Tablets for Children ▣ 696
Demazin Nasal Decongestant/ Antihistamine Repetabs Tablets & Syrup ▣ 697
Dexatrim ▣ 733
Dimetane-DC Cough Syrup 1857
Dimetapp Elixir ▣ 673
Dimetapp DM Elixir ▣ 674
Dimetapp Extentabs ▣ 674
Dimetapp Plus Caplets ▣ 675
Dimetapp Tablets ▣ 675
Entex Capsules 1623
Entex LA Tablets 1623
Entex Liquid 1623
4-Way Cold Tablets 750
Hycomine Syrup 927
Naldecon CX Adult Liquid ▣ 521
Naldecon DX Adult Liquid ▣ 521
Naldecon DX Children's Syrup ▣ 522
Naldecon DX Pediatric Drops ▣ 522
Naldecon EX Children's Syrup ▣ 522
Naldecon EX Pediatric Drops ▣ 523
Naldecon Syrup, Tablets, Pediatric Drops and Pediatric Syrup 709
Nolamine Tablets 838
Nolex LA Tablets 838
Ornade Spansule Capsules 2221
Orthoxicol Cough Syrup ▣ 668
Propagest 839
Pyrroxate Capsules ▣ 669
Robitussin-CF ▣ 676
Ru-Tuss II Capsules 693
Ru-Tuss with Hydrocodone 694
Ru-Tuss Tablets 693
Sine-Off Sinus Medicine Tablets-Aspirin Formula ▣ 722
Sinulin 840
St. Joseph Cold Tablets for Children ▣ 704
Tavist-D Tablets 2035
Triaminic Allergy Tablets ▣ 688
Triaminic Chewables ▣ 688
Triaminic Cold Tablets ▣ 688
Triaminic Expectorant ▣ 688
Triaminic Expectorant w/Codeine 1996
Triaminic Expectorant DH 1995
Triaminic Oral Infant Drops 1996
Triaminic Syrup ▣ 689
Triaminic-12 Tablets ▣ 690
Triaminic-DM Syrup ▣ 689
Triaminicin Tablets ▣ 690
Triaminicol Multi-Symptom Cold Tablets ▣ 691
Triaminicol Multi-Symptom Relief ▣ 691
Tuss-Ornade Liquid 2242
Tuss-Ornade Spansule Capsules 2242
Tylenol Cold Medication, Effervescent Tablets 1369

Pirbuterol Acetate (Combined effects on cardiovascular system may be deleterious). Products include:

Maxair Inhaler 1311

Protriptyline Hydrochloride (Epinephrine effects may be potentiated). Products include:

Vivactil Tablets 1567

Pseudoephedrine Hydrochloride (Combined effects on cardiovascular system may be deleterious). Products include:

Actifed Capsules .... ⊞ 539
Actifed Plus Caplets .... ⊞ 539
Actifed Plus Tablets .... ⊞ 540
Actifed with Codeine Cough Syrup.. 752
Actifed Syrup .... ⊞ 540
Actifed Tablets .... ⊞ 540
Actifed 12-Hour Capsules .... ⊞ 539
Advil Cold & Sinus Caplets (formerly CoAdvil) 2416
Allerest .... ⊞ 559
Anatuss LA Tablets 1359
Benadryl Decongestant Elixir .... ⊞ 635
Benadryl Decongestant .... ⊞ 635
Benadryl Plus .... ⊞ 636
Benadryl Plus Nighttime .... ⊞ 637
Benylin Decongestant .... ⊞ 638
Brexin L.A. Capsules 2078
Bromfed Capsules (Timed Release) 1615
Bromfed Syrup .... ⊞ 628
Bromfed 1615
CoAdvil .... ⊞ 748
Allergy-Sinus Comtrex Multi-Symptom Allergy Sinus Formula Tablets & Caplets 746
Cough Formula Comtrex 746
Comtrex Multi-Symptom Cold Reliever Tablets/Caplets/Liqui-Gels/Liquid 745
Day-Night Comtrex 747
Non-Drowsy Comtrex 747
Congess 994
Congestac Caplets .... ⊞ 617
Contac Jr. Children's Cold Medicine .... ⊞ 712
Contac Nighttime Cold Medicine .... ⊞ 713
Contac Sinus Caplets Maximum Strength Non-Drowsy Formula .... ⊞ 710
Contac Sinus Tablets Maximum Strength Non-Drowsy Formula .... ⊞ 710
Deconamine 663
Deconsal II Tablets 559
Dimacol Caplets .... ⊞ 672
Dimetane-DX Cough Syrup 1858
Dorcol Children's Cough Syrup .... ⊞ 685
Dorcol Children's Decongestant Liquid .... ⊞ 685
Dorcol Children's Liquid Cold Formula .... ⊞ 686
Maximum Strength Dristan Decongestant/Analgesic Coated Caplets .... ⊞ 750
No Drowsiness Dristan Cold Nasal Decongestant/Analgesic Coated Caplets 2420
Dristan Sinus Caplets 2419
Sinus Excedrin Analgesic, Decongestant Tablets & Caplets .... ⊞ 533
Fedahist Gyrocaps 2145
Fedahist Timecaps 2145
Guaifed 1615
Guaifed Syrup .... ⊞ 629
Isoclor Expectorant 982
Isoclor Timesule Capsules .... ⊞ 561
Kronofed-A 970
Medi-Flu Caplet, Liquid .... ⊞ 640
Novafed A Capsules 1342
Novafed Capsules 1342
Novahistine DH 1342
Novahistine DMX .... ⊞ 595
Novahistine Expectorant 1343
Nucofed Capsules 2219
Nucofed Expectorant 2219
Nucofed Pediatric Expectorant 2220
Nucofed Syrup 2219
Ornex Caplets .... ⊞ 618
PediaCare Allergy Relief Formula Liquid 1362
PediaCare Cough-Cold Formula Liquid 1362
PediaCare Infants' Oral Decongestant Drops 1362
PediaCare Night Rest Cough-Cold Formula Liquid 1362
PediaCare 6-12 Cough-Cold Formula Chewable Tablets 1362
Robitussin-DAC Syrup 1875
Robitussin-PE .... ⊞ 677
Rondec 1975
Rondec-DM 1976
Rondec-TR Tablet 1975
Ru-Tuss DE Tablets 694
Ryna .... ⊞ 741
Seldane-D Extended-Release Tablets 1350
Sinarest .... ⊞ 562
Sine-Aid Maximum Strength Sinus Headache Caplets 1365
Sine-Aid Maximum Strength Sinus Headache Tablets 1365
Sine-Off Maximum Strength Allergy/Sinus Formula Caplets .... ⊞ 721
Sine-Off Maximum Strength No Drowsiness Formula Caplets .... ⊞ 722
Singlet Tablets .... ⊞ 598
Sinutab Maximum Strength .... ⊞ 641
Sinutab Maximum Strength Without Drowsiness Tablets & Caplets .... ⊞ 642
Sinutab Regular Strength Without Drowsiness Formula .... ⊞ 641
St. Joseph Nighttime Cold Medicine .... ⊞ 705
Sudafed Children's Liquid .... ⊞ 543
Sudafed Cough Syrup .... ⊞ 543
Sudafed Plus Liquid .... ⊞ 544
Sudafed Plus Tablets .... ⊞ 545
Sudafed Sinus Caplets .... ⊞ 545
Sudafed Sinus Tablets .... ⊞ 545
Sudafed Tablets, 30 mg .... ⊞ 544
Sudafed Tablets, Adult Strength, 60 mg .... ⊞ 544
Sudafed 12 Hour Capsules .... ⊞ 545
TheraFlu Flu and Cold Medicine .... ⊞ 687
Triaminic Nite Light .... ⊞ 689
Tylenol Allergy Sinus Medication Caplets and Gelcaps, Maximum Strength 1372
Children's Tylenol Cold Liquid Formula and Chewable Tablets 1368
Tylenol Cold & Flu Hot Medication, Packets 1369
Tylenol Cold & Flu No Drowsiness Hot Medication, Packets 1371
Tylenol Cold Medication Caplets and Tablets 1370
Tylenol Cold Medication No Drowsiness Formula Caplets 1370
Tylenol Cold Night Time Medication Liquid 1371
Tylenol Cough Medication Liquid with Decongestant, Maximum Strength 1372
Tylenol, Maximum Strength, Sinus Medication Gelcaps, Caplets and Tablets 1373
Ursinus Inlay-Tabs .... ⊞ 691
Vicks Children's NyQuil .... ⊞ 664
Vicks Daycare .... ⊞ 660
Vicks Formula 44D Decongestant Cough Medicine .... ⊞ 662
Vicks Formula 44M Multi-Symptom Cough Medicine .... ⊞ 662
Vicks NyQuil Nighttime Colds Medicine-Original & Cherry Flavor .... ⊞ 664
Vicks Pediatric Formula 44 Cough & Congestion Medicine .... ⊞ 663
Vicks Pediatric Formula 44m Multi-Symptom Cough & Cold Medicine .... ⊞ 663

Pseudoephedrine Sulfate (Combined effects on cardiovascular system may be deleterious). Products include:

Afrin Tablets .... ⊞ 693
Chlor-Trimeton Decongestant .... ⊞ 694
Disophrol Chronotab Sustained-Action Tablets .... ⊞ 698
Drixoral Antihistamine/Nasal Decongestant Syrup .... ⊞ 698
Drixoral Non-Drowsy Formula .... ⊞ 699
Drixoral Plus Extended-Release Tablets .... ⊞ 699
Drixoral Sinus .... ⊞ 700
Drixoral Sustained-Action Tablets ⊞ 698
Sinutab Allergy Formula Sustained Action Tablets .... ⊞ 640
Trinalin Repetabs Tablets 1170

Terbutaline Sulfate (Combined effects on cardiovascular system may be deleterious). Products include:

Brethaire Inhaler 1024
Brethine Ampuls 1026
Brethine Tablets 1026
Bricanyl Injection 1324
Bricanyl Tablets 1325

Thyroxine Sodium (Epinephrine effects may be potentiated).

No products indexed under this heading.

Trimipramine Maleate (Epinephrine effects may be potentiated). Products include:

Surmontil Capsules 2524

Tripelennamine Hydrochloride (Epinephrine effects may be potentiated). Products include:

PBZ Tablets & Elixir 1037
PBZ-SR Tablets 1037

Tripelennamine Preparations (Epinephrine effects may be potentiated).

SWEEN CREAM

(Benzethonium Chloride, Lanolin Oil) 2286
No interactions described in labeling.

SWEEN PREP, PROTECTIVE SKIN BARRIER

(Chloroxylenol) 2287
No interactions described in labeling.

SWEEN-A-PEEL, WAFER SKIN PROTECTANT

(Methylbenzethonium Chloride) 2286
No interactions described in labeling.

SYLLACT POWDER

(Psyllium Preparations) .... ⊞ 741
No interactions described in labeling.

SYMMETREL CAPSULES & SYRUP

(Amantadine Hydrochloride) 936
May interact with central nervous system stimulants, anticholinergics, and certain other agents. Compounds in these categories include:

Amphetamine Resins (Caution is advised when concurrently administered). Products include:

Biphetamine Capsules 973

Atropine Sulfate (May require reduction in dosage of either drug). Products include:

Arco-Lase Plus Tablets 607
Atropine Sulfate Sterile Ophthalmic Solution and S.O.P. Sterile Ophthalmic Ointment .... ⊙ 239
Donnagel .... ⊞ 675
Donnagel-PG 1858
Donnatal 1858
Donnatal Extentabs 1859
Donnatal Tablets 1858
Donnazyme Tablets 1860
Isopto Atropine .... ⊙ 218
Lomotil 2174
Motofen Tablets 836
Ru-Tuss Tablets 693
Urised Tablets 2396

Belladonna Alkaloids (May require reduction in dosage of either drug). Products include:

Bellergal-S Tablets 1998
Hyland's Bed Wetting Tablets .... ⊞ 728
Hyland's Teething Tablets .... ⊞ 728
Kinesed Tablets 2272

Benztropine Mesylate (May require reduction in dosage of either drug). Products include:

Cogentin 1435

Biperiden (May require reduction in dosage of either drug). Products include:

Akineton 1171

Clidinium Bromide (May require reduction in dosage of either drug). Products include:

Librax Capsules 1929
Quarzan Capsules 1937

Dextroamphetamine Sulfate (Caution is advised when concurrently administered). Products include:

Dexedrine 2206

Dicyclomine Hydrochloride (May require reduction in dosage of either drug). Products include:

Bentyl 1322

Ethopropazine Hydrochloride (May require reduction in dosage of either drug).

Glycopyrrolate (May require reduction in dosage of either drug). Products include:

Robinul Forte Tablets 1873
Robinul Injectable 1873
Robinul Tablets 1873

Hyoscyamine (May require reduction in dosage of either drug). Products include:

Cystospaz Tablets 2395
Urised Tablets 2396

Hyoscyamine Sulfate (May require reduction in dosage of either drug). Products include:

Arco-Lase Plus Tablets 607
Cystospaz-M Capsules 2395
Donnagel .... ⊞ 675
Donnagel-PG 1858
Donnatal 1858
Donnatal Extentabs 1859
Donnatal Tablets 1858
Donnazyme Tablets 1860
Kutrase Capsules 2146
Levsin/Levsinex 2147
Ru-Tuss Tablets 693

Ipratropium Bromide (May require reduction in dosage of either drug). Products include:

Atrovent Inhalation Aerosol 675

Mepenzolate Bromide (May require reduction in dosage of either drug). Products include:

Cantil Tablets 1326

Methamphetamine Hydrochloride (Caution is advised when concurrently administered). Products include:

Desoxyn Gradumet Tablets 514

Methylphenidate Hydrochloride (Caution is advised when concurrently administered). Products include:

Ritalin 880

Oxybutynin Chloride (May require reduction in dosage of either drug). Products include:

Ditropan 1332

Pemoline (Caution is advised when concurrently administered). Products include:

Cylert Tablets 510

Procyclidine Hydrochloride (May require reduction in dosage of either drug). Products include:

Kemadrin Tablets 771

Propantheline Bromide (May require reduction in dosage of either drug). Products include:

Pro-Banthine Tablets 2141

Scopolamine Hydrobromide (May require reduction in dosage of either drug). Products include:

Donnagel .... ⊞ 675
Donnagel-PG 1858
Donnatal 1858
Donnatal Extentabs 1859
Donnatal Tablets 1858
Donnazyme Tablets 1860
Isopto Hyoscine .... ⊙ 222
Murocoll-2 Sterile Ophthalmic Solution .... ⊙ 261
Ru-Tuss Tablets 693

Tridihexethyl Chloride (May require reduction in dosage of either drug).

No products indexed under this heading.

Trihexyphenidyl Hydrochloride (May require reduction in dosage of either drug). Products include:

Artane ... 1195

SYNACORT CREAMS 1%, 2.5%
(Hydrocortisone) ... 2296
No interactions described in labeling.

SYNALAR CREAMS 0.025%, 0.01%
(Fluocinolone Acetonide) ... 2296
No interactions described in labeling.

SYNALAR OINTMENT 0.025%
(Fluocinolone Acetonide) ... 2296
No interactions described in labeling.

SYNALAR TOPICAL SOLUTION 0.01%
(Fluocinolone Acetonide) ... 2296
No interactions described in labeling.

SYNALAR-HP CREAM 0.2%
(Fluocinolone Acetonide) ... 2296
No interactions described in labeling.

SYNALGOS-DC CAPSULES
(Dihydrocodeine Bitartrate, Aspirin) .. 2525
May interact with narcotic analgesics, general anesthetics, tranquilizers, hypnotics and sedatives, and central nervous system depressants. Compounds in these categories include:

Alcohol (Additive CNS depression).

Alfentanil Hydrochloride (Additive CNS depression). Products include:

Alfenta Injection ... 1131

Alprazolam (Additive CNS depression). Products include:

Xanax Tablets ... 2367

Aprobarbital (Additive CNS depression). Products include:

Alurate Elixir ... 1883

Buprenorphine (Additive CNS depression).

No products indexed under this heading.

Buspirone Hydrochloride (Additive CNS depression). Products include:

BuSpar ... 1401

Butabarbital (Additive CNS depression). Products include:

Pyridium Plus ... 1764

Butalbital (Additive CNS depression). Products include:

Esgic-Plus Tablets ... 1002
Esgic Tablets & Capsules ... 1001
Fioricet Tablets ... 2006
Fiorinal Capsules ... 2007
Fiorinal with Codeine Capsules ... 2008
Fiorinal Tablets ... 2007
Phrenilin ... 838
Sedapap Tablets 50 mg/650 mg .. 1360

Chlordiazepoxide (Additive CNS depression). Products include:

Libritabs Tablets ... 1930
Limbitrol ... 1933
Menrium Tablets ... 1934

Chlordiazepoxide Hydrochloride (Additive CNS depression). Products include:

Librax Capsules ... 1929
Librium Capsules ... 1931
Librium Injectable ... 1932

Chlorpromazine (Additive CNS depression). Products include:

Thorazine ... 2234

Chlorprothixene (Additive CNS depression). Products include:

Taractan Tablets ... 1920

Chlorprothixene Hydrochloride (Additive CNS depression). Products include:

Taractan ... 1920

Clorazepate Dipotassium (Additive CNS depression). Products include:

Tranxene ... 556

Codeine (Additive CNS depression). Products include:

Calcidrine Syrup ... 506

Codeine Phosphate (Additive CNS depression). Products include:

Actifed with Codeine Cough Syrup.. 752
Cheracol Cough Syrup ... 1853
Codimal PH Syrup ... 846
Dimetane-DC Cough Syrup ... 1857
Empirin with Codeine Phosphate Nos. 2, 3 & 4 ... 764
Fiorinal with Codeine Capsules ... 2008
Isoclor Expectorant ... 982
Naldecon CX Adult Liquid ... ▣ 521
Novahistine DH ... 1342
Novahistine Expectorant ... 1343
Nucofed Capsules ... 2219
Nucofed Expectorant ... 2219
Nucofed Pediatric Expectorant ... 2220
Nucofed Syrup ... 2219
Phenaphen with Codeine Capsules 1865
Phenaphen-650 with Codeine Tablets ... 1866
Phenergan with Codeine ... 2497
Phenergan VC with Codeine ... 2501
Robitussin A-C Syrup ... 1875
Robitussin-DAC Syrup ... 1875
Ryna ... ▣ 741
Soma Compound w/Codeine Tablets ... 2390
Triaminic Expectorant w/Codeine .. 1996
Tussi-Organidin Liquid ... 2391
Tylenol with Codeine ... 1381

Codeine Polistirex (Additive CNS depression).

No products indexed under this heading.

Dezocine (Additive CNS depression).

Diazepam (Additive CNS depression). Products include:

Valium Injectable ... 1937
Valium Tablets ... 1939
Valrelease Capsules ... 1923

Droperidol (Additive CNS depression). Products include:

Inapsine Injection ... 1140
Innovar Injection ... 1141

Enflurane (Additive CNS depression). Products include:

Ethrane ... 599

Estazolam (Additive CNS depression). Products include:

ProSom Tablets ... 554

Ethchlorvynol (Additive CNS depression). Products include:

Placidyl Capsules ... 553

Ethinamate (Additive CNS depression).

No products indexed under this heading.

Fentanyl (Additive CNS depression). Products include:

Duragesic Transdermal System ... 1133

Fentanyl Citrate (Additive CNS depression). Products include:

Innovar Injection ... 1141
Sublimaze Injection ... 1146

Fluphenazine Decanoate (Additive CNS depression). Products include:

Prolixin Decanoate ... 1795

Fluphenazine Enanthate (Additive CNS depression). Products include:

Prolixin Enanthate ... 1796

Fluphenazine Hydrochloride (Additive CNS depression). Products include:

Prolixin Elixir ... 1793
Prolixin Injection ... 1791
Prolixin Oral Concentrate ... 1792
Prolixin Tablets ... 1793

Flurazepam Hydrochloride (Additive CNS depression). Products include:

Dalmane Capsules ... 1927

Glutethimide (Additive CNS depression).

No products indexed under this heading.

Haloperidol (Additive CNS depression). Products include:

Haldol Injection, Tablets and Concentrate ... 1373

Haloperidol Decanoate (Additive CNS depression). Products include:

Haldol Decanoate ... 1375

Hydrocodone Bitartrate (Additive CNS depression). Products include:

Anexsia 5/500 Tablets ... 2196
Anexsia 7.5/650 Tablets ... 2197
Azdone Tablets ... 844
Codiclear DH Syrup ... 845
Codimal DH Syrup ... 846
Damason-P ... 1356
Hycodan Syrup, Tablets ... 927
Hycomine Compound Tablets ... 929
Hycomine Syrup ... 927
Hycotuss Expectorant Syrup ... 930
Hydrocet Capsules ... 835
Lortab ASA Tablets ... 2414
Lortab ... 2412
Ru-Tuss with Hydrocodone ... 694
Triaminic Expectorant DH ... 1995
Vicodin Tablets ... 1187
Vicodin ES Tablets ... 1189
Zydone Capsules ... 941

Hydrocodone Polistirex (Additive CNS depression). Products include:

Tussionex Extended-Release Suspension ... 988

Hydroxyzine Hydrochloride (Additive CNS depression). Products include:

Atarax Tablets & Syrup ... 1941
Marax Tablets & DF Syrup ... 1954
Vistaril Intramuscular Solution ... 1970

Isoflurane (Additive CNS depression). Products include:

Forane ... 600

Ketamine Hydrochloride (Additive CNS depression). Products include:

Ketalar ... 1726

Levorphanol Tartrate (Additive CNS depression). Products include:

Levo-Dromoran ... 1906

Lorazepam (Additive CNS depression). Products include:

Ativan Injection ... 2432
Ativan Tablets ... 2434

Loxapine Hydrochloride (Additive CNS depression). Products include:

Loxitane ... 1213

Loxapine Succinate (Additive CNS depression). Products include:

Loxitane Capsules ... 1213

Meperidine Hydrochloride (Additive CNS depression). Products include:

Demerol ... 2047
Mepergan Injection ... 2479

Mephobarbital (Additive CNS depression). Products include:

Mebaral Tablets ... 2061

Meprobamate (Additive CNS depression). Products include:

Deprol Tablets ... 2382
Equagesic Tablets ... 2451
Miltown Tablets ... 2386
PMB 200 and PMB 400 ... 2504

Mesoridazine (Additive CNS depression). Products include:

Serentil ... 686

Methadone Hydrochloride (Additive CNS depression). Products include:

Dolophine Hydrochloride Ampoules & Vials ... 1260
Dolophine Hydrochloride Tablets ... 1261
Methadone Hydrochloride Diskets .. 1284
Methadone Hydrochloride Oral Solution & Tablets ... 1987

Methohexital Sodium (Additive CNS depression). Products include:

Brevital Sodium Vials ... 1248

Methoxyflurane (Additive CNS depression).

No products indexed under this heading.

Midazolam Hydrochloride (Additive CNS depression). Products include:

Versed Injection ... 1924

Molindone Hydrochloride (Additive CNS depression). Products include:

Moban Tablets & Concentrate ... 932

Morphine Sulfate (Additive CNS depression). Products include:

Astramorph/PF Injection, USP (Preservative-Free) ... 618
Duramorph ... 960
Infumorph 200 and Infumorph 500 Sterile Solutions ... 962
MS Contin Tablets ... 1814
MSIR ... 1817
Oramorph SR (Morphine Sulfate Sustained Release Tablets) ... 1988
Roxanol ... 1991

Opium Alkaloids (Additive CNS depression). Products include:

B & O No. 15A & No. 16A Supprettes ... 2395
Pantopon Injectable ... 1911

Oxazepam (Additive CNS depression). Products include:

Serax Capsules ... 2522
Serax Tablets ... 2522

Oxycodone Hydrochloride (Additive CNS depression). Products include:

Percocet Tablets ... 950
Percodan ... 951
Roxicodone Tablets, Oral Solution & Intensol (Oxycodone) ... 1992
Tylox Capsules ... 1382

Pentobarbital Sodium (Additive CNS depression). Products include:

Nembutal Sodium Capsules ... 534
Nembutal Sodium Solution ... 536
Nembutal Sodium Suppositories ... 538

Perphenazine (Additive CNS depression). Products include:

Etrafon ... 2087
Triavil Tablets ... 1556
Trilafon ... 2123

Phenobarbital (Additive CNS depression). Products include:

Arco-Lase Plus Tablets ... 607
Bellergal-S Tablets ... 1998
Bronkolixir ... ▣ 761
Bronkotabs Tablets ... ▣ 762
Donnatal ... 1858
Donnatal Extentabs ... 1859
Donnatal Tablets ... 1858
Donnazyme Tablets ... 1860
Kinesed Tablets ... 2272
Phenobarbital Elixir and Tablets ... 1293
Primatene Tablets-P Formula ... 2421
Quadrinal Tablets ... 1183
Tedral SA ... 1765

Prazepam (Additive CNS depression). Products include:

Centrax ... 1693

Prochlorperazine (Additive CNS depression). Products include:

Compazine ... 2201

Promethazine Hydrochloride (Additive CNS depression). Products include:

Mepergan Injection ... 2479
Phenergan with Codeine ... 2497
Phenergan with Dextromethorphan 2499
Phenergan Injection ... 2493
Phenergan Suppositories ... 2496
Phenergan Syrup ... 2495
Phenergan Tablets ... 2496
Phenergan VC ... 2500
Phenergan VC with Codeine ... 2501

Propofol (Additive CNS depression). Products include:
- Diprivan Injection 2267

Propoxyphene Hydrochloride (Additive CNS depression). Products include:
- Darvon 1256
- Wygesic Tablets 2540

Propoxyphene Napsylate (Additive CNS depression). Products include:
- Darvon-N/Darvocet-N 1254

Quazepam (Additive CNS depression). Products include:
- Doral Tablets 2383

Secobarbital Sodium (Additive CNS depression). Products include:
- Seconal Sodium Pulvules 1296

Sufentanil Citrate (Additive CNS depression). Products include:
- Sufenta Injection 1147

Temazepam (Additive CNS depression). Products include:
- Restoril Capsules 2023

Thiamylal Sodium (Additive CNS depression). Products include:
- Surital Ampoules, Steri-Vials 1764

Thioridazine Hydrochloride (Additive CNS depression). Products include:
- Mellaril 2011

Thiothixene (Additive CNS depression). Products include:
- Navane Capsules and Concentrate 1954
- Navane Intramuscular 1956

Triazolam (Additive CNS depression). Products include:
- Halcion Tablets 2340

Trifluoperazine Hydrochloride (Additive CNS depression). Products include:
- Stelazine 2226

SYNAREL NASAL SOLUTION
(Nafarelin Acetate) 2300
No interactions described in labeling.

SYNEMOL CREAM 0.025%
(Fluocinolone Acetonide) 2296
No interactions described in labeling.

SYNKAYVITE INJECTION
(Menadiol Sodium Diphosphate) 1919
May interact with oral anticoagulants. Compounds in this category include:

Dicumarol (Decreased sensitivity to oral anticoagulants). Products include:
- Dicumarol Tablets 516

Warfarin Sodium (Decreased sensitivity to oral anticoagulants). Products include:
- Coumadin Injection & Tablets 944
- Panwarfin Tablets 547

SYNKAYVITE TABLETS
(Menadiol Sodium Diphosphate) 1920
May interact with oral anticoagulants. Compounds in this category include:

Dicumarol (Decreased sensitivity to oral anticoagulants). Products include:
- Dicumarol Tablets 516

Warfarin Sodium (Decreased sensitivity to oral anticoagulants). Products include:
- Coumadin Injection & Tablets 944
- Panwarfin Tablets 547

SYNTHROID INJECTION
(Levothyroxine Sodium) 695
May interact with oral anticoagulants, insulin, oral hypoglycemic agents, estrogens, oral contraceptives, and certain other agents. Compounds in these categories include:

Chlorotrianisene (Patients without a functioning thyroid gland who are on thyroid replacement therapy may need to increase their thyroid dose if estrogen is given). Products include:
- TACE 12 and 25 mg 1353

Chlorpropamide (Initiating thyroid replacement therapy may cause increases in hypoglycemic requirements). Products include:
- Diabinese Tablets 1775

Cholestyramine (Impairs absorption of thyroid hormones). Products include:
- Cholybar 1705
- Questran Light 711
- Questran Powder 710

Dicumarol (Increased catabolism of vitamin K-dependent clotting factors, compensatory increases in clotting factor synthesis are impaired). Products include:
- Dicumarol Tablets 516

Dienestrol (Patients without a functioning thyroid gland who are on thyroid replacement therapy may need to increase their thyroid dose if estrogen is given). Products include:
- Ortho Dienestrol Cream 1664

Diethylstilbestrol (Patients without a functioning thyroid gland who are on thyroid replacement therapy may need to increase their thyroid dose if estrogen is given). Products include:
- Diethylstilbestrol Tablets 1258

Estradiol (Patients without a functioning thyroid gland who are on thyroid replacement therapy may need to increase their thyroid dose if estrogen is given). Products include:
- Emcyt Capsules 1161
- Estrace 1385
- Estrace Vaginal Cream 1388
- Estraderm Transdermal System 866

Estrogens, Conjugated (Patients without a functioning thyroid gland who are on thyroid replacement therapy may need to increase their thyroid dose if estrogen is given). Products include:
- Mediatric Capsules 2476
- PMB 200 and PMB 400 2504
- Premarin Intravenous 2508
- Premarin with Methyltestosterone .. 2515
- Premarin Tablets 2510
- Premarin Vaginal Cream 2512

Estrogens, Esterified (Patients without a functioning thyroid gland who are on thyroid replacement therapy may need to increase their thyroid dose if estrogen is given). Products include:
- Estratest 2245
- Menrium Tablets 1934

Estropipate (Patients without a functioning thyroid gland who are on thyroid replacement therapy may need to increase their thyroid dose if estrogen is given). Products include:
- Ogen 540

Ethinyl Estradiol (Patients without a functioning thyroid gland who are on thyroid replacement therapy may need to increase their thyroid dose if estrogen is given). Products include:
- Brevicon 2304
- Demulen 2161
- Estinyl Tablets 2085
- Jenest-28 Tablets 1636
- Levlen/Tri-Levlen 665
- Lo/Ovral Tablets 2471
- Lo/Ovral-28 Tablets 2476
- Loestrin 1728
- Modicon 1667
- Nordette-21 Tablets 2481
- Nordette-28 Tablets 2483
- Norethin 2133
- Norinyl 2304
- Norlestrin 1746
- Ortho-Cyclen Tablets 1658
- Ortho-Novum 1667
- Ovcon 1391
- Ovral Tablets 2490
- Ovral-28 Tablets 2491
- Levlen/Tri-Levlen 665
- Tri-Norinyl 2304
- Triphasil-21 Tablets 2527
- Triphasil-28 Tablets 2532

Ethynodiol Diacetate (Patients without a functioning thyroid gland who are on thyroid replacement therapy may need to increase their thyroid dose if estrogen is given). Products include:
- Demulen 2161

Glipizide (Initiating thyroid replacement therapy may cause increases in hypoglycemic requirements). Products include:
- Glucotrol 1952

Glyburide (Initiating thyroid replacement therapy may cause increases in hypoglycemic requirements). Products include:
- DiaBeta 1091
- Micronase Tablets 2350

Insulin, Human (Initiating thyroid replacement therapy may cause increases in insulin requirements).
- No products indexed under this heading.

Insulin, Human Isophane Suspension (Initiating thyroid replacement therapy may cause increases in insulin requirements). Products include:
- Humulin N, 100 Units 1270

Insulin, Human NPH (Initiating thyroid replacement therapy may cause increases in insulin requirements). Products include:
- Insulatard NPH Human 1627
- Novolin N 1627
- Novolin N PenFill Cartridges 1628
- Novolin N Prefilled 1628

Insulin, Human Regular (Initiating thyroid replacement therapy may cause increases in insulin requirements). Products include:
- Humulin BR, 100 Units 1268
- Humulin R, 100 Units 1272
- Novolin R 1627
- Novolin R PenFill Cartridges 1628
- Novolin R Prefilled 1629
- Velosulin Human 1628

Insulin, Human, Zinc Suspension (Initiating thyroid replacement therapy may cause increases in insulin requirements). Products include:
- Humulin L, 100 Units 1268
- Humulin U, 100 Units 1272
- Novolin L 1627

Insulin, NPH (Initiating thyroid replacement therapy may cause increases in insulin requirements). Products include:
- NPH, 40 & 100 Units 1273
- Beef NPH, 100 Units 1274
- Pork NPH, 100 Units 1275
- Insulatard NPH 1626
- NPH Insulin 1626
- NPH Purified Pork Isophane Insulin 1626

Insulin, Regular (Initiating thyroid replacement therapy may cause increases in insulin requirements). Products include:
- Regular, 40 & 100 Units 1273
- Beef Regular, 100 Units 1275
- Pork Regular, 100 Units 1275
- Pork Regular (Concentrated), 500 Units 1276
- Regular Insulin 1625
- Regular Purified Pork Insulin 1626
- Velosulin 1627

Insulin, Zinc Crystals (Initiating thyroid replacement therapy may cause increases in insulin requirements). Products include:
- NPH, 40 & 100 Units 1273

Insulin, Zinc Suspension (Initiating thyroid replacement therapy may cause increases in insulin requirements). Products include:
- Lente, 40 & 100 Units 1272
- Protamine, Zinc, 40 & 100 Units.... 1273
- Lente Iletin I 1272
- Beef Lente, 100 Units 1274
- Beef Protamine Zinc, 100 Units 1274
- Pork Lente, 100 Units 1275
- Pork, Protamine, Zinc, 100 Units.... 1275
- Lente Insulin 1626
- Lente Purified Pork Insulin 1626
- Semilente Insulin 1625
- Ultralente Insulin 1626

Levonorgestrel (Patients without a functioning thyroid gland who are on thyroid replacement therapy may need to increase their thyroid dose if estrogen is given). Products include:
- Levlen/Tri-Levlen 665
- Nordette-21 Tablets 2481
- Nordette-28 Tablets 2483
- Norplant System 2484
- Levlen/Tri-Levlen 665
- Triphasil-21 Tablets 2527
- Triphasil-28 Tablets 2532

Mestranol (Patients without a functioning thyroid gland who are on thyroid replacement therapy may need to increase their thyroid dose if estrogen is given). Products include:
- Enovid 2161
- Norethin 2133
- Norinyl 2304
- Ortho-Novum 1667

Norethindrone (Patients without a functioning thyroid gland who are on thyroid replacement therapy may need to increase their thyroid dose if estrogen is given). Products include:
- Brevicon 2304
- Jenest-28 Tablets 1636
- Micronor Tablets 1667
- Modicon 1667
- Norethin 2133
- Norinyl 2304
- Norlutin 1755
- Nor-Q D Tablets 2304
- Ortho-Novum 1667
- Ovcon 1391
- Tri-Norinyl 2304

Norethynodrel (Patients without a functioning thyroid gland who are on thyroid replacement therapy may need to increase their thyroid dose if estrogen is given). Products include:
- Enovid 2161

Norgestimate (Patients without a functioning thyroid gland who are on thyroid replacement therapy may need to increase their thyroid dose if estrogen is given). Products include:
- Ortho-Cyclen Tablets 1658

Norgestrel (Patients without a functioning thyroid gland who are on thyroid replacement therapy may need to increase their thyroid dose if estrogen is given). Products include:
- Lo/Ovral Tablets 2471
- Lo/Ovral-28 Tablets 2476
- Ovral Tablets 2490
- Ovral-28 Tablets 2491
- Ovrette Tablets 2492

Polyestradiol Phosphate (Patients without a functioning thyroid gland who are on thyroid replacement therapy may need to increase their thyroid dose if estrogen is given). Products include:
- Estradurin 2452

Quinestrol (Patients without a functioning thyroid gland who are on thyroid replacement therapy may need to increase their thyroid dose if estrogen is given). Products include:
- Estrovis 1721

Tolazamide (Initiating thyroid replacement therapy may cause increases in hypoglycemic requirements). Products include:
- Tolinase Tablets ... 2365

Tolbutamide (Initiating thyroid replacement therapy may cause increases in hypoglycemic requirements). Products include:
- Orinase Tablets ... 2354

Warfarin Sodium (Increased catabolism of vitamin K-dependent clotting factors, compensatory increases in clotting factor synthesis are impaired). Products include:
- Coumadin Injection & Tablets ... 944
- Panwarfin Tablets ... 547

Food Interactions

Soybean formula, children's (May cause excessive fecal loss).

SYNTHROID TABLETS
(Levothyroxine Sodium) ... 695
See **Synthroid Injection**

SYNTOCINON INJECTION
(Oxytocin (Injection)) ... 2032
May interact with vasopressors and certain other agents. Compounds in these categories include:

Cyclopropane (Modifies cardiovascular effects resulting in hypotension).

Dopamine Hydrochloride (Potential for severe hypertension following prophylactic administration of a vasoconstrictor in conjunction with caudal block anesthesia). Products include:
- Intropin Injection ... 930

Epinephrine Hydrochloride (Potential for severe hypertension following prophylactic administration of a vasoconstrictor in conjunction with caudal block anesthesia). Products include:
- Adrenalin Chloride Solution 1:100 & 1:1,000 ... 1689
- Epifrin ... ⊙ 244
- Glaucon ... ⊙ 218

Metaraminol Bitartrate (Potential for severe hypertension following prophylactic administration of a vasoconstrictor in conjunction with caudal block anesthesia). Products include:
- Aramine Injection ... 1424

Methoxamine Hydrochloride (Potential for severe hypertension following prophylactic administration of a vasoconstrictor in conjunction with caudal block anesthesia). Products include:
- Vasoxyl Injection ... 819

Norepinephrine Bitartrate (Potential for severe hypertension following prophylactic administration of a vasoconstrictor in conjunction with caudal block anesthesia). Products include:
- Levophed Bitartrate Injection ... 2054

Phenylephrine Hydrochloride (Potential for severe hypertension following prophylactic administration of a vasoconstrictor in conjunction with caudal block anesthesia). Products include:
- AK-Dilate Solution 2.5% and 10% ... ⊙ 203
- Atrohist Sprinkle Capsules ... 558
- Cerose-DM ... 2443
- Codimal ... 846
- Comhist LA Capsules ... 1618
- Congespirin For Children Aspirin Free Chewable Cold Tablets ... 748
- Cyclomydril ... ⊙ 216
- Deconsal Sprinkle Capsules ... 559
- Dimetane Decongestant ... ⊞ 673
- Dristan Decongestant/Antihistamine/ Analgesic Coated Caplets ... ⊞ 749
- Dristan Cold Nasal Decongestant/ Antihistamine/ Analgesic Coated Tablets ... 2419
- Dristan Advanced Formula Decongestant/Antihistamine/ Analgesic Tablets ... ⊞ 749
- Dristan Nasal Spray, Menthol ... 2419
- Dristan Nasal Spray, Regular and Regular with Metered Pump ... 2419
- Entex Capsules ... 1623
- Entex Liquid ... 1623
- Sinus Excedrin Analgesic, Decongestant Tablets & Caplets ... 750
- Extendryl ... 994
- 4-Way Fast Acting Nasal Spray - Original Formula (regular & mentholated) & Metered Spray Pump (regular) ... 751
- Hycomine Compound Tablets ... 929
- Murocoll-2 Sterile Ophthalmic Solution ... ⊙ 261
- Mydfrin 2.5% ... ⊙ 224
- Naldecon Syrup, Tablets, Pediatric Drops and Pediatric Syrup ... 709
- Neo-Synephrine Hydrochloride 1% Carpuject ... 2063
- Neo-Synephrine Hydrochloride 1% Injection ... 2063
- Neo-Synephrine Hydrochloride (Ophthalmic) ... 2064
- Neo-Synephrine ... ⊞ 759
- Nōstril Nasal Decongestant ... ⊞ 520
- Novahistine Elixir ... ⊞ 596
- Phenergan VC ... 2500
- Phenergan VC with Codeine ... 2501
- Prefrin Liquifilm Vasoconstrictor and Lubricant Eye Drops ... ⊙ 254
- Prefrin-A ... ⊙ 255
- Quelidrine Syrup ... 556
- Relief Vasoconstrictor and Lubricant Eye Drops ... ⊙ 256
- Robitussin Night Relief ... ⊞ 677
- Ru-Tuss with Hydrocodone ... 694
- Ru-Tuss Tablets ... 693
- Vasosulf ... ⊙ 279
- Vicks Sinex ... ⊞ 665
- Zincfrin ... ⊙ 230

SYNTOCINON NASAL SPRAY
(Oxytocin (Nasal Spray)) ... 2033
No interactions described in labeling.

SYPRINE CAPSULES
(Trientine Hydrochloride) ... 1546
No interactions described in labeling.

TACE 12 MG CAPSULES
(Chlorotrianisene) ... 1353
May interact with progestins. Compounds in this category include:

Medroxyprogesterone Acetate (Potential adverse effects on carbohydrate and lipid metabolism). Products include:
- Amen ... 833
- Cycrin Tablets ... 2449
- Depo-Provera Sterile Aqueous Suspension ... 2336
- Provera Tablets ... 2356

Megestrol Acetate (Potential adverse effects on carbohydrate and lipid metabolism). Products include:
- Megace Tablets ... 732

Norgestimate (Potential adverse effects on carbohydrate and lipid metabolism). Products include:
- Ortho-Cyclen Tablets ... 1658

TACE 25 MG CAPSULES
(Chlorotrianisene) ... 1353
See **TACE 12 mg Capsules**

T-PHYL (UNIPHYL) 200 MG TABLETS
(Theophylline Anhydrous) ... 1820
May interact with macrolide antibiotics, sympathomimetic bronchodilators, and certain other agents. Compounds in these categories include:

Albuterol (Toxic synergism). Products include:
- Proventil Inhalation Aerosol ... 2117
- Ventolin Inhalation Aerosol and Refill ... 583

Albuterol Sulfate (Toxic synergism). Products include:
- Proventil Repetabs Tablets ... 2120
- Proventil Solutions for Inhalation 0.5% and 0.083% ... 2118
- Proventil Syrup ... 2119
- Proventil Tablets ... 2120
- Ventolin ... 583

Bitolterol Mesylate (Toxic synergism). Products include:
- Tornalate ... 2074

Cimetidine (Increases serum theophylline levels). Products include:
- Tagamet Tablets ... 2228

Cimetidine Hydrochloride (Increases serum theophylline levels). Products include:
- Tagamet ... 2228

Ephedrine Hydrochloride (Toxic synergism). Products include:
- Amesec ... ⊞ 682
- Primatene Tablets-M Formula ... 2421
- Primatene Tablets-P Formula ... 2421
- Primatene Tablets-Regular Formula ... 2421
- Quadrinal Tablets ... 1183
- Quelidrine Syrup ... 556
- Tedral SA ... 1765

Ephedrine Sulfate (Toxic synergism). Products include:
- Bronkaid Tablets ... ⊞ 757
- Bronkolixir ... ⊞ 761
- Bronkotabs Tablets ... ⊞ 762
- Marax Tablets & DF Syrup ... 1954
- Pazo Hemorrhoid Ointment & Suppositories ... 752
- Vicks Vatronol Nose Drops ... ⊞ 666

Ephedrine Tannate (Toxic synergism). Products include:
- Rynatuss ... 2388

Epinephrine (Toxic synergism). Products include:
- Ana-Kit Anaphylaxis Emergency Treatment Kit ... 1100
- Bronkaid Mist ... ⊞ 757
- EpiPen ... 843
- Marcaine Hydrochloride 0.5% with Epinephrine 1:200,000 (as bitartrate) ... 958
- Marcaine Hydrochloride with Epinephrine 1:200,000 ... 2055
- Primatene Mist ... 2420
- Sus-Phrine Injection ... 1006
- Xylocaine with Epinephrine Injections ... 637

Epinephrine Hydrochloride (Toxic synergism). Products include:
- Adrenalin Chloride Solution 1:100 & 1:1,000 ... 1689
- Epifrin ... ⊙ 244
- Glaucon ... ⊙ 218

Erythromycin (Increases serum theophylline levels). Products include:
- A/T/S Topical Gel and Topical Solution ... 1089
- AK-Mycin Ointment ... ⊙ 204
- Benzamycin Topical Gel ... 907
- E-Mycin Tablets ... 688
- ETS-2% ... 1685
- ERYC ... 1720
- Erycette (erythromycin 2%) Topical Solution ... 1678
- Ery-Tab Tablets ... 521
- Erythromycin Base Filmtab ... 525
- Erythromycin Delayed-Release Capsules, USP ... 526
- Ilotycin Ophthalmic Ointment ... 915
- PCE Dispertab Tablets ... 549
- Pediazole ... 1973
- T-Stat 2.0% Topical Solution and Pads ... 2409
- Theramycin Z Topical Solution 2% ... 1410

Erythromycin Estolate (Increases serum theophylline levels). Products include:
- Ilosone ... 913

Erythromycin Ethylsuccinate (Increases serum theophylline levels). Products include:
- E.E.S. ... 522
- EryPed ... 519
- Pediazole ... 1973

Erythromycin Gluceptate (Increases serum theophylline levels). Products include:
- Ilotycin Gluceptate, IV, Vials ... 915

Erythromycin Stearate (Increases serum theophylline levels). Products include:
- Erythrocin Stearate Filmtab ... 523

Ethylnorepinephrine Hydrochloride (Toxic synergism). Products include:
- Bronkephrine Injection ... 2042

Isoetharine (Toxic synergism). Products include:
- Arm-a-Med Isoetharine Inhalation Solution, USP ... 616
- Bronkometer Aerosol ... 2042
- Bronkosol Solution ... 2042

Isoproterenol Hydrochloride (Toxic synergism). Products include:
- Isuprel Hydrochloride Injection 1:5000 ... 2050
- Isuprel Hydrochloride Mistometer .. 2051
- Isuprel Hydrochloride Solution 1:200 & 1:100 ... 2052
- Norisodrine Aerotrol ... 540

Lithium Carbonate (Increased lithium excretion). Products include:
- Eskalith ... 2214
- Lithane Tablets ... 1596
- Lithium Carbonate Capsules & Tablets ... 1984
- Lithobid Tablets ... 870

Metaproterenol Sulfate (Toxic synergism). Products include:
- Alupent ... 674
- Arm-a-Med Metaproterenol Sulfate Inhalation Solution, USP ... 617
- Metaprel Inhalation Aerosol Bronchodilator ... 2014
- Metaprel Inhalation Solution ... 2015
- Metaprel ... 2015
- Metaproterenol Sulfate Inhalation Solution, USP ... 912

Pirbuterol Acetate (Toxic synergism). Products include:
- Maxair Inhaler ... 1311

Propranolol Hydrochloride (Propranolol effects antagonized). Products include:
- Inderal ... 2459
- Inderal LA Long Acting Capsules ... 2461
- Inderide Tablets ... 2463
- Inderide LA Long Acting Capsules .. 2465

Terbutaline Sulfate (Toxic synergism). Products include:
- Brethaire Inhaler ... 1024
- Brethine Ampuls ... 1026
- Brethine Tablets ... 1026
- Bricanyl Injection ... 1324
- Bricanyl Tablets ... 1325

Troleandomycin (Increases serum theophylline levels). Products include:
- Tao Capsules ... 1963

T-STAT 2.0% TOPICAL SOLUTION AND PADS
(Erythromycin) ... 2409
May interact with:

Concomitant Topical Acne Therapy (Possible cumulative irritant effect).

TACARYL CHEWABLE TABLETS
(Methdilazine) ... 2409
May interact with central nervous system depressants, monoamine oxidase inhibitors, thiazides, oral

contraceptives, progestins, and certain other agents. Compounds in these categories include:

Alcohol (Additive effect).

Alfentanil Hydrochloride (Additive effect). Products include:
Alfenta Injection ... 1131

Alprazolam (Additive effect). Products include:
Xanax Tablets ... 2367

Aprobarbital (Additive effect). Products include:
Alurate Elixir ... 1883

Bendroflumethiazide (Anticholinergic effects of phenothiazines may be prolonged and intensified). Products include:
Corzide Tablets ... 702
Naturetin Tablets ... 1789
Rauzide Tablets ... 1804

Buprenorphine (Additive effect).
No products indexed under this heading.

Buspirone Hydrochloride (Additive effect). Products include:
BuSpar ... 1401

Butabarbital (Additive effect). Products include:
Pyridium Plus ... 1764

Butalbital (Additive effect). Products include:
Esgic-Plus Tablets ... 1002
Esgic Tablets & Capsules ... 1001
Fioricet Tablets ... 2006
Fiorinal Capsules ... 2007
Fiorinal with Codeine Capsules ... 2008
Fiorinal Tablets ... 2007
Phrenilin ... 838
Sedapap Tablets 50 mg/650 mg .. 1360

Chlordiazepoxide (Additive effect). Products include:
Libritabs Tablets ... 1930
Limbitrol ... 1933
Menrium Tablets ... 1934

Chlordiazepoxide Hydrochloride (Additive effect). Products include:
Librax Capsules ... 1929
Librium Capsules ... 1931
Librium Injectable ... 1932

Chlorothiazide (Anticholinergic effects of phenothiazines may be prolonged and intensified). Products include:
Aldoclor Tablets ... 1413
Diupres Tablets ... 1461
Diuril Oral ... 1464

Chlorothiazide Sodium (Anticholinergic effects of phenothiazines may be prolonged and intensified). Products include:
Diuril Sodium Intravenous ... 1463

Chlorpromazine (Additive effect). Products include:
Thorazine ... 2234

Chlorprothixene (Additive effect). Products include:
Taractan Tablets ... 1920

Chlorprothixene Hydrochloride (Additive effect). Products include:
Taractan ... 1920

Clorazepate Dipotassium (Additive effect). Products include:
Tranxene ... 556

Codeine (Additive effect). Products include:
Calcidrine Syrup ... 506

Codeine Phosphate (Additive effect). Products include:
Actifed with Codeine Cough Syrup.. 752
Cheracol Cough Syrup ... 1853
Codimal PH Syrup ... 846
Dimetane-DC Cough Syrup ... 1857
Empirin with Codeine Phosphate Nos. 2, 3 & 4 ... 764
Fiorinal with Codeine Capsules ... 2008
Isoclor Expectorant ... 982
Naldecon CX Adult Liquid ... ◘ 521
Novahistine DH ... 1342
Novahistine Expectorant ... 1343
Nucofed Capsules ... 2219
Nucofed Expectorant ... 2219
Nucofed Pediatric Expectorant ... 2220
Nucofed Syrup ... 2219
Phenaphen with Codeine Capsules 1865
Phenaphen-650 with Codeine Tablets ... 1866
Phenergan with Codeine ... 2497
Phenergan VC with Codeine ... 2501
Robitussin A-C Syrup ... 1875
Robitussin-DAC Syrup ... 1875
Ryna ... ◘ 741
Soma Compound w/Codeine Tablets ... 2390
Triaminic Expectorant w/Codeine .. 1996
Tussi-Organidin Liquid ... 2391
Tylenol with Codeine ... 1381

Codeine Polistirex (Additive effect).
No products indexed under this heading.

Dezocine (Additive effect).

Diazepam (Additive effect). Products include:
Valium Injectable ... 1937
Valium Tablets ... 1939
Valrelease Capsules ... 1923

Droperidol (Additive effect). Products include:
Inapsine Injection ... 1140
Innovar Injection ... 1141

Enflurane (Additive effect). Products include:
Ethrane ... 599

Epinephrine Hydrochloride (Phenothiazines may block and even reverse some actions of epinephrine). Products include:
Adrenalin Chloride Solution 1:100 & 1:1,000 ... 1689
Epifrin ... ⊙ 244
Glaucon ... ⊙ 218

Estazolam (Additive effect). Products include:
ProSom Tablets ... 554

Ethchlorvynol (Additive effect). Products include:
Placidyl Capsules ... 553

Ethinamate (Additive effect).
No products indexed under this heading.

Ethinyl Estradiol (Effects of phenothiazines potentiated). Products include:
Brevicon ... 2304
Demulen ... 2161
Estinyl Tablets ... 2085
Jenest-28 Tablets ... 1636
Levlen/Tri-Levlen ... 665
Lo/Ovral Tablets ... 2471
Lo/Ovral-28 Tablets ... 2476
Loestrin ... 1728
Modicon ... 1667
Nordette-21 Tablets ... 2481
Nordette-28 Tablets ... 2483
Norethin ... 2133
Norinyl ... 2304
Norlestrin ... 1746
Ortho-Cyclen Tablets ... 1658
Ortho-Novum ... 1667
Ovcon ... 1391
Ovral Tablets ... 2490
Ovral-28 Tablets ... 2491
Levlen/Tri-Levlen ... 665
Tri-Norinyl ... 2304
Triphasil-21 Tablets ... 2527
Triphasil-28 Tablets ... 2532

Ethynodiol Diacetate (Effects of phenothiazines potentiated). Products include:
Demulen ... 2161

Fentanyl (Additive effect). Products include:
Duragesic Transdermal System ... 1133

Fentanyl Citrate (Additive effect). Products include:
Innovar Injection ... 1141
Sublimaze Injection ... 1146

Fluphenazine Decanoate (Additive effect). Products include:
Prolixin Decanoate ... 1795

Fluphenazine Enanthate (Additive effect). Products include:
Prolixin Enanthate ... 1796

Fluphenazine Hydrochloride (Additive effect). Products include:
Prolixin Elixir ... 1793
Prolixin Injection ... 1791
Prolixin Oral Concentrate ... 1792
Prolixin Tablets ... 1793

Flurazepam Hydrochloride (Additive effect). Products include:
Dalmane Capsules ... 1927

Furazolidone (Possible hypotension and extrapyramidal reactions). Products include:
Furoxone ... 1855

Glutethimide (Additive effect).
No products indexed under this heading.

Haloperidol (Additive effect). Products include:
Haldol Injection, Tablets and Concentrate ... 1373

Haloperidol Decanoate (Additive effect). Products include:
Haldol Decanoate ... 1375

Hydrochlorothiazide (Anticholinergic effects of phenothiazines may be prolonged and intensified). Products include:
Aldactazide ... 2150
Aldoril Tablets ... 1418
Apresazide Capsules ... 854
Apresoline-Esidrix Tablets ... 857
Capozide ... 2258
Dyazide Capsules ... 2208
Esidrix Tablets ... 863
Esimil Tablets ... 864
HydroDIURIL Tablets ... 1484
Hydropres Tablets ... 1485
Inderide Tablets ... 2463
Inderide LA Long Acting Capsules .. 2465
Lopressor HCT Tablets ... 1034
Maxzide ... 1215
Moduretic Tablets ... 1510
Normozide Tablets ... 2112
Oretic Tablets ... 544
Oreticyl ... 545
Prinzide Tablets ... 1540
Ser-Ap-Es Tablets ... 881
Serpasil-Esidrix Tablets ... 886
Timolide Tablets ... 1547
Trandate HCT Tablets ... 579
Vaseretic Tablets ... 1559
Zestoretic ... 2274

Hydrocodone Bitartrate (Additive effect). Products include:
Anexsia 5/500 Tablets ... 2196
Anexsia 7.5/650 Tablets ... 2197
Azdône Tablets ... 844
Codiclear DH Syrup ... 845
Codimal DH Syrup ... 846
Damason-P ... 1356
Hycodan Syrup, Tablets ... 927
Hycomine Compound Tablets ... 929
Hycomine Syrup ... 927
Hycotuss Expectorant Syrup ... 930
Hydrocet Capsules ... 835
Lortab ASA Tablets ... 2414
Lortab ... 2412
Ru-Tuss with Hydrocodone ... 694
Triaminic Expectorant DH ... 1995
Vicodin Tablets ... 1187
Vicodin ES Tablets ... 1189
Zydone Capsules ... 941

Hydrocodone Polistirex (Additive effect). Products include:
Tussionex Extended-Release Suspension ... 988

Hydroflumethiazide (Anticholinergic effects of phenothiazines may be prolonged and intensified). Products include:
Diucardin Tablets ... 2450
Saluron ... 718
Salutensin/Salutensin-Demi ... 719

Hydroxyzine Hydrochloride (Additive effect). Products include:
Atarax Tablets & Syrup ... 1941
Marax Tablets & DF Syrup ... 1954
Vistaril Intramuscular Solution ... 1970

Isocarboxazid (Possible hypotension and extrapyramidal reactions). Products include:
Marplan Tablets ... 1906

Isoflurane (Additive effect). Products include:
Forane ... 600

Ketamine Hydrochloride (Additive effect). Products include:
Ketalar ... 1726

Levonorgestrel (Effects of phenothiazines potentiated). Products include:
Levlen/Tri-Levlen ... 665
Nordette-21 Tablets ... 2481
Nordette-28 Tablets ... 2483
Norplant System ... 2484
Levlen/Tri-Levlen ... 665
Triphasil-21 Tablets ... 2527
Triphasil-28 Tablets ... 2532

Levorphanol Tartrate (Additive effect). Products include:
Levo-Dromoran ... 1906

Lorazepam (Additive effect). Products include:
Ativan Injection ... 2432
Ativan Tablets ... 2434

Loxapine Hydrochloride (Additive effect). Products include:
Loxitane ... 1213

Loxapine Succinate (Additive effect). Products include:
Loxitane Capsules ... 1213

Medroxyprogesterone Acetate (Effects of phenothiazines potentiated). Products include:
Amen ... 833
Cycrin Tablets ... 2449
Depo-Provera Sterile Aqueous Suspension ... 2336
Provera Tablets ... 2356

Megestrol Acetate (Effects of phenothiazines potentiated). Products include:
Megace Tablets ... 732

Meperidine Hydrochloride (Additive effect). Products include:
Demerol ... 2047
Mepergan Injection ... 2479

Mephobarbital (Additive effect). Products include:
Mebaral Tablets ... 2061

Meprobamate (Additive effect). Products include:
Deprol Tablets ... 2382
Equagesic Tablets ... 2451
Miltown Tablets ... 2386
PMB 200 and PMB 400 ... 2504

Mesoridazine (Additive effect). Products include:
Serentil ... 686

Mestranol (Effects of phenothiazines potentiated). Products include:
Enovid ... 2161
Norethin ... 2133
Norinyl ... 2304
Ortho-Novum ... 1667

Methadone Hydrochloride (Additive effect). Products include:
Dolophine Hydrochloride Ampoules & Vials ... 1260
Dolophine Hydrochloride Tablets ... 1261
Methadone Hydrochloride Diskets .. 1284
Methadone Hydrochloride Oral Solution & Tablets ... 1987

Methohexital Sodium (Additive effect). Products include:
Brevital Sodium Vials ... 1248

Methoxyflurane (Additive effect).
No products indexed under this heading.

Methyclothiazide (Anticholinergic effects of phenothiazines may be prolonged and intensified). Products include:
Enduron Tablets ... 517
Enduronyl ... 518

Midazolam Hydrochloride (Additive effect). Products include:
- Versed Injection ... 1924

Molindone Hydrochloride (Additive effect). Products include:
- Moban Tablets & Concentrate ... 932

Morphine Sulfate (Additive effect). Products include:
- Astramorph/PF Injection, USP (Preservative-Free) ... 618
- Duramorph ... 960
- Infumorph 200 and Infumorph 500 Sterile Solutions ... 962
- MS Contin Tablets ... 1814
- MSIR ... 1817
- Oramorph SR (Morphine Sulfate Sustained Release Tablets) ... 1988
- Roxanol ... 1991

Norethindrone (Effects of phenothiazines potentiated). Products include:
- Brevicon ... 2304
- Jenest-28 Tablets ... 1636
- Micronor Tablets ... 1667
- Modicon ... 1667
- Norethin ... 2133
- Norinyl ... 2304
- Norlutin ... 1755
- Nor-Q D Tablets ... 2304
- Ortho-Novum ... 1667
- Ovcon ... 1391
- Tri-Norinyl ... 2304

Norethynodrel (Effects of phenothiazines potentiated). Products include:
- Enovid ... 2161

Norgestimate (Effects of phenothiazines potentiated). Products include:
- Ortho-Cyclen Tablets ... 1658

Norgestrel (Effects of phenothiazines potentiated). Products include:
- Lo/Ovral Tablets ... 2471
- Lo/Ovral-28 Tablets ... 2476
- Ovral Tablets ... 2490
- Ovral-28 Tablets ... 2491
- Ovrette Tablets ... 2492

Nylidrin Hydrochloride (Effects of phenothiazines potentiated).
- No products indexed under this heading.

Opium Alkaloids (Additive effect). Products include:
- B & O No. 15A & No. 16A Supprettes ... 2395
- Pantopon Injectable ... 1911

Oxazepam (Additive effect). Products include:
- Serax Capsules ... 2522
- Serax Tablets ... 2522

Oxycodone Hydrochloride (Additive effect). Products include:
- Percocet Tablets ... 950
- Percodan ... 951
- Roxicodone Tablets, Oral Solution & Intensol (Oxycodone) ... 1992
- Tylox Capsules ... 1382

Pentobarbital Sodium (Additive effect). Products include:
- Nembutal Sodium Capsules ... 534
- Nembutal Sodium Solution ... 536
- Nembutal Sodium Suppositories ... 538

Perphenazine (Additive effect). Products include:
- Etrafon ... 2087
- Triavil Tablets ... 1556
- Trilafon ... 2123

Phenelzine Sulfate (Possible hypotension and extrapyramidal reactions). Products include:
- Nardil ... 1742

Phenobarbital (Additive effect). Products include:
- Arco-Lase Plus Tablets ... 607
- Bellergal-S Tablets ... 1998
- Bronkolixir ... ▣ 761
- Bronkotabs Tablets ... ▣ 762
- Donnatal ... 1858
- Donnatal Extentabs ... 1859
- Donnatal Tablets ... 1858
- Donnazyme Tablets ... 1860
- Kinesed Tablets ... 2272
- Phenobarbital Elixir and Tablets ... 1293
- Primatene Tablets-P Formula ... 2421
- Quadrinal Tablets ... 1183
- Tedral SA ... 1765

Polythiazide (Anticholinergic effects of phenothiazines may be prolonged and intensified). Products include:
- Minizide Capsules ... 1779
- Renese Tablets ... 1785
- Renese-R Tablets ... 1786

Prazepam (Additive effect). Products include:
- Centrax ... 1693

Probenecid (Effects of phenothiazines potentiated). Products include:
- Benemid Tablets ... 1426
- ColBENEMID Tablets ... 1436
- Wycillin Injection and Probenecid Tablets ... 2539

Prochlorperazine (Additive effect). Products include:
- Compazine ... 2201

Promethazine Hydrochloride (Additive effect). Products include:
- Mepergan Injection ... 2479
- Phenergan with Codeine ... 2497
- Phenergan with Dextromethorphan ... 2499
- Phenergan Injection ... 2493
- Phenergan Suppositories ... 2496
- Phenergan Syrup ... 2495
- Phenergan Tablets ... 2496
- Phenergan VC ... 2500
- Phenergan VC with Codeine ... 2501

Propofol (Additive effect). Products include:
- Diprivan Injection ... 2267

Propoxyphene Hydrochloride (Additive effect). Products include:
- Darvon ... 1256
- Wygesic Tablets ... 2540

Propoxyphene Napsylate (Additive effect). Products include:
- Darvon-N/Darvocet-N ... 1254

Quazepam (Additive effect). Products include:
- Doral Tablets ... 2383

Reserpine (Effects of phenothiazines potentiated). Products include:
- Diupres Tablets ... 1461
- Hydromox R Tablets ... 1209
- Hydropres Tablets ... 1485
- Renese-R Tablets ... 1786
- Salutensin/Salutensin-Demi ... 719
- Ser-Ap-Es Tablets ... 881
- Serpasil Tablets ... 883
- Serpasil-Apresoline Tablets ... 884
- Serpasil-Esidrix Tablets ... 886

Secobarbital Sodium (Additive effect). Products include:
- Seconal Sodium Pulvules ... 1296

Selegiline Hydrochloride (Possible hypotension and extrapyramidal reactions). Products include:
- Eldepryl ... 2250

Sufentanil Citrate (Additive effect). Products include:
- Sufenta Injection ... 1147

Temazepam (Additive effect). Products include:
- Restoril Capsules ... 2023

Thiamylal Sodium (Additive effect). Products include:
- Surital Ampoules, Steri-Vials ... 1764

Thioridazine Hydrochloride (Additive effect). Products include:
- Mellaril ... 2011

Thiothixene (Additive effect). Products include:
- Navane Capsules and Concentrate ... 1954
- Navane Intramuscular ... 1956

Tranylcypromine Sulfate (Possible hypotension and extrapyramidal reactions). Products include:
- Parnate Tablets ... 2222

Triazolam (Additive effect). Products include:
- Halcion Tablets ... 2340

Trifluoperazine Hydrochloride (Additive effect). Products include:
- Stelazine ... 2226

TACARYL SYRUP & TABLETS
(Methdilazine Hydrochloride) ... 2409
See **Tacaryl Chewable Tablets**

TAGAMET INJECTION
(Cimetidine) ... 2228
May interact with oral anticoagulants, tricyclic antidepressants, antacids, and certain other agents. Compounds in these categories include:

Aluminum Carbonate Gel (Simultaneous administration is not recommended, since antacids may interfere with the absorption of cimetidine). Products include:
- Basaljel ... 2438

Aluminum Hydroxide (Simultaneous administration is not recommended, since antacids may interfere with the absorption of cimetidine). Products include:
- Cama Arthritis Pain Reliever ... ▣ 685
- Gaviscon Extra Strength Relief Formula Liquid Antacid ... ▣ 594
- Gaviscon Extra Strength Relief Formula Antacid Tablets ... ▣ 594
- Gaviscon Liquid Antacid ... ▣ 594
- Gelusil Liquid & Tablets ... ▣ 639
- Extra Strength Maalox Plus Suspension ... 1850
- Maalox TC Suspension ... 1851
- Maalox Plus Tablets ... ▣ 655
- Extra Strength Maalox Plus Tablets ... 1850
- Nephrox Suspension ... ▣ 563
- WinGel Liquid & Tablets ... ▣ 761

Aluminum Hydroxide Gel (Simultaneous administration is not recommended, since antacids may interfere with the absorption of cimetidine). Products include:
- ALternaGEL Liquid ... 1154
- Aludrox Oral Suspension ... 2428
- Amphojel Suspension ... 2429
- Amphojel Suspension without Flavor ... 2429
- Mylanta Liquid ... 1155
- Mylanta Double Strength Liquid ... 1155

Aluminum Hydroxide Gel, Dried (Simultaneous administration is not recommended, since antacids may interfere with the absorption of cimetidine). Products include:
- Alu-Tab/Alu-Cap ... 1309
- Amphojel Tablets ... 2429
- Ascriptin A/D Caplets ... 1850
- Regular Strength Ascriptin Tablets ... 1850
- Gaviscon Antacid Tablets ... ▣ 593
- Gaviscon-2 Antacid Tablets ... ▣ 594
- Mylanta Tablets ... 1155
- Mylanta Double Strength Tablets ... 1155

Aminophylline (Reduced hepatic metabolism of aminophylline; increased blood levels). Products include:
- Amesec ... ▣ 682
- Aminophyllin Tablets ... 2153

Amitriptyline Hydrochloride (Reduced hepatic metabolism of tricyclic antidepressant; increased blood levels). Products include:
- Elavil ... 2269
- Endep Tablets ... 1927
- Etrafon ... 2087
- Limbitrol ... 1933
- Triavil Tablets ... 1556

Amoxapine (Reduced hepatic metabolism of tricyclic antidepressant; increased blood levels). Products include:
- Asendin Tablets ... 1196

Chlordiazepoxide (Reduced hepatic metabolism of chlordiazepoxide; increased blood levels). Products include:
- Libritabs Tablets ... 1930
- Limbitrol ... 1933
- Menrium Tablets ... 1934

Chlordiazepoxide Hydrochloride (Reduced hepatic metabolism of chlordiazepoxide; increased blood levels). Products include:
- Librax Capsules ... 1929
- Librium Capsules ... 1931
- Librium Injectable ... 1932

Clomipramine Hydrochloride (Reduced hepatic metabolism of tricyclic antidepressant; increased blood levels). Products include:
- Anafranil Capsules ... 650

Desipramine Hydrochloride (Reduced hepatic metabolism of tricyclic antidepressant; increased blood levels). Products include:
- Norpramin Tablets ... 1340

Diazepam (Reduced hepatic metabolism of diazepam; increased blood levels). Products include:
- Valium Injectable ... 1937
- Valium Tablets ... 1939
- Valrelease Capsules ... 1923

Dicumarol (Increased blood levels; dosage adjustment may be necessary). Products include:
- Dicumarol Tablets ... 516

Dihydroxyaluminum Sodium Carbonate (Simultaneous administration is not recommended, since antacids may interfere with the absorption of cimetidine). Products include:
- Rolaids ... ▣ 743

Doxepin Hydrochloride (Reduced hepatic metabolism of tricyclic antidepressant; increased blood levels). Products include:
- Sinequan ... 1960

Dyphylline (Reduced hepatic metabolism of dyphylline; increased blood levels). Products include:
- Dilor ... 2079
- Dilor-G Tablets & Liquid ... 2079
- Lufyllin Elixir ... 2384
- Lufyllin & Lufyllin-400 Tablets ... 2384
- Lufyllin-GG Elixir & Tablets ... 2385

Imipramine Hydrochloride (Reduced hepatic metabolism of tricyclic antidepressant; increased blood levels). Products include:
- Tofranil Ampuls ... 1038
- Tofranil Tablets ... 1039

Imipramine Pamoate (Reduced hepatic metabolism of tricyclic antidepressant; increased blood levels). Products include:
- Tofranil-PM Capsules ... 1041

Lidocaine Hydrochloride (Reduced hepatic metabolism of lidocaine; increased blood levels). Products include:
- Anestacon Solution ... 2394
- Bactine Antiseptic/Anesthetic First Aid Spray ... ▣ 624
- Decadron Phosphate with Xylocaine Injection, Sterile ... 1451
- Xylocaine Injections ... 637
- Xylocaine Injections for Ventricular Arrhythmias ... 639
- Xylocaine 2% Jelly ... 643
- 4% Xylocaine-MPF Sterile Solution ... 641
- Xylocaine 2% Viscous Solution ... 646

Magaldrate (Simultaneous administration is not recommended, since antacids may interfere with the absorption of cimetidine). Products include:
- Riopan Antacid Chew Tablets ... ▣ 754
- Riopan Antacid Chew Tablets in Rollpacks ... ▣ 754
- Riopan Antacid Suspension ... 2421
- Riopan Antacid Swallow Tablets ... 2421
- Riopan Plus Chew Tablets ... 2422
- Riopan Plus Chew Tablets in Rollpack ... 2422
- Riopan Plus 2 Chew Tablets, Mint Flavor, Cherry Flavor ... 2422
- Riopan Plus Suspension ... 2422

Riopan Plus 2 Suspension, Mint Flavor, Cherry Flavor 2422

Magnesium Hydroxide (Simultaneous administration is not recommended, since antacids may interfere with the absorption of cimetidine). Products include:
- Aludrox Oral Suspension 2428
- Ascriptin A/D Caplets 1850
- Regular Strength Ascriptin Tablets 1850
- Di-Gel Antacid/Anti-Gas 697
- Gelusil Liquid & Tablets 639
- Haley's M-O, Regular & Flavored 569
- Extra Strength Maalox Plus Suspension 1850
- Maalox TC Suspension 1851
- Maalox Plus Tablets 655
- Extra Strength Maalox Plus Tablets 1850
- Mylanta Liquid 1155
- Mylanta Tablets 1155
- Mylanta Double Strength Liquid 1155
- Mylanta Double Strength Tablets 1155
- Concentrated Phillips' Milk of Magnesia 573
- Phillips' Milk of Magnesia Liquid 572
- Phillips' Milk of Magnesia Tablets 573
- WinGel Liquid & Tablets 761

Magnesium Oxide (Simultaneous administration is not recommended, since antacids may interfere with the absorption of cimetidine). Products include:
- Bayer Plus Aspirin Tablets 567
- Beelith Tablets 659
- Bufferin Analgesic Tablets and Caplets 524
- Cama Arthritis Pain Reliever 685
- Mag-Ox 400 673
- Uro-Mag 673

Maprotiline Hydrochloride (Reduced hepatic metabolism of tricyclic antidepressant; increased blood levels). Products include:
- Ludiomil Tablets 874

Metronidazole (Reduced hepatic metabolism of metronidazole; increased blood levels). Products include:
- Flagyl I.V. RTU 2131
- Flagyl Tablets 2170
- MetroGel 903
- Protostat Tablets 1674

Nortriptyline Hydrochloride (Reduced hepatic metabolism of tricyclic antidepressant; increased blood levels). Products include:
- Pamelor 2019

Phenytoin (Reduced hepatic metabolism of phenytoin; increased blood levels). Products include:
- Dilantin Infatabs 1710
- Dilantin-30 Pediatric/Dilantin-125 Suspension 1713

Phenytoin Sodium (Reduced hepatic metabolism of phenytoin; increased blood levels). Products include:
- Dilantin Kapseals 1708
- Dilantin Parenteral 1712
- Dilantin with Phenobarbital Kapseals 1715

Propranolol Hydrochloride (Reduced hepatic metabolism of propranolol; increased blood levels). Products include:
- Inderal 2459
- Inderal LA Long Acting Capsules 2461
- Inderide Tablets 2463
- Inderide LA Long Acting Capsules 2465

Protriptyline Hydrochloride (Reduced hepatic metabolism of tricyclic antidepressant; increased blood levels). Products include:
- Vivactil Tablets 1567

Theophylline (Reduced hepatic metabolism of theophylline; increased blood levels). Products include:
- Bronkaid Tablets 757
- Bronkolixir 761
- Bronkotabs Tablets 762
- Constant-T Tablets 1029
- Marax Tablets & DF Syrup 1954
- Primatene Tablets 2421
- Quibron Capsules 713
- Quibron-T 714
- Quibron-T/SR 716
- Theolair Liquid 1317
- Theo-Organidin Elixir 2391

Theophylline Anhydrous (Reduced hepatic metabolism of theophylline; increased blood levels). Products include:
- Aerolate 994
- Primatene Tablets-M Formula 753
- Primatene Tablets-Regular Formula 2421
- Respbid Tablets 684
- Slo-bid Gyrocaps 1847
- T-PHYL (Uniphyl) 200 mg Tablets 1820
- Tedral SA 1765
- Theo-24 2179
- Theo-Dur Sprinkle 1168
- Theo-Dur Extended-Release Tablets 1166
- Theolair Tablets 1317
- Theolair-SR Tablets 1319
- TheoX Extended-Release Tablets 841
- Uniphyl 400 mg Tablets 1823

Theophylline Sodium Glycinate (Reduced hepatic metabolism of theophylline; increased blood levels). Products include:
- Asbron G 1997

Trimipramine Maleate (Reduced hepatic metabolism of tricyclic antidepressant; increased blood levels). Products include:
- Surmontil Capsules 2524

Warfarin Sodium (Increased blood levels; dosage adjustment may be necessary). Products include:
- Coumadin Injection & Tablets 944
- Panwarfin Tablets 547

TAGAMET LIQUID
(Cimetidine) 2228
See **Tagamet Injection**

TAGAMET TABLETS
(Cimetidine) 2228
See **Tagamet Injection**

TALACEN
(Pentazocine Hydrochloride) 2070
May interact with narcotic analgesics, central nervous system depressants, and certain other agents. Compounds in these categories include:

Alcohol (Potential for increased CNS depressant effects).

Alfentanil Hydrochloride (Potential for withdrawal symptoms; additive CNS depressant effects). Products include:
- Alfenta Injection 1131

Alprazolam (Additive CNS depressant effects). Products include:
- Xanax Tablets 2367

Aprobarbital (Additive CNS depressant effects). Products include:
- Alurate Elixir 1883

Buprenorphine (Potential for withdrawal symptoms; additive CNS depressant effects).
No products indexed under this heading.

Buspirone Hydrochloride (Additive CNS depressant effects). Products include:
- BuSpar 1401

Butabarbital (Additive CNS depressant effects). Products include:
- Pyridium Plus 1764

Butalbital (Additive CNS depressant effects). Products include:
- Esgic-Plus Tablets 1002
- Esgic Tablets & Capsules 1001
- Fioricet Tablets 2006
- Fiorinal Capsules 2007
- Fiorinal with Codeine Capsules 2008
- Fiorinal Tablets 2007
- Phrenilin 838
- Sedapap Tablets 50 mg/650 mg 1360

Chlordiazepoxide (Additive CNS depressant effects). Products include:
- Libritabs Tablets 1930
- Limbitrol 1933
- Menrium Tablets 1934

Chlordiazepoxide Hydrochloride (Additive CNS depressant effects). Products include:
- Librax Capsules 1929
- Librium Capsules 1931
- Librium Injectable 1932

Chlorpromazine (Additive CNS depressant effects). Products include:
- Thorazine 2234

Chlorprothixene (Additive CNS depressant effects). Products include:
- Taractan Tablets 1920

Chlorprothixene Hydrochloride (Additive CNS depressant effects). Products include:
- Taractan 1920

Clorazepate Dipotassium (Additive CNS depressant effects). Products include:
- Tranxene 556

Codeine (Potential for withdrawal symptoms; additive CNS depressant effects). Products include:
- Calcidrine Syrup 506

Codeine Phosphate (Potential for withdrawal symptoms; additive CNS depressant effects). Products include:
- Actifed with Codeine Cough Syrup 752
- Cheracol Cough Syrup 1853
- Codimal PH Syrup 846
- Dimetane-DC Cough Syrup 1857
- Empirin with Codeine Phosphate Nos. 2, 3 & 4 764
- Fiorinal with Codeine Capsules 2008
- Isoclor Expectorant 982
- Naldecon CX Adult Liquid 521
- Novahistine DH 1342
- Novahistine Expectorant 1343
- Nucofed Capsules 2219
- Nucofed Expectorant 2219
- Nucofed Pediatric Expectorant 2220
- Nucofed Syrup 2219
- Phenaphen with Codeine Capsules 1865
- Phenaphen-650 with Codeine Tablets 1866
- Phenergan with Codeine 2497
- Phenergan VC with Codeine 2501
- Robitussin A-C Syrup 1875
- Robitussin-DAC Syrup 1875
- Ryna 741
- Soma Compound w/Codeine Tablets 2390
- Triaminic Expectorant w/Codeine 1996
- Tussi-Organidin Liquid 2391
- Tylenol with Codeine 1381

Codeine Polistirex (Potential for withdrawal symptoms; additive CNS depressant effects).
No products indexed under this heading.

Dezocine (Potential for withdrawal symptoms).

Diazepam (Additive CNS depressant effects). Products include:
- Valium Injectable 1937
- Valium Tablets 1939
- Valrelease Capsules 1923

Diphenoxylate Hydrochloride (Potential for withdrawal symptoms). Products include:
- Lomotil 2174

Droperidol (Additive CNS depressant effects). Products include:
- Inapsine Injection 1140
- Innovar Injection 1141

Enflurane (Additive CNS depressant effects). Products include:
- Ethrane 599

Estazolam (Potential for withdrawal symptoms; additive CNS depressant effects). Products include:
- ProSom Tablets 554

Ethchlorvynol (Additive CNS depressant effects). Products include:
- Placidyl Capsules 553

Ethinamate (Additive CNS depressant effects).
No products indexed under this heading.

Fentanyl (Potential for withdrawal symptoms). Products include:
- Duragesic Transdermal System 1133

Fentanyl Citrate (Potential for withdrawal symptoms; additive CNS depressant effects). Products include:
- Innovar Injection 1141
- Sublimaze Injection 1146

Fluphenazine Decanoate (Additive CNS depressant effects). Products include:
- Prolixin Decanoate 1795

Fluphenazine Enanthate (Additive CNS depressant effects). Products include:
- Prolixin Enanthate 1796

Fluphenazine Hydrochloride (Additive CNS depressant effects). Products include:
- Prolixin Elixir 1793
- Prolixin Injection 1791
- Prolixin Oral Concentrate 1792
- Prolixin Tablets 1793

Flurazepam Hydrochloride (Additive CNS depressant effects). Products include:
- Dalmane Capsules 1927

Glutethimide (Additive CNS depressant effects).
No products indexed under this heading.

Haloperidol (Additive CNS depressant effects). Products include:
- Haldol Injection, Tablets and Concentrate 1373

Haloperidol Decanoate (Additive CNS depressant effects). Products include:
- Haldol Decanoate 1375

Hydrocodone Bitartrate (Potential for withdrawal symptoms; additive CNS depressant effects). Products include:
- Anexsia 5/500 Tablets 2196
- Anexsia 7.5/650 Tablets 2197
- Azdōne Tablets 844
- Codiclear DH Syrup 845
- Codimal DH Syrup 846
- Damason-P 1356
- Hycodan Syrup, Tablets 927
- Hycomine Compound Tablets 929
- Hycomine Syrup 927
- Hycotuss Expectorant Syrup 930
- Hydrocet Capsules 835
- Lortab ASA Tablets 2414
- Lortab 2412
- Ru-Tuss with Hydrocodone 694
- Triaminic Expectorant DH 1995
- Vicodin Tablets 1187
- Vicodin ES Tablets 1189
- Zydone Capsules 941

Hydrocodone Polistirex (Potential for withdrawal symptoms; additive CNS depressant effects). Products include:
- Tussionex Extended-Release Suspension 988

Hydroxyzine Hydrochloride (Additive CNS depressant effects). Products include:
- Atarax Tablets & Syrup 1941
- Marax Tablets & DF Syrup 1954
- Vistaril Intramuscular Solution 1970

Isoflurane (Additive CNS depressant effects). Products include:
- Forane 600

Ketamine Hydrochloride (Additive CNS depressant effects). Products include:
- Ketalar ... 1726

Levorphanol Tartrate (Potential for withdrawal symptoms; additive CNS depressant effects). Products include:
- Levo-Dromoran ... 1906

Lorazepam (Additive CNS depressant effects). Products include:
- Ativan Injection ... 2432
- Ativan Tablets ... 2434

Loxapine Hydrochloride (Additive CNS depressant effects). Products include:
- Loxitane ... 1213

Loxapine Succinate (Additive CNS depressant effects). Products include:
- Loxitane Capsules ... 1213

Meperidine Hydrochloride (Potential for withdrawal symptoms; additive CNS depressant effects). Products include:
- Demerol ... 2047
- Mepergan Injection ... 2479

Mephobarbital (Additive CNS depressant effects). Products include:
- Mebaral Tablets ... 2061

Meprobamate (Additive CNS depressant effects). Products include:
- Deprol Tablets ... 2382
- Equagesic Tablets ... 2451
- Miltown Tablets ... 2386
- PMB 200 and PMB 400 ... 2504

Mesoridazine (Additive CNS depressant effects). Products include:
- Serentil ... 686

Methadone Hydrochloride (Potential for withdrawal symptoms; additive CNS depressant effects). Products include:
- Dolophine Hydrochloride Ampoules & Vials ... 1260
- Dolophine Hydrochloride Tablets ... 1261
- Methadone Hydrochloride Diskets .. 1284
- Methadone Hydrochloride Oral Solution & Tablets ... 1987

Methohexital Sodium (Additive CNS depressant effects). Products include:
- Brevital Sodium Vials ... 1248

Methoxyflurane (Additive CNS depressant effects).
- No products indexed under this heading.

Midazolam Hydrochloride (Additive CNS depressant effects). Products include:
- Versed Injection ... 1924

Molindone Hydrochloride (Additive CNS depressant effects). Products include:
- Moban Tablets & Concentrate ... 932

Morphine Sulfate (Potential for withdrawal symptoms; additive CNS depressant effects). Products include:
- Astramorph/PF Injection, USP (Preservative-Free) ... 618
- Duramorph ... 960
- Infumorph 200 and Infumorph 500 Sterile Solutions ... 962
- MS Contin Tablets ... 1814
- MSIR ... 1817
- Oramorph SR (Morphine Sulfate Sustained Release Tablets) ... 1988
- Roxanol ... 1991

Opium Alkaloids (Potential for withdrawal symptoms; additive CNS depressant effects). Products include:
- B & O No. 15A & No. 16A Supprettes ... 2395
- Pantopon Injectable ... 1911

Oxazepam (Additive CNS depressant effects). Products include:
- Serax Capsules ... 2522
- Serax Tablets ... 2522

Oxycodone Hydrochloride (Potential for withdrawal symptoms; additive CNS depressant effects). Products include:
- Percocet Tablets ... 950
- Percodan ... 951
- Roxicodone Tablets, Oral Solution & Intensol (Oxycodone) ... 1992
- Tylox Capsules ... 1382

Paregoric (Potential for withdrawal symptoms). Products include:
- Donnagel-PG ... 1858

Pentobarbital Sodium (Additive CNS depressant effects). Products include:
- Nembutal Sodium Capsules ... 534
- Nembutal Sodium Solution ... 536
- Nembutal Sodium Suppositories ... 538

Perphenazine (Additive CNS depressant effects). Products include:
- Etrafon ... 2087
- Triavil Tablets ... 1556
- Trilafon ... 2123

Phenobarbital (Additive CNS depressant effects). Products include:
- Arco-Lase Plus Tablets ... 607
- Bellergal-S Tablets ... 1998
- Bronkolixir ... ▣ 761
- Bronkotabs Tablets ... ▣ 762
- Donnatal ... 1858
- Donnatal Extentabs ... 1859
- Donnatal Tablets ... 1858
- Donnazyme Tablets ... 1860
- Kinesed Tablets ... 2272
- Phenobarbital Elixir and Tablets ... 1293
- Primatene Tablets-P Formula ... 2421
- Quadrinal Tablets ... 1183
- Tedral SA ... 1765

Prazepam (Additive CNS depressant effects). Products include:
- Centrax ... 1693

Prochlorperazine (Additive CNS depressant effects). Products include:
- Compazine ... 2201

Promethazine Hydrochloride (Potential for withdrawal symptoms; additive CNS depressant effects). Products include:
- Mepergan Injection ... 2479
- Phenergan with Codeine ... 2497
- Phenergan with Dextromethorphan 2499
- Phenergan Injection ... 2493
- Phenergan Suppositories ... 2496
- Phenergan Syrup ... 2495
- Phenergan Tablets ... 2496
- Phenergan VC ... 2500
- Phenergan VC with Codeine ... 2501

Propofol (Additive CNS depressant effects). Products include:
- Diprivan Injection ... 2267

Propoxyphene Hydrochloride (Potential for withdrawal symptoms; additive CNS depressant effects). Products include:
- Darvon ... 1256
- Wygesic Tablets ... 2540

Propoxyphene Napsylate (Potential for withdrawal symptoms; additive CNS depressant effects). Products include:
- Darvon-N/Darvocet-N ... 1254

Quazepam (Additive CNS depressant effects). Products include:
- Doral Tablets ... 2383

Secobarbital Sodium (Potential for withdrawal symptoms; additive CNS depressant effects). Products include:
- Seconal Sodium Pulvules ... 1296

Sufentanil Citrate (Potential for withdrawal symptoms; additive CNS depressant effects). Products include:
- Sufenta Injection ... 1147

Temazepam (Potential for withdrawal symptoms; additive CNS depressant effects). Products include:
- Restoril Capsules ... 2023

Thiamylal Sodium (Potential for withdrawal symptoms; additive CNS depressant effects). Products include:
- Surital Ampoules, Steri-Vials ... 1764

Thioridazine Hydrochloride (Potential for withdrawal symptoms; additive CNS depressant effects). Products include:
- Mellaril ... 2011

Thiothixene (Potential for withdrawal symptoms; additive CNS depressant effects). Products include:
- Navane Capsules and Concentrate 1954
- Navane Intramuscular ... 1956

Triazolam (Potential for withdrawal symptoms; additive CNS depressant effects). Products include:
- Halcion Tablets ... 2340

Trifluoperazine Hydrochloride (Potential for withdrawal symptoms; additive CNS depressant effects). Products include:
- Stelazine ... 2226

TALWIN AMPULS
(Pentazocine Lactate) ... 2071
May interact with narcotic analgesics, general anesthetics, preanesthetic medications, central nervous system depressants, and certain other agents. Compounds in these categories include:

Alcohol (Potential for increased CNS depressant effects).

Alfentanil Hydrochloride (Potential for withdrawal symptoms; may produce additive CNS depression). Products include:
- Alfenta Injection ... 1131

Alprazolam (May produce additive CNS depression). Products include:
- Xanax Tablets ... 2367

Aprobarbital (May produce additive CNS depression). Products include:
- Alurate Elixir ... 1883

Buprenorphine (Potential for withdrawal symptoms; may produce additive CNS depression).
- No products indexed under this heading.

Buspirone Hydrochloride (May produce additive CNS depression). Products include:
- BuSpar ... 1401

Butabarbital (May produce additive CNS depression). Products include:
- Pyridium Plus ... 1764

Butalbital (May produce additive CNS depression). Products include:
- Esgic-Plus Tablets ... 1002
- Esgic Tablets & Capsules ... 1001
- Fioricet Tablets ... 2006
- Fiorinal Capsules ... 2007
- Fiorinal with Codeine Capsules ... 2008
- Fiorinal Tablets ... 2007
- Phrenilin ... 838
- Sedapap Tablets 50 mg/650 mg .. 1360

Chlordiazepoxide (May produce additive CNS depression). Products include:
- Libritabs Tablets ... 1930
- Limbitrol ... 1933
- Menrium Tablets ... 1934

Chlordiazepoxide Hydrochloride (May produce additive CNS depression). Products include:
- Librax Capsules ... 1929
- Librium Capsules ... 1931
- Librium Injectable ... 1932

Chlorpromazine (May produce additive CNS depression). Products include:
- Thorazine ... 2234

Chlorprothixene (May produce additive CNS depression). Products include:
- Taractan Tablets ... 1920

Chlorprothixene Hydrochloride (May produce additive CNS depression). Products include:
- Taractan ... 1920

Clorazepate Dipotassium (May produce additive CNS depression). Products include:
- Tranxene ... 556

Codeine (Potential for withdrawal symptoms; may produce additive CNS depression). Products include:
- Calcidrine Syrup ... 506

Codeine Phosphate (Potential for withdrawal symptoms; may produce additive CNS depression). Products include:
- Actifed with Codeine Cough Syrup.. 752
- Cheracol Cough Syrup ... 1853
- Codimal PH Syrup ... 846
- Dimetane-DC Cough Syrup ... 1857
- Empirin with Codeine Phosphate Nos. 2, 3 & 4 ... 764
- Fiorinal with Codeine Capsules ... 2008
- Isoclor Expectorant ... 982
- Naldecon CX Adult Liquid ... ▣ 521
- Novahistine DH ... 1342
- Novahistine Expectorant ... 1343
- Nucofed Capsules ... 2219
- Nucofed Expectorant ... 2219
- Nucofed Pediatric Expectorant ... 2220
- Nucofed Syrup ... 2219
- Phenaphen with Codeine Capsules 1865
- Phenaphen-650 with Codeine Tablets ... 1866
- Phenergan with Codeine ... 2497
- Phenergan VC with Codeine ... 2501
- Robitussin A-C Syrup ... 1875
- Robitussin-DAC Syrup ... 1875
- Ryna ... ▣ 741
- Soma Compound w/Codeine Tablets ... 2390
- Triaminic Expectorant w/Codeine .. 1996
- Tussi-Organidin Liquid ... 2391
- Tylenol with Codeine ... 1381

Codeine Polistirex (Potential for withdrawal symptoms; may produce additive CNS depression).
- No products indexed under this heading.

Dezocine (Potential for withdrawal symptoms).

Diazepam (May produce additive CNS depressant effects). Products include:
- Valium Injectable ... 1937
- Valium Tablets ... 1939
- Valrelease Capsules ... 1923

Droperidol (May produce additive CNS depressant effects). Products include:
- Inapsine Injection ... 1140
- Innovar Injection ... 1141

Enflurane (May produce additive CNS depressant effects). Products include:
- Ethrane ... 599

Estazolam (Potential for withdrawal symptoms; may produce additive CNS depression). Products include:
- ProSom Tablets ... 554

Ethchlorvynol (May produce additive CNS depression). Products include:
- Placidyl Capsules ... 553

Ethinamate (May produce additive CNS depression).
- No products indexed under this heading.

Fentanyl (Potential for withdrawal symptoms). Products include:
- Duragesic Transdermal System ... 1133

Fentanyl Citrate (Potential for withdrawal symptoms; may produce additive CNS depressant effects). Products include:
- Innovar Injection ... 1141
- Sublimaze Injection ... 1146

Fluphenazine Decanoate (May produce additive CNS depression). Products include:
- Prolixin Decanoate ... 1795

Fluphenazine Enanthate (May produce additive CNS depression). Products include:
- Prolixin Enanthate ... 1796

Fluphenazine Hydrochloride (May produce additive CNS depression). Products include:
- Prolixin Elixir ... 1793
- Prolixin Injection ... 1791
- Prolixin Oral Concentrate ... 1792
- Prolixin Tablets ... 1793

Flurazepam Hydrochloride (May produce additive CNS depression). Products include:
- Dalmane Capsules ... 1927

Glutethimide (May produce additive CNS depression).
- No products indexed under this heading.

Haloperidol (May produce additive CNS depression). Products include:
- Haldol Injection, Tablets and Concentrate ... 1373

Haloperidol Decanoate (May produce additive CNS depression). Products include:
- Haldol Decanoate ... 1375

Hydrocodone Bitartrate (Potential for withdrawal symptoms; may produce additive CNS depression). Products include:
- Anexsia 5/500 Tablets ... 2196
- Anexsia 7.5/650 Tablets ... 2197
- Azdōne Tablets ... 844
- Codiclear DH Syrup ... 845
- Codimal DH Syrup ... 846
- Damason-P ... 1356
- Hycodan Syrup, Tablets ... 927
- Hycomine Compound Tablets ... 929
- Hycomine Syrup ... 927
- Hycotuss Expectorant Syrup ... 930
- Hydrocet Capsules ... 835
- Lortab ASA Tablets ... 2414
- Lortab ... 2412
- Ru-Tuss with Hydrocodone ... 694
- Triaminic Expectorant DH ... 1995
- Vicodin Tablets ... 1187
- Vicodin ES Tablets ... 1189
- Zydone Capsules ... 941

Hydrocodone Polistirex (Potential for withdrawal symptoms; may produce additive CNS depression). Products include:
- Tussionex Extended-Release Suspension ... 988

Hydroxyzine Hydrochloride (May produce additive CNS depressant effects). Products include:
- Atarax Tablets & Syrup ... 1941
- Marax Tablets & DF Syrup ... 1954
- Vistaril Intramuscular Solution ... 1970

Isoflurane (May produce additive CNS depressant effects). Products include:
- Forane ... 600

Ketamine Hydrochloride (May produce additive CNS depressant effects). Products include:
- Ketalar ... 1726

Levorphanol Tartrate (Potential for withdrawal symptoms; may produce additive CNS depression). Products include:
- Levo-Dromoran ... 1906

Lorazepam (May produce additive CNS depressant effects). Products include:
- Ativan Injection ... 2432
- Ativan Tablets ... 2434

Loxapine Hydrochloride (May produce additive CNS depression). Products include:
- Loxitane ... 1213

Loxapine Succinate (May produce additive CNS depression). Products include:
- Loxitane Capsules ... 1213

Meperidine Hydrochloride (Potential for withdrawal symptoms; may produce additive CNS depressant effects). Products include:
- Demerol ... 2047
- Mepergan Injection ... 2479

Mephobarbital (May produce additive CNS depression). Products include:
- Mebaral Tablets ... 2061

Meprobamate (May produce additive CNS depression). Products include:
- Deprol Tablets ... 2382
- Equagesic Tablets ... 2451
- Miltown Tablets ... 2386
- PMB 200 and PMB 400 ... 2504

Mesoridazine (May produce additive CNS depression). Products include:
- Serentil ... 686

Methadone Hydrochloride (Potential for withdrawal symptoms; may produce additive CNS depression). Products include:
- Dolophine Hydrochloride Ampoules & Vials ... 1260
- Dolophine Hydrochloride Tablets ... 1261
- Methadone Hydrochloride Diskets ... 1284
- Methadone Hydrochloride Oral Solution & Tablets ... 1987

Methohexital Sodium (May produce additive CNS depressant effects). Products include:
- Brevital Sodium Vials ... 1248

Methoxyflurane (Potential for withdrawal symptoms; may produce additive CNS depression).
- No products indexed under this heading.

Midazolam Hydrochloride (May produce additive CNS depression). Products include:
- Versed Injection ... 1924

Molindone Hydrochloride (May produce additive CNS depression). Products include:
- Moban Tablets & Concentrate ... 932

Morphine Sulfate (Potential for withdrawal symptoms; may produce additive CNS depressant effects). Products include:
- Astramorph/PF Injection, USP (Preservative-Free) ... 618
- Duramorph ... 960
- Infumorph 200 and Infumorph 500 Sterile Solutions ... 962
- MS Contin Tablets ... 1814
- MSIR ... 1817
- Oramorph SR (Morphine Sulfate Sustained Release Tablets) ... 1988
- Roxanol ... 1991

Opium Alkaloids (Potential for withdrawal symptoms; may produce additive CNS depressant effects). Products include:
- B & O No. 15A & No. 16A Supprettes ... 2395
- Pantopon Injectable ... 1911

Oxazepam (May produce additive CNS depression). Products include:
- Serax Capsules ... 2522
- Serax Tablets ... 2522

Oxycodone Hydrochloride (Potential for withdrawal symptoms; may produce additive CNS depression). Products include:
- Percocet Tablets ... 950
- Percodan ... 951
- Roxicodone Tablets, Oral Solution & Intensol (Oxycodone) ... 1992
- Tylox Capsules ... 1382

Pentobarbital Sodium (Potential for withdrawal symptoms; may produce additive CNS depression). Products include:
- Nembutal Sodium Capsules ... 534
- Nembutal Sodium Solution ... 536
- Nembutal Sodium Suppositories ... 538

Perphenazine (May produce additive CNS depression). Products include:
- Etrafon ... 2087
- Triavil Tablets ... 1556
- Trilafon ... 2123

Phenobarbital (May produce additive CNS depression). Products include:
- Arco-Lase Plus Tablets ... 607
- Bellergal-S Tablets ... 1998
- Bronkolixir ... ▣ 761
- Bronkotabs Tablets ... ▣ 762
- Donnatal ... 1858
- Donnatal Extentabs ... 1859
- Donnatal Tablets ... 1858
- Donnazyme Tablets ... 1860
- Kinesed Tablets ... 2272
- Phenobarbital Elixir and Tablets ... 1293
- Primatene Tablets-P Formula ... 2421
- Quadrinal Tablets ... 1183
- Tedral SA ... 1765

Prazepam (May produce additive CNS depression). Products include:
- Centrax ... 1693

Prochlorperazine (May produce additive CNS depression). Products include:
- Compazine ... 2201

Promethazine Hydrochloride (May produce additive CNS depressant effects). Products include:
- Mepergan Injection ... 2479
- Phenergan with Codeine ... 2497
- Phenergan with Dextromethorphan ... 2499
- Phenergan Injection ... 2493
- Phenergan Suppositories ... 2496
- Phenergan Syrup ... 2495
- Phenergan Tablets ... 2496
- Phenergan VC ... 2500
- Phenergan VC with Codeine ... 2501

Propofol (May produce additive CNS depressant effects). Products include:
- Diprivan Injection ... 2267

Propoxyphene Hydrochloride (Potential for withdrawal symptoms; may produce additive CNS depressant effects). Products include:
- Darvon ... 1256
- Wygesic Tablets ... 2540

Propoxyphene Napsylate (Potential for withdrawal symptoms; may produce additive CNS depressant effects). Products include:
- Darvon-N/Darvocet-N ... 1254

Secobarbital Sodium (May produce additive CNS depressant effects). Products include:
- Seconal Sodium Pulvules ... 1296

Sufentanil Citrate (Potential for withdrawal symptoms; may produce additive CNS depressant effects). Products include:
- Sufenta Injection ... 1147

Temazepam (May produce additive CNS depressant effects). Products include:
- Restoril Capsules ... 2023

Thiamylal Sodium (Potential for withdrawal symptoms; may produce additive CNS depressant effects). Products include:
- Surital Ampoules, Steri-Vials ... 1764

Thioridazine Hydrochloride (May produce additive CNS depressant effects). Products include:
- Mellaril ... 2011

Thiothixene (May produce additive CNS depressant effects). Products include:
- Navane Capsules and Concentrate ... 1954
- Navane Intramuscular ... 1956

Triazolam (May produce additive CNS depressant effects). Products include:
- Halcion Tablets ... 2340

Trifluoperazine Hydrochloride (May produce additive CNS depressant effects). Products include:
- Stelazine ... 2226

TALWIN CARPUJECT
(Pentazocine Lactate) ... 2071
- See **Talwin Ampuls**

TALWIN COMPOUND
(Pentazocine Hydrochloride, Aspirin) 2072
May interact with narcotic analgesics, oral anticoagulants, and certain other agents. Compounds in these categories include:

Alcohol (Potential for increased CNS depressant effects).

Alfentanil Hydrochloride (Potential for withdrawal symptoms). Products include:
- Alfenta Injection ... 1131

Buprenorphine (Potential for withdrawal symptoms).
- No products indexed under this heading.

Codeine (Potential for withdrawal symptoms). Products include:
- Calcidrine Syrup ... 506

Codeine Phosphate (Potential for withdrawal symptoms). Products include:
- Actifed with Codeine Cough Syrup ... 752
- Cheracol Cough Syrup ... 1853
- Codimal PH Syrup ... 846
- Dimetane-DC Cough Syrup ... 1857
- Empirin with Codeine Phosphate Nos. 2, 3 & 4 ... 764
- Fiorinal with Codeine Capsules ... 2008
- Isoclor Expectorant ... 982
- Naldecon CX Adult Liquid ... ▣ 521
- Novahistine DH ... 1342
- Novahistine Expectorant ... 1343
- Nucofed Capsules ... 2219
- Nucofed Expectorant ... 2219
- Nucofed Pediatric Expectorant ... 2220
- Nucofed Syrup ... 2219
- Phenaphen with Codeine Capsules ... 1865
- Phenaphen-650 with Codeine Tablets ... 1866
- Phenergan with Codeine ... 2497
- Phenergan VC with Codeine ... 2501
- Robitussin A-C Syrup ... 1875
- Robitussin-DAC Syrup ... 1875
- Ryna ... ▣ 741
- Soma Compound w/Codeine Tablets ... 2390
- Triaminic Expectorant w/Codeine ... 1996
- Tussi-Organidin Liquid ... 2391
- Tylenol with Codeine ... 1381

Codeine Polistirex (Potential for withdrawal symptoms).
- No products indexed under this heading.

Dezocine (Potential for withdrawal symptoms).

Dicumarol (Effects of aspirin may be deleterious in conjunction with anticoagulant therapy). Products include:
- Dicumarol Tablets ... 516

Fentanyl (Potential for withdrawal symptoms). Products include:
- Duragesic Transdermal System ... 1133

Fentanyl Citrate (Potential for withdrawal symptoms). Products include:
- Innovar Injection ... 1141
- Sublimaze Injection ... 1146

Hydrocodone Bitartrate (Potential for withdrawal symptoms). Products include:
- Anexsia 5/500 Tablets ... 2196
- Anexsia 7.5/650 Tablets ... 2197
- Azdōne Tablets ... 844
- Codiclear DH Syrup ... 845
- Codimal DH Syrup ... 846
- Damason-P ... 1356

Hycodan Syrup, Tablets ... 927
Hycomine Compound Tablets ... 929
Hycomine Syrup ... 927
Hycotuss Expectorant Syrup ... 930
Hydrocet Capsules ... 835
Lortab ASA Tablets ... 2414
Lortab ... 2412
Ru-Tuss with Hydrocodone ... 694
Triaminic Expectorant DH ... 1995
Vicodin Tablets ... 1187
Vicodin ES Tablets ... 1189
Zydone Capsules ... 941

Hydrocodone Polistirex (Potential for withdrawal symptoms). Products include:
Tussionex Extended-Release Suspension ... 988

Levorphanol Tartrate (Potential for withdrawal symptoms). Products include:
Levo-Dromoran ... 1906

Meperidine Hydrochloride (Potential for withdrawal symptoms). Products include:
Demerol ... 2047
Mepergan Injection ... 2479

Methadone Hydrochloride (Potential for withdrawal symptoms). Products include:
Dolophine Hydrochloride Ampoules & Vials ... 1260
Dolophine Hydrochloride Tablets ... 1261
Methadone Hydrochloride Diskets ... 1284
Methadone Hydrochloride Oral Solution & Tablets ... 1987

Morphine Sulfate (Potential for withdrawal symptoms). Products include:
Astramorph/PF Injection, USP (Preservative-Free) ... 618
Duramorph ... 960
Infumorph 200 and Infumorph 500 Sterile Solutions ... 962
MS Contin Tablets ... 1814
MSIR ... 1817
Oramorph SR (Morphine Sulfate Sustained Release Tablets) ... 1988
Roxanol ... 1991

Opium Alkaloids (Potential for withdrawal symptoms). Products include:
B & O No. 15A & No. 16A Supprettes ... 2395
Pantopon Injectable ... 1911

Oxycodone Hydrochloride (Potential for withdrawal symptoms). Products include:
Percocet Tablets ... 950
Percodan ... 951
Roxicodone Tablets, Oral Solution & Intensol (Oxycodone) ... 1992
Tylox Capsules ... 1382

Propoxyphene Hydrochloride (Potential for withdrawal symptoms). Products include:
Darvon ... 1256
Wygesic Tablets ... 2540

Propoxyphene Napsylate (Potential for withdrawal symptoms). Products include:
Darvon-N/Darvocet-N ... 1254

Sufentanil Citrate (Potential for withdrawal symptoms). Products include:
Sufenta Injection ... 1147

Warfarin Sodium (Effects of aspirin may be deleterious in conjunction with anticoagulant therapy). Products include:
Coumadin Injection & Tablets ... 944
Panwarfin Tablets ... 547

TALWIN INJECTION
(Pentazocine Lactate) ... 2071
See **Talwin Ampuls**

TALWIN NX
(Pentazocine Hydrochloride, Naloxone Hydrochloride) ... 2073
May interact with narcotic analgesics, central nervous system depressants, and certain other agents. Compounds in these categories include:

Alcohol (May increase CNS depression).

Alfentanil Hydrochloride (Potential for withdrawal symptoms). Products include:
Alfenta Injection ... 1131

Alprazolam (Additive CNS depressant properties). Products include:
Xanax Tablets ... 2367

Aprobarbital (Additive CNS depressant properties). Products include:
Alurate Elixir ... 1883

Buprenorphine (Potential for withdrawal symptoms).
No products indexed under this heading.

Buspirone Hydrochloride (Additive CNS depressant properties). Products include:
BuSpar ... 1401

Butabarbital (Additive CNS depressant properties). Products include:
Pyridium Plus ... 1764

Butalbital (Additive CNS depressant properties). Products include:
Esgic-Plus Tablets ... 1002
Esgic Tablets & Capsules ... 1001
Fioricet Tablets ... 2006
Fiorinal Capsules ... 2007
Fiorinal with Codeine Capsules ... 2008
Fiorinal Tablets ... 2007
Phrenilin ... 838
Sedapap Tablets 50 mg/650 mg ... 1360

Chlordiazepoxide (Additive CNS depressant properties). Products include:
Libritabs Tablets ... 1930
Limbitrol ... 1933
Menrium Tablets ... 1934

Chlordiazepoxide Hydrochloride (Additive CNS depressant properties). Products include:
Librax Capsules ... 1929
Librium Capsules ... 1931
Librium Injectable ... 1932

Chlorpromazine (Additive CNS depressant properties). Products include:
Thorazine ... 2234

Chlorprothixene (Additive CNS depressant properties). Products include:
Taractan Tablets ... 1920

Chlorprothixene Hydrochloride (Additive CNS depressant properties). Products include:
Taractan ... 1920

Clorazepate Dipotassium (Additive CNS depressant properties). Products include:
Tranxene ... 556

Codeine (Potential for withdrawal symptoms). Products include:
Calcidrine Syrup ... 506

Codeine Phosphate (Potential for withdrawal symptoms). Products include:
Actifed with Codeine Cough Syrup ... 752
Cheracol Cough Syrup ... 1853
Codimal PH Syrup ... 846
Dimetane-DC Cough Syrup ... 1857
Empirin with Codeine Phosphate Nos. 2, 3 & 4 ... 764
Fiorinal with Codeine Capsules ... 2008
Isoclor Expectorant ... 982
Naldecon CX Adult Liquid ... ■ 521
Novahistine DH ... 1342
Novahistine Expectorant ... 1343
Nucofed Capsules ... 2219
Nucofed Expectorant ... 2219
Nucofed Pediatric Expectorant ... 2220
Nucofed Syrup ... 2219
Phenaphen with Codeine Capsules ... 1865
Phenaphen-650 with Codeine Tablets ... 1866
Phenergan with Codeine ... 2497
Phenergan VC with Codeine ... 2501
Robitussin A-C Syrup ... 1875
Robitussin-DAC Syrup ... 1875
Ryna ... ■ 741
Soma Compound w/Codeine Tablets ... 2390
Triaminic Expectorant w/Codeine ... 1996
Tussi-Organidin Liquid ... 2391
Tylenol with Codeine ... 1381

Codeine Polistirex (Potential for withdrawal symptoms).
No products indexed under this heading.

Dezocine (Potential for withdrawal symptoms).

Diazepam (Additive CNS depressant properties). Products include:
Valium Injectable ... 1937
Valium Tablets ... 1939
Valrelease Capsules ... 1923

Droperidol (Additive CNS depressant properties). Products include:
Inapsine Injection ... 1140
Innovar Injection ... 1141

Enflurane (Additive CNS depressant properties). Products include:
Ethrane ... 599

Estazolam (Potential for withdrawal symptoms). Products include:
ProSom Tablets ... 554

Ethchlorvynol (Additive CNS depressant properties). Products include:
Placidyl Capsules ... 553

Ethinamate (Additive CNS depressant properties).
No products indexed under this heading.

Fentanyl (Potential for withdrawal symptoms). Products include:
Duragesic Transdermal System ... 1133

Fentanyl Citrate (Potential for withdrawal symptoms). Products include:
Innovar Injection ... 1141
Sublimaze Injection ... 1146

Fluphenazine Decanoate (Additive CNS depressant properties). Products include:
Prolixin Decanoate ... 1795

Fluphenazine Enanthate (Additive CNS depressant properties). Products include:
Prolixin Enanthate ... 1796

Fluphenazine Hydrochloride (Additive CNS depressant properties). Products include:
Prolixin Elixir ... 1793
Prolixin Injection ... 1791
Prolixin Oral Concentrate ... 1792
Prolixin Tablets ... 1793

Flurazepam Hydrochloride (Additive CNS depressant properties). Products include:
Dalmane Capsules ... 1927

Glutethimide (Additive CNS depressant properties).
No products indexed under this heading.

Haloperidol (Additive CNS depressant properties). Products include:
Haldol Injection, Tablets and Concentrate ... 1373

Haloperidol Decanoate (Additive CNS depressant properties). Products include:
Haldol Decanoate ... 1375

Hydrocodone Bitartrate (Potential for withdrawal symptoms). Products include:
Anexsia 5/500 Tablets ... 2196
Anexsia 7.5/650 Tablets ... 2197
Azdōne Tablets ... 844
Codiclear DH Syrup ... 845
Codimal DH Syrup ... 846
Damason-P ... 1356
Hycodan Syrup, Tablets ... 927
Hycomine Compound Tablets ... 929
Hycomine Syrup ... 927
Hycotuss Expectorant Syrup ... 930
Hydrocet Capsules ... 835
Lortab ASA Tablets ... 2414
Lortab ... 2412
Ru-Tuss with Hydrocodone ... 694
Triaminic Expectorant DH ... 1995
Vicodin Tablets ... 1187
Vicodin ES Tablets ... 1189
Zydone Capsules ... 941

Hydrocodone Polistirex (Potential for withdrawal symptoms). Products include:
Tussionex Extended-Release Suspension ... 988

Hydroxyzine Hydrochloride (Additive CNS depressant properties). Products include:
Atarax Tablets & Syrup ... 1941
Marax Tablets & DF Syrup ... 1954
Vistaril Intramuscular Solution ... 1970

Isoflurane (Additive CNS depressant properties). Products include:
Forane ... 600

Ketamine Hydrochloride (Additive CNS depressant properties). Products include:
Ketalar ... 1726

Levorphanol Tartrate (Potential for withdrawal symptoms). Products include:
Levo-Dromoran ... 1906

Lorazepam (Additive CNS depressant properties). Products include:
Ativan Injection ... 2432
Ativan Tablets ... 2434

Loxapine Hydrochloride (Additive CNS depressant properties). Products include:
Loxitane ... 1213

Loxapine Succinate (Additive CNS depressant properties). Products include:
Loxitane Capsules ... 1213

Meperidine Hydrochloride (Potential for withdrawal symptoms). Products include:
Demerol ... 2047
Mepergan Injection ... 2479

Mephobarbital (Additive CNS depressant properties). Products include:
Mebaral Tablets ... 2061

Meprobamate (Additive CNS depressant properties). Products include:
Deprol Tablets ... 2382
Equagesic Tablets ... 2451
Miltown Tablets ... 2386
PMB 200 and PMB 400 ... 2504

Mesoridazine (Additive CNS depressant properties). Products include:
Serentil ... 686

Methadone Hydrochloride (Potential for withdrawal symptoms). Products include:
Dolophine Hydrochloride Ampoules & Vials ... 1260
Dolophine Hydrochloride Tablets ... 1261
Methadone Hydrochloride Diskets ... 1284
Methadone Hydrochloride Oral Solution & Tablets ... 1987

Methohexital Sodium (Additive CNS depressant properties). Products include:
Brevital Sodium Vials ... 1248

Methoxyflurane (Additive CNS depressant properties).
No products indexed under this heading.

Midazolam Hydrochloride (Additive CNS depressant properties). Products include:
Versed Injection ... 1924

Molindone Hydrochloride (Additive CNS depressant properties). Products include:
Moban Tablets & Concentrate ... 932

Morphine Sulfate (Potential for withdrawal symptoms). Products include:
- Astramorph/PF Injection, USP (Preservative-Free) 618
- Duramorph 960
- Infumorph 200 and Infumorph 500 Sterile Solutions 962
- MS Contin Tablets 1814
- MSIR 1817
- Oramorph SR (Morphine Sulfate Sustained Release Tablets) 1988
- Roxanol 1991

Opium Alkaloids (Potential for withdrawal symptoms). Products include:
- B & O No. 15A & No. 16A Supprettes 2395
- Pantopon Injectable 1911

Oxazepam (Additive CNS depressant properties). Products include:
- Serax Capsules 2522
- Serax Tablets 2522

Oxycodone Hydrochloride (Potential for withdrawal symptoms). Products include:
- Percocet Tablets 950
- Percodan 951
- Roxicodone Tablets, Oral Solution & Intensol (Oxycodone) 1992
- Tylox Capsules 1382

Pentobarbital Sodium (Additive CNS depressant properties). Products include:
- Nembutal Sodium Capsules 534
- Nembutal Sodium Solution 536
- Nembutal Sodium Suppositories 538

Perphenazine (Additive CNS depressant properties). Products include:
- Etrafon 2087
- Triavil Tablets 1556
- Trilafon 2123

Phenobarbital (Additive CNS depressant properties). Products include:
- Arco-Lase Plus Tablets 607
- Bellergal-S Tablets 1998
- Bronkolixir ▣ 761
- Bronkotabs Tablets ▣ 762
- Donnatal 1858
- Donnatal Extentabs 1859
- Donnatal Tablets 1858
- Donnazyme Tablets 1860
- Kinesed Tablets 2272
- Phenobarbital Elixir and Tablets 1293
- Primatene Tablets-P Formula 2421
- Quadrinal Tablets 1183
- Tedral SA 1765

Prazepam (Additive CNS depressant properties). Products include:
- Centrax 1693

Prochlorperazine (Additive CNS depressant properties). Products include:
- Compazine 2201

Promethazine Hydrochloride (Additive CNS depressant properties). Products include:
- Mepergan Injection 2479
- Phenergan with Codeine 2497
- Phenergan with Dextromethorphan 2499
- Phenergan Injection 2493
- Phenergan Suppositories 2496
- Phenergan Syrup 2495
- Phenergan Tablets 2496
- Phenergan VC 2500
- Phenergan VC with Codeine 2501

Propofol (Potential for withdrawal symptoms). Products include:
- Diprivan Injection 2267

Propoxyphene Hydrochloride (Potential for withdrawal symptoms). Products include:
- Darvon 1256
- Wygesic Tablets 2540

Propoxyphene Napsylate (Potential for withdrawal symptoms). Products include:
- Darvon-N/Darvocet-N 1254

Quazepam (Potential for withdrawal symptoms). Products include:
- Doral Tablets 2383

Secobarbital Sodium (Potential for withdrawal symptoms). Products include:
- Seconal Sodium Pulvules 1296

Sufentanil Citrate (Potential for withdrawal symptoms). Products include:
- Sufenta Injection 1147

Temazepam (Additive CNS depressant properties). Products include:
- Restoril Capsules 2023

Thiamylal Sodium (Additive CNS depressant properties). Products include:
- Surital Ampoules, Steri-Vials 1764

Thioridazine Hydrochloride (Additive CNS depressant properties). Products include:
- Mellaril 2011

Thiothixene (Additive CNS depressant properties). Products include:
- Navane Capsules and Concentrate 1954
- Navane Intramuscular 1956

Triazolam (Additive CNS depressant properties). Products include:
- Halcion Tablets 2340

Trifluoperazine Hydrochloride (Additive CNS depressant properties). Products include:
- Stelazine 2226

TAMBOCOR TABLETS

(Flecainide Acetate) 1315

May interact with beta blockers and certain other agents. Compounds in these categories include:

Acebutolol Hydrochloride (Possibility of additive negative inotropic effects). Products include:
- Sectral Capsules 2520

Amiodarone Hydrochloride (Increases plasma levels by two-fold or more; reduction of flecainide dose by 50% is recommended). Products include:
- Cordarone Tablets 2446

Atenolol (Possibility of additive negative inotropic effects). Products include:
- Tenoretic Tablets 1105
- Tenormin Tablets and I.V. Injection 1107

Betaxolol Hydrochloride (Possibility of additive negative inotropic effects). Products include:
- Betoptic Sterile Ophthalmic Solution 569
- Betoptic S Sterile Ophthalmic Suspension 570
- Kerlone Tablets 2172

Carbamazepine (A 30% increase in the rate of flecainide elimination). Products include:
- Tegretol Chewable Tablets 654
- Tegretol Suspension 656
- Tegretol Tablets 654

Carteolol Hydrochloride (Possibility of additive negative inotropic effects). Products include:
- Cartrol Tablets 507

Cimetidine (Increases flecainide plasma levels and half-life). Products include:
- Tagamet Tablets 2228

Cimetidine Hydrochloride (Increases flecainide plasma levels and half-life). Products include:
- Tagamet 2228

Digoxin (Concurrent administration increases plasma digoxin levels by a 13% +/− 19%). Products include:
- Lanoxicaps 772
- Lanoxin Elixir Pediatric 775
- Lanoxin Injection 778
- Lanoxin Injection Pediatric 781
- Lanoxin Tablets 783

Disopyramide Phosphate (Concurrent administration is not recommended). Products include:
- Norpace 2177

Esmolol Hydrochloride (Possibility of additive negative inotropic effects). Products include:
- Brevibloc Injection 942

Labetalol Hydrochloride (Possibility of additive negative inotropic effects). Products include:
- Normodyne Injection 2108
- Normodyne Tablets 2110
- Normozide Tablets 2112
- Trandate HCT Tablets 579
- Trandate Injection 577
- Trandate Tablets 579

Metoprolol Tartrate (Possibility of additive negative inotropic effects). Products include:
- Lopressor Ampuls 1032
- Lopressor HCT Tablets 1034
- Lopressor Tablets 1032

Nadolol (Possibility of additive negative inotropic effects). Products include:
- Corgard Tablets 701
- Corzide Tablets 702

Penbutolol Sulfate (Possibility of additive negative inotropic effects). Products include:
- Levatol 1832

Phenobarbital (A 30% increase in the rate of flecainide elimination). Products include:
- Arco-Lase Plus Tablets 607
- Bellergal-S Tablets 1998
- Bronkolixir ▣ 761
- Bronkotabs Tablets ▣ 762
- Donnatal 1858
- Donnatal Extentabs 1859
- Donnatal Tablets 1858
- Donnazyme Tablets 1860
- Kinesed Tablets 2272
- Phenobarbital Elixir and Tablets 1293
- Primatene Tablets-P Formula 2421
- Quadrinal Tablets 1183
- Tedral SA 1765

Phenytoin (A 30% increase in the rate of flecainide elimination). Products include:
- Dilantin Infatabs 1710
- Dilantin-30 Pediatric/Dilantin-125 Suspension 1713

Phenytoin Sodium (A 30% increase in the rate of flecainide elimination). Products include:
- Dilantin Kapseals 1708
- Dilantin Parenteral 1712
- Dilantin with Phenobarbital Kapseals 1715

Pindolol (Possibility of additive negative inotropic effects). Products include:
- Visken Tablets 2036

Propranolol Hydrochloride (Possibility of additive negative inotropic effects). Products include:
- Inderal 2459
- Inderal LA Long Acting Capsules 2461
- Inderide Tablets 2463
- Inderide LA Long Acting Capsules 2465

Timolol Maleate (Possibility of additive negative inotropic effects). Products include:
- Blocadren Tablets 1429
- Timolide Tablets 1547
- Timoptic in Ocudose 1552
- Timoptic Sterile Ophthalmic Solution 1550

Verapamil Hydrochloride (Concurrent administration is not recommended). Products include:
- Calan SR Caplets 2157
- Calan Tablets 2155
- Isoptin Injectable 1177
- Isoptin Oral Tablets 1179
- Isoptin SR Sustained Release Tablets 1181
- Verelan Capsules 1243
- Verelan Capsules 2535

TAO CAPSULES

(Troleandomycin) 1963

May interact with antimigraine drugs, xanthine bronchodilators, and certain other agents. Compounds in these categories include:

Aminophylline (Elevated serum concentrations of theophylline). Products include:
- Amesec ▣ 682
- Aminophyllin Tablets 2153

Dihydroergotamine Mesylate (May induce ischemic reactions). Products include:
- D.H.E. 45 Injection 2003

Dyphylline (Elevated serum concentrations of theophylline). Products include:
- Dilor 2079
- Dilor-G Tablets & Liquid 2079
- Lufyllin Elixir 2384
- Lufyllin & Lufyllin-400 Tablets 2384
- Lufyllin-GG Elixir & Tablets 2385

Ergotamine Tartrate (May induce ischemic reactions). Products include:
- Bellergal-S Tablets 1998
- Cafergot/Cafergot P-B 1999
- Ergostat 1719
- Medihaler Ergotamine Aerosol 1312
- Wigraine Tablets & Suppositories 1645

Metoclopramide Hydrochloride (May induce ischemic reactions). Products include:
- Reglan 1869

Theophylline (Elevated serum concentrations of theophylline). Products include:
- Bronkaid Tablets ▣ 757
- Bronkolixir ▣ 761
- Bronkotabs Tablets ▣ 762
- Constant-T Tablets 1029
- Marax Tablets & DF Syrup 1954
- Primatene Tablets 2421
- Quibron Capsules 713
- Quibron-T 714
- Quibron-T/SR 716
- Theolair Liquid 1317
- Theo-Organidin Elixir 2391

Theophylline Anhydrous (Elevated serum concentrations of theophylline). Products include:
- Aerolate 994
- Primatene Tablets-M Formula ▣ 753
- Primatene Tablets-Regular Formula 2421
- Respbid Tablets 684
- Slo-bid Gyrocaps 1847
- T-PHYL (Uniphyl) 200 mg Tablets 1820
- Tedral SA 1765
- Theo-24 2179
- Theo-Dur Sprinkle 1168
- Theo-Dur Extended-Release Tablets 1166
- Theolair Tablets 1317
- Theolair-SR Tablets 1319
- TheoX Extended-Release Tablets 841
- Uniphyl 400 mg Tablets 1823

Theophylline Calcium Salicylate (Elevated serum concentrations of theophylline). Products include:
- Quadrinal Tablets 1183

Theophylline Sodium Glycinate (Elevated serum concentrations of theophylline). Products include:
- Asbron G 1997

TAPAZOLE TABLETS

(Methimazole) 1298

May interact with anticoagulants. Compounds in this category include:

Dicumarol (Activity of anticoagulant may be potentiated). Products include:
- Dicumarol Tablets 516

Heparin Calcium (Activity of anticoagulant may be potentiated). Products include:
- Calciparine Injection 925

Heparin Sodium (Activity of anticoagulant may be potentiated). Products include:
Heparin Lock Flush Solution 2456
Heparin Sodium Vials 1264
Heparin Sodium Injection 2457
Heparin Sodium Injection, USP, Sterile Solution 2342

Warfarin Sodium (Activity of anticoagulant may be potentiated). Products include:
Coumadin Injection & Tablets 944
Panwarfin Tablets 547

TARACTAN CONCENTRATE
(Chlorprothixene Lactate, Chlorprothixene Hydrochloride) 1920
May interact with barbiturates, narcotic analgesics, anticholinergics, psychotropics, anticonvulsants, and certain other agents. Compounds in these categories include:

Alfentanil Hydrochloride (Additive effects). Products include:
Alfenta Injection 1131

Alprazolam (Altered absorption, metabolism, or therapeutic activity). Products include:
Xanax Tablets 2367

Amitriptyline Hydrochloride (Altered absorption, metabolism, or therapeutic activity). Products include:
Elavil 2269
Endep Tablets 1927
Etrafon 2087
Limbitrol 1933
Triavil Tablets 1556

Amoxapine (Altered absorption, metabolism, or therapeutic activity). Products include:
Asendin Tablets 1196

Aprobarbital (Additive effects). Products include:
Alurate Elixir 1883

Atropine Sulfate (Additive anticholinergic effects). Products include:
Arco-Lase Plus Tablets 607
Atropine Sulfate Sterile Ophthalmic Solution and S.O.P. Sterile Ophthalmic Ointment ⊙ 239
Donnagel ▣ 675
Donnagel-PG 1858
Donnatal 1858
Donnatal Extentabs 1859
Donnatal Tablets 1858
Donnazyme Tablets 1860
Isopto Atropine ⊙ 218
Lomotil 2174
Motofen Tablets 836
Ru-Tuss Tablets 693
Urised Tablets 2396

Belladonna Alkaloids (Additive anticholinergic effects). Products include:
Bellergal-S Tablets 1998
Hyland's Bed Wetting Tablets ▣ 728
Hyland's Teething Tablets ▣ 728
Kinesed Tablets 2272

Benztropine Mesylate (Additive anticholinergic effects). Products include:
Cogentin 1435

Biperiden (Additive anticholinergic effects). Products include:
Akineton 1171

Buprenorphine (Additive effects).
No products indexed under this heading.

Buspirone Hydrochloride (Altered absorption, metabolism, or therapeutic activity). Products include:
BuSpar 1401

Butabarbital (Additive effects). Products include:
Pyridium Plus 1764

Butalbital (Additive effects). Products include:
Esgic-Plus Tablets 1002
Esgic Tablets & Capsules 1001
Fioricet Tablets 2006
Fiorinal Capsules 2007
Fiorinal with Codeine Capsules 2008
Fiorinal Tablets 2007
Phrenilin 838
Sedapap Tablets 50 mg/650 mg 1360

Carbamazepine (Convulsive threshold lowered). Products include:
Tegretol Chewable Tablets 654
Tegretol Suspension 656
Tegretol Tablets 654

Chlordiazepoxide (Altered absorption, metabolism, or therapeutic activity). Products include:
Libritabs Tablets 1930
Limbitrol 1933
Menrium Tablets 1934

Chlordiazepoxide Hydrochloride (Altered absorption, metabolism, or therapeutic activity). Products include:
Librax Capsules 1929
Librium Capsules 1931
Librium Injectable 1932

Chlorpromazine (Altered absorption, metabolism, or therapeutic activity). Products include:
Thorazine 2234

Clidinium Bromide (Additive anticholinergic effects). Products include:
Librax Capsules 1929
Quarzan Capsules 1937

Clorazepate Dipotassium (Altered absorption, metabolism, or therapeutic activity). Products include:
Tranxene 556

Codeine (Additive effects). Products include:
Calcidrine Syrup 506

Codeine Phosphate (Additive effects). Products include:
Actifed with Codeine Cough Syrup 752
Cheracol Cough Syrup 1853
Codimal PH Syrup 846
Dimetane-DC Cough Syrup 1857
Empirin with Codeine Phosphate Nos. 2, 3 & 4 764
Fiorinal with Codeine Capsules 2008
Isoclor Expectorant 982
Naldecon CX Adult Liquid ▣ 521
Novahistine DH 1342
Novahistine Expectorant 1343
Nucofed Capsules 2219
Nucofed Expectorant 2219
Nucofed Pediatric Expectorant 2220
Nucofed Syrup 2219
Phenaphen with Codeine Capsules 1865
Phenaphen-650 with Codeine Tablets 1866
Phenergan with Codeine 2497
Phenergan VC with Codeine 2501
Robitussin A-C Syrup 1875
Robitussin-DAC Syrup 1875
Ryna ▣ 741
Soma Compound w/Codeine Tablets 2390
Triaminic Expectorant w/Codeine 1996
Tussi-Organidin Liquid 2391
Tylenol with Codeine 1381

Codeine Polistirex (Additive effects).
No products indexed under this heading.

Desipramine Hydrochloride (Altered absorption, metabolism, or therapeutic activity). Products include:
Norpramin Tablets 1340

Dezocine (Additive effects).

Diazepam (Altered absorption, metabolism, or therapeutic activity). Products include:
Valium Injectable 1937
Valium Tablets 1939
Valrelease Capsules 1923

Dicyclomine Hydrochloride (Additive anticholinergic effects). Products include:
Bentyl 1322

Divalproex Sodium (Convulsive threshold lowered). Products include:
Depakote 512

Doxepin Hydrochloride (Altered absorption, metabolism, or therapeutic activity). Products include:
Sinequan 1960

Droperidol (Altered absorption, metabolism, or therapeutic activity). Products include:
Inapsine Injection 1140
Innovar Injection 1141

Epinephrine Hydrochloride (Paradoxical lowering of blood pressure). Products include:
Adrenalin Chloride Solution 1:100 & 1:1,000 1689
Epifrin ⊙ 244
Glaucon ⊙ 218

Ethopropazine Hydrochloride (Additive anticholinergic effects).

Ethosuximide (Convulsive threshold lowered). Products include:
Zarontin Capsules 1768
Zarontin Syrup 1769

Ethotoin (Convulsive threshold lowered). Products include:
Peganone Tablets 551

Fentanyl (Additive effects). Products include:
Duragesic Transdermal System 1133

Fentanyl Citrate (Additive effects). Products include:
Innovar Injection 1141
Sublimaze Injection 1146

Fluphenazine Decanoate (Altered absorption, metabolism, or therapeutic activity). Products include:
Prolixin Decanoate 1795

Fluphenazine Enanthate (Altered absorption, metabolism, or therapeutic activity). Products include:
Prolixin Enanthate 1796

Fluphenazine Hydrochloride (Altered absorption, metabolism, or therapeutic activity). Products include:
Prolixin Elixir 1793
Prolixin Injection 1791
Prolixin Oral Concentrate 1792
Prolixin Tablets 1793

Glycopyrrolate (Additive anticholinergic effects). Products include:
Robinul Forte Tablets 1873
Robinul Injectable 1873
Robinul Tablets 1873

Haloperidol (Altered absorption, metabolism, or therapeutic activity). Products include:
Haldol Injection, Tablets and Concentrate 1373

Haloperidol Decanoate (Altered absorption, metabolism, or therapeutic activity). Products include:
Haldol Decanoate 1375

Hydrocodone Bitartrate (Additive effects). Products include:
Anexsia 5/500 Tablets 2196
Anexsia 7.5/650 Tablets 2197
Azdōne Tablets 844
Codiclear DH Syrup 845
Codimal DH Syrup 846
Damason-P 1356
Hycodan Syrup, Tablets 927
Hycomine Compound Tablets 929
Hycomine Syrup 927
Hycotuss Expectorant Syrup 930
Hydrocet Capsules 835
Lortab ASA Tablets 2414
Lortab 2412
Ru-Tuss with Hydrocodone 694
Triaminic Expectorant DH 1995
Vicodin Tablets 1187
Vicodin ES Tablets 1189
Zydone Capsules 941

Hydrocodone Polistirex (Additive effects). Products include:
Tussionex Extended-Release Suspension 988

Hydroxyzine Hydrochloride (Altered absorption, metabolism, or therapeutic activity). Products include:
Atarax Tablets & Syrup 1941
Marax Tablets & DF Syrup 1954
Vistaril Intramuscular Solution 1970

Hyoscyamine (Additive anticholinergic effects). Products include:
Cystospaz Tablets 2395
Urised Tablets 2396

Hyoscyamine Sulfate (Additive anticholinergic effects). Products include:
Arco-Lase Plus Tablets 607
Cystospaz-M Capsules 2395
Donnagel ▣ 675
Donnagel-PG 1858
Donnatal 1858
Donnatal Extentabs 1859
Donnatal Tablets 1858
Donnazyme Tablets 1860
Kutrase Capsules 2146
Levsin/Levsinex 2147
Ru-Tuss Tablets 693

Imipramine Hydrochloride (Altered absorption, metabolism, or therapeutic activity). Products include:
Tofranil Ampuls 1038
Tofranil Tablets 1039

Imipramine Pamoate (Altered absorption, metabolism, or therapeutic activity). Products include:
Tofranil-PM Capsules 1041

Ipratropium Bromide (Additive anticholinergic effects). Products include:
Atrovent Inhalation Aerosol 675

Isocarboxazid (Altered absorption, metabolism, or therapeutic activity). Products include:
Marplan Tablets 1906

Levorphanol Tartrate (Additive effects). Products include:
Levo-Dromoran 1906

Lithium Carbonate (Altered absorption, metabolism, or therapeutic activity). Products include:
Eskalith 2214
Lithane Tablets 1596
Lithium Carbonate Capsules & Tablets 1984
Lithobid Tablets 870

Lithium Citrate (Altered absorption, metabolism, or therapeutic activity). Products include:
Cibalith-S 870

Lorazepam (Altered absorption, metabolism, or therapeutic activity). Products include:
Ativan Injection 2432
Ativan Tablets 2434

Loxapine Hydrochloride (Altered absorption, metabolism, or therapeutic activity). Products include:
Loxitane 1213

Maprotiline Hydrochloride (Altered absorption, metabolism, or therapeutic activity). Products include:
Ludiomil Tablets 874

Mepenzolate Bromide (Additive anticholinergic effects). Products include:
Cantil Tablets 1326

Meperidine Hydrochloride (Additive effects). Products include:
Demerol 2047
Mepergan Injection 2479

Mephenytoin (Convulsive threshold lowered). Products include:
Mesantoin Tablets 2013

(▣ Described in PDR For Nonprescription Drugs)

(⊙ Described in PDR For Ophthalmology)

Mephobarbital (Additive effects). Products include:
- Mebaral Tablets 2061

Meprobamate (Altered absorption, metabolism, or therapeutic activity). Products include:
- Deprol Tablets 2382
- Equagesic Tablets 2451
- Miltown Tablets 2386
- PMB 200 and PMB 400 2504

Mesoridazine (Altered absorption, metabolism, or therapeutic activity). Products include:
- Serentil 686

Methadone Hydrochloride (Additive effects). Products include:
- Dolophine Hydrochloride Ampoules & Vials 1260
- Dolophine Hydrochloride Tablets 1261
- Methadone Hydrochloride Diskets 1284
- Methadone Hydrochloride Oral Solution & Tablets 1987

Methsuximide (Convulsive threshold lowered). Products include:
- Celontin 1692

Midazolam Hydrochloride (Altered absorption, metabolism, or therapeutic activity). Products include:
- Versed Injection 1924

Molindone Hydrochloride (Altered absorption, metabolism, or therapeutic activity). Products include:
- Moban Tablets & Concentrate 932

Morphine Sulfate (Additive effects). Products include:
- Astramorph/PF Injection, USP (Preservative-Free) 618
- Duramorph 960
- Infumorph 200 and Infumorph 500 Sterile Solutions 962
- MS Contin Tablets 1814
- MSIR 1817
- Oramorph SR (Morphine Sulfate Sustained Release Tablets) 1988
- Roxanol 1991

Nortriptyline Hydrochloride (Altered absorption, metabolism, or therapeutic activity). Products include:
- Pamelor 2019

Opium Alkaloids (Additive effects). Products include:
- B & O No. 15A & No. 16A Supprettes 2395
- Pantopon Injectable 1911

Oxazepam (Altered absorption, metabolism, or therapeutic activity). Products include:
- Serax Capsules 2522
- Serax Tablets 2522

Oxybutynin Chloride (Additive anticholinergic effects). Products include:
- Ditropan 1332

Oxycodone Hydrochloride (Additive effects). Products include:
- Percocet Tablets 950
- Percodan 951
- Roxicodone Tablets, Oral Solution & Intensol (Oxycodone) 1992
- Tylox Capsules 1382

Oxyphenonium Bromide (Additive anticholinergic effects).

Paramethadione (Convulsive threshold lowered). Products include:
- Paradione Capsules 548

Pentobarbital Sodium (Additive effects). Products include:
- Nembutal Sodium Capsules 534
- Nembutal Sodium Solution 536
- Nembutal Sodium Suppositories 538

Perphenazine (Altered absorption, metabolism, or therapeutic activity). Products include:
- Etrafon 2087
- Triavil Tablets 1556
- Trilafon 2123

Phenacemide (Convulsive threshold lowered). Products include:
- Phenurone Tablets 552

Phenelzine Sulfate (Altered absorption, metabolism, or therapeutic activity). Products include:
- Nardil 1742

Phenobarbital (Additive effects; convulsive threshold lowered). Products include:
- Arco-Lase Plus Tablets 607
- Bellergal-S Tablets 1998
- Bronkolixir .... ▣ 761
- Bronkotabs Tablets .... ▣ 762
- Donnatal 1858
- Donnatal Extentabs 1859
- Donnatal Tablets 1858
- Donnazyme Tablets 1860
- Kinesed Tablets 2272
- Phenobarbital Elixir and Tablets 1293
- Primatene Tablets-P Formula 2421
- Quadrinal Tablets 1183
- Tedral SA 1765

Phensuximide (Convulsive threshold lowered). Products include:
- Milontin Kapseals 1741

Phenylephrine Hydrochloride (Paradoxical lowering of blood pressure). Products include:
- AK-Dilate Solution 2.5% and 10% .... ⊙ 203
- Atrohist Sprinkle Capsules 558
- Cerose-DM 2443
- Codimal 846
- Comhist LA Capsules 1618
- Congespirin For Children Aspirin Free Chewable Cold Tablets 748
- Cyclomydril .... ⊙ 216
- Deconsal Sprinkle Capsules 559
- Dimetane Decongestant .... ▣ 673
- Dristan Decongestant/Antihistamine/ Analgesic Coated Caplets .... ▣ 749
- Dristan Cold Nasal Decongestant/ Antihistamine/ Analgesic Coated Tablets 2419
- Dristan Advanced Formula Decongestant/Antihistamine/ Analgesic Tablets .... ▣ 749
- Dristan Nasal Spray, Menthol 2419
- Dristan Nasal Spray, Regular and Regular with Metered Pump 2419
- Entex Capsules 1623
- Entex Liquid 1623
- Sinus Excedrin Analgesic, Decongestant Tablets & Caplets 750
- Extendryl 994
- 4-Way Fast Acting Nasal Spray - Original Formula (regular & mentholated) & Metered Spray Pump (regular) 751
- Hycomine Compound Tablets 929
- Murocoll-2 Sterile Ophthalmic Solution .... ⊙ 261
- Mydfrin 2.5% .... ⊙ 224
- Naldecon Syrup, Tablets, Pediatric Drops and Pediatric Syrup 709
- Neo-Synephrine Hydrochloride 1% Carpuject 2063
- Neo-Synephrine Hydrochloride 1% Injection 2063
- Neo-Synephrine Hydrochloride (Ophthalmic) 2064
- Neo-Synephrine .... ▣ 759
- Nōstril Nasal Decongestant .... ▣ 520
- Novahistine Elixir .... ▣ 596
- Phenergan VC 2500
- Phenergan VC with Codeine 2501
- Prefrin Liquifilm Vasoconstrictor and Lubricant Eye Drops .... ⊙ 254
- Prefrin-A .... ⊙ 255
- Quelidrine Syrup 556
- Relief Vasoconstrictor and Lubricant Eye Drops .... ⊙ 256
- Robitussin Night Relief .... ▣ 677
- Ru-Tuss with Hydrocodone 694
- Ru-Tuss Tablets 693
- Vasosulf .... ⊙ 279
- Vicks Sinex .... ▣ 665
- Zincfrin .... ⊙ 230

Phenytoin (Convulsive threshold lowered). Products include:
- Dilantin Infatabs 1710
- Dilantin-30 Pediatric/Dilantin-125 Suspension 1713

Phenytoin Sodium (Convulsive threshold lowered). Products include:
- Dilantin Kapseals 1708
- Dilantin Parenteral 1712
- Dilantin with Phenobarbital Kapseals 1715

Prazepam (Altered absorption, metabolism, or therapeutic activity). Products include:
- Centrax 1693

Primidone (Convulsive threshold lowered). Products include:
- Mysoline 2480

Prochlorperazine (Altered absorption, metabolism, or therapeutic activity). Products include:
- Compazine 2201

Procyclidine Hydrochloride (Additive anticholinergic effects). Products include:
- Kemadrin Tablets 771

Promethazine Hydrochloride (Altered absorption, metabolism, or therapeutic activity). Products include:
- Mepergan Injection 2479
- Phenergan with Codeine 2497
- Phenergan with Dextromethorphan 2499
- Phenergan Injection 2493
- Phenergan Suppositories 2496
- Phenergan Syrup 2495
- Phenergan Tablets 2496
- Phenergan VC 2500
- Phenergan VC with Codeine 2501

Propantheline Bromide (Additive anticholinergic effects). Products include:
- Pro-Banthīne Tablets 2141

Propoxyphene Hydrochloride (Additive effects). Products include:
- Darvon 1256
- Wygesic Tablets 2540

Propoxyphene Napsylate (Additive effects). Products include:
- Darvon-N/Darvocet-N 1254

Protriptyline Hydrochloride (Altered absorption, metabolism, or therapeutic activity). Products include:
- Vivactil Tablets 1567

Scopolamine Hydrobromide (Additive anticholinergic effects). Products include:
- Donnagel .... ▣ 675
- Donnagel-PG 1858
- Donnatal 1858
- Donnatal Extentabs 1859
- Donnatal Tablets 1858
- Donnazyme Tablets 1860
- Isopto Hyoscine .... ⊙ 222
- Murocoll-2 Sterile Ophthalmic Solution .... ⊙ 261
- Ru-Tuss Tablets 693

Scopolamine Preparations (Additive anticholinergic effects). Products include:
- Transderm Scōp Transdermal Therapeutic System 887

Secobarbital Sodium (Additive effects). Products include:
- Seconal Sodium Pulvules 1296

Sufentanil Citrate (Additive effects). Products include:
- Sufenta Injection 1147

Thiamylal Sodium (Additive effects). Products include:
- Surital Ampoules, Steri-Vials 1764

Thioridazine Hydrochloride (Altered absorption, metabolism, or therapeutic activity). Products include:
- Mellaril 2011

Thiothixene (Altered absorption, metabolism, or therapeutic activity). Products include:
- Navane Capsules and Concentrate 1954
- Navane Intramuscular 1956

Tranylcypromine Sulfate (Altered absorption, metabolism, or therapeutic activity). Products include:
- Parnate Tablets 2222

Tridihexethyl Chloride (Additive anticholinergic effects).
- No products indexed under this heading.

Trifluoperazine Hydrochloride (Altered absorption, metabolism, or therapeutic activity). Products include:
- Stelazine 2226

Trihexyphenidyl Hydrochloride (Additive anticholinergic effects). Products include:
- Artane 1195

Trimethadione (Convulsive threshold lowered). Products include:
- Tridione 557

Trimipramine Maleate (Altered absorption, metabolism, or therapeutic activity). Products include:
- Surmontil Capsules 2524

Valproic Acid (Convulsive threshold lowered). Products include:
- Depakene Capsules & Syrup 511

TARACTAN INJECTABLE
(Chlorprothixene) 1920
See **Taractan Concentrate**

TARACTAN TABLETS
(Chlorprothixene) 1920
See **Taractan Concentrate**

TAVIST SYRUP
(Clemastine Fumarate) 2033
May interact with central nervous system depressants, hypnotics and sedatives, tranquilizers, monoamine oxidase inhibitors, and certain other agents. Compounds in these categories include:

Alcohol (Additive effects).

Alfentanil Hydrochloride (Additive effects). Products include:
- Alfenta Injection 1131

Alprazolam (Additive effects). Products include:
- Xanax Tablets 2367

Aprobarbital (Additive effects). Products include:
- Alurate Elixir 1883

Buprenorphine (Additive effects).
- No products indexed under this heading.

Buspirone Hydrochloride (Additive effects). Products include:
- BuSpar 1401

Butabarbital (Additive effects). Products include:
- Pyridium Plus 1764

Butalbital (Additive effects). Products include:
- Esgic-Plus Tablets 1002
- Esgic Tablets & Capsules 1001
- Fioricet Tablets 2006
- Fiorinal Capsules 2007
- Fiorinal with Codeine Capsules 2008
- Fiorinal Tablets 2007
- Phrenilin 838
- Sedapap Tablets 50 mg/650 mg 1360

Chlordiazepoxide (Additive effects). Products include:
- Libritabs Tablets 1930
- Limbitrol 1933
- Menrium Tablets 1934

Chlordiazepoxide Hydrochloride (Additive effects). Products include:
- Librax Capsules 1929
- Librium Capsules 1931
- Librium Injectable 1932

(▣ Described in PDR For Nonprescription Drugs) (⊙ Described in PDR For Ophthalmology)

Chlorpromazine (Additive effects). Products include:
Thorazine ... 2234

Chlorprothixene (Additive effects). Products include:
Taractan Tablets ... 1920

Chlorprothixene Hydrochloride (Additive effects). Products include:
Taractan ... 1920

Chlorprothixene Lactate (Additive effects). Products include:
Taractan Concentrate ... 1920

Clorazepate Dipotassium (Additive effects). Products include:
Tranxene ... 556

Codeine (Additive effects). Products include:
Calcidrine Syrup ... 506

Codeine Phosphate (Additive effects). Products include:
Actifed with Codeine Cough Syrup.. 752
Cheracol Cough Syrup ... 1853
Codimal PH Syrup ... 846
Dimetane-DC Cough Syrup ... 1857
Empirin with Codeine Phosphate Nos. 2, 3 & 4 ... 764
Fiorinal with Codeine Capsules ... 2008
Isoclor Expectorant ... 982
Naldecon CX Adult Liquid ... 521
Novahistine DH ... 1342
Novahistine Expectorant ... 1343
Nucofed Capsules ... 2219
Nucofed Expectorant ... 2219
Nucofed Pediatric Expectorant ... 2220
Nucofed Syrup ... 2219
Phenaphen with Codeine Capsules 1865
Phenaphen-650 with Codeine Tablets ... 1866
Phenergan with Codeine ... 2497
Phenergan VC with Codeine ... 2501
Robitussin A-C Syrup ... 1875
Robitussin-DAC Syrup ... 1875
Ryna ... 741
Soma Compound w/Codeine Tablets ... 2390
Triaminic Expectorant w/Codeine .. 1996
Tussi-Organidin Liquid ... 2391
Tylenol with Codeine ... 1381

Codeine Polistirex (Additive effects).
No products indexed under this heading.

Dezocine (Additive effects).

Diazepam (Additive effects). Products include:
Valium Injectable ... 1937
Valium Tablets ... 1939
Valrelease Capsules ... 1923

Droperidol (Additive effects). Products include:
Inapsine Injection ... 1140
Innovar Injection ... 1141

Enflurane (Additive effects). Products include:
Ethrane ... 599

Estazolam (Additive effects). Products include:
ProSom Tablets ... 554

Ethchlorvynol (Additive effects). Products include:
Placidyl Capsules ... 553

Ethinamate (Additive effects).
No products indexed under this heading.

Fentanyl (Additive effects). Products include:
Duragesic Transdermal System ... 1133

Fentanyl Citrate (Additive effects). Products include:
Innovar Injection ... 1141
Sublimaze Injection ... 1146

Fluphenazine Decanoate (Additive effects). Products include:
Prolixin Decanoate ... 1795

Fluphenazine Enanthate (Additive effects). Products include:
Prolixin Enanthate ... 1796

Fluphenazine Hydrochloride (Additive effects). Products include:
Prolixin Elixir ... 1793
Prolixin Injection ... 1791
Prolixin Oral Concentrate ... 1792
Prolixin Tablets ... 1793

Flurazepam Hydrochloride (Additive effects). Products include:
Dalmane Capsules ... 1927

Furazolidone (Prolongs anticholinergic effects of Tavist). Products include:
Furoxone ... 1855

Glutethimide (Additive effects).
No products indexed under this heading.

Haloperidol (Additive effects). Products include:
Haldol Injection, Tablets and Concentrate ... 1373

Haloperidol Decanoate (Additive effects). Products include:
Haldol Decanoate ... 1375

Hydrocodone Bitartrate (Additive effects). Products include:
Anexsia 5/500 Tablets ... 2196
Anexsia 7.5/650 Tablets ... 2197
Azdone Tablets ... 844
Codiclear DH Syrup ... 845
Codimal DH Syrup ... 846
Damason-P ... 1356
Hycodan Syrup, Tablets ... 927
Hycomine Compound Tablets ... 929
Hycomine Syrup ... 927
Hycotuss Expectorant Syrup ... 930
Hydrocet Capsules ... 835
Lortab ASA Tablets ... 2414
Lortab ... 2412
Ru-Tuss with Hydrocodone ... 694
Triaminic Expectorant DH ... 1995
Vicodin Tablets ... 1187
Vicodin ES Tablets ... 1189
Zydone Capsules ... 941

Hydrocodone Polistirex (Additive effects). Products include:
Tussionex Extended-Release Suspension ... 988

Hydroxyzine Hydrochloride (Additive effects). Products include:
Atarax Tablets & Syrup ... 1941
Marax Tablets & DF Syrup ... 1954
Vistaril Intramuscular Solution ... 1970

Isocarboxazid (Prolongs anticholinergic effects of Tavist). Products include:
Marplan Tablets ... 1906

Isoflurane (Additive effects). Products include:
Forane ... 600

Ketamine Hydrochloride (Additive effects). Products include:
Ketalar ... 1726

Levorphanol Tartrate (Additive effects). Products include:
Levo-Dromoran ... 1906

Lorazepam (Additive effects). Products include:
Ativan Injection ... 2432
Ativan Tablets ... 2434

Loxapine Hydrochloride (Additive effects). Products include:
Loxitane ... 1213

Loxapine Succinate (Additive effects). Products include:
Loxitane Capsules ... 1213

Meperidine Hydrochloride (Additive effects). Products include:
Demerol ... 2047
Mepergan Injection ... 2479

Mephobarbital (Additive effects). Products include:
Mebaral Tablets ... 2061

Meprobamate (Additive effects). Products include:
Deprol Tablets ... 2382
Equagesic Tablets ... 2451
Miltown Tablets ... 2386
PMB 200 and PMB 400 ... 2504

Mesoridazine (Additive effects). Products include:
Serentil ... 686

Methadone Hydrochloride (Additive effects). Products include:
Dolophine Hydrochloride Ampoules & Vials ... 1260
Dolophine Hydrochloride Tablets ... 1261
Methadone Hydrochloride Diskets .. 1284
Methadone Hydrochloride Oral Solution & Tablets ... 1987

Methohexital Sodium (Additive effects). Products include:
Brevital Sodium Vials ... 1248

Methoxyflurane (Additive effects).
No products indexed under this heading.

Midazolam Hydrochloride (Additive effects). Products include:
Versed Injection ... 1924

Molindone Hydrochloride (Additive effects). Products include:
Moban Tablets & Concentrate ... 932

Morphine Sulfate (Additive effects). Products include:
Astramorph/PF Injection, USP (Preservative-Free) ... 618
Duramorph ... 960
Infumorph 200 and Infumorph 500 Sterile Solutions ... 962
MS Contin Tablets ... 1814
MSIR ... 1817
Oramorph SR (Morphine Sulfate Sustained Release Tablets) ... 1988
Roxanol ... 1991

Opium Alkaloids (Additive effects). Products include:
B & O No. 15A & No. 16A Supprettes ... 2395
Pantopon Injectable ... 1911

Oxazepam (Additive effects). Products include:
Serax Capsules ... 2522
Serax Tablets ... 2522

Oxycodone Hydrochloride (Additive effects). Products include:
Percocet Tablets ... 950
Percodan ... 951
Roxicodone Tablets, Oral Solution & Intensol (Oxycodone) ... 1992
Tylox Capsules ... 1382

Pentobarbital Sodium (Additive effects). Products include:
Nembutal Sodium Capsules ... 534
Nembutal Sodium Solution ... 536
Nembutal Sodium Suppositories ... 538

Perphenazine (Additive effects). Products include:
Etrafon ... 2087
Triavil Tablets ... 1556
Trilafon ... 2123

Phenelzine Sulfate (Prolongs anticholinergic effects of Tavist). Products include:
Nardil ... 1742

Phenobarbital (Additive effects). Products include:
Arco-Lase Plus Tablets ... 607
Bellergal-S Tablets ... 1998
Bronkolixir ... 761
Bronkotabs Tablets ... 762
Donnatal ... 1858
Donnatal Extentabs ... 1859
Donnatal Tablets ... 1858
Donnazyme Tablets ... 1860
Kinesed Tablets ... 2272
Phenobarbital Elixir and Tablets ... 1293
Primatene Tablets-P Formula ... 2421
Quadrinal Tablets ... 1183
Tedral SA ... 1765

Prazepam (Additive effects). Products include:
Centrax ... 1693

Prochlorperazine (Additive effects). Products include:
Compazine ... 2201

Promethazine Hydrochloride (Additive effects). Products include:
Mepergan Injection ... 2479
Phenergan with Codeine ... 2497
Phenergan with Dextromethorphan 2499
Phenergan Injection ... 2493
Phenergan Suppositories ... 2496
Phenergan Syrup ... 2495
Phenergan Tablets ... 2496
Phenergan VC ... 2500
Phenergan VC with Codeine ... 2501

Propofol (Additive effects). Products include:
Diprivan Injection ... 2267

Propoxyphene Hydrochloride (Additive effects). Products include:
Darvon ... 1256
Wygesic Tablets ... 2540

Propoxyphene Napsylate (Additive effects). Products include:
Darvon-N/Darvocet-N ... 1254

Quazepam (Additive effects). Products include:
Doral Tablets ... 2383

Secobarbital Sodium (Additive effects). Products include:
Seconal Sodium Pulvules ... 1296

Selegiline Hydrochloride (Prolongs anticholinergic effects of Tavist). Products include:
Eldepryl ... 2250

Sufentanil Citrate (Additive effects). Products include:
Sufenta Injection ... 1147

Temazepam (Additive effects). Products include:
Restoril Capsules ... 2023

Thiamylal Sodium (Additive effects). Products include:
Surital Ampoules, Steri-Vials ... 1764

Thioridazine Hydrochloride (Additive effects). Products include:
Mellaril ... 2011

Thiothixene (Additive effects). Products include:
Navane Capsules and Concentrate 1954
Navane Intramuscular ... 1956

Tranylcypromine Sulfate (Prolongs anticholinergic effects of Tavist). Products include:
Parnate Tablets ... 2222

Triazolam (Additive effects). Products include:
Halcion Tablets ... 2340

Trifluoperazine Hydrochloride (Additive effects). Products include:
Stelazine ... 2226

TAVIST TABLETS
(Clemastine Fumarate) ... 2035
May interact with monoamine oxidase inhibitors, central nervous system depressants, hypnotics and sedatives, tranquilizers, and certain other agents. Compounds in these categories include:

Alcohol (Additive effects).

Alfentanil Hydrochloride (Additive effects). Products include:
Alfenta Injection ... 1131

Alprazolam (Additive effects). Products include:
Xanax Tablets ... 2367

Aprobarbital (Additive effects). Products include:
Alurate Elixir ... 1883

Buprenorphine (Additive effects).
No products indexed under this heading.

Buspirone Hydrochloride (Additive effects). Products include:
BuSpar ... 1401

Butabarbital (Additive effects). Products include:
Pyridium Plus ... 1764

Butalbital (Additive effects). Products include:
Esgic-Plus Tablets ... 1002
Esgic Tablets & Capsules ... 1001
Fioricet Tablets ... 2006
Fiorinal Capsules ... 2007
Fiorinal with Codeine Capsules ... 2008
Fiorinal Tablets ... 2007
Phrenilin ... 838
Sedapap Tablets 50 mg/650 mg .. 1360

Chlordiazepoxide (Additive effects). Products include:
- Libritabs Tablets 1930
- Limbitrol 1933
- Menrium Tablets 1934

Chlordiazepoxide Hydrochloride (Additive effects). Products include:
- Librax Capsules 1929
- Librium Capsules 1931
- Librium Injectable 1932

Chlorpromazine (Additive effects). Products include:
- Thorazine 2234

Chlorprothixene (Additive effects). Products include:
- Taractan Tablets 1920

Chlorprothixene Hydrochloride (Additive effects). Products include:
- Taractan 1920

Chlorprothixene Lactate (Additive effects). Products include:
- Taractan Concentrate 1920

Clorazepate Dipotassium (Additive effects). Products include:
- Tranxene 556

Codeine (Additive effects). Products include:
- Calcidrine Syrup 506

Codeine Phosphate (Additive effects). Products include:
- Actifed with Codeine Cough Syrup 752
- Cheracol Cough Syrup 1853
- Codimal PH Syrup 846
- Dimetane-DC Cough Syrup 1857
- Empirin with Codeine Phosphate Nos. 2, 3 & 4 764
- Fiorinal with Codeine Capsules 2008
- Isoclor Expectorant 982
- Naldecon CX Adult Liquid 521
- Novahistine DH 1342
- Novahistine Expectorant 1343
- Nucofed Capsules 2219
- Nucofed Expectorant 2219
- Nucofed Pediatric Expectorant 2220
- Nucofed Syrup 2219
- Phenaphen with Codeine Capsules 1865
- Phenaphen-650 with Codeine Tablets 1866
- Phenergan with Codeine 2497
- Phenergan VC with Codeine 2501
- Robitussin A-C Syrup 1875
- Robitussin-DAC Syrup 1875
- Ryna 741
- Soma Compound w/Codeine Tablets 2390
- Triaminic Expectorant w/Codeine 1996
- Tussi-Organidin Liquid 2391
- Tylenol with Codeine 1381

Codeine Polistirex (Additive effects).
- No products indexed under this heading.

Dezocine (Additive effects).

Diazepam (Additive effects). Products include:
- Valium Injectable 1937
- Valium Tablets 1939
- Valrelease Capsules 1923

Droperidol (Additive effects). Products include:
- Inapsine Injection 1140
- Innovar Injection 1141

Enflurane (Additive effects). Products include:
- Ethrane 599

Estazolam (Additive effects). Products include:
- ProSom Tablets 554

Ethchlorvynol (Additive effects). Products include:
- Placidyl Capsules 553

Ethinamate (Additive effects).
- No products indexed under this heading.

Fentanyl (Additive effects). Products include:
- Duragesic Transdermal System 1133

Fentanyl Citrate (Additive effects). Products include:
- Innovar Injection 1141
- Sublimaze Injection 1146

Fluphenazine Decanoate (Additive effects). Products include:
- Prolixin Decanoate 1795

Fluphenazine Enanthate (Additive effects). Products include:
- Prolixin Enanthate 1796

Fluphenazine Hydrochloride (Additive effects). Products include:
- Prolixin Elixir 1793
- Prolixin Injection 1791
- Prolixin Oral Concentrate 1792
- Prolixin Tablets 1793

Flurazepam Hydrochloride (Additive effects). Products include:
- Dalmane Capsules 1927

Furazolidone (Prolongs anticholinergic effects of Tavist; concurrent use is contraindicated). Products include:
- Furoxone 1855

Glutethimide (Additive effects).
- No products indexed under this heading.

Haloperidol (Additive effects). Products include:
- Haldol Injection, Tablets and Concentrate 1373

Haloperidol Decanoate (Additive effects). Products include:
- Haldol Decanoate 1375

Hydrocodone Bitartrate (Additive effects). Products include:
- Anexsia 5/500 Tablets 2196
- Anexsia 7.5/650 Tablets 2197
- Azdone Tablets 844
- Codiclear DH Syrup 845
- Codimal DH Syrup 846
- Damason-P 1356
- Hycodan Syrup, Tablets 927
- Hycomine Compound Tablets 929
- Hycomine Syrup 927
- Hycotuss Expectorant Syrup 930
- Hydrocet Capsules 835
- Lortab ASA Tablets 2414
- Lortab 2412
- Ru-Tuss with Hydrocodone 694
- Triaminic Expectorant DH 1995
- Vicodin Tablets 1187
- Vicodin ES Tablets 1189
- Zydone Capsules 941

Hydrocodone Polistirex (Additive effects). Products include:
- Tussionex Extended-Release Suspension 988

Hydroxyzine Hydrochloride (Additive effects). Products include:
- Atarax Tablets & Syrup 1941
- Marax Tablets & DF Syrup 1954
- Vistaril Intramuscular Solution 1970

Isocarboxazid (Prolongs anticholinergic effects of Tavist; concurrent use is contraindicated). Products include:
- Marplan Tablets 1906

Isoflurane (Additive effects). Products include:
- Forane 600

Ketamine Hydrochloride (Additive effects). Products include:
- Ketalar 1726

Levorphanol Tartrate (Additive effects). Products include:
- Levo-Dromoran 1906

Lorazepam (Additive effects). Products include:
- Ativan Injection 2432
- Ativan Tablets 2434

Loxapine Hydrochloride (Additive effects). Products include:
- Loxitane 1213

Loxapine Succinate (Additive effects). Products include:
- Loxitane Capsules 1213

Meperidine Hydrochloride (Additive effects). Products include:
- Demerol 2047
- Mepergan Injection 2479

Mephobarbital (Additive effects). Products include:
- Mebaral Tablets 2061

Meprobamate (Additive effects). Products include:
- Deprol Tablets 2382
- Equagesic Tablets 2451
- Miltown Tablets 2386
- PMB 200 and PMB 400 2504

Mesoridazine (Additive effects). Products include:
- Serentil 686

Methadone Hydrochloride (Additive effects). Products include:
- Dolophine Hydrochloride Ampoules & Vials 1260
- Dolophine Hydrochloride Tablets 1261
- Methadone Hydrochloride Diskets 1284
- Methadone Hydrochloride Oral Solution & Tablets 1987

Methohexital Sodium (Additive effects). Products include:
- Brevital Sodium Vials 1248

Methoxyflurane (Additive effects).
- No products indexed under this heading.

Midazolam Hydrochloride (Additive effects). Products include:
- Versed Injection 1924

Molindone Hydrochloride (Additive effects). Products include:
- Moban Tablets & Concentrate 932

Morphine Sulfate (Additive effects). Products include:
- Astramorph/PF Injection, USP (Preservative-Free) 618
- Duramorph 960
- Infumorph 200 and Infumorph 500 Sterile Solutions 962
- MS Contin Tablets 1814
- MSIR 1817
- Oramorph SR (Morphine Sulfate Sustained Release Tablets) 1988
- Roxanol 1991

Opium Alkaloids (Additive effects). Products include:
- B & O No. 15A & No. 16A Supprettes 2395
- Pantopon Injectable 1911

Oxazepam (Additive effects). Products include:
- Serax Capsules 2522
- Serax Tablets 2522

Oxycodone Hydrochloride (Additive effects). Products include:
- Percocet Tablets 950
- Percodan 951
- Roxicodone Tablets, Oral Solution & Intensol (Oxycodone) 1992
- Tylox Capsules 1382

Pentobarbital Sodium (Additive effects). Products include:
- Nembutal Sodium Capsules 534
- Nembutal Sodium Solution 536
- Nembutal Sodium Suppositories 538

Perphenazine (Additive effects). Products include:
- Etrafon 2087
- Triavil Tablets 1556
- Trilafon 2123

Phenelzine Sulfate (Prolongs anticholinergic effects of Tavist; concurrent use is contraindicated). Products include:
- Nardil 1742

Phenobarbital (Additive effects). Products include:
- Arco-Lase Plus Tablets 607
- Bellergal-S Tablets 1998
- Bronkolixir 761
- Bronkotabs Tablets 762
- Donnatal 1858
- Donnatal Extentabs 1859
- Donnatal Tablets 1858
- Donnazyme Tablets 1860
- Kinesed Tablets 2272
- Phenobarbital Elixir and Tablets 1293
- Primatene Tablets-P Formula 2421
- Quadrinal Tablets 1183
- Tedral SA 1765

Prazepam (Additive effects). Products include:
- Centrax 1693

Prochlorperazine (Additive effects). Products include:
- Compazine 2201

Promethazine Hydrochloride (Additive effects). Products include:
- Mepergan Injection 2479
- Phenergan with Codeine 2497
- Phenergan with Dextromethorphan 2499
- Phenergan Injection 2493
- Phenergan Suppositories 2496
- Phenergan Syrup 2495
- Phenergan Tablets 2496
- Phenergan VC 2500
- Phenergan VC with Codeine 2501

Propofol (Additive effects). Products include:
- Diprivan Injection 2267

Propoxyphene Hydrochloride (Additive effects). Products include:
- Darvon 1256
- Wygesic Tablets 2540

Propoxyphene Napsylate (Additive effects). Products include:
- Darvon-N/Darvocet-N 1254

Quazepam (Additive effects). Products include:
- Doral Tablets 2383

Secobarbital Sodium (Additive effects). Products include:
- Seconal Sodium Pulvules 1296

Selegiline Hydrochloride (Prolongs anticholinergic effects of Tavist; concurrent use is contraindicated). Products include:
- Eldepryl 2250

Sufentanil Citrate (Additive effects). Products include:
- Sufenta Injection 1147

Temazepam (Additive effects). Products include:
- Restoril Capsules 2023

Thiamylal Sodium (Additive effects). Products include:
- Surital Ampoules, Steri-Vials 1764

Thioridazine Hydrochloride (Additive effects). Products include:
- Mellaril 2011

Thiothixene (Additive effects). Products include:
- Navane Capsules and Concentrate 1954
- Navane Intramuscular 1956

Tranylcypromine Sulfate (Prolongs anticholinergic effects of Tavist; concurrent use is contraindicated). Products include:
- Parnate Tablets 2222

Triazolam (Additive effects). Products include:
- Halcion Tablets 2340

Trifluoperazine Hydrochloride (Additive effects). Products include:
- Stelazine 2226

TAVIST-1 TABLETS

(Clemastine Fumarate) 2035

See **Tavist Tablets**

TAVIST-D TABLETS

(Clemastine Fumarate, Phenylpropanolamine Hydrochloride) 2035

May interact with monoamine oxidase inhibitors, central nervous system depressants, hypnotics and sedatives, tranquilizers, veratrum alkaloids, and certain other agents. Compounds in these categories include:

Alcohol (Additive effects).

Alfentanil Hydrochloride (Additive effects). Products include:
- Alfenta Injection 1131

Alprazolam (Additive effects). Products include:
- Xanax Tablets 2367

Aprobarbital (Additive effects). Products include:
- Alurate Elixir ... 1883

Buprenorphine (Additive effects).
- No products indexed under this heading.

Buspirone Hydrochloride (Additive effects). Products include:
- BuSpar ... 1401

Butabarbital (Additive effects). Products include:
- Pyridium Plus ... 1764

Butalbital (Additive effects). Products include:
- Esgic-Plus Tablets ... 1002
- Esgic Tablets & Capsules ... 1001
- Fioricet Tablets ... 2006
- Fiorinal Capsules ... 2007
- Fiorinal with Codeine Capsules ... 2008
- Fiorinal Tablets ... 2007
- Phrenilin ... 838
- Sedapap Tablets 50 mg/650 mg ... 1360

Chlordiazepoxide (Additive effects). Products include:
- Libritabs Tablets ... 1930
- Limbitrol ... 1933
- Menrium Tablets ... 1934

Chlordiazepoxide Hydrochloride (Additive effects). Products include:
- Librax Capsules ... 1929
- Librium Capsules ... 1931
- Librium Injectable ... 1932

Chlorpromazine (Additive effects). Products include:
- Thorazine ... 2234

Chlorprothixene (Additive effects). Products include:
- Taractan Tablets ... 1920

Chlorprothixene Hydrochloride (Additive effects). Products include:
- Taractan ... 1920

Chlorprothixene Lactate (Additive effects). Products include:
- Taractan Concentrate ... 1920

Clorazepate Dipotassium (Additive effects). Products include:
- Tranxene ... 556

Codeine (Additive effects). Products include:
- Calcidrine Syrup ... 506

Codeine Phosphate (Additive effects). Products include:
- Actifed with Codeine Cough Syrup ... 752
- Cheracol Cough Syrup ... 1853
- Codimal PH Syrup ... 846
- Dimetane-DC Cough Syrup ... 1857
- Empirin with Codeine Phosphate Nos. 2, 3 & 4 ... 764
- Fiorinal with Codeine Capsules ... 2008
- Isoclor Expectorant ... 982
- Naldecon CX Adult Liquid ... ▣ 521
- Novahistine DH ... 1342
- Novahistine Expectorant ... 1343
- Nucofed Capsules ... 2219
- Nucofed Expectorant ... 2219
- Nucofed Pediatric Expectorant ... 2220
- Nucofed Syrup ... 2219
- Phenaphen with Codeine Capsules 1865
- Phenaphen-650 with Codeine Tablets ... 1866
- Phenergan with Codeine ... 2497
- Phenergan VC with Codeine ... 2501
- Robitussin A-C Syrup ... 1875
- Robitussin-DAC Syrup ... 1875
- Ryna ... ▣ 741
- Soma Compound w/Codeine Tablets ... 2390
- Triaminic Expectorant w/Codeine ... 1996
- Tussi-Organidin Liquid ... 2391
- Tylenol with Codeine ... 1381

Codeine Polistirex (Additive effects).
- No products indexed under this heading.

Cryptenamine Preparations (Reduced antihypertensive effects).

Dezocine (Additive effects).

Diazepam (Additive effects). Products include:
- Valium Injectable ... 1937
- Valium Tablets ... 1939
- Valrelease Capsules ... 1923

Droperidol (Additive effects). Products include:
- Inapsine Injection ... 1140
- Innovar Injection ... 1141

Enflurane (Additive effects). Products include:
- Ethrane ... 599

Estazolam (Additive effects). Products include:
- ProSom Tablets ... 554

Ethchlorvynol (Additive effects). Products include:
- Placidyl Capsules ... 553

Ethinamate (Additive effects).
- No products indexed under this heading.

Fentanyl (Additive effects). Products include:
- Duragesic Transdermal System ... 1133

Fentanyl Citrate (Additive effects). Products include:
- Innovar Injection ... 1141
- Sublimaze Injection ... 1146

Fluphenazine Decanoate (Additive effects). Products include:
- Prolixin Decanoate ... 1795

Fluphenazine Enanthate (Additive effects). Products include:
- Prolixin Enanthate ... 1796

Fluphenazine Hydrochloride (Additive effects). Products include:
- Prolixin Elixir ... 1793
- Prolixin Injection ... 1791
- Prolixin Oral Concentrate ... 1792
- Prolixin Tablets ... 1793

Flurazepam Hydrochloride (Additive effects). Products include:
- Dalmane Capsules ... 1927

Furazolidone (Concurrent administration is contraindicated; prolongs and intensifies the anticholinergic effects of antihistamines and potentiates the pressor effects of sympathomimetics). Products include:
- Furoxone ... 1855

Glutethimide (Additive effects).
- No products indexed under this heading.

Haloperidol (Additive effects). Products include:
- Haldol Injection, Tablets and Concentrate ... 1373

Haloperidol Decanoate (Additive effects). Products include:
- Haldol Decanoate ... 1375

Hydrocodone Bitartrate (Additive effects). Products include:
- Anexsia 5/500 Tablets ... 2196
- Anexsia 7.5/650 Tablets ... 2197
- Azdone Tablets ... 844
- Codiclear DH Syrup ... 845
- Codimal DH Syrup ... 846
- Damason-P ... 1356
- Hycodan Syrup, Tablets ... 927
- Hycomine Compound Tablets ... 929
- Hycomine Syrup ... 927
- Hycotuss Expectorant Syrup ... 930
- Hydrocet Capsules ... 835
- Lortab ASA Tablets ... 2414
- Lortab ... 2412
- Ru-Tuss with Hydrocodone ... 694
- Triaminic Expectorant DH ... 1995
- Vicodin Tablets ... 1187
- Vicodin ES Tablets ... 1189
- Zydone Capsules ... 941

Hydrocodone Polistirex (Additive effects). Products include:
- Tussionex Extended-Release Suspension ... 988

Hydroxyzine Hydrochloride (Additive effects). Products include:
- Atarax Tablets & Syrup ... 1941
- Marax Tablets & DF Syrup ... 1954
- Vistaril Intramuscular Solution ... 1970

Isocarboxazid (Concurrent administration is contraindicated; prolongs and intensifies the anticholinergic effects of antihistamines and potentiates the pressor effects of sympathomimetics). Products include:
- Marplan Tablets ... 1906

Isoflurane (Additive effects). Products include:
- Forane ... 600

Ketamine Hydrochloride (Additive effects). Products include:
- Ketalar ... 1726

Levorphanol Tartrate (Additive effects). Products include:
- Levo-Dromoran ... 1906

Lorazepam (Additive effects). Products include:
- Ativan Injection ... 2432
- Ativan Tablets ... 2434

Loxapine Hydrochloride (Additive effects). Products include:
- Loxitane ... 1213

Loxapine Succinate (Additive effects). Products include:
- Loxitane Capsules ... 1213

Mecamylamine Hydrochloride (Reduced antihypertensive effects). Products include:
- Inversine Tablets ... 1492

Meperidine Hydrochloride (Additive effects). Products include:
- Demerol ... 2047
- Mepergan Injection ... 2479

Mephobarbital (Additive effects). Products include:
- Mebaral Tablets ... 2061

Meprobamate (Additive effects). Products include:
- Deprol Tablets ... 2382
- Equagesic Tablets ... 2451
- Miltown Tablets ... 2386
- PMB 200 and PMB 400 ... 2504

Mesoridazine (Additive effects). Products include:
- Serentil ... 686

Methadone Hydrochloride (Additive effects). Products include:
- Dolophine Hydrochloride Ampoules & Vials ... 1260
- Dolophine Hydrochloride Tablets ... 1261
- Methadone Hydrochloride Diskets ... 1284
- Methadone Hydrochloride Oral Solution & Tablets ... 1987

Methohexital Sodium (Additive effects). Products include:
- Brevital Sodium Vials ... 1248

Methoxyflurane (Additive effects).
- No products indexed under this heading.

Methyldopa (Reduced antihypertensive effects). Products include:
- Aldoclor Tablets ... 1413
- Aldomet Oral ... 1415
- Aldoril Tablets ... 1418

Methyldopate Hydrochloride (Reduced antihypertensive effects). Products include:
- Aldomet Ester HCl Injection ... 1417

Midazolam Hydrochloride (Additive effects). Products include:
- Versed Injection ... 1924

Molindone Hydrochloride (Additive effects). Products include:
- Moban Tablets & Concentrate ... 932

Morphine Sulfate (Additive effects). Products include:
- Astramorph/PF Injection, USP (Preservative-Free) ... 618
- Duramorph ... 960
- Infumorph 200 and Infumorph 500 Sterile Solutions ... 962
- MS Contin Tablets ... 1814
- MSIR ... 1817
- Oramorph SR (Morphine Sulfate Sustained Release Tablets) ... 1988
- Roxanol ... 1991

Opium Alkaloids (Additive effects). Products include:
- B & O No. 15A & No. 16A Supprettes ... 2395
- Pantopon Injectable ... 1911

Oxazepam (Additive effects). Products include:
- Serax Capsules ... 2522
- Serax Tablets ... 2522

Oxycodone Hydrochloride (Additive effects). Products include:
- Percocet Tablets ... 950
- Percodan ... 951
- Roxicodone Tablets, Oral Solution & Intensol (Oxycodone) ... 1992
- Tylox Capsules ... 1382

Pentobarbital Sodium (Additive effects). Products include:
- Nembutal Sodium Capsules ... 534
- Nembutal Sodium Solution ... 536
- Nembutal Sodium Suppositories ... 538

Perphenazine (Additive effects). Products include:
- Etrafon ... 2087
- Triavil Tablets ... 1556
- Trilafon ... 2123

Phenelzine Sulfate (Concurrent administration is contraindicated; prolongs and intensifies the anticholinergic effects of antihistamines and potentiates the pressor effects of sympathomimetics). Products include:
- Nardil ... 1742

Phenobarbital (Additive effects). Products include:
- Arco-Lase Plus Tablets ... 607
- Bellergal-S Tablets ... 1998
- Bronkolixir ... ▣ 761
- Bronkotabs Tablets ... ▣ 762
- Donnatal ... 1858
- Donnatal Extentabs ... 1859
- Donnatal Tablets ... 1858
- Donnazyme Tablets ... 1860
- Kinesed Tablets ... 2272
- Phenobarbital Elixir and Tablets ... 1293
- Primatene Tablets-P Formula ... 2421
- Quadrinal Tablets ... 1183
- Tedral SA ... 1765

Prazepam (Additive effects). Products include:
- Centrax ... 1693

Prochlorperazine (Additive effects). Products include:
- Compazine ... 2201

Promethazine Hydrochloride (Additive effects). Products include:
- Mepergan Injection ... 2479
- Phenergan with Codeine ... 2497
- Phenergan with Dextromethorphan 2499
- Phenergan Injection ... 2493
- Phenergan Suppositories ... 2496
- Phenergan Syrup ... 2495
- Phenergan Tablets ... 2496
- Phenergan VC ... 2500
- Phenergan VC with Codeine ... 2501

Propofol (Additive effects). Products include:
- Diprivan Injection ... 2267

Propoxyphene Hydrochloride (Additive effects). Products include:
- Darvon ... 1256
- Wygesic Tablets ... 2540

Propoxyphene Napsylate (Additive effects). Products include:
- Darvon-N/Darvocet-N ... 1254

Quazepam (Additive effects). Products include:
- Doral Tablets ... 2383

Reserpine (Reduced antihypertensive effects). Products include:
- Diupres Tablets ... 1461
- Hydromox R Tablets ... 1209
- Hydropres Tablets ... 1485
- Renese-R Tablets ... 1786
- Salutensin/Salutensin-Demi ... 719
- Ser-Ap-Es Tablets ... 881
- Serpasil Tablets ... 883
- Serpasil-Apresoline Tablets ... 884
- Serpasil-Esidrix Tablets ... 886

Secobarbital Sodium (Additive effects). Products include:
- Seconal Sodium Pulvules ... 1296

Selegiline Hydrochloride (Concurrent administration is contraindicated; prolongs and intensifies the anticholinergic effects of antihistamines and potentiates the pressor effects of sympathomimetics). Products include:
- Eldepryl ... 2250

Sufentanil Citrate (Additive effects). Products include:
- Sufenta Injection ... 1147

Temazepam (Additive effects). Products include:
- Restoril Capsules ... 2023

Thiamylal Sodium (Additive effects). Products include:
- Surital Ampoules, Steri-Vials ... 1764

Thioridazine Hydrochloride (Additive effects). Products include:
- Mellaril ... 2011

Thiothixene (Additive effects). Products include:
- Navane Capsules and Concentrate 1954
- Navane Intramuscular ... 1956

Tranylcypromine Sulfate (Concurrent administration is contraindicated; prolongs and intensifies the anticholinergic effects of antihistamines and potentiates the pressor effects of sympathomimetics). Products include:
- Parnate Tablets ... 2222

Triazolam (Additive effects). Products include:
- Halcion Tablets ... 2340

Trifluoperazine Hydrochloride (Additive effects). Products include:
- Stelazine ... 2226

TAZICEF FOR INJECTION
(Ceftazidime) ... 2231
May interact with aminoglycosides and certain other agents. Compounds in these categories include:

Amikacin Sulfate (Nephrotoxicity). Products include:
- Amikin Injectable ... 602

Bumetanide (Nephrotoxicity). Products include:
- Bumex ... 1895

Ethacrynic Acid (Nephrotoxicity). Products include:
- Edecrin Tablets ... 1468

Furosemide (Nephrotoxicity). Products include:
- Lasix ... 1093

Gentamicin Sulfate (Nephrotoxicity). Products include:
- Garamycin Injectable ... 2093
- Garamycin Ophthalmic ... ◉ 305
- Genoptic Liquifilm Sterile Ophthalmic Solution ... ◉ 247
- Genoptic S.O.P. Sterile Ophthalmic Ointment ... ◉ 247
- Gentacidin Ointment ... ◉ 273
- Gentacidin Solution ... ◉ 273
- Gentak Ointment & Solution ... ◉ 208
- G-myticin Creme and Ointment 0.1% ... 1770
- Pred-G Liquifilm Sterile Ophthalmic Suspension ... ◉ 252
- Pred-G S.O.P. Sterile Ophthalmic Ointment ... ◉ 253

Kanamycin Sulfate (Nephrotoxicity). Products include:
- Kantrex Injection ... 601
- Kantrex Pediatric Injection ... 601

Streptomycin Sulfate (Nephrotoxicity).
- No products indexed under this heading.

Tobramycin Sulfate (Nephrotoxicity). Products include:
- Nebcin Vials, Hyporets & ADD-Vantage ... 1286

TAZIDIME VIALS, FASPAK & ADD-VANTAGE
(Ceftazidime) ... 1299
May interact with aminoglycosides and certain other agents. Compounds in these categories include:

Amikacin Sulfate (Potential for nephrotoxicity and ototoxicity; monitor renal function). Products include:
- Amikin Injectable ... 602

Furosemide (Nephrotoxicity). Products include:
- Lasix ... 1093

Gentamicin Sulfate (Potential for nephrotoxicity and ototoxicity; monitor renal function). Products include:
- Garamycin Injectable ... 2093
- Garamycin Ophthalmic ... ◉ 305
- Genoptic Liquifilm Sterile Ophthalmic Solution ... ◉ 247
- Genoptic S.O.P. Sterile Ophthalmic Ointment ... ◉ 247
- Gentacidin Ointment ... ◉ 273
- Gentacidin Solution ... ◉ 273
- Gentak Ointment & Solution ... ◉ 208
- G-myticin Creme and Ointment 0.1% ... 1770
- Pred-G Liquifilm Sterile Ophthalmic Suspension ... ◉ 252
- Pred-G S.O.P. Sterile Ophthalmic Ointment ... ◉ 253

Kanamycin Sulfate (Potential for nephrotoxicity and ototoxicity; monitor renal function). Products include:
- Kantrex Injection ... 601
- Kantrex Pediatric Injection ... 601

Streptomycin Sulfate (Potential for nephrotoxicity and ototoxicity; monitor renal function).
- No products indexed under this heading.

Tobramycin (Potential for nephrotoxicity and ototoxicity; monitor renal function). Products include:
- TobraDex Ophthalmic Suspension and Ointment ... ◉ 228
- Tobrex Ophthalmic Ointment and Solution ... 572

Tobramycin Sulfate (Potential for nephrotoxicity and ototoxicity; monitor renal function). Products include:
- Nebcin Vials, Hyporets & ADD-Vantage ... 1286

TEARS NATURALE II LUBRICANT EYE DROPS
(Dextran 70, Hydroxypropyl Methylcellulose) ... 572
No interactions described in labeling.

TEARS NATURALE FREE
(Dextran 70, Hydroxypropyl Methylcellulose) ... 572
No interactions described in labeling.

TEARS PLUS LUBRICANT OPHTHALMIC SOLUTION
(Polyvinyl Alcohol, Povidone) ... ◉ 256
No interactions described in labeling.

TEARS RENEWED OINTMENT
(Petrolatum, White) ... ◉ 209
No interactions described in labeling.

TEARS RENEWED SOLUTION
(Dextran 70) ... ◉ 209
No interactions described in labeling.

TECNU POISON OAK-N-IVY CLEANER
(Alkanes, mixed) ... ■ 732
No interactions described in labeling.

TEDRAL SA
(Theophylline Anhydrous, Ephedrine Hydrochloride, Phenobarbital) ... 1765
No interactions described in labeling.

TEGISON CAPSULES
(Etretinate) ... 1881
May interact with:

Vitamin A (Additive toxic effects). Products include:
- Aquasol A Vitamin A Capsules, USP ... 615
- Aquasol A Parenteral, USP ... 615
- Bugs Bunny Children's Chewable Vitamins (Sugar Free) ... ■ 625
- Bugs Bunny With Extra C Children's Chewable Vitamins (Sugar Free) ... ■ 626
- Bugs Bunny/Flintstones ... ■ 625
- Flintstones Children's Chewable Vitamins With Extra C ... ■ 626
- Flintstones Children's Chewable Vitamins Plus Iron ... ■ 625
- Lazer Creme ... 1770
- Myadec ... ■ 640
- Natalins Rx ... 1391
- Natalins Tablets ... 1391
- Ocuvite Vitamin and Mineral Supplement ... ◉ 312
- One-A-Day Essential Vitamins ... ■ 627
- One-A-Day Maximum Formula Vitamins and Minerals ... ■ 627
- One-A-Day Plus Extra C Vitamins ... ■ 627
- Stressgard Stress Formula Vitamins ... ■ 628
- Tri-Vi-Flor 1.0 mg Vitamins with Fluoride Chewable Tablets ... 1400
- Tri-Vi-Flor Drops ... 1400
- Tri-Vi-Sol Vitamin Drops ... ■ 614
- Tri-Vi-Sol Vitamin Drops with Iron ■ 614
- Vicon Forte Capsules ... 2416
- Vicon Plus ... ■ 682
- Vi-Daylin ADC Vitamins Drops ... 1980
- Vi-Daylin ADC Vitamins + Iron Drops ... 1980
- Vi-Daylin/F ADC Vitamins Drops With Fluoride ... 1981
- Vi-Daylin/F ADC Vitamins + Iron Drops With Fluoride ... 1981
- Vi-Zac ... ■ 682
- Within Women's Formula Multivitamin with Calcium, Extra Iron and Zinc ... ■ 628
- Zymacap Capsules ... ■ 670

Food Interactions

Dairy products (Increases absorption of etretinate).

Diet, high-lipid (Increases absorption of etretinate).

TEGRETOL CHEWABLE TABLETS
(Carbamazepine) ... 654
See **Tegretol Tablets**

TEGRETOL SUSPENSION
(Carbamazepine) ... 656
May interact with monoamine oxidase inhibitors, xanthine bronchodilators, calcium channel blockers, lithium preparations, oral contraceptives, anticonvulsants, and certain other agents. Compounds in these categories include:

Aminophylline (Half-life of theophylline significantly shortened). Products include:
- Amesec ... ■ 682
- Aminophyllin Tablets ... 2153

Bepridil Hydrochloride (Possible carbamazepine toxicity). Products include:
- Vascor (200, 300 and 400 mg) Tablets ... 1383

Cimetidine (Possible carbamazepine toxicity). Products include:
- Tagamet Tablets ... 2228

Cimetidine Hydrochloride (Possible carbamazepine toxicity). Products include:
- Tagamet ... 2228

Diltiazem Hydrochloride (Possible carbamazepine toxicity). Products include:
- Cardizem Tablets-30 mg, 60 mg, 90 mg and 120 mg ... 1329
- Cardizem SR Capsules-60 mg, 90 mg and 120 mg ... 1327

Divalproex Sodium (Combination therapy may alter thyroid function; valproic acid serum levels may be reduced). Products include:
- Depakote ... 512

Doxycycline Calcium (Half-life of doxycycline significantly shortened).
- No products indexed under this heading.

Doxycycline Hyclate (Half-life of doxycycline significantly shortened). Products include:
- Doryx Capsules ... 1717
- Vibramycin Hyclate Capsules ... 1787
- Vibramycin Hyclate Intravenous ... 1968
- Vibra-Tabs Film Coated Tablets ... 1787

Doxycycline Monohydrate (Half-life of doxycycline significantly shortened). Products include:
- Monodox Capsules ... 1630
- Vibramycin Monohydrate for Oral Suspension ... 1787

Dyphylline (Half-life of theophylline significantly shortened). Products include:
- Dilor ... 2079
- Dilor-G Tablets & Liquid ... 2079
- Lufyllin Elixir ... 2384
- Lufyllin & Lufyllin-400 Tablets ... 2384
- Lufyllin-GG Elixir & Tablets ... 2385

Erythromycin (Possible carbamazepine toxicity). Products include:
- A/T/S Topical Gel and Topical Solution ... 1089
- AK-Mycin Ointment ... ◉ 204
- Benzamycin Topical Gel ... 907
- E-Mycin Tablets ... 688
- ETS-2% ... 1685
- ERYC ... 1720
- Erycette (erythromycin 2%) Topical Solution ... 1678
- Ery-Tab Tablets ... 521
- Erythromycin Base Filmtab ... 525
- Erythromycin Delayed-Release Capsules, USP ... 526
- Ilotycin Ophthalmic Ointment ... 915
- PCE Dispertab Tablets ... 549
- Pediazole ... 1973
- T-Stat 2.0% Topical Solution and Pads ... 2409
- Theramycin Z Topical Solution 2% 1410

Erythromycin Estolate (Possible carbamazepine toxicity). Products include:
- Ilosone ... 913

Erythromycin Ethylsuccinate (Possible carbamazepine toxicity). Products include:
- E.E.S. ... 522
- EryPed ... 519
- Pediazole ... 1973

Erythromycin Gluceptate (Possible carbamazepine toxicity). Products include:
- Ilotycin Gluceptate, IV, Vials ... 915

Erythromycin Lactobionate (Possible carbamazepine toxicity).
- No products indexed under this heading.

Erythromycin Stearate (Possible carbamazepine toxicity). Products include:
- Erythrocin Stearate Filmtab ... 523

Ethinyl Estradiol (Potential for breakthrough bleeding; reliability of oral contraceptives may be adversely affected). Products include:
- Brevicon ... 2304
- Demulen ... 2161
- Estinyl Tablets ... 2085
- Jenest-28 Tablets ... 1636
- Levlen/Tri-Levlen ... 665
- Lo/Ovral Tablets ... 2471
- Lo/Ovral-28 Tablets ... 2476
- Loestrin ... 1728
- Modicon ... 1667
- Nordette-21 Tablets ... 2481
- Nordette-28 Tablets ... 2483
- Norethin ... 2133
- Norinyl ... 2304
- Norlestrin ... 1746

Ortho-Cyclen Tablets 1658
Ortho-Novum 1667
Ovcon 1391
Ovral Tablets 2490
Ovral-28 Tablets 2491
Levlen/Tri-Levlen 665
Tri-Norinyl 2304
Triphasil-21 Tablets 2527
Triphasil-28 Tablets 2532

Ethosuximide (Combination therapy may alter thyroid function). Products include:
Zarontin Capsules 1768
Zarontin Syrup 1769

Ethotoin (Combination therapy may alter thyroid function). Products include:
Peganone Tablets 551

Ethynodiol Diacetate (Potential for breakthrough bleeding; reliability of oral contraceptives may be adversely affected). Products include:
Demulen 2161

Felodipine (Possible carbamazepine toxicity). Products include:
Plendil Extended-Release Tablets 1526

Furazolidone (Concurrent use contraindicated). Products include:
Furoxone 1855

Haloperidol (Haloperidol serum levels may be reduced). Products include:
Haldol Injection, Tablets and Concentrate 1373

Haloperidol Decanoate (Haloperidol serum levels may be reduced). Products include:
Haldol Decanoate 1375

Isocarboxazid (Concurrent use contraindicated). Products include:
Marplan Tablets 1906

Isoniazid (Possible carbamazepine toxicity). Products include:
INH Tablets 868
Rifamate Capsules 1347

Isradipine (Possible carbamazepine toxicity). Products include:
DynaCirc Capsules 2004

Levonorgestrel (Potential for breakthrough bleeding; reliability of oral contraceptives may be adversely affected). Products include:
Levlen/Tri-Levlen 665
Nordette-21 Tablets 2481
Nordette-28 Tablets 2483
Norplant System 2484
Levlen/Tri-Levlen 665
Triphasil-21 Tablets 2527
Triphasil-28 Tablets 2532

Lithium Carbonate (Increased risk of neurotoxic side effects). Products include:
Eskalith 2214
Lithane Tablets 1596
Lithium Carbonate Capsules & Tablets 1984
Lithobid Tablets 870

Lithium Citrate (Increased risk of neurotoxic side effects). Products include:
Cibalith-S 870

Mephenytoin (Combination therapy may alter thyroid function). Products include:
Mesantoin Tablets 2013

Mestranol (Potential for breakthrough bleeding; reliability of oral contraceptives may be adversely affected). Products include:
Enovid 2161
Norethin 2133
Norinyl 2304
Ortho-Novum 1667

Methsuximide (Combination therapy may alter thyroid function). Products include:
Celontin 1692

Nicardipine Hydrochloride (Possible carbamazepine toxicity). Products include:
Cardene Capsules 2290

Nifedipine (Possible carbamazepine toxicity). Products include:
Adalat Capsules (10 mg and 20 mg) 1587
Procardia Capsules 1781
Procardia XL Tablets 1783

Nimodipine (Possible carbamazepine toxicity). Products include:
Nimotop Capsules 1607

Norethindrone (Potential for breakthrough bleeding; reliability of oral contraceptives may be adversely affected). Products include:
Brevicon 2304
Jenest-28 Tablets 1636
Micronor Tablets 1667
Modicon 1667
Norethin 2133
Norinyl 2304
Norlutin 1755
Nor-Q D Tablets 2304
Ortho-Novum 1667
Ovcon 1391
Tri-Norinyl 2304

Norethynodrel (Potential for breakthrough bleeding; reliability of oral contraceptives may be adversely affected). Products include:
Enovid 2161

Norgestimate (Potential for breakthrough bleeding; reliability of oral contraceptives may be adversely affected). Products include:
Ortho-Cyclen Tablets 1658

Norgestrel (Potential for breakthrough bleeding; reliability of oral contraceptives may be adversely affected). Products include:
Lo/Ovral Tablets 2471
Lo/Ovral-28 Tablets 2476
Ovral Tablets 2490
Ovral-28 Tablets 2491
Ovrette Tablets 2492

Paramethadione (Combination therapy may alter thyroid function). Products include:
Paradione Capsules 548

Phenacemide (Combination therapy may alter thyroid function). Products include:
Phenurone Tablets 552

Phenelzine Sulfate (Concurrent use contraindicated). Products include:
Nardil 1742

Phenobarbital (Combination therapy may alter thyroid function; marked lowering of serum levels of Tegretol). Products include:
Arco-Lase Plus Tablets 607
Bellergal-S Tablets 1998
Bronkolixir .... ■ 761
Bronkotabs Tablets .... ■ 762
Donnatal 1858
Donnatal Extentabs 1859
Donnatal Tablets 1858
Donnazyme Tablets 1860
Kinesed Tablets 2272
Phenobarbital Elixir and Tablets 1293
Primatene Tablets-P Formula 2421
Quadrinal Tablets 1183
Tedral SA 1765

Phensuximide (Combination therapy may alter thyroid function). Products include:
Milontin Kapseals 1741

Phenytoin (Combination therapy may alter thyroid function; marked lowering of serum levels of Tegretol; phenytoin half-life significantly shortened). Products include:
Dilantin Infatabs 1710
Dilantin-30 Pediatric/Dilantin-125 Suspension 1713

Phenytoin Sodium (Combination therapy may alter thyroid function; marked lowering of serum levels of Tegretol; phenytoin half-life significantly shortened). Products include:
Dilantin Kapseals 1708
Dilantin Parenteral 1712
Dilantin with Phenobarbital Kapseals 1715

Primidone (Combination therapy may alter thyroid function; marked lowering of serum levels of Tegretol). Products include:
Mysoline 2480

Propoxyphene Hydrochloride (Possible carbamazepine toxicity). Products include:
Darvon 1256
Wygesic Tablets 2540

Propoxyphene Napsylate (Possible carbamazepine toxicity). Products include:
Darvon-N/Darvocet-N 1254

Selegiline Hydrochloride (Concurrent use contraindicated). Products include:
Eldepryl 2250

Theophylline (Half-life of theophylline significantly shortened). Products include:
Bronkaid Tablets .... ■ 757
Bronkolixir .... ■ 761
Bronkotabs Tablets .... ■ 762
Constant-T Tablets 1029
Marax Tablets & DF Syrup 1954
Primatene Tablets 2421
Quibron Capsules 713
Quibron-T 714
Quibron-T/SR 716
Theolair Liquid 1317
Theo-Organidin Elixir 2391

Theophylline Anhydrous (Half-life of theophylline significantly shortened). Products include:
Aerolate 994
Primatene Tablets-M Formula .... ■ 753
Primatene Tablets-Regular Formula 2421
Respbid Tablets 684
Slo-bid Gyrocaps 1847
T-PHYL (Uniphyl) 200 mg Tablets 1820
Tedral SA 1765
Theo-24 2179
Theo-Dur Sprinkle 1168
Theo-Dur Extended-Release Tablets 1166
Theolair Tablets 1317
Theolair-SR Tablets 1319
TheoX Extended-Release Tablets 841
Uniphyl 400 mg Tablets 1823

Theophylline Calcium Salicylate (Half-life of theophylline significantly shortened). Products include:
Quadrinal Tablets 1183

Theophylline Sodium Glycinate (Half-life of theophylline significantly shortened). Products include:
Asbron G 1997

Tranylcypromine Sulfate (Concurrent use contraindicated). Products include:
Parnate Tablets 2222

Trimethadione (Combination therapy may alter thyroid function). Products include:
Tridione 557

Valproic Acid (Combination therapy may alter thyroid function; valproic acid serum levels may be reduced). Products include:
Depakene Capsules & Syrup 511

Verapamil Hydrochloride (Possible carbamazepine toxicity). Products include:
Calan SR Caplets 2157
Calan Tablets 2155
Isoptin Injectable 1177
Isoptin Oral Tablets 1179
Isoptin SR Sustained Release Tablets 1181
Verelan Capsules 1243
Verelan Capsules 2535

Warfarin Sodium (Half-life of warfarin significantly shortened). Products include:
Coumadin Injection & Tablets 944
Panwarfin Tablets 547

TEGRETOL TABLETS
(Carbamazepine) 654
May interact with calcium channel blockers, anticonvulsants, oral contraceptives, lithium preparations, xanthine bronchodilators, monoamine oxidase inhibitors, and certain other agents. Compounds in these categories include:

Aminophylline (Half-life significantly shortened when administered concurrently with Tegretol). Products include:
Amesec .... ■ 682
Aminophyllin Tablets 2153

Bepridil Hydrochloride (Elevated plasma levels of carbamazepine). Products include:
Vascor (200, 300 and 400 mg) Tablets 1383

Cimetidine (Elevated plasma levels of carbamazepine). Products include:
Tagamet Tablets 2228

Cimetidine Hydrochloride (Elevated plasma levels of carbamazepine). Products include:
Tagamet 2228

Diltiazem Hydrochloride (Elevated plasma levels of carbamazepine). Products include:
Cardizem Tablets-30 mg, 60 mg, 90 mg and 120 mg 1329
Cardizem SR Capsules-60 mg, 90 mg and 120 mg 1327

Divalproex Sodium (Alterations of thyroid function; valproic acid serum levels may be reduced). Products include:
Depakote 512

Doxycycline Calcium (Half-life significantly shortened when administered concurrently with Tegretol).
No products indexed under this heading.

Doxycycline Hyclate (Half-life significantly shortened when administered concurrently with Tegretol). Products include:
Doryx Capsules 1717
Vibramycin Hyclate Capsules 1787
Vibramycin Hyclate Intravenous 1968
Vibra-Tabs Film Coated Tablets 1787

Doxycycline Monohydrate (Half-life significantly shortened when administered concurrently with Tegretol). Products include:
Monodox Capsules 1630
Vibramycin Monohydrate for Oral Suspension 1787

Dyphylline (Half-life significantly shortened when administered concurrently with Tegretol). Products include:
Dilor 2079
Dilor-G Tablets & Liquid 2079
Lufyllin Elixir 2384
Lufyllin & Lufyllin-400 Tablets 2384
Lufyllin-GG Elixir & Tablets 2385

Erythromycin (Elevated plasma levels of carbamazepine). Products include:
A/T/S Topical Gel and Topical Solution 1089
AK-Mycin Ointment .... ⊙ 204
Benzamycin Topical Gel 907
E-Mycin Tablets 688
ETS-2% 1685
ERYC 1720
Erycette (erythromycin 2%) Topical Solution 1678
Ery-Tab Tablets 521
Erythromycin Base Filmtab 525
Erythromycin Delayed-Release Capsules, USP 526

Ilotycin Ophthalmic Ointment........... 915
PCE Dispertab Tablets 549
Pediazole... 1973
T-Stat 2.0% Topical Solution and Pads 2409
Theramycin Z Topical Solution 2% 1410

Erythromycin Estolate (Elevated plasma levels of carbamazepine). Products include:
Ilosone 913

Erythromycin Ethylsuccinate (Elevated plasma levels of carbamazepine). Products include:
E.E.S. 522
EryPed 519
Pediazole 1973

Erythromycin Gluceptate (Elevated plasma levels of carbamazepine). Products include:
Ilotycin Gluceptate, IV, Vials 915

Erythromycin Lactobionate (Elevated plasma levels of carbamazepine).
No products indexed under this heading.

Erythromycin Stearate (Elevated plasma levels of carbamazepine). Products include:
Erythrocin Stearate Filmtab 523

Ethinyl Estradiol (Breakthrough bleeding may occur). Products include:
Brevicon.. 2304
Demulen 2161
Estinyl Tablets.................................... 2085
Jenest-28 Tablets 1636
Levlen/Tri-Levlen 665
Lo/Ovral Tablets 2471
Lo/Ovral-28 Tablets............................ 2476
Loestrin 1728
Modicon.. 1667
Nordette-21 Tablets........................... 2481
Nordette-28 Tablets........................... 2483
Norethin.. 2133
Norinyl 2304
Norlestrin 1746
Ortho-Cyclen Tablets 1658
Ortho-Novum....................................... 1667
Ovcon 1391
Ovral Tablets....................................... 2490
Ovral-28 Tablets 2491
Levlen/Tri-Levlen 665
Tri-Norinyl... 2304
Triphasil-21 Tablets 2527
Triphasil-28 Tablets............................ 2532

Ethosuximide (Alterations of thyroid function). Products include:
Zarontin Capsules 1768
Zarontin Syrup 1769

Ethotoin (Alterations of thyroid function). Products include:
Peganone Tablets 551

Ethynodiol Diacetate (Breakthrough bleeding may occur). Products include:
Demulen 2161

Felodipine (Elevated plasma levels of carbamazepine). Products include:
Plendil Extended-Release Tablets.... 1526

Furazolidone (Concurrent use is contraindicated). Products include:
Furoxone 1855

Haloperidol (Haloperidol serum levels may be reduced when administered with Tegretol). Products include:
Haldol Injection, Tablets and Concentrate 1373

Haloperidol Decanoate (Haloperidol serum levels may be reduced when administered with Tegretol). Products include:
Haldol Decanoate............................... 1375

Isocarboxazid (Concurrent use is contraindicated). Products include:
Marplan Tablets 1906

Isoniazid (Elevated plasma levels of carbamazepine). Products include:
INH Tablets 868

Rifamate Capsules 1347

Isradipine (Elevated plasma levels of carbamazepine). Products include:
DynaCirc Capsules 2004

Levonorgestrel (Breakthrough bleeding may occur). Products include:
Levlen/Tri-Levlen................................ 665
Nordette-21 Tablets........................... 2481
Nordette-28 Tablets........................... 2483
Norplant System 2484
Levlen/Tri-Levlen................................ 665
Triphasil-21 Tablets............................ 2527
Triphasil-28 Tablets............................ 2532

Lithium Carbonate (Increased risk of neurotoxic effects). Products include:
Eskalith 2214
Lithane Tablets.................................... 1596
Lithium Carbonate Capsules & Tablets 1984
Lithobid Tablets 870

Lithium Citrate (Increased risk of neurotoxic effects). Products include:
Cibalith-S... 870

Mephenytoin (Alterations of thyroid function). Products include:
Mesantoin Tablets............................... 2013

Mestranol (Breakthrough bleeding may occur). Products include:
Enovid... 2161
Norethin.. 2133
Norinyl 2304
Ortho-Novum....................................... 1667

Methsuximide (Alterations of thyroid function). Products include:
Celontin 1692

Nicardipine Hydrochloride (Elevated plasma levels of carbamazepine). Products include:
Cardene Capsules 2290

Nifedipine (Elevated plasma levels of carbamazepine). Products include:
Adalat Capsules (10 mg and 20 mg) 1587
Procardia Capsules............................. 1781
Procardia XL Tablets 1783

Nimodipine (Elevated plasma levels of carbamazepine). Products include:
Nimotop Capsules 1607

Norethindrone (Breakthrough bleeding may occur). Products include:
Brevicon.. 2304
Jenest-28 Tablets 1636
Micronor Tablets 1667
Modicon.. 1667
Norethin.. 2133
Norinyl 2304
Norlutin 1755
Nor-Q D Tablets 2304
Ortho-Novum....................................... 1667
Ovcon 1391
Tri-Norinyl... 2304

Norethindrone Acetate (Breakthrough bleeding may occur). Products include:
Aygestin Tablets.................................. 2437
Loestrin 1728
Norlestrin 1746
Norlutate 1754

Norethynodrel (Breakthrough bleeding may occur). Products include:
Enovid 2161

Norgestimate (Breakthrough bleeding may occur). Products include:
Ortho-Cyclen Tablets 1658

Norgestrel (Breakthrough bleeding may occur). Products include:
Lo/Ovral Tablets 2471
Lo/Ovral-28 Tablets............................ 2476
Ovral Tablets 2490
Ovral-28 Tablets 2491
Ovrette Tablets.................................... 2492

Paramethadione (Alterations of thyroid function). Products include:
Paradione Capsules 548

Phenacemide (Alterations of thyroid function). Products include:
Phenurone Tablets 552

Phenelzine Sulfate (Concurrent use is contraindicated). Products include:
Nardil 1742

Phenobarbital (Marked lowering of serum levels of Tegretol; alterations of thyroid function). Products include:
Arco-Lase Plus Tablets 607
Bellergal-S Tablets 1998
Bronkolixir ....▣ 761
Bronkotabs Tablets.............................▣ 762
Donnatal 1858
Donnatal Extentabs............................ 1859
Donnatal Tablets 1858
Donnazyme Tablets 1860
Kinesed Tablets 2272
Phenobarbital Elixir and Tablets........ 1293
Primatene Tablets-P Formula............ 2421
Quadrinal Tablets 1183
Tedral SA 1765

Phensuximide (Alterations of thyroid function). Products include:
Milontin Kapseals............................... 1741

Phenytoin (Marked lowering of serum levels of Tegretol; half-life of phenytoin significantly shortened when administered concurrently with Tegretol; alterations of thyroid function). Products include:
Dilantin Infatabs................................. 1710
Dilantin-30 Pediatric/Dilantin-125 Suspension 1713

Phenytoin Sodium (Marked lowering of serum levels of Tegretol; half-life of phenytoin significantly shortened when administered concurrently with Tegretol; alterations of thyroid function). Products include:
Dilantin Kapseals 1708
Dilantin Parenteral 1712
Dilantin with Phenobarbital Kapseals 1715

Primidone (Marked lowering of serum levels of Tegretol; alterations of thyroid function). Products include:
Mysoline.. 2480

Propoxyphene Hydrochloride (Elevated plasma levels of carbamazepine). Products include:
Darvon 1256
Wygesic Tablets 2540

Propoxyphene Napsylate (Elevated plasma levels of carbamazepine). Products include:
Darvon-N/Darvocet-N 1254

Selegiline Hydrochloride (Concurrent use is contraindicated). Products include:
Eldepryl 2250

Theophylline (Half-life significantly shortened when administered concurrently with Tegretol). Products include:
Bronkaid Tablets ....▣ 757
Bronkolixir ....▣ 761
Bronkotabs Tablets.............................▣ 762
Constant-T Tablets 1029
Marax Tablets & DF Syrup................. 1954
Primatene Tablets............................... 2421
Quibron Capsules 713
Quibron-T 714
Quibron-T/SR 716
Theolair Liquid 1317
Theo-Organidin Elixir 2391

Theophylline Anhydrous (Half-life significantly shortened when administered concurrently with Tegretol). Products include:
Aerolate 994
Primatene Tablets-M Formula ....▣ 753
Primatene Tablets-Regular Formula 2421

Respbid Tablets 684
Slo-bid Gyrocaps 1847
T-PHYL (Uniphyl) 200 mg Tablets 1820
Tedral SA 1765
Theo-24 2179
Theo-Dur Sprinkle 1168
Theo-Dur Extended-Release Tablets 1166
Theolair Tablets 1317
Theolair-SR Tablets............................. 1319
TheoX Extended-Release Tablets 841
Uniphyl 400 mg Tablets..................... 1823

Theophylline Calcium Salicylate (Half-life significantly shortened when administered concurrently with Tegretol). Products include:
Quadrinal Tablets 1183

Theophylline Sodium Glycinate (Half-life significantly shortened when administered concurrently with Tegretol). Products include:
Asbron G 1997

Tranylcypromine Sulfate (Concurrent use is contraindicated). Products include:
Parnate Tablets 2222

Trimethadione (Alterations of thyroid function). Products include:
Tridione 557

Valproic Acid (Alterations of thyroid function; valproic acid serum levels may be reduced). Products include:
Depakene Capsules & Syrup.............. 511

Verapamil Hydrochloride (Elevated plasma levels of carbamazepine). Products include:
Calan SR Caplets 2157
Calan Tablets...................................... 2155
Isoptin Injectable 1177
Isoptin Oral Tablets 1179
Isoptin SR Sustained Release Tablets 1181
Verelan Capsules 1243
Verelan Capsules 2535

Warfarin Sodium (Half-life significantly shortened when administered concurrently with Tegretol). Products include:
Coumadin Injection & Tablets 944
Panwarfin Tablets 547

TEGRIN FOR PSORIASIS LOTION, CREAM & SOAP
(Allantoin, Coal Tar) ....▣ 518
No interactions described in labeling.

TEGRIN MEDICATED SHAMPOO
(Coal Tar)..▣ 518
No interactions described in labeling.

TELDRIN TIMED-RELEASE ALLERGY CAPSULES, 12 MG.
(Chlorpheniramine Maleate)................2192

Food Interactions
Beverages, alcoholic (Avoid concurrent use).

TEMARIL TABLETS, SYRUP AND SPANSULE SUSTAINED RELEASE CAPSULES
(Trimeprazine Tartrate) 1085
May interact with monoamine oxidase inhibitors, thiazides, narcotic analgesics, oral contraceptives, central nervous system depressants, and certain other agents. Compounds in these categories include:

Alcohol (Additive CNS depressant effect).

Alfentanil Hydrochloride (CNS depressant and analgesic effects potentiated). Products include:
Alfenta Injection 1131

Alprazolam (Additive CNS depressant effect). Products include:
Xanax Tablets 2367

Aprobarbital (Additive CNS depressant effect). Products include:
Alurate Elixir 1883

Atropine Nitrate, Methyl (Action of atropine intensified and prolonged).
No products indexed under this heading.

Atropine Sulfate (Action of atropine intensified and prolonged). Products include:
Arco-Lase Plus Tablets 607
Atropine Sulfate Sterile Ophthalmic Solution and S.O.P. Sterile Ophthalmic Ointment ◉ 239
Donnagel ▣ 675
Donnagel-PG 1858
Donnatal 1858
Donnatal Extentabs 1859
Donnatal Tablets 1858
Donnazyme Tablets 1860
Isopto Atropine ◉ 218
Lomotil 2174
Motofen Tablets 836
Ru-Tuss Tablets 693
Urised Tablets 2396

Bendroflumethiazide (Anticholinergic effects of Temaril prolonged and intensified). Products include:
Corzide Tablets 702
Naturetin Tablets 1789
Rauzide Tablets 1804

Buprenorphine (CNS depressant and analgesic effects potentiated).
No products indexed under this heading.

Buspirone Hydrochloride (Additive CNS depressant effect). Products include:
BuSpar 1401

Butabarbital (Additive CNS depressant effect). Products include:
Pyridium Plus 1764

Butalbital (Additive CNS depressant effect). Products include:
Esgic-Plus Tablets 1002
Esgic Tablets & Capsules 1001
Fioricet Tablets 2006
Fiorinal Capsules 2007
Fiorinal with Codeine Capsules 2008
Fiorinal Tablets 2007
Phrenilin 838
Sedapap Tablets 50 mg/650 mg 1360

Chlordiazepoxide (Additive CNS depressant effect). Products include:
Libritabs Tablets 1930
Limbitrol 1933
Menrium Tablets 1934

Chlordiazepoxide Hydrochloride (Additive CNS depressant effect). Products include:
Librax Capsules 1929
Librium Capsules 1931
Librium Injectable 1932

Chlorothiazide (Anticholinergic effects of Temaril prolonged and intensified). Products include:
Aldoclor Tablets 1413
Diupres Tablets 1461
Diuril Oral 1464

Chlorothiazide Sodium (Anticholinergic effects of Temaril prolonged and intensified). Products include:
Diuril Sodium Intravenous 1463

Chlorpromazine (Additive CNS depressant effect). Products include:
Thorazine 2234

Chlorprothixene (Additive CNS depressant effect). Products include:
Taractan Tablets 1920

Chlorprothixene Hydrochloride (Additive CNS depressant effect). Products include:
Taractan 1920

Chlorprothixene Lactate (Additive CNS depressant effect). Products include:
Taractan Concentrate 1920

Clorazepate Dipotassium (Additive CNS depressant effect). Products include:
Tranxene 556

Codeine (CNS depressant and analgesic effects potentiated). Products include:
Calcidrine Syrup 506

Codeine Phosphate (CNS depressant and analgesic effects potentiated). Products include:
Actifed with Codeine Cough Syrup 752
Cheracol Cough Syrup 1853
Codimal PH Syrup 846
Dimetane-DC Cough Syrup 1857
Empirin with Codeine Phosphate Nos. 2, 3 & 4 764
Fiorinal with Codeine Capsules 2008
Isoclor Expectorant 982
Naldecon CX Adult Liquid ▣ 521
Novahistine DH 1342
Novahistine Expectorant 1343
Nucofed Capsules 2219
Nucofed Expectorant 2219
Nucofed Pediatric Expectorant 2220
Nucofed Syrup 2219
Phenaphen with Codeine Capsules 1865
Phenaphen-650 with Codeine Tablets 1866
Phenergan with Codeine 2497
Phenergan VC with Codeine 2501
Robitussin A-C Syrup 1875
Robitussin-DAC Syrup 1875
Ryna ▣ 741
Soma Compound w/Codeine Tablets 2390
Triaminic Expectorant w/Codeine 1996
Tussi-Organidin Liquid 2391
Tylenol with Codeine 1381

Codeine Polistirex (CNS depressant and analgesic effects potentiated).
No products indexed under this heading.

Dezocine (CNS depressant and analgesic effects potentiated).

Diazepam (Additive CNS depressant effect). Products include:
Valium Injectable 1937
Valium Tablets 1939
Valrelease Capsules 1923

Droperidol (Additive CNS depressant effect). Products include:
Inapsine Injection 1140
Innovar Injection 1141

Enflurane (Additive CNS depressant effect). Products include:
Ethrane 599

Epinephrine (Possible blockage or reversal of pressor effect). Products include:
Ana-Kit Anaphylaxis Emergency Treatment Kit 1100
Bronkaid Mist ▣ 757
EpiPen 843
Marcaine Hydrochloride 0.5% with Epinephrine 1:200,000 (as bitartrate) 958
Marcaine Hydrochloride with Epinephrine 1:200,000 2055
Primatene Mist 2420
Sus-Phrine Injection 1006
Xylocaine with Epinephrine Injections 637

Estazolam (CNS depressant and analgesic effects potentiated). Products include:
ProSom Tablets 554

Ethchlorvynol (Additive CNS depressant effect). Products include:
Placidyl Capsules 553

Ethinamate (Additive CNS depressant effect).
No products indexed under this heading.

Ethinyl Estradiol (Potentiates phenothiazine effects). Products include:
Brevicon 2304
Demulen 2161
Estinyl Tablets 2085
Jenest-28 Tablets 1636
Levlen/Tri-Levlen 665
Lo/Ovral Tablets 2471
Lo/Ovral-28 Tablets 2476
Loestrin 1728
Modicon 1667
Nordette-21 Tablets 2481
Nordette-28 Tablets 2483
Norethin 2133
Norinyl 2304
Norlestrin 1746
Ortho-Cyclen Tablets 1658
Ortho-Novum 1667
Ovcon 1391
Ovral Tablets 2490
Ovral-28 Tablets 2491
Levlen/Tri-Levlen 665
Tri-Norinyl 2304
Triphasil-21 Tablets 2527
Triphasil-28 Tablets 2532

Ethynodiol Diacetate (Potentiates phenothiazine effects). Products include:
Demulen 2161

Fentanyl (CNS depressant and analgesic effects potentiated). Products include:
Duragesic Transdermal System 1133

Fentanyl Citrate (CNS depressant and analgesic effects potentiated). Products include:
Innovar Injection 1141
Sublimaze Injection 1146

Fluphenazine Decanoate (Additive CNS depressant effect). Products include:
Prolixin Decanoate 1795

Fluphenazine Enanthate (Additive CNS depressant effect). Products include:
Prolixin Enanthate 1796

Fluphenazine Hydrochloride (Additive CNS depressant effect). Products include:
Prolixin Elixir 1793
Prolixin Injection 1791
Prolixin Oral Concentrate 1792
Prolixin Tablets 1793

Flurazepam Hydrochloride (Additive CNS depressant effect). Products include:
Dalmane Capsules 1927

Furazolidone (Anticholinergic effects of Temaril prolonged and intensified; hypertension and extrapyramidal reactions). Products include:
Furoxone 1855

Glutethimide (Additive CNS depressant effect).
No products indexed under this heading.

Haloperidol (Additive CNS depressant effect). Products include:
Haldol Injection, Tablets and Concentrate 1373

Haloperidol Decanoate (Additive CNS depressant effect). Products include:
Haldol Decanoate 1375

Hydrochlorothiazide (Anticholinergic effects of Temaril prolonged and intensified). Products include:
Aldactazide 2150
Aldoril Tablets 1418
Apresazide Capsules 854
Apresoline-Esidrix Tablets 857
Capozide 2258
Dyazide Capsules 2208
Esidrix Tablets 863
Esimil Tablets 864
HydroDIURIL Tablets 1484
Hydropres Tablets 1485
Inderide Tablets 2463
Inderide LA Long Acting Capsules 2465
Lopressor HCT Tablets 1034
Maxzide 1215
Moduretic Tablets 1510
Normozide Tablets 2112
Oretic Tablets 544
Oreticyl 545
Prinzide Tablets 1540
Ser-Ap-Es Tablets 881
Serpasil-Esidrix Tablets 886
Timolide Tablets 1547
Trandate HCT Tablets 579
Vaseretic Tablets 1559
Zestoretic 2274

Hydrocodone Bitartrate (CNS depressant and analgesic effects potentiated). Products include:
Anexsia 5/500 Tablets 2196
Anexsia 7.5/650 Tablets 2197
Azdōne Tablets 844
Codiclear DH Syrup 845
Codimal DH Syrup 846
Damason-P 1356
Hycodan Syrup, Tablets 927
Hycomine Compound Tablets 929
Hycomine Syrup 927
Hycotuss Expectorant Syrup 930
Hydrocet Capsules 835
Lortab ASA Tablets 2414
Lortab 2412
Ru-Tuss with Hydrocodone 694
Triaminic Expectorant DH 1995
Vicodin Tablets 1187
Vicodin ES Tablets 1189
Zydone Capsules 941

Hydrocodone Polistirex (CNS depressant and analgesic effects potentiated). Products include:
Tussionex Extended-Release Suspension 988

Hydroflumethiazide (Anticholinergic effects of Temaril prolonged and intensified). Products include:
Diucardin Tablets 2450
Saluron 718
Salutensin/Salutensin-Demi 719

Hydroxyzine Hydrochloride (Additive CNS depressant effect). Products include:
Atarax Tablets & Syrup 1941
Marax Tablets & DF Syrup 1954
Vistaril Intramuscular Solution 1970

Isocarboxazid (Anticholinergic effects of Temaril prolonged and intensified; hypertension and extrapyramidal reactions). Products include:
Marplan Tablets 1906

Isoflurane (Additive CNS depressant effect). Products include:
Forane 600

Ketamine Hydrochloride (CNS depressant and analgesic effects potentiated). Products include:
Ketalar 1726

Levonorgestrel (Potentiates phenothiazine effects). Products include:
Levlen/Tri-Levlen 665
Nordette-21 Tablets 2481
Nordette-28 Tablets 2483
Norplant System 2484
Levlen/Tri-Levlen 665
Triphasil-21 Tablets 2527
Triphasil-28 Tablets 2532

Levorphanol Tartrate (CNS depressant and analgesic effects potentiated). Products include:
Levo-Dromoran 1906

Lorazepam (Additive CNS depressant effect). Products include:
Ativan Injection 2432
Ativan Tablets 2434

Loxapine Hydrochloride (Additive CNS depressant effect). Products include:
Loxitane 1213

Loxapine Succinate (CNS depressant and analgesic effects potentiated). Products include:
Loxitane Capsules 1213

Meperidine Hydrochloride (CNS depressant and analgesic effects potentiated). Products include:
Demerol 2047
Mepergan Injection 2479

Mephobarbital (Additive CNS depressant effect). Products include:
Mebaral Tablets 2061

Meprobamate (Additive CNS depressant effect). Products include:
Deprol Tablets 2382
Equagesic Tablets 2451

Miltown Tablets ... 2386
PMB 200 and PMB 400 ... 2504

Mesoridazine (Additive CNS depressant effect). Products include:
Serentil ... 686

Mestranol (Potentiates phenothiazine effects). Products include:
Enovid ... 2161
Norethin ... 2133
Norinyl ... 2304
Ortho-Novum ... 1667

Methadone Hydrochloride (CNS depressant and analgesic effects potentiated). Products include:
Dolophine Hydrochloride Ampoules & Vials ... 1260
Dolophine Hydrochloride Tablets ... 1261
Methadone Hydrochloride Diskets ... 1284
Methadone Hydrochloride Oral Solution & Tablets ... 1987

Methohexital Sodium (Additive CNS depressant effect). Products include:
Brevital Sodium Vials ... 1248

Methoxyflurane (Additive CNS depressant effect).
No products indexed under this heading.

Methyclothiazide (Anticholinergic effects of Temaril prolonged and intensified). Products include:
Enduron Tablets ... 517
Enduronyl ... 518

Midazolam Hydrochloride (Additive CNS depressant effect). Products include:
Versed Injection ... 1924

Molindone Hydrochloride (Additive CNS depressant effect). Products include:
Moban Tablets & Concentrate ... 932

Morphine Sulfate (CNS depressant and analgesic effects potentiated). Products include:
Astramorph/PF Injection, USP (Preservative-Free) ... 618
Duramorph ... 960
Infumorph 200 and Infumorph 500 Sterile Solutions ... 962
MS Contin Tablets ... 1814
MSIR ... 1817
Oramorph SR (Morphine Sulfate Sustained Release Tablets) ... 1988
Roxanol ... 1991

Norethindrone (Potentiates phenothiazine effects). Products include:
Brevicon ... 2304
Jenest-28 Tablets ... 1636
Micronor Tablets ... 1667
Modicon ... 1667
Norethin ... 2133
Norinyl ... 2304
Norlutin ... 1755
Nor-Q D Tablets ... 2304
Ortho-Novum ... 1667
Ovcon ... 1391
Tri-Norinyl ... 2304

Norethynodrel (Potentiates phenothiazine effects). Products include:
Enovid ... 2161

Norgestimate (Potentiates phenothiazine effects). Products include:
Ortho-Cyclen Tablets ... 1658

Norgestrel (Potentiates phenothiazine effects). Products include:
Lo/Ovral Tablets ... 2471
Lo/Ovral-28 Tablets ... 2476
Ovral Tablets ... 2490
Ovral-28 Tablets ... 2491
Ovrette Tablets ... 2492

Nylidrin Hydrochloride (Potentiates phenothiazine effects).
No products indexed under this heading.

Opium Alkaloids (CNS depressant and analgesic effects potentiated). Products include:
B & O No. 15A & No. 16A Supprettes ... 2395
Pantopon Injectable ... 1911

Oxazepam (Additive CNS depressant effect). Products include:
Serax Capsules ... 2522
Serax Tablets ... 2522

Oxycodone Hydrochloride (CNS depressant and analgesic effects potentiated). Products include:
Percocet Tablets ... 950
Percodan ... 951
Roxicodone Tablets, Oral Solution & Intensol (Oxycodone) ... 1992
Tylox Capsules ... 1382

Pentobarbital Sodium (Additive CNS depressant effect). Products include:
Nembutal Sodium Capsules ... 534
Nembutal Sodium Solution ... 536
Nembutal Sodium Suppositories ... 538

Perphenazine (Additive CNS depressant effect). Products include:
Etrafon ... 2087
Triavil Tablets ... 1556
Trilafon ... 2123

Phenelzine Sulfate (Anticholinergic effects of Temaril prolonged and intensified; hypertension and extrapyramidal reactions). Products include:
Nardil ... 1742

Phenobarbital (Additive CNS depressant effect). Products include:
Arco-Lase Plus Tablets ... 607
Bellergal-S Tablets ... 1998
Bronkolixir ... ⊡ 761
Bronkotabs Tablets ... ⊡ 762
Donnatal ... 1858
Donnatal Extentabs ... 1859
Donnatal Tablets ... 1858
Donnazyme Tablets ... 1860
Kinesed Tablets ... 2272
Phenobarbital Elixir and Tablets ... 1293
Primatene Tablets-P Formula ... 2421
Quadrinal Tablets ... 1183
Tedral SA ... 1765

Polythiazide (Anticholinergic effects of Temaril prolonged and intensified). Products include:
Minizide Capsules ... 1779
Renese Tablets ... 1785
Renese-R Tablets ... 1786

Prazepam (Additive CNS depressant effect). Products include:
Centrax ... 1693

Prochlorperazine (Additive CNS depressant effect). Products include:
Compazine ... 2201

Progesterone (Potentiates phenothiazine effects).
No products indexed under this heading.

Promethazine Hydrochloride (Additive CNS depressant effect). Products include:
Mepergan Injection ... 2479
Phenergan with Codeine ... 2497
Phenergan with Dextromethorphan ... 2499
Phenergan Injection ... 2493
Phenergan Suppositories ... 2496
Phenergan Syrup ... 2495
Phenergan Tablets ... 2496
Phenergan VC ... 2500
Phenergan VC with Codeine ... 2501

Propofol (CNS depressant and analgesic effects potentiated). Products include:
Diprivan Injection ... 2267

Propoxyphene Hydrochloride (CNS depressant and analgesic effects potentiated). Products include:
Darvon ... 1256
Wygesic Tablets ... 2540

Propoxyphene Napsylate (CNS depressant and analgesic effects potentiated). Products include:
Darvon-N/Darvocet-N ... 1254

Quazepam (CNS depressant and analgesic effects potentiated). Products include:
Doral Tablets ... 2383

Reserpine (Potentiates phenothiazine effects). Products include:
Diupres Tablets ... 1461
Hydromox R Tablets ... 1209
Hydropres Tablets ... 1485
Renese-R Tablets ... 1786
Salutensin/Salutensin-Demi ... 719
Ser-Ap-Es Tablets ... 881
Serpasil Tablets ... 883
Serpasil-Apresoline Tablets ... 884
Serpasil-Esidrix Tablets ... 886

Secobarbital Sodium (CNS depressant and analgesic effects potentiated). Products include:
Seconal Sodium Pulvules ... 1296

Selegiline Hydrochloride (Anticholinergic effects of Temaril prolonged and intensified; hypertension and extrapyramidal reactions). Products include:
Eldepryl ... 2250

Sufentanil Citrate (CNS depressant and analgesic effects potentiated). Products include:
Sufenta Injection ... 1147

Temazepam (Additive CNS depressant effect). Products include:
Restoril Capsules ... 2023

Thiamylal Sodium (Additive CNS depressant effect). Products include:
Surital Ampoules, Steri-Vials ... 1764

Thioridazine Hydrochloride (Additive CNS depressant effect). Products include:
Mellaril ... 2011

Thiothixene (Additive CNS depressant effect). Products include:
Navane Capsules and Concentrate ... 1954
Navane Intramuscular ... 1956

Tranylcypromine Sulfate (Anticholinergic effects of Temaril prolonged and intensified; hypertension and extrapyramidal reactions). Products include:
Parnate Tablets ... 2222

Triazolam (Additive CNS depressant effect). Products include:
Halcion Tablets ... 2340

Trifluoperazine Hydrochloride (Additive CNS depressant effect). Products include:
Stelazine ... 2226

TEMOVATE CREAM
(Clobetasol Propionate) ... 1056
No interactions described in labeling.

TEMOVATE OINTMENT
(Clobetasol Propionate) ... 1056
No interactions described in labeling.

TEMOVATE SCALP APPLICATION
(Clobetasol Propionate) ... 1056
No interactions described in labeling.

TEMPRA, ACETAMINOPHEN
(Acetaminophen) ... ⊡ 613
May interact with oral anticoagulants and certain other agents. Compounds in these categories include:

Chloramphenicol (Enhanced elimination of chloramphenicol). Products include:
AK-Chlor Sterile Ophthalmic Ointment & Solution ... ◉ 201
Chloromycetin Cream, 1% ... 1694
Chloromycetin Hydrocortisone Ophthalmic ... 1694
Chloromycetin Kapseals ... 1695
Chloromycetin Ophthalmic Ointment, 1% ... 1696
Chloromycetin Ophthalmic Solution ... 1696
Chloromycetin Otic ... 1697
Chloroptic S.O.P. ... ◉ 243
Chloroptic Sterile Ophthalmic Solution ... ◉ 243
Ophthochlor Ophthalmic Solution ... ◉ 300
Ophthocort ... ◉ 301

Chloramphenicol Palmitate (Enhanced elimination of chloramphenicol). Products include:
Chloromycetin Palmitate, Oral Suspension ... 1697

Chloramphenicol Sodium Succinate (Enhanced elimination of chloramphenicol). Products include:
Chloromycetin Sodium Succinate ... 1698

Dicumarol (The effect of orally administered anticoagulant potentiated). Products include:
Dicumarol Tablets ... 516

Warfarin Sodium (The effect of orally administered anticoagulant potentiated). Products include:
Coumadin Injection & Tablets ... 944
Panwarfin Tablets ... 547

TENEX TABLETS
(Guanfacine Hydrochloride) ... 1875
May interact with central nervous system depressants. Compounds in this category include:

Alfentanil Hydrochloride (Potential for increased sedation). Products include:
Alfenta Injection ... 1131

Alprazolam (Potential for increased sedation). Products include:
Xanax Tablets ... 2367

Aprobarbital (Potential for increased sedation). Products include:
Alurate Elixir ... 1883

Buprenorphine (Potential for increased sedation).
No products indexed under this heading.

Buspirone Hydrochloride (Potential for increased sedation). Products include:
BuSpar ... 1401

Butabarbital (Potential for increased sedation). Products include:
Pyridium Plus ... 1764

Butalbital (Potential for increased sedation). Products include:
Esgic-Plus Tablets ... 1002
Esgic Tablets & Capsules ... 1001
Fioricet Tablets ... 2006
Fiorinal Capsules ... 2007
Fiorinal with Codeine Capsules ... 2008
Fiorinal Tablets ... 2007
Phrenilin ... 838
Sedapap Tablets 50 mg/650 mg ... 1360

Chlordiazepoxide (Potential for increased sedation). Products include:
Libritabs Tablets ... 1930
Limbitrol ... 1933
Menrium Tablets ... 1934

Chlordiazepoxide Hydrochloride (Potential for increased sedation). Products include:
Librax Capsules ... 1929
Librium Capsules ... 1931
Librium Injectable ... 1932

Chlorpromazine (Potential for increased sedation). Products include:
Thorazine ... 2234

Chlorprothixene (Potential for increased sedation). Products include:
Taractan Tablets ... 1920

Chlorprothixene Hydrochloride (Potential for increased sedation). Products include:
Taractan ... 1920

Clorazepate Dipotassium (Potential for increased sedation). Products include:
Tranxene ... 556

Codeine (Potential for increased sedation). Products include:
Calcidrine Syrup ... 506

Codeine Phosphate (Potential for increased sedation). Products include:
- Actifed with Codeine Cough Syrup.. 752
- Cheracol Cough Syrup 1853
- Codimal PH Syrup 846
- Dimetane-DC Cough Syrup 1857
- Empirin with Codeine Phosphate Nos. 2, 3 & 4 764
- Fiorinal with Codeine Capsules 2008
- Isoclor Expectorant 982
- Naldecon CX Adult Liquid ⊞ 521
- Novahistine DH 1342
- Novahistine Expectorant 1343
- Nucofed Capsules 2219
- Nucofed Expectorant 2219
- Nucofed Pediatric Expectorant 2220
- Nucofed Syrup 2219
- Phenaphen with Codeine Capsules 1865
- Phenaphen-650 with Codeine Tablets 1866
- Phenergan with Codeine 2497
- Phenergan VC with Codeine 2501
- Robitussin A-C Syrup 1875
- Robitussin-DAC Syrup 1875
- Ryna ⊞ 741
- Soma Compound w/Codeine Tablets 2390
- Triaminic Expectorant w/Codeine .. 1996
- Tussi-Organidin Liquid 2391
- Tylenol with Codeine 1381

Codeine Polistirex (Potential for increased sedation).
- No products indexed under this heading.

Dezocine (Potential for increased sedation).

Diazepam (Potential for increased sedation). Products include:
- Valium Injectable 1937
- Valium Tablets 1939
- Valrelease Capsules 1923

Droperidol (Potential for increased sedation). Products include:
- Inapsine Injection 1140
- Innovar Injection 1141

Enflurane (Potential for increased sedation). Products include:
- Ethrane 599

Estazolam (Potential for increased sedation). Products include:
- ProSom Tablets 554

Ethchlorvynol (Potential for increased sedation). Products include:
- Placidyl Capsules 553

Ethinamate (Potential for increased sedation).
- No products indexed under this heading.

Fentanyl (Potential for increased sedation). Products include:
- Duragesic Transdermal System 1133

Fentanyl Citrate (Potential for increased sedation). Products include:
- Innovar Injection 1141
- Sublimaze Injection 1146

Fluphenazine Decanoate (Potential for increased sedation). Products include:
- Prolixin Decanoate 1795

Fluphenazine Enanthate (Potential for increased sedation). Products include:
- Prolixin Enanthate 1796

Fluphenazine Hydrochloride (Potential for increased sedation). Products include:
- Prolixin Elixir 1793
- Prolixin Injection 1791
- Prolixin Oral Concentrate 1792
- Prolixin Tablets 1793

Flurazepam Hydrochloride (Potential for increased sedation). Products include:
- Dalmane Capsules 1927

Glutethimide (Potential for increased sedation).
- No products indexed under this heading.

Haloperidol (Potential for increased sedation). Products include:
- Haldol Injection, Tablets and Concentrate 1373

Haloperidol Decanoate (Potential for increased sedation). Products include:
- Haldol Decanoate 1375

Hydrocodone Bitartrate (Potential for increased sedation). Products include:
- Anexsia 5/500 Tablets 2196
- Anexsia 7.5/650 Tablets 2197
- Azdone Tablets 844
- Codiclear DH Syrup 845
- Codimal DH Syrup 846
- Damason-P 1356
- Hycodan Syrup, Tablets 927
- Hycomine Compound Tablets 929
- Hycomine Syrup 927
- Hycotuss Expectorant Syrup 930
- Hydrocet Capsules 835
- Lortab ASA Tablets 2414
- Lortab 2412
- Ru-Tuss with Hydrocodone 694
- Triaminic Expectorant DH 1995
- Vicodin Tablets 1187
- Vicodin ES Tablets 1189
- Zydone Capsules 941

Hydrocodone Polistirex (Potential for increased sedation). Products include:
- Tussionex Extended-Release Suspension 988

Hydroxyzine Hydrochloride (Potential for increased sedation). Products include:
- Atarax Tablets & Syrup 1941
- Marax Tablets & DF Syrup 1954
- Vistaril Intramuscular Solution 1970

Isoflurane (Potential for increased sedation). Products include:
- Forane 600

Ketamine Hydrochloride (Potential for increased sedation). Products include:
- Ketalar 1726

Levorphanol Tartrate (Potential for increased sedation). Products include:
- Levo-Dromoran 1906

Lorazepam (Potential for increased sedation). Products include:
- Ativan Injection 2432
- Ativan Tablets 2434

Loxapine Hydrochloride (Potential for increased sedation). Products include:
- Loxitane 1213

Loxapine Succinate (Potential for increased sedation). Products include:
- Loxitane Capsules 1213

Meperidine Hydrochloride (Potential for increased sedation). Products include:
- Demerol 2047
- Mepergan Injection 2479

Mephobarbital (Potential for increased sedation). Products include:
- Mebaral Tablets 2061

Meprobamate (Potential for increased sedation). Products include:
- Deprol Tablets 2382
- Equagesic Tablets 2451
- Miltown Tablets 2386
- PMB 200 and PMB 400 2504

Mesoridazine (Potential for increased sedation). Products include:
- Serentil 686

Methadone Hydrochloride (Potential for increased sedation). Products include:
- Dolophine Hydrochloride Ampoules & Vials 1260
- Dolophine Hydrochloride Tablets 1261
- Methadone Hydrochloride Diskets .. 1284
- Methadone Hydrochloride Oral Solution & Tablets 1987

Methohexital Sodium (Potential for increased sedation). Products include:
- Brevital Sodium Vials 1248

Methoxyflurane (Potential for increased sedation).
- No products indexed under this heading.

Midazolam Hydrochloride (Potential for increased sedation). Products include:
- Versed Injection 1924

Molindone Hydrochloride (Potential for increased sedation). Products include:
- Moban Tablets & Concentrate 932

Morphine Sulfate (Potential for increased sedation). Products include:
- Astramorph/PF Injection, USP (Preservative-Free) 618
- Duramorph 960
- Infumorph 200 and Infumorph 500 Sterile Solutions 962
- MS Contin Tablets 1814
- MSIR 1817
- Oramorph SR (Morphine Sulfate Sustained Release Tablets) 1988
- Roxanol 1991

Opium Alkaloids (Potential for increased sedation). Products include:
- B & O No. 15A & No. 16A Supprettes 2395
- Pantopon Injectable 1911

Oxazepam (Potential for increased sedation). Products include:
- Serax Capsules 2522
- Serax Tablets 2522

Oxycodone Hydrochloride (Potential for increased sedation). Products include:
- Percocet Tablets 950
- Percodan 951
- Roxicodone Tablets, Oral Solution & Intensol (Oxycodone) 1992
- Tylox Capsules 1382

Pentobarbital Sodium (Potential for increased sedation). Products include:
- Nembutal Sodium Capsules 534
- Nembutal Sodium Solution 536
- Nembutal Sodium Suppositories 538

Perphenazine (Potential for increased sedation). Products include:
- Etrafon 2087
- Triavil Tablets 1556
- Trilafon 2123

Phenobarbital (Potential for increased sedation; concurrent administration may result in significant reductions in elimination half-life and plasma concentration). Products include:
- Arco-Lase Plus Tablets 607
- Bellergal-S Tablets 1998
- Bronkolixir ⊞ 761
- Bronkotabs Tablets ⊞ 762
- Donnatal 1858
- Donnatal Extentabs 1859
- Donnatal Tablets 1858
- Donnazyme Tablets 1860
- Kinesed Tablets 2272
- Phenobarbital Elixir and Tablets 1293
- Primatene Tablets-P Formula 2421
- Quadrinal Tablets 1183
- Tedral SA 1765

Phenytoin (Concurrent administration may result in significant reductions in elimination half-life and plasma concentration). Products include:
- Dilantin Infatabs 1710
- Dilantin-30 Pediatric/Dilantin-125 Suspension 1713

Phenytoin Sodium (Concurrent administration may result in significant reductions in elimination half-life and plasma concentration). Products include:
- Dilantin Kapseals 1708
- Dilantin Parenteral 1712
- Dilantin with Phenobarbital Kapseals 1715

Prazepam (Potential for increased sedation). Products include:
- Centrax 1693

Prochlorperazine (Potential for increased sedation). Products include:
- Compazine 2201

Promethazine Hydrochloride (Potential for increased sedation). Products include:
- Mepergan Injection 2479
- Phenergan with Codeine 2497
- Phenergan with Dextromethorphan 2499
- Phenergan Injection 2493
- Phenergan Suppositories 2496
- Phenergan Syrup 2495
- Phenergan Tablets 2496
- Phenergan VC 2500
- Phenergan VC with Codeine 2501

Propofol (Potential for increased sedation). Products include:
- Diprivan Injection 2267

Propoxyphene Hydrochloride (Potential for increased sedation). Products include:
- Darvon 1256
- Wygesic Tablets 2540

Propoxyphene Napsylate (Potential for increased sedation). Products include:
- Darvon-N/Darvocet-N 1254

Quazepam (Potential for increased sedation). Products include:
- Doral Tablets 2383

Secobarbital Sodium (Potential for increased sedation). Products include:
- Seconal Sodium Pulvules 1296

Sufentanil Citrate (Potential for increased sedation). Products include:
- Sufenta Injection 1147

Temazepam (Potential for increased sedation). Products include:
- Restoril Capsules 2023

Thiamylal Sodium (Potential for increased sedation). Products include:
- Surital Ampoules, Steri-Vials 1764

Thioridazine Hydrochloride (Potential for increased sedation). Products include:
- Mellaril 2011

Thiothixene (Potential for increased sedation). Products include:
- Navane Capsules and Concentrate 1954
- Navane Intramuscular 1956

Triazolam (Potential for increased sedation). Products include:
- Halcion Tablets 2340

Trifluoperazine Hydrochloride (Potential for increased sedation). Products include:
- Stelazine 2226

TEN-K CONTROLLED-RELEASE TABLETS
(Potassium Chloride) 2282
May interact with potassium sparing diuretics. Compounds in this category include:

Amiloride Hydrochloride (Can produce severe hyperkalemia). Products include:
- Midamor Tablets 1508
- Moduretic Tablets 1510

Spironolactone (Can produce severe hyperkalemia). Products include:
- Aldactazide 2150
- Aldactone 2152

Triamterene (Can produce severe hyperkalemia). Products include:
- Dyazide Capsules 2208
- Dyrenium Capsules 2210
- Maxzide 1215

TENORETIC TABLETS
(Atenolol, Chlorthalidone) 1105
May interact with antihypertensives, catecholamine depleting drugs, lithium preparations, insulin, corticosteroids, cardiac glycosides, and certain other agents. Compounds in these categories include:

Acebutolol Hydrochloride (Potentiated). Products include:
Sectral Capsules 2520

Benazepril Hydrochloride (Potentiated). Products include:
Lotensin Tablets 872

Bendroflumethiazide (Potentiated). Products include:
Corzide Tablets 702
Naturetin Tablets 1789
Rauzide Tablets 1804

Betamethasone Acetate (Potential for hypokalemia). Products include:
Celestone Soluspan Suspension 2081

Betamethasone Sodium Phosphate (Potential for hypokalemia). Products include:
Celestone Soluspan Suspension 2081

Betaxolol Hydrochloride (Potentiated). Products include:
Betoptic Sterile Ophthalmic Solution 569
Betoptic S Sterile Ophthalmic Suspension 570
Kerlone Tablets 2172

Captopril (Potentiated). Products include:
Capoten 2255
Capozide 2258

Carteolol Hydrochloride (Potentiated). Products include:
Cartrol Tablets 507

Chlorothiazide (Potentiated). Products include:
Aldoclor Tablets 1413
Diupres Tablets 1461
Diuril Oral 1464

Chlorothiazide Sodium (Potentiated). Products include:
Diuril Sodium Intravenous 1463

Clonidine (Tenoretic should be discontinued several days before the gradual withdrawal of clonidine). Products include:
Catapres-TTS 677

Clonidine Hydrochloride (Tenoretic should be discontinued several days before the gradual withdrawal of clonidine). Products include:
Catapres Tablets 676
Combipres Tablets 678

Cortisone Acetate (Potential for hypokalemia). Products include:
Cortone Acetate Sterile Suspension 1437
Cortone Acetate Tablets 1439

Deserpidine (Hypotension/bradycardia). Products include:
Enduronyl 518
Harmonyl Tablets 528
Oreticyl 545

Deslanoside (Hypokalemia induced by Tenoretic therapy can sensitize or exaggerate the response of the heart to the toxic effects of digitalis).
No products indexed under this heading.

Dexamethasone (Potential for hypokalemia). Products include:
AK-Trol Ointment & Suspension ⊙ 207
Decadron Elixir 1445
Decadron Tablets 1447
Decaspray Topical Aerosol 1459
Dexacidin ⊙ 272
Maxidex Sterile Ophthalmic Suspension ⊙ 223
Maxitrol Ophthalmic Ointment/Suspension ⊙ 223
TobraDex Ophthalmic Suspension and Ointment ⊙ 228

Dexamethasone Acetate (Potential for hypokalemia). Products include:
Dalalone D.P. Injectable 999
Decadron-LA Sterile Suspension 1457

Dexamethasone Sodium Phosphate (Potential for hypokalemia). Products include:
AK-Dex ⊙ 203
Decadron Phosphate Respihaler 1454
Decadron Phosphate Sterile Ophthalmic Ointment 1453
Decadron Phosphate Sterile Ophthalmic Solution 1453
Decadron Phosphate Topical Cream 1455
Decadron Phosphate Turbinaire 1456
Maxidex Sterile Ophthalmic Ointment ⊙ 222
NeoDecadron Sterile Ophthalmic Ointment 1517
NeoDecadron Sterile Ophthalmic Solution 1518
NeoDecadron Topical Cream 1518

Diazoxide (Potentiated). Products include:
Hyperstat I.V. Injection 2095
Proglycem 649

Digitoxin (Hypokalemia induced by Tenoretic therapy can sensitize or exaggerate the response of the heart to the toxic effects of digitalis). Products include:
Crystodigin Tablets 1253

Digoxin (Hypokalemia induced by Tenoretic therapy can sensitize or exaggerate the response of the heart to the toxic effects of digitalis). Products include:
Lanoxicaps 772
Lanoxin Elixir Pediatric 775
Lanoxin Injection 778
Lanoxin Injection Pediatric 781
Lanoxin Tablets 783

Doxazosin Mesylate (Potentiated). Products include:
Cardura Tablets 1941

Enalapril Maleate (Potentiated). Products include:
Vaseretic Tablets 1559
Vasotec Tablets 1564

Enalaprilat (Potentiated). Products include:
Vasotec I.V. 1562

Esmolol Hydrochloride (Potentiated). Products include:
Brevibloc Injection 942

Felodipine (Potentiated). Products include:
Plendil Extended-Release Tablets 1526

Fosinopril Sodium (Potentiated). Products include:
Monopril Tablets 1406

Furosemide (Potentiated). Products include:
Lasix 1093

Guanabenz Acetate (Potentiated). Products include:
Wytensin Tablets 2542

Guanethidine Monosulfate (Potentiated). Products include:
Esimil Tablets 864
Ismelin Tablets 869

Hydralazine Hydrochloride (Potentiated). Products include:
Apresazide Capsules 854
Apresoline Hydrochloride Parenteral (Ampuls) 856
Apresoline Hydrochloride Tablets 855
Apresoline-Esidrix Tablets 857
Ser-Ap-Es Tablets 881
Serpasil-Apresoline Tablets 884

Hydrochlorothiazide (Potentiated). Products include:
Aldactazide 2150
Aldoril Tablets 1418
Apresazide Capsules 854
Apresoline-Esidrix Tablets 857
Capozide 2258
Dyazide Capsules 2208
Esidrix Tablets 863
Esimil Tablets 864
HydroDIURIL Tablets 1484
Hydropres Tablets 1485
Inderide Tablets 2463
Inderide LA Long Acting Capsules 2465
Lopressor HCT Tablets 1034
Maxzide 1215
Moduretic Tablets 1510
Normozide Tablets 2112
Oretic Tablets 544
Oreticyl 545
Prinzide Tablets 1540
Ser-Ap-Es Tablets 881
Serpasil-Esidrix Tablets 886
Timolide Tablets 1547
Trandate HCT Tablets 579
Vaseretic Tablets 1559
Zestoretic 2274

Hydrocortisone (Potential for hypokalemia). Products include:
AK-Spore H.C. ⊙ 206
Bactine Hydrocortisone Anti-Itch Cream ▣ 625
CaldeCORT Anti-Itch Hydrocortisone Spray ▣ 560
Carmol HC Cream 1% 2296
Cortaid Spray ▣ 735
Cortenema 2244
Cortisporin Ointment 758
Cortisporin Ophthalmic Ointment Sterile 758
Cortisporin Ophthalmic Suspension Sterile 759
Cortisporin Otic Solution Sterile 760
Cortisporin Otic Suspension Sterile 760
Cortizone-5 Creme & Ointment ▣ 732
Dermolate Anti-Itch Cream ▣ 697
Eldecort Cream 1.0% 1113
Eldecort Cream 1.0% and 2.5% 1113
Fungoid HC Creme 1770
Hydrocortone Tablets 1482
Hytone 909
LazerSporin-C Solution 1770
Massengill Medicated Soft Cloth Towelettes 2192
Nutracort Cream & Lotion 1684
PediOtic Suspension Sterile 797
Synacort Creams 1%, 2.5% 2296
Vanoxide-HC Acne Lotion 911
Vioform-Hydrocortisone Cream and Mild Cream 889
Vioform-Hydrocortisone Ointment 889
VōSoL HC Otic Solution 2392
Vytone Cream 1% 911

Hydrocortisone Acetate (Potential for hypokalemia). Products include:
Analpram-HC Rectal Cream 1% and 2.5% 970
Anusol-HC Cream 1690
Anusol-HC Suppositories 1691
Caldecort ▣ 560
Carmol HC Cream 1% 2296
Chloromycetin Hydrocortisone Ophthalmic 1694
Coly-Mycin S Otic w/Neomycin & Hydrocortisone 1708
Cortaid ▣ 735
Cortef Feminine Itch Cream ▣ 735
Corticaine ▣ 682
Cortifoam 1827
Cortisporin Cream 757
Epifoam 1828
Gynecort 5 Creme ▣ 556
Hydrocortone Acetate Sterile Suspension 1479
Lanacort 5 Creme and Ointment ▣ 557
Mantadil Cream 789
Ophthocort ⊙ 301
Orabase HCA Oral Paste 890
Pramosone Cream, Lotion & Ointment 971
ProctoCream-HC 1834
Proctofoam-HC 1835

Hydrocortisone Sodium Phosphate (Potential for hypokalemia). Products include:
Hydrocortone Phosphate Injection, Sterile 1481

Hydrocortisone Sodium Succinate (Potential for hypokalemia). Products include:
Solu-Cortef Sterile Powder 2361

Hydroflumethiazide (Potentiated). Products include:
Diucardin Tablets 2450
Saluron 718
Salutensin/Salutensin-Demi 719

Indapamide (Potentiated). Products include:
Lozol Tablets 1843

Insulin, Human (Insulin requirements in diabetic patients may be altered).
No products indexed under this heading.

Insulin, Human Isophane Suspension (Insulin requirements in diabetic patients may be altered). Products include:
Humulin N, 100 Units 1270

Insulin, Human NPH (Insulin requirements in diabetic patients may be altered). Products include:
Insulatard NPH Human 1627
Novolin N 1627
Novolin N PenFill Cartridges 1628
Novolin N Prefilled 1628

Insulin, Human Regular (Insulin requirements in diabetic patients may be altered). Products include:
Humulin BR, 100 Units 1268
Humulin R, 100 Units 1272
Novolin R 1627
Novolin R PenFill Cartridges 1628
Novolin R Prefilled 1629
Velosulin Human 1628

Insulin, Human, Zinc Suspension (Insulin requirements in diabetic patients may be altered). Products include:
Humulin L, 100 Units 1268
Humulin U, 100 Units 1272
Novolin L 1627

Insulin, NPH (Insulin requirements in diabetic patients may be altered). Products include:
NPH, 40 & 100 Units 1273
Beef NPH, 100 Units 1274
Pork NPH, 100 Units 1275
Insulatard NPH 1626
NPH Insulin 1626
NPH Purified Pork Isophane Insulin 1626

Insulin, Regular (Insulin requirements in diabetic patients may be altered). Products include:
Regular, 40 & 100 Units 1273
Beef Regular, 100 Units 1275
Pork Regular, 100 Units 1275
Pork Regular (Concentrated), 500 Units 1276
Regular Insulin 1625
Regular Purified Pork Insulin 1626
Velosulin 1627

Insulin, Zinc Crystals (Insulin requirements in diabetic patients may be altered). Products include:
NPH, 40 & 100 Units 1273

Insulin, Zinc Suspension (Insulin requirements in diabetic patients may be altered). Products include:
Lente, 40 & 100 Units 1272
Protamine, Zinc, 40 & 100 Units 1273
Lente Iletin I 1272
Beef Lente, 100 Units 1274
Beef Protamine Zinc, 100 Units 1274
Pork Lente, 100 Units 1275
Pork, Protamine, Zinc, 100 Units 1275
Lente Insulin 1626
Lente Purified Pork Insulin 1626
Semilente Insulin 1625
Ultralente Insulin 1626

Isradipine (Potentiated). Products include:
DynaCirc Capsules 2004

Labetalol Hydrochloride (Potentiated). Products include:
Normodyne Injection 2108
Normodyne Tablets 2110
Normozide Tablets 2112
Trandate HCT Tablets 579
Trandate Injection 577
Trandate Tablets 579

Lisinopril (Potentiated). Products include:
Prinivil Tablets 1538
Prinzide Tablets 1540

Zestoretic ... 2274
Zestril Tablets ... 2277

Lithium Carbonate (Reduced renal clearance; lithium toxicity). Products include:
Eskalith ... 2214
Lithane Tablets ... 1596
Lithium Carbonate Capsules & Tablets ... 1984
Lithobid Tablets ... 870

Lithium Citrate (Reduced renal clearance; lithium toxicity). Products include:
Cibalith-S ... 870

Mecamylamine Hydrochloride (Potentiated). Products include:
Inversine Tablets ... 1492

Methyclothiazide (Potentiated). Products include:
Enduron Tablets ... 517
Enduronyl ... 518

Methyldopa (Potentiated). Products include:
Aldoclor Tablets ... 1413
Aldomet Oral ... 1415
Aldoril Tablets ... 1418

Methyldopate Hydrochloride (Potentiated). Products include:
Aldomet Ester HCl Injection ... 1417

Methylprednisolone Acetate (Potential for hypokalemia). Products include:
Depo-Medrol Sterile Aqueous Suspension ... 2334

Methylprednisolone Sodium Succinate (Potential for hypokalemia). Products include:
Solu-Medrol Sterile Powder ... 2363

Metolazone (Potentiated). Products include:
Diulo ... 2129
Mykrox ½ mg Tablets ... 984
Zaroxolyn Tablets ... 989

Metoprolol Tartrate (Potentiated). Products include:
Lopressor Ampuls ... 1032
Lopressor HCT Tablets ... 1034
Lopressor Tablets ... 1032

Metyrosine (Potentiated). Products include:
Demser Capsules ... 1460

Minoxidil (Potentiated). Products include:
Loniten Tablets ... 2346
Rogaine Topical Solution ... 2357

Nadolol (Potentiated). Products include:
Corgard Tablets ... 701
Corzide Tablets ... 702

Nicardipine Hydrochloride (Potentiated). Products include:
Cardene Capsules ... 2290

Nitroglycerin (Potentiated). Products include:
Deponit NTG Transdermal Delivery System ... 2143
Minitran Transdermal Delivery System ... 1312
Nitro-Bid Ointment ... 1339
Nitro-Bid Capsules ... 1338
Nitrodisc ... 2176
Nitro-Dur (nitroglycerin) Transdermal Infusion System ... 1164
Nitrogard Tablets ... 1004
Nitrolingual Spray ... 1846
Nitrostat Tablets ... 1743
Transderm-Nitro Transdermal Therapeutic System ... 2283

Norepinephrine Bitartrate (Decreased arterial responsiveness to norepinephrine). Products include:
Levophed Bitartrate Injection ... 2054

Penbutolol Sulfate (Potentiated). Products include:
Levatol ... 1832

Phenoxybenzamine Hydrochloride (Potentiated). Products include:
Dibenzyline Capsules ... 2207

Phentolamine Mesylate (Potentiated). Products include:
Regitine ... 878

Pindolol (Potentiated). Products include:
Visken Tablets ... 2036

Polythiazide (Potentiated). Products include:
Minizide Capsules ... 1779
Renese Tablets ... 1785
Renese-R Tablets ... 1786

Prazosin Hydrochloride (Potentiated). Products include:
Minipress Capsules ... 1778
Minizide Capsules ... 1779

Prednisolone Acetate (Potential for hypokalemia). Products include:
AK-Cide Sterile Ophthalmic Ointment & Suspension ... ◉ 202
Blephamide Liquifilm Sterile Ophthalmic Suspension ... 586
Blephamide S.O.P. Sterile Ophthalmic Ointment ... 586
Cetapred Ointment ... ◉ 220
⅛% Econopred & 1% Econopred Plus ... ◉ 217
Isopto Cetapred Suspension ... ◉ 220
Metimyd ... ◉ 306
Poly-Pred Liquifilm ... ◉ 250
Pred Forte ... ◉ 252
Pred Mild ... ◉ 254
Pred-G Liquifilm Sterile Ophthalmic Suspension ... ◉ 252
Pred-G S.O.P. Sterile Ophthalmic Ointment ... ◉ 253
Vasocidin Ointment ... ◉ 275

Prednisolone Sodium Phosphate (Potential for hypokalemia). Products include:
AK-Pred ... ◉ 205
Hydeltrasol Injection, Sterile ... 1476
Inflamase ... ◉ 274
Pediapred Oral Liquid ... 987
Vasocidin Ophthalmic Solution ... ◉ 276

Prednisolone Tebutate (Potential for hypokalemia). Products include:
Hydeltra-T.B.A. Sterile Suspension 1478

Prednisone (Potential for hypokalemia). Products include:
Deltasone Tablets ... 2332

Propranolol Hydrochloride (Potentiated). Products include:
Inderal ... 2459
Inderal LA Long Acting Capsules ... 2461
Inderide Tablets ... 2463
Inderide LA Long Acting Capsules ... 2465

Ramipril (Potentiated). Products include:
Altace Capsules ... 1086

Rauwolfia Serpentina (Hypotension/bradycardia). Products include:
Raudixin Tablets ... 1803
Rauzide Tablets ... 1804

Rescinnamine (Hypotension/bradycardia).
No products indexed under this heading.

Reserpine (Hypotension/bradycardia). Products include:
Diupres Tablets ... 1461
Hydromox R Tablets ... 1209
Hydropres Tablets ... 1485
Renese-R Tablets ... 1786
Salutensin/Salutensin-Demi ... 719
Ser-Ap-Es Tablets ... 881
Serpasil Tablets ... 883
Serpasil-Apresoline Tablets ... 884
Serpasil-Esidrix Tablets ... 886

Sodium Nitroprusside (Potentiated). Products include:
Nipride I.V. Infusion ... 1909

Terazosin Hydrochloride (Potentiated). Products include:
Hytrin Tablets ... 529

Timolol Maleate (Potentiated). Products include:
Blocadren Tablets ... 1429
Timolide Tablets ... 1547
Timoptic in Ocudose ... 1552
Timoptic Sterile Ophthalmic Solution ... 1550

Triamcinolone (Potential for hypokalemia).
No products indexed under this heading.

Triamcinolone Acetonide (Potential for hypokalemia). Products include:
Aristocort A ... 1010
Azmacort Inhaler ... 1837
Kenalog Cream, Lotion & Ointment 2401
Kenalog-10 Injection ... 2402
Kenalog-40 Injection ... 2403
Kenalog in Orabase ... 604
Kenalog Spray ... 2401
Mycolog II Cream and Ointment ... 2407
Mytrex Cream & Ointment ... 2080
Nasacort Nasal Inhaler ... 1844

Triamcinolone Diacetate (Potential for hypokalemia). Products include:
Aristocort Suspension ... 1008

Triamcinolone Hexacetonide (Potential for hypokalemia). Products include:
Aristospan Suspension ... 1011

Trimethaphan Camsylate (Potentiated). Products include:
Arfonad Ampuls ... 1887

Tubocurarine Chloride (Increased responsiveness to tubocurarine).
No products indexed under this heading.

TENORMIN TABLETS AND I.V. INJECTION
(Atenolol) ... 1107
May interact with catecholamine depleting drugs and certain other agents. Compounds in these categories include:

Clonidine (Discontinue beta blocker before gradually withdrawing clonidine). Products include:
Catapres-TTS ... 677

Clonidine Hydrochloride (Discontinue beta blocker before gradually withdrawing clonidine). Products include:
Catapres Tablets ... 676
Combipres Tablets ... 678

Deserpidine (Additive effect; hypotension and/or bradycardia). Products include:
Enduronyl ... 518
Harmonyl Tablets ... 528
Oreticyl ... 545

Rauwolfia Serpentina (Additive effect; hypotension and/or bradycardia). Products include:
Raudixin Tablets ... 1803
Rauzide Tablets ... 1804

Rescinnamine (Additive effect; hypotension and/or bradycardia).
No products indexed under this heading.

Reserpine (Additive effect; hypotension and/or bradycardia). Products include:
Diupres Tablets ... 1461
Hydromox R Tablets ... 1209
Hydropres Tablets ... 1485
Renese-R Tablets ... 1786
Salutensin/Salutensin-Demi ... 719
Ser-Ap-Es Tablets ... 881
Serpasil Tablets ... 883
Serpasil-Apresoline Tablets ... 884
Serpasil-Esidrix Tablets ... 886

Verapamil Hydrochloride (Potential for serious adverse effects in patients with severe cardiomyopathy, congestive heart failure, or recent myocardial infarction when both drugs are given by intravenous route). Products include:
Calan SR Caplets ... 2157
Calan Tablets ... 2155
Isoptin Injectable ... 1177
Isoptin Oral Tablets ... 1179
Isoptin SR Sustained Release Tablets ... 1181
Verelan Capsules ... 1243
Verelan Capsules ... 2535

TENSILON INJECTABLE
(Edrophonium Chloride) ... 1123
No interactions described in labeling.

TENUATE DOSPAN CONTROLLED-RELEASE TABLETS
(Diethylpropion Hydrochloride) ... 1354
See **Tenuate Immediate-release Tablets**

TENUATE IMMEDIATE-RELEASE TABLETS
(Diethylpropion Hydrochloride) ... 1354
May interact with insulin, monoamine oxidase inhibitors, general anesthetics, vasopressors, antihypertensives, phenothiazines, and certain other agents. Compounds in these categories include:

Acebutolol Hydrochloride (Possible interference with antihypertensive drugs). Products include:
Sectral Capsules ... 2520

Alcohol (Adverse interactions).

Atenolol (Possible interference with antihypertensive drugs). Products include:
Tenoretic Tablets ... 1105
Tenormin Tablets and I.V. Injection 1107

Benazepril Hydrochloride (Possible interference with antihypertensive drugs). Products include:
Lotensin Tablets ... 872

Bendroflumethiazide (Possible interference with antihypertensive drugs). Products include:
Corzide Tablets ... 702
Naturetin Tablets ... 1789
Rauzide Tablets ... 1804

Betaxolol Hydrochloride (Possible interference with antihypertensive drugs). Products include:
Betoptic Sterile Ophthalmic Solution ... 569
Betoptic S Sterile Ophthalmic Suspension ... 570
Kerlone Tablets ... 2172

Captopril (Possible interference with antihypertensive drugs). Products include:
Capoten ... 2255
Capozide ... 2258

Carteolol Hydrochloride (Possible interference with antihypertensive drugs). Products include:
Cartrol Tablets ... 507

Chlorothiazide (Possible interference with antihypertensive drugs). Products include:
Aldoclor Tablets ... 1413
Diupres Tablets ... 1461
Diuril Oral ... 1464

Chlorothiazide Sodium (Possible interference with antihypertensive drugs). Products include:
Diuril Sodium Intravenous ... 1463

Chlorpromazine (Concurrent use may antagonize anorectic effect). Products include:
Thorazine ... 2234

Chlorthalidone (Possible interference with antihypertensive drugs). Products include:
Combipres Tablets ... 678
Tenoretic Tablets ... 1105
Thalitone Tablets ... 687

Clonidine (Possible interference with antihypertensive drugs). Products include:
Catapres-TTS ... 677

Clonidine Hydrochloride (Possible interference with antihypertensive drugs). Products include:
- Catapres Tablets ... 676
- Combipres Tablets ... 678

Deserpidine (Possible interference with antihypertensive drugs). Products include:
- Enduronyl ... 518
- Harmonyl Tablets ... 528
- Oreticyl ... 545

Diazoxide (Possible interference with antihypertensive drugs). Products include:
- Hyperstat I.V. Injection ... 2095
- Proglycem ... 649

Dopamine Hydrochloride (Possible additive pressor effects). Products include:
- Intropin Injection ... 930

Doxazosin Mesylate (Possible interference with antihypertensive drugs). Products include:
- Cardura Tablets ... 1941

Enalapril Maleate (Possible interference with antihypertensive drugs). Products include:
- Vaseretic Tablets ... 1559
- Vasotec Tablets ... 1564

Enalaprilat (Possible interference with antihypertensive drugs). Products include:
- Vasotec I.V. ... 1562

Enflurane (Concurrent use may result in arrhythmias). Products include:
- Ethrane ... 599

Epinephrine (Possible additive pressor effects). Products include:
- Ana-Kit Anaphylaxis Emergency Treatment Kit ... 1100
- Bronkaid Mist ... ▣ 757
- EpiPen ... 843
- Marcaine Hydrochloride 0.5% with Epinephrine 1:200,000 (as bitartrate) ... 958
- Marcaine Hydrochloride with Epinephrine 1:200,000 ... 2055
- Primatene Mist ... 2420
- Sus-Phrine Injection ... 1006
- Xylocaine with Epinephrine Injections ... 637

Epinephrine Hydrochloride (Possible additive pressor effects). Products include:
- Adrenalin Chloride Solution 1:100 & 1:1,000 ... 1689
- Epifrin ... ◉ 244
- Glaucon ... ◉ 218

Esmolol Hydrochloride (Possible interference with antihypertensive drugs). Products include:
- Brevibloc Injection ... 942

Felodipine (Possible interference with antihypertensive drugs). Products include:
- Plendil Extended-Release Tablets ... 1526

Fluphenazine Decanoate (Concurrent use may antagonize anorectic effect). Products include:
- Prolixin Decanoate ... 1795

Fluphenazine Enanthate (Concurrent use may antagonize anorectic effect). Products include:
- Prolixin Enanthate ... 1796

Fluphenazine Hydrochloride (Concurrent use may antagonize anorectic effect). Products include:
- Prolixin Elixir ... 1793
- Prolixin Injection ... 1791
- Prolixin Oral Concentrate ... 1792
- Prolixin Tablets ... 1793

Fosinopril Sodium (Possible interference with antihypertensive drugs). Products include:
- Monopril Tablets ... 1406

Furazolidone (Contraindication; hypertensive crises may result). Products include:
- Furoxone ... 1855

Furosemide (Possible interference with antihypertensive drugs). Products include:
- Lasix ... 1093

Guanabenz Acetate (Possible interference with antihypertensive drugs). Products include:
- Wytensin Tablets ... 2542

Guanethidine Monosulfate (Decreased hypotensive effect of guanethidine). Products include:
- Esimil Tablets ... 864
- Ismelin Tablets ... 869

Hydralazine Hydrochloride (Possible interference with antihypertensive drugs). Products include:
- Apresazide Capsules ... 854
- Apresoline Hydrochloride Parenteral (Ampuls) ... 856
- Apresoline Hydrochloride Tablets ... 855
- Apresoline-Esidrix Tablets ... 857
- Ser-Ap-Es Tablets ... 881
- Serpasil-Apresoline Tablets ... 884

Hydrochlorothiazide (Possible interference with antihypertensive drugs). Products include:
- Aldactazide ... 2150
- Aldoril Tablets ... 1418
- Apresazide Capsules ... 854
- Apresoline-Esidrix Tablets ... 857
- Capozide ... 2258
- Dyazide Capsules ... 2208
- Esidrix Tablets ... 863
- Esimil Tablets ... 864
- HydroDIURIL Tablets ... 1484
- Hydropres Tablets ... 1485
- Inderide Tablets ... 2463
- Inderide LA Long Acting Capsules ... 2465
- Lopressor HCT Tablets ... 1034
- Maxzide ... 1215
- Moduretic Tablets ... 1510
- Normozide Tablets ... 2112
- Oretic Tablets ... 544
- Oreticyl ... 545
- Prinzide Tablets ... 1540
- Ser-Ap-Es Tablets ... 881
- Serpasil-Esidrix Tablets ... 886
- Timolide Tablets ... 1547
- Trandate HCT Tablets ... 579
- Vaseretic Tablets ... 1559
- Zestoretic ... 2274

Hydroflumethiazide (Possible interference with antihypertensive drugs). Products include:
- Diucardin Tablets ... 2450
- Saluron ... 718
- Salutensin/Salutensin-Demi ... 719

Indapamide (Possible interference with antihypertensive drugs). Products include:
- Lozol Tablets ... 1843

Insulin, Human (Insulin requirements may be altered).
- No products indexed under this heading.

Insulin, Human Isophane Suspension (Insulin requirements may be altered). Products include:
- Humulin N, 100 Units ... 1270

Insulin, Human NPH (Insulin requirements may be altered). Products include:
- Insulatard NPH Human ... 1627
- Novolin N ... 1627
- Novolin N PenFill Cartridges ... 1628
- Novolin N Prefilled ... 1628

Insulin, Human Regular (Insulin requirements may be altered). Products include:
- Humulin BR, 100 Units ... 1268
- Humulin R, 100 Units ... 1272
- Novolin R ... 1627
- Novolin R PenFill Cartridges ... 1628
- Novolin R Prefilled ... 1629
- Velosulin Human ... 1628

Insulin, Human, Zinc Suspension (Insulin requirements may be altered). Products include:
- Humulin L, 100 Units ... 1268
- Humulin U, 100 Units ... 1272
- Novolin L ... 1627

Insulin, NPH (Insulin requirements may be altered). Products include:
- NPH, 40 & 100 Units ... 1273
- Beef NPH, 100 Units ... 1274
- Pork NPH, 100 Units ... 1275
- Insulatard NPH ... 1626
- NPH Insulin ... 1626
- NPH Purified Pork Isophane Insulin ... 1626

Insulin, Regular (Insulin requirements may be altered). Products include:
- Regular, 40 & 100 Units ... 1273
- Beef Regular, 100 Units ... 1275
- Pork Regular, 100 Units ... 1275
- Pork Regular (Concentrated), 500 Units ... 1276
- Regular Insulin ... 1625
- Regular Purified Pork Insulin ... 1626
- Velosulin ... 1627

Insulin, Zinc Crystals (Insulin requirements may be altered). Products include:
- NPH, 40 & 100 Units ... 1273

Insulin, Zinc Suspension (Insulin requirements may be altered). Products include:
- Lente, 40 & 100 Units ... 1272
- Protamine, Zinc, 40 & 100 Units ... 1273
- Lente Iletin I ... 1272
- Beef Lente, 100 Units ... 1274
- Beef Protamine Zinc, 100 Units ... 1274
- Pork Lente, 100 Units ... 1275
- Pork, Protamine, Zinc, 100 Units ... 1275
- Lente Insulin ... 1626
- Lente Purified Pork Insulin ... 1626
- Semilente Insulin ... 1625
- Ultralente Insulin ... 1626

Isocarboxazid (Contraindication; hypertensive crises may result). Products include:
- Marplan Tablets ... 1906

Isoflurane (Concurrent use may result in arrhythmias). Products include:
- Forane ... 600

Isradipine (Possible interference with antihypertensive drugs). Products include:
- DynaCirc Capsules ... 2004

Ketamine Hydrochloride (Concurrent use may result in arrhythmias). Products include:
- Ketalar ... 1726

Labetalol Hydrochloride (Possible interference with antihypertensive drugs). Products include:
- Normodyne Injection ... 2108
- Normodyne Tablets ... 2110
- Normozide Tablets ... 2112
- Trandate HCT Tablets ... 579
- Trandate Injection ... 577
- Trandate Tablets ... 579

Lisinopril (Possible interference with antihypertensive drugs). Products include:
- Prinivil Tablets ... 1538
- Prinzide Tablets ... 1540
- Zestoretic ... 2274
- Zestril Tablets ... 2277

Mecamylamine Hydrochloride (Possible interference with antihypertensive drugs). Products include:
- Inversine Tablets ... 1492

Mesoridazine (Concurrent use may antagonize anorectic effect). Products include:
- Serentil ... 686

Metaraminol Bitartrate (Possible additive pressor effects). Products include:
- Aramine Injection ... 1424

Methohexital Sodium (Concurrent use may result in arrhythmias). Products include:
- Brevital Sodium Vials ... 1248

Methoxamine Hydrochloride (Possible additive pressor effects). Products include:
- Vasoxyl Injection ... 819

Methoxyflurane (Concurrent use may result in arrhythmias).
- No products indexed under this heading.

Methyclothiazide (Possible interference with antihypertensive drugs). Products include:
- Enduron Tablets ... 517
- Enduronyl ... 518

Methyldopa (Possible interference with antihypertensive drugs). Products include:
- Aldoclor Tablets ... 1413
- Aldomet Oral ... 1415
- Aldoril Tablets ... 1418

Methyldopate Hydrochloride (Possible interference with antihypertensive drugs). Products include:
- Aldomet Ester HCl Injection ... 1417

Metolazone (Possible interference with antihypertensive drugs). Products include:
- Diulo ... 2129
- Mykrox ½ mg Tablets ... 984
- Zaroxolyn Tablets ... 989

Metoprolol Tartrate (Possible interference with antihypertensive drugs). Products include:
- Lopressor Ampuls ... 1032
- Lopressor HCT Tablets ... 1034
- Lopressor Tablets ... 1032

Metyrosine (Possible interference with antihypertensive drugs). Products include:
- Demser Capsules ... 1460

Minoxidil (Possible interference with antihypertensive drugs). Products include:
- Loniten Tablets ... 2346
- Rogaine Topical Solution ... 2357

Nadolol (Possible interference with antihypertensive drugs). Products include:
- Corgard Tablets ... 701
- Corzide Tablets ... 702

Nicardipine Hydrochloride (Possible interference with antihypertensive drugs). Products include:
- Cardene Capsules ... 2290

Nitroglycerin (Possible interference with antihypertensive drugs). Products include:
- Deponit NTG Transdermal Delivery System ... 2143
- Minitran Transdermal Delivery System ... 1312
- Nitro-Bid Ointment ... 1339
- Nitro-Bid Capsules ... 1338
- Nitrodisc ... 2176
- Nitro-Dur (nitroglycerin) Transdermal Infusion System ... 1164
- Nitrogard Tablets ... 1004
- Nitrolingual Spray ... 1846
- Nitrostat Tablets ... 1743
- Transderm-Nitro Transdermal Therapeutic System ... 2283

Norepinephrine Bitartrate (Possible additive pressor effects). Products include:
- Levophed Bitartrate Injection ... 2054

Penbutolol Sulfate (Possible interference with antihypertensive drugs). Products include:
- Levatol ... 1832

Perphenazine (Concurrent use may antagonize anorectic effect). Products include:
- Etrafon ... 2087
- Triavil Tablets ... 1556
- Trilafon ... 2123

Phenelzine Sulfate (Contraindication; hypertensive crises may result). Products include:
- Nardil ... 1742

Phenoxybenzamine Hydrochloride (Possible interference with antihypertensive drugs). Products include:
- Dibenzyline Capsules ... 2207

Phentolamine Mesylate (Possible interference with antihypertensive drugs). Products include:
Regitine ... 878

Pindolol (Possible interference with antihypertensive drugs). Products include:
Visken Tablets ... 2036

Polythiazide (Possible interference with antihypertensive drugs). Products include:
Minizide Capsules ... 1779
Renese Tablets ... 1785
Renese-R Tablets ... 1786

Prazosin Hydrochloride (Possible interference with antihypertensive drugs). Products include:
Minipress Capsules ... 1778
Minizide Capsules ... 1779

Prochlorperazine (Concurrent use may antagonize anorectic effect). Products include:
Compazine ... 2201

Promethazine Hydrochloride (Concurrent use may antagonize anorectic effect). Products include:
Mepergan Injection ... 2479
Phenergan with Codeine ... 2497
Phenergan with Dextromethorphan 2499
Phenergan Injection ... 2493
Phenergan Suppositories ... 2496
Phenergan Syrup ... 2495
Phenergan Tablets ... 2496
Phenergan VC ... 2500
Phenergan VC with Codeine ... 2501

Propofol (Concurrent use may result in arrhythmias). Products include:
Diprivan Injection ... 2267

Propranolol Hydrochloride (Possible interference with antihypertensive drugs). Products include:
Inderal ... 2459
Inderal LA Long Acting Capsules ... 2461
Inderide Tablets ... 2463
Inderide LA Long Acting Capsules .. 2465

Ramipril (Possible interference with antihypertensive drugs). Products include:
Altace Capsules ... 1086

Rauwolfia Serpentina (Possible interference with antihypertensive drugs). Products include:
Raudixin Tablets ... 1803
Rauzide Tablets ... 1804

Rescinnamine (Possible interference with antihypertensive drugs).
No products indexed under this heading.

Reserpine (Possible interference with antihypertensive drugs). Products include:
Diupres Tablets ... 1461
Hydromox R Tablets ... 1209
Hydropres Tablets ... 1485
Renese-R Tablets ... 1786
Salutensin/Salutensin-Demi ... 719
Ser-Ap-Es Tablets ... 881
Serpasil Tablets ... 883
Serpasil-Apresoline Tablets ... 884
Serpasil-Esidrix Tablets ... 886

Selegiline Hydrochloride (Contraindication; hypertensive crises may result). Products include:
Eldepryl ... 2250

Sodium Nitroprusside (Possible interference with antihypertensive drugs). Products include:
Nipride I.V. Infusion ... 1909

Terazosin Hydrochloride (Possible interference with antihypertensive drugs). Products include:
Hytrin Tablets ... 529

Thioridazine Hydrochloride (Concurrent use may antagonize anorectic effect). Products include:
Mellaril ... 2011

Timolol Maleate (Possible interference with antihypertensive drugs). Products include:
Blocadren Tablets ... 1429
Timolide Tablets ... 1547
Timoptic in Ocudose ... 1552
Timoptic Sterile Ophthalmic Solution ... 1550

Tranylcypromine Sulfate (Contraindication; hypertensive crises may result). Products include:
Parnate Tablets ... 2222

Trifluoperazine Hydrochloride (Concurrent use may antagonize anorectic effect). Products include:
Stelazine ... 2226

Trimethaphan Camsylate (Possible interference with antihypertensive drugs). Products include:
Arfonad Ampuls ... 1887

TERAZOL 3 VAGINAL CREAM
(Terconazole) ... 1676
No interactions described in labeling.

TERAZOL 3 VAGINAL SUPPOSITORIES
(Terconazole) ... 1677
No interactions described in labeling.

TERAZOL 7 VAGINAL CREAM
(Terconazole) ... 1677
No interactions described in labeling.

TERRA-CORTRIL OPHTHALMIC SUSPENSION
(Oxytetracycline Hydrochloride, Hydrocortisone Acetate) ... 1963
No interactions described in labeling.

TERRAMYCIN CAPSULES
(Oxytetracycline) ... 1786
May interact with oral anticoagulants, penicillins, and antacids containing aluminum, calcium and magnesium. Compounds in these categories include:

Aluminum Carbonate Gel (Impaired tetracycline absorption). Products include:
Basaljel ... 2438

Aluminum Hydroxide (Impaired tetracycline absorption). Products include:
Cama Arthritis Pain Reliever ... ▣ 685
Gaviscon Extra Strength Relief Formula Liquid Antacid ... ▣ 594
Gaviscon Extra Strength Relief Formula Antacid Tablets ... ▣ 594
Gaviscon Liquid Antacid ... ▣ 594
Gelusil Liquid & Tablets ... ▣ 639
Extra Strength Maalox Plus Suspension ... 1850
Maalox TC Suspension ... 1851
Maalox Plus Tablets ... ▣ 655
Extra Strength Maalox Plus Tablets 1850
Nephrox Suspension ... ▣ 563
WinGel Liquid & Tablets ... ▣ 761

Aluminum Hydroxide Gel (Impaired tetracycline absorption). Products include:
ALternaGEL Liquid ... 1154
Aludrox Oral Suspension ... 2428
Amphojel Suspension ... 2429
Amphojel Suspension without Flavor ... 2429
Mylanta Liquid ... 1155
Mylanta Double Strength Liquid ... 1155

Aluminum Hydroxide Gel, Dried (Impaired tetracycline absorption). Products include:
Alu-Tab/Alu-Cap ... 1309
Amphojel Tablets ... 2429
Ascriptin A/D Caplets ... 1850
Regular Strength Ascriptin Tablets 1850
Gaviscon Antacid Tablets ... ▣ 593
Gaviscon-2 Antacid Tablets ... ▣ 594
Mylanta Tablets ... 1155
Mylanta Double Strength Tablets ... 1155

Amoxicillin (Interference with bactericidal action of penicillin). Products include:
Amoxil ... 2193
Augmentin Tablets, Powder for Oral Suspension, and Chewable Tablets ... 2198

Ampicillin Sodium (Interference with bactericidal action of penicillin). Products include:
Unasyn ... 1965

Azlocillin Sodium (Interference with bactericidal action of penicillin).
No products indexed under this heading.

Bacampicillin Hydrochloride (Interference with bactericidal action of penicillin). Products include:
Spectrobid Tablets & Powder for Oral Suspension ... 1961

Carbenicillin Disodium (Interference with bactericidal action of penicillin).

Carbenicillin Indanyl Sodium (Interference with bactericidal action of penicillin). Products include:
Geocillin Tablets ... 1951

Dicumarol (Decreased anticoagulant dosage). Products include:
Dicumarol Tablets ... 516

Dihydroxyaluminum Sodium Carbonate (Impaired tetracycline absorption). Products include:
Rolaids ... ▣ 743

Magaldrate (Impaired tetracycline absorption). Products include:
Riopan Antacid Chew Tablets ... ▣ 754
Riopan Antacid Chew Tablets in Rollpacks ... ▣ 754
Riopan Antacid Suspension ... 2421
Riopan Antacid Swallow Tablets ... 2421
Riopan Plus Chew Tablets ... 2422
Riopan Plus Chew Tablets in Rollpack ... 2422
Riopan Plus 2 Chew Tablets, Mint Flavor, Cherry Flavor ... 2422
Riopan Plus Suspension ... 2422
Riopan Plus 2 Suspension, Mint Flavor, Cherry Flavor ... 2422

Magnesium Hydroxide (Impaired tetracycline absorption). Products include:
Aludrox Oral Suspension ... 2428
Ascriptin A/D Caplets ... 1850
Regular Strength Ascriptin Tablets 1850
Di-Gel Antacid/Anti-Gas ... ▣ 697
Gelusil Liquid & Tablets ... ▣ 639
Haley's M-O, Regular & Flavored .. ▣ 569
Extra Strength Maalox Plus Suspension ... 1850
Maalox TC Suspension ... 1851
Maalox Plus Tablets ... ▣ 655
Extra Strength Maalox Plus Tablets 1850
Mylanta Liquid ... 1155
Mylanta Tablets ... 1155
Mylanta Double Strength Liquid ... 1155
Mylanta Double Strength Tablets ... 1155
Concentrated Phillips' Milk of Magnesia ... ▣ 573
Phillips' Milk of Magnesia Liquid ... ▣ 572
Phillips' Milk of Magnesia Tablets ... ▣ 573
WinGel Liquid & Tablets ... ▣ 761

Magnesium Oxide (Impaired tetracycline absorption). Products include:
Bayer Plus Aspirin Tablets ... ▣ 567
Beelith Tablets ... 659
Bufferin Analgesic Tablets and Caplets ... ▣ 524
Cama Arthritis Pain Reliever ... ▣ 685
Mag-Ox 400 ... 673
Uro-Mag ... 673

Mezlocillin Sodium (Interference with bactericidal action of penicillin). Products include:
Mezlin ... 1597
Mezlin Pharmacy Bulk Package ... 1599

Nafcillin Sodium (Interference with bactericidal action of penicillin). Products include:
Unipen ... 2533

Penicillin G Potassium (Interference with bactericidal action of penicillin). Products include:
Pfizerpen for Injection ... 1957

Penicillin G Procaine (Interference with bactericidal action of penicillin). Products include:
Bicillin C-R Injection ... 2438
Bicillin C-R 900/300 Injection ... 2440
Pfizerpen-AS Aqueous Suspension 1959
Wycillin Injection ... 2537
Wycillin Injection and Probenecid Tablets ... 2539

Penicillin G Sodium (Interference with bactericidal action of penicillin).
No products indexed under this heading.

Penicillin G, Benzathine (Interference with bactericidal action of penicillin). Products include:
Bicillin C-R Injection ... 2438
Bicillin C-R 900/300 Injection ... 2440
Bicillin L-A Injection ... 2442

Penicillin V Potassium (Interference with bactericidal action of penicillin).
No products indexed under this heading.

Ticarcillin Disodium (Interference with bactericidal action of penicillin). Products include:
Ticar for Injection ... 2236
Timentin for Injection ... 2239

Warfarin Sodium (Decreased anticoagulant dosage). Products include:
Coumadin Injection & Tablets ... 944
Panwarfin Tablets ... 547

Food Interactions

Dairy products (Interferes with absorption).

Food, unspecified (Interferes with absorption).

TERRAMYCIN INTRAMUSCULAR SOLUTION
(Oxytetracycline) ... 1964
May interact with anticoagulants, penicillins, and certain other agents. Compounds in these categories include:

Amoxicillin (Interference with penicillin's bactericidal action). Products include:
Amoxil ... 2193
Augmentin Tablets, Powder for Oral Suspension, and Chewable Tablets ... 2198

Ampicillin Sodium (Interference with penicillin's bactericidal action). Products include:
Unasyn ... 1965

Azlocillin Sodium (Interference with penicillin's bactericidal action).
No products indexed under this heading.

Bacampicillin Hydrochloride (Interference with penicillin's bactericidal action). Products include:
Spectrobid Tablets & Powder for Oral Suspension ... 1961

Carbenicillin Disodium (Interference with penicillin's bactericidal action).

Carbenicillin Indanyl Sodium (Interference with penicillin's bactericidal action). Products include:
Geocillin Tablets ... 1951

Dicumarol (Depressed plasma prothrombin activity; downward adjustment of anticoagulant dosage may be necessary). Products include:
Dicumarol Tablets ... 516

Heparin Calcium (Depressed plasma prothrombin activity; downward adjustment of anticoagulant dosage may be necessary). Products include:

- Calciparine Injection ... 925

Heparin Sodium (Depressed plasma prothrombin activity; downward adjustment of anticoagulant dosage may be necessary). Products include:

- Heparin Lock Flush Solution ... 2456
- Heparin Sodium Vials ... 1264
- Heparin Sodium Injection ... 2457
- Heparin Sodium Injection, USP, Sterile Solution ... 2342

Mezlocillin Sodium (Interference with penicillin's bactericidal action). Products include:

- Mezlin ... 1597
- Mezlin Pharmacy Bulk Package ... 1599

Nafcillin Sodium (Interference with penicillin's bactericidal action). Products include:

- Unipen ... 2533

Other Potentially Hepatotoxic Drugs (Should not be prescribed concomitantly).

Penicillin G Potassium (Interference with penicillin's bactericidal action). Products include:

- Pfizerpen for Injection ... 1957

Penicillin G Procaine (Interference with penicillin's bactericidal action). Products include:

- Bicillin C-R Injection ... 2438
- Bicillin C-R 900/300 Injection ... 2440
- Pfizerpen-AS Aqueous Suspension ... 1959
- Wycillin Injection ... 2537
- Wycillin Injection and Probenecid Tablets ... 2539

Penicillin G Sodium (Interference with penicillin's bactericidal action).

- No products indexed under this heading.

Penicillin G, Benzathine (Interference with penicillin's bactericidal action). Products include:

- Bicillin C-R Injection ... 2438
- Bicillin C-R 900/300 Injection ... 2440
- Bicillin L-A Injection ... 2442

Penicillin (Repository) (Interference with penicillin's bactericidal action). Products include:

- Bicillin C-R Injection ... 2438
- Bicillin C-R 900/300 Injection ... 2440
- Bicillin L-A Injection ... 2442

Penicillin V Potassium (Interference with penicillin's bactericidal action).

- No products indexed under this heading.

Ticarcillin Disodium (Interference with penicillin's bactericidal action). Products include:

- Ticar for Injection ... 2236
- Timentin for Injection ... 2239

Warfarin Sodium (Depressed plasma prothrombin activity; downward adjustment of anticoagulant dosage may be necessary). Products include:

- Coumadin Injection & Tablets ... 944
- Panwarfin Tablets ... 547

TERRAMYCIN WITH POLYMYXIN B SULFATE OPHTHALMIC OINTMENT

(Oxytetracycline Hydrochloride, Polymyxin B Sulfate) ... 1965
No interactions described in labeling.

TESLAC TABLETS

(Testolactone) ... 741
May interact with oral anticoagulants. Compounds in this category include:

Dicumarol (Increased effects of oral anticoagulant). Products include:

- Dicumarol Tablets ... 516

Warfarin Sodium (Increased effects of oral anticoagulant). Products include:

- Coumadin Injection & Tablets ... 944
- Panwarfin Tablets ... 547

TESSALON PERLES

(Benzonatate) ... 1006
No interactions described in labeling.

TESTRED CAPSULES

(Methyltestosterone) ... 1124
May interact with oral anticoagulants, insulin, and certain other agents. Compounds in these categories include:

Dicumarol (Decreased need for anticoagulants). Products include:

- Dicumarol Tablets ... 516

Insulin, Human (Possibly decreased insulin requirements).

- No products indexed under this heading.

Insulin, Human Isophane Suspension (Possibly decreased insulin requirements). Products include:

- Humulin N, 100 Units ... 1270

Insulin, Human NPH (Possibly decreased insulin requirements). Products include:

- Insulatard NPH Human ... 1627
- Novolin N ... 1627
- Novolin N PenFill Cartridges ... 1628
- Novolin N Prefilled ... 1628

Insulin, Human Regular (Possibly decreased insulin requirements). Products include:

- Humulin BR, 100 Units ... 1268
- Humulin R, 100 Units ... 1272
- Novolin R ... 1627
- Novolin R PenFill Cartridges ... 1628
- Novolin R Prefilled ... 1629
- Velosulin Human ... 1628

Insulin, Human, Zinc Suspension (Possibly decreased insulin requirements). Products include:

- Humulin L, 100 Units ... 1268
- Humulin U, 100 Units ... 1272
- Novolin L ... 1627

Insulin, NPH (Possibly decreased insulin requirements). Products include:

- NPH, 40 & 100 Units ... 1273
- Beef NPH, 100 Units ... 1274
- Pork NPH, 100 Units ... 1275
- Insulatard NPH ... 1626
- NPH Insulin ... 1626
- NPH Purified Pork Isophane Insulin ... 1626

Insulin, Regular (Possibly decreased insulin requirements). Products include:

- Regular, 40 & 100 Units ... 1273
- Beef Regular, 100 Units ... 1275
- Pork Regular, 100 Units ... 1275
- Pork Regular (Concentrated), 500 Units ... 1276
- Regular Insulin ... 1625
- Regular Purified Pork Insulin ... 1626
- Velosulin ... 1627

Insulin, Zinc Crystals (Possibly decreased insulin requirements). Products include:

- NPH, 40 & 100 Units ... 1273

Insulin, Zinc Suspension (Possibly decreased insulin requirements). Products include:

- Lente, 40 & 100 Units ... 1272
- Protamine, Zinc, 40 & 100 Units ... 1273
- Lente Iletin I ... 1272
- Beef Lente, 100 Units ... 1274
- Beef Protamine Zinc, 100 Units ... 1274
- Pork Lente, 100 Units ... 1275
- Pork, Protamine, Zinc, 100 Units ... 1275
- Lente Insulin ... 1626
- Lente Purified Pork Insulin ... 1626
- Semilente Insulin ... 1625
- Ultralente Insulin ... 1626

Oxyphenbutazone (Elevated serum levels of oxyphenbutazone).

Warfarin Sodium (Decreased need for anticoagulants). Products include:

- Coumadin Injection & Tablets ... 944
- Panwarfin Tablets ... 547

TETANUS & DIPHTHERIA TOXOIDS, ADSORBED PUROGENATED

(Tetanus & Diphtheria Toxoids Adsorbed (For Adult Use)) ... 1237
No interactions described in labeling.

TETANUS TOXOID, ADSORBED PUROGENATED

(Tetanus Toxoid, Adsorbed) ... 1238
May interact with immunosuppressive agents and certain other agents. Compounds in these categories include:

Azathioprine (Concurrent use should be avoided). Products include:

- Imuran ... 768

Cyclosporine (Concurrent use should be avoided). Products include:

- Sandimmune ... 2024

Immune Globulin (Human) (Concurrent use should be avoided). Products include:

- MICRhoGAM Rh_0(D) Immune Globulin (Human) ... 1650
- RhoGAM Rh_0(D) Immune Globulin (Human) ... 1651

Immune Globulin Intravenous (Human) (Concurrent use should be avoided). Products include:

- Gamimune N Immune Globulin Intravenous (Human) ... 1572
- Gammagard Immune Globulin, Intravenous (Human) ... 658
- Iveegam ... 1129
- Sandoglobulin I.V. ... 2027

Muromonab-CD3 (Concurrent use should be avoided). Products include:

- Orthoclone OKT3 Sterile Solution ... 1645

THALITONE TABLETS

(Chlorthalidone) ... 687
May interact with cardiac glycosides, ganglionic blocking agents, insulin, antihypertensives, oral hypoglycemic agents, lithium preparations, corticosteroids, narcotic analgesics, barbiturates, and certain other agents. Compounds in these categories include:

Acebutolol Hydrochloride (Potentiated or additive action). Products include:

- Sectral Capsules ... 2520

ACTH (Potential for hypokalemia).

- No products indexed under this heading.

Alcohol (Orthostatic hypotension may be aggravated; increased chances of dizziness).

Alfentanil Hydrochloride (Aggravates orthostatic hypotension). Products include:

- Alfenta Injection ... 1131

Aprobarbital (Aggravates orthostatic hypotension). Products include:

- Alurate Elixir ... 1883

Atenolol (Potentiated or additive action). Products include:

- Tenoretic Tablets ... 1105
- Tenormin Tablets and I.V. Injection ... 1107

Benazepril Hydrochloride (Potentiated or additive action). Products include:

- Lotensin Tablets ... 872

Bendroflumethiazide (Potentiated). Products include:

- Corzide Tablets ... 702
- Naturetin Tablets ... 1789
- Rauzide Tablets ... 1804

Betamethasone Acetate (Potential for hypokalemia). Products include:

- Celestone Soluspan Suspension ... 2081

Betamethasone Sodium Phosphate (Potential for hypokalemia). Products include:

- Celestone Soluspan Suspension ... 2081

Betaxolol Hydrochloride (Potentiated or additive action). Products include:

- Betoptic Sterile Ophthalmic Solution ... 569
- Betoptic S Sterile Ophthalmic Suspension ... 570
- Kerlone Tablets ... 2172

Buprenorphine (Aggravates orthostatic hypotension).

- No products indexed under this heading.

Butabarbital (Aggravates orthostatic hypotension). Products include:

- Pyridium Plus ... 1764

Butalbital (Aggravates orthostatic hypotension). Products include:

- Esgic-Plus Tablets ... 1002
- Esgic Tablets & Capsules ... 1001
- Fioricet Tablets ... 2006
- Fiorinal Capsules ... 2007
- Fiorinal with Codeine Capsules ... 2008
- Fiorinal Tablets ... 2007
- Phrenilin ... 838
- Sedapap Tablets 50 mg/650 mg ... 1360

Captopril (Potentiated or additive action). Products include:

- Capoten ... 2255
- Capozide ... 2258

Carteolol Hydrochloride (Potentiated or additive action). Products include:

- Cartrol Tablets ... 507

Chlorothiazide (Potentiated or additive action). Products include:

- Aldoclor Tablets ... 1413
- Diupres Tablets ... 1461
- Diuril Oral ... 1464

Chlorothiazide Sodium (Potentiated or additive action). Products include:

- Diuril Sodium Intravenous ... 1463

Chlorpropamide (Higher dosage oral hypoglycemic agents may be required). Products include:

- Diabinese Tablets ... 1775

Clonidine (Potentiated or additive action). Products include:

- Catapres-TTS ... 677

Clonidine Hydrochloride (Potentiated or additive action). Products include:

- Catapres Tablets ... 676
- Combipres Tablets ... 678

Codeine (Aggravates orthostatic hypotension). Products include:

- Calcidrine Syrup ... 506

Codeine Phosphate (Aggravates orthostatic hypotension). Products include:

- Actifed with Codeine Cough Syrup ... 752
- Cheracol Cough Syrup ... 1853
- Codimal PH Syrup ... 846
- Dimetane-DC Cough Syrup ... 1857
- Empirin with Codeine Phosphate Nos. 2, 3 & 4 ... 764
- Fiorinal with Codeine Capsules ... 2008
- Isoclor Expectorant ... 982
- Naldecon CX Adult Liquid ... ▣ 521
- Novahistine DH ... 1342
- Novahistine Expectorant ... 1343
- Nucofed Capsules ... 2219

Nucofed Expectorant 2219
Nucofed Pediatric Expectorant 2220
Nucofed Syrup 2219
Phenaphen with Codeine Capsules 1865
Phenaphen-650 with Codeine Tablets 1866
Phenergan with Codeine 2497
Phenergan VC with Codeine 2501
Robitussin A-C Syrup 1875
Robitussin-DAC Syrup 1875
Ryna .... ▣ 741
Soma Compound w/Codeine Tablets 2390
Triaminic Expectorant w/Codeine .. 1996
Tussi-Organidin Liquid 2391
Tylenol with Codeine 1381

Codeine Polistirex (Aggravates orthostatic hypotension).
No products indexed under this heading.

Cortisone Acetate (Potential for hypokalemia). Products include:
Cortone Acetate Sterile Suspension 1437
Cortone Acetate Tablets 1439

Deserpidine (Potentiated). Products include:
Enduronyl 518
Harmonyl Tablets 528
Oreticyl 545

Deslanoside (May exaggerate metabolic effects of hypokalemia, especially with reference to myocardial activity).
No products indexed under this heading.

Dexamethasone (Potential for hypokalemia). Products include:
AK-Trol Ointment & Suspension .... ◉ 207
Decadron Elixir 1445
Decadron Tablets 1447
Decaspray Topical Aerosol 1459
Dexacidin .... ◉ 272
Maxidex Sterile Ophthalmic Suspension .... ◉ 223
Maxitrol Ophthalmic Ointment/Suspension .... ◉ 223
TobraDex Ophthalmic Suspension and Ointment .... ◉ 228

Dexamethasone Acetate (Potential for hypokalemia). Products include:
Dalalone D.P. Injectable 999
Decadron-LA Sterile Suspension 1457

Dexamethasone Sodium Phosphate (Potential for hypokalemia). Products include:
AK-Dex .... ◉ 203
Decadron Phosphate Respihaler 1454
Decadron Phosphate Sterile Ophthalmic Ointment 1453
Decadron Phosphate Sterile Ophthalmic Solution 1453
Decadron Phosphate Topical Cream 1455
Decadron Phosphate Turbinaire 1456
Maxidex Sterile Ophthalmic Ointment .... ◉ 222
NeoDecadron Sterile Ophthalmic Ointment 1517
NeoDecadron Sterile Ophthalmic Solution 1518
NeoDecadron Topical Cream 1518

Dezocine (Aggravates orthostatic hypotension).

Diazoxide (Potentiated or additive action). Products include:
Hyperstat I.V. Injection 2095
Proglycem 649

Digitoxin (May exaggerate metabolic effects of hypokalemia, especially with reference to myocardial activity). Products include:
Crystodigin Tablets 1253

Digoxin (May exaggerate metabolic effects of hypokalemia, especially with reference to myocardial activity). Products include:
Lanoxicaps 772
Lanoxin Elixir Pediatric 775
Lanoxin Injection 778
Lanoxin Injection Pediatric 781
Lanoxin Tablets 783

Doxazosin Mesylate (Potentiated or additive action). Products include:
Cardura Tablets 1941

Enalapril Maleate (Potentiated or additive action). Products include:
Vaseretic Tablets 1559
Vasotec Tablets 1564

Enalaprilat (Potentiated or additive action). Products include:
Vasotec I.V. 1562

Esmolol Hydrochloride (Potentiated or additive action). Products include:
Brevibloc Injection 942

Felodipine (Potentiated or additive action). Products include:
Plendil Extended-Release Tablets 1526

Fentanyl (Aggravates orthostatic hypotension). Products include:
Duragesic Transdermal System 1133

Fentanyl Citrate (Aggravates orthostatic hypotension). Products include:
Innovar Injection 1141
Sublimaze Injection 1146

Fosinopril Sodium (Potentiated or additive action). Products include:
Monopril Tablets 1406

Furosemide (Potentiated or additive action). Products include:
Lasix 1093

Glipizide (Higher dosage oral hypoglycemic agents may be required). Products include:
Glucotrol 1952

Glyburide (Higher dosage oral hypoglycemic agents may be required). Products include:
DiaBeta 1091
Micronase Tablets 2350

Guanabenz Acetate (Potentiated or additive action). Products include:
Wytensin Tablets 2542

Guanethidine Monosulfate (Potentiated). Products include:
Esimil Tablets 864
Ismelin Tablets 869

Hydralazine Hydrochloride (Potentiated or additive action). Products include:
Apresazide Capsules 854
Apresoline Hydrochloride Parenteral (Ampuls) 856
Apresoline Hydrochloride Tablets .. 855
Apresoline-Esidrix Tablets 857
Ser-Ap-Es Tablets 881
Serpasil-Apresoline Tablets 884

Hydrochlorothiazide (Potentiated). Products include:
Aldactazide 2150
Aldoril Tablets 1418
Apresazide Capsules 854
Apresoline-Esidrix Tablets 857
Capozide 2258
Dyazide Capsules 2208
Esidrix Tablets 863
Esimil Tablets 864
HydroDIURIL Tablets 1484
Hydropres Tablets 1485
Inderide Tablets 2463
Inderide LA Long Acting Capsules .. 2465
Lopressor HCT Tablets 1034
Maxzide 1215
Moduretic Tablets 1510
Normozide Tablets 2112
Oretic Tablets 544
Oreticyl 545
Prinzide Tablets 1540
Ser-Ap-Es Tablets 881
Serpasil-Esidrix Tablets 886
Timolide Tablets 1547
Trandate HCT Tablets 579
Vaseretic Tablets 1559
Zestoretic 2274

Hydrocodone Bitartrate (Aggravates orthostatic hypotension). Products include:
Anexsia 5/500 Tablets 2196
Anexsia 7.5/650 Tablets 2197
Azdone Tablets 844
Codiclear DH Syrup 845
Codimal DH Syrup 846
Damason-P 1356
Hycodan Syrup, Tablets 927
Hycomine Compound Tablets 929
Hycomine Syrup 927
Hycotuss Expectorant Syrup 930
Hydrocet Capsules 835
Lortab ASA Tablets 2414
Lortab 2412
Ru-Tuss with Hydrocodone 694
Triaminic Expectorant DH 1995
Vicodin Tablets 1187
Vicodin ES Tablets 1189
Zydone Capsules 941

Hydrocodone Polistirex (Aggravates orthostatic hypotension). Products include:
Tussionex Extended-Release Suspension 988

Hydrocortisone (Potential for hypokalemia). Products include:
AK-Spore H.C. .... ◉ 206
Bactine Hydrocortisone Anti-Itch Cream .... ▣ 625
CaldeCORT Anti-Itch Hydrocortisone Spray .... ▣ 560
Carmol HC Cream 1% 2296
Cortaid Spray .... ▣ 735
Cortenema 2244
Cortisporin Ointment 758
Cortisporin Ophthalmic Ointment Sterile 758
Cortisporin Ophthalmic Suspension Sterile 759
Cortisporin Otic Solution Sterile 760
Cortisporin Otic Suspension Sterile 760
Cortizone-5 Creme & Ointment .... ▣ 732
Dermolate Anti-Itch Cream .... ▣ 697
Eldecort Cream 1.0% 1113
Eldecort Cream 1.0% and 2.5% 1113
Fungoid HC Creme 1770
Hydrocortone Tablets 1482
Hytone 909
LazerSporin-C Solution 1770
Massengill Medicated Soft Cloth Towelettes 2192
Nutracort Cream & Lotion 1684
PediOtic Suspension Sterile 797
Synacort Creams 1%, 2.5% 2296
Vanoxide-HC Acne Lotion 911
Vioform-Hydrocortisone Cream and Mild Cream 889
Vioform-Hydrocortisone Ointment .. 889
VōSoL HC Otic Solution 2392
Vytone Cream 1% 911

Hydrocortisone Acetate (Potential for hypokalemia). Products include:
Analpram-HC Rectal Cream 1% and 2.5% 970
Anusol-HC Cream 1690
Anusol-HC Suppositories 1691
Caldecort .... ▣ 560
Carmol HC Cream 1% 2296
Chloromycetin Hydrocortisone Ophthalmic 1694
Coly-Mycin S Otic w/Neomycin & Hydrocortisone 1708
Cortaid .... ▣ 735
Cortef Feminine Itch Cream .... ▣ 735
Corticaine .... ▣ 682
Cortifoam 1827
Cortisporin Cream 757
Epifoam 1828
Gynecort 5 Creme .... ▣ 556
Hydrocortone Acetate Sterile Suspension 1479
Lanacort 5 Creme and Ointment .. ▣ 557
Mantadil Cream 789
Ophthocort .... ◉ 301
Orabase HCA Oral Paste 890
Pramosone Cream, Lotion & Ointment 971
ProctoCream-HC 1834
Proctofoam-HC 1835

Hydrocortisone Sodium Phosphate (Potential for hypokalemia). Products include:
Hydrocortone Phosphate Injection, Sterile 1481

Hydrocortisone Sodium Succinate (Potential for hypokalemia). Products include:
Solu-Cortef Sterile Powder 2361

Hydroflumethiazide (Potentiated or additive action). Products include:
Diucardin Tablets 2450
Saluron 718
Salutensin/Salutensin-Demi 719

Indapamide (Potentiated or additive action). Products include:
Lozol Tablets 1843

Insulin, Human (Insulin requirements may change).
No products indexed under this heading.

Insulin, Human Isophane Suspension (Insulin requirements may change). Products include:
Humulin N, 100 Units 1270

Insulin, Human NPH (Insulin requirements may change). Products include:
Insulatard NPH Human 1627
Novolin N 1627
Novolin N PenFill Cartridges 1628
Novolin N Prefilled 1628

Insulin, Human Regular (Insulin requirements may change). Products include:
Humulin BR, 100 Units 1268
Humulin R, 100 Units 1272
Novolin R 1627
Novolin R PenFill Cartridges 1628
Novolin R Prefilled 1629
Velosulin Human 1628

Insulin, Human, Zinc Suspension (Insulin requirements may change). Products include:
Humulin L, 100 Units 1268
Humulin U, 100 Units 1272
Novolin L 1627

Insulin, NPH (Insulin requirements may change). Products include:
NPH, 40 & 100 Units 1273
Beef NPH, 100 Units 1274
Pork NPH, 100 Units 1275
Insulatard NPH 1626
NPH Insulin 1626
NPH Purified Pork Isophane Insulin 1626

Insulin, Regular (Insulin requirements may change). Products include:
Regular, 40 & 100 Units 1273
Beef Regular, 100 Units 1275
Pork Regular, 100 Units 1275
Pork Regular (Concentrated), 500 Units 1276
Regular Insulin 1625
Regular Purified Pork Insulin 1626
Velosulin 1627

Insulin, Zinc Crystals (Insulin requirements may change). Products include:
NPH, 40 & 100 Units 1273

Insulin, Zinc Suspension (Insulin requirements may change). Products include:
Lente, 40 & 100 Units 1272
Protamine, Zinc, 40 & 100 Units 1273
Lente Iletin I 1272
Beef Lente, 100 Units 1274
Beef Protamine Zinc, 100 Units 1274
Pork Lente, 100 Units 1275
Pork, Protamine, Zinc, 100 Units 1275
Lente Insulin 1626
Lente Purified Pork Insulin 1626
Semilente Insulin 1625
Ultralente Insulin 1626

Isradipine (Potentiated or additive action). Products include:
DynaCirc Capsules 2004

Labetalol Hydrochloride (Potentiated or additive action). Products include:
Normodyne Injection 2108
Normodyne Tablets 2110
Normozide Tablets 2112
Trandate HCT Tablets 579
Trandate Injection 577
Trandate Tablets 579

Levorphanol Tartrate (Aggravates orthostatic hypotension). Products include:
Levo-Dromoran 1906

Lisinopril (Potentiated or additive action). Products include:
Prinivil Tablets 1538
Prinzide Tablets 1540

Zestoretic ... 2274
Zestril Tablets ... 2277

Lithium Carbonate (Increased risk of lithium toxicity). Products include:
Eskalith ... 2214
Lithane Tablets ... 1596
Lithium Carbonate Capsules & Tablets ... 1984
Lithobid Tablets ... 870

Lithium Citrate (Increased risk of lithium toxicity). Products include:
Cibalith-S ... 870

Mecamylamine Hydrochloride (Potentiated). Products include:
Inversine Tablets ... 1492

Meperidine Hydrochloride (Aggravates orthostatic hypotension). Products include:
Demerol ... 2047
Mepergan Injection ... 2479

Mephobarbital (Aggravates orthostatic hypotension). Products include:
Mebaral Tablets ... 2061

Methadone Hydrochloride (Aggravates orthostatic hypotension). Products include:
Dolophine Hydrochloride Ampoules & Vials ... 1260
Dolophine Hydrochloride Tablets ... 1261
Methadone Hydrochloride Diskets ... 1284
Methadone Hydrochloride Oral Solution & Tablets ... 1987

Methyclothiazide (Potentiated or additive action). Products include:
Enduron Tablets ... 517
Enduronyl ... 518

Methyldopa (Potentiated or additive action). Products include:
Aldoclor Tablets ... 1413
Aldomet Oral ... 1415
Aldoril Tablets ... 1418

Methyldopate Hydrochloride (Potentiated or additive action). Products include:
Aldomet Ester HCl Injection ... 1417

Methylprednisolone Acetate (Potential for hypokalemia). Products include:
Depo-Medrol Sterile Aqueous Suspension ... 2334

Methylprednisolone Sodium Succinate (Potential for hypokalemia). Products include:
Solu-Medrol Sterile Powder ... 2363

Metolazone (Potentiated or additive action). Products include:
Diulo ... 2129
Mykrox ½ mg Tablets ... 984
Zaroxolyn Tablets ... 989

Metoprolol Tartrate (Potentiated or additive action). Products include:
Lopressor Ampuls ... 1032
Lopressor HCT Tablets ... 1034
Lopressor Tablets ... 1032

Metyrosine (Potentiated or additive action). Products include:
Demser Capsules ... 1460

Minoxidil (Potentiated or additive action). Products include:
Loniten Tablets ... 2346
Rogaine Topical Solution ... 2357

Morphine Sulfate (Aggravates orthostatic hypotension). Products include:
Astramorph/PF Injection, USP (Preservative-Free) ... 618
Duramorph ... 960
Infumorph 200 and Infumorph 500 Sterile Solutions ... 962
MS Contin Tablets ... 1814
MSIR ... 1817
Oramorph SR (Morphine Sulfate Sustained Release Tablets) ... 1988
Roxanol ... 1991

Nadolol (Potentiated or additive action). Products include:
Corgard Tablets ... 701
Corzide Tablets ... 702

Nicardipine Hydrochloride (Potentiated or additive action). Products include:
Cardene Capsules ... 2290

Nitroglycerin (Potentiated or additive action). Products include:
Deponit NTG Transdermal Delivery System ... 2143
Minitran Transdermal Delivery System ... 1312
Nitro-Bid Ointment ... 1339
Nitro-Bid Capsules ... 1338
Nitrodisc ... 2176
Nitro-Dur (nitroglycerin) Transdermal Infusion System ... 1164
Nitrogard Tablets ... 1004
Nitrolingual Spray ... 1846
Nitrostat Tablets ... 1743
Transderm-Nitro Transdermal Therapeutic System ... 2283

Norepinephrine Bitartrate (Decreased arterial responsiveness). Products include:
Levophed Bitartrate Injection ... 2054

Opium Alkaloids (Aggravates orthostatic hypotension). Products include:
B & O No. 15A & No. 16A Supprettes ... 2395
Pantopon Injectable ... 1911

Oxycodone Hydrochloride (Aggravates orthostatic hypotension). Products include:
Percocet Tablets ... 950
Percodan ... 951
Roxicodone Tablets, Oral Solution & Intensol (Oxycodone) ... 1992
Tylox Capsules ... 1382

Penbutolol Sulfate (Potentiated or additive action). Products include:
Levatol ... 1832

Pentobarbital Sodium (Aggravates orthostatic hypotension). Products include:
Nembutal Sodium Capsules ... 534
Nembutal Sodium Solution ... 536
Nembutal Sodium Suppositories ... 538

Phenobarbital (Aggravates orthostatic hypotension). Products include:
Arco-Lase Plus Tablets ... 607
Bellergal-S Tablets ... 1998
Bronkolixir ... ▣ 761
Bronkotabs Tablets ... ▣ 762
Donnatal ... 1858
Donnatal Extentabs ... 1859
Donnatal Tablets ... 1858
Donnazyme Tablets ... 1860
Kinesed Tablets ... 2272
Phenobarbital Elixir and Tablets ... 1293
Primatene Tablets-P Formula ... 2421
Quadrinal Tablets ... 1183
Tedral SA ... 1765

Phenoxybenzamine Hydrochloride (Potentiated or additive action). Products include:
Dibenzyline Capsules ... 2207

Phentolamine Mesylate (Potentiated or additive action). Products include:
Regitine ... 878

Pindolol (Potentiated or additive action). Products include:
Visken Tablets ... 2036

Polythiazide (Potentiated or additive action). Products include:
Minizide Capsules ... 1779
Renese Tablets ... 1785
Renese-R Tablets ... 1786

Prazosin Hydrochloride (Potentiated). Products include:
Minipress Capsules ... 1778
Minizide Capsules ... 1779

Prednisolone Acetate (Potential for hypokalemia). Products include:
AK-Cide Sterile Ophthalmic Ointment & Suspension ... ⊙ 202
Blephamide Liquifilm Sterile Ophthalmic Suspension ... 586
Blephamide S.O.P. Sterile Ophthalmic Ointment ... 586
Cetapred Ointment ... ⊙ 220
⅛% Econopred & 1% Econopred Plus ... ⊙ 217
Isopto Cetapred Suspension ... ⊙ 220
Metimyd ... ⊙ 306
Poly-Pred Liquifilm ... ⊙ 250
Pred Forte ... ⊙ 252
Pred Mild ... ⊙ 254
Pred-G Liquifilm Sterile Ophthalmic Suspension ... ⊙ 252
Pred-G S.O.P. Sterile Ophthalmic Ointment ... ⊙ 253
Vasocidin Ointment ... ⊙ 275

Prednisolone Sodium Phosphate (Potential for hypokalemia). Products include:
AK-Pred ... ⊙ 205
Hydeltrasol Injection, Sterile ... 1476
Inflamase ... ⊙ 274
Pediapred Oral Liquid ... 987
Vasocidin Ophthalmic Solution ... ⊙ 276

Prednisolone Tebutate (Potential for hypokalemia). Products include:
Hydeltra-T.B.A. Sterile Suspension 1478

Prednisone (Potential for hypokalemia). Products include:
Deltasone Tablets ... 2332

Propoxyphene Hydrochloride (Aggravates orthostatic hypotension). Products include:
Darvon ... 1256
Wygesic Tablets ... 2540

Propoxyphene Napsylate (Aggravates orthostatic hypotension). Products include:
Darvon-N/Darvocet-N ... 1254

Propranolol Hydrochloride (Potentiated or additive action). Products include:
Inderal ... 2459
Inderal LA Long Acting Capsules ... 2461
Inderide Tablets ... 2463
Inderide LA Long Acting Capsules ... 2465

Ramipril (Potentiated or additive action). Products include:
Altace Capsules ... 1086

Rauwolfia Serpentina (Potentiated). Products include:
Raudixin Tablets ... 1803
Rauzide Tablets ... 1804

Rescinnamine (Potentiated).
No products indexed under this heading.

Reserpine (Potentiated). Products include:
Diupres Tablets ... 1461
Hydromox R Tablets ... 1209
Hydropres Tablets ... 1485
Renese-R Tablets ... 1786
Salutensin/Salutensin-Demi ... 719
Ser-Ap-Es Tablets ... 881
Serpasil Tablets ... 883
Serpasil-Apresoline Tablets ... 884
Serpasil-Esidrix Tablets ... 886

Secobarbital Sodium (Aggravates orthostatic hypotension). Products include:
Seconal Sodium Pulvules ... 1296

Sodium Nitroprusside (Potentiated or additive action). Products include:
Nipride I.V. Infusion ... 1909

Sufentanil Citrate (Aggravates orthostatic hypotension). Products include:
Sufenta Injection ... 1147

Terazosin Hydrochloride (Potentiated or additive action). Products include:
Hytrin Tablets ... 529

Thiamylal Sodium (Aggravates orthostatic hypotension). Products include:
Surital Ampoules, Steri-Vials ... 1764

Timolol Maleate (Potentiated or additive action). Products include:
Blocadren Tablets ... 1429
Timolide Tablets ... 1547
Timoptic in Ocudose ... 1552
Timoptic Sterile Ophthalmic Solution ... 1550

Tolazamide (Higher dosage oral hypoglycemic agents may be required). Products include:
Tolinase Tablets ... 2365

Tolbutamide (Higher dosage oral hypoglycemic agents may be required). Products include:
Orinase Tablets ... 2354

Triamcinolone (Potential for hypokalemia).
No products indexed under this heading.

Triamcinolone Acetonide (Potential for hypokalemia). Products include:
Aristocort A ... 1010
Azmacort Inhaler ... 1837
Kenalog Cream, Lotion & Ointment 2401
Kenalog-10 Injection ... 2402
Kenalog-40 Injection ... 2403
Kenalog in Orabase ... 604
Kenalog Spray ... 2401
Mycolog II Cream and Ointment ... 2407
Mytrex Cream & Ointment ... 2080
Nasacort Nasal Inhaler ... 1844

Triamcinolone Diacetate (Potential for hypokalemia). Products include:
Aristocort Suspension ... 1008

Triamcinolone Hexacetonide (Potential for hypokalemia). Products include:
Aristospan Suspension ... 1011

Trimethaphan Camsylate (Potentiated). Products include:
Arfonad Ampuls ... 1887

Tubocurarine Chloride (Increased responsiveness to tubocurarine).
No products indexed under this heading.

THEO-24
(Theophylline Anhydrous) ... 2179
May interact with macrolide antibiotics, sympathomimetic bronchodilators, oral contraceptives, and certain other agents. Compounds in these categories include:

Albuterol (Increased toxicity). Products include:
Proventil Inhalation Aerosol ... 2117
Ventolin Inhalation Aerosol and Refill ... 583

Albuterol Sulfate (Increased toxicity). Products include:
Proventil Repetabs Tablets ... 2120
Proventil Solutions for Inhalation 0.5% and 0.083% ... 2118
Proventil Syrup ... 2119
Proventil Tablets ... 2120
Ventolin ... 583

Allopurinol (Elevated theophylline serum levels with high dose of allopurinol). Products include:
Zyloprim Tablets ... 830

Bitolterol Mesylate (Increased toxicity). Products include:
Tornalate ... 2074

Carbamazepine (Decreases serum theophylline levels). Products include:
Tegretol Chewable Tablets ... 654
Tegretol Suspension ... 656
Tegretol Tablets ... 654

Cimetidine (Elevated theophylline serum levels). Products include:
Tagamet Tablets ... 2228

Cimetidine Hydrochloride (Elevated theophylline serum levels). Products include:
Tagamet ... 2228

Ciprofloxacin Hydrochloride (Increases serum theophylline levels). Products include:
Ciloxan Sterile Ophthalmic Solution ... ⊙ 214
Cipro I.V. ... 1592
Cipro Tablets ... 1589

Ephedrine Hydrochloride (Increased toxicity). Products include:
- Amesec ▣ 682
- Primatene Tablets-M Formula 2421
- Primatene Tablets-P Formula 2421
- Primatene Tablets-Regular Formula 2421
- Quadrinal Tablets 1183
- Quelidrine Syrup 556
- Tedral SA 1765

Ephedrine Sulfate (Increased toxicity). Products include:
- Bronkaid Tablets ▣ 757
- Bronkolixir ▣ 761
- Bronkotabs Tablets ▣ 762
- Marax Tablets & DF Syrup 1954
- Pazo Hemorrhoid Ointment & Suppositories 752
- Vicks Vatronol Nose Drops ▣ 666

Ephedrine Tannate (Increased toxicity). Products include:
- Rynatuss 2388

Epinephrine (Increased toxicity). Products include:
- Ana-Kit Anaphylaxis Emergency Treatment Kit 1100
- Bronkaid Mist ▣ 757
- EpiPen 843
- Marcaine Hydrochloride 0.5% with Epinephrine 1:200,000 (as bitartrate) 958
- Marcaine Hydrochloride with Epinephrine 1:200,000 2055
- Primatene Mist 2420
- Sus-Phrine Injection 1006
- Xylocaine with Epinephrine Injections 637

Epinephrine Bitartrate (Increased toxicity). Products include:
- AsthmaHaler Mist Epinephrine Bitartrate Bronchodilator ▣ 616
- Bronkaid Mist Suspension ▣ 757
- Primatene Mist Suspension 2421

Epinephrine Hydrochloride (Increased toxicity). Products include:
- Adrenalin Chloride Solution 1:100 & 1:1,000 1689
- Epifrin ⊙ 244
- Glaucon ⊙ 218

Erythromycin (Elevated theophylline serum levels). Products include:
- A/T/S Topical Gel and Topical Solution 1089
- AK-Mycin Ointment ⊙ 204
- Benzamycin Topical Gel 907
- E-Mycin Tablets 688
- ETS-2% 1685
- ERYC 1720
- Erycette (erythromycin 2%) Topical Solution 1678
- Ery-Tab Tablets 521
- Erythromycin Base Filmtab 525
- Erythromycin Delayed-Release Capsules, USP 526
- Ilotycin Ophthalmic Ointment 915
- PCE Dispertab Tablets 549
- Pediazole 1973
- T-Stat 2.0% Topical Solution and Pads 2409
- Theramycin Z Topical Solution 2% 1410

Erythromycin Estolate (Elevated theophylline serum levels). Products include:
- Ilosone 913

Erythromycin Ethylsuccinate (Elevated theophylline serum levels). Products include:
- E.E.S. 522
- EryPed 519
- Pediazole 1973

Erythromycin Gluceptate (Elevated theophylline serum levels). Products include:
- Ilotycin Gluceptate, IV, Vials 915

Erythromycin Stearate (Elevated theophylline serum levels). Products include:
- Erythrocin Stearate Filmtab 523

Ethinyl Estradiol (Elevated theophylline serum levels). Products include:
- Brevicon 2304
- Demulen 2161
- Estinyl Tablets 2085
- Jenest-28 Tablets 1636
- Levlen/Tri-Levlen 665
- Lo/Ovral Tablets 2471
- Lo/Ovral-28 Tablets 2476
- Loestrin 1728
- Modicon 1667
- Nordette-21 Tablets 2481
- Nordette-28 Tablets 2483
- Norethin 2133
- Norinyl 2304
- Norlestrin 1746
- Ortho-Cyclen Tablets 1658
- Ortho-Novum 1667
- Ovcon 1391
- Ovral Tablets 2490
- Ovral-28 Tablets 2491
- Levlen/Tri-Levlen 665
- Tri-Norinyl 2304
- Triphasil-21 Tablets 2527
- Triphasil-28 Tablets 2532

Ethylnorepinephrine Hydrochloride (Increased toxicity). Products include:
- Bronkephrine Injection 2042

Ethynodiol Diacetate (Elevated theophylline serum levels). Products include:
- Demulen 2161

Halothane (May produce sinus tachycardia or ventricular arrhythmias). Products include:
- Fluothane 2453

Isoetharine (Increased toxicity). Products include:
- Arm-a-Med Isoetharine Inhalation Solution, USP 616
- Bronkometer Aerosol 2042
- Bronkosol Solution 2042

Isoproterenol Hydrochloride (Increased toxicity). Products include:
- Isuprel Hydrochloride Injection 1:5000 2050
- Isuprel Hydrochloride Mistometer 2051
- Isuprel Hydrochloride Solution 1:200 & 1:100 2052
- Norisodrine Aerotrol 540

Levonorgestrel (Elevated theophylline serum levels). Products include:
- Levlen/Tri-Levlen 665
- Nordette-21 Tablets 2481
- Nordette-28 Tablets 2483
- Norplant System 2484
- Levlen/Tri-Levlen 665
- Triphasil-21 Tablets 2527
- Triphasil-28 Tablets 2532

Lithium Carbonate (Increased renal excretion of lithium carbonate). Products include:
- Eskalith 2214
- Lithane Tablets 1596
- Lithium Carbonate Capsules & Tablets 1984
- Lithobid Tablets 870

Mestranol (Elevated theophylline serum levels). Products include:
- Enovid 2161
- Norethin 2133
- Norinyl 2304
- Ortho-Novum 1667

Metaproterenol Sulfate (Increased toxicity). Products include:
- Alupent 674
- Arm-a-Med Metaproterenol Sulfate Inhalation Solution, USP 617
- Metaprel Inhalation Aerosol Bronchodilator 2014
- Metaprel Inhalation Solution 2015
- Metaprel 2015
- Metaproterenol Sulfate Inhalation Solution, USP 912

Norethindrone (Elevated theophylline serum levels). Products include:
- Brevicon 2304
- Jenest-28 Tablets 1636
- Micronor Tablets 1667
- Modicon 1667
- Norethin 2133
- Norinyl 2304
- Norlutin 1755
- Nor-Q D Tablets 2304
- Ortho-Novum 1667
- Ovcon 1391
- Tri-Norinyl 2304

Norethynodrel (Elevated theophylline serum levels). Products include:
- Enovid 2161

Norgestimate (Elevated theophylline serum levels). Products include:
- Ortho-Cyclen Tablets 1658

Norgestrel (Elevated theophylline serum levels). Products include:
- Lo/Ovral Tablets 2471
- Lo/Ovral-28 Tablets 2476
- Ovral Tablets 2490
- Ovral-28 Tablets 2491
- Ovrette Tablets 2492

Phenobarbital (Decreases serum theophylline levels). Products include:
- Arco-Lase Plus Tablets 607
- Bellergal-S Tablets 1998
- Bronkolixir ▣ 761
- Bronkotabs Tablets ▣ 762
- Donnatal 1858
- Donnatal Extentabs 1859
- Donnatal Tablets 1858
- Donnazyme Tablets 1860
- Kinesed Tablets 2272
- Phenobarbital Elixir and Tablets 1293
- Primatene Tablets-P Formula 2421
- Quadrinal Tablets 1183
- Tedral SA 1765

Phenytoin (Decreased theophylline and phenytoin serum levels). Products include:
- Dilantin Infatabs 1710
- Dilantin-30 Pediatric/Dilantin-125 Suspension 1713

Phenytoin Sodium (Decreased theophylline and phenytoin serum levels). Products include:
- Dilantin Kapseals 1708
- Dilantin Parenteral 1712
- Dilantin with Phenobarbital Kapseals 1715

Pirbuterol Acetate (Increased toxicity). Products include:
- Maxair Inhaler 1311

Propranolol Hydrochloride (Increased serum theophylline levels). Products include:
- Inderal 2459
- Inderal LA Long Acting Capsules 2461
- Inderide Tablets 2463
- Inderide LA Long Acting Capsules 2465

Rifampin (Decreased serum theophylline levels). Products include:
- Rifadin 1345
- Rifamate Capsules 1347
- Rimactane Capsules 879

Terbutaline Sulfate (Increased toxicity). Products include:
- Brethaire Inhaler 1024
- Brethine Ampuls 1026
- Brethine Tablets 1026
- Bricanyl Injection 1324
- Bricanyl Tablets 1325

Troleandomycin (Elevated theophylline serum levels). Products include:
- Tao Capsules 1963

Food Interactions

Diet, high-lipid (May result in a significant increase in peak serum level).

THEO-DUR SPRINKLE

(Theophylline Anhydrous) 1168

May interact with macrolide antibiotics, sympathomimetic bronchodilators, and certain other agents. Compounds in these categories include:

Albuterol (Toxic synergism may occur). Products include:
- Proventil Inhalation Aerosol 2117
- Ventolin Inhalation Aerosol and Refill 583

Albuterol Sulfate (Toxic synergism may occur). Products include:
- Proventil Repetabs Tablets 2120
- Proventil Solutions for Inhalation 0.5% and 0.083% 2118
- Proventil Syrup 2119
- Proventil Tablets 2120
- Ventolin 583

Bitolterol Mesylate (Toxic synergism may occur). Products include:
- Tornalate 2074

Cimetidine (Increased theophylline blood levels). Products include:
- Tagamet Tablets 2228

Ephedrine (Toxic synergism may occur).

Ephedrine Hydrochloride (Toxic synergism may occur). Products include:
- Amesec ▣ 682
- Primatene Tablets-M Formula 2421
- Primatene Tablets-P Formula 2421
- Primatene Tablets-Regular Formula 2421
- Quadrinal Tablets 1183
- Quelidrine Syrup 556
- Tedral SA 1765

Ephedrine Sulfate (Toxic synergism may occur). Products include:
- Bronkaid Tablets ▣ 757
- Bronkolixir ▣ 761
- Bronkotabs Tablets ▣ 762
- Marax Tablets & DF Syrup 1954
- Pazo Hemorrhoid Ointment & Suppositories 752
- Vicks Vatronol Nose Drops ▣ 666

Ephedrine Tannate (Toxic synergism may occur). Products include:
- Rynatuss 2388

Epinephrine (Toxic synergism may occur). Products include:
- Ana-Kit Anaphylaxis Emergency Treatment Kit 1100
- Bronkaid Mist ▣ 757
- EpiPen 843
- Marcaine Hydrochloride 0.5% with Epinephrine 1:200,000 (as bitartrate) 958
- Marcaine Hydrochloride with Epinephrine 1:200,000 2055
- Primatene Mist 2420
- Sus-Phrine Injection 1006
- Xylocaine with Epinephrine Injections 637

Epinephrine Hydrochloride (Toxic synergism may occur). Products include:
- Adrenalin Chloride Solution 1:100 & 1:1,000 1689
- Epifrin ⊙ 244
- Glaucon ⊙ 218

Erythromycin (Increased theophylline blood levels). Products include:
- A/T/S Topical Gel and Topical Solution 1089
- AK-Mycin Ointment ⊙ 204
- Benzamycin Topical Gel 907
- E-Mycin Tablets 688
- ETS-2% 1685
- ERYC 1720
- Erycette (erythromycin 2%) Topical Solution 1678
- Ery-Tab Tablets 521
- Erythromycin Base Filmtab 525
- Erythromycin Delayed-Release Capsules, USP 526
- Ilotycin Ophthalmic Ointment 915
- PCE Dispertab Tablets 549
- Pediazole 1973
- T-Stat 2.0% Topical Solution and Pads 2409
- Theramycin Z Topical Solution 2% 1410

Erythromycin Estolate (Increased theophylline blood levels). Products include:
- Ilosone 913

Erythromycin Ethylsuccinate (Increased theophylline blood levels). Products include:
- E.E.S. 522
- EryPed 519
- Pediazole 1973

Erythromycin Gluceptate (Increased theophylline blood levels). Products include:
- Ilotycin Gluceptate, IV, Vials 915

Erythromycin Stearate (Increased theophylline blood levels). Products include:
- Erythrocin Stearate Filmtab 523

Ethylnorepinephrine Hydrochloride (Toxic synergism may occur). Products include:
- Bronkephrine Injection 2042

Isoetharine (Toxic synergism may occur). Products include:
- Arm-a-Med Isoetharine Inhalation Solution, USP 616
- Bronkometer Aerosol 2042
- Bronkosol Solution 2042

Isoproterenol Hydrochloride (Toxic synergism may occur). Products include:
- Isuprel Hydrochloride Injection 1:5000 2050
- Isuprel Hydrochloride Mistometer 2051
- Isuprel Hydrochloride Solution 1:200 & 1:100 2052
- Norisodrine Aerotrol 540

Lithium Carbonate (Increased excretion of lithium carbonate). Products include:
- Eskalith 2214
- Lithane Tablets 1596
- Lithium Carbonate Capsules & Tablets 1984
- Lithobid Tablets 870

Metaproterenol Sulfate (Toxic synergism may occur). Products include:
- Alupent 674
- Arm-a-Med Metaproterenol Sulfate Inhalation Solution, USP 617
- Metaprel Inhalation Aerosol Bronchodilator 2014
- Metaprel Inhalation Solution 2015
- Metaprel 2015
- Metaproterenol Sulfate Inhalation Solution, USP 912

Pirbuterol Acetate (Toxic synergism may occur). Products include:
- Maxair Inhaler 1311

Propranolol Hydrochloride (Antagonism of propranolol effect; increased theophylline serum concentrations). Products include:
- Inderal 2459
- Inderal LA Long Acting Capsules 2461
- Inderide Tablets 2463
- Inderide LA Long Acting Capsules 2465

Terbutaline Sulfate (Toxic synergism may occur). Products include:
- Brethaire Inhaler 1024
- Brethine Ampuls 1026
- Brethine Tablets 1026
- Bricanyl Injection 1324
- Bricanyl Tablets 1325

Troleandomycin (Increased theophylline blood levels). Products include:
- Tao Capsules 1963

Food Interactions

Food, unspecified (Food ingestion may affect the bioavailability).

THEO-DUR EXTENDED-RELEASE TABLETS

(Theophylline Anhydrous) 1166

May interact with macrolide antibiotics, oral contraceptives, sympathomimetic bronchodilators, and certain other agents. Compounds in these categories include:

Albuterol (Potential for toxic synergism). Products include:
- Proventil Inhalation Aerosol 2117
- Ventolin Inhalation Aerosol and Refill 583

Albuterol Sulfate (Potential for toxic synergism). Products include:
- Proventil Repetabs Tablets 2120
- Proventil Solutions for Inhalation 0.5% and 0.083% 2118
- Proventil Syrup 2119
- Proventil Tablets 2120
- Ventolin 583

Allopurinol (Increased serum theophylline levels at high dose of allopurinol). Products include:
- Zyloprim Tablets 830

Bitolterol Mesylate (Potential for toxic synergism). Products include:
- Tornalate 2074

Cimetidine (Increases serum theophylline levels). Products include:
- Tagamet Tablets 2228

Cimetidine Hydrochloride (Increases serum theophylline levels). Products include:
- Tagamet 2228

Ciprofloxacin Hydrochloride (Increases serum theophylline levels). Products include:
- Ciloxan Sterile Ophthalmic Solution ⊙ 214
- Cipro I.V. 1592
- Cipro Tablets 1589

Ephedrine Hydrochloride (Potential for toxic synergism). Products include:
- Amesec ⊞ 682
- Primatene Tablets-M Formula 2421
- Primatene Tablets-P Formula 2421
- Primatene Tablets-Regular Formula 2421
- Quadrinal Tablets 1183
- Quelidrine Syrup 556
- Tedral SA 1765

Ephedrine Sulfate (Potential for toxic synergism). Products include:
- Bronkaid Tablets ⊞ 757
- Bronkolixir ⊞ 761
- Bronkotabs Tablets ⊞ 762
- Marax Tablets & DF Syrup 1954
- Pazo Hemorrhoid Ointment & Suppositories 752
- Vicks Vatronol Nose Drops ⊞ 666

Ephedrine Tannate (Potential for toxic synergism). Products include:
- Rynatuss 2388

Epinephrine (Potential for toxic synergism). Products include:
- Ana-Kit Anaphylaxis Emergency Treatment Kit 1100
- Bronkaid Mist ⊞ 757
- EpiPen 843
- Marcaine Hydrochloride 0.5% with Epinephrine 1:200,000 (as bitartrate) 958
- Marcaine Hydrochloride with Epinephrine 1:200,000 2055
- Primatene Mist 2420
- Sus-Phrine Injection 1006
- Xylocaine with Epinephrine Injections 637

Epinephrine Hydrochloride (Potential for toxic synergism). Products include:
- Adrenalin Chloride Solution 1:100 & 1:1,000 1689
- Epifrin ⊙ 244
- Glaucon ⊙ 218

Erythromycin (Increases serum theophylline levels). Products include:
- A/T/S Topical Gel and Topical Solution 1089
- AK-Mycin Ointment ⊙ 204
- Benzamycin Topical Gel 907
- E-Mycin Tablets 688
- ETS-2% 1685
- ERYC 1720
- Erycette (erythromycin 2%) Topical Solution 1678
- Ery-Tab Tablets 521
- Erythromycin Base Filmtab 525
- Erythromycin Delayed-Release Capsules, USP 526
- Ilotycin Ophthalmic Ointment 915
- PCE Dispertab Tablets 549
- Pediazole 1973
- T-Stat 2.0% Topical Solution and Pads 2409
- Theramycin Z Topical Solution 2% 1410

Erythromycin Estolate (Increases serum theophylline levels). Products include:
- Ilosone 913

Erythromycin Ethylsuccinate (Increases serum theophylline levels). Products include:
- E.E.S. 522
- EryPed 519
- Pediazole 1973

Erythromycin Gluceptate (Increases serum theophylline levels). Products include:
- Ilotycin Gluceptate, IV, Vials 915

Erythromycin Stearate (Increases serum theophylline levels). Products include:
- Erythrocin Stearate Filmtab 523

Ethinyl Estradiol (Increases serum theophylline levels). Products include:
- Brevicon 2304
- Demulen 2161
- Estinyl Tablets 2085
- Jenest-28 Tablets 1636
- Levlen/Tri-Levlen 665
- Lo/Ovral Tablets 2471
- Lo/Ovral-28 Tablets 2476
- Loestrin 1728
- Modicon 1667
- Nordette-21 Tablets 2481
- Nordette-28 Tablets 2483
- Norethin 2133
- Norinyl 2304
- Norlestrin 1746
- Ortho-Cyclen Tablets 1658
- Ortho-Novum 1667
- Ovcon 1391
- Ovral Tablets 2490
- Ovral-28 Tablets 2491
- Levlen/Tri-Levlen 665
- Tri-Norinyl 2304
- Triphasil-21 Tablets 2527
- Triphasil-28 Tablets 2532

Ethylnorepinephrine Hydrochloride (Potential for toxic synergism). Products include:
- Bronkephrine Injection 2042

Ethynodiol Diacetate (Increases serum theophylline levels). Products include:
- Demulen 2161

Isoetharine (Potential for toxic synergism). Products include:
- Arm-a-Med Isoetharine Inhalation Solution, USP 616
- Bronkometer Aerosol 2042
- Bronkosol Solution 2042

Isoproterenol Hydrochloride (Potential for toxic synergism). Products include:
- Isuprel Hydrochloride Injection 1:5000 2050
- Isuprel Hydrochloride Mistometer 2051
- Isuprel Hydrochloride Solution 1:200 & 1:100 2052
- Norisodrine Aerotrol 540

Levonorgestrel (Increases serum theophylline levels). Products include:
- Levlen/Tri-Levlen 665
- Nordette-21 Tablets 2481
- Nordette-28 Tablets 2483
- Norplant System 2484
- Levlen/Tri-Levlen 665
- Triphasil-21 Tablets 2527
- Triphasil-28 Tablets 2532

Lithium Carbonate (Increased renal excretion of lithium). Products include:
- Eskalith 2214
- Lithane Tablets 1596
- Lithium Carbonate Capsules & Tablets 1984
- Lithobid Tablets 870

Mestranol (Increases serum theophylline levels). Products include:
- Enovid 2161
- Norethin 2133
- Norinyl 2304
- Ortho-Novum 1667

Metaproterenol Sulfate (Potential for toxic synergism). Products include:
- Alupent 674
- Arm-a-Med Metaproterenol Sulfate Inhalation Solution, USP 617
- Metaprel Inhalation Aerosol Bronchodilator 2014
- Metaprel Inhalation Solution 2015
- Metaprel 2015
- Metaproterenol Sulfate Inhalation Solution, USP 912

Norethindrone (Increases serum theophylline levels). Products include:
- Brevicon 2304
- Jenest-28 Tablets 1636
- Micronor Tablets 1667
- Modicon 1667
- Norethin 2133
- Norinyl 2304
- Norlutin 1755
- Nor-Q D Tablets 2304
- Ortho-Novum 1667
- Ovcon 1391
- Tri-Norinyl 2304

Norethynodrel (Increases serum theophylline levels). Products include:
- Enovid 2161

Norgestimate (Increases serum theophylline levels). Products include:
- Ortho-Cyclen Tablets 1658

Norgestrel (Increases serum theophylline levels). Products include:
- Lo/Ovral Tablets 2471
- Lo/Ovral-28 Tablets 2476
- Ovral Tablets 2490
- Ovral-28 Tablets 2491
- Ovrette Tablets 2492

Phenytoin (Decreased theophylline and phenytoin levels). Products include:
- Dilantin Infatabs 1710
- Dilantin-30 Pediatric/Dilantin-125 Suspension 1713

Phenytoin Sodium (Decreased theophylline and phenytoin levels). Products include:
- Dilantin Kapseals 1708
- Dilantin Parenteral 1712
- Dilantin with Phenobarbital Kapseals 1715

Pirbuterol Acetate (Potential for toxic synergism). Products include:
- Maxair Inhaler 1311

Propranolol Hydrochloride (Increases serum theophylline levels). Products include:
- Inderal 2459
- Inderal LA Long Acting Capsules 2461
- Inderide Tablets 2463
- Inderide LA Long Acting Capsules 2465

Rifampin (Decreased serum theophylline levels). Products include:
- Rifadin 1345
- Rifamate Capsules 1347
- Rimactane Capsules 879

Terbutaline Sulfate (Potential for toxic synergism). Products include:
- Brethaire Inhaler 1024
- Brethine Ampuls 1026
- Brethine Tablets 1026
- Bricanyl Injection 1324
- Bricanyl Tablets 1325

Troleandomycin (Increases serum theophylline levels). Products include:
- Tao Capsules 1963

Food Interactions

Food, unspecified (May influence absorption of theophylline from a 100 mg dosage form).

THEOLAIR LIQUID

(Theophylline Anhydrous) 1317

May interact with oral contraceptives, sympathomimetic bronchodilators, macrolide antibiotics, and certain other agents. Compounds in these categories include:

Albuterol (Potential for toxic synergism). Products include:
- Proventil Inhalation Aerosol 2117
- Ventolin Inhalation Aerosol and Refill 583

Albuterol Sulfate (Potential for toxic synergism). Products include:
- Proventil Repetabs Tablets 2120
- Proventil Solutions for Inhalation 0.5% and 0.083% 2118
- Proventil Syrup 2119
- Proventil Tablets 2120
- Ventolin 583

Allopurinol (Increases serum theophylline levels when high dose of allopurinol is used). Products include:
- Zyloprim Tablets 830

Bitolterol Mesylate (Potential for toxic synergism). Products include:
- Tornalate 2074

Cimetidine (Increases serum theophylline levels). Products include:
- Tagamet Tablets 2228

Cimetidine Hydrochloride (Increases serum theophylline levels). Products include:
- Tagamet 2228

Ciprofloxacin (Increases serum theophylline levels).
- No products indexed under this heading.

Ciprofloxacin Hydrochloride (Increases serum theophylline levels). Products include:
- Ciloxan Sterile Ophthalmic Solution .... ⊙ 214
- Cipro I.V. 1592
- Cipro Tablets 1589

Ephedrine Hydrochloride (Potential for toxic synergism). Products include:
- Amesec .... ⊞ 682
- Primatene Tablets-M Formula 2421
- Primatene Tablets-P Formula 2421
- Primatene Tablets-Regular Formula 2421
- Quadrinal Tablets 1183
- Quelidrine Syrup 556
- Tedral SA 1765

Ephedrine Sulfate (Potential for toxic synergism). Products include:
- Bronkaid Tablets .... ⊞ 757
- Bronkolixir .... ⊞ 761
- Bronkotabs Tablets .... ⊞ 762
- Marax Tablets & DF Syrup 1954
- Pazo Hemorrhoid Ointment & Suppositories 752
- Vicks Vatronol Nose Drops .... ⊞ 666

Ephedrine Tannate (Potential for toxic synergism). Products include:
- Rynatuss 2388

Epinephrine (Potential for toxic synergism). Products include:
- Ana-Kit Anaphylaxis Emergency Treatment Kit 1100
- Bronkaid Mist .... ⊞ 757
- EpiPen 843
- Marcaine Hydrochloride 0.5% with Epinephrine 1:200,000 (as bitartrate) 958
- Marcaine Hydrochloride with Epinephrine 1:200,000 2055
- Primatene Mist 2420
- Sus-Phrine Injection 1006
- Xylocaine with Epinephrine Injections 637

Epinephrine Hydrochloride (Potential for toxic synergism). Products include:
- Adrenalin Chloride Solution 1:100 & 1:1,000 1689
- Epifrin .... ⊙ 244
- Glaucon .... ⊙ 218

Erythromycin (Increases serum theophylline levels). Products include:
- A/T/S Topical Gel and Topical Solution 1089
- AK-Mycin Ointment .... ⊙ 204
- Benzamycin Topical Gel 907
- E-Mycin Tablets 688
- ETS-2% 1685
- ERYC 1720
- Erycette (erythromycin 2%) Topical Solution 1678
- Ery-Tab Tablets 521
- Erythromycin Base Filmtab 525
- Erythromycin Delayed-Release Capsules, USP 526
- Ilotycin Ophthalmic Ointment 915
- PCE Dispertab Tablets 549
- Pediazole 1973
- T-Stat 2.0% Topical Solution and Pads 2409
- Theramycin Z Topical Solution 2% 1410

Erythromycin Estolate (Increases serum theophylline levels). Products include:
- Ilosone 913

Erythromycin Ethylsuccinate (Increases serum theophylline levels). Products include:
- E.E.S. 522
- EryPed 519
- Pediazole 1973

Erythromycin Gluceptate (Increases serum theophylline levels). Products include:
- Ilotycin Gluceptate, IV, Vials 915

Erythromycin Stearate (Increases serum theophylline levels). Products include:
- Erythrocin Stearate Filmtab 523

Ethinyl Estradiol (Increases serum theophylline levels). Products include:
- Brevicon 2304
- Demulen 2161
- Estinyl Tablets 2085
- Jenest-28 Tablets 1636
- Levlen/Tri-Levlen 665
- Lo/Ovral Tablets 2471
- Lo/Ovral-28 Tablets 2476
- Loestrin 1728
- Modicon 1667
- Nordette-21 Tablets 2481
- Nordette-28 Tablets 2483
- Norethin 2133
- Norinyl 2304
- Norlestrin 1746
- Ortho-Cyclen Tablets 1658
- Ortho-Novum 1667
- Ovcon 1391
- Ovral Tablets 2490
- Ovral-28 Tablets 2491
- Levlen/Tri-Levlen 665
- Tri-Norinyl 2304
- Triphasil-21 Tablets 2527
- Triphasil-28 Tablets 2532

Ethylnorepinephrine Hydrochloride (Potential for toxic synergism). Products include:
- Bronkephrine Injection 2042

Ethynodiol Diacetate (Increases serum theophylline levels). Products include:
- Demulen 2161

Isoetharine (Potential for toxic synergism). Products include:
- Arm-a-Med Isoetharine Inhalation Solution, USP 616
- Bronkometer Aerosol 2042
- Bronkosol Solution 2042

Isoproterenol Hydrochloride (Potential for toxic synergism). Products include:
- Isuprel Hydrochloride Injection 1:5000 2050
- Isuprel Hydrochloride Mistometer .. 2051
- Isuprel Hydrochloride Solution 1:200 & 1:100 2052
- Norisodrine Aerotrol 540

Levonorgestrel (Increases serum theophylline levels). Products include:
- Levlen/Tri-Levlen 665
- Nordette-21 Tablets 2481
- Nordette-28 Tablets 2483
- Norplant System 2484
- Levlen/Tri-Levlen 665
- Triphasil-21 Tablets 2527
- Triphasil-28 Tablets 2532

Lithium Carbonate (Increased renal excretion of lithium). Products include:
- Eskalith 2214
- Lithane Tablets 1596
- Lithium Carbonate Capsules & Tablets 1984
- Lithobid Tablets 870

Mestranol (Increases serum theophylline levels). Products include:
- Enovid 2161
- Norethin 2133
- Norinyl 2304
- Ortho-Novum 1667

Metaproterenol Sulfate (Potential for toxic synergism). Products include:
- Alupent 674
- Arm-a-Med Metaproterenol Sulfate Inhalation Solution, USP 617
- Metaprel Inhalation Aerosol Bronchodilator 2014
- Metaprel Inhalation Solution 2015
- Metaprel 2015
- Metaproterenol Sulfate Inhalation Solution, USP 912

Norethindrone (Increases serum theophylline levels). Products include:
- Brevicon 2304
- Jenest-28 Tablets 1636
- Micronor Tablets 1667
- Modicon 1667
- Norethin 2133
- Norinyl 2304
- Norlutin 1755
- Nor-Q D Tablets 2304
- Ortho-Novum 1667
- Ovcon 1391
- Tri-Norinyl 2304

Norethynodrel (Increases serum theophylline levels). Products include:
- Enovid 2161

Norgestimate (Increases serum theophylline levels). Products include:
- Ortho-Cyclen Tablets 1658

Norgestrel (Increases serum theophylline levels). Products include:
- Lo/Ovral Tablets 2471
- Lo/Ovral-28 Tablets 2476
- Ovral Tablets 2490
- Ovral-28 Tablets 2491
- Ovrette Tablets 2492

Phenytoin (Decreased theophylline and phenytoin serum levels). Products include:
- Dilantin Infatabs 1710
- Dilantin-30 Pediatric/Dilantin-125 Suspension 1713

Phenytoin Sodium (Decreased theophylline and phenytoin serum levels). Products include:
- Dilantin Kapseals 1708
- Dilantin Parenteral 1712
- Dilantin with Phenobarbital Kapseals 1715

Pirbuterol Acetate (Potential for toxic synergism). Products include:
- Maxair Inhaler 1311

Propranolol Hydrochloride (Increases serum theophylline levels). Products include:
- Inderal 2459
- Inderal LA Long Acting Capsules 2461
- Inderide Tablets 2463
- Inderide LA Long Acting Capsules .. 2465

Rifampin (Decreases serum theophylline levels). Products include:
- Rifadin 1345
- Rifamate Capsules 1347
- Rimactane Capsules 879

Terbutaline Sulfate (Potential for toxic synergism). Products include:
- Brethaire Inhaler 1024
- Brethine Ampuls 1026
- Brethine Tablets 1026
- Bricanyl Injection 1324
- Bricanyl Tablets 1325

Troleandomycin (Increases serum theophylline levels). Products include:
- Tao Capsules 1963

THEOLAIR TABLETS
(Theophylline Anhydrous) 1317

See **Theolair Liquid**

THEOLAIR-SR TABLETS
(Theophylline Anhydrous) 1319

May interact with sympathomimetic bronchodilators, macrolide antibiotics, oral contraceptives, and certain other agents. Compounds in these categories include:

Albuterol (Potential for toxic synergism). Products include:
- Proventil Inhalation Aerosol 2117
- Ventolin Inhalation Aerosol and Refill 583

Albuterol Sulfate (Potential for toxic synergism). Products include:
- Proventil Repetabs Tablets 2120
- Proventil Solutions for Inhalation 0.5% and 0.083% 2118
- Proventil Syrup 2119
- Proventil Tablets 2120
- Ventolin 583

Allopurinol (Increases serum theophylline levels when high dose of allopurinol is used). Products include:
- Zyloprim Tablets 830

Bitolterol Mesylate (Potential for toxic synergism). Products include:
- Tornalate 2074

Cimetidine (Increases serum theophylline levels). Products include:
- Tagamet Tablets 2228

Cimetidine Hydrochloride (Increases serum theophylline levels). Products include:
- Tagamet 2228

Ciprofloxacin (Increases serum theophylline levels).
- No products indexed under this heading.

Ciprofloxacin Hydrochloride (Increases serum theophylline levels). Products include:
- Ciloxan Sterile Ophthalmic Solution .... ⊙ 214
- Cipro I.V. 1592
- Cipro Tablets 1589

Ephedrine Hydrochloride (Potential for toxic synergism). Products include:
- Amesec .... ⊞ 682
- Primatene Tablets-M Formula 2421
- Primatene Tablets-P Formula 2421
- Primatene Tablets-Regular Formula 2421
- Quadrinal Tablets 1183
- Quelidrine Syrup 556
- Tedral SA 1765

Ephedrine Sulfate (Potential for toxic synergism). Products include:
- Bronkaid Tablets .... ⊞ 757
- Bronkolixir .... ⊞ 761
- Bronkotabs Tablets .... ⊞ 762
- Marax Tablets & DF Syrup 1954
- Pazo Hemorrhoid Ointment & Suppositories 752
- Vicks Vatronol Nose Drops .... ⊞ 666

Ephedrine Tannate (Potential for toxic synergism). Products include:
- Rynatuss 2388

Epinephrine (Potential for toxic synergism). Products include:
- Ana-Kit Anaphylaxis Emergency Treatment Kit 1100
- Bronkaid Mist .... ⊞ 757
- EpiPen 843
- Marcaine Hydrochloride 0.5% with Epinephrine 1:200,000 (as bitartrate) 958
- Marcaine Hydrochloride with Epinephrine 1:200,000 2055
- Primatene Mist 2420
- Sus-Phrine Injection 1006
- Xylocaine with Epinephrine Injections 637

Epinephrine Hydrochloride (Potential for toxic synergism). Products include:
- Adrenalin Chloride Solution 1:100 & 1:1,000 1689
- Epifrin .... ⊙ 244
- Glaucon .... ⊙ 218

Erythromycin (Increases serum theophylline levels). Products include:
A/T/S Topical Gel and Topical Solution ... 1089
AK-Mycin Ointment ... ⊙ 204
Benzamycin Topical Gel ... 907
E-Mycin Tablets ... 688
ETS-2% ... 1685
ERYC ... 1720
Erycette (erythromycin 2%) Topical Solution ... 1678
Ery-Tab Tablets ... 521
Erythromycin Base Filmtab ... 525
Erythromycin Delayed-Release Capsules, USP ... 526
Ilotycin Ophthalmic Ointment ... 915
PCE Dispertab Tablets ... 549
Pediazole ... 1973
T-Stat 2.0% Topical Solution and Pads ... 2409
Theramycin Z Topical Solution 2% 1410

Erythromycin Estolate (Increases serum theophylline levels). Products include:
Ilosone ... 913

Erythromycin Ethylsuccinate (Increases serum theophylline levels). Products include:
E.E.S. ... 522
EryPed ... 519
Pediazole ... 1973

Erythromycin Gluceptate (Increases serum theophylline levels). Products include:
Ilotycin Gluceptate, IV, Vials ... 915

Erythromycin Stearate (Increases serum theophylline levels). Products include:
Erythrocin Stearate Filmtab ... 523

Ethinyl Estradiol (Increases serum theophylline levels). Products include:
Brevicon ... 2304
Demulen ... 2161
Estinyl Tablets ... 2085
Jenest-28 Tablets ... 1636
Levlen/Tri-Levlen ... 665
Lo/Ovral Tablets ... 2471
Lo/Ovral-28 Tablets ... 2476
Loestrin ... 1728
Modicon ... 1667
Nordette-21 Tablets ... 2481
Nordette-28 Tablets ... 2483
Norethin ... 2133
Norinyl ... 2304
Norlestrin ... 1746
Ortho-Cyclen Tablets ... 1658
Ortho-Novum ... 1667
Ovcon ... 1391
Ovral Tablets ... 2490
Ovral-28 Tablets ... 2491
Levlen/Tri-Levlen ... 665
Tri-Norinyl ... 2304
Triphasil-21 Tablets ... 2527
Triphasil-28 Tablets ... 2532

Ethylnorepinephrine Hydrochloride (Potential for toxic synergism). Products include:
Bronkephrine Injection ... 2042

Ethynodiol Diacetate (Increases serum theophylline levels). Products include:
Demulen ... 2161

Isoetharine (Potential for toxic synergism). Products include:
Arm-a-Med Isoetharine Inhalation Solution, USP ... 616
Bronkometer Aerosol ... 2042
Bronkosol Solution ... 2042

Isoproterenol Hydrochloride (Potential for toxic synergism). Products include:
Isuprel Hydrochloride Injection 1:5000 ... 2050
Isuprel Hydrochloride Mistometer .. 2051
Isuprel Hydrochloride Solution 1:200 & 1:100 ... 2052
Norisodrine Aerotrol ... 540

Levonorgestrel (Increases serum theophylline levels). Products include:
Levlen/Tri-Levlen ... 665
Nordette-21 Tablets ... 2481
Nordette-28 Tablets ... 2483
Norplant System ... 2484
Levlen/Tri-Levlen ... 665
Triphasil-21 Tablets ... 2527
Triphasil-28 Tablets ... 2532

Mestranol (Increases serum theophylline levels). Products include:
Enovid ... 2161
Norethin ... 2133
Norinyl ... 2304
Ortho-Novum ... 1667

Metaproterenol Sulfate (Potential for toxic synergism). Products include:
Alupent ... 674
Arm-a-Med Metaproterenol Sulfate Inhalation Solution, USP ... 617
Metaprel Inhalation Aerosol Bronchodilator ... 2014
Metaprel Inhalation Solution ... 2015
Metaprel ... 2015
Metaproterenol Sulfate Inhalation Solution, USP ... 912

Norethindrone (Increases serum theophylline levels). Products include:
Brevicon ... 2304
Jenest-28 Tablets ... 1636
Micronor Tablets ... 1667
Modicon ... 1667
Norethin ... 2133
Norinyl ... 2304
Norlutin ... 1755
Nor-Q D Tablets ... 2304
Ortho-Novum ... 1667
Ovcon ... 1391
Tri-Norinyl ... 2304

Norethynodrel (Increases serum theophylline levels). Products include:
Enovid ... 2161

Norgestimate (Increases serum theophylline levels). Products include:
Ortho-Cyclen Tablets ... 1658

Norgestrel (Increases serum theophylline levels). Products include:
Lo/Ovral Tablets ... 2471
Lo/Ovral-28 Tablets ... 2476
Ovral Tablets ... 2490
Ovral-28 Tablets ... 2491
Ovrette Tablets ... 2492

Phenytoin (Decreased theophylline and phenytoin serum levels). Products include:
Dilantin Infatabs ... 1710
Dilantin-30 Pediatric/Dilantin-125 Suspension ... 1713

Phenytoin Sodium (Decreased theophylline and phenytoin serum levels). Products include:
Dilantin Kapseals ... 1708
Dilantin Parenteral ... 1712
Dilantin with Phenobarbital Kapseals ... 1715

Pirbuterol Acetate (Potential for toxic synergism). Products include:
Maxair Inhaler ... 1311

Propranolol Hydrochloride (Increased serum theophylline levels). Products include:
Inderal ... 2459
Inderal LA Long Acting Capsules ... 2461
Inderide Tablets ... 2463
Inderide LA Long Acting Capsules .. 2465

Rifampin (Decreases serum theophylline levels). Products include:
Rifadin ... 1345
Rifamate Capsules ... 1347
Rimactane Capsules ... 879

Terbutaline Sulfate (Potential for toxic synergism). Products include:
Brethaire Inhaler ... 1024
Brethine Ampuls ... 1026
Brethine Tablets ... 1026
Bricanyl Injection ... 1324
Bricanyl Tablets ... 1325

Troleandomycin (Increases serum theophylline levels). Products include:
Tao Capsules ... 1963

Food Interactions

Diet, high-lipid (Potential for plasma concentration levels of 40-60% of those noted in the fasted state and delay in the time to peak plasma level).

THEO-ORGANIDIN ELIXIR
(Theophylline Anhydrous, Iodinated Glycerol) ... 2391
May interact with sympathomimetic bronchodilators, antithyroid agents, and certain other agents. Compounds in these categories include:

Albuterol (Toxic synergism-CNS stimulation). Products include:
Proventil Inhalation Aerosol ... 2117
Ventolin Inhalation Aerosol and Refill ... 583

Albuterol Sulfate (Toxic synergism-CNS stimulation). Products include:
Proventil Repetabs Tablets ... 2120
Proventil Solutions for Inhalation 0.5% and 0.083% ... 2118
Proventil Syrup ... 2119
Proventil Tablets ... 2120
Ventolin ... 583

Bitolterol Mesylate (Toxic synergism-CNS stimulation). Products include:
Tornalate ... 2074

Ephedrine Hydrochloride (Toxic synergism-CNS stimulation). Products include:
Amesec ... ▣ 682
Primatene Tablets-M Formula ... 2421
Primatene Tablets-P Formula ... 2421
Primatene Tablets-Regular Formula ... 2421
Quadrinal Tablets ... 1183
Quelidrine Syrup ... 556
Tedral SA ... 1765

Ephedrine Sulfate (Toxic synergism-CNS stimulation). Products include:
Bronkaid Tablets ... ▣ 757
Bronkolixir ... ▣ 761
Bronkotabs Tablets ... ▣ 762
Marax Tablets & DF Syrup ... 1954
Pazo Hemorrhoid Ointment & Suppositories ... 752
Vicks Vatronol Nose Drops ... ▣ 666

Ephedrine Tannate (Toxic synergism-CNS stimulation). Products include:
Rynatuss ... 2388

Epinephrine (Toxic synergism-CNS stimulation). Products include:
Ana-Kit Anaphylaxis Emergency Treatment Kit ... 1100
Bronkaid Mist ... ▣ 757
EpiPen ... 843
Marcaine Hydrochloride 0.5% with Epinephrine 1:200,000 (as bitartrate) ... 958
Marcaine Hydrochloride with Epinephrine 1:200,000 ... 2055
Primatene Mist ... 2420
Sus-Phrine Injection ... 1006
Xylocaine with Epinephrine Injections ... 637

Epinephrine Hydrochloride (Toxic synergism-CNS stimulation). Products include:
Adrenalin Chloride Solution 1:100 & 1:1,000 ... 1689
Epifrin ... ⊙ 244
Glaucon ... ⊙ 218

Ethylnorepinephrine Hydrochloride (Toxic synergism-CNS stimulation). Products include:
Bronkephrine Injection ... 2042

Isoetharine (Toxic synergism-CNS stimulation). Products include:
Arm-a-Med Isoetharine Inhalation Solution, USP ... 616
Bronkometer Aerosol ... 2042
Bronkosol Solution ... 2042

Isoproterenol Hydrochloride (Toxic synergism-CNS stimulation). Products include:
Isuprel Hydrochloride Injection 1:5000 ... 2050
Isuprel Hydrochloride Mistometer .. 2051
Isuprel Hydrochloride Solution 1:200 & 1:100 ... 2052
Norisodrine Aerotrol ... 540

Lithium Carbonate (Hypothyroid effect of lithium potentiated). Products include:
Eskalith ... 2214
Lithane Tablets ... 1596
Lithium Carbonate Capsules & Tablets ... 1984
Lithobid Tablets ... 870

Lithium Citrate (Hypothyroid effect of lithium potentiated). Products include:
Cibalith-S ... 870

Metaproterenol Sulfate (Toxic synergism-CNS stimulation). Products include:
Alupent ... 674
Arm-a-Med Metaproterenol Sulfate Inhalation Solution, USP ... 617
Metaprel Inhalation Aerosol Bronchodilator ... 2014
Metaprel Inhalation Solution ... 2015
Metaprel ... 2015
Metaproterenol Sulfate Inhalation Solution, USP ... 912

Methimazole (Hypothyroid effect of antithyroid drugs potentiated). Products include:
Tapazole Tablets ... 1298

Pirbuterol Acetate (Toxic synergism-CNS stimulation). Products include:
Maxair Inhaler ... 1311

Propylthiouracil (Hypothyroid effect of antithyroid drugs potentiated).
No products indexed under this heading.

Terbutaline Sulfate (Toxic synergism-CNS stimulation). Products include:
Brethaire Inhaler ... 1024
Brethine Ampuls ... 1026
Brethine Tablets ... 1026
Bricanyl Injection ... 1324
Bricanyl Tablets ... 1325

THEOX EXTENDED-RELEASE TABLETS
(Theophylline Anhydrous) ... 841
May interact with macrolide antibiotics, oral contraceptives, sympathomimetic bronchodilators, and certain other agents. Compounds in these categories include:

Albuterol (Potential for toxic synergism). Products include:
Proventil Inhalation Aerosol ... 2117
Ventolin Inhalation Aerosol and Refill ... 583

Albuterol Sulfate (Potential for toxic synergism). Products include:
Proventil Repetabs Tablets ... 2120
Proventil Solutions for Inhalation 0.5% and 0.083% ... 2118
Proventil Syrup ... 2119
Proventil Tablets ... 2120
Ventolin ... 583

Allopurinol (Increased serum theophylline levels at high dose of allopurinol). Products include:
Zyloprim Tablets ... 830

Bitolterol Mesylate (Potential for toxic synergism). Products include:
Tornalate ... 2074

Cimetidine (Increases serum theophylline levels). Products include:
Tagamet Tablets ... 2228

(▣ Described in PDR For Nonprescription Drugs) (⊙ Described in PDR For Ophthalmology)

Cimetidine Hydrochloride (Increases serum theophylline levels). Products include:
- Tagamet ... 2228

Ciprofloxacin (Increases serum theophylline levels).
- No products indexed under this heading.

Ciprofloxacin Hydrochloride (Increases serum theophylline levels). Products include:
- Ciloxan Sterile Ophthalmic Solution ... ⊙ 214
- Cipro I.V. ... 1592
- Cipro Tablets ... 1589

Ephedrine Hydrochloride (Potential for toxic synergism). Products include:
- Amesec ... ▣ 682
- Primatene Tablets-M Formula ... 2421
- Primatene Tablets-P Formula ... 2421
- Primatene Tablets-Regular Formula ... 2421
- Quadrinal Tablets ... 1183
- Quelidrine Syrup ... 556
- Tedral SA ... 1765

Ephedrine Sulfate (Potential for toxic synergism). Products include:
- Bronkaid Tablets ... ▣ 757
- Bronkolixir ... ▣ 761
- Bronkotabs Tablets ... ▣ 762
- Marax Tablets & DF Syrup ... 1954
- Pazo Hemorrhoid Ointment & Suppositories ... 752
- Vicks Vatronol Nose Drops ... ▣ 666

Ephedrine Tannate (Potential for toxic synergism). Products include:
- Rynatuss ... 2388

Epinephrine (Potential for toxic synergism). Products include:
- Ana-Kit Anaphylaxis Emergency Treatment Kit ... 1100
- Bronkaid Mist ... ▣ 757
- EpiPen ... 843
- Marcaine Hydrochloride 0.5% with Epinephrine 1:200,000 (as bitartrate) ... 958
- Marcaine Hydrochloride with Epinephrine 1:200,000 ... 2055
- Primatene Mist ... 2420
- Sus-Phrine Injection ... 1006
- Xylocaine with Epinephrine Injections ... 637

Epinephrine Hydrochloride (Potential for toxic synergism). Products include:
- Adrenalin Chloride Solution 1:100 & 1:1,000 ... 1689
- Epifrin ... ⊙ 244
- Glaucon ... ⊙ 218

Erythromycin (Increases serum theophylline levels). Products include:
- A/T/S Topical Gel and Topical Solution ... 1089
- AK-Mycin Ointment ... ⊙ 204
- Benzamycin Topical Gel ... 907
- E-Mycin Tablets ... 688
- ETS-2% ... 1685
- ERYC ... 1720
- Erycette (erythromycin 2%) Topical Solution ... 1678
- Ery-Tab Tablets ... 521
- Erythromycin Base Filmtab ... 525
- Erythromycin Delayed-Release Capsules, USP ... 526
- Ilotycin Ophthalmic Ointment ... 915
- PCE Dispertab Tablets ... 549
- Pediazole ... 1973
- T-Stat 2.0% Topical Solution and Pads ... 2409
- Theramycin Z Topical Solution 2% 1410

Erythromycin Estolate (Increases serum theophylline levels). Products include:
- Ilosone ... 913

Erythromycin Ethylsuccinate (Increases serum theophylline levels). Products include:
- E.E.S. ... 522
- EryPed ... 519
- Pediazole ... 1973

Erythromycin Gluceptate (Increases serum theophylline levels). Products include:
- Ilotycin Gluceptate, IV, Vials ... 915

Erythromycin Stearate (Increases serum theophylline levels). Products include:
- Erythrocin Stearate Filmtab ... 523

Ethinyl Estradiol (Increases serum theophylline levels). Products include:
- Brevicon ... 2304
- Demulen ... 2161
- Estinyl Tablets ... 2085
- Jenest-28 Tablets ... 1636
- Levlen/Tri-Levlen ... 665
- Lo/Ovral Tablets ... 2471
- Lo/Ovral-28 Tablets ... 2476
- Loestrin ... 1728
- Modicon ... 1667
- Nordette-21 Tablets ... 2481
- Nordette-28 Tablets ... 2483
- Norethin ... 2133
- Norinyl ... 2304
- Norlestrin ... 1746
- Ortho-Cyclen Tablets ... 1658
- Ortho-Novum ... 1667
- Ovcon ... 1391
- Ovral Tablets ... 2490
- Ovral-28 Tablets ... 2491
- Levlen/Tri-Levlen ... 665
- Tri-Norinyl ... 2304
- Triphasil-21 Tablets ... 2527
- Triphasil-28 Tablets ... 2532

Ethylnorepinephrine Hydrochloride (Potential for toxic synergism). Products include:
- Bronkephrine Injection ... 2042

Ethynodiol Diacetate (Increases serum theophylline levels). Products include:
- Demulen ... 2161

Isoetharine (Potential for toxic synergism). Products include:
- Arm-a-Med Isoetharine Inhalation Solution, USP ... 616
- Bronkometer Aerosol ... 2042
- Bronkosol Solution ... 2042

Isoproterenol Hydrochloride (Potential for toxic synergism). Products include:
- Isuprel Hydrochloride Injection 1:5000 ... 2050
- Isuprel Hydrochloride Mistometer .. 2051
- Isuprel Hydrochloride Solution 1:200 & 1:100 ... 2052
- Norisodrine Aerotrol ... 540

Levonorgestrel (Increases serum theophylline levels). Products include:
- Levlen/Tri-Levlen ... 665
- Nordette-21 Tablets ... 2481
- Nordette-28 Tablets ... 2483
- Norplant System ... 2484
- Levlen/Tri-Levlen ... 665
- Triphasil-21 Tablets ... 2527
- Triphasil-28 Tablets ... 2532

Lithium Carbonate (Increased renal excretion of lithium). Products include:
- Eskalith ... 2214
- Lithane Tablets ... 1596
- Lithium Carbonate Capsules & Tablets ... 1984
- Lithobid Tablets ... 870

Mestranol (Increases serum theophylline levels). Products include:
- Enovid ... 2161
- Norethin ... 2133
- Norinyl ... 2304
- Ortho-Novum ... 1667

Metaproterenol Sulfate (Potential for toxic synergism). Products include:
- Alupent ... 674
- Arm-a-Med Metaproterenol Sulfate Inhalation Solution, USP ... 617
- Metaprel Inhalation Aerosol Bronchodilator ... 2014
- Metaprel Inhalation Solution ... 2015
- Metaprel ... 2015
- Metaproterenol Sulfate Inhalation Solution, USP ... 912

Norethindrone (Increases serum theophylline levels). Products include:
- Brevicon ... 2304
- Jenest-28 Tablets ... 1636
- Micronor Tablets ... 1667
- Modicon ... 1667
- Norethin ... 2133
- Norinyl ... 2304
- Norlutin ... 1755
- Nor-Q D Tablets ... 2304
- Ortho-Novum ... 1667
- Ovcon ... 1391
- Tri-Norinyl ... 2304

Norethynodrel (Increases serum theophylline levels). Products include:
- Enovid ... 2161

Norgestimate (Increases serum theophylline levels). Products include:
- Ortho-Cyclen Tablets ... 1658

Norgestrel (Increases serum theophylline levels). Products include:
- Lo/Ovral Tablets ... 2471
- Lo/Ovral-28 Tablets ... 2476
- Ovral Tablets ... 2490
- Ovral-28 Tablets ... 2491
- Ovrette Tablets ... 2492

Phenytoin (Decreased theophylline and phenytoin levels). Products include:
- Dilantin Infatabs ... 1710
- Dilantin-30 Pediatric/Dilantin-125 Suspension ... 1713

Phenytoin Sodium (Decreased theophylline and phenytoin levels). Products include:
- Dilantin Kapseals ... 1708
- Dilantin Parenteral ... 1712
- Dilantin with Phenobarbital Kapseals ... 1715

Pirbuterol Acetate (Potential for toxic synergism). Products include:
- Maxair Inhaler ... 1311

Propranolol Hydrochloride (Increases serum theophylline levels). Products include:
- Inderal ... 2459
- Inderal LA Long Acting Capsules 2461
- Inderide Tablets ... 2463
- Inderide LA Long Acting Capsules .. 2465

Rifampin (Decreased serum theophylline levels). Products include:
- Rifadin ... 1345
- Rifamate Capsules ... 1347
- Rimactane Capsules ... 879

Terbutaline Sulfate (Potential for toxic synergism). Products include:
- Brethaire Inhaler ... 1024
- Brethine Ampuls ... 1026
- Brethine Tablets ... 1026
- Bricanyl Injection ... 1324
- Bricanyl Tablets ... 1325

Troleandomycin (Increases serum theophylline levels). Products include:
- Tao Capsules ... 1963

Food Interactions

Diet, high-lipid (May result in a somewhat higher C_{max} and delayed T_{max}, and a somewhat greater extent of absorption when compared to taking in the fasting state).

THERA-COMBEX H-P KAPSEALS (Vitamin B Complex With Vitamin C) ... ▣ 642

No interactions described in labeling.

THERACYS BCG LIVE (INTRAVESICAL) (BCG, Live (Intravesical)) ... 898

May interact with immunosuppressive agents and certain other agents. Compounds in these categories include:

Azathioprine (May impair the response to TheraCys or increase the risk of osteomyelitis or disseminated BCG infection). Products include:
- Imuran ... 768

Bone Marrow Depressants, unspecified (May impair the response to TheraCys or increase the risk of osteomyelitis or disseminated BCG infection).

Cyclosporine (May impair the response to TheraCys or increase the risk of osteomyelitis or disseminated BCG infection). Products include:
- Sandimmune ... 2024

Immune Globulin (Human) (May impair the response to TheraCys or increase the risk of osteomyelitis or disseminated BCG infection). Products include:
- MICRhoGAM $Rh_o(D)$ Immune Globulin (Human) ... 1650
- RhoGAM $Rh_o(D)$ Immune Globulin (Human) ... 1651

Immune Globulin Intravenous (Human) (May impair the response to TheraCys or increase the risk of osteomyelitis or disseminated BCG infection). Products include:
- Gamimune N Immune Globulin Intravenous (Human) ... 1572
- Gammagard Immune Globulin, Intravenous (Human) ... 658
- Iveegam ... 1129
- Sandoglobulin I.V. ... 2027

Muromonab-CD3 (May impair the response to TheraCys or increase the risk of osteomyelitis or disseminated BCG infection). Products include:
- Orthoclone OKT3 Sterile Solution .. 1645

THERAFLU FLU AND COLD MEDICINE (Acetaminophen, Chlorpheniramine Maleate, Pseudoephedrine Hydrochloride) ... ▣ 687

May interact with antihypertensives, antidepressant drugs, and certain other agents. Compounds in these categories include:

Acebutolol Hydrochloride (Concurrent use not recommended). Products include:
- Sectral Capsules ... 2520

Alcohol (Concurrent use not recommended).

Amitriptyline Hydrochloride (Concurrent use not recommended). Products include:
- Elavil ... 2269
- Endep Tablets ... 1927
- Etrafon ... 2087
- Limbitrol ... 1933
- Triavil Tablets ... 1556

Amoxapine (Concurrent use not recommended). Products include:
- Asendin Tablets ... 1196

Atenolol (Concurrent use not recommended). Products include:
- Tenoretic Tablets ... 1105
- Tenormin Tablets and I.V. Injection 1107

Benazepril Hydrochloride (Concurrent use not recommended). Products include:
- Lotensin Tablets ... 872

Bendroflumethiazide (Concurrent use not recommended). Products include:
- Corzide Tablets ... 702
- Naturetin Tablets ... 1789
- Rauzide Tablets ... 1804

Betaxolol Hydrochloride (Concurrent use not recommended). Products include:
- Betoptic Sterile Ophthalmic Solution ... 569
- Betoptic S Sterile Ophthalmic Suspension ... 570
- Kerlone Tablets ... 2172

Bupropion Hydrochloride (Concurrent use not recommended). Products include:
- Wellbutrin Tablets ... 821

Captopril (Concurrent use not recommended). Products include:
- Capoten ... 2255
- Capozide ... 2258

Carteolol Hydrochloride (Concurrent use not recommended). Products include:
- Cartrol Tablets ... 507

Clonidine (Concurrent use not recommended). Products include:
- Catapres-TTS ... 677

Clonidine Hydrochloride (Concurrent use not recommended). Products include:
- Catapres Tablets ... 676
- Combipres Tablets ... 678

Deserpidine (Concurrent use not recommended). Products include:
- Enduronyl ... 518
- Harmonyl Tablets ... 528
- Oreticyl ... 545

Desipramine Hydrochloride (Concurrent use not recommended). Products include:
- Norpramin Tablets ... 1340

Diazoxide (Concurrent use not recommended). Products include:
- Hyperstat I.V. Injection ... 2095
- Proglycem ... 649

Doxazosin Mesylate (Concurrent use not recommended). Products include:
- Cardura Tablets ... 1941

Doxepin Hydrochloride (Concurrent use not recommended). Products include:
- Sinequan ... 1960

Enalapril Maleate (Concurrent use not recommended). Products include:
- Vaseretic Tablets ... 1559
- Vasotec Tablets ... 1564

Enalaprilat (Concurrent use not recommended). Products include:
- Vasotec I.V. ... 1562

Esmolol Hydrochloride (Concurrent use not recommended). Products include:
- Brevibloc Injection ... 942

Felodipine (Concurrent use not recommended). Products include:
- Plendil Extended-Release Tablets ... 1526

Fluoxetine Hydrochloride (Concurrent use not recommended). Products include:
- Prozac Pulvules ... 920

Fosinopril Sodium (Concurrent use not recommended). Products include:
- Monopril Tablets ... 1406

Guanabenz Acetate (Concurrent use not recommended). Products include:
- Wytensin Tablets ... 2542

Guanethidine Monosulfate (Concurrent use not recommended). Products include:
- Esimil Tablets ... 864
- Ismelin Tablets ... 869

Hydralazine Hydrochloride (Concurrent use not recommended). Products include:
- Apresazide Capsules ... 854
- Apresoline Hydrochloride Parenteral (Ampuls) ... 856
- Apresoline Hydrochloride Tablets ... 855
- Apresoline-Esidrix Tablets ... 857
- Ser-Ap-Es Tablets ... 881
- Serpasil-Apresoline Tablets ... 884

Imipramine Hydrochloride (Concurrent use not recommended). Products include:
- Tofranil Ampuls ... 1038
- Tofranil Tablets ... 1039

Imipramine Pamoate (Concurrent use not recommended). Products include:
- Tofranil-PM Capsules ... 1041

Isocarboxazid (Concurrent use not recommended). Products include:
- Marplan Tablets ... 1906

Isradipine (Concurrent use not recommended). Products include:
- DynaCirc Capsules ... 2004

Labetalol Hydrochloride (Concurrent use not recommended). Products include:
- Normodyne Injection ... 2108
- Normodyne Tablets ... 2110
- Normozide Tablets ... 2112
- Trandate HCT Tablets ... 579
- Trandate Injection ... 577
- Trandate Tablets ... 579

Lisinopril (Concurrent use not recommended). Products include:
- Prinivil Tablets ... 1538
- Prinzide Tablets ... 1540
- Zestoretic ... 2274
- Zestril Tablets ... 2277

Maprotiline Hydrochloride (Concurrent use not recommended). Products include:
- Ludiomil Tablets ... 874

Mecamylamine Hydrochloride (Concurrent use not recommended). Products include:
- Inversine Tablets ... 1492

Methyldopa (Concurrent use not recommended). Products include:
- Aldoclor Tablets ... 1413
- Aldomet Oral ... 1415
- Aldoril Tablets ... 1418

Methyldopate Hydrochloride (Concurrent use not recommended). Products include:
- Aldomet Ester HCl Injection ... 1417

Metoprolol Tartrate (Concurrent use not recommended). Products include:
- Lopressor Ampuls ... 1032
- Lopressor HCT Tablets ... 1034
- Lopressor Tablets ... 1032

Metyrosine (Concurrent use not recommended). Products include:
- Demser Capsules ... 1460

Minoxidil (Concurrent use not recommended). Products include:
- Loniten Tablets ... 2346
- Rogaine Topical Solution ... 2357

Nadolol (Concurrent use not recommended). Products include:
- Corgard Tablets ... 701
- Corzide Tablets ... 702

Nicardipine Hydrochloride (Concurrent use not recommended). Products include:
- Cardene Capsules ... 2290

Nitroglycerin (Concurrent use not recommended). Products include:
- Deponit NTG Transdermal Delivery System ... 2143
- Minitran Transdermal Delivery System ... 1312
- Nitro-Bid Ointment ... 1339
- Nitro-Bid Capsules ... 1338
- Nitrodisc ... 2176
- Nitro-Dur (nitroglycerin) Transdermal Infusion System ... 1164
- Nitrogard Tablets ... 1004
- Nitrolingual Spray ... 1846
- Nitrostat Tablets ... 1743
- Transderm-Nitro Transdermal Therapeutic System ... 2283

Nortriptyline Hydrochloride (Concurrent use not recommended). Products include:
- Pamelor ... 2019

Penbutolol Sulfate (Concurrent use not recommended). Products include:
- Levatol ... 1832

Phenelzine Sulfate (Concurrent use not recommended). Products include:
- Nardil ... 1742

Phenoxybenzamine Hydrochloride (Concurrent use not recommended). Products include:
- Dibenzyline Capsules ... 2207

Phentolamine Mesylate (Concurrent use not recommended). Products include:
- Regitine ... 878

Pindolol (Concurrent use not recommended). Products include:
- Visken Tablets ... 2036

Prazosin Hydrochloride (Concurrent use not recommended). Products include:
- Minipress Capsules ... 1778
- Minizide Capsules ... 1779

Propranolol Hydrochloride (Concurrent use not recommended). Products include:
- Inderal ... 2459
- Inderal LA Long Acting Capsules ... 2461
- Inderide Tablets ... 2463
- Inderide LA Long Acting Capsules ... 2465

Protriptyline Hydrochloride (Concurrent use not recommended). Products include:
- Vivactil Tablets ... 1567

Ramipril (Concurrent use not recommended). Products include:
- Altace Capsules ... 1086

Rauwolfia Serpentina (Concurrent use not recommended). Products include:
- Raudixin Tablets ... 1803
- Rauzide Tablets ... 1804

Rescinnamine (Concurrent use not recommended).
- No products indexed under this heading.

Reserpine (Concurrent use not recommended). Products include:
- Diupres Tablets ... 1461
- Hydromox R Tablets ... 1209
- Hydropres Tablets ... 1485
- Renese-R Tablets ... 1786
- Salutensin/Salutensin-Demi ... 719
- Ser-Ap-Es Tablets ... 881
- Serpasil Tablets ... 883
- Serpasil-Apresoline Tablets ... 884
- Serpasil-Esidrix Tablets ... 886

Sodium Nitroprusside (Concurrent use not recommended). Products include:
- Nipride I.V. Infusion ... 1909

Terazosin Hydrochloride (Concurrent use not recommended). Products include:
- Hytrin Tablets ... 529

Timolol Maleate (Concurrent use not recommended). Products include:
- Blocadren Tablets ... 1429
- Timolide Tablets ... 1547
- Timoptic in Ocudose ... 1552
- Timoptic Sterile Ophthalmic Solution ... 1550

Tranylcypromine Sulfate (Concurrent use not recommended). Products include:
- Parnate Tablets ... 2222

Trazodone Hydrochloride (Concurrent use not recommended). Products include:
- Desyrel and Desyrel Dividose ... 1404

Trimethaphan Camsylate (Concurrent use not recommended). Products include:
- Arfonad Ampuls ... 1887

Trimipramine Maleate (Concurrent use not recommended). Products include:
- Surmontil Capsules ... 2524

THERA-GESIC
(Methyl Salicylate, Menthol) ... 1614
No interactions described in labeling.

THERAGOLD - THE GOLD LOTION
(Methyl Salicylate, Menthol, Camphor) ... (OTC) 508
No interactions described in labeling.

THERAGRAN HEMATINIC TABLETS
(Vitamins with Minerals, Therapeutic, Ferrous Fumarate) ... 605
May interact with oral anticoagulants, tetracyclines, and certain other agents. Compounds in these categories include:

Cholestyramine (Decreased absorption of fat-soluble vitamins). Products include:
- Cholybar ... 1705
- Questran Light ... 711
- Questran Powder ... 710

Colchicine (Impaired cyanocobalamin absorption). Products include:
- ColBENEMID Tablets ... 1436
- Colchicine Ampoules ... 1252

Colestipol Hydrochloride (Decreased bioavailability of niacin). Products include:
- Colestid Granules ... 2328

Cycloserine (Antagonism of pyridoxine hydrochloride). Products include:
- Seromycin Pulvules ... 1298

Demeclocycline Hydrochloride (Interference with absorption of oral tetracyclines). Products include:
- Declomycin Capsules, Tablets ... 1199

Dicumarol (Hypoprothrombinemic effect decreased). Products include:
- Dicumarol Tablets ... 516

Doxycycline Calcium (Interference with absorption of oral tetracyclines).
- No products indexed under this heading.

Doxycycline Hyclate (Interference with absorption of oral tetracyclines). Products include:
- Doryx Capsules ... 1717
- Vibramycin Hyclate Capsules ... 1787
- Vibramycin Hyclate Intravenous ... 1968
- Vibra-Tabs Film Coated Tablets ... 1787

Doxycycline Monohydrate (Interference with absorption of oral tetracyclines). Products include:
- Monodox Capsules ... 1630
- Vibramycin Monohydrate for Oral Suspension ... 1787

Hydralazine Hydrochloride (Antagonism of pyridoxine hydrochloride). Products include:
- Apresazide Capsules ... 854
- Apresoline Hydrochloride Parenteral (Ampuls) ... 856
- Apresoline Hydrochloride Tablets ... 855
- Apresoline-Esidrix Tablets ... 857
- Ser-Ap-Es Tablets ... 881
- Serpasil-Apresoline Tablets ... 884

Isoniazid (Antagonism of pyridoxine hydrochloride). Products include:
- INH Tablets ... 868
- Rifamate Capsules ... 1347

Levodopa (Pyridoxine hydrochloride may act as antagonist). Products include:
- Larodopa Tablets ... 1905
- Sinemet Tablets ... 952

Sinemet CR Tablets 953

Methacycline Hydrochloride (Interference with absorption of oral tetracyclines).
No products indexed under this heading.

Methotrexate Sodium (Interference with folic acid absorption). Products include:
- Methotrexate Tablets, Parenteral, LPF Parenteral 1217
- Rheumatrex Methotrexate Dose Pack 1234

Mineral Oil (Decreased absorption of fat-soluble vitamins). Products include:
- AKWA Tears Ointment .... ⊙ 208
- Agoral .... ⊞ 634
- Aqua Care Cream .... ⊞ 616
- Aqua Care Lotion .... ⊞ 616
- Aquaphor Antibiotic Formula 662
- Aquaphor Healing Ointment, Original Formula 662
- Aquaphor Natural Healing Formula 662
- Complex 15 Hand & Body Moisturizing Cream .... ⊞ 694
- Complex 15 Hand & Body Moisturizing Lotion .... ⊞ 695
- Complex 15 Moisturizing Face Cream .... ⊞ 695
- Duolube Eye Ointment .... ⊙ 258
- Duratears Naturale .... ⊙ 216
- Eucerin Dry Skin Care Lotion 662
- Eucerin Moisturizing Creme (Unscented) 662
- Eucerin Dry Skin Care Lotion (Fragrace-free) .... ⊞ 514
- Fleet Mineral Oil Enema 992
- Fleet Relief 993
- Haley's M-O, Regular & Flavored .. ⊞ 569
- Keri Lotion - Original Formula .... ⊞ 535
- Lacri-Lube NP Lubricant Ophthalmic Ointment .... ⊙ 249
- Lacri-Lube S.O.P. Sterile Ophthalmic Ointment .... ⊙ 249
- Nephrox Suspension .... ⊞ 563
- Nivea Bath Silk Bath Oil .... ⊞ 514
- Nivea Bath Silk Bath & Shower Gel (Extra-Dry Skin) .... ⊞ 514
- Nivea Moisturizing Creme .... ⊞ 514
- Nivea Moisturizing Lotion (Original Formula) .... ⊞ 514
- Nivea Moisturizing Oil .... ⊞ 515
- Nivea Skin Oil .... ⊞ 515
- Nivea Sun After Sun Lotion .... ⊞ 515
- Nutraderm Cream & Lotion 1684
- pHisoDerm For Baby .... ⊞ 761
- pHisoDerm Skin Cleanser and Conditioner - Regular and Oily .... ⊞ 760
- Refresh P.M. Lubricant Ophthalmic Ointment .... ⊙ 256
- Replens .... ⊞ 556
- Tears Renewed Ointment .... ⊙ 209
- Theraplex ClearLotion 1410

Minocycline Hydrochloride (Interference with absorption of oral tetracyclines). Products include:
- Minocin Intravenous 1221
- Minocin Oral Suspension 1224
- Minocin Pellet-Filled Capsules 1222

Neomycin, oral (Impaired cyanocobalamin absorption).

Oxytetracycline (Interference with absorption of oral tetracyclines). Products include:
- Terramycin Intramuscular Solution 1964
- Urobiotic-250 Capsules 1968

Oxytetracycline Hydrochloride (Interference with absorption of oral tetracyclines). Products include:
- Terra-Cortril Ophthalmic Suspension 1963
- Terramycin Capsules 1786
- Terramycin Intramuscular Solution 1964
- Terramycin with Polymyxin B Sulfate Ophthalmic Ointment 1965

Penicillamine (Antagonism of pyridoxine hydrochloride). Products include:
- Cuprimine Capsules 1442
- Depen Titratable Tablets 2379

Phenytoin (Interference with folic acid absorption). Products include:
- Dilantin Infatabs 1710
- Dilantin-30 Pediatric/Dilantin-125 Suspension 1713

Phenytoin Sodium (Interference with folic acid absorption). Products include:
- Dilantin Kapseals 1708
- Dilantin Parenteral 1712
- Dilantin with Phenobarbital Kapseals 1715

Pyrimethamine (Interference with folic acid absorption). Products include:
- Daraprim Tablets 761
- Fansidar Tablets 1896

Tetracycline Hydrochloride (Interference with absorption of oral tetracyclines). Products include:
- Achromycin V Capsules 1193
- Achromycin Ophthalmic Ointment 1% .... ⊙ 307
- Achromycin Ophthalmic Suspension 1% .... ⊙ 308
- Topicycline for Topical Solution 1856

Warfarin Sodium (Hypoprothrombinemic effect decreased). Products include:
- Coumadin Injection & Tablets 944
- Panwarfin Tablets 547

THERAGRAN LIQUID
(Multivitamins) .... ⊞ 727
No interactions described in labeling.

THERAGRAN STRESS FORMULA
(Vitamins, Multiple, Ferrous Fumarate) .... ⊞ 727
No interactions described in labeling.

THERAGRAN TABLETS
(Multivitamins) .... ⊞ 727
No interactions described in labeling.

THERAGRAN-M TABLETS
(Multivitamins with Minerals) .... ⊞ 727
No interactions described in labeling.

THERAMYCIN Z TOPICAL SOLUTION 2%
(Erythromycin) 1410
No interactions described in labeling.

THERAPEUTIC GOLD - THE GOLD LOTION
(Methyl Salicylate, Menthol, Camphor) .... ⊞ 508
No interactions described in labeling.

THERAPEUTIC MINERAL ICE PAIN RELIEVING GEL
(Menthol) 752
No interactions described in labeling.

THERAPEUTIC MINERAL ICE EXERCISE FORMULA, PAIN RELIEVING GEL
(Menthol) .... ⊞ 538
No interactions described in labeling.

THERAPLEX CLEARLOTION
(Mineral Oil) 1410
No interactions described in labeling.

THERAPLEX EMOLLIENT
(Petrolatum) 1411
No interactions described in labeling.

THERAPLEX HYDROLOTION
(Petrolatum) 1411
No interactions described in labeling.

THERAPLEX T SHAMPOO
(Coal Tar) 1411
No interactions described in labeling.

THERAPLEX Z SHAMPOO
(Zinc Pyrithione) 1411
No interactions described in labeling.

THERMOTABS
(Potassium Chloride, Sodium Chloride) .... ⊞ 619
No interactions described in labeling.

THEROXIDE 5% AND 10%
(Benzoyl Peroxide) 1411
No interactions described in labeling.

THEROXIDE WASH
(Benzoyl Peroxide) 1411
No interactions described in labeling.

THIOGUANINE TABLETS, TABLOID BRAND
(Thioguanine) 815
May interact with cytotoxic drugs and certain other agents. Compounds in these categories include:

Bleomycin Sulfate (Combination therapy may produce hepatic disease). Products include:
- Blenoxane 724

Busulfan (Potential for esophageal varices associated with abnormal liver function tests). Products include:
- Myleran Tablets 790

Daunorubicin Hydrochloride (Combination therapy may produce hepatic disease). Products include:
- Cerubidine 2443

Doxorubicin Hydrochloride (Combination therapy may produce hepatic disease). Products include:
- Adriamycin PFS 561
- Adriamycin RDF 562
- Doxorubicin Hydrochloride for Injection, USP 622
- Doxorubicin Hydrochloride Injection, USP 848
- Rubex 739

Fluorouracil (Combination therapy may produce hepatic disease). Products include:
- Efudex 1880
- Fluoroplex Topical Solution & Cream 1% 1082
- Fluorouracil Injection 1897

Hydroxyurea (Combination therapy may produce hepatic disease). Products include:
- Hydrea Capsules 728

Mercaptopurine (Complete cross-resistance). Products include:
- Purinethol Tablets 800

Methotrexate Sodium (Combination therapy may produce hepatic disease). Products include:
- Methotrexate Tablets, Parenteral, LPF Parenteral 1217
- Rheumatrex Methotrexate Dose Pack 1234

Mitotane (Combination therapy may produce hepatic disease). Products include:
- Lysodren 731

Mitoxantrone Hydrochloride (Combination therapy may produce hepatic disease). Products include:
- Novantrone for Injection Concentrate 1226

Procarbazine Hydrochloride (Combination therapy may produce hepatic disease). Products include:
- Matulane Capsules 1907

Tamoxifen Citrate (Combination therapy may produce hepatic disease). Products include:
- Nolvadex Tablets 1102

Vincristine Sulfate (Combination therapy may produce hepatic disease). Products include:
- Oncovin Solution Vials & Hyporets 1288

THIOSULFIL FORTE TABLETS
(Sulfamethizole) 2526
May interact with oral anticoagulants, oral hypoglycemic agents, hydantoin anticonvulsants, para-aminobenzoic acid based local anesthetics, and certain other agents. Compounds in these categories include:

Chlorpropamide (Potentiated effects). Products include:
- Diabinese Tablets 1775

Dicumarol (Potentiated effects). Products include:
- Dicumarol Tablets 516

Ethotoin (Potentiated effects). Products include:
- Peganone Tablets 551

Glipizide (Potentiated effects). Products include:
- Glucotrol 1952

Glyburide (Potentiated effects). Products include:
- DiaBeta 1091
- Micronase Tablets 2350

Mephenytoin (Potentiated effects). Products include:
- Mesantoin Tablets 2013

Methenamine Mandelate (An insoluble precipitate may form in acidic urine). Products include:
- Mandelamine 1738
- Uroqid-Acid 661

Phenytoin (Prolonged half-life; potentiated effects). Products include:
- Dilantin Infatabs 1710
- Dilantin-30 Pediatric/Dilantin-125 Suspension 1713

Phenytoin Sodium (Prolonged half-life; potentiated effects). Products include:
- Dilantin Kapseals 1708
- Dilantin Parenteral 1712
- Dilantin with Phenobarbital Kapseals 1715

Procaine Hydrochloride (Antagonizes the effects of sulfonamides and therefore decreases their effectiveness). Products include:
- Novocain Hydrochloride for Spinal Anesthesia 2065

Tetracaine Hydrochloride (Antagonizes the effects of sulfonamides and therefore decreases their effectiveness). Products include:
- Cetacaine Topical Anesthetic 850
- Pontocaine Hydrochloride for Spinal Anesthesia 2069

Tolazamide (Potentiated effects). Products include:
- Tolinase Tablets 2365

Tolbutamide (Prolonged half-life; potentiated effects). Products include:
- Orinase Tablets 2354

Warfarin Sodium (Prolonged half-life; potentiated effects). Products include:
- Coumadin Injection & Tablets 944
- Panwarfin Tablets 547

THIOTEPA PARENTERAL
(Thiotepa) 1240
May interact with nitrogen-mustard-type alkylating agents and certain other agents. Compounds in these categories include:

Bone Marrow Depressants, unspecified (Avoid concurrent use).

Chlorambucil (Intensified toxicity). Products include:
- Leukeran Tablets 788

Cyclophosphamide (Intensified toxicity). Products include:
- Cytoxan for Injection 726
- Neosar for Injection 566

Estramustine Phosphate Sodium (Intensified toxicity). Products include:
- Emcyt Capsules 1161

Mechlorethamine Hydrochloride (Intensified toxicity). Products include:
- Mustargen 1514

Melphalan (Intensified toxicity). Products include:
- Alkeran Tablets 754

THORAZINE AMPULS
(Chlorpromazine) 2234
See **Thorazine Concentrate**

THORAZINE CONCENTRATE
(Chlorpromazine) 2234
May interact with central nervous system depressants, oral anticoagulants, anticonvulsants, thiazides, and certain other agents. Compounds in these categories include:

Alfentanil Hydrochloride (Prolonged and intensified action of CNS depressants). Products include:
- Alfenta Injection 1131

Alprazolam (Prolonged and intensified action of CNS depressants). Products include:
- Xanax Tablets 2367

Aprobarbital (Prolonged and intensified action of CNS depressants). Products include:
- Alurate Elixir 1883

Atropine Nitrate, Methyl (Use with caution).
No products indexed under this heading.

Atropine Sulfate (Use with caution). Products include:
- Arco-Lase Plus Tablets 607
- Atropine Sulfate Sterile Ophthalmic Solution and S.O.P. Sterile Ophthalmic Ointment .... ◉ 239
- Donnagel .... ⊞ 675
- Donnagel-PG 1858
- Donnatal 1858
- Donnatal Extentabs 1859
- Donnatal Tablets 1858
- Donnazyme Tablets 1860
- Isopto Atropine .... ◉ 218
- Lomotil 2174
- Motofen Tablets 836
- Ru-Tuss Tablets 693
- Urised Tablets 2396

Bendroflumethiazide (Orthostatic hypotension that may occur with chlorpromazine may be accentuated). Products include:
- Corzide Tablets 702
- Naturetin Tablets 1789
- Rauzide Tablets 1804

Buprenorphine (Prolonged and intensified action of CNS depressants).
No products indexed under this heading.

Buspirone Hydrochloride (Prolonged and intensified action of CNS depressants). Products include:
- BuSpar 1401

Butabarbital (Prolonged and intensified action of CNS depressants). Products include:
- Pyridium Plus 1764

Butalbital (Prolonged and intensified action of CNS depressants). Products include:
- Esgic-Plus Tablets 1002
- Esgic Tablets & Capsules 1001
- Fioricet Tablets 2006
- Fiorinal Capsules 2007
- Fiorinal with Codeine Capsules 2008
- Fiorinal Tablets 2007
- Phrenilin 838
- Sedapap Tablets 50 mg/650 mg .. 1360

Carbamazepine (Chlorpromazine may lower convulsive threshold; dosage adjustments of anticonvulsants may be necessary). Products include:
- Tegretol Chewable Tablets 654
- Tegretol Suspension 656
- Tegretol Tablets 654

Carmustine (BCNU) (Antiemetic action of chlorpromazine may obscure vomiting as a sign of toxicity). Products include:
- BiCNU 723

Chlordiazepoxide (Prolonged and intensified action of CNS depressants). Products include:
- Libritabs Tablets 1930
- Limbitrol 1933
- Menrium Tablets 1934

Chlordiazepoxide Hydrochloride (Prolonged and intensified action of CNS depressants). Products include:
- Librax Capsules 1929
- Librium Capsules 1931
- Librium Injectable 1932

Chlorothiazide (Orthostatic hypotension that may occur with chlorpromazine may be accentuated). Products include:
- Aldoclor Tablets 1413
- Diupres Tablets 1461
- Diuril Oral 1464

Chlorothiazide Sodium (Orthostatic hypotension that may occur with chlorpromazine may be accentuated). Products include:
- Diuril Sodium Intravenous 1463

Chlorprothixene (Prolonged and intensified action of CNS depressants). Products include:
- Taractan Tablets 1920

Chlorprothixene Hydrochloride (Prolonged and intensified action of CNS depressants). Products include:
- Taractan 1920

Clorazepate Dipotassium (Prolonged and intensified action of CNS depressants). Products include:
- Tranxene 556

Codeine (Prolonged and intensified action of CNS depressants). Products include:
- Calcidrine Syrup 506

Codeine Phosphate (Prolonged and intensified action of CNS depressants). Products include:
- Actifed with Codeine Cough Syrup.. 752
- Cheracol Cough Syrup 1853
- Codimal PH Syrup 846
- Dimetane-DC Cough Syrup 1857
- Empirin with Codeine Phosphate Nos. 2, 3 & 4 764
- Fiorinal with Codeine Capsules 2008
- Isoclor Expectorant 982
- Naldecon CX Adult Liquid .... ⊞ 521
- Novahistine DH 1342
- Novahistine Expectorant 1343
- Nucofed Capsules 2219
- Nucofed Expectorant 2219
- Nucofed Pediatric Expectorant 2220
- Nucofed Syrup 2219
- Phenaphen with Codeine Capsules 1865
- Phenaphen-650 with Codeine Tablets 1866
- Phenergan with Codeine 2497
- Phenergan VC with Codeine 2501
- Robitussin A-C Syrup 1875
- Robitussin-DAC Syrup 1875
- Ryna .... ⊞ 741
- Soma Compound w/Codeine Tablets 2390
- Triaminic Expectorant w/Codeine .. 1996
- Tussi-Organidin Liquid 2391
- Tylenol with Codeine 1381

Codeine Polistirex (Prolonged and intensified action of CNS depressants).
No products indexed under this heading.

Dezocine (Prolonged and intensified action of CNS depressants).

Diazepam (Prolonged and intensified action of CNS depressants). Products include:
- Valium Injectable 1937
- Valium Tablets 1939
- Valrelease Capsules 1923

Dicumarol (Effects diminished). Products include:
- Dicumarol Tablets 516

Divalproex Sodium (Chlorpromazine may lower convulsive threshold; dosage adjustments of anticonvulsants may be necessary). Products include:
- Depakote 512

Droperidol (Prolonged and intensified action of CNS depressants). Products include:
- Inapsine Injection 1140
- Innovar Injection 1141

Enflurane (Prolonged and intensified action of CNS depressants). Products include:
- Ethrane 599

Estazolam (Prolonged and intensified action of CNS depressants). Products include:
- ProSom Tablets 554

Estramustine Phosphate Sodium (Antiemetic action of chlorpromazine may obscure vomiting as a sign of toxicity). Products include:
- Emcyt Capsules 1161

Ethchlorvynol (Prolonged and intensified action of CNS depressants). Products include:
- Placidyl Capsules 553

Ethinamate (Prolonged and intensified action of CNS depressants).
No products indexed under this heading.

Ethosuximide (Chlorpromazine may lower convulsive threshold; dosage adjustments of anticonvulsants may be necessary). Products include:
- Zarontin Capsules 1768
- Zarontin Syrup 1769

Ethotoin (Chlorpromazine may lower convulsive threshold; dosage adjustments of anticonvulsants may be necessary). Products include:
- Peganone Tablets 551

Fentanyl (Prolonged and intensified action of CNS depressants). Products include:
- Duragesic Transdermal System 1133

Fentanyl Citrate (Prolonged and intensified action of CNS depressants). Products include:
- Innovar Injection 1141
- Sublimaze Injection 1146

Fluphenazine Decanoate (Prolonged and intensified action of CNS depressants). Products include:
- Prolixin Decanoate 1795

Fluphenazine Enanthate (Prolonged and intesnified action of CNS depressants). Products include:
- Prolixin Enanthate 1796

Fluphenazine Hydrochloride (Prolonged and intensified action of CNS depressants). Products include:
- Prolixin Elixir 1793
- Prolixin Injection 1791
- Prolixin Oral Concentrate 1792
- Prolixin Tablets 1793

Flurazepam Hydrochloride (Prolonged and intensified action of CNS depressants). Products include:
- Dalmane Capsules 1927

Glutethimide (Prolonged and intensified action of CNS depressants).
No products indexed under this heading.

Guanethidine Monosulfate (Antihypertensive effect of guanethidine and related compounds may be counteracted). Products include:
- Esimil Tablets 864
- Ismelin Tablets 869

Haloperidol (Prolonged and intensified action of CNS depressants). Products include:
- Haldol Injection, Tablets and Concentrate 1373

Haloperidol Decanoate (Prolonged and intensified action of CNS depressants). Products include:
- Haldol Decanoate 1375

Hydrochlorothiazide (Orthostatic hypotension that may occur with chlorpromazine may be accentuated). Products include:
- Aldactazide 2150
- Aldoril Tablets 1418
- Apresazide Capsules 854
- Apresoline-Esidrix Tablets 857
- Capozide 2258
- Dyazide Capsules 2208
- Esidrix Tablets 863
- Esimil Tablets 864
- HydroDIURIL Tablets 1484
- Hydropres Tablets 1485
- Inderide Tablets 2463
- Inderide LA Long Acting Capsules .. 2465
- Lopressor HCT Tablets 1034
- Maxzide 1215
- Moduretic Tablets 1510
- Normozide Tablets 2112
- Oretic Tablets 544
- Oreticyl 545
- Prinzide Tablets 1540
- Ser-Ap-Es Tablets 881
- Serpasil-Esidrix Tablets 886
- Timolide Tablets 1547
- Trandate HCT Tablets 579
- Vaseretic Tablets 1559
- Zestoretic 2274

Hydrocodone Bitartrate (Prolonged and intensified action of CNS depressants). Products include:
- Anexsia 5/500 Tablets 2196
- Anexsia 7.5/650 Tablets 2197
- Azdōne Tablets 844
- Codiclear DH Syrup 845
- Codimal DH Syrup 846
- Damason-P 1356
- Hycodan Syrup, Tablets 927
- Hycomine Compound Tablets 929
- Hycomine Syrup 927
- Hycotuss Expectorant Syrup 930
- Hydrocet Capsules 835
- Lortab ASA Tablets 2414
- Lortab 2412
- Ru-Tuss with Hydrocodone 694
- Triaminic Expectorant DH 1995
- Vicodin Tablets 1187
- Vicodin ES Tablets 1189
- Zydone Capsules 941

Hydrocodone Polistirex (Prolonged and intensified action of CNS depressants). Products include:
- Tussionex Extended-Release Suspension 988

Hydroflumethiazide (Orthostatic hypotension that may occur with chlorpromazine may be accentuated). Products include:
- Diucardin Tablets 2450
- Saluron 718
- Salutensin/Salutensin-Demi 719

Hydroxyurea (Antiemetic action of chlorpromazine may obscure vomiting as a sign of toxicity). Products include:
- Hydrea Capsules 728

Hydroxyzine Hydrochloride (Prolonged and intensified action of CNS depressants). Products include:
- Atarax Tablets & Syrup 1941
- Marax Tablets & DF Syrup 1954
- Vistaril Intramuscular Solution 1970

Isoflurane (Prolonged and intensified action of CNS depressants). Products include:
- Forane 600

Ketamine Hydrochloride (Prolonged and intensified action of CNS depressants). Products include:
Ketalar 1726

Levorphanol Tartrate (Prolonged and intensified action of CNS depressants). Products include:
Levo-Dromoran 1906

Lorazepam (Prolonged and intensified action of CNS depressants). Products include:
Ativan Injection 2432
Ativan Tablets 2434

Loxapine Hydrochloride (Prolonged and intensified action of CNS depressants). Products include:
Loxitane 1213

Loxapine Succinate (Prolonged and intensified action of CNS depressants). Products include:
Loxitane Capsules 1213

Mechlorethamine Hydrochloride (Antiemetic action of chlorpromazine may obscure vomiting as a sign of toxicity). Products include:
Mustargen 1514

Melphalan (Antiemetic action of chlorpromazine may obscure vomiting as a sign of toxicity). Products include:
Alkeran Tablets 754

Meperidine Hydrochloride (Prolonged and intensified action of CNS depressants). Products include:
Demerol 2047
Mepergan Injection 2479

Mephenytoin (Chlorpromazine may lower convulsive threshold; dosage adjustments of anticonvulsants may be necessary). Products include:
Mesantoin Tablets 2013

Mephobarbital (Prolonged and intensified action of CNS depressants). Products include:
Mebaral Tablets 2061

Meprobamate (Prolonged and intensified action of CNS depressants). Products include:
Deprol Tablets 2382
Equagesic Tablets 2451
Miltown Tablets 2386
PMB 200 and PMB 400 2504

Mesoridazine (Prolonged and intensified action of CNS depressants). Products include:
Serentil 686

Methadone Hydrochloride (Prolonged and intensified action of CNS depressants). Products include:
Dolophine Hydrochloride Ampoules & Vials 1260
Dolophine Hydrochloride Tablets 1261
Methadone Hydrochloride Diskets 1284
Methadone Hydrochloride Oral Solution & Tablets 1987

Methohexital Sodium (Prolonged and intensified action of CNS depressants). Products include:
Brevital Sodium Vials 1248

Methoxyflurane (Prolonged and intensified action of CNS depressants).
No products indexed under this heading.

Methsuximide (Chlorpromazine may lower convulsive threshold; dosage adjustments of anticonvulsants may be necessary). Products include:
Celontin 1692

Methyclothiazide (Orthostatic hypotension that may occur with chlorpromazine may be accentuated). Products include:
Enduron Tablets 517
Enduronyl 518

Metrizamide (Chlorpromazine may lower convulsive threshold; avoid concurrent use).

Midazolam Hydrochloride (Prolonged and intensified action of CNS depressants). Products include:
Versed Injection 1924

Molindone Hydrochloride (Prolonged and intensified action of CNS depressants). Products include:
Moban Tablets & Concentrate 932

Morphine Sulfate (Prolonged and intensified action of CNS depressants). Products include:
Astramorph/PF Injection, USP (Preservative-Free) 618
Duramorph 960
Infumorph 200 and Infumorph 500 Sterile Solutions 962
MS Contin Tablets 1814
MSIR 1817
Oramorph SR (Morphine Sulfate Sustained Release Tablets) 1988
Roxanol 1991

Opium Alkaloids (Prolonged and intensified action of CNS depressants). Products include:
B & O No. 15A & No. 16A Supprettes 2395
Pantopon Injectable 1911

Oxazepam (Prolonged and intensified action of CNS depressants). Products include:
Serax Capsules 2522
Serax Tablets 2522

Oxycodone Hydrochloride (Prolonged and intensified action of CNS depressants). Products include:
Percocet Tablets 950
Percodan 951
Roxicodone Tablets, Oral Solution & Intensol (Oxycodone) 1992
Tylox Capsules 1382

Paramethadione (Chlorpromazine may lower convulsive threshold; dosage adjustments of anticonvulsants may be necessary). Products include:
Paradione Capsules 548

Pentobarbital Sodium (Prolonged and intensified action of CNS depressants). Products include:
Nembutal Sodium Capsules 534
Nembutal Sodium Solution 536
Nembutal Sodium Suppositories 538

Perphenazine (Prolonged and intensified action of CNS depressants). Products include:
Etrafon 2087
Triavil Tablets 1556
Trilafon 2123

Phenacemide (Chlorpromazine may lower convulsive threshold; dosage adjustments of anticonvulsants may be necessary). Products include:
Phenurone Tablets 552

Phenobarbital (Chlorpromazine may lower convulsive threshold and does not potentiate anticonvulsant action of barbiturates). Products include:
Arco-Lase Plus Tablets 607
Bellergal-S Tablets 1998
Bronkolixir .... ⊞ 761
Bronkotabs Tablets .... ⊞ 762
Donnatal 1858
Donnatal Extentabs 1859
Donnatal Tablets 1858
Donnazyme Tablets 1860
Kinesed Tablets 2272
Phenobarbital Elixir and Tablets 1293
Primatene Tablets-P Formula 2421
Quadrinal Tablets 1183
Tedral SA 1765

Phensuximide (Chlorpromazine may lower convulsive threshold; dosage adjustments of anticonvulsants may be necessary). Products include:
Milontin Kapseals 1741

Phenytoin (Phenytoin toxicity may be precipitated). Products include:
Dilantin Infatabs 1710
Dilantin-30 Pediatric/Dilantin-125 Suspension 1713

Phenytoin Sodium (Phenytoin toxicity may be precipitated). Products include:
Dilantin Kapseals 1708
Dilantin Parenteral 1712
Dilantin with Phenobarbital Kapseals 1715

Polythiazide (Orthostatic hypotension that may occur with chlorpromazine may be accentuated). Products include:
Minizide Capsules 1779
Renese Tablets 1785
Renese-R Tablets 1786

Prazepam (Prolonged and intensified action of CNS depressants). Products include:
Centrax 1693

Primidone (Chlorpromazine may lower convulsive threshold; dosage adjustments of anticonvulsants may be necessary). Products include:
Mysoline 2480

Prochlorperazine (Prolonged and intensified action of CNS depressants). Products include:
Compazine 2201

Promethazine Hydrochloride (Prolonged and intensified action of CNS depressants). Products include:
Mepergan Injection 2479
Phenergan with Codeine 2497
Phenergan with Dextromethorphan 2499
Phenergan Injection 2493
Phenergan Suppositories 2496
Phenergan Syrup 2495
Phenergan Tablets 2496
Phenergan VC 2500
Phenergan VC with Codeine 2501

Propofol (Prolonged and intensified action of CNS depressants). Products include:
Diprivan Injection 2267

Propoxyphene Hydrochloride (Prolonged and intensified action of CNS depressants). Products include:
Darvon 1256
Wygesic Tablets 2540

Propoxyphene Napsylate (Prolonged and intensified action of CNS depressants). Products include:
Darvon-N/Darvocet-N 1254

Propranolol Hydrochloride (Concomitant administration results in increased plasma levels of both drugs). Products include:
Inderal 2459
Inderal LA Long Acting Capsules 2461
Inderide Tablets 2463
Inderide LA Long Acting Capsules 2465

Secobarbital Sodium (Prolonged and intensified action of CNS depressants). Products include:
Seconal Sodium Pulvules 1296

Sufentanil Citrate (Prolonged and intensified action of CNS depressants). Products include:
Sufenta Injection 1147

Temazepam (Prolonged and intensified action of CNS depressants). Products include:
Restoril Capsules 2023

Thiamylal Sodium (Prolonged and intensified action of CNS depressants). Products include:
Surital Ampoules, Steri-Vials 1764

Thioridazine Hydrochloride (Prolonged and intensified action of CNS depressants). Products include:
Mellaril 2011

Thiothixene (Prolonged and intensified action of CNS depressants). Products include:
Navane Capsules and Concentrate 1954
Navane Intramuscular 1956

Triazolam (Prolonged and intensified action of CNS depressants). Products include:
Halcion Tablets 2340

Trifluoperazine Hydrochloride (Prolonged and intensified action of CNS depressants). Products include:
Stelazine 2226

Trimethadione (Chlorpromazine may lower convulsive threshold; dosage adjustments of anticonvulsants may be necessary). Products include:
Tridione 557

Valproic Acid (Chlorpromazine may lower convulsive threshold; dosage adjustments of anticonvulsants may be necessary). Products include:
Depakene Capsules & Syrup 511

Warfarin Sodium (Effect of oral anticoagulants diminished). Products include:
Coumadin Injection & Tablets 944
Panwarfin Tablets 547

THORAZINE MULTIPLE-DOSE VIALS
(Chlorpromazine) 2234
See **Thorazine Concentrate**

THORAZINE SPANSULE CAPSULES
(Chlorpromazine) 2234
See **Thorazine Concentrate**

THORAZINE SUPPOSITORIES
(Chlorpromazine) 2234
See **Thorazine Concentrate**

THORAZINE SYRUP
(Chlorpromazine) 2234
See **Thorazine Concentrate**

THORAZINE TABLETS
(Chlorpromazine) 2234
See **Thorazine Concentrate**

THROMBOGEN TOPICAL THROMBIN, USP
(Thrombin) 1153
No interactions described in labeling.

THROMBOGEN TOPICAL THROMBIN, USP, SPRAY KIT
(Thrombin) 1153
No interactions described in labeling.

THROMBOGEN TOPICAL THROMBIN, USP, TRANSFER NEEDLE
(Thrombin) 1153
No interactions described in labeling.

THROMBOSTAT
(Thrombin) 1765
No interactions described in labeling.

TICAR FOR INJECTION
(Ticarcillin Disodium) 2236
May interact with:

Probenecid (Concurrent administration prolongs serum levels of ticarcillin). Products include:
Benemid Tablets 1426
ColBENEMID Tablets 1436
Wycillin Injection and Probenecid Tablets 2539

TICE BCG VACCINE, USP
(BCG Vaccine) 1632
May interact with immunosuppressive agents and certain other agents.

Compounds in these categories include:

Azathioprine (May interfere with development of immune response). Products include:
- Imuran 768

Cyclosporine (May interfere with development of immune response). Products include:
- Sandimmune 2024

Immune Globulin (Human) (May interfere with development of immune response). Products include:
- MICRhoGAM Rh_0(D) Immune Globulin (Human) 1650
- RhoGAM Rh_0(D) Immune Globulin (Human) 1651

Immune Globulin Intravenous (Human) (May interfere with development of immune response). Products include:
- Gamimune N Immune Globulin Intravenous (Human) 1572
- Gammagard Immune Globulin, Intravenous (Human) 658
- Iveegam 1129
- Sandoglobulin I.V. 2027

Muromonab-CD3 (May interfere with development of immune response). Products include:
- Orthoclone OKT3 Sterile Solution .. 1645

TIGAN CAPSULES
(Trimethobenzamide Hydrochloride) 2239
May interact with phenothiazines, barbiturates, belladona products, and certain other agents. Compounds in these categories include:

Alcohol (May result in an adverse drug interaction).

Aprobarbital (Exercise caution in recent recipients of barbiturates). Products include:
- Alurate Elixir 1883

Atropine Sulfate (Exercise caution in recent recipients of belladonna derivatives). Products include:
- Arco-Lase Plus Tablets 607
- Atropine Sulfate Sterile Ophthalmic Solution and S.O.P. Sterile Ophthalmic Ointment .... ⊙ 239
- Donnagel .... ▣ 675
- Donnagel-PG 1858
- Donnatal 1858
- Donnatal Extentabs 1859
- Donnatal Tablets 1858
- Donnazyme Tablets 1860
- Isopto Atropine .... ⊙ 218
- Lomotil 2174
- Motofen Tablets 836
- Ru-Tuss Tablets 693
- Urised Tablets 2396

Belladonna Alkaloids (Exercise caution in recent recipients of belladonna derivatives). Products include:
- Bellergal-S Tablets 1998
- Hyland's Bed Wetting Tablets .... ▣ 728
- Hyland's Teething Tablets .... ▣ 728
- Kinesed Tablets 2272

Butabarbital (Exercise caution in recent recipients of barbiturates). Products include:
- Pyridium Plus 1764

Butalbital (Exercise caution in recent recipients of barbiturates). Products include:
- Esgic-Plus Tablets 1002
- Esgic Tablets & Capsules 1001
- Fioricet Tablets 2006
- Fiorinal Capsules 2007
- Fiorinal with Codeine Capsules 2008
- Fiorinal Tablets 2007
- Phrenilin 838
- Sedapap Tablets 50 mg/650 mg .. 1360

Chlorpromazine (Exercise caution in recent recipients of phenothiazines). Products include:
- Thorazine 2234

Fluphenazine Decanoate (Exercise caution in recent recipients of phenothiazines). Products include:
- Prolixin Decanoate 1795

Fluphenazine Enanthate (Exercise caution in recent recipients of phenothiazines). Products include:
- Prolixin Enanthate 1796

Fluphenazine Hydrochloride (Exercise caution in recent recipients of phenothiazines). Products include:
- Prolixin Elixir 1793
- Prolixin Injection 1791
- Prolixin Oral Concentrate 1792
- Prolixin Tablets 1793

Hyoscyamine (Exercise caution in recent recipients of belladonna derivatives). Products include:
- Cystospaz Tablets 2395
- Urised Tablets 2396

Hyoscyamine Sulfate (Exercise caution in recent recipients of belladonna derivatives). Products include:
- Arco-Lase Plus Tablets 607
- Cystospaz-M Capsules 2395
- Donnagel .... ▣ 675
- Donnagel-PG 1858
- Donnatal 1858
- Donnatal Extentabs 1859
- Donnatal Tablets 1858
- Donnazyme Tablets 1860
- Kutrase Capsules 2146
- Levsin/Levsinex 2147
- Ru-Tuss Tablets 693

Mephobarbital (Exercise caution in recent recipients of barbiturates). Products include:
- Mebaral Tablets 2061

Mesoridazine (Exercise caution in recent recipients of phenothiazines). Products include:
- Serentil 686

Pentobarbital Sodium (Exercise caution in recent recipients of barbiturates). Products include:
- Nembutal Sodium Capsules 534
- Nembutal Sodium Solution 536
- Nembutal Sodium Suppositories 538

Perphenazine (Exercise caution in recent recipients of phenothiazines). Products include:
- Etrafon 2087
- Triavil Tablets 1556
- Trilafon 2123

Phenobarbital (Exercise caution in recent recipients of barbiturates). Products include:
- Arco-Lase Plus Tablets 607
- Bellergal-S Tablets 1998
- Bronkolixir .... ▣ 761
- Bronkotabs Tablets .... ▣ 762
- Donnatal 1858
- Donnatal Extentabs 1859
- Donnatal Tablets 1858
- Donnazyme Tablets 1860
- Kinesed Tablets 2272
- Phenobarbital Elixir and Tablets 1293
- Primatene Tablets-P Formula 2421
- Quadrinal Tablets 1183
- Tedral SA 1765

Prochlorperazine (Exercise caution in recent recipients of phenothiazines). Products include:
- Compazine 2201

Promethazine Hydrochloride (Exercise caution in recent recipients of phenothiazines). Products include:
- Mepergan Injection 2479
- Phenergan with Codeine 2497
- Phenergan with Dextromethorphan 2499
- Phenergan Injection 2493
- Phenergan Suppositories 2496
- Phenergan Syrup 2495
- Phenergan Tablets 2496
- Phenergan VC 2500
- Phenergan VC with Codeine 2501

Scopolamine Hydrobromide (Exercise caution in recent recipients of belladonna derivatives). Products include:
- Donnagel .... ▣ 675
- Donnagel-PG 1858
- Donnatal 1858
- Donnatal Extentabs 1859
- Donnatal Tablets 1858
- Donnazyme Tablets 1860
- Isopto Hyoscine .... ⊙ 222
- Murocoll-2 Sterile Ophthalmic Solution .... ⊙ 261
- Ru-Tuss Tablets 693

Scopolamine Preparations (Exercise caution in recent recipients of belladonna derivatives). Products include:
- Transderm Scōp Transdermal Therapeutic System 887

Secobarbital Sodium (Exercise caution in recent recipients of barbiturates). Products include:
- Seconal Sodium Pulvules 1296

Thiamylal Sodium (Exercise caution in recent recipients of barbiturates). Products include:
- Surital Ampoules, Steri-Vials 1764

Thioridazine Hydrochloride (Exercise caution in recent recipients of phenothiazines). Products include:
- Mellaril 2011

Trifluoperazine Hydrochloride (Exercise caution in recent recipients of phenothiazines). Products include:
- Stelazine 2226

TIGAN INJECTABLE
(Trimethobenzamide Hydrochloride) 2239
See **Tigan Capsules**

TIGAN SUPPOSITORIES
(Trimethobenzamide Hydrochloride) 2239
See **Tigan Capsules**

TIMENTIN FOR INJECTION
(Ticarcillin Disodium, Clavulanate Potassium) 2239
May interact with:

Probenecid (Increases serum concentration and prolongs half-life of ticarcillin). Products include:
- Benemid Tablets 1426
- ColBENEMID Tablets 1436
- Wycillin Injection and Probenecid Tablets 2539

TIMOLIDE TABLETS
(Timolol Maleate, Hydrochlorothiazide) 1547
May interact with insulin, corticosteroids, antihypertensives, catecholamine depleting drugs, non-steroidal anti-inflammatory agents, lithium preparations, cardiac glycosides, and certain other agents. Compounds in these categories include:

Acebutolol Hydrochloride (Potentiated). Products include:
- Sectral Capsules 2520

ACTH (Hypokalemia).
- No products indexed under this heading.

Atenolol (Potentiated). Products include:
- Tenoretic Tablets 1105
- Tenormin Tablets and I.V. Injection 1107

Benazepril Hydrochloride (Potentiated). Products include:
- Lotensin Tablets 872

Bendroflumethiazide (Potentiated). Products include:
- Corzide Tablets 702
- Naturetin Tablets 1789
- Rauzide Tablets 1804

Betamethasone Acetate (Hypokalemia). Products include:
- Celestone Soluspan Suspension 2081

Betamethasone Sodium Phosphate (Hypokalemia). Products include:
- Celestone Soluspan Suspension 2081

Betaxolol Hydrochloride (Potentiated). Products include:
- Betoptic Sterile Ophthalmic Solution 569
- Betoptic S Sterile Ophthalmic Suspension 570
- Kerlone Tablets 2172

Captopril (Potentiated). Products include:
- Capoten 2255
- Capozide 2258

Carteolol Hydrochloride (Potentiated). Products include:
- Cartrol Tablets 507

Chlorothiazide (Potentiated). Products include:
- Aldoclor Tablets 1413
- Diupres Tablets 1461
- Diuril Oral 1464

Chlorothiazide Sodium (Potentiated). Products include:
- Diuril Sodium Intravenous 1463

Chlorthalidone (Potentiated). Products include:
- Combipres Tablets 678
- Tenoretic Tablets 1105
- Thalitone Tablets 687

Clonidine (Potentiated). Products include:
- Catapres-TTS 677

Clonidine Hydrochloride (Potentiated). Products include:
- Catapres Tablets 676
- Combipres Tablets 678

Cortisone Acetate (Hypokalemia). Products include:
- Cortone Acetate Sterile Suspension 1437
- Cortone Acetate Tablets 1439

Deslanoside (Hypokalemia can lead to increased cardiac toxicity of digitalis).
- No products indexed under this heading.

Dexamethasone (Hypokalemia). Products include:
- AK-Trol Ointment & Suspension .... ⊙ 207
- Decadron Elixir 1445
- Decadron Tablets 1447
- Decaspray Topical Aerosol 1459
- Dexacidin .... ⊙ 272
- Maxidex Sterile Ophthalmic Suspension .... ⊙ 223
- Maxitrol Ophthalmic Ointment/Suspension .... ⊙ 223
- TobraDex Ophthalmic Suspension and Ointment .... ⊙ 228

Dexamethasone Acetate (Hypokalemia). Products include:
- Dalalone D.P. Injectable 999
- Decadron-LA Sterile Suspension 1457

Dexamethasone Sodium Phosphate (Hypokalemia). Products include:
- AK-Dex .... ⊙ 203
- Decadron Phosphate Respihaler 1454
- Decadron Phosphate Sterile Ophthalmic Ointment 1453
- Decadron Phosphate Sterile Ophthalmic Solution 1453
- Decadron Phosphate Topical Cream 1455
- Decadron Phosphate Turbinaire 1456
- Maxidex Sterile Ophthalmic Ointment .... ⊙ 222
- NeoDecadron Sterile Ophthalmic Ointment 1517
- NeoDecadron Sterile Ophthalmic Solution 1518
- NeoDecadron Topical Cream 1518

Diazoxide (Potentiated). Products include:
- Hyperstat I.V. Injection 2095
- Proglycem 649

Diclofenac Sodium (Reduced diuretic, natriuretic, and antihypertensive effects of Timolide). Products include:
- Voltaren Ophthalmic Sterile Ophthalmic Solution .... ⊙ 268
- Voltaren Tablets 1042

Digitoxin (Hypokalemia can lead to increased cardiac toxicity of digitalis). Products include:
Crystodigin Tablets 1253

Digoxin (Hypokalemia can lead to increased cardiac toxicity of digitalis). Products include:
Lanoxicaps 772
Lanoxin Elixir Pediatric 775
Lanoxin Injection 778
Lanoxin Injection Pediatric 781
Lanoxin Tablets 783

Diltiazem Hydrochloride (Left ventricular failure and AV conduction disturbances). Products include:
Cardizem Tablets-30 mg, 60 mg, 90 mg and 120 mg 1329
Cardizem SR Capsules-60 mg, 90 mg and 120 mg 1327

Doxazosin Mesylate (Potentiated). Products include:
Cardura Tablets 1941

Enalapril Maleate (Potentiated). Products include:
Vaseretic Tablets 1559
Vasotec Tablets 1564

Enalaprilat (Potentiated). Products include:
Vasotec I.V. 1562

Esmolol Hydrochloride (Potentiated). Products include:
Brevibloc Injection 942

Etodolac (Reduced diuretic, natriuretic, and antihypertensive effects of Timolide). Products include:
Lodine Capsules 2468

Felodipine (Potentiated). Products include:
Plendil Extended-Release Tablets 1526

Fenoprofen Calcium (Reduced diuretic, natriuretic, and antihypertensive effects of Timolide). Products include:
Nalfon Pulvules & Tablets 919

Flurbiprofen (Reduced diuretic, natriuretic, and antihypertensive effects of Timolide). Products include:
Ansaid Tablets 2319

Fosinopril Sodium (Potentiated). Products include:
Monopril Tablets 1406

Furosemide (Potentiated). Products include:
Lasix 1093

Guanabenz Acetate (Potentiated). Products include:
Wytensin Tablets 2542

Guanethidine Monosulfate (Potentiated). Products include:
Esimil Tablets 864
Ismelin Tablets 869

Hydralazine Hydrochloride (Potentiated). Products include:
Apresazide Capsules 854
Apresoline Hydrochloride Parenteral (Ampuls) 856
Apresoline Hydrochloride Tablets 855
Apresoline-Esidrix Tablets 857
Ser-Ap-Es Tablets 881
Serpasil-Apresoline Tablets 884

Hydrocortisone (Hypokalemia). Products include:
AK-Spore H.C. ◉ 206
Bactine Hydrocortisone Anti-Itch Cream ◼ 625
CaldeCORT Anti-Itch Hydrocortisone Spray ◼ 560
Carmol HC Cream 1% 2296
Cortaid Spray ◼ 735
Cortenema 2244
Cortisporin Ointment 758
Cortisporin Ophthalmic Ointment Sterile 758
Cortisporin Ophthalmic Suspension Sterile 759
Cortisporin Otic Solution Sterile 760
Cortisporin Otic Suspension Sterile 760
Cortizone-5 Creme & Ointment ◼ 732
Dermolate Anti-Itch Cream ◼ 697
Eldecort Cream 1.0% 1113
Eldecort Cream 1.0% and 2.5% 1113
Fungoid HC Creme 1770
Hydrocortone Tablets 1482
Hytone 909
LazerSporin-C Solution 1770
Massengill Medicated Soft Cloth Towelettes 2192
Nutracort Cream & Lotion 1684
PediOtic Suspension Sterile 797
Synacort Creams 1%, 2.5% 2296
Vanoxide-HC Acne Lotion 911
Vioform-Hydrocortisone Cream and Mild Cream 889
Vioform-Hydrocortisone Ointment 889
VōSoL HC Otic Solution 2392
Vytone Cream 1% 911

Hydrocortisone Acetate (Hypokalemia). Products include:
Analpram-HC Rectal Cream 1% and 2.5% 970
Anusol-HC Cream 1690
Anusol-HC Suppositories 1691
Caldecort ◼ 560
Carmol HC Cream 1% 2296
Chloromycetin Hydrocortisone Ophthalmic 1694
Coly-Mycin S Otic w/Neomycin & Hydrocortisone 1708
Cortaid ◼ 735
Cortef Feminine Itch Cream ◼ 735
Corticaine ◼ 682
Cortifoam 1827
Cortisporin Cream 757
Epifoam 1828
Gynecort 5 Creme ◼ 556
Hydrocortone Acetate Sterile Suspension 1479
Lanacort 5 Creme and Ointment ◼ 557
Mantadil Cream 789
Ophthocort ◉ 301
Orabase HCA Oral Paste 890
Pramosone Cream, Lotion & Ointment 971
ProctoCream-HC 1834
Proctofoam-HC 1835

Hydrocortisone Sodium Phosphate (Hypokalemia). Products include:
Hydrocortone Phosphate Injection, Sterile 1481

Hydrocortisone Sodium Succinate (Hypokalemia). Products include:
Solu-Cortef Sterile Powder 2361

Hydroflumethiazide (Potentiated). Products include:
Diucardin Tablets 2450
Saluron 718
Salutensin/Salutensin-Demi 719

Ibuprofen (Reduced diuretic, natriuretic, and antihypertensive effects of Timolide). Products include:
Advil Cold & Sinus Caplets (formerly CoAdvil) 2416
Advil Ibuprofen Tablets and Caplets 2416
Children's Advil Suspension 2426
CoAdvil ◼ 748
Dristan Sinus Caplets 2419
Haltran Tablets ◼ 668
Ibuprofen ◼ 631
Medipren ibuprofen Caplets and Tablets 1362
Midol 200 Cramp Relief Formula ◼ 570
Motrin Tablets 2351
Motrin IB Caplets and Tablets ◼ 736
Nuprin Ibuprofen/Analgesic Tablets & Caplets 752
PediaProfen Suspension 1363
Rufen Tablets 691
Trendar Ibuprofen Tablets ◼ 756

Indapamide (Potentiated). Products include:
Lozol Tablets 1843

Indomethacin (Reduced diuretic, natriuretic, and antihypertensive effects of Timolide). Products include:
Indocin 1487

Indomethacin Sodium Trihydrate (Reduced diuretic, natriuretic, and antihypertensive effects of Timolide). Products include:
Indocin I.V. 1490

Insulin, Human (Insulin requirements may be altered).
No products indexed under this heading.

Insulin, Human Isophane Suspension (Insulin requirements may be altered). Products include:
Humulin N, 100 Units 1270

Insulin, Human NPH (Insulin requirements may be altered). Products include:
Insulatard NPH Human 1627
Novolin N 1627
Novolin N PenFill Cartridges 1628
Novolin N Prefilled 1628

Insulin, Human Regular (Insulin requirements may be altered). Products include:
Humulin BR, 100 Units 1268
Humulin R, 100 Units 1272
Novolin R 1627
Novolin R PenFill Cartridges 1628
Novolin R Prefilled 1629
Velosulin Human 1628

Insulin, Human, Zinc Suspension (Insulin requirements may be altered). Products include:
Humulin L, 100 Units 1268
Humulin U, 100 Units 1272
Novolin L 1627

Insulin, NPH (Insulin requirements may be altered). Products include:
NPH, 40 & 100 Units 1273
Beef NPH, 100 Units 1274
Pork NPH, 100 Units 1275
Insulatard NPH 1626
NPH Insulin 1626
NPH Purified Pork Isophane Insulin 1626

Insulin, Regular (Insulin requirements may be altered). Products include:
Regular, 40 & 100 Units 1273
Beef Regular, 100 Units 1275
Pork Regular, 100 Units 1275
Pork Regular (Concentrated), 500 Units 1276
Regular Insulin 1625
Regular Purified Pork Insulin 1626
Velosulin 1627

Insulin, Zinc Crystals (Insulin requirements may be altered). Products include:
NPH, 40 & 100 Units 1273

Insulin, Zinc Suspension (Insulin requirements may be altered). Products include:
Lente, 40 & 100 Units 1272
Protamine, Zinc, 40 & 100 Units 1273
Lente Iletin I 1272
Beef Lente, 100 Units 1274
Beef Protamine Zinc, 100 Units 1274
Pork Lente, 100 Units 1275
Pork, Protamine, Zinc, 100 Units 1275
Lente Insulin 1626
Lente Purified Pork Insulin 1626
Semilente Insulin 1625
Ultralente Insulin 1626

Isradipine (Potentiated). Products include:
DynaCirc Capsules 2004

Ketoprofen (Reduced diuretic, natriuretic, and antihypertensive effects of Timolide). Products include:
Orudis Capsules 2488

Ketorolac Tromethamine (Reduced diuretic, natriuretic, and antihypertensive effects of Timolide). Products include:
Toradol IM Injection 2302

Labetalol Hydrochloride (Potentiated). Products include:
Normodyne Injection 2108
Normodyne Tablets 2110
Normozide Tablets 2112
Trandate HCT Tablets 579
Trandate Injection 577
Trandate Tablets 579

Lisinopril (Potentiated). Products include:
Prinivil Tablets 1538
Prinzide Tablets 1540
Zestoretic 2274
Zestril Tablets 2277

Lithium Carbonate (High risk of lithium toxicity). Products include:
Eskalith 2214
Lithane Tablets 1596
Lithium Carbonate Capsules & Tablets 1984
Lithobid Tablets 870

Lithium Citrate (High risk of lithium toxicity). Products include:
Cibalith-S 870

Mecamylamine Hydrochloride (Potentiated). Products include:
Inversine Tablets 1492

Meclofenamate Sodium (Reduced diuretic, natriuretic, and antihypertensive effects of Timolide). Products include:
Meclomen Capsules 1739

Mefenamic Acid (Reduced diuretic, natriuretic, and antihypertensive effects of Timolide). Products include:
Ponstel 1758

Methyclothiazide (Potentiated). Products include:
Enduron Tablets 517
Enduronyl 518

Methyldopa (Potentiated). Products include:
Aldoclor Tablets 1413
Aldomet Oral 1415
Aldoril Tablets 1418

Methyldopate Hydrochloride (Potentiated). Products include:
Aldomet Ester HCl Injection 1417

Methylprednisolone (Hypokalemia). Products include:
Medrol 2348

Methylprednisolone Acetate (Hypokalemia). Products include:
Depo-Medrol Sterile Aqueous Suspension 2334

Methylprednisolone Sodium Succinate (Hypokalemia). Products include:
Solu-Medrol Sterile Powder 2363

Metolazone (Potentiated). Products include:
Diulo 2129
Mykrox ½ mg Tablets 984
Zaroxolyn Tablets 989

Metoprolol Tartrate (Potentiated). Products include:
Lopressor Ampuls 1032
Lopressor HCT Tablets 1034
Lopressor Tablets 1032

Metyrosine (Potentiated). Products include:
Demser Capsules 1460

Minoxidil (Potentiated). Products include:
Loniten Tablets 2346
Rogaine Topical Solution 2357

Nadolol (Potentiated). Products include:
Corgard Tablets 701
Corzide Tablets 702

Naproxen (Reduced diuretic, natriuretic, and antihypertensive effects of Timolide). Products include:
Naprosyn 2297

Naproxen Sodium (Reduced diuretic, natriuretic, and antihypertensive effects of Timolide). Products include:
Anaprox and Anaprox DS Tablets 2288

Nicardipine Hydrochloride (Potentiated). Products include:
Cardene Capsules 2290

Nifedipine (Hypotension). Products include:
Adalat Capsules (10 mg and 20 mg) 1587
Procardia Capsules 1781
Procardia XL Tablets 1783

Nitroglycerin (Potentiated). Products include:
- Deponit NTG Transdermal Delivery System ... 2143
- Minitran Transdermal Delivery System ... 1312
- Nitro-Bid Ointment ... 1339
- Nitro-Bid Capsules ... 1338
- Nitrodisc ... 2176
- Nitro-Dur (nitroglycerin) Transdermal Infusion System ... 1164
- Nitrogard Tablets ... 1004
- Nitrolingual Spray ... 1846
- Nitrostat Tablets ... 1743
- Transderm-Nitro Transdermal Therapeutic System ... 2283

Norepinephrine Bitartrate (Decreased arterial responsiveness to norepinephrine). Products include:
- Levophed Bitartrate Injection ... 2054

Penbutolol Sulfate (Potentiated). Products include:
- Levatol ... 1832

Phenoxybenzamine Hydrochloride (Potentiated). Products include:
- Dibenzyline Capsules ... 2207

Phentolamine Mesylate (Potentiated). Products include:
- Regitine ... 878

Phenylbutazone (Reduced diuretic, natriuretic, and antihypertensive effects of Timolide). Products include:
- Butazolidin Capsules & Tablets ... 1027

Pindolol (Potentiated). Products include:
- Visken Tablets ... 2036

Piroxicam (Reduced diuretic, natriuretic, and antihypertensive effects of Timolide). Products include:
- Feldene Capsules ... 1777

Polythiazide (Potentiated). Products include:
- Minizide Capsules ... 1779
- Renese Tablets ... 1785
- Renese-R Tablets ... 1786

Prazosin Hydrochloride (Potentiated). Products include:
- Minipress Capsules ... 1778
- Minizide Capsules ... 1779

Prednisolone Acetate (Hypokalemia). Products include:
- AK-Cide Sterile Ophthalmic Ointment & Suspension ... ◉ 202
- Blephamide Liquifilm Sterile Ophthalmic Suspension ... 586
- Blephamide S.O.P. Sterile Ophthalmic Ointment ... 586
- Cetapred Ointment ... ◉ 220
- ⅛% Econopred & 1% Econopred Plus ... ◉ 217
- Isopto Cetapred Suspension ... ◉ 220
- Metimyd ... ◉ 306
- Poly-Pred Liquifilm ... ◉ 250
- Pred Forte ... ◉ 252
- Pred Mild ... ◉ 254
- Pred-G Liquifilm Sterile Ophthalmic Suspension ... ◉ 252
- Pred-G S.O.P. Sterile Ophthalmic Ointment ... ◉ 253
- Vasocidin Ointment ... ◉ 275

Prednisolone Sodium Phosphate (Hypokalemia). Products include:
- AK-Pred ... ◉ 205
- Hydeltrasol Injection, Sterile ... 1476
- Inflamase ... ◉ 274
- Pediapred Oral Liquid ... 987
- Vasocidin Ophthalmic Solution ... ◉ 276

Prednisolone Tebutate (Hypokalemia). Products include:
- Hydeltra-T.B.A. Sterile Suspension 1478

Prednisone (Hypokalemia). Products include:
- Deltasone Tablets ... 2332

Propranolol Hydrochloride (Potentiated). Products include:
- Inderal ... 2459
- Inderal LA Long Acting Capsules ... 2461
- Inderide Tablets ... 2463
- Inderide LA Long Acting Capsules .. 2465

Ramipril (Potentiated). Products include:
- Altace Capsules ... 1086

Rauwolfia Serpentina (Potentiated; hypotension; marked bradycardia). Products include:
- Raudixin Tablets ... 1803
- Rauzide Tablets ... 1804

Rescinnamine (Potentiated; hypotension; marked bradycardia).
- No products indexed under this heading.

Reserpine (Potentiated; hypotension; marked bradycardia). Products include:
- Diupres Tablets ... 1461
- Hydromox R Tablets ... 1209
- Hydropres Tablets ... 1485
- Renese-R Tablets ... 1786
- Salutensin/Salutensin-Demi ... 719
- Ser-Ap-Es Tablets ... 881
- Serpasil Tablets ... 883
- Serpasil-Apresoline Tablets ... 884
- Serpasil-Esidrix Tablets ... 886

Sodium Nitroprusside (Potentiated). Products include:
- Nipride I.V. Infusion ... 1909

Sulindac (Reduced diuretic, natriuretic, and antihypertensive effects of Timolide). Products include:
- Clinoril Tablets ... 1433

Terazosin Hydrochloride (Potentiation of other antihypertensives). Products include:
- Hytrin Tablets ... 529

Tolmetin Sodium (Reduced diuretic, natriuretic, and antihypertensive effects of Timolide). Products include:
- Tolectin (200, 400 and 600 mg) .. 1379

Triamcinolone (Hypokalemia).
- No products indexed under this heading.

Triamcinolone Acetonide (Hypokalemia). Products include:
- Aristocort A ... 1010
- Azmacort Inhaler ... 1837
- Kenalog Cream, Lotion & Ointment 2401
- Kenalog-10 Injection ... 2402
- Kenalog-40 Injection ... 2403
- Kenalog in Orabase ... 604
- Kenalog Spray ... 2401
- Mycolog II Cream and Ointment ... 2407
- Mytrex Cream & Ointment ... 2080
- Nasacort Nasal Inhaler ... 1844

Triamcinolone Diacetate (Hypokalemia). Products include:
- Aristocort Suspension ... 1008

Triamcinolone Hexacetonide (Hypokalemia). Products include:
- Aristospan Suspension ... 1011

Trimethaphan Camsylate (Potentiated). Products include:
- Arfonad Ampuls ... 1887

Tubocurarine Chloride (Increased responsiveness to tubocurarine).
- No products indexed under this heading.

Verapamil Hydrochloride (Left ventricular failure and AV conduction disturbances). Products include:
- Calan SR Caplets ... 2157
- Calan Tablets ... 2155
- Isoptin Injectable ... 1177
- Isoptin Oral Tablets ... 1179
- Isoptin SR Sustained Release Tablets ... 1181
- Verelan Capsules ... 1243
- Verelan Capsules ... 2535

TIMOPTIC IN OCUDOSE
(Timolol Maleate) ... 1552
May interact with general anesthetics, beta blockers, catecholamine depleting drugs, calcium channel blockers, cardiac glycosides, and certain other agents. Compounds in these categories include:

Acebutolol Hydrochloride (Additive effect). Products include:
- Sectral Capsules ... 2520

Atenolol (Additive effect). Products include:
- Tenoretic Tablets ... 1105
- Tenormin Tablets and I.V. Injection 1107

Bepridil Hydrochloride (Atrioventricular conduction disturbances; left ventricular failure; hypotension). Products include:
- Vascor (200, 300 and 400 mg) Tablets ... 1383

Betaxolol Hydrochloride (Additive effect). Products include:
- Betoptic Sterile Ophthalmic Solution ... 569
- Betoptic S Sterile Ophthalmic Suspension ... 570
- Kerlone Tablets ... 2172

Carteolol Hydrochloride (Additive effect). Products include:
- Cartrol Tablets ... 507

Deslanoside (Prolonged AV conduction time).
- No products indexed under this heading.

Digitoxin (Prolonged AV conduction time). Products include:
- Crystodigin Tablets ... 1253

Digoxin (Prolonged AV conduction time). Products include:
- Lanoxicaps ... 772
- Lanoxin Elixir Pediatric ... 775
- Lanoxin Injection ... 778
- Lanoxin Injection Pediatric ... 781
- Lanoxin Tablets ... 783

Diltiazem Hydrochloride (Atrioventricular conduction disturbances; left ventricular failure; hypotension). Products include:
- Cardizem Tablets-30 mg, 60 mg, 90 mg and 120 mg ... 1329
- Cardizem SR Capsules-60 mg, 90 mg and 120 mg ... 1327

Enflurane (Protracted severe hypotension). Products include:
- Ethrane ... 599

Epinephrine (Mydriasis). Products include:
- Ana-Kit Anaphylaxis Emergency Treatment Kit ... 1100
- Bronkaid Mist ... ▣ 757
- EpiPen ... 843
- Marcaine Hydrochloride 0.5% with Epinephrine 1:200,000 (as bitartrate) ... 958
- Marcaine Hydrochloride with Epinephrine 1:200,000 ... 2055
- Primatene Mist ... 2420
- Sus-Phrine Injection ... 1006
- Xylocaine with Epinephrine Injections ... 637

Esmolol Hydrochloride (Additive effect). Products include:
- Brevibloc Injection ... 942

Felodipine (Atrioventricular conduction disturbances; left ventricular failure; hypotension). Products include:
- Plendil Extended-Release Tablets ... 1526

Isoflurane (Protracted severe hypotension). Products include:
- Forane ... 600

Isradipine (Atrioventricular conduction disturbances; left ventricular failure; hypotension). Products include:
- DynaCirc Capsules ... 2004

Labetalol Hydrochloride (Additive effect). Products include:
- Normodyne Injection ... 2108
- Normodyne Tablets ... 2110
- Normozide Tablets ... 2112
- Trandate HCT Tablets ... 579
- Trandate Injection ... 577
- Trandate Tablets ... 579

Methohexital Sodium (Protracted severe hypotension). Products include:
- Brevital Sodium Vials ... 1248

Methoxyflurane (Protracted severe hypotension).
- No products indexed under this heading.

Metoprolol Tartrate (Additive effect). Products include:
- Lopressor Ampuls ... 1032
- Lopressor HCT Tablets ... 1034
- Lopressor Tablets ... 1032

Nadolol (Additive effect). Products include:
- Corgard Tablets ... 701
- Corzide Tablets ... 702

Nicardipine Hydrochloride (Atrioventricular conduction disturbances; left ventricular failure; hypotension). Products include:
- Cardene Capsules ... 2290

Nifedipine (Atrioventricular conduction disturbances; left ventricular failure; hypotension). Products include:
- Adalat Capsules (10 mg and 20 mg) ... 1587
- Procardia Capsules ... 1781
- Procardia XL Tablets ... 1783

Nimodipine (Atrioventricular conduction disturbances; left ventricular failure; hypotension). Products include:
- Nimotop Capsules ... 1607

Penbutolol Sulfate (Additive effect). Products include:
- Levatol ... 1832

Pindolol (Additive effect). Products include:
- Visken Tablets ... 2036

Propofol (Protracted severe hypotension). Products include:
- Diprivan Injection ... 2267

Propranolol Hydrochloride (Additive effect). Products include:
- Inderal ... 2459
- Inderal LA Long Acting Capsules ... 2461
- Inderide Tablets ... 2463
- Inderide LA Long Acting Capsules .. 2465

Rauwolfia Serpentina (Hypotension; marked bradycardia). Products include:
- Raudixin Tablets ... 1803
- Rauzide Tablets ... 1804

Rescinnamine (Hypotension; marked bradycardia).
- No products indexed under this heading.

Reserpine (Hypotension; marked bradycardia). Products include:
- Diupres Tablets ... 1461
- Hydromox R Tablets ... 1209
- Hydropres Tablets ... 1485
- Renese-R Tablets ... 1786
- Salutensin/Salutensin-Demi ... 719
- Ser-Ap-Es Tablets ... 881
- Serpasil Tablets ... 883
- Serpasil-Apresoline Tablets ... 884
- Serpasil-Esidrix Tablets ... 886

Verapamil Hydrochloride (Atrioventricular conduction disturbances; left ventricular failure; hypotension). Products include:
- Calan SR Caplets ... 2157
- Calan Tablets ... 2155
- Isoptin Injectable ... 1177
- Isoptin Oral Tablets ... 1179
- Isoptin SR Sustained Release Tablets ... 1181
- Verelan Capsules ... 1243
- Verelan Capsules ... 2535

TIMOPTIC STERILE OPHTHALMIC SOLUTION
(Timolol Maleate) ... 1550
May interact with general anesthetics, beta blockers, catecholamine depleting drugs, calcium channel blockers, cardiac glycosides, and

certain other agents. Compounds in these categories include:

Acebutolol Hydrochloride (Potential for additive effects). Products include:
Sectral Capsules 2520

Atenolol (Potential for additive effects). Products include:
Tenoretic Tablets 1105
Tenormin Tablets and I.V. Injection 1107

Bepridil Hydrochloride (Possible atrioventricular conduction disturbances; left ventricular failure; hypotension). Products include:
Vascor (200, 300 and 400 mg) Tablets 1383

Betaxolol Hydrochloride (Potential for additive effects). Products include:
Betoptic Sterile Ophthalmic Solution 569
Betoptic S Sterile Ophthalmic Suspension 570
Kerlone Tablets 2172

Carteolol Hydrochloride (Potential for additive effects). Products include:
Cartrol Tablets 507

Deslanoside (Prolonged AV conduction time).
No products indexed under this heading.

Digitoxin (Prolonged AV conduction time). Products include:
Crystodigin Tablets 1253

Digoxin (Prolonged AV conduction time). Products include:
Lanoxicaps 772
Lanoxin Elixir Pediatric 775
Lanoxin Injection 778
Lanoxin Injection Pediatric 781
Lanoxin Tablets 783

Diltiazem Hydrochloride (Possible atrioventricular conduction disturbances; left ventricular failure; hypotension). Products include:
Cardizem Tablets-30 mg, 60 mg, 90 mg and 120 mg 1329
Cardizem SR Capsules-60 mg, 90 mg and 120 mg 1327

Enflurane (Protracted severe hypotension). Products include:
Ethrane 599

Epinephrine (Mydriasis). Products include:
Ana-Kit Anaphylaxis Emergency Treatment Kit 1100
Bronkaid Mist .... ▣ 757
EpiPen 843
Marcaine Hydrochloride 0.5% with Epinephrine 1:200,000 (as bitartrate) 958
Marcaine Hydrochloride with Epinephrine 1:200,000 2055
Primatene Mist 2420
Sus-Phrine Injection 1006
Xylocaine with Epinephrine Injections 637

Esmolol Hydrochloride (Potential for additive effects). Products include:
Brevibloc Injection 942

Felodipine (Possible atrioventricular conduction disturbances; left ventricular failure; hypotension). Products include:
Plendil Extended-Release Tablets 1526

Isoflurane (Protracted severe hypotension). Products include:
Forane 600

Isradipine (Possible atrioventricular conduction disturbances; left ventricular failure; hypotension). Products include:
DynaCirc Capsules 2004

Labetalol Hydrochloride (Potential for additive effects). Products include:
Normodyne Injection 2108
Normodyne Tablets 2110
Normozide Tablets 2112
Trandate HCT Tablets 579
Trandate Injection 577
Trandate Tablets 579

Methohexital Sodium (Protracted severe hypotension). Products include:
Brevital Sodium Vials 1248

Methoxyflurane (Protracted severe hypotension).
No products indexed under this heading.

Metoprolol Tartrate (Potential for additive effects). Products include:
Lopressor Ampuls 1032
Lopressor HCT Tablets 1034
Lopressor Tablets 1032

Nadolol (Potential for additive effects). Products include:
Corgard Tablets 701
Corzide Tablets 702

Nicardipine Hydrochloride (Possible atrioventricular conduction disturbances; left ventricular failure; hypotension). Products include:
Cardene Capsules 2290

Nifedipine (Possible atrioventricular conduction disturbances; left ventricular failure; hypotension). Products include:
Adalat Capsules (10 mg and 20 mg) 1587
Procardia Capsules 1781
Procardia XL Tablets 1783

Nimodipine (Possible atrioventricular conduction disturbances; left ventricular failure; hypotension). Products include:
Nimotop Capsules 1607

Penbutolol Sulfate (Potential for additive effects). Products include:
Levatol 1832

Pindolol (Potential for additive effects). Products include:
Visken Tablets 2036

Propofol (Protracted severe hypotension). Products include:
Diprivan Injection 2267

Propranolol Hydrochloride (Potential for additive effects). Products include:
Inderal 2459
Inderal LA Long Acting Capsules 2461
Inderide Tablets 2463
Inderide LA Long Acting Capsules .. 2465

Rauwolfia Serpentina (Hypotension; marked bradycardia). Products include:
Raudixin Tablets 1803
Rauzide Tablets 1804

Rescinnamine (Hypotension; marked bradycardia).
No products indexed under this heading.

Reserpine (Hypotension; marked bradycardia). Products include:
Diupres Tablets 1461
Hydromox R Tablets 1209
Hydropres Tablets 1485
Renese-R Tablets 1786
Salutensin/Salutensin-Demi 719
Ser-Ap-Es Tablets 881
Serpasil Tablets 883
Serpasil-Apresoline Tablets 884
Serpasil-Esidrix Tablets 886

Verapamil Hydrochloride (Possible atrioventricular conduction disturbances; left ventricular failure; hypotension). Products include:
Calan SR Caplets 2157
Calan Tablets 2155
Isoptin Injectable 1177
Isoptin Oral Tablets 1179
Isoptin SR Sustained Release Tablets 1181
Verelan Capsules 1243
Verelan Capsules 2535

TINACTIN AEROSOL LIQUID 1%
(Tolnaftate) .... ▣ 706
No interactions described in labeling.

TINACTIN AEROSOL POWDER 1%
(Tolnaftate) .... ▣ 706
No interactions described in labeling.

TINACTIN ANTIFUNGAL CREAM, SOLUTION & POWDER 1%
(Tolnaftate) .... ▣ 706
No interactions described in labeling.

TINACTIN JOCK ITCH CREAM 1%
(Tolnaftate) .... ▣ 706
No interactions described in labeling.

TINACTIN JOCK ITCH SPRAY POWDER 1%
(Tolnaftate) .... ▣ 706
No interactions described in labeling.

TING ANTIFUNGAL CREAM
(Tolnaftate) .... ▣ 562
No interactions described in labeling.

TING ANTIFUNGAL POWDER
(Tolnaftate) .... ▣ 562
No interactions described in labeling.

TING ANTIFUNGAL SPRAY LIQUID
(Tolnaftate) .... ▣ 562
No interactions described in labeling.

TING ANTIFUNGAL SPRAY POWDER
(Tolnaftate) .... ▣ 562
No interactions described in labeling.

TOBRADEX OPHTHALMIC SUSPENSION AND OINTMENT
(Dexamethasone, Tobramycin) .... ⊙ 228
May interact with aminoglycosides. Compounds in this category include:

Amikacin Sulfate (Monitor the total serum concentration if administered with systemic aminoglycosides). Products include:
Amikin Injectable 602

Gentamicin Sulfate (Monitor the total serum concentration if administered with systemic aminoglycosides). Products include:
Garamycin Injectable 2093
Garamycin Ophthalmic .... ⊙ 305
Genoptic Liquifilm Sterile Ophthalmic Solution .... ⊙ 247
Genoptic S.O.P. Sterile Ophthalmic Ointment .... ⊙ 247
Gentacidin Ointment .... ⊙ 273
Gentacidin Solution .... ⊙ 273
Gentak Ointment & Solution .... ⊙ 208
G-myticin Creme and Ointment 0.1% 1770
Pred-G Liquifilm Sterile Ophthalmic Suspension .... ⊙ 252
Pred-G S.O.P. Sterile Ophthalmic Ointment .... ⊙ 253

Kanamycin Sulfate (Monitor the total serum concentration if administered with systemic aminoglycosides). Products include:
Kantrex Injection 601
Kantrex Pediatric Injection 601

Streptomycin Sulfate (Monitor the total serum concentration if administered with systemic aminoglycosides).
No products indexed under this heading.

Tobramycin Sulfate (Monitor the total serum concentration if administered with systemic aminoglycosides). Products include:
Nebcin Vials, Hyporets & ADD-Vantage 1286

TOBREX OPHTHALMIC OINTMENT AND SOLUTION
(Tobramycin) 572
May interact with aminoglycosides. Compounds in this category include:

Amikacin Sulfate (Total serum concentration should be monitored if administered concomitantly with systemic aminoglycosides). Products include:
Amikin Injectable 602

Gentamicin Sulfate (Total serum concentration should be monitored if administered concomitantly with systemic aminoglycosides). Products include:
Garamycin Injectable 2093
Garamycin Ophthalmic .... ⊙ 305
Genoptic Liquifilm Sterile Ophthalmic Solution .... ⊙ 247
Genoptic S.O.P. Sterile Ophthalmic Ointment .... ⊙ 247
Gentacidin Ointment .... ⊙ 273
Gentacidin Solution .... ⊙ 273
Gentak Ointment & Solution .... ⊙ 208
G-myticin Creme and Ointment 0.1% 1770
Pred-G Liquifilm Sterile Ophthalmic Suspension .... ⊙ 252
Pred-G S.O.P. Sterile Ophthalmic Ointment .... ⊙ 253

Kanamycin Sulfate (Total serum concentration should be monitored if administered concomitantly with systemic aminoglycosides). Products include:
Kantrex Injection 601
Kantrex Pediatric Injection 601

Streptomycin Sulfate (Total serum concentration should be monitored if administered concomitantly with systemic aminoglycosides).
No products indexed under this heading.

Tobramycin Sulfate (Total serum concentration should be monitored if administered concomitantly with systemic aminoglycosides). Products include:
Nebcin Vials, Hyporets & ADD-Vantage 1286

TODAY VAGINAL CONTRACEPTIVE SPONGE
(Nonoxynol-9) 2422
No interactions described in labeling.

TOFRANIL AMPULS
(Imipramine Hydrochloride) 1038
May interact with monoamine oxidase inhibitors, anticholinergics, belladona products, central nervous system depressants, sympathomimetic aerosol bronchodilators, thyroid preparations, and certain other agents. Compounds in these categories include:

Albuterol (Potentiated). Products include:
Proventil Inhalation Aerosol 2117
Ventolin Inhalation Aerosol and Refill 583

Albuterol Sulfate (Potentiated). Products include:
Proventil Repetabs Tablets 2120
Proventil Solutions for Inhalation 0.5% and 0.083% 2118
Proventil Syrup 2119
Proventil Tablets 2120
Ventolin 583

Alcohol (Tofranil may enhance alcohol's CNS depressant effects).

Alfentanil Hydrochloride (Potentiated). Products include:
- Alfenta Injection ... 1131

Alprazolam (Potentiated). Products include:
- Xanax Tablets ... 2367

Aprobarbital (Potentiated). Products include:
- Alurate Elixir ... 1883

Atropine Sulfate (Atropine-like effects may become more pronounced). Products include:
- Arco-Lase Plus Tablets ... 607
- Atropine Sulfate Sterile Ophthalmic Solution and S.O.P. Sterile Ophthalmic Ointment ... ⊙ 239
- Donnagel ... ◘ 675
- Donnagel-PG ... 1858
- Donnatal ... 1858
- Donnatal Extentabs ... 1859
- Donnatal Tablets ... 1858
- Donnazyme Tablets ... 1860
- Isopto Atropine ... ⊙ 218
- Lomotil ... 2174
- Motofen Tablets ... 836
- Ru-Tuss Tablets ... 693
- Urised Tablets ... 2396

Belladonna Alkaloids (Atropine-like effects may become more pronounced). Products include:
- Bellergal-S Tablets ... 1998
- Hyland's Bed Wetting Tablets ... ◘ 728
- Hyland's Teething Tablets ... ◘ 728
- Kinesed Tablets ... 2272

Benztropine Mesylate (Atropine-like effects may become more pronounced). Products include:
- Cogentin ... 1435

Biperiden (Atropine-like effects may become more pronounced). Products include:
- Akineton ... 1171

Buprenorphine (Potentiated).
- No products indexed under this heading.

Buspirone Hydrochloride (Potentiated). Products include:
- BuSpar ... 1401

Butabarbital (Potentiated). Products include:
- Pyridium Plus ... 1764

Butalbital (Potentiated). Products include:
- Esgic-Plus Tablets ... 1002
- Esgic Tablets & Capsules ... 1001
- Fioricet Tablets ... 2006
- Fiorinal Capsules ... 2007
- Fiorinal with Codeine Capsules ... 2008
- Fiorinal Tablets ... 2007
- Phrenilin ... 838
- Sedapap Tablets 50 mg/650 mg .. 1360

Chlordiazepoxide (Potentiated). Products include:
- Libritabs Tablets ... 1930
- Limbitrol ... 1933
- Menrium Tablets ... 1934

Chlordiazepoxide Hydrochloride (Potentiated). Products include:
- Librax Capsules ... 1929
- Librium Capsules ... 1931
- Librium Injectable ... 1932

Chlorpromazine (Potentiated). Products include:
- Thorazine ... 2234

Chlorprothixene (Potentiated). Products include:
- Taractan Tablets ... 1920

Chlorprothixene Hydrochloride (Potentiated). Products include:
- Taractan ... 1920

Cimetidine (Plasma concentration of imipramine may increase). Products include:
- Tagamet Tablets ... 2228

Cimetidine Hydrochloride (Plasma concentration of imipramine may increase). Products include:
- Tagamet ... 2228

Clidinium Bromide (Atropine-like effects may become more pronounced). Products include:
- Librax Capsules ... 1929
- Quarzan Capsules ... 1937

Clonidine (Imipramine may block clonidine's effect). Products include:
- Catapres-TTS ... 677

Clonidine Hydrochloride (Imipramine may block clonidine's effect). Products include:
- Catapres Tablets ... 676
- Combipres Tablets ... 678

Clorazepate Dipotassium (Potentiated). Products include:
- Tranxene ... 556

Codeine (Potentiated). Products include:
- Calcidrine Syrup ... 506

Codeine Phosphate (Potentiated). Products include:
- Actifed with Codeine Cough Syrup.. 752
- Cheracol Cough Syrup ... 1853
- Codimal PH Syrup ... 846
- Dimetane-DC Cough Syrup ... 1857
- Empirin with Codeine Phosphate Nos. 2, 3 & 4 ... 764
- Fiorinal with Codeine Capsules ... 2008
- Isoclor Expectorant ... 982
- Naldecon CX Adult Liquid ... ◘ 521
- Novahistine DH ... 1342
- Novahistine Expectorant ... 1343
- Nucofed Capsules ... 2219
- Nucofed Expectorant ... 2219
- Nucofed Pediatric Expectorant ... 2220
- Nucofed Syrup ... 2219
- Phenaphen with Codeine Capsules 1865
- Phenaphen-650 with Codeine Tablets ... 1866
- Phenergan with Codeine ... 2497
- Phenergan VC with Codeine ... 2501
- Robitussin A-C Syrup ... 1875
- Robitussin-DAC Syrup ... 1875
- Ryna ... ◘ 741
- Soma Compound w/Codeine Tablets ... 2390
- Triaminic Expectorant w/Codeine .. 1996
- Tussi-Organidin Liquid ... 2391
- Tylenol with Codeine ... 1381

Codeine Polistirex (Potentiated).
- No products indexed under this heading.

Dezocine (Potentiated).

Diazepam (Potentiated). Products include:
- Valium Injectable ... 1937
- Valium Tablets ... 1939
- Valrelease Capsules ... 1923

Dicyclomine Hydrochloride (Atropine-like effects may become more pronounced). Products include:
- Bentyl ... 1322

Dobutamine Hydrochloride (Potentiated). Products include:
- Dobutrex Solution Vials ... 1259

Dopamine Hydrochloride (Potentiated). Products include:
- Intropin Injection ... 930

Droperidol (Potentiated). Products include:
- Inapsine Injection ... 1140
- Innovar Injection ... 1141

Enflurane (Potentiated). Products include:
- Ethrane ... 599

Ephedrine Hydrochloride (Potentiated). Products include:
- Amesec ... ◘ 682
- Primatene Tablets-M Formula ... 2421
- Primatene Tablets-P Formula ... 2421
- Primatene Tablets-Regular Formula ... 2421
- Quadrinal Tablets ... 1183
- Quelidrine Syrup ... 556
- Tedral SA ... 1765

Ephedrine Sulfate (Potentiated). Products include:
- Bronkaid Tablets ... ◘ 757
- Bronkolixir ... ◘ 761
- Bronkotabs Tablets ... ◘ 762
- Marax Tablets & DF Syrup ... 1954
- Pazo Hemorrhoid Ointment & Suppositories ... 752
- Vicks Vatronol Nose Drops ... ◘ 666

Ephedrine Tannate (Potentiated). Products include:
- Rynatuss ... 2388

Epinephrine (Potentiated). Products include:
- Ana-Kit Anaphylaxis Emergency Treatment Kit ... 1100
- Bronkaid Mist ... ◘ 757
- EpiPen ... 843
- Marcaine Hydrochloride 0.5% with Epinephrine 1:200,000 (as bitartrate) ... 958
- Marcaine Hydrochloride with Epinephrine 1:200,000 ... 2055
- Primatene Mist ... 2420
- Sus-Phrine Injection ... 1006
- Xylocaine with Epinephrine Injections ... 637

Epinephrine Bitartrate (Potentiated). Products include:
- AsthmaHaler Mist Epinephrine Bitartrate Bronchodilator ... ◘ 616
- Bronkaid Mist Suspension ... ◘ 757
- Primatene Mist Suspension ... 2421

Epinephrine Hydrochloride (Potentiated). Products include:
- Adrenalin Chloride Solution 1:100 & 1:1,000 ... 1689
- Epifrin ... ⊙ 244
- Glaucon ... ⊙ 218

Estazolam (Potentiated). Products include:
- ProSom Tablets ... 554

Ethchlorvynol (Potentiated). Products include:
- Placidyl Capsules ... 553

Ethinamate (Potentiated).
- No products indexed under this heading.

Fentanyl (Potentiated). Products include:
- Duragesic Transdermal System ... 1133

Fentanyl Citrate (Potentiated). Products include:
- Innovar Injection ... 1141
- Sublimaze Injection ... 1146

Fluphenazine Decanoate (Potentiated). Products include:
- Prolixin Decanoate ... 1795

Fluphenazine Enanthate (Potentiated). Products include:
- Prolixin Enanthate ... 1796

Fluphenazine Hydrochloride (Potentiated). Products include:
- Prolixin Elixir ... 1793
- Prolixin Injection ... 1791
- Prolixin Oral Concentrate ... 1792
- Prolixin Tablets ... 1793

Flurazepam Hydrochloride (Potentiated). Products include:
- Dalmane Capsules ... 1927

Furazolidone (Hyperpyretic crises or severe convulsive seizures may occur). Products include:
- Furoxone ... 1855

Glutethimide (Potentiated).
- No products indexed under this heading.

Glycopyrrolate (Atropine-like effects may become more pronounced). Products include:
- Robinul Forte Tablets ... 1873
- Robinul Injectable ... 1873
- Robinul Tablets ... 1873

Guanethidine Monosulfate (Imipramine may block guanethidine's effect). Products include:
- Esimil Tablets ... 864
- Ismelin Tablets ... 869

Haloperidol (Potentiated). Products include:
- Haldol Injection, Tablets and Concentrate ... 1373

Haloperidol Decanoate (Potentiated). Products include:
- Haldol Decanoate ... 1375

Hydrocodone Bitartrate (Potentiated). Products include:
- Anexsia 5/500 Tablets ... 2196
- Anexsia 7.5/650 Tablets ... 2197
- Azdōne Tablets ... 844
- Codiclear DH Syrup ... 845
- Codimal DH Syrup ... 846
- Damason-P ... 1356
- Hycodan Syrup, Tablets ... 927
- Hycomine Compound Tablets ... 929
- Hycomine Syrup ... 927
- Hycotuss Expectorant Syrup ... 930
- Hydrocet Capsules ... 835
- Lortab ASA Tablets ... 2414
- Lortab ... 2412
- Ru-Tuss with Hydrocodone ... 694
- Triaminic Expectorant DH ... 1995
- Vicodin Tablets ... 1187
- Vicodin ES Tablets ... 1189
- Zydone Capsules ... 941

Hydrocodone Polistirex (Potentiated). Products include:
- Tussionex Extended-Release Suspension ... 988

Hydroxyzine Hydrochloride (Potentiated). Products include:
- Atarax Tablets & Syrup ... 1941
- Marax Tablets & DF Syrup ... 1954
- Vistaril Intramuscular Solution ... 1970

Hyoscyamine (Atropine-like effects may become more pronounced). Products include:
- Cystospaz Tablets ... 2395
- Urised Tablets ... 2396

Hyoscyamine Sulfate (Atropine-like effects may become more pronounced). Products include:
- Arco-Lase Plus Tablets ... 607
- Cystospaz-M Capsules ... 2395
- Donnagel ... ◘ 675
- Donnagel-PG ... 1858
- Donnatal ... 1858
- Donnatal Extentabs ... 1859
- Donnatal Tablets ... 1858
- Donnazyme Tablets ... 1860
- Kutrase Capsules ... 2146
- Levsin/Levsinex ... 2147
- Ru-Tuss Tablets ... 693

Ipratropium Bromide (Atropine-like effects may become more pronounced). Products include:
- Atrovent Inhalation Aerosol ... 675

Isocarboxazid (Hyperpyretic crises or severe convulsive seizures may occur). Products include:
- Marplan Tablets ... 1906

Isoflurane (Potentiated). Products include:
- Forane ... 600

Isoproterenol Hydrochloride (Potentiated). Products include:
- Isuprel Hydrochloride Injection 1:5000 ... 2050
- Isuprel Hydrochloride Mistometer .. 2051
- Isuprel Hydrochloride Solution 1:200 & 1:100 ... 2052
- Norisodrine Aerotrol ... 540

Ketamine Hydrochloride (Potentiated). Products include:
- Ketalar ... 1726

Levorphanol Tartrate (Potentiated). Products include:
- Levo-Dromoran ... 1906

Levothyroxine Sodium (Possibility of cardiovascular toxicity). Products include:
- Levothroid Tablets ... 1003
- Levoxine Tablets ... 904
- Synthroid ... 695

Liothyronine Sodium (Possibility of cardiovascular toxicity). Products include:
- Cytomel Tablets ... 2203

Liotrix (Possibility of cardiovascular toxicity). Products include:
- Euthroid ... 1724

Lorazepam (Potentiated). Products include:
- Ativan Injection ... 2432
- Ativan Tablets ... 2434

(◘ Described in PDR For Nonprescription Drugs) (⊙ Described in PDR For Ophthalmology)

Loxapine Hydrochloride (Potentiated). Products include:
Loxitane 1213

Loxapine Succinate (Potentiated). Products include:
Loxitane Capsules 1213

Mepenzolate Bromide (Atropine-like effects may become more pronounced). Products include:
Cantil Tablets 1326

Meperidine Hydrochloride (Potentiated). Products include:
Demerol 2047
Mepergan Injection 2479

Mephobarbital (Potentiated). Products include:
Mebaral Tablets 2061

Meprobamate (Potentiated). Products include:
Deprol Tablets 2382
Equagesic Tablets 2451
Miltown Tablets 2386
PMB 200 and PMB 400 2504

Mesoridazine (Potentiated). Products include:
Serentil 686

Metaproterenol Sulfate (Potentiated). Products include:
Alupent 674
Arm-a-Med Metaproterenol Sulfate Inhalation Solution, USP 617
Metaprel Inhalation Aerosol Bronchodilator 2014
Metaprel Inhalation Solution 2015
Metaprel 2015
Metaproterenol Sulfate Inhalation Solution, USP 912

Metaraminol Bitartrate (Potentiated). Products include:
Aramine Injection 1424

Methadone Hydrochloride (Potentiated). Products include:
Dolophine Hydrochloride Ampoules & Vials 1260
Dolophine Hydrochloride Tablets 1261
Methadone Hydrochloride Diskets 1284
Methadone Hydrochloride Oral Solution & Tablets 1987

Methohexital Sodium (Potentiated). Products include:
Brevital Sodium Vials 1248

Methoxamine Hydrochloride (Potentiated). Products include:
Vasoxyl Injection 819

Methoxyflurane (Potentiated).
No products indexed under this heading.

Methylphenidate Hydrochloride (May inhibit the metabolism of imipramine hydrochloride). Products include:
Ritalin 880

Midazolam Hydrochloride (Potentiated). Products include:
Versed Injection 1924

Molindone Hydrochloride (Potentiated). Products include:
Moban Tablets & Concentrate 932

Morphine Sulfate (Potentiated). Products include:
Astramorph/PF Injection, USP (Preservative-Free) 618
Duramorph 960
Infumorph 200 and Infumorph 500 Sterile Solutions 962
MS Contin Tablets 1814
MSIR 1817
Oramorph SR (Morphine Sulfate Sustained Release Tablets) 1988
Roxanol 1991

Norepinephrine Bitartrate (Potentiated). Products include:
Levophed Bitartrate Injection 2054

Opium Alkaloids (Potentiated). Products include:
B & O No. 15A & No. 16A Supprettes 2395
Pantopon Injectable 1911

Oxazepam (Potentiated). Products include:
Serax Capsules 2522
Serax Tablets 2522

Oxybutynin Chloride (Atropine-like effects may become more pronounced). Products include:
Ditropan 1332

Oxycodone Hydrochloride (Potentiated). Products include:
Percocet Tablets 950
Percodan 951
Roxicodone Tablets, Oral Solution & Intensol (Oxycodone) 1992
Tylox Capsules 1382

Pentobarbital Sodium (Potentiated). Products include:
Nembutal Sodium Capsules 534
Nembutal Sodium Solution 536
Nembutal Sodium Suppositories 538

Perphenazine (Potentiated). Products include:
Etrafon 2087
Triavil Tablets 1556
Trilafon 2123

Phenelzine Sulfate (Hyperpyretic crises or severe convulsive seizures may occur). Products include:
Nardil 1742

Phenobarbital (Potentiated). Products include:
Arco-Lase Plus Tablets 607
Bellergal-S Tablets 1998
Bronkolixir .... ◘ 761
Bronkotabs Tablets .... ◘ 762
Donnatal 1858
Donnatal Extentabs 1859
Donnatal Tablets 1858
Donnazyme Tablets 1860
Kinesed Tablets 2272
Phenobarbital Elixir and Tablets 1293
Primatene Tablets-P Formula 2421
Quadrinal Tablets 1183
Tedral SA 1765

Phenylephrine Hydrochloride (Potentiated). Products include:
AK-Dilate Solution 2.5% and 10% .... ⊙ 203
Atrohist Sprinkle Capsules 558
Cerose-DM 2443
Codimal 846
Comhist LA Capsules 1618
Congespirin For Children Aspirin Free Chewable Cold Tablets 748
Cyclomydril .... ⊙ 216
Deconsal Sprinkle Capsules 559
Dimetane Decongestant .... ◘ 673
Dristan Decongestant/Antihistamine/ Analgesic Coated Caplets .... ◘ 749
Dristan Cold Nasal Decongestant/ Antihistamine/ Analgesic Coated Tablets 2419
Dristan Advanced Formula Decongestant/Antihistamine/ Analgesic Tablets .... ◘ 749
Dristan Nasal Spray, Menthol 2419
Dristan Nasal Spray, Regular and Regular with Metered Pump 2419
Entex Capsules 1623
Entex Liquid 1623
Sinus Excedrin Analgesic, Decongestant Tablets & Caplets 750
Extendryl 994
4-Way Fast Acting Nasal Spray - Original Formula (regular & mentholated) & Metered Spray Pump (regular) 751
Hycomine Compound Tablets 929
Murocoll-2 Sterile Ophthalmic Solution .... ⊙ 261
Mydfrin 2.5% .... ⊙ 224
Naldecon Syrup, Tablets, Pediatric Drops and Pediatric Syrup 709
Neo-Synephrine Hydrochloride 1% Carpuject 2063
Neo-Synephrine Hydrochloride 1% Injection 2063
Neo-Synephrine Hydrochloride (Ophthalmic) 2064
Neo-Synephrine .... ◘ 759
Nōstril Nasal Decongestant .... ◘ 520
Novahistine Elixir .... ◘ 596
Phenergan VC 2500
Phenergan VC with Codeine 2501
Prefrin Liquifilm Vasoconstrictor and Lubricant Eye Drops .... ⊙ 254
Prefrin-A .... ⊙ 255
Quelidrine Syrup 556
Relief Vasoconstrictor and Lubricant Eye Drops .... ⊙ 256
Robitussin Night Relief .... ◘ 677
Ru-Tuss with Hydrocodone 694
Ru-Tuss Tablets 693
Vasosulf .... ⊙ 279
Vicks Sinex .... ◘ 665
Zincfrin .... ⊙ 230

Phenylephrine Tannate (Potentiated). Products include:
Rynatan 2387
Rynatuss 2388

Phenylpropanolamine Hydrochloride (Potentiated). Products include:
A.R.M. Allergy Relief Medicine Caplets .... ◘ 615
Acutrim .... ◘ 548
Allerest .... ◘ 559
BC Cold Powder .... ◘ 517
Cheracol Plus Head Cold/Cough Formula .... ◘ 667
Codimal Expectorant 846
Comtrex Multi-Symptom Cold Reliever Tablets/Caplets/Liqui-Gels/Liquid 745
Contac Continuous Action Decongestant/Antihistamine Capsules ◘ 710
Contac Maximum Strength Continuous Action Decongestant/ Antihistamine Caplets .... ◘ 709
Contac Severe Cold and Flu Formula Caplets .... ◘ 711
Coricidin 'D' Decongestant Tablets .... ◘ 695
Coricidin Demilets Tablets for Children .... ◘ 696
Demazin Nasal Decongestant/ Antihistamine Repetabs Tablets & Syrup .... ◘ 697
Dexatrim .... ◘ 733
Dimetane-DC Cough Syrup 1857
Dimetapp Elixir .... ◘ 673
Dimetapp DM Elixir .... ◘ 674
Dimetapp Extentabs .... ◘ 674
Dimetapp Plus Caplets .... ◘ 675
Dimetapp Tablets .... ◘ 675
Entex Capsules 1623
Entex LA Tablets 1623
Entex Liquid 1623
4-Way Cold Tablets 750
Hycomine Syrup 927
Naldecon CX Adult Liquid .... ◘ 521
Naldecon DX Adult Liquid .... ◘ 521
Naldecon DX Children's Syrup .... ◘ 522
Naldecon DX Pediatric Drops .... ◘ 522
Naldecon EX Children's Syrup .... ◘ 522
Naldecon EX Pediatric Drops .... ◘ 523
Naldecon Syrup, Tablets, Pediatric Drops and Pediatric Syrup 709
Nolamine Tablets 838
Nolex LA Tablets 838
Ornade Spansule Capsules 2221
Orthoxicol Cough Syrup .... ◘ 668
Propagest 839
Pyrroxate Capsules .... ◘ 669
Robitussin-CF .... ◘ 676
Ru-Tuss II Capsules 693
Ru-Tuss with Hydrocodone 694
Ru-Tuss Tablets 693
Sine-Off Sinus Medicine Tablets-Aspirin Formula .... ◘ 722
Sinulin 840
St. Joseph Cold Tablets for Children .... ◘ 704
Tavist-D Tablets 2035
Triaminic Allergy Tablets .... ◘ 688
Triaminic Chewables .... ◘ 688
Triaminic Cold Tablets .... ◘ 688
Triaminic Expectorant .... ◘ 688
Triaminic Expectorant w/Codeine 1996
Triaminic Expectorant DH 1995
Triaminic Oral Infant Drops 1996
Triaminic Syrup .... ◘ 689
Triaminic-12 Tablets .... ◘ 690
Triaminic-DM Syrup .... ◘ 689
Triaminicin Tablets .... ◘ 690
Triaminicol Multi-Symptom Cold Tablets .... ◘ 691
Triaminicol Multi-Symptom Relief ◘ 691
Tuss-Ornade Liquid 2242
Tuss-Ornade Spansule Capsules 2242
Tylenol Cold Medication, Effervescent Tablets 1369

Pirbuterol Acetate (Potentiated). Products include:
Maxair Inhaler 1311

Prazepam (Potentiated). Products include:
Centrax 1693

Prochlorperazine (Potentiated). Products include:
Compazine 2201

Procyclidine Hydrochloride (Atropine-like effects may become more pronounced). Products include:
Kemadrin Tablets 771

Promethazine Hydrochloride (Potentiated). Products include:
Mepergan Injection 2479
Phenergan with Codeine 2497
Phenergan with Dextromethorphan 2499
Phenergan Injection 2493
Phenergan Suppositories 2496
Phenergan Syrup 2495
Phenergan Tablets 2496
Phenergan VC 2500
Phenergan VC with Codeine 2501

Propantheline Bromide (Atropine-like effects may become more pronounced). Products include:
Pro-Banthīne Tablets 2141

Propofol (Potentiated). Products include:
Diprivan Injection 2267

Propoxyphene Hydrochloride (Potentiated). Products include:
Darvon 1256
Wygesic Tablets 2540

Propoxyphene Napsylate (Potentiated). Products include:
Darvon-N/Darvocet-N 1254

Pseudoephedrine Hydrochloride (Potentiated). Products include:
Actifed Capsules .... ◘ 539
Actifed Plus Caplets .... ◘ 539
Actifed Plus Tablets .... ◘ 540
Actifed with Codeine Cough Syrup 752
Actifed Syrup .... ◘ 540
Actifed Tablets .... ◘ 540
Actifed 12-Hour Capsules .... ◘ 539
Advil Cold & Sinus Caplets (formerly CoAdvil) 2416
Allerest .... ◘ 559
Anatuss LA Tablets 1359
Benadryl Decongestant Elixir .... ◘ 635
Benadryl Decongestant .... ◘ 635
Benadryl Plus .... ◘ 636
Benadryl Plus Nighttime .... ◘ 637
Benylin Decongestant .... ◘ 638
Brexin L.A. Capsules 2078
Bromfed Capsules (Timed Release) 1615
Bromfed Syrup .... ◘ 628
Bromfed 1615
CoAdvil .... ◘ 748
Allergy-Sinus Comtrex Multi-Symptom Allergy Sinus Formula Tablets & Caplets 746
Cough Formula Comtrex 746
Comtrex Multi-Symptom Cold Reliever Tablets/Caplets/Liqui-Gels/Liquid 745
Day-Night Comtrex 747
Non-Drowsy Comtrex 747
Congess 994
Congestac Caplets .... ◘ 617
Contac Jr. Children's Cold Medicine .... ◘ 712
Contac Nighttime Cold Medicine .... ◘ 713
Contac Sinus Caplets Maximum Strength Non-Drowsy Formula .... ◘ 710
Contac Sinus Tablets Maximum Strength Non-Drowsy Formula .... ◘ 710
Deconamine 663
Deconsal II Tablets 559
Dimacol Caplets .... ◘ 672
Dimetane-DX Cough Syrup 1858
Dorcol Children's Cough Syrup .... ◘ 685
Dorcol Children's Decongestant Liquid .... ◘ 685
Dorcol Children's Liquid Cold Formula .... ◘ 686
Maximum Strength Dristan Decongestant/Analgesic Coated Caplets .... ◘ 750
No Drowsiness Dristan Cold Nasal Decongestant/Analgesic Coated Caplets 2420
Dristan Sinus Caplets 2419

Sinus Excedrin Analgesic, Decongestant Tablets & Caplets ▣ 533
Fedahist Gyrocaps 2145
Fedahist Timecaps 2145
Guaifed 1615
Guaifed Syrup ▣ 629
Isoclor Expectorant 982
Isoclor Timesule Capsules ▣ 561
Kronofed-A 970
Medi-Flu Caplet, Liquid ▣ 640
Novafed A Capsules 1342
Novafed Capsules 1342
Novahistine DH 1342
Novahistine DMX ▣ 595
Novahistine Expectorant 1343
Nucofed Capsules 2219
Nucofed Expectorant 2219
Nucofed Pediatric Expectorant 2220
Nucofed Syrup 2219
Ornex Caplets ▣ 618
PediaCare Allergy Relief Formula Liquid 1362
PediaCare Cough-Cold Formula Liquid 1362
PediaCare Infants' Oral Decongestant Drops 1362
PediaCare Night Rest Cough-Cold Formula Liquid 1362
PediaCare 6-12 Cough-Cold Formula Chewable Tablets 1362
Robitussin-DAC Syrup 1875
Robitussin-PE ▣ 677
Rondec 1975
Rondec-DM 1976
Rondec-TR Tablet 1975
Ru-Tuss DE Tablets 694
Ryna ▣ 741
Seldane-D Extended-Release Tablets 1350
Sinarest ▣ 562
Sine-Aid Maximum Strength Sinus Headache Caplets 1365
Sine-Aid Maximum Strength Sinus Headache Tablets 1365
Sine-Off Maximum Strength Allergy/Sinus Formula Caplets ▣ 721
Sine-Off Maximum Strength No Drowsiness Formula Caplets ▣ 722
Singlet Tablets ▣ 598
Sinutab Maximum Strength ▣ 641
Sinutab Maximum Strength Without Drowsiness Tablets & Caplets ▣ 642
Sinutab Regular Strength Without Drowsiness Formula ▣ 641
St. Joseph Nighttime Cold Medicine ▣ 705
Sudafed Children's Liquid ▣ 543
Sudafed Cough Syrup ▣ 543
Sudafed Plus Liquid ▣ 544
Sudafed Plus Tablets ▣ 545
Sudafed Sinus Caplets ▣ 545
Sudafed Sinus Tablets ▣ 545
Sudafed Tablets, 30 mg ▣ 544
Sudafed Tablets, Adult Strength, 60 mg ▣ 544
Sudafed 12 Hour Capsules ▣ 545
TheraFlu Flu and Cold Medicine ▣ 687
Triaminic Nite Light ▣ 689
Tylenol Allergy Sinus Medication Caplets and Gelcaps, Maximum Strength 1372
Children's Tylenol Cold Liquid Formula and Chewable Tablets 1368
Tylenol Cold & Flu Hot Medication, Packets 1369
Tylenol Cold & Flu No Drowsiness Hot Medication, Packets 1371
Tylenol Cold Medication Caplets and Tablets 1370
Tylenol Cold Medication No Drowsiness Formula Caplets 1370
Tylenol Cold Night Time Medication Liquid 1371
Tylenol Cough Medication Liquid with Decongestant, Maximum Strength 1372
Tylenol, Maximum Strength, Sinus Medication Gelcaps, Caplets and Tablets 1373
Ursinus Inlay-Tabs ▣ 691
Vicks Children's NyQuil ▣ 664
Vicks Daycare ▣ 660
Vicks Formula 44D Decongestant Cough Medicine ▣ 662
Vicks Formula 44M Multi-Symptom Cough Medicine ▣ 662
Vicks NyQuil Nighttime Colds Medicine-Original & Cherry Flavor ▣ 664
Vicks Pediatric Formula 44 Cough & Congestion Medicine ▣ 663
Vicks Pediatric Formula 44m Multi-Symptom Cough & Cold Medicine ▣ 663

Pseudoephedrine Sulfate (Potentiated). Products include:
Afrin Tablets ▣ 693
Chlor-Trimeton Decongestant ▣ 694
Disophrol Chronotab Sustained-Action Tablets ▣ 698
Drixoral Antihistamine/Nasal Decongestant Syrup ▣ 698
Drixoral Non-Drowsy Formula ▣ 699
Drixoral Plus Extended-Release Tablets ▣ 699
Drixoral Sinus ▣ 700
Drixoral Sustained-Action Tablets ▣ 698
Sinutab Allergy Formula Sustained Action Tablets ▣ 640
Trinalin Repetabs Tablets 1170

Quazepam (Potentiated). Products include:
Doral Tablets 2383

Scopolamine Hydrobromide (Atropine-like effects may become more pronounced). Products include:
Donnagel ▣ 675
Donnagel-PG 1858
Donnatal 1858
Donnatal Extentabs 1859
Donnatal Tablets 1858
Donnazyme Tablets 1860
Isopto Hyoscine ⊙ 222
Murocoll-2 Sterile Ophthalmic Solution ⊙ 261
Ru-Tuss Tablets 693

Scopolamine Preparations (Atropine-like effects may become more prnounced). Products include:
Transderm Scōp Transdermal Therapeutic System 887

Secobarbital Sodium (Potentiated). Products include:
Seconal Sodium Pulvules 1296

Selegiline Hydrochloride (Hyperpyretic crises or severe convulsive seizures may occur). Products include:
Eldepryl 2250

Sufentanil Citrate (Potentiated). Products include:
Sufenta Injection 1147

Temazepam (Potentiated). Products include:
Restoril Capsules 2023

Terbutaline Sulfate (Potentiated). Products include:
Brethaire Inhaler 1024
Brethine Ampuls 1026
Brethine Tablets 1026
Bricanyl Injection 1324
Bricanyl Tablets 1325

Thiamylal Sodium (Potentiated). Products include:
Surital Ampoules, Steri-Vials 1764

Thioridazine Hydrochloride (Potentiated). Products include:
Mellaril 2011

Thiothixene (Potentiated). Products include:
Navane Capsules and Concentrate 1954
Navane Intramuscular 1956

Thyroglobulin (Possibility of cardiovascular toxicity). Products include:
Proloid Tablets 1761

Thyroid (Possibility of cardiovascular toxicity). Products include:
S-P-T "Liquid" Capsules 995

Thyroxine Sodium (Possibility of cardiovascular toxicity).
No products indexed under this heading.

Tranylcypromine Sulfate (Hyperpyretic crises or severe convulsive seizures may occur). Products include:
Parnate Tablets 2222

Triazolam (Potentiated). Products include:
Halcion Tablets 2340

Tridihexethyl Chloride (Atropine-like effects may become more pronounced).
No products indexed under this heading.

Trifluoperazine Hydrochloride (Potentiated). Products include:
Stelazine 2226

Trihexyphenidyl Hydrochloride (Atropine-like effects may become more pronounced). Products include:
Artane 1195

TOFRANIL TABLETS

(Imipramine Hydrochloride) 1039
May interact with monoamine oxidase inhibitors, central nervous system depressants, thyroid preparations, sympathomimetic aerosol bronchodilators, anticholinergics, and certain other agents. Compounds in these categories include:

Albuterol (Potentiated). Products include:
Proventil Inhalation Aerosol 2117
Ventolin Inhalation Aerosol and Refill 583

Albuterol Sulfate (Potentiated). Products include:
Proventil Repetabs Tablets 2120
Proventil Solutions for Inhalation 0.5% and 0.083% 2118
Proventil Syrup 2119
Proventil Tablets 2120
Ventolin 583

Alcohol (Enhanced CNS depressant effects of alcohol).

Alfentanil Hydrochloride (May potentiate the CNS depressant effect). Products include:
Alfenta Injection 1131

Alprazolam (May potentiate the CNS depressant effect). Products include:
Xanax Tablets 2367

Aprobarbital (May potentiate the CNS depressant effect). Products include:
Alurate Elixir 1883

Atropine Sulfate (Atropine-like effects may become more pronounced). Products include:
Arco-Lase Plus Tablets 607
Atropine Sulfate Sterile Ophthalmic Solution and S.O.P. Sterile Ophthalmic Ointment ⊙ 239
Donnagel ▣ 675
Donnagel-PG 1858
Donnatal 1858
Donnatal Extentabs 1859
Donnatal Tablets 1858
Donnazyme Tablets 1860
Isopto Atropine ⊙ 218
Lomotil 2174
Motofen Tablets 836
Ru-Tuss Tablets 693
Urised Tablets 2396

Belladonna Alkaloids (Atropine-like effects may become more pronounced). Products include:
Bellergal-S Tablets 1998
Hyland's Bed Wetting Tablets ▣ 728
Hyland's Teething Tablets ▣ 728
Kinesed Tablets 2272

Benztropine Mesylate (Atropine-like effects may become more pronounced). Products include:
Cogentin 1435

Biperiden (Atropine-like effects may become more pronounced). Products include:
Akineton 1171

Buprenorphine (May potentiate the CNS depressant effect).
No products indexed under this heading.

Buspirone Hydrochloride (May potentiate the CNS depressant effect). Products include:
BuSpar 1401

Butabarbital (May potentiate the CNS depressant effect). Products include:
Pyridium Plus 1764

Butalbital (May potentiate the CNS depressant effect). Products include:
Esgic-Plus Tablets 1002
Esgic Tablets & Capsules 1001
Fioricet Tablets 2006
Fiorinal Capsules 2007
Fiorinal with Codeine Capsules 2008
Fiorinal Tablets 2007
Phrenilin 838
Sedapap Tablets 50 mg/650 mg 1360

Chlordiazepoxide (May potentiate the CNS depressant effect). Products include:
Libritabs Tablets 1930
Limbitrol 1933
Menrium Tablets 1934

Chlordiazepoxide Hydrochloride (May potentiate the CNS depressant effect). Products include:
Librax Capsules 1929
Librium Capsules 1931
Librium Injectable 1932

Chlorpromazine (May potentiate the CNS depressant effect). Products include:
Thorazine 2234

Chlorprothixene (May potentiate the CNS depressant effect). Products include:
Taractan Tablets 1920

Chlorprothixene Hydrochloride (May potentiate the CNS depressant effect). Products include:
Taractan 1920

Cimetidine (Increased plasma concentration of imipramine may potentiate the CNS depressant effect). Products include:
Tagamet Tablets 2228

Cimetidine Hydrochloride (Increased plasma concentration of imipramine may potentiate the CNS depressant effect). Products include:
Tagamet 2228

Clidinium Bromide (Atropine-like effects may become more pronounced). Products include:
Librax Capsules 1929
Quarzan Capsules 1937

Clonidine (Imipramine may block clonidine's effect). Products include:
Catapres-TTS 677

Clonidine Hydrochloride (Imipramine may block clonidine's effect). Products include:
Catapres Tablets 676
Combipres Tablets 678

Clorazepate Dipotassium (May potentiate the CNS depressant effect). Products include:
Tranxene 556

Codeine (May potentiate the CNS depressant effect). Products include:
Calcidrine Syrup 506

Codeine Phosphate (May potentiate the CNS depressant effect). Products include:
Actifed with Codeine Cough Syrup 752
Cheracol Cough Syrup 1853
Codimal PH Syrup 846
Dimetane-DC Cough Syrup 1857
Empirin with Codeine Phosphate Nos. 2, 3 & 4 764
Fiorinal with Codeine Capsules 2008
Isoclor Expectorant 982
Naldecon CX Adult Liquid ▣ 521
Novahistine DH 1342
Novahistine Expectorant 1343
Nucofed Capsules 2219
Nucofed Expectorant 2219
Nucofed Pediatric Expectorant 2220
Nucofed Syrup 2219

Phenaphen with Codeine Capsules 1865
Phenaphen-650 with Codeine Tablets 1866
Phenergan with Codeine 2497
Phenergan VC with Codeine 2501
Robitussin A-C Syrup 1875
Robitussin-DAC Syrup 1875
Ryna ◙ 741
Soma Compound w/Codeine Tablets 2390
Triaminic Expectorant w/Codeine .. 1996
Tussi-Organidin Liquid 2391
Tylenol with Codeine 1381

Codeine Polistirex (May potentiate the CNS depressant effect).
No products indexed under this heading.

Dezocine (May potentiate the CNS depressant effect).

Diazepam (May potentiate the CNS depressant effect). Products include:
Valium Injectable 1937
Valium Tablets 1939
Valrelease Capsules 1923

Dicyclomine Hydrochloride (Atropine-like effects may become more pronounced). Products include:
Bentyl 1322

Dobutamine Hydrochloride (Potentiated). Products include:
Dobutrex Solution Vials 1259

Dopamine Hydrochloride (Potentiated). Products include:
Intropin Injection 930

Droperidol (May potentiate the CNS depressant effect). Products include:
Inapsine Injection 1140
Innovar Injection 1141

Enflurane (May potentiate the CNS depressant effect). Products include:
Ethrane 599

Ephedrine Hydrochloride (Potentiated). Products include:
Amesec ◙ 682
Primatene Tablets-M Formula 2421
Primatene Tablets-P Formula 2421
Primatene Tablets-Regular Formula 2421
Quadrinal Tablets 1183
Quelidrine Syrup 556
Tedral SA 1765

Ephedrine Sulfate (Potentiated). Products include:
Bronkaid Tablets ◙ 757
Bronkolixir ◙ 761
Bronkotabs Tablets ◙ 762
Marax Tablets & DF Syrup 1954
Pazo Hemorrhoid Ointment & Suppositories 752
Vicks Vatronol Nose Drops ◙ 666

Ephedrine Tannate (Potentiated). Products include:
Rynatuss 2388

Epinephrine (Potentiated). Products include:
Ana-Kit Anaphylaxis Emergency Treatment Kit 1100
Bronkaid Mist ◙ 757
EpiPen 843
Marcaine Hydrochloride 0.5% with Epinephrine 1:200,000 (as bitartrate) 958
Marcaine Hydrochloride with Epinephrine 1:200,000 2055
Primatene Mist 2420
Sus-Phrine Injection 1006
Xylocaine with Epinephrine Injections 637

Epinephrine Bitartrate (Potentiated). Products include:
AsthmaHaler Mist Epinephrine Bitartrate Bronchodilator ◙ 616
Bronkaid Mist Suspension ◙ 757
Primatene Mist Suspension 2421

Epinephrine Hydrochloride (Potentiated). Products include:
Adrenalin Chloride Solution 1:100 & 1:1,000 1689
Epifrin ◎ 244
Glaucon ◎ 218

Estazolam (May potentiate the CNS depressant effect). Products include:
ProSom Tablets 554

Ethchlorvynol (May potentiate the CNS depressant effect). Products include:
Placidyl Capsules 553

Ethinamate (May potentiate the CNS depressant effect).
No products indexed under this heading.

Fentanyl (May potentiate the CNS depressant effect). Products include:
Duragesic Transdermal System 1133

Fentanyl Citrate (May potentiate the CNS depressant effect). Products include:
Innovar Injection 1141
Sublimaze Injection 1146

Fluphenazine Decanoate (May potentiate the CNS depressant effect). Products include:
Prolixin Decanoate 1795

Fluphenazine Enanthate (May potentiate the CNS depressant effect). Products include:
Prolixin Enanthate 1796

Fluphenazine Hydrochloride (May potentiate the CNS depressant effect). Products include:
Prolixin Elixir 1793
Prolixin Injection 1791
Prolixin Oral Concentrate 1792
Prolixin Tablets 1793

Flurazepam Hydrochloride (May potentiate the CNS depressant effect). Products include:
Dalmane Capsules 1927

Furazolidone (Concomitant use is contraindicated; hyperpyretic crises or severe convulsive seizures may occur). Products include:
Furoxone 1855

Glutethimide (May potentiate the CNS depressant effect).
No products indexed under this heading.

Glycopyrrolate (Atropine-like effects may become more pronounced). Products include:
Robinul Forte Tablets 1873
Robinul Injectable 1873
Robinul Tablets 1873

Guanethidine Monosulfate (Imipramine may block guanethidine's effect). Products include:
Esimil Tablets 864
Ismelin Tablets 869

Haloperidol (May potentiate the CNS depressant effect). Products include:
Haldol Injection, Tablets and Concentrate 1373

Haloperidol Decanoate (May potentiate the CNS depressant effect). Products include:
Haldol Decanoate 1375

Hydrocodone Bitartrate (May potentiate the CNS depressant effect). Products include:
Anexsia 5/500 Tablets 2196
Anexsia 7.5/650 Tablets 2197
Azdōne Tablets 844
Codiclear DH Syrup 845
Codimal DH Syrup 846
Damason-P 1356
Hycodan Syrup, Tablets 927
Hycomine Compound Tablets 929
Hycomine Syrup 927
Hycotuss Expectorant Syrup 930
Hydrocet Capsules 835
Lortab ASA Tablets 2414
Lortab 2412
Ru-Tuss with Hydrocodone 694
Triaminic Expectorant DH 1995
Vicodin Tablets 1187
Vicodin ES Tablets 1189
Zydone Capsules 941

Hydrocodone Polistirex (May potentiate the CNS depressant effect). Products include:
Tussionex Extended-Release Suspension 988

Hydroxyzine Hydrochloride (May potentiate the CNS depressant effect). Products include:
Atarax Tablets & Syrup 1941
Marax Tablets & DF Syrup 1954
Vistaril Intramuscular Solution 1970

Hyoscyamine (Atropine-like effects may become more pronounced). Products include:
Cystospaz Tablets 2395
Urised Tablets 2396

Hyoscyamine Sulfate (Atropine-like effects may become more pronounced). Products include:
Arco-Lase Plus Tablets 607
Cystospaz-M Capsules 2395
Donnagel ◙ 675
Donnagel-PG 1858
Donnatal 1858
Donnatal Extentabs 1859
Donnatal Tablets 1858
Donnazyme Tablets 1860
Kutrase Capsules 2146
Levsin/Levsinex 2147
Ru-Tuss Tablets 693

Ipratropium Bromide (Atropine-like effects may become more pronounced). Products include:
Atrovent Inhalation Aerosol 675

Isocarboxazid (Concomitant use is contraindicated; hyperpyretic crises or severe convulsive seizures may occur). Products include:
Marplan Tablets 1906

Isoflurane (May potentiate the CNS depressant effect). Products include:
Forane 600

Isoproterenol Hydrochloride (Potentiated). Products include:
Isuprel Hydrochloride Injection 1:5000 2050
Isuprel Hydrochloride Mistometer .. 2051
Isuprel Hydrochloride Solution 1:200 & 1:100 2052
Norisodrine Aerotrol 540

Ketamine Hydrochloride (May potentiate the CNS depressant effect). Products include:
Ketalar 1726

Levorphanol Tartrate (May potentiate the CNS depressant effect). Products include:
Levo-Dromoran 1906

Levothyroxine Sodium (Potential for cardiovascular toxicity). Products include:
Levothroid Tablets 1003
Levoxine Tablets 904
Synthroid 695

Liothyronine Sodium (Potential for cardiovascular toxicity). Products include:
Cytomel Tablets 2203

Liotrix (Potential for cardiovascular toxicity). Products include:
Euthroid 1724

Lorazepam (May potentiate the CNS depressant effect). Products include:
Ativan Injection 2432
Ativan Tablets 2434

Loxapine Hydrochloride (May potentiate the CNS depressant effect). Products include:
Loxitane 1213

Loxapine Succinate (May potentiate the CNS depressant effect). Products include:
Loxitane Capsules 1213

Mepenzolate Bromide (Atropine-like effects may become more pronounced). Products include:
Cantil Tablets 1326

Meperidine Hydrochloride (May potentiate the CNS depressant effect). Products include:
Demerol 2047
Mepergan Injection 2479

Mephobarbital (May potentiate the CNS depressant effect). Products include:
Mebaral Tablets 2061

Meprobamate (May potentiate the CNS depressant effect). Products include:
Deprol Tablets 2382
Equagesic Tablets 2451
Miltown Tablets 2386
PMB 200 and PMB 400 2504

Mesoridazine (May potentiate the CNS depressant effect). Products include:
Serentil 686

Metaproterenol Sulfate (Potentiated). Products include:
Alupent 674
Arm-a-Med Metaproterenol Sulfate Inhalation Solution, USP 617
Metaprel Inhalation Aerosol Bronchodilator 2014
Metaprel Inhalation Solution 2015
Metaprel 2015
Metaproterenol Sulfate Inhalation Solution, USP 912

Metaraminol Bitartrate (Potentiated). Products include:
Aramine Injection 1424

Methadone Hydrochloride (May potentiate the CNS depressant effect). Products include:
Dolophine Hydrochloride Ampoules & Vials 1260
Dolophine Hydrochloride Tablets 1261
Methadone Hydrochloride Diskets .. 1284
Methadone Hydrochloride Oral Solution & Tablets 1987

Methohexital Sodium (May potentiate the CNS depressant effect). Products include:
Brevital Sodium Vials 1248

Methoxamine Hydrochloride (Potentiated). Products include:
Vasoxyl Injection 819

Methoxyflurane (May potentiate the CNS depressant effect).
No products indexed under this heading.

Methylphenidate Hydrochloride (May inhibit the metabolism of imipramine). Products include:
Ritalin 880

Midazolam Hydrochloride (May potentiate the CNS depressant effect). Products include:
Versed Injection 1924

Molindone Hydrochloride (May potentiate the CNS depressant effect). Products include:
Moban Tablets & Concentrate 932

Morphine Sulfate (May potentiate the CNS depressant effect). Products include:
Astramorph/PF Injection, USP (Preservative-Free) 618
Duramorph 960
Infumorph 200 and Infumorph 500 Sterile Solutions 962
MS Contin Tablets 1814
MSIR 1817
Oramorph SR (Morphine Sulfate Sustained Release Tablets) 1988
Roxanol 1991

Norepinephrine Bitartrate (Potentiated). Products include:
Levophed Bitartrate Injection 2054

Opium Alkaloids (May potentiate the CNS depressant effect). Products include:
B & O No. 15A & No. 16A Supprettes 2395
Pantopon Injectable 1911

(◙ Described in PDR For Nonprescription Drugs) (◎ Described in PDR For Ophthalmology)

Oxazepam (May potentiate the CNS depressant effect). Products include:

Serax Capsules ... 2522
Serax Tablets ... 2522

Oxybutynin Chloride (Atropine-like effects may become more pronounced). Products include:

Ditropan ... 1332

Oxycodone Hydrochloride (May potentiate the CNS depressant effect). Products include:

Percocet Tablets ... 950
Percodan ... 951
Roxicodone Tablets, Oral Solution & Intensol (Oxycodone) ... 1992
Tylox Capsules ... 1382

Pentobarbital Sodium (May potentiate the CNS depressant effect). Products include:

Nembutal Sodium Capsules ... 534
Nembutal Sodium Solution ... 536
Nembutal Sodium Suppositories ... 538

Perphenazine (May potentiate the CNS depressant effect). Products include:

Etrafon ... 2087
Triavil Tablets ... 1556
Trilafon ... 2123

Phenelzine Sulfate (Concomitant use is contraindicated; hyperpyretic crises or severe convulsive seizures may occur). Products include:

Nardil ... 1742

Phenobarbital (May potentiate the CNS depressant effect). Products include:

Arco-Lase Plus Tablets ... 607
Bellergal-S Tablets ... 1998
Bronkolixir ... ■ 761
Bronkotabs Tablets ... ■ 762
Donnatal ... 1858
Donnatal Extentabs ... 1859
Donnatal Tablets ... 1858
Donnazyme Tablets ... 1860
Kinesed Tablets ... 2272
Phenobarbital Elixir and Tablets ... 1293
Primatene Tablets-P Formula ... 2421
Quadrinal Tablets ... 1183
Tedral SA ... 1765

Phenylephrine Bitartrate (Potentiated).

No products indexed under this heading.

Phenylephrine Hydrochloride (Potentiated). Products include:

AK-Dilate Solution 2.5% and 10% ... ◉ 203
Atrohist Sprinkle Capsules ... 558
Cerose-DM ... 2443
Codimal ... 846
Comhist LA Capsules ... 1618
Congespirin For Children Aspirin Free Chewable Cold Tablets ... 748
Cyclomydril ... ◉ 216
Deconsal Sprinkle Capsules ... 559
Dimetane Decongestant ... ■ 673
Dristan Decongestant/Antihistamine/ Analgesic Coated Caplets ... ■ 749
Dristan Cold Nasal Decongestant/ Antihistamine/ Analgesic Coated Tablets ... 2419
Dristan Advanced Formula Decongestant/Antihistamine/ Analgesic Tablets ... ■ 749
Dristan Nasal Spray, Menthol ... 2419
Dristan Nasal Spray, Regular and Regular with Metered Pump ... 2419
Entex Capsules ... 1623
Entex Liquid ... 1623
Sinus Excedrin Analgesic, Decongestant Tablets & Caplets ... 750
Extendryl ... 994
4-Way Fast Acting Nasal Spray - Original Formula (regular & mentholated) & Metered Spray Pump (regular) ... 751
Hycomine Compound Tablets ... 929
Murocoll-2 Sterile Ophthalmic Solution ... ◉ 261
Mydfrin 2.5% ... ◉ 224
Naldecon Syrup, Tablets, Pediatric Drops and Pediatric Syrup ... 709
Neo-Synephrine Hydrochloride 1% Carpuject ... 2063
Neo-Synephrine Hydrochloride 1% Injection ... 2063
Neo-Synephrine Hydrochloride (Ophthalmic) ... 2064
Neo-Synephrine ... ■ 759
Nōstril Nasal Decongestant ... ■ 520
Novahistine Elixir ... ■ 596
Phenergan VC ... 2500
Phenergan VC with Codeine ... 2501
Prefrin Liquifilm Vasoconstrictor and Lubricant Eye Drops ... ◉ 254
Prefrin-A ... ◉ 255
Quelidrine Syrup ... 556
Relief Vasoconstrictor and Lubricant Eye Drops ... ◉ 256
Robitussin Night Relief ... ■ 677
Ru-Tuss with Hydrocodone ... 694
Ru-Tuss Tablets ... 693
Vasosulf ... ◉ 279
Vicks Sinex ... ■ 665
Zincfrin ... ◉ 230

Phenylephrine Tannate (Potentiated). Products include:

Rynatan ... 2387
Rynatuss ... 2388

Phenylpropanolamine Hydrochloride (Potentiated). Products include:

A.R.M. Allergy Relief Medicine Caplets ... ■ 615
Acutrim ... ■ 548
Allerest ... ■ 559
BC Cold Powder ... ■ 517
Cheracol Plus Head Cold/Cough Formula ... ■ 667
Codimal Expectorant ... 846
Comtrex Multi-Symptom Cold Reliever Tablets/Caplets/Liqui-Gels/Liquid ... 745
Contac Continuous Action Decongestant/Antihistamine Capsules ■ 710
Contac Maximum Strength Continuous Action Decongestant/ Antihistamine Caplets ... ■ 709
Contac Severe Cold and Flu Formula Caplets ... ■ 711
Coricidin 'D' Decongestant Tablets ... ■ 695
Coricidin Demilets Tablets for Children ... ■ 696
Demazin Nasal Decongestant/ Antihistamine Repetabs Tablets & Syrup ... ■ 697
Dexatrim ... ■ 733
Dimetane-DC Cough Syrup ... 1857
Dimetapp Elixir ... ■ 673
Dimetapp DM Elixir ... ■ 674
Dimetapp Extentabs ... ■ 674
Dimetapp Plus Caplets ... ■ 675
Dimetapp Tablets ... ■ 675
Entex Capsules ... 1623
Entex LA Tablets ... 1623
Entex Liquid ... 1623
4-Way Cold Tablets ... 750
Hycomine Syrup ... 927
Naldecon CX Adult Liquid ... ■ 521
Naldecon DX Adult Liquid ... ■ 521
Naldecon DX Children's Syrup ... ■ 522
Naldecon DX Pediatric Drops ... ■ 522
Naldecon EX Children's Syrup ... ■ 522
Naldecon EX Pediatric Drops ... ■ 523
Naldecon Syrup, Tablets, Pediatric Drops and Pediatric Syrup ... 709
Nolamine Tablets ... 838
Nolex LA Tablets ... 838
Ornade Spansule Capsules ... 2221
Orthoxicol Cough Syrup ... ■ 668
Propagest ... 839
Pyrroxate Capsules ... ■ 669
Robitussin-CF ... ■ 676
Ru-Tuss II Capsules ... 693
Ru-Tuss with Hydrocodone ... 694
Ru-Tuss Tablets ... 693
Sine-Off Sinus Medicine Tablets-Aspirin Formula ... ■ 722
Sinulin ... 840
St. Joseph Cold Tablets for Children ... ■ 704
Tavist-D Tablets ... 2035
Triaminic Allergy Tablets ... ■ 688
Triaminic Chewables ... ■ 688
Triaminic Cold Tablets ... ■ 688
Triaminic Expectorant ... ■ 688
Triaminic Expectorant w/Codeine ... 1996
Triaminic Expectorant DH ... 1995
Triaminic Oral Infant Drops ... 1996
Triaminic Syrup ... ■ 689
Triaminic-12 Tablets ... ■ 690
Triaminic-DM Syrup ... ■ 689
Triaminicin Tablets ... ■ 690
Triaminicol Multi-Symptom Cold Tablets ... ■ 691
Triaminicol Multi-Symptom Relief ■ 691
Tuss-Ornade Liquid ... 2242
Tuss-Ornade Spansule Capsules ... 2242
Tylenol Cold Medication, Effervescent Tablets ... 1369

Pirbuterol Acetate (Potentiated). Products include:

Maxair Inhaler ... 1311

Prazepam (May potentiate the CNS depressant effect). Products include:

Centrax ... 1693

Prochlorperazine (May potentiate the CNS depressant effect). Products include:

Compazine ... 2201

Procyclidine Hydrochloride (Atropine-like effects may become more pronounced). Products include:

Kemadrin Tablets ... 771

Promethazine Hydrochloride (May potentiate the CNS depressant effect). Products include:

Mepergan Injection ... 2479
Phenergan with Codeine ... 2497
Phenergan with Dextromethorphan 2499
Phenergan Injection ... 2493
Phenergan Suppositories ... 2496
Phenergan Syrup ... 2495
Phenergan Tablets ... 2496
Phenergan VC ... 2500
Phenergan VC with Codeine ... 2501

Propantheline Bromide (Atropine-like effects may become more pronounced). Products include:

Pro-Banthīne Tablets ... 2141

Propofol (May potentiate the CNS depressant effect). Products include:

Diprivan Injection ... 2267

Propoxyphene Hydrochloride (May potentiate the CNS depressant effect). Products include:

Darvon ... 1256
Wygesic Tablets ... 2540

Propoxyphene Napsylate (May potentiate the CNS depressant effect). Products include:

Darvon-N/Darvocet-N ... 1254

Pseudoephedrine Hydrochloride (Potentiated). Products include:

Actifed Capsules ... ■ 539
Actifed Plus Caplets ... ■ 539
Actifed Plus Tablets ... ■ 540
Actifed with Codeine Cough Syrup.. 752
Actifed Syrup ... ■ 540
Actifed Tablets ... ■ 540
Actifed 12-Hour Capsules ... ■ 539
Advil Cold & Sinus Caplets (formerly CoAdvil) ... 2416
Allerest ... ■ 559
Anatuss LA Tablets ... 1359
Benadryl Decongestant Elixir ... ■ 635
Benadryl Decongestant ... ■ 635
Benadryl Plus ... ■ 636
Benadryl Plus Nighttime ... ■ 637
Benylin Decongestant ... ■ 638
Brexin L.A. Capsules ... 2078
Bromfed Capsules (Timed Release) ... 1615
Bromfed Syrup ... ■ 628
Bromfed ... 1615
CoAdvil ... ■ 748
Allergy-Sinus Comtrex Multi-Symptom Allergy Sinus Formula Tablets & Caplets ... 746
Cough Formula Comtrex ... 746
Comtrex Multi-Symptom Cold Reliever Tablets/Caplets/Liqui-Gels/Liquid ... 745
Day-Night Comtrex ... 747
Non-Drowsy Comtrex ... 747
Congess ... 994
Congestac Caplets ... ■ 617
Contac Jr. Children's Cold Medicine ... ■ 712
Contac Nighttime Cold Medicine ... ■ 713
Contac Sinus Caplets Maximum Strength Non-Drowsy Formula ... ■ 710
Contac Sinus Tablets Maximum Strength Non-Drowsy Formula ... ■ 710
Deconamine ... 663
Deconsal II Tablets ... 559
Dimacol Caplets ... ■ 672
Dimetane-DX Cough Syrup ... 1858
Dorcol Children's Cough Syrup ... ■ 685
Dorcol Children's Decongestant Liquid ... ■ 685
Dorcol Children's Liquid Cold Formula ... ■ 686
Maximum Strength Dristan Decongestant/Analgesic Coated Caplets ... ■ 750
No Drowsiness Dristan Cold Nasal Decongestant/Analgesic Coated Caplets ... 2420
Dristan Sinus Caplets ... 2419
Sinus Excedrin Analgesic, Decongestant Tablets & Caplets ... ■ 533
Fedahist Gyrocaps ... 2145
Fedahist Timecaps ... 2145
Guaifed ... 1615
Guaifed Syrup ... ■ 629
Isoclor Expectorant ... 982
Isoclor Timesule Capsules ... ■ 561
Kronofed-A ... 970
Medi-Flu Caplet, Liquid ... ■ 640
Novafed A Capsules ... 1342
Novafed Capsules ... 1342
Novahistine DH ... 1342
Novahistine DMX ... ■ 595
Novahistine Expectorant ... 1343
Nucofed Capsules ... 2219
Nucofed Expectorant ... 2219
Nucofed Pediatric Expectorant ... 2220
Nucofed Syrup ... 2219
Ornex Caplets ... ■ 618
PediaCare Allergy Relief Formula Liquid ... 1362
PediaCare Cough-Cold Formula Liquid ... 1362
PediaCare Infants' Oral Decongestant Drops ... 1362
PediaCare Night Rest Cough-Cold Formula Liquid ... 1362
PediaCare 6-12 Cough-Cold Formula Chewable Tablets ... 1362
Robitussin-DAC Syrup ... 1875
Robitussin-PE ... ■ 677
Rondec ... 1975
Rondec-DM ... 1976
Rondec-TR Tablet ... 1975
Ru-Tuss DE Tablets ... 694
Ryna ... ■ 741
Seldane-D Extended-Release Tablets ... 1350
Sinarest ... ■ 562
Sine-Aid Maximum Strength Sinus Headache Caplets ... 1365
Sine-Aid Maximum Strength Sinus Headache Tablets ... 1365
Sine-Off Maximum Strength Allergy/Sinus Formula Caplets ... ■ 721
Sine-Off Maximum Strength No Drowsiness Formula Caplets ... ■ 722
Singlet Tablets ... ■ 598
Sinutab Maximum Strength ... ■ 641
Sinutab Maximum Strength Without Drowsiness Tablets & Caplets ... ■ 642
Sinutab Regular Strength Without Drowsiness Formula ... ■ 641
St. Joseph Nighttime Cold Medicine ... ■ 705
Sudafed Children's Liquid ... ■ 543
Sudafed Cough Syrup ... ■ 543
Sudafed Plus Liquid ... ■ 544
Sudafed Plus Tablets ... ■ 545
Sudafed Sinus Caplets ... ■ 545
Sudafed Sinus Tablets ... ■ 545
Sudafed Tablets, 30 mg ... ■ 544
Sudafed Tablets, Adult Strength, 60 mg ... ■ 544
Sudafed 12 Hour Capsules ... ■ 545
TheraFlu Flu and Cold Medicine ... ■ 687
Triaminic Nite Light ... ■ 689
Tylenol Allergy Sinus Medication Caplets and Gelcaps, Maximum Strength ... 1372
Children's Tylenol Cold Liquid Formula and Chewable Tablets ... 1368
Tylenol Cold & Flu Hot Medication, Packets ... 1369
Tylenol Cold & Flu No Drowsiness Hot Medication, Packets ... 1371
Tylenol Cold Medication Caplets and Tablets ... 1370
Tylenol Cold Medication No Drowsiness Formula Caplets ... 1370
Tylenol Cold Night Time Medication Liquid ... 1371

Tylenol Cough Medication Liquid with Decongestant, Maximum Strength ... 1372
Tylenol, Maximum Strength, Sinus Medication Gelcaps, Caplets and Tablets ... 1373
Ursinus Inlay-Tabs ... ⊞ 691
Vicks Children's NyQuil ... ⊞ 664
Vicks Daycare ... ⊞ 660
Vicks Formula 44D Decongestant Cough Medicine ... ⊞ 662
Vicks Formula 44M Multi-Symptom Cough Medicine ... ⊞ 662
Vicks NyQuil Nighttime Colds Medicine-Original & Cherry Flavor ... ⊞ 664
Vicks Pediatric Formula 44 Cough & Congestion Medicine ... ⊞ 663
Vicks Pediatric Formula 44m Multi-Symptom Cough & Cold Medicine ... ⊞ 663

Pseudoephedrine Sulfate (Potentiated). Products include:
Afrin Tablets ... ⊞ 693
Chlor-Trimeton Decongestant ... ⊞ 694
Disophrol Chronotab Sustained-Action Tablets ... ⊞ 698
Drixoral Antihistamine/Nasal Decongestant Syrup ... ⊞ 698
Drixoral Non-Drowsy Formula ... ⊞ 699
Drixoral Plus Extended-Release Tablets ... ⊞ 699
Drixoral Sinus ... ⊞ 700
Drixoral Sustained-Action Tablets ⊞ 698
Sinutab Allergy Formula Sustained Action Tablets ... ⊞ 640
Trinalin Repetabs Tablets ... 1170

Quazepam (May potentiate the CNS depressant effect). Products include:
Doral Tablets ... 2383

Scopolamine Hydrobromide (Atropine-like effects may become more pronounced). Products include:
Donnagel ... ⊞ 675
Donnagel-PG ... 1858
Donnatal ... 1858
Donnatal Extentabs ... 1859
Donnatal Tablets ... 1858
Donnazyme Tablets ... 1860
Isopto Hyoscine ... ◉ 222
Murocoll-2 Sterile Ophthalmic Solution ... ◉ 261
Ru-Tuss Tablets ... 693

Scopolamine Preparations (Atropine-like effects may become more pronounced). Products include:
Transderm Scōp Transdermal Therapeutic System ... 887

Secobarbital Sodium (May potentiate the CNS depressant effect). Products include:
Seconal Sodium Pulvules ... 1296

Selegiline Hydrochloride (Concomitant use is contraindicated; hyperpyretic crises or severe convulsive seizures may occur). Products include:
Eldepryl ... 2250

Sufentanil Citrate (May potentiate the CNS depressant effect). Products include:
Sufenta Injection ... 1147

Temazepam (May potentiate the CNS depressant effect). Products include:
Restoril Capsules ... 2023

Terbutaline Sulfate (Potentiated). Products include:
Brethaire Inhaler ... 1024
Brethine Ampuls ... 1026
Brethine Tablets ... 1026
Bricanyl Injection ... 1324
Bricanyl Tablets ... 1325

Thiamylal Sodium (May potentiate the CNS depressant effect). Products include:
Surital Ampules, Steri-Vials ... 1764

Thioridazine Hydrochloride (May potentiate the CNS depressant effect). Products include:
Mellaril ... 2011

Thiothixene (May potentiate the CNS depressant effect). Products include:
Navane Capsules and Concentrate 1954
Navane Intramuscular ... 1956

Thyroglobulin (Potential for cardiovascular toxicity). Products include:
Proloid Tablets ... 1761

Thyroid (Potential for cardiovascular toxicity). Products include:
S-P-T "Liquid" Capsules ... 995

Thyroxine (Potential for cardiovascular toxicity).
No products indexed under this heading.

Thyroxine Sodium (Potential for cardiovascular toxicity).
No products indexed under this heading.

Tranylcypromine Sulfate (Concomitant use is contraindicated; hyperpyretic crises or severe convulsive seizures may occur). Products include:
Parnate Tablets ... 2222

Triazolam (May potentiate the CNS depressant effect). Products include:
Halcion Tablets ... 2340

Tridihexethyl Chloride (Atropine-like effects may become more pronounced).
No products indexed under this heading.

Trifluoperazine Hydrochloride (May potentiate the CNS depressant effect). Products include:
Stelazine ... 2226

Trihexyphenidyl Hydrochloride (Atropine-like effects may become more pronounced). Products include:
Artane ... 1195

TOFRANIL-PM CAPSULES

(Imipramine Pamoate) ... 1041
May interact with anticholinergics, sympathomimetic aerosol bronchodilators, central nervous system depressants, monoamine oxidase inhibitors, thyroid preparations, and certain other agents. Compounds in these categories include:

Albuterol (Potentiation of catecholamine effects). Products include:
Proventil Inhalation Aerosol ... 2117
Ventolin Inhalation Aerosol and Refill ... 583

Albuterol Sulfate (Potentiation of catecholamine effects). Products include:
Proventil Repetabs Tablets ... 2120
Proventil Solutions for Inhalation 0.5% and 0.083% ... 2118
Proventil Syrup ... 2119
Proventil Tablets ... 2120
Ventolin ... 583

Alfentanil Hydrochloride (Potentiation of CNS depressants). Products include:
Alfenta Injection ... 1131

Alprazolam (Potentiation of CNS depressants). Products include:
Xanax Tablets ... 2367

Aprobarbital (Potentiation of CNS depressants). Products include:
Alurate Elixir ... 1883

Atropine Sulfate (Atropine-like effects may become more pronounced). Products include:
Arco-Lase Plus Tablets ... 607
Atropine Sulfate Sterile Ophthalmic Solution and S.O.P. Sterile Ophthalmic Ointment ... ◉ 239
Donnagel ... ⊞ 675
Donnagel-PG ... 1858
Donnatal ... 1858
Donnatal Extentabs ... 1859
Donnatal Tablets ... 1858
Donnazyme Tablets ... 1860
Isopto Atropine ... ◉ 218
Lomotil ... 2174
Motofen Tablets ... 836
Ru-Tuss Tablets ... 693
Urised Tablets ... 2396

Belladonna Alkaloids (Atropine-like effects may become more pronounced). Products include:
Bellergal-S Tablets ... 1998
Hyland's Bed Wetting Tablets ... ⊞ 728
Hyland's Teething Tablets ... ⊞ 728
Kinesed Tablets ... 2272

Benztropine Mesylate (Atropine-like effects may become more pronounced). Products include:
Cogentin ... 1435

Biperiden (Atropine-like effects may become more pronounced). Products include:
Akineton ... 1171

Buprenorphine (Potentiation of CNS depressants).
No products indexed under this heading.

Buspirone Hydrochloride (Potentiation of CNS depressants). Products include:
BuSpar ... 1401

Butabarbital (Potentiation of CNS depressants). Products include:
Pyridium Plus ... 1764

Butalbital (Potentiation of CNS depressants). Products include:
Esgic-Plus Tablets ... 1002
Esgic Tablets & Capsules ... 1001
Fioricet Tablets ... 2006
Fiorinal Capsules ... 2007
Fiorinal with Codeine Capsules ... 2008
Fiorinal Tablets ... 2007
Phrenilin ... 838
Sedapap Tablets 50 mg/650 mg .. 1360

Chlordiazepoxide (Potentiation of CNS depressants). Products include:
Libritabs Tablets ... 1930
Limbitrol ... 1933
Menrium Tablets ... 1934

Chlordiazepoxide Hydrochloride (Potentiation of CNS depressants). Products include:
Librax Capsules ... 1929
Librium Capsules ... 1931
Librium Injectable ... 1932

Chlorpromazine (Potentiation of CNS depressants). Products include:
Thorazine ... 2234

Chlorprothixene (Potentiation of CNS depressants). Products include:
Taractan Tablets ... 1920

Chlorprothixene Hydrochloride (Potentiation of CNS depressants). Products include:
Taractan ... 1920

Cimetidine (Plasma levels of imipramine elevated). Products include:
Tagamet Tablets ... 2228

Cimetidine Hydrochloride (Plasma levels of imipramine elevated). Products include:
Tagamet ... 2228

Clidinium Bromide (Atropine-like effects may become more pronounced). Products include:
Librax Capsules ... 1929
Quarzan Capsules ... 1937

Clorazepate Dipotassium (Potentiation of CNS depressants). Products include:
Tranxene ... 556

Codeine (Potentiation of CNS depressants). Products include:
Calcidrine Syrup ... 506

Codeine Phosphate (Potentiation of CNS depressants). Products include:
Actifed with Codeine Cough Syrup.. 752
Cheracol Cough Syrup ... 1853
Codimal PH Syrup ... 846
Dimetane-DC Cough Syrup ... 1857
Empirin with Codeine Phosphate Nos. 2, 3 & 4 ... 764
Fiorinal with Codeine Capsules ... 2008
Isoclor Expectorant ... 982
Naldecon CX Adult Liquid ... ⊞ 521
Novahistine DH ... 1342
Novahistine Expectorant ... 1343
Nucofed Capsules ... 2219
Nucofed Expectorant ... 2219
Nucofed Pediatric Expectorant ... 2220
Nucofed Syrup ... 2219
Phenaphen with Codeine Capsules 1865
Phenaphen-650 with Codeine Tablets ... 1866
Phenergan with Codeine ... 2497
Phenergan VC with Codeine ... 2501
Robitussin A-C Syrup ... 1875
Robitussin-DAC Syrup ... 1875
Ryna ... ⊞ 741
Soma Compound w/Codeine Tablets ... 2390
Triaminic Expectorant w/Codeine .. 1996
Tussi-Organidin Liquid ... 2391
Tylenol with Codeine ... 1381

Codeine Polistirex (Potentiation of CNS depressants).
No products indexed under this heading.

Dezocine (Potentiation of CNS depressants).

Diazepam (Potentiation of CNS depressants). Products include:
Valium Injectable ... 1937
Valium Tablets ... 1939
Valrelease Capsules ... 1923

Dicyclomine Hydrochloride (Atropine-like effects may become more pronounced). Products include:
Bentyl ... 1322

Dobutamine Hydrochloride (Potentiation of catecholamine effects). Products include:
Dobutrex Solution Vials ... 1259

Dopamine Hydrochloride (Potentiation of catecholamine effects). Products include:
Intropin Injection ... 930

Droperidol (Potentiation of CNS depressants). Products include:
Inapsine Injection ... 1140
Innovar Injection ... 1141

Enflurane (Potentiation of CNS depressants). Products include:
Ethrane ... 599

Ephedrine Hydrochloride (Potentiation of catecholamine effects). Products include:
Amesec ... ⊞ 682
Primatene Tablets-M Formula ... 2421
Primatene Tablets-P Formula ... 2421
Primatene Tablets-Regular Formula ... 2421
Quadrinal Tablets ... 1183
Quelidrine Syrup ... 556
Tedral SA ... 1765

Ephedrine Sulfate (Potentiation of catecholamine effects). Products include:
Bronkaid Tablets ... ⊞ 757
Bronkolixir ... ⊞ 761
Bronkotabs Tablets ... ⊞ 762
Marax Tablets & DF Syrup ... 1954
Pazo Hemorrhoid Ointment & Suppositories ... 752
Vicks Vatronol Nose Drops ... ⊞ 666

Ephedrine Tannate (Potentiation of catecholamine effects). Products include:
Rynatuss ... 2388

Epinephrine (Potentiation of catecholamine effects). Products include:
Ana-Kit Anaphylaxis Emergency Treatment Kit ... 1100
Bronkaid Mist ... ⊞ 757
EpiPen ... 843
Marcaine Hydrochloride 0.5% with Epinephrine 1:200,000 (as bitartrate) ... 958
Marcaine Hydrochloride with Epinephrine 1:200,000 ... 2055
Primatene Mist ... 2420
Sus-Phrine Injection ... 1006
Xylocaine with Epinephrine Injections ... 637

Epinephrine Bitartrate (Potentiation of catecholamine effects). Products include:
- AsthmaHaler Mist Epinephrine Bitartrate Bronchodilator ▣ 616
- Bronkaid Mist Suspension ▣ 757
- Primatene Mist Suspension 2421

Epinephrine Hydrochloride (Potentiation of catecholamine effects). Products include:
- Adrenalin Chloride Solution 1:100 & 1:1,000 1689
- Epifrin ◉ 244
- Glaucon ◉ 218

Estazolam (Potentiation of CNS depressants). Products include:
- ProSom Tablets 554

Ethchlorvynol (Potentiation of CNS depressants). Products include:
- Placidyl Capsules 553

Ethinamate (Potentiation of CNS depressants).
- No products indexed under this heading.

Ethopropazine Hydrochloride (Atropine-like effects may become more pronounced).

Fentanyl (Potentiation of CNS depressants). Products include:
- Duragesic Transdermal System 1133

Fentanyl Citrate (Potentiation of CNS depressants). Products include:
- Innovar Injection 1141
- Sublimaze Injection 1146

Fluphenazine Decanoate (Potentiation of CNS depressants). Products include:
- Prolixin Decanoate 1795

Fluphenazine Enanthate (Potentiation of CNS depressants). Products include:
- Prolixin Enanthate 1796

Fluphenazine Hydrochloride (Potentiation of CNS depressants). Products include:
- Prolixin Elixir 1793
- Prolixin Injection 1791
- Prolixin Oral Concentrate 1792
- Prolixin Tablets 1793

Flurazepam Hydrochloride (Potentiation of CNS depressants). Products include:
- Dalmane Capsules 1927

Furazolidone (Concomitant use is contraindicated). Products include:
- Furoxone 1855

Glutethimide (Potentiation of CNS depressants).
- No products indexed under this heading.

Glycopyrrolate (Atropine-like effects may become more pronounced). Products include:
- Robinul Forte Tablets 1873
- Robinul Injectable 1873
- Robinul Tablets 1873

Haloperidol (Potentiation of CNS depressants). Products include:
- Haldol Injection, Tablets and Concentrate 1373

Haloperidol Decanoate (Potentiation of CNS depressants). Products include:
- Haldol Decanoate 1375

Hydrocodone Bitartrate (Potentiation of CNS depressants). Products include:
- Anexsia 5/500 Tablets 2196
- Anexsia 7.5/650 Tablets 2197
- Azdōne Tablets 844
- Codiclear DH Syrup 845
- Codimal DH Syrup 846
- Damason-P 1356
- Hycodan Syrup, Tablets 927
- Hycomine Compound Tablets 929
- Hycomine Syrup 927
- Hycotuss Expectorant Syrup 930
- Hydrocet Capsules 835
- Lortab ASA Tablets 2414
- Lortab 2412
- Ru-Tuss with Hydrocodone 694
- Triaminic Expectorant DH 1995
- Vicodin Tablets 1187
- Vicodin ES Tablets 1189
- Zydone Capsules 941

Hydrocodone Polistirex (Potentiation of CNS depressants). Products include:
- Tussionex Extended-Release Suspension 988

Hydroxyzine Hydrochloride (Potentiation of CNS depressants). Products include:
- Atarax Tablets & Syrup 1941
- Marax Tablets & DF Syrup 1954
- Vistaril Intramuscular Solution 1970

Hyoscyamine (Atropine-like effects may become more pronounced). Products include:
- Cystospaz Tablets 2395
- Urised Tablets 2396

Hyoscyamine Sulfate (Atropine-like effects may become more pronounced). Products include:
- Arco-Lase Plus Tablets 607
- Cystospaz-M Capsules 2395
- Donnagel ▣ 675
- Donnagel-PG 1858
- Donnatal 1858
- Donnatal Extentabs 1859
- Donnatal Tablets 1858
- Donnazyme Tablets 1860
- Kutrase Capsules 2146
- Levsin/Levsinex 2147
- Ru-Tuss Tablets 693

Ipratropium Bromide (Atropine-like effects may become more pronounced). Products include:
- Atrovent Inhalation Aerosol 675

Isocarboxazid (Concomitant use is contraindicated). Products include:
- Marplan Tablets 1906

Isoflurane (Potentiation of CNS depressants). Products include:
- Forane 600

Isoproterenol Hydrochloride (Potentiation of catecholamine effects). Products include:
- Isuprel Hydrochloride Injection 1:5000 2050
- Isuprel Hydrochloride Mistometer 2051
- Isuprel Hydrochloride Solution 1:200 & 1:100 2052
- Norisodrine Aerotrol 540

Ketamine Hydrochloride (Potentiation of CNS depressants). Products include:
- Ketalar 1726

Levorphanol Tartrate (Potentiation of CNS depressants). Products include:
- Levo-Dromoran 1906

Levothyroxine Sodium (Possibility of cardiovascular toxicity). Products include:
- Levothroid Tablets 1003
- Levoxine Tablets 904
- Synthroid 695

Liothyronine Sodium (Possibility of cardiovascular toxicity). Products include:
- Cytomel Tablets 2203

Liotrix (Possibility of cardiovascular toxicity). Products include:
- Euthroid 1724

Lorazepam (Potentiation of CNS depressants). Products include:
- Ativan Injection 2432
- Ativan Tablets 2434

Loxapine Hydrochloride (Potentiation of CNS depressants). Products include:
- Loxitane 1213

Loxapine Succinate (Potentiation of CNS depressants). Products include:
- Loxitane Capsules 1213

Mepenzolate Bromide (Atropine-like effects may become more pronounced). Products include:
- Cantil Tablets 1326

Meperidine Hydrochloride (Potentiation of CNS depressants). Products include:
- Demerol 2047
- Mepergan Injection 2479

Mephobarbital (Potentiation of CNS depressants). Products include:
- Mebaral Tablets 2061

Meprobamate (Potentiation of CNS depressants). Products include:
- Deprol Tablets 2382
- Equagesic Tablets 2451
- Miltown Tablets 2386
- PMB 200 and PMB 400 2504

Mesoridazine (Potentiation of CNS depressants). Products include:
- Serentil 686

Metaproterenol Sulfate (Potentiation of catecholamine effects). Products include:
- Alupent 674
- Arm-a-Med Metaproterenol Sulfate Inhalation Solution, USP 617
- Metaprel Inhalation Aerosol Bronchodilator 2014
- Metaprel Inhalation Solution 2015
- Metaprel 2015
- Metaproterenol Sulfate Inhalation Solution, USP 912

Metaraminol Bitartrate (Potentiation of catecholamine effects). Products include:
- Aramine Injection 1424

Methadone Hydrochloride (Potentiation of CNS depressants). Products include:
- Dolophine Hydrochloride Ampoules & Vials 1260
- Dolophine Hydrochloride Tablets 1261
- Methadone Hydrochloride Diskets 1284
- Methadone Hydrochloride Oral Solution & Tablets 1987

Methohexital Sodium (Potentiation of CNS depressants). Products include:
- Brevital Sodium Vials 1248

Methoxamine Hydrochloride (Potentiation of catecholamine effects). Products include:
- Vasoxyl Injection 819

Methoxyflurane (Potentiation of CNS depressants).
- No products indexed under this heading.

Methylphenidate Hydrochloride (Metabolism of imipramine may be inhibited). Products include:
- Ritalin 880

Midazolam Hydrochloride (Potentiation of CNS depressants). Products include:
- Versed Injection 1924

Molindone Hydrochloride (Potentiation of CNS depressants). Products include:
- Moban Tablets & Concentrate 932

Morphine Sulfate (Potentiation of CNS depressants). Products include:
- Astramorph/PF Injection, USP (Preservative-Free) 618
- Duramorph 960
- Infumorph 200 and Infumorph 500 Sterile Solutions 962
- MS Contin Tablets 1814
- MSIR 1817
- Oramorph SR (Morphine Sulfate Sustained Release Tablets) 1988
- Roxanol 1991

Norepinephrine Bitartrate (Potentiation of catecholamine effects). Products include:
- Levophed Bitartrate Injection 2054

Opium Alkaloids (Potentiation of catecholamine effects). Products include:
- B & O No. 15A & No. 16A Supprettes 2395
- Pantopon Injectable 1911

Oxazepam (Potentiation of CNS depressants). Products include:
- Serax Capsules 2522
- Serax Tablets 2522

Oxybutynin Chloride (Atropine-like effects may become more pronounced). Products include:
- Ditropan 1332

Oxycodone Hydrochloride (Potentiation of CNS depressants). Products include:
- Percocet Tablets 950
- Percodan 951
- Roxicodone Tablets, Oral Solution & Intensol (Oxycodone) 1992
- Tylox Capsules 1382

Oxyphenonium Bromide (Atropine-like effects may become more pronounced).

Pentobarbital Sodium (Potentiation of CNS depressants). Products include:
- Nembutal Sodium Capsules 534
- Nembutal Sodium Solution 536
- Nembutal Sodium Suppositories 538

Perphenazine (Potentiation of CNS depressants). Products include:
- Etrafon 2087
- Triavil Tablets 1556
- Trilafon 2123

Phenelzine Sulfate (Concomitant use is contraindicated). Products include:
- Nardil 1742

Phenobarbital (Potentiation of CNS depressants). Products include:
- Arco-Lase Plus Tablets 607
- Bellergal-S Tablets 1998
- Bronkolixir ▣ 761
- Bronkotabs Tablets ▣ 762
- Donnatal 1858
- Donnatal Extentabs 1859
- Donnatal Tablets 1858
- Donnazyme Tablets 1860
- Kinesed Tablets 2272
- Phenobarbital Elixir and Tablets 1293
- Primatene Tablets-P Formula 2421
- Quadrinal Tablets 1183
- Tedral SA 1765

Phenylephrine Bitartrate (Potentiation of catecholamine effects).
- No products indexed under this heading.

Phenylephrine Hydrochloride (Potentiation of catecholamine effects). Products include:
- AK-Dilate Solution 2.5% and 10% ◉ 203
- Atrohist Sprinkle Capsules 558
- Cerose-DM 2443
- Codimal 846
- Comhist LA Capsules 1618
- Congespirin For Children Aspirin Free Chewable Cold Tablets 748
- Cyclomydril ◉ 216
- Deconsal Sprinkle Capsules 559
- Dimetane Decongestant ▣ 673
- Dristan Decongestant/Antihistamine/ Analgesic Coated Caplets ▣ 749
- Dristan Cold Nasal Decongestant/ Antihistamine/ Analgesic Coated Tablets 2419
- Dristan Advanced Formula Decongestant/Antihistamine/ Analgesic Tablets ▣ 749
- Dristan Nasal Spray, Menthol 2419
- Dristan Nasal Spray, Regular and Regular with Metered Pump 2419
- Entex Capsules 1623
- Entex Liquid 1623
- Sinus Excedrin Analgesic, Decongestant Tablets & Caplets 750
- Extendryl 994
- 4-Way Fast Acting Nasal Spray - Original Formula (regular & mentholated) & Metered Spray Pump (regular) 751

Hycomine Compound Tablets 929
Murocoll-2 Sterile Ophthalmic Solution .... ⊙ 261
Mydfrin 2.5% .... ⊙ 224
Naldecon Syrup, Tablets, Pediatric Drops and Pediatric Syrup 709
Neo-Synephrine Hydrochloride 1% Carpuject 2063
Neo-Synephrine Hydrochloride 1% Injection 2063
Neo-Synephrine Hydrochloride (Ophthalmic) 2064
Neo-Synephrine .... ▣ 759
Nōstril Nasal Decongestant .... ▣ 520
Novahistine Elixir .... ▣ 596
Phenergan VC 2500
Phenergan VC with Codeine 2501
Prefrin Liquifilm Vasoconstrictor and Lubricant Eye Drops .... ⊙ 254
Prefrin-A .... ⊙ 255
Quelidrine Syrup 556
Relief Vasoconstrictor and Lubricant Eye Drops .... ⊙ 256
Robitussin Night Relief .... ▣ 677
Ru-Tuss with Hydrocodone 694
Ru-Tuss Tablets 693
Vasosulf .... ⊙ 279
Vicks Sinex .... ▣ 665
Zincfrin .... ⊙ 230

Phenylephrine Tannate (Potentiation of catecholamine effects). Products include:
Rynatan 2387
Rynatuss 2388

Phenylpropanolamine Hydrochloride (Potentiation of catecholamine effects). Products include:
A.R.M. Allergy Relief Medicine Caplets .... ▣ 615
Acutrim .... ▣ 548
Allerest .... ▣ 559
BC Cold Powder .... ▣ 517
Cheracol Plus Head Cold/Cough Formula .... ▣ 667
Codimal Expectorant 846
Comtrex Multi-Symptom Cold Reliever Tablets/Caplets/Liqui-Gels/Liquid 745
Contac Continuous Action Decongestant/Antihistamine Capsules ▣ 710
Contac Maximum Strength Continuous Action Decongestant/Antihistamine Caplets .... ▣ 709
Contac Severe Cold and Flu Formula Caplets .... ▣ 711
Coricidin 'D' Decongestant Tablets .... ▣ 695
Coricidin Demilets Tablets for Children .... ▣ 696
Demazin Nasal Decongestant/Antihistamine Repetabs Tablets & Syrup .... ▣ 697
Dexatrim .... ▣ 733
Dimetane-DC Cough Syrup 1857
Dimetapp Elixir .... ▣ 673
Dimetapp DM Elixir .... ▣ 674
Dimetapp Extentabs .... ▣ 674
Dimetapp Plus Caplets .... ▣ 675
Dimetapp Tablets .... ▣ 675
Entex Capsules 1623
Entex LA Tablets 1623
Entex Liquid 1623
4-Way Cold Tablets 750
Hycomine Syrup 927
Naldecon CX Adult Liquid .... ▣ 521
Naldecon DX Adult Liquid .... ▣ 521
Naldecon DX Children's Syrup .... ▣ 522
Naldecon DX Pediatric Drops .... ▣ 522
Naldecon EX Children's Syrup .... ▣ 522
Naldecon EX Pediatric Drops .... ▣ 523
Naldecon Syrup, Tablets, Pediatric Drops and Pediatric Syrup 709
Nolamine Tablets 838
Nolex LA Tablets 838
Ornade Spansule Capsules 2221
Orthoxicol Cough Syrup .... ▣ 668
Propagest 839
Pyrroxate Capsules .... ▣ 669
Robitussin-CF .... ▣ 676
Ru-Tuss II Capsules 693
Ru-Tuss with Hydrocodone 694
Ru-Tuss Tablets 693
Sine-Off Sinus Medicine Tablets-Aspirin Formula .... ▣ 722
Sinulin 840
St. Joseph Cold Tablets for Children .... ▣ 704
Tavist-D Tablets 2035
Triaminic Allergy Tablets .... ▣ 688
Triaminic Chewables .... ▣ 688
Triaminic Cold Tablets .... ▣ 688
Triaminic Expectorant .... ▣ 688
Triaminic Expectorant w/Codeine 1996
Triaminic Expectorant DH 1995
Triaminic Oral Infant Drops 1996
Triaminic Syrup .... ▣ 689
Triaminic-12 Tablets .... ▣ 690
Triaminic-DM Syrup .... ▣ 689
Triaminicin Tablets .... ▣ 690
Triaminicol Multi-Symptom Cold Tablets .... ▣ 691
Triaminicol Multi-Symptom Relief ▣ 691
Tuss-Ornade Liquid 2242
Tuss-Ornade Spansule Capsules 2242
Tylenol Cold Medication, Effervescent Tablets 1369

Pirbuterol Acetate (Potentiation of catecholamine effects). Products include:
Maxair Inhaler 1311

Prazepam (Potentiation of CNS depressants). Products include:
Centrax 1693

Prochlorperazine (Potentiation of CNS depressants). Products include:
Compazine 2201

Procyclidine Hydrochloride (Atropine-like effects may become more pronounced). Products include:
Kemadrin Tablets 771

Promethazine Hydrochloride (Potentiation of CNS depressants). Products include:
Mepergan Injection 2479
Phenergan with Codeine 2497
Phenergan with Dextromethorphan 2499
Phenergan Injection 2493
Phenergan Suppositories 2496
Phenergan Syrup 2495
Phenergan Tablets 2496
Phenergan VC 2500
Phenergan VC with Codeine 2501

Propantheline Bromide (Atropine-like effects may become more pronounced). Products include:
Pro-Banthīne Tablets 2141

Propofol (Potentiation of CNS depressants). Products include:
Diprivan Injection 2267

Propoxyphene Hydrochloride (Potentiation of CNS depressants). Products include:
Darvon 1256
Wygesic Tablets 2540

Propoxyphene Napsylate (Potentiation of CNS depressants). Products include:
Darvon-N/Darvocet-N 1254

Pseudoephedrine Hydrochloride (Potentiation of catecholamine effects). Products include:
Actifed Capsules .... ▣ 539
Actifed Plus Caplets .... ▣ 539
Actifed Plus Tablets .... ▣ 540
Actifed with Codeine Cough Syrup 752
Actifed Syrup .... ▣ 540
Actifed Tablets .... ▣ 540
Actifed 12-Hour Capsules .... ▣ 539
Advil Cold & Sinus Caplets (formerly CoAdvil) 2416
Allerest .... ▣ 559
Anatuss LA Tablets 1359
Benadryl Decongestant Elixir .... ▣ 635
Benadryl Decongestant .... ▣ 635
Benadryl Plus .... ▣ 636
Benadryl Plus Nighttime .... ▣ 637
Benylin Decongestant .... ▣ 638
Brexin L.A. Capsules 2078
Bromfed Capsules (Timed Release) 1615
Bromfed Syrup .... ▣ 628
Bromfed 1615
CoAdvil .... ▣ 748
Allergy-Sinus Comtrex Multi-Symptom Allergy Sinus Formula Tablets & Caplets 746
Cough Formula Comtrex 746
Comtrex Multi-Symptom Cold Reliever Tablets/Caplets/Liqui-Gels/Liquid 745
Day-Night Comtrex 747
Non-Drowsy Comtrex 747
Congess 994
Congestac Caplets .... ▣ 617
Contac Jr. Children's Cold Medicine .... ▣ 712
Contac Nighttime Cold Medicine .... ▣ 713
Contac Sinus Caplets Maximum Strength Non-Drowsy Formula .... ▣ 710
Contac Sinus Tablets Maximum Strength Non-Drowsy Formula .... ▣ 710
Deconamine 663
Deconsal II Tablets 559
Dimacol Caplets .... ▣ 672
Dimetane-DX Cough Syrup 1858
Dorcol Children's Cough Syrup .... ▣ 685
Dorcol Children's Decongestant Liquid .... ▣ 685
Dorcol Children's Liquid Cold Formula .... ▣ 686
Maximum Strength Dristan Decongestant/Analgesic Coated Caplets .... ▣ 750
No Drowsiness Dristan Cold Nasal Decongestant/Analgesic Coated Caplets 2420
Dristan Sinus Caplets 2419
Sinus Excedrin Analgesic, Decongestant Tablets & Caplets .... ▣ 533
Fedahist Gyrocaps 2145
Fedahist Timecaps 2145
Guaifed 1615
Guaifed Syrup .... ▣ 629
Isoclor Expectorant 982
Isoclor Timesule Capsules .... ▣ 561
Kronofed-A 970
Medi-Flu Caplet, Liquid .... ▣ 640
Novafed A Capsules 1342
Novafed Capsules 1342
Novahistine DH 1342
Novahistine DMX .... ▣ 595
Novahistine Expectorant 1343
Nucofed Capsules 2219
Nucofed Expectorant 2219
Nucofed Pediatric Expectorant 2220
Nucofed Syrup 2219
Ornex Caplets .... ▣ 618
PediaCare Allergy Relief Formula Liquid 1362
PediaCare Cough-Cold Formula Liquid 1362
PediaCare Infants' Oral Decongestant Drops 1362
PediaCare Night Rest Cough-Cold Formula Liquid 1362
PediaCare 6-12 Cough-Cold Formula Chewable Tablets 1362
Robitussin-DAC Syrup 1875
Robitussin-PE .... ▣ 677
Rondec 1975
Rondec-DM 1976
Rondec-TR Tablet 1975
Ru-Tuss DE Tablets 694
Ryna .... ▣ 741
Seldane-D Extended-Release Tablets 1350
Sinarest .... ▣ 562
Sine-Aid Maximum Strength Sinus Headache Caplets 1365
Sine-Aid Maximum Strength Sinus Headache Tablets 1365
Sine-Off Maximum Strength Allergy/Sinus Formula Caplets .... ▣ 721
Sine-Off Maximum Strength No Drowsiness Formula Caplets .... ▣ 722
Singlet Tablets .... ▣ 598
Sinutab Maximum Strength .... ▣ 641
Sinutab Maximum Strength Without Drowsiness Tablets & Caplets .... ▣ 642
Sinutab Regular Strength Without Drowsiness Formula .... ▣ 641
St. Joseph Nighttime Cold Medicine .... ▣ 705
Sudafed Children's Liquid .... ▣ 543
Sudafed Cough Syrup .... ▣ 543
Sudafed Plus Liquid .... ▣ 544
Sudafed Plus Tablets .... ▣ 545
Sudafed Sinus Caplets .... ▣ 545
Sudafed Sinus Tablets .... ▣ 545
Sudafed Tablets, 30 mg .... ▣ 544
Sudafed Tablets, Adult Strength, 60 mg .... ▣ 544
Sudafed 12 Hour Capsules .... ▣ 545
TheraFlu Flu and Cold Medicine .... ▣ 687
Triaminic Nite Light .... ▣ 689
Tylenol Allergy Sinus Medication Caplets and Gelcaps, Maximum Strength 1372
Children's Tylenol Cold Liquid Formula and Chewable Tablets 1368
Tylenol Cold & Flu Hot Medication, Packets 1369
Tylenol Cold & Flu No Drowsiness Hot Medication, Packets 1371
Tylenol Cold Medication Caplets and Tablets 1370
Tylenol Cold Medication No Drowsiness Formula Caplets 1370
Tylenol Cold Night Time Medication Liquid 1371
Tylenol Cough Medication Liquid with Decongestant, Maximum Strength 1372
Tylenol, Maximum Strength, Sinus Medication Gelcaps, Caplets and Tablets 1373
Ursinus Inlay-Tabs .... ▣ 691
Vicks Children's NyQuil .... ▣ 664
Vicks Daycare .... ▣ 660
Vicks Formula 44D Decongestant Cough Medicine .... ▣ 662
Vicks Formula 44M Multi-Symptom Cough Medicine .... ▣ 662
Vicks NyQuil Nighttime Colds Medicine-Original & Cherry Flavor .... ▣ 664
Vicks Pediatric Formula 44 Cough & Congestion Medicine .... ▣ 663
Vicks Pediatric Formula 44m Multi-Symptom Cough & Cold Medicine .... ▣ 663

Pseudoephedrine Sulfate (Potentiation of catecholamine effects). Products include:
Afrin Tablets .... ▣ 693
Chlor-Trimeton Decongestant .... ▣ 694
Disophrol Chronotab Sustained-Action Tablets .... ▣ 698
Drixoral Antihistamine/Nasal Decongestant Syrup .... ▣ 698
Drixoral Non-Drowsy Formula .... ▣ 699
Drixoral Plus Extended-Release Tablets .... ▣ 699
Drixoral Sinus .... ▣ 700
Drixoral Sustained-Action Tablets ▣ 698
Sinutab Allergy Formula Sustained Action Tablets .... ▣ 640
Trinalin Repetabs Tablets 1170

Quazepam (Potentiation of CNS depressants). Products include:
Doral Tablets 2383

Scopolamine Hydrobromide (Atropine-like effects may become more pronounced). Products include:
Donnagel .... ▣ 675
Donnagel-PG 1858
Donnatal 1858
Donnatal Extentabs 1859
Donnatal Tablets 1858
Donnazyme Tablets 1860
Isopto Hyoscine .... ⊙ 222
Murocoll-2 Sterile Ophthalmic Solution .... ⊙ 261
Ru-Tuss Tablets 693

Scopolamine Preparations (Atropine-like effects may become more pronounced). Products include:
Transderm Scōp Transdermal Therapeutic System 887

Secobarbital Sodium (Potentiation of CNS depressants). Products include:
Seconal Sodium Pulvules 1296

Selegiline Hydrochloride (Concomitant use is contraindicated). Products include:
Eldepryl 2250

Sufentanil Citrate (Potentiation of CNS depressants). Products include:
Sufenta Injection 1147

Temazepam (Potentiation of CNS depressants). Products include:
Restoril Capsules 2023

Terbutaline Sulfate (Potentiation of catecholamine effects). Products include:
Brethaire Inhaler 1024
Brethine Ampuls 1026
Brethine Tablets 1026
Bricanyl Injection 1324
Bricanyl Tablets 1325

Thiamylal Sodium (Potentiation of CNS depressants). Products include:
Surital Ampoules, Steri-Vials 1764

Thioridazine Hydrochloride (Potentiation of CNS depressants). Products include:
- Mellaril 2011

Thiothixene (Potentiation of CNS depressants). Products include:
- Navane Capsules and Concentrate 1954
- Navane Intramuscular 1956

Thyroglobulin (Possibility of cardiovascular toxicity). Products include:
- Proloid Tablets 1761

Thyroid (Possibility of cardiovascular toxicity). Products include:
- S-P-T "Liquid" Capsules 995

Thyroxine (Possibility of cardiovascular toxicity).
- No products indexed under this heading.

Thyroxine Sodium (Possibility of cardiovascular toxicity).
- No products indexed under this heading.

Tranylcypromine Sulfate (Concomitant use is contraindicated). Products include:
- Parnate Tablets 2222

Triazolam (Potentiation of CNS depressants). Products include:
- Halcion Tablets 2340

Tridihexethyl Chloride (Atropine-like effects may become more pronounced).
- No products indexed under this heading.

Trifluoperazine Hydrochloride (Potentiation of CNS depressants). Products include:
- Stelazine 2226

Trihexyphenidyl Hydrochloride (Atropine-like effects may become more pronounced). Products include:
- Artane 1195

TOLECTIN (200, 400 AND 600 MG)
(Tolmetin Sodium) 1379
May interact with oral anticoagulants and certain other agents. Compounds in these categories include:

Dicumarol (Increased prothrombin time and bleeding). Products include:
- Dicumarol Tablets 516

Methotrexate Sodium (Reduced tubular secretion of methotrexate in an animal model). Products include:
- Methotrexate Tablets, Parenteral, LPF Parenteral 1217
- Rheumatrex Methotrexate Dose Pack 1234

Warfarin Sodium (Increased prothrombin time and bleeding). Products include:
- Coumadin Injection & Tablets 944
- Panwarfin Tablets 547

Food Interactions

Dairy products (Decreases total tolmetin bioavailability by 16%).

Meal, unspecified (Decreases total tolmetin bioavailability by 16%; reduces peak plasma concentrations by 50%).

TOLINASE TABLETS
(Tolazamide) 2365
May interact with non-steroidal anti-inflammatory agents, salicylates, sulfonamides, oral anticoagulants, beta blockers, monoamine oxidase inhibitors, thiazides, oral contraceptives, estrogens, corticosteroids, phenothiazines, thyroid preparations, calcium channel blockers, sympathomimetic aerosol bronchodilators, and certain other agents. Compounds in these categories include:

Acebutolol Hydrochloride (Hypoglycemic action potentiated). Products include:
- Sectral Capsules 2520

Albuterol (Hyperglycemia). Products include:
- Proventil Inhalation Aerosol 2117
- Ventolin Inhalation Aerosol and Refill 583

Albuterol Sulfate (Hyperglycemia). Products include:
- Proventil Repetabs Tablets 2120
- Proventil Solutions for Inhalation 0.5% and 0.083% 2118
- Proventil Syrup 2119
- Proventil Tablets 2120
- Ventolin 583

Aspirin (Hypoglycemic action potentiated). Products include:
- Alka-Seltzer Effervescent Antacid and Pain Reliever 1568
- Alka-Seltzer Extra Strength Effervescent Antacid and Pain Reliever 1570
- Alka-Seltzer (Flavored) Effervescent Antacid and Pain Reliever 1569
- Alka-Seltzer Plus Cold Medicine .... ■ 623
- Alka-Seltzer Plus Night-Time Cold Medicine .... ■ 623
- Alka Seltzer Plus Sinus Allergy Medicine .... ■ 624
- Anacin Coated Analgesic Caplets 2417
- Anacin Coated Analgesic Tablets 2417
- Anacin Maximum Strength Analgesic Coated Tablets 2417
- Maximum Strength Arthritis Pain Formula By the Makers of Anacin Analgesic Tablets and Caplets 2418
- Arthritis Pain Formula by the Makers of Anacin Analgesic Tablets and Caplets .... ■ 747
- Arthritis Strength BC Powder .... ■ 516
- Ascriptin A/D Caplets 1850
- Regular Strength Ascriptin Tablets 1850
- Azdone Tablets 844
- BC Powder .... ■ 517
- BC Cold Powder .... ■ 517
- Children's Bayer Chewable Aspirin .... ■ 564
- Genuine Bayer Aspirin Tablets & Caplets .... ■ 564
- Maximum Bayer Aspirin Tablets & Caplets .... ■ 566
- Bayer Plus Aspirin Tablets .... ■ 567
- Therapy Bayer Aspirin Caplets ...... ■ 568
- 8 Hour Bayer Timed-Release Aspirin .... ■ 566
- Arthritis Strength Bufferin Analgesic Caplets 744
- Extra Strength Bufferin Analgesic Tablets 745
- Bufferin Analgesic Tablets and Caplets 743
- Cama Arthritis Pain Reliever .... ■ 685
- Damason-P 1356
- Easprin 1719
- Ecotrin Enteric Coated Aspirin Maximum Strength Tablets and Caplets 2189
- Ecotrin Enteric Coated Aspirin Regular Strength Tablets and Caplets 2189
- Empirin Aspirin .... ■ 541
- Empirin with Codeine Phosphate Nos. 2, 3 & 4 764
- Equagesic Tablets 2451
- Excedrin Extra-Strength Analgesic Tablets & Caplets 749
- 4-Way Cold Tablets 750
- Fiorinal Capsules 2007
- Fiorinal with Codeine Capsules 2008
- Fiorinal Tablets 2007
- Lortab ASA Tablets 2414
- Momentum Muscular Backache Formula .... ■ 751
- Norgesic 1314
- Norwich Extra-Strength Aspirin ...... ■ 546
- Norwich Regular Strength Aspirin ■ 547
- P-A-C Analgesic Tablets .... ■ 669
- Percodan 951
- Robaxisal Tablets 1872
- Sine-Off Sinus Medicine Tablets-Aspirin Formula .... ■ 722
- Soma Compound w/Codeine Tablets 2390
- Soma Compound Tablets 2389
- St. Joseph Adult Chewable Aspirin (81 mg.) .... ■ 703
- Synalgos-DC Capsules 2525
- Talwin Compound 2072
- Ursinus Inlay-Tabs .... ■ 691
- Vanquish Analgesic Caplets .... ■ 574
- Zorprin Tablets 698

Atenolol (Hypoglycemic action potentiated). Products include:
- Tenoretic Tablets 1105
- Tenormin Tablets and I.V. Injection 1107

Bendroflumethiazide (Hyperglycemia; loss of control). Products include:
- Corzide Tablets 702
- Naturetin Tablets 1789
- Rauzide Tablets 1804

Bepridil Hydrochloride (Hyperglycemia). Products include:
- Vascor (200, 300 and 400 mg) Tablets 1383

Betamethasone Acetate (Hyperglycemia; loss of control). Products include:
- Celestone Soluspan Suspension 2081

Betamethasone Sodium Phosphate (Hyperglycemia; loss of control). Products include:
- Celestone Soluspan Suspension 2081

Betaxolol Hydrochloride (Hypoglycemic action potentiated). Products include:
- Betoptic Sterile Ophthalmic Solution 569
- Betoptic S Sterile Ophthalmic Suspension 570
- Kerlone Tablets 2172

Carteolol Hydrochloride (Hypoglycemic action potentiated). Products include:
- Cartrol Tablets 507

Chloramphenicol (Hypoglycemic action potentiated). Products include:
- AK-Chlor Sterile Ophthalmic Ointment & Solution .... ⊙ 201
- Chloromycetin Cream, 1% 1694
- Chloromycetin Hydrocortisone Ophthalmic 1694
- Chloromycetin Kapseals 1695
- Chloromycetin Ophthalmic Ointment, 1% 1696
- Chloromycetin Ophthalmic Solution 1696
- Chloromycetin Otic 1697
- Chloroptic S.O.P. .... ⊙ 243
- Chloroptic Sterile Ophthalmic Solution .... ⊙ 243
- Ophthochlor Ophthalmic Solution ⊙ 300
- Ophthocort .... ⊙ 301

Chloramphenicol Palmitate (Hypoglycemic action potentiated). Products include:
- Chloromycetin Palmitate, Oral Suspension 1697

Chloramphenicol Sodium Succinate (Hypoglycemic action potentiated). Products include:
- Chloromycetin Sodium Succinate 1698

Chlorothiazide (Hyperglycemia; loss of control). Products include:
- Aldoclor Tablets 1413
- Diupres Tablets 1461
- Diuril Oral 1464

Chlorothiazide Sodium (Hyperglycemia; loss of control). Products include:
- Diuril Sodium Intravenous 1463

Chlorotrianisene (Hyperglycemia; loss of control). Products include:
- TACE 12 and 25 mg 1353

Chlorpromazine (Hyperglycemia; loss of control). Products include:
- Thorazine 2234

Chlorpropamide (Severe hypoglycemia). Products include:
- Diabinese Tablets 1775

Choline Magnesium Trisalicylate (Severe hypoglycemia). Products include:
- Trilisate 1822

Cortisone Acetate (Hyperglycemia; loss of control). Products include:
- Cortone Acetate Sterile Suspension 1437
- Cortone Acetate Tablets 1439

Dexamethasone (Hyperglycemia; loss of control). Products include:
- AK-Trol Ointment & Suspension .... ⊙ 207
- Decadron Elixir 1445
- Decadron Tablets 1447
- Decaspray Topical Aerosol 1459
- Dexacidin .... ⊙ 272
- Maxidex Sterile Ophthalmic Suspension .... ⊙ 223
- Maxitrol Ophthalmic Ointment/Suspension .... ⊙ 223
- TobraDex Ophthalmic Suspension and Ointment .... ⊙ 228

Dexamethasone Acetate (Hyperglycemia; loss of control). Products include:
- Dalalone D.P. Injectable 999
- Decadron-LA Sterile Suspension 1457

Dexamethasone Sodium Phosphate (Hyperglycemia; loss of control). Products include:
- AK-Dex .... ⊙ 203
- Decadron Phosphate Respihaler 1454
- Decadron Phosphate Sterile Ophthalmic Ointment 1453
- Decadron Phosphate Sterile Ophthalmic Solution 1453
- Decadron Phosphate Topical Cream 1455
- Decadron Phosphate Turbinaire 1456
- Maxidex Sterile Ophthalmic Ointment .... ⊙ 222
- NeoDecadron Sterile Ophthalmic Ointment 1517
- NeoDecadron Sterile Ophthalmic Solution 1518
- NeoDecadron Topical Cream 1518

Diclofenac Sodium (Severe hypoglycemia). Products include:
- Voltaren Ophthalmic Sterile Ophthalmic Solution .... ⊙ 268
- Voltaren Tablets 1042

Dicumarol (Hypoglycemic action potentiated). Products include:
- Dicumarol Tablets 516

Dienestrol (Hyperglycemia; loss of control). Products include:
- Ortho Dienestrol Cream 1664

Diethylstilbestrol (Hyperglycemia; loss of control). Products include:
- Diethylstilbestrol Tablets 1258

Diflunisal (Hypoglycemic action potentiated). Products include:
- Dolobid Tablets 1465

Diltiazem Hydrochloride (Hyperglycemia). Products include:
- Cardizem Tablets-30 mg, 60 mg, 90 mg and 120 mg 1329
- Cardizem SR Capsules-60 mg, 90 mg and 120 mg 1327

Dobutamine Hydrochloride (Hyperglycemia). Products include:
- Dobutrex Solution Vials 1259

Dopamine Hydrochloride (Hyperglycemia). Products include:
- Intropin Injection 930

Ephedrine Hydrochloride (Hyperglycemia). Products include:
- Amesec .... ■ 682
- Primatene Tablets-M Formula 2421
- Primatene Tablets-P Formula 2421
- Primatene Tablets-Regular Formula 2421
- Quadrinal Tablets 1183
- Quelidrine Syrup 556
- Tedral SA 1765

Ephedrine Sulfate (Hyperglycemia). Products include:
- Bronkaid Tablets .... ■ 757
- Bronkolixir .... ■ 761
- Bronkotabs Tablets .... ■ 762
- Marax Tablets & DF Syrup 1954
- Pazo Hemorrhoid Ointment & Suppositories 752
- Vicks Vatronol Nose Drops .... ■ 666

Ephedrine Tannate (Hyperglycemia). Products include:
Rynatuss 2388

Epinephrine (Hyperglycemia). Products include:
Ana-Kit Anaphylaxis Emergency Treatment Kit 1100
Bronkaid Mist ▣ 757
EpiPen 843
Marcaine Hydrochloride 0.5% with Epinephrine 1:200,000 (as bitartrate) 958
Marcaine Hydrochloride with Epinephrine 1:200,000 2055
Primatene Mist 2420
Sus-Phrine Injection 1006
Xylocaine with Epinephrine Injections 637

Epinephrine Bitartrate (Hyperglycemia). Products include:
AsthmaHaler Mist Epinephrine Bitartrate Bronchodilator ▣ 616
Bronkaid Mist Suspension ▣ 757
Primatene Mist Suspension 2421

Epinephrine Hydrochloride (Hyperglycemia). Products include:
Adrenalin Chloride Solution 1:100 & 1:1,000 1689
Epifrin ⊙ 244
Glaucon ⊙ 218

Esmolol Hydrochloride (Hypoglycemic action potentiated). Products include:
Brevibloc Injection 942

Estradiol (Hyperglycemia; loss of control). Products include:
Emcyt Capsules 1161
Estrace 1385
Estrace Vaginal Cream 1388
Estraderm Transdermal System 866

Estrogens, Conjugated (Hyperglycemia; loss of control). Products include:
Mediatric Capsules 2476
PMB 200 and PMB 400 2504
Premarin Intravenous 2508
Premarin with Methyltestosterone 2515
Premarin Tablets 2510
Premarin Vaginal Cream 2512

Estrogens, Esterified (Hyperglycemia; loss of control). Products include:
Estratest 2245
Menrium Tablets 1934

Estropipate (Hyperglycemia; loss of control). Products include:
Ogen 540

Ethinyl Estradiol (Hyperglycemia; loss of control). Products include:
Brevicon 2304
Demulen 2161
Estinyl Tablets 2085
Jenest-28 Tablets 1636
Levlen/Tri-Levlen 665
Lo/Ovral Tablets 2471
Lo/Ovral-28 Tablets 2476
Loestrin 1728
Modicon 1667
Nordette-21 Tablets 2481
Nordette-28 Tablets 2483
Norethin 2133
Norinyl 2304
Norlestrin 1746
Ortho-Cyclen Tablets 1658
Ortho-Novum 1667
Ovcon 1391
Ovral Tablets 2490
Ovral-28 Tablets 2491
Levlen/Tri-Levlen 665
Tri-Norinyl 2304
Triphasil-21 Tablets 2527
Triphasil-28 Tablets 2532

Ethynodiol Diacetate (Hyperglycemia; loss of control). Products include:
Demulen 2161

Etodolac (Severe hypoglycemia). Products include:
Lodine Capsules 2468

Felodipine (Hyperglycemia). Products include:
Plendil Extended-Release Tablets 1526

Fenoprofen Calcium (Hypoglycemic action potentiated). Products include:
Nalfon Pulvules & Tablets 919

Fluphenazine Decanoate (Hyperglycemia; loss of control). Products include:
Prolixin Decanoate 1795

Fluphenazine Enanthate (Hyperglycemia; loss of control). Products include:
Prolixin Enanthate 1796

Fluphenazine Hydrochloride (Hyperglycemia; loss of control). Products include:
Prolixin Elixir 1793
Prolixin Injection 1791
Prolixin Oral Concentrate 1792
Prolixin Tablets 1793

Flurbiprofen (Severe hypoglycemia potentiated). Products include:
Ansaid Tablets 2319

Furazolidone (Hypoglycemic action potentiated). Products include:
Furoxone 1855

Glipizide (Severe hypoglycemia). Products include:
Glucotrol 1952

Glyburide (Severe hypoglycemia). Products include:
DiaBeta 1091
Micronase Tablets 2350

Hydrochlorothiazide (Hyperglycemia; loss of control). Products include:
Aldactazide 2150
Aldoril Tablets 1418
Apresazide Capsules 854
Apresoline-Esidrix Tablets 857
Capozide 2258
Dyazide Capsules 2208
Esidrix Tablets 863
Esimil Tablets 864
HydroDIURIL Tablets 1484
Hydropres Tablets 1485
Inderide Tablets 2463
Inderide LA Long Acting Capsules 2465
Lopressor HCT Tablets 1034
Maxzide 1215
Moduretic Tablets 1510
Normozide Tablets 2112
Oretic Tablets 544
Oreticyl 545
Prinzide Tablets 1540
Ser-Ap-Es Tablets 881
Serpasil-Esidrix Tablets 886
Timolide Tablets 1547
Trandate HCT Tablets 579
Vaseretic Tablets 1559
Zestoretic 2274

Hydrocortisone (Hyperglycemia; loss of control). Products include:
AK-Spore H.C. ⊙ 206
Bactine Hydrocortisone Anti-Itch Cream ▣ 625
CaldeCORT Anti-Itch Hydrocortisone Spray ▣ 560
Carmol HC Cream 1% 2296
Cortaid Spray ▣ 735
Cortenema 2244
Cortisporin Ointment 758
Cortisporin Ophthalmic Ointment Sterile 758
Cortisporin Ophthalmic Suspension Sterile 759
Cortisporin Otic Solution Sterile 760
Cortisporin Otic Suspension Sterile 760
Cortizone-5 Creme & Ointment ▣ 732
Dermolate Anti-Itch Cream ▣ 697
Eldecort Cream 1.0% 1113
Eldecort Cream 1.0% and 2.5% 1113
Fungoid HC Creme 1770
Hydrocortone Tablets 1482
Hytone 909
LazerSporin-C Solution 1770
Massengill Medicated Soft Cloth Towelettes 2192
Nutracort Cream & Lotion 1684
PediOtic Suspension Sterile 797
Synacort Creams 1%, 2.5% 2296
Vanoxide-HC Acne Lotion 911
Vioform-Hydrocortisone Cream and Mild Cream 889
Vioform-Hydrocortisone Ointment 889
VōSoL HC Otic Solution 2392
Vytone Cream 1% 911

Hydrocortisone Acetate (Hyperglycemia; loss of control). Products include:
Analpram-HC Rectal Cream 1% and 2.5% 970
Anusol-HC Cream 1690
Anusol-HC Suppositories 1691
Caldecort ▣ 560
Carmol HC Cream 1% 2296
Chloromycetin Hydrocortisone Ophthalmic 1694
Coly-Mycin S Otic w/Neomycin & Hydrocortisone 1708
Cortaid ▣ 735
Cortef Feminine Itch Cream ▣ 735
Corticaine ▣ 682
Cortifoam 1827
Cortisporin Cream 757
Epifoam 1828
Gynecort 5 Creme ▣ 556
Hydrocortone Acetate Sterile Suspension 1479
Lanacort 5 Creme and Ointment ▣ 557
Mantadil Cream 789
Ophthocort ⊙ 301
Orabase HCA Oral Paste 890
Pramosone Cream, Lotion & Ointment 971
ProctoCream-HC 1834
Proctofoam-HC 1835

Hydrocortisone Sodium Phosphate (Hyperglycemia; loss of control). Products include:
Hydrocortone Phosphate Injection, Sterile 1481

Hydrocortisone Sodium Succinate (Hyperglycemia; loss of control). Products include:
Solu-Cortef Sterile Powder 2361

Hydroflumethiazide (Hypoglycemic action potentiated; hyperglycemia; loss of control). Products include:
Diucardin Tablets 2450
Saluron 718
Salutensin/Salutensin-Demi 719

Ibuprofen (Hypoglycemic action potentiated). Products include:
Advil Cold & Sinus Caplets (formerly CoAdvil) 2416
Advil Ibuprofen Tablets and Caplets 2416
Children's Advil Suspension 2426
CoAdvil ▣ 748
Dristan Sinus Caplets 2419
Haltran Tablets ▣ 668
Ibuprofen ▣ 631
Medipren ibuprofen Caplets and Tablets 1362
Midol 200 Cramp Relief Formula ▣ 570
Motrin Tablets 2351
Motrin IB Caplets and Tablets ▣ 736
Nuprin Ibuprofen/Analgesic Tablets & Caplets 752
PediaProfen Suspension 1363
Rufen Tablets 691
Trendar Ibuprofen Tablets ▣ 756

Indomethacin (Hypoglycemic action potentiated). Products include:
Indocin 1487

Indomethacin Sodium Trihydrate (Hypoglycemic action potentiated). Products include:
Indocin I.V. 1490

Isocarboxazid (Hypoglycemic action potentiated). Products include:
Marplan Tablets 1906

Isoniazid (Hyperglycemia). Products include:
INH Tablets 868
Rifamate Capsules 1347

Isoproterenol Hydrochloride (Hyperglycemia). Products include:
Isuprel Hydrochloride Injection 1:5000 2050
Isuprel Hydrochloride Mistometer 2051
Isuprel Hydrochloride Solution 1:200 & 1:100 2052

Norisodrine Aerotrol 540

Isradipine (Hyperglycemia). Products include:
DynaCirc Capsules 2004

Ketoprofen (Hypoglycemic action potentiated). Products include:
Orudis Capsules 2488

Ketorolac Tromethamine (Severe hypoglycemia). Products include:
Toradol IM Injection 2302

Labetalol Hydrochloride (Hypoglycemic action potentiated). Products include:
Normodyne Injection 2108
Normodyne Tablets 2110
Normozide Tablets 2112
Trandate HCT Tablets 579
Trandate Injection 577
Trandate Tablets 579

Levonorgestrel (Hyperglycemia; loss of control). Products include:
Levlen/Tri-Levlen 665
Nordette-21 Tablets 2481
Nordette-28 Tablets 2483
Norplant System 2484
Levlen/Tri-Levlen 665
Triphasil-21 Tablets 2527
Triphasil-28 Tablets 2532

Levothyroxine Sodium (Hyperglycemia; loss of control). Products include:
Levothroid Tablets 1003
Levoxine Tablets 904
Synthroid 695

Liothyronine Sodium (Hyperglycemia; loss of control). Products include:
Cytomel Tablets 2203

Liotrix (Hyperglycemia; loss of control). Products include:
Euthroid 1724

Magnesium Salicylate (Hypoglycemic action potentiated). Products include:
Doan's - Extra-Strength Analgesic ▣ 549
Doan's - Regular Strength Analgesic ▣ 549
Mobigesic Analgesic Tablets ▣ 507

Meclofenamate Sodium (Hypoglycemic action potentiated). Products include:
Meclomen Capsules 1739

Mefenamic Acid (Hypoglycemic action potentiated). Products include:
Ponstel 1758

Mesoridazine (Hyperglycemia; loss of control). Products include:
Serentil 686

Mestranol (Hyperglycemia; loss of control). Products include:
Enovid 2161
Norethin 2133
Norinyl 2304
Ortho-Novum 1667

Metaproterenol Sulfate (Hyperglycemia). Products include:
Alupent 674
Arm-a-Med Metaproterenol Sulfate Inhalation Solution, USP 617
Metaprel Inhalation Aerosol Bronchodilator 2014
Metaprel Inhalation Solution 2015
Metaprel 2015
Metaproterenol Sulfate Inhalation Solution, USP 912

Metaraminol Bitartrate (Hyperglycemia). Products include:
Aramine Injection 1424

Methoxamine Hydrochloride (Hyperglycemia). Products include:
Vasoxyl Injection 819

Methyclothiazide (Hyperglycemia; loss of control). Products include:
Enduron Tablets 517
Enduronyl 518

(▣ Described in PDR For Nonprescription Drugs) (⊙ Described in PDR For Ophthalmology)

Methylprednisolone (Hyperglycemia; loss of control). Products include:
- Medrol 2348

Methylprednisolone Acetate (Hyperglycemia; loss of control). Products include:
- Depo-Medrol Sterile Aqueous Suspension 2334

Methylprednisolone Sodium Succinate (Hyperglycemia; loss of control). Products include:
- Solu-Medrol Sterile Powder 2363

Metoprolol Tartrate (Hypoglycemic action potentiated). Products include:
- Lopressor Ampuls 1032
- Lopressor HCT Tablets 1034
- Lopressor Tablets 1032

Miconazole (Hypoglycemia). Products include:
- Monistat I.V. 1143

Miconazole Nitrate (Hypoglycemia). Products include:
- Micatin .... ⊡ 632
- Micatin for Jock Itch .... ⊡ 633
- Monistat Dual-Pak 1657
- Monistat 3 Vaginal Suppositories 1657
- Monistat-Derm (miconazole nitrate) Cream 1679

Nadolol (Hypoglycemic action potentiated). Products include:
- Corgard Tablets 701
- Corzide Tablets 702

Naproxen (Hypoglycemic action potentiated). Products include:
- Naprosyn 2297

Naproxen Sodium (Hypoglycemic action potentiated). Products include:
- Anaprox and Anaprox DS Tablets 2288

Nicardipine Hydrochloride (Hyperglycemia). Products include:
- Cardene Capsules 2290

Nicotinic Acid (Hyperglycemia; loss of control). Products include:
- Niacor Tablets 2376
- Nicobid 1846
- Nicolar Tablets 1846
- Nicotinex Elixir .... ⊡ 563
- Slo-Niacin Tablets 2376

Nifedipine (Hyperglycemia). Products include:
- Adalat Capsules (10 mg and 20 mg) 1587
- Procardia Capsules 1781
- Procardia XL Tablets 1783

Nimodipine (Hyperglycemia). Products include:
- Nimotop Capsules 1607

Norepinephrine Bitartrate (Hyperglycemia). Products include:
- Levophed Bitartrate Injection 2054

Norethindrone (Hyperglycemia; loss of control). Products include:
- Brevicon 2304
- Jenest-28 Tablets 1636
- Micronor Tablets 1667
- Modicon 1667
- Norethin 2133
- Norinyl 2304
- Norlutin 1755
- Nor-Q D Tablets 2304
- Ortho-Novum 1667
- Ovcon 1391
- Tri-Norinyl 2304

Norethynodrel (Hyperglycemia; loss of control). Products include:
- Enovid 2161

Norgestimate (Hyperglycemia; loss of control). Products include:
- Ortho-Cyclen Tablets 1658

Norgestrel (Hyperglycemia; loss of control). Products include:
- Lo/Ovral Tablets 2471
- Lo/Ovral-28 Tablets 2476
- Ovral Tablets 2490
- Ovral-28 Tablets 2491
- Ovrette Tablets 2492

Penbutolol Sulfate (Hypoglycemic action potentiated). Products include:
- Levatol 1832

Perphenazine (Hyperglycemia; loss of control). Products include:
- Etrafon 2087
- Triavil Tablets 1556
- Trilafon 2123

Phenelzine Sulfate (Hypoglycemic action potentiated). Products include:
- Nardil 1742

Phenylbutazone (Hypoglycemic action potentiated). Products include:
- Butazolidin Capsules & Tablets 1027

Phenylephrine Bitartrate (Hyperglycemia).
- No products indexed under this heading.

Phenylephrine Hydrochloride (Hyperglycemia). Products include:
- AK-Dilate Solution 2.5% and 10% .... ⊙ 203
- Atrohist Sprinkle Capsules 558
- Cerose-DM 2443
- Codimal 846
- Comhist LA Capsules 1618
- Congespirin For Children Aspirin Free Chewable Cold Tablets 748
- Cyclomydril .... ⊙ 216
- Deconsal Sprinkle Capsules 559
- Dimetane Decongestant .... ⊡ 673
- Dristan Decongestant/Antihistamine/ Analgesic Coated Caplets .... ⊡ 749
- Dristan Cold Nasal Decongestant/ Antihistamine/ Analgesic Coated Tablets 2419
- Dristan Advanced Formula Decongestant/Antihistamine/ Analgesic Tablets .... ⊡ 749
- Dristan Nasal Spray, Menthol 2419
- Dristan Nasal Spray, Regular and Regular with Metered Pump 2419
- Entex Capsules 1623
- Entex Liquid 1623
- Sinus Excedrin Analgesic, Decongestant Tablets & Caplets 750
- Extendryl 994
- 4-Way Fast Acting Nasal Spray - Original Formula (regular & mentholated) & Metered Spray Pump (regular) 751
- Hycomine Compound Tablets 929
- Murocoll-2 Sterile Ophthalmic Solution .... ⊙ 261
- Mydfrin 2.5% .... ⊙ 224
- Naldecon Syrup, Tablets, Pediatric Drops and Pediatric Syrup 709
- Neo-Synephrine Hydrochloride 1% Carpuject 2063
- Neo-Synephrine Hydrochloride 1% Injection 2063
- Neo-Synephrine Hydrochloride (Ophthalmic) 2064
- Neo-Synephrine .... ⊡ 759
- Nōstril Nasal Decongestant .... ⊡ 520
- Novahistine Elixir .... ⊡ 596
- Phenergan VC 2500
- Phenergan VC with Codeine 2501
- Prefrin Liquifilm Vasoconstrictor and Lubricant Eye Drops .... ⊙ 254
- Prefrin-A .... ⊙ 255
- Quelidrine Syrup 556
- Relief Vasoconstrictor and Lubricant Eye Drops .... ⊙ 256
- Robitussin Night Relief .... ⊡ 677
- Ru-Tuss with Hydrocodone 694
- Ru-Tuss Tablets 693
- Vasosulf .... ⊙ 279
- Vicks Sinex .... ⊡ 665
- Zincfrin .... ⊙ 230

Phenylephrine Tannate (Hyperglycemia). Products include:
- Rynatan 2387
- Rynatuss 2388

Phenylpropanolamine Hydrochloride (Hyperglycemia). Products include:
- A.R.M. Allergy Relief Medicine Caplets .... ⊡ 615
- Acutrim .... ⊡ 548
- Allerest .... ⊡ 559
- BC Cold Powder .... ⊡ 517
- Cheracol Plus Head Cold/Cough Formula .... ⊡ 667
- Codimal Expectorant 846
- Comtrex Multi-Symptom Cold Reliever Tablets/Caplets/Liqui-Gels/Liquid 745
- Contac Continuous Action Decongestant/Antihistamine Capsules .... ⊡ 710
- Contac Maximum Strength Continuous Action Decongestant/ Antihistamine Caplets .... ⊡ 709
- Contac Severe Cold and Flu Formula Caplets .... ⊡ 711
- Coricidin 'D' Decongestant Tablets .... ⊡ 695
- Coricidin Demilets Tablets for Children .... ⊡ 696
- Demazin Nasal Decongestant/ Antihistamine Repetabs Tablets & Syrup .... ⊡ 697
- Dexatrim .... ⊡ 733
- Dimetane-DC Cough Syrup 1857
- Dimetapp Elixir .... ⊡ 673
- Dimetapp DM Elixir .... ⊡ 674
- Dimetapp Extentabs .... ⊡ 674
- Dimetapp Plus Caplets .... ⊡ 675
- Dimetapp Tablets .... ⊡ 675
- Entex Capsules 1623
- Entex LA Tablets 1623
- Entex Liquid 1623
- 4-Way Cold Tablets 750
- Hycomine Syrup 927
- Naldecon CX Adult Liquid .... ⊡ 521
- Naldecon DX Adult Liquid .... ⊡ 521
- Naldecon DX Children's Syrup .... ⊡ 522
- Naldecon DX Pediatric Drops .... ⊡ 522
- Naldecon EX Children's Syrup .... ⊡ 522
- Naldecon EX Pediatric Drops .... ⊡ 523
- Naldecon Syrup, Tablets, Pediatric Drops and Pediatric Syrup 709
- Nolamine Tablets 838
- Nolex LA Tablets 838
- Ornade Spansule Capsules 2221
- Orthoxicol Cough Syrup .... ⊡ 668
- Propagest 839
- Pyrroxate Capsules .... ⊡ 669
- Robitussin-CF .... ⊡ 676
- Ru-Tuss II Capsules 693
- Ru-Tuss with Hydrocodone 694
- Ru-Tuss Tablets 693
- Sine-Off Sinus Medicine Tablets-Aspirin Formula .... ⊡ 722
- Sinulin 840
- St. Joseph Cold Tablets for Children .... ⊡ 704
- Tavist-D Tablets 2035
- Triaminic Allergy Tablets .... ⊡ 688
- Triaminic Chewables .... ⊡ 688
- Triaminic Cold Tablets .... ⊡ 688
- Triaminic Expectorant .... ⊡ 688
- Triaminic Expectorant w/Codeine 1996
- Triaminic Expectorant DH 1995
- Triaminic Oral Infant Drops 1996
- Triaminic Syrup .... ⊡ 689
- Triaminic-12 Tablets .... ⊡ 690
- Triaminic-DM Syrup .... ⊡ 689
- Triaminicin Tablets .... ⊡ 690
- Triaminicol Multi-Symptom Cold Tablets .... ⊡ 691
- Triaminicol Multi-Symptom Relief ⊡ 691
- Tuss-Ornade Liquid 2242
- Tuss-Ornade Spansule Capsules 2242
- Tylenol Cold Medication, Effervescent Tablets 1369

Phenytoin (Hyperglycemia; loss of control). Products include:
- Dilantin Infatabs 1710
- Dilantin-30 Pediatric/Dilantin-125 Suspension 1713

Phenytoin Sodium (Hyperglycemia; loss of control). Products include:
- Dilantin Kapseals 1708
- Dilantin Parenteral 1712
- Dilantin with Phenobarbital Kapseals 1715

Pindolol (Hypoglycemic action potentiated). Products include:
- Visken Tablets 2036

Pirbuterol Acetate (Hyperglycemia). Products include:
- Maxair Inhaler 1311

Piroxicam (Hypoglycemic action potentiated). Products include:
- Feldene Capsules 1777

Polyestradiol Phosphate (Hyperglycemia; loss of control). Products include:
- Estradurin 2452

Polythiazide (Hyperglycemia; loss of control). Products include:
- Minizide Capsules 1779
- Renese Tablets 1785
- Renese-R Tablets 1786

Prednisolone Acetate (Hyperglycemia; loss of control). Products include:
- AK-Cide Sterile Ophthalmic Ointment & Suspension .... ⊙ 202
- Blephamide Liquifilm Sterile Ophthalmic Suspension 586
- Blephamide S.O.P. Sterile Ophthalmic Ointment 586
- Cetapred Ointment .... ⊙ 220
- ⅛% Econopred & 1% Econopred Plus .... ⊙ 217
- Isopto Cetapred Suspension .... ⊙ 220
- Metimyd .... ⊙ 306
- Poly-Pred Liquifilm .... ⊙ 250
- Pred Forte .... ⊙ 252
- Pred Mild .... ⊙ 254
- Pred-G Liquifilm Sterile Ophthalmic Suspension .... ⊙ 252
- Pred-G S.O.P. Sterile Ophthalmic Ointment .... ⊙ 253
- Vasocidin Ointment .... ⊙ 275

Prednisolone Sodium Phosphate (Hyperglycemia; loss of control). Products include:
- AK-Pred .... ⊙ 205
- Hydeltrasol Injection, Sterile 1476
- Inflamase .... ⊙ 274
- Pediapred Oral Liquid 987
- Vasocidin Ophthalmic Solution .... ⊙ 276

Prednisolone Tebutate (Hyperglycemia; loss of control). Products include:
- Hydeltra-T.B.A. Sterile Suspension 1478

Prednisone (Hyperglycemia; loss of control). Products include:
- Deltasone Tablets 2332

Probenecid (Hypoglycemic action potentiated). Products include:
- Benemid Tablets 1426
- ColBENEMID Tablets 1436
- Wycillin Injection and Probenecid Tablets 2539

Prochlorperazine (Hyperglycemia; loss of control). Products include:
- Compazine 2201

Promethazine Hydrochloride (Hyperglycemia; loss of control). Products include:
- Mepergan Injection 2479
- Phenergan with Codeine 2497
- Phenergan with Dextromethorphan 2499
- Phenergan Injection 2493
- Phenergan Suppositories 2496
- Phenergan Syrup 2495
- Phenergan Tablets 2496
- Phenergan VC 2500
- Phenergan VC with Codeine 2501

Propranolol Hydrochloride (Hypoglycemic action potentiated). Products include:
- Inderal 2459
- Inderal LA Long Acting Capsules 2461
- Inderide Tablets 2463
- Inderide LA Long Acting Capsules 2465

Pseudoephedrine Hydrochloride (Hyperglycemia). Products include:
- Actifed Capsules .... ⊡ 539
- Actifed Plus Caplets .... ⊡ 539
- Actifed Plus Tablets .... ⊡ 540
- Actifed with Codeine Cough Syrup 752
- Actifed Syrup .... ⊡ 540
- Actifed Tablets .... ⊡ 540
- Actifed 12-Hour Capsules .... ⊡ 539
- Advil Cold & Sinus Caplets (formerly CoAdvil) 2416
- Allerest .... ⊡ 559
- Anatuss LA Tablets 1359
- Benadryl Decongestant Elixir .... ⊡ 635
- Benadryl Decongestant .... ⊡ 635
- Benadryl Plus .... ⊡ 636
- Benadryl Plus Nighttime .... ⊡ 637
- Benylin Decongestant .... ⊡ 638

Brexin L.A. Capsules ... 2078
Bromfed Capsules (Timed Release) ... 1615
Bromfed Syrup ... ▣ 628
Bromfed ... 1615
CoAdvil ... ▣ 748
Allergy-Sinus Comtrex Multi-Symptom Allergy Sinus Formula Tablets & Caplets ... 746
Cough Formula Comtrex ... 746
Comtrex Multi-Symptom Cold Reliever Tablets/Caplets/Liqui-Gels/Liquid ... 745
Day-Night Comtrex ... 747
Non-Drowsy Comtrex ... 747
Congess ... 994
Congestac Caplets ... ▣ 617
Contac Jr. Children's Cold Medicine ... ▣ 712
Contac Nighttime Cold Medicine ... ▣ 713
Contac Sinus Caplets Maximum Strength Non-Drowsy Formula ... ▣ 710
Contac Sinus Tablets Maximum Strength Non-Drowsy Formula ... ▣ 710
Deconamine ... 663
Deconsal II Tablets ... 559
Dimacol Caplets ... ▣ 672
Dimetane-DX Cough Syrup ... 1858
Dorcol Children's Cough Syrup ... ▣ 685
Dorcol Children's Decongestant Liquid ... ▣ 685
Dorcol Children's Liquid Cold Formula ... ▣ 686
Maximum Strength Dristan Decongestant/Analgesic Coated Caplets ... ▣ 750
No Drowsiness Dristan Cold Nasal Decongestant/Analgesic Coated Caplets ... 2420
Dristan Sinus Caplets ... 2419
Sinus Excedrin Analgesic, Decongestant Tablets & Caplets ... ▣ 533
Fedahist Gyrocaps ... 2145
Fedahist Timecaps ... 2145
Guaifed ... 1615
Guaifed Syrup ... ▣ 629
Isoclor Expectorant ... 982
Isoclor Timesule Capsules ... ▣ 561
Kronofed-A ... 970
Medi-Flu Caplet, Liquid ... ▣ 640
Novafed A Capsules ... 1342
Novafed Capsules ... 1342
Novahistine DH ... 1342
Novahistine DMX ... ▣ 595
Novahistine Expectorant ... 1343
Nucofed Capsules ... 2219
Nucofed Expectorant ... 2219
Nucofed Pediatric Expectorant ... 2220
Nucofed Syrup ... 2219
Ornex Caplets ... ▣ 618
PediaCare Allergy Relief Formula Liquid ... 1362
PediaCare Cough-Cold Formula Liquid ... 1362
PediaCare Infants' Oral Decongestant Drops ... 1362
PediaCare Night Rest Cough-Cold Formula Liquid ... 1362
PediaCare 6-12 Cough-Cold Formula Chewable Tablets ... 1362
Robitussin-DAC Syrup ... 1875
Robitussin-PE ... ▣ 677
Rondec ... 1975
Rondec-DM ... 1976
Rondec-TR Tablet ... 1975
Ru-Tuss DE Tablets ... 694
Ryna ... ▣ 741
Seldane-D Extended-Release Tablets ... 1350
Sinarest ... ▣ 562
Sine-Aid Maximum Strength Sinus Headache Caplets ... 1365
Sine-Aid Maximum Strength Sinus Headache Tablets ... 1365
Sine-Off Maximum Strength Allergy/Sinus Formula Caplets ... ▣ 721
Sine-Off Maximum Strength No Drowsiness Formula Caplets ... ▣ 722
Singlet Tablets ... ▣ 598
Sinutab Maximum Strength ... ▣ 641
Sinutab Maximum Strength Without Drowsiness Tablets & Caplets ... ▣ 642
Sinutab Regular Strength Without Drowsiness Formula ... ▣ 641
St. Joseph Nighttime Cold Medicine ... ▣ 705
Sudafed Children's Liquid ... ▣ 543
Sudafed Cough Syrup ... ▣ 543
Sudafed Plus Liquid ... ▣ 544
Sudafed Plus Tablets ... ▣ 545
Sudafed Sinus Caplets ... ▣ 545
Sudafed Sinus Tablets ... ▣ 545
Sudafed Tablets, 30 mg ... ▣ 544
Sudafed Tablets, Adult Strength, 60 mg ... ▣ 544
Sudafed 12 Hour Capsules ... ▣ 545
TheraFlu Flu and Cold Medicine ... ▣ 687
Triaminic Nite Light ... ▣ 689
Tylenol Allergy Sinus Medication Caplets and Gelcaps, Maximum Strength ... 1372
Children's Tylenol Cold Liquid Formula and Chewable Tablets ... 1368
Tylenol Cold & Flu Hot Medication, Packets ... 1369
Tylenol Cold & Flu No Drowsiness Hot Medication, Packets ... 1371
Tylenol Cold Medication Caplets and Tablets ... 1370
Tylenol Cold Medication No Drowsiness Formula Caplets ... 1370
Tylenol Cold Night Time Medication Liquid ... 1371
Tylenol Cough Medication Liquid with Decongestant, Maximum Strength ... 1372
Tylenol, Maximum Strength, Sinus Medication Gelcaps, Caplets and Tablets ... 1373
Ursinus Inlay-Tabs ... ▣ 691
Vicks Children's NyQuil ... ▣ 664
Vicks Daycare ... ▣ 660
Vicks Formula 44D Decongestant Cough Medicine ... ▣ 662
Vicks Formula 44M Multi-Symptom Cough Medicine ... ▣ 662
Vicks NyQuil Nighttime Colds Medicine-Original & Cherry Flavor ... ▣ 664
Vicks Pediatric Formula 44 Cough & Congestion Medicine ... ▣ 663
Vicks Pediatric Formula 44m Multi-Symptom Cough & Cold Medicine ... ▣ 663

Pseudoephedrine Sulfate (Hyperglycemia). Products include:
Afrin Tablets ... ▣ 693
Chlor-Trimeton Decongestant ... ▣ 694
Disophrol Chronotab Sustained-Action Tablets ... ▣ 698
Drixoral Antihistamine/Nasal Decongestant Syrup ... ▣ 698
Drixoral Non-Drowsy Formula ... ▣ 699
Drixoral Plus Extended-Release Tablets ... ▣ 699
Drixoral Sinus ... ▣ 700
Drixoral Sustained-Action Tablets ▣ 698
Sinutab Allergy Formula Sustained Action Tablets ... ▣ 640
Trinalin Repetabs Tablets ... 1170

Quinestrol (Hyperglycemia; loss of control). Products include:
Estrovis ... 1721

Salsalate (Hypoglycemic action potentiated). Products include:
Disalcid ... 1310
Mono-Gesic Tablets ... 846
Salflex ... 839

Selegiline Hydrochloride (Hypoglycemic action potentiated). Products include:
Eldepryl ... 2250

Sulfamethizole (Hypoglycemic action potentiated). Products include:
Thiosulfil Forte Tablets ... 2526
Urobiotic-250 Capsules ... 1968

Sulfamethoxazole (Hypoglycemic action potentiated). Products include:
Azo Gantanol Tablets ... 1887
Bactrim DS Tablets ... 1891
Bactrim I.V. Infusion ... 1889
Bactrim ... 1891
Gantanol ... 1899
Septra ... 813
Septra I.V. Infusion ... 808
Septra I.V. Infusion ADD-Vantage Vials ... 810
Septra ... 813

Sulfasalazine (Hypoglycemic action potentiated). Products include:
Azulfidine Tablets, EN-tabs, Oral Suspension ... 1157

Sulfinpyrazone (Hypoglycemic action potentiated). Products include:
Anturane ... 853

Sulfisoxazole (Hypoglycemic action potentiated). Products include:
Azo Gantrisin Tablets ... 1888
Gantrisin Tablets ... 1901
Pediazole ... 1973

Sulfisoxazole Diolamine (Hypoglycemic action potentiated). Products include:
Gantrisin Ophthalmic Ointment/Solution ... 1900

Sulindac (Hypoglycemic action potentiated). Products include:
Clinoril Tablets ... 1433

Terbutaline Sulfate (Hyperglycemia). Products include:
Brethaire Inhaler ... 1024
Brethine Ampuls ... 1026
Brethine Tablets ... 1026
Bricanyl Injection ... 1324
Bricanyl Tablets ... 1325

Thioridazine Hydrochloride (Hyperglycemia; loss of control). Products include:
Mellaril ... 2011

Thyroglobulin (Hyperglycemia; loss of control). Products include:
Proloid Tablets ... 1761

Thyroid (Hyperglycemia; loss of control). Products include:
S-P-T "Liquid" Capsules ... 995

Thyroxine (Hyperglycemia; loss of control).
No products indexed under this heading.

Thyroxine Sodium (Hyperglycemia; loss of control).
No products indexed under this heading.

Timolol Maleate (Hypoglycemic action potentiated). Products include:
Blocadren Tablets ... 1429
Timolide Tablets ... 1547
Timoptic in Ocudose ... 1552
Timoptic Sterile Ophthalmic Solution ... 1550

Tolbutamide (Severe hypoglycemia). Products include:
Orinase Tablets ... 2354

Tolmetin Sodium (Severe hypoglycemia). Products include:
Tolectin (200, 400 and 600 mg) .. 1379

Tranylcypromine Sulfate (Severe hypoglycemia). Products include:
Parnate Tablets ... 2222

Triamcinolone (Hyperglycemia; loss of control).
No products indexed under this heading.

Triamcinolone Acetonide (Hyperglycemia; loss of control). Products include:
Aristocort A ... 1010
Azmacort Inhaler ... 1837
Kenalog Cream, Lotion & Ointment 2401
Kenalog-10 Injection ... 2402
Kenalog-40 Injection ... 2403
Kenalog in Orabase ... 604
Kenalog Spray ... 2401
Mycolog II Cream and Ointment ... 2407
Mytrex Cream & Ointment ... 2080
Nasacort Nasal Inhaler ... 1844

Triamcinolone Diacetate (Hyperglycemia; loss of control). Products include:
Aristocort Suspension ... 1008

Triamcinolone Hexacetonide (Hyperglycemia; loss of control). Products include:
Aristospan Suspension ... 1011

Trifluoperazine Hydrochloride (Hyperglycemia; loss of control). Products include:
Stelazine ... 2226

Verapamil Hydrochloride (Hyperglycemia). Products include:
Calan SR Caplets ... 2157
Calan Tablets ... 2155
Isoptin Injectable ... 1177
Isoptin Oral Tablets ... 1179
Isoptin SR Sustained Release Tablets ... 1181
Verelan Capsules ... 1243
Verelan Capsules ... 2535

Warfarin Sodium (Hypoglycemic action potentiated). Products include:
Coumadin Injection & Tablets ... 944
Panwarfin Tablets ... 547

TONOCARD TABLETS
(Tocainide Hydrochloride) ... 1554
May interact with:

Lidocaine Hydrochloride (Increased incidence of adverse reactions such as seizure). Products include:
Anestacon Solution ... 2394
Bactine Antiseptic/Anesthetic First Aid Spray ... ▣ 624
Decadron Phosphate with Xylocaine Injection, Sterile ... 1451
Xylocaine Injections ... 637
Xylocaine Injections for Ventricular Arrhythmias ... 639
Xylocaine 2% Jelly ... 643
4% Xylocaine-MPF Sterile Solution 641
Xylocaine 2% Viscous Solution ... 646

Metoprolol Tartrate (Additive effects on wedge pressure and cardiac index). Products include:
Lopressor Ampuls ... 1032
Lopressor HCT Tablets ... 1034
Lopressor Tablets ... 1032

TOPICORT CREAM
(Desoximetasone) ... 1098
No interactions described in labeling.

TOPICORT GEL
(Desoximetasone) ... 1098
No interactions described in labeling.

TOPICORT LP
(Desoximetasone) ... 1098
No interactions described in labeling.

TOPICORT OINTMENT
(Desoximetasone) ... 1098
No interactions described in labeling.

TOPICYCLINE FOR TOPICAL SOLUTION
(Tetracycline Hydrochloride) ... 1856
No interactions described in labeling.

TORADOL IM INJECTION
(Ketorolac Tromethamine) ... 2302
May interact with diuretics, salicylates, non-steroidal anti-inflammatory agents, and certain other agents. Compounds in these categories include:

Alcohol (Increased risk of peptic ulceration and bleeding).

Amiloride Hydrochloride (Renal toxicity; may precipitate overt renal failure). Products include:
Midamor Tablets ... 1508
Moduretic Tablets ... 1510

Aspirin (Protein-binding is affected by salicylate). Products include:
Alka-Seltzer Effervescent Antacid and Pain Reliever ... 1568
Alka-Seltzer Extra Strength Effervescent Antacid and Pain Reliever ... 1570
Alka-Seltzer (Flavored) Effervescent Antacid and Pain Reliever ... 1569
Alka-Seltzer Plus Cold Medicine ... ▣ 623
Alka-Seltzer Plus Night-Time Cold Medicine ... ▣ 623
Alka Seltzer Plus Sinus Allergy Medicine ... ▣ 624
Anacin Coated Analgesic Caplets ... 2417

Anacin Coated Analgesic Tablets 2417
Anacin Maximum Strength Analgesic Coated Tablets 2417
Maximum Strength Arthritis Pain Formula By the Makers of Anacin Analgesic Tablets and Caplets 2418
Arthritis Pain Formula by the Makers of Anacin Analgesic Tablets and Caplets .... ▣ 747
Arthritis Strength BC Powder .... ▣ 516
Ascriptin A/D Caplets 1850
Regular Strength Ascriptin Tablets 1850
Azdōne Tablets 844
BC Powder .... ▣ 517
BC Cold Powder .... ▣ 517
Children's Bayer Chewable Aspirin .... ▣ 564
Genuine Bayer Aspirin Tablets & Caplets .... ▣ 564
Maximum Bayer Aspirin Tablets & Caplets .... ▣ 566
Bayer Plus Aspirin Tablets .... ▣ 567
Therapy Bayer Aspirin Caplets .... ▣ 568
8 Hour Bayer Timed-Release Aspirin .... ▣ 566
Arthritis Strength Bufferin Analgesic Caplets 744
Extra Strength Bufferin Analgesic Tablets 745
Bufferin Analgesic Tablets and Caplets 743
Cama Arthritis Pain Reliever .... ▣ 685
Damason-P 1356
Easprin 1719
Ecotrin Enteric Coated Aspirin Maximum Strength Tablets and Caplets 2189
Ecotrin Enteric Coated Aspirin Regular Strength Tablets and Caplets 2189
Empirin Aspirin .... ▣ 541
Empirin with Codeine Phosphate Nos. 2, 3 & 4 764
Equagesic Tablets 2451
Excedrin Extra-Strength Analgesic Tablets & Caplets 749
4-Way Cold Tablets 750
Fiorinal Capsules 2007
Fiorinal with Codeine Capsules 2008
Fiorinal Tablets 2007
Lortab ASA Tablets 2414
Momentum Muscular Backache Formula .... ▣ 751
Norgesic 1314
Norwich Extra-Strength Aspirin .... ▣ 546
Norwich Regular Strength Aspirin ▣ 547
P-A-C Analgesic Tablets .... ▣ 669
Percodan 951
Robaxisal Tablets 1872
Sine-Off Sinus Medicine Tablets-Aspirin Formula .... ▣ 722
Soma Compound w/Codeine Tablets 2390
Soma Compound Tablets 2389
St. Joseph Adult Chewable Aspirin (81 mg.) .... ▣ 703
Synalgos-DC Capsules 2525
Talwin Compound 2072
Ursinus Inlay-Tabs .... ▣ 691
Vanquish Analgesic Caplets .... ▣ 574
Zorprin Tablets 698

Bendroflumethiazide (Renal toxicity; may precipitate overt renal failure). Products include:
Corzide Tablets 702
Naturetin Tablets 1789
Rauzide Tablets 1804

Bumetanide (Renal toxicity; may precipitate overt renal failure). Products include:
Bumex 1895

Chlorothiazide (Renal toxicity; may precipitate overt renal failure). Products include:
Aldoclor Tablets 1413
Diupres Tablets 1461
Diuril Oral 1464

Chlorothiazide Sodium (Renal toxicity; may precipitate overt renal failure). Products include:
Diuril Sodium Intravenous 1463

Chlorthalidone (Renal toxicity; may precipitate overt renal failure). Products include:
Combipres Tablets 678
Tenoretic Tablets 1105
Thalitone Tablets 687

Choline Magnesium Trisalicylate (Protein-binding is affected by salicylate). Products include:
Trilisate 1822

Diclofenac Sodium (Potential for additive side effects). Products include:
Voltaren Ophthalmic Sterile Ophthalmic Solution .... ◉ 268
Voltaren Tablets 1042

Diflunisal (Protein-binding is affected by salicylate). Products include:
Dolobid Tablets 1465

Ethacrynic Acid (Renal toxicity; may precipitate overt renal failure). Products include:
Edecrin Tablets 1468

Etodolac (Potential for additive side effects). Products include:
Lodine Capsules 2468

Fenoprofen Calcium (Potential for additive side effects). Products include:
Nalfon Pulvules & Tablets 919

Flurbiprofen (Potential for additive side effects). Products include:
Ansaid Tablets 2319

Furosemide (Renal toxicity; may precipitate overt renal failure). Products include:
Lasix 1093

Hydrochlorothiazide (Renal toxicity; may precipitate overt renal failure). Products include:
Aldactazide 2150
Aldoril Tablets 1418
Apresazide Capsules 854
Apresoline-Esidrix Tablets 857
Capozide 2258
Dyazide Capsules 2208
Esidrix Tablets 863
Esimil Tablets 864
HydroDIURIL Tablets 1484
Hydropres Tablets 1485
Inderide Tablets 2463
Inderide LA Long Acting Capsules .. 2465
Lopressor HCT Tablets 1034
Maxzide 1215
Moduretic Tablets 1510
Normozide Tablets 2112
Oretic Tablets 544
Oreticyl 545
Prinzide Tablets 1540
Ser-Ap-Es Tablets 881
Serpasil-Esidrix Tablets 886
Timolide Tablets 1547
Trandate HCT Tablets 579
Vaseretic Tablets 1559
Zestoretic 2274

Hydroflumethiazide (Renal toxicity; may precipitate overt renal failure). Products include:
Diucardin Tablets 2450
Saluron 718
Salutensin/Salutensin-Demi 719

Ibuprofen (Potential for additive side effects). Products include:
Advil Cold & Sinus Caplets (formerly CoAdvil) 2416
Advil Ibuprofen Tablets and Caplets 2416
Children's Advil Suspension 2426
CoAdvil .... ▣ 748
Dristan Sinus Caplets 2419
Haltran Tablets .... ▣ 668
Ibuprofen .... ▣ 631
Medipren ibuprofen Caplets and Tablets 1362
Midol 200 Cramp Relief Formula .. ▣ 570
Motrin Tablets 2351
Motrin IB Caplets and Tablets .... ▣ 736
Nuprin Ibuprofen/Analgesic Tablets & Caplets 752
PediaProfen Suspension 1363
Rufen Tablets 691
Trendar Ibuprofen Tablets .... ▣ 756

Indapamide (Renal toxicity; may precipitate overt renal failure). Products include:
Lozol Tablets 1843

Indomethacin (Potential for additive side effects). Products include:
Indocin 1487

Indomethacin Sodium Trihydrate (Potential for additive side effects). Products include:
Indocin I.V. 1490

Ketoprofen (Potential for additive side effects). Products include:
Orudis Capsules 2488

Magnesium Salicylate (Protein-binding is affected by salicylate). Products include:
Doan's - Extra-Strength Analgesic ▣ 549
Doan's - Regular Strength Analgesic .... ▣ 549
Mobigesic Analgesic Tablets .... ▣ 507

Meclofenamate Sodium (Potential for additive side effects). Products include:
Meclomen Capsules 1739

Mefenamic Acid (Potential for additive side effects). Products include:
Ponstel 1758

Methyclothiazide (Renal toxicity; may precipitate overt renal failure). Products include:
Enduron Tablets 517
Enduronyl 518

Metolazone (Renal toxicity; may precipitate overt renal failure). Products include:
Diulo 2129
Mykrox ½ mg Tablets 984
Zaroxolyn Tablets 989

Naproxen (Potential for additive side effects). Products include:
Naprosyn 2297

Naproxen Sodium (Potential for additive side effects). Products include:
Anaprox and Anaprox DS Tablets 2288

Phenylbutazone (Potential for additive side effects). Products include:
Butazolidin Capsules & Tablets 1027

Piroxicam (Potential for additive side effects). Products include:
Feldene Capsules 1777

Polythiazide (Renal toxicity; may precipitate overt renal failure). Products include:
Minizide Capsules 1779
Renese Tablets 1785
Renese-R Tablets 1786

Salsalate (Protein-binding is affected by salicylate). Products include:
Disalcid 1310
Mono-Gesic Tablets 846
Salflex 839

Spironolactone (Renal toxicity; may precipitate overt renal failure). Products include:
Aldactazide 2150
Aldactone 2152

Sulindac (Potential for additive side effects). Products include:
Clinoril Tablets 1433

Tolmetin Sodium (Potential for additive side effects). Products include:
Tolectin (200, 400 and 600 mg) .. 1379

Triamterene (Renal toxicity; may precipitate overt renal failure). Products include:
Dyazide Capsules 2208
Dyrenium Capsules 2210
Maxzide 1215

TORECAN INJECTION (THIETHYLPERAZINE MALATE)
(Thiethylperazine Maleate) 1993
May interact with central nervous system depressants, belladona products, and certain other agents. Compounds in these categories include:

Alcohol (Potentiated).

Alfentanil Hydrochloride (Potentiated). Products include:
Alfenta Injection 1131

Alprazolam (Potentiated). Products include:
Xanax Tablets 2367

Aprobarbital (Potentiated). Products include:
Alurate Elixir 1883

Atropine Sulfate (Potentiated). Products include:
Arco-Lase Plus Tablets 607
Atropine Sulfate Sterile Ophthalmic Solution and S.O.P. Sterile Ophthalmic Ointment .... ◉ 239
Donnagel .... ▣ 675
Donnagel-PG 1858
Donnatal 1858
Donnatal Extentabs 1859
Donnatal Tablets 1858
Donnazyme Tablets 1860
Isopto Atropine .... ◉ 218
Lomotil 2174
Motofen Tablets 836
Ru-Tuss Tablets 693
Urised Tablets 2396

Belladonna Alkaloids (Potentiated). Products include:
Bellergal-S Tablets 1998
Hyland's Bed Wetting Tablets .... ▣ 728
Hyland's Teething Tablets .... ▣ 728
Kinesed Tablets 2272

Buprenorphine (Potentiated).
No products indexed under this heading.

Buspirone Hydrochloride (Potentiated). Products include:
BuSpar 1401

Butabarbital (Potentiated). Products include:
Pyridium Plus 1764

Butalbital (Potentiated). Products include:
Esgic-Plus Tablets 1002
Esgic Tablets & Capsules 1001
Fioricet Tablets 2006
Fiorinal Capsules 2007
Fiorinal with Codeine Capsules 2008
Fiorinal Tablets 2007
Phrenilin 838
Sedapap Tablets 50 mg/650 mg .. 1360

Chlordiazepoxide (Potentiated). Products include:
Libritabs Tablets 1930
Limbitrol 1933
Menrium Tablets 1934

Chlordiazepoxide Hydrochloride (Potentiated). Products include:
Librax Capsules 1929
Librium Capsules 1931
Librium Injectable 1932

Chlorpromazine (Potentiated). Products include:
Thorazine 2234

Chlorprothixene (Potentiated). Products include:
Taractan Tablets 1920

Chlorprothixene Hydrochloride (Potentiated). Products include:
Taractan 1920

Clorazepate Dipotassium (Potentiated). Products include:
Tranxene 556

Codeine (Potentiated). Products include:
Calcidrine Syrup 506

Codeine Phosphate (Potentiated). Products include:
Actifed with Codeine Cough Syrup .. 752
Cheracol Cough Syrup 1853
Codimal PH Syrup 846
Dimetane-DC Cough Syrup 1857
Empirin with Codeine Phosphate Nos. 2, 3 & 4 764
Fiorinal with Codeine Capsules 2008
Isoclor Expectorant 982
Naldecon CX Adult Liquid .... ▣ 521
Novahistine DH 1342

Novahistine Expectorant ... 1343
Nucofed Capsules ... 2219
Nucofed Expectorant ... 2219
Nucofed Pediatric Expectorant ... 2220
Nucofed Syrup ... 2219
Phenaphen with Codeine Capsules 1865
Phenaphen-650 with Codeine Tablets ... 1866
Phenergan with Codeine ... 2497
Phenergan VC with Codeine ... 2501
Robitussin A-C Syrup ... 1875
Robitussin-DAC Syrup ... 1875
Ryna ... ▣ 741
Soma Compound w/Codeine Tablets ... 2390
Triaminic Expectorant w/Codeine .. 1996
Tussi-Organidin Liquid ... 2391
Tylenol with Codeine ... 1381

Codeine Polistirex (Potentiated).
No products indexed under this heading.

Dezocine (Potentiated).

Diazepam (Potentiated). Products include:
Valium Injectable ... 1937
Valium Tablets ... 1939
Valrelease Capsules ... 1923

Droperidol (Potentiated). Products include:
Inapsine Injection ... 1140
Innovar Injection ... 1141

Enflurane (Potentiated). Products include:
Ethrane ... 599

Epinephrine Hydrochloride (Reversed epinephrine effect). Products include:
Adrenalin Chloride Solution 1:100 & 1:1,000 ... 1689
Epifrin ... ⊙ 244
Glaucon ... ⊙ 218

Estazolam (Potentiated). Products include:
ProSom Tablets ... 554

Ethchlorvynol (Potentiated). Products include:
Placidyl Capsules ... 553

Ethinamate (Potentiated).
No products indexed under this heading.

Fentanyl (Potentiated). Products include:
Duragesic Transdermal System ... 1133

Fentanyl Citrate (Potentiated). Products include:
Innovar Injection ... 1141
Sublimaze Injection ... 1146

Fluphenazine Decanoate (Potentiated). Products include:
Prolixin Decanoate ... 1795

Fluphenazine Enanthate (Potentiated). Products include:
Prolixin Enanthate ... 1796

Fluphenazine Hydrochloride (Potentiated). Products include:
Prolixin Elixir ... 1793
Prolixin Injection ... 1791
Prolixin Oral Concentrate ... 1792
Prolixin Tablets ... 1793

Flurazepam Hydrochloride (Potentiated). Products include:
Dalmane Capsules ... 1927

Glutethimide (Potentiated).
No products indexed under this heading.

Haloperidol (Potentiated). Products include:
Haldol Injection, Tablets and Concentrate ... 1373

Haloperidol Decanoate (Potentiated). Products include:
Haldol Decanoate ... 1375

Hydrocodone Bitartrate (Potentiated). Products include:
Anexsia 5/500 Tablets ... 2196
Anexsia 7.5/650 Tablets ... 2197
Azdōne Tablets ... 844
Codiclear DH Syrup ... 845
Codimal DH Syrup ... 846
Damason-P ... 1356
Hycodan Syrup, Tablets ... 927
Hycomine Compound Tablets ... 929
Hycomine Syrup ... 927
Hycotuss Expectorant Syrup ... 930
Hydrocet Capsules ... 835
Lortab ASA Tablets ... 2414
Lortab ... 2412
Ru-Tuss with Hydrocodone ... 694
Triaminic Expectorant DH ... 1995
Vicodin Tablets ... 1187
Vicodin ES Tablets ... 1189
Zydone Capsules ... 941

Hydrocodone Polistirex (Potentiated). Products include:
Tussionex Extended-Release Suspension ... 988

Hydroxyzine Hydrochloride (Potentiated). Products include:
Atarax Tablets & Syrup ... 1941
Marax Tablets & DF Syrup ... 1954
Vistaril Intramuscular Solution ... 1970

Hyoscyamine (Potentiated). Products include:
Cystospaz Tablets ... 2395
Urised Tablets ... 2396

Hyoscyamine Sulfate (Potentiated). Products include:
Arco-Lase Plus Tablets ... 607
Cystospaz-M Capsules ... 2395
Donnagel ... ▣ 675
Donnagel-PG ... 1858
Donnatal ... 1858
Donnatal Extentabs ... 1859
Donnatal Tablets ... 1858
Donnazyme Tablets ... 1860
Kutrase Capsules ... 2146
Levsin/Levsinex ... 2147
Ru-Tuss Tablets ... 693

Isoflurane (Potentiated). Products include:
Forane ... 600

Ketamine Hydrochloride (Potentiated). Products include:
Ketalar ... 1726

Levorphanol Tartrate (Potentiated). Products include:
Levo-Dromoran ... 1906

Lorazepam (Potentiated). Products include:
Ativan Injection ... 2432
Ativan Tablets ... 2434

Loxapine Hydrochloride (Potentiated). Products include:
Loxitane ... 1213

Loxapine Succinate (Potentiated). Products include:
Loxitane Capsules ... 1213

Meperidine Hydrochloride (Potentiated). Products include:
Demerol ... 2047
Mepergan Injection ... 2479

Mephobarbital (Potentiated). Products include:
Mebaral Tablets ... 2061

Meprobamate (Potentiated). Products include:
Deprol Tablets ... 2382
Equagesic Tablets ... 2451
Miltown Tablets ... 2386
PMB 200 and PMB 400 ... 2504

Mesoridazine (Potentiated). Products include:
Serentil ... 686

Methadone Hydrochloride (Potentiated). Products include:
Dolophine Hydrochloride Ampoules & Vials ... 1260
Dolophine Hydrochloride Tablets ... 1261
Methadone Hydrochloride Diskets .. 1284
Methadone Hydrochloride Oral Solution & Tablets ... 1987

Methohexital Sodium (Potentiated). Products include:
Brevital Sodium Vials ... 1248

Methoxyflurane (Potentiated).
No products indexed under this heading.

Midazolam Hydrochloride (Potentiated). Products include:
Versed Injection ... 1924

Molindone Hydrochloride (Potentiated). Products include:
Moban Tablets & Concentrate ... 932

Morphine Sulfate (Potentiated). Products include:
Astramorph/PF Injection, USP (Preservative-Free) ... 618
Duramorph ... 960
Infumorph 200 and Infumorph 500 Sterile Solutions ... 962
MS Contin Tablets ... 1814
MSIR ... 1817
Oramorph SR (Morphine Sulfate Sustained Release Tablets) ... 1988
Roxanol ... 1991

Opium Alkaloids (Potentiated). Products include:
B & O No. 15A & No. 16A Supprettes ... 2395
Pantopon Injectable ... 1911

Oxazepam (Potentiated). Products include:
Serax Capsules ... 2522
Serax Tablets ... 2522

Oxycodone Hydrochloride (Potentiated). Products include:
Percocet Tablets ... 950
Percodan ... 951
Roxicodone Tablets, Oral Solution & Intensol (Oxycodone) ... 1992
Tylox Capsules ... 1382

Pentobarbital Sodium (Potentiated). Products include:
Nembutal Sodium Capsules ... 534
Nembutal Sodium Solution ... 536
Nembutal Sodium Suppositories ... 538

Perphenazine (Potentiated). Products include:
Etrafon ... 2087
Triavil Tablets ... 1556
Trilafon ... 2123

Phenobarbital (Potentiated). Products include:
Arco-Lase Plus Tablets ... 607
Bellergal-S Tablets ... 1998
Bronkolixir ... ▣ 761
Bronkotabs Tablets ... ▣ 762
Donnatal ... 1858
Donnatal Extentabs ... 1859
Donnatal Tablets ... 1858
Donnazyme Tablets ... 1860
Kinesed Tablets ... 2272
Phenobarbital Elixir and Tablets ... 1293
Primatene Tablets-P Formula ... 2421
Quadrinal Tablets ... 1183
Tedral SA ... 1765

Prazepam (Potentiated). Products include:
Centrax ... 1693

Prochlorperazine (Potentiated). Products include:
Compazine ... 2201

Promethazine Hydrochloride (Potentiated). Products include:
Mepergan Injection ... 2479
Phenergan with Codeine ... 2497
Phenergan with Dextromethorphan 2499
Phenergan Injection ... 2493
Phenergan Suppositories ... 2496
Phenergan Syrup ... 2495
Phenergan Tablets ... 2496
Phenergan VC ... 2500
Phenergan VC with Codeine ... 2501

Propofol (Potentiated). Products include:
Diprivan Injection ... 2267

Propoxyphene Hydrochloride (Potentiated). Products include:
Darvon ... 1256
Wygesic Tablets ... 2540

Propoxyphene Napsylate (Potentiated). Products include:
Darvon-N/Darvocet-N ... 1254

Quazepam (Potentiated). Products include:
Doral Tablets ... 2383

Scopolamine Hydrobromide (Potentiated). Products include:
Donnagel ... ▣ 675
Donnagel-PG ... 1858
Donnatal ... 1858
Donnatal Extentabs ... 1859
Donnatal Tablets ... 1858
Donnazyme Tablets ... 1860
Isopto Hyoscine ... ⊙ 222
Murocoll-2 Sterile Ophthalmic Solution ... ⊙ 261
Ru-Tuss Tablets ... 693

Scopolamine Preparations (Potentiated). Products include:
Transderm Scōp Transdermal Therapeutic System ... 887

Secobarbital Sodium (Potentiated). Products include:
Seconal Sodium Pulvules ... 1296

Sufentanil Citrate (Potentiated). Products include:
Sufenta Injection ... 1147

Temazepam (Potentiated). Products include:
Restoril Capsules ... 2023

Thiamylal Sodium (Potentiated). Products include:
Surital Ampoules, Steri-Vials ... 1764

Thioridazine Hydrochloride (Potentiated). Products include:
Mellaril ... 2011

Thiothixene (Potentiated). Products include:
Navane Capsules and Concentrate 1954
Navane Intramuscular ... 1956

Triazolam (Potentiated). Products include:
Halcion Tablets ... 2340

Trifluoperazine Hydrochloride (Potentiated). Products include:
Stelazine ... 2226

TORECAN SUPPOSITORIES (THIETHYLPERAZINE MALEATE)
(Thiethylperazine Maleate) ... 1993
See **Torecan Injection (Thiethylperazine Malate)**

TORECAN TABLETS (THIETHYLPERAZINE MALEATE)
(Thiethylperazine Maleate) ... 1993
See **Torecan Injection (Thiethylperazine Malate)**

TORNALATE
(Bitolterol Mesylate) ... 2074
May interact with sympathomimetic bronchodilators and sympathomimetic aerosol bronchodilators. Compounds in these categories include:

Albuterol (Potential for deleterious cardiovascular effects; concomitant use should be avoided). Products include:
Proventil Inhalation Aerosol ... 2117
Ventolin Inhalation Aerosol and Refill ... 583

Albuterol Sulfate (Potential for deleterious cardiovascular effects). Products include:
Proventil Repetabs Tablets ... 2120
Proventil Solutions for Inhalation 0.5% and 0.083% ... 2118
Proventil Syrup ... 2119
Proventil Tablets ... 2120
Ventolin ... 583

Ephedrine Hydrochloride (Potential for deleterious cardiovascular effects). Products include:
Amesec ... ▣ 682
Primatene Tablets-M Formula ... 2421
Primatene Tablets-P Formula ... 2421
Primatene Tablets-Regular Formula ... 2421
Quadrinal Tablets ... 1183
Quelidrine Syrup ... 556
Tedral SA ... 1765

Ephedrine Sulfate (Potential for deleterious cardiovascular effects). Products include:
Bronkaid Tablets ... ▣ 757
Bronkolixir ... ▣ 761
Bronkotabs Tablets ... ▣ 762
Marax Tablets & DF Syrup ... 1954

Pazo Hemorrhoid Ointment & Suppositories.... 752
Vicks Vatronol Nose Drops .... ▣ 666

Ephedrine Tannate (Potential for deleterious cardiovascular effects). Products include:
Rynatuss 2388

Epinephrine (Potential for deleterious cardiovascular effects). Products include:
Ana-Kit Anaphylaxis Emergency Treatment Kit 1100
Bronkaid Mist .... ▣ 757
EpiPen 843
Marcaine Hydrochloride 0.5% with Epinephrine 1:200,000 (as bitartrate) 958
Marcaine Hydrochloride with Epinephrine 1:200,000 2055
Primatene Mist 2420
Sus-Phrine Injection 1006
Xylocaine with Epinephrine Injections.... 637

Epinephrine Bitartrate (Potential for deleterious cardiovascular effects). Products include:
AsthmaHaler Mist Epinephrine Bitartrate Bronchodilator .... ▣ 616
Bronkaid Mist Suspension .... ▣ 757
Primatene Mist Suspension.... 2421

Epinephrine Hydrochloride (Potential for deleterious cardiovascular effects). Products include:
Adrenalin Chloride Solution 1:100 & 1:1,000 1689
Epifrin.... ⊙ 244
Glaucon .... ⊙ 218

Ethylnorepinephrine Hydrochloride (Potential for deleterious cardiovascular effects). Products include:
Bronkephrine Injection 2042

Isoetharine (Potential for deleterious cardiovascular effects; concomitant use should be avoided). Products include:
Arm-a-Med Isoetharine Inhalation Solution, USP.... 616
Bronkometer Aerosol.... 2042
Bronkosol Solution 2042

Isoproterenol Hydrochloride (Potential for deleterious cardiovascular effects; concomitant use should be avoided). Products include:
Isuprel Hydrochloride Injection 1:5000 2050
Isuprel Hydrochloride Mistometer .. 2051
Isuprel Hydrochloride Solution 1:200 & 1:100 2052
Norisodrine Aerotrol.... 540

Metaproterenol Sulfate (Potential for deleterious cardiovascular effects; concomitant use should be avoided). Products include:
Alupent.... 674
Arm-a-Med Metaproterenol Sulfate Inhalation Solution, USP 617
Metaprel Inhalation Aerosol Bronchodilator 2014
Metaprel Inhalation Solution.... 2015
Metaprel 2015
Metaproterenol Sulfate Inhalation Solution, USP.... 912

Pirbuterol Acetate (Potential for deleterious cardiovascular effects; concomitant use should be avoided). Products include:
Maxair Inhaler.... 1311

Terbutaline Sulfate (Potential for deleterious cardiovascular effects; concomitant use should be avoided). Products include:
Brethaire Inhaler 1024
Brethine Ampuls 1026
Brethine Tablets.... 1026
Bricanyl Injection.... 1324
Bricanyl Tablets 1325

TOTAL FORMULA-2 (MULTIVITAMIN/ MULTIMINERAL)

(Vitamins with Minerals).... 2377
No interactions described in labeling.

TRACRIUM INJECTION

(Atracurium Besylate).... 817
May interact with aminoglycosides, muscle relaxants, and certain other agents. Compounds in these categories include:

Amikacin Sulfate (Enhances neuromuscular blocking action of Tracrium). Products include:
Amikin Injectable 602

Baclofen (Synergistic or antagonist effect). Products include:
Lioresal Tablets 1031

Carisoprodol (Synergistic or antagonist effect). Products include:
Soma Compound w/Codeine Tablets.... 2390
Soma Compound Tablets.... 2389
Soma Tablets.... 2388

Chlorzoxazone (Synergistic or antagonist effect). Products include:
Paraflex Caplets.... 1378
Parafon Forte DSC Caplets 1379

Cyclobenzaprine Hydrochloride (Synergistic or antagonist effect). Products include:
Flexeril Tablets 1471

Dantrolene Sodium (Synergistic or antagonist effect). Products include:
Dantrium Capsules 1619
Dantrium Intravenous 1620

DOXACURIUM CHLORIDE (Synergistic or antagonist effect). Products include:
Nuromax Injection.... 794

Enflurane (Enhances neuromuscular blocking action of Tracrium). Products include:
Ethrane.... 599

Gentamicin Sulfate (Enhances neuromuscular blocking action of Tracrium). Products include:
Garamycin Injectable 2093
Garamycin Ophthalmic .... ⊙ 305
Genoptic Liquifilm Sterile Ophthalmic Solution .... ⊙ 247
Genoptic S.O.P. Sterile Ophthalmic Ointment.... ⊙ 247
Gentacidin Ointment .... ⊙ 273
Gentacidin Solution.... ⊙ 273
Gentak Ointment & Solution.... ⊙ 208
G-myticin Creme and Ointment 0.1%.... 1770
Pred-G Liquifilm Sterile Ophthalmic Suspension .... ⊙ 252
Pred-G S.O.P. Sterile Ophthalmic Ointment.... ⊙ 253

Halothane (Enhances neuromuscular blocking action of Tracrium). Products include:
Fluothane 2453

Isoflurane (Enhances neuromuscular blocking action of Tracrium). Products include:
Forane.... 600

Kanamycin Sulfate (Enhances neuromuscular blocking action of Tracrium). Products include:
Kantrex Injection 601
Kantrex Pediatric Injection.... 601

Lithium Carbonate (Enhances neuromuscular blocking action of Tracrium). Products include:
Eskalith 2214
Lithane Tablets 1596
Lithium Carbonate Capsules & Tablets 1984
Lithobid Tablets 870

Lithium Citrate (Enhances neuromuscular blocking action of Tracrium). Products include:
Cibalith-S.... 870

Magnesium Salts (Enhances neuromuscular blocking action of Tracrium).

Metaxalone (Synergistic or antagonist effect). Products include:
Skelaxin 840

Methocarbamol (Synergistic or antagonist effect). Products include:
Robaxin Injectable.... 1871
Robaxin Tablets 1872
Robaxisal Tablets.... 1872

Metocurine Iodide (Synergistic or antagonist effect). Products include:
Metubine Iodide Vials.... 1285

Orphenadrine Citrate (Synergistic or antagonist effect). Products include:
Norflex 1314
Norgesic.... 1314

Pancuronium Bromide Injection (Synergistic or antagonist effect).
No products indexed under this heading.

Polymyxin Preparations (Enhances neuromuscular blocking action of Tracrium).

Procainamide (Enhances neuromuscular blocking action of Tracrium).

Quinidine Gluconate (Enhances neuromuscular blocking action of Tracrium). Products include:
Quinaglute Dura-Tabs Tablets 663

Quinidine Polygalacturonate (Enhances neuromuscular blocking action of Tracrium). Products include:
Cardioquin Tablets 1812

Quinidine Sulfate (Enhances neuromuscular blocking action of Tracrium). Products include:
Quinidex Extentabs.... 1868

Streptomycin Sulfate (Enhances neuromuscular blocking action of Tracrium).
No products indexed under this heading.

Succinylcholine Chloride (Increases neuromuscular blockade induced by Tracrium). Products include:
Anectine.... 755

Tobramycin (Enhances neuromuscular blocking action of Tracrium). Products include:
TobraDex Ophthalmic Suspension and Ointment.... ⊙ 228
Tobrex Ophthalmic Ointment and Solution 572

Tobramycin Sulfate (Enhances neuromuscular blocking action of Tracrium). Products include:
Nebcin Vials, Hyporets & ADD-Vantage 1286

Vecuronium Bromide (Synergistic or antagonist effect). Products include:
Norcuron 1642

TRANCOPAL CAPLETS

(Chlormezanone) 2075
May interact with central nervous system depressants and certain other agents. Compounds in these categories include:

Alcohol (Possible additive effects).

Alfentanil Hydrochloride (Possible additive effects). Products include:
Alfenta Injection 1131

Alprazolam (Possible additive effects). Products include:
Xanax Tablets 2367

Aprobarbital (Possible additive effects). Products include:
Alurate Elixir 1883

Buprenorphine (Possible additive effects).
No products indexed under this heading.

Buspirone Hydrochloride (Possible additive effects). Products include:
BuSpar 1401

Butabarbital (Possible additive effects). Products include:
Pyridium Plus 1764

Butalbital (Possible additive effects). Products include:
Esgic-Plus Tablets 1002
Esgic Tablets & Capsules.... 1001
Fioricet Tablets.... 2006
Fiorinal Capsules 2007
Fiorinal with Codeine Capsules 2008
Fiorinal Tablets.... 2007
Phrenilin 838
Sedapap Tablets 50 mg/650 mg .. 1360

Chlordiazepoxide (Possible additive effects). Products include:
Libritabs Tablets 1930
Limbitrol 1933
Menrium Tablets 1934

Chlordiazepoxide Hydrochloride (Possible additive effects). Products include:
Librax Capsules 1929
Librium Capsules.... 1931
Librium Injectable 1932

Chlorpromazine (Possible additive effects). Products include:
Thorazine 2234

Chlorprothixene (Possible additive effects). Products include:
Taractan Tablets 1920

Chlorprothixene Hydrochloride (Possible additive effects). Products include:
Taractan 1920

Clorazepate Dipotassium (Possible additive effects). Products include:
Tranxene 556

Codeine (Possible additive effects). Products include:
Calcidrine Syrup.... 506

Codeine Phosphate (Possible additive effects). Products include:
Actifed with Codeine Cough Syrup.. 752
Cheracol Cough Syrup.... 1853
Codimal PH Syrup.... 846
Dimetane-DC Cough Syrup 1857
Empirin with Codeine Phosphate Nos. 2, 3 & 4.... 764
Fiorinal with Codeine Capsules 2008
Isoclor Expectorant.... 982
Naldecon CX Adult Liquid .... ▣ 521
Novahistine DH.... 1342
Novahistine Expectorant.... 1343
Nucofed Capsules 2219
Nucofed Expectorant 2219
Nucofed Pediatric Expectorant 2220
Nucofed Syrup 2219
Phenaphen with Codeine Capsules 1865
Phenaphen-650 with Codeine Tablets 1866
Phenergan with Codeine.... 2497
Phenergan VC with Codeine 2501
Robitussin A-C Syrup.... 1875
Robitussin-DAC Syrup 1875
Ryna .... ▣ 741
Soma Compound w/Codeine Tablets 2390
Triaminic Expectorant w/Codeine .. 1996
Tussi-Organidin Liquid 2391
Tylenol with Codeine 1381

Codeine Polistirex (Possible additive effects).
No products indexed under this heading.

Dezocine (Possible additive effects).

Diazepam (Possible additive effects). Products include:
Valium Injectable 1937
Valium Tablets 1939
Valrelease Capsules 1923

Droperidol (Possible additive effects). Products include:
- Inapsine Injection ... 1140
- Innovar Injection ... 1141

Enflurane (Possible additive effects). Products include:
- Ethrane ... 599

Estazolam (Possible additive effects). Products include:
- ProSom Tablets ... 554

Ethchlorvynol (Possible additive effects). Products include:
- Placidyl Capsules ... 553

Ethinamate (Possible additive effects).
- No products indexed under this heading.

Fentanyl (Possible additive effects). Products include:
- Duragesic Transdermal System ... 1133

Fentanyl Citrate (Possible additive effects). Products include:
- Innovar Injection ... 1141
- Sublimaze Injection ... 1146

Fluphenazine Decanoate (Possible additive effects). Products include:
- Prolixin Decanoate ... 1795

Fluphenazine Enanthate (Possible additive effects). Products include:
- Prolixin Enanthate ... 1796

Fluphenazine Hydrochloride (Possible additive effects). Products include:
- Prolixin Elixir ... 1793
- Prolixin Injection ... 1791
- Prolixin Oral Concentrate ... 1792
- Prolixin Tablets ... 1793

Flurazepam Hydrochloride (Possible additive effects). Products include:
- Dalmane Capsules ... 1927

Glutethimide (Possible additive effects).
- No products indexed under this heading.

Haloperidol (Possible additive effects). Products include:
- Haldol Injection, Tablets and Concentrate ... 1373

Haloperidol Decanoate (Possible additive effects). Products include:
- Haldol Decanoate ... 1375

Hydrocodone Bitartrate (Possible additive effects). Products include:
- Anexsia 5/500 Tablets ... 2196
- Anexsia 7.5/650 Tablets ... 2197
- Azdone Tablets ... 844
- Codiclear DH Syrup ... 845
- Codimal DH Syrup ... 846
- Damason-P ... 1356
- Hycodan Syrup, Tablets ... 927
- Hycomine Compound Tablets ... 929
- Hycomine Syrup ... 927
- Hycotuss Expectorant Syrup ... 930
- Hydrocet Capsules ... 835
- Lortab ASA Tablets ... 2414
- Lortab ... 2412
- Ru-Tuss with Hydrocodone ... 694
- Triaminic Expectorant DH ... 1995
- Vicodin Tablets ... 1187
- Vicodin ES Tablets ... 1189
- Zydone Capsules ... 941

Hydrocodone Polistirex (Possible additive effects). Products include:
- Tussionex Extended-Release Suspension ... 988

Hydroxyzine Hydrochloride (Possible additive effects). Products include:
- Atarax Tablets & Syrup ... 1941
- Marax Tablets & DF Syrup ... 1954
- Vistaril Intramuscular Solution ... 1970

Isoflurane (Possible additive effects). Products include:
- Forane ... 600

Ketamine Hydrochloride (Possible additive effects). Products include:
- Ketalar ... 1726

Levorphanol Tartrate (Possible additive effects). Products include:
- Levo-Dromoran ... 1906

Lorazepam (Possible additive effects). Products include:
- Ativan Injection ... 2432
- Ativan Tablets ... 2434

Loxapine Hydrochloride (Possible additive effects). Products include:
- Loxitane ... 1213

Loxapine Succinate (Possible additive effects). Products include:
- Loxitane Capsules ... 1213

Meperidine Hydrochloride (Possible additive effects). Products include:
- Demerol ... 2047
- Mepergan Injection ... 2479

Mephobarbital (Possible additive effects). Products include:
- Mebaral Tablets ... 2061

Meprobamate (Possible additive effects). Products include:
- Deprol Tablets ... 2382
- Equagesic Tablets ... 2451
- Miltown Tablets ... 2386
- PMB 200 and PMB 400 ... 2504

Mesoridazine (Possible additive effects). Products include:
- Serentil ... 686

Methadone Hydrochloride (Possible additive effects). Products include:
- Dolophine Hydrochloride Ampoules & Vials ... 1260
- Dolophine Hydrochloride Tablets ... 1261
- Methadone Hydrochloride Diskets ... 1284
- Methadone Hydrochloride Oral Solution & Tablets ... 1987

Methohexital Sodium (Possible additive effects). Products include:
- Brevital Sodium Vials ... 1248

Methoxyflurane (Possible additive effects).
- No products indexed under this heading.

Midazolam Hydrochloride (Possible additive effects). Products include:
- Versed Injection ... 1924

Molindone Hydrochloride (Possible additive effects). Products include:
- Moban Tablets & Concentrate ... 932

Morphine Sulfate (Possible additive effects). Products include:
- Astramorph/PF Injection, USP (Preservative-Free) ... 618
- Duramorph ... 960
- Infumorph 200 and Infumorph 500 Sterile Solutions ... 962
- MS Contin Tablets ... 1814
- MSIR ... 1817
- Oramorph SR (Morphine Sulfate Sustained Release Tablets) ... 1988
- Roxanol ... 1991

Opium Alkaloids (Possible additive effects). Products include:
- B & O No. 15A & No. 16A Supprettes ... 2395
- Pantopon Injectable ... 1911

Oxazepam (Possible additive effects). Products include:
- Serax Capsules ... 2522
- Serax Tablets ... 2522

Oxycodone Hydrochloride (Possible additive effects). Products include:
- Percocet Tablets ... 950
- Percodan ... 951
- Roxicodone Tablets, Oral Solution & Intensol (Oxycodone) ... 1992
- Tylox Capsules ... 1382

Pentobarbital Sodium (Possible additive effects). Products include:
- Nembutal Sodium Capsules ... 534
- Nembutal Sodium Solution ... 536
- Nembutal Sodium Suppositories ... 538

Perphenazine (Possible additive effects). Products include:
- Etrafon ... 2087
- Triavil Tablets ... 1556
- Trilafon ... 2123

Phenobarbital (Possible additive effects). Products include:
- Arco-Lase Plus Tablets ... 607
- Bellergal-S Tablets ... 1998
- Bronkolixir ... ▣ 761
- Bronkotabs Tablets ... ▣ 762
- Donnatal ... 1858
- Donnatal Extentabs ... 1859
- Donnatal Tablets ... 1858
- Donnazyme Tablets ... 1860
- Kinesed Tablets ... 2272
- Phenobarbital Elixir and Tablets ... 1293
- Primatene Tablets-P Formula ... 2421
- Quadrinal Tablets ... 1183
- Tedral SA ... 1765

Prazepam (Possible additive effects). Products include:
- Centrax ... 1693

Prochlorperazine (Possible additive effects). Products include:
- Compazine ... 2201

Promethazine Hydrochloride (Possible additive effects). Products include:
- Mepergan Injection ... 2479
- Phenergan with Codeine ... 2497
- Phenergan with Dextromethorphan ... 2499
- Phenergan Injection ... 2493
- Phenergan Suppositories ... 2496
- Phenergan Syrup ... 2495
- Phenergan Tablets ... 2496
- Phenergan VC ... 2500
- Phenergan VC with Codeine ... 2501

Propofol (Possible additive effects). Products include:
- Diprivan Injection ... 2267

Propoxyphene Hydrochloride (Possible additive effects). Products include:
- Darvon ... 1256
- Wygesic Tablets ... 2540

Propoxyphene Napsylate (Possible additive effects). Products include:
- Darvon-N/Darvocet-N ... 1254

Quazepam (Possible additive effects). Products include:
- Doral Tablets ... 2383

Secobarbital Sodium (Possible additive effects). Products include:
- Seconal Sodium Pulvules ... 1296

Sufentanil Citrate (Possible additive effects). Products include:
- Sufenta Injection ... 1147

Temazepam (Possible additive effects). Products include:
- Restoril Capsules ... 2023

Thiamylal Sodium (Possible additive effects). Products include:
- Surital Ampoules, Steri-Vials ... 1764

Thioridazine Hydrochloride (Possible additive effects). Products include:
- Mellaril ... 2011

Thiothixene (Possible additive effects). Products include:
- Navane Capsules and Concentrate ... 1954
- Navane Intramuscular ... 1956

Triazolam (Possible additive effects). Products include:
- Halcion Tablets ... 2340

Trifluoperazine Hydrochloride (Possible additive effects). Products include:
- Stelazine ... 2226

TRANDATE HCT TABLETS (Labetalol Hydrochloride, Hydrochlorothiazide) ... 579

May interact with tricyclic antidepressants, sympathomimetic bronchodilators, para-aminobenzoic acid based local anesthetics, antihypertensives, insulin, lithium preparations, non-steroidal anti-inflammatory agents, oral hypoglycemic agents, and certain other agents. Compounds in these categories include:

Acebutolol Hydrochloride (Potentiation of antihypertensive effects). Products include:
- Sectral Capsules ... 2520

Albuterol (Blunting of bronchodilator effects). Products include:
- Proventil Inhalation Aerosol ... 2117
- Ventolin Inhalation Aerosol and Refill ... 583

Albuterol Sulfate (Blunting of bronchodilator effects). Products include:
- Proventil Repetabs Tablets ... 2120
- Proventil Solutions for Inhalation 0.5% and 0.083% ... 2118
- Proventil Syrup ... 2119
- Proventil Tablets ... 2120
- Ventolin ... 583

Amitriptyline Hydrochloride (Concurrent administration may produce tremor). Products include:
- Elavil ... 2269
- Endep Tablets ... 1927
- Etrafon ... 2087
- Limbitrol ... 1933
- Triavil Tablets ... 1556

Amoxapine (Concurrent administration may produce tremor). Products include:
- Asendin Tablets ... 1196

Atenolol (Potentiation of antihypertensive effects). Products include:
- Tenoretic Tablets ... 1105
- Tenormin Tablets and I.V. Injection 1107

Benazepril Hydrochloride (Potentiation of antihypertensive effects). Products include:
- Lotensin Tablets ... 872

Bendroflumethiazide (Potentiation of antihypertensive effects). Products include:
- Corzide Tablets ... 702
- Naturetin Tablets ... 1789
- Rauzide Tablets ... 1804

Betaxolol Hydrochloride (Potentiation of antihypertensive effects). Products include:
- Betoptic Sterile Ophthalmic Solution ... 569
- Betoptic S Sterile Ophthalmic Suspension ... 570
- Kerlone Tablets ... 2172

Bitolterol Mesylate (Blunting of bronchodilator effects). Products include:
- Tornalate ... 2074

Captopril (Potentiation of antihypertensive effects). Products include:
- Capoten ... 2255
- Capozide ... 2258

Carteolol Hydrochloride (Potentiation of antihypertensive effects). Products include:
- Cartrol Tablets ... 507

Chlorothiazide (Potentiation of antihypertensive effects). Products include:
- Aldoclor Tablets ... 1413
- Diupres Tablets ... 1461
- Diuril Oral ... 1464

Chlorothiazide Sodium (Potentiation of antihypertensive effects). Products include:
- Diuril Sodium Intravenous ... 1463

Chlorpropamide (Beta-blockade reduces the release of insulin in response to hyperglycemia; adjust the dose of antidiabetic drugs). Products include:
- Diabinese Tablets ... 1775

Chlorthalidone (Potentiation of antihypertensive effects). Products include:

Combipres Tablets ... 678
Tenoretic Tablets ... 1105
Thalitone Tablets ... 687

Cimetidine (Increases the bioavailability of labetalol). Products include:

Tagamet Tablets ... 2228

Cimetidine Hydrochloride (Increases the bioavailability of labetalol). Products include:

Tagamet ... 2228

Clomipramine Hydrochloride (Concurrent administration may produce tremor). Products include:

Anafranil Capsules ... 650

Clonidine (Potentiation of antihypertensive effects). Products include:

Catapres-TTS ... 677

Clonidine Hydrochloride (Potentiation of antihypertensive effects). Products include:

Catapres Tablets ... 676
Combipres Tablets ... 678

Deserpidine (Potentiation of antihypertensive effects). Products include:

Enduronyl ... 518
Harmonyl Tablets ... 528
Oreticyl ... 545

Desipramine Hydrochloride (Concurrent administration may produce tremor). Products include:

Norpramin Tablets ... 1340

Diazoxide (Potentiation of antihypertensive effects). Products include:

Hyperstat I.V. Injection ... 2095
Proglycem ... 649

Diclofenac Sodium (Antihypertensive and diuretic effects may be reduced). Products include:

Voltaren Ophthalmic Sterile Ophthalmic Solution ... ⊙ 268
Voltaren Tablets ... 1042

Doxazosin Mesylate (Potentiation of antihypertensive effects). Products include:

Cardura Tablets ... 1941

Doxepin Hydrochloride (Concurrent administration may produce tremor). Products include:

Sinequan ... 1960

Enalapril Maleate (Potentiation of antihypertensive effects). Products include:

Vaseretic Tablets ... 1559
Vasotec Tablets ... 1564

Enalaprilat (Potentiation of antihypertensive effects). Products include:

Vasotec I.V. ... 1562

Ephedrine Hydrochloride (Blunting of bronchodilator effects). Products include:

Amesec ... ⊡ 682
Primatene Tablets-M Formula ... 2421
Primatene Tablets-P Formula ... 2421
Primatene Tablets-Regular Formula ... 2421
Quadrinal Tablets ... 1183
Quelidrine Syrup ... 556
Tedral SA ... 1765

Ephedrine Sulfate (Blunting of bronchodilator effects). Products include:

Bronkaid Tablets ... ⊡ 757
Bronkolixir ... ⊡ 761
Bronkotabs Tablets ... ⊡ 762
Marax Tablets & DF Syrup ... 1954
Pazo Hemorrhoid Ointment & Suppositories ... 752
Vicks Vatronol Nose Drops ... ⊡ 666

Ephedrine Tannate (Blunting of bronchodilator effects). Products include:

Rynatuss ... 2388

Epinephrine (Blunting of bronchodilator effects). Products include:

Ana-Kit Anaphylaxis Emergency Treatment Kit ... 1100
Bronkaid Mist ... ⊡ 757
EpiPen ... 843
Marcaine Hydrochloride 0.5% with Epinephrine 1:200,000 (as bitartrate) ... 958
Marcaine Hydrochloride with Epinephrine 1:200,000 ... 2055
Primatene Mist ... 2420
Sus-Phrine Injection ... 1006
Xylocaine with Epinephrine Injections ... 637

Epinephrine Hydrochloride (Blunting of bronchodilator effects). Products include:

Adrenalin Chloride Solution 1:100 & 1:1,000 ... 1689
Epifrin ... ⊙ 244
Glaucon ... ⊙ 218

Esmolol Hydrochloride (Potentiation of antihypertensive effects). Products include:

Brevibloc Injection ... 942

Ethylnorepinephrine Hydrochloride (Blunting of bronchodilator effects). Products include:

Bronkephrine Injection ... 2042

Etodolac (Antihypertensive and diuretic effects may be reduced). Products include:

Lodine Capsules ... 2468

Felodipine (Potentiation of antihypertensive effects). Products include:

Plendil Extended-Release Tablets ... 1526

Fenoprofen Calcium (Antihypertensive and diuretic effects may be reduced). Products include:

Nalfon Pulvules & Tablets ... 919

Flurbiprofen (Antihypertensive and diuretic effects may be reduced). Products include:

Ansaid Tablets ... 2319

Fosinopril Sodium (Potentiation of antihypertensive effects). Products include:

Monopril Tablets ... 1406

Furosemide (Potentiation of antihypertensive effects). Products include:

Lasix ... 1093

Glipizide (Beta-blockade reduces the release of insulin in response to hyperglycemia; adjust the dose of antidiabetic drugs). Products include:

Glucotrol ... 1952

Glyburide (Beta-blockade reduces the release of insulin in response to hyperglycemia). Products include:

DiaBeta ... 1091
Micronase Tablets ... 2350

Guanabenz Acetate (Potentiation of antihypertensive effects). Products include:

Wytensin Tablets ... 2542

Guanethidine Monosulfate (Potentiation of antihypertensive effects). Products include:

Esimil Tablets ... 864
Ismelin Tablets ... 869

Halothane (Synergism has been shown between halothane anesthesia and IV labetalol). Products include:

Fluothane ... 2453

Hydralazine Hydrochloride (Potentiation of antihypertensive effects). Products include:

Apresazide Capsules ... 854
Apresoline Hydrochloride Parenteral (Ampuls) ... 856
Apresoline Hydrochloride Tablets ... 855
Apresoline-Esidrix Tablets ... 857
Ser-Ap-Es Tablets ... 881
Serpasil-Apresoline Tablets ... 884

Hydroflumethiazide (Potentiation of antihypertensive effects). Products include:

Diucardin Tablets ... 2450
Saluron ... 718
Salutensin/Salutensin-Demi ... 719

Ibuprofen (Antihypertensive and diuretic effects may be reduced). Products include:

Advil Cold & Sinus Caplets (formerly CoAdvil) ... 2416
Advil Ibuprofen Tablets and Caplets ... 2416
Children's Advil Suspension ... 2426
CoAdvil ... ⊡ 748
Dristan Sinus Caplets ... 2419
Haltran Tablets ... ⊡ 668
Ibuprofen ... ⊡ 631
Medipren ibuprofen Caplets and Tablets ... 1362
Midol 200 Cramp Relief Formula .. ⊡ 570
Motrin Tablets ... 2351
Motrin IB Caplets and Tablets ... ⊡ 736
Nuprin Ibuprofen/Analgesic Tablets & Caplets ... 752
PediaProfen Suspension ... 1363
Rufen Tablets ... 691
Trendar Ibuprofen Tablets ... ⊡ 756

Imipramine Hydrochloride (Concurrent administration may produce tremor). Products include:

Tofranil Ampuls ... 1038
Tofranil Tablets ... 1039

Imipramine Pamoate (Concurrent administration may produce tremor). Products include:

Tofranil-PM Capsules ... 1041

Indapamide (Potentiation of antihypertensive effects). Products include:

Lozol Tablets ... 1843

Indomethacin (Antihypertensive and diuretic effects may be reduced). Products include:

Indocin ... 1487

Indomethacin Sodium Trihydrate (Antihypertensive and diuretic effects may be reduced). Products include:

Indocin I.V. ... 1490

Insulin, Human (Altered insulin requirement).

No products indexed under this heading.

Insulin, Human Isophane Suspension (Altered insulin requirement). Products include:

Humulin N, 100 Units ... 1270

Insulin, Human NPH (Altered insulin requirement). Products include:

Insulatard NPH Human ... 1627
Novolin N ... 1627
Novolin N PenFill Cartridges ... 1628
Novolin N Prefilled ... 1628

Insulin, Human Regular (Altered insulin requirement). Products include:

Humulin BR, 100 Units ... 1268
Humulin R, 100 Units ... 1272
Novolin R ... 1627
Novolin R PenFill Cartridges ... 1628
Novolin R Prefilled ... 1629
Velosulin Human ... 1628

Insulin, Human, Zinc Suspension (Altered insulin requirement). Products include:

Humulin L, 100 Units ... 1268
Humulin U, 100 Units ... 1272
Novolin L ... 1627

Insulin, NPH (Altered insulin requirement). Products include:

NPH, 40 & 100 Units ... 1273
Beef NPH, 100 Units ... 1274
Pork NPH, 100 Units ... 1275
Insulatard NPH ... 1626
NPH Insulin ... 1626
NPH Purified Pork Isophane Insulin ... 1626

Insulin, Regular (Altered insulin requirement). Products include:

Regular, 40 & 100 Units ... 1273
Beef Regular, 100 Units ... 1275
Pork Regular, 100 Units ... 1275
Pork Regular (Concentrated), 500 Units ... 1276
Regular Insulin ... 1625
Regular Purified Pork Insulin ... 1626
Velosulin ... 1627

Insulin, Zinc Crystals (Altered insulin requirement). Products include:

NPH, 40 & 100 Units ... 1273

Insulin, Zinc Suspension (Altered insulin requirement). Products include:

Lente, 40 & 100 Units ... 1272
Protamine, Zinc, 40 & 100 Units ... 1273
Lente Iletin I ... 1272
Beef Lente, 100 Units ... 1274
Beef Protamine Zinc, 100 Units ... 1274
Pork Lente, 100 Units ... 1275
Pork, Protamine, Zinc, 100 Units ... 1275
Lente Insulin ... 1626
Lente Purified Pork Insulin ... 1626
Semilente Insulin ... 1625
Ultralente Insulin ... 1626

Isoetharine (Blunting of bronchodilator effects). Products include:

Arm-a-Med Isoetharine Inhalation Solution, USP ... 616
Bronkometer Aerosol ... 2042
Bronkosol Solution ... 2042

Isoproterenol Hydrochloride (Blunting of bronchodilator effects). Products include:

Isuprel Hydrochloride Injection 1:5000 ... 2050
Isuprel Hydrochloride Mistometer .. 2051
Isuprel Hydrochloride Solution 1:200 & 1:100 ... 2052
Norisodrine Aerotrol ... 540

Isradipine (Potentiation of antihypertensive effects). Products include:

DynaCirc Capsules ... 2004

Ketoprofen (Antihypertensive and diuretic effects may be reduced). Products include:

Orudis Capsules ... 2488

Ketorolac Tromethamine (Antihypertensive and diuretic effects may be reduced). Products include:

Toradol IM Injection ... 2302

Lisinopril (Potentiation of antihypertensive effects). Products include:

Prinivil Tablets ... 1538
Prinzide Tablets ... 1540
Zestoretic ... 2274
Zestril Tablets ... 2277

Lithium Carbonate (Increased lithium toxicity). Products include:

Eskalith ... 2214
Lithane Tablets ... 1596
Lithium Carbonate Capsules & Tablets ... 1984
Lithobid Tablets ... 870

Lithium Citrate (Increased lithium toxicity). Products include:

Cibalith-S ... 870

Maprotiline Hydrochloride (Concurrent administration may produce tremor). Products include:

Ludiomil Tablets ... 874

Mecamylamine Hydrochloride (Potentiation of antihypertensive effects). Products include:

Inversine Tablets ... 1492

Meclofenamate Sodium (Antihypertensive and diuretic effects may be reduced). Products include:

Meclomen Capsules ... 1739

Metaproterenol Sulfate (Blunting of bronchodilator effects). Products include:

Alupent ... 674
Arm-a-Med Metaproterenol Sulfate Inhalation Solution, USP ... 617
Metaprel Inhalation Aerosol Bronchodilator ... 2014
Metaprel Inhalation Solution ... 2015
Metaprel ... 2015

(⊡ Described in PDR For Nonprescription Drugs) (⊙ Described in PDR For Ophthalmology)

Metaproterenol Sulfate Inhalation Solution, USP 912

Methyclothiazide (Potentiation of antihypertensive effects). Products include:
Enduron Tablets 517
Enduronyl 518

Methyldopa (Potentiation of antihypertensive effects). Products include:
Aldoclor Tablets 1413
Aldomet Oral 1415
Aldoril Tablets 1418

Methyldopate Hydrochloride (Potentiation of antihypertensive effects). Products include:
Aldomet Ester HCl Injection 1417

Metolazone (Potentiation of antihypertensive effects). Products include:
Diulo 2129
Mykrox ½ mg Tablets 984
Zaroxolyn Tablets 989

Metoprolol Tartrate (Potentiation of antihypertensive effects). Products include:
Lopressor Ampuls 1032
Lopressor HCT Tablets 1034
Lopressor Tablets 1032

Metyrosine (Potentiation of antihypertensive effects). Products include:
Demser Capsules 1460

Minoxidil (Potentiation of antihypertensive effects). Products include:
Loniten Tablets 2346
Rogaine Topical Solution 2357

Nadolol (Potentiation of antihypertensive effects). Products include:
Corgard Tablets 701
Corzide Tablets 702

Naproxen (Antihypertensive and diuretic effects may be reduced). Products include:
Naprosyn 2297

Naproxen Sodium (Antihypertensive and diuretic effects may be reduced). Products include:
Anaprox and Anaprox DS Tablets 2288

Nicardipine Hydrochloride (Potentiation of antihypertensive effects). Products include:
Cardene Capsules 2290

Nitroglycerin (Potentiation of antihypertensive effects; labetalol blunts reflex tachycardia produced by nitroglycerine). Products include:
Deponit NTG Transdermal Delivery System 2143
Minitran Transdermal Delivery System 1312
Nitro-Bid Ointment 1339
Nitro-Bid Capsules 1338
Nitrodisc 2176
Nitro-Dur (nitroglycerin) Transdermal Infusion System 1164
Nitrogard Tablets 1004
Nitrolingual Spray 1846
Nitrostat Tablets 1743
Transderm-Nitro Transdermal Therapeutic System 2283

Nortriptyline Hydrochloride (Concurrent administration may produce tremor). Products include:
Pamelor 2019

Penbutolol Sulfate (Potentiation of antihypertensive effects). Products include:
Levatol 1832

Phenoxybenzamine Hydrochloride (Potentiation of antihypertensive effects). Products include:
Dibenzyline Capsules 2207

Phentolamine Mesylate (Potentiation of antihypertensive effects). Products include:
Regitine 878

Phenylbutazone (Antihypertensive and diuretic effects may be reduced). Products include:
Butazolidin Capsules & Tablets 1027

Pindolol (Potentiation of antihypertensive effects). Products include:
Visken Tablets 2036

Pirbuterol Acetate (Blunting of bronchodilator effects). Products include:
Maxair Inhaler 1311

Piroxicam (Antihypertensive and diuretic effects may be reduced). Products include:
Feldene Capsules 1777

Polythiazide (Potentiation of antihypertensive effects). Products include:
Minizide Capsules 1779
Renese Tablets 1785
Renese-R Tablets 1786

Prazosin Hydrochloride (Potentiation of antihypertensive effects). Products include:
Minipress Capsules 1778
Minizide Capsules 1779

Propranolol Hydrochloride (Potentiation of antihypertensive effects). Products include:
Inderal 2459
Inderal LA Long Acting Capsules 2461
Inderide Tablets 2463
Inderide LA Long Acting Capsules 2465

Protriptyline Hydrochloride (Concurrent administration may produce tremor). Products include:
Vivactil Tablets 1567

Ramipril (Potentiation of antihypertensive effects). Products include:
Altace Capsules 1086

Rauwolfia Serpentina (Potentiation of antihypertensive effects). Products include:
Raudixin Tablets 1803
Rauzide Tablets 1804

Rescinnamine (Potentiation of antihypertensive effects).
No products indexed under this heading.

Reserpine (Potentiation of antihypertensive effects). Products include:
Diupres Tablets 1461
Hydromox R Tablets 1209
Hydropres Tablets 1485
Renese-R Tablets 1786
Salutensin/Salutensin-Demi 719
Ser-Ap-Es Tablets 881
Serpasil Tablets 883
Serpasil-Apresoline Tablets 884
Serpasil-Esidrix Tablets 886

Sodium Nitroprusside (Potentiation of antihypertensive effects). Products include:
Nipride I.V. Infusion 1909

Sulindac (Antihypertensive and diuretic effects may be reduced). Products include:
Clinoril Tablets 1433

Terazosin Hydrochloride (Potentiation of antihypertensive effects). Products include:
Hytrin Tablets 529

Terbutaline Sulfate (Blunting of bronchodilator effects). Products include:
Brethaire Inhaler 1024
Brethine Ampuls 1026
Brethine Tablets 1026
Bricanyl Injection 1324
Bricanyl Tablets 1325

Timolol Maleate (Potentiation of antihypertensive effects). Products include:
Blocadren Tablets 1429
Timolide Tablets 1547
Timoptic in Ocudose 1552
Timoptic Sterile Ophthalmic Solution 1550

Tolazamide (Beta-blockade reduces the release of insulin in response to hyperglycemia; adjust the dose of antidiabetic drugs). Products include:
Tolinase Tablets 2365

Tolbutamide (Beta-blockade reduces the release of insulin in response to hyperglycemia; adjust the dose of antidiabetic drugs). Products include:
Orinase Tablets 2354

Tolmetin Sodium (Antihypertensive and diuretic effects may be reduced). Products include:
Tolectin (200, 400 and 600 mg) 1379

Trimethaphan Camsylate (Potentiation of antihypertensive effects). Products include:
Arfonad Ampuls 1887

Trimipramine Maleate (Concurrent administration may produce tremor). Products include:
Surmontil Capsules 2524

Tubocurarine Chloride (Increased responsiveness to tubocurarine).
No products indexed under this heading.

Verapamil Hydrochloride (Exercise caution if used concomitantly). Products include:
Calan SR Caplets 2157
Calan Tablets 2155
Isoptin Injectable 1177
Isoptin Oral Tablets 1179
Isoptin SR Sustained Release Tablets 1181
Verelan Capsules 1243
Verelan Capsules 2535

TRANDATE INJECTION
(Labetalol Hydrochloride) 577
May interact with tricyclic antidepressants, sympathomimetic bronchodilators, oral hypoglycemic agents, insulin, and certain other agents. Compounds in these categories include:

Albuterol (Blunting of bronchodilator effects). Products include:
Proventil Inhalation Aerosol 2117
Ventolin Inhalation Aerosol and Refill 583

Albuterol Sulfate (Blunting of bronchodilator effects). Products include:
Proventil Repetabs Tablets 2120
Proventil Solutions for Inhalation 0.5% and 0.083% 2118
Proventil Syrup 2119
Proventil Tablets 2120
Ventolin 583

Amitriptyline Hydrochloride (Concurrent administration may produce tremor). Products include:
Elavil 2269
Endep Tablets 1927
Etrafon 2087
Limbitrol 1933
Triavil Tablets 1556

Amoxapine (Concurrent administration may produce tremor). Products include:
Asendin Tablets 1196

Bitolterol Mesylate (Blunting of bronchodilator effects). Products include:
Tornalate 2074

Chlorpropamide (Beta-blockade reduces the release of insulin in response to hyperglycemia; dose of antidiabetic drugs need to be adjusted). Products include:
Diabinese Tablets 1775

Cimetidine (Increases bioavailability by altering hepatic metabolism of labetalol). Products include:
Tagamet Tablets 2228

Cimetidine Hydrochloride (Increases bioavailability by altering hepatic metabolism of labetalol). Products include:
Tagamet 2228

Clomipramine Hydrochloride (Concurrent administration may produce tremor). Products include:
Anafranil Capsules 650

Desipramine Hydrochloride (Concurrent administration may produce tremor). Products include:
Norpramin Tablets 1340

Doxepin Hydrochloride (Concurrent administration may produce tremor). Products include:
Sinequan 1960

Ephedrine Hydrochloride (Blunting of bronchodilator effects). Products include:
Amesec .... ▣ 682
Primatene Tablets-M Formula 2421
Primatene Tablets-P Formula 2421
Primatene Tablets-Regular Formula 2421
Quadrinal Tablets 1183
Quelidrine Syrup 556
Tedral SA 1765

Ephedrine Sulfate (Blunting of bronchodilator effects). Products include:
Bronkaid Tablets .... ▣ 757
Bronkolixir .... ▣ 761
Bronkotabs Tablets .... ▣ 762
Marax Tablets & DF Syrup 1954
Pazo Hemorrhoid Ointment & Suppositories 752
Vicks Vatronol Nose Drops .... ▣ 666

Ephedrine Tannate (Blunting of bronchodilator effects). Products include:
Rynatuss 2388

Epinephrine (Blunting of bronchodilator effects). Products include:
Ana-Kit Anaphylaxis Emergency Treatment Kit 1100
Bronkaid Mist .... ▣ 757
EpiPen 843
Marcaine Hydrochloride 0.5% with Epinephrine 1:200,000 (as bitartrate) 958
Marcaine Hydrochloride with Epinephrine 1:200,000 2055
Primatene Mist 2420
Sus-Phrine Injection 1006
Xylocaine with Epinephrine Injections 637

Epinephrine Bitartrate (Blunting of bronchodilator effects). Products include:
AsthmaHaler Mist Epinephrine Bitartrate Bronchodilator .... ▣ 616
Bronkaid Mist Suspension .... ▣ 757
Primatene Mist Suspension 2421

Epinephrine Hydrochloride (Blunting of bronchodilator effects). Products include:
Adrenalin Chloride Solution 1:100 & 1:1,000 1689
Epifrin .... ⊙ 244
Glaucon .... ⊙ 218

Ethylnorepinephrine Hydrochloride (Blunting of bronchodilator effects). Products include:
Bronkephrine Injection 2042

Glipizide (Beta-blockade reduces the release of insulin in response to hyperglycemia; dose of antidiabetic drugs need to be adjusted). Products include:
Glucotrol 1952

Glyburide (Beta-blockade reduces the release of insulin in response to hyperglycemia; dose of antidiabetic drugs need to be adjusted). Products include:
DiaBeta 1091
Micronase Tablets 2350

Halothane (Synergism has been shown between halothane anesthesia and IV labetalol). Products include:
- Fluothane 2453

Imipramine Hydrochloride (Concurrent administration may produce tremor). Products include:
- Tofranil Ampuls 1038
- Tofranil Tablets 1039

Imipramine Pamoate (Concurrent administration may produce tremor). Products include:
- Tofranil-PM Capsules 1041

Insulin, Human (Beta-blockade reduces the release of insulin in response to hyperglycemia).
- No products indexed under this heading.

Insulin, Human Isophane Suspension (Beta-blockade reduces the release of insulin in response to hyperglycemia). Products include:
- Humulin N, 100 Units 1270

Insulin, Human NPH (Beta-blockade reduces the release of insulin in response to hyperglycemia). Products include:
- Insulatard NPH Human 1627
- Novolin N 1627
- Novolin N PenFill Cartridges 1628
- Novolin N Prefilled 1628

Insulin, Human Regular (Beta-blockade reduces the release of insulin in response to hyperglycemia). Products include:
- Humulin BR, 100 Units 1268
- Humulin R, 100 Units 1272
- Novolin R 1627
- Novolin R PenFill Cartridges 1628
- Novolin R Prefilled 1629
- Velosulin Human 1628

Insulin, Human, Zinc Suspension (Beta-blockade reduces the release of insulin in response to hyperglycemia). Products include:
- Humulin L, 100 Units 1268
- Humulin U, 100 Units 1272
- Novolin L 1627

Insulin, NPH (Beta-blockade reduces the release of insulin in response to hyperglycemia). Products include:
- NPH, 40 & 100 Units 1273
- Beef NPH, 100 Units 1274
- Pork NPH, 100 Units 1275
- Insulatard NPH 1626
- NPH Insulin 1626
- NPH Purified Pork Isophane Insulin 1626

Insulin, Regular (Beta-blockade reduces the release of insulin in response to hyperglycemia). Products include:
- Regular, 40 & 100 Units 1273
- Beef Regular, 100 Units 1275
- Pork Regular, 100 Units 1275
- Pork Regular (Concentrated), 500 Units 1276
- Regular Insulin 1625
- Regular Purified Pork Insulin 1626
- Velosulin 1627

Insulin, Zinc Crystals (Beta-blockade reduces the release of insulin in response to hyperglycemia). Products include:
- NPH, 40 & 100 Units 1273

Insulin, Zinc Suspension (Beta-blockade reduces the release of insulin in response to hyperglycemia). Products include:
- Lente, 40 & 100 Units 1272
- Protamine, Zinc, 40 & 100 Units 1273
- Lente Iletin I 1272
- Beef Lente, 100 Units 1274
- Beef Protamine Zinc, 100 Units 1274
- Pork Lente, 100 Units 1275
- Pork, Protamine, Zinc, 100 Units 1275
- Lente Insulin 1626
- Lente Purified Pork Insulin 1626
- Semilente Insulin 1625
- Ultralente Insulin 1626

Isoetharine (Blunting of bronchodilator effects). Products include:
- Arm-a-Med Isoetharine Inhalation Solution, USP 616
- Bronkometer Aerosol 2042
- Bronkosol Solution 2042

Isoproterenol Hydrochloride (Blunting of bronchodilator effects). Products include:
- Isuprel Hydrochloride Injection 1:5000 2050
- Isuprel Hydrochloride Mistometer 2051
- Isuprel Hydrochloride Solution 1:200 & 1:100 2052
- Norisodrine Aerotrol 540

Maprotiline Hydrochloride (Concurrent administration may produce tremor). Products include:
- Ludiomil Tablets 874

Metaproterenol Sulfate (Blunting of bronchodilator effects). Products include:
- Alupent 674
- Arm-a-Med Metaproterenol Sulfate Inhalation Solution, USP 617
- Metaprel Inhalation Aerosol Bronchodilator 2014
- Metaprel Inhalation Solution 2015
- Metaprel 2015
- Metaproterenol Sulfate Inhalation Solution, USP 912

Nitroglycerin (Labetalol blunts reflex tachycardia produced by nitroglycerine; additional antihypertensive effects may occur). Products include:
- Deponit NTG Transdermal Delivery System 2143
- Minitran Transdermal Delivery System 1312
- Nitro-Bid Ointment 1339
- Nitro-Bid Capsules 1338
- Nitrodisc 2176
- Nitro-Dur (nitroglycerin) Transdermal Infusion System 1164
- Nitrogard Tablets 1004
- Nitrolingual Spray 1846
- Nitrostat Tablets 1743
- Transderm-Nitro Transdermal Therapeutic System 2283

Nortriptyline Hydrochloride (Concurrent administration may produce tremor). Products include:
- Pamelor 2019

Pirbuterol Acetate (Blunting of bronchodilator effects). Products include:
- Maxair Inhaler 1311

Protriptyline Hydrochloride (Concurrent administration may produce tremor). Products include:
- Vivactil Tablets 1567

Terbutaline Sulfate (Blunting of bronchodilator effects). Products include:
- Brethaire Inhaler 1024
- Brethine Ampuls 1026
- Brethine Tablets 1026
- Bricanyl Injection 1324
- Bricanyl Tablets 1325

Tolazamide (Beta-blockade reduces the release of insulin in response to hyperglycemia; dose of antidiabetic drugs need to be adjusted). Products include:
- Tolinase Tablets 2365

Tolbutamide (Beta-blockade reduces the release of insulin in response to hyperglycemia; dose of antidiabetic drugs need to be adjusted). Products include:
- Orinase Tablets 2354

Trimipramine Maleate (Concurrent administration may produce tremor). Products include:
- Surmontil Capsules 2524

Verapamil Hydrochloride (Exercise caution if used concomitantly). Products include:
- Calan SR Caplets 2157
- Calan Tablets 2155
- Isoptin Injectable 1177
- Isoptin Oral Tablets 1179
- Isoptin SR Sustained Release Tablets 1181
- Verelan Capsules 1243
- Verelan Capsules 2535

TRANDATE TABLETS
(Labetalol Hydrochloride) 579

See **Trandate HCT Tablets**

TRANSDERM SCŌP TRANSDERMAL THERAPEUTIC SYSTEM
(Scopolamine Preparations) 887

May interact with anticholinergics, belladona products, antihistamines, tricyclic antidepressants, and certain other agents. Compounds in these categories include:

Alcohol (Effect unspecified).

Amitriptyline Hydrochloride (Effect unspecified). Products include:
- Elavil 2269
- Endep Tablets 1927
- Etrafon 2087
- Limbitrol 1933
- Triavil Tablets 1556

Amoxapine (Effect unspecified). Products include:
- Asendin Tablets 1196

Astemizole (Effect unspecified). Products include:
- Hismanal Tablets 1138

Atropine Sulfate (Effect unspecified). Products include:
- Arco-Lase Plus Tablets 607
- Atropine Sulfate Sterile Ophthalmic Solution and S.O.P. Sterile Ophthalmic Ointment ◉ 239
- Donnagel ▣ 675
- Donnagel-PG 1858
- Donnatal 1858
- Donnatal Extentabs 1859
- Donnatal Tablets 1858
- Donnazyme Tablets 1860
- Isopto Atropine ◉ 218
- Lomotil 2174
- Motofen Tablets 836
- Ru-Tuss Tablets 693
- Urised Tablets 2396

Azatadine Maleate (Effect unspecified). Products include:
- Optimine Tablets 2115
- Trinalin Repetabs Tablets 1170

Belladonna Alkaloids (Effect unspecified). Products include:
- Bellergal-S Tablets 1998
- Hyland's Bed Wetting Tablets ▣ 728
- Hyland's Teething Tablets ▣ 728
- Kinesed Tablets 2272

Benztropine Mesylate (Effect unspecified). Products include:
- Cogentin 1435

Biperiden (Effect unspecified). Products include:
- Akineton 1171

Bromodiphenhydramine Hydrochloride (Effect unspecified).
- No products indexed under this heading.

Brompheniramine Maleate (Effect unspecified). Products include:
- Alka Seltzer Plus Sinus Allergy Medicine ▣ 624
- Atrohist Sprinkle Capsules 558
- Bromfed Capsules (Timed Release) 1615
- Bromfed Syrup ▣ 628
- Bromfed 1615
- Dimetane Decongestant ▣ 673
- Dimetane ▣ 672
- Dimetane-DC Cough Syrup 1857
- Dimetane-DX Cough Syrup 1858
- Dimetapp Elixir ▣ 673
- Dimetapp DM Elixir ▣ 674
- Dimetapp Extentabs ▣ 674
- Dimetapp Plus Caplets ▣ 675
- Dimetapp Tablets ▣ 675
- Drixoral Antihistamine/Nasal Decongestant Syrup ▣ 698

Chlorpheniramine Maleate (Effect unspecified). Products include:
- A.R.M. Allergy Relief Medicine Caplets ▣ 615
- Alka-Seltzer Plus Cold Medicine ▣ 623
- Allerest ▣ 559
- Ana-Kit Anaphylaxis Emergency Treatment Kit 1100
- BC Cold Powder Multi-Symptom Formula ▣ 517
- Brexin L.A. Capsules 2078
- Cerose-DM 2443
- Cheracol Plus Head Cold/Cough Formula ▣ 667
- Chlor-Trimeton Allergy Syrup, Tablets & Long-Acting Repetabs Tablets ▣ 693
- Chlor-Trimeton Decongestant ▣ 694
- Comhist LA Capsules 1618
- Allergy-Sinus Comtrex Multi-Symptom Allergy Sinus Formula Tablets & Caplets 746
- Comtrex Multi-Symptom Cold Reliever Tablets/Caplets/Liqui-Gels/Liquid 745
- Day-Night Comtrex 747
- Contac Continuous Action Decongestant/Antihistamine Capsules ▣ 710
- Contac Maximum Strength Continuous Action Decongestant/Antihistamine Caplets ▣ 709
- Contac Severe Cold and Flu Formula Caplets ▣ 711
- Coricidin 'D' Decongestant Tablets ▣ 695
- Coricidin Demilets Tablets for Children ▣ 696
- Coricidin Tablets ▣ 695
- Deconamine 663
- Demazin Nasal Decongestant/Antihistamine Repetabs Tablets & Syrup ▣ 697
- Dorcol Children's Liquid Cold Formula ▣ 686
- Dristan Decongestant/Antihistamine/ Analgesic Coated Caplets ▣ 749
- Dristan Cold Nasal Decongestant/Antihistamine/ Analgesic Coated Tablets 2419
- Dristan Advanced Formula Decongestant/Antihistamine/ Analgesic Tablets ▣ 749
- Extendryl 994
- 4-Way Cold Tablets 750
- Fedahist Gyrocaps 2145
- Fedahist Timecaps 2145
- Hycomine Compound Tablets 929
- Isoclor Timesule Capsules ▣ 561
- Kronofed-A 970
- Medi-Flu Caplet, Liquid ▣ 640
- Naldecon Syrup, Tablets, Pediatric Drops and Pediatric Syrup 709
- Nolamine Tablets 838
- Novafed A Capsules 1342
- Novahistine DH 1342
- Novahistine Elixir ▣ 596
- Ornade Spansule Capsules 2221
- Orthoxicol Cough Syrup ▣ 668
- PediaCare Allergy Relief Formula Liquid 1362
- PediaCare Cough-Cold Formula Liquid 1362
- PediaCare Night Rest Cough-Cold Formula Liquid 1362
- PediaCare 6-12 Cough-Cold Formula Chewable Tablets 1362
- Pyrroxate Capsules ▣ 669
- Quelidrine Syrup 556
- Ru-Tuss II Capsules 693
- Ru-Tuss Tablets 693
- Ryna ▣ 741
- Sinarest Tablets & Extra Strength Tablets ▣ 562
- Sine-Off Maximum Strength Allergy/Sinus Formula Caplets ▣ 721
- Sine-Off Sinus Medicine Tablets-Aspirin Formula ▣ 722
- Singlet Tablets ▣ 598
- Sinulin 840
- Sinutab Maximum Strength ▣ 641
- St. Joseph Nighttime Cold Medicine ▣ 705
- Sudafed Plus Liquid ▣ 544
- Sudafed Plus Tablets ▣ 545
- Teldrin Timed-Release Allergy Capsules, 12 mg 2192
- TheraFlu Flu and Cold Medicine ▣ 687
- Triaminic Allergy Tablets ▣ 688
- Triaminic Chewables ▣ 688

(▣ Described in PDR For Nonprescription Drugs) (◉ Described in PDR For Ophthalmology)

Triaminic Cold Tablets ▣ 688
Triaminic Nite Light ▣ 689
Triaminic Syrup ▣ 689
Triaminic-12 Tablets ▣ 690
Triaminicin Tablets ▣ 690
Triaminicol Multi-Symptom Cold Tablets ▣ 691
Triaminicol Multi-Symptom Relief ▣ 691
Tylenol Allergy Sinus Medication Caplets and Gelcaps, Maximum Strength 1372
Children's Tylenol Cold Liquid Formula and Chewable Tablets 1368
Tylenol Cold & Flu Hot Medication, Packets 1369
Tylenol Cold Medication Caplets and Tablets 1370
Tylenol Cold Medication, Effervescent Tablets 1369
Vicks Children's NyQuil ▣ 664
Vicks Formula 44 Cough Medicine ▣ 661
Vicks Formula 44M Multi-Symptom Cough Medicine ▣ 662
Vicks Pediatric Formula 44m Multi-Symptom Cough & Cold Medicine ▣ 663

Chlorpheniramine Polistirex (Effect unspecified). Products include:
Tussionex Extended-Release Suspension 988

Chlorpheniramine Tannate (Effect unspecified). Products include:
Rynatan 2387
Rynatuss 2388

Clemastine Fumarate (Effect unspecified). Products include:
Tavist Syrup 2033
Tavist Tablets 2035
Tavist-D Tablets 2035

Clidinium Bromide (Effect unspecified). Products include:
Librax Capsules 1929
Quarzan Capsules 1937

Clomipramine Hydrochloride (Effect unspecified). Products include:
Anafranil Capsules 650

Cyproheptadine Hydrochloride (Effect unspecified). Products include:
Periactin 1525

Desipramine Hydrochloride (Effect unspecified). Products include:
Norpramin Tablets 1340

Dexchlorpheniramine Maleate (Effect unspecified). Products include:
Polaramine 2116

Dicyclomine Hydrochloride (Effect unspecified). Products include:
Bentyl 1322

Diphenhydramine Citrate (Effect unspecified). Products include:
Alka-Seltzer Plus Night-Time Cold Medicine ▣ 623
Bufferin AF Nite Time Analgesic/Sleeping Aid Caplets 744
Excedrin P.M. Analgesic/Sleeping Aid Tablets, Caplets and Liquid 749

Diphenylpyraline Hydrochloride (Effect unspecified).
No products indexed under this heading.

Doxepin Hydrochloride (Effect unspecified). Products include:
Sinequan 1960

Glycopyrrolate (Effect unspecified). Products include:
Robinul Forte Tablets 1873
Robinul Injectable 1873
Robinul Tablets 1873

Hyoscyamine (Effect unspecified). Products include:
Cystospaz Tablets 2395
Urised Tablets 2396

Hyoscyamine Sulfate (Effect unspecified). Products include:
Arco-Lase Plus Tablets 607
Cystospaz-M Capsules 2395
Donnagel ▣ 675
Donnagel-PG 1858
Donnatal 1858
Donnatal Extentabs 1859
Donnatal Tablets 1858
Donnazyme Tablets 1860
Kutrase Capsules 2146
Levsin/Levsinex 2147
Ru-Tuss Tablets 693

Imipramine Hydrochloride (Effect unspecified). Products include:
Tofranil Ampuls 1038
Tofranil Tablets 1039

Imipramine Pamoate (Effect unspecified). Products include:
Tofranil-PM Capsules 1041

Ipratropium Bromide (Effect unspecified). Products include:
Atrovent Inhalation Aerosol 675

Maprotiline Hydrochloride (Effect unspecified). Products include:
Ludiomil Tablets 874

Meclizine Hydrochloride (Effect unspecified). Products include:
Antivert, Antivert/25 Tablets, Antivert/25 Chewable Tablets & Antivert/50 Tablets 1940
Bonine Tablets 1773

Mepenzolate Bromide (Effect unspecified). Products include:
Cantil Tablets 1326

Methdilazine Hydrochloride (Effect unspecified). Products include:
Tacaryl Syrup & Tablets 2409

Nortriptyline Hydrochloride (Effect unspecified). Products include:
Pamelor 2019

Oxybutynin Chloride (Effect unspecified). Products include:
Ditropan 1332

Procyclidine Hydrochloride (Effect unspecified). Products include:
Kemadrin Tablets 771

Promethazine Hydrochloride (Effect unspecified). Products include:
Mepergan Injection 2479
Phenergan with Codeine 2497
Phenergan with Dextromethorphan 2499
Phenergan Injection 2493
Phenergan Suppositories 2496
Phenergan Syrup 2495
Phenergan Tablets 2496
Phenergan VC 2500
Phenergan VC with Codeine 2501

Propantheline Bromide (Effect unspecified). Products include:
Pro-Banthīne Tablets 2141

Protriptyline Hydrochloride (Effect unspecified). Products include:
Vivactil Tablets 1567

Pyrilamine Maleate (Effect unspecified). Products include:
Codimal 846
4-Way Fast Acting Nasal Spray - Original Formula (regular & mentholated) & Metered Spray Pump (regular) 751
Maximum Strength Midol Multi-Symptom Menstrual Formula ▣ 571
Maximum Strength Midol PMS Premenstrual Syndrome Formula ▣ 570
Regular Strength Midol Multi-Symptom Menstrual Formula ▣ 570
Prefrin-A ⊙ 255
Prēmsyn PMS Capsules & Caplets ▣ 547
Primatene Tablets-M Formula 2421
Robitussin Night Relief ▣ 677
Ru-Tuss with Hydrocodone 694
Triaminic Expectorant DH 1995
Triaminic Oral Infant Drops 1996

Pyrilamine Tannate (Effect unspecified). Products include:
Rynatan 2387

Terfenadine (Effect unspecified). Products include:
Seldane Tablets 1349
Seldane-D Extended-Release Tablets 1350

Tridihexethyl Chloride (Effect unspecified).
No products indexed under this heading.

Trihexyphenidyl Hydrochloride (Effect unspecified). Products include:
Artane 1195

Trimeprazine Tartrate (Effect unspecified). Products include:
Temaril Tablets, Syrup and Spansule Sustained Release Capsules 1085

Trimipramine Maleate (Effect unspecified). Products include:
Surmontil Capsules 2524

Tripelennamine Hydrochloride (Effect unspecified). Products include:
PBZ Tablets & Elixir 1037
PBZ-SR Tablets 1037

Triprolidine Hydrochloride (Effect unspecified). Products include:
Actidil ▣ 538
Actifed Capsules ▣ 539
Actifed Plus Caplets ▣ 539
Actifed Plus Tablets ▣ 540
Actifed with Codeine Cough Syrup 752
Actifed Syrup ▣ 540
Actifed Tablets ▣ 540
Actifed 12-Hour Capsules ▣ 539

TRANSDERM-NITRO TRANSDERMAL THERAPEUTIC SYSTEM
(Nitroglycerin) 2283
May interact with calcium channel blockers and vasodilators. Compounds in these categories include:

Bepridil Hydrochloride (Potential for marked symptomatic hypotension). Products include:
Vascor (200, 300 and 400 mg) Tablets 1383

Diazoxide (Additive vasodilating effects). Products include:
Hyperstat I.V. Injection 2095
Proglycem 649

Diltiazem Hydrochloride (Potential for marked symptomatic hypotension). Products include:
Cardizem Tablets-30 mg, 60 mg, 90 mg and 120 mg 1329
Cardizem SR Capsules-60 mg, 90 mg and 120 mg 1327

Felodipine (Potential for marked symptomatic hypotension). Products include:
Plendil Extended-Release Tablets 1526

Hydralazine Hydrochloride (Additive vasodilating effects). Products include:
Apresazide Capsules 854
Apresoline Hydrochloride Parenteral (Ampuls) 856
Apresoline Hydrochloride Tablets 855
Apresoline-Esidrix Tablets 857
Ser-Ap-Es Tablets 881
Serpasil-Apresoline Tablets 884

Isradipine (Potential for marked symptomatic hypotension). Products include:
DynaCirc Capsules 2004

Minoxidil (Additive vasodilating effects). Products include:
Loniten Tablets 2346
Rogaine Topical Solution 2357

Nicardipine Hydrochloride (Potential for marked symptomatic hypotension). Products include:
Cardene Capsules 2290

Nifedipine (Potential for marked symptomatic hypotension). Products include:
Adalat Capsules (10 mg and 20 mg) 1587
Procardia Capsules 1781
Procardia XL Tablets 1783

Nimodipine (Potential for marked symptomatic hypotension). Products include:
Nimotop Capsules 1607

Verapamil Hydrochloride (Potential for marked symptomatic hypotension). Products include:
Calan SR Caplets 2157
Calan Tablets 2155
Isoptin Injectable 1177
Isoptin Oral Tablets 1179
Isoptin SR Sustained Release Tablets 1181
Verelan Capsules 1243
Verelan Capsules 2535

TRANS-PLANTAR
(Salicylic Acid) 2315
No interactions described in labeling.

TRANS-VER-SAL WART REMOVER DERMAL PATCH DELIVERY SYSTEM
(Salicylic Acid) 2315
No interactions described in labeling.

TRANXENE T-TAB TABLETS
(Clorazepate Dipotassium) 556
May interact with central nervous system depressants, monoamine oxidase inhibitors, antidepressant drugs, narcotic analgesics, and certain other agents. Compounds in these categories include:

Alcohol (Increased effects, prolonged sleeping time).

Alfentanil Hydrochloride (Increased effects, prolonged sleeping time, potentiates action). Products include:
Alfenta Injection 1131

Alprazolam (Increased effects, prolonged sleeping time). Products include:
Xanax Tablets 2367

Amitriptyline Hydrochloride (Potentiates action). Products include:
Elavil 2269
Endep Tablets 1927
Etrafon 2087
Limbitrol 1933
Triavil Tablets 1556

Amoxapine (Potentiates action). Products include:
Asendin Tablets 1196

Aprobarbital (Increased effects, prolonged sleeping time). Products include:
Alurate Elixir 1883

Buprenorphine (Increased effects, prolonged sleeping time, potentiates action).
No products indexed under this heading.

Bupropion Hydrochloride (Potentiates action). Products include:
Wellbutrin Tablets 821

Buspirone Hydrochloride (Increased effects, prolonged sleeping time). Products include:
BuSpar 1401

Butabarbital (Increased effects, prolonged sleeping time). Products include:
Pyridium Plus 1764

Butalbital (Increased effects, prolonged sleeping time). Products include:
Esgic-Plus Tablets 1002
Esgic Tablets & Capsules 1001
Fioricet Tablets 2006
Fiorinal Capsules 2007
Fiorinal with Codeine Capsules 2008
Fiorinal Tablets 2007
Phrenilin 838

Sedapap Tablets 50 mg/650 mg .. 1360

Chlordiazepoxide (Increased effects, prolonged sleeping time). Products include:
- Libritabs Tablets ... 1930
- Limbitrol ... 1933
- Menrium Tablets ... 1934

Chlordiazepoxide Hydrochloride (Increased effects, prolonged sleeping time). Products include:
- Librax Capsules ... 1929
- Librium Capsules ... 1931
- Librium Injectable ... 1932

Chlorpromazine (Increased inhibitory effects). Products include:
- Thorazine ... 2234

Chlorprothixene (Increased effects, prolonged sleeping time, potentiates action). Products include:
- Taractan Tablets ... 1920

Chlorprothixene Hydrochloride (Increased effects, prolonged sleeping time, potentiates action). Products include:
- Taractan ... 1920

Codeine (Increased effects, prolonged sleeping time, potentiates action). Products include:
- Calcidrine Syrup ... 506

Codeine Phosphate (Increased effects, prolonged sleeping time, potentiates action). Products include:
- Actifed with Codeine Cough Syrup.. 752
- Cheracol Cough Syrup ... 1853
- Codimal PH Syrup ... 846
- Dimetane-DC Cough Syrup ... 1857
- Empirin with Codeine Phosphate Nos. 2, 3 & 4 ... 764
- Fiorinal with Codeine Capsules ... 2008
- Isoclor Expectorant ... 982
- Naldecon CX Adult Liquid ... ◼ 521
- Novahistine DH ... 1342
- Novahistine Expectorant ... 1343
- Nucofed Capsules ... 2219
- Nucofed Expectorant ... 2219
- Nucofed Pediatric Expectorant ... 2220
- Nucofed Syrup ... 2219
- Phenaphen with Codeine Capsules 1865
- Phenaphen-650 with Codeine Tablets ... 1866
- Phenergan with Codeine ... 2497
- Phenergan VC with Codeine ... 2501
- Robitussin A-C Syrup ... 1875
- Robitussin-DAC Syrup ... 1875
- Ryna ... ◼ 741
- Soma Compound w/Codeine Tablets ... 2390
- Triaminic Expectorant w/Codeine .. 1996
- Tussi-Organidin Liquid ... 2391
- Tylenol with Codeine ... 1381

Codeine Polistirex (Increased effects, prolonged sleeping time, potentiates action).
- No products indexed under this heading.

Desipramine Hydrochloride (Potentiates action). Products include:
- Norpramin Tablets ... 1340

Dezocine (Increased effects, prolonged sleeping time, potentiates action).

Diazepam (Increased effects, prolonged sleeping time). Products include:
- Valium Injectable ... 1937
- Valium Tablets ... 1939
- Valrelease Capsules ... 1923

Doxepin Hydrochloride (Potentiates action). Products include:
- Sinequan ... 1960

Droperidol (Increased effects, prolonged sleeping time). Products include:
- Inapsine Injection ... 1140
- Innovar Injection ... 1141

Enflurane (Increased effects, prolonged sleeping time). Products include:
- Ethrane ... 599

Estazolam (Increased effects, prolonged sleeping time, potentiates action). Products include:
- ProSom Tablets ... 554

Ethchlorvynol (Increased effects, prolonged sleeping time). Products include:
- Placidyl Capsules ... 553

Ethinamate (Increased effects, prolonged sleeping time).
- No products indexed under this heading.

Fentanyl (Increased effects, prolonged sleeping time, potentiates action). Products include:
- Duragesic Transdermal System ... 1133

Fentanyl Citrate (Increased effects, prolonged sleeping time, potentiates action). Products include:
- Innovar Injection ... 1141
- Sublimaze Injection ... 1146

Fluoxetine Hydrochloride (Potentiates action). Products include:
- Prozac Pulvules ... 920

Fluphenazine Decanoate (Increased effects, prolonged sleeping time). Products include:
- Prolixin Decanoate ... 1795

Fluphenazine Enanthate (Increased effects, prolonged sleeping time). Products include:
- Prolixin Enanthate ... 1796

Fluphenazine Hydrochloride (Increased effects, prolonged sleeping time). Products include:
- Prolixin Elixir ... 1793
- Prolixin Injection ... 1791
- Prolixin Oral Concentrate ... 1792
- Prolixin Tablets ... 1793

Flurazepam Hydrochloride (Increased effects, prolonged sleeping time). Products include:
- Dalmane Capsules ... 1927

Furazolidone (Potentiates action). Products include:
- Furoxone ... 1855

Glutethimide (Increased effects, prolonged sleeping time).
- No products indexed under this heading.

Haloperidol (Increased effects, prolonged sleeping time). Products include:
- Haldol Injection, Tablets and Concentrate ... 1373

Haloperidol Decanoate (Increased effects, prolonged sleeping time). Products include:
- Haldol Decanoate ... 1375

Hydrocodone Bitartrate (Increased effects, prolonged sleeping time, potentiates action). Products include:
- Anexsia 5/500 Tablets ... 2196
- Anexsia 7.5/650 Tablets ... 2197
- Azdone Tablets ... 844
- Codiclear DH Syrup ... 845
- Codimal DH Syrup ... 846
- Damason-P ... 1356
- Hycodan Syrup, Tablets ... 927
- Hycomine Compound Tablets ... 929
- Hycomine Syrup ... 927
- Hycotuss Expectorant Syrup ... 930
- Hydrocet Capsules ... 835
- Lortab ASA Tablets ... 2414
- Lortab ... 2412
- Ru-Tuss with Hydrocodone ... 694
- Triaminic Expectorant DH ... 1995
- Vicodin Tablets ... 1187
- Vicodin ES Tablets ... 1189
- Zydone Capsules ... 941

Hydrocodone Polistirex (Increased effects, prolonged sleeping time, potentiates action). Products include:
- Tussionex Extended-Release Suspension ... 988

Hydroxyzine Hydrochloride (Increased effects, prolonged sleeping time). Products include:
- Atarax Tablets & Syrup ... 1941
- Marax Tablets & DF Syrup ... 1954
- Vistaril Intramuscular Solution ... 1970

Imipramine Hydrochloride (Potentiates action). Products include:
- Tofranil Ampuls ... 1038
- Tofranil Tablets ... 1039

Imipramine Pamoate (Potentiates action). Products include:
- Tofranil-PM Capsules ... 1041

Isocarboxazid (Potentiates action). Products include:
- Marplan Tablets ... 1906

Isoflurane (Increased effects, prolonged sleeping time). Products include:
- Forane ... 600

Ketamine Hydrochloride (Increased effects, prolonged sleeping time, potentiates action). Products include:
- Ketalar ... 1726

Levorphanol Tartrate (Increased effects, prolonged sleeping time, potentiates action). Products include:
- Levo-Dromoran ... 1906

Lorazepam (Increased effects, prolonged sleeping time). Products include:
- Ativan Injection ... 2432
- Ativan Tablets ... 2434

Loxapine Hydrochloride (Increased effects, prolonged sleeping time). Products include:
- Loxitane ... 1213

Loxapine Succinate (Increased effects, prolonged sleeping time, potentiates action). Products include:
- Loxitane Capsules ... 1213

Maprotiline Hydrochloride (Potentiates action). Products include:
- Ludiomil Tablets ... 874

Meperidine Hydrochloride (Increased effects, prolonged sleeping time, potentiates action). Products include:
- Demerol ... 2047
- Mepergan Injection ... 2479

Mephobarbital (Increased effects, prolonged sleeping time). Products include:
- Mebaral Tablets ... 2061

Meprobamate (Increased effects, prolonged sleeping time). Products include:
- Deprol Tablets ... 2382
- Equagesic Tablets ... 2451
- Miltown Tablets ... 2386
- PMB 200 and PMB 400 ... 2504

Mesoridazine (Increased effects, prolonged sleeping time). Products include:
- Serentil ... 686

Methadone Hydrochloride (Increased effects, prolonged sleeping time, potentiates action). Products include:
- Dolophine Hydrochloride Ampoules & Vials ... 1260
- Dolophine Hydrochloride Tablets ... 1261
- Methadone Hydrochloride Diskets .. 1284
- Methadone Hydrochloride Oral Solution & Tablets ... 1987

Methohexital Sodium (Increased effects, prolonged sleeping time). Products include:
- Brevital Sodium Vials ... 1248

Methoxyflurane (Increased effects, prolonged sleeping time).
- No products indexed under this heading.

Midazolam Hydrochloride (Increased effects, prolonged sleeping time). Products include:
- Versed Injection ... 1924

Molindone Hydrochloride (Increased effects, prolonged sleeping time). Products include:
- Moban Tablets & Concentrate ... 932

Morphine Sulfate (Increased effects, prolonged sleeping time, potentiates action). Products include:
- Astramorph/PF Injection, USP (Preservative-Free) ... 618
- Duramorph ... 960
- Infumorph 200 and Infumorph 500 Sterile Solutions ... 962
- MS Contin Tablets ... 1814
- MSIR ... 1817
- Oramorph SR (Morphine Sulfate Sustained Release Tablets) ... 1988
- Roxanol ... 1991

Nortriptyline Hydrochloride (Potentiates action). Products include:
- Pamelor ... 2019

Opium Alkaloids (Increased effects, prolonged sleeping time, potentiates action). Products include:
- B & O No. 15A & No. 16A Supprettes ... 2395
- Pantopon Injectable ... 1911

Oxazepam (Increased effects, prolonged sleeping time). Products include:
- Serax Capsules ... 2522
- Serax Tablets ... 2522

Oxycodone Hydrochloride (Increased effects, prolonged sleeping time, potentiates action). Products include:
- Percocet Tablets ... 950
- Percodan ... 951
- Roxicodone Tablets, Oral Solution & Intensol (Oxycodone) ... 1992
- Tylox Capsules ... 1382

Pentobarbital Sodium (Increased effects, prolonged sleeping time). Products include:
- Nembutal Sodium Capsules ... 534
- Nembutal Sodium Solution ... 536
- Nembutal Sodium Suppositories ... 538

Perphenazine (Increased effects, prolonged sleeping time). Products include:
- Etrafon ... 2087
- Triavil Tablets ... 1556
- Trilafon ... 2123

Phenelzine Sulfate (Potentiates action). Products include:
- Nardil ... 1742

Phenobarbital (Increased effects, prolonged sleeping time). Products include:
- Arco-Lase Plus Tablets ... 607
- Bellergal-S Tablets ... 1998
- Bronkolixir ... ◼ 761
- Bronkotabs Tablets ... ◼ 762
- Donnatal ... 1858
- Donnatal Extentabs ... 1859
- Donnatal Tablets ... 1858
- Donnazyme Tablets ... 1860
- Kinesed Tablets ... 2272
- Phenobarbital Elixir and Tablets ... 1293
- Primatene Tablets-P Formula ... 2421
- Quadrinal Tablets ... 1183
- Tedral SA ... 1765

Phenothiazine Derivatives (Potentiates action).

Prazepam (Increased effects, prolonged sleeping time). Products include:
- Centrax ... 1693

Prochlorperazine (Increased inhibitory effects). Products include:
- Compazine ... 2201

Promethazine Hydrochloride (Increased effects, prolonged sleeping time). Products include:
- Mepergan Injection ... 2479
- Phenergan with Codeine ... 2497
- Phenergan with Dextromethorphan 2499

Phenergan Injection ... 2493
Phenergan Suppositories ... 2496
Phenergan Syrup ... 2495
Phenergan Tablets ... 2496
Phenergan VC ... 2500
Phenergan VC with Codeine ... 2501

Propofol (Increased effects, prolonged sleeping time, potentiates action). Products include:
Diprivan Injection ... 2267

Propoxyphene Hydrochloride (Increased effects, prolonged sleeping time, potentiates action). Products include:
Darvon ... 1256
Wygesic Tablets ... 2540

Propoxyphene Napsylate (Increased effects, prolonged sleeping time, potentiates action). Products include:
Darvon-N/Darvocet-N ... 1254

Protriptyline Hydrochloride (Potentiates action). Products include:
Vivactil Tablets ... 1567

Quazepam (Increased effects, prolonged sleeping time, potentiates action). Products include:
Doral Tablets ... 2383

Secobarbital Sodium (Increased effects, prolonged sleeping time, potentiates action). Products include:
Seconal Sodium Pulvules ... 1296

Selegiline Hydrochloride (Potentiates action). Products include:
Eldepryl ... 2250

Sufentanil Citrate (Increased effects, prolonged sleeping time, potentiates action). Products include:
Sufenta Injection ... 1147

Temazepam (Increased effects, prolonged sleeping time). Products include:
Restoril Capsules ... 2023

Thiamylal Sodium (Increased effects, prolonged sleeping time). Products include:
Surital Ampoules, Steri-Vials ... 1764

Thioridazine Hydrochloride (Increased effects, prolonged sleeping time). Products include:
Mellaril ... 2011

Thiothixene (Increased effects, prolonged sleeping time). Products include:
Navane Capsules and Concentrate 1954
Navane Intramuscular ... 1956

Tranylcypromine Sulfate (Potentiates action). Products include:
Parnate Tablets ... 2222

Trazodone Hydrochloride (Potentiates action). Products include:
Desyrel and Desyrel Dividose ... 1404

Triazolam (Increased effects, prolonged sleeping time). Products include:
Halcion Tablets ... 2340

Trifluoperazine Hydrochloride (Increased effects, prolonged sleeping time). Products include:
Stelazine ... 2226

Trimipramine Maleate (Potentiates action). Products include:
Surmontil Capsules ... 2524

TRANXENE-SD HALF STRENGTH TABLETS
(Clorazepate Dipotassium) ... 556
See **Tranxene T-TAB Tablets**

TRANXENE-SD TABLETS
(Clorazepate Dipotassium) ... 556
See **Tranxene T-TAB Tablets**

TRAVASE OINTMENT
(Sutilains) ... 697
May interact with:

Benzalkonium Chloride (May render substrate indifferent to enzyme activity in vitro). Products include:
Amino-Cerv ... 1613
Bactine Antiseptic/Anesthetic First Aid Spray ... ▣ 624
Enuclene ... ◉ 232
Fungoid Tincture ... 1770
Ionil T Shampoo ... 1683
Zephiran ... ▣ 762

Hexachlorophene (May render substrate indifferent to enzyme activity in vitro). Products include:
pHisoHex ... 2066

Iodine Preparations (May render substrate indifferent to enzyme activity in vitro). Products include:
Ethiodol ... 2560
One-A-Day Maximum Formula Vitamins and Minerals ... ▣ 627
Pima Syrup ... 994
Ponaris Nasal Mucosal Emollient ... 1131
STUART PRENATAL Tablets ... ▣ 731
The Stuart Formula Tablets ... ▣ 581

Nitrofurazone (May render substrate indifferent to enzyme activity in vitro). Products include:
Furacin Soluble Dressing ... 1854
Furacin Topical Cream ... 1854
Furacin Topical Solution 0.2% ... 1855

Thimerosal (Interferes directly with enzyme activity to a slight degree in vitro).
No products indexed under this heading.

TRECATOR-SC TABLETS
(Ethionamide) ... 2527
May interact with antituberculosis drugs. Compounds in this category include:

Cycloserine (Convulsions; the adverse effects of other antituberculous drugs intensified). Products include:
Seromycin Pulvules ... 1298

Ethambutol Hydrochloride (The adverse effects of other antituberculous drugs intensified). Products include:
Myambutol Tablets ... 1225

Isoniazid (The adverse effects of other antituberculous drugs intensified). Products include:
INH Tablets ... 868
Rifamate Capsules ... 1347

Rifampin (The adverse effects of other antituberculous drugs intensified). Products include:
Rifadin ... 1345
Rifamate Capsules ... 1347
Rimactane Capsules ... 879

TRENDAR IBUPROFEN TABLETS
(Ibuprofen) ... ▣ 756
May interact with aspirin and acetaminophen containing products. Compounds in this category include:

Acetaminophen (Product labeling recommends physician's supervision for concurrent administration of these drugs). Products include:
Acetaminophen Uniserts Suppositories ... 2374
Actifed Plus Caplets ... ▣ 539
Actifed Plus Tablets ... ▣ 540
Alka-Seltzer Advanced Formula Antacid & Non-Aspirin Pain Reliever ... ▣ 620
Allerest ... ▣ 559
Aspirin Free Anacin Maximum Strength Acetaminophen Film Coated Caplets ... 2417
Aspirin Free Anacin Maximum Strength Acetaminophen Film Coated Tablets ... 2417
Anacin-3 Regular Strength Acetaminophen Film Coated Tablets ▣ 746
Anexsia 5/500 Tablets ... 2196
Anexsia 7.5/650 Tablets ... 2197
Benadryl Plus ... ▣ 636
Benadryl Plus Nighttime ... ▣ 637
Bufferin AF Nite Time Analgesic/Sleeping Aid Caplets ... 744
Allergy-Sinus Comtrex Multi-Symptom Allergy Sinus Formula Tablets & Caplets ... 746
Cough Formula Comtrex ... 746
Comtrex Multi-Symptom Cold Reliever Tablets/Caplets/Liqui-Gels/Liquid ... 745
Day-Night Comtrex ... 747
Non-Drowsy Comtrex ... 747
Congespirin For Children Aspirin Free Chewable Cold Tablets ... 748
Contac Cough & Sore Throat Formula ... ▣ 712
Contac Jr. Children's Cold Medicine ... ▣ 712
Contac Nighttime Cold Medicine ... ▣ 713
Contac Severe Cold and Flu Formula Caplets ... ▣ 711
Contac Sinus Caplets Maximum Strength Non-Drowsy Formula ... ▣ 710
Contac Sinus Tablets Maximum Strength Non-Drowsy Formula ... ▣ 710
Coricidin 'D' Decongestant Tablets ... ▣ 695
Coricidin Demilets Tablets for Children ... ▣ 696
Coricidin Tablets ... ▣ 695
Darvon-N/Darvocet-N ... 1254
Datril Extra-Strength Analgesic Tablets ... 748
Dimetapp Plus Caplets ... ▣ 675
Dorcol Children's Fever & Pain Reducer ... ▣ 686
Dristan Decongestant/Antihistamine/ Analgesic Coated Caplets ... ▣ 749
Dristan Cold Nasal Decongestant/ Antihistamine/ Analgesic Coated Tablets ... 2419
Dristan Advanced Formula Decongestant/Antihistamine/ Analgesic Tablets ... ▣ 749
Maximum Strength Dristan Decongestant/Analgesic Coated Caplets ... ▣ 750
No Drowsiness Dristan Cold Nasal Decongestant/Analgesic Coated Caplets ... 2420
Drixoral Plus Extended-Release Tablets ... ▣ 699
Drixoral Sinus ... ▣ 700
Esgic-Plus Tablets ... 1002
Esgic Tablets & Capsules ... 1001
Aspirin Free Excedrin Analgesic Caplets ... 748
Excedrin Extra-Strength Analgesic Tablets & Caplets ... 749
Excedrin P.M. Analgesic/Sleeping Aid Tablets, Caplets and Liquid ... 749
Sinus Excedrin Analgesic, Decongestant Tablets & Caplets ... 750
4-Way Cold Tablets ... 750
Feverall Sprinkle Caps ... 2374
Feverall Suppositories ... 2374
Fioricet Tablets ... 2006
Hycomine Compound Tablets ... 929
Hydrocet Capsules ... 835
Isocom Capsules ... 1629
Liquiprin ... ▣ 618
Lortab ... 2412
Lurline PMS Tablets ... 972
Medi-Flu Caplet, Liquid ... ▣ 640
Maximum Strength Midol Multi-Symptom Menstrual Formula ... ▣ 571
Maximum Strength Midol PMS Premenstrual Syndrome Formula ... ▣ 570
Regular Strength Midol Multi-Symptom Menstrual Formula ... ▣ 570
Midrin Capsules ... 836
Ornex Caplets ... ▣ 618
Children's Panadol Chewable Tablets, Liquid, Infants' Drops ... ▣ 571
Junior Strength Panadol ... ▣ 571
Maximum Strength Panadol Tablets and Caplets ... ▣ 572
Percocet Tablets ... 950
Percogesic Analgesic Tablets ... ▣ 660
Phenaphen with Codeine Capsules 1865
Phenaphen-650 with Codeine Tablets ... 1866
Phrenilin ... 838
Prēmsyn PMS Capsules & Caplets ▣ 547
Pyrroxate Capsules ... ▣ 669
Robitussin Night Relief ... ▣ 677
Sedapap Tablets 50 mg/650 mg .. 1360
Sinarest ... ▣ 562
Sine-Aid Maximum Strength Sinus Headache Caplets ... 1365
Sine-Aid Maximum Strength Sinus Headache Tablets ... 1365
Sine-Off Maximum Strength Allergy/Sinus Formula Caplets ... ▣ 721
Sine-Off Maximum Strength No Drowsiness Formula Caplets ... ▣ 722
Singlet Tablets ... ▣ 598
Sinulin ... 840
Sinutab Maximum Strength ... ▣ 641
Sinutab Maximum Strength Without Drowsiness Tablets & Caplets ... ▣ 642
Sinutab Regular Strength Without Drowsiness Formula ... ▣ 641
Sominex Pain Relief Formula ... ▣ 723
St. Joseph Aspirin-Free Fever Reducer for Children Chewable Tablets, Liquid & Infant Drops ... ▣ 704
St. Joseph Cold Tablets for Children ... ▣ 704
St. Joseph Nighttime Cold Medicine ... ▣ 705
Sudafed Sinus Caplets ... ▣ 545
Sudafed Sinus Tablets ... ▣ 545
Talacen ... 2070
Tempra, Acetaminophen ... ▣ 613
TheraFlu Flu and Cold Medicine ... ▣ 687
Triaminicin Tablets ... ▣ 690
Tylenol acetaminophen Children's Chewable Tablets & Elixir ... 1366
Tylenol Allergy Sinus Medication Caplets and Gelcaps, Maximum Strength ... 1372
Tylenol with Codeine ... 1381
Children's Tylenol Cold Liquid Formula and Chewable Tablets ... 1368
Tylenol Cold & Flu Hot Medication, Packets ... 1369
Tylenol Cold & Flu No Drowsiness Hot Medication, Packets ... 1371
Tylenol Cold Medication Caplets and Tablets ... 1370
Tylenol Cold Medication, Effervescent Tablets ... 1369
Tylenol Cold Medication No Drowsiness Formula Caplets ... 1370
Tylenol Cold Night Time Medication Liquid ... 1371
Tylenol Cough Medication Liquid, Maximum Strength ... 1372
Tylenol Cough Medication Liquid with Decongestant, Maximum Strength ... 1372
Tylenol, Extra Strength, acetaminophen Adult Liquid Pain Reliever .. 1367
Tylenol, Extra Strength, acetaminophen Gelcaps, Caplets, Tablets ... 1367
Tylenol, Infants' Drops ... 1366
Tylenol, Junior Strength, acetaminophen Coated Caplets, Grape and Fruit Chewable Tablets ... 1366
Tylenol, Maximum Strength, Sinus Medication Gelcaps, Caplets and Tablets ... 1373
Tylenol, Regular Strength, acetaminophen Tablets and Caplets ... 1367
Tylenol PM, Extra Strength Caplets and Tablets ... 1368
Tylox Capsules ... 1382
Unisom Dual Relief Nighttime Sleep Aid/Analgesic ... 1774
Vanquish Analgesic Caplets ... ▣ 574
Vicks Daycare ... ▣ 660
Vicks Formula 44M Multi-Symptom Cough Medicine ... ▣ 662
Vicks NyQuil Nighttime Colds Medicine-Original & Cherry Flavor ... ▣ 664
Vicodin Tablets ... 1187
Vicodin ES Tablets ... 1189
Wygesic Tablets ... 2540
Zydone Capsules ... 941

Aspirin (Product labeling recommends physician's supervision for concurrent administration of these drugs). Products include:
Alka-Seltzer Effervescent Antacid and Pain Reliever ... 1568
Alka-Seltzer Extra Strength Effervescent Antacid and Pain Reliever ... 1570

Alka-Seltzer (Flavored) Effervescent Antacid and Pain Reliever 1569
Alka-Seltzer Plus Cold Medicine .... ▣ 623
Alka-Seltzer Plus Night-Time Cold Medicine .... ▣ 623
Alka Seltzer Plus Sinus Allergy Medicine .... ▣ 624
Anacin Coated Analgesic Caplets 2417
Anacin Coated Analgesic Tablets 2417
Anacin Maximum Strength Analgesic Coated Tablets 2417
Maximum Strength Arthritis Pain Formula By the Makers of Anacin Analgesic Tablets and Caplets 2418
Arthritis Pain Formula by the Makers of Anacin Analgesic Tablets and Caplets .... ▣ 747
Arthritis Strength BC Powder .... ▣ 516
Ascriptin A/D Caplets 1850
Regular Strength Ascriptin Tablets 1850
Azdōne Tablets 844
BC Powder .... ▣ 517
BC Cold Powder .... ▣ 517
Children's Bayer Chewable Aspirin .... ▣ 564
Genuine Bayer Aspirin Tablets & Caplets .... ▣ 564
Maximum Bayer Aspirin Tablets & Caplets .... ▣ 566
Bayer Plus Aspirin Tablets .... ▣ 567
Therapy Bayer Aspirin Caplets .... ▣ 568
8 Hour Bayer Timed-Release Aspirin .... ▣ 566
Arthritis Strength Bufferin Analgesic Caplets 744
Extra Strength Bufferin Analgesic Tablets 745
Bufferin Analgesic Tablets and Caplets 743
Cama Arthritis Pain Reliever .... ▣ 685
Damason-P 1356
Easprin 1719
Ecotrin Enteric Coated Aspirin Maximum Strength Tablets and Caplets 2189
Ecotrin Enteric Coated Aspirin Regular Strength Tablets and Caplets 2189
Empirin Aspirin .... ▣ 541
Empirin with Codeine Phosphate Nos. 2, 3 & 4 764
Equagesic Tablets 2451
Excedrin Extra-Strength Analgesic Tablets & Caplets 749
4-Way Cold Tablets 750
Fiorinal Capsules 2007
Fiorinal with Codeine Capsules 2008
Fiorinal Tablets 2007
Lortab ASA Tablets 2414
Momentum Muscular Backache Formula .... ▣ 751
Norgesic 1314
Norwich Extra-Strength Aspirin .... ▣ 546
Norwich Regular Strength Aspirin ▣ 547
P-A-C Analgesic Tablets .... ▣ 669
Percodan 951
Robaxisal Tablets 1872
Sine-Off Sinus Medicine Tablets-Aspirin Formula .... ▣ 722
Soma Compound w/Codeine Tablets 2390
Soma Compound Tablets 2389
St. Joseph Adult Chewable Aspirin (81 mg.) .... ▣ 703
Synalgos-DC Capsules 2525
Talwin Compound 2072
Ursinus Inlay-Tabs .... ▣ 691
Vanquish Analgesic Caplets .... ▣ 574
Zorprin Tablets 698

TRENTAL
(Pentoxifylline) 1099
May interact with anticoagulants and antihypertensives. Compounds in these categories include:

Acebutolol Hydrochloride (May require to reduce the dosage of antihypertensive). Products include:
Sectral Capsules 2520
Atenolol (May require to reduce the dosage of antihypertensive). Products include:
Tenoretic Tablets 1105
Tenormin Tablets and I.V. Injection 1107
Benazepril Hydrochloride (May require to reduce the dosage of antihypertensive). Products include:
Lotensin Tablets 872
Bendroflumethiazide (May require to reduce the dosage of antihypertensive). Products include:
Corzide Tablets 702
Naturetin Tablets 1789
Rauzide Tablets 1804
Betaxolol Hydrochloride (May require to reduce the dosage of antihypertensive). Products include:
Betoptic Sterile Ophthalmic Solution 569
Betoptic S Sterile Ophthalmic Suspension 570
Kerlone Tablets 2172
Captopril (May require to reduce the dosage of antihypertensive). Products include:
Capoten 2255
Capozide 2258
Carteolol Hydrochloride (May require to reduce the dosage of antihypertensive). Products include:
Cartrol Tablets 507
Chlorothiazide (May require to reduce the dosage of antihypertensive). Products include:
Aldoclor Tablets 1413
Diupres Tablets 1461
Diuril Oral 1464
Chlorothiazide Sodium (May require to reduce the dosage of antihypertensive). Products include:
Diuril Sodium Intravenous 1463
Chlorthalidone (May require to reduce the dosage of antihypertensive). Products include:
Combipres Tablets 678
Tenoretic Tablets 1105
Thalitone Tablets 687
Clonidine (May require to reduce the dosage of antihypertensive). Products include:
Catapres-TTS 677
Clonidine Hydrochloride (May require to reduce the dosage of antihypertensive). Products include:
Catapres Tablets 676
Combipres Tablets 678
Deserpidine (May require to reduce the dosage of antihypertensive). Products include:
Enduronyl 518
Harmonyl Tablets 528
Oreticyl 545
Diazoxide (May require to reduce the dosage of antihypertensive). Products include:
Hyperstat I.V. Injection 2095
Proglycem 649
Dicumarol (Bleeding; prolonged prothrombin time). Products include:
Dicumarol Tablets 516
Doxazosin Mesylate (May require to reduce the dosage of antihypertensive). Products include:
Cardura Tablets 1941
Enalapril Maleate (May require to reduce the dosage of antihypertensive). Products include:
Vaseretic Tablets 1559
Vasotec Tablets 1564
Enalaprilat (May require to reduce the dosage of antihypertensive). Products include:
Vasotec I.V. 1562
Esmolol Hydrochloride (May require to reduce the dosage of antihypertensive). Products include:
Brevibloc Injection 942
Felodipine (May require to reduce the dosage of antihypertensive). Products include:
Plendil Extended-Release Tablets 1526
Fosinopril Sodium (May require to reduce the dosage of antihypertensive). Products include:
Monopril Tablets 1406
Furosemide (May require to reduce the dosage of antihypertensive). Products include:
Lasix 1093
Guanabenz Acetate (May require to reduce the dosage of antihypertensive). Products include:
Wytensin Tablets 2542
Guanethidine Monosulfate (May require to reduce the dosage of antihypertensive). Products include:
Esimil Tablets 864
Ismelin Tablets 869
Heparin Calcium (Bleeding; prolonged prothrombin time). Products include:
Calciparine Injection 925
Heparin Sodium (Bleeding; prolonged prothrombin time). Products include:
Heparin Lock Flush Solution 2456
Heparin Sodium Vials 1264
Heparin Sodium Injection 2457
Heparin Sodium Injection, USP, Sterile Solution 2342
Hydralazine Hydrochloride (May require to reduce the dosage of antihypertensive). Products include:
Apresazide Capsules 854
Apresoline Hydrochloride Parenteral (Ampuls) 856
Apresoline Hydrochloride Tablets .. 855
Apresoline-Esidrix Tablets 857
Ser-Ap-Es Tablets 881
Serpasil-Apresoline Tablets 884
Hydrochlorothiazide (May require to reduce the dosage of antihypertensive). Products include:
Aldactazide 2150
Aldoril Tablets 1418
Apresazide Capsules 854
Apresoline-Esidrix Tablets 857
Capozide 2258
Dyazide Capsules 2208
Esidrix Tablets 863
Esimil Tablets 864
HydroDIURIL Tablets 1484
Hydropres Tablets 1485
Inderide Tablets 2463
Inderide LA Long Acting Capsules .. 2465
Lopressor HCT Tablets 1034
Maxzide 1215
Moduretic Tablets 1510
Normozide Tablets 2112
Oretic Tablets 544
Oreticyl 545
Prinzide Tablets 1540
Ser-Ap-Es Tablets 881
Serpasil-Esidrix Tablets 886
Timolide Tablets 1547
Trandate HCT Tablets 579
Vaseretic Tablets 1559
Zestoretic 2274
Hydroflumethiazide (May require to reduce the dosage of antihypertensive). Products include:
Diucardin Tablets 2450
Saluron 718
Salutensin/Salutensin-Demi 719
Indapamide (May require to reduce the dosage of antihypertensive). Products include:
Lozol Tablets 1843
Isradipine (May require to reduce the dosage of antihypertensive). Products include:
DynaCirc Capsules 2004
Labetalol Hydrochloride (May require to reduce the dosage of antihypertensive). Products include:
Normodyne Injection 2108
Normodyne Tablets 2110
Normozide Tablets 2112
Trandate HCT Tablets 579
Trandate Injection 577
Trandate Tablets 579
Lisinopril (May require to reduce the dosage of antihypertensive). Products include:
Prinivil Tablets 1538
Prinzide Tablets 1540
Zestoretic 2274
Zestril Tablets 2277
Mecamylamine Hydrochloride (May require to reduce the dosage of antihypertensive). Products include:
Inversine Tablets 1492
Methyclothiazide (May require to reduce the dosage of antihypertensive). Products include:
Enduron Tablets 517
Enduronyl 518
Methyldopa (May require to reduce the dosage of antihypertensive). Products include:
Aldoclor Tablets 1413
Aldomet Oral 1415
Aldoril Tablets 1418
Methyldopate Hydrochloride (May require to reduce the dosage of antihypertensive). Products include:
Aldomet Ester HCl Injection 1417
Metolazone (May require to reduce the dosage of antihypertensive). Products include:
Diulo 2129
Mykrox ½ mg Tablets 984
Zaroxolyn Tablets 989
Metoprolol Tartrate (May require to reduce the dosage of antihypertensive). Products include:
Lopressor Ampuls 1032
Lopressor HCT Tablets 1034
Lopressor Tablets 1032
Metyrosine (May require to reduce the dosage of antihypertensive). Products include:
Demser Capsules 1460
Minoxidil (May require to reduce the dosage of antihypertensive). Products include:
Loniten Tablets 2346
Rogaine Topical Solution 2357
Nadolol (May require to reduce the dosage of antihypertensive). Products include:
Corgard Tablets 701
Corzide Tablets 702
Nicardipine Hydrochloride (May require to reduce the dosage of antihypertensive). Products include:
Cardene Capsules 2290
Nitroglycerin (May require to reduce the dosage of antihypertensive). Products include:
Deponit NTG Transdermal Delivery System 2143
Minitran Transdermal Delivery System 1312
Nitro-Bid Ointment 1339
Nitro-Bid Capsules 1338
Nitrodisc 2176
Nitro-Dur (nitroglycerin) Transdermal Infusion System 1164
Nitrogard Tablets 1004
Nitrolingual Spray 1846
Nitrostat Tablets 1743
Transderm-Nitro Transdermal Therapeutic System 2283
Penbutolol Sulfate (May require to reduce the dosage of antihypertensive). Products include:
Levatol 1832
Phenoxybenzamine Hydrochloride (May require to reduce the dosage of antihypertensive). Products include:
Dibenzyline Capsules 2207
Phentolamine Mesylate (May require to reduce the dosage of antihypertensive). Products include:
Regitine 878
Pindolol (May require to reduce the dosage of antihypertensive). Products include:
Visken Tablets 2036
Polythiazide (May require to reduce the dosage of antihypertensive). Products include:
Minizide Capsules 1779
Renese Tablets 1785
Renese-R Tablets 1786

Prazosin Hydrochloride (May require to reduce the dosage of antihypertensive). Products include:
Minipress Capsules 1778
Minizide Capsules 1779

Propranolol Hydrochloride (May require to reduce the dosage of antihypertensive). Products include:
Inderal 2459
Inderal LA Long Acting Capsules 2461
Inderide Tablets 2463
Inderide LA Long Acting Capsules 2465

Ramipril (May require to reduce the dosage of antihypertensive). Products include:
Altace Capsules 1086

Rauwolfia Serpentina (May require to reduce the dosage of antihypertensive). Products include:
Raudixin Tablets 1803
Rauzide Tablets 1804

Rescinnamine (May require to reduce the dosage of antihypertensive).
No products indexed under this heading.

Reserpine (May require to reduce the dosage of antihypertensive). Products include:
Diupres Tablets 1461
Hydromox R Tablets 1209
Hydropres Tablets 1485
Renese-R Tablets 1786
Salutensin/Salutensin-Demi 719
Ser-Ap-Es Tablets 881
Serpasil Tablets 883
Serpasil-Apresoline Tablets 884
Serpasil-Esidrix Tablets 886

Sodium Nitroprusside (May require to reduce the dosage of antihypertensive). Products include:
Nipride I.V. Infusion 1909

Terazosin Hydrochloride (May require to reduce the dosage of antihypertensive). Products include:
Hytrin Tablets 529

Timolol Maleate (May require to reduce the dosage of antihypertensive). Products include:
Blocadren Tablets 1429
Timolide Tablets 1547
Timoptic in Ocudose 1552
Timoptic Sterile Ophthalmic Solution 1550

Trimethaphan Camsylate (May require to reduce the dosage of antihypertensive). Products include:
Arfonad Ampuls 1887

Warfarin Sodium (Bleeding; prolonged prothrombin time). Products include:
Coumadin Injection & Tablets 944
Panwarfin Tablets 547

Food Interactions

Food, unspecified (Delays absorption but does not affect total absorption).

TREXAN TABLETS

(Naltrexone Hydrochloride) 937
May interact with narcotic analgesics and certain other agents. Compounds in these categories include:

Alfentanil Hydrochloride (Trexan blocks the pharmacologic effect of exogenously administered opioids). Products include:
Alfenta Injection 1131

Buprenorphine (Trexan blocks the pharmacologic effect of exogenously administered opioids).
No products indexed under this heading.

Codeine (Trexan blocks the pharmacologic effect of exogenously administered opioids). Products include:
Calcidrine Syrup 506

Codeine Phosphate (Trexan blocks the pharmacologic effect of exogenously administered opioids). Products include:
Actifed with Codeine Cough Syrup 752
Cheracol Cough Syrup 1853
Codimal PH Syrup 846
Dimetane-DC Cough Syrup 1857
Empirin with Codeine Phosphate Nos. 2, 3 & 4 764
Fiorinal with Codeine Capsules 2008
Isoclor Expectorant 982
Naldecon CX Adult Liquid 521
Novahistine DH 1342
Novahistine Expectorant 1343
Nucofed Capsules 2219
Nucofed Expectorant 2219
Nucofed Pediatric Expectorant 2220
Nucofed Syrup 2219
Phenaphen with Codeine Capsules 1865
Phenaphen-650 with Codeine Tablets 1866
Phenergan with Codeine 2497
Phenergan VC with Codeine 2501
Robitussin A-C Syrup 1875
Robitussin-DAC Syrup 1875
Ryna 741
Soma Compound w/Codeine Tablets 2390
Triaminic Expectorant w/Codeine 1996
Tussi-Organidin Liquid 2391
Tylenol with Codeine 1381

Codeine Polistirex (Trexan blocks the pharmacologic effect of exogenously administered opioids).
No products indexed under this heading.

Dezocine (Trexan blocks the pharmacologic effect of exogenously administered opioids).

Diphenoxylate Hydrochloride (Trexan interferes with the action of narcotic containing drug products). Products include:
Lomotil 2174

Fentanyl (Trexan blocks the pharmacologic effect of exogenously administered opioids). Products include:
Duragesic Transdermal System 1133

Fentanyl Citrate (Trexan blocks the pharmacologic effect of exogenously administered opioids). Products include:
Innovar Injection 1141
Sublimaze Injection 1146

Hydrocodone Bitartrate (Trexan blocks the pharmacologic effect of exogenously administered opioids). Products include:
Anexsia 5/500 Tablets 2196
Anexsia 7.5/650 Tablets 2197
Azdone Tablets 844
Codiclear DH Syrup 845
Codimal DH Syrup 846
Damason-P 1356
Hycodan Syrup, Tablets 927
Hycomine Compound Tablets 929
Hycomine Syrup 927
Hycotuss Expectorant Syrup 930
Hydrocet Capsules 835
Lortab ASA Tablets 2414
Lortab 2412
Ru-Tuss with Hydrocodone 694
Triaminic Expectorant DH 1995
Vicodin Tablets 1187
Vicodin ES Tablets 1189
Zydone Capsules 941

Hydrocodone Polistirex (Trexan blocks the pharmacologic effect of exogenously administered opioids). Products include:
Tussionex Extended-Release Suspension 988

Levorphanol Tartrate (Trexan blocks the pharmacologic effect of exogenously administered opioids). Products include:
Levo-Dromoran 1906

Meperidine Hydrochloride (Trexan blocks the pharmacologic effect of exogenously administered opioids). Products include:
Demerol 2047
Mepergan Injection 2479

Methadone Hydrochloride (Trexan blocks the pharmacologic effect of exogenously administered opioids). Products include:
Dolophine Hydrochloride Ampoules & Vials 1260
Dolophine Hydrochloride Tablets 1261
Methadone Hydrochloride Diskets 1284
Methadone Hydrochloride Oral Solution & Tablets 1987

Morphine Sulfate (Trexan blocks the pharmacologic effect of exogenously administered opioids). Products include:
Astramorph/PF Injection, USP (Preservative-Free) 618
Duramorph 960
Infumorph 200 and Infumorph 500 Sterile Solutions 962
MS Contin Tablets 1814
MSIR 1817
Oramorph SR (Morphine Sulfate Sustained Release Tablets) 1988
Roxanol 1991

Opium Alkaloids (Trexan blocks the pharmacologic effect of exogenously administered opioids). Products include:
B & O No. 15A & No. 16A Supprettes 2395
Pantopon Injectable 1911

Oxycodone Hydrochloride (Trexan blocks the pharmacologic effect of exogenously administered opioids). Products include:
Percocet Tablets 950
Percodan 951
Roxicodone Tablets, Oral Solution & Intensol (Oxycodone) 1992
Tylox Capsules 1382

Paregoric (Trexan interferes with the action of narcotic containing drug products). Products include:
Donnagel-PG 1858

Propoxyphene Hydrochloride (Trexan blocks the pharmacologic effect of exogenously administered opioids). Products include:
Darvon 1256
Wygesic Tablets 2540

Propoxyphene Napsylate (Trexan blocks the pharmacologic effect of exogenously administered opioids). Products include:
Darvon-N/Darvocet-N 1254

Sufentanil Citrate (Trexan blocks the pharmacologic effect of exogenously administered opioids). Products include:
Sufenta Injection 1147

Thioridazine Hydrochloride (Potential for lethargy and somnolence). Products include:
Mellaril 2011

TRIAMINIC ALLERGY TABLETS

(Chlorpheniramine Maleate, Phenylpropanolamine Hydrochloride) 688
May interact with monoamine oxidase inhibitors, hypnotics and sedatives, tranquilizers, and certain other agents. Compounds in these categories include:

Alcohol (Increased drowsiness effect).

Alprazolam (Increased drowsiness effect). Products include:
Xanax Tablets 2367

Buspirone Hydrochloride (Increased drowsiness effect). Products include:
BuSpar 1401

Chlordiazepoxide (Increased drowsiness effect). Products include:
Libritabs Tablets 1930
Limbitrol 1933
Menrium Tablets 1934

Chlordiazepoxide Hydrochloride (Increased drowsiness effect). Products include:
Librax Capsules 1929
Librium Capsules 1931
Librium Injectable 1932

Chlorpromazine (Increased drowsiness effect). Products include:
Thorazine 2234

Chlorprothixene (Increased drowsiness effect). Products include:
Taractan Tablets 1920

Chlorprothixene Hydrochloride (Increased drowsiness effect). Products include:
Taractan 1920

Clorazepate Dipotassium (Increased drowsiness effect). Products include:
Tranxene 556

Diazepam (Increased drowsiness effect). Products include:
Valium Injectable 1937
Valium Tablets 1939
Valrelease Capsules 1923

Droperidol (Increased drowsiness effect). Products include:
Inapsine Injection 1140
Innovar Injection 1141

Estazolam (Increased drowsiness effect). Products include:
ProSom Tablets 554

Ethchlorvynol (Increased drowsiness effect). Products include:
Placidyl Capsules 553

Ethinamate (Increased drowsiness effect).
No products indexed under this heading.

Fluphenazine Decanoate (Increased drowsiness effect). Products include:
Prolixin Decanoate 1795

Fluphenazine Enanthate (Increased drowsiness effect). Products include:
Prolixin Enanthate 1796

Fluphenazine Hydrochloride (Increased drowsiness effect). Products include:
Prolixin Elixir 1793
Prolixin Injection 1791
Prolixin Oral Concentrate 1792
Prolixin Tablets 1793

Flurazepam Hydrochloride (Increased drowsiness effect). Products include:
Dalmane Capsules 1927

Furazolidone (Concomitant administration is not recommended). Products include:
Furoxone 1855

Glutethimide (Increased drowsiness effect).
No products indexed under this heading.

Haloperidol (Increased drowsiness effect). Products include:
Haldol Injection, Tablets and Concentrate 1373

Haloperidol Decanoate (Increased drowsiness effect). Products include:
Haldol Decanoate 1375

Hydroxyzine Hydrochloride (Increased drowsiness effect). Products include:
Atarax Tablets & Syrup 1941
Marax Tablets & DF Syrup 1954
Vistaril Intramuscular Solution 1970

Isocarboxazid (Concomitant administration is not recommended). Products include:
Marplan Tablets 1906

Lorazepam (Increased drowsiness effect). Products include:
Ativan Injection 2432
Ativan Tablets 2434

Loxapine Hydrochloride (Increased drowsiness effect). Products include:
Loxitane 1213

Loxapine Succinate (Increased drowsiness effect). Products include:
Loxitane Capsules 1213

Meprobamate (Increased drowsiness effect). Products include:
Deprol Tablets 2382
Equagesic Tablets 2451
Miltown Tablets 2386
PMB 200 and PMB 400 2504

Mesoridazine Besylate (Increased drowsiness effect).

Midazolam Hydrochloride (Increased drowsiness effect). Products include:
Versed Injection 1924

Molindone Hydrochloride (Increased drowsiness effect). Products include:
Moban Tablets & Concentrate 932

Oxazepam (Increased drowsiness effect). Products include:
Serax Capsules 2522
Serax Tablets 2522

Perphenazine (Increased drowsiness effect). Products include:
Etrafon 2087
Triavil Tablets 1556
Trilafon 2123

Phenelzine Sulfate (Concomitant administration is not recommended). Products include:
Nardil 1742

Prazepam (Increased drowsiness effect). Products include:
Centrax 1693

Prochlorperazine (Increased drowsiness effect). Products include:
Compazine 2201

Promethazine Hydrochloride (Increased drowsiness effect). Products include:
Mepergan Injection 2479
Phenergan with Codeine 2497
Phenergan with Dextromethorphan 2499
Phenergan Injection 2493
Phenergan Suppositories 2496
Phenergan Syrup 2495
Phenergan Tablets 2496
Phenergan VC 2500
Phenergan VC with Codeine 2501

Propofol (Increased drowsiness effect). Products include:
Diprivan Injection 2267

Quazepam (Increased drowsiness effect). Products include:
Doral Tablets 2383

Secobarbital Sodium (Increased drowsiness effect). Products include:
Seconal Sodium Pulvules 1296

Selegiline Hydrochloride (Concomitant administration is not recommended). Products include:
Eldepryl 2250

Temazepam (Increased drowsiness effect). Products include:
Restoril Capsules 2023

Thioridazine Hydrochloride (Increased drowsiness effect). Products include:
Mellaril 2011

Thiothixene (Increased drowsiness effect). Products include:
Navane Capsules and Concentrate 1954
Navane Intramuscular 1956

Tranylcypromine Sulfate (Concomitant administration is not recommended). Products include:
Parnate Tablets 2222

Triazolam (Increased drowsiness effect). Products include:
Halcion Tablets 2340

Trifluoperazine Hydrochloride (Increased drowsiness effect). Products include:
Stelazine 2226

TRIAMINIC CHEWABLES

(Chlorpheniramine Maleate, Phenylpropanolamine Hydrochloride) ▣ 688

May interact with hypnotics and sedatives, tranquilizers, and certain other agents. Compounds in these categories include:

Alcohol (Increases drowsiness effect).

Alprazolam (Increases drowsiness effect). Products include:
Xanax Tablets 2367

Antidepressant Medications, unspecified (Increases drowsiness effect).

Blood Pressure Medications, unspecified (Increases drowsiness effect).
No products indexed under this heading.

Buspirone Hydrochloride (Increases drowsiness effect). Products include:
BuSpar 1401

Chlordiazepoxide (Increases drowsiness effect). Products include:
Libritabs Tablets 1930
Limbitrol 1933
Menrium Tablets 1934

Chlordiazepoxide Hydrochloride (Increases drowsiness effect). Products include:
Librax Capsules 1929
Librium Capsules 1931
Librium Injectable 1932

Chlorpromazine (Increases drowsiness effect). Products include:
Thorazine 2234

Chlorprothixene (Increases drowsiness effect). Products include:
Taractan Tablets 1920

Chlorprothixene Hydrochloride (Increases drowsiness effect). Products include:
Taractan 1920

Clorazepate Dipotassium (Increases drowsiness effect). Products include:
Tranxene 556

Diazepam (Increases drowsiness effect). Products include:
Valium Injectable 1937
Valium Tablets 1939
Valrelease Capsules 1923

Droperidol (Increases drowsiness effect). Products include:
Inapsine Injection 1140
Innovar Injection 1141

Estazolam (Increases drowsiness effect). Products include:
ProSom Tablets 554

Ethchlorvynol (Increases drowsiness effect). Products include:
Placidyl Capsules 553

Ethinamate (Increases drowsiness effect).
No products indexed under this heading.

Fluphenazine Decanoate (Increases drowsiness effect). Products include:
Prolixin Decanoate 1795

Fluphenazine Enanthate (Increases drowsiness effect). Products include:
Prolixin Enanthate 1796

Fluphenazine Hydrochloride (Increases drowsiness effect). Products include:
Prolixin Elixir 1793
Prolixin Injection 1791
Prolixin Oral Concentrate 1792
Prolixin Tablets 1793

Flurazepam Hydrochloride (Increases drowsiness effect). Products include:
Dalmane Capsules 1927

Glutethimide (Increases drowsiness effect).
No products indexed under this heading.

Haloperidol (Increases drowsiness effect). Products include:
Haldol Injection, Tablets and Concentrate 1373

Haloperidol Decanoate (Increases drowsiness effect). Products include:
Haldol Decanoate 1375

Hydroxyzine Hydrochloride (Increases drowsiness effect). Products include:
Atarax Tablets & Syrup 1941
Marax Tablets & DF Syrup 1954
Vistaril Intramuscular Solution 1970

Lorazepam (Increases drowsiness effect). Products include:
Ativan Injection 2432
Ativan Tablets 2434

Loxapine Hydrochloride (Increases drowsiness effect). Products include:
Loxitane 1213

Loxapine Succinate (Increases drowsiness effect). Products include:
Loxitane Capsules 1213

Meprobamate (Increases drowsiness effect). Products include:
Deprol Tablets 2382
Equagesic Tablets 2451
Miltown Tablets 2386
PMB 200 and PMB 400 2504

Mesoridazine Besylate (Increases drowsiness effect).

Midazolam Hydrochloride (Increases drowsiness effect). Products include:
Versed Injection 1924

Molindone Hydrochloride (Increases drowsiness effect). Products include:
Moban Tablets & Concentrate 932

Oxazepam (Increases drowsiness effect). Products include:
Serax Capsules 2522
Serax Tablets 2522

Perphenazine (Increases drowsiness effect). Products include:
Etrafon 2087
Triavil Tablets 1556
Trilafon 2123

Prazepam (Increases drowsiness effect). Products include:
Centrax 1693

Prochlorperazine (Increases drowsiness effect). Products include:
Compazine 2201

Promethazine Hydrochloride (Increases drowsiness effect). Products include:
Mepergan Injection 2479
Phenergan with Codeine 2497
Phenergan with Dextromethorphan 2499
Phenergan Injection 2493
Phenergan Suppositories 2496
Phenergan Syrup 2495
Phenergan Tablets 2496
Phenergan VC 2500
Phenergan VC with Codeine 2501

Propofol (Increases drowsiness effect). Products include:
Diprivan Injection 2267

Quazepam (Increases drowsiness effect). Products include:
Doral Tablets 2383

Secobarbital Sodium (Increases drowsiness effect). Products include:
Seconal Sodium Pulvules 1296

Temazepam (Increases drowsiness effect). Products include:
Restoril Capsules 2023

Thioridazine Hydrochloride (Increases drowsiness effect). Products include:
Mellaril 2011

Thiothixene (Increases drowsiness effect). Products include:
Navane Capsules and Concentrate 1954
Navane Intramuscular 1956

Triazolam (Increases drowsiness effect). Products include:
Halcion Tablets 2340

Trifluoperazine Hydrochloride (Increases drowsiness effect). Products include:
Stelazine 2226

TRIAMINIC COLD TABLETS

(Phenylpropanolamine Hydrochloride, Chlorpheniramine Maleate) ▣ 688

May interact with monoamine oxidase inhibitors, central nervous system depressants, hypnotics and sedatives, tranquilizers, and certain other agents. Compounds in these categories include:

Alcohol (Potentiation of sedative effects of antihistamines).

Alfentanil Hydrochloride (Potentiation of sedative effects of antihistamines). Products include:
Alfenta Injection 1131

Alprazolam (Potentiation of sedative effects of antihistamines). Products include:
Xanax Tablets 2367

Aprobarbital (Potentiation of sedative effects of antihistamines). Products include:
Alurate Elixir 1883

Buprenorphine (Potentiation of sedative effects of antihistamines).
No products indexed under this heading.

Buspirone Hydrochloride (Potentiation of sedative effects of antihistamines). Products include:
BuSpar 1401

Butabarbital (Potentiation of sedative effects of antihistamines). Products include:
Pyridium Plus 1764

Butalbital (Potentiation of sedative effects of antihistamines). Products include:
Esgic-Plus Tablets 1002
Esgic Tablets & Capsules 1001
Fioricet Tablets 2006
Fiorinal Capsules 2007
Fiorinal with Codeine Capsules 2008
Fiorinal Tablets 2007
Phrenilin 838
Sedapap Tablets 50 mg/650 mg 1360

Chlordiazepoxide (Potentiation of sedative effects of antihistamines). Products include:
Libritabs Tablets 1930
Limbitrol 1933
Menrium Tablets 1934

Chlordiazepoxide Hydrochloride (Potentiation of sedative effects of antihistamines). Products include:
Librax Capsules 1929
Librium Capsules 1931
Librium Injectable 1932

Chlorpromazine (Potentiation of sedative effects of antihistamines). Products include:
Thorazine ... 2234

Chlorprothixene (Potentiation of sedative effects of antihistamines). Products include:
Taractan Tablets ... 1920

Chlorprothixene Hydrochloride (Potentiation of sedative effects of antihistamines). Products include:
Taractan ... 1920

Clorazepate Dipotassium (Potentiation of sedative effects of antihistamines). Products include:
Tranxene ... 556

Codeine (Potentiation of sedative effects of antihistamines). Products include:
Calcidrine Syrup ... 506

Codeine Phosphate (Potentiation of sedative effects of antihistamines). Products include:
Actifed with Codeine Cough Syrup.. 752
Cheracol Cough Syrup ... 1853
Codimal PH Syrup ... 846
Dimetane-DC Cough Syrup ... 1857
Empirin with Codeine Phosphate Nos. 2, 3 & 4 ... 764
Fiorinal with Codeine Capsules ... 2008
Isoclor Expectorant ... 982
Naldecon CX Adult Liquid ... ▣ 521
Novahistine DH ... 1342
Novahistine Expectorant ... 1343
Nucofed Capsules ... 2219
Nucofed Expectorant ... 2219
Nucofed Pediatric Expectorant ... 2220
Nucofed Syrup ... 2219
Phenaphen with Codeine Capsules 1865
Phenaphen-650 with Codeine Tablets ... 1866
Phenergan with Codeine ... 2497
Phenergan VC with Codeine ... 2501
Robitussin A-C Syrup ... 1875
Robitussin-DAC Syrup ... 1875
Ryna ... ▣ 741
Soma Compound w/Codeine Tablets ... 2390
Triaminic Expectorant w/Codeine .. 1996
Tussi-Organidin Liquid ... 2391
Tylenol with Codeine ... 1381

Codeine Polistirex (Potentiation of sedative effects of antihistamines).
No products indexed under this heading.

Dezocine (Potentiation of sedative effects of antihistamines).

Diazepam (Potentiation of sedative effects of antihistamines). Products include:
Valium Injectable ... 1937
Valium Tablets ... 1939
Valrelease Capsules ... 1923

Droperidol (Potentiation of sedative effects of antihistamines). Products include:
Inapsine Injection ... 1140
Innovar Injection ... 1141

Enflurane (Potentiation of sedative effects of antihistamines). Products include:
Ethrane ... 599

Estazolam (Potentiation of sedative effects of antihistamines). Products include:
ProSom Tablets ... 554

Ethchlorvynol (Potentiation of sedative effects of antihistamines). Products include:
Placidyl Capsules ... 553

Ethinamate (Potentiation of sedative effects of antihistamines).
No products indexed under this heading.

Fentanyl (Potentiation of sedative effects of antihistamines). Products include:
Duragesic Transdermal System ... 1133

Fentanyl Citrate (Potentiation of sedative effects of antihistamines). Products include:
Innovar Injection ... 1141
Sublimaze Injection ... 1146

Fluphenazine Decanoate (Potentiation of sedative effects of antihistamines). Products include:
Prolixin Decanoate ... 1795

Fluphenazine Enanthate (Potentiation of sedative effects of antihistamines). Products include:
Prolixin Enanthate ... 1796

Fluphenazine Hydrochloride (Potentiation of sedative effects of antihistamines). Products include:
Prolixin Elixir ... 1793
Prolixin Injection ... 1791
Prolixin Oral Concentrate ... 1792
Prolixin Tablets ... 1793

Flurazepam Hydrochloride (Potentiation of sedative effects of antihistamines). Products include:
Dalmane Capsules ... 1927

Furazolidone (Contraindicated). Products include:
Furoxone ... 1855

Glutethimide (Potentiation of sedative effects of antihistamines).
No products indexed under this heading.

Haloperidol (Potentiation of sedative effects of antihistamines). Products include:
Haldol Injection, Tablets and Concentrate ... 1373

Haloperidol Decanoate (Potentiation of sedative effects of antihistamines). Products include:
Haldol Decanoate ... 1375

Hydrocodone Bitartrate (Potentiation of sedative effects of antihistamines). Products include:
Anexsia 5/500 Tablets ... 2196
Anexsia 7.5/650 Tablets ... 2197
Azdone Tablets ... 844
Codiclear DH Syrup ... 845
Codimal DH Syrup ... 846
Damason-P ... 1356
Hycodan Syrup, Tablets ... 927
Hycomine Compound Tablets ... 929
Hycomine Syrup ... 927
Hycotuss Expectorant Syrup ... 930
Hydrocet Capsules ... 835
Lortab ASA Tablets ... 2414
Lortab ... 2412
Ru-Tuss with Hydrocodone ... 694
Triaminic Expectorant DH ... 1995
Vicodin Tablets ... 1187
Vicodin ES Tablets ... 1189
Zydone Capsules ... 941

Hydrocodone Polistirex (Potentiation of sedative effects of antihistamines). Products include:
Tussionex Extended-Release Suspension ... 988

Hydroxyzine Hydrochloride (Potentiation of sedative effects of antihistamines). Products include:
Atarax Tablets & Syrup ... 1941
Marax Tablets & DF Syrup ... 1954
Vistaril Intramuscular Solution ... 1970

Isocarboxazid (Contraindicated). Products include:
Marplan Tablets ... 1906

Isoflurane (Potentiation of sedative effects of antihistamines). Products include:
Forane ... 600

Ketamine Hydrochloride (Potentiation of sedative effects of antihistamines). Products include:
Ketalar ... 1726

Levorphanol Tartrate (Potentiation of sedative effects of antihistamines). Products include:
Levo-Dromoran ... 1906

Lorazepam (Potentiation of sedative effects of antihistamines). Products include:
Ativan Injection ... 2432
Ativan Tablets ... 2434

Loxapine Hydrochloride (Potentiation of sedative effects of antihistamines). Products include:
Loxitane ... 1213

Loxapine Succinate (Potentiation of sedative effects of antihistamines). Products include:
Loxitane Capsules ... 1213

Meperidine Hydrochloride (Potentiation of sedative effects of antihistamines). Products include:
Demerol ... 2047
Mepergan Injection ... 2479

Mephobarbital (Potentiation of sedative effects of antihistamines). Products include:
Mebaral Tablets ... 2061

Meprobamate (Potentiation of sedative effects of antihistamines). Products include:
Deprol Tablets ... 2382
Equagesic Tablets ... 2451
Miltown Tablets ... 2386
PMB 200 and PMB 400 ... 2504

Mesoridazine (Potentiation of sedative effects of antihistamines). Products include:
Serentil ... 686

Mesoridazine Besylate (Potentiation of sedative effects of antihistamines).

Methadone Hydrochloride (Potentiation of sedative effects of antihistamines). Products include:
Dolophine Hydrochloride Ampoules & Vials ... 1260
Dolophine Hydrochloride Tablets ... 1261
Methadone Hydrochloride Diskets .. 1284
Methadone Hydrochloride Oral Solution & Tablets ... 1987

Methohexital Sodium (Potentiation of sedative effects of antihistamines). Products include:
Brevital Sodium Vials ... 1248

Methoxyflurane (Potentiation of sedative effects of antihistamines).
No products indexed under this heading.

Midazolam Hydrochloride (Potentiation of sedative effects of antihistamines). Products include:
Versed Injection ... 1924

Molindone Hydrochloride (Potentiation of sedative effects of antihistamines). Products include:
Moban Tablets & Concentrate ... 932

Morphine Sulfate (Potentiation of sedative effects of antihistamines). Products include:
Astramorph/PF Injection, USP (Preservative-Free) ... 618
Duramorph ... 960
Infumorph 200 and Infumorph 500 Sterile Solutions ... 962
MS Contin Tablets ... 1814
MSIR ... 1817
Oramorph SR (Morphine Sulfate Sustained Release Tablets) ... 1988
Roxanol ... 1991

Opium Alkaloids (Potentiation of sedative effects of antihistamines). Products include:
B & O No. 15A & No. 16A Supprettes ... 2395
Pantopon Injectable ... 1911

Oxazepam (Potentiation of sedative effects of antihistamines). Products include:
Serax Capsules ... 2522
Serax Tablets ... 2522

Oxycodone Hydrochloride (Potentiation of sedative effects of antihistamines). Products include:
Percocet Tablets ... 950
Percodan ... 951
Roxicodone Tablets, Oral Solution & Intensol (Oxycodone) ... 1992
Tylox Capsules ... 1382

Pentobarbital Sodium (Potentiation of sedative effects of antihistamines). Products include:
Nembutal Sodium Capsules ... 534
Nembutal Sodium Solution ... 536
Nembutal Sodium Suppositories ... 538

Perphenazine (Potentiation of sedative effects of antihistamines). Products include:
Etrafon ... 2087
Triavil Tablets ... 1556
Trilafon ... 2123

Phenelzine Sulfate (Contraindicated). Products include:
Nardil ... 1742

Phenobarbital (Potentiation of sedative effects of antihistamines). Products include:
Arco-Lase Plus Tablets ... 607
Bellergal-S Tablets ... 1998
Bronkolixir ... ▣ 761
Bronkotabs Tablets ... ▣ 762
Donnatal ... 1858
Donnatal Extentabs ... 1859
Donnatal Tablets ... 1858
Donnazyme Tablets ... 1860
Kinesed Tablets ... 2272
Phenobarbital Elixir and Tablets ... 1293
Primatene Tablets-P Formula ... 2421
Quadrinal Tablets ... 1183
Tedral SA ... 1765

Prazepam (Potentiation of sedative effects of antihistamines). Products include:
Centrax ... 1693

Prochlorperazine (Potentiation of sedative effects of antihistamines). Products include:
Compazine ... 2201

Promethazine Hydrochloride (Potentiation of sedative effects of antihistamines). Products include:
Mepergan Injection ... 2479
Phenergan with Codeine ... 2497
Phenergan with Dextromethorphan 2499
Phenergan Injection ... 2493
Phenergan Suppositories ... 2496
Phenergan Syrup ... 2495
Phenergan Tablets ... 2496
Phenergan VC ... 2500
Phenergan VC with Codeine ... 2501

Propofol (Potentiation of sedative effects of antihistamines). Products include:
Diprivan Injection ... 2267

Propoxyphene Hydrochloride (Potentiation of sedative effects of antihistamines). Products include:
Darvon ... 1256
Wygesic Tablets ... 2540

Propoxyphene Napsylate (Potentiation of sedative effects of antihistamines). Products include:
Darvon-N/Darvocet-N ... 1254

Quazepam (Potentiation of sedative effects of antihistamines). Products include:
Doral Tablets ... 2383

Secobarbital Sodium (Potentiation of sedative effects of antihistamines). Products include:
Seconal Sodium Pulvules ... 1296

Selegiline Hydrochloride (Contraindicated). Products include:
Eldepryl ... 2250

Sufentanil Citrate (Potentiation of sedative effects of antihistamines). Products include:
Sufenta Injection ... 1147

Temazepam (Potentiation of sedative effects of antihistamines). Products include:
Restoril Capsules ... 2023

Thiamylal Sodium (Potentiation of sedative effects of antihistamines). Products include:
Surital Ampoules, Steri-Vials ... 1764

Thioridazine Hydrochloride (Potentiation of sedative effects of antihistamines). Products include:
Mellaril ... 2011
Thiothixene (Potentiation of sedative effects of antihistamines). Products include:
Navane Capsules and Concentrate 1954
Navane Intramuscular ... 1956
Tranylcypromine Sulfate (Contraindicated). Products include:
Parnate Tablets ... 2222
Triazolam (Potentiation of sedative effects of antihistamines). Products include:
Halcion Tablets ... 2340
Trifluoperazine Hydrochloride (Potentiation of sedative effects of antihistamines). Products include:
Stelazine ... 2226

TRIAMINIC EXPECTORANT
(Phenylpropanolamine Hydrochloride, Guaifenesin) ... ▣ 688
May interact with:

Antidepressant Medications, unspecified (Effect not specified).
Blood Pressure Medications, unspecified (Effect not specified).
No products indexed under this heading.

TRIAMINIC EXPECTORANT W/CODEINE
(Codeine Phosphate, Phenylpropanolamine Hydrochloride, Guaifenesin) ... 1996
May interact with antihypertensives and antidepressant drugs. Compounds in these categories include:

Acebutolol Hydrochloride (Effect not specified). Products include:
Sectral Capsules ... 2520
Amitriptyline Hydrochloride (Effect not specified). Products include:
Elavil ... 2269
Endep Tablets ... 1927
Etrafon ... 2087
Limbitrol ... 1933
Triavil Tablets ... 1556
Amoxapine (Effect not specified). Products include:
Asendin Tablets ... 1196
Atenolol (Effect not specified). Products include:
Tenoretic Tablets ... 1105
Tenormin Tablets and I.V. Injection 1107
Benazepril Hydrochloride (Effect not specified). Products include:
Lotensin Tablets ... 872
Betaxolol Hydrochloride (Effect not specified). Products include:
Betoptic Sterile Ophthalmic Solution ... 569
Betoptic S Sterile Ophthalmic Suspension ... 570
Kerlone Tablets ... 2172
Bupropion Hydrochloride (Effect not specified). Products include:
Wellbutrin Tablets ... 821
Captopril (Effect not specified). Products include:
Capoten ... 2255
Capozide ... 2258
Carteolol Hydrochloride (Effect not specified). Products include:
Cartrol Tablets ... 507
Clonidine (Effect not specified). Products include:
Catapres-TTS ... 677
Clonidine Hydrochloride (Effect not specified). Products include:
Catapres Tablets ... 676
Combipres Tablets ... 678
Deserpidine (Effect not specified). Products include:
Enduronyl ... 518
Harmonyl Tablets ... 528
Oreticyl ... 545
Desipramine Hydrochloride (Effect not specified). Products include:
Norpramin Tablets ... 1340
Diazoxide (Effect not specified). Products include:
Hyperstat I.V. Injection ... 2095
Proglycem ... 649
Doxazosin Mesylate (Effect not specified). Products include:
Cardura Tablets ... 1941
Doxepin Hydrochloride (Effect not specified). Products include:
Sinequan ... 1960
Enalapril Maleate (Effect not specified). Products include:
Vaseretic Tablets ... 1559
Vasotec Tablets ... 1564
Enalaprilat (Effect not specified). Products include:
Vasotec I.V. ... 1562
Esmolol Hydrochloride (Effect not specified). Products include:
Brevibloc Injection ... 942
Felodipine (Effect not specified). Products include:
Plendil Extended-Release Tablets ... 1526
Fluoxetine Hydrochloride (Effect not specified). Products include:
Prozac Pulvules ... 920
Fosinopril Sodium (Effect not specified). Products include:
Monopril Tablets ... 1406
Furazolidone (Contraindicated). Products include:
Furoxone ... 1855
Guanabenz Acetate (Effect not specified). Products include:
Wytensin Tablets ... 2542
Guanethidine Monosulfate (Effect not specified). Products include:
Esimil Tablets ... 864
Ismelin Tablets ... 869
Hydralazine Hydrochloride (Effect not specified). Products include:
Apresazide Capsules ... 854
Apresoline Hydrochloride Parenteral (Ampuls) ... 856
Apresoline Hydrochloride Tablets .. 855
Apresoline-Esidrix Tablets ... 857
Ser-Ap-Es Tablets ... 881
Serpasil-Apresoline Tablets ... 884
Imipramine Hydrochloride (Effect not specified). Products include:
Tofranil Ampuls ... 1038
Tofranil Tablets ... 1039
Imipramine Pamoate (Effect not specified). Products include:
Tofranil-PM Capsules ... 1041
Isocarboxazid (Effect not specified). Products include:
Marplan Tablets ... 1906
Isradipine (Effect not specified). Products include:
DynaCirc Capsules ... 2004
Labetalol Hydrochloride (Effect not specified). Products include:
Normodyne Injection ... 2108
Normodyne Tablets ... 2110
Normozide Tablets ... 2112
Trandate HCT Tablets ... 579
Trandate Injection ... 577
Trandate Tablets ... 579
Lisinopril (Effect not specified). Products include:
Prinivil Tablets ... 1538
Prinzide Tablets ... 1540
Zestoretic ... 2274
Zestril Tablets ... 2277
Maprotiline Hydrochloride (Effect not specified). Products include:
Ludiomil Tablets ... 874
Mecamylamine Hydrochloride (Effect not specified). Products include:
Inversine Tablets ... 1492
Methyclothiazide (Effect not specified). Products include:
Enduron Tablets ... 517
Enduronyl ... 518
Methyldopa (Effect not specified). Products include:
Aldoclor Tablets ... 1413
Aldomet Oral ... 1415
Aldoril Tablets ... 1418
Methyldopate Hydrochloride (Effect not specified). Products include:
Aldomet Ester HCl Injection ... 1417
Metoprolol Tartrate (Effect not specified). Products include:
Lopressor Ampuls ... 1032
Lopressor HCT Tablets ... 1034
Lopressor Tablets ... 1032
Metyrosine (Effect not specified). Products include:
Demser Capsules ... 1460
Minoxidil (Effect not specified). Products include:
Loniten Tablets ... 2346
Rogaine Topical Solution ... 2357
Nadolol (Effect not specified). Products include:
Corgard Tablets ... 701
Corzide Tablets ... 702
Nicardipine Hydrochloride (Effect not specified). Products include:
Cardene Capsules ... 2290
Nitroglycerin (Effect not specified). Products include:
Deponit NTG Transdermal Delivery System ... 2143
Minitran Transdermal Delivery System ... 1312
Nitro-Bid Ointment ... 1339
Nitro-Bid Capsules ... 1338
Nitrodisc ... 2176
Nitro-Dur (nitroglycerin) Transdermal Infusion System ... 1164
Nitrogard Tablets ... 1004
Nitrolingual Spray ... 1846
Nitrostat Tablets ... 1743
Transderm-Nitro Transdermal Therapeutic System ... 2283
Nortriptyline Hydrochloride (Effect not specified). Products include:
Pamelor ... 2019
Penbutolol Sulfate (Effect not specified). Products include:
Levatol ... 1832
Phenelzine Sulfate (Effect not specified). Products include:
Nardil ... 1742
Phenoxybenzamine Hydrochloride (Effect not specified). Products include:
Dibenzyline Capsules ... 2207
Phentolamine Mesylate (Effect not specified). Products include:
Regitine ... 878
Pindolol (Effect not specified). Products include:
Visken Tablets ... 2036
Polythiazide (Effect not specified). Products include:
Minizide Capsules ... 1779
Renese Tablets ... 1785
Renese-R Tablets ... 1786
Prazosin Hydrochloride (Effect not specified). Products include:
Minipress Capsules ... 1778
Minizide Capsules ... 1779
Propranolol Hydrochloride (Effect not specified). Products include:
Inderal ... 2459
Inderal LA Long Acting Capsules ... 2461
Inderide Tablets ... 2463
Inderide LA Long Acting Capsules .. 2465
Protriptyline Hydrochloride (Effect not specified). Products include:
Vivactil Tablets ... 1567
Ramipril (Effect not specified). Products include:
Altace Capsules ... 1086
Rauwolfia Serpentina (Effect not specified). Products include:
Raudixin Tablets ... 1803
Rauzide Tablets ... 1804
Rescinnamine (Effect not specified).
No products indexed under this heading.
Reserpine (Effect not specified). Products include:
Diupres Tablets ... 1461
Hydromox R Tablets ... 1209
Hydropres Tablets ... 1485
Renese-R Tablets ... 1786
Salutensin/Salutensin-Demi ... 719
Ser-Ap-Es Tablets ... 881
Serpasil Tablets ... 883
Serpasil-Apresoline Tablets ... 884
Serpasil-Esidrix Tablets ... 886
Sodium Nitroprusside (Effect not specified). Products include:
Nipride I.V. Infusion ... 1909
Terazosin Hydrochloride (Effect not specified). Products include:
Hytrin Tablets ... 529
Timolol Maleate (Effect not specified). Products include:
Blocadren Tablets ... 1429
Timolide Tablets ... 1547
Timoptic in Ocudose ... 1552
Timoptic Sterile Ophthalmic Solution ... 1550
Tranylcypromine Sulfate (Effect not specified). Products include:
Parnate Tablets ... 2222
Trazodone Hydrochloride (Effect not specified). Products include:
Desyrel and Desyrel Dividose ... 1404
Trimethaphan Camsylate (Effect not specified). Products include:
Arfonad Ampuls ... 1887
Trimipramine Maleate (Effect not specified). Products include:
Surmontil Capsules ... 2524

TRIAMINIC EXPECTORANT DH
(Hydrocodone Bitartrate, Phenylpropanolamine Hydrochloride, Pheniramine Maleate, Pyrilamine Maleate, Guaifenesin) ... 1995
May interact with monoamine oxidase inhibitors, central nervous system depressants, phenothiazines, tricyclic antidepressants, veratrum alkaloids, and certain other agents. Compounds in these categories include:

Alcohol (Potentiation of sedative effects).
Alfentanil Hydrochloride (Potentiation of sedative effects). Products include:
Alfenta Injection ... 1131
Alprazolam (Potentiation of sedative effects). Products include:
Xanax Tablets ... 2367
Amitriptyline Hydrochloride (Potentiation of sedative effects). Products include:
Elavil ... 2269
Endep Tablets ... 1927
Etrafon ... 2087
Limbitrol ... 1933
Triavil Tablets ... 1556
Amoxapine (Potentiation of sedative effects). Products include:
Asendin Tablets ... 1196
Aprobarbital (Potentiation of sedative effects). Products include:
Alurate Elixir ... 1883

Atenolol (Reduced antihypertensive effects). Products include:
- Tenoretic Tablets ... 1105
- Tenormin Tablets and I.V. Injection 1107

Buprenorphine (Potentiation of sedative effects).
- No products indexed under this heading.

Buspirone Hydrochloride (Potentiation of sedative effects). Products include:
- BuSpar ... 1401

Butabarbital (Potentiation of sedative effects). Products include:
- Pyridium Plus ... 1764

Butalbital (Potentiation of sedative effects). Products include:
- Esgic-Plus Tablets ... 1002
- Esgic Tablets & Capsules ... 1001
- Fioricet Tablets ... 2006
- Fiorinal Capsules ... 2007
- Fiorinal with Codeine Capsules ... 2008
- Fiorinal Tablets ... 2007
- Phrenilin ... 838
- Sedapap Tablets 50 mg/650 mg .. 1360

Captopril (Reduced antihypertensive effects). Products include:
- Capoten ... 2255
- Capozide ... 2258

Chlordiazepoxide (Potentiation of sedative effects). Products include:
- Libritabs Tablets ... 1930
- Limbitrol ... 1933
- Menrium Tablets ... 1934

Chlordiazepoxide Hydrochloride (Potentiation of sedative effects). Products include:
- Librax Capsules ... 1929
- Librium Capsules ... 1931
- Librium Injectable ... 1932

Chlorpromazine (Potentiation of sedative effects). Products include:
- Thorazine ... 2234

Chlorprothixene (Potentiation of sedative effects). Products include:
- Taractan Tablets ... 1920

Chlorprothixene Hydrochloride (Potentiation of sedative effects). Products include:
- Taractan ... 1920

Chlorprothixene Lactate (Potentiation of sedative effects). Products include:
- Taractan Concentrate ... 1920

Clomipramine Hydrochloride (Potentiation of sedative effects). Products include:
- Anafranil Capsules ... 650

Clonidine Hydrochloride (Reduced antihypertensive effects). Products include:
- Catapres Tablets ... 676
- Combipres Tablets ... 678

Clorazepate Dipotassium (Potentiation of sedative effects). Products include:
- Tranxene ... 556

Codeine (Potentiation of sedative effects). Products include:
- Calcidrine Syrup ... 506

Codeine Phosphate (Potentiation of sedative effects). Products include:
- Actifed with Codeine Cough Syrup.. 752
- Cheracol Cough Syrup ... 1853
- Codimal PH Syrup ... 846
- Dimetane-DC Cough Syrup ... 1857
- Empirin with Codeine Phosphate Nos. 2, 3 & 4 ... 764
- Fiorinal with Codeine Capsules ... 2008
- Isoclor Expectorant ... 982
- Naldecon CX Adult Liquid ... ▣ 521
- Novahistine DH ... 1342
- Novahistine Expectorant ... 1343
- Nucofed Capsules ... 2219
- Nucofed Expectorant ... 2219
- Nucofed Pediatric Expectorant ... 2220
- Nucofed Syrup ... 2219
- Phenaphen with Codeine Capsules 1865
- Phenaphen-650 with Codeine Tablets ... 1866
- Phenergan with Codeine ... 2497
- Phenergan VC with Codeine ... 2501
- Robitussin A-C Syrup ... 1875
- Robitussin-DAC Syrup ... 1875
- Ryna ... ▣ 741
- Soma Compound w/Codeine Tablets ... 2390
- Triaminic Expectorant w/Codeine .. 1996
- Tussi-Organidin Liquid ... 2391
- Tylenol with Codeine ... 1381

Codeine Polistirex (Potentiation of sedative effects).
- No products indexed under this heading.

Cryptenamine Preparations (Reduced antihypertensive effects).

Deserpidine (Reduced antihypertensive effects). Products include:
- Enduronyl ... 518
- Harmonyl Tablets ... 528
- Oreticyl ... 545

Desipramine Hydrochloride (Potentiation of sedative effects). Products include:
- Norpramin Tablets ... 1340

Dezocine (Potentiation of sedative effects).

Diazepam (Potentiation of sedative effects). Products include:
- Valium Injectable ... 1937
- Valium Tablets ... 1939
- Valrelease Capsules ... 1923

Doxepin Hydrochloride (Potentiation of sedative effects). Products include:
- Sinequan ... 1960

Droperidol (Potentiation of sedative effects). Products include:
- Inapsine Injection ... 1140
- Innovar Injection ... 1141

Enflurane (Potentiation of sedative effects). Products include:
- Ethrane ... 599

Estazolam (Potentiation of sedative effects). Products include:
- ProSom Tablets ... 554

Ethchlorvynol (Potentiation of sedative effects). Products include:
- Placidyl Capsules ... 553

Ethinamate (Potentiation of sedative effects).
- No products indexed under this heading.

Fentanyl (Potentiation of sedative effects). Products include:
- Duragesic Transdermal System ... 1133

Fentanyl Citrate (Potentiation of sedative effects). Products include:
- Innovar Injection ... 1141
- Sublimaze Injection ... 1146

Fluphenazine Decanoate (Potentiation of sedative effects). Products include:
- Prolixin Decanoate ... 1795

Fluphenazine Enanthate (Potentiation of sedative effects). Products include:
- Prolixin Enanthate ... 1796

Fluphenazine Hydrochloride (Potentiation of sedative effects). Products include:
- Prolixin Elixir ... 1793
- Prolixin Injection ... 1791
- Prolixin Oral Concentrate ... 1792
- Prolixin Tablets ... 1793

Flurazepam Hydrochloride (Potentiation of sedative effects). Products include:
- Dalmane Capsules ... 1927

Furazolidone (Contraindicated; potentiates anticholinergic and pressor effects). Products include:
- Furoxone ... 1855

Glutethimide (Potentiation of sedative effects).
- No products indexed under this heading.

Haloperidol (Potentiation of sedative effects). Products include:
- Haldol Injection, Tablets and Concentrate ... 1373

Haloperidol Decanoate (Potentiation of sedative effects). Products include:
- Haldol Decanoate ... 1375

Hydrocodone Polistirex (Potentiation of sedative effects). Products include:
- Tussionex Extended-Release Suspension ... 988

Hydroxyzine Hydrochloride (Potentiation of sedative effects). Products include:
- Atarax Tablets & Syrup ... 1941
- Marax Tablets & DF Syrup ... 1954
- Vistaril Intramuscular Solution ... 1970

Imipramine Hydrochloride (Potentiation of sedative effects). Products include:
- Tofranil Ampuls ... 1038
- Tofranil Tablets ... 1039

Imipramine Pamoate (Potentiation of sedative effects). Products include:
- Tofranil-PM Capsules ... 1041

Isocarboxazid (Contraindicated; potentiates anticholinergic and pressor effects). Products include:
- Marplan Tablets ... 1906

Isoflurane (Potentiation of sedative effects). Products include:
- Forane ... 600

Ketamine Hydrochloride (Potentiation of sedative effects). Products include:
- Ketalar ... 1726

Levorphanol Tartrate (Potentiation of sedative effects). Products include:
- Levo-Dromoran ... 1906

Lorazepam (Potentiation of sedative effects). Products include:
- Ativan Injection ... 2432
- Ativan Tablets ... 2434

Loxapine Hydrochloride (Potentiation of sedative effects). Products include:
- Loxitane ... 1213

Loxapine Succinate (Potentiation of sedative effects). Products include:
- Loxitane Capsules ... 1213

Maprotiline Hydrochloride (Potentiation of sedative effects). Products include:
- Ludiomil Tablets ... 874

Mecamylamine Hydrochloride (Reduced antihypertensive effects). Products include:
- Inversine Tablets ... 1492

Meperidine Hydrochloride (Potentiation of sedative effects). Products include:
- Demerol ... 2047
- Mepergan Injection ... 2479

Mephobarbital (Potentiation of sedative effects). Products include:
- Mebaral Tablets ... 2061

Meprobamate (Potentiation of sedative effects). Products include:
- Deprol Tablets ... 2382
- Equagesic Tablets ... 2451
- Miltown Tablets ... 2386
- PMB 200 and PMB 400 ... 2504

Mesoridazine (Potentiation of sedative effects). Products include:
- Serentil ... 686

Methadone Hydrochloride (Potentiation of sedative effects). Products include:
- Dolophine Hydrochloride Ampoules & Vials ... 1260
- Dolophine Hydrochloride Tablets ... 1261
- Methadone Hydrochloride Diskets .. 1284
- Methadone Hydrochloride Oral Solution & Tablets ... 1987

Methohexital Sodium (Potentiation of sedative effects). Products include:
- Brevital Sodium Vials ... 1248

Methoxyflurane (Potentiation of sedative effects).
- No products indexed under this heading.

Methyclothiazide (Reduced antihypertensive effects). Products include:
- Enduron Tablets ... 517
- Enduronyl ... 518

Methyldopa (Reduced antihypertensive effects). Products include:
- Aldoclor Tablets ... 1413
- Aldomet Oral ... 1415
- Aldoril Tablets ... 1418

Methyldopate Hydrochloride (Reduced antihypertensive effects). Products include:
- Aldomet Ester HCl Injection ... 1417

Midazolam Hydrochloride (Potentiation of sedative effects). Products include:
- Versed Injection ... 1924

Minoxidil (Reduced antihypertensive effects). Products include:
- Loniten Tablets ... 2346
- Rogaine Topical Solution ... 2357

Molindone Hydrochloride (Potentiation of sedative effects). Products include:
- Moban Tablets & Concentrate ... 932

Morphine Sulfate (Potentiation of sedative effects). Products include:
- Astramorph/PF Injection, USP (Preservative-Free) ... 618
- Duramorph ... 960
- Infumorph 200 and Infumorph 500 Sterile Solutions ... 962
- MS Contin Tablets ... 1814
- MSIR ... 1817
- Oramorph SR (Morphine Sulfate Sustained Release Tablets) ... 1988
- Roxanol ... 1991

Nortriptyline Hydrochloride (Potentiation of sedative effects). Products include:
- Pamelor ... 2019

Opium Alkaloids (Potentiation of sedative effects). Products include:
- B & O No. 15A & No. 16A Supprettes ... 2395
- Pantopon Injectable ... 1911

Oxazepam (Potentiation of sedative effects). Products include:
- Serax Capsules ... 2522
- Serax Tablets ... 2522

Oxycodone Hydrochloride (Potentiation of sedative effects). Products include:
- Percocet Tablets ... 950
- Percodan ... 951
- Roxicodone Tablets, Oral Solution & Intensol (Oxycodone) ... 1992
- Tylox Capsules ... 1382

Pentobarbital Sodium (Potentiation of sedative effects). Products include:
- Nembutal Sodium Capsules ... 534
- Nembutal Sodium Solution ... 536
- Nembutal Sodium Suppositories ... 538

Perphenazine (Potentiation of sedative effects). Products include:
- Etrafon ... 2087
- Triavil Tablets ... 1556
- Trilafon ... 2123

Phenelzine Sulfate (Contraindicated; potentiates anticholinergic and pressor effects). Products include:
- Nardil ... 1742

Phenobarbital (Potentiation of sedative effects). Products include:
- Arco-Lase Plus Tablets ... 607
- Bellergal-S Tablets ... 1998
- Bronkolixir ... ▣ 761
- Bronkotabs Tablets ... ▣ 762

Donnatal ... 1858
Donnatal Extentabs ... 1859
Donnatal Tablets ... 1858
Donnazyme Tablets ... 1860
Kinesed Tablets ... 2272
Phenobarbital Elixir and Tablets ... 1293
Primatene Tablets-P Formula ... 2421
Quadrinal Tablets ... 1183
Tedral SA ... 1765

Prazepam (Potentiation of sedative effects). Products include:
Centrax ... 1693

Prochlorperazine (Potentiation of sedative effects). Products include:
Compazine ... 2201

Promethazine Hydrochloride (Potentiation of sedative effects). Products include:
Mepergan Injection ... 2479
Phenergan with Codeine ... 2497
Phenergan with Dextromethorphan 2499
Phenergan Injection ... 2493
Phenergan Suppositories ... 2496
Phenergan Syrup ... 2495
Phenergan Tablets ... 2496
Phenergan VC ... 2500
Phenergan VC with Codeine ... 2501

Propofol (Potentiation of sedative effects). Products include:
Diprivan Injection ... 2267

Propoxyphene Hydrochloride (Potentiation of sedative effects). Products include:
Darvon ... 1256
Wygesic Tablets ... 2540

Propoxyphene Napsylate (Potentiation of sedative effects). Products include:
Darvon-N/Darvocet-N ... 1254

Protriptyline Hydrochloride (Potentiation of sedative effects). Products include:
Vivactil Tablets ... 1567

Quazepam (Potentiation of sedative effects). Products include:
Doral Tablets ... 2383

Rauwolfia Serpentina (Reduced antihypertensive effects). Products include:
Raudixin Tablets ... 1803
Rauzide Tablets ... 1804

Rescinnamine (Reduced antihypertensive effects).
No products indexed under this heading.

Reserpine (Reduced antihypertensive effects). Products include:
Diupres Tablets ... 1461
Hydromox R Tablets ... 1209
Hydropres Tablets ... 1485
Renese-R Tablets ... 1786
Salutensin/Salutensin-Demi ... 719
Ser-Ap-Es Tablets ... 881
Serpasil Tablets ... 883
Serpasil-Apresoline Tablets ... 884
Serpasil-Esidrix Tablets ... 886

Secobarbital Sodium (Potentiation of sedative effects). Products include:
Seconal Sodium Pulvules ... 1296

Selegiline Hydrochloride (Contraindicated; potentiates anticholinergic and pressor effects). Products include:
Eldepryl ... 2250

Sufentanil Citrate (Potentiation of sedative effects). Products include:
Sufenta Injection ... 1147

Temazepam (Potentiation of sedative effects). Products include:
Restoril Capsules ... 2023

Thiamylal Sodium (Potentiation of sedative effects). Products include:
Surital Ampoules, Steri-Vials ... 1764

Thioridazine Hydrochloride (Potentiation of sedative effects). Products include:
Mellaril ... 2011

Thiothixene (Potentiation of sedative effects). Products include:
Navane Capsules and Concentrate 1954
Navane Intramuscular ... 1956

Tranylcypromine Sulfate (Contraindicated; potentiates anticholinergic and pressor effects). Products include:
Parnate Tablets ... 2222

Triazolam (Potentiation of sedative effects). Products include:
Halcion Tablets ... 2340

Trifluoperazine Hydrochloride (Potentiation of sedative effects). Products include:
Stelazine ... 2226

Trimipramine Maleate (Potentiation of sedative effects). Products include:
Surmontil Capsules ... 2524

TRIAMINIC NITE LIGHT
(Chlorpheniramine Maleate, Dextromethorphan Hydrobromide, Pseudoephedrine Hydrochloride) ... ▣ 689
May interact with antidepressant drugs, hypnotics and sedatives, tranquilizers, antihypertensives, and certain other agents. Compounds in these categories include:

Acebutolol Hydrochloride (Concurrent use is not recommended unless directed by physician). Products include:
Sectral Capsules ... 2520

Alcohol (May increrase drowsiness effect).

Alprazolam (May increase drowsiness effect). Products include:
Xanax Tablets ... 2367

Amitriptyline Hydrochloride (Concurrent use is not recommended unless directed by physician). Products include:
Elavil ... 2269
Endep Tablets ... 1927
Etrafon ... 2087
Limbitrol ... 1933
Triavil Tablets ... 1556

Amoxapine (Concurrent use is not recommended unless directed by physician). Products include:
Asendin Tablets ... 1196

Atenolol (Concurrent use is not recommended unless directed by physician). Products include:
Tenoretic Tablets ... 1105
Tenormin Tablets and I.V. Injection 1107

Benazepril Hydrochloride (Concurrent use is not recommended unless directed by physician). Products include:
Lotensin Tablets ... 872

Bendroflumethiazide (Concurrent use is not recommended unless directed by physician). Products include:
Corzide Tablets ... 702
Naturetin Tablets ... 1789
Rauzide Tablets ... 1804

Betaxolol Hydrochloride (Concurrent use is not recommended unless directed by physician). Products include:
Betoptic Sterile Ophthalmic Solution ... ◉ 569
Betoptic S Sterile Ophthalmic Suspension ... ◉ 570
Kerlone Tablets ... 2172

Bupropion Hydrochloride (Concurrent use is not recommended unless directed by physician). Products include:
Wellbutrin Tablets ... 821

Buspirone Hydrochloride (May increase drowsiness effect). Products include:
BuSpar ... 1401

Captopril (Concurrent use is not recommended unless directed by physician). Products include:
Capoten ... 2255
Capozide ... 2258

Carteolol Hydrochloride (Concurrent use is not recommended unless directed by physician). Products include:
Cartrol Tablets ... 507

Chlordiazepoxide (May increase drowsiness effect). Products include:
Libritabs Tablets ... 1930
Limbitrol ... 1933
Menrium Tablets ... 1934

Chlordiazepoxide Hydrochloride (May increase drowsiness effect). Products include:
Librax Capsules ... 1929
Librium Capsules ... 1931
Librium Injectable ... 1932

Chlorothiazide (Concurrent use is not recommended unless directed by physician). Products include:
Aldoclor Tablets ... 1413
Diupres Tablets ... 1461
Diuril Oral ... 1464

Chlorothiazide Sodium (Concurrent use is not recommended unless directed by physician). Products include:
Diuril Sodium Intravenous ... 1463

Chlorpromazine (May increase drowsiness effect). Products include:
Thorazine ... 2234

Chlorprothixene (May increase drowsiness effect). Products include:
Taractan Tablets ... 1920

Chlorprothixene Hydrochloride (May increase drowsiness effect). Products include:
Taractan ... 1920

Chlorthalidone (Concurrent use is not recommended unless directed by physician). Products include:
Combipres Tablets ... 678
Tenoretic Tablets ... 1105
Thalitone Tablets ... 687

Clonidine (Concurrent use is not recommended unless directed by physician). Products include:
Catapres-TTS ... 677

Clonidine Hydrochloride (Concurrent use is not recommended unless directed by physician). Products include:
Catapres Tablets ... 676
Combipres Tablets ... 678

Clorazepate Dipotassium (May increase drowsiness effect). Products include:
Tranxene ... 556

Deserpidine (Concurrent use is not recommended unless directed by physician). Products include:
Enduronyl ... 518
Harmonyl Tablets ... 528
Oreticyl ... 545

Desipramine Hydrochloride (Concurrent use is not recommended unless directed by physician). Products include:
Norpramin Tablets ... 1340

Diazepam (May increase drowsiness effect). Products include:
Valium Injectable ... 1937
Valium Tablets ... 1939
Valrelease Capsules ... 1923

Diazoxide (Concurrent use is not recommended unless directed by physician). Products include:
Hyperstat I.V. Injection ... 2095
Proglycem ... 649

Doxazosin Mesylate (Concurrent use is not recommended unless directed by physician). Products include:
Cardura Tablets ... 1941

Doxepin Hydrochloride (Concurrent use is not recommended unless directed by physician). Products include:
Sinequan ... 1960

Droperidol (May increase drowsiness effect). Products include:
Inapsine Injection ... 1140
Innovar Injection ... 1141

Enalapril Maleate (Concurrent use is not recommended unless directed by physician). Products include:
Vaseretic Tablets ... 1559
Vasotec Tablets ... 1564

Enalaprilat (Concurrent use is not recommended unless directed by physician). Products include:
Vasotec I.V. ... 1562

Esmolol Hydrochloride (Concurrent use is not recommended unless directed by physician). Products include:
Brevibloc Injection ... 942

Estazolam (May increase drowsiness effect). Products include:
ProSom Tablets ... 554

Ethchlorvynol (May increase drowsiness effect). Products include:
Placidyl Capsules ... 553

Ethinamate (May increase drowsiness effect).
No products indexed under this heading.

Felodipine (Concurrent use is not recommended unless directed by physician). Products include:
Plendil Extended-Release Tablets ... 1526

Fluoxetine Hydrochloride (Concurrent use is not recommended unless directed by physician). Products include:
Prozac Pulvules ... 920

Fluphenazine Decanoate (May increase drowsiness effect). Products include:
Prolixin Decanoate ... 1795

Fluphenazine Enanthate (May increase drowsiness effect). Products include:
Prolixin Enanthate ... 1796

Fluphenazine Hydrochloride (May increase drowsiness effect). Products include:
Prolixin Elixir ... 1793
Prolixin Injection ... 1791
Prolixin Oral Concentrate ... 1792
Prolixin Tablets ... 1793

Flurazepam Hydrochloride (May increase drowsiness effect). Products include:
Dalmane Capsules ... 1927

Fosinopril Sodium (Concurrent use is not recommended unless directed by physician). Products include:
Monopril Tablets ... 1406

Furosemide (Concurrent use is not recommended unless directed by physician). Products include:
Lasix ... 1093

Glutethimide (May increase drowsiness effect).
No products indexed under this heading.

Guanabenz Acetate (Concurrent use is not recommended unless directed by physician). Products include:
Wytensin Tablets ... 2542

Guanethidine Monosulfate (Concurrent use is not recommended unless directed by physician). Products include:
Esimil Tablets ... 864
Ismelin Tablets ... 869

Haloperidol (May increase drowsiness effect). Products include:
- Haldol Injection, Tablets and Concentrate ... 1373

Haloperidol Decanoate (May increase drowsiness effect). Products include:
- Haldol Decanoate ... 1375

Hydralazine Hydrochloride (Concurrent use is not recommended unless directed by physician). Products include:
- Apresazide Capsules ... 854
- Apresoline Hydrochloride Parenteral (Ampuls) ... 856
- Apresoline Hydrochloride Tablets .. 855
- Apresoline-Esidrix Tablets ... 857
- Ser-Ap-Es Tablets ... 881
- Serpasil-Apresoline Tablets ... 884

Hydrochlorothiazide (Concurrent use is not recommended unless directed by physician). Products include:
- Aldactazide ... 2150
- Aldoril Tablets ... 1418
- Apresazide Capsules ... 854
- Apresoline-Esidrix Tablets ... 857
- Capozide ... 2258
- Dyazide Capsules ... 2208
- Esidrix Tablets ... 863
- Esimil Tablets ... 864
- HydroDIURIL Tablets ... 1484
- Hydropres Tablets ... 1485
- Inderide Tablets ... 2463
- Inderide LA Long Acting Capsules .. 2465
- Lopressor HCT Tablets ... 1034
- Maxzide ... 1215
- Moduretic Tablets ... 1510
- Normozide Tablets ... 2112
- Oretic Tablets ... 544
- Oreticyl ... 545
- Prinzide Tablets ... 1540
- Ser-Ap-Es Tablets ... 881
- Serpasil-Esidrix Tablets ... 886
- Timolide Tablets ... 1547
- Trandate HCT Tablets ... 579
- Vaseretic Tablets ... 1559
- Zestoretic ... 2274

Hydroflumethiazide (Concurrent use is not recommended unless directed by physician). Products include:
- Diucardin Tablets ... 2450
- Saluron ... 718
- Salutensin/Salutensin-Demi ... 719

Hydroxyzine Hydrochloride (May increase drowsiness effect). Products include:
- Atarax Tablets & Syrup ... 1941
- Marax Tablets & DF Syrup ... 1954
- Vistaril Intramuscular Solution ... 1970

Imipramine Hydrochloride (Concurrent use is not recommended unless directed by physician). Products include:
- Tofranil Ampuls ... 1038
- Tofranil Tablets ... 1039

Imipramine Pamoate (Concurrent use is not recommended unless directed by physician). Products include:
- Tofranil-PM Capsules ... 1041

Indapamide (Concurrent use is not recommended unless directed by physician). Products include:
- Lozol Tablets ... 1843

Isocarboxazid (Concurrent use is not recommended unless directed by physician). Products include:
- Marplan Tablets ... 1906

Isradipine (Concurrent use is not recommended unless directed by physician). Products include:
- DynaCirc Capsules ... 2004

Labetalol Hydrochloride (Concurrent use is not recommended unless directed by physician). Products include:
- Normodyne Injection ... 2108
- Normodyne Tablets ... 2110
- Normozide Tablets ... 2112
- Trandate HCT Tablets ... 579
- Trandate Injection ... 577
- Trandate Tablets ... 579

Lisinopril (Concurrent use is not recommended unless directed by physician). Products include:
- Prinivil Tablets ... 1538
- Prinzide Tablets ... 1540
- Zestoretic ... 2274
- Zestril Tablets ... 2277

Lorazepam (May increase drowsiness effect). Products include:
- Ativan Injection ... 2432
- Ativan Tablets ... 2434

Loxapine Hydrochloride (May increase drowsiness effect). Products include:
- Loxitane ... 1213

Loxapine Succinate (May increase drowsiness effect). Products include:
- Loxitane Capsules ... 1213

Maprotiline Hydrochloride (Concurrent use is not recommended unless directed by physician). Products include:
- Ludiomil Tablets ... 874

Mecamylamine Hydrochloride (Concurrent use is not recommended unless directed by physician). Products include:
- Inversine Tablets ... 1492

Meprobamate (May increase drowsiness effect). Products include:
- Deprol Tablets ... 2382
- Equagesic Tablets ... 2451
- Miltown Tablets ... 2386
- PMB 200 and PMB 400 ... 2504

Mesoridazine Besylate (May increase drowsiness effect).

Methyclothiazide (Concurrent use is not recommended unless directed by physician). Products include:
- Enduron Tablets ... 517
- Enduronyl ... 518

Methyldopa (Concurrent use is not recommended unless directed by physician). Products include:
- Aldoclor Tablets ... 1413
- Aldomet Oral ... 1415
- Aldoril Tablets ... 1418

Methyldopate Hydrochloride (Concurrent use is not recommended unless directed by physician). Products include:
- Aldomet Ester HCl Injection ... 1417

Metolazone (Concurrent use is not recommended unless directed by physician). Products include:
- Diulo ... 2129
- Mykrox ½ mg Tablets ... 984
- Zaroxolyn Tablets ... 989

Metoprolol Tartrate (Concurrent use is not recommended unless directed by physician). Products include:
- Lopressor Ampuls ... 1032
- Lopressor HCT Tablets ... 1034
- Lopressor Tablets ... 1032

Metyrosine (Concurrent use is not recommended unless directed by physician). Products include:
- Demser Capsules ... 1460

Midazolam Hydrochloride (May increase drowsiness effect). Products include:
- Versed Injection ... 1924

Minoxidil (Concurrent use is not recommended unless directed by physician). Products include:
- Loniten Tablets ... 2346
- Rogaine Topical Solution ... 2357

Molindone Hydrochloride (May increase drowsiness effect). Products include:
- Moban Tablets & Concentrate ... 932

Nadolol (Concurrent use is not recommended unless directed by physician). Products include:
- Corgard Tablets ... 701
- Corzide Tablets ... 702

Nicardipine Hydrochloride (Concurrent use is not recommended unless directed by physician). Products include:
- Cardene Capsules ... 2290

Nitroglycerin (Concurrent use is not recommended unless directed by physician). Products include:
- Deponit NTG Transdermal Delivery System ... 2143
- Minitran Transdermal Delivery System ... 1312
- Nitro-Bid Ointment ... 1339
- Nitro-Bid Capsules ... 1338
- Nitrodisc ... 2176
- Nitro-Dur (nitroglycerin) Transdermal Infusion System ... 1164
- Nitrogard Tablets ... 1004
- Nitrolingual Spray ... 1846
- Nitrostat Tablets ... 1743
- Transderm-Nitro Transdermal Therapeutic System ... 2283

Nortriptyline Hydrochloride (Concurrent use is not recommended unless directed by physician). Products include:
- Pamelor ... 2019

Oxazepam (May increase drowsiness effect). Products include:
- Serax Capsules ... 2522
- Serax Tablets ... 2522

Penbutolol Sulfate (Concurrent use is not recommended unless directed by physician). Products include:
- Levatol ... 1832

Perphenazine (May increase drowsiness effect). Products include:
- Etrafon ... 2087
- Triavil Tablets ... 1556
- Trilafon ... 2123

Phenelzine Sulfate (Concurrent use is not recommended unless directed by physician). Products include:
- Nardil ... 1742

Phenoxybenzamine Hydrochloride (Concurrent use is not recommended unless directed by physician). Products include:
- Dibenzyline Capsules ... 2207

Phentolamine Mesylate (Concurrent use is not recommended unless directed by physician). Products include:
- Regitine ... 878

Pindolol (Concurrent use is not recommended unless directed by physician). Products include:
- Visken Tablets ... 2036

Polythiazide (Concurrent use is not recommended unless directed by physician). Products include:
- Minizide Capsules ... 1779
- Renese Tablets ... 1785
- Renese-R Tablets ... 1786

Prazepam (May increase drowsiness effect). Products include:
- Centrax ... 1693

Prazosin Hydrochloride (Concurrent use is not recommended unless directed by physician). Products include:
- Minipress Capsules ... 1778
- Minizide Capsules ... 1779

Prochlorperazine (May increase drowsiness effect). Products include:
- Compazine ... 2201

Promethazine Hydrochloride (May increase drowsiness effect). Products include:
- Mepergan Injection ... 2479
- Phenergan with Codeine ... 2497
- Phenergan with Dextromethorphan 2499
- Phenergan Injection ... 2493
- Phenergan Suppositories ... 2496
- Phenergan Syrup ... 2495
- Phenergan Tablets ... 2496
- Phenergan VC ... 2500
- Phenergan VC with Codeine ... 2501

Propofol (May increase drowsiness effect). Products include:
- Diprivan Injection ... 2267

Propranolol Hydrochloride (Concurrent use is not recommended unless directed by physician). Products include:
- Inderal ... 2459
- Inderal LA Long Acting Capsules ... 2461
- Inderide Tablets ... 2463
- Inderide LA Long Acting Capsules .. 2465

Protriptyline Hydrochloride (Concurrent use is not recommended unless directed by physician). Products include:
- Vivactil Tablets ... 1567

Quazepam (May increase drowsiness effect). Products include:
- Doral Tablets ... 2383

Ramipril (Concurrent use is not recommended unless directed by physician). Products include:
- Altace Capsules ... 1086

Rauwolfia Serpentina (Concurrent use is not recommended unless directed by physician). Products include:
- Raudixin Tablets ... 1803
- Rauzide Tablets ... 1804

Rescinnamine (Concurrent use is not recommended unless directed by physician).
- No products indexed under this heading.

Reserpine (Concurrent use is not recommended unless directed by physician). Products include:
- Diupres Tablets ... 1461
- Hydromox R Tablets ... 1209
- Hydropres Tablets ... 1485
- Renese-R Tablets ... 1786
- Salutensin/Salutensin-Demi ... 719
- Ser-Ap-Es Tablets ... 881
- Serpasil Tablets ... 883
- Serpasil-Apresoline Tablets ... 884
- Serpasil-Esidrix Tablets ... 886

Secobarbital Sodium (May increase drowsiness effect). Products include:
- Seconal Sodium Pulvules ... 1296

Sodium Nitroprusside (Concurrent use is not recommended unless directed by physician). Products include:
- Nipride I.V. Infusion ... 1909

Temazepam (May increase drowsiness effect). Products include:
- Restoril Capsules ... 2023

Terazosin Hydrochloride (Concurrent use is not recommended unless directed by physician). Products include:
- Hytrin Tablets ... 529

Thioridazine Hydrochloride (May increase drowsiness effect). Products include:
- Mellaril ... 2011

Thiothixene (May increase drowsiness effect). Products include:
- Navane Capsules and Concentrate 1954
- Navane Intramuscular ... 1956

Timolol Maleate (Concurrent use is not recommended unless directed by physician). Products include:
- Blocadren Tablets ... 1429
- Timolide Tablets ... 1547
- Timoptic in Ocudose ... 1552
- Timoptic Sterile Ophthalmic Solution ... 1550

Tranylcypromine Sulfate (Concurrent use is not recommended unless directed by physician). Products include:
- Parnate Tablets ... 2222

Trazodone Hydrochloride (Concurrent use is not recommended unless directed by physician). Products include:
- Desyrel and Desyrel Dividose ... 1404

Triazolam (May increase drowsiness effect). Products include:
- Halcion Tablets ... 2340

Trifluoperazine Hydrochloride (May increase drowsiness effect). Products include:
- Stelazine ... 2226

Trimethaphan Camsylate (Concurrent use is not recommended unless directed by physician). Products include:
- Arfonad Ampuls ... 1887

Trimipramine Maleate (Concurrent use is not recommended unless directed by physician). Products include:
- Surmontil Capsules ... 2524

TRIAMINIC ORAL INFANT DROPS
(Phenylpropanolamine Hydrochloride, Pheniramine Maleate, Pyrilamine Maleate) ... 1996

May interact with monoamine oxidase inhibitors, central nervous system depressants, veratrum alkaloids, hypnotics and sedatives, tranquilizers, and certain other agents. Compounds in these categories include:

Alcohol (Potentiation of sedative effects).

Alfentanil Hydrochloride (Potentiation of sedative effects). Products include:
- Alfenta Injection ... 1131

Alprazolam (Potentiation of sedative effects). Products include:
- Xanax Tablets ... 2367

Aprobarbital (Potentiation of sedative effects). Products include:
- Alurate Elixir ... 1883

Buprenorphine (Potentiation of sedative effects).
- No products indexed under this heading.

Buspirone Hydrochloride (Potentiation of sedative effects). Products include:
- BuSpar ... 1401

Butabarbital (Potentiation of sedative effects). Products include:
- Pyridium Plus ... 1764

Butalbital (Potentiation of sedative effects). Products include:
- Esgic-Plus Tablets ... 1002
- Esgic Tablets & Capsules ... 1001
- Fioricet Tablets ... 2006
- Fiorinal Capsules ... 2007
- Fiorinal with Codeine Capsules ... 2008
- Fiorinal Tablets ... 2007
- Phrenilin ... 838
- Sedapap Tablets 50 mg/650 mg ... 1360

Chlordiazepoxide (Potentiation of sedative effects). Products include:
- Libritabs Tablets ... 1930
- Limbitrol ... 1933
- Menrium Tablets ... 1934

Chlordiazepoxide Hydrochloride (Potentiation of sedative effects). Products include:
- Librax Capsules ... 1929
- Librium Capsules ... 1931
- Librium Injectable ... 1932

Chlorpromazine (Potentiation of sedative effects). Products include:
- Thorazine ... 2234

Chlorprothixene (Potentiation of sedative effects). Products include:
- Taractan Tablets ... 1920

Chlorprothixene Hydrochloride (Potentiation of sedative effects). Products include:
- Taractan ... 1920

Chlorprothixene Lactate (Potentiation of sedative effects). Products include:
- Taractan Concentrate ... 1920

Clorazepate Dipotassium (Potentiation of sedative effects). Products include:
- Tranxene ... 556

Codeine (Potentiation of sedative effects). Products include:
- Calcidrine Syrup ... 506

Codeine Phosphate (Potentiation of sedative effects). Products include:
- Actifed with Codeine Cough Syrup.. 752
- Cheracol Cough Syrup ... 1853
- Codimal PH Syrup ... 846
- Dimetane-DC Cough Syrup ... 1857
- Empirin with Codeine Phosphate Nos. 2, 3 & 4 ... 764
- Fiorinal with Codeine Capsules ... 2008
- Isoclor Expectorant ... 982
- Naldecon CX Adult Liquid ... ◘ 521
- Novahistine DH ... 1342
- Novahistine Expectorant ... 1343
- Nucofed Capsules ... 2219
- Nucofed Expectorant ... 2219
- Nucofed Pediatric Expectorant ... 2220
- Nucofed Syrup ... 2219
- Phenaphen with Codeine Capsules ... 1865
- Phenaphen-650 with Codeine Tablets ... 1866
- Phenergan with Codeine ... 2497
- Phenergan VC with Codeine ... 2501
- Robitussin A-C Syrup ... 1875
- Robitussin-DAC Syrup ... 1875
- Ryna ... ◘ 741
- Soma Compound w/Codeine Tablets ... 2390
- Triaminic Expectorant w/Codeine .. 1996
- Tussi-Organidin Liquid ... 2391
- Tylenol with Codeine ... 1381

Codeine Polistirex (Potentiation of sedative effects).
- No products indexed under this heading.

Cryptenamine Preparations (Reduced antihypertensive effects).

Deserpidine (Reduced antihypertensive effects). Products include:
- Enduronyl ... 518
- Harmonyl Tablets ... 528
- Oreticyl ... 545

Dezocine (Potentiation of sedative effects).

Diazepam (Potentiation of sedative effects). Products include:
- Valium Injectable ... 1937
- Valium Tablets ... 1939
- Valrelease Capsules ... 1923

Droperidol (Potentiation of sedative effects). Products include:
- Inapsine Injection ... 1140
- Innovar Injection ... 1141

Enflurane (Potentiation of sedative effects). Products include:
- Ethrane ... 599

Estazolam (Potentiation of sedative effects). Products include:
- ProSom Tablets ... 554

Ethchlorvynol (Potentiation of sedative effects). Products include:
- Placidyl Capsules ... 553

Ethinamate (Potentiation of sedative effects).
- No products indexed under this heading.

Fentanyl (Potentiation of sedative effects). Products include:
- Duragesic Transdermal System ... 1133

Fentanyl Citrate (Potentiation of sedative effects). Products include:
- Innovar Injection ... 1141
- Sublimaze Injection ... 1146

Fluphenazine Decanoate (Potentiation of sedative effects). Products include:
- Prolixin Decanoate ... 1795

Fluphenazine Enanthate (Potentiation of sedative effects). Products include:
- Prolixin Enanthate ... 1796

Fluphenazine Hydrochloride (Potentiation of sedative effects). Products include:
- Prolixin Elixir ... 1793
- Prolixin Injection ... 1791
- Prolixin Oral Concentrate ... 1792
- Prolixin Tablets ... 1793

Flurazepam Hydrochloride (Potentiation of sedative effects). Products include:
- Dalmane Capsules ... 1927

Furazolidone (Contraindicated; potentiates anticholinergic and pressor effects). Products include:
- Furoxone ... 1855

Glutethimide (Potentiation of sedative effects).
- No products indexed under this heading.

Haloperidol (Potentiation of sedative effects). Products include:
- Haldol Injection, Tablets and Concentrate ... 1373

Haloperidol Decanoate (Potentiation of sedative effects). Products include:
- Haldol Decanoate ... 1375

Hydrocodone Bitartrate (Potentiation of sedative effects). Products include:
- Anexsia 5/500 Tablets ... 2196
- Anexsia 7.5/650 Tablets ... 2197
- Azdōne Tablets ... 844
- Codiclear DH Syrup ... 845
- Codimal DH Syrup ... 846
- Damason-P ... 1356
- Hycodan Syrup, Tablets ... 927
- Hycomine Compound Tablets ... 929
- Hycomine Syrup ... 927
- Hycotuss Expectorant Syrup ... 930
- Hydrocet Capsules ... 835
- Lortab ASA Tablets ... 2414
- Lortab ... 2412
- Ru-Tuss with Hydrocodone ... 694
- Triaminic Expectorant DH ... 1995
- Vicodin Tablets ... 1187
- Vicodin ES Tablets ... 1189
- Zydone Capsules ... 941

Hydrocodone Polistirex (Potentiation of sedative effects). Products include:
- Tussionex Extended-Release Suspension ... 988

Hydroxyzine Hydrochloride (Potentiation of sedative effects). Products include:
- Atarax Tablets & Syrup ... 1941
- Marax Tablets & DF Syrup ... 1954
- Vistaril Intramuscular Solution ... 1970

Isocarboxazid (Contraindicated; potentiates anticholinergic and pressor effects). Products include:
- Marplan Tablets ... 1906

Isoflurane (Potentiation of sedative effects). Products include:
- Forane ... 600

Ketamine Hydrochloride (Potentiation of sedative effects). Products include:
- Ketalar ... 1726

Levorphanol Tartrate (Potentiation of sedative effects). Products include:
- Levo-Dromoran ... 1906

Lorazepam (Potentiation of sedative effects). Products include:
- Ativan Injection ... 2432
- Ativan Tablets ... 2434

Loxapine Hydrochloride (Potentiation of sedative effects). Products include:
- Loxitane ... 1213

Loxapine Succinate (Potentiation of sedative effects). Products include:
- Loxitane Capsules ... 1213

Mecamylamine Hydrochloride (Reduced antihypertensive effects). Products include:
- Inversine Tablets ... 1492

Meperidine Hydrochloride (Potentiation of sedative effects). Products include:
- Demerol ... 2047
- Mepergan Injection ... 2479

Mephobarbital (Potentiation of sedative effects). Products include:
- Mebaral Tablets ... 2061

Meprobamate (Potentiation of sedative effects). Products include:
- Deprol Tablets ... 2382
- Equagesic Tablets ... 2451
- Miltown Tablets ... 2386
- PMB 200 and PMB 400 ... 2504

Mesoridazine (Potentiation of sedative effects). Products include:
- Serentil ... 686

Mesoridazine Besylate (Potentiation of sedative effects).

Methadone Hydrochloride (Potentiation of sedative effects). Products include:
- Dolophine Hydrochloride Ampoules & Vials ... 1260
- Dolophine Hydrochloride Tablets ... 1261
- Methadone Hydrochloride Diskets .. 1284
- Methadone Hydrochloride Oral Solution & Tablets ... 1987

Methohexital Sodium (Potentiation of sedative effects). Products include:
- Brevital Sodium Vials ... 1248

Methoxyflurane (Potentiation of sedative effects).
- No products indexed under this heading.

Methyldopa (Reduced antihypertensive effects). Products include:
- Aldoclor Tablets ... 1413
- Aldomet Oral ... 1415
- Aldoril Tablets ... 1418

Methyldopate Hydrochloride (Reduced antihypertensive effects). Products include:
- Aldomet Ester HCl Injection ... 1417

Midazolam Hydrochloride (Potentiation of sedative effects). Products include:
- Versed Injection ... 1924

Molindone Hydrochloride (Potentiation of sedative effects). Products include:
- Moban Tablets & Concentrate ... 932

Morphine Sulfate (Potentiation of sedative effects). Products include:
- Astramorph/PF Injection, USP (Preservative-Free) ... 618
- Duramorph ... 960
- Infumorph 200 and Infumorph 500 Sterile Solutions ... 962
- MS Contin Tablets ... 1814
- MSIR ... 1817
- Oramorph SR (Morphine Sulfate Sustained Release Tablets) ... 1988
- Roxanol ... 1991

Opium Alkaloids (Potentiation of sedative effects). Products include:
- B & O No. 15A & No. 16A Supprettes ... 2395
- Pantopon Injectable ... 1911

Oxazepam (Potentiation of sedative effects). Products include:
- Serax Capsules ... 2522
- Serax Tablets ... 2522

Oxycodone Hydrochloride (Potentiation of sedative effects). Products include:
- Percocet Tablets ... 950
- Percodan ... 951
- Roxicodone Tablets, Oral Solution & Intensol (Oxycodone) ... 1992
- Tylox Capsules ... 1382

Pentobarbital Sodium (Potentiation of sedative effects). Products include:
- Nembutal Sodium Capsules ... 534
- Nembutal Sodium Solution ... 536
- Nembutal Sodium Suppositories ... 538

Perphenazine (Potentiation of sedative effects). Products include:
Etrafon 2087
Triavil Tablets 1556
Trilafon 2123

Phenelzine Sulfate (Contraindicated; potentiates anticholinergic and pressor effects). Products include:
Nardil 1742

Phenobarbital (Potentiation of sedative effects). Products include:
Arco-Lase Plus Tablets 607
Bellergal-S Tablets 1998
Bronkolixir ▣ 761
Bronkotabs Tablets ▣ 762
Donnatal 1858
Donnatal Extentabs 1859
Donnatal Tablets 1858
Donnazyme Tablets 1860
Kinesed Tablets 2272
Phenobarbital Elixir and Tablets 1293
Primatene Tablets-P Formula 2421
Quadrinal Tablets 1183
Tedral SA 1765

Prazepam (Potentiation of sedative effects). Products include:
Centrax 1693

Prochlorperazine (Potentiation of sedative effects). Products include:
Compazine 2201

Promethazine Hydrochloride (Potentiation of sedative effects). Products include:
Mepergan Injection 2479
Phenergan with Codeine 2497
Phenergan with Dextromethorphan 2499
Phenergan Injection 2493
Phenergan Suppositories 2496
Phenergan Syrup 2495
Phenergan Tablets 2496
Phenergan VC 2500
Phenergan VC with Codeine 2501

Propofol (Potentiation of sedative effects). Products include:
Diprivan Injection 2267

Propoxyphene Hydrochloride (Potentiation of sedative effects). Products include:
Darvon 1256
Wygesic Tablets 2540

Propoxyphene Napsylate (Potentiation of sedative effects). Products include:
Darvon-N/Darvocet-N 1254

Quazepam (Potentiation of sedative effects). Products include:
Doral Tablets 2383

Rauwolfia Serpentina (Reduced antihypertensive effect of antihypertensives). Products include:
Raudixin Tablets 1803
Rauzide Tablets 1804

Rescinnamine (Reduced antihypertensive effect of antihypertensives).
No products indexed under this heading.

Reserpine (Reduced antihypertensive effects). Products include:
Diupres Tablets 1461
Hydromox R Tablets 1209
Hydropres Tablets 1485
Renese-R Tablets 1786
Salutensin/Salutensin-Demi 719
Ser-Ap-Es Tablets 881
Serpasil Tablets 883
Serpasil-Apresoline Tablets 884
Serpasil-Esidrix Tablets 886

Secobarbital Sodium (Potentiation of sedative effects). Products include:
Seconal Sodium Pulvules 1296

Selegiline Hydrochloride (Contraindicated; potentiates anticholinergic and pressor effects). Products include:
Eldepryl 2250

Sufentanil Citrate (Potentiation of sedative effects). Products include:
Sufenta Injection 1147

Temazepam (Potentiation of sedative effects). Products include:
Restoril Capsules 2023

Thiamylal Sodium (Potentiation of sedative effects). Products include:
Surital Ampoules, Steri-Vials 1764

Thioridazine Hydrochloride (Potentiation of sedative effects). Products include:
Mellaril 2011

Thiothixene (Potentiation of sedative effects). Products include:
Navane Capsules and Concentrate 1954
Navane Intramuscular 1956

Tranylcypromine Sulfate (Contraindicated; potentiates anticholinergic and pressor effects). Products include:
Parnate Tablets 2222

Triazolam (Potentiation of sedative effects). Products include:
Halcion Tablets 2340

Trifluoperazine Hydrochloride (Potentiation of sedative effects). Products include:
Stelazine 2226

TRIAMINIC SYRUP
(Phenylpropanolamine Hydrochloride, Chlorpheniramine Maleate) ▣ 689
May interact with monoamine oxidase inhibitors, central nervous system depressants, and certain other agents. Compounds in these categories include:

Alcohol (Potentiation of sedative effects of antihistamines).

Alfentanil Hydrochloride (Potentiation of sedative effects of antihistamines). Products include:
Alfenta Injection 1131

Alprazolam (Potentiation of sedative effects of antihistamines). Products include:
Xanax Tablets 2367

Aprobarbital (Potentiation of sedative effects of antihistamines). Products include:
Alurate Elixir 1883

Buprenorphine (Potentiation of sedative effects of antihistamines).
No products indexed under this heading.

Buspirone Hydrochloride (Potentiation of sedative effects of antihistamines). Products include:
BuSpar 1401

Butabarbital (Potentiation of sedative effects of antihistamines). Products include:
Pyridium Plus 1764

Butalbital (Potentiation of sedative effects of antihistamines). Products include:
Esgic-Plus Tablets 1002
Esgic Tablets & Capsules 1001
Fioricet Tablets 2006
Fiorinal Capsules 2007
Fiorinal with Codeine Capsules 2008
Fiorinal Tablets 2007
Phrenilin 838
Sedapap Tablets 50 mg/650 mg 1360

Chlordiazepoxide (Potentiation of sedative effects of antihistamines). Products include:
Libritabs Tablets 1930
Limbitrol 1933
Menrium Tablets 1934

Chlordiazepoxide Hydrochloride (Potentiation of sedative effects of antihistamines). Products include:
Librax Capsules 1929
Librium Capsules 1931
Librium Injectable 1932

Chlorpromazine (Potentiation of sedative effects of antihistamines). Products include:
Thorazine 2234

Chlorprothixene (Potentiation of sedative effects of antihistamines). Products include:
Taractan Tablets 1920

Chlorprothixene Hydrochloride (Potentiation of sedative effects of antihistamines). Products include:
Taractan 1920

Chlorprothixene Lactate (Potentiation of sedative effects of antihistamines). Products include:
Taractan Concentrate 1920

Clorazepate Dipotassium (Potentiation of sedative effects of antihistamines). Products include:
Tranxene 556

Codeine (Potentiation of sedative effects of antihistamines). Products include:
Calcidrine Syrup 506

Codeine Phosphate (Potentiation of sedative effects of antihistamines). Products include:
Actifed with Codeine Cough Syrup 752
Cheracol Cough Syrup 1853
Codimal PH Syrup 846
Dimetane-DC Cough Syrup 1857
Empirin with Codeine Phosphate Nos. 2, 3 & 4 764
Fiorinal with Codeine Capsules 2008
Isoclor Expectorant 982
Naldecon CX Adult Liquid ▣ 521
Novahistine DH 1342
Novahistine Expectorant 1343
Nucofed Capsules 2219
Nucofed Expectorant 2219
Nucofed Pediatric Expectorant 2220
Nucofed Syrup 2219
Phenaphen with Codeine Capsules 1865
Phenaphen-650 with Codeine Tablets 1866
Phenergan with Codeine 2497
Phenergan VC with Codeine 2501
Robitussin A-C Syrup 1875
Robitussin-DAC Syrup 1875
Ryna ▣ 741
Soma Compound w/Codeine Tablets 2390
Triaminic Expectorant w/Codeine 1996
Tussi-Organidin Liquid 2391
Tylenol with Codeine 1381

Codeine Polistirex (Potentiation of sedative effects of antihistamines).
No products indexed under this heading.

Dezocine (Potentiation of sedative effects of antihistamines).

Diazepam (Potentiation of sedative effects of antihistamines). Products include:
Valium Injectable 1937
Valium Tablets 1939
Valrelease Capsules 1923

Droperidol (Potentiation of sedative effects of antihistamines). Products include:
Inapsine Injection 1140
Innovar Injection 1141

Enflurane (Potentiation of sedative effects of antihistamines). Products include:
Ethrane 599

Estazolam (Potentiation of sedative effects of antihistamines). Products include:
ProSom Tablets 554

Ethchlorvynol (Potentiation of sedative effects of antihistamines). Products include:
Placidyl Capsules 553

Ethinamate (Potentiation of sedative effects of antihistamines).
No products indexed under this heading.

Fentanyl (Potentiation of sedative effects of antihistamines). Products include:
Duragesic Transdermal System 1133

Fentanyl Citrate (Potentiation of sedative effects of antihistamines). Products include:
Innovar Injection 1141
Sublimaze Injection 1146

Fluphenazine Decanoate (Potentiation of sedative effects of antihistamines). Products include:
Prolixin Decanoate 1795

Fluphenazine Enanthate (Potentiation of sedative effects of antihistamines). Products include:
Prolixin Enanthate 1796

Fluphenazine Hydrochloride (Potentiation of sedative effects of antihistamines). Products include:
Prolixin Elixir 1793
Prolixin Injection 1791
Prolixin Oral Concentrate 1792
Prolixin Tablets 1793

Flurazepam Hydrochloride (Potentiation of sedative effects of antihistamines). Products include:
Dalmane Capsules 1927

Furazolidone (Contraindicated). Products include:
Furoxone 1855

Glutethimide (Potentiation of sedative effects of antihistamines).
No products indexed under this heading.

Haloperidol (Potentiation of sedative effects of antihistamines). Products include:
Haldol Injection, Tablets and Concentrate 1373

Haloperidol Decanoate (Potentiation of sedative effects of antihistamines). Products include:
Haldol Decanoate 1375

Hydrocodone Bitartrate (Potentiation of sedative effects of antihistamines). Products include:
Anexsia 5/500 Tablets 2196
Anexsia 7.5/650 Tablets 2197
Azdone Tablets 844
Codiclear DH Syrup 845
Codimal DH Syrup 846
Damason-P 1356
Hycodan Syrup, Tablets 927
Hycomine Compound Tablets 929
Hycomine Syrup 927
Hycotuss Expectorant Syrup 930
Hydrocet Capsules 835
Lortab ASA Tablets 2414
Lortab 2412
Ru-Tuss with Hydrocodone 694
Triaminic Expectorant DH 1995
Vicodin Tablets 1187
Vicodin ES Tablets 1189
Zydone Capsules 941

Hydrocodone Polistirex (Potentiation of sedative effects of antihistamines). Products include:
Tussionex Extended-Release Suspension 988

Hydroxyzine Hydrochloride (Potentiation of sedative effects of antihistamines). Products include:
Atarax Tablets & Syrup 1941
Marax Tablets & DF Syrup 1954
Vistaril Intramuscular Solution 1970

Isocarboxazid (Contraindicated). Products include:
Marplan Tablets 1906

Isoflurane (Potentiation of sedative effects of antihistamines). Products include:
Forane 600

Ketamine Hydrochloride (Potentiation of sedative effects of antihistamines). Products include:
Ketalar 1726

Levorphanol Tartrate (Potentiation of sedative effects of antihistamines). Products include:
Levo-Dromoran ... 1906

Lorazepam (Potentiation of sedative effects of antihistamines). Products include:
Ativan Injection ... 2432
Ativan Tablets ... 2434

Loxapine Hydrochloride (Potentiation of sedative effects of antihistamines). Products include:
Loxitane ... 1213

Loxapine Succinate (Potentiation of sedative effects of antihistamines). Products include:
Loxitane Capsules ... 1213

Meperidine Hydrochloride (Potentiation of sedative effects of antihistamines). Products include:
Demerol ... 2047
Mepergan Injection ... 2479

Mephobarbital (Potentiation of sedative effects of antihistamines). Products include:
Mebaral Tablets ... 2061

Meprobamate (Potentiation of sedative effects of antihistamines). Products include:
Deprol Tablets ... 2382
Equagesic Tablets ... 2451
Miltown Tablets ... 2386
PMB 200 and PMB 400 ... 2504

Mesoridazine (Potentiation of sedative effects of antihistamines). Products include:
Serentil ... 686

Methadone Hydrochloride (Potentiation of sedative effects of antihistamines). Products include:
Dolophine Hydrochloride Ampoules & Vials ... 1260
Dolophine Hydrochloride Tablets ... 1261
Methadone Hydrochloride Diskets ... 1284
Methadone Hydrochloride Oral Solution & Tablets ... 1987

Methohexital Sodium (Potentiation of sedative effects of antihistamines). Products include:
Brevital Sodium Vials ... 1248

Methoxyflurane (Potentiation of sedative effects of antihistamines).
No products indexed under this heading.

Midazolam Hydrochloride (Potentiation of sedative effects of antihistamines). Products include:
Versed Injection ... 1924

Molindone Hydrochloride (Potentiation of sedative effects of antihistamines). Products include:
Moban Tablets & Concentrate ... 932

Morphine Sulfate (Potentiation of sedative effects of antihistamines). Products include:
Astramorph/PF Injection, USP (Preservative-Free) ... 618
Duramorph ... 960
Infumorph 200 and Infumorph 500 Sterile Solutions ... 962
MS Contin Tablets ... 1814
MSIR ... 1817
Oramorph SR (Morphine Sulfate Sustained Release Tablets) ... 1988
Roxanol ... 1991

Opium Alkaloids (Potentiation of sedative effects of antihistamines). Products include:
B & O No. 15A & No. 16A Supprettes ... 2395
Pantopon Injectable ... 1911

Oxazepam (Potentiation of sedative effects of antihistamines). Products include:
Serax Capsules ... 2522
Serax Tablets ... 2522

Oxycodone Hydrochloride (Potentiation of sedative effects of antihistamines). Products include:
Percocet Tablets ... 950
Percodan ... 951
Roxicodone Tablets, Oral Solution & Intensol (Oxycodone) ... 1992
Tylox Capsules ... 1382

Pentobarbital Sodium (Potentiation of sedative effects of antihistamines). Products include:
Nembutal Sodium Capsules ... 534
Nembutal Sodium Solution ... 536
Nembutal Sodium Suppositories ... 538

Perphenazine (Potentiation of sedative effects of antihistamines). Products include:
Etrafon ... 2087
Triavil Tablets ... 1556
Trilafon ... 2123

Phenelzine Sulfate (Contraindicated). Products include:
Nardil ... 1742

Phenobarbital (Potentiation of sedative effects of antihistamines). Products include:
Arco-Lase Plus Tablets ... 607
Bellergal-S Tablets ... 1998
Bronkolixir ... 761
Bronkotabs Tablets ... 762
Donnatal ... 1858
Donnatal Extentabs ... 1859
Donnatal Tablets ... 1858
Donnazyme Tablets ... 1860
Kinesed Tablets ... 2272
Phenobarbital Elixir and Tablets ... 1293
Primatene Tablets-P Formula ... 2421
Quadrinal Tablets ... 1183
Tedral SA ... 1765

Prazepam (Potentiation of sedative effects of antihistamines). Products include:
Centrax ... 1693

Prochlorperazine (Potentiation of sedative effects of antihistamines). Products include:
Compazine ... 2201

Promethazine Hydrochloride (Potentiation of sedative effects of antihistamines). Products include:
Mepergan Injection ... 2479
Phenergan with Codeine ... 2497
Phenergan with Dextromethorphan 2499
Phenergan Injection ... 2493
Phenergan Suppositories ... 2496
Phenergan Syrup ... 2495
Phenergan Tablets ... 2496
Phenergan VC ... 2500
Phenergan VC with Codeine ... 2501

Propofol (Potentiation of sedative effects of antihistamines). Products include:
Diprivan Injection ... 2267

Propoxyphene Hydrochloride (Potentiation of sedative effects of antihistamines). Products include:
Darvon ... 1256
Wygesic Tablets ... 2540

Propoxyphene Napsylate (Potentiation of sedative effects of antihistamines). Products include:
Darvon-N/Darvocet-N ... 1254

Quazepam (Potentiation of sedative effects of antihistamines). Products include:
Doral Tablets ... 2383

Secobarbital Sodium (Potentiation of sedative effects of antihistamines). Products include:
Seconal Sodium Pulvules ... 1296

Selegiline Hydrochloride (Contraindicated). Products include:
Eldepryl ... 2250

Sufentanil Citrate (Potentiation of sedative effects of antihistamines). Products include:
Sufenta Injection ... 1147

Temazepam (Potentiation of sedative effects of antihistamines). Products include:
Restoril Capsules ... 2023

Thiamylal Sodium (Potentiation of sedative effects of antihistamines). Products include:
Surital Ampoules, Steri-Vials ... 1764

Thioridazine Hydrochloride (Potentiation of sedative effects of antihistamines). Products include:
Mellaril ... 2011

Thiothixene (Potentiation of sedative effects of antihistamines). Products include:
Navane Capsules and Concentrate 1954
Navane Intramuscular ... 1956

Tranylcypromine Sulfate (Contraindicated). Products include:
Parnate Tablets ... 2222

Triazolam (Potentiation of sedative effects of antihistamines). Products include:
Halcion Tablets ... 2340

Trifluoperazine Hydrochloride (Potentiation of sedative effects of antihistamines). Products include:
Stelazine ... 2226

TRIAMINIC-12 TABLETS
(Phenylpropanolamine Hydrochloride, Chlorpheniramine Maleate) ... 690
May interact with monoamine oxidase inhibitors, hypnotics and sedatives, tranquilizers, and certain other agents. Compounds in these categories include:

Alcohol (Increases the drowsiness effect).

Alprazolam (Increases the drowsiness effect). Products include:
Xanax Tablets ... 2367

Buspirone Hydrochloride (Increases the drowsiness effect). Products include:
BuSpar ... 1401

Chlordiazepoxide (Increases the drowsiness effect). Products include:
Libritabs Tablets ... 1930
Limbitrol ... 1933
Menrium Tablets ... 1934

Chlordiazepoxide Hydrochloride (Increases the drowsiness effect). Products include:
Librax Capsules ... 1929
Librium Capsules ... 1931
Librium Injectable ... 1932

Chlorpromazine (Increases the drowsiness effect). Products include:
Thorazine ... 2234

Chlorprothixene (Increases the drowsiness effect). Products include:
Taractan Tablets ... 1920

Chlorprothixene Hydrochloride (Increases the drowsiness effect). Products include:
Taractan ... 1920

Clorazepate Dipotassium (Increases the drowsiness effect). Products include:
Tranxene ... 556

Diazepam (Increases the drowsiness effect). Products include:
Valium Injectable ... 1937
Valium Tablets ... 1939
Valrelease Capsules ... 1923

Droperidol (Increases the drowsiness effect). Products include:
Inapsine Injection ... 1140
Innovar Injection ... 1141

Estazolam (Increases the drowsiness effect). Products include:
ProSom Tablets ... 554

Ethchlorvynol (Increases the drowsiness effect). Products include:
Placidyl Capsules ... 553

Ethinamate (Increases the drowsiness effect).
No products indexed under this heading.

Fluphenazine Decanoate (Increases the drowsiness effect). Products include:
Prolixin Decanoate ... 1795

Fluphenazine Enanthate (Increases the drowsiness effect). Products include:
Prolixin Enanthate ... 1796

Fluphenazine Hydrochloride (Increases the drowsiness effect). Products include:
Prolixin Elixir ... 1793
Prolixin Injection ... 1791
Prolixin Oral Concentrate ... 1792
Prolixin Tablets ... 1793

Flurazepam Hydrochloride (Increases the drowsiness effect). Products include:
Dalmane Capsules ... 1927

Furazolidone (Use cautiously). Products include:
Furoxone ... 1855

Glutethimide (Increases the drowsiness effect).
No products indexed under this heading.

Haloperidol (Increases the drowsiness effect). Products include:
Haldol Injection, Tablets and Concentrate ... 1373

Haloperidol Decanoate (Increases the drowsiness effect). Products include:
Haldol Decanoate ... 1375

Hydroxyzine Hydrochloride (Increases the drowsiness effect). Products include:
Atarax Tablets & Syrup ... 1941
Marax Tablets & DF Syrup ... 1954
Vistaril Intramuscular Solution ... 1970

Isocarboxazid (Use cautiously). Products include:
Marplan Tablets ... 1906

Lorazepam (Increases the drowsiness effect). Products include:
Ativan Injection ... 2432
Ativan Tablets ... 2434

Loxapine Hydrochloride (Increases the drowsiness effect). Products include:
Loxitane ... 1213

Loxapine Succinate (Increases the drowsiness effect). Products include:
Loxitane Capsules ... 1213

Meprobamate (Increases the drowsiness effect). Products include:
Deprol Tablets ... 2382
Equagesic Tablets ... 2451
Miltown Tablets ... 2386
PMB 200 and PMB 400 ... 2504

Mesoridazine (Increases the drowsiness effect). Products include:
Serentil ... 686

Midazolam Hydrochloride (Increases the drowsiness effect). Products include:
Versed Injection ... 1924

Molindone Hydrochloride (Increases the drowsiness effect). Products include:
Moban Tablets & Concentrate ... 932

Oxazepam (Increases the drowsiness effect). Products include:
Serax Capsules ... 2522
Serax Tablets ... 2522

Perphenazine (Increases the drowsiness effect). Products include:
Etrafon ... 2087
Triavil Tablets ... 1556
Trilafon ... 2123

Phenelzine Sulfate (Use cautiously). Products include:
Nardil ... 1742

Prazepam (Increases the drowsiness effect). Products include:
Centrax ... 1693

Prochlorperazine (Increases the drowsiness effect). Products include:
Compazine ... 2201

Promethazine Hydrochloride (Increases the drowsiness effect). Products include:
Mepergan Injection ... 2479
Phenergan with Codeine ... 2497
Phenergan with Dextromethorphan 2499
Phenergan Injection ... 2493
Phenergan Suppositories ... 2496
Phenergan Syrup ... 2495
Phenergan Tablets ... 2496
Phenergan VC ... 2500
Phenergan VC with Codeine ... 2501

Propofol (Increases the drowsiness effect). Products include:
Diprivan Injection ... 2267

Quazepam (Increases the drowsiness effect). Products include:
Doral Tablets ... 2383

Secobarbital Sodium (Increases the drowsiness effect). Products include:
Seconal Sodium Pulvules ... 1296

Selegiline Hydrochloride (Use cautiously). Products include:
Eldepryl ... 2250

Temazepam (Increases the drowsiness effect). Products include:
Restoril Capsules ... 2023

Thioridazine Hydrochloride (Increases the drowsiness effect). Products include:
Mellaril ... 2011

Thiothixene (Increases the drowsiness effect). Products include:
Navane Capsules and Concentrate 1954
Navane Intramuscular ... 1956

Tranylcypromine Sulfate (Use cautiously). Products include:
Parnate Tablets ... 2222

Triazolam (Increases the drowsiness effect). Products include:
Halcion Tablets ... 2340

Trifluoperazine Hydrochloride (Increases the drowsiness effect). Products include:
Stelazine ... 2226

TRIAMINIC-DM SYRUP
(Phenylpropanolamine Hydrochloride, Dextromethorphan Hydrobromide) ... ▣ 689
May interact with monoamine oxidase inhibitors. Compounds in this category include:

Furazolidone (Contraindicated). Products include:
Furoxone ... 1855

Isocarboxazid (Contraindicated). Products include:
Marplan Tablets ... 1906

Phenelzine Sulfate (Contraindicated). Products include:
Nardil ... 1742

Selegiline Hydrochloride (Contraindicated). Products include:
Eldepryl ... 2250

Tranylcypromine Sulfate (Contraindicated). Products include:
Parnate Tablets ... 2222

TRIAMINICIN TABLETS
(Acetaminophen, Chlorpheniramine Maleate, Phenylpropanolamine Hydrochloride) ... ▣ 690
May interact with antihypertensives, antidepressant drugs, tranquilizers, hypnotics and sedatives, and certain other agents. Compounds in these categories include:

Acebutolol Hydrochloride (Concurrent use not recommended). Products include:
Sectral Capsules ... 2520

Alcohol (Increases drowsiness).

Alprazolam (Concurrent use not recommended). Products include:
Xanax Tablets ... 2367

Amitriptyline Hydrochloride (Concurrent use not recommended). Products include:
Elavil ... 2269
Endep Tablets ... 1927
Etrafon ... 2087
Limbitrol ... 1933
Triavil Tablets ... 1556

Amoxapine (Concurrent use not recommended). Products include:
Asendin Tablets ... 1196

Atenolol (Concurrent use not recommended). Products include:
Tenoretic Tablets ... 1105
Tenormin Tablets and I.V. Injection 1107

Benazepril Hydrochloride (Concurrent use not recommended). Products include:
Lotensin Tablets ... 872

Betaxolol Hydrochloride (Concurrent use not recommended). Products include:
Betoptic Sterile Ophthalmic Solution ... 569
Betoptic S Sterile Ophthalmic Suspension ... 570
Kerlone Tablets ... 2172

Bupropion Hydrochloride (Concurrent use not recommended). Products include:
Wellbutrin Tablets ... 821

Buspirone Hydrochloride (Concurrent use not recommended). Products include:
BuSpar ... 1401

Captopril (Concurrent use not recommended). Products include:
Capoten ... 2255
Capozide ... 2258

Carteolol Hydrochloride (Concurrent use not recommended). Products include:
Cartrol Tablets ... 507

Chlordiazepoxide (Concurrent use not recommended). Products include:
Libritabs Tablets ... 1930
Limbitrol ... 1933
Menrium Tablets ... 1934

Chlordiazepoxide Hydrochloride (Concurrent use not recommended). Products include:
Librax Capsules ... 1929
Librium Capsules ... 1931
Librium Injectable ... 1932

Chlorpromazine (Concurrent use not recommended). Products include:
Thorazine ... 2234

Chlorprothixene (Concurrent use not recommended). Products include:
Taractan Tablets ... 1920

Chlorprothixene Hydrochloride (Concurrent use not recommended). Products include:
Taractan ... 1920

Clonidine (Concurrent use not recommended). Products include:
Catapres-TTS ... 677

Clonidine Hydrochloride (Concurrent use not recommended). Products include:
Catapres Tablets ... 676
Combipres Tablets ... 678

Clorazepate Dipotassium (Concurrent use not recommended). Products include:
Tranxene ... 556

Deserpidine (Concurrent use not recommended). Products include:
Enduronyl ... 518
Harmonyl Tablets ... 528
Oreticyl ... 545

Desipramine Hydrochloride (Concurrent use not recommended). Products include:
Norpramin Tablets ... 1340

Diazepam (Concurrent use not recommended). Products include:
Valium Injectable ... 1937
Valium Tablets ... 1939
Valrelease Capsules ... 1923

Diazoxide (Concurrent use not recommended). Products include:
Hyperstat I.V. Injection ... 2095
Proglycem ... 649

Doxazosin Mesylate (Concurrent use not recommended). Products include:
Cardura Tablets ... 1941

Doxepin Hydrochloride (Concurrent use not recommended). Products include:
Sinequan ... 1960

Droperidol (Concurrent use not recommended). Products include:
Inapsine Injection ... 1140
Innovar Injection ... 1141

Enalapril Maleate (Concurrent use not recommended). Products include:
Vaseretic Tablets ... 1559
Vasotec Tablets ... 1564

Enalaprilat (Concurrent use not recommended). Products include:
Vasotec I.V. ... 1562

Esmolol Hydrochloride (Concurrent use not recommended). Products include:
Brevibloc Injection ... 942

Estazolam (Concurrent use not recommended). Products include:
ProSom Tablets ... 554

Ethchlorvynol (Concurrent use not recommended). Products include:
Placidyl Capsules ... 553

Ethinamate (Concurrent use not recommended).
No products indexed under this heading.

Felodipine (Concurrent use not recommended). Products include:
Plendil Extended-Release Tablets ... 1526

Fluoxetine Hydrochloride (Concurrent use not recommended). Products include:
Prozac Pulvules ... 920

Fluphenazine Decanoate (Concurrent use not recommended). Products include:
Prolixin Decanoate ... 1795

Fluphenazine Enanthate (Concurrent use not recommended). Products include:
Prolixin Enanthate ... 1796

Fluphenazine Hydrochloride (Concurrent use not recommended). Products include:
Prolixin Elixir ... 1793
Prolixin Injection ... 1791
Prolixin Oral Concentrate ... 1792
Prolixin Tablets ... 1793

Flurazepam Hydrochloride (Concurrent use not recommended). Products include:
Dalmane Capsules ... 1927

Fosinopril Sodium (Concurrent use not recommended). Products include:
Monopril Tablets ... 1406

Glutethimide (Concurrent use not recommended).
No products indexed under this heading.

Guanabenz Acetate (Concurrent use not recommended). Products include:
Wytensin Tablets ... 2542

Guanethidine Monosulfate (Concurrent use not recommended). Products include:
Esimil Tablets ... 864
Ismelin Tablets ... 869

Haloperidol (Concurrent use not recommended). Products include:
Haldol Injection, Tablets and Concentrate ... 1373

Haloperidol Decanoate (Concurrent use not recommended). Products include:
Haldol Decanoate ... 1375

Hydralazine Hydrochloride (Concurrent use not recommended). Products include:
Apresazide Capsules ... 854
Apresoline Hydrochloride Parenteral (Ampuls) ... 856
Apresoline Hydrochloride Tablets .. 855
Apresoline-Esidrix Tablets ... 857
Ser-Ap-Es Tablets ... 881
Serpasil-Apresoline Tablets ... 884

Hydroxyzine Hydrochloride (Concurrent use not recommended). Products include:
Atarax Tablets & Syrup ... 1941
Marax Tablets & DF Syrup ... 1954
Vistaril Intramuscular Solution ... 1970

Imipramine Hydrochloride (Concurrent use not recommended). Products include:
Tofranil Ampuls ... 1038
Tofranil Tablets ... 1039

Imipramine Pamoate (Concurrent use not recommended). Products include:
Tofranil-PM Capsules ... 1041

Indapamide (Concurrent use not recommended). Products include:
Lozol Tablets ... 1843

Isocarboxazid (Concurrent use not recommended). Products include:
Marplan Tablets ... 1906

Isradipine (Concurrent use not recommended). Products include:
DynaCirc Capsules ... 2004

Labetalol Hydrochloride (Concurrent use not recommended). Products include:
Normodyne Injection ... 2108
Normodyne Tablets ... 2110
Normozide Tablets ... 2112
Trandate HCT Tablets ... 579
Trandate Injection ... 577
Trandate Tablets ... 579

Lisinopril (Concurrent use not recommended). Products include:
Prinivil Tablets ... 1538
Prinzide Tablets ... 1540
Zestoretic ... 2274
Zestril Tablets ... 2277

Lorazepam (Concurrent use not recommended). Products include:
Ativan Injection ... 2432
Ativan Tablets ... 2434

Loxapine Hydrochloride (Concurrent use not recommended). Products include:
Loxitane ... 1213

Loxapine Succinate (Concurrent use not recommended). Products include:
Loxitane Capsules ... 1213

Maprotiline Hydrochloride (Concurrent use not recommended). Products include:
Ludiomil Tablets ... 874

Mecamylamine Hydrochloride (Concurrent use not recommended). Products include:
Inversine Tablets ... 1492

Meprobamate (Concurrent use not recommended). Products include:
Deprol Tablets ... 2382
Equagesic Tablets ... 2451
Miltown Tablets ... 2386
PMB 200 and PMB 400 ... 2504

Mesoridazine Besylate (Concurrent use not recommended).

Methyldopa (Concurrent use not recommended). Products include:
- Aldoclor Tablets 1413
- Aldomet Oral 1415
- Aldoril Tablets 1418

Methyldopate Hydrochloride (Concurrent use not recommended). Products include:
- Aldomet Ester HCl Injection 1417

Metoprolol Tartrate (Concurrent use not recommended). Products include:
- Lopressor Ampuls 1032
- Lopressor HCT Tablets 1034
- Lopressor Tablets 1032

Metyrosine (Concurrent use not recommended). Products include:
- Demser Capsules 1460

Midazolam Hydrochloride (Concurrent use not recommended). Products include:
- Versed Injection 1924

Minoxidil (Concurrent use not recommended). Products include:
- Loniten Tablets 2346
- Rogaine Topical Solution 2357

Molindone Hydrochloride (Concurrent use not recommended). Products include:
- Moban Tablets & Concentrate 932

Nadolol (Concurrent use not recommended). Products include:
- Corgard Tablets 701
- Corzide Tablets 702

Nicardipine Hydrochloride (Concurrent use not recommended). Products include:
- Cardene Capsules 2290

Nitroglycerin (Concurrent use not recommended). Products include:
- Deponit NTG Transdermal Delivery System 2143
- Minitran Transdermal Delivery System 1312
- Nitro-Bid Ointment 1339
- Nitro-Bid Capsules 1338
- Nitrodisc 2176
- Nitro-Dur (nitroglycerin) Transdermal Infusion System 1164
- Nitrogard Tablets 1004
- Nitrolingual Spray 1846
- Nitrostat Tablets 1743
- Transderm-Nitro Transdermal Therapeutic System 2283

Nortriptyline Hydrochloride (Concurrent use not recommended). Products include:
- Pamelor 2019

Oxazepam (Concurrent use not recommended). Products include:
- Serax Capsules 2522
- Serax Tablets 2522

Penbutolol Sulfate (Concurrent use not recommended). Products include:
- Levatol 1832

Perphenazine (Concurrent use not recommended). Products include:
- Etrafon 2087
- Triavil Tablets 1556
- Trilafon 2123

Phenelzine Sulfate (Concurrent use not recommended). Products include:
- Nardil 1742

Phenoxybenzamine Hydrochloride (Concurrent use not recommended). Products include:
- Dibenzyline Capsules 2207

Phentolamine Mesylate (Concurrent use not recommended). Products include:
- Regitine 878

Pindolol (Concurrent use not recommended). Products include:
- Visken Tablets 2036

Prazepam (Concurrent use not recommended). Products include:
- Centrax 1693

Prazosin Hydrochloride (Concurrent use not recommended). Products include:
- Minipress Capsules 1778
- Minizide Capsules 1779

Prochlorperazine (Concurrent use not recommended). Products include:
- Compazine 2201

Promethazine Hydrochloride (Concurrent use not recommended). Products include:
- Mepergan Injection 2479
- Phenergan with Codeine 2497
- Phenergan with Dextromethorphan 2499
- Phenergan Injection 2493
- Phenergan Suppositories 2496
- Phenergan Syrup 2495
- Phenergan Tablets 2496
- Phenergan VC 2500
- Phenergan VC with Codeine 2501

Propofol (Concurrent use not recommended). Products include:
- Diprivan Injection 2267

Propranolol Hydrochloride (Concurrent use not recommended). Products include:
- Inderal 2459
- Inderal LA Long Acting Capsules 2461
- Inderide Tablets 2463
- Inderide LA Long Acting Capsules .. 2465

Protriptyline Hydrochloride (Concurrent use not recommended). Products include:
- Vivactil Tablets 1567

Quazepam (Concurrent use not recommended). Products include:
- Doral Tablets 2383

Ramipril (Concurrent use not recommended). Products include:
- Altace Capsules 1086

Rauwolfia Serpentina (Concurrent use not recommended). Products include:
- Raudixin Tablets 1803
- Rauzide Tablets 1804

Rescinnamine (Concurrent use not recommended).
- No products indexed under this heading.

Reserpine (Concurrent use not recommended). Products include:
- Diupres Tablets 1461
- Hydromox R Tablets 1209
- Hydropres Tablets 1485
- Renese-R Tablets 1786
- Salutensin/Salutensin-Demi 719
- Ser-Ap-Es Tablets 881
- Serpasil Tablets 883
- Serpasil-Apresoline Tablets 884
- Serpasil-Esidrix Tablets 886

Secobarbital Sodium (Concurrent use not recommended). Products include:
- Seconal Sodium Pulvules 1296

Sodium Nitroprusside (Concurrent use not recommended). Products include:
- Nipride I.V. Infusion 1909

Temazepam (Concurrent use not recommended). Products include:
- Restoril Capsules 2023

Terazosin Hydrochloride (Concurrent use not recommended). Products include:
- Hytrin Tablets 529

Thioridazine Hydrochloride (Concurrent use not recommended). Products include:
- Mellaril 2011

Thiothixene (Concurrent use not recommended). Products include:
- Navane Capsules and Concentrate 1954
- Navane Intramuscular 1956

Timolol Maleate (Concurrent use not recommended). Products include:
- Blocadren Tablets 1429
- Timolide Tablets 1547
- Timoptic in Ocudose 1552
- Timoptic Sterile Ophthalmic Solution 1550

Tranylcypromine Sulfate (Concurrent use not recommended). Products include:
- Parnate Tablets 2222

Trazodone Hydrochloride (Concurrent use not recommended). Products include:
- Desyrel and Desyrel Dividose 1404

Triazolam (Concurrent use not recommended). Products include:
- Halcion Tablets 2340

Trifluoperazine Hydrochloride (Concurrent use not recommended). Products include:
- Stelazine 2226

Trimethaphan Camsylate (Concurrent use not recommended). Products include:
- Arfonad Ampuls 1887

Trimipramine Maleate (Concurrent use not recommended). Products include:
- Surmontil Capsules 2524

TRIAMINICOL MULTI-SYMPTOM COLD TABLETS
(Phenylpropanolamine Hydrochloride, Chlorpheniramine Maleate, Dextromethorphan Hydrobromide) .... ▣ 691
May interact with hypnotics and sedatives, tranquilizers, antihypertensives, antidepressant drugs, and certain other agents. Compounds in these categories include:

Acebutolol Hydrochloride (Effect not specified). Products include:
- Sectral Capsules 2520

Alcohol (May increase the drowsiness effect).

Alprazolam (May increase the drowsiness effect). Products include:
- Xanax Tablets 2367

Amitriptyline Hydrochloride (Effect not specified). Products include:
- Elavil 2269
- Endep Tablets 1927
- Etrafon 2087
- Limbitrol 1933
- Triavil Tablets 1556

Amoxapine (Effect not specified). Products include:
- Asendin Tablets 1196

Atenolol (Effect not specified). Products include:
- Tenoretic Tablets 1105
- Tenormin Tablets and I.V. Injection 1107

Benazepril Hydrochloride (Effect not specified). Products include:
- Lotensin Tablets 872

Bendroflumethiazide (Effect not specified). Products include:
- Corzide Tablets 702
- Naturetin Tablets 1789
- Rauzide Tablets 1804

Betaxolol Hydrochloride (Effect not specified). Products include:
- Betoptic Sterile Ophthalmic Solution 569
- Betoptic S Sterile Ophthalmic Suspension 570
- Kerlone Tablets 2172

Bupropion Hydrochloride (Effect not specified). Products include:
- Wellbutrin Tablets 821

Buspirone Hydrochloride (May increase the drowsiness effect). Products include:
- BuSpar 1401

Captopril (Effect not specified). Products include:
- Capoten 2255
- Capozide 2258

Carteolol Hydrochloride (Effect not specified). Products include:
- Cartrol Tablets 507

Chlordiazepoxide (May increase the drowsiness effect). Products include:
- Libritabs Tablets 1930
- Limbitrol 1933
- Menrium Tablets 1934

Chlordiazepoxide Hydrochloride (May increase the drowsiness effect). Products include:
- Librax Capsules 1929
- Librium Capsules 1931
- Librium Injectable 1932

Chlorothiazide (Effect not specified). Products include:
- Aldoclor Tablets 1413
- Diupres Tablets 1461
- Diuril Oral 1464

Chlorothiazide Sodium (Effect not specified). Products include:
- Diuril Sodium Intravenous 1463

Chlorpromazine (May increase the drowsiness effect). Products include:
- Thorazine 2234

Chlorprothixene (May increase the drowsiness effect). Products include:
- Taractan Tablets 1920

Chlorprothixene Hydrochloride (May increase the drowsiness effect). Products include:
- Taractan 1920

Chlorthalidone (Effect not specified). Products include:
- Combipres Tablets 678
- Tenoretic Tablets 1105
- Thalitone Tablets 687

Clonidine (Effect not specified). Products include:
- Catapres-TTS 677

Clonidine Hydrochloride (Effect not specified). Products include:
- Catapres Tablets 676
- Combipres Tablets 678

Clorazepate Dipotassium (May increase the drowsiness effect). Products include:
- Tranxene 556

Deserpidine (Effect not specified). Products include:
- Enduronyl 518
- Harmonyl Tablets 528
- Oreticyl 545

Desipramine Hydrochloride (Effect not specified). Products include:
- Norpramin Tablets 1340

Diazepam (May increase the drowsiness effect). Products include:
- Valium Injectable 1937
- Valium Tablets 1939
- Valrelease Capsules 1923

Diazoxide (Effect not specified). Products include:
- Hyperstat I.V. Injection 2095
- Proglycem 649

Doxazosin Mesylate (Effect not specified). Products include:
- Cardura Tablets 1941

Doxepin Hydrochloride (Effect not specified). Products include:
- Sinequan 1960

Droperidol (May increase the drowsiness effect). Products include:
- Inapsine Injection 1140
- Innovar Injection 1141

Enalapril Maleate (Effect not specified). Products include:
- Vaseretic Tablets 1559
- Vasotec Tablets 1564

Enalaprilat (Effect not specified). Products include:
- Vasotec I.V. 1562

Esmolol Hydrochloride (Effect not specified). Products include:
- Brevibloc Injection 942

Estazolam (May increase the drowsiness effect). Products include:
- ProSom Tablets 554

Ethchlorvynol (May increase the drowsiness effect). Products include:
- Placidyl Capsules 553

Ethinamate (May increase the drowsiness effect).
- No products indexed under this heading.

Felodipine (Effect not specified). Products include:
- Plendil Extended-Release Tablets 1526

Fluoxetine Hydrochloride (Effect not specified). Products include:
- Prozac Pulvules 920

Fluphenazine Decanoate (May increase the drowsiness effect). Products include:
- Prolixin Decanoate 1795

Fluphenazine Enanthate (May increase the drowsiness effect). Products include:
- Prolixin Enanthate 1796

Fluphenazine Hydrochloride (May increase the drowsiness effect). Products include:
- Prolixin Elixir 1793
- Prolixin Injection 1791
- Prolixin Oral Concentrate 1792
- Prolixin Tablets 1793

Flurazepam Hydrochloride (May increase the drowsiness effect). Products include:
- Dalmane Capsules 1927

Fosinopril Sodium (Effect not specified). Products include:
- Monopril Tablets 1406

Furosemide (Effect not specified). Products include:
- Lasix 1093

Glutethimide (May increase the drowsiness effect).
- No products indexed under this heading.

Guanabenz Acetate (Effect not specified). Products include:
- Wytensin Tablets 2542

Guanethidine Monosulfate (Effect not specified). Products include:
- Esimil Tablets 864
- Ismelin Tablets 869

Haloperidol (May increase the drowsiness effect). Products include:
- Haldol Injection, Tablets and Concentrate 1373

Haloperidol Decanoate (May increase the drowsiness effect). Products include:
- Haldol Decanoate 1375

Hydralazine Hydrochloride (Effect not specified). Products include:
- Apresazide Capsules 854
- Apresoline Hydrochloride Parenteral (Ampuls) 856
- Apresoline Hydrochloride Tablets 855
- Apresoline-Esidrix Tablets 857
- Ser-Ap-Es Tablets 881
- Serpasil-Apresoline Tablets 884

Hydrochlorothiazide (Effect not specified). Products include:
- Aldactazide 2150
- Aldoril Tablets 1418
- Apresazide Capsules 854
- Apresoline-Esidrix Tablets 857
- Capozide 2258
- Dyazide Capsules 2208
- Esidrix Tablets 863
- Esimil Tablets 864
- HydroDIURIL Tablets 1484
- Hydropres Tablets 1485
- Inderide Tablets 2463
- Inderide LA Long Acting Capsules 2465
- Lopressor HCT Tablets 1034
- Maxzide 1215
- Moduretic Tablets 1510
- Normozide Tablets 2112
- Oretic Tablets 544
- Oreticyl 545
- Prinzide Tablets 1540
- Ser-Ap-Es Tablets 881
- Serpasil-Esidrix Tablets 886
- Timolide Tablets 1547
- Trandate HCT Tablets 579
- Vaseretic Tablets 1559
- Zestoretic 2274

Hydroflumethiazide (Effect not specified). Products include:
- Diucardin Tablets 2450
- Saluron 718
- Salutensin/Salutensin-Demi 719

Hydroxyzine Hydrochloride (May increase the drowsiness effect). Products include:
- Atarax Tablets & Syrup 1941
- Marax Tablets & DF Syrup 1954
- Vistaril Intramuscular Solution 1970

Imipramine Hydrochloride (Effect not specified). Products include:
- Tofranil Ampuls 1038
- Tofranil Tablets 1039

Imipramine Pamoate (Effect not specified). Products include:
- Tofranil-PM Capsules 1041

Indapamide (Effect not specified). Products include:
- Lozol Tablets 1843

Isocarboxazid (Effect not specified). Products include:
- Marplan Tablets 1906

Isradipine (Effect not specified). Products include:
- DynaCirc Capsules 2004

Labetalol Hydrochloride (Effect not specified). Products include:
- Normodyne Injection 2108
- Normodyne Tablets 2110
- Normozide Tablets 2112
- Trandate HCT Tablets 579
- Trandate Injection 577
- Trandate Tablets 579

Lisinopril (Effect not specified). Products include:
- Prinivil Tablets 1538
- Prinzide Tablets 1540
- Zestoretic 2274
- Zestril Tablets 2277

Lorazepam (May increase the drowsiness effect). Products include:
- Ativan Injection 2432
- Ativan Tablets 2434

Loxapine Hydrochloride (May increase the drowsiness effect). Products include:
- Loxitane 1213

Loxapine Succinate (May increase the drowsiness effect). Products include:
- Loxitane Capsules 1213

Maprotiline Hydrochloride (Effect not specified). Products include:
- Ludiomil Tablets 874

Mecamylamine Hydrochloride (Effect not specified). Products include:
- Inversine Tablets 1492

Meprobamate (May increase the drowsiness effect). Products include:
- Deprol Tablets 2382
- Equagesic Tablets 2451
- Miltown Tablets 2386
- PMB 200 and PMB 400 2504

Mesoridazine (May increase the drowsiness effect). Products include:
- Serentil 686

Methyclothiazide (Effect not specified). Products include:
- Enduron Tablets 517
- Enduronyl 518

Methyldopa (Effect not specified). Products include:
- Aldoclor Tablets 1413
- Aldomet Oral 1415
- Aldoril Tablets 1418

Methyldopate Hydrochloride (Effect not specified). Products include:
- Aldomet Ester HCl Injection 1417

Metolazone (Effect not specified). Products include:
- Diulo 2129
- Mykrox ½ mg Tablets 984
- Zaroxolyn Tablets 989

Metoprolol Tartrate (Effect not specified). Products include:
- Lopressor Ampuls 1032
- Lopressor HCT Tablets 1034
- Lopressor Tablets 1032

Metyrosine (Effect not specified). Products include:
- Demser Capsules 1460

Midazolam Hydrochloride (May increase the drowsiness effect). Products include:
- Versed Injection 1924

Minoxidil (Effect not specified). Products include:
- Loniten Tablets 2346
- Rogaine Topical Solution 2357

Molindone Hydrochloride (May increase the drowsiness effect). Products include:
- Moban Tablets & Concentrate 932

Nadolol (Effect not specified). Products include:
- Corgard Tablets 701
- Corzide Tablets 702

Nicardipine Hydrochloride (Effect not specified). Products include:
- Cardene Capsules 2290

Nitroglycerin (Effect not specified). Products include:
- Deponit NTG Transdermal Delivery System 2143
- Minitran Transdermal Delivery System 1312
- Nitro-Bid Ointment 1339
- Nitro-Bid Capsules 1338
- Nitrodisc 2176
- Nitro-Dur (nitroglycerin) Transdermal Infusion System 1164
- Nitrogard Tablets 1004
- Nitrolingual Spray 1846
- Nitrostat Tablets 1743
- Transderm-Nitro Transdermal Therapeutic System 2283

Nortriptyline Hydrochloride (Effect not specified). Products include:
- Pamelor 2019

Oxazepam (May increase the drowsiness effect). Products include:
- Serax Capsules 2522
- Serax Tablets 2522

Penbutolol Sulfate (Effect not specified). Products include:
- Levatol 1832

Perphenazine (May increase the drowsiness effect). Products include:
- Etrafon 2087
- Triavil Tablets 1556
- Trilafon 2123

Phenelzine Sulfate (Effect not specified). Products include:
- Nardil 1742

Phenoxybenzamine Hydrochloride (Effect not specified). Products include:
- Dibenzyline Capsules 2207

Phentolamine Mesylate (Effect not specified). Products include:
- Regitine 878

Pindolol (Effect not specified). Products include:
- Visken Tablets 2036

Polythiazide (Effect not specified). Products include:
- Minizide Capsules 1779
- Renese Tablets 1785
- Renese-R Tablets 1786

Prazepam (May increase the drowsiness effect). Products include:
- Centrax 1693

Prazosin Hydrochloride (Effect not specified). Products include:
- Minipress Capsules 1778
- Minizide Capsules 1779

Prochlorperazine (May increase the drowsiness effect). Products include:
- Compazine 2201

Promethazine Hydrochloride (May increase the drowsiness effect). Products include:
- Mepergan Injection 2479
- Phenergan with Codeine 2497
- Phenergan with Dextromethorphan 2499
- Phenergan Injection 2493
- Phenergan Suppositories 2496
- Phenergan Syrup 2495
- Phenergan Tablets 2496
- Phenergan VC 2500
- Phenergan VC with Codeine 2501

Propofol (May increase the drowsiness effect). Products include:
- Diprivan Injection 2267

Propranolol Hydrochloride (Effect not specified). Products include:
- Inderal 2459
- Inderal LA Long Acting Capsules 2461
- Inderide Tablets 2463
- Inderide LA Long Acting Capsules 2465

Protriptyline Hydrochloride (Effect not specified). Products include:
- Vivactil Tablets 1567

Quazepam (May increase the drowsiness effect). Products include:
- Doral Tablets 2383

Ramipril (Effect not specified). Products include:
- Altace Capsules 1086

Rauwolfia Serpentina (Effect not specified). Products include:
- Raudixin Tablets 1803
- Rauzide Tablets 1804

Rescinnamine (Effect not specified).
- No products indexed under this heading.

Reserpine (Effect not specified). Products include:
- Diupres Tablets 1461
- Hydromox R Tablets 1209
- Hydropres Tablets 1485
- Renese-R Tablets 1786
- Salutensin/Salutensin-Demi 719
- Ser-Ap-Es Tablets 881
- Serpasil Tablets 883
- Serpasil-Apresoline Tablets 884
- Serpasil-Esidrix Tablets 886

Secobarbital Sodium (May increase the drowsiness effect). Products include:
- Seconal Sodium Pulvules 1296

Sodium Nitroprusside (Effect not specified). Products include:
- Nipride I.V. Infusion 1909

Temazepam (May increase the drowsiness effect). Products include:
- Restoril Capsules 2023

Terazosin Hydrochloride (Effect not specified). Products include:
- Hytrin Tablets 529

Thioridazine Hydrochloride (May increase the drowsiness effect). Products include:
- Mellaril 2011

Thiothixene (May increase the drowsiness effect). Products include:
- Navane Capsules and Concentrate 1954
- Navane Intramuscular 1956

Timolol Maleate (Effect not specified). Products include:
- Blocadren Tablets 1429
- Timolide Tablets 1547
- Timoptic in Ocudose 1552

Timoptic Sterile Ophthalmic Solution 1550

Tranylcypromine Sulfate (Effect not specified). Products include:
Parnate Tablets 2222

Trazodone Hydrochloride (Effect not specified). Products include:
Desyrel and Desyrel Dividose 1404

Triazolam (May increase the drowsiness effect). Products include:
Halcion Tablets 2340

Trifluoperazine Hydrochloride (May increase the drowsiness effect). Products include:
Stelazine 2226

Trimethaphan Camsylate (Effect not specified). Products include:
Arfonad Ampuls 1887

Trimipramine Maleate (Effect not specified). Products include:
Surmontil Capsules 2524

TRIAMINICOL MULTI-SYMPTOM RELIEF

(Phenylpropanolamine Hydrochloride, Chlorpheniramine Maleate, Dextromethorphan Hydrobromide) ▣ 691

May interact with monoamine oxidase inhibitors and central nervous system depressants. Compounds in these categories include:

Alcohol (Potentiation of sedative effects).

Alfentanil Hydrochloride (Potentiation of sedative effects). Products include:
Alfenta Injection 1131

Alprazolam (Potentiation of sedative effects). Products include:
Xanax Tablets 2367

Aprobarbital (Potentiation of sedative effects). Products include:
Alurate Elixir 1883

Buprenorphine (Potentiation of sedative effects).
No products indexed under this heading.

Buspirone Hydrochloride (Potentiation of sedative effects). Products include:
BuSpar 1401

Butabarbital (Potentiation of sedative effects). Products include:
Pyridium Plus 1764

Butalbital (Potentiation of sedative effects). Products include:
Esgic-Plus Tablets 1002
Esgic Tablets & Capsules 1001
Fioricet Tablets 2006
Fiorinal Capsules 2007
Fiorinal with Codeine Capsules 2008
Fiorinal Tablets 2007
Phrenilin 838
Sedapap Tablets 50 mg/650 mg 1360

Chlordiazepoxide (Potentiation of sedative effects). Products include:
Libritabs Tablets 1930
Limbitrol 1933
Menrium Tablets 1934

Chlordiazepoxide Hydrochloride (Potentiation of sedative effects). Products include:
Librax Capsules 1929
Librium Capsules 1931
Librium Injectable 1932

Chlorpromazine (Potentiation of sedative effects). Products include:
Thorazine 2234

Chlorprothixene (Potentiation of sedative effects). Products include:
Taractan Tablets 1920

Chlorprothixene Hydrochloride (Potentiation of sedative effects). Products include:
Taractan 1920

Clorazepate Dipotassium (Potentiation of sedative effects). Products include:
Tranxene 556

Codeine (Potentiation of sedative effects). Products include:
Calcidrine Syrup 506

Codeine Phosphate (Potentiation of sedative effects). Products include:
Actifed with Codeine Cough Syrup 752
Cheracol Cough Syrup 1853
Codimal PH Syrup 846
Dimetane-DC Cough Syrup 1857
Empirin with Codeine Phosphate Nos. 2, 3 & 4 764
Fiorinal with Codeine Capsules 2008
Isoclor Expectorant 982
Naldecon CX Adult Liquid ▣ 521
Novahistine DH 1342
Novahistine Expectorant 1343
Nucofed Capsules 2219
Nucofed Expectorant 2219
Nucofed Pediatric Expectorant 2220
Nucofed Syrup 2219
Phenaphen with Codeine Capsules 1865
Phenaphen-650 with Codeine Tablets 1866
Phenergan with Codeine 2497
Phenergan VC with Codeine 2501
Robitussin A-C Syrup 1875
Robitussin-DAC Syrup 1875
Ryna ▣ 741
Soma Compound w/Codeine Tablets 2390
Triaminic Expectorant w/Codeine 1996
Tussi-Organidin Liquid 2391
Tylenol with Codeine 1381

Codeine Polistirex (Potentiation of sedative effects).
No products indexed under this heading.

Dezocine (Potentiation of sedative effects).

Diazepam (Potentiation of sedative effects). Products include:
Valium Injectable 1937
Valium Tablets 1939
Valrelease Capsules 1923

Droperidol (Potentiation of sedative effects). Products include:
Inapsine Injection 1140
Innovar Injection 1141

Enflurane (Potentiation of sedative effects). Products include:
Ethrane 599

Estazolam (Potentiation of sedative effects). Products include:
ProSom Tablets 554

Ethchlorvynol (Potentiation of sedative effects). Products include:
Placidyl Capsules 553

Ethinamate (Potentiation of sedative effects).
No products indexed under this heading.

Fentanyl (Potentiation of sedative effects). Products include:
Duragesic Transdermal System 1133

Fentanyl Citrate (Potentiation of sedative effects). Products include:
Innovar Injection 1141
Sublimaze Injection 1146

Fluphenazine Decanoate (Potentiation of sedative effects). Products include:
Prolixin Decanoate 1795

Fluphenazine Enanthate (Potentiation of sedative effects). Products include:
Prolixin Enanthate 1796

Fluphenazine Hydrochloride (Potentiation of sedative effects). Products include:
Prolixin Elixir 1793
Prolixin Injection 1791
Prolixin Oral Concentrate 1792
Prolixin Tablets 1793

Flurazepam Hydrochloride (Potentiation of sedative effects). Products include:
Dalmane Capsules 1927

Furazolidone (Contraindicated). Products include:
Furoxone 1855

Glutethimide (Potentiation of sedative effects).
No products indexed under this heading.

Haloperidol (Potentiation of sedative effects). Products include:
Haldol Injection, Tablets and Concentrate 1373

Haloperidol Decanoate (Potentiation of sedative effects). Products include:
Haldol Decanoate 1375

Hydrocodone Bitartrate (Potentiation of sedative effects). Products include:
Anexsia 5/500 Tablets 2196
Anexsia 7.5/650 Tablets 2197
Azdone Tablets 844
Codiclear DH Syrup 845
Codimal DH Syrup 846
Damason-P 1356
Hycodan Syrup, Tablets 927
Hycomine Compound Tablets 929
Hycomine Syrup 927
Hycotuss Expectorant Syrup 930
Hydrocet Capsules 835
Lortab ASA Tablets 2414
Lortab 2412
Ru-Tuss with Hydrocodone 694
Triaminic Expectorant DH 1995
Vicodin Tablets 1187
Vicodin ES Tablets 1189
Zydone Capsules 941

Hydrocodone Polistirex (Potentiation of sedative effects). Products include:
Tussionex Extended-Release Suspension 988

Hydroxyzine Hydrochloride (Potentiation of sedative effects). Products include:
Atarax Tablets & Syrup 1941
Marax Tablets & DF Syrup 1954
Vistaril Intramuscular Solution 1970

Isocarboxazid (Contraindicated). Products include:
Marplan Tablets 1906

Isoflurane (Potentiation of sedative effects). Products include:
Forane 600

Ketamine Hydrochloride (Potentiation of sedative effects). Products include:
Ketalar 1726

Levorphanol Tartrate (Potentiation of sedative effects). Products include:
Levo-Dromoran 1906

Lorazepam (Potentiation of sedative effects). Products include:
Ativan Injection 2432
Ativan Tablets 2434

Loxapine Hydrochloride (Potentiation of sedative effects). Products include:
Loxitane 1213

Loxapine Succinate (Potentiation of sedative effects). Products include:
Loxitane Capsules 1213

Meperidine Hydrochloride (Potentiation of sedative effects). Products include:
Demerol 2047
Mepergan Injection 2479

Mephobarbital (Potentiation of sedative effects). Products include:
Mebaral Tablets 2061

Meprobamate (Potentiation of sedative effects). Products include:
Deprol Tablets 2382
Equagesic Tablets 2451
Miltown Tablets 2386
PMB 200 and PMB 400 2504

Mesoridazine (Potentiation of sedative effects). Products include:
Serentil 686

Methadone Hydrochloride (Potentiation of sedative effects). Products include:
Dolophine Hydrochloride Ampoules & Vials 1260
Dolophine Hydrochloride Tablets 1261
Methadone Hydrochloride Diskets 1284
Methadone Hydrochloride Oral Solution & Tablets 1987

Methohexital Sodium (Potentiation of sedative effects). Products include:
Brevital Sodium Vials 1248

Methoxyflurane (Potentiation of sedative effects).
No products indexed under this heading.

Midazolam Hydrochloride (Potentiation of sedative effects). Products include:
Versed Injection 1924

Molindone Hydrochloride (Potentiation of sedative effects). Products include:
Moban Tablets & Concentrate 932

Morphine Sulfate (Potentiation of sedative effects). Products include:
Astramorph/PF Injection, USP (Preservative-Free) 618
Duramorph 960
Infumorph 200 and Infumorph 500 Sterile Solutions 962
MS Contin Tablets 1814
MSIR 1817
Oramorph SR (Morphine Sulfate Sustained Release Tablets) 1988
Roxanol 1991

Opium Alkaloids (Potentiation of sedative effects). Products include:
B & O No. 15A & No. 16A Supprettes 2395
Pantopon Injectable 1911

Oxazepam (Potentiation of sedative effects). Products include:
Serax Capsules 2522
Serax Tablets 2522

Oxycodone Hydrochloride (Potentiation of sedative effects). Products include:
Percocet Tablets 950
Percodan 951
Roxicodone Tablets, Oral Solution & Intensol (Oxycodone) 1992
Tylox Capsules 1382

Pentobarbital Sodium (Potentiation of sedative effects). Products include:
Nembutal Sodium Capsules 534
Nembutal Sodium Solution 536
Nembutal Sodium Suppositories 538

Perphenazine (Potentiation of sedative effects). Products include:
Etrafon 2087
Triavil Tablets 1556
Trilafon 2123

Phenelzine Sulfate (Contraindicated). Products include:
Nardil 1742

Phenobarbital (Potentiation of sedative effects). Products include:
Arco-Lase Plus Tablets 607
Bellergal-S Tablets 1998
Bronkolixir ▣ 761
Bronkotabs Tablets ▣ 762
Donnatal 1858
Donnatal Extentabs 1859
Donnatal Tablets 1858
Donnazyme Tablets 1860
Kinesed Tablets 2272
Phenobarbital Elixir and Tablets 1293
Primatene Tablets-P Formula 2421
Quadrinal Tablets 1183
Tedral SA 1765

Prazepam (Potentiation of sedative effects). Products include:
Centrax 1693

(▣ Described in PDR For Nonprescription Drugs) (◉ Described in PDR For Ophthalmology)

Prochlorperazine (Potentiation of sedative effects). Products include:
- Compazine ... 2201

Promethazine Hydrochloride (Potentiation of sedative effects). Products include:
- Mepergan Injection ... 2479
- Phenergan with Codeine ... 2497
- Phenergan with Dextromethorphan 2499
- Phenergan Injection ... 2493
- Phenergan Suppositories ... 2496
- Phenergan Syrup ... 2495
- Phenergan Tablets ... 2496
- Phenergan VC ... 2500
- Phenergan VC with Codeine ... 2501

Propofol (Potentiation of sedative effects). Products include:
- Diprivan Injection ... 2267

Propoxyphene Hydrochloride (Potentiation of sedative effects). Products include:
- Darvon ... 1256
- Wygesic Tablets ... 2540

Propoxyphene Napsylate (Potentiation of sedative effects). Products include:
- Darvon-N/Darvocet-N ... 1254

Quazepam (Potentiation of sedative effects). Products include:
- Doral Tablets ... 2383

Secobarbital Sodium (Potentiation of sedative effects). Products include:
- Seconal Sodium Pulvules ... 1296

Selegiline Hydrochloride (Contraindicated). Products include:
- Eldepryl ... 2250

Sufentanil Citrate (Potentiation of sedative effects). Products include:
- Sufenta Injection ... 1147

Temazepam (Potentiation of sedative effects). Products include:
- Restoril Capsules ... 2023

Thiamylal Sodium (Potentiation of sedative effects). Products include:
- Surital Ampoules, Steri-Vials ... 1764

Thioridazine Hydrochloride (Potentiation of sedative effects). Products include:
- Mellaril ... 2011

Thiothixene (Potentiation of sedative effects). Products include:
- Navane Capsules and Concentrate 1954
- Navane Intramuscular ... 1956

Tranylcypromine Sulfate (Contraindicated). Products include:
- Parnate Tablets ... 2222

Triazolam (Potentiation of sedative effects). Products include:
- Halcion Tablets ... 2340

Trifluoperazine Hydrochloride (Potentiation of sedative effects). Products include:
- Stelazine ... 2226

TRIAVIL TABLETS

(Perphenazine, Amitriptyline Hydrochloride) ... 1556

May interact with thyroid preparations, antihistamines, monoamine oxidase inhibitors, para-aminobenzoic acid based local anesthetics, anticonvulsants, central nervous system depressants, anticholinergics, sympathomimetic aerosol bronchodilators, neuromuscular blocking agents, barbiturates, and certain other agents. Compounds in these categories include:

Albuterol (Close supervision and careful dosage adjustment required). Products include:
- Proventil Inhalation Aerosol ... 2117
- Ventolin Inhalation Aerosol and Refill ... 583

Albuterol Sulfate (Close supervision and careful dosage adjustment required). Products include:
- Proventil Repetabs Tablets ... 2120
- Proventil Solutions for Inhalation 0.5% and 0.083% ... 2118
- Proventil Syrup ... 2119
- Proventil Tablets ... 2120
- Ventolin ... 583

Alcohol (Potentiated; contraindication).

Alfentanil Hydrochloride (Potentiated). Products include:
- Alfenta Injection ... 1131

Alprazolam (Potentiated). Products include:
- Xanax Tablets ... 2367

Aprobarbital (Potentiated). Products include:
- Alurate Elixir ... 1883

Astemizole (Potentiated). Products include:
- Hismanal Tablets ... 1138

Atropine Sulfate (Potentiated; hyperpyrexia; paralytic ileus). Products include:
- Arco-Lase Plus Tablets ... 607
- Atropine Sulfate Sterile Ophthalmic Solution and S.O.P. Sterile Ophthalmic Ointment ... ⊙ 239
- Donnagel ... ◘ 675
- Donnagel-PG ... 1858
- Donnatal ... 1858
- Donnatal Extentabs ... 1859
- Donnatal Tablets ... 1858
- Donnazyme Tablets ... 1860
- Isopto Atropine ... ⊙ 218
- Lomotil ... 2174
- Motofen Tablets ... 836
- Ru-Tuss Tablets ... 693
- Urised Tablets ... 2396

Azatadine Maleate (Potentiated). Products include:
- Optimine Tablets ... 2115
- Trinalin Repetabs Tablets ... 1170

Belladonna Alkaloids (Hyperpyrexia; paralytic ileus). Products include:
- Bellergal-S Tablets ... 1998
- Hyland's Bed Wetting Tablets ... ◘ 728
- Hyland's Teething Tablets ... ◘ 728
- Kinesed Tablets ... 2272

Benztropine Mesylate (Hyperpyrexia; paralytic ileus). Products include:
- Cogentin ... 1435

Biperiden (Hyperpyrexia; paralytic ileus). Products include:
- Akineton ... 1171

Bromodiphenhydramine Hydrochloride (Potentiated).
- No products indexed under this heading.

Brompheniramine Maleate (Potentiated). Products include:
- Alka Seltzer Plus Sinus Allergy Medicine ... ◘ 624
- Atrohist Sprinkle Capsules ... 558
- Bromfed Capsules (Timed Release) ... 1615
- Bromfed Syrup ... ◘ 628
- Bromfed ... 1615
- Dimetane Decongestant ... ◘ 673
- Dimetane ... ◘ 672
- Dimetane-DC Cough Syrup ... 1857
- Dimetane-DX Cough Syrup ... 1858
- Dimetapp Elixir ... ◘ 673
- Dimetapp DM Elixir ... ◘ 674
- Dimetapp Extentabs ... ◘ 674
- Dimetapp Plus Caplets ... ◘ 675
- Dimetapp Tablets ... ◘ 675
- Drixoral Antihistamine/Nasal Decongestant Syrup ... ◘ 698

Buprenorphine (Potentiated).
- No products indexed under this heading.

Buspirone Hydrochloride (Potentiated). Products include:
- BuSpar ... 1401

Butabarbital (Potentiated). Products include:
- Pyridium Plus ... 1764

Butalbital (Potentiated). Products include:
- Esgic-Plus Tablets ... 1002
- Esgic Tablets & Capsules ... 1001
- Fioricet Tablets ... 2006
- Fiorinal Capsules ... 2007
- Fiorinal with Codeine Capsules ... 2008
- Fiorinal Tablets ... 2007
- Phrenilin ... 838
- Sedapap Tablets 50 mg/650 mg .. 1360

Carbamazepine (Increased anticonvulsant dosage may be necessary). Products include:
- Tegretol Chewable Tablets ... 654
- Tegretol Suspension ... 656
- Tegretol Tablets ... 654

Chlordiazepoxide (Potentiated). Products include:
- Libritabs Tablets ... 1930
- Limbitrol ... 1933
- Menrium Tablets ... 1934

Chlordiazepoxide Hydrochloride (Potentiated). Products include:
- Librax Capsules ... 1929
- Librium Capsules ... 1931
- Librium Injectable ... 1932

Chlorpheniramine Maleate (Potentiated). Products include:
- A.R.M. Allergy Relief Medicine Caplets ... ◘ 615
- Alka-Seltzer Plus Cold Medicine ... ◘ 623
- Allerest ... ◘ 559
- Ana-Kit Anaphylaxis Emergency Treatment Kit ... 1100
- BC Cold Powder Multi-Symptom Formula ... ◘ 517
- Brexin L.A. Capsules ... 2078
- Cerose-DM ... 2443
- Cheracol Plus Head Cold/Cough Formula ... ◘ 667
- Chlor-Trimeton Allergy Syrup, Tablets & Long-Acting Repetabs Tablets ... ◘ 693
- Chlor-Trimeton Decongestant ... ◘ 694
- Comhist LA Capsules ... 1618
- Allergy-Sinus Comtrex Multi-Symptom Allergy Sinus Formula Tablets & Caplets ... 746
- Comtrex Multi-Symptom Cold Reliever Tablets/Caplets/Liqui-Gels/Liquid ... 745
- Day-Night Comtrex ... 747
- Contac Continuous Action Decongestant/Antihistamine Capsules ◘ 710
- Contac Maximum Strength Continuous Action Decongestant/Antihistamine Caplets ... ◘ 709
- Contac Severe Cold and Flu Formula Caplets ... ◘ 711
- Coricidin 'D' Decongestant Tablets ... ◘ 695
- Coricidin Demilets Tablets for Children ... ◘ 696
- Coricidin Tablets ... ◘ 695
- Deconamine ... 663
- Demazin Nasal Decongestant/Antihistamine Repetabs Tablets & Syrup ... ◘ 697
- Dorcol Children's Liquid Cold Formula ... ◘ 686
- Dristan Decongestant/Antihistamine/ Analgesic Coated Caplets ... ◘ 749
- Dristan Cold Nasal Decongestant/Antihistamine/ Analgesic Coated Tablets ... 2419
- Dristan Advanced Formula Decongestant/Antihistamine/Analgesic Tablets ... ◘ 749
- Extendryl ... 994
- 4-Way Cold Tablets ... 750
- Fedahist Gyrocaps ... 2145
- Fedahist Timecaps ... 2145
- Hycomine Compound Tablets ... 929
- Isoclor Timesule Capsules ... ◘ 561
- Kronofed-A ... 970
- Medi-Flu Caplet, Liquid ... ◘ 640
- Naldecon Syrup, Tablets, Pediatric Drops and Pediatric Syrup ... 709
- Nolamine Tablets ... 838
- Novafed A Capsules ... 1342
- Novahistine DH ... 1342
- Novahistine Elixir ... ◘ 596
- Ornade Spansule Capsules ... 2221
- Orthoxicol Cough Syrup ... ◘ 668
- PediaCare Allergy Relief Formula Liquid ... 1362
- PediaCare Cough-Cold Formula Liquid ... 1362
- PediaCare Night Rest Cough-Cold Formula Liquid ... 1362
- PediaCare 6-12 Cough-Cold Formula Chewable Tablets ... 1362
- Pyrroxate Capsules ... ◘ 669
- Quelidrine Syrup ... 556
- Ru-Tuss II Capsules ... 693
- Ru-Tuss Tablets ... 693
- Ryna ... ◘ 741
- Sinarest Tablets & Extra Strength Tablets ... ◘ 562
- Sine-Off Maximum Strength Allergy/Sinus Formula Caplets ... ◘ 721
- Sine-Off Sinus Medicine Tablets-Aspirin Formula ... ◘ 722
- Singlet Tablets ... ◘ 598
- Sinulin ... 840
- Sinutab Maximum Strength ... ◘ 641
- St. Joseph Nighttime Cold Medicine ... ◘ 705
- Sudafed Plus Liquid ... ◘ 544
- Sudafed Plus Tablets ... ◘ 545
- Teldrin Timed-Release Allergy Capsules, 12 mg ... 2192
- TheraFlu Flu and Cold Medicine ... ◘ 687
- Triaminic Allergy Tablets ... ◘ 688
- Triaminic Chewables ... ◘ 688
- Triaminic Cold Tablets ... ◘ 688
- Triaminic Nite Light ... ◘ 689
- Triaminic Syrup ... ◘ 689
- Triaminic-12 Tablets ... ◘ 690
- Triaminicin Tablets ... ◘ 690
- Triaminicol Multi-Symptom Cold Tablets ... ◘ 691
- Triaminicol Multi-Symptom Relief ◘ 691
- Tylenol Allergy Sinus Medication Caplets and Gelcaps, Maximum Strength ... 1372
- Children's Tylenol Cold Liquid Formula and Chewable Tablets ... 1368
- Tylenol Cold & Flu Hot Medication, Packets ... 1369
- Tylenol Cold Medication Caplets and Tablets ... 1370
- Tylenol Cold Medication, Effervescent Tablets ... 1369
- Vicks Children's NyQuil ... ◘ 664
- Vicks Formula 44 Cough Medicine ... ◘ 661
- Vicks Formula 44M Multi-Symptom Cough Medicine ... ◘ 662
- Vicks Pediatric Formula 44m Multi-Symptom Cough & Cold Medicine ... ◘ 663

Chlorpheniramine Polistirex (Potentiated). Products include:
- Tussionex Extended-Release Suspension ... 988

Chlorpheniramine Tannate (Potentiated). Products include:
- Rynatan ... 2387
- Rynatuss ... 2388

Chlorpromazine (Potentiated; hyperpyrexia). Products include:
- Thorazine ... 2234

Chlorprothixene (Potentiated; hyperpyrexia). Products include:
- Taractan Tablets ... 1920

Chlorprothixene Hydrochloride (Potentiated; hyperpyrexia). Products include:
- Taractan ... 1920

Cimetidine (Increased frequency and severity of side effects). Products include:
- Tagamet Tablets ... 2228

Cimetidine Hydrochloride (Increased frequency and severity of side effects). Products include:
- Tagamet ... 2228

Clemastine Fumarate (Potentiated). Products include:
- Tavist Syrup ... 2033
- Tavist Tablets ... 2035
- Tavist-D Tablets ... 2035

Clidinium Bromide (Hyperpyrexia; paralytic ileus). Products include:
- Librax Capsules ... 1929
- Quarzan Capsules ... 1937

Clorazepate Dipotassium (Potentiated). Products include:
- Tranxene ... 556

Clozapine (Potentiated; hyperpyrexia). Products include:
Clozaril Tablets ... 2000

Codeine (Potentiated). Products include:
Calcidrine Syrup ... 506

Codeine Phosphate (Potentiated). Products include:
Actifed with Codeine Cough Syrup.. 752
Cheracol Cough Syrup ... 1853
Codimal PH Syrup ... 846
Dimetane-DC Cough Syrup ... 1857
Empirin with Codeine Phosphate Nos. 2, 3 & 4 ... 764
Fiorinal with Codeine Capsules ... 2008
Isoclor Expectorant ... 982
Naldecon CX Adult Liquid ... ND 521
Novahistine DH ... 1342
Novahistine Expectorant ... 1343
Nucofed Capsules ... 2219
Nucofed Expectorant ... 2219
Nucofed Pediatric Expectorant ... 2220
Nucofed Syrup ... 2219
Phenaphen with Codeine Capsules 1865
Phenaphen-650 with Codeine Tablets ... 1866
Phenergan with Codeine ... 2497
Phenergan VC with Codeine ... 2501
Robitussin A-C Syrup ... 1875
Robitussin-DAC Syrup ... 1875
Ryna ... ND 741
Soma Compound w/Codeine Tablets ... 2390
Triaminic Expectorant w/Codeine .. 1996
Tussi-Organidin Liquid ... 2391
Tylenol with Codeine ... 1381

Codeine Polistirex (Potentiated).
No products indexed under this heading.

Cyproheptadine Hydrochloride (Potentiated). Products include:
Periactin ... 1525

Deserpidine (Antihypertensive effect of deserpidine blocked). Products include:
Enduronyl ... 518
Harmonyl Tablets ... 528
Oreticyl ... 545

Dexchlorpheniramine Maleate (Potentiated). Products include:
Polaramine ... 2116

Dezocine (Potentiated).

Diazepam (Potentiated). Products include:
Valium Injectable ... 1937
Valium Tablets ... 1939
Valrelease Capsules ... 1923

Dicyclomine Hydrochloride (Hyperpyrexia; paralytic ileus). Products include:
Bentyl ... 1322

Diphenhydramine Citrate (Potentiated). Products include:
Alka-Seltzer Plus Night-Time Cold Medicine ... ND 623
Bufferin AF Nite Time Analgesic/Sleeping Aid Caplets ... 744
Excedrin P.M. Analgesic/Sleeping Aid Tablets, Caplets and Liquid.... 749

Diphenhydramine Hydrochloride (Potentiated). Products include:
Benadryl Anti-Itch Cream ... ND 635
Benadryl Capsules ... 1691
Benadryl Decongestant Elixir ... ND 635
Benadryl Decongestant ... ND 635
Benadryl Elixir ... ND 636
Benadryl Kapseals ... 1691
Benadryl 25 Kapseals ... ND 636
Benadryl Parenteral ... 1692
Benadryl Plus ... ND 636
Benadryl Plus Nighttime ... ND 637
Benadryl Spray, Maximum Strength ... ND 637
Benadryl Spray, Regular Strength ND 637
Benadryl Steri-Vials, Ampoules, and Steri-Dose Syringe ... 1692
Benadryl 25 Tablets ... ND 636
Benylin Cough Syrup ... ND 637
Benylin Decongestant ... ND 638
Caladryl Cream, Lotion, Spray ... ND 638
Miles Nervine Nighttime Sleep-Aid ND 627
Nytol Tablets ... ND 517
Sleep-ettes-D Tablets ... ND 653
Sleep-eze 3 Tablets ... ND 755
Sleepinal Night-time Sleep Aid Capsules ... ND 734
Sominex Caplets and Tablets ... ND 722
Sominex Liquid ... ND 723
Sominex Pain Relief Formula ... ND 723
Tylenol Cold Night Time Medication Liquid ... 1371
Tylenol PM, Extra Strength Caplets and Tablets ... 1368
Unisom Dual Relief Nighttime Sleep Aid/Analgesic ... 1774
Ziradryl Lotion ... ND 643

Diphenylpyraline Hydrochloride (Potentiated).
No products indexed under this heading.

Disulfiram (Delerium). Products include:
Antabuse Tablets ... 2429

Divalproex Sodium (Increased anticonvulsant dosage may be necessary). Products include:
Depakote ... 512

Dobutamine Hydrochloride (Close supervision and careful dosage adjustment required). Products include:
Dobutrex Solution Vials ... 1259

Dopamine Hydrochloride (Close supervision and careful dosage adjustment required). Products include:
Intropin Injection ... 930

Droperidol (Potentiated). Products include:
Inapsine Injection ... 1140
Innovar Injection ... 1141

Enflurane (Potentiated). Products include:
Ethrane ... 599

Ephedrine (Close supervision and careful dosage adjustment required).

Ephedrine Hydrochloride (Close supervision and careful dosage adjustment required). Products include:
Amesec ... ND 682
Primatene Tablets-M Formula ... 2421
Primatene Tablets-P Formula ... 2421
Primatene Tablets-Regular Formula ... 2421
Quadrinal Tablets ... 1183
Quelidrine Syrup ... 556
Tedral SA ... 1765

Ephedrine Sulfate (Close supervision and careful dosage adjustment required). Products include:
Bronkaid Tablets ... ND 757
Bronkolixir ... ND 761
Bronkotabs Tablets ... ND 762
Marax Tablets & DF Syrup ... 1954
Pazo Hemorrhoid Ointment & Suppositories ... 752
Vicks Vatronol Nose Drops ... ND 666

Ephedrine Tannate (Close supervision and careful dosage adjustment required). Products include:
Rynatuss ... 2388

Epinephrine (Close supervision and careful dosage adjustment required). Products include:
Ana-Kit Anaphylaxis Emergency Treatment Kit ... 1100
Bronkaid Mist ... ND 757
EpiPen ... 843
Marcaine Hydrochloride 0.5% with Epinephrine 1:200,000 (as bitartrate) ... 958
Marcaine Hydrochloride with Epinephrine 1:200,000 ... 2055
Primatene Mist ... 2420
Sus-Phrine Injection ... 1006
Xylocaine with Epinephrine Injections ... 637

Epinephrine Bitartrate (Close supervision and careful dosage adjustment required). Products include:
AsthmaHaler Mist Epinephrine Bitartrate Bronchodilator ... ND 616
Bronkaid Mist Suspension ... ND 757
Primatene Mist Suspension ... 2421

Epinephrine Hydrochloride (Close supervision and careful dosage adjustment required). Products include:
Adrenalin Chloride Solution 1:100 & 1:1,000 ... 1689
Epifrin ... ⊙ 244
Glaucon ... ⊙ 218

Estazolam (Potentiated). Products include:
ProSom Tablets ... 554

Ethchlorvynol (Potentiated; transient delirium). Products include:
Placidyl Capsules ... 553

Ethinamate (Potentiated).
No products indexed under this heading.

Ethopropazine Hydrochloride (Hyperpyrexia; paralytic ileus).

Ethosuximide (Increased anticonvulsant dosage may be necessary). Products include:
Zarontin Capsules ... 1768
Zarontin Syrup ... 1769

Ethotoin (Increased anticonvulsant dosage may be necessary). Products include:
Peganone Tablets ... 551

Fentanyl (Potentiated). Products include:
Duragesic Transdermal System ... 1133

Fentanyl Citrate (Potentiated). Products include:
Innovar Injection ... 1141
Sublimaze Injection ... 1146

Fluphenazine Decanoate (Potentiated; hyperpyrexia). Products include:
Prolixin Decanoate ... 1795

Fluphenazine Enanthate (Potentiated; hyperpyrexia). Products include:
Prolixin Enanthate ... 1796

Fluphenazine Hydrochloride (Potentiated; hyperpyrexia). Products include:
Prolixin Elixir ... 1793
Prolixin Injection ... 1791
Prolixin Oral Concentrate ... 1792
Prolixin Tablets ... 1793

Flurazepam Hydrochloride (Potentiated). Products include:
Dalmane Capsules ... 1927

Furazolidone (Concomitant administration is contraindicated; hyperpyretic crises and severe convulsions have occurred). Products include:
Furoxone ... 1855

Glutethimide (Potentiated).
No products indexed under this heading.

Glycopyrrolate (Hyperpyrexia; paralytic ileus). Products include:
Robinul Forte Tablets ... 1873
Robinul Injectable ... 1873
Robinul Tablets ... 1873

Guanethidine Monosulfate (Antihypertensive effect of guanethidine). Products include:
Esimil Tablets ... 864
Ismelin Tablets ... 869

Haloperidol (Potentiated; hyperpyrexia). Products include:
Haldol Injection, Tablets and Concentrate ... 1373

Haloperidol Decanoate (Potentiated; hyperpyrexia). Products include:
Haldol Decanoate ... 1375

Hydrocodone Bitartrate (Potentiated). Products include:
Anexsia 5/500 Tablets ... 2196
Anexsia 7.5/650 Tablets ... 2197
Azdōne Tablets ... 844
Codiclear DH Syrup ... 845
Codimal DH Syrup ... 846
Damason-P ... 1356
Hycodan Syrup, Tablets ... 927
Hycomine Compound Tablets ... 929
Hycomine Syrup ... 927
Hycotuss Expectorant Syrup ... 930
Hydrocet Capsules ... 835
Lortab ASA Tablets ... 2414
Lortab ... 2412
Ru-Tuss with Hydrocodone ... 694
Triaminic Expectorant DH ... 1995
Vicodin Tablets ... 1187
Vicodin ES Tablets ... 1189
Zydone Capsules ... 941

Hydrocodone Polistirex (Potentiated). Products include:
Tussionex Extended-Release Suspension ... 988

Hydroxyzine Hydrochloride (Potentiated). Products include:
Atarax Tablets & Syrup ... 1941
Marax Tablets & DF Syrup ... 1954
Vistaril Intramuscular Solution ... 1970

Hyoscyamine (Hyperpyrexia; paralytic ileus). Products include:
Cystospaz Tablets ... 2395
Urised Tablets ... 2396

Hyoscyamine Sulfate (Hyperpyrexia; paralytic ileus). Products include:
Arco-Lase Plus Tablets ... 607
Cystospaz-M Capsules ... 2395
Donnagel ... ND 675
Donnagel-PG ... 1858
Donnatal ... 1858
Donnatal Extentabs ... 1859
Donnatal Tablets ... 1858
Donnazyme Tablets ... 1860
Kutrase Capsules ... 2146
Levsin/Levsinex ... 2147
Ru-Tuss Tablets ... 693

Ipratropium Bromide (Hyperpyrexia; paralytic ileus). Products include:
Atrovent Inhalation Aerosol ... 675

Isocarboxazid (Concomitant administration is contraindicated; hyperpyretic crises and severe convulsions have occurred). Products include:
Marplan Tablets ... 1906

Isoflurane (Potentiated; contraindication). Products include:
Forane ... 600

Isoproterenol Hydrochloride (Close supervision and careful dosage adjustment required). Products include:
Isuprel Hydrochloride Injection 1:5000 ... 2050
Isuprel Hydrochloride Mistometer .. 2051
Isuprel Hydrochloride Solution 1:200 & 1:100 ... 2052
Norisodrine Aerotrol ... 540

Ketamine Hydrochloride (Potentiated). Products include:
Ketalar ... 1726

Levorphanol Tartrate (Potentiated). Products include:
Levo-Dromoran ... 1906

Levothyroxine Sodium (Close supervision is indicated). Products include:
Levothroid Tablets ... 1003
Levoxine Tablets ... 904
Synthroid ... 695

Liothyronine Sodium (Close supervision is indicated). Products include:
Cytomel Tablets ... 2203

Lithium Carbonate (Hyperpyrexia). Products include:
Eskalith ... 2214
Lithane Tablets ... 1596
Lithium Carbonate Capsules & Tablets ... 1984
Lithobid Tablets ... 870

Lithium Citrate (Hyperpyrexia). Products include:
Cibalith-S ... 870

Lorazepam (Potentiated; contraindication). Products include:
Ativan Injection ... 2432
Ativan Tablets ... 2434

Loxapine Hydrochloride (Potentiated; hyperpyrexia). Products include:
- Loxitane ... 1213

Loxapine Succinate (Potentiated). Products include:
- Loxitane Capsules ... 1213

Mepenzolate Bromide (Hyperpyrexia; paralytic ileus). Products include:
- Cantil Tablets ... 1326

Meperidine Hydrochloride (Potentiated). Products include:
- Demerol ... 2047
- Mepergan Injection ... 2479

Mephenytoin (Increased anticonvulsant dosage may be necessary). Products include:
- Mesantoin Tablets ... 2013

Mephobarbital (Potentiated). Products include:
- Mebaral Tablets ... 2061

Meprobamate (Potentiated). Products include:
- Deprol Tablets ... 2382
- Equagesic Tablets ... 2451
- Miltown Tablets ... 2386
- PMB 200 and PMB 400 ... 2504

Mesoridazine (Potentiated; hyperpyrexia; contraindication). Products include:
- Serentil ... 686

Metaproterenol Sulfate (Close supervision and careful dosage adjustment required). Products include:
- Alupent ... 674
- Arm-a-Med Metaproterenol Sulfate Inhalation Solution, USP ... 617
- Metaprel Inhalation Aerosol Bronchodilator ... 2014
- Metaprel Inhalation Solution ... 2015
- Metaprel ... 2015
- Metaproterenol Sulfate Inhalation Solution, USP ... 912

Metaraminol Bitartrate (Close supervision and careful dosage adjustment required). Products include:
- Aramine Injection ... 1424

Methadone Hydrochloride (Potentiated). Products include:
- Dolophine Hydrochloride Ampoules & Vials ... 1260
- Dolophine Hydrochloride Tablets ... 1261
- Methadone Hydrochloride Diskets .. 1284
- Methadone Hydrochloride Oral Solution & Tablets ... 1987

Methdilazine Hydrochloride (Potentiated). Products include:
- Tacaryl Syrup & Tablets ... 2409

Methohexital Sodium (Potentiated). Products include:
- Brevital Sodium Vials ... 1248

Methoxamine Hydrochloride (Close supervision and careful dosage adjustment required). Products include:
- Vasoxyl Injection ... 819

Methoxyflurane (Potentiated).
- No products indexed under this heading.

Methsuximide (Increased anticonvulsant dosage may be necessary). Products include:
- Celontin ... 1692

Midazolam Hydrochloride (Potentiated). Products include:
- Versed Injection ... 1924

Molindone Hydrochloride (Potentiated; hyperpyrexia). Products include:
- Moban Tablets & Concentrate ... 932

Morphine Sulfate (Potentiated). Products include:
- Astramorph/PF Injection, USP (Preservative-Free) ... 618
- Duramorph ... 960
- Infumorph 200 and Infumorph 500 Sterile Solutions ... 962
- MS Contin Tablets ... 1814
- MSIR ... 1817
- Oramorph SR (Morphine Sulfate Sustained Release Tablets) ... 1988
- Roxanol ... 1991

Norepinephrine Bitartrate (Close supervision and careful dosage adjustment required). Products include:
- Levophed Bitartrate Injection ... 2054

Opium Alkaloids (Potentiated). Products include:
- B & O No. 15A & No. 16A Supprettes ... 2395
- Pantopon Injectable ... 1911

Oxazepam (Potentiated). Products include:
- Serax Capsules ... 2522
- Serax Tablets ... 2522

Oxybutynin Chloride (Hyperpyrexia; paralytic ileus). Products include:
- Ditropan ... 1332

Oxycodone Hydrochloride (Potentiated). Products include:
- Percocet Tablets ... 950
- Percodan ... 951
- Roxicodone Tablets, Oral Solution & Intensol (Oxycodone) ... 1992
- Tylox Capsules ... 1382

Paramethadione (Increased anticonvulsant dosage may be necessary). Products include:
- Paradione Capsules ... 548

Pentobarbital Sodium (Potentiated). Products include:
- Nembutal Sodium Capsules ... 534
- Nembutal Sodium Solution ... 536
- Nembutal Sodium Suppositories ... 538

Phenacemide (Increased anticonvulsant dosage may be necessary). Products include:
- Phenurone Tablets ... 552

Phenelzine Sulfate (Concomitant administration is contraindicated; hyperpyretic crises and severe convulsions have occurred). Products include:
- Nardil ... 1742

Phenobarbital (Potentiated; increased anticonvulsant dosage may be necessary). Products include:
- Arco-Lase Plus Tablets ... 607
- Bellergal-S Tablets ... 1998
- Bronkolixir ... ▣ 761
- Bronkotabs Tablets ... ▣ 762
- Donnatal ... 1858
- Donnatal Extentabs ... 1859
- Donnatal Tablets ... 1858
- Donnazyme Tablets ... 1860
- Kinesed Tablets ... 2272
- Phenobarbital Elixir and Tablets ... 1293
- Primatene Tablets-P Formula ... 2421
- Quadrinal Tablets ... 1183
- Tedral SA ... 1765

Phensuximide (Increased anticonvulsant dosage may be necessary). Products include:
- Milontin Kapseals ... 1741

Phenylephrine Bitartrate (Close supervision and careful dosage adjustment required).
- No products indexed under this heading.

Phenylephrine Hydrochloride (Close supervision and careful dosage adjustment required). Products include:
- AK-Dilate Solution 2.5% and 10% ... ⊙ 203
- Atrohist Sprinkle Capsules ... 558
- Cerose-DM ... 2443
- Codimal ... 846
- Comhist LA Capsules ... 1618
- Congespirin For Children Aspirin Free Chewable Cold Tablets ... 748
- Cyclomydril ... ⊙ 216
- Deconsal Sprinkle Capsules ... 559
- Dimetane Decongestant ... ▣ 673
- Dristan Decongestant/Antihistamine/ Analgesic Coated Caplets ... ▣ 749
- Dristan Cold Nasal Decongestant/ Antihistamine/ Analgesic Coated Tablets ... 2419
- Dristan Advanced Formula Decongestant/Antihistamine/ Analgesic Tablets ... ▣ 749
- Dristan Nasal Spray, Menthol ... 2419
- Dristan Nasal Spray, Regular and Regular with Metered Pump ... 2419
- Entex Capsules ... 1623
- Entex Liquid ... 1623
- Sinus Excedrin Analgesic, Decongestant Tablets & Caplets ... 750
- Extendryl ... 994
- 4-Way Fast Acting Nasal Spray - Original Formula (regular & mentholated) & Metered Spray Pump (regular) ... 751
- Hycomine Compound Tablets ... 929
- Murocoll-2 Sterile Ophthalmic Solution ... ⊙ 261
- Mydfrin 2.5% ... ⊙ 224
- Naldecon Syrup, Tablets, Pediatric Drops and Pediatric Syrup ... 709
- Neo-Synephrine Hydrochloride 1% Carpuject ... 2063
- Neo-Synephrine Hydrochloride 1% Injection ... 2063
- Neo-Synephrine Hydrochloride (Ophthalmic) ... 2064
- Neo-Synephrine ... ▣ 759
- Nōstril Nasal Decongestant ... ▣ 520
- Novahistine Elixir ... ▣ 596
- Phenergan VC ... 2500
- Phenergan VC with Codeine ... 2501
- Prefrin Liquifilm Vasoconstrictor and Lubricant Eye Drops ... ⊙ 254
- Prefrin-A ... ⊙ 255
- Quelidrine Syrup ... 556
- Relief Vasoconstrictor and Lubricant Eye Drops ... ⊙ 256
- Robitussin Night Relief ... ▣ 677
- Ru-Tuss with Hydrocodone ... 694
- Ru-Tuss Tablets ... 693
- Vasosulf ... ⊙ 279
- Vicks Sinex ... ▣ 665
- Zincfrin ... ⊙ 230

Phenylephrine Tannate (Close supervision and careful dosage adjustment required). Products include:
- Rynatan ... 2387
- Rynatuss ... 2388

Phenylpropanolamine Hydrochloride (Close supervision and careful dosage adjustment required). Products include:
- A.R.M. Allergy Relief Medicine Caplets ... ▣ 615
- Acutrim ... ▣ 548
- Allerest ... ▣ 559
- BC Cold Powder ... ▣ 517
- Cheracol Plus Head Cold/Cough Formula ... ▣ 667
- Codimal Expectorant ... 846
- Comtrex Multi-Symptom Cold Reliever Tablets/Caplets/Liqui-Gels/Liquid ... 745
- Contac Continuous Action Decongestant/Antihistamine Capsules ▣ 710
- Contac Maximum Strength Continuous Action Decongestant/ Antihistamine Caplets ... ▣ 709
- Contac Severe Cold and Flu Formula Caplets ... ▣ 711
- Coricidin 'D' Decongestant Tablets ... ▣ 695
- Coricidin Demilets Tablets for Children ... ▣ 696
- Demazin Nasal Decongestant/ Antihistamine Repetabs Tablets & Syrup ... ▣ 697
- Dexatrim ... ▣ 733
- Dimetane-DC Cough Syrup ... 1857
- Dimetapp Elixir ... ▣ 673
- Dimetapp DM Elixir ... ▣ 674
- Dimetapp Extentabs ... ▣ 674
- Dimetapp Plus Caplets ... ▣ 675
- Dimetapp Tablets ... ▣ 675
- Entex Capsules ... 1623
- Entex LA Tablets ... 1623
- Entex Liquid ... 1623
- 4-Way Cold Tablets ... 750
- Hycomine Syrup ... 927
- Naldecon CX Adult Liquid ... ▣ 521
- Naldecon DX Adult Liquid ... ▣ 521
- Naldecon DX Children's Syrup ... ▣ 522
- Naldecon DX Pediatric Drops ... ▣ 522
- Naldecon EX Children's Syrup ... ▣ 522
- Naldecon EX Pediatric Drops ... ▣ 523
- Naldecon Syrup, Tablets, Pediatric Drops and Pediatric Syrup ... 709
- Nolamine Tablets ... 838
- Nolex LA Tablets ... 838
- Ornade Spansule Capsules ... 2221
- Orthoxicol Cough Syrup ... ▣ 668
- Propagest ... 839
- Pyrroxate Capsules ... ▣ 669
- Robitussin-CF ... ▣ 676
- Ru-Tuss II Capsules ... 693
- Ru-Tuss with Hydrocodone ... 694
- Ru-Tuss Tablets ... 693
- Sine-Off Sinus Medicine Tablets-Aspirin Formula ... ▣ 722
- Sinulin ... 840
- St. Joseph Cold Tablets for Children ... ▣ 704
- Tavist-D Tablets ... 2035
- Triaminic Allergy Tablets ... ▣ 688
- Triaminic Chewables ... ▣ 688
- Triaminic Cold Tablets ... ▣ 688
- Triaminic Expectorant ... ▣ 688
- Triaminic Expectorant w/Codeine .. 1996
- Triaminic Expectorant DH ... 1995
- Triaminic Oral Infant Drops ... 1996
- Triaminic Syrup ... ▣ 689
- Triaminic-12 Tablets ... ▣ 690
- Triaminic-DM Syrup ... ▣ 689
- Triaminicin Tablets ... ▣ 690
- Triaminicol Multi-Symptom Cold Tablets ... ▣ 691
- Triaminicol Multi-Symptom Relief ▣ 691
- Tuss-Ornade Liquid ... 2242
- Tuss-Ornade Spansule Capsules ... 2242
- Tylenol Cold Medication, Effervescent Tablets ... 1369

Phenytoin (Increased anticonvulsant dosage may be necessary). Products include:
- Dilantin Infatabs ... 1710
- Dilantin-30 Pediatric/Dilantin-125 Suspension ... 1713

Phenytoin Sodium (Increased anticonvulsant dosage may be necessary). Products include:
- Dilantin Kapseals ... 1708
- Dilantin Parenteral ... 1712
- Dilantin with Phenobarbital Kapseals ... 1715

Pimozide (Hyperpyrexia). Products include:
- Orap Tablets ... 1020

Pirbuterol Acetate (Close supervision and careful dosage adjustment required). Products include:
- Maxair Inhaler ... 1311

Prazepam (Potentiated). Products include:
- Centrax ... 1693

Prazosin Hydrochloride (Antihypertensive effect of prazosin blocked). Products include:
- Minipress Capsules ... 1778
- Minizide Capsules ... 1779

Primidone (Increased anticonvulsant dosage may be necessary). Products include:
- Mysoline ... 2480

Prochlorperazine (Potentiated; hyperpyrexia). Products include:
- Compazine ... 2201

Procyclidine Hydrochloride (Hyperpyrexia; paralytic ileus). Products include:
- Kemadrin Tablets ... 771

Promethazine Hydrochloride (Potentiated; hyperpyrexia). Products include:
- Mepergan Injection ... 2479
- Phenergan with Codeine ... 2497
- Phenergan with Dextromethorphan 2499
- Phenergan Injection ... 2493
- Phenergan Suppositories ... 2496
- Phenergan Syrup ... 2495
- Phenergan Tablets ... 2496
- Phenergan VC ... 2500
- Phenergan VC with Codeine ... 2501

Propantheline Bromide (Hyperpyrexia; paralytic ileus). Products include:
- Pro-Banthīne Tablets ... 2141

(▣ Described in PDR For Nonprescription Drugs)

(⊙ Described in PDR For Ophthalmology)

Propofol (Potentiated). Products include:
- Diprivan Injection 2267

Propoxyphene Hydrochloride (Potentiated). Products include:
- Darvon 1256
- Wygesic Tablets 2540

Propoxyphene Napsylate (Potentiated). Products include:
- Darvon-N/Darvocet-N 1254

Pseudoephedrine Hydrochloride (Close supervision and careful dosage adjustment required). Products include:
- Actifed Capsules ◼ 539
- Actifed Plus Caplets ◼ 539
- Actifed Plus Tablets ◼ 540
- Actifed with Codeine Cough Syrup 752
- Actifed Syrup ◼ 540
- Actifed Tablets ◼ 540
- Actifed 12-Hour Capsules ◼ 539
- Advil Cold & Sinus Caplets (formerly CoAdvil) 2416
- Allerest ◼ 559
- Anatuss LA Tablets 1359
- Benadryl Decongestant Elixir ◼ 635
- Benadryl Decongestant ◼ 635
- Benadryl Plus ◼ 636
- Benadryl Plus Nighttime ◼ 637
- Benylin Decongestant ◼ 638
- Brexin L.A. Capsules 2078
- Bromfed Capsules (Timed Release) 1615
- Bromfed Syrup ◼ 628
- Bromfed 1615
- CoAdvil ◼ 748
- Allergy-Sinus Comtrex Multi-Symptom Allergy Sinus Formula Tablets & Caplets 746
- Cough Formula Comtrex 746
- Comtrex Multi-Symptom Cold Reliever Tablets/Caplets/Liqui-Gels/Liquid 745
- Day-Night Comtrex 747
- Non-Drowsy Comtrex 747
- Congess 994
- Congestac Caplets ◼ 617
- Contac Jr. Children's Cold Medicine ◼ 712
- Contac Nighttime Cold Medicine ◼ 713
- Contac Sinus Caplets Maximum Strength Non-Drowsy Formula ◼ 710
- Contac Sinus Tablets Maximum Strength Non-Drowsy Formula ◼ 710
- Deconamine 663
- Deconsal II Tablets 559
- Dimacol Caplets ◼ 672
- Dimetane-DX Cough Syrup 1858
- Dorcol Children's Cough Syrup ◼ 685
- Dorcol Children's Decongestant Liquid ◼ 685
- Dorcol Children's Liquid Cold Formula ◼ 686
- Maximum Strength Dristan Decongestant/Analgesic Coated Caplets ◼ 750
- No Drowsiness Dristan Cold Nasal Decongestant/Analgesic Coated Caplets 2420
- Dristan Sinus Caplets 2419
- Sinus Excedrin Analgesic, Decongestant Tablets & Caplets ◼ 533
- Fedahist Gyrocaps 2145
- Fedahist Timecaps 2145
- Guaifed 1615
- Guaifed Syrup ◼ 629
- Isoclor Expectorant 982
- Isoclor Timesule Capsules ◼ 561
- Kronofed-A 970
- Medi-Flu Caplet, Liquid ◼ 640
- Novafed A Capsules 1342
- Novafed Capsules 1342
- Novahistine DH 1342
- Novahistine DMX ◼ 595
- Novahistine Expectorant 1343
- Nucofed Capsules 2219
- Nucofed Expectorant 2219
- Nucofed Pediatric Expectorant 2220
- Nucofed Syrup 2219
- Ornex Caplets ◼ 618
- PediaCare Allergy Relief Formula Liquid 1362
- PediaCare Cough-Cold Formula Liquid 1362
- PediaCare Infants' Oral Decongestant Drops 1362
- PediaCare Night Rest Cough-Cold Formula Liquid 1362
- PediaCare 6-12 Cough-Cold Formula Chewable Tablets 1362
- Robitussin-DAC Syrup 1875
- Robitussin-PE ◼ 677
- Rondec 1975
- Rondec-DM 1976
- Rondec-TR Tablet 1975
- Ru-Tuss DE Tablets 694
- Ryna ◼ 741
- Seldane-D Extended-Release Tablets 1350
- Sinarest ◼ 562
- Sine-Aid Maximum Strength Sinus Headache Caplets 1365
- Sine-Aid Maximum Strength Sinus Headache Tablets 1365
- Sine-Off Maximum Strength Allergy/Sinus Formula Caplets ◼ 721
- Sine-Off Maximum Strength No Drowsiness Formula Caplets ◼ 722
- Singlet Tablets ◼ 598
- Sinutab Maximum Strength ◼ 641
- Sinutab Maximum Strength Without Drowsiness Tablets & Caplets ◼ 642
- Sinutab Regular Strength Without Drowsiness Formula ◼ 641
- St. Joseph Nighttime Cold Medicine ◼ 705
- Sudafed Children's Liquid ◼ 543
- Sudafed Cough Syrup ◼ 543
- Sudafed Plus Liquid ◼ 544
- Sudafed Plus Tablets ◼ 545
- Sudafed Sinus Caplets ◼ 545
- Sudafed Sinus Tablets ◼ 545
- Sudafed Tablets, 30 mg ◼ 544
- Sudafed Tablets, Adult Strength, 60 mg ◼ 544
- Sudafed 12 Hour Capsules ◼ 545
- TheraFlu Flu and Cold Medicine ◼ 687
- Triaminic Nite Light ◼ 689
- Tylenol Allergy Sinus Medication Caplets and Gelcaps, Maximum Strength 1372
- Children's Tylenol Cold Liquid Formula and Chewable Tablets 1368
- Tylenol Cold & Flu Hot Medication, Packets 1369
- Tylenol Cold & Flu No Drowsiness Hot Medication, Packets 1371
- Tylenol Cold Medication Caplets and Tablets 1370
- Tylenol Cold Medication No Drowsiness Formula Caplets 1370
- Tylenol Cold Night Time Medication Liquid 1371
- Tylenol Cough Medication Liquid with Decongestant, Maximum Strength 1372
- Tylenol, Maximum Strength, Sinus Medication Gelcaps, Caplets and Tablets 1373
- Ursinus Inlay-Tabs ◼ 691
- Vicks Children's NyQuil ◼ 664
- Vicks Daycare ◼ 660
- Vicks Formula 44D Decongestant Cough Medicine ◼ 662
- Vicks Formula 44M Multi-Symptom Cough Medicine ◼ 662
- Vicks NyQuil Nighttime Colds Medicine-Original & Cherry Flavor ◼ 664
- Vicks Pediatric Formula 44 Cough & Congestion Medicine ◼ 663
- Vicks Pediatric Formula 44m Multi-Symptom Cough & Cold Medicine ◼ 663

Pseudoephedrine Sulfate (Close supervision and careful dosage adjustment required). Products include:
- Afrin Tablets ◼ 693
- Chlor-Trimeton Decongestant ◼ 694
- Disophrol Chronotab Sustained-Action Tablets ◼ 698
- Drixoral Antihistamine/Nasal Decongestant Syrup ◼ 698
- Drixoral Non-Drowsy Formula ◼ 699
- Drixoral Plus Extended-Release Tablets ◼ 699
- Drixoral Sinus ◼ 700
- Drixoral Sustained-Action Tablets ◼ 698
- Sinutab Allergy Formula Sustained Action Tablets ◼ 640
- Trinalin Repetabs Tablets 1170

Pyrilamine Maleate (Potentiated). Products include:
- Codimal 846
- 4-Way Fast Acting Nasal Spray - Original Formula (regular & mentholated) & Metered Spray Pump (regular) 751
- Maximum Strength Midol Multi-Symptom Menstrual Formula ◼ 571
- Maximum Strength Midol PMS Premenstrual Syndrome Formula ◼ 570
- Regular Strength Midol Multi-Symptom Menstrual Formula ◼ 570
- Prefrin-A ◉ 255
- Prēmsyn PMS Capsules & Caplets ◼ 547
- Primatene Tablets-M Formula 2421
- Robitussin Night Relief ◼ 677
- Ru-Tuss with Hydrocodone 694
- Triaminic Expectorant DH 1995
- Triaminic Oral Infant Drops 1996

Pyrilamine Tannate (Potentiated). Products include:
- Rynatan 2387

Quazepam (Potentiated). Products include:
- Doral Tablets 2383

Rauwolfia Serpentina (Antihypertensive effect of rauwolfia serpentina blocked). Products include:
- Raudixin Tablets 1803
- Rauzide Tablets 1804

Rescinnamine (Antihypertensive effect of rescinnamine blocked).
- No products indexed under this heading.

Reserpine (Antihypertensive effect of reserpine blocked). Products include:
- Diupres Tablets 1461
- Hydromox R Tablets 1209
- Hydropres Tablets 1485
- Renese-R Tablets 1786
- Salutensin/Salutensin-Demi 719
- Ser-Ap-Es Tablets 881
- Serpasil Tablets 883
- Serpasil-Apresoline Tablets 884
- Serpasil-Esidrix Tablets 886

Scopolamine Hydrobromide (Hyperpyrexia; paralytic ileus). Products include:
- Donnagel ◼ 675
- Donnagel-PG 1858
- Donnatal 1858
- Donnatal Extentabs 1859
- Donnatal Tablets 1858
- Donnazyme Tablets 1860
- Isopto Hyoscine ◉ 222
- Murocoll-2 Sterile Ophthalmic Solution ◉ 261
- Ru-Tuss Tablets 693

Scopolamine Preparations (Hyperpyrexia; paralytic ileus). Products include:
- Transderm Scōp Transdermal Therapeutic System 887

Secobarbital Sodium (Potentiated). Products include:
- Seconal Sodium Pulvules 1296

Selegiline Hydrochloride (Concomitant administration is contraindicated; hyperpyretic crises and severe convulsions have occurred). Products include:
- Eldepryl 2250

Sufentanil Citrate (Potentiated). Products include:
- Sufenta Injection 1147

Temazepam (Potentiated). Products include:
- Restoril Capsules 2023

Terazosin Hydrochloride (Antihypertensive effect of terazosin blocked). Products include:
- Hytrin Tablets 529

Terbutaline Sulfate (Close supervision and careful dosage adjustment required). Products include:
- Brethaire Inhaler 1024
- Brethine Ampuls 1026
- Brethine Tablets 1026
- Bricanyl Injection 1324
- Bricanyl Tablets 1325

Terfenadine (Potentiated). Products include:
- Seldane Tablets 1349
- Seldane-D Extended-Release Tablets 1350

Thiamylal Sodium (Potentiated). Products include:
- Surital Ampoules, Steri-Vials 1764

Thioridazine Hydrochloride (Potentiated; hyperpyrexia). Products include:
- Mellaril 2011

Thiothixene (Potentiated; hyperpyrexia). Products include:
- Navane Capsules and Concentrate 1954
- Navane Intramuscular 1956

Thyroid (Close supervision is indicated). Products include:
- S-P-T "Liquid" Capsules 995

Thyroxine (Close supervision is indicated).
- No products indexed under this heading.

Thyroxine Sodium (Close supervision is indicated).
- No products indexed under this heading.

Tranylcypromine Sulfate (Concomitant administration is contraindicated; hyperpyretic crises and severe convulsions have occurred). Products include:
- Parnate Tablets 2222

Triazolam (Potentiated). Products include:
- Halcion Tablets 2340

Tridihexethyl Chloride (Hyperpyrexia; paralytic ileus).
- No products indexed under this heading.

Trifluoperazine Hydrochloride (Potentiated; hyperpyrexia). Products include:
- Stelazine 2226

Trihexyphenidyl Hydrochloride (Hyperpyrexia; paralytic ileus). Products include:
- Artane 1195

Trimeprazine Tartrate (Potentiated). Products include:
- Temaril Tablets, Syrup and Spansule Sustained Release Capsules 1085

Trimethadione (Increased anticonvulsant dosage may be necessary). Products include:
- Tridione 557

Tripelennamine Hydrochloride (Potentiated). Products include:
- PBZ Tablets & Elixir 1037
- PBZ-SR Tablets 1037

Triprolidine Hydrochloride (Potentiated). Products include:
- Actidil ◼ 538
- Actifed Capsules ◼ 539
- Actifed Plus Caplets ◼ 539
- Actifed Plus Tablets ◼ 540
- Actifed with Codeine Cough Syrup 752
- Actifed Syrup ◼ 540
- Actifed Tablets ◼ 540
- Actifed 12-Hour Capsules ◼ 539

Valproic Acid (Increased anticonvulsant dosage may be necessary). Products include:
- Depakene Capsules & Syrup 511

TRIDESILON CREME 0.05%
(Desonide) 1611
No interactions described in labeling.

TRIDESILON OINTMENT 0.05%
(Desonide) 1611
No interactions described in labeling.

TRIDIL AMPULS & VIALS
(Nitroglycerin) 939
May interact with vasodilators and

(◼ Described in PDR For Nonprescription Drugs) (◉ Described in PDR For Ophthalmology)

certain other agents. Compounds in these categories include:

Diazoxide (Additive vasodilating effects). Products include:
- Hyperstat I.V. Injection 2095
- Proglycem 649

Heparin Calcium (Concurrent administration requires higher doses of heparin; close monitoring of the PTI is required when therapy with nitroglycerin is terminated). Products include:
- Calciparine Injection 925

Heparin Sodium (Concurrent administration requires higher doses of heparin; close monitoring of the PTI is required when therapy with nitroglycerin is terminated). Products include:
- Heparin Lock Flush Solution 2456
- Heparin Sodium Vials 1264
- Heparin Sodium Injection 2457
- Heparin Sodium Injection, USP, Sterile Solution 2342

Hydralazine Hydrochloride (Additive vasodilating effects). Products include:
- Apresazide Capsules 854
- Apresoline Hydrochloride Parenteral (Ampuls) 856
- Apresoline Hydrochloride Tablets 855
- Apresoline-Esidrix Tablets 857
- Ser-Ap-Es Tablets 881
- Serpasil-Apresoline Tablets 884

Minoxidil (Additive vasodilating effects). Products include:
- Loniten Tablets 2346
- Rogaine Topical Solution 2357

TRIDIONE CAPSULES
(Trimethadione) 557

Concurrent therapy with drugs known to cause toxic effects similar to those of the oxazolidinediones should be avoided or used with extreme caution .

TRIDIONE DULCET TABLETS
(Trimethadione) 557
No interactions described in labeling.

TRIDIONE SOLUTION
(Trimethadione) 557
No interactions described in labeling.

TRI-IMMUNOL DIPHTHERIA & TETANUS TOXOIDS & PERTUSSIS VACCINE, ADSORBED
(Diphtheria & Tetanus Toxoids w/Pertussis Vaccine Combined, Aluminum Phosphate Adsorbed) 1241
May interact with corticosteroids, antineoplastics, and cytotoxic drugs. Compounds in these categories include:

Altretamine (Aberrant responses to active immunization procedures). Products include:
- Hexalen Capsules 2316

Asparaginase (Aberrant responses to active immunization procedures). Products include:
- Elspar 1470

Betamethasone Acetate (Aberrant responses to active immunization procedures). Products include:
- Celestone Soluspan Suspension 2081

Betamethasone Sodium Phosphate (Aberrant responses to active immunization procedures). Products include:
- Celestone Soluspan Suspension 2081

Bleomycin Sulfate (Aberrant responses to active immunization procedures). Products include:
- Blenoxane 724

Busulfan (Aberrant responses to active immunization procedures). Products include:
- Myleran Tablets 790

Carboplatin (Aberrant responses to active immunization procedures). Products include:
- Paraplatin for Injection 735

Carmustine (BCNU) (Aberrant responses to active immunization procedures). Products include:
- BiCNU 723

Chlorambucil (Aberrant responses to active immunization procedures). Products include:
- Leukeran Tablets 788

Cisplatin (Aberrant responses to active immunization procedures). Products include:
- Platinol 737
- Platinol-AQ Injection 738

Cortisone Acetate (Aberrant responses to active immunization procedures). Products include:
- Cortone Acetate Sterile Suspension 1437
- Cortone Acetate Tablets 1439

Cyclophosphamide (Aberrant responses to active immunization procedures). Products include:
- Cytoxan for Injection 726
- Neosar for Injection 566

Dacarbazine (Aberrant responses to active immunization procedures). Products include:
- DTIC-Dome 1595

Daunorubicin Hydrochloride (Aberrant responses to active immunization procedures). Products include:
- Cerubidine 2443

Dexamethasone (Aberrant responses to active immunization procedures). Products include:
- AK-Trol Ointment & Suspension ⊙ 207
- Decadron Elixir 1445
- Decadron Tablets 1447
- Decaspray Topical Aerosol 1459
- Dexacidin ⊙ 272
- Maxidex Sterile Ophthalmic Suspension ⊙ 223
- Maxitrol Ophthalmic Ointment/Suspension ⊙ 223
- TobraDex Ophthalmic Suspension and Ointment ⊙ 228

Dexamethasone Acetate (Aberrant responses to active immunization procedures). Products include:
- Dalalone D.P. Injectable 999
- Decadron-LA Sterile Suspension 1457

Dexamethasone Sodium Phosphate (Aberrant responses to active immunization procedures). Products include:
- AK-Dex ⊙ 203
- Decadron Phosphate Respihaler 1454
- Decadron Phosphate Sterile Ophthalmic Ointment 1453
- Decadron Phosphate Sterile Ophthalmic Solution 1453
- Decadron Phosphate Topical Cream 1455
- Decadron Phosphate Turbinaire 1456
- Maxidex Sterile Ophthalmic Ointment ⊙ 222
- NeoDecadron Sterile Ophthalmic Ointment 1517
- NeoDecadron Sterile Ophthalmic Solution 1518
- NeoDecadron Topical Cream 1518

Doxorubicin Hydrochloride (Aberrant responses to active immunization procedures). Products include:
- Adriamycin PFS 561
- Adriamycin RDF 562
- Doxorubicin Hydrochloride for Injection, USP 622
- Doxorubicin Hydrochloride Injection, USP 848
- Rubex 739

Estramustine Phosphate Sodium (Aberrant responses to active immunization procedures). Products include:
- Emcyt Capsules 1161

Etoposide (Aberrant responses to active immunization procedures). Products include:
- VePesid Capsules and Injection 741

Floxuridine (Aberrant responses to active immunization procedures). Products include:
- Sterile FUDR 1898

Fluorouracil (Aberrant responses to active immunization procedures). Products include:
- Efudex 1880
- Fluoroplex Topical Solution & Cream 1% 1082
- Fluorouracil Injection 1897

Flutamide (Abberrant responses to active immunization procedures). Products include:
- Eulexin Capsules 2089

Hydrocortisone (Aberrant responses to active immunization procedures). Products include:
- AK-Spore H.C. ⊙ 206
- Bactine Hydrocortisone Anti-Itch Cream [ND] 625
- CaldeCORT Anti-Itch Hydrocortisone Spray [ND] 560
- Carmol HC Cream 1% 2296
- Cortaid Spray [ND] 735
- Cortenema 2244
- Cortisporin Ointment 758
- Cortisporin Ophthalmic Ointment Sterile 758
- Cortisporin Ophthalmic Suspension Sterile 759
- Cortisporin Otic Solution Sterile 760
- Cortisporin Otic Suspension Sterile 760
- Cortizone-5 Creme & Ointment [ND] 732
- Dermolate Anti-Itch Cream [ND] 697
- Eldecort Cream 1.0% 1113
- Eldecort Cream 1.0% and 2.5% 1113
- Fungoid HC Creme 1770
- Hydrocortone Tablets 1482
- Hytone 909
- LazerSporin-C Solution 1770
- Massengill Medicated Soft Cloth Towelettes 2192
- Nutracort Cream & Lotion 1684
- PediOtic Suspension Sterile 797
- Synacort Creams 1%, 2.5% 2296
- Vanoxide-HC Acne Lotion 911
- Vioform-Hydrocortisone Cream and Mild Cream 889
- Vioform-Hydrocortisone Ointment 889
- VōSoL HC Otic Solution 2392
- Vytone Cream 1% 911

Hydrocortisone Acetate (Aberrant responses to active immunization procedures). Products include:
- Analpram-HC Rectal Cream 1% and 2.5% 970
- Anusol-HC Cream 1690
- Anusol-HC Suppositories 1691
- Caldecort [ND] 560
- Carmol HC Cream 1% 2296
- Chloromycetin Hydrocortisone Ophthalmic 1694
- Coly-Mycin S Otic w/Neomycin & Hydrocortisone 1708
- Cortaid [ND] 735
- Cortef Feminine Itch Cream [ND] 735
- Corticaine [ND] 682
- Cortifoam 1827
- Cortisporin Cream 757
- Epifoam 1828
- Gynecort 5 Creme [ND] 556
- Hydrocortone Acetate Sterile Suspension 1479
- Lanacort 5 Creme and Ointment [ND] 557
- Mantadil Cream 789
- Ophthocort ⊙ 301
- Orabase HCA Oral Paste 890
- Pramosone Cream, Lotion & Ointment 971
- ProctoCream-HC 1834
- Proctofoam-HC 1835

Hydrocortisone Sodium Phosphate (Aberrant responses to active immunization procedures). Products include:
- Hydrocortone Phosphate Injection, Sterile 1481

Hydrocortisone Sodium Succinate (Aberrant responses to active immunization procedures). Products include:
- Solu-Cortef Sterile Powder 2361

Hydroxyurea (Aberrant responses to active immunization procedures). Products include:
- Hydrea Capsules 728

Ifosfamide (Aberrant responses to active immunization procedures). Products include:
- IFEX 729

Interferon alfa-2A, Recombinant (Aberrant responses to active immunization procedures). Products include:
- Roferon-A Injection 1916

Interferon alfa-2B, Recombinant (Aberrant responses to active immunization procedures). Products include:
- Intron A 2097

Levamisole Hydrochloride (Aberrant responses to active immunization procedures). Products include:
- Ergamisol Tablets 1136

Lomustine (CCNU) (Aberrant responses to active immunization procedures). Products include:
- CeeNU 725

Mechlorethamine Hydrochloride (Aberrant responses to active immunization procedures). Products include:
- Mustargen 1514

Megestrol Acetate (Aberrant responses to active immunization procedures). Products include:
- Megace Tablets 732

Melphalan (Aberrant responses to active immunization procedures). Products include:
- Alkeran Tablets 754

Mercaptopurine (Aberrant responses to active immunization procedures). Products include:
- Purinethol Tablets 800

Methotrexate Sodium (Aberrant responses to active immunization procedures). Products include:
- Methotrexate Tablets, Parenteral, LPF Parenteral 1217
- Rheumatrex Methotrexate Dose Pack 1234

Methylprednisolone Acetate (Aberrant responses to active immunization procedures). Products include:
- Depo-Medrol Sterile Aqueous Suspension 2334

Methylprednisolone Sodium Succinate (Aberrant responses to active immunization procedures). Products include:
- Solu-Medrol Sterile Powder 2363

Mitomycin (Mitomycin-C) (Aberrant responses to active immunization procedures). Products include:
- Mutamycin 733

Mitotane (Aberrant responses to active immunization procedures). Products include:
- Lysodren 731

Mitoxantrone Hydrochloride (Aberrant responses to active immunization procedures). Products include:
- Novantrone for Injection Concentrate 1226

Prednisolone Acetate (Aberrant responses to active immunization procedures). Products include:
- AK-Cide Sterile Ophthalmic Ointment & Suspension ⊛ 202
- Blephamide Liquifilm Sterile Ophthalmic Suspension 586
- Blephamide S.O.P. Sterile Ophthalmic Ointment 586
- Cetapred Ointment ⊛ 220
- ⅛% Econopred & 1% Econopred Plus ⊛ 217
- Isopto Cetapred Suspension ⊛ 220
- Metimyd ⊛ 306
- Poly-Pred Liquifilm ⊛ 250
- Pred Forte ⊛ 252
- Pred Mild ⊛ 254
- Pred-G Liquifilm Sterile Ophthalmic Suspension ⊛ 252
- Pred-G S.O.P. Sterile Ophthalmic Ointment ⊛ 253
- Vasocidin Ointment ⊛ 275

Prednisolone Sodium Phosphate (Aberrant responses to active immunization procedures). Products include:
- AK-Pred ⊛ 205
- Hydeltrasol Injection, Sterile 1476
- Inflamase ⊛ 274
- Pediapred Oral Liquid 987
- Vasocidin Ophthalmic Solution ⊛ 276

Prednisolone Tebutate (Aberrant responses to active immunization procedures). Products include:
- Hydeltra-T.B.A. Sterile Suspension 1478

Prednisone (Aberrant responses to active immunization procedures). Products include:
- Deltasone Tablets 2332

Procarbazine Hydrochloride (Aberrant responses to active immunization procedures). Products include:
- Matulane Capsules 1907

Streptozocin (Aberrant responses to active immunization procedures). Products include:
- Zanosar Sterile Powder 2371

Tamoxifen Citrate (Aberrant responses to active immunization procedures). Products include:
- Nolvadex Tablets 1102

Thioguanine (Aberrant responses to active immunization procedures). Products include:
- Thioguanine Tablets, Tabloid Brand 815

Thiotepa (Aberrant responses to active immunization procedures). Products include:
- Thiotepa Parenteral 1240

Triamcinolone (Aberrant responses to active immunization procedures).
- No products indexed under this heading.

Triamcinolone Acetonide (Aberrant responses to active immunization procedures). Products include:
- Aristocort A 1010
- Azmacort Inhaler 1837
- Kenalog Cream, Lotion & Ointment 2401
- Kenalog-10 Injection 2402
- Kenalog-40 Injection 2403
- Kenalog in Orabase 604
- Kenalog Spray 2401
- Mycolog II Cream and Ointment 2407
- Mytrex Cream & Ointment 2080
- Nasacort Nasal Inhaler 1844

Triamcinolone Diacetate (Aberrant responses to active immunization procedures). Products include:
- Aristocort Suspension 1008

Triamcinolone Hexacetonide (Aberrant responses to active immunization procedures). Products include:
- Aristospan Suspension 1011

Vincristine Sulfate (Aberrant responses to active immunization procedures). Products include:
- Oncovin Solution Vials & Hyporets 1288

TRILAFON CONCENTRATE
(Perphenazine) 2123

May interact with central nervous system depressants, anticonvulsants, and certain other agents. Compounds in these categories include:

Alcohol (Additive effects; hypotension).

Alfentanil Hydrochloride (Potentiation of both drugs). Products include:
- Alfenta Injection 1131

Alprazolam (Potentiation of both drugs). Products include:
- Xanax Tablets 2367

Aprobarbital (Potentiation of both drugs). Products include:
- Alurate Elixir 1883

Atropine Sulfate (Additive anticholinergic effects). Products include:
- Arco-Lase Plus Tablets 607
- Atropine Sulfate Sterile Ophthalmic Solution and S.O.P. Sterile Ophthalmic Ointment ⊛ 239
- Donnagel ▣ 675
- Donnagel-PG 1858
- Donnatal 1858
- Donnatal Extentabs 1859
- Donnatal Tablets 1858
- Donnazyme Tablets 1860
- Isopto Atropine ⊛ 218
- Lomotil 2174
- Motofen Tablets 836
- Ru-Tuss Tablets 693
- Urised Tablets 2396

Buprenorphine (Potentiation of both drugs).
- No products indexed under this heading.

Buspirone Hydrochloride (Potentiation of both drugs). Products include:
- BuSpar 1401

Butabarbital (Potentiation of both drugs). Products include:
- Pyridium Plus 1764

Butalbital (Potentiation of both drugs). Products include:
- Esgic-Plus Tablets 1002
- Esgic Tablets & Capsules 1001
- Fioricet Tablets 2006
- Fiorinal Capsules 2007
- Fiorinal with Codeine Capsules 2008
- Fiorinal Tablets 2007
- Phrenilin 838
- Sedapap Tablets 50 mg/650 mg 1360

Carbamazepine (Increased dosage of anticonvulsant may be required). Products include:
- Tegretol Chewable Tablets 654
- Tegretol Suspension 656
- Tegretol Tablets 654

Chlordiazepoxide (Potentiation of both drugs). Products include:
- Libritabs Tablets 1930
- Limbitrol 1933
- Menrium Tablets 1934

Chlordiazepoxide Hydrochloride (Potentiation of both drugs). Products include:
- Librax Capsules 1929
- Librium Capsules 1931
- Librium Injectable 1932

Chlorpromazine (Potentiation of both drugs). Products include:
- Thorazine 2234

Chlorprothixene (Potentiation of both drugs). Products include:
- Taractan Tablets 1920

Chlorprothixene Hydrochloride (Potentiation of both drugs). Products include:
- Taractan 1920

Clorazepate Dipotassium (Potentiation of both drugs). Products include:
- Tranxene 556

Codeine (Potentiation of both drugs). Products include:
- Calcidrine Syrup 506

Codeine Phosphate (Potentiation of both drugs). Products include:
- Actifed with Codeine Cough Syrup 752
- Cheracol Cough Syrup 1853
- Codimal PH Syrup 846
- Dimetane-DC Cough Syrup 1857
- Empirin with Codeine Phosphate Nos. 2, 3 & 4 764
- Fiorinal with Codeine Capsules 2008
- Isoclor Expectorant 982
- Naldecon CX Adult Liquid ▣ 521
- Novahistine DH 1342
- Novahistine Expectorant 1343
- Nucofed Capsules 2219
- Nucofed Expectorant 2219
- Nucofed Pediatric Expectorant 2220
- Nucofed Syrup 2219
- Phenaphen with Codeine Capsules 1865
- Phenaphen-650 with Codeine Tablets 1866
- Phenergan with Codeine 2497
- Phenergan VC with Codeine 2501
- Robitussin A-C Syrup 1875
- Robitussin-DAC Syrup 1875
- Ryna ▣ 741
- Soma Compound w/Codeine Tablets 2390
- Triaminic Expectorant w/Codeine 1996
- Tussi-Organidin Liquid 2391
- Tylenol with Codeine 1381

Codeine Polistirex (Potentiation of both drugs).
- No products indexed under this heading.

Dezocine (Potentiation of both drugs).

Diazepam (Potentiation of both drugs). Products include:
- Valium Injectable 1937
- Valium Tablets 1939
- Valrelease Capsules 1923

Divalproex Sodium (Increased dosage of anticonvulsant may be required). Products include:
- Depakote 512

Droperidol (Potentiation of both drugs). Products include:
- Inapsine Injection 1140
- Innovar Injection 1141

Enflurane (Potentiation of both drugs). Products include:
- Ethrane 599

Epinephrine (Action of epinephrine blocked and partially reversed). Products include:
- Ana-Kit Anaphylaxis Emergency Treatment Kit 1100
- Bronkaid Mist ▣ 757
- EpiPen 843
- Marcaine Hydrochloride 0.5% with Epinephrine 1:200,000 (as bitartrate) 958
- Marcaine Hydrochloride with Epinephrine 1:200,000 2055
- Primatene Mist 2420
- Sus-Phrine Injection 1006
- Xylocaine with Epinephrine Injections 637

Epinephrine Bitartrate (Action of epinephrine blocked and partially reversed). Products include:
- AsthmaHaler Mist Epinephrine Bitartrate Bronchodilator ▣ 616
- Bronkaid Mist Suspension ▣ 757
- Primatene Mist Suspension 2421

Estazolam (Potentiation of both drugs). Products include:
- ProSom Tablets 554

Ethchlorvynol (Potentiation of both drugs). Products include:
- Placidyl Capsules 553

Ethinamate (Potentiation of both drugs).
- No products indexed under this heading.

Ethosuximide (Increased dosage of anticonvulsant may be required). Products include:
- Zarontin Capsules 1768
- Zarontin Syrup 1769

Ethotoin (Increased dosage of anticonvulsant may be required). Products include:
- Peganone Tablets 551

Fentanyl (Potentiation of both drugs). Products include:
- Duragesic Transdermal System 1133

Fentanyl Citrate (Potentiation of both drugs). Products include:
- Innovar Injection 1141
- Sublimaze Injection 1146

Fluphenazine Decanoate (Potentiation of both drugs). Products include:
- Prolixin Decanoate 1795

Fluphenazine Enanthate (Potentiation of both drugs). Products include:
- Prolixin Enanthate 1796

Fluphenazine Hydrochloride (Potentiation of both drugs). Products include:
- Prolixin Elixir 1793
- Prolixin Injection 1791
- Prolixin Oral Concentrate 1792
- Prolixin Tablets 1793

Flurazepam Hydrochloride (Potentiation of both drugs). Products include:
- Dalmane Capsules 1927

Glutethimide (Potentiation of both drugs).
- No products indexed under this heading.

Haloperidol (Potentiation of both drugs). Products include:
- Haldol Injection, Tablets and Concentrate 1373

Haloperidol Decanoate (Potentiation of both drugs). Products include:
- Haldol Decanoate 1375

Hydrocodone Bitartrate (Potentiation of both drugs). Products include:
- Anexsia 5/500 Tablets 2196
- Anexsia 7.5/650 Tablets 2197
- Azdone Tablets 844
- Codiclear DH Syrup 845
- Codimal DH Syrup 846
- Damason-P 1356
- Hycodan Syrup, Tablets 927
- Hycomine Compound Tablets 929
- Hycomine Syrup 927
- Hycotuss Expectorant Syrup 930
- Hydrocet Capsules 835
- Lortab ASA Tablets 2414
- Lortab 2412
- Ru-Tuss with Hydrocodone 694
- Triaminic Expectorant DH 1995
- Vicodin Tablets 1187
- Vicodin ES Tablets 1189
- Zydone Capsules 941

Hydrocodone Polistirex (Potentiation of both drugs). Products include:
- Tussionex Extended-Release Suspension 988

Hydroxyzine Hydrochloride (Potentiation of both drugs). Products include:
- Atarax Tablets & Syrup 1941
- Marax Tablets & DF Syrup 1954
- Vistaril Intramuscular Solution 1970

Isoflurane (Potentiation of both drugs). Products include:
- Forane 600

Ketamine Hydrochloride (Potentiation of both drugs). Products include:
- Ketalar 1726

Levorphanol Tartrate (Potentiation of both drugs). Products include:
- Levo-Dromoran 1906

Lorazepam (Potentiation of both drugs). Products include:
Ativan Injection 2432
Ativan Tablets 2434
Loxapine Hydrochloride (Potentiation of both drugs). Products include:
Loxitane 1213
Loxapine Succinate (Potentiation of both drugs). Products include:
Loxitane Capsules 1213
Meperidine Hydrochloride (Potentiation of both drugs). Products include:
Demerol 2047
Mepergan Injection 2479
Mephenytoin (Increased dosage of anticonvulsant may be required). Products include:
Mesantoin Tablets 2013
Mephobarbital (Potentiation of both drugs). Products include:
Mebaral Tablets 2061
Meprobamate (Potentiation of both drugs). Products include:
Deprol Tablets 2382
Equagesic Tablets 2451
Miltown Tablets 2386
PMB 200 and PMB 400 2504
Mesoridazine (Potentiation of both drugs). Products include:
Serentil 686
Methadone Hydrochloride (Potentiation of both drugs). Products include:
Dolophine Hydrochloride Ampoules & Vials 1260
Dolophine Hydrochloride Tablets 1261
Methadone Hydrochloride Diskets 1284
Methadone Hydrochloride Oral Solution & Tablets 1987
Methohexital Sodium (Potentiation of both drugs). Products include:
Brevital Sodium Vials 1248
Methoxyflurane (Potentiation of both drugs).
No products indexed under this heading.
Methsuximide (Increased dosage of anticonvulsant may be required). Products include:
Celontin 1692
Midazolam Hydrochloride (Potentiation of both drugs). Products include:
Versed Injection 1924
Molindone Hydrochloride (Potentiation of both drugs). Products include:
Moban Tablets & Concentrate 932
Morphine Sulfate (Potentiation of both drugs). Products include:
Astramorph/PF Injection, USP (Preservative-Free) 618
Duramorph 960
Infumorph 200 and Infumorph 500 Sterile Solutions 962
MS Contin Tablets 1814
MSIR 1817
Oramorph SR (Morphine Sulfate Sustained Release Tablets) 1988
Roxanol 1991
Opium Alkaloids (Potentiation of both drugs). Products include:
B & O No. 15A & No. 16A Supprettes 2395
Pantopon Injectable 1911
Oxazepam (Potentiation of both drugs). Products include:
Serax Capsules 2522
Serax Tablets 2522
Oxycodone Hydrochloride (Potentiation of both drugs). Products include:
Percocet Tablets 950
Percodan 951
Roxicodone Tablets, Oral Solution & Intensol (Oxycodone) 1992
Tylox Capsules 1382
Paramethadione (Increased dosage of anticonvulsant may be required). Products include:
Paradione Capsules 548
Pentobarbital Sodium (Potentiation of both drugs). Products include:
Nembutal Sodium Capsules 534
Nembutal Sodium Solution 536
Nembutal Sodium Suppositories 538
Phenacemide (Increased dosage of anticonvulsant may be required). Products include:
Phenurone Tablets 552
Phenobarbital (Increased dosage of anticonvulsant may be required; potentiation of both drugs). Products include:
Arco-Lase Plus Tablets 607
Bellergal-S Tablets 1998
Bronkolixir ▣ 761
Bronkotabs Tablets ▣ 762
Donnatal 1858
Donnatal Extentabs 1859
Donnatal Tablets 1858
Donnazyme Tablets 1860
Kinesed Tablets 2272
Phenobarbital Elixir and Tablets 1293
Primatene Tablets-P Formula 2421
Quadrinal Tablets 1183
Tedral SA 1765
Phensuximide (Increased dosage of anticonvulsant may be required). Products include:
Milontin Kapseals 1741
Phenytoin (Increased dosage of anticonvulsant may be required). Products include:
Dilantin Infatabs 1710
Dilantin-30 Pediatric/Dilantin-125 Suspension 1713
Phenytoin Sodium (Increased dosage of anticonvulsant may be required). Products include:
Dilantin Kapseals 1708
Dilantin Parenteral 1712
Dilantin with Phenobarbital Kapseals 1715
Prazepam (Potentiation of both drugs). Products include:
Centrax 1693
Primidone (Increased dosage of anticonvulsant may be required). Products include:
Mysoline 2480
Prochlorperazine (Potentiation of both drugs). Products include:
Compazine 2201
Promethazine Hydrochloride (Potentiation of both drugs). Products include:
Mepergan Injection 2479
Phenergan with Codeine 2497
Phenergan with Dextromethorphan 2499
Phenergan Injection 2493
Phenergan Suppositories 2496
Phenergan Syrup 2495
Phenergan Tablets 2496
Phenergan VC 2500
Phenergan VC with Codeine 2501
Propofol (Potentiation of both drugs). Products include:
Diprivan Injection 2267
Propoxyphene Hydrochloride (Potentiation of both drugs). Products include:
Darvon 1256
Wygesic Tablets 2540
Propoxyphene Napsylate (Potentiation of both drugs). Products include:
Darvon-N/Darvocet-N 1254
Quazepam (Potentiation of both drugs). Products include:
Doral Tablets 2383
Secobarbital Sodium (Potentiation of both drugs). Products include:
Seconal Sodium Pulvules 1296
Sufentanil Citrate (Potentiation of both drugs). Products include:
Sufenta Injection 1147
Temazepam (Potentiation of both drugs). Products include:
Restoril Capsules 2023
Thiamylal Sodium (Potentiation of both drugs). Products include:
Surital Ampoules, Steri-Vials 1764
Thioridazine Hydrochloride (Potentiation of both drugs). Products include:
Mellaril 2011
Thiothixene (Potentiation of both drugs). Products include:
Navane Capsules and Concentrate 1954
Navane Intramuscular 1956
Triazolam (Potentiation of both drugs). Products include:
Halcion Tablets 2340
Trifluoperazine Hydrochloride (Potentiation of both drugs). Products include:
Stelazine 2226
Trimethadione (Increased dosage of anticonvulsant may be required). Products include:
Tridione 557
Valproic Acid (Increased dosage of anticonvulsant may be required). Products include:
Depakene Capsules & Syrup 511

TRILAFON INJECTION
(Perphenazine) 2123
See **Trilafon Concentrate**

TRILAFON TABLETS
(Perphenazine) 2123
See **Trilafon Concentrate**

TRI-LEVLEN 21 TABLETS
(Levonorgestrel, Ethinyl Estradiol) 665
See **Levlen 21 Tablets**

TRI-LEVLEN 28 TABLETS
(Levonorgestrel, Ethinyl Estradiol) 665
See **Levlen 21 Tablets**

TRILISATE LIQUID
(Choline Magnesium Trisalicylate) 1822
May interact with corticosteroids, oral anticoagulants, oral hypoglycemic agents, insulin, carbonic anhydrase inhibitors, and certain other agents. Compounds in these categories include:

Acetazolamide (Competition for protein binding sites). Products include:
Diamox Parenteral 1200
Diamox Parenteral ⊙ 308
Diamox Sequels (Sustained Release) 1201
Diamox Sequels (Sustained Release) ⊙ 310
Diamox Tablets 1200
Diamox Tablets ⊙ 308
Alcohol (Increased risk of gastrointestinal ulceration).
Allopurinol (Decreased efficacy of uricosuric agents). Products include:
Zyloprim Tablets 830
Betamethasone Acetate (Reduces plasma salicylate levels by increasing renal elimination). Products include:
Celestone Soluspan Suspension 2081
Betamethasone Sodium Phosphate (Reduces plasma salicylate levels by increasing renal elimination). Products include:
Celestone Soluspan Suspension 2081
Chlorpropamide (Enhanced hypoglycemic effect). Products include:
Diabinese Tablets 1775
Cortisone Acetate (Reduces plasma salicylate levels by increasing renal elimination). Products include:
Cortone Acetate Sterile Suspension 1437
Cortone Acetate Tablets 1439
Dexamethasone (Reduces plasma salicylate levels by increasing renal elimination). Products include:
AK-Trol Ointment & Suspension ⊙ 207
Decadron Elixir 1445
Decadron Tablets 1447
Decaspray Topical Aerosol 1459
Dexacidin ⊙ 272
Maxidex Sterile Ophthalmic Suspension ⊙ 223
Maxitrol Ophthalmic Ointment/Suspension ⊙ 223
TobraDex Ophthalmic Suspension and Ointment ⊙ 228
Dexamethasone Acetate (Reduces plasma salicylate levels by increasing renal elimination). Products include:
Dalalone D.P. Injectable 999
Decadron-LA Sterile Suspension 1457
Dexamethasone Sodium Phosphate (Reduces plasma salicylate levels by increasing renal elimination). Products include:
AK-Dex ⊙ 203
Decadron Phosphate Respihaler 1454
Decadron Phosphate Sterile Ophthalmic Ointment 1453
Decadron Phosphate Sterile Ophthalmic Solution 1453
Decadron Phosphate Topical Cream 1455
Decadron Phosphate Turbinaire 1456
Maxidex Sterile Ophthalmic Ointment ⊙ 222
NeoDecadron Sterile Ophthalmic Ointment 1517
NeoDecadron Sterile Ophthalmic Solution 1518
NeoDecadron Topical Cream 1518
Dichlorphenamide (Competition for protein binding sites). Products include:
Daranide Tablets 1445
Dicumarol (Potential exists for increased levels of unbound anticoagulant with the concurrent use). Products include:
Dicumarol Tablets 516
Divalproex Sodium (Competition for protein binding sites). Products include:
Depakote 512
Glipizide (Enhanced hypoglycemic effect). Products include:
Glucotrol 1952
Glyburide (Enhanced hypoglycemic effect). Products include:
DiaBeta 1091
Micronase Tablets 2350
Heparin Calcium (Use cautiously). Products include:
Calciparine Injection 925
Heparin Sodium (Use cautiously). Products include:
Heparin Lock Flush Solution 2456
Heparin Sodium Vials 1264
Heparin Sodium Injection 2457
Heparin Sodium Injection, USP, Sterile Solution 2342
Hydrocortisone (Reduces plasma salicylate levels by increasing renal elimination). Products include:
AK-Spore H.C. ⊙ 206
Bactine Hydrocortisone Anti-Itch Cream ▣ 625
CaldeCORT Anti-Itch Hydrocortisone Spray ▣ 560
Carmol HC Cream 1% 2296
Cortaid Spray ▣ 735
Cortenema 2244
Cortisporin Ointment 758
Cortisporin Ophthalmic Ointment Sterile 758
Cortisporin Ophthalmic Suspension Sterile 759
Cortisporin Otic Solution Sterile 760

(▣ Described in PDR For Nonprescription Drugs)

(⊙ Described in PDR For Ophthalmology)

Cortisporin Otic Suspension Sterile ... 760
Cortizone-5 Creme & Ointment ... ⊞ 732
Dermolate Anti-Itch Cream ... ⊞ 697
Eldecort Cream 1.0% ... 1113
Eldecort Cream 1.0% and 2.5% ... 1113
Fungoid HC Creme ... 1770
Hydrocortone Tablets ... 1482
Hytone ... 909
LazerSporin-C Solution ... 1770
Massengill Medicated Soft Cloth Towelettes ... 2192
Nutracort Cream & Lotion ... 1684
PediOtic Suspension Sterile ... 797
Synacort Creams 1%, 2.5% ... 2296
Vanoxide-HC Acne Lotion ... 911
Vioform-Hydrocortisone Cream and Mild Cream ... 889
Vioform-Hydrocortisone Ointment .. 889
VōSoL HC Otic Solution ... 2392
Vytone Cream 1% ... 911

Hydrocortisone Acetate (Reduces plasma salicylate levels by increasing renal elimination). Products include:

Analpram-HC Rectal Cream 1% and 2.5% ... 970
Anusol-HC Cream ... 1690
Anusol-HC Suppositories ... 1691
Caldecort ... ⊞ 560
Carmol HC Cream 1% ... 2296
Chloromycetin Hydrocortisone Ophthalmic ... 1694
Coly-Mycin S Otic w/Neomycin & Hydrocortisone ... 1708
Cortaid ... ⊞ 735
Cortef Feminine Itch Cream ... ⊞ 735
Corticaine ... ⊞ 682
Cortifoam ... 1827
Cortisporin Cream ... 757
Epifoam ... 1828
Gynecort 5 Creme ... ⊞ 556
Hydrocortone Acetate Sterile Suspension ... 1479
Lanacort 5 Creme and Ointment .. ⊞ 557
Mantadil Cream ... 789
Ophthocort ... ⊙ 301
Orabase HCA Oral Paste ... 890
Pramosone Cream, Lotion & Ointment ... 971
ProctoCream-HC ... 1834
Proctofoam-HC ... 1835

Hydrocortisone Sodium Phosphate (Reduces plasma salicylate levels by increasing renal elimination). Products include:

Hydrocortone Phosphate Injection, Sterile ... 1481

Hydrocortisone Sodium Succinate (Reduces plasma salicylate levels by increasing renal elimination). Products include:

Solu-Cortef Sterile Powder ... 2361

Insulin, Human (Insulin-treated diabetics on high doses of salicylates should be monitored for enhanced hypoglycemic response).

No products indexed under this heading.

Insulin, Human Isophane Suspension (Insulin-treated diabetics on high doses of salicylates should be monitored for enhanced hypoglycemic response). Products include:

Humulin N, 100 Units ... 1270

Insulin, Human NPH (Insulin-treated diabetics on high doses of salicylates should be monitored for enhanced hypoglycemic response). Products include:

Insulatard NPH Human ... 1627
Novolin N ... 1627
Novolin N PenFill Cartridges ... 1628
Novolin N Prefilled ... 1628

Insulin, Human Regular (Insulin-treated diabetics on high doses of salicylates should be monitored for enhanced hypoglycemic response). Products include:

Humulin BR, 100 Units ... 1268
Humulin R, 100 Units ... 1272
Novolin R ... 1627
Novolin R PenFill Cartridges ... 1628
Novolin R Prefilled ... 1629
Velosulin Human ... 1628

Insulin, Human, Zinc Suspension (Insulin-treated diabetics on high doses of salicylates should be monitored for enhanced hypoglycemic response). Products include:

Humulin L, 100 Units ... 1268
Humulin U, 100 Units ... 1272
Novolin L ... 1627

Insulin, NPH (Insulin-treated diabetics on high doses of salicylates should be monitored for enhanced hypoglycemic response). Products include:

NPH, 40 & 100 Units ... 1273
Beef NPH, 100 Units ... 1274
Pork NPH, 100 Units ... 1275
Insulatard NPH ... 1626
NPH Insulin ... 1626
NPH Purified Pork Isophane Insulin ... 1626

Insulin, Regular (Insulin-treated diabetics on high doses of salicylates should be monitored for enhanced hypoglycemic response). Products include:

Regular, 40 & 100 Units ... 1273
Beef Regular, 100 Units ... 1275
Pork Regular, 100 Units ... 1275
Pork Regular (Concentrated), 500 Units ... 1276
Regular Insulin ... 1625
Regular Purified Pork Insulin ... 1626
Velosulin ... 1627

Insulin, Zinc Crystals (Insulin-treated diabetics on high doses of salicylates should be monitored for enhanced hypoglycemic response). Products include:

NPH, 40 & 100 Units ... 1273

Insulin, Zinc Suspension (Insulin-treated diabetics on high doses of salicylates should be monitored for enhanced hypoglycemic response). Products include:

Lente, 40 & 100 Units ... 1272
Protamine, Zinc, 40 & 100 Units 1273
Lente Iletin I ... 1272
Beef Lente, 100 Units ... 1274
Beef Protamine Zinc, 100 Units ... 1274
Pork Lente, 100 Units ... 1275
Pork, Protamine, Zinc, 100 Units 1275
Lente Insulin ... 1626
Lente Purified Pork Insulin ... 1626
Semilente Insulin ... 1625
Ultralente Insulin ... 1626

Methazolamide (Competition for protein binding sites). Products include:

Neptazane Tablets ... ⊙ 311

Methotrexate Sodium (Increased methotrexate effects). Products include:

Methotrexate Tablets, Parenteral, LPF Parenteral ... 1217
Rheumatrex Methotrexate Dose Pack ... 1234

Methylprednisolone (Increased risk of gastrointestinal ulceration). Products include:

Medrol ... 2348

Methylprednisolone Acetate (Reduces plasma salicylate levels by increasing renal elimination). Products include:

Depo-Medrol Sterile Aqueous Suspension ... 2334

Methylprednisolone Sodium Succinate (Reduces plasma salicylate levels by increasing renal elimination). Products include:

Solu-Medrol Sterile Powder ... 2363

Phenylbutazone (Increased risk of gastrointestinal ulceration). Products include:

Butazolidin Capsules & Tablets ... 1027

Phenytoin (Competition for protein binding sites). Products include:

Dilantin Infatabs ... 1710
Dilantin-30 Pediatric/Dilantin-125 Suspension ... 1713

Phenytoin Sodium (Competition for protein binding sites). Products include:

Dilantin Kapseals ... 1708
Dilantin Parenteral ... 1712
Dilantin with Phenobarbital Kapseals ... 1715

Prednisolone Acetate (Reduces plasma salicylate levels by increasing renal elimination). Products include:

AK-Cide Sterile Ophthalmic Ointment & Suspension ... ⊙ 202
Blephamide Liquifilm Sterile Ophthalmic Suspension ... 586
Blephamide S.O.P. Sterile Ophthalmic Ointment ... 586
Cetapred Ointment ... ⊙ 220
⅛% Econopred & 1% Econopred Plus ... ⊙ 217
Isopto Cetapred Suspension ... ⊙ 220
Metimyd ... ⊙ 306
Poly-Pred Liquifilm ... ⊙ 250
Pred Forte ... ⊙ 252
Pred Mild ... ⊙ 254
Pred-G Liquifilm Sterile Ophthalmic Suspension ... ⊙ 252
Pred-G S.O.P. Sterile Ophthalmic Ointment ... ⊙ 253
Vasocidin Ointment ... ⊙ 275

Prednisolone Sodium Phosphate (Reduces plasma salicylate levels by increasing renal elimination). Products include:

AK-Pred ... ⊙ 205
Hydeltrasol Injection, Sterile ... 1476
Inflamase ... ⊙ 274
Pediapred Oral Liquid ... 987
Vasocidin Ophthalmic Solution ... ⊙ 276

Prednisolone Tebutate (Reduces plasma salicylate levels by increasing renal elimination). Products include:

Hydeltra-T.B.A. Sterile Suspension 1478

Prednisone (Reduces plasma salicylate levels by increasing renal elimination). Products include:

Deltasone Tablets ... 2332

Probenecid (Decreased efficacy of uricosuric agents). Products include:

Benemid Tablets ... 1426
ColBENEMID Tablets ... 1436
Wycillin Injection and Probenecid Tablets ... 2539

Sulfinpyrazone (Decreased efficacy of uricosuric agents). Products include:

Anturane ... 853

Tolazamide (Enhanced hypoglycemic effect). Products include:

Tolinase Tablets ... 2365

Tolbutamide (Enhanced hypoglycemic effect). Products include:

Orinase Tablets ... 2354

Triamcinolone (Reduces plasma salicylate levels by increasing renal elimination).

No products indexed under this heading.

Triamcinolone Acetonide (Reduces plasma salicylate levels by increasing renal elimination). Products include:

Aristocort A ... 1010
Azmacort Inhaler ... 1837
Kenalog Cream, Lotion & Ointment 2401
Kenalog-10 Injection ... 2402
Kenalog-40 Injection ... 2403
Kenalog in Orabase ... 604
Kenalog Spray ... 2401
Mycolog II Cream and Ointment ... 2407
Mytrex Cream & Ointment ... 2080
Nasacort Nasal Inhaler ... 1844

Triamcinolone Diacetate (Reduces plasma salicylate levels by increasing renal elimination). Products include:

Aristocort Suspension ... 1008

Triamcinolone Hexacetonide (Reduces plasma salicylate levels by increasing renal elimination). Products include:

Aristospan Suspension ... 1011

Valproic Acid (Competition for protein binding sites). Products include:

Depakene Capsules & Syrup ... 511

Warfarin Sodium (Potential exists for increased levels of unbound anticoagulant with the concurrent use). Products include:

Coumadin Injection & Tablets ... 944
Panwarfin Tablets ... 547

Food Interactions

Food that lowers urinary pH (Decreases urinary salicylate excretion & increases plasma levels).

Food that raises urinary pH (Enhance renal salicylate clearance & diminishes plasma salicylate concentration).

TRILISATE TABLETS

(Choline Magnesium Trisalicylate) 1822

See **Trilisate Liquid**

TRIMPEX TABLETS

(Trimethoprim) ... 1922

May interact with:

Phenytoin (Possible excessive phenytoin effect). Products include:

Dilantin Infatabs ... 1710
Dilantin-30 Pediatric/Dilantin-125 Suspension ... 1713

Phenytoin Sodium (Possible excessive phenytoin effect). Products include:

Dilantin Kapseals ... 1708
Dilantin Parenteral ... 1712
Dilantin with Phenobarbital Kapseals ... 1715

TRINALIN REPETABS TABLETS

(Azatadine Maleate, Pseudoephedrine Sulfate) ... 1170

May interact with monoamine oxidase inhibitors, tricyclic antidepressants, barbiturates, central nervous system depressants, veratrum alkaloids, antacids, oral anticoagulants, beta blockers, and certain other agents. Compounds in these categories include:

Acebutolol Hydrochloride (Effect not specified). Products include:

Sectral Capsules ... 2520

Alcohol (Additive effect).

Alfentanil Hydrochloride (Additive effect). Products include:

Alfenta Injection ... 1131

Alprazolam (Additive effect). Products include:

Xanax Tablets ... 2367

Aluminum Carbonate Gel (Increased rate of absorption of pseudoephedrine). Products include:

Basaljel ... 2438

Aluminum Hydroxide (Increased rate of absorption of pseudoephedrine). Products include:

Cama Arthritis Pain Reliever ... ⊞ 685
Gaviscon Extra Strength Relief Formula Liquid Antacid ... ⊞ 594
Gaviscon Extra Strength Relief Formula Antacid Tablets ... ⊞ 594
Gaviscon Liquid Antacid ... ⊞ 594
Gelusil Liquid & Tablets ... ⊞ 639
Extra Strength Maalox Plus Suspension ... 1850
Maalox TC Suspension ... 1851
Maalox Plus Tablets ... ⊞ 655
Extra Strength Maalox Plus Tablets 1850
Nephrox Suspension ... ⊞ 563
WinGel Liquid & Tablets ... ⊞ 761

Aluminum Hydroxide Gel (Increased rate of absorption of pseudoephedrine). Products include:

ALternaGEL Liquid ... 1154
Aludrox Oral Suspension ... 2428
Amphojel Suspension ... 2429
Amphojel Suspension without Flavor ... 2429

(⊞ Described in PDR For Nonprescription Drugs)

(⊙ Described in PDR For Ophthalmology)

Mylanta Liquid ... 1155
Mylanta Double Strength Liquid ... 1155

Aluminum Hydroxide Gel, Dried (Increased rate of absorption of pseudoephedrine). Products include:
Alu-Tab/Alu-Cap ... 1309
Amphojel Tablets ... 2429
Ascriptin A/D Caplets ... 1850
Regular Strength Ascriptin Tablets 1850
Gaviscon Antacid Tablets ... ■ 593
Gaviscon-2 Antacid Tablets ... ■ 594
Mylanta Tablets ... 1155
Mylanta Double Strength Tablets ... 1155

Amitriptyline Hydrochloride (Additive effect). Products include:
Elavil ... 2269
Endep Tablets ... 1927
Etrafon ... 2087
Limbitrol ... 1933
Triavil Tablets ... 1556

Amoxapine (Additive effect). Products include:
Asendin Tablets ... 1196

Aprobarbital (Additive effect). Products include:
Alurate Elixir ... 1883

Atenolol (Effect not specified). Products include:
Tenoretic Tablets ... 1105
Tenormin Tablets and I.V. Injection 1107

Betaxolol Hydrochloride (Effect not specified). Products include:
Betoptic Sterile Ophthalmic Solution ... 569
Betoptic S Sterile Ophthalmic Suspension ... 570
Kerlone Tablets ... 2172

Buprenorphine (Additive effect).
No products indexed under this heading.

Buspirone Hydrochloride (Additive effect). Products include:
BuSpar ... 1401

Butabarbital (Additive effect). Products include:
Pyridium Plus ... 1764

Butalbital (Additive effect). Products include:
Esgic-Plus Tablets ... 1002
Esgic Tablets & Capsules ... 1001
Fioricet Tablets ... 2006
Fiorinal Capsules ... 2007
Fiorinal with Codeine Capsules ... 2008
Fiorinal Tablets ... 2007
Phrenilin ... 838
Sedapap Tablets 50 mg/650 mg .. 1360

Carteolol Hydrochloride (Effect not specified). Products include:
Cartrol Tablets ... 507

Chlordiazepoxide (Additive effect). Products include:
Libritabs Tablets ... 1930
Limbitrol ... 1933
Menrium Tablets ... 1934

Chlordiazepoxide Hydrochloride (Additive effect). Products include:
Librax Capsules ... 1929
Librium Capsules ... 1931
Librium Injectable ... 1932

Chlorpromazine (Additive effect). Products include:
Thorazine ... 2234

Chlorprothixene (Additive effect). Products include:
Taractan Tablets ... 1920

Chlorprothixene Hydrochloride (Additive effect). Products include:
Taractan ... 1920

Clomipramine Hydrochloride (Additive effect). Products include:
Anafranil Capsules ... 650

Clorazepate Dipotassium (Additive effect). Products include:
Tranxene ... 556

Codeine (Additive effect). Products include:
Calcidrine Syrup ... 506

Codeine Phosphate (Additive effect). Products include:
Actifed with Codeine Cough Syrup.. 752
Cheracol Cough Syrup ... 1853
Codimal PH Syrup ... 846
Dimetane-DC Cough Syrup ... 1857
Empirin with Codeine Phosphate Nos. 2, 3 & 4 ... 764
Fiorinal with Codeine Capsules ... 2008
Isoclor Expectorant ... 982
Naldecon CX Adult Liquid ... ■ 521
Novahistine DH ... 1342
Novahistine Expectorant ... 1343
Nucofed Capsules ... 2219
Nucofed Expectorant ... 2219
Nucofed Pediatric Expectorant ... 2220
Nucofed Syrup ... 2219
Phenaphen with Codeine Capsules 1865
Phenaphen-650 with Codeine Tablets ... 1866
Phenergan with Codeine ... 2497
Phenergan VC with Codeine ... 2501
Robitussin A-C Syrup ... 1875
Robitussin-DAC Syrup ... 1875
Ryna ... ■ 741
Soma Compound w/Codeine Tablets ... 2390
Triaminic Expectorant w/Codeine .. 1996
Tussi-Organidin Liquid ... 2391
Tylenol with Codeine ... 1381

Codeine Polistirex (Additive effect).
No products indexed under this heading.

Cryptenamine Preparations (Antihypertensive effects of veratrum alkaloids reduced).

Desipramine Hydrochloride (Additive effect). Products include:
Norpramin Tablets ... 1340

Deslanoside (Increased ectopic pacemaker activity).
No products indexed under this heading.

Dezocine (Additive effect).

Diazepam (Additive effect). Products include:
Valium Injectable ... 1937
Valium Tablets ... 1939
Valrelease Capsules ... 1923

Dicumarol (Action of oral anticoagulants inhibited). Products include:
Dicumarol Tablets ... 516

Digitoxin (Increased ectopic pacemaker activity). Products include:
Crystodigin Tablets ... 1253

Digoxin (Increased ectopic pacemaker activity). Products include:
Lanoxicaps ... 772
Lanoxin Elixir Pediatric ... 775
Lanoxin Injection ... 778
Lanoxin Injection Pediatric ... 781
Lanoxin Tablets ... 783

Dihydroxyaluminum Sodium Carbonate (Increased rate of absorption of pseudoephedrine). Products include:
Rolaids ... ■ 743

Doxepin Hydrochloride (Additive effect). Products include:
Sinequan ... 1960

Droperidol (Additive effect). Products include:
Inapsine Injection ... 1140
Innovar Injection ... 1141

Enflurane (Additive effect). Products include:
Ethrane ... 599

Esmolol Hydrochloride (Effect not specified). Products include:
Brevibloc Injection ... 942

Estazolam (Additive effect). Products include:
ProSom Tablets ... 554

Ethchlorvynol (Additive effect). Products include:
Placidyl Capsules ... 553

Ethinamate (Additive effect).
No products indexed under this heading.

Fentanyl (Additive effect). Products include:
Duragesic Transdermal System ... 1133

Fentanyl Citrate (Additive effect). Products include:
Innovar Injection ... 1141
Sublimaze Injection ... 1146

Fluphenazine Decanoate (Additive effect). Products include:
Prolixin Decanoate ... 1795

Fluphenazine Enanthate (Additive effect). Products include:
Prolixin Enanthate ... 1796

Fluphenazine Hydrochloride (Additive effect). Products include:
Prolixin Elixir ... 1793
Prolixin Injection ... 1791
Prolixin Oral Concentrate ... 1792
Prolixin Tablets ... 1793

Flurazepam Hydrochloride (Additive effect). Products include:
Dalmane Capsules ... 1927

Furazolidone (Hypertensive crisis; effects of antihistamines prolonged and intensified; concurrent use is contraindicated). Products include:
Furoxone ... 1855

Glutethimide (Additive effect).
No products indexed under this heading.

Haloperidol (Additive effect). Products include:
Haldol Injection, Tablets and Concentrate ... 1373

Haloperidol Decanoate (Additive effect). Products include:
Haldol Decanoate ... 1375

Hydrocodone Bitartrate (Additive effect). Products include:
Anexsia 5/500 Tablets ... 2196
Anexsia 7.5/650 Tablets ... 2197
Azdone Tablets ... 844
Codiclear DH Syrup ... 845
Codimal DH Syrup ... 846
Damason-P ... 1356
Hycodan Syrup, Tablets ... 927
Hycomine Compound Tablets ... 929
Hycomine Syrup ... 927
Hycotuss Expectorant Syrup ... 930
Hydrocet Capsules ... 835
Lortab ASA Tablets ... 2414
Lortab ... 2412
Ru-Tuss with Hydrocodone ... 694
Triaminic Expectorant DH ... 1995
Vicodin Tablets ... 1187
Vicodin ES Tablets ... 1189
Zydone Capsules ... 941

Hydrocodone Polistirex (Additive effect). Products include:
Tussionex Extended-Release Suspension ... 988

Hydroxyzine Hydrochloride (Additive effect). Products include:
Atarax Tablets & Syrup ... 1941
Marax Tablets & DF Syrup ... 1954
Vistaril Intramuscular Solution ... 1970

Imipramine Hydrochloride (Additive effect). Products include:
Tofranil Ampuls ... 1038
Tofranil Tablets ... 1039

Imipramine Pamoate (Additive effect). Products include:
Tofranil-PM Capsules ... 1041

Isocarboxazid (Hypertensive crisis; effects of antihistamines prolonged and intensified; concurrent use is contraindicated). Products include:
Marplan Tablets ... 1906

Isoflurane (Additive effect). Products include:
Forane ... 600

Kaolin (Decreased rate of absorption of pseudoephedrine). Products include:
Donnagel ... ■ 675
Donnagel-PG ... 1858

Ketamine Hydrochloride (Additive effect). Products include:
Ketalar ... 1726

Labetalol Hydrochloride (Effect not specified). Products include:
Normodyne Injection ... 2108
Normodyne Tablets ... 2110
Normozide Tablets ... 2112
Trandate HCT Tablets ... 579
Trandate Injection ... 577
Trandate Tablets ... 579

Levorphanol Tartrate (Additive effect). Products include:
Levo-Dromoran ... 1906

Lorazepam (Additive effect). Products include:
Ativan Injection ... 2432
Ativan Tablets ... 2434

Loxapine Hydrochloride (Additive effect). Products include:
Loxitane ... 1213

Loxapine Succinate (Additive effect). Products include:
Loxitane Capsules ... 1213

Magaldrate (Increased rate of absorption of pseudoephedrine). Products include:
Riopan Antacid Chew Tablets ... ■ 754
Riopan Antacid Chew Tablets in Rollpacks ... ■ 754
Riopan Antacid Suspension ... 2421
Riopan Antacid Swallow Tablets ... 2421
Riopan Plus Chew Tablets ... 2422
Riopan Plus Chew Tablets in Rollpack ... 2422
Riopan Plus 2 Chew Tablets, Mint Flavor, Cherry Flavor ... 2422
Riopan Plus Suspension ... 2422
Riopan Plus 2 Suspension, Mint Flavor, Cherry Flavor ... 2422

Magnesium Hydroxide (Increased rate of absorption of pseudoephedrine). Products include:
Aludrox Oral Suspension ... 2428
Ascriptin A/D Caplets ... 1850
Regular Strength Ascriptin Tablets 1850
Di-Gel Antacid/Anti-Gas ... ■ 697
Gelusil Liquid & Tablets ... ■ 639
Haley's M-O, Regular & Flavored .. ■ 569
Extra Strength Maalox Plus Suspension ... 1850
Maalox TC Suspension ... 1851
Maalox Plus Tablets ... ■ 655
Extra Strength Maalox Plus Tablets 1850
Mylanta Liquid ... 1155
Mylanta Tablets ... 1155
Mylanta Double Strength Liquid ... 1155
Mylanta Double Strength Tablets ... 1155
Concentrated Phillips' Milk of Magnesia ... ■ 573
Phillips' Milk of Magnesia Liquid ... ■ 572
Phillips' Milk of Magnesia Tablets ■ 573
WinGel Liquid & Tablets ... ■ 761

Magnesium Oxide (Increased rate of absorption of pseudoephedrine). Products include:
Bayer Plus Aspirin Tablets ... ■ 567
Beelith Tablets ... 659
Bufferin Analgesic Tablets and Caplets ... ■ 524
Cama Arthritis Pain Reliever ... ■ 685
Mag-Ox 400 ... 673
Uro-Mag ... 673

Maprotiline Hydrochloride (Additive effect). Products include:
Ludiomil Tablets ... 874

Mecamylamine Hydrochloride (Antihypertensive effects of mecamylamine reduced). Products include:
Inversine Tablets ... 1492

Meperidine Hydrochloride (Additive effect). Products include:
Demerol ... 2047
Mepergan Injection ... 2479

Mephobarbital (Additive effect). Products include:
Mebaral Tablets ... 2061

Meprobamate (Additive effect). Products include:
Deprol Tablets ... 2382
Equagesic Tablets ... 2451
Miltown Tablets ... 2386
PMB 200 and PMB 400 ... 2504

(■ Described in PDR For Nonprescription Drugs)

(⊙ Described in PDR For Ophthalmology)

Mesoridazine (Additive effect). Products include:
- Serentil 686

Methadone Hydrochloride (Additive effect). Products include:
- Dolophine Hydrochloride Ampoules & Vials 1260
- Dolophine Hydrochloride Tablets 1261
- Methadone Hydrochloride Diskets 1284
- Methadone Hydrochloride Oral Solution & Tablets 1987

Methohexital Sodium (Additive effect). Products include:
- Brevital Sodium Vials 1248

Methoxyflurane (Additive effect).
- No products indexed under this heading.

Methyldopa (Antihypertensive effects of methyldopa reduced). Products include:
- Aldoclor Tablets 1413
- Aldomet Oral 1415
- Aldoril Tablets 1418

Methyldopate Hydrochloride (Antihypertensive effects of methyldopa reduced). Products include:
- Aldomet Ester HCl Injection 1417

Metoprolol Tartrate (Not specified). Products include:
- Lopressor Ampuls 1032
- Lopressor HCT Tablets 1034
- Lopressor Tablets 1032

Midazolam Hydrochloride (Additive effect). Products include:
- Versed Injection 1924

Molindone Hydrochloride (Additive effect). Products include:
- Moban Tablets & Concentrate 932

Morphine Sulfate (Additive effect). Products include:
- Astramorph/PF Injection, USP (Preservative-Free) 618
- Duramorph 960
- Infumorph 200 and Infumorph 500 Sterile Solutions 962
- MS Contin Tablets 1814
- MSIR 1817
- Oramorph SR (Morphine Sulfate Sustained Release Tablets) 1988
- Roxanol 1991

Nadolol (Effect not specified). Products include:
- Corgard Tablets 701
- Corzide Tablets 702

Nortriptyline Hydrochloride (Additive effect). Products include:
- Pamelor 2019

Opium Alkaloids (Additive effect). Products include:
- B & O No. 15A & No. 16A Supprettes 2395
- Pantopon Injectable 1911

Oxazepam (Additive effect). Products include:
- Serax Capsules 2522
- Serax Tablets 2522

Oxycodone Hydrochloride (Additive effect). Products include:
- Percocet Tablets 950
- Percodan 951
- Roxicodone Tablets, Oral Solution & Intensol (Oxycodone) 1992
- Tylox Capsules 1382

Penbutolol Sulfate (Effect not specified). Products include:
- Levatol 1832

Pentobarbital Sodium (Additive effect). Products include:
- Nembutal Sodium Capsules 534
- Nembutal Sodium Solution 536
- Nembutal Sodium Suppositories 538

Perphenazine (Additive effect). Products include:
- Etrafon 2087
- Triavil Tablets 1556
- Trilafon 2123

Phenelzine Sulfate (Hypertensive crisis; effects of antihistamines prolonged and intensified; concurrent use is contraindicated). Products include:
- Nardil 1742

Phenobarbital (Additive effect). Products include:
- Arco-Lase Plus Tablets 607
- Bellergal-S Tablets 1998
- Bronkolixir .... ■ 761
- Bronkotabs Tablets .... ■ 762
- Donnatal 1858
- Donnatal Extentabs 1859
- Donnatal Tablets 1858
- Donnazyme Tablets 1860
- Kinesed Tablets 2272
- Phenobarbital Elixir and Tablets 1293
- Primatene Tablets-P Formula 2421
- Quadrinal Tablets 1183
- Tedral SA 1765

Pindolol (Effect not specified). Products include:
- Visken Tablets 2036

Prazepam (Additive effect). Products include:
- Centrax 1693

Prochlorperazine (Additive effect). Products include:
- Compazine 2201

Promethazine Hydrochloride (Additive effect). Products include:
- Mepergan Injection 2479
- Phenergan with Codeine 2497
- Phenergan with Dextromethorphan 2499
- Phenergan Injection 2493
- Phenergan Suppositories 2496
- Phenergan Syrup 2495
- Phenergan Tablets 2496
- Phenergan VC 2500
- Phenergan VC with Codeine 2501

Propofol (Additive effect). Products include:
- Diprivan Injection 2267

Propoxyphene Hydrochloride (Additive effect). Products include:
- Darvon 1256
- Wygesic Tablets 2540

Propoxyphene Napsylate (Additive effect). Products include:
- Darvon-N/Darvocet-N 1254

Propranolol Hydrochloride (Effect not specified). Products include:
- Inderal 2459
- Inderal LA Long Acting Capsules 2461
- Inderide Tablets 2463
- Inderide LA Long Acting Capsules 2465

Protriptyline Hydrochloride (Additive effect). Products include:
- Vivactil Tablets 1567

Quazepam (Additive effect). Products include:
- Doral Tablets 2383

Reserpine (Antihypertensive effects of reserpine reduced). Products include:
- Diupres Tablets 1461
- Hydromox R Tablets 1209
- Hydropres Tablets 1485
- Renese-R Tablets 1786
- Salutensin/Salutensin-Demi 719
- Ser-Ap-Es Tablets 881
- Serpasil Tablets 883
- Serpasil-Apresoline Tablets 884
- Serpasil-Esidrix Tablets 886

Secobarbital Sodium (Additive effect). Products include:
- Seconal Sodium Pulvules 1296

Selegiline Hydrochloride (Hypertensive crisis; effects of antihistamines prolonged and intensified; concurrent use is contraindicated). Products include:
- Eldepryl 2250

Sufentanil Citrate (Additive effect). Products include:
- Sufenta Injection 1147

Temazepam (Additive effect). Products include:
- Restoril Capsules 2023

Thiamylal Sodium (Additive effect). Products include:
- Surital Ampoules, Steri-Vials 1764

Thioridazine Hydrochloride (Additive effect). Products include:
- Mellaril 2011

Thiothixene (Additive effect). Products include:
- Navane Capsules and Concentrate 1954
- Navane Intramuscular 1956

Timolol Maleate (Effect not specified). Products include:
- Blocadren Tablets 1429
- Timolide Tablets 1547
- Timoptic in Ocudose 1552
- Timoptic Sterile Ophthalmic Solution 1550

Tranylcypromine Sulfate (Hypertensive crisis; effects of antihistamines prolonged and intensified; concurrent use is contraindicated). Products include:
- Parnate Tablets 2222

Triazolam (Additive effect). Products include:
- Halcion Tablets 2340

Trifluoperazine Hydrochloride (Additive effect). Products include:
- Stelazine 2226

Trimipramine Maleate (Additive effect). Products include:
- Surmontil Capsules 2524

Warfarin Sodium (Action of oral anticoagulants inhibited). Products include:
- Coumadin Injection & Tablets 944
- Panwarfin Tablets 547

TRI-NORINYL 21-DAY TABLETS
(Norethindrone, Ethinyl Estradiol) 2304
See **Brevicon 21-Day Tablets**

TRI-NORINYL 28-DAY TABLETS
(Norethindrone, Ethinyl Estradiol) 2304
See **Brevicon 21-Day Tablets**

TRINSICON CAPSULES
(Vitamins with Iron) 2415
No interactions described in labeling.

TRIPHASIL-21 TABLETS
(Levonorgestrel, Ethinyl Estradiol) 2527
May interact with barbiturates and certain other agents. Compounds in these categories include:

Ampicillin Sodium (Reduced efficacy; increased incidence of breakthrough bleeding). Products include:
- Unasyn 1965

Aprobarbital (Reduced efficacy; increased incidence of breakthrough bleeding). Products include:
- Alurate Elixir 1883

Butabarbital (Reduced efficacy; increased incidence of breakthrough bleeding). Products include:
- Pyridium Plus 1764

Butalbital (Reduced efficacy; increased incidence of breakthrough bleeding). Products include:
- Esgic-Plus Tablets 1002
- Esgic Tablets & Capsules 1001
- Fioricet Tablets 2006
- Fiorinal Capsules 2007
- Fiorinal with Codeine Capsules 2008
- Fiorinal Tablets 2007
- Phrenilin 838
- Sedapap Tablets 50 mg/650 mg 1360

Mephobarbital (Reduced efficacy; increased incidence of breakthrough bleeding). Products include:
- Mebaral Tablets 2061

Oxytetracycline (Reduced efficacy; increased incidence of breakthrough bleeding). Products include:
- Terramycin Intramuscular Solution 1964
- Urobiotic-250 Capsules 1968

Oxytetracycline Hydrochloride (Reduced efficacy; increased incidence of breakthrough bleeding). Products include:
- Terra-Cortril Ophthalmic Suspension 1963
- Terramycin Capsules 1786
- Terramycin Intramuscular Solution 1964
- Terramycin with Polymyxin B Sulfate Ophthalmic Ointment 1965

Pentobarbital Sodium (Reduced efficacy; increased incidence of breakthroughbleeding). Products include:
- Nembutal Sodium Capsules 534
- Nembutal Sodium Solution 536
- Nembutal Sodium Suppositories 538

Phenobarbital (Reduced efficacy; increased incidence of breakthrough bleeding). Products include:
- Arco-Lase Plus Tablets 607
- Bellergal-S Tablets 1998
- Bronkolixir .... ■ 761
- Bronkotabs Tablets .... ■ 762
- Donnatal 1858
- Donnatal Extentabs 1859
- Donnatal Tablets 1858
- Donnazyme Tablets 1860
- Kinesed Tablets 2272
- Phenobarbital Elixir and Tablets 1293
- Primatene Tablets-P Formula 2421
- Quadrinal Tablets 1183
- Tedral SA 1765

Phenylbutazone (Reduced efficacy; increased incidence of breakthrough bleeding). Products include:
- Butazolidin Capsules & Tablets 1027

Phenytoin Sodium (Reduced efficacy; increased incidence of breakthrough bleeding). Products include:
- Dilantin Kapseals 1708
- Dilantin Parenteral 1712
- Dilantin with Phenobarbital Kapseals 1715

Rifampin (Reduced efficacy; increased incidence of breakthrough bleeding). Products include:
- Rifadin 1345
- Rifamate Capsules 1347
- Rimactane Capsules 879

Secobarbital Sodium (Reduced efficacy; increased incidence of breakthrough bleeding). Products include:
- Seconal Sodium Pulvules 1296

Tetracycline Hydrochloride (Reduced efficacy; increased incidence of breakthrough bleeding). Products include:
- Achromycin V Capsules 1193
- Achromycin Ophthalmic Ointment 1% .... ◉ 307
- Achromycin Ophthalmic Suspension 1% .... ◉ 308
- Topicycline for Topical Solution 1856

Thiamylal Sodium (Reduced efficacy; increased incidence of breakthrough bleeding). Products include:
- Surital Ampoules, Steri-Vials 1764

TRIPHASIL-28 TABLETS
(Levonorgestrel, Ethinyl Estradiol) 2532
See **Triphasil-21 Tablets**

TRISORALEN TABLETS
(Trioxsalen) 1125
No interactions described in labeling.

TRI-VI-FLOR 1.0 MG VITAMINS WITH FLUORIDE CHEWABLE TABLETS
(Vitamins with Fluoride) 1400
No interactions described in labeling.

TRI-VI-FLOR 0.25 MG VITAMINS WITH FLUORIDE DROPS
(Vitamins with Fluoride) 1400
No interactions described in labeling.

TRI-VI-FLOR 0.5 MG VITAMINS WITH FLUORIDE DROPS
(Vitamins with Fluoride) 1400
No interactions described in labeling.

TRI-VI-FLOR 0.25 MG VITAMINS WITH IRON AND FLUORIDE DROPS
(Vitamins with Fluoride, Ferrous Sulfate) 1401
No interactions described in labeling.

TRI-VI-SOL VITAMIN DROPS
(Vitamins A & D, Vitamin C) .... ▣ 614
No interactions described in labeling.

TRI-VI-SOL VITAMIN DROPS WITH IRON
(Vitamins with Iron) .... ▣ 614
No interactions described in labeling.

TROBICIN STERILE POWDER
(Spectinomycin Hydrochloride) 2366
No interactions described in labeling.

TRONOLANE ANESTHETIC CREAM FOR HEMORRHOIDS
(Pramoxine Hydrochloride) .... ▣ 681
No interactions described in labeling.

TRONOTHANE HYDROCHLORIDE CREAM
(Pramoxine Hydrochloride) 558
No interactions described in labeling.

TROPAMINE
(Amino Acid Preparations, Nutritional Supplement) 1358
May interact with monoamine oxidase inhibitors. Compounds in this category include:

Furazolidone (Tropamine contraindicated). Products include:
Furoxone 1855

Isocarboxazid (Tropamine contraindicated). Products include:
Marplan Tablets 1906

Phenelzine Sulfate (Tropamine contraindicated). Products include:
Nardil 1742

Selegiline Hydrochloride (Tropamine contraindicated). Products include:
Eldepryl 2250

Tranylcypromine Sulfate (Tropamine contraindicated). Products include:
Parnate Tablets 2222

TROPH-IRON LIQUID
(Vitamins with Iron) .... ▣ 619
May interact with tetracyclines. Compounds in this category include:

Demeclocycline Hydrochloride (Interference with absorption of tetracycline). Products include:
Declomycin Capsules, Tablets 1199

Doxycycline Calcium (Interference with absorption of tetracycline).
No products indexed under this heading.

Doxycycline Hyclate (Interference with absorption of tetracycline). Products include:
Doryx Capsules 1717
Vibramycin Hyclate Capsules 1787
Vibramycin Hyclate Intravenous 1968
Vibra-Tabs Film Coated Tablets 1787

Doxycycline Monohydrate (Interference with absorption of tetracycline). Products include:
Monodox Capsules 1630
Vibramycin Monohydrate for Oral Suspension 1787

Methacycline Hydrochloride (Interference with absorption of tetracycline).
No products indexed under this heading.

Minocycline Hydrochloride (Interference with absorption of tetracycline). Products include:
Minocin Intravenous 1221
Minocin Oral Suspension 1224
Minocin Pellet-Filled Capsules 1222

Oxytetracycline Hydrochloride (Interference with absorption of tetracycline). Products include:
Terra-Cortril Ophthalmic Suspension 1963
Terramycin Capsules 1786
Terramycin Intramuscular Solution 1964
Terramycin with Polymyxin B Sulfate Ophthalmic Ointment 1965

Tetracycline Hydrochloride (Interference with absorption of tetracycline). Products include:
Achromycin V Capsules 1193
Achromycin Ophthalmic Ointment 1% .... ◉ 307
Achromycin Ophthalmic Suspension 1% .... ◉ 308
Topicycline for Topical Solution 1856

TROPHITE LIQUID
(Vitamin B_1, Vitamin B_{12}) .... ▣ 619
No interactions described in labeling.

TROPICACYL
(Tropicamide) .... ◉ 209
No interactions described in labeling.

TRYSUL VAGINAL CREAM
(Sulfathiazole, Sulfacetamide, Sulfabenzamide) 2081
No interactions described in labeling.

TUBERCULIN, OLD, TINE TEST
(Diagnostic aid) 2549
May interact with corticosteroids and immunosuppressive agents. Compounds in these categories include:

Azathioprine (Reactivity to the test may be suppressed). Products include:
Imuran 768

Betamethasone Acetate (Reactivity to the test may be suppressed). Products include:
Celestone Soluspan Suspension 2081

Betamethasone Sodium Phosphate (Reactivity to the test may be suppressed). Products include:
Celestone Soluspan Suspension 2081

Cortisone Acetate (Reactivity to the test may be suppressed). Products include:
Cortone Acetate Sterile Suspension 1437
Cortone Acetate Tablets 1439

Cyclosporine (Reactivity to the test may be suppressed). Products include:
Sandimmune 2024

Desoximetasone (Reactivity to the test may be suppressed). Products include:
Topicort 1098

Dexamethasone Acetate (Reactivity to the test may be suppressed). Products include:
Dalalone D.P. Injectable 999
Decadron-LA Sterile Suspension 1457

Dexamethasone Sodium Phosphate (Reactivity to the test may be suppressed). Products include:
AK-Dex .... ◉ 203
Decadron Phosphate Respihaler 1454
Decadron Phosphate Sterile Ophthalmic Ointment 1453
Decadron Phosphate Sterile Ophthalmic Solution 1453
Decadron Phosphate Topical Cream 1455
Decadron Phosphate Turbinaire 1456
Maxidex Sterile Ophthalmic Ointment .... ◉ 222
NeoDecadron Sterile Ophthalmic Ointment 1517
NeoDecadron Sterile Ophthalmic Solution 1518
NeoDecadron Topical Cream 1518

Hydrocortisone (Reactivity to the test may be suppressed). Products include:
AK-Spore H.C. .... ◉ 206
Bactine Hydrocortisone Anti-Itch Cream .... ▣ 625
CaldeCORT Anti-Itch Hydrocortisone Spray .... ▣ 560
Carmol HC Cream 1% 2296
Cortaid Spray .... ▣ 735
Cortenema 2244
Cortisporin Ointment 758
Cortisporin Ophthalmic Ointment Sterile 758
Cortisporin Ophthalmic Suspension Sterile 759
Cortisporin Otic Solution Sterile 760
Cortisporin Otic Suspension Sterile 760
Cortizone-5 Creme & Ointment .... ▣ 732
Dermolate Anti-Itch Cream .... ▣ 697
Eldecort Cream 1.0% 1113
Eldecort Cream 1.0% and 2.5% 1113
Fungoid HC Creme 1770
Hydrocortone Tablets 1482
Hytone 909
LazerSporin-C Solution 1770
Massengill Medicated Soft Cloth Towelettes 2192
Nutracort Cream & Lotion 1684
PediOtic Suspension Sterile 797
Synacort Creams 1%, 2.5% 2296
Vanoxide-HC Acne Lotion 911
Vioform-Hydrocortisone Cream and Mild Cream 889
Vioform-Hydrocortisone Ointment 889
VōSoL HC Otic Solution 2392
Vytone Cream 1% 911

Hydrocortisone Acetate (Reactivity to the test may be suppressed). Products include:
Analpram-HC Rectal Cream 1% and 2.5% 970
Anusol-HC Cream 1690
Anusol-HC Suppositories 1691
Caldecort .... ▣ 560
Carmol HC Cream 1% 2296
Chloromycetin Hydrocortisone Ophthalmic 1694
Coly-Mycin S Otic w/Neomycin & Hydrocortisone 1708
Cortaid .... ▣ 735
Cortef Feminine Itch Cream .... ▣ 735
Corticaine .... ▣ 682
Cortifoam 1827
Cortisporin Cream 757
Epifoam 1828
Gynecort 5 Creme .... ▣ 556
Hydrocortone Acetate Sterile Suspension 1479
Lanacort 5 Creme and Ointment .... ▣ 557
Mantadil Cream 789
Ophthocort .... ◉ 301
Orabase HCA Oral Paste 890
Pramosone Cream, Lotion & Ointment 971
ProctoCream-HC 1834
Proctofoam-HC 1835

Hydrocortisone Sodium Phosphate (Reactivity to the test may be suppressed). Products include:
Hydrocortone Phosphate Injection, Sterile 1481

Hydrocortisone Sodium Succinate (Reactivity to the test may be suppressed). Products include:
Solu-Cortef Sterile Powder 2361

Immune Globulin (Human) (Reactivity to the test may be suppressed). Products include:
MICRhoGAM Rh_0(D) Immune Globulin (Human) 1650
RhoGAM Rh_0(D) Immune Globulin (Human) 1651

Immune Globulin Intravenous (Human) (Reactivity to the test may be suppressed). Products include:
Gamimune N Immune Globulin Intravenous (Human) 1572
Gammagard Immune Globulin, Intravenous (Human) 658
Iveegam 1129
Sandoglobulin I.V. 2027

Methylprednisolone Acetate (Reactivity to the test may be suppressed). Products include:
Depo-Medrol Sterile Aqueous Suspension 2334

Methylprednisolone Sodium Succinate (Reactivity to the test may be suppressed). Products include:
Solu-Medrol Sterile Powder 2363

Muromonab-CD3 (Reactivity to the test may be suppressed). Products include:
Orthoclone OKT3 Sterile Solution .. 1645

Prednisolone Acetate (Reactivity to the test may be suppressed). Products include:
AK-Cide Sterile Ophthalmic Ointment & Suspension .... ◉ 202
Blephamide Liquifilm Sterile Ophthalmic Suspension 586
Blephamide S.O.P. Sterile Ophthalmic Ointment 586
Cetapred Ointment .... ◉ 220
⅛% Econopred & 1% Econopred Plus .... ◉ 217
Isopto Cetapred Suspension .... ◉ 220
Metimyd .... ◉ 306
Poly-Pred Liquifilm .... ◉ 250
Pred Forte .... ◉ 252
Pred Mild .... ◉ 254
Pred-G Liquifilm Sterile Ophthalmic Suspension .... ◉ 252
Pred-G S.O.P. Sterile Ophthalmic Ointment .... ◉ 253
Vasocidin Ointment .... ◉ 275

Prednisolone Sodium Phosphate (Reactivity to the test may be suppressed). Products include:
AK-Pred .... ◉ 205
Hydeltrasol Injection, Sterile 1476
Inflamase .... ◉ 274
Pediapred Oral Liquid 987
Vasocidin Ophthalmic Solution .... ◉ 276

Prednisolone Tebutate (Reactivity to the test may be suppressed). Products include:
Hydeltra-T.B.A. Sterile Suspension 1478

Prednisone (Reactivity to the test may be suppressed). Products include:
Deltasone Tablets 2332

Triamcinolone (Reactivity to the test may be suppressed).
No products indexed under this heading.

Triamcinolone Acetonide (Reactivity to the test may be suppressed). Products include:
Aristocort A 1010
Azmacort Inhaler 1837
Kenalog Cream, Lotion & Ointment 2401
Kenalog-10 Injection 2402
Kenalog-40 Injection 2403
Kenalog in Orabase 604
Kenalog Spray 2401
Mycolog II Cream and Ointment 2407
Mytrex Cream & Ointment 2080
Nasacort Nasal Inhaler 1844

Triamcinolone Diacetate (Reactivity to the test may be suppressed). Products include:
Aristocort Suspension 1008

Triamcinolone Hexacetonide (Reactivity to the test may be suppressed). Products include:
Aristospan Suspension 1011

TUCKS CREAM
(Petrolatum, White, Witch Hazel) .... ◘ 643
No interactions described in labeling.

TUCKS PREMOISTENED PADS
(Glycerin, Witch Hazel)....... ◘ 642
No interactions described in labeling.

TUCKS TAKE-ALONGS
(Glycerin, Witch Hazel)....... ◘ 642
No interactions described in labeling.

TUMS ANTACID TABLETS
(Calcium Carbonate, Precipitated) .. ◘ 725
No interactions described in labeling.

TUMS E-X ANTACID TABLETS
(Calcium Carbonate, Precipitated) .. ◘ 725
No interactions described in labeling.

TUMS LIQUID EXTRA-STRENGTH ANTACID
(Calcium Carbonate) .... ◘ 726
No interactions described in labeling.

TUMS LIQUID EXTRA-STRENGTH ANTACID WITH SIMETHICONE
(Simethicone, Calcium Carbonate) .. ◘ 726
No interactions described in labeling.

TUSSIONEX EXTENDED-RELEASE SUSPENSION
(Hydrocodone Polistirex, Chlorpheniramine Polistirex) 988
May interact with central nervous system depressants, antihistamines, monoamine oxidase inhibitors, tricyclic antidepressants, and certain other agents. Compounds in these categories include:

Alcohol (Additive CNS depression).

Alfentanil Hydrochloride (Additive CNS depression). Products include:
Alfenta Injection 1131

Alprazolam (Additive CNS depression). Products include:
Xanax Tablets 2367

Amitriptyline Hydrochloride (Effect of either agent may be increased). Products include:
Elavil 2269
Endep Tablets 1927
Etrafon 2087
Limbitrol 1933
Triavil Tablets 1556

Amoxapine (Effect of either agent may be increased). Products include:
Asendin Tablets 1196

Aprobarbital (Additive CNS depression). Products include:
Alurate Elixir 1883

Astemizole (Additive CNS depression). Products include:
Hismanal Tablets 1138

Azatadine Maleate (Additive CNS depression). Products include:
Optimine Tablets 2115
Trinalin Repetabs Tablets 1170

Bromodiphenhydramine Hydrochloride (Additive CNS depression).
No products indexed under this heading.

Brompheniramine Maleate (Additive CNS depression). Products include:
Alka Seltzer Plus Sinus Allergy Medicine .... ◘ 624
Atrohist Sprinkle Capsules 558
Bromfed Capsules (Timed Release) 1615
Bromfed Syrup .... ◘ 628
Bromfed 1615
Dimetane Decongestant .... ◘ 673
Dimetane .... ◘ 672
Dimetane-DC Cough Syrup 1857
Dimetane-DX Cough Syrup 1858
Dimetapp Elixir .... ◘ 673
Dimetapp DM Elixir .... ◘ 674
Dimetapp Extentabs .... ◘ 674
Dimetapp Plus Caplets .... ◘ 675
Dimetapp Tablets .... ◘ 675
Drixoral Antihistamine/Nasal Decongestant Syrup .... ◘ 698

Buprenorphine (Additive CNS depression).
No products indexed under this heading.

Buspirone Hydrochloride (Additive CNS depression). Products include:
BuSpar 1401

Butabarbital (Additive CNS depression). Products include:
Pyridium Plus 1764

Butalbital (Additive CNS depression). Products include:
Esgic-Plus Tablets 1002
Esgic Tablets & Capsules 1001
Fioricet Tablets 2006
Fiorinal Capsules 2007
Fiorinal with Codeine Capsules 2008
Fiorinal Tablets 2007
Phrenilin 838
Sedapap Tablets 50 mg/650 mg .. 1360

Chlordiazepoxide (Additive CNS depression). Products include:
Libritabs Tablets 1930
Limbitrol 1933
Menrium Tablets 1934

Chlordiazepoxide Hydrochloride (Additive CNS depression). Products include:
Librax Capsules 1929
Librium Capsules 1931
Librium Injectable 1932

Chlorpheniramine Maleate (Additive CNS depression). Products include:
A.R.M. Allergy Relief Medicine Caplets .... ◘ 615
Alka-Seltzer Plus Cold Medicine .... ◘ 623
Allerest .... ◘ 559
Ana-Kit Anaphylaxis Emergency Treatment Kit 1100
BC Cold Powder Multi-Symptom Formula .... ◘ 517
Brexin L.A. Capsules 2078
Cerose-DM 2443
Cheracol Plus Head Cold/Cough Formula .... ◘ 667
Chlor-Trimeton Allergy Syrup, Tablets & Long-Acting Repetabs Tablets .... ◘ 693
Chlor-Trimeton Decongestant .... ◘ 694
Comhist LA Capsules 1618
Allergy-Sinus Comtrex Multi-Symptom Allergy Sinus Formula Tablets & Caplets 746
Comtrex Multi-Symptom Cold Reliever Tablets/Caplets/Liqui-Gels/Liquid 745
Day-Night Comtrex 747
Contac Continuous Action Decongestant/Antihistamine Capsules ◘ 710
Contac Maximum Strength Continuous Action Decongestant/Antihistamine Caplets .... ◘ 709
Contac Severe Cold and Flu Formula Caplets .... ◘ 711
Coricidin 'D' Decongestant Tablets .... ◘ 695
Coricidin Demilets Tablets for Children .... ◘ 696
Coricidin Tablets .... ◘ 695
Deconamine 663
Demazin Nasal Decongestant/Antihistamine Repetabs Tablets & Syrup .... ◘ 697
Dorcol Children's Liquid Cold Formula .... ◘ 686
Dristan Decongestant/Antihistamine/ Analgesic Coated Caplets .... ◘ 749
Dristan Cold Nasal Decongestant/ Antihistamine/ Analgesic Coated Tablets 2419
Dristan Advanced Formula Decongestant/Antihistamine/ Analgesic Tablets .... ◘ 749
Extendryl 994
4-Way Cold Tablets 750
Fedahist Gyrocaps 2145
Fedahist Timecaps 2145
Hycomine Compound Tablets 929
Isoclor Timesule Capsules .... ◘ 561
Kronofed-A 970
Medi-Flu Caplet, Liquid .... ◘ 640
Naldecon Syrup, Tablets, Pediatric Drops and Pediatric Syrup 709
Nolamine Tablets 838
Novafed A Capsules 1342
Novahistine DH 1342
Novahistine Elixir .... ◘ 596
Ornade Spansule Capsules 2221
Orthoxicol Cough Syrup .... ◘ 668
PediaCare Allergy Relief Formula Liquid 1362
PediaCare Cough-Cold Formula Liquid 1362
PediaCare Night Rest Cough-Cold Formula Liquid 1362
PediaCare 6-12 Cough-Cold Formula Chewable Tablets 1362
Pyrroxate Capsules .... ◘ 669
Quelidrine Syrup 556
Ru-Tuss II Capsules 693
Ru-Tuss Tablets 693
Ryna .... ◘ 741
Sinarest Tablets & Extra Strength Tablets .... ◘ 562
Sine-Off Maximum Strength Allergy/Sinus Formula Caplets .... ◘ 721
Sine-Off Sinus Medicine Tablets-Aspirin Formula .... ◘ 722
Singlet Tablets .... ◘ 598
Sinulin 840
Sinutab Maximum Strength .... ◘ 641
St. Joseph Nighttime Cold Medicine .... ◘ 705
Sudafed Plus Liquid .... ◘ 544
Sudafed Plus Tablets .... ◘ 545
Teldrin Timed-Release Allergy Capsules, 12 mg 2192
TheraFlu Flu and Cold Medicine .... ◘ 687
Triaminic Allergy Tablets .... ◘ 688
Triaminic Chewables .... ◘ 688
Triaminic Cold Tablets .... ◘ 688
Triaminic Nite Light .... ◘ 689
Triaminic Syrup .... ◘ 689
Triaminic-12 Tablets .... ◘ 690
Triaminicin Tablets .... ◘ 690
Triaminicol Multi-Symptom Cold Tablets .... ◘ 691
Triaminicol Multi-Symptom Relief ◘ 691
Tylenol Allergy Sinus Medication Caplets and Gelcaps, Maximum Strength 1372
Children's Tylenol Cold Liquid Formula and Chewable Tablets 1368
Tylenol Cold & Flu Hot Medication, Packets 1369
Tylenol Cold Medication Caplets and Tablets 1370
Tylenol Cold Medication, Effervescent Tablets 1369
Vicks Children's NyQuil .... ◘ 664
Vicks Formula 44 Cough Medicine .... ◘ 661
Vicks Formula 44M Multi-Symptom Cough Medicine .... ◘ 662
Vicks Pediatric Formula 44m Multi-Symptom Cough & Cold Medicine .... ◘ 663

Chlorpheniramine Tannate (Additive CNS depression). Products include:
Rynatan 2387
Rynatuss 2388

Chlorpromazine (Additive CNS depression). Products include:
Thorazine 2234

Chlorprothixene (Additive CNS depression). Products include:
Taractan Tablets 1920

Chlorprothixene Hydrochloride (Additive CNS depression). Products include:
Taractan 1920

Clemastine Fumarate (Additive CNS depression). Products include:
Tavist Syrup 2033
Tavist Tablets 2035
Tavist-D Tablets 2035

Clomipramine Hydrochloride (Effect of either agent may be increased). Products include:
Anafranil Capsules 650

Clorazepate Dipotassium (Additive CNS depression). Products include:
Tranxene 556

Codeine (Additive CNS depression). Products include:
Calcidrine Syrup 506

Codeine Phosphate (Additive CNS depression). Products include:
Actifed with Codeine Cough Syrup.. 752
Cheracol Cough Syrup 1853
Codimal PH Syrup 846
Dimetane-DC Cough Syrup 1857
Empirin with Codeine Phosphate Nos. 2, 3 & 4 764
Fiorinal with Codeine Capsules 2008
Isoclor Expectorant 982
Naldecon CX Adult Liquid .... ◘ 521
Novahistine DH 1342
Novahistine Expectorant 1343
Nucofed Capsules 2219
Nucofed Expectorant 2219
Nucofed Pediatric Expectorant 2220
Nucofed Syrup 2219
Phenaphen with Codeine Capsules 1865
Phenaphen-650 with Codeine Tablets 1866
Phenergan with Codeine 2497
Phenergan VC with Codeine 2501
Robitussin A-C Syrup 1875
Robitussin-DAC Syrup 1875
Ryna .... ◘ 741
Soma Compound w/Codeine Tablets 2390
Triaminic Expectorant w/Codeine .. 1996
Tussi-Organidin Liquid 2391
Tylenol with Codeine 1381

Codeine Polistirex (Additive CNS depression).
No products indexed under this heading.

Cyproheptadine Hydrochloride (Additive CNS depression). Products include:
Periactin 1525

Desipramine Hydrochloride (Effect of either agent may be increased). Products include:
Norpramin Tablets 1340

Dexchlorpheniramine Maleate (Additive CNS depression). Products include:
Polaramine 2116

Dezocine (Additive CNS depression).

Diazepam (Additive CNS depression). Products include:
Valium Injectable 1937
Valium Tablets 1939
Valrelease Capsules 1923

Diphenhydramine Citrate (Additive CNS depression). Products include:
Alka-Seltzer Plus Night-Time Cold Medicine .... ◘ 623
Bufferin AF Nite Time Analgesic/ Sleeping Aid Caplets 744
Excedrin P.M. Analgesic/Sleeping Aid Tablets, Caplets and Liquid 749

Diphenhydramine Hydrochloride (Additive CNS depression). Products include:
Benadryl Anti-Itch Cream .... ◘ 635
Benadryl Capsules 1691
Benadryl Decongestant Elixir .... ◘ 635
Benadryl Decongestant .... ◘ 635
Benadryl Elixir .... ◘ 636
Benadryl Kapseals 1691
Benadryl 25 Kapseals .... ◘ 636
Benadryl Parenteral 1692

Benadryl Plus ■ 636
Benadryl Plus Nighttime ■ 637
Benadryl Spray, Maximum Strength ■ 637
Benadryl Spray, Regular Strength ■ 637
Benadryl Steri-Vials, Ampoules, and Steri-Dose Syringe 1692
Benadryl 25 Tablets ■ 636
Benylin Cough Syrup ■ 637
Benylin Decongestant ■ 638
Caladryl Cream, Lotion, Spray ■ 638
Miles Nervine Nighttime Sleep-Aid ■ 627
Nytol Tablets ■ 517
Sleep-ettes-D Tablets ■ 653
Sleep-eze 3 Tablets ■ 755
Sleepinal Night-time Sleep Aid Capsules ■ 734
Sominex Caplets and Tablets ■ 722
Sominex Liquid ■ 723
Sominex Pain Relief Formula ■ 723
Tylenol Cold Night Time Medication Liquid 1371
Tylenol PM, Extra Strength Caplets and Tablets 1368
Unisom Dual Relief Nighttime Sleep Aid/Analgesic 1774
Ziradryl Lotion ■ 643

Diphenylpyraline Hydrochloride (Additive CNS depression).
No products indexed under this heading.

Doxepin Hydrochloride (Effect of either agent may be increased). Products include:
Sinequan 1960

Droperidol (Additive CNS depression). Products include:
Inapsine Injection 1140
Innovar Injection 1141

Enflurane (Additive CNS depression). Products include:
Ethrane 599

Estazolam (Additive CNS depression). Products include:
ProSom Tablets 554

Ethchlorvynol (Additive CNS depression). Products include:
Placidyl Capsules 553

Ethinamate (Additive CNS depression).
No products indexed under this heading.

Fentanyl (Additive CNS depression). Products include:
Duragesic Transdermal System 1133

Fentanyl Citrate (Additive CNS depression). Products include:
Innovar Injection 1141
Sublimaze Injection 1146

Fluphenazine Decanoate (Additive CNS depression). Products include:
Prolixin Decanoate 1795

Fluphenazine Enanthate (Additive CNS depression). Products include:
Prolixin Enanthate 1796

Fluphenazine Hydrochloride (Additive CNS depression). Products include:
Prolixin Elixir 1793
Prolixin Injection 1791
Prolixin Oral Concentrate 1792
Prolixin Tablets 1793

Flurazepam Hydrochloride (Additive CNS depression). Products include:
Dalmane Capsules 1927

Furazolidone (Effect of either agent may be increased). Products include:
Furoxone 1855

Glutethimide (Additive CNS depression).
No products indexed under this heading.

Haloperidol (Additive CNS depression). Products include:
Haldol Injection, Tablets and Concentrate 1373

Haloperidol Decanoate (Additive CNS depression). Products include:
Haldol Decanoate 1375

Hydrocodone Bitartrate (Additive CNS depression). Products include:
Anexsia 5/500 Tablets 2196
Anexsia 7.5/650 Tablets 2197
Azdone Tablets 844
Codiclear DH Syrup 845
Codimal DH Syrup 846
Damason-P 1356
Hycodan Syrup, Tablets 927
Hycomine Compound Tablets 929
Hycomine Syrup 927
Hycotuss Expectorant Syrup 930
Hydrocet Capsules 835
Lortab ASA Tablets 2414
Lortab 2412
Ru-Tuss with Hydrocodone 694
Triaminic Expectorant DH 1995
Vicodin Tablets 1187
Vicodin ES Tablets 1189
Zydone Capsules 941

Hydroxyzine Hydrochloride (Additive CNS depression). Products include:
Atarax Tablets & Syrup 1941
Marax Tablets & DF Syrup 1954
Vistaril Intramuscular Solution 1970

Imipramine Hydrochloride (Effect of either agent may be increased). Products include:
Tofranil Ampuls 1038
Tofranil Tablets 1039

Imipramine Pamoate (Effect of either agent may be increased). Products include:
Tofranil-PM Capsules 1041

Isocarboxazid (Effect of either agent may be increased). Products include:
Marplan Tablets 1906

Isoflurane (Additive CNS depression). Products include:
Forane 600

Ketamine Hydrochloride (Additive CNS depression). Products include:
Ketalar 1726

Levorphanol Tartrate (Additive CNS depression). Products include:
Levo-Dromoran 1906

Lorazepam (Additive CNS depression). Products include:
Ativan Injection 2432
Ativan Tablets 2434

Loxapine Hydrochloride (Additive CNS depression). Products include:
Loxitane 1213

Loxapine Succinate (Additive CNS depression). Products include:
Loxitane Capsules 1213

Maprotiline Hydrochloride (Effect of either agent may be increased). Products include:
Ludiomil Tablets 874

Meperidine Hydrochloride (Additive CNS depression). Products include:
Demerol 2047
Mepergan Injection 2479

Mephobarbital (Additive CNS depression). Products include:
Mebaral Tablets 2061

Meprobamate (Additive CNS depression). Products include:
Deprol Tablets 2382
Equagesic Tablets 2451
Miltown Tablets 2386
PMB 200 and PMB 400 2504

Mesoridazine (Additive CNS depression). Products include:
Serentil 686

Methadone Hydrochloride (Additive CNS depression). Products include:
Dolophine Hydrochloride Ampoules & Vials 1260
Dolophine Hydrochloride Tablets 1261
Methadone Hydrochloride Diskets 1284
Methadone Hydrochloride Oral Solution & Tablets 1987

Methdilazine Hydrochloride (Additive CNS depression). Products include:
Tacaryl Syrup & Tablets 2409

Methohexital Sodium (Additive CNS depression). Products include:
Brevital Sodium Vials 1248

Methoxyflurane (Additive CNS depression).
No products indexed under this heading.

Midazolam Hydrochloride (Additive CNS depression). Products include:
Versed Injection 1924

Molindone Hydrochloride (Additive CNS depression). Products include:
Moban Tablets & Concentrate 932

Morphine Sulfate (Additive CNS depression). Products include:
Astramorph/PF Injection, USP (Preservative-Free) 618
Duramorph 960
Infumorph 200 and Infumorph 500 Sterile Solutions 962
MS Contin Tablets 1814
MSIR 1817
Oramorph SR (Morphine Sulfate Sustained Release Tablets) 1988
Roxanol 1991

Nortriptyline Hydrochloride (Effect of either agent may be increased). Products include:
Pamelor 2019

Opium Alkaloids (Additive CNS depression). Products include:
B & O No. 15A & No. 16A Supprettes 2395
Pantopon Injectable 1911

Oxazepam (Additive CNS depression). Products include:
Serax Capsules 2522
Serax Tablets 2522

Oxycodone Hydrochloride (Additive CNS depression). Products include:
Percocet Tablets 950
Percodan 951
Roxicodone Tablets, Oral Solution & Intensol (Oxycodone) 1992
Tylox Capsules 1382

Pentobarbital Sodium (Additive CNS depression). Products include:
Nembutal Sodium Capsules 534
Nembutal Sodium Solution 536
Nembutal Sodium Suppositories 538

Perphenazine (Additive CNS depression). Products include:
Etrafon 2087
Triavil Tablets 1556
Trilafon 2123

Phenelzine Sulfate (Effect of either agent may be increased). Products include:
Nardil 1742

Phenobarbital (Additive CNS depression). Products include:
Arco-Lase Plus Tablets 607
Bellergal-S Tablets 1998
Bronkolixir ■ 761
Bronkotabs Tablets ■ 762
Donnatal 1858
Donnatal Extentabs 1859
Donnatal Tablets 1858
Donnazyme Tablets 1860
Kinesed Tablets 2272
Phenobarbital Elixir and Tablets 1293
Primatene Tablets-P Formula 2421
Quadrinal Tablets 1183
Tedral SA 1765

Prazepam (Additive CNS depression). Products include:
Centrax 1693

Prochlorperazine (Additive CNS depression). Products include:
Compazine 2201

Promethazine Hydrochloride (Additive CNS depression). Products include:
Mepergan Injection 2479
Phenergan with Codeine 2497
Phenergan with Dextromethorphan 2499
Phenergan Injection 2493
Phenergan Suppositories 2496
Phenergan Syrup 2495
Phenergan Tablets 2496
Phenergan VC 2500
Phenergan VC with Codeine 2501

Propofol (Additive CNS depression). Products include:
Diprivan Injection 2267

Propoxyphene Hydrochloride (Additive CNS depression). Products include:
Darvon 1256
Wygesic Tablets 2540

Propoxyphene Napsylate (Additive CNS depression). Products include:
Darvon-N/Darvocet-N 1254

Protriptyline Hydrochloride (Effect of either agent may be increased). Products include:
Vivactil Tablets 1567

Pyrilamine Maleate (Additive CNS depression). Products include:
Codimal 846
4-Way Fast Acting Nasal Spray - Original Formula (regular & mentholated) & Metered Spray Pump (regular) 751
Maximum Strength Midol Multi-Symptom Menstrual Formula ■ 571
Maximum Strength Midol PMS Premenstrual Syndrome Formula ■ 570
Regular Strength Midol Multi-Symptom Menstrual Formula ■ 570
Prefrin-A ◉ 255
Prēmsyn PMS Capsules & Caplets ■ 547
Primatene Tablets-M Formula 2421
Robitussin Night Relief ■ 677
Ru-Tuss with Hydrocodone 694
Triaminic Expectorant DH 1995
Triaminic Oral Infant Drops 1996

Pyrilamine Tannate (Additive CNS depression). Products include:
Rynatan 2387

Quazepam (Additive CNS depression). Products include:
Doral Tablets 2383

Secobarbital Sodium (Additive CNS depression). Products include:
Seconal Sodium Pulvules 1296

Selegiline Hydrochloride (Effect of either agent may be increased). Products include:
Eldepryl 2250

Sufentanil Citrate (Additive CNS depression). Products include:
Sufenta Injection 1147

Temazepam (Additive CNS depression). Products include:
Restoril Capsules 2023

Terfenadine (Additive CNS depression). Products include:
Seldane Tablets 1349
Seldane-D Extended-Release Tablets 1350

Thiamylal Sodium (Additive CNS depression). Products include:
Surital Ampoules, Steri-Vials 1764

Thioridazine Hydrochloride (Additive CNS depression). Products include:
Mellaril 2011

Thiothixene (Additive CNS depression). Products include:
Navane Capsules and Concentrate 1954
Navane Intramuscular 1956

Tranylcypromine Sulfate (Effect of either agent may be increased). Products include:
Parnate Tablets 2222

Triazolam (Additive CNS depression). Products include:
Halcion Tablets 2340

Trifluoperazine Hydrochloride (Additive CNS depression). Products include:
- Stelazine ... 2226

Trimeprazine Tartrate (Additive CNS depression). Products include:
- Temaril Tablets, Syrup and Spansule Sustained Release Capsules 1085

Trimipramine Maleate (Effect of either agent may be increased). Products include:
- Surmontil Capsules ... 2524

Tripelennamine Hydrochloride (Additive CNS depression). Products include:
- PBZ Tablets & Elixir ... 1037
- PBZ-SR Tablets ... 1037

Triprolidine Hydrochloride (Additive CNS depression). Products include:
- Actidil ... ◘ 538
- Actifed Capsules ... ◘ 539
- Actifed Plus Caplets ... ◘ 539
- Actifed Plus Tablets ... ◘ 540
- Actifed with Codeine Cough Syrup .. 752
- Actifed Syrup ... ◘ 540
- Actifed Tablets ... ◘ 540
- Actifed 12-Hour Capsules ... ◘ 539

TUSSI-ORGANIDIN DM LIQUID

(Iodinated Glycerol, Dextromethorphan Hydrobromide) ... 2392
May interact with antithyroid agents and lithium preparations. Compounds in these categories include:

Lithium Carbonate (Hypothyroid effect of lithium potentiated). Products include:
- Eskalith ... 2214
- Lithane Tablets ... 1596
- Lithium Carbonate Capsules & Tablets ... 1984
- Lithobid Tablets ... 870

Lithium Citrate (Hypothyroid effect of lithium potentiated). Products include:
- Cibalith-S ... 870

Methimazole (Hypothyroid effect of antithyroid drugs potentiated). Products include:
- Tapazole Tablets ... 1298

Propylthiouracil (Hypothyroid effect of antithyroid drugs potentiated).
- No products indexed under this heading.

TUSSI-ORGANIDIN LIQUID

(Iodinated Glycerol, Codeine Phosphate) ... 2391
May interact with lithium preparations and antithyroid agents. Compounds in these categories include:

Lithium Carbonate (Potentiation of hypothyroid effect of lithium). Products include:
- Eskalith ... 2214
- Lithane Tablets ... 1596
- Lithium Carbonate Capsules & Tablets ... 1984
- Lithobid Tablets ... 870

Lithium Citrate (Potentiation of hypothyroid effect of lithium). Products include:
- Cibalith-S ... 870

Methimazole (Potentiation of hypothyroid effects of antithyroid drugs). Products include:
- Tapazole Tablets ... 1298

Propylthiouracil (Potentiation of hypothyroid effects of antithyroid drugs).
- No products indexed under this heading.

TUSS-ORNADE LIQUID

(Caramiphen Edisylate, Phenylpropanolamine Hydrochloride) ... 2242
May interact with monoamine oxidase inhibitors and certain other agents. Compounds in these categories include:

Amphetamine Resins (Concurrent use should be avoided). Products include:
- Biphetamine Capsules ... 973

Benzphetamine Hydrochloride (Concurrent use should be avoided). Products include:
- Didrex Tablets ... 2338

Dextroamphetamine Sulfate (Concurrent use should be avoided). Products include:
- Dexedrine ... 2206

Furazolidone (Contraindication). Products include:
- Furoxone ... 1855

Isocarboxazid (Contraindication). Products include:
- Marplan Tablets ... 1906

Methamphetamine Hydrochloride (Concurrent use should be avoided). Products include:
- Desoxyn Gradumet Tablets ... 514

Phenelzine Sulfate (Contraindication). Products include:
- Nardil ... 1742

Phenylpropanolamine Containing Anorectics (Concurrent use should be avoided).

Selegiline Hydrochloride (Contraindication). Products include:
- Eldepryl ... 2250

Tranylcypromine Sulfate (Contraindication). Products include:
- Parnate Tablets ... 2222

TUSS-ORNADE SPANSULE CAPSULES

(Caramiphen Edisylate, Phenylpropanolamine Hydrochloride) ... 2242
May interact with monoamine oxidase inhibitors and certain other agents. Compounds in these categories include:

Amphetamine Resins (Concurrent use should be avoided). Products include:
- Biphetamine Capsules ... 973

Benzphetamine Hydrochloride (Concurrent use should be avoided). Products include:
- Didrex Tablets ... 2338

Dextroamphetamine Sulfate (Concurrent use should be avoided). Products include:
- Dexedrine ... 2206

Furazolidone (Contraindication). Products include:
- Furoxone ... 1855

Isocarboxazid (Contraindication). Products include:
- Marplan Tablets ... 1906

Methamphetamine Hydrochloride (Concurrent use should be avoided). Products include:
- Desoxyn Gradumet Tablets ... 514

Phenelzine Sulfate (Contraindication). Products include:
- Nardil ... 1742

Phenylpropanolamine Containing Anorectics (Concurrent use should be avoided).

Selegiline Hydrochloride (Contraindication). Products include:
- Eldepryl ... 2250

Tranylcypromine Sulfate (Contraindication). Products include:
- Parnate Tablets ... 2222

TYLENOL ACETAMINOPHEN CHILDREN'S CHEWABLE TABLETS & ELIXIR

(Acetaminophen) ... 1366
No interactions described in labeling.

TYLENOL ALLERGY SINUS MEDICATION CAPLETS AND GELCAPS, MAXIMUM STRENGTH

(Acetaminophen, Chlorpheniramine Maleate, Pseudoephedrine Hydrochloride) ... 1372
May interact with antidepressant drugs, antihypertensives, and certain other agents. Compounds in these categories include:

Acebutolol Hydrochloride (Effects not specified). Products include:
- Sectral Capsules ... 2520

Alcohol (Increases the drowsiness effect).

Amitriptyline Hydrochloride (Effects not specified). Products include:
- Elavil ... 2269
- Endep Tablets ... 1927
- Etrafon ... 2087
- Limbitrol ... 1933
- Triavil Tablets ... 1556

Amoxapine (Effects not specified). Products include:
- Asendin Tablets ... 1196

Atenolol (Effects not specified). Products include:
- Tenoretic Tablets ... 1105
- Tenormin Tablets and I.V. Injection 1107

Benazepril Hydrochloride (Effects not specified). Products include:
- Lotensin Tablets ... 872

Betaxolol Hydrochloride (Effects not specified). Products include:
- Betoptic Sterile Ophthalmic Solution ... 569
- Betoptic S Sterile Ophthalmic Suspension ... 570
- Kerlone Tablets ... 2172

Bupropion Hydrochloride (Effects not specified). Products include:
- Wellbutrin Tablets ... 821

Captopril (Effects not specified). Products include:
- Capoten ... 2255
- Capozide ... 2258

Carteolol Hydrochloride (Effects not specified). Products include:
- Cartrol Tablets ... 507

Clonidine (Effects not specified). Products include:
- Catapres-TTS ... 677

Clonidine Hydrochloride (Effects not specified). Products include:
- Catapres Tablets ... 676
- Combipres Tablets ... 678

Deserpidine (Effects not specified). Products include:
- Enduronyl ... 518
- Harmonyl Tablets ... 528
- Oreticyl ... 545

Desipramine Hydrochloride (Effects not specified). Products include:
- Norpramin Tablets ... 1340

Diazoxide (Effects not specified). Products include:
- Hyperstat I.V. Injection ... 2095
- Proglycem ... 649

Doxazosin Mesylate (Effects not specified). Products include:
- Cardura Tablets ... 1941

Doxepin Hydrochloride (Effects not specified). Products include:
- Sinequan ... 1960

Enalapril Maleate (Effects not specified). Products include:
- Vaseretic Tablets ... 1559
- Vasotec Tablets ... 1564

Enalaprilat (Effects not specified). Products include:
- Vasotec I.V. ... 1562

Esmolol Hydrochloride (Effects not specified). Products include:
- Brevibloc Injection ... 942

Felodipine (Effects not specified). Products include:
- Plendil Extended-Release Tablets 1526

Fluoxetine Hydrochloride (Effects not specified). Products include:
- Prozac Pulvules ... 920

Fosinopril Sodium (Effects not specified). Products include:
- Monopril Tablets ... 1406

Guanabenz Acetate (Effects not specified). Products include:
- Wytensin Tablets ... 2542

Guanethidine Monosulfate (Effects not specified). Products include:
- Esimil Tablets ... 864
- Ismelin Tablets ... 869

Hydralazine Hydrochloride (Effects not specified). Products include:
- Apresazide Capsules ... 854
- Apresoline Hydrochloride Parenteral (Ampuls) ... 856
- Apresoline Hydrochloride Tablets .. 855
- Apresoline-Esidrix Tablets ... 857
- Ser-Ap-Es Tablets ... 881
- Serpasil-Apresoline Tablets ... 884

Imipramine Hydrochloride (Effects not specified). Products include:
- Tofranil Ampuls ... 1038
- Tofranil Tablets ... 1039

Imipramine Pamoate (Effects not specified). Products include:
- Tofranil-PM Capsules ... 1041

Indapamide (Effects not specified). Products include:
- Lozol Tablets ... 1843

Isocarboxazid (Effects not specified). Products include:
- Marplan Tablets ... 1906

Isradipine (Effects not specified). Products include:
- DynaCirc Capsules ... 2004

Labetalol Hydrochloride (Effects not specified). Products include:
- Normodyne Injection ... 2108
- Normodyne Tablets ... 2110
- Normozide Tablets ... 2112
- Trandate HCT Tablets ... 579
- Trandate Injection ... 577
- Trandate Tablets ... 579

Lisinopril (Effects not specified). Products include:
- Prinivil Tablets ... 1538
- Prinzide Tablets ... 1540
- Zestoretic ... 2274
- Zestril Tablets ... 2277

Maprotiline Hydrochloride (Effects not specified). Products include:
- Ludiomil Tablets ... 874

Mecamylamine Hydrochloride (Effects not specified). Products include:
- Inversine Tablets ... 1492

Methyldopa (Effects not specified). Products include:
- Aldoclor Tablets ... 1413
- Aldomet Oral ... 1415
- Aldoril Tablets ... 1418

Methyldopate Hydrochloride (Effects not specified). Products include:
Aldomet Ester HCl Injection 1417
Metoprolol Tartrate (Effects not specified). Products include:
Lopressor Ampuls 1032
Lopressor HCT Tablets 1034
Lopressor Tablets 1032
Metyrosine (Effects not specified). Products include:
Demser Capsules 1460
Minoxidil (Effects not specified). Products include:
Loniten Tablets 2346
Rogaine Topical Solution 2357
Nadolol (Effects not specified). Products include:
Corgard Tablets 701
Corzide Tablets 702
Nicardipine Hydrochloride (Effects not specified). Products include:
Cardene Capsules 2290
Nitroglycerin (Effects not specified). Products include:
Deponit NTG Transdermal Delivery System 2143
Minitran Transdermal Delivery System 1312
Nitro-Bid Ointment 1339
Nitro-Bid Capsules 1338
Nitrodisc 2176
Nitro-Dur (nitroglycerin) Transdermal Infusion System 1164
Nitrogard Tablets 1004
Nitrolingual Spray 1846
Nitrostat Tablets 1743
Transderm-Nitro Transdermal Therapeutic System 2283
Nortriptyline Hydrochloride (Effects not specified). Products include:
Pamelor 2019
Penbutolol Sulfate (Effects not specified). Products include:
Levatol 1832
Phenelzine Sulfate (Effects not specified). Products include:
Nardil 1742
Phenoxybenzamine Hydrochloride (Effects not specified). Products include:
Dibenzyline Capsules 2207
Phentolamine Mesylate (Effects not specified). Products include:
Regitine 878
Pindolol (Effects not specified). Products include:
Visken Tablets 2036
Prazosin Hydrochloride (Effects not specified). Products include:
Minipress Capsules 1778
Minizide Capsules 1779
Propranolol Hydrochloride (Effects not specified). Products include:
Inderal 2459
Inderal LA Long Acting Capsules 2461
Inderide Tablets 2463
Inderide LA Long Acting Capsules 2465
Protriptyline Hydrochloride (Effects not specified). Products include:
Vivactil Tablets 1567
Ramipril (Effects not specified). Products include:
Altace Capsules 1086
Rauwolfia Serpentina (Effects not specified). Products include:
Raudixin Tablets 1803
Rauzide Tablets 1804
Rescinnamine (Effects not specified).
No products indexed under this heading.
Reserpine (Effects not specified). Products include:
Diupres Tablets 1461
Hydromox R Tablets 1209
Hydropres Tablets 1485
Renese-R Tablets 1786
Salutensin/Salutensin-Demi 719
Ser-Ap-Es Tablets 881
Serpasil Tablets 883
Serpasil-Apresoline Tablets 884
Serpasil-Esidrix Tablets 886
Sodium Nitroprusside (Effects not specified). Products include:
Nipride I.V. Infusion 1909
Terazosin Hydrochloride (Effects not specified). Products include:
Hytrin Tablets 529
Timolol Maleate (Effects not specified). Products include:
Blocadren Tablets 1429
Timolide Tablets 1547
Timoptic in Ocudose 1552
Timoptic Sterile Ophthalmic Solution 1550
Tranylcypromine Sulfate (Effects not specified). Products include:
Parnate Tablets 2222
Trazodone Hydrochloride (Effects not specified). Products include:
Desyrel and Desyrel Dividose 1404
Trimethaphan Camsylate (Effects not specified). Products include:
Arfonad Ampuls 1887
Trimipramine Maleate (Effects not specified). Products include:
Surmontil Capsules 2524

TYLENOL WITH CODEINE PHOSPHATE ELIXIR (Acetaminophen, Codeine Phosphate) 1381
May interact with central nervous system depressants, anticholinergics, neuromuscular blocking agents, narcotic analgesics, and certain other agents. Compounds in these categories include:

Alcohol (Additive CNS depression).
Alfentanil Hydrochloride (Additive CNS depression). Products include:
Alfenta Injection 1131
Alprazolam (Additive CNS depression). Products include:
Xanax Tablets 2367
Aprobarbital (Additive CNS depression). Products include:
Alurate Elixir 1883
Atropine Sulfate (May produce paralytic ileus). Products include:
Arco-Lase Plus Tablets 607
Atropine Sulfate Sterile Ophthalmic Solution and S.O.P. Sterile Ophthalmic Ointment .... ⊙ 239
Donnagel .... ▣ 675
Donnagel-PG 1858
Donnatal 1858
Donnatal Extentabs 1859
Donnatal Tablets 1858
Donnazyme Tablets 1860
Isopto Atropine .... ⊙ 218
Lomotil 2174
Motofen Tablets 836
Ru-Tuss Tablets 693
Urised Tablets 2396
Belladonna Alkaloids (May produce paralytic ileus). Products include:
Bellergal-S Tablets 1998
Hyland's Bed Wetting Tablets .... ▣ 728
Hyland's Teething Tablets .... ▣ 728
Kinesed Tablets 2272
Benztropine Mesylate (May produce paralytic ileus). Products include:
Cogentin 1435
Biperiden (May produce paralytic ileus). Products include:
Akineton 1171
Buprenorphine (Additive CNS depression).
No products indexed under this heading.
Buspirone Hydrochloride (Additive CNS depression). Products include:
BuSpar 1401
Butabarbital (Additive CNS depression). Products include:
Pyridium Plus 1764
Butalbital (Additive CNS depression). Products include:
Esgic-Plus Tablets 1002
Esgic Tablets & Capsules 1001
Fioricet Tablets 2006
Fiorinal Capsules 2007
Fiorinal with Codeine Capsules 2008
Fiorinal Tablets 2007
Phrenilin 838
Sedapap Tablets 50 mg/650 mg 1360
Chlordiazepoxide (Additive CNS depression). Products include:
Libritabs Tablets 1930
Limbitrol 1933
Menrium Tablets 1934
Chlordiazepoxide Hydrochloride (Additive CNS depression). Products include:
Librax Capsules 1929
Librium Capsules 1931
Librium Injectable 1932
Chlorpromazine (Additive CNS depression). Products include:
Thorazine 2234
Chlorprothixene (Additive CNS depression). Products include:
Taractan Tablets 1920
Chlorprothixene Hydrochloride (Additive CNS depression). Products include:
Taractan 1920
Clidinium Bromide (May produce paralytic ileus). Products include:
Librax Capsules 1929
Quarzan Capsules 1937
Clorazepate Dipotassium (Additive CNS depression). Products include:
Tranxene 556
Clozapine (Additive CNS depression). Products include:
Clozaril Tablets 2000
Codeine (Additive CNS depression). Products include:
Calcidrine Syrup 506
Codeine Polistirex (Additive CNS depression).
No products indexed under this heading.
Dezocine (Additive CNS depression).
Diazepam (Additive CNS depression). Products include:
Valium Injectable 1937
Valium Tablets 1939
Valrelease Capsules 1923
Dicyclomine Hydrochloride (May produce paralytic ileus). Products include:
Bentyl 1322
Droperidol (Additive CNS depression). Products include:
Inapsine Injection 1140
Innovar Injection 1141
Enflurane (Additive CNS depression). Products include:
Ethrane 599
Estazolam (Additive CNS depression). Products include:
ProSom Tablets 554
Ethchlorvynol (Additive CNS depression). Products include:
Placidyl Capsules 553
Ethinamate (Additive CNS depression).
No products indexed under this heading.
Ethopropazine Hydrochloride (May produce paralytic ileus).
Fentanyl (Additive CNS depression). Products include:
Duragesic Transdermal System 1133
Fentanyl Citrate (Additive CNS depression). Products include:
Innovar Injection 1141
Sublimaze Injection 1146
Fluphenazine Decanoate (Additive CNS depression). Products include:
Prolixin Decanoate 1795
Fluphenazine Enanthate (Additive CNS depression). Products include:
Prolixin Enanthate 1796
Fluphenazine Hydrochloride (Additive CNS depression). Products include:
Prolixin Elixir 1793
Prolixin Injection 1791
Prolixin Oral Concentrate 1792
Prolixin Tablets 1793
Flurazepam Hydrochloride (Additive CNS depression). Products include:
Dalmane Capsules 1927
Glutethimide (Additive CNS depression).
No products indexed under this heading.
Glycopyrrolate (May produce paralytic ileus). Products include:
Robinul Forte Tablets 1873
Robinul Injectable 1873
Robinul Tablets 1873
Haloperidol (Additive CNS depression). Products include:
Haldol Injection, Tablets and Concentrate 1373
Haloperidol Decanoate (Additive CNS depression). Products include:
Haldol Decanoate 1375
Hydrocodone Bitartrate (Additive CNS depression). Products include:
Anexsia 5/500 Tablets 2196
Anexsia 7.5/650 Tablets 2197
Azdone Tablets 844
Codiclear DH Syrup 845
Codimal DH Syrup 846
Damason-P 1356
Hycodan Syrup, Tablets 927
Hycomine Compound Tablets 929
Hycomine Syrup 927
Hycotuss Expectorant Syrup 930
Hydrocet Capsules 835
Lortab ASA Tablets 2414
Lortab 2412
Ru-Tuss with Hydrocodone 694
Triaminic Expectorant DH 1995
Vicodin Tablets 1187
Vicodin ES Tablets 1189
Zydone Capsules 941
Hydrocodone Polistirex (Additive CNS depression). Products include:
Tussionex Extended-Release Suspension 988
Hydroxyzine Hydrochloride (Additive CNS depression). Products include:
Atarax Tablets & Syrup 1941
Marax Tablets & DF Syrup 1954
Vistaril Intramuscular Solution 1970
Hyoscyamine (May produce paralytic ileus). Products include:
Cystospaz Tablets 2395
Urised Tablets 2396
Hyoscyamine Sulfate (May produce paralytic ileus). Products include:
Arco-Lase Plus Tablets 607
Cystospaz-M Capsules 2395
Donnagel .... ▣ 675
Donnagel-PG 1858
Donnatal 1858
Donnatal Extentabs 1859
Donnatal Tablets 1858
Donnazyme Tablets 1860
Kutrase Capsules 2146

Levsin/Levsinex 2147
Ru-Tuss Tablets 693

Ipratropium Bromide (May produce paralytic ileus). Products include:
Atrovent Inhalation Aerosol 675

Isoflurane (Additive CNS depression). Products include:
Forane 600

Ketamine Hydrochloride (Additive CNS depression). Products include:
Ketalar 1726

Levorphanol Tartrate (Additive CNS depression). Products include:
Levo-Dromoran 1906

Lithium Carbonate (Additive CNS depression). Products include:
Eskalith 2214
Lithane Tablets 1596
Lithium Carbonate Capsules & Tablets 1984
Lithobid Tablets 870

Lithium Citrate (Additive CNS depression). Products include:
Cibalith-S 870

Lorazepam (Additive CNS depression). Products include:
Ativan Injection 2432
Ativan Tablets 2434

Loxapine Hydrochloride (Additive CNS depression). Products include:
Loxitane 1213

Loxapine Succinate (Additive CNS depression). Products include:
Loxitane Capsules 1213

Maprotiline Hydrochloride (May result in increased effects). Products include:
Ludiomil Tablets 874

Mepenzolate Bromide (May produce paralytic ileus). Products include:
Cantil Tablets 1326

Meperidine Hydrochloride (Additive CNS depression). Products include:
Demerol 2047
Mepergan Injection 2479

Mephobarbital (Additive CNS depression). Products include:
Mebaral Tablets 2061

Meprobamate (Additive CNS depression). Products include:
Deprol Tablets 2382
Equagesic Tablets 2451
Miltown Tablets 2386
PMB 200 and PMB 400 2504

Mesoridazine (Additive CNS depression). Products include:
Serentil 686

Methadone Hydrochloride (Additive CNS depression). Products include:
Dolophine Hydrochloride Ampoules & Vials 1260
Dolophine Hydrochloride Tablets 1261
Methadone Hydrochloride Diskets 1284
Methadone Hydrochloride Oral Solution & Tablets 1987

Methohexital Sodium (Additive CNS depression). Products include:
Brevital Sodium Vials 1248

Methoxyflurane (Additive CNS depression).
No products indexed under this heading.

Midazolam Hydrochloride (Additive CNS depression). Products include:
Versed Injection 1924

Molindone Hydrochloride (Additive CNS depression). Products include:
Moban Tablets & Concentrate 932

Morphine Sulfate (Additive CNS depression). Products include:
Astramorph/PF Injection, USP (Preservative-Free) 618
Duramorph 960
Infumorph 200 and Infumorph 500 Sterile Solutions 962
MS Contin Tablets 1814
MSIR 1817
Oramorph SR (Morphine Sulfate Sustained Release Tablets) 1988
Roxanol 1991

Opium Alkaloids (Additive CNS depression). Products include:
B & O No. 15A & No. 16A Supprettes 2395
Pantopon Injectable 1911

Oxazepam (Additive CNS depression). Products include:
Serax Capsules 2522
Serax Tablets 2522

Oxybutynin Chloride (May produce paralytic ileus). Products include:
Ditropan 1332

Oxycodone Hydrochloride (Additive CNS depression). Products include:
Percocet Tablets 950
Percodan 951
Roxicodone Tablets, Oral Solution & Intensol (Oxycodone) 1992
Tylox Capsules 1382

Oxyphenonium Bromide (May produce paralytic ileus).

Pentobarbital Sodium (Additive CNS depression). Products include:
Nembutal Sodium Capsules 534
Nembutal Sodium Solution 536
Nembutal Sodium Suppositories 538

Perphenazine (Additive CNS depression). Products include:
Etrafon 2087
Triavil Tablets 1556
Trilafon 2123

Phenobarbital (Additive CNS depression). Products include:
Arco-Lase Plus Tablets 607
Bellergal-S Tablets 1998
Bronkolixir ..... ▣ 761
Bronkotabs Tablets ..... ▣ 762
Donnatal 1858
Donnatal Extentabs 1859
Donnatal Tablets 1858
Donnazyme Tablets 1860
Kinesed Tablets 2272
Phenobarbital Elixir and Tablets 1293
Primatene Tablets-P Formula 2421
Quadrinal Tablets 1183
Tedral SA 1765

Pimozide (Additive CNS depression). Products include:
Orap Tablets 1020

Prazepam (Additive CNS depression). Products include:
Centrax 1693

Prochlorperazine (Additive CNS depression). Products include:
Compazine 2201

Procyclidine Hydrochloride (May produce paralytic ileus). Products include:
Kemadrin Tablets 771

Promethazine Hydrochloride (Additive CNS depression). Products include:
Mepergan Injection 2479
Phenergan with Codeine 2497
Phenergan with Dextromethorphan 2499
Phenergan Injection 2493
Phenergan Suppositories 2496
Phenergan Syrup 2495
Phenergan Tablets 2496
Phenergan VC 2500
Phenergan VC with Codeine 2501

Propantheline Bromide (May produce paralytic ileus). Products include:
Pro-Banthine Tablets 2141

Propofol (Additive CNS depression). Products include:
Diprivan Injection 2267

Propoxyphene Hydrochloride (Additive CNS depression). Products include:
Darvon 1256
Wygesic Tablets 2540

Propoxyphene Napsylate (Additive CNS depression). Products include:
Darvon-N/Darvocet-N 1254

Quazepam (Additive CNS depression). Products include:
Doral Tablets 2383

Scopolamine Hydrobromide (May produce paralytic ileus). Products include:
Donnagel ..... ▣ 675
Donnagel-PG 1858
Donnatal 1858
Donnatal Extentabs 1859
Donnatal Tablets 1858
Donnazyme Tablets 1860
Isopto Hyoscine ..... ◉ 222
Murocoll-2 Sterile Ophthalmic Solution ..... ◉ 261
Ru-Tuss Tablets 693

Scopolamine Preparations (May produce paralytic ileus). Products include:
Transderm Scōp Transdermal Therapeutic System 887

Secobarbital Sodium (Additive CNS depression). Products include:
Seconal Sodium Pulvules 1296

Sufentanil Citrate (Additive CNS depression). Products include:
Sufenta Injection 1147

Temazepam (Additive CNS depression). Products include:
Restoril Capsules 2023

Thiamylal Sodium (Additive CNS depression). Products include:
Surital Ampoules, Steri-Vials 1764

Thioridazine Hydrochloride (Additive CNS depression). Products include:
Mellaril 2011

Thiothixene (Additive CNS depression). Products include:
Navane Capsules and Concentrate 1954
Navane Intramuscular 1956

Triazolam (Additive CNS depression). Products include:
Halcion Tablets 2340

Tridihexethyl Chloride (May produce paralytic ileus).
No products indexed under this heading.

Trifluoperazine Hydrochloride (Additive CNS depression). Products include:
Stelazine 2226

Trihexyphenidyl Hydrochloride (May produce paralytic ileus). Products include:
Artane 1195

TYLENOL WITH CODEINE PHOSPHATE TABLETS
(Acetaminophen, Codeine Phosphate) 1381
See **Tylenol with Codeine Phosphate Elixir**

CHILDREN'S TYLENOL COLD LIQUID FORMULA AND CHEWABLE TABLETS
(Acetaminophen, Chlorpheniramine Maleate, Pseudoephedrine Hydrochloride) 1368
May interact with antidepressant drugs and antihypertensives. Compounds in these categories include:

Acebutolol Hydrochloride (Concurrent administration is recommended under the advice and supervision of a physician). Products include:
Sectral Capsules 2520

Amitriptyline Hydrochloride (Concurrent administration is recommended under the advice and supervision of a physician). Products include:
Elavil 2269
Endep Tablets 1927
Etrafon 2087
Limbitrol 1933
Triavil Tablets 1556

Amoxapine (Concurrent administration is recommended under the advice and supervision of a physician). Products include:
Asendin Tablets 1196

Atenolol (Concurrent administration is recommended under the advice and supervision of a physician). Products include:
Tenoretic Tablets 1105
Tenormin Tablets and I.V. Injection 1107

Benazepril Hydrochloride (Concurrent administration is recommended under the advice and supervision of a physician). Products include:
Lotensin Tablets 872

Betaxolol Hydrochloride (Concurrent administration is recommended under the advice and supervision of a physician). Products include:
Betoptic Sterile Ophthalmic Solution 569
Betoptic S Sterile Ophthalmic Suspension 570
Kerlone Tablets 2172

Bupropion Hydrochloride (Concurrent administration is recommended under the advice and supervision of a physician). Products include:
Wellbutrin Tablets 821

Captopril (Concurrent administration is recommended under the advice and supervision of a physician). Products include:
Capoten 2255
Capozide 2258

Carteolol Hydrochloride (Concurrent administration is recommended under the advice and supervision of a physician). Products include:
Cartrol Tablets 507

Clonidine (Concurrent administration is recommended under the advice and supervision of a physician). Products include:
Catapres-TTS 677

Clonidine Hydrochloride (Concurrent administration is recommended under the advice and supervision of a physician). Products include:
Catapres Tablets 676
Combipres Tablets 678

Deserpidine (Concurrent administration is recommended under the advice and supervision of a physician). Products include:
Enduronyl 518
Harmonyl Tablets 528
Oreticyl 545

Desipramine Hydrochloride (Concurrent administration is recommended under the advice and supervision of a physician). Products include:
Norpramin Tablets 1340

Diazoxide (Concurrent administration is recommended under the advice and supervision of a physician). Products include:
Hyperstat I.V. Injection 2095
Proglycem 649

Doxazosin Mesylate (Concurrent administration is recommended under the advice and supervision of a physician). Products include:
Cardura Tablets ... 1941
Doxepin Hydrochloride (Concurrent administration is recommended under the advice and supervision of a physician). Products include:
Sinequan ... 1960
Enalapril Maleate (Concurrent administration is recommended under the advice and supervision of a physician). Products include:
Vaseretic Tablets ... 1559
Vasotec Tablets ... 1564
Enalaprilat (Concurrent administration is recommended under the advice and supervision of a physician). Products include:
Vasotec I.V. ... 1562
Esmolol Hydrochloride (Concurrent administration is recommended under the advice and supervision of a physician). Products include:
Brevibloc Injection ... 942
Felodipine (Concurrent administration is recommended under the advice and supervision of a physician). Products include:
Plendil Extended-Release Tablets ... 1526
Fluoxetine Hydrochloride (Concurrent administration is recommended under the advice and supervision of a physician). Products include:
Prozac Pulvules ... 920
Fosinopril Sodium (Concurrent administration is recommended under the advice and supervision of a physician). Products include:
Monopril Tablets ... 1406
Guanabenz Acetate (Concurrent administration is recommended under the advice and supervision of a physician). Products include:
Wytensin Tablets ... 2542
Guanethidine Monosulfate (Concurrent administration is recommended under the advice and supervision of a physician). Products include:
Esimil Tablets ... 864
Ismelin Tablets ... 869
Hydralazine Hydrochloride (Concurrent administration is recommended under the advice and supervision of a physician). Products include:
Apresazide Capsules ... 854
Apresoline Hydrochloride Parenteral (Ampuls) ... 856
Apresoline Hydrochloride Tablets .. 855
Apresoline-Esidrix Tablets ... 857
Ser-Ap-Es Tablets ... 881
Serpasil-Apresoline Tablets ... 884
Imipramine Hydrochloride (Concurrent administration is recommended under the advice and supervision of a physician). Products include:
Tofranil Ampuls ... 1038
Tofranil Tablets ... 1039
Imipramine Pamoate (Concurrent administration is recommended under the advice and supervision of a physician). Products include:
Tofranil-PM Capsules ... 1041
Indapamide (Concurrent administration is recommended under the advice and supervision of a physician). Products include:
Lozol Tablets ... 1843
Isocarboxazid (Concurrent administration is recommended under the advice and supervision of a physician). Products include:
Marplan Tablets ... 1906
Isradipine (Concurrent administration is recommended under the advice and supervision of a physician). Products include:
DynaCirc Capsules ... 2004
Labetalol Hydrochloride (Concurrent administration is recommended under the advice and supervision of a physician). Products include:
Normodyne Injection ... 2108
Normodyne Tablets ... 2110
Normozide Tablets ... 2112
Trandate HCT Tablets ... 579
Trandate Injection ... 577
Trandate Tablets ... 579
Lisinopril (Concurrent administration is recommended under the advice and supervision of a physician). Products include:
Prinivil Tablets ... 1538
Prinzide Tablets ... 1540
Zestoretic ... 2274
Zestril Tablets ... 2277
Maprotiline Hydrochloride (Concurrent administration is recommended under the advice and supervision of a physician). Products include:
Ludiomil Tablets ... 874
Mecamylamine Hydrochloride (Concurrent administration is recommended under the advice and supervision of a physician). Products include:
Inversine Tablets ... 1492
Methyldopa (Concurrent administration is recommended under the advice and supervision of a physician). Products include:
Aldoclor Tablets ... 1413
Aldomet Oral ... 1415
Aldoril Tablets ... 1418
Methyldopate Hydrochloride (Concurrent administration is recommended under the advice and supervision of a physician). Products include:
Aldomet Ester HCl Injection ... 1417
Metoprolol Tartrate (Concurrent administration is recommended under the advice and supervision of a physician). Products include:
Lopressor Ampuls ... 1032
Lopressor HCT Tablets ... 1034
Lopressor Tablets ... 1032
Metyrosine (Concurrent administration is recommended under the advice and supervision of a physician). Products include:
Demser Capsules ... 1460
Minoxidil (Concurrent administration is recommended under the advice and supervision of a physician). Products include:
Loniten Tablets ... 2346
Rogaine Topical Solution ... 2357
Nadolol (Concurrent administration is recommended under the advice and supervision of a physician). Products include:
Corgard Tablets ... 701
Corzide Tablets ... 702
Nicardipine Hydrochloride (Concurrent administration is recommended under the advice and supervision of a physician). Products include:
Cardene Capsules ... 2290
Nitroglycerin (Concurrent administration is recommended under the advice and supervision of a physician). Products include:
Deponit NTG Transdermal Delivery System ... 2143
Minitran Transdermal Delivery System ... 1312
Nitro-Bid Ointment ... 1339
Nitro-Bid Capsules ... 1338
Nitrodisc ... 2176
Nitro-Dur (nitroglycerin) Transdermal Infusion System ... 1164
Nitrogard Tablets ... 1004
Nitrolingual Spray ... 1846
Nitrostat Tablets ... 1743
Transderm-Nitro Transdermal Therapeutic System ... 2283
Nortriptyline Hydrochloride (Concurrent administration is recommended under the advice and supervision of a physician). Products include:
Pamelor ... 2019
Penbutolol Sulfate (Concurrent administration is recommended under the advice and supervision of a physician). Products include:
Levatol ... 1832
Phenelzine Sulfate (Concurrent administration is recommended under the advice and supervision of a physician). Products include:
Nardil ... 1742
Phenoxybenzamine Hydrochloride (Concurrent administration is recommended under the advice and supervision of a physician). Products include:
Dibenzyline Capsules ... 2207
Phentolamine Mesylate (Concurrent administration is recommended under the advice and supervision of a physician). Products include:
Regitine ... 878
Pindolol (Concurrent administration is recommended under the advice and supervision of a physician). Products include:
Visken Tablets ... 2036
Prazosin Hydrochloride (Concurrent administration is recommended under the advice and supervision of a physician). Products include:
Minipress Capsules ... 1778
Minizide Capsules ... 1779
Propranolol Hydrochloride (Concurrent administration is recommended under the advice and supervision of a physician). Products include:
Inderal ... 2459
Inderal LA Long Acting Capsules ... 2461
Inderide Tablets ... 2463
Inderide LA Long Acting Capsules .. 2465
Protriptyline Hydrochloride (Concurrent administration is recommended under the advice and supervision of a physician). Products include:
Vivactil Tablets ... 1567
Ramipril (Concurrent administration is recommended under the advice and supervision of a physician). Products include:
Altace Capsules ... 1086
Rauwolfia Serpentina (Concurrent administration is recommended under the advice and supervision of a physician). Products include:
Raudixin Tablets ... 1803
Rauzide Tablets ... 1804
Rescinnamine (Concurrent administration is recommended under the advice and supervision of a physician).
No products indexed under this heading.
Reserpine (Concurrent administration is recommended under the advice and supervision of a physician). Products include:
Diupres Tablets ... 1461
Hydromox R Tablets ... 1209
Hydropres Tablets ... 1485
Renese-R Tablets ... 1786
Salutensin/Salutensin-Demi ... 719
Ser-Ap-Es Tablets ... 881
Serpasil Tablets ... 883
Serpasil-Apresoline Tablets ... 884
Serpasil-Esidrix Tablets ... 886
Sodium Nitroprusside (Concurrent administration is recommended under the advice and supervision of a physician). Products include:
Nipride I.V. Infusion ... 1909
Terazosin Hydrochloride (Concurrent administration is recommended under the advice and supervision of a physician). Products include:
Hytrin Tablets ... 529
Timolol Maleate (Concurrent administration is recommended under the advice and supervision of a physician). Products include:
Blocadren Tablets ... 1429
Timolide Tablets ... 1547
Timoptic in Ocudose ... 1552
Timoptic Sterile Ophthalmic Solution ... 1550
Tranylcypromine Sulfate (Concurrent administration is recommended under the advice and supervision of a physician). Products include:
Parnate Tablets ... 2222
Trazodone Hydrochloride (Concurrent administration is recommended under the advice and supervision of a physician). Products include:
Desyrel and Desyrel Dividose ... 1404
Trimethaphan Camsylate (Concurrent administration is recommended under the advice and supervision of a physician). Products include:
Arfonad Ampuls ... 1887
Trimipramine Maleate (Concurrent administration is recommended under the advice and supervision of a physician). Products include:
Surmontil Capsules ... 2524

TYLENOL COLD & FLU HOT MEDICATION, PACKETS
(Acetaminophen, Chlorpheniramine Maleate, Pseudoephedrine Hydrochloride, Dextromethorphan Hydrobromide) ... 1369
May interact with antihypertensives, antidepressant drugs, and certain other agents. Compounds in these categories include:

Acebutolol Hydrochloride (Effect not specified). Products include:
Sectral Capsules ... 2520
Alcohol (Increases drowsiness effect).
Amitriptyline Hydrochloride (Effect not specified). Products include:
Elavil ... 2269
Endep Tablets ... 1927
Etrafon ... 2087
Limbitrol ... 1933
Triavil Tablets ... 1556
Amoxapine (Effect not specified). Products include:
Asendin Tablets ... 1196
Atenolol (Effect not specified). Products include:
Tenoretic Tablets ... 1105
Tenormin Tablets and I.V. Injection 1107
Benazepril Hydrochloride (Effect not specified). Products include:
Lotensin Tablets ... 872
Betaxolol Hydrochloride (Effect not specified). Products include:
Betoptic Sterile Ophthalmic Solution ... 569
Betoptic S Sterile Ophthalmic Suspension ... 570
Kerlone Tablets ... 2172
Bupropion Hydrochloride (Effect not specified). Products include:
Wellbutrin Tablets ... 821

Captopril (Effect not specified). Products include:
Capoten 2255
Capozide 2258
Carteolol Hydrochloride (Effect not specified). Products include:
Cartrol Tablets 507
Clonidine (Effect not specified). Products include:
Catapres-TTS........ 677
Clonidine Hydrochloride (Effect not specified). Products include:
Catapres Tablets 676
Combipres Tablets 678
Deserpidine (Effect not specified). Products include:
Enduronyl 518
Harmonyl Tablets 528
Oreticyl........ 545
Desipramine Hydrochloride (Effect not specified). Products include:
Norpramin Tablets 1340
Diazoxide (Effect not specified). Products include:
Hyperstat I.V. Injection 2095
Proglycem........ 649
Doxazosin Mesylate (Effect not specified). Products include:
Cardura Tablets 1941
Doxepin Hydrochloride (Effect not specified). Products include:
Sinequan 1960
Enalapril Maleate (Effect not specified). Products include:
Vaseretic Tablets 1559
Vasotec Tablets 1564
Enalaprilat (Effect not specified). Products include:
Vasotec I.V........ 1562
Esmolol Hydrochloride (Effect not specified). Products include:
Brevibloc Injection........ 942
Felodipine (Effect not specified). Products include:
Plendil Extended-Release Tablets.... 1526
Fluoxetine Hydrochloride (Effect not specified). Products include:
Prozac Pulvules 920
Fosinopril Sodium (Effect not specified). Products include:
Monopril Tablets 1406
Guanabenz Acetate (Effect not specified). Products include:
Wytensin Tablets 2542
Guanethidine Monosulfate (Effect not specified). Products include:
Esimil Tablets 864
Ismelin Tablets 869
Hydralazine Hydrochloride (Effect not specified). Products include:
Apresazide Capsules 854
Apresoline Hydrochloride Parenteral (Ampuls)........ 856
Apresoline Hydrochloride Tablets .. 855
Apresoline-Esidrix Tablets........ 857
Ser-Ap-Es Tablets 881
Serpasil-Apresoline Tablets........ 884
Imipramine Hydrochloride (Effect not specified). Products include:
Tofranil Ampuls 1038
Tofranil Tablets 1039
Imipramine Pamoate (Effect not specified). Products include:
Tofranil-PM Capsules........ 1041
Isocarboxazid (Effect not specified). Products include:
Marplan Tablets........ 1906
Isradipine (Effect not specified). Products include:
DynaCirc Capsules 2004
Labetalol Hydrochloride (Effect not specified). Products include:
Normodyne Injection 2108
Normodyne Tablets 2110
Normozide Tablets 2112
Trandate HCT Tablets........ 579
Trandate Injection 577
Trandate Tablets 579
Lisinopril (Effect not specified). Products include:
Prinivil Tablets 1538
Prinzide Tablets 1540
Zestoretic 2274
Zestril Tablets........ 2277
Maprotiline Hydrochloride (Effect not specified). Products include:
Ludiomil Tablets........ 874
Mecamylamine Hydrochloride (Effect not specified). Products include:
Inversine Tablets 1492
Methyldopa (Effect not specified). Products include:
Aldoclor Tablets........ 1413
Aldomet Oral 1415
Aldoril Tablets........ 1418
Methyldopate Hydrochloride (Effect not specified). Products include:
Aldomet Ester HCl Injection 1417
Metoprolol Tartrate (Effect not specified). Products include:
Lopressor Ampuls........ 1032
Lopressor HCT Tablets........ 1034
Lopressor Tablets 1032
Metyrosine (Effect not specified). Products include:
Demser Capsules........ 1460
Minoxidil (Effect not specified). Products include:
Loniten Tablets........ 2346
Rogaine Topical Solution 2357
Nadolol (Effect not specified). Products include:
Corgard Tablets 701
Corzide Tablets 702
Nicardipine Hydrochloride (Effect not specified). Products include:
Cardene Capsules 2290
Nitroglycerin (Effect not specified). Products include:
Deponit NTG Transdermal Delivery System 2143
Minitran Transdermal Delivery System 1312
Nitro-Bid Ointment 1339
Nitro-Bid Capsules 1338
Nitrodisc 2176
Nitro-Dur (nitroglycerin) Transdermal Infusion System 1164
Nitrogard Tablets........ 1004
Nitrolingual Spray 1846
Nitrostat Tablets 1743
Transderm-Nitro Transdermal Therapeutic System 2283
Nortriptyline Hydrochloride (Effect not specified). Products include:
Pamelor 2019
Penbutolol Sulfate (Effect not specified). Products include:
Levatol 1832
Phenelzine Sulfate (Effect not specified). Products include:
Nardil 1742
Phenoxybenzamine Hydrochloride (Effect not specified). Products include:
Dibenzyline Capsules........ 2207
Phentolamine Mesylate (Effect not specified). Products include:
Regitine 878
Pindolol (Effect not specified). Products include:
Visken Tablets........ 2036
Prazosin Hydrochloride (Effect not specified). Products include:
Minipress Capsules........ 1778
Minizide Capsules 1779
Propranolol Hydrochloride (Effect not specified). Products include:
Inderal 2459
Inderal LA Long Acting Capsules 2461
Inderide Tablets 2463
Inderide LA Long Acting Capsules .. 2465
Protriptyline Hydrochloride (Effect not specified). Products include:
Vivactil Tablets 1567
Ramipril (Effect not specified). Products include:
Altace Capsules 1086
Rauwolfia Serpentina (Effect not specified). Products include:
Raudixin Tablets........ 1803
Rauzide Tablets 1804
Rescinnamine (Effect not specified).
No products indexed under this heading.
Reserpine (Effect not specified). Products include:
Diupres Tablets 1461
Hydromox R Tablets........ 1209
Hydropres Tablets........ 1485
Renese-R Tablets........ 1786
Salutensin/Salutensin-Demi 719
Ser-Ap-Es Tablets 881
Serpasil Tablets 883
Serpasil-Apresoline Tablets........ 884
Serpasil-Esidrix Tablets........ 886
Sodium Nitroprusside (Effect not specified). Products include:
Nipride I.V. Infusion 1909
Terazosin Hydrochloride (Effect not specified). Products include:
Hytrin Tablets 529
Timolol Maleate (Effect not specified). Products include:
Blocadren Tablets 1429
Timolide Tablets........ 1547
Timoptic in Ocudose 1552
Timoptic Sterile Ophthalmic Solution........ 1550
Tranylcypromine Sulfate (Effect not specified). Products include:
Parnate Tablets 2222
Trazodone Hydrochloride (Effect not specified). Products include:
Desyrel and Desyrel Dividose........ 1404
Trimethaphan Camsylate (Effect not specified). Products include:
Arfonad Ampuls........ 1887
Trimipramine Maleate (Effect not specified). Products include:
Surmontil Capsules........ 2524

TYLENOL COLD & FLU NO DROWSINESS HOT MEDICATION, PACKETS
(Acetaminophen, Dextromethorphan Hydrobromide, Pseudoephedrine Hydrochloride) 1371
May interact with antihypertensives, antidepressant drugs, and certain other agents. Compounds in these categories include:

Acebutolol Hydrochloride (Effect not specified). Products include:
Sectral Capsules 2520
Alcohol (May increase drowsiness effect).
Amitriptyline Hydrochloride (Effect not specified). Products include:
Elavil 2269
Endep Tablets 1927
Etrafon 2087
Limbitrol 1933
Triavil Tablets 1556
Amoxapine (Effect not specified). Products include:
Asendin Tablets 1196
Atenolol (Effect not specified). Products include:
Tenoretic Tablets........ 1105
Tenormin Tablets and I.V. Injection 1107
Benazepril Hydrochloride (Effect not specified). Products include:
Lotensin Tablets........ 872
Betaxolol Hydrochloride (Effect not specified). Products include:
Betoptic Sterile Ophthalmic Solution........ 569
Betoptic S Sterile Ophthalmic Suspension........ 570
Kerlone Tablets........ 2172
Bupropion Hydrochloride (Effect not specified). Products include:
Wellbutrin Tablets 821
Captopril (Effect not specified). Products include:
Capoten 2255
Capozide 2258
Carteolol Hydrochloride (Effect not specified). Products include:
Cartrol Tablets 507
Clonidine (Effect not specified). Products include:
Catapres-TTS........ 677
Clonidine Hydrochloride (Effect not specified). Products include:
Catapres Tablets 676
Combipres Tablets 678
Deserpidine (Effect not specified). Products include:
Enduronyl 518
Harmonyl Tablets 528
Oreticyl........ 545
Desipramine Hydrochloride (Effect not specified). Products include:
Norpramin Tablets 1340
Diazoxide (Effect not specified). Products include:
Hyperstat I.V. Injection 2095
Proglycem........ 649
Doxazosin Mesylate (Effect not specified). Products include:
Cardura Tablets 1941
Doxepin Hydrochloride (Effect not specified). Products include:
Sinequan 1960
Enalapril Maleate (Effect not specified). Products include:
Vaseretic Tablets 1559
Vasotec Tablets 1564
Enalaprilat (Effect not specified). Products include:
Vasotec I.V........ 1562
Esmolol Hydrochloride (Effect not specified). Products include:
Brevibloc Injection........ 942
Felodipine (Effect not specified). Products include:
Plendil Extended-Release Tablets.... 1526
Fluoxetine Hydrochloride (Effect not specified). Products include:
Prozac Pulvules 920
Fosinopril Sodium (Effect not specified). Products include:
Monopril Tablets 1406
Guanabenz Acetate (Effect not specified). Products include:
Wytensin Tablets 2542
Guanethidine Monosulfate (Effect not specified). Products include:
Esimil Tablets 864
Ismelin Tablets 869
Hydralazine Hydrochloride (Effect not specified). Products include:
Apresazide Capsules 854
Apresoline Hydrochloride Parenteral (Ampuls)........ 856
Apresoline Hydrochloride Tablets .. 855
Apresoline-Esidrix Tablets........ 857
Ser-Ap-Es Tablets 881
Serpasil-Apresoline Tablets........ 884
Imipramine Hydrochloride (Effect not specified). Products include:
Tofranil Ampuls 1038
Tofranil Tablets 1039
Imipramine Pamoate (Effect not specified). Products include:
Tofranil-PM Capsules........ 1041
Indapamide (Effect not specified). Products include:
Lozol Tablets........ 1843
Isocarboxazid (Effect not specified). Products include:
Marplan Tablets 1906

Isradipine (Effect not specified). Products include:
DynaCirc Capsules ... 2004
Labetalol Hydrochloride (Effect not specified). Products include:
Normodyne Injection ... 2108
Normodyne Tablets ... 2110
Normozide Tablets ... 2112
Trandate HCT Tablets ... 579
Trandate Injection ... 577
Trandate Tablets ... 579
Lisinopril (Effect not specified). Products include:
Prinivil Tablets ... 1538
Prinzide Tablets ... 1540
Zestoretic ... 2274
Zestril Tablets ... 2277
Maprotiline Hydrochloride (Effect not specified). Products include:
Ludiomil Tablets ... 874
Mecamylamine Hydrochloride (Effect not specified). Products include:
Inversine Tablets ... 1492
Methyldopa (Effect not specified). Products include:
Aldoclor Tablets ... 1413
Aldomet Oral ... 1415
Aldoril Tablets ... 1418
Metoprolol Tartrate (Effect not specified). Products include:
Lopressor Ampuls ... 1032
Lopressor HCT Tablets ... 1034
Lopressor Tablets ... 1032
Metyrosine (Effect not specified). Products include:
Demser Capsules ... 1460
Minoxidil (Effect not specified). Products include:
Loniten Tablets ... 2346
Rogaine Topical Solution ... 2357
Nadolol (Effect not specified). Products include:
Corgard Tablets ... 701
Corzide Tablets ... 702
Nicardipine Hydrochloride (Effect not specified). Products include:
Cardene Capsules ... 2290
Nitroglycerin (Effect not specified). Products include:
Deponit NTG Transdermal Delivery System ... 2143
Minitran Transdermal Delivery System ... 1312
Nitro-Bid Ointment ... 1339
Nitro-Bid Capsules ... 1338
Nitrodisc ... 2176
Nitro-Dur (nitroglycerin) Transdermal Infusion System ... 1164
Nitrogard Tablets ... 1004
Nitrolingual Spray ... 1846
Nitrostat Tablets ... 1743
Transderm-Nitro Transdermal Therapeutic System ... 2283
Nortriptyline Hydrochloride (Effect not specified). Products include:
Pamelor ... 2019
Penbutolol Sulfate (Effect not specified). Products include:
Levatol ... 1832
Phenelzine Sulfate (Effect not specified). Products include:
Nardil ... 1742
Phenoxybenzamine Hydrochloride (Effect not specified). Products include:
Dibenzyline Capsules ... 2207
Phentolamine Mesylate (Effect not specified). Products include:
Regitine ... 878
Pindolol (Effect not specified). Products include:
Visken Tablets ... 2036
Prazosin Hydrochloride (Effect not specified). Products include:
Minipress Capsules ... 1778
Minizide Capsules ... 1779
Propranolol Hydrochloride (Effect not specified). Products include:
Inderal ... 2459
Inderal LA Long Acting Capsules ... 2461
Inderide Tablets ... 2463
Inderide LA Long Acting Capsules ... 2465
Protriptyline Hydrochloride (Effect not specified). Products include:
Vivactil Tablets ... 1567
Ramipril (Effect not specified). Products include:
Altace Capsules ... 1086
Rauwolfia Serpentina (Effect not specified). Products include:
Raudixin Tablets ... 1803
Rauzide Tablets ... 1804
Rescinnamine (Effect not specified).
No products indexed under this heading.
Reserpine (Effect not specified). Products include:
Diupres Tablets ... 1461
Hydromox R Tablets ... 1209
Hydropres Tablets ... 1485
Renese-R Tablets ... 1786
Salutensin/Salutensin-Demi ... 719
Ser-Ap-Es Tablets ... 881
Serpasil Tablets ... 883
Serpasil-Apresoline Tablets ... 884
Serpasil-Esidrix Tablets ... 886
Sodium Nitroprusside (Effect not specified). Products include:
Nipride I.V. Infusion ... 1909
Terazosin Hydrochloride (Effect not specified). Products include:
Hytrin Tablets ... 529
Timolol Maleate (Effect not specified). Products include:
Blocadren Tablets ... 1429
Timolide Tablets ... 1547
Timoptic in Ocudose ... 1552
Timoptic Sterile Ophthalmic Solution ... 1550
Tranylcypromine Sulfate (Effect not specified). Products include:
Parnate Tablets ... 2222
Trazodone Hydrochloride (Effect not specified). Products include:
Desyrel and Desyrel Dividose ... 1404
Trimethaphan Camsylate (Effect not specified). Products include:
Arfonad Ampuls ... 1887
Trimipramine Maleate (Effect not specified). Products include:
Surmontil Capsules ... 2524

TYLENOL COLD MEDICATION CAPLETS AND TABLETS
(Acetaminophen, Chlorpheniramine Maleate, Pseudoephedrine Hydrochloride, Dextromethorphan Hydrobromide) ... 1370
May interact with antidepressant drugs, antihypertensives, and certain other agents. Compounds in these categories include:

Acebutolol Hydrochloride (Concurrent use is not recommended unless directed by a physician). Products include:
Sectral Capsules ... 2520
Alcohol (May increase drowsiness).
Amitriptyline Hydrochloride (Concurrent use is not recommended unless directed by a physician). Products include:
Elavil ... 2269
Endep Tablets ... 1927
Etrafon ... 2087
Limbitrol ... 1933
Triavil Tablets ... 1556
Amoxapine (Concurrent use is not recommended unless directed by a physician). Products include:
Asendin Tablets ... 1196
Atenolol (Concurrent use is not recommended unless directed by a physician). Products include:
Tenoretic Tablets ... 1105
Tenormin Tablets and I.V. Injection 1107
Benazepril Hydrochloride (Concurrent use is not recommended unless directed by a physician). Products include:
Lotensin Tablets ... 872
Betaxolol Hydrochloride (Concurrent use is not recommended unless directed by a physician). Products include:
Betoptic Sterile Ophthalmic Solution ... 569
Betoptic S Sterile Ophthalmic Suspension ... 570
Kerlone Tablets ... 2172
Bupropion Hydrochloride (Concurrent use is not recommended unless directed by a physician). Products include:
Wellbutrin Tablets ... 821
Captopril (Concurrent use is not recommended unless directed by a physician). Products include:
Capoten ... 2255
Capozide ... 2258
Carteolol Hydrochloride (Concurrent use is not recommended unless directed by a physician). Products include:
Cartrol Tablets ... 507
Clonidine (Concurrent use is not recommended unless directed by a physician). Products include:
Catapres-TTS ... 677
Clonidine Hydrochloride (Concurrent use is not recommended unless directed by a physician). Products include:
Catapres Tablets ... 676
Combipres Tablets ... 678
Deserpidine (Concurrent use is not recommended unless directed by a physician). Products include:
Enduronyl ... 518
Harmonyl Tablets ... 528
Oreticyl ... 545
Desipramine Hydrochloride (Concurrent use is not recommended unless directed by a physician). Products include:
Norpramin Tablets ... 1340
Diazoxide (Concurrent use is not recommended unless directed by a physician). Products include:
Hyperstat I.V. Injection ... 2095
Proglycem ... 649
Doxazosin Mesylate (Concurrent use is not recommended unless directed by a physician). Products include:
Cardura Tablets ... 1941
Doxepin Hydrochloride (Concurrent use is not recommended unless directed by a physician). Products include:
Sinequan ... 1960
Enalapril Maleate (Concurrent use is not recommended unless directed by a physician). Products include:
Vaseretic Tablets ... 1559
Vasotec Tablets ... 1564
Enalaprilat (Concurrent use is not recommended unless directed by a physician). Products include:
Vasotec I.V. ... 1562
Esmolol Hydrochloride (Concurrent use is not recommended unless directed by a physician). Products include:
Brevibloc Injection ... 942
Felodipine (Concurrent use is not recommended unless directed by a physician). Products include:
Plendil Extended-Release Tablets ... 1526
Fluoxetine Hydrochloride (Concurrent use is not recommended unless directed by a physician). Products include:
Prozac Pulvules ... 920
Fosinopril Sodium (Concurrent use is not recommended unless directed by a physician). Products include:
Monopril Tablets ... 1406
Guanabenz Acetate (Concurrent use is not recommended unless directed by a physician). Products include:
Wytensin Tablets ... 2542
Guanethidine Monosulfate (Concurrent use is not recommended unless directed by a physician). Products include:
Esimil Tablets ... 864
Ismelin Tablets ... 869
Hydralazine Hydrochloride (Concurrent use is not recommended unless directed by a physician). Products include:
Apresazide Capsules ... 854
Apresoline Hydrochloride Parenteral (Ampuls) ... 856
Apresoline Hydrochloride Tablets ... 855
Apresoline-Esidrix Tablets ... 857
Ser-Ap-Es Tablets ... 881
Serpasil-Apresoline Tablets ... 884
Imipramine Hydrochloride (Concurrent use is not recommended unless directed by a physician). Products include:
Tofranil Ampuls ... 1038
Tofranil Tablets ... 1039
Imipramine Pamoate (Concurrent use is not recommended unless directed by a physician). Products include:
Tofranil-PM Capsules ... 1041
Isocarboxazid (Concurrent use is not recommended unless directed by a physician). Products include:
Marplan Tablets ... 1906
Isradipine (Concurrent use is not recommended unless directed by a physician). Products include:
DynaCirc Capsules ... 2004
Labetalol Hydrochloride (Concurrent use is not recommended unless directed by a physician). Products include:
Normodyne Injection ... 2108
Normodyne Tablets ... 2110
Normozide Tablets ... 2112
Trandate HCT Tablets ... 579
Trandate Injection ... 577
Trandate Tablets ... 579
Lisinopril (Concurrent use is not recommended unless directed by a physician). Products include:
Prinivil Tablets ... 1538
Prinzide Tablets ... 1540
Zestoretic ... 2274
Zestril Tablets ... 2277
Maprotiline Hydrochloride (Concurrent use is not recommended unless directed by a physician). Products include:
Ludiomil Tablets ... 874
Mecamylamine Hydrochloride (Concurrent use is not recommended unless directed by a physician). Products include:
Inversine Tablets ... 1492
Methyclothiazide (Concurrent use is not recommended unless directed by a physician). Products include:
Enduron Tablets ... 517
Enduronyl ... 518

Methyldopa (Concurrent use is not recommended unless directed by a physician). Products include:
Aldoclor Tablets ... 1413
Aldomet Oral ... 1415
Aldoril Tablets ... 1418
Methyldopate Hydrochloride (Concurrent use is not recommended unless directed by a physician). Products include:
Aldomet Ester HCl Injection ... 1417
Metoprolol Tartrate (Concurrent use is not recommended unless directed by a physician). Products include:
Lopressor Ampuls ... 1032
Lopressor HCT Tablets ... 1034
Lopressor Tablets ... 1032
Metyrosine (Concurrent use is not recommended unless directed by a physician). Products include:
Demser Capsules ... 1460
Minoxidil (Concurrent use is not recommended unless directed by a physician). Products include:
Loniten Tablets ... 2346
Rogaine Topical Solution ... 2357
Nadolol (Concurrent use is not recommended unless directed by a physician). Products include:
Corgard Tablets ... 701
Corzide Tablets ... 702
Nicardipine Hydrochloride (Concurrent use is not recommended unless directed by a physician). Products include:
Cardene Capsules ... 2290
Nitroglycerin (Concurrent use is not recommended unless directed by a physician). Products include:
Deponit NTG Transdermal Delivery System ... 2143
Minitran Transdermal Delivery System ... 1312
Nitro-Bid Ointment ... 1339
Nitro-Bid Capsules ... 1338
Nitrodisc ... 2176
Nitro-Dur (nitroglycerin) Transdermal Infusion System ... 1164
Nitrogard Tablets ... 1004
Nitrolingual Spray ... 1846
Nitrostat Tablets ... 1743
Transderm-Nitro Transdermal Therapeutic System ... 2283
Nortriptyline Hydrochloride (Concurrent use is not recommended unless directed by a physician). Products include:
Pamelor ... 2019
Penbutolol Sulfate (Concurrent use is not recommended unless directed by a physician). Products include:
Levatol ... 1832
Phenelzine Sulfate (Concurrent use is not recommended unless directed by a physician). Products include:
Nardil ... 1742
Phenoxybenzamine Hydrochloride (Concurrent use is not recommended unless directed by a physician). Products include:
Dibenzyline Capsules ... 2207
Phentolamine Mesylate (Concurrent use is not recommended unless directed by a physician). Products include:
Regitine ... 878
Pindolol (Concurrent use is not recommended unless directed by a physician). Products include:
Visken Tablets ... 2036
Polythiazide (Concurrent use is not recommended unless directed by a physician). Products include:
Minizide Capsules ... 1779
Renese Tablets ... 1785
Renese-R Tablets ... 1786
Prazosin Hydrochloride (Concurrent use is not recommended unless directed by a physician). Products include:
Minipress Capsules ... 1778
Minizide Capsules ... 1779
Propranolol Hydrochloride (Concurrent use is not recommended unless directed by a physician). Products include:
Inderal ... 2459
Inderal LA Long Acting Capsules ... 2461
Inderide Tablets ... 2463
Inderide LA Long Acting Capsules .. 2465
Protriptyline Hydrochloride (Concurrent use is not recommended unless directed by a physician). Products include:
Vivactil Tablets ... 1567
Ramipril (Concurrent use is not recommended unless directed by a physician). Products include:
Altace Capsules ... 1086
Rauwolfia Serpentina (Concurrent use is not recommended unless directed by a physician). Products include:
Raudixin Tablets ... 1803
Rauzide Tablets ... 1804
Rescinnamine (Concurrent use is not recommended unless directed by a physician).
No products indexed under this heading.
Reserpine (Concurrent use is not recommended unless directed by a physician). Products include:
Diupres Tablets ... 1461
Hydromox R Tablets ... 1209
Hydropres Tablets ... 1485
Renese-R Tablets ... 1786
Salutensin/Salutensin-Demi ... 719
Ser-Ap-Es Tablets ... 881
Serpasil Tablets ... 883
Serpasil-Apresoline Tablets ... 884
Serpasil-Esidrix Tablets ... 886
Sodium Nitroprusside (Concurrent use is not recommended unless directed by a physician). Products include:
Nipride I.V. Infusion ... 1909
Terazosin Hydrochloride (Concurrent use is not recommended unless directed by a physician). Products include:
Hytrin Tablets ... 529
Timolol Maleate (Concurrent use is not recommended unless directed by a physician). Products include:
Blocadren Tablets ... 1429
Timolide Tablets ... 1547
Timoptic in Ocudose ... 1552
Timoptic Sterile Ophthalmic Solution ... 1550
Tranylcypromine Sulfate (Concurrent use is not recommended unless directed by a physician). Products include:
Parnate Tablets ... 2222
Trazodone Hydrochloride (Concurrent use is not recommended unless directed by a physician). Products include:
Desyrel and Desyrel Dividose ... 1404
Trimethaphan Camsylate (Concurrent use is not recommended unless directed by a physician). Products include:
Arfonad Ampuls ... 1887
Trimipramine Maleate (Concurrent use is not recommended unless directed by a physician). Products include:
Surmontil Capsules ... 2524

TYLENOL COLD MEDICATION, EFFERVESCENT TABLETS
(Acetaminophen, Phenylpropanolamine Hydrochloride, Chlorpheniramine Maleate) ... 1369
May interact with antihypertensives, antidepressant drugs, and certain other agents. Compounds in these categories include:
Acebutolol Hydrochloride (Effect not specified). Products include:
Sectral Capsules ... 2520
Alcohol (Increases drowsiness effect).
Amitriptyline Hydrochloride (Effect not specified). Products include:
Elavil ... 2269
Endep Tablets ... 1927
Etrafon ... 2087
Limbitrol ... 1933
Triavil Tablets ... 1556
Amoxapine (Effect not specified). Products include:
Asendin Tablets ... 1196
Atenolol (Effect not specified). Products include:
Tenoretic Tablets ... 1105
Tenormin Tablets and I.V. Injection 1107
Benazepril Hydrochloride (Effect not specified). Products include:
Lotensin Tablets ... 872
Betaxolol Hydrochloride (Effect not specified). Products include:
Betoptic Sterile Ophthalmic Solution ... 569
Betoptic S Sterile Ophthalmic Suspension ... 570
Kerlone Tablets ... 2172
Bupropion Hydrochloride (Effect not specified). Products include:
Wellbutrin Tablets ... 821
Captopril (Effect not specified). Products include:
Capoten ... 2255
Capozide ... 2258
Carteolol Hydrochloride (Effect not specified). Products include:
Cartrol Tablets ... 507
Clonidine (Effect not specified). Products include:
Catapres-TTS ... 677
Clonidine Hydrochloride (Effect not specified). Products include:
Catapres Tablets ... 676
Combipres Tablets ... 678
Deserpidine (Effect not specified). Products include:
Enduronyl ... 518
Harmonyl Tablets ... 528
Oreticyl ... 545
Desipramine Hydrochloride (Effect not specified). Products include:
Norpramin Tablets ... 1340
Diazoxide (Effect not specified). Products include:
Hyperstat I.V. Injection ... 2095
Proglycem ... 649
Doxazosin Mesylate (Effect not specified). Products include:
Cardura Tablets ... 1941
Doxepin Hydrochloride (Effect not specified). Products include:
Sinequan ... 1960
Enalapril Maleate (Effect not specified). Products include:
Vaseretic Tablets ... 1559
Vasotec Tablets ... 1564
Enalaprilat (Effect not specified). Products include:
Vasotec I.V. ... 1562
Esmolol Hydrochloride (Effect not specified). Products include:
Brevibloc Injection ... 942
Felodipine (Effect not specified). Products include:
Plendil Extended-Release Tablets ... 1526
Fluoxetine Hydrochloride (Effect not specified). Products include:
Prozac Pulvules ... 920
Fosinopril Sodium (Effect not specified). Products include:
Monopril Tablets ... 1406
Guanabenz Acetate (Effect not specified). Products include:
Wytensin Tablets ... 2542
Guanethidine Monosulfate (Effect not specified). Products include:
Esimil Tablets ... 864
Ismelin Tablets ... 869
Hydralazine Hydrochloride (Effect not specified). Products include:
Apresazide Capsules ... 854
Apresoline Hydrochloride Parenteral (Ampuls) ... 856
Apresoline Hydrochloride Tablets .. 855
Apresoline-Esidrix Tablets ... 857
Ser-Ap-Es Tablets ... 881
Serpasil-Apresoline Tablets ... 884
Imipramine Hydrochloride (Effect not specified). Products include:
Tofranil Ampuls ... 1038
Tofranil Tablets ... 1039
Imipramine Pamoate (Effect not specified). Products include:
Tofranil-PM Capsules ... 1041
Isocarboxazid (Effect not specified). Products include:
Marplan Tablets ... 1906
Isradipine (Effect not specified). Products include:
DynaCirc Capsules ... 2004
Labetalol Hydrochloride (Effect not specified). Products include:
Normodyne Injection ... 2108
Normodyne Tablets ... 2110
Normozide Tablets ... 2112
Trandate HCT Tablets ... 579
Trandate Injection ... 577
Trandate Tablets ... 579
Lisinopril (Effect not specified). Products include:
Prinivil Tablets ... 1538
Prinzide Tablets ... 1540
Zestoretic ... 2274
Zestril Tablets ... 2277
Maprotiline Hydrochloride (Effect not specified). Products include:
Ludiomil Tablets ... 874
Mecamylamine Hydrochloride (Effect not specified). Products include:
Inversine Tablets ... 1492
Methyldopa (Effect not specified). Products include:
Aldoclor Tablets ... 1413
Aldomet Oral ... 1415
Aldoril Tablets ... 1418
Methyldopate Hydrochloride (Effect not specified). Products include:
Aldomet Ester HCl Injection ... 1417
Metoprolol Tartrate (Effect not specified). Products include:
Lopressor Ampuls ... 1032
Lopressor HCT Tablets ... 1034
Lopressor Tablets ... 1032
Metyrosine (Effect not specified). Products include:
Demser Capsules ... 1460
Minoxidil (Effect not specified). Products include:
Loniten Tablets ... 2346
Rogaine Topical Solution ... 2357
Nadolol (Effect not specified). Products include:
Corgard Tablets ... 701
Corzide Tablets ... 702
Nicardipine Hydrochloride (Effect not specified). Products include:
Cardene Capsules ... 2290

Nitroglycerin (Effect not specified). Products include:
- Deponit NTG Transdermal Delivery System ... 2143
- Minitran Transdermal Delivery System ... 1312
- Nitro-Bid Ointment ... 1339
- Nitro-Bid Capsules ... 1338
- Nitrodisc ... 2176
- Nitro-Dur (nitroglycerin) Transdermal Infusion System ... 1164
- Nitrogard Tablets ... 1004
- Nitrolingual Spray ... 1846
- Nitrostat Tablets ... 1743
- Transderm-Nitro Transdermal Therapeutic System ... 2283

Nortriptyline Hydrochloride (Effect not specified). Products include:
- Pamelor ... 2019

Penbutolol Sulfate (Effect not specified). Products include:
- Levatol ... 1832

Phenelzine Sulfate (Effect not specified). Products include:
- Nardil ... 1742

Phenoxybenzamine Hydrochloride (Effect not specified). Products include:
- Dibenzyline Capsules ... 2207

Phentolamine Mesylate (Effect not specified). Products include:
- Regitine ... 878

Pindolol (Effect not specified). Products include:
- Visken Tablets ... 2036

Prazosin Hydrochloride (Effect not specified). Products include:
- Minipress Capsules ... 1778
- Minizide Capsules ... 1779

Propranolol Hydrochloride (Effect not specified). Products include:
- Inderal ... 2459
- Inderal LA Long Acting Capsules ... 2461
- Inderide Tablets ... 2463
- Inderide LA Long Acting Capsules .. 2465

Protriptyline Hydrochloride (Effect not specified). Products include:
- Vivactil Tablets ... 1567

Ramipril (Effect not specified). Products include:
- Altace Capsules ... 1086

Rauwolfia Serpentina (Effect not specified). Products include:
- Raudixin Tablets ... 1803
- Rauzide Tablets ... 1804

Rescinnamine (Effect not specified).
- No products indexed under this heading.

Reserpine (Effect not specified). Products include:
- Diupres Tablets ... 1461
- Hydromox R Tablets ... 1209
- Hydropres Tablets ... 1485
- Renese-R Tablets ... 1786
- Salutensin/Salutensin-Demi ... 719
- Ser-Ap-Es Tablets ... 881
- Serpasil Tablets ... 883
- Serpasil-Apresoline Tablets ... 884
- Serpasil-Esidrix Tablets ... 886

Sodium Nitroprusside (Effect not specified). Products include:
- Nipride I.V. Infusion ... 1909

Terazosin Hydrochloride (Effect not specified). Products include:
- Hytrin Tablets ... 529

Timolol Maleate (Effect not specified). Products include:
- Blocadren Tablets ... 1429
- Timolide Tablets ... 1547
- Timoptic in Ocudose ... 1552
- Timoptic Sterile Ophthalmic Solution ... 1550

Tranylcypromine Sulfate (Effect not specified). Products include:
- Parnate Tablets ... 2222

Trazodone Hydrochloride (Effect not specified). Products include:
- Desyrel and Desyrel Dividose ... 1404

Trimethaphan Camsylate (Effect not specified). Products include:
- Arfonad Ampuls ... 1887

Trimipramine Maleate (Effect not specified). Products include:
- Surmontil Capsules ... 2524

TYLENOL COLD MEDICATION NO DROWSINESS FORMULA CAPLETS

(Acetaminophen, Pseudoephedrine Hydrochloride, Dextromethorphan Hydrobromide) ... 1370

May interact with antidepressant drugs, antihypertensives, and certain other agents. Compounds in these categories include:

Acebutolol Hydrochloride (Concurrent use is not recommended unless directed by a physician). Products include:
- Sectral Capsules ... 2520

Alcohol (Effects not specified).

Amitriptyline Hydrochloride (Concurrent use is not recommended unless directed by a physician). Products include:
- Elavil ... 2269
- Endep Tablets ... 1927
- Etrafon ... 2087
- Limbitrol ... 1933
- Triavil Tablets ... 1556

Amoxapine (Concurrent use is not recommended unless directed by a physician). Products include:
- Asendin Tablets ... 1196

Atenolol (Concurrent use is not recommended unless directed by a physician). Products include:
- Tenoretic Tablets ... 1105
- Tenormin Tablets and I.V. Injection 1107

Benazepril Hydrochloride (Concurrent use is not recommended unless directed by a physician). Products include:
- Lotensin Tablets ... 872

Betaxolol Hydrochloride (Concurrent use is not recommended unless directed by a physician). Products include:
- Betoptic Sterile Ophthalmic Solution ... 569
- Betoptic S Sterile Ophthalmic Suspension ... 570
- Kerlone Tablets ... 2172

Bupropion Hydrochloride (Concurrent use is not recommended unless directed by a physician). Products include:
- Wellbutrin Tablets ... 821

Captopril (Concurrent use is not recommended unless directed by a physician). Products include:
- Capoten ... 2255
- Capozide ... 2258

Carteolol Hydrochloride (Concurrent use is not recommended unless directed by a physician). Products include:
- Cartrol Tablets ... 507

Clonidine (Concurrent use is not recommended unless directed by a physician). Products include:
- Catapres-TTS ... 677

Clonidine Hydrochloride (Concurrent use is not recommended unless directed by a physician). Products include:
- Catapres Tablets ... 676
- Combipres Tablets ... 678

Deserpidine (Concurrent use is not recommended unless directed by a physician). Products include:
- Enduronyl ... 518
- Harmonyl Tablets ... 528
- Oreticyl ... 545

Desipramine Hydrochloride (Concurrent use is not recommended unless directed by a physician). Products include:
- Norpramin Tablets ... 1340

Diazoxide (Concurrent use is not recommended unless directed by a physician). Products include:
- Hyperstat I.V. Injection ... 2095
- Proglycem ... 649

Doxazosin Mesylate (Concurrent use is not recommended unless directed by a physician). Products include:
- Cardura Tablets ... 1941

Doxepin Hydrochloride (Concurrent use is not recommended unless directed by a physician). Products include:
- Sinequan ... 1960

Enalapril Maleate (Concurrent use is not recommended unless directed by a physician). Products include:
- Vaseretic Tablets ... 1559
- Vasotec Tablets ... 1564

Enalaprilat (Concurrent use is not recommended unless directed by a physician). Products include:
- Vasotec I.V. ... 1562

Esmolol Hydrochloride (Concurrent use is not recommended unless directed by a physician). Products include:
- Brevibloc Injection ... 942

Felodipine (Concurrent use is not recommended unless directed by a physician). Products include:
- Plendil Extended-Release Tablets ... 1526

Fluoxetine Hydrochloride (Concurrent use is not recommended unless directed by a physician). Products include:
- Prozac Pulvules ... 920

Fosinopril Sodium (Concurrent use is not recommended unless directed by a physician). Products include:
- Monopril Tablets ... 1406

Guanabenz Acetate (Concurrent use is not recommended unless directed by a physician). Products include:
- Wytensin Tablets ... 2542

Guanethidine Monosulfate (Concurrent use is not recommended unless directed by a physician). Products include:
- Esimil Tablets ... 864
- Ismelin Tablets ... 869

Hydralazine Hydrochloride (Concurrent use is not recommended unless directed by a physician). Products include:
- Apresazide Capsules ... 854
- Apresoline Hydrochloride Parenteral (Ampuls) ... 856
- Apresoline Hydrochloride Tablets .. 855
- Apresoline-Esidrix Tablets ... 857
- Ser-Ap-Es Tablets ... 881
- Serpasil-Apresoline Tablets ... 884

Imipramine Hydrochloride (Concurrent use is not recommended unless directed by a physician). Products include:
- Tofranil Ampuls ... 1038
- Tofranil Tablets ... 1039

Imipramine Pamoate (Concurrent use is not recommended unless directed by a physician). Products include:
- Tofranil-PM Capsules ... 1041

Isocarboxazid (Concurrent use is not recommended unless directed by a physician). Products include:
- Marplan Tablets ... 1906

Isradipine (Concurrent use is not recommended unless directed by a physician). Products include:
- DynaCirc Capsules ... 2004

Labetalol Hydrochloride (Concurrent use is not recommended unless directed by a physician). Products include:
- Normodyne Injection ... 2108
- Normodyne Tablets ... 2110
- Normozide Tablets ... 2112
- Trandate HCT Tablets ... 579
- Trandate Injection ... 577
- Trandate Tablets ... 579

Lisinopril (Concurrent use is not recommended unless directed by a physician). Products include:
- Prinivil Tablets ... 1538
- Prinzide Tablets ... 1540
- Zestoretic ... 2274
- Zestril Tablets ... 2277

Maprotiline Hydrochloride (Concurrent use is not recommended unless directed by a physician). Products include:
- Ludiomil Tablets ... 874

Mecamylamine Hydrochloride (Concurrent use is not recommended unless directed by a physician). Products include:
- Inversine Tablets ... 1492

Methyldopa (Concurrent use is not recommended unless directed by a physician). Products include:
- Aldoclor Tablets ... 1413
- Aldomet Oral ... 1415
- Aldoril Tablets ... 1418

Methyldopate Hydrochloride (Concurrent use is not recommended unless directed by a physician). Products include:
- Aldomet Ester HCl Injection ... 1417

Metoprolol Tartrate (Concurrent use is not recommended unless directed by a physician). Products include:
- Lopressor Ampuls ... 1032
- Lopressor HCT Tablets ... 1034
- Lopressor Tablets ... 1032

Metyrosine (Concurrent use is not recommended unless directed by a physician). Products include:
- Demser Capsules ... 1460

Minoxidil (Concurrent use is not recommended unless directed by a physician). Products include:
- Loniten Tablets ... 2346
- Rogaine Topical Solution ... 2357

Nadolol (Concurrent use is not recommended unless directed by a physician). Products include:
- Corgard Tablets ... 701
- Corzide Tablets ... 702

Nicardipine Hydrochloride (Concurrent use is not recommended unless directed by a physician). Products include:
- Cardene Capsules ... 2290

Nitroglycerin (Concurrent use is not recommended unless directed by a physician). Products include:
- Deponit NTG Transdermal Delivery System ... 2143
- Minitran Transdermal Delivery System ... 1312
- Nitro-Bid Ointment ... 1339
- Nitro-Bid Capsules ... 1338
- Nitrodisc ... 2176
- Nitro-Dur (nitroglycerin) Transdermal Infusion System ... 1164
- Nitrogard Tablets ... 1004
- Nitrolingual Spray ... 1846
- Nitrostat Tablets ... 1743
- Transderm-Nitro Transdermal Therapeutic System ... 2283

Nortriptyline Hydrochloride (Concurrent use is not recommended unless directed by a physician). Products include:
- Pamelor ... 2019

Penbutolol Sulfate (Concurrent use is not recommended unless directed by a physician). Products include:
- Levatol 1832

Phenelzine Sulfate (Concurrent use is not recommended unless directed by a physician). Products include:
- Nardil 1742

Phenoxybenzamine Hydrochloride (Concurrent use is not recommended unless directed by a physician). Products include:
- Dibenzyline Capsules 2207

Phentolamine Mesylate (Concurrent use is not recommended unless directed by a physician). Products include:
- Regitine 878

Pindolol (Concurrent use is not recommended unless directed by a physician). Products include:
- Visken Tablets 2036

Prazosin Hydrochloride (Concurrent use is not recommended unless directed by a physician). Products include:
- Minipress Capsules 1778
- Minizide Capsules 1779

Propranolol Hydrochloride (Concurrent use is not recommended unless directed by a physician). Products include:
- Inderal 2459
- Inderal LA Long Acting Capsules 2461
- Inderide Tablets 2463
- Inderide LA Long Acting Capsules .. 2465

Protriptyline Hydrochloride (Concurrent use is not recommended unless directed by a physician). Products include:
- Vivactil Tablets 1567

Ramipril (Concurrent use is not recommended unless directed by a physician). Products include:
- Altace Capsules 1086

Rauwolfia Serpentina (Concurrent use is not recommended unless directed by a physician). Products include:
- Raudixin Tablets 1803
- Rauzide Tablets 1804

Rescinnamine (Concurrent use is not recommended unless directed by a physician).
- No products indexed under this heading.

Reserpine (Concurrent use is not recommended unless directed by a physician). Products include:
- Diupres Tablets 1461
- Hydromox R Tablets 1209
- Hydropres Tablets 1485
- Renese-R Tablets 1786
- Salutensin/Salutensin-Demi 719
- Ser-Ap-Es Tablets 881
- Serpasil Tablets 883
- Serpasil-Apresoline Tablets 884
- Serpasil-Esidrix Tablets 886

Sodium Nitroprusside (Concurrent use is not recommended unless directed by a physician). Products include:
- Nipride I.V. Infusion 1909

Terazosin Hydrochloride (Concurrent use is not recommended unless directed by a physician). Products include:
- Hytrin Tablets 529

Timolol Maleate (Concurrent use is not recommended unless directed by a physician). Products include:
- Blocadren Tablets 1429
- Timolide Tablets 1547
- Timoptic in Ocudose 1552
- Timoptic Sterile Ophthalmic Solution 1550

Tranylcypromine Sulfate (Concurrent use is not recommended unless directed by a physician). Products include:
- Parnate Tablets 2222

Trazodone Hydrochloride (Concurrent use is not recommended unless directed by a physician). Products include:
- Desyrel and Desyrel Dividose 1404

Trimethaphan Camsylate (Concurrent use is not recommended unless directed by a physician). Products include:
- Arfonad Ampuls 1887

Trimipramine Maleate (Concurrent use is not recommended unless directed by a physician). Products include:
- Surmontil Capsules 2524

TYLENOL COLD NIGHT TIME MEDICATION LIQUID
(Acetaminophen, Chlorpheniramine Maleate, Pseudoephedrine Hydrochloride, Dextromethorphan Hydrobromide) 1371
May interact with antidepressant drugs, antihypertensives, hypnotics and sedatives, tranquilizers, and certain other agents. Compounds in these categories include:

Acebutolol Hydrochloride (Concurrent use is not recommended unless directed by a physician). Products include:
- Sectral Capsules 2520

Alcohol (May increase drowsiness).

Alprazolam (Increases drowsiness effect). Products include:
- Xanax Tablets 2367

Amitriptyline Hydrochloride (Concurrent use is not recommended unless directed by a physician). Products include:
- Elavil 2269
- Endep Tablets 1927
- Etrafon 2087
- Limbitrol 1933
- Triavil Tablets 1556

Amoxapine (Concurrent use is not recommended unless directed by a physician). Products include:
- Asendin Tablets 1196

Atenolol (Concurrent use is not recommended unless directed by a physician). Products include:
- Tenoretic Tablets 1105
- Tenormin Tablets and I.V. Injection 1107

Benazepril Hydrochloride (Concurrent use is not recommended unless directed by a physician). Products include:
- Lotensin Tablets 872

Betaxolol Hydrochloride (Concurrent use is not recommended unless directed by a physician). Products include:
- Betoptic Sterile Ophthalmic Solution 569
- Betoptic S Sterile Ophthalmic Suspension 570
- Kerlone Tablets 2172

Bupropion Hydrochloride (Concurrent use is not recommended unless directed by a physician). Products include:
- Wellbutrin Tablets 821

Buspirone Hydrochloride (Increases drowsiness effect). Products include:
- BuSpar 1401

Captopril (Concurrent use is not recommended unless directed by a physician). Products include:
- Capoten 2255
- Capozide 2258

Carteolol Hydrochloride (Concurrent use is not recommended unless directed by a physician). Products include:
- Cartrol Tablets 507

Chlordiazepoxide (Increases drowsiness effect). Products include:
- Libritabs Tablets 1930
- Limbitrol 1933
- Menrium Tablets 1934

Chlordiazepoxide Hydrochloride (Increases drowsiness effect). Products include:
- Librax Capsules 1929
- Librium Capsules 1931
- Librium Injectable 1932

Chlorpromazine (Increases drowsiness effect). Products include:
- Thorazine 2234

Chlorprothixene (Increases drowsiness effect). Products include:
- Taractan Tablets 1920

Chlorprothixene Hydrochloride (Increases drowsiness effect). Products include:
- Taractan 1920

Clonidine (Concurrent use is not recommended unless directed by a physician). Products include:
- Catapres-TTS 677

Clonidine Hydrochloride (Concurrent use is not recommended unless directed by a physician). Products include:
- Catapres Tablets 676
- Combipres Tablets 678

Clorazepate Dipotassium (Increases drowsiness effect). Products include:
- Tranxene 556

Deserpidine (Concurrent use is not recommended unless directed by a physician). Products include:
- Enduronyl 518
- Harmonyl Tablets 528
- Oreticyl 545

Desipramine Hydrochloride (Concurrent use is not recommended unless directed by a physician). Products include:
- Norpramin Tablets 1340

Diazepam (Increases drowsiness effect). Products include:
- Valium Injectable 1937
- Valium Tablets 1939
- Valrelease Capsules 1923

Diazoxide (Concurrent use is not recommended unless directed by a physician). Products include:
- Hyperstat I.V. Injection 2095
- Proglycem 649

Doxazosin Mesylate (Concurrent use is not recommended unless directed by a physician). Products include:
- Cardura Tablets 1941

Doxepin Hydrochloride (Concurrent use is not recommended unless directed by a physician). Products include:
- Sinequan 1960

Droperidol (Increases drowsiness effect). Products include:
- Inapsine Injection 1140
- Innovar Injection 1141

Enalapril Maleate (Concurrent use is not recommended unless directed by a physician). Products include:
- Vaseretic Tablets 1559
- Vasotec Tablets 1564

Enalaprilat (Concurrent use is not recommended unless directed by a physician). Products include:
- Vasotec I.V. 1562

Esmolol Hydrochloride (Concurrent use is not recommended unless directed by a physician). Products include:
- Brevibloc Injection 942

Estazolam (Increases drowsiness effect). Products include:
- ProSom Tablets 554

Ethchlorvynol (Increases drowsiness effect). Products include:
- Placidyl Capsules 553

Ethinamate (Increases drowsiness effect).
- No products indexed under this heading.

Felodipine (Concurrent use is not recommended unless directed by a physician). Products include:
- Plendil Extended-Release Tablets 1526

Fluoxetine Hydrochloride (Concurrent use is not recommended unless directed by a physician). Products include:
- Prozac Pulvules 920

Fluphenazine Decanoate (Increases drowsiness effect). Products include:
- Prolixin Decanoate 1795

Fluphenazine Enanthate (Increases drowsiness effect). Products include:
- Prolixin Enanthate 1796

Fluphenazine Hydrochloride (Increases drowsiness effect). Products include:
- Prolixin Elixir 1793
- Prolixin Injection 1791
- Prolixin Oral Concentrate 1792
- Prolixin Tablets 1793

Flurazepam Hydrochloride (Increases drowsiness effect). Products include:
- Dalmane Capsules 1927

Fosinopril Sodium (Concurrent use is not recommended unless directed by a physician). Products include:
- Monopril Tablets 1406

Glutethimide (Increases drowsiness effect).
- No products indexed under this heading.

Guanabenz Acetate (Concurrent use is not recommended unless directed by a physician). Products include:
- Wytensin Tablets 2542

Guanethidine Monosulfate (Concurrent use is not recommended unless directed by a physician). Products include:
- Esimil Tablets 864
- Ismelin Tablets 869

Haloperidol (Increases drowsiness effect). Products include:
- Haldol Injection, Tablets and Concentrate 1373

Haloperidol Decanoate (Increases drowsiness effect). Products include:
- Haldol Decanoate 1375

Hydralazine Hydrochloride (Concurrent use is not recommended unless directed by a physician). Products include:
- Apresazide Capsules 854
- Apresoline Hydrochloride Parenteral (Ampuls) 856
- Apresoline Hydrochloride Tablets .. 855
- Apresoline-Esidrix Tablets 857
- Ser-Ap-Es Tablets 881
- Serpasil-Apresoline Tablets 884

Hydroxyzine Hydrochloride (Increases drowsiness effect). Products include:
- Atarax Tablets & Syrup 1941
- Marax Tablets & DF Syrup 1954
- Vistaril Intramuscular Solution 1970

Imipramine Hydrochloride (Concurrent use is not recommended unless directed by a physician). Products include:
Tofranil Ampuls ... 1038
Tofranil Tablets ... 1039

Imipramine Pamoate (Concurrent use is not recommended unless directed by a physician). Products include:
Tofranil-PM Capsules ... 1041

Isocarboxazid (Concurrent use is not recommended unless directed by a physician). Products include:
Marplan Tablets ... 1906

Isradipine (Concurrent use is not recommended unless directed by a physician). Products include:
DynaCirc Capsules ... 2004

Labetalol Hydrochloride (Concurrent use is not recommended unless directed by a physician). Products include:
Normodyne Injection ... 2108
Normodyne Tablets ... 2110
Normozide Tablets ... 2112
Trandate HCT Tablets ... 579
Trandate Injection ... 577
Trandate Tablets ... 579

Lisinopril (Concurrent use is not recommended unless directed by a physician). Products include:
Prinivil Tablets ... 1538
Prinzide Tablets ... 1540
Zestoretic ... 2274
Zestril Tablets ... 2277

Lorazepam (Increases drowsiness effect). Products include:
Ativan Injection ... 2432
Ativan Tablets ... 2434

Loxapine Hydrochloride (Increases drowsiness effect). Products include:
Loxitane ... 1213

Loxapine Succinate (Increases drowsiness effect). Products include:
Loxitane Capsules ... 1213

Maprotiline Hydrochloride (Concurrent use is not recommended unless directed by a physician). Products include:
Ludiomil Tablets ... 874

Mecamylamine Hydrochloride (Concurrent use is not recommended unless directed by a physician). Products include:
Inversine Tablets ... 1492

Meprobamate (Increases drowsiness effect). Products include:
Deprol Tablets ... 2382
Equagesic Tablets ... 2451
Miltown Tablets ... 2386
PMB 200 and PMB 400 ... 2504

Mesoridazine Besylate (Increases drowsiness effect).

Methyldopa (Concurrent use is not recommended unless directed by a physician). Products include:
Aldoclor Tablets ... 1413
Aldomet Oral ... 1415
Aldoril Tablets ... 1418

Methyldopate Hydrochloride (Concurrent use is not recommended unless directed by a physician). Products include:
Aldomet Ester HCl Injection ... 1417

Metoprolol Tartrate (Concurrent use is not recommended unless directed by a physician). Products include:
Lopressor Ampuls ... 1032
Lopressor HCT Tablets ... 1034
Lopressor Tablets ... 1032

Metyrosine (Concurrent use is not recommended unless directed by a physician). Products include:
Demser Capsules ... 1460

Midazolam Hydrochloride (Increases drowsiness effect). Products include:
Versed Injection ... 1924

Minoxidil (Concurrent use is not recommended unless directed by a physician). Products include:
Loniten Tablets ... 2346
Rogaine Topical Solution ... 2357

Molindone Hydrochloride (Increases drowsiness effect). Products include:
Moban Tablets & Concentrate ... 932

Nadolol (Concurrent use is not recommended unless directed by a physician). Products include:
Corgard Tablets ... 701
Corzide Tablets ... 702

Nicardipine Hydrochloride (Concurrent use is not recommended unless directed by a physician). Products include:
Cardene Capsules ... 2290

Nitroglycerin (Concurrent use is not recommended unless directed by a physician). Products include:
Deponit NTG Transdermal Delivery System ... 2143
Minitran Transdermal Delivery System ... 1312
Nitro-Bid Ointment ... 1339
Nitro-Bid Capsules ... 1338
Nitrodisc ... 2176
Nitro-Dur (nitroglycerin) Transdermal Infusion System ... 1164
Nitrogard Tablets ... 1004
Nitrolingual Spray ... 1846
Nitrostat Tablets ... 1743
Transderm-Nitro Transdermal Therapeutic System ... 2283

Nortriptyline Hydrochloride (Concurrent use is not recommended unless directed by a physician). Products include:
Pamelor ... 2019

Oxazepam (Increases drowsiness effect). Products include:
Serax Capsules ... 2522
Serax Tablets ... 2522

Penbutolol Sulfate (Concurrent use is not recommended unless directed by a physician). Products include:
Levatol ... 1832

Perphenazine (Increases drowsiness effect). Products include:
Etrafon ... 2087
Triavil Tablets ... 1556
Trilafon ... 2123

Phenelzine Sulfate (Concurrent use is not recommended unless directed by a physician). Products include:
Nardil ... 1742

Phenoxybenzamine Hydrochloride (Concurrent use is not recommended unless directed by a physician). Products include:
Dibenzyline Capsules ... 2207

Phentolamine Mesylate (Concurrent use is not recommended unless directed by a physician). Products include:
Regitine ... 878

Pindolol (Concurrent use is not recommended unless directed by a physician). Products include:
Visken Tablets ... 2036

Prazepam (Increases drowsiness effect). Products include:
Centrax ... 1693

Prazosin Hydrochloride (Concurrent use is not recommended unless directed by a physician). Products include:
Minipress Capsules ... 1778
Minizide Capsules ... 1779

Prochlorperazine (Increases drowsiness effect). Products include:
Compazine ... 2201

Promethazine Hydrochloride (Increases drowsiness effect). Products include:
Mepergan Injection ... 2479
Phenergan with Codeine ... 2497
Phenergan with Dextromethorphan ... 2499
Phenergan Injection ... 2493
Phenergan Suppositories ... 2496
Phenergan Syrup ... 2495
Phenergan Tablets ... 2496
Phenergan VC ... 2500
Phenergan VC with Codeine ... 2501

Propofol (Increases drowsiness effect). Products include:
Diprivan Injection ... 2267

Propranolol Hydrochloride (Concurrent use is not recommended unless directed by a physician). Products include:
Inderal ... 2459
Inderal LA Long Acting Capsules ... 2461
Inderide Tablets ... 2463
Inderide LA Long Acting Capsules ... 2465

Protriptyline Hydrochloride (Concurrent use is not recommended unless directed by a physician). Products include:
Vivactil Tablets ... 1567

Quazepam (Increases drowsiness effect). Products include:
Doral Tablets ... 2383

Ramipril (Concurrent use is not recommended unless directed by a physician). Products include:
Altace Capsules ... 1086

Rauwolfia Serpentina (Concurrent use is not recommended unless directed by a physician). Products include:
Raudixin Tablets ... 1803
Rauzide Tablets ... 1804

Rescinnamine (Concurrent use is not recommended unless directed by a physician).
No products indexed under this heading.

Reserpine (Concurrent use is not recommended unless directed by a physician). Products include:
Diupres Tablets ... 1461
Hydromox R Tablets ... 1209
Hydropres Tablets ... 1485
Renese-R Tablets ... 1786
Salutensin/Salutensin-Demi ... 719
Ser-Ap-Es Tablets ... 881
Serpasil Tablets ... 883
Serpasil-Apresoline Tablets ... 884
Serpasil-Esidrix Tablets ... 886

Secobarbital Sodium (Increases drowsiness effect). Products include:
Seconal Sodium Pulvules ... 1296

Sodium Nitroprusside (Concurrent use is not recommended unless directed by a physician). Products include:
Nipride I.V. Infusion ... 1909

Temazepam (Increases drowsiness effect). Products include:
Restoril Capsules ... 2023

Terazosin Hydrochloride (Concurrent use is not recommended unless directed by a physician). Products include:
Hytrin Tablets ... 529

Thioridazine Hydrochloride (Increases drowsiness effect). Products include:
Mellaril ... 2011

Thiothixene (Increases drowsiness effect). Products include:
Navane Capsules and Concentrate ... 1954
Navane Intramuscular ... 1956

Timolol Maleate (Concurrent use is not recommended unless directed by a physician). Products include:
Blocadren Tablets ... 1429
Timolide Tablets ... 1547
Timoptic in Ocudose ... 1552
Timoptic Sterile Ophthalmic Solution ... 1550

Tranylcypromine Sulfate (Concurrent use is not recommended unless directed by a physician). Products include:
Parnate Tablets ... 2222

Trazodone Hydrochloride (Concurrent use is not recommended unless directed by a physician). Products include:
Desyrel and Desyrel Dividose ... 1404

Triazolam (Increases drowsiness effect). Products include:
Halcion Tablets ... 2340

Trifluoperazine Hydrochloride (Increases drowsiness effect). Products include:
Stelazine ... 2226

Trimethaphan Camsylate (Concurrent use is not recommended unless directed by a physician). Products include:
Arfonad Ampuls ... 1887

Trimipramine Maleate (Concurrent use is not recommended unless directed by a physician). Products include:
Surmontil Capsules ... 2524

TYLENOL COUGH MEDICATION LIQUID, MAXIMUM STRENGTH
(Dextromethorphan Hydrobromide, Acetaminophen) ... 1372
No interactions described in labeling.

TYLENOL COUGH MEDICATION LIQUID WITH DECONGESTANT, MAXIMUM STRENGTH
(Dextromethorphan Hydrobromide, Acetaminophen, Pseudoephedrine Hydrochloride) ... 1372
May interact with:

Antidepressant Medications, unspecified (Effect not specified).

Antihypertensive agents, unspecified (Effect not specified).

TYLENOL, EXTRA STRENGTH, ACETAMINOPHEN ADULT LIQUID PAIN RELIEVER
(Acetaminophen) ... 1367
No interactions described in labeling.

TYLENOL, EXTRA STRENGTH, ACETAMINOPHEN GELCAPS, CAPLETS, TABLETS
(Acetaminophen) ... 1367
No interactions described in labeling.

TYLENOL, INFANTS' DROPS
(Acetaminophen) ... 1366
No interactions described in labeling.

TYLENOL, JUNIOR STRENGTH, ACETAMINOPHEN COATED CAPLETS, GRAPE AND FRUIT CHEWABLE TABLETS
(Acetaminophen) ... 1366
No interactions described in labeling.

TYLENOL, MAXIMUM STRENGTH, SINUS MEDICATION GELCAPS, CAPLETS AND TABLETS
(Acetaminophen, Pseudoephedrine Hydrochloride) 1373
May interact with:

Antidepressant Medications, unspecified (Effect not specified).

Blood Pressure Medications, unspecified (Effect not specified).
No products indexed under this heading.

TYLENOL, REGULAR STRENGTH, ACETAMINOPHEN TABLETS AND CAPLETS
(Acetaminophen) 1367
No interactions described in labeling.

TYLENOL PM, EXTRA STRENGTH CAPLETS AND TABLETS
(Acetaminophen, Diphenhydramine Hydrochloride) 1368
May interact with hypnotics and sedatives, tranquilizers, and certain other agents. Compounds in these categories include:

Alcohol (Effect not specified).

Alprazolam (Effect not specified). Products include:
Xanax Tablets 2367

Buspirone Hydrochloride (Effect not specified). Products include:
BuSpar 1401

Chlordiazepoxide (Effect not specified). Products include:
Libritabs Tablets 1930
Limbitrol 1933
Menrium Tablets 1934

Chlordiazepoxide Hydrochloride (Effect not specified). Products include:
Librax Capsules 1929
Librium Capsules 1931
Librium Injectable 1932

Chlorpromazine (Effect not specified). Products include:
Thorazine 2234

Chlorprothixene (Effect not specified). Products include:
Taractan Tablets 1920

Chlorprothixene Hydrochloride (Effect not specified). Products include:
Taractan 1920

Clorazepate Dipotassium (Effect not specified). Products include:
Tranxene 556

Diazepam (Effect not specified). Products include:
Valium Injectable 1937
Valium Tablets 1939
Valrelease Capsules 1923

Droperidol (Effect not specified). Products include:
Inapsine Injection 1140
Innovar Injection 1141

Estazolam (Effect not specified). Products include:
ProSom Tablets 554

Ethchlorvynol (Effect not specified). Products include:
Placidyl Capsules 553

Ethinamate (Effect not specified).
No products indexed under this heading.

Fluphenazine Decanoate (Effect not specified). Products include:
Prolixin Decanoate 1795

Fluphenazine Enanthate (Effect not specified). Products include:
Prolixin Enanthate 1796

Fluphenazine Hydrochloride (Effect not specified). Products include:
Prolixin Elixir 1793
Prolixin Injection 1791
Prolixin Oral Concentrate 1792
Prolixin Tablets 1793

Flurazepam Hydrochloride (Effect not specified). Products include:
Dalmane Capsules 1927

Glutethimide (Effect not specified).
No products indexed under this heading.

Haloperidol (Effect not specified). Products include:
Haldol Injection, Tablets and Concentrate 1373

Haloperidol Decanoate (Effect not specified). Products include:
Haldol Decanoate 1375

Hydroxyzine Hydrochloride (Effect not specified). Products include:
Atarax Tablets & Syrup 1941
Marax Tablets & DF Syrup 1954
Vistaril Intramuscular Solution 1970

Lorazepam (Effect not specified). Products include:
Ativan Injection 2432
Ativan Tablets 2434

Loxapine Hydrochloride (Effect not specified). Products include:
Loxitane 1213

Loxapine Succinate (Effect not specified). Products include:
Loxitane Capsules 1213

Meprobamate (Effect not specified). Products include:
Deprol Tablets 2382
Equagesic Tablets 2451
Miltown Tablets 2386
PMB 200 and PMB 400 2504

Mesoridazine Besylate (Effect not specified).

Midazolam Hydrochloride (Effect not specified). Products include:
Versed Injection 1924

Molindone Hydrochloride (Effect not specified). Products include:
Moban Tablets & Concentrate 932

Oxazepam (Effect not specified). Products include:
Serax Capsules 2522
Serax Tablets 2522

Perphenazine (Effect not specified). Products include:
Etrafon 2087
Triavil Tablets 1556
Trilafon 2123

Prazepam (Effect not specified). Products include:
Centrax 1693

Prochlorperazine (Effect not specified). Products include:
Compazine 2201

Promethazine Hydrochloride (Effect not specified). Products include:
Mepergan Injection 2479
Phenergan with Codeine 2497
Phenergan with Dextromethorphan 2499
Phenergan Injection 2493
Phenergan Suppositories 2496
Phenergan Syrup 2495
Phenergan Tablets 2496
Phenergan VC 2500
Phenergan VC with Codeine 2501

Propofol (Effect not specified). Products include:
Diprivan Injection 2267

Quazepam (Effect not specified). Products include:
Doral Tablets 2383

Secobarbital Sodium (Effect not specified). Products include:
Seconal Sodium Pulvules 1296

Temazepam (Effect not specified). Products include:
Restoril Capsules 2023

Thioridazine Hydrochloride (Effect not specified). Products include:
Mellaril 2011

Thiothixene (Effect not specified). Products include:
Navane Capsules and Concentrate 1954
Navane Intramuscular 1956

Triazolam (Effect not specified). Products include:
Halcion Tablets 2340

Trifluoperazine Hydrochloride (Effect not specified). Products include:
Stelazine 2226

TYLOX CAPSULES
(Oxycodone Hydrochloride, Acetaminophen) 1382
May interact with anticholinergics, central nervous system depressants, neuromuscular blocking agents, narcotic analgesics, phenothiazines, general anesthetics, hypnotics and sedatives, tranquilizers, and certain other agents. Compounds in these categories include:

Alcohol (Additive CNS depression).

Alfentanil Hydrochloride (Additive CNS depression). Products include:
Alfenta Injection 1131

Alprazolam (Additive CNS depression). Products include:
Xanax Tablets 2367

Aprobarbital (Additive CNS depression). Products include:
Alurate Elixir 1883

Atropine Sulfate (May produce paralytic ileus). Products include:
Arco-Lase Plus Tablets 607
Atropine Sulfate Sterile Ophthalmic Solution and S.O.P. Sterile Ophthalmic Ointment ◉ 239
Donnagel ▣ 675
Donnagel-PG 1858
Donnatal 1858
Donnatal Extentabs 1859
Donnatal Tablets 1858
Donnazyme Tablets 1860
Isopto Atropine ◉ 218
Lomotil 2174
Motofen Tablets 836
Ru-Tuss Tablets 693
Urised Tablets 2396

Belladonna Alkaloids (May produce paralytic ileus). Products include:
Bellergal-S Tablets 1998
Hyland's Bed Wetting Tablets ▣ 728
Hyland's Teething Tablets ▣ 728
Kinesed Tablets 2272

Benztropine Mesylate (May produce paralytic ileus). Products include:
Cogentin 1435

Biperiden (May produce paralytic ileus). Products include:
Akineton 1171

Buprenorphine (Additive CNS depression).
No products indexed under this heading.

Buspirone Hydrochloride (Additive CNS depression). Products include:
BuSpar 1401

Butabarbital (Additive CNS depression). Products include:
Pyridium Plus 1764

Butalbital (Additive CNS depression). Products include:
Esgic-Plus Tablets 1002
Esgic Tablets & Capsules 1001
Fioricet Tablets 2006
Fiorinal Capsules 2007
Fiorinal with Codeine Capsules 2008
Fiorinal Tablets 2007
Phrenilin 838
Sedapap Tablets 50 mg/650 mg 1360

Chlordiazepoxide (Additive CNS depression). Products include:
Libritabs Tablets 1930
Limbitrol 1933
Menrium Tablets 1934

Chlordiazepoxide Hydrochloride (Additive CNS depression). Products include:
Librax Capsules 1929
Librium Capsules 1931
Librium Injectable 1932

Chlorpromazine (Additive CNS depression). Products include:
Thorazine 2234

Chlorprothixene (Additive CNS depression). Products include:
Taractan Tablets 1920

Chlorprothixene Hydrochloride (Additive CNS depression). Products include:
Taractan 1920

Chlorprothixene Lactate (Additive CNS depression). Products include:
Taractan Concentrate 1920

Clidinium Bromide (May produce paralytic ileus). Products include:
Librax Capsules 1929
Quarzan Capsules 1937

Clorazepate Dipotassium (Additive CNS depression). Products include:
Tranxene 556

Clozapine (Additive CNS depression). Products include:
Clozaril Tablets 2000

Codeine (Additive CNS depression). Products include:
Calcidrine Syrup 506

Codeine Phosphate (Additive CNS depression). Products include:
Actifed with Codeine Cough Syrup 752
Cheracol Cough Syrup 1853
Codimal PH Syrup 846
Dimetane-DC Cough Syrup 1857
Empirin with Codeine Phosphate Nos. 2, 3 & 4 764
Fiorinal with Codeine Capsules 2008
Isoclor Expectorant 982
Naldecon CX Adult Liquid ▣ 521
Novahistine DH 1342
Novahistine Expectorant 1343
Nucofed Capsules 2219
Nucofed Expectorant 2219
Nucofed Pediatric Expectorant 2220
Nucofed Syrup 2219
Phenaphen with Codeine Capsules 1865
Phenaphen-650 with Codeine Tablets 1866
Phenergan with Codeine 2497
Phenergan VC with Codeine 2501
Robitussin A-C Syrup 1875
Robitussin-DAC Syrup 1875
Ryna ▣ 741
Soma Compound w/Codeine Tablets 2390
Triaminic Expectorant w/Codeine 1996
Tussi-Organidin Liquid 2391
Tylenol with Codeine 1381

Codeine Polistirex (Additive CNS depression).
No products indexed under this heading.

Dezocine (Additive CNS depression).

Diazepam (Additive CNS depression). Products include:
Valium Injectable 1937
Valium Tablets 1939
Valrelease Capsules 1923

Dicyclomine Hydrochloride (May produce paralytic ileus). Products include:
Bentyl 1322

Droperidol (Additive CNS depression). Products include:
Inapsine Injection 1140
Innovar Injection 1141

Enflurane (Additive CNS depression). Products include:
Ethrane ... 599
Estazolam (Additive CNS depression). Products include:
ProSom Tablets ... 554
Ethchlorvynol (Additive CNS depression). Products include:
Placidyl Capsules ... 553
Ethinamate (Additive CNS depression).
No products indexed under this heading.
Fentanyl (Additive CNS depression). Products include:
Duragesic Transdermal System ... 1133
Fentanyl Citrate (Additive CNS depression). Products include:
Innovar Injection ... 1141
Sublimaze Injection ... 1146
Fluphenazine Decanoate (Additive CNS depression). Products include:
Prolixin Decanoate ... 1795
Fluphenazine Enanthate (Additive CNS depression). Products include:
Prolixin Enanthate ... 1796
Fluphenazine Hydrochloride (Additive CNS depression). Products include:
Prolixin Elixir ... 1793
Prolixin Injection ... 1791
Prolixin Oral Concentrate ... 1792
Prolixin Tablets ... 1793
Flurazepam Hydrochloride (Additive CNS depression). Products include:
Dalmane Capsules ... 1927
Glutethimide (Additive CNS depression).
No products indexed under this heading.
Glycopyrrolate (May produce paralytic ileus). Products include:
Robinul Forte Tablets ... 1873
Robinul Injectable ... 1873
Robinul Tablets ... 1873
Haloperidol (Additive CNS depression). Products include:
Haldol Injection, Tablets and Concentrate ... 1373
Haloperidol Decanoate (Additive CNS depression). Products include:
Haldol Decanoate ... 1375
Hydrocodone Bitartrate (Additive CNS depression). Products include:
Anexsia 5/500 Tablets ... 2196
Anexsia 7.5/650 Tablets ... 2197
Azdone Tablets ... 844
Codiclear DH Syrup ... 845
Codimal DH Syrup ... 846
Damason-P ... 1356
Hycodan Syrup, Tablets ... 927
Hycomine Compound Tablets ... 929
Hycomine Syrup ... 927
Hycotuss Expectorant Syrup ... 930
Hydrocet Capsules ... 835
Lortab ASA Tablets ... 2414
Lortab ... 2412
Ru-Tuss with Hydrocodone ... 694
Triaminic Expectorant DH ... 1995
Vicodin Tablets ... 1187
Vicodin ES Tablets ... 1189
Zydone Capsules ... 941
Hydrocodone Polistirex (Additive CNS depression). Products include:
Tussionex Extended-Release Suspension ... 988
Hydroxyzine Hydrochloride (Additive CNS depression). Products include:
Atarax Tablets & Syrup ... 1941
Marax Tablets & DF Syrup ... 1954
Vistaril Intramuscular Solution ... 1970
Hyoscyamine (May produce paralytic ileus). Products include:
Cystospaz Tablets ... 2395
Urised Tablets ... 2396
Hyoscyamine Sulfate (May produce paralytic ileus). Products include:
Arco-Lase Plus Tablets ... 607
Cystospaz-M Capsules ... 2395
Donnagel ... ▣ 675
Donnagel-PG ... 1858
Donnatal ... 1858
Donnatal Extentabs ... 1859
Donnatal Tablets ... 1858
Donnazyme Tablets ... 1860
Kutrase Capsules ... 2146
Levsin/Levsinex ... 2147
Ru-Tuss Tablets ... 693
Ipratropium Bromide (May produce paralytic ileus). Products include:
Atrovent Inhalation Aerosol ... 675
Isoflurane (Additive CNS depression). Products include:
Forane ... 600
Ketamine Hydrochloride (Additive CNS depression). Products include:
Ketalar ... 1726
Levorphanol Tartrate (Additive CNS depression). Products include:
Levo-Dromoran ... 1906
Lithium Carbonate (Additive CNS depression). Products include:
Eskalith ... 2214
Lithane Tablets ... 1596
Lithium Carbonate Capsules & Tablets ... 1984
Lithobid Tablets ... 870
Lithium Citrate (Additive CNS depression). Products include:
Cibalith-S ... 870
Lorazepam (Additive CNS depression). Products include:
Ativan Injection ... 2432
Ativan Tablets ... 2434
Loxapine Hydrochloride (Additive CNS depression). Products include:
Loxitane ... 1213
Loxapine Succinate (Additive CNS depression). Products include:
Loxitane Capsules ... 1213
Mepenzolate Bromide (May produce paralytic ileus). Products include:
Cantil Tablets ... 1326
Meperidine Hydrochloride (Additive CNS depression). Products include:
Demerol ... 2047
Mepergan Injection ... 2479
Mephobarbital (Additive CNS depression). Products include:
Mebaral Tablets ... 2061
Meprobamate (Additive CNS depression). Products include:
Deprol Tablets ... 2382
Equagesic Tablets ... 2451
Miltown Tablets ... 2386
PMB 200 and PMB 400 ... 2504
Mesoridazine (Additive CNS depression). Products include:
Serentil ... 686
Methadone Hydrochloride (Additive CNS depression). Products include:
Dolophine Hydrochloride Ampoules & Vials ... 1260
Dolophine Hydrochloride Tablets ... 1261
Methadone Hydrochloride Diskets ... 1284
Methadone Hydrochloride Oral Solution & Tablets ... 1987
Methohexital Sodium (Additive CNS depression). Products include:
Brevital Sodium Vials ... 1248
Methoxyflurane (Additive CNS depression).
No products indexed under this heading.
Midazolam Hydrochloride (Additive CNS depression). Products include:
Versed Injection ... 1924
Molindone Hydrochloride (Additive CNS depression). Products include:
Moban Tablets & Concentrate ... 932
Morphine Sulfate (Additive CNS depression). Products include:
Astramorph/PF Injection, USP (Preservative-Free) ... 618
Duramorph ... 960
Infumorph 200 and Infumorph 500 Sterile Solutions ... 962
MS Contin Tablets ... 1814
MSIR ... 1817
Oramorph SR (Morphine Sulfate Sustained Release Tablets) ... 1988
Roxanol ... 1991
Opium Alkaloids (Additive CNS depression). Products include:
B & O No. 15A & No. 16A Supprettes ... 2395
Pantopon Injectable ... 1911
Oxazepam (Additive CNS depression). Products include:
Serax Capsules ... 2522
Serax Tablets ... 2522
Oxybutynin Chloride (May produce paralytic ileus). Products include:
Ditropan ... 1332
Pentobarbital Sodium (Additive CNS depression). Products include:
Nembutal Sodium Capsules ... 534
Nembutal Sodium Solution ... 536
Nembutal Sodium Suppositories ... 538
Perphenazine (Additive CNS depression). Products include:
Etrafon ... 2087
Triavil Tablets ... 1556
Trilafon ... 2123
Phenobarbital (Additive CNS depression). Products include:
Arco-Lase Plus Tablets ... 607
Bellergal-S Tablets ... 1998
Bronkolixir ... ▣ 761
Bronkotabs Tablets ... ▣ 762
Donnatal ... 1858
Donnatal Extentabs ... 1859
Donnatal Tablets ... 1858
Donnazyme Tablets ... 1860
Kinesed Tablets ... 2272
Phenobarbital Elixir and Tablets ... 1293
Primatene Tablets-P Formula ... 2421
Quadrinal Tablets ... 1183
Tedral SA ... 1765
Pimozide (Additive CNS depression). Products include:
Orap Tablets ... 1020
Prazepam (Additive CNS depression). Products include:
Centrax ... 1693
Prochlorperazine (Additive CNS depression). Products include:
Compazine ... 2201
Procyclidine Hydrochloride (May produce paralytic ileus). Products include:
Kemadrin Tablets ... 771
Promethazine Hydrochloride (Additive CNS depression). Products include:
Mepergan Injection ... 2479
Phenergan with Codeine ... 2497
Phenergan with Dextromethorphan ... 2499
Phenergan Injection ... 2493
Phenergan Suppositories ... 2496
Phenergan Syrup ... 2495
Phenergan Tablets ... 2496
Phenergan VC ... 2500
Phenergan VC with Codeine ... 2501
Propantheline Bromide (May produce paralytic ileus). Products include:
Pro-Banthine Tablets ... 2141
Propofol (Additive CNS depression). Products include:
Diprivan Injection ... 2267
Propoxyphene Hydrochloride (Additive CNS depression). Products include:
Darvon ... 1256
Wygesic Tablets ... 2540
Propoxyphene Napsylate (Additive CNS depression). Products include:
Darvon-N/Darvocet-N ... 1254
Quazepam (Additive CNS depression). Products include:
Doral Tablets ... 2383
Scopolamine Hydrobromide (May produce paralytic ileus). Products include:
Donnagel ... ▣ 675
Donnagel-PG ... 1858
Donnatal ... 1858
Donnatal Extentabs ... 1859
Donnatal Tablets ... 1858
Donnazyme Tablets ... 1860
Isopto Hyoscine ... ◉ 222
Murocoll-2 Sterile Ophthalmic Solution ... ◉ 261
Ru-Tuss Tablets ... 693
Scopolamine Preparations (May produce paralytic ileus). Products include:
Transderm Scōp Transdermal Therapeutic System ... 887
Secobarbital Sodium (Additive CNS depression). Products include:
Seconal Sodium Pulvules ... 1296
Sufentanil Citrate (Additive CNS depression). Products include:
Sufenta Injection ... 1147
Temazepam (Additive CNS depression). Products include:
Restoril Capsules ... 2023
Thiamylal Sodium (Additive CNS depression). Products include:
Surital Ampoules, Steri-Vials ... 1764
Thioridazine Hydrochloride (Additive CNS depression). Products include:
Mellaril ... 2011
Thiothixene (Additive CNS depression). Products include:
Navane Capsules and Concentrate ... 1954
Navane Intramuscular ... 1956
Triazolam (Additive CNS depression). Products include:
Halcion Tablets ... 2340
Tridihexethyl Chloride (May produce paralytic ileus).
No products indexed under this heading.
Trifluoperazine Hydrochloride (Additive CNS depression). Products include:
Stelazine ... 2226
Trihexyphenidyl Hydrochloride (May produce paralytic ileus). Products include:
Artane ... 1195

TYPHOID VACCINE
(Typhoid Vaccine) ... 2533
No interactions described in labeling.

ULTRA MIDE 25
(Moisturizing formula) ... ▣ 510
No interactions described in labeling.

ULTRA SLIM-FAST
(Nutritional Supplement) ... ▣ 707
No interactions described in labeling.

ULTRACEF CAPSULES, TABLETS & ORAL SUSPENSION
(Cefadroxil Monohydrate) ... 722
No interactions described in labeling.

ULTRALENTE INSULIN
(Insulin, Zinc Suspension) ... 1626
No interactions described in labeling.

ULTRAVATE CREAM 0.05%
(Halobetasol Propionate) 2410
No interactions described in labeling.

ULTRAVATE OINTMENT 0.05%
(Halobetasol Propionate) 2411
No interactions described in labeling.

UNASYN
(Ampicillin Sodium, Sulbactam Sodium)..1965
May interact with aminoglycosides and certain other agents. Compounds in these categories include:

Allopurinol (Increased incidence of rash). Products include:
Zyloprim Tablets 830

Amikacin Sulfate (In vitro inactivation of aminoglycosides when reconstituted with Unasyn). Products include:
Amikin Injectable 602

Gentamicin Sulfate (In vitro inactivation of aminoglycosides when reconstituted with Unasyn). Products include:
Garamycin Injectable 2093
Garamycin Ophthalmic .... ⊙ 305
Genoptic Liquifilm Sterile Ophthalmic Solution .... ⊙ 247
Genoptic S.O.P. Sterile Ophthalmic Ointment .... ⊙ 247
Gentacidin Ointment .... ⊙ 273
Gentacidin Solution.......................... ⊙ 273
Gentak Ointment & Solution........... ⊙ 208
G-myticin Creme and Ointment 0.1% 1770
Pred-G Liquifilm Sterile Ophthalmic Suspension .... ⊙ 252
Pred-G S.O.P. Sterile Ophthalmic Ointment .... ⊙ 253

Kanamycin Sulfate (In vitro inactivation of aminoglycosides when reconstituted with Unasyn). Products include:
Kantrex Injection 601
Kantrex Pediatric Injection.................. 601

Probenecid (Increased and prolonged blood levels of ampicillin and sulbactam). Products include:
Benemid Tablets 1426
ColBENEMID Tablets 1436
Wycillin Injection and Probenecid Tablets 2539

Streptomycin Sulfate (In vitro inactivation of aminoglycosides when reconstituted with Unasyn).
No products indexed under this heading.

Tobramycin Sulfate (In vitro inactivation of aminoglycosides when reconstituted with Unasyn). Products include:
Nebcin Vials, Hyporets & ADD-Vantage 1286

UNICAP JR CHEWABLE TABLETS
(Multivitamins) ....⊡ 738
No interactions described in labeling.

UNICAP M TABLETS
(Multivitamins with Minerals) ....⊡ 738
No interactions described in labeling.

UNICAP PLUS IRON VITAMIN FORMULA TABLETS
(Vitamins with Iron) ....⊡ 738
No interactions described in labeling.

UNICAP SOFTGEL CAPSULES & TABLETS
(Multivitamins) ....⊡ 738
No interactions described in labeling.

UNICAP SR. TABLETS
(Multivitamins with Minerals) ....⊡ 738
No interactions described in labeling.

UNICAP T TABLETS
(Vitamins with Minerals) ....⊡ 739
No interactions described in labeling.

UNIPEN CAPSULES
(Nafcillin Sodium) 2533
No interactions described in labeling.

UNIPEN INJECTION
(Nafcillin Sodium) 2533
No interactions described in labeling.

UNIPEN POWDER FOR ORAL SOLUTION
(Nafcillin Sodium) 2533
No interactions described in labeling.

UNIPEN TABLETS
(Nafcillin Sodium) 2533
No interactions described in labeling.

UNIPHYL 400 MG TABLETS
(Theophylline Anhydrous)...................1823
May interact with macrolide antibiotics, sympathomimetic bronchodilators, oral contraceptives, and certain other agents. Compounds in these categories include:

Albuterol (Toxic synergism). Products include:
Proventil Inhalation Aerosol 2117
Ventolin Inhalation Aerosol and Refill 583

Albuterol Sulfate (Toxic synergism). Products include:
Proventil Repetabs Tablets 2120
Proventil Solutions for Inhalation 0.5% and 0.083%.......................... 2118
Proventil Syrup................................... 2119
Proventil Tablets 2120
Ventolin 583

Allopurinol (Increases serum theophylline levels). Products include:
Zyloprim Tablets 830

Bitolterol Mesylate (Toxic synergism). Products include:
Tornalate.. 2074

Cimetidine (Increases serum theophylline levels). Products include:
Tagamet Tablets 2228

Cimetidine Hydrochloride (Increases serum theophylline levels). Products include:
Tagamet.. 2228

Ciprofloxacin Hydrochloride (Increases serum theophylline levels). Products include:
Ciloxan Sterile Ophthalmic Solution.. ⊙ 214
Cipro I.V. 1592
Cipro Tablets..................................... 1589

Ephedrine Hydrochloride (Toxic synergism). Products include:
Amesec ....⊡ 682
Primatene Tablets-M Formula 2421
Primatene Tablets-P Formula........... 2421
Primatene Tablets-Regular Formula 2421
Quadrinal Tablets 1183
Quelidrine Syrup 556
Tedral SA 1765

Ephedrine Sulfate (Toxic synergism). Products include:
Bronkaid Tablets ....⊡ 757
Bronkolixir ....⊡ 761
Bronkotabs Tablets...........................⊡ 762
Marax Tablets & DF Syrup................ 1954
Pazo Hemorrhoid Ointment & Suppositories...................................... 752
Vicks Vatronol Nose Drops ....⊡ 666

Ephedrine Tannate (Toxic synergism). Products include:
Rynatuss 2388

Epinephrine (Toxic synergism). Products include:
Ana-Kit Anaphylaxis Emergency Treatment Kit 1100
Bronkaid Mist ....⊡ 757
EpiPen 843
Marcaine Hydrochloride 0.5% with Epinephrine 1:200,000 (as bitartrate) 958
Marcaine Hydrochloride with Epinephrine 1:200,000 2055
Primatene Mist 2420
Sus-Phrine Injection 1006
Xylocaine with Epinephrine Injections.. 637

Epinephrine Hydrochloride (Toxic synergism). Products include:
Adrenalin Chloride Solution 1:100 & 1:1,000 1689
Epifrin... ⊙ 244
Glaucon .... ⊙ 218

Erythromycin (Increases serum theophylline levels). Products include:
A/T/S Topical Gel and Topical Solution 1089
AK-Mycin Ointment.......................... ⊙ 204
Benzamycin Topical Gel 907
E-Mycin Tablets 688
ETS-2% 1685
ERYC 1720
Erycette (erythromycin 2%) Topical Solution 1678
Ery-Tab Tablets 521
Erythromycin Base Filmtab 525
Erythromycin Delayed-Release Capsules, USP................................... 526
Ilotycin Ophthalmic Ointment........... 915
PCE Dispertab Tablets 549
Pediazole... 1973
T-Stat 2.0% Topical Solution and Pads 2409
Theramycin Z Topical Solution 2% 1410

Erythromycin Estolate (Increases serum theophylline levels). Products include:
Ilosone 913

Erythromycin Ethylsuccinate (Increases serum theophylline levels). Products include:
E.E.S. 522
EryPed 519
Pediazole 1973

Erythromycin Gluceptate (Increases serum theophylline levels). Products include:
Ilotycin Gluceptate, IV, Vials 915

Erythromycin Stearate (Increases serum theophylline levels). Products include:
Erythrocin Stearate Filmtab 523

Ethinyl Estradiol (Increases serum theophylline levels). Products include:
Brevicon... 2304
Demulen 2161
Estinyl Tablets................................... 2085
Jenest-28 Tablets 1636
Levlen/Tri-Levlen 665
Lo/Ovral Tablets 2471
Lo/Ovral-28 Tablets........................... 2476
Loestrin 1728
Modicon... 1667
Nordette-21 Tablets........................... 2481
Nordette-28 Tablets........................... 2483
Norethin... 2133
Norinyl 2304
Norlestrin 1746
Ortho-Cyclen Tablets 1658
Ortho-Novum..................................... 1667
Ovcon 1391
Ovral Tablets 2490
Ovral-28 Tablets 2491
Levlen/Tri-Levlen................................. 665
Tri-Norinyl... 2304
Triphasil-21 Tablets........................... 2527
Triphasil-28 Tablets........................... 2532

Ethylnorepinephrine Hydrochloride (Toxic synergism). Products include:
Bronkephrine Injection 2042

Ethynodiol Diacetate (Increases serum theophylline levels). Products include:
Demulen 2161

Influenza Virus Vaccine (Decreased theophylline clearance). Products include:
Flu-Imune Influenza Virus Vaccine .. 1204

Isoetharine (Toxic synergism). Products include:
Arm-a-Med Isoetharine Inhalation Solution, USP..................................... 616
Bronkometer Aerosol......................... 2042
Bronkosol Solution 2042

Isoproterenol Hydrochloride (Toxic synergism). Products include:
Isuprel Hydrochloride Injection 1:5000 2050
Isuprel Hydrochloride Mistometer .. 2051
Isuprel Hydrochloride Solution 1:200 & 1:100 2052
Norisodrine Aerotrol........................... 540

Levonorgestrel (Increases serum theophylline levels). Products include:
Levlen/Tri-Levlen................................. 665
Nordette-21 Tablets........................... 2481
Nordette-28 Tablets........................... 2483
Norplant System 2484
Levlen/Tri-Levlen................................. 665
Triphasil-21 Tablets........................... 2527
Triphasil-28 Tablets........................... 2532

Lithium Carbonate (Increased lithium excretion). Products include:
Eskalith 2214
Lithane Tablets.................................. 1596
Lithium Carbonate Capsules & Tablets 1984
Lithobid Tablets 870

Mestranol (Increases serum theophylline levels). Products include:
Enovid.. 2161
Norethin... 2133
Norinyl 2304
Ortho-Novum..................................... 1667

Metaproterenol Sulfate (Toxic synergism). Products include:
Alupent.. 674
Arm-a-Med Metaproterenol Sulfate Inhalation Solution, USP 617
Metaprel Inhalation Aerosol Bronchodilator 2014
Metaprel Inhalation Solution 2015
Metaprel 2015
Metaproterenol Sulfate Inhalation Solution, USP..................................... 912

Norethindrone (Increases serum theophylline levels). Products include:
Brevicon... 2304
Jenest-28 Tablets 1636
Micronor Tablets 1667
Modicon... 1667
Norethin... 2133
Norinyl 2304
Norlutin 1755
Nor-Q D Tablets 2304
Ortho-Novum..................................... 1667
Ovcon 1391
Tri-Norinyl... 2304

Norethynodrel (Increases serum theophylline levels). Products include:
Enovid.. 2161

Norfloxacin (Increased serum theophylline levels). Products include:
Chibroxin Sterile Ophthalmic Solution.. 1431
Noroxin Tablets 1519

Norgestimate (Increases serum theophylline levels). Products include:
Ortho-Cyclen Tablets 1658

Norgestrel (Increases serum theophylline levels). Products include:
Lo/Ovral Tablets 2471
Lo/Ovral-28 Tablets........................... 2476
Ovral Tablets 2490
Ovral-28 Tablets 2491
Ovrette Tablets 2492

Phenytoin (Decreased theophylline and phenytoin serum levels). Products include:
Dilantin Infatabs................................ 1710
Dilantin-30 Pediatric/Dilantin-125 Suspension 1713

(⊡ Described in PDR For Nonprescription Drugs) (⊙ Described in PDR For Ophthalmology)

Phenytoin Sodium (Decreased theophylline and phenytoin serum levels). Products include:
Dilantin Kapseals ... 1708
Dilantin Parenteral ... 1712
Dilantin with Phenobarbital Kapseals ... 1715

Pirbuterol Acetate (Toxic synergism). Products include:
Maxair Inhaler ... 1311

Propranolol Hydrochloride (Increased serum theophylline levels). Products include:
Inderal ... 2459
Inderal LA Long Acting Capsules ... 2461
Inderide Tablets ... 2463
Inderide LA Long Acting Capsules ... 2465

Rifampin (Decreases serum theophylline levels). Products include:
Rifadin ... 1345
Rifamate Capsules ... 1347
Rimactane Capsules ... 879

Terbutaline Sulfate (Toxic synergism). Products include:
Brethaire Inhaler ... 1024
Brethine Ampuls ... 1026
Brethine Tablets ... 1026
Bricanyl Injection ... 1324
Bricanyl Tablets ... 1325

Troleandomycin (Increases serum theophylline levels). Products include:
Tao Capsules ... 1963

Food Interactions

Diet, high-lipid (Affects the bioavailability of theophylline).

UNISOM DUAL RELIEF NIGHTTIME SLEEP AID/ANALGESIC
(Diphenhydramine Hydrochloride, Acetaminophen) ... 1774
May interact with monoamine oxidase inhibitors, central nervous system depressants, and certain other agents. Compounds in these categories include:

Alcohol (Heightened CNS depressant effect of antihistamines).

Alfentanil Hydrochloride (Heightened CNS depressant effect of antihistamines). Products include:
Alfenta Injection ... 1131

Alprazolam (Heightened CNS depressant effect of antihistamines). Products include:
Xanax Tablets ... 2367

Aprobarbital (Heightened CNS depressant effect of antihistamines). Products include:
Alurate Elixir ... 1883

Buprenorphine (Heightened CNS depressant effect of antihistamines).
No products indexed under this heading.

Buspirone Hydrochloride (Heightened CNS depressant effect of antihistamines). Products include:
BuSpar ... 1401

Butabarbital (Heightened CNS depressant effect of antihistamines). Products include:
Pyridium Plus ... 1764

Butalbital (Heightened CNS depressant effect of antihistamines). Products include:
Esgic-Plus Tablets ... 1002
Esgic Tablets & Capsules ... 1001
Fioricet Tablets ... 2006
Fiorinal Capsules ... 2007
Fiorinal with Codeine Capsules ... 2008
Fiorinal Tablets ... 2007
Phrenilin ... 838
Sedapap Tablets 50 mg/650 mg ... 1360

Chlordiazepoxide (Heightened CNS depressant effect of antihistamines). Products include:
Libritabs Tablets ... 1930
Limbitrol ... 1933
Menrium Tablets ... 1934

Chlordiazepoxide Hydrochloride (Heightened CNS depressant effect of antihistamines). Products include:
Librax Capsules ... 1929
Librium Capsules ... 1931
Librium Injectable ... 1932

Chlorpromazine (Heightened CNS depressant effect of antihistamines). Products include:
Thorazine ... 2234

Chlorprothixene (Heightened CNS depressant effect of antihistamines). Products include:
Taractan Tablets ... 1920

Chlorprothixene Hydrochloride (Heightened CNS depressant effect of antihistamines). Products include:
Taractan ... 1920

Chlorprothixene Lactate (Heightened CNS depressant effect of antihistamines). Products include:
Taractan Concentrate ... 1920

Clorazepate Dipotassium (Heightened CNS depressant effect of antihistamines). Products include:
Tranxene ... 556

Codeine (Heightened CNS depressant effect of antihistamines). Products include:
Calcidrine Syrup ... 506

Codeine Phosphate (Heightened CNS depressant effect of antihistamines). Products include:
Actifed with Codeine Cough Syrup ... 752
Cheracol Cough Syrup ... 1853
Codimal PH Syrup ... 846
Dimetane-DC Cough Syrup ... 1857
Empirin with Codeine Phosphate Nos. 2, 3 & 4 ... 764
Fiorinal with Codeine Capsules ... 2008
Isoclor Expectorant ... 982
Naldecon CX Adult Liquid ... ▣ 521
Novahistine DH ... 1342
Novahistine Expectorant ... 1343
Nucofed Capsules ... 2219
Nucofed Expectorant ... 2219
Nucofed Pediatric Expectorant ... 2220
Nucofed Syrup ... 2219
Phenaphen with Codeine Capsules ... 1865
Phenaphen-650 with Codeine Tablets ... 1866
Phenergan with Codeine ... 2497
Phenergan VC with Codeine ... 2501
Robitussin A-C Syrup ... 1875
Robitussin-DAC Syrup ... 1875
Ryna ... ▣ 741
Soma Compound w/Codeine Tablets ... 2390
Triaminic Expectorant w/Codeine ... 1996
Tussi-Organidin Liquid ... 2391
Tylenol with Codeine ... 1381

Codeine Polistirex (Heightened CNS depressant effect of antihistamines).
No products indexed under this heading.

Dezocine (Heightened CNS depressant effect of antihistamines).

Diazepam (Heightened CNS depressant effect of antihistamines). Products include:
Valium Injectable ... 1937
Valium Tablets ... 1939
Valrelease Capsules ... 1923

Droperidol (Heightened CNS depressant effect of antihistamines). Products include:
Inapsine Injection ... 1140
Innovar Injection ... 1141

Enflurane (Heightened CNS depressant effect of antihistamines). Products include:
Ethrane ... 599

Estazolam (Heightened CNS depressant effect of antihistamines). Products include:
ProSom Tablets ... 554

Ethchlorvynol (Heightened CNS depressant effect of antihistamines). Products include:
Placidyl Capsules ... 553

Ethinamate (Heightened CNS depressant effect of antihistamines).
No products indexed under this heading.

Fentanyl (Heightened CNS depressant effect of antihistamines). Products include:
Duragesic Transdermal System ... 1133

Fentanyl Citrate (Heightened CNS depressant effect of antihistamines). Products include:
Innovar Injection ... 1141
Sublimaze Injection ... 1146

Fluphenazine Decanoate (Heightened CNS depressant effect of antihistamines). Products include:
Prolixin Decanoate ... 1795

Fluphenazine Enanthate (Heightened CNS depressant effect of antihistamines). Products include:
Prolixin Enanthate ... 1796

Fluphenazine Hydrochloride (Heightened CNS depressant effect of antihistamines). Products include:
Prolixin Elixir ... 1793
Prolixin Injection ... 1791
Prolixin Oral Concentrate ... 1792
Prolixin Tablets ... 1793

Flurazepam Hydrochloride (Heightened CNS depressant effect of antihistamines). Products include:
Dalmane Capsules ... 1927

Furazolidone (Prolonged and intensified anticholinergic effects of antihistamines). Products include:
Furoxone ... 1855

Glutethimide (Heightened CNS depressant effect of antihistamines).
No products indexed under this heading.

Haloperidol (Heightened CNS depressant effect of antihistamines). Products include:
Haldol Injection, Tablets and Concentrate ... 1373

Haloperidol Decanoate (Heightened CNS depressant effect of antihistamines). Products include:
Haldol Decanoate ... 1375

Hydrocodone Bitartrate (Heightened CNS depressant effect of antihistamines). Products include:
Anexsia 5/500 Tablets ... 2196
Anexsia 7.5/650 Tablets ... 2197
Azdōne Tablets ... 844
Codiclear DH Syrup ... 845
Codimal DH Syrup ... 846
Damason-P ... 1356
Hycodan Syrup, Tablets ... 927
Hycomine Compound Tablets ... 929
Hycomine Syrup ... 927
Hycotuss Expectorant Syrup ... 930
Hydrocet Capsules ... 835
Lortab ASA Tablets ... 2414
Lortab ... 2412
Ru-Tuss with Hydrocodone ... 694
Triaminic Expectorant DH ... 1995
Vicodin Tablets ... 1187
Vicodin ES Tablets ... 1189
Zydone Capsules ... 941

Hydrocodone Polistirex (Heightened CNS depressant effect of antihistamines). Products include:
Tussionex Extended-Release Suspension ... 988

Hydroxyzine Hydrochloride (Heightened CNS depressant effect of antihistamines). Products include:
Atarax Tablets & Syrup ... 1941
Marax Tablets & DF Syrup ... 1954
Vistaril Intramuscular Solution ... 1970

Isocarboxazid (Prolonged and intensified anticholinergic effects of antihistamines). Products include:
Marplan Tablets ... 1906

Isoflurane (Heightened CNS depressant effect of antihistamines). Products include:
Forane ... 600

Ketamine Hydrochloride (Heightened CNS depressant effect of antihistamines). Products include:
Ketalar ... 1726

Levorphanol Tartrate (Heightened CNS depressant effect of antihistamines). Products include:
Levo-Dromoran ... 1906

Lorazepam (Heightened CNS depressant effect of antihistamines). Products include:
Ativan Injection ... 2432
Ativan Tablets ... 2434

Loxapine Hydrochloride (Heightened CNS depressant effect of antihistamines). Products include:
Loxitane ... 1213

Loxapine Succinate (Heightened CNS depressant effect of antihistamines). Products include:
Loxitane Capsules ... 1213

Meperidine Hydrochloride (Heightened CNS depressant effect of antihistamines). Products include:
Demerol ... 2047
Mepergan Injection ... 2479

Mephobarbital (Heightened CNS depressant effect of antihistamines). Products include:
Mebaral Tablets ... 2061

Meprobamate (Heightened CNS depressant effect of antihistamines). Products include:
Deprol Tablets ... 2382
Equagesic Tablets ... 2451
Miltown Tablets ... 2386
PMB 200 and PMB 400 ... 2504

Mesoridazine (Heightened CNS depressant effect of antihistamines). Products include:
Serentil ... 686

Methadone Hydrochloride (Heightened CNS depressant effect of antihistamines). Products include:
Dolophine Hydrochloride Ampoules & Vials ... 1260
Dolophine Hydrochloride Tablets ... 1261
Methadone Hydrochloride Diskets ... 1284
Methadone Hydrochloride Oral Solution & Tablets ... 1987

Methohexital Sodium (Heightened CNS depressant effect of antihistamines). Products include:
Brevital Sodium Vials ... 1248

Methoxyflurane (Heightened CNS depressant effect of antihistamines).
No products indexed under this heading.

Midazolam Hydrochloride (Heightened CNS depressant effect of antihistamines). Products include:
Versed Injection ... 1924

Molindone Hydrochloride (Heightened CNS depressant effect of antihistamines). Products include:
Moban Tablets & Concentrate ... 932

Morphine Sulfate (Heightened CNS depressant effect of antihistamines). Products include:
Astramorph/PF Injection, USP (Preservative-Free) ... 618
Duramorph ... 960
Infumorph 200 and Infumorph 500 Sterile Solutions ... 962
MS Contin Tablets ... 1814
MSIR ... 1817
Oramorph SR (Morphine Sulfate Sustained Release Tablets) ... 1988
Roxanol ... 1991

Opium Alkaloids (Heightened CNS depressant effect of antihistamines). Products include:
B & O No. 15A & No. 16A Supprettes ... 2395
Pantopon Injectable ... 1911

Oxazepam (Heightened CNS depressant effect of antihistamines). Products include:
Serax Capsules 2522
Serax Tablets 2522

Oxycodone Hydrochloride (Heightened CNS depressant effect of antihistamines). Products include:
Percocet Tablets 950
Percodan 951
Roxicodone Tablets, Oral Solution & Intensol (Oxycodone) 1992
Tylox Capsules 1382

Pentobarbital Sodium (Heightened CNS depressant effect of antihistamines). Products include:
Nembutal Sodium Capsules 534
Nembutal Sodium Solution 536
Nembutal Sodium Suppositories 538

Perphenazine (Heightened CNS depressant effect of antihistamines). Products include:
Etrafon 2087
Triavil Tablets 1556
Trilafon 2123

Phenelzine Sulfate (Prolonged and intensified anticholinergic effects of antihistamines). Products include:
Nardil 1742

Phenobarbital (Heightened CNS depressant effect of antihistamines). Products include:
Arco-Lase Plus Tablets 607
Bellergal-S Tablets 1998
Bronkolixir .... ▣ 761
Bronkotabs Tablets .... ▣ 762
Donnatal 1858
Donnatal Extentabs 1859
Donnatal Tablets 1858
Donnazyme Tablets 1860
Kinesed Tablets 2272
Phenobarbital Elixir and Tablets 1293
Primatene Tablets-P Formula 2421
Quadrinal Tablets 1183
Tedral SA 1765

Prazepam (Heightened CNS depressant effect of antihistamines). Products include:
Centrax 1693

Prochlorperazine (Heightened CNS depressant effect of antihistamines). Products include:
Compazine 2201

Promethazine Hydrochloride (Heightened CNS depressant effect of antihistamines). Products include:
Mepergan Injection 2479
Phenergan with Codeine 2497
Phenergan with Dextromethorphan 2499
Phenergan Injection 2493
Phenergan Suppositories 2496
Phenergan Syrup 2495
Phenergan Tablets 2496
Phenergan VC 2500
Phenergan VC with Codeine 2501

Propofol (Heightened CNS depressant effect of antihistamines). Products include:
Diprivan Injection 2267

Propoxyphene Hydrochloride (Heightened CNS depressant effect of antihistamines). Products include:
Darvon 1256
Wygesic Tablets 2540

Propoxyphene Napsylate (Heightened CNS depressant effect of antihistamines). Products include:
Darvon-N/Darvocet-N 1254

Quazepam (Heightened CNS depressant effect of antihistamines). Products include:
Doral Tablets 2383

Secobarbital Sodium (Heightened CNS depressant effect of antihistamines). Products include:
Seconal Sodium Pulvules 1296

Selegiline Hydrochloride (Prolonged and intensified anticholinergic effects of antihistamines). Products include:
Eldepryl 2250

Sufentanil Citrate (Heightened CNS depressant effect of antihistamines). Products include:
Sufenta Injection 1147

Temazepam (Heightened CNS depressant effect of antihistamines). Products include:
Restoril Capsules 2023

Thiamylal Sodium (Heightened CNS depressant effect of antihistamines). Products include:
Surital Ampoules, Steri-Vials 1764

Thioridazine Hydrochloride (Heightened CNS depressant effect of antihistamines). Products include:
Mellaril 2011

Thiothixene (Heightened CNS depressant effect of antihistamines). Products include:
Navane Capsules and Concentrate 1954
Navane Intramuscular 1956

Tranylcypromine Sulfate (Prolonged and intensified anticholinergic effects of antihistamines). Products include:
Parnate Tablets 2222

Triazolam (Heightened CNS depressant effect of antihistamines). Products include:
Halcion Tablets 2340

Trifluoperazine Hydrochloride (Heightened CNS depressant effect of antihistamines). Products include:
Stelazine 2226

UNISOM NIGHTTIME SLEEP AID

(Doxylamine Succinate) 1774
May interact with:

Alcohol (Use Unisom cautiously).

UREACIN LOTION & CREME

(Urea Preparations) 1771
No interactions described in labeling.

URECHOLINE INJECTION

(Bethanechol Chloride) 1558
See **Urecholine Tablets**

URECHOLINE TABLETS

(Bethanechol Chloride) 1558
May interact with ganglionic blocking agents. Compounds in this category include:

Mecamylamine Hydrochloride (Critical fall in blood pressure). Products include:
Inversine Tablets 1492

Trimethaphan Camsylate (Critical fall in blood pressure). Products include:
Arfonad Ampuls 1887

URISED TABLETS

(Atropine Sulfate, Hyoscyamine, Methenamine, Phenyl Salicylate) 2396
May interact with sulfonamides. Compounds in this category include:

Sulfamethizole (Mutual antagonism; concurrent use should be avoided since insoluble precipitate may form in the urine). Products include:
Thiosulfil Forte Tablets 2526
Urobiotic-250 Capsules 1968

Sulfamethoxazole (Mutual antagonism; concurrent use should be avoided since insoluble precipitate may form in the urine). Products include:
Azo Gantanol Tablets 1887
Bactrim DS Tablets 1891
Bactrim I.V. Infusion 1889
Bactrim 1891
Gantanol 1899
Septra 813
Septra I.V. Infusion 808
Septra I.V. Infusion ADD-Vantage Vials 810
Septra 813

Sulfasalazine (Mutual antagonism; concurrent use should be avoided since insoluble precipitate may form in the urine). Products include:
Azulfidine Tablets, EN-tabs, Oral Suspension 1157

Sulfinpyrazone (Mutual antagonism; concurrent use should be avoided since insoluble precipitate may form in the urine). Products include:
Anturane 853

Sulfisoxazole (Mutual antagonism; concurrent use should be avoided since insoluble precipitate may form in the urine). Products include:
Azo Gantrisin Tablets 1888
Gantrisin Tablets 1901
Pediazole 1973

Sulfisoxazole Diolamine (Mutual antagonism; concurrent use should be avoided since insoluble precipitate may form in the urine). Products include:
Gantrisin Ophthalmic Ointment/Solution 1900

URISPAS TABLETS

(Flavoxate Hydrochloride) 2242
No interactions described in labeling.

UROBIOTIC-250 CAPSULES

(Oxytetracycline Hydrochloride, Sulfamethizole, Phenazopyridine Hydrochloride) 1968
May interact with:

Aluminum Hydroxide (Decreases absorption of Urobiotic). Products include:
Cama Arthritis Pain Reliever .... ▣ 685
Gaviscon Extra Strength Relief Formula Liquid Antacid .... ▣ 594
Gaviscon Extra Strength Relief Formula Antacid Tablets .... ▣ 594
Gaviscon Liquid Antacid .... ▣ 594
Gelusil Liquid & Tablets .... ▣ 639
Extra Strength Maalox Plus Suspension 1850
Maalox TC Suspension 1851
Maalox Plus Tablets .... ▣ 655
Extra Strength Maalox Plus Tablets 1850
Nephrox Suspension .... ▣ 563
WinGel Liquid & Tablets .... ▣ 761

Aluminum Hydroxide Gel (Decreases absorption of Urobiotic). Products include:
ALternaGEL Liquid 1154
Aludrox Oral Suspension 2428
Amphojel Suspension 2429
Amphojel Suspension without Flavor 2429
Mylanta Liquid 1155
Mylanta Double Strength Liquid 1155

Aluminum Hydroxide Gel, Dried (Decreases absorption of Urobiotic). Products include:
Alu-Tab/Alu-Cap 1309
Amphojel Tablets 2429
Ascriptin A/D Caplets 1850
Regular Strength Ascriptin Tablets 1850
Gaviscon Antacid Tablets .... ▣ 593
Gaviscon-2 Antacid Tablets .... ▣ 594
Mylanta Tablets 1155
Mylanta Double Strength Tablets 1155

URO-MAG

(Magnesium Oxide) 673
No interactions described in labeling.

UROQID-ACID TABLETS

(Methenamine Mandelate, Sodium Acid Phosphate) 661
May interact with sulfonamides, thiazides, carbonic anhydrase inhibitors, antacids, urinary alkalizing agents, catecholamine depleting drugs, corticosteroids, salicylates, and certain other agents. Compounds in these categories include:

Acetazolamide (Reduces effectiveness of methenamine). Products include:
Diamox Parenteral 1200
Diamox Parenteral .... ⊙ 308
Diamox Sequels (Sustained Release) 1201
Diamox Sequels (Sustained Release) .... ⊙ 310
Diamox Tablets 1200
Diamox Tablets .... ⊙ 308

ACTH (Hypernatremia).
No products indexed under this heading.

Aluminum Carbonate Gel (Reduces effectiveness of methenamine). Products include:
Basaljel 2438

Aluminum Hydroxide (Reduces effectiveness of methenamine). Products include:
Cama Arthritis Pain Reliever .... ▣ 685
Gaviscon Extra Strength Relief Formula Liquid Antacid .... ▣ 594
Gaviscon Extra Strength Relief Formula Antacid Tablets .... ▣ 594
Gaviscon Liquid Antacid .... ▣ 594
Gelusil Liquid & Tablets .... ▣ 639
Extra Strength Maalox Plus Suspension 1850
Maalox TC Suspension 1851
Maalox Plus Tablets .... ▣ 655
Extra Strength Maalox Plus Tablets 1850
Nephrox Suspension .... ▣ 563
WinGel Liquid & Tablets .... ▣ 761

Aluminum Hydroxide Gel (Reduces effectiveness of methenamine). Products include:
ALternaGEL Liquid 1154
Aludrox Oral Suspension 2428
Amphojel Suspension 2429
Amphojel Suspension without Flavor 2429
Mylanta Liquid 1155
Mylanta Double Strength Liquid 1155

Aluminum Hydroxide Gel, Dried (Reduces effectiveness of methenamine). Products include:
Alu-Tab/Alu-Cap 1309
Amphojel Tablets 2429
Ascriptin A/D Caplets 1850
Regular Strength Ascriptin Tablets 1850
Gaviscon Antacid Tablets .... ▣ 593
Gaviscon-2 Antacid Tablets .... ▣ 594
Mylanta Tablets 1155
Mylanta Double Strength Tablets 1155

Aspirin (Increased serum salicylate levels; possible toxicity). Products include:
Alka-Seltzer Effervescent Antacid and Pain Reliever 1568
Alka-Seltzer Extra Strength Effervescent Antacid and Pain Reliever 1570
Alka-Seltzer (Flavored) Effervescent Antacid and Pain Reliever 1569
Alka-Seltzer Plus Cold Medicine .... ▣ 623
Alka-Seltzer Plus Night-Time Cold Medicine .... ▣ 623
Alka Seltzer Plus Sinus Allergy Medicine .... ▣ 624
Anacin Coated Analgesic Caplets 2417
Anacin Coated Analgesic Tablets 2417
Anacin Maximum Strength Analgesic Coated Tablets 2417
Maximum Strength Arthritis Pain Formula By the Makers of Anacin Analgesic Tablets and Caplets 2418
Arthritis Pain Formula by the Makers of Anacin Analgesic Tablets and Caplets .... ▣ 747

Arthritis Strength BC Powder ▣ 516
Ascriptin A/D Caplets 1850
Regular Strength Ascriptin Tablets 1850
Azdōne Tablets 844
BC Powder ▣ 517
BC Cold Powder ▣ 517
Children's Bayer Chewable Aspirin ▣ 564
Genuine Bayer Aspirin Tablets & Caplets ▣ 564
Maximum Bayer Aspirin Tablets & Caplets ▣ 566
Bayer Plus Aspirin Tablets ▣ 567
Therapy Bayer Aspirin Caplets ▣ 568
8 Hour Bayer Timed-Release Aspirin ▣ 566
Arthritis Strength Bufferin Analgesic Caplets 744
Extra Strength Bufferin Analgesic Tablets 745
Bufferin Analgesic Tablets and Caplets 743
Cama Arthritis Pain Reliever ▣ 685
Damason-P 1356
Easprin 1719
Ecotrin Enteric Coated Aspirin Maximum Strength Tablets and Caplets 2189
Ecotrin Enteric Coated Aspirin Regular Strength Tablets and Caplets 2189
Empirin Aspirin ▣ 541
Empirin with Codeine Phosphate Nos. 2, 3 & 4 764
Equagesic Tablets 2451
Excedrin Extra-Strength Analgesic Tablets & Caplets 749
4-Way Cold Tablets 750
Fiorinal Capsules 2007
Fiorinal with Codeine Capsules 2008
Fiorinal Tablets 2007
Lortab ASA Tablets 2414
Momentum Muscular Backache Formula ▣ 751
Norgesic 1314
Norwich Extra-Strength Aspirin ▣ 546
Norwich Regular Strength Aspirin ▣ 547
P-A-C Analgesic Tablets ▣ 669
Percodan 951
Robaxisal Tablets 1872
Sine-Off Sinus Medicine Tablets-Aspirin Formula ▣ 722
Soma Compound w/Codeine Tablets 2390
Soma Compound Tablets 2389
St. Joseph Adult Chewable Aspirin (81 mg.) ▣ 703
Synalgos-DC Capsules 2525
Talwin Compound 2072
Ursinus Inlay-Tabs ▣ 691
Vanquish Analgesic Caplets ▣ 574
Zorprin Tablets 698

Bendroflumethiazide (Reduces effectiveness of methenamine). Products include:
Corzide Tablets 702
Naturetin Tablets 1789
Rauzide Tablets 1804

Betamethasone Acetate (Hypernatremia). Products include:
Celestone Soluspan Suspension 2081

Betamethasone Sodium Phosphate (Hypernatremia). Products include:
Celestone Soluspan Suspension 2081

Chlorothiazide (Reduces effectiveness of methenamine). Products include:
Aldoclor Tablets 1413
Diupres Tablets 1461
Diuril Oral 1464

Chlorothiazide Sodium (Reduces effectiveness of methenamine). Products include:
Diuril Sodium Intravenous 1463

Choline Magnesium Trisalicylate (Increased serum salicylate levels; possible toxicity). Products include:
Trilisate 1822

Cortisone Acetate (Hypernatremia). Products include:
Cortone Acetate Sterile Suspension 1437
Cortone Acetate Tablets 1439

Deserpidine (Hypernatremia). Products include:
Enduronyl 518
Harmonyl Tablets 528
Oreticyl 545

Desoxycorticosterone Acetate (Hypernatremia).

Dexamethasone (Hypernatremia). Products include:
AK-Trol Ointment & Suspension ⊙ 207
Decadron Elixir 1445
Decadron Tablets 1447
Decaspray Topical Aerosol 1459
Dexacidin ⊙ 272
Maxidex Sterile Ophthalmic Suspension ⊙ 223
Maxitrol Ophthalmic Ointment/Suspension ⊙ 223
TobraDex Ophthalmic Suspension and Ointment ⊙ 228

Dexamethasone Acetate (Hypernatremia). Products include:
Dalalone D.P. Injectable 999
Decadron-LA Sterile Suspension 1457

Dexamethasone Sodium Phosphate (Hypernatremia). Products include:
AK-Dex ⊙ 203
Decadron Phosphate Respihaler 1454
Decadron Phosphate Sterile Ophthalmic Ointment 1453
Decadron Phosphate Sterile Ophthalmic Solution 1453
Decadron Phosphate Topical Cream 1455
Decadron Phosphate Turbinaire 1456
Maxidex Sterile Ophthalmic Ointment ⊙ 222
NeoDecadron Sterile Ophthalmic Ointment 1517
NeoDecadron Sterile Ophthalmic Solution 1518
NeoDecadron Topical Cream 1518

Diazoxide (Hypernatremia). Products include:
Hyperstat I.V. Injection 2095
Proglycem 649

Dichlorphenamide (Reduces effectiveness of methenamine). Products include:
Daranide Tablets 1445

Diflunisal (Increased serum salicylate levels; possible toxicity). Products include:
Dolobid Tablets 1465

Dihydroxyaluminum Sodium Carbonate (Reduces effectiveness of methenamine). Products include:
Rolaids ▣ 743

Guanethidine Monosulfate (Hypernatremia). Products include:
Esimil Tablets 864
Ismelin Tablets 869

Hydralazine Hydrochloride (Hypernatremia). Products include:
Apresazide Capsules 854
Apresoline Hydrochloride Parenteral (Ampuls) 856
Apresoline Hydrochloride Tablets 855
Apresoline-Esidrix Tablets 857
Ser-Ap-Es Tablets 881
Serpasil-Apresoline Tablets 884

Hydrochlorothiazide (Reduces effectiveness of methenamine). Products include:
Aldactazide 2150
Aldoril Tablets 1418
Apresazide Capsules 854
Apresoline-Esidrix Tablets 857
Capozide 2258
Dyazide Capsules 2208
Esidrix Tablets 863
Esimil Tablets 864
HydroDIURIL Tablets 1484
Hydropres Tablets 1485
Inderide Tablets 2463
Inderide LA Long Acting Capsules 2465
Lopressor HCT Tablets 1034
Maxzide 1215
Moduretic Tablets 1510
Normozide Tablets 2112
Oretic Tablets 544
Oreticyl 545
Prinzide Tablets 1540
Ser-Ap-Es Tablets 881
Serpasil-Esidrix Tablets 886
Timolide Tablets 1547
Trandate HCT Tablets 579
Vaseretic Tablets 1559
Zestoretic 2274

Hydrocortisone (Hypernatremia). Products include:
AK-Spore H.C. ⊙ 206
Bactine Hydrocortisone Anti-Itch Cream ▣ 625
CaldeCORT Anti-Itch Hydrocortisone Spray ▣ 560
Carmol HC Cream 1% 2296
Cortaid Spray ▣ 735
Cortenema 2244
Cortisporin Ointment 758
Cortisporin Ophthalmic Ointment Sterile 758
Cortisporin Ophthalmic Suspension Sterile 759
Cortisporin Otic Solution Sterile 760
Cortisporin Otic Suspension Sterile 760
Cortizone-5 Creme & Ointment ▣ 732
Dermolate Anti-Itch Cream ▣ 697
Eldecort Cream 1.0% 1113
Eldecort Cream 1.0% and 2.5% 1113
Fungoid HC Creme 1770
Hydrocortone Tablets 1482
Hytone 909
LazerSporin-C Solution 1770
Massengill Medicated Soft Cloth Towelettes 2192
Nutracort Cream & Lotion 1684
PediOtic Suspension Sterile 797
Synacort Creams 1%, 2.5% 2296
Vanoxide-HC Acne Lotion 911
Vioform-Hydrocortisone Cream and Mild Cream 889
Vioform-Hydrocortisone Ointment 889
VōSoL HC Otic Solution 2392
Vytone Cream 1% 911

Hydrocortisone Acetate (Hypernatremia). Products include:
Analpram-HC Rectal Cream 1% and 2.5% 970
Anusol-HC Cream 1690
Anusol-HC Suppositories 1691
Caldecort ▣ 560
Carmol HC Cream 1% 2296
Chloromycetin Hydrocortisone Ophthalmic 1694
Coly-Mycin S Otic w/Neomycin & Hydrocortisone 1708
Cortaid ▣ 735
Cortef Feminine Itch Cream ▣ 735
Corticaine ▣ 682
Cortifoam 1827
Cortisporin Cream 757
Epifoam 1828
Gynecort 5 Creme ▣ 556
Hydrocortone Acetate Sterile Suspension 1479
Lanacort 5 Creme and Ointment ▣ 557
Mantadil Cream 789
Ophthocort ⊙ 301
Orabase HCA Oral Paste 890
Pramosone Cream, Lotion & Ointment 971
ProctoCream-HC 1834
Proctofoam-HC 1835

Hydrocortisone Sodium Phosphate (Hypernatremia). Products include:
Hydrocortone Phosphate Injection, Sterile 1481

Hydrocortisone Sodium Succinate (Hypernatremia). Products include:
Solu-Cortef Sterile Powder 2361

Hydroflumethiazide (Reduces effectiveness of methenamine). Products include:
Diucardin Tablets 2450
Saluron 718
Salutensin/Salutensin-Demi 719

Magaldrate (Reduces effectiveness of methenamine). Products include:
Riopan Antacid Chew Tablets ▣ 754
Riopan Antacid Chew Tablets in Rollpacks ▣ 754
Riopan Antacid Suspension 2421
Riopan Antacid Swallow Tablets 2421
Riopan Plus Chew Tablets 2422
Riopan Plus Chew Tablets in Rollpack 2422
Riopan Plus 2 Chew Tablets, Mint Flavor, Cherry Flavor 2422
Riopan Plus Suspension 2422
Riopan Plus 2 Suspension, Mint Flavor, Cherry Flavor 2422

Magnesium Hydroxide (Reduces effectiveness of methenamine). Products include:
Aludrox Oral Suspension 2428
Ascriptin A/D Caplets 1850
Regular Strength Ascriptin Tablets 1850
Di-Gel Antacid/Anti-Gas ▣ 697
Gelusil Liquid & Tablets ▣ 639
Haley's M-O, Regular & Flavored ▣ 569
Extra Strength Maalox Plus Suspension 1850
Maalox TC Suspension 1851
Maalox Plus Tablets ▣ 655
Extra Strength Maalox Plus Tablets 1850
Mylanta Liquid 1155
Mylanta Tablets 1155
Mylanta Double Strength Liquid 1155
Mylanta Double Strength Tablets 1155
Concentrated Phillips' Milk of Magnesia ▣ 573
Phillips' Milk of Magnesia Liquid ▣ 572
Phillips' Milk of Magnesia Tablets ▣ 573
WinGel Liquid & Tablets ▣ 761

Magnesium Oxide (Reduces effectiveness of methenamine). Products include:
Bayer Plus Aspirin Tablets ▣ 567
Beelith Tablets 659
Bufferin Analgesic Tablets and Caplets ▣ 524
Cama Arthritis Pain Reliever ▣ 685
Mag-Ox 400 673
Uro-Mag 673

Magnesium Salicylate (Increased serum salicylate levels; possible toxicity). Products include:
Doan's - Extra-Strength Analgesic ▣ 549
Doan's - Regular Strength Analgesic ▣ 549
Mobigesic Analgesic Tablets ▣ 507

Methazolamide (Reduces effectiveness of methenamine). Products include:
Neptazane Tablets ⊙ 311

Methyclothiazide (Reduces effectiveness of methenamine). Products include:
Enduron Tablets 517
Enduronyl 518

Methyldopa (Hypernatremia). Products include:
Aldoclor Tablets 1413
Aldomet Oral 1415
Aldoril Tablets 1418

Methyldopate Hydrochloride (Hypernatremia). Products include:
Aldomet Ester HCl Injection 1417

Methylprednisolone Acetate (Hypernatremia). Products include:
Depo-Medrol Sterile Aqueous Suspension 2334

Methylprednisolone Sodium Succinate (Hypernatremia). Products include:
Solu-Medrol Sterile Powder 2363

Polythiazide (Reduces effectiveness of methenamine). Products include:
Minizide Capsules 1779
Renese Tablets 1785
Renese-R Tablets 1786

Potassium Citrate (Reduces effectiveness of methenamine). Products include:
Alka-Seltzer Effervescent Antacid 1570
K-Lyte 707
Polycitra Syrup 2424
Polycitra-K 2424
Polycitra-LC—Sugar-Free 2424
Ricelyte, Rice-Based Oral Electrolyte Maintenance Solution ▣ 613

Prednisolone Acetate (Hypernatremia). Products include:
AK-Cide Sterile Ophthalmic Ointment & Suspension ⊙ 202
Blephamide Liquifilm Sterile Ophthalmic Suspension 586
Blephamide S.O.P. Sterile Ophthalmic Ointment 586

Cetapred Ointment ◉ 220
⅛ % Econopred & 1 % Econopred Plus ◉ 217
Isopto Cetapred Suspension ◉ 220
Metimyd ◉ 306
Poly-Pred Liquifilm ◉ 250
Pred Forte ◉ 252
Pred Mild ◉ 254
Pred-G Liquifilm Sterile Ophthalmic Suspension ◉ 252
Pred-G S.O.P. Sterile Ophthalmic Ointment ◉ 253
Vasocidin Ointment ◉ 275

Prednisolone Sodium Phosphate (Hypernatremia). Products include:
AK-Pred ◉ 205
Hydeltrasol Injection, Sterile 1476
Inflamase ◉ 274
Pediapred Oral Liquid 987
Vasocidin Ophthalmic Solution ◉ 276

Prednisolone Tebutate (Hypernatremia). Products include:
Hydeltra-T.B.A. Sterile Suspension 1478

Prednisone (Hypernatremia). Products include:
Deltasone Tablets 2332

Rauwolfia Serpentina (Hypernatremia). Products include:
Raudixin Tablets 1803
Rauzide Tablets 1804

Rescinnamine (Hypernatremia).
No products indexed under this heading.

Reserpine (Hypernatremia). Products include:
Diupres Tablets 1461
Hydromox R Tablets 1209
Hydropres Tablets 1485
Renese-R Tablets 1786
Salutensin/Salutensin-Demi 719
Ser-Ap-Es Tablets 881
Serpasil Tablets 883
Serpasil-Apresoline Tablets 884
Serpasil-Esidrix Tablets 886

Salsalate (Increased salicylate levels; possible toxicity). Products include:
Disalcid 1310
Mono-Gesic Tablets 846
Salflex 839

Sodium Bicarbonate (Reduces effectiveness of methenamine). Products include:
Alka-Seltzer Advanced Formula Antacid & Non-Aspirin Pain Reliever ▣ 620
Alka-Seltzer Effervescent Antacid ▣ 622
Alka-Seltzer Effervescent Antacid and Pain Reliever 1568
Alka-Seltzer Extra Strength Effervescent Antacid and Pain Reliever ▣ 623
Alka-Seltzer (Flavored) Effervescent Antacid and Pain Reliever ▣ 621
Arm & Hammer Pure Baking Soda ▣ 548
Ceo-Two Rectal Suppositories 671
Citrocarbonate Antacid ▣ 668
Massengill Liquid Concentrate 2191
NuLYTELY 699

Sodium Citrate (Reduces effectiveness of methenamine). Products include:
Alka-Seltzer Effervescent Antacid 1570
Alka-Seltzer Extra Strength Effervescent Antacid and Pain Reliever 1570
Alka-Seltzer (Flavored) Effervescent Antacid and Pain Reliever 1569
Bicitra—Sugar-Free 2423
Citrocarbonate Antacid ▣ 668
Polycitra 2424
Ricelyte, Rice-Based Oral Electrolyte Maintenance Solution ▣ 613

Sulfamethizole (Increased risk of crystalluria). Products include:
Thiosulfil Forte Tablets 2526
Urobiotic-250 Capsules 1968

Sulfamethoxazole (Increased risk of crystalluria). Products include:
Azo Gantanol Tablets 1887
Bactrim DS Tablets 1891
Bactrim I.V. Infusion 1889
Bactrim 1891
Gantanol 1899
Septra 813
Septra I.V. Infusion 808
Septra I.V. Infusion ADD-Vantage Vials 810
Septra 813

Sulfasalazine (Increased risk of crystalluria). Products include:
Azulfidine Tablets, EN-tabs, Oral Suspension 1157

Sulfinpyrazone (Increased risk of crystalluria). Products include:
Anturane 853

Sulfisoxazole (Increased risk of crystalluria). Products include:
Azo Gantrisin Tablets 1888
Gantrisin Tablets 1901
Pediazole 1973

Sulfisoxazole Diolamine (Increased risk of crystalluria). Products include:
Gantrisin Ophthalmic Ointment/Solution 1900

Triamcinolone (Hypernatremia).
No products indexed under this heading.

Triamcinolone Acetonide (Hypernatremia). Products include:
Aristocort A 1010
Azmacort Inhaler 1837
Kenalog Cream, Lotion & Ointment 2401
Kenalog-10 Injection 2402
Kenalog-40 Injection 2403
Kenalog in Orabase 604
Kenalog Spray 2401
Mycolog II Cream and Ointment 2407
Mytrex Cream & Ointment 2080
Nasacort Nasal Inhaler 1844

Triamcinolone Diacetate (Hypernatremia). Products include:
Aristocort Suspension 1008

Triamcinolone Hexacetonide (Hypernatremia). Products include:
Aristospan Suspension 1011

Food Interactions

Dairy products (Concurrent use should be avoided or restricted to assure an acidic pH).

Fruits, unspecified (Concurrent use should be avoided or restricted to assure an acidic pH).

UROQID-ACID NO. 2 TABLETS
(Methenamine Mandelate, Sodium Phosphate, Monobasic) 661
See **Uroqid-Acid Tablets**

URSINUS INLAY-TABS
(Aspirin, Pseudoephedrine Hydrochloride) ▣ 691
May interact with oral anticoagulants and certain other agents. Compounds in these categories include:

Antiarthritic Drugs, unspecified (Effect not specified).

Antidepressant Medications, unspecified (Effect not specified).

Antidiabetic Drugs, unspecified (Effect not specified).

Antihypertensive agents, unspecified (Effect not specified).

Dicumarol (Effect not specified). Products include:
Dicumarol Tablets 516

Warfarin Sodium (Effect not specified). Products include:
Coumadin Injection & Tablets 944
Panwarfin Tablets 547

VAGISEC MEDICATED LIQUID DOUCHE CONCENTRATE
(Antiseptics) 2143
No interactions described in labeling.

VAGISEC PLUS SUPPOSITORIES
(Antiseptics) 2143
No interactions described in labeling.

VAGISIL CREME
(Benzocaine) ▣ 557
No interactions described in labeling.

VAGISIL FEMININE POWDER
(Corn Starch) ▣ 558
No interactions described in labeling.

VAGISTAT
(Tioconazole) 1397
May interact with:

Rubber or latex products (The Vagistat ointment base may interact with rubber or latex products, such as condoms or vaginal contraceptive diaphragms; therefore, use of such products within 72 hours following treatment is not recommended).

VALIUM INJECTABLE
(Diazepam) 1937
May interact with barbiturates, anticonvulsants, phenothiazines, narcotic analgesics, monoamine oxidase inhibitors, tricyclic antidepressants, central nervous system depressants, and certain other agents. Compounds in these categories include:

Alcohol (Increased depression/apnea; hypotension/muscular weakness).

Alfentanil Hydrochloride (Potentiated action of Valium; increased depression/apnea). Products include:
Alfenta Injection 1131

Alprazolam (Increased depression/apnea). Products include:
Xanax Tablets 2367

Amitriptyline Hydrochloride (Potentiated action of Valium). Products include:
Elavil 2269
Endep Tablets 1927
Etrafon 2087
Limbitrol 1933
Triavil Tablets 1556

Amoxapine (Potentiated action of Valium). Products include:
Asendin Tablets 1196

Aprobarbital (Increased depression/apnea; hypotension/muscular weakness; potentiated action of Valium). Products include:
Alurate Elixir 1883

Buprenorphine (Potentiated action of Valium; increased depression/apnea).
No products indexed under this heading.

Buspirone Hydrochloride (Increased depression/apnea). Products include:
BuSpar 1401

Butabarbital (Increased depression/apnea; hypotension/muscular weakness; potentiated action of Valium). Products include:
Pyridium Plus 1764

Butalbital (Increased depression/apnea; hypotension/muscular weakness; potentiated action of Valium). Products include:
Esgic-Plus Tablets 1002
Esgic Tablets & Capsules 1001
Fioricet Tablets 2006
Fiorinal Capsules 2007
Fiorinal with Codeine Capsules 2008
Fiorinal Tablets 2007
Phrenilin 838
Sedapap Tablets 50 mg/650 mg 1360

Carbamazepine (Potentiated action of Valium). Products include:
Tegretol Chewable Tablets 654
Tegretol Suspension 656
Tegretol Tablets 654

Chlordiazepoxide (Potentiated action of Valium; increased depression/apnea). Products include:
Libritabs Tablets 1930
Limbitrol 1933
Menrium Tablets 1934

Chlordiazepoxide Hydrochloride (Potentiated action of Valium; increased depression/apnea). Products include:
Librax Capsules 1929
Librium Capsules 1931
Librium Injectable 1932

Chlorpromazine (Potentiated action of Valium; increased depression/apnea). Products include:
Thorazine 2234

Chlorprothixene (Potentiated action of Valium; increased depression/apnea). Products include:
Taractan Tablets 1920

Chlorprothixene Hydrochloride (Potentiated action of Valium; increased depression/apnea). Products include:
Taractan 1920

Cimetidine (Delayed Valium clearance). Products include:
Tagamet Tablets 2228

Cimetidine Hydrochloride (Delayed Valium clearance). Products include:
Tagamet 2228

Clomipramine Hydrochloride (Potentiated action of Valium). Products include:
Anafranil Capsules 650

Clorazepate Dipotassium (Increased depression/apnea). Products include:
Tranxene 556

Codeine (Potentiated action of Valium; increased depression/apnea). Products include:
Calcidrine Syrup 506

Codeine Phosphate (Potentiated action of Valium; increased depression/apnea). Products include:
Actifed with Codeine Cough Syrup 752
Cheracol Cough Syrup 1853
Codimal PH Syrup 846
Dimetane-DC Cough Syrup 1857
Empirin with Codeine Phosphate Nos. 2, 3 & 4 764
Fiorinal with Codeine Capsules 2008
Isoclor Expectorant 982
Naldecon CX Adult Liquid ▣ 521
Novahistine DH 1342
Novahistine Expectorant 1343
Nucofed Capsules 2219
Nucofed Expectorant 2219
Nucofed Pediatric Expectorant 2220
Nucofed Syrup 2219
Phenaphen with Codeine Capsules 1865
Phenaphen-650 with Codeine Tablets 1866
Phenergan with Codeine 2497
Phenergan VC with Codeine 2501
Robitussin A-C Syrup 1875
Robitussin-DAC Syrup 1875
Ryna ▣ 741
Soma Compound w/Codeine Tablets 2390
Triaminic Expectorant w/Codeine 1996
Tussi-Organidin Liquid 2391
Tylenol with Codeine 1381

Codeine Polistirex (Potentiated action of Valium; increased depression/apnea).
No products indexed under this heading.

Desipramine Hydrochloride (Potentiated action of Valium). Products include:
Norpramin Tablets 1340

(▣ Described in PDR For Nonprescription Drugs) (◉ Described in PDR For Ophthalmology)

Dezocine (Potentiated action of Valium; increased depression/apnea).

Divalproex Sodium (Potentiated action of Valium). Products include:
- Depakote 512

Doxepin Hydrochloride (Potentiated action of Valium). Products include:
- Sinequan 1960

Droperidol (Increased depression/apnea). Products include:
- Inapsine Injection 1140
- Innovar Injection 1141

Enflurane (Increased depression/apnea). Products include:
- Ethrane 599

Estazolam (Potentiated action of Valium; increased depression/apnea). Products include:
- ProSom Tablets 554

Ethchlorvynol (Increased depression/apnea). Products include:
- Placidyl Capsules 553

Ethinamate (Increased depression/apnea).
- No products indexed under this heading.

Ethosuximide (Potentiated action of Valium). Products include:
- Zarontin Capsules 1768
- Zarontin Syrup 1769

Ethotoin (Potentiated action of Valium). Products include:
- Peganone Tablets 551

Fentanyl (Potentiated action of Valium; increased depression/apnea). Products include:
- Duragesic Transdermal System 1133

Fentanyl Citrate (Potentiated action of Valium; increased depression/apnea). Products include:
- Innovar Injection 1141
- Sublimaze Injection 1146

Fluphenazine Decanoate (Potentiated action of Valium; increased depression/apnea). Products include:
- Prolixin Decanoate 1795

Fluphenazine Enanthate (Potentiated action of Valium; increased depression/apnea). Products include:
- Prolixin Enanthate 1796

Fluphenazine Hydrochloride (Potentiated action of Valium; increased depression/apnea). Products include:
- Prolixin Elixir 1793
- Prolixin Injection 1791
- Prolixin Oral Concentrate 1792
- Prolixin Tablets 1793

Flurazepam Hydrochloride (Increased depression/apnea). Products include:
- Dalmane Capsules 1927

Furazolidone (Potentiated action of Valium). Products include:
- Furoxone 1855

Glutethimide (Increased depression/apnea).
- No products indexed under this heading.

Haloperidol (Increased depression/apnea). Products include:
- Haldol Injection, Tablets and Concentrate 1373

Haloperidol Decanoate (Increased depression/apnea). Products include:
- Haldol Decanoate 1375

Hydrocodone Bitartrate (Potentiated action of Valium; increased depression/apnea). Products include:
- Anexsia 5/500 Tablets 2196
- Anexsia 7.5/650 Tablets 2197
- Azdōne Tablets 844
- Codiclear DH Syrup 845
- Codimal DH Syrup 846
- Damason-P 1356
- Hycodan Syrup, Tablets 927
- Hycomine Compound Tablets 929
- Hycomine Syrup 927
- Hycotuss Expectorant Syrup 930
- Hydrocet Capsules 835
- Lortab ASA Tablets 2414
- Lortab 2412
- Ru-Tuss with Hydrocodone 694
- Triaminic Expectorant DH 1995
- Vicodin Tablets 1187
- Vicodin ES Tablets 1189
- Zydone Capsules 941

Hydrocodone Polistirex (Potentiated action of Valium; increased depression/apnea). Products include:
- Tussionex Extended-Release Suspension 988

Hydroxyzine Hydrochloride (Increased depression/apnea). Products include:
- Atarax Tablets & Syrup 1941
- Marax Tablets & DF Syrup 1954
- Vistaril Intramuscular Solution 1970

Imipramine Hydrochloride (Potentiated action of Valium). Products include:
- Tofranil Ampuls 1038
- Tofranil Tablets 1039

Imipramine Pamoate (Potentiated action of Valium). Products include:
- Tofranil-PM Capsules 1041

Isocarboxazid (Potentiated action of Valium). Products include:
- Marplan Tablets 1906

Isoflurane (Increased depression/apnea). Products include:
- Forane 600

Ketamine Hydrochloride (Potentiated action of Valium; increased depression/apnea). Products include:
- Ketalar 1726

Levorphanol Tartrate (Potentiated action of Valium; increased depression/apnea). Products include:
- Levo-Dromoran 1906

Lorazepam (Increased depression/apnea). Products include:
- Ativan Injection 2432
- Ativan Tablets 2434

Loxapine Hydrochloride (Increased depression/apnea). Products include:
- Loxitane 1213

Loxapine Succinate (Potentiated action of Valium; increased depression/apnea). Products include:
- Loxitane Capsules 1213

Maprotiline Hydrochloride (Potentiated action of Valium). Products include:
- Ludiomil Tablets 874

Meperidine Hydrochloride (Potentiated action of Valium; increased depression/apnea). Products include:
- Demerol 2047
- Mepergan Injection 2479

Mephenytoin (Potentiated action of Valium). Products include:
- Mesantoin Tablets 2013

Mephobarbital (Increased depression/apnea; hypotension/muscular weakness; potentiated action of Valium). Products include:
- Mebaral Tablets 2061

Meprobamate (Increased depression/apnea). Products include:
- Deprol Tablets 2382
- Equagesic Tablets 2451
- Miltown Tablets 2386
- PMB 200 and PMB 400 2504

Mesoridazine (Potentiated action of Valium; increased depression/apnea). Products include:
- Serentil 686

Methadone Hydrochloride (Potentiated action of Valium; increased depression/apnea). Products include:
- Dolophine Hydrochloride Ampoules & Vials 1260
- Dolophine Hydrochloride Tablets 1261
- Methadone Hydrochloride Diskets 1284
- Methadone Hydrochloride Oral Solution & Tablets 1987

Methohexital Sodium (Increased depression/apnea). Products include:
- Brevital Sodium Vials 1248

Methoxyflurane (Increased depression/apnea).
- No products indexed under this heading.

Methsuximide (Potentiated action of Valium). Products include:
- Celontin 1692

Midazolam Hydrochloride (Increased depression/apnea; potentiated action of Valium). Products include:
- Versed Injection 1924

Molindone Hydrochloride (Increased depression/apnea). Products include:
- Moban Tablets & Concentrate 932

Morphine Sulfate (Potentiated action of Valium; increased depression/apnea). Products include:
- Astramorph/PF Injection, USP (Preservative-Free) 618
- Duramorph 960
- Infumorph 200 and Infumorph 500 Sterile Solutions 962
- MS Contin Tablets 1814
- MSIR 1817
- Oramorph SR (Morphine Sulfate Sustained Release Tablets) 1988
- Roxanol 1991

Nortriptyline Hydrochloride (Potentiated action of Valium). Products include:
- Pamelor 2019

Opium Alkaloids (Potentiated action of Valium; increased depression/apnea). Products include:
- B & O No. 15A & No. 16A Supprettes 2395
- Pantopon Injectable 1911

Oxazepam (Increased depression/apnea). Products include:
- Serax Capsules 2522
- Serax Tablets 2522

Oxycodone Hydrochloride (Potentiated action of Valium; increased depression/apnea). Products include:
- Percocet Tablets 950
- Percodan 951
- Roxicodone Tablets, Oral Solution & Intensol (Oxycodone) 1992
- Tylox Capsules 1382

Paramethadione (Potentiated action of Valium). Products include:
- Paradione Capsules 548

Pentobarbital Sodium (Increased depression/apnea; hypotension/muscular weakness; potentiated action of Valium). Products include:
- Nembutal Sodium Capsules 534
- Nembutal Sodium Solution 536
- Nembutal Sodium Suppositories 538

Perphenazine (Potentiated action of Valium; increased depression/apnea). Products include:
- Etrafon 2087
- Triavil Tablets 1556
- Trilafon 2123

Phenacemide (Potentiated action of Valium). Products include:
- Phenurone Tablets 552

Phenelzine Sulfate (Potentiated action of Valium). Products include:
- Nardil 1742

Phenobarbital (Increased depression/apnea; hypotension/muscular weakness; potentiated action of Valium). Products include:
- Arco-Lase Plus Tablets 607
- Bellergal-S Tablets 1998
- Bronkolixir .... ▣ 761
- Bronkotabs Tablets .... ▣ 762
- Donnatal 1858
- Donnatal Extentabs 1859
- Donnatal Tablets 1858
- Donnazyme Tablets 1860
- Kinesed Tablets 2272
- Phenobarbital Elixir and Tablets 1293
- Primatene Tablets-P Formula 2421
- Quadrinal Tablets 1183
- Tedral SA 1765

Phensuximide (Potentiated action of Valium). Products include:
- Milontin Kapseals 1741

Phenytoin (Potentiated action of Valium). Products include:
- Dilantin Infatabs 1710
- Dilantin-30 Pediatric/Dilantin-125 Suspension 1713

Phenytoin Sodium (Potentiated action of Valium). Products include:
- Dilantin Kapseals 1708
- Dilantin Parenteral 1712
- Dilantin with Phenobarbital Kapseals 1715

Prazepam (Increased depression/apnea). Products include:
- Centrax 1693

Primidone (Potentiated action of Valium). Products include:
- Mysoline 2480

Prochlorperazine (Potentiated action of Valium; increased depression/apnea). Products include:
- Compazine 2201

Promethazine Hydrochloride (Potentiated action of Valium; increased depression/apnea). Products include:
- Mepergan Injection 2479
- Phenergan with Codeine 2497
- Phenergan with Dextromethorphan 2499
- Phenergan Injection 2493
- Phenergan Suppositories 2496
- Phenergan Syrup 2495
- Phenergan Tablets 2496
- Phenergan VC 2500
- Phenergan VC with Codeine 2501

Propofol (Potentiated action of Valium; increased depression/apnea). Products include:
- Diprivan Injection 2267

Propoxyphene Hydrochloride (Potentiated action of Valium; increased depression/apnea). Products include:
- Darvon 1256
- Wygesic Tablets 2540

Propoxyphene Napsylate (Potentiated action of Valium; increased depression/apnea). Products include:
- Darvon-N/Darvocet-N 1254

Protriptyline Hydrochloride (Potentiated action of Valium). Products include:
- Vivactil Tablets 1567

Quazepam (Potentiated action of Valium; increased depression/apnea). Products include:
- Doral Tablets 2383

Secobarbital Sodium (Increased depression/apnea; hypotension/muscular weakness; potentiated action of Valium). Products include:
- Seconal Sodium Pulvules 1296

Selegiline Hydrochloride (Potentiated action of Valium). Products include:
- Eldepryl 2250

Sufentanil Citrate (Potentiated action of Valium; increased depression/apnea). Products include:
- Sufenta Injection ... 1147

Temazepam (Increased depression/apnea). Products include:
- Restoril Capsules ... 2023

Thiamylal Sodium (Increased depression/apnea; hypotension/muscular weakness; potentiated action of Valium). Products include:
- Surital Ampoules, Steri-Vials ... 1764

Thioridazine Hydrochloride (Potentiated action of Valium; increased depression/apnea). Products include:
- Mellaril ... 2011

Thiothixene (Increased depression/apnea). Products include:
- Navane Capsules and Concentrate 1954
- Navane Intramuscular ... 1956

Tranylcypromine Sulfate (Potentiated action of Valium). Products include:
- Parnate Tablets ... 2222

Triazolam (Increased depression/apnea). Products include:
- Halcion Tablets ... 2340

Trifluoperazine Hydrochloride (Potentiated action of Valium; increased depression/apnea). Products include:
- Stelazine ... 2226

Trimethadione (Potentiated action of Valium). Products include:
- Tridione ... 557

Trimipramine Maleate (Potentiated action of Valium). Products include:
- Surmontil Capsules ... 2524

Valproic Acid (Potentiated action of Valium). Products include:
- Depakene Capsules & Syrup ... 511

VALIUM TABLETS

(Diazepam) ... 1939

May interact with anticonvulsants, phenothiazines, narcotic analgesics, barbiturates, monoamine oxidase inhibitors, tricyclic antidepressants, central nervous system depressants, and certain other agents. Compounds in these categories include:

Alcohol (Simultaneous use of alcohol not recommended).

Alfentanil Hydrochloride (Potentiated action of Valium; concurrent use not recommended). Products include:
- Alfenta Injection ... 1131

Alprazolam (Concurrent use not recommended). Products include:
- Xanax Tablets ... 2367

Amitriptyline Hydrochloride (Potentiated action of Valium). Products include:
- Elavil ... 2269
- Endep Tablets ... 1927
- Etrafon ... 2087
- Limbitrol ... 1933
- Triavil Tablets ... 1556

Amoxapine (Potentiated action of Valium). Products include:
- Asendin Tablets ... 1196

Aprobarbital (Potentiated action of Valium; concurrent use not recommended). Products include:
- Alurate Elixir ... 1883

Buprenorphine (Potentiated action of Valium; concurrent use not recommended).
- No products indexed under this heading.

Buspirone Hydrochloride (Concurrent use not recommended). Products include:
- BuSpar ... 1401

Butabarbital (Potentiated action of Valium; concurrent use not recommended). Products include:
- Pyridium Plus ... 1764

Butalbital (Potentiated action of Valium; concurrent use not recommended). Products include:
- Esgic-Plus Tablets ... 1002
- Esgic Tablets & Capsules ... 1001
- Fioricet Tablets ... 2006
- Fiorinal Capsules ... 2007
- Fiorinal with Codeine Capsules ... 2008
- Fiorinal Tablets ... 2007
- Phrenilin ... 838
- Sedapap Tablets 50 mg/650 mg .. 1360

Carbamazepine (Increase in dosage may be required). Products include:
- Tegretol Chewable Tablets ... 654
- Tegretol Suspension ... 656
- Tegretol Tablets ... 654

Chlordiazepoxide (Potentiated action of Valium; concurrent use not recommended). Products include:
- Libritabs Tablets ... 1930
- Limbitrol ... 1933
- Menrium Tablets ... 1934

Chlordiazepoxide Hydrochloride (Potentiated action of Valium; concurrent use not recommended). Products include:
- Librax Capsules ... 1929
- Librium Capsules ... 1931
- Librium Injectable ... 1932

Chlorpromazine (Potentiated action of Valium; concurrent use not recommended). Products include:
- Thorazine ... 2234

Chlorprothixene (Concurrent use not recommended). Products include:
- Taractan Tablets ... 1920

Chlorprothixene Hydrochloride (Concurrent use not recommended). Products include:
- Taractan ... 1920

Cimetidine (Delayed Valium clearance). Products include:
- Tagamet Tablets ... 2228

Cimetidine Hydrochloride (Delayed Valium clearance). Products include:
- Tagamet ... 2228

Clomipramine Hydrochloride (Potentiated action of Valium). Products include:
- Anafranil Capsules ... 650

Clorazepate Dipotassium (Concurrent use not recommended). Products include:
- Tranxene ... 556

Codeine (Potentiated action of Valium; concurrent use not recommended). Products include:
- Calcidrine Syrup ... 506

Codeine Phosphate (Potentiated action of Valium; concurrent use not recommended). Products include:
- Actifed with Codeine Cough Syrup.. 752
- Cheracol Cough Syrup ... 1853
- Codimal PH Syrup ... 846
- Dimetane-DC Cough Syrup ... 1857
- Empirin with Codeine Phosphate Nos. 2, 3 & 4 ... 764
- Fiorinal with Codeine Capsules ... 2008
- Isoclor Expectorant ... 982
- Naldecon CX Adult Liquid ... ▣ 521
- Novahistine DH ... 1342
- Novahistine Expectorant ... 1343
- Nucofed Capsules ... 2219
- Nucofed Expectorant ... 2219
- Nucofed Pediatric Expectorant ... 2220
- Nucofed Syrup ... 2219
- Phenaphen with Codeine Capsules 1865
- Phenaphen-650 with Codeine Tablets ... 1866
- Phenergan with Codeine ... 2497
- Phenergan VC with Codeine ... 2501
- Robitussin A-C Syrup ... 1875
- Robitussin-DAC Syrup ... 1875
- Ryna ... ▣ 741
- Soma Compound w/Codeine Tablets ... 2390
- Triaminic Expectorant w/Codeine .. 1996
- Tussi-Organidin Liquid ... 2391
- Tylenol with Codeine ... 1381

Codeine Polistirex (Potentiated action of Valium; concurrent use not recommended).
- No products indexed under this heading.

Desipramine Hydrochloride (Potentiated action of Valium). Products include:
- Norpramin Tablets ... 1340

Dezocine (Potentiated action of Valium; concurrent use not recommended).

Divalproex Sodium (Increase in dosage may be required). Products include:
- Depakote ... 512

Doxepin Hydrochloride (Potentiated action of Valium). Products include:
- Sinequan ... 1960

Droperidol (Concurrent use not recommended). Products include:
- Inapsine Injection ... 1140
- Innovar Injection ... 1141

Enflurane (Concurrent use not recommended). Products include:
- Ethrane ... 599

Estazolam (Potentiated action of Valium; concurrent use not recommended). Products include:
- ProSom Tablets ... 554

Ethchlorvynol (Concurrent use not recommended). Products include:
- Placidyl Capsules ... 553

Ethinamate (Concurrent use not recommended).
- No products indexed under this heading.

Ethosuximide (Increase in dosage may be required). Products include:
- Zarontin Capsules ... 1768
- Zarontin Syrup ... 1769

Ethotoin (Increase in dosage may be required). Products include:
- Peganone Tablets ... 551

Fentanyl (Potentiated action of Valium; concurrent use not recommended). Products include:
- Duragesic Transdermal System ... 1133

Fentanyl Citrate (Potentiated action of Valium; concurrent use not recommended). Products include:
- Innovar Injection ... 1141
- Sublimaze Injection ... 1146

Fluphenazine Decanoate (Potentiated action of Valium; concurrent use not recommended). Products include:
- Prolixin Decanoate ... 1795

Fluphenazine Enanthate (Potentiated action of Valium; concurrent use not recommended). Products include:
- Prolixin Enanthate ... 1796

Fluphenazine Hydrochloride (Potentiated action of Valium; concurrent use not recommended). Products include:
- Prolixin Elixir ... 1793
- Prolixin Injection ... 1791
- Prolixin Oral Concentrate ... 1792
- Prolixin Tablets ... 1793

Flurazepam Hydrochloride (Concurrent use not recommended). Products include:
- Dalmane Capsules ... 1927

Furazolidone (Potentiated action of Valium). Products include:
- Furoxone ... 1855

Glutethimide (Concurrent use not recommended).
- No products indexed under this heading.

Haloperidol (Concurrent use not recommended). Products include:
- Haldol Injection, Tablets and Concentrate ... 1373

Haloperidol Decanoate (Concurrent use not recommended). Products include:
- Haldol Decanoate ... 1375

Hydrocodone Bitartrate (Potentiated action of Valium; concurrent use not recommended). Products include:
- Anexsia 5/500 Tablets ... 2196
- Anexsia 7.5/650 Tablets ... 2197
- Azdone Tablets ... 844
- Codiclear DH Syrup ... 845
- Codimal DH Syrup ... 846
- Damason-P ... 1356
- Hycodan Syrup, Tablets ... 927
- Hycomine Compound Tablets ... 929
- Hycomine Syrup ... 927
- Hycotuss Expectorant Syrup ... 930
- Hydrocet Capsules ... 835
- Lortab ASA Tablets ... 2414
- Lortab ... 2412
- Ru-Tuss with Hydrocodone ... 694
- Triaminic Expectorant DH ... 1995
- Vicodin Tablets ... 1187
- Vicodin ES Tablets ... 1189
- Zydone Capsules ... 941

Hydrocodone Polistirex (Potentiated action of Valium; concurrent use not recommended). Products include:
- Tussionex Extended-Release Suspension ... 988

Hydroxyzine Hydrochloride (Concurrent use not recommended). Products include:
- Atarax Tablets & Syrup ... 1941
- Marax Tablets & DF Syrup ... 1954
- Vistaril Intramuscular Solution ... 1970

Imipramine Hydrochloride (Potentiated action of Valium). Products include:
- Tofranil Ampuls ... 1038
- Tofranil Tablets ... 1039

Imipramine Pamoate (Potentiated action of Valium). Products include:
- Tofranil-PM Capsules ... 1041

Isocarboxazid (Potentiated action of Valium). Products include:
- Marplan Tablets ... 1906

Isoflurane (Concurrent use not recommended). Products include:
- Forane ... 600

Ketamine Hydrochloride (Potentiated action of Valium; concurrent use not recommended). Products include:
- Ketalar ... 1726

Levorphanol Tartrate (Potentiated action of Valium; concurrent use not recommended). Products include:
- Levo-Dromoran ... 1906

Lorazepam (Potentiated action of Valium; concurrent use not recommended). Products include:
- Ativan Injection ... 2432
- Ativan Tablets ... 2434

Loxapine Hydrochloride (Potentiated action of Valium; concurrent use not recommended). Products include:
- Loxitane ... 1213

Loxapine Succinate (Potentiated action of Valium; concurrent use not recommended). Products include:
- Loxitane Capsules ... 1213

Maprotiline Hydrochloride (Potentiated action of Valium). Products include:
- Ludiomil Tablets ... 874

Meperidine Hydrochloride (Potentiated action of Valium; concurrent use not recommended). Products include:
- Demerol ... 2047

Mepergan Injection 2479

Mephenytoin (Increase in dosage may be required). Products include:

Mesantoin Tablets 2013

Mephobarbital (Potentiated action of Valium; concurrent use not recommended). Products include:

Mebaral Tablets 2061

Meprobamate (Concurrent use not recommended). Products include:

Deprol Tablets 2382
Equagesic Tablets 2451
Miltown Tablets 2386
PMB 200 and PMB 400 2504

Mesoridazine (Potentiated action of Valium; concurrent use not recommended). Products include:

Serentil 686

Methadone Hydrochloride (Potentiated action of Valium; concurrent use not recommended). Products include:

Dolophine Hydrochloride Ampoules & Vials 1260
Dolophine Hydrochloride Tablets 1261
Methadone Hydrochloride Diskets 1284
Methadone Hydrochloride Oral Solution & Tablets 1987

Methohexital Sodium (Concurrent use not recommended). Products include:

Brevital Sodium Vials 1248

Methoxyflurane (Concurrent use not recommended).

No products indexed under this heading.

Methsuximide (Increase in dosage may be required). Products include:

Celontin 1692

Midazolam Hydrochloride (Potentiated action of Valium; concurrent use not recommended). Products include:

Versed Injection 1924

Molindone Hydrochloride (Concurrent use not recommended). Products include:

Moban Tablets & Concentrate 932

Morphine Sulfate (Potentiated action of Valium; concurrent use not recommended). Products include:

Astramorph/PF Injection, USP (Preservative-Free) 618
Duramorph 960
Infumorph 200 and Infumorph 500 Sterile Solutions 962
MS Contin Tablets 1814
MSIR 1817
Oramorph SR (Morphine Sulfate Sustained Release Tablets) 1988
Roxanol 1991

Nortriptyline Hydrochloride (Potentiated action of Valium). Products include:

Pamelor 2019

Opium Alkaloids (Potentiated action of Valium; concurrent use not recommended). Products include:

B & O No. 15A & No. 16A Supprettes 2395
Pantopon Injectable 1911

Oxazepam (Concurrent use not recommended). Products include:

Serax Capsules 2522
Serax Tablets 2522

Oxycodone Hydrochloride (Potentiated action of Valium; concurrent use not recommended). Products include:

Percocet Tablets 950
Percodan 951
Roxicodone Tablets, Oral Solution & Intensol (Oxycodone) 1992
Tylox Capsules 1382

Paramethadione (Increase in dosage may be required). Products include:

Paradione Capsules 548

Pentobarbital Sodium (Potentiated action of Valium; concurrent use not recommended). Products include:

Nembutal Sodium Capsules 534
Nembutal Sodium Solution 536
Nembutal Sodium Suppositories 538

Perphenazine (Potentiated action of Valium; concurrent use not recommended). Products include:

Etrafon 2087
Triavil Tablets 1556
Trilafon 2123

Phenacemide (Increase in dosage may be required). Products include:

Phenurone Tablets 552

Phenelzine Sulfate (Potentiated action of Valium). Products include:

Nardil 1742

Phenobarbital (Increase in dosage may be required; concurrent use not recommended). Products include:

Arco-Lase Plus Tablets 607
Bellergal-S Tablets 1998
Bronkolixir .... ▣ 761
Bronkotabs Tablets .... ▣ 762
Donnatal 1858
Donnatal Extentabs 1859
Donnatal Tablets 1858
Donnazyme Tablets 1860
Kinesed Tablets 2272
Phenobarbital Elixir and Tablets 1293
Primatene Tablets-P Formula 2421
Quadrinal Tablets 1183
Tedral SA 1765

Phensuximide (Increase in dosage may be required). Products include:

Milontin Kapseals 1741

Phenytoin (Increase in dosage may be required). Products include:

Dilantin Infatabs 1710
Dilantin-30 Pediatric/Dilantin-125 Suspension 1713

Phenytoin Sodium (Increase in dosage may be required). Products include:

Dilantin Kapseals 1708
Dilantin Parenteral 1712
Dilantin with Phenobarbital Kapseals 1715

Prazepam (Concurrent use not recommended). Products include:

Centrax 1693

Primidone (Increase in dosage may be required). Products include:

Mysoline 2480

Prochlorperazine (Potentiated action of Valium; concurrent use not recommended). Products include:

Compazine 2201

Promethazine Hydrochloride (Potentiated action of Valium; concurrent use not recommended). Products include:

Mepergan Injection 2479
Phenergan with Codeine 2497
Phenergan with Dextromethorphan 2499
Phenergan Injection 2493
Phenergan Suppositories 2496
Phenergan Syrup 2495
Phenergan Tablets 2496
Phenergan VC 2500
Phenergan VC with Codeine 2501

Propofol (Potentiated action of Valium; concurrent use not recommended). Products include:

Diprivan Injection 2267

Propoxyphene Hydrochloride (Potentiated action of Valium; concurrent use not recommended). Products include:

Darvon 1256
Wygesic Tablets 2540

Propoxyphene Napsylate (Potentiated action of Valium; concurrent use not recommended). Products include:

Darvon-N/Darvocet-N 1254

Protriptyline Hydrochloride (Potentiated action of Valium). Products include:

Vivactil Tablets 1567

Quazepam (Potentiated action of Valium; concurrent use not recommended). Products include:

Doral Tablets 2383

Secobarbital Sodium (Potentiated action of Valium; concurrent use not recommended). Products include:

Seconal Sodium Pulvules 1296

Selegiline Hydrochloride (Potentiated action of Valium). Products include:

Eldepryl 2250

Sufentanil Citrate (Potentiated action of Valium; concurrent use not recommended). Products include:

Sufenta Injection 1147

Temazepam (Concurrent use not recommended). Products include:

Restoril Capsules 2023

Thiamylal Sodium (Potentiated action of Valium; concurrent use not recommended). Products include:

Surital Ampoules, Steri-Vials 1764

Thioridazine Hydrochloride (Potentiated action of Valium; concurrent use not recommended). Products include:

Mellaril 2011

Thiothixene (Concurrent use not recommended). Products include:

Navane Capsules and Concentrate 1954
Navane Intramuscular 1956

Tranylcypromine Sulfate (Potentiated action of Valium). Products include:

Parnate Tablets 2222

Triazolam (Concurrent use not recommended). Products include:

Halcion Tablets 2340

Trifluoperazine Hydrochloride (Potentiated action of Valium; concurrent use not recommended). Products include:

Stelazine 2226

Trimethadione (Increase in dosage may be required). Products include:

Tridione 557

Trimipramine Maleate (Potentiated action of Valium). Products include:

Surmontil Capsules 2524

Valproic Acid (Increase in dosage may be required). Products include:

Depakene Capsules & Syrup 511

VALPIN 50 TABLETS

(Anisotropine Methylbromide) 941

No interactions described in labeling.

VALRELEASE CAPSULES

(Diazepam) 1923

May interact with phenothiazines, narcotic analgesics, barbiturates, monoamine oxidase inhibitors, tricyclic antidepressants, and certain other agents. Compounds in these categories include:

Alcohol (Potentiates action of diazepam).

Alfentanil Hydrochloride (Potentiates action of diazepam). Products include:

Alfenta Injection 1131

Amitriptyline Hydrochloride (Potentiates action of diazepam). Products include:

Elavil 2269
Endep Tablets 1927
Etrafon 2087
Limbitrol 1933
Triavil Tablets 1556

Amoxapine (Potentiates action of diazepam). Products include:

Asendin Tablets 1196

Aprobarbital (Potentiates action of diazepam). Products include:

Alurate Elixir 1883

Buprenorphine (Potentiates action of diazepam).

No products indexed under this heading.

Butabarbital (Potentiates action of diazepam). Products include:

Pyridium Plus 1764

Butalbital (Potentiates action of diazepam). Products include:

Esgic-Plus Tablets 1002
Esgic Tablets & Capsules 1001
Fioricet Tablets 2006
Fiorinal Capsules 2007
Fiorinal with Codeine Capsules 2008
Fiorinal Tablets 2007
Phrenilin 838
Sedapap Tablets 50 mg/650 mg .. 1360

Chlorpromazine (Potentiates action of diazepam). Products include:

Thorazine 2234

Cimetidine (Delays clearance of diazepam). Products include:

Tagamet Tablets 2228

Cimetidine Hydrochloride (Delays clearance of diazepam). Products include:

Tagamet 2228

Clomipramine Hydrochloride (Potentiates action of diazepam). Products include:

Anafranil Capsules 650

Codeine (Potentiates action of diazepam). Products include:

Calcidrine Syrup 506

Codeine Phosphate (Potentiates action of diazepam). Products include:

Actifed with Codeine Cough Syrup .. 752
Cheracol Cough Syrup 1853
Codimal PH Syrup 846
Dimetane-DC Cough Syrup 1857
Empirin with Codeine Phosphate Nos. 2, 3 & 4 764
Fiorinal with Codeine Capsules 2008
Isoclor Expectorant 982
Naldecon CX Adult Liquid .... ▣ 521
Novahistine DH 1342
Novahistine Expectorant 1343
Nucofed Capsules 2219
Nucofed Expectorant 2219
Nucofed Pediatric Expectorant 2220
Nucofed Syrup 2219
Phenaphen with Codeine Capsules 1865
Phenaphen-650 with Codeine Tablets 1866
Phenergan with Codeine 2497
Phenergan VC with Codeine 2501
Robitussin A-C Syrup 1875
Robitussin-DAC Syrup 1875
Ryna .... ▣ 741
Soma Compound w/Codeine Tablets 2390
Triaminic Expectorant w/Codeine .. 1996
Tussi-Organidin Liquid 2391
Tylenol with Codeine 1381

Codeine Polistirex (Potentiates action of diazepam).

No products indexed under this heading.

Desipramine Hydrochloride (Potentiates action of diazepam). Products include:

Norpramin Tablets 1340

Dezocine (Potentiates action of diazepam).

Doxepin Hydrochloride (Potentiates action of diazepam). Products include:

Sinequan 1960

Fentanyl (Potentiates action of diazepam). Products include:

Duragesic Transdermal System 1133

Fentanyl Citrate (Potentiates action of diazepam). Products include:
- Innovar Injection 1141
- Sublimaze Injection 1146

Fluphenazine Decanoate (Potentiates action of diazepam). Products include:
- Prolixin Decanoate 1795

Fluphenazine Enanthate (Potentiates action of diazepam). Products include:
- Prolixin Enanthate 1796

Fluphenazine Hydrochloride (Potentiates action of diazepam). Products include:
- Prolixin Elixir 1793
- Prolixin Injection 1791
- Prolixin Oral Concentrate 1792
- Prolixin Tablets 1793

Furazolidone (Potentiates action of diazepam). Products include:
- Furoxone 1855

Hydrocodone Bitartrate (Potentiates action of diazepam). Products include:
- Anexsia 5/500 Tablets 2196
- Anexsia 7.5/650 Tablets 2197
- Azdōne Tablets 844
- Codiclear DH Syrup 845
- Codimal DH Syrup 846
- Damason-P 1356
- Hycodan Syrup, Tablets 927
- Hycomine Compound Tablets 929
- Hycomine Syrup 927
- Hycotuss Expectorant Syrup 930
- Hydrocet Capsules 835
- Lortab ASA Tablets 2414
- Lortab 2412
- Ru-Tuss with Hydrocodone 694
- Triaminic Expectorant DH 1995
- Vicodin Tablets 1187
- Vicodin ES Tablets 1189
- Zydone Capsules 941

Hydrocodone Polistirex (Potentiates action of diazepam). Products include:
- Tussionex Extended-Release Suspension 988

Imipramine Hydrochloride (Potentiates action of diazepam). Products include:
- Tofranil Ampuls 1038
- Tofranil Tablets 1039

Imipramine Pamoate (Potentiates action of diazepam). Products include:
- Tofranil-PM Capsules 1041

Isocarboxazid (Potentiates action of diazepam). Products include:
- Marplan Tablets 1906

Levorphanol Tartrate (Potentiates action of diazepam). Products include:
- Levo-Dromoran 1906

Maprotiline Hydrochloride (Potentiates action of diazepam). Products include:
- Ludiomil Tablets 874

Meperidine Hydrochloride (Potentiates action of diazepam). Products include:
- Demerol 2047
- Mepergan Injection 2479

Mephobarbital (Potentiates action of diazepam). Products include:
- Mebaral Tablets 2061

Mesoridazine (Potentiates action of diazepam). Products include:
- Serentil 686

Methadone Hydrochloride (Potentiates action of diazepam). Products include:
- Dolophine Hydrochloride Ampoules & Vials 1260
- Dolophine Hydrochloride Tablets 1261
- Methadone Hydrochloride Diskets 1284
- Methadone Hydrochloride Oral Solution & Tablets 1987

Morphine Sulfate (Potentiates action of diazepam). Products include:
- Astramorph/PF Injection, USP (Preservative-Free) 618
- Duramorph 960
- Infumorph 200 and Infumorph 500 Sterile Solutions 962
- MS Contin Tablets 1814
- MSIR 1817
- Oramorph SR (Morphine Sulfate Sustained Release Tablets) 1988
- Roxanol 1991

Nortriptyline Hydrochloride (Potentiates action of diazepam). Products include:
- Pamelor 2019

Opium Alkaloids (Potentiates action of diazepam). Products include:
- B & O No. 15A & No. 16A Supprettes 2395
- Pantopon Injectable 1911

Oxycodone Hydrochloride (Potentiates action of diazepam). Products include:
- Percocet Tablets 950
- Percodan 951
- Roxicodone Tablets, Oral Solution & Intensol (Oxycodone) 1992
- Tylox Capsules 1382

Pentobarbital Sodium (Potentiates action of diazepam). Products include:
- Nembutal Sodium Capsules 534
- Nembutal Sodium Solution 536
- Nembutal Sodium Suppositories 538

Perphenazine (Potentiates action of diazepam). Products include:
- Etrafon 2087
- Triavil Tablets 1556
- Trilafon 2123

Phenelzine Sulfate (Potentiates action of diazepam). Products include:
- Nardil 1742

Phenobarbital (Potentiates action of diazepam). Products include:
- Arco-Lase Plus Tablets 607
- Bellergal-S Tablets 1998
- Bronkolixir ..... ⊞ 761
- Bronkotabs Tablets ..... ⊞ 762
- Donnatal 1858
- Donnatal Extentabs 1859
- Donnatal Tablets 1858
- Donnazyme Tablets 1860
- Kinesed Tablets 2272
- Phenobarbital Elixir and Tablets 1293
- Primatene Tablets-P Formula 2421
- Quadrinal Tablets 1183
- Tedral SA 1765

Prochlorperazine (Potentiates action of diazepam). Products include:
- Compazine 2201

Promethazine Hydrochloride (Potentiates action of diazepam). Products include:
- Mepergan Injection 2479
- Phenergan with Codeine 2497
- Phenergan with Dextromethorphan 2499
- Phenergan Injection 2493
- Phenergan Suppositories 2496
- Phenergan Syrup 2495
- Phenergan Tablets 2496
- Phenergan VC 2500
- Phenergan VC with Codeine 2501

Propoxyphene Hydrochloride (Potentiates action of diazepam). Products include:
- Darvon 1256
- Wygesic Tablets 2540

Propoxyphene Napsylate (Potentiates action of diazepam). Products include:
- Darvon-N/Darvocet-N 1254

Protriptyline Hydrochloride (Potentiates action of diazepam). Products include:
- Vivactil Tablets 1567

Secobarbital Sodium (Potentiates action of diazepam). Products include:
- Seconal Sodium Pulvules 1296

Selegiline Hydrochloride (Potentiates action of diazepam). Products include:
- Eldepryl 2250

Sufentanil Citrate (Potentiates action of diazepam). Products include:
- Sufenta Injection 1147

Thiamylal Sodium (Potentiates action of diazepam). Products include:
- Surital Ampoules, Steri-Vials 1764

Thioridazine Hydrochloride (Potentiates action of diazepam). Products include:
- Mellaril 2011

Tranylcypromine Sulfate (Potentiates action of diazepam). Products include:
- Parnate Tablets 2222

Trifluoperazine Hydrochloride (Potentiates action of diazepam). Products include:
- Stelazine 2226

Trimipramine Maleate (Potentiates action of diazepam). Products include:
- Surmontil Capsules 2524

VANCENASE AQ NASAL SPRAY 0.042%

(Beclomethasone Dipropionate) 2127
No interactions described in labeling.

VANCENASE NASAL INHALER

(Betamethasone Dipropionate) 2126
May interact with:

Prednisone (Increased likelihood of HPA suppression). Products include:
- Deltasone Tablets 2332

VANCERIL INHALER

(Betamethasone Dipropionate) 2128
No interactions described in labeling.

VANCOCIN HCL, ORAL SOLUTION & PULVULES

(Vancomycin Hydrochloride) 1304
May interact with aminoglycosides and ototoxic drugs. Compounds in these categories include:

Amikacin Sulfate (Concurrent use may result in increased ototoxicity and/or nephrotoxicity). Products include:
- Amikin Injectable 602

Cisplatin (Concurrent use may result in increased ototoxicity and/or nephrotoxicity). Products include:
- Platinol 737
- Platinol-AQ Injection 738

Gentamicin Sulfate (Concurrent use may result in increased ototoxicity and/or nephrotoxicity). Products include:
- Garamycin Injectable 2093
- Garamycin Ophthalmic ..... ◉ 305
- Genoptic Liquifilm Sterile Ophthalmic Solution ..... ◉ 247
- Genoptic S.O.P. Sterile Ophthalmic Ointment ..... ◉ 247
- Gentacidin Ointment ..... ◉ 273
- Gentacidin Solution ..... ◉ 273
- Gentak Ointment & Solution ..... ◉ 208
- G-myticin Creme and Ointment 0.1% 1770
- Pred-G Liquifilm Sterile Ophthalmic Suspension ..... ◉ 252
- Pred-G S.O.P. Sterile Ophthalmic Ointment ..... ◉ 253

Kanamycin Sulfate (Concurrent use may result in increased ototoxicity and/or nephrotoxicity). Products include:
- Kantrex Injection 601
- Kantrex Pediatric Injection 601

Streptomycin Sulfate (Concurrent use may result in increased ototoxicity and/or nephrotoxicity).
- No products indexed under this heading.

Tobramycin Sulfate (Concurrent use may result in increased ototoxicity and/or nephrotoxicity). Products include:
- Nebcin Vials, Hyporets & ADD-Vantage 1286

VANCOCIN HCL, VIALS & ADD-VANTAGE

(Vancomycin Hydrochloride) 1302
May interact with aminoglycosides, general anesthetics, and certain other agents. Compounds in these categories include:

Amikacin Sulfate (Concurrent use may result in increased ototoxicity). Products include:
- Amikin Injectable 602

Amphotericin B (Concurrent and/or sequential use requires careful monitoring due to increased potential for nephrotoxicity and/or neurotoxicity). Products include:
- Fungizone Cream, Lotion and Ointment 2261
- Fungizone Intravenous 2262

Bacitracin Zinc (Concurrent and/or sequential use requires careful monitoring due to increased potential for nephrotoxicity and/or neurotoxicity). Products include:
- AK-Poly-Bac Ointment ..... ◉ 205
- AK-Spore H.C. Ointment ..... ◉ 206
- AK-Spore Ointment ..... ◉ 205
- Aquaphor Antibiotic Formula 662
- Cortisporin Ointment 758
- Cortisporin Ophthalmic Ointment Sterile 758
- Neosporin Ointment 793
- Maximum Strength Neosporin Ointment 793
- Neosporin Ophthalmic Ointment Sterile 793
- Polysporin Ointment ..... ⊞ 543
- Polysporin Ophthalmic Ointment Sterile 798
- Polysporin Powder ..... ⊞ 543
- Polysporin Spray ..... ⊞ 543

Cisplatin (Concurrent and/or sequential use requires careful monitoring due to increased potential for nephrotoxicity and/or neurotoxicity). Products include:
- Platinol 737
- Platinol-AQ Injection 738

Colistin Sulfate (Concurrent and/or sequential use requires careful monitoring due to increased potential for nephrotoxicity and/or neurotoxicity). Products include:
- Coly-Mycin S For Oral Suspension 1708
- Coly-Mycin S Otic w/Neomycin & Hydrocortisone 1708

Enflurane (Concomitant administration has been associated with erythema and histamine-like flushing). Products include:
- Ethrane 599

Gentamicin Sulfate (Concurrent use may result in increased ototoxicity). Products include:
- Garamycin Injectable 2093
- Garamycin Ophthalmic ..... ◉ 305
- Genoptic Liquifilm Sterile Ophthalmic Solution ..... ◉ 247
- Genoptic S.O.P. Sterile Ophthalmic Ointment ..... ◉ 247
- Gentacidin Ointment ..... ◉ 273
- Gentacidin Solution ..... ◉ 273
- Gentak Ointment & Solution ..... ◉ 208

G-myticin Creme and Ointment 0.1% 1770
Pred-G Liquifilm Sterile Ophthalmic Suspension ..... ◉ 252
Pred-G S.O.P. Sterile Ophthalmic Ointment ..... ◉ 253

Isoflurane (Concomitant administration has been associated with erythema and histamine-like flushing). Products include:
Forane 600

Kanamycin Sulfate (Concurrent use may result in increased ototoxicity). Products include:
Kantrex Injection 601
Kantrex Pediatric Injection 601

Ketamine Hydrochloride (Concomitant administration has been associated with erythema and histamine-like flushing). Products include:
Ketalar 1726

Methohexital Sodium (Concomitant administration has been associated with erythema and histamine-like flushing). Products include:
Brevital Sodium Vials 1248

Methoxyflurane (Concomitant administration has been associated with erythema and histamine-like flushing).
No products indexed under this heading.

Polymyxin B Sulfate (Concurrent and/or sequential use requires careful monitoring due to increased potential for nephrotoxicity and/or neurotoxicity). Products include:
AK-Poly-Bac Ointment ..... ◉ 205
AK-Spore H.C. ..... ◉ 206
AK-Spore ..... ◉ 205
AK-Trol Ointment & Suspension ..... ◉ 207
Aquaphor Antibiotic Formula 662
Bactine First Aid Antibiotic Ointment ..... ▣ 625
Campho-Phenique Triple Antibiotic Ointment Plus Pain Reliever ▣ 758
Cortisporin Cream 757
Cortisporin Ointment 758
Cortisporin Ophthalmic Ointment Sterile 758
Cortisporin Ophthalmic Suspension Sterile 759
Cortisporin Otic Solution Sterile 760
Cortisporin Otic Suspension Sterile 760
Dexacidin ..... ◉ 272
Lanabiotic Ointment ..... ▣ 556
LazerSporin-C Solution 1770
Maxitrol Ophthalmic Ointment/Suspension ..... ◉ 223
Mycitracin ..... ▣ 737
Neosporin Cream 792
Neosporin G.U. Irrigant Sterile 793
Neosporin Ointment 793
Maximum Strength Neosporin Ointment 793
Neosporin Ophthalmic Ointment Sterile 793
Neosporin Ophthalmic Solution Sterile 794
Ophthocort ..... ◉ 301
PediOtic Suspension Sterile 797
Polymyxin B Sulfate, Aerosporin Brand Sterile Powder 798
Poly-Pred Liquifilm ..... ◉ 250
Polysporin Ointment ..... ▣ 543
Polysporin Ophthalmic Ointment Sterile 798
Polysporin Powder ..... ▣ 543
Polysporin Spray ..... ▣ 543
Polytrim Ophthalmic Solution Sterile 588
Terramycin with Polymyxin B Sulfate Ophthalmic Ointment 1965

Propofol (Concomitant administration has been associated with erythema and histamine-like flushing). Products include:
Diprivan Injection 2267

Streptomycin Sulfate (Concurrent use may result in increased ototoxicity).
No products indexed under this heading.

Tobramycin (Concurrent use may result in increased ototoxicity). Products include:
TobraDex Ophthalmic Suspension and Ointment ..... ◉ 228
Tobrex Ophthalmic Ointment and Solution 572

Tobramycin Sulfate (Concurrent use may result in increased ototoxicity). Products include:
Nebcin Vials, Hyporets & ADD-Vantage 1286

VANOXIDE-HC ACNE LOTION
(Benzoyl Peroxide, Hydrocortisone) .. 911
No interactions described in labeling.

VANQUISH ANALGESIC CAPLETS
(Acetaminophen, Aspirin, Caffeine) ▣ 574
May interact with oral anticoagulants and certain other agents. Compounds in these categories include:

Antiarthritic Drugs, unspecified (Effect not specified).

Dicumarol (Concurrent use requires caution). Products include:
Dicumarol Tablets 516

Warfarin Sodium (Concurrent use requires caution). Products include:
Coumadin Injection & Tablets 944
Panwarfin Tablets 547

VASCOR (200, 300 AND 400 MG) TABLETS
(Bepridil Hydrochloride) 1383
May interact with type 1 antiarrhythmic drugs, tricyclic antidepressants, cardiac glycosides, and certain other agents. Compounds in these categories include:

Amitriptyline Hydrochloride (Potential for exaggeration of the QT interval prolongation). Products include:
Elavil 2269
Endep Tablets 1927
Etrafon 2087
Limbitrol 1933
Triavil Tablets 1556

Amoxapine (Potential for exaggeration of the QT interval prolongation). Products include:
Asendin Tablets 1196

Clomipramine Hydrochloride (Potential for exaggeration of the QT interval prolongation). Products include:
Anafranil Capsules 650

Desipramine Hydrochloride (Potential for exaggeration of the QT interval prolongation). Products include:
Norpramin Tablets 1340

Deslanoside (Cardiac glycosides could exaggerate the depression of AV nodal conduction).
No products indexed under this heading.

Digitoxin (Cardiac glycosides could exaggerate the depression of AV nodal conduction). Products include:
Crystodigin Tablets 1253

Digoxin (May be associated with modest increases in steady-state serum digoxin concentrations; cardiac glycosides could exaggerate the depression of AV nodal conduction). Products include:
Lanoxicaps 772
Lanoxin Elixir Pediatric 775
Lanoxin Injection 778
Lanoxin Injection Pediatric 781
Lanoxin Tablets 783

Disopyramide Phosphate (Potential for exaggeration of the QT interval prolongation). Products include:
Norpace 2177

Doxepin Hydrochloride (Potential for exaggeration of the QT interval prolongation). Products include:
Sinequan 1960

Imipramine Hydrochloride (Potential for exaggeration of the QT interval prolongation). Products include:
Tofranil Ampuls 1038
Tofranil Tablets 1039

Imipramine Pamoate (Potential for exaggeration of the QT interval prolongation). Products include:
Tofranil-PM Capsules 1041

Maprotiline Hydrochloride (Potential for exaggeration of the QT interval prolongation). Products include:
Ludiomil Tablets 874

Moricizine Hydrochloride (Potential for exaggeration of the QT interval prolongation). Products include:
Ethmozine Tablets 946

Nortriptyline Hydrochloride (Potential for exaggeration of the QT interval prolongation). Products include:
Pamelor 2019

Procainamide Hydrochloride (Potential for exaggeration of the QT interval prolongation). Products include:
Procan SR Tablets 1760
Pronestyl Capsules and Tablets 1800
Pronestyl Injection 1798
Pronestyl-SR Tablets 1801

Propafenone Hydrochloride (Potential for exaggeration of the QT interval prolongation). Products include:
Rythmol Tablets 1184

Protriptyline Hydrochloride (Potential for exaggeration of the QT interval prolongation). Products include:
Vivactil Tablets 1567

Quinidine Gluconate (Potential for exaggeration of the QT interval prolongation). Products include:
Quinaglute Dura-Tabs Tablets 663

Quinidine Polygalacturonate (Potential for exaggeration of the QT interval prolongation). Products include:
Cardioquin Tablets 1812

Quinidine Sulfate (Potential for exaggeration of the QT interval prolongation). Products include:
Quinidex Extentabs 1868

Trimipramine Maleate (Potential for exaggeration of the QT interval prolongation). Products include:
Surmontil Capsules 2524

VASERETIC TABLETS
(Enalapril Maleate, Hydrochlorothiazide) 1559
May interact with insulin, potassium-depleting corticosteroids, diuretics, potassium sparing diuretics, barbiturates, narcotic analgesics, oral hypoglycemic agents, antihypertensives, corticosteroids, nondepolarizing neuromuscular blocking agents, lithium preparations, non-steroidal anti-inflammatory agents, cardiac glycosides, and certain other agents. Compounds in these categories include:

Acebutolol Hydrochloride (Additive effect or potentiation). Products include:
Sectral Capsules 2520

ACTH (Intensifed electrolyte depletion, particularly hypokalemia).
No products indexed under this heading.

Alcohol (Potentiation of orthostatic hypotension may occur).

Alfentanil Hydrochloride (Potentiation of orthostatic hypotension may occur). Products include:
Alfenta Injection 1131

Amiloride Hydrochloride (Significant increases in serum potassium; excessive hypotension). Products include:
Midamor Tablets 1508
Moduretic Tablets 1510

Aprobarbital (Potentiation of orthostatic hypotension may occur). Products include:
Alurate Elixir 1883

Atenolol (Additive effect or potentiation). Products include:
Tenoretic Tablets 1105
Tenormin Tablets and I.V. Injection 1107

Atracurium Besylate (Increased responsiveness to muscle relaxant). Products include:
Tracrium Injection 817

Benazepril Hydrochloride (Additive effect or potentiation). Products include:
Lotensin Tablets 872

Bendroflumethiazide (Additive effect or potentiation; excessive hypotension). Products include:
Corzide Tablets 702
Naturetin Tablets 1789
Rauzide Tablets 1804

Betamethasone Acetate (Intensified electrolyte depletion, particularly hypokalemia). Products include:
Celestone Soluspan Suspension 2081

Betamethasone Sodium Phosphate (Intensified electrolyte depletion, particularly hypokalemia). Products include:
Celestone Soluspan Suspension 2081

Betaxolol Hydrochloride (Additive effect or potentiation). Products include:
Betoptic Sterile Ophthalmic Solution 569
Betoptic S Sterile Ophthalmic Suspension 570
Kerlone Tablets 2172

Bumetanide (Excessive hypotension). Products include:
Bumex 1895

Buprenorphine (Potentiation of orthostatic hypotension may occur).
No products indexed under this heading.

Butabarbital (Potentiation of orthostatic hypotension may occur). Products include:
Pyridium Plus 1764

Butalbital (Potentiation of orthostatic hypotension may occur). Products include:
Esgic-Plus Tablets 1002
Esgic Tablets & Capsules 1001
Fioricet Tablets 2006
Fiorinal Capsules 2007
Fiorinal with Codeine Capsules 2008
Fiorinal Tablets 2007
Phrenilin 838
Sedapap Tablets 50 mg/650 mg .. 1360

Captopril (Additive effect or potentiation). Products include:
Capoten 2255
Capozide 2258

Carteolol Hydrochloride (Additive effect or potentiation). Products include:
Cartrol Tablets 507

Chlorothiazide (Additive effect or potentiation; excessive hypotension). Products include:
Aldoclor Tablets 1413
Diupres Tablets 1461
Diuril Oral 1464

Chlorothiazide Sodium (Additive effect or potentiation; excessive hypotension). Products include:
Diuril Sodium Intravenous 1463

Chlorpropamide (Dosage adjustment of hypoglycemic may be required). Products include:
Diabinese Tablets 1775

Chlorthalidone (Additive effect or potentiation; significant increases in serum potassium; excessive hypotension). Products include:
Combipres Tablets 678
Tenoretic Tablets 1105
Thalitone Tablets 687

Clonidine (Additive effect or potentiation). Products include:
Catapres-TTS 677

Clonidine Hydrochloride (Additive effect or potentiation). Products include:
Catapres Tablets 676
Combipres Tablets 678

Codeine (Potentiation of orthostatic hypotension may occur). Products include:
Calcidrine Syrup 506

Codeine Phosphate (Potentiation of orthostatic hypotension may occur). Products include:
Actifed with Codeine Cough Syrup 752
Cheracol Cough Syrup 1853
Codimal PH Syrup 846
Dimetane-DC Cough Syrup 1857
Empirin with Codeine Phosphate Nos. 2, 3 & 4 764
Fiorinal with Codeine Capsules 2008
Isoclor Expectorant 982
Naldecon CX Adult Liquid ▣ 521
Novahistine DH 1342
Novahistine Expectorant 1343
Nucofed Capsules 2219
Nucofed Expectorant 2219
Nucofed Pediatric Expectorant 2220
Nucofed Syrup 2219
Phenaphen with Codeine Capsules 1865
Phenaphen-650 with Codeine Tablets 1866
Phenergan with Codeine 2497
Phenergan VC with Codeine 2501
Robitussin A-C Syrup 1875
Robitussin-DAC Syrup 1875
Ryna ▣ 741
Soma Compound w/Codeine Tablets 2390
Triaminic Expectorant w/Codeine 1996
Tussi-Organidin Liquid 2391
Tylenol with Codeine 1381

Codeine Polistirex (Potentiation of orthostatic hypotension may occur).
No products indexed under this heading.

Cortisone Acetate (Intensified electrolyte depletion, particularly hypokalemia). Products include:
Cortone Acetate Sterile Suspension 1437
Cortone Acetate Tablets 1439

Deserpidine (Additive effect or potentiation). Products include:
Enduronyl 518
Harmonyl Tablets 528
Oreticyl 545

Deslanoside (Hypokalemia produced by hydrochlorothiazide may exaggerate the response of the heart to the digitalis toxicity).
No products indexed under this heading.

Dexamethasone (Intensified electrolyte depletion, particularly hypokalemia). Products include:
AK-Trol Ointment & Suspension ⊙ 207
Decadron Elixir 1445
Decadron Tablets 1447
Decaspray Topical Aerosol 1459
Dexacidin ⊙ 272
Maxidex Sterile Ophthalmic Suspension ⊙ 223
Maxitrol Ophthalmic Ointment/Suspension ⊙ 223
TobraDex Ophthalmic Suspension and Ointment ⊙ 228

Dexamethasone Acetate (Intensified electrolyte depletion, particularly hypokalemia). Products include:
Dalalone D.P. Injectable 999
Decadron-LA Sterile Suspension 1457

Dexamethasone Sodium Phosphate (Intensified electrolyte depletion, particularly hypokalemia). Products include:
AK-Dex ⊙ 203
Decadron Phosphate Respihaler 1454
Decadron Phosphate Sterile Ophthalmic Ointment 1453
Decadron Phosphate Sterile Ophthalmic Solution 1453
Decadron Phosphate Topical Cream 1455
Decadron Phosphate Turbinaire 1456
Maxidex Sterile Ophthalmic Ointment ⊙ 222
NeoDecadron Sterile Ophthalmic Ointment 1517
NeoDecadron Sterile Ophthalmic Solution 1518
NeoDecadron Topical Cream 1518

Dezocine (Potentiation of orthostatic hypotension may occur).

Diazoxide (Additive effect or potentiation). Products include:
Hyperstat I.V. Injection 2095
Proglycem 649

Diclofenac Sodium (Reduced diuretic, natriuretic, and antihypertensive effects of Vaseretic). Products include:
Voltaren Ophthalmic Sterile Ophthalmic Solution ⊙ 268
Voltaren Tablets 1042

Digitoxin (Hypokalemia produced by hydrochlorothiazide may exaggerate the response of the heart to the digitalis toxicity). Products include:
Crystodigin Tablets 1253

Digoxin (Hypokalemia produced by hydrochlorothiazide may exaggerate the response of the heart to the digitalis toxicity). Products include:
Lanoxicaps 772
Lanoxin Elixir Pediatric 775
Lanoxin Injection 778
Lanoxin Injection Pediatric 781
Lanoxin Tablets 783

Doxazosin Mesylate (Additive effect or potentiation). Products include:
Cardura Tablets 1941

Enalaprilat (Additive effect or potentiation). Products include:
Vasotec I.V. 1562

Esmolol Hydrochloride (Additive effect or potentiation). Products include:
Brevibloc Injection 942

Ethacrynic Acid (Excessive hypotension). Products include:
Edecrin Tablets 1468

Etodolac (Reduced diuretic, natriuretic, and antihypertensive effects of Vaseretic). Products include:
Lodine Capsules 2468

Felodipine (Additive effect or potentiation). Products include:
Plendil Extended-Release Tablets 1526

Fenoprofen Calcium (Reduced diuretic, natriuretic, and antihypertensive effects of Vaseretic). Products include:
Nalfon Pulvules & Tablets 919

Fentanyl (Potentiation of orthostatic hypotension may occur). Products include:
Duragesic Transdermal System 1133

Fentanyl Citrate (Potentiation of orthostatic hypotension may occur). Products include:
Innovar Injection 1141
Sublimaze Injection 1146

Flurbiprofen (Reduced diuretic, natriuretic, and antihypertensive effects of Vaseretic). Products include:
Ansaid Tablets 2319

Fosinopril Sodium (Additive effect or potentiation). Products include:
Monopril Tablets 1406

Furosemide (Additive effect or potentiation; excessive hypotension). Products include:
Lasix 1093

Glipizide (Dosage adjustment of hypoglycemic may be required). Products include:
Glucotrol 1952

Glyburide (Dosage adjustment of hypoglycemic may be required). Products include:
DiaBeta 1091
Micronase Tablets 2350

Guanabenz Acetate (Additive effect or potentiation). Products include:
Wytensin Tablets 2542

Guanethidine Monosulfate (Additive effect or potentiation). Products include:
Esimil Tablets 864
Ismelin Tablets 869

Hydralazine Hydrochloride (Additive effect or potentiation). Products include:
Apresazide Capsules 854
Apresoline Hydrochloride Parenteral (Ampuls) 856
Apresoline Hydrochloride Tablets 855
Apresoline-Esidrix Tablets 857
Ser-Ap-Es Tablets 881
Serpasil-Apresoline Tablets 884

Hydrocodone Bitartrate (Potentiation of orthostatic hypotension may occur). Products include:
Anexsia 5/500 Tablets 2196
Anexsia 7.5/650 Tablets 2197
Azdone Tablets 844
Codiclear DH Syrup 845
Codimal DH Syrup 846
Damason-P 1356
Hycodan Syrup, Tablets 927
Hycomine Compound Tablets 929
Hycomine Syrup 927
Hycotuss Expectorant Syrup 930
Hydrocet Capsules 835
Lortab ASA Tablets 2414
Lortab 2412
Ru-Tuss with Hydrocodone 694
Triaminic Expectorant DH 1995
Vicodin Tablets 1187
Vicodin ES Tablets 1189
Zydone Capsules 941

Hydrocodone Polistirex (Potentiation of orthostatic hypotension may occur). Products include:
Tussionex Extended-Release Suspension 988

Hydrocortisone (Intensified electrolyte depletion, particularly hypokalemia). Products include:
AK-Spore H.C. ⊙ 206
Bactine Hydrocortisone Anti-Itch Cream ▣ 625
CaldeCORT Anti-Itch Hydrocortisone Spray ▣ 560
Carmol HC Cream 1% 2296
Cortaid Spray ▣ 735
Cortenema 2244
Cortisporin Ointment 758
Cortisporin Ophthalmic Ointment Sterile 758
Cortisporin Ophthalmic Suspension Sterile 759
Cortisporin Otic Solution Sterile 760
Cortisporin Otic Suspension Sterile 760
Cortizone-5 Creme & Ointment ▣ 732
Dermolate Anti-Itch Cream ▣ 697
Eldecort Cream 1.0% 1113
Eldecort Cream 1.0% and 2.5% 1113
Fungoid HC Creme 1770
Hydrocortone Tablets 1482
Hytone 909
LazerSporin-C Solution 1770
Massengill Medicated Soft Cloth Towelettes 2192
Nutracort Cream & Lotion 1684
PediOtic Suspension Sterile 797
Synacort Creams 1%, 2.5% 2296
Vanoxide-HC Acne Lotion 911
Vioform-Hydrocortisone Cream and Mild Cream 889
Vioform-Hydrocortisone Ointment 889
VōSoL HC Otic Solution 2392
Vytone Cream 1% 911

Hydrocortisone Acetate (Intensified electrolyte depletion, particularly hypokalemia). Products include:
Analpram-HC Rectal Cream 1% and 2.5% 970
Anusol-HC Cream 1690
Anusol-HC Suppositories 1691
Caldecort ▣ 560
Carmol HC Cream 1% 2296
Chloromycetin Hydrocortisone Ophthalmic 1694
Coly-Mycin S Otic w/Neomycin & Hydrocortisone 1708
Cortaid ▣ 735
Cortef Feminine Itch Cream ▣ 735
Corticaine ▣ 682
Cortifoam 1827
Cortisporin Cream 757
Epifoam 1828
Gynecort 5 Creme ▣ 556
Hydrocortone Acetate Sterile Suspension 1479
Lanacort 5 Creme and Ointment ▣ 557
Mantadil Cream 789
Ophthocort ⊙ 301
Orabase HCA Oral Paste 890
Pramosone Cream, Lotion & Ointment 971
ProctoCream-HC 1834
Proctofoam-HC 1835

Hydrocortisone Sodium Phosphate (Intensified electrolyte depletion, particularly hypokalemia). Products include:
Hydrocortone Phosphate Injection, Sterile 1481

Hydrocortisone Sodium Succinate (Intensified electrolyte depletion, particularly hypokalemia). Products include:
Solu-Cortef Sterile Powder 2361

Hydroflumethiazide (Additive effect or potentiation; excessive hypotension). Products include:
Diucardin Tablets 2450
Saluron 718
Salutensin/Salutensin-Demi 719

Ibuprofen (Reduced diuretic, natriuretic, and antihypertensive effects of Vaseretic). Products include:
Advil Cold & Sinus Caplets (formerly CoAdvil) 2416
Advil Ibuprofen Tablets and Caplets 2416
Children's Advil Suspension 2426
CoAdvil ▣ 748
Dristan Sinus Caplets 2419
Haltran Tablets ▣ 668
Ibuprofen ▣ 631
Medipren ibuprofen Caplets and Tablets 1362
Midol 200 Cramp Relief Formula ▣ 570
Motrin Tablets 2351
Motrin IB Caplets and Tablets ▣ 736
Nuprin Ibuprofen/Analgesic Tablets & Caplets 752
PediaProfen Suspension 1363
Rufen Tablets 691
Trendar Ibuprofen Tablets ▣ 756

Indapamide (Potentiation; excessive hypotension). Products include:
Lozol Tablets 1843

Indomethacin (Reduced diuretic, natriuretic, and antihypertensive effects of Vaseretic). Products include:
Indocin 1487

Indomethacin Sodium Trihydrate (Reduced diuretic, natriuretic, and antihypertensive effects of Vaseretic). Products include:

Indocin I.V. 1490

Insulin, Human (Dosage adjustments of insulin may be required).

No products indexed under this heading.

Insulin, Human Isophane Suspension (Dosage adjustments of insulin may be required). Products include:

Humulin N, 100 Units 1270

Insulin, Human NPH (Dosage adjustments of insulin may be required). Products include:

Insulatard NPH Human 1627
Novolin N 1627
Novolin N PenFill Cartridges 1628
Novolin N Prefilled 1628

Insulin, Human Regular (Dosage adjustments of insulin may be required). Products include:

Humulin BR, 100 Units 1268
Humulin R, 100 Units 1272
Novolin R 1627
Novolin R PenFill Cartridges 1628
Novolin R Prefilled 1629
Velosulin Human 1628

Insulin, Human, Zinc Suspension (Dosage adjustments of insulin may be required). Products include:

Humulin L, 100 Units 1268
Humulin U, 100 Units 1272
Novolin L 1627

Insulin, NPH (Dosage adjustments of insulin may be required). Products include:

NPH, 40 & 100 Units 1273
Beef NPH, 100 Units 1274
Pork NPH, 100 Units 1275
Insulatard NPH 1626
NPH Insulin 1626
NPH Purified Pork Isophane Insulin 1626

Insulin, Regular (Dosage adjustments of insulin may be required). Products include:

Regular, 40 & 100 Units 1273
Beef Regular, 100 Units 1275
Pork Regular, 100 Units 1275
Pork Regular (Concentrated), 500 Units 1276
Regular Insulin 1625
Regular Purified Pork Insulin 1626
Velosulin 1627

Insulin, Zinc Crystals (Dosage adjustments of insulin may be required). Products include:

NPH, 40 & 100 Units 1273

Insulin, Zinc Suspension (Dosage adjustments of insulin may be required). Products include:

Lente, 40 & 100 Units 1272
Protamine, Zinc, 40 & 100 Units 1273
Lente Iletin I 1272
Beef Lente, 100 Units 1274
Beef Protamine Zinc, 100 Units 1274
Pork Lente, 100 Units 1275
Pork, Protamine, Zinc, 100 Units 1275
Lente Insulin 1626
Lente Purified Pork Insulin 1626
Semilente Insulin 1625
Ultralente Insulin 1626

Isradipine (Additive effect or potentiation). Products include:

DynaCirc Capsules 2004

Ketoprofen (Reduced diuretic, natriuretic, and antihypertensive effects of Vaseretic). Products include:

Orudis Capsules 2488

Ketorolac Tromethamine (Reduced diuretic, natriuretic, and antihypertensive effects of Vaseretic). Products include:

Toradol IM Injection 2302

Labetalol Hydrochloride (Additive effect or potentiation). Products include:

Normodyne Injection 2108
Normodyne Tablets 2110
Normozide Tablets 2112
Trandate HCT Tablets 579
Trandate Injection 577
Trandate Tablets 579

Levorphanol Tartrate (Potentiation of orthostatic hypotension may occur). Products include:

Levo-Dromoran 1906

Lisinopril (Additive effect or potentiation). Products include:

Prinivil Tablets 1538
Prinzide Tablets 1540
Zestoretic 2274
Zestril Tablets 2277

Lithium Carbonate (High risk of lithium toxicity; frequent monitoring of lithium serum levels is recommended). Products include:

Eskalith 2214
Lithane Tablets 1596
Lithium Carbonate Capsules & Tablets 1984
Lithobid Tablets 870

Lithium Citrate (High risk of lithium toxicity; frequent monitoring of lithium serum levels is recommended). Products include:

Cibalith-S 870

Mecamylamine Hydrochloride (Additive effect or potentiation). Products include:

Inversine Tablets 1492

Meclofenamate Sodium (Reduced diuretic, natriuretic, and antihypertensive effects of Vaseretic). Products include:

Meclomen Capsules 1739

Mefenamic Acid (Reduced diuretic, natriuretic, and antihypertensive effects of Vaseretic). Products include:

Ponstel 1758

Meperidine Hydrochloride (Potentiation of orthostatic hypotension may occur). Products include:

Demerol 2047
Mepergan Injection 2479

Mephobarbital (Potentiation of orthostatic hypotension may occur). Products include:

Mebaral Tablets 2061

Methadone Hydrochloride (Potentiation of orthostatic hypotension may occur). Products include:

Dolophine Hydrochloride Ampoules & Vials 1260
Dolophine Hydrochloride Tablets 1261
Methadone Hydrochloride Diskets 1284
Methadone Hydrochloride Oral Solution & Tablets 1987

Methyclothiazide (Additive effect or potentiation; excessive hypotension). Products include:

Enduron Tablets 517
Enduronyl 518

Methyldopa (Additive effect or potentiation). Products include:

Aldoclor Tablets 1413
Aldomet Oral 1415
Aldoril Tablets 1418

Methyldopate Hydrochloride (Additive effect or potentiation). Products include:

Aldomet Ester HCl Injection 1417

Methylprednisolone Acetate (Intensified electrolyte depletion, particularly hypokalemia). Products include:

Depo-Medrol Sterile Aqueous Suspension 2334

Methylprednisolone Sodium Succinate (Intensified electrolyte depletion, particularly hypokalemia). Products include:

Solu-Medrol Sterile Powder 2363

Metocurine Iodide (Increased responsiveness to muscle relaxant). Products include:

Metubine Iodide Vials 1285

Metolazone (Additive effect or potentiation; excessive hypotension). Products include:

Diulo 2129
Mykrox ½ mg Tablets 984
Zaroxolyn Tablets 989

Metoprolol Tartrate (Additive effect or potentiation). Products include:

Lopressor Ampuls 1032
Lopressor HCT Tablets 1034
Lopressor Tablets 1032

Metyrosine (Additive effect or potentiation). Products include:

Demser Capsules 1460

Minoxidil (Additive effect or potentiation). Products include:

Loniten Tablets 2346
Rogaine Topical Solution 2357

Morphine Sulfate (Potentiation of orthostatic hypotension may occur). Products include:

Astramorph/PF Injection, USP (Preservative-Free) 618
Duramorph 960
Infumorph 200 and Infumorph 500 Sterile Solutions 962
MS Contin Tablets 1814
MSIR 1817
Oramorph SR (Morphine Sulfate Sustained Release Tablets) 1988
Roxanol 1991

Nadolol (Additive effect or potentiation). Products include:

Corgard Tablets 701
Corzide Tablets 702

Naproxen (Reduced diuretic, natriuretic, and antihypertensive effects of Vaseretic). Products include:

Naprosyn 2297

Naproxen Sodium (Reduced diuretic, natriuretic, and antihypertensive effects of Vaseretic). Products include:

Anaprox and Anaprox DS Tablets 2288

Nicardipine Hydrochloride (Additive effect or potentiation). Products include:

Cardene Capsules 2290

Nitroglycerin (Additive effect or potentiation). Products include:

Deponit NTG Transdermal Delivery System 2143
Minitran Transdermal Delivery System 1312
Nitro-Bid Ointment 1339
Nitro-Bid Capsules 1338
Nitrodisc 2176
Nitro-Dur (nitroglycerin) Transdermal Infusion System 1164
Nitrogard Tablets 1004
Nitrolingual Spray 1846
Nitrostat Tablets 1743
Transderm-Nitro Transdermal Therapeutic System 2283

Norepinephrine Bitartrate (Decreased reponse to pressor amines). Products include:

Levophed Bitartrate Injection 2054

Opium Alkaloids (Potentiation of orthostatic hypotension may occur). Products include:

B & O No. 15A & No. 16A Supprettes 2395
Pantopon Injectable 1911

Oxycodone Hydrochloride (Potentiation of orthostatic hypotension may occur). Products include:

Percocet Tablets 950
Percodan 951
Roxicodone Tablets, Oral Solution & Intensol (Oxycodone) 1992
Tylox Capsules 1382

Pancuronium Bromide Injection (Increased responsiveness to muscle relaxant).

No products indexed under this heading.

Penbutolol Sulfate (Additive effect or potentiation). Products include:

Levatol 1832

Pentobarbital Sodium (Potentiation of orthostatic hypotension may occur). Products include:

Nembutal Sodium Capsules 534
Nembutal Sodium Solution 536
Nembutal Sodium Suppositories 538

Phenobarbital (Potentiation of orthostatic hypotension may occur). Products include:

Arco-Lase Plus Tablets 607
Bellergal-S Tablets 1998
Bronkolixir .... ▣ 761
Bronkotabs Tablets .... ▣ 762
Donnatal 1858
Donnatal Extentabs 1859
Donnatal Tablets 1858
Donnazyme Tablets 1860
Kinesed Tablets 2272
Phenobarbital Elixir and Tablets 1293
Primatene Tablets-P Formula 2421
Quadrinal Tablets 1183
Tedral SA 1765

Phenoxybenzamine Hydrochloride (Additive effect or potentiation). Products include:

Dibenzyline Capsules 2207

Phentolamine Mesylate (Additive effect or potentiation). Products include:

Regitine 878

Phenylbutazone (Reduced diuretic, natriuretic, and antihypertensive effects of Vaseretic). Products include:

Butazolidin Capsules & Tablets 1027

Pindolol (Additive effect or potentiation). Products include:

Visken Tablets 2036

Piroxicam (Reduced diuretic, natriuretic, and antihypertensive effects of Vaseretic). Products include:

Feldene Capsules 1777

Polythiazide (Additive effect or potentiation; excessive hypotension). Products include:

Minizide Capsules 1779
Renese Tablets 1785
Renese-R Tablets 1786

Potassium Acid Phosphate (Significant increases in serum potassium). Products include:

K-Phos M.F. Tablets 659
K-Phos Original Formula 'Sodium Free' Tablets 660
K-Phos No. 2 Tablets 659

Potassium Bicarbonate (Significant increases in serum potassium). Products include:

Alka-Seltzer Advanced Formula Antacid & Non-Aspirin Pain Reliever .... ▣ 620
Alka-Seltzer Effervescent Antacid ▣ 622
K-Lyte 707
Klorvess Effervescent Granules 2010
Klorvess Effervescent Tablets 2011

Potassium Chloride (Significant increases in serum potassium). Products include:

Chlor-3 Condiment 994
K-Dur Microburst Release System (potassium chloride, USP) E.R. Tablets 1163
K-Lor Powder Packets 531
K-Lyte 707
K-Norm Capsules 982
K-Tab Filmtab 532
Kato Potassium Supplement 1114
Klor-Con 8/Klor-Con 10 Extended-release Tablets 2374
Klorvess Effervescent Granules 2010
Klorvess Effervescent Tablets 2011
Klorvess 10% Liquid 2010
Klotrix 708

Kolyum Liquid ... 983
Micro-K ... 1863
Micro-K LS Packets ... 1864
NuLYTELY ... 699
Oral Rehydration Salts, Citrate ... 1150
Rum-K Syrup ... 995
Slow-K Tablets ... 2281
Ten-K Controlled-Release Tablets ... 2282
Thermotabs ... ▣ 619

Potassium Citrate (Significant increases in serum potassium). Products include:
Alka-Seltzer Effervescent Antacid .. 1570
K-Lyte ... 707
Polycitra Syrup ... 2424
Polycitra-K ... 2424
Polycitra-LC—Sugar-Free ... 2424
Ricelyte, Rice-Based Oral Electrolyte Maintenance Solution ... ▣ 613

Potassium Gluconate (Significant increases in serum potassium). Products include:
Kolyum Liquid ... 983

Potassium Phosphate, Dibasic (Significant increases in serum potassium). Products include:
Neutra-Phos ... 2423

Potassium Phosphate, Monobasic (Significant increases in serum potassium). Products include:
K-Phos M.F. Tablets ... 659
K-Phos Neutral Tablets ... 660
Neutra-Phos ... 2423

Prazosin Hydrochloride (Potentiation). Products include:
Minipress Capsules ... 1778
Minizide Capsules ... 1779

Prednisolone Acetate (Intensified electrolyte depletion, particularly hypokalemia). Products include:
AK-Cide Sterile Ophthalmic Ointment & Suspension ... ◉ 202
Blephamide Liquifilm Sterile Ophthalmic Suspension ... 586
Blephamide S.O.P. Sterile Ophthalmic Ointment ... 586
Cetapred Ointment ... ◉ 220
⅛% Econopred & 1% Econopred Plus ... ◉ 217
Isopto Cetapred Suspension ... ◉ 220
Metimyd ... ◉ 306
Poly-Pred Liquifilm ... ◉ 250
Pred Forte ... ◉ 252
Pred Mild ... ◉ 254
Pred-G Liquifilm Sterile Ophthalmic Suspension ... ◉ 252
Pred-G S.O.P. Sterile Ophthalmic Ointment ... ◉ 253
Vasocidin Ointment ... ◉ 275

Prednisolone Sodium Phosphate (Intensified electrolyte depletion, particularly hypokalemia). Products include:
AK-Pred ... ◉ 205
Hydeltrasol Injection, Sterile ... 1476
Inflamase ... ◉ 274
Pediapred Oral Liquid ... 987
Vasocidin Ophthalmic Solution ... ◉ 276

Prednisolone Tebutate (Intensified electrolyte depletion, particularly hypokalemia). Products include:
Hydeltra-T.B.A. Sterile Suspension 1478

Prednisone (Intensified electrolyte depletion, particularly hypokalemia). Products include:
Deltasone Tablets ... 2332

Propoxyphene Hydrochloride (Potentiation of orthostatic hypotension may occur). Products include:
Darvon ... 1256
Wygesic Tablets ... 2540

Propoxyphene Napsylate (Potentiation of orthostatic hypotension may occur). Products include:
Darvon-N/Darvocet-N ... 1254

Propranolol Hydrochloride (Additive effect or potentiation). Products include:
Inderal ... 2459
Inderal LA Long Acting Capsules ... 2461
Inderide Tablets ... 2463
Inderide LA Long Acting Capsules .. 2465

Ramipril (Additive effect or potentiation). Products include:
Altace Capsules ... 1086

Rauwolfia Serpentina (Additive effect or potentiation). Products include:
Raudixin Tablets ... 1803
Rauzide Tablets ... 1804

Rescinnamine (Additive effect or potentiation).
No products indexed under this heading.

Reserpine (Additive effect or potentiation). Products include:
Diupres Tablets ... 1461
Hydromox R Tablets ... 1209
Hydropres Tablets ... 1485
Renese-R Tablets ... 1786
Salutensin/Salutensin-Demi ... 719
Ser-Ap-Es Tablets ... 881
Serpasil Tablets ... 883
Serpasil-Apresoline Tablets ... 884
Serpasil-Esidrix Tablets ... 886

Secobarbital Sodium (Potentiation of orthostatic hypotension may occur). Products include:
Seconal Sodium Pulvules ... 1296

Sodium Nitroprusside (Additive effect or potentiation). Products include:
Nipride I.V. Infusion ... 1909

Spironolactone (Significant increases in serum potassium; excessive hypotension). Products include:
Aldactazide ... 2150
Aldactone ... 2152

Sufentanil Citrate (Potentiation of orthostatic hypotension may occur). Products include:
Sufenta Injection ... 1147

Sulindac (Reduced diuretic, natriuretic, and antihypertensive effects of Vaseretic). Products include:
Clinoril Tablets ... 1433

Terazosin Hydrochloride (Additive effect or potentiation). Products include:
Hytrin Tablets ... 529

Thiamylal Sodium (Potentiation of orthostatic hypotension may occur). Products include:
Surital Ampoules, Steri-Vials ... 1764

Timolol Maleate (Additive effect or potentiation). Products include:
Blocadren Tablets ... 1429
Timolide Tablets ... 1547
Timoptic in Ocudose ... 1552
Timoptic Sterile Ophthalmic Solution ... 1550

Tolazamide (Dosage adjustment of hypoglycemic may be required). Products include:
Tolinase Tablets ... 2365

Tolbutamide (Dosage adjustment of hypoglycemic may be required). Products include:
Orinase Tablets ... 2354

Tolmetin Sodium (Reduced diuretic, natriuretic, and antihypertensive effects of Vaseretic). Products include:
Tolectin (200, 400 and 600 mg) .. 1379

Triamcinolone (Intensified electrolyte depletion, particularly hypokalemia).
No products indexed under this heading.

Triamcinolone Acetonide (Intensified electrolyte depletion, particularly hypokalemia). Products include:
Aristocort A ... 1010
Azmacort Inhaler ... 1837
Kenalog Cream, Lotion & Ointment 2401
Kenalog-10 Injection ... 2402
Kenalog-40 Injection ... 2403
Kenalog in Orabase ... 604
Kenalog Spray ... 2401
Mycolog II Cream and Ointment ... 2407
Mytrex Cream & Ointment ... 2080
Nasacort Nasal Inhaler ... 1844

Triamcinolone Diacetate (Intensified electrolyte depletion, particularly hypokalemia). Products include:
Aristocort Suspension ... 1008

Triamcinolone Hexacetonide (Intensified electrolyte depletion, particularly hypokalemia). Products include:
Aristospan Suspension ... 1011

Triamterene (Significant increases potentiation; excessive hypotension). Products include:
Dyazide Capsules ... 2208
Dyrenium Capsules ... 2210
Maxzide ... 1215

Trimethaphan Camsylate (Additive effect or potentiation). Products include:
Arfonad Ampuls ... 1887

Vecuronium Bromide (Increased responsiveness to muscle relaxant). Products include:
Norcuron ... 1642

VASOCIDIN OINTMENT
(Prednisolone Acetate, Sulfacetamide Sodium) ... ◉ 275
No interactions described in labeling.

VASOCIDIN OPHTHALMIC SOLUTION
(Prednisolone Sodium Phosphate, Sulfacetamide Sodium) ... ◉ 276
May interact with silver preparations and para-aminobenzoic acid based local anesthetics. Compounds in these categories include:

Procaine Hydrochloride (May antagonize the actions of sulfonamides). Products include:
Novocain Hydrochloride for Spinal Anesthesia ... 2065

Silver Nitrate (Incompatible).
No products indexed under this heading.

Tetracaine Hydrochloride (May antagonize the actions of sulfonamides). Products include:
Cetacaine Topical Anesthetic ... 850
Pontocaine Hydrochloride for Spinal Anesthesia ... 2069

VASOCON-A
(Antazoline Phosphate, Naphazoline Hydrochloride) ... ◉ 278
May interact with monoamine oxidase inhibitors, tricyclic antidepressants, and certain other agents. Compounds in these categories include:

Amitriptyline Hydrochloride (May potentiate the pressor effect of naphazoline). Products include:
Elavil ... 2269
Endep Tablets ... 1927
Etrafon ... 2087
Limbitrol ... 1933
Triavil Tablets ... 1556

Amoxapine (May potentiate the pressor effect of naphazoline). Products include:
Asendin Tablets ... 1196

Clomipramine Hydrochloride (May potentiate the pressor effect of naphazoline). Products include:
Anafranil Capsules ... 650

Desipramine Hydrochloride (May potentiate the pressor effect of naphazoline). Products include:
Norpramin Tablets ... 1340

Doxepin Hydrochloride (May potentiate the pressor effect of naphazoline). Products include:
Sinequan ... 1960

Furazolidone (Severe hypertensive crisis). Products include:
Furoxone ... 1855

Imipramine Hydrochloride (May potentiate the pressor effect of naphazoline). Products include:
Tofranil Ampuls ... 1038
Tofranil Tablets ... 1039

Imipramine Pamoate (May potentiate the pressor effect of naphazoline). Products include:
Tofranil-PM Capsules ... 1041

Isocarboxazid (Severe hypertensive crisis). Products include:
Marplan Tablets ... 1906

Maprotiline Hydrochloride (May potentiate the pressor effect of naphazoline). Products include:
Ludiomil Tablets ... 874

Nortriptyline Hydrochloride (May potentiate the pressor effect of naphazoline). Products include:
Pamelor ... 2019

Phenelzine Sulfate (Severe hypertensive crisis). Products include:
Nardil ... 1742

Protriptyline Hydrochloride (May potentiate the pressor effect of naphazoline). Products include:
Vivactil Tablets ... 1567

Selegiline Hydrochloride (Severe hypertensive crisis). Products include:
Eldepryl ... 2250

Tranylcypromine Sulfate (Severe hypertensive crisis). Products include:
Parnate Tablets ... 2222

Trimipramine Maleate (May potentiate the pressor effect of naphazoline). Products include:
Surmontil Capsules ... 2524

VASOSULF
(Phenylephrine Hydrochloride, Sulfacetamide Sodium) ... ◉ 279
May interact with silver preparations. Compounds in this category include:

Silver Nitrate (Incompatible).

VASOTEC I.V.
(Enalaprilat) ... 1562
May interact with diuretics, potassium sparing diuretics, potassium-depleting corticosteroids, lithium preparations, and certain other agents. Compounds in these categories include:

Amiloride Hydrochloride (Potential for excessive hypotension and significant hyperkalemia). Products include:
Midamor Tablets ... 1508
Moduretic Tablets ... 1510

Bendroflumethiazide (Potential for excessive hypotension). Products include:
Corzide Tablets ... 702
Naturetin Tablets ... 1789
Rauzide Tablets ... 1804

Bumetanide (Potential for excessive hypotension). Products include:
Bumex ... 1895

Chlorothiazide (Potential for excessive hypotension). Products include:
Aldoclor Tablets ... 1413
Diupres Tablets ... 1461
Diuril Oral ... 1464

Chlorothiazide Sodium (Potential for excessive hypotension). Products include:
Diuril Sodium Intravenous ... 1463

Chlorthalidone (Potential for excessive hypotension). Products include:
Combipres Tablets ... 678
Tenoretic Tablets ... 1105
Thalitone Tablets ... 687

Ethacrynic Acid (Potential for excessive hypotension). Products include:
- Edecrin Tablets ... 1468

Furosemide (Potential for excessive hypotension). Products include:
- Lasix ... 1093

Hydrochlorothiazide (Potential for excessive hypotension). Products include:
- Aldactazide ... 2150
- Aldoril Tablets ... 1418
- Apresazide Capsules ... 854
- Apresoline-Esidrix Tablets ... 857
- Capozide ... 2258
- Dyazide Capsules ... 2208
- Esidrix Tablets ... 863
- Esimil Tablets ... 864
- HydroDIURIL Tablets ... 1484
- Hydropres Tablets ... 1485
- Inderide Tablets ... 2463
- Inderide LA Long Acting Capsules .. 2465
- Lopressor HCT Tablets ... 1034
- Maxzide ... 1215
- Moduretic Tablets ... 1510
- Normozide Tablets ... 2112
- Oretic Tablets ... 544
- Oreticyl ... 545
- Prinzide Tablets ... 1540
- Ser-Ap-Es Tablets ... 881
- Serpasil-Esidrix Tablets ... 886
- Timolide Tablets ... 1547
- Trandate HCT Tablets ... 579
- Vaseretic Tablets ... 1559
- Zestoretic ... 2274

Hydroflumethiazide (Potential for excessive hypotension). Products include:
- Diucardin Tablets ... 2450
- Saluron ... 718
- Salutensin/Salutensin-Demi ... 719

Indapamide (Potential for excessive hypotension). Products include:
- Lozol Tablets ... 1843

Lithium Carbonate (Potential for reversible lithium toxicity; monitor lithium levels frequently). Products include:
- Eskalith ... 2214
- Lithane Tablets ... 1596
- Lithium Carbonate Capsules & Tablets ... 1984
- Lithobid Tablets ... 870

Lithium Citrate (Potential for reversible lithium toxicity; monitor lithium levels frequently). Products include:
- Cibalith-S ... 870

Methyclothiazide (Potential for excessive hypotension). Products include:
- Enduron Tablets ... 517
- Enduronyl ... 518

Metolazone (Potential for excessive hypotension). Products include:
- Diulo ... 2129
- Mykrox ½ mg Tablets ... 984
- Zaroxolyn Tablets ... 989

Polythiazide (Potential for excessive hypotension). Products include:
- Minizide Capsules ... 1779
- Renese Tablets ... 1785
- Renese-R Tablets ... 1786

Potassium Acid Phosphate (Potential for significant hyperkalemia). Products include:
- K-Phos M.F. Tablets ... 659
- K-Phos Original Formula 'Sodium Free' Tablets ... 660
- K-Phos No. 2 Tablets ... 659

Potassium Bicarbonate (Potential for significant hyperkalemia). Products include:
- Alka-Seltzer Advanced Formula Antacid & Non-Aspirin Pain Reliever ... ◘ 620
- Alka-Seltzer Effervescent Antacid ◘ 622
- K-Lyte ... 707
- Klorvess Effervescent Granules ... 2010
- Klorvess Effervescent Tablets ... 2011

Potassium Chloride (Potential for significant hyperkalemia). Products include:
- Chlor-3 Condiment ... 994
- K-Dur Microburst Release System (potassium chloride, USP) E.R. Tablets ... 1163
- K-Lor Powder Packets ... 531
- K-Lyte ... 707
- K-Norm Capsules ... 982
- K-Tab Filmtab ... 532
- Kato Potassium Supplement ... 1114
- Klor-Con 8/Klor-Con 10 Extended-release Tablets ... 2374
- Klorvess Effervescent Granules ... 2010
- Klorvess Effervescent Tablets ... 2011
- Klorvess 10% Liquid ... 2010
- Klotrix ... 708
- Kolyum Liquid ... 983
- Micro-K ... 1863
- Micro-K LS Packets ... 1864
- NuLYTELY ... 699
- Oral Rehydration Salts, Citrate ... 1150
- Rum-K Syrup ... 995
- Slow-K Tablets ... 2281
- Ten-K Controlled-Release Tablets ... 2282
- Thermotabs ... ◘ 619

Potassium Citrate (Potential for significant hyperkalemia). Products include:
- Alka-Seltzer Effervescent Antacid .. 1570
- K-Lyte ... 707
- Polycitra Syrup ... 2424
- Polycitra-K ... 2424
- Polycitra-LC—Sugar-Free ... 2424
- Ricelyte, Rice-Based Oral Electrolyte Maintenance Solution ... ◘ 613

Potassium Gluconate (Potential for significant hyperkalemia). Products include:
- Kolyum Liquid ... 983

Potassium Phosphate, Dibasic (Potential for significant hyperkalemia). Products include:
- Neutra-Phos ... 2423

Potassium Phosphate, Monobasic (Potential for significant hyperkalemia). Products include:
- K-Phos M.F. Tablets ... 659
- K-Phos Neutral Tablets ... 660
- Neutra-Phos ... 2423

Spironolactone (Potential for excessive hypotension and significant hyperkalemia). Products include:
- Aldactazide ... 2150
- Aldactone ... 2152

Triamterene (Potential for excessive hypotension and significant hyperkalemia). Products include:
- Dyazide Capsules ... 2208
- Dyrenium Capsules ... 2210
- Maxzide ... 1215

VASOTEC TABLETS
(Enalapril Maleate) ... 1564

May interact with diuretics, thiazides, potassium-depleting corticosteroids, lithium preparations, and certain other agents. Compounds in these categories include:

Amiloride Hydrochloride (Significant increases in serum potassium; excessive hypotension). Products include:
- Midamor Tablets ... 1508
- Moduretic Tablets ... 1510

Bendroflumethiazide (Attenuated potassium loss; excessive hypotension). Products include:
- Corzide Tablets ... 702
- Naturetin Tablets ... 1789
- Rauzide Tablets ... 1804

Bumetanide (Excessive hypotension). Products include:
- Bumex ... 1895

Chlorothiazide (Attenuated potassium loss; excessive hypotension). Products include:
- Aldoclor Tablets ... 1413
- Diupres Tablets ... 1461
- Diuril Oral ... 1464

Chlorothiazide Sodium (Attenuated potassium loss; excessive hypotension). Products include:
- Diuril Sodium Intravenous ... 1463

Chlorthalidone (Significant increases in serum potassium; excessive hypotension). Products include:
- Combipres Tablets ... 678
- Tenoretic Tablets ... 1105
- Thalitone Tablets ... 687

Ethacrynic Acid (Excessive hypotension). Products include:
- Edecrin Tablets ... 1468

Furosemide (Excessive hypotension). Products include:
- Lasix ... 1093

Hydrochlorothiazide (Attenuated potassium loss; excessive hypotension). Products include:
- Aldactazide ... 2150
- Aldoril Tablets ... 1418
- Apresazide Capsules ... 854
- Apresoline-Esidrix Tablets ... 857
- Capozide ... 2258
- Dyazide Capsules ... 2208
- Esidrix Tablets ... 863
- Esimil Tablets ... 864
- HydroDIURIL Tablets ... 1484
- Hydropres Tablets ... 1485
- Inderide Tablets ... 2463
- Inderide LA Long Acting Capsules .. 2465
- Lopressor HCT Tablets ... 1034
- Maxzide ... 1215
- Moduretic Tablets ... 1510
- Normozide Tablets ... 2112
- Oretic Tablets ... 544
- Oreticyl ... 545
- Prinzide Tablets ... 1540
- Ser-Ap-Es Tablets ... 881
- Serpasil-Esidrix Tablets ... 886
- Timolide Tablets ... 1547
- Trandate HCT Tablets ... 579
- Vaseretic Tablets ... 1559
- Zestoretic ... 2274

Hydroflumethiazide (Attenuated potassium loss; excessive hypotension). Products include:
- Diucardin Tablets ... 2450
- Saluron ... 718
- Salutensin/Salutensin-Demi ... 719

Indapamide (Excessive hypotension). Products include:
- Lozol Tablets ... 1843

Lithium Carbonate (Potential for reversible lithium toxicity; frequent monitoring of serum lithium levels is recommended). Products include:
- Eskalith ... 2214
- Lithane Tablets ... 1596
- Lithium Carbonate Capsules & Tablets ... 1984
- Lithobid Tablets ... 870

Lithium Citrate (Potential for reversible lithium toxicity; frequent monitoring of serum lithium levels is recommended). Products include:
- Cibalith-S ... 870

Methyclothiazide (Attenuated potassium loss; excessive hypotension). Products include:
- Enduron Tablets ... 517
- Enduronyl ... 518

Metolazone (Excessive hypotension). Products include:
- Diulo ... 2129
- Mykrox ½ mg Tablets ... 984
- Zaroxolyn Tablets ... 989

Polythiazide (Attenuated potassium loss; excessive hypotension). Products include:
- Minizide Capsules ... 1779
- Renese Tablets ... 1785
- Renese-R Tablets ... 1786

Potassium Acid Phosphate (Significant increases in serum potassium). Products include:
- K-Phos M.F. Tablets ... 659
- K-Phos Original Formula 'Sodium Free' Tablets ... 660
- K-Phos No. 2 Tablets ... 659

Potassium Bicarbonate (Significant increases in serum potassium). Products include:
- Alka-Seltzer Advanced Formula Antacid & Non-Aspirin Pain Reliever ... ◘ 620
- Alka-Seltzer Effervescent Antacid ◘ 622
- K-Lyte ... 707
- Klorvess Effervescent Granules ... 2010
- Klorvess Effervescent Tablets ... 2011

Potassium Chloride (Significant increases in serum potassium). Products include:
- Chlor-3 Condiment ... 994
- K-Dur Microburst Release System (potassium chloride, USP) E.R. Tablets ... 1163
- K-Lor Powder Packets ... 531
- K-Lyte ... 707
- K-Norm Capsules ... 982
- K-Tab Filmtab ... 532
- Kato Potassium Supplement ... 1114
- Klor-Con 8/Klor-Con 10 Extended-release Tablets ... 2374
- Klorvess Effervescent Granules ... 2010
- Klorvess Effervescent Tablets ... 2011
- Klorvess 10% Liquid ... 2010
- Klotrix ... 708
- Kolyum Liquid ... 983
- Micro-K ... 1863
- Micro-K LS Packets ... 1864
- NuLYTELY ... 699
- Oral Rehydration Salts, Citrate ... 1150
- Rum-K Syrup ... 995
- Slow-K Tablets ... 2281
- Ten-K Controlled-Release Tablets ... 2282
- Thermotabs ... ◘ 619

Potassium Citrate (Significant increases in serum potassium). Products include:
- Alka-Seltzer Effervescent Antacid .. 1570
- K-Lyte ... 707
- Polycitra Syrup ... 2424
- Polycitra-K ... 2424
- Polycitra-LC—Sugar-Free ... 2424
- Ricelyte, Rice-Based Oral Electrolyte Maintenance Solution ... ◘ 613

Potassium Gluconate (Significant increases in serum potassium). Products include:
- Kolyum Liquid ... 983

Potassium Phosphate, Dibasic (Significant increases in serum potassium). Products include:
- Neutra-Phos ... 2423

Potassium Phosphate, Monobasic (Significant increases in serum potassium). Products include:
- K-Phos M.F. Tablets ... 659
- K-Phos Neutral Tablets ... 660
- Neutra-Phos ... 2423

Spironolactone (Significant increases in serum potassium; excessive hypotension). Products include:
- Aldactazide ... 2150
- Aldactone ... 2152

Triamterene (Significant increases in serum potassium; excessive hypotension). Products include:
- Dyazide Capsules ... 2208
- Dyrenium Capsules ... 2210
- Maxzide ... 1215

VASOXYL INJECTION
(Methoxamine Hydrochloride) ... 819

May interact with monoamine oxidase inhibitors, tricyclic antidepressants, and certain other agents. Compounds in these categories include:

Amitriptyline Hydrochloride (Potentiation of pressor effect). Products include:
- Elavil ... 2269
- Endep Tablets ... 1927
- Etrafon ... 2087
- Limbitrol ... 1933
- Triavil Tablets ... 1556

Amoxapine (Potentiation of pressor effect). Products include:
- Asendin Tablets ... 1196

Clomipramine Hydrochloride (Potentiation of pressor effect). Products include:
- Anafranil Capsules ... 650

Desipramine Hydrochloride (Potentiation of pressor effect). Products include:
- Norpramin Tablets ... 1340

Doxepin Hydrochloride (Potentiation of pressor effect). Products include:
- Sinequan ... 1960

Ergonovine Maleate (Potentiation of pressor effect).

Ergot Alkaloids (Hydrogenated) (Potentiation of pressor effect).

Ergotamine Tartrate (Potentiation of pressor effect). Products include:
- Bellergal-S Tablets ... 1998
- Cafergot/Cafergot P-B ... 1999
- Ergostat ... 1719
- Medihaler Ergotamine Aerosol ... 1312
- Wigraine Tablets & Suppositories .. 1645

Furazolidone (Potentiation of pressor effect). Products include:
- Furoxone ... 1855

Imipramine Hydrochloride (Potentiation of pressor effect). Products include:
- Tofranil Ampuls ... 1038
- Tofranil Tablets ... 1039

Imipramine Pamoate (Potentiation of pressor effect). Products include:
- Tofranil-PM Capsules ... 1041

Isocarboxazid (Potentiation of pressor effect). Products include:
- Marplan Tablets ... 1906

Maprotiline Hydrochloride (Potentiation of pressor effect). Products include:
- Ludiomil Tablets ... 874

Methylergonovine Maleate (Potentiation of pressor effect). Products include:
- Methergine ... 2016

Nortriptyline Hydrochloride (Potentiation of pressor effect). Products include:
- Pamelor ... 2019

Phenelzine Sulfate (Potentiation of pressor effect). Products include:
- Nardil ... 1742

Protriptyline Hydrochloride (Potentiation of pressor effect). Products include:
- Vivactil Tablets ... 1567

Selegiline Hydrochloride (Potentiation of pressor effect). Products include:
- Eldepryl ... 2250

Tranylcypromine Sulfate (Potentiation of pressor effect). Products include:
- Parnate Tablets ... 2222

Trimipramine Maleate (Potentiation of pressor effect). Products include:
- Surmontil Capsules ... 2524

Vasopressin (Potentiation of pressor effect). Products include:
- Pitressin Synthetic, Ampoules ... 1758

VELBAN VIALS
(Vinblastine Sulfate) ... 1305
May interact with:

Mitomycin (Mitomycin-C) (Acute shortness of breath; severe bronchospasm). Products include:
- Mutamycin ... 733

Phenytoin (Reduced blood levels of phenytoin and increased seizure activity). Products include:
- Dilantin Infatabs ... 1710
- Dilantin-30 Pediatric/Dilantin-125 Suspension ... 1713

Phenytoin Sodium (Reduced blood levels of phenytoin and increased seizure activity). Products include:
- Dilantin Kapseals ... 1708
- Dilantin Parenteral ... 1712
- Dilantin with Phenobarbital Kapseals ... 1715

VELOSEF CAPSULES AND FOR ORAL SUSPENSION
(Cephradine) ... 606
May interact with aminoglycosides, loop diuretics, and certain other agents. Compounds in these categories include:

Amikacin Sulfate (Increased possibility of nephrotoxicity). Products include:
- Amikin Injectable ... 602

Bumetanide (Enhanced possibility for renal toxicity). Products include:
- Bumex ... 1895

Colistin Sulfate (Increased possibility of nephrotoxicity). Products include:
- Coly-Mycin S For Oral Suspension .. 1708
- Coly-Mycin S Otic w/Neomycin & Hydrocortisone ... 1708

Ethacrynic Acid (Enhanced possibility for renal toxicity). Products include:
- Edecrin Tablets ... 1468

Furosemide (Enhanced possibility for renal toxicity). Products include:
- Lasix ... 1093

Gentamicin Sulfate (Increased possibility of nephrotoxicity). Products include:
- Garamycin Injectable ... 2093
- Garamycin Ophthalmic ... ◉ 305
- Genoptic Liquifilm Sterile Ophthalmic Solution ... ◉ 247
- Genoptic S.O.P. Sterile Ophthalmic Ointment ... ◉ 247
- Gentacidin Ointment ... ◉ 273
- Gentacidin Solution ... ◉ 273
- Gentak Ointment & Solution ... ◉ 208
- G-myticin Creme and Ointment 0.1% ... 1770
- Pred-G Liquifilm Sterile Ophthalmic Suspension ... ◉ 252
- Pred-G S.O.P. Sterile Ophthalmic Ointment ... ◉ 253

Kanamycin Sulfate (Increased possibility of nephrotoxicity). Products include:
- Kantrex Injection ... 601
- Kantrex Pediatric Injection ... 601

Polymyxin B Sulfate (Increased possibility of nephrotoxicity). Products include:
- AK-Poly-Bac Ointment ... ◉ 205
- AK-Spore H.C. ... ◉ 206
- AK-Spore ... ◉ 205
- AK-Trol Ointment & Suspension ... ◉ 207
- Aquaphor Antibiotic Formula ... 662
- Bactine First Aid Antibiotic Ointment ... ▣ 625
- Campho-Phenique Triple Antibiotic Ointment Plus Pain Reliever ▣ 758
- Cortisporin Cream ... 757
- Cortisporin Ointment ... 758
- Cortisporin Ophthalmic Ointment Sterile ... 758
- Cortisporin Ophthalmic Suspension Sterile ... 759
- Cortisporin Otic Solution Sterile ... 760
- Cortisporin Otic Suspension Sterile 760
- Dexacidin ... ◉ 272
- Lanabiotic Ointment ... ▣ 556
- LazerSporin-C Solution ... 1770
- Maxitrol Ophthalmic Ointment/Suspension ... ◉ 223
- Mycitracin ... ▣ 737
- Neosporin Cream ... 792
- Neosporin G.U. Irrigant Sterile ... 793
- Neosporin Ointment ... 793
- Maximum Strength Neosporin Ointment ... 793
- Neosporin Ophthalmic Ointment Sterile ... 793
- Neosporin Ophthalmic Solution Sterile ... 794
- Ophthocort ... ◉ 301
- PediOtic Suspension Sterile ... 797
- Polymyxin B Sulfate, Aerosporin Brand Sterile Powder ... 798
- Poly-Pred Liquifilm ... ◉ 250
- Polysporin Ointment ... ▣ 543
- Polysporin Ophthalmic Ointment Sterile ... 798
- Polysporin Powder ... ▣ 543
- Polysporin Spray ... ▣ 543
- Polytrim Ophthalmic Solution Sterile ... 588
- Terramycin with Polymyxin B Sulfate Ophthalmic Ointment ... 1965

Polymyxin Preparations (Increased possibility of nephrotoxicity).

Probenecid (Increased possibility of nephrotoxicity). Products include:
- Benemid Tablets ... 1426
- ColBENEMID Tablets ... 1436
- Wycillin Injection and Probenecid Tablets ... 2539

Streptomycin Sulfate (Increased possibility of nephrotoxicity).
- No products indexed under this heading.

Tobramycin (Increased possibility of nephrotoxicity). Products include:
- TobraDex Ophthalmic Suspension and Ointment ... ◉ 228
- Tobrex Ophthalmic Ointment and Solution ... 572

Tobramycin Sulfate (Increased possibility of nephrotoxicity). Products include:
- Nebcin Vials, Hyporets & ADD-Vantage ... 1286

Trichlormethiazide (Enhanced possibility for renal toxicity).
- No products indexed under this heading.

Vancomycin Hydrochloride (Increased possibility of nephrotoxicity). Products include:
- Vancocin HCl, Oral Solution & Pulvules ... 1304
- Vancocin HCl, Vials & ADD-Vantage ... 1302

VELOSULIN
(Insulin, Regular) ... 1627
No interactions described in labeling.

VELOSULIN HUMAN
(Insulin, Human Regular) ... 1628
No interactions described in labeling.

VENTOLIN INHALATION AEROSOL AND REFILL
(Albuterol) ... 583
May interact with sympathomimetic bronchodilators, monoamine oxidase inhibitors, tricyclic antidepressants, beta blockers, and certain other agents. Compounds in these categories include:

Acebutolol Hydrochloride (Beta receptor blocking agents and albuterol inhibit effect of each other). Products include:
- Sectral Capsules ... 2520

Amitriptyline Hydrochloride (Action of albuterol on vascular system may be potentiated). Products include:
- Elavil ... 2269
- Endep Tablets ... 1927
- Etrafon ... 2087
- Limbitrol ... 1933
- Triavil Tablets ... 1556

Amoxapine (Action of albuterol on vascular system may be potentiated). Products include:
- Asendin Tablets ... 1196

Atenolol (Beta receptor blocking agents and albuterol inhibit effect of each other). Products include:
- Tenoretic Tablets ... 1105
- Tenormin Tablets and I.V. Injection 1107

Betaxolol Hydrochloride (Beta receptor blocking agents and albuterol inhibit effect of each other). Products include:
- Betoptic Sterile Ophthalmic Solution ... 569
- Betoptic S Sterile Ophthalmic Suspension ... 570
- Kerlone Tablets ... 2172

Bitolterol Mesylate (Sympathomimetic aerosol bronchodilators should not be used concomitantly with albuterol, may have additive effects). Products include:
- Tornalate ... 2074

Carteolol Hydrochloride (Beta receptor blocking agents and albuterol inhibit effect of each other). Products include:
- Cartrol Tablets ... 507

Clomipramine Hydrochloride (Action of albuterol on vascular system may be potentiated). Products include:
- Anafranil Capsules ... 650

Desipramine Hydrochloride (Action of albuterol on vascular system may be potentiated). Products include:
- Norpramin Tablets ... 1340

Doxepin Hydrochloride (Action of albuterol on vascular system may be potentiated). Products include:
- Sinequan ... 1960

Ephedrine Hydrochloride (Sympathomimetic aerosol bronchodilators should not be used concomitantly with albuterol, may have additive effects). Products include:
- Amesec ... ▣ 682
- Primatene Tablets-M Formula ... 2421
- Primatene Tablets-P Formula ... 2421
- Primatene Tablets-Regular Formula ... 2421
- Quadrinal Tablets ... 1183
- Quelidrine Syrup ... 556
- Tedral SA ... 1765

Ephedrine Sulfate (Sympathomimetic aerosol bronchodilators should not be used concomitantly with albuterol, may have additive effects). Products include:
- Bronkaid Tablets ... ▣ 757
- Bronkolixir ... ▣ 761
- Bronkotabs Tablets ... ▣ 762
- Marax Tablets & DF Syrup ... 1954
- Pazo Hemorrhoid Ointment & Suppositories ... 752
- Vicks Vatronol Nose Drops ... ▣ 666

Ephedrine Tannate (Sympathomimetic aerosol bronchodilators should not be used concomitantly with albuterol, may have additive effects). Products include:
- Rynatuss ... 2388

Epinephrine (Sympathomimetic aerosol bronchodilators should not be used concomitantly with albuterol, may have additive effects). Products include:
- Ana-Kit Anaphylaxis Emergency Treatment Kit ... 1100
- Bronkaid Mist ... ▣ 757
- EpiPen ... 843
- Marcaine Hydrochloride 0.5% with Epinephrine 1:200,000 (as bitartrate) ... 958
- Marcaine Hydrochloride with Epinephrine 1:200,000 ... 2055
- Primatene Mist ... 2420
- Sus-Phrine Injection ... 1006
- Xylocaine with Epinephrine Injections ... 637

Epinephrine Hydrochloride (Sympathomimetic aerosol bronchodilators should not be used concomitantly with albuterol). Products include:
- Adrenalin Chloride Solution 1:100 & 1:1,000 ... 1689
- Epifrin ... ◉ 244

Glaucon ◉ 218

Esmolol Hydrochloride (Beta receptor blocking agents and albuterol inhibit effect of each other). Products include:
Brevibloc Injection 942

Ethylnorepinephrine Hydrochloride (Sympathomimetic aerosol bronchodilators should not be used concomitantly with albuterol, may have additive effects). Products include:
Bronkephrine Injection 2042

Furazolidone (Action of albuterol on vascular system may be potentiated). Products include:
Furoxone 1855

Imipramine Hydrochloride (Action of albuterol on vascular system may be potentiated). Products include:
Tofranil Ampuls 1038
Tofranil Tablets 1039

Imipramine Pamoate (Action of albuterol on vascular system may be potentiated). Products include:
Tofranil-PM Capsules 1041

Isocarboxazid (Action of albuterol on vascular system may be potentiated). Products include:
Marplan Tablets 1906

Isoetharine (Sympathomimetic aerosol bronchodilators should not be used concomitantly with albuterol, may have additive effects). Products include:
Arm-a-Med Isoetharine Inhalation Solution, USP 616
Bronkometer Aerosol 2042
Bronkosol Solution 2042

Isoproterenol Hydrochloride (Sympathomimetic aerosol bronchodilators should not be used concomitantly with albuterol). Products include:
Isuprel Hydrochloride Injection 1:5000 2050
Isuprel Hydrochloride Mistometer .. 2051
Isuprel Hydrochloride Solution 1:200 & 1:100 2052
Norisodrine Aerotrol 540

Labetalol Hydrochloride (Beta receptor blocking agents and albuterol inhibit effect of each other). Products include:
Normodyne Injection 2108
Normodyne Tablets 2110
Normozide Tablets 2112
Trandate HCT Tablets 579
Trandate Injection 577
Trandate Tablets 579

Maprotiline Hydrochloride (Action of albuterol on vascular system may be potentiated). Products include:
Ludiomil Tablets 874

Metaproterenol Sulfate (Sympathomimetic aerosol bronchodilators should not be used concomitantly with albuterol, may have additive effects). Products include:
Alupent 674
Arm-a-Med Metaproterenol Sulfate Inhalation Solution, USP 617
Metaprel Inhalation Aerosol Bronchodilator 2014
Metaprel Inhalation Solution 2015
Metaprel 2015
Metaproterenol Sulfate Inhalation Solution, USP 912

Metoprolol Tartrate (Beta receptor blocking agents and albuterol inhibit effect of each other). Products include:
Lopressor Ampuls 1032
Lopressor HCT Tablets 1034
Lopressor Tablets 1032

Nadolol (Beta receptor blocking agents and albuterol inhibit effect of each other). Products include:
Corgard Tablets 701
Corzide Tablets 702

Nortriptyline Hydrochloride (Action of albuterol on vascular system may be potentiated). Products include:
Pamelor 2019

Penbutolol Sulfate (Beta receptor blocking agents and albuterol inhibit effect of each other). Products include:
Levatol 1832

Phenelzine Sulfate (Action of albuterol on vascular system may be potentiated). Products include:
Nardil 1742

Pindolol (Beta receptor blocking agents and albuterol inhibit effect of each other). Products include:
Visken Tablets 2036

Pirbuterol Acetate (Sympathomimetic aerosol bronchodilators should not be used concomitantly with albuterol, may have additive effects). Products include:
Maxair Inhaler 1311

Propranolol Hydrochloride (Beta receptor blocking agents and albuterol inhibit effect of each other). Products include:
Inderal 2459
Inderal LA Long Acting Capsules 2461
Inderide Tablets 2463
Inderide LA Long Acting Capsules .. 2465

Protriptyline Hydrochloride (Action of albuterol on vascular system may be potentiated). Products include:
Vivactil Tablets 1567

Selegiline Hydrochloride (Action of albuterol on vascular system may be potentiated). Products include:
Eldepryl 2250

Terbutaline Sulfate (Sympathomimetic aerosol bronchodilators should not be used concomitantly with albuterol, may have additive effects). Products include:
Brethaire Inhaler 1024
Brethine Ampuls 1026
Brethine Tablets 1026
Bricanyl Injection 1324
Bricanyl Tablets 1325

Timolol Maleate (Beta receptor blocking agents and albuterol inhibit effect of each other). Products include:
Blocadren Tablets 1429
Timolide Tablets 1547
Timoptic in Ocudose 1552
Timoptic Sterile Ophthalmic Solution 1550

Tranylcypromine Sulfate (Action of albuterol on vascular system may be potentiated). Products include:
Parnate Tablets 2222

Trimipramine Maleate (Action of albuterol on vascular system may be potentiated). Products include:
Surmontil Capsules 2524

VENTOLIN INHALATION SOLUTION
(Albuterol Sulfate) 583
See **Ventolin Inhalation Aerosol and Refill**

VENTOLIN ROTACAPS FOR INHALATION
(Albuterol Sulfate) 583
See **Ventolin Inhalation Aerosol and Refill**

VENTOLIN SYRUP
(Albuterol Sulfate) 583
May interact with monoamine oxidase inhibitors, beta blockers, tricyclic antidepressants, sympathomimetic aerosal brochodilators, and certain other agents. Compounds in these categories include:

Acebutolol Hydrochloride (Beta receptor blocking agents and albuterol inhibit effect of each other). Products include:
Sectral Capsules 2520

Albuterol (Concomitant use of albuterol with oral sympathomimetic agents is not recommended due to potential for cardiovascular toxicity). Products include:
Proventil Inhalation Aerosol 2117
Ventolin Inhalation Aerosol and Refill 583

Amitriptyline Hydrochloride (Action of albuterol on vascular system may be potentiated). Products include:
Elavil 2269
Endep Tablets 1927
Etrafon 2087
Limbitrol 1933
Triavil Tablets 1556

Amoxapine (Action of albuterol on vascular system may be potentiated). Products include:
Asendin Tablets 1196

Atenolol (Beta receptor blocking agents and albuterol inhibit effect of each other). Products include:
Tenoretic Tablets 1105
Tenormin Tablets and I.V. Injection 1107

Betaxolol Hydrochloride (Beta receptor blocking agents and albuterol inhibit effect of each other). Products include:
Betoptic Sterile Ophthalmic Solution 569
Betoptic S Sterile Ophthalmic Suspension 570
Kerlone Tablets 2172

Carteolol Hydrochloride (Beta receptor blocking agents and albuterol inhibit effect of each other). Products include:
Cartrol Tablets 507

Clomipramine Hydrochloride (Action of albuterol on vascular system may be potentiated). Products include:
Anafranil Capsules 650

Desipramine Hydrochloride (Action of albuterol on vascular system may be potentiated). Products include:
Norpramin Tablets 1340

Dobutamine Hydrochloride (Concomitant use of albuterol with oral sympathomimetic agents is not recommended due to potential for cardiovascular toxicity). Products include:
Dobutrex Solution Vials 1259

Dopamine Hydrochloride (Concomitant use of albuterol with oral sympathomimetic agents is not recommended due to potential for cardiovascular toxicity). Products include:
Intropin Injection 930

Doxepin Hydrochloride (Action of albuterol on vascular system may be potentiated). Products include:
Sinequan 1960

Ephedrine Hydrochloride (Concomitant use of albuterol with oral sympathomimetic agents is not recommended due to potential for cardiovascular toxicity). Products include:
Amesec ▣ 682
Primatene Tablets-M Formula 2421
Primatene Tablets-P Formula 2421
Primatene Tablets-Regular Formula 2421
Quadrinal Tablets 1183
Quelidrine Syrup 556
Tedral SA 1765

Ephedrine Sulfate (Concomitant use of albuterol with oral sympathomimetic agents is not recommended due to potential for cardiovascular toxicity). Products include:
Bronkaid Tablets ▣ 757
Bronkolixir ▣ 761
Bronkotabs Tablets ▣ 762
Marax Tablets & DF Syrup 1954
Pazo Hemorrhoid Ointment & Suppositories 752
Vicks Vatronol Nose Drops ▣ 666

Ephedrine Tannate (Concomitant use of albuterol with oral sympathomimetic agents is not recommended due to potential for cardiovascular toxicity). Products include:
Rynatuss 2388

Epinephrine Hydrochloride (Concomitant use of albuterol with oral sympathomimetic agents is not recommended due to potential for cardiovascular toxicity). Products include:
Adrenalin Chloride Solution 1:100 & 1:1,000 1689
Epifrin ◉ 244
Glaucon ◉ 218

Esmolol Hydrochloride (Beta receptor blocking agents and albuterol inhibit effect of each other). Products include:
Brevibloc Injection 942

Furazolidone (Action of albuterol on vascular system may be potentiated). Products include:
Furoxone 1855

Imipramine Hydrochloride (Action of albuterol on vascular system may be potentiated). Products include:
Tofranil Ampuls 1038
Tofranil Tablets 1039

Imipramine Pamoate (Action of albuterol on vascular system may be potentiated). Products include:
Tofranil-PM Capsules 1041

Isocarboxazid (Action of albuterol on vascular system may be potentiated). Products include:
Marplan Tablets 1906

Isoproterenol Hydrochloride (Concomitant use of albuterol with oral sympathomimetic agents is not recommended due to potential for cardiovascular toxicity). Products include:
Isuprel Hydrochloride Injection 1:5000 2050
Isuprel Hydrochloride Mistometer .. 2051
Isuprel Hydrochloride Solution 1:200 & 1:100 2052
Norisodrine Aerotrol 540

Labetalol Hydrochloride (Beta receptor blocking agents and albuterol inhibit effect of each other). Products include:
Normodyne Injection 2108
Normodyne Tablets 2110
Normozide Tablets 2112
Trandate HCT Tablets 579
Trandate Injection 577
Trandate Tablets 579

Maprotiline Hydrochloride (Action of albuterol on vascular system may be potentiated). Products include:
Ludiomil Tablets 874

Metaproterenol Sulfate (Concomitant use of albuterol with oral sympathomimetic agents is not recommended due to potential for cardiovascular toxicity). Products include:
Alupent 674

Arm-a-Med Metaproterenol Sulfate Inhalation Solution, USP 617
Metaprel Inhalation Aerosol Bronchodilator 2014
Metaprel Inhalation Solution 2015
Metaprel 2015
Metaproterenol Sulfate Inhalation Solution, USP 912

Metaraminol Bitartrate (Concomitant use of albuterol with oral sympathomimetic agents is not recommended due to potential for cardiovascular toxicity). Products include:
Aramine Injection 1424

Methoxamine Hydrochloride (Concomitant use of albuterol with oral sympathomimetic agents is not recommended due to potential for cardiovascular toxicity). Products include:
Vasoxyl Injection 819

Metoprolol Tartrate (Beta receptor blocking agents and albuterol inhibit effect of each other). Products include:
Lopressor Ampuls 1032
Lopressor HCT Tablets 1034
Lopressor Tablets 1032

Nadolol (Beta receptor blocking agents and albuterol inhibit effect of each other). Products include:
Corgard Tablets 701
Corzide Tablets 702

Norepinephrine Bitartrate (Concomitant use of albuterol with oral sympathomimetic agents is not recommended due to potential for cardiovascular toxicity). Products include:
Levophed Bitartrate Injection 2054

Nortriptyline Hydrochloride (Action of albuterol on vascular system may be potentiated). Products include:
Pamelor 2019

Penbutolol Sulfate (Beta receptor blocking agents and albuterol inhibit effect of each other). Products include:
Levatol 1832

Phenelzine Sulfate (Action of albuterol on vascular system may be potentiated). Products include:
Nardil 1742

Phenylephrine Bitartrate (Concomitant use of albuterol with oral sympathomimetic agents is not recommended due to potential for cardiovascular toxicity).
No products indexed under this heading.

Phenylephrine Hydrochloride (Concomitant use of albuterol with oral sympathomimetic agents is not recommended due to potential for cardiovascular toxicity). Products include:
AK-Dilate Solution 2.5% and 10% .... ⊙ 203
Atrohist Sprinkle Capsules 558
Cerose-DM 2443
Codimal 846
Comhist LA Capsules 1618
Congespirin For Children Aspirin Free Chewable Cold Tablets 748
Cyclomydril .... ⊙ 216
Deconsal Sprinkle Capsules 559
Dimetane Decongestant .... ▣ 673
Dristan Decongestant/Antihistamine/ Analgesic Coated Caplets .... ▣ 749
Dristan Cold Nasal Decongestant/ Antihistamine/ Analgesic Coated Tablets 2419
Dristan Advanced Formula Decongestant/Antihistamine/ Analgesic Tablets .... ▣ 749
Dristan Nasal Spray, Menthol 2419
Dristan Nasal Spray, Regular and Regular with Metered Pump 2419
Entex Capsules 1623
Entex Liquid 1623
Sinus Excedrin Analgesic, Decongestant Tablets & Caplets 750
Extendryl 994
4-Way Fast Acting Nasal Spray - Original Formula (regular & mentholated) & Metered Spray Pump (regular) 751
Hycomine Compound Tablets 929
Murocoll-2 Sterile Ophthalmic Solution .... ⊙ 261
Mydfrin 2.5% .... ⊙ 224
Naldecon Syrup, Tablets, Pediatric Drops and Pediatric Syrup 709
Neo-Synephrine Hydrochloride 1% Carpuject 2063
Neo-Synephrine Hydrochloride 1% Injection 2063
Neo-Synephrine Hydrochloride (Ophthalmic) 2064
Neo-Synephrine .... ▣ 759
Nōstril Nasal Decongestant .... ▣ 520
Novahistine Elixir .... ▣ 596
Phenergan VC 2500
Phenergan VC with Codeine 2501
Prefrin Liquifilm Vasoconstrictor and Lubricant Eye Drops .... ⊙ 254
Prefrin-A .... ⊙ 255
Quelidrine Syrup 556
Relief Vasoconstrictor and Lubricant Eye Drops .... ⊙ 256
Robitussin Night Relief .... ▣ 677
Ru-Tuss with Hydrocodone 694
Ru-Tuss Tablets 693
Vasosulf .... ⊙ 279
Vicks Sinex .... ▣ 665
Zincfrin .... ⊙ 230

Phenylephrine Tannate (Concomitant use of albuterol with oral sympathomimetic agents is not recommended due to potential for cardiovascular toxicity). Products include:
Rynatan 2387
Rynatuss 2388

Phenylpropanolamine Hydrochloride (Concomitant use of albuterol with oral sympathomimetic agents is not recommended due to potential for cardiovascular toxicity). Products include:
A.R.M. Allergy Relief Medicine Caplets .... ▣ 615
Acutrim .... ▣ 548
Allerest .... ▣ 559
BC Cold Powder .... ▣ 517
Cheracol Plus Head Cold/Cough Formula .... ▣ 667
Codimal Expectorant 846
Comtrex Multi-Symptom Cold Reliever Tablets/Caplets/Liqui-Gels/Liquid 745
Contac Continuous Action Decongestant/Antihistamine Capsules ▣ 710
Contac Maximum Strength Continuous Action Decongestant/ Antihistamine Caplets .... ▣ 709
Contac Severe Cold and Flu Formula Caplets .... ▣ 711
Coricidin 'D' Decongestant Tablets .... ▣ 695
Coricidin Demilets Tablets for Children .... ▣ 696
Demazin Nasal Decongestant/ Antihistamine Repetabs Tablets & Syrup .... ▣ 697
Dexatrim .... ▣ 733
Dimetane-DC Cough Syrup 1857
Dimetapp Elixir .... ▣ 673
Dimetapp DM Elixir .... ▣ 674
Dimetapp Extentabs .... ▣ 674
Dimetapp Plus Caplets .... ▣ 675
Dimetapp Tablets .... ▣ 675
Entex Capsules 1623
Entex LA Tablets 1623
Entex Liquid 1623
4-Way Cold Tablets 750
Hycomine Syrup 927
Naldecon CX Adult Liquid .... ▣ 521
Naldecon DX Adult Liquid .... ▣ 521
Naldecon DX Children's Syrup .... ▣ 522
Naldecon DX Pediatric Drops .... ▣ 522
Naldecon EX Children's Syrup .... ▣ 522
Naldecon EX Pediatric Drops .... ▣ 523
Naldecon Syrup, Tablets, Pediatric Drops and Pediatric Syrup 709
Nolamine Tablets 838
Nolex LA Tablets 838
Ornade Spansule Capsules 2221
Orthoxicol Cough Syrup .... ▣ 668
Propagest 839
Pyrroxate Capsules .... ▣ 669
Robitussin-CF .... ▣ 676
Ru-Tuss II Capsules 693
Ru-Tuss with Hydrocodone 694
Ru-Tuss Tablets 693
Sine-Off Sinus Medicine Tablets-Aspirin Formula .... ▣ 722
Sinulin 840
St. Joseph Cold Tablets for Children .... ▣ 704
Tavist-D Tablets 2035
Triaminic Allergy Tablets .... ▣ 688
Triaminic Chewables .... ▣ 688
Triaminic Cold Tablets .... ▣ 688
Triaminic Expectorant .... ▣ 688
Triaminic Expectorant w/Codeine 1996
Triaminic Expectorant DH 1995
Triaminic Oral Infant Drops 1996
Triaminic Syrup .... ▣ 689
Triaminic-12 Tablets .... ▣ 690
Triaminic-DM Syrup .... ▣ 689
Triaminicin Tablets .... ▣ 690
Triaminicol Multi-Symptom Cold Tablets .... ▣ 691
Triaminicol Multi-Symptom Relief ▣ 691
Tuss-Ornade Liquid 2242
Tuss-Ornade Spansule Capsules 2242
Tylenol Cold Medication, Effervescent Tablets 1369

Pindolol (Beta receptor blocking agents and albuterol inhibit effect of each other). Products include:
Visken Tablets 2036

Pirbuterol Acetate (Concomitant use of albuterol with oral sympathomimetic agents is not recommended due to potential for cardiovascular toxicity). Products include:
Maxair Inhaler 1311

Propranolol Hydrochloride (Beta receptor blocking agents and albuterol inhibit effect of each other). Products include:
Inderal 2459
Inderal LA Long Acting Capsules 2461
Inderide Tablets 2463
Inderide LA Long Acting Capsules 2465

Protriptyline Hydrochloride (Action of albuterol on vascular system may be potentiated). Products include:
Vivactil Tablets 1567

Pseudoephedrine Hydrochloride (Concomitant use of albuterol with oral sympathomimetic agents is not recommended due to potential for cardiovascular toxicity). Products include:
Actifed Capsules .... ▣ 539
Actifed Plus Caplets .... ▣ 539
Actifed Plus Tablets .... ▣ 540
Actifed with Codeine Cough Syrup 752
Actifed Syrup .... ▣ 540
Actifed Tablets .... ▣ 540
Actifed 12-Hour Capsules .... ▣ 539
Advil Cold & Sinus Caplets (formerly CoAdvil) 2416
Allerest .... ▣ 559
Anatuss LA Tablets 1359
Benadryl Decongestant Elixir .... ▣ 635
Benadryl Decongestant .... ▣ 635
Benadryl Plus .... ▣ 636
Benadryl Plus Nighttime .... ▣ 637
Benylin Decongestant .... ▣ 638
Brexin L.A. Capsules 2078
Bromfed Capsules (Timed Release) 1615
Bromfed Syrup .... ▣ 628
Bromfed 1615
CoAdvil .... ▣ 748
Allergy-Sinus Comtrex Multi-Symptom Allergy Sinus Formula Tablets & Caplets 746
Cough Formula Comtrex 746
Comtrex Multi-Symptom Cold Reliever Tablets/Caplets/Liqui-Gels/Liquid 745
Day-Night Comtrex 747
Non-Drowsy Comtrex 747
Congess 994
Congestac Caplets .... ▣ 617
Contac Jr. Children's Cold Medicine .... ▣ 712
Contac Nighttime Cold Medicine .... ▣ 713
Contac Sinus Caplets Maximum Strength Non-Drowsy Formula .... ▣ 710
Contac Sinus Tablets Maximum Strength Non-Drowsy Formula .... ▣ 710
Deconamine 663
Deconsal II Tablets 559
Dimacol Caplets .... ▣ 672
Dimetane-DX Cough Syrup 1858
Dorcol Children's Cough Syrup .... ▣ 685
Dorcol Children's Decongestant Liquid .... ▣ 685
Dorcol Children's Liquid Cold Formula .... ▣ 686
Maximum Strength Dristan Decongestant/Analgesic Coated Caplets .... ▣ 750
No Drowsiness Dristan Cold Nasal Decongestant/Analgesic Coated Caplets 2420
Dristan Sinus Caplets 2419
Sinus Excedrin Analgesic, Decongestant Tablets & Caplets .... ▣ 533
Fedahist Gyrocaps 2145
Fedahist Timecaps 2145
Guaifed 1615
Guaifed Syrup .... ▣ 629
Isoclor Expectorant 982
Isoclor Timesule Capsules .... ▣ 561
Kronofed-A 970
Medi-Flu Caplet, Liquid .... ▣ 640
Novafed A Capsules 1342
Novafed Capsules 1342
Novahistine DH 1342
Novahistine DMX .... ▣ 595
Novahistine Expectorant 1343
Nucofed Capsules 2219
Nucofed Expectorant 2219
Nucofed Pediatric Expectorant 2220
Nucofed Syrup 2219
Ornex Caplets .... ▣ 618
PediaCare Allergy Relief Formula Liquid 1362
PediaCare Cough-Cold Formula Liquid 1362
PediaCare Infants' Oral Decongestant Drops 1362
PediaCare Night Rest Cough-Cold Formula Liquid 1362
PediaCare 6-12 Cough-Cold Formula Chewable Tablets 1362
Robitussin-DAC Syrup 1875
Robitussin-PE .... ▣ 677
Rondec 1975
Rondec-DM 1976
Rondec-TR Tablet 1975
Ru-Tuss DE Tablets 694
Ryna .... ▣ 741
Seldane-D Extended-Release Tablets 1350
Sinarest .... ▣ 562
Sine-Aid Maximum Strength Sinus Headache Caplets 1365
Sine-Aid Maximum Strength Sinus Headache Tablets 1365
Sine-Off Maximum Strength Allergy/Sinus Formula Caplets .... ▣ 721
Sine-Off Maximum Strength No Drowsiness Formula Caplets .... ▣ 722
Singlet Tablets .... ▣ 598
Sinutab Maximum Strength .... ▣ 641
Sinutab Maximum Strength Without Drowsiness Tablets & Caplets .... ▣ 642
Sinutab Regular Strength Without Drowsiness Formula .... ▣ 641
St. Joseph Nighttime Cold Medicine .... ▣ 705
Sudafed Children's Liquid .... ▣ 543
Sudafed Cough Syrup .... ▣ 543
Sudafed Plus Liquid .... ▣ 544
Sudafed Plus Tablets .... ▣ 545
Sudafed Sinus Caplets .... ▣ 545
Sudafed Sinus Tablets .... ▣ 545
Sudafed Tablets, 30 mg .... ▣ 544
Sudafed Tablets, Adult Strength, 60 mg .... ▣ 544
Sudafed 12 Hour Capsules .... ▣ 545
TheraFlu Flu and Cold Medicine .... ▣ 687
Triaminic Nite Light .... ▣ 689
Tylenol Allergy Sinus Medication Caplets and Gelcaps, Maximum Strength 1372
Children's Tylenol Cold Liquid Formula and Chewable Tablets 1368
Tylenol Cold & Flu Hot Medication, Packets 1369
Tylenol Cold & Flu No Drowsiness Hot Medication, Packets 1371
Tylenol Cold Medication Caplets and Tablets 1370

Tylenol Cold Medication No Drowsiness Formula Caplets ... 1370
Tylenol Cold Night Time Medication Liquid ... 1371
Tylenol Cough Medication Liquid with Decongestant, Maximum Strength ... 1372
Tylenol, Maximum Strength, Sinus Medication Gelcaps, Caplets and Tablets ... 1373
Ursinus Inlay-Tabs ... ▣ 691
Vicks Children's NyQuil ... ▣ 664
Vicks Daycare ... ▣ 660
Vicks Formula 44D Decongestant Cough Medicine ... ▣ 662
Vicks Formula 44M Multi-Symptom Cough Medicine ... ▣ 662
Vicks NyQuil Nighttime Colds Medicine-Original & Cherry Flavor ... ▣ 664
Vicks Pediatric Formula 44 Cough & Congestion Medicine ... ▣ 663
Vicks Pediatric Formula 44m Multi-Symptom Cough & Cold Medicine ... ▣ 663

Pseudoephedrine Sulfate (Concomitant use of albuterol with oral sympathomimetic agents is not recommended due to potential for cardiovascular toxicity). Products include:
Afrin Tablets ... ▣ 693
Chlor-Trimeton Decongestant ... ▣ 694
Disophrol Chronotab Sustained-Action Tablets ... ▣ 698
Drixoral Antihistamine/Nasal Decongestant Syrup ... ▣ 698
Drixoral Non-Drowsy Formula ... ▣ 699
Drixoral Plus Extended-Release Tablets ... ▣ 699
Drixoral Sinus ... ▣ 700
Drixoral Sustained-Action Tablets ▣ 698
Sinutab Allergy Formula Sustained Action Tablets ... ▣ 640
Trinalin Repetabs Tablets ... 1170

Selegiline Hydrochloride (Action of albuterol on vascular system may be potentiated). Products include:
Eldepryl ... 2250

Terbutaline Sulfate (Concomitant use of albuterol with oral sympathomimetic agents is not recommended due to potential for cardiovascular toxicity). Products include:
Brethaire Inhaler ... 1024
Brethine Ampuls ... 1026
Brethine Tablets ... 1026
Bricanyl Injection ... 1324
Bricanyl Tablets ... 1325

Timolol Maleate (Beta receptor blocking agents and albuterol inhibit effect of each other). Products include:
Blocadren Tablets ... 1429
Timolide Tablets ... 1547
Timoptic in Ocudose ... 1552
Timoptic Sterile Ophthalmic Solution ... 1550

Tranylcypromine Sulfate (Action of albuterol on vascular system may be potentiated). Products include:
Parnate Tablets ... 2222

Trimipramine Maleate (Action of albuterol on vascular system may be potentiated). Products include:
Surmontil Capsules ... 2524

VENTOLIN TABLETS
(Albuterol Sulfate) ... 583
See **Ventolin Syrup**

VEPESID CAPSULES AND INJECTION
(Etoposide) ... 741
May interact with antineoplastics. Compounds in this category include:

Altretamine (Concomitant administration may result rarely in leukemia). Products include:
Hexalen Capsules ... 2316

Asparaginase (Concomitant administration may result rarely in leukemia). Products include:
Elspar ... 1470

Bleomycin Sulfate (Concomitant administration may result rarely in leukemia). Products include:
Blenoxane ... 724

Busulfan (Concomitant administration may result rarely in leukemia). Products include:
Myleran Tablets ... 790

Carboplatin (Concomitant administration may result rarely in leukemia). Products include:
Paraplatin for Injection ... 735

Carmustine (BCNU) (Concomitant administration may result rarely in leukemia). Products include:
BiCNU ... 723

Chlorambucil (Concomitant administration may result rarely in leukemia). Products include:
Leukeran Tablets ... 788

Cisplatin (Concomitant administration may result rarely in leukemia). Products include:
Platinol ... 737
Platinol-AQ Injection ... 738

Cyclophosphamide (Concomitant administration may result rarely in leukemia). Products include:
Cytoxan for Injection ... 726
Neosar for Injection ... 566

Dacarbazine (Concomitant administration may result rarely in leukemia). Products include:
DTIC-Dome ... 1595

Daunorubicin Hydrochloride (Concomitant administration may result rarely in leukemia). Products include:
Cerubidine ... 2443

Doxorubicin Hydrochloride (Concomitant administration may result rarely in leukemia). Products include:
Adriamycin PFS ... 561
Adriamycin RDF ... 562
Doxorubicin Hydrochloride for Injection, USP ... 622
Doxorubicin Hydrochloride Injection, USP ... 848
Rubex ... 739

Estramustine Phosphate Sodium (Concomitant administration may result rarely in leukemia). Products include:
Emcyt Capsules ... 1161

Floxuridine (Concomitant administration may result rarely in leukemia). Products include:
Sterile FUDR ... 1898

Fluorouracil (Concomitant administration may result rarely in leukemia). Products include:
Efudex ... 1880
Fluoroplex Topical Solution & Cream 1% ... 1082
Fluorouracil Injection ... 1897

Flutamide (Concomitant administration may result rarely in leukemia). Products include:
Eulexin Capsules ... 2089

Hydroxyurea (Concomitant administration may result rarely in leukemia). Products include:
Hydrea Capsules ... 728

Ifosfamide (Concomitant administration may result rarely in leukemia). Products include:
IFEX ... 729

Interferon alfa-2A, Recombinant (Concomitant administration may result rarely in leukemia). Products include:
Roferon-A Injection ... 1916

Interferon alfa-2B, Recombinant (Concomitant administration may result rarely in leukemia). Products include:
Intron A ... 2097

Levamisole Hydrochloride (Concomitant administration may result rarely in leukemia). Products include:
Ergamisol Tablets ... 1136

Lomustine (CCNU) (Concomitant administration may result rarely in leukemia). Products include:
CeeNU ... 725

Mechlorethamine Hydrochloride (Concomitant administration may result rarely in leukemia). Products include:
Mustargen ... 1514

Megestrol Acetate (Concomitant administration may result rarely in leukemia). Products include:
Megace Tablets ... 732

Melphalan (Concomitant administration may result rarely in leukemia). Products include:
Alkeran Tablets ... 754

Mercaptopurine (Concomitant administration may result rarely in leukemia). Products include:
Purinethol Tablets ... 800

Methotrexate Sodium (Concomitant administration may result rarely in leukemia). Products include:
Methotrexate Tablets, Parenteral, LPF Parenteral ... 1217
Rheumatrex Methotrexate Dose Pack ... 1234

Mitomycin (Mitomycin-C) (Concomitant administration may result rarely in leukemia). Products include:
Mutamycin ... 733

Mitotane (Concomitant administration may result rarely in leukemia). Products include:
Lysodren ... 731

Mitoxantrone Hydrochloride (Concomitant administration may result rarely in leukemia). Products include:
Novantrone for Injection Concentrate ... 1226

Procarbazine Hydrochloride (Concomitant administration may result rarely in leukemia). Products include:
Matulane Capsules ... 1907

Streptozocin (Concomitant administration may result rarely in leukemia). Products include:
Zanosar Sterile Powder ... 2371

Tamoxifen Citrate (Concomitant administration may result rarely in leukemia). Products include:
Nolvadex Tablets ... 1102

Thioguanine (Concomitant administration may result rarely in leukemia). Products include:
Thioguanine Tablets, Tabloid Brand ... 815

Thiotepa (Concomitant administration may result rarely in leukemia). Products include:
Thiotepa Parenteral ... 1240

Vincristine Sulfate (Concomitant administration may result rarely in leukemia). Products include:
Oncovin Solution Vials & Hyporets 1288

VERELAN CAPSULES
(Verapamil Hydrochloride) ... 1243
May interact with antihypertensives, beta blockers, diuretics, inhalant anesthetics, nondepolarizing neuromuscular blocking agents, vasodilators, ACE inhibitors, lithium preparations, alpha adrenergic blockers, cardiac glycosides, and certain other agents. Compounds in these categories include:

Acebutolol Hydrochloride (Additive negative effects on heart rate, AV conduction and/or cardiac contractility). Products include:
Sectral Capsules ... 2520

Amiloride Hydrochloride (Additive effect on lowering blood pressure). Products include:
Midamor Tablets ... 1508
Moduretic Tablets ... 1510

Atenolol (Additive negative effects on heart rate, AV conduction and/or cardiac contractility). Products include:
Tenoretic Tablets ... 1105
Tenormin Tablets and I.V. Injection 1107

Atracurium Besylate (Verapamil may potentiate the activity of neuromuscular blocking agents). Products include:
Tracrium Injection ... 817

Benazepril Hydrochloride (Additive effect on lowering blood pressure). Products include:
Lotensin Tablets ... 872

Bendroflumethiazide (Additive effect on lowering blood pressure). Products include:
Corzide Tablets ... 702
Naturetin Tablets ... 1789
Rauzide Tablets ... 1804

Betaxolol Hydrochloride (Additive effect on lowering blood pressure). Products include:
Betoptic Sterile Ophthalmic Solution ... 569
Betoptic S Sterile Ophthalmic Suspension ... 570
Kerlone Tablets ... 2172

Bumetanide (Additive effect on lowering blood pressure). Products include:
Bumex ... 1895

Captopril (Additive effect on lowering blood pressure). Products include:
Capoten ... 2255
Capozide ... 2258

Carbamazepine (Increased carbamazepine concentrations). Products include:
Tegretol Chewable Tablets ... 654
Tegretol Suspension ... 656
Tegretol Tablets ... 654

Carteolol Hydrochloride (Additive negative effects on heart rate, AV conduction and/or cardiac contractility). Products include:
Cartrol Tablets ... 507

Chlorothiazide (Additive effect on lowering blood pressure). Products include:
Aldoclor Tablets ... 1413
Diupres Tablets ... 1461
Diuril Oral ... 1464

Chlorothiazide Sodium (Additive effect on lowering blood pressure). Products include:
Diuril Sodium Intravenous ... 1463

Chlorthalidone (Additive effect on lowering blood pressure). Products include:
Combipres Tablets ... 678
Tenoretic Tablets ... 1105
Thalitone Tablets ... 687

Cimetidine (Possible reduced verapamil clearance). Products include:
Tagamet Tablets ... 2228

Cimetidine Hydrochloride (Possible reduced verapamil clearance). Products include:
Tagamet ... 2228

Clonidine (Additive effect on lowering blood pressure). Products include:
Catapres-TTS ... 677

Clonidine Hydrochloride (Additive effect on lowering blood pressure; adverse effects on cardiac function). Products include:
Catapres Tablets ... 676
Combipres Tablets ... 678

Cyclosporine (Increased serum levels of cyclosporine). Products include:
Sandimmune ... 2024

Deserpidine (Additive effect on lowering blood pressure). Products include:
Enduronyl ... 518
Harmonyl Tablets ... 528
Oreticyl ... 545

Deslanoside (Chronic verapamil treatment can increase serum digoxin levels and this can result in digitalis toxicity).
No products indexed under this heading.

Diazoxide (Additive negative effects on heart rate, AV conduction and/or cardiac contractility). Products include:
Hyperstat I.V. Injection ... 2095
Proglycem ... 649

Digitoxin (Chronic verapamil treatment can increase serum digoxin levels and this can result in digitalis toxicity). Products include:
Crystodigin Tablets ... 1253

Digoxin (Chronic verapamil treatment can increase serum digoxin levels and this can result in digitalis toxicity). Products include:
Lanoxicaps ... 772
Lanoxin Elixir Pediatric ... 775
Lanoxin Injection ... 778
Lanoxin Injection Pediatric ... 781
Lanoxin Tablets ... 783

Disopyramide Phosphate (Should not be administered within 48 hours before or 24 hours after verapamil administration). Products include:
Norpace ... 2177

Doxazosin Mesylate (May result in a reduction in blood pressure that is excessive in some patients). Products include:
Cardura Tablets ... 1941

Enalapril Maleate (Additive effect on lowering blood pressure). Products include:
Vaseretic Tablets ... 1559
Vasotec Tablets ... 1564

Enalaprilat (Additive effect on lowering blood pressure). Products include:
Vasotec I.V. ... 1562

Enflurane (Potential for excessive cardiovascular depression). Products include:
Ethrane ... 599

Esmolol Hydrochloride (Additive negative effects on heart rate, AV conduction and/or cardiac contractility). Products include:
Brevibloc Injection ... 942

Ethacrynic Acid (Additive effect on lowering blood pressure). Products include:
Edecrin Tablets ... 1468

Felodipine (Additive effect on lowering blood pressure). Products include:
Plendil Extended-Release Tablets ... 1526

Flecainide Acetate (Additive effects on myocardial contractility, AV conduction, and repolarization). Products include:
Tambocor Tablets ... 1315

Fosinopril Sodium (Additive effect on lowering blood pressure). Products include:
Monopril Tablets ... 1406

Furosemide (Additive effect on lowering blood pressure). Products include:
Lasix ... 1093

Guanabenz Acetate (Additive effect on lowering blood pressure). Products include:
Wytensin Tablets ... 2542

Guanethidine Monosulfate (Additive effect on lowering blood pressure). Products include:
Esimil Tablets ... 864
Ismelin Tablets ... 869

Halothane (Potential for excessive cardiovascular depression). Products include:
Fluothane ... 2453

Hydralazine Hydrochloride (Additive effect on lowering blood pressure; adverse effects on cardiac function). Products include:
Apresazide Capsules ... 854
Apresoline Hydrochloride Parenteral (Ampuls) ... 856
Apresoline Hydrochloride Tablets ... 855
Apresoline-Esidrix Tablets ... 857
Ser-Ap-Es Tablets ... 881
Serpasil-Apresoline Tablets ... 884

Hydrochlorothiazide (Additive effect on lowering blood pressure). Products include:
Aldactazide ... 2150
Aldoril Tablets ... 1418
Apresazide Capsules ... 854
Apresoline-Esidrix Tablets ... 857
Capozide ... 2258
Dyazide Capsules ... 2208
Esidrix Tablets ... 863
Esimil Tablets ... 864
HydroDIURIL Tablets ... 1484
Hydropres Tablets ... 1485
Inderide Tablets ... 2463
Inderide LA Long Acting Capsules ... 2465
Lopressor HCT Tablets ... 1034
Maxzide ... 1215
Moduretic Tablets ... 1510
Normozide Tablets ... 2112
Oretic Tablets ... 544
Oreticyl ... 545
Prinzide Tablets ... 1540
Ser-Ap-Es Tablets ... 881
Serpasil-Esidrix Tablets ... 886
Timolide Tablets ... 1547
Trandate HCT Tablets ... 579
Vaseretic Tablets ... 1559
Zestoretic ... 2274

Hydroflumethiazide (Additive effect on lowering blood pressure). Products include:
Diucardin Tablets ... 2450
Saluron ... 718
Salutensin/Salutensin-Demi ... 719

Indapamide (Additive effect on lowering blood pressure). Products include:
Lozol Tablets ... 1843

Isoflurane (Potential for excessive cardiovascular depression). Products include:
Forane ... 600

Isradipine (Additive effect on lowering blood pressure). Products include:
DynaCirc Capsules ... 2004

Labetalol Hydrochloride (Additive negative effects on heart rate, AV conduction and/or cardiac contractility). Products include:
Normodyne Injection ... 2108
Normodyne Tablets ... 2110
Normozide Tablets ... 2112
Trandate HCT Tablets ... 579
Trandate Injection ... 577
Trandate Tablets ... 579

Lisinopril (Additive effect on lowering blood pressure). Products include:
Prinivil Tablets ... 1538
Prinzide Tablets ... 1540
Zestoretic ... 2274
Zestril Tablets ... 2277

Lithium Carbonate (May result in lowering of serum lithium levels and increased sensitivity to the effects of lithium). Products include:
Eskalith ... 2214
Lithane Tablets ... 1596
Lithium Carbonate Capsules & Tablets ... 1984
Lithobid Tablets ... 870

Lithium Citrate (May result in lowering of serum lithium levels and increased sensitivity to the effects of lithium). Products include:
Cibalith-S ... 870

Mecamylamine Hydrochloride (Additive effect on lowering blood pressure). Products include:
Inversine Tablets ... 1492

Methoxyflurane (Potential for excessive cardiovascular depression).
No products indexed under this heading.

Methyclothiazide (Additive effect on lowering blood pressure). Products include:
Enduron Tablets ... 517
Enduronyl ... 518

Methyldopa (Additive effect on lowering blood pressure). Products include:
Aldoclor Tablets ... 1413
Aldomet Oral ... 1415
Aldoril Tablets ... 1418

Methyldopate Hydrochloride (Additive effect on lowering blood pressure). Products include:
Aldomet Ester HCl Injection ... 1417

Metocurine Iodide (Verapamil may potentiate the activity of neuromuscular blocking agents). Products include:
Metubine Iodide Vials ... 1285

Metolazone (Additive effect on lowering blood pressure). Products include:
Diulo ... 2129
Mykrox ½ mg Tablets ... 984
Zaroxolyn Tablets ... 989

Metoprolol Tartrate (Additive negative effects on heart rate, AV conduction and/or cardiac contractility; a decrease in metoprolol clearance). Products include:
Lopressor Ampuls ... 1032
Lopressor HCT Tablets ... 1034
Lopressor Tablets ... 1032

Metyrosine (Additive effect on lowering blood pressure). Products include:
Demser Capsules ... 1460

Minoxidil (Additive effect on lowering blood pressure). Products include:
Loniten Tablets ... 2346
Rogaine Topical Solution ... 2357

Nadolol (Additive negative effects on heart rate, AV conduction and/or cardiac contractility). Products include:
Corgard Tablets ... 701
Corzide Tablets ... 702

Nicardipine Hydrochloride (Additive effect on lowering blood pressure). Products include:
Cardene Capsules ... 2290

Pancuronium Bromide Injection (Verapamil may potentiate the activity of neuromuscular blocking agents).
No products indexed under this heading.

Penbutolol Sulfate (Additive negative effects on heart rate, AV conduction and/or cardiac contractility). Products include:
Levatol ... 1832

Phenobarbital (Increases verapamil clearance). Products include:
Arco-Lase Plus Tablets ... 607
Bellergal-S Tablets ... 1998
Bronkolixir ... ▣ 761
Bronkotabs Tablets ... ▣ 762
Donnatal ... 1858
Donnatal Extentabs ... 1859
Donnatal Tablets ... 1858
Donnazyme Tablets ... 1860
Kinesed Tablets ... 2272
Phenobarbital Elixir and Tablets ... 1293
Primatene Tablets-P Formula ... 2421
Quadrinal Tablets ... 1183
Tedral SA ... 1765

Phenoxybenzamine Hydrochloride (Additive effect on lowering blood pressure). Products include:
Dibenzyline Capsules ... 2207

Phentolamine Mesylate (Additive effect on lowering blood pressure). Products include:
Regitine ... 878

Pindolol (Additive negative effects on heart rate, AV conduction and/or cardiac contractility). Products include:
Visken Tablets ... 2036

Polythiazide (Additive effect on lowering blood pressure). Products include:
Minizide Capsules ... 1779
Renese Tablets ... 1785
Renese-R Tablets ... 1786

Prazosin Hydrochloride (May result in a reduction in blood pressure that is excessive in some patients). Products include:
Minipress Capsules ... 1778
Minizide Capsules ... 1779

Propranolol Hydrochloride (Additive negative effects on heart rate, AV conduction and/or cardiac contractility). Products include:
Inderal ... 2459
Inderal LA Long Acting Capsules ... 2461
Inderide Tablets ... 2463
Inderide LA Long Acting Capsules ... 2465

Quinidine Gluconate (Hypotension (in patients with hypertrophic cardiomyopathy); increased quinidine levels). Products include:
Quinaglute Dura-Tabs Tablets ... 663

Quinidine Polygalacturonate (Hypotension (in patients with hypertrophic cardiomyopathy); increased quinidine levels). Products include:
Cardioquin Tablets ... 1812

Quinidine Sulfate (Hypotension (in patients with hypertrophic cardiomyopathy); increased quinidine levels). Products include:
Quinidex Extentabs ... 1868

Ramipril (Additive effect on lowering blood pressure). Products include:
Altace Capsules ... 1086

Rauwolfia Serpentina (Additive effect on lowering blood pressure). Products include:
Raudixin Tablets ... 1803
Rauzide Tablets ... 1804

Rescinnamine (Additive effect on lowering blood pressure).
No products indexed under this heading.

Reserpine (Additive effect on lowering blood pressure). Products include:
Diupres Tablets ... 1461
Hydromox R Tablets ... 1209
Hydropres Tablets ... 1485
Renese-R Tablets ... 1786
Salutensin/Salutensin-Demi ... 719
Ser-Ap-Es Tablets ... 881

Serpasil Tablets ... 883
Serpasil-Apresoline Tablets ... 884
Serpasil-Esidrix Tablets ... 886

Rifampin (Reduced verapamil bioavailability). Products include:
Rifadin ... 1345
Rifamate Capsules ... 1347
Rimactane Capsules ... 879

Sodium Nitroprusside (Additive effect on lowering blood pressure). Products include:
Nipride I.V. Infusion ... 1909

Spironolactone (Additive effect on lowering blood pressure). Products include:
Aldactazide ... 2150
Aldactone ... 2152

Succinylcholine Chloride (Verapamil may potentiate the activity of neuromuscular blocking agents). Products include:
Anectine ... 755

Terazosin Hydrochloride (May result in a reduction in blood preesure that is excessive in some patients). Products include:
Hytrin Tablets ... 529

Timolol Maleate (Additive negative effects on heart rate, AV conduction and/or cardiac contractility). Products include:
Blocadren Tablets ... 1429
Timolide Tablets ... 1547
Timoptic in Ocudose ... 1552
Timoptic Sterile Ophthalmic Solution ... 1550

Triamterene (Additive effect on lowering blood pressure). Products include:
Dyazide Capsules ... 2208
Dyrenium Capsules ... 2210
Maxzide ... 1215

Trimethaphan Camsylate (Additive effect on lowering blood pressure). Products include:
Arfonad Ampuls ... 1887

Vecuronium Bromide (Verapamil prolongs recovery from the neuromuscular blockade; may potentiate the activity of neuromuscular blocking agents). Products include:
Norcuron ... 1642

VERMOX CHEWABLE TABLETS
(Mebendazole) ... 1149
No interactions described in labeling.

VERSED INJECTION
(Midazolam Hydrochloride) ... 1924
May interact with narcotic analgesics, barbiturates, tranquilizers, inhalant anesthetics, central nervous system depressants, and certain other agents. Compounds in these categories include:

Alcohol (May increase risk of underventilation and prolong drug effect).

Alfentanil Hydrochloride (Versed accentuated by premedication). Products include:
Alfenta Injection ... 1131

Alprazolam (Versed accentuated by premedication). Products include:
Xanax Tablets ... 2367

Aprobarbital (Versed accentuated by premedication). Products include:
Alurate Elixir ... 1883

Buprenorphine (Versed accentuated by premedication).
No products indexed under this heading.

Buspirone Hydrochloride (Versed accentuated by premedication). Products include:
BuSpar ... 1401

Butabarbital (Versed accentuated by premedication). Products include:
Pyridium Plus ... 1764

Butalbital (Versed accentuated by premedication). Products include:
Esgic-Plus Tablets ... 1002
Esgic Tablets & Capsules ... 1001
Fioricet Tablets ... 2006
Fiorinal Capsules ... 2007
Fiorinal with Codeine Capsules ... 2008
Fiorinal Tablets ... 2007
Phrenilin ... 838
Sedapap Tablets 50 mg/650 mg ... 1360

Chlordiazepoxide (Versed accentuated by premedication). Products include:
Libritabs Tablets ... 1930
Limbitrol ... 1933
Menrium Tablets ... 1934

Chlordiazepoxide Hydrochloride (Versed accentuated by premedication). Products include:
Librax Capsules ... 1929
Librium Capsules ... 1931
Librium Injectable ... 1932

Chlorpromazine (Versed accentuated by premedication). Products include:
Thorazine ... 2234

Chlorprothixene (Versed accentuated by premedication). Products include:
Taractan Tablets ... 1920

Chlorprothixene Hydrochloride (Versed accentuated by premedication). Products include:
Taractan ... 1920

Clorazepate Dipotassium (Versed accentuated by premedication). Products include:
Tranxene ... 556

Codeine (Versed accentuated by premedication). Products include:
Calcidrine Syrup ... 506

Codeine Phosphate (Versed accentuated by premedication). Products include:
Actifed with Codeine Cough Syrup ... 752
Cheracol Cough Syrup ... 1853
Codimal PH Syrup ... 846
Dimetane-DC Cough Syrup ... 1857
Empirin with Codeine Phosphate Nos. 2, 3 & 4 ... 764
Fiorinal with Codeine Capsules ... 2008
Isoclor Expectorant ... 982
Naldecon CX Adult Liquid ... ■ 521
Novahistine DH ... 1342
Novahistine Expectorant ... 1343
Nucofed Capsules ... 2219
Nucofed Expectorant ... 2219
Nucofed Pediatric Expectorant ... 2220
Nucofed Syrup ... 2219
Phenaphen with Codeine Capsules ... 1865
Phenaphen-650 with Codeine Tablets ... 1866
Phenergan with Codeine ... 2497
Phenergan VC with Codeine ... 2501
Robitussin A-C Syrup ... 1875
Robitussin-DAC Syrup ... 1875
Ryna ... ■ 741
Soma Compound w/Codeine Tablets ... 2390
Triaminic Expectorant w/Codeine ... 1996
Tussi-Organidin Liquid ... 2391
Tylenol with Codeine ... 1381

Codeine Polistirex (Versed accentuated by premedication).
No products indexed under this heading.

Dezocine (Versed accentuated by premedication).

Diazepam (Versed accentuated by premedication). Products include:
Valium Injectable ... 1937
Valium Tablets ... 1939
Valrelease Capsules ... 1923

Droperidol (Versed accentuated by premedication). Products include:
Inapsine Injection ... 1140
Innovar Injection ... 1141

Enflurane (Reduced amount of inhalant required). Products include:
Ethrane ... 599

Estazolam (Versed accentuated by premedication). Products include:
ProSom Tablets ... 554

Ethchlorvynol (Versed accentuated by premedication). Products include:
Placidyl Capsules ... 553

Ethinamate (Versed accentuated by premedication).
No products indexed under this heading.

Fentanyl (Versed accentuated by premedication). Products include:
Duragesic Transdermal System ... 1133

Fentanyl Citrate (Versed accentuated by premedication). Products include:
Innovar Injection ... 1141
Sublimaze Injection ... 1146

Fluphenazine Decanoate (Versed accentuated by premedication). Products include:
Prolixin Decanoate ... 1795

Fluphenazine Enanthate (Versed accentuated by premedication). Products include:
Prolixin Enanthate ... 1796

Fluphenazine Hydrochloride (Versed accentuated by premedication). Products include:
Prolixin Elixir ... 1793
Prolixin Injection ... 1791
Prolixin Oral Concentrate ... 1792
Prolixin Tablets ... 1793

Flurazepam Hydrochloride (Versed accentuated by premedication). Products include:
Dalmane Capsules ... 1927

Glutethimide (Versed accentuated by premedication).
No products indexed under this heading.

Haloperidol (Versed accentuated by premedication). Products include:
Haldol Injection, Tablets and Concentrate ... 1373

Haloperidol Decanoate (Versed accentuated by premedication). Products include:
Haldol Decanoate ... 1375

Halothane (Reduced amount of inhalant required). Products include:
Fluothane ... 2453

Hydrocodone Bitartrate (Versed accentuated by premedication). Products include:
Anexsia 5/500 Tablets ... 2196
Anexsia 7.5/650 Tablets ... 2197
Azdone Tablets ... 844
Codiclear DH Syrup ... 845
Codimal DH Syrup ... 846
Damason-P ... 1356
Hycodan Syrup, Tablets ... 927
Hycomine Compound Tablets ... 929
Hycomine Syrup ... 927
Hycotuss Expectorant Syrup ... 930
Hydrocet Capsules ... 835
Lortab ASA Tablets ... 2414
Lortab ... 2412
Ru-Tuss with Hydrocodone ... 694
Triaminic Expectorant DH ... 1995
Vicodin Tablets ... 1187
Vicodin ES Tablets ... 1189
Zydone Capsules ... 941

Hydrocodone Polistirex (Versed accentuated by premedication). Products include:
Tussionex Extended-Release Suspension ... 988

Hydroxyzine Hydrochloride (Versed accentuated by premedication). Products include:
Atarax Tablets & Syrup ... 1941
Marax Tablets & DF Syrup ... 1954
Vistaril Intramuscular Solution ... 1970

Isoflurane (Reduced amount of inhalant required). Products include:
Forane ... 600

Ketamine Hydrochloride (Versed accentuated by premedication). Products include:
Ketalar ... 1726

Levorphanol Tartrate (Versed accentuated by premedication). Products include:
Levo-Dromoran ... 1906

Lorazepam (Versed accentuated by premedication). Products include:
Ativan Injection ... 2432
Ativan Tablets ... 2434

Loxapine Hydrochloride (Versed accentuated by premedication). Products include:
Loxitane ... 1213

Loxapine Succinate (Versed accentuated by premedication). Products include:
Loxitane Capsules ... 1213

Meperidine Hydrochloride (Versed accentuated by premedication). Products include:
Demerol ... 2047
Mepergan Injection ... 2479

Mephobarbital (Versed accentuated by premedication). Products include:
Mebaral Tablets ... 2061

Meprobamate (Versed accentuated by premedication). Products include:
Deprol Tablets ... 2382
Equagesic Tablets ... 2451
Miltown Tablets ... 2386
PMB 200 and PMB 400 ... 2504

Mesoridazine (Versed accentuated by premedication). Products include:
Serentil ... 686

Methadone Hydrochloride (Versed accentuated by premedication). Products include:
Dolophine Hydrochloride Ampoules & Vials ... 1260
Dolophine Hydrochloride Tablets ... 1261
Methadone Hydrochloride Diskets ... 1284
Methadone Hydrochloride Oral Solution & Tablets ... 1987

Methohexital Sodium (Reduced amount of inhalant required). Products include:
Brevital Sodium Vials ... 1248

Methoxyflurane (Reduced amount of inhalant required).
No products indexed under this heading.

Molindone Hydrochloride (Versed accentuated by premedication). Products include:
Moban Tablets & Concentrate ... 932

Morphine Sulfate (Versed accentuated by premedication). Products include:
Astramorph/PF Injection, USP (Preservative-Free) ... 618
Duramorph ... 960
Infumorph 200 and Infumorph 500 Sterile Solutions ... 962
MS Contin Tablets ... 1814
MSIR ... 1817
Oramorph SR (Morphine Sulfate Sustained Release Tablets) ... 1988
Roxanol ... 1991

Opium Alkaloids (Versed accentuated by premedication). Products include:
B & O No. 15A & No. 16A Supprettes ... 2395
Pantopon Injectable ... 1911

Oxazepam (Versed accentuated by premedication). Products include:
Serax Capsules ... 2522
Serax Tablets ... 2522

Oxycodone Hydrochloride (Versed accentuated by premedication). Products include:
- Percocet Tablets 950
- Percodan 951
- Roxicodone Tablets, Oral Solution & Intensol (Oxycodone) 1992
- Tylox Capsules 1382

Pentobarbital Sodium (Versed accentuated by premedication). Products include:
- Nembutal Sodium Capsules 534
- Nembutal Sodium Solution 536
- Nembutal Sodium Suppositories 538

Perphenazine (Versed accentuated by premedication). Products include:
- Etrafon 2087
- Triavil Tablets 1556
- Trilafon 2123

Phenobarbital (Versed accentuated by premedication). Products include:
- Arco-Lase Plus Tablets 607
- Bellergal-S Tablets 1998
- Bronkolixir .... ■ 761
- Bronkotabs Tablets .... ■ 762
- Donnatal 1858
- Donnatal Extentabs 1859
- Donnatal Tablets 1858
- Donnazyme Tablets 1860
- Kinesed Tablets 2272
- Phenobarbital Elixir and Tablets 1293
- Primatene Tablets-P Formula 2421
- Quadrinal Tablets 1183
- Tedral SA 1765

Prazepam (Versed accentuated by premedication). Products include:
- Centrax 1693

Prochlorperazine (Versed accentuated by premedication). Products include:
- Compazine 2201

Promethazine Hydrochloride (Versed accentuated by premedication). Products include:
- Mepergan Injection 2479
- Phenergan with Codeine 2497
- Phenergan with Dextromethorphan 2499
- Phenergan Injection 2493
- Phenergan Suppositories 2496
- Phenergan Syrup 2495
- Phenergan Tablets 2496
- Phenergan VC 2500
- Phenergan VC with Codeine 2501

Propofol (Versed accentuated by premedication). Products include:
- Diprivan Injection 2267

Propoxyphene Hydrochloride (Versed accentuated by premedication). Products include:
- Darvon 1256
- Wygesic Tablets 2540

Propoxyphene Napsylate (Versed accentuated by premedication). Products include:
- Darvon-N/Darvocet-N 1254

Quazepam (Versed accentuated by premedication). Products include:
- Doral Tablets 2383

Secobarbital Sodium (Versed accentuated by premedication). Products include:
- Seconal Sodium Pulvules 1296

Sufentanil Citrate (Versed accentuated by premedication). Products include:
- Sufenta Injection 1147

Temazepam (Versed accentuated by premedication). Products include:
- Restoril Capsules 2023

Thiamylal Sodium (Versed accentuated by premedication). Products include:
- Surital Ampoules, Steri-Vials 1764

Thioridazine Hydrochloride (Versed accentuated by premedication). Products include:
- Mellaril 2011

Thiothixene (Versed accentuated by premedication). Products include:
- Navane Capsules and Concentrate 1954
- Navane Intramuscular 1956

Triazolam (Versed accentuated by premedication). Products include:
- Halcion Tablets 2340

Trifluoperazine Hydrochloride (Versed accentuated by premedication). Products include:
- Stelazine 2226

VIBRAMYCIN HYCLATE CAPSULES

(Doxycycline Hyclate) 1787

May interact with oral anticoagulants, penicillins, and antacids containing aluminum, calcium and magnesium. Compounds in these categories include:

Aluminum Carbonate Gel (Concomitant therapy may impair oral absorption of tetracycline). Products include:
- Basaljel 2438

Aluminum Hydroxide (Concomitant therapy may impair oral absorption of tetracycline). Products include:
- Cama Arthritis Pain Reliever .... ■ 685
- Gaviscon Extra Strength Relief Formula Liquid Antacid .... ■ 594
- Gaviscon Extra Strength Relief Formula Antacid Tablets .... ■ 594
- Gaviscon Liquid Antacid .... ■ 594
- Gelusil Liquid & Tablets .... ■ 639
- Extra Strength Maalox Plus Suspension 1850
- Maalox TC Suspension 1851
- Maalox Plus Tablets .... ■ 655
- Extra Strength Maalox Plus Tablets 1850
- Nephrox Suspension .... ■ 563
- WinGel Liquid & Tablets .... ■ 761

Aluminum Hydroxide Gel (Concomitant therapy may impair oral absorption of tetracycline). Products include:
- ALternaGEL Liquid 1154
- Aludrox Oral Suspension 2428
- Amphojel Suspension 2429
- Amphojel Suspension without Flavor 2429
- Mylanta Liquid 1155
- Mylanta Double Strength Liquid 1155

Aluminum Hydroxide Gel, Dried (Concomitant therapy may impair oral absorption of tetracycline). Products include:
- Alu-Tab/Alu-Cap 1309
- Amphojel Tablets 2429
- Ascriptin A/D Caplets 1850
- Regular Strength Ascriptin Tablets 1850
- Gaviscon Antacid Tablets .... ■ 593
- Gaviscon-2 Antacid Tablets .... ■ 594
- Mylanta Tablets 1155
- Mylanta Double Strength Tablets 1155

Amoxicillin (Bacteriostatic drugs may interfere with bactericidal action of penicillin). Products include:
- Amoxil 2193
- Augmentin Tablets, Powder for Oral Suspension, and Chewable Tablets 2198

Ampicillin Sodium (Bacteriostatic drugs may interfere with bactericidal action of penicillin). Products include:
- Unasyn 1965

Azlocillin Sodium (Bacteriostatic drugs may interfere with bactericidal action of penicillin).
- No products indexed under this heading.

Bacampicillin Hydrochloride (Bacteriostatic drugs may interfere with bactericidal action of penicillin). Products include:
- Spectrobid Tablets & Powder for Oral Suspension 1961

Carbenicillin Disodium (Bacteriostatic drugs may interfere with bactericidal action of penicillin).

Carbenicillin Indanyl Sodium (Bacteriostatic drugs may interfere with bactericidal action of penicillin). Products include:
- Geocillin Tablets 1951

Dicumarol (Depressed plasma prothrombin activity; may require downward adjustment of the anticoagulant dosage). Products include:
- Dicumarol Tablets 516

Dihydroxyaluminum Sodium Carbonate (Concomitant therapy may impair oral absorption of tetracycline). Products include:
- Rolaids .... ■ 743

Magaldrate (Concomitant therapy may impair oral absorption of tetracycline). Products include:
- Riopan Antacid Chew Tablets .... ■ 754
- Riopan Antacid Chew Tablets in Rollpacks .... ■ 754
- Riopan Antacid Suspension 2421
- Riopan Antacid Swallow Tablets 2421
- Riopan Plus Chew Tablets 2422
- Riopan Plus Chew Tablets in Rollpack 2422
- Riopan Plus 2 Chew Tablets, Mint Flavor, Cherry Flavor 2422
- Riopan Plus Suspension 2422
- Riopan Plus 2 Suspension, Mint Flavor, Cherry Flavor 2422

Magnesium Hydroxide (Concomitant therapy may impair oral absorption of tetracycline). Products include:
- Aludrox Oral Suspension 2428
- Ascriptin A/D Caplets 1850
- Regular Strength Ascriptin Tablets 1850
- Di-Gel Antacid/Anti-Gas .... ■ 697
- Gelusil Liquid & Tablets .... ■ 639
- Haley's M-O, Regular & Flavored .... ■ 569
- Extra Strength Maalox Plus Suspension 1850
- Maalox TC Suspension 1851
- Maalox Plus Tablets .... ■ 655
- Extra Strength Maalox Plus Tablets 1850
- Mylanta Liquid 1155
- Mylanta Tablets 1155
- Mylanta Double Strength Liquid 1155
- Mylanta Double Strength Tablets 1155
- Concentrated Phillips' Milk of Magnesia .... ■ 573
- Phillips' Milk of Magnesia Liquid .... ■ 572
- Phillips' Milk of Magnesia Tablets .... ■ 573
- WinGel Liquid & Tablets .... ■ 761

Magnesium Oxide (Concomitant therapy may impair oral absorption of tetracycline). Products include:
- Bayer Plus Aspirin Tablets .... ■ 567
- Beelith Tablets 659
- Bufferin Analgesic Tablets and Caplets .... ■ 524
- Cama Arthritis Pain Reliever .... ■ 685
- Mag-Ox 400 673
- Uro-Mag 673

Mezlocillin Sodium (Bacteriostatic drugs may interfere with bactericidal action of penicillin). Products include:
- Mezlin 1597
- Mezlin Pharmacy Bulk Package 1599

Nafcillin Sodium (Bacteriostatic drugs may interfere with bactericidal action of penicillin). Products include:
- Unipen 2533

Penicillin G Potassium (Bacteriostatic drugs may interfere with bactericidal action of penicillin). Products include:
- Pfizerpen for Injection 1957

Penicillin G Procaine (Bacteriostatic drugs may interfere with bactericidal action of penicillin). Products include:
- Bicillin C-R Injection 2438
- Bicillin C-R 900/300 Injection 2440
- Pfizerpen-AS Aqueous Suspension 1959
- Wycillin Injection 2537
- Wycillin Injection and Probenecid Tablets 2539

Penicillin G Sodium (Bacteriostatic drugs may interfere with bactericidal action of penicillin).
- No products indexed under this heading.

Penicillin G, Benzathine (Bacteriostatic drugs may interfere with bactericidal action of penicillin). Products include:
- Bicillin C-R Injection 2438
- Bicillin C-R 900/300 Injection 2440
- Bicillin L-A Injection 2442

Penicillin (Repository) (Bacteriostatic drugs may interfere with bactericidal action of penicillin). Products include:
- Bicillin C-R Injection 2438
- Bicillin C-R 900/300 Injection 2440
- Bicillin L-A Injection 2442

Penicillin V Potassium (Bacteriostatic drugs may interfere with bactericidal action of penicillin).
- No products indexed under this heading.

Ticarcillin Disodium (Bacteriostatic drugs may interfere with bactericidal action of penicillin). Products include:
- Ticar for Injection 2236
- Timentin for Injection 2239

Warfarin Sodium (Depressed plasma prothrombin activity; may require downward adjustment of the anticoagulant dosage). Products include:
- Coumadin Injection & Tablets 944
- Panwarfin Tablets 547

VIBRAMYCIN HYCLATE INTRAVENOUS

(Doxycycline Hyclate) 1968

May interact with anticoagulants and penicillins. Compounds in these categories include:

Amoxicillin (Interference with bactericidal action of penicillin). Products include:
- Amoxil 2193
- Augmentin Tablets, Powder for Oral Suspension, and Chewable Tablets 2198

Ampicillin Sodium (Interference with bactericidal action of penicillin). Products include:
- Unasyn 1965

Azlocillin Sodium (Interference with bactericidal action of penicillin).
- No products indexed under this heading.

Bacampicillin Hydrochloride (Interference with bactericidal action of penicillin). Products include:
- Spectrobid Tablets & Powder for Oral Suspension 1961

Carbenicillin Disodium (Interference with bactericidal action of penicillin).

Carbenicillin Indanyl Sodium (Interference with bactericidal action of penicillin). Products include:
- Geocillin Tablets 1951

Dicumarol (Depressed plasma prothrombin activity; downward adjustment of anticoagulant dosage may be necessary). Products include:
- Dicumarol Tablets 516

Heparin Calcium (Depressed plasma prothrombin activity; downward adjustment of anticoagulant dosage may be necessary). Products include:
- Calciparine Injection 925

Heparin Sodium (Depressed plasma prothrombin activity; downward adjustment of anticoagulant dosage may be necessary). Products include:
Heparin Lock Flush Solution 2456
Heparin Sodium Vials 1264
Heparin Sodium Injection 2457
Heparin Sodium Injection, USP, Sterile Solution 2342

Mezlocillin Sodium (Interference with bactericidal action of penicillin). Products include:
Mezlin 1597
Mezlin Pharmacy Bulk Package 1599

Nafcillin Sodium (Interference with bactericidal action of penicillin). Products include:
Unipen 2533

Penicillin G Potassium (Interference with bactericidal action of penicillin). Products include:
Pfizerpen for Injection 1957

Penicillin G Procaine (Interference with bactericidal action of penicillin). Products include:
Bicillin C-R Injection 2438
Bicillin C-R 900/300 Injection 2440
Pfizerpen-AS Aqueous Suspension 1959
Wycillin Injection 2537
Wycillin Injection and Probenecid Tablets 2539

Penicillin G Sodium (Interference with bactericidal action of penicillin).
No products indexed under this heading.

Penicillin G, Benzathine (Interference with bactericidal action of penicillin). Products include:
Bicillin C-R Injection 2438
Bicillin C-R 900/300 Injection 2440
Bicillin L-A Injection 2442

Penicillin (Repository) (Interference with bactericidal action of penicillin). Products include:
Bicillin C-R Injection 2438
Bicillin C-R 900/300 Injection 2440
Bicillin L-A Injection 2442

Penicillin V Potassium (Interference with bactericidal action of penicillin).
No products indexed under this heading.

Ticarcillin Disodium (Interference with bactericidal action of penicillin). Products include:
Ticar for Injection 2236
Timentin for Injection 2239

Warfarin Sodium (Depressed plasma prothrombin activity; downward adjustment of anticoagulant dosage may be necessary). Products include:
Coumadin Injection & Tablets 944
Panwarfin Tablets 547

VIBRAMYCIN MONOHYDRATE FOR ORAL SUSPENSION
(Doxycycline Monohydrate) 1787
See **Vibramycin Hyclate Capsules**

VIBRA-TABS FILM COATED TABLETS
(Doxycycline Hyclate) 1787
See **Vibramycin Hyclate Capsules**

VICKS CHILDREN'S COUGH SYRUP
(Dextromethorphan Hydrobromide, Guaifenesin) ▣ 660
No interactions described in labeling.

VICKS COUGH SILENCERS COUGH DROPS
(Benzocaine, Dextromethorphan Hydrobromide) ▣ 660
No interactions described in labeling.

VICKS DAYCARE DAYTIME COLD MEDICINE CAPLETS
(Acetaminophen, Dextromethorphan Hydrobromide, Pseudoephedrine Hydrochloride, Guaifenesin) ▣ 660
May interact with antihypertensives and antidepressant drugs. Compounds in these categories include:

Acebutolol Hydrochloride (Effect not specified). Products include:
Sectral Capsules 2520

Amitriptyline Hydrochloride (Effect not specified). Products include:
Elavil 2269
Endep Tablets 1927
Etrafon 2087
Limbitrol 1933
Triavil Tablets 1556

Amoxapine (Effect not specified). Products include:
Asendin Tablets 1196

Atenolol (Effect not specified). Products include:
Tenoretic Tablets 1105
Tenormin Tablets and I.V. Injection 1107

Benazepril Hydrochloride (Effect not specified). Products include:
Lotensin Tablets 872

Betaxolol Hydrochloride (Effect not specified). Products include:
Betoptic Sterile Ophthalmic Solution 569
Betoptic S Sterile Ophthalmic Suspension 570
Kerlone Tablets 2172

Bupropion Hydrochloride (Effect not specified). Products include:
Wellbutrin Tablets 821

Captopril (Effect not specified). Products include:
Capoten 2255
Capozide 2258

Carteolol Hydrochloride (Effect not specified). Products include:
Cartrol Tablets 507

Clonidine (Effect not specified). Products include:
Catapres-TTS 677

Clonidine Hydrochloride (Effect not specified). Products include:
Catapres Tablets 676
Combipres Tablets 678

Deserpidine (Effect not specified). Products include:
Enduronyl 518
Harmonyl Tablets 528
Oreticyl 545

Desipramine Hydrochloride (Effect not specified). Products include:
Norpramin Tablets 1340

Diazoxide (Effect not specified). Products include:
Hyperstat I.V. Injection 2095
Proglycem 649

Doxazosin Mesylate (Effect not specified). Products include:
Cardura Tablets 1941

Doxepin Hydrochloride (Effect not specified). Products include:
Sinequan 1960

Enalapril Maleate (Effect not specified). Products include:
Vaseretic Tablets 1559
Vasotec Tablets 1564

Enalaprilat (Effect not specified). Products include:
Vasotec I.V. 1562

Esmolol Hydrochloride (Effect not specified). Products include:
Brevibloc Injection 942

Felodipine (Effect not specified). Products include:
Plendil Extended-Release Tablets 1526

Fluoxetine Hydrochloride (Effect not specified). Products include:
Prozac Pulvules 920

Fosinopril Sodium (Effect not specified). Products include:
Monopril Tablets 1406

Guanabenz Acetate (Effect not specified). Products include:
Wytensin Tablets 2542

Guanethidine Monosulfate (Effect not specified). Products include:
Esimil Tablets 864
Ismelin Tablets 869

Hydralazine Hydrochloride (Effect not specified). Products include:
Apresazide Capsules 854
Apresoline Hydrochloride Parenteral (Ampuls) 856
Apresoline Hydrochloride Tablets 855
Apresoline-Esidrix Tablets 857
Ser-Ap-Es Tablets 881
Serpasil-Apresoline Tablets 884

Imipramine Hydrochloride (Effect not specified). Products include:
Tofranil Ampuls 1038
Tofranil Tablets 1039

Imipramine Pamoate (Effect not specified). Products include:
Tofranil-PM Capsules 1041

Indapamide (Effect not specified). Products include:
Lozol Tablets 1843

Isocarboxazid (Effect not specified). Products include:
Marplan Tablets 1906

Isradipine (Effect not specified). Products include:
DynaCirc Capsules 2004

Labetalol Hydrochloride (Effect not specified). Products include:
Normodyne Injection 2108
Normodyne Tablets 2110
Normozide Tablets 2112
Trandate HCT Tablets 579
Trandate Injection 577
Trandate Tablets 579

Lisinopril (Effect not specified). Products include:
Prinivil Tablets 1538
Prinzide Tablets 1540
Zestoretic 2274
Zestril Tablets 2277

Maprotiline Hydrochloride (Effect not specified). Products include:
Ludiomil Tablets 874

Mecamylamine Hydrochloride (Effect not specified). Products include:
Inversine Tablets 1492

Methyldopa (Effect not specified). Products include:
Aldoclor Tablets 1413
Aldomet Oral 1415
Aldoril Tablets 1418

Methyldopate Hydrochloride (Effect not specified). Products include:
Aldomet Ester HCl Injection 1417

Metoprolol Tartrate (Effect not specified). Products include:
Lopressor Ampuls 1032
Lopressor HCT Tablets 1034
Lopressor Tablets 1032

Metyrosine (Effect not specified). Products include:
Demser Capsules 1460

Minoxidil (Effect not specified). Products include:
Loniten Tablets 2346
Rogaine Topical Solution 2357

Nadolol (Effect not specified). Products include:
Corgard Tablets 701
Corzide Tablets 702

Nicardipine Hydrochloride (Effect not specified). Products include:
Cardene Capsules 2290

Nitroglycerin (Effect not specified). Products include:
Deponit NTG Transdermal Delivery System 2143
Minitran Transdermal Delivery System 1312
Nitro-Bid Ointment 1339
Nitro-Bid Capsules 1338
Nitrodisc 2176
Nitro-Dur (nitroglycerin) Transdermal Infusion System 1164
Nitrogard Tablets 1004
Nitrolingual Spray 1846
Nitrostat Tablets 1743
Transderm-Nitro Transdermal Therapeutic System 2283

Nortriptyline Hydrochloride (Effect not specified). Products include:
Pamelor 2019

Penbutolol Sulfate (Effect not specified). Products include:
Levatol 1832

Phenelzine Sulfate (Effect not specified). Products include:
Nardil 1742

Phenoxybenzamine Hydrochloride (Effect not specified). Products include:
Dibenzyline Capsules 2207

Phentolamine Mesylate (Effect not specified). Products include:
Regitine 878

Pindolol (Effect not specified). Products include:
Visken Tablets 2036

Prazosin Hydrochloride (Effect not specified). Products include:
Minipress Capsules 1778
Minizide Capsules 1779

Propranolol Hydrochloride (Effect not specified). Products include:
Inderal 2459
Inderal LA Long Acting Capsules 2461
Inderide Tablets 2463
Inderide LA Long Acting Capsules 2465

Protriptyline Hydrochloride (Effect not specified). Products include:
Vivactil Tablets 1567

Ramipril (Effect not specified). Products include:
Altace Capsules 1086

Rauwolfia Serpentina (Effect not specified). Products include:
Raudixin Tablets 1803
Rauzide Tablets 1804

Rescinnamine (Effect not specified).
No products indexed under this heading.

Reserpine (Effect not specified). Products include:
Diupres Tablets 1461
Hydromox R Tablets 1209
Hydropres Tablets 1485
Renese-R Tablets 1786
Salutensin/Salutensin-Demi 719
Ser-Ap-Es Tablets 881
Serpasil Tablets 883
Serpasil-Apresoline Tablets 884
Serpasil-Esidrix Tablets 886

Sodium Nitroprusside (Effect not specified). Products include:
Nipride I.V. Infusion 1909

Terazosin Hydrochloride (Effect not specified). Products include:
Hytrin Tablets 529

Timolol Maleate (Effect not specified). Products include:
Blocadren Tablets 1429
Timolide Tablets 1547
Timoptic in Ocudose 1552
Timoptic Sterile Ophthalmic Solution 1550

Tranylcypromine Sulfate (Effect not specified). Products include:
Parnate Tablets 2222

Trazodone Hydrochloride (Effect not specified). Products include:
- Desyrel and Desyrel Dividose 1404

Trimethaphan Camsylate (Effect not specified). Products include:
- Arfonad Ampuls 1887

Trimipramine Maleate (Effect not specified). Products include:
- Surmontil Capsules 2524

VICKS DAYCARE DAYTIME COLD MEDICINE LIQUID
(Acetaminophen, Dextromethorphan Hydrobromide, Pseudoephedrine Hydrochloride, Guaifenesin) .... ▣ 660
See **Vicks Daycare Daytime Cold Medicine Caplets**

VICKS FORMULA 44 COUGH CONTROL DISCS
(Benzocaine, Dextromethorphan Hydrobromide) .... ▣ 661
No interactions described in labeling.

VICKS FORMULA 44 COUGH MEDICINE
(Chlorpheniramine Maleate, Dextromethorphan Hydrobromide) ▣ 661
May interact with hypnotics and sedatives, tranquilizers, and certain other agents. Compounds in these categories include:

Alcohol (May increase drowsiness effect).

Alprazolam (Effect not specified). Products include:
- Xanax Tablets 2367

Buspirone Hydrochloride (Effect not specified). Products include:
- BuSpar 1401

Chlordiazepoxide (Effect not specified). Products include:
- Libritabs Tablets 1930
- Limbitrol 1933
- Menrium Tablets 1934

Chlordiazepoxide Hydrochloride (Effect not specified). Products include:
- Librax Capsules 1929
- Librium Capsules 1931
- Librium Injectable 1932

Chlorpromazine (Effect not specified). Products include:
- Thorazine 2234

Chlorprothixene (Effect not specified). Products include:
- Taractan Tablets 1920

Chlorprothixene Hydrochloride (Effect not specified). Products include:
- Taractan 1920

Clorazepate Dipotassium (Effect not specified). Products include:
- Tranxene 556

Diazepam (Effect not specified). Products include:
- Valium Injectable 1937
- Valium Tablets 1939
- Valrelease Capsules 1923

Droperidol (Effect not specified). Products include:
- Inapsine Injection 1140
- Innovar Injection 1141

Estazolam (Effect not specified). Products include:
- ProSom Tablets 554

Ethchlorvynol (Effect not specified). Products include:
- Placidyl Capsules 553

Ethinamate (Effect not specified).
No products indexed under this heading.

Fluphenazine Decanoate (Effect not specified). Products include:
- Prolixin Decanoate 1795

Fluphenazine Enanthate (Effect not specified). Products include:
- Prolixin Enanthate 1796

Fluphenazine Hydrochloride (Effect not specified). Products include:
- Prolixin Elixir 1793
- Prolixin Injection 1791
- Prolixin Oral Concentrate 1792
- Prolixin Tablets 1793

Flurazepam Hydrochloride (Effect not specified). Products include:
- Dalmane Capsules 1927

Glutethimide (Effect not specified).
No products indexed under this heading.

Haloperidol (Effect not specified). Products include:
- Haldol Injection, Tablets and Concentrate 1373

Haloperidol Decanoate (Effect not specified). Products include:
- Haldol Decanoate 1375

Hydroxyzine Hydrochloride (Effect not specified). Products include:
- Atarax Tablets & Syrup 1941
- Marax Tablets & DF Syrup 1954
- Vistaril Intramuscular Solution 1970

Lorazepam (Effect not specified). Products include:
- Ativan Injection 2432
- Ativan Tablets 2434

Loxapine Hydrochloride (Effect not specified). Products include:
- Loxitane 1213

Loxapine Succinate (Effect not specified). Products include:
- Loxitane Capsules 1213

Meprobamate (Effect not specified). Products include:
- Deprol Tablets 2382
- Equagesic Tablets 2451
- Miltown Tablets 2386
- PMB 200 and PMB 400 2504

Mesoridazine Besylate (Effect not specified).

Midazolam Hydrochloride (Effect not specified). Products include:
- Versed Injection 1924

Molindone Hydrochloride (Effect not specified). Products include:
- Moban Tablets & Concentrate 932

Oxazepam (Effect not specified). Products include:
- Serax Capsules 2522
- Serax Tablets 2522

Perphenazine (Effect not specified). Products include:
- Etrafon 2087
- Triavil Tablets 1556
- Trilafon 2123

Prazepam (Effect not specified). Products include:
- Centrax 1693

Prochlorperazine (Effect not specified). Products include:
- Compazine 2201

Promethazine Hydrochloride (Effect not specified). Products include:
- Mepergan Injection 2479
- Phenergan with Codeine 2497
- Phenergan with Dextromethorphan 2499
- Phenergan Injection 2493
- Phenergan Suppositories 2496
- Phenergan Syrup 2495
- Phenergan Tablets 2496
- Phenergan VC 2500
- Phenergan VC with Codeine 2501

Propofol (Effect not specified). Products include:
- Diprivan Injection 2267

Quazepam (Effect not specified). Products include:
- Doral Tablets 2383

Secobarbital Sodium (Effect not specified). Products include:
- Seconal Sodium Pulvules 1296

Temazepam (Effect not specified). Products include:
- Restoril Capsules 2023

Thioridazine Hydrochloride (Effect not specified). Products include:
- Mellaril 2011

Thiothixene (Effect not specified). Products include:
- Navane Capsules and Concentrate 1954
- Navane Intramuscular 1956

Triazolam (Effect not specified). Products include:
- Halcion Tablets 2340

Trifluoperazine Hydrochloride (Effect not specified). Products include:
- Stelazine 2226

VICKS FORMULA 44D DECONGESTANT COUGH MEDICINE
(Dextromethorphan Hydrobromide, Guaifenesin, Pseudoephedrine Hydrochloride) .... ▣ 662
May interact with antihypertensives and antidepressant drugs. Compounds in these categories include:

Acebutolol Hydrochloride (Concurrent use not recommended). Products include:
- Sectral Capsules 2520

Amitriptyline Hydrochloride (Concurrent use not recommended). Products include:
- Elavil 2269
- Endep Tablets 1927
- Etrafon 2087
- Limbitrol 1933
- Triavil Tablets 1556

Amoxapine (Concurrent use not recommended). Products include:
- Asendin Tablets 1196

Atenolol (Concurrent use not recommended). Products include:
- Tenoretic Tablets 1105
- Tenormin Tablets and I.V. Injection 1107

Benazepril Hydrochloride (Concurrent use not recommended). Products include:
- Lotensin Tablets 872

Betaxolol Hydrochloride (Concurrent use not recommended). Products include:
- Betoptic Sterile Ophthalmic Solution .... ⊙ 569
- Betoptic S Sterile Ophthalmic Suspension .... ⊙ 570
- Kerlone Tablets 2172

Bupropion Hydrochloride (Concurrent use not recommended). Products include:
- Wellbutrin Tablets 821

Captopril (Concurrent use not recommended). Products include:
- Capoten 2255
- Capozide 2258

Carteolol Hydrochloride (Concurrent use not recommended). Products include:
- Cartrol Tablets 507

Clonidine (Concurrent use not recommended). Products include:
- Catapres-TTS 677

Clonidine Hydrochloride (Concurrent use not recommended). Products include:
- Catapres Tablets 676
- Combipres Tablets 678

Deserpidine (Concurrent use not recommended). Products include:
- Enduronyl 518
- Harmonyl Tablets 528
- Oreticyl 545

Desipramine Hydrochloride (Concurrent use not recommended). Products include:
- Norpramin Tablets 1340

Diazoxide (Concurrent use not recommended). Products include:
- Hyperstat I.V. Injection 2095
- Proglycem 649

Doxazosin Mesylate (Concurrent use not recommended). Products include:
- Cardura Tablets 1941

Doxepin Hydrochloride (Concurrent use not recommended). Products include:
- Sinequan 1960

Enalapril Maleate (Concurrent use not recommended). Products include:
- Vaseretic Tablets 1559
- Vasotec Tablets 1564

Enalaprilat (Concurrent use not recommended). Products include:
- Vasotec I.V. 1562

Esmolol Hydrochloride (Concurrent use not recommended). Products include:
- Brevibloc Injection 942

Felodipine (Concurrent use not recommended). Products include:
- Plendil Extended-Release Tablets 1526

Fluoxetine Hydrochloride (Concurrent use not recommended). Products include:
- Prozac Pulvules 920

Fosinopril Sodium (Concurrent use not recommended). Products include:
- Monopril Tablets 1406

Guanabenz Acetate (Concurrent use not recommended). Products include:
- Wytensin Tablets 2542

Guanethidine Monosulfate (Concurrent use not recommended). Products include:
- Esimil Tablets 864
- Ismelin Tablets 869

Hydralazine Hydrochloride (Concurrent use not recommended). Products include:
- Apresazide Capsules 854
- Apresoline Hydrochloride Parenteral (Ampuls) 856
- Apresoline Hydrochloride Tablets .. 855
- Apresoline-Esidrix Tablets 857
- Ser-Ap-Es Tablets 881
- Serpasil-Apresoline Tablets 884

Imipramine Hydrochloride (Concurrent use not recommended). Products include:
- Tofranil Ampuls 1038
- Tofranil Tablets 1039

Imipramine Pamoate (Concurrent use not recommended). Products include:
- Tofranil-PM Capsules 1041

Indapamide (Concurrent use not recommended). Products include:
- Lozol Tablets 1843

Isocarboxazid (Concurrent use not recommended). Products include:
- Marplan Tablets 1906

Isradipine (Concurrent use not recommended). Products include:
- DynaCirc Capsules 2004

Labetalol Hydrochloride (Concurrent use not recommended). Products include:
- Normodyne Injection 2108
- Normodyne Tablets 2110
- Normozide Tablets 2112
- Trandate HCT Tablets 579
- Trandate Injection 577
- Trandate Tablets 579

Lisinopril (Concurrent use not recommended). Products include:
- Prinivil Tablets 1538

Prinzide Tablets 1540
Zestoretic 2274
Zestril Tablets 2277

Maprotiline Hydrochloride (Concurrent use not recommended). Products include:
Ludiomil Tablets 874

Mecamylamine Hydrochloride (Concurrent use not recommended). Products include:
Inversine Tablets 1492

Methyldopa (Concurrent use not recommended). Products include:
Aldoclor Tablets 1413
Aldomet Oral 1415
Aldoril Tablets 1418

Methyldopate Hydrochloride (Concurrent use not recommended). Products include:
Aldomet Ester HCl Injection 1417

Metoprolol Tartrate (Concurrent use not recommended). Products include:
Lopressor Ampuls 1032
Lopressor HCT Tablets 1034
Lopressor Tablets 1032

Metyrosine (Concurrent use not recommended). Products include:
Demser Capsules 1460

Minoxidil (Concurrent use not recommended). Products include:
Loniten Tablets 2346
Rogaine Topical Solution 2357

Nadolol (Concurrent use not recommended). Products include:
Corgard Tablets 701
Corzide Tablets 702

Nicardipine Hydrochloride (Concurrent use not recommended). Products include:
Cardene Capsules 2290

Nitroglycerin (Concurrent use not recommended). Products include:
Deponit NTG Transdermal Delivery System 2143
Minitran Transdermal Delivery System 1312
Nitro-Bid Ointment 1339
Nitro-Bid Capsules 1338
Nitrodisc 2176
Nitro-Dur (nitroglycerin) Transdermal Infusion System 1164
Nitrogard Tablets 1004
Nitrolingual Spray 1846
Nitrostat Tablets 1743
Transderm-Nitro Transdermal Therapeutic System 2283

Nortriptyline Hydrochloride (Concurrent use not recommended). Products include:
Pamelor 2019

Penbutolol Sulfate (Concurrent use not recommended). Products include:
Levatol 1832

Phenelzine Sulfate (Concurrent use not recommended). Products include:
Nardil 1742

Phenoxybenzamine Hydrochloride (Concurrent use not recommended). Products include:
Dibenzyline Capsules 2207

Phentolamine Mesylate (Concurrent use not recommended). Products include:
Regitine 878

Pindolol (Concurrent use not recommended). Products include:
Visken Tablets 2036

Prazosin Hydrochloride (Concurrent use not recommended). Products include:
Minipress Capsules 1778
Minizide Capsules 1779

Propranolol Hydrochloride (Concurrent use not recommended). Products include:
Inderal 2459
Inderal LA Long Acting Capsules 2461
Inderide Tablets 2463
Inderide LA Long Acting Capsules 2465

Protriptyline Hydrochloride (Concurrent use not recommended). Products include:
Vivactil Tablets 1567

Ramipril (Concurrent use not recommended). Products include:
Altace Capsules 1086

Rauwolfia Serpentina (Concurrent use not recommended). Products include:
Raudixin Tablets 1803
Rauzide Tablets 1804

Rescinnamine (Concurrent use not recommended).
No products indexed under this heading.

Reserpine (Concurrent use not recommended). Products include:
Diupres Tablets 1461
Hydromox R Tablets 1209
Hydropres Tablets 1485
Renese-R Tablets 1786
Salutensin/Salutensin-Demi 719
Ser-Ap-Es Tablets 881
Serpasil Tablets 883
Serpasil-Apresoline Tablets 884
Serpasil-Esidrix Tablets 886

Sodium Nitroprusside (Concurrent use not recommended). Products include:
Nipride I.V. Infusion 1909

Terazosin Hydrochloride (Concurrent use not recommended). Products include:
Hytrin Tablets 529

Timolol Maleate (Concurrent use not recommended). Products include:
Blocadren Tablets 1429
Timolide Tablets 1547
Timoptic in Ocudose 1552
Timoptic Sterile Ophthalmic Solution 1550

Tranylcypromine Sulfate (Concurrent use not recommended). Products include:
Parnate Tablets 2222

Trazodone Hydrochloride (Concurrent use not recommended). Products include:
Desyrel and Desyrel Dividose 1404

Trimethaphan Camsylate (Concurrent use not recommended). Products include:
Arfonad Ampuls 1887

Trimipramine Maleate (Concurrent use not recommended). Products include:
Surmontil Capsules 2524

VICKS FORMULA 44M MULTI-SYMPTOM COUGH MEDICINE
(Acetaminophen, Dextromethorphan Hydrobromide, Chlorpheniramine Maleate, Pseudoephedrine Hydrochloride) 662
May interact with antihypertensives, antidepressant drugs, hypnotics and sedatives, tranquilizers, and certain other agents. Compounds in these categories include:

Acebutolol Hydrochloride (Concurrent use not recommended). Products include:
Sectral Capsules 2520

Alcohol (Increases the drowsiness effect).

Alprazolam (Increases the drowsiness effect). Products include:
Xanax Tablets 2367

Amitriptyline Hydrochloride (Concurrent use not recommended). Products include:
Elavil 2269
Endep Tablets 1927
Etrafon 2087
Limbitrol 1933
Triavil Tablets 1556

Amoxapine (Concurrent use not recommended). Products include:
Asendin Tablets 1196

Atenolol (Concurrent use not recommended). Products include:
Tenoretic Tablets 1105
Tenormin Tablets and I.V. Injection 1107

Benazepril Hydrochloride (Concurrent use not recommended). Products include:
Lotensin Tablets 872

Betaxolol Hydrochloride (Concurrent use not recommended). Products include:
Betoptic Sterile Ophthalmic Solution 569
Betoptic S Sterile Ophthalmic Suspension 570
Kerlone Tablets 2172

Bupropion Hydrochloride (Concurrent use not recommended). Products include:
Wellbutrin Tablets 821

Buspirone Hydrochloride (Increases the drowsiness effect). Products include:
BuSpar 1401

Captopril (Concurrent use not recommended). Products include:
Capoten 2255
Capozide 2258

Carteolol Hydrochloride (Concurrent use not recommended). Products include:
Cartrol Tablets 507

Chlordiazepoxide (Increases the drowsiness effect). Products include:
Libritabs Tablets 1930
Limbitrol 1933
Menrium Tablets 1934

Chlordiazepoxide Hydrochloride (Increases the drowsiness effect). Products include:
Librax Capsules 1929
Librium Capsules 1931
Librium Injectable 1932

Chlorpromazine (Increases the drowsiness effect). Products include:
Thorazine 2234

Chlorprothixene (Increases the drowsiness effect). Products include:
Taractan Tablets 1920

Chlorprothixene Hydrochloride (Increases the drowsiness effect). Products include:
Taractan 1920

Clonidine (Concurrent use not recommended). Products include:
Catapres-TTS 677

Clonidine Hydrochloride (Concurrent use not recommended). Products include:
Catapres Tablets 676
Combipres Tablets 678

Clorazepate Dipotassium (Increases the drowsiness effect). Products include:
Tranxene 556

Deserpidine (Concurrent use not recommended). Products include:
Enduronyl 518
Harmonyl Tablets 528
Oreticyl 545

Desipramine Hydrochloride (Concurrent use not recommended). Products include:
Norpramin Tablets 1340

Diazepam (Increases the drowsiness effect). Products include:
Valium Injectable 1937
Valium Tablets 1939
Valrelease Capsules 1923

Diazoxide (Concurrent use not recommended). Products include:
Hyperstat I.V. Injection 2095
Proglycem 649

Doxazosin Mesylate (Concurrent use not recommended). Products include:
Cardura Tablets 1941

Doxepin Hydrochloride (Concurrent use not recommended). Products include:
Sinequan 1960

Droperidol (Increases the drowsiness effect). Products include:
Inapsine Injection 1140
Innovar Injection 1141

Enalapril Maleate (Concurrent use not recommended). Products include:
Vaseretic Tablets 1559
Vasotec Tablets 1564

Enalaprilat (Concurrent use not recommended). Products include:
Vasotec I.V. 1562

Esmolol Hydrochloride (Concurrent use not recommended). Products include:
Brevibloc Injection 942

Estazolam (Increases the drowsiness effect). Products include:
ProSom Tablets 554

Ethchlorvynol (Increases the drowsiness effect). Products include:
Placidyl Capsules 553

Ethinamate (Increases the drowsiness effect).
No products indexed under this heading.

Felodipine (Concurrent use not recommended). Products include:
Plendil Extended-Release Tablets 1526

Fluoxetine Hydrochloride (Concurrent use not recommended). Products include:
Prozac Pulvules 920

Fluphenazine Decanoate (Increases the drowsiness effect). Products include:
Prolixin Decanoate 1795

Fluphenazine Enanthate (Increases the drowsiness effect). Products include:
Prolixin Enanthate 1796

Fluphenazine Hydrochloride (Increases the drowsiness effect). Products include:
Prolixin Elixir 1793
Prolixin Injection 1791
Prolixin Oral Concentrate 1792
Prolixin Tablets 1793

Flurazepam Hydrochloride (Increases the drowsiness effect). Products include:
Dalmane Capsules 1927

Fosinopril Sodium (Concurrent use not recommended). Products include:
Monopril Tablets 1406

Glutethimide (Increases the drowsiness effect).
No products indexed under this heading.

Guanabenz Acetate (Concurrent use not recommended). Products include:
Wytensin Tablets 2542

Guanethidine Monosulfate (Concurrent use not recommended). Products include:
Esimil Tablets 864
Ismelin Tablets 869

Haloperidol (Increases the drowsiness effect). Products include:
Haldol Injection, Tablets and Concentrate 1373

Haloperidol Decanoate (Increases the drowsiness effect). Products include:
Haldol Decanoate 1375

Hydralazine Hydrochloride (Concurrent use not recommended). Products include:
- Apresazide Capsules 854
- Apresoline Hydrochloride Parenteral (Ampuls) 856
- Apresoline Hydrochloride Tablets .. 855
- Apresoline-Esidrix Tablets 857
- Ser-Ap-Es Tablets 881
- Serpasil-Apresoline Tablets 884

Hydroxyzine Hydrochloride (Increases the drowsiness effect). Products include:
- Atarax Tablets & Syrup 1941
- Marax Tablets & DF Syrup 1954
- Vistaril Intramuscular Solution 1970

Imipramine Hydrochloride (Concurrent use not recommended). Products include:
- Tofranil Ampuls 1038
- Tofranil Tablets 1039

Imipramine Pamoate (Concurrent use not recommended). Products include:
- Tofranil-PM Capsules 1041

Indapamide (Concurrent use not recommended). Products include:
- Lozol Tablets 1843

Isocarboxazid (Concurrent use not recommended). Products include:
- Marplan Tablets 1906

Isradipine (Concurrent use not recommended). Products include:
- DynaCirc Capsules 2004

Labetalol Hydrochloride (Concurrent use not recommended). Products include:
- Normodyne Injection 2108
- Normodyne Tablets 2110
- Normozide Tablets 2112
- Trandate HCT Tablets 579
- Trandate Injection 577
- Trandate Tablets 579

Lisinopril (Concurrent use not recommended). Products include:
- Prinivil Tablets 1538
- Prinzide Tablets 1540
- Zestoretic 2274
- Zestril Tablets 2277

Lorazepam (Increases the drowsiness effect). Products include:
- Ativan Injection 2432
- Ativan Tablets 2434

Loxapine Hydrochloride (Increases the drowsiness effect). Products include:
- Loxitane 1213

Loxapine Succinate (Increases the drowsiness effect). Products include:
- Loxitane Capsules 1213

Maprotiline Hydrochloride (Concurrent use not recommended). Products include:
- Ludiomil Tablets 874

Mecamylamine Hydrochloride (Concurrent use not recommended). Products include:
- Inversine Tablets 1492

Meprobamate (Increases the drowsiness effect). Products include:
- Deprol Tablets 2382
- Equagesic Tablets 2451
- Miltown Tablets 2386
- PMB 200 and PMB 400 2504

Mesoridazine (Concurrent use not recommended). Products include:
- Serentil 686

Methyldopa (Concurrent use not recommended). Products include:
- Aldoclor Tablets 1413
- Aldomet Oral 1415
- Aldoril Tablets 1418

Methyldopate Hydrochloride (Concurrent use not recommended). Products include:
- Aldomet Ester HCl Injection 1417

Metoprolol Tartrate (Concurrent use not recommended). Products include:
- Lopressor Ampuls 1032
- Lopressor HCT Tablets 1034
- Lopressor Tablets 1032

Metyrosine (Concurrent use not recommended). Products include:
- Demser Capsules 1460

Midazolam Hydrochloride (Increases the drowsiness effect). Products include:
- Versed Injection 1924

Minoxidil (Concurrent use not recommended). Products include:
- Loniten Tablets 2346
- Rogaine Topical Solution 2357

Molindone Hydrochloride (Increases the drowsiness effect). Products include:
- Moban Tablets & Concentrate 932

Nadolol (Concurrent use not recommended). Products include:
- Corgard Tablets 701
- Corzide Tablets 702

Nicardipine Hydrochloride (Concurrent use not recommended). Products include:
- Cardene Capsules 2290

Nitroglycerin (Concurrent use not recommended). Products include:
- Deponit NTG Transdermal Delivery System 2143
- Minitran Transdermal Delivery System 1312
- Nitro-Bid Ointment 1339
- Nitro-Bid Capsules 1338
- Nitrodisc 2176
- Nitro-Dur (nitroglycerin) Transdermal Infusion System 1164
- Nitrogard Tablets 1004
- Nitrolingual Spray 1846
- Nitrostat Tablets 1743
- Transderm-Nitro Transdermal Therapeutic System 2283

Nortriptyline Hydrochloride (Concurrent use not recommended). Products include:
- Pamelor 2019

Oxazepam (Increases the drowsiness effect). Products include:
- Serax Capsules 2522
- Serax Tablets 2522

Penbutolol Sulfate (Concurrent use not recommended). Products include:
- Levatol 1832

Perphenazine (Increases the drowsiness effect). Products include:
- Etrafon 2087
- Triavil Tablets 1556
- Trilafon 2123

Phenelzine Sulfate (Concurrent use not recommended). Products include:
- Nardil 1742

Phenoxybenzamine Hydrochloride (Concurrent use not recommended). Products include:
- Dibenzyline Capsules 2207

Phentolamine Mesylate (Concurrent use not recommended). Products include:
- Regitine 878

Pindolol (Concurrent use not recommended). Products include:
- Visken Tablets 2036

Prazepam (Increases the drowsiness effect). Products include:
- Centrax 1693

Prazosin Hydrochloride (Concurrent use not recommended). Products include:
- Minipress Capsules 1778
- Minizide Capsules 1779

Prochlorperazine (Increases the drowsiness effect). Products include:
- Compazine 2201

Promethazine Hydrochloride (Increases the drowsiness effect). Products include:
- Mepergan Injection 2479
- Phenergan with Codeine 2497
- Phenergan with Dextromethorphan 2499
- Phenergan Injection 2493
- Phenergan Suppositories 2496
- Phenergan Syrup 2495
- Phenergan Tablets 2496
- Phenergan VC 2500
- Phenergan VC with Codeine 2501

Propofol (Increases the drowsiness effect). Products include:
- Diprivan Injection 2267

Propranolol Hydrochloride (Concurrent use not recommended). Products include:
- Inderal 2459
- Inderal LA Long Acting Capsules 2461
- Inderide Tablets 2463
- Inderide LA Long Acting Capsules .. 2465

Protriptyline Hydrochloride (Concurrent use not recommended). Products include:
- Vivactil Tablets 1567

Quazepam (Increases the drowsiness effect). Products include:
- Doral Tablets 2383

Ramipril (Concurrent use not recommended). Products include:
- Altace Capsules 1086

Rauwolfia Serpentina (Concurrent use not recommended). Products include:
- Raudixin Tablets 1803
- Rauzide Tablets 1804

Rescinnamine (Concurrent use not recommended).
- No products indexed under this heading.

Reserpine (Concurrent use not recommended). Products include:
- Diupres Tablets 1461
- Hydromox R Tablets 1209
- Hydropres Tablets 1485
- Renese-R Tablets 1786
- Salutensin/Salutensin-Demi 719
- Ser-Ap-Es Tablets 881
- Serpasil Tablets 883
- Serpasil-Apresoline Tablets 884
- Serpasil-Esidrix Tablets 886

Secobarbital Sodium (Increases the drowsiness effect). Products include:
- Seconal Sodium Pulvules 1296

Sodium Nitroprusside (Concurrent use not recommended). Products include:
- Nipride I.V. Infusion 1909

Temazepam (Increases the drowsiness effect). Products include:
- Restoril Capsules 2023

Terazosin Hydrochloride (Concurrent use not recommended). Products include:
- Hytrin Tablets 529

Thioridazine Hydrochloride (Increases the drowsiness effect). Products include:
- Mellaril 2011

Thiothixene (Increases the drowsiness effect). Products include:
- Navane Capsules and Concentrate 1954
- Navane Intramuscular 1956

Timolol Maleate (Concurrent use not recommended). Products include:
- Blocadren Tablets 1429
- Timolide Tablets 1547
- Timoptic in Ocudose 1552
- Timoptic Sterile Ophthalmic Solution 1550

Tranylcypromine Sulfate (Concurrent use not recommended). Products include:
- Parnate Tablets 2222

Trazodone Hydrochloride (Concurrent use not recommended). Products include:
- Desyrel and Desyrel Dividose 1404

Triazolam (Increases the drowsiness effect). Products include:
- Halcion Tablets 2340

Trifluoperazine Hydrochloride (Increases the drowsiness effect). Products include:
- Stelazine 2226

Trimethaphan Camsylate (Concurrent use not recommended). Products include:
- Arfonad Ampuls 1887

Trimipramine Maleate (Concurrent use not recommended). Products include:
- Surmontil Capsules 2524

VICKS INHALER

(Camphor, Desoxyephedrine-Levo, Menthol) .... ■ 664

No interactions described in labeling.

VICKS NYQUIL NIGHTTIME COLD MEDICINE-ORIGINAL & CHERRY FLAVOR

(Acetaminophen, Dextromethorphan Hydrobromide, Doxylamine Succinate, Pseudoephedrine Hydrochloride) .... ■ 664

May interact with antihypertensives, antidepressant drugs, hypnotics and sedatives, tranquilizers, and certain other agents. Compounds in these categories include:

Acebutolol Hydrochloride (Concurrent use not recommended). Products include:
- Sectral Capsules 2520

Alcohol (Do not use concomitantly).

Alprazolam (Concurrent use not recommended). Products include:
- Xanax Tablets 2367

Amitriptyline Hydrochloride (Concurrent use not recommended). Products include:
- Elavil 2269
- Endep Tablets 1927
- Etrafon 2087
- Limbitrol 1933
- Triavil Tablets 1556

Amoxapine (Concurrent use not recommended). Products include:
- Asendin Tablets 1196

Atenolol (Concurrent use not recommended). Products include:
- Tenoretic Tablets 1105
- Tenormin Tablets and I.V. Injection 1107

Benazepril Hydrochloride (Concurrent use not recommended). Products include:
- Lotensin Tablets 872

Betaxolol Hydrochloride (Concurrent use not recommended). Products include:
- Betoptic Sterile Ophthalmic Solution 569
- Betoptic S Sterile Ophthalmic Suspension 570
- Kerlone Tablets 2172

Bupropion Hydrochloride (Concurrent use not recommended). Products include:
- Wellbutrin Tablets 821

Buspirone Hydrochloride (Concurrent use not recommended). Products include:
- BuSpar 1401

Captopril (Concurrent use not recommended). Products include:
- Capoten 2255
- Capozide 2258

Carteolol Hydrochloride (Concurrent use not recommended). Products include:
Cartrol Tablets ... 507

Chlordiazepoxide (Concurrent use not recommended). Products include:
Libritabs Tablets ... 1930
Limbitrol ... 1933
Menrium Tablets ... 1934

Chlordiazepoxide Hydrochloride (Concurrent use not recommended). Products include:
Librax Capsules ... 1929
Librium Capsules ... 1931
Librium Injectable ... 1932

Chlorpromazine (Concurrent use not recommended). Products include:
Thorazine ... 2234

Chlorprothixene (Concurrent use not recommended). Products include:
Taractan Tablets ... 1920

Chlorprothixene Hydrochloride (Concurrent use not recommended). Products include:
Taractan ... 1920

Clonidine (Concurrent use not recommended). Products include:
Catapres-TTS ... 677

Clonidine Hydrochloride (Concurrent use not recommended). Products include:
Catapres Tablets ... 676
Combipres Tablets ... 678

Clorazepate Dipotassium (Concurrent use not recommended). Products include:
Tranxene ... 556

Deserpidine (Concurrent use not recommended). Products include:
Enduronyl ... 518
Harmonyl Tablets ... 528
Oreticyl ... 545

Desipramine Hydrochloride (Concurrent use not recommended). Products include:
Norpramin Tablets ... 1340

Diazepam (Concurrent use not recommended). Products include:
Valium Injectable ... 1937
Valium Tablets ... 1939
Valrelease Capsules ... 1923

Diazoxide (Concurrent use not recommended). Products include:
Hyperstat I.V. Injection ... 2095
Proglycem ... 649

Doxazosin Mesylate (Concurrent use not recommended). Products include:
Cardura Tablets ... 1941

Doxepin Hydrochloride (Concurrent use not recommended). Products include:
Sinequan ... 1960

Droperidol (Concurrent use not recommended). Products include:
Inapsine Injection ... 1140
Innovar Injection ... 1141

Enalapril Maleate (Concurrent use not recommended). Products include:
Vaseretic Tablets ... 1559
Vasotec Tablets ... 1564

Enalaprilat (Concurrent use not recommended). Products include:
Vasotec I.V. ... 1562

Esmolol Hydrochloride (Concurrent use not recommended). Products include:
Brevibloc Injection ... 942

Estazolam (Concurrent use not recommended). Products include:
ProSom Tablets ... 554

Ethchlorvynol (Concurrent use not recommended). Products include:
Placidyl Capsules ... 553

Ethinamate (Concurrent use not recommended).
No products indexed under this heading.

Felodipine (Concurrent use not recommended). Products include:
Plendil Extended-Release Tablets ... 1526

Fluoxetine Hydrochloride (Concurrent use not recommended). Products include:
Prozac Pulvules ... 920

Fluphenazine Decanoate (Concurrent use not recommended). Products include:
Prolixin Decanoate ... 1795

Fluphenazine Enanthate (Concurrent use not recommended). Products include:
Prolixin Enanthate ... 1796

Fluphenazine Hydrochloride (Concurrent use not recommended). Products include:
Prolixin Elixir ... 1793
Prolixin Injection ... 1791
Prolixin Oral Concentrate ... 1792
Prolixin Tablets ... 1793

Flurazepam Hydrochloride (Concurrent use not recommended). Products include:
Dalmane Capsules ... 1927

Fosinopril Sodium (Concurrent use not recommended). Products include:
Monopril Tablets ... 1406

Glutethimide (Concurrent use not recommended).
No products indexed under this heading.

Guanabenz Acetate (Concurrent use not recommended). Products include:
Wytensin Tablets ... 2542

Guanethidine Monosulfate (Concurrent use not recommended). Products include:
Esimil Tablets ... 864
Ismelin Tablets ... 869

Haloperidol (Concurrent use not recommended). Products include:
Haldol Injection, Tablets and Concentrate ... 1373

Haloperidol Decanoate (Concurrent use not recommended). Products include:
Haldol Decanoate ... 1375

Hydralazine Hydrochloride (Concurrent use not recommended). Products include:
Apresazide Capsules ... 854
Apresoline Hydrochloride Parenteral (Ampuls) ... 856
Apresoline Hydrochloride Tablets ... 855
Apresoline-Esidrix Tablets ... 857
Ser-Ap-Es Tablets ... 881
Serpasil-Apresoline Tablets ... 884

Hydroxyzine Hydrochloride (Concurrent use not recommended). Products include:
Atarax Tablets & Syrup ... 1941
Marax Tablets & DF Syrup ... 1954
Vistaril Intramuscular Solution ... 1970

Imipramine Hydrochloride (Concurrent use not recommended). Products include:
Tofranil Ampuls ... 1038
Tofranil Tablets ... 1039

Imipramine Pamoate (Concurrent use not recommended). Products include:
Tofranil-PM Capsules ... 1041

Indapamide (Concurrent use not recommended). Products include:
Lozol Tablets ... 1843

Isocarboxazid (Concurrent use not recommended). Products include:
Marplan Tablets ... 1906

Isradipine (Concurrent use not recommended). Products include:
DynaCirc Capsules ... 2004

Labetalol Hydrochloride (Concurrent use not recommended). Products include:
Normodyne Injection ... 2108
Normodyne Tablets ... 2110
Normozide Tablets ... 2112
Trandate HCT Tablets ... 579
Trandate Injection ... 577
Trandate Tablets ... 579

Lisinopril (Concurrent use not recommended). Products include:
Prinivil Tablets ... 1538
Prinzide Tablets ... 1540
Zestoretic ... 2274
Zestril Tablets ... 2277

Lorazepam (Concurrent use not recommended). Products include:
Ativan Injection ... 2432
Ativan Tablets ... 2434

Loxapine Hydrochloride (Concurrent use not recommended). Products include:
Loxitane ... 1213

Loxapine Succinate (Concurrent use not recommended). Products include:
Loxitane Capsules ... 1213

Maprotiline Hydrochloride (Concurrent use not recommended). Products include:
Ludiomil Tablets ... 874

Mecamylamine Hydrochloride (Concurrent use not recommended). Products include:
Inversine Tablets ... 1492

Meprobamate (Concurrent use not recommended). Products include:
Deprol Tablets ... 2382
Equagesic Tablets ... 2451
Miltown Tablets ... 2386
PMB 200 and PMB 400 ... 2504

Mesoridazine (Concurrent use not recommended). Products include:
Serentil ... 686

Methyldopa (Concurrent use not recommended). Products include:
Aldoclor Tablets ... 1413
Aldomet Oral ... 1415
Aldoril Tablets ... 1418

Methyldopate Hydrochloride (Concurrent use not recommended). Products include:
Aldomet Ester HCl Injection ... 1417

Metoprolol Tartrate (Concurrent use not recommended). Products include:
Lopressor Ampuls ... 1032
Lopressor HCT Tablets ... 1034
Lopressor Tablets ... 1032

Metyrosine (Concurrent use not recommended). Products include:
Demser Capsules ... 1460

Midazolam Hydrochloride (Concurrent use not recommended). Products include:
Versed Injection ... 1924

Minoxidil (Concurrent use not recommended). Products include:
Loniten Tablets ... 2346
Rogaine Topical Solution ... 2357

Molindone Hydrochloride (Concurrent use not recommended). Products include:
Moban Tablets & Concentrate ... 932

Nadolol (Concurrent use not recommended). Products include:
Corgard Tablets ... 701
Corzide Tablets ... 702

Nicardipine Hydrochloride (Concurrent use not recommended). Products include:
Cardene Capsules ... 2290

Nitroglycerin (Concurrent use not recommended). Products include:
Deponit NTG Transdermal Delivery System ... 2143
Minitran Transdermal Delivery System ... 1312
Nitro-Bid Ointment ... 1339
Nitro-Bid Capsules ... 1338
Nitrodisc ... 2176
Nitro-Dur (nitroglycerin) Transdermal Infusion System ... 1164
Nitrogard Tablets ... 1004
Nitrolingual Spray ... 1846
Nitrostat Tablets ... 1743
Transderm-Nitro Transdermal Therapeutic System ... 2283

Nortriptyline Hydrochloride (Concurrent use not recommended). Products include:
Pamelor ... 2019

Oxazepam (Concurrent use not recommended). Products include:
Serax Capsules ... 2522
Serax Tablets ... 2522

Penbutolol Sulfate (Concurrent use not recommended). Products include:
Levatol ... 1832

Perphenazine (Concurrent use not recommended). Products include:
Etrafon ... 2087
Triavil Tablets ... 1556
Trilafon ... 2123

Phenelzine Sulfate (Concurrent use not recommended). Products include:
Nardil ... 1742

Phenoxybenzamine Hydrochloride (Concurrent use not recommended). Products include:
Dibenzyline Capsules ... 2207

Phentolamine Mesylate (Concurrent use not recommended). Products include:
Regitine ... 878

Pindolol (Concurrent use not recommended). Products include:
Visken Tablets ... 2036

Prazepam (Concurrent use not recommended). Products include:
Centrax ... 1693

Prazosin Hydrochloride (Concurrent use not recommended). Products include:
Minipress Capsules ... 1778
Minizide Capsules ... 1779

Prochlorperazine (Concurrent use not recommended). Products include:
Compazine ... 2201

Promethazine Hydrochloride (Concurrent use not recommended). Products include:
Mepergan Injection ... 2479
Phenergan with Codeine ... 2497
Phenergan with Dextromethorphan 2499
Phenergan Injection ... 2493
Phenergan Suppositories ... 2496
Phenergan Syrup ... 2495
Phenergan Tablets ... 2496
Phenergan VC ... 2500
Phenergan VC with Codeine ... 2501

Propofol (Concurrent use not recommended). Products include:
Diprivan Injection ... 2267

Propranolol Hydrochloride (Concurrent use not recommended). Products include:
Inderal ... 2459
Inderal LA Long Acting Capsules ... 2461
Inderide Tablets ... 2463
Inderide LA Long Acting Capsules .. 2465

Protriptyline Hydrochloride (Concurrent use not recommended). Products include:
Vivactil Tablets ... 1567

Quazepam (Concurrent use not recommended). Products include:
Doral Tablets ... 2383

Ramipril (Concurrent use not recommended). Products include:
- Altace Capsules ... 1086

Rauwolfia Serpentina (Concurrent use not recommended). Products include:
- Raudixin Tablets ... 1803
- Rauzide Tablets ... 1804

Rescinnamine (Concurrent use not recommended).
- No products indexed under this heading.

Reserpine (Concurrent use not recommended). Products include:
- Diupres Tablets ... 1461
- Hydromox R Tablets ... 1209
- Hydropres Tablets ... 1485
- Renese-R Tablets ... 1786
- Salutensin/Salutensin-Demi ... 719
- Ser-Ap-Es Tablets ... 881
- Serpasil Tablets ... 883
- Serpasil-Apresoline Tablets ... 884
- Serpasil-Esidrix Tablets ... 886

Secobarbital Sodium (Concurrent use not recommended). Products include:
- Seconal Sodium Pulvules ... 1296

Sodium Nitroprusside (Concurrent use not recommended). Products include:
- Nipride I.V. Infusion ... 1909

Temazepam (Concurrent use not recommended). Products include:
- Restoril Capsules ... 2023

Terazosin Hydrochloride (Concurrent use not recommended). Products include:
- Hytrin Tablets ... 529

Thioridazine Hydrochloride (Concurrent use not recommended). Products include:
- Mellaril ... 2011

Thiothixene (Concurrent use not recommended). Products include:
- Navane Capsules and Concentrate ... 1954
- Navane Intramuscular ... 1956

Timolol Maleate (Concurrent use not recommended). Products include:
- Blocadren Tablets ... 1429
- Timolide Tablets ... 1547
- Timoptic in Ocudose ... 1552
- Timoptic Sterile Ophthalmic Solution ... 1550

Tranylcypromine Sulfate (Concurrent use not recommended). Products include:
- Parnate Tablets ... 2222

Trazodone Hydrochloride (Concurrent use not recommended). Products include:
- Desyrel and Desyrel Dividose ... 1404

Triazolam (Concurrent use not recommended). Products include:
- Halcion Tablets ... 2340

Trifluoperazine Hydrochloride (Concurrent use not recommended). Products include:
- Stelazine ... 2226

Trimethaphan Camsylate (Concurrent use not recommended). Products include:
- Arfonad Ampuls ... 1887

Trimipramine Maleate (Concurrent use not recommended). Products include:
- Surmontil Capsules ... 2524

VICKS SINEX DECONGESTANT NASAL SPRAY
(Cetylpyridinium Chloride, Phenylephrine Hydrochloride) ... ▣ 665
No interactions described in labeling.

VICKS SINEX DECONGESTANT NASAL ULTRA FINE MIST
(Cetylpyridinium Chloride, Phenylephrine Hydrochloride) ... ▣ 665
No interactions described in labeling.

VICKS SINEX LONG-ACTING DECONGESTANT NASAL SPRAY
(Oxymetazoline Hydrochloride) ... ▣ 665
No interactions described in labeling.

VICKS SINEX LONG-ACTING DECONGESTANT NASAL ULTRA FINE MIST
(Oxymetazoline Hydrochloride) ... ▣ 665
No interactions described in labeling.

VICKS THROAT LOZENGES
(Benzocaine, Cetylpyridinium Chloride) ... ▣ 665
No interactions described in labeling.

VICKS VAPORUB
(Menthol, Camphor, Eucalyptus, Oil of) ... ▣ 666
No interactions described in labeling.

VICKS VAPOSTEAM
(Camphor, Eucalyptus, Oil of, Menthol) ... ▣ 666
No interactions described in labeling.

VICKS VATRONOL NOSE DROPS
(Ephedrine Sulfate) ... ▣ 666
No interactions described in labeling.

VICODIN TABLETS
(Hydrocodone Bitartrate, Acetaminophen) ... 1187
May interact with tricyclic antidepressants, monoamine oxidase inhibitors, anticholinergics, neuromuscular blocking agents, central nervous system depressants, narcotic analgesics, and certain other agents. Compounds in these categories include:

Alcohol (Additive CNS depression).

Alfentanil Hydrochloride (Additive CNS depression). Products include:
- Alfenta Injection ... 1131

Alprazolam (Additive CNS depression). Products include:
- Xanax Tablets ... 2367

Amitriptyline Hydrochloride (Additive CNS depression; increased effects). Products include:
- Elavil ... 2269
- Endep Tablets ... 1927
- Etrafon ... 2087
- Limbitrol ... 1933
- Triavil Tablets ... 1556

Amoxapine (Additive CNS depression; increased effects). Products include:
- Asendin Tablets ... 1196

Aprobarbital (Additive CNS depression). Products include:
- Alurate Elixir ... 1883

Atropine Sulfate (Paralytic ileus). Products include:
- Arco-Lase Plus Tablets ... 607
- Atropine Sulfate Sterile Ophthalmic Solution and S.O.P. Sterile Ophthalmic Ointment ... ⊙ 239
- Donnagel ... ▣ 675
- Donnagel-PG ... 1858
- Donnatal ... 1858
- Donnatal Extentabs ... 1859
- Donnatal Tablets ... 1858
- Donnazyme Tablets ... 1860
- Isopto Atropine ... ⊙ 218
- Lomotil ... 2174
- Motofen Tablets ... 836
- Ru-Tuss Tablets ... 693
- Urised Tablets ... 2396

Belladonna Alkaloids (Paralytic ileus). Products include:
- Bellergal-S Tablets ... 1998
- Hyland's Bed Wetting Tablets ... ▣ 728
- Hyland's Teething Tablets ... ▣ 728
- Kinesed Tablets ... 2272

Benztropine Mesylate (Paralytic ileus). Products include:
- Cogentin ... 1435

Biperiden (Paralytic ileus). Products include:
- Akineton ... 1171

Buprenorphine (Additive CNS depression).
- No products indexed under this heading.

Buspirone Hydrochloride (Additive CNS depression). Products include:
- BuSpar ... 1401

Butabarbital (Additive CNS depression). Products include:
- Pyridium Plus ... 1764

Butalbital (Additive CNS depression). Products include:
- Esgic-Plus Tablets ... 1002
- Esgic Tablets & Capsules ... 1001
- Fioricet Tablets ... 2006
- Fiorinal Capsules ... 2007
- Fiorinal with Codeine Capsules ... 2008
- Fiorinal Tablets ... 2007
- Phrenilin ... 838
- Sedapap Tablets 50 mg/650 mg ... 1360

Chlordiazepoxide (Additive CNS depression). Products include:
- Libritabs Tablets ... 1930
- Limbitrol ... 1933
- Menrium Tablets ... 1934

Chlordiazepoxide Hydrochloride (Additive CNS depression). Products include:
- Librax Capsules ... 1929
- Librium Capsules ... 1931
- Librium Injectable ... 1932

Chlorpromazine (Additive CNS depression). Products include:
- Thorazine ... 2234

Chlorprothixene (Additive CNS depression). Products include:
- Taractan Tablets ... 1920

Chlorprothixene Hydrochloride (Additive CNS depression). Products include:
- Taractan ... 1920

Clidinium Bromide (Paralytic ileus). Products include:
- Librax Capsules ... 1929
- Quarzan Capsules ... 1937

Clomipramine Hydrochloride (Additive CNS depression; increased effects). Products include:
- Anafranil Capsules ... 650

Clorazepate Dipotassium (Additive CNS depression; paralytic ileus). Products include:
- Tranxene ... 556

Clozapine (Additive CNS depression). Products include:
- Clozaril Tablets ... 2000

Codeine (Additive CNS depression). Products include:
- Calcidrine Syrup ... 506

Codeine Phosphate (Additive CNS depression). Products include:
- Actifed with Codeine Cough Syrup ... 752
- Cheracol Cough Syrup ... 1853
- Codimal PH Syrup ... 846
- Dimetane-DC Cough Syrup ... 1857
- Empirin with Codeine Phosphate Nos. 2, 3 & 4 ... 764
- Fiorinal with Codeine Capsules ... 2008
- Isoclor Expectorant ... 982
- Naldecon CX Adult Liquid ... ▣ 521
- Novahistine DH ... 1342
- Novahistine Expectorant ... 1343
- Nucofed Capsules ... 2219
- Nucofed Expectorant ... 2219
- Nucofed Pediatric Expectorant ... 2220
- Nucofed Syrup ... 2219
- Phenaphen with Codeine Capsules ... 1865
- Phenaphen-650 with Codeine Tablets ... 1866
- Phenergan with Codeine ... 2497
- Phenergan VC with Codeine ... 2501
- Robitussin A-C Syrup ... 1875
- Robitussin-DAC Syrup ... 1875
- Ryna ... ▣ 741
- Soma Compound w/Codeine Tablets ... 2390
- Triaminic Expectorant w/Codeine ... 1996
- Tussi-Organidin Liquid ... 2391
- Tylenol with Codeine ... 1381

Codeine Polistirex (Additive CNS depression).
- No products indexed under this heading.

Desipramine Hydrochloride (Additive CNS depression; increased effects). Products include:
- Norpramin Tablets ... 1340

Dezocine (Additive CNS depression).

Diazepam (Additive CNS depression). Products include:
- Valium Injectable ... 1937
- Valium Tablets ... 1939
- Valrelease Capsules ... 1923

Dicyclomine Hydrochloride (Paralytic ileus). Products include:
- Bentyl ... 1322

Doxepin Hydrochloride (Additive CNS depression; increased effects). Products include:
- Sinequan ... 1960

Droperidol (Additive CNS depression). Products include:
- Inapsine Injection ... 1140
- Innovar Injection ... 1141

Enflurane (Additive CNS depression). Products include:
- Ethrane ... 599

Estazolam (Additive CNS depression). Products include:
- ProSom Tablets ... 554

Ethchlorvynol (Additive CNS depression). Products include:
- Placidyl Capsules ... 553

Ethinamate (Additive CNS depression).
- No products indexed under this heading.

Ethopropazine Hydrochloride (Paralytic ileus).

Fentanyl (Additive CNS depression). Products include:
- Duragesic Transdermal System ... 1133

Fentanyl Citrate (Additive CNS depression). Products include:
- Innovar Injection ... 1141
- Sublimaze Injection ... 1146

Fluphenazine Decanoate (Additive CNS depression). Products include:
- Prolixin Decanoate ... 1795

Fluphenazine Enanthate (Additive CNS depression). Products include:
- Prolixin Enanthate ... 1796

Fluphenazine Hydrochloride (Additive CNS depression). Products include:
- Prolixin Elixir ... 1793
- Prolixin Injection ... 1791
- Prolixin Oral Concentrate ... 1792
- Prolixin Tablets ... 1793

Flurazepam Hydrochloride (Additive CNS depression). Products include:
- Dalmane Capsules ... 1927

Furazolidone (Increased effects). Products include:
- Furoxone ... 1855

Glutethimide (Additive CNS depression).
- No products indexed under this heading.

Glycopyrrolate (Paralytic ileus). Products include:
- Robinul Forte Tablets ... 1873

Robinul Injectable ... 1873
Robinul Tablets ... 1873

Haloperidol (Additive CNS depression). Products include:
Haldol Injection, Tablets and Concentrate ... 1373

Haloperidol Decanoate (Additive CNS depression). Products include:
Haldol Decanoate ... 1375

Hydrocodone Polistirex (Additive CNS depression). Products include:
Tussionex Extended-Release Suspension ... 988

Hydroxyzine Hydrochloride (Additive CNS depression). Products include:
Atarax Tablets & Syrup ... 1941
Marax Tablets & DF Syrup ... 1954
Vistaril Intramuscular Solution ... 1970

Hyoscyamine (Paralytic ileus). Products include:
Cystospaz Tablets ... 2395
Urised Tablets ... 2396

Hyoscyamine Sulfate (Paralytic ileus). Products include:
Arco-Lase Plus Tablets ... 607
Cystospaz-M Capsules ... 2395
Donnagel ... ▣ 675
Donnagel-PG ... 1858
Donnatal ... 1858
Donnatal Extentabs ... 1859
Donnatal Tablets ... 1858
Donnazyme Tablets ... 1860
Kutrase Capsules ... 2146
Levsin/Levsinex ... 2147
Ru-Tuss Tablets ... 693

Imipramine Hydrochloride (Additive CNS depression; increased effects). Products include:
Tofranil Ampuls ... 1038
Tofranil Tablets ... 1039

Imipramine Pamoate (Additive CNS depression; increased effects). Products include:
Tofranil-PM Capsules ... 1041

Ipratropium Bromide (Paralytic ileus). Products include:
Atrovent Inhalation Aerosol ... 675

Isocarboxazid (Increased effects). Products include:
Marplan Tablets ... 1906

Isoflurane (Additive CNS depression). Products include:
Forane ... 600

Ketamine Hydrochloride (Additive CNS depression). Products include:
Ketalar ... 1726

Levorphanol Tartrate (Additive CNS depression). Products include:
Levo-Dromoran ... 1906

Lithium Carbonate (Additive CNS depression). Products include:
Eskalith ... 2214
Lithane Tablets ... 1596
Lithium Carbonate Capsules & Tablets ... 1984
Lithobid Tablets ... 870

Lithium Citrate (Additive CNS depression). Products include:
Cibalith-S ... 870

Lorazepam (Additive CNS depression). Products include:
Ativan Injection ... 2432
Ativan Tablets ... 2434

Loxapine Hydrochloride (Additive CNS depression). Products include:
Loxitane ... 1213

Loxapine Succinate (Additive CNS depression). Products include:
Loxitane Capsules ... 1213

Maprotiline Hydrochloride (Additive CNS depression; increased effects). Products include:
Ludiomil Tablets ... 874

Mepenzolate Bromide (Paralytic ileus). Products include:
Cantil Tablets ... 1326

Meperidine Hydrochloride (Additive CNS depression). Products include:
Demerol ... 2047
Mepergan Injection ... 2479

Mephobarbital (Additive CNS depression). Products include:
Mebaral Tablets ... 2061

Meprobamate (Additive CNS depression). Products include:
Deprol Tablets ... 2382
Equagesic Tablets ... 2451
Miltown Tablets ... 2386
PMB 200 and PMB 400 ... 2504

Mesoridazine (Additive CNS depression). Products include:
Serentil ... 686

Mesoridazine Besylate (Additive CNS depression).

Methadone Hydrochloride (Additive CNS depression). Products include:
Dolophine Hydrochloride Ampoules & Vials ... 1260
Dolophine Hydrochloride Tablets ... 1261
Methadone Hydrochloride Diskets ... 1284
Methadone Hydrochloride Oral Solution & Tablets ... 1987

Methohexital Sodium (Additive CNS depression). Products include:
Brevital Sodium Vials ... 1248

Methoxyflurane (Additive CNS depression).
No products indexed under this heading.

Midazolam Hydrochloride (Additive CNS depression). Products include:
Versed Injection ... 1924

Molindone Hydrochloride (Additive CNS depression). Products include:
Moban Tablets & Concentrate ... 932

Morphine Sulfate (Additive CNS depression). Products include:
Astramorph/PF Injection, USP (Preservative-Free) ... 618
Duramorph ... 960
Infumorph 200 and Infumorph 500 Sterile Solutions ... 962
MS Contin Tablets ... 1814
MSIR ... 1817
Oramorph SR (Morphine Sulfate Sustained Release Tablets) ... 1988
Roxanol ... 1991

Nortriptyline Hydrochloride (Additive CNS depression; increased effects). Products include:
Pamelor ... 2019

Opium Alkaloids (Additive CNS depression). Products include:
B & O No. 15A & No. 16A Supprettes ... 2395
Pantopon Injectable ... 1911

Oxazepam (Additive CNS depression). Products include:
Serax Capsules ... 2522
Serax Tablets ... 2522

Oxybutynin Chloride (Paralytic ileus). Products include:
Ditropan ... 1332

Oxycodone Hydrochloride (Additive CNS depression). Products include:
Percocet Tablets ... 950
Percodan ... 951
Roxicodone Tablets, Oral Solution & Intensol (Oxycodone) ... 1992
Tylox Capsules ... 1382

Oxyphenonium Bromide (Paralytic ileus).

Pentobarbital Sodium (Additive CNS depression). Products include:
Nembutal Sodium Capsules ... 534
Nembutal Sodium Solution ... 536
Nembutal Sodium Suppositories ... 538

Perphenazine (Additive CNS depression). Products include:
Etrafon ... 2087
Triavil Tablets ... 1556
Trilafon ... 2123

Phenelzine Sulfate (Increased effects). Products include:
Nardil ... 1742

Phenobarbital (Additive CNS depression). Products include:
Arco-Lase Plus Tablets ... 607
Bellergal-S Tablets ... 1998
Bronkolixir ... ▣ 761
Bronkotabs Tablets ... ▣ 762
Donnatal ... 1858
Donnatal Extentabs ... 1859
Donnatal Tablets ... 1858
Donnazyme Tablets ... 1860
Kinesed Tablets ... 2272
Phenobarbital Elixir and Tablets ... 1293
Primatene Tablets-P Formula ... 2421
Quadrinal Tablets ... 1183
Tedral SA ... 1765

Pimozide (Additive CNS depression). Products include:
Orap Tablets ... 1020

Prazepam (Additive CNS depression). Products include:
Centrax ... 1693

Prochlorperazine (Additive CNS depression). Products include:
Compazine ... 2201

Procyclidine Hydrochloride (Paralytic ileus). Products include:
Kemadrin Tablets ... 771

Promethazine Hydrochloride (Additive CNS depression). Products include:
Mepergan Injection ... 2479
Phenergan with Codeine ... 2497
Phenergan with Dextromethorphan 2499
Phenergan Injection ... 2493
Phenergan Suppositories ... 2496
Phenergan Syrup ... 2495
Phenergan Tablets ... 2496
Phenergan VC ... 2500
Phenergan VC with Codeine ... 2501

Propantheline Bromide (Paralytic ileus). Products include:
Pro-Banthīne Tablets ... 2141

Propofol (Additive CNS depression). Products include:
Diprivan Injection ... 2267

Propoxyphene Hydrochloride (Additive CNS depression). Products include:
Darvon ... 1256
Wygesic Tablets ... 2540

Propoxyphene Napsylate (Additive CNS depression). Products include:
Darvon-N/Darvocet-N ... 1254

Protriptyline Hydrochloride (Additive CNS depression; increased effects). Products include:
Vivactil Tablets ... 1567

Quazepam (Additive CNS depression). Products include:
Doral Tablets ... 2383

Scopolamine Hydrobromide (Paralytic ileus). Products include:
Donnagel ... ▣ 675
Donnagel-PG ... 1858
Donnatal ... 1858
Donnatal Extentabs ... 1859
Donnatal Tablets ... 1858
Donnazyme Tablets ... 1860
Isopto Hyoscine ... ⊙ 222
Murocoll-2 Sterile Ophthalmic Solution ... ⊙ 261
Ru-Tuss Tablets ... 693

Scopolamine Preparations (Paralytic ileus). Products include:
Transderm Scōp Transdermal Therapeutic System ... 887

Secobarbital Sodium (Additive CNS depression). Products include:
Seconal Sodium Pulvules ... 1296

Selegiline Hydrochloride (Increased effects). Products include:
Eldepryl ... 2250

Sufentanil Citrate (Additive CNS depression). Products include:
Sufenta Injection ... 1147

Temazepam (Additive CNS depression). Products include:
Restoril Capsules ... 2023

Thiamylal Sodium (Additive CNS depression). Products include:
Surital Ampoules, Steri-Vials ... 1764

Thiothixene (Additive CNS depression). Products include:
Navane Capsules and Concentrate 1954
Navane Intramuscular ... 1956

Tranylcypromine Sulfate (Increased effects). Products include:
Parnate Tablets ... 2222

Triazolam (Additive CNS depression). Products include:
Halcion Tablets ... 2340

Tridihexethyl Chloride (Paralytic ileus).
No products indexed under this heading.

Trifluoperazine Hydrochloride (Additive CNS depression). Products include:
Stelazine ... 2226

Trihexyphenidyl Hydrochloride (Paralytic ileus). Products include:
Artane ... 1195

Trimipramine Maleate (Additive CNS depression; increased effects). Products include:
Surmontil Capsules ... 2524

VICODIN ES TABLETS
(Hydrocodone Bitartrate, Acetaminophen) ... 1189
May interact with central nervous system depressants, narcotic analgesics, psychotropics, tranquilizers, monoamine oxidase inhibitors, tricyclic antidepressants, anticholinergics, and certain other agents. Compounds in these categories include:

Alcohol (Additive CNS depression).

Alfentanil Hydrochloride (Additive CNS depression; the dose of one or both agents should be reduced). Products include:
Alfenta Injection ... 1131

Alprazolam (Additive CNS depression; the dose of one or both agents should be reduced). Products include:
Xanax Tablets ... 2367

Amitriptyline Hydrochloride (Additive CNS depression; the dose of one or both agents should be reduced; increased effect of either hydrocodone or antidepressant). Products include:
Elavil ... 2269
Endep Tablets ... 1927
Etrafon ... 2087
Limbitrol ... 1933
Triavil Tablets ... 1556

Amoxapine (Additive CNS depression; the dose of one or both agents should be reduced; increased effect of either hydrocodone or antidepressant). Products include:
Asendin Tablets ... 1196

Aprobarbital (Additive CNS depression; the dose of one or both agents should be reduced). Products include:
Alurate Elixir ... 1883

Atropine Sulfate (May produce paralytic ileus). Products include:
Arco-Lase Plus Tablets ... 607
Atropine Sulfate Sterile Ophthalmic Solution and S.O.P. Sterile Ophthalmic Ointment ... ⊙ 239
Donnagel ... ▣ 675
Donnagel-PG ... 1858
Donnatal ... 1858
Donnatal Extentabs ... 1859

Donnatal Tablets ... 1858
Donnazyme Tablets ... 1860
Isopto Atropine ... ⊙ 218
Lomotil ... 2174
Motofen Tablets ... 836
Ru-Tuss Tablets ... 693
Urised Tablets ... 2396

Belladonna Alkaloids (May produce paralytic ileus). Products include:
Bellergal-S Tablets ... 1998
Hyland's Bed Wetting Tablets ... ▣ 728
Hyland's Teething Tablets ... ▣ 728
Kinesed Tablets ... 2272

Benztropine Mesylate (May produce paralytic ileus). Products include:
Cogentin ... 1435

Biperiden (May produce paralytic ileus). Products include:
Akineton ... 1171

Buprenorphine (Additive CNS depression; the dose of one or both agents should be reduced).
No products indexed under this heading.

Buspirone Hydrochloride (Additive CNS depression; the dose of one or both agents should be reduced). Products include:
BuSpar ... 1401

Butabarbital (Additive CNS depression; the dose of one or both agents should be reduced). Products include:
Pyridium Plus ... 1764

Butalbital (Additive CNS depression; the dose of one or both agents should be reduced). Products include:
Esgic-Plus Tablets ... 1002
Esgic Tablets & Capsules ... 1001
Fioricet Tablets ... 2006
Fiorinal Capsules ... 2007
Fiorinal with Codeine Capsules ... 2008
Fiorinal Tablets ... 2007
Phrenilin ... 838
Sedapap Tablets 50 mg/650 mg .. 1360

Chlordiazepoxide (Additive CNS depression; the dose of one or both agents should be reduced). Products include:
Libritabs Tablets ... 1930
Limbitrol ... 1933
Menrium Tablets ... 1934

Chlordiazepoxide Hydrochloride (Additive CNS depression; the dose of one or both agents should be reduced). Products include:
Librax Capsules ... 1929
Librium Capsules ... 1931
Librium Injectable ... 1932

Chlorpromazine (Additive CNS depression; the dose of one or both agents should be reduced). Products include:
Thorazine ... 2234

Chlorprothixene (Additive CNS depression; the dose of one or both agents should be reduced). Products include:
Taractan Tablets ... 1920

Chlorprothixene Hydrochloride (Additive CNS depression; the dose of one or both agents should be reduced). Products include:
Taractan ... 1920

Clidinium Bromide (May produce paralytic ileus). Products include:
Librax Capsules ... 1929
Quarzan Capsules ... 1937

Clomipramine Hydrochloride (Additive CNS depression; the dose of one or both agents should be reduced; increased effect of either hydrocodone or antidepressant). Products include:
Anafranil Capsules ... 650

Clorazepate Dipotassium (Additive CNS depression; the dose of one or both agents should be reduced). Products include:
Tranxene ... 556

Codeine (Additive CNS depression; the dose of one or both agents should be reduced). Products include:
Calcidrine Syrup ... 506

Codeine Phosphate (Additive CNS depression; the dose of one or both agents should be reduced). Products include:
Actifed with Codeine Cough Syrup.. 752
Cheracol Cough Syrup ... 1853
Codimal PH Syrup ... 846
Dimetane-DC Cough Syrup ... 1857
Empirin with Codeine Phosphate Nos. 2, 3 & 4 ... 764
Fiorinal with Codeine Capsules ... 2008
Isoclor Expectorant ... 982
Naldecon CX Adult Liquid ... ▣ 521
Novahistine DH ... 1342
Novahistine Expectorant ... 1343
Nucofed Capsules ... 2219
Nucofed Expectorant ... 2219
Nucofed Pediatric Expectorant ... 2220
Nucofed Syrup ... 2219
Phenaphen with Codeine Capsules 1865
Phenaphen-650 with Codeine Tablets ... 1866
Phenergan with Codeine ... 2497
Phenergan VC with Codeine ... 2501
Robitussin A-C Syrup ... 1875
Robitussin-DAC Syrup ... 1875
Ryna ... ▣ 741
Soma Compound w/Codeine Tablets ... 2390
Triaminic Expectorant w/Codeine .. 1996
Tussi-Organidin Liquid ... 2391
Tylenol with Codeine ... 1381

Codeine Polistirex (Additive CNS depression; the dose of one or both agents should be reduced).
No products indexed under this heading.

Desipramine Hydrochloride (Additive CNS depression; the dose of one or both agents should be reduced; increased effect of either hydrocodone or antidepressant). Products include:
Norpramin Tablets ... 1340

Dezocine (Additive CNS depression; the dose of one or both agents should be reduced).

Diazepam (Additive CNS depression; the dose of one or both agents should be reduced). Products include:
Valium Injectable ... 1937
Valium Tablets ... 1939
Valrelease Capsules ... 1923

Dicyclomine Hydrochloride (May produce paralytic ileus). Products include:
Bentyl ... 1322

Doxepin Hydrochloride (Additive CNS depression; the dose of one or both agents should be reduced; increased effect of either hydrocodone or antidepressant). Products include:
Sinequan ... 1960

Droperidol (Additive CNS depression; the dose of one or both agents should be reduced). Products include:
Inapsine Injection ... 1140
Innovar Injection ... 1141

Enflurane (Additive CNS depression; the dose of one or both agents should be reduced). Products include:
Ethrane ... 599

Estazolam (Additive CNS depression; the dose of one or both agents should be reduced). Products include:
ProSom Tablets ... 554

Ethchlorvynol (Additive CNS depression; the dose of one or both agents should be reduced). Products include:
Placidyl Capsules ... 553

Ethinamate (Additive CNS depression; the dose of one or both agents should be reduced).
No products indexed under this heading.

Fentanyl (Additive CNS depression; the dose of one or both agents should be reduced). Products include:
Duragesic Transdermal System ... 1133

Fentanyl Citrate (Additive CNS depression; the dose of one or both agents should be reduced). Products include:
Innovar Injection ... 1141
Sublimaze Injection ... 1146

Fluphenazine Decanoate (Additive CNS depression; the dose of one or both agents should be reduced). Products include:
Prolixin Decanoate ... 1795

Fluphenazine Enanthate (Additive CNS depression; the dose of one or both agents should be reduced). Products include:
Prolixin Enanthate ... 1796

Fluphenazine Hydrochloride (Additive CNS depression; the dose of one or both agents should be reduced). Products include:
Prolixin Elixir ... 1793
Prolixin Injection ... 1791
Prolixin Oral Concentrate ... 1792
Prolixin Tablets ... 1793

Flurazepam Hydrochloride (Additive CNS depression; the dose of one or both agents should be reduced). Products include:
Dalmane Capsules ... 1927

Furazolidone (Additive CNS depression; the dose of one or both agents should be reduced; increased effect of either hydrocodone or MAO inhibitor). Products include:
Furoxone ... 1855

Glutethimide (Additive CNS depression; the dose of one or both agents should be reduced).
No products indexed under this heading.

Glycopyrrolate (May produce paralytic ileus). Products include:
Robinul Forte Tablets ... 1873
Robinul Injectable ... 1873
Robinul Tablets ... 1873

Haloperidol (Additive CNS depression; the dose of one or both agents should be reduced). Products include:
Haldol Injection, Tablets and Concentrate ... 1373

Haloperidol Decanoate (Additive CNS depression; the dose of one or both agents should be reduced). Products include:
Haldol Decanoate ... 1375

Hydrocodone Polistirex (Additive CNS depression; the dose of one or both agents should be reduced). Products include:
Tussionex Extended-Release Suspension ... 988

Hydroxyzine Hydrochloride (Additive CNS depression; the dose of one or both agents should be reduced). Products include:
Atarax Tablets & Syrup ... 1941
Marax Tablets & DF Syrup ... 1954
Vistaril Intramuscular Solution ... 1970

Hyoscyamine (May produce paralytic ileus). Products include:
Cystospaz Tablets ... 2395
Urised Tablets ... 2396

Hyoscyamine Sulfate (May produce paralytic ileus). Products include:
Arco-Lase Plus Tablets ... 607
Cystospaz-M Capsules ... 2395
Donnagel ... ▣ 675
Donnagel-PG ... 1858
Donnatal ... 1858
Donnatal Extentabs ... 1859
Donnatal Tablets ... 1858
Donnazyme Tablets ... 1860
Kutrase Capsules ... 2146
Levsin/Levsinex ... 2147
Ru-Tuss Tablets ... 693

Imipramine Hydrochloride (Additive CNS depression; the dose of one or both agents should be reduced; increased effect of either hydrocodone or antidepressant). Products include:
Tofranil Ampuls ... 1038
Tofranil Tablets ... 1039

Imipramine Pamoate (Additive CNS depression; the dose of one or both agents should be reduced; increased effect of either hydrocodone or antidepressant). Products include:
Tofranil-PM Capsules ... 1041

Ipratropium Bromide (May produce paralytic ileus). Products include:
Atrovent Inhalation Aerosol ... 675

Isocarboxazid (Additive CNS depression; the dose of one or both agents should be reduced; increased effect of either hydrocodone or MAO inhibitor). Products include:
Marplan Tablets ... 1906

Isoflurane (Additive CNS depression; the dose of one or both agents should be reduced). Products include:
Forane ... 600

Ketamine Hydrochloride (Additive CNS depression; the dose of one or both agents should be reduced). Products include:
Ketalar ... 1726

Levorphanol Tartrate (Additive CNS depression; the dose of one or both agents should be reduced). Products include:
Levo-Dromoran ... 1906

Lithium Carbonate (Additive CNS depression; the dose of one or both agents should be reduced). Products include:
Eskalith ... 2214
Lithane Tablets ... 1596
Lithium Carbonate Capsules & Tablets ... 1984
Lithobid Tablets ... 870

Lithium Citrate (Additive CNS depression; the dose of one or both agents should be reduced). Products include:
Cibalith-S ... 870

Lorazepam (Additive CNS depression; the dose of one or both agents should be reduced). Products include:
Ativan Injection ... 2432
Ativan Tablets ... 2434

Loxapine Hydrochloride (Additive CNS depression; the dose of one or both agents should be reduced). Products include:
Loxitane ... 1213

Loxapine Succinate (Additive CNS depression; the dose of one or both agents should be reduced). Products include:
Loxitane Capsules ... 1213

Maprotiline Hydrochloride (Additive CNS depression; the dose of one or both agents should be reduced; increased effect of either hydrocodone or antidepressant). Products include:
Ludiomil Tablets 874

Mepenzolate Bromide (May produce paralytic ileus). Products include:
Cantil Tablets 1326

Meperidine Hydrochloride (Additive CNS depression; the dose of one or both agents should be reduced). Products include:
Demerol 2047
Mepergan Injection 2479

Mephobarbital (Additive CNS depression; the dose of one or both agents should be reduced). Products include:
Mebaral Tablets 2061

Meprobamate (Additive CNS depression; the dose of one or both agents should be reduced). Products include:
Deprol Tablets 2382
Equagesic Tablets 2451
Miltown Tablets 2386
PMB 200 and PMB 400 2504

Mesoridazine (Additive CNS depression; the dose of one or both agents should be reduced). Products include:
Serentil 686

Mesoridazine Besylate (Additive CNS depression; the dose of one or both agents should be reduced).

Methadone Hydrochloride (Additive CNS depression; the dose of one or both agents should be reduced). Products include:
Dolophine Hydrochloride Ampoules & Vials 1260
Dolophine Hydrochloride Tablets 1261
Methadone Hydrochloride Diskets 1284
Methadone Hydrochloride Oral Solution & Tablets 1987

Methohexital Sodium (Additive CNS depression; the dose of one or both agents should be reduced). Products include:
Brevital Sodium Vials 1248

Methoxyflurane (Additive CNS depression; the dose of one or both agents should be reduced).
No products indexed under this heading.

Midazolam Hydrochloride (Additive CNS depression; the dose of one or both agents should be reduced). Products include:
Versed Injection 1924

Molindone Hydrochloride (Additive CNS depression; the dose of one or both agents should be reduced). Products include:
Moban Tablets & Concentrate 932

Morphine Sulfate (Additive CNS depression; the dose of one or both agents should be reduced). Products include:
Astramorph/PF Injection, USP (Preservative-Free) 618
Duramorph 960
Infumorph 200 and Infumorph 500 Sterile Solutions 962
MS Contin Tablets 1814
MSIR 1817
Oramorph SR (Morphine Sulfate Sustained Release Tablets) 1988
Roxanol 1991

Nortriptyline Hydrochloride (Additive CNS depression; the dose of one or both agents should be reduced; increased effect of either hydrocodone or antidepressant). Products include:
Pamelor 2019

Opium Alkaloids (Additive CNS depression; the dose of one or both agents should be reduced). Products include:
B & O No. 15A & No. 16A Supprettes 2395
Pantopon Injectable 1911

Oxazepam (Additive CNS depression; the dose of one or both agents should be reduced). Products include:
Serax Capsules 2522
Serax Tablets 2522

Oxybutynin Chloride (May produce paralytic ileus). Products include:
Ditropan 1332

Oxycodone Hydrochloride (Additive CNS depression; the dose of one or both agents should be reduced). Products include:
Percocet Tablets 950
Percodan 951
Roxicodone Tablets, Oral Solution & Intensol (Oxycodone) 1992
Tylox Capsules 1382

Pentobarbital Sodium (Additive CNS depression; the dose of one or both agents should be reduced). Products include:
Nembutal Sodium Capsules 534
Nembutal Sodium Solution 536
Nembutal Sodium Suppositories 538

Perphenazine (Additive CNS depression; the dose of one or both agents should be reduced). Products include:
Etrafon 2087
Triavil Tablets 1556
Trilafon 2123

Phenelzine Sulfate (Additive CNS depression; the dose of one or both agents should be reduced; increased effect of either hydrocodone or MAO inhibitor). Products include:
Nardil 1742

Phenobarbital (Additive CNS depression; the dose of one or both agents should be reduced). Products include:
Arco-Lase Plus Tablets 607
Bellergal-S Tablets 1998
Bronkolixir .... ⊡ 761
Bronkotabs Tablets .... ⊡ 762
Donnatal 1858
Donnatal Extentabs 1859
Donnatal Tablets 1858
Donnazyme Tablets 1860
Kinesed Tablets 2272
Phenobarbital Elixir and Tablets 1293
Primatene Tablets-P Formula 2421
Quadrinal Tablets 1183
Tedral SA 1765

Prazepam (Additive CNS depression; the dose of one or both agents should be reduced). Products include:
Centrax 1693

Prochlorperazine (Additive CNS depression; the dose of one or both agents should be reduced). Products include:
Compazine 2201

Procyclidine Hydrochloride (May produce paralytic ileus). Products include:
Kemadrin Tablets 771

Promethazine Hydrochloride (Additive CNS depression; the dose of one or both agents should be reduced). Products include:
Mepergan Injection 2479
Phenergan with Codeine 2497
Phenergan with Dextromethorphan 2499
Phenergan Injection 2493
Phenergan Suppositories 2496
Phenergan Syrup 2495
Phenergan Tablets 2496
Phenergan VC 2500
Phenergan VC with Codeine 2501

Propantheline Bromide (May produce paralytic ileus). Products include:
Pro-Banthīne Tablets 2141

Propofol (Additive CNS depression; the dose of one or both agents should be reduced). Products include:
Diprivan Injection 2267

Propoxyphene Hydrochloride (Additive CNS depression; the dose of one or both agents should be reduced). Products include:
Darvon 1256
Wygesic Tablets 2540

Propoxyphene Napsylate (Additive CNS depression; the dose of one or both agents should be reduced). Products include:
Darvon-N/Darvocet-N 1254

Protriptyline Hydrochloride (Additive CNS depression; the dose of one or both agents should be reduced; increased effect of either hydrocodone or antidepressant). Products include:
Vivactil Tablets 1567

Quazepam (Additive CNS depression; the dose of one or both agents should be reduced). Products include:
Doral Tablets 2383

Scopolamine Hydrobromide (May produce paralytic ileus). Products include:
Donnagel .... ⊡ 675
Donnagel-PG 1858
Donnatal 1858
Donnatal Extentabs 1859
Donnatal Tablets 1858
Donnazyme Tablets 1860
Isopto Hyoscine .... ◉ 222
Murocoll-2 Sterile Ophthalmic Solution .... ◉ 261
Ru-Tuss Tablets 693

Scopolamine Preparations (May produce paralytic ileus). Products include:
Transderm Scōp Transdermal Therapeutic System 887

Secobarbital Sodium (Additive CNS depression; the dose of one or both agents should be reduced). Products include:
Seconal Sodium Pulvules 1296

Selegiline Hydrochloride (Additive CNS depression; the dose of one or both agents should be reduced; increased effect of either hydrocodone or MAO inhibitor). Products include:
Eldepryl 2250

Sufentanil Citrate (Additive CNS depression; the dose of one or both agents should be reduced). Products include:
Sufenta Injection 1147

Temazepam (Additive CNS depression; the dose of one or both agents should be reduced). Products include:
Restoril Capsules 2023

Thiamylal Sodium (Additive CNS depression; the dose of one or both agents should be reduced). Products include:
Surital Ampoules, Steri-Vials 1764

Thioridazine Hydrochloride (Additive CNS depression; the dose of one or both agents sjould be reduced). Products include:
Mellaril 2011

Thiothixene (Additive CNS depression; the dose of one or both agents should be reduced). Products include:
Navane Capsules and Concentrate 1954
Navane Intramuscular 1956

Tranylcypromine Sulfate (Additive CNS depression; the dose of one or both agents should be reduced; increased effect of either hydrocodone or MAO inhibitor). Products include:
Parnate Tablets 2222

Triazolam (Additive CNS depression; the dose of one or both agents should be reduced). Products include:
Halcion Tablets 2340

Tridihexethyl Chloride (May produce paralytic ileus).
No products indexed under this heading.

Trifluoperazine Hydrochloride (Additive CNS depression; the dose of one or both agents should be reduced). Products include:
Stelazine 2226

Trihexyphenidyl Hydrochloride (May produce paralytic ileus). Products include:
Artane 1195

Trimipramine Maleate (Additive CNS depression; the dose of one or both agents should be reduced; increased effect of either hydrocodone or antidepressant). Products include:
Surmontil Capsules 2524

VICON FORTE CAPSULES
(Vitamins with Minerals, Therapeutic) 2416
No interactions described in labeling.

VICON PLUS
(Vitamins with Minerals) .... ⊡ 682
No interactions described in labeling.

VICON-C
(Vitamins with Minerals) .... ⊡ 682
No interactions described in labeling.

VI-DAYLIN ADC VITAMINS DROPS
(Vitamin B Complex With Vitamin C, Vitamin C) 1980
No interactions described in labeling.

VI-DAYLIN ADC VITAMINS + IRON DROPS
(Vitamins with Iron) 1980
No interactions described in labeling.

VI-DAYLIN MULTIVITAMIN DROPS
(Vitamins A & D) 1980
No interactions described in labeling.

VI-DAYLIN MULTIVITAMIN + IRON DROPS
(Vitamins with Iron) 1981
No interactions described in labeling.

VI-DAYLIN/F ADC VITAMINS DROPS WITH FLUORIDE
(Vitamins with Fluoride) 1981
No interactions described in labeling.

VI-DAYLIN/F ADC VITAMINS + IRON DROPS WITH FLUORIDE
(Vitamins with Fluoride, Ferrous Sulfate) 1981
No interactions described in labeling.

VI-DAYLIN/F MULTIVITAMIN DROPS WITH FLUORIDE
(Vitamins with Fluoride) 1981
No interactions described in labeling.

VI-DAYLIN/F MULTIVITAMIN + IRON DROPS WITH FLUORIDE
(Ferrous Sulfate, Vitamins with Fluoride) 1981
No interactions described in labeling.

VI-DAYLIN MULTIVITAMIN CHEWABLE TABLETS
(Vitamins A & D) 1982
No interactions described in labeling.

VI-DAYLIN MULTIVITAMIN + IRON CHEWABLE TABLETS
(Vitamins with Iron) 1982
No interactions described in labeling.

VI-DAYLIN/F MULTIVITAMIN CHEWABLE TABLETS WITH FLUORIDE
(Vitamins with Fluoride) 1982
No interactions described in labeling.

VI-DAYLIN/F MULTIVITAMIN + IRON CHEWABLE TABLETS WITH FLUORIDE
(Ferrous Fumarate, Vitamins with Fluoride) 1982
No interactions described in labeling.

VI-DAYLIN MULTIVITAMIN LIQUID
(Vitamins A & D) 1982
No interactions described in labeling.

VI-DAYLIN MULTIVITAMIN + IRON LIQUID
(Vitamins with Iron) 1983
No interactions described in labeling.

VIOFORM CREAM & OINTMENT
(Clioquinol) 889
No interactions described in labeling.

VIOFORM-HYDROCORTISON- E CREAM AND MILD CREAM
(Clioquinol, Hydrocortisone) 889
No interactions described in labeling.

VIOFORM-HYDROCORTISON- E OINTMENT
(Clioquinol, Hydrocortisone) 889
No interactions described in labeling.

VIOKASE POWDER
(Pancrelipase) 1877
No interactions described in labeling.

VIOKASE TABLETS
(Pancrelipase) 1877
No interactions described in labeling.

VIRA-A FOR INJECTION
(Vidarabine) 1766
May interact with:

Allopurinol (May interfere with Vira-A metabolism). Products include:
- Zyloprim Tablets 830

VIRA-A OPHTHALMIC OINTMENT, 3%
(Vidarabine) 1767
No interactions described in labeling.

VIRANOL GEL
(Salicylic Acid) 591
No interactions described in labeling.

VIRAZOLE
(Ribavirin) 1126
No interactions described in labeling.

VIROPTIC OPHTHALMIC SOLUTION, 1% STERILE
(Trifluridine) 820
No interactions described in labeling.

VISCOAT STERILE VISCOELASTIC OPHTHALMIC
(Sodium Chrondroitin Sulfate, Sodium Hyaluronate) .... ⊛ 235
No interactions described in labeling.

VISINE A.C. EYE DROPS
(Tetrahydrozoline Hydrochloride, Zinc Sulfate) .... ⊛ 303
No interactions described in labeling.

VISINE EXTRA EYE DROPS
(Tetrahydrozoline Hydrochloride) .. ⊛ 303
No interactions described in labeling.

VISINE EYE DROPS
(Tetrahydrozoline Hydrochloride) .. ⊛ 303
No interactions described in labeling.

VISINE L.R. EYE DROPS
(Oxymetazoline Hydrochloride) .... ⊛ 303
No interactions described in labeling.

VISKEN TABLETS
(Pindolol) 2036
May interact with general anesthetics, insulin, oral hypoglycemic agents, catecholamine depleting drugs, and certain other agents. Compounds in these categories include:

Chlorpropamide (Altered dosage requirements). Products include:
- Diabinese Tablets 1775

Deserpidine (Additive effect). Products include:
- Enduronyl 518
- Harmonyl Tablets 528
- Oreticyl 545

Enflurane (Risks of general anesthesia increased). Products include:
- Ethrane 599

Glipizide (Altered dosage requirements). Products include:
- Glucotrol 1952

Glyburide (Altered dosage requirements). Products include:
- DiaBeta 1091
- Micronase Tablets 2350

Insulin, Human (Altered insulin requirements).
No products indexed under this heading.

Insulin, Human Isophane Suspension (Altered insulin requirements). Products include:
- Humulin N, 100 Units 1270

Insulin, Human NPH (Altered insulin requirements). Products include:
- Insulatard NPH Human 1627
- Novolin N 1627
- Novolin N PenFill Cartridges 1628
- Novolin N Prefilled 1628

Insulin, Human Regular (Altered insulin requirements). Products include:
- Humulin BR, 100 Units 1268
- Humulin R, 100 Units 1272
- Novolin R 1627
- Novolin R PenFill Cartridges 1628
- Novolin R Prefilled 1629
- Velosulin Human 1628

Insulin, Human, Zinc Suspension (Altered insulin requirements). Products include:
- Humulin L, 100 Units 1268
- Humulin U, 100 Units 1272
- Novolin L 1627

Insulin, NPH (Altered insulin requirements). Products include:
- NPH, 40 & 100 Units 1273
- Beef NPH, 100 Units 1274
- Pork NPH, 100 Units 1275
- Insulatard NPH 1626
- NPH Insulin 1626
- NPH Purified Pork Isophane Insulin 1626

Insulin, Regular (Altered insulin requirements). Products include:
- Regular, 40 & 100 Units 1273
- Beef Regular, 100 Units 1275
- Pork Regular, 100 Units 1275
- Pork Regular (Concentrated), 500 Units 1276
- Regular Insulin 1625
- Regular Purified Pork Insulin 1626
- Velosulin 1627

Insulin, Zinc Crystals (Altered insulin requirements). Products include:
- NPH, 40 & 100 Units 1273

Insulin, Zinc Suspension (Altered insulin requirements). Products include:
- Lente, 40 & 100 Units 1272
- Protamine, Zinc, 40 & 100 Units 1273
- Lente Iletin I 1272
- Beef Lente, 100 Units 1274
- Beef Protamine Zinc, 100 Units 1274
- Pork Lente, 100 Units 1275
- Pork, Protamine, Zinc, 100 Units 1275
- Lente Insulin 1626
- Lente Purified Pork Insulin 1626
- Semilente Insulin 1625
- Ultralente Insulin 1626

Isoflurane (Risks of general anesthesia increased). Products include:
- Forane 600

Ketamine Hydrochloride (Risks of general anesthesia increased). Products include:
- Ketalar 1726

Methohexital Sodium (Risks of general anesthesia increased). Products include:
- Brevital Sodium Vials 1248

Methoxyflurane (Risks of general anesthesia increased).
No products indexed under this heading.

Propofol (Risks of general anesthesia increased). Products include:
- Diprivan Injection 2267

Rauwolfia Serpentina (Additive effect). Products include:
- Raudixin Tablets 1803
- Rauzide Tablets 1804

Rescinnamine (Additive effect).
No products indexed under this heading.

Reserpine (Additive effect). Products include:
- Diupres Tablets 1461
- Hydromox R Tablets 1209
- Hydropres Tablets 1485
- Renese-R Tablets 1786
- Salutensin/Salutensin-Demi 719
- Ser-Ap-Es Tablets 881
- Serpasil Tablets 883
- Serpasil-Apresoline Tablets 884
- Serpasil-Esidrix Tablets 886

Thioridazine Hydrochloride (Increased serum levels of both drugs). Products include:
- Mellaril 2011

Tolazamide (Altered dosage requirements). Products include:
- Tolinase Tablets 2365

Tolbutamide (Altered dosage requirements). Products include:
- Orinase Tablets 2354

VISTARIL CAPSULES
(Hydroxyzine Pamoate) 1789
May interact with barbiturates, preanesthetic medications, narcotic analgesics, central nervous system depressants, hypnotics and sedatives, benzodiazepines, and certain other agents. Compounds in these categories include:

Alcohol (Increased effect of alcohol).

Alfentanil Hydrochloride (Potentiation of narcotics). Products include:
- Alfenta Injection 1131

Alprazolam (Potentiation of CNS depression). Products include:
- Xanax Tablets 2367

Aprobarbital (Potentiation of barbiturates). Products include:
- Alurate Elixir 1883

Buprenorphine (Potentiation of narcotics).
No products indexed under this heading.

Buspirone Hydrochloride (Potentiation of CNS depression). Products include:
- BuSpar 1401

Butabarbital (Potentiation of barbiturates). Products include:
- Pyridium Plus 1764

Butalbital (Potentiation of barbiturates). Products include:
- Esgic-Plus Tablets 1002
- Esgic Tablets & Capsules 1001
- Fioricet Tablets 2006
- Fiorinal Capsules 2007
- Fiorinal with Codeine Capsules 2008
- Fiorinal Tablets 2007
- Phrenilin 838
- Sedapap Tablets 50 mg/650 mg .. 1360

Chlordiazepoxide (Potentiation of CNS depression). Products include:
- Libritabs Tablets 1930
- Limbitrol 1933
- Menrium Tablets 1934

Chlordiazepoxide Hydrochloride (Potentiation of CNS depression). Products include:
- Librax Capsules 1929
- Librium Capsules 1931
- Librium Injectable 1932

Chlorpromazine (Potentiation of CNS depression). Products include:
- Thorazine 2234

Chlorprothixene (Potentiation of CNS depression). Products include:
- Taractan Tablets 1920

Chlorprothixene Hydrochloride (Potentiation of CNS depression). Products include:
- Taractan 1920

Chlorprothixene Lactate (Potentiation of CNS depression). Products include:
- Taractan Concentrate 1920

Clorazepate Dipotassium (Potentiation of CNS depression). Products include:
- Tranxene 556

Codeine (Potentiation of CNS depression). Products include:
- Calcidrine Syrup 506

Codeine Phosphate (Potentiation of narcotics). Products include:
- Actifed with Codeine Cough Syrup .. 752
- Cheracol Cough Syrup 1853
- Codimal PH Syrup 846
- Dimetane-DC Cough Syrup 1857
- Empirin with Codeine Phosphate Nos. 2, 3 & 4 764
- Fiorinal with Codeine Capsules 2008
- Isoclor Expectorant 982
- Naldecon CX Adult Liquid .... ▣ 521
- Novahistine DH 1342
- Novahistine Expectorant 1343
- Nucofed Capsules 2219
- Nucofed Expectorant 2219
- Nucofed Pediatric Expectorant 2220
- Nucofed Syrup 2219
- Phenaphen with Codeine Capsules 1865
- Phenaphen-650 with Codeine Tablets 1866
- Phenergan with Codeine 2497
- Phenergan VC with Codeine 2501
- Robitussin A-C Syrup 1875

Robitussin-DAC Syrup 1875
Ryna .... ⊞ 741
Soma Compound w/Codeine Tablets 2390
Triaminic Expectorant w/Codeine .. 1996
Tussi-Organidin Liquid 2391
Tylenol with Codeine 1381

Codeine Polistirex (Potentiation of narcotics).
No products indexed under this heading.

Dezocine (Potentiation of narcotics).

Diazepam (Potentiation of CNS depression). Products include:
Valium Injectable 1937
Valium Tablets 1939
Valrelease Capsules 1923

Droperidol (Potentiation of CNS depression). Products include:
Inapsine Injection 1140
Innovar Injection 1141

Enflurane (Potentiation of CNS depression). Products include:
Ethrane 599

Epinephrine (Pressor action counteracted). Products include:
Ana-Kit Anaphylaxis Emergency Treatment Kit 1100
Bronkaid Mist .... ⊞ 757
EpiPen 843
Marcaine Hydrochloride 0.5% with Epinephrine 1:200,000 (as bitartrate) 958
Marcaine Hydrochloride with Epinephrine 1:200,000 2055
Primatene Mist 2420
Sus-Phrine Injection 1006
Xylocaine with Epinephrine Injections 637

Estazolam (Potentiation of CNS depression). Products include:
ProSom Tablets 554

Ethchlorvynol (Potentiation of CNS depression). Products include:
Placidyl Capsules 553

Ethinamate (Potentiation of CNS depression).
No products indexed under this heading.

Fentanyl (Potentiation of narcotics). Products include:
Duragesic Transdermal System 1133

Fentanyl Citrate (Potentiation of narcotics). Products include:
Innovar Injection 1141
Sublimaze Injection 1146

Fluphenazine Decanoate (Potentiation of CNS depression). Products include:
Prolixin Decanoate 1795

Fluphenazine Enanthate (Potentiation of CNS depression). Products include:
Prolixin Enanthate 1796

Fluphenazine Hydrochloride (Potentiation of CNS depression). Products include:
Prolixin Elixir 1793
Prolixin Injection 1791
Prolixin Oral Concentrate 1792
Prolixin Tablets 1793

Flurazepam Hydrochloride (Potentiation of CNS depression). Products include:
Dalmane Capsules 1927

Glutethimide (Potentiation of CNS depression).
No products indexed under this heading.

Haloperidol (Potentiation of CNS depression). Products include:
Haldol Injection, Tablets and Concentrate 1373

Haloperidol Decanoate (Potentiation of CNS depression). Products include:
Haldol Decanoate 1375

Hydrocodone Bitartrate (Potentiation of narcotics). Products include:
Anexsia 5/500 Tablets 2196
Anexsia 7.5/650 Tablets 2197
Azdone Tablets 844
Codiclear DH Syrup 845
Codimal DH Syrup 846
Damason-P 1356
Hycodan Syrup, Tablets 927
Hycomine Compound Tablets 929
Hycomine Syrup 927
Hycotuss Expectorant Syrup 930
Hydrocet Capsules 835
Lortab ASA Tablets 2414
Lortab 2412
Ru-Tuss with Hydrocodone 694
Triaminic Expectorant DH 1995
Vicodin Tablets 1187
Vicodin ES Tablets 1189
Zydone Capsules 941

Hydrocodone Polistirex (Potentiation of narcotics). Products include:
Tussionex Extended-Release Suspension 988

Hydroxyzine Hydrochloride (Potentiation of narcotics). Products include:
Atarax Tablets & Syrup 1941
Marax Tablets & DF Syrup 1954
Vistaril Intramuscular Solution 1970

Isoflurane (Potentiation of CNS depression). Products include:
Forane 600

Ketamine Hydrochloride (Potentiation of CNS depression). Products include:
Ketalar 1726

Levorphanol Tartrate (Potentiation of narcotics). Products include:
Levo-Dromoran 1906

Lorazepam (Potentiation of CNS depression). Products include:
Ativan Injection 2432
Ativan Tablets 2434

Loxapine Hydrochloride (Potentiation of CNS depression). Products include:
Loxitane 1213

Loxapine Succinate (Potentiation of CNS depression). Products include:
Loxitane Capsules 1213

Meperidine Hydrochloride (Potentiation of meperidine). Products include:
Demerol 2047
Mepergan Injection 2479

Mephobarbital (Potentiation of barbiturates). Products include:
Mebaral Tablets 2061

Meprobamate (Potentiation of CNS depression). Products include:
Deprol Tablets 2382
Equagesic Tablets 2451
Miltown Tablets 2386
PMB 200 and PMB 400 2504

Mesoridazine (Potentiation of CNS depression). Products include:
Serentil 686

Methadone Hydrochloride (Potentiation of narcotics). Products include:
Dolophine Hydrochloride Ampoules & Vials 1260
Dolophine Hydrochloride Tablets 1261
Methadone Hydrochloride Diskets .. 1284
Methadone Hydrochloride Oral Solution & Tablets 1987

Methohexital Sodium (Potentiation of CNS depression). Products include:
Brevital Sodium Vials 1248

Methoxyflurane (Potentiation of CNS depression).
No products indexed under this heading.

Midazolam Hydrochloride (Potentiation of CNS depression). Products include:
Versed Injection 1924

Molindone Hydrochloride (Potentiation of CNS depression). Products include:
Moban Tablets & Concentrate 932

Morphine Sulfate (Potentiation of narcotics). Products include:
Astramorph/PF Injection, USP (Preservative-Free) 618
Duramorph 960
Infumorph 200 and Infumorph 500 Sterile Solutions 962
MS Contin Tablets 1814
MSIR 1817
Oramorph SR (Morphine Sulfate Sustained Release Tablets) 1988
Roxanol 1991

Opium Alkaloids (Potentiation of narcotics). Products include:
B & O No. 15A & No. 16A Supprettes 2395
Pantopon Injectable 1911

Oxazepam (Potentiation of CNS depression). Products include:
Serax Capsules 2522
Serax Tablets 2522

Oxycodone Hydrochloride (Potentiation of narcotics). Products include:
Percocet Tablets 950
Percodan 951
Roxicodone Tablets, Oral Solution & Intensol (Oxycodone) 1992
Tylox Capsules 1382

Pentobarbital Sodium (Potentiation of barbiturates). Products include:
Nembutal Sodium Capsules 534
Nembutal Sodium Solution 536
Nembutal Sodium Suppositories 538

Perphenazine (Potentiation of CNS depression). Products include:
Etrafon 2087
Triavil Tablets 1556
Trilafon 2123

Phenobarbital (Potentiation of barbiturates). Products include:
Arco-Lase Plus Tablets 607
Bellergal-S Tablets 1998
Bronkolixir .... ⊞ 761
Bronkotabs Tablets .... ⊞ 762
Donnatal 1858
Donnatal Extentabs 1859
Donnatal Tablets 1858
Donnazyme Tablets 1860
Kinesed Tablets 2272
Phenobarbital Elixir and Tablets 1293
Primatene Tablets-P Formula 2421
Quadrinal Tablets 1183
Tedral SA 1765

Prazepam (Potentiation of CNS depression). Products include:
Centrax 1693

Prochlorperazine (Potentiation of CNS depression). Products include:
Compazine 2201

Promethazine Hydrochloride (Potentiation of CNS depression). Products include:
Mepergan Injection 2479
Phenergan with Codeine 2497
Phenergan with Dextromethorphan 2499
Phenergan Injection 2493
Phenergan Suppositories 2496
Phenergan Syrup 2495
Phenergan Tablets 2496
Phenergan VC 2500
Phenergan VC with Codeine 2501

Propofol (Potentiation of narcotics). Products include:
Diprivan Injection 2267

Propoxyphene Hydrochloride (Potentiation of narcotics). Products include:
Darvon 1256
Wygesic Tablets 2540

Propoxyphene Napsylate (Potentiation of narcotics). Products include:
Darvon-N/Darvocet-N 1254

Quazepam (Potentiation of CNS depression). Products include:
Doral Tablets 2383

Secobarbital Sodium (Potentiation of barbiturates). Products include:
Seconal Sodium Pulvules 1296

Sufentanil Citrate (Potentiation of narcotics). Products include:
Sufenta Injection 1147

Temazepam (Potentiation of CNS depression). Products include:
Restoril Capsules 2023

Thiamylal Sodium (Potentiation of barbiturates). Products include:
Surital Ampoules, Steri-Vials 1764

Thioridazine Hydrochloride (Potentiation of CNS depression). Products include:
Mellaril 2011

Thiothixene (Potentiation of barbiturates). Products include:
Navane Capsules and Concentrate 1954
Navane Intramuscular 1956

Triazolam (Potentiation of CNS depression). Products include:
Halcion Tablets 2340

Trifluoperazine Hydrochloride (Potentiation of CNS depression). Products include:
Stelazine 2226

VISTARIL INTRAMUSCULAR SOLUTION
(Hydroxyzine Hydrochloride) 1970
May interact with central nervous system depressants, narcotic analgesics, barbiturates, and certain other agents. Compounds in these categories include:

Alcohol (May be potentiated).

Alfentanil Hydrochloride (May be potentiated; dosage should be decreased by up to 50%; rare potential for cardiac arrest and death). Products include:
Alfenta Injection 1131

Alprazolam (May be potentiated; dosage should be decreased by up to 50%; rare potential for cardiac arrest and death). Products include:
Xanax Tablets 2367

Aprobarbital (May be potentiated; dosage should be decreased by up to 50%; rare potential for cardiac arrest and death). Products include:
Alurate Elixir 1883

Buprenorphine (May be potentiated; dosage should be decreased by up to 50%; rare potential for cardiac arrest and death).
No products indexed under this heading.

Buspirone Hydrochloride (May be potentiated; dosage should be decreased by up to 50%; rare potential for cardiac arrest and death). Products include:
BuSpar 1401

Butabarbital (May be potentiated; dosage should be decreased by up to 50%; rare potential for cardiac arrest and death). Products include:
Pyridium Plus 1764

Butalbital (May be potentiated; dosage should be decreased by up to 50%; rare potential for cardiac arrest and death). Products include:
Esgic-Plus Tablets 1002
Esgic Tablets & Capsules 1001
Fioricet Tablets 2006
Fiorinal Capsules 2007

Fiorinal with Codeine Capsules 2008
Fiorinal Tablets 2007
Phrenilin 838
Sedapap Tablets 50 mg/650 mg .. 1360

Chlordiazepoxide (May be potentiated; dosage should be decreased by up to 50%; rare potential for cardiac arrest and death). Products include:
Libritabs Tablets 1930
Limbitrol 1933
Menrium Tablets 1934

Chlordiazepoxide Hydrochloride (May be potentiated; dosage should be decreased by up to 50%; rare potential for cardiac arrest and death). Products include:
Librax Capsules 1929
Librium Capsules 1931
Librium Injectable 1932

Chlorpromazine (May be potentiated; dosage should be decreased by up to 50%; rare potential for cardiac arrest and death). Products include:
Thorazine 2234

Chlorprothixene (May be potentiated; dosage should be decreased by up to 50%; rare potential for cardiac arrest and death). Products include:
Taractan Tablets 1920

Chlorprothixene Hydrochloride (May be potentiated; dosage should be decreased by up to 50%; rare potential for cardiac arrest and death). Products include:
Taractan 1920

Clorazepate Dipotassium (May be potentiated; dosage should be decreased by up to 50%; rare potential for cardiac arrest and death). Products include:
Tranxene 556

Codeine (May be potentiated; dosage should be decreased by up to 50%; rare potential for cardiac arrest and death). Products include:
Calcidrine Syrup 506

Codeine Phosphate (May be potentiated; dosage should be decreased by up to 50%; rare potential for cardiac arrest and death). Products include:
Actifed with Codeine Cough Syrup.. 752
Cheracol Cough Syrup 1853
Codimal PH Syrup 846
Dimetane-DC Cough Syrup 1857
Empirin with Codeine Phosphate Nos. 2, 3 & 4 764
Fiorinal with Codeine Capsules 2008
Isoclor Expectorant 982
Naldecon CX Adult Liquid .... ▣ 521
Novahistine DH 1342
Novahistine Expectorant 1343
Nucofed Capsules 2219
Nucofed Expectorant 2219
Nucofed Pediatric Expectorant 2220
Nucofed Syrup 2219
Phenaphen with Codeine Capsules 1865
Phenaphen-650 with Codeine Tablets 1866
Phenergan with Codeine 2497
Phenergan VC with Codeine 2501
Robitussin A-C Syrup 1875
Robitussin-DAC Syrup 1875
Ryna .... ▣ 741
Soma Compound w/Codeine Tablets 2390
Triaminic Expectorant w/Codeine .. 1996
Tussi-Organidin Liquid 2391
Tylenol with Codeine 1381

Codeine Polistirex (May be potentiated; dosage should be decreased by up to 50%; rare potential for cardiac arrest and death).
No products indexed under this heading.

Dezocine (May be potentiated; dosage should be decreased by up to 50%; rare potential for cardiac arrest and death).

Diazepam (May be potentiated; dosage should be decreased by up to 50%; rare potential for cardiac arrest and death). Products include:
Valium Injectable 1937
Valium Tablets 1939
Valrelease Capsules 1923

Droperidol (May be potentiated; dosage should be decreased by up to 50%; rare potential for cardiac arrest and death). Products include:
Inapsine Injection 1140
Innovar Injection 1141

Enflurane (May be potentiated; dosage should be decreased by up to 50%; rare potential for cardiac arrest and death). Products include:
Ethrane 599

Estazolam (May be potentiated; dosage should be decreased by up to 50%; rare potential for cardiac arrest and death). Products include:
ProSom Tablets 554

Ethchlorvynol (May be potentiated; dosage should be decreased by up to 50%; rare potential for cardiac arrest and death). Products include:
Placidyl Capsules 553

Ethinamate (May be potentiated; dosage should be decreased by up to 50%; rare potential for cardiac arrest and death).
No products indexed under this heading.

Fentanyl (May be potentiated; dosage should be decreased by up to 50%; rare potential for cardiac arrest and death). Products include:
Duragesic Transdermal System 1133

Fentanyl Citrate (May be potentiated; dosage should be decreased by up to 50%; rare potential for cardiac arrest and death). Products include:
Innovar Injection 1141
Sublimaze Injection 1146

Fluphenazine Decanoate (May be potentiated; dosage should be decreased by up to 50%; rare potential for cardiac arrest and death). Products include:
Prolixin Decanoate 1795

Fluphenazine Enanthate (May be potentiated; dosage should be decreased by up to 50%; rare potential for cardiac arrest and death). Products include:
Prolixin Enanthate 1796

Fluphenazine Hydrochloride (May be potentiated; dosage should be decreased by up to 50%; rare potential for cardiac arrest and death). Products include:
Prolixin Elixir 1793
Prolixin Injection 1791
Prolixin Oral Concentrate 1792
Prolixin Tablets 1793

Flurazepam Hydrochloride (May be potentiated; dosage should be decreased by up to 50%; rare potential for cardiac arrest and death). Products include:
Dalmane Capsules 1927

Glutethimide (May be potentiated; dosage should be decreased by up to 50%; rare potential for cardiac arrest and death).
No products indexed under this heading.

Haloperidol (May be potentiated; dosage should be decreased by up to 50%; rare potential for cardiac arrest and death). Products include:
Haldol Injection, Tablets and Concentrate 1373

Haloperidol Decanoate (May be potentiated; dosage should be decreased by up to 50%; rare potential for cardiac arrest and death). Products include:
Haldol Decanoate 1375

Hydrocodone Bitartrate (May be potentiated; dosage should be decreased by up to 50%; rare potential for cardiac arrest and death). Products include:
Anexsia 5/500 Tablets 2196
Anexsia 7.5/650 Tablets 2197
Azdone Tablets 844
Codiclear DH Syrup 845
Codimal DH Syrup 846
Damason-P 1356
Hycodan Syrup, Tablets 927
Hycomine Compound Tablets 929
Hycomine Syrup 927
Hycotuss Expectorant Syrup 930
Hydrocet Capsules 835
Lortab ASA Tablets 2414
Lortab 2412
Ru-Tuss with Hydrocodone 694
Triaminic Expectorant DH 1995
Vicodin Tablets 1187
Vicodin ES Tablets 1189
Zydone Capsules 941

Hydrocodone Polistirex (May be potentiated; dosage should be decreased by up to 50%; rare potential for cardiac arrest and death). Products include:
Tussionex Extended-Release Suspension 988

Isoflurane (May be potentiated; dosage should be decreased by up to 50%; rare potential for cardiac arrest and death). Products include:
Forane 600

Ketamine Hydrochloride (May be potentiated; dosage should be decreased by up to 50%; rare potential for cardiac arrest and death). Products include:
Ketalar 1726

Levorphanol Tartrate (May be potentiated; dosage should be decreased by up to 50%; rare potential for cardiac arrest and death). Products include:
Levo-Dromoran 1906

Lorazepam (May be potentiated; dosage should be decreased by up to 50%; rare potential for cardiac arrest and death). Products include:
Ativan Injection 2432
Ativan Tablets 2434

Loxapine Hydrochloride (May be potentiated; dosage should be decreased by up to 50%; rare potential for cardiac arrest and death). Products include:
Loxitane 1213

Loxapine Succinate (May be potentiated; dosage should be decreased by up to 50%; rare potential for cardiac arrest and death). Products include:
Loxitane Capsules 1213

Meperidine Hydrochloride (May be potentiated; dosage should be decreased by up to 50%; rare potential for cardiac arrest and death). Products include:
Demerol 2047
Mepergan Injection 2479

Mephobarbital (May be potentiated; dosage should be decreased by up to 50%; rare potential for cardiac arrest and death). Products include:
Mebaral Tablets 2061

Meprobamate (May be potentiated; dosage should be decreased by up to 50%; rare potential for cardiac arrest and death). Products include:
Deprol Tablets 2382
Equagesic Tablets 2451
Miltown Tablets 2386
PMB 200 and PMB 400 2504

Mesoridazine (May be potentiated; dosage should be decreased by up to 50%; rare potential for cardiac arrest and death). Products include:
Serentil 686

Methadone Hydrochloride (May be potentiated; dosage should be decreased by up to 50%; rare potential for cardiac arrest and death). Products include:
Dolophine Hydrochloride Ampoules & Vials 1260
Dolophine Hydrochloride Tablets .. 1261
Methadone Hydrochloride Diskets .. 1284
Methadone Hydrochloride Oral Solution & Tablets 1987

Methohexital Sodium (May be potentiated; dosage should be decreased by up to 50%; rare potential for cardiac arrest and death). Products include:
Brevital Sodium Vials 1248

Methoxyflurane (May be potentiated; dosage should be decreased by up to 50%; rare potential for cardiac arrest and death).
No products indexed under this heading.

Midazolam Hydrochloride (May be potentiated; dosage should be decreased by up to 50%; rare potential for cardiac arrest and death). Products include:
Versed Injection 1924

Molindone Hydrochloride (May be potentiated; dosage should be decreased by up to 50%; rare potential for cardiac arrest and death). Products include:
Moban Tablets & Concentrate 932

Morphine Sulfate (May be potentiated; dosage should be decreased by up to 50%; rare potential for cardiac arrest and death). Products include:
Astramorph/PF Injection, USP (Preservative-Free) 618
Duramorph 960
Infumorph 200 and Infumorph 500 Sterile Solutions 962
MS Contin Tablets 1814
MSIR 1817
Oramorph SR (Morphine Sulfate Sustained Release Tablets) 1988
Roxanol 1991

Opium Alkaloids (May be potentiated; dosage should be decreased by up to 50%; rare potential for cardiac arrest and death). Products include:
B & O No. 15A & No. 16A Supprettes 2395
Pantopon Injectable 1911

Oxazepam (May be potentiated; dosage should be decreased by up to 50%; rare potential for cardiac arrest and death). Products include:
Serax Capsules 2522
Serax Tablets 2522

Oxycodone Hydrochloride (May be potentiated; dosage should be decreased by up to 50%; rare potential for cardiac arrest and death). Products include:
Percocet Tablets 950
Percodan 951
Roxicodone Tablets, Oral Solution & Intensol (Oxycodone) 1992
Tylox Capsules 1382

Pentobarbital Sodium (May be potentiated; dosage should be decreased by up to 50%; rare potential for cardiac arrest and death). Products include:
Nembutal Sodium Capsules 534
Nembutal Sodium Solution 536
Nembutal Sodium Suppositories 538

Perphenazine (May be potentiated; dosage should be decreased by up to 50%; rare potential for cardiac arrest and death). Products include:
Etrafon 2087
Triavil Tablets 1556
Trilafon 2123

Phenobarbital (May be potentiated; dosage should be decreased by up to 50%; rare potential for cardiac arrest and death). Products include:
Arco-Lase Plus Tablets 607
Bellergal-S Tablets 1998
Bronkolixir .... ▣ 761
Bronkotabs Tablets .... ▣ 762
Donnatal 1858
Donnatal Extentabs 1859
Donnatal Tablets 1858
Donnazyme Tablets 1860
Kinesed Tablets 2272
Phenobarbital Elixir and Tablets 1293
Primatene Tablets-P Formula 2421
Quadrinal Tablets 1183
Tedral SA 1765

Prazepam (May be potentiated; dosage should be decreased by up to 50%; rare potential for cardiac arrest and death). Products include:
Centrax 1693

Prochlorperazine (May be potentiated; dosage should be decreased by up to 50%; rare potential for cardiac arrest and death). Products include:
Compazine 2201

Promethazine Hydrochloride (May be potentiated; dosage should be decreased by up to 50%; rare potential for cardiac arrest and death). Products include:
Mepergan Injection 2479
Phenergan with Codeine 2497
Phenergan with Dextromethorphan 2499
Phenergan Injection 2493
Phenergan Suppositories 2496
Phenergan Syrup 2495
Phenergan Tablets 2496
Phenergan VC 2500
Phenergan VC with Codeine 2501

Propofol (May be potentiated; dosage should be decreased by up to 50%; rare potential for cardiac arrest and death). Products include:
Diprivan Injection 2267

Propoxyphene Hydrochloride (May be potentiated; dosage should be decreased by up to 50%; rare potential for cardiac arrest and death). Products include:
Darvon 1256
Wygesic Tablets 2540

Propoxyphene Napsylate (May be potentiated; dosage should be decreased by up to 50%; rare potential for cardiac arrest and death). Products include:
Darvon-N/Darvocet-N 1254

Quazepam (May be potentiated; dosage should be decreased by up to 50%; rare potential for cardiac arrest and death). Products include:
Doral Tablets 2383

Secobarbital Sodium (May be potentiated; dosage should be decreased by up to 50%; rare potential for cardiac arrest and death). Products include:
Seconal Sodium Pulvules 1296

Sufentanil Citrate (May be potentiated; dosage should be decreased by up to 50%; rare potential for cardiac arrest and death). Products include:
Sufenta Injection 1147

Temazepam (May be potentiated; dosage should be decreased by up to 50%; rare potential for cardiac arrest and death). Products include:
Restoril Capsules 2023

Thiamylal Sodium (May be potentiated; dosage should be decreased by up to 50%; rare potential for cardiac arrest and death). Products include:
Surital Ampoules, Steri-Vials 1764

Thioridazine Hydrochloride (May be potentiated; dosage should be decreased by up to 50%; rare potential for cardiac arrest and death). Products include:
Mellaril 2011

Thiothixene (May be potentiated; dosage should be decreased by up to 50%; rare potential for cardiac arrest and death). Products include:
Navane Capsules and Concentrate 1954
Navane Intramuscular 1956

Triazolam (May be potentiated; dosage should be decreased by up to 50%; rare potential for cardiac arrest and death). Products include:
Halcion Tablets 2340

Trifluoperazine Hydrochloride (May be potentiated; dosage should be decreased by up to 50%; rare potential for cardiac arrest and death). Products include:
Stelazine 2226

VISTARIL ORAL SUSPENSION
(Hydroxyzine Pamoate) 1789
See **Vistaril Capsules**

VITAL HIGH NITROGEN NUTRITIONALLY COMPLETE PARTIALLY HYDROLYZED DIET
(Nutritional Supplement) 1983
No interactions described in labeling.

VIVACTIL TABLETS
(Protriptyline Hydrochloride) 1567
May interact with monoamine oxidase inhibitors, thyroid preparations, para-aminobenzoic acid based local anesthetics, anticholinergics, sympathomimetic aerosol bronchodilators, neuromuscular blocking agents, barbiturates, central nervous system depressants, and certain other agents. Compounds in these categories include:

Albuterol (Close supervision and careful adjustment of dosages required). Products include:
Proventil Inhalation Aerosol 2117
Ventolin Inhalation Aerosol and Refill 583

Albuterol Sulfate (Close supervision and careful adjustment of dosages required). Products include:
Proventil Repetabs Tablets 2120
Proventil Solutions for Inhalation 0.5% and 0.083% 2118
Proventil Syrup 2119
Proventil Tablets 2120
Ventolin 583

Alcohol (Enhanced response to alcohol; potentiation).

Alfentanil Hydrochloride (Enhanced response to CNS depressants). Products include:
Alfenta Injection 1131

Alprazolam (Enhanced response to CNS depressants). Products include:
Xanax Tablets 2367

Aprobarbital (Enhanced response to barbiturates). Products include:
Alurate Elixir 1883

Atropine Sulfate (Close supervision and careful adjustment of dosages required; hyperpyrexia). Products include:
Arco-Lase Plus Tablets 607
Atropine Sulfate Sterile Ophthalmic Solution and S.O.P. Sterile Ophthalmic Ointment .... ⊙ 239
Donnagel .... ▣ 675
Donnagel-PG 1858
Donnatal 1858
Donnatal Extentabs 1859
Donnatal Tablets 1858
Donnazyme Tablets 1860
Isopto Atropine .... ⊙ 218
Lomotil 2174
Motofen Tablets 836
Ru-Tuss Tablets 693
Urised Tablets 2396

Belladonna Alkaloids (Close supervision and careful adjustment of dosages required; hyperpyrexia). Products include:
Bellergal-S Tablets 1998
Hyland's Bed Wetting Tablets .... ▣ 728
Hyland's Teething Tablets .... ▣ 728
Kinesed Tablets 2272

Benztropine Mesylate (Close supervision and careful adjustment of dosages required; hyperpyrexia). Products include:
Cogentin 1435

Biperiden (Close supervision and careful adjustment of dosages required; hyperpyrexia). Products include:
Akineton 1171

Buprenorphine (Enhanced response to CNS depressants).
No products indexed under this heading.

Buspirone Hydrochloride (Enhanced response to CNS depressants). Products include:
BuSpar 1401

Butabarbital (Enhanced response to barbiturates). Products include:
Pyridium Plus 1764

Butalbital (Enhanced response to barbiturates). Products include:
Esgic-Plus Tablets 1002
Esgic Tablets & Capsules 1001
Fioricet Tablets 2006
Fiorinal Capsules 2007
Fiorinal with Codeine Capsules 2008
Fiorinal Tablets 2007
Phrenilin 838
Sedapap Tablets 50 mg/650 mg .. 1360

Chlordiazepoxide (Enhanced response to CNS depressants). Products include:
Libritabs Tablets 1930
Limbitrol 1933
Menrium Tablets 1934

Chlordiazepoxide Hydrochloride (Enhanced response to CNS depressants). Products include:
Librax Capsules 1929
Librium Capsules 1931
Librium Injectable 1932

Chlorpromazine (Enhanced response to CNS depressants; hyperpyrexia). Products include:
Thorazine 2234

Chlorprothixene (Enhanced response to CNS depressants). Products include:
Taractan Tablets 1920

Chlorprothixene Hydrochloride (Enhanced response to CNS depressants). Products include:
Taractan 1920

Cimetidine (Increased frequency and severity of side effects, particularly anticholinergic). Products include:
Tagamet Tablets 2228

Cimetidine Hydrochloride (Increased frequency and severity of side effects, particularly anticholinergic). Products include:
Tagamet 2228

Clidinium Bromide (Close supervision and careful adjustment of dosages required; hyperpyrexia). Products include:
Librax Capsules 1929
Quarzan Capsules 1937

Clorazepate Dipotassium (Enhanced response to CNS depressants). Products include:
Tranxene 556

Clozapine (Enhanced response to CNS depressants). Products include:
Clozaril Tablets 2000

Codeine (Enhanced response to CNS depressants). Products include:
Calcidrine Syrup 506

Codeine Phosphate (Enhanced response to CNS depressants). Products include:
Actifed with Codeine Cough Syrup.. 752
Cheracol Cough Syrup 1853
Codimal PH Syrup 846
Dimetane-DC Cough Syrup 1857
Empirin with Codeine Phosphate Nos. 2, 3 & 4 764
Fiorinal with Codeine Capsules 2008
Isoclor Expectorant 982
Naldecon CX Adult Liquid .... ▣ 521
Novahistine DH 1342
Novahistine Expectorant 1343
Nucofed Capsules 2219
Nucofed Expectorant 2219
Nucofed Pediatric Expectorant 2220
Nucofed Syrup 2219
Phenaphen with Codeine Capsules 1865
Phenaphen-650 with Codeine Tablets 1866
Phenergan with Codeine 2497
Phenergan VC with Codeine 2501
Robitussin A-C Syrup 1875
Robitussin-DAC Syrup 1875
Ryna .... ▣ 741
Soma Compound w/Codeine Tablets 2390
Triaminic Expectorant w/Codeine .. 1996
Tussi-Organidin Liquid 2391
Tylenol with Codeine 1381

Codeine Polistirex (Enhanced response to CNS depressants).
No products indexed under this heading.

Deserpidine (Antihypertensive effects blocked). Products include:
Enduronyl 518
Harmonyl Tablets 528
Oreticyl 545

Dezocine (Enhanced response to CNS depressants).

Diazepam (Enhanced response to CNS depressants). Products include:
Valium Injectable 1937
Valium Tablets 1939
Valrelease Capsules 1923

Dicyclomine Hydrochloride (Close supervision and careful adjustment of dosages required; hyperpyrexia). Products include:
Bentyl 1322

Dobutamine Hydrochloride (Close supervision and careful adjustment of dosages required). Products include:
Dobutrex Solution Vials 1259

Dopamine Hydrochloride (Close supervision and careful adjustment of dosages required). Products include:
Intropin Injection 930

Droperidol (Enhanced response to CNS depressants). Products include:
Inapsine Injection 1140
Innovar Injection 1141

Enflurane (Enhanced response to CNS depressants). Products include:
Ethrane 599

Ephedrine Hydrochloride (Close supervision and careful adjustment of dosages required). Products include:
Amesec .... ▣ 682
Primatene Tablets-M Formula 2421
Primatene Tablets-P Formula 2421
Primatene Tablets-Regular Formula 2421
Quadrinal Tablets 1183
Quelidrine Syrup 556
Tedral SA 1765

Ephedrine Sulfate (Close supervision and careful adjustment of dosages required). Products include:
- Bronkaid Tablets ▣ 757
- Bronkolixir ▣ 761
- Bronkotabs Tablets ▣ 762
- Marax Tablets & DF Syrup 1954
- Pazo Hemorrhoid Ointment & Suppositories 752
- Vicks Vatronol Nose Drops ▣ 666

Ephedrine Tannate (Close supervision and careful adjustment of dosages required). Products include:
- Rynatuss 2388

Epinephrine (Close supervision and careful adjustment of dosages required). Products include:
- Ana-Kit Anaphylaxis Emergency Treatment Kit 1100
- Bronkaid Mist ▣ 757
- EpiPen 843
- Marcaine Hydrochloride 0.5% with Epinephrine 1:200,000 (as bitartrate) 958
- Marcaine Hydrochloride with Epinephrine 1:200,000 2055
- Primatene Mist 2420
- Sus-Phrine Injection 1006
- Xylocaine with Epinephrine Injections 637

Epinephrine Bitartrate (Close supervision and careful adjustment of dosages required). Products include:
- AsthmaHaler Mist Epinephrine Bitartrate Bronchodilator ▣ 616
- Bronkaid Mist Suspension ▣ 757
- Primatene Mist Suspension 2421

Epinephrine Hydrochloride (Close supervision and careful adjustment of dosages required). Products include:
- Adrenalin Chloride Solution 1:100 & 1:1,000 1689
- Epifrin ⊙ 244
- Glaucon ⊙ 218

Estazolam (Enhanced response to CNS depressants). Products include:
- ProSom Tablets 554

Ethchlorvynol (Enhanced response to CNS depressants). Products include:
- Placidyl Capsules 553

Ethinamate (Enhanced response to CNS depressants).
- No products indexed under this heading.

Ethopropazine Hydrochloride (Close supervision and careful adjustment of dosages required; hyperpyrexia).

Fentanyl (Enhanced response to CNS depressants). Products include:
- Duragesic Transdermal System 1133

Fentanyl Citrate (Enhanced response to CNS depressants). Products include:
- Innovar Injection 1141
- Sublimaze Injection 1146

Fluphenazine Decanoate (Enhanced response to CNS depressants; hyperpyrexia). Products include:
- Prolixin Decanoate 1795

Fluphenazine Enanthate (Enhanced response to CNS depressants; hyperpyrexia). Products include:
- Prolixin Enanthate 1796

Fluphenazine Hydrochloride (Enhanced response to CNS depressants; hyperpyrexia). Products include:
- Prolixin Elixir 1793
- Prolixin Injection 1791
- Prolixin Oral Concentrate 1792
- Prolixin Tablets 1793

Flurazepam Hydrochloride (Enhanced response to CNS depressants). Products include:
- Dalmane Capsules 1927

Furazolidone (Contraindication; hyperpyretic crises; severe convulsions; death). Products include:
- Furoxone 1855

Glutethimide (Enhanced response to CNS depressants).
- No products indexed under this heading.

Glycopyrrolate (Close supervision and careful adjustment of dosages required; hyperpyrexia). Products include:
- Robinul Forte Tablets 1873
- Robinul Injectable 1873
- Robinul Tablets 1873

Guanethidine Monosulfate (Antihypertensive effects of guanethidine blocked). Products include:
- Esimil Tablets 864
- Ismelin Tablets 869

Haloperidol (Enhanced response to CNS depressants; hyperpyrexia). Products include:
- Haldol Injection, Tablets and Concentrate 1373

Haloperidol Decanoate (Enhanced response to CNS depressants; hyperpyrexia). Products include:
- Haldol Decanoate 1375

Hydrocodone Bitartrate (Enhanced response to CNS depressants). Products include:
- Anexsia 5/500 Tablets 2196
- Anexsia 7.5/650 Tablets 2197
- Azdone Tablets 844
- Codiclear DH Syrup 845
- Codimal DH Syrup 846
- Damason-P 1356
- Hycodan Syrup, Tablets 927
- Hycomine Compound Tablets 929
- Hycomine Syrup 927
- Hycotuss Expectorant Syrup 930
- Hydrocet Capsules 835
- Lortab ASA Tablets 2414
- Lortab 2412
- Ru-Tuss with Hydrocodone 694
- Triaminic Expectorant DH 1995
- Vicodin Tablets 1187
- Vicodin ES Tablets 1189
- Zydone Capsules 941

Hydrocodone Polistirex (Enhanced response to CNS depressants). Products include:
- Tussionex Extended-Release Suspension 988

Hydroxyzine Hydrochloride (Enhanced response to CNS depressants). Products include:
- Atarax Tablets & Syrup 1941
- Marax Tablets & DF Syrup 1954
- Vistaril Intramuscular Solution 1970

Hyoscyamine (Close supervision and careful adjustment of dosages required; hyperpyrexia). Products include:
- Cystospaz Tablets 2395
- Urised Tablets 2396

Hyoscyamine Sulfate (Close supervision and careful adjustment of dosages required; hyperpyrexia). Products include:
- Arco-Lase Plus Tablets 607
- Cystospaz-M Capsules 2395
- Donnagel ▣ 675
- Donnagel-PG 1858
- Donnatal 1858
- Donnatal Extentabs 1859
- Donnatal Tablets 1858
- Donnazyme Tablets 1860
- Kutrase Capsules 2146
- Levsin/Levsinex 2147
- Ru-Tuss Tablets 693

Ipratropium Bromide (Close supervision and careful adjustment of dosages required; hyperpyrexia). Products include:
- Atrovent Inhalation Aerosol 675

Isocarboxazid (Contraindication; hyperpyretic crises; severe convulsions; death). Products include:
- Marplan Tablets 1906

Isoflurane (Enhanced response to CNS depressants). Products include:
- Forane 600

Isoproterenol Hydrochloride (Close supervision and careful adjustment of dosages required). Products include:
- Isuprel Hydrochloride Injection 1:5000 2050
- Isuprel Hydrochloride Mistometer 2051
- Isuprel Hydrochloride Solution 1:200 & 1:100 2052
- Norisodrine Aerotrol 540

Ketamine Hydrochloride (Enhanced response to CNS depressants). Products include:
- Ketalar 1726

Levorphanol Tartrate (Enhanced response to CNS depressants). Products include:
- Levo-Dromoran 1906

Levothyroxine Sodium (Arrhythmias). Products include:
- Levothroid Tablets 1003
- Levoxine Tablets 904
- Synthroid 695

Liothyronine Sodium (Arrhythmias). Products include:
- Cytomel Tablets 2203

Liotrix (Arrhythmias). Products include:
- Euthroid 1724

Lithium Carbonate (Hyperpyrexia). Products include:
- Eskalith 2214
- Lithane Tablets 1596
- Lithium Carbonate Capsules & Tablets 1984
- Lithobid Tablets 870

Lithium Citrate (Hyperpyrexia). Products include:
- Cibalith-S 870

Lorazepam (Enhanced response to CNS depressants). Products include:
- Ativan Injection 2432
- Ativan Tablets 2434

Loxapine Hydrochloride (Enhanced response to CNS depressants; hyperpyrexia). Products include:
- Loxitane 1213

Loxapine Succinate (Enhanced response to CNS depressants). Products include:
- Loxitane Capsules 1213

Mepenzolate Bromide (Close supervision and careful adjustment of dosages required; hyperpyrexia). Products include:
- Cantil Tablets 1326

Meperidine Hydrochloride (Enhanced response to CNS depressants). Products include:
- Demerol 2047
- Mepergan Injection 2479

Mephobarbital (Enhanced response to barbiturates). Products include:
- Mebaral Tablets 2061

Meprobamate (Enhanced response to CNS depressants). Products include:
- Deprol Tablets 2382
- Equagesic Tablets 2451
- Miltown Tablets 2386
- PMB 200 and PMB 400 2504

Mesoridazine (Enhanced response to CNS depressants; hyperpyrexia). Products include:
- Serentil 686

Metaproterenol Sulfate (Close supervision and careful adjustment of dosages required). Products include:
- Alupent 674
- Arm-a-Med Metaproterenol Sulfate Inhalation Solution, USP 617
- Metaprel Inhalation Aerosol Bronchodilator 2014
- Metaprel Inhalation Solution 2015
- Metaprel 2015
- Metaproterenol Sulfate Inhalation Solution, USP 912

Metaraminol Bitartrate (Close supervision and careful adjustment of dosages required). Products include:
- Aramine Injection 1424

Methadone Hydrochloride (Enhanced response to CNS depressants). Products include:
- Dolophine Hydrochloride Ampoules & Vials 1260
- Dolophine Hydrochloride Tablets 1261
- Methadone Hydrochloride Diskets 1284
- Methadone Hydrochloride Oral Solution & Tablets 1987

Methohexital Sodium (Enhanced response to CNS depressants). Products include:
- Brevital Sodium Vials 1248

Methoxamine Hydrochloride (Close supervision and careful adjustment of dosages required). Products include:
- Vasoxyl Injection 819

Methoxyflurane (Enhanced response to CNS depressants).
- No products indexed under this heading.

Midazolam Hydrochloride (Enhanced response to CNS depressants). Products include:
- Versed Injection 1924

Molindone Hydrochloride (Enhanced response to CNS depressants; hyperpyrexia). Products include:
- Moban Tablets & Concentrate 932

Morphine Sulfate (Enhanced response to CNS depressants). Products include:
- Astramorph/PF Injection, USP (Preservative-Free) 618
- Duramorph 960
- Infumorph 200 and Infumorph 500 Sterile Solutions 962
- MS Contin Tablets 1814
- MSIR 1817
- Oramorph SR (Morphine Sulfate Sustained Release Tablets) 1988
- Roxanol 1991

Norepinephrine Bitartrate (Close supervision and careful adjustment of dosages required). Products include:
- Levophed Bitartrate Injection 2054

Opium Alkaloids (Enhanced response to CNS depressants). Products include:
- B & O No. 15A & No. 16A Supprettes 2395
- Pantopon Injectable 1911

Oxazepam (Enhanced response to CNS depressants). Products include:
- Serax Capsules 2522
- Serax Tablets 2522

Oxybutynin Chloride (Close supervision and careful adjustment of dosages required; hyperpyrexia). Products include:
- Ditropan 1332

Oxycodone Hydrochloride (Enhanced response to CNS depressants). Products include:
- Percocet Tablets 950
- Percodan 951
- Roxicodone Tablets, Oral Solution & Intensol (Oxycodone) 1992
- Tylox Capsules 1382

Pentobarbital Sodium (Enhanced response to barbiturates). Products include:
- Nembutal Sodium Capsules 534
- Nembutal Sodium Solution 536
- Nembutal Sodium Suppositories 538

Perphenazine (Enhanced response to CNS depressants; hyperpyrexia). Products include:
- Etrafon 2087

(▣ Described in PDR For Nonprescription Drugs)

(⊙ Described in PDR For Ophthalmology)

Triavil Tablets ... 1556
Trilafon ... 2123

Phenelzine Sulfate (Contraindication; hyperpyretic crises; severe convulsions; death). Products include:
Nardil ... 1742

Phenobarbital (Enhanced response to barbiturates). Products include:
Arco-Lase Plus Tablets ... 607
Bellergal-S Tablets ... 1998
Bronkolixir ... ▣ 761
Bronkotabs Tablets ... ▣ 762
Donnatal ... 1858
Donnatal Extentabs ... 1859
Donnatal Tablets ... 1858
Donnazyme Tablets ... 1860
Kinesed Tablets ... 2272
Phenobarbital Elixir and Tablets ... 1293
Primatene Tablets-P Formula ... 2421
Quadrinal Tablets ... 1183
Tedral SA ... 1765

Phenylephrine Bitartrate (Close supervision and careful adjustment of dosages required).
No products indexed under this heading.

Phenylephrine Hydrochloride (Close supervision and careful adjustment of dosages required). Products include:
AK-Dilate Solution 2.5% and 10% ... ⊙ 203
Atrohist Sprinkle Capsules ... 558
Cerose-DM ... 2443
Codimal ... 846
Comhist LA Capsules ... 1618
Congespirin For Children Aspirin Free Chewable Cold Tablets ... 748
Cyclomydril ... ⊙ 216
Deconsal Sprinkle Capsules ... 559
Dimetane Decongestant ... ▣ 673
Dristan Decongestant/Antihistamine/ Analgesic Coated Caplets ... ▣ 749
Dristan Cold Nasal Decongestant/ Antihistamine/ Analgesic Coated Tablets ... 2419
Dristan Advanced Formula Decongestant/Antihistamine/ Analgesic Tablets ... ▣ 749
Dristan Nasal Spray, Menthol ... 2419
Dristan Nasal Spray, Regular and Regular with Metered Pump ... 2419
Entex Capsules ... 1623
Entex Liquid ... 1623
Sinus Excedrin Analgesic, Decongestant Tablets & Caplets ... 750
Extendryl ... 994
4-Way Fast Acting Nasal Spray - Original Formula (regular & mentholated) & Metered Spray Pump (regular) ... 751
Hycomine Compound Tablets ... 929
Murocoll-2 Sterile Ophthalmic Solution ... ⊙ 261
Mydfrin 2.5% ... ⊙ 224
Naldecon Syrup, Tablets, Pediatric Drops and Pediatric Syrup ... 709
Neo-Synephrine Hydrochloride 1% Carpuject ... 2063
Neo-Synephrine Hydrochloride 1% Injection ... 2063
Neo-Synephrine Hydrochloride (Ophthalmic) ... 2064
Neo-Synephrine ... ▣ 759
Nôstril Nasal Decongestant ... ▣ 520
Novahistine Elixir ... ▣ 596
Phenergan VC ... 2500
Phenergan VC with Codeine ... 2501
Prefrin Liquifilm Vasoconstrictor and Lubricant Eye Drops ... ⊙ 254
Prefrin-A ... ⊙ 255
Quelidrine Syrup ... 556
Relief Vasoconstrictor and Lubricant Eye Drops ... ⊙ 256
Robitussin Night Relief ... ▣ 677
Ru-Tuss with Hydrocodone ... 694
Ru-Tuss Tablets ... 693
Vasosulf ... ⊙ 279
Vicks Sinex ... ▣ 665
Zincfrin ... ⊙ 230

Phenylephrine Tannate (Close supervision and careful adjustment of dosages required). Products include:
Rynatan ... 2387
Rynatuss ... 2388

Phenylpropanolamine Hydrochloride (Close supervision and careful adjustment of dosages required). Products include:
A.R.M. Allergy Relief Medicine Caplets ... ▣ 615
Acutrim ... ▣ 548
Allerest ... ▣ 559
BC Cold Powder ... ▣ 517
Cheracol Plus Head Cold/Cough Formula ... ▣ 667
Codimal Expectorant ... 846
Comtrex Multi-Symptom Cold Reliever Tablets/Caplets/Liqui-Gels/Liquid ... 745
Contac Continuous Action Decongestant/Antihistamine Capsules ▣ 710
Contac Maximum Strength Continuous Action Decongestant/ Antihistamine Caplets ... ▣ 709
Contac Severe Cold and Flu Formula Caplets ... ▣ 711
Coricidin 'D' Decongestant Tablets ... ▣ 695
Coricidin Demilets Tablets for Children ... ▣ 696
Demazin Nasal Decongestant/ Antihistamine Repetabs Tablets & Syrup ... ▣ 697
Dexatrim ... ▣ 733
Dimetane-DC Cough Syrup ... 1857
Dimetapp Elixir ... ▣ 673
Dimetapp DM Elixir ... ▣ 674
Dimetapp Extentabs ... ▣ 674
Dimetapp Plus Caplets ... ▣ 675
Dimetapp Tablets ... ▣ 675
Entex Capsules ... 1623
Entex LA Tablets ... 1623
Entex Liquid ... 1623
4-Way Cold Tablets ... 750
Hycomine Syrup ... 927
Naldecon CX Adult Liquid ... ▣ 521
Naldecon DX Adult Liquid ... ▣ 521
Naldecon DX Children's Syrup ... ▣ 522
Naldecon DX Pediatric Drops ... ▣ 522
Naldecon EX Children's Syrup ... ▣ 522
Naldecon EX Pediatric Drops ... ▣ 523
Naldecon Syrup, Tablets, Pediatric Drops and Pediatric Syrup ... 709
Nolamine Tablets ... 838
Nolex LA Tablets ... 838
Ornade Spansule Capsules ... 2221
Orthoxicol Cough Syrup ... ▣ 668
Propagest ... 839
Pyrroxate Capsules ... ▣ 669
Robitussin-CF ... ▣ 676
Ru-Tuss II Capsules ... 693
Ru-Tuss with Hydrocodone ... 694
Ru-Tuss Tablets ... 693
Sine-Off Sinus Medicine Tablets-Aspirin Formula ... ▣ 722
Sinulin ... 840
St. Joseph Cold Tablets for Children ... ▣ 704
Tavist-D Tablets ... 2035
Triaminic Allergy Tablets ... ▣ 688
Triaminic Chewables ... ▣ 688
Triaminic Cold Tablets ... ▣ 688
Triaminic Expectorant ... ▣ 688
Triaminic Expectorant w/Codeine ... 1996
Triaminic Expectorant DH ... 1995
Triaminic Oral Infant Drops ... 1996
Triaminic Syrup ... ▣ 689
Triaminic-12 Tablets ... ▣ 690
Triaminic-DM Syrup ... ▣ 689
Triaminicin Tablets ... ▣ 690
Triaminicol Multi-Symptom Cold Tablets ... ▣ 691
Triaminicol Multi-Symptom Relief ▣ 691
Tuss-Ornade Liquid ... 2242
Tuss-Ornade Spansule Capsules ... 2242
Tylenol Cold Medication, Effervescent Tablets ... 1369

Pimozide (Hyperpyrexia). Products include:
Orap Tablets ... 1020

Pirbuterol Acetate (Close supervision and careful adjustment of dosages required). Products include:
Maxair Inhaler ... 1311

Prazepam (Enhanced response to CNS depressants). Products include:
Centrax ... 1693

Prazosin Hydrochloride (Antihypertensive effects blocked). Products include:
Minipress Capsules ... 1778
Minizide Capsules ... 1779

Prochlorperazine (Enhanced response to CNS depressants; hyperpyrexia). Products include:
Compazine ... 2201

Procyclidine Hydrochloride (Close supervision and careful adjustment of dosages; hyperpyrexia). Products include:
Kemadrin Tablets ... 771

Promethazine Hydrochloride (Enhanced response to CNS depressants; hyperpyrexia). Products include:
Mepergan Injection ... 2479
Phenergan with Codeine ... 2497
Phenergan with Dextromethorphan 2499
Phenergan Injection ... 2493
Phenergan Suppositories ... 2496
Phenergan Syrup ... 2495
Phenergan Tablets ... 2496
Phenergan VC ... 2500
Phenergan VC with Codeine ... 2501

Propantheline Bromide (Close supervision and careful adjustment of dosages required; hyperpyrexia). Products include:
Pro-Banthīne Tablets ... 2141

Propofol (Enhanced response to CNS depressants). Products include:
Diprivan Injection ... 2267

Propoxyphene Hydrochloride (Enhanced response to CNS depressants). Products include:
Darvon ... 1256
Wygesic Tablets ... 2540

Propoxyphene Napsylate (Enhanced response to CNS depressants). Products include:
Darvon-N/Darvocet-N ... 1254

Pseudoephedrine Hydrochloride (Close supervision and careful adjustment of dosages required). Products include:
Actifed Capsules ... ▣ 539
Actifed Plus Caplets ... ▣ 539
Actifed Plus Tablets ... ▣ 540
Actifed with Codeine Cough Syrup.. 752
Actifed Syrup ... ▣ 540
Actifed Tablets ... ▣ 540
Actifed 12-Hour Capsules ... ▣ 539
Advil Cold & Sinus Caplets (formerly CoAdvil) ... 2416
Allerest ... ▣ 559
Anatuss LA Tablets ... 1359
Benadryl Decongestant Elixir ... ▣ 635
Benadryl Decongestant ... ▣ 635
Benadryl Plus ... ▣ 636
Benadryl Plus Nighttime ... ▣ 637
Benylin Decongestant ... ▣ 638
Brexin L.A. Capsules ... 2078
Bromfed Capsules (Timed Release) ... 1615
Bromfed Syrup ... ▣ 628
Bromfed ... 1615
CoAdvil ... ▣ 748
Allergy-Sinus Comtrex Multi-Symptom Allergy Sinus Formula Tablets & Caplets ... 746
Cough Formula Comtrex ... 746
Comtrex Multi-Symptom Cold Reliever Tablets/Caplets/Liqui-Gels/Liquid ... 745
Day-Night Comtrex ... 747
Non-Drowsy Comtrex ... 747
Congess ... 994
Congestac Caplets ... ▣ 617
Contac Jr. Children's Cold Medicine ... ▣ 712
Contac Nighttime Cold Medicine ... ▣ 713
Contac Sinus Caplets Maximum Strength Non-Drowsy Formula ... ▣ 710
Contac Sinus Tablets Maximum Strength Non-Drowsy Formula ... ▣ 710
Deconamine ... 663
Deconsal II Tablets ... 559
Dimacol Caplets ... ▣ 672
Dimetane-DX Cough Syrup ... 1858
Dorcol Children's Cough Syrup ... ▣ 685
Dorcol Children's Decongestant Liquid ... ▣ 685
Dorcol Children's Liquid Cold Formula ... ▣ 686
Maximum Strength Dristan Decongestant/Analgesic Coated Caplets ... ▣ 750
No Drowsiness Dristan Cold Nasal Decongestant/Analgesic Coated Caplets ... 2420
Dristan Sinus Caplets ... 2419
Sinus Excedrin Analgesic, Decongestant Tablets & Caplets ... ▣ 533
Fedahist Gyrocaps ... 2145
Fedahist Timecaps ... 2145
Guaifed ... 1615
Guaifed Syrup ... ▣ 629
Isoclor Expectorant ... 982
Isoclor Timesule Capsules ... ▣ 561
Kronofed-A ... 970
Medi-Flu Caplet, Liquid ... ▣ 640
Novafed A Capsules ... 1342
Novafed Capsules ... 1342
Novahistine DH ... 1342
Novahistine DMX ... ▣ 595
Novahistine Expectorant ... 1343
Nucofed Capsules ... 2219
Nucofed Expectorant ... 2219
Nucofed Pediatric Expectorant ... 2220
Nucofed Syrup ... 2219
Ornex Caplets ... ▣ 618
PediaCare Allergy Relief Formula Liquid ... 1362
PediaCare Cough-Cold Formula Liquid ... 1362
PediaCare Infants' Oral Decongestant Drops ... 1362
PediaCare Night Rest Cough-Cold Formula Liquid ... 1362
PediaCare 6-12 Cough-Cold Formula Chewable Tablets ... 1362
Robitussin-DAC Syrup ... 1875
Robitussin-PE ... ▣ 677
Rondec ... 1975
Rondec-DM ... 1976
Rondec-TR Tablet ... 1975
Ru-Tuss DE Tablets ... 694
Ryna ... ▣ 741
Seldane-D Extended-Release Tablets ... 1350
Sinarest ... ▣ 562
Sine-Aid Maximum Strength Sinus Headache Caplets ... 1365
Sine-Aid Maximum Strength Sinus Headache Tablets ... 1365
Sine-Off Maximum Strength Allergy/Sinus Formula Caplets ... ▣ 721
Sine-Off Maximum Strength No Drowsiness Formula Caplets ... ▣ 722
Singlet Tablets ... ▣ 598
Sinutab Maximum Strength ... ▣ 641
Sinutab Maximum Strength Without Drowsiness Tablets & Caplets ... ▣ 642
Sinutab Regular Strength Without Drowsiness Formula ... ▣ 641
St. Joseph Nighttime Cold Medicine ... ▣ 705
Sudafed Children's Liquid ... ▣ 543
Sudafed Cough Syrup ... ▣ 543
Sudafed Plus Liquid ... ▣ 544
Sudafed Plus Tablets ... ▣ 545
Sudafed Sinus Caplets ... ▣ 545
Sudafed Sinus Tablets ... ▣ 545
Sudafed Tablets, 30 mg ... ▣ 544
Sudafed Tablets, Adult Strength, 60 mg ... ▣ 544
Sudafed 12 Hour Capsules ... ▣ 545
TheraFlu Flu and Cold Medicine ... ▣ 687
Triaminic Nite Light ... ▣ 689
Tylenol Allergy Sinus Medication Caplets and Gelcaps, Maximum Strength ... 1372
Children's Tylenol Cold Liquid Formula and Chewable Tablets ... 1368
Tylenol Cold & Flu Hot Medication, Packets ... 1369
Tylenol Cold & Flu No Drowsiness Hot Medication, Packets ... 1371
Tylenol Cold Medication Caplets and Tablets ... 1370
Tylenol Cold Medication No Drowsiness Formula Caplets ... 1370
Tylenol Cold Night Time Medication Liquid ... 1371
Tylenol Cough Medication Liquid with Decongestant, Maximum Strength ... 1372
Tylenol, Maximum Strength, Sinus Medication Gelcaps, Caplets and Tablets ... 1373
Ursinus Inlay-Tabs ... ▣ 691
Vicks Children's NyQuil ... ▣ 664
Vicks Daycare ... ▣ 660
Vicks Formula 44D Decongestant Cough Medicine ... ▣ 662

(▣ Described in PDR For Nonprescription Drugs)

(⊙ Described in PDR For Ophthalmology)

Vicks Formula 44M Multi-Symptom Cough Medicine ▣ 662
Vicks NyQuil Nighttime Colds Medicine-Original & Cherry Flavor ▣ 664
Vicks Pediatric Formula 44 Cough & Congestion Medicine ▣ 663
Vicks Pediatric Formula 44m Multi-Symptom Cough & Cold Medicine ▣ 663

Pseudoephedrine Sulfate (Close supervision and careful adjustment of dosages required). Products include:
Afrin Tablets ▣ 693
Chlor-Trimeton Decongestant ▣ 694
Disophrol Chronotab Sustained-Action Tablets ▣ 698
Drixoral Antihistamine/Nasal Decongestant Syrup ▣ 698
Drixoral Non-Drowsy Formula ▣ 699
Drixoral Plus Extended-Release Tablets ▣ 699
Drixoral Sinus ▣ 700
Drixoral Sustained-Action Tablets ▣ 698
Sinutab Allergy Formula Sustained Action Tablets ▣ 640
Trinalin Repetabs Tablets 1170

Quazepam (Enhanced response to CNS depressants). Products include:
Doral Tablets 2383

Rauwolfia Serpentina (Antihypertensive effects blocked). Products include:
Raudixin Tablets 1803
Rauzide Tablets 1804

Rescinnamine (Antihypertensive effects blocked).
No products indexed under this heading.

Reserpine (Antihypertensive effects blocked). Products include:
Diupres Tablets 1461
Hydromox R Tablets 1209
Hydropres Tablets 1485
Renese-R Tablets 1786
Salutensin/Salutensin-Demi 719
Ser-Ap-Es Tablets 881
Serpasil Tablets 883
Serpasil-Apresoline Tablets 884
Serpasil-Esidrix Tablets 886

Scopolamine Hydrobromide (Close supervision and careful adjustment of dosages required; hyperpyrexia). Products include:
Donnagel ▣ 675
Donnagel-PG 1858
Donnatal 1858
Donnatal Extentabs 1859
Donnatal Tablets 1858
Donnazyme Tablets 1860
Isopto Hyoscine ⊙ 222
Murocoll-2 Sterile Ophthalmic Solution ⊙ 261
Ru-Tuss Tablets 693

Scopolamine Preparations (Close supervision and careful adjustment of dosages required; hyperpyrexia). Products include:
Transderm Scōp Transdermal Therapeutic System 887

Secobarbital Sodium (Enhanced response to barbiturates). Products include:
Seconal Sodium Pulvules 1296

Selegiline Hydrochloride (Contraindication; hyperpyretic crises; severe convulsions; death). Products include:
Eldepryl 2250

Sufentanil Citrate (Enhanced response to CNS depressants). Products include:
Sufenta Injection 1147

Temazepam (Enhanced response to CNS depressants). Products include:
Restoril Capsules 2023

Terazosin Hydrochloride (Antihypertensive effects of guanadrel blocked). Products include:
Hytrin Tablets 529

Terbutaline Sulfate (Close supervision and careful adjustment of dosages required). Products include:
Brethaire Inhaler 1024
Brethine Ampuls 1026
Brethine Tablets 1026
Bricanyl Injection 1324
Bricanyl Tablets 1325

Thiamylal Sodium (Enhanced response to barbiturates; hyperpyrexia). Products include:
Surital Ampoules, Steri-Vials 1764

Thioridazine Hydrochloride (Enhanced response to CNS depressants; hyperpyrexia). Products include:
Mellaril 2011

Thiothixene (Enhanced response to CNS depressants; hyperpyrexia). Products include:
Navane Capsules and Concentrate 1954
Navane Intramuscular 1956

Thyroglobulin (Arrhythmias). Products include:
Proloid Tablets 1761

Thyroid (Arrhythmias). Products include:
S-P-T "Liquid" Capsules 995

Thyroxine (Arrhythmias).
No products indexed under this heading.

Thyroxine Sodium (Arrhythmias).
No products indexed under this heading.

Tranylcypromine Sulfate (Contraindication; hyperpyretic crises; severe convulsions; death). Products include:
Parnate Tablets 2222

Triazolam (Enhanced response to CNS depressants). Products include:
Halcion Tablets 2340

Tridihexethyl Chloride (Close supervision and careful adjustment of dosages required; hyperpyrexia).
No products indexed under this heading.

Trifluoperazine Hydrochloride (Enhanced response to CNS depressants; hyperpyrexia). Products include:
Stelazine 2226

Trihexyphenidyl Hydrochloride (Close supervision and careful adjustment of dosages required; hyperpyrexia). Products include:
Artane 1195

VIVARIN STIMULANT TABLETS
(Caffeine) ▣ 726
May interact with:

Use of caffeine should be lowered or avoided if used concurrently with drugs to treat psychological problems, kidney trouble, or heart ailments ().

Food Interactions

Beverages, caffeine-containing (May cause nervousness, irritability, sleeplessness, and occasionally, rapid heart beat).

Food, caffeine containing (May cause nervousness, irritability, sleeplessness, and occasionally, rapid heart beat).

VI-ZAC
(Vitamins with Minerals) ▣ 682
No interactions described in labeling.

VOLTAREN OPHTHALMIC STERILE OPHTHALMIC SOLUTION
(Diclofenac Sodium) ⊙ 268
No interactions described in labeling.

VOLTAREN TABLETS
(Diclofenac Sodium) 1042
May interact with oral anticoagulants, oral hypoglycemic agents, diuretics, lithium preparations, potassium sparing diuretics, insulin, and certain other agents. Compounds in these categories include:

Amiloride Hydrochloride (Potential for increased serum potassium levels; Voltaren can inhibit diuretic activity). Products include:
Midamor Tablets 1508
Moduretic Tablets 1510

Aspirin (Lowers plasma concentrations, peak plasma levels, and AUC values). Products include:
Alka-Seltzer Effervescent Antacid and Pain Reliever 1568
Alka-Seltzer Extra Strength Effervescent Antacid and Pain Reliever 1570
Alka-Seltzer (Flavored) Effervescent Antacid and Pain Reliever 1569
Alka-Seltzer Plus Cold Medicine ▣ 623
Alka-Seltzer Plus Night-Time Cold Medicine ▣ 623
Alka Seltzer Plus Sinus Allergy Medicine ▣ 624
Anacin Coated Analgesic Caplets 2417
Anacin Coated Analgesic Tablets 2417
Anacin Maximum Strength Analgesic Coated Tablets 2417
Maximum Strength Arthritis Pain Formula By the Makers of Anacin Analgesic Tablets and Caplets 2418
Arthritis Pain Formula by the Makers of Anacin Analgesic Tablets and Caplets ▣ 747
Arthritis Strength BC Powder ▣ 516
Ascriptin A/D Caplets 1850
Regular Strength Ascriptin Tablets 1850
Azdōne Tablets 844
BC Powder ▣ 517
BC Cold Powder ▣ 517
Children's Bayer Chewable Aspirin ▣ 564
Genuine Bayer Aspirin Tablets & Caplets ▣ 564
Maximum Bayer Aspirin Tablets & Caplets ▣ 566
Bayer Plus Aspirin Tablets ▣ 567
Therapy Bayer Aspirin Caplets ▣ 568
8 Hour Bayer Timed-Release Aspirin ▣ 566
Arthritis Strength Bufferin Analgesic Caplets 744
Extra Strength Bufferin Analgesic Tablets 745
Bufferin Analgesic Tablets and Caplets 743
Cama Arthritis Pain Reliever ▣ 685
Damason-P 1356
Easprin 1719
Ecotrin Enteric Coated Aspirin Maximum Strength Tablets and Caplets 2189
Ecotrin Enteric Coated Aspirin Regular Strength Tablets and Caplets 2189
Empirin Aspirin ▣ 541
Empirin with Codeine Phosphate Nos. 2, 3 & 4 764
Equagesic Tablets 2451
Excedrin Extra-Strength Analgesic Tablets & Caplets 749
4-Way Cold Tablets 750
Fiorinal Capsules 2007
Fiorinal with Codeine Capsules 2008
Fiorinal Tablets 2007
Lortab ASA Tablets 2414
Momentum Muscular Backache Formula ▣ 751
Norgesic 1314
Norwich Extra-Strength Aspirin ▣ 546
Norwich Regular Strength Aspirin ▣ 547
P-A-C Analgesic Tablets ▣ 669
Percodan 951
Robaxisal Tablets 1872
Sine-Off Sinus Medicine Tablets-Aspirin Formula ▣ 722
Soma Compound w/Codeine Tablets 2390
Soma Compound Tablets 2389
St. Joseph Adult Chewable Aspirin (81 mg.) ▣ 703
Synalgos-DC Capsules 2525
Talwin Compound 2072
Ursinus Inlay-Tabs ▣ 691
Vanquish Analgesic Caplets ▣ 574
Zorprin Tablets 698

Aspirin, Enteric Coated (Lowers plasma concentrations, peak plasma levels, and AUC values). Products include:
Therapy Bayer Aspirin Caplets ▣ 568
Ecotrin 2189

Bendroflumethiazide (Voltaren can inhibit diuretic activity). Products include:
Corzide Tablets 702
Naturetin Tablets 1789
Rauzide Tablets 1804

Bumetanide (Voltaren can inhibit diuretic activity). Products include:
Bumex 1895

Chlorothiazide (Voltaren can inhibit diuretic activity). Products include:
Aldoclor Tablets 1413
Diupres Tablets 1461
Diuril Oral 1464

Chlorothiazide Sodium (Voltaren can inhibit diuretic activity). Products include:
Diuril Sodium Intravenous 1463

Chlorpropamide (Diclofenac may alter a diabetic patient's response to oral hypoglycemic agents). Products include:
Diabinese Tablets 1775

Chlorthalidone (Voltaren can inhibit diuretic activity). Products include:
Combipres Tablets 678
Tenoretic Tablets 1105
Thalitone Tablets 687

Cyclosporine (Voltaren through renal prostaglandins may cause increased toxicity of cyclosporine). Products include:
Sandimmune 2024

Dicumarol (Concurrent therapy requires close monitoring of patients for anticoagulant dosage). Products include:
Dicumarol Tablets 516

Digoxin (Voltaren through renal prostaglandins may cause increased toxicity of digoxin). Products include:
Lanoxicaps 772
Lanoxin Elixir Pediatric 775
Lanoxin Injection 778
Lanoxin Injection Pediatric 781
Lanoxin Tablets 783

Ethacrynic Acid (Voltaren can inhibit diuretic activity). Products include:
Edecrin Tablets 1468

Furosemide (Voltaren can inhibit diuretic activity). Products include:
Lasix 1093

Glipizide (Diclofenac may alter a diabetic patient's response to oral hypoglycemic agents). Products include:
Glucotrol 1952

Glyburide (Diclofenac may alter a diabetic patient's response to oral hypoglycemic agents). Products include:
DiaBeta 1091
Micronase Tablets 2350

Hydrochlorothiazide (Voltaren can inhibit diuretic activity). Products include:
Aldactazide 2150
Aldoril Tablets 1418
Apresazide Capsules 854
Apresoline-Esidrix Tablets 857
Capozide 2258
Dyazide Capsules 2208
Esidrix Tablets 863
Esimil Tablets 864
HydroDIURIL Tablets 1484
Hydropres Tablets 1485
Inderide Tablets 2463
Inderide LA Long Acting Capsules 2465
Lopressor HCT Tablets 1034

- Maxzide 1215
- Moduretic Tablets 1510
- Normozide Tablets 2112
- Oretic Tablets 544
- Oreticyl 545
- Prinzide Tablets 1540
- Ser-Ap-Es Tablets 881
- Serpasil-Esidrix Tablets 886
- Timolide Tablets 1547
- Trandate HCT Tablets 579
- Vaseretic Tablets 1559
- Zestoretic 2274

Hydroflumethiazide (Voltaren can inhibit diuretic activity). Products include:
- Diucardin Tablets 2450
- Saluron 718
- Salutensin/Salutensin-Demi 719

Indapamide (Voltaren can inhibit diuretic activity). Products include:
- Lozol Tablets 1843

Insulin, Human (Diclofenac may alter a diabetic patient's response to insulin).
- No products indexed under this heading.

Insulin, Human Isophane Suspension (Diclofenac may alter a diabetic patient's response to insulin). Products include:
- Humulin N, 100 Units 1270

Insulin, Human NPH (Diclofenac may alter a diabetic patient's response to insulin). Products include:
- Insulatard NPH Human 1627
- Novolin N 1627
- Novolin N PenFill Cartridges 1628
- Novolin N Prefilled 1628

Insulin, Human Regular (Diclofenac may alter a diabetic patient's response to insulin). Products include:
- Humulin BR, 100 Units 1268
- Humulin R, 100 Units 1272
- Novolin R 1627
- Novolin R PenFill Cartridges 1628
- Novolin R Prefilled 1629
- Velosulin Human 1628

Insulin, Human, Zinc Suspension (Diclofenac may alter a diabetic patient's response to insulin). Products include:
- Humulin L, 100 Units 1268
- Humulin U, 100 Units 1272
- Novolin L 1627

Insulin, NPH (Diclofenac may alter a diabetic patient's response to insulin). Products include:
- NPH, 40 & 100 Units 1273
- Beef NPH, 100 Units 1274
- Pork NPH, 100 Units 1275
- Insulatard NPH 1626
- NPH Insulin 1626
- NPH Purified Pork Isophane Insulin 1626

Insulin, Regular (Diclofenac may alter a diabetic patient's response to insulin). Products include:
- Regular, 40 & 100 Units 1273
- Beef Regular, 100 Units 1275
- Pork Regular, 100 Units 1275
- Pork Regular (Concentrated), 500 Units 1276
- Regular Insulin 1625
- Regular Purified Pork Insulin 1626
- Velosulin 1627

Insulin, Zinc Crystals (Diclofenac may alter a diabetic patient's response to insulin). Products include:
- NPH, 40 & 100 Units 1273

Insulin, Zinc Suspension (Diclofenac may alter a diabetic patient's response to insulin). Products include:
- Lente, 40 & 100 Units 1272
- Protamine, Zinc, 40 & 100 Units 1273
- Lente Iletin I 1272
- Beef Lente, 100 Units 1274
- Beef Protamine Zinc, 100 Units 1274
- Pork Lente, 100 Units 1275
- Pork, Protamine, Zinc, 100 Units 1275
- Lente Insulin 1626
- Lente Purified Pork Insulin 1626
- Semilente Insulin 1625
- Ultralente Insulin 1626

Lithium Carbonate (Decreased lithium renal clearance and increased lithium plasma levels). Products include:
- Eskalith 2214
- Lithane Tablets 1596
- Lithium Carbonate Capsules & Tablets 1984
- Lithobid Tablets 870

Lithium Citrate (Decreased lithium renal clearance and increased lithium plasma levels). Products include:
- Cibalith-S 870

Methotrexate Sodium (Voltaren through renal prostaglandins may cause increased toxicity of methotrexate). Products include:
- Methotrexate Tablets, Parenteral, LPF Parenteral 1217
- Rheumatrex Methotrexate Dose Pack 1234

Methyclothiazide (Voltaren can inhibit diuretic activity). Products include:
- Enduron Tablets 517
- Enduronyl 518

Metolazone (Voltaren can inhibit diuretic activity). Products include:
- Diulo 2129
- Mykrox ½ mg Tablets 984
- Zaroxolyn Tablets 989

Polythiazide (Voltaren can inhibit diuretic activity). Products include:
- Minizide Capsules 1779
- Renese Tablets 1785
- Renese-R Tablets 1786

Spironolactone (Potential for increased serum potassium levels; Voltaren can inhibit diuretic activity). Products include:
- Aldactazide 2150
- Aldactone 2152

Tolazamide (Diclofenac may alter a diabetic patient's response to oral hypoglycemic agents). Products include:
- Tolinase Tablets 2365

Tolbutamide (Diclofenac may alter a diabetic patient's response to oral hypoglycemic agents). Products include:
- Orinase Tablets 2354

Triamterene (Potential for increased serum potassium levels; Voltaren can inhibit diuretic activity). Products include:
- Dyazide Capsules 2208
- Dyrenium Capsules 2210
- Maxzide 1215

Warfarin Sodium (Concurrent therapy requires close monitoring of patients for anticoagulant dosage). Products include:
- Coumadin Injection & Tablets 944
- Panwarfin Tablets 547

VONTROL TABLETS
(Diphenidol) 2243
No interactions described in labeling.

VŌSOL HC OTIC SOLUTION
(Acetic Acid, Hydrocortisone) 2392
No interactions described in labeling.

VŌSOL OTIC SOLUTION
(Acetic Acid) 2392
No interactions described in labeling.

VYTONE CREAM 1%
(Hydrocortisone, Iodoquinol) 911
No interactions described in labeling.

WELLBUTRIN TABLETS
(Bupropion Hydrochloride) 821
May interact with drugs affecting hepatic drug metabolizing enzyme systems, monoamine oxidase inhibitors, drugs which lower seizure threshold, and certain other agents. Compounds in these categories include:

Alcohol (Concurrent alcohol consumption should be avoided or minimized).

Alprazolam (Concurrent therapy should be undertaken with extreme caution). Products include:
- Xanax Tablets 2367

Amitriptyline Hydrochloride (Concurrent therapy should be undertaken with extreme caution). Products include:
- Elavil 2269
- Endep Tablets 1927
- Etrafon 2087
- Limbitrol 1933
- Triavil Tablets 1556

Amoxapine (Concurrent therapy should be undertaken with extreme caution). Products include:
- Asendin Tablets 1196

Carbamazepine (Concurrent therapy may affect metabolism of bupropion). Products include:
- Tegretol Chewable Tablets 654
- Tegretol Suspension 656
- Tegretol Tablets 654

Chlordiazepoxide (Concurrent therapy should be undertaken with extreme caution). Products include:
- Libritabs Tablets 1930
- Limbitrol 1933
- Menrium Tablets 1934

Chlordiazepoxide Hydrochloride (Concurrent therapy should be undertaken with extreme caution). Products include:
- Librax Capsules 1929
- Librium Capsules 1931
- Librium Injectable 1932

Chlorpromazine (Concurrent therapy should be undertaken with extreme caution). Products include:
- Thorazine 2234

Cimetidine (Concurrent therapy may affect metabolism of bupropion). Products include:
- Tagamet Tablets 2228

Cimetidine Hydrochloride (Concurrent therapy may affect metabolism of bupropion). Products include:
- Tagamet 2228

Desipramine Hydrochloride (Concurrent therapy should be undertaken with extreme caution). Products include:
- Norpramin Tablets 1340

Diazepam (Concurrent therapy should be undertaken with extreme caution). Products include:
- Valium Injectable 1937
- Valium Tablets 1939
- Valrelease Capsules 1923

Doxepin Hydrochloride (Concurrent therapy should be undertaken with extreme caution). Products include:
- Sinequan 1960

Fluoxetine Hydrochloride (Concurrent therapy should be undertaken with extreme caution). Products include:
- Prozac Pulvules 920

Fluphenazine Decanoate (Concurrent therapy should be undertaken with extreme caution). Products include:
- Prolixin Decanoate 1795

Fluphenazine Enanthate (Concurrent therapy should be undertaken with extreme caution). Products include:
- Prolixin Enanthate 1796

Fluphenazine Hydrochloride (Concurrent therapy should be undertaken with extreme caution). Products include:
- Prolixin Elixir 1793
- Prolixin Injection 1791
- Prolixin Oral Concentrate 1792
- Prolixin Tablets 1793

Furazolidone (Concurrent administration is contraindicated). Products include:
- Furoxone 1855

Haloperidol (Concurrent therapy should be undertaken with extreme caution). Products include:
- Haldol Injection, Tablets and Concentrate 1373

Haloperidol Decanoate (Concurrent therapy should be undertaken with extreme caution). Products include:
- Haldol Decanoate 1375

Imipramine Hydrochloride (Concurrent therapy should be undertaken with extreme caution). Products include:
- Tofranil Ampuls 1038
- Tofranil Tablets 1039

Imipramine Pamoate (Concurrent therapy should be undertaken with extreme caution). Products include:
- Tofranil-PM Capsules 1041

Isocarboxazid (Concurrent administration is contraindicated). Products include:
- Marplan Tablets 1906

Levodopa (Potential for higher incidence of adverse experiences). Products include:
- Larodopa Tablets 1905
- Sinemet Tablets 952
- Sinemet CR Tablets 953

Lorazepam (Concurrent therapy should be undertaken with extreme caution). Products include:
- Ativan Injection 2432
- Ativan Tablets 2434

Maprotiline Hydrochloride (Concurrent therapy should be undertaken with extreme caution). Products include:
- Ludiomil Tablets 874

Mesoridazine (Concurrent therapy should be undertaken with extreme caution). Products include:
- Serentil 686

Nortriptyline Hydrochloride (Concurrent therapy should be undertaken with extreme caution). Products include:
- Pamelor 2019

Oxazepam (Concurrent therapy should be undertaken with extreme caution). Products include:
- Serax Capsules 2522
- Serax Tablets 2522

Perphenazine (Concurrent therapy should be undertaken with extreme caution). Products include:
- Etrafon 2087
- Triavil Tablets 1556
- Trilafon 2123

Phenelzine Sulfate (Concurrent administration is contraindicated). Products include:
- Nardil 1742

Phenobarbital (Concurrent therapy may affect metabolism of bupropion). Products include:
- Arco-Lase Plus Tablets 607
- Bellergal-S Tablets 1998
- Bronkolixir ▣ 761
- Bronkotabs Tablets ▣ 762
- Donnatal 1858
- Donnatal Extentabs 1859
- Donnatal Tablets 1858
- Donnazyme Tablets 1860
- Kinesed Tablets 2272
- Phenobarbital Elixir and Tablets 1293

(▣ Described in PDR For Nonprescription Drugs) (◉ Described in PDR For Ophthalmology)

Primatene Tablets-P Formula 2421
Quadrinal Tablets 1183
Tedral SA 1765

Phenytoin (Concurrent therapy may affect metabolism of bupropion). Products include:
Dilantin Infatabs 1710
Dilantin-30 Pediatric/Dilantin-125 Suspension 1713

Phenytoin Sodium (Concurrent therapy may affect metabolism of bupropion). Products include:
Dilantin Kapseals 1708
Dilantin Parenteral 1712
Dilantin with Phenobarbital Kapseals 1715

Prazepam (Concurrent therapy should be undertaken with extreme caution). Products include:
Centrax 1693

Prochlorperazine (Concurrent therapy should be undertaken with extreme caution). Products include:
Compazine 2201

Promethazine Hydrochloride (Concurrent therapy should be undertaken with extreme caution). Products include:
Mepergan Injection 2479
Phenergan with Codeine 2497
Phenergan with Dextromethorphan 2499
Phenergan Injection 2493
Phenergan Suppositories 2496
Phenergan Syrup 2495
Phenergan Tablets 2496
Phenergan VC 2500
Phenergan VC with Codeine 2501

Protriptyline Hydrochloride (Concurrent therapy should be undertaken with extreme caution). Products include:
Vivactil Tablets 1567

Selegiline Hydrochloride (Concurrent administration is contraindicated). Products include:
Eldepryl 2250

Thioridazine Hydrochloride (Concurrent therapy should be undertaken with extreme caution). Products include:
Mellaril 2011

Tranylcypromine Sulfate (Concurrent administration is contraindicated). Products include:
Parnate Tablets 2222

Trazodone Hydrochloride (Concurrent therapy should be undertaken with extreme caution). Products include:
Desyrel and Desyrel Dividose 1404

Trifluoperazine Hydrochloride (Concurrent therapy should be undertaken with extreme caution). Products include:
Stelazine 2226

Trimipramine Maleate (Concurrent therapy should be undertaken with extreme caution). Products include:
Surmontil Capsules 2524

WELLCOME LANOLINE
(Lanolin) .... ■ 546
No interactions described in labeling.

WESTCORT CREAM 0.2%
(Hydrocortisone Valerate) 2411
No interactions described in labeling.

WESTCORT OINTMENT 0.2%
(Hydrocortisone Valerate) 2411
No interactions described in labeling.

WIGRAINE TABLETS & SUPPOSITORIES
(Ergotamine Tartrate, Caffeine) 1645
No interactions described in labeling.

WINGEL LIQUID & TABLETS
(Aluminum Hydroxide, Magnesium Hydroxide) .... ■ 761
May interact with tetracyclines. Compounds in this category include:

Demeclocycline Hydrochloride (Concurrent use with any form of tetracycline is not recommended). Products include:
Declomycin Capsules, Tablets 1199

Doxycycline Calcium (Concurrent use with any form of tetracycline is not recommended).
No products indexed under this heading.

Doxycycline Hyclate (Concurrent use with any form of tetracycline is not recommended). Products include:
Doryx Capsules 1717
Vibramycin Hyclate Capsules 1787
Vibramycin Hyclate Intravenous 1968
Vibra-Tabs Film Coated Tablets 1787

Doxycycline Monohydrate (Concurrent use with any form of tetracycline is not recommended). Products include:
Monodox Capsules 1630
Vibramycin Monohydrate for Oral Suspension 1787

Methacycline Hydrochloride (Concurrent use with any form of tetracycline is not recommended).
No products indexed under this heading.

Minocycline Hydrochloride (Concurrent use with any form of tetracycline is not recommended). Products include:
Minocin Intravenous 1221
Minocin Oral Suspension 1224
Minocin Pellet-Filled Capsules 1222

Oxytetracycline Hydrochloride (Concurrent use with any form of tetracycline is not recommended). Products include:
Terra-Cortril Ophthalmic Suspension 1963
Terramycin Capsules 1786
Terramycin Intramuscular Solution 1964
Terramycin with Polymyxin B Sulfate Ophthalmic Ointment 1965

Tetracycline Hydrochloride (Concurrent use with any form of tetracycline is not recommended). Products include:
Achromycin V Capsules 1193
Achromycin Ophthalmic Ointment 1% .... ⊚ 307
Achromycin Ophthalmic Suspension 1% .... ⊚ 308
Topicycline for Topical Solution 1856

WINSTROL TABLETS
(Stanozolol) 2075
May interact with oral anticoagulants. Compounds in this category include:

Dicumarol (Increased sensitivity to anticoagulants). Products include:
Dicumarol Tablets 516

Warfarin Sodium (Increased sensitivity to anticoagulants). Products include:
Coumadin Injection & Tablets 944
Panwarfin Tablets 547

WITHIN WOMEN'S FORMULA MULTIVITAMIN WITH CALCIUM, EXTRA IRON AND ZINC
(Multivitamins with Minerals) .... ■ 628
No interactions described in labeling.

WYANOIDS RELIEF FACTOR HEMORRHOIDAL SUPPOSITORIES
(Belladonna Alkaloids, Ephedrine Sulfate) 2537
No interactions described in labeling.

WYCILLIN INJECTION
(Penicillin G Procaine) 2537
No interactions described in labeling.

WYGESIC TABLETS
(Propoxyphene Hydrochloride, Acetaminophen) 2540
May interact with central nervous system depressants, antidepressant drugs, oral anticoagulants, anticonvulsants, tranquilizers, and certain other agents. Compounds in these categories include:

Alcohol (Additive effects).

Alfentanil Hydrochloride (Additive effects). Products include:
Alfenta Injection 1131

Alprazolam (Additive effects). Products include:
Xanax Tablets 2367

Amitriptyline Hydrochloride (Propoxyphene may slow the metabolism of antidepressants). Products include:
Elavil 2269
Endep Tablets 1927
Etrafon 2087
Limbitrol 1933
Triavil Tablets 1556

Amoxapine (Propoxyphene may slow the metabolism of antidepressants). Products include:
Asendin Tablets 1196

Aprobarbital (Additive effects). Products include:
Alurate Elixir 1883

Buprenorphine (Additive effects).
No products indexed under this heading.

Bupropion Hydrochloride (Propoxyphene may slow the metabolism of antidepressants). Products include:
Wellbutrin Tablets 821

Buspirone Hydrochloride (Additive effects). Products include:
BuSpar 1401

Butabarbital (Additive effects). Products include:
Pyridium Plus 1764

Butalbital (Additive effects). Products include:
Esgic-Plus Tablets 1002
Esgic Tablets & Capsules 1001
Fioricet Tablets 2006
Fiorinal Capsules 2007
Fiorinal with Codeine Capsules 2008
Fiorinal Tablets 2007
Phrenilin 838
Sedapap Tablets 50 mg/650 mg .. 1360

Carbamazepine (Propoxyphene may slow the metabolism of anticonvulsants). Products include:
Tegretol Chewable Tablets 654
Tegretol Suspension 656
Tegretol Tablets 654

Chlordiazepoxide (Additive effects). Products include:
Libritabs Tablets 1930
Limbitrol 1933
Menrium Tablets 1934

Chlordiazepoxide Hydrochloride (Additive effects). Products include:
Librax Capsules 1929
Librium Capsules 1931
Librium Injectable 1932

Chlorpromazine (Additive effects). Products include:
Thorazine 2234

Chlorprothixene (Additive effects). Products include:
Taractan Tablets 1920

Chlorprothixene Hydrochloride (Additive effects). Products include:
Taractan 1920

Clorazepate Dipotassium (Additive effects). Products include:
Tranxene 556

Codeine (Additive effects). Products include:
Calcidrine Syrup 506

Codeine Phosphate (Additive effects). Products include:
Actifed with Codeine Cough Syrup.. 752
Cheracol Cough Syrup 1853
Codimal PH Syrup 846
Dimetane-DC Cough Syrup 1857
Empirin with Codeine Phosphate Nos. 2, 3 & 4 764
Fiorinal with Codeine Capsules 2008
Isoclor Expectorant 982
Naldecon CX Adult Liquid .... ■ 521
Novahistine DH 1342
Novahistine Expectorant 1343
Nucofed Capsules 2219
Nucofed Expectorant 2219
Nucofed Pediatric Expectorant 2220
Nucofed Syrup 2219
Phenaphen with Codeine Capsules 1865
Phenaphen-650 with Codeine Tablets 1866
Phenergan with Codeine 2497
Phenergan VC with Codeine 2501
Robitussin A-C Syrup 1875
Robitussin-DAC Syrup 1875
Ryna .... ■ 741
Soma Compound w/Codeine Tablets 2390
Triaminic Expectorant w/Codeine .. 1996
Tussi-Organidin Liquid 2391
Tylenol with Codeine 1381

Codeine Polistirex (Additive effects).
No products indexed under this heading.

Desipramine Hydrochloride (Propoxyphene may slow the metabolism of antidepressants). Products include:
Norpramin Tablets 1340

Dezocine (Additive effects).

Diazepam (Additive effects). Products include:
Valium Injectable 1937
Valium Tablets 1939
Valrelease Capsules 1923

Dicumarol (Propoxyphene may slow the metabolism of warfarin-like drug). Products include:
Dicumarol Tablets 516

Divalproex Sodium (Propoxyphene may slow the metabolism of anticonvulsants). Products include:
Depakote 512

Doxepin Hydrochloride (Propoxyphene may slow the metabolism of antidepressants). Products include:
Sinequan 1960

Droperidol (Additive effects). Products include:
Inapsine Injection 1140
Innovar Injection 1141

Enflurane (Additive effects). Products include:
Ethrane 599

Estazolam (Additive effects). Products include:
ProSom Tablets 554

Ethchlorvynol (Additive effects). Products include:
Placidyl Capsules 553

Ethinamate (Additive effects).
No products indexed under this heading.

Ethosuximide (Propoxyphene may slow the metabolism of anticonvulsants). Products include:
Zarontin Capsules 1768
Zarontin Syrup 1769

Ethotoin (Propoxyphene may slow the metabolism of anticonvulsants). Products include:
Peganone Tablets ... 551
Fentanyl (Additive effects). Products include:
Duragesic Transdermal System ... 1133
Fentanyl Citrate (Additive effects). Products include:
Innovar Injection ... 1141
Sublimaze Injection ... 1146
Fluoxetine Hydrochloride (Propoxyphene may slow the metabolism of antidepressants). Products include:
Prozac Pulvules ... 920
Fluphenazine Decanoate (Additive effects). Products include:
Prolixin Decanoate ... 1795
Fluphenazine Enanthate (Additive effects). Products include:
Prolixin Enanthate ... 1796
Fluphenazine Hydrochloride (Additive effects). Products include:
Prolixin Elixir ... 1793
Prolixin Injection ... 1791
Prolixin Oral Concentrate ... 1792
Prolixin Tablets ... 1793
Flurazepam Hydrochloride (Additive effects). Products include:
Dalmane Capsules ... 1927
Glutethimide (Additive effects).
No products indexed under this heading.
Haloperidol (Additive effects). Products include:
Haldol Injection, Tablets and Concentrate ... 1373
Haloperidol Decanoate (Additive effects). Products include:
Haldol Decanoate ... 1375
Hydrocodone Bitartrate (Additive effects). Products include:
Anexsia 5/500 Tablets ... 2196
Anexsia 7.5/650 Tablets ... 2197
Azdone Tablets ... 844
Codiclear DH Syrup ... 845
Codimal DH Syrup ... 846
Damason-P ... 1356
Hycodan Syrup, Tablets ... 927
Hycomine Compound Tablets ... 929
Hycomine Syrup ... 927
Hycotuss Expectorant Syrup ... 930
Hydrocet Capsules ... 835
Lortab ASA Tablets ... 2414
Lortab ... 2412
Ru-Tuss with Hydrocodone ... 694
Triaminic Expectorant DH ... 1995
Vicodin Tablets ... 1187
Vicodin ES Tablets ... 1189
Zydone Capsules ... 941
Hydrocodone Polistirex (Additive effects). Products include:
Tussionex Extended-Release Suspension ... 988
Hydroxyzine Hydrochloride (Additive effects). Products include:
Atarax Tablets & Syrup ... 1941
Marax Tablets & DF Syrup ... 1954
Vistaril Intramuscular Solution ... 1970
Imipramine Hydrochloride (Propoxyphene may slow the metabolism of antidepressants). Products include:
Tofranil Ampuls ... 1038
Tofranil Tablets ... 1039
Imipramine Pamoate (Propoxyphene may slow the metabolism of antidepressants). Products include:
Tofranil-PM Capsules ... 1041
Isocarboxazid (Propoxyphene may slow the metabolism of antidepressants). Products include:
Marplan Tablets ... 1906
Isoflurane (Additive effects). Products include:
Forane ... 600
Ketamine Hydrochloride (Additive effects). Products include:
Ketalar ... 1726
Levorphanol Tartrate (Additive effects). Products include:
Levo-Dromoran ... 1906
Lorazepam (Additive effects). Products include:
Ativan Injection ... 2432
Ativan Tablets ... 2434
Loxapine Hydrochloride (Additive effects). Products include:
Loxitane ... 1213
Loxapine Succinate (Additive effects). Products include:
Loxitane Capsules ... 1213
Maprotiline Hydrochloride (Propoxyphene may slow the metabolism of antidepressants). Products include:
Ludiomil Tablets ... 874
Meperidine Hydrochloride (Additive effects). Products include:
Demerol ... 2047
Mepergan Injection ... 2479
Mephenytoin (Propoxyphene may slow the metabolism of anticonvulsants). Products include:
Mesantoin Tablets ... 2013
Mephobarbital (Additive effects). Products include:
Mebaral Tablets ... 2061
Meprobamate (Additive effects). Products include:
Deprol Tablets ... 2382
Equagesic Tablets ... 2451
Miltown Tablets ... 2386
PMB 200 and PMB 400 ... 2504
Mesoridazine (Additive effects). Products include:
Serentil ... 686
Mesoridazine Besylate (Additive effects).
Methadone Hydrochloride (Additive effects). Products include:
Dolophine Hydrochloride Ampoules & Vials ... 1260
Dolophine Hydrochloride Tablets ... 1261
Methadone Hydrochloride Diskets ... 1284
Methadone Hydrochloride Oral Solution & Tablets ... 1987
Methohexital Sodium (Additive effects). Products include:
Brevital Sodium Vials ... 1248
Methoxyflurane (Additive effects).
No products indexed under this heading.
Methsuximide (Propoxyphene may slow the metabolism of anticonvulsants). Products include:
Celontin ... 1692
Midazolam Hydrochloride (Additive effects). Products include:
Versed Injection ... 1924
Molindone Hydrochloride (Additive effects). Products include:
Moban Tablets & Concentrate ... 932
Morphine Sulfate (Additive effects). Products include:
Astramorph/PF Injection, USP (Preservative-Free) ... 618
Duramorph ... 960
Infumorph 200 and Infumorph 500 Sterile Solutions ... 962
MS Contin Tablets ... 1814
MSIR ... 1817
Oramorph SR (Morphine Sulfate Sustained Release Tablets) ... 1988
Roxanol ... 1991
Nortriptyline Hydrochloride (Propoxyphene may slow the metabolism of antidepressants). Products include:
Pamelor ... 2019
Opium Alkaloids (Additive effects). Products include:
B & O No. 15A & No. 16A Supprettes ... 2395
Pantopon Injectable ... 1911
Oxazepam (Additive effects). Products include:
Serax Capsules ... 2522
Serax Tablets ... 2522
Oxycodone Hydrochloride (Additive effects). Products include:
Percocet Tablets ... 950
Percodan ... 951
Roxicodone Tablets, Oral Solution & Intensol (Oxycodone) ... 1992
Tylox Capsules ... 1382
Paramethadione (Propoxyphene may slow the metabolism of anticonvulsants). Products include:
Paradione Capsules ... 548
Pentobarbital Sodium (Additive effects). Products include:
Nembutal Sodium Capsules ... 534
Nembutal Sodium Solution ... 536
Nembutal Sodium Suppositories ... 538
Perphenazine (Additive effects). Products include:
Etrafon ... 2087
Triavil Tablets ... 1556
Trilafon ... 2123
Phenacemide (Propoxyphene may slow the metabolism of anticonvulsants). Products include:
Phenurone Tablets ... 552
Phenelzine Sulfate (Propoxyphene may slow the metabolism of antidepressants). Products include:
Nardil ... 1742
Phenobarbital (Additive effects; propoxyphene may slow the metabolism of anticonvulsants). Products include:
Arco-Lase Plus Tablets ... 607
Bellergal-S Tablets ... 1998
Bronkolixir ... 761
Bronkotabs Tablets ... 762
Donnatal ... 1858
Donnatal Extentabs ... 1859
Donnatal Tablets ... 1858
Donnazyme Tablets ... 1860
Kinesed Tablets ... 2272
Phenobarbital Elixir and Tablets ... 1293
Primatene Tablets-P Formula ... 2421
Quadrinal Tablets ... 1183
Tedral SA ... 1765
Phensuximide (Propoxyphene may slow the metabolism of anticonvulsants). Products include:
Milontin Kapseals ... 1741
Phenytoin (Propoxyphene may slow the metabolism of anticonvulsants). Products include:
Dilantin Infatabs ... 1710
Dilantin-30 Pediatric/Dilantin-125 Suspension ... 1713
Phenytoin Sodium (Propoxyphene may slow the metabolism of anticonvulsants). Products include:
Dilantin Kapseals ... 1708
Dilantin Parenteral ... 1712
Dilantin with Phenobarbital Kapseals ... 1715
Prazepam (Additive effects). Products include:
Centrax ... 1693
Primidone (Propoxyphene may slow the metabolism of anticonvulsants). Products include:
Mysoline ... 2480
Prochlorperazine (Additive effects). Products include:
Compazine ... 2201
Promethazine Hydrochloride (Additive effects). Products include:
Mepergan Injection ... 2479
Phenergan with Codeine ... 2497
Phenergan with Dextromethorphan ... 2499
Phenergan Injection ... 2493
Phenergan Suppositories ... 2496
Phenergan Syrup ... 2495
Phenergan Tablets ... 2496
Phenergan VC ... 2500
Phenergan VC with Codeine ... 2501
Propofol (Additive effects). Products include:
Diprivan Injection ... 2267
Propoxyphene Napsylate (Additive effects). Products include:
Darvon-N/Darvocet-N ... 1254
Protriptyline Hydrochloride (Propoxyphene may slow the metabolism of antidepressants). Products include:
Vivactil Tablets ... 1567
Quazepam (Additive effects). Products include:
Doral Tablets ... 2383
Secobarbital Sodium (Additive effects). Products include:
Seconal Sodium Pulvules ... 1296
Sufentanil Citrate (Additive effects). Products include:
Sufenta Injection ... 1147
Temazepam (Additive effects). Products include:
Restoril Capsules ... 2023
Thiamylal Sodium (Additive effects). Products include:
Surital Ampoules, Steri-Vials ... 1764
Thioridazine Hydrochloride (Additive effects). Products include:
Mellaril ... 2011
Thiothixene (Additive effects). Products include:
Navane Capsules and Concentrate 1954
Navane Intramuscular ... 1956
Tranylcypromine Sulfate (Propoxyphene may slow the metabolism of antidepressants). Products include:
Parnate Tablets ... 2222
Trazodone Hydrochloride (Propoxyphene may slow the metabolism of antidepressants). Products include:
Desyrel and Desyrel Dividose ... 1404
Triazolam (Additive effects). Products include:
Halcion Tablets ... 2340
Trifluoperazine Hydrochloride (Additive effects). Products include:
Stelazine ... 2226
Trimethadione (Propoxyphene may slow the metabolism of anticonvulsants). Products include:
Tridione ... 557
Trimipramine Maleate (Propoxyphene may slow the metabolism of antidepressants). Products include:
Surmontil Capsules ... 2524
Valproic Acid (Propoxyphene may slow the metabolism of anticonvulsants). Products include:
Depakene Capsules & Syrup ... 511
Warfarin Sodium (Propoxyphene may slow the metabolism of warfarin-like drug). Products include:
Coumadin Injection & Tablets ... 944
Panwarfin Tablets ... 547

WYTENSIN TABLETS
(Guanabenz Acetate) ... 2542
May interact with central nervous system depressants and certain other agents. Compounds in these categories include:

Alcohol (Tolerance for alcohol may be diminished).
Alfentanil Hydrochloride (Potential for increased sedation). Products include:
Alfenta Injection ... 1131
Alprazolam (Potential for increased sedation). Products include:
Xanax Tablets ... 2367
Aprobarbital (Potential for increased sedation). Products include:
Alurate Elixir ... 1883
Buprenorphine (Potential for increased sedation).
No products indexed under this heading.

Buspirone Hydrochloride (Potential for increased sedation). Products include:
- BuSpar ... 1401

Butabarbital (Potential for increased sedation). Products include:
- Pyridium Plus ... 1764

Butalbital (Potential for increased sedation). Products include:
- Esgic-Plus Tablets ... 1002
- Esgic Tablets & Capsules ... 1001
- Fioricet Tablets ... 2006
- Fiorinal Capsules ... 2007
- Fiorinal with Codeine Capsules ... 2008
- Fiorinal Tablets ... 2007
- Phrenilin ... 838
- Sedapap Tablets 50 mg/650 mg .. 1360

Chlordiazepoxide (Potential for increased sedation). Products include:
- Libritabs Tablets ... 1930
- Limbitrol ... 1933
- Menrium Tablets ... 1934

Chlordiazepoxide Hydrochloride (Potential for increased sedation). Products include:
- Librax Capsules ... 1929
- Librium Capsules ... 1931
- Librium Injectable ... 1932

Chlorpromazine (Potential for increased sedation). Products include:
- Thorazine ... 2234

Chlorprothixene (Potential for increased sedation). Products include:
- Taractan Tablets ... 1920

Chlorprothixene Hydrochloride (Potential for increased sedation). Products include:
- Taractan ... 1920

Clorazepate Dipotassium (Potential for increased sedation). Products include:
- Tranxene ... 556

Codeine (Potential for increased sedation). Products include:
- Calcidrine Syrup ... 506

Codeine Phosphate (Potential for increased sedation). Products include:
- Actifed with Codeine Cough Syrup.. 752
- Cheracol Cough Syrup ... 1853
- Codimal PH Syrup ... 846
- Dimetane-DC Cough Syrup ... 1857
- Empirin with Codeine Phosphate Nos. 2, 3 & 4 ... 764
- Fiorinal with Codeine Capsules ... 2008
- Isoclor Expectorant ... 982
- Naldecon CX Adult Liquid ... ▣ 521
- Novahistine DH ... 1342
- Novahistine Expectorant ... 1343
- Nucofed Capsules ... 2219
- Nucofed Expectorant ... 2219
- Nucofed Pediatric Expectorant ... 2220
- Nucofed Syrup ... 2219
- Phenaphen with Codeine Capsules 1865
- Phenaphen-650 with Codeine Tablets ... 1866
- Phenergan with Codeine ... 2497
- Phenergan VC with Codeine ... 2501
- Robitussin A-C Syrup ... 1875
- Robitussin-DAC Syrup ... 1875
- Ryna ... ▣ 741
- Soma Compound w/Codeine Tablets ... 2390
- Triaminic Expectorant w/Codeine .. 1996
- Tussi-Organidin Liquid ... 2391
- Tylenol with Codeine ... 1381

Codeine Polistirex (Potential for increased sedation).
- No products indexed under this heading.

Dezocine (Potential for increased sedation).

Diazepam (Potential for increased sedation). Products include:
- Valium Injectable ... 1937
- Valium Tablets ... 1939
- Valrelease Capsules ... 1923

Droperidol (Potential for increased sedation). Products include:
- Inapsine Injection ... 1140
- Innovar Injection ... 1141

Enflurane (Potential for increased sedation). Products include:
- Ethrane ... 599

Estazolam (Potential for increased sedation). Products include:
- ProSom Tablets ... 554

Ethchlorvynol (Potential for increased sedation). Products include:
- Placidyl Capsules ... 553

Ethinamate (Potential for increased sedation).
- No products indexed under this heading.

Fentanyl (Potential for increased sedation). Products include:
- Duragesic Transdermal System ... 1133

Fentanyl Citrate (Potential for increased sedation). Products include:
- Innovar Injection ... 1141
- Sublimaze Injection ... 1146

Fluphenazine Decanoate (Potential for increased sedation). Products include:
- Prolixin Decanoate ... 1795

Fluphenazine Enanthate (Potential for increased sedation). Products include:
- Prolixin Enanthate ... 1796

Fluphenazine Hydrochloride (Potential for increased sedation). Products include:
- Prolixin Elixir ... 1793
- Prolixin Injection ... 1791
- Prolixin Oral Concentrate ... 1792
- Prolixin Tablets ... 1793

Flurazepam Hydrochloride (Potential for increased sedation). Products include:
- Dalmane Capsules ... 1927

Glutethimide (Potential for increased sedation).
- No products indexed under this heading.

Haloperidol (Potential for increased sedation). Products include:
- Haldol Injection, Tablets and Concentrate ... 1373

Haloperidol Decanoate (Potential for increased sedation). Products include:
- Haldol Decanoate ... 1375

Hydrochlorothiazide (Partially additive effects in patients not responding adequately to either drug alone). Products include:
- Aldactazide ... 2150
- Aldoril Tablets ... 1418
- Apresazide Capsules ... 854
- Apresoline-Esidrix Tablets ... 857
- Capozide ... 2258
- Dyazide Capsules ... 2208
- Esidrix Tablets ... 863
- Esimil Tablets ... 864
- HydroDIURIL Tablets ... 1484
- Hydropres Tablets ... 1485
- Inderide Tablets ... 2463
- Inderide LA Long Acting Capsules .. 2465
- Lopressor HCT Tablets ... 1034
- Maxzide ... 1215
- Moduretic Tablets ... 1510
- Normozide Tablets ... 2112
- Oretic Tablets ... 544
- Oreticyl ... 545
- Prinzide Tablets ... 1540
- Ser-Ap-Es Tablets ... 881
- Serpasil-Esidrix Tablets ... 886
- Timolide Tablets ... 1547
- Trandate HCT Tablets ... 579
- Vaseretic Tablets ... 1559
- Zestoretic ... 2274

Hydrocodone Bitartrate (Potential for increased sedation). Products include:
- Anexsia 5/500 Tablets ... 2196
- Anexsia 7.5/650 Tablets ... 2197
- Azdōne Tablets ... 844
- Codiclear DH Syrup ... 845
- Codimal DH Syrup ... 846
- Damason-P ... 1356
- Hycodan Syrup, Tablets ... 927
- Hycomine Compound Tablets ... 929
- Hycomine Syrup ... 927
- Hycotuss Expectorant Syrup ... 930
- Hydrocet Capsules ... 835
- Lortab ASA Tablets ... 2414
- Lortab ... 2412
- Ru-Tuss with Hydrocodone ... 694
- Triaminic Expectorant DH ... 1995
- Vicodin Tablets ... 1187
- Vicodin ES Tablets ... 1189
- Zydone Capsules ... 941

Hydrocodone Polistirex (Potential for increased sedation). Products include:
- Tussionex Extended-Release Suspension ... 988

Hydroxyzine Hydrochloride (Potential for increased sedation). Products include:
- Atarax Tablets & Syrup ... 1941
- Marax Tablets & DF Syrup ... 1954
- Vistaril Intramuscular Solution ... 1970

Isoflurane (Potential for increased sedation). Products include:
- Forane ... 600

Ketamine Hydrochloride (Potential for increased sedation). Products include:
- Ketalar ... 1726

Levorphanol Tartrate (Potential for increased sedation). Products include:
- Levo-Dromoran ... 1906

Lorazepam (Potential for increased sedation). Products include:
- Ativan Injection ... 2432
- Ativan Tablets ... 2434

Loxapine Hydrochloride (Potential for increased sedation). Products include:
- Loxitane ... 1213

Loxapine Succinate (Potential for increased sedation). Products include:
- Loxitane Capsules ... 1213

Meperidine Hydrochloride (Potential for increased sedation). Products include:
- Demerol ... 2047
- Mepergan Injection ... 2479

Mephobarbital (Potential for increased sedation). Products include:
- Mebaral Tablets ... 2061

Meprobamate (Potential for increased sedation). Products include:
- Deprol Tablets ... 2382
- Equagesic Tablets ... 2451
- Miltown Tablets ... 2386
- PMB 200 and PMB 400 ... 2504

Mesoridazine (Potential for increased sedation). Products include:
- Serentil ... 686

Methadone Hydrochloride (Potential for increased sedation). Products include:
- Dolophine Hydrochloride Ampoules & Vials ... 1260
- Dolophine Hydrochloride Tablets ... 1261
- Methadone Hydrochloride Diskets .. 1284
- Methadone Hydrochloride Oral Solution & Tablets ... 1987

Methohexital Sodium (Potential for increased sedation). Products include:
- Brevital Sodium Vials ... 1248

Methoxyflurane (Potential for increased sedation).
- No products indexed under this heading.

Midazolam Hydrochloride (Potential for increased sedation). Products include:
- Versed Injection ... 1924

Molindone Hydrochloride (Potential for increased sedation). Products include:
- Moban Tablets & Concentrate ... 932

Morphine Sulfate (Potential for increased sedation). Products include:
- Astramorph/PF Injection, USP (Preservative-Free) ... 618
- Duramorph ... 960
- Infumorph 200 and Infumorph 500 Sterile Solutions ... 962
- MS Contin Tablets ... 1814
- MSIR ... 1817
- Oramorph SR (Morphine Sulfate Sustained Release Tablets) ... 1988
- Roxanol ... 1991

Opium Alkaloids (Potential for increased sedation). Products include:
- B & O No. 15A & No. 16A Supprettes ... 2395
- Pantopon Injectable ... 1911

Oxazepam (Potential for increased sedation). Products include:
- Serax Capsules ... 2522
- Serax Tablets ... 2522

Oxycodone Hydrochloride (Potential for increased sedation). Products include:
- Percocet Tablets ... 950
- Percodan ... 951
- Roxicodone Tablets, Oral Solution & Intensol (Oxycodone) ... 1992
- Tylox Capsules ... 1382

Pentobarbital Sodium (Potential for increased sedation). Products include:
- Nembutal Sodium Capsules ... 534
- Nembutal Sodium Solution ... 536
- Nembutal Sodium Suppositories ... 538

Perphenazine (Potential for increased sedation). Products include:
- Etrafon ... 2087
- Triavil Tablets ... 1556
- Trilafon ... 2123

Phenobarbital (Potential for increased sedation). Products include:
- Arco-Lase Plus Tablets ... 607
- Bellergal-S Tablets ... 1998
- Bronkolixir ... ▣ 761
- Bronkotabs Tablets ... ▣ 762
- Donnatal ... 1858
- Donnatal Extentabs ... 1859
- Donnatal Tablets ... 1858
- Donnazyme Tablets ... 1860
- Kinesed Tablets ... 2272
- Phenobarbital Elixir and Tablets ... 1293
- Primatene Tablets-P Formula ... 2421
- Quadrinal Tablets ... 1183
- Tedral SA ... 1765

Prazepam (Potential for increased sedation). Products include:
- Centrax ... 1693

Prochlorperazine (Potential for increased sedation). Products include:
- Compazine ... 2201

Promethazine Hydrochloride (Potential for increased sedation). Products include:
- Mepergan Injection ... 2479
- Phenergan with Codeine ... 2497
- Phenergan with Dextromethorphan 2499
- Phenergan Injection ... 2493
- Phenergan Suppositories ... 2496
- Phenergan Syrup ... 2495
- Phenergan Tablets ... 2496
- Phenergan VC ... 2500
- Phenergan VC with Codeine ... 2501

Propofol (Potential for increased sedation). Products include:
- Diprivan Injection ... 2267

Propoxyphene Hydrochloride (Potential for increased sedation). Products include:
- Darvon ... 1256
- Wygesic Tablets ... 2540

Propoxyphene Napsylate (Potential for increased sedation). Products include:
- Darvon-N/Darvocet-N ... 1254

Quazepam (Potential for increased sedation). Products include:
Doral Tablets 2383
Secobarbital Sodium (Potential for increased sedation). Products include:
Seconal Sodium Pulvules 1296
Sufentanil Citrate (Potential for increased sedation). Products include:
Sufenta Injection 1147
Temazepam (Potential for increased sedation). Products include:
Restoril Capsules 2023
Thiamylal Sodium (Potential for increased sedation). Products include:
Surital Ampoules, Steri-Vials 1764
Thioridazine Hydrochloride (Potential for increased sedation). Products include:
Mellaril 2011
Thiothixene (Potential for increased sedation). Products include:
Navane Capsules and Concentrate 1954
Navane Intramuscular 1956
Triazolam (Potential for increased sedation). Products include:
Halcion Tablets 2340
Trifluoperazine Hydrochloride (Potential for increased sedation). Products include:
Stelazine 2226

X-SEB SHAMPOO
(Salicylic Acid) .... ▣ 510
No interactions described in labeling.

X-SEB PLUS CONDITIONING SHAMPOO
(Salicylic Acid, Pyrithione Zinc) .... ▣ 510
No interactions described in labeling.

X-SEB T SHAMPOO
(Coal Tar, Ethyl Alcohol, Salicylic Acid) .... ▣ 510
No interactions described in labeling.

X-SEB T PLUS CONDITIONING SHAMPOO
(Coal Tar, Salicylic Acid, Menthol) .. ▣ 510
No interactions described in labeling.

XANAX TABLETS
(Alprazolam) 2367
May interact with central nervous system depressants, anticonvulsants, antihistamines, oral contraceptives, and certain other agents. Compounds in these categories include:

Alcohol (Additive CNS depressant effects).
Alfentanil Hydrochloride (Additive CNS depressant effects). Products include:
Alfenta Injection 1131
Aprobarbital (Additive CNS depressant effects). Products include:
Alurate Elixir 1883
Astemizole (Additive CNS depressant effects). Products include:
Hismanal Tablets 1138
Azatadine Maleate (Additive CNS depressant effects). Products include:
Optimine Tablets 2115
Trinalin Repetabs Tablets 1170
Bromodiphenhydramine Hydrochloride (Additive CNS depressant effects).
No products indexed under this heading.
Brompheniramine Maleate (Additive CNS depressant effects). Products include:
Alka Seltzer Plus Sinus Allergy Medicine .... ▣ 624
Atrohist Sprinkle Capsules 558
Bromfed Capsules (Timed Release) 1615
Bromfed Syrup .... ▣ 628
Bromfed 1615
Dimetane Decongestant .... ▣ 673
Dimetane .... ▣ 672
Dimetane-DC Cough Syrup 1857
Dimetane-DX Cough Syrup 1858
Dimetapp Elixir .... ▣ 673
Dimetapp DM Elixir .... ▣ 674
Dimetapp Extentabs .... ▣ 674
Dimetapp Plus Caplets .... ▣ 675
Dimetapp Tablets .... ▣ 675
Drixoral Antihistamine/Nasal Decongestant Syrup .... ▣ 698
Buprenorphine (Additive CNS depressant effects).
No products indexed under this heading.
Buspirone Hydrochloride (Additive CNS depressant effects). Products include:
BuSpar 1401
Butabarbital (Additive CNS depressant effects). Products include:
Pyridium Plus 1764
Butalbital (Additive CNS depressant effects). Products include:
Esgic-Plus Tablets 1002
Esgic Tablets & Capsules 1001
Fioricet Tablets 2006
Fiorinal Capsules 2007
Fiorinal with Codeine Capsules 2008
Fiorinal Tablets 2007
Phrenilin 838
Sedapap Tablets 50 mg/650 mg .. 1360
Carbamazepine (Additive CNS depressant effects). Products include:
Tegretol Chewable Tablets 654
Tegretol Suspension 656
Tegretol Tablets 654
Chlordiazepoxide (Additive CNS depressant effects). Products include:
Libritabs Tablets 1930
Limbitrol 1933
Menrium Tablets 1934
Chlordiazepoxide Hydrochloride (Additive CNS depressant effects). Products include:
Librax Capsules 1929
Librium Capsules 1931
Librium Injectable 1932
Chlorpheniramine Maleate (Additive CNS depressant effects). Products include:
A.R.M. Allergy Relief Medicine Caplets .... ▣ 615
Alka-Seltzer Plus Cold Medicine .... ▣ 623
Allerest .... ▣ 559
Ana-Kit Anaphylaxis Emergency Treatment Kit 1100
BC Cold Powder Multi-Symptom Formula .... ▣ 517
Brexin L.A. Capsules 2078
Cerose-DM 2443
Cheracol Plus Head Cold/Cough Formula .... ▣ 667
Chlor-Trimeton Allergy Syrup, Tablets & Long-Acting Repetabs Tablets .... ▣ 693
Chlor-Trimeton Decongestant .... ▣ 694
Comhist LA Capsules 1618
Allergy-Sinus Comtrex Multi-Symptom Allergy Sinus Formula Tablets & Caplets 746
Comtrex Multi-Symptom Cold Reliever Tablets/Caplets/Liqui-Gels/Liquid 745
Day-Night Comtrex 747
Contac Continuous Action Decongestant/Antihistamine Capsules ▣ 710
Contac Maximum Strength Continuous Action Decongestant/Antihistamine Caplets .... ▣ 709
Contac Severe Cold and Flu Formula Caplets .... ▣ 711
Coricidin 'D' Decongestant Tablets .... ▣ 695
Coricidin Demilets Tablets for Children .... ▣ 696
Coricidin Tablets .... ▣ 695
Deconamine 663
Demazin Nasal Decongestant/Antihistamine Repetabs Tablets & Syrup .... ▣ 697
Dorcol Children's Liquid Cold Formula .... ▣ 686
Dristan Decongestant/Antihistamine/ Analgesic Coated Caplets .... ▣ 749
Dristan Cold Nasal Decongestant/Antihistamine/ Analgesic Coated Tablets 2419
Dristan Advanced Formula Decongestant/Antihistamine/Analgesic Tablets .... ▣ 749
Extendryl 994
4-Way Cold Tablets 750
Fedahist Gyrocaps 2145
Fedahist Timecaps 2145
Hycomine Compound Tablets 929
Isoclor Timesule Capsules .... ▣ 561
Kronofed-A 970
Medi-Flu Caplet, Liquid .... ▣ 640
Naldecon Syrup, Tablets, Pediatric Drops and Pediatric Syrup 709
Nolamine Tablets 838
Novafed A Capsules 1342
Novahistine DH 1342
Novahistine Elixir .... ▣ 596
Ornade Spansule Capsules 2221
Orthoxicol Cough Syrup .... ▣ 668
PediaCare Allergy Relief Formula Liquid 1362
PediaCare Cough-Cold Formula Liquid 1362
PediaCare Night Rest Cough-Cold Formula Liquid 1362
PediaCare 6-12 Cough-Cold Formula Chewable Tablets 1362
Pyrroxate Capsules .... ▣ 669
Quelidrine Syrup 556
Ru-Tuss II Capsules 693
Ru-Tuss Tablets 693
Ryna .... ▣ 741
Sinarest Tablets & Extra Strength Tablets .... ▣ 562
Sine-Off Maximum Strength Allergy/Sinus Formula Caplets .... ▣ 721
Sine-Off Sinus Medicine Tablets-Aspirin Formula .... ▣ 722
Singlet Tablets .... ▣ 598
Sinulin 840
Sinutab Maximum Strength .... ▣ 641
St. Joseph Nighttime Cold Medicine .... ▣ 705
Sudafed Plus Liquid .... ▣ 544
Sudafed Plus Tablets .... ▣ 545
Teldrin Timed-Release Allergy Capsules, 12 mg 2192
TheraFlu Flu and Cold Medicine .... ▣ 687
Triaminic Allergy Tablets .... ▣ 688
Triaminic Chewables .... ▣ 688
Triaminic Cold Tablets .... ▣ 688
Triaminic Nite Light .... ▣ 689
Triaminic Syrup .... ▣ 689
Triaminic-12 Tablets .... ▣ 690
Triaminicin Tablets .... ▣ 690
Triaminicol Multi-Symptom Cold Tablets .... ▣ 691
Triaminicol Multi-Symptom Relief ▣ 691
Tylenol Allergy Sinus Medication Caplets and Gelcaps, Maximum Strength 1372
Children's Tylenol Cold Liquid Formula and Chewable Tablets 1368
Tylenol Cold & Flu Hot Medication, Packets 1369
Tylenol Cold Medication Caplets and Tablets 1370
Tylenol Cold Medication, Effervescent Tablets 1369
Vicks Children's NyQuil .... ▣ 664
Vicks Formula 44 Cough Medicine .... ▣ 661
Vicks Formula 44M Multi-Symptom Cough Medicine .... ▣ 662
Vicks Pediatric Formula 44m Multi-Symptom Cough & Cold Medicine .... ▣ 663
Chlorpheniramine Polistirex (Additive CNS depressant effects). Products include:
Tussionex Extended-Release Suspension 988
Chlorpheniramine Tannate (Additive CNS depressant effects). Products include:
Rynatan 2387
Rynatuss 2388
Chlorpromazine (Additive CNS depressant effects). Products include:
Thorazine 2234
Chlorprothixene (Additive CNS depressant effects). Products include:
Taractan Tablets 1920
Chlorprothixene Hydrochloride (Additive CNS depressant effects). Products include:
Taractan 1920
Cimetidine (Delayed clearance of alprazolam). Products include:
Tagamet Tablets 2228
Cimetidine Hydrochloride (Delayed clearance of alprazolam). Products include:
Tagamet 2228
Clemastine Fumarate (Additive CNS depressant effects). Products include:
Tavist Syrup 2033
Tavist Tablets 2035
Tavist-D Tablets 2035
Clorazepate Dipotassium (Additive CNS depressant effects). Products include:
Tranxene 556
Codeine (Additive CNS depressant effects). Products include:
Calcidrine Syrup 506
Codeine Phosphate (Additive CNS depressant effects). Products include:
Actifed with Codeine Cough Syrup.. 752
Cheracol Cough Syrup 1853
Codimal PH Syrup 846
Dimetane-DC Cough Syrup 1857
Empirin with Codeine Phosphate Nos. 2, 3 & 4 764
Fiorinal with Codeine Capsules 2008
Isoclor Expectorant 982
Naldecon CX Adult Liquid .... ▣ 521
Novahistine DH 1342
Novahistine Expectorant 1343
Nucofed Capsules 2219
Nucofed Expectorant 2219
Nucofed Pediatric Expectorant 2220
Nucofed Syrup 2219
Phenaphen with Codeine Capsules 1865
Phenaphen-650 with Codeine Tablets 1866
Phenergan with Codeine 2497
Phenergan VC with Codeine 2501
Robitussin A-C Syrup 1875
Robitussin-DAC Syrup 1875
Ryna .... ▣ 741
Soma Compound w/Codeine Tablets 2390
Triaminic Expectorant w/Codeine .. 1996
Tussi-Organidin Liquid 2391
Tylenol with Codeine 1381
Codeine Polistirex (Additive CNS depressant effects).
No products indexed under this heading.
Cyproheptadine Hydrochloride (Additive CNS depressant effects). Products include:
Periactin 1525
Desipramine Hydrochloride (Increased steady state-plasma concentrations). Products include:
Norpramin Tablets 1340
Dexchlorpheniramine Maleate (Additive CNS depressant effects). Products include:
Polaramine 2116
Dezocine (Additive CNS depressant effects).
Diazepam (Additive CNS depressant effects). Products include:
Valium Injectable 1937
Valium Tablets 1939
Valrelease Capsules 1923

Diphenhydramine Citrate (Additive CNS depressant effects). Products include:
- Alka-Seltzer Plus Night-Time Cold Medicine ND 623
- Bufferin AF Nite Time Analgesic/Sleeping Aid Caplets 744
- Excedrin P.M. Analgesic/Sleeping Aid Tablets, Caplets and Liquid 749

Diphenhydramine Hydrochloride (Additive CNS depressant effects). Products include:
- Benadryl Anti-Itch Cream ND 635
- Benadryl Capsules 1691
- Benadryl Decongestant Elixir ND 635
- Benadryl Decongestant ND 635
- Benadryl Elixir ND 636
- Benadryl Kapseals 1691
- Benadryl 25 Kapseals ND 636
- Benadryl Parenteral 1692
- Benadryl Plus ND 636
- Benadryl Plus Nighttime ND 637
- Benadryl Spray, Maximum Strength ND 637
- Benadryl Spray, Regular Strength ND 637
- Benadryl Steri-Vials, Ampoules, and Steri-Dose Syringe 1692
- Benadryl 25 Tablets ND 636
- Benylin Cough Syrup ND 637
- Benylin Decongestant ND 638
- Caladryl Cream, Lotion, Spray ND 638
- Miles Nervine Nighttime Sleep-Aid ND 627
- Nytol Tablets ND 517
- Sleep-ettes-D Tablets ND 653
- Sleep-eze 3 Tablets ND 755
- Sleepinal Night-time Sleep Aid Capsules ND 734
- Sominex Caplets and Tablets ND 722
- Sominex Liquid ND 723
- Sominex Pain Relief Formula ND 723
- Tylenol Cold Night Time Medication Liquid 1371
- Tylenol PM, Extra Strength Caplets and Tablets 1368
- Unisom Dual Relief Nighttime Sleep Aid/Analgesic 1774
- Ziradryl Lotion ND 643

Diphenylpyraline Hydrochloride (Additive CNS depressant effects).
- No products indexed under this heading.

Divalproex Sodium (Additive CNS depressant effects). Products include:
- Depakote 512

Droperidol (Additive CNS depressant effects). Products include:
- Inapsine Injection 1140
- Innovar Injection 1141

Enflurane (Additive CNS depressant effects). Products include:
- Ethrane 599

Estazolam (Additive CNS depressant effects). Products include:
- ProSom Tablets 554

Ethchlorvynol (Additive CNS depressant effects). Products include:
- Placidyl Capsules 553

Ethinamate (Additive CNS depressant effects).
- No products indexed under this heading.

Ethinyl Estradiol (Delayed clearance of alprazolam). Products include:
- Brevicon 2304
- Demulen 2161
- Estinyl Tablets 2085
- Jenest-28 Tablets 1636
- Levlen/Tri-Levlen 665
- Lo/Ovral Tablets 2471
- Lo/Ovral-28 Tablets 2476
- Loestrin 1728
- Modicon 1667
- Nordette-21 Tablets 2481
- Nordette-28 Tablets 2483
- Norethin 2133
- Norinyl 2304
- Norlestrin 1746
- Ortho-Cyclen Tablets 1658
- Ortho-Novum 1667
- Ovcon 1391
- Ovral Tablets 2490
- Ovral-28 Tablets 2491
- Levlen/Tri-Levlen 665
- Tri-Norinyl 2304
- Triphasil-21 Tablets 2527
- Triphasil-28 Tablets 2532

Ethosuximide (Additive CNS depressant effects). Products include:
- Zarontin Capsules 1768
- Zarontin Syrup 1769

Ethotoin (Additive CNS depressant effects). Products include:
- Peganone Tablets 551

Ethynodiol Diacetate (Delayed clearance of alprazolam). Products include:
- Demulen 2161

Fentanyl (Additive CNS depressant effects). Products include:
- Duragesic Transdermal System 1133

Fentanyl Citrate (Additive CNS depressant effects). Products include:
- Innovar Injection 1141
- Sublimaze Injection 1146

Fluphenazine Decanoate (Additive CNS depressant effects). Products include:
- Prolixin Decanoate 1795

Fluphenazine Enanthate (Additive CNS depressant effects). Products include:
- Prolixin Enanthate 1796

Fluphenazine Hydrochloride (Additive CNS depressant effects). Products include:
- Prolixin Elixir 1793
- Prolixin Injection 1791
- Prolixin Oral Concentrate 1792
- Prolixin Tablets 1793

Flurazepam Hydrochloride (Additive CNS depressant effects). Products include:
- Dalmane Capsules 1927

Glutethimide (Additive CNS depressant effects).
- No products indexed under this heading.

Haloperidol (Additive CNS depressant effects). Products include:
- Haldol Injection, Tablets and Concentrate 1373

Haloperidol Decanoate (Additive CNS depressant effects). Products include:
- Haldol Decanoate 1375

Hydrocodone Bitartrate (Additive CNS depressant effects). Products include:
- Anexsia 5/500 Tablets 2196
- Anexsia 7.5/650 Tablets 2197
- Azdone Tablets 844
- Codiclear DH Syrup 845
- Codimal DH Syrup 846
- Damason-P 1356
- Hycodan Syrup, Tablets 927
- Hycomine Compound Tablets 929
- Hycomine Syrup 927
- Hycotuss Expectorant Syrup 930
- Hydrocet Capsules 835
- Lortab ASA Tablets 2414
- Lortab 2412
- Ru-Tuss with Hydrocodone 694
- Triaminic Expectorant DH 1995
- Vicodin Tablets 1187
- Vicodin ES Tablets 1189
- Zydone Capsules 941

Hydrocodone Polistirex (Additive CNS depressant effects). Products include:
- Tussionex Extended-Release Suspension 988

Hydroxyzine Hydrochloride (Additive CNS depressant effects). Products include:
- Atarax Tablets & Syrup 1941
- Marax Tablets & DF Syrup 1954
- Vistaril Intramuscular Solution 1970

Imipramine Hydrochloride (Increased steady state-plasma concentrations). Products include:
- Tofranil Ampuls 1038
- Tofranil Tablets 1039

Imipramine Pamoate (Increased steady state-plasma concentrations). Products include:
- Tofranil-PM Capsules 1041

Isoflurane (Additive CNS depressant effects). Products include:
- Forane 600

Ketamine Hydrochloride (Additive CNS depressant effects). Products include:
- Ketalar 1726

Levonorgestrel (Delayed clearance of alprazolam). Products include:
- Levlen/Tri-Levlen 665
- Nordette-21 Tablets 2481
- Nordette-28 Tablets 2483
- Norplant System 2484
- Levlen/Tri-Levlen 665
- Triphasil-21 Tablets 2527
- Triphasil-28 Tablets 2532

Levorphanol Tartrate (Additive CNS depressant effects). Products include:
- Levo-Dromoran 1906

Lorazepam (Additive CNS depressant effects). Products include:
- Ativan Injection 2432
- Ativan Tablets 2434

Loxapine Hydrochloride (Additive CNS depressant effects). Products include:
- Loxitane 1213

Loxapine Succinate (Additive CNS depressant effects). Products include:
- Loxitane Capsules 1213

Meperidine Hydrochloride (Additive CNS depressant effects). Products include:
- Demerol 2047
- Mepergan Injection 2479

Mephenytoin (Additive CNS depressant effects). Products include:
- Mesantoin Tablets 2013

Mephobarbital (Additive CNS depressant effects). Products include:
- Mebaral Tablets 2061

Meprobamate (Additive CNS depressant effects). Products include:
- Deprol Tablets 2382
- Equagesic Tablets 2451
- Miltown Tablets 2386
- PMB 200 and PMB 400 2504

Mesoridazine (Additive CNS depressant effects). Products include:
- Serentil 686

Mesoridazine Besylate (Additive CNS depressant effects).

Mestranol (Delayed clearance of alprazolam). Products include:
- Enovid 2161
- Norethin 2133
- Norinyl 2304
- Ortho-Novum 1667

Methadone Hydrochloride (Additive CNS depressant effects). Products include:
- Dolophine Hydrochloride Ampoules & Vials 1260
- Dolophine Hydrochloride Tablets 1261
- Methadone Hydrochloride Diskets 1284
- Methadone Hydrochloride Oral Solution & Tablets 1987

Methdilazine Hydrochloride (Additive CNS depressant effects). Products include:
- Tacaryl Syrup & Tablets 2409

Methohexital Sodium (Additive CNS depressant effects). Products include:
- Brevital Sodium Vials 1248

Methoxyflurane (Additive CNS depressant effects).
- No products indexed under this heading.

Methsuximide (Additive CNS depressant effects). Products include:
- Celontin 1692

Midazolam Hydrochloride (Additive CNS depressant effects). Products include:
- Versed Injection 1924

Molindone Hydrochloride (Additive CNS depressant effects). Products include:
- Moban Tablets & Concentrate 932

Morphine Sulfate (Additive CNS depressant effects). Products include:
- Astramorph/PF Injection, USP (Preservative-Free) 618
- Duramorph 960
- Infumorph 200 and Infumorph 500 Sterile Solutions 962
- MS Contin Tablets 1814
- MSIR 1817
- Oramorph SR (Morphine Sulfate Sustained Release Tablets) 1988
- Roxanol 1991

Norethindrone (Delayed clearance of alprazolam). Products include:
- Brevicon 2304
- Jenest-28 Tablets 1636
- Micronor Tablets 1667
- Modicon 1667
- Norethin 2133
- Norinyl 2304
- Norlutin 1755
- Nor-Q D Tablets 2304
- Ortho-Novum 1667
- Ovcon 1391
- Tri-Norinyl 2304

Norethynodrel (Delayed clearance of alprazolam). Products include:
- Enovid 2161

Norgestimate (Delayed clearance of alprazolam). Products include:
- Ortho-Cyclen Tablets 1658

Norgestrel (Delayed clearance of alprazolam). Products include:
- Lo/Ovral Tablets 2471
- Lo/Ovral-28 Tablets 2476
- Ovral Tablets 2490
- Ovral-28 Tablets 2491
- Ovrette Tablets 2492

Opium Alkaloids (Additive CNS depressant effects). Products include:
- B & O No. 15A & No. 16A Supprettes 2395
- Pantopon Injectable 1911

Oxazepam (Additive CNS depressant effects). Products include:
- Serax Capsules 2522
- Serax Tablets 2522

Oxycodone Hydrochloride (Additive CNS depressant effects). Products include:
- Percocet Tablets 950
- Percodan 951
- Roxicodone Tablets, Oral Solution & Intensol (Oxycodone) 1992
- Tylox Capsules 1382

Paramethadione (Additive CNS depressant effects). Products include:
- Paradione Capsules 548

Pentobarbital Sodium (Additive CNS depressant effects). Products include:
- Nembutal Sodium Capsules 534
- Nembutal Sodium Solution 536
- Nembutal Sodium Suppositories 538

Perphenazine (Additive CNS depressant effects). Products include:
- Etrafon 2087
- Triavil Tablets 1556
- Trilafon 2123

Phenacemide (Additive CNS depressant effects). Products include:
- Phenurone Tablets 552

Phenobarbital (Additive CNS depressant effects). Products include:
- Arco-Lase Plus Tablets 607
- Bellergal-S Tablets 1998
- Bronkolixir ND 761

Bronkotabs Tablets ▣ 762
Donnatal 1858
Donnatal Extentabs 1859
Donnatal Tablets 1858
Donnazyme Tablets 1860
Kinesed Tablets 2272
Phenobarbital Elixir and Tablets 1293
Primatene Tablets-P Formula 2421
Quadrinal Tablets 1183
Tedral SA 1765

Phensuximide (Additive CNS depressant effects). Products include:
Milontin Kapseals 1741

Phenytoin (Additive CNS depressant effects). Products include:
Dilantin Infatabs 1710
Dilantin-30 Pediatric/Dilantin-125 Suspension 1713

Phenytoin Sodium (Additive CNS depressant effects). Products include:
Dilantin Kapseals 1708
Dilantin Parenteral 1712
Dilantin with Phenobarbital Kapseals 1715

Prazepam (Additive CNS depressant effects). Products include:
Centrax 1693

Primidone (Additive CNS depressant effects). Products include:
Mysoline 2480

Prochlorperazine (Additive CNS depressant effects). Products include:
Compazine 2201

Promethazine Hydrochloride (Additive CNS depressant effects). Products include:
Mepergan Injection 2479
Phenergan with Codeine 2497
Phenergan with Dextromethorphan 2499
Phenergan Injection 2493
Phenergan Suppositories 2496
Phenergan Syrup 2495
Phenergan Tablets 2496
Phenergan VC 2500
Phenergan VC with Codeine 2501

Propofol (Additive CNS depressant effects). Products include:
Diprivan Injection 2267

Propoxyphene Hydrochloride (Additive CNS depressant effects). Products include:
Darvon 1256
Wygesic Tablets 2540

Propoxyphene Napsylate (Additive CNS depressant effects). Products include:
Darvon-N/Darvocet-N 1254

Pyrilamine Maleate (Additive CNS depressant effects). Products include:
Codimal 846
4-Way Fast Acting Nasal Spray - Original Formula (regular & mentholated) & Metered Spray Pump (regular) 751
Maximum Strength Midol Multi-Symptom Menstrual Formula ▣ 571
Maximum Strength Midol PMS Premenstrual Syndrome Formula ▣ 570
Regular Strength Midol Multi-Symptom Menstrual Formula ▣ 570
Prefrin-A ⊙ 255
Prēmsyn PMS Capsules & Caplets ▣ 547
Primatene Tablets-M Formula 2421
Robitussin Night Relief ▣ 677
Ru-Tuss with Hydrocodone 694
Triaminic Expectorant DH 1995
Triaminic Oral Infant Drops 1996

Pyrilamine Tannate (Additive CNS depressant effects). Products include:
Rynatan 2387

Quazepam (Additive CNS depressant effects). Products include:
Doral Tablets 2383

Secobarbital Sodium (Additive CNS depressant effects). Products include:
Seconal Sodium Pulvules 1296

Sufentanil Citrate (Additive CNS depressant effects). Products include:
Sufenta Injection 1147

Temazepam (Additive CNS depressant effects). Products include:
Restoril Capsules 2023

Terfenadine (Additive CNS depressant effects). Products include:
Seldane Tablets 1349
Seldane-D Extended-Release Tablets 1350

Thiamylal Sodium (Additive CNS depressant effects). Products include:
Surital Ampoules, Steri-Vials 1764

Thioridazine Hydrochloride (Additive CNS depressant effects). Products include:
Mellaril 2011

Thiothixene (Additive CNS depressant effects). Products include:
Navane Capsules and Concentrate 1954
Navane Intramuscular 1956

Triazolam (Additive CNS depressant effects). Products include:
Halcion Tablets 2340

Trifluoperazine Hydrochloride (Additive CNS depressant effects). Products include:
Stelazine 2226

Trimeprazine Tartrate (Additive CNS depressant effects). Products include:
Temaril Tablets, Syrup and Spansule Sustained Release Capsules 1085

Trimethadione (Additive CNS depressant effects). Products include:
Tridione 557

Tripelennamine Hydrochloride (Additive CNS depressant effects). Products include:
PBZ Tablets & Elixir 1037
PBZ-SR Tablets 1037

Triprolidine Hydrochloride (Additive CNS depressant effects). Products include:
Actidil ▣ 538
Actifed Capsules ▣ 539
Actifed Plus Caplets ▣ 539
Actifed Plus Tablets ▣ 540
Actifed with Codeine Cough Syrup 752
Actifed Syrup ▣ 540
Actifed Tablets ▣ 540
Actifed 12-Hour Capsules ▣ 539

Valproic Acid (Additive CNS depressant effects). Products include:
Depakene Capsules & Syrup 511

XERAC AC
(Aluminum Chloride) 1773
No interactions described in labeling.

XERAC BP5 & BP10
(Benzoyl Peroxide) 1773
No interactions described in labeling.

XYLOCAINE INJECTIONS
(Lidocaine Hydrochloride) 637
See **Xylocaine with Epinephrine Injections**

XYLOCAINE WITH EPINEPHRINE INJECTIONS
(Lidocaine Hydrochloride, Epinephrine) 637
May interact with monoamine oxidase inhibitors, tricyclic antidepressants, phenothiazines, butyrophenones, and certain other agents. Compounds in these categories include:

Amitriptyline Hydrochloride (Potential for severe, prolonged hypertension). Products include:
Elavil 2269
Endep Tablets 1927
Etrafon 2087
Limbitrol 1933
Triavil Tablets 1556

Amoxapine (Potential for severe, prolonged hypertension). Products include:
Asendin Tablets 1196

Chlorpromazine (Reduces or reverses the pressor effect of epinephrine). Products include:
Thorazine 2234

Clomipramine Hydrochloride (Potential for severe, prolonged hypertension). Products include:
Anafranil Capsules 650

Desipramine Hydrochloride (Potential for severe, prolonged hypertension). Products include:
Norpramin Tablets 1340

Doxepin Hydrochloride (Potential for severe, prolonged hypertension). Products include:
Sinequan 1960

Ergonovine Maleate (Potential for severe, persistent hypertension or cerebrovascular accidents).

Fluphenazine Decanoate (Reduces or reverses the pressor effect of epinephrine). Products include:
Prolixin Decanoate 1795

Fluphenazine Enanthate (Reduces or reverses the pressor effect of epinephrine). Products include:
Prolixin Enanthate 1796

Fluphenazine Hydrochloride (Reduces or reverses the pressor effect of epinephrine). Products include:
Prolixin Elixir 1793
Prolixin Injection 1791
Prolixin Oral Concentrate 1792
Prolixin Tablets 1793

Furazolidone (Potential for severe, prolonged hypertension). Products include:
Furoxone 1855

Haloperidol (Reduces or reverses the pressor effect of epinephrine). Products include:
Haldol Injection, Tablets and Concentrate 1373

Haloperidol Decanoate (Reduces or reverses the pressor effect of epinephrine). Products include:
Haldol Decanoate 1375

Imipramine Hydrochloride (Potential for severe, prolonged hypertension). Products include:
Tofranil Ampuls 1038
Tofranil Tablets 1039

Imipramine Pamoate (Potential for severe, prolonged hypertension). Products include:
Tofranil-PM Capsules 1041

Isocarboxazid (Potential for severe, prolonged hypertension). Products include:
Marplan Tablets 1906

Maprotiline Hydrochloride (Potential for severe, prolonged hypertension). Products include:
Ludiomil Tablets 874

Mesoridazine Besylate (Reduces or reverses the pressor effect of epinephrine).

Methylergonovine Maleate (Potential for severe, persistent hypertension or cerebrovascular accidents). Products include:
Methergine 2016

Nortriptyline Hydrochloride (Potential for severe, prolonged hypertension). Products include:
Pamelor 2019

Perphenazine (Reduces or reverses the pressor effect of epinephrine). Products include:
Etrafon 2087
Triavil Tablets 1556
Trilafon 2123

Phenelzine Sulfate (Potential for severe, prolonged hypertension). Products include:
Nardil 1742

Prochlorperazine (Reduces or reverses the pressor effect of epinephrine). Products include:
Compazine 2201

Promethazine Hydrochloride (Reduces or reverses the pressor effect of epinephrine). Products include:
Mepergan Injection 2479
Phenergan with Codeine 2497
Phenergan with Dextromethorphan 2499
Phenergan Injection 2493
Phenergan Suppositories 2496
Phenergan Syrup 2495
Phenergan Tablets 2496
Phenergan VC 2500
Phenergan VC with Codeine 2501

Protriptyline Hydrochloride (Potential for severe, prolonged hypertension). Products include:
Vivactil Tablets 1567

Selegiline Hydrochloride (Potential for severe, prolonged hypertension). Products include:
Eldepryl 2250

Thioridazine Hydrochloride (Reduces or reverses the pressor effect of epinephrine). Products include:
Mellaril 2011

Tranylcypromine Sulfate (Potential for severe, prolonged hypertension). Products include:
Parnate Tablets 2222

Trifluoperazine Hydrochloride (Reduces or reverses the pressor effect of epinephrine). Products include:
Stelazine 2226

Trimipramine Maleate (Potential for severe, prolonged hypertension). Products include:
Surmontil Capsules 2524

XYLOCAINE INJECTIONS FOR VENTRICULAR ARRHYTHMIAS
(Lidocaine Hydrochloride) 639
May interact with cardiac glycosides, beta blockers, and certain other agents. Compounds in these categories include:

Acebutolol Hydrochloride (Concomitant use may reduce lidocaine clearance). Products include:
Sectral Capsules 2520

Atenolol (Concomitant use may reduce lidocaine clearance). Products include:
Tenoretic Tablets 1105
Tenormin Tablets and I.V. Injection 1107

Betaxolol Hydrochloride (Concomitant use may reduce lidocaine clearance). Products include:
Betoptic Sterile Ophthalmic Solution 569
Betoptic S Sterile Ophthalmic Suspension 570
Kerlone Tablets 2172

Cimetidine (Concomitant use may reduce lidocaine clearance). Products include:
Tagamet Tablets 2228

Cimetidine Hydrochloride (Concomitant use may reduce lidocaine clearance). Products include:
Tagamet 2228

Deslanoside (Use lidocaine cautiously in patients with digitalis toxicity accompanied by atrioventricular block).
No products indexed under this heading.

Digitoxin (Use lidocaine cautiously in patients with digitalis toxicity accompanied by atrioventricular block). Products include:
Crystodigin Tablets ... 1253
Digoxin (Use lidocaine cautiously in patients with digitalis toxicity accompanied by atrioventricular block). Products include:
Lanoxicaps ... 772
Lanoxin Elixir Pediatric ... 775
Lanoxin Injection ... 778
Lanoxin Injection Pediatric ... 781
Lanoxin Tablets ... 783
Esmolol Hydrochloride (Concomitant use may reduce lidocaine clearance). Products include:
Brevibloc Injection ... 942
Labetalol Hydrochloride (Concomitant use may reduce lidocaine clearance). Products include:
Normodyne Injection ... 2108
Normodyne Tablets ... 2110
Normozide Tablets ... 2112
Trandate HCT Tablets ... 579
Trandate Injection ... 577
Trandate Tablets ... 579
Metoprolol Tartrate (Concomitant use may reduce lidocaine clearance). Products include:
Lopressor Ampuls ... 1032
Lopressor HCT Tablets ... 1034
Lopressor Tablets ... 1032
Nadolol (Concomitant use may reduce lidocaine clearance). Products include:
Corgard Tablets ... 701
Corzide Tablets ... 702
Penbutolol Sulfate (Concomitant use may reduce lidocaine clearance). Products include:
Levatol ... 1832
Pindolol (Concomitant use may reduce lidocaine clearance). Products include:
Visken Tablets ... 2036
Propranolol Hydrochloride (Concomitant use may reduce lidocaine clearance). Products include:
Inderal ... 2459
Inderal LA Long Acting Capsules ... 2461
Inderide Tablets ... 2463
Inderide LA Long Acting Capsules ... 2465
Timolol Maleate (Concomitant use may reduce lidocaine clearance). Products include:
Blocadren Tablets ... 1429
Timolide Tablets ... 1547
Timoptic in Ocudose ... 1552
Timoptic Sterile Ophthalmic Solution ... 1550
Tocainide Hydrochloride (Concomitant use may cause an increased incidence of adverse reactions including seizure). Products include:
Tonocard Tablets ... 1554

XYLOCAINE 2% JELLY
(Lidocaine Hydrochloride) ... 643

Food Interactions

Food, unspecified (Topical anesthesia may impair swallowing and thus enhance the danger of aspiration; avoid food ingestion for 60 minutes).

XYLOCAINE OINTMENT 2.5%
(Lidocaine Base) ... ▣ 508
No interactions described in labeling.

XYLOCAINE 5% OINTMENT
(Lidocaine) ... 644

Food Interactions

Food, unspecified (Food should not be ingested for 60 minutes following usage; danger of biting trauma and aspiration).

XYLOCAINE 10% ORAL SPRAY
(Lidocaine) ... 645

Food Interactions

Food, unspecified (Food should not be ingested for 60 minutes following usage; danger of biting trauma and aspiration).

4% XYLOCAINE-MPF STERILE SOLUTION
(Lidocaine Hydrochloride) ... 641
May interact with (with epinephrine solutions only), general anesthetics, monoamine oxidase inhibitors, tricyclic antidepressants, and phenothiazines. Compounds in these categories include:

Amitriptyline Hydrochloride (Severe, prolonged hypotension or hypertension). Products include:
Elavil ... 2269
Endep Tablets ... 1927
Etrafon ... 2087
Limbitrol ... 1933
Triavil Tablets ... 1556
Amoxapine (Severe, prolonged hypotension or hypertension). Products include:
Asendin Tablets ... 1196
Chlorpromazine (Severe, prolonged hypotension or hypertension). Products include:
Thorazine ... 2234
Clomipramine Hydrochloride (Severe, prolonged hypotension or hypertension). Products include:
Anafranil Capsules ... 650
Desipramine Hydrochloride (Severe, prolonged hypotension or hypertension). Products include:
Norpramin Tablets ... 1340
Doxepin Hydrochloride (Severe, prolonged hypotension or hypertension). Products include:
Sinequan ... 1960
Enflurane (Cardiac arrhythmias may result). Products include:
Ethrane ... 599
Fluphenazine Decanoate (Severe, prolonged hypotension or hypertension). Products include:
Prolixin Decanoate ... 1795
Fluphenazine Enanthate (Severe, prolonged hypotension or hypertension). Products include:
Prolixin Enanthate ... 1796
Fluphenazine Hydrochloride (Severe, prolonged hypotension or hypertension). Products include:
Prolixin Elixir ... 1793
Prolixin Injection ... 1791
Prolixin Oral Concentrate ... 1792
Prolixin Tablets ... 1793
Furazolidone (Severe, prolonged hypotension or hypertension). Products include:
Furoxone ... 1855
Imipramine Hydrochloride (Severe, prolonged hypotension or hypertension). Products include:
Tofranil Ampuls ... 1038
Tofranil Tablets ... 1039
Imipramine Pamoate (Severe, prolonged hypotension or hypertension). Products include:
Tofranil-PM Capsules ... 1041
Isocarboxazid (Severe, prolonged hypotension or hypertension). Products include:
Marplan Tablets ... 1906
Isoflurane (Cardiac arrhythmias may result). Products include:
Forane ... 600
Maprotiline Hydrochloride (Severe, prolonged hypotension or hypertension). Products include:
Ludiomil Tablets ... 874
Mesoridazine (Severe, prolonged hypotension or hypertension). Products include:
Serentil ... 686
Methohexital Sodium (Cardiac arrhythmias may result). Products include:
Brevital Sodium Vials ... 1248
Methoxyflurane (Cardiac arrhythmias may result).
No products indexed under this heading.
Nortriptyline Hydrochloride (Severe, prolonged hypotension or hypertension). Products include:
Pamelor ... 2019
Perphenazine (Severe, prolonged hypotension or hypertension). Products include:
Etrafon ... 2087
Triavil Tablets ... 1556
Trilafon ... 2123
Phenelzine Sulfate (Severe, prolonged hypotension or hypertension). Products include:
Nardil ... 1742
Prochlorperazine (Severe, prolonged hypotension or hypertension). Products include:
Compazine ... 2201
Promethazine Hydrochloride (Severe, prolonged hypotension or hypertension). Products include:
Mepergan Injection ... 2479
Phenergan with Codeine ... 2497
Phenergan with Dextromethorphan 2499
Phenergan Injection ... 2493
Phenergan Suppositories ... 2496
Phenergan Syrup ... 2495
Phenergan Tablets ... 2496
Phenergan VC ... 2500
Phenergan VC with Codeine ... 2501
Propofol (Cardiac arrhythmias may result). Products include:
Diprivan Injection ... 2267
Protriptyline Hydrochloride (Severe, prolonged hypotension or hypertension). Products include:
Vivactil Tablets ... 1567
Selegiline Hydrochloride (Severe, prolonged hypotension or hypertension). Products include:
Eldepryl ... 2250
Thioridazine Hydrochloride (Severe, prolonged hypotension or hypertension). Products include:
Mellaril ... 2011
Tranylcypromine Sulfate (Severe, prolonged hypotension or hypertension). Products include:
Parnate Tablets ... 2222
Trifluoperazine Hydrochloride (Severe, prolonged hypotension or hypertension). Products include:
Stelazine ... 2226
Trimipramine Maleate (Severe, prolonged hypotension or hypertension). Products include:
Surmontil Capsules ... 2524

Food Interactions

Food, unspecified (Topical anesthesia may impair swallowing and thus enhance the danger of aspiration; food should not be ingested for 60 minutes).

XYLOCAINE 2% VISCOUS SOLUTION
(Lidocaine Hydrochloride) ... 646

Food Interactions

Food, unspecified (Topical anesthesia may impair swallowing and thus enhance the danger of aspiration; avoid food ingestion for 60 minutes).

YELLOLAX
(Phenolphthalein, Yellow, Homeopathic Medications) ... ▣ 590
No interactions described in labeling.

YOCON
(Yohimbine Hydrochloride) ... 1686
May interact with tricyclic antidepressants. Compounds in this category include:

Amitriptyline Hydrochloride (Should not be used together). Products include:
Elavil ... 2269
Endep Tablets ... 1927
Etrafon ... 2087
Limbitrol ... 1933
Triavil Tablets ... 1556
Amoxapine (Should not be used together). Products include:
Asendin Tablets ... 1196
Clomipramine Hydrochloride (Should not be used together). Products include:
Anafranil Capsules ... 650
Desipramine Hydrochloride (Should not be used together). Products include:
Norpramin Tablets ... 1340
Doxepin Hydrochloride (Should not be used together). Products include:
Sinequan ... 1960
Imipramine Hydrochloride (Should not be used together). Products include:
Tofranil Ampuls ... 1038
Tofranil Tablets ... 1039
Imipramine Pamoate (Should not be used together). Products include:
Tofranil-PM Capsules ... 1041
Maprotiline Hydrochloride (Should not be used together). Products include:
Ludiomil Tablets ... 874
Nortriptyline Hydrochloride (Should not be used together). Products include:
Pamelor ... 2019
Protriptyline Hydrochloride (Should not be used together). Products include:
Vivactil Tablets ... 1567
Trimipramine Maleate (Should not be used together). Products include:
Surmontil Capsules ... 2524

YODOXIN
(Iodoquinol) ... 1072
No interactions described in labeling.

YOHIMEX TABLETS
(Yohimbine Hydrochloride) ... 1190
May interact with tricyclic antidepressants, neuromuscular blocking agents, and certain other agents. Compounds in these categories include:

Amitriptyline Hydrochloride (Do not use concomitantly). Products include:
Elavil ... 2269
Endep Tablets ... 1927
Etrafon ... 2087
Limbitrol ... 1933
Triavil Tablets ... 1556
Amoxapine (Do not use concomitantly). Products include:
Asendin Tablets ... 1196
Chlorpromazine (Do not use concomitantly). Products include:
Thorazine ... 2234
Chlorprothixene (Do not use concomitantly). Products include:
Taractan Tablets ... 1920

Chlorprothixene Hydrochloride (Do not use concomitantly). Products include:
- Taractan ... 1920

Clomipramine Hydrochloride (Do not use concomitantly). Products include:
- Anafranil Capsules ... 650

Clozapine (Do not use concomitantly). Products include:
- Clozaril Tablets ... 2000

Desipramine Hydrochloride (Do not use concomitantly). Products include:
- Norpramin Tablets ... 1340

Doxepin Hydrochloride (Do not use concomitantly). Products include:
- Sinequan ... 1960

Fluoxetine Hydrochloride (Do not use concomitantly). Products include:
- Prozac Pulvules ... 920

Fluphenazine Decanoate (Do not use concomitantly). Products include:
- Prolixin Decanoate ... 1795

Fluphenazine Enanthate (Do not use concomitantly). Products include:
- Prolixin Enanthate ... 1796

Fluphenazine Hydrochloride (Do not use concomitantly). Products include:
- Prolixin Elixir ... 1793
- Prolixin Injection ... 1791
- Prolixin Oral Concentrate ... 1792
- Prolixin Tablets ... 1793

Haloperidol (Do not use concomitantly). Products include:
- Haldol Injection, Tablets and Concentrate ... 1373

Haloperidol Decanoate (Do not use concomitantly). Products include:
- Haldol Decanoate ... 1375

Imipramine Hydrochloride (Do not use concomitantly). Products include:
- Tofranil Ampuls ... 1038
- Tofranil Tablets ... 1039

Imipramine Pamoate (Do not use concomitantly). Products include:
- Tofranil-PM Capsules ... 1041

Lithium Carbonate (Do not use concomitantly). Products include:
- Eskalith ... 2214
- Lithane Tablets ... 1596
- Lithium Carbonate Capsules & Tablets ... 1984
- Lithobid Tablets ... 870

Lithium Citrate (Do not use concomitantly). Products include:
- Cibalith-S ... 870

Loxapine Hydrochloride (Do not use concomitantly). Products include:
- Loxitane ... 1213

Loxapine Succinate (Do not use concomitantly). Products include:
- Loxitane Capsules ... 1213

Maprotiline Hydrochloride (Do not use concomitantly). Products include:
- Ludiomil Tablets ... 874

Mesoridazine (Do not use concomitantly). Products include:
- Serentil ... 686

Molindone Hydrochloride (Do not use concomitantly). Products include:
- Moban Tablets & Concentrate ... 932

Nortriptyline Hydrochloride (Do not use concomitantly). Products include:
- Pamelor ... 2019

Perphenazine (Do not use concomitantly). Products include:
- Etrafon ... 2087
- Triavil Tablets ... 1556
- Trilafon ... 2123

Pimozide (Do not use concomitantly). Products include:
- Orap Tablets ... 1020

Prochlorperazine (Do not use concomitantly). Products include:
- Compazine ... 2201

Promethazine Hydrochloride (Do not use concomitantly). Products include:
- Mepergan Injection ... 2479
- Phenergan with Codeine ... 2497
- Phenergan with Dextromethorphan 2499
- Phenergan Injection ... 2493
- Phenergan Suppositories ... 2496
- Phenergan Syrup ... 2495
- Phenergan Tablets ... 2496
- Phenergan VC ... 2500
- Phenergan VC with Codeine ... 2501

Protriptyline Hydrochloride (Do not use concomitantly). Products include:
- Vivactil Tablets ... 1567

Thioridazine Hydrochloride (Do not use concomitantly). Products include:
- Mellaril ... 2011

Thiothixene (Do not use concomitantly). Products include:
- Navane Capsules and Concentrate 1954
- Navane Intramuscular ... 1956

Trazodone Hydrochloride (Do not use concomitantly). Products include:
- Desyrel and Desyrel Dividose ... 1404

Trifluoperazine Hydrochloride (Do not use concomitantly). Products include:
- Stelazine ... 2226

Trimipramine Maleate (Do not use concomitantly). Products include:
- Surmontil Capsules ... 2524

YUTOPAR INTRAVENOUS INJECTION
(Ritodrine Hydrochloride) ... 647
May interact with corticosteroids, general anesthetics, anticholinergics, sympathomimetic aerosol bronchodilators, beta blockers, and certain other agents. Compounds in these categories include:

Acebutolol Hydrochloride (Inhibition of Yutopar's action). Products include:
- Sectral Capsules ... 2520

Albuterol (Possible additive effects). Products include:
- Proventil Inhalation Aerosol ... 2117
- Ventolin Inhalation Aerosol and Refill ... 583

Albuterol Sulfate (Possible additive effects). Products include:
- Proventil Repetabs Tablets ... 2120
- Proventil Solutions for Inhalation 0.5% and 0.083% ... 2118
- Proventil Syrup ... 2119
- Proventil Tablets ... 2120
- Ventolin ... 583

Atenolol (Inhibition of Yutopar's action). Products include:
- Tenoretic Tablets ... 1105
- Tenormin Tablets and I.V. Injection 1107

Atropine Sulfate (Systemic hypertension exaggerated). Products include:
- Arco-Lase Plus Tablets ... 607
- Atropine Sulfate Sterile Ophthalmic Solution and S.O.P. Sterile Ophthalmic Ointment ... ◉ 239
- Donnagel ... ⊞ 675
- Donnagel-PG ... 1858
- Donnatal ... 1858
- Donnatal Extentabs ... 1859
- Donnatal Tablets ... 1858
- Donnazyme Tablets ... 1860
- Isopto Atropine ... ◉ 218
- Lomotil ... 2174
- Motofen Tablets ... 836
- Ru-Tuss Tablets ... 693
- Urised Tablets ... 2396

Belladonna Alkaloids (Systemic hypertension exaggerated). Products include:
- Bellergal-S Tablets ... 1998
- Hyland's Bed Wetting Tablets ... ⊞ 728
- Hyland's Teething Tablets ... ⊞ 728
- Kinesed Tablets ... 2272

Benztropine Mesylate (Systemic hypertension exaggerated). Products include:
- Cogentin ... 1435

Betamethasone Acetate (Maternal pulmonary edema; maternal death). Products include:
- Celestone Soluspan Suspension ... 2081

Betamethasone Sodium Phosphate (Maternal pulmonary edema; maternal death). Products include:
- Celestone Soluspan Suspension ... 2081

Betaxolol Hydrochloride (Inhibition of Yutopar's action). Products include:
- Betoptic Sterile Ophthalmic Solution ... 569
- Betoptic S Sterile Ophthalmic Suspension ... 570
- Kerlone Tablets ... 2172

Biperiden (Systemic hypertension exaggerated). Products include:
- Akineton ... 1171

Carteolol Hydrochloride (Inhibition of Yutopar's action). Products include:
- Cartrol Tablets ... 507

Clidinium Bromide (Systemic hypertension exaggerated). Products include:
- Librax Capsules ... 1929
- Quarzan Capsules ... 1937

Cortisone Acetate (Maternal pulmonary edema; maternal death). Products include:
- Cortone Acetate Sterile Suspension ... 1437
- Cortone Acetate Tablets ... 1439

Dexamethasone Acetate (Maternal pulmonary edema; maternal death). Products include:
- Dalalone D.P. Injectable ... 999
- Decadron-LA Sterile Suspension ... 1457

Dexamethasone Sodium Phosphate (Maternal pulmonary edema; maternal death). Products include:
- AK-Dex ... ◉ 203
- Decadron Phosphate Respihaler ... 1454
- Decadron Phosphate Sterile Ophthalmic Ointment ... 1453
- Decadron Phosphate Sterile Ophthalmic Solution ... 1453
- Decadron Phosphate Topical Cream ... 1455
- Decadron Phosphate Turbinaire ... 1456
- Maxidex Sterile Ophthalmic Ointment ... ◉ 222
- NeoDecadron Sterile Ophthalmic Ointment ... 1517
- NeoDecadron Sterile Ophthalmic Solution ... 1518
- NeoDecadron Topical Cream ... 1518

Diazoxide (Potentiates Yutopar's cardiovascular effects, particularly cardiac arrhythmia or hypotension). Products include:
- Hyperstat I.V. Injection ... 2095
- Proglycem ... 649

Dicyclomine Hydrochloride (Systemic hypertension exaggerated). Products include:
- Bentyl ... 1322

Dobutamine Hydrochloride (Possible additive effects). Products include:
- Dobutrex Solution Vials ... 1259

Dopamine Hydrochloride (Possible additive effects). Products include:
- Intropin Injection ... 930

Enflurane (Potentiates Yutopar's cardiovascular effects, particularly cardiac arrhythmia or hypotension). Products include:
- Ethrane ... 599

Ephedrine Hydrochloride (Possible additive effects). Products include:
- Amesec ... ⊞ 682
- Primatene Tablets-M Formula ... 2421
- Primatene Tablets-P Formula ... 2421
- Primatene Tablets-Regular Formula ... 2421
- Quadrinal Tablets ... 1183
- Quelidrine Syrup ... 556
- Tedral SA ... 1765

Ephedrine Sulfate (Possible additive effects). Products include:
- Bronkaid Tablets ... ⊞ 757
- Bronkolixir ... ⊞ 761
- Bronkotabs Tablets ... ⊞ 762
- Marax Tablets & DF Syrup ... 1954
- Pazo Hemorrhoid Ointment & Suppositories ... 752
- Vicks Vatronol Nose Drops ... ⊞ 666

Ephedrine Tannate (Possible additive effects). Products include:
- Rynatuss ... 2388

Epinephrine (Possible additive effects). Products include:
- Ana-Kit Anaphylaxis Emergency Treatment Kit ... 1100
- Bronkaid Mist ... ⊞ 757
- EpiPen ... 843
- Marcaine Hydrochloride 0.5% with Epinephrine 1:200,000 (as bitartrate) ... 958
- Marcaine Hydrochloride with Epinephrine 1:200,000 ... 2055
- Primatene Mist ... 2420
- Sus-Phrine Injection ... 1006
- Xylocaine with Epinephrine Injections ... 637

Epinephrine Bitartrate (Possible additive effects). Products include:
- AsthmaHaler Mist Epinephrine Bitartrate Bronchodilator ... ⊞ 616
- Bronkaid Mist Suspension ... ⊞ 757
- Primatene Mist Suspension ... 2421

Epinephrine Hydrochloride (Possible additive effects). Products include:
- Adrenalin Chloride Solution 1:100 & 1:1,000 ... 1689
- Epifrin ... ◉ 244
- Glaucon ... ◉ 218

Esmolol Hydrochloride (Inhibition of Yutopar's action). Products include:
- Brevibloc Injection ... 942

Glycopyrrolate (Systemic hypertension exaggerated). Products include:
- Robinul Forte Tablets ... 1873
- Robinul Injectable ... 1873
- Robinul Tablets ... 1873

Hydrocortisone (Maternal pulmonary edema; maternal death). Products include:
- AK-Spore H.C. ... ◉ 206
- Bactine Hydrocortisone Anti-Itch Cream ... ⊞ 625
- CaldeCORT Anti-Itch Hydrocortisone Spray ... ⊞ 560
- Carmol HC Cream 1% ... 2296
- Cortaid Spray ... ⊞ 735
- Cortenema ... 2244
- Cortisporin Ointment ... 758
- Cortisporin Ophthalmic Ointment Sterile ... 758
- Cortisporin Ophthalmic Suspension Sterile ... 759
- Cortisporin Otic Solution Sterile ... 760
- Cortisporin Otic Suspension Sterile 760
- Cortizone-5 Creme & Ointment ... ⊞ 732
- Dermolate Anti-Itch Cream ... ⊞ 697
- Eldecort Cream 1.0% ... 1113
- Eldecort Cream 1.0% and 2.5% ... 1113
- Fungoid HC Creme ... 1770
- Hydrocortone Tablets ... 1482

Hytone ... 909
LazerSporin-C Solution ... 1770
Massengill Medicated Soft Cloth Towelettes ... 2192
Nutracort Cream & Lotion ... 1684
PediOtic Suspension Sterile ... 797
Synacort Creams 1%, 2.5% ... 2296
Vanoxide-HC Acne Lotion ... 911
Vioform-Hydrocortisone Cream and Mild Cream ... 889
Vioform-Hydrocortisone Ointment ... 889
VōSoL HC Otic Solution ... 2392
Vytone Cream 1% ... 911

Hydrocortisone Acetate (Maternal pulmonary edema; maternal death). Products include:
Analpram-HC Rectal Cream 1% and 2.5% ... 970
Anusol-HC Cream ... 1690
Anusol-HC Suppositories ... 1691
Caldecort ... ▣ 560
Carmol HC Cream 1% ... 2296
Chloromycetin Hydrocortisone Ophthalmic ... 1694
Coly-Mycin S Otic w/Neomycin & Hydrocortisone ... 1708
Cortaid ... ▣ 735
Cortef Feminine Itch Cream ... ▣ 735
Corticaine ... ▣ 682
Cortifoam ... 1827
Cortisporin Cream ... 757
Epifoam ... 1828
Gynecort 5 Creme ... ▣ 556
Hydrocortone Acetate Sterile Suspension ... 1479
Lanacort 5 Creme and Ointment ... ▣ 557
Mantadil Cream ... 789
Ophthocort ... ⊙ 301
Orabase HCA Oral Paste ... 890
Pramosone Cream, Lotion & Ointment ... 971
ProctoCream-HC ... 1834
Proctofoam-HC ... 1835

Hydrocortisone Sodium Phosphate (Maternal pulmonary edema; maternal death). Products include:
Hydrocortone Phosphate Injection, Sterile ... 1481

Hydrocortisone Sodium Succinate (Maternal pulmonary edema; maternal death). Products include:
Solu-Cortef Sterile Powder ... 2361

Hyoscyamine (Systemic hypertension exaggerated). Products include:
Cystospaz Tablets ... 2395
Urised Tablets ... 2396

Hyoscyamine Sulfate (Systemic hypertension exaggerated). Products include:
Arco-Lase Plus Tablets ... 607
Cystospaz-M Capsules ... 2395
Donnagel ... ▣ 675
Donnagel-PG ... 1858
Donnatal ... 1858
Donnatal Extentabs ... 1859
Donnatal Tablets ... 1858
Donnazyme Tablets ... 1860
Kutrase Capsules ... 2146
Levsin/Levsinex ... 2147
Ru-Tuss Tablets ... 693

Ipratropium Bromide (Systemic hypertension exaggerated). Products include:
Atrovent Inhalation Aerosol ... 675

Isoflurane (Potentiates Yutopar's cardiovascular effects, particularly cardiac arrhythmia or hypotension). Products include:
Forane ... 600

Isoproterenol Hydrochloride (Possible additive effects). Products include:
Isuprel Hydrochloride Injection 1:5000 ... 2050
Isuprel Hydrochloride Mistometer ... 2051
Isuprel Hydrochloride Solution 1:200 & 1:100 ... 2052
Norisodrine Aerotrol ... 540

Labetalol Hydrochloride (Inhibition of Yutopar's action). Products include:
Normodyne Injection ... 2108
Normodyne Tablets ... 2110
Normozide Tablets ... 2112
Trandate HCT Tablets ... 579
Trandate Injection ... 577
Trandate Tablets ... 579

Magnesium Sulfate (Potentiates Yutopar's cardiovascular effects, particularly cardiac arrhythmia or hypotension hypotension). Products include:
Eldertonic ... 1359
Vicon Forte Capsules ... 2416
Vicon Plus ... ▣ 682
Vicon-C ... ▣ 682

Mepenzolate Bromide (Systemic hypertension exaggerated). Products include:
Cantil Tablets ... 1326

Meperidine Hydrochloride (Potentiates Yutopar's cardiovascular effects, particularly cardiac arrhythmia or hypotension). Products include:
Demerol ... 2047
Mepergan Injection ... 2479

Metaproterenol Sulfate (Possible additive effects). Products include:
Alupent ... 674
Arm-a-Med Metaproterenol Sulfate Inhalation Solution, USP ... 617
Metaprel Inhalation Aerosol Bronchodilator ... 2014
Metaprel Inhalation Solution ... 2015
Metaprel ... 2015
Metaproterenol Sulfate Inhalation Solution, USP ... 912

Metaraminol Bitartrate (Possible additive effects). Products include:
Aramine Injection ... 1424

Methohexital Sodium (Potentiates Yutopar's cardiovascular effects, particularly cardiac arrhythmia or hypotension). Products include:
Brevital Sodium Vials ... 1248

Methoxamine Hydrochloride (Possible addictive effects). Products include:
Vasoxyl Injection ... 819

Methoxyflurane (Potentiates Yutopar's cardiovascular effects, particularly cardiac arrhythmia or hypotension).
No products indexed under this heading.

Methylprednisolone Acetate (Maternal pulmonary edema; maternal death). Products include:
Depo-Medrol Sterile Aqueous Suspension ... 2334

Methylprednisolone Sodium Succinate (Maternal pulmonary edema; maternal death). Products include:
Solu-Medrol Sterile Powder ... 2363

Metoprolol Tartrate (Inhibition of Yutopar's action). Products include:
Lopressor Ampuls ... 1032
Lopressor HCT Tablets ... 1034
Lopressor Tablets ... 1032

Nadolol (Inhibition of Yutopar's action). Products include:
Corgard Tablets ... 701
Corzide Tablets ... 702

Norepinephrine Bitartrate (Possible additive effects). Products include:
Levophed Bitartrate Injection ... 2054

Oxybutynin Chloride (Systemic hypertension exaggerated). Products include:
Ditropan ... 1332

Penbutolol Sulfate (Inhibition of Yutopar's action). Products include:
Levatol ... 1832

Phenylephrine Bitartrate (Possible additive effects).
No products indexed under this heading.

Phenylephrine Hydrochloride (Possible additive effects). Products include:
AK-Dilate Solution 2.5% and 10% ... ⊙ 203
Atrohist Sprinkle Capsules ... 558
Cerose-DM ... 2443
Codimal ... 846
Comhist LA Capsules ... 1618
Congespirin For Children Aspirin Free Chewable Cold Tablets ... 748
Cyclomydril ... ⊙ 216
Deconsal Sprinkle Capsules ... 559
Dimetane Decongestant ... ▣ 673
Dristan Decongestant/Antihistamine/ Analgesic Coated Caplets ... ▣ 749
Dristan Cold Nasal Decongestant/ Antihistamine/ Analgesic Coated Tablets ... 2419
Dristan Advanced Formula Decongestant/Antihistamine/ Analgesic Tablets ... ▣ 749
Dristan Nasal Spray, Menthol ... 2419
Dristan Nasal Spray, Regular and Regular with Metered Pump ... 2419
Entex Capsules ... 1623
Entex Liquid ... 1623
Sinus Excedrin Analgesic, Decongestant Tablets & Caplets ... 750
Extendryl ... 994
4-Way Fast Acting Nasal Spray - Original Formula (regular & mentholated) & Metered Spray Pump (regular) ... 751
Hycomine Compound Tablets ... 929
Murocoll-2 Sterile Ophthalmic Solution ... ⊙ 261
Mydfrin 2.5% ... ⊙ 224
Naldecon Syrup, Tablets, Pediatric Drops and Pediatric Syrup ... 709
Neo-Synephrine Hydrochloride 1% Carpuject ... 2063
Neo-Synephrine Hydrochloride 1% Injection ... 2063
Neo-Synephrine Hydrochloride (Ophthalmic) ... 2064
Neo-Synephrine ... ▣ 759
Nōstril Nasal Decongestant ... ▣ 520
Novahistine Elixir ... ▣ 596
Phenergan VC ... 2500
Phenergan VC with Codeine ... 2501
Prefrin Liquifilm Vasoconstrictor and Lubricant Eye Drops ... ⊙ 254
Prefrin-A ... ⊙ 255
Quelidrine Syrup ... 556
Relief Vasoconstrictor and Lubricant Eye Drops ... ⊙ 256
Robitussin Night Relief ... ▣ 677
Ru-Tuss with Hydrocodone ... 694
Ru-Tuss Tablets ... 693
Vasosulf ... ⊙ 279
Vicks Sinex ... ▣ 665
Zincfrin ... ⊙ 230

Phenylephrine Tannate (Possible additive effects). Products include:
Rynatan ... 2387
Rynatuss ... 2388

Phenylpropanolamine Hydrochloride (Possible additive effects). Products include:
A.R.M. Allergy Relief Medicine Caplets ... ▣ 615
Acutrim ... ▣ 548
Allerest ... ▣ 559
BC Cold Powder ... ▣ 517
Cheracol Plus Head Cold/Cough Formula ... ▣ 667
Codimal Expectorant ... 846
Comtrex Multi-Symptom Cold Reliever Tablets/Caplets/Liqui-Gels/Liquid ... 745
Contac Continuous Action Decongestant/Antihistamine Capsules ▣ 710
Contac Maximum Strength Continuous Action Decongestant/ Antihistamine Caplets ... ▣ 709
Contac Severe Cold and Flu Formula Caplets ... ▣ 711
Coricidin 'D' Decongestant Tablets ... ▣ 695
Coricidin Demilets Tablets for Children ... ▣ 696
Demazin Nasal Decongestant/ Antihistamine Repetabs Tablets & Syrup ... ▣ 697
Dexatrim ... ▣ 733
Dimetane-DC Cough Syrup ... 1857
Dimetapp Elixir ... ▣ 673
Dimetapp DM Elixir ... ▣ 674
Dimetapp Extentabs ... ▣ 674
Dimetapp Plus Caplets ... ▣ 675
Dimetapp Tablets ... ▣ 675
Entex Capsules ... 1623
Entex LA Tablets ... 1623
Entex Liquid ... 1623
4-Way Cold Tablets ... 750
Hycomine Syrup ... 927
Naldecon CX Adult Liquid ... ▣ 521
Naldecon DX Adult Liquid ... ▣ 521
Naldecon DX Children's Syrup ... ▣ 522
Naldecon DX Pediatric Drops ... ▣ 522
Naldecon EX Children's Syrup ... ▣ 522
Naldecon EX Pediatric Drops ... ▣ 523
Naldecon Syrup, Tablets, Pediatric Drops and Pediatric Syrup ... 709
Nolamine Tablets ... 838
Nolex LA Tablets ... 838
Ornade Spansule Capsules ... 2221
Orthoxicol Cough Syrup ... ▣ 668
Propagest ... 839
Pyrroxate Capsules ... ▣ 669
Robitussin-CF ... ▣ 676
Ru-Tuss II Capsules ... 693
Ru-Tuss with Hydrocodone ... 694
Ru-Tuss Tablets ... 693
Sine-Off Sinus Medicine Tablets-Aspirin Formula ... ▣ 722
Sinulin ... 840
St. Joseph Cold Tablets for Children ... ▣ 704
Tavist-D Tablets ... 2035
Triaminic Allergy Tablets ... ▣ 688
Triaminic Chewables ... ▣ 688
Triaminic Cold Tablets ... ▣ 688
Triaminic Expectorant ... ▣ 688
Triaminic Expectorant w/Codeine ... 1996
Triaminic Expectorant DH ... 1995
Triaminic Oral Infant Drops ... 1996
Triaminic Syrup ... ▣ 689
Triaminic-12 Tablets ... ▣ 690
Triaminic-DM Syrup ... ▣ 689
Triaminicin Tablets ... ▣ 690
Triaminicol Multi-Symptom Cold Tablets ... ▣ 691
Triaminicol Multi-Symptom Relief ▣ 691
Tuss-Ornade Liquid ... 2242
Tuss-Ornade Spansule Capsules ... 2242
Tylenol Cold Medication, Effervescent Tablets ... 1369

Pindolol (Inhibition of Yutopar's action). Products include:
Visken Tablets ... 2036

Pirbuterol Acetate (Possible additive effects). Products include:
Maxair Inhaler ... 1311

Prednisolone Acetate (Maternal pulmonary edema; maternal death). Products include:
AK-Cide Sterile Ophthalmic Ointment & Suspension ... ⊙ 202
Blephamide Liquifilm Sterile Ophthalmic Suspension ... 586
Blephamide S.O.P. Sterile Ophthalmic Ointment ... 586
Cetapred Ointment ... ⊙ 220
⅛% Econopred & 1% Econopred Plus ... ⊙ 217
Isopto Cetapred Suspension ... ⊙ 220
Metimyd ... ⊙ 306
Poly-Pred Liquifilm ... ⊙ 250
Pred Forte ... ⊙ 252
Pred Mild ... ⊙ 254
Pred-G Liquifilm Sterile Ophthalmic Suspension ... ⊙ 252
Pred-G S.O.P. Sterile Ophthalmic Ointment ... ⊙ 253
Vasocidin Ointment ... ⊙ 275

Prednisolone Sodium Phosphate (Maternal pulmonary edema; maternal death). Products include:
AK-Pred ... ⊙ 205
Hydeltrasol Injection, Sterile ... 1476
Inflamase ... ⊙ 274
Pediapred Oral Liquid ... 987
Vasocidin Ophthalmic Solution ... ⊙ 276

Prednisolone Tebutate (Maternal pulmonary edema; maternal death). Products include:
Hydeltra-T.B.A. Sterile Suspension 1478

Prednisone (Maternal pulmonary edema; maternal death). Products include:
Deltasone Tablets ... 2332

Procyclidine Hydrochloride (Systemic hypertension exaggerated). Products include:
Kemadrin Tablets 771

Propantheline Bromide (Systemic hypertension exaggerated). Products include:
Pro-Banthīne Tablets 2141

Propofol (Potentiates Yutopar's cardiovascular effects, particularly cardiac arrhythymia or hypotension). Products include:
Diprivan Injection 2267

Propranolol Hydrochloride (Inhibition of Yutopar's action). Products include:
Inderal 2459
Inderal LA Long Acting Capsules 2461
Inderide Tablets 2463
Inderide LA Long Acting Capsules 2465

Pseudoephedrine Hydrochloride (Possible additive effects). Products include:
Actifed Capsules ▣ 539
Actifed Plus Caplets ▣ 539
Actifed Plus Tablets ▣ 540
Actifed with Codeine Cough Syrup 752
Actifed Syrup ▣ 540
Actifed Tablets ▣ 540
Actifed 12-Hour Capsules ▣ 539
Advil Cold & Sinus Caplets (formerly CoAdvil) 2416
Allerest ▣ 559
Anatuss LA Tablets 1359
Benadryl Decongestant Elixir ▣ 635
Benadryl Decongestant ▣ 635
Benadryl Plus ▣ 636
Benadryl Plus Nighttime ▣ 637
Benylin Decongestant ▣ 638
Brexin L.A. Capsules 2078
Bromfed Capsules (Timed Release) 1615
Bromfed Syrup ▣ 628
Bromfed 1615
CoAdvil ▣ 748
Allergy-Sinus Comtrex Multi-Symptom Allergy Sinus Formula Tablets & Caplets 746
Cough Formula Comtrex 746
Comtrex Multi-Symptom Cold Reliever Tablets/Caplets/Liqui-Gels/Liquid 745
Day-Night Comtrex 747
Non-Drowsy Comtrex 747
Congess 994
Congestac Caplets ▣ 617
Contac Jr. Children's Cold Medicine ▣ 712
Contac Nighttime Cold Medicine ▣ 713
Contac Sinus Caplets Maximum Strength Non-Drowsy Formula ▣ 710
Contac Sinus Tablets Maximum Strength Non-Drowsy Formula ▣ 710
Deconamine 663
Deconsal II Tablets 559
Dimacol Caplets ▣ 672
Dimetane-DX Cough Syrup 1858
Dorcol Children's Cough Syrup ▣ 685
Dorcol Children's Decongestant Liquid ▣ 685
Dorcol Children's Liquid Cold Formula ▣ 686
Maximum Strength Dristan Decongestant/Analgesic Coated Caplets ▣ 750
No Drowsiness Dristan Cold Nasal Decongestant/Analgesic Coated Caplets 2420
Dristan Sinus Caplets 2419
Sinus Excedrin Analgesic, Decongestant Tablets & Caplets ▣ 533
Fedahist Gyrocaps 2145
Fedahist Timecaps 2145
Guaifed 1615
Guaifed Syrup ▣ 629
Isoclor Expectorant 982
Isoclor Timesule Capsules ▣ 561
Kronofed-A 970
Medi-Flu Caplet, Liquid ▣ 640
Novafed A Capsules 1342
Novafed Capsules 1342
Novahistine DH 1342
Novahistine DMX ▣ 595
Novahistine Expectorant 1343
Nucofed Capsules 2219
Nucofed Expectorant 2219
Nucofed Pediatric Expectorant 2220
Nucofed Syrup 2219
Ornex Caplets ▣ 618
PediaCare Allergy Relief Formula Liquid 1362
PediaCare Cough-Cold Formula Liquid 1362
PediaCare Infants' Oral Decongestant Drops 1362
PediaCare Night Rest Cough-Cold Formula Liquid 1362
PediaCare 6-12 Cough-Cold Formula Chewable Tablets 1362
Robitussin-DAC Syrup 1875
Robitussin-PE ▣ 677
Rondec 1975
Rondec-DM 1976
Rondec-TR Tablet 1975
Ru-Tuss DE Tablets 694
Ryna ▣ 741
Seldane-D Extended-Release Tablets 1350
Sinarest ▣ 562
Sine-Aid Maximum Strength Sinus Headache Caplets 1365
Sine-Aid Maximum Strength Sinus Headache Tablets 1365
Sine-Off Maximum Strength Allergy/Sinus Formula Caplets ▣ 721
Sine-Off Maximum Strength No Drowsiness Formula Caplets ▣ 722
Singlet Tablets ▣ 598
Sinutab Maximum Strength ▣ 641
Sinutab Maximum Strength Without Drowsiness Tablets & Caplets ▣ 642
Sinutab Regular Strength Without Drowsiness Formula ▣ 641
St. Joseph Nighttime Cold Medicine ▣ 705
Sudafed Children's Liquid ▣ 543
Sudafed Cough Syrup ▣ 543
Sudafed Plus Liquid ▣ 544
Sudafed Plus Tablets ▣ 545
Sudafed Sinus Caplets ▣ 545
Sudafed Sinus Tablets ▣ 545
Sudafed Tablets, 30 mg ▣ 544
Sudafed Tablets, Adult Strength, 60 mg ▣ 544
Sudafed 12 Hour Capsules ▣ 545
TheraFlu Flu and Cold Medicine ▣ 687
Triaminic Nite Light ▣ 689
Tylenol Allergy Sinus Medication Caplets and Gelcaps, Maximum Strength 1372
Children's Tylenol Cold Liquid Formula and Chewable Tablets 1368
Tylenol Cold & Flu Hot Medication, Packets 1369
Tylenol Cold & Flu No Drowsiness Hot Medication, Packets 1371
Tylenol Cold Medication Caplets and Tablets 1370
Tylenol Cold Medication No Drowsiness Formula Caplets 1370
Tylenol Cold Night Time Medication Liquid 1371
Tylenol Cough Medication Liquid with Decongestant, Maximum Strength 1372
Tylenol, Maximum Strength, Sinus Medication Gelcaps, Caplets and Tablets 1373
Ursinus Inlay-Tabs ▣ 691
Vicks Children's NyQuil ▣ 664
Vicks Daycare ▣ 660
Vicks Formula 44D Decongestant Cough Medicine ▣ 662
Vicks Formula 44M Multi-Symptom Cough Medicine ▣ 662
Vicks NyQuil Nighttime Colds Medicine-Original & Cherry Flavor ▣ 664
Vicks Pediatric Formula 44 Cough & Congestion Medicine ▣ 663
Vicks Pediatric Formula 44m Multi-Symptom Cough & Cold Medicine ▣ 663

Pseudoephedrine Sulfate (Possible additive effects). Products include:
Afrin Tablets ▣ 693
Chlor-Trimeton Decongestant ▣ 694
Disophrol Chronotab Sustained-Action Tablets ▣ 698
Drixoral Antihistamine/Nasal Decongestant Syrup ▣ 698
Drixoral Non-Drowsy Formula ▣ 699
Drixoral Plus Extended-Release Tablets ▣ 699
Drixoral Sinus ▣ 700
Drixoral Sustained-Action Tablets ▣ 698
Sinutab Allergy Formula Sustained Action Tablets ▣ 640
Trinalin Repetabs Tablets 1170

Scopolamine Hydrobromide (Systemic hypertension exaggerated). Products include:
Donnagel ▣ 675
Donnagel-PG 1858
Donnatal 1858
Donnatal Extentabs 1859
Donnatal Tablets 1858
Donnazyme Tablets 1860
Isopto Hyoscine ⊙ 222
Murocoll-2 Sterile Ophthalmic Solution ⊙ 261
Ru-Tuss Tablets 693

Scopolamine Preparations (Systemic hypertension exaggerated). Products include:
Transderm Scōp Transdermal Therapeutic System 887

Terbutaline Sulfate (Possible additive effects). Products include:
Brethaire Inhaler 1024
Brethine Ampuls 1026
Brethine Tablets 1026
Bricanyl Injection 1324
Bricanyl Tablets 1325

Timolol Maleate (Inhibition of Yutopar's action). Products include:
Blocadren Tablets 1429
Timolide Tablets 1547
Timoptic in Ocudose 1552
Timoptic Sterile Ophthalmic Solution 1550

Triamcinolone (Maternal pulmonary edema; maternal death).
No products indexed under this heading.

Triamcinolone Acetonide (Maternal pulmonary edema; maternal death). Products include:
Aristocort A 1010
Azmacort Inhaler 1837
Kenalog Cream, Lotion & Ointment 2401
Kenalog-10 Injection 2402
Kenalog-40 Injection 2403
Kenalog in Orabase 604
Kenalog Spray 2401
Mycolog II Cream and Ointment 2407
Mytrex Cream & Ointment 2080
Nasacort Nasal Inhaler 1844

Triamcinolone Diacetate (Maternal pulmonary edema; maternal death). Products include:
Aristocort Suspension 1008

Triamcinolone Hexacetonide (Maternal pulmonary edema; maternal death). Products include:
Aristospan Suspension 1011

Tridihexethyl Chloride (Systemic hypertension exaggerated).
No products indexed under this heading.

Trihexyphenidyl Hydrochloride (Systemic hypertension exaggerated). Products include:
Artane 1195

YUTOPAR TABLETS
(Ritodrine Hydrochloride) 647
See **Yutopar Intravenous Injection**

Z-BEC TABLETS
(Multivitamins, Zinc Sulfate) ▣ 678
No interactions described in labeling.

ZANOSAR STERILE POWDER
(Streptozocin) 2371
May interact with:

Nephrotoxic Drugs (Concomitant or combination use should be avoided).

ZANTAC INJECTION AND ZANTAC INJECTION PREMIXED
(Ranitidine Hydrochloride) 1063
May interact with:

Warfarin Sodium (Potential for increased or decreased prothrombin time; doses of ranitidine up to 400 mg per day had no effect on prothrombin time or warfarin clearance). Products include:
Coumadin Injection & Tablets 944
Panwarfin Tablets 547

ZANTAC SYRUP
(Ranitidine Hydrochloride) 1065
See **Zantac 150 & 300 Tablets**

ZANTAC 150 & 300 TABLETS
(Ranitidine Hydrochloride) 1065
May interact with:

Warfarin Sodium (Potential for increased or decreased prothrombin time; doses of ranitidine up to 400 mg per day had no effect on prothrombin time or warfarin clearance). Products include:
Coumadin Injection & Tablets 944
Panwarfin Tablets 547

ZARONTIN CAPSULES
(Ethosuximide) 1768
May interact with:

Divalproex Sodium (Valproic acid may increase or decrease ethosuximide levels). Products include:
Depakote 512

Phenytoin (Ethosuximide may elevate phenytoin serum levels). Products include:
Dilantin Infatabs 1710
Dilantin-30 Pediatric/Dilantin-125 Suspension 1713

Phenytoin Sodium (Ethosuximide may elevate phenytoin serum levels). Products include:
Dilantin Kapseals 1708
Dilantin Parenteral 1712
Dilantin with Phenobarbital Kapseals 1715

Valproic Acid (Valproic acid may increase or decrease ethosuximide levels). Products include:
Depakene Capsules & Syrup 511

ZARONTIN SYRUP
(Ethosuximide) 1769
May interact with:

Divalproex Sodium (Valproic acid may increase or decrease ethosuximide levels). Products include:
Depakote 512

Phenytoin (Ethosuximide may elevate phenytoin serum levels). Products include:
Dilantin Infatabs 1710
Dilantin-30 Pediatric/Dilantin-125 Suspension 1713

Phenytoin Sodium (Ethosuximide may elevate phenytoin serum levels). Products include:
Dilantin Kapseals 1708
Dilantin Parenteral 1712
Dilantin with Phenobarbital Kapseals 1715

Valproic Acid (Valproic acid may increase or decrease ethosuximide levels). Products include:
Depakene Capsules & Syrup 511

ZAROXOLYN TABLETS
(Metolazone) 989
May interact with loop diuretics, antihypertensives, barbiturates, narcotic analgesics, cardiac glycosides, corticosteroids, lithium preparations,

salicylates, non-steroidal anti-inflammatory agents, oral hypoglycemic agents, insulin, and certain other agents. Compounds in these categories include:

Acebutolol Hydrochloride (Excessive hypotension may result especially during initial therapy). Products include:
- Sectral Capsules ... 2520

ACTH (May increase the risk of hypokalemia and increase salt and water retention).
- No products indexed under this heading.

Alcohol (Hypotensive effect may be potentiated).

Alfentanil Hydrochloride (Hypotensive effect may be potentiated). Products include:
- Alfenta Injection ... 1131

Aprobarbital (Hypotensive effect may be potentiated). Products include:
- Alurate Elixir ... 1883

Aspirin (Increases the antihypertensive effect). Products include:
- Alka-Seltzer Effervescent Antacid and Pain Reliever ... 1568
- Alka-Seltzer Extra Strength Effervescent Antacid and Pain Reliever ... 1570
- Alka-Seltzer (Flavored) Effervescent Antacid and Pain Reliever ... 1569
- Alka-Seltzer Plus Cold Medicine ... ■ 623
- Alka-Seltzer Plus Night-Time Cold Medicine ... ■ 623
- Alka Seltzer Plus Sinus Allergy Medicine ... ■ 624
- Anacin Coated Analgesic Caplets ... 2417
- Anacin Coated Analgesic Tablets ... 2417
- Anacin Maximum Strength Analgesic Coated Tablets ... 2417
- Maximum Strength Arthritis Pain Formula By the Makers of Anacin Analgesic Tablets and Caplets ... 2418
- Arthritis Pain Formula by the Makers of Anacin Analgesic Tablets and Caplets ... ■ 747
- Arthritis Strength BC Powder ... ■ 516
- Ascriptin A/D Caplets ... 1850
- Regular Strength Ascriptin Tablets 1850
- Azdone Tablets ... 844
- BC Powder ... ■ 517
- BC Cold Powder ... ■ 517
- Children's Bayer Chewable Aspirin ... ■ 564
- Genuine Bayer Aspirin Tablets & Caplets ... ■ 564
- Maximum Bayer Aspirin Tablets & Caplets ... ■ 566
- Bayer Plus Aspirin Tablets ... ■ 567
- Therapy Bayer Aspirin Caplets ... ■ 568
- 8 Hour Bayer Timed-Release Aspirin ... ■ 566
- Arthritis Strength Bufferin Analgesic Caplets ... 744
- Extra Strength Bufferin Analgesic Tablets ... 745
- Bufferin Analgesic Tablets and Caplets ... 743
- Cama Arthritis Pain Reliever ... ■ 685
- Damason-P ... 1356
- Easprin ... 1719
- Ecotrin Enteric Coated Aspirin Maximum Strength Tablets and Caplets ... 2189
- Ecotrin Enteric Coated Aspirin Regular Strength Tablets and Caplets ... 2189
- Empirin Aspirin ... ■ 541
- Empirin with Codeine Phosphate Nos. 2, 3 & 4 ... 764
- Equagesic Tablets ... 2451
- Excedrin Extra-Strength Analgesic Tablets & Caplets ... 749
- 4-Way Cold Tablets ... 750
- Fiorinal Capsules ... 2007
- Fiorinal with Codeine Capsules ... 2008
- Fiorinal Tablets ... 2007
- Lortab ASA Tablets ... 2414
- Momentum Muscular Backache Formula ... ■ 751
- Norgesic ... 1314
- Norwich Extra-Strength Aspirin ... ■ 546
- Norwich Regular Strength Aspirin ■ 547
- P-A-C Analgesic Tablets ... ■ 669
- Percodan ... 951
- Robaxisal Tablets ... 1872
- Sine-Off Sinus Medicine Tablets-Aspirin Formula ... ■ 722
- Soma Compound w/Codeine Tablets ... 2390
- Soma Compound Tablets ... 2389
- St. Joseph Adult Chewable Aspirin (81 mg.) ... ■ 703
- Synalgos-DC Capsules ... 2525
- Talwin Compound ... 2072
- Ursinus Inlay-Tabs ... ■ 691
- Vanquish Analgesic Caplets ... ■ 574
- Zorprin Tablets ... 698

Atenolol (Excessive hypotension may result especially during initial therapy). Products include:
- Tenoretic Tablets ... 1105
- Tenormin Tablets and I.V. Injection 1107

Benazepril Hydrochloride (Excessive hypotension may result especially during initial therapy). Products include:
- Lotensin Tablets ... 872

Bendroflumethiazide (Excessive hypotension may result especially during initial therapy). Products include:
- Corzide Tablets ... 702
- Naturetin Tablets ... 1789
- Rauzide Tablets ... 1804

Betamethasone Acetate (May increase the risk of hypokalemia and increase salt and water retention). Products include:
- Celestone Soluspan Suspension ... 2081

Betamethasone Sodium Phosphate (May increase the risk of hypokalemia and increase salt and water retention). Products include:
- Celestone Soluspan Suspension ... 2081

Betaxolol Hydrochloride (Excessive hypotension may result especially during initial therapy). Products include:
- Betoptic Sterile Ophthalmic Solution ... 569
- Betoptic S Sterile Ophthalmic Suspension ... 570
- Kerlone Tablets ... 2172

Bumetanide (May result in large or prolonged losses of fluids and electrolytes). Products include:
- Bumex ... 1895

Buprenorphine (Hypotensive effect may be potentiated).
- No products indexed under this heading.

Butabarbital (Hypotensive effect may be potentiated). Products include:
- Pyridium Plus ... 1764

Butalbital (Hypotensive effect may be potentiated). Products include:
- Esgic-Plus Tablets ... 1002
- Esgic Tablets & Capsules ... 1001
- Fioricet Tablets ... 2006
- Fiorinal Capsules ... 2007
- Fiorinal with Codeine Capsules ... 2008
- Fiorinal Tablets ... 2007
- Phrenilin ... 838
- Sedapap Tablets 50 mg/650 mg ... 1360

Captopril (Excessive hypotension may result especially during initial therapy). Products include:
- Capoten ... 2255
- Capozide ... 2258

Carteolol Hydrochloride (Excessive hypotension may result especially during initial therapy). Products include:
- Cartrol Tablets ... 507

Chlorothiazide (Excessive hypotension may result especially during initial therapy). Products include:
- Aldoclor Tablets ... 1413
- Diupres Tablets ... 1461
- Diuril Oral ... 1464

Chlorothiazide Sodium (Excessive hypotension may result especially during initial therapy). Products include:
- Diuril Sodium Intravenous ... 1463

Chlorpropamide (Blood glucose concentration may be raised). Products include:
- Diabinese Tablets ... 1775

Chlorthalidone (Excessive hypotension may result especially during initial therapy). Products include:
- Combipres Tablets ... 678
- Tenoretic Tablets ... 1105
- Thalitone Tablets ... 687

Choline Magnesium Trisalicylate (Increases the antihypertensive effect). Products include:
- Trilisate ... 1822

Clonidine (Excessive hypotension may result especially during initial therapy). Products include:
- Catapres-TTS ... 677

Clonidine Hydrochloride (Excessive hypotension may result especially during initial therapy). Products include:
- Catapres Tablets ... 676
- Combipres Tablets ... 678

Codeine (Hypotensive effect may be potentiated). Products include:
- Calcidrine Syrup ... 506

Codeine Phosphate (Hypotensive effect may be potentiated). Products include:
- Actifed with Codeine Cough Syrup ... 752
- Cheracol Cough Syrup ... 1853
- Codimal PH Syrup ... 846
- Dimetane-DC Cough Syrup ... 1857
- Empirin with Codeine Phosphate Nos. 2, 3 & 4 ... 764
- Fiorinal with Codeine Capsules ... 2008
- Isoclor Expectorant ... 982
- Naldecon CX Adult Liquid ... ■ 521
- Novahistine DH ... 1342
- Novahistine Expectorant ... 1343
- Nucofed Capsules ... 2219
- Nucofed Expectorant ... 2219
- Nucofed Pediatric Expectorant ... 2220
- Nucofed Syrup ... 2219
- Phenaphen with Codeine Capsules 1865
- Phenaphen-650 with Codeine Tablets ... 1866
- Phenergan with Codeine ... 2497
- Phenergan VC with Codeine ... 2501
- Robitussin A-C Syrup ... 1875
- Robitussin-DAC Syrup ... 1875
- Ryna ... ■ 741
- Soma Compound w/Codeine Tablets ... 2390
- Triaminic Expectorant w/Codeine ... 1996
- Tussi-Organidin Liquid ... 2391
- Tylenol with Codeine ... 1381

Codeine Polistirex (Hypotensive effect may be potentiated).
- No products indexed under this heading.

Cortisone Acetate (May increase the risk of hypokalemia and increase salt and water retention). Products include:
- Cortone Acetate Sterile Suspension ... 1437
- Cortone Acetate Tablets ... 1439

Deserpidine (Excessive hypotension may result especially during initial therapy). Products include:
- Enduronyl ... 518
- Harmonyl Tablets ... 528
- Oreticyl ... 545

Deslanoside (Hypokalemia induced by diuretic may increase the sensitivity of the myocardium to digitalis therapy).
- No products indexed under this heading.

Dexamethasone (May increase the risk of hypokalemia and increase salt and water retention). Products include:
- AK-Trol Ointment & Suspension ... ⊚ 207
- Decadron Elixir ... 1445
- Decadron Tablets ... 1447
- Decaspray Topical Aerosol ... 1459
- Dexacidin ... ⊚ 272
- Maxidex Sterile Ophthalmic Suspension ... ⊚ 223
- Maxitrol Ophthalmic Ointment/Suspension ... ⊚ 223
- TobraDex Ophthalmic Suspension and Ointment ... ⊚ 228

Dexamethasone Acetate (May increase the risk of hypokalemia and increase salt and water retention). Products include:
- Dalalone D.P. Injectable ... 999
- Decadron-LA Sterile Suspension ... 1457

Dexamethasone Sodium Phosphate (May increase the risk of hypokalemia and increase salt and water retention). Products include:
- AK-Dex ... ⊚ 203
- Decadron Phosphate Respihaler ... 1454
- Decadron Phosphate Sterile Ophthalmic Ointment ... 1453
- Decadron Phosphate Sterile Ophthalmic Solution ... 1453
- Decadron Phosphate Topical Cream ... 1455
- Decadron Phosphate Turbinaire ... 1456
- Maxidex Sterile Ophthalmic Ointment ... ⊚ 222
- NeoDecadron Sterile Ophthalmic Ointment ... 1517
- NeoDecadron Sterile Ophthalmic Solution ... 1518
- NeoDecadron Topical Cream ... 1518

Dezocine (Hypotensive effect may be potentiated).

Diazoxide (Excessive hypotension may result especially during initial therapy). Products include:
- Hyperstat I.V. Injection ... 2095
- Proglycem ... 649

Diclofenac Sodium (Increases the antihypertensive effect). Products include:
- Voltaren Ophthalmic Sterile Ophthalmic Solution ... ⊚ 268
- Voltaren Tablets ... 1042

Diflunisal (Increases the antihypertensive effect). Products include:
- Dolobid Tablets ... 1465

Digitoxin (Hypokalemia induced by diuretic may increase the sensitivity of the myocardium to digitalis therapy). Products include:
- Crystodigin Tablets ... 1253

Digoxin (Hypokalemia induced by diuretic may increase the sensitivity of the myocardium to digitalis therapy). Products include:
- Lanoxicaps ... 772
- Lanoxin Elixir Pediatric ... 775
- Lanoxin Injection ... 778
- Lanoxin Injection Pediatric ... 781
- Lanoxin Tablets ... 783

Doxazosin Mesylate (Excessive hypotension may result especially during initial therapy). Products include:
- Cardura Tablets ... 1941

Enalapril Maleate (Excessive hypotension may result especially during initial therapy). Products include:
- Vaseretic Tablets ... 1559
- Vasotec Tablets ... 1564

Enalaprilat (Excessive hypotension may result especially during initial therapy). Products include:
- Vasotec I.V. ... 1562

Esmolol Hydrochloride (Excessive hypotension may result especially during initial therapy). Products include:
- Brevibloc Injection ... 942

Ethacrynic Acid (May result in large or prolonged losses of fluids and electrolytes). Products include:
- Edecrin Tablets ... 1468

Etodolac (Increases the antihypertensive effect). Products include:
- Lodine Capsules 2468

Felodipine (Excessive hypotension may result especially during initial therapy). Products include:
- Plendil Extended-Release Tablets 1526

Fenoprofen Calcium (Increases the antihypertensive effect). Products include:
- Nalfon Pulvules & Tablets 919

Fentanyl (Hypotensive effect may be potentiated). Products include:
- Duragesic Transdermal System 1133

Fentanyl Citrate (Hypotensive effect may be potentiated). Products include:
- Innovar Injection 1141
- Sublimaze Injection 1146

Flurbiprofen (Increases the antihypertensive effect). Products include:
- Ansaid Tablets 2319

Fosinopril Sodium (Excessive hypotension may result especially during initial therapy). Products include:
- Monopril Tablets 1406

Furosemide (May result in large or prolonged losses of fluids and electrolytes; excessive hypotension may result especially during initial therapy). Products include:
- Lasix 1093

Glipizide (Blood glucose concentration may be raised). Products include:
- Glucotrol 1952

Glyburide (Blood glucose concentration may be raised). Products include:
- DiaBeta 1091
- Micronase Tablets 2350

Guanabenz Acetate (Excessive hypotension may result especially during initial therapy). Products include:
- Wytensin Tablets 2542

Guanethidine Monosulfate (Excessive hypotension may result especially during initial therapy). Products include:
- Esimil Tablets 864
- Ismelin Tablets 869

Hydralazine Hydrochloride (Excessive hypotension may result especially during initial therapy). Products include:
- Apresazide Capsules 854
- Apresoline Hydrochloride Parenteral (Ampuls) 856
- Apresoline Hydrochloride Tablets .. 855
- Apresoline-Esidrix Tablets 857
- Ser-Ap-Es Tablets 881
- Serpasil-Apresoline Tablets 884

Hydrochlorothiazide (Excessive hypotension may result especially during initial therapy). Products include:
- Aldactazide 2150
- Aldoril Tablets 1418
- Apresazide Capsules 854
- Apresoline-Esidrix Tablets 857
- Capozide 2258
- Dyazide Capsules 2208
- Esidrix Tablets 863
- Esimil Tablets 864
- HydroDIURIL Tablets 1484
- Hydropres Tablets 1485
- Inderide Tablets 2463
- Inderide LA Long Acting Capsules .. 2465
- Lopressor HCT Tablets 1034
- Maxzide 1215
- Moduretic Tablets 1510
- Normozide Tablets 2112
- Oretic Tablets 544
- Oreticyl 545
- Prinzide Tablets 1540
- Ser-Ap-Es Tablets 881
- Serpasil-Esidrix Tablets 886
- Timolide Tablets 1547
- Trandate HCT Tablets 579
- Vaseretic Tablets 1559
- Zestoretic 2274

Hydrocodone Bitartrate (Hypotensive effect may be potentiated). Products include:
- Anexsia 5/500 Tablets 2196
- Anexsia 7.5/650 Tablets 2197
- Azdone Tablets 844
- Codiclear DH Syrup 845
- Codimal DH Syrup 846
- Damason-P 1356
- Hycodan Syrup, Tablets 927
- Hycomine Compound Tablets 929
- Hycomine Syrup 927
- Hycotuss Expectorant Syrup 930
- Hydrocet Capsules 835
- Lortab ASA Tablets 2414
- Lortab 2412
- Ru-Tuss with Hydrocodone 694
- Triaminic Expectorant DH 1995
- Vicodin Tablets 1187
- Vicodin ES Tablets 1189
- Zydone Capsules 941

Hydrocodone Polistirex (Hypotensive effect may be potentiated). Products include:
- Tussionex Extended-Release Suspension 988

Hydrocortisone (May increase the risk of hypokalemia and increase salt and water retention). Products include:
- AK-Spore H.C. .... ⊙ 206
- Bactine Hydrocortisone Anti-Itch Cream .... ▣ 625
- CaldeCORT Anti-Itch Hydrocortisone Spray .... ▣ 560
- Carmol HC Cream 1% 2296
- Cortaid Spray .... ▣ 735
- Cortenema 2244
- Cortisporin Ointment 758
- Cortisporin Ophthalmic Ointment Sterile 758
- Cortisporin Ophthalmic Suspension Sterile 759
- Cortisporin Otic Solution Sterile 760
- Cortisporin Otic Suspension Sterile 760
- Cortizone-5 Creme & Ointment .... ▣ 732
- Dermolate Anti-Itch Cream .... ▣ 697
- Eldecort Cream 1.0% 1113
- Eldecort Cream 1.0% and 2.5% 1113
- Fungoid HC Creme 1770
- Hydrocortone Tablets 1482
- Hytone 909
- LazerSporin-C Solution 1770
- Massengill Medicated Soft Cloth Towelettes 2192
- Nutracort Cream & Lotion 1684
- PediOtic Suspension Sterile 797
- Synacort Creams 1%, 2.5% 2296
- Vanoxide-HC Acne Lotion 911
- Vioform-Hydrocortisone Cream and Mild Cream 889
- Vioform-Hydrocortisone Ointment .. 889
- VōSoL HC Otic Solution 2392
- Vytone Cream 1% 911

Hydrocortisone Acetate (May increase the risk of hypokalemia and increase salt and water retention). Products include:
- Analpram-HC Rectal Cream 1% and 2.5% 970
- Anusol-HC Cream 1690
- Anusol-HC Suppositories 1691
- Caldecort .... ▣ 560
- Carmol HC Cream 1% 2296
- Chloromycetin Hydrocortisone Ophthalmic 1694
- Coly-Mycin S Otic w/Neomycin & Hydrocortisone 1708
- Cortaid .... ▣ 735
- Cortef Feminine Itch Cream .... ▣ 735
- Corticaine .... ▣ 682
- Cortifoam 1827
- Cortisporin Cream 757
- Epifoam 1828
- Gynecort 5 Creme .... ▣ 556
- Hydrocortone Acetate Sterile Suspension 1479
- Lanacort 5 Creme and Ointment .. ▣ 557
- Mantadil Cream 789
- Ophthocort .... ⊙ 301
- Orabase HCA Oral Paste 890
- Pramosone Cream, Lotion & Ointment 971
- ProctoCream-HC 1834
- Proctofoam-HC 1835

Hydrocortisone Sodium Phosphate (May increase the risk of hypokalemia and increase salt and water retention). Products include:
- Hydrocortone Phosphate Injection, Sterile 1481

Hydrocortisone Sodium Succinate (May increase the risk of hypokalemia and increase salt and water retention). Products include:
- Solu-Cortef Sterile Powder 2361

Hydroflumethiazide (Excessive hypotension may result especially during initial therapy). Products include:
- Diucardin Tablets 2450
- Saluron 718
- Salutensin/Salutensin-Demi 719

Ibuprofen (Increases the antihypertensive effect). Products include:
- Advil Cold & Sinus Caplets (formerly CoAdvil) 2416
- Advil Ibuprofen Tablets and Caplets 2416
- Children's Advil Suspension 2426
- CoAdvil .... ▣ 748
- Dristan Sinus Caplets 2419
- Haltran Tablets .... ▣ 668
- Ibuprofen .... ▣ 631
- Medipren ibuprofen Caplets and Tablets 1362
- Midol 200 Cramp Relief Formula .. ▣ 570
- Motrin Tablets 2351
- Motrin IB Caplets and Tablets .... ▣ 736
- Nuprin Ibuprofen/Analgesic Tablets & Caplets 752
- PediaProfen Suspension 1363
- Rufen Tablets 691
- Trendar Ibuprofen Tablets .... ▣ 756

Indapamide (Excessive hypotension may result especially during initial therapy). Products include:
- Lozol Tablets 1843

Indomethacin (Increases the antihypertensive effect). Products include:
- Indocin 1487

Indomethacin Sodium Trihydrate (Increases the antihypertensive effect). Products include:
- Indocin I.V. 1490

Insulin, Human (Blood glucose concentration may be raised).
- No products indexed under this heading.

Insulin, Human Isophane Suspension (Blood glucose concentration may be raised). Products include:
- Humulin N, 100 Units 1270

Insulin, Human NPH (Blood glucose concentration may be raised). Products include:
- Insulatard NPH Human 1627
- Novolin N 1627
- Novolin N PenFill Cartridges 1628
- Novolin N Prefilled 1628

Insulin, Human Regular (Blood glucose concentration may be raised). Products include:
- Humulin BR, 100 Units 1268
- Humulin R, 100 Units 1272
- Novolin R 1627
- Novolin R PenFill Cartridges 1628
- Novolin R Prefilled 1629
- Velosulin Human 1628

Insulin, Human, Zinc Suspension (Blood glucose concentration may be raised). Products include:
- Humulin L, 100 Units 1268
- Humulin U, 100 Units 1272
- Novolin L 1627

Insulin, NPH (Blood glucose concentration may be raised). Products include:
- NPH, 40 & 100 Units 1273
- Beef NPH, 100 Units 1274
- Pork NPH, 100 Units 1275
- Insulatard NPH 1626
- NPH Insulin 1626
- NPH Purified Pork Isophane Insulin 1626

Insulin, Regular (Blood glucose concentration may be raised). Products include:
- Regular, 40 & 100 Units 1273
- Beef Regular, 100 Units 1275
- Pork Regular, 100 Units 1275
- Pork Regular (Concentrated), 500 Units 1276
- Regular Insulin 1625
- Regular Purified Pork Insulin 1626
- Velosulin 1627

Insulin, Zinc Crystals (Blood glucose concentration may be raised). Products include:
- NPH, 40 & 100 Units 1273

Insulin, Zinc Suspension (Blood glucose concentration may be raised). Products include:
- Lente, 40 & 100 Units 1272
- Protamine, Zinc, 40 & 100 Units 1273
- Lente Iletin I 1272
- Beef Lente, 100 Units 1274
- Beef Protamine Zinc, 100 Units 1274
- Pork Lente, 100 Units 1275
- Pork, Protamine, Zinc, 100 Units 1275
- Lente Insulin 1626
- Lente Purified Pork Insulin 1626
- Semilente Insulin 1625
- Ultralente Insulin 1626

Isradipine (Excessive hypotension may result especially during initial therapy). Products include:
- DynaCirc Capsules 2004

Ketoprofen (Increases the antihypertensive effect). Products include:
- Orudis Capsules 2488

Ketorolac Tromethamine (Increases the antihypertensive effect). Products include:
- Toradol IM Injection 2302

Labetalol Hydrochloride (Excessive hypotension may result especially during initial therapy). Products include:
- Normodyne Injection 2108
- Normodyne Tablets 2110
- Normozide Tablets 2112
- Trandate HCT Tablets 579
- Trandate Injection 577
- Trandate Tablets 579

Levorphanol Tartrate (Hypotensive effect may be potentiated). Products include:
- Levo-Dromoran 1906

Lisinopril (Excessive hypotension may result especially during initial therapy). Products include:
- Prinivil Tablets 1538
- Prinzide Tablets 1540
- Zestoretic 2274
- Zestril Tablets 2277

Lithium Carbonate (Serum lithium levels may increase). Products include:
- Eskalith 2214
- Lithane Tablets 1596
- Lithium Carbonate Capsules & Tablets 1984
- Lithobid Tablets 870

Lithium Citrate (Serum lithium levels may increase). Products include:
- Cibalith-S 870

Magnesium Salicylate (Increases the antihypertensive effect). Products include:
- Doan's - Extra-Strength Analgesic ▣ 549
- Doan's - Regular Strength Analgesic .... ▣ 549
- Mobigesic Analgesic Tablets .... ▣ 507

Mecamylamine Hydrochloride (Excessive hypotension may result especially during initial therapy). Products include:
- Inversine Tablets 1492

Meclofenamate Sodium (Increases the antihypertensive effect). Products include:
- Meclomen Capsules 1739

Mefenamic Acid (Increases the antihypertensive effect). Products include:

Ponstel 1758

Meperidine Hydrochloride (Hypotensive effect may be potentiated). Products include:

Demerol 2047
Mepergan Injection 2479

Mephobarbital (Hypotensive effect may be potentiated). Products include:

Mebaral Tablets 2061

Methadone Hydrochloride (Hypotensive effect may be potentiated). Products include:

Dolophine Hydrochloride Ampoules & Vials 1260
Dolophine Hydrochloride Tablets 1261
Methadone Hydrochloride Diskets .. 1284
Methadone Hydrochloride Oral Solution & Tablets 1987

Methenamine (Efficacy of methenamine may be decreased). Products include:

Urised Tablets 2396

Methenamine Hippurate (Efficacy of methenamine may be decreased). Products include:

Hiprex Tablets 1333
Urex Tablets 1321

Methenamine Mandelate (Efficacy of methenamine may be decreased). Products include:

Mandelamine 1738
Uroqid-Acid 661

Methyclothiazide (Excessive hypotension may result especially during initial therapy). Products include:

Enduron Tablets 517
Enduronyl 518

Methyldopa (Excessive hypotension may result especially during initial therapy). Products include:

Aldoclor Tablets 1413
Aldomet Oral 1415
Aldoril Tablets 1418

Methyldopate Hydrochloride (Excessive hypotension may result especially during initial therapy). Products include:

Aldomet Ester HCl Injection 1417

Methylprednisolone Acetate (May increase the risk of hypokalemia and increase salt and water retention). Products include:

Depo-Medrol Sterile Aqueous Suspension 2334

Methylprednisolone Sodium Succinate (May increase the risk of hypokalemia and increase salt and water retention). Products include:

Solu-Medrol Sterile Powder 2363

Metoprolol Tartrate (Excessive hypotension may result especially during initial therapy). Products include:

Lopressor Ampuls 1032
Lopressor HCT Tablets 1034
Lopressor Tablets 1032

Metyrosine (Excessive hypotension may result especially during initial therapy). Products include:

Demser Capsules 1460

Minoxidil (Excessive hypotension may result especially during initial therapy). Products include:

Loniten Tablets 2346
Rogaine Topical Solution 2357

Morphine Sulfate (Hypotensive effect may be potentiated). Products include:

Astramorph/PF Injection, USP (Preservative-Free) 618
Duramorph 960
Infumorph 200 and Infumorph 500 Sterile Solutions 962
MS Contin Tablets 1814
MSIR 1817
Oramorph SR (Morphine Sulfate Sustained Release Tablets) 1988
Roxanol 1991

Nadolol (Excessive hypotension may result especially during initial therapy). Products include:

Corgard Tablets 701
Corzide Tablets 702

Naproxen (Increases the antihypertensive effect). Products include:

Naprosyn 2297

Naproxen Sodium (Increases the antihypertensive effect). Products include:

Anaprox and Anaprox DS Tablets 2288

Nicardipine Hydrochloride (Excessive hypotension may result especially during initial therapy). Products include:

Cardene Capsules 2290

Nitroglycerin (Excessive hypotension may result especially during initial therapy). Products include:

Deponit NTG Transdermal Delivery System 2143
Minitran Transdermal Delivery System 1312
Nitro-Bid Ointment 1339
Nitro-Bid Capsules 1338
Nitrodisc 2176
Nitro-Dur (nitroglycerin) Transdermal Infusion System 1164
Nitrogard Tablets 1004
Nitrolingual Spray 1846
Nitrostat Tablets 1743
Transderm-Nitro Transdermal Therapeutic System 2283

Norepinephrine Bitartrate (Arterial responsiveness to norepinephrine may be decreased). Products include:

Levophed Bitartrate Injection 2054

Opium Alkaloids (Hypotensive effect may be potentiated). Products include:

B & O No. 15A & No. 16A Supprettes 2395
Pantopon Injectable 1911

Oxycodone Hydrochloride (Hypotensive effect may be potentiated). Products include:

Percocet Tablets 950
Percodan 951
Roxicodone Tablets, Oral Solution & Intensol (Oxycodone) 1992
Tylox Capsules 1382

Penbutolol Sulfate (Excessive hypotension may result especially during initial therapy). Products include:

Levatol 1832

Pentobarbital Sodium (Hypotensive effect may be potentiated). Products include:

Nembutal Sodium Capsules 534
Nembutal Sodium Solution 536
Nembutal Sodium Suppositories...... 538

Phenobarbital (Hypotensive effect may be potentiated). Products include:

Arco-Lase Plus Tablets 607
Bellergal-S Tablets 1998
Bronkolixir .... □ 761
Bronkotabs Tablets .... □ 762
Donnatal 1858
Donnatal Extentabs 1859
Donnatal Tablets 1858
Donnazyme Tablets 1860
Kinesed Tablets 2272
Phenobarbital Elixir and Tablets 1293
Primatene Tablets-P Formula 2421
Quadrinal Tablets 1183
Tedral SA 1765

Phenoxybenzamine Hydrochloride (Excessive hypotension may result especially during initial therapy). Products include:

Dibenzyline Capsules 2207

Phentolamine Mesylate (Excessive hypotension may result especially during initial therapy). Products include:

Regitine 878

Phenylbutazone (Increases the antihypertensive effect). Products include:

Butazolidin Capsules & Tablets 1027

Pindolol (Excessive hypotension may result especially during initial therapy). Products include:

Visken Tablets 2036

Piroxicam (Increases the antihypertensive effect). Products include:

Feldene Capsules 1777

Polythiazide (Excessive hypotension may result especially during initial therapy). Products include:

Minizide Capsules 1779
Renese Tablets 1785
Renese-R Tablets 1786

Prazosin Hydrochloride (Excessive hypotension may result especially during initial therapy). Products include:

Minipress Capsules 1778
Minizide Capsules 1779

Prednisolone Acetate (May increase the risk of hypokalemia and increase salt and water retention). Products include:

AK-Cide Sterile Ophthalmic Ointment & Suspension .... ⊙ 202
Blephamide Liquifilm Sterile Ophthalmic Suspension 586
Blephamide S.O.P. Sterile Ophthalmic Ointment 586
Cetapred Ointment .... ⊙ 220
⅛% Econopred & 1% Econopred Plus .... ⊙ 217
Isopto Cetapred Suspension .... ⊙ 220
Metimyd .... ⊙ 306
Poly-Pred Liquifilm .... ⊙ 250
Pred Forte .... ⊙ 252
Pred Mild .... ⊙ 254
Pred-G Liquifilm Sterile Ophthalmic Suspension .... ⊙ 252
Pred-G S.O.P. Sterile Ophthalmic Ointment .... ⊙ 253
Vasocidin Ointment .... ⊙ 275

Prednisolone Sodium Phosphate (May increase the risk of hypokalemia and increase salt and water retention). Products include:

AK-Pred .... ⊙ 205
Hydeltrasol Injection, Sterile 1476
Inflamase .... ⊙ 274
Pediapred Oral Liquid 987
Vasocidin Ophthalmic Solution ...... ⊙ 276

Prednisolone Tebutate (May increase the risk of hypokalemia and increase salt and water retention). Products include:

Hydeltra-T.B.A. Sterile Suspension 1478

Prednisone (May increase the risk of hypokalemia and increase salt and water retention). Products include:

Deltasone Tablets 2332

Propoxyphene Hydrochloride (Hypotensive effect may be potentiated). Products include:

Darvon 1256
Wygesic Tablets 2540

Propoxyphene Napsylate (Hypotensive effect may be potentiated). Products include:

Darvon-N/Darvocet-N 1254

Propranolol Hydrochloride (Excessive hypotension may result especially during initial therapy). Products include:

Inderal 2459
Inderal LA Long Acting Capsules 2461
Inderide Tablets 2463
Inderide LA Long Acting Capsules .. 2465

Ramipril (Excessive hypotension may result especially during initial therapy). Products include:

Altace Capsules 1086

Rauwolfia Serpentina (Excessive hypotension may result especially during initial therapy). Products include:

Raudixin Tablets 1803
Rauzide Tablets 1804

Rescinnamine (Excessive hypotension may result especially during initial therapy).

No products indexed under this heading.

Reserpine (Excessive hypotension may result especially during initial therapy). Products include:

Diupres Tablets 1461
Hydromox R Tablets 1209
Hydropres Tablets 1485
Renese-R Tablets 1786
Salutensin/Salutensin-Demi 719
Ser-Ap-Es Tablets 881
Serpasil Tablets 883
Serpasil-Apresoline Tablets 884
Serpasil-Esidrix Tablets 886

Salsalate (Increases the antihypertensive effect). Products include:

Disalcid 1310
Mono-Gesic Tablets 846
Salflex 839

Secobarbital Sodium (Hypotensive effect may be potentiated). Products include:

Seconal Sodium Pulvules 1296

Sodium Nitroprusside (Excessive hypotension may result especially during initial therapy). Products include:

Nipride I.V. Infusion 1909

Sufentanil Citrate (Hypotensive effect may be potentiated). Products include:

Sufenta Injection 1147

Sulindac (Increases the antihypertensive effect). Products include:

Clinoril Tablets 1433

Terazosin Hydrochloride (Excessive hypotension may result especially during initial therapy). Products include:

Hytrin Tablets 529

Thiamylal Sodium (Hypotensive effect may be potentiated). Products include:

Surital Ampoules, Steri-Vials 1764

Timolol Maleate (Excessive hypotension may result especially during initial therapy). Products include:

Blocadren Tablets 1429
Timolide Tablets 1547
Timoptic in Ocudose 1552
Timoptic Sterile Ophthalmic Solution 1550

Tolazamide (Blood glucose concentration may be raised). Products include:

Tolinase Tablets 2365

Tolbutamide (Blood glucose concentration may be raised). Products include:

Orinase Tablets 2354

Tolmetin Sodium (Increases the antihypertensive effect). Products include:

Tolectin (200, 400 and 600 mg) .. 1379

Triamcinolone (May increase the risk of hypokalemia and increase salt and water retention).

No products indexed under this heading.

Triamcinolone Acetonide (May increase the risk of hypokalemia and increase salt and water retention). Products include:

Aristocort A 1010
Azmacort Inhaler 1837
Kenalog Cream, Lotion & Ointment 2401
Kenalog-10 Injection 2402
Kenalog-40 Injection 2403
Kenalog in Orabase 604
Kenalog Spray 2401
Mycolog II Cream and Ointment 2407

Mytrex Cream & Ointment 2080
Nasacort Nasal Inhaler 1844

Triamcinolone Diacetate (May increase the risk of hypokalemia and increase salt and water retention). Products include:
Aristocort Suspension 1008

Triamcinolone Hexacetonide (May increase the risk of hypokalemia and increase salt and water retention). Products include:
Aristospan Suspension 1011

Trimethaphan Camsylate (Excessive hypotension may result especially during initial therapy). Products include:
Arfonad Ampuls 1887

Tubocurarine Chloride (Neuromuscular blocking effects of curariform drugs may be enhanced).
No products indexed under this heading.

ZEFAZONE STERILE POWDER
(Cefmetazole Sodium) 2372
May interact with aminoglycosides and certain other agents. Compounds in these categories include:

Alcohol (Disulfiram-like reactions characterized by flushing, sweating, headache, and tachycardia).

Amikacin Sulfate (Nephrotoxicity possible with concomitant use). Products include:
Amikin Injectable 602

Gentamicin Sulfate (Nephrotoxicity possible with concomitant use). Products include:
Garamycin Injectable 2093
Garamycin Ophthalmic .... ⊙ 305
Genoptic Liquifilm Sterile Ophthalmic Solution .... ⊙ 247
Genoptic S.O.P. Sterile Ophthalmic Ointment .... ⊙ 247
Gentacidin Ointment .... ⊙ 273
Gentacidin Solution .... ⊙ 273
Gentak Ointment & Solution .... ⊙ 208
G-myticin Creme and Ointment 0.1% 1770
Pred-G Liquifilm Sterile Ophthalmic Suspension .... ⊙ 252
Pred-G S.O.P. Sterile Ophthalmic Ointment .... ⊙ 253

Kanamycin Sulfate (Nephrotoxicity possible with concomitant use). Products include:
Kantrex Injection 601
Kantrex Pediatric Injection 601

Streptomycin Sulfate (Nephrotoxicity possible with concomitant use).
No products indexed under this heading.

Tobramycin (Nephrotoxicity possible with concomitant use). Products include:
TobraDex Ophthalmic Suspension and Ointment .... ⊙ 228
Tobrex Ophthalmic Ointment and Solution 572

Tobramycin Sulfate (Nephrotoxicity possible with concomitant use). Products include:
Nebcin Vials, Hyporets & ADD-Vantage 1286

ZENATE TABLETS
(Vitamin Preparation With Folic Acid or its Derivatives) 2250
No interactions described in labeling.

ZEPHIRAN CHLORIDE AQUEOUS SOLUTION
(Benzalkonium Chloride) .... ⊡ 762
No interactions described in labeling.

ZEPHIRAN CHLORIDE SPRAY
(Benzalkonium Chloride) .... ⊡ 762
No interactions described in labeling.

ZEPHIRAN CHLORIDE TINTED TINCTURE
(Benzalkonium Chloride) .... ⊡ 762
No interactions described in labeling.

ZESTORETIC
(Lisinopril, Hydrochlorothiazide) 2274
May interact with diuretics, non-steroidal anti-inflammatory agents, potassium sparing diuretics, potassium-depleting corticosteroids, barbiturates, narcotic analgesics, oral hypoglycemic agents, insulin, antihypertensives, corticosteroids, lithium preparations, nondepolarizing neuromuscular blocking agents, and certain other agents. Compounds in these categories include:

Acebutolol Hydrochloride (Additive effects). Products include:
Sectral Capsules 2520

ACTH (Intensifies electrolyte depletion).
No products indexed under this heading.

Alcohol (Potentiates orthostatic hypotension).

Alfentanil Hydrochloride (Potentiates orthostatic hypotension). Products include:
Alfenta Injection 1131

Amiloride Hydrochloride (Potential for hyperkalemia; additive antihypertensive effect). Products include:
Midamor Tablets 1508
Moduretic Tablets 1510

Aprobarbital (Potentiates orthostatic hypotension). Products include:
Alurate Elixir 1883

Atenolol (Additive effects). Products include:
Tenoretic Tablets 1105
Tenormin Tablets and I.V. Injection 1107

Atracurium Besylate (Increased responsiveness to the muscle relaxant). Products include:
Tracrium Injection 817

Benazepril Hydrochloride (Additive effects). Products include:
Lotensin Tablets 872

Bendroflumethiazide (Additive effects; additive antihypertensive effect). Products include:
Corzide Tablets 702
Naturetin Tablets 1789
Rauzide Tablets 1804

Betamethasone Acetate (Intensifies electrolyte depletion). Products include:
Celestone Soluspan Suspension 2081

Betamethasone Sodium Phosphate (Intensifies electrolyte depletion). Products include:
Celestone Soluspan Suspension 2081

Betaxolol Hydrochloride (Additive effects). Products include:
Betoptic Sterile Ophthalmic Solution 569
Betoptic S Sterile Ophthalmic Suspension 570
Kerlone Tablets 2172

Bumetanide (Additive antihypertensive effect). Products include:
Bumex 1895

Buprenorphine (Potentiates orthostatic hypotension).
No products indexed under this heading.

Butabarbital (Potentiates orthostatic hypotension). Products include:
Pyridium Plus 1764

Butalbital (Potentiates orthostatic hypotension). Products include:
Esgic-Plus Tablets 1002
Esgic Tablets & Capsules 1001
Fioricet Tablets 2006
Fiorinal Capsules 2007
Fiorinal with Codeine Capsules 2008
Fiorinal Tablets 2007
Phrenilin 838
Sedapap Tablets 50 mg/650 mg .. 1360

Captopril (Additive effects). Products include:
Capoten 2255
Capozide 2258

Carteolol Hydrochloride (Additive effects). Products include:
Cartrol Tablets 507

Chlorothiazide (Additive effects; additive antihypertensive effect). Products include:
Aldoclor Tablets 1413
Diupres Tablets 1461
Diuril Oral 1464

Chlorothiazide Sodium (Additive effects; additive antihypertensive effect). Products include:
Diuril Sodium Intravenous 1463

Chlorpropamide (Dosage adjustment of the antidiabetic may be required). Products include:
Diabinese Tablets 1775

Chlorthalidone (Additive effects; additive antihypertensive effect). Products include:
Combipres Tablets 678
Tenoretic Tablets 1105
Thalitone Tablets 687

Clonidine (Additive effects). Products include:
Catapres-TTS 677

Clonidine Hydrochloride (Additive effects). Products include:
Catapres Tablets 676
Combipres Tablets 678

Codeine (Potentiates orthostatic hypotension). Products include:
Calcidrine Syrup 506

Codeine Phosphate (Potentiates orthostatic hypotension). Products include:
Actifed with Codeine Cough Syrup .. 752
Cheracol Cough Syrup 1853
Codimal PH Syrup 846
Dimetane-DC Cough Syrup 1857
Empirin with Codeine Phosphate Nos. 2, 3 & 4 764
Fiorinal with Codeine Capsules 2008
Isoclor Expectorant 982
Naldecon CX Adult Liquid .... ⊡ 521
Novahistine DH 1342
Novahistine Expectorant 1343
Nucofed Capsules 2219
Nucofed Expectorant 2219
Nucofed Pediatric Expectorant 2220
Nucofed Syrup 2219
Phenaphen with Codeine Capsules 1865
Phenaphen-650 with Codeine Tablets 1866
Phenergan with Codeine 2497
Phenergan VC with Codeine 2501
Robitussin A-C Syrup 1875
Robitussin-DAC Syrup 1875
Ryna .... ⊡ 741
Soma Compound w/Codeine Tablets 2390
Triaminic Expectorant w/Codeine .. 1996
Tussi-Organidin Liquid 2391
Tylenol with Codeine 1381

Codeine Polistirex (Potentiates orthostatic hypotension).
No products indexed under this heading.

Cortisone Acetate (Intensifies electrolyte depletion). Products include:
Cortone Acetate Sterile Suspension 1437
Cortone Acetate Tablets 1439

Deserpidine (Additive effects). Products include:
Enduronyl 518
Harmonyl Tablets 528
Oreticyl 545

Dexamethasone (Intensifies electrolyte depletion). Products include:
AK-Trol Ointment & Suspension .... ⊙ 207
Decadron Elixir 1445
Decadron Tablets 1447
Decaspray Topical Aerosol 1459
Dexacidin .... ⊙ 272
Maxidex Sterile Ophthalmic Suspension .... ⊙ 223
Maxitrol Ophthalmic Ointment/Suspension .... ⊙ 223
TobraDex Ophthalmic Suspension and Ointment .... ⊙ 228

Dexamethasone Acetate (Intensifies electrolyte depletion). Products include:
Dalalone D.P. Injectable 999
Decadron-LA Sterile Suspension 1457

Dexamethasone Sodium Phosphate (Intensifies electrolyte depletion). Products include:
AK-Dex .... ⊙ 203
Decadron Phosphate Respihaler 1454
Decadron Phosphate Sterile Ophthalmic Ointment 1453
Decadron Phosphate Sterile Ophthalmic Solution 1453
Decadron Phosphate Topical Cream 1455
Decadron Phosphate Turbinaire 1456
Maxidex Sterile Ophthalmic Ointment .... ⊙ 222
NeoDecadron Sterile Ophthalmic Ointment 1517
NeoDecadron Sterile Ophthalmic Solution 1518
NeoDecadron Topical Cream 1518

Dezocine (Potentiates orthostatic hypotension).

Diazoxide (Additive effects). Products include:
Hyperstat I.V. Injection 2095
Proglycem 649

Diclofenac Sodium (Reduces antihypertensive effects). Products include:
Voltaren Ophthalmic Sterile Ophthalmic Solution .... ⊙ 268
Voltaren Tablets 1042

Doxazosin Mesylate (Additive effects). Products include:
Cardura Tablets 1941

Enalapril Maleate (Additive effects). Products include:
Vaseretic Tablets 1559
Vasotec Tablets 1564

Enalaprilat (Additive effects). Products include:
Vasotec I.V. 1562

Esmolol Hydrochloride (Additive effects). Products include:
Brevibloc Injection 942

Ethacrynic Acid (Additive antihypertensive effect). Products include:
Edecrin Tablets 1468

Etodolac (Reduces antihypertensive effects). Products include:
Lodine Capsules 2468

Felodipine (Additive effects). Products include:
Plendil Extended-Release Tablets 1526

Fenoprofen Calcium (Reduces antihypertensive effects). Products include:
Nalfon Pulvules & Tablets 919

Fentanyl (Potentiates orthostatic hypotension). Products include:
Duragesic Transdermal System 1133

Fentanyl Citrate (Potentiates orthostatic hypotension). Products include:
Innovar Injection 1141
Sublimaze Injection 1146

Flurbiprofen (Reduces antihypertensive effects). Products include:
- Ansaid Tablets 2319

Fosinopril Sodium (Additive effects). Products include:
- Monopril Tablets 1406

Furosemide (Additive effects; additive antihypertensive effect). Products include:
- Lasix 1093

Glipizide (Dosage adjustment of the antidiabetic may be required). Products include:
- Glucotrol 1952

Glyburide (Dosage adjustment of the antidiabetic may be required). Products include:
- DiaBeta 1091
- Micronase Tablets 2350

Guanabenz Acetate (Additive effects). Products include:
- Wytensin Tablets 2542

Guanethidine Monosulfate (Additive effects). Products include:
- Esimil Tablets 864
- Ismelin Tablets 869

Hydralazine Hydrochloride (Additive effects). Products include:
- Apresazide Capsules 854
- Apresoline Hydrochloride Parenteral (Ampuls) 856
- Apresoline Hydrochloride Tablets .. 855
- Apresoline-Esidrix Tablets 857
- Ser-Ap-Es Tablets 881
- Serpasil-Apresoline Tablets 884

Hydrocodone Bitartrate (Potentiates orthostatic hypotension). Products include:
- Anexsia 5/500 Tablets 2196
- Anexsia 7.5/650 Tablets 2197
- Azdone Tablets 844
- Codiclear DH Syrup 845
- Codimal DH Syrup 846
- Damason-P 1356
- Hycodan Syrup, Tablets 927
- Hycomine Compound Tablets 929
- Hycomine Syrup 927
- Hycotuss Expectorant Syrup 930
- Hydrocet Capsules 835
- Lortab ASA Tablets 2414
- Lortab 2412
- Ru-Tuss with Hydrocodone 694
- Triaminic Expectorant DH 1995
- Vicodin Tablets 1187
- Vicodin ES Tablets 1189
- Zydone Capsules 941

Hydrocodone Polistirex (Potentiates orthostatic hypotension). Products include:
- Tussionex Extended-Release Suspension 988

Hydrocortisone (Intensifies electrolyte depletion). Products include:
- AK-Spore H.C. .... ◉ 206
- Bactine Hydrocortisone Anti-Itch Cream .... ⊡ 625
- CaldeCORT Anti-Itch Hydrocortisone Spray .... ⊡ 560
- Carmol HC Cream 1% 2296
- Cortaid Spray .... ⊡ 735
- Cortenema 2244
- Cortisporin Ointment 758
- Cortisporin Ophthalmic Ointment Sterile 758
- Cortisporin Ophthalmic Suspension Sterile 759
- Cortisporin Otic Solution Sterile 760
- Cortisporin Otic Suspension Sterile 760
- Cortizone-5 Creme & Ointment ...... ⊡ 732
- Dermolate Anti-Itch Cream .... ⊡ 697
- Eldecort Cream 1.0% 1113
- Eldecort Cream 1.0% and 2.5% 1113
- Fungoid HC Creme 1770
- Hydrocortone Tablets 1482
- Hytone 909
- LazerSporin-C Solution 1770
- Massengill Medicated Soft Cloth Towelettes 2192
- Nutracort Cream & Lotion 1684
- PediOtic Suspension Sterile 797
- Synacort Creams 1%, 2.5% 2296
- Vanoxide-HC Acne Lotion 911
- Vioform-Hydrocortisone Cream and Mild Cream 889
- Vioform-Hydrocortisone Ointment .. 889
- VōSoL HC Otic Solution 2392
- Vytone Cream 1% 911

Hydrocortisone Acetate (Intensifies electrolyte depletion). Products include:
- Analpram-HC Rectal Cream 1% and 2.5% 970
- Anusol-HC Cream 1690
- Anusol-HC Suppositories 1691
- Caldecort .... ⊡ 560
- Carmol HC Cream 1% 2296
- Chloromycetin Hydrocortisone Ophthalmic 1694
- Coly-Mycin S Otic w/Neomycin & Hydrocortisone 1708
- Cortaid .... ⊡ 735
- Cortef Feminine Itch Cream .... ⊡ 735
- Corticaine .... ⊡ 682
- Cortifoam 1827
- Cortisporin Cream 757
- Epifoam 1828
- Gynecort 5 Creme .... ⊡ 556
- Hydrocortone Acetate Sterile Suspension 1479
- Lanacort 5 Creme and Ointment .. ⊡ 557
- Mantadil Cream 789
- Ophthocort .... ◉ 301
- Orabase HCA Oral Paste 890
- Pramosone Cream, Lotion & Ointment 971
- ProctoCream-HC 1834
- Proctofoam-HC 1835

Hydrocortisone Sodium Phosphate (Intensifies electrolyte depletion). Products include:
- Hydrocortone Phosphate Injection, Sterile 1481

Hydrocortisone Sodium Succinate (Intensifies electrolyte depletion). Products include:
- Solu-Cortef Sterile Powder 2361

Hydroflumethiazide (Additive effects; additive antihypertensive effect). Products include:
- Diucardin Tablets 2450
- Saluron 718
- Salutensin/Salutensin-Demi 719

Ibuprofen (Reduces antihypertensive effects). Products include:
- Advil Cold & Sinus Caplets (formerly CoAdvil) 2416
- Advil Ibuprofen Tablets and Caplets 2416
- Children's Advil Suspension 2426
- CoAdvil .... ⊡ 748
- Dristan Sinus Caplets 2419
- Haltran Tablets .... ⊡ 668
- Ibuprofen .... ⊡ 631
- Medipren ibuprofen Caplets and Tablets 1362
- Midol 200 Cramp Relief Formula .. ⊡ 570
- Motrin Tablets 2351
- Motrin IB Caplets and Tablets .... ⊡ 736
- Nuprin Ibuprofen/Analgesic Tablets & Caplets 752
- PediaProfen Suspension 1363
- Rufen Tablets 691
- Trendar Ibuprofen Tablets .... ⊡ 756

Indapamide (Additive effects; additive antihypertensive effect). Products include:
- Lozol Tablets 1843

Indomethacin (Reduces antihypertensive effects). Products include:
- Indocin 1487

Indomethacin Sodium Trihydrate (Reduces antihypertensive effects). Products include:
- Indocin I.V. 1490

Insulin, Human (Dosage adjustment of the antidiabetic may be required).
- No products indexed under this heading.

Insulin, Human Isophane Suspension (Dosage adjustment of the antidiabetic may be required). Products include:
- Humulin N, 100 Units 1270

Insulin, Human NPH (Dosage adjustment of the antidiabetic may be required). Products include:
- Insulatard NPH Human 1627
- Novolin N 1627
- Novolin N PenFill Cartridges 1628
- Novolin N Prefilled 1628

Insulin, Human Regular (Dosage adjustment of the antidiabetic may be required). Products include:
- Humulin BR, 100 Units 1268
- Humulin R, 100 Units 1272
- Novolin R 1627
- Novolin R PenFill Cartridges 1628
- Novolin R Prefilled 1629
- Velosulin Human 1628

Insulin, Human, Zinc Suspension (Dosage adjustment of the antidiabetic may be required). Products include:
- Humulin L, 100 Units 1268
- Humulin U, 100 Units 1272
- Novolin L 1627

Insulin, NPH (Dosage adjustment of the antidiabetic may be required). Products include:
- NPH, 40 & 100 Units 1273
- Beef NPH, 100 Units 1274
- Pork NPH, 100 Units 1275
- Insulatard NPH 1626
- NPH Insulin 1626
- NPH Purified Pork Isophane Insulin 1626

Insulin, Regular (Dosage adjustment of the antidiabetic may be required). Products include:
- Regular, 40 & 100 Units 1273
- Beef Regular, 100 Units 1275
- Pork Regular, 100 Units 1275
- Pork Regular (Concentrated), 500 Units 1276
- Regular Insulin 1625
- Regular Purified Pork Insulin 1626
- Velosulin 1627

Insulin, Zinc Crystals (Dosage adjustment of the antidiabetic may be required). Products include:
- NPH, 40 & 100 Units 1273

Insulin, Zinc Suspension (Dosage adjustment of the antidiabetic may be required). Products include:
- Lente, 40 & 100 Units 1272
- Protamine, Zinc, 40 & 100 Units 1273
- Lente Iletin I 1272
- Beef Lente, 100 Units 1274
- Beef Protamine Zinc, 100 Units 1274
- Pork Lente, 100 Units 1275
- Pork, Protamine, Zinc, 100 Units 1275
- Lente Insulin 1626
- Lente Purified Pork Insulin 1626
- Semilente Insulin 1625
- Ultralente Insulin 1626

Isradipine (Additive effects). Products include:
- DynaCirc Capsules 2004

Ketoprofen (Reduces antihypertensive effects). Products include:
- Orudis Capsules 2488

Ketorolac Tromethamine (Reduces antihypertensive effects). Products include:
- Toradol IM Injection 2302

Labetalol Hydrochloride (Additive effects). Products include:
- Normodyne Injection 2108
- Normodyne Tablets 2110
- Normozide Tablets 2112
- Trandate HCT Tablets 579
- Trandate Injection 577
- Trandate Tablets 579

Levorphanol Tartrate (Potentiates orthostatic hypotension). Products include:
- Levo-Dromoran 1906

Lithium Carbonate (Reduced renal clearance of lithium resulting in lithium toxicity). Products include:
- Eskalith 2214
- Lithane Tablets 1596
- Lithium Carbonate Capsules & Tablets 1984
- Lithobid Tablets 870

Lithium Citrate (Reduced renal clearance of lithium resulting in lithium toxicity). Products include:
- Cibalith-S 870

Mecamylamine Hydrochloride (Additive effects). Products include:
- Inversine Tablets 1492

Meclofenamate Sodium (Reduces antihypertensive effects). Products include:
- Meclomen Capsules 1739

Mefenamic Acid (Reduces antihypertensive effects). Products include:
- Ponstel 1758

Meperidine Hydrochloride (Potentiates orthostatic hypotension). Products include:
- Demerol 2047
- Mepergan Injection 2479

Mephobarbital (Potentiates orthostatic hypotension). Products include:
- Mebaral Tablets 2061

Methadone Hydrochloride (Potentiates orthostatic hypotension). Products include:
- Dolophine Hydrochloride Ampoules & Vials 1260
- Dolophine Hydrochloride Tablets 1261
- Methadone Hydrochloride Diskets .. 1284
- Methadone Hydrochloride Oral Solution & Tablets 1987

Methyclothiazide (Additive effects; additive antihypertensive effect). Products include:
- Enduron Tablets 517
- Enduronyl 518

Methyldopa (Additive effects). Products include:
- Aldoclor Tablets 1413
- Aldomet Oral 1415
- Aldoril Tablets 1418

Methyldopate Hydrochloride (Additive effects). Products include:
- Aldomet Ester HCl Injection 1417

Methylprednisolone Acetate (Intensifies electrolyte depletion). Products include:
- Depo-Medrol Sterile Aqueous Suspension 2334

Methylprednisolone Sodium Succinate (Intensifies electrolyte depletion). Products include:
- Solu-Medrol Sterile Powder 2363

Metocurine Iodide (Increased responsiveness to the muscle relaxant). Products include:
- Metubine Iodide Vials 1285

Metolazone (Additive effects; additive antihypertensive effect). Products include:
- Diulo 2129
- Mykrox ½ mg Tablets 984
- Zaroxolyn Tablets 989

Metoprolol Tartrate (Additive effects). Products include:
- Lopressor Ampuls 1032
- Lopressor HCT Tablets 1034
- Lopressor Tablets 1032

Metyrosine (Additive effects). Products include:
- Demser Capsules 1460

Minoxidil (Additive effects). Products include:
- Loniten Tablets 2346
- Rogaine Topical Solution 2357

Morphine Sulfate (Potentiates orthostatic hypotension). Products include:
- Astramorph/PF Injection, USP (Preservative-Free) 618
- Duramorph 960
- Infumorph 200 and Infumorph 500 Sterile Solutions 962
- MS Contin Tablets 1814
- MSIR 1817
- Oramorph SR (Morphine Sulfate Sustained Release Tablets) 1988
- Roxanol 1991

Nadolol (Additive effects). Products include:
- Corgard Tablets 701
- Corzide Tablets 702

(⊡ Described in PDR For Nonprescription Drugs) (◉ Described in PDR For Ophthalmology)

Naproxen (Reduces antihypertensive effects). Products include:
- Naprosyn 2297

Naproxen Sodium (Reduces antihypertensive effects). Products include:
- Anaprox and Anaprox DS Tablets 2288

Nicardipine Hydrochloride (Additive effects). Products include:
- Cardene Capsules 2290

Nitroglycerin (Additive effects). Products include:
- Deponit NTG Transdermal Delivery System 2143
- Minitran Transdermal Delivery System 1312
- Nitro-Bid Ointment 1339
- Nitro-Bid Capsules 1338
- Nitrodisc 2176
- Nitro-Dur (nitroglycerin) Transdermal Infusion System 1164
- Nitrogard Tablets 1004
- Nitrolingual Spray 1846
- Nitrostat Tablets 1743
- Transderm-Nitro Transdermal Therapeutic System 2283

Norepinephrine Bitartrate (Possible decreased response to pressor amines). Products include:
- Levophed Bitartrate Injection 2054

Opium Alkaloids (Potentiates orthostatic hypotension). Products include:
- B & O No. 15A & No. 16A Supprettes 2395
- Pantopon Injectable 1911

Oxycodone Hydrochloride (Potentiates orthostatic hypotension). Products include:
- Percocet Tablets 950
- Percodan 951
- Roxicodone Tablets, Oral Solution & Intensol (Oxycodone) 1992
- Tylox Capsules 1382

Pancuronium Bromide Injection (Increased responsiveness to the muscle relaxant).
- No products indexed under this heading.

Penbutolol Sulfate (Additive effects). Products include:
- Levatol 1832

Pentobarbital Sodium (Potentiates orthostatic hypotension). Products include:
- Nembutal Sodium Capsules 534
- Nembutal Sodium Solution 536
- Nembutal Sodium Suppositories 538

Phenobarbital (Potentiates orthostatic hypotension). Products include:
- Arco-Lase Plus Tablets 607
- Bellergal-S Tablets 1998
- Bronkolixir ⊞ 761
- Bronkotabs Tablets ⊞ 762
- Donnatal 1858
- Donnatal Extentabs 1859
- Donnatal Tablets 1858
- Donnazyme Tablets 1860
- Kinesed Tablets 2272
- Phenobarbital Elixir and Tablets 1293
- Primatene Tablets-P Formula 2421
- Quadrinal Tablets 1183
- Tedral SA 1765

Phenoxybenzamine Hydrochloride (Additive effects). Products include:
- Dibenzyline Capsules 2207

Phentolamine Mesylate (Additive effects). Products include:
- Regitine 878

Phenylbutazone (Reduces antihypertensive effects). Products include:
- Butazolidin Capsules & Tablets 1027

Pindolol (Additive effects). Products include:
- Visken Tablets 2036

Piroxicam (Reduces antihypertensive effects). Products include:
- Feldene Capsules 1777

Polythiazide (Additive effects; additive antihypertensive effect). Products include:
- Minizide Capsules 1779
- Renese Tablets 1785
- Renese-R Tablets 1786

Potassium Acid Phosphate (Potential for hyperkalemia). Products include:
- K-Phos M.F. Tablets 659
- K-Phos Original Formula 'Sodium Free' Tablets 660
- K-Phos No. 2 Tablets 659

Potassium Bicarbonate (Potential for hyperkalemia). Products include:
- Alka-Seltzer Advanced Formula Antacid & Non-Aspirin Pain Reliever ⊞ 620
- Alka-Seltzer Effervescent Antacid ⊞ 622
- K-Lyte 707
- Klorvess Effervescent Granules 2010
- Klorvess Effervescent Tablets 2011

Potassium Chloride (Potential for hyperkalemia). Products include:
- Chlor-3 Condiment 994
- K-Dur Microburst Release System (potassium chloride, USP) E.R. Tablets 1163
- K-Lor Powder Packets 531
- K-Lyte 707
- K-Norm Capsules 982
- K-Tab Filmtab 532
- Kato Potassium Supplement 1114
- Klor-Con 8/Klor-Con 10 Extended-release Tablets 2374
- Klorvess Effervescent Granules 2010
- Klorvess Effervescent Tablets 2011
- Klorvess 10% Liquid 2010
- Klotrix 708
- Kolyum Liquid 983
- Micro-K 1863
- Micro-K LS Packets 1864
- NuLYTELY 699
- Oral Rehydration Salts, Citrate 1150
- Rum-K Syrup 995
- Slow-K Tablets 2281
- Ten-K Controlled-Release Tablets 2282
- Thermotabs ⊞ 619

Potassium Citrate (Potential for hyperkalemia). Products include:
- Alka-Seltzer Effervescent Antacid 1570
- K-Lyte 707
- Polycitra Syrup 2424
- Polycitra-K 2424
- Polycitra-LC—Sugar-Free 2424
- Ricelyte, Rice-Based Oral Electrolyte Maintenance Solution ⊞ 613

Potassium Gluconate (Potential for hyperkalemia). Products include:
- Kolyum Liquid 983

Potassium Phosphate, Dibasic (Potential for hyperkalemia). Products include:
- Neutra-Phos 2423

Potassium Phosphate, Monobasic (Potential for hyperkalemia). Products include:
- K-Phos M.F. Tablets 659
- K-Phos Neutral Tablets 660
- Neutra-Phos 2423

Prazosin Hydrochloride (Additive effects). Products include:
- Minipress Capsules 1778
- Minizide Capsules 1779

Prednisolone Acetate (Intensifies electrolyte depletion). Products include:
- AK-Cide Sterile Ophthalmic Ointment & Suspension ◎ 202
- Blephamide Liquifilm Sterile Ophthalmic Suspension 586
- Blephamide S.O.P. Sterile Ophthalmic Ointment 586
- Cetapred Ointment ◎ 220
- ⅛% Econopred & 1% Econopred Plus ◎ 217
- Isopto Cetapred Suspension ◎ 220
- Metimyd ◎ 306
- Poly-Pred Liquifilm ◎ 250
- Pred Forte ◎ 252
- Pred Mild ◎ 254
- Pred-G Liquifilm Sterile Ophthalmic Suspension ◎ 252
- Pred-G S.O.P. Sterile Ophthalmic Ointment ◎ 253
- Vasocidin Ointment ◎ 275

Prednisolone Sodium Phosphate (Intensifies electrolyte depletion). Products include:
- AK-Pred ◎ 205
- Hydeltrasol Injection, Sterile 1476
- Inflamase ◎ 274
- Pediapred Oral Liquid 987
- Vasocidin Ophthalmic Solution ◎ 276

Prednisolone Tebutate (Intensifies electrolyte depletion). Products include:
- Hydeltra-T.B.A. Sterile Suspension 1478

Prednisone (Intensifies electrolyte depletion). Products include:
- Deltasone Tablets 2332

Propoxyphene Hydrochloride (Potentiates orthostatic hypotension). Products include:
- Darvon 1256
- Wygesic Tablets 2540

Propoxyphene Napsylate (Potentiates orthostatic hypotension). Products include:
- Darvon-N/Darvocet-N 1254

Propranolol Hydrochloride (Additive effects). Products include:
- Inderal 2459
- Inderal LA Long Acting Capsules 2461
- Inderide Tablets 2463
- Inderide LA Long Acting Capsules 2465

Ramipril (Additive effects). Products include:
- Altace Capsules 1086

Rauwolfia Serpentina (Additive effects). Products include:
- Raudixin Tablets 1803
- Rauzide Tablets 1804

Rescinnamine (Additive effects).
- No products indexed under this heading.

Reserpine (Additive effects). Products include:
- Diupres Tablets 1461
- Hydromox R Tablets 1209
- Hydropres Tablets 1485
- Renese-R Tablets 1786
- Salutensin/Salutensin-Demi 719
- Ser-Ap-Es Tablets 881
- Serpasil Tablets 883
- Serpasil-Apresoline Tablets 884
- Serpasil-Esidrix Tablets 886

Secobarbital Sodium (Potentiates orthostatic hypotension). Products include:
- Seconal Sodium Pulvules 1296

Sodium Nitroprusside (Additive effects). Products include:
- Nipride I.V. Infusion 1909

Spironolactone (Potential for hyperkalemia; additive antihypertensive effect). Products include:
- Aldactazide 2150
- Aldactone 2152

Sufentanil Citrate (Potentiates orthostatic hypotension). Products include:
- Sufenta Injection 1147

Sulindac (Reduces antihypertensive effects). Products include:
- Clinoril Tablets 1433

Terazosin Hydrochloride (Additive effects). Products include:
- Hytrin Tablets 529

Thiamylal Sodium (Potentiates orthostatic hypotension). Products include:
- Surital Ampoules, Steri-Vials 1764

Timolol Maleate (Additive effects). Products include:
- Blocadren Tablets 1429
- Timolide Tablets 1547
- Timoptic in Ocudose 1552
- Timoptic Sterile Ophthalmic Solution 1550

Tolazamide (Dosage adjustment of the antidiabetic may be required). Products include:
- Tolinase Tablets 2365

Tolbutamide (Dosage adjustment of the antidiabetic may be required). Products include:
- Orinase Tablets 2354

Tolmetin Sodium (Reduces antihypertensive effects). Products include:
- Tolectin (200, 400 and 600 mg) 1379

Triamcinolone (Intensifies electrolyte depletion).
- No products indexed under this heading.

Triamcinolone Acetonide (Intensifies electrolyte depletion). Products include:
- Aristocort A 1010
- Azmacort Inhaler 1837
- Kenalog Cream, Lotion & Ointment 2401
- Kenalog-10 Injection 2402
- Kenalog-40 Injection 2403
- Kenalog in Orabase 604
- Kenalog Spray 2401
- Mycolog II Cream and Ointment 2407
- Mytrex Cream & Ointment 2080
- Nasacort Nasal Inhaler 1844

Triamcinolone Diacetate (Intensifies electrolyte depletion). Products include:
- Aristocort Suspension 1008

Triamcinolone Hexacetonide (Intensifies electrolyte depletion). Products include:
- Aristospan Suspension 1011

Triamterene (Potential for hyperkalemia; additive antihypertensive effect). Products include:
- Dyazide Capsules 2208
- Dyrenium Capsules 2210
- Maxzide 1215

Trimethaphan Camsylate (Additive effects). Products include:
- Arfonad Ampuls 1887

Vecuronium Bromide (Increased responsiveness to the muscle relaxant). Products include:
- Norcuron 1642

ZESTRIL TABLETS
(Lisinopril) 2277

May interact with diuretics, potassium sparing diuretics, potassium-depleting corticosteroids, thiazides, lithium preparations, and certain other agents. Compounds in these categories include:

Amiloride Hydrochloride (Potential for significant hyperkalemia; possibility of excessive reduction in blood pressure). Products include:
- Midamor Tablets 1508
- Moduretic Tablets 1510

Bendroflumethiazide (Thiazide-induced potassium loss attenuated; possibility of excessive reduction in blood pressure). Products include:
- Corzide Tablets 702
- Naturetin Tablets 1789
- Rauzide Tablets 1804

Bumetanide (Possibility of excessive reduction in blood pressure). Products include:
- Bumex 1895

Chlorothiazide (Thiazide-induced potassium loss attenuated; possibility of excessive reduction in blood pressure). Products include:
- Aldoclor Tablets 1413
- Diupres Tablets 1461
- Diuril Oral 1464

Chlorothiazide Sodium (Thiazide-induced potassium loss attenuated; possibility of excessive reduction in blood pressure). Products include:
- Diuril Sodium Intravenous 1463

Chlorthalidone (Possibility of excessive reduction in blood pressure). Products include:
- Combipres Tablets ... 678
- Tenoretic Tablets ... 1105
- Thalitone Tablets ... 687

Ethacrynic Acid (Possibility of excessive reduction in blood pressure). Products include:
- Edecrin Tablets ... 1468

Furosemide (Possibility of excessive reduction in blood pressure). Products include:
- Lasix ... 1093

Hydrochlorothiazide (Thiazide-induced potassium loss attenuated; possibility of excessive reduction in blood pressure). Products include:
- Aldactazide ... 2150
- Aldoril Tablets ... 1418
- Apresazide Capsules ... 854
- Apresoline-Esidrix Tablets ... 857
- Capozide ... 2258
- Dyazide Capsules ... 2208
- Esidrix Tablets ... 863
- Esimil Tablets ... 864
- HydroDIURIL Tablets ... 1484
- Hydropres Tablets ... 1485
- Inderide Tablets ... 2463
- Inderide LA Long Acting Capsules ... 2465
- Lopressor HCT Tablets ... 1034
- Maxzide ... 1215
- Moduretic Tablets ... 1510
- Normozide Tablets ... 2112
- Oretic Tablets ... 544
- Oreticyl ... 545
- Prinzide Tablets ... 1540
- Ser-Ap-Es Tablets ... 881
- Serpasil-Esidrix Tablets ... 886
- Timolide Tablets ... 1547
- Trandate HCT Tablets ... 579
- Vaseretic Tablets ... 1559
- Zestoretic ... 2274

Hydroflumethiazide (Thiazide-induced potassium loss attenuated; possibility of excessive reduction in blood pressure). Products include:
- Diucardin Tablets ... 2450
- Saluron ... 718
- Salutensin/Salutensin-Demi ... 719

Indapamide (Possibility of excessive reduction in blood pressure). Products include:
- Lozol Tablets ... 1843

Indomethacin (Reduces antihypertensive effect). Products include:
- Indocin ... 1487

Indomethacin Sodium Trihydrate (Reduces antihypertensive effect). Products include:
- Indocin I.V. ... 1490

Lithium Carbonate (Possibility of lithium toxicity—serum lithium levels should be monitored frequently). Products include:
- Eskalith ... 2214
- Lithane Tablets ... 1596
- Lithium Carbonate Capsules & Tablets ... 1984
- Lithobid Tablets ... 870

Lithium Citrate (Possibility of lithium toxicity—serum lithium levels should be monitored frequently). Products include:
- Cibalith-S ... 870

Methyclothiazide (Thiazide-induced potassium loss attenuated; possibility of excessive reduction in blood pressure). Products include:
- Enduron Tablets ... 517
- Enduronyl ... 518

Metolazone (Possibility of excessive reduction in blood pressure). Products include:
- Diulo ... 2129
- Mykrox ½ mg Tablets ... 984
- Zaroxolyn Tablets ... 989

Polythiazide (Thiazide-induced potassium loss attenuated; possibility of excessive reduction in blood pressure). Products include:
- Minizide Capsules ... 1779
- Renese Tablets ... 1785
- Renese-R Tablets ... 1786

Potassium Acid Phosphate (Potential for significant hyperkalemia). Products include:
- K-Phos M.F. Tablets ... 659
- K-Phos Original Formula 'Sodium Free' Tablets ... 660
- K-Phos No. 2 Tablets ... 659

Potassium Bicarbonate (Potential for significant hyperkalemia). Products include:
- Alka-Seltzer Advanced Formula Antacid & Non-Aspirin Pain Reliever ... ◘ 620
- Alka-Seltzer Effervescent Antacid ◘ 622
- K-Lyte ... 707
- Klorvess Effervescent Granules ... 2010
- Klorvess Effervescent Tablets ... 2011

Potassium Chloride (Potential for significant hyperkalemia). Products include:
- Chlor-3 Condiment ... 994
- K-Dur Microburst Release System (potassium chloride, USP) E.R. Tablets ... 1163
- K-Lor Powder Packets ... 531
- K-Lyte ... 707
- K-Norm Capsules ... 982
- K-Tab Filmtab ... 532
- Kato Potassium Supplement ... 1114
- Klor-Con 8/Klor-Con 10 Extended-release Tablets ... 2374
- Klorvess Effervescent Granules ... 2010
- Klorvess Effervescent Tablets ... 2011
- Klorvess 10% Liquid ... 2010
- Klotrix ... 708
- Kolyum Liquid ... 983
- Micro-K ... 1863
- Micro-K LS Packets ... 1864
- NuLYTELY ... 699
- Oral Rehydration Salts, Citrate ... 1150
- Rum-K Syrup ... 995
- Slow-K Tablets ... 2281
- Ten-K Controlled-Release Tablets ... 2282
- Thermotabs ... ◘ 619

Potassium Citrate (Potential for significant hyperkalemia). Products include:
- Alka-Seltzer Effervescent Antacid ... 1570
- K-Lyte ... 707
- Polycitra Syrup ... 2424
- Polycitra-K ... 2424
- Polycitra-LC—Sugar-Free ... 2424
- Ricelyte, Rice-Based Oral Electrolyte Maintenance Solution ... ◘ 613

Potassium Gluconate (Potential for significant hyperkalemia). Products include:
- Kolyum Liquid ... 983

Potassium Phosphate, Dibasic (Potential for significant hyperkalemia). Products include:
- Neutra-Phos ... 2423

Potassium Phosphate, Monobasic (Potential for significant hyperkalemia). Products include:
- K-Phos M.F. Tablets ... 659
- K-Phos Neutral Tablets ... 660
- Neutra-Phos ... 2423

Spironolactone (Potential for significant hyperkalemia; possibility of excessive reduction in blood pressure). Products include:
- Aldactazide ... 2150
- Aldactone ... 2152

Triamterene (Potential for significant hyperkalemia; possibility of excessive reduction in blood pressure). Products include:
- Dyazide Capsules ... 2208
- Dyrenium Capsules ... 2210
- Maxzide ... 1215

ZETAR EMULSION
(Coal Tar, Oxytetracycline, Oxytetracycline Hydrochloride) ... 911
No interactions described in labeling.

ZILABRACE ORAL ANALGESIC GEL
(Benzocaine) ... ◘ 768
No interactions described in labeling.

ZILACTIN MEDICATED GEL
(Tannic Acid) ... ◘ 768
No interactions described in labeling.

ZILACTOL MEDICATED LIQUID
(Tannic Acid) ... ◘ 768
No interactions described in labeling.

ZILADENT ORAL ANALGESIC GEL
(Benzocaine) ... ◘ 768
No interactions described in labeling.

ZINACEF
(Cefuroxime Sodium) ... 1066
May interact with aminoglycosides and certain other agents. Compounds in these categories include:

Amikacin Sulfate (Concomitant administration may produce nephrotoxicity). Products include:
- Amikin Injectable ... 602

Gentamicin Sulfate (Concomitant administration may produce nephrotoxicity). Products include:
- Garamycin Injectable ... 2093
- Garamycin Ophthalmic ... ⊙ 305
- Genoptic Liquifilm Sterile Ophthalmic Solution ... ⊙ 247
- Genoptic S.O.P. Sterile Ophthalmic Ointment ... ⊙ 247
- Gentacidin Ointment ... ⊙ 273
- Gentacidin Solution ... ⊙ 273
- Gentak Ointment & Solution ... ⊙ 208
- G-myticin Creme and Ointment 0.1% ... 1770
- Pred-G Liquifilm Sterile Ophthalmic Suspension ... ⊙ 252
- Pred-G S.O.P. Sterile Ophthalmic Ointment ... ⊙ 253

Kanamycin Sulfate (Concomitant administration may produce nephrotoxicity). Products include:
- Kantrex Injection ... 601
- Kantrex Pediatric Injection ... 601

Probenecid (Concurrent administration of probenecid decreases renal clearance and increases peak serum levels of cefuroxime). Products include:
- Benemid Tablets ... 1426
- ColBENEMID Tablets ... 1436
- Wycillin Injection and Probenecid Tablets ... 2539

Streptomycin Sulfate (Concomitant administration may produce nephrotoxicity).
- No products indexed under this heading.

Tobramycin Sulfate (Concomitant administration may produce nephrotoxicity). Products include:
- Nebcin Vials, Hyporets & ADD-Vantage ... 1286

ZINCFRIN
(Phenylephrine Hydrochloride, Zinc Sulfate) ... ⊙ 230
No interactions described in labeling.

ZINCON DANDRUFF SHAMPOO
(Zinc Pyrithione) ... ◘ 590
No interactions described in labeling.

ZIRADRYL LOTION
(Diphenhydramine Hydrochloride, Zinc Oxide) ... ◘ 643
No interactions described in labeling.

ZOFRAN INJECTION
(Ondansetron Hydrochloride) ... 1069
May interact with drugs affecting hepatic drug metabolizing enzyme systems. Compounds in this category include:

Carbamazepine (Inducers or inhibitors of these enzymes may change the clearance and hence, the half-life). Products include:
- Tegretol Chewable Tablets ... 654
- Tegretol Suspension ... 656
- Tegretol Tablets ... 654

Cimetidine (Inducers or inhibitors of these enzymes may change the clearance and hence, the half-life). Products include:
- Tagamet Tablets ... 2228

Cimetidine Hydrochloride (Inducers or inhibitors of these enzymes may change the clearance and hence, the half-life). Products include:
- Tagamet ... 2228

Phenobarbital (Inducers or inhibitors of these enzymes may change the clearance and hence, the half-life). Products include:
- Arco-Lase Plus Tablets ... 607
- Bellergal-S Tablets ... 1998
- Bronkolixir ... ◘ 761
- Bronkotabs Tablets ... ◘ 762
- Donnatal ... 1858
- Donnatal Extentabs ... 1859
- Donnatal Tablets ... 1858
- Donnazyme Tablets ... 1860
- Kinesed Tablets ... 2272
- Phenobarbital Elixir and Tablets ... 1293
- Primatene Tablets-P Formula ... 2421
- Quadrinal Tablets ... 1183
- Tedral SA ... 1765

Phenytoin (Inducers or inhibitors of these enzymes may change the clearance and hence, the half-life). Products include:
- Dilantin Infatabs ... 1710
- Dilantin-30 Pediatric/Dilantin-125 Suspension ... 1713

Phenytoin Sodium (Inducers or inhibitors of these enzymes may change the clearance and hence, the half-life). Products include:
- Dilantin Kapseals ... 1708
- Dilantin Parenteral ... 1712
- Dilantin with Phenobarbital Kapseals ... 1715

ZOLADEX
(Goserelin Acetate Implant) ... 1110
No interactions described in labeling.

ZOLYSE
(Alpha Chymotrypsin) ... ⊙ 236
No interactions described in labeling.

ZORPRIN TABLETS
(Aspirin) ... 698
May interact with oral anticoagulants, oral hypoglycemic agents, insulin, antigout agents, non-steroidal anti-inflammatory agents, urinary alkalizing agents, and certain other agents. Compounds in these categories include:

Alcohol (Increased risk of gastrointestinal bleeding).

Allopurinol (Possible antagonism of uricosurics). Products include:
- Zyloprim Tablets ... 830

Betamethasone Dipropionate (Increased risk of gastrointestinal ulceration). Products include:
- Alphatrex Cream, Ointment & Lotion ... 2076
- Diprolene ... 2083
- Lotrisone Cream ... 2103
- Maxivate Cream, Lotion & Ointment 0.05% ... 2406
- Psorion Cream 0.05% ... 1121

Betamethasone Sodium Phosphate (Increased risk of gastrointestinal ulceration). Products include:
- Celestone Soluspan Suspension ... 2081

Chlorpropamide (Concomitant use not recommended; potentiation of hypoglycemic effect). Products include:
- Diabinese Tablets 1775

Diclofenac Sodium (May alter clinical efficacy of both drugs; may increase the risk of gastrointestinal ulceration). Products include:
- Voltaren Ophthalmic Sterile Ophthalmic Solution .... ◉ 268
- Voltaren Tablets 1042

Dicumarol (Depressed platelet aggregation; increased bleeding time). Products include:
- Dicumarol Tablets 516

Etodolac (May alter clinical efficacy of both drugs; may increase the risk of gastrointestinal ulceration). Products include:
- Lodine Capsules 2468

Fenoprofen Calcium (May alter clinical efficacy of both drugs; may increase the risk of gastrointestinal ulceration). Products include:
- Nalfon Pulvules & Tablets 919

Flurbiprofen (May alter clinical efficacy of both drugs; may increase the risk of gastrointestinal ulceration). Products include:
- Ansaid Tablets 2319

Glipizide (Concomitant use not recommended; potentiation of hypoglycemic effect). Products include:
- Glucotrol 1952

Glyburide (Concomitant use not recommended; potentiation of hypoglycemic effect). Products include:
- DiaBeta 1091
- Micronase Tablets 2350

Ibuprofen (May alter clinical efficacy of both drugs; may increase the risk of gastrointestinal ulceration). Products include:
- Advil Cold & Sinus Caplets (formerly CoAdvil) 2416
- Advil Ibuprofen Tablets and Caplets 2416
- Children's Advil Suspension 2426
- CoAdvil .... ▣ 748
- Dristan Sinus Caplets 2419
- Haltran Tablets .... ▣ 668
- Ibuprofen .... ▣ 631
- Medipren ibuprofen Caplets and Tablets 1362
- Midol 200 Cramp Relief Formula .. ▣ 570
- Motrin Tablets 2351
- Motrin IB Caplets and Tablets .... ▣ 736
- Nuprin Ibuprofen/Analgesic Tablets & Caplets 752
- PediaProfen Suspension 1363
- Rufen Tablets 691
- Trendar Ibuprofen Tablets .... ▣ 756

Indomethacin (May alter clinical efficacy of both drugs; may increase the risk of gastrointestinal ulceration). Products include:
- Indocin 1487

Indomethacin Sodium Trihydrate (May alter clinical efficacy of both drugs; may increase the risk of gastrointestinal ulceration). Products include:
- Indocin I.V. 1490

Insulin, Human (May alter insulin requirements).
- No products indexed under this heading.

Insulin, Human Isophane Suspension (May alter insulin requirements). Products include:
- Humulin N, 100 Units 1270

Insulin, Human NPH (May alter insulin requirements). Products include:
- Insulatard NPH Human 1627
- Novolin N 1627
- Novolin N PenFill Cartridges 1628
- Novolin N Prefilled 1628

Insulin, Human Regular (May alter insulin requirements). Products include:
- Humulin BR, 100 Units 1268
- Humulin R, 100 Units 1272
- Novolin R 1627
- Novolin R PenFill Cartridges 1628
- Novolin R Prefilled 1629
- Velosulin Human 1628

Insulin, Human, Zinc Suspension (May alter insulin requirements). Products include:
- Humulin L, 100 Units 1268
- Humulin U, 100 Units 1272
- Novolin L 1627

Insulin, NPH (May alter insulin requirements). Products include:
- NPH, 40 & 100 Units 1273
- Beef NPH, 100 Units 1274
- Pork NPH, 100 Units 1275
- Insulatard NPH 1626
- NPH Insulin 1626
- NPH Purified Pork Isophane Insulin 1626

Insulin, Regular (May alter insulin requirements). Products include:
- Regular, 40 & 100 Units 1273
- Beef Regular, 100 Units 1275
- Pork Regular, 100 Units 1275
- Pork Regular (Concentrated), 500 Units 1276
- Regular Insulin 1625
- Regular Purified Pork Insulin 1626
- Velosulin 1627

Insulin, Zinc Crystals (May alter insulin requirements). Products include:
- NPH, 40 & 100 Units 1273

Insulin, Zinc Suspension (May alter insulin requirements). Products include:
- Lente, 40 & 100 Units 1272
- Protamine, Zinc, 40 & 100 Units 1273
- Lente Iletin I 1272
- Beef Lente, 100 Units 1274
- Beef Protamine Zinc, 100 Units 1274
- Pork Lente, 100 Units 1275
- Pork, Protamine, Zinc, 100 Units 1275
- Lente Insulin 1626
- Lente Purified Pork Insulin 1626
- Semilente Insulin 1625
- Ultralente Insulin 1626

Ketoprofen (May alter clinical efficacy of both drugs; may increase the risk of gastrointestinal ulceration). Products include:
- Orudis Capsules 2488

Ketorolac Tromethamine (May alter clinical efficacy of both drugs; may increase the risk of gastrointestinal ulceration). Products include:
- Toradol IM Injection 2302

Meclofenamate Sodium (May alter clinical efficacy of both drugs; may increase the risk of gastrointestinal ulceration). Products include:
- Meclomen Capsules 1739

Mefenamic Acid (May alter clinical efficacy of both drugs; may increase the risk of gastrointestinal ulceration). Products include:
- Ponstel 1758

Methotrexate Sodium (Enhanced methotrexate activity; increased toxicity). Products include:
- Methotrexate Tablets, Parenteral, LPF Parenteral 1217
- Rheumatrex Methotrexate Dose Pack 1234

Naproxen (May alter clinical efficacy of both drugs; may increase the risk of gastrointestinal ulceration). Products include:
- Naprosyn 2297

Naproxen Sodium (May alter clinical efficacy of both drugs; may increase the risk of gastrointestinal ulceration). Products include:
- Anaprox and Anaprox DS Tablets 2288

Phenobarbital (Decreased serum concentration of salicylates). Products include:
- Arco-Lase Plus Tablets 607
- Bellergal-S Tablets 1998
- Bronkolixir .... ▣ 761
- Bronkotabs Tablets .... ▣ 762
- Donnatal 1858
- Donnatal Extentabs 1859
- Donnatal Tablets 1858
- Donnazyme Tablets 1860
- Kinesed Tablets 2272
- Phenobarbital Elixir and Tablets 1293
- Primatene Tablets-P Formula 2421
- Quadrinal Tablets 1183
- Tedral SA 1765

Phenylbutazone (May alter clinical efficacy of both drugs; may increase the risk of gastrointestinal ulceration). Products include:
- Butazolidin Capsules & Tablets 1027

Piroxicam (May alter clinical efficacy of both drugs; may increase the risk of gastrointestinal ulceration). Products include:
- Feldene Capsules 1777

Potassium Citrate (May decrease serum concentration of salicylates). Products include:
- Alka-Seltzer Effervescent Antacid .. 1570
- K-Lyte 707
- Polycitra Syrup 2424
- Polycitra-K 2424
- Polycitra-LC—Sugar-Free 2424
- Ricelyte, Rice-Based Oral Electrolyte Maintenance Solution .... ▣ 613

Probenecid (Possible antagonism of uricosurics). Products include:
- Benemid Tablets 1426
- ColBENEMID Tablets 1436
- Wycillin Injection and Probenecid Tablets 2539

Sodium Citrate (May decrease serum concentration of salicylates). Products include:
- Alka-Seltzer Effervescent Antacid .. 1570
- Alka-Seltzer Extra Strength Effervescent Antacid and Pain Reliever 1570
- Alka-Seltzer (Flavored) Effervescent Antacid and Pain Reliever 1569
- Bicitra—Sugar-Free 2423
- Citrocarbonate Antacid .... ▣ 668
- Polycitra 2424
- Ricelyte, Rice-Based Oral Electrolyte Maintenance Solution .... ▣ 613

Spironolactone (Decreased sodium excretion). Products include:
- Aldactazide 2150
- Aldactone 2152

Sulfinpyrazone (Possible antagonism of uricosurics). Products include:
- Anturane 853

Sulindac (May alter clinical efficacy of both drugs; may increase the risk of gastrointestinal ulceration). Products include:
- Clinoril Tablets 1433

Tolazamide (Concomitant use not recommended; potentiation of hypoglycemic effect). Products include:
- Tolinase Tablets 2365

Tolbutamide (Concomitant use not recommended; potentiation of hypoglycemic effect). Products include:
- Orinase Tablets 2354

Tolmetin Sodium (May alter clinical efficacy of both drugs; may increase the risk of gastrointestinal ulceration). Products include:
- Tolectin (200, 400 and 600 mg) .. 1379

Warfarin Sodium (Depressed platelet aggregation; increased bleeding time). Products include:
- Coumadin Injection & Tablets 944
- Panwarfin Tablets 547

ZOSTRIX
(Capsaicin) 1045
No interactions described in labeling.

ZOSTRIX-HP TOPICAL ANALGESIC CREAM
(Capsaicin) 1045
No interactions described in labeling.

ZOVIRAX CAPSULES
(Acyclovir) 824
May interact with:

Nephrotoxic Drugs (Increased risk of renal dysfunction).

Probenecid (Increases mean half-life and the AUC when co-administered with intravenous acyclovir). Products include:
- Benemid Tablets 1426
- ColBENEMID Tablets 1436
- Wycillin Injection and Probenecid Tablets 2539

ZOVIRAX OINTMENT 5%
(Acyclovir) 827
No interactions described in labeling.

ZOVIRAX STERILE POWDER
(Acyclovir Sodium) 828
May interact with cytotoxic drugs and certain other agents. Compounds in these categories include:

Bleomycin Sulfate (Use with caution in patients who have manifested prior neurologic reactions to cytotoxic drugs). Products include:
- Blenoxane 724

Daunorubicin Hydrochloride (Use with caution in patients who have manifested prior neurologic reactions to cytotoxic drugs). Products include:
- Cerubidine 2443

Doxorubicin Hydrochloride (Use with caution in patients who have manifested prior neurologic reactions to cytotoxic drugs). Products include:
- Adriamycin PFS 561
- Adriamycin RDF 562
- Doxorubicin Hydrochloride for Injection, USP 622
- Doxorubicin Hydrochloride Injection, USP 848
- Rubex 739

Fluorouracil (Use with caution in patients who have manifested prior neurologic reactions to cytotoxic drugs). Products include:
- Efudex 1880
- Fluoroplex Topical Solution & Cream 1% 1082
- Fluorouracil Injection 1897

Hydroxyurea (Use with caution in patients who have manifested prior neurologic reactions to cytotoxic drugs). Products include:
- Hydrea Capsules 728

Interferon alfa-2A, Recombinant (Concomitant administration requires caution). Products include:
- Roferon-A Injection 1916

Interferon alfa-2B, Recombinant (Concomitant administration requires caution). Products include:
- Intron A 2097

Methotrexate Sodium (Use with caution in patients who have manifested prior neurologic reactions to cytotoxic drugs; use with caution in patients receiving intrathecal methotrexate). Products include:
- Methotrexate Tablets, Parenteral, LPF Parenteral 1217
- Rheumatrex Methotrexate Dose Pack 1234

Mitotane (Use with caution in patients who have manifested prior neurologic reactions to cytotoxic drugs). Products include:
Lysodren ... 731
Mitoxantrone Hydrochloride (Use with caution in patients who have manifested prior neurologic reactions to cytotoxic drugs). Products include:
Novantrone for Injection Concentrate ... 1226
Probenecid (Increases mean half-life of Zovirax). Products include:
Benemid Tablets ... 1426
ColBENEMID Tablets ... 1436
Wycillin Injection and Probenecid Tablets ... 2539
Procarbazine Hydrochloride (Use with caution in patients who have manifested prior neurologic reactions to cytotoxic drugs). Products include:
Matulane Capsules ... 1907
Tamoxifen Citrate (Use with caution in patients who have manifested prior neurologic reactions to cytotoxic drugs). Products include:
Nolvadex Tablets ... 1102
Vincristine Sulfate (Use with caution in patients who have manifested prior neurologic reactions to cytotoxic drugs). Products include:
Oncovin Solution Vials & Hyporets 1288

ZOVIRAX SUSPENSION
(Acyclovir) ... 824
See **Zovirax Capsules**

ZOVIRAX TABLETS
(Acyclovir) ... 824
See **Zovirax Capsules**

ZYDONE CAPSULES
(Acetaminophen, Hydrocodone Bitartrate) ... 941
May interact with narcotic analgesics, neuromuscular blocking agents, monoamine oxidase inhibitors, anticholinergics, tricyclic antidepressants, tranquilizers, central nervous system depressants, and certain other agents. Compounds in these categories include:

Alcohol (Additive CNS depression).
Alfentanil Hydrochloride (Additive CNS depression). Products include:
Alfenta Injection ... 1131
Alprazolam (Additive CNS depression). Products include:
Xanax Tablets ... 2367
Amitriptyline Hydrochloride (Increased effect of antidepressant or hydrocodone; additive CNS depression). Products include:
Elavil ... 2269
Endep Tablets ... 1937
Etrafon ... 2087
Limbitrol ... 1933
Triavil Tablets ... 1556
Amoxapine (Increased effect of antidepressant or hydrocodone; additive CNS depression). Products include:
Asendin Tablets ... 1196
Aprobarbital (Additive CNS depression). Products include:
Alurate Elixir ... 1883
Atropine Sulfate (Paralytic ileus). Products include:
Arco-Lase Plus Tablets ... 607
Atropine Sulfate Sterile Ophthalmic Solution and S.O.P. Sterile Ophthalmic Ointment ... ◉ 239
Donnagel ... ■ 675
Donnagel-PG ... 1858
Donnatal ... 1858
Donnatal Extentabs ... 1859
Donnatal Tablets ... 1858
Donnazyme Tablets ... 1860
Isopto Atropine ... ◉ 218
Lomotil ... 2174
Motofen Tablets ... 836
Ru-Tuss Tablets ... 693
Urised Tablets ... 2396
Belladonna Alkaloids (Paralytic ileus). Products include:
Bellergal-S Tablets ... 1998
Hyland's Bed Wetting Tablets ... ■ 728
Hyland's Teething Tablets ... ■ 728
Kinesed Tablets ... 2272
Benztropine Mesylate (Paralytic ileus). Products include:
Cogentin ... 1435
Biperiden (Paralytic ileus). Products include:
Akineton ... 1171
Buprenorphine (Additive CNS depression).
No products indexed under this heading.
Buspirone Hydrochloride (Additive CNS depression). Products include:
BuSpar ... 1401
Butabarbital (Additive CNS depression). Products include:
Pyridium Plus ... 1764
Butalbital (Additive CNS depression). Products include:
Esgic-Plus Tablets ... 1002
Esgic Tablets & Capsules ... 1001
Fioricet Tablets ... 2006
Fiorinal Capsules ... 2007
Fiorinal with Codeine Capsules ... 2008
Fiorinal Tablets ... 2007
Phrenilin ... 838
Sedapap Tablets 50 mg/650 mg .. 1360
Chlordiazepoxide (Additive CNS depression). Products include:
Libritabs Tablets ... 1930
Limbitrol ... 1933
Menrium Tablets ... 1934
Chlordiazepoxide Hydrochloride (Additive CNS depression). Products include:
Librax Capsules ... 1929
Librium Capsules ... 1931
Librium Injectable ... 1932
Chlorpromazine (Additive CNS depression). Products include:
Thorazine ... 2234
Chlorprothixene (Additive CNS depression). Products include:
Taractan Tablets ... 1920
Chlorprothixene Hydrochloride (Additive CNS depression). Products include:
Taractan ... 1920
Chlorprothixene Lactate (Additive CNS depression). Products include:
Taractan Concentrate ... 1920
Clidinium Bromide (Paralytic ileus). Products include:
Librax Capsules ... 1929
Quarzan Capsules ... 1937
Clomipramine Hydrochloride (Increased effect of antidepressant or hydrocodone; additive CNS depression). Products include:
Anafranil Capsules ... 650
Clorazepate Dipotassium (Additive CNS depression). Products include:
Tranxene ... 556
Clozapine (Additive CNS depression). Products include:
Clozaril Tablets ... 2000
Codeine (Additive CNS depression). Products include:
Calcidrine Syrup ... 506
Codeine Phosphate (Additive CNS depression). Products include:
Actifed with Codeine Cough Syrup.. 752
Cheracol Cough Syrup ... 1853
Codimal PH Syrup ... 846
Dimetane-DC Cough Syrup ... 1857
Empirin with Codeine Phosphate Nos. 2, 3 & 4 ... 764
Fiorinal with Codeine Capsules ... 2008
Isoclor Expectorant ... 982
Naldecon CX Adult Liquid ... ■ 521
Novahistine DH ... 1342
Novahistine Expectorant ... 1343
Nucofed Capsules ... 2219
Nucofed Expectorant ... 2219
Nucofed Pediatric Expectorant ... 2220
Nucofed Syrup ... 2219
Phenaphen with Codeine Capsules 1865
Phenaphen-650 with Codeine Tablets ... 1866
Phenergan with Codeine ... 2497
Phenergan VC with Codeine ... 2501
Robitussin A-C Syrup ... 1875
Robitussin-DAC Syrup ... 1875
Ryna ... ■ 741
Soma Compound w/Codeine Tablets ... 2390
Triaminic Expectorant w/Codeine .. 1996
Tussi-Organidin Liquid ... 2391
Tylenol with Codeine ... 1381
Codeine Polistirex (Additive CNS depression).
No products indexed under this heading.
Desipramine Hydrochloride (Increased effect of antidepressant or hydrocodone; additive CNS depression). Products include:
Norpramin Tablets ... 1340
Dezocine (Additive CNS depression).
Diazepam (Additive CNS depression). Products include:
Valium Injectable ... 1937
Valium Tablets ... 1939
Valrelease Capsules ... 1923
Dicyclomine Hydrochloride (Paralytic ileus). Products include:
Bentyl ... 1322
Doxepin Hydrochloride (Increased effect of antidepressant or hydrocodone; additive CNS depression). Products include:
Sinequan ... 1960
Droperidol (Additive CNS depression). Products include:
Inapsine Injection ... 1140
Innovar Injection ... 1141
Enflurane (Additive CNS depression). Products include:
Ethrane ... 599
Estazolam (Additive CNS depression). Products include:
ProSom Tablets ... 554
Ethchlorvynol (Additive CNS depression). Products include:
Placidyl Capsules ... 553
Ethinamate (Additive CNS depression).
No products indexed under this heading.
Ethopropazine Hydrochloride (Paralytic ileus).
Fentanyl (Additive CNS depression). Products include:
Duragesic Transdermal System ... 1133
Fentanyl Citrate (Additive CNS depression). Products include:
Innovar Injection ... 1141
Sublimaze Injection ... 1146
Fluphenazine Decanoate (Additive CNS depression). Products include:
Prolixin Decanoate ... 1795
Fluphenazine Enanthate (Additive CNS depression). Products include:
Prolixin Enanthate ... 1796
Fluphenazine Hydrochloride (Additive CNS depression). Products include:
Prolixin Elixir ... 1793
Prolixin Injection ... 1791
Prolixin Oral Concentrate ... 1792
Prolixin Tablets ... 1793
Flurazepam Hydrochloride (Additive CNS depression). Products include:
Dalmane Capsules ... 1927
Furazolidone (Increased effect of hydrocodone or antidepressant; additive CNS depression). Products include:
Furoxone ... 1855
Glutethimide (Additive CNS depression).
No products indexed under this heading.
Glycopyrrolate (Paralytic ileus). Products include:
Robinul Forte Tablets ... 1873
Robinul Injectable ... 1873
Robinul Tablets ... 1873
Haloperidol (Additive CNS depression). Products include:
Haldol Injection, Tablets and Concentrate ... 1373
Haloperidol Decanoate (Additive CNS depression). Products include:
Haldol Decanoate ... 1375
Hydrocodone Polistirex (Additive CNS depression). Products include:
Tussionex Extended-Release Suspension ... 988
Hydroxyzine Hydrochloride (Additive CNS depression). Products include:
Atarax Tablets & Syrup ... 1941
Marax Tablets & DF Syrup ... 1954
Vistaril Intramuscular Solution ... 1970
Hyoscyamine (Paralytic ileus). Products include:
Cystospaz Tablets ... 2395
Urised Tablets ... 2396
Hyoscyamine Sulfate (Paralytic ileus). Products include:
Arco-Lase Plus Tablets ... 607
Cystospaz-M Capsules ... 2395
Donnagel ... ■ 675
Donnagel-PG ... 1858
Donnatal ... 1858
Donnatal Extentabs ... 1859
Donnatal Tablets ... 1858
Donnazyme Tablets ... 1860
Kutrase Capsules ... 2146
Levsin/Levsinex ... 2147
Ru-Tuss Tablets ... 693
Imipramine Hydrochloride (Increased effect of antidepressant or hydrocodone; additive CNS depression). Products include:
Tofranil Ampuls ... 1038
Tofranil Tablets ... 1039
Imipramine Pamoate (Increased effect of antidepressant or hydrocodone; additive CNS depression). Products include:
Tofranil-PM Capsules ... 1041
Ipratropium Bromide (Paralytic ileus). Products include:
Atrovent Inhalation Aerosol ... 675
Isocarboxazid (Increased effect of hydrocodone or antidepressant; additive CNS depression). Products include:
Marplan Tablets ... 1906
Isoflurane (Additive CNS depression). Products include:
Forane ... 600
Ketamine Hydrochloride (Additive CNS depression). Products include:
Ketalar ... 1726
Levorphanol Tartrate (Additive CNS depression). Products include:
Levo-Dromoran ... 1906
Lithium Carbonate (Additive CNS depression). Products include:
Eskalith ... 2214
Lithane Tablets ... 1596
Lithium Carbonate Capsules & Tablets ... 1984
Lithobid Tablets ... 870

Lithium Citrate (Additive CNS depression). Products include:
Cibalith-S 870
Lorazepam (Additive CNS depression). Products include:
Ativan Injection 2432
Ativan Tablets 2434
Loxapine Hydrochloride (Additive CNS depression). Products include:
Loxitane 1213
Loxapine Succinate (Additive CNS depression). Products include:
Loxitane Capsules 1213
Maprotiline Hydrochloride (Increased effect of antidepressant or hydrocodone; additive CNS depressant). Products include:
Ludiomil Tablets 874
Mepenzolate Bromide (Paralytic ileus). Products include:
Cantil Tablets 1326
Meperidine Hydrochloride (Additive CNS depression). Products include:
Demerol 2047
Mepergan Injection 2479
Mephobarbital (Additive CNS depression). Products include:
Mebaral Tablets 2061
Meprobamate (Additive CNS depression). Products include:
Deprol Tablets 2382
Equagesic Tablets 2451
Miltown Tablets 2386
PMB 200 and PMB 400 2504
Mesoridazine (Additive CNS depression). Products include:
Serentil 686
Methadone Hydrochloride (Additive CNS depression). Products include:
Dolophine Hydrochloride Ampoules & Vials 1260
Dolophine Hydrochloride Tablets 1261
Methadone Hydrochloride Diskets 1284
Methadone Hydrochloride Oral Solution & Tablets 1987
Methohexital Sodium (Additive CNS depression). Products include:
Brevital Sodium Vials 1248
Methoxyflurane (Additive CNS depression).
No products indexed under this heading.
Midazolam Hydrochloride (Additive CNS depression). Products include:
Versed Injection 1924
Molindone Hydrochloride (Additive CNS depression). Products include:
Moban Tablets & Concentrate 932
Morphine Sulfate (Additive CNS depression). Products include:
Astramorph/PF Injection, USP (Preservative-Free) 618
Duramorph 960
Infumorph 200 and Infumorph 500 Sterile Solutions 962
MS Contin Tablets 1814
MSIR 1817
Oramorph SR (Morphine Sulfate Sustained Release Tablets) 1988
Roxanol 1991
Nortriptyline Hydrochloride (Increased effect of antidepressant or hydrocodone; additive CNS depression). Products include:
Pamelor 2019
Opium Alkaloids (Additive CNS depression). Products include:
B & O No. 15A & No. 16A Supprettes 2395
Pantopon Injectable 1911
Oxazepam (Additive CNS depression). Products include:
Serax Capsules 2522
Serax Tablets 2522
Oxybutynin Chloride (Paralytic ileus). Products include:
Ditropan 1332
Oxycodone Hydrochloride (Additive CNS depression). Products include:
Percocet Tablets 950
Percodan 951
Roxicodone Tablets, Oral Solution & Intensol (Oxycodone) 1992
Tylox Capsules 1382
Oxyphenonium Bromide (Paralytic ileus).
Pentobarbital Sodium (Additive CNS depression). Products include:
Nembutal Sodium Capsules 534
Nembutal Sodium Solution 536
Nembutal Sodium Suppositories 538
Perphenazine (Additive CNS depression). Products include:
Etrafon 2087
Triavil Tablets 1556
Trilafon 2123
Phenelzine Sulfate (Increased effect of hydrocodone or antidepressant; additive CNS depression). Products include:
Nardil 1742
Phenobarbital (Additive CNS depression). Products include:
Arco-Lase Plus Tablets 607
Bellergal-S Tablets 1998
Bronkolixir ..... ▣ 761
Bronkotabs Tablets ..... ▣ 762
Donnatal 1858
Donnatal Extentabs 1859
Donnatal Tablets 1858
Donnazyme Tablets 1860
Kinesed Tablets 2272
Phenobarbital Elixir and Tablets 1293
Primatene Tablets-P Formula 2421
Quadrinal Tablets 1183
Tedral SA 1765
Pimozide (Additive CNS depression). Products include:
Orap Tablets 1020
Prazepam (Additive CNS depression). Products include:
Centrax 1693
Prochlorperazine (Additive CNS depression). Products include:
Compazine 2201
Procyclidine Hydrochloride (Paralytic ileus). Products include:
Kemadrin Tablets 771
Promethazine Hydrochloride (Additive CNS depression). Products include:
Mepergan Injection 2479
Phenergan with Codeine 2497
Phenergan with Dextromethorphan 2499
Phenergan Injection 2493
Phenergan Suppositories 2496
Phenergan Syrup 2495
Phenergan Tablets 2496
Phenergan VC 2500
Phenergan VC with Codeine 2501
Propantheline Bromide (Paralytic ileus). Products include:
Pro-Banthīne Tablets 2141
Propofol (Additive CNS depression). Products include:
Diprivan Injection 2267
Propoxyphene Hydrochloride (Additive CNS depression). Products include:
Darvon 1256
Wygesic Tablets 2540
Propoxyphene Napsylate (Additive CNS depression). Products include:
Darvon-N/Darvocet-N 1254
Protriptyline Hydrochloride (Increased effect of antidepressant or hydrocodone; additive CNS depression). Products include:
Vivactil Tablets 1567
Quazepam (Additive CNS depression). Products include:
Doral Tablets 2383
Scopolamine Hydrobromide (Paralytic ileus). Products include:
Donnagel ..... ▣ 675
Donnagel-PG 1858
Donnatal 1858
Donnatal Extentabs 1859
Donnatal Tablets 1858
Donnazyme Tablets 1860
Isopto Hyoscine ..... ◉ 222
Murocoll-2 Sterile Ophthalmic Solution ..... ◉ 261
Ru-Tuss Tablets 693
Secobarbital Sodium (Additive CNS depression). Products include:
Seconal Sodium Pulvules 1296
Selegiline Hydrochloride (Increased effect of hydrocodone or antidepressant; additive CNS depression). Products include:
Eldepryl 2250
Sufentanil Citrate (Additive CNS depression). Products include:
Sufenta Injection 1147
Temazepam (Additive CNS depression). Products include:
Restoril Capsules 2023
Thiamylal Sodium (Additive CNS depression). Products include:
Surital Ampoules, Steri-Vials 1764
Thioridazine Hydrochloride (Additive CNS depression). Products include:
Mellaril 2011
Thiothixene (Additive CNS depression). Products include:
Navane Capsules and Concentrate 1954
Navane Intramuscular 1956
Tranylcypromine Sulfate (Increased effect of hydrocodone or antidepressant; additive CNS depression). Products include:
Parnate Tablets 2222
Triazolam (Additive CNS depression). Products include:
Halcion Tablets 2340
Tridihexethyl Chloride (Paralytic ileus).
No products indexed under this heading.
Trifluoperazine Hydrochloride (Additive CNS depression). Products include:
Stelazine 2226
Trihexyphenidyl Hydrochloride (Paralytic ileus). Products include:
Artane 1195
Trimipramine Maleate (Increased effect of antidepressant or hydrocodone; additive CNS depression). Products include:
Surmontil Capsules 2524

ZYLOPRIM TABLETS
(Allopurinol) 830
May interact with antigout agents, thiazides, and certain other agents. Compounds in these categories include:

Amoxicillin (Increased frequency of skin rash). Products include:
Amoxil 2193
Augmentin Tablets, Powder for Oral Suspension, and Chewable Tablets 2198
Ampicillin Sodium (Increased frequency of skin rash). Products include:
Unasyn 1965
Azathioprine (Enhanced therapeutic response). Products include:
Imuran 768
Bendroflumethiazide (May enhance allopurinol toxicity). Products include:
Corzide Tablets 702
Naturetin Tablets 1789
Rauzide Tablets 1804
Chlorothiazide (May enhance allopurinol toxicity). Products include:
Aldoclor Tablets 1413
Diupres Tablets 1461
Diuril Oral 1464
Chlorothiazide Sodium (May enhance allopurinol toxicity). Products include:
Diuril Sodium Intravenous 1463
Chlorpropamide (Prolonged half-life). Products include:
Diabinese Tablets 1775
Cyclophosphamide (Enhanced bone marrow suppression). Products include:
Cytoxan for Injection 726
Neosar for Injection 566
Dicumarol (Prolonged half-life). Products include:
Dicumarol Tablets 516
Hydrochlorothiazide (May enhance allopurinol toxicity). Products include:
Aldactazide 2150
Aldoril Tablets 1418
Apresazide Capsules 854
Apresoline-Esidrix Tablets 857
Capozide 2258
Dyazide Capsules 2208
Esidrix Tablets 863
Esimil Tablets 864
HydroDIURIL Tablets 1484
Hydropres Tablets 1485
Inderide Tablets 2463
Inderide LA Long Acting Capsules .. 2465
Lopressor HCT Tablets 1034
Maxzide 1215
Moduretic Tablets 1510
Normozide Tablets 2112
Oretic Tablets 544
Oreticyl 545
Prinzide Tablets 1540
Ser-Ap-Es Tablets 881
Serpasil-Esidrix Tablets 886
Timolide Tablets 1547
Trandate HCT Tablets 579
Vaseretic Tablets 1559
Zestoretic 2274
Hydroflumethiazide (May enhance allopurinol toxicity). Products include:
Diucardin Tablets 2450
Saluron 718
Salutensin/Salutensin-Demi 719
Mercaptopurine (Enhanced therapeutic response). Products include:
Purinethol Tablets 800
Methyclothiazide (May enhance allopurinol toxicity). Products include:
Enduron Tablets 517
Enduronyl 518
Polythiazide (May enhance allopurinol toxicity). Products include:
Minizide Capsules 1779
Renese Tablets 1785
Renese-R Tablets 1786
Probenecid (Decreased excretion of oxypurines and increased excretion of urinary uric acid). Products include:
Benemid Tablets 1426
ColBENEMID Tablets 1436
Wycillin Injection and Probenecid Tablets 2539
Sulfinpyrazone (Decreased excretion of oxypurines and increased excretion of urinary uric acid). Products include:
Anturane 853
Tolbutamide (Metabolism of tolbutamide may be affected). Products include:
Orinase Tablets 2354

ZYMACAP CAPSULES
(Vitamins, Multiple) ..... ▣ 670
No interactions described in labeling.

ZYMASE CAPSULES
(Pancrelipase) 1645
No interactions described in labeling.

NOTES

SECTION 2

Food Interactions Cross-Reference

In this section, food interactions cited in the preceding index are cross-referenced by dietary item. Under each food heading is an alphabetical list, by brand name, of all products citing an interaction with the item. A brief summary of results follows each brand, along with the page number of the product's labeling. All page numbers refer to the 1992 editions of PDR® and PDR For Ophthalmology® and the 1991 edition of PDR For Nonprescription Drugs®. Symbols denoting the subsidiary PDR volumes appear in the bottom margin.

Content of this section is limited to only those food interactions cited in official prescribing information as published by PDR.

Anchovies

Parnate Tablets (Potential for hypertensive crisis).......... 2222

Avocados

Parnate Tablets (Potential for hypertensive crisis).......... 2222

Bananas

Matulane Capsules (Concurrent use should be avoided).......... 1907

Parnate Tablets (Potential for hypertensive crisis).......... 2222

Beans, broad

Furoxone Oral Suspension (Concurrent and/or sequential intake must be avoided).......... 1855

Marplan Tablets (Hypertensive reactions).......... 1906

Nardil (Concurrent and/or sequential intake must be avoided).......... 1742

Parnate Tablets (Potential for hypertensive crisis).......... 2222

Beans, Fava

Furoxone Oral Suspension (Concurrent and/or sequential intake must be avoided).......... 1855

Nardil (Concurrent and/or sequential intake must be avoided).......... 1742

Parnate Tablets (Potential for hypertensive crisis).......... 2222

Beer, alcohol-free

Marplan Tablets (Hypertensive reactions).......... 1906

Nardil (Concurrent and/or sequential intake must be avoided).......... 1742

Parnate Tablets (Potential for hypertensive crisis).......... 2222

Beer, reduced-alcohol

Marplan Tablets (Hypertensive reactions).......... 1906

Nardil (Concurrent and/or sequential intake must be avoided).......... 1742

Beer, unspecified

Furoxone Oral Suspension (Concurrent and/or sequential intake must be avoided).......... 1855

Marplan Tablets (Hypertensive reactions).......... 1906

Nardil (Concurrent and/or sequential intake must be avoided).......... 1742

Parnate Tablets (Potential for hypertensive crisis).......... 2222

Beverages, alcoholic (see also under Alcohol; Beer, unspecified; Wine products; Wine, Chianti; Wine, unspecified)

Protostat Tablets (Alcoholic beverages should not be consumed during and for at least one day after therapy).......... 1674

Teldrin Timed-Release Allergy Capsules, 12 mg. (Avoid concurrent use).......... 2192

Beverages, caffeine-containing

Marplan Tablets (Hypertensive reactions).......... 1906

Nardil (Excessive caffeine intake should be avoided).......... 1742

No Doz Fast Acting Alertness Aid Tablets (May cause sleeplessness, irritability, nervousness and rapid heart beat).......... 751

No Doz Maximum Strength Caplets (May cause sleeplessness, irritability, nervousness and rapid heart beat).......... 751

Respbid Tablets (Avoid large quantities; increased side effects).......... 684

Vivarin Stimulant Tablets (May cause nervousness, irritability, sleeplessness, and occasionally, rapid heart beat).. ▣ 726

Bologna, Lebanon

Nardil (Concurrent and/or sequential intake must be avoided).......... 1742

Bran, unspecified

Neo-Calglucon Syrup (Large quantities of phytic acid found in bran interfere with absorption of calcium).......... 2018

Broccoli (see under Diet high in vitamin K)

Caviar

Parnate Tablets (Potential for hypertensive crisis).......... 2222

Cereals, whole

Neo-Calglucon Syrup (Large quantities of phytic acid found in whole cereals interfere with absorption of calcium).......... 2018

Cheese, aged

Matulane Capsules (Concurrent use should be avoided).......... 1907

Nardil (Concurrent and/or sequential intake must be avoided).......... 1742

Parnate Tablets (Potential for hypertensive crisis).......... 2222

Cheese, strong, unpasteurized

Furoxone Oral Suspension (Concurrent and/or sequential intake must be avoided).......... 1855

Parnate Tablets (Potential for hypertensive crisis).......... 2222

Cheese, unspecified

Marplan Tablets (Hypertensive reactions).......... 1906

Nardil (Concurrent and/or sequential intake must be avoided).......... 1742

Parnate Tablets (Potential for hypertensive crisis).......... 2222

Chocolate

Nardil (Concurrent and/or sequential intake must be avoided).......... 1742

Parnate Tablets (Potential for hypertensive crisis).......... 2222

Respbid Tablets (Eating large quantity of chocolate increases theophylline side effects).......... 684

Coffee (see under Beverages, caffeine-containing)

Cola

Respbid Tablets (Drinking large quantity of cola increases theophylline side effects).......... 684

Cream, sour

Parnate Tablets (Potential for hypertensive crisis).......... 2222

Dairy products

Accutane Capsules (Increases oral absorption of isotretinoin).......... 1878

Achromycin V Capsules (Interferes with absorption of oral forms of tetracycline) ... 1193
Declomycin Capsules, Tablets (Interferes with absorption) ... 1199
Emcyt Capsules (Impairs the absorption of Emcyt) ... 1161
Fero-Folic-500 Filmtab (Ingestion of milk inhibits iron absorption) .. 527
Luride Drops (Incompatibility of fluoride with dairy foods results in the formation of poorly absorbed calcium fluoride) ... 889
Luride Lozi-Tabs Tablets (Incompatibility of fluoride with dairy foods results in the formation of poorly absorbed calcium fluoride) ... 890
Minocin Pellet-Filled Capsules (The peak plasma concentrations were slightly decreased (11.2%) and delayed by 1 hour) ... 1222
Nalfon Pulvules & Tablets (Peak blood levels are delayed and diminished) ... 919
Neo-Calglucon Syrup (Phosphorus from milk and other dairy products interferes with the absorption of calcium) ... 2018
Tegison Capsules (Increases absorption of etretinate) ... 1881
Terramycin Capsules (Interferes with absorption) ... 1786
Tolectin (200, 400 and 600 mg) (Decreases total tolmetin bioavailability by 16%) ... 1379
Uroqid-Acid Tablets (Concurrent use should be avoided or restricted to assure an acidic pH) ... 661

Diet high in protein

Sinemet Tablets (Levodopa competes with certain amino acids, the absorption of levodopa may be impaired in some patients on a high protein diet) 952

Diet high in vitamin K

Coumadin Injection & Tablets (Decreased prothrombin time) 944
Dicumarol Tablets (Decreased prothrombin time response) ... 516
Panwarfin Tablets (Decreased prothrombin time response) ... 547

Diet, high-lipid

Respbid Tablets (Reduced plasma concentration levels; delay in time of peak plasma levels) ... 684
Slo-bid Gyrocaps (Decreases in the rate of absorption, but with no significant difference in the extent of absorption) ... 1847
Tegison Capsules (Increases absorption of etretinate) ... 1881
Theo-24 (May result in a significant increase in peak serum level) ... 2179
Theolair-SR Tablets (Potential for plasma concentration levels of 40-60% of those noted in the fasted state and delay in the time to peak plasma level) ... 1319
TheoX Extended-Release Tablets (May result in a somewhat higher C_{max} and delayed T_{max}, and a somewhat greater extent of absorption when compared to taking in the fasting state) ... 841
Uniphyl 400 mg Tablets (Affects the bioavailability of theophylline) ... 1823

Diet, potassium-rich

Midamor Tablets (Potential for rapid increases in serum potassium levels) ... 1508
Moduretic Tablets (Potential for rapid increases in serum potassium levels) ... 1510

Eggs

Fero-Folic-500 Filmtab (Ingestion of eggs inhibits iron absorption) .. 527

Figs, canned

Parnate Tablets (Potential for hypertensive crisis) ... 2222

Fish, smoked

Nardil (Concurrent and/or sequential intake must be avoided) ... 1742

Food having a pH greater than 5.5

Creon Capsules (Dissolves the protective enteric coating) ... 2245

Food that lowers urinary pH

Disalcid Capsules (Decreases urinary excretion and increases plasma levels) ... 1310
Mono-Gesic Tablets (Decreases urinary excretion and increases plasma levels) ... 846
Trilisate Liquid (Decrease urinary salicylate excretion & increases plasma levels) ... 1822

Food that raises urinary pH

Disalcid Capsules (Increases renal clearance and urinary excretion of salicylic acid) ... 1310
Mandelamine Granules (Acidic urine is essential for antibacterial activity; restrict alkalinizing food) 1738
Mono-Gesic Tablets (Increases renal clearance and urinary excretion of salicylic acid) ... 846
Trilisate Liquid (Enhance renal salicylate clearance & diminishes plasma salicylate concentration).. 1822

Food with high concentration of dopamine

Furoxone Oral Suspension (Concurrent and/or sequential intake must be avoided) ... 1855
Nardil (Concurrent and/or sequential intake must be avoided) ... 1742

Food with high concentration of tyramine

Eldepryl (Potential for "cheese reaction" if attention is not paid to the dose dependent nature of selegine's selectivity) ... 2250
Furoxone Oral Suspension (Concurrent and/or sequential intake must be avoided) ... 1855
Matulane Capsules (Concurrent use should be avoided) ... 1907
Nardil (Concurrent and/or sequential intake must be avoided) ... 1742
Parnate Tablets (Potential for hypertensive crisis) ... 2222

Food, caffeine containing

Marplan Tablets (Hypertensive reactions) ... 1906
No Doz Fast Acting Alertness Aid Tablets (May cause sleeplessness, irritability, nervousness and rapid heart beat) ... 751
No Doz Maximum Strength Caplets (May cause sleeplessness, irritability, nervousness and rapid heart beat) ... 751
Vivarin Stimulant Tablets (May cause nervousness, irritability, sleeplessness, and occasionally, rapid heart beat).. ⊞ 726

Food, calcium-rich

Emcyt Capsules (Impairs the absorption of Emcyt) ... 1161

Food, unspecified

Accutane Capsules (Increases oral absorption of isotretinoin) ... 1878
Achromycin V Capsules (Interferes with absorption of oral forms of tetracycline) ... 1193
Altace Capsules (The rate of absorption is reduced not the extent of absorption) ... 1086
Ansaid Tablets (Alters the rate of absorption but does not affect the extent of drug availability) ... 2319
Apresazide Capsules (Enhances gastrointestinal absorption of hydrochlorothiazide) ... 854
Apresoline Hydrochloride Tablets (Results in higher plasma levels) 855
Apresoline-Esidrix Tablets (Enhances gastrointestinal absorption of hydrochlorothiazide; results in higher plasma levels of hydralazine) ... 857
Azdōne Tablets (Slightly delays the absorption of aspirin) ... 844
BuSpar (Food may decrease presystemic clearance of buspirone) ... 1401
Calan SR Caplets (Produces decreased bioavailability (AUC) but a narrower peak-to-trough ratio) ... 2157
Capoten (Reduces absorption by about 30 to 40 percent) ... 2255
Ceftin Tablets (Absorption is greater when taken after food) 575
Children's Advil Suspension (Peak plasma levels are somewhat lower (up to 30%) and the time to reach peak levels is slightly prolonged (up to 30 min.)) ... 2426
Cipro Tablets (Delays the absorption of the drug resulting in peak concentrations that are closer to 2 hours after dosing) 1589
Clinoril Tablets (The peak plasma concentrations of biologically active sulfide metabolite is delayed slightly in the presence of food) ... 1433
Constant-T Tablets (Food ingestion may influence the absorption characteristics) ... 1029
Cytotec (Diminishes maximum plasma concentrations) ... 2159
Declomycin Capsules, Tablets (Interferes with absorption) ... 1199
Desyrel and Desyrel Dividose (Food may affect the bioavailability including amount of drug absorbed and peak plasma levels) ... 1404
Dyclone 0.5% and 1% Topical Solutions, USP (Topical anesthesia may impair swallowing and thus enhance the danger of aspiration; food should not be ingested for 60 minutes).. 626
DynaCirc Capsules (Coadministration significantly increases the time to peak by about an hour with no effect on AUC) ... 2004
DynaCirc Capsules (Coadministration significantly increases the time to peak by about an hour with no effect on AUC) ... 2004
Erythromycin Delayed-Release Capsules, USP (Lowers the blood levels of systemically available erythromycin) ... 526
Esimil Tablets (Enhances gastrointestinal absorption of hydrochlorothiazide) ... 864
Floxin Tablets (Concurrent intake should be avoided) ... 1652
Glucotrol (Delays absorption by about 40 minutes) ... 1952
GoLYTELY (For best results, no solid food should be consumed during 3 to 4 hour period before drinking solution) ... 699
Isoptin SR Sustained Release Tablets (Produces decreased bioavailability (AUC) but a narrower peak to trough ratio) 1181
Lodine Capsules (Reduces the peak concentration reached by approximately one-half and increases the time-to-peak concentration by 1.4 to 3.8 hours) ... 2468
Macrodantin Capsules (Increases bioavailability of Macrodantin) ... 1624
Meclomen Capsules (Decreases in rate and the extent of absorption) ... 1739
Methotrexate Tablets, Parenteral, LPF Parenteral (Delays absorption and reduces peak concentration) ... 1217
Monopril Tablets (Rate of absorption may be slowed by the presence of food in the GI tract; the extent of absorption is not affected) ... 1406
Motrin Tablets (A reduction in the rate of absorption but no appreciable decrease in the extent of absorption) ... 2351
Noroxin Tablets (The presence of food may decrease the absorption) ... 1519
NuLYTELY (Solid food should not be given for at least two hours before the solution is given) ... 699
Orudis Capsules (Slows rate of absorption resulting in delayed and reduced peak concentrations) ... 2488
PediaProfen Suspension (The peak levels are somewhat lower (up to 30%) and the time to reach peak levels is slightly prolonged (up to 30 min.) although the extent of absorption is unchanged) ... 1363
Pepcid Oral Suspension (Bioavailability may be slightly increased by antacids) ... 1524
Procardia XL Tablets (Presence of food slightly alters the early rate of drug absorption) ... 1783
Prozac Pulvules (May delay absorption of fluoxetine inconsequentially) ... 920
Quibron-T/SR (May influence absorption) ... 716
Rythmol Tablets (Increased peak blood level and bioavailability in a single dose study) ... 1184
Salflex (Slows the absorption) ... 839
Sectral Capsules (Slightly decreases absorption and peak concentration) ... 2520
Ser-Ap-Es Tablets (Concomitant administration enhances gastrointestinal absorption of hydrochlorothiazide and results in higher plasma levels of hydralazine) ... 881
Serpasil-Apresoline Tablets (Concomitant administration enhances gastrointestinal absorption of hydrochlorothiazide and results in higher plasma levels of hydralazine) ... 884
Serpasil-Esidrix Tablets (Enhances gastrointestinal absorption of hydrochlorothiazide) ... 886
Sinemet CR Tablets (Increases the extent of availability and peak concentrations of levodopa) ... 953
Spectrobid Tablets & Powder for Oral Suspension (Spectrobid oral suspension absorption is affected by food) ... 1961
Terramycin Capsules (Interferes with absorption) ... 1786
Theo-Dur Sprinkle (Food ingestion may affect the bioavailability) ... 1168
Theo-Dur Extended-Release Tablets (May influence absorption of theophylline from a 100 mg dosage form) ... 1166
Trental (Delays absorption but does not affect total absorption) 1099
Xylocaine 2% Jelly (Topical anesthesia may impair swallowing and thus enhance the danger of aspiration; avoid food ingestion for 60 minutes) ... 643
Xylocaine 5% Ointment (Food should not be ingested for 60 minutes following usage; danger of biting trauma and aspiration) .. 644
Xylocaine 10% Oral Spray (Food should not be ingested for 60 minutes following usage; danger of biting trauma and aspiration) .. 645
4% Xylocaine-MPF Sterile Solution (Topical anesthesia may impair swallowing and thus enhance the danger of aspiration; food should not be ingested for 60 minutes) .. 641
Xylocaine 2% Viscous Solution (Topical anesthesia may impair swallowing and thus enhance the danger of aspiration; avoid food ingestion for 60 minutes) ... 646

Fruit juices, unspecified

Dexedrine Elixir (Lowers blood levels and efficacy) ... 2206

Fruits, unspecified

Uroqid-Acid Tablets (Concurrent use should be avoided or

restricted to assure an acidic pH) 661

Grapefruit juice, doubly concentrated

Plendil Extended-Release Tablets (Increases bioavailability more than two-fold) 1526

Herring, pickled

Furoxone Oral Suspension (Concurrent and/or sequential intake must be avoided) 1855
Marplan Tablets (Hypertensive reactions) 1906
Nardil (Concurrent and/or sequential intake must be avoided) 1742
Parnate Tablets (Potential for hypertensive crisis) 2222

Liqueurs

Parnate Tablets (Potential for hypertensive crisis) 2222

Liver

Nardil (Concurrent and/or sequential intake must be avoided) 1742
Parnate Tablets (Potential for hypertensive crisis) 2222

Liver, chicken

Furoxone Oral Suspension (Concurrent and/or sequential intake must be avoided) 1855
Marplan Tablets (Hypertensive reactions) 1906

Meal with dairy products

Minocin Pellet-Filled Capsules (The peak plasma concentrations were slightly decreased (11.2%) and delayed by 1 hour) 1222

Meal, high in bran fiber

Lanoxicaps (Reduces the amount of digoxin from an oral dose) 772
Lanoxin Tablets (The amount of digoxin from an oral dose may be reduced) 783

Meal, unspecified

ERYC (Optimum blood levels are obtained on a fasting stomach; administration is preferable one-half hour pre- or two hours post-meal) 1720
Ethmozine Tablets (Administration 30 minutes after a meal delays the rate of absorption but the extent of absorption is not altered) 946
Hismanal Tablets (Reduces the absorption by 60%) 1138
Lanoxicaps (The rate of absorption is slowed) 772
Lanoxin Tablets (Slows the rate of absorption) 783
Nalfon Pulvules & Tablets (Peak blood levels are delayed and diminished) 919
PCE Dispertab Tablets (Optimal blood levels are obtained when PCE is given in the fasting state) 549
Rufen Tablets (Reduces the rate of absorption but no appreciable decrease in the extent of absorption) 691
Tolectin (200, 400 and 600 mg) (Decreases total tolmetin bioavailability by 16%; reduces peak plasma concentrations by 50%) 1379

Meat extracts

Nardil (Concurrent and/or sequential intake must be avoided) 1742
Parnate Tablets (Potential for hypertensive crisis) 2222

Meat prepared with tenderizers

Parnate Tablets (Potential for hypertensive crisis) 2222

Meat, unspecified

Nardil (Concurrent and/or sequential intake must be avoided) 1742

Milk

(see under Dairy products)

Milk products

(see under Dairy products)

Pepperoni

Nardil (Concurrent and/or sequential intake must be avoided) 1742

Raisins

Parnate Tablets (Potential for hypertensive crisis) 2222

Rhubarb

Neo-Calglucon Syrup (Large quantities of oxalic acid found in rhubarb interfere with absorption of calcium) 2018

Salami, hard

Nardil (Concurrent and/or sequential intake must be avoided) 1742

Salami, Genoa

Nardil (Concurrent and/or sequential intake must be avoided) 1742

Sauerkraut

Nardil (Concurrent and/or sequential intake must be avoided) 1742
Parnate Tablets (Potential for hypertensive crisis) 2222

Sausage, dry

Nardil (Concurrent and/or sequential intake must be avoided) 1742

Sherry

Parnate Tablets (Potential for hypertensive crisis) 2222

Soy sauce

Parnate Tablets (Potential for hypertensive crisis) 2222

Soybean formula, children's

Euthroid (May cause excessive fecal loss) 1724
Proloid Tablets (May cause excessive fecal loss) 1761
Synthroid Injection (May cause excessive fecal loss) 695

Spinach

Neo-Calglucon Syrup (Large quantities of oxalic acid found in spinach interfere with absorption of calcium) 2018

Tea

(see under Beverages, caffeine-containing)

Vegetables, green leafy

Coumadin Injection & Tablets (Large amounts of green leafy vegetables may affect Coumadin therapy) 944

Wine products

Marplan Tablets (Hypertensive reactions) 1906
Nardil (Concurrent and/or sequential intake must be avoided) 1742

Wine, unspecified

Furoxone Oral Suspension (Concurrent and/or sequential intake must be avoided) 1855
Marplan Tablets (Hypertensive reactions) 1906
Matulane Capsules (Concurrent use should be avoided) 1907
Nardil (Concurrent and/or sequential intake must be avoided) 1742

Wine, Chianti

Parnate Tablets (Potential for hypertensive crisis) 2222

Yeast extract

Furoxone Oral Suspension (Concurrent and/or sequential intake must be avoided) 1855
Marplan Tablets (Hypertensive reactions) 1906
Nardil (Concurrent and/or sequential intake must be avoided) 1742
Parnate Tablets (Potential for hypertensive crisis) 2222

Yeast, brewer's

Nardil (Concurrent and/or sequential intake must be avoided) 1742

Yogurt

Matulane Capsules (Concurrent use should be avoided) 1907
Nardil (Concurrent and/or sequential intake must be avoided) 1742
Parnate Tablets (Potential for hypertensive crisis) 2222

NOTES

SECTION 3

Side Effects Index

Presented in this section is an alphabetical list of all side effects reported in the Adverse Reactions section of the product descriptions in PDR® and its companion volumes. Below each side-effect heading is an alphabetical list, by brand name, of all products citing the reaction. If noted in the underlying text, incidence of the side effect is shown in parentheses immediately after the brand name. Products citing an incidence of 3% or more are marked with the symbol (▲) at their left. All page numbers refer to the 1992 editions of PDR® and PDR For Ophthalmology® and the 1991 edition of PDR For Nonprescription Drugs®. Symbols denoting the subsidiary PDR volumes appear in the bottom margin.

The Index lists only side effects noted in official prescribing information as published by PDR. The listings are restricted to reactions occurring at recommended dosages in the general patient population. Precautions to be taken under special circumstances are not included, nor are the effects of overdosage.

A

A-V block

Blocadren Tablets (Less than 1%) 1429
Brethaire Inhaler 1024
Calan SR Caplets (0.8% to 1.2%) 2157
Calan Tablets 2155
Cardizem Tablets-30 mg, 60 mg, 90 mg and 120 mg (Less than 1%) 1329
▲ Cardizem SR Capsules-60 mg, 90 mg and 120 mg (0.6-7.6%) 1327
Cartrol Tablets 507
Catapres Tablets (Rare) 676
Catapres-TTS (Rare) 677
Combipres Tablets (Rare) 678
Corgard Tablets 701
Corzide Tablets 702
Ethmozine Tablets (1.6%) 946
Inderide Tablets 2463
Inderide LA Long Acting Capsules 2465
Isoptin Injectable (Rare) 1177
Isoptin Oral Tablets (0.8 to 1.2%) 1179
Isoptin SR Sustained Release Tablets (0.8% to 1.2%) 1181
Kerlone Tablets 2172
Lanoxicaps 772
Lanoxin Elixir Pediatric (Common) 775
Lanoxin Injection (Common) 778
Lanoxin Injection Pediatric (Common) 781
Lanoxin Tablets (Common) 783
Levatol 1832
Lopressor HCT Tablets 1034
Mexitil Capsules (Less than 1% or about 2 in 1,000) 680
Normodyne Tablets 2110
Normozide Tablets 2112
Norpace (Less than 1%) 2177
Pepcid (Infrequent) 1524
Permax Tablets (Infrequent) 1291
Prostigmin Injectable 1120
Prostigmin Tablets 1121
Quinidex Extentabs 1868
▲ Rythmol Tablets (0.8 to 4.5%) 1184
Sectral Capsules 2520
Tagamet (Rare) 2228
Tambocor Tablets 1315
Tegretol Chewable Tablets 654
Tegretol Suspension 656
Tegretol Tablets 654
Tenoretic Tablets 1105
Timolide Tablets 1547
Tonocard Tablets (Less than 1%) 1554
Verelan Capsules (0.8 to 1.2%) 1243
Visken Tablets 2036
Wytensin Tablets (Very rare) 2542
Zantac Injection and Zantac Injection Premixed (Rare) 1063
Zantac (Rare) 1065

A-V block, first-degree

Calan SR Caplets (1.2%) 2157
Calan Tablets 2155
Cardizem Tablets-30 mg, 60 mg, 90 mg and 120 mg (Less than 1%) 1329
▲ Cardizem SR Capsules-60 mg, 90 mg and 120 mg (1.8%-7.6%) 1327
Corgard Tablets (Single instance) 701
Corzide Tablets (Single instance) 702
Isoptin Oral Tablets (1.2%) 1179
Isoptin SR Sustained Release Tablets 1181
Prozac Pulvules (Rare) 920
Rythmol Tablets 1184
Verelan Capsules (1.2%) 1243

A-V block, intensification of

Blocadren Tablets 1429
Cartrol Tablets 507
Corgard Tablets 701
Corzide Tablets 702
Inderal 2459
Inderal LA Long Acting Capsules 2461
Inderide Tablets 2463
Inderide LA Long Acting Capsules 2465
Kerlone Tablets 2172
Levatol 1832
Sectral Capsules 2520
Trandate HCT/Trandate 579

A-V block, second-degree

Blocadren Tablets (Less than 1%) 1429
Calan SR Caplets (0.8%) 2157
Calan Tablets (0.8%) 2155
Cardizem Tablets-30 mg, 60 mg, 90 mg and 120 mg (Less than 1%) 1329
Cardizem SR Capsules-60 mg, 90 mg and 120 mg (0.6%) 1327
Isoptin Oral Tablets (0.8%) 1179
Isoptin SR Sustained Release Tablets (0.8%) 1181
Verelan Capsules (0.8% to 1.2%) 1243

A-V block, third-degree

Blocadren Tablets (Less than 1%) 1429
Calan SR Caplets (0.8%) 2157
Calan Tablets (0.8%) 2155
Cardizem Tablets-30 mg, 60 mg, 90 mg and 120 mg (Less than 1%) 1329
Corgard Tablets 701
Corzide Tablets (Single instance) 702
Isoptin Oral Tablets (0.8%) 1179
Isoptin SR Sustained Release Tablets (0.8%) 1181
Verelan Capsules (0.8% to 1.2%) 1243

A-V conduction, prolongation

Isoptin Injectable 1177
Sensorcaine 631
Sensorcaine-MPF Spinal 634

A-V conduction changes, unspecified

Elavil 2269

A-V fistula, clotted

Atgam Sterile Solution (More than 1% but less than 5%) 2320

A-V shunt, thrombosis of (see under Thrombosis of vascular access)

Abdominal adhesion

Lippes Loop Intrauterine Double-S 1654
ParaGard T380A Intrauterine Copper Contraceptive 411

Abdominal bloating

AeroBid Inhaler System (Less than 1%) 995
Atromid-S Capsules 2435
Brevicon 2304
Colyte 1826
Corgard Tablets (1 to 5 of 1000 patients) 701
Cortenema 2244
Corzide Tablets (1 to 5 of 1000 patients) 702
Demulen 2161
DiaBeta (1.8%) 1091
Diulo 2129
Enovid 2161
Estraderm Transdermal System 866
Estradurin 2452
Estratest 2245
Estrovis 1721
▲ GoLYTELY (Up to 50%) 699
Jenest-28 Tablets 1636
Levlen/Tri-Levlen 665
Loestrin 1728
Menrium Tablets 1934
Metrodin (urofollitropin for injection) 2182
Midamor Tablets (Less than or equal to 1%) 1508
Mitrolan Chewable Tablets (Occasional) 1878
Moduretic Tablets (Less than or equal to 1%) 1510
Mycelex-G 100 mg Vaginal Tablets (Rare) 1606

Mycelex-G 500 mg Vaginal Tablets (Rare) ... 1606
Mykrox ½ mg Tablets (Less than 2%) ... 984
Naturetin Tablets (Occasional) ... 1789
Norethin ... 2133
Norinyl ... 2304
Norlestrin ... 1746
▲ Norpace (3 to 9%) ... 2177
Nor-Q D Tablets ... 2304
▲ NuLYTELY (Up to 50% of patients) ... 699
Ogen ... 540
Ortho-Cyclen Tablets ... 1658
PMB 200 and PMB 400 ... 2504
Pergonal (menotropins for injection, USP) ... 2184
Premarin Intravenous ... 2508
Premarin with Methyltestosterone ... 2515
Premarin Tablets ... 2510
Premarin Vaginal Cream ... 2512
Prilosec Delayed-Release Capsules (Less than 1%) ... 1530
Rauzide Tablets ... 1804
Roferon-A Injection (Less than 1%) ... 1916
Sandostatin Injection (Less than 1%) ... 2029
TACE 12 and 25 mg ... 1353
▲ Trental (0.6% to 9.0%) ... 1099
Levlen/Tri-Levlen ... 665
Tri-Norinyl ... 2304
Valpin 50 Tablets ... 941
Zaroxolyn Tablets ... 989

Abdominal discomfort (see also under Distress, gastrointestinal; Distress, abdominal)

Aquasol A Vitamin A Capsules, USP ... 615
Aquasol A Parenteral, USP ... 615
Arfonad Ampuls ... 1887
Brevibloc Injection ... 942
BuSpar (2%) ... 1401
▲ Butazolidin Capsules & Tablets (3-9%) ... 1027
Carafate Tablets (Less than 0.5%) ... 1326
Cephulac Syrup ... 1331
Children's Advil Suspension (Less than 3%) ... 2426
Cipro I.V. (1.7%) ... 1592
Cipro Tablets (1.7%) ... 1589
▲ Clozaril Tablets (4%) ... 2000
Corgard Tablets (1 to 5 of 1000 patients) ... 701
Corzide Tablets (1 to 5 of 1000 patients) ... 702
Crystodigin Tablets ... 1253
Cytoxan for Injection ... 726
Dalgan Injection (Less than 1%) ... 620
Desferal Vials ... 862
▲ E.E.S. (Most frequent) ... 522
▲ EryPed 200 & EryPed 400 Granules (Most frequent) ... 519
Feldene Capsules ... 1777
Flagyl I.V. ... 2131
Fleet Bisacodyl Enema ... 991
Fleet Prep Kits ... 993
Hyperstat I.V. Injection ... 2095
Imodium Capsules ... 1139
K-Dur Microburst Release System (potassium chloride, USP) E.R. Tablets ... 1163
▲ K-Lyte (Among most common) ... 707
▲ Klor-Con 8/Klor-Con 10 Extended-release Tablets (Among most common) ... 2374
Klorvess Effervescent Granules ... 2010
Klorvess Effervescent Tablets ... 2011
Klorvess 10% Liquid ... 2010
▲ Kolyum Liquid (Among most common) ... 983
Lomotil ... 2174
Modane Tablets ... ▣ 503
Motrin Tablets (Less than 3%) ... 2351
Mykrox ½ mg Tablets (Less than 2%) ... 984
Papaverine Hydrochloride Vials and Ampoules ... 1290
Parlodel ... 2020
PediaProfen Suspension (Less than 3%) ... 1363
Pediazole ... 1973
Pepcid (Infrequent) ... 1524
▲ Rowasa (8.10%) ... 2248
▲ Sandimmune (Up to 7%) ... 2024
▲ Serophene (clomiphene citrate tablets, USP) (Approximately 1 in 15 patients) ... 2186
▲ Slow-K Tablets (Among most common) ... 2281
▲ Ten-K Controlled-Release Tablets (Among most common) ... 2282
Tenuate ... 1354
Tonocard Tablets (Less than 1%) ... 1554
▲ Trental (4%) ... 1099
▲ Visken Tablets (4%) ... 2036
Wytensin Tablets (3% or less) ... 2542

Abdominal distention

Aldoclor Tablets ... 1413
Aldomet Ester HCl Injection ... 1417
Aldomet Oral ... 1415
Aldoril Tablets ... 1418
Aristocort Suspension ... 1008
Aristospan Suspension ... 1011
Butazolidin Capsules & Tablets (Less than 1%) ... 1027
Celestone Soluspan Suspension ... 2081
▲ Cephulac Syrup (20%) ... 1331
Children's Advil Suspension (Less than 3%) ... 2426
Clozaril Tablets (Less than 1%) ... 2000
Colestid Granules (1 in 30 to 1 in 100 patients) ... 2328
Cortone Acetate Sterile Suspension ... 1437
Cortone Acetate Tablets ... 1439
Cyclogyl ... ⊚ 215
Dalalone D.P. Injectable ... 999
Decadron Elixir ... 1445
Decadron Phosphate Injection ... 1449
Decadron Phosphate Respihaler ... 1454
Decadron Phosphate Turbinaire ... 1456
Decadron Phosphate with Xylocaine Injection, Sterile ... 1451
Decadron Tablets ... 1447
Decadron-LA Sterile Suspension ... 1457
Deltasone Tablets ... 2332
Depo-Medrol Sterile Aqueous Suspension ... 2334
Duragesic Transdermal System (Less than 1%) ... 1133
Enrich Liquid Nutrition with Fiber ... 1971
Ensure Liquid Nutrition ... 1971
Ensure Plus High Calorie Liquid Nutrition ... 1971
Hydeltrasol Injection, Sterile ... 1476
Hydeltra-T.B.A. Sterile Suspension ... 1478
Hydrocortone Acetate Sterile Suspension ... 1479
Hydrocortone Phosphate Injection, Sterile ... 1481
Hydrocortone Tablets ... 1482
Imodium Capsules ... 1139
Indocin I.V. (1% to 3%) ... 1490
Intron A (1% or less) ... 2097
Kenalog-10 Injection ... 2402
Kenalog-40 Injection ... 2403
Medrol ... 2348
▲ Metrodin (urofollitropin for injection) (Approximately 20%) ... 2182
Monopril Tablets (0.2 to 1.0%) ... 1406
Motrin Tablets (Less than 3%) ... 2351
Osmolite Isotonic Liquid Nutrition ... 1972
Osmolite HN High Nitrogen Isotonic Liquid Nutrition ... 1972
Pediapred Oral Liquid ... 987
PediaProfen Suspension (Less than 3%) ... 1363
Permax Tablets (Infrequent) ... 1291
Prozac Pulvules (Rare) ... 920
Pulmocare Specialized Nutrition for Pulmonary Patients ... 1975
Serophene (clomiphene citrate tablets, USP) ... 2186
Solu-Cortef Sterile Powder ... 2361
Solu-Medrol Sterile Powder ... 2363
▲ Trental (4.0%) ... 1099
Unasyn (Less than 1%) ... 1965
Voltaren Tablets (1-3%) ... 1042

Abdominal mass

Demulen ... 2161
Enovid ... 2161
Estratest ... 2245

Abdominal pain/cramps

Actigall Capsules ... 2280
▲ Actimmune (8%) ... 1046
▲ AeroBid Inhaler System (3-9%) ... 995
Aldactazide ... 2150
Aldactone ... 2152
Aldoclor Tablets ... 1413
Aldoril Tablets ... 1418
Altace Capsules (Less than 1%) ... 1086
Aminohippurate Sodium Injection ... 1421
▲ Anafranil Capsules (11% to 13%) ... 650
▲ Anaprox and Anaprox DS Tablets (3-9%) ... 2288
Ancef Injection ... 2194
Ancobon Capsules ... 1886
▲ Ansaid Tablets (3-9%) ... 2319
Aralen Hydrochloride Injection ... 2038
Aralen Phosphate with Primaquine Phosphate Tablets ... 2040
Aralen Phosphate Tablets ... 2039
Asendin Tablets (Less than 1%) ... 1196
Atabrine Hydrochloride Tablets ... 2041
Atgam Sterile Solution (Less than 5%) ... 2320
Azactam for Injection (Less than 1%) ... 2252
Azdōne Tablets ... 844
Azo Gantanol Tablets ... 1887
Azo Gantrisin Tablets ... 1888
Azulfidine Tablets, EN-tabs, Oral Suspension (Rare) ... 1157
BAL in Oil Ampules ... 661
Bactrim DS Tablets ... 1891
Bactrim I.V. Infusion ... 1889
Bactrim ... 1891
Bentyl ... 1322
Blocadren Tablets ... 1429
Bretylol Injection (1 in 1000) ... 923
Brevicon ... 2304
Brevital Sodium Vials ... 1248
Bumex (0.2%) ... 1895
▲ Butazolidin Capsules & Tablets (3-9%) ... 1027
Calciparine Injection ... 925
Capoten (About 0.5 to 2%) ... 2255
Capozide (0.5 to 2%) ... 2258
Cardioquin Tablets ... 1812
Cardura Tablets (0%) ... 1941
Carnitor ... 2188
Cartrol Tablets (1.3%) ... 507
Ceftin Tablets ... 575
Celontin (Frequent) ... 1692
Centrax ... 1693
▲ Cephulac Syrup (20%) ... 1331
Ceptaz for Injection (One in 416 patients) ... 1057
▲ CHEMET (succimer) Capsules (5.2 to 15.7%) ... 1361
Children's Advil Suspension (Less than 1%) ... 2426
Chronulac Syrup ... 1332
Cibacalcin Double-chambered Syringes (Few) ... 859
Cipro I.V. (1% or less) ... 1592
Cipro Tablets (1.7%) ... 1589
Cleocin HCl Capsules ... 2322
Cleocin Pediatric Flavored Granules ... 2324
Cleocin Phosphate Injection ... 2325
Cleocin T Topical ... 2327
▲ Clinoril Tablets (10%) ... 1433
ColBENEMID Tablets ... 1436
Colchicine Ampoules ... 1252
Colestid Granules (1 in 30 to 1 in 100) ... 2328
Colyte ... 1826
Cordarone Tablets (1 to 3%) ... 2446
Corzide Tablets ... 702
Cosmegen Injection ... 1440
Coumadin Injection & Tablets (Infrequent) ... 944
Creon Capsules ... 2245
Crystodigin Tablets ... 1253
Cytosar-U Sterile Powder (Less frequent) ... 2329
▲ Cytotec (13-20%) ... 2159
Cytovene Sterile Powder (1% or less) ... 2292
Cytoxan for Injection ... 726
DDAVP Injection (Infrequent) ... 1840
DDAVP (2%) ... 1841
Dalgan Injection (Less than 1%) ... 620
Dalmane Capsules (Rare) ... 1927
Damason-P ... 1356
Dantrium Capsules (Less frequent) ... 1619
Dapsone USP ... 1130
Darvon-N/Darvocet-N ... 1254
Darvon ... 1256
Darvon-N Suspension & Tablets ... 1254
Demser Capsules (Infrequent) ... 1460
Demulen ... 2161
Depakene Capsules & Syrup ... 511
Depakote ... 512
Diapid Nasal Spray (Infrequent) ... 2003
Dicumarol Tablets ... 516
Diethylstilbestrol Tablets ... 1258
Diflucan Injection and Tablets (1.7% in 4048 patients) ... 1948
Dilaudid-HP Injection ... 1175
▲ Dipentum Capsules (1.1% to 10.1%) ... 1160
Diprivan Injection (Greater than 1%) ... 2267
Disalcid ... 1310
Diucardin Tablets ... 2450
Diuril Sodium Intravenous ... 1463
Doral Tablets ... 2383
▲ Duragesic Transdermal System (3% to 10%) ... 1133
Duvoid Tablets ... 1853
Dyazide Capsules ... 2208
▲ E.E.S. (Most frequent) ... 522
▲ E-Mycin Tablets (Most frequent) ... 688
Edecrin ... 1468
▲ Eldepryl (4 of 49 patients) ... 2250
Elspar ... 1470
Empirin with Codeine Phosphate Nos. 2, 3 & 4 ... 764
Enduron Tablets ... 517
Enduronyl ... 518
Engerix-B Unit-Dose Vials (Less than 1%) ... 2213
Enlon Injection ... 598
Enovid ... 2161
Enrich Liquid Nutrition with Fiber ... 1971
Ensure Liquid Nutrition ... 1971
Ensure Plus High Calorie Liquid Nutrition ... 1971
▲ Ergamisol Tablets (2 to 5%) ... 1136
▲ ERYC (Among most frequent) ... 1720
▲ EryPed (Among most frequent) ... 519
▲ Ery-Tab Tablets (Among most frequent) ... 521
▲ Erythrocin Stearate Filmtab (Among most frequent) ... 523
▲ Erythromycin Base Filmtab (Among most frequent) ... 525
▲ Erythromycin Delayed-Release Capsules, USP (Among most frequent) ... 526
Esidrix Tablets ... 863
Esimil Tablets ... 864
Eskalith ... 2214
Estinyl Tablets ... 2085
Estrace ... 1385
Estrace Vaginal Cream ... 1388
Estraderm Transdermal System ... 866
Estradurin ... 2452
Estratest ... 2245
Estrovis ... 1721
▲ Ethmozine Tablets (2%-5%) ... 946
Exna Tablets ... 1862
Sterile FUDR ... 1898
Fansidar Tablets ... 1896
Feldene Capsules (1 to 3%) ... 1777
▲ Fiorinal with Codeine Capsules (3.7%) ... 2008
Flagyl Tablets ... 2170
Fleet Bisacodyl Enema ... 991
Fleet Prep Kits ... 993
Floropryl Sterile Ophthalmic Ointment (Rare) ... 1473
Fortaz (1 in 416) ... 1060
Gamimune N Immune Globulin Intravenous (Human) ... 1572
Gantanol ... 1899
Gantrisin Ophthalmic Ointment/Solution ... 1900
Gantrisin ... 1901
Gastrocrom Capsules (2 of 87 patients) ... 974
Geocillin Tablets ... 1951
GoLYTELY (Infrequent) ... 699
Hismanal Tablets (1.4%) ... 1138
Humatin Capsules ... 1726
Humorsol Sterile Ophthalmic Solution (Rare) ... 1475
HydroDIURIL Tablets ... 1484
Hydromox R Tablets ... 1209
Hydromox Tablets ... 1208
Hylorel Tablets (1.7%) ... 975
Hytrin Tablets (At least 1%) ... 529
▲ Idamycin for Injection (73%) ... 564
▲ Ilosone (Most frequent) ... 913
Imferon ... 976
Imodium Capsules ... 1139
Imuran (Rare) ... 768
Inderal ... 2459
Inderal LA Long Acting Capsules ... 2461
Inderide Tablets ... 2463
Inderide LA Long Acting Capsules ... 2465
Indocin (Greater than 1%) ... 1487
Inocor Lactate Injection (0.4%) ... 2048
▲ Intron A (Up to 21%) ... 2097
IOPIDINE ... ⊚ 232
Isopto Carbachol ... ⊚ 219
Jenest-28 Tablets ... 1636
K-Dur Microburst Release System (potassium chloride, USP) E.R. Tablets ... 1163
▲ K-Lor Powder Packets (Most common) ... 531
Keflex Pulvules, Oral Suspension & Pediatric Drops ... 916
Keftab Tablets ... 917

▲ Klor-Con 8/Klor-Con 10 Extended-release Tablets (Among most common) 2374
▲ Klotrix (Most common) 708
Ku-Zyme HP Capsules 2147
▲ Lamprene Capsules (40-50%) 1030
Lanoxicaps (Very rare) 772
Lanoxin Elixir Pediatric (Very rare) 775
Lanoxin Injection (Very rare) 778
Lanoxin Injection Pediatric (Very rare) 781
Lanoxin Tablets (Very rare) 783
▲ Lariam Tablets (Among most frequent) 1904
Larodopa Tablets (Relatively frequent) 1905
Lasix Tablets and Injection 1093
Levlen/Tri-Levlen 665
Lioresal Tablets (Rare) 1031
▲ Lodine Capsules (3-9%) 2468
Lo/Ovral Tablets 2471
Lo/Ovral-28 Tablets 2476
Loestrin 1728
▲ Lopid Capsules and Tablets (9.8%) 1736
Lopressor Ampuls (Less than 1%) 1032
Lopressor HCT Tablets 1034
Lopressor Tablets (Less than 1%) 1032
Lorelco Tablets 1333
Lortab ASA Tablets 2414
Lozol Tablets (Less than 5%) 1843
Ludiomil Tablets (Rare) 874
MS Contin Tablets (Infrequent) 1814
MSIR (Infrequent) 1817
Macrodantin Capsules (Less common) 1624
Marax Tablets & DF Syrup (Frequent, on empty stomach) 1954
Matulane Capsules 1907
Maxair Inhaler (Less than 1%) 1311
▲ Meclomen Capsules (3-9%) 1739
Mediatric Capsules 2476
Menrium Tablets 1934
Mestinon Injectable 1115
Mestinon 1116
Methadone Hydrochloride Diskets 1284
Metopirone Tablets 876
▲ Metrodin (urofollitropin for injection) (Approximately 20%) 2182
▲ Mevacor Tablets (5.7%) 1505
Mexitil Capsules (1.2%) 680
Miacalcin Injection 2017
Micro-K 1863
▲ Micro-K LS Packets (Most common) 1864
Micronor Tablets 1667
Midamor Tablets (Between 1% and 3%) 1508
Minipress Capsules (Less than 1%) 1778
Minizide Capsules (Rare) 1779
MIOSTAT ⊙ 233
Modane Plus Tablets ▣ 504
Modane Tablets ▣ 503
Modicon 1667
Moduretic Tablets (Greater than 1%, less than 3%) 1510
Monopril Tablets (0.2 to 1.0%) 1406
Motrin Tablets (Less than 1%) 2351
Myambutol Tablets 1225
Mycelex-G 100 mg Vaginal Tablets (Rare) 1606
Mycelex-G 500 mg Vaginal Tablets (Rare) 1606
Mykrox ½ mg Tablets (Less than 2%) 984
Myochrysine Injection 1516
Nalfon Pulvules & Tablets (2%) 919
▲ Naprosyn (3 to 9%) 2297
Naturetin Tablets (Common) 1789
NebuPent for Inhalation Solution (Greater than 1%, up to 5%) 1017
NegGram 2062
Neo-Calglucon Syrup 2018
Neosar for Injection (Less frequent) 566
Nipride I.V. Infusion 1909
Nitro-Bid IV (Less than 1%) 1338
Nitrostat IV (Less than 1%) 1744
Nizoral Tablets (1.2%) 1145
Nolvadex Tablets (1%) 1102
Nordette-21 Tablets 2481
Nordette-28 Tablets 2483
Norethin 2133
Norinyl 2304
Norlestrin 1746
Normodyne Tablets 2110
Normozide Tablets 2112
Noroxin Tablets (0.3% to 1%) 1519
▲ Norpace (3 to 9%) 2177
Norpramin Tablets 1340
Nor-Q D Tablets 2304
Novantrone for Injection Concentrate (B 9 to 15%) 1226
Nullo Deodorant Tablets (1 case) ▣ 547
NuLYTELY (Less frequent) 699
Ogen 540
▲ Omnipaque (Less than 0.1 to 7%) 2552
Oncovin Solution Vials & Hyporets 1288
Oramorph SR (Morphine Sulfate Sustained Release Tablets) (Less frequent) 1988
Oretic Tablets 544
Oreticyl 545
Ornade Spansule Capsules 2221
Ortho Dienestrol Cream 1664
Ortho-Cyclen Tablets 1658
Ortho-Novum 1667
▲ Orudis Capsules (Greater than 3%) 2488
Osmolite Isotonic Liquid Nutrition 1972
Osmolite HN High Nitrogen Isotonic Liquid Nutrition 1972
Ovcon 1391
Ovral Tablets 2490
Ovral-28 Tablets 2491
Ovrette Tablets 2492
▲ PCE Dispertab Tablets (Among most frequent) 549
PMB 200 and PMB 400 2504
Pamelor 2019
Panwarfin Tablets 547
Paradione Capsules 548
▲ Parlodel (4%) 2020
Parnate Tablets 2222
Pavabid Capsules (Rare) 1344
Pavabid HP Capsulets (Rare) 1344
PediaProfen Suspension (Less than 3%) 1363
Pediazole 1973
Peptavlon 2563
Pergonal (menotropins for injection, USP) 2184
Peri-Colace (Exceedingly small) 1409
▲ Permax Tablets (5.8%) 1291
Phenaphen with Codeine Capsules 1865
Phenaphen-650 with Codeine Tablets 1866
Pitressin Synthetic, Ampoules 1758
Plaquenil Sulfate Tablets 2067
Plendil Extended-Release Tablets (0.3%) 1526
Pondimin Tablets 1867
Ponstel 1758
Premarin Intravenous 2508
Premarin with Methyltestosterone 2515
Premarin Tablets 2510
Premarin Vaginal Cream 2512
Prilosec Delayed-Release Capsules (0.4 to 5.2%) 1530
Primaxin I.M. 1532
Primaxin I.V. (Less than 0.2%) 1535
Prinivil Tablets (1% or less) 1538
Prinzide Tablets (0.3 to 1%) 1540
Procan SR Tablets (Common) 1760
Procardia Capsules (2% or less) 1781
Procardia XL Tablets (Less than 3%) 1783
Proglycem (Frequent) 649
▲ Pronestyl Capsules and Tablets (3-4%) 1800
Pronestyl Injection 1798
▲ Pronestyl-SR Tablets (3 to 4%) 1801
ProSom Tablets (1%) 554
▲ Prostigmin Injectable (Most common) 1120
Prostigmin Tablets 1121
Protostat Tablets (Occasional) 1674
▲ Prozac Pulvules (3.4%) 920
Pulmocare Specialized Nutrition for Pulmonary Patients 1975
Quinaglute Dura-Tabs Tablets 663
▲ Quinidex Extentabs (Among most frequent) 1868
Rauzide Tablets 1804
Recombivax HB (Less than 1%) 1544
Renese Tablets 1785
▲ Retrovir (3.2%) 802
▲ Ridaura Capsules (14%) 2224
Rifadin (Some patients) 1345
Rimactane Capsules 879
Ritalin 880
Rocephin Injectable Vials, ADD-Vantage (Rare) 1914
▲ Roferon-A Injection (15%) 1916
▲ Rowasa (3.0 to 8.10%) 2248
Rufen Tablets (1 to 3%) 691
Rythmol Tablets (0.8 to 1.9%) 1184
Salflex 839
▲ Sandostatin Injection (6.7%) 2029
Sansert Tablets 2031
Sectral Capsules (Up to 2%) 2520
Septra 813
Septra I.V. Infusion 808
Septra I.V. Infusion ADD-Vantage Vials 810
Septra 813
Serpasil-Esidrix Tablets 886
Sinemet Tablets 952
Sinemet CR Tablets 953
Solganal Suspension (Rare) 2122
Stilphostrol Tablets and Ampuls 1609
▲ Suprax (3%) 1235
Surmontil Capsules 2524
TACE 12 and 25 mg 1353
Talwin Injection (Rare) 2071
▲ Tambocor Tablets (3.3%) 1315
Tao Capsules (Most frequent) 1963
Tazicef for Injection (Less than 2%; 1 in 416 patients) 2231
Tazidime Vials, Faspak & ADD-Vantage (1 in 416) 1299
▲ Tegison Capsules (25-50%) 1881
Tegretol Chewable Tablets 654
Tegretol Suspension 656
Tegretol Tablets 654
Tenex Tablets (Less than 3%) 1875
Tensilon Injectable 1123
▲ Terazol 3 Vaginal Cream (3.4%) 1676
▲ TheraCys BCG Live (Intravesical) (2.7% to 6.3%) 898
Thiosulfil Forte Tablets 2526
Tofranil Ampuls 1038
Tofranil Tablets 1039
Tofranil-PM Capsules 1041
▲ Tolectin (200, 400 and 600 mg) (3 to 9%) 1379
Tonocard Tablets (Less than 1%) 1554
Trandate HCT/Trandate 579
▲ Trexan Tablets (Greater than 10%) 937
Tridione 557
Levlen/Tri-Levlen 665
Trinalin Repetabs Tablets 1170
Tri-Norinyl 2304
Triphasil-21 Tablets (Occasional) 2527
Triphasil-28 Tablets 2532
Tylenol with Codeine 1381
Urecholine 1558
▲ Vascor (200, 300 and 400 mg) Tablets (3.02%) 1383
Vaseretic Tablets (0.5% to 2.0%) 1559
Vasotec I.V. 1562
Vasotec Tablets (0.5% to 1%) 1564
Velban Vials 1305
VePesid Capsules and Injection (Infrequent) 741
Vermox Chewable Tablets 1149
Vivactil Tablets 1567
▲ Voltaren Tablets (3% to 9%) 1042
Wygesic Tablets 2540
Yodoxin 1072
Zantac Injection and Zantac Injection Premixed 1063
Zantac 1065
Zarontin Capsules (Frequent) 1768
Zarontin Syrup (Frequent) 1769
Zaroxolyn Tablets (Less than 2%) 989
Zestoretic (0.3 to 1.0%) 2274
Zestril Tablets (Less than 1%) 2277
Zinacef 1066
Zovirax Sterile Powder (Less than 1%) 828
Zyloprim Tablets (Less than 1%) 830

Abortion
Amen 833
Methotrexate Tablets, Parenteral, LPF Parenteral 1217
Metrodin (urofollitropin for injection) (3 reported) 2182
Nicorette 1335
Permax Tablets (Infrequent) 1291
Prozac Pulvules (Rare) 920
Rheumatrex Methotrexate Dose Pack 1234

Abortion, septic
Lippes Loop Intrauterine Double-S 1654
ParaGard T380A Intrauterine Copper Contraceptive 411

Abortion, spontaneous
Accutane Capsules 1878
Demulen 2161
Depo-Provera Sterile Aqueous Suspension 2336
Enovid 2161
Lippes Loop Intrauterine Double-S 1654
Lupron Depot 7.5 mg 2311
ParaGard T380A Intrauterine Copper Contraceptive 411
▲ Parlodel (11%) 2020
Syntocinon Injection 2032
Vermox Chewable Tablets 1149

Abscess
Aramine Injection 1424
Aristocort Suspension 1008
Aristospan Suspension 1011
BAL in Oil Ampules (Occasional) 661
Capastat Sulfate Vials 1250
Celestone Soluspan Suspension 2081
Cortone Acetate Sterile Suspension 1437
Cytosar-U Sterile Powder 2329
Dalalone D.P. Injectable 999
Decadron Phosphate Injection 1449
Decadron Phosphate with Xylocaine Injection, Sterile 1451
Decadron-LA Sterile Suspension 1457
Deltasone Tablets 2332
Depo-Medrol Sterile Aqueous Suspension 2334
Depo-Provera Sterile Aqueous Suspension 2336
Sterile FUDR 1898
Gelfoam Sterile Sponge 2338
Hydeltrasol Injection, Sterile 1476
Hydeltra-T.B.A. Sterile Suspension 1478
Hydrocortone Acetate Sterile Suspension 1479
Hydrocortone Phosphate Injection, Sterile 1481
Imferon 976
Intron A (Less than 1%) 2097
Kenalog-10 Injection 2402
Kenalog-40 Injection 2403
Omnipaque (0.1%) 2552
ParaGard T380A Intrauterine Copper Contraceptive 411
Pentam 300 Injection 1018
Permax Tablets (Infrequent) 1291
Plague Vaccine (Rare) 1584
▲ Sandimmune (4.4 to 5.3%) 2024
Solu-Cortef Sterile Powder 2361
Solu-Medrol Sterile Powder 2363

Abscess, periesophageal
Ethamolin (0.1% to 0.4%) 1829

Abscess, periodontal
Ansaid Tablets (Less than 1%) 2319
NebuPent for Inhalation Solution (1% or less) 1017
Permax Tablets (Infrequent) 1291

Abscess, tubo-ovarian
ParaGard T380A Intrauterine Copper Contraceptive 411

Abuse
Astramorph/PF Injection, USP (Preservative-Free) 618
Fiorinal with Codeine Capsules 2008
Miltown Tablets 2386

Accommodation, impaired
AK-Cide Sterile Ophthalmic Ointment & Suspension (Occasional) ⊙ 202
Anafranil Capsules (Infrequent) 650
Aralen Hydrochloride Injection 2038
Aralen Phosphate with Primaquine Phosphate Tablets (Occasional) 2040
Aralen Phosphate Tablets 2039
Arfonad Ampuls 1887
Asendin Tablets (Less than 1%) 1196
Atrovent Inhalation Aerosol (About 1 in 100) 675
Elavil 2269
Endep Tablets 1927
Equagesic Tablets 2451
Etrafon 2087
Limbitrol 1933
Ludiomil Tablets (Rare) 874
Metimyd ⊙ 306
Micronase Tablets 2350
Norpramin Tablets 1340
PMB 200 and PMB 400 2504
Pamelor 2019
Plaquenil Sulfate Tablets 2067
Protopam Chloride for Injection 2518
Surmontil Capsules 2524
Tofranil Ampuls 1038
Tofranil Tablets 1039
Tofranil-PM Capsules 1041
Transderm Scōp Transdermal Therapeutic System 887
Triavil Tablets 1556
Urispas Tablets 2242
Vasocidin Ointment (Occasional) ⊙ 275
Vasocidin Ophthalmic Solution (Occasional) ⊙ 276

Vivactil Tablets 1567
Zantac Injection and Zantac Injection Premixed (Rare) 1063
Zantac (Rare) 1065

Accommodation, paresis
Diphtheria and Tetanus Toxoids and Pertussis Vaccine Adsorbed USP (For Pediatric Use) 892

Accommodation, spasm
Pilagan ⊙ 250
Tensilon Injectable 1123

Aches
Atgam Sterile Solution (At least 1 patient and less than 5% of total patients) 2320
Cartrol Tablets 507
Cipro I.V. (1% or less) 1592
Cipro Tablets (Less than 1%) 1589
Corgard Tablets 701
Corzide Tablets 702
Cytotec (Infrequent) 2159
Eldepryl (1 of 49 patients) 2250
Humorsol Sterile Ophthalmic Solution 1475
Hydropres Tablets 1485
Inderal 2459
Inderal LA Long Acting Capsules 2461
Inderide Tablets 2463
Inderide LA Long Acting Capsules 2465
Kerlone Tablets 2172
Koro-Flex Arcing Spring Diaphragm 2142
Koromex Coil Spring Diaphragm 2142
Levatol 1832
Lysodren (Infrequent) 731
Methadone Hydrochloride Diskets 1284
Midamor Tablets (Less than or equal to 1%) 1508
Normodyne Tablets 2110
Normozide Tablets 2112
Pergonal (menotropins for injection, USP) 2184
Recombivax HB (Less than 1%) 1544
Rogaine Topical Solution (2.59%) 2357
Sectral Capsules 2520
Tenoretic Tablets 1105
Tenormin Tablets and I.V. Injection 1107
Teslac Tablets 741
Timoptic in Ocudose 1552
Timoptic Sterile Ophthalmic Solution 1550
Trandate HCT/Trandate 579
Trexan Tablets (Less than 1%) 937
Trilafon 2123
Visken Tablets 2036
Wytensin Tablets (3% or less) 2542

Aches, joints (see under Arthralgia)

Acidosis
Children's Advil Suspension (Less than 1%) 2426
Cipro I.V. (1% or less) 1592
Cipro Tablets (Less than 1%) 1589
Dyazide Capsules 2208
IFEX (Rare) 729
Indocin I.V. (Less than 3%) 1490
Kerlone Tablets (Less than 2%) 2172
Minocin Oral Suspension 1224
Motrin Tablets (Less than 1%) 2351
PediaProfen Suspension (Less than 1%) 1363
Permax Tablets (Rare) 1291
Proglycem (Infrequent) 649
Rufen Tablets (Less than 1%) 691
Terramycin Capsules 1786

Acidosis, hypochloremic metabolic
Sandimmune (Occasional) 2024

Acidosis, metabolic
Butazolidin Capsules & Tablets (Less than 1%) 1027
Corzide Tablets 702
Daranide Tablets 1445
Diamox Parenteral (Occasional) 1200
Diamox Sequels (Sustained Release) 1201
Diamox Tablets (Occasional) 1200
INH Tablets 868
▲IFEX (31%) 729
Nardil (Less frequent) 1742
Naturetin Tablets (Occasional) 1789
NegGram (Rare) 2062
Rauzide Tablets (Occasional) 1804
Rifamate Capsules 1347
Sensorcaine 631
Sensorcaine-MPF Spinal 634
VePesid Capsules and Injection 741

Acidosis, renal tubular
Fungizone Intravenous (Common) 2262
IFEX (1 episode) 729
Zanosar Sterile Powder 2371

Acne (see under Acneiform eruptions)

Acne, adolescent, flare-up of
Theo-Organidin Elixir 2391
Tussi-Organidin DM Liquid 2392
Tussi-Organidin Liquid 2391

Acneiform eruptions
Aclovate Cream 1053
AeroBid Inhaler System (1-3%) 995
Alphatrex Cream, Ointment & Lotion (Infrequent) 2076
Amen (Few cases) 833
Anadrol-50 Tablets 2287
Anafranil Capsules (Up to 2%) 650
Analpram-HC Rectal Cream 1% and 2.5% 970
Android 1111
Antabuse Tablets (Small number of patients) 2429
Anusol-HC Cream (Infrequent) 1690
Aristocort A (Infrequent) 1010
Betatrex Cream, Ointment & Lotion 2077
Brevicon 2304
BuSpar (Rare) 1401
Carmol HC Cream 1% (Infrequent) 2296
Cortifoam 1827
Cortisporin Cream 757
Cortisporin Ointment 758
Cortisporin Otic Solution Sterile 760
Cortisporin Otic Suspension Sterile 760
Cosmegen Injection 1440
Cutivate Cream 0.05% 1054
Cutivate Ointment 0.005% (Infrequent to more frequent) 1054
Cyclocort Lotion (Infrequent) 1198
Cycrin Tablets (A few cases) 2449
Danocrine Capsules 2046
Dantrium Capsules (Less frequent) 1619
Decadron Phosphate Topical Cream 1455
Decaspray Topical Aerosol 1459
Depo-Provera Sterile Aqueous Suspension (Few cases) 2336
DesOwen Cream, Ointment and Lotion (Infrequent) 1682
Diprolene (Infrequent) 2083
Eldecort Cream 1.0% (Infrequent) 1113
Eldecort Cream 1.0% and 2.5% (Infrequent) 1113
Elocon (Infrequent) 2084
Eskalith 2214
Estratest 2245
Florone/Florone E 908
Halog (Infrequent) 2399
Halotestin Tablets 2341
Hytone 909
Intron A (1% or less) 2097
Jenest-28 Tablets 1636
Kenalog Cream, Lotion & Ointment (Infrequent) 2401
Kenalog-10 Injection 2402
Kenalog-40 Injection 2403
Lamprene Capsules (Less than 1%) 1030
Levlen/Tri-Levlen 665
Lidex (Infrequent) 2296
Loestrin 1728
Lotrisone Cream (Infrequent) 2103
Mantadil Cream 789
Maxivate Cream, Lotion & Ointment 0.05% 2406
Metandren Linguets and Tablets 875
Methotrexate Tablets, Parenteral, LPF Parenteral 1217
Micronor Tablets 1667
Modicon 1667
Mycolog II Cream and Ointment (1%) 2407
Mytrex Cream & Ointment (Single case) 2080
NeoDecadron Topical Cream 1518
Neo-Synalar Cream (Infrequent) 2296
Nimotop Capsules (Up to 1.4%) 1607
Norinyl 2304
Norlestrin 1746
Norplant System 2484
Nor-Q D Tablets 2304
Ortho-Cyclen Tablets 1658
Ortho-Novum 1667
Paradione Capsules 548
PediOtic Suspension Sterile 797
Pentaspan Injection 949
Pepcid (Infrequent) 1524
Permax Tablets (Infrequent) 1291
Pramosone Cream, Lotion & Ointment 971
Premarin with Methyltestosterone 2515
ProctoCream-HC (Infrequent) 1834
Proctofoam-HC 1835
ProSom Tablets (Rare) 554
Provera Tablets (A few cases) 2356
Prozac Pulvules (Infrequent) 920
Psorcon Ointment 0.05% 909
Psorion Cream 0.05% (Infrequent) 1121
Retrovir Capsules (Less than 5%) 802
Retrovir I.V. Infusion (Less than 5%) 805
Retrovir Syrup (Less than 5%) 802
Rheumatrex Methotrexate Dose Pack 1234
Rowasa 2248
▲Sandimmune (1 to 8%) 2024
Synacort Creams 1%, 2.5% (Infrequent) 2296
Synalar (Infrequent) 2296
▲Synarel Nasal Solution (13% of patients) 2300
Synemol Cream 0.025% (Infrequent) 2296
Temovate 1056
Testred Capsules 1124
Topicort (Infrequent) 1098
Trexan Tablets (Less than 1%) 937
Tridesilon Creme 0.05% 1611
Tridesilon Ointment 0.05% 1611
Tridione 557
Levlen/Tri-Levlen 665
Tri-Norinyl 2304
Ultravate Cream 0.05% (Infrequent) 2410
Ultravate Ointment 0.05% (Less frequent) 2411
Vanoxide-HC Acne Lotion 911
Vioform-Hydrocortisone Cream and Mild Cream 889
Vioform-Hydrocortisone Ointment 889
Vytone Cream 1% 911
Wellbutrin Tablets (Rare) 821
Westcort 2411
Winstrol Tablets 2075
Yodoxin 1072

Acneiform reactions
Elocon Lotion 0.1% (2 in 209 patients) 2084
Haldol Decanoate 1375
Haldol Injection, Tablets and Concentrate 1373

Adams-Stokes syndrome
Isuprel Hydrochloride Injection 1:5000 2050

Adenitis
Asendin Tablets 1196
Clinoril Tablets 1433
Dolobid Tablets (Less than 1 in 100) 1465
Ludiomil Tablets 874
Norpramin Tablets (Rare) 1340
Pamelor (Rare) 2019
Pneumovax 23 (Rare) 1528
Pnu-Imune 23 Pneumococcal Vaccine Polyvalent (Rare) 1233
Surmontil Capsules 2524
Tofranil Ampuls 1038
Tofranil Tablets 1039
Tofranil-PM Capsules 1041
Vivactil Tablets (Rare) 1567

Adenomas, benign
Demulen 2161
Enovid 2161
Norethin 2133

Adenomas, endocrine system
Permax Tablets (Infrequent) 1291

Adenopathy
Deprol Tablets 2382
Equagesic Tablets 2451
Miltown Tablets 2386
PMB 200 and PMB 400 2504
Tegretol Chewable Tablets 654
Tegretol Suspension 656
Tegretol Tablets 654
Tetanus Toxoid, Adsorbed Purogenated 1238

Adenopathy, inguinal
Zovirax (0.3%) 824

Adhesion
Hemopad Absorbable Collagen Hemostat 627
INSTAT Collagen Absorbable Hemostat 1151
Lippes Loop Intrauterine Double-S 1654

Adnexal enlargement
Norplant System 2484

Adrenal insufficiency
Beclovent Inhalation Aerosol and Refill 572
Beconase AQ Nasal Spray 574
Beconase Inhalation Aerosol & Refill 574
Cortifoam 1827
Dicumarol Tablets 516
Heparin Lock Flush Solution 2456
Heparin Sodium Vials 1264
Heparin Sodium Injection 2457
Heparin Sodium Injection, USP, Sterile Solution 2342
Motrin Tablets 2351
Panwarfin Tablets 547

Adrenocortical suppression
Depo-Medrol Sterile Aqueous Suspension 2334
Kenalog in Orabase 604
Medrol 2348
Nasacort Nasal Inhaler 1844
Solu-Cortef Sterile Powder 2361
Solu-Medrol Sterile Powder 2363

Adrenocortical unresponsiveness, secondary
Aristospan Suspension (Intra-articular) 1011
Celestone Soluspan Suspension 2081
Cortenema 2244
Cortone Acetate Sterile Suspension 1437
Cortone Acetate Tablets 1439
Decadron Elixir 1445
Decadron Phosphate Injection 1449
Decadron Phosphate Respihaler 1454
Decadron Phosphate Turbinaire 1456
Decadron Phosphate with Xylocaine Injection, Sterile 1451
Decadron Tablets 1447
Decadron-LA Sterile Suspension 1457
Deltasone Tablets 2332
Hydeltrasol Injection, Sterile 1476
Hydeltra-T.B.A. Sterile Suspension 1478
Hydrocortone Acetate Sterile Suspension 1479
Hydrocortone Phosphate Injection, Sterile 1481
Hydrocortone Tablets 1482
Kenalog-10 Injection 2402
Kenalog-40 Injection 2403

Afibrinogenemia
Oxytocin Injection 2492
Pitocin Injection, Ampoules, Steri-Dose Syringes 1757
Syntocinon Injection 2032

Aftertaste
Antabuse Tablets (Small number of patients) 2429
Placidyl Capsules 553
VePesid Capsules and Injection (Infrequent) 741

Ageusia
▲AeroBid Inhaler System (3-9%) 995
Anafranil Capsules (Infrequent) 650
Bentyl 1322
Cantil Tablets 1326
Capoten (Approximately 2 to 4 of 100 patients) 2255
Capozide (Approximately 2 to 4 of 100 patients) 2258
Clinoril Tablets (Less than 1 in 100) 1433
Darbid Tablets 2205
▲Depen Titratable Tablets (12%) 2379
▲Didronel I.V. Infusion (5%) 1307
Donnatal 1858
Donnatal Extentabs 1859
Donnatal Tablets 1858
Donnazyme Tablets 1860
Elavil 2269
Flexeril Tablets (Less than 1%) 1471
Intron A (1 patient) 2097
Kerlone Tablets (Less than 2%) 2172

Kinesed Tablets 2272
Levsin/Levsinex 2147
Lorelco Tablets 1333
Nasalide Nasal Solution 0.025% (5% or less) 2299
NebuPent for Inhalation Solution (1% or less) 1017
Nolvadex Tablets (Infrequent) 1102
Platinol 737
Platinol-AQ Injection 738
Pro-Banthīne Tablets 2141
Proglycem (Frequent) 649
Prozac Pulvules (Rare) 920
Robinul Forte Tablets 1873
Robinul Injectable 1873
Robinul Tablets 1873
Tapazole Tablets 1298
Valpin 50 Tablets 941
Zyloprim Tablets (Less than 1%) 830

Aggression

A.P.L. 2431
Anafranil Capsules (Up to 2%) 650
Celontin 1692
Depakene Capsules & Syrup 511
Depakote 512
Halcion Tablets 2340
Intron A (1% or less) 2097
Prilosec Delayed-Release Capsules (Less than 1%) 1530
Seromycin Pulvules 1298
Ventolin (1%) 583
Zarontin Capsules 1768
Zarontin Syrup 1769

Agitation

Akineton 1171
Alurate Elixir (Less than 1 in 100) 1883
Amoxil (Rare) 2193
Anafranil Capsules (Up to 3%) 650
Artane 1195
Atgam Sterile Solution (At least 1 patient and less than 5% of total patients) 2320
Ativan Tablets (Less frequent) 2434
Augmentin Tablets, Powder for Oral Suspension, and Chewable Tablets (Rare) 2198
Bontril Slow-Release 834
Brevibloc Injection (2%) 942
Butazolidin Capsules & Tablets (Less than 1%) 1027
Butisol Sodium Elixir & Tablets (Less than 1 in 100) 2377
Cardura Tablets (0.5% to 1%) 1941
Catapres Tablets (About 3 in 100 patients) 676
▲ Catapres-TTS (3%) 677
▲ Clozaril Tablets (4%) 2000
Combipres Tablets (About 3%) 678
Compazine 2201
Demerol 2047
Desyrel and Desyrel Dividose 1404
Dexedrine 2206
Dilaudid-HP Injection 1175
Dilor 2079
Diprivan Injection (Less than 1%) 2267
Dolophine Hydrochloride Ampoules & Vials 1260
Dolophine Hydrochloride Tablets 1261
Donnatal (In elderly patients) 1858
Donnatal Extentabs (In elderly patients) 1859
Donnatal Tablets (In elderly patients) 1858
Donnazyme Tablets (In elderly patients) 1860
Doral Tablets 2383
Duragesic Transdermal System (1% or greater) 1133
Eldepryl 2250
Elspar 1470
▲ Eminase (Less than 10%) 2211
Engerix-B Unit-Dose Vials (Less than 1%) 2213
Ethmozine Tablets (Less than 2%) 946
Fiorinal with Codeine Capsules (Infrequent) 2008
Flexeril Tablets (Less than 1%) 1471
Halcion Tablets 2340
Haldol Decanoate 1375
Haldol Injection, Tablets and Concentrate 1373
Intron A (Up to 1%) 2097
Keflex Pulvules, Oral Suspension & Pediatric Drops 916
Keftab Tablets 917
Kinesed Tablets 2272
Larodopa Tablets (Relatively frequent) 1905
Leukeran Tablets (Rare) 788
Loxitane 1213
▲ Lozol Tablets (Greater than or equal to 5%) 1843
Ludiomil Tablets (2%) 874
Lufyllin & Lufyllin-400 Tablets 2384
Lufyllin-GG Elixir & Tablets 2385
MS Contin Tablets (Infrequent) 1814
MSIR (Infrequent) 1817
Mebaral Tablets (Less than 1 in 100) 2061
Mellaril 2011
Mepergan Injection 2479
Methadone Hydrochloride Diskets 1284
Methadone Hydrochloride Oral Solution & Tablets 1987
Nardil (Uncommon) 1742
Navane Capsules and Concentrate 1954
Navane Intramuscular 1956
Nembutal Sodium Capsules (Less than 1%) 534
Nembutal Sodium Solution (Less than 1%) 536
Nembutal Sodium Suppositories (Less than 1%) 538
Norflex 1314
Norgesic 1314
Norpramin Tablets 1340
Norzine 1818
Omnipaque (Occasional) 2552
Oramorph SR (Morphine Sulfate Sustained Release Tablets) (Less frequent) 1988
Pamelor 2019
Pantopon Injectable 1911
Parnate Tablets 2222
Pepcid (Infrequent) 1524
Permax Tablets (Infrequent) 1291
Pfizerpen-AS Aqueous Suspension (Approximately 1 in 500) 1959
Phenobarbital Elixir and Tablets (Less than 1 in 100 patients) 1293
Plegine Tablets 2504
Pondimin Tablets 1867
ProSom Tablets (Infrequent) 554
Prozac Pulvules (Frequent) 920
Reglan 1869
Roxanol 1991
Seconal Sodium Pulvules (Less than 1 in 100) 1296
Serentil 686
Sinemet Tablets 952
Sinemet CR Tablets 953
Soma Compound w/Codeine Tablets (Infrequent or rare) 2390
Soma Compound Tablets (Infrequent or rare) 2389
Soma Tablets 2388
Stadol (Less than 1%) 721
Stelazine 2226
Surmontil Capsules 2524
Tagamet 2228
Taractan 1920
Tegretol Chewable Tablets 654
Tegretol Suspension 656
Tegretol Tablets 654
Tenex Tablets 1875
Thorazine 2234
Tofranil Ampuls 1038
Tofranil Tablets 1039
Tofranil-PM Capsules 1041
Tonocard Tablets (Less than 1%) 1554
Torecan 1993
Trental 1099
Ventolin (1%) 583
Versed Injection (Less than 1%) 1924
Vivactil Tablets 1567
▲ Wellbutrin Tablets (31.9%) 821
Xanax Tablets (2.9%) 2367
Zantac Injection and Zantac Injection Premixed 1063
Zantac (Rare) 1065
Zovirax Sterile Powder 828

Agranulocytopenia

Sterile FUDR (Remote possibility) 1898
INH Tablets 868
Rauzide Tablets 1804

Agranulocytosis

Actifed with Codeine Cough Syrup 752
Aldactazide (A few cases) 2150
Aldactone (A few cases) 2152
Aldoclor Tablets 1413
Aldoril Tablets 1418
Altace Capsules (Rare to more frequent) 1086
Amoxil 2193
Anaprox and Anaprox DS Tablets (Less than 1%) 2288
Ancobon Capsules 1886
Anturane (Rare) 853
Apresazide Capsules (Less frequent) 854
Apresoline Hydrochloride Parenteral (Ampuls) 856
Apresoline Hydrochloride Tablets (Less frequent) 855
Apresoline-Esidrix Tablets 857
Asendin Tablets (Less than 1%) 1196
Atromid-S Capsules 2435
Augmentin Tablets, Powder for Oral Suspension, and Chewable Tablets 2198
Azo Gantanol Tablets 1887
Azo Gantrisin Tablets 1888
Azulfidine Tablets, EN-tabs, Oral Suspension (Rare) 1157
Bactrim DS Tablets (Rare) 1891
Bactrim I.V. Infusion (Rare) 1889
Bactrim (Rare) 1891
Benadryl Capsules 1691
Benadryl Injection 1692
Blocadren Tablets 1429
Butazolidin Capsules & Tablets (Less than 1%) 1027
Capoten 2255
Capozide 2258
Cardioquin Tablets 1812
Cartrol Tablets 507
Cefotan 2265
Ceftin Tablets 575
Ceptaz for Injection (Very rare) 1057
Children's Advil Suspension (Less than 1%) 2426
Cipro I.V. 1592
Cipro Tablets 1589
Claforan Sterile Injection (Less than 1%) 1089
Cleocin HCl Capsules 2322
Cleocin Pediatric Flavored Granules 2324
Cleocin Phosphate Injection 2325
Clinoril Tablets (Less than 1%) 1433
Clozaril Tablets (1%) 2000
ColBENEMID Tablets 1436
Colchicine Ampoules 1252
Combipres Tablets 678
Comhist LA Capsules 1618
Compazine 2201
Corgard Tablets 701
Corzide Tablets 702
Cosmegen Injection 1440
Cuprimine Capsules 1442
▲ Cytadren Tablets (4 out of 27) 861
Dapsone USP 1130
Daranide Tablets 1445
Deconamine 663
Depen Titratable Tablets 2379
Deprol Tablets (Rare) 2382
DiaBeta 1091
Diabinese Tablets 1775
Diamox Parenteral 1200
Diamox Sequels (Sustained Release) 1201
Diamox Tablets 1200
Dilantin Infatabs (Occasional) 1710
Dilantin Kapseals (Occasional) 1708
Dilantin Parenteral (Occasional) 1712
Dilantin-30 Pediatric/Dilantin-125 Suspension (Occasional) 1713
Dilantin with Phenobarbital Kapseals (Occasional) 1715
Dimetane-DC Cough Syrup 1857
Dimetane-DX Cough Syrup 1858
Diucardin Tablets 2450
Diulo 2129
Diupres Tablets 1461
Diuril Oral Suspension 1464
Diuril Sodium Intravenous 1463
Diuril Tablets 1464
Dolobid Tablets (Less than 1 in 100) 1465
Dyazide Capsules 2208
Edecrin 1468
Elavil 2269
Endep Tablets 1927
Enduron Tablets 517
Enduronyl 518
Equagesic Tablets 2451
Ergamisol Tablets (One patient) 1136
Esidrix Tablets 863
Esimil Tablets 864
Etrafon 2087
Exna Tablets 1862
FML-S Sterile Ophthalmic Suspension ⊙ 246
Fansidar Tablets 1896
Floxin Tablets 1652
Fluorouracil Injection 1897
Fortaz (Very rare) 1060
Fungizone Intravenous 2262
Gantanol 1899
Gantrisin Ophthalmic Ointment/Solution 1900
Gantrisin 1901
Garamycin Injectable 2093
Glucotrol 1952
Haldol Decanoate (Rare) 1375
Haldol Injection, Tablets and Concentrate 1373
HydroDIURIL Tablets 1484
Hydromox R Tablets 1209
Hydromox Tablets 1208
Hydropres Tablets 1485
INH Tablets 868
Inderal 2459
Inderal LA Long Acting Capsules 2461
Inderide Tablets 2463
Inderide LA Long Acting Capsules 2465
Indocin Capsules (Less than 1%) 1487
Indocin I.V. (Less than 1%) 1490
Indocin (Less than 1%) 1487
Kefurox Vials, Faspak & ADD-Vantage 1277
Kerlone Tablets 2172
Larodopa Tablets (Rare) 1905
Lasix (Rare) 1093
Levatol 1832
Librax Capsules (Occasional) 1929
Libritabs Tablets (Occasional) 1930
Librium Capsules (Occasional) 1931
Librium Injectable (Occasional) 1932
Limbitrol 1933
Lincocin 2344
Lopressor Ampuls (Rare) 1032
Lopressor HCT Tablets 1034
Lopressor Tablets (Rare) 1032
Lotensin Tablets (Rare) 872
Loxitane (Rare) 1213
Lozol Tablets 1843
Ludiomil Tablets 874
Macrodantin Capsules 1624
Maxzide 1215
Meclomen Capsules (Less than 1%) 1739
Mellaril 2011
Menrium Tablets (Occasional) 1934
Mepergan Injection (1 instance) 2479
Mesantoin Tablets 2013
Mexitil Capsules (About 1 in 1,000) 680
Micronase Tablets 2350
Miltown Tablets 2386
Minizide Capsules 1779
Moduretic Tablets 1510
Monopril Tablets (0.2 to 1.0%) 1406
Motrin Tablets (Less than 1%) 2351
Mustargen (Relatively infrequent) 1514
Mykrox ½ mg Tablets 984
Nalfon Pulvules & Tablets (Less than 1%) 919
Naprosyn (Less than 1%) 2297
Naturetin Tablets 1789
Navane Capsules and Concentrate 1954
Navane Intramuscular 1956
Neptazane Tablets ⊙ 311
Normodyne Tablets 2110
Normozide Tablets 2112
Norpace (Rare) 2177
Norpramin Tablets 1340
Norzine 1818
Optimine Tablets 2115
Oretic Tablets 544
Oreticyl 545
Orinase Tablets 2354
Ornade Spansule Capsules 2221
Orudis Capsules (Less than 1%) 2488
PBZ Tablets & Elixir 1037
PBZ-SR Tablets 1037
PMB 200 and PMB 400 2504
Pamelor 2019
Paradione Capsules 548
Parnate Tablets 2222
PediaProfen Suspension (Less than 1%) 1363
Pediazole 1973
Pepcid (Rare) 1524
Periactin 1525
Phenergan with Codeine (1 case) 2497
Phenergan with Dextromethorphan (1 case) 2499
Phenergan Injection 2493
Phenergan Suppositories (1 case) 2496
Phenergan Syrup (1 case) 2495
Phenergan Tablets (1 case) 2496
Phenergan VC (1 case) 2500
Phenergan VC with Codeine (1 case) 2501
Plaquenil Sulfate Tablets 2067
Polaramine 2116
Ponstel (Occasional) 1758
Prilosec Delayed-Release Capsules (One case) 1530

Primaxin I.M. 1532
Primaxin I.V. (Less than 0.2%) 1535
Prinzide Tablets (Rare) 1540
Procan SR Tablets 1760
Prolixin Decanoate 1795
Prolixin Elixir 1793
Prolixin Enanthate 1796
Prolixin Injection 1791
Prolixin Oral Concentrate 1792
Prolixin Tablets 1793
Pronestyl Capsules and Tablets (Approximately 0.5%) 1800
Pronestyl Injection (Approximately 0.5%) 1798
Pronestyl-SR Tablets (0.5%) 1801
ProSom Tablets (Rare) 554
Quinaglute Dura-Tabs Tablets 663
Quinamm Tablets 1344
Quinidex Extentabs 1868
Rauzide Tablets 1804
Reglan (A few cases) 1869
Renese Tablets 1785
Renese-R Tablets 1786
Ridaura Capsules (Less than 0.1%) 2224
Rifamate Capsules 1347
Rufen Tablets (Less than 1%) 691
Ru-Tuss II Capsules 693
Ru-Tuss Tablets 693
Rythmol Tablets (Less than 1%) 1184
SSD RP Cream 690
Saluron 718
Salutensin/Salutensin-Demi 719
Sectral Capsules 2520
Septra 813
Septra I.V. Infusion 808
Septra I.V. Infusion ADD-Vantage Vials (Rare) 810
Septra 813
Ser-Ap-Es Tablets 881
Serax Capsules 2522
Serax Tablets 2522
Serentil 686
Serpasil-Apresoline Tablets 884
Serpasil-Esidrix Tablets 886
Silvadene Cream 1% 1352
Sinemet Tablets (Rare) 952
Sinemet CR Tablets 953
Sinequan (Occasional) 1960
Solganal Suspension (Rare) 2122
Spectrobid Tablets & Powder for Oral Suspension 1961
Stelazine 2226
Sultrin (One case) 1675
Surmontil Capsules 2524
Tacaryl 2409
Tagamet (Approximately 3 per 1,000,000) 2228
Talacen (Rare) 2070
Tapazole Tablets 1298
Taractan (Very rare) 1920
Tavist Syrup 2033
Tavist Tablets 2035
Tavist-D Tablets 2035
Tegretol Chewable Tablets (Very low incidence) 654
Tegretol Suspension (Very low incidence) 656
Tegretol Tablets (Very low incidence) 654
Temaril Tablets, Syrup and Spansule Sustained Release Capsules 1085
Tenoretic Tablets 1105
Tenormin Tablets and I.V. Injection 1107
Tenuate 1354
Thalitone Tablets 687
Thiosulfil Forte Tablets 2526
Thorazine 2234
Timolide Tablets 1547
Timoptic in Ocudose 1552
Timoptic Sterile Ophthalmic Solution 1550
Tofranil Ampuls 1038
Tofranil Tablets 1039
Tofranil-PM Capsules 1041
Tolectin (200, 400 and 600 mg) (Less than 1%) 1379
Tolinase Tablets 2365
Tonocard Tablets (Less than 1%) 1554
Torecan 1993
Trandate HCT/Trandate 579
Triaminic Expectorant DH 1995
Triaminic Oral Infant Drops 1996
Triavil Tablets 1556
Tridione 557
Trilafon 2123
Trinalin Repetabs Tablets 1170
Unasyn 1965
Urobiotic-250 Capsules 1968
Vascor (200, 300 and 400 mg) Tablets 1383
Vaseretic Tablets 1559
Visken Tablets 2036
Vivactil Tablets 1567
Voltaren Tablets (Rare) 1042
Zantac Injection and Zantac Injection Premixed (Rare) 1063
Zantac (Rare) 1065
Zarontin Capsules 1768
Zarontin Syrup 1769
Zaroxolyn Tablets 989
Zefazone Sterile Powder 2372
Zestoretic (Rare) 2274
Zestril Tablets (Rare) 2277
Zinacef 1066
Zyloprim Tablets (Less than 1%) 830

Airway obstruction

Ativan Injection (5 patients) 2432
Capoten 2255
Capozide 2258
Diprivan Injection (Less than 1%) 2267
Fiorinal with Codeine Capsules 2008
Versed Injection (Less than 1%) 1924

Airway resistance

Demerol 2047
Versed Injection (Less than 1%) 1924

Akathisia

BuSpar 1401
▲ Clozaril Tablets (3%) 2000
Compazine 2201
Desyrel and Desyrel Dividose 1404
Ethmozine Tablets (Less than 2%) 946
Etrafon 2087
Feldene Capsules (Less than 1%) 1777
Haldol Decanoate (Less frequent) 1375
Haldol Injection, Tablets and Concentrate 1373
Inapsine Injection 1140
Innovar Injection 1141
Loxitane 1213
Ludiomil Tablets (Rare) 874
Marplan Tablets (Rare) 1906
Mellaril 2011
Moban Tablets & Concentrate 932
Navane Capsules and Concentrate 1954
Navane Intramuscular 1956
Norzine 1818
Orap Tablets (Less frequent) 1020
Permax Tablets (1.6%) 1291
Prolixin Decanoate 1795
Prolixin Elixir 1793
Prolixin Enanthate 1796
Prolixin Injection 1791
▲ Prolixin Oral Concentrate (Among most frequent) 1792
Prolixin Tablets 1793
Prozac Pulvules (Infrequent) 920
Reglan 1869
Serentil 686
Stelazine 2226
Sublimaze Injection 1146
Taractan (Common) 1920
Temaril Tablets, Syrup and Spansule Sustained Release Capsules 1085
Torecan 1993
Triavil Tablets 1556
Trilafon 2123
Vascor (200, 300 and 400 mg) Tablets (0.5 to 2.0%) 1383
Wellbutrin Tablets (1.5%) 821
Xanax Tablets (1.6% to 3.0%) 2367
Zofran Injection 1069

Akinesia

Cardura Tablets (1%) 1941
▲ Clozaril Tablets (4%) 2000
Loxitane 1213
Mellaril 2011
Moban Tablets & Concentrate 932
Norzine 1818
Orap Tablets 1020
Permax Tablets (1.1%) 1291
Serentil 686
Torecan 1993
▲ Wellbutrin Tablets (8.0%) 821

Albuminuria

Amikin Injectable 602
Anafranil Capsules (Rare) 650
Asbron G 1997
Calcijex Calcitriol Injection 506
Calderol Capsules 1635
Choledyl SA Tablets 1704
Cibalith-S 870
Cipro I.V. (1% or less) 1592
Cipro Tablets 1589
Constant-T Tablets 1029
Dapsone USP 1130
Dilor 2079
Dopram Injectable 1860
Eskalith 2214
Floxin Tablets (More than or equal to 1.0%) 1652
Lamprene Capsules (Less than 1%) 1030
Lithane Tablets 1596
Lithium Carbonate Capsules & Tablets 1984
Lithobid Tablets 870
Lufyllin & Lufyllin-400 Tablets 2384
Lufyllin-GG Elixir & Tablets 2385
Lysodren (Infrequent) 731
Paradione Capsules 548
Polymyxin B Sulfate, Aerosporin Brand Sterile Powder 798
Proglycem 649
Prozac Pulvules (Rare) 920
Quadrinal Tablets 1183
Quibron-T/SR 716
Rocaltrol Capsules 1913
Solganal Suspension 2122
T-PHYL (Uniphyl) 200 mg Tablets 1820
Tegretol Chewable Tablets 654
Tegretol Suspension 656
Tegretol Tablets 654
Theo-Dur Sprinkle 1168
Tridione 557
Uniphyl 400 mg Tablets 1823
Xanax Tablets (Less than 1%) 2367
Zyloprim Tablets (Less than 1%) 830

Alcohol, increased sensitivity to

Ativan Injection 2432
Catapres Tablets 676
Catapres-TTS 677
Combipres Tablets 678
Nicotinex Elixir ▣ 563
Parlodel (Less than 1%) 2020

Aldosterone synthesis, suppression

Calciparine Injection 925
Heparin Lock Flush Solution 2456
Heparin Sodium Vials 1264
Heparin Sodium Injection 2457
Heparin Sodium Injection, USP, Sterile Solution 2342

Alice in Wonderland syndrome

Sansert Tablets 2031

Alkalosis

Anadrol-50 Tablets 2287
Ancef Injection 2194
Bicitra—Sugar-Free 2423
CeeNU (Small percentage) 725
Depen Titratable Tablets (Few) 2379
Glucotrol 1952
Kefurox Vials, Faspak & ADD-Vantage (1 in 50) 1277
Lioresal Tablets 1031
Netromycin Injection 100 mg/ml (15 of 1000 patients) 2104
Polycitra Syrup 2424
Polycitra-K 2424
Polycitra-LC—Sugar-Free 2424
▲ Tazidime Vials, Faspak & ADD-Vantage (1 in 23) 1299
Trobicin Sterile Powder 2366

Alkalosis, metabolic

Indocin I.V. (Less than 3%) 1490

Allergic contact dermatitis

Aclovate Cream 1053
AK-Taine ◉ 207
Alcaine ◉ 210
Analpram-HC Rectal Cream 1% and 2.5% 970
Anusol-HC Cream (Infrequent) 1690
Anusol-HC Suppositories 1691
Benzac 5 & 10 Gel 1682
Benzac AC 1681
Benzac 1682
5 Benzagel (5% benzoyl peroxide) & 10 Benzagel (10% benzoyl peroxide), Acne Gels, Microgel Formula 907
▲ Catapres-TTS (19 in 100) 677
Cerumenex Drops 1813
Cortisporin Cream 757
Cortisporin Ointment 758
Cortisporin Otic Solution Sterile 760
Cortisporin Otic Suspension Sterile 760
Cutivate Cream 0.05% 1054
Cutivate Ointment 0.005% (Infrequent to more frequent) 1054
Cyclocort Lotion (Infrequent) 1198
Decadron Phosphate Topical Cream 1455
Decaspray Topical Aerosol 1459
DesOwen Cream, Ointment and Lotion (Infrequent) 1682
Diprolene (Infrequent) 2083
Efudex 1880
Eldecort Cream 1.0% (Infrequent) 1113
Eldecort Cream 1.0% and 2.5% (Infrequent) 1113
Elocon Lotion 0.1% 2084
Florone/Florone E 908
Fluoracaine ◉ 208
Fluoroplex Topical Solution & Cream 1% 1082
Fungizone Cream, Lotion and Ointment (Rare) 2261
Hytone 909
Locoid Cream, Ointment and Topical Solution (Infrequent) 970
Mantadil Cream 789
Monistat Dual-Pak 1657
NeoDecadron Topical Cream 1518
Nutracort Cream & Lotion (Infrequent) 1684
Ophthetic ◉ 249
Orabase HCA Oral Paste (Infrequent) 890
PediOtic Suspension Sterile 797
Pramosone Cream, Lotion & Ointment 971
Psorcon Ointment 0.05% 909
Psorion Cream 0.05% (Infrequent) 1121
Retin-A (tretinoin) Cream/Gel/Liquid (Rare) 1680
▲ Rogaine Topical Solution (7.36%) 2357
Synacort Creams 1%, 2.5% (Infrequent) 2296
Synalar (Infrequent) 2296
Temovate 1056
Topicort (Infrequent) 1098
Ultravate Cream 0.05% (Infrequent) 2410
Ultravate Ointment 0.05% (Less frequent) 2411
Vanoxide-HC Acne Lotion (Among most frequent) 911
Vioform-Hydrocortisone Cream and Mild Cream 889
Vioform-Hydrocortisone Ointment 889
Vytone Cream 1% 911
Westcort 2411

Allergic reactions

Abbokinase 503
Abbokinase Open-Cath 505
Adipex-P Tablets and Capsules 1019
Alka-Seltzer Plus Cold Medicine ▣ 623
Alka-Seltzer Plus Night-Time Cold Medicine ▣ 623
Alkeran Tablets 754
Americaine Hemorrhoidal Ointment ▣ 558
▲ Anafranil Capsules (3% to 7%) 650
Anaprox and Anaprox DS Tablets 2288
Anbesol 2417
▲ Anestacon Solution (Among most common) 2394
AquaMEPHYTON Injection 1422
Aquasol A Parenteral, USP (Rare) 615
Atromid-S Capsules 2435
Atropine Sulfate Sterile Ophthalmic Solution and S.O.P. Sterile Ophthalmic Ointment ◉ 239
Attenuvax (Rare) 1424
Augmentin Tablets, Powder for Oral Suspension, and Chewable Tablets 2198
Azdōne Tablets 844
Azo Gantrisin Tablets 1888
▲ Bactrim DS Tablets (Among most common) 1891
▲ Bactrim I.V. Infusion (Among most common) 1889
Bactrim (Among most common) 1891
Benemid Tablets 1426
Bentyl 1322
Berocca Plus Tablets (Possible) 1894
Berocca Tablets (Possible) 1893
Betoptic Sterile Ophthalmic Solution (Small numbers of patients) 569
Betoptic S Sterile Ophthalmic Suspension (Small numbers of patients) 570
Biavax II 1427
Bicillin L-A Injection 2442
Brevital Sodium Vials 1248
BuSpar (Rare) 1401

Calcimar Injection, Synthetic (A few cases) 1839
Cantil Tablets 1326
Carbocaine Hydrochloride 3% Injection (Rare) 956
Carbocaine Hydrochloride Injection 2043
Carbocaine Hydrochloride 2% with Neo-Cobefrin (Rare) 956
Cardene Capsules (Rare) 2290
Catapres Tablets 676
▲ Catapres-TTS (5 of 101 patients) 677
Cefol Filmtab 509
Ceftin Tablets 575
Ceptaz for Injection 1057
Cetacaine Topical Anesthetic 850
Children's Advil Suspension (Less than 1%) 2426
Chloromycetin Hydrocortisone Ophthalmic 1694
Chloromycetin Ophthalmic Ointment, 1% 1696
Cipro I.V. (1% or less) 1592
Cipro Tablets 1589
Clear by Design Medicated Acne Gel ▣ 709
Clear By Design Medicated Cleansing Pads ▣ 709
Cogentin Injection 1435
ColBENEMID Tablets 1436
Colyte 1826
Compazine 2201
Cortisporin Cream (1%) 757
Cortisporin Ointment (1%) 758
Cortisporin Otic Solution Sterile (0.09%) 760
Cortisporin Otic Suspension Sterile (0.09% to 1%) 760
Creon Capsules (Less frequent) 2245
Cystospaz 2395
Cytadren Tablets (Rare) 861
CytoGam (Rare) 891
Cytomel Tablets (Rare) 2203
Damason-P 1356
Danocrine Capsules 2046
Darbid Tablets 2205
Depen Titratable Tablets (Rare) 2379
Depo-Medrol Sterile Aqueous Suspension 2334
Deprol Tablets 2382
Desquam-E Gel (10 to 25 patients per 1,000) 2397
Desquam-X Gel (10 to 25 patients per 1,000) 2397
Desquam-X 5 Wash (10 to 25 patients per 1,000) 2397
Desquam-X 10 Bar (10 to 25 patients per 1,000) 2397
Desquam-X 10 Wash (10 to 25 patients per 1,000) 2397
Desyrel and Desyrel Dividose (Less than 1%) 1404
DiaBeta (1.5%) 1091
Didrex Tablets 2338
Digibind (Rare) 762
Diphtheria and Tetanus Toxoids and Pertussis Vaccine Adsorbed USP (For Pediatric Use) 892
Donnatal 1858
Donnatal Extentabs 1859
Donnatal Tablets 1858
Donnazyme Tablets 1860
Drithocreme (Very few instances) 590
Dritho-Scalp (Very few instances) 591
Duranest Injections 624
Dyclone 0.5% and 1% Topical Solutions, USP 626
E.E.S. 522
E-Mycin Tablets 688
Elspar 1470
Emete-con Intramuscular/Intravenous 1950
Eminase (0.2%) 2211
Empirin with Codeine Phosphate Nos. 2, 3 & 4 764
Epifrin ⊙ 244
Epogen for Injection 591
Ergamisol Tablets 1136
Ergotrate Maleate Ampoules 1263
ERYC 1720
EryPed 200 & EryPed 400 Granules 519
Ery-Tab Tablets 521
Erythrocin Stearate Filmtab 523
Eurax Cream & Lotion 2398
Sterile FUDR (Remote possibility) 1898
Factrel (Rare) 2561
Fero-Folic-500 Filmtab 527
Fiberall Fiber Wafers-Fruit & Nut 851
Fiorinal with Codeine Capsules 2008
Flu-Imune Influenza Virus Vaccine (Rare) 1204
Fluorouracil Injection 1897
Fortaz 1060
Fungizone Intravenous 2262
Furacin Topical Solution 0.2% 1855
Gamimune N Immune Globulin Intravenous (Human) 1572
Gamulin Rh, Rh_0(D) Immune Globulin (Human) (Infrequent) 610
Gantanol 1899
Gantrisin 1901
Geref (sermorelin acetate for injection) (One patient) 2560
Glucagon for Injection Vials and Emergency Kit 1263
Halcion Tablets (Rare) 2340
Hemopad Absorbable Collagen Hemostat 627
Herplex Liquifilm ⊙ 248
Hibiclens Antimicrobial Skin Cleanser 2271
Hibistat (Very rare) 2272
Humulin 70/30, 100 Units 1267
Humulin BR, 100 Units 1268
Humulin L, 100 Units 1268
Humulin U, 100 Units 1272
Hurricaine Topical Anesthetic Aerosol Spray, 2 oz (Rare) 672
Hurricaine Topical (Rare) 672
Iberet-Folic-500 Filmtab 527
IFEX (Less than 1%) 729
Beef Regular, 100 Units 1275
Ilosone 913
Ilotycin Gluceptate, IV, Vials 915
Inderide Tablets 2463
INSTAT Collagen Absorbable Hemostat 1151
IOPIDINE ⊙ 232
Keflex Pulvules, Oral Suspension & Pediatric Drops 916
Keftab Tablets 917
Kerlone Tablets (Less than 2%) 2172
Kinesed Tablets 2272
Koāte-HP Antihemophilic Factor (Human) 1581
Koāte-HS Antihemophilic Factor (Human) 1580
Konakion Injection 1903
Kutrase Capsules 2146
Larobec Tablets 1905
Leucovorin Calcium Tablets, Wellcovorin Brand 787
Levsin/Levsinex 2147
Loniten Tablets 2346
Lortab ASA Tablets 2414
Luroscrub Antimicrobial Skin Cleanser 912
M-M-R II 1494
M-R-VAX II 1496
Marcaine Hydrochloride 0.5% with Epinephrine 1:200,000 (as bitartrate) 958
Marcaine Hydrochloride with Epinephrine 1:200,000 (Rare) 2055
Marcaine Hydrochloride Injection (Rare) 2055
Marcaine Spinal (Rare) 2058
Matulane Capsules 1907
May-Vita Elixir 1359
Meclan (meclocycline sulfosalicylate) Cream 1679
Medrol 2348
Mefoxin 1498
▲ Mesnex Injection (17%) 733
Metamucil 1806
Metandren Linguets and Tablets 875
Metimyd ⊙ 306
Metubine Iodide Vials 1285
Mezlin 1597
Miacalcin Injection (A few cases) 2017
Micronase Tablets (1.5%) 2350
Miltown Tablets 2386
Minocin Oral Suspension 1224
Modane Plus Tablets ▣ 504
Modane Tablets ▣ 503
Monoclate-P Factor VIII:C, Pasteurized, Antihemophilic Factor (Human) 612
Motrin Tablets (Less than 1%) 2351
Mumpsvax (Extremely rare) 1513
Mydriacyl ⊙ 225
Myochrysine Injection 1516
Naprosyn 2297
Natacyn (One case) ⊙ 227
NebuPent for Inhalation Solution (1% or less) 1017
NeoDecadron Sterile Ophthalmic Ointment 1517
NeoDecadron Sterile Ophthalmic Solution 1518
Neosporin Cream (1%) 792
Neosporin G.U. Irrigant Sterile 793
Neosporin Ointment (1%) 793
Nescaine/Nescaine MPF (Rare) 629
Nicobid 1846
Nicorette (Rare) 1335
Niferex-PN Tablets 847
Nitrodisc (Extremely rare) 2176
▲ Nizoral 2% Cream (5%) 1143
Novafed A Capsules 1342
Novocain Hydrochloride for Spinal Anesthesia 2065
NuLYTELY 699
Ocusert Pilo-20 and Pilo-40 Ocular Therapeutic Systems (Uncommon) ⊙ 256
Omnipaque 2552
Oncovin Solution Vials & Hyporets (Rare) 1288
OptiPranolol Sterile Ophthalmic Solution (A small number of patients) ⊙ 261
Orinase Tablets (1.1%) 2354
Orudis Capsules (Less than 1%) 2488
PBZ Tablets & Elixir 1037
PBZ-SR Tablets 1037
PCE Dispertab Tablets 549
PMB 200 and PMB 400 2504
Pamelor 2019
Pancrease Capsules 1377
Pancrease MT Capsules (Less frequent) 1378
Paraflex Caplets (Rare) 1378
Parafon Forte DSC Caplets (Rare) 1379
ParaGard T380A Intrauterine Copper Contraceptive 411
Paraplatin for Injection (2%) 735
PediaProfen Suspension (Less than 1%) 1363
Pediazole 1973
PediOtic Suspension Sterile (0.09% to 1%) 797
Peptavlon 2563
Perdiem Fiber Granules (Rare) 1852
Perdiem Granules (Rare) 1852
Pergonal (menotropins for injection, USP) 2184
Peridex (Rare) 1808
Phenaphen with Codeine Capsules 1865
Phenaphen-650 with Codeine Tablets 1866
Phenergan Injection 2493
Phenobarbital Elixir and Tablets 1293
Pitressin Synthetic, Ampoules 1758
Pontocaine Hydrochloride for Spinal Anesthesia 2069
Pramilet FA 1974
Pre-Pen (Rare) 2148
Pro-Banthīne Tablets 2141
Procrit for Injection 1647
ProHIBiT Haemophilus b Conjugate Vaccine (Diphtheria Toxoid Conjugate) (Infrequent) 896
Prolixin Oral Concentrate 1792
Pronestyl Injection 1798
Propine with C Cap Compliance Cap (Infrequent) ⊙ 255
ProSom Tablets (Infrequent) 554
Prostigmin Injectable 1120
Prostigmin Tablets 1121
Protropin 1049
Prozac Pulvules (1.2%) 920
Quarzan Capsules 1937
Rauzide Tablets 1804
Retrovir Capsules 802
Retrovir I.V. Infusion 805
Retrovir Syrup 802
Robinul Forte Tablets 1873
Robinul Injectable 1873
Robinul Tablets 1873
Rogaine Topical Solution (1.27%) 2357
Rowasa 2248
SSD RP Cream 690
Sandimmune (2% or less) 2024
Secretin-Ferring 2547
Selsun Rx 2.5% Selenium Sulfide Lotion, USP 1977
Sensorcaine (Rare) 631
Sensorcaine-MPF Spinal (Rare) 634
▲ Septra (Among most common) 813
▲ Septra I.V. Infusion (Most common) 808
▲ Septra I.V. Infusion ADD-Vantage Vials (Most common) 810
▲ Septra (Among most common) 813
Seromycin Pulvules 1298
Serpasil-Apresoline Tablets 884
Serpasil-Esidrix Tablets 886
Silvadene Cream 1% 1352
Sinequan (Occasional) 1960
Slo-Niacin Tablets 2376
Solu-Cortef Sterile Powder 2361
Soma Compound w/Codeine Tablets 2390
Soma Compound Tablets 2389
Sotradecol (Sodium Tetradecyl Sulfate Injection) 964
Stelazine (Occasional) 2226
Sultrin (Frequent) 1675
Suprax 1235
Synkayvite Tablets 1920
Tagamet (Rare) 2228
Talacen 2070
▲ Tazicef for Injection (Most common) 2231
Terra-Cortril Ophthalmic Suspension 1963
Terramycin Intramuscular Solution 1964
Terramycin with Polymyxin B Sulfate Ophthalmic Ointment (Rare) 1965
Theragran Hematinic Tablets 605
Thiosulfil Forte Tablets 2526
Thorazine (Occasional) 2234
THROMBOGEN Topical Thrombin, USP 1153
THROMBOGEN Topical Thrombin, USP, Spray Kit 1153
THROMBOGEN Topical Thrombin, USP, Transfer Needle 1153
Thrombostat 1765
Tigan 2239
Tolinase Tablets (0.4%) 2365
Tracrium Injection 817
Trinsicon Capsules 2415
Tronolane Anesthetic Cream for Hemorrhoids ▣ 681
Tropicacyl ⊙ 209
Tylenol with Codeine 1381
Tylox Capsules 1382
Ultracef Capsules, Tablets & Oral Suspension 722
Urobiotic-250 Capsules (Rare) 1968
Valpin 50 Tablets 941
Vasocidin Ophthalmic Solution ⊙ 276
VePesid Capsules and Injection (1 to 2%) 741
Vibramycin Hyclate Intravenous 1968
Voltaren Tablets 1042
▲ Xanax Tablets (3.8%) 2367
Xylocaine Injections (Extremely rare) 637
Xylocaine Injections for Ventricular Arrhythmias (Extremely rare) 639
Xylocaine 2% Jelly (Extremely rare) 643
Xylocaine 5% Ointment 644
Xylocaine 10% Oral Spray (Extremely rare) 645
4% Xylocaine-MPF Sterile Solution (Extremely rare) 641
Xylocaine 2% Viscous Solution 646
Yutopar Tablets 647
Zefazone Sterile Powder 2372
Zenate Tablets 2250
Zorprin Tablets 698

Allergic sensitization

▲ AK-Trol Ointment & Suspension (Most often) ⊙ 207
▲ Alferon N Injection (18%) 1809
Atropine Sulfate Sterile Ophthalmic Solution and S.O.P. Sterile Ophthalmic Ointment ⊙ 239
▲ Blephamide (Most often) 586
▲ Cetapred Ointment (Most often) ⊙ 220
Chloroptic S.O.P. ⊙ 243
▲ Cortisporin Otic Suspension Sterile (Most often) 760
Desquam-E Gel (10 to 25 per 1,000) 2397
Desquam-X Gel (10 to 25 per 1,000) 2397
Desquam-X 5 Wash (10 to 25 per 1,000) 2397
Desquam-X 10 Bar (10 to 25 per 1,000) 2397
Desquam-X 10 Wash (10 to 25 per 1,000) 2397
▲ Dexacidin (Most often) ⊙ 272
▲ FML-S Sterile Ophthalmic Suspension (Among most often) ⊙ 246
▲ Isopto Cetapred Suspension (Most often) ⊙ 220
Leucovorin Calcium for Injection, Wellcovorin Brand 786
Leucovorin Calcium Injection 1210
Leucovorin Calcium Tablets 1212
▲ Maxitrol Ophthalmic Ointment/Suspension (Most often) ⊙ 223
Ophthocort ⊙ 301

- ▲ Poly-Pred Liquifilm (Most often) ◉ 250
- Pramet FA 1974
- ▲ Pred-G Liquifilm Sterile Ophthalmic Suspension (Most often) ◉ 252
- Pred-G S.O.P. Sterile Ophthalmic Ointment ◉ 253
- ▲ Vasocidin Ointment (Most often) ◉ 275
- ▲ Vasocidin Ophthalmic Solution (Most often) ◉ 276
- ▲ Vasosulf (Most often) ◉ 279

Allergic vasospastic reactions

- Calciparine Injection 925
- Heparin Lock Flush Solution 2456
- Heparin Sodium Injection 2457

Allergy (see under Allergic reactions)

Alopecia

- ▲ Adriamycin PFS (Most cases) 561
- Adriamycin RDF (Occurs in most cases) 562
- Alkeran Tablets 754
- Amen (Few cases) 833
- Aminophyllin Tablets 2153
- Anadrol-50 Tablets 2287
- Anafranil Capsules (Infrequent) 650
- Anaprox and Anaprox DS Tablets (Less than 1%) 2288
- Ansaid Tablets (Less than 1%) 2319
- Aquasol A Vitamin A Capsules, USP 615
- Aquasol A Parenteral, USP 615
- Aralen Phosphate Tablets 2039
- Asendin Tablets (Very rare) 1196
- Atromid-S Capsules (Less frequent) 2435
- Atrovent Inhalation Aerosol (Less than 1 in 100) 675
- Azulfidine Tablets, EN-tabs, Oral Suspension (Rare) 1157
- Benemid Tablets 1426
- Betoptic Sterile Ophthalmic Solution (Rare) 569
- Betoptic S Sterile Ophthalmic Suspension (Rare) 570
- Blenoxane 724
- Blocadren Tablets (Less than 1%) 1429
- Brevicon 2304
- BuSpar (Infrequent) 1401
- Calan SR Caplets (1% or less) 2157
- Calan Tablets (1% or less) 2155
- Calciparine Injection 925
- Capoten (About 0.5 to 2%) 2255
- Capozide (0.5 to 2%) 2258
- Cardizem Tablets-30 mg, 60 mg, 90 mg and 120 mg (Infrequent) 1329
- Cardizem SR Capsules-60 mg, 90 mg and 120 mg (Infrequent) 1327
- Cardura Tablets (Less than 0.5% of 3960 patients) 1941
- Cartrol Tablets 507
- Catapres Tablets 676
- Catapres-TTS (2 in 1,000) 677
- CeeNU (Infrequent) 725
- ▲ Cerubidine (In most patients) 2443
- Children's Advil Suspension (Less than 1%) 2426
- Choledyl Pediatric Elixir 1702
- Choledyl Tablets 1700
- Cibalith-S 870
- Clinoril Tablets (Less than 1%) 1433
- ColBENEMID Tablets 1436
- Combipres Tablets (About 2 in 1,000) 678
- Cordarone Tablets (Less than 1%) 2446
- Corgard Tablets (Infrequent) 701
- Corzide Tablets (Infrequent) 702
- Cosmegen Injection 1440
- Coumadin Injection & Tablets (Infrequent) 944
- Cuprimine Capsules (Rare) 1442
- Cycrin Tablets (A few cases) 2449
- Cytosar-U Sterile Powder (Less frequent) 2329
- Cytotec (Infrequent) 2159
- Cytovene Sterile Powder (1% or less) 2292
- Cytoxan for Injection (Frequent) 726
- DTIC-Dome 1595
- Danocrine Capsules 2046
- Demulen 2161
- Depakene Capsules & Syrup 511
- Depakote 512
- Depen Titratable Tablets (Rare) 2379
- Depo-Provera Sterile Aqueous Suspension (Few cases) 2336
- Desyrel and Desyrel Dividose 1404
- Dicumarol Tablets (Infrequent) 516
- Diethylstilbestrol Tablets 1258
- Dipentum Capsules (Rare) 1160
- ▲ Doxorubicin Hydrochloride for Injection, USP (Most cases) 622
- ▲ Doxorubicin Hydrochloride Injection, USP (Most cases) 848
- Efudex 1880
- Elavil 2269
- Eldepryl (0 of 49 patients) 2250
- Emcyt Capsules (1%) 1161
- Endep Tablets 1927
- Enovid 2161
- ▲ Ergamisol Tablets (3 to 22%) 1136
- Esimil Tablets 864
- Eskalith 2214
- Estinyl Tablets 2085
- Estrace 1385
- Estrace Vaginal Cream 1388
- Estradurin 2452
- Estratest 2245
- Estrovis 1721
- Etrafon 2087
- Sterile FUDR 1898
- Feldene Capsules (Less than 1%) 1777
- Flexeril Tablets (Rare) 1471
- Fluorouracil Injection (Substantial number of cases) 1897
- Garamycin Injectable 2093
- Haldol Decanoate (Isolated cases) 1375
- Haldol Injection, Tablets and Concentrate (Isolated cases) 1373
- Heparin Lock Flush Solution 2456
- Heparin Sodium Vials 1264
- Heparin Sodium Injection 2457
- Heparin Sodium Injection, USP, Sterile Solution 2342
- Hexalen Capsules (Less than 1%) 2316
- Hydrea Capsules (Very rare) 728
- ▲ Idamycin for Injection (77%) 564
- ▲ IFEX (83%) 729
- Imuran (Less than 1%) 768
- Inderal (Rare) 2459
- Inderal LA Long Acting Capsules (Rare) 2461
- Inderide Tablets (Rare) 2463
- Inderide LA Long Acting Capsules (Rare) 2465
- Indocin Capsules (Less than 1%) 1487
- Indocin I.V. (Less than 1%) 1490
- Indocin (Less than 1%) 1487
- ▲ Intron A (8% to 31%) 2097
- Ismelin Tablets 869
- Isoptin Oral Tablets (Less than 1%) 1179
- Isoptin SR Sustained Release Tablets (Less than 1%) 1181
- Jenest-28 Tablets 1636
- Kerlone Tablets 2172
- Klonopin Tablets 1902
- Lariam Tablets (Less than 1%) 1904
- Larodopa Tablets (Rare) 1905
- Leukine for IV Infusion 1127
- Levatol 1832
- Levlen/Tri-Levlen 665
- Levothroid Tablets 1003
- Limbitrol 1933
- Lithane Tablets 1596
- Lithium Carbonate Capsules & Tablets 1984
- Lithobid Tablets 870
- Lodine Capsules (Less than 1%) 2468
- Lo/Ovral Tablets 2471
- Lo/Ovral-28 Tablets 2476
- Loestrin 1728
- Lopid Capsules and Tablets 1736
- Lopressor Ampuls (Rare) 1032
- Lopressor HCT Tablets 1034
- Lopressor Tablets (Rare) 1032
- Loxitane 1213
- Ludiomil Tablets 874
- ▲ Lupron Depot 3.75 mg (Among most frequent) 2312
- Lupron Depot 7.5 mg 2311
- Lupron Injection (Less than 5%) 2310
- Macrodantin Capsules 1624
- Matulane Capsules 1907
- Maxair Inhaler (Less than 1%) 1311
- Meclomen Capsules (Rare) 1739
- Mediatric Capsules 2476
- Megace Tablets 732
- Menrium Tablets 1934
- Mesantoin Tablets 2013
- Methotrexate Tablets, Parenteral, LPF Parenteral (1 to 3%) 1217
- Metrodin (urofollitropin for injection) 2182
- Mevacor Tablets 1505
- Mexitil Capsules (About 4 in 1,000) 680
- Micronor Tablets 1667
- Midamor Tablets (Less than or equal to 1%) 1508
- Milontin Kapseals 1741
- Minipress Capsules (Less than 1%) 1778
- Minizide Capsules (Rare) 1779
- Modicon 1667
- Moduretic Tablets 1510
- Motrin Tablets (Less than 1%) 2351
- Mustargen (Infrequent) 1514
- ▲ Mutamycin (Frequent) 733
- Myleran Tablets (Rare) 790
- Myochrysine Injection 1516
- Nalfon Pulvules & Tablets (Less than 1%) 919
- Naprosyn (Less than 1%) 2297
- Neosar for Injection (Common) 566
- ▲ Neupogen for Injection (18%) 595
- Niclocide Chewable Tablets 1607
- Nizoral 2% Shampoo (Less than 1%) 1144
- Nordette-21 Tablets 2481
- Nordette-28 Tablets 2483
- Norethin 2133
- Norinyl 2304
- Norlestrin 1746
- Norlutate 1754
- Norlutin 1755
- Normodyne Tablets 2110
- Normozide Tablets 2112
- Norplant System 2484
- Norpramin Tablets 1340
- Nor-Q D Tablets 2304
- ▲ Novantrone for Injection Concentrate (22 to 37%) 1226
- Ogen 540
- ▲ Oncovin Solution Vials & Hyporets (Most common) 1288
- Ortho Dienestrol Cream 1664
- Ortho-Cyclen Tablets 1658
- Ortho-Novum 1667
- Orudis Capsules (Less than 1%) 2488
- Ovcon 1391
- Ovral Tablets 2490
- Ovral-28 Tablets 2491
- Ovrette Tablets 2492
- PMB 200 and PMB 400 2504
- Pamelor 2019
- Panwarfin Tablets (Infrequent) 547
- Paradione Capsules 548
- Paraplatin for Injection (2%) 735
- Parlodel (Less than 1%) 2020
- PediaProfen Suspension (Less than 1%) 1363
- Pepcid (Infrequent) 1524
- Permax Tablets (Infrequent) 1291
- Plaquenil Sulfate Tablets 2067
- Platinol (Infrequent) 737
- Platinol-AQ Injection (Infrequent) 738
- Premarin Intravenous 2508
- Premarin with Methyltestosterone 2515
- Premarin Tablets 2510
- Premarin Vaginal Cream 2512
- Prilosec Delayed-Release Capsules (Less than 1%) 1530
- Procardia XL Tablets (1% or less) 1783
- Proglycem 649
- Prokine for I.V. Infusion 1096
- Provera Tablets (A few cases) 2356
- Prozac Pulvules (Infrequent) 920
- Quibron-T 714
- Respbid Tablets 684
- Rheumatrex Methotrexate Dose Pack (1% to 3%) 1234
- Ridaura Capsules (Rare) 2224
- Ritalin (A few instances) 880
- ▲ Roferon-A Injection (8% to 22%) 1916
- Rogaine Topical Solution 2357
- Rowasa (0.86%) 2248
- ▲ Rubex (Most cases) 739
- Rufen Tablets (Less than 1%) 691
- Rythmol Tablets (Less than 1%) 1184
- Sandostatin Injection (Less than 1%) 2029
- Sectral Capsules 2520
- Seldane Tablets 1349
- Seldane-D Extended-Release Tablets 1350
- Selsun Rx 2.5% Selenium Sulfide Lotion, USP 1977
- Serophene (clomiphene citrate tablets, USP) (Less than 1 in 100 patients) 2186
- Sinemet Tablets 952
- Sinemet CR Tablets 953
- Sinequan (Occasional) 1960
- Slo-bid Gyrocaps 1847
- Solganal Suspension 2122
- Stilphostrol Tablets and Ampuls 1609
- Surmontil Capsules 2524
- TACE 12 and 25 mg 1353
- Tagamet (Rare) 2228
- Tapazole Tablets 1298
- ▲ Tegison Capsules (Less than 75%) 1881
- Tegretol Chewable Tablets 654
- Tegretol Suspension 656
- Tegretol Tablets 654
- Temovate Scalp Application (1 of 294 patients) 1056
- Tenex Tablets 1875
- Tenoretic Tablets 1105
- Tenormin Tablets and I.V. Injection 1107
- Tenuate 1354
- Teslac Tablets (Rare) 741
- Theo-24 2179
- Theo-Dur Extended-Release Tablets 1166
- Theolair 1317
- Theolair-SR Tablets 1319
- ▲ TheoX Extended-Release Tablets (Among most consistent) 841
- Thiotepa Parenteral (1 case) 1240
- Timolide Tablets 1547
- Timoptic in Ocudose 1552
- Timoptic Sterile Ophthalmic Solution 1550
- Tofranil Ampuls 1038
- Tofranil Tablets 1039
- Tofranil-PM Capsules 1041
- Tonocard Tablets (Less than 1%) 1554
- Trandate HCT/Trandate 579
- Trexan Tablets (Less than 1%) 937
- Triavil Tablets 1556
- Tridione 557
- Levlen/Tri-Levlen 665
- Tri-Norinyl 2304
- Triphasil-21 Tablets 2527
- Triphasil-28 Tablets 2532
- Uniphyl 400 mg Tablets 1823
- Vaseretic Tablets 1559
- Vasotec I.V. 1562
- Vasotec Tablets (0.5% to 1%) 1564
- Velban Vials (Common) 1305
- ▲ VePesid Capsules and Injection (Up to 66%) 741
- Verelan Capsules (Less than 1%) 1243
- Visken Tablets 2036
- Vivactil Tablets 1567
- Voltaren Tablets (Less than 1%) 1042
- Wellbutrin Tablets (Infrequent) 821
- Winstrol Tablets 2075
- Zantac Injection and Zantac Injection Premixed (Rare No incidence data in labeling) 1063
- Zantac (Rare) 1065
- Zovirax 824
- Zyloprim Tablets (Less than 1%) 830

Alopecia, hereditaria

- Android 1111
- Estratest 2245
- Metandren Linguets and Tablets 875
- Testred Capsules 1124

Alpha-glutamyl transferase, elevation

- Eulexin Capsules 2089

Alveolalgia

- Hemopad Absorbable Collagen Hemostat 627
- INSTAT Collagen Absorbable Hemostat 1151

Alveolitis

- Cordarone Tablets 2446
- Cuprimine Capsules 1442
- Depen Titratable Tablets (Rare) 2379
- Prozac Pulvules (Rare) 920

Alveolitis, allergic

- Depen Titratable Tablets (Rare) 2379

Alveolitis, fibrosing

- Azulfidine Tablets, EN-tabs, Oral Suspension 1157
- Rowasa 2248
- Tonocard Tablets (Less than 1%) 1554

Amblyopia

- Butazolidin Capsules & Tablets (Less than 1%) 1027
- Cardizem Tablets-30 mg, 60 mg, 90 mg and 120 mg (Less than 1%) 1329
- Cardizem SR Capsules-60 mg, 90 mg and 120 mg (Less than 1%) 1327
- Children's Advil Suspension (Less than 1%) 2426
- Diprivan Injection (Less than 1%) 2267
- Ditropan 1332

Duragesic Transdermal System (Less than 1%) 1133
Marplan Tablets (One case) 1906
Motrin Tablets (Less than 1%) 2351
Niacor Tablets 2376
Nicolar Tablets 1846
Omnipaque 2552
PediaProfen Suspension (Less than 1%) 1363
Prozac Pulvules (Infrequent) 920
Retrovir Capsules (Less than 5%) 802
Retrovir I.V. Infusion (Less than 5%) 805
Retrovir Syrup (Less than 5%) 802
Rufen Tablets (Less than 1%) 691
Voltaren Tablets (Less than 1%) 1042
Zyloprim Tablets (Less than 1%) 830

Amenorrhea

Aldactazide 2150
Aldactone 2152
Aldoclor Tablets 1413
Aldomet Ester HCl Injection 1417
Aldomet Oral 1415
Aldoril Tablets 1418
Amen 833
Anadrol-50 Tablets 2287
Anafranil Capsules (Up to 1%) 650
Android 1111
Aygestin Tablets 2437
Brevicon 2304
BuSpar (Rare) 1401
Compazine 2201
Cycrin Tablets 2449
Cytoxan for Injection (Reported in a number of patients) 726
Danocrine Capsules (Occasional) 2046
Demulen 2161
Depakene Capsules & Syrup 511
Depakote 512
Depo-Provera Sterile Aqueous Suspension 2336
Diethylstilbestrol Tablets 1258
Enovid 2161
Estinyl Tablets 2085
Estrace 1385
Estrace Vaginal Cream 1388
▲Estratest (Among most common) 2245
Estrovis 1721
Etrafon 2087
Halotestin Tablets 2341
Jenest-28 Tablets 1636
Levlen/Tri-Levlen 665
Lo/Ovral Tablets 2471
Lo/Ovral-28 Tablets 2476
Loestrin 1728
Loxitane (Rare) 1213
Mediatric Capsules 2476
Mellaril 2011
Menrium Tablets 1934
▲Metandren Linguets and Tablets (Most common) 875
Micronor Tablets 1667
Moban Tablets & Concentrate (Infrequent) 932
Modicon 1667
Mustargen 1514
Navane Capsules and Concentrate 1954
Navane Intramuscular 1956
Neosar for Injection (Reported in a number of patients) 566
▲Nolvadex Tablets (16.3%) 1102
Nordette-21 Tablets 2481
Nordette-28 Tablets 2483
Norethin 2133
Norinyl 2304
Norlestrin 1746
Norlutate 1754
Norlutin 1755
▲Norplant System (9.4%) 2484
Nor-Q D Tablets 2304
Ogen 540
Ortho Dienestrol Cream 1664
Ortho-Cyclen Tablets 1658
Ortho-Novum 1667
Ovcon 1391
Ovral Tablets 2490
Ovral-28 Tablets 2491
Ovrette Tablets 2492
PMB 200 and PMB 400 2504
ParaGard T380A Intrauterine Copper Contraceptive 411
Permax Tablets (Rare) 1291
Premarin Intravenous 2508
Premarin with Methyltestosterone 2515
Premarin Vaginal Cream 2512
Prolixin Oral Concentrate 1792
Provera Tablets 2356
Prozac Pulvules (Infrequent) 920
Reglan 1869
Stelazine 2226
TACE 12 and 25 mg 1353
Testred Capsules 1124
Thiotepa Parenteral 1240
Thorazine 2234
Trilafon 2123
Levlen/Tri-Levlen 665
Tri-Norinyl 2304
Triphasil-21 Tablets 2527
Triphasil-28 Tablets 2532

Amnesia

Altace Capsules 1086
Ansaid Tablets (1-3%) 2319
Ativan Tablets 2434
Cardizem Tablets-30 mg, 60 mg, 90 mg and 120 mg (Less than 1%) 1329
Cardizem SR Capsules-60 mg, 90 mg and 120 mg (Less than 1%) 1327
Cardura Tablets (Less than 0.5% of 3960 patients) 1941
Clozaril Tablets (Less than 1%) 2000
Doral Tablets 2383
Duragesic Transdermal System (1% or greater) 1133
Ergamisol Tablets (1%) 1136
Halcion Tablets 2340
▲Intron A (Up to 14%) 2097
Kerlone Tablets (Less than 2%) 2172
Klonopin Tablets 1902
Omnipaque 2552
Orudis Capsules (Less than 1%) 2488
Permax Tablets (Frequent) 1291
ProSom Tablets (Infrequent) 554
Prozac Pulvules (Infrequent) 920
Roferon-A Injection (Less than 0.5%) 1916
Serax Capsules 2522
Serax Tablets 2522
Tambocor Tablets (Less than 1%) 1315
Tegison Capsules (Less than 1%) 1881
Tenex Tablets 1875
Versed Injection (Less than 1%) 1924
Xanax Tablets 2367
Zyloprim Tablets (Less than 1%) 830

Amnesia, traveler's

Halcion Tablets 2340

Amputation, gangrene of the extremities-induced

Heparin Lock Flush Solution 2456
Heparin Sodium Injection 2457

Analgesia, reversal

Narcan Injection 933

Anaphylactic reactions

Adriamycin RDF 562
Aldoclor Tablets 1413
Aldoril Tablets 1418
Anaprox and Anaprox DS Tablets (Less than 1%) 2288
Ancef Injection 2194
Ansaid Tablets (Rare) 2319
Antivenin (Black Widow Spider) 1422
AquaMEPHYTON Injection 1422
Atgam Sterile Solution (At least 1 patient and less than 5% of total patients) 2320
Augmentin Tablets, Powder for Oral Suspension, and Chewable Tablets 2198
Azo Gantanol Tablets 1887
Azulfidine Tablets, EN-tabs, Oral Suspension (Rare) 1157
Benemid Tablets 1426
Biavax II 1427
Bicillin C-R Injection 2438
Bicillin L-A Injection 2442
Capozide 2258
Cefotan 2265
Chloromycetin Kapseals 1695
Chloromycetin Palmitate, Oral Suspension 1697
Chloromycetin Sodium Succinate 1698
Cipro I.V. (1% or less) 1592
Cipro Tablets 1589
Cleocin HCl Capsules 2322
Cleocin Pediatric Flavored Granules 2324
Cleocin Phosphate Injection 2325
Compazine Ampuls 2201
Corzide Tablets (Occasional) 702
Cytosar-U Sterile Powder (Less frequent) 2329
Cytoxan for Injection (Rare) 726
Deltasone Tablets (Rare) 2332
Depo-Provera Sterile Aqueous Suspension (Occasional) 2336
Deprol Tablets (Rare) 2382
Desferal Vials 862
Digibind 762
Diphtheria and Tetanus Toxoids and Pertussis Vaccine Adsorbed USP (For Pediatric Use) (Rare) 892
Diucardin Tablets 2450
Diulo 2129
Diupres Tablets 1461
Diuril Oral Suspension 1464
Diuril Sodium Intravenous 1463
Diuril Tablets 1464
Dobutrex Solution Vials 1259
Dolobid Tablets (Less than 1 in 100) 1465
Doryx Capsules 1717
Duranest Injections 624
Dyclone 0.5% and 1% Topical Solutions, USP 626
Easprin 1719
Elspar 1470
Eminase (0.2%) 2211
Enduron Tablets 517
ERYC 1720
Etrafon 2087
Factrel (One case) 2561
Feldene Capsules (Less than 1%) 1777
Floxin Tablets 1652
Gamimune N Immune Globulin Intravenous (Human) 1572
Gammagard Immune Globulin, Intravenous (Human) (Possible) 658
Gammar, Immune Globulin (Human) U.S.P. (Rare) 609
Gammar-IV, Immune Globulin Intravenous (Human) 610
Garamycin Injectable 2093
Geocillin Tablets 1951
Halotestin Tablets 2341
Heparin Lock Flush Solution 2456
Heparin Sodium Injection 2457
Heparin Sodium Injection, USP, Sterile Solution 2342
Hep-B-Gammagee (Rare) 1474
HydroDIURIL Tablets 1484
Hydropres Tablets 1485
HyperHep Hepatitis B Immune Globulin (Human) (Rare) 1575
Hyskon Hysteroscopy Fluid (Rare) 1162
Imferon (.0.2% to 0.3%) 976
Inderide Tablets 2463
Inderide LA Long Acting Capsules 2465
Intal Inhaler (Infrequent) 979
Kenalog-10 Injection 2402
Kenalog-40 Injection 2403
Kinesed Tablets 2272
Konakion Injection 1903
Levatol 1832
Lincocin 2344
Lozol Tablets 1843
Lupron Injection 2310
M-M-R II 1494
Macrodantin Capsules 1624
Marcaine Spinal (Rare) 2058
Meclan (meclocycline sulfosalicylate) Cream 1679
Medrol 2348
Mefoxin Premixed Intravenous Solution 1500
Meruvax II 1503
Metandren Linguets and Tablets (Rare) 875
Mezlin 1597
Mezlin Pharmacy Bulk Package 1599
Mintezol 1510
Moduretic Tablets 1510
Mykrox ½ mg Tablets 984
Naprosyn (Less than 1%) 2297
Nasalcrom Nasal Solution (1 in 430) 986
Naturetin Tablets (Occasional) 1789
Neosar for Injection (Rare) 566
Nescaine/Nescaine MPF 629
Norflex (Rare) 1314
Normodyne Injection 2108
Normodyne Tablets 2110
Normozide Tablets 2112
Noroxin Tablets (Occasional) 1519
Omnipaque 2552
Orthoclone OKT3 Sterile Solution (One patient) 1645
Orudis Capsules (Less than 1%) 2488
Oxytocin Injection 2492
Paraflex Caplets (Extremely rare) 1378
Parafon Forte DSC Caplets (Extremely rare) 1379
Pediazole 1973
Pfizerpen for Injection (Occasional) 1957
Pfizerpen-AS Aqueous Suspension 1959
Phenergan Injection 2493
Pipracil 1230
Pitocin Injection, Ampoules, Steri-Dose Syringes 1757
Pitressin Synthetic, Ampoules 1758
Platinol (Occasional) 737
Platinol-AQ Injection (Occasional) 738
Premarin with Methyltestosterone (Rare) 2515
Primaxin I.M. 1532
Primaxin I.V. 1535
Prinzide Tablets 1540
ProHIBiT Haemophilus b Conjugate Vaccine (Diphtheria Toxoid Conjugate) 896
Pronestyl Injection 1798
Protamine Sulfate Ampoules & Vials 1295
Quarzan Capsules 1937
Rauzide Tablets 1804
Ridaura Capsules 2224
Robaxin Injectable 1871
Rowasa 2248
Salutensin/Salutensin-Demi 719
Sandimmune I.V. Ampuls for Infusion (Rare) 2024
Sensorcaine 631
Sensorcaine-MPF Spinal 634
Solu-Cortef Sterile Powder 2361
Solu-Medrol Sterile Powder 2363
Soma Compound w/Codeine Tablets 2390
Spectrobid Tablets & Powder for Oral Suspension (Occasional) 1961
Stelazine 2226
Streptase for Infusion 635
Syntocinon Injection 2032
Talacen (One instance) 2070
Tao Capsules 1963
Taractan 1920
Temaril Tablets, Syrup and Spansule Sustained Release Capsules 1085
Terramycin Capsules 1786
Terramycin Intramuscular Solution 1964
Thorazine 2234
Timentin for Injection 2239
Timolide Tablets 1547
Tracrium Injection (Rare) 817
Trandate HCT Tablets 579
Trandate Injection 577
Trandate Tablets 579
Triavil Tablets 1556
Tri-Immunol Diphtheria & Tetanus Toxoids & Pertussis Vaccine, Adsorbed (Rare) 1241
Trilafon 2123
Trobicin Sterile Powder 2366
Unasyn 1965
Unipen 2533
Valpin 50 Tablets 941
Vaseretic Tablets 1559
Vibramycin Hyclate Intravenous 1968
Vibra-Tabs Film Coated Tablets 1787
Wycillin Injection 2537
Xylocaine 2% Jelly (Extremely rare) 643
Xylocaine 10% Oral Spray (Extremely rare) 645
4% Xylocaine-MPF Sterile Solution (Extremely rare) 641
Yutopar Tablets 647
Zaroxolyn Tablets 989
Zestoretic 2274
Zoladex 1110
Zorprin Tablets 698

Anaphylactic shock

Achromycin V Capsules 1193
Actifed with Codeine Cough Syrup 752
Aquasol A Parenteral, USP 615
Azdōne Tablets 844
Benadryl Capsules 1691
Benadryl Injection 1692
Butazolidin Capsules & Tablets (Less than 1%) 1027
Calcimar Injection, Synthetic (A few cases) 1839
CytoGam 891
Damason-P 1356
Declomycin Capsules, Tablets 1199
Deconamine 663
Disalcid 1310
Eminase (0.1%) 2211
Empirin with Codeine Phosphate Nos. 2, 3 & 4 764
Ethamolin 1829
Fiorinal with Codeine Capsules 2008
Hep-B-Gammagee 1474
Hyperab Rabies Immune Globulin (Human) (Rare) 1574
Hyper-Tet Tetanus Immune Globulin (Human) (Few cases) 1576

Lortab ASA Tablets 2414
Miacalcin Injection (A few cases) 2017
Myochrysine Injection 1516
Optimine Tablets 2115
Ornade Spansule Capsules 2221
PBZ Tablets & Elixir 1037
PBZ-SR Tablets 1037
Periactin 1525
Plague Vaccine (Rare) 1584
Polaramine 2116
Protamine Sulfate Ampoules & Vials 1295
Ru-Tuss II Capsules 693
Salflex 839
Solganal Suspension 2122
Soma Compound w/Codeine Tablets 2390
Soma Compound Tablets 2389
Soma Tablets 2388
Sotradecol (Sodium Tetradecyl Sulfate Injection) 964
Streptase for Infusion (0.1%) 635
Tavist Syrup 2033
Tavist Tablets 2035
Tavist-D Tablets 2035
Triaminic Expectorant DH 1995
Triaminic Oral Infant Drops 1996
Trinalin Repetabs Tablets 1170
Yutopar (Infrequent) 647
Zorprin Tablets 698

Anaphylactoid reactions

Achromycin V Capsules 1193
Amoxil 2193
Android (Rare) 1111
Aquasol A Parenteral, USP (One case) 615
Aristospan Suspension (Intra-articular) 1011
Attenuvax 1424
Biavax II 1427
Calciparine Injection (Rare) 925
Carbocaine Hydrochloride Injection (Rare) 2043
Cefizox Injection 1012
Cerubidine 2443
Compazine 2201
Cortone Acetate Sterile Suspension 1437
Cycrin Tablets 2449
Decadron Phosphate Injection 1449
Decadron Phosphate with Xylocaine Injection, Sterile 1451
Decadron-LA Sterile Suspension 1457
Depo-Medrol Sterile Aqueous Suspension (Rare) 2334
Digibind 762
Eminase (0.2%) 2211
Estratest (Rare) 2245
Fansidar Tablets 1896
Fungizone Intravenous 2262
Gamimune N Immune Globulin Intravenous (Human) (Very rare) 1572
Gammar-IV, Immune Globulin Intravenous (Human) (Rare) 610
Gantrisin Ophthalmic Ointment/Solution 1900
Heparin Sodium Vials (Rare) 1264
Hespan Injection 948
Hydeltrasol Injection, Sterile 1476
Hydeltra-T.B.A. Sterile Suspension 1478
Hydrocortone Acetate Sterile Suspension 1479
Hydrocortone Phosphate Injection, Sterile 1481
Leucovorin Calcium Injection 1210
Leucovorin Calcium Tablets 1212
M-M-R II 1494
M-R-VAX II 1496
Marcaine Hydrochloride with Epinephrine 1:200,000 2055
Marcaine Hydrochloride Injection 2055
Meruvax II 1503
Methotrexate Tablets, Parenteral, LPF Parenteral (A few cases) 1217
Mezlin 1597
Monocid Injection (Less than 1%) 2217
Mumpsvax 1513
Myambutol Tablets 1225
NegGram (Rare) 2062
Noroxin Tablets (Occasional) 1519
Novocain Hydrochloride for Spinal Anesthesia 2065
Omnipaque 2552
Pantopon Injectable 1911
Pneumovax 23 (Rare) 1528
Pnu-Imune 23 Pneumococcal Vaccine Polyvalent (Rare) 1233
Prolixin Decanoate 1795
Prolixin Enanthate 1796
Prolixin Oral Concentrate 1792
Protamine Sulfate Ampoules & Vials 1295
Provera Tablets 2356
Pyridium (One case) 1763
Pyridium Plus (One case) 1764
Rheumatrex Methotrexate Dose Pack (A few cases) 1234
Sandoglobulin I.V. 2027
Stelazine Concentrate 2226
Streptase for Infusion 635
Tacaryl 2409
Testred Capsules (Rare) 1124
Tetanus Toxoid, Adsorbed Purogenated 1238
Thiosulfil Forte Tablets 2526
Tolectin (200, 400 and 600 mg) (Less than 1%) 1379
Trandate HCT Tablets (Rare) 579
Trandate Injection (Rare) 577
Trandate Tablets (Rare) 579
Vancocin HCl, Vials & ADD-Vantage 1302
Voltaren Tablets (Less than 1%) 1042
Xylocaine Injections (Extremely rare) 637
Xylocaine 5% Ointment 644

Anaphylaxis

Achromycin V Capsules 1193
Adriamycin PFS 561
Adriamycin RDF 562
Amen (Occasional) 833
Ancef Injection 2194
Antivenin (Crotalidae) Polyvalent 2430
AquaMEPHYTON Injection 1422
Atgam Sterile Solution (Less than 1%) 2320
Attenuvax 1424
Augmentin Tablets, Powder for Oral Suspension, and Chewable Tablets 2198
Axid Pulvules (Rare) 1246
Azactam for Injection (Less than 1%) 2252
Azo Gantrisin Tablets 1888
Azulfidine Tablets, EN-tabs, Oral Suspension 1157
Bactrim DS Tablets 1891
Bactrim I.V. Infusion 1889
Bactrim 1891
Benemid Tablets 1426
Bentyl 1322
Biavax II 1427
Bicillin C-R Injection 2438
Bicillin C-R 900/300 Injection 2440
Blenoxane 724
Cantil Tablets 1326
Ceclor Pulvules & Suspension (Rare) 1251
Ceftin Tablets 575
Ceptaz for Injection (Rare) 1057
Children's Advil Suspension (Less than 1%) 2426
Chloromycetin Kapseals 1695
Chloromycetin Palmitate, Oral Suspension 1697
Chloromycetin Sodium Succinate 1698
Clinoril Tablets 1433
ColBENEMID Tablets 1436
Cycrin Tablets 2449
CytoGam 891
Cytosar-U Sterile Powder 2329
Cytotec (Infrequent) 2159
Darbid Tablets 2205
Declomycin Capsules, Tablets 1199
Depo-Provera Sterile Aqueous Suspension (Occasional) 2336
Deprol Tablets 2382
Diamox 1200
Diflucan Injection and Tablets (Rare) 1948
Digibind 762
Diprivan Injection (Rare) 2267
Donnatal 1858
Donnatal Extentabs 1859
Donnatal Tablets 1858
Donnazyme Tablets 1860
Doryx Capsules 1717
Doxorubicin Hydrochloride for Injection, USP 622
Doxorubicin Hydrochloride Injection, USP 848
Dyazide Capsules 2208
Dyrenium Capsules 2210
E.E.S. 522
E-Mycin Tablets 688
Easprin 1719
Elspar 1470
Engerix-B Unit-Dose Vials 2213
Equagesic Tablets (Rare) 2451
Ergamisol Tablets (Less frequent) 1136
ERYC 1720
EryPed 519
Ery-Tab Tablets 521
Erythrocin Stearate Filmtab 523
Erythromycin Base Filmtab 525
Erythromycin Delayed-Release Capsules, USP 526
Sterile FUDR (Remote possibility) 1898
Feldene Capsules (Less than 1%) 1777
Flexeril Tablets 1471
Flu-Imune Influenza Virus Vaccine (Rare) 1204
Fluorescite (Very rare) ⊙ 217
Fluorouracil Injection 1897
Fortaz (Very rare) 1060
Gamimune N Immune Globulin Intravenous (Human) (Rare) 1572
Gammar, Immune Globulin (Human) U.S.P. 609
Gantanol 1899
Gantrisin 1901
Hep-B-Gammagee 1474
Beef Regular, 100 Units 1275
Ilosone 913
Ilotycin Gluceptate, IV, Vials 915
Imferon 976
Indocin Capsules (Less than 1%) 1487
Indocin I.V. (Less than 1%) 1490
Indocin (Less than 1%) 1487
Insulatard NPH 1626
Insulatard NPH Human 1627
Intal Capsules (Less than 1 in 100,000 patients) 978
Intal Inhaler (Infrequent) 979
Intal Nebulizer Solution (Rare) 980
Intron A 2097
Keflex Pulvules, Oral Suspension & Pediatric Drops 916
Keftab Tablets 917
Kefurox Vials, Faspak & ADD-Vantage (Rare) 1277
Kefzol Vials, Faspak & ADD-Vantage 1279
Kinesed Tablets 2272
Lincocin 2344
Lomotil 2174
Lopid Capsules and Tablets 1736
Lutrepulse for Injection 1655
M-M-R II 1494
M-R-VAX II 1496
Macrodantin Capsules 1624
Mandol Vials, Faspak & ADD-Vantage 1281
Maxzide 1215
Mefoxin 1498
Mefoxin Premixed Intravenous Solution 1500
Meruvax II 1503
Mevacor Tablets (Rare) 1505
Mezlin 1597
Miltown Tablets (Rare) 2386
Minocin Intravenous 1221
Minocin Oral Suspension 1224
Minocin Pellet-Filled Capsules 1222
Mintezol 1510
Mixtard 70/30 1627
Mixtard Human 70/30 1628
Monistat I.V. (Rare) 1143
Monodox Capsules 1630
Motofen Tablets 836
Motrin Tablets (Less than 1%) 2351
Mumpsvax 1513
Mustargen 1514
Nalfon Pulvules & Tablets (Less than 1%) 919
Nasalcrom Nasal Solution (1 case) 986
Navane Capsules and Concentrate (Rare) 1954
Navane Intramuscular (Rare) 1956
Neptazane Tablets ⊙ 311
Nizoral Tablets (Rare) 1145
Oncovin Solution Vials & Hyporets (Rare) 1288
Orthoclone OKT3 Sterile Solution (1 patient) 1645
Orudis Capsules 2488
PCE Dispertab Tablets 549
PMB 200 and PMB 400 2504
PediaProfen Suspension (Less than 1%) 1363
Pediazole 1973
Pepcid (Infrequent) 1524
Pfizerpen for Injection 1957
Pfizerpen-AS Aqueous Suspension 1959
Pitressin Synthetic, Ampoules 1758
Pontocaine Hydrochloride for Spinal Anesthesia 2069
Pro-Banthine Tablets 2141
Proloprim Tablets (Rare) 799
Prostigmin Injectable 1120
Prostigmin Tablets 1121
Protamine Sulfate Ampoules & Vials 1295
Provera Tablets 2356
Quarzan Capsules 1937
Recombivax HB (Less than 1%) 1544
Retrovir Capsules (One patient) 802
Retrovir I.V. Infusion (One patient) 805
Retrovir Syrup (One patient) 802
Robinul Forte Tablets 1873
Robinul Injectable 1873
Robinul Tablets 1873
Rocephin Injectable Vials, ADD-Vantage (Rare) 1914
Rubex 739
Rufen Tablets (Less than 1%) 691
Seldane Tablets 1349
Seldane-D Extended-Release Tablets 1350
Septra 813
Septra I.V. Infusion 808
Septra I.V. Infusion ADD-Vantage Vials 810
Septra 813
Suprax 1235
Tagamet (Rare) 2228
Tao Capsules 1963
Terramycin Capsules 1786
Terramycin Intramuscular Solution 1964
Tetanus Toxoid, Adsorbed Purogenated 1238
Trimpex Tablets (Rare) 1922
Trobicin Sterile Powder (Few cases) 2366
Valpin 50 Tablets 941
Vancocin HCl, Oral Solution & Pulvules (Infrequent) 1304
Vancocin HCl, Vials & ADD-Vantage (Infrequent) 1302
Velosulin (Allergic reaction to insulin) 1627
Velosulin Human (Allergic reaction to insulin) 1628
Vibramycin 1787
Voltaren Tablets (Rare) 1042
Wycillin Injection (Severe & fatal) 2537
Zantac Injection and Zantac Injection Premixed (Rare) 1063
Zantac (Rare) 1065
Zefazone Sterile Powder 2372
Zinacef (Rare) 1066

Androgen excess, signs or symptoms of

A.P.L. 2431
Danocrine Capsules 2046

Anemia
(see also under Aplastic anemia; Hypoplastic anemia; Megaloblastic anemia)

Accutane Capsules (Less than 1%) 1878
Adalat Capsules (10 mg and 20 mg) (Less than 0.5%) 1587
Adriamycin RDF 562
Amikin Injectable (Rare) 602
Amoxil 2193
Anadrol-50 Tablets 2287
Anafranil Capsules (Up to 2%) 650
Ancobon Capsules 1886
Ansaid Tablets (Rare) 2319
Anturane (Rare) 853
Atgam Sterile Solution (Less than 5%) 2320
Atromid-S Capsules 2435
Augmentin Tablets, Powder for Oral Suspension, and Chewable Tablets 2198
Azactam for Injection (Less than 1%) 2252
Azo Gantrisin Tablets 1888
Azulfidine Tablets, EN-tabs, Oral Suspension 1157
Benemid Tablets 1426
BiCNU (Less frequent) 723
Butazolidin Capsules & Tablets (Less than 1%) 1027
Capoten 2255
Capozide 2258
CeeNU 725
Cefizox Injection (Rare) 1012
Children's Advil Suspension (Less than 1%) 2426
Cholybar 1705
Cipro Tablets (Less than 1%) 1589
Clinoril Tablets (Less than 1%) 1433

Clozaril Tablets (Less than 1%) 2000
ColBENEMID Tablets 1436
Cosmegen Injection 1440
▲Cytosar-U Sterile Powder (Among most frequent) 2329
Cytotec (Infrequent) 2159
Cytovene Sterile Powder (2%) 2292
Cytoxan for Injection 726
DTIC-Dome 1595
Dalgan Injection (Less than 1%) 620
Daraprim Tablets 761
Demser Capsules (Rare) 1460
Demulen 2161
Depakene Capsules & Syrup 511
Depakote Tablets 512
Desyrel and Desyrel Dividose (Less than 1%) 1404
Dipentum Capsules (Rare) 1160
Eldepryl (0 of 49 patients) 2250
Empirin with Codeine Phosphate Nos. 2, 3 & 4 764
Enovid 2161
▲Ergamisol Tablets (Up to 6%) 1136
Esimil Tablets 864
▲Eulexin Capsules (6%) 2089
▲Sterile FUDR (Among more common) 1898
Feldene Capsules (1-3%) 1777
Fluorouracil Injection 1897
Ganite Injection 1016
Garamycin Injectable 2093
Geocillin Tablets 1951
Haldol Decanoate 1375
Haldol Injection, Tablets and Concentrate 1373
Hydrea Capsules 728
Indocin Capsules (Less than 1%) 1487
Indocin I.V. (Less than 1%) 1490
Indocin (Less than 1%) 1487
Intal Capsules (Less than 1 in 100,000 patients) 978
Intal Inhaler (Rare) 979
Intal Nebulizer Solution (Rare) 980
Intron A (1 patient) 2097
Ismelin Tablets 869
Klonopin Tablets 1902
Lamprene Capsules (Less than 1%) 1030
Lasix 1093
Lincocin (Rare) 2344
Lippes Loop Intrauterine Double-S.. 1654
Lodine Capsules (Less than 1%) 2468
Lopid Capsules and Tablets (Rare) 1736
▲Lupron Depot 3.75 mg (Among most frequent) 2312
Lupron Depot 7.5 mg 2311
Lupron Injection 2310
▲Matulane Capsules (Frequent) 1907
Mefoxin 1498
Mefoxin Premixed Intravenous Solution 1500
Mellaril 2011
Mesantoin Tablets (Uncommon) 2013
Methotrexate Tablets, Parenteral, LPF Parenteral 1217
Micronase Tablets 2350
Monopril Tablets (0.2 to 1.0%) 1406
Motrin Tablets (Less than 1%) 2351
Myleran Tablets 790
Nebcin Vials, Hyporets & ADD-Vantage 1286
NebuPent for Inhalation Solution (Greater than 1%, up to 5%) 1017
Neosar for Injection (Occasional) 566
Netromycin Injection 100 mg/ml (Fewer than 1 per 1000 patients) 2104
Nimotop Capsules (Less than 1%) 1607
Norethin 2133
Omnipaque (0.3%) 2552
Oncovin Solution Vials & Hyporets 1288
Orinase Tablets 2354
Orudis Capsules (Less than 1%) 2488
ParaGard T380A Intrauterine Copper Contraceptive 411
▲Paraplatin for Injection (21% to 90%) 735
Parnate Tablets 2222
Pentam 300 Injection (Moderate 1.2%) 1018
Permax Tablets (1.1%) 1291
Platinol 737
Plendil Extended-Release Tablets (0.5% to 1.5%) 1526
Prilosec Delayed-Release Capsules 1530
Prinivil Tablets 1538
Procardia Capsules (Less than 0.5%) 1781
Prostin VR Pediatric Sterile Solution (Less than 1%) 2355
Prozac Pulvules (Infrequent) 920
Purinethol Tablets (Frequent) 800
Questran Powder 710
▲Retrovir (3% to 30%) 802
Rheumatrex Methotrexate Dose Pack 1234
Ridaura Capsules (3.1%) 2224
Ritalin 880
Rocephin Injectable Vials, ADD-Vantage (Less than 1%) 1914
Rogaine Topical Solution 2357
Rythmol Tablets (Less than 1%) 1184
Sandimmune (2% or less) 2024
Serentil 686
Sinemet Tablets (Rare) 952
Spectrobid Tablets & Powder for Oral Suspension 1961
Stelazine 2226
Tegretol Suspension 656
Temaril Tablets, Syrup and Spansule Sustained Release Capsules 1085
▲TheraCys BCG Live (Intravesical) (Up to 20.5%) 898
Thiotepa Parenteral 1240
Ticar for Injection 2236
Tonocard Tablets (Less than 1%) .. 1554
Vaseretic Tablets (Less than 1%) .. 1559
Vasotec I.V. (Less than 0.1%) 1562
Velban Vials 1305
▲VePesid Capsules and Injection (33%) 741
Virazole 1126
Wellbutrin Tablets (Rare) 821
Zestoretic 2274
Zestril Tablets 2277
Zoladex (1% to 5%) 1110
Zovirax Sterile Powder (Less than 1%) 828
Zyloprim Tablets (Less than 1%) 830

Anemia, aplastic (see under Aplastic anemia)

Anemia, dilutional

Prolastin Alpha$_1$-Proteinase Inhibitor (Human) 1585

Anemia, glucose-6-phosphate dehydrogenase deficiency

Aralen Phosphate with Primaquine Phosphate Tablets 2040
Macrodantin Capsules 1624
Plaquenil Sulfate Tablets 2067

Anemia, Heinz-body

▲Azulfidine Tablets, EN-tabs, Oral Suspension (3 to 4%) 1157

Anemia, hypoplastic (see under Hypoplastic anemia)

Anemia, iron deficiency

Anadrol-50 Tablets 2287
Ansaid Tablets (Less than 1%) 2319
Azdone Tablets (Infrequent) 844
Damason-P (Infrequent) 1356
Empirin with Codeine Phosphate Nos. 2, 3 & 4 (Infrequent) 764
Fiorinal with Codeine Capsules 2008
Prozac Pulvules (Rare) 920
Questran Light 711
Zorprin Tablets 698

Anemia, microangiopathic hemolytic

Mutamycin 733
Sandimmune 2024

Anemia, nonhemolytic

Sinemet CR Tablets 953

Anemia, normochromic

▲Fungizone Intravenous (Among most common) 2262

Anemia, normocytic

▲Fungizone Intravenous (Among most common) 2262

Anemia, sideroblastic

Cuprimine Capsules 1442
Depen Titratable Tablets 2379
INH Tablets 868

Anesthesia, persistent

Marcaine Hydrochloride with Epinephrine 1:200,000 2055
Marcaine Hydrochloride Injection 2055

Anesthetic effect

Lithium Carbonate Capsules & Tablets 1984
Sensorcaine 631
Sensorcaine-MPF Spinal 634
Tonocard Tablets (Less than 1%) .. 1554
Versed Injection 1924

Anetoderma

Cuprimine Capsules (Rare) 1442
Depen Titratable Tablets 2379

Aneurysm

Anafranil Capsules (Rare) 650

Anger

BuSpar (2%) 1401
Desyrel and Desyrel Dividose (Greater than 1%) 1404
Valium Injectable 1937
Valrelease Capsules (Infrequent) 1923

Angiitis

Esidrix Tablets 863
Esimil Tablets 864
Indocin Capsules (Less than 1%) 1487
Indocin I.V. (Less than 1%) 1490
Indocin (Less than 1%) 1487
Timolide Tablets 1547
Trandate HCT Tablets 579
Zyloprim Tablets (Less than 1%) 830

Angina

Adalat Capsules (10 mg and 20 mg) (1 in 8 patients) 1587
Apresoline Hydrochloride Parenteral (Ampuls) 856
Arfonad Ampuls 1887
Atromid-S Capsules 2435
Bretylol Injection (1-2 in 1000) 923
▲Cardene Capsules (5.6%) 2290
Cardizem Tablets-30 mg, 60 mg, 90 mg and 120 mg (Less than 1%) 1329
Cardizem SR Capsules-60 mg, 90 mg and 120 mg (Less than 1%) 1327
Clozaril Tablets (1%) 2000
Dobutrex Solution Vials (1 to 3%).. 1259
Ergamisol Tablets 1136
Esimil Tablets 864
Sterile FUDR (Remote possibility) .. 1898
Fluorouracil Injection 1897
Harmonyl Tablets 528
Hyperstat I.V. Injection 2095
▲Intropin Injection (Among most frequent) 930
Ismelin Tablets 869
Isuprel Hydrochloride Injection 1:5000 2050
Isuprel Hydrochloride Mistometer .. 2051
Isuprel Hydrochloride Solution 1:200 & 1:100 2052
Loniten Tablets 2346
▲Lupron Depot 3.75 mg (Among most frequent) 2312
Lupron Depot 7.5 mg (Less than 5%) 2311
Lupron Injection (Less than 5%) 2310
Mexitil Capsules (1.7% or about 3 in 1,000) 680
Monopril Tablets (0.2 to 1.0%) 1406
Normodyne Tablets 2110
▲Omnipaque (1 to 8%) 2552
OptiPranolol Sterile Ophthalmic Solution (A small number of patients) ...... ⊙ 261
Ornade Spansule Capsules 2221
Pitressin Synthetic, Ampoules 1758
Prilosec Delayed-Release Capsules (Less than 1%) 1530
Procardia XL Tablets (1% or less).. 1783
Proventil Inhalation Aerosol 2117
Proventil Repetabs Tablets 2120
Proventil Syrup 2119
Proventil Tablets 2120
Quinamm Tablets 1344
Raudixin Tablets 1803
Rauzide Tablets 1804
Renese-R Tablets 1786
Ritalin 880
Rogaine Topical Solution 2357
Ru-Tuss II Capsules 693
▲Rythmol Tablets (1.2 to 4.6%) 1184
Ser-Ap-Es Tablets 881
Serpasil Tablets 883
Serpasil-Apresoline Tablets 884
Serpasil-Esidrix Tablets 886
Sus-Phrine Injection 1006
Tonocard Tablets (Less than 1%) .. 1554
Trental (0.3% to 1.1%) 1099
Trinalin Repetabs Tablets 1170
Tuss-Ornade Liquid 2242
Tuss-Ornade Spansule Capsules 2242
Ventolin 583
Zofran Injection (Rare) 1069

Angina, crescendo

Deponit NTG Transdermal Delivery System 2143
Minitran Transdermal Delivery System (2%) 1312
Nitrodisc (Uncommon) 2176
Nitro-Dur (nitroglycerin) Transdermal Infusion System (Uncommon) 1164
Nitrogard Tablets (Uncommon) 1004
Transderm-Nitro Transdermal Therapeutic System (2%) 2283
Tridil Ampuls & Vials (Uncommon) 939

Angina, increased

Deponit NTG Transdermal Delivery System (2%) 2143
Nitro-Bid IV 1338
Transderm-Nitro Transdermal Therapeutic System (2%) 2283
▲Vascor (200, 300 and 400 mg) Tablets (4.5%) 1383

Angina pectoris

Altace Capsules (Less than 1%) 1086
Ansaid Tablets (Less than 1%) 2319
Apresazide Capsules (Common) 854
Apresoline Hydrochloride Tablets (Common) 855
Apresoline-Esidrix Tablets 857
Brethaire Inhaler 1024
Calan SR Caplets (1% or less) 2157
Calan Tablets (1% or less) 2155
Capoten (2 to 3 of 1000 patients) 2255
Capozide (2 to 3 of 1000 patients) 2258
Cardura Tablets (Less than 0.5% of 3960 patients) 1941
Cartrol Tablets (Less common) 507
Cipro I.V. (1% or less) 1592
Cipro Tablets (Less than 1%) 1589
Diupres Tablets 1461
Dobutrex Solution Vials (1 to 3%).. 1259
Eldepryl 2250
Esimil Tablets 864
Hydropres Tablets 1485
Ismelin Tablets 869
Isoptin Oral Tablets (Less than 1%) 1179
Isoptin SR Sustained Release Tablets (Less than 1%) 1181
Kerlone Tablets (Less than 2%) 2172
Lotensin Tablets 872
Micronor Tablets 1667
Midamor Tablets (Less than or equal to 1%) 1508
Modicon 1667
Moduretic Tablets (Less than or equal to 1%) 1510
Normodyne Injection 2108
Ortho-Novum 1667
Permax Tablets (Infrequent) 1291
Persantine Tablets (Rare) 683
Plendil Extended-Release Tablets (0.5% to 1.5%) 1526
Prinivil Tablets (1% or less) 1538
Prinzide Tablets 1540
Prozac Pulvules (Infrequent) 920
Salutensin/Salutensin-Demi 719
Ser-Ap-Es Tablets 881
Serpasil-Apresoline Tablets 884
Tambocor Tablets (Less than 1%) 1315
Timolide Tablets 1547
Timoptic in Ocudose 1552
Timoptic Sterile Ophthalmic Solution 1550
Vaseretic Tablets 1559
Vasotec I.V. 1562
Verelan Capsules (Less than 1%) .. 1243
Zestoretic 2274
Zestril Tablets (Less than 1%) 2277

Angina pectoris, aggravation

Aldoclor Tablets 1413
Aldomet Ester HCl Injection 1417
Aldomet Oral 1415
Aldoril Tablets 1418
Blocadren Tablets (Less than 1%) 1429
Eldepryl 2250
Feldene Capsules (Less than 1%) .. 1777
Tenoretic Tablets 1105

Angina pectoris, exacerbation of, post-abrupt discontinuation

Normodyne Tablets 2110

Angioedema (see also under Edema, angioneurotic)

Alurate Elixir 1883
Amen 833
Bactrim DS Tablets 1891
Bactrim I.V. Infusion 1889
Bactrim 1891
Beclovent Inhalation Aerosol and Refill 572
Beconase AQ Nasal Spray 574
Beconase Inhalation Aerosol & Refill 574
Butisol Sodium Elixir & Tablets 2377
Capoten (1 in 1,000 patients) 2255
Capozide (Approximately 1 in 1000 patients) 2258
Cardioquin Tablets 1812
Catapres Tablets 676
Ceptaz for Injection (Very rare) 1057
Children's Advil Suspension (Less than 1%) 2426
Chloromycetin Kapseals 1695
Chloromycetin Sodium Succinate 1698
Cipro I.V. (1% or less) 1592
Cipro Tablets 1589
Didronel Tablets (Rare) 1621
Disalcid 1310
Easprin 1719
Eskalith 2214
Feldene Capsules (Less than 1%) 1777
Fortaz (Very rare) 1060
Gammar, Immune Globulin (Human) U.S.P. 609
Hep-B-Gammagee 1474
Beef Regular, 100 Units 1275
Indocin (Less than 1%) 1487
Insulatard NPH 1626
Insulatard NPH Human 1627
Intal Capsules (Less than 1 in 10,000 patients) 978
Intal Inhaler 979
Keflex Pulvules, Oral Suspension & Pediatric Drops 916
Keftab Tablets 917
Macrodantin Capsules 1624
Mebaral Tablets 2061
Mintezol 1510
Mixtard 70/30 1627
Mixtard Human 70/30 1628
Motrin Tablets 2351
Nalfon Pulvules & Tablets 919
Nasalcrom Nasal Solution 986
NegGram 2062
Nembutal Sodium Capsules 534
Nembutal Sodium Solution 536
Nembutal Sodium Suppositories 538
Noroxin Tablets 1519
PediaProfen Suspension (Less than 1%) 1363
Phenobarbital Elixir and Tablets (Less than 1 in 100 patients) 1293
Prinivil Tablets (0.1%) 1538
Proventil Inhalation Aerosol (Rare) 2117
Prozac Pulvules 920
Quinaglute Dura-Tabs Tablets 663
Quinidex Extentabs 1868
Recombivax HB (Less than 1%) 1544
Reglan 1869
Ridaura Capsules 2224
Robaxisal Tablets 1872
Rufen Tablets 691
Seconal Sodium Pulvules (Less than 1 in 100) 1296
Seldane Tablets 1349
Septra 813
Septra I.V. Infusion 808
Septra I.V. Infusion ADD-Vantage Vials 810
Septra 813
Soma Compound w/Codeine Tablets 2390
Soma Compound Tablets 2389
Trental (Less than 1%) 1099
Ultracef Capsules, Tablets & Oral Suspension 722
Vancenase Nasal Inhaler (Rare) 2126
Vanceril Inhaler 2128
Vaseretic Tablets (0.6%) 1559
Vasotec I.V. (0.5 to 1%) 1562
Vasotec Tablets (0.5% to 1%) 1564
Velosulin 1627
Velosulin Human 1628
Ventolin 583
Voltaren Tablets (Less than 1%) 1042
Zestril Tablets (0.1%) 2277
Zorprin Tablets 698

Angioedema, extremities

Altace Capsules 1086
Capoten (1 in 1000 patients) 2255
Capozide (Approximately 1 in 1000 patients) 2258
Lotensin Tablets 872
Monopril Tablets 1406
Prinivil Tablets 1538
Prinzide Tablets (Rare) 1540
Vaseretic Tablets 1559
Vasotec I.V. 1562
Vasotec Tablets 1564
Zestoretic (Rare) 2274
Zestril Tablets 2277

Angioedema, face

Altace Capsules 1086
Capoten (1 in 1000 patients) 2255
Capozide (Approximately 1 in 1000 patients) 2258
Lotensin Tablets (0.5%) 872
Monopril Tablets 1406
Prinivil Tablets 1538
Prinzide Tablets (Rare) 1540
Vaseretic Tablets 1559
Vasotec I.V. 1562
Vasotec Tablets 1564
Zestoretic (Rare) 2274
Zestril Tablets 2277

Angioedema, glottis

Altace Capsules 1086
Capoten (Approximately 1 in 1000 patients) 2255
Capozide (Approximately 1 in 1000 patients) 2258
Lotensin Tablets 872
Monopril Tablets 1406
Prinivil Tablets 1538
Prinzide Tablets (Rare) 1540
Vaseretic Tablets 1559
Vasotec I.V. 1562
Vasotec Tablets 1564
Zestoretic (Rare) 2274
Zestril Tablets 2277

Angioedema, larynx

Altace Capsules 1086
Capoten (Approximately 1 in 1000 patients) 2255
Capozide (Approximately 1 in 1000 patients) 2258
Lotensin Tablets 872
Monopril Tablets 1406
Prinivil Tablets 1538
Prinzide Tablets (Rare) 1540
Vaseretic Tablets 1559
Vasotec I.V. 1562
Vasotec Tablets 1564
Zestoretic (Rare) 2274
Zestril Tablets 2277

Angioedema, lips

Altace Capsules 1086
Capoten (Approximately 1 in 1000 patients) 2255
Capozide (Approximately 1 in 1000 patients) 2258
Lotensin Tablets (0.5%) 872
Monopril Tablets 1406
Prinivil Tablets 1538
Prinzide Tablets (Rare) 1540
Vaseretic Tablets 1559
Vasotec I.V. 1562
Vasotec Tablets 1564
Zestoretic (Rare) 2274
Zestril Tablets 2277

Angioedema, mucous membranes of the mouth

Capoten (1 in 1000 patients) 2255
Capozide (Approximately 1 in 1000 patients) 2258

Angioedema of tongue

Altace Capsules 1086
Capoten (Approximately 1 in 1000 patients) 2255
Capozide (Approximately 1 in 1000 patients) 2258
Catapres-TTS (One case) 677
Lotensin Tablets 872
Monopril Tablets 1406
Prinivil Tablets 1538
Prinzide Tablets (Rare) 1540
Vaseretic Tablets 1559
Vasotec I.V. 1562
Vasotec Tablets 1564
Zestoretic (Rare) 2274
Zestril Tablets 2277

Anhidrosis

Cogentin 1435

Anisocoria

Anafranil Capsules (Up to 2%) 650
Betoptic Sterile Ophthalmic Solution (Small numbers of patients) 569
Betoptic S Sterile Ophthalmic Suspension (Small numbers of patients) 570

Ankylosing spondylosis

Lupron Depot 7.5 mg 2311
Lupron Injection 2310

Anorexia

Achromycin V Capsules 1193
Actifed with Codeine Cough Syrup 752
▲ Actimmune (3%) 1046
Adriamycin PFS (Occasional) 561
Adriamycin RDF (Occasional) 562
Aldactazide 2150
Aldoclor Tablets 1413
Aldoril Tablets 1418
▲ Alferon N Injection (45% to 68%) 1809
Altace Capsules (Less than 1%) 1086
▲ Anafranil Capsules (12% to 22%) 650
Ancef Injection 2194
Ancobon Capsules 1886
Apresazide Capsules (Common) 854
Apresoline Hydrochloride Parenteral (Ampuls) 856
Apresoline Hydrochloride Tablets (Common) 855
Apresoline-Esidrix Tablets 857
Aquasol A Vitamin A Capsules, USP 615
Aquasol A Parenteral, USP 615
Aralen Hydrochloride Injection 2038
Aralen Phosphate with Primaquine Phosphate Tablets 2040
Aralen Phosphate Tablets 2039
Arfonad Ampuls 1887
Asendin Tablets (Very rare) 1196
Atabrine Hydrochloride Tablets 2041
Atrohist Sprinkle Capsules 558
Azo Gantanol Tablets 1887
Azo Gantrisin Tablets 1888
▲ Azulfidine Tablets, EN-tabs, Oral Suspension (Approximately one-third of patients) 1157
▲ Bactrim DS Tablets (Among most common) 1891
▲ Bactrim I.V. Infusion (Among most common) 1889
▲ Bactrim (Among most common) 1891
Benadryl Capsules 1691
Benadryl Injection 1692
Benemid Tablets 1426
Bentyl 1322
Blenoxane (Common) 724
Brevibloc Injection (Less than 1%) 942
BuSpar (Infrequent) 1401
Calcijex Calcitriol Injection 506
Calderol Capsules 1635
Capoten (About 0.5 to 2%) 2255
Capozide (0.5 to 2%) 2258
Cardizem Tablets-30 mg, 60 mg, 90 mg and 120 mg (Less than 1%) 1329
Cardizem SR Capsules-60 mg, 90 mg and 120 mg (Less than 1%) 1327
Cardura Tablets (Less than 0.5% of 3960 patients) 1941
Catapres Tablets (About 1 in 100 patients) 676
Catapres-TTS (1%) 677
Celontin (Frequent) 1692
Cholybar (Less frequent) 1705
Cibacalcin Double-chambered Syringes (Few) 859
Cibalith-S 870
Cipro I.V. (1% or less) 1592
Cipro Tablets (Less than 1%) 1589
Clinoril Tablets (Greater than 1%) 1433
Clozaril Tablets (1%) 2000
ColBENEMID Tablets 1436
Colestid Granules (1-3 patients in 1,000) 2328
Combipres Tablets (About 1%) 678
Comhist LA Capsules 1618
Compazine Ampuls 2201
▲ Cordarone Tablets (4 to 9%) 2446
Corgard Tablets (1 to 5 of 1000 patients) 701
Corzide Tablets (1 to 5 of 1000 patients) 702
Cosmegen Injection 1440
Crystodigin Tablets 1253
Cuprimine Capsules 1442
Cylert Tablets 510
▲ Cytadren Tablets (1 in 8) 861
▲ Cytosar-U Sterile Powder (Among most frequent) 2329
Cytovene Sterile Powder (1% or less) 2292
Cytoxan for Injection 726
▲ DTIC-Dome (90% with the initial few doses) 1595
Dalmane Capsules (Rare) 1927
Dantrium Capsules (Less frequent) 1619
Daranide Tablets (Among the most common effects) 1445
Daraprim Tablets 761
Declomycin Capsules, Tablets 1199
Deconamine 663
Depakene Capsules & Syrup 511
Depakote 512
▲ Depen Titratable Tablets (17%) 2379
Dexedrine 2206
Diabinese Tablets (Less than 2%) 1775
Diamox Parenteral 1200
Diamox Sequels (Sustained Release) 1201
Diamox Tablets 1200
Dilaudid-HP Injection 1175
Dimetane-DC Cough Syrup 1857
Dimetane-DX Cough Syrup 1858
Dipentum Capsules (1.3%) 1160
Diphtheria and Tetanus Toxoids and Pertussis Vaccine Adsorbed USP (For Pediatric Use) (Frequent) 892
Diucardin Tablets 2450
Diulo 2129
Diupres Tablets 1461
Diuril Oral Suspension 1464
Diuril Sodium Intravenous 1463
Diuril Tablets 1464
Dolobid Tablets (Less than 1 in 100) 1465
Dolophine Hydrochloride Ampoules & Vials 1260
Dolophine Hydrochloride Tablets 1261
Doral Tablets 2383
Doryx Capsules 1717
Doxorubicin Hydrochloride for Injection, USP (Occasional) 622
Doxorubicin Hydrochloride Injection, USP (Occasional) 848
▲ Duragesic Transdermal System (3% to 10%) 1133
▲ E.E.S. (Among most frequent) 522
Edecrin 1468
Elavil 2269
Eldepryl 2250
Elspar 1470
▲ Emcyt Capsules (4%) 1161
Emete-con Intramuscular/Intravenous 1950
Endep Tablets 1927
Enduron Tablets 517
Enduronyl 518
Engerix-B Unit-Dose Vials (Less than 1%) 2213
▲ Ergamisol Tablets (2 to 6%) 1136
▲ ERYC (Among most frequent) 1720
▲ EryPed (Among most frequent) 519
▲ Ery-Tab Tablets (Among most frequent) 521
▲ Erythrocin Stearate Filmtab (Among most frequent) 523
▲ Erythromycin Base Filmtab (Among most frequent) 525
▲ Erythromycin Delayed-Release Capsules, USP (Among most frequent) 526
Esidrix Tablets 863
Esimil Tablets 864
Eskalith 2214
Ethmozine Tablets (Less than 2%) 946
Etrafon 2087
Eulexin Capsules 2089
Exna Tablets 1862
Sterile FUDR 1898
Fedahist Gyrocaps 2145
Fedahist Timecaps 2145
Feldene Capsules (1 to 3%) 1777
Fiorinal with Codeine Capsules 2008
Flagyl Tablets 2170
Flexeril Tablets (Less than 1%) 1471
Fluorouracil Injection (Common) 1897
▲ Fungizone Intravenous (Among most common) 2262
Gantanol 1899
Gantrisin Ophthalmic Ointment/Solution 1900
Gantrisin 1901
Geocillin Tablets 1951
Halcion Tablets 2340
Haldol Decanoate 1375
Haldol Injection, Tablets and Concentrate 1373

Harmonyl Tablets 528
Hexalen Capsules (1%) 2316
HibTITER 1206
Hydrea Capsules 728
HydroDIURIL Tablets 1484
Hydromox R Tablets 1209
Hydromox Tablets 1208
Hydropres Tablets 1485
▲ Hylorel Tablets (18.7%) 975
Hyperstat I.V. Injection 2095
INH Tablets 868
IFEX (Less than 1%) 729
Inderide Tablets 2463
Inderide LA Long Acting Capsules 2465
Indocin (Less than 1%) 1487
Inocor Lactate Injection (0.4%) 2048
▲ Intron A (1% to 41%) 2097
Inversine Tablets 1492
Kayexalate 2053
Kefzol Vials, Faspak & ADD-Vantage 1279
Kerlone Tablets (Less than 2%) 2172
Ketalar 1726
Klonopin Tablets 1902
Lamprene Capsules (Less than 1%) 1030
Lanoxicaps (Common) 772
Lanoxin Elixir Pediatric (Common) 775
Lanoxin Injection (Common) 778
Lanoxin Injection Pediatric (Common) 781
Lanoxin Tablets (Common) 783
▲ Lariam Tablets (Among most frequent) 1904
Larodopa Tablets (Relatively frequent) 1905
Lasix 1093
Leukine for IV Infusion 1127
Limbitrol 1933
Lioresal Tablets (Rare) 1031
Lithane Tablets 1596
Lithium Carbonate Capsules & Tablets 1984
Lithobid Tablets 870
Lodine Capsules (Less than 1%) 2468
Lomotil 2174
Lopressor HCT Tablets (1 in 100 patients) 1034
Lorelco Tablets 1333
Lozol Tablets (Less than 5%) 1843
Lupron Depot 7.5 mg (Less than 5%) 2311
▲ Lupron Injection (5% or more) 2310
Lysodren 731
MS Contin Tablets (Infrequent) 1814
MSIR (Infrequent) 1817
▲ Macrodantin Capsules (Most often) 1624
▲ Marplan Tablets (Among most frequent) 1906
Maxair Inhaler (Less than 1%) 1311
Maxzide 1215
Meclomen Capsules (Greater than 1%) 1739
Mellaril 2011
Methadone Hydrochloride Diskets 1284
Methadone Hydrochloride Oral Solution & Tablets 1987
Methotrexate Tablets, Parenteral, LPF Parenteral (Less common) 1217
Mevacor Tablets 1505
▲ Midamor Tablets (3% to 8%) 1508
Milontin Kapseals (Frequent) 1741
Minizide Capsules 1779
Minocin Intravenous 1221
Minocin Oral Suspension 1224
Minocin Pellet-Filled Capsules 1222
Mintezol 1510
Mithracin 1602
▲ Moduretic Tablets (3% to 8%) 1510
Monistat I.V. 1143
Monodox Capsules 1630
Motofen Tablets 836
Mustargen 1514
▲ Mutamycin (14%) 733
Myambutol Tablets 1225
Mykrox ½ mg Tablets 984
Myleran Tablets 790
Myochrysine Injection 1516
Mysoline (Occasional) 2480
Naldecon Syrup, Tablets, Pediatric Drops and Pediatric Syrup 709
Nalfon Pulvules & Tablets (Less than 1%) 919
Naturetin Tablets (Common) 1789
Navane Capsules and Concentrate 1954
Navane Intramuscular 1956
Neo-Calglucon Syrup 2018
Neosar for Injection (Common) 566
Neptazane Tablets ⊙ 311
▲ Neupogen for Injection (9%) 595
▲ Niclocide Chewable Tablets (3.4%) 1607
Nicorette (1.1%) 1335
Nolvadex Tablets (1%) 1102
Normodyne Injection 2108
Normodyne Tablets 2110
Normozide Tablets 2112
Norpace (1 to 3%) 2177
Norpramin Tablets 1340
Norzine 1818
Novafed A Capsules 1342
Novahistine DH 1342
Novahistine Elixir ◙ 596
Oncovin Solution Vials & Hyporets 1288
Optimine Tablets 2115
Oramorph SR (Morphine Sulfate Sustained Release Tablets) (Less frequent) 1988
Orap Tablets 1020
Oretic Tablets 544
Oreticyl 545
Ornade Spansule Capsules 2221
Orudis Capsules (Greater than 1%) 2488
PBZ Tablets & Elixir 1037
PBZ-SR Tablets 1037
▲ PCE Dispertab Tablets (Among most frequent) 549
Pamelor 2019
Papaverine Hydrochloride Vials and Ampoules 1290
Paradione Capsules 548
▲ Parlodel (4%) 2020
Parnate Tablets 2222
Pavabid Capsules (Rare) 1344
Pavabid HP Capsules (Rare) 1344
Pediazole 1973
▲ Pentam 300 Injection (5.9%) 1018
Pepcid (Infrequent) 1524
Periactin 1525
▲ Permax Tablets (4.8%) 1291
▲ Phenurone Tablets (5%) 552
PhosLo Tablets 700
Plaquenil Sulfate Tablets 2067
Platinol 737
Platinol-AQ Injection 738
Polaramine 2116
Ponstel (Less frequent) 1758
Potaba (Infrequent) 1071
Prilosec Delayed-Release Capsules (Less than 1%) 1530
Prinivil Tablets (1% or less) 1538
Prinzide Tablets 1540
▲ Procan SR Tablets (3-4%) 1760
Proglycem (Frequent) 649
▲ ProHIBiT Haemophilus b Conjugate Vaccine (Diphtheria Toxoid Conjugate) (16.1%) 896
Prokine for I.V. Infusion 1096
▲ Pronestyl Capsules and Tablets (3-4%) 1800
Pronestyl Injection 1798
▲ Pronestyl-SR Tablets (3 to 4%) 1801
Protostat Tablets 1674
Proventil Syrup (Children 2-6: 1%) 2119
▲ Prozac Pulvules (8.7%) 920
Purinethol Tablets (Uncommon) 800
Quadrinal Tablets 1183
Questran Light (Less frequent) 711
Questran Powder 710
▲ Quinidex Extentabs (Among most frequent) 1868
Raudixin Tablets 1803
Rauzide Tablets 1804
Renese Tablets 1785
Renese-R Tablets 1786
Restoril Capsules (1-2%) 2023
▲ Retrovir Capsules (11%) 802
▲ Retrovir I.V. Infusion (11%) 805
▲ Retrovir Syrup (11%) 802
Rheumatrex Methotrexate Dose Pack (Less common) 1234
▲ Ridaura Capsules (3 to 9%) 2224
Rifadin (Some patients) 1345
Rifamate Capsules (Some patients) 1347
Rimactane Capsules 879
Ritalin 880
Rocaltrol Capsules 1913
▲ Roferon-A Injection (46% to 65%) 1916
Rondec 1975
Rondec-DM 1976
Rondec-TR Tablet 1975
Roxanol 1991
Rubex (Occasional) 739
Ru-Tuss II Capsules 693
Ru-Tuss with Hydrocodone 694
Ru-Tuss Tablets 693
Rythmol Tablets (0.5 to 1.7%) 1184
Saluron 718
Salutensin/Salutensin-Demi 719
Sandimmune (2% or less) 2024
Sandostatin Injection (Less than 1%) 2029
Sectral Capsules 2520
▲ Seldane-D Extended-Release Tablets (3.7%) 1350
▲ Septra (Among most common) 813
▲ Septra I.V. Infusion (Most common) 808
▲ Septra I.V. Infusion ADD-Vantage Vials (Most common) 810
▲ Septra (Among most common) 813
Ser-Ap-Es Tablets 881
Serentil 686
Serpasil Tablets 883
Serpasil-Apresoline Tablets 884
Serpasil-Esidrix Tablets 886
Sinemet Tablets (Less frequent) 952
Sinemet CR Tablets (1.2%) 953
Sinequan 1960
Sodium Polystyrene Sulfonate Suspension 1993
Solganal Suspension (Rare) 2122
Stelazine 2226
Stilphostrol Tablets and Ampuls 1609
Surmontil Capsules 2524
Symmetrel Capsules & Syrup (1-5%) 936
Tacaryl 2409
Talacen (Rare) 2070
Talwin Compound (Rare) 2072
Talwin Nx 2073
Tambocor Tablets (1-3%) 1315
Tapazole Tablets 1298
Tavist Syrup 2033
Tavist Tablets 2035
Tavist-D Tablets 2035
Tegretol Chewable Tablets 654
Tegretol Suspension 656
Tegretol Tablets 654
Temaril Tablets, Syrup and Spansule Sustained Release Capsules 1085
Tenoretic Tablets 1105
Terramycin Capsules 1786
Terramycin Intramuscular Solution 1964
Teslac Tablets 741
Thalitone Tablets 687
▲ TheraCys BCG Live (Intravesical) (Up to 10.7%) 898
Thioguanine Tablets, Tabloid Brand 815
Thiosulfil Forte Tablets 2526
Thiotepa Parenteral 1240
Timolide Tablets 1547
Timoptic in Ocudose 1552
Timoptic Sterile Ophthalmic Solution 1550
Tofranil Ampuls 1038
Tofranil Tablets 1039
Tofranil-PM Capsules 1041
▲ Tonocard Tablets (1.2-11.3%) 1554
Torecan 1993
Trandate HCT Tablets 579
Trandate Injection 577
Trental (Less than 1%) 1099
Triaminic Expectorant DH 1995
Triaminic Oral Infant Drops 1996
Triavil Tablets 1556
Tridione 557
Tri-Immunol Diphtheria & Tetanus Toxoids & Pertussis Vaccine, Adsorbed 1241
Trilafon (Occasional) 2123
Trilisate (Less than 1%) 1822
Trinalin Repetabs Tablets 1170
Tuss-Ornade Liquid 2242
Tuss-Ornade Spansule Capsules 2242
▲ Vascor (200, 300 and 400 mg) Tablets (3.02 to 6.82%) 1383
Vaseretic Tablets 1559
Vasotec I.V. 1562
Vasotec Tablets (0.5% to 1.0%) 1564
Velban Vials 1305
Ventolin Syrup (1% of children) 583
▲ VePesid Capsules and Injection (10 to 13%) 741
Vibramycin Hyclate Capsules 1787
Vibramycin Hyclate Intravenous 1968
Vibramycin 1787
Vira-A for Injection 1766
Vivactil Tablets 1567
▲ Wellbutrin Tablets (18.3%) 821
Xanax Tablets 2367
Zarontin Capsules (Frequent) 1768
Zarontin Syrup (Frequent) 1769
Zaroxolyn Tablets 989
Zestoretic 2274
Zestril Tablets (Less than 1%) 2277
▲ Zoladex (5%) 1110
Zovirax Capsules (0.3%) 824
Zovirax Sterile Powder (Less than 1%) 828
Zovirax (0.3%) 824
Zyloprim Tablets (Less than 1%) 830

Anorgasmia

Anafranil Capsules (Rare) 650
Eldepryl 2250
Nardil (Common) 1742

Anosmia

Cipro I.V. (1% or less) 1592
Cipro Tablets 1589
Decadron Phosphate Turbinaire 1456
Ergamisol Tablets (1%) 1136
NebuPent for Inhalation Solution (1% or less) 1017
Vaseretic Tablets 1559
Vasotec I.V. 1562
Vasotec Tablets 1564

Anotia, fetal

Accutane Capsules 1878

Antibodies development, persistent

Epogen for Injection 591
Geref (sermorelin acetate for injection) (Approximately 1 in 4 patients) 2560
Procrit for Injection 1647
Protropin (B 30%) 1049

Anticholinergic syndrome

Anafranil Capsules (Rare) 650

Antidiuretic effect

Actibine 900
Dayto Himbin Tablets and Liquid 905
Demerol 2047
MS Contin Tablets (Infrequent) 1814
MSIR 1817
Mepergan Injection 2479
Methadone Hydrochloride Diskets 1284
Oramorph SR (Morphine Sulfate Sustained Release Tablets) (Less frequent) 1988
Phenergan with Codeine 2497
Phenergan VC with Codeine 2501
Yohimex Tablets 1190

Antimitochondrial antibodies

Normodyne Tablets 2110
Normozide Tablets 2112
Trandate HCT/Trandate 579

Antithrombin, decrease

Brevicon 2304
Estrace 1385
Estrace Vaginal Cream 1388
Estratest 2245
Micronor Tablets 1667
Modicon 1667
Norinyl 2304
Ortho-Novum 1667
Tri-Norinyl 28-Day Tablets 2304

Anuria

Azo Gantanol Tablets 1887
Azo Gantrisin Tablets 1888
Azulfidine Tablets, EN-tabs, Oral Suspension (Rare) 1157
Bactrim DS Tablets 1891
Bactrim I.V. Infusion 1889
Bactrim 1891
Butazolidin Capsules & Tablets (Less than 1%) 1027
Deprol Tablets (Rare) 2382
Equagesic Tablets 2451
Fansidar Tablets 1896
Fungizone Intravenous 2262
Gantanol 1899
Gantrisin Ophthalmic Ointment/Solution 1900
Gantrisin 1901
Miltown Tablets (Rare) 2386
Nalfon Pulvules & Tablets (Less than 1%) 919
Omnipaque (Rare) 2552
PMB 200 and PMB 400 (Rare) 2504
Pediazole 1973
Primaxin I.M. 1532
Primaxin I.V. (Less than 0.2%) 1535
Prostin VR Pediatric Sterile Solution (Less than 1%) 2355
Septra 813
Septra I.V. Infusion 808
Septra I.V. Infusion ADD-Vantage Vials 810
Septra 813
Thiosulfil Forte Tablets 2526

(◙ Described in PDR For Nonprescription Drugs) Incidence data in parenthesis; ▲ 3% or more (⊙ Described in PDR For Ophthalmology)

Zanosar Sterile Powder 2371
Zovirax Sterile Powder (Less than 1%) 828

Anxiety

Actifed with Codeine Cough Syrup 752
Actigall Capsules 2280
▲Adrenalin Chloride Solution 1:100 & 1:1,000 (Often) 1689
AeroBid Inhaler System (1-3%) 995
Altace Capsules 1086
Alurate Elixir (Less than 1 in 100) 1883
Amoxil (Rare) 2193
▲Anafranil Capsules (2% to 9%) 650
Ana-Kit Anaphylaxis Emergency Treatment Kit 1100
Android 1111
Anexsia 5/500 Tablets 2196
Anexsia 7.5/650 Tablets 2197
Ansaid Tablets (1-3%) 2319
Apresazide Capsules (Less frequent) 854
Apresoline Hydrochloride Parenteral (Ampuls) 856
Apresoline Hydrochloride Tablets (Less frequent) 855
Apresoline-Esidrix Tablets 857
Arm-a-Med Isoetharine Inhalation Solution, USP 616
Asendin Tablets (Greater than 1%) 1196
Astramorph/PF Injection, USP (Preservative-Free) 618
Atrohist Sprinkle Capsules 558
Augmentin Tablets, Powder for Oral Suspension, and Chewable Tablets (Rare) 2198
Azdōne Tablets 844
Azo Gantrisin Tablets 1888
BAL in Oil Ampules 661
Brethine Ampuls (Less than 0.5%) 1026
Bretylol Injection (1 in 1000) 923
Brevibloc Injection (Less than 1%) 942
Brevital Sodium Vials 1248
Bronkometer Aerosol 2042
Bronkosol Solution 2042
Butisol Sodium Elixir & Tablets (Less than 1 in 100) 2377
Carbocaine Hydrochloride Injection 2043
Cardene Capsules (Rare) 2290
Cartrol Tablets (Less common) 507
Catapres Tablets 676
Catapres-TTS 677
Cholybar 1705
Cipro I.V. (1% or less) 1592
Clozaril Tablets (1%) 2000
Colestid Granules (Fewer than 1 in 1,000) 2328
Combipres Tablets 678
Cytotec (Infrequent) 2159
Dalgan Injection (Less than 1%) 620
Damason-P 1356
Danocrine Capsules (Rare) 2046
Deconamine 663
Deconsal 559
Demser Capsules 1460
Deprol Tablets 2382
Dilaudid Cough Syrup 1174
Dilaudid 1173
Diprivan Injection (Less than 1%) 2267
Doral Tablets 2383
▲Duragesic Transdermal System (3% to 10%) 1133
Duramorph 960
Elavil 2269
Eldepryl (1 of 49 patients) 2250
Emcyt Capsules (1%) 1161
Endep Tablets 1927
EpiPen 843
Ergamisol Tablets (1%) 1136
Estratest 2245
Ethmozine Tablets (0.3-less than 2%) 946
Etrafon 2087
Eulexin Capsules (1%) 2089
Fedahist Gyrocaps 2145
Fedahist Timecaps 2145
Fiorinal with Codeine Capsules 2008
Flexeril Tablets (Less than 1%) 1471
Floxin Tablets (Less than 1%) 1652
Gamimune N Immune Globulin Intravenous (Human) 1572
Gastrocrom Capsules (Infrequent) 974
Haldol Decanoate 1375
Haldol Injection, Tablets and Concentrate 1373
Halotestin Tablets 2341
Hycodan Syrup, Tablets 927
Hycomine Compound Tablets 929
Hycomine Syrup 927
Hycotuss Expectorant Syrup 930
Hydrocet Capsules 835
Hyperstat I.V. Injection 2095
Hytrin Tablets 529
Inapsine Injection 1140
Indocin (Less than 1%) 1487
Infumorph 200 and Infumorph 500 Sterile Solutions 962
Innovar Injection 1141
▲Intron A (Up to 5%) 2097
K-Lyte 707
Lariam Tablets 1904
Larodopa Tablets (Relatively frequent) 1905
Levophed Bitartrate Injection 2054
Lortab ASA Tablets 2414
Lortab 2412
Lotensin Tablets 872
▲Lozol Tablets (Greater than or equal to 5%) 1843
▲Ludiomil Tablets (3%) 874
▲Lupron Depot 3.75 mg (Among most frequent) 2312
Lupron Depot 7.5 mg 2311
▲Lupron Injection (Greater than 5%) 2310
Marcaine Hydrochloride with Epinephrine 1:200,000 2055
Marcaine Hydrochloride Injection 2055
Marcaine Spinal 2058
▲Marinol (Dronabinol) Capsules (16%) 1985
Maxair Inhaler (Less than 1%) 1311
Maxzide 1215
Mebaral Tablets (Less than 1 in 100) 2061
Metandren Linguets and Tablets 875
Methadone Hydrochloride Diskets 1284
Mevacor Tablets 1505
Murocoll-2 Sterile Ophthalmic Solution ⊙ 261
Mykrox ½ mg Tablets (Less than 2%) 984
Nardil (Less frequent) 1742
NebuPent for Inhalation Solution (1% or less) 1017
Nembutal Sodium Capsules (Less than 1%) 534
Nembutal Sodium Solution (Less than 1%) 536
Nembutal Sodium Suppositories (Less than 1%) 538
Nescaine/Nescaine MPF 629
Norpramin Tablets 1340
Novafed A Capsules 1342
Novafed Capsules 1342
Novahistine DH 1342
Novahistine DMX ▣ 595
Novahistine Elixir ▣ 596
Novahistine Expectorant 1343
Omnipaque 2552
OptiPranolol Sterile Ophthalmic Solution (A small number of patients) ⊙ 261
Orap Tablets 1020
Pamelor 2019
Parlodel 2020
Parnate Tablets 2222
Pentaspan Injection 949
Pepcid (Infrequent) 1524
▲Permax Tablets (6.4%) 1291
Pfizerpen-AS Aqueous Suspension (Approximately 1 in 500) 1959
Phenergan VC 2500
Phenergan VC with Codeine 2501
Phenobarbital Elixir and Tablets (Less than 1 in 100 patients) 1293
Plendil Extended-Release Tablets (0.5% to 1.5%) 1526
Pondimin Tablets 1867
Premarin with Methyltestosterone 2515
Prilosec Delayed-Release Capsules (Less than 1%) 1530
Procardia XL Tablets (1% or less) 1783
Proglycem 649
ProSom Tablets (Frequent) 554
▲Prozac Pulvules (9.4%) 920
Questran Light 711
Questran Powder 710
Reglan 1869
Retrovir Capsules (Less than 5%) 802
Retrovir I.V. Infusion (Less than 5%) 805
Retrovir Syrup (Less than 5%) 802
Roferon-A Injection (Less than 3%) 1916
Rogaine Topical Solution (0.36%) 2357
Ru-Tuss DE Tablets 694
Rythmol Tablets (0.7 to 2.0%) 1184
Sandimmune (Rare) 2024
Sandostatin Injection (Less than 1%) 2029
Seconal Sodium Pulvules (Less than 1 in 100) 1296
Sectral Capsules (Up to 2%) 2520
Seldane-D Extended-Release Tablets 1350
Sensorcaine 631
Sensorcaine-MPF Spinal 634
Ser-Ap-Es Tablets 881
Serpasil-Apresoline Tablets 884
Sinemet Tablets 952
Sinemet CR Tablets 953
Surmontil Capsules 2524
Sus-Phrine Injection 1006
Symmetrel Capsules & Syrup (1-5%) 936
Tagamet 2228
Tambocor Tablets (1-3%) 1315
Tegison Capsules (Less than 1%) 1881
Tenex Tablets 1875
Tenuate 1354
Testred Capsules 1124
Timoptic in Ocudose 1552
Timoptic Sterile Ophthalmic Solution 1550
Tofranil Ampuls 1038
Tofranil Tablets 1039
Tofranil-PM Capsules 1041
Tonocard Tablets (1.1-1.5%) 1554
Trental (Less than 1%) 1099
▲Trexan Tablets (Greater than 10%) 937
Triavil Tablets 1556
Trinalin Repetabs Tablets 1170
Tussionex Extended-Release Suspension 988
Vascor (200, 300 and 400 mg) Tablets (0.5 to 2.0%) 1383
Vasoxyl Injection 819
Versed Injection (Less than 1%) 1924
Vicodin Tablets 1187
Vicodin ES Tablets 1189
Visken Tablets (2% or fewer patients) 2036
Vivactil Tablets 1567
Voltaren Tablets (Less than 1%) 1042
▲Wellbutrin Tablets (3.1%) 821
Wytensin Tablets (3% or less) 2542
▲Xanax Tablets (16.6%) 2367
Xylocaine Injections 637
▲Yutopar (5 to 6% with IV administration) 647
Zoladex (1% to 5%) 1110
Zydone Capsules 941

Anxiety, paradoxical

Diupres Tablets 1461
Halcion Tablets 2340
Hydropres Tablets 1485
Raudixin Tablets 1803
Rauzide Tablets 1804
Renese-R Tablets 1786
Salutensin/Salutensin-Demi 719
Ser-Ap-Es Tablets 881
Serpasil Tablets 883
Serpasil-Apresoline Tablets 884
Serpasil-Esidrix Tablets 886
Valium Injectable 1937
Valium Tablets 1939
Valrelease Capsules 1923
Vivactil Tablets 1567

Apathy

Anafranil Capsules (Infrequent) 650
Bactrim DS Tablets 1891
Bactrim I.V. Infusion 1889
Bactrim 1891
BuSpar (Infrequent) 1401
Doral Tablets 2383
Eldepryl 2250
Fansidar Tablets 1896
Gantanol 1899
Gantrisin 1901
Intron A (1 patient) 2097
Lanoxicaps 772
Lanoxin Elixir Pediatric 775
Lanoxin Injection 778
Lanoxin Injection Pediatric 781
Lanoxin Tablets 783
Permax Tablets (Infrequent) 1291
Prilosec Delayed-Release Capsules (Less than 1%) 1530
ProSom Tablets (Infrequent) 554
Prozac Pulvules (Infrequent) 920
Roferon-A Injection (Less than 1%) 1916
Septra 813
Septra I.V. Infusion 808
Septra I.V. Infusion ADD-Vantage Vials 810
Septra 813
Tambocor Tablets (Less than 1%) 1315

Apgar score, low

Syntocinon Injection 2032

Aphasia

Anafranil Capsules (Rare) 650
Duragesic Transdermal System (Less than 1%) 1133
Intron A (2 patients) 2097
Methotrexate Tablets, Parenteral, LPF Parenteral 1217
Omnipaque (Rare) 2552
Rheumatrex Methotrexate Dose Pack 1234
Roferon-A Injection (Less than 0.5%) 1916
Wellbutrin Tablets (Rare) 821

Aphonia

BuSpar (Rare) 1401
Klonopin Tablets 1902
Roferon-A Injection (Less than 0.5%) 1916

Aplasia, red cell

Cuprimine Capsules 1442
Depen Titratable Tablets 2379
Ridaura Capsules (Less than 1%) 2224
Tolinase Tablets 2365

Aplasia, unspecified

Atgam Sterile Solution (Less than 5%) 2320

Aplasia cutis, fetal

Tapazole Tablets (Rare) 1298

Aplastic anemia

AK-Chlor Sterile Ophthalmic Ointment & Solution ⊙ 201
Aldactazide 2150
Aldoclor Tablets 1413
Aldoril Tablets 1418
Anaprox and Anaprox DS Tablets (Rare) 2288
Ancobon Capsules 1886
Ansaid Tablets (Rare) 2319
Anturane 853
Apresazide Capsules 854
Apresoline-Esidrix Tablets 857
Atabrine Hydrochloride Tablets 2041
Azo Gantanol Tablets 1887
Azo Gantrisin Tablets 1888
Azulfidine Tablets, EN-tabs, Oral Suspension (Rare) 1157
Bactrim DS Tablets (Rare) 1891
Bactrim I.V. Infusion (Rare) 1889
Bactrim (Rare) 1891
Butazolidin Capsules & Tablets (Less than 1%) 1027
Capozide 2258
Ceftin Tablets 575
Ceptaz for Injection 1057
Chloromycetin Hydrocortisone Ophthalmic 1694
Chloromycetin Kapseals 1695
Chloromycetin Ophthalmic Ointment, 1% 1696
Chloromycetin Ophthalmic Solution 1696
Chloromycetin Otic 1697
Chloromycetin Palmitate, Oral Suspension 1697
Chloromycetin Sodium Succinate 1698
Chloroptic Sterile Ophthalmic Solution (Rare) ⊙ 243
Clinoril Tablets (Less than 1 in 100) 1433
Colchicine Ampoules 1252
Combipres Tablets 678
Compazine 2201
Corzide Tablets 702
Cosmegen Injection 1440
Cuprimine Capsules 1442
Cylert Tablets (Isolated reports) 510
Cytovene Sterile Powder (2%) 2292
Dapsone USP 1130
Depakote Sprinkle Capsules 512
Depen Titratable Tablets 2379
DiaBeta 1091
Diabinese Tablets 1775
Diamox Parenteral 1200
Diamox Sequels (Sustained Release) 1201
Diamox Tablets 1200
Diucardin Tablets 2450
Diulo 2129
Diupres Tablets 1461
Diuril Oral Suspension 1464
Diuril Sodium Intravenous 1463
Diuril Tablets 1464
Dyazide Capsules 2208

Eminase (Less than 1%) 2211
Enduron Tablets 517
Enduronyl 518
Equagesic Tablets 2451
Esidrix Tablets 863
Esimil Tablets 864
Exna Tablets 1862
FML-S Sterile Ophthalmic Suspension ◉ 246
Fansidar Tablets 1896
Feldene Capsules (Less than 1%) 1777
Fortaz 1060
Gantanol 1899
Gantrisin Ophthalmic Ointment/Solution 1900
Gantrisin 1901
Glucotrol 1952
▲ Hexalen Capsules (13% to 33%) 2316
HydroDIURIL Tablets 1484
Hydromox R Tablets 1209
Hydromox Tablets 1208
Hydropres Tablets 1485
INH Tablets 868
Inderide Tablets 2463
Inderide LA Long Acting Capsules 2465
Indocin Capsules (Less than 1%) 1487
Indocin I.V. (Less than 1%) 1490
Indocin (Less than 1%) 1487
Kefurox Vials, Faspak & ADD-Vantage 1277
Lasix (Rare) 1093
Lopressor HCT Tablets 1034
Lozol Tablets 1843
Macrodantin Capsules (Rare) 1624
Maxzide 1215
Mellaril 2011
Mesantoin Tablets (Uncommon) 2013
Micronase Tablets 2350
Midamor Tablets (Rare) 1508
Miltown Tablets 2386
Minizide Capsules 1779
Moduretic Tablets 1510
Monopril Tablets (0.2 to 1.0%) 1406
Mykrox ½ mg Tablets 984
Myochrysine Injection 1516
Nalfon Pulvules & Tablets (Less than 1%) 919
Naprosyn Suspension (Rare) 2297
Naturetin Tablets 1789
Norflex (Very rare) 1314
Norgesic (1 case) 1314
Normozide Tablets 2112
Norzine 1818
Ophthochlor Ophthalmic Solution ◉ 300
Ophthocort ◉ 301
Oretic Tablets 544
Oreticyl 545
PBZ Tablets & Elixir 1037
PBZ-SR Tablets 1037
PMB 200 and PMB 400 2504
Paradione Capsules 548
PediaProfen Suspension (Less than 1%) 1363
Pediazole 1973
Phenurone Tablets (2%) 552
Plaquenil Sulfate Tablets 2067
Prinzide Tablets 1540
Prozac Pulvules 920
Rauzide Tablets 1804
Renese Tablets 1785
▲ Retrovir Capsules (3% to 29%) 802
▲ Retrovir I.V. Infusion (1% to 45%) 805
▲ Retrovir Syrup (3% to 29%) 802
Ridaura Capsules (Less than 0.1%) 2224
Rifamate Capsules 1347
Rufen Tablets (Less than 1%) 691
Rythmol Tablets (Less than 1%) 1184
SSD RP Cream 690
Saluron 718
Salutensin/Salutensin-Demi 719
Septra 813
Septra I.V. Infusion 808
Septra I.V. Infusion ADD-Vantage Vials (Rare) 810
Septra 813
Ser-Ap-Es Tablets 881
Serentil 686
Serpasil-Esidrix Tablets 886
Silvadene Cream 1% 1352
Solganal Suspension (Rare) 2122
Stelazine 2226
Suprax 1235
Tagamet (A few cases) 2228
Tapazole Tablets 1298
Tegretol Chewable Tablets (Very low incidence) 654
Tegretol Suspension (Very low incidence) 656
Tegretol Tablets (Very low incidence) 654
Tenoretic Tablets 1105
Thalitone Tablets 687
Thiosulfil Forte Tablets 2526
Thorazine 2234
Timolide Tablets 1547
Torecan 1993
Trandate HCT Tablets 579
Trental (Rare) 1099
Tridione 557
Urobiotic-250 Capsules 1968
Vaseretic Tablets 1559
Voltaren Tablets (Rare) 1042
Zantac Injection and Zantac Injection Premixed (Rare) 1063
Zantac (Rare) 1065
Zaroxolyn Tablets 989
Zefazone Sterile Powder 2372
Zestoretic 2274
Zinacef 1066
Zovirax Sterile Powder (Less than 1%) 828
Zyloprim Tablets (Less than 1%) 830

Apnea

▲ Alfenta Injection (7%) 1131
Alurate Elixir (Less than 1 in 100) 1883
Amikin Injectable 602
Anectine 755
▲ Atgam Sterile Solution (More than 1% to 10%) 2320
Bentyl 1322
Brevital Sodium Vials 1248
Butisol Sodium Elixir & Tablets (Less than 1 in 100) 2377
Carbocaine Hydrochloride Injection 2043
Coly-Mycin M Parenteral 1706
Demerol 2047
Desyrel and Desyrel Dividose 1404
Dilaudid-HP Injection 1175
Diphtheria and Tetanus Toxoids and Pertussis Vaccine Adsorbed USP (For Pediatric Use) 892
Diprivan Injection (Greater than 1%) 2267
▲ Duragesic Transdermal System (3% to 10%) 1133
Ethmozine Tablets (Less than 2%) 946
▲ Exosurf Neonatal for Intratracheal Suspension (33% to 62%) 765
Indocin I.V. (Less than 3%) 1490
▲ Innovar Injection (Most common) 1141
Ketalar 1726
MS Contin Tablets 1814
MSIR 1817
Marcaine Hydrochloride with Epinephrine 1:200,000 2055
Marcaine Hydrochloride Injection 2055
Mebaral Tablets (Less than 1 in 100) 2061
Metubine Iodide Vials 1285
Nembutal Sodium Capsules (Less than 1%) 534
Nembutal Sodium Solution (Less than 1%) 536
Nembutal Sodium Suppositories (Less than 1%) 538
Nescaine/Nescaine MPF 629
Netromycin Injection 100 mg/ml 2104
Norcuron 1642
Nuromax Injection 794
Omnipaque (0.3%) 2552
Oramorph SR (Morphine Sulfate Sustained Release Tablets) 1988
Permax Tablets (Infrequent) 1291
Phenobarbital Elixir and Tablets (Less than 1 in 100 patients) 1293
Polymyxin B Sulfate, Aerosporin Brand Sterile Powder 798
▲ Prostin VR Pediatric Sterile Solution (10-12%) 2355
Prozac Pulvules (Rare) 920
Rythmol Tablets (Less than 1%) 1184
Seconal Sodium Pulvules (Less than 1 in 100) 1296
Sensorcaine 631
Sensorcaine-MPF Spinal 634
Stadol (Less than 1%) 721
Sublimaze Injection 1146
Sufenta Injection (Less than 1%) 1147
Surital Ampoules, Steri-Vials 1764
▲ Survanta Beractant Intratracheal Suspension (46.1 to 65.4%) 1978
Talwin Injection 2071
Thiotepa Parenteral (1 case) 1240
Tri-Immunol Diphtheria & Tetanus Toxoids & Pertussis Vaccine, Adsorbed (Rare) 1241
▲ Versed Injection (15.4%) 1924
Virazole 1126

Apnea, neonatal

Sinequan (One case) 1960
Survanta Beractant Intratracheal Suspension (Less than 1%) 1978

Appetite, changes

▲ AeroBid Inhaler System (3-9%) 995
Amen 833
Ansaid Tablets (Less than 1%) 2319
Asendin Tablets (Greater than 1%) 1196
Ativan Tablets (Less frequent) 2434
Brevicon 2304
BuSpar (Infrequent) 1401
Children's Advil Suspension (Less than 3%) 2426
Compazine 2201
Cortifoam 1827
Cortone Acetate Sterile Suspension 1437
Cortone Acetate Tablets 1439
Cycrin Tablets 2449
Cytotec (Infrequent) 2159
Dalalone D.P. Injectable 999
Danocrine Capsules (Rare) 2046
Decadron Elixir 1445
Decadron Phosphate Injection 1449
Decadron Phosphate Respihaler 1454
Decadron Phosphate Turbinaire 1456
Decadron Phosphate with Xylocaine Injection, Sterile 1451
Decadron Tablets 1447
Decadron-LA Sterile Suspension 1457
Demulen 2161
Depakene Capsules & Syrup 511
Depakote 512
Depo-Provera Sterile Aqueous Suspension 2336
Desyrel and Desyrel Dividose (Greater than 1%) 1404
Diabinese Tablets (Less than 2%) 1775
Eldepryl 2250
Enovid 2161
Etrafon 2087
Floxin Tablets (1% to 3%) 1652
Garamycin Injectable 2093
▲ Hismanal Tablets (3.9%) 1138
Hydeltrasol Injection, Sterile 1476
Hydeltra-T.B.A. Sterile Suspension 1478
Hydrocortone Acetate Sterile Suspension 1479
Hydrocortone Phosphate Injection, Sterile 1481
Hydrocortone Tablets 1482
Jenest-28 Tablets 1636
Klonopin Tablets 1902
Levlen/Tri-Levlen 665
Lo/Ovral Tablets 2471
Lo/Ovral-28 Tablets 2476
Loestrin 1728
▲ Lupron Depot 3.75 mg (Among most frequent) 2312
Maxzide 1215
Megace Tablets 732
Mexitil Capsules (2.6%) 680
Micronor Tablets 1667
Midamor Tablets (Between 1% and 3%) 1508
Modicon 1667
Moduretic Tablets (Less than or equal to 1%) 1510
Monopril Tablets (0.2 to 1.0%) 1406
Motrin Tablets (Less than 3%) 2351
Navane Capsules and Concentrate 1954
Navane Intramuscular 1956
Nordette-21 Tablets 2481
Nordette-28 Tablets 2483
Norethin 2133
Norinyl 2304
Norlestrin 1746
Norlutate 1754
Norlutin 1755
Normozide Tablets (Less than 1%) 2112
Norplant System 2484
Nor-Q D Tablets 2304
Ogen 540
Omnipaque (Less than 0.1%) 2552
▲ Orap Tablets (5%) 1020
Ortho-Cyclen Tablets 1658
Ortho-Novum 1667
Orudis Capsules (Less than 1%) 2488
Ovcon 1391
Ovral Tablets 2490
Ovral-28 Tablets 2491
Ovrette Tablets 2492
PediaProfen Suspension (Less than 3%) 1363
Permax Tablets (Infrequent) 1291
Prolixin Decanoate 1795
Prolixin Elixir 1793
Prolixin Enanthate 1796
Prolixin Injection 1791
Prolixin Oral Concentrate 1792
Prolixin Tablets 1793
▲ Proventil Syrup (3 of 100) 2119
Provera Tablets 2356
Prozac Pulvules (Frequent) 920
Quadrinal Tablets 1183
Recombivax HB (Less than 1%) 1544
Rufen Tablets (Less than 1-3%) 691
Seldane Tablets (0.5%) 1349
Seldane-D Extended-Release Tablets 1350
Stelazine (Occasional) 2226
Tacaryl 2409
▲ Tegison Capsules (25-50%) 1881
Temaril Tablets, Syrup and Spansule Sustained Release Capsules 1085
Thorazine (Sometimes) 2234
Trandate HCT Tablets (Less than 1% in 208 patients) 579
▲ Trexan Tablets (Less than 10%) 937
Trilafon 2123
Levlen/Tri-Levlen 665
Tri-Norinyl 2304
Triphasil-21 Tablets 2527
Triphasil-28 Tablets 2532
▲ Ventolin Syrup (3%) 583
Voltaren Tablets (Less than 1%) 1042
▲ Wellbutrin Tablets (3.7%) 821

Appetite, decreased

IPOL Poliovirus Vaccine Inactivated 894
▲ NebuPent for Inhalation Solution (53 to 72%) 1017
ProSom Tablets (Infrequent) 554

Appetite, increased

▲ Anafranil Capsules (Up to 11%) 650
Cardura Tablets (Less than 0.5% of 3960 patients) 1941
Clozaril Tablets (Less than 1%) 2000
Fiorinal with Codeine Capsules 2008
Intron A (1% or less) 2097
Kerlone Tablets (Less than 2%) 2172
ProSom Tablets (Infrequent) 554
Vascor (200, 300 and 400 mg) Tablets (0.5 to 2.0%) 1383
▲ Xanax Tablets (32.7%) 2367

Appetite, loss of (see also under Anorexia)

▲ CHEMET (succimer) Capsules (12 to 20.9%) 1361
HibTITER (23 of 1,118 vaccinations) 1206
Miacalcin Injection 2017

Apprehension

Adenocard Injection (Less than 1%) 1007
Ana-Kit Anaphylaxis Emergency Treatment Kit 1100
▲ Anestacon Solution (Among most common) 2394
Antivenin (Crotalidae) Polyvalent 2430
Cardioquin Tablets 1812
Dalmane Capsules 1927
Dilaudid-HP Injection 1175
Dopram Injectable 1860
Duranest Injections 624
Dyclone 0.5% and 1% Topical Solutions, USP 626
Edecrin 1468
EpiPen Jr. 843
Hyperstat I.V. Injection 2095
Limbitrol 1933
MS Contin Tablets (Infrequent) 1814
MSIR (Infrequent) 1817
Matulane Capsules 1907
Nipride I.V. Infusion 1909
Nitro-Bid IV (Less than 1%) 1338
Nitrostat IV (Less than 1%) 1744
Omnipaque (Occasional) 2552
Oramorph SR (Morphine Sulfate Sustained Release Tablets) (Less frequent) 1988
Quinaglute Dura-Tabs Tablets 663
Quinamm Tablets 1344
Quinidex Extentabs 1868
▲ Xylocaine Injections (Among most common) 637
Xylocaine Injections for Ventricular Arrhythmias 639
Xylocaine 2% Jelly 643
Xylocaine 5% Ointment 644
Xylocaine 10% Oral Spray 645
4% Xylocaine-MPF Sterile Solution 641
Xylocaine 2% Viscous Solution 646

Apraxia
Anafranil Capsules (Rare) ... 650
Eldepryl ... 2250

Arachnoiditis
Depo-Medrol Sterile Aqueous Suspension ... 2334
Gelfoam Sterile Sponge ... 2338
Marcaine Spinal ... 2058
Methotrexate Tablets, Parenteral, LPF Parenteral ... 1217
Nescaine/Nescaine MPF ... 629
Novocain Hydrochloride for Spinal Anesthesia ... 2065
Pontocaine Hydrochloride for Spinal Anesthesia ... 2069
Rheumatrex Methotrexate Dose Pack ... 1234

Areflexia
Omnipaque ... 2552
Platinol ... 737
Platinol-AQ Injection ... 738

Argumentativeness
Versed Injection (Less than 1%) ... 1924

Arm, stiffness of
Engerix-B Unit-Dose Vials (Less than 1%) ... 2213

Arrhythmia, exacerbation of
Cordarone Tablets ... 2446

Arrhythmias
Abbokinase (Occasionally) ... 503
Adenocard Injection ... 1007
Adriamycin PFS ... 561
Adriamycin RDF ... 562
Alfenta Injection (2%) ... 1131
Altace Capsules (Less than 1%) ... 1086
Aminophyllin Tablets ... 2153
Anafranil Capsules (Infrequent) ... 650
Ana-Kit Anaphylaxis Emergency Treatment Kit ... 1100
Anectine ... 755
Ansaid Tablets (Less than 1%) ... 2319
Aramine Injection ... 1424
Atgam Sterile Solution (At least 1 patient and less than 5% of total patients) ... 2320
Atrohist Sprinkle Capsules ... 558
Atromid-S Capsules ... 2435
Betagan ... ⊙ 239
Blocadren Tablets (Greater than 1.1%) ... 1429
Bretylol Injection (1-2 in 1000) ... 923
Calcijex Calcitriol Injection ... 506
Calderol Capsules ... 1635
Capoten (Rare) ... 2255
Carbocaine Hydrochloride Injection ... 2043
Cardizem Tablets-30 mg, 60 mg, 90 mg and 120 mg (Less than 1%) ... 1329
Cardizem SR Capsules-60 mg, 90 mg and 120 mg (Less than 1%) ... 1327
Cardura Tablets (1%) ... 1941
Cartrol Tablets (Less common) ... 507
Catapres Tablets (Rare) ... 676
Catapres-TTS (Rare) ... 677
CHEMET (succimer) Capsules (Up to 1.8%) ... 1361
Children's Advil Suspension (Less than 1%) ... 2426
Choledyl SA Tablets ... 1704
Cibalith-S ... 870
Cipro I.V. (1% or less) ... 1592
Clinoril Tablets (Rare) ... 1433
Clozaril Tablets ... 2000
Combipres Tablets (Rare) ... 678
Compazine ... 2201
Cordarone Tablets (1 to 3%) ... 2446
Cytotec (Infrequent) ... 2159
Cytovene Sterile Powder (1% or less) ... 2292
Dalgan Injection (Less than 1%) ... 620
Deconamine ... 663
Deconsal ... 559
Deprol Tablets ... 2382
Desyrel and Desyrel Dividose ... 1404
Dimetane-DC Cough Syrup ... 1857
Dimetane-DX Cough Syrup ... 1858
Diprivan Injection (Less than 1%) ... 2267
Diupres Tablets ... 1461
Dopram Injectable ... 1860
Doxorubicin Hydrochloride for Injection, USP ... 622
Doxorubicin Hydrochloride Injection, USP ... 848
Duragesic Transdermal System (1% or greater) ... 1133
Dyazide Capsules ... 2208
E.E.S. (Occasional reports) ... 522
Elavil ... 2269
Eldepryl ... 2250
▲ Eminase (38%) ... 2211
Endep Tablets ... 1927
Enduronyl ... 518
Enlon Injection ... 598
EpiPen Jr. ... 843
Equagesic Tablets ... 2451
EryPed (Occasional reports) ... 519
Ery-Tab Tablets (Occasional reports) ... 521
Erythrocin Stearate Filmtab (Occasional reports) ... 523
Erythromycin Base Filmtab (Occasional reports) ... 525
Erythromycin Delayed-Release Capsules, USP (Occasional reports) ... 526
Eskalith ... 2214
Ethrane ... 599
Etrafon ... 2087
Fedahist Gyrocaps ... 2145
Fedahist Timecaps ... 2145
Flexeril Tablets (Less than 1%) ... 1471
Fluothane ... 2453
Forane ... 600
Fungizone Intravenous ... 2262
Glaucon ... ⊙ 218
Harmonyl Tablets ... 528
Hydropres Tablets ... 1485
Hytrin Tablets (At least 1%) ... 529
Idamycin for Injection ... 564
Indocin Capsules (Less than 1%) ... 1487
Indocin I.V. (Less than 1%) ... 1490
Indocin (Less than 1%) ... 1487
▲ Inocor Lactate Injection (3%) ... 2048
Intron A (Less than 1%) ... 2097
Isopto Carbachol ... ⊙ 219
K-Lyte ... 707
Kenalog-10 Injection ... 2402
Kenalog-40 Injection ... 2403
Kerlone Tablets (Less than 2%) ... 2172
Ketalar ... 1726
Klorvess Effervescent Granules ... 2010
Klorvess Effervescent Tablets ... 2011
Klorvess 10% Liquid ... 2010
Lanoxicaps ... 772
Lanoxin Elixir Pediatric ... 775
Lanoxin Injection ... 778
Lanoxin Injection Pediatric ... 781
Lanoxin Tablets ... 783
Levo-Dromoran (Infrequent) ... 1906
Levophed Bitartrate Injection ... 2054
Limbitrol ... 1933
Lithane Tablets ... 1596
Lithium Carbonate Capsules & Tablets ... 1984
Lithobid Tablets ... 870
Lodine Capsules (Less than 1%) ... 2468
Lorelco Tablets ... 1333
Ludiomil Tablets (Rare) ... 874
Lufyllin & Lufyllin-400 Tablets ... 2384
Lufyllin-GG Elixir & Tablets ... 2385
▲ Lupron Depot 3.75 mg (Among most frequent) ... 2312
Lupron Depot 7.5 mg (Less than 5%) ... 2311
Lupron Injection (Less than 5%) ... 2310
Marax Tablets & DF Syrup ... 1954
▲ Marplan Tablets (Among most frequent) ... 1906
Mellaril ... 2011
Midamor Tablets (Less than or equal to 1%) ... 1508
Miltown Tablets ... 2386
Moban Tablets & Concentrate ... 932
Moduretic Tablets (Greater than 1%, less than 3%) ... 1510
Monopril Tablets (0.2 to 1.0%) ... 1406
Motrin Tablets (Less than 1%) ... 2351
Murocoll-2 Sterile Ophthalmic Solution ... ⊙ 261
Mydfrin 2.5% ... ⊙ 224
Naldecon Syrup, Tablets, Pediatric Drops and Pediatric Syrup ... 709
Navane Capsules and Concentrate ... 1954
Navane Intramuscular ... 1956
Neo-Synephrine Hydrochloride 1% Carpuject (Rare) ... 2063
Neo-Synephrine Hydrochloride 1% Injection (Rare) ... 2063
Niacor Tablets ... 2376
Nicolar Tablets ... 1846
Norpramin Tablets ... 1340
Novafed A Capsules ... 1342
Novafed Capsules ... 1342
Novahistine DH ... 1342
Novahistine DMX ... ▣ 595
Novahistine Elixir ... ▣ 596
Novahistine Expectorant ... 1343
▲ Novantrone for Injection Concentrate (3 to 4%) ... 1226
Omnipaque (2%) ... 2552
Orap Tablets ... 1020
Oreticyl ... 545
Orudis Capsules (Less than 1%) ... 2488
OSM_GLYN ... ⊙ 234
Oxytocin Injection ... 2492
PCE Dispertab Tablets (Occasional reports) ... 549
PMB 200 and PMB 400 ... 2504
Pamelor ... 2019
Parlodel (Less than 1%) ... 2020
PediaProfen Suspension (Less than 1%) ... 1363
Pentam 300 Injection ... 1018
Pepcid (Infrequent) ... 1524
Permax Tablets (1.1%) ... 1291
Pfizerpen for Injection ... 1957
Pitocin Injection, Ampoules, Steri-Dose Syringes ... 1757
Pitressin Synthetic, Ampoules ... 1758
Plendil Extended-Release Tablets (0.5% to 1.5%) ... 1526
Prinzide Tablets ... 1540
Priscoline Hydrochloride Ampuls ... 877
Procardia XL Tablets (1% or less) ... 1783
Propine with C Cap Compliance Cap ... ⊙ 255
ProSom Tablets (Rare) ... 554
Prostigmin Injectable ... 1120
Prostigmin Tablets ... 1121
Prozac Pulvules (Infrequent) ... 920
Raudixin Tablets ... 1803
Rauzide Tablets ... 1804
Regitine ... 878
Renese-R Tablets ... 1786
Ritalin ... 880
Rocaltrol Capsules ... 1913
Roferon-A Injection (Less than 3%) ... 1916
Rondec ... 1975
Rondec-DM ... 1976
Rondec-TR Tablet ... 1975
Rubex ... 739
Rufen Tablets (Less than 1%) ... 691
Rum-K Syrup ... 995
Seldane Tablets (Rare) ... 1349
Seldane-D Extended-Release Tablets (Rare) ... 1350
Sensorcaine ... 631
Sensorcaine-MPF Spinal ... 634
Ser-Ap-Es Tablets ... 881
Serpasil Tablets ... 883
Serpasil-Apresoline Tablets ... 884
Serpasil-Esidrix Tablets ... 886
Slo-bid Gyrocaps ... 1847
Sodium Polystyrene Sulfonate Suspension ... 1993
Solu-Medrol Sterile Powder ... 2363
Stelazine ... 2226
Sufenta Injection (Less than 1%) ... 1147
Surmontil Capsules ... 2524
Sus-Phrine Injection ... 1006
Syntocinon Injection ... 2032
Tegretol Chewable Tablets ... 654
Tegretol Suspension ... 656
Tegretol Tablets ... 654
Tensilon Injectable ... 1123
Tenuate ... 1354
Timolide Tablets (Less than 1%) ... 1547
Timoptic in Ocudose ... 1552
Timoptic Sterile Ophthalmic Solution ... 1550
Tofranil Ampuls ... 1038
Tofranil Tablets ... 1039
Tofranil-PM Capsules ... 1041
Trental (1.7%) ... 1099
Triavil Tablets ... 1556
Trilafon ... 2123
Trinalin Repetabs Tablets ... 1170
Uniphyl 400 mg Tablets ... 1823
Vascor (200, 300 and 400 mg) Tablets (About 2.4%) ... 1383
Vaseretic Tablets ... 1559
Vasotec Tablets (0.5% to 1.0%) ... 1564
Vivactil Tablets ... 1567
▲ Wellbutrin Tablets (5.3%) ... 821
Wytensin Tablets (3% or less) ... 2542
Yutopar (1% (with oral administration)) ... 647
Zantac Injection and Zantac Injection Premixed (Rare) ... 1063
Zantac (Rare) ... 1065
Zestoretic ... 2274
Zoladex (1% to 5%) ... 1110

Arrhythmias, preexisting, worsening of
Aminophyllin Tablets ... 2153
▲ Rythmol Tablets (4.7%) ... 1184
Slo-bid Gyrocaps ... 1847

Arrhythmias, supraventricular
Ethmozine Tablets (Less than 2%) ... 946

Arterial insufficiency
Blocadren Tablets ... 1429
Inderal ... 2459
Inderal LA Long Acting Capsules ... 2461
Inderide Tablets ... 2463
Inderide LA Long Acting Capsules ... 2465
Lopressor Ampuls (1%) ... 1032
Lopressor HCT Tablets ... 1034
Lopressor Tablets (1%) ... 1032
Timolide Tablets ... 1547
Timoptic in Ocudose ... 1552
Timoptic Sterile Ophthalmic Solution ... 1550

Arterial occlusion
Metrodin (urofollitropin for injection) ... 2182
Serophene (clomiphene citrate tablets, USP) ... 2186

Arteriostenosis
Aralen Phosphate with Primaquine Phosphate Tablets ... 2040

Arteritis
Azo Gantrisin Tablets ... 1888

Arteritis, temporal, aggravation of
Butazolidin Capsules & Tablets ... 1027

Arthralgia
▲ Accutane Capsules (Approximately 16%) ... 1878
Actigall Capsules ... 2280
Actimmune (2%) ... 1046
Aldoclor Tablets ... 1413
Aldomet Ester HCl Injection ... 1417
Aldomet Oral ... 1415
Aldoril Tablets ... 1418
▲ Alferon N Injection (1% to 16%) ... 1809
Altace Capsules (Less than 1%) ... 1086
Amikin Injectable (Rare) ... 602
Anafranil Capsules (Up to 3%) ... 650
Antivenin (Crotalidae) Polyvalent ... 2430
Apresazide Capsules (Less frequent) ... 854
Apresoline Hydrochloride Parenteral (Ampuls) ... 856
Apresoline Hydrochloride Tablets (Less frequent) ... 855
Apresoline-Esidrix Tablets ... 857
▲ Atgam Sterile Solution (More than 1% to 10%; 1 in 2 patients) ... 2320
Atromid-S Capsules ... 2435
Augmentin Tablets, Powder for Oral Suspension, and Chewable Tablets ... 2198
Azo Gantanol Tablets ... 1887
Azo Gantrisin Tablets ... 1888
Azulfidine Tablets, EN-tabs, Oral Suspension (Rare) ... 1157
Bactrim DS Tablets ... 1891
Bactrim I.V. Infusion ... 1889
Bactrim ... 1891
Biavax II ... 1427
Bicillin C-R Injection ... 2438
Bicillin C-R 900/300 Injection ... 2440
Bicillin L-A Injection ... 2442
Blocadren Tablets (Less than 1%) ... 1429
BuSpar (Infrequent) ... 1401
Butazolidin Capsules & Tablets (Less than 1%) ... 1027
Calan SR Caplets (1% or less) ... 2157
Calan Tablets (1% or less) ... 2155
Calciparine Injection ... 925
▲ Capoten (About 4 to 7 of 100) ... 2255
Capozide ... 2258
Cardene Capsules (Rare) ... 2290
Cardura Tablets (1%) ... 1941
Cartrol Tablets (1.2%) ... 507
Catapres Tablets (About 6 in 1,000 patients) ... 676
Catapres-TTS (6 per 1,000) ... 677
Ceclor Pulvules & Suspension ... 1251
Centrax ... 1693
Cholybar ... 1705
Cipro I.V. (1% or less) ... 1592
Cipro Tablets (Less than 1%) ... 1589
Clinoril Tablets (Less than 1 in 100) ... 1433
Clozaril Tablets (Less than 1%) ... 2000
Colestid Granules (Less than 1 in 1,000) ... 2328
Combipres Tablets (About 6 in 1,000) ... 678

Coumadin Injection & Tablets 944
Cuprimine Capsules 1442
Cytotec (Infrequent) 2159
Danocrine Capsules 2046
Depen Titratable Tablets 2379
Dilantin Infatabs 1710
Dilantin Kapseals 1708
Dilantin-30 Pediatric/Dilantin-125 Suspension 1713
Dilantin with Phenobarbital Kapseals 1715
▲Dipentum Capsules (4.0%) 1160
Diulo 2129
Dolobid Tablets (Less than 1 in 100) 1465
Elspar 1470
▲Eminase (Less than 10%) 2211
Engerix-B Unit-Dose Vials (Less than 1%) 2213
▲Epogen for Injection (Up to 11.0%) 591
▲Ergamisol Tablets (2 to 5%) 1136
Eskalith 2214
Fansidar Tablets 1896
Feldene Capsules (Occasional) 1777
Flagyl Tablets 2170
Floxin Tablets (Less than 1%) 1652
▲Fungizone Intravenous (Among most common) 2262
Furoxone 1855
Gamimune N Immune Globulin Intravenous (Human) 1572
Gantanol 1899
Gantrisin Ophthalmic Ointment/Solution 1900
Gantrisin 1901
Garamycin Injectable 2093
Gastrocrom Capsules (Infrequent) .. 974
Hismanal Tablets (1.2%) 1138
Hylorel Tablets (1.7%) 975
Hyskon Hysteroscopy Fluid (Rare) .. 1162
Hytrin Tablets (1%) 529
Imferon 976
Imuran (Less than 1%) 768
Intal Capsules (Less than 1 in 10,000 patients) 978
Intal Nebulizer Solution 980
▲Intron A (Up to 19%) 2097
Isoptin Oral Tablets (Less than 1%) 1179
Isoptin SR Sustained Release Tablets (Less than 1%) 1181
K-Phos M.F. Tablets 659
K-Phos Neutral Tablets 660
K-Phos Original Formula 'Sodium Free' Tablets (Less frequent) 660
K-Phos No. 2 Tablets 659
Keflex Pulvules, Oral Suspension & Pediatric Drops 916
Keftab Tablets 917
Kenalog-10 Injection (Occasional) .. 2402
Kenalog-40 Injection 2403
▲Kerlone Tablets (3.1%) 2172
Koro-Flex Arcing Spring Diaphragm 2142
Koromex Coil Spring Diaphragm 2142
Lopid Capsules and Tablets 1736
Lotensin Tablets 872
Lupron Depot 7.5 mg 2311
Lupron Injection (Less than 5%) 2310
M-M-R II 1494
M-R-VAX II 1496
Macrodantin Capsules 1624
Matulane Capsules 1907
Meruvax II 1503
Methotrexate Tablets, Parenteral, LPF Parenteral (Rare) 1217
Metrodin (urofollitropin for injection) 2182
Mevacor Tablets (Rare) 1505
Mexitil Capsules (1.7%) 680
Micronase Tablets 2350
Midamor Tablets (Less than or equal to 1%) 1508
Minipress Capsules 1778
Moduretic Tablets (Less than or equal to 1%) 1510
Monopril Tablets (0.2 to 1.0%) 1406
Myambutol Tablets 1225
▲Mykrox ½ mg Tablets (3.1%) 984
Myochrysine Injection 1516
Nasalcrom Nasal Solution 986
NebuPent for Inhalation Solution (1% or less) 1017
NegGram 2062
Noroxin Tablets 1519
Ortho Diaphragm Kit 1664
Orthoclone OKT3 Sterile Solution .. 1645
Ortho-White Diaphragm Kit-Flat Spring 1664
Pediazole 1973
Pepcid (Infrequent) 1524
Pergonal (menotropins for injection, USP) 2184
Permax Tablets (1.6%) 1291
Pfizerpen for Injection 1957
Pfizerpen-AS Aqueous Suspension 1959
Phenobarbital Elixir and Tablets (Rare) 1293
Plague Vaccine 1584
Plendil Extended-Release Tablets (0.5% to 1.5%) 1526
Pneumovax 23 (Rare) 1528
Pnu-Imune 23 Pneumococcal Vaccine Polyvalent (Rare to infrequent) 1233
Prilosec Delayed-Release Capsules (Less than 1%) 1530
Prinivil Tablets (1% or less) 1538
Prinzide Tablets 1540
Procan SR Tablets (Common) 1760
Procardia Capsules (2% or less) 1781
Procardia XL Tablets (Less than 3%) 1783
▲Procrit for Injection (Up to 11%) 1647
Pronestyl Capsules and Tablets 1800
Pronestyl Injection 1798
Pronestyl-SR Tablets 1801
ProSom Tablets (Rare) 554
Prostigmin Injectable 1120
Prostigmin Tablets 1121
Protostat Tablets 1674
Prozac Pulvules (1.2%) 920
Quadrinal Tablets 1183
Questran Powder 710
Quinidex Extentabs 1868
Recombivax HB (Less than 1%) 1544
Retrovir Capsules (Less than 5%) .. 802
Retrovir I.V. Infusion (Less than 5%) 805
Retrovir Syrup (Less than 5%) 802
Rheumatrex Methotrexate Dose Pack (Rare) 1234
Ritalin 880
▲Roferon-A Injection (5% to 24%) .. 1916
Rowasa (2.09%) 2248
Rythmol Tablets (0.2 to 1.0%) 1184
Sandimmune (Rare) 2024
Sandostatin Injection (Less than 1%) 2029
Sansert Tablets 2031
Sectral Capsules 2520
Septra 813
Septra I.V. Infusion 808
Septra I.V. Infusion ADD-Vantage Vials 810
Septra 813
Ser-Ap-Es Tablets 881
Serpasil-Apresoline Tablets 884
Solatene Capsules (Rare) 1881
Solganal Suspension 2122
Solu-Medrol Sterile Powder 2363
Synarel Nasal Solution (Less than 1%) 2300
Tagamet (Rare) 2228
Tambocor Tablets (Less than 1%) 1315
Tapazole Tablets 1298
▲Tegison Capsules (50-75%) 1881
Tegretol Chewable Tablets 654
Tegretol Suspension 656
Tegretol Tablets 654
Tenex Tablets 1875
▲TheraCys BCG Live (Intravesical) (1.0% to 7.1%) 898
Thiosulfil Forte Tablets 2526
Timentin for Injection 2239
Timolide Tablets 1547
Timoptic in Ocudose 1552
Timoptic Sterile Ophthalmic Solution 1550
▲Tonocard Tablets (Less than 1%-4.7%) 1554
▲Trexan Tablets (Greater than 10%) 937
Tri-Immunol Diphtheria & Tetanus Toxoids & Pertussis Vaccine, Adsorbed 1241
Uroqid-Acid 661
Vaseretic Tablets (0.5% to 2.0%) 1559
Vasotec I.V. 1562
Vasotec Tablets (0.5% to 1%) 1564
Velosef Capsules and for Oral Suspension (Few) 606
Verelan Capsules (Less than 1%) .. 1243
▲Visken Tablets (7%) 2036
Wellbutrin Tablets 821
Wycillin Injection 2537
Zantac Injection and Zantac Injection Premixed (Rare) 1063
Zantac (Rare) 1065
Zaroxolyn Tablets 989
Zefazone Sterile Powder 2372
Zestoretic 2274
Zestril Tablets (Less than 1%) 2277
Zyloprim Tablets (Less than 1%) 830

Arthralgia, migratory

Aquasol A Vitamin A Capsules, USP 615
Aquasol A Parenteral, USP 615

Arthralgia, monoarticular

Recombivax HB (Less than 1%) 1544

Arthritis

Accutane Capsules (Less than 1%) 1878
Adalat Capsules (10 mg and 20 mg) (Less than 0.5%) 1587
Altace Capsules (Less than 1%) 1086
Augmentin Tablets, Powder for Oral Suspension, and Chewable Tablets 2198
Benemid Tablets 1426
Biavax II (Rare) 1427
Bumex (0.2%) 1895
Cardura Tablets (1%) 1941
Cartrol Tablets (Rare) 507
Ceclor Pulvules & Suspension 1251
Cholybar 1705
Clinoril Tablets (Less than 1 in 100) 1433
ColBENEMID Tablets 1436
Colestid Granules (Less than 1 in 1,000) 2328
Dolobid Tablets (Less than 1 in 100) 1465
Engerix-B Unit-Dose Vials 2213
Hytrin Tablets (At least 1%) 529
Imferon 976
Intron A (Less than 1%) 2097
Keflex Pulvules, Oral Suspension & Pediatric Drops 916
Keftab Tablets 917
Lotensin Tablets 872
M-M-R II 1494
M-R-VAX II 1496
Meruvax II (Rare) 1503
Mevacor Tablets (Rare) 1505
Monopril Tablets (0.2 to 1.0%) 1406
Norethin 2133
Noroxin Tablets 1519
OptiPranolol Sterile Ophthalmic Solution (A small number of patients) .... ◉ 261
Orthoclone OKT3 Sterile Solution .. 1645
Permax Tablets (Infrequent) 1291
Pneumovax 23 1528
Pnu-Imune 23 Pneumococcal Vaccine Polyvalent (Rare) 1233
Prinivil Tablets (1% or less) 1538
Prinzide Tablets 1540
Procan SR Tablets (Common) 1760
Procardia Capsules (Less than 0.5%) 1781
Pronestyl Capsules and Tablets 1800
Pronestyl Injection 1798
Pronestyl-SR Tablets 1801
ProSom Tablets (Infrequent) 554
Prozac Pulvules (Infrequent) 920
Questran Light 711
Questran Powder 710
▲TheraCys BCG Live (Intravesical) (1.0% to 7.1%) 898
▲Tonocard Tablets (4.7%) 1554
Vascor (200, 300 and 400 mg) Tablets (0.5 to 2.0%) 1383
Vaseretic Tablets 1559
Vasotec I.V. 1562
Vasotec Tablets 1564
▲Wellbutrin Tablets (3.1%) 821
Zestoretic 2274
Zestril Tablets 2277

Arthritis, acute gouty, precipitation of

Benemid Tablets 1426

Arthritis, migratory

Elavil 2269

Arthropathy, Charcot-like

Aristospan Suspension (Intra-articular) 1011
Celestone Soluspan Suspension 2081
Dalalone D.P. Injectable 999
Decadron Phosphate Injection 1449
Decadron Phosphate with Xylocaine Injection, Sterile 1451
Decadron-LA Sterile Suspension 1457
Depo-Medrol Sterile Aqueous Suspension 2334
Hydeltrasol Injection, Sterile 1476
Hydeltra-T.B.A. Sterile Suspension 1478
Hydrocortone Acetate Sterile Suspension 1479
Kenalog-10 Injection 2402
Kenalog-40 Injection 2403

Arthropathy, unspecified

Kerlone Tablets (Less than 2%) 2172

Arthrosis

Anafranil Capsules (Infrequent) 650
▲Intron A (1% to 5%) 2097

Ascaris, appearance in mouth and nose

Mintezol 1510

Ascites

Cosmegen Injection 1440
Hyskon Hysteroscopy Fluid (Rare) .. 1162
Inocor Lactate Injection (1 case) 2048
Lutrepulse for Injection (Rare) 1655
Serophene (clomiphene citrate tablets, USP) 2186

Aseptic meningitis syndrome

Children's Advil Suspension (Less than 1%) 2426
Clinoril Tablets (Less than 1 in 100) 1433
Motrin Tablets (Less than 1%) 2351
Omnipaque (Less than 0.01%) 2552
Orthoclone OKT3 Sterile Solution .. 1645
PediaProfen Suspension (Less than 1%) 1363
Rufen Tablets (Less than 1%) 691
Trimpex Tablets (Rare) 1922

Aseptic necrosis of femoral/humeral heads

Aristospan Suspension (Intra-articular) 1011
Celestone Soluspan Suspension 2081
Cortenema 2244
Cortone Acetate Sterile Suspension 1437
Cortone Acetate Tablets 1439
Decadron Elixir 1445
Decadron Phosphate Injection 1449
Decadron Phosphate Respihaler 1454
Decadron Phosphate Turbinaire 1456
Decadron Phosphate with Xylocaine Injection, Sterile 1451
Decadron Tablets 1447
Decadron-LA Sterile Suspension 1457
Deltasone Tablets 2332
Depo-Medrol Sterile Aqueous Suspension 2334
Hydeltrasol Injection, Sterile 1476
Hydeltra-T.B.A. Sterile Suspension 1478
Hydrocortone Acetate Sterile Suspension 1479
Hydrocortone Phosphate Injection, Sterile 1481
Hydrocortone Tablets 1482

Aspermatogenesis

Velban Vials 1305

Asphyxia

Bentyl 1322
Compazine 2201
Navane Intramuscular 1956
Stelazine 2226
Taractan 1920
Thorazine 2234

Aspiration

Compazine 2201

Asterixis

Bumex (0.1%) 1895
Ceptaz for Injection 1057
Depakene Capsules & Syrup 511
Depakote 512
Dilantin Infatabs (Rare) 1710
Dilantin Kapseals (Rare) 1708
Dilantin Parenteral (Rare) 1712
Dilantin-30 Pediatric/Dilantin-125 Suspension (Rare) 1713
Dilantin with Phenobarbital Kapseals (Rare) 1715
Gelfoam Sterile Sponge 2338
Omnipaque 2552

Asthenia

Accutane Capsules 1878
▲Adalat Capsules (10 mg and 20 mg) (About 10% to 12%) 1587
AeroBid Inhaler System (1-3%) 995
Albalon Solution with Liquifilm .... ◉ 238

Aldactazide 2150
Aldoclor Tablets 1413
Aldomet Ester HCl Injection 1417
Aldomet Oral 1415
Aldoril Tablets 1418
Altace Capsules (2.0%) 1086
Amicar Syrup, Tablets, and Injection 1194
Anafranil Capsules (Up to 2%) 650
Ana-Kit Anaphylaxis Emergency Treatment Kit 1100
Anatuss LA Tablets 1359
Ancobon Capsules 1886
Ansaid Tablets (1-3%) 2319
Apresazide Capsules 854
Apresoline-Esidrix Tablets 857
Arfonad Ampuls 1887
Arm-a-Med Isoetharine Inhalation Solution, USP 616
Artane 1195
Asendin Tablets (Greater than 1%) 1196
Atgam Sterile Solution (Less than 1%) 2320
▲ Ativan Tablets (4.2%) 2434
Atrohist Sprinkle Capsules 558
Atromid-S Capsules (Less often) 2435
Azactam for Injection (Less than 1%) 2252
Azdōne Tablets 844
BAL in Oil Ampules 661
Bactrim DS Tablets 1891
Bactrim I.V. Infusion 1889
Bactrim 1891
▲ Bentyl (7%) 1322
Blocadren Tablets (0.6%) 1429
Brevibloc Injection (Less than 1%) 942
Bronkometer Aerosol 2042
Bronkosol Solution 2042
Bumex (0.2%) 1895
BuSpar (2%) 1401
Butazolidin Capsules & Tablets (Less than 1%) 1027
Cafergot/Cafergot P-B 1999
Calcijex Calcitriol Injection 506
Calderol Capsules 1635
Cantil Tablets 1326
Capoten 2255
Capozide 2258
Carbocaine Hydrochloride Injection 2043
▲ Cardene Capsules (4.2-5.8%) 2290
Cardilate Oral/Sublingual Tablets 757
Cardizem Tablets-30 mg, 60 mg, 90 mg and 120 mg (1.2%) 1329
▲ Cardizem SR Capsules-60 mg, 90 mg and 120 mg (2.8-5%) 1327
Cardura Tablets (1%) 1941
▲ Cartrol Tablets (0.5-7.1%) 507
Catapres Tablets (About 10 in 100 patients) 676
▲ Catapres-TTS (10%) 677
▲ Centrax (7.7%) 1693
Cibacalcin Double-chambered Syringes (Rare) 859
Cipro I.V. (1% or less) 1592
Cipro Tablets (Less than 1%) 1589
Clinoril Tablets (Less than 1 in 100) 1433
Clozaril Tablets (1%) 2000
Cogentin 1435
ColBENEMID Tablets 1436
Colestid Granules (1-3 patients in 1,000) 2328
▲ Combipres Tablets (About 10%) 678
Cortone Acetate Sterile Suspension 1437
Cortone Acetate Tablets 1439
Corzide Tablets (Not uncommon) 702
Cytotec (Infrequent) 2159
DDAVP (Up to 2%) 1841
Dalmane Capsules 1927
Damason-P (Occasional) 1356
Danocrine Capsules 2046
▲ Dantrium Capsules (Among most frequent) 1619
Dapsone USP 1130
Daranide Tablets 1445
Darbid Tablets 2205
Darvon-N/Darvocet-N 1254
Darvon 1256
Darvon-N Suspension & Tablets 1254
Decadron Elixir 1445
Decadron Phosphate Respihaler 1454
Decadron Phosphate Turbinaire 1456
Decadron Phosphate with Xylocaine Injection, Sterile 1451
Deconamine 663
Deconsal 559
Demerol 2047
Depakene Capsules & Syrup 511
Depakote 512
Depen Titratable Tablets 2379
Deprol Tablets 2382
Desyrel and Desyrel Dividose 1404
Dilatrate-SR 1827
Dilaudid-HP Injection 1175
Dimetane-DC Cough Syrup 1857
Dimetane-DX Cough Syrup 1858
Ditropan 1332
Diucardin Tablets 2450
Diulo 2129
Diupres Tablets 1461
Diuril Oral Suspension 1464
Diuril Sodium Intravenous 1463
Diuril Tablets 1464
Dolobid Tablets (Less than 1 in 100) 1465
Dolophine Hydrochloride Ampoules & Vials 1260
Dolophine Hydrochloride Tablets 1261
Donnatal 1858
Donnatal Extentabs 1859
Donnatal Tablets 1858
Donnazyme Tablets 1860
Doral Tablets 2383
▲ Duragesic Transdermal System (10% or more) 1133
Dyazide Capsules 2208
DynaCirc Capsules (1.2%) 2004
Dyrenium Capsules (Rare) 2210
Elavil 2269
Eldepryl 2250
Emete-con Intramuscular/Intravenous 1950
Empirin with Codeine Phosphate Nos. 2, 3 & 4 (Occasional) 764
Endep Tablets 1927
Enduron Tablets 517
Enduronyl 518
Engerix-B Unit-Dose Vials (Less than 1%) 2213
Enlon Injection 598
EpiPen 843
▲ Epogen for Injection (7.0% to 11%) 591
Equagesic Tablets 2451
Ergamisol Tablets (10 patients) 1136
Esidrix Tablets 863
Esimil Tablets 864
Eskalith 2214
▲ Ethmozine Tablets (2%-5%) 946
Etrafon 2087
Exna Tablets 1862
Sterile FUDR 1898
Fansidar Tablets 1896
Fedahist Gyrocaps 2145
Fedahist Timecaps 2145
Feldene Capsules (Less than 1%) 1777
▲ Fiorinal with Codeine Capsules (Among most common) 2008
Flagyl Tablets 2170
Flexeril Tablets (Less than 1%) 1471
Floxin Tablets (Less than 1%) 1652
Gantanol 1899
Gantrisin 1901
Halcion Tablets (Rare) 2340
Humatrope Vials (Infrequent) 1266
Hydeltrasol Injection, Sterile 1476
HydroDIURIL Tablets 1484
Hydromox R Tablets 1209
Hydromox Tablets 1208
Hydropres Tablets 1485
Hyperstat I.V. Injection (2%) 2095
▲ Hytrin Tablets (1.6% to 11.3%) 529
INH Tablets 868
Imferon 976
Inderal 2459
Inderal LA Long Acting Capsules 2461
Inderide Tablets 2463
Inderide LA Long Acting Capsules 2465
▲ Intron A (4% to 24%) 2097
Inversine Tablets 1492
Ismelin Tablets 869
Isordil (Occasional) 2467
Isuprel Hydrochloride Injection 1:5000 2050
Isuprel Hydrochloride Mistometer 2051
Isuprel Hydrochloride Solution 1:200 & 1:100 2052
K-Lyte 707
K-Phos M.F. Tablets 659
K-Phos Neutral Tablets 660
K-Phos No. 2 Tablets 659
▲ Kerlone Tablets (7.1%) 2172
Kinesed Tablets 2272
Koro-Flex Arcing Spring Diaphragm 2142
Koromex Coil Spring Diaphragm 2142
Kutrase Capsules 2146
Lanoxicaps 772
Lanoxin Elixir Pediatric 775
Lanoxin Injection 778
Lanoxin Injection Pediatric 781
Lanoxin Tablets 783
Lariam Tablets (Less than 1%) 1904
Larodopa Tablets (Relatively frequent) 1905
Lasix 1093
▲ Leukine for IV Infusion (Among most frequent) 1127
Levatol (1.6%) 1832
Levsin/Levsinex 2147
Limbitrol 1933
▲ Lioresal Tablets (5-15%) 1031
Lodine Capsules (More than 1% but less than 3%) 2468
Lopid Capsules and Tablets 1736
Lopressor HCT Tablets 1034
Lortab ASA Tablets (Occasional) 2414
Lotensin Tablets 872
Loxitane 1213
▲ Lozol Tablets (Greater than or equal to 5%) 1843
▲ Ludiomil Tablets (4%) 874
▲ Lupron Depot 7.5 mg (5.4%) 2311
Lupron Injection (5% or more) 2310
MS Contin Tablets 1814
MSIR (Infrequent) 1817
Macrodantin Capsules (Less frequent) 1624
Marcaine Hydrochloride with Epinephrine 1:200,000 2055
Marcaine Hydrochloride Injection 2055
Marcaine Spinal 2058
Marplan Tablets 1906
Matulane Capsules 1907
Maxair Inhaler (Less than 1%) 1311
Maxzide 1215
Medihaler Ergotamine Aerosol 1312
Mepergan Injection 2479
Mestinon Injectable 1115
Mestinon 1116
Methadone Hydrochloride Diskets 1284
Methadone Hydrochloride Oral Solution & Tablets 1987
Mevacor Tablets (Rare) 1505
▲ Mexitil Capsules (1.9% to 5%) 680
Micronor Tablets 1667
Midamor Tablets (Between 1% and 3%) 1508
▲ Minipress Capsules (6.5%) 1778
▲ Minizide Capsules (6.5%) 1779
Mithracin 1602
Modane Plus Tablets ⊞ 504
Modane Tablets ⊞ 503
Modicon 1667
▲ Moduretic Tablets (3% to 8%) 1510
Monopril Tablets (0.2 to 1.0%) 1406
Mulvidren-F Softab Tablets 2273
Mustargen 1514
Mykrox ½ mg Tablets (Less than 2%) 984
Myleran Tablets 790
Myochrysine Injection 1516
Naldecon Syrup, Tablets, Pediatric Drops and Pediatric Syrup 709
▲ Nalfon Pulvules & Tablets (5.4%) 919
Naphcon Forte ⊙ 226
Nardil (Common) 1742
Naturetin Tablets (Common) 1789
Navane Capsules and Concentrate 1954
Navane Intramuscular 1956
NegGram 2062
▲ Neupogen for Injection (4%) 595
Niclocide Chewable Tablets 1607
Nicorette 1335
Nitro-Bid IV (Less than 1%) 1338
Nitro-Bid Ointment 1339
Nitro-Bid Capsules 1338
Nitrolingual Spray 1846
Nitrostat IV 1744
Nitrostat Tablets (Occasional) 1743
Norflex 1314
Norgesic 1314
Normodyne Tablets (1%) 2110
Normozide Tablets (1%) 2112
Norpramin Tablets 1340
Novafed A Capsules 1342
Novafed Capsules 1342
Novahistine DH 1342
Novahistine DMX ⊞ 595
Novahistine Elixir ⊞ 596
Novahistine Expectorant 1343
Nucofed Capsules 2219
Nucofed Expectorant 2219
Nucofed Pediatric Expectorant 2220
Nucofed Syrup 2219
Omnipaque 2552
OptiPranolol Sterile Ophthalmic Solution (A small number of patients) ⊙ 261
Oramorph SR (Morphine Sulfate Sustained Release Tablets) 1988
Orap Tablets 1020
Oretic Tablets 544
Oreticyl 545
Ornade Spansule Capsules 2221
Ortho Diaphragm Kit 1664
Ortho-Novum 1667
Ortho-White Diaphragm Kit-Flat Spring 1664
PMB 200 and PMB 400 2504
Pamelor 2019
Pantopon Injectable 1911
▲ Paraplatin for Injection (11%) 735
Parlodel 2020
Parnate Tablets 2222
Pentaspan Injection 949
Pepcid (Infrequent) 1524
Peritrate (Occasional) 1756
▲ Permax Tablets (4.2%) 1291
Pfizerpen-AS Aqueous Suspension (Approximately 1 in 500) 1959
Phenergan with Codeine 2497
Phenergan VC 2500
Phenergan VC with Codeine 2501
Plaquenil Sulfate Tablets 2067
Plendil Extended-Release Tablets (0.1%) 1526
Pneumovax 23 1528
Polycitra Syrup 2424
Polycitra-K 2424
Polycitra-LC—Sugar-Free 2424
Pondimin Tablets 1867
Prilosec Delayed-Release Capsules (0.2 to 1.3%) 1530
Primaxin I.M. 1532
Primaxin I.V. (Less than 0.2%) 1535
Prinivil Tablets (1.3%) 1538
Prinzide Tablets (1.8%) 1540
Pro-Banthīne Tablets 2141
Procan SR Tablets (Occasional) 1760
▲ Procardia XL Tablets (Less than 3% to 12%) 1783
▲ Procrit for Injection (7% to 11%) 1647
Proglycem 649
Prokine for I.V. Infusion 1096
Pronestyl Capsules and Tablets 1800
Pronestyl Injection 1798
Pronestyl-SR Tablets (Occasional) 1801
▲ ProSom Tablets (11%) 554
Prostigmin Injectable 1120
Prostigmin Tablets 1121
Protostat Tablets 1674
Proventil Repetabs Tablets (2%) 2120
Proventil Syrup (Less than 1 of 100) 2119
Proventil Tablets (2%) 2120
▲ Prozac Pulvules (4.4%) 920
Quadrinal Tablets 1183
Quarzan Capsules 1937
Rauzide Tablets 1804
Recombivax HB (Equal to or greater than 1%) 1544
Regitine 878
Renese Tablets 1785
Renese-R Tablets 1786
Restoril Capsules (1-2%) 2023
▲ Retrovir Capsules (19%) 802
▲ Retrovir I.V. Infusion (19%) 805
▲ Retrovir Syrup (19%) 802
Rifamate Capsules 1347
Robinul Forte Tablets 1873
Robinul Injectable 1873
Robinul Tablets 1873
Rocaltrol Capsules 1913
Roferon-A Injection (Less than 0.5%) 1916
Rondec 1975
Rondec-DM 1976
Rondec-TR Tablet 1975
Rowasa (0.12 to 1.2%) 2248
Roxanol 1991
Rum-K Syrup 995
Ru-Tuss DE Tablets 694
Rythmol Tablets (0.6 to 2.6%) 1184
Saluron 718
Salutensin/Salutensin-Demi 719
Sandimmune (Rare) 2024
Sandostatin Injection (1.0%) 2029
Sanorex Tablets 2030
Sansert Tablets 2031
Scleromate (Rare) 1685
Seldane Tablets (0.6%) 1349
Seldane-D Extended-Release Tablets 1350
Septra 813
Septra I.V. Infusion 808
Septra I.V. Infusion ADD-Vantage Vials 810
Septra 813
Ser-Ap-Es Tablets 881
Serentil 686
Serpasil-Esidrix Tablets 886

Sinemet Tablets 952
Sinemet CR Tablets 953
Sinequan (Occasional) 1960
Solganal Suspension (Rare) 2122
Soma Compound w/Codeine Tablets (Very rare) 2390
Soma Compound Tablets (Very rare) 2389
Soma Tablets 2388
Sorbitrate 1103
Surmontil Capsules 2524
Sus-Phrine Injection 1006
Symmetrel Capsules & Syrup (0.1-1%) 936
Synarel Nasal Solution (Less than 1%) 2300
Talacen (Infrequent) 2070
Talwin Injection (Infrequent) 2071
Talwin Compound (Infrequent) 2072
Talwin Injection (Infrequent) 2071
Talwin Nx (Infrequent) 2073
▲ Tambocor Tablets (4.9%) 1315
Taractan 1920
▲ Tenex Tablets (10%) 1875
Tenoretic Tablets 1105
Tensilon Injectable 1123
Thalitone Tablets 687
Timolide Tablets (1.9%) 1547
Timoptic in Ocudose 1552
Timoptic Sterile Ophthalmic Solution 1550
Tofranil Ampuls 1038
Tofranil Tablets 1039
Tofranil-PM Capsules 1041
▲ Tolectin (200, 400 and 600 mg) (3 to 9%) 1379
Tolinase Tablets (Infrequently) 2365
Tonocard Tablets (Less than 1%) 1554
Toradol IM Injection (1% or less) 2302
Trancopal Caplets 2075
Trandate HCT/Trandate (1% in 208 patients) 579
Triavil Tablets 1556
Trinalin Repetabs Tablets 1170
Trobicin Sterile Powder 2366
Tuss-Ornade Liquid 2242
Tuss-Ornade Spansule Capsules 2242
Uroqid-Acid (Less frequent) 661
Valpin 50 Tablets 941
▲ Vascor (200, 300 and 400 mg) Tablets (0.5 to 13.95%) 1383
Vaseretic Tablets (2.4%) 1559
Vasocon-A ◉ 278
Vasotec I.V. 1562
Vasotec Tablets (1.1% to 1.6%) 1564
Velban Vials 1305
Ventolin (Less than 1 of 100) 583
Versed Injection (Less than 1%) 1924
▲ Visken Tablets (4%) 2036
Vivactil Tablets 1567
Wygesic Tablets 2540
▲ Wytensin Tablets (10%) 2542
▲ Xanax Tablets (7.1%) 2367
Yutopar (1 to 3% (with IV administration)) 647
Zaroxolyn Tablets 989
Zestoretic (1.8%) 2274
Zestril Tablets (1.3%) 2277
Zovirax (1.2%) 824
Zyloprim Tablets (Less than 1%) 830

Asthma, allergic

Flu-Imune Influenza Virus Vaccine (Rare) 1204

Asthma, bronchial

Ansaid Tablets (Less than 1%) 2319
Cholybar 1705
Cuprimine Capsules 1442
Decadron Phosphate Turbinaire 1456
Depen Titratable Tablets 2379
Exna Tablets 1862
Lortab ASA Tablets 2414
Norzine 1818
Permax Tablets (Infrequent) 1291
Pronestyl Capsules and Tablets 1800
Pronestyl Injection 1798
Prozac Pulvules (Infrequent) 920
Questran Light 711
Soma Compound Tablets 2389
Toradol IM Injection (1% or less) 2302
Vaseretic Tablets 1559
Vasotec I.V. 1562
Zyloprim Tablets (Less than 1%) 830

Asthmatic episodes

Alupent (1 to 4%) 674
Azdōne Tablets 844
Betoptic Sterile Ophthalmic Solution (Rare) 569
Betoptic S Sterile Ophthalmic Suspension (Rare) 570
Butazolidin Capsules & Tablets 1027
Calciparine Injection (Rare) 925
Cardioquin Tablets 1812
Compazine 2201
Damason-P 1356
Dobutrex Solution Vials 1259
Duragesic Transdermal System (Less than 1%) 1133
Duvoid Tablets 1853
Easprin 1719
Eldepryl 2250
Empirin with Codeine Phosphate Nos. 2, 3 & 4 764
Engerix-B Unit-Dose Vials 2213
Equagesic Tablets 2451
Esimil Tablets 864
Etrafon 2087
Harmonyl Tablets 528
Heparin Lock Flush Solution 2456
Heparin Sodium Vials (Rare) 1264
Heparin Sodium Injection 2457
Heparin Sodium Injection, USP, Sterile Solution 2342
Indocin Capsules (Less than 1%) 1487
Indocin I.V. (Less than 1%) 1490
Indocin (Less than 1%) 1487
Ismelin Tablets 869
Isopto Carbachol ◉ 219
Lodine Capsules (Less than 1%) 2468
Lotensin Tablets 872
Meclan (meclocycline sulfosalicylate) Cream 1679
Mellaril 2011
Minocin Oral Suspension 1224
Nubain Injection (Less than 1%) 934
Omnipaque 2552
Oreticyl 545
Phenergan Injection 2493
Phenergan Tablets 2496
Plague Vaccine (Rare) 1584
Prolixin Decanoate 1795
Prolixin Elixir 1793
Prolixin Enanthate 1796
Prolixin Injection 1791
Prolixin Oral Concentrate 1792
Prolixin Tablets 1793
Pronestyl Injection 1798
ProSom Tablets (Infrequent) 554
Questran Powder 710
Quinaglute Dura-Tabs Tablets 663
Quinamm Tablets 1344
Quinidex Extentabs 1868
Robaxisal Tablets 1872
Rowasa 2248
Scleromate (Rare) 1685
Serentil 686
Soma Compound w/Codeine Tablets (Rare) 2390
Soma Compound Tablets (Rare) 2389
Soma Tablets 2388
Sotradecol (Sodium Tetradecyl Sulfate Injection) 964
Stelazine 2226
Tacaryl 2409
Taractan 1920
Temaril Tablets, Syrup and Spansule Sustained Release Capsules 1085
Terramycin Intramuscular Solution 1964
Thorazine 2234
Torecan 1993
Triavil Tablets 1556
Trilafon 2123
Trilisate (Rare) 1822
Urecholine 1558
Viokase 1877
Voltaren Tablets (Less than 1%) 1042

Asystole

Adenocard Injection 1007
Alfenta Injection 1131
Brevibloc Injection (2 Patients) 942
Cardioquin Tablets 1812
Enlon Injection 598
Isoptin Injectable (In extreme cases) 1177
Omnipaque (Less than 0.4%) 2552
Quinaglute Dura-Tabs Tablets 663
Zantac Injection and Zantac Injection Premixed (Rare) 1063

Asystole, ventricular

Procan SR Tablets (Common) 1760
Pronestyl Capsules and Tablets 1800
▲ Pronestyl Injection (More common) 1798
Pronestyl-SR Tablets 1801

Ataxia

AK-Pentolate ◉ 204
Aldactazide 2150
Aldactone 2152
Alurate Elixir (Less than 1 in 100) 1883
Anafranil Capsules (Infrequent) 650
Ancobon Capsules 1886
Ansaid Tablets (Less than 1%) 2319
Asendin Tablets (Greater than 1%) 1196
Attenuvax (Rare) 1424
Azo Gantanol Tablets 1887
Azo Gantrisin Tablets 1888
Azulfidine Tablets, EN-tabs, Oral Suspension (Rare) 1157
Bactrim DS Tablets 1891
Bactrim I.V. Infusion 1889
Bactrim 1891
Betagan (Rare) ◉ 239
BuSpar (1%) 1401
Butisol Sodium Elixir & Tablets (Less than 1 in 100) 2377
Capoten 2255
Capozide 2258
Cardura Tablets (1%) 1941
CeeNU 725
Celontin (Frequent) 1692
▲ Centrax (5%) 1693
Cibalith-S 870
Cipro I.V. (1% or less) 1592
Cipro Tablets (Less than 1%) 1589
Clozaril Tablets (1%) 2000
▲ Cordarone Tablets (4 to 9%) 2446
Cyclogyl (Common) ◉ 215
Cyclomydril ◉ 216
Cytovene Sterile Powder (1% or less) 2292
Dalalone D.P. Injectable 999
Dalmane Capsules 1927
Daranide Tablets 1445
Decadron-LA Sterile Suspension (Low) 1457
Demerol 2047
Depakene Capsules & Syrup 511
Depakote 512
Deprol Tablets 2382
Desyrel and Desyrel Dividose (Greater than 1%) 1404
▲ Dilantin Infatabs (Among most common) 1710
▲ Dilantin Kapseals (Among most common) 1708
▲ Dilantin Parenteral (Among most common) 1712
▲ Dilantin-30 Pediatric/Dilantin-125 Suspension (Among most common) 1713
Dilantin with Phenobarbital Kapseals (Common) 1715
Doral Tablets 2383
Elavil 2269
Endep Tablets 1927
Equagesic Tablets 2451
Ergamisol Tablets (Up to 2%) 1136
Eskalith 2214
Ethmozine Tablets (Less than 2%) 946
Etrafon 2087
Fansidar Tablets 1896
Flagyl I.V. 2131
Flagyl Tablets 2170
Flexeril Tablets (Less than 1%) 1471
Gantanol 1899
Gantrisin Ophthalmic Ointment/Solution 1900
Gantrisin 1901
▲ Halcion Tablets (4.6%) 2340
Hexalen Capsules 2316
Intron A (2 patients) 2097
▲ Klonopin Tablets (30%) 1902
Larodopa Tablets (Relatively frequent) 1905
Leukeran Tablets (Rare) 788
Levsin/Levsinex 2147
Librax Capsules 1929
Libritabs Tablets 1930
Librium Capsules (Some patients) 1931
Librium Injectable 1932
Limbitrol 1933
Lioresal Tablets 1031
Lithane Tablets 1596
Lithium Carbonate Capsules & Tablets 1984
Lithobid Tablets 870
Ludiomil Tablets (Rare) 874
M-M-R II (Rare) 1494
M-R-VAX II (Rare) 1496
Marplan Tablets (Rare) 1906
Matulane Capsules 1907
Mebaral Tablets (Less than 1 in 100) 2061
Menrium Tablets (Particularly in elderly and debilitated) 1934
Mepergan Injection 2479
Mesantoin Tablets 2013
Methotrexate Tablets, Parenteral, LPF Parenteral 1217
Milontin Kapseals 1741
Miltown Tablets 2386
▲ Mysoline (Among most frequent) 2480
Nardil (Less frequent) 1742
Nembutal Sodium Capsules (Less than 1%) 534
Nembutal Sodium Solution (Less than 1%) 536
Nembutal Sodium Suppositories (Less than 1%) 538
Norpramin Tablets 1340
Oncovin Solution Vials & Hyporets 1288
PBZ-SR Tablets 1037
PMB 200 and PMB 400 (Rare) 2504
Pamelor 2019
Pantopon Injectable 1911
Parlodel 2020
Pediazole 1973
Peganone Tablets (Rare) 551
Permax Tablets (1.6%) 1291
Phenergan Injection 2493
Phenergan Tablets 2496
Phenobarbital Elixir and Tablets (Less than 1 in 100 patients) 1293
Placidyl Capsules 553
Plaquenil Sulfate Tablets 2067
Polymyxin B Sulfate, Aerosporin Brand Sterile Powder 798
Pondimin Tablets 1867
Procardia XL Tablets (1% or less) 1783
ProSom Tablets (Rare) 554
Protostat Tablets 1674
Prozac Pulvules (Infrequent) 920
Quinidex Extentabs 1868
Restoril Capsules (Less than 1%) 2023
Rheumatrex Methotrexate Dose Pack 1234
Rifadin 1345
Rifamate Capsules 1347
Rimactane Capsules 879
Robaxin Injectable 1871
Roferon-A Injection (Less than 1%) 1916
Ru-Tuss with Hydrocodone 694
Ru-Tuss Tablets 693
Rythmol Tablets (0.3 to 1.6%) 1184
Sansert Tablets 2031
Seconal Sodium Pulvules (Less than 1 in 100) 1296
Septra 813
Septra I.V. Infusion 808
Septra I.V. Infusion ADD-Vantage Vials 810
Septra 813
Serax Capsules (Rare) 2522
Serax Tablets (Rare) 2522
Serentil 686
Sinemet Tablets 952
Sinequan (Infrequent) 1960
Soma Compound w/Codeine Tablets 2390
Soma Compound Tablets 2389
Soma Tablets 2388
Surmontil Capsules 2524
Symmetrel Capsules & Syrup (1-5%) 936
Tacaryl 2409
Tambocor Tablets (1-3%) 1315
Taractan 1920
Temaril Tablets, Syrup and Spansule Sustained Release Capsules 1085
Thiosulfil Forte Tablets 2526
Tofranil Ampuls 1038
Tofranil Tablets 1039
Tofranil-PM Capsules 1041
▲ Tonocard Tablets (0.2-10.8%) 1554
Tranxene 556
Triavil Tablets 1556
Trilafon 2123
Tuss-Ornade Liquid 2242
Tuss-Ornade Spansule Capsules 2242
Valium Injectable (Among most common) 1937
Valium Tablets (Among most common) 1939
▲ Valrelease Capsules (Among most common) 1923
Vaseretic Tablets 1559
Vasotec I.V. 1562
Vasotec Tablets (0.5% to 1.0%) 1564
Versed Injection (Less than 1%) 1924
Vira-A for Injection 1766
Vivactil Tablets 1567
Wellbutrin Tablets (Frequent) 821

Wytensin Tablets (3% or less) 2542
Yohimex Tablets 1190
Zarontin Capsules 1768
Zarontin Syrup 1769

Ateleclasis

Dalgan Injection (Less than 1%) 620
Metrodin (urofollitropin for injection) 2182

Athetosis

Versed Injection (Less than 1%) 1924

Atrial arrhythmias

Adalat Capsules (10 mg and 20 mg) (1 in 150 patients) 1587
Asendin Tablets (Very rare) 1196
Hyperstat I.V. Injection 2095
Mexitil Capsules (1 in 1,000) 680
Streptase for Infusion 635

Atrial contractions, premature

Brethaire Inhaler 1024
Diprivan Injection (Less than 1%) .. 2267
Emete-con Intramuscular/Intravenous 1950
▲Omnipaque (6.5%) 2552
Sodium Polystyrene Sulfonate Suspension 1993

Atrial depression

Dilantin Parenteral 1712

Atrial flutter

Anafranil Capsules (Rare) 650
Cipro Tablets (Less than 1%) 1589
Ethmozine Tablets (Less than 2%) 946
Rythmol Tablets (Less than 1%) 1184
Tenormin Tablets and I.V. Injection (1.6%) 1107

Atrial tachycardia

Vaseretic Tablets 1559

Atrioventricular dissociation

Calan SR Caplets (1% or less) 2157
Calan Tablets (1% or less) 2155
Isoptin Oral Tablets (Less than 1%) 1179
Isoptin SR Sustained Release Tablets (Less than 1%) 1181
Lanoxicaps (Common) 772
Lanoxin Elixir Pediatric (Common).. 775
Lanoxin Injection (Common) 778
Lanoxin Injection Pediatric (Common) 781
Lanoxin Tablets (Common) 783
Rythmol Tablets (Less than 1%) 1184
Verelan Capsules (Less than 1%) .. 1243

Atrioventricular dysfunction

Wytensin Tablets (Very rare) 2542

Atrophy

Antivenin (Crotalidae) Polyvalent 2430
Celestone Soluspan Suspension 2081
Cuprimine Capsules 1442
Dalalone D.P. Injectable 999
Imferon 976
Solu-Cortef Sterile Powder 2361
Solu-Medrol Sterile Powder 2363

Atrophy, acute yellow

Solganal Suspension 2122

Atrophy, cutaneous

Aristospan Suspension (Intra-articular) 1011
Celestone Soluspan Suspension 2081
Cortone Acetate Sterile Suspension 1437
Decadron Phosphate Injection 1449
Decadron Phosphate with Xylocaine Injection, Sterile 1451
Decadron-LA Sterile Suspension 1457
Depen Titratable Tablets (Rare) 2379
Depo-Medrol Sterile Aqueous Suspension 2334
Hydeltrasol Injection, Sterile 1476
Hydeltra-T.B.A. Sterile Suspension 1478
Hydrocortone Acetate Sterile Suspension 1479
Hydrocortone Phosphate Injection, Sterile 1481
Kenalog-10 Injection 2402
Kenalog-40 Injection 2403

Atrophy, subcutaneous

Aristospan Suspension (Intra-articular) 1011
Carmol HC Cream 1% 2296
Cortone Acetate Sterile Suspension 1437
Dalalone D.P. Injectable 999
Decadron Phosphate Injection 1449
Decadron Phosphate with Xylocaine Injection, Sterile 1451
Decadron-LA Sterile Suspension 1457
Depo-Medrol Sterile Aqueous Suspension 2334
Garamycin Injectable (Rare) 2093
Hydeltrasol Injection, Sterile 1476
Hydeltra-T.B.A. Sterile Suspension 1478
Hydrocortone Acetate Sterile Suspension 1479
Hydrocortone Phosphate Injection, Sterile 1481
Kenalog-10 Injection 2402
Kenalog-40 Injection 2403
Lidex 2296
Neo-Synalar Cream 2296
Solu-Cortef Sterile Powder 2361
Solu-Medrol Sterile Powder 2363
Synacort Creams 1%, 2.5% 2296
Synalar 2296

Atypical measles

Attenuvax 1424

Auditory acuity, decrease

▲Capastat Sulfate Vials (Approximately 11%) 1250
Cardioquin Tablets 1812
Desferal Vials 862
Ganite Injection 1016
Quinaglute Dura-Tabs Tablets 663
Quinidex Extentabs 1868

Auditory canals, small or absent, fetal

Accutane Capsules 1878

Auditory disturbances

Aralen Hydrochloride Injection 2038
Aralen Phosphate with Primaquine Phosphate Tablets 2040
Aralen Phosphate Tablets 2039
Demulen 2161
Enovid 2161
Norethin 2133
▲Wellbutrin Tablets (5.3%) 821

Autonomic deficit, persistent

Duranest Injections 624
Nescaine/Nescaine MPF 629
Stelazine 2226
Xylocaine Injections (Rare) 637

Awareness, altered

▲Tonocard Tablets (1.5-11.0%) 1554

Awareness, heightened

Demser Capsules 1460
▲Marinol (Dronabinol) Capsules (24%) 1985

Azoospermia

ColBENEMID Tablets 1436
Cytoxan for Injection (Reported in a number of patients) 726
Matulane Capsules 1907
Mustargen 1514
Neosar for Injection (Reported in a number of patients) 566

Azotemia

Amikin Injectable 602
Ancobon Capsules 1886
BiCNU 723
▲Bumex (10.6%) 1895
CeeNU 725
Children's Advil Suspension (Less than 1%) 2426
Cleocin HCl Capsules 2322
Cleocin Pediatric Flavored Granules 2324
Cleocin Phosphate Injection 2325
Diuril Sodium Intravenous 1463
Dyrenium Capsules (Rare) 2210
Elspar (Frequent) 1470
Fungizone Intravenous (Common) .. 2262
HydroDIURIL Tablets 1484
Hydropres Tablets 1485
▲Indocin I.V. (41% of infants) 1490
Intropin Injection (Infrequent) 930
Lincocin 2344
Methotrexate Tablets, Parenteral, LPF Parenteral 1217
Minocin Oral Suspension 1224
Motrin Tablets (Less than 1%) 2351
Nalfon Pulvules & Tablets (Less than 1%) 919
Oncovin Solution Vials & Hyporets 1288
PediaProfen Suspension (Less than 1%) 1363
Polymyxin B Sulfate, Aerosporin Brand Sterile Powder 798
Prinivil Tablets (1% or less) 1538
Prinzide Tablets 1540
Proglycem 649
Rauzide Tablets 1804
Rheumatrex Methotrexate Dose Pack 1234
Rufen Tablets (Less than 1%) 691
Tegretol Chewable Tablets 654
Tegretol Suspension 656
Tegretol Tablets 654
Terramycin Capsules 1786
Thalitone Tablets 687
Vancocin HCl, Oral Solution & Pulvules 1304
Vancocin HCl, Vials & ADD-Vantage 1302
Vaseretic Tablets 1559
Voltaren Tablets (Less than 1%) 1042
Zanosar Sterile Powder 2371
Zestoretic 2274
Zestril Tablets (Less than 1%) 2277
Zyloprim Tablets (Less than 1%).... 830

ADH syndrome, inappropriate

Aminophyllin Tablets 2153
Asbron G 1997
Asendin Tablets (Less than 1%) 1196
Choledyl Pediatric Elixir 1702
Choledyl Tablets 1700
Choledyl SA Tablets 1704
Constant-T Tablets 1029
Desyrel and Desyrel Dividose 1404
DiaBeta 1091
Diabinese Tablets (Rare) 1775
Elavil 2269
Endep Tablets 1927
Etrafon 2087
Flexeril Tablets (Rare) 1471
Glucotrol 1952
Limbitrol 1933
Lufyllin & Lufyllin-400 Tablets 2384
Lufyllin-GG Elixir & Tablets 2385
Marplan Tablets 1906
Methadone Hydrochloride Oral Solution & Tablets 1987
Micronase Tablets 2350
Norpramin Tablets 1340
Oncovin Solution Vials & Hyporets (Rare) 1288
Orinase Tablets 2354
Pamelor 2019
Parnate Tablets 2222
Permax Tablets (Infrequent) 1291
Platinol 737
Platinol-AQ Injection 738
Prozac Pulvules 920
Quadrinal Tablets 1183
Quibron Capsules 713
Quibron-T 714
Quibron-T/SR 716
Respbid Tablets 684
Roxanol 1991
Rythmol Tablets (Less than 1%) 1184
Slo-bid Gyrocaps 1847
Surmontil Capsules 2524
T-PHYL (Uniphyl) 200 mg Tablets 1820
Tegretol Chewable Tablets 654
Tegretol Suspension 656
Tegretol Tablets 654
Theo-24 2179
Theo-Dur Sprinkle 1168
Theo-Dur Extended-Release Tablets 1166
Theolair 1317
Theolair-SR Tablets 1319
▲TheoX Extended-Release Tablets (Among most consistent) 841
Tofranil Ampuls 1038
Tofranil Tablets 1039
Tofranil-PM Capsules 1041
Tolinase Tablets 2365
Triavil Tablets 1556
Trilafon 2123
Uniphyl 400 mg Tablets 1823
Velban Vials 1305
Vivactil Tablets 1567

ANA, positive

Adalat Capsules (10 mg and 20 mg) (Less than 0.5%) 1587
Aldoclor Tablets 1413
Aldomet Ester HCl Injection 1417
Aldomet Oral 1415
Aldoril Tablets 1418
Capoten 2255
Capozide 2258
Elavil 2269
Feldene Capsules (Less than 1%) .. 1777
Mevacor Tablets (Rare) 1505
Mexitil Capsules (About 2 in 1,000) 680
Minipress Capsules 1778
Monopril Tablets (0.2 to 1.0%) 1406
Normodyne Tablets 2110
Normozide Tablets 2112
Prinivil Tablets (1% or less) 1538
Prinzide Tablets 1540
Procan SR Tablets 1760
Procardia Capsules (Less than 0.5%) 1781
Pronestyl Capsules and Tablets 1800
Pronestyl Injection 1798
Pronestyl-SR Tablets 1801
Rythmol Tablets (0.7%) 1184
Tenoretic Tablets 1105
Tenormin Tablets and I.V. Injection 1107
Tonocard Tablets (Less than 1%) .. 1554
Trandate HCT/Trandate 579
Vaseretic Tablets 1559
Vasotec I.V. 1562
Vasotec Tablets 1564
Zestoretic 2274
Zestril Tablets 2277

B

Babinski's phenomenon, bilateral

Dopram Injectable 1860

Backache

Actigall Capsules 2280
Actimmune (2%) 1046
Adenocard Injection (Less than 1%) 1007
▲Alferon N Injection (1% to 4%) 1809
Amen 833
▲Anafranil Capsules (Up to 6%) 650
▲Atgam Sterile Solution (More than 1% to 10%) 2320
Carafate Tablets (Less than 0.5%) 1326
Carbocaine Hydrochloride Injection 2043
Cardura Tablets (Less than 0.5% of 3960 patients) 1941
Cartrol Tablets (2.1%) 507
▲CHEMET (succimer) Capsules (5.2 to 15.7%) 1361
Cholybar 1705
Cipro I.V. (1% or less) 1592
Cipro Tablets (Less than 1%) 1589
Clozaril Tablets (1%) 2000
Cycrin Tablets 2449
▲CytoGam (Less than 5.0%) 891
Cytotec (Infrequent) 2159
Danocrine Capsules 2046
Dantrium Capsules (Less frequent) 1619
Demulen 2161
Depo-Provera Sterile Aqueous Suspension 2336
Duranest Injections 624
Eldepryl (1 of 49 patients) 2250
Engerix-B Unit-Dose Vials (Less than 1%) 2213
Enovid 2161
Gamimune N Immune Globulin Intravenous (Human) 1572
Gammagard Immune Globulin, Intravenous (Human) (Occasional) 658
Gammar-IV, Immune Globulin Intravenous (Human) 610
Gelfoam Sterile Sponge 2338
Hylorel Tablets (1.5%) 975
Hyperstat I.V. Injection 2095
Hytrin Tablets (2.4%) 529
Imferon 976
▲Intron A (Up to 19%) 2097
Lippes Loop Intrauterine Double-S.. 1654
Marcaine Hydrochloride with Epinephrine 1:200,000 2055
Marcaine Hydrochloride Injection.... 2055
Marcaine Spinal 2058
Methotrexate Tablets, Parenteral, LPF Parenteral 1217
Midamor Tablets (Less than or equal to 1%) 1508
Moduretic Tablets (Less than or equal to 1%) 1510
Mykrox ½ mg Tablets (Less than 2%) 984
Nescaine/Nescaine MPF 629
Niclocide Chewable Tablets 1607
Norethin 2133
Norlutate 1754
Norlutin 1755
Normozide Tablets 2112
▲Omnipaque (1.3 to about 8%) 2552
Oncovin Solution Vials & Hyporets 1288

ParaGard T380A Intrauterine Copper Contraceptive 411
Permax Tablets (1.6%) 1291
Plendil Extended-Release Tablets..... 1526
Prilosec Delayed-Release Capsules (1.1%) 1530
Prinivil Tablets (0.5%) 1538
Prinzide Tablets (0.3% to 1%) 1540
Procardia XL Tablets (1% or less).. 1783
ProSom Tablets (2%) 554
Protamine Sulfate Ampoules & Vials 1295
Provera Tablets 2356
Prozac Pulvules (2.0%) 920
Questran Light 711
Questran Powder 710
Recombivax HB (Less than 1%) 1544
Retrovir Capsules (Less than 5%) 802
Retrovir I.V. Infusion (Less than 5%) 805
Retrovir Syrup (Less than 5%) 802
Rheumatrex Methotrexate Dose Pack 1234
Rogaine Topical Solution (2.59%).. 2357
Rowasa (1.35%) 2248
Sandostatin Injection (Less than 1%) 2029
Sansert Tablets 2031
Sectral Capsules (Up to 2%) 2520
Sensorcaine 631
Sensorcaine-MPF Spinal 634
Sinemet CR Tablets (1.6%) 953
Stilphostrol Tablets and Ampuls 1609
Vancocin HCl, Vials & ADD-Vantage (Infrequent) 1302
Vaseretic Tablets (0.5% to 2.0%) 1559
▲Xylocaine Injections (3%) 637
Zestoretic (0.3 to 1%) 2274
Zestril Tablets (0.5%) 2277

Bacteremia
Ethamolin 1829
Retrovir 802

Bacteriuria
Sinemet CR Tablets (1% or greater) 953

Baldness, male pattern (see under Alopecia, hereditaria)

Bartter's syndrome
Capastat Sulfate Vials (1 patient) 1250

Basophils, increase
Primaxin I.M. 1532
Primaxin I.V. 1535
Rocephin Injectable Vials, ADD-Vantage (Rare) 1914
Unasyn 1965
Zefazone Sterile Powder 2372

Behavior, hypochondriacal
Celontin 1692

Behavior, inappropriate
Artane 1195
Ativan Injection (Occasional) 2432
Halcion Tablets 2340
Hydromox R Tablets 1209
Xanax Tablets (Rare) 2367

Behavior, violent
Prozac Pulvules 920

Behavioral changes
Akineton 1171
AK-Pentolate ..... ⊙ 204
Amoxil (Rare) 2193
Augmentin Tablets, Powder for Oral Suspension, and Chewable Tablets (Rare) 2198
Catapres Tablets 676
Catapres-TTS 677
Combipres Tablets 678
Corgard Tablets (Approximately 6 of 1000 patients) 701
Corzide Tablets (Approximately 6 of 1000 patients) 702
Cyclogyl ..... ⊙ 215
Cyclomydril ..... ⊙ 216
Cytotec (Infrequent) 2159
Eldepryl 2250
Gastrocrom Capsules (Infrequent).. 974
▲Klonopin Tablets (25%) 1902
Methotrexate Tablets, Parenteral, LPF Parenteral 1217
Mydriacyl ..... ⊙ 225
Rheumatrex Methotrexate Dose Pack 1234
Rifadin 1345
Timoptic in Ocudose 1552
Timoptic Sterile Ophthalmic Solution 1550
Torecan 1993
Tropicacyl ..... ⊙ 209
Vascor (200, 300 and 400 mg) Tablets (0.5 to 2.0%) 1383

Behavioral deterioration
Depakene Capsules & Syrup 511
Depakote 512

Bell's palsy
Aldoclor Tablets 1413
Aldomet Ester HCl Injection 1417
Aldomet Oral 1415
Aldoril Tablets 1418
Engerix-B Unit-Dose Vials 2213
Flexeril Tablets (Rare) 1471
Permax Tablets (Rare) 1291
Recombivax HB 1544
Sandostatin Injection (Less than 1%) 2029

Benzyl alcohol, sensitivity to
AquaMEPHYTON Injection 1422
Cytosar-U Sterile Powder 2329
Depo-Medrol Sterile Aqueous Suspension 2334
Lincocin Sterile Solution 2344
Nuromax Injection 794
Protropin 1049
Septra I.V. Infusion 808
Septra I.V. Infusion ADD-Vantage Vials 810
Tracrium Injection 817
Trobicin Sterile Powder 2366

Bigeminy
Diprivan Injection (Less than 1%) .. 2267
Versed Injection (Less than 1%) 1924

Bile duct "sludge", presence of metabolites
Clinoril Tablets (Rare) 1433

Biliary atresia
Cholybar (One case) 1705

Biliary sclerosis
Sterile FUDR 1898

Biliary stasis
Compazine 2201
Mellaril 2011
Norzine 1818
Serentil 686
Stelazine 2226
Taractan 1920
Torecan 1993
Triavil Tablets 1556
Trilafon 2123

Biliary tract spasm
Mepergan Injection 2479
Oramorph SR (Morphine Sulfate Sustained Release Tablets) (Less frequent) 1988

Biliary tree, calcification
Cholybar (Occasional) 1705

Bilirubinemia
Intron A (Less than 1%) 2097

Bilirubinuria
INH Tablets 868
Imuran 768
Primaxin I.M. 1532
Primaxin I.V. 1535
Rifamate Capsules 1347

Birth defects
Aygestin Tablets 2437
Celontin 1692
Centrax Capsules 1693
Coumadin Injection & Tablets 944
Cuprimine Capsules 1442
Demulen 2161
Depakene Capsules & Syrup (Multiple reports) 511
Depakote (Multiple reports) 512
Depen Titratable Tablets 2379
Dicumarol Tablets 516
Dilantin Infatabs 1710
Dilantin Kapseals 1708
Dilantin Parenteral 1712
Dilantin-30 Pediatric/Dilantin-125 Suspension 1713
Dilantin with Phenobarbital Kapseals 1715
Encare Vaginal Contraceptive Suppositories ..... ▣ 733
Enovid 2161
Klonopin Tablets 1902
Lo/Ovral Tablets 2471
Lo/Ovral-28 Tablets 2476
Loestrin 1728
Mediatric Capsules 2476
Mesantoin Tablets 2013
Metrodin (urofollitropin for injection) (4 incidents) 2182
Milontin Kapseals 1741
Mysoline 2480
Nolvadex Tablets 1102
Nordette-21 Tablets 2481
Nordette-28 Tablets 2483
Norethin 2133
Ortho Dienestrol Cream 1664
Ovral Tablets 2490
Ovral-28 Tablets 2491
Ovrette Tablets 2492
Panwarfin Tablets 547
Paradione Capsules (Multiple reports) 548
Peganone Tablets (Multiple reports) 551
Pergonal (menotropins for injection, USP) (1.7%) 2184
Phenurone Tablets (Multiple reports) 552
Premarin Intravenous 2508
Premarin with Methyltestosterone .. 2515
Premarin Vaginal Cream 2512
Quadrinal Tablets 1183
Serophene (clomiphene citrate tablets, USP) (2.5%) 2186
Tridione 557
Triphasil-21 Tablets 2527
Triphasil-28 Tablets 2532
Zarontin Capsules 1768
Zarontin Syrup 1769

Birth weight, low
Cytosar-U Sterile Powder (Up to 5 infants) 2329
Dexedrine 2206
Easprin 1719
Sectral Capsules 2520

Births, multiple
A.P.L. 2431
Metrodin (urofollitropin for injection) 2182
▲Pergonal (menotropins for injection, USP) (20%) 2184
Profasi (human chorionic gonadotropin, USP) 2186
▲Serophene (clomiphene citrate tablets, USP) (Less than 1% to 10%) 2186

Blackout spells
Cibalith-S 870
Eskalith 2214
Lithane Tablets 1596
Lithium Carbonate Capsules & Tablets 1984
Lithobid Tablets 870
▲Lupron Depot 3.75 mg (Among most frequent) 2312
Lupron Depot 7.5 mg 2311
Lupron Injection (Less than 5%) 2310

Bladder, dysfunction
Depo-Medrol Sterile Aqueous Suspension 2334
Gelfoam Sterile Sponge 2338
▲TheraCys BCG Live (Intravesical) (Up to 5.4%) 898

Bladder, irritability
IFEX 729
Winstrol Tablets 2075

Bladder, loss of control
Anadrol-50 Tablets 2287
Duranest Injections 624
Nescaine/Nescaine MPF 629
Trilafon 2123
Xylocaine Injections 637

Bladder, neurogenic
Gelfoam Sterile Sponge 2338

Bladder, spasms
Lasix 1093
▲Lupron Depot 3.75 mg (Among most frequent) 2312
Lupron Depot 7.5 mg 2311
Lupron Injection (Less than 5%) 2310
Midamor Tablets (Less than or equal to 1%) 1508
Moduretic Tablets 1510

Blanching
Catapres-TTS (1 of 101 patients) .. 677

Blebs, filtering (ocular)
Decadron Phosphate Sterile Ophthalmic Ointment (Rare) 1453
Decadron Phosphate Sterile Ophthalmic Solution (Rare) 1453
⅛% Econopred & 1% Econopred Plus (Rare) ..... ⊙ 217
Inflamase (Rare) ..... ⊙ 274
Maxidex Sterile Ophthalmic Ointment (Rare) ..... ⊙ 222
Vasocidin Ophthalmic Solution ..... ⊙ 276

Bleeding
Abbokinase 503
Abbokinase Open-Cath 505
▲Activase (Most common complication) 1047
Adriamycin PFS 561
Adriamycin RDF 562
Alka-Seltzer Effervescent Antacid and Pain Reliever 1568
Aplitest (tuberculin PPD, multiple-puncture device) (Infrequent) 2551
Azdone Tablets (Occasional) 844
BiCNU 723
Calciparine Injection (Chief complication) 925
Capastat Sulfate Vials 1250
CeeNU 725
Cefotan 2265
Ceftin Tablets 575
Ceptaz for Injection 1057
Children's Advil Suspension (Less than 1%) 2426
Condylox (Less than 5%) 1630
Coumadin Injection & Tablets 944
▲Cytosar-U Sterile Powder (Among most frequent) 2329
Cytovene Sterile Powder (1% or less) 2292
Damason-P (Occasional) 1356
Debrisan 1150
Depakene Capsules & Syrup 511
Depakote Tablets 512
Depen Titratable Tablets 2379
Dicumarol Tablets 516
Diupres Tablets 1461
Elspar 1470
▲Eminase (14.6% to 14.8%) 2211
Sterile FUDR 1898
Fluorouracil Injection 1897
Fortaz 1060
Halotestin Tablets 2341
Heparin Lock Flush Solution 2456
Heparin Sodium Vials 1264
Heparin Sodium Injection 2457
Heparin Sodium Injection, USP, Sterile Solution 2342
Hydropres Tablets 1485
▲Idamycin for Injection (63%) 564
Imuran (2 cases) 768
Leukine for IV Infusion 1127
Motrin Tablets (Less than 1%) 2351
Mustargen 1514
▲Novantrone for Injection Concentrate (20 to 37%) 1226
PPD Tine Test 2548
Panwarfin Tablets 547
▲Paraplatin for Injection (5%) 735
PediaProfen Suspension (Less than 1%) 1363
Pitocin Injection, Ampoules, Steri-Dose Syringes 1757
Priscoline Hydrochloride Ampuls 877
Proglycem 649
Prokine for I.V. Infusion 1096
Pronestyl Capsules and Tablets 1800
Pronestyl Injection 1798
Pronestyl-SR Tablets 1801
Prostin VR Pediatric Sterile Solution (Less than 1%) 2355
Prozac Pulvules (Infrequent) 920
Quadrinal Tablets 1183
Retrovir 802
Rufen Tablets (Less than 1%) 691
Soma Compound w/Codeine Tablets 2390
Streptase for Infusion 635
Suprax 1235
Testred Capsules 1124
Tonocard Tablets 1554
Travase Ointment 697
Tuberculin, Old, Tine Test 2549

(▣ Described in PDR For Nonprescription Drugs) Incidence data in parenthesis; ▲ 3% or more (⊙ Described in PDR For Ophthalmology)

Winstrol Tablets 2075
Wyanoids Relief Factor Hemorrhoidal Suppositories 2537
Zefazone Sterile Powder 2372
Zinacef 1066

Bleeding, at invaded sites
Eminase 2211

Bleeding, at site of administration
Eminase 2211
Intron A (1% or less) 2097

Bleeding, breakthrough
Amen 833
Aygestin Tablets 2437
Brevicon 2304
Cycrin Tablets 2449
Demulen 2161
Depo-Provera Sterile Aqueous Suspension 2336
Diethylstilbestrol Tablets 1258
Enovid 2161
Estinyl Tablets 2085
Estrace 1385
Estrace Vaginal Cream 1388
Estraderm Transdermal System 866
Estratest 2245
Estrovis 1721
Jenest-28 Tablets 1636
Levlen/Tri-Levlen 665
Lo/Ovral Tablets 2471
Lo/Ovral-28 Tablets 2476
Loestrin 1728
Mediatric Capsules 2476
Megace Tablets 732
Menrium Tablets 1934
Micronor Tablets 1667
Modicon 1667
Nordette-21 Tablets 2481
Nordette-28 Tablets 2483
Norethin 2133
Norinyl 2304
Norlestrin 1746
Norlutate 1754
Norlutin 1755
Nor-Q D Tablets 2304
Ogen 540
Ortho Dienestrol Cream 1664
Ortho-Cyclen Tablets 1658
Ortho-Novum 1667
Ovral Tablets 2490
Ovral-28 Tablets 2491
Ovrette Tablets 2492
PMB 200 and PMB 400 2504
Premarin Intravenous 2508
Premarin with Methyltestosterone 2515
Premarin Tablets 2510
Premarin Vaginal Cream 2512
Provera Tablets 2356
TACE 12 and 25 mg 1353
Levlen/Tri-Levlen 665
Tri-Norinyl 2304
Triphasil-21 Tablets 2527
Triphasil-28 Tablets 2532

Bleeding, dental
Accutane Capsules (Less than 1%) 1878
Activase 1047
Anafranil Capsules (Rare) 650
Cholybar 1705
Danocrine Capsules (Rare) 2046
Eminase (1%) 2211
Mustargen 1514
Paradione Capsules 548
Questran Light 711
Questran Powder 710
Retrovir Capsules (Less than 5%) 802
Retrovir I.V. Infusion (Less than 5%) 805
Retrovir Syrup (Less than 5%) 802
Roferon-A Injection (Less than 3%) 1916
▲ Tegison Capsules (1-10%) 1881
Tridione 557

Bleeding, gastrointestinal
Abbokinase 503
Abbokinase Open-Cath 505
Actimmune (Rare) 1046
▲ Activase (5%) 1047
Aldactazide 2150
Aldactone 2152
Anaprox and Anaprox DS Tablets (Rare) 2288
Ancobon Capsules 1886
Ansaid Tablets 2319
Atgam Sterile Solution (Less than 5%) 2320
Atromid-S Capsules 2435
Azactam for Injection (Less than 1%) 2252
Azo Gantrisin Tablets 1888
Genuine Bayer Aspirin Tablets & Caplets ▣ 564
Bayer Plus Aspirin Tablets ▣ 567
Therapy Bayer Aspirin Caplets ▣ 568
Bufferin Analgesic Tablets and Caplets 743
Butazolidin Capsules & Tablets (1-4%) 1027
Children's Advil Suspension (Less than 1%) 2426
Cholybar 1705
Cipro I.V. (Less than 1%) 1592
Cipro Tablets (Less than 1%) 1589
Clinoril Tablets (Less than 1%) 1433
Colestid Granules (Fewer than 1 in 500) 2328
Cortone Acetate Sterile Suspension 1437
Cortone Acetate Tablets 1439
Cytotec (Infrequent) 2159
Dantrium Capsules (Less frequent) 1619
Decadron Phosphate Respihaler 1454
Decadron Phosphate Turbinaire 1456
Demulen 2161
Disalcid 1310
Dolobid Tablets (Less than 1 in 100) 1465
Doxorubicin Hydrochloride Injection, USP 848
Easprin 1719
Ecotrin 2189
Edecrin 1468
Eldepryl 2250
Emcyt Capsules (1%) 1161
Eminase (2%) 2211
Empirin with Codeine Phosphate Nos. 2, 3 & 4 (Occasional) 764
Enovid 2161
Ergamisol Tablets 1136
Sterile FUDR 1898
Feldene Capsules (Less than 1%) 1777
Fluorouracil Injection 1897
Fulvicin P/G Tablets (Rare) 2090
Fulvicin P/G 165 & 330 Tablets (Rare) 2091
Fulvicin-U/F Tablets (Rare) 2092
Heparin Lock Flush Solution 2456
Heparin Sodium Injection 2457
Indocin Capsules (Less than 1%) 1487
▲ Indocin I.V. (3% to 9%) 1490
Indocin (Less than 1%) 1487
Intron A (1 patient) 2097
K-Dur Microburst Release System (potassium chloride, USP) E.R. Tablets 1163
K-Norm Capsules 982
K-Tab Filmtab 532
Klor-Con 8/Klor-Con 10 Extended-release Tablets 2374
Klotrix 708
Lamprene Capsules (Less than 1%) 1030
Larodopa Tablets (Rare) 1905
Leukine for IV Infusion 1127
Lodine Capsules 2468
Lorelco Tablets 1333
▲ Lupron Depot 3.75 mg (Among most frequent) 2312
Lupron Depot 7.5 mg 2311
Lupron Injection (Less than 5%) 2310
Meclomen Capsules (Less than 1%) 1739
Methotrexate Tablets, Parenteral, LPF Parenteral 1217
Mexitil Capsules (About 7 in 10,000) 680
Micro-K 1863
Micro-K LS Packets 1864
Midamor Tablets (Less than or equal to 1%) 1508
Moduretic Tablets (Less than or equal to 1%) 1510
Motrin Tablets (Less than 1%) 2351
Mustargen 1514
Nalfon Pulvules & Tablets (Less than 1%) 919
Naprosyn (Rare) 2297
Nimotop Capsules (Less than 1%) 1607
Norgesic (Rare) 1314
▲ Novantrone for Injection Concentrate (2 to 16%) 1226
Orudis Capsules (Less than 1%) 2488
Paraflex Caplets (Rare) 1378
Parafon Forte DSC Caplets (Rare) 1379
Parlodel (Less than 1%) 2020
PediaProfen Suspension (Less than 1%) 1363
Ponstel 1758
Priscoline Hydrochloride Ampuls 877
Procardia XL Tablets (Less than 1%) 1783
Prokine for I.V. Infusion 1096
Prozac Pulvules 920
Questran Light 711
Questran Powder 710
Raudixin Tablets 1803
Rauzide Tablets 1804
Rheumatrex Methotrexate Dose Pack 1234
Ridaura Capsules (0.1 to 1%) 2224
Rubex 739
Rufen Tablets (Less than 1%) 691
Salflex 839
Sandimmune (Rare) 2024
Sandostatin Injection (Less than 1%) 2029
Sinemet Tablets (Rare) 952
Sinemet CR Tablets 953
Slow-K Tablets 2281
Solu-Cortef Sterile Powder 2361
Solu-Medrol Sterile Powder 2363
Soma Compound Tablets 2389
St. Joseph Adult Chewable Aspirin (81 mg.) ▣ 703
Streptase for Infusion (0.3 to 6.2%) 635
Ten-K Controlled-Release Tablets 2282
Tolectin (200, 400 and 600 mg) (Less than 1%) 1379
Toradol IM Injection (Approximately 1% to 4%) 2302
Voltaren Tablets (1-3%) 1042
Wellbutrin Tablets (Rare) 821
Zorprin Tablets (Some patients) 698

Bleeding, genitourinary tract
Abbokinase 503
▲ Activase (4%) 1047
Eminase 2211
Streptase for Infusion (0.3 to 6.2%) 635

Bleeding, gingival (see under Bleeding, dental)

Bleeding, in immediate coronary catheterization
▲ Eminase (13.3%) 2211

Bleeding, in patients not undergoing coronary catheterization
▲ Eminase (3%) 2211

Bleeding, internal
Eminase 2211

Bleeding, intracranial
Abbokinase 503
Abbokinase Open-Cath 505
Activase (0.4% to 1.3%) 1047
Elspar 1470
Eminase (1%) 2211
▲ Indocin I.V. (3% to 9%) 1490
Streptase for Infusion (0.3 to 6.2%) 635
▲ Survanta Beractant Intratracheal Suspension (24.1 to 48.1%) 1978

Bleeding, menstrual, frequent onsets
▲ Norplant System (7.6%) 2484

Bleeding, menstrual, prolonged episodes
▲ Norplant System (27.6%) 2484

Bleeding, mouth
Eminase (1%) 2211

Bleeding, mucosal
Quadrinal Tablets 1183
Unasyn (Less than 1%) 1965
Vancenase Nasal Inhaler (2 per 100 patients) 2126

Bleeding, nasal (see under Epistaxis)

Bleeding, nonpuncture site
▲ Eminase (10.2%) 2211

Bleeding, pericardial
Activase 1047
Eminase 2211

Bleeding, postmenopausal
Aldactazide 2150
Aldactone 2152

Bleeding, puncture site
▲ Eminase (Up to 5.7%) 2211

Bleeding, renal-pelvic
Cipro I.V. (1% or less) 1592
Cipro Tablets (Less than 1%) 1589

Bleeding, retroperitoneal
Streptase for Infusion (0.3 to 6.2%) 635

Bleeding, superficial
Abbokinase 503
Abbokinase Open-Cath 505
Activase 1047
Eminase 2211
Sandostatin Injection (Less than 1%) 2029

Bleeding, Upper GI (see under Bleeding, gastrointestinal)

Bleeding, uterine, irregularities
Lodine Capsules (Less than 1%) 2468

Bleeding, uterine
Anafranil Capsules (Infrequent) 650
Ansaid Tablets (Less than 1%) 2319
Cytotec 2159
Dicumarol Tablets 516
Estrace 1385
Estrace Vaginal Cream 1388
Estratest 2245
Intron A (1% or less) 2097
Mediatric Capsules 2476
PMB 200 and PMB 400 2504
Panwarfin Tablets 547
Permax Tablets (Infrequent) 1291
Premarin Intravenous 2508
Premarin with Methyltestosterone 2515
Premarin Tablets 2510
Premarin Vaginal Cream 2512
Prozac Pulvules (Rare) 920
Serophene (clomiphene citrate tablets, USP) (Less than 1 in 100 patients) 2186
Syntocinon Nasal Spray 2033

Bleeding, vaginal
Abbokinase 503
Abbokinase Open-Cath 505
Anafranil Capsules (Infrequent) 650
Ansaid Tablets (Less than 1%) 2319
Brevicon 2304
Clinoril Tablets (Less than 1%) 1433
Coumadin Injection & Tablets 944
Danocrine Capsules 2046
Demulen 2161
Enovid 2161
Ergamisol Tablets (Less frequent) 1136
Estratest 2245
Indocin Capsules (Less than 1%) 1487
Indocin I.V. (Less than 1%) 1490
Indocin (Less than 1%) 1487
Lo/Ovral Tablets 2471
Lo/Ovral-28 Tablets 2476
Micronor Tablets 1667
Modicon 1667
Nolvadex Tablets (Less frequent) 1102
Norinyl 2304
Ortho-Novum 1667
Ovral Tablets 2490
Ovral-28 Tablets 2491
Ovrette Tablets 2492
Paradione Capsules 548
Permax Tablets (Infrequent) 1291
Premarin Tablets 2510
Prozac Pulvules 920
Synarel Nasal Solution 2300
Tridione 557
Tri-Norinyl 28-Day Tablets 2304
Triphasil-21 Tablets 2527
Triphasil-28 Tablets 2532
Voltaren Tablets (Less than 1%) 1042
Zarontin Capsules 1768
Zarontin Syrup 1769

Bleeding diathesis
Cipro I.V. (Rare) 1592
Cipro Tablets (Less than 0.1%) 1589

Bleeding irregularities
BuSpar (Rare) 1401
Cycrin Tablets 2449
Demulen 2161
Enovid 2161
Estrace 1385
Estrace Vaginal Cream 1388

Loestrin 1728
Meclomen Capsules 1739
▲ Norplant System (7.6%) 2484
Ovcon 1391
Premarin Tablets 2510
Quadrinal Tablets 1183

Bleeding syndrome
Mithracin 1602

Bleeding tendencies due to hypoprothrombinemia
Cholybar (Less frequent) 1705
Questran Powder 710

Bleeding time, prolongation
Anaprox and Anaprox DS Tablets (Less than 3%) 2288
Cardizem Tablets-30 mg, 60 mg, 90 mg and 120 mg 1329
Cardizem SR Capsules-60 mg, 90 mg and 120 mg (Less than 1%) 1327
Children's Advil Suspension 2426
Depakene Capsules & Syrup 511
Depakote Tablets 512
Easprin 1719
Fiorinal with Codeine Capsules 2008
Hespan Injection 948
Lodine Capsules (Less than 1%) 2468
Metandren Linguets and Tablets 875
Mithracin 1602
Motrin Tablets 2351
Ocufen ⊙ 237
Procardia XL Tablets (Some patients) 1783
Prozac Pulvules (Rare) 920
Timentin for Injection 2239
Tolectin (200, 400 and 600 mg) 1379

Blepharitis
Anafranil Capsules (Rare) 650
NebuPent for Inhalation Solution (1% or less) 1017
OptiPranolol Sterile Ophthalmic Solution (A small number of patients) ⊙ 261
Prozac Pulvules (Rare) 920
Timoptic in Ocudose 1552
Timoptic Sterile Ophthalmic Solution 1550

Blepharoconjunctivitis
▲ Betagan (About 1 in 20 patients) ⊙ 239
Cyclogyl ⊙ 215

Blepharoptosis (see also under Ptosis, eyelids)
Betagan ⊙ 239

Blepharospasm
Anafranil Capsules (Up to 2%) 650
Eldepryl 2250
Larodopa Tablets (Infrequent) 1905
Parlodel 2020
Sinemet Tablets 952
Sinemet CR Tablets 953

Blind spot, enlargement
Cibalith-S 870
Eskalith 2214
Lithane Tablets 1596
Lithobid Tablets 870

Blindness
Aristospan Suspension (Intra-articular) (Rare) 1011
Brevicon (Rare) 2304
Celestone Soluspan Suspension 2081
Cibalith-S 870
Cortone Acetate Sterile Suspension 1437
Dalalone D.P. Injectable 999
Decadron Phosphate Injection (Rare) 1449
Decadron Phosphate with Xylocaine Injection, Sterile (Rare) 1451
Decadron-LA Sterile Suspension (Rare) 1457
Depo-Medrol Sterile Aqueous Suspension 2334
Eskalith 2214
Hydeltrasol Injection, Sterile (Rare) 1476
Hydeltra-T.B.A. Sterile Suspension (Rare) 1478
Hydrocortone Acetate Sterile Suspension (Rare) 1479
Hydrocortone Phosphate Injection, Sterile (Rare) 1481
Kenalog-10 Injection (Rare) 2402
Lithane Tablets 1596
Lithobid Tablets 870
Micronor Tablets 1667
Modicon 1667
Norinyl (Rare) 2304
Oncovin Solution Vials & Hyporets 1288
Ortho-Novum 1667
Permax Tablets (Rare) 1291
Surgicel 1151
Tri-Norinyl 28-Day Tablets (Rare) 2304

Blindness, cerebral
Platinol 737
Platinol-AQ Injection 738

Blindness, night (see under Nyctalopia)

Blindness, transient
Adalat Capsules (10 mg and 20 mg) (Less than 0.5%) 1587

Blindness, transient cortical
Oncovin Solution Vials & Hyporets 1288
Procardia Capsules (Less than 0.5%) 1781
VePesid Capsules and Injection 741

Blistering
BuSpar (Infrequent) 1401
Doxorubicin Hydrochloride Injection, USP 848
Icy Hot ▣ 659
Lotrimin 2102
Lotrisone Cream 2103
Mycelex 1% Cream and Topical Solution 1% 1604
Retin-A (tretinoin) Cream/Gel/Liquid 1680
Rubex 739
Surgicel 1151

Bloated feeling (see under Bloating)

Bloating
Bentyl 1322
Cantil Tablets 1326
Children's Advil Suspension (Less than 3%) 2426
Colyte 1826
Darbid Tablets 2205
Dipentum Capsules (1.5%) 1160
Donnatal 1858
Donnatal Extentabs 1859
Donnatal Tablets 1858
Donnazyme Tablets 1860
Estinyl Tablets 2085
Estrace 1385
Estrace Vaginal Cream 1388
▲ GoLYTELY (Up to 50%) 699
Indocin Capsules (Less than 1%) 1487
Indocin I.V. (Less than 1%) 1490
Indocin (Less than 1%) 1487
Kinesed Tablets 2272
Levsin/Levsinex 2147
▲ Limbitrol (Among most frequent) 1933
Lo/Ovral Tablets 2471
Lo/Ovral-28 Tablets 2476
Loestrin 1728
Mediatric Capsules 2476
Metrodin (urofollitropin for injection) 2182
Micronor Tablets 1667
Modicon 1667
Motrin Tablets (Less than 3%) 2351
Nordette-21 Tablets 2481
Nordette-28 Tablets 2483
▲ Norpace (3 to 9%) 2177
Orinase Tablets (1.4%) 2354
Ortho Dienestrol Cream 1664
Ortho-Novum 1667
Ovcon 1391
Ovral Tablets 2490
Ovral-28 Tablets 2491
Ovrette Tablets 2492
PediaProfen Suspension (Less than 3%) 1363
Premarin Vaginal Cream 2512
Pro-Banthīne Tablets 2141
Quarzan Capsules 1937
Robinul Forte Tablets 1873
Robinul Injectable 1873
Robinul Tablets 1873
Rowasa (1.47%) 2248
Rufen Tablets (1 to 3%) 691
Stilphostrol Tablets and Ampuls 1609
TACE 12 and 25 mg 1353
Triphasil-21 Tablets 2527
Triphasil-28 Tablets 2532
Valpin 50 Tablets 941
Yutopar (Infrequent) 647

Blood dyscrasias
AK-Chlor Sterile Ophthalmic Ointment & Solution ⊙ 201
Anturane (Rare) 853
Apresazide Capsules (Less frequent) 854
Apresoline Hydrochloride Parenteral (Ampuls) 856
Apresoline Hydrochloride Tablets (Less frequent) 855
Apresoline-Esidrix Tablets 857
Aralen Hydrochloride Injection 2038
Aralen Phosphate Tablets 2039
Azo Gantanol Tablets 1887
Bactrim DS Tablets (Rare) 1891
Bactrim I.V. Infusion (Rare) 1889
Bactrim (Rare) 1891
Butazolidin Capsules & Tablets 1027
Celontin 1692
Chloromycetin Hydrocortisone Ophthalmic 1694
Chloromycetin Kapseals 1695
Chloromycetin Ophthalmic Ointment, 1% 1696
Chloromycetin Ophthalmic Solution 1696
Chloromycetin Otic 1697
Chloromycetin Palmitate, Oral Suspension 1697
Chloromycetin Sodium Succinate 1698
Chloroptic Sterile Ophthalmic Solution (Rare) ⊙ 243
Compazine 2201
Dapsone USP 1130
Diamox Parenteral 1200
Diamox Sequels (Sustained Release) 1201
Diamox Tablets 1200
Elase-Chloromycetin Ointment 1015
Esimil Tablets 864
Fansidar Tablets 1896
Ismelin Tablets 869
Leukine for IV Infusion 1127
Librax Capsules 1929
Libritabs Tablets (Occasional) 1930
Librium Capsules (Occasional) 1931
Maxzide Tablets 1215
Menrium Tablets 1934
Mesantoin Tablets 2013
Mexitil Capsules 680
Milontin Kapseals 1741
Myochrysine Injection (Rare) 1516
Ophthochlor Ophthalmic Solution ⊙ 300
Ophthocort ⊙ 301
Pediazole 1973
Plaquenil Sulfate Tablets 2067
Procan SR Tablets 1760
Prokine for I.V. Infusion 1096
Prolixin Decanoate 1795
Prolixin Enanthate 1796
Prolixin Oral Concentrate 1792
Pronestyl Capsules and Tablets 1800
Pronestyl Injection 1798
Pronestyl-SR Tablets 1801
Prozac Pulvules (Rare) 920
Ridaura Capsules 2224
SSD RP Cream 690
Septra 813
Septra I.V. Infusion 808
Septra I.V. Infusion ADD-Vantage Vials (Rare) 810
Septra 813
Ser-Ap-Es Tablets 881
Serax Capsules 2522
Serax Tablets 2522
Serpasil-Apresoline Tablets 884
Silvadene Cream 1% 1352
Solganal Suspension (Rare) 2122
Stelazine 2226
Tambocor Tablets (Extremely rare) 1315
Thiosulfil Forte Tablets 2526
Tigan 2239
Tonocard Tablets 1554
Triavil Tablets 1556
Urobiotic-250 Capsules 1968
Zarontin Capsules 1768
Zarontin Syrup 1769

Blood glucose, elevation (see under Hyperglycinemia)

Blood glucose, reduction (see under Hypoglycemia)

Blood loss, increase (see under Bleeding)

Blood pressure, changes
Arm-a-Med Isoetharine Inhalation Solution, USP 616
Asendin Tablets 1196
Bronkephrine Injection 2042
Bronkometer Aerosol 2042
Bronkosol Solution 2042
Bufferin Analgesic Tablets and Caplets 743
DDAVP Injection (Infrequent) 1840
Dantrium Capsules (Less frequent) 1619
Desoxyn Gradumet Tablets 514
Loxitane 1213
Marcaine Hydrochloride 0.5% with Epinephrine 1:200,000 (as bitartrate) 958
Mellaril 2011
Metaprel Inhalation Aerosol Bronchodilator 2014
Norisodrine Aerotrol 540
Orap Tablets 1020
Paradione Capsules 548
Pontocaine Hydrochloride for Spinal Anesthesia 2069
Prolixin Decanoate 1795
Prolixin Elixir 1793
Prolixin Enanthate 1796
Prolixin Injection 1791
Prolixin Oral Concentrate 1792
Prolixin Tablets 1793
Ritalin 880
Sandimmune 2024
Sensorcaine 631
Sensorcaine-MPF Spinal 634
Stelazine 2226
Tridil Ampuls & Vials 939
Tridione 557
Trilafon 2123
▲ Yutopar (80 to 100% with IV administration) 647

Blood pressure, elevation (see under Hypertension)

Blood pressure, reduction (see under Hypotension)

Blood urea levels, increase
Ceptaz for Injection (Occasional) 1057
Fortaz (Occasional) 1060
Inderide Tablets 2463
Normodyne Tablets (Rare) 2110
Normozide Tablets (Rare) 2112
▲ Paraplatin for Injection (22%) 735
Trandate HCT Tablets 579

Blood urea nitrogen levels, increase (see under BUN levels, elevation)

Blurred vision
Achromycin V Capsules 1193
Actifed with Codeine Cough Syrup 752
Adalat Capsules (10 mg and 20 mg) (2% or less) 1587
Adenocard Injection (Less than 1%) 1007
AeroBid Inhaler System (1-3%) 995
Akineton 1171
Albalon Solution with Liquifilm ⊙ 238
Alfenta Injection (2%) 1131
▲ Alferon N Injection (3% to 6%) 1809
Ana-Kit Anaphylaxis Emergency Treatment Kit 1100
▲ Anestacon Solution (Among most common) 2394
Antivert, Antivert/25 Tablets, Antivert/25 Chewable Tablets & Antivert/50 Tablets (Rare) 1940
Aralen Hydrochloride Injection 2038
Aralen Phosphate with Primaquine Phosphate Tablets (Occasional) 2040
Aralen Phosphate Tablets 2039
Arco-Lase Plus Tablets 607
▲ Artane (30% to 50%) 1195
▲ Asendin Tablets (7%) 1196
Atabrine Hydrochloride Tablets 2041
Ativan Injection (Occasional) 2432
Atrohist Sprinkle Capsules 558
Atromid-S Capsules 2435
Atrovent Inhalation Aerosol (1.2%) 675
B & O No. 15A & No. 16A Supprettes 2395
Bellergal-S Tablets (Rare) 1998
Benadryl Capsules 1691
Benadryl Injection 1692
▲ Bentyl (27%) 1322
Betoptic Sterile Ophthalmic Solution (Small numbers of patients) 569
Betoptic S Sterile Ophthalmic Suspension (Small numbers of patients) 570
Bonine Tablets (Rare) 1773

Bontril Slow-Release 834
Brexin L.A. Capsules 2078
Bromfed 1615
BuSpar (2%) 1401
Butazolidin Capsules & Tablets (Less than 1%) 1027
Calan SR Caplets (1% or less) 2157
Calan Tablets (1% or less) 2155
Cantil Tablets 1326
Capoten 2255
Capozide 2258
Carbocaine Hydrochloride 3% Injection 956
Carbocaine Hydrochloride Injection 2043
Carbocaine Hydrochloride 2% with Neo-Cobefrin 956
Cardene Capsules (Rare) 2290
Cardioquin Tablets 1812
Cartrol Tablets (Less common) 507
Catapres Tablets 676
Catapres-TTS 677
Celontin 1692
Centrax 1693
Children's Advil Suspension (Less than 1%) 2426
Cibalith-S 870
Cipro I.V. (1% or less) 1592
Cipro Tablets (Less than 1%) 1589
Clinoril Tablets (Less than 1 in 100) 1433
Codimal 846
Cogentin 1435
Combipres Tablets 678
Comhist LA Capsules 1618
Compazine 2201
Corgard Tablets (1 to 5 of 1000 patients) 701
Corzide Tablets (1 to 5 of 1000 patients) 702
Cyclogyl ◉ 215
Cystospaz 2395
Dalgan Injection (Less than 1%) 620
Dalmane Capsules (Rare) 1927
Dapsone USP 1130
Darbid Tablets 2205
Decadron Phosphate Sterile Ophthalmic Ointment 1453
Decadron Phosphate Sterile Ophthalmic Solution 1453
Decadron Phosphate with Xylocaine Injection, Sterile 1451
Declomycin Capsules, Tablets 1199
Deconamine 663
Deprol Tablets 2382
Desferal Vials 862
Desyrel and Desyrel Dividose (Greater than 1%) 1404
Dilaudid-HP Injection 1175
Dipentum Capsules (Rare) 1160
Ditropan 1332
Diucardin Tablets 2450
Diulo 2129
Diupres Tablets 1461
Dolobid Tablets (Less than 1 in 100) 1465
Donnagel (Rare) ▣ 675
Donnagel-PG (Rare) 1858
Donnatal 1858
Donnatal Extentabs 1859
Donnatal Tablets 1858
Donnazyme Tablets 1860
Dorcol Children's Liquid Cold Formula (Occasional) ▣ 686
Duranest Injections 624
Dyclone 0.5% and 1% Topical Solutions, USP 626
Edecrin 1468
Elavil 2269
Eldepryl 2250
Emete-con Intramuscular/Intravenous 1950
Endep Tablets 1927
Enduron Tablets 517
Ergamisol Tablets (1 to 2%) 1136
Esimil Tablets 864
Eskalith 2214
Estrace 1385
Estrace Vaginal Cream 1388
▲ Ethmozine Tablets (0.3%-5%) 946
Etrafon 2087
Fedahist Gyrocaps 2145
Fedahist Timecaps 2145
Feldene Capsules (Less than 1%) 1777
Flexeril Tablets (1% to 3%) 1471
Floropryl Sterile Ophthalmic Ointment 1473
Fungizone Intravenous 2262
Haldol Decanoate 1375
Haldol Injection, Tablets and Concentrate 1373
Humorsol Sterile Ophthalmic Solution 1475
Hycomine Compound Tablets 929
Hycomine Syrup 927
Hycotuss Expectorant Syrup 930
HydroDIURIL Tablets 1484
Hydropres Tablets 1485
Hyperstat I.V. Injection 2095
Hytrin Tablets (0.6% to 1.6%) 529
Indocin (Less than 1%) 1487
Innovar Injection 1141
Intron A (1% or less) 2097
Inversine Tablets 1492
IOPIDINE ◉ 232
Ismelin Tablets 869
Isoptin Oral Tablets (Less than 1%) 1179
Isoptin SR Sustained Release Tablets (Less than 1%) 1181
Kemadrin Tablets 771
Kinesed Tablets 2272
Kutrase Capsules 2146
Lacrisert Sterile Ophthalmic Insert 1493
Lanoxicaps 772
Lanoxin Elixir Pediatric 775
Lanoxin Injection 778
Lanoxin Injection Pediatric 781
Lanoxin Tablets 783
Larodopa Tablets (Infrequent) 1905
Lasix 1093
Levsin/Levsinex 2147
Librax Capsules 1929
Librium Injectable (Isolated instances) 1932
▲ Limbitrol (Among most frequent) 1933
Lioresal Tablets 1031
Lithane Tablets 1596
Lithium Carbonate Capsules & Tablets 1984
Lithobid Tablets 870
Lodine Capsules (More than 1% but less than 3%) 2468
Lopid Capsules and Tablets 1736
Lopressor Ampuls 1032
Lopressor HCT Tablets (1 in 100 patients) 1034
Lopressor Tablets 1032
Lorelco Tablets 1333
Loxitane 1213
Lozol Tablets (Less than 5%) 1843
▲ Ludiomil Tablets (4%) 874
Lupron Depot 7.5 mg 2311
Lupron Injection (Less than 5%) 2310
Lysodren (Infrequent) 731
MS Contin Tablets (Infrequent) 1814
MSIR (Infrequent) 1817
Marcaine Hydrochloride 0.5% with Epinephrine 1:200,000 (as bitartrate) 958
Marcaine Hydrochloride with Epinephrine 1:200,000 2055
Marcaine Hydrochloride Injection 2055
Marcaine Spinal 2058
▲ Marplan Tablets (Among most frequent) 1906
Meclomen Capsules (Rare) 1739
Mellaril 2011
Mepergan Injection (Occasional) 2479
Methotrexate Tablets, Parenteral, LPF Parenteral 1217
Mevacor Tablets (1.5%) 1505
▲ Mexitil Capsules (5.7% to 7.5%) 680
Micronase Tablets 2350
Minipress Capsules (1-4%) 1778
Minizide Capsules 1779
Minocin Intravenous 1221
Mintezol 1510
Moban Tablets & Concentrate (Occasional) 932
Moduretic Tablets 1510
Motofen Tablets (Less frequent) 836
Motrin Tablets (Less than 1%) 2351
Mutamycin 733
Mydriacyl ◉ 225
Naldecon Syrup, Tablets, Pediatric Drops and Pediatric Syrup 709
Nalfon Pulvules & Tablets (2.2%) 919
Naphcon Forte ◉ 226
Nardil (Less common) 1742
Navane Capsules and Concentrate 1954
Navane Intramuscular 1956
NebuPent for Inhalation Solution (1% or less) 1017
Nescaine/Nescaine MPF 629
Netromycin Injection 100 mg/ml (Fewer than 1 of 1000 patients) 2104
Norflex 1314
Norgesic 1314
Normozide Tablets 2112
▲ Norpace (3 to 9%) 2177
Norpramin Tablets 1340
Norzine 1818
Novafed A Capsules 1342
Novocain Hydrochloride for Spinal Anesthesia 2065
Nubain Injection (Less than 1%) 934
Omnipaque (Less than 0.3 to 2%) 2552
Optimine Tablets 2115
OptiPranolol Sterile Ophthalmic Solution (A small number of patients) ◉ 261
Oramorph SR (Morphine Sulfate Sustained Release Tablets) (Less frequent) 1988
Orap Tablets 1020
Ornade Spansule Capsules 2221
Ovcon 1391
PBZ Tablets & Elixir 1037
PBZ-SR Tablets 1037
Pamelor 2019
Parnate Tablets 2222
PediaProfen Suspension (Less than 1%) 1363
Periactin 1525
Phenergan with Codeine (Occasional) 2497
Phenergan with Dextromethorphan (Occasional) 2499
Phenergan Injection 2493
Phenergan Suppositories (Occasional) 2496
Phenergan Syrup (Occasional) 2495
Phenergan Tablets (Occasional) 2496
Phenergan VC (Occasional) 2500
Phenergan VC with Codeine (Occasional) 2501
Phospholine Iodide ◉ 315
Pilagan ◉ 250
Placidyl Capsules 553
Plaquenil Sulfate Tablets 2067
Platinol 737
Platinol-AQ Injection 738
Plegine Tablets 2504
Plendil Extended-Release Tablets (0.5% or greater) 1526
Polaramine 2116
Pondimin Tablets 1867
Ponstel 1758
Pontocaine Hydrochloride for Spinal Anesthesia 2069
Prinivil Tablets (1% or less) 1538
Prinzide Tablets (0.3 to 1%) 1540
Pro-Banthīne Tablets 2141
Procardia Capsules (2% or less) 1781
Proglycem 649
Prolixin Decanoate 1795
Prolixin Elixir 1793
Prolixin Enanthate 1796
Prolixin Injection 1791
Prolixin Oral Concentrate 1792
Prolixin Tablets 1793
Protopam Chloride for Injection 2518
Pyridium Plus 1764
Quarzan Capsules (Among most frequent) 1937
Quelidrine Syrup 556
Quinaglute Dura-Tabs Tablets 663
Quinamm Tablets 1344
Quinidex Extentabs 1868
Rauzide Tablets 1804
Rēv-Eyes Ophthalmic Eyedrops 0.5% (Less frequently) ◉ 312
Rheumatrex Methotrexate Dose Pack 1234
Robaxin Injectable 1871
Robaxin Tablets 1872
Robaxisal Tablets 1872
Robinul Forte Tablets 1873
Robinul Injectable 1873
Robinul Tablets 1873
Rufen Tablets (Less than 1%) 691
Ru-Tuss II Capsules 693
Ru-Tuss with Hydrocodone 694
Ru-Tuss Tablets 693
▲ Rythmol Tablets (0.6 to 5.7%) 1184
Salutensin/Salutensin-Demi 719
Seldane-D Extended-Release Tablets (1.1%) 1350
Sensorcaine 631
Sensorcaine-MPF Spinal 634
Ser-Ap-Es Tablets 881
Serax Capsules 2522
Serax Tablets 2522
Serentil 686
Serophene (clomiphene citrate tablets, USP) (Occasionally) 2186
Sinemet Tablets 952
Sinemet CR Tablets 953
Sinequan 1960
Stadol (Less than 1%) 721
Stelazine 2226
Sublimaze Injection 1146
Surmontil Capsules 2524
Tacaryl 2409
Talacen (Infrequent) 2070
Talwin Injection 2071
Talwin Compound (Infrequent) 2072
Talwin Injection 2071
Talwin Nx 2073
▲ Tambocor Tablets (15.9%) 1315
Tavist Syrup 2033
Tavist Tablets 2035
Tavist-D Tablets 2035
Tegretol Chewable Tablets 654
Tegretol Suspension 656
Tegretol Tablets 654
Temaril Tablets, Syrup and Spansule Sustained Release Capsules 1085
Tenex Tablets 1875
Tenuate 1354
Tigan 2239
Timolide Tablets 1547
Tofranil Ampuls 1038
Tofranil Tablets 1039
Tofranil-PM Capsules 1041
▲ Tonocard Tablets (1.3-10.0%) 1554
Torecan 1993
Trandate HCT Tablets 579
Transderm Scōp Transdermal Therapeutic System 887
Tranxene (Less common) 556
Trental (2.3%) 1099
Trexan Tablets (Less than 1%) 937
Triaminic Cold Tablets ▣ 688
Triaminic Expectorant DH 1995
Triaminic Oral Infant Drops 1996
Triaminic Syrup (Occasional) ▣ 689
Triaminicol Multi-Symptom Relief ▣ 691
Triavil Tablets 1556
Trilafon (Occasional) 2123
Trinalin Repetabs Tablets 1170
Tropicacyl ◉ 209
Urised Tablets 2396
Urispas Tablets 2242
Valium Injectable 1937
Valium Tablets (Infrequent) 1939
Valpin 50 Tablets 941
Valrelease Capsules (Infrequent) 1923
Vascor (200, 300 and 400 mg) Tablets (0.5 to 2.0%) 1383
Vasocon-A ◉ 278
Vasosulf ◉ 279
Vasotec I.V. 1562
Verelan Capsules (1% or less) 1243
Versed Injection (Less than 1%) 1924
Vivactil Tablets 1567
Voltaren Tablets (Less than 1%) 1042
Vontrol Tablets 2243
▲ Wellbutrin Tablets (14.6%) 821
Wytensin Tablets (3% or less) 2542
▲ Xanax Tablets (6.2% to 21%) 2367
▲ Xylocaine Injections (Among most common) 637
Xylocaine Injections for Ventricular Arrhythmias 639
Xylocaine 2% Jelly 643
Xylocaine 5% Ointment 644
Xylocaine 10% Oral Spray 645
4% Xylocaine-MPF Sterile Solution 641
Xylocaine 2% Viscous Solution 646
Zantac Injection and Zantac Injection Premixed (Rare) 1063
Zantac (Rare) 1065
Zestoretic (0.3 to 1%) 2274
Zestril Tablets (Less than 1%) 2277

Blurred vision, transient (see also under Blurred vision)

Aldoclor Tablets 1413
Aldoril Tablets 1418
Apresazide Capsules 854
Apresoline-Esidrix Tablets 857
Capozide 2258
Diucardin Tablets 2450
Diulo 2129
Diupres Tablets 1461
Diuril Oral Suspension 1464
Diuril Sodium Intravenous 1463
Diuril Tablets 1464
Dyazide Capsules 2208
Esidrix Tablets 863
Esimil Tablets 864
HydroDIURIL Tablets 1484
Inderide Tablets 2463
Inderide LA Long Acting Capsules 2465
Lopressor HCT Tablets 1034
Maxzide 1215
Mykrox ½ mg Tablets 984
Naturetin Tablets (Occasional) 1789
Peptavlon 2563
Rauzide Tablets 1804

Ser-Ap-Es Tablets 881
Serpasil-Esidrix Tablets 886
Vaseretic Tablets 1559
Zaroxolyn Tablets 989

Body odor

Carnitor 2188
Retrovir Capsules (Less than 5%) .. 802
Retrovir I.V. Infusion (Less than 5%) 805
Retrovir Syrup (Less than 5%) 802
Wellbutrin Tablets (Rare) 821

Bone density, changes

▲ Lupron Depot 3.75 mg (13.5%) 2312

Bone disorders

Accutane Capsules 1878
Intron A (Less than 5%) 2097

Bone fractures

Kenalog-10 Injection 2402
Kenalog-40 Injection 2403

Bone marrow depression

▲ Adriamycin PFS (High incidence) 561
▲ Adriamycin RDF (High incidence) 562
Aldoclor Tablets 1413
Aldomet Ester HCl Injection 1417
Aldomet Oral 1415
Aldoril Tablets 1418
Altace Capsules (Rare to more frequent) 1086
Anafranil Capsules (Rare) 650
Azdone Tablets 844
Butazolidin Capsules & Tablets (Less than 1%) 1027
Cetamide Ointment ..... ⊙ 220
Chloromycetin Kapseals 1695
Chloromycetin Palmitate, Oral Suspension 1697
Chloromycetin Sodium Succinate 1698
Chloroptic Sterile Ophthalmic Solution (Three cases) ..... ⊙ 243
Clinoril Tablets (Less than 1%) 1433
Clozaril Tablets 2000
Colchicine Ampoules 1252
Cuprimine Capsules 1442
Damason-P (Occasional) 1356
Depen Titratable Tablets 2379
Diamox 1200
▲ Doxorubicin Hydrochloride for Injection, USP (High incidence) 622
Doxorubicin Hydrochloride Injection, USP 848
Elavil 2269
Elspar (Rare) 1470
Endep Tablets 1927
FML-S Sterile Ophthalmic Suspension ..... ⊙ 246
Feldene Capsules (Less than 1%) .. 1777
Flexeril Tablets (Rare) 1471
Indocin Capsules (Less than 1%) 1487
Indocin I.V. (Less than 1%) 1490
Indocin (Less than 1%) 1487
Limbitrol 1933
Lortab ASA Tablets (Occasional) 2414
Lotensin Tablets (Rare) 872
Ludiomil Tablets 874
Mefoxin 1498
Mefoxin Premixed Intravenous Solution 1500
Methotrexate Tablets, Parenteral, LPF Parenteral 1217
Metopirone Tablets (Rare) 876
Neptazane Tablets ..... ⊙ 311
Norpramin Tablets 1340
Oncovin Solution Vials & Hyporets 1288
Pamelor 2019
Prinivil Tablets (Rare) 1538
Prinzide Tablets (Rare) 1540
Procan SR Tablets 1760
Pronestyl Capsules and Tablets (Approximately 0.5%) 1800
Pronestyl Injection (Approximately 0.5%) 1798
Pronestyl-SR Tablets (0.5%) 1801
Rheumatrex Methotrexate Dose Pack 1234
Rubex 739
Sinequan (Occasional) 1960
Surmontil Capsules 2524
Tegretol Chewable Tablets 654
Tegretol Suspension 656
Tegretol Tablets 654
Tenuate 1354
Thiotepa Parenteral 1240
Tofranil Ampuls 1038
Tofranil Tablets 1039
Tofranil-PM Capsules 1041
Tonocard Tablets (Less than 1%) .. 1554
Triavil Tablets 1556
Vaseretic Tablets (Rare) 1559
Vasotec I.V. (Rare) 1562
Vasotec Tablets (Rare) 1564
Vivactil Tablets 1567
Zestoretic (Rare) 2274
Zestril Tablets (Rare) 2277

Bone marrow dysplasia

BiCNU 723
CeeNU 725

Bone marrow hyperplasia

Ponstel (Occasional) 1758

Bone marrow hypoplasia

AK-Chlor Sterile Ophthalmic Ointment & Solution ..... ⊙ 201
Chloromycetin Ophthalmic Ointment, 1% 1696
Chloromycetin Ophthalmic Solution 1696
Chloromycetin Otic 1697
Lopid Capsules and Tablets (Rare) 1736
Ophthochlor Ophthalmic Solution ..... ⊙ 300
Ophthocort ..... ⊙ 301
Zantac Injection and Zantac Injection Premixed (Rare) 1063
Zantac (Rare) 1065

Bone marrow suppression

▲ Alkeran Tablets (Most common) 754
▲ BiCNU (Most common) 723
▲ CeeNU (Most common) 725
▲ Cerubidine (All patients) 2443
Chloroptic S.O.P. ..... ⊙ 243
▲ Cytosar-U Sterile Powder (Among most frequent) 2329
Depakene Capsules & Syrup 511
Depakote 512
Dilantin Infatabs 1710
Dilantin Kapseals 1708
Dilantin Parenteral 1712
Dilantin-30 Pediatric/Dilantin-125 Suspension 1713
Dilantin with Phenobarbital Kapseals 1715
Empirin with Codeine Phosphate Nos. 2, 3 & 4 (Occasional) 764
Etrafon 2087
Fiorinal Capsules (Single case) 2007
Fiorinal with Codeine Capsules (Single case) 2008
Fiorinal Tablets (Single case) 2007
Imuran 768
▲ Leukeran Tablets (Frequent) 788
Milontin Kapseals 1741
Paraplatin for Injection 735
▲ Purinethol Tablets (Frequent) 800
Zarontin Capsules 1768
Zarontin Syrup 1769

Borborygmi

Duvoid Tablets 1853
Peptavlon 2563
Urecholine 1558

Bowel, loss of control

Duranest Injections 624
Nescaine/Nescaine MPF 629
Xylocaine Injections 637

Bowel disease, inflammatory, exacerbation of

Butazolidin Capsules & Tablets 1027

Bowel dysfunction

Depo-Medrol Sterile Aqueous Suspension 2334
Gelfoam Sterile Sponge 2338

Bowel frequency, increase

Diapid Nasal Spray (Infrequent) 2003
Esimil Tablets 864
Sterile FUDR 1898
▲ Hylorel Tablets (4.9%) 975
Ismelin Tablets 869
Modane Plus Tablets ..... ▣ 504
Modane Tablets ..... ▣ 503

Bowel habits, changes

▲ Seldane Tablets (7.6%) 1349
Seldane-D Extended-Release Tablets 1350

Bowel syndrome, irritable

Anafranil Capsules (Infrequent) 650

Bowels, perforation

Cortone Acetate Sterile Suspension 1437
Cortone Acetate Tablets 1439
Decadron Elixir 1445
Decadron Phosphate Injection 1449
Decadron Phosphate Respihaler 1454
Decadron Phosphate Turbinaire 1456
Decadron Phosphate with Xylocaine Injection, Sterile 1451
Decadron Tablets 1447
Decadron-LA Sterile Suspension 1457
Hydeltrasol Injection, Sterile 1476
Hydeltra-T.B.A. Sterile Suspension 1478
Hydrocortone Acetate Sterile Suspension 1479
Hydrocortone Phosphate Injection, Sterile 1481
Hydrocortone Tablets 1482
Indocin I.V. (1% to 3%) 1490

Brachial plexus neuropathies

Diphtheria and Tetanus Toxoids and Pertussis Vaccine Adsorbed USP (For Pediatric Use) 892

Bradycardia

Akineton 1171
Aldoclor Tablets 1413
Aldomet Ester HCl Injection 1417
Aldomet Oral 1415
Aldoril Tablets 1418
▲ Alfenta Injection (14%) 1131
Alurate Elixir (Less than 1 in 100) 1883
Anafranil Capsules (Infrequent) 650
Anectine 755
▲ Anestacon Solution (Among most common) 2394
Antilirium Injectable 998
Atgam Sterile Solution (At least 1 patient and less than 5% of total patients) 2320
Betoptic Sterile Ophthalmic Solution (Rare) 569
Betoptic S Sterile Ophthalmic Suspension (Rare) 570
▲ Blocadren Tablets (5% to 9.1%) 1429
Bretylol Injection (1-2 in 1000) 923
Brevibloc Injection (Less than 1%) 942
BuSpar (Rare) 1401
Butisol Sodium Elixir & Tablets (Less than 1 in 100) 2377
Cafergot/Cafergot P-B 1999
Calan SR Caplets (1.4%) 2157
Calan Tablets (1.4%) 2155
Carbocaine Hydrochloride Injection 2043
Cardizem Tablets-30 mg, 60 mg, 90 mg and 120 mg (Less than 1%) 1329
▲ Cardizem SR Capsules-60 mg, 90 mg and 120 mg (1.5-6%) 1327
Cartrol Tablets (0.0%) 507
Catapres Tablets (About 5 in 1,000 patients) 676
Catapres-TTS (5 per 1,000) 677
Clozaril Tablets (Less than 1%) 2000
Combipres Tablets (About 5 in 1,000) 678
Cordarone Tablets (Uncommon) 2446
▲ Corgard Tablets (Common) 701
Corzide Tablets (Common) 702
D.H.E. 45 Injection 2003
Decadron Phosphate with Xylocaine Injection, Sterile 1451
Demerol 2047
Desyrel and Desyrel Dividose 1404
Dilaudid-HP Injection 1175
Diprivan Injection (Greater than 1%) 2267
Diupres Tablets 1461
Dolophine Hydrochloride Ampoules & Vials 1260
Dolophine Hydrochloride Tablets 1261
Duranest Injections 624
Dyclone 0.5% and 1% Topical Solutions, USP 626
Enduronyl 518
Enlon Injection 598
Esimil Tablets 864
Eskalith 2214
Ethmozine Tablets (Less than 2%) 946
Etrafon 2087
Floropryl Sterile Ophthalmic Ointment (Rare) 1473
Harmonyl Tablets 528
Humorsol Sterile Ophthalmic Solution (Rare) 1475
Hydropres Tablets 1485
Hyperstat I.V. Injection 2095
Inderal 2459
Inderal LA Long Acting Capsules 2461
Inderide Tablets 2463
Inderide LA Long Acting Capsules .. 2465
Indocin I.V. (Less than 3%) 1490
Innovar Injection 1141
Intron A (Less than 1%) 2097
Intropin Injection (Infrequent) 930
IOPIDINE ..... ⊙ 232
Ismelin Tablets 869
Isoptin Injectable (1.2%) 1177
Isoptin Oral Tablets (1.4%) 1179
Isoptin SR Sustained Release Tablets (1.4%) 1181
▲ Kerlone Tablets (5.8% to 8.8%) 2172
Ketalar 1726
Lariam Tablets (Less than 1%) 1904
Levophed Bitartrate Injection 2054
Lippes Loop Intrauterine Double-S .. 1654
▲ Lopressor Ampuls (3%) 1032
▲ Lopressor HCT Tablets (6 in 100 patients) 1034
▲ Lopressor Tablets (3%) 1032
MS Contin Tablets (Infrequent) 1814
MSIR (Infrequent) 1817
Marcaine Hydrochloride with Epinephrine 1:200,000 2055
Marcaine Hydrochloride Injection 2055
Marcaine Spinal 2058
Mebaral Tablets (Less than 1 in 100) 2061
Mepergan Injection 2479
Methadone Hydrochloride Diskets .. 1284
Methadone Hydrochloride Oral Solution & Tablets 1987
Mexitil Capsules (About 4 in 1,000) 680
Midamor Tablets 1508
Miochol with locare Steri-Tags, Miochol System Pak and Miochol System Pak Plus (Rare) ..... ⊙ 274
Motrin Tablets (Less than 1%) 2351
Myochrysine Injection 1516
Nembutal Sodium Capsules (Less than 1%) 534
Nembutal Sodium Solution (Less than 1%) 536
Nembutal Sodium Suppositories (Less than 1%) 538
Neo-Synephrine Hydrochloride 1% Carpuject 2063
Neo-Synephrine Hydrochloride 1% Injection 2063
Nescaine/Nescaine MPF 629
Nimotop Capsules (Up to 1.0%) 1607
Nipride I.V. Infusion 1909
Normodyne Injection 2108
Normodyne Tablets (Rare) 2110
Normozide Tablets (Rare) 2112
Novocain Hydrochloride for Spinal Anesthesia 2065
Nubain Injection (Less than 1%) 934
Omnipaque (Less than 0.4 to 1.0%) 2552
OptiPranolol Sterile Ophthalmic Solution (A small number of patients) ..... ⊙ 261
Oramorph SR (Morphine Sulfate Sustained Release Tablets) (Less frequent) 1988
Oreticyl 545
Oxytocin Injection 2492
Pantopon Injectable 1911
ParaGard T380A Intrauterine Copper Contraceptive 411
Parlodel (Less than 1%) 2020
Permax Tablets (Infrequent) 1291
Phenergan with Codeine 2497
Phenergan Injection 2493
Phenergan Tablets 2496
Phenergan VC with Codeine 2501
Phenobarbital Elixir and Tablets (Less than 1 in 100 patients) 1293
Prilosec Delayed-Release Capsules (Less than 1%) 1530
Prinivil Tablets 1538
Prinzide Tablets 1540
Prostigmin Injectable 1120
Prostigmin Tablets 1121
▲ Prostin VR Pediatric Sterile Solution (7%) 2355
Protamine Sulfate Ampoules & Vials 1295
Prozac Pulvules (Rare) 920
Raudixin Tablets 1803
Rauzide Tablets 1804
Reglan 1869
Renese-R Tablets 1786
Robaxin Injectable 1871
Roxanol 1991
Rythmol Tablets (0.5 to 1.5%) 1184
Salutensin/Salutensin-Demi 719

Seconal Sodium Pulvules (Less than 1 in 100) 1296
Sectral Capsules (Up to 2%) 2520
Sensorcaine 631
Sensorcaine-MPF Spinal 634
Ser-Ap-Es Tablets 881
Serpasil Tablets 883
Serpasil-Apresoline Tablets 884
Serpasil-Esidrix Tablets 886
Solganal Suspension 2122
Sublimaze Injection 1146
▲ Sufenta Injection (3%) 1147
Tacaryl 2409
Tagamet (Rare) 2228
Tambocor Tablets (Less than 1%) 1315
Taractan 1920
Temaril Tablets, Syrup and Spansule Sustained Release Capsules 1085
Tenex Tablets (Less than 3%) 1875
▲ Tenoretic Tablets (3%) 1105
▲ Tenormin Tablets and I.V. Injection (3 to 18%) 1107
Tensilon Injectable 1123
Timolide Tablets (1.2%) 1547
Timoptic in Ocudose 1552
Timoptic Sterile Ophthalmic Solution 1550
Tonocard Tablets (0.4-1.8%) 1554
Tracrium Injection 817
Trandate HCT Tablets (Rare) 579
Trandate Injection (Rare) 577
Trandate Tablets (Rare) 579
Trilafon 2123
Valium Injectable 1937
Vancocin HCl, Vials & ADD-Vantage 1302
Vascor (200, 300 and 400 mg) Tablets 1383
Vaseretic Tablets 1559
Vasotec I.V. 1562
Vasotec Tablets 1564
Verelan Capsules (1.4%) 1243
Visken Tablets (2% or fewer patients) 2036
Xylocaine Injections 637
Xylocaine Injections for Ventricular Arrhythmias 639
Xylocaine 2% Jelly 643
Xylocaine 5% Ointment 644
Xylocaine 10% Oral Spray 645
4% Xylocaine-MPF Sterile Solution 641
Xylocaine 2% Viscous Solution 646
Zantac Injection and Zantac Injection Premixed (Rare) 1063
Zantac (Rare) 1065
Zestoretic 2274
Zestril Tablets 2277
Zyloprim Tablets (Less than 1%) 830

Bradycardia, fetal
Carbocaine Hydrochloride Injection 2043
Duranest Injections 624
Nescaine/Nescaine MPF 629
Sensorcaine 631
Sensorcaine-MPF Spinal 634
Syntocinon Injection 2032
▲ Xylocaine Injections (20% to 30%) 637

Bradycardia, neonatal
Diupres Tablets 1461
Hydropres Tablets 1485
Normodyne Tablets (Rare) 2110
Oxytocin Injection 2492
Pitocin Injection, Ampoules, Steri-Dose Syringes 1757
Syntocinon Injection 2032
Tenoretic Tablets 1105
Tenormin Tablets and I.V. Injection 1107
Trandate HCT Tablets 579
Trandate Injection 577
Trandate Tablets 579

Bradycardia, paradoxical
Nitro-Bid IV 1338

Bradycardia, severe
Eskalith 2214

Bradycardia, symptomatic
Kerlone Tablets (0.8% to 1.9%) 2172

Bradycardia, transient
Medihaler Ergotamine Aerosol 1312
▲ Survanta Beractant Intratracheal Suspension (11.9%) 1978
Wigraine Tablets & Suppositories 1645

Bradycardia with nodal escape rhythms
Isoptin SR Sustained Release Tablets 1181
Verelan Capsules 1243

Bradykinesia
Eldepryl 2250
Reglan 1869
Taractan 1920
▲ Wellbutrin Tablets (8.0%) 821

Bradykinetic episodes
Larodopa Tablets (Infrequent) 1905
Sinemet Tablets (Less frequent) 952
Sinemet CR Tablets 953

Bradypnea
Prostin VR Pediatric Sterile Solution (Less than 1%) 2355

Brain, compression
Gelfoam Sterile Sponge 2338

Brain syndrome, chronic
Prozac Pulvules (Rare) 920

Breast carcinoma
Aldactazide 2150
Aldactone 2152
Demulen 2161
Enovid 2161
Estratest 2245
Jenest-28 Tablets 1636
Norethin 2133
Permax Tablets (Infrequent) 1291
Protostat Tablets 1674

Breast changes, unspecified
Brevicon 2304
Demulen 2161
▲ Emcyt Capsules (10 to 66%) 1161
Enovid 2161
Jenest-28 Tablets 1636
Lo/Ovral Tablets 2471
Lo/Ovral-28 Tablets 2476
Loestrin 1728
Micronor Tablets 1667
Modicon 1667
Nordette-21 Tablets 2481
Nordette-28 Tablets 2483
Norinyl 2304
Norlestrin 1746
Nor-Q D Tablets 2304
Ortho-Novum 1667
Ovral Tablets 2490
Ovral-28 Tablets 2491
Ovrette Tablets 2492
Proglycem 649
Rogaine Topical Solution (0.47%) 2357
Tri-Norinyl 2304
Triphasil-21 Tablets 2527
Triphasil-28 Tablets 2532

Breast engorgement
Anafranil Capsules (Rare) 650
Desyrel and Desyrel Dividose 1404
Haldol Decanoate 1375
Haldol Injection, Tablets and Concentrate 1373
Mellaril 2011
Permax Tablets (Rare) 1291
Rauzide Tablets 1804
Ser-Ap-Es Tablets 881
Serpasil Tablets 883
Serpasil-Apresoline Tablets 884
Serpasil-Esidrix Tablets 886
Synarel Nasal Solution (Less than 1%) 2300
Zoladex (1% to 5%) 1110

Breast enlargement
Aldoclor Tablets 1413
Aldomet Ester HCl Injection 1417
Aldomet Oral 1415
Aldoril Tablets 1418
Anafranil Capsules (Up to 2%) 650
Asendin Tablets (Less than 1%) 1196
Brevicon 2304
Demser Capsules (Infrequent) 1460
Demulen 2161
Depakene Capsules & Syrup (Rare) 511
Depakote 512
Desyrel and Desyrel Dividose 1404
Diethylstilbestrol Tablets 1258
Elavil 2269
▲ Emcyt Capsules (60%) 1161
Endep Tablets 1927
Enovid 2161
Estinyl Tablets 2085
Estrace 1385
Estrace Vaginal Cream 1388
Estraderm Transdermal System 866
Estradurin 2452
Estratest 2245
Estrovis 1721
Etrafon 2087
Flexeril Tablets (Rare) 1471
Indocin Capsules (Less than 1%) 1487
Indocin I.V. (Less than 1%) 1490
Indocin (Less than 1%) 1487
Jenest-28 Tablets 1636
Levlen/Tri-Levlen 665
Limbitrol 1933
Loestrin 1728
Ludiomil Tablets 874
Mediatric Capsules 2476
Menrium Tablets 1934
Micronor Tablets 1667
Modicon 1667
Navane Capsules and Concentrate 1954
Navane Intramuscular 1956
Norethin 2133
Norinyl 2304
Norlestrin 1746
Norpramin Tablets 1340
Nor-Q D Tablets 2304
Ogen 540
Ortho Dienestrol Cream 1664
Ortho-Cyclen Tablets 1658
Ortho-Novum 1667
Ovcon 1391
PMB 200 and PMB 400 2504
Pamelor 2019
Premarin Intravenous 2508
Premarin with Methyltestosterone 2515
Premarin Tablets 2510
Premarin Vaginal Cream 2512
ProSom Tablets (Rare) 554
Prozac Pulvules (Rare) 920
Raudixin Tablets 1803
Sinequan 1960
Stilphostrol Tablets and Ampuls 1609
Surmontil Capsules 2524
TACE 12 and 25 mg 1353
Taractan 1920
Thorazine 2234
Tofranil Ampuls 1038
Tofranil Tablets 1039
Tofranil-PM Capsules 1041
Triavil Tablets 1556
Trilafon 2123
Levlen/Tri-Levlen 665
Tri-Norinyl 2304
Triphasil-21 Tablets 2527
Triphasil-28 Tablets 2532
Vivactil Tablets 1567

Breast fibroadenosis
Anafranil Capsules (Rare) 650
Kerlone Tablets (Less than 2%) 2172

Breast fibrocystic
Micronor Tablets 1667
Modicon 1667
Ortho-Novum 1667
Permax Tablets (Infrequent) 1291
Prozac Pulvules (Infrequent) 920

Breast milk, maternal, excreted in
Adalat Capsules (10 mg and 20 mg) 1587
Aldactazide 2150
Aldactone 2152
Aldoclor Tablets 1413
Aldomet Ester HCl Injection 1417
Aldomet Oral 1415
Aldoril Tablets 1418
Alfenta Injection 1131
Anatuss LA Tablets 1359
Ansaid Tablets 2319
Asendin Tablets 1196
Astramorph/PF Injection, USP (Preservative-Free) 618
Atromid-S Capsules 2435
Augmentin Tablets, Powder for Oral Suspension, and Chewable Tablets 2198
Axid Pulvules 1246
Azactam for Injection 2252
Azo Gantanol Tablets 1887
Azo Gantrisin Tablets 1888
Azulfidine Tablets, EN-tabs, Oral Suspension 1157
Bactrim DS Tablets 1891
Bactrim I.V. Infusion 1889
Bactrim 1891
Bentyl 1322
Biavax II 1427
Bicillin C-R Injection 2438
Bicillin C-R 900/300 Injection 2440
Bicillin L-A Injection 2442
Biltricide 1589
Bricanyl Injection 1324
Bricanyl Tablets 1325
Butazolidin Capsules & Tablets 1027
Butisol Sodium Elixir & Tablets 2377
Calan SR Caplets 2157
Calan Tablets 2155
Capoten 2255
Capozide 2258
Cardioquin Tablets 1812
Cardizem Tablets-30 mg, 60 mg, 90 mg and 120 mg 1329
Cardizem SR Capsules-60 mg, 90 mg and 120 mg 1327
Catapres Tablets 676
Catapres-TTS 677
Cefizox Injection 1012
Cefotan 2265
Ceftin Tablets 575
Ceptaz for Injection 1057
Choledyl Pediatric Elixir 1702
Choledyl Tablets 1700
Cibalith-S 870
Cipro I.V. 1592
Cipro Tablets 1589
Cleocin HCl Capsules 2322
Cleocin Pediatric Flavored Granules 2324
Cleocin Phosphate Injection 2325
Clozaril Tablets (Less than 1%) 2000
Combipres Tablets 678
Compazine 2201
Cordarone Tablets 2446
Corgard Tablets 701
Cortone Acetate Sterile Suspension 1437
Cortone Acetate Tablets 1439
Corzide Tablets 702
Coumadin Injection & Tablets 944
Cycrin Tablets 2449
Cytotec 2159
Damason-P 1356
Dapsone USP 1130
Daraprim Tablets 761
Decadron Elixir 1445
Decadron Phosphate Injection 1449
Decadron Phosphate Respihaler 1454
Decadron Phosphate Turbinaire 1456
Decadron Phosphate with Xylocaine Injection, Sterile 1451
Decadron Tablets 1447
Decadron-LA Sterile Suspension 1457
Deconamine 663
Demerol 2047
Demulen 2161
Deprol Tablets 2382
Desoxyn Gradumet Tablets 514
Desyrel and Desyrel Dividose 1404
Dexedrine 2206
Diabinese Tablets 1775
Dicumarol Tablets 516
Didrex Tablets 2338
Dilantin Infatabs 1710
Dilantin Kapseals 1708
Dilantin Parenteral 1712
Dilantin-30 Pediatric/Dilantin-125 Suspension 1713
Dilantin with Phenobarbital Kapseals 1715
Diprivan Injection 2267
Disalcid 1310
Diucardin Tablets 2450
Diulo 2129
Diupres Tablets 1461
Diuril Oral Suspension 1464
Diuril Sodium Intravenous 1463
Diuril Tablets 1464
Dolobid Tablets 1465
Doral Tablets 2383
Doryx Capsules 1717
Duragesic Transdermal System 1133
Duramorph 960
Dyazide Capsules 2208
Dyrenium Capsules 2210
E.E.S. 522
ETS-2% 1685
Elavil 2269
Empirin with Codeine Phosphate Nos. 2, 3 & 4 764
Endep Tablets 1927
Enduron Tablets 517
Enduronyl 518
Enovid 2161
Equagesic Tablets 2451
ERYC 1720
EryPed 200 & EryPed 400 Granules 519
Ery-Tab Tablets 521
Erythrocin Stearate Filmtab 523
Esgic-Plus Tablets 1002

Esidrix Tables ... 863
Eskalith ... 2214
Ethmozine Tablets ... 946
Fansidar Tablets ... 1896
Fedahist Gyrocaps ... 2145
Fedahist Timecaps ... 2145
Fioricet Tablets ... 2006
Fiorinal Capsules ... 2007
Fiorinal with Codeine Capsules ... 2008
Fiorinal Tablets ... 2007
Flagyl I.V. ... 2131
Flagyl Tablets ... 2170
Fortaz ... 1060
Gantanol ... 1899
Gantrisin Ophthalmic Ointment/Solution ... 1900
Gantrisin ... 1901
Halcion Tablets ... 2340
Haldol Decanoate ... 1375
Haldol Injection, Tablets and Concentrate ... 1373
Harmonyl Tablets ... 528
Hydeltrasol Injection, Sterile ... 1476
Hydeltra-T.B.A. Sterile Suspension ... 1478
Hydrocortone Acetate Sterile Suspension ... 1479
Hydrocortone Phosphate Injection, Sterile ... 1481
Hydrocortone Tablets ... 1482
HydroDIURIL Tablets ... 1484
Hydromox R Tablets ... 1209
Hydromox Tablets ... 1208
Hydropres Tablets ... 1485
Hylorel Tablets ... 975
INH Tablets ... 868
Ilosone ... 913
Inderal ... 2459
Inderal LA Long Acting Capsules ... 2461
Inderide Tablets ... 2463
Inderide LA Long Acting Capsules ... 2465
Indocin ... 1487
Inversine Tablets ... 1492
Isoptin Injectable ... 1177
Isoptin Oral Tablets ... 1179
Isoptin SR Sustained Release Tablets ... 1181
Jenest-28 Tablets ... 1636
Kefurox Vials, Faspak & ADD-Vantage ... 1277
Konakion Injection ... 1903
Kutrase Capsules ... 2146
Lamprene Capsules ... 1030
Lanoxicaps ... 772
Lanoxin Elixir Pediatric ... 775
Lanoxin Injection ... 778
Lanoxin Injection Pediatric ... 781
Lanoxin Tablets ... 783
Lasix ... 1093
Levsin/Levsinex ... 2147
Lincocin ... 2344
Lithane Tablets ... 1596
Lithium Carbonate Capsules & Tablets ... 1984
Lithobid Tablets ... 870
Lo/Ovral Tablets ... 2471
Lo/Ovral-28 Tablets ... 2476
Lomotil ... 2174
Loniten Tablets ... 2346
Lopressor Ampuls ... 1032
Lopressor HCT Tablets ... 1034
Lopressor Tablets ... 1032
Lortab ASA Tablets ... 2414
Lozol Tablets ... 1843
Ludiomil Tablets ... 874
Lufyllin & Lufyllin-400 Tablets ... 2384
Lufyllin-GG Elixir & Tablets ... 2385
MS Contin Tablets ... 1814
MSIR Oral Solution ... 1817
Marinol (Dronabinol) Capsules ... 1985
Mepergan Injection ... 2479
Meruvax$_{11}$ ... 1503
Methergine ... 2016
Mezlin ... 1597
Midamor Tablets ... 1508
Miltown Tablets ... 2386
Minizide Capsules ... 1779
Minocin Oral Suspension ... 1224
Minocin Pellet-Filled Capsules ... 1222
Moduretic Tablets ... 1510
Monocid Injection ... 2217
Monodox Capsules ... 1630
Mono-Gesic Tablets ... 846
Mykrox ½ mg Tablets ... 984
Myochrysine Injection ... 1516
Mysoline ... 2480
Naprosyn ... 2297
Naturetin Tablets ... 1789
Nordette-21 Tablets ... 2481
Nordette-28 Tablets ... 2483
Norethin ... 2133
Norlutate ... 1754
Norlutin ... 1755
Normodyne Injection ... 2108
Normodyne Tablets ... 2110
Normozide Tablets ... 2112
Norpace ... 2177
Norplant System ... 2484
Novahistine DH ... 1342
Novahistine Expectorant ... 1343
Nucofed Capsules ... 2219
Nucofed Expectorant ... 2219
Nucofed Pediatric Expectorant ... 2220
Nucofed Syrup ... 2219
Oramorph SR (Morphine Sulfate Sustained Release Tablets) ... 1988
Oretic Tablets ... 544
Oreticyl Tablets ... 545
Ovral Tablets ... 2490
Ovral-28 Tablets ... 2491
Ovrette Tablets ... 2492
PCE Dispertab Tablets ... 549
PMB 200 and PMB 400 ... 2504
Panwarfin Tablets ... 547
Pediazole ... 1973
Persantine Tablets ... 683
Pfizerpen for Injection ... 1957
Pfizerpen-AS Aqueous Suspension ... 1959
Phenergan with Codeine ... 2497
Phenergan VC with Codeine ... 2501
Phenobarbital Elixir and Tablets ... 1293
Prinzide Tablets ... 1540
Procan SR Tablets ... 1760
Proloprim Tablets ... 799
Pronestyl Capsules and Tablets ... 1800
Pronestyl Injection ... 1798
Pronestyl-SR Tablets ... 1801
Protostat Tablets ... 1674
Prozac Pulvules ... 920
Quadrinal Tablets ... 1183
Quarzan Capsules ... 1937
Quibron Capsules ... 713
Quibron-T ... 714
Quinaglute Dura-Tabs Tablets ... 663
Quinamm Tablets ... 1344
Quinidex Extentabs ... 1868
Raudixin Tablets ... 1803
Rauzide Tablets ... 1804
Reglan ... 1869
Renese Tablets ... 1785
Renese-R Tablets ... 1786
Ridaura Capsules ... 2224
Rifamate Capsules ... 1347
Rimactane Capsules ... 879
Robaxisal Tablets ... 1872
Rocaltrol Capsules ... 1913
Rocephin Injectable Vials, ADD-Vantage ... 1914
Rogaine Topical Solution ... 2357
Roxanol ... 1991
Salflex ... 839
Saluron ... 718
Salutensin/Salutensin-Demi ... 719
Sandimmune ... 2024
Sectral Capsules ... 2520
Septra ... 813
Ser-Ap-Es Tablets ... 881
Seromycin Pulvules ... 1298
Serpasil Tablets ... 883
Serpasil-Apresoline Tablets ... 884
Serpasil-Esidrix Tablets ... 886
Slo-bid Gyrocaps ... 1847
Solganal Suspension ... 2122
Soma Compound w/Codeine Tablets ... 2390
Soma Compound Tablets ... 2389
Soma Tablets ... 2388
Spectrobid Tablets & Powder for Oral Suspension ... 1961
Stelazine ... 2226
Symmetrel Capsules & Syrup ... 936
Syntocinon Injection ... 2032
Tagamet ... 2228
Tambocor Tablets ... 1315
Tavist Syrup ... 2033
Tazicef for Injection ... 2231
Tegretol Chewable Tablets ... 654
Tegretol Suspension ... 656
Tegretol Tablets ... 654
Tenoretic Tablets ... 1105
Tenormin Tablets and I.V. Injection ... 1107
Tenuate ... 1354
Terramycin Capsules ... 1786
Thalitone Tablets ... 687
Theolair ... 1317
Theolair-SR Tablets ... 1319
Thiosulfil Forte Tablets ... 2526
Thorazine ... 2234
Timolide Tablets ... 1547
Timoptic in Ocudose ... 1552
Tolectin (200, 400 and 600 mg) ... 1379
Trandate HCT/Trandate ... 579
Tranxene ... 556
Trental ... 1099
Trilisate ... 1822
Trimpex Tablets ... 1922
Triphasil-21 Tablets ... 2527
Triphasil-28 Tablets ... 2532
Tylenol with Codeine ... 1381
Uniphyl 400 mg Tablets ... 1823
Vanceril Inhaler ... 2128
Vancocin HCl, Oral Solution & Pulvules ... 1304
Vancocin HCl, Vials & ADD-Vantage ... 1302
Vascor (200, 300 and 400 mg) Tablets ... 1383
Vaseretic Tablets ... 1559
Velosef Capsules and for Oral Suspension ... 606
Vibramycin Hyclate Capsules ... 1787
Vibramycin Hyclate Intravenous ... 1968
Vibramycin ... 1787
Vicodin ES Tablets ... 1189
Visken Tablets ... 2036
Voltaren Tablets ... 1042
Wygesic Tablets ... 2540
Xanax Tablets ... 2367
Zantac Injection and Zantac Injection Premixed ... 1063
Zantac ... 1065
Zestoretic ... 2274
Zinacef ... 1066
Zorprin Tablets ... 698
Zovirax Sterile Powder ... 828
Zyloprim Tablets ... 830

Breast pain

Anafranil Capsules (Up to 1%) ... 650
Cardura Tablets (Less than 0.5% of 3960 patients) ... 1941
Clozaril Tablets (Less than 1%) ... 2000
Lupron Depot 7.5 mg ... 2311
Procardia XL Tablets (1% or less) ... 1783
Prozac Pulvules (Infrequent) ... 920

Breast secretion

Brevicon ... 2304
Danocrine Capsules (Rare) ... 2046
Demulen ... 2161
Diethylstilbestrol Tablets ... 1258
Enovid ... 2161
Estinyl Tablets ... 2085
Estrace ... 1385
Estrace Vaginal Cream ... 1388
Estradurin ... 2452
Estratest ... 2245
Estrovis ... 1721
Jenest-28 Tablets ... 1636
Levlen/Tri-Levlen ... 665
Loestrin ... 1728
Mediatric Capsules ... 2476
Menrium Tablets ... 1934
Micronor Tablets ... 1667
Modicon ... 1667
Norethin ... 2133
Norinyl ... 2304
Norlestrin ... 1746
Norplant System ... 2484
Nor-Q D Tablets ... 2304
Ogen ... 540
Ortho Dienestrol Cream ... 1664
Ortho-Cyclen Tablets ... 1658
Ortho-Novum ... 1667
Ovcon ... 1391
PMB 200 and PMB 400 ... 2504
Premarin Intravenous ... 2508
Premarin with Methyltestosterone ... 2515
Premarin Vaginal Cream ... 2512
Stilphostrol Tablets and Ampuls ... 1609
Levlen/Tri-Levlen ... 665
Tri-Norinyl ... 2304

Breast size reduction

Danocrine Capsules ... 2046
▲ Synarel Nasal Solution (10% of patients) ... 2300

Breast tenderness

Amen (Rare) ... 833
Azactam for Injection (Less than 1%) ... 2252
Brevicon ... 2304
Bumex (0.1%) ... 1895
Cycrin Tablets (Rare) ... 2449
Demulen ... 2161
Depo-Provera Sterile Aqueous Suspension (Few instances) ... 2336
Diethylstilbestrol Tablets ... 1258
▲ Emcyt Capsules (66%) ... 1161
Enovid ... 2161
Estinyl Tablets ... 2085
Estraderm Transdermal System ... 866
Estradurin ... 2452
Estratest ... 2245
Estrovis ... 1721
Indocin Capsules (Less than 1%) ... 1487
Indocin I.V. (Less than 1%) ... 1490
Indocin (Less than 1%) ... 1487
Jenest-28 Tablets ... 1636
Levlen/Tri-Levlen ... 665
Lo/Ovral Tablets ... 2471
Lo/Ovral-28 Tablets ... 2476
Loniten Tablets (Less than 1%) ... 2346
Lupron Depot 7.5 mg ... 2311
▲ Lupron Injection (5% or more) ... 2310
Mediatric Capsules ... 2476
Menrium Tablets ... 1934
Metrodin (urofollitropin for injection) ... 2182
Micronor Tablets ... 1667
Modicon ... 1667
Norethin ... 2133
Norinyl ... 2304
Ogen ... 540
Ortho Dienestrol Cream ... 1664
Ortho-Cyclen Tablets ... 1658
Ortho-Novum ... 1667
Ovral Tablets ... 2490
Ovral-28 Tablets ... 2491
Ovrette Tablets ... 2492
PMB 200 and PMB 400 ... 2504
Premarin Intravenous ... 2508
Premarin with Methyltestosterone ... 2515
Premarin Tablets ... 2510
Premarin Vaginal Cream ... 2512
Provera Tablets ... 2356
Serophene (clomiphene citrate tablets, USP) (1 in 50 patients) ... 2186
Stilphostrol Tablets and Ampuls ... 1609
TACE 12 and 25 mg ... 1353
Levlen/Tri-Levlen ... 665
Tri-Norinyl ... 2304
Triphasil-21 Tablets ... 2527
Triphasil-28 Tablets ... 2532
Zoladex (1% to 5%) ... 1110

Breath, shortness

Adalat Capsules (10 mg and 20 mg) (2% or less) ... 1587
▲ Adenocard Injection (12%) ... 1007
AeroBid Inhaler System (Less than 1%) ... 995
Azo Gantrisin Tablets ... 1888
Bretylol Injection (1 in 1000) ... 923
BuSpar (Infrequent) ... 1401
Calciparine Injection ... 925
Cholybar ... 1705
Cibacalcin Double-chambered Syringes (Rare) ... 859
Clozaril Tablets (1%) ... 2000
Colestid Granules (1–3 patients in 1,000) ... 2328
Contac Nighttime Cold Medicine ... ▣ 713
Coumadin Injection & Tablets ... 944
Cytosar-U Sterile Powder (Less frequent) ... 2329
Dalmane Capsules (Rare) ... 1927
Desyrel and Desyrel Dividose (Less than 1%) ... 1404
Dimetane-DC Cough Syrup ... 1857
Dimetane-DX Cough Syrup ... 1858
Dipentum Capsules (Rare) ... 1160
Dobutrex Solution Vials (1 to 3%) ... 1259
DynaCirc Capsules (0.5% to 1%) ... 2004
Eldepryl ... 2250
Empirin with Codeine Phosphate Nos. 2, 3 & 4 ... 764
Epogen for Injection (0.14% to 14%) ... 591
Gamimune N Immune Globulin Intravenous (Human) ... 1572
Guaifed ... 1615
Humulin 70/30, 100 Units (Less common) ... 1267
Humulin BR, 100 Units (Less common) ... 1268
Humulin L, 100 Units (Less common) ... 1268
Humulin U, 100 Units (Less common) ... 1272
Insulatard NPH ... 1626
Insulatard NPH Human ... 1627
IOPIDINE ... ◉ 232
K-Lyte ... 707
K-Phos M.F. Tablets ... 659
K-Phos Neutral Tablets ... 660
K-Phos Original Formula 'Sodium Free' Tablets (Less frequent) ... 660
K-Phos No. 2 Tablets ... 659
Klonopin Tablets ... 1902
▲ Lopressor Ampuls (3%) ... 1032
Lopressor HCT Tablets ... 1034
▲ Lopressor Tablets (3%) ... 1032
Maxzide ... 1215

Micronor Tablets 1667
Midamor Tablets (Less than or equal to 1%) 1508
Mixtard 70/30 1627
Mixtard Human 70/30 1628
Modicon 1667
Moduretic Tablets 1510
▲ NebuPent for Inhalation Solution (53 to 72%) 1017
Norpace (1 to 3%) 2177
Oncovin Solution Vials & Hyporets 1288
Ortho-Novum 1667
Parlodel (Less than 1%) 2020
Peptavlon 2563
▲ Phenaphen with Codeine Capsules (Among most frequent) 1865
▲ Phenaphen-650 with Codeine Tablets (Among most frequent) 1866
Procardia Capsules (2%) 1781
▲ Procrit for Injection (0.14% to 14%) 1647
Quadrinal Tablets 1183
Questran Light 711
Questran Powder 710
Rifadin 1345
Sandostatin Injection (Less than 1%) 2029
Septra (Rare) 813
Septra I.V. Infusion (Rare) 808
Septra I.V. Infusion ADD-Vantage Vials 810
Septra (Rare) 813
Soma Compound Tablets 2389
Stilphostrol Tablets and Ampuls 1609
Trexan Tablets (Less than 1%) 937
Tylenol with Codeine 1381
Uroqid-Acid (Less frequent) 661
Velban Vials 1305
Velosulin 1627
Velosulin Human 1628
Wellbutrin Tablets (Infrequent) 821

Breathing, difficult (see under Dyspnea)

Breathing, irregular
Anexsia 5/500 Tablets 2196
Anexsia 7.5/650 Tablets 2197
Azdōne Tablets 844
Damason-P 1356
Dilaudid Cough Syrup 1174
Dilaudid 1173
Dilaudid-HP Injection 1175
Hydrocet Capsules 835
Larodopa Tablets (Infrequent) 1905
Lortab ASA Tablets 2414
Lortab 2412
Nicorette 1335
Quadrinal Tablets 1183
Sinemet CR Tablets 953
Vicodin Tablets 1187
Vicodin ES Tablets 1189
Zydone Capsules 941

Breathing, labored (see under Dyspnea)

Breathing, shallow (see under Hypopnea)

Breathing, stertorous
Duragesic Transdermal System (Less than 1%) 1133

Bromsulphalein retention, increase (see under BSP retention, increase)

Bronchial constriction
Pitressin Synthetic, Ampoules 1758

Bronchial obstruction
Blocadren Tablets 1429
Timoptic in Ocudose 1552
Timoptic Sterile Ophthalmic Solution 1550

Bronchial secretion, decreased
Atrovent Inhalation Aerosol (About 1 in 100) 675
Cyclogyl ⊙ 215
Cyclomydril ⊙ 216

Bronchial secretions, increase
Klonopin Tablets 1902
Mestinon Injectable 1115
Mestinon 1116
Prostigmin Injectable 1120
Prostigmin Tablets 1121
Tensilon Injectable 1123

Bronchial secretions, thickening
Actifed with Codeine Cough Syrup 752
▲ Benadryl Capsules (Among most frequent) 1691
▲ Benadryl Injection (Among most frequent) 1692
Betoptic Sterile Ophthalmic Solution (Rare) 569
Betoptic S Sterile Ophthalmic Suspension (Rare) 570
Comhist LA Capsules 1618
Deconamine 663
▲ Dimetane-DC Cough Syrup (Most frequent) 1857
Dimetane-DX Cough Syrup (Among most frequent) 1858
Dorcol Children's Liquid Cold Formula ▣ 686
Optimine Tablets (Among most frequent) 2115
Ornade Spansule Capsules 2221
PBZ Tablets & Elixir (Among most frequent) 1037
PBZ-SR Tablets (Among most frequent) 1037
Periactin 1525
Polaramine 2116
Ru-Tuss II Capsules 693
Ru-Tuss with Hydrocodone 694
Ru-Tuss Tablets 693
Tacaryl 2409
Tavist Syrup (Among most frequent) 2033
▲ Tavist Tablets (Among most frequent) 2035
▲ Tavist-D Tablets (Among most frequent) 2035
Temaril Tablets, Syrup and Spansule Sustained Release Capsules 1085
Triaminic Cold Tablets ▣ 688
Triaminic Expectorant DH 1995
▲ Triaminic Oral Infant Drops (Among most frequent) 1996
Triaminic Syrup ▣ 689
Triaminicol Multi-Symptom Relief ▣ 691
▲ Trinalin Repetabs Tablets (Among most frequent) 1170

Bronchiolitis
Cuprimine Capsules 1442
Depen Titratable Tablets 2379
▲ Proventil Solutions for Inhalation 0.5% and 0.083% (4%) 2118
Solganal Suspension 2122

Bronchiolitis, obliterative
Depen Titratable Tablets (Rare) 2379

Bronchitis
Anafranil Capsules (Infrequent) 650
Ansaid Tablets (Less than 1%) 2319
Cartrol Tablets (Less common) 507
Clozaril Tablets (Less than 1%) 2000
Cytotec (Infrequent) 2159
Hytrin Tablets 529
Kerlone Tablets (Less than 2%) 2172
Lodine Capsules (Less than 1%) 2468
Lotensin Tablets 872
OptiPranolol Sterile Ophthalmic Solution (A small number of patients) ⊙ 261
Permax Tablets (Infrequent) 1291
Plendil Extended-Release Tablets (0.5% to 1.5%) 1526
Prinivil Tablets (1% or less) 1538
Prinzide Tablets (0.3 to 1%) 1540
Prozac Pulvules (Frequent) 920
Ridaura Capsules (Rare) 2224
▲ Rogaine Topical Solution (7.16%) 2357
Vaseretic Tablets 1559
Vasotec I.V. 1562
▲ Ventolin Inhalation Solution (4%) 583
Wellbutrin Tablets (Infrequent) 821
Zestoretic (0.3 to 1%) 2274
Zestril Tablets (Less than 1%) 2277

Bronchoconstriction
Enlon Injection 598
Platinol 737
Platinol-AQ Injection 738
Tensilon Injectable 1123
Urecholine 1558

Bronchoconstriction, paradoxical
Alupent 674
Arm-a-Med Metaproterenol Sulfate Inhalation Solution, USP 617
Maxair Inhaler 1311

Bronchospasm
Abbokinase (Rare) 503
Abbokinase Open-Cath (Rare) 505
Actimmune (Rare) 1046
Alfenta Injection (Less than 1%) 1131
▲ Anafranil Capsules (2% to 7%) 650
Axid Pulvules (Rare) 1246
Azactam for Injection (Less than 1%) 2252
Beclovent Inhalation Aerosol and Refill (Rare) 572
Beconase AQ Nasal Spray (Rare) 574
Beconase Inhalation Aerosol & Refill (Rare) 574
Betagan ⊙ 239
Betoptic Sterile Ophthalmic Solution (Rare) 569
Betoptic S Sterile Ophthalmic Suspension (Rare) 570
Blocadren Tablets (0.6%) 1429
Brevibloc Injection (Less than 1%) 942
Brevital Sodium Vials 1248
Calcimar Injection, Synthetic (A few cases) 1839
Capoten 2255
Capozide 2258
Cardura Tablets (Less than 0.5% of 3960 patients) 1941
Cartrol Tablets (Rare) 507
Ceftin Tablets (One case) 575
Ceptaz for Injection (Rare) 1057
Children's Advil Suspension (Less than 1%) 2426
Cipro Tablets (Less than 1%) 1589
Clinoril Tablets (Less than 1 in 100) 1433
Corgard Tablets (1 in 1000 patients) 701
Corzide Tablets (Approximately 1 of 1000 patients) 702
Cytotec (Infrequent) 2159
Deprol Tablets (Rare) 2382
Dilaudid-HP Injection 1175
Dipentum Capsules (Rare) 1160
Diprivan Injection (Less than 1%) 2267
Disalcid 1310
Dobutrex Solution Vials (Occasionally) 1259
Dolobid Tablets (Less than 1 in 100) 1465
Dopram Injectable 1860
Eminase 2211
Engerix-B Unit-Dose Vials 2213
Equagesic Tablets (Rare) 2451
Factrel (Rare) 2561
Feldene Capsules (Less than 1%) 1777
Fluorescite (Very rare) ⊙ 217
Fortaz (Very rare) 1060
Fungizone Intravenous 2262
Haldol Decanoate 1375
Haldol Injection, Tablets and Concentrate 1373
Hismanal Tablets (Less frequent) 1138
Imferon 976
Inapsine Injection 1140
Inderal 2459
Inderal LA Long Acting Capsules 2461
Inderide Tablets 2463
Inderide LA Long Acting Capsules 2465
Innovar Injection 1141
Intal Capsules (Less than 1 in 10,000 patients) 978
Intal Inhaler (Frequent) 979
Intal Nebulizer Solution 980
Intron A (Less than 1%) 2097
Isoptin Injectable (Rare) 1177
Kerlone Tablets (Less than 2%) 2172
Lopressor HCT Tablets (Fewer than 1 in 100) 1034
Lutrepulse for Injection 1655
Metubine Iodide Vials 1285
Miacalcin Injection (A few cases) 2017
Miltown Tablets (Rare) 2386
Monopril Tablets (0.2 to 1.0%) 1406
Motrin Tablets (Less than 1%) 2351
▲ NebuPent for Inhalation Solution (15%) 1017
Norcuron (Rare) 1642
Normodyne Tablets 2110
Normozide Tablets (Less than 1%) 2112
Nuromax Injection 794
Omnipaque 2552
Oncovin Solution Vials & Hyporets 1288
Orudis Capsules (Less than 1%) 2488
PMB 200 and PMB 400 (Rare) 2504
Paraplatin for Injection (Rare) 735
PediaProfen Suspension (Less than 1%) 1363
Pentam 300 Injection (1 patient) 1018
Pepcid (Infrequent) 1524
Pilocar ⊙ 275
Pilostat Sterile Ophthalmic Solution 0.5%, 1%, 2%, 3%, 4%, 5%, 6% (Extremely rare) ⊙ 263
Prostigmin Injectable 1120
Prostigmin Tablets 1121
▲ Proventil Solutions for Inhalation 0.5% and 0.083% (8%) 2118
Recombivax HB (Less than 1%) 1544
Reglan (A few cases) 1869
Rocephin Injectable Vials, ADD-Vantage (Rare) 1914
Roferon-A Injection (Less than 1%) 1916
Rufen Tablets (Less than 1%) 691
Salflex 839
Seldane Tablets 1349
Seldane-D Extended-Release Tablets 1350
Streptase for Infusion 635
Sufenta Injection (Less than 1%) 1147
Surital Ampoules, Steri-Vials 1764
Tambocor Tablets (Less than 1%) 1315
Tenormin Tablets and I.V. Injection (1.2%) 1107
Timolide Tablets (1.6%) 1547
Timoptic in Ocudose 1552
Timoptic Sterile Ophthalmic Solution 1550
Tornalate (Less than 1%) 2074
Tracrium Injection 817
Trandate HCT Tablets (Less than 1% in 208 patients) 579
Trandate Injection 577
Trandate Tablets 579
Vancenase Nasal Inhaler (Rare) 2126
Vanceril Inhaler (Rare) 2128
Vaseretic Tablets 1559
Vasotec I.V. 1562
Vasotec Tablets (0.5% to 1%) 1564
Velban Vials 1305
Ventolin (Rare) 583
VePesid Capsules and Injection (0.7 to 2%) 741
Versed Injection (Less than 1%) 1924
Voltaren Tablets 1042
Zantac Injection and Zantac Injection Premixed 1063
Zantac (Rare) 1065
Zofran Injection (Rare) 1069
Zorprin Tablets 698
Zyloprim Tablets (Less than 1%) 830

Bronchospasm, exacerbation of
Brethine Ampuls 1026
Brethine Tablets 1026

Bronchospasm, paradoxical
Alupent 674
Metaprel Inhalation Aerosol Bronchodilator 2014
Proventil Inhalation Aerosol 2117

Browache
Epifrin ⊙ 244
Floropryl Sterile Ophthalmic Ointment 1473
Humorsol Sterile Ophthalmic Solution 1475
Murocoll-2 Sterile Ophthalmic Solution (Frequent) ⊙ 261
OptiPranolol Sterile Ophthalmic Solution (A small number of patients) ⊙ 261
Phospholine Iodide ⊙ 315
▲ Rēv-Eyes Ophthalmic Eyedrops 0.5% (10% to 40%) ⊙ 312
Vasosulf ⊙ 279

Bruising
Accutane Capsules (Less than 1%) 1878
Anafranil Capsules (Rare) 650
Azdōne Tablets 844
BuSpar (Infrequent) 1401
Calan SR Caplets (1% or less) 2157
Calan Tablets (1% or less) 2155
Clozaril Tablets (Less than 1%) 2000
Coumadin Injection & Tablets 944
Damason-P (Occasional) 1356
Depakene Capsules & Syrup 511
Depakote 512
▲ Emcyt Capsules (3%) 1161
Eminase 2211
Empirin with Codeine Phosphate Nos. 2, 3 & 4 764
Feldene Capsules (Less than 1%) 1777
Isoptin Oral Tablets (Less than 1%) 1179
Isoptin SR Sustained Release Tablets (Less than 1%) 1181
Lortab ASA Tablets (Occasional) 2414

Maxair Inhaler (Less than 1%) 1311
Nalfon Pulvules & Tablets (Less than 1%) 919
Plendil Extended-Release Tablets (0.5% to 1.5%) 1526
Pronestyl Capsules and Tablets 1800
Pronestyl Injection 1798
Pronestyl-SR Tablets 1801
Quadrinal Tablets 1183
Q-vel Muscle Relaxant Pain Reliever .... ▣ 552
Rythmol Tablets (Less than 1%) 1184
Sandostatin Injection (Less than 1%) 2029
▲ Tegison Capsules (25-50%) 1881
Tegretol Chewable Tablets 654
Tegretol Suspension 656
Tegretol Tablets 654
Tonocard Tablets 1554
Verelan Capsules (Less than 1%) .. 1243
Voltaren Tablets (Rare) 1042

Bruxism

Eldepryl 2250
Larodopa Tablets (Relatively frequent) 1905
Sinemet Tablets 952
Sinemet CR Tablets 953
Wellbutrin Tablets (Infrequent) 821

Buccal-lingual-masticatory syndrome

Prozac Pulvules 920

Buccoglossal syndrome

Prozac Pulvules (Infrequent) 920

Bucking

Diprivan Injection (Greater than 1%) 2267

Budd-Chiari syndrome

Brevicon 2304
Demulen 2161
Enovid 2161
Levlen/Tri-Levlen 665
Loestrin 1728
Norethin 2133
Norinyl 2304
Norlestrin 1746
Nor-Q D Tablets 2304
Levlen/Tri-Levlen 665
Tri-Norinyl 2304

Bulbus oculi, perforation

AK-Dex .... ◉ 203
AK-Pred .... ◉ 205
Blephamide 586
Dexacidin .... ◉ 272
FML Forte Liquifilm .... ◉ 245
FML Liquifilm .... ◉ 244
FML S.O.P. .... ◉ 245
FML-S Sterile Ophthalmic Suspension .... ◉ 246
Fluor-Op Ophthalmic Suspension .... ◉ 272
Inflamase .... ◉ 274
Isopto Cetapred Suspension .... ◉ 220
Maxidex Sterile Ophthalmic Ointment .... ◉ 222
Maxidex Sterile Ophthalmic Suspension .... ◉ 223
Maxitrol Ophthalmic Ointment/Suspension .... ◉ 223
Pred Forte .... ◉ 252
Pred Mild .... ◉ 254
TobraDex Ophthalmic Suspension and Ointment .... ◉ 228
Vasocidin Ointment .... ◉ 275
Vasocidin Ophthalmic Solution .... ◉ 276

Bullae

NegGram 2062

Bundle branch block

Anafranil Capsules (Rare) 650
Cardizem Tablets-30 mg, 60 mg, 90 mg and 120 mg (Less than 1%) 1329
Cardizem SR Capsules-60 mg, 90 mg and 120 mg (Less than 1%) 1327
Prozac Pulvules (Rare) 920
Rythmol Tablets (0.3 to 1.9%) 1184
▲ Tenormin Tablets and I.V. Injection (6.6%) 1107
Tonocard Tablets (Less than 1%) .. 1554
Yutopar 647

Burning

Aclovate (1 in 100 patients) 1053
Adsorbonac 2% and 5% .... ◉ 210
Afrin .... ▣ 692
Alcaine .... ◉ 210
Alphatrex Cream, Ointment & Lotion (Infrequent) 2076
Americaine Anesthetic Lubricant 972
Americaine Otic Topical Anesthetic Ear Drops 973
Analpram-HC Rectal Cream 1% and 2.5% 970
Anusol Ointment .... ▣ 634
Anusol-HC Cream (Infrequent) 1690
Anusol-HC Suppositories 1691
Aristocort A (Infrequent) 1010
Bactroban Ointment (1.5%) 2200
Benoquin Cream 20% (Occasional) 1112
Betatrex Cream, Ointment & Lotion 2077
BiCNU 723
Brevibloc Injection (Less than 1%) 942
Caladryl Cream, Lotion, Spray ...... ▣ 638
Calciparine Injection 925
Carmol HC Cream 1% (Infrequent) 2296
▲ Catapres-TTS (3 of 101 patients) .. 677
Chloromycetin Ophthalmic Ointment, 1% (Occasional) 1696
Chloromycetin Otic 1697
Clear by Design Medicated Acne Gel .... ▣ 709
▲ Condylox (64% to 78%) 1630
Cortisporin Cream 757
Cortisporin Ointment 758
Cortisporin Otic Solution Sterile 760
Cortisporin Otic Suspension Sterile 760
Cutivate Cream 0.05% (0.6%) 1054
Cutivate Ointment 0.005% (0.6%) 1054
Decadron Phosphate Injection 1449
Decadron Phosphate Topical Cream 1455
Decaspray Topical Aerosol 1459
DesOwen Cream, Ointment and Lotion (Infrequent) 1682
▲ Diprivan Injection (10% or greater) 2267
Dristan Long Lasting Nasal Spray, Regular and Regular with Metered Dose Pump 2419
Dristan Nasal Spray, Regular and Regular with Metered Pump 2419
Elase-Chloromycetin Ointment 1015
Eldecort Cream 1.0% (Infrequent) 1113
Eldecort Cream 1.0% and 2.5% (Infrequent) 1113
Eldepryl 2250
▲ Elimite (permethrin) 5% Cream (10%) 1082
Elocon (1 of 319 patients) 2084
▲ Exelderm Cream 1.0% (3%) 2398
Exelderm Solution 1.0% (Approximately 1%) 2399
4-Way Fast Acting Nasal Spray - Original Formula (regular & mentholated) & Metered Spray Pump (regular) 751
4-Way Long Lasting Nasal Spray & Metered Spray Pump 751
Fleet Bisacodyl Enema 991
Fleet Prep Kits 993
Florone/Florone E 908
Floropryl Sterile Ophthalmic Ointment 1473
Floxin Tablets (Less than 1%) 1652
Fluoroplex Topical Solution & Cream 1% 1082
Garamycin Injectable 2093
Garamycin Ophthalmic Ointment—Sterile .... ◉ 305
Gentak Ointment & Solution (Occasional) .... ◉ 208
Glaucon .... ◉ 218
Halotex Cream & Solution (0.8 to 1.7%) 2400
Heparin Lock Flush Solution 2456
Heparin Sodium Vials 1264
Heparin Sodium Injection 2457
Heparin Sodium Injection, USP, Sterile Solution 2342
Humorsol Sterile Ophthalmic Solution 1475
Hydeltrasol Injection, Sterile 1476
Hydrocortone Phosphate Injection, Sterile 1481
Hytone 909
Inflamase (Rare) .... ◉ 274
Intal Inhaler (Infrequent) 979
▲ Intron A (20%) 2097
IOPIDINE .... ◉ 232
Kenalog Cream, Lotion & Ointment (Infrequent) 2401
Lidex (Infrequent) 2296
Locoid Cream, Ointment and Topical Solution (Infrequent) 970
Lotrimin 2102
Lotrisone Cream (Infrequent) 2103
Maxidex Sterile Ophthalmic Ointment (Rare) .... ◉ 222
Maxivate Cream, Lotion & Ointment 0.05% 2406
Monistat-Derm (miconazole nitrate) Cream (Isolated reports) 1679
Mycelex 1% Cream and Topical Solution 1% 1604
Mycelex-G 1% Vaginal Cream (0.5%) 1605
Mycolog II Cream and Ointment (Infrequent) 2407
Mytrex Cream & Ointment (Infrequent) 2080
▲ Naftin Gel 1% (5.0%) 1084
NeoDecadron Topical Cream 1518
Neo-Synalar Cream (Infrequent) 2296
Nubain Injection (Less than 1%) 934
Nutracort Cream & Lotion (Infrequent) 1684
▲ Ocufen (Among most frequent) .. ◉ 237
Omnipaque (Less than or equal to 1%) 2552
Ophthetic (Occasional) .... ◉ 249
Orabase HCA Oral Paste (Infrequent) 890
Otic Tridesilon Solution 0.05% (Infrequent) 1612
Oxistat Cream (1.4%) 1055
Oxy-5 and Oxy-10 Tinted and Vanishing Formulas with Sorboxyl .... ▣ 719
Panafil (Occasional) 1995
PediOtic Suspension Sterile 797
Phospholine Iodide .... ◉ 315
Polytrim Ophthalmic Solution Sterile 588
Pramosone Cream, Lotion & Ointment 971
Pred-G Liquifilm Sterile Ophthalmic Suspension .... ◉ 252
ProctoCream-HC (Infrequent) 1834
▲ Profenal Sterile Ophthalmic Solution (Among most frequent).. ◉ 234
Psorcon Ointment 0.05% 909
Psorion Cream 0.05% (Infrequent) 1121
▲ Rēv-Eyes Ophthalmic Eyedrops 0.5% (Approximately 50%) .... ◉ 312
Rowasa (0.61%) 2248
Sodium Sulamyd 2122
▲ Spectazole (econazole nitrate) Cream (3%) 1681
Surgicel (Occasional) 1151
Synacort Creams 1%, 2.5% (Infrequent) 2296
Synalar (Infrequent) 2296
Temovate (2 of 366 patients) 1056
Terazol 3 Vaginal Suppositories 1677
Topicort (Infrequent) 1098
Trexan Tablets (Less than 1%) 937
Tridesilon Creme 0.05% (Infrequent) 1611
Tridesilon Ointment 0.05% (Infrequent) 1611
▲ Ultravate Cream 0.05% (4%) 2410
Ultravate Ointment 0.05% (1.6%) 2411
▲ Vagistat (Approximately 6%) 1397
Vanoxide-HC Acne Lotion 911
Vioform-Hydrocortisone Cream and Mild Cream 889
Vioform-Hydrocortisone Ointment .. 889
▲ Viroptic Ophthalmic Solution, 1% Sterile (4.6%) 820
VōSol (Occasional) 2392
Vytone Cream 1% 911
Westcort 2411
Zantac Injection and Zantac Injection Premixed 1063
▲ Zovirax Ointment 5% (28.3%) 827

Burning, at injection site

▲ Ativan Injection (17%) 2432
Attenuvax 1424
Biavax II 1427
BiCNU 723
Brevibloc Injection (Less than 1%) 942
▲ Cefizox Injection (1 to 5%) 1012
Ceredase Injection 1052
Cipro I.V. (1% or less) 1592
DDAVP Injection (Occasional) 1840
Doxorubicin Hydrochloride Injection, USP 848
Inocor Lactate Injection (0.2%) 2048
M-M-R II 1494
M-R-VAX II 1496
Meruvax II 1503
Monocid Injection (Greater than 1%) 2217
Mumpsvax 1513
Rubex 739
Timentin for Injection 2239
Versed Injection (Less than 1%) 1924

Burning, local

Aci-Jel Therapeutic Vaginal Jelly (Occasional cases) 1652
Americaine Anesthetic Lubricant 972
Calciparine Injection 925
▲ Chibroxin Sterile Ophthalmic Solution (Most frequent) 1431
▲ Condylox (64% to 78%) 1630
Cyclocort Lotion (Infrequent) 1198
▲ Efudex (Among most frequent) 1880
▲ Elimite (permethrin) 5% Cream (10%) 1082
Mumpsvax 1513
▲ Naftin Cream 1% (6%) 1084
Selsun Rx 2.5% Selenium Sulfide Lotion, USP 1977
Spectazole (econazole nitrate) Cream 1681

Burning, mild

Lactinol-E Creme 1770
Mycelex-G 100 mg Vaginal Tablets (6 in 1,116 patients) 1606
Mycelex-G 500 mg Vaginal Tablets (6 in 1,116 patients) 1606

Burning, sexual partner

Mycelex-G 100 mg Vaginal Tablets (Rare) 1606
Mycelex-G 500 mg Vaginal Tablets (Rare) 1606
Today Vaginal Contraceptive Sponge 2422

Burning, vaginal (see under Vaginal burning)

Burning, vulvovaginal (see under Vaginal burning)

Burning sensation

▲ A/T/S Topical Gel and Topical Solution (17 out of 90) 1089
AVC 1322
Aclovate Ointment (2 of 366 patients) 1053
Adenocard Injection (Less than 1%) 1007
Adriamycin PFS 561
Adriamycin RDF 562
BAL in Oil Ampules 661
Chloromycetin Cream, 1% 1694
Chloromycetin Ophthalmic Solution 1696
Cyclogyl .... ◉ 215
Decadron Phosphate Sterile Ophthalmic Ointment (Rare) 1453
Decadron Phosphate Sterile Ophthalmic Solution (Rare) 1453
Dopram Injectable 1860
ETS-2% 1685
Erycette (erythromycin 2%) Topical Solution 1678
Fungizone Cream, Lotion and Ointment 2261
Gamimune N Immune Globulin Intravenous (Human) 1572
Idamycin for Injection 564
Loprox Cream 1% and Lotion 1% (1 out of 514) 1095
Mutamycin 733
Ophthochlor Ophthalmic Solution .... ◉ 300
Peptavlon 2563
Pondimin Tablets 1867
Quadrinal Tablets 1183
SSD 694
SSD RP Cream (Infrequent) 690
Sandostatin Injection (Less than 1%) 2029
Scleromate 1685
Silvadene Cream 1% (2.2%) 1352
Stilphostrol Tablets and Ampuls 1609
T-Stat 2.0% Topical Solution and Pads 2409
Temovate (2 of 366 patients) 1056
Theramycin Z Topical Solution 2% 1410
▲ Topicycline for Topical Solution (About 33%) 1856
Vagistat (Less than 1%) 1397
Ventolin (Less than 1%) 583
Vira-A Ophthalmic Ointment, 3% 1767
Zilactin Medicated Gel .... ▣ 768
Ziradryl Lotion .... ▣ 643

Bursitis
- Permax Tablets (1.6%) 1291
- Prozac Pulvules (Infrequent) 920

BBB+ Major Axis Deviation
- ▲ Tenormin Tablets and I.V. Injection (6.6%) 1107

BCG infection, disseminated
- BCG Vaccine, USP (Tice) (1 per 10,000,000 vaccinees) 1632
- Tice BCG Vaccine, USP (1 per 10,000,000 vaccines) 1632

BEI, increase
- Aygestin Tablets 2437

BSP retention
- Atromid-S Capsules 2435
- Capastat Sulfate Vials 1250
- Sterile FUDR 1898
- Hydrea Capsules 728
- Synkayvite Injection 1919
- Synkayvite Tablets 1920

BSP retention, increase
- Anadrol-50 Tablets 2287
- Estratest 2245
- Mithracin 1602
- Parafon Forte DSC Caplets 1379
- Rifadin 1345
- Rifamate Capsules 1347
- Rimactane Capsules 879
- Serophene (clomiphene citrate tablets, USP) (Approximately 10% to 20% of patients) 2186
- Winstrol Tablets 2075

BUN levels, changes
- Aristocort Suspension 1008
- Aristospan Suspension 1011
- Celestone Soluspan Suspension 2081
- Cortenema 2244
- Cortifoam 1827
- Cortone Acetate Sterile Suspension 1437
- Cortone Acetate Tablets 1439
- Dalalone D.P. Injectable 999
- Decadron Elixir 1445
- Decadron Phosphate Injection 1449
- Decadron Phosphate Respihaler 1454
- Decadron Phosphate Turbinaire 1456
- Decadron Phosphate with Xylocaine Injection, Sterile 1451
- Decadron Tablets 1447
- Decadron-LA Sterile Suspension 1457
- Deltasone Tablets 2332
- Doral Tablets (Less than 1%) 2383
- Hydeltrasol Injection, Sterile 1476
- Imuran (Less than 1%) 768
- Intron A (Up to 1%) 2097
- Kenalog-10 Injection 2402
- Kenalog-40 Injection 2403
- ▲ Roferon-A Injection (4%) 1916
- Sinemet Tablets 952
- Solu-Cortef Sterile Powder 2361
- Solu-Medrol Sterile Powder 2363
- Vasotec I.V. (0.5 to 1%) 1562
- Vasotec Tablets (0.5% to 1%) 1564

BUN levels, decrease
- Cipro I.V. (Infrequent) 1592

BUN levels, elevation
- Achromycin V Capsules 1193
- Aldactone 2152
- Aldoclor Tablets 1413
- Aldomet Ester HCl Injection 1417
- Aldomet Oral 1415
- Aldoril Tablets 1418
- Altace Capsules (Less than 1% to 3%) 1086
- Ancef Injection 2194
- Ancobon Capsules 1886
- Azo Gantrisin Tablets 1888
- Bactrim DS Tablets 1891
- Bactrim I.V. Infusion 1889
- Bactrim 1891
- Blocadren Tablets 1429
- Bufferin Analgesic Tablets and Caplets 743
- Calcijex Calcitriol Injection 506
- Calderol Capsules 1635
- ▲ Capastat Sulfate Vials (36%) 1250
- Capoten 2255
- Capozide 2258
- Ceclor Pulvules & Suspension (Less than 1 in 500) 1251
- Cefizox Injection (Occasional) 1012
- ▲ Cefobid Intravenous/Intramuscular (1 in 16) 1943
- ▲ Cefobid Pharmacy Bulk Package - Not for Direct Infusion (1 in 16) 1945
- Ceftin Tablets 575
- Ceptaz for Injection (Occasional) 1057
- Children's Advil Suspension (Occasional) 2426
- ▲ Cipro I.V. (Among most frequent) 1592
- Cipro Tablets (0.9%) 1589
- Claforan Sterile Injection (Occasional) 1089
- Corzide Tablets 702
- Cytotec (Infrequent) 2159
- Cytovene Sterile Powder (1% or less) 2292
- Declomycin Capsules, Tablets 1199
- Didronel I.V. Infusion 1307
- Diulo 2129
- Dopram Injectable 1860
- Doryx Capsules 1717
- Dyazide Capsules 2208
- Dyrenium Capsules (Rare) 2210
- Ecotrin 2189
- Esimil Tablets 864
- Eulexin Capsules 2089
- Feldene Capsules (1 to 3%) 1777
- Fortaz (Occasional) 1060
- Fungizone Intravenous 2262
- ▲ Ganite Injection (12.5%) 1016
- Glucotrol 1952
- ▲ Hexalen Capsules (1% to 9%) 2316
- Hydrea Capsules (Occasional) 728
- IFEX 729
- Indocin Capsules (Less than 1%) 1487
- ▲ Indocin I.V. (41% of infants) 1490
- Indocin (Less than 1%) 1487
- Intron A (1 patient) 2097
- Ismelin Tablets 869
- Keftab Tablets 917
- Kefurox Vials, Faspak & ADD-Vantage 1277
- Kefzol Vials, Faspak & ADD-Vantage 1279
- Larodopa Tablets (Rare) 1905
- Loniten Tablets 2346
- Lorelco Tablets 1333
- Lotensin Tablets (Less than 0.1%) 872
- Lozol Tablets (Less than 5%) 1843
- ▲ Lupron Depot 3.75 mg (Among most frequent) 2312
- Lupron Depot 7.5 mg 2311
- Lupron Injection (Less than 5%) 2310
- Mandol Vials, Faspak & ADD-Vantage 1281
- Maxzide 1215
- Mefoxin 1498
- Mefoxin Premixed Intravenous Solution 1500
- Mezlin 1597
- Mezlin Pharmacy Bulk Package 1599
- Minocin Intravenous 1221
- Minocin Oral Suspension 1224
- Minocin Pellet-Filled Capsules 1222
- Mithracin 1602
- Monocid Injection (Occasional) 2217
- Monodox Capsules 1630
- Monopril Tablets 1406
- Motrin Tablets (Occasional) 2351
- Mykrox ½ mg Tablets 984
- Nebcin Vials, Hyporets & ADD-Vantage 1286
- Netromycin Injection 100 mg/ml 2104
- ▲ Normodyne Injection (8%) 2108
- Noroxin Tablets (Less frequent) 1519
- Norpace (1%) 2177
- ▲ Orudis Capsules (Greater than 3%) 2488
- Parlodel 2020
- PediaProfen Suspension (Occasional) 1363
- Pipracil 1230
- Platinol 737
- Platinol-AQ Injection 738
- Polymyxin B Sulfate, Aerosporin Brand Sterile Powder 798
- Primaxin I.M. 1532
- Primaxin I.V. 1535
- Prinivil Tablets (2%) 1538
- Prinzide Tablets 1540
- Procardia XL Tablets (Rare) 1783
- Proloprim Tablets 799
- Rauzide Tablets 1804
- Rifadin 1345
- Rifamate Capsules 1347
- Rimactane Capsules 879
- Rocaltrol Capsules 1913
- Rocephin Injectable Vials, ADD-Vantage (1.2%) 1914
- Sansert Tablets 2031
- Septra 813
- Septra I.V. Infusion 808
- Septra I.V. Infusion ADD-Vantage Vials 810
- Septra 813
- Sinemet CR Tablets 953
- Suprax (Less than 2%) 1235
- Tazicef for Injection (Occasional) 2231
- Tazidime Vials, Faspak & ADD-Vantage (Occasionally) 1299
- ▲ Tegison Capsules (1-10%) 1881
- Tegretol Chewable Tablets 654
- Tegretol Suspension 656
- Tegretol Tablets 654
- Terramycin Capsules 1786
- Terramycin Intramuscular Solution 1964
- Timentin for Injection 2239
- Tolectin (200, 400 and 600 mg) (1 to 3%) 1379
- ▲ Trandate Injection (8 of 100 patients) 577
- Trilisate (Less than 1%) 1822
- Trimpex Tablets 1922
- Trobicin Sterile Powder 2366
- Unasyn 1965
- Vancocin HCl, Oral Solution & Pulvules (Rare) 1304
- Vancocin HCl, Vials & ADD-Vantage (A few dozen cases) 1302
- Vaseretic Tablets (About 0.6%) 1559
- Velosef Capsules and for Oral Suspension 606
- Vibramycin Hyclate Capsules 1787
- Vibramycin Hyclate Intravenous 1968
- Vibramycin 1787
- Vira-A for Injection 1766
- Zaroxolyn Tablets 989
- Zefazone Sterile Powder 2372
- Zestoretic 2274
- Zestril Tablets (About 2%) 2277
- Zinacef 1066
- Zovirax Sterile Powder 828

C

Cachexia
- Intron A (Less than 1%) 2097
- Permax Tablets (Rare) 1291

Calcification, ectopic
- Calcijex Calcitriol Injection 506
- Rocaltrol Capsules 1913

Calcium retention
- Android 1111
- Capozide 2258
- Estratest 2245
- Halotestin Tablets 2341
- Inderide Tablets 2463
- ▲ Lupron Depot 3.75 mg (Among most frequent) 2312
- Lupron Injection (Less than 5%) 2310
- Premarin with Methyltestosterone 2515
- Testred Capsules 1124

Cancer, breast
- Brevicon 2304
- Micronor Tablets 1667
- Modicon 1667
- Norinyl 2304
- Ortho-Novum 1667
- Tri-Norinyl 28-Day Tablets 2304

Cancer, cervical
- Demulen 2161
- Diethylstilbestrol Tablets 1258
- Enovid 2161
- Estratest 2245
- Jenest-28 Tablets 1636
- Mediatric Capsules (Extremely rare) 2476
- Micronor Tablets 1667
- Modicon 1667
- Norethin 2133
- Ortho-Novum 1667
- PMB 200 and PMB 400 2504
- Permax Tablets (Infrequent) 1291
- Premarin Intravenous 2508
- Premarin with Methyltestosterone 2515
- Premarin Vaginal Cream 2512

Cancer, vaginal
- Diethylstilbestrol Tablets 1258
- Estratest 2245
- Mediatric Capsules (Extremely rare) 2476
- PMB 200 and PMB 400 2504
- Premarin Intravenous 2508
- Premarin with Methyltestosterone 2515
- Premarin Vaginal Cream 2512

Candidiasis
- ▲ AeroBid Inhaler System (3-9%) 995
- Beconase Inhalation Aerosol & Refill (Rare) 574
- Ceptaz for Injection (Fewer than 1%) 1057
- Cipro I.V. (1% or less) 1592
- Cipro Tablets (Less than 1%) 1589
- Flagyl I.V. 2131
- Flagyl Tablets 2170
- Fortaz (Less than 1%) 1060
- Pipracil 1230
- Primaxin I.M. 1532
- Primaxin I.V. (Less than 0.2%) 1535
- Suprax (Less than 2%) 1235
- Tazicef for Injection (Less than 1%) 2231
- Unasyn (Less than 1%) 1965
- Zefazone Sterile Powder 2372

Candidiasis, esophageal
- Prilosec Delayed-Release Capsules (Less than 1%) 1530

Candidiasis, mouth (see under Candidiasis, oral)

Candidiasis, nasal
- Nasacort Nasal Inhaler (Rare) 1844
- Vancenase Nasal Inhaler (Rare) 2126

Candidiasis, oral
- Ancef Injection 2194
- Azmacort Inhaler (A few cases) 1837
- Ceptaz for Injection 1057
- Cipro I.V. (1% or less) 1592
- Cipro Tablets (Less than 1%) 1589
- Fortaz (Less than 1%) 1060
- Fulvicin P/G Tablets 2090
- Fulvicin P/G 165 & 330 Tablets 2091
- Fulvicin-U/F Tablets 2092
- Grifulvin V (griseofulvin microsize) Tablets/Suspension (Occasional) 1678
- Grisactin (Occasional) 2454
- Grisactin Ultra Tablets (Occasional) 2455
- Gris-PEG Tablets, 125 mg & 250 mg (Occasional) 1083
- Kefzol Vials, Faspak & ADD-Vantage 1279

Candidiasis, pharynx
- Azmacort Inhaler (A few cases) 1837
- Nasacort Nasal Inhaler (Rare) 1844
- Vancenase Nasal Inhaler (Rare) 2126

Candidiasis, vaginal (see under Vaginal candidiasis)

Candiduria
- Cipro I.V. (1% or less) 1592
- Cipro Tablets 1589
- Floxin Tablets (More than or equal to 1.0%) 1652

Capillary fragility
- AeroBid Inhaler System (1-3%) 995

Carbohydrate tolerance, decrease
- Aristocort Suspension 1008
- Aristospan Suspension 1011
- Brevicon 2304
- Celestone Soluspan Suspension 2081
- Cortenema 2244
- Cortone Acetate Sterile Suspension 1437
- Cortone Acetate Tablets 1439
- Dalalone D.P. Injectable 999
- Decadron Elixir 1445
- Decadron Phosphate Injection 1449
- Decadron Phosphate Respihaler 1454
- Decadron Phosphate Turbinaire 1456
- Decadron Phosphate with Xylocaine Injection, Sterile 1451
- Decadron Tablets 1447
- Decadron-LA Sterile Suspension 1457
- Deltasone Tablets 2332
- Demulen 2161
- Depo-Medrol Sterile Aqueous Suspension 2334
- Diethylstilbestrol Tablets 1258
- Enovid 2161
- Estinyl Tablets 2085
- Estrace 1385
- Estrace Vaginal Cream 1388
- Estradurin 2452
- Estratest 2245
- Estrovis 1721
- Hydeltrasol Injection, Sterile 1476
- Hydeltra-T.B.A. Sterile Suspension 1478

Hydrocortone Acetate Sterile Suspension 1479
Hydrocortone Phosphate Injection, Sterile 1481
Hydrocortone Tablets 1482
Jenest-28 Tablets 1636
Kenalog-10 Injection 2402
Kenalog-40 Injection 2403
Levlen/Tri-Levlen 665
Lo/Ovral Tablets 2471
Lo/Ovral-28 Tablets 2476
Loestrin 1728
Mediatric Capsules 2476
Medrol 2348
Menrium Tablets 1934
Micronor Tablets 1667
Modicon 1667
Nordette-21 Tablets 2481
Nordette-28 Tablets 2483
Norethin 2133
Norinyl 2304
Norlestrin 1746
Nor-Q D Tablets 2304
Ogen 540
Ortho Dienestrol Cream 1664
Ortho-Cyclen Tablets 1658
Ortho-Novum 1667
Ovcon 1391
Ovral Tablets 2490
Ovral-28 Tablets 2491
Ovrette Tablets 2492
PMB 200 and PMB 400 2504
Premarin Intravenous 2508
Premarin with Methyltestosterone 2515
Premarin Tablets 2510
Premarin Vaginal Cream 2512
Solu-Cortef Sterile Powder 2361
Solu-Medrol Sterile Powder 2363
Stilphostrol Tablets and Ampuls 1609
TACE 12 and 25 mg 1353
Levlen/Tri-Levlen 665
Tri-Norinyl 2304
Triphasil-21 Tablets 2527
Triphasil-28 Tablets 2532

Carcinoma
Demulen 2161
Diethylstilbestrol Tablets 1258
Enovid 2161
Permax Tablets (Infrequent) 1291

Carcinoma, bile duct
Demulen 2161
Enovid 2161
Norethin 2133

Carcinoma, ear
Lupron Depot 7.5 mg 2311
Lupron Injection (Less than 5%) 2310

Carcinoma, endometrial
Demulen 2161
Enovid 2161
Estrace 1385
Estrace Vaginal Cream 1388
Estraderm Transdermal System 866
Estratest 2245
Estrovis 1721
Levlen/Tri-Levlen 665
Mediatric Capsules 2476
Menrium Tablets 1934
Micronor Tablets 1667
Modicon 1667
Nolvadex Tablets (Isolated cases) 1102
Norethin 2133
Ortho Dienestrol Cream 1664
Ortho-Novum 1667
Ovcon 1391
Premarin Intravenous 2508
Premarin with Methyltestosterone 2515
Premarin Tablets 2510
Premarin Vaginal Cream 2512
Levlen/Tri-Levlen 665

Carcinoma, renal pelvis
Cytoxan for Injection (One case) 726
Neosar for Injection (One case) 566

Carcinoma, skin
Lupron Depot 7.5 mg 2311
Lupron Injection (Less than 5%) 2310
Permax Tablets (Infrequent) 1291

Cardiac abnormalities
Adriamycin RDF 562
AK-Con ◉ 202
AK-Con-A ◉ 203
Albalon Solution with Liquifilm ◉ 238
Albalon-A Liquifilm (Rare) ◉ 238
Clozaril Tablets (1%) 2000
Cordarone Tablets (Infrequent) 2446
Floropryl Sterile Ophthalmic Ointment (Rare) 1473
Humorsol Sterile Ophthalmic Solution 1475
Marax Tablets & DF Syrup 1954
Naphcon Forte ◉ 226
Naphcon-A Ophthalmic Solution 571
Neosar for Injection 566
Nicorette 1335
Novantrone for Injection Concentrate 1226
Opcon-A Ophthalmic Solution ◉ 262
Pergonal (menotropins for injection, USP) (One report) 2184
Phospholine Iodide ◉ 315
Platinol (Infrequent) 737
Platinol-AQ Injection (Infrequent) 738
Sansert Tablets 2031
Sinemet Tablets (Less frequent) 952
Sinemet CR Tablets 953
Tri-Immunol Diphtheria & Tetanus Toxoids & Pertussis Vaccine, Adsorbed 1241
Vasocon-A ◉ 278

Cardiac anomalies
Cibalith-S 870
Eskalith 2214
Lithane Tablets 1596
Lithium Carbonate Capsules & Tablets 1984
Lithobid Tablets 870
Norinyl 2304
Tri-Norinyl 2304

Cardiac arrest
AK-Fluor Injection 10% and 25% ◉ 204
Anafranil Capsules (Infrequent) 650
Ancobon Capsules 1886
Anectine 755
▲Anestacon Solution (Among most common) 2394
AquaMEPHYTON Injection 1422
Arm-a-Med Metaproterenol Sulfate Inhalation Solution, USP 617
Blocadren Tablets (Less than 1%) 1429
Capoten 2255
Capozide 2258
Carbocaine Hydrochloride Injection 2043
Compazine 2201
Decadron Phosphate with Xylocaine Injection, Sterile 1451
Demerol 2047
Desyrel and Desyrel Dividose 1404
Dilaudid 1173
Dilaudid-HP Injection 1175
Dolophine Hydrochloride Ampoules & Vials 1260
Dolophine Hydrochloride Tablets 1261
Dyclone 0.5% and 1% Topical Solutions, USP 626
Enlon Injection (Isolated instances) 598
Ethmozine Tablets (Less than 2%) 946
Etrafon 2087
Fluorescite ◉ 217
Fluothane 2453
Fungizone Intravenous 2262
Innovar Injection 1141
Intron A (Less than 1%) 2097
Isuprel Hydrochloride Mistometer (Several instances) 2051
Isuprel Hydrochloride Solution 1:200 & 1:100 (Several instances) 2052
K-Lor Powder Packets 531
K-Norm Capsules 982
K-Tab Filmtab 532
Klor-Con 8/Klor-Con 10 Extended-release Tablets 2374
Klorvess Effervescent Granules 2010
Klorvess Effervescent Tablets 2011
Klorvess 10% Liquid 2010
Kolyum Liquid 983
MS Contin Tablets 1814
MSIR 1817
Marcaine Hydrochloride 0.5% with Epinephrine 1:200,000 (as bitartrate) 958
Marcaine Hydrochloride with Epinephrine 1:200,000 2055
Marcaine Hydrochloride Injection 2055
Marcaine Spinal 2058
Mellaril (Rare) 2011
Mepergan Injection 2479
Metaprel Inhalation Aerosol Bronchodilator (Several cases) 2014
Metaprel Inhalation Solution (Several cases) 2015
Methadone Hydrochloride Diskets 1284
Methadone Hydrochloride Oral Solution & Tablets 1987
Micro-K 1863
Micro-K LS Packets 1864
Monopril Tablets (0.2 to 1.0%) 1406
Narcan Injection 933
Navane Intramuscular 1956
Nescaine/Nescaine MPF 629
Nicorette 1335
Norzine (Rare) 1818
Novocain Hydrochloride for Spinal Anesthesia 2065
Omnipaque 2552
Oramorph SR (Morphine Sulfate Sustained Release Tablets) (Less frequent) 1988
Permax Tablets (Infrequent) 1291
Pfizerpen for Injection 1957
Pitressin Synthetic, Ampoules 1758
Pontocaine Hydrochloride for Spinal Anesthesia 2069
Prolixin Decanoate 1795
Prolixin Enanthate 1796
Prolixin Oral Concentrate 1792
Prostigmin Injectable 1120
Prostigmin Tablets 1121
Prostin VR Pediatric Sterile Solution (1%) 2355
Proventil Inhalation Aerosol 2117
Roxanol 1991
Rythmol Tablets (Less than 1%) 1184
Sensorcaine 631
Sensorcaine-MPF Spinal 634
Serentil 686
Slow-K Tablets 2281
Stelazine 2226
Sublimaze Injection 1146
Tacaryl 2409
▲Tambocor Tablets (5.1%) 1315
Taractan 1920
Temaril Tablets, Syrup and Spansule Sustained Release Capsules 1085
Tenormin Tablets and I.V. Injection (1.6%) 1107
Thorazine 2234
Timolide Tablets 1547
Timoptic in Ocudose 1552
Timoptic Sterile Ophthalmic Solution 1550
Torecan 1993
Tracrium Injection 817
Trilafon 2123
Vancocin HCl, Vials & ADD-Vantage 1302
Vaseretic Tablets 1559
Vasotec I.V. 1562
Vasotec Tablets (0.5% to 1.0%) 1564
Virazole 1126
Xylocaine Injections 637
Xylocaine Injections for Ventricular Arrhythmias 639
Xylocaine 2% Jelly 643
Xylocaine 5% Ointment 644
Xylocaine 10% Oral Spray 645
4% Xylocaine-MPF Sterile Solution 641
Xylocaine 2% Viscous Solution 646

Cardiac arrhythmias (see under Arrhythmias)

Cardiac asystole (see under Asystole)

Cardiac collapse
Oculinum for Injecton (2 patients) 587

Cardiac death
▲Ethmozine Tablets (2%-5%) 946

Cardiac dysrhythmias (see under Arrhythmias)

Cardiac enzymes, elevation
Cytotec (Infrequent) 2159

Cardiac failure
Adriamycin PFS 561
Anafranil Capsules (Rare) 650
Blocadren Tablets 1429
Corgard Tablets 701
Corzide Tablets 702
Fungizone Intravenous 2262
Levatol 1832
Normodyne Tablets 2110
Omnipaque (Less than 0.4%) 2552
Paraplatin for Injection 735
Tenoretic Tablets 1105
Timolide Tablets (Less than 1%) 1547
Timoptic in Ocudose 1552
Timoptic Sterile Ophthalmic Solution 1550
Trandate HCT Tablets 579
Trandate Injection 577

Cardiac output, decrease
Carbocaine Hydrochloride Injection 2043
Digibind (Few instances) 762
Marcaine Hydrochloride with Epinephrine 1:200,000 2055
Marcaine Hydrochloride Injection 2055
Marcaine Spinal 2058
Pitressin Synthetic, Ampoules 1758
Pronestyl Capsules and Tablets 1800
Pronestyl Injection 1798
Protamine Sulfate Ampoules & Vials 1295
Sensorcaine 631
Sensorcaine-MPF Spinal 634
Tensilon Injectable 1123

Cardiac rhythms, disturbances
Capoten 2255
Capozide 2258
Daraprim Tablets 761
Prinivil Tablets (1% or less) 1538
Prinzide Tablets 1540
Vaseretic Tablets 1559
Vasotec I.V. 1562
Vasotec Tablets 1564
Zestoretic 2274
Zestril Tablets 2277

Cardiac rupture
▲Eminase (Less than 10%) 2211

Cardiac standstill
Enlon Injection 598

Cardiac stimulation, unspecified
Fiorinal with Codeine Capsules 2008

Cardiac tamponade
Loniten Tablets 2346
Zovirax Sterile Powder (Less than 1%) 828

Cardiac toxicity
Adriamycin PFS 561
Adriamycin RDF 562
Cerubidine 2443
Cytoxan for Injection 726
Doxorubicin Hydrochloride for Injection, USP 622
Doxorubicin Hydrochloride Injection, USP (Uncommon) 848
Idamycin for Injection (Common) 564
IFEX (Less than 1%) 729
Lanoxicaps 772
Lanoxin Elixir Pediatric 775
Lanoxin Injection 778
Lanoxin Injection Pediatric 781
Lanoxin Tablets 783
Neosar for Injection 566
Roferon-A Injection (Less than 3%) 1916
Rubex (Uncommon) 739
TheraCys BCG Live (Intravesical) (Up to 2.7%) 898

Cardialgia (see under Heartburn)

Cardiodynia (see under Heartburn)

Cardiogenic shock
Mexitil Capsules (1 in 1,000) 680
Tenormin Tablets and I.V. Injection (0.4%) 1107
Tonocard Tablets (Less than 1%) 1554

Cardiomegaly
Cytosar-U Sterile Powder 2329
Tonocard Tablets (Less than 1%) 1554

Cardiomyopathy
Adriamycin PFS 561
Adriamycin RDF 562
Biphetamine Capsules (Isolated reports) 973
BuSpar (Rare) 1401
Cytosar-U Sterile Powder 2329
Dexedrine (Isolated reports) 2206
Didrex Tablets (Isolated reports) 2338
Doxorubicin Hydrochloride Injection, USP 848
Idamycin for Injection 564
Intron A (1 patient) 2097
Novantrone for Injection Concentrate 1226

Retrovir (0.8%) 802
Roferon-A Injection (Rare) 1916
Rubex 739

Cardiopulmonary arrest
Cipro I.V. (1% or less) 1592
Cipro Tablets (Less than 1%) 1589

Cardiorespiratory arrest
Brevital Sodium Vials 1248
Monistat I.V. (Several reports) 1143

Cardiorespiratory collapse
Mydriacyl ⊙ 225
Tropicacyl ⊙ 209

Cardiospasm
Lodine Capsules (Less than 1%) 2468
Prostin VR Pediatric Sterile Solution (Less than 1%) 2355

Cardiovascular abnormalities, fetal
Accutane Capsules 1878
Anaprox and Anaprox DS Tablets 2288
Clinoril Tablets 1433
Dolobid Tablets 1465
Naprosyn 2297
Voltaren Tablets 1042

Cardiovascular collapse
▲ Anestacon Solution (Among most common) 2394
Aralen Hydrochloride Injection 2038
Atrohist Sprinkle Capsules 558
Cipro I.V. (1% or less) 1592
Cipro Tablets 1589
Deconamine 663
Deconsal 559
Dilantin Parenteral 1712
Duranest Injections 624
Dyclone 0.5% and 1% Topical Solutions, USP 626
Fedahist Gyrocaps 2145
Fedahist Timecaps 2145
Imferon 976
Marcaine Spinal 2058
Naldecon Syrup, Tablets, Pediatric Drops and Pediatric Syrup 709
Nescaine/Nescaine MPF 629
Noroxin Tablets 1519
Novafed A Capsules 1342
Novafed Capsules 1342
Novahistine DH 1342
Novahistine DMX ▣ 595
Novahistine Elixir ▣ 596
Novahistine Expectorant 1343
Ru-Tuss DE Tablets 694
Seldane-D Extended-Release Tablets 1350
Tegretol Chewable Tablets 654
Trinalin Repetabs Tablets 1170
Valium Injectable 1937
Xylocaine Injections 637
Xylocaine Injections for Ventricular Arrhythmias 639
Xylocaine 2% Jelly 643
Xylocaine 5% Ointment 644
Xylocaine 10% Oral Spray 645
Xylocaine 2% Viscous Solution 646

Cardiovascular depression
Nardil (Less frequent) 1742

Cardiovascular disorders
Ansaid Tablets (Less than 1%) 2319
Diapid Nasal Spray 2003
Larodopa Tablets 1905
Lincocin (Rare) 2344
Metaprel Inhalation Aerosol Bronchodilator 2014
▲ Novantrone for Injection Concentrate (11 to 26%) 1226
▲ Paraplatin for Injection (6%) 735
Phospholine Iodide ⊙ 315
Seldane-D Extended-Release Tablets (Rare) 1350
Sinequan (Occasional) 1960
Tegretol Tablets 654
Ventolin Rotacaps for Inhalation (Less than 1%) 583
Xylocaine Injections for Ventricular Arrhythmias 639

Carotid sinus hypersensitivity
Aldoclor Tablets 1413
Aldomet Ester HCl Injection 1417
Aldomet Oral 1415
Aldoril Tablets 1418

Carpal tunnel syndrome
Danocrine Capsules (Rare) 2046
Megace Tablets 732

Carpopedal spasm
Compazine 2201
Stelazine 2226
Thorazine 2234
Triavil Tablets 1556

Catalepsy
Anafranil Capsules (Rare) 650

Cataracts
Accutane Capsules 1878
Aristocort Suspension 1008
Brevicon 2304
Children's Advil Suspension (Less than 1%) 2426
Cortisporin Ophthalmic Ointment Sterile 758
Cortisporin Ophthalmic Suspension Sterile 759
Danocrine Capsules (Rare) 2046
Demulen 2161
Doral Tablets 2383
Enovid 2161
Haldol Decanoate 1375
Haldol Injection, Tablets and Concentrate 1373
Hyperstat I.V. Injection 2095
Jenest-28 Tablets 1636
Kerlone Tablets (Less than 2%) 2172
Levlen/Tri-Levlen 665
Lo/Ovral Tablets 2471
Lo/Ovral-28 Tablets 2476
Loestrin 1728
Lopid Capsules and Tablets 1736
Maxidex Sterile Ophthalmic Suspension ⊙ 223
Micronor Tablets 1667
Minipress Capsules (A few reports) 1778
Minizide Capsules (Rare) 1779
Modicon 1667
Motrin Tablets (Less than 1%) 2351
Myleran Tablets (Rare) 790
Nolvadex Tablets 1102
Nordette-21 Tablets 2481
Nordette-28 Tablets 2483
Norethin 2133
Norinyl 2304
Norlestrin 1746
Nor-Q D Tablets 2304
Orap Tablets 1020
Ortho-Cyclen Tablets 1658
Ortho-Novum 1667
Ovcon 1391
Ovral Tablets 2490
Ovral-28 Tablets 2491
Ovrette Tablets 2492
PediaProfen Suspension (Less than 1%) 1363
Permax Tablets (Rare) 1291
Proglycem 649
Prozac Pulvules (Rare) 920
Rufen Tablets (Less than 1%) 691
Solu-Cortef Sterile Powder 2361
Solu-Medrol Sterile Powder 2363
Levlen/Tri-Levlen 665
Tri-Norinyl 2304
Triphasil-21 Tablets 2527
Triphasil-28 Tablets 2532

Cataracts, posterior subcapsular
AK-Cide Sterile Ophthalmic Ointment & Suspension ⊙ 202
AK-Dex ⊙ 203
AK-Pred ⊙ 205
AK-Spore H.C. ⊙ 206
AK-Trol Ointment & Suspension ⊙ 207
Aristospan Suspension 1011
Blephamide 586
Celestone Soluspan Suspension 2081
Cetapred Ointment ⊙ 220
Chloromycetin Hydrocortisone Ophthalmic 1694
Cortenema 2244
Cortifoam (Following long-term use) 1827
Cortone Acetate Sterile Suspension 1437
Cortone Acetate Tablets 1439
Dalalone D.P. Injectable 999
Decadron Elixir 1445
Decadron Phosphate Injection 1449
Decadron Phosphate Respihaler 1454
Decadron Phosphate Sterile Ophthalmic Ointment 1453
Decadron Phosphate Sterile Ophthalmic Solution 1453
Decadron Phosphate Turbinaire 1456
Decadron Phosphate with Xylocaine Injection, Sterile 1451
Decadron Tablets 1447
Decadron-LA Sterile Suspension 1457
Deltasone Tablets 2332
Depo-Medrol Sterile Aqueous Suspension 2334
Dexacidin ⊙ 272
⅛% Econopred & 1% Econopred Plus ⊙ 217
FML Forte Liquifilm ⊙ 245
FML Liquifilm ⊙ 244
FML S.O.P. ⊙ 245
FML-S Sterile Ophthalmic Suspension ⊙ 246
Fluor-Op Ophthalmic Suspension ⊙ 272
HMS Liquifilm (Rare) ⊙ 247
Hydeltrasol Injection, Sterile 1476
Hydeltra-T.B.A. Sterile Suspension 1478
Hydrocortone Acetate Sterile Suspension 1479
Hydrocortone Phosphate Injection, Sterile 1481
Hydrocortone Tablets 1482
Inflamase ⊙ 274
Isopto Cetapred Suspension ⊙ 220
Kenalog-10 Injection 2402
Kenalog-40 Injection 2403
Maxidex Sterile Ophthalmic Ointment ⊙ 222
Maxitrol Ophthalmic Ointment/Suspension ⊙ 223
Metimyd ⊙ 306
NeoDecadron Sterile Ophthalmic Ointment 1517
NeoDecadron Sterile Ophthalmic Solution 1518
Ophthocort ⊙ 301
Pediapred Oral Liquid 987
Poly-Pred Liquifilm ⊙ 250
Pred Forte ⊙ 252
Pred Mild ⊙ 254
Pred-G Liquifilm Sterile Ophthalmic Suspension ⊙ 252
Pred-G S.O.P. Sterile Ophthalmic Ointment ⊙ 253
Terra-Cortril Ophthalmic Suspension 1963
TobraDex Ophthalmic Suspension and Ointment ⊙ 228
Vasocidin Ointment ⊙ 275
Vasocidin Ophthalmic Solution ⊙ 276

Catatonia
Blocadren Tablets 1429
Cartrol Tablets 507
Compazine 2201
Corgard Tablets 701
Corzide Tablets 702
Etrafon 2087
Haldol Decanoate 1375
Haldol Injection, Tablets and Concentrate 1373
Inderal 2459
Inderal LA Long Acting Capsules 2461
Inderide Tablets 2463
Inderide LA Long Acting Capsules 2465
Kerlone Tablets 2172
Levatol 1832
Lopressor HCT Tablets 1034
Normodyne Tablets 2110
Normozide Tablets 2112
Orap Tablets 1020
Phenergan Injection 2493
Phenergan Tablets 2496
Prolixin Decanoate 1795
Prolixin Enanthate 1796
Prolixin Oral Concentrate 1792
Sectral Capsules 2520
Stelazine 2226
Tacaryl 2409
Taractan 1920
Temaril Tablets, Syrup and Spansule Sustained Release Capsules 1085
Tenoretic Tablets 1105
Tenormin Tablets and I.V. Injection 1107
Thorazine (Rare) 2234
Timolide Tablets 1547
Timoptic in Ocudose 1552
Timoptic Sterile Ophthalmic Solution 1550
Trandate HCT/Trandate 579
Triavil Tablets 1556
Trilafon 2123
Visken Tablets 2036

Cauda equine syndrome
Gelfoam Sterile Sponge 2338
Omnipaque (Rare) 2552

Cell granuloma
Gelfoam Sterile Sponge 2338

Cells in urine
Amikin Injectable 602
Garamycin Injectable 2093
Neosar for Injection 566
Netromycin Injection 100 mg/ml 2104

Cellulitis
Adriamycin PFS 561
Adriamycin RDF 562
Anafranil Capsules (Infrequent) 650
Doxorubicin Hydrochloride for Injection, USP (Occasional) 622
Hyperstat I.V. Injection 2095
Oncovin Solution Vials & Hyporets 1288
Permax Tablets (Infrequent) 1291
Prozac Pulvules (Rare) 920
Velban Vials 1305

Cellulitis, at injection site
▲ Cefizox Injection (1 to 5%) 1012
Cytosar-U Sterile Powder (Less frequent) 2329
Doxorubicin Hydrochloride Injection, USP 848
Imferon 976
Mutamycin 733
Rubex 739

Central retinal artery occlusion
Sus-Phrine Injection 1006

Cephalic flocculation, increase
Prolixin Decanoate 1795
Prolixin Elixir 1793
Prolixin Enanthate 1796
Prolixin Injection 1791
Prolixin Oral Concentrate 1792
Prolixin Tablets 1793

Cephalin flocculation test, positive
Cuprimine Capsules 1442
Depen Titratable Tablets (Few reports) 2379

Cerebellar dysfunction
Cytosar-U Sterile Powder (With experimental doses) 2329
▲ Idamycin for Injection (4%) 564

Cerebellar malformation, fetal
Accutane Capsules 1878

Cerebellar syndrome, acute
Ergamisol Tablets 1136
Sterile FUDR (Remote possibility) 1898
Fluorouracil Injection 1897

Cerebral abnormalities, fetal
Accutane Capsules 1878

Cerebral arterial insufficiency, symptoms
Tegretol Chewable Tablets 654
Tegretol Suspension 656
Tegretol Tablets 654

Cerebral arteritis
Blenoxane (Rare) 724
Platinol 737
Platinol-AQ Injection (Rare) 738

Cerebral bleeding (see under Cerebral hemorrhage)

Cerebral hemorrhage
Anafranil Capsules (Rare) 650
Brevicon 2304
Demulen 2161
Enovid 2161
Jenest-28 Tablets 1636
Levlen/Tri-Levlen 665
Lo/Ovral Tablets 2471
Lo/Ovral-28 Tablets 2476
Loestrin 1728
Lopid Capsules and Tablets 1736
Micronor Tablets 1667
Modicon 1667
Nordette-21 Tablets 2481
Nordette-28 Tablets 2483
Norethin 2133
Norinyl 2304
Norlestrin 1746
Nor-Q D Tablets 2304
Ortho-Cyclen Tablets 1658
Ortho-Novum 1667
Ovral Tablets 2490
Ovral-28 Tablets 2491
Ovrette Tablets 2492
Permax Tablets (Rare) 1291
Prostin VR Pediatric Sterile Solution (Less than 1%) 2355

Rifadin 1345
Levlen/Tri-Levlen 665
Tri-Norinyl 2304
Triphasil-21 Tablets 2527
Triphasil-28 Tablets 2532

Cerebral hypoxia

Carbocaine 956

Cerebral infarction

Hyperstat I.V. Injection 2095
Omnipaque (Less than 0.3 to 1.6%) 2552

Cerebral ischemia

Hyperstat I.V. Injection 2095
Isordil 2467
Nitro-Bid Ointment 1339
Permax Tablets (Infrequent) 1291
Prozac Pulvules (Rare) 920
Timolide Tablets 1547
Timoptic in Ocudose 1552
Timoptic Sterile Ophthalmic Solution 1550

Cerebral thrombosis

Amen 833
Brevicon 2304
Cipro I.V. (1% or less) 1592
Cipro Tablets (Less than 1%) 1589
Cycrin Tablets 2449
DDAVP Injection (Rare) 1840
Demulen 2161
Enovid 2161
Jenest-28 Tablets 1636
Levlen/Tri-Levlen 665
Lo/Ovral Tablets 2471
Lo/Ovral-28 Tablets 2476
Loestrin 1728
Micronor Tablets 1667
Modicon 1667
Nordette-21 Tablets 2481
Nordette-28 Tablets 2483
Norethin 2133
Norinyl 2304
Norlestrin 1746
Norlutate 1754
Norlutin 1755
Nor-Q D Tablets 2304
Ortho-Cyclen Tablets 1658
Ortho-Novum 1667
Ovral Tablets 2490
Ovral-28 Tablets 2491
Ovrette Tablets 2492
Provera Tablets 2356
Stilphostrol Tablets and Ampuls 1609
Levlen/Tri-Levlen 665
Tri-Norinyl 2304
Triphasil-21 Tablets 2527
Triphasil-28 Tablets 2532

Cerebral vascular spasm

Norzine (Occasional) 1818
Torecan (Occasional case) 1993

Cerebrospinal fluid proteins, changes

Compazine 2201
Etrafon 2087
Navane Capsules and Concentrate 1954
Navane Intramuscular 1956
Polymyxin B Sulfate, Aerosporin Brand Sterile Powder 798
Prolixin Decanoate 1795
Prolixin Enanthate 1796
Prolixin Oral Concentrate 1792
Stelazine 2226
Taractan 1920
Thorazine 2234
Triavil Tablets 1556
Trilafon 2123

Cerebrospinal fluid rhinorrhea

Parlodel (A few cases) 2020

Cerebrovascular accident

Ansaid Tablets (Less than 1%) 2319
Betagan ⊙ 239
Blenoxane 724
Blocadren Tablets (Less than 1%) 1429
BuSpar (Rare) 1401
Calan SR Caplets (1% or less) 2157
Calan Tablets (1% or less) 2155
Capoten 2255
Capozide 2258
Cardura Tablets (Less than 0.5% of 3960 patients) 1941
Demulen 2161
Emcyt Capsules (2%) 1161
Enovid 2161
Epogen for Injection (0.4%) 591
Isoptin Oral Tablets (Less than 1%) 1179
Isoptin SR Sustained Release Tablets (Less than 1%) 1181
Metrodin (urofollitropin for injection) 2182
Monopril Tablets (0.2 to 1.0%) 1406
NebuPent for Inhalation Solution (1% or less) 1017
Nicorette 1335
Paraplatin for Injection 735
Permax Tablets (Infrequent) 1291
Platinol (Rare) 737
Platinol-AQ Injection (Rare) 738
Prinivil Tablets (1% or less) 1538
Prinzide Tablets 1540
Procrit for Injection (0.4%) 1647
Prozac Pulvules 920
Tenex Tablets 1875
Timolide Tablets 1547
Timoptic in Ocudose 1552
Timoptic Sterile Ophthalmic Solution 1550
Tonocard Tablets 1554
Vaseretic Tablets 1559
Vasotec I.V. 1562
Vasotec Tablets (0.5% to 1%) 1564
Velban Vials 1305
Verelan Capsules (Less than 1%) 1243
Zestoretic 2274
Zestril Tablets 2277
Zoladex (1% to 5%) 1110

Cerebrovascular disorders

Aldoclor Tablets 1413
Aldomet Ester HCl Injection 1417
Aldomet Oral 1415
Aldoril Tablets 1418
Brevicon 2304
Cycrin Tablets (Occasional) 2449
Demulen 2161
Enovid 2161
Ethmozine Tablets (Less than 2%) 946
Jenest-28 Tablets 1636
Kerlone Tablets (Less than 2%) 2172
Levlen/Tri-Levlen 665
Loestrin 1728
Micronor Tablets 1667
Modicon 1667
Norinyl 2304
Ortho-Novum 1667
Ovcon 1391
Levlen/Tri-Levlen 665
Tri-Norinyl 28-Day Tablets 2304

Cerebrovascular insufficiency

Capoten 2255
Capozide 2258

Cervical disorders (see under Cervical irregularities)

Cervical erosion, changes

Amen 833
Aygestin Tablets 2437
Brevicon 2304
Cycrin Tablets 2449
Demulen 2161
Depo-Provera Sterile Aqueous Suspension 2336
Diethylstilbestrol Tablets 1258
Enovid 2161
Estraderm Transdermal System 866
Estratest 2245
Estrovis 1721
Jenest-28 Tablets 1636
Levlen/Tri-Levlen 665
Lippes Loop Intrauterine Double-S 1654
Lo/Ovral Tablets 2471
Lo/Ovral-28 Tablets 2476
Loestrin 1728
Mediatric Capsules 2476
Menrium Tablets 1934
Micronor Tablets 1667
Modicon 1667
Nordette-21 Tablets 2481
Nordette-28 Tablets 2483
Norethin 2133
Norinyl 2304
Norlestrin 1746
Norlutate 1754
Norlutin 1755
Nor-Q D Tablets 2304
Ortho Dienestrol Cream 1664
Ortho-Cyclen Tablets 1658
Ortho-Novum 1667
Ovral Tablets 2490
Ovral-28 Tablets 2491
Ovrette Tablets 2492
PMB 200 and PMB 400 2504
Premarin Intravenous 2508
Premarin with Methyltestosterone 2515
Premarin Vaginal Cream 2512
Provera Tablets 2356
TACE 12 and 25 mg 1353
Levlen/Tri-Levlen 665
Tri-Norinyl 2304
Triphasil-21 Tablets 2527
Triphasil-28 Tablets 2532

Cervical irregularities

Demulen 2161
Enovid 2161
Estrace 1385
Estrace Vaginal Cream 1388
Ovcon 1391
TACE 12 and 25 mg 1353

Cervical secretion, changes

Amen 833
Aygestin Tablets 2437
Brevicon 2304
Cycrin Tablets 2449
Demulen 2161
Diethylstilbestrol Tablets 1258
Enovid 2161
Estinyl Tablets 2085
Estraderm Transdermal System 866
Estratest 2245
Estrovis 1721
Jenest-28 Tablets 1636
Levlen/Tri-Levlen 665
Lo/Ovral Tablets 2471
Lo/Ovral-28 Tablets 2476
Mediatric Capsules 2476
Menrium Tablets 1934
Micronor Tablets 1667
Modicon 1667
Nordette-21 Tablets 2481
Nordette-28 Tablets 2483
Norethin 2133
Norinyl 2304
Norlutate 1754
Norlutin 1755
Nor-Q D Tablets 2304
Ogen 540
Ortho Dienestrol Cream 1664
Ortho-Cyclen Tablets 1658
Ortho-Novum 1667
Ovral Tablets 2490
Ovral-28 Tablets 2491
Ovrette Tablets 2492
PMB 200 and PMB 400 2504
Premarin Intravenous 2508
Premarin with Methyltestosterone 2515
Premarin Tablets 2510
Premarin Vaginal Cream 2512
Provera Tablets 2356
TACE 12 and 25 mg 1353
Levlen/Tri-Levlen 665
Tri-Norinyl 2304
Triphasil-21 Tablets 2527
Triphasil-28 Tablets 2532

Cervicitis

Norplant System 2484

Chafing, genital

Condylox (Less than 5%) 1630

Change in blood glucose levels (see under Insulin reaction)

Character changes

Seromycin Pulvules 1298

Charcot's syndrome

Atromid-S Capsules 2435
Calan SR Caplets (1% or less) 2157
Calan Tablets (1% or less) 2155
Isoptin Oral Tablets (Less than 1%) 1179
Isoptin SR Sustained Release Tablets (Less than 1%) 1181
Timolide Tablets 1547
Timoptic in Ocudose 1552
Timoptic Sterile Ophthalmic Solution 1550
Tonocard Tablets (Less than 1%) 1554

Cheek puffing

Compazine 2201
Haldol Decanoate 1375
Moban Tablets & Concentrate 932
Navane Intramuscular 1956
Orap Tablets 1020
Phenobarbital Elixir and Tablets 1293
Prolixin Decanoate 1795
Prolixin Enanthate 1796
Prolixin Oral Concentrate 1792
Stelazine 2226
Thorazine 2234

Cheilitis

▲ Accutane Capsules (More than 90%) 1878
Anafranil Capsules (Rare) 650
Cosmegen Injection 1440
▲ Tegison Capsules (Less than 75%) 1881

Cheilitis, actinic

▲ Tegison Capsules (Greater than 75%) 1881

Cheilosis

Cuprimine Capsules (Rare) 1442
Depen Titratable Tablets (Rare) 2379

Cheilosis, monilial

Lamprene Capsules (Less than 1%) 1030

Chemosis

Chibroxin Sterile Ophthalmic Solution 1431
Profenal Sterile Ophthalmic Solution (Less than 0.5%) ⊙ 234
▲ Rēv-Eyes Ophthalmic Eyedrops 0.5% (10% to 40%) ⊙ 312

Chest congestion

Klonopin Tablets 1902
▲ NebuPent for Inhalation Solution (10 to 23%) 1017
Roferon-A Injection (Less than 3%) 1916

Chest pain

Accutane Capsules 1878
Adenocard Injection (Less than 1%) 1007
▲ AeroBid Inhaler System (3-9%) 995
▲ Alferon N Injection (6% to 10%) 1809
Altace Capsules (Less than 1%) 1086
▲ Anafranil Capsules (4% to 7%) 650
Ancobon Capsules 1886
▲ Atgam Sterile Solution (More than 1% to 10%; 1 in 15 patients) 2320
Azactam for Injection (1 patient) 2252
Blenoxane (Rare) 724
Blocadren Tablets (0.6%) 1429
Brevibloc Injection (Less than 1%) 942
Bumex (0.1%) 1895
BuSpar (Frequent) 1401
Calan SR Caplets (1% or less) 2157
Calan Tablets (1% or less) 2155
Calciparine Injection 925
Capoten (Approximately 1 of 100 patients) 2255
Capozide (Approximately 1 of 100 patients) 2258
Cardene Capsules (Rare) 2290
Cardura Tablets (2%) 1941
Cartrol Tablets (0.4-2.2%) 507
Cipro I.V. (1% or less) 1592
Cipro Tablets (Less than 1%) 1589
Clinoril Tablets (Less than 1 in 100) 1433
Clozaril Tablets (1%) 2000
Coumadin Injection & Tablets 944
Cytosar-U Sterile Powder (Less frequent) 2329
Cytotec (Infrequent) 2159
Dalgan Injection (Less than 1%) 620
Dalmane Capsules 1927
Desyrel and Desyrel Dividose (Less than 1%) 1404
Dipentum Capsules (Rare) 1160
Diprivan Injection (Less than 1%) 2267
Diulo 2129
Dobutrex Solution Vials (1 to 3%) 1259
Dolobid Tablets (Rare) 1465
Dopram Injectable 1860
Duragesic Transdermal System (1% or greater) 1133
DynaCirc Capsules (2.4%) 2004
E.E.S. (Isolated reports) 522
Emcyt Capsules (1%) 1161
▲ Eminase (Less than 10%) 2211
▲ Epogen for Injection (7.0%) 591
Ergamisol Tablets (Less than 1%) 1136
EryPed (Isolated reports) 519
Ery-Tab Tablets (Isolated reports) 521
Erythrocin Stearate Filmtab (Isolated reports) 523
Erythromycin Base Filmtab (Isolated reports) 525
Erythromycin Delayed-Release Capsules, USP (Isolated reports) 526
Esimil Tablets 864
▲ Ethmozine Tablets (2%-5%) 946
Fiorinal with Codeine Capsules 2008

Flexeril Tablets (Rare) ... 1471
Floxin Tablets (1% to 3%) ... 1652
Gamimune N Immune Globulin Intravenous (Human) ... 1572
Halcion Tablets ... 2340
▲Hylorel Tablets (27.9%) ... 975
Hytrin Tablets (At least 1%) ... 529
Idamycin for Injection ... 564
Imferon ... 976
Indocin (Less than 1%) ... 1487
Inocor Lactate Injection (0.2%) ... 2048
▲Intron A (Up to 28%) ... 2097
Ismelin Tablets ... 869
Isoptin Oral Tablets (Less than 1%) ... 1179
Isoptin SR Sustained Release Tablets (Less than 1%) ... 1181
▲Kerlone Tablets (2.4% to 7.1%) ... 2172
Levatol (2.4%) ... 1832
Lioresal Tablets (Rare) ... 1031
Lorelco Tablets ... 1333
Macrodantin Capsules ... 1624
Maxair Inhaler (Less than 1%) ... 1311
Maxzide ... 1215
Methergine (Rare) ... 2016
Methotrexate Tablets, Parenteral, LPF Parenteral (Less common) ... 1217
Mevacor Tablets ... 1505
▲Mexitil Capsules (2.6% to 7.5%) .. 680
Micronor Tablets ... 1667
Midamor Tablets (Less than or equal to 1%) ... 1508
Modicon ... 1667
Moduretic Tablets (Less than or equal to 1%) ... 1510
Monopril Tablets (0.2 to 1.0%) ... 1406
Mykrox ½ mg Tablets (2.7%) ... 984
▲NebuPent for Inhalation Solution (10 to 23%) ... 1017
▲Neupogen for Injection (5%) ... 595
Norpace (1 to 3%) ... 2177
Novantrone for Injection Concentrate ... 1226
Omnipaque (1%) ... 2552
Orap Tablets ... 1020
▲Orthoclone OKT3 Sterile Solution (14%) ... 1645
Ortho-Novum ... 1667
PCE Dispertab Tablets (Isolated reports) ... 549
Peganone Tablets ... 551
Pentaspan Injection ... 949
Perdiem Fiber Granules ... 1852
Perdiem Granules ... 1852
▲Permax Tablets (3.7%) ... 1291
Plendil Extended-Release Tablets (0.1%) ... 1526
Pondimin Tablets ... 1867
Prilosec Delayed-Release Capsules (Less than 1%) ... 1530
Prinivil Tablets (1% or less) ... 1538
Prinzide Tablets (0.3 to 1%) ... 1540
Procardia XL Tablets (Less than 3%) ... 1783
▲Procrit for Injection (7%) ... 1647
Proglycem (Rare) ... 649
Pronestyl Capsules and Tablets ... 1800
Pronestyl Injection ... 1798
ProSom Tablets (1%) ... 554
Proventil Syrup (Less than 1 of 100) ... 2119
Provocholine for Inhalation ... 1911
Prozac Pulvules (1.3%) ... 920
Retrovir Capsules (Less than 5%) .. 802
Retrovir I.V. Infusion (Less than 5%) ... 805
Retrovir Syrup (Less than 5%) ... 802
Rheumatrex Methotrexate Dose Pack (Less common) ... 1234
Roferon-A Injection (Less than 3% to 4%) ... 1916
Rogaine Topical Solution (1.53%) .. 2357
Rythmol Tablets (0.5 to 1.8%) ... 1184
Sandimmune (Rare) ... 2024
Sandostatin Injection (Less than 1%) ... 2029
Sansert Tablets ... 2031
Sectral Capsules (2%) ... 2520
Sinemet CR Tablets (1.0%) ... 953
Stilphostrol Tablets and Ampuls ... 1609
▲Tambocor Tablets (5.4%) ... 1315
Tegison Capsules (Less than 1%) .. 1881
Tenex Tablets (Less than 3%) ... 1875
Timolide Tablets (Less than 1%) ... 1547
Timoptic in Ocudose ... 1552
Timoptic Sterile Ophthalmic Solution ... 1550
Tolectin (200, 400 and 600 mg) (1 to 3%) ... 1379
Tonocard Tablets (0.4-1.6%) ... 1554
Trental (0.3% to 1.1%) ... 1099
Unasyn (Less than 1%) ... 1965
Valium Injectable ... 1937
Vancocin HCl, Vials & ADD-Vantage (Infrequent) ... 1302
Vaseretic Tablets (0.5% to 2.0%) ... 1559
Vasotec I.V. ... 1562
Vasotec Tablets (0.5% to 1%) ... 1564
Ventolin Syrup (Less than 1 of 100 patients) ... 583
Verelan Capsules (Less than 1%) .. 1243
Virazole ... 1126
▲Visken Tablets (3%) ... 2036
Voltaren Tablets (Less than 1%) ... 1042
Wellbutrin Tablets (Infrequent) ... 821
Wytensin Tablets (3% or less) ... 2542
▲Xanax Tablets (10.6%) ... 2367
Yutopar (1 to 2% (with IV administration)) ... 647
Zaroxolyn Tablets ... 989
Zestoretic (0.3 to 1.0%) ... 2274
Zestril Tablets (1.3%) ... 2277
Zofran Injection (Rare) ... 1069
Zoladex (1% to 5%) ... 1110
Zovirax Sterile Powder (Less than 1%) ... 828

Chest tightness

Actifed with Codeine Cough Syrup.. 752
▲Adenocard Injection (7%) ... 1007
AeroBid Inhaler System (1-3%) ... 995
▲Alfenta Injection (17%) ... 1131
Benadryl Capsules ... 1691
Benadryl Injection ... 1692
Cibacalcin Double-chambered Syringes (Rare) ... 859
Comhist LA Capsules ... 1618
Deconamine ... 663
Diapid Nasal Spray ... 2003
Dimetane-DC Cough Syrup ... 1857
Dimetane-DX Cough Syrup ... 1858
Dopram Injectable ... 1860
Eskalith ... 2214
Furoxone (Rare) ... 1855
Gamimune N Immune Globulin Intravenous (Human) ... 1572
Geref (sermorelin acetate for injection) ... 2560
Hyperstat I.V. Injection ... 2095
Hyskon Hysteroscopy Fluid (Rare) .. 1162
Micronor Tablets ... 1667
Modicon ... 1667
Optimine Tablets ... 2115
Ornade Spansule Capsules ... 2221
Ortho-Novum ... 1667
PBZ Tablets & Elixir ... 1037
PBZ-SR Tablets ... 1037
Perdiem Fiber Granules ... 1852
Perdiem Granules ... 1852
Periactin ... 1525
Polaramine ... 2116
Quadrinal Tablets ... 1183
Ru-Tuss II Capsules ... 693
Ru-Tuss with Hydrocodone ... 694
Ru-Tuss Tablets ... 693
Sandoglobulin I.V. (Less than 1%).. 2027
Sansert Tablets ... 2031
Sublimaze Injection ... 1146
▲Sufenta Injection (3%) ... 1147
Tacaryl ... 2409
Tavist Syrup ... 2033
Tavist Tablets ... 2035
Tavist-D Tablets ... 2035
Temaril Tablets, Syrup and Spansule Sustained Release Capsules ... 1085
Tornalate (Less than 1%) ... 2074
Triaminic Expectorant DH ... 1995
Triaminic Oral Infant Drops ... 1996
Trinalin Repetabs Tablets ... 1170
Tussionex Extended-Release Suspension ... 988
Tuss-Ornade Liquid ... 2242
Tuss-Ornade Spansule Capsules ... 2242
Velosef Capsules and for Oral Suspension ... 606
Yutopar (1 to 2% with IV administration) ... 647

Chewing movements

Compazine ... 2201
Etrafon ... 2087
Haldol Decanoate ... 1375
Haldol Injection, Tablets and Concentrate ... 1373
Mellaril ... 2011
Navane Capsules and Concentrate ... 1954
Navane Intramuscular ... 1956
Orap Tablets ... 1020
Prolixin Decanoate ... 1795
Prolixin Enanthate ... 1796
Prolixin Oral Concentrate ... 1792
Serentil ... 686
Stelazine ... 2226
Taractan ... 1920
Thorazine ... 2234
Triavil Tablets ... 1556
Trilafon ... 2123

Chills

Abbokinase ... 503
Abbokinase Open-Cath ... 505
Actifed with Codeine Cough Syrup.. 752
▲Actimmune (14%) ... 1046
Adalat Capsules (10 mg and 20 mg) (2% or less) ... 1587
Adriamycin PFS (Occasional) ... 561
Adriamycin RDF (Occasional) ... 562
AeroBid Inhaler System (1-3%) ... 995
▲Alferon N Injection (2% to 87%) ... 1809
Anadrol-50 Tablets ... 2287
Anafranil Capsules (Up to 2%) ... 650
Anaprox and Anaprox DS Tablets (Less than 1%) ... 2288
Ansaid Tablets (Less than 1%) ... 2319
Apresazide Capsules (Less frequent) ... 854
Apresoline Hydrochloride Parenteral (Ampuls) ... 856
Apresoline Hydrochloride Tablets (Less frequent) ... 855
Apresoline-Esidrix Tablets ... 857
Arfonad Ampuls ... 1887
▲Atgam Sterile Solution (1 in 2 to 1 in 7 patients; 16%) ... 2320
Azo Gantanol Tablets ... 1887
Bactrim DS Tablets ... 1891
Bactrim I.V. Infusion ... 1889
Bactrim ... 1891
Benadryl Capsules ... 1691
Benadryl Injection ... 1692
Bicillin C-R Injection ... 2438
Bicillin C-R 900/300 Injection ... 2440
Bicillin L-A Injection ... 2442
▲Blenoxane (Frequent) ... 724
Calciparine Injection ... 925
Carbocaine Hydrochloride Injection 2043
Ceredase Injection ... 1052
Cerubidine (Rare) ... 2443
▲CHEMET (succimer) Capsules (5.2 to 15.7%) ... 1361
Children's Advil Suspension (Less than 1%) ... 2426
Cibacalcin Double-chambered Syringes (Rare) ... 859
Cipro I.V. (1% or less) ... 1592
Cipro Tablets (Less than 1%) ... 1589
Clinoril Tablets (Less than 1 in 100) ... 1433
▲CytoGam (Less than 5.0%) ... 891
Cytovene Sterile Powder (1% or less) ... 2292
DDAVP (Up to 2%) ... 1841
Dalgan Injection (Less than 1%) ... 620
Danocrine Capsules (Rare) ... 2046
Dantrium Capsules (Less frequent) 1619
Deconamine ... 663
Deprol Tablets (Rare) ... 2382
Dilaudid-HP Injection ... 1175
Dipentum Capsules (Rare) ... 1160
Diphtheria & Tetanus Toxoids, Adsorbed Purogenated (Mild) ... 1202
Diulo ... 2129
Dolobid Tablets (Less than 1 in 100) ... 1465
Doxorubicin Hydrochloride for Injection, USP (Occasional) ... 622
Doxorubicin Hydrochloride Injection, USP (Occasional) ... 848
Edecrin ... 1468
Eldepryl ... 2250
Elspar ... 1470
Emete-con Intramuscular/Intravenous ... 1950
▲Eminase (Less than 10%) ... 2211
Engerix-B Unit-Dose Vials (Less than 1%) ... 2213
Equagesic Tablets (Rare) ... 2451
Ergamisol Tablets (5 patients) ... 1136
Fansidar Tablets ... 1896
Floxin Tablets (Less than 1%) ... 1652
Fungizone Intravenous (Infrequent) 2262
Gamimune N Immune Globulin Intravenous (Human) ... 1572
Gammagard Immune Globulin, Intravenous (Human) (Occasional) ... 658
Gammar-IV, Immune Globulin Intravenous (Human) ... 610
Gantanol ... 1899
Gantrisin Ophthalmic Ointment/Solution ... 1900
Gantrisin ... 1901
Heparin Lock Flush Solution ... 2456
▲Heparin Sodium Vials (Among most common) ... 1264
Heparin Sodium Injection ... 2457
Heparin Sodium Injection, USP, Sterile Solution ... 2342
Hespan Injection ... 948
Hydrea Capsules ... 728
Imferon ... 976
Inapsine Injection ... 1140
Innovar Injection ... 1141
▲Intron A (45% to 46%) ... 2097
Konÿne 80 Factor IX Complex ... 1571
Konÿne-HT Factor IX Complex ... 1583
▲Lariam Tablets (Among most frequent) ... 1904
▲Leukine for IV Infusion (Among most frequent) ... 1127
Lodine Capsules (Greater than or equal to 1%) ... 2468
Lupron Depot 7.5 mg (Less than 5%) ... 2311
Lupron Injection (Less than 5%) ... 2310
MS Contin Tablets (Infrequent) ... 1814
MSIR (Infrequent) ... 1817
Macrodantin Capsules ... 1624
Marcaine Hydrochloride 0.5% with Epinephrine 1:200,000 (as bitartrate) ... 958
Marcaine Hydrochloride with Epinephrine 1:200,000 ... 2055
Marcaine Hydrochloride Injection ... 2055
Matulane Capsules ... 1907
Methadone Hydrochloride Diskets .. 1284
Methotrexate Tablets, Parenteral, LPF Parenteral (Frequent) ... 1217
Metrodin (urofollitropin for injection) (Less than 1 in 50) ... 2182
Mevacor Tablets (Rare) ... 1505
Miltown Tablets (Rare) ... 2386
Mintezol ... 1510
▲Monistat I.V. (10%) ... 1143
Monoclate-P Factor VIII:C, Pasteurized, Antihemophilic Factor (Human) .. 612
Motrin Tablets (Less than 1%) ... 2351
Mykrox ½ mg Tablets ... 984
Naprosyn (Less than 1%) ... 2297
▲NebuPent for Inhalation Solution (10 to 23%) ... 1017
Nizoral Tablets (Less than 1%) ... 1145
Omnipaque ... 2552
Optimine Tablets ... 2115
Oramorph SR (Morphine Sulfate Sustained Release Tablets) (Less frequent) ... 1988
Ornade Spansule Capsules ... 2221
▲Orthoclone OKT3 Sterile Solution (59%) ... 1645
Orudis Capsules (Less than 1%) ... 2488
PBZ Tablets & Elixir ... 1037
PBZ-SR Tablets ... 1037
PMB 200 and PMB 400 (Rare) ... 2504
Parnate Tablets ... 2222
PediaProfen Suspension (Less than 1%) ... 1363
Pediazole ... 1973
Pentaspan Injection ... 949
Peptavlon ... 2563
Pergonal (menotropins for injection, USP) ... 2184
Periactin ... 1525
Permax Tablets (1.1%) ... 1291
Pfizerpen for Injection ... 1957
Pfizerpen-AS Aqueous Suspension 1959
Polaramine ... 2116
Pondimin Tablets ... 1867
Pontocaine Hydrochloride for Spinal Anesthesia ... 2069
Priscoline Hydrochloride Ampuls ... 877
Procan SR Tablets (Common) ... 1760
Procardia Capsules (2% or less) ... 1781
Pronestyl Capsules and Tablets ... 1800
Pronestyl Injection ... 1798
Pronestyl-SR Tablets ... 1801
ProSom Tablets (Infrequent) ... 554
Prozac Pulvules (Frequent) ... 920
Recombivax HB (Less than 1%) ... 1544
Retrovir Capsules (Less than 5%).. 802
Retrovir I.V. Infusion (Less than 5%) ... 805
Retrovir Syrup (Less than 5%) ... 802
Rheumatrex Methotrexate Dose Pack (Frequent) ... 1234
Rifadin ... 1345
Rocephin Injectable Vials, ADD-Vantage (Less than 1%) ... 1914
▲Roferon-A Injection (41% to 64%) 1916
Rubex (Occasional) ... 739
Rufen Tablets (Less than 1%) ... 691
Ru-Tuss II Capsules ... 693

Sandoglobulin I.V. (Less than 1%) 2027
Sandostatin Injection (Less than 1%) 2029
Sensorcaine 631
Sensorcaine-MPF Spinal 634
Septra 813
Septra I.V. Infusion 808
Septra I.V. Infusion ADD-Vantage Vials 810
Septra 813
Ser-Ap-Es Tablets 881
Serpasil-Apresoline Tablets 884
Sinequan (Occasional) 1960
Staphage Lysate (SPL) 905
Sublimaze Injection 1146
Sufenta Injection (Less than 1%) 1147
Talacen (Rare) 2070
Talwin Injection (Rare) 2071
Talwin Compound (Rare) 2072
Talwin Injection (Rare) 2071
Talwin Nx (Rare) 2073
Tavist Syrup 2033
Tavist Tablets 2035
Tavist-D Tablets 2035
Tegretol Chewable Tablets 654
Tegretol Suspension 656
Tegretol Tablets 654
Terazol 3 Vaginal Suppositories (1.8% of 284 patients) 1677
Terazol 7 Vaginal Cream (0.4% of 521 patients) 1677
Tessalon Perles 1006
Tetanus & Diphtheria Toxoids, Adsorbed Purogenated (Rare) 1237
Tetanus Toxoid, Adsorbed Purogenated 1238
▲ TheraCys BCG Live (Intravesical) (2.6% to 33.9%) 898
Thiosulfil Forte Tablets 2526
Timentin for Injection 2239
Tonocard Tablets (Less than 1%) 1554
▲ Trexan Tablets (Less than 10%) 937
Triaminic Expectorant DH 1995
Triaminic Oral Infant Drops 1996
Trinalin Repetabs Tablets 1170
Trobicin Sterile Powder 2366
Unasyn (Less than 1%) 1965
Vancocin HCl, Oral Solution & Pulvules (Infrequent) 1304
Vancocin HCl, Vials & ADD-Vantage (Infrequent) 1302
VePesid Capsules and Injection (0.7 to 2%) 741
Versed Injection (Less than 1%) 1924
Wellbutrin Tablets (1.2%) 821
Wycillin Injection 2537
Yodoxin 1072
Yutopar (1 to 3% with IV administration) 647
Zaroxolyn Tablets 989
Zoladex (1% to 5%) 1110
Zyloprim Tablets (Less than 1%) 830

Chloasma
Amen 833
Anafranil Capsules (Rare) 650
Aygestin Tablets 2437
Demulen 2161
Diethylstilbestrol Tablets 1258
Enovid 2161
Estinyl Tablets 2085
Estrace 1385
Estrace Vaginal Cream 1388
Estradurin 2452
Estratest 2245
Estrovis 1721
Lo/Ovral Tablets 2471
Lo/Ovral-28 Tablets 2476
Mediatric Capsules 2476
Menrium Tablets 1934
Nordette-21 Tablets 2481
Nordette-28 Tablets 2483
Norethin 2133
Norlestrin 1746
Norlutate 1754
Norlutin 1755
Ogen 540
Ortho Dienestrol Cream 1664
Ovcon 1391
Ovral Tablets 2490
Ovral-28 Tablets 2491
Ovrette Tablets 2492
PMB 200 and PMB 400 2504
Premarin Intravenous 2508
Premarin with Methyltestosterone 2515
Premarin Tablets 2510
Premarin Vaginal Cream 2512
Stilphostrol Tablets and Ampuls 1609
Synarel Nasal Solution (Less than 1%) 2300
TACE 12 and 25 mg 1353
Triphasil-21 Tablets 2527
Triphasil-28 Tablets 2532

Chloride retention
Anadrol-50 Tablets 2287
Butazolidin Capsules & Tablets (Less than 1%) 1027
Estratest 2245
Halotestin Tablets 2341
Premarin with Methyltestosterone 2515
Testred Capsules 1124

Choking sensation
Hyperstat I.V. Injection 2095

Cholangiocarcinoma
Fiorinal with Codeine Capsules 2008

Cholecystectomy, prolongation of drainage
Surgicel 1151

Cholecystitis
Actigall Capsules 2280
Ansaid Tablets (Less than 1%) 2319
Colestid Granules (Fewer than 1 in 500) 2328
Lopid Capsules and Tablets 1736
Permax Tablets (Rare) 1291
Prozac Pulvules (Rare) 920
Trental (Less than 1%) 1099

Cholecystitis, acalculus
Sterile FUDR 1898

Cholelithiasis
Atromid-S Capsules 2435
Colestid Granules (Fewer than 1 in 500) 2328
Lopid Capsules and Tablets 1736
Parafon Forte DSC Caplets 1379
Permax Tablets (Infrequent) 1291
Prozac Pulvules (Rare) 920
Sandostatin Injection (Less than 1%) 2029

Cholestasis
Capoten (Rare) 2255
Capozide (Rare) 2258
Ceftin Tablets 575
Ceptaz for Injection 1057
Clinoril Tablets (Less than 1%) 1433
Dolobid Tablets (Less than 1 in 100) 1465
Flexeril Tablets (Less than 1%) 1471
Fortaz 1060
Keftab Tablets 917
Mintezol 1510
NegGram (Rare) 2062
Normozide Tablets 2112
Procardia XL Tablets 1783
Rythmol Tablets (0.1%) 1184
Suprax 1235
Tagamet (Rare) 2228
Tambocor Tablets (Rare) 1315
Trandate Tablets 579
Zefazone Sterile Powder 2372
Zinacef 1066

Cholestasis, intrahepatic
Cuprimine Capsules (Rare) 1442
Depen Titratable Tablets (Rare) 2379

Cholestatic hepatic injury
Axid Pulvules (Rare) 1246
Coumadin Injection & Tablets (Infrequent) 944

Cholinergic reactions
Anafranil Capsules (Rare) 650
Enlon Injection 598
Tensilon Injectable 1123

Chondrodystrophy
Prozac Pulvules (Rare) 920

Chorea
Demulen 2161
Diethylstilbestrol Tablets 1258
Dilantin Infatabs (Rare) 1710
Dilantin Kapseals (Rare) 1708
Dilantin Parenteral (Rare) 1712
Dilantin-30 Pediatric/Dilantin-125 Suspension (Rare) 1713
Dilantin with Phenobarbital Kapseals (Rare) 1715
Dilaudid-HP Injection 1175
Eldepryl 2250
Enovid 2161
Estinyl Tablets 2085
Estrace 1385
Estrace Vaginal Cream 1388
Estradurin 2452
Estratest 2245
Estrovis 1721
Etrafon 2087
Inversine Tablets 1492
Klonopin Tablets 1902
Larodopa Tablets (Frequent) 1905
Levlen/Tri-Levlen 665
Lo/Ovral Tablets 2471
Lo/Ovral-28 Tablets 2476
Mediatric Capsules 2476
Menrium Tablets 1934
Mesantoin Tablets 2013
Nordette-21 Tablets 2481
Nordette-28 Tablets 2483
Norethin 2133
Norlestrin 1746
Ogen 540
Ortho Dienestrol Cream 1664
Ovcon 1391
Ovral Tablets 2490
Ovral-28 Tablets 2491
Ovrette Tablets 2492
PMB 200 and PMB 400 2504
Premarin Intravenous 2508
Premarin with Methyltestosterone 2515
Premarin Tablets 2510
Premarin Vaginal Cream 2512
▲ Sinemet Tablets (Among most common) 952
Sinemet CR Tablets 953
Stilphostrol Tablets and Ampuls 1609
TACE 12 and 25 mg 1353
Trilafon Concentrate 2123
Levlen/Tri-Levlen 665
Triphasil-21 Tablets 2527
Triphasil-28 Tablets 2532

Choreoathetotic movements
Aldoclor Tablets 1413
Aldomet Ester HCl Injection 1417
Aldomet Oral 1415
Aldoril Tablets 1418
Anafranil Capsules (Rare) 650
Cibalith-S 870
Eskalith 2214
Lithane Tablets 1596
Lithium Carbonate Capsules & Tablets 1984
Lithobid Tablets 870
Loxitane 1213
Mellaril 2011
Permax Tablets (Frequent) 1291
Prolixin Decanoate 1795
Prolixin Enanthate 1796
Prolixin Oral Concentrate 1792
Reglan 1869
Taractan 1920
Triavil Tablets 1556

Chromatopsia
Anafranil Capsules (Rare) 650

Chromosomal abnormalities
Imuran 768
Metrodin (urofollitropin for injection) (3 incidents) 2182
Mustargen 1514
Roferon-A Injection 1916

Chrysiasis
Solganal Suspension 2122

Ciliary injection
Isopto Carbachol ◉ 219

Ciliary redness
Floropryl Sterile Ophthalmic Ointment 1473
Humorsol Sterile Ophthalmic Solution 1475
Phospholine Iodide ◉ 315

Ciliary spasm
Isopto Carbachol ◉ 219
Isopto Carpine ◉ 219
Ocusert Pilo-20 and Pilo-40 Ocular Therapeutic Systems ◉ 256
Pilocar ◉ 275
Pilopine HS Gel ◉ 227
Pilostat Sterile Ophthalmic Solution 0.5%, 1%, 2%, 3%, 4%, 5%, 6% ◉ 263

Cinchonism
Cardioquin Tablets 1812
Quinaglute Dura-Tabs Tablets 663
Quinamm Tablets 1344
Quinidex Extentabs 1868
Tonocard Tablets (Less than 1%) 1554

Circulatory collapse
Protamine Sulfate Ampoules & Vials 1295

Circulatory collapse, peripheral
Cibalith-S 870
Eskalith 2214
Lithane Tablets 1596
Lithium Carbonate Capsules & Tablets 1984
Lithobid Tablets 870
Phenobarbital Elixir and Tablets 1293

Circulatory depression
Brevital Sodium Vials 1248
Demerol 2047
Dilaudid 1173
Dilaudid-HP Injection 1175
Dolophine Hydrochloride Ampoules & Vials 1260
Dolophine Hydrochloride Tablets 1261
MS Contin Tablets 1814
MSIR 1817
Mepergan Injection 2479
Methadone Hydrochloride Diskets 1284
Oramorph SR (Morphine Sulfate Sustained Release Tablets) 1988
Phenergan with Codeine 2497
Phenergan VC with Codeine 2501
Talwin Injection 2071

Circulatory failure
Aminophyllin Tablets 2153
Asbron G 1997
Choledyl Pediatric Elixir 1702
Choledyl Tablets 1700
Choledyl SA Tablets 1704
Constant-T Tablets 1029
Dilaudid 1173
Dilor 2079
Etrafon 2087
Lufyllin & Lufyllin-400 Tablets 2384
Lufyllin-GG Elixir & Tablets 2385
Metubine Iodide Vials 1285
Quadrinal Tablets 1183
Quibron Capsules 713
Quibron-T 714
Quibron-T/SR 716
Respbid Tablets 684
Slo-bid Gyrocaps 1847
Surital Ampoules, Steri-Vials 1764
T-PHYL (Uniphyl) 200 mg Tablets 1820
Theo-24 2179
Theo-Dur Sprinkle 1168
Theo-Dur Extended-Release Tablets 1166
Theolair 1317
Theolair-SR Tablets 1319
▲ TheoX Extended-Release Tablets (Among most consistent) 841
Trilafon (Extremely rare) 2123
Uniphyl 400 mg Tablets 1823

Circulatory overload
Hespan Injection 948
Pentaspan Injection 949

Cirrhosis, hepatic (see under Cirrhosis of liver)

Cirrhosis of liver
Cordarone Tablets (Rare) 2446
Methotrexate Tablets, Parenteral, LPF Parenteral 1217
Papaverine Hydrochloride Vials and Ampoules (Rare) 1290
Rheumatrex Methotrexate Dose Pack 1234

Clamminess
BuSpar 1401
Desyrel and Desyrel Dividose 1404
IOPIDINE ◉ 232
▲ Nubain Injection (9%) 934
Sanorex Tablets 2030
▲ Stadol (6%) 721
▲ Tegison Capsules (1-10%) 1881

Claudication
Blocadren Tablets 1429
Calan SR Caplets (1% or less) 2157
Calan Tablets (1% or less) 2155
Isoptin Oral Tablets 1179
Isoptin SR Sustained Release Tablets (Less than 1%) 1181
Monopril Tablets (0.2 to 1.0%) 1406
Timolide Tablets 1547
Timoptic in Ocudose 1552
Timoptic Sterile Ophthalmic Solution 1550
Tonocard Tablets (Less than 1%) 1554

Verelan Capsules (Less than 1%) .. 1243
Visken Tablets (2% or fewer patients) 2036

Claudication, intermittent (see under Charcot's syndrome)

Claustrophobia
BuSpar (Rare) 1401
Roferon-A Injection (Less than 1%) 1916

Climacteric, onset masked
Cycrin Tablets 2449
Demulen 2161
Enovid 2161

Clitoral hypertrophy
Amen (A few cases) 833
Danocrine Capsules (Rare) 2046

Clitoris, enlargement (see under Clitoromegaly)

Clitoromegaly
Anadrol-50 Tablets 2287
Android 1111
Estratest 2245
Halotestin Tablets 2341
Metandren Linguets and Tablets 875
Premarin with Methyltestosterone (Among most common) 2515
Testred Capsules 1124
Winstrol Tablets 2075

Clonic movements of whole limbs
Cibalith-S 870
Diprivan Injection (Greater than 1%) 2267
Eskalith 2214
Lithane Tablets 1596
Lithium Carbonate Capsules & Tablets 1984
Lithobid Tablets 870

Clonus
Dopram Injectable 1860

Clot formation in renal pelvis
Cytoxan for Injection 726

Clotting time, prolongation
Hespan Injection 948
Hyskon Hysteroscopy Fluid (Rare) .. 1162
Mithracin 1602

Coagulation, dysfunction
Children's Advil Suspension 2426
Cordarone Tablets (1 to 3%) 2446
Depakote Sprinkle Capsules 512
Elspar 1470
Estratest 2245
Fungizone Intravenous 2262
IFEX (Less than 1%) 729
Lo/Ovral Tablets 2471
Lo/Ovral-28 Tablets 2476
Mediatric Capsules 2476
Nimotop Capsules (Less than 1%) 1607
Ovral Tablets 2490
Ovral-28 Tablets 2491
Ovrette Tablets 2492
PMB 200 and PMB 400 2504
Premarin Intravenous 2508
Premarin with Methyltestosterone .. 2515
Premarin Tablets 2510
Premarin Vaginal Cream 2512
Tegison Capsules (Less than 1%) .. 1881

Coagulation defects, neonatal
Dilantin Infatabs 1710
Dilantin Kapseals 1708
Dilantin Parenteral 1712
Dilantin-30 Pediatric/Dilantin-125 Suspension 1713
Dilantin with Phenobarbital Kapseals 1715

Coagulation tests, altered results
Cycrin Tablets 2449
Eminase 2211

Cochlear lesion
Diphtheria and Tetanus Toxoids and Pertussis Vaccine Adsorbed USP (For Pediatric Use) 892

Cognitive dysfunction
Anaprox and Anaprox DS Tablets 2288
Doral Tablets 2383
Floxin Tablets (Less than 1%) 1652

Methotrexate Tablets, Parenteral, LPF Parenteral 1217
Naprosyn (Rare) 2297
Rheumatrex Methotrexate Dose Pack 1234

Cogwheel rigidity
BuSpar (Rare) 1401
Compazine 2201
Eskalith 2214
Prolixin Decanoate 1795
Prolixin Enanthate 1796
Reglan 1869
Stelazine 2226
Taractan 1920
Thorazine 2234

Cold, reduced tolerance
Parlodel (Less than 1%) 2020

Coldness of extremities
▲Blocadren Tablets (8%) 1429
Cibalith-S 870
Eskalith (A few reports) 2214
Kerlone Tablets (1.9%) 2172
Lithane Tablets 1596
Lithium Carbonate Capsules & Tablets (A single report) 1984
Lithobid Tablets 870
Lopressor Ampuls (1%) 1032
Lopressor HCT Tablets 1034
Lopressor Tablets (1%) 1032
Mykrox ½ mg Tablets (Less than 2%) 984
Parlodel 2020
Sansert Tablets 2031
▲Tenoretic Tablets (Up to 12%) 1105
▲Tenormin Tablets and I.V. Injection (Up to 12%) 1107
Timolide Tablets 1547
Timoptic in Ocudose 1552
Timoptic Sterile Ophthalmic Solution 1550
Tonocard Tablets (Less than 1%) .. 1554
Visken Tablets (2% or fewer patients) 2036

Cold sensations
BuSpar (Rare) 1401
Diprivan Injection (Less than 1%) .. 2267
Duranest Injections 624
Dyclone 0.5% and 1% Topical Solutions, USP 626
Versed Injection (Less than 1%) 1924
▲Xylocaine Injections (Among most common) 637
Xylocaine Injections for Ventricular Arrhythmias 639
Xylocaine 2% Jelly 643
Xylocaine 5% Ointment 644
Xylocaine 10% Oral Spray 645
4% Xylocaine-MPF Sterile Solution 641
Xylocaine 2% Viscous Solution 646

Cold sore, non-herpetic
Intron A (Less than 1%) 2097
Trexan Tablets (Less than 1%) 937

Colds, susceptibility
Diupres Tablets 1461
Hydropres Tablets 1485
Hytrin Tablets (At least 1%) 529
Lopid Capsules and Tablets 1736
Prinzide Tablets (0.3% to 1%) 1540
Rowasa 2248
Salutensin/Salutensin-Demi 719
Zestoretic (0.3 to 1%) 2274

Colic
Duvoid Tablets 1853
Feldene Capsules (Less than 1%) .. 1777
Solganal Suspension (Rare) 2122
Urecholine 1558

Colic, biliary
Cholybar (One case) 1705
Questran Light (1 patient) 711
Questran Powder 710

Colitis
Aldoclor Tablets 1413
Aldomet Ester HCl Injection 1417
Aldomet Oral 1415
Aldoril Tablets 1418
Anafranil Capsules (Infrequent) 650
Anaprox and Anaprox DS Tablets (Less than 3%) 2288
Ancef Injection 2194
Brevicon 2304
Ceftin Tablets 575
Ceptaz for Injection 1057

Claforan Sterile Injection (1.4%) 1089
Cleocin HCl Capsules 2322
Cleocin Pediatric Flavored Granules 2324
Cleocin Phosphate Injection 2325
Cleocin T Topical 2327
Clinoril Tablets (Less than 1%) 1433
Compazine Ampuls 2201
Demulen 2161
Enovid 2161
Fortaz 1060
Furoxone 1855
Jenest-28 Tablets 1636
Keftab Tablets 917
Kefurox Vials, Faspak & ADD-Vantage 1277
Levlen/Tri-Levlen 665
Lincocin 2344
Lodine Capsules (Less than 1%) 2468
Loestrin 1728
Lopid Capsules and Tablets 1736
Meclomen Capsules (Less than 1%) 1739
Micronor Tablets 1667
Modicon 1667
Naprosyn (Less than 1%) 2297
NebuPent for Inhalation Solution (1% or less) 1017
Norethin 2133
Norinyl 2304
Norlestrin 1746
Nor-Q D Tablets 2304
Ortho-Cyclen Tablets 1658
Ortho-Novum 1667
Permax Tablets (Rare) 1291
Prozac Pulvules (Rare) 920
Rocephin Injectable Vials, ADD-Vantage (Rare) 1914
Rowasa 2248
Solganal Suspension 2122
Tazicef for Injection 2231
Levlen/Tri-Levlen 665
Tri-Norinyl 2304
Voltaren Tablets (Rare) 1042
Wellbutrin Tablets (Rare) 821
Zinacef 1066

Colitis, ischemic
Blocadren Tablets 1429
Cartrol Tablets 507
Normozide Tablets 2112
Tenoretic Tablets 1105
Tenormin Tablets and I.V. Injection 1107
Trandate HCT/Trandate 579
Visken Tablets 2036

Colitis, necrotizing
Cytosar-U Sterile Powder (With experimental doses) 2329
Doxorubicin Hydrochloride Injection, USP 848
Rubex 739

Colitis, pseudomembranous (see under Pseudomembranous colitis)

Colitis, ulcerative
Ancobon Capsules 1886
Indocin (Less than 1%) 1487
Orudis Capsules (Less than 1%) 2488

Collapse
AK-Dilate Solution 2.5% and 10% (Rare) .... ⊚ 203
Antivenin (Crotalidae) Polyvalent 2430
Cardilate Oral/Sublingual Tablets (Occasional) 757
Dilatrate-SR (Occasional) 1827
Diphtheria and Tetanus Toxoids and Pertussis Vaccine Adsorbed USP (For Pediatric Use) (Infrequent) 892
Isordil (Occasional) 2467
Mintezol 1510
Nitro-Bid Ointment 1339
Nitrolingual Spray 1846
Norpramin Tablets (One report) 1340
Pantopon Injectable 1911
Peritrate (Occasional) 1756
Sorbitrate (Occasional) 1103
Tegretol Chewable Tablets 654
Tegretol Suspension 656
Tegretol Tablets 654
Tofranil Ampuls 1038
Tofranil Tablets 1039
Tofranil-PM Capsules 1041

Colon, cancer
Protostat Tablets 1674

Colon, dilatation
Artane (Rare) 1195
Phenergan with Codeine 2497
Phenergan VC with Codeine 2501

Colon, irritable
BuSpar (Infrequent) 1401
Compazine 2201
Prilosec Delayed-Release Capsules (Less than 1%) 1530

Colon, motility, increase
Phenergan with Codeine 2497
Phenergan VC with Codeine 2501

Colon, transverse, presence of "pasty mass"
Cholybar (One case) 1705

Color perception, disturbed
Cardioquin Tablets 1812
Children's Advil Suspension (Less than 1%) 2426
Motrin Tablets 2351
NegGram (Infrequent) 2062
PediaProfen Suspension (Less than 1%) 1363
Platinol 737
Platinol-AQ Injection 738
Quinaglute Dura-Tabs Tablets 663
Quinamm Tablets 1344
Quinidex Extentabs 1868
Rufen Tablets (Less than 1%) 691
Zefazone Sterile Powder 2372

Coma
Aminophyllin Tablets 2153
Anafranil Capsules (Infrequent) 650
Children's Advil Suspension (Less than 1%) 2426
Cibalith-S 870
Compazine 2201
Cyclogyl .... ⊚ 215
Cyclomydril .... ⊚ 216
Cytosar-U Sterile Powder 2329
Cytovene Sterile Powder (1% or less) 2292
Dalmane Capsules 1927
Depakene Capsules & Syrup (Rare) 511
Depakote (Rare) 512
Elavil 2269
Elspar 1470
Eskalith 2214
Ethmozine Tablets (Less than 2%) 946
IFEX (Occasional) 729
Indocin Capsules (Less than 1%) 1487
Indocin I.V. (Less than 1%) 1490
Indocin (Less than 1%) 1487
Intron A (Less than 1%) 2097
Isopto Atropine .... ⊚ 218
Klonopin Tablets 1902
Lithane Tablets 1596
Lithium Carbonate Capsules & Tablets 1984
Lithobid Tablets 870
Marplan Tablets (Rare) 1906
Matulane Capsules 1907
Motrin Tablets (Less than 1%) 2351
Nardil (Less frequent) 1742
Omnipaque (Several instances) 2552
Oncovin Solution Vials & Hyporets 1288
Orthoclone OKT3 Sterile Solution .. 1645
Oxytocin Injection 2492
Pantopon Injectable 1911
PediaProfen Suspension (Less than 1%) 1363
Permax Tablets (Infrequent) 1291
Pfizerpen for Injection 1957
PhosLo Tablets 700
Prozac Pulvules (Rare) 920
Roferon-A Injection (Less than 1%) 1916
Rufen Tablets (Less than 1%) 691
Ru-Tuss Tablets 693
Rythmol Tablets (Less than 1%) 1184
Seromycin Pulvules 1298
Syntocinon Injection 2032
Tigan 2239
Tonocard Tablets (Less than 1%) .. 1554
Triavil Tablets 1556
Vasocon-A .... ⊚ 278
Wellbutrin Tablets 821
Zovirax Sterile Powder 828

Coma, hepatic (see under Hepatic coma)

Coma, hyperosmolar non-ketonic
Hyperstat I.V. Injection 2095
OSM_GLYN .... ⊚ 234

Proglycem 649

Coma, hypoglycemic

Tapazole Tablets 1298

Conduction delay, intraventricular

Rythmol Tablets (0.2 to 1.1%) 1184

Conduction disturbances

Adalat Capsules (10 mg and 20 mg) (Fewer than 0.5%) 1587
Blocadren Tablets 1429
Capoten (Rare) 2255
Catapres Tablets (Rare) 676
Catapres-TTS (Rare) 677
Combipres Tablets (Rare) 678
Corgard Tablets (1 in 100 patients) 701
Corzide Tablets (About 1 of 100 patients) 702
Desyrel and Desyrel Dividose 1404
Dilantin Parenteral 1712
▲ Eminase (38%) 2211
Ethmozine Tablets (1.6%) 946
Intropin Injection (Infrequent) 930
Mexitil Capsules (2 in 1,000) 680
Procardia Capsules (Less than 0.5%) 1781
Procardia XL Tablets (Fewer than 0.5%) 1783
▲ Rythmol Tablets (0.2 to 4.0%) 1184
Tonocard Tablets (0.0-1.5%) 1554

Confusion

Actifed with Codeine Cough Syrup 752
Actimmune (Rare) 1046
Aldactazide 2150
Aldactone 2152
Aldoclor Tablets 1413
Aldomet Ester HCl Injection 1417
Aldomet Oral 1415
Aldoril Tablets 1418
Alfenta Injection (Less than 1%) 1131
Alferon N Injection (One patient to 3%) 1809
Alurate Elixir (Less than 1 in 100) 1883
Amoxil (Rare) 2193
Anafranil Capsules (2% to 3%) 650
Ancobon Capsules 1886
▲ Anestacon Solution (Among most common) 2394
Ansaid Tablets (Less than 1%) 2319
Artane 1195
Asendin Tablets (Greater than 1%) 1196
Atgam Sterile Solution (Less than 5%) 2320
Ativan Injection (1.3%) 2432
Augmentin Tablets, Powder for Oral Suspension, and Chewable Tablets (Rare) 2198
Axid Pulvules (Rare) 1246
Azactam for Injection (Less than 1%) 2252
Azdōne Tablets 844
Benadryl Capsules 1691
Benadryl Injection 1692
Bentyl 1322
Blenoxane (1%) 724
Bretylol Injection (1 in 1000) 923
Brevibloc Injection (2%) 942
BuSpar (2%) 1401
Butazolidin Capsules & Tablets (Less than 1%) 1027
Butisol Sodium Elixir & Tablets (Less than 1 in 100) 2377
Calan SR Caplets (1% or less) 2157
Calan Tablets (1% or less) 2155
Cantil Tablets 1326
Capoten 2255
Capozide 2258
Cardene Capsules (Rare) 2290
Cardioquin Tablets 1812
Cardura Tablets (Less than 0.5% of 3960 patients) 1941
Ceclor Pulvules & Suspension (Rare) 1251
Celontin 1692
Centrax (Less frequent) 1693
Children's Advil Suspension (Less than 1%) 2426
Chloromycetin Kapseals 1695
Chloromycetin Palmitate, Oral Suspension 1697
Chloromycetin Sodium Succinate 1698
Cibalith-S 870
Cipro I.V. (1% or less) 1592
Cipro Tablets 1589
▲ Clozaril Tablets (3%) 2000
Cogentin 1435
Cytovene Sterile Powder (1% or less) 2292
Dalgan Injection (Less than 1%) 620
Dalmane Capsules (Rare) 1927
Dantrium Capsules (Less frequent) 1619
Daranide Tablets 1445
Darbid Tablets 2205
Deconamine 663
Demser Capsules 1460
Desyrel and Desyrel Dividose (Greater than 1%) 1404
Diamox Parenteral (Occasional) 1200
Diamox Sequels (Sustained Release) (Occasional) 1201
Diamox Tablets (Occasional) 1200
▲ Dilantin Infatabs (Among most common) 1710
▲ Dilantin Kapseals (Among most common) 1708
▲ Dilantin Parenteral (Among most common) 1712
▲ Dilantin-30 Pediatric/Dilantin-125 Suspension (Among most common) 1713
▲ Dilantin with Phenobarbital Kapseals (Among most common) 1715
Dilaudid Cough Syrup 1174
Dilaudid 1173
Diprivan Injection (Less than 1%) 2267
Dolobid Tablets (Less than 1 in 100) 1465
Doral Tablets 2383
▲ Duragesic Transdermal System (10% or more) 1133
Duranest Injections 624
Dyclone 0.5% and 1% Topical Solutions, USP 626
E.E.S. (Isolated reports) 522
Easprin 1719
Edecrin 1468
Elavil 2269
▲ Eldepryl (3 of 49 patients) 2250
Elspar 1470
Empirin with Codeine Phosphate Nos. 2, 3 & 4 764
Endep Tablets 1927
Ergamisol Tablets (Less frequent) 1136
EryPed (Isolated reports) 519
Ery-Tab Tablets (Isolated reports) 521
Erythrocin Stearate Filmtab (Isolated reports) 523
Erythromycin Base Filmtab (Isolated reports) 525
Erythromycin Delayed-Release Capsules, USP (Isolated reports) 526
Esgic-Plus Tablets 1002
Esgic Tablets & Capsules 1001
Eskalith 2214
Ethmozine Tablets (Less than 2%) 946
Etrafon 2087
Eulexin Capsules (1%) 2089
Sterile FUDR (Remote possibility) 1898
Feldene Capsules (Less than 1%) 1777
Fioricet Tablets 2006
Flagyl I.V. 2131
Flagyl Tablets 2170
Floxin Tablets 1652
Fluorouracil Injection 1897
Fulvicin P/G Tablets 2090
Fulvicin P/G 165 & 330 Tablets 2091
Fulvicin-U/F Tablets 2092
Ganite Injection 1016
Garamycin Injectable 2093
Grifulvin V (griseofulvin microsize) Tablets/Suspension (Occasional) 1678
Grisactin (Occasional) 2454
Grisactin Ultra Tablets (Occasional) 2455
Gris-PEG Tablets, 125 mg & 250 mg (Occasional) 1083
Halcion Tablets (Less than 1%) 2340
Haldol Decanoate 1375
Haldol Injection, Tablets and Concentrate 1373
Humulin 70/30, 100 Units 1267
Humulin BR, 100 Units 1268
Humulin L, 100 Units 1268
Humulin U, 100 Units 1272
▲ Hylorel Tablets (14.8%) 975
Hyperstat I.V. Injection 2095
▲ IFEX (Among most common) 729
Indocin (Less than 1%) 1487
▲ Intron A (Up to 12%) 2097
ISMOTIC ◉ 233
Isoptin Oral Tablets (Less than 1%) 1179
Isoptin SR Sustained Release Tablets (Less than 1%) 1181
K-Lyte 707
K-Phos M.F. Tablets 659
K-Phos Neutral Tablets 660
K-Phos Original Formula 'Sodium Free' Tablets (Less frequent) 660
K-Phos No. 2 Tablets 659
Keflex Pulvules, Oral Suspension & Pediatric Drops 916
Keftab Tablets 917
Kerlone Tablets (Less than 2%) 2172
Klonopin Tablets 1902
Klorvess Effervescent Granules 2010
Klorvess Effervescent Tablets 2011
Klorvess 10% Liquid 2010
Lariam Tablets 1904
Larodopa Tablets (Relatively frequent) 1905
Leukeran Tablets (Rare) 788
Levsin/Levsinex 2147
Librax Capsules 1929
Libritabs Tablets 1930
Librium Capsules (Some patients) 1931
Librium Injectable 1932
Limbitrol (Less common) 1933
▲ Lioresal Tablets (1-11%) 1031
Lithane Tablets 1596
Lithium Carbonate Capsules & Tablets 1984
Lithobid Tablets 870
Lodine Capsules (Less than 1%) 2468
Lomotil 2174
Lopid Capsules and Tablets 1736
Lopressor 1032
Lortab ASA Tablets 2414
Loxitane 1213
Ludiomil Tablets (Rare) 874
▲ Marplan Tablets (Among most frequent) 1906
Matulane Capsules 1907
Maxair Inhaler (Less than 1%) 1311
Mebaral Tablets (Less than 1 in 100) 2061
Mellaril 2011
Menrium Tablets (Particularly in elderly and debilitated) 1934
Methadone Hydrochloride Oral Solution & Tablets 1987
Methotrexate Tablets, Parenteral, LPF Parenteral 1217
Mexitil Capsules (1.9% to 2.6%) 680
Midamor Tablets (Less than or equal to 1%) 1508
Miltown Tablets 2386
Moduretic Tablets (Less than or equal to 1%) 1510
Mono-Gesic Tablets 846
Monopril Tablets (0.2 to 1.0%) 1406
Motofen Tablets (1 in 200 to 1 in 600) 836
Motrin Tablets (Less than 1%) 2351
Mutamycin 733
Myambutol Tablets 1225
Myochrysine Injection (Rare) 1516
Nalfon Pulvules & Tablets (1.4%) 919
Nebcin Vials, Hyporets & ADD-Vantage 1286
NebuPent for Inhalation Solution (1% or less) 1017
Nembutal Sodium Capsules (Less than 1%) 534
Nembutal Sodium Solution (Less than 1%) 536
Nembutal Sodium Suppositories (Less than 1%) 538
Neptazane Tablets ◉ 311
Nicorette 1335
Nipride I.V. Infusion 1909
Norgesic (Infrequent) 1314
Noroxin Tablets 1519
Norpramin Tablets 1340
Norzine 1818
Nubain Injection (Less than 1%) 934
Omnipaque (Rare) 2552
Optimine Tablets 2115
Oramorph SR (Morphine Sulfate Sustained Release Tablets) 1988
Ornade Spansule Capsules 2221
Orthoclone OKT3 Sterile Solution 1645
Orudis Capsules (Less than 1%) 2488
OSM_GLYN ◉ 234
PBZ Tablets & Elixir 1037
PBZ-SR Tablets 1037
PCE Dispertab Tablets (Isolated reports) 549
Pamelor 2019
Parlodel 2020
PediaProfen Suspension (Less than 1%) 1363
Pentam 300 Injection (1.7%) 1018
Pepcid (Infrequent) 1524
Periactin 1525
▲ Permax Tablets (11.1%) 1291
Pfizerpen-AS Aqueous Suspension (Approximately 1 in 500) 1959
Phenergan with Codeine (Rare) 2497
Phenergan with Dextromethorphan (Rare) 2499
Phenergan Suppositories (Rare) 2496
Phenergan Syrup (Rare) 2495
Phenergan VC (Rare) 2500
Phenergan VC with Codeine (Rare) 2501
Phenobarbital Elixir and Tablets (Less than 1 in 100 patients) 1293
PhosLo Tablets 700
Phrenilin 838
Polaramine 2116
Polycitra Syrup 2424
Polycitra-K 2424
Polycitra-LC—Sugar-Free 2424
Pondimin Tablets 1867
Prilosec Delayed-Release Capsules (Less than 1%) 1530
Primaxin I.M. 1532
Primaxin I.V. (Less than 0.2%) 1535
Prinivil Tablets (1% or less) 1538
Prinzide Tablets 1540
Pro-Banthīne Tablets 2141
Procan SR Tablets (Infrequent) 1760
ProSom Tablets (2%) 554
Protostat Tablets 1674
Prozac Pulvules 920
Quadrinal Tablets 1183
Quarzan Capsules 1937
Quinaglute Dura-Tabs Tablets 663
Quinamm Tablets 1344
Quinidex Extentabs 1868
Reglan 1869
Renese-R Tablets 1786
Restoril Capsules (2-3%) 2023
Retrovir Capsules (Less than 5%) 802
Retrovir I.V. Infusion (Less than 5%) 805
Retrovir Syrup (Less than 5%) 802
Rheumatrex Methotrexate Dose Pack 1234
Rifadin 1345
Rifamate Capsules 1347
Rimactane Capsules 879
Robinul Forte Tablets 1873
Robinul Injectable 1873
Robinul Tablets 1873
▲ Roferon-A Injection (8%) 1916
Roxanol 1991
Roxicodone Tablets, Oral Solution & Intensol (Oxycodone) 1992
Rufen Tablets (Less than 1%) 691
Ru-Tuss II Capsules 693
Rythmol Tablets (Less than 1%) 1184
Sandimmune (2% or less) 2024
Seconal Sodium Pulvules (Less than 1 in 100) 1296
Sedapap Tablets 50 mg/650 mg 1360
Seldane Tablets 1349
Seldane-D Extended-Release Tablets 1350
Serentil 686
Seromycin Pulvules 1298
Sinemet Tablets 952
▲ Sinemet CR Tablets (3.7%) 953
Sinequan (Infrequent) 1960
Soma Compound w/Codeine Tablets (Very rare) 2390
Soma Compound Tablets (Very rare) 2389
Soma Tablets 2388
Stadol (1%) 721
Surmontil Capsules 2524
Symmetrel Capsules & Syrup (1-5%) 936
Tagamet (Occasional) 2228
Talacen 2070
Talwin Injection 2071
Talwin Compound 2072
Talwin Injection 2071
Talwin Nx 2073
Tambocor Tablets (Less than 1%) 1315
Tavist Syrup 2033
Tavist Tablets 2035
Tavist-D Tablets 2035
Tegretol Chewable Tablets 654
Tegretol Suspension 656
Tegretol Tablets 654
Tenex Tablets (Less than 3%) 1875
Timolide Tablets (Less than 1%) 1547
Timoptic in Ocudose 1552
Timoptic Sterile Ophthalmic Solution 1550
Tofranil Ampuls 1038
Tofranil Tablets 1039
Tofranil-PM Capsules 1041
▲ Tonocard Tablets (2.1-11.2%) 1554
Torecan 1993
Trancopal Caplets 2075
Transderm Scōp Transdermal Therapeutic System (Infrequent) 887

Tranxene (Less common) 556
Trental (Less than 1%) 1099
Trexan Tablets (Less than 1%) 937
Triaminic Expectorant DH 1995
Triaminic Oral Infant Drops 1996
Triavil Tablets 1556
Trilisate (Rare) 1822
Trinalin Repetabs Tablets 1170
Urispas Tablets 2242
Uroqid-Acid (Less frequent) 661
Valium Injectable 1937
Valium Tablets (Infrequent) 1939
Valpin 50 Tablets 941
Valrelease Capsules (Occasional) 1923
Vaseretic Tablets 1559
Vasotec I.V. 1562
Vasotec Tablets (0.5% to 1%) 1564
Verelan Capsules (Less than 1%) 1243
Versed Injection (Less than 1%) 1924
Vira-A for Injection 1766
Vivactil Tablets 1567
Vontrol Tablets (Approximately 1 in 350) 2243
▲ Wellbutrin Tablets (8.4%) 821
▲ Xanax Tablets (9.9% to 10.4%) 2367
▲ Xylocaine Injections (Among most common) 637
Xylocaine Injections for Ventricular Arrhythmias 639
Xylocaine 2% Jelly 643
Xylocaine 5% Ointment 644
Xylocaine 10% Oral Spray 645
4% Xylocaine-MPF Sterile Solution 641
Xylocaine 2% Viscous Solution 646
Zantac Injection and Zantac Injection Premixed (Rare) 1063
Zantac (Rare) 1065
Zestoretic 2274
Zestril Tablets 2277
Zovirax Capsules 824
Zovirax Sterile Powder 828
Zovirax 824
Zyloprim Tablets (Less than 1%) 830

Confusion, mental (see under Confusion)

Confusion, nocturnal
Trilafon 2123

Confusional state (see under Confusion)

Congelation
Eldepryl 2250
Ethyl Chloride, U.S.P. 1022
Fluori-Methane 1022
Fluro-Ethyl 1023

Congenital anomalies
Amen 833
Aygestin Tablets 2437
Cycrin Tablets 2449
Demulen 2161
Depo-Provera Sterile Aqueous Suspension 2336
Diabinese Tablets 1775
Diethylstilbestrol Tablets 1258
Enovid 2161
Estrovis 1721
Halcion Tablets 2340
Levlen/Tri-Levlen 665
Lo/Ovral Tablets 2471
Lo/Ovral-28 Tablets 2476
Loestrin 1728
Menrium Tablets 1934
Methotrexate Tablets, Parenteral, LPF Parenteral 1217
Metrodin (urofollitropin for injection) 2182
Nordette-21 Tablets 2481
Nordette-28 Tablets 2483
Norethin 2133
Norlestrin 1746
Ogen 540
Ortho Dienestrol Cream 1664
Ovral Tablets 2490
Ovral-28 Tablets 2491
Ovrette Tablets 2492
PMB 200 and PMB 400 2504
▲ Parlodel (3.3%) 2020
Pergonal (menotropins for injection, USP) 2184
Permax Tablets 1291
Premarin Intravenous 2508
Premarin with Methyltestosterone 2515
Premarin Tablets 2510
Provera Tablets 2356
Rheumatrex Methotrexate Dose Pack 1234
Serophene (clomiphene citrate tablets, USP) 2186
Levlen/Tri-Levlen 665
Triphasil-21 Tablets 2527
Triphasil-28 Tablets 2532
Xanax Tablets 2367

Congenital malformation
Ativan Injection 2432
Ativan Tablets 2434
Cytosar-U Sterile Powder 2329
Dalmane Capsules 1927
Deprol Tablets 2382
Dilantin Infatabs 1710
Dilantin Kapseals 1708
Dilantin Parenteral 1712
Dilantin-30 Pediatric/Dilantin-125 Suspension 1713
Dilantin with Phenobarbital Kapseals 1715
Doral Tablets 2383
Equagesic Tablets 2451
Halcion Tablets 2340
Librax Capsules 1929
Libritabs Tablets 1930
Librium Capsules 1931
Librium Injectable 1932
Limbitrol 1933
Miltown Tablets 2386
PMB 200 and PMB 400 2504
ProSom Tablets 554
Quinamm Tablets 1344
Restoril Capsules 2023
Tegretol Chewable Tablets 654
Tegretol Suspension 656
Tegretol Tablets 654
Tofranil Ampuls 1038
Tofranil Tablets 1039
Tofranil-PM Capsules 1041
Tranxene 556
Valium Injectable 1937
Valium Tablets 1939
Valrelease Capsules 1923
Versed Injection 1924

Congestion
Adalat Capsules (10 mg and 20 mg) (2% or less) 1587
▲ AeroBid Inhaler System (3-9%) 995
BuSpar (Infrequent) 1401
Halcion Tablets (Rare) 2340
Omnipaque (0.3%) 2552
Procardia Capsules (2% or less) 1781

Congestion, nasal (see under Nasal congestion)

Congestive heart failure
Adalat Capsules (10 mg and 20 mg) (About 2%) 1587
Adriamycin PFS 561
Adriamycin RDF 562
Aldoclor Tablets 1413
Aldomet Ester HCl Injection 1417
Aldomet Oral 1415
Aldoril Tablets 1418
Aminohippurate Sodium Injection 1421
Anaprox and Anaprox DS Tablets (Less than 1%) 2288
Android 1111
Aristocort Suspension 1008
Aristospan Suspension 1011
Atgam Sterile Solution (At least 1 patient and less than 5% of total patients) 2320
Betagan ◉ 239
Betoptic Sterile Ophthalmic Solution (Rare) 569
Betoptic S Sterile Ophthalmic Suspension (Rare) 570
BuSpar (Rare) 1401
Butazolidin Capsules & Tablets (Less than 1%) 1027
Calan SR Caplets (1.8%) 2157
Calan Tablets (1.8%) 2155
Capoten (2 to 3 of 1000 patients) 2255
Capozide (2 to 3 of 1000 patients) 2258
Cardizem Tablets-30 mg, 60 mg, 90 mg and 120 mg (Less than 1%) 1329
Cardizem SR Capsules-60 mg, 90 mg and 120 mg (Less than 1%) 1327
Catapres Tablets (Rare) 676
Catapres-TTS (Rare) 677
Celestone Soluspan Suspension 2081
Cerubidine 2443
Children's Advil Suspension (Less than 1%) 2426
Clinoril Tablets (Less than 1%) 1433
Combipres Tablets (Rare) 678
Cordarone Tablets (1 to 3%) 2446
Cortenema 2244
Cortone Acetate Sterile Suspension 1437
Cortone Acetate Tablets 1439
Dalalone D.P. Injectable 999
Decadron Elixir 1445
Decadron Phosphate Injection 1449
Decadron Phosphate Respihaler 1454
Decadron Phosphate Turbinaire 1456
Decadron Phosphate with Xylocaine Injection, Sterile 1451
Decadron Tablets 1447
Decadron-LA Sterile Suspension 1457
Deltasone Tablets 2332
Depo-Medrol Sterile Aqueous Suspension 2334
Digibind (Few instances) 762
Diupres Tablets 1461
Doxorubicin Hydrochloride for Injection, USP 622
Doxorubicin Hydrochloride Injection, USP 848
▲ Emcyt Capsules (3%) 1161
Esimil Tablets 864
▲ Ethmozine Tablets (1%-5%) 946
Feldene Capsules (Less than 1%) 1777
Hydeltrasol Injection, Sterile 1476
Hydeltra-T.B.A. Sterile Suspension 1478
Hydrocortone Acetate Sterile Suspension 1479
Hydrocortone Phosphate Injection, Sterile 1481
Hydrocortone Tablets 1482
Hydropres Tablets 1485
Idamycin for Injection 564
Inderal 2459
Inderal LA Long Acting Capsules 2461
Inderide Tablets 2463
Inderide LA Long Acting Capsules 2465
Indocin Capsules (Less than 1%) 1487
Indocin I.V. (Less than 1%) 1490
Indocin (Less than 1%) 1487
Ismelin Tablets 869
Isoptin Oral Tablets (1.8%) 1179
Isoptin SR Sustained Release Tablets (1.8%) 1181
Kenalog-10 Injection 2402
Kenalog-40 Injection 2403
Kerlone Tablets 2172
Lodine Capsules (Less than 1%) 2468
Lopressor Ampuls (1%) 1032
Lopressor HCT Tablets 1034
Lopressor Tablets (1%) 1032
▲ Lupron Depot 3.75 mg (Among most frequent) 2312
Lupron Depot 7.5 mg 2311
▲ Lupron Injection (5% or more) 2310
Medrol 2348
Mexitil Capsules (Less than 1%) 680
Motrin Tablets (Less than 1%) 2351
Mutamycin (Rare) 733
Naprosyn (Less than 1%) 2297
Neosar for Injection 566
Nicorette 1335
Nimotop Capsules (Less than 1%) 1607
Normodyne Injection 2108
Normodyne Tablets 2110
Norpace (1 to 3%) 2177
▲ Novantrone for Injection Concentrate (0 to 5%) 1226
Orudis Capsules (Less than 1%) 2488
Pediapred Oral Liquid 987
PediaProfen Suspension (Less than 1%) 1363
Permax Tablets (Frequent) 1291
Premarin with Methyltestosterone 2515
Procardia Capsules (Approximately 2%) 1781
Procardia XL Tablets (About 1 patient in 15) 1783
Proglycem 649
Prostin VR Pediatric Sterile Solution (Less than 1%) 2355
Retrovir (0.8%) 802
Roferon-A Injection (Less than 1%) 1916
Rubex 739
Rufen Tablets (Less than 1%) 691
▲ Rythmol Tablets (0.8 to 3.7%) 1184
Salutensin/Salutensin-Demi 719
Sandostatin Injection (Less than 1%) 2029
Seromycin Pulvules 1298
Solu-Cortef Sterile Powder 2361
Solu-Medrol Sterile Powder 2363
Symmetrel Capsules & Syrup (0.1-1%) 936
▲ Tambocor Tablets (Approximately 5%) 1315
Tegretol Chewable Tablets 654
Tegretol Suspension 656
Tegretol Tablets 654
Tenex Tablets 1875
Tofranil Ampuls 1038
Tofranil Tablets 1039
Tofranil-PM Capsules 1041
Tolectin (200, 400 and 600 mg) (Less than 1%) 1379
▲ Tonocard Tablets (4.0%) 1554
Vascor (200, 300 and 400 mg) Tablets (About 1%) 1383
Vasotec I.V. 1562
Verelan Capsules (1.8%) 1243
Voltaren Tablets (Less than 1%) 1042
▲ Zoladex (5%) 1110

Conjunctiva, progressive pigmentation
Serentil 686
Torecan 1993

Conjunctiva, sensitization
Akarpine Ophthalmic Solution (Occasional) ◉ 201

Conjunctiva, suffusion
Amicar Syrup, Tablets, and Injection (Occasional) 1194
Arfonad Ampuls 1887
BiCNU 723

Conjunctiva, thickening
Floropryl Sterile Ophthalmic Ointment 1473
Humorsol Sterile Ophthalmic Solution 1475
Phospholine Iodide ◉ 315

Conjunctival blanching
IOPIDINE (0.4%) ◉ 232

Conjunctival chemosis
Natacyn ◉ 227

Conjunctival deposits
Epifrin ◉ 244
Propine with C Cap Compliance Cap ◉ 255
Solganal Suspension 2122

Conjunctival erythema
Cortisporin Ophthalmic Ointment Sterile 758
Cortisporin Ophthalmic Suspension Sterile 759
Ocusert Pilo-20 and Pilo-40 Ocular Therapeutic Systems ◉ 256

Conjunctival hyperemia
AK-Spore H.C. ◉ 206
AK-Spore ◉ 205
Alcaine ◉ 210
▲ Ciloxan Sterile Ophthalmic Solution (Less than 10%) ◉ 214
Epifrin ◉ 244
Fluoracaine ◉ 208
Natacyn (One case) ◉ 227
Ophthetic ◉ 249
Phospholine Iodide ◉ 315
Pilagan ◉ 250

Conjunctival injection
Azo Gantanol Tablets 1887
Azo Gantrisin Tablets 1888
Azulfidine Tablets, EN-tabs, Oral Suspension 1157
Bactrim DS Tablets 1891
Bactrim I.V. Infusion 1889
Bactrim 1891
Diupres Tablets 1461
Enduronyl 518
Fansidar Tablets 1896
Gantanol 1899
Gantrisin Ophthalmic Ointment/Solution 1900
Gantrisin 1901
Harmonyl Tablets 528
Hydropres Tablets 1485
Isopto Carbachol ◉ 219
Mintezol 1510
Opticrom 4% 986
Oreticyl 545
Pediazole 1973
Pepcid (Infrequent) 1524
Raudixin Tablets 1803
Rauzide Tablets 1804
▲ Rēv-Eyes Ophthalmic Eyedrops 0.5% (80%) ◉ 312
Salutensin/Salutensin-Demi 719
Septra 813
Septra I.V. Infusion 808

Septra I.V. Infusion ADD-Vantage Vials 810
Septra 813
Ser-Ap-Es Tablets 881
Serpasil Tablets 883
Serpasil-Apresoline Tablets 884
Serpasil-Esidrix Tablets 886
Thiosulfil Forte Tablets 2526

Conjunctival irritation
Ocusert Pilo-20 and Pilo-40 Ocular Therapeutic Systems ⊙ 256

Conjunctival microhemorrhage
IOPIDINE ⊙ 232

Conjunctival vascular congestion
Isopto Atropine ⊙ 218
Isopto Carpine ⊙ 219
Isopto Homatropine ⊙ 221
Isopto Hyoscine ⊙ 222
Pilocar ⊙ 275
Pilopine HS Gel ⊙ 227
Pilostat Sterile Ophthalmic Solution 0.5%, 1%, 2%, 3%, 4%, 5%, 6% ⊙ 263

Conjunctivitis
▲ Accutane Capsules (About 2 in 5) 1878
Adriamycin PFS (Rare) 561
Adriamycin RDF (Rare) 562
Anafranil Capsules (Up to 1%) 650
Ansaid Tablets (Less than 1%) 2319
Apresazide Capsules (Less frequent) 854
Apresoline Hydrochloride Parenteral (Ampuls) 856
Apresoline Hydrochloride Tablets (Less frequent) 855
Apresoline-Esidrix Tablets 857
BAL in Oil Ampules 661
Bretylol Injection (1 in 1000) 923
BuSpar (Infrequent) 1401
Cardura Tablets (1%) 1941
Cartrol Tablets (Less common) 507
Children's Advil Suspension (Less than 1%) 2426
Clinoril Tablets (Less than 1 in 100) 1433
Cyclogyl ⊙ 215
Cytosar-U Sterile Powder (Less frequent) 2329
Cytotec (Infrequent) 2159
DDAVP (Up to 2%) 1841
Diapid Nasal Spray (Infrequent) 2003
Doxorubicin Hydrochloride for Injection, USP (Rare) 622
Doxorubicin Hydrochloride Injection, USP (Rare) 848
Engerix-B Unit-Dose Vials 2213
Ergamisol Tablets (Less than 1 to 2%) 1136
Hismanal Tablets (1.2%) 1138
Hytrin Tablets (At least 1%) 529
Intron A (Up to 1%) 2097
Kerlone Tablets (Less than 2%) 2172
Lodine Capsules (Less than 1%) 2468
Lorelco Tablets 1333
M-M-R II 1494
Meclomen Capsules (Rare) 1739
Mesantoin Tablets 2013
Motrin Tablets (Less than 1%) 2351
Myochrysine Injection (Rare) 1516
NebuPent for Inhalation Solution (1% or less) 1017
Neosporin Ophthalmic Ointment Sterile 793
Neosporin Ophthalmic Solution Sterile 794
▲ Novantrone for Injection Concentrate (0 to 5%) 1226
OptiPranolol Sterile Ophthalmic Solution (A small number of patients) ⊙ 261
Orudis Capsules (Less than 1%) 2488
PediaProfen Suspension (Less than 1%) 1363
Permax Tablets (Infrequent) 1291
Proventil Syrup (Children 2-6: 1%) 2119
Prozac Pulvules (Infrequent) 920
▲ Ridaura Capsules (3 to 9%) 2224
Rifadin (Occasional) 1345
Rimactane Capsules 879
Robaxin Injectable 1871
Robaxin Tablets 1872
Rocaltrol Capsules 1913
Roferon-A Injection (Less than 3%) 1916
Rogaine Topical Solution (1.17%) 2357
Rubex (Rare) 739
Rufen Tablets (Less than 1%) 691
Sandimmune (2% or less) 2024
Sectral Capsules (Up to 2%) 2520
Ser-Ap-Es Tablets 881
Serpasil-Apresoline Tablets 884
Solganal Suspension (Rare) 2122
▲ Tegison Capsules (10-25%) 1881
Tegretol Chewable Tablets 654
Tegretol Suspension 656
Tegretol Tablets 654
Tenex Tablets 1875
Timoptic in Ocudose 1552
Timoptic Sterile Ophthalmic Solution 1550
Trental (Less than 1%) 1099
Vaseretic Tablets 1559
Vasotec I.V. 1562
Vasotec Tablets 1564
Ventolin Syrup (1% of children) 583
Vira-A Ophthalmic Ointment, 3% 1767
Virazole 1126
Zyloprim Tablets (Less than 1%) 830

Conjunctivitis, calcific
Calcijex Calcitriol Injection 506
Calderol Capsules 1635

Conjunctivitis, exudative
Rifamate Capsules (Occasional) 1347
Rimactane Capsules 879

Conjunctivitis, follicular
Atropine Sulfate Sterile Ophthalmic Solution and S.O.P. Sterile Ophthalmic Ointment ⊙ 239
Isopto Atropine ⊙ 218
Isopto Homatropine ⊙ 221
Isopto Hyoscine ⊙ 222
Propine with C Cap Compliance Cap (Infrequent) ⊙ 255

Conjunctivitis, hemorrhagic
Anafranil Capsules (Rare) 650
Cytosar-U Sterile Powder (With experimental doses) 2329

Conjunctivitis sicca
Orudis Capsules (Less than 1%) 2488

Consciousness, disorders
Hexalen Capsules 2316

Consciousness, loss of
▲ Anestacon Solution (Among most common) 2394
Carbocaine Hydrochloride 3% Injection 956
Carbocaine Hydrochloride Injection 2043
Carbocaine Hydrochloride 2% with Neo-Cobefrin 956
Cipro I.V. (1% or less) 1592
Cipro Tablets 1589
Decadron Phosphate with Xylocaine Injection, Sterile 1451
Duranest Injections 624
Dyclone 0.5% and 1% Topical Solutions, USP 626
Fiorinal with Codeine Capsules 2008
Humulin 70/30, 100 Units 1267
Humulin BR, 100 Units 1268
Humulin L, 100 Units 1268
Humulin U, 100 Units 1272
Hyperstat I.V. Injection 2095
Intron A (Less than 1%) 2097
Marcaine Hydrochloride 0.5% with Epinephrine 1:200,000 (as bitartrate) 958
Marcaine Hydrochloride with Epinephrine 1:200,000 2055
Marcaine Hydrochloride Injection 2055
Marcaine Spinal 2058
Mexitil Capsules (Less than 1% or about 6 in 10,000) 680
Nescaine/Nescaine MPF 629
Noroxin Tablets 1519
Novocain Hydrochloride for Spinal Anesthesia 2065
Pontocaine Hydrochloride for Spinal Anesthesia 2069
Prostigmin Injectable 1120
Prostigmin Tablets 1121
Sensorcaine (Rare) 631
Sensorcaine-MPF Spinal (Rare) 634
Stelazine 2226
▲ Xylocaine Injections (Among most common) 637
Xylocaine Injections for Ventricular Arrhythmias 639
Xylocaine 2% Jelly 643
Xylocaine 5% Ointment 644
Xylocaine 10% Oral Spray 645
4% Xylocaine-MPF Sterile Solution 641
Xylocaine 2% Viscous Solution 646

Constipation
Actifed with Codeine Cough Syrup 752
Actigall Capsules 2280
Adalat Capsules (10 mg and 20 mg) (2% or less) 1587
Adipex-P Tablets and Capsules 1019
AeroBid Inhaler System (1-3%) 995
Akineton 1171
Aldoclor Tablets 1413
Aldomet Ester HCl Injection 1417
Aldomet Oral 1415
Aldoril Tablets 1418
Alferon N Injection (One patient) 1809
Alka-Seltzer Advanced Formula Antacid & Non-Aspirin Pain Reliever ▣ 620
Allbee C-800 Plus Iron Tablets ▣ 670
Altace Capsules (Less than 1%) 1086
ALternaGEL Liquid 1154
Alu-Cap Capsules 1309
Alurate Elixir (Less than 1 in 100) 1883
Alu-Tab Tablets 1309
▲ Anafranil Capsules (22% to 47%) 650
▲ Anaprox and Anaprox DS Tablets (3-9%) 2288
Anexsia 5/500 Tablets 2196
Anexsia 7.5/650 Tablets 2197
Ansaid Tablets (1-3%) 2319
Apresazide Capsules (Less frequent) 854
Apresoline Hydrochloride Tablets (Less frequent) 855
Apresoline-Esidrix Tablets 857
Arfonad Ampuls 1887
Artane 1195
▲ Asendin Tablets (12%) 1196
Astramorph/PF Injection, USP (Preservative-Free) 618
Atrovent Inhalation Aerosol (Less than 1 in 100) 675
Azdone Tablets 844
B & O No. 15A & No. 16A Supprettes 2395
Basaljel 2438
Benadryl Capsules 1691
Benadryl Injection 1692
Bentyl 1322
Biphetamine Capsules 973
Bontril Slow-Release 834
Brevibloc Injection (Less than 1%) 942
BuSpar (1%) 1401
Butazolidin Capsules & Tablets (Less than 1%) 1027
Butisol Sodium Elixir & Tablets (Less than 1 in 100) 2377
▲ Calan SR Caplets (7.3%) 2157
▲ Calan Tablets (7.3%) 2155
Calcidrine Syrup 506
Calcijex Calcitriol Injection 506
Calderol Capsules 1635
Cantil Tablets 1326
Capoten (0.5 to 2%) 2255
Capozide (0.5 to 2%) 2258
Carafate Tablets (2%) 1326
Cardene Capsules (0.6%) 2290
Cardizem Tablets-30 mg, 60 mg, 90 mg and 120 mg (Less than 1%) 1329
Cardizem SR Capsules-60 mg, 90 mg and 120 mg (1.6%) 1327
Cardura Tablets (1%) 1941
Cartrol Tablets (Rare) 507
Catapres Tablets (About 10 in 100 patients) 676
Catapres-TTS (1 of 101 patients) 677
Celontin (Frequent) 1692
Cheracol Cough Syrup 1853
Children's Advil Suspension (Less than 3%) 2426
▲ Cholybar (Most common) 1705
Cipro I.V. (1% or less) 1592
Cipro Tablets 1589
▲ Clinoril Tablets (3-9%) 1433
▲ Clozaril Tablets (More than 5 to 14%) 2000
Codiclear DH Syrup 845
Cogentin 1435
▲ Colestid Granules (1 in 10) 2328
▲ Combipres Tablets (About 10%) 678
Comhist LA Capsules 1618
Compazine 2201
▲ Cordarone Tablets (4 to 9%) 2446
Corgard Tablets (1 to 5 of 1000 patients) 701
Corzide Tablets (1 to 5 of 1000 patients) 702
Cystospaz 2395
Cytotec (1.1%) 2159
Dalgan Injection (Less than 1%) 620
Dalmane Capsules 1927
Danocrine Capsules 2046
Dantrium Capsules (Less frequent) 1619
Daranide Tablets 1445
Darbid Tablets 2205
Darvon-N/Darvocet-N 1254
Darvon 1256
Darvon-N Suspension & Tablets 1254
Deconamine 663
Demerol 2047
Depakene Capsules & Syrup 511
Depakote 512
Desoxyn Gradumet Tablets 514
Desyrel and Desyrel Dividose (Greater than 1%) 1404
Dexedrine 2206
Dilantin Infatabs 1710
Dilantin Kapseals 1708
Dilantin Parenteral 1712
Dilantin-30 Pediatric/Dilantin-125 Suspension 1713
Dilantin with Phenobarbital Kapseals 1715
Dilaudid Cough Syrup 1174
Dilaudid 1173
Dilaudid-HP Injection 1175
Dimetane-DC Cough Syrup 1857
Dimetane-DX Cough Syrup 1858
Ditropan 1332
Diucardin Tablets 2450
Diulo 2129
Diupres Tablets 1461
Diuril Oral Suspension 1464
Diuril Sodium Intravenous 1463
Diuril Tablets 1464
Dolobid Tablets (Greater than 1 in 100) 1465
Dolophine Hydrochloride Ampoules & Vials 1260
Dolophine Hydrochloride Tablets 1261
Donnatal 1858
Donnatal Extentabs 1859
Donnatal Tablets 1858
Donnazyme Tablets 1860
Doral Tablets 2383
▲ Duragesic Transdermal System (10% or more) 1133
Duramorph 960
Dyazide Capsules 2208
DynaCirc Capsules (0.5% to 1%) 2004
Elavil 2269
Eldepryl 2250
▲ Empirin with Codeine Phosphate Nos. 2, 3 & 4 (Among most frequent) 764
Endep Tablets 1927
Enduron Tablets 517
Enduronyl 518
Engerix-B Unit-Dose Vials (Less than 1%) 2213
Ergamisol Tablets (2 to 3%) 1136
Esidrix Tablets 863
Esimil Tablets 864
Etrafon 2087
Exna Tablets 1862
Fastin Capsules 2216
Feldene Capsules (1 to 3%) 1777
Feosol Capsules 2191
Feosol Elixir (Occasional) 2191
Feosol Tablets (Occasional) 2191
Fiorinal with Codeine Capsules 2008
Flagyl I.V. 2131
Flagyl Tablets 2170
Flexeril Tablets (1% to 3%) 1471
Floxin Tablets (Less than 1%) 1652
Ganite Injection 1016
Glucotrol (1 in 100) 1952
Halcion Tablets (Rare) 2340
Haldol Decanoate 1375
Haldol Injection, Tablets and Concentrate 1373
Hycodan Syrup, Tablets 927
Hycomine Syrup 927
Hydrea Capsules 728
HydroDIURIL Tablets 1484
Hydromox R Tablets 1209
Hydromox Tablets 1208
Hydropres Tablets 1485
▲ Hylorel Tablets (21.0%) 975
Hyperstat I.V. Injection 2095
Hytrin Tablets (At least 1%) 529
IFEX (Less than 1%) 729
Imodium Capsules 1139
Inderal 2459
Inderal LA Long Acting Capsules 2461
Inderide Tablets 2463
Inderide LA Long Acting Capsules 2465
Indocin Capsules (Greater than 1%) 1487

Indocin I.V. (1% to 3%) 1490
Indocin (Greater than 1%) 1487
Infumorph 200 and Infumorph 500 Sterile Solutions (Frequent) 962
▲ Intron A (Up to 10%) 2097
Inversine Tablets 1492
Ionamin Capsules 981
▲ Isoptin Oral Tablets (7.3%) 1179
▲ Isoptin SR Sustained Release Tablets (7.3%) 1181
Kayexalate 2053
Kemadrin Tablets 771
Kerlone Tablets (Less than 2%) 2172
Kinesed Tablets 2272
Klonopin Tablets 1902
Lamprene Capsules (Less than 1%) 1030
Larodopa Tablets (Infrequent) 1905
Lasix 1093
Levsin/Levsinex 2147
Librax Capsules (Infrequent) 1929
Libritabs Tablets (Isolated cases) 1930
Librium Capsules (Isolated cases) 1931
Librium Injectable (Isolated instances) 1932
▲ Limbitrol (Among most frequent) 1933
▲ Lioresal Tablets (2-6%) 1031
Lodine Capsules (More than 1% but less than 3%) 2468
Lopid Capsules and Tablets (1.4%) 1736
Lopressor Ampuls (1%) 1032
Lopressor HCT Tablets (1 in 100 patients) 1034
Lopressor Tablets (1%) 1032
Lortab ASA Tablets 2414
Lortab 2412
Lotensin Tablets 872
Loxitane 1213
Lozol Tablets (Less than 5%) 1843
▲ Ludiomil Tablets (6%) 874
Lupron Depot 7.5 mg 2311
▲ Lupron Injection (5% or more) 2310
▲ MS Contin Tablets (Among most frequent) 1814
▲ MSIR (Among most frequent) 1817
▲ Marplan Tablets (Among most frequent) 1906
Matulane Capsules 1907
Maxzide 1215
Mebaral Tablets (Less than 1 in 100) 2061
Meclomen Capsules (Greater than 1%) 1739
Mellaril 2011
Menrium Tablets (Rare) 1934
Mepergan Injection 2479
Methadone Hydrochloride Diskets 1284
Methadone Hydrochloride Oral Solution & Tablets 1987
▲ Mevacor Tablets (4.9%) 1505
▲ Mexitil Capsules (4%) 680
Midamor Tablets (Between 1% and 3%) 1508
Minipress Capsules (1-4%) 1778
Minizide Capsules (Rare) 1779
Moban Tablets & Concentrate (Occasional) 932
Moduretic Tablets (Less than or equal to 1%) 1510
Monopril Tablets (0.2 to 1.0%) 1406
Motofen Tablets (1 in 300) 836
Motrin Tablets (Less than 3%) 2351
Mykrox ½ mg Tablets (Less than 2%) 984
▲ Nalfon Pulvules & Tablets (7%) 919
▲ Naprosyn (3 to 9%) 2297
Nardil (Common) 1742
Naturetin Tablets (Occasional) 1789
Navane Capsules and Concentrate 1954
Navane Intramuscular 1956
Nembutal Sodium Capsules (Less than 1%) 534
Nembutal Sodium Solution (Less than 1%) 536
Nembutal Sodium Suppositories (Less than 1%) 538
Neo-Calglucon Syrup 2018
▲ Neupogen for Injection (5%) 595
Niclocide Chewable Tablets 1607
Nicorette 1335
Norflex 1314
Norgesic 1314
Normozide Tablets (Less than 1%) 2112
Noroxin Tablets (0.3% to 1%) 1519
▲ Norpace (11%) 2177
Norpramin Tablets 1340
Novahistine DH 1342
Novahistine Expectorant 1343
Nucofed Capsules 2219
Nucofed Expectorant 2219
Nucofed Pediatric Expectorant 2220
Nucofed Syrup 2219
Oncovin Solution Vials & Hyporets 1288
Optimine Tablets 2115
▲ Oramorph SR (Morphine Sulfate Sustained Release Tablets) (Among most frequent) 1988
Orap Tablets 1020
Oretic Tablets 544
Oreticyl 545
Ornade Spansule Capsules 2221
▲ Orudis Capsules (Greater than 3%) 2488
PBZ Tablets & Elixir 1037
PBZ-SR Tablets 1037
Pamelor 2019
Pantopon Injectable 1911
Papaverine Hydrochloride Vials and Ampoules 1290
▲ Paraplatin for Injection (6%) 735
▲ Parlodel (3-14%) 2020
Parnate Tablets 2222
Pavabid Capsules (Rare) 1344
Pavabid HP Capsulets (Rare) 1344
PediaProfen Suspension (Less than 3%) 1363
Pepcid (1.2%) 1524
Percocet Tablets 950
Percodan 951
Periactin 1525
▲ Permax Tablets (10.6%) 1291
Phenaphen with Codeine Capsules 1865
Phenaphen-650 with Codeine Tablets 1866
Phenergan with Codeine 2497
Phenergan VC with Codeine 2501
Phenobarbital Elixir and Tablets (Less than 1 in 100 patients) 1293
PhosLo Tablets 700
Plegine Tablets 2504
Plendil Extended-Release Tablets (0.1%) 1526
Polaramine 2116
Pondimin Tablets 1867
Ponstel (Less frequent) 1758
Prelu-2 Capsules 683
Prilosec Delayed-Release Capsules (0.9 to 1.5%) 1530
Prinivil Tablets (1% or less) 1538
Prinzide Tablets (0.3% to 1%) 1540
Pro-Banthīne Tablets 2141
Procardia Capsules (2% or less) 1781
▲ Procardia XL Tablets (3.3%) 1783
Prolixin Decanoate 1795
Prolixin Elixir 1793
Prolixin Enanthate 1796
Prolixin Injection 1791
Prolixin Oral Concentrate 1792
Prolixin Tablets 1793
ProSom Tablets (Frequent) 554
Protostat Tablets 1674
▲ Prozac Pulvules (4.5%) 920
Quarzan Capsules (Among most frequent) 1937
Quelidrine Syrup 556
▲ Questran Light (Most common) 711
Questran Powder 710
Rauzide Tablets 1804
Renese Tablets 1785
▲ Retrovir Capsules (6.4%) 802
Retrovir I.V. Infusion (Less than 5%) 805
▲ Retrovir Syrup (6.4%) 802
Ridaura Capsules (1 to 3%) 2224
Robaxisal Tablets 1872
Robinul Forte Tablets 1873
Robinul Injectable 1873
Robinul Tablets 1873
Robitussin A-C Syrup 1875
Robitussin-DAC Syrup 1875
Rocaltrol Capsules 1913
Roferon-A Injection (Less than 3%) 1916
Rowasa (0.98%) 2248
Roxanol 1991
Roxicodone Tablets, Oral Solution & Intensol (Oxycodone) 1992
Rufen Tablets (1 to 3%) 691
Ru-Tuss II Capsules 693
Ru-Tuss with Hydrocodone 694
Ru-Tuss Tablets 693
Ryna ..... ▣ 741
▲ Rythmol Tablets (2.0 to 7.2%) 1184
Saluron 718
Salutensin/Salutensin-Demi 719
Sandimmune (Rare) 2024
Sandostatin Injection (Less than 1%) 2029
▲ Sanorex Tablets (Among most common) 2030
Sansert Tablets 2031
Seconal Sodium Pulvules (Less than 1 in 100) 1296
▲ Sectral Capsules (4%) 2520
Ser-Ap-Es Tablets 881
Serentil 686
Serpasil-Apresoline Tablets 884
Serpasil-Esidrix Tablets 886
Sinemet Tablets 952
Sinemet CR Tablets (0.2%) 953
Sinequan 1960
Sodium Polystyrene Sulfonate Suspension 1993
Soma Compound w/Codeine Tablets 2390
Soma Compound Tablets 2389
Stelazine 2226
Surmontil Capsules 2524
Symmetrel Capsules & Syrup (1-5%) 936
Synalgos-DC Capsules 2525
Tacaryl 2409
Talacen (Infrequent) 2070
Talwin Injection (Infrequent) 2071
Talwin Compound (Infrequent) 2072
Talwin Injection (Infrequent) 2071
Talwin Nx 2073
▲ Tambocor Tablets (4.4%) 1315
Taractan (Occasional) 1920
Tavist Syrup 2033
Tavist Tablets 2035
Tavist-D Tablets 2035
Tegison Capsules (Less than 1%) 1881
Tegretol Chewable Tablets 654
Tegretol Suspension 656
Tegretol Tablets 654
Temaril Tablets, Syrup and Spansule Sustained Release Capsules 1085
Tenex Tablets (1%) 1875
Tenoretic Tablets 1105
Tenuate 1354
Tessalon Perles 1006
Thalitone Tablets 687
TheraCys BCG Live (Intravesical) (Up to 0.9%) 898
Theragran Hematinic Tablets 605
Thorazine 2234
Timolide Tablets (Less than 1%) 1547
Tofranil Ampuls 1038
Tofranil Tablets 1039
Tofranil-PM Capsules 1041
Tolectin (200, 400 and 600 mg) (1 to 3%) 1379
Tonocard Tablets (Less than 1%) 1554
Toradol IM Injection (1% or less) 2302
Trandate HCT Tablets (Less than 1% in 208 patients) 579
Trental (Less than 1%) 1099
▲ Trexan Tablets (Less than 10%) 937
Triaminic Expectorant w/Codeine 1996
▲ Triaminic Expectorant DH (Among most frequent) 1995
Triaminic Oral Infant Drops 1996
Triavil Tablets 1556
Trilafon (Occasional) 2123
▲ Trilisate (Less than 20%) 1822
Trinalin Repetabs Tablets 1170
Trinsicon Capsules (Rare) 2415
Troph-Iron Liquid (Occasional) ..... ▣ 619
Tussionex Extended-Release Suspension 988
Tussi-Organidin Liquid 2391
Tuss-Ornade Liquid 2242
Tuss-Ornade Spansule Capsules 2242
Tylenol with Codeine 1381
Tylox Capsules 1382
Valium Injectable 1937
Valium Tablets (Infrequent) 1939
Valpin 50 Tablets 941
Valrelease Capsules (Occasional) 1923
Vascor (200, 300 and 400 mg) Tablets (0.5 to 2.84%) 1383
Vaseretic Tablets (0.5% to 2.0%) 1559
Vasotec I.V. (0.5 to 1%) 1562
Vasotec Tablets (0.5% to 1%) 1564
▲ Velban Vials (Among most common) 1305
VePesid Capsules and Injection (Infrequent) 741
▲ Verelan Capsules (7.3%) 1243
Vicodin Tablets 1187
Vicodin ES Tablets 1189
Vivactil Tablets 1567
▲ Voltaren Tablets (3% to 9%) 1042
▲ Wellbutrin Tablets (26.0%) 821
Wygesic Tablets 2540
Wytensin Tablets (3% or less) 2542
▲ Xanax Tablets (10.4% to 26.2%) 2367
Yutopar (Infrequent) 647
Zantac Injection and Zantac Injection Premixed 1063
Zantac 1065
Zaroxolyn Tablets 989
Zestoretic (0.3 to 1%) 2274
Zestril Tablets (Less than 1%) 2277
▲ Zofran Injection (11%) 1069
Zoladex (1% to 5%) 1110
Zovirax (0.9%) 824
Zydone Capsules 941

Constriction, pupillary (see under Miosis)

Constriction, pupils (see under Miosis)

Contact lenses, intolerance

Accutane Capsules 1878
Brevicon 2304
Demulen 2161
Diethylstilbestrol Tablets 1258
Enovid 2161
Estinyl Tablets 2085
Estrace 1385
Estrace Vaginal Cream 1388
Estraderm Transdermal System 866
Estradurin 2452
Estratest 2245
Estrovis 1721
Jenest-28 Tablets 1636
Levlen/Tri-Levlen 665
Lo/Ovral Tablets 2471
Lo/Ovral-28 Tablets 2476
Loestrin 1728
Mediatric Capsules 2476
Menrium Tablets 1934
Micronor Tablets 1667
Modicon 1667
Nordette-21 Tablets 2481
Nordette-28 Tablets 2483
Norethin 2133
Norinyl 2304
Norlestrin 1746
Nor-Q D Tablets 2304
Ogen 540
Ortho Dienestrol Cream 1664
Ortho-Cyclen Tablets 1658
Ortho-Novum 1667
Ovcon 1391
Ovral Tablets 2490
Ovral-28 Tablets 2491
Ovrette Tablets 2492
PMB 200 and PMB 400 2504
Premarin Intravenous 2508
Premarin with Methyltestosterone 2515
Premarin Tablets 2510
Premarin Vaginal Cream 2512
Stilphostrol Tablets and Ampuls 1609
TACE 12 and 25 mg 1353
Levlen/Tri-Levlen 665
Tri-Norinyl 2304

Contact lens staining

Pyridium 1763
Pyridium Plus 1764

Convulsions

Actifed with Codeine Cough Syrup 752
AK-Fluor Injection 10% and 25% ..... ⊙ 204
Altace Capsules 1086
Amicar Syrup, Tablets, and Injection (Two cases) 1194
Anafranil Capsules (Infrequent) 650
Ana-Kit Anaphylaxis Emergency Treatment Kit (Occasional) 1100
▲ Anestacon Solution (Among most common) 2394
Ansaid Tablets (Less than 1%) 2319
Antilirium Injectable 998
Aralen Hydrochloride Injection 2038
Aristocort Suspension 1008
Aristospan Suspension 1011
Astramorph/PF Injection, USP (Preservative-Free) 618
Atabrine Hydrochloride Tablets (Rare) 2041
Atarax Tablets & Syrup 1941
Atrohist Sprinkle Capsules 558
Attenuvax (Rare) 1424
Azo Gantanol Tablets 1887
Azo Gantrisin Tablets 1888
Azulfidine Tablets, EN-tabs, Oral Suspension (Rare) 1157
Bactrim DS Tablets 1891
Bactrim I.V. Infusion 1889
Bactrim 1891
Benadryl Capsules 1691
Benadryl Injection 1692
Biavax II (Rare) 1427
Brevital Sodium Vials 1248

Carbocaine Hydrochloride 3% Injection 956
Carbocaine Hydrochloride Injection 2043
Carbocaine Hydrochloride 2% with Neo-Cobefrin 956
Celestone Soluspan Suspension 2081
Clinoril Tablets (Less than 1%) 1433
▲ Clozaril Tablets (3%) 2000
Comhist LA Capsules 1618
Compazine 2201
Constant-T Tablets 1029
Cortenema (Rare) 2244
Cortone Acetate Sterile Suspension 1437
Cortone Acetate Tablets 1439
Dalalone D.P. Injectable 999
Daraprim Tablets 761
Decadron Elixir 1445
Decadron Phosphate Injection 1449
Decadron Phosphate Respihaler 1454
Decadron Phosphate Turbinaire 1456
Decadron Phosphate with Xylocaine Injection, Sterile 1451
Decadron Tablets 1447
Decadron-LA Sterile Suspension 1457
Deconamine 663
Deconsal 559
Deltasone Tablets 2332
Demerol 2047
Depo-Medrol Sterile Aqueous Suspension 2334
Diamox Parenteral (Occasional) 1200
Diamox Sequels (Sustained Release) 1201
Diamox Tablets (Occasional) 1200
Dimetane-DC Cough Syrup 1857
Dimetane-DX Cough Syrup 1858
Diphtheria and Tetanus Toxoids and Pertussis Vaccine Adsorbed USP (For Pediatric Use) (Infrequent) 892
Diprivan Injection 2267
Dopram Injectable 1860
Duramorph 960
Duranest Injections 624
Dyclone 0.5% and 1% Topical Solutions, USP 626
Enlon Injection 598
Ergamisol Tablets (Less frequent) 1136
Fansidar Tablets 1896
Fedahist Gyrocaps 2145
Fedahist Timecaps 2145
Flexeril Tablets (Less than 1%) 1471
Floxin Tablets 1652
Fluorescite ⊙ 217
Fungizone Intravenous 2262
Gantanol 1899
Gantrisin Ophthalmic Ointment/Solution 1900
Gantrisin 1901
Garamycin Injectable 2093
HibTITER 1206
Hismanal Tablets (Isolated cases) 1138
Humulin 70/30, 100 Units 1267
Humulin BR, 100 Units 1268
Humulin L, 100 Units 1268
Humulin U, 100 Units 1272
Hydeltrasol Injection, Sterile 1476
Hydeltra-T.B.A. Sterile Suspension 1478
Hydrea Capsules (Extremely rare) 728
Hydrocortone Acetate Sterile Suspension 1479
Hydrocortone Phosphate Injection, Sterile 1481
Hydrocortone Tablets 1482
Hyperstat I.V. Injection 2095
Hyskon Hysteroscopy Fluid (Rare) 1162
INH Tablets (Uncommon) 868
Imferon 976
Indocin Capsules (Less than 1%) 1487
Indocin I.V. (Less than 1%) 1490
Indocin (Less than 1%) 1487
Infumorph 200 and Infumorph 500 Sterile Solutions 962
Inversine Tablets 1492
Kenalog-10 Injection 2402
Kenalog-40 Injection 2403
Kinesed Tablets 2272
Kwell Cream (Rare) 1830
Kwell Lotion (Rare) 1831
Kwell Shampoo (Rare) 1832
Larodopa Tablets (Rare) 1905
Leukeran Tablets (Rare) 788
Lopid Capsules and Tablets 1736
Lufyllin-GG Elixir & Tablets 2385
M-M-R II (Rare) 1494
M-R-VAX II (Rare) 1496
Marcaine Hydrochloride 0.5% with Epinephrine 1:200,000 (as bitartrate) 958
Marcaine Hydrochloride with Epinephrine 1:200,000 2055
Marcaine Hydrochloride Injection 2055
Marcaine Spinal 2058
Matulane Capsules 1907
Medrol 2348
Methotrexate Tablets, Parenteral, LPF Parenteral 1217
Mexitil Capsules (About 2 in 1,000) 680
Mintezol 1510
Naldecon Syrup, Tablets, Pediatric Drops and Pediatric Syrup 709
Nardil (Less frequent) 1742
NegGram (Rare) 2062
Nescaine/Nescaine MPF 629
Netromycin Injection 100 mg/ml 2104
Nicorette 1335
Noroxin Tablets 1519
Norzine 1818
Novafed A Capsules 1342
Novafed Capsules 1342
Novahistine DH 1342
Novahistine DMX ▣ 595
Novahistine Elixir ▣ 596
Novahistine Expectorant 1343
Novocain Hydrochloride for Spinal Anesthesia 2065
Omnipaque (Less than 0.1 to 0.3%) 2552
Oncovin Solution Vials & Hyporets (A few patients) 1288
Optimine Tablets 2115
Ornade Spansule Capsules 2221
Oxytocin Injection 2492
PBZ Tablets & Elixir 1037
PBZ-SR Tablets 1037
Pediapred Oral Liquid 987
Pediazole 1973
Periactin 1525
Permax Tablets (Infrequent) 1291
Pfizerpen for Injection 1957
Phenergan with Codeine 2497
Phenergan VC with Codeine 2501
Pitocin Injection, Ampoules, Steri-Dose Syringes 1757
Plaquenil Sulfate Tablets 2067
Polaramine 2116
Pontocaine Hydrochloride for Spinal Anesthesia 2069
Procan SR Tablets (Infrequent) 1760
Prostigmin Injectable 1120
Prostigmin Tablets 1121
Prozac Pulvules (Infrequent) 920
Rheumatrex Methotrexate Dose Pack 1234
Rifamate Capsules (Uncommon) 1347
Rondec 1975
Rondec-DM 1976
Rondec-TR Tablet 1975
Ru-Tuss DE Tablets 694
Ru-Tuss II Capsules 693
▲ Sandimmune (1 to 5%) 2024
Sandostatin Injection (Less than 1%) 2029
Seldane-D Extended-Release Tablets 1350
Sensorcaine (0.1%) 631
Sensorcaine-MPF Spinal (0.1%) 634
Septra 813
Septra I.V. Infusion 808
Septra I.V. Infusion ADD-Vantage Vials 810
Septra 813
Seromycin Pulvules 1298
Sinemet Tablets 952
Sinemet CR Tablets 953
Slo-bid Gyrocaps 1847
Solu-Cortef Sterile Powder 2361
Solu-Medrol Sterile Powder 2363
Stelazine 2226
Symmetrel Capsules & Syrup (Less than 0.1%) 936
Tambocor Tablets (Less than 1%) 1315
Taractan 1920
Tavist Syrup 2033
Tavist Tablets 2035
Tavist-D Tablets 2035
Tensilon Injectable 1123
Tenuate 1354
Thiosulfil Forte Tablets 2526
Ticar for Injection (With very high doses) 2236
Tigan 2239
Tofranil Ampuls 1038
Tofranil Tablets 1039
Tonocard Tablets (Less than 1%) 1554
Torecan 1993
Triaminic Expectorant DH 1995
Triaminic Oral Infant Drops 1996
Tri-Immunol Diphtheria & Tetanus Toxoids & Pertussis Vaccine, Adsorbed (1 per 1,750) 1241
Trinalin Repetabs Tablets 1170
Velban Vials 1305
Vistaril Capsules (Rare) 1789
Vistaril Intramuscular Solution (Rare) 1970
Vistaril Oral Suspension (Rare) 1789
Voltaren Tablets (Less than 1%) 1042
▲ Xylocaine Injections (Among most common) 637
Xylocaine Injections for Ventricular Arrhythmias 639
Xylocaine 2% Jelly 643
Xylocaine 5% Ointment 644
Xylocaine 10% Oral Spray 645
4% Xylocaine-MPF Sterile Solution 641
Xylocaine 2% Viscous Solution 646
Zovirax Sterile Powder 828

Convulsions, clonic

Aminophyllin Tablets 2153
Asbron G 1997
Choledyl Pediatric Elixir 1702
Choledyl Tablets 1700
Choledyl SA Tablets 1704
Cocaine Hydrochloride Topical Solution 620
Dilor 2079
Lufyllin & Lufyllin-400 Tablets 2384
Lufyllin-GG Elixir & Tablets 2385
M-M-R II (Rare) 1494
Quadrinal Tablets 1183
Quibron Capsules 713
Quibron-T 714
Quibron-T/SR 716
Respbid Tablets 684
Seromycin Pulvules 1298
Slo-bid Gyrocaps 1847
T-PHYL (Uniphyl) 200 mg Tablets 1820
Theo-24 2179
Theo-Dur Sprinkle 1168
Theo-Dur Extended-Release Tablets 1166
Theolair 1317
Theolair-SR Tablets 1319
▲ TheoX Extended-Release Tablets (Among most consistent) 841
Uniphyl 400 mg Tablets 1823

Convulsions, epileptiform

Atabrine Hydrochloride Tablets 2041

Convulsions, grand mal

Compazine 2201
Stelazine 2226
Triavil Tablets 1556

Convulsions, major

Compazine Ampuls 2201
Dilantin Parenteral 1712
Methotrexate Tablets, Parenteral, LPF Parenteral (Occasional) 1217
Rheumatrex Methotrexate Dose Pack (Occasional) 1234
Seromycin Pulvules 1298

Convulsions, spinal

Omnipaque (Unusual) 2552

Convulsions, tonic generalized

Aminophyllin Tablets 2153
Asbron G 1997
Choledyl Pediatric Elixir 1702
Choledyl Tablets 1700
Choledyl SA Tablets 1704
Cocaine Hydrochloride Topical Solution 620
Dilor 2079
Lufyllin & Lufyllin-400 Tablets 2384
Lufyllin-GG Elixir & Tablets 2385
Quadrinal Tablets 1183
Quibron Capsules 713
Quibron-T 714
Quibron-T/SR 716
Respbid Tablets 684
Slo-bid Gyrocaps 1847
T-PHYL (Uniphyl) 200 mg Tablets 1820
Theo-24 2179
Theo-Dur Sprinkle 1168
Theo-Dur Extended-Release Tablets 1166
Theolair 1317
Theolair-SR Tablets 1319
▲ TheoX Extended-Release Tablets (Among most consistent) 841
Uniphyl 400 mg Tablets 1823

Coombs' test, positive

Aldoclor Tablets 1413
Aldomet Ester HCl Injection 1417
Aldomet Oral 1415
Aldoril Tablets 1418
Azactam for Injection 2252
Catapres Tablets 676
Catapres-TTS 677
Ceclor Pulvules & Suspension (Less than 1 in 200) 1251
Cefizox Injection (Some patients) 1012
Cefobid Intravenous/Intramuscular (1 in 60) 1943
Cefobid Pharmacy Bulk Package - Not for Direct Infusion (1 in 60) 1945
Cefotan (1 in 250) 2265
Ceftin Tablets (0.4%) 575
Ceptaz for Injection (One in 23) 1057
Children's Advil Suspension (Less than 1%) 2426
Claforan Sterile Injection (Less than 1%) 1089
Combipres Tablets 678
▲ Fortaz (1 in 23) 1060
Kefurox Vials, Faspak & ADD-Vantage (Less than 1 in 250) 1277
Kefzol Vials, Faspak & ADD-Vantage 1279
Larodopa Tablets 1905
Mandol Vials, Faspak & ADD-Vantage 1281
Mefoxin 1498
Mefoxin Premixed Intravenous Solution 1500
Mezlin 1597
Mezlin Pharmacy Bulk Package 1599
Monocid Injection (Less than 1%) 2217
Motrin Tablets (Less than 1%) 2351
PediaProfen Suspension (Less than 1%) 1363
Pipracil (Less frequent) 1230
Platinol 737
Platinol-AQ Injection 738
Ponstel 1758
Primaxin I.M. 1532
Primaxin I.V. 1535
Procan SR Tablets (Rare) 1760
Procardia XL Tablets 1783
Rufen Tablets (Less than 1%) 691
Sinemet Tablets 952
Sinemet CR Tablets 953
Suprax 1235
▲ Tazicef for Injection (1 in 23 patients) 2231
▲ Tazidime Vials, Faspak & ADD-Vantage (1 in 23) 1299
Zefazone Sterile Powder 2372
Zinacef (Less than 1 in 250 patients) 1066

Coordination, disturbed (see under Coordination, impaired)

Coordination, impaired

▲ Actifed with Codeine Cough Syrup (Among most frequent) 752
Anafranil Capsules (Infrequent) 650
Atrovent Inhalation Aerosol (Less than 1 in 100) 675
▲ Benadryl Capsules (Among most frequent) 1691
▲ Benadryl Injection (Among most frequent) 1692
Cibalith-S 870
Clozaril Tablets (Less than 1%) 2000
▲ Cordarone Tablets (4 to 9%) 2446
Deconamine 663
Dilantin Infatabs 1710
Dilantin Kapseals 1708
Dilantin-30 Pediatric/Dilantin-125 Suspension 1713
Dilantin with Phenobarbital Kapseals 1715
Dimetane-DX Cough Syrup 1858
Duragesic Transdermal System (1% or greater) 1133
Ethmozine Tablets (Less than 2%) 946
▲ Halcion Tablets (4.6%) 2340
Intron A (Less than 1%) 2097
Lioresal Tablets 1031
Lithium Carbonate Capsules & Tablets 1984
Lithobid Tablets 870
Marinol (Dronabinol) Capsules 1985
▲ Mexitil Capsules (9.4% to 10.2%) 680
▲ Optimine Tablets (Among most frequent) 2115
Ornade Spansule Capsules 2221
PBZ Tablets & Elixir (Among most frequent) 1037

PBZ-SR Tablets (Among most frequent) 1037
Pamelor 2019
Periactin 1525
Polaramine 2116
▲ ProSom Tablets (4%) 554
Roferon-A Injection (Less than 0.5%) 1916
Ru-Tuss II Capsules 693
▲ Tavist Syrup (Among most frequent) 2033
▲ Tavist Tablets (Among most frequent) 2035
▲ Tavist-D Tablets (Among most frequent) 2035
Tegretol Chewable Tablets 654
Tegretol Suspension 656
Tegretol Tablets 654
Tofranil Ampuls 1038
Tofranil Tablets 1039
Tofranil-PM Capsules 1041
Tonocard Tablets (0.0-1.2%) 1554
▲ Triaminic Expectorant DH (Among most frequent) 1995
▲ Triaminic Oral Infant Drops (Among most frequent) 1996
Triavil Tablets 1556
▲ Trinalin Repetabs Tablets (Among most frequent) 1170
Voltaren Tablets (Rare) 1042
▲ Xanax Tablets (40.1%) 2367

Coordination, lack of (see under Ataxia)

Coordination difficulty (see under Coordination, impaired)

Cornea, discoloration

Mellaril 2011
Norzine 1818
Serentil 686
Torecan 1993

Cornea, fungal infections

AK-Cide Sterile Ophthalmic Ointment & Suspension .... ⊙ 202
AK-Dex .... ⊙ 203
AK-Pred .... ⊙ 205
AK-Spore H.C. .... ⊙ 206
AK-Trol Ointment & Suspension .... ⊙ 207
Metimyd .... ⊙ 306
NeoDecadron Sterile Ophthalmic Ointment 1517
NeoDecadron Sterile Ophthalmic Solution 1518
Pred Mild .... ⊙ 254
Pred-G Liquifilm Sterile Ophthalmic Suspension .... ⊙ 252
Terra-Cortril Ophthalmic Suspension 1963
TobraDex Ophthalmic Suspension and Ointment .... ⊙ 228

Cornea, gray, ground-glass appearance

Alcaine .... ⊙ 210

Cornea, opacities

▲ Accutane Capsules (5 in 72) 1878
AK-Taine .... ⊙ 207
Alcaine .... ⊙ 210
Ansaid Tablets (Less than 1%) 2319
Fluoracaine .... ⊙ 208
Mellaril 2011
Ophthetic .... ⊙ 249
Plaquenil Sulfate Tablets 2067
Prolixin Decanoate 1795
Prolixin Elixir 1793
Prolixin Enanthate 1796
Prolixin Injection 1791
Prolixin Tablets 1793
Serentil 686
Tacaryl 2409
Torecan 1993

Cornea, sensitization

Akarpine Ophthalmic Solution (Occasional) .... ⊙ 201

Cornea, white crystalline precipitates, presence of

▲ Ciloxan Sterile Ophthalmic Solution (Approximately 17%) .... ⊙ 214

Corneal abrasion

Ocusert Pilo-20 and Pilo-40 Ocular Therapeutic Systems .... ⊙ 256

Corneal changes

Aralen Phosphate with Primaquine Phosphate Tablets 2040
Aralen Phosphate Tablets 2039
Azulfidine Tablets, EN-tabs, Oral Suspension 1157
Cocaine Hydrochloride Topical Solution 620
Nolvadex Tablets 1102
Plaquenil Sulfate Tablets 2067
Prozac Pulvules (Rare) 920
▲ Tegison Capsules (10-25%) 1881

Corneal clouding

▲ CHEMET (succimer) Capsules (1.0 to 3.7%) 1361
Cocaine Hydrochloride Topical Solution 620
Herplex Liquifilm (Occasional) .... ⊙ 248
Miochol with Iocare Steri-Tags, Miochol System Pak and Miochol System Pak Plus (Infrequent) .... ⊙ 274
MIOSTAT (Occasional) .... ⊙ 233

Corneal curvature, steepening

Brevicon 2304
Demulen 2161
Diethylstilbestrol Tablets 1258
Enovid 2161
Estinyl Tablets 2085
Estraderm Transdermal System 866
Estradurin 2452
Estratest 2245
Estrovis 1721
Jenest-28 Tablets 1636
Levlen/Tri-Levlen 665
Lo/Ovral Tablets 2471
Lo/Ovral-28 Tablets 2476
Loestrin 1728
Mediatric Capsules 2476
Micronor Tablets 1667
Modicon 1667
Nordette-21 Tablets 2481
Nordette-28 Tablets 2483
Norethin 2133
Norinyl 2304
Norlestrin 1746
Nor-Q D Tablets 2304
Ogen 540
Ortho Dienestrol Cream 1664
Ortho-Cyclen Tablets 1658
Ortho-Novum 1667
Ovral Tablets 2490
Ovral-28 Tablets 2491
Ovrette Tablets 2492
PMB 200 and PMB 400 2504
Premarin Intravenous 2508
Premarin with Methyltestosterone 2515
Premarin Tablets 2510
Premarin Vaginal Cream 2512
Stilphostrol Tablets and Ampuls 1609
TACE 12 and 25 mg 1353
Levlen/Tri-Levlen 665
Tri-Norinyl 2304
Triphasil-21 Tablets 2527
Triphasil-28 Tablets 2532

Corneal decompensation

AMVISC Plus .... ⊙ 323
BSS (15 mL & 30 mL) Sterile Irrigation Solution .... ⊙ 230
BSS (250 mL) Sterile Irrigation Solution .... ⊙ 231
BSS (500 mL) Sterile Irrigation Solution .... ⊙ 231
BSS PLUS (500 mL) Sterile Irrigation Solution .... ⊙ 231
Healon (Rare) .... ⊙ 279
Miochol with Iocare Steri-Tags, Miochol System Pak and Miochol System Pak Plus (Infrequent) .... ⊙ 274

Corneal deposits

Atabrine Hydrochloride Tablets 2041
Compazine 2201
Cordarone Tablets 2446
Epifrin .... ⊙ 244
Indocin (Less than 1%) 1487
Plaquenil Sulfate Tablets 2067
Prolixin Oral Concentrate 1792
Propine with C Cap Compliance Cap .... ⊙ 255
Ridaura Capsules (Less than 1%) 2224
Solganal Suspension 2122
Stelazine 2226
Taractan 1920
Thorazine 2234
Trilafon 2123

Corneal infiltrate

Ciloxan Sterile Ophthalmic Solution (Less than 1%) .... ⊙ 214

Corneal pitting

Cocaine Hydrochloride Topical Solution 620

Corneal punctate, defects

Herplex Liquifilm (Occasional) .... ⊙ 248

Corneal punctate staining

Ophthocort .... ⊙ 301

Corneal punctate keratitis

Betoptic Sterile Ophthalmic Solution (Rare) 569
Betoptic S Sterile Ophthalmic Suspension (Rare) 570

Corneal sensitivity, decrease

Betagan (A small number of patients) .... ⊙ 239
Betoptic Sterile Ophthalmic Solution (Small numbers of patients) 569
Betoptic S Sterile Ophthalmic Suspension (Small numbers of patients) 570
Plaquenil Sulfate Tablets 2067
Timoptic in Ocudose 1552
Timoptic Sterile Ophthalmic Solution 1550

Corneal staining

Ciloxan Sterile Ophthalmic Solution (Less than 1%) .... ⊙ 214
Mydriacyl .... ⊙ 225
Tropicacyl .... ⊙ 209

Corneal stippling

Herplex Liquifilm (Occasional) .... ⊙ 248

Corneal toxicity

Cytosar-U Sterile Powder (With experimental doses) 2329

Corneal ulceration

Cocaine Hydrochloride Topical Solution 620
Oculinum for Injecton 587

Coronary artery disease, aggravation

Oncovin Solution Vials & Hyporets 1288
Tegretol Chewable Tablets 654
Tegretol Suspension 656
Tegretol Tablets 654
Vasotec I.V. 1562

Coronary thrombosis

Demulen 2161
Enovid 2161
Levlen/Tri-Levlen 665
Lo/Ovral Tablets 2471
Lo/Ovral-28 Tablets 2476
Micronor Tablets 1667
Modicon 1667
Nordette-21 Tablets 2481
Nordette-28 Tablets 2483
Norethin 2133
Ortho-Novum 1667
Ovral Tablets 2490
Ovral-28 Tablets 2491
Ovrette Tablets 2492
Stilphostrol Tablets and Ampuls 1609
Levlen/Tri-Levlen 665
Triphasil-21 Tablets 2527
Triphasil-28 Tablets 2532

Cortical lens opacities, scattered punctate

Tegretol Chewable Tablets 654
Tegretol Suspension 656
Tegretol Tablets 654

Cortical proliferation of long bones

Prostin VR Pediatric Sterile Solution 2355

Coryza

Quadrinal Tablets 1183

Costovertebral pain

Benemid Tablets 1426
ColBENEMID Tablets 1436

Cough

Actigall Capsules 2280
▲ Adalat Capsules (10 mg and 20 mg) (6%) 1587
▲ AeroBid Inhaler System (3-9%) 995
Alferon N Injection (One patient) 1809
▲ Altace Capsules (Almost 12%) 1086
Alupent (1 to 4%) 674
▲ Anafranil Capsules (4% to 6%) 650
Antivenin (Crotalidae) Polyvalent 2430
Atgam Sterile Solution (Less than 5%) 2320
▲ Atrovent Inhalation Aerosol (5.9%) 675
Azmacort Inhaler 1837
Azo Gantrisin Tablets 1888
Blocadren Tablets 1429
Capoten (0.5 to 2%) 2255
Capozide (0.5 to 2%) 2258
Cardura Tablets (Less than 0.5% of 3960 patients) 1941
Cartrol Tablets (Less common) 507
Cerose-DM 2443
▲ CHEMET (succimer) Capsules (0.7 to 3.7%) 1361
Clozaril Tablets (Less than 1%) 2000
▲ Cordarone Tablets (2% to 7%) 2446
Corgard Tablets (1 to 5 of 1000 patients) 701
Corzide Tablets (1 to 5 of 1000 patients) 702
Decadron Phosphate Respihaler 1454
Depen Titratable Tablets 2379
Diapid Nasal Spray 2003
Diprivan Injection (Greater than 1%) 2267
Dopram Injectable 1860
DynaCirc Capsules (0.5% to 1%) 2004
▲ Epogen for Injection (18%) 591
▲ Ergamisol Tablets (3 to 5%) 1136
Ethmozine Tablets (Less than 2%) 946
Floxin Tablets (Less than 1%) 1652
▲ Hylorel Tablets (26.9%) 975
Hyperstat I.V. Injection 2095
Hyskon Hysteroscopy Fluid (Rare) 1162
Hytrin Tablets (At least 1%) 529
Intal Capsules (Less than 1 in 10,000 patients to 1 in 5 patients) 978
Intal Inhaler (Frequent) 979
Intal Nebulizer Solution 980
▲ Intron A (Up to 31%) 2097
Kerlone Tablets (Less than 2%) 2172
Levatol (2.1%) 1832
Lotensin Tablets (1.9%) 872
▲ Lupron Depot 3.75 mg (Among most frequent) 2312
Lupron Depot 7.5 mg 2311
Lupron Injection (Less than 5%) 2310
Macrodantin Capsules (Common) 1624
Matulane Capsules 1907
Maxair Inhaler (1.2%) 1311
Metaprel Inhalation Aerosol Bronchodilator (1 to 4%) 2014
Methotrexate Tablets, Parenteral, LPF Parenteral (Less common) 1217
Midamor Tablets (Between 1% and 3%) 1508
Moduretic Tablets 1510
Monopril Tablets 1406
Mumpsvax 1513
Mykrox ½ mg Tablets (Less than 2%) 984
Nasalcrom Nasal Solution 986
▲ NebuPent for Inhalation Solution (38%) 1017
▲ Neupogen for Injection (6%) 595
Nicorette 1335
▲ Nolvadex Tablets (6%) 1102
▲ Novantrone for Injection Concentrate (9 to 13%) 1226
Omnipaque (0.2% or less) 2552
OptiPranolol Sterile Ophthalmic Solution (A small number of patients) .... ⊙ 261
Plendil Extended-Release Tablets 1526
Prilosec Delayed-Release Capsules 1530
▲ Prinivil Tablets (2.9% to 4.5%) 1538
▲ Prinzide Tablets (3.9%) 1540
▲ Procardia XL Tablets (1% or less to 6%) 1783
▲ Procrit for Injection (18%) 1647
ProSom Tablets (Infrequent) 554
▲ Proventil Solutions for Inhalation 0.5% and 0.083% (4%) 2118
Proventil Syrup (Less than 1 of 100) 2119
Prozac Pulvules (1.6%) 920
Quadrinal Tablets 1183
Recombivax HB (Less than 1%) 1544
Retrovir Capsules (Less than 5%) 802
Retrovir I.V. Infusion (Less than 5%) 805

Retrovir Syrup (Less than 5%) 802
Rheumatrex Methotrexate Dose Pack (Less common) 1234
▲ Roferon-A Injection (27%) 1916
Sectral Capsules (1%) 2520
Seldane Tablets (2.5%) 1349
Seldane-D Extended-Release Tablets (1.6%) 1350
Septra (Rare) 813
Septra I.V. Infusion (Rare) 808
Septra I.V. Infusion ADD-Vantage Vials 810
Septra (Rare) 813
Sinemet CR Tablets 953
Tegison Capsules (Less than 1%) 1881
Timolide Tablets 1547
Timoptic in Ocudose 1552
Timoptic Sterile Ophthalmic Solution 1550
▲ Tornalate (4%) 2074
Trexan Tablets (Less than 1%) 937
Valium Injectable 1937
Vascor (200, 300 and 400 mg) Tablets (0.5 to 2.0%) 1383
▲ Vaseretic Tablets (3.5%) 1559
Vasotec I.V. 1562
Vasotec Tablets (1.3% to 2.2%) 1564
▲ Ventolin (2% to 5%) 583
Versed Injection (1.3%) 1924
▲ Zestoretic (3.9%) 2274
Zestril Tablets (2.9%) 2277

Cough, productive

Permax Tablets (Frequent) 1291

Cough reflex, depression

Astramorph/PF Injection, USP (Preservative-Free) 618
Compazine 2201
Duramorph 960
Infumorph 200 and Infumorph 500 Sterile Solutions 962
Stelazine 2226
Thorazine 2234

Cramping

Adalat Capsules (10 mg and 20 mg) (2% or less) 1587
Aldactazide 2150
Aldactone 2152
Aldoclor Tablets 1413
Aldoril Tablets 1418
Alferon N Injection (One patient) 1809
Amicar Syrup, Tablets, and Injection (Occasional) 1194
Aminohippurate Sodium Injection 1421
Capozide 2258
▲ Cephulac Syrup (20%) 1331
Clinoril Tablets (Greater than 1%) 1433
Combipres Tablets 678
Corzide Tablets 702
Coumadin Injection & Tablets (Infrequent) 944
▲ Creon Capsules (Among most frequent) 2245
Cytotec (0.6%) 2159
Diucardin Tablets 2450
Diupres Tablets 1461
Diuril Oral Suspension 1464
Diuril Sodium Intravenous 1463
Diuril Tablets 1464
Enduron Tablets 517
Enduronyl 518
Esidrix Tablets 863
Esimil Tablets 864
Exna Tablets 1862
Sterile FUDR 1898
▲ Fungizone Intravenous (Among most common) 2262
HydroDIURIL Tablets 1484
Hydromox R Tablets 1209
Hydromox Tablets 1208
Hydropres Tablets 1485
Inderide Tablets 2463
Inderide LA Long Acting Capsules 2465
Lasix Oral Solution 1093
Lippes Loop Intrauterine Double-S 1654
Lopressor HCT Tablets 1034
Maxzide 1215
Modane Tablets ▣ 503
Moduretic Tablets 1510
Monistat Dual-Pak (2%) 1657
Monistat 3 Vaginal Suppositories (2%) 1657
Mycelex-G 100 mg Vaginal Tablets (Rare) 1606
Mycelex-G 500 mg Vaginal Tablets (Rare) 1606
Normozide Tablets 2112
Nubain Injection (Less than 1%) 934
Oramorph SR (Morphine Sulfate Sustained Release Tablets) (Less frequent) 1988
Oretic Tablets 544
Oreticyl 545
ParaGard T380A Intrauterine Copper Contraceptive 411
Prinzide Tablets 1540
Rifamate Capsules 1347
Saluron 718
Salutensin/Salutensin-Demi 719
▲ Sandimmune (Up to 4%) 2024
Scleromate 1685
Serpasil-Esidrix Tablets 886
Tenoretic Tablets 1105
Thalitone Tablets 687
Timolide Tablets 1547
Trandate HCT Tablets 579
Vaseretic Tablets 1559
Zarontin Capsules (Frequent) 1768
Zarontin Syrup (Frequent) 1769
Zestoretic (0.3 to 1.0%) 2274

Cramping, abdominal (see under Abdominal pain/cramps)

Cramping, muscular

▲ Adalat Capsules (10 mg and 20 mg) (2% or less to 8%) 1587
Alferon N Injection (1%) 1809
Anadrol-50 Tablets 2287
Apresazide Capsules (Less frequent) 854
Apresoline Hydrochloride Parenteral (Ampuls) 856
Apresoline Hydrochloride Tablets (Less frequent) 855
Apresoline-Esidrix Tablets 857
Atromid-S Capsules (Less often) 2435
Brethine Ampuls (Less than 0.5%) 1026
Brethine Tablets 1026
Bricanyl Injection 1324
Bricanyl Tablets 1325
Bumex (1.1%) 1895
BuSpar (Infrequent) 1401
Calan SR Caplets (1% or less) 2157
Calan Tablets (1% or less) 2155
Cardizem Tablets-30 mg, 60 mg, 90 mg and 120 mg 1329
Cardizem SR Capsules-60 mg, 90 mg and 120 mg (Less than 1%) 1327
Cardura Tablets (1%) 1941
Cartrol Tablets (2.6%) 507
Corzide Tablets 702
▲ CytoGam (Less than 5.0%) 891
Cytotec (Infrequent) 2159
Dalgan Injection (Less than 1%) 620
Danocrine Capsules 2046
Diapid Nasal Spray (Infrequent) 2003
Dipentum Capsules (Rare) 1160
Diucardin Tablets 2450
Diulo 2129
Diuril Sodium Intravenous 1463
Dolobid Tablets (Rare) 1465
Dyazide Capsules 2208
Eldepryl 2250
Isoptin Oral Tablets (Less than 1%) 1179
Isoptin SR Sustained Release Tablets (Less than 1%) 1181
K-Phos M.F. Tablets 659
K-Phos Neutral Tablets 660
K-Phos Original Formula 'Sodium Free' Tablets (Less frequent) 660
K-Phos No. 2 Tablets 659
Kerlone Tablets 2172
▲ Lozol Tablets (Greater than or equal to 5%) 1843
Maxzide 1215
Mestinon Injectable 1115
Mestinon 1116
Mevacor Tablets (1.1%) 1505
Midamor Tablets (Between 1% and 3%) 1508
Moduretic Tablets (Less than or equal to 1%) 1510
Monopril Tablets (0.2 to 1.0%) 1406
▲ Mykrox ½ mg Tablets (5.8%) 984
Nimotop Capsules (Up to 1.4%) 1607
Normodyne Tablets 2110
Normozide Tablets 2112
Omnipaque (Unusual) 2552
Parlodel (Less than 1%) 2020
Plendil Extended-Release Tablets 1526
Prilosec Delayed-Release Capsules (Less than 1%) 1530
Prinivil Tablets (0.6%) 1538
Prinzide Tablets (2%) 1540
Procardia Capsules (2% or less) 1781
▲ Procardia XL Tablets (8%) 1783
Prostigmin Injectable 1120
Prostigmin Tablets 1121
▲ Proventil (3%) 2120
Raudixin Tablets 1803
Rauzide Tablets 1804
Rythmol Tablets (Less than 1%) 1184
Sandostatin Injection (Less than 1%) 2029
Ser-Ap-Es Tablets 881
Serpasil Tablets 883
Serpasil-Apresoline Tablets 884
Sinemet Tablets 952
Sinemet CR Tablets (0.8%) 953
▲ Tegison Capsules (25-50%) 1881
Thalitone Tablets 687
Tigan 2239
Timolide Tablets 1547
Tonocard Tablets (Less than 1%) 1554
Trandate HCT/Trandate 579
Uroqid-Acid (Less frequent) 661
Vaseretic Tablets (2.7%) 1559
Vasotec I.V. 1562
Vasotec Tablets (0.5% to 1%) 1564
Ventolin (1%) 583
Verelan Capsules (Less than 1%) 1243
▲ Visken Tablets (3%) 2036
Xanax Tablets (2.4%) 2367
Zaroxolyn Tablets 989
Zestoretic (2.0%) 2274
Zestril Tablets (0.6%) 2277

Cramps, abdominal (see under Abdominal pain/cramps)

Cramps, lower limbs

Anafranil Capsules (Infrequent) 650
Catapres-TTS (3 Per 1,000) 677
Combipres Tablets (About 3 in 1,000) 678
Desferal Vials 862
DynaCirc Capsules (0.5% to 1%) 2004
▲ Emcyt Capsules (8%) 1161
Gammagard Immune Globulin, Intravenous (Human) (Occasional) 658
▲ Hylorel Tablets (21.1% to 25.6%) 975
Intron A (Up to 5%) 2097
Kerlone Tablets (Less than 2%) 2172
Methergine (Rare) 2016
Normozide Tablets (1%) 2112
Oxsoralen-Ultra Capsule 1117
Procardia XL Tablets (Less than 3%) 1783
Sandostatin Injection (Less than 1%) 2029
Tegretol Chewable Tablets 654
Tegretol Suspension 656
Tegretol Tablets 654
Tenex Tablets (Less than 3%) 1875
Trandate HCT Tablets (1% in 208 patients) 579

Cramps, pelvic

Cytotec (0.6%) 2159

Cranial nerve, dysfunction

IFEX (Less frequent) 729

Cranial nerve deficit, fetal

Accutane Capsules 1878

Cranial sensations, unspecified

Methotrexate Tablets, Parenteral, LPF Parenteral 1217
Rheumatrex Methotrexate Dose Pack 1234

Craniofacial deformities

Prinivil Tablets 1538
Prinzide Tablets 1540
Vaseretic Tablets 1559
Vasotec I.V. 1562
Vasotec Tablets 1564
Zestoretic 2274
Zestril Tablets 2277

Creatinine, increase (see under Serum creatinine, elevation)

Creatinine clearance, decrease

Bumex (0.3%) 1895
Children's Advil Suspension (Less than 1%) 2426
Disalcid 1310
Eskalith 2214
IFEX 729
Kefurox Vials, Faspak & ADD-Vantage 1277
Mandol Vials, Faspak & ADD-Vantage 1281
Motrin Tablets (Less than 1%) 2351
Netromycin Injection 100 mg/ml 2104
PediaProfen Suspension (Less than 1%) 1363
Platinol 737
Platinol-AQ Injection 738
Proglycem 649
Rufen Tablets (Less than 1%) 691
Salflex 839
Trobicin Sterile Powder 2366
Zinacef 1066

Creatinine phosphokinase, increase

Anadrol-50 Tablets 2287
Lopid Capsules and Tablets 1736
Lorelco Tablets 1333
▲ Mevacor Tablets (11%) 1505
Normozide Tablets (Less than 1%) 2112
Orap Tablets 1020
Parlodel 2020
Prolixin Decanoate 1795
Prolixin Elixir 1793
Prolixin Enanthate 1796
Prolixin Injection 1791
Prolixin Oral Concentrate 1792
Prolixin Tablets 1793
Trandate HCT Tablets (Less than 1% in 208 patients) 579
Winstrol Tablets (no incidence data in labeling) 2075

Cretinism, fetal

Tapazole Tablets 1298

Crohn's disease

Demulen 2161
Enovid 2161
Norethin 2133

Crohn's disease, exacerbation

Butazolidin Capsules & Tablets (Less than 1%) 1027

Crying

Ativan Injection (1.3%) 2432
Dalgan Injection (Less than 1%) 620
Diphtheria and Tetanus Toxoids and Pertussis Vaccine Adsorbed USP (For Pediatric Use) (1 in 100 doses) 892
HibTITER (38 of 1,118 vaccinations) 1206
IPOL Poliovirus Vaccine Inactivated 894
Nubain Injection (Less than 1%) 934
ProHIBiT Haemophilus b Conjugate Vaccine (Diphtheria Toxoid Conjugate) (1.2% or less) 896
Tri-Immunol Diphtheria & Tetanus Toxoids & Pertussis Vaccine, Adsorbed 1241

Crystalluria

Ancobon Capsules 1886
Azo Gantrisin Tablets 1888
Azulfidine Tablets, EN-tabs, Oral Suspension (Rare) 1157
Bactrim DS Tablets 1891
Bactrim I.V. Infusion 1889
Bactrim 1891
Cipro I.V. (1% or less) 1592
Cipro Tablets 1589
Clinoril Tablets (Less than 1 in 100) 1433
Dantrium Capsules (Less frequent) 1619
Demser Capsules (A few patients) 1460
Diamox 1200
Floxin Tablets 1652
Mintezol 1510
Neptazane Tablets ◉ 311
Septra 813
Septra I.V. Infusion 808
Septra I.V. Infusion ADD-Vantage Vials 810
Septra 813
Thiosulfil Forte Tablets 2526
Urobiotic-250 Capsules 1968

Cushingoid state (see under Cushing's syndrome)

Cushing's syndrome

Aclovate 1053
Alphatrex Cream, Ointment & Lotion 2076
Aristospan Suspension (Intra-articular) 1011

- Beconase Inhalation Aerosol & Refill 574
- Celestone Soluspan Suspension 2081
- Cortenema 2244
- Cortone Acetate Sterile Suspension 1437
- Cortone Acetate Tablets 1439
- Cutivate Cream 0.05% 1054
- Cutivate Ointment 0.005% 1054
- ▲ Cytadren Tablets (2 out of 3) 861
- Dalalone D.P. Injectable 999
- Decadron Elixir 1445
- Decadron Phosphate Injection 1449
- Decadron Phosphate Respihaler 1454
- Decadron Phosphate Turbinaire 1456
- Decadron Phosphate with Xylocaine Injection, Sterile 1451
- Decadron Tablets 1447
- Decadron-LA Sterile Suspension 1457
- Deltasone Tablets 2332
- Depo-Medrol Sterile Aqueous Suspension 2334
- Diprolene 2083
- Hydeltrasol Injection, Sterile 1476
- Hydeltra-T.B.A. Sterile Suspension 1478
- Hydrocortone Acetate Sterile Suspension 1479
- Hydrocortone Phosphate Injection, Sterile 1481
- Hydrocortone Tablets 1482
- Kenalog-10 Injection 2402
- Kenalog-40 Injection 2403
- Maxivate Cream, Lotion & Ointment 0.05% 2406
- Medrol 2348
- Nasalide Nasal Solution 0.025% (With excessive dose) 2299
- Pediapred Oral Liquid 987
- Solu-Cortef Sterile Powder 2361
- Solu-Medrol Sterile Powder 2363
- Temovate 1056
- Ultravate Cream 0.05% 2410
- Ultravate Ointment 0.05% 2411

Cutaneous tenderness
- Oxsoralen-Ultra Capsule 1117

Cyanide toxicity
- Nipride I.V. Infusion 1909

Cyanosis
- Americaine Anesthetic Lubricant 972
- Americaine Otic Topical Anesthetic Ear Drops 973
- Anafranil Capsules (Rare) 650
- Antivenin (Crotalidae) Polyvalent 2430
- AquaMEPHYTON Injection 1422
- Azo Gantrisin Tablets 1888
- ▲ Azulfidine Tablets, EN-tabs, Oral Suspension (3 to 4%) 1157
- Calciparine Injection 925
- Chloromycetin Kapseals 1695
- Chloromycetin Palmitate, Oral Suspension 1697
- Chloromycetin Sodium Succinate 1698
- Clozaril Tablets (Less than 1%) 2000
- Diupres Tablets 1461
- Ethrane 599
- Harmonyl Tablets 528
- Heparin Sodium Vials 1264
- Heparin Sodium Injection, USP, Sterile Solution 2342
- Hydropres Tablets 1485
- Hyskon Hysteroscopy Fluid (Rare) 1162
- Intron A (Less than 1%) 2097
- Mephyton Tablets (Rare) 1503
- NebuPent for Inhalation Solution (1% or less) 1017
- Omnipaque 2552
- Permax Tablets (Infrequent) 1291
- Primaxin I.M. 1532
- Primaxin I.V. (Less than 0.2%) 1535
- Roferon-A Injection (Less than 1%) 1916
- Ser-Ap-Es Tablets 881
- Serpasil Tablets 883
- Serpasil-Apresoline Tablets 884
- Serpasil-Esidrix Tablets 886

Cyanosis, hand
- Intron A (1% or less) 2097

Cycloplegia
- Alcaine ◉ 210
- Arfonad Ampuls 1887
- Bentyl 1322
- Cantil Tablets 1326
- Darbid Tablets 2205
- Ditropan 1332
- Donnatal 1858
- Donnatal Extentabs 1859
- Donnatal Tablets 1858
- Donnazyme Tablets 1860
- Kinesed Tablets 2272
- Kutrase Capsules 2146
- Levsin/Levsinex 2147
- Pro-Banthīne Tablets 2141
- Quarzan Capsules 1937
- Robinul Forte Tablets 1873
- Robinul Injectable 1873
- Robinul Tablets 1873
- Valpin 50 Tablets 941

Cylindruria
- Cipro I.V. (1% or less) 1592
- Cipro Tablets 1589
- Floxin Tablets 1652
- Garamycin Injectable 2093
- Nebcin Vials, Hyporets & ADD-Vantage 1286
- Netromycin Injection 100 mg/ml 2104
- Polymyxin B Sulfate, Aerosporin Brand Sterile Powder 798

Cyst
- Anafranil Capsules (Infrequent) 650

Cyst, renal
- Anafranil Capsules (Rare) 650

Cystic masses in the pelvis
- Lippes Loop Intrauterine Double-S 1654
- ParaGard T380A Intrauterine Copper Contraceptive 411

Cystitis
- Amen 833
- Anafranil Capsules (Up to 2%) 650
- Brevicon 2304
- Children's Advil Suspension (Less than 1%) 2426
- Cycrin Tablets 2449
- Demulen 2161
- Depo-Provera Sterile Aqueous Suspension 2336
- Diethylstilbestrol Tablets 1258
- Enovid 2161
- Estrace 1385
- Estrace Vaginal Cream 1388
- Estratest 2245
- Estrovis 1721
- Flagyl I.V. 2131
- Flagyl Tablets 2170
- Jenest-28 Tablets 1636
- Kerlone Tablets (Less than 2%) 2172
- Lamprene Capsules (Less than 1%) 1030
- Leukeran Tablets 788
- Levlen/Tri-Levlen 665
- Lodine Capsules (Less than 1%) 2468
- Lo/Ovral Tablets 2471
- Lo/Ovral-28 Tablets 2476
- Loestrin 1728
- Mediatric Capsules 2476
- Menrium Tablets 1934
- Methotrexate Tablets, Parenteral, LPF Parenteral 1217
- Micronor Tablets 1667
- Modicon 1667
- Motrin Tablets (Less than 1%) 2351
- Nalfon Pulvules & Tablets (Less than 1%) 919
- Neosar for Injection 566
- Nordette-21 Tablets 2481
- Nordette-28 Tablets 2483
- Norethin 2133
- Norinyl 2304
- Norlestrin 1746
- Norlutate 1754
- Norlutin 1755
- Nor-Q D Tablets 2304
- Ogen 540
- Ortho Dienestrol Cream 1664
- Ortho-Cyclen Tablets 1658
- Ortho-Novum 1667
- Ovcon 1391
- Ovral Tablets 2490
- Ovral-28 Tablets 2491
- Ovrette Tablets 2492
- PMB 200 and PMB 400 2504
- PediaProfen Suspension (Less than 1%) 1363
- Permax Tablets (Infrequent) 1291
- Premarin Intravenous 2508
- Premarin with Methyltestosterone 2515
- Premarin Vaginal Cream 2512
- Protostat Tablets 1674
- Provera Tablets 2356
- Prozac Pulvules (Infrequent) 920
- Rheumatrex Methotrexate Dose Pack 1234
- Rimso-50 1836
- Rufen Tablets (Less than 1%) 691
- ▲ TheraCys BCG Live (Intravesical) (Up to 29.5%) 898
- Thiotepa Parenteral 1240
- Levlen/Tri-Levlen 665
- Tri-Norinyl 2304
- Triphasil-21 Tablets 2527
- Triphasil-28 Tablets 2532
- Wellbutrin Tablets (Rare) 821

Cystitis, hemorrhagic
- Adriamycin RDF 562
- Cipro I.V. (1% or less) 1592
- Cytoxan for Injection 726
- IFEX 729
- Lysodren (Infrequent) 731
- Neosar for Injection 566
- Thiotepa Parenteral 1240

Cystitis, intercurrent
- Mycelex-G 1% Vaginal Cream (0.5%) 1605

Cystitis, non-hemorrhagic
- Cytoxan for Injection 726

Cystitis, viral
- Retrovir (0.8%) 802

Cystitis-like syndrome (see under Cystitis)

Cytarabine syndrome
- Cytosar-U Sterile Powder 2329

cAMP, elevation
- ▲ Yutopar (80 to 100% with IV administration) 647

CHF (see under Congestive heart failure)

CNS abnormalities, fetal
- Accutane Capsules 1878
- Elavil 2269
- Oxytocin Injection 2492
- Sensorcaine 631

CNS damage
- Pitocin Injection, Ampoules, Steri-Dose Syringes 1757
- Tri-Immunol Diphtheria & Tetanus Toxoids & Pertussis Vaccine, Adsorbed (1 per 330,000) 1241

CNS damage, permanent
- Oxytocin Injection 2492
- Syntocinon Injection 2032

CNS depression
- Actifed with Codeine Cough Syrup 752
- AK-Taine (Exceedingly rare) ◉ 207
- Alurate Elixir (Less than 1 in 100) 1883
- Ana-Kit Anaphylaxis Emergency Treatment Kit 1100
- Ansaid Tablets (1-3%) 2319
- Ativan Injection 2432
- Atrohist Sprinkle Capsules 558
- Butisol Sodium Elixir & Tablets (Less than 1 in 100) 2377
- Carbocaine Hydrochloride Injection 2043
- Children's Advil Suspension (Less than 1%) 2426
- Cocaine Hydrochloride Topical Solution 620
- Deconamine 663
- Deconsal 559
- Depakote Sprinkle Capsules 512
- Dilantin Parenteral 1712
- Fedahist Gyrocaps 2145
- Fedahist Timecaps 2145
- ▲ Klonopin Tablets (Most frequent) 1902
- ▲ Lysodren (40%) 731
- Mebaral Tablets (Less than 1 in 100) 2061
- Motrin Tablets (Less than 1%) 2351
- Naldecon Syrup, Tablets, Pediatric Drops and Pediatric Syrup 709
- Naphcon-A Ophthalmic Solution 571
- Naprosyn (Less than 1%) 2297
- Nembutal Sodium Capsules (Less than 1%) 534
- Nembutal Sodium Solution (Less than 1%) 536
- Nembutal Sodium Suppositories (Less than 1%) 538
- Novafed A Capsules 1342
- Novafed Capsules 1342
- Novahistine DH 1342
- Novahistine DMX ▣ 595
- Novahistine Elixir ▣ 596
- Novahistine Expectorant 1343
- PediaProfen Suspension (Less than 1%) 1363
- Phenergan with Codeine 2497
- Phenergan VC with Codeine 2501
- Phenobarbital Elixir and Tablets (Less than 1 in 100 patients) 1293
- Pontocaine Hydrochloride for Spinal Anesthesia 2069
- Prozac Pulvules (Rare) 920
- Ru-Tuss DE Tablets 694
- Seconal Sodium Pulvules (Less than 1 in 100) 1296
- Seldane-D Extended-Release Tablets 1350
- Triaminic Expectorant DH 1995
- Triaminic Oral Infant Drops 1996
- Trinalin Repetabs Tablets 1170
- ▲ Xanax Tablets (13.8% to 13.9%) 2367
- Xylocaine Injections 637
- Xylocaine Injections for Ventricular Arrhythmias 639

CNS depression, neonatal
- Hydromox R Tablets 1209
- ProSom Tablets 554
- Versed Injection 1924

CNS reactions
- Anestacon Solution (Among most comon) 2394
- Attenuvax 1424
- Biavax II 1427
- BuSpar 1401
- Compazine 2201
- Danocrine Capsules 2046
- Deprol Tablets (One case) 2382
- Desyrel and Desyrel Dividose (Greater than 1%) 1404
- Diupres Tablets 1461
- Dorcol Children's Cough Syrup ▣ 685
- Dorcol Children's Decongestant Liquid ▣ 685
- Dorcol Children's Liquid Cold Formula (Occasional) ▣ 686
- Harmonyl Tablets 528
- Hexalen Capsules 2316
- Hydrocet Capsules 835
- Hydropres Tablets 1485
- Intron A (2 patients) 2097
- Lanoxicaps 772
- Lanoxin Elixir Pediatric 775
- Lanoxin Injection 778
- Lanoxin Injection Pediatric 781
- Lanoxin Tablets 783
- Lariam Tablets 1904
- Leukine for IV Infusion 1127
- Marax Tablets & DF Syrup (Rare) 1954
- Noroxin Tablets 1519
- ▲ Novantrone for Injection Concentrate (30 to 34%) 1226
- Omnipaque (Rare) 2552
- Orap Tablets 1020
- Orudis Capsules (Less than 1%) 2488
- ▲ Paraplatin for Injection (5%) 735
- Rauzide Tablets 1804
- Roferon-A Injection (Less than 3%) 1916
- SSD RP Cream 690
- Sandostatin Injection (Less than 1%) 2029
- Silvadene Cream 1% 1352
- Stelazine 2226
- Triaminic Cold Tablets ▣ 688
- Triaminic Expectorant ▣ 688
- Triaminic Syrup (Occasional) ▣ 689
- Triaminicol Multi-Symptom Relief ▣ 691

CNS stimulation
- Adipex-P Tablets and Capsules 1019
- AK-Taine (Exceedingly rare) ◉ 207
- Anadrol-50 Tablets 2287
- Ansaid Tablets (1-3%) 2319
- Brethaire Inhaler 1024
- Carbocaine Hydrochloride Injection 2043
- Choledyl Pediatric Elixir 1702
- Choledyl Tablets 1700
- ▲ Cipro I.V. (Among most frequent) 1592
- Cipro Tablets 1589
- Cocaine Hydrochloride Topical Solution 620
- Deconamine 663
- Dilor-G Tablets & Liquid 2079
- Kwell Cream (Rare) 1830
- Kwell Lotion (Rare) 1831
- Kwell Shampoo (Rare) 1832
- Lufyllin-GG Elixir & Tablets 2385
- Norisodrine Aerotrol 540
- Noroxin Tablets 1519

Pontocaine Hydrochloride for Spinal Anesthesia 2069
Proventil Inhalation Aerosol 2117
Prozac Pulvules (Infrequent) 920
Rondec 1975
Rondec-DM 1976
Rondec-TR Tablet 1975
Tedral SA 1765
Theo-Organidin Elixir 2391
Triaminic-DM Syrup ▣ 689
Ventolin 583
Xylocaine Injections 637

CNS stimulation, paradoxical
Doral Tablets 2383
Halcion Tablets 2340
Libritabs Tablets 1930
Librium Capsules 1931
Restoril Capsules (Less than 0.5%) 2023

CNS toxicity
Cytosar-U Sterile Powder 2329
▲IFEX (12%) 729
Marcaine Spinal 2058
Parlodel 2020

CNS, unresponsiveness, unspecified
▲Cipro I.V. (Among most frequent) 1592

CPK, elevation
Accutane Capsules (1 in 5 to 1 in 10) 1878
Atromid-S Capsules 2435
Cardizem Tablets-30 mg, 60 mg, 90 mg and 120 mg (Less than 1%) 1329
Cardizem SR Capsules-60 mg, 90 mg and 120 mg (Less than 1%) 1327
Catapres-TTS (Rare) 677
Danocrine Capsules 2046
Lopid Capsules and Tablets 1736
▲Mevacor Tablets (11%) 1505
Nardil (Less frequent) 1742
Procardia XL Tablets (Rare) 1783
Prolixin Decanoate 1795
Prolixin Enanthate 1796
Sandostatin Injection (Less than 1%) 2029
Sinemet Tablets 952
▲Tegison Capsules (1-10%) 1881
Winstrol Tablets 2075

D

Deafness
Amikin Injectable 602
Anafranil Capsules (Infrequent) 650
Aralen Hydrochloride Injection (A few cases) 2038
Aralen Phosphate Tablets (A few cases) 2039
Cytotec (Infrequent) 2159
Diupres Tablets 1461
Edecrin 1468
Enduronyl 518
Harmonyl Tablets 528
Hibiclens Antimicrobial Skin Cleanser 2271
Hibistat 2272
Hydropres Tablets 1485
Indocin Capsules (Less than 1%) 1487
Indocin I.V. (Less than 1%) 1490
Indocin (Less than 1%) 1487
Kerlone Tablets (Less than 2%) 2172
Legatrin ▣ 556
Lodine Capsules (Less than 1%) 2468
M-M-R II 1494
Permax Tablets (Infrequent) 1291
Plaquenil Sulfate Tablets 2067
Platinol (Rare) 737
Platinol-AQ Injection (Rare) 738
Prozac Pulvules (Rare) 920
Quinamm Tablets 1344
Q-vel Muscle Relaxant Pain Reliever ▣ 552
Raudixin Tablets 1803
Rauzide Tablets 1804
Renese-R Tablets 1786
Salutensin/Salutensin-Demi 719
Ser-Ap-Es Tablets 881
Serpasil Tablets 883
Serpasil-Apresoline Tablets 884
Serpasil-Esidrix Tablets 886

Deafness, transient
ERYC (A few cases) 1720
Oreticyl 545

Death, fetal
Oxytocin Injection 2492
Prinivil Tablets 1538
Prinzide Tablets 1540
Sensorcaine 631
Syntocinon Injection 2032
Vaseretic Tablets 1559
Vasotec I.V. 1562
Vasotec Tablets 1564
Zestoretic 2274
Zestril Tablets 2277

Death, sudden
Haldol Decanoate 1375
Norpramin Tablets (One report) 1340
Rheumatrex Methotrexate Dose Pack (Rare) 1234
Thorazine 2234

Deep tendon reflexes, loss
Oncovin Solution Vials & Hyporets 1288
Plaquenil Sulfate Tablets 2067
Velban Vials 1305

Defecate, desire to
Aminohippurate Sodium Injection 1421
Dopram Injectable 1860
Peptavlon 2563

Dehydration
Anafranil Capsules (Infrequent) 650
Bumex (0.1%) 1895
Capoten 2255
Capozide 2258
Cibalith-S 870
Cytotec (Rare) 2159
Diapid Nasal Spray 2003
Dilor 2079
Eskalith 2214
Intron A (Less than 1%) 2097
Klonopin Tablets 1902
Lithane Tablets 1596
Lithium Carbonate Capsules & Tablets 1984
Lithobid Tablets 870
Methotrexate Tablets, Parenteral, LPF Parenteral 1217
Moduretic Tablets (Less than or equal to 1%) 1510
Permax Tablets (Infrequent) 1291
Prinzide Tablets 1540
Prozac Pulvules (Rare) 920
Rheumatrex Methotrexate Dose Pack 1234
Zestril Tablets 2277

Delirium
Anafranil Capsules (Infrequent) 650
Ativan Injection (1.3%) 2432
Brevital Sodium Vials 1248
Cardioquin Tablets 1812
Catapres Tablets 676
Catapres-TTS 677
Chloromycetin Kapseals 1695
Chloromycetin Palmitate, Oral Suspension 1697
Chloromycetin Sodium Succinate 1698
Combipres Tablets 678
Dalgan Injection (Less than 1%) 620
▲Dilantin with Phenobarbital Kapseals (Among most common) 1715
Diprivan Injection (Less than 1%) 2267
Innovar Injection 1141
Kinesed Tablets 2272
Nardil (Less frequent) 1742
Pantopon Injectable 1911
Phenobarbital Elixir and Tablets 1293
PhosLo Tablets 700
Quinaglute Dura-Tabs Tablets 663
Quinidex Extentabs 1868
Ru-Tuss Tablets 693
Surital Ampoules, Steri-Vials 1764
Wellbutrin Tablets 821

Delivery complications, unspecified
Advil Cold & Sinus Caplets (formerly CoAdvil) 2416
Advil Ibuprofen Tablets and Caplets 2416
Alka-Seltzer Effervescent Antacid and Pain Reliever 1568
Alka-Seltzer Extra Strength Effervescent Antacid and Pain Reliever 1570
Alka-Seltzer (Flavored) Effervescent Antacid and Pain Reliever 1569
Alka-Seltzer Plus Cold Medicine ▣ 623
Alka-Seltzer Plus Night-Time Cold Medicine ▣ 623
Alka Seltzer Plus Sinus Allergy Medicine ▣ 624
Anacin 2417
Anacin Maximum Strength Analgesic Coated Tablets 2417
Maximum Strength Arthritis Pain Formula By the Makers of Anacin Analgesic Tablets and Caplets 2418
Ascriptin A/D Caplets 1850
Regular Strength Ascriptin Tablets 1850
BC Powder ▣ 517
BC Cold Powder ▣ 517
Children's Bayer Chewable Aspirin ▣ 564
Genuine Bayer Aspirin Tablets & Caplets ▣ 564
Maximum Bayer Aspirin Tablets & Caplets ▣ 566
Bayer Plus Aspirin Tablets ▣ 567
Therapy Bayer Aspirin Caplets ▣ 568
8 Hour Bayer Timed-Release Aspirin ▣ 566
Cama Arthritis Pain Reliever ▣ 685
Dristan Sinus Caplets 2419
Ecotrin 2189
Empirin Aspirin ▣ 541
Empirin with Codeine Phosphate Nos. 2, 3 & 4 764
Fiorinal with Codeine Capsules 2008
Marcaine Hydrochloride with Epinephrine 1:200,000 2055
Marcaine Hydrochloride Injection 2055
Medipren ibuprofen Caplets and Tablets 1362
Midol 200 Cramp Relief Formula ▣ 570
Norwich Extra-Strength Aspirin ▣ 546
Norwich Regular Strength Aspirin ▣ 547
Sensorcaine 631
Sensorcaine-MPF Spinal 634
Sine-Off Sinus Medicine Tablets-Aspirin Formula ▣ 722
Soma Compound w/Codeine Tablets 2390
Soma Compound Tablets 2389
Ursinus Inlay-Tabs ▣ 691
Vanquish Analgesic Caplets ▣ 574

Delusions
Anafranil Capsules (Infrequent) 650
Artane (Rare) 1195
Clozaril Tablets (Less than 1%) 2000
Dalgan Injection (Less than 1%) 620
Desyrel and Desyrel Dividose (Less than 1%) 1404
Elavil 2269
Eldepryl 2250
Endep Tablets 1927
Etrafon 2087
Flexeril Tablets (Rare) 1471
Halcion Tablets 2340
Larodopa Tablets (Relatively frequent) 1905
Limbitrol 1933
Ludiomil Tablets (Rare) 874
▲Lupron Depot 3.75 mg (Among most frequent) 2312
Norpramin Tablets 1340
Nubain Injection (Less than 1%) 934
Pamelor 2019
Parlodel 2020
Permax Tablets (Infrequent) 1291
Prozac Pulvules (Infrequent) 920
Sinemet Tablets 952
Sinemet CR Tablets 953
Surmontil Capsules 2524
Tofranil Ampuls 1038
Tofranil Tablets 1039
Tofranil-PM Capsules 1041
Triavil Tablets 1556
Vivactil Tablets 1567
Wellbutrin Tablets (1.2%) 821

Dementia
Larodopa Tablets (Infrequent) 1905
Methotrexate Tablets, Parenteral, LPF Parenteral 1217
Quinidex Extentabs 1868
Rheumatrex Methotrexate Dose Pack 1234
Sinemet Tablets 952
Sinemet CR Tablets 953

Dental caries
Anafranil Capsules (Infrequent) 650
Eskalith 2214
Tegison Capsules (Less than 1%) 1881

Dependence, drug
Adipex-P Tablets and Capsules 1019
Alfenta Injection 1131
Anexsia 5/500 Tablets 2196
Anexsia 7.5/650 Tablets 2197
Astramorph/PF Injection, USP (Preservative-Free) 618
B & O No. 15A & No. 16A Supprettes 2395
Biphetamine Capsules 973
Correctol Laxative Tablets ▣ 696
Dalmane Capsules 1927
Damason-P 1356
Darvon-N/Darvocet-N 1254
Darvon 1256
Darvon-N Suspension & Tablets 1254
Demerol 2047
Dexedrine 2206
Dilaudid Cough Syrup 1174
Dilaudid 1173
Dolophine Hydrochloride Tablets 1261
Duragesic Transdermal System (Less than 1%) 1133
Duramorph 960
Equagesic Tablets 2451
Evac-U-Gen Mild Laxative ▣ 739
Ex-Lax Chocolated Laxative ▣ 686
Ex-Lax Pills, Unflavored ▣ 686
Extra Gentle Ex-Lax ▣ 687
Fioricet Tablets 2006
Fiorinal Capsules 2007
Fiorinal with Codeine Capsules 2008
Fiorinal Tablets 2007
Gentle Nature Natural Vegetable Laxative ▣ 687
Hycodan Syrup, Tablets 927
Hycomine Compound Tablets 929
Hycomine Syrup 927
Hycotuss Expectorant Syrup 930
Ionamin Capsules 981
Isordil 2467
Libritabs Tablets 1930
Librium Capsules 1931
Librium Injectable 1932
Limbitrol 1933
Lortab ASA Tablets 2414
Lortab 2412
MS Contin Tablets 1814
MSIR 1817
Mepergan Injection 2479
Methadone Hydrochloride Diskets 1284
Methadone Hydrochloride Oral Solution & Tablets 1987
Modane Plus Tablets ▣ 504
Modane Tablets ▣ 503
Nature's Remedy Natural Vegetable Laxative ▣ 719
Nembutal Sodium Capsules 534
Nembutal Sodium Solution 536
Nembutal Sodium Suppositories 538
Numorphan Hydrochloride Injection 935
Numorphan Suppositories 935
Oramorph SR (Morphine Sulfate Sustained Release Tablets) 1988
PMB 200 and PMB 400 2504
Pantopon Injectable 1911
Percocet Tablets 950
Percodan 951
Phenaphen with Codeine Capsules 1865
Phenaphen-650 with Codeine Tablets 1866
Phenergan with Codeine 2497
Phenergan VC with Codeine 2501
Phenobarbital Elixir and Tablets 1293
Placidyl Capsules 553
Prelu-2 Capsules 683
Restoril Capsules 2023
Ritalin Tablets 880
Roxanol 1991
Roxicodone Tablets, Oral Solution & Intensol (Oxycodone) 1992
Sanorex Tablets 2030
Seconal Sodium Pulvules 1296
Sublimaze Injection 1146
Synalgos-DC Capsules 2525
Talwin Injection 2071
Talwin Compound 2072
Talwin Injection 2071
Talwin Nx 2073
Tranxene 556
Triaminic Expectorant DH 1995
Tylenol with Codeine 1381
Tylox Capsules 1382
Valium Injectable 1937
Valium Tablets 1939
Valrelease Capsules 1923
Wygesic Tablets 2540
Yellolax ▣ 590
Zydone Capsules 941

Dependence, physical
Alurate Elixir 1883
Codiclear DH Syrup 845

Codimal DH Syrup 846
Dexedrine 2206
Doral Tablets 2383
Esgic-Plus Tablets 1002
Fiorinal Capsules (Less frequent) 2007
Fiorinal with Codeine Capsules 2008
Fiorinal Tablets (Less frequent) 2007
Hycomine Compound Tablets 929
Hycomine Syrup 927
Hycotuss Expectorant Syrup 930
Infumorph 200 and Infumorph 500 Sterile Solutions 962
Kinesed Tablets 2272
Klonopin Tablets 1902
Libritabs Tablets 1930
MS Contin Tablets 1814
MSIR 1817
Mebaral Tablets 2061
Methadone Hydrochloride Diskets 1284
Methadone Hydrochloride Oral Solution & Tablets 1987
Miltown Tablets 2386
Oramorph SR (Morphine Sulfate Sustained Release Tablets) 1988
Peri-Colace (Exceedingly small) 1409
Quadrinal Tablets 1183
Roxanol 1991
Seconal Sodium Pulvules 1296
Serax Capsules 2522
Serax Tablets 2522
Sorbitrate 1103
Talacen 2070
Talwin Injection 2071
Talwin Nx 2073
Tylenol with Codeine 1381
Tylox Capsules 1382
Versed Injection 1924
Vicodin ES Tablets 1189
Zydone Capsules 941

Dependence, psychic (see under Dependence, psychological)

Dependence, psychological

Alurate Elixir 1883
Anexsia 5/500 Tablets 2196
Anexsia 7.5/650 Tablets 2197
Azdone Tablets 844
Biphetamine Capsules 973
Damason-P 1356
Darvon-N/Darvocet-N 1254
Darvon 1256
Darvon-N Suspension & Tablets 1254
Demerol 2047
Desoxyn Gradumet Tablets 514
Dexedrine 2206
Dilaudid 1173
Dolophine Hydrochloride Tablets 1261
Duragesic Transdermal System (Less than 1%) 1133
Fastin Capsules 2216
Fiorinal with Codeine Capsules 2008
Hycodan Syrup, Tablets 927
Hydrocet Capsules 835
Infumorph 200 and Infumorph 500 Sterile Solutions 962
Ionamin Capsules 981
Kinesed Tablets 2272
Klonopin Tablets 1902
Libritabs Tablets 1930
Lortab ASA Tablets 2414
Lortab 2412
MS Contin Tablets 1814
MSIR 1817
Mebaral Tablets 2061
Methadone Hydrochloride Diskets 1284
Methadone Hydrochloride Oral Solution & Tablets 1987
Miltown Tablets 2386
Nembutal Sodium Capsules 534
Nembutal Sodium Solution 536
Nembutal Sodium Suppositories 538
Oramorph SR (Morphine Sulfate Sustained Release Tablets) 1988
Placidyl Capsules 553
Roxanol 1991
Roxicodone Tablets, Oral Solution & Intensol (Oxycodone) 1992
Sanorex Tablets 2030
Serax Capsules 2522
Serax Tablets 2522
Talacen 2070
Talwin Nx 2073
Tenuate 1354
Tussionex Extended-Release Suspension 988
Tylox Capsules 1382
Vicodin Tablets 1187
Vicodin ES Tablets 1189
Zydone Capsules 941

Depersonalization

Anafranil Capsules (2%) 650
BuSpar (Infrequent) 1401
Cardura Tablets (Less than 0.5% of 3960 patients) 1941
Cipro I.V. (1% or less) 1592
Cipro Tablets (Less than 1%) 1589
Duragesic Transdermal System (Less than 1%) 1133
Halcion Tablets 2340
Indocin (Less than 1%) 1487
Nubain Injection (Less than 1%) 934
Omnipaque 2552
Prozac Pulvules (Infrequent) 920
Tambocor Tablets (Less than 1%) 1315
Wellbutrin Tablets (Infrequent) 821
Xanax Tablets 2367

Depilation (see under Epilation)

Depression (see also under Depression, mental)

A.P.L. 2431
Accutane Capsules (Some patients) 1878
Actigall Capsules 2280
▲ Actimmune (3%) 1046
Adalat Capsules (10 mg and 20 mg) (Less than 0.5%) 1587
AeroBid Inhaler System (1-3%) 995
Aldoclor Tablets 1413
Aldomet Ester HCI Injection 1417
Aldomet Oral 1415
Aldoril Tablets 1418
Alferon N Injection (One patient to 3%) 1809
Altace Capsules 1086
▲ Anafranil Capsules (Up to 5%) 650
Anaprox and Anaprox DS Tablets (Less than 3%) 2288
Android 1111
▲ Anestacon Solution (Among most common) 2394
Ansaid Tablets (1-3%) 2319
Apresazide Capsules (Less frequent) 854
Apresoline Hydrochloride Parenteral (Ampuls) 856
Apresoline Hydrochloride Tablets (Less frequent) 855
Apresoline-Esidrix Tablets 857
Aristospan Suspension (Intra-articular) 1011
Astramorph/PF Injection, USP (Preservative-Free) 618
Ativan Injection (1.3%) 2432
Ativan Tablets (Less frequent) 2434
Azo Gantrisin Tablets 1888
Bactrim DS Tablets 1891
Bactrim I.V. Infusion 1889
Bactrim 1891
Betagan ◉ 239
Betoptic Sterile Ophthalmic Solution (Rare) 569
Betoptic S Sterile Ophthalmic Suspension (Rare) 570
Blocadren Tablets 1429
Brevibloc Injection (Less than 1%) 942
Brevicon 2304
BuSpar (2%) 1401
Capoten 2255
Capozide 2258
Carbocaine 956
Cardene Capsules (Rare) 2290
Cardizem Tablets-30 mg, 60 mg, 90 mg and 120 mg (Less than 1%) 1329
Cardizem SR Capsules-60 mg, 90 mg and 120 mg (Less than 1%) 1327
Cardura Tablets (1%) 1941
Cartrol Tablets (Less common) 507
Children's Advil Suspension (Less than 1%) 2426
Cipro I.V. (1% or less) 1592
Cipro Tablets (Less than 1%) 1589
Clinoril Tablets (Less than 1%) 1433
Clozaril Tablets (1%) 2000
Cogentin 1435
Cylert Tablets 510
DDAVP 1841
Dalgan Injection (Less than 1%) 620
Dalmane Capsules (Rare) 1927
Danocrine Capsules 2046
Daranide Tablets 1445
Daraprim Tablets (Rare) 761
Demser Capsules 1460
Diethylstilbestrol Tablets 1258
Dilaudid-HP Injection 1175
Dipentum Capsules (1.5%) 1160
Diprivan Injection (Less than 1%) 2267
Dolobid Tablets (Less than 1 in 100) 1465
Doral Tablets 2383
▲ Duragesic Transdermal System (3% to 10%) 1133
DynaCirc Capsules (0.5% to 1%) 2004
Eldepryl 2250
Elspar 1470
Ergamisol Tablets (1 to 2%) 1136
Esgic Tablets & Capsules 1001
Estinyl Tablets 2085
Estrace 1385
Estrace Vaginal Cream 1388
Estratest 2245
Ethmozine Tablets (Less than 2%) 946
Eulexin Capsules (1%) 2089
Feldene Capsules (Less than 1%) 1777
Fioricet Tablets 2006
Fiorinal with Codeine Capsules 2008
Flagyl I.V. 2131
Flagyl Tablets 2170
Floxin Tablets (Less than 1%) 1652
Gantanol 1899
Gantrisin 1901
Garamycin Injectable 2093
Gastrocrom Capsules (Infrequent) 974
Halcion Tablets (Less frequent) 2340
Haldol Decanoate 1375
Haldol Injection, Tablets and Concentrate 1373
Halotestin Tablets 2341
Harmonyl Tablets 528
Hismanal Tablets (Less frequent) 1138
Hydropres Tablets 1485
Hylorel Tablets (1.9%) 975
Hytrin Tablets (0.3%) 529
Indocin (Greater than 1%) 1487
▲ Intron A (Up to 28%) 2097
Isoptin Injectable (Few) 1177
Kerlone Tablets (0.8%) 2172
Klonopin Tablets 1902
Lamprene Capsules (Less than 1%) 1030
Lariam Tablets 1904
Larodopa Tablets (Infrequent) 1905
Levatol (0.6%) 1832
Lioresal Tablets 1031
Lodine Capsules (More than 1% but less than 3%) 2468
Lomotil 2174
Lopid Capsules and Tablets 1736
▲ Lopressor Ampuls (5%) 1032
▲ Lopressor HCT Tablets (5 in 100) 1034
▲ Lopressor Tablets (5%) 1032
Lozol Tablets (Less than 5%) 1843
Lupron Depot 7.5 mg 2311
Lupron Injection (Less than 5%) 2310
MS Contin Tablets (Infrequent) 1814
MSIR (Infrequent) 1817
Marcaine Hydrochloride 0.5% with Epinephrine 1:200,000 (as bitartrate) 958
Marcaine Hydrochloride with Epinephrine 1:200,000 2055
Marcaine Hydrochloride Injection 2055
Marcaine Spinal 2058
▲ Marinol (Dronabinol) Capsules (7%) 1985
Matulane Capsules 1907
Maxair Inhaler (Less than 1%) 1311
Maxzide 1215
Mebaral Tablets 2061
Meclomen Capsules (Rare) 1739
Mesantoin Tablets 2013
Metandren Linguets and Tablets 875
Mevacor Tablets 1505
Mexitil Capsules (2.4%) 680
Micronor Tablets 1667
Midamor Tablets (Less than or equal to 1%) 1508
Minipress Capsules (1-4%) 1778
Minizide Capsules (Rare) 1779
Mithracin 1602
Moban Tablets & Concentrate (Less frequent) 932
Modicon 1667
Moduretic Tablets (Less than or equal to 1%) 1510
Motofen Tablets 836
Motrin Tablets (Less than 1%) 2351
Mykrox ½ mg Tablets (Less than 2%) 984
Nalfon Pulvules & Tablets (Less than 1%) 919
NebuPent for Inhalation Solution (1% or less) 1017
Neptazane Tablets ◉ 311
Nescaine/Nescaine MPF 629
Nicorette 1335
Nimotop Capsules (Up to 1.4%) 1607
Nolvadex Tablets (1.9%) 1102
Norinyl 2304
Noroxin Tablets (0.3% to 1%) 1519
Nor-Q D Tablets 2304
Omnipaque 2552
OptiPranolol Sterile Ophthalmic Solution (A small number of patients) ◉ 261
Oramorph SR (Morphine Sulfate Sustained Release Tablets) (Less frequent) 1988
Ortho-Novum 1667
Orudis Capsules (Greater than 1%) 2488
Ovcon 1391
Oxsoralen-Ultra Capsule 1117
Parlodel 2020
PediaProfen Suspension (Less than 1%) 1363
Pepcid (Infrequent) 1524
▲ Permax Tablets (3.2%) 1291
Phrenilin 838
Plendil Extended-Release Tablets (0.5% to 1.5%) 1526
Pondimin Tablets 1867
Pregnyl 1644
Prilosec Delayed-Release Capsules (Less than 1%) 1530
Prinivil Tablets (1% or less) 1538
Prinzide Tablets (0.3% to 1%) 1540
Procardia Capsules (Less than 0.5%) 1781
Procardia XL Tablets (1% or less) 1783
Profasi (human chorionic gonadotropin, USP) 2186
Protostat Tablets 1674
Quadrinal Tablets 1183
Quinidex Extentabs 1868
Raudixin Tablets 1803
Rauzide Tablets 1804
Reglan (Less frequent) 1869
Renese-R Tablets 1786
Retrovir Capsules (Less than 5%) 802
Retrovir I.V. Infusion (Less than 5%) 805
Retrovir Syrup (Less than 5%) 802
Rogaine Topical Solution (0.36%) 2357
Rufen Tablets (Less than 1%) 691
Rythmol Tablets (Less than 1%) 1184
Sandimmune (Rare) 2024
Sandostatin Injection (Less than 1%) 2029
Sanorex Tablets 2030
Sectral Capsules (2%) 2520
Sedapap Tablets 50 mg/650 mg 1360
Seldane Tablets 1349
Seldane-D Extended-Release Tablets 1350
Sensorcaine 631
Sensorcaine-MPF Spinal 634
Septra 813
Septra I.V. Infusion 808
Septra I.V. Infusion ADD-Vantage Vials 810
Septra 813
Ser-Ap-Es Tablets 881
Serophene (clomiphene citrate tablets, USP) (Less than 1 in 100 patients) 2186
Serpasil-Apresoline Tablets 884
Serpasil-Esidrix Tablets 886
Sinemet Tablets 952
Sinemet CR Tablets (2.2%) 953
Stilphostrol Tablets and Ampuls 1609
Symmetrel Capsules & Syrup (1-5%) 936
▲ Synarel Nasal Solution (5% of patients) 2300
Tagamet 2228
Talacen (Infrequent) 2070
Talwin Injection (Infrequent) 2071
Talwin Compound (Infrequent) 2072
Talwin Injection 2071
Talwin Nx 2073
Tambocor Tablets (1-3%) 1315
Tegison Capsules (Less than 1%) 1881
Tegretol Chewable Tablets 654
Tegretol Suspension 656
Tegretol Tablets 654
Tenex Tablets (Less than 3%) 1875
▲ Tenoretic Tablets (0.6 to 12%) 1105
▲ Tenormin Tablets and I.V. Injection (0.6 to 12%) 1107
Tenuate 1354
Testred Capsules 1124
Timolide Tablets 1547
Timoptic in Ocudose 1552
Timoptic Sterile Ophthalmic Solution 1550

Tolectin (200, 400 and 600 mg) (1 to 3%) 1379
Tonocard Tablets (Less than 1%) 1554
Toradol IM Injection (1% or less) 2302
Trancopal Caplets 2075
Tranxene 556
▲ Trexan Tablets (Less than 10%) 937
Tri-Norinyl 28-Day Tablets 2304
Valium Injectable 1937
Valium Tablets (Infrequent) 1939
Valrelease Capsules (Occasional) 1923
Vascor (200, 300 and 400 mg) Tablets 1383
Vaseretic Tablets 1559
Vasotec I.V. 1562
Vasotec Tablets (0.5% to 1%) 1564
Velban Vials 1305
Voltaren Tablets (Less than 1%) 1042
Vontrol Tablets 2243
Wellbutrin Tablets (Frequent) 821
Winstrol Tablets 2075
Wytensin Tablets (3% or less) 2542
▲ Xanax Tablets (13.8% to 13.9%) 2367
Zantac Injection and Zantac Injection Premixed (Rare) 1063
Zantac (Rare) 1065
Zaroxolyn Tablets 989
Zestoretic (0.3 to 1%) 2274
Zestril Tablets (Less than 1%) 2277
Zoladex (1% to 5%) 1110
Zyloprim Tablets (Less than 1%) 830

Depression, circulatory

Innovar Injection 1141
Methadone Hydrochloride Oral Solution & Tablets 1987
Oramorph SR (Morphine Sulfate Sustained Release Tablets) 1988
Roxanol 1991
Sublimaze Injection 1146

Depression, mental

Aldomet Ester HCl Injection 1417
Amen 833
Android 1111
Aygestin Tablets 2437
Azo Gantanol Tablets 1887
Azulfidine Tablets, EN-tabs, Oral Suspension (Rare) 1157
Blocadren Tablets 1429
Brevicon 2304
Cartrol Tablets 507
Catapres Tablets (About 1 in 100 patients) 676
Catapres-TTS (1%) 677
Celontin 1692
Chloromycetin Kapseals 1695
Chloromycetin Palmitate, Oral Suspension 1697
Chloromycetin Sodium Succinate 1698
Combipres Tablets (About 1%) 678
Corgard Tablets 701
Corzide Tablets 702
Cycrin Tablets 2449
Dantrium Capsules (Less frequent) 1619
Demulen 2161
Depakene Capsules & Syrup 511
Depakote Tablets 512
Depo-Medrol Sterile Aqueous Suspension 2334
Depo-Provera Sterile Aqueous Suspension 2336
Diulo 2129
Diupres Tablets 1461
Enduronyl 518
Enovid 2161
Esgic-Plus Tablets 1002
Esgic Tablets & Capsules 1001
Esimil Tablets 864
Estradurin 2452
Estratest 2245
Estrovis 1721
Fansidar Tablets 1896
Flexeril Tablets (Less than 1%) 1471
Gantrisin Ophthalmic Ointment/Solution 1900
Hydrocortone Acetate Sterile Suspension 1479
Hydropres Tablets 1485
Hylorel Tablets (1.9%) 975
Inapsine Injection 1140
Inderal 2459
Inderal LA Long Acting Capsules 2461
Inderide Tablets 2463
Inderide LA Long Acting Capsules 2465
Innovar Injection 1141
Ismelin Tablets 869
Isoptin Injectable 1177
Jenest-28 Tablets 1636
Kerlone Tablets 2172
Levatol 1832
Levlen/Tri-Levlen 665
Lo/Ovral Tablets 2471
Lo/Ovral-28 Tablets 2476
Loestrin 1728
Lopressor HCT Tablets 1034
Mediatric Capsules 2476
Menrium Tablets 1934
Micronor Tablets 1667
Modicon 1667
Nizoral Tablets (Rare) 1145
Nordette-21 Tablets 2481
Nordette-28 Tablets 2483
Norethin 2133
Norinyl 2304
Norlestrin 1746
Norlutate 1754
Norlutin 1755
Normodyne Tablets 2110
Normozide Tablets 2112
Nor-Q D Tablets 2304
Ogen 540
Oreticyl 545
Ortho Dienestrol Cream 1664
Ortho-Cyclen Tablets 1658
Ortho-Novum 1667
Ovral Tablets 2490
Ovral-28 Tablets 2491
Ovrette Tablets 2492
PMB 200 and PMB 400 2504
Pediazole 1973
Pfizerpen-AS Aqueous Suspension (Approximately 1 in 500) 1959
Premarin Intravenous 2508
Premarin with Methyltestosterone 2515
Premarin Tablets 2510
Premarin Vaginal Cream 2512
Prinivil Tablets (Less than 1%) 1538
Procan SR Tablets (Occasional) 1760
Pronestyl Capsules and Tablets 1800
Pronestyl Injection 1798
Pronestyl-SR Tablets (Occasional) 1801
ProSom Tablets (2%) 554
Provera Tablets 2356
Quadrinal Tablets 1183
Reglan 1869
Ritalin Tablets 880
▲ Roferon-A Injection (16%) 1916
Salutensin/Salutensin-Demi 719
Sectral Capsules 2520
Serpasil Tablets 883
Stilphostrol Tablets and Ampuls 1609
Sublimaze Injection 1146
TACE 12 and 25 mg 1353
Tenoretic Tablets 1105
Tenormin Tablets and I.V. Injection 1107
Thiosulfil Forte Tablets 2526
Tigan 2239
Timoptic in Ocudose 1552
Timoptic Sterile Ophthalmic Solution 1550
Trandate HCT/Trandate 579
Trecator-SC Tablets 2527
Levlen/Tri-Levlen 665
Tri-Norinyl 2304
Triphasil-21 Tablets 2527
Triphasil-28 Tablets 2532
Visken Tablets 2036
Zantac Injection and Zantac Injection Premixed (Rare) 1063
Zantac (Rare) 1065
Zarontin Capsules (Rare) 1768
Zarontin Syrup (Rare) 1769
Zaroxolyn Tablets 989
Zoladex (1% to 5%) 1110

Depression, mood (see under Depression, mental)

Depression, respiratory

Actifed with Codeine Cough Syrup 752
▲ Alfenta Injection (Most common) 1131
Anectine 755
▲ Anestacon Solution (Among most common) 2394
Anexsia 5/500 Tablets 2196
Anexsia 7.5/650 Tablets 2197
Aralen Hydrochloride Injection 2038
Arfonad Ampuls 1887
Astramorph/PF Injection, USP (Preservative-Free) 618
Azdōne Tablets 844
Brevital Sodium Vials 1248
Clozaril Tablets (Rare) 2000
Codiclear DH Syrup 845
Dalgan Injection (Less than 1%) 620
Damason-P 1356
Demerol 2047
Dilaudid Cough Syrup 1174
Dilaudid 1173
Dilaudid-HP Injection 1175
Dolophine Hydrochloride Ampoules & Vials 1260
Dolophine Hydrochloride Tablets 1261
Doral Tablets 2383
Duramorph 960
Duranest Injections 624
Dyclone 0.5% and 1% Topical Solutions, USP 626
▲ Empirin with Codeine Phosphate Nos. 2, 3 & 4 (Among most frequent) 764
Ethrane 599
Forane 600
Garamycin Injectable 2093
Hycodan Syrup, Tablets 927
Hycomine Compound Tablets 929
Hycomine Syrup 927
Hycotuss Expectorant Syrup 930
Hydrocet Capsules 835
Infumorph 200 and Infumorph 500 Sterile Solutions 962
▲ Innovar Injection (Most common) 1141
Ketalar 1726
Klonopin Tablets 1902
Levo-Dromoran (Infrequent) 1906
Lortab ASA Tablets 2414
Lortab 2412
MS Contin Tablets 1814
MSIR 1817
Marcaine Hydrochloride with Epinephrine 1:200,000 2055
Marcaine Hydrochloride Injection 2055
Mepergan Injection 2479
Methadone Hydrochloride Diskets 1284
Methadone Hydrochloride Oral Solution & Tablets 1987
Nardil (Less frequent) 1742
Nubain Injection (Less than 1%) 934
Numorphan Hydrochloride Injection 935
Numorphan Suppositories 935
Oramorph SR (Morphine Sulfate Sustained Release Tablets) 1988
Pantopon Injectable 1911
Percocet Tablets 950
Phenaphen with Codeine Capsules 1865
Phenaphen-650 with Codeine Tablets 1866
Phenergan with Codeine 2497
Phenergan VC with Codeine 2501
Phenobarbital Elixir and Tablets 1293
Prostigmin Injectable 1120
Prostigmin Tablets 1121
Prostin VR Pediatric Sterile Solution (Less than 1%) 2355
Roxanol 1991
Scleromate (Rare) 1685
▲ Sublimaze Injection (Most common) 1146
▲ Sufenta Injection (Most common) 1147
Surital Ampoules, Steri-Vials 1764
Survanta Beractant Intratracheal Suspension 1978
Talacen (Rare) 2070
Talwin Injection (Infrequent) 2071
Talwin Compound 2072
Talwin Injection (Infrequent) 2071
Talwin Nx (Rare) 2073
Tussionex Extended-Release Suspension 988
Tylenol with Codeine 1381
Tylox Capsules 1382
Valium Injectable 1937
Versed Injection 1924
Vicodin Tablets 1187
Vicodin ES Tablets 1189
Xylocaine Injections 637
Xylocaine Injections for Ventricular Arrhythmias 639
Xylocaine 2% Jelly 643
Xylocaine 5% Ointment 644
Xylocaine 10% Oral Spray 645
4% Xylocaine-MPF Sterile Solution 641
Zydone Capsules 941

Depression, respiratory, neonatal

Anexsia 5/500 Tablets 2196
Anexsia 7.5/650 Tablets 2197
Astramorph/PF Injection, USP (Preservative-Free) 618
Damason-P 1356
Demerol 2047
Dilaudid Cough Syrup 1174
Dilaudid 1173
Dolophine Hydrochloride Tablets 1261
Duramorph 960
Fiorinal with Codeine Capsules 2008
Hycodan Syrup, Tablets 927
Hycomine Compound Tablets 929
Hycomine Syrup 927
Hycotuss Expectorant Syrup 930
Lortab ASA Tablets 2414
Lortab 2412
MS Contin Tablets 1814
MSIR 1817
Mepergan Injection 2479
Methadone Hydrochloride Oral Solution & Tablets 1987
Nubain Injection 934
Oramorph SR (Morphine Sulfate Sustained Release Tablets) 1988
Percocet Tablets 950
Quadrinal Tablets 1183
Roxanol 1991
Tracrium Injection 817
Trandate HCT Tablets 579
Trandate Injection 577
Trandate Tablets 579
Tussionex Extended-Release Suspension 988
Tylenol with Codeine 1381
Tylox Capsules 1382
Vicodin Tablets 1187
Vicodin ES Tablets 1189
Zydone Capsules 941

Depressive reactions

Renese-R Tablets 1786
Soma Compound w/Codeine Tablets (Infrequent or rare) 2390
Soma Compound Tablets (Infrequent or rare) 2389
Soma Tablets 2388

Dermal creases

Doxorubicin Hydrochloride for Injection, USP (A few cases) 622
Doxorubicin Hydrochloride Injection, USP (A few cases) 848
Rubex 739

Dermatitis

Achromycin Ophthalmic Ointment 1% ⊙ 307
Achromycin Ophthalmic Suspension 1% ⊙ 308
Adalat Capsules (10 mg and 20 mg) (2% or less) 1587
Altace Capsules 1086
Anafranil Capsules (Up to 2%) 650
Atrohist Sprinkle Capsules (Very rare) 558
Atropine Sulfate Sterile Ophthalmic Solution and S.O.P. Sterile Ophthalmic Ointment ⊙ 239
Aureomycin Ophthalmic Ointment 1.0% ⊙ 308
Benemid Tablets 1426
Benoquin Cream 20% (Occasional) 1112
Cerumenex Drops (1% of 2,700 patients) 1813
Clozaril Tablets (Less than 1%) 2000
ColBENEMID Tablets 1436
Colestid Granules (Fewer than 1 in 1,000) 2328
Colyte 1826
Coumadin Injection & Tablets (Infrequent) 944
Cytotec (Infrequent) 2159
Daraprim Tablets (Rare) 761
Dicumarol Tablets (Infrequent) 516
Dilantin Infatabs 1710
Dilantin Kapseals 1708
Dilantin-30 Pediatric/Dilantin-125 Suspension (Rare) 1713
Dilantin with Phenobarbital Kapseals (Rare) 1715
Diulo 2129
Efudex 1880
▲ Ergamisol Tablets (8 to 23%) 1136
Esimil Tablets 864
Sterile FUDR 1898
Fedahist Gyrocaps (Very rare) 2145
Fedahist Timecaps (Rare) 2145
Fluorouracil Injection (Substantial number of cases) 1897
GoLYTELY (Isolated cases) 699
Halcion Tablets (Rare) 2340
Hibistat Germicidal Hand Rinse (Rare) 2272
IFEX (Less than 1%) 729
▲ Intron A (8%) 2097
Ismelin Tablets 869
Kinesed Tablets 2272
Lincocin (Rare) 2344
Lopid Capsules and Tablets 1736
Lotensin Tablets 872
Loxitane 1213
Lupron Depot 7.5 mg (Less than 5%) 2311

- ▲ Lupron Injection (5% or more) 2310
- Matulane Capsules 1907
- Maxair Inhaler (Less than 1%) 1311
- Mellaril (Infrequent) 2011
- Methotrexate Tablets, Parenteral, LPF Parenteral (1 to 3%) 1217
- Myambutol Tablets 1225
- Mykrox ½ mg Tablets 984
- Myochrysine Injection 1516
- Naldecon Syrup, Tablets, Pediatric Drops and Pediatric Syrup (Very rare) 709
- Naprosyn (Less than 1%) 2297
- Nitro-Dur (nitroglycerin) Transdermal Infusion System 1164
- Norplant System 2484
- Novafed A Capsules (Rare) 1342
- Novahistine DH (Rare) 1342
- Novahistine Elixir (Rare) ▣ 596
- NuLYTELY 699
- pHisoHex 2066
- Panwarfin Tablets (Infrequent) 547
- Phenergan Injection 2493
- Phenergan Tablets 2496
- Pro-Banthīne Tablets 2141
- Procardia Capsules (2% or Less) 1781
- Proglycem 649
- Rheumatrex Methotrexate Dose Pack (1% to 3%) 1234
- ▲ Ridaura Capsules (Second most common) 2224
- ▲ Rogaine Topical Solution (7.36%) 2357
- Solganal Suspension 2122
- Tacaryl 2409
- Talwin Injection 2071
- Talwin Nx 2073
- Taractan (Infrequent) 1920
- Temaril Tablets, Syrup and Spansule Sustained Release Capsules 1085
- Temovate Scalp Application (1 of 294 patients) 1056
- Tenex Tablets (Less than 3%) 1875
- Theo-Organidin Elixir 2391
- Travase Ointment 697
- Tussi-Organidin DM Liquid 2392
- Tussi-Organidin Liquid 2391
- Urispas Tablets 2242
- Urobiotic-250 Capsules (Rare) 1968
- Voltaren Tablets (Less than 1%) 1042
- ▲ Xanax Tablets (3.8%) 2367
- Zaroxolyn Tablets 989

Dermatitis, allergic

- Alphatrex Cream, Ointment & Lotion (Infrequent) 2076
- Antabuse Tablets (Small number of patients) 2429
- Aristocort A (Infrequent) 1010
- Betatrex Cream, Ointment & Lotion 2077
- Cortone Acetate Sterile Suspension 1437
- Cortone Acetate Tablets 1439
- Decadron Elixir 1445
- Decadron Phosphate Injection 1449
- Decadron Phosphate Respihaler 1454
- Decadron Phosphate Turbinaire 1456
- Decadron Phosphate with Xylocaine Injection, Sterile 1451
- Decadron Tablets 1447
- Decadron-LA Sterile Suspension 1457
- Elocon (Infrequent) 2084
- Epifoam 1828
- Halog (Infrequent) 2399
- Hydeltrasol Injection, Sterile 1476
- Hydeltra-T.B.A. Sterile Suspension 1478
- Hydrocortone Acetate Sterile Suspension 1479
- Hydrocortone Phosphate Injection, Sterile 1481
- Hydrocortone Tablets 1482
- Kenalog Cream, Lotion & Ointment (Infrequent) 2401
- Lanacane Creme ▣ 556
- Lidex (Infrequent) 2296
- Lotrisone Cream (Infrequent) 2103
- Monistat-Derm (miconazole nitrate) Cream (Isolated reports) 1679
- Mycolog II Cream and Ointment (Infrequent) 2407
- Mytrex Cream & Ointment (Infrequent) 2080
- Neo-Synalar Cream (Infrequent) 2296
- Otic Tridesilon Solution 0.05% (Infrequent) 1612
- Persa-Gel 1680
- ProctoCream-HC (Infrequent) 1834
- Proctofoam-HC 1835
- Serophene (clomiphene citrate tablets, USP) (Less than 1 in 100 patients) 2186
- Temovate Scalp Application (Infrequent) 1056
- Theroxide 1411
- Topicycline for Topical Solution (One case) 1856
- Tridesilon Creme 0.05% (Infrequent) 1611
- Tridesilon Ointment 0.05% (Infrequent) 1611
- Vagisil Creme ▣ 557

Dermatitis, bullous

- Chloromycetin Cream, 1% 1694
- Chloromycetin Otic 1697
- Chloroptic Sterile Ophthalmic Solution ⊙ 243
- Deprol Tablets (Rare) 2382
- Dilantin Infatabs 1710
- Dilantin Kapseals 1708
- Dilantin Parenteral 1712
- Dilantin-30 Pediatric/Dilantin-125 Suspension 1713
- Dilantin with Phenobarbital Kapseals 1715
- Elase-Chloromycetin Ointment 1015
- Equagesic Tablets (Rare) 2451
- Miltown Tablets (Rare) 2386
- PMB 200 and PMB 400 (Rare) 2504
- Solganal Suspension (Occasional) 2122
- Zyloprim Tablets (Less than 1%) 830

Dermatitis, contact

- Americaine Anesthetic Lubricant 972
- Americaine Otic Topical Anesthetic Ear Drops 973
- Atabrine Hydrochloride Tablets 2041
- Bactroban Ointment (Less than 1%) 2200
- BenzaShave Medicated Shave Cream 5% and 10% 1409
- Capitrol Shampoo 2396
- Cleocin T Topical 2327
- Compazine 2201
- Cortisporin Otic Suspension Sterile 760
- Eldopaque Forte 4% Cream (Occasional) 1114
- Eldoquin Forte 4% Cream (Occasional) 1114
- Furacin Soluble Dressing (Approximately 1%) 1854
- Furacin Topical Cream (Approximately 1%) 1854
- Furacin Topical Solution 0.2% 1855
- Maxivate Cream, Lotion & Ointment 0.05% 2406
- Meclan (meclocycline sulfosalicylate) Cream (One report) 1679
- Mellaril 2011
- Navane Capsules and Concentrate 1954
- Navane Intramuscular 1956
- Norzine 1818
- ProctoCream-HC (Infrequent) 1834
- Prozac Pulvules (Infrequent) 920
- Serentil 686
- Solaquin Forte 4% Cream (Occasional) 1122
- Solaquin Forte 4% Gel (Occasional) 1123
- Temovate Scalp Application (Infrequent) 1056
- Theroxide 1411
- Thorazine 2234
- Torecan 1993

Dermatitis, eczematoid

- Isopto Atropine ⊙ 218
- Isopto Homatropine ⊙ 221
- Isopto Hyoscine ⊙ 222
- Symmetrel Capsules & Syrup (Less than 0.1%) 936
- Zyloprim Tablets (Less than 1%) 830

Dermatitis, erythematous

- Phenobarbital Elixir and Tablets 1293

Dermatitis, exfoliative

- Achromycin V Capsules (Uncommon) 1193
- Adalat Capsules (10 mg and 20 mg) (Less than 0.5%) 1587
- Alurate Elixir 1883
- Ansaid Tablets (Rare) 2319
- Atabrine Hydrochloride Tablets 2041
- Augmentin Tablets, Powder for Oral Suspension, and Chewable Tablets (Occasional case) 2198
- Axid Pulvules 1246
- Azactam for Injection (Less than 1%) 2252
- Azo Gantanol Tablets 1887
- Azo Gantrisin Tablets 1888
- Azulfidine Tablets, EN-tabs, Oral Suspension (Rare) 1157
- Bactrim DS Tablets 1891
- Bactrim I.V. Infusion 1889
- Bactrim 1891
- Bicillin C-R Injection 2438
- Bicillin C-R 900/300 Injection 2440
- Bicillin L-A Injection 2442
- Butisol Sodium Elixir & Tablets (Less than 1 in 100) 2377
- Capoten 2255
- Capozide 2258
- Cardilate Oral/Sublingual Tablets (Occasional) 757
- Cardizem Tablets-30 mg, 60 mg, 90 mg and 120 mg (Infrequent) 1329
- Cardizem SR Capsules-60 mg, 90 mg and 120 mg (Less than 1%) 1327
- Cipro I.V. (1% or less) 1592
- Cipro Tablets 1589
- Clinoril Tablets 1433
- Compazine 2201
- Corzide Tablets 702
- Cuprimine Capsules 1442
- Declomycin Capsules, Tablets (Uncommon) 1199
- Depen Titratable Tablets 2379
- Deprol Tablets (Rare) 2382
- Diabinese Tablets 1775
- Dilantin Infatabs 1710
- Dilantin Kapseals 1708
- Dilantin Parenteral 1712
- Dilantin-30 Pediatric/Dilantin-125 Suspension 1713
- Dilantin with Phenobarbital Kapseals 1715
- Dilatrate-SR (Occasional) 1827
- Dolobid Tablets (Less than 1 in 100) 1465
- Doryx Capsules 1717
- Duragesic Transdermal System (Less than 1%) 1133
- Equagesic Tablets (Rare) 2451
- Ergamisol Tablets (Less frequent) 1136
- Etrafon 2087
- Fansidar Tablets 1896
- Feldene Capsules (Less than 1%) 1777
- Fiorinal with Codeine Capsules 2008
- Floxin Tablets 1652
- Gantanol 1899
- Gantrisin Ophthalmic Ointment/Solution 1900
- Gantrisin 1901
- Indocin Capsules (Less than 1%) 1487
- Indocin I.V. (Less than 1%) 1490
- Indocin (Less than 1%) 1487
- Intal Capsules (Less than 1 in 100,000 patients) 978
- Intal Inhaler (Rare) 979
- Intal Nebulizer Solution (Rare) 980
- Isordil (Occasional) 2467
- Lasix 1093
- Lopid Capsules and Tablets 1736
- Macrodantin Capsules (Rare) 1624
- Mebaral Tablets (Less than 1 in 100) 2061
- Meclomen Capsules (Less than 1%) 1739
- Mefoxin 1498
- Mefoxin Premixed Intravenous Solution 1500
- Mellaril 2011
- Mesantoin Tablets (Rare) 2013
- Mexitil Capsules (Rare) 680
- Miltown Tablets (Rare) 2386
- Minocin Intravenous (Uncommon) 1221
- Minocin Oral Suspension (Uncommon) 1224
- Minocin Pellet-Filled Capsules (Uncommon) 1222
- Monodox Capsules (Uncommon) 1630
- Monopril Tablets (0.2 to 1.0%) 1406
- Myochrysine Injection 1516
- Nalfon Pulvules & Tablets (Less than 1%) 919
- Nasalcrom Nasal Solution (Rare) 986
- Naturetin Tablets (Occasional) 1789
- Navane Capsules and Concentrate 1954
- Navane Intramuscular 1956
- Nembutal Sodium Capsules (Less than 1%) 534
- Nembutal Sodium Solution 536
- Nitro-Bid IV 1338
- Nitro-Bid Ointment 1339
- Nitro-Bid Capsules 1338
- Nitrolingual Spray 1846
- Nitrostat IV (Occasional) 1744
- Noroxin Tablets 1519
- Norzine 1818
- Orudis Capsules (Less than 1%) 2488
- PMB 200 and PMB 400 (Rare) 2504
- Pediazole 1973
- Pfizerpen for Injection 1957
- Pfizerpen-AS Aqueous Suspension 1959
- Phenobarbital Elixir and Tablets (Less than 1 in 100 patients) 1293
- Plaquenil Sulfate Tablets 2067
- Procardia XL Tablets 1783
- Prolixin Decanoate 1795
- Prolixin Elixir 1793
- Prolixin Enanthate 1796
- Prolixin Injection 1791
- Prolixin Oral Concentrate 1792
- Prolixin Tablets 1793
- Proloprim Tablets (Rare) 799
- Rauzide Tablets 1804
- Rifamate Capsules 1347
- Ritalin 880
- SSD RP Cream 690
- Seconal Sodium Pulvules (Less than 1 in 100) 1296
- Septra 813
- Septra I.V. Infusion 808
- Septra I.V. Infusion ADD-Vantage Vials 810
- Septra 813
- Serentil 686
- Silvadene Cream 1% 1352
- Solganal Suspension (Occasional) 2122
- Sorbitrate (Occasional) 1103
- Spectrobid Tablets & Powder for Oral Suspension (Occasional) 1961
- Stelazine (Occasional) 2226
- Tagamet (Very rare) 2228
- Tambocor Tablets (Less than 1%) 1315
- Taractan 1920
- Tegretol Chewable Tablets 654
- Tegretol Suspension 656
- Tegretol Tablets 654
- Tenex Tablets 1875
- Terramycin Capsules (Uncommon) 1786
- Terramycin Intramuscular Solution (Uncommon) 1964
- Thiosulfil Forte Tablets 2526
- Thorazine 2234
- Tonocard Tablets (Less than 1%) 1554
- Torecan 1993
- Triavil Tablets 1556
- Tridione 557
- Trilafon 2123
- Trimpex Tablets (Rare) 1922
- Unasyn (Occasional) 1965
- Vancocin HCl, Oral Solution & Pulvules (Infrequent) 1304
- Vancocin HCl, Vials & ADD-Vantage (Infrequent) 1302
- Vaseretic Tablets 1559
- Vasosulf ⊙ 279
- Vasotec I.V. 1562
- Vasotec Tablets 1564
- Vibramycin Hyclate Capsules (Uncommon) 1787
- Vibramycin Hyclate Intravenous (Uncommon) 1968
- Vibramycin (Uncommon) 1787
- Voltaren Tablets (Rare) 1042
- Wellbutrin Tablets 821
- Wycillin Injection 2537
- Zyloprim Tablets (Less than 1%) 830

Dermatitis, eyelid

- OptiPranolol Sterile Ophthalmic Solution (A small number of patients) ⊙ 261

Dermatitis, fungal

- Permax Tablets (Infrequent) 1291
- Prozac Pulvules (Rare) 920

Dermatitis, gold-induced

- Ridaura Capsules 2224
- Solganal Suspension 2122

Dermatitis, lichenoides

- Intron A (1% or less) 2097

Dermatitis, maculopapular

- Chloromycetin Cream, 1% 1694
- Chloromycetin Otic 1697
- Chloroptic S.O.P. ⊙ 243
- Chloroptic Sterile Ophthalmic Solution ⊙ 243
- Elase-Chloromycetin Ointment 1015
- Solganal Suspension (Occasional) 2122

Dermatitis, perioral

- Aclovate Cream 1053

Alphatrex Cream, Ointment & Lotion (Infrequent) 2076
Analpram-HC Rectal Cream 1% and 2.5% 970
Anusol-HC Cream (Infrequent) 1690
Aristocort A (Infrequent) 1010
Betatrex Cream, Ointment & Lotion 2077
Carmol HC Cream 1% (Infrequent) 2296
Cortisporin Cream 757
Cortisporin Ointment 758
Cortisporin Otic Solution Sterile 760
Cortisporin Otic Suspension Sterile 760
Cutivate Cream 0.05% 1054
Cutivate Ointment 0.005% 1054
Cyclocort Lotion (Infrequent) 1198
Decadron Phosphate Topical Cream 1455
Decaspray Topical Aerosol 1459
DesOwen Cream, Ointment and Lotion (Infrequent) 1682
Diprolene (Infrequent) 2083
Eldecort Cream 1.0% (Infrequent) 1113
Eldecort Cream 1.0% and 2.5% (Infrequent) 1113
Elocon (Infrequent) 2084
Epifoam 1828
Florone/Florone E 908
Halog (Infrequent) 2399
Hytone 909
Kenalog Cream, Lotion & Ointment (Infrequent) 2401
Lidex (Infrequent) 2296
Locoid Cream, Ointment and Topical Solution (Infrequent) 970
Lotrisone Cream (Infrequent) 2103
Maxivate Cream, Lotion & Ointment 0.05% 2406
Mycolog II Cream and Ointment (Infrequent) 2407
Mytrex Cream & Ointment (Infrequent) 2080
NeoDecadron Topical Cream 1518
Neo-Synalar Cream (Infrequent) 2296
Nutracort Cream & Lotion (Infrequent) 1684
Orabase HCA Oral Paste (Infrequent) 890
PediOtic Suspension Sterile 797
Pramosone Cream, Lotion & Ointment 971
ProctoCream-HC (Infrequent) 1834
Proctofoam-HC 1835
Psorcon Ointment 0.05% 909
Psorion Cream 0.05% (Infrequent) 1121
Synacort Creams 1%, 2.5% (Infrequent) 2296
Synalar (Infrequent) 2296
Temovate 1056
Topicort (Infrequent) 1098
Tridesilon Creme 0.05% (Infrequent) 1611
Tridesilon Ointment 0.05% (Infrequent) 1611
Ultravate Cream 0.05% (Infrequent) 2410
Ultravate Ointment 0.05% (Less frequent) 2411
Vanoxide-HC Acne Lotion 911
Vioform-Hydrocortisone Cream and Mild Cream 889
Vioform-Hydrocortisone Ointment 889
Vytone Cream 1% 911
Westcort 2411

Dermatitis, photosensitive
Anaprox and Anaprox DS Tablets (Less than 3%) 2288
▲ Cordarone Tablets (4 to 9%) 2446
Intal Capsules (Less than 1 in 100,000 patients) 978
Intal Nebulizer Solution (Rare) 980

Dermatitis, purpuric
Dilantin Infatabs 1710
Dilantin Kapseals 1708
Dilantin Parenteral 1712
Dilantin-30 Pediatric/Dilantin-125 Suspension 1713
Dilantin with Phenobarbital Kapseals 1715

Dermatitis, radiation recall
Methotrexate Tablets, Parenteral, LPF Parenteral 1217
Rheumatrex Methotrexate Dose Pack 1234
VePesid Capsules and Injection (Single case) 741

Dermatitis, vesicular bullous (see under Dermatitis, bullous)

Dermatologic reactions, unspecified
Atgam Sterile Solution (1 in 8 patients) 2320
Ativan Tablets (Less frequent) 2434
Bentyl 1322
Capoten 2255
Capozide 2258
Clinoril Tablets (Less than 1 in 100) 1433
Darbid Tablets 2205
Depen Titratable Tablets (Rare) 2379
▲ Idamycin for Injection (46%) 564
Intron A (2 patients) 2097
Kerlone Tablets (Less than 2%) 2172
Kutrase Capsules 2146
Levsin/Levsinex 2147
Metrodin (urofollitropin for injection) 2182
Monopril Tablets (0.2 to 1.0%) 1406
Nicorette 1335
Norflex (Rare) 1314
Norgesic (Rare) 1314
SSD RP Cream 690
Silvadene Cream 1% 1352
Solu-Cortef Sterile Powder 2361
Solu-Medrol Sterile Powder 2363
Vaseretic Tablets 1559
▲ Xanax Tablets (Greater than 3%) 2367

Dermatomyositis
Cuprimine Capsules (Rare) 1442
Depen Titratable Tablets (Rare) 2379

Dermatomyositis, exacerbation of
Actimmune (Rare) 1046

Descemetitis
AK-Taine ⊙ 207
Alcaine (Occasional) ⊙ 210
Fluoracaine (Sometimes) ⊙ 208
Ophthetic ⊙ 249

Desquamation
A/T/S Topical Gel and Topical Solution 1089
Cytosar-U Sterile Powder (Rare) 2329
ETS-2% 1685
Erycette (erythromycin 2%) Topical Solution 1678
Feldene Capsules (Less than 1%) 1777
NebuPent for Inhalation Solution (1% or less) 1017
T-Stat 2.0% Topical Solution and Pads 2409
Theramycin Z Topical Solution 2% 1410
Vagistat (Less than 1%) 1397

Diabetes (see under Diabetes mellitus)

Diabetes insipidus, nephrogenic
Declomycin Capsules, Tablets 1199
Eskalith (Some reports) 2214
Lithane Tablets 1596
Zanosar Sterile Powder (Two cases) 2371

Diabetes mellitus
Anafranil Capsules (Infrequent) 650
Aristocort Suspension 1008
Aristospan Suspension (Intralesional) 1011
Celestone Soluspan Suspension 2081
Dalalone D.P. Injectable 999
Dyazide Capsules 2208
Hydeltra-T.B.A. Sterile Suspension 1478
Kerlone Tablets (Less than 2%) 2172
▲ Lupron Depot 3.75 mg (Among most frequent) 2312
Lupron Depot 7.5 mg (Less than 5%) 2311
Lupron Injection (Less than 5%) 2310
Maxzide 1215
Methotrexate Tablets, Parenteral, LPF Parenteral 1217
Permax Tablets (Infrequent) 1291
Rheumatrex Methotrexate Dose Pack 1234
Thalitone Tablets 687

Diabetes mellitus, increase
Hydrocortone Phosphate Injection, Sterile 1481
Intron A (1% or less) 2097
Medrol 2348

Diabetes mellitus, precipitation of latent
Aristospan Suspension (Intra-articular) 1011
Capozide 2258
Cortenema 2244
Cortone Acetate Sterile Suspension 1437
Cortone Acetate Tablets 1439
Decadron Elixir 1445
Decadron Phosphate Injection 1449
Decadron Phosphate Respihaler 1454
Decadron Phosphate Turbinaire 1456
Decadron Phosphate with Xylocaine Injection, Sterile 1451
Decadron Tablets 1447
Decadron-LA Sterile Suspension 1457
Deltasone Tablets 2332
Depo-Medrol Sterile Aqueous Suspension 2334
Hydeltrasol Injection, Sterile 1476
Hydrocortone Acetate Sterile Suspension 1479
Hydrocortone Tablets 1482
Kenalog-10 Injection 2402
Kenalog-40 Injection 2403
Orudis Capsules (Less than 1%) 2488
Pediapred Oral Liquid 987
Prinzide Tablets 1540
Rauzide Tablets 1804
Solu-Cortef Sterile Powder 2361
Solu-Medrol Sterile Powder 2363
Vaseretic Tablets 1559
Zestoretic 2274

Dialysis encephalopathy
ALternaGEL Liquid 1154
Aludrox Oral Suspension 2428
Amphojel 2429
Basaljel 2438
Gelusil Liquid & Tablets ■ 639
Maalox Plus Extra Strength 1850
Mylanta 1155
Mylanta • Double Strength 1155
Rolaids ■ 743

Dialysis osteomalacia, results in, or worsening of
ALternaGEL Liquid 1154
Aludrox Oral Suspension 2428
Amphojel 2429
Basaljel 2438
Gelusil Liquid & Tablets ■ 639
Maalox Plus Extra Strength 1850
Mylanta 1155
Mylanta • Double Strength 1155
Rolaids ■ 743

Diaphoresis
Accutane Capsules (Less than 1%) 1878
Actifed with Codeine Cough Syrup 752
Actigall Capsules 2280
Adalat Capsules (10 mg and 20 mg) (2% or less) 1587
Adenocard Injection (Less than 1%) 1007
AeroBid Inhaler System (1-3%) 995
AK-Dilate Solution 2.5% and 10% (Rare) ⊙ 203
Albalon Solution with Liquifilm ⊙ 238
Alferon N Injection (One patient to 3%) 1809
Altace Capsules (Less than 1%) 1086
▲ Anafranil Capsules (9% to 29%) 650
Ana-Kit Anaphylaxis Emergency Treatment Kit 1100
Anaprox and Anaprox DS Tablets (Less than 3%) 2288
Ansaid Tablets (Less than 1%) 2319
AquaMEPHYTON Injection 1422
Aristocort Suspension 1008
Aristospan Suspension 1011
Asendin Tablets (Greater than 1%) 1196
Atgam Sterile Solution (At least 1 patient and less than 5% of total patients) 2320
Atromid-S Capsules 2435
Axid Pulvules (1%) 1246
Azactam for Injection (Less than 1%) 2252
Azdōne Tablets 844
BAL in Oil Ampules 661
Baron-X Tablets 650
Benadryl Capsules 1691
Benadryl Injection 1692
Blocadren Tablets (Less than 1%) 1429
Bontril Slow-Release 834
Brethine Ampuls (0.0 to 2.4%) 1026
Brethine Tablets 1026
Bretylol Injection (1 in 1000) 923
▲ Brevibloc Injection (12%) 942
Bricanyl Injection 1324
Bricanyl Tablets 1325
Bumex (0.1%) 1895
BuSpar (1%) 1401
Calan SR Caplets (1% or less) 2157
Calan Tablets (1% or less) 2155
Capoten 2255
Capozide 2258
Carbocaine Hydrochloride 3% Injection 956
Carbocaine Hydrochloride Injection 2043
Carbocaine Hydrochloride 2% with Neo-Cobefrin 956
Cardilate Oral/Sublingual Tablets (Occasional) 757
Cardura Tablets (0.5% to 1%) 1941
Cartrol Tablets (0.7-1.0%) 507
Celestone Soluspan Suspension 2081
Centrax (Less frequent) 1693
Cibalith-S 870
Cipro I.V. (1% or less) 1592
Clinoril Tablets (Less than 1 in 100) 1433
▲ Clozaril Tablets (More than 5 to 6%) 2000
Compazine 2201
Corgard Tablets (1 to 5 of 1000 patients) 701
Cortenema 2244
Cortifoam 1827
Cortone Acetate Sterile Suspension 1437
Cortone Acetate Tablets 1439
Corzide Tablets (1 to 5 of 1000 patients) 702
Cytotec (Infrequent) 2159
Dalalone D.P. Injectable 999
Dalgan Injection (Less than 1%) 620
Dalmane Capsules (Rare) 1927
Damason-P 1356
Danocrine Capsules 2046
Dantrium Capsules (Less frequent) 1619
Decadron Elixir 1445
Decadron Phosphate Injection 1449
Decadron Phosphate Respihaler 1454
Decadron Phosphate Turbinaire 1456
Decadron Phosphate with Xylocaine Injection, Sterile 1451
Decadron Tablets 1447
Decadron-LA Sterile Suspension 1457
Deconamine 663
Deltasone Tablets 2332
Demerol 2047
Depo-Medrol Sterile Aqueous Suspension 2334
Desyrel and Desyrel Dividose (Greater than 1%) 1404
Didrex Tablets 2338
Dilatrate-SR 1827
Dilaudid-HP Injection 1175
Diprivan Injection (Less than 1%) 2267
Dolobid Tablets (Less than 1 in 100) 1465
▲ Dolophine Hydrochloride Ampoules & Vials (Among most frequent) 1260
▲ Dolophine Hydrochloride Tablets (Among most frequent) 1261
Dopram Injectable 1860
▲ Duragesic Transdermal System (10% or more) 1133
Easprin 1719
Elavil 2269
Eldepryl 2250
Emete-con Intramuscular/Intravenous 1950
▲ Eminase (Less than 10%) 2211
Empirin with Codeine Phosphate Nos. 2, 3 & 4 764
Endep Tablets 1927
Engerix-B Unit-Dose Vials (Less than 1%) 2213
Enlon Injection 598
▲ Ethmozine Tablets (2%-5%) 946
Etrafon 2087
Feldene Capsules (Less than 1%) 1777
Flexeril Tablets (Less than 1%) 1471
Floropryl Sterile Ophthalmic Ointment (Rare) 1473
Floxin Tablets (Less than 1%) 1652
Haldol Decanoate 1375
Haldol Injection, Tablets and Concentrate 1373
Humorsol Sterile Ophthalmic Solution (Rare) 1475
Humulin 70/30, 100 Units 1267
Humulin BR, 100 Units 1268

Humulin L, 100 Units (Less common) 1268
Humulin U, 100 Units 1272
Hydeltrasol Injection, Sterile 1476
Hydeltra-T.B.A. Sterile Suspension 1478
Hydrocortone Acetate Sterile Suspension 1479
Hydrocortone Phosphate Injection, Sterile 1481
Hydrocortone Tablets 1482
Hyperstat I.V. Injection 2095
Hytrin Tablets (At least 1%) 529
Imferon 976
Indocin (Less than 1%) 1487
Innovar Injection 1141
Insulatard NPH 1626
Insulatard NPH Human 1627
▲Intron A (2% to 21%) 2097
Isoptin Injectable (Few) 1177
Isoptin Oral Tablets (Less than 1%) 1179
Isoptin SR Sustained Release Tablets (Less than 1%) 1181
Isordil (Occasional) 2467
Isuprel Hydrochloride Injection 1:5000 2050
Isuprel Hydrochloride Mistometer 2051
Isuprel Hydrochloride Solution 1:200 & 1:100 2052
Kenalog-10 Injection 2402
Kenalog-40 Injection 2403
Kerlone Tablets (Less than 2%) 2172
Larodopa Tablets (Infrequent) 1905
Levatol (1.6%) 1832
Levo-Dromoran (Rare) 1906
Levophed Bitartrate Injection 2054
Limbitrol 1933
Lioresal Tablets 1031
Lithobid Tablets 870
Lodine Capsules (Less than 1%) 2468
Lopressor HCT Tablets (1 in 100 patients) 1034
Lorelco Tablets 1333
Lortab ASA Tablets 2414
Lotensin Tablets 872
Loxitane 1213
Ludiomil Tablets 874
▲Lupron Depot 7.5 mg (58.9%) 2311
▲MS Contin Tablets (Among most frequent) 1814
▲MSIR (Among most frequent) 1817
Marax Tablets & DF Syrup 1954
Marcaine Hydrochloride with Epinephrine 1:200,000 (Rare) 2055
Marcaine Hydrochloride Injection (Rare) 2055
Marcaine Spinal (Rare) 2058
Matulane Capsules 1907
Medrol 2348
Mellaril 2011
▲Mepergan Injection (Among most frequent) 2479
Mephyton Tablets (Rare) 1503
Mestinon Injectable 1115
Mestinon 1116
▲Methadone Hydrochloride Diskets (Among most frequent) 1284
Methadone Hydrochloride Oral Solution & Tablets 1987
Methergine (Rare) 2016
Methotrexate Tablets, Parenteral, LPF Parenteral 1217
Mexitil Capsules (Less than 1% or about 6 in 1,000) 680
Minipress Capsules 1778
Minizide Capsules 1779
Miochol with Iocare Steri-Tags, Miochol System Pak and Miochol System Pak Plus (Rare) ⊙ 274
MIOSTAT ⊙ 233
Mixtard 70/30 1627
Mixtard Human 70/30 1628
Moban Tablets & Concentrate 932
Modane Plus Tablets ▣ 504
Modane Tablets ▣ 503
Moduretic Tablets (Less than or equal to 1%) 1510
Mono-Gesic Tablets 846
Monopril Tablets (0.2 to 1.0%) 1406
Murocoll-2 Sterile Ophthalmic Solution ⊙ 261
Myochrysine Injection 1516
▲Nalfon Pulvules & Tablets (4.6%) 919
Naphcon Forte ⊙ 226
Naprosyn (Less than 3%) 2297
Narcan Injection 933
Nardil (Less common) 1742
Navane Capsules and Concentrate 1954
Navane Intramuscular 1956
Nescaine/Nescaine MPF 629
Niclocide Chewable Tablets 1607
Nimotop Capsules (Less than 1%) 1607
Nipride I.V. Infusion 1909
Nitro-Bid Ointment 1339
Nitrolingual Spray 1846
▲Normodyne Injection (4%) 2108
Normodyne Tablets (Less than 1%) 2110
Normozide Tablets (Less than 1%) 2112
Norpramin Tablets 1340
▲Nubain Injection (9%) 934
Nucofed Capsules 2219
Nucofed Expectorant 2219
Nucofed Pediatric Expectorant 2220
Nucofed Syrup 2219
Omnipaque (Less than 0.1%) 2552
Optimine Tablets 2115
▲Oramorph SR (Morphine Sulfate Sustained Release Tablets) (Among most frequent) 1988
Orap Tablets 1020
Ornade Spansule Capsules 2221
Orudis Capsules (Less than 1%) 2488
Pamelor 2019
Pantopon Injectable 1911
Papaverine Hydrochloride Vials and Ampoules 1290
Pavabid Capsules (Rare) 1344
Pavabid HP Capsulets (Rare) 1344
Pediapred Oral Liquid 987
Peptavlon 2563
Periactin 1525
Peritrate (Occasional) 1756
Permax Tablets (2.1%) 1291
Phenergan with Codeine 2497
Phenergan VC with Codeine 2501
Pilocar (Extremely rare) ⊙ 275
Pilostat Sterile Ophthalmic Solution 0.5%, 1%, 2%, 3%, 4%, 5%, 6% (Extremely rare) ⊙ 263
Pitressin Synthetic, Ampoules 1758
Plegine Tablets 2504
Polaramine 2116
Pondimin Tablets 1867
Ponstel 1758
Prinivil Tablets (1% or less) 1538
Prinzide Tablets 1540
Procardia Capsules (2% or less) 1781
Procardia XL Tablets (1% or less) 1783
Prolixin Decanoate 1795
Prolixin Elixir 1793
Prolixin Enanthate 1796
Prolixin Injection 1791
Prolixin Oral Concentrate 1792
Prolixin Tablets 1793
ProSom Tablets (Infrequent) 554
Prostigmin Injectable 1120
Prostigmin Tablets 1121
Proventil Syrup (Less than 1 of 100) 2119
▲Prozac Pulvules (8.4%) 920
Quadrinal Tablets 1183
Quinamm Tablets 1344
Recombivax HB (Less than 1%) 1544
▲Retrovir Capsules (5%) 802
▲Retrovir I.V. Infusion (5%) 805
▲Retrovir Syrup (5%) 802
Rheumatrex Methotrexate Dose Pack 1234
Rocephin Injectable Vials, ADD-Vantage (Occasional) 1914
▲Roferon-A Injection (7% to 8%) 1916
▲Roxanol (Among most frequent) 1991
Ru-Tuss II Capsules 693
Rythmol Tablets (0.6 to 1.4%) 1184
Sandoglobulin I.V. (Less than 1%) 2027
Sanorex Tablets 2030
Seldane Tablets 1349
Seldane-D Extended-Release Tablets 1350
Sensorcaine (Rare) 631
Sensorcaine-MPF Spinal (Rare) 634
Sinemet Tablets 952
Sinemet CR Tablets 953
Sinequan (Occasional) 1960
Solganal Suspension 2122
Solu-Cortef Sterile Powder 2361
Solu-Medrol Sterile Powder 2363
Sorbitrate (Occasional) 1103
▲Stadol (6%) 721
Stelazine 2226
Sublimaze Injection 1146
Surmontil Capsules 2524
Talacen 2070
Talwin Injection 2071
Talwin Compound 2072
Talwin Injection 2071
Talwin Nx 2073
Tambocor Tablets (1-3%) 1315
Tavist Syrup 2033
Tavist Tablets 2035
Tavist-D Tablets 2035
▲Tegison Capsules (1-10%) 1881
Tegretol Chewable Tablets 654
Tegretol Suspension 656
Tegretol Tablets 654
Tenex Tablets (Less than 3%) 1875
Tensilon Injectable 1123
Tenuate 1354
Thorazine 2234
Timolide Tablets 1547
Timoptic in Ocudose 1552
Timoptic Sterile Ophthalmic Solution 1550
Tofranil Ampuls 1038
Tofranil Tablets 1039
Tofranil-PM Capsules 1041
▲Tonocard Tablets (2.3-5.1%) 1554
Toradol IM Injection (1% to 3%) 2302
▲Trandate Injection (4 of 100 patients) 577
Trandate Tablets (Less than 1% of 227 patients) 579
Triaminic Expectorant DH 1995
Triaminic Oral Infant Drops 1996
Triavil Tablets 1556
Trilafon 2123
Trinalin Repetabs Tablets 1170
Urecholine 1558
Vascor (200, 300 and 400 mg) Tablets (0.5 to 2.0%) 1383
Vaseretic Tablets 1559
Vasocon-A ⊙ 278
Vasotec I.V. 1562
Vasotec Tablets 1564
Vasoxyl Injection 819
Velosulin 1627
Velosulin Human 1628
Verelan Capsules (Less than 1%) 1243
Vivactil Tablets 1567
Voltaren Tablets (Less than 1%) 1042
▲Wellbutrin Tablets (22.3%) 821
▲Xanax Tablets (15.1%) 2367
Yocon (Common) 1686
Yutopar (Infrequent) 647
Zestoretic 2274
Zestril Tablets 2277
▲Zoladex (6%) 1110
Zovirax Sterile Powder (Less than 1%) 828

Diaphoresis, nocturnal

▲NebuPent for Inhalation Solution (10 to 23%) 1017
Roferon-A Injection 1916
Sandimmune (Rare) 2024

Diaphragm, paralyzed

Survanta Beractant Intratracheal Suspension 1978

Diarrhea

Accutane Capsules 1878
Achromycin V Capsules 1193
Actifed with Codeine Cough Syrup 752
Actigall Capsules (Less than 1%) 2280
▲Actimmune (14%) 1046
Adalat Capsules (10 mg and 20 mg) (2% or less) 1587
Adipex-P Tablets and Capsules 1019
Adriamycin PFS (Occasional) 561
Adriamycin RDF (Occasional) 562
▲AeroBid Inhaler System (10%) 995
Aldactazide 2150
Aldactone 2152
Aldoclor Tablets 1413
Aldomet Ester HCl Injection 1417
Aldomet Oral 1415
Aldoril Tablets 1418
▲Alferon N Injection (2% to 6%) 1809
Alkeran Tablets (Infrequent) 754
Allbee C-800 Plus Iron Tablets ▣ 670
Altace Capsules (Less than 1%) 1086
Amicar Syrup, Tablets, and Injection (Occasional) 1194
Aminophyllin Tablets 2153
Amoxil 2193
Anadrol-50 Tablets 2287
▲Anafranil Capsules (7% to 13%) 650
Anaprox and Anaprox DS Tablets (Less than 3%) 2288
Ancef Injection 2194
Ancobon Capsules 1886
▲Ansaid Tablets (3-9%) 2319
Apresazide Capsules (Common) 854
Apresoline Hydrochloride Parenteral (Ampuls) 856
Apresoline Hydrochloride Tablets (Common) 855
Apresoline-Esidrix Tablets 857
Aralen Hydrochloride Injection 2038
Aralen Phosphate Tablets 2039
Arfonad Ampuls (Occasional) 1887
Asbron G 1997
Asendin Tablets (Less than 1%) 1196
Atabrine Hydrochloride Tablets 2041
▲Atgam Sterile Solution (At least 1 patient to 10%) 2320
Atromid-S Capsules 2435
Attenuvax (Rare) 1424
▲Augmentin Tablets, Powder for Oral Suspension, and Chewable Tablets (9%) 2198
Azactam for Injection (1-1.3%) 2252
Azo Gantanol Tablets 1887
Azo Gantrisin Tablets 1888
Azulfidine Tablets, EN-tabs, Oral Suspension (Rare) 1157
Bactrim DS Tablets 1891
Bactrim I.V. Infusion 1889
Bactrim 1891
Benadryl Capsules 1691
Benadryl Injection 1692
Biavax II 1427
Biphetamine Capsules 973
Blocadren Tablets (Less than 1%) 1429
Bontril Slow-Release 834
Bretylol Injection (1 in 1000) 923
Bumex (0.1%) 1895
BuSpar (2%) 1401
Butazolidin Capsules & Tablets (Less than 1%) 1027
Calan SR Caplets (1% or less) 2157
Calan Tablets (1% or less) 2155
Capoten (0.5 to 2%) 2255
Capozide (0.5 to 2%) 2258
Carafate Tablets (Less than 0.5%) 1326
▲Cardioquin Tablets (Frequent) 1812
Cardizem Tablets-30 mg, 60 mg, 90 mg and 120 mg (Less than 1%) 1329
Cardizem SR Capsules-60 mg, 90 mg and 120 mg (Less than 1%) 1327
Cardura Tablets (2%) 1941
Carnitor 2188
Cartrol Tablets (2.1-4.4%) 507
Ceclor Pulvules & Suspension (1 in 70) 1251
Cefizox Injection (Occasional) 1012
▲Cefobid Intravenous/Intramuscular (1 in 30) 1943
▲Cefobid Pharmacy Bulk Package - Not for Direct Infusion (1 in 30) 1945
Cefotan (1 in 80) 2265
▲Ceftin Tablets (3.5%) 575
Celontin (Frequent) 1692
Cephulac Syrup 1331
Ceptaz for Injection (One in 78 patients) 1057
Cerubidine (Occasional) 2443
▲CHEMET (succimer) Capsules (12 to 20.9%) 1361
Children's Advil Suspension (Less than 3%) 2426
Chloromycetin Kapseals 1695
Chloromycetin Palmitate, Oral Suspension 1697
Chloromycetin Sodium Succinate 1698
Choledyl Pediatric Elixir 1702
Choledyl Tablets 1700
Choledyl SA Tablets 1704
Cholybar (Less frequent) 1705
Chromagen Capsules 2078
Chronulac Syrup 1332
Cibacalcin Double-chambered Syringes (Few) 859
Cibalith-S 870
Cipro I.V. (1% or less) 1592
Cipro Tablets (2.3%) 1589
Claforan Sterile Injection (1.4%) 1089
Cleocin HCl Capsules 2322
Cleocin Pediatric Flavored Granules 2324
Cleocin Phosphate Injection 2325
Cleocin T Topical 2327
▲Clinoril Tablets (3-9%) 1433
Clozaril Tablets (2%) 2000
ColBENEMID Tablets 1436
Colchicine Ampoules 1252
Colestid Granules (1 in 30 to 1 in 100 patients) 2328
Combipres Tablets 678
Comhist LA Capsules 1618
Constant-T Tablets 1029
Corgard Tablets (1 to 5 of 1000 patients) 701
Corzide Tablets (1 to 5 of 1000 patients) 702
Cosmegen Injection 1440
Coumadin Injection & Tablets (Infrequent) 944
▲Creon Capsules (Among most frequent) 2245

Crystodigin Tablets 1253
Cuprimine Capsules 1442
Cyklokapron Tablets and Injection 1159
▲Cytosar-U Sterile Powder (Among most frequent) 2329
▲Cytotec (14-40%) 2159
Cytovene Sterile Powder (1% or less) 2292
Cytoxan for Injection 726
DTIC-Dome (Rare) 1595
Dalgan Injection (Less than 1%) 620
Dalmane Capsules 1927
▲Dantrium Capsules (Among most frequent) 1619
Daraprim Tablets (Rare) 761
Declomycin Capsules, Tablets 1199
Deconamine 663
▲Demser Capsules (10%) 1460
Depakene Capsules & Syrup 511
Depakote 512
▲Depen Titratable Tablets (17%) 2379
Deprol Tablets 2382
Desferal Vials 862
Desoxyn Gradumet Tablets 514
Desyrel and Desyrel Dividose (Greater than 1%) 1404
Dexedrine 2206
Diabinese Tablets (Less than 2%) 1775
Diamox Parenteral 1200
Diamox Sequels (Sustained Release) 1201
Diamox Tablets 1200
Dicumarol Tablets (Infrequent) 516
Didrex Tablets 2338
Didronel Tablets 1621
Diflucan Injection and Tablets (1.5% in 4048 patients) 1948
Dilaudid-HP Injection 1175
Dilor 2079
Dimetane-DC Cough Syrup 1857
Dimetane-DX Cough Syrup 1858
▲Dipentum Capsules (5.9% to 11.1%) 1160
Diprivan Injection (Less than 1%) 2267
Disalcid 1310
Diucardin Tablets 2450
Diulo 2129
Diupres Tablets 1461
Diuril Oral Suspension 1464
Diuril Sodium Intravenous 1463
Diuril Tablets 1464
▲Dolobid Tablets (3% to 9%) 1465
Dopram Injectable 1860
Doral Tablets 2383
Doryx Capsules (Infrequent) 1717
Doxorubicin Hydrochloride for Injection, USP (Occasional) 622
Doxorubicin Hydrochloride Injection, USP (Occasional) 848
▲Duragesic Transdermal System (3% to 10%) 1133
Duricef 1405
Duvoid Tablets 1853
Dyazide Capsules 2208
DynaCirc Capsules (1.1%) 2004
Dyrenium Capsules (Rare) 2210
▲E.E.S. (Most frequent) 522
E-Mycin Tablets (Infrequent) 688
Easprin 1719
Edecrin 1468
Elavil 2269
Eldepryl (1 of 49 patients) 2250
▲Emcyt Capsules (12%) 1161
Endep Tablets 1927
Enduron Tablets 517
Enduronyl 518
Engerix-B Unit-Dose Vials (Less than 1%) 2213
Enlon Injection 598
Enrich Liquid Nutrition with Fiber 1971
Ensure Liquid Nutrition 1971
Ensure Plus High Calorie Liquid Nutrition 1971
▲Epogen for Injection (0.11 to 16%) 591
Equagesic Tablets 2451
▲Ergamisol Tablets (9 to 52%) 1136
▲ERYC (Among most frequent) 1720
▲EryPed (Among most frequent) 519
▲Ery-Tab Tablets (Among most frequent) 521
▲Erythrocin Stearate Filmtab (Among most frequent) 523
▲Erythromycin Base Filmtab (Among most frequent) 525
▲Erythromycin Delayed-Release Capsules, USP (Among most frequent) 526
Esidrix Tablets 863
Esimil Tablets 864
Eskalith 2214
▲Ethmozine Tablets (2%-5%) 946
Etrafon 2087
▲Eulexin Capsules (12% with LHRH-agonist) 2089
Exna Tablets 1862
▲Sterile FUDR (Among more common) 1898
Fansidar Tablets 1896
Fastin Capsules 2216
Feldene Capsules (1 to 3%) 1777
Feosol Capsules 2191
Feosol Elixir (Occasional) 2191
Feosol Tablets (Occasional) 2191
Fiorinal with Codeine Capsules 2008
Flagyl I.V. 2131
Flagyl Tablets 2170
Flexeril Tablets (Less than 1%) 1471
Floropryl Sterile Ophthalmic Ointment (Rare) 1473
Floxin Tablets (1% to 4%) 1652
Fluorouracil Injection (Common) 1897
Fortaz (1 in 78 patients) 1060
Fulvicin P/G Tablets 2090
Fulvicin P/G 165 & 330 Tablets 2091
Fulvicin-U/F Tablets 2092
▲Fungizone Intravenous (Among most common) 2262
Ganite Injection 1016
Gantanol 1899
Gantrisin Ophthalmic Ointment/Solution 1900
Gantrisin 1901
▲Gastrocrom Capsules (4 of 87 patients) 974
Geocillin Tablets 1951
Glucotrol (1 in 70) 1952
Grifulvin V (griseofulvin microsize) Tablets/Suspension (Occasional) 1678
Grisactin (Occasional) 2454
Grisactin Ultra Tablets (Occasional) 2455
Gris-PEG Tablets, 125 mg & 250 mg (Occasional) 1083
Guaifed 1615
Halcion Tablets (Rare) 2340
Haldol Decanoate 1375
Haldol Injection, Tablets and Concentrate 1373
Harmonyl Tablets 528
HibTITER (2 of 1,118 vaccinations) 1206
Hismanal Tablets (1.8%) 1138
Humatin Capsules 1726
Humorsol Sterile Ophthalmic Solution (Rare) 1475
Hydrea Capsules 728
HydroDIURIL Tablets 1484
Hydromox R Tablets 1209
Hydromox Tablets 1208
Hydropres Tablets 1485
Hyperstat I.V. Injection 2095
Hytrin Tablets (At least 1%) 529
▲Idamycin for Injection (73%) 564
IFEX (Less than 1%) 729
Ilosone (Infrequent) 913
Imferon 976
Imuran (Less than 1%) 768
Inderal 2459
Inderal LA Long Acting Capsules 2461
Inderide Tablets 2463
Inderide LA Long Acting Capsules 2465
Indocin Capsules (Greater than 1%) 1487
Indocin I.V. (1% to 3%) 1490
Indocin (Greater than 1%) 1487
▲Intron A (2% to 45%) 2097
Ionamin Capsules 981
IOPIDINE ⊙ 232
Ismelin Tablets 869
Isoptin Oral Tablets (Less than 1%) 1179
Isoptin SR Sustained Release Tablets (Less than 1%) 1181
Isopto Carbachol ⊙ 219
K-Dur Microburst Release System (potassium chloride, USP) E.R. Tablets 1163
▲K-Lor Powder Packets (Most common) 531
▲K-Lyte (Among most common) 707
▲K-Norm Capsules (Among most common) 982
K-Phos M.F. Tablets 659
K-Phos Neutral Tablets 660
K-Phos Original Formula 'Sodium Free' Tablets 660
K-Phos No. 2 Tablets 659
▲K-Tab Filmtab (Most common) 532
Kato Potassium Supplement 1114
Kayexalate (Occasional) 2053
▲Keflex Pulvules, Oral Suspension & Pediatric Drops (Most frequent) 916
▲Keftab Tablets (Most frequent) 917
Kefurox Vials, Faspak & ADD-Vantage (1 in 220) 1277
Kefzol Vials, Faspak & ADD-Vantage 1279
Kerlone Tablets (1.9% to 2.0%) 2172
Klonopin Tablets 1902
▲Klor-Con 8/Klor-Con 10 Extended-release Tablets (Among most common) 2374
Klorvess Effervescent Granules 2010
Klorvess Effervescent Tablets 2011
Klorvess 10% Liquid 2010
▲Klotrix (Most common) 708
▲Kolyum Liquid (Among most common) 983
Koro-Flex Arcing Spring Diaphragm 2142
Koromex Coil Spring Diaphragm 2142
Ku-Zyme HP Capsules 2147
▲Lamprene Capsules (40-50%) 1030
Lanoxicaps (Less common) 772
Lanoxin Elixir Pediatric (Less common) 775
Lanoxin Injection (Less common) 778
Lanoxin Injection Pediatric (Less common) 781
Lanoxin Tablets (Less common) 783
▲Lariam Tablets (Among most frequent) 1904
Larodopa Tablets (Infrequent) 1905
Lasix 1093
Legatrin ▣ 556
Leukeran Tablets (Infrequent) 788
Leukine for IV Infusion 1127
▲Levatol (3.3%) 1832
Limbitrol 1933
Lincocin 2344
Lioresal Tablets (Rare) 1031
Lithane Tablets 1596
Lithium Carbonate Capsules & Tablets 1984
Lithobid Tablets 870
▲Lodine Capsules (3-9%) 2468
▲Lopid Capsules and Tablets (7.2%) 1736
▲Lopressor Ampuls (5%) 1032
Lopressor HCT Tablets (1 in 100 patients) 1034
▲Lopressor Tablets (5%) 1032
Lorelco Tablets 1333
Lozol Tablets (Less than 5%) 1843
Ludiomil Tablets (Rare) 874
Lufyllin & Lufyllin-400 Tablets 2384
Lufyllin-GG Elixir & Tablets 2385
Lupron Depot 7.5 mg (Less than 5%) 2311
Lupron Injection (Less than 5%) 2310
▲Lysodren (80%) 731
M-M-R II 1494
M-R-VAX II 1496
MS Contin Tablets (Infrequent) 1814
MSIR (Infrequent) 1817
Maalox TC Suspension (Mild) 1851
Macrodantin Capsules (Less common) 1624
Maxair Inhaler (Less than 1%) 1311
Maxzide 1215
▲Meclomen Capsules (10-33%) 1739
Mefoxin 1498
Mefoxin Premixed Intravenous Solution 1500
Mellaril 2011
Meruvax II 1503
▲Mesnex Injection (83%) 733
Mestinon Injectable 1115
Mestinon 1116
Methadone Hydrochloride Diskets 1284
Methergine (Rare) 2016
Methotrexate Tablets, Parenteral, LPF Parenteral (1 to 3%) 1217
Metrodin (urofollitropin for injection) 2182
▲Mevacor Tablets (5.5%) 1505
▲Mexitil Capsules (5.2%) 680
Mezlin 1597
Mezlin Pharmacy Bulk Package 1599
Micro-K 1863
▲Micro-K LS Packets (Most common) 1864
▲Midamor Tablets (3% to 8%) 1508
Miltown Tablets 2386
Minipress Capsules (1-4%) 1778
Minizide Capsules (Rare) 1779
Minocin Intravenous 1221
Minocin Oral Suspension 1224
Minocin Pellet-Filled Capsules (Infrequent) 1222
Mintezol 1510
Mithracin 1602
Modane Plus Tablets ▣ 504
Modane Tablets ▣ 503
Moduretic Tablets (Greater than 1%, less than 3%) 1510
Monistat I.V. 1143
Monocid Injection (Less than 1%) 2217
Monodox Capsules (Infrequent) 1630
Mono-Gesic Tablets 846
Monopril Tablets 1406
Motrin Tablets (Less than 3%) 2351
Mumpsvax 1513
Mustargen 1514
Mutamycin 733
Mycostatin Oral Suspension (Occasional) 605
Mycostatin Oral Tablets (Occasional) 605
Mycostatin Pastilles (Occasional) 734
Mykrox ½ mg Tablets (Less than 2%) 984
Myochrysine Injection 1516
Nalfon Pulvules & Tablets (1.8%) 919
Naprosyn (Less than 3%) 2297
Naturetin Tablets (Occasional) 1789
Navane Capsules and Concentrate 1954
Navane Intramuscular 1956
Nebcin Vials, Hyporets & ADD-Vantage 1286
NebuPent for Inhalation Solution (Greater than 1%, up to 5%) 1017
NegGram 2062
Neosar for Injection (Less freequent) 566
Netromycin Injection 100 mg/ml (Fewer than 1 of 1000 patients) 2104
▲Neupogen for Injection (14%) 595
Niclocide Chewable Tablets (1.6%) 1607
Nicorette 1335
▲Nimotop Capsules (Up to 4.2%) 1607
Nizoral Tablets (Less than 1%) 1145
Normodyne Tablets (Less than 1%) 2110
Normozide Tablets (Less than 1%) 2112
Noroxin Tablets (Less frequent) 1519
Norpace (1 to 3%) 2177
Norpramin Tablets 1340
▲Novantrone for Injection Concentrate (18 to 47%) 1226
Nullo Deodorant Tablets (Few cases) ▣ 547
Nystatin, USP for Extemporaneous Preparation of Oral Suspension (Occasional) 1685
▲Omnipaque (0.1 to 42%) 2552
Oncovin Solution Vials & Hyporets 1288
Optimine Tablets 2115
Oramorph SR (Morphine Sulfate Sustained Release Tablets) (Less frequent) 1988
Orap Tablets 1020
Oretic Tablets 544
Oreticyl 545
Ornade Spansule Capsules 2221
Ortho Diaphragm Kit 1664
▲Orthoclone OKT3 Sterile Solution (14%) 1645
Ortho-White Diaphragm Kit-Flat Spring 1664
▲Orudis Capsules (Greater than 3%) 2488
Osmolite Isotonic Liquid Nutrition 1972
Osmolite HN High Nitrogen Isotonic Liquid Nutrition 1972
PBZ Tablets & Elixir 1037
PBZ-SR Tablets 1037
▲PCE Dispertab Tablets (Among most frequent) 549
PMB 200 and PMB 400 2504
Pamelor 2019
Panwarfin Tablets (Infrequent) 547
Papaverine Hydrochloride Vials and Ampoules 1290
▲Paraplatin for Injection (6%) 735
Parlodel (0.4-3%) 2020
Parnate Tablets 2222
Pavabid Capsules (Rare) 1344
Pavabid HP Capsulets (Rare) 1344
PediaProfen Suspension (Less than 3%) 1363
Pediazole (Infrequent) 1973
PedvaxHIB (One case) 1521
Peganone Tablets 551
Pentam 300 Injection (1 patient) 1018
Pentaspan Injection 949
Pepcid (1.7%) 1524
Pergonal (menotropins for injection, USP) 2184
Periactin 1525
Peri-Colace (Exceedingly small) 1409

(▣ Described in PDR For Nonprescription Drugs) Incidence data in parenthesis; ▲ 3% or more (⊙ Described in PDR For Ophthalmology)

▲ Permax Tablets (6.4%) 1291
Persantine Tablets 683
Pilocar (Extremely rare) ⊙ 275
Pilostat Sterile Ophthalmic Solution 0.5%, 1%, 2%, 3%, 4%, 5%, 6% (Extremely rare) ⊙ 263
Pipracil (2%) 1230
Plaquenil Sulfate Tablets 2067
Plegine Tablets 2504
Plendil Extended-Release Tablets (0.1%) 1526
Polaramine 2116
Pondimin Tablets (Among most common) 1867
▲ Ponstel (Approximately 5%) 1758
Prelu-2 Capsules 683
Prilosec Delayed-Release Capsules (1.9 to 3.7%) 1530
Primaxin I.M. (0.6%) 1532
Primaxin I.V. (1.8%) 1535
▲ Prinivil Tablets (2.6% to 3.2%) 1538
Prinzide Tablets (2.5%) 1540
Priscoline Hydrochloride Ampuls 877
▲ Procan SR Tablets (3-4%) 1760
Procardia Capsules (2% or less) 1781
Procardia XL Tablets (Less than 3%) 1783
▲ Procrit for Injection (0.11% to 16%) 1647
Proglycem (Frequent) 649
ProHIBiT Haemophilus b Conjugate Vaccine (Diphtheria Toxoid Conjugate) (1.2% or less) 896
Prokine for I.V. Infusion 1096
▲ Pronestyl Capsules and Tablets (3-4%) 1800
Pronestyl Injection 1798
▲ Pronestyl-SR Tablets (3 to 4%) 1801
Prostigmin Injectable 1120
Prostigmin Tablets 1121
Prostin VR Pediatric Sterile Solution (2%) 2355
Protostat Tablets (Occasional) 1674
▲ Prozac Pulvules (12.3%) 920
Pulmocare Specialized Nutrition for Pulmonary Patients 1975
Purinethol Tablets (Occasional) 800
Quadrinal Tablets 1183
Questran Light (Less frequent) 711
Questran Powder 710
Quibron Capsules 713
Quibron-T 714
Quibron-T/SR 716
Quinaglute Dura-Tabs Tablets 663
▲ Quinidex Extentabs (Among most frequent) 1868
Q-vel Muscle Relaxant Pain Reliever ▣ 552
Raudixin Tablets 1803
Rauzide Tablets 1804
Recombivax HB (Equal to or greater than 1%) 1544
Regitine 878
Reglan 1869
Renese Tablets 1785
Renese-R Tablets 1786
Respbid Tablets 684
Restoril Capsules (1-2%) 2023
▲ Retrovir Capsules (0.8% to 12%) 802
▲ Retrovir I.V. Infusion (12%) 805
▲ Retrovir Syrup (0.8% to 12%) 802
Rheumatrex Methotrexate Dose Pack (1% to 3%) 1234
▲ Ridaura Capsules (42.5%) 2224
Rifadin (Some patients) 1345
Rifamate Capsules (Some patients) 1347
Rimactane Capsules 879
Robaxisal Tablets 1872
Robitussin-DM ▣ 676
Rocephin Injectable Vials, ADD-Vantage (2.7%) 1914
▲ Roferon-A Injection (29% to 42%) 1916
▲ Rogaine Topical Solution (4.33%) 2357
Rondec 1975
Rondec-DM 1976
Rondec-TR Tablet 1975
Rowasa (2.09 to 3.0%) 2248
Rubex (Occasional) 739
Rufen Tablets (1 to 3%) 691
Rum-K Syrup 995
Ru-Tuss II Capsules 693
Ru-Tuss with Hydrocodone 694
Ru-Tuss Tablets 693
▲ Rythmol Tablets (0 to 5.7%) 1184
Salflex 839
Saluron 718
Salutensin/Salutensin-Demi 719
▲ Sandimmune (Less than 1 to 8%) 2024
▲ Sandostatin Injection (6.9%) 2029
Sanorex Tablets 2030
Sansert Tablets 2031
▲ Sectral Capsules (4%) 2520
Septra 813
Septra I.V. Infusion 808
Septra I.V. Infusion ADD-Vantage Vials 810
Septra 813
Ser-Ap-Es Tablets 881
Serpasil Tablets 883
Serpasil-Apresoline Tablets 884
Serpasil-Esidrix Tablets 886
Sinemet Tablets 952
Sinemet CR Tablets (1.2%) 953
Sinequan 1960
Slo-bid Gyrocaps 1847
▲ Slow-K Tablets (Among most common) 2281
Sodium Polystyrene Sulfonate Suspension (Occasional) 1993
Solganal Suspension (Rare) 2122
Soma Compound w/Codeine Tablets 2390
Soma Compound Tablets 2389
▲ Spectrobid Tablets & Powder for Oral Suspension (2%-4%) 1961
▲ Suprax (16%) 1235
Surmontil Capsules 2524
T-PHYL (Uniphyl) 200 mg Tablets 1820
Tacaryl 2409
Tagamet (Approximately 1 in 100) 2228
Talacen (Rare) 2070
Talwin Injection (Rare) 2071
Talwin Compound (Rare) 2072
Talwin Injection (Rare) 2071
Talwin Nx 2073
Tambocor Tablets (1-3%) 1315
Tao Capsules (Infrequent) 1963
Tavist Syrup 2033
Tavist Tablets 2035
Tavist-D Tablets 2035
Tazicef for Injection (Less than 2%; 1 in 78 patients) 2231
Tazidime Vials, Faspak & ADD-Vantage (1 in 78) 1299
Tegison Capsules (Less than 1%) 1881
Tegretol Chewable Tablets 654
Tegretol Suspension 656
Tegretol Tablets 654
Temaril Tablets, Syrup and Spansule Sustained Release Capsules 1085
Tenex Tablets (Less than 3%) 1875
▲ Ten-K Controlled-Release Tablets (Among most common) 2282
▲ Tenoretic Tablets (Up to 3%) 1105
▲ Tenormin Tablets and I.V. Injection (2 to 3%) 1107
Tensilon Injectable 1123
Tenuate 1354
Terramycin Capsules 1786
Terramycin Intramuscular Solution 1964
Thalitone Tablets 687
Theo-24 2179
Theo-Dur Sprinkle 1168
Theo-Dur Extended-Release Tablets 1166
Theolair 1317
Theolair-SR Tablets 1319
▲ TheoX Extended-Release Tablets (Among most consistent) 841
▲ TheraCys BCG Live (Intravesical) (Up to 6.3%) 898
Theragran Hematinic Tablets 605
Thiosulfil Forte Tablets 2526
Tigan 2239
Timentin for Injection 2239
Timolide Tablets (Less than 1%) 1547
Timoptic in Ocudose 1552
Timoptic Sterile Ophthalmic Solution 1550
Tofranil Ampuls 1038
Tofranil Tablets 1039
Tofranil-PM Capsules 1041
▲ Tolectin (200, 400 and 600 mg) (3 to 9%) 1379
▲ Tonocard Tablets (0.0-6.8%) 1554
Toradol IM Injection (1% to 3%) 2302
Trandate HCT/Trandate 579
▲ Trental (3.4%) 1099
▲ Trexan Tablets (Less than 10%) 937
Triaminic Expectorant DH 1995
Triaminic Oral Infant Drops 1996
Triavil Tablets 1556
Trilafon (Occasional) 2123
▲ Trilisate (Less than 20%) 1822
Trinalin Repetabs Tablets 1170
Trinsicon Capsules (Rare) 2415
Troph-Iron Liquid (Occasional) ▣ 619
Tuss-Ornade Liquid 2242
Tuss-Ornade Spansule Capsules 2242
Ultracef Capsules, Tablets & Oral Suspension 722
▲ Unasyn (3%) 1965
Unipen 2533
Uniphyl 400 mg Tablets 1823
Urecholine 1558
Urobiotic-250 Capsules (Rare) 1968
Uroqid-Acid 661
▲ Vascor (200, 300 and 400 mg) Tablets (6.82 to 10.87%) 1383
Vaseretic Tablets (2.1%) 1559
Vasotec I.V. 1562
Vasotec Tablets (1.4% to 2.1%) 1564
Velban Vials 1305
Ventolin (Less than or equal to 1%) 583
▲ VePesid Capsules and Injection (1 to 13%) 741
Verelan Capsules (Less than 1%) 1243
Vermox Chewable Tablets 1149
Vibramycin Hyclate Capsules (Infrequent) 1787
Vibramycin Hyclate Intravenous 1968
Vibramycin (Infrequent) 1787
Viokase 1877
Vira-A for Injection 1766
Visken Tablets (2% or fewer patients) 2036
Vivactil Tablets 1567
▲ Voltaren Tablets (3% to 9%) 1042
▲ Wellbutrin Tablets (6.8%) 821
Wigraine Tablets & Suppositories 1645
Winstrol Tablets 2075
Wytensin Tablets (3% or less) 2542
▲ Xanax Tablets (10.1% to 20.6%) 2367
Yodoxin 1072
Yutopar (Infrequent) 647
Zanosar Sterile Powder (Some patients) 2371
Zantac Injection and Zantac Injection Premixed 1063
Zantac 1065
Zarontin Capsules (Frequent) 1768
Zarontin Syrup (Frequent) 1769
Zaroxolyn Tablets 989
▲ Zefazone Sterile Powder (3.6%) 2372
Zestoretic (2.5%) 2274
▲ Zestril Tablets (3.2%) 2277
Zinacef (1 in 220 patients) 1066
▲ Zofran Injection (22%) 1069
Zoladex (1% to 5%) 1110
Zovirax (0.3% to 2.7%) 824
Zyloprim Tablets (Less than 1%) 830

Diarrhea, bloody

Ansaid Tablets (Less than 1%) 2319
Azulfidine Tablets, EN-tabs, Oral Suspension 1157
Cleocin HCl Capsules 2322
Cleocin Pediatric Flavored Granules 2324
Cleocin Phosphate Injection 2325
Pipracil (Less frequent) 1230
Prozac Pulvules (Rare) 920
Rowasa 2248
Voltaren Tablets (Less than 1%) 1042

Diplopia

Actifed with Codeine Cough Syrup 752
AK-NaCl 5% Ointment & Solution ⊙ 204
Anafranil Capsules (Infrequent) 650
▲ Anestacon Solution (Among most common) 2394
Ativan Injection (Occasional) 2432
Azactam for Injection (Less than 1%) 2252
Benadryl Capsules 1691
Benadryl Injection 1692
Bentyl 1322
Betagan ⊙ 239
Blocadren Tablets 1429
Brevicon (Rare) 2304
Cardioquin Tablets 1812
Children's Advil Suspension (Less than 1%) 2426
Cipro I.V. (1% or less) 1592
Cipro Tablets (Less than 1%) 1589
Cycrin Tablets 2449
Dalgan Injection (Less than 1%) 620
Dalmane Capsules 1927
Dantrium Capsules (Less frequent) 1619
Deconamine 663
Demulen 2161
Depakene Capsules & Syrup 511
Depakote 512
Depen Titratable Tablets 2379
Desyrel and Desyrel Dividose 1404
Dilaudid-HP Injection 1175
Diprivan Injection (Less than 1%) 2267
Duranest Injections 624
Dyclone 0.5% and 1% Topical Solutions, USP 626
Eldepryl 2250
Enlon Injection 598
Enovid 2161
Ethmozine Tablets (Less than 2%) 946
Flexeril Tablets (Less than 1%) 1471
Fungizone Intravenous 2262
Indocin (Less than 1%) 1487
Ketalar 1726
Klonopin Tablets 1902
Larodopa Tablets (Infrequent) 1905
Levlen/Tri-Levlen 665
Lioresal Tablets 1031
Lysodren (Infrequent) 731
MS Contin Tablets (Infrequent) 1814
MSIR (Infrequent) 1817
Matulane Capsules 1907
Mesantoin Tablets 2013
Micronor Tablets 1667
Modicon 1667
Motrin Tablets (Less than 1%) 2351
Mysoline (Occasional) 2480
Nalfon Pulvules & Tablets (Less than 1%) 919
NegGram (Infrequent) 2062
Norinyl (Rare) 2304
Novahistine DH 1342
Novahistine Elixir ▣ 596
Nuromax Injection 794
Oculinum for Injecton (Less than 1%) 587
Omnipaque 2552
Optimine Tablets 2115
Oramorph SR (Morphine Sulfate Sustained Release Tablets) (Less frequent) 1988
Ornade Spansule Capsules 2221
Ortho-Novum 1667
PBZ Tablets & Elixir 1037
PBZ-SR Tablets 1037
Paradione Capsules 548
PediaProfen Suspension (Less than 1%) 1363
Peganone Tablets 551
Periactin 1525
Permax Tablets (2.1%) 1291
Phenergan Injection 2493
Phenergan Tablets 2496
Proglycem 649
ProSom Tablets (Rare) 554
Protopam Chloride for Injection 2518
Prozac Pulvules (Rare) 920
Quinaglute Dura-Tabs Tablets 663
Quinamm Tablets 1344
Quinidex Extentabs 1868
Robaxin Injectable 1871
Rondec 1975
Rondec-DM 1976
Rondec-TR Tablet 1975
Rufen Tablets (Less than 1%) 691
Ru-Tuss II Capsules 693
Serax Capsules 2522
Serax Tablets 2522
Serophene (clomiphene citrate tablets, USP) 2186
Sinemet Tablets 952
Soma Compound w/Codeine Tablets (Very rare) 2390
Soma Compound Tablets (Very rare) 2389
Soma Tablets 2388
Stadol (Less than 1%) 721
Tacaryl 2409
Talwin Injection 2071
Tambocor Tablets (1-3%) 1315
Tavist Syrup 2033
Tavist Tablets 2035
Tavist-D Tablets 2035
▲ Tegison Capsules (10-25%) 1881
Tegretol Chewable Tablets 654
Tegretol Suspension 656
Tegretol Tablets 654
Temaril Tablets, Syrup and Spansule Sustained Release Capsules 1085
Tensilon Injectable 1123
Timolide Tablets 1547
Timoptic in Ocudose 1552
Timoptic Sterile Ophthalmic Solution 1550
Tonocard Tablets (Less than 1%) 1554
Tranxene 556
Triaminic Expectorant DH 1995
Triaminic Oral Infant Drops 1996
Tridione 557
Levlen/Tri-Levlen 665

Tri-Norinyl 28-Day Tablets (Rare) .. 2304
Valium Injectable ... 1937
Valium Tablets (Infrequent) ... 1939
Valrelease Capsules (Occasional) ... 1923
Versed Injection (Less than 1%) ... 1924
Voltaren Tablets (Less than 1%) ... 1042
Wellbutrin Tablets (Rare) ... 821
Xanax Tablets ... 2367
▲ Xylocaine Injections (Less than 1% to among most common) ... 637
Xylocaine Injections for Ventricular Arrhythmias ... 639
Xylocaine 2% Jelly ... 643
Xylocaine 5% Ointment ... 644
Xylocaine 10% Oral Spray ... 645
4% Xylocaine-MPF Sterile Solution ... 641
Xylocaine 2% Viscous Solution ... 646

Dipsesis

Aldactone ... 2152
Alferon N Injection (1%) ... 1809
Anafranil Capsules (Up to 2%) ... 650
Anaprox and Anaprox DS Tablets (Less than 3%) ... 2288
Azdōne Tablets ... 844
Cardizem Tablets-30 mg, 60 mg, 90 mg and 120 mg (Less than 1%) ... 1329
Cardizem SR Capsules-60 mg, 90 mg and 120 mg (Less than 1%) 1327
Cardura Tablets (Less than 0.5% of 3960 patients) ... 1941
Cibalith-S ... 870
Corzide Tablets ... 702
Cytotec (Infrequent) ... 2159
Damason-P ... 1356
Diapid Nasal Spray ... 2003
Easprin ... 1719
Emcyt Capsules (1%) ... 1161
Empirin with Codeine Phosphate Nos. 2, 3 & 4 ... 764
Eskalith ... 2214
Flexeril Tablets (Less than 1%) ... 1471
Floxin Tablets (Less than 1%) ... 1652
Intron A (1% or less) ... 2097
ISMOTIC (Very rare) ... ⊙ 233
K-Phos M.F. Tablets ... 659
K-Phos Neutral Tablets ... 660
K-Phos No. 2 Tablets ... 659
Lithane Tablets ... 1596
Lithium Carbonate Capsules & Tablets ... 1984
Lithobid Tablets ... 870
Lodine Capsules (Less than 1%) ... 2468
Lortab ASA Tablets ... 2414
▲ Lupron Depot 3.75 mg (Among most frequent) ... 2312
Maxzide ... 1215
Midamor Tablets (Less than or equal to 1%) ... 1508
Moduretic Tablets (Less than or equal to 1%) ... 1510
Naprosyn (Less than 3%) ... 2297
Neo-Calglucon Syrup ... 2018
Orap Tablets ... 1020
Orudis Capsules (Less than 1%) ... 2488
Permax Tablets (Infrequent) ... 1291
Prinzide Tablets ... 1540
ProSom Tablets (Infrequent) ... 554
Prozac Pulvules (Infrequent) ... 920
Rauzide Tablets ... 1804
Taractan ... 1920
▲ Tegison Capsules (50-75%) ... 1881
Tenoretic Tablets ... 1105
Thalitone Tablets ... 687
Tonocard Tablets (Less than 1%) .. 1554
Toradol IM Injection (1% or less) ... 2302
Trental (Less than 1%) ... 1099
▲ Trexan Tablets (Less than 10%) ... 937
Uroqid-Acid (Less frequent) ... 661
Vaseretic Tablets ... 1559
Zestoretic ... 2274
Zovirax Sterile Powder (Less than 1%) ... 828

Discoloration, injection site

Diprivan Injection (Less than 1%) .. 2267

Discomfort, chest

Brethine Ampuls (1.3 to 1.5%) ... 1026
Primaxin I.M. ... 1532
Primaxin I.V. (Less than 0.2%) ... 1535
Prinivil Tablets ... 1538
Prinzide Tablets (0.3 to 1%) ... 1540
Proventil (Less than 1%) ... 2120
Recombivax HB (Less than 1%) ... 1544
Timentin for Injection ... 2239
Tornalate (0.5%) ... 2074
Ventolin Tablets (Less than 1 of 100 patients) ... 583
Zestoretic (0.3 to 1.0%) ... 2274
Zestril Tablets (0.3% to 1%) ... 2277

Discomfort, general

AVC ... 1322
Coumadin Injection & Tablets ... 944
Epifrin ... ⊙ 244
Eskalith ... 2214
IOPIDINE ... ⊙ 232
Kenalog-10 Injection ... 2402
Lithane Tablets ... 1596
Lithium Carbonate Capsules & Tablets ... 1984
Omnipaque (Less than or equal to 1%) ... 2552
Papaverine Hydrochloride Vials and Ampoules ... 1290
Pilopine HS Gel ... ⊙ 227
Zovirax Ointment 5% ... 827

Discomfort, local

Albalon Solution with Liquifilm ... ⊙ 238
▲ Chibroxin Sterile Ophthalmic Solution (Most frequent) ... 1431
▲ Ciloxan Sterile Ophthalmic Solution (Among most frequent) .. ⊙ 214
Naphcon Forte ... ⊙ 226
OptiPranolol Sterile Ophthalmic Solution (A small number of patients) ... ⊙ 261
Vasocon-A ... ⊙ 278

Discomfort at injection site

Azactam for Injection (1.9%) ... 2252
Cefotan (1 in 500) ... 2265
Ceredase Injection ... 1052
Diprivan Injection (Less than 1%) .. 2267
MICRhoGAM Rh_o(D) Immune Globulin (Human) ... 1650
▲ Monocid Injection (5.7%) ... 2217
Oncovin Solution Vials & Hyporets 1288
PPD Tine Test ... 2548
RhoGAM Rh_o(D) Immune Globulin (Human) ... 1651
Tuberculin, Old, Tine Test ... 2549

Discontinuation syndrome

Catapres Tablets (About 1 in 100 patients) ... 676
Catapres-TTS (1%) ... 677
Combipres Tablets (About 1%) ... 678

Disorientation

Actimmune (Rare) ... 1046
Akineton ... 1171
AK-Pentolate ... ⊙ 204
Apresazide Capsules (Less frequent) ... 854
Apresoline Hydrochloride Parenteral (Ampuls) ... 856
Apresoline Hydrochloride Tablets (Less frequent) ... 855
Apresoline-Esidrix Tablets ... 857
Asendin Tablets (Less than 1%) ... 1196
Atgam Sterile Solution (Less than 5%) ... 2320
Ativan Tablets (Less frequent) ... 2434
Azo Gantrisin Tablets ... 1888
CeeNU ... 725
Cyclogyl (Common) ... ⊙ 215
Cyclomydril ... ⊙ 216
Dalmane Capsules ... 1927
Daranide Tablets ... 1445
Demerol ... 2047
Demser Capsules ... 1460
Desyrel and Desyrel Dividose (Greater than 1%) ... 1404
Dilaudid-HP Injection ... 1175
Dolobid Tablets (Less than 1 in 100) ... 1465
Dolophine Hydrochloride Ampoules & Vials ... 1260
Dolophine Hydrochloride Tablets ... 1261
Dopram Injectable ... 1860
Elavil ... 2269
Eldepryl ... 2250
Endep Tablets ... 1927
Etrafon ... 2087
Sterile FUDR (Remote possibility) .. 1898
Fiorinal with Codeine Capsules ... 2008
Flexeril Tablets (Less than 1%) ... 1471
Fluorouracil Injection ... 1897
Halcion Tablets ... 2340
Hydrea Capsules (Extremely rare) .. 728
IFEX (Less frequent) ... 729
ISMOTIC ... ⊙ 233
Ludiomil Tablets (Rare) ... 874
MS Contin Tablets (Infrequent) ... 1814
MSIR (Infrequent) ... 1817
Mepergan Injection ... 2479
Methadone Hydrochloride Diskets .. 1284
Methadone Hydrochloride Oral Solution & Tablets ... 1987
Myambutol Tablets ... 1225
Nalfon Pulvules & Tablets (Less than 1%) ... 919
Nebcin Vials, Hyporets & ADD-Vantage ... 1286
Netromycin Injection 100 mg/ml (1 of 1000 patients) ... 2104
Norpramin Tablets ... 1340
Oculinum for Injecton ... 587
Omnipaque (Rare) ... 2552
Oramorph SR (Morphine Sulfate Sustained Release Tablets) (Less frequent) ... 1988
Orthoclone OKT3 Sterile Solution .. 1645
OSM_GLYN ... ⊙ 234
Pamelor ... 2019
Phenergan with Codeine ... 2497
Phenergan with Dextromethorphan 2499
Phenergan Suppositories ... 2496
Phenergan Syrup ... 2495
Phenergan VC ... 2500
Phenergan VC with Codeine ... 2501
Roxanol ... 1991
Seldane-D Extended-Release Tablets (1.1%) ... 1350
Ser-Ap-Es Tablets ... 881
Serax Capsules ... 2522
Serax Tablets ... 2522
Seromycin Pulvules ... 1298
Serpasil-Apresoline Tablets ... 884
Sinemet CR Tablets ... 953
Sinequan (Infrequent) ... 1960
Soma Compound w/Codeine Tablets (Very rare) ... 2390
Soma Compound Tablets (Very rare) ... 2389
Soma Tablets ... 2388
Surmontil Capsules ... 2524
Tagamet ... 2228
Talacen ... 2070
Talwin Injection ... 2071
Talwin Compound ... 2072
Talwin Injection ... 2071
Talwin Nx ... 2073
Tigan ... 2239
Timoptic in Ocudose ... 1552
Timoptic Sterile Ophthalmic Solution ... 1550
Tofranil Ampuls ... 1038
Tofranil Tablets ... 1039
Tofranil-PM Capsules ... 1041
▲ Tonocard Tablets (2.1-11.2%) ... 1554
Trandate HCT Tablets ... 579
Trexan Tablets (Less than 1%) ... 937
Triavil Tablets ... 1556
Vivactil Tablets ... 1567
Voltaren Tablets (Rare) ... 1042
Vontrol Tablets (Approximately 1 in 350) ... 2243

Disorientation, place

AK-Pentolate ... ⊙ 204
Blocadren Tablets ... 1429
Cartrol Tablets ... 507
Corgard Tablets ... 701
Corzide Tablets ... 702
Cyclogyl (Common) ... ⊙ 215
Cyclomydril ... ⊙ 216
Inderal ... 2459
Inderal LA Long Acting Capsules ... 2461
Inderide Tablets ... 2463
Inderide LA Long Acting Capsules .. 2465
Kerlone Tablets ... 2172
Levatol ... 1832
Lopressor HCT Tablets ... 1034
Normodyne Tablets ... 2110
Normozide Tablets ... 2112
Sectral Capsules ... 2520
Tenoretic Tablets ... 1105
Tenormin Tablets and I.V. Injection 1107
Timolide Tablets ... 1547
Timoptic in Ocudose ... 1552
Timoptic Sterile Ophthalmic Solution ... 1550
Trandate HCT/Trandate ... 579
Visken Tablets ... 2036

Disorientation, time

AK-Pentolate ... ⊙ 204
Blocadren Tablets ... 1429
Cartrol Tablets ... 507
Corgard Tablets ... 701
Corzide Tablets ... 702
Cyclogyl (Common) ... ⊙ 215
Cyclomydril ... ⊙ 216
Inderal ... 2459
Inderal LA Long Acting Capsules ... 2461
Inderide Tablets ... 2463
Inderide LA Long Acting Capsules .. 2465
Kerlone Tablets ... 2172
Levatol ... 1832
Lopressor HCT Tablets ... 1034
Normodyne Tablets ... 2110
Normozide Tablets ... 2112
Sectral Capsules ... 2520
Tenoretic Tablets ... 1105
Tenormin Tablets and I.V. Injection 1107
Timolide Tablets ... 1547
Timoptic in Ocudose ... 1552
Timoptic Sterile Ophthalmic Solution ... 1550
Trandate HCT/Trandate ... 579
Visken Tablets ... 2036

Distention, abdominal (see under Abdominal distention)

Distress, abdominal

Atromid-S Capsules (Less frequent) ... 2435
Augmentin Tablets, Powder for Oral Suspension, and Chewable Tablets (Less frequent) ... 2198
▲ Butazolidin Capsules & Tablets (3-9%) ... 1027
Ceredase Injection ... 1052
Cholybar (Less frequent) ... 1705
Colestid Granules ... 2328
Duvoid Tablets ... 1853
EryPed 200 & EryPed 400 Granules ... 519
Ery-Tab Tablets ... 521
Erythrocin Stearate Filmtab ... 523
Factrel (Rare) ... 2561
Hylorel Tablets (1.7%) ... 975
Indocin (Greater than 1%) ... 1487
IOPIDINE ... ⊙ 232
▲ K-Lor Powder Packets (Most common) ... 531
▲ K-Tab Filmtab (Most common) ... 532
▲ Methotrexate Tablets, Parenteral, LPF Parenteral (Among most frequent) ... 1217
Mexitil Capsules (1.2%) ... 680
▲ Niclocide Chewable Tablets (3.4%) ... 1607
Norplant System ... 2484
Pediazole ... 1973
▲ Persantine Tablets (6.1%) ... 683
Protostat Tablets ... 1674
Questran Light (Less frequent) ... 711
Questran Powder ... 710
▲ Rheumatrex Methotrexate Dose Pack (Among most frequent) ... 1234
Rufen Tablets (Less than 3%) ... 691
Rum-K Syrup ... 995
▲ Seldane Tablets (7.6%) ... 1349
Seldane-D Extended-Release Tablets ... 1350
Senna X-Prep Bowel Evacuant Liquid ... 1073
Sinemet Tablets ... 952
Talacen (Rare) ... 2070
Talwin Compound (Rare) ... 2072
Talwin Nx (Rare) ... 2073
▲ Xanax Tablets (18.3%) ... 2367
Zantac Injection and Zantac Injection Premixed ... 1063
Zantac ... 1065

Distress, epigastric

Actifed with Codeine Cough Syrup.. 752
Aerolate ... 994
Aminophyllin Tablets ... 2153
Aralen Phosphate with Primaquine Phosphate Tablets ... 2040
Asbron G ... 1997
Asendin Tablets (Less than 1%) ... 1196
Atgam Sterile Solution (Less than 1% to less than 5%) ... 2320
▲ Benadryl Capsules (Among most frequent) ... 1691
▲ Benadryl Injection (Among most frequent) ... 1692
Butazolidin Capsules & Tablets ... 1027
Cafergot/Cafergot P-B ... 1999
Celontin (Frequent) ... 1692
▲ Children's Advil Suspension (3-9%) ... 2426
Choledyl Pediatric Elixir ... 1702
Choledyl Tablets ... 1700
Choledyl SA Tablets ... 1704
Cibacalcin Double-chambered Syringes (Few) ... 859
Cipro I.V. (1% or less) ... 1592
Combipres Tablets ... 678
Comhist LA Capsules ... 1618
Constant-T Tablets ... 1029
Cuprimine Capsules ... 1442
D.H.E. 45 Injection ... 2003

Deconamine 663
▲ Depen Titratable Tablets (17%) 2379
Dilor 2079
Dimetane-DC Cough Syrup 1857
Dimetane-DX Cough Syrup 1858
Dipentum Capsules (Rare) 1160
Diulo 2129
Elavil 2269
Endep Tablets 1927
Equagesic Tablets 2451
Ergostat 1719
Etrafon 2087
▲ Feldene Capsules (3 to 9%) 1777
Flagyl I.V. 2131
Flagyl Tablets 2170
Fulvicin P/G Tablets 2090
Fulvicin P/G 165 & 330 Tablets 2091
Fulvicin-U/F Tablets 2092
▲ Fungizone Intravenous (Among most common) 2262
Geocillin Tablets 1951
Grifulvin V (griseofulvin microsize) Tablets/Suspension (Occasional) 1678
Grisactin (Occasional) 2454
Grisactin Ultra Tablets (Occasional) 2455
Gris-PEG Tablets, 125 mg & 250 mg (Occasional) 1083
INH Tablets 868
Inderal 2459
Inderal LA Long Acting Capsules 2461
Inderide Tablets 2463
Inderide LA Long Acting Capsules 2465
▲ Indocin (3% to 9%) 1487
Isuprel Hydrochloride Mistometer 2051
Isuprel Hydrochloride Solution 1:200 & 1:100 2052
Kemadrin Tablets 771
▲ Lamprene Capsules (40-50%) 1030
Limbitrol 1933
Ludiomil Tablets 874
Lufyllin & Lufyllin-400 Tablets 2384
Lufyllin-GG Elixir & Tablets 2385
Medihaler Ergotamine Aerosol 1312
▲ Mexitil Capsules (41%) 680
Micronase Tablets (1.8%) 2350
Mintezol 1510
MIOSTAT ⊙ 233
Motofen Tablets (1 in 100) 836
▲ Motrin Tablets (3-9%) 2351
Norpramin Tablets 1340
▲ Optimine Tablets (Among most frequent) 2115
Ornade Spansule Capsules 2221
PBZ Tablets & Elixir (Among most frequent) 1037
PBZ-SR Tablets (Among most frequent) 1037
Pamelor 2019
▲ PediaProfen Suspension (3-9%) 1363
Periactin 1525
Phenergan VC 2500
Phenergan VC with Codeine 2501
Pima Syrup 994
Polaramine 2116
Proloprim Tablets 799
Protostat Tablets (Occasional) 1674
Proventil Syrup (Less than 1 of 100) 2119
Quadrinal Tablets 1183
Quibron Capsules 713
Quibron-T 714
Quibron-T/SR 716
Quinamm Tablets 1344
Respbid Tablets 684
Rifadin (Some patients) 1345
Rifamate Capsules (Some patients) 1347
Rimactane Capsules 879
▲ Rufen Tablets (3-9%) 691
Ru-Tuss II Capsules 693
Ru-Tuss with Hydrocodone 694
Ru-Tuss Tablets 693
Slo-bid Gyrocaps 1847
Soma Compound w/Codeine Tablets 2390
Soma Compound Tablets 2389
Soma Tablets 2388
Spectrobid Tablets & Powder for Oral Suspension (2%) 1961
Surmontil Capsules 2524
T-PHYL (Uniphyl) 200 mg Tablets 1820
Tacaryl 2409
Tapazole Tablets 1298
▲ Tavist Syrup (Among most frequent) 2033
▲ Tavist Tablets (Among most frequent) 2035
▲ Tavist-D Tablets (Among most frequent) 2035
Tedral SA 1765
Temaril Tablets, Syrup and Spansule Sustained Release Capsules 1085
Theo-24 2179
Theo-Dur Sprinkle 1168
Theo-Dur Extended-Release Tablets 1166
Theolair 1317
Theolair-SR Tablets 1319
▲ TheoX Extended-Release Tablets (Among most consistent) 841
Timentin for Injection 2239
Tofranil Ampuls 1038
Tofranil Tablets 1039
Tofranil-PM Capsules 1041
Tolinase Tablets (1%) 2365
Triaminic Expectorant DH (Among most frequent) 1995
▲ Triaminic Oral Infant Drops (Among most frequent) 1996
Triavil Tablets 1556
▲ Trilisate (Less than 20%) 1822
Trimpex Tablets 1922
▲ Trinalin Repetabs Tablets (Among most frequent) 1170
Uniphyl 400 mg Tablets 1823
Ventolin Syrup (Less than 1 of 100 patients) 583
Vivactil Tablets 1567
Wigraine Tablets & Suppositories 1645
Wytensin Tablets (3% or less) 2542
Yutopar (Infrequent) 647
Zarontin Capsules (Frequent) 1768
Zarontin Syrup (Frequent) 1769
Zaroxolyn Tablets 989
Zefazone Sterile Powder 2372

Distress, gastric (see under Distress, gastrointestinal)

Distress, gastrointestinal

AeroBid Inhaler System (1-3%) 995
AK-Fluor Injection 10% and 25% ⊙ 204
Alferon N Injection (One patient) 1809
Allbee C-800 Plus Iron Tablets ▣ 670
Alupent (1 to 4%) 674
Atrovent Inhalation Aerosol (2.4%) 675
▲ Azulfidine Tablets, EN-tabs, Oral Suspension (Approximately one-third of patients) 1157
Biltricide 1589
Bumex (0.1%) 1895
BuSpar (2%) 1401
Calan SR Caplets (1% or less) 2157
Calan Tablets (1% or less) 2155
Capoten 2255
Carafate Tablets (Less than 0.5%) 1326
Celontin (Frequent) 1692
Centrax (Less frequent) 1693
Ceredase Injection 1052
Choledyl Pediatric Elixir 1702
Choledyl Tablets 1700
▲ Clinoril Tablets (10%) 1433
Colestid Granules 2328
Coly-Mycin M Parenteral 1706
Corgard Tablets (1 to 5 of 1000 patients) 701
Corzide Tablets (1 to 5 of 1000 patients) 702
Cuprimine Capsules 1442
Desyrel and Desyrel Dividose (Greater than 1%) 1404
DiaBeta (1.8%) 1091
Dilantin with Phenobarbital Kapseals 1715
Dilor-G Tablets & Liquid 2079
▲ Dolobid Tablets (3% to 9%) 1465
Duvoid Tablets 1853
DynaCirc Capsules (1.7%) 2004
▲ Emcyt Capsules (11%) 1161
Enduronyl Forte Tablets 518
Esimil Tablets 864
Fastin Capsules 2216
Feldene Capsules (1 to 3%) 1777
Feosol Elixir (Occasional) 2191
Feosol Tablets (Occasional) 2191
Fiorinal with Codeine Capsules 2008
Flexeril Tablets (Less than 1%) 1471
Floxin Tablets (1% to 3%) 1652
Fluorescite ⊙ 217
Hydergine 2010
Iberet Filmtab 531
Imodium Capsules 1139
▲ Imuran (Approximately 12%) 768
ISMOTIC (Very rare) ⊙ 233
Isoptin Injectable (0.6%) 1177
Isoptin Oral Tablets (Less than 1%) 1179
Isoptin SR Sustained Release Tablets (Less than 1%) 1181
K-Dur Microburst Release System (potassium chloride, USP) E.R. Tablets 1163
▲ K-Norm Capsules (Among most common) 982
Kato Potassium Supplement 1114
Klotrix 708
▲ Lactaid (Most frequent) 1191
Larodopa Tablets 1905
Lasix Tablets and Injection 1093
Lopid Capsules and Tablets 1736
Lopressor Ampuls (1%) 1032
Lopressor HCT Tablets (1 in 100 patients) 1034
Lopressor Tablets (1%) 1032
Lupron Depot 7.5 mg 2311
▲ Lysodren (80%) 731
Mandelamine (Occasional) 1738
Metaprel Inhalation Aerosol Bronchodilator (1 to 4%) 2014
Midamor Tablets (Between 1% and 3%) 1508
Minipress Capsules (Less than 1%) 1778
Minizide Capsules (Rare) 1779
Moduretic Tablets (Greater than 1%, less than 3%) 1510
Nardil (Common) 1742
Neosar for Injection (Less frequent) 566
Nicobid 1846
▲ Nicorette (9.6%) 1335
Normozide Tablets 2112
Nullo Deodorant Tablets (1 case) ▣ 547
Nystatin, USP for Extemporaneous Preparation of Oral Suspension (Occasional) 1685
Omnipaque (Less than or equal to 1%) 2552
Orap Tablets 1020
Paradione Capsules 548
Peri-Colace (Exceedingly small) 1409
Peritrate 1756
▲ Phenurone Tablets (8%) 552
Placidyl Capsules 553
Ponstel 1758
Prelu-2 Capsules 683
Pyridium (Occasional) 1763
Robaxisal Tablets 1872
Roferon-A Injection (Less than 1%) 1916
▲ Sandostatin Injection (6.7%) 2029
Sanorex Tablets 2030
Scleromate (Rare) 1685
Sedapap Tablets 50 mg/650 mg (Less frequent) 1360
Sodium Polystyrene Sulfonate Suspension 1993
Taractan 1920
Tegretol Chewable Tablets 654
Tegretol Suspension 656
Tegretol Tablets 654
Tenuate 1354
Timolide Tablets (Less than 1%) 1547
Timoptic in Ocudose 1552
Timoptic Sterile Ophthalmic Solution 1550
▲ Tolectin (200, 400 and 600 mg) (3 to 9%) 1379
Tridione 557
Verelan Capsules (Less than 1%) 1243
Zarontin Capsules (Frequent) 1768
Zarontin Syrup (Frequent) 1769
Zorprin Tablets 698
Zovirax 824

Distress, precordial (see under Distress, epigastric)

Distress, stomach (see under Distress, gastrointestinal)

Distress, upper GI (see under Distress, epigastric)

Disturbances, emotional (see under Emotional disturbances)

Disturbances, gastrointestinal (see under Distress, gastrointestinal)

Disulfiram-like reactions

DiaBeta (Very rare) 1091
Diabinese Tablets 1775
Furoxone (Rare) 1855
Glucotrol 1952
Micronase Tablets (Rare) 2350
Orinase Tablets 2354
Tolinase Tablets 2365

Diuresis

Azo Gantanol Tablets (Rare) 1887
Azo Gantrisin Tablets (Rare) 1888
Azulfidine Tablets, EN-tabs, Oral Suspension (Rare) 1157
Bactrim DS Tablets (Rare) 1891
Bactrim I.V. Infusion (Rare) 1889
Bactrim (Rare) 1891
Cholybar 1705
Fansidar Tablets (Rare) 1896
Fiorinal with Codeine Capsules (Infrequent) 2008
Gantanol (Rare) 1899
Gantrisin Ophthalmic Ointment/Solution 1900
Gantrisin (Rare) 1901
Pediazole (Rare) 1973
Quadrinal Tablets 1183
Questran Light 711
Questran Powder 710
Septra (Rare) 813
Septra I.V. Infusion (Rare) 808
Septra I.V. Infusion ADD-Vantage Vials (Rare) 810
Septra (Rare) 813
Thiosulfil Forte Tablets (Rare) 2526
Tonocard Tablets (Less than 1%) 1554

Diuresis, potentiation of

Aminophyllin Tablets 2153
Asbron G 1997
Choledyl Tablets 1700
Choledyl Pediatric Elixir 1702
Choledyl SA Tablets 1704
Constant-T Tablets 1029
Lufyllin & Lufyllin-400 Tablets 2384
Lufyllin-GG Elixir & Tablets 2385
Marax Tablets & DF Syrup 1954
Quibron Capsules 713
Quibron-T 714
Quibron-T/SR 716
Respbid Tablets 684
Slo-bid Gyrocaps 1847
T-PHYL (Uniphyl) 200 mg Tablets 1820
Theo-24 2179
Theo-Dur Extended-Release Tablets 1166
Theo-Dur Sprinkle 1168
Theolair 1317
Theolair-SR Tablets 1319
▲ TheoX Extended-Release Tablets (Among most consistent) 841
Uniphyl 400 mg Tablets 1823

Diverticulitis

Cholybar 1705
Questran Light 711
Questran Powder 710

Dizziness

A.R.M. Allergy Relief Medicine Caplets ▣ 615
Accutane Capsules 1878
Actibine 900
Actifed Capsules ▣ 539
Actifed Plus Caplets ▣ 539
Actifed Plus Tablets (At higher doses) ▣ 540
▲ Actifed with Codeine Cough Syrup (Among most frequent) 752
Actifed Syrup ▣ 540
Actifed Tablets ▣ 540
Actifed 12-Hour Capsules ▣ 539
Acutrim ▣ 548
▲ Adalat Capsules (10 mg and 20 mg) (About 10% to 27%) 1587
Adenocard Injection (1%) 1007
Adipex-P Tablets and Capsules 1019
Advil Cold & Sinus Caplets (formerly CoAdvil) 2416
▲ AeroBid Inhaler System (3-9%) 995
Aerolate 994
Afrin Tablets ▣ 693
Albalon Solution with Liquifilm ⊙ 238
Aldactazide 2150
Aldoclor Tablets 1413
Aldomet Ester HCl Injection 1417
Aldomet Oral 1415
Aldoril Tablets 1418
▲ Alfenta Injection (3%) 1131
▲ Alferon N Injection (4% to 9%) 1809
Alka-Seltzer Plus Cold Medicine ▣ 623
Alka-Seltzer Plus Night-Time Cold Medicine ▣ 623
Allerest ▣ 559
Altace Capsules (2.2%) 1086
Alupent (1 to 4%) 674

Alurate Elixir (Less than 1 in 100) 1883
Amen 833
Amicar Syrup, Tablets, and Injection (Occasional) 1194
Amoxil (Rare) 2193
▲ Anafranil Capsules (41% to 54%) 650
Ana-Kit Anaphylaxis Emergency Treatment Kit 1100
▲ Anaprox and Anaprox DS Tablets (3-9%) 2288
Anatuss LA Tablets 1359
▲ Anestacon Solution (Among most common) 2394
▲ Anexsia 5/500 Tablets (Among most frequent) 2196
Ansaid Tablets (1-3%) 2319
Apresazide Capsules (Less frequent) 854
Apresoline Hydrochloride Parenteral (Ampuls) 856
Apresoline Hydrochloride Tablets (Less frequent) 855
Apresoline-Esidrix Tablets 857
AquaMEPHYTON Injection 1422
Arm-a-Med Isoetharine Inhalation Solution, USP 616
▲ Artane (30% to 50%) 1195
Asendin Tablets (Greater than 1%) 1196
Atabrine Hydrochloride Tablets 2041
Atgam Sterile Solution (Less than 1% to less than 5%) 2320
Ativan Injection (Occasional) 2432
▲ Ativan Tablets (6.9%) 2434
Atrohist Sprinkle Capsules 558
Atromid-S Capsules (Less often) 2435
Atrovent Inhalation Aerosol (2.4%) 675
Augmentin Tablets, Powder for Oral Suspension, and Chewable Tablets (Rare) 2198
Azactam for Injection (Less than 1%) 2252
▲ Azdōne Tablets (Among most frequent) 844
Azo Gantrisin Tablets 1888
B & O No. 15A & No. 16A Supprettes 2395
Baron-X Tablets 650
▲ 8 Hour Bayer Timed-Release Aspirin (Among most frequent) ▣ 566
▲ Benadryl Capsules (Among most frequent) 1691
Benadryl Decongestant Elixir ▣ 635
Benadryl Decongestant ▣ 635
▲ Benadryl Kapseals (Among most frequent) 1691
▲ Benadryl Parenteral (Among most frequent) 1692
Benadryl Plus ▣ 636
Benadryl Plus Nighttime ▣ 637
▲ Benadryl Steri-Vials, Ampoules, and Steri-Dose Syringe (Among most frequent) 1692
Benemid Tablets 1426
▲ Bentyl (29%) 1322
Benylin Decongestant ▣ 638
Betagan (Rare) ◉ 239
Betoptic Sterile Ophthalmic Solution (Rare) 569
Betoptic S Sterile Ophthalmic Suspension (Rare) 570
Biavax II 1427
Biltricide 1589
Biphetamine Capsules 973
Blocadren Tablets (2.3%) 1429
Bontril Slow-Release 834
▲ Brethine Ampuls (1.3 to 10.2%) 1026
Bretylol Injection (7 in 1000) 923
▲ Brevibloc Injection (3% to 12%) 942
Brevicon 2304
Brexin L.A. Capsules 2078
Bricanyl Injection (Common) 1324
Bricanyl Tablets (Common) 1325
Bromfed 1615
Bronkephrine Injection 2042
Bronkometer Aerosol 2042
Bronkosol Solution 2042
Arthritis Strength Bufferin Analgesic Caplets 744
Bumex (1.1%) 1895
▲ BuSpar (12%) 1401
Butisol Sodium Elixir & Tablets (Less than 1 in 100) 2377
▲ Calan SR Caplets (3.3%) 2157
▲ Calan Tablets (3.3%) 2155
Cama Arthritis Pain Reliever ▣ 685
Cantil Tablets 1326
Capoten (0.5 to 2%) 2255
Capozide (0.5 to 2%) 2258
Carafate Tablets (Less than 0.5%) 1326
Carbocaine Hydrochloride 3% Injection 956
Carbocaine Hydrochloride Injection 2043
Carbocaine Hydrochloride 2% with Neo-Cobefrin 956
▲ Cardene Capsules (4.0-6.9%) 2290
Cardilate Oral/Sublingual Tablets 757
Cardizem Tablets-30 mg, 60 mg, 90 mg and 120 mg (1.5%) 1329
▲ Cardizem SR Capsules-60 mg, 90 mg and 120 mg (3.4-7%) 1327
▲ Cardura Tablets (Up to 23%) 1941
Cartrol Tablets (Less common) 507
Catapres Tablets (About 16 in 100 patients) 676
Catapres-TTS (2 of 101 patients) 677
Ceclor Pulvules & Suspension (Rare) 1251
Ceftin Tablets (Less than 0.2%) 575
Celontin (Frequent) 1692
▲ Centrax (8.7%) 1693
Ceptaz for Injection (Fewer than 1%) 1057
Cerose-DM 2443
▲ CHEMET (succimer) Capsules (1.0 to 12.7%) 1361
▲ Children's Advil Suspension (3-9%) 2426
Chlor-Trimeton Decongestant ▣ 694
Cholybar 1705
Cibacalcin Double-chambered Syringes (Rare) 859
Cibalith-S 870
Cipro I.V. (1% or less) 1592
Cipro Tablets (Less than 1%) 1589
▲ Clinoril Tablets (3-9%) 1433
▲ Clozaril Tablets (More than 5 to 19%) 2000
Codiclear DH Syrup 845
Codimal 846
ColBENEMID Tablets 1436
Colestid Granules (1 in 300) 2328
Coly-Mycin M Parenteral 1706
▲ Combipres Tablets (About 16%) 678
Comhist LA Capsules 1618
Compazine 2201
Allergy-Sinus Comtrex Multi-Symptom Allergy Sinus Formula Tablets & Caplets 746
Cough Formula Comtrex (At higher doses) 746
Comtrex Multi-Symptom Cold Reliever Tablets/Caplets/Liqui-Gels/Liquid- 745
Day-Night Comtrex 747
Non-Drowsy Comtrex 747
Condylox (Less than 5%) 1630
Contac Continuous Action Decongestant/Antihistamine Capsules ▣ 710
Contac Jr. Children's Cold Medicine ▣ 712
Contac Maximum Strength Continuous Action Decongestant/Antihistamine Caplets ▣ 709
Contac Nighttime Cold Medicine ▣ 713
Contac Severe Cold and Flu Formula Caplets ▣ 711
Contac Sinus Caplets Maximum Strength Non-Drowsy Formula ▣ 710
Contac Sinus Tablets Maximum Strength Non-Drowsy Formula ▣ 710
▲ Cordarone Tablets (4 to 9%) 2446
Corgard Tablets (2 in 100 patients) 701
Coricidin 'D' Decongestant Tablets ▣ 695
Coricidin Demilets Tablets for Children ▣ 696
Corzide Tablets (Approximately 2 of 100 patients) 702
Cycrin Tablets 2449
Cyklokapron Tablets and Injection 1159
Cylert Tablets 510
Cystospaz 2395
▲ Cytadren Tablets (5%) 861
Cytosar-U Sterile Powder (Less frequent) 2329
Cytotec (Infrequent) 2159
Cytovene Sterile Powder (1% or less) 2292
DDAVP (Up to 3%) 1841
Dalgan Injection (1 to less than 3%) 620
Dalmane Capsules 1927
▲ Damason-P (Among most frequent) 1356
Danocrine Capsules 2046
▲ Dantrium Capsules (Among most frequent) 1619
Daranide Tablets 1445
Darbid Tablets 2205
▲ Darvon-N/Darvocet-N (Among most frequent) 1254
▲ Darvon (Among most frequent) 1256
▲ Darvon-N Suspension & Tablets (Among most frequent) 1254
Dayto Himbin Tablets and Liquid 905
Decadron Phosphate with Xylocaine Injection, Sterile 1451
Deconamine 663
Deconsal 559
Demazin Nasal Decongestant/ Antihistamine Repetabs Tablets & Syrup ▣ 697
Demerol 2047
Demulen 2161
Depakene Capsules & Syrup 511
Depakote 512
Depo-Provera Sterile Aqueous Suspension (Occasional) 2336
Deprol Tablets 2382
Desoxyn Gradumet Tablets (Rare) 514
Desyrel and Desyrel Dividose (Greater than 1%) 1404
Dexatrim ▣ 733
Dexedrine 2206
Didrex Tablets 2338
Diethylstilbestrol Tablets 1258
Dilantin Infatabs 1710
Dilantin Kapseals 1708
Dilantin Parenteral 1712
Dilantin-30 Pediatric/Dilantin-125 Suspension 1713
Dilantin with Phenobarbital Kapseals 1715
▲ Dilatrate-SR (2-36%) 1827
Dilaudid Cough Syrup 1174
Dilaudid 1173
Dilaudid-HP Injection 1175
Dimacol Caplets ▣ 672
Dimetane Decongestant ▣ 673
▲ Dimetane-DC Cough Syrup (Most frequent) 1857
Dimetane-DX Cough Syrup (Among most frequent) 1858
Dimetapp Elixir ▣ 673
Dimetapp Extentabs ▣ 674
Dimetapp Plus Caplets ▣ 675
Dimetapp Tablets ▣ 675
Dipentum Capsules (1 out of 441 patients) 1160
Diprivan Injection (Greater than 1%) 2267
Disophrol Chronotab Sustained-Action Tablets ▣ 698
Ditropan 1332
Diucardin Tablets 2450
Diulo 2129
Diupres Tablets 1461
Diuril Oral Suspension 1464
Diuril Sodium Intravenous 1463
Diuril Tablets 1464
Dolobid Tablets (Greater than 1 in 100) 1465
▲ Dolophine Hydrochloride Ampoules & Vials (Among most frequent) 1260
▲ Dolophine Hydrochloride Tablets (Among most frequent) 1261
Donnagel (Rare) ▣ 675
Donnatal 1858
Donnatal Extentabs 1859
Donnatal Tablets 1858
Donnazyme Tablets 1860
Dopram Injectable 1860
Doral Tablets (1.5%) 2383
Dorcol Children's Cough Syrup ▣ 685
Dorcol Children's Decongestant Liquid ▣ 685
Dorcol Children's Liquid Cold Formula (Occasional) ▣ 686
Dristan Cold Nasal Decongestant/ Antihistamine/ Analgesic Coated Tablets 2419
Dristan Sinus Caplets 2419
Drixoral Antihistamine/Nasal Decongestant Syrup ▣ 698
Drixoral Plus Extended-Release Tablets ▣ 699
Drixoral Sinus ▣ 700
Drixoral Sustained-Action Tablets ▣ 698
▲ Duragesic Transdermal System (3% to 10%) 1133
Duranest Injections 624
Duvoid Tablets 1853
Dyazide Capsules 2208
Dyclone 0.5% and 1% Topical Solutions, USP 626
▲ DynaCirc Capsules (1.6% to 7.3%) 2004
Dyrenium Capsules (Rare) 2210
E.E.S. (Isolated reports) 522
Easprin 1719
Ecotrin 2189
Elavil 2269
▲ Eldepryl (7 of 49 patients) 2250
Emete-con Intramuscular/Intravenous 1950
▲ Eminase (Less than 10%) 2211
▲ Empirin with Codeine Phosphate Nos. 2, 3 & 4 (Among most frequent) 764
Endep Tablets 1927
Enduron Tablets 517
Enduronyl 518
▲ Engerix-B Unit-Dose Vials (1% to 10%) 2213
Enovid 2161
EpiPen 843
▲ Epogen for Injection (7.0% to 9.0%) 591
Equagesic Tablets 2451
▲ Ergamisol Tablets (3 to 4%) 1136
EryPed (Isolated reports) 519
Ery-Tab Tablets (Isolated reports) 521
Erythrocin Stearate Filmtab (Isolated reports) 523
Erythromycin Base Filmtab (Isolated reports) 525
Erythromycin Delayed-Release Capsules, USP (Isolated reports) 526
▲ Esgic-Plus Tablets (Among most frequent) 1002
▲ Esgic Tablets & Capsules (Among most frequent) 1001
Esidrix Tablets 863
Esimil Tablets 864
Eskalith 2214
Estinyl Tablets 2085
Estrace 1385
Estrace Vaginal Cream 1388
Estraderm Transdermal System 866
Estradurin 2452
Estratest 2245
Estrovis 1721
▲ Ethmozine Tablets (0.3%-20%) 946
Etrafon 2087
Sinus Excedrin Analgesic, Decongestant Tablets & Caplets 750
Exna Tablets 1862
4-Way Cold Tablets 750
Fastin Capsules 2216
Fedahist Gyrocaps 2145
Fedahist Timecaps 2145
Feldene Capsules (1 to 3%) 1777
▲ Fioricet Tablets (Among most frequent) 2006
▲ Fiorinal Capsules (Among most frequent) 2007
Fiorinal with Codeine Capsules (2.6%) 2008
▲ Fiorinal Tablets (Among most frequent) 2007
Flagyl I.V. 2131
Flagyl Tablets 2170
▲ Flexeril Tablets (3% to 11%) 1471
Floxin Tablets (1% to 5%) 1652
Fortaz (Less than 1%) 1060
Fulvicin P/G Tablets 2090
Fulvicin P/G 165 & 330 Tablets 2091
Fulvicin-U/F Tablets 2092
Gamimune N Immune Globulin Intravenous (Human) 1572
Gantrisin (Rare) 1901
Garamycin Injectable 2093
Gastrocrom Capsules (Infrequent) 974
Glucotrol (1 in 50) 1952
Grifulvin V (griseofulvin microsize) Tablets/Suspension (Occasional) 1678
Grisactin (Occasional) 2454
Grisactin Ultra Tablets (Occasional) 2455
Gris-PEG Tablets, 125 mg & 250 mg (Occasional) 1083
Guaifed 1615
▲ Halcion Tablets (7.8%) 2340
Harmonyl Tablets 528
Hexalen Capsules 2316
Hismanal Tablets (2.0%) 1138
Hycodan Syrup, Tablets 927
Hycomine Compound Tablets 929
Hycomine Syrup 927
Hycotuss Expectorant Syrup 930
Hydrea Capsules (Extremely rare) 728
Hydrocet Capsules 835
HydroDIURIL Tablets 1484
Hydromox R Tablets 1209

Hydromox Tablets 1208
Hydropres Tablets 1485
Hyperstat I.V. Injection (2%) 2095
▲Hytrin Tablets (3.1% to 19.3%) 529
IFEX (Less frequent) 729
Imodium Capsules 1139
Inapsine Injection 1140
Inderide Tablets 2463
Inderide LA Long Acting Capsules 2465
▲Indocin (3% to 9%) 1487
Infumorph 200 and Infumorph 500 Sterile Solutions 962
Innovar Injection 1141
Intal Capsules (Less than 1 in 10,000 patients) 978
Intal Inhaler (Infrequent) 979
Intal Nebulizer Solution 980
▲Intron A (7% to 24%) 2097
Inversine Tablets 1492
Ismelin Tablets 869
ISMOTIC (Very rare) ⊙ 233
Isoclor Timesule Capsules ⊡ 561
Isoptin Injectable (1.2%) 1177
▲Isoptin Oral Tablets (3.3%) 1179
▲Isoptin SR Sustained Release Tablets (3.3%) 1181
Isordil (Occasional) 2467
Isuprel Hydrochloride Injection 1:5000 2050
Isuprel Hydrochloride Mistometer 2051
Isuprel Hydrochloride Solution 1:200 & 1:100 2052
Jenest-28 Tablets 1636
K-Phos M.F. Tablets 659
K-Phos Neutral Tablets 660
K-Phos Original Formula 'Sodium Free' Tablets (Less frequent) 660
K-Phos No. 2 Tablets 659
Keflex Pulvules, Oral Suspension & Pediatric Drops 916
Keftab Tablets 917
Kemadrin Tablets 771
▲Kerlone Tablets (4.5% to 14.8%) 2172
Kinesed Tablets 2272
Koro-Flex Arcing Spring Diaphragm 2142
Koromex Coil Spring Diaphragm 2142
Kwell Cream (Rare) 1830
Kwell Lotion (Rare) 1831
Kwell Shampoo (Rare) 1832
Lamprene Capsules (Less than 1%) 1030
Lanoxicaps 772
Lanoxin Elixir Pediatric 775
Lanoxin Injection 778
Lanoxin Injection Pediatric 781
Lanoxin Tablets 783
▲Lariam Tablets (Among most frequent) 1904
Larodopa Tablets (Relatively frequent) 1905
Lasix 1093
▲Levatol (4.9%) 1832
Levlen/Tri-Levlen 665
Levo-Dromoran (Common) 1906
Levsin/Levsinex 2147
▲Limbitrol (Among most frequent) 1933
▲Lioresal Tablets (5-15%) 1031
Lithane Tablets 1596
Lithium Carbonate Capsules & Tablets 1984
Lithobid Tablets 870
▲Lodine Capsules (3-9%) 2468
Lo/Ovral Tablets 2471
Lo/Ovral-28 Tablets 2476
Loestrin 1728
Lomotil 2174
Lopid Capsules and Tablets 1736
▲Lopressor Ampuls (10%) 1032
▲Lopressor HCT Tablets (10 in 100 patients) 1034
▲Lopressor Tablets (10%) 1032
Lorelco Tablets 1333
Lortab ASA Tablets 2414
▲Lortab (Among most frequent) 2412
▲Lotensin Tablets (3.3%) 872
Loxitane 1213
▲Lozol Tablets (Greater than or equal to 5%) 1843
▲Ludiomil Tablets (8%) 874
Lupron Depot 7.5 mg 2311
▲Lupron Injection (5% or more) 2310
▲Lysodren (15%) 731
M-M-R II 1494
M-R-VAX II 1496
▲MS Contin Tablets (Among most frequent) 1814
▲MSIR (Among most frequent) 1817
Macrodantin Capsules (Less frequent) 1624
Marax Tablets & DF Syrup 1954
Marcaine Hydrochloride 0.5% with Epinephrine 1:200,000 (as bitartrate) 958
Marcaine Hydrochloride with Epinephrine 1:200,000 (Rare) 2055
Marcaine Hydrochloride Injection (Rare) 2055
Marcaine Spinal (Rare) 2058
Marinol (Dronabinol) Capsules 1985
▲Marplan Tablets (Among most frequent) 1906
Matulane Capsules 1907
Maxair Inhaler (1.2%) 1311
Maxzide 1215
Mebaral Tablets (Less than 1 in 100) 2061
▲Meclomen Capsules (3-9%) 1739
Mediatric Capsules 2476
Medi-Flu Caplet, Liquid ⊡ 640
Menrium Tablets 1934
▲Mepergan Injection (Among most frequent) 2479
Mephyton Tablets (Rare) 1503
Meruvax II 1503
Mesantoin Tablets 2013
Metaprel Inhalation Aerosol Bronchodilator (1 to 4%) 2014
▲Methadone Hydrochloride Diskets (Among most frequent) 1284
Methadone Hydrochloride Oral Solution & Tablets 1987
Methergine (Rare) 2016
Methotrexate Tablets, Parenteral, LPF Parenteral (Frequent; 1 to 3%) 1217
Metopirone Tablets 876
Mevacor Tablets (2.0%) 1505
▲Mexitil Capsules (18.9% to 26.4%) 680
Micronor Tablets 1667
Midamor Tablets (Between 1% and 3%) 1508
Midrin Capsules 836
Milontin Kapseals 1741
Miltown Tablets 2386
▲Minipress Capsules (10.3%) 1778
▲Minizide Capsules (10.3%) 1779
Minocin Intravenous 1221
Minocin Oral Suspension 1224
Minocin Pellet-Filled Capsules 1222
Mintezol 1510
Modane Plus Tablets ⊡ 504
Modane Tablets ⊡ 503
Modicon 1667
▲Moduretic Tablets (3% to 8%) 1510
Monopril Tablets 1406
Motofen Tablets (1 in 20) 836
▲Motrin Tablets (3-9%) 2351
Myambutol Tablets 1225
▲Mykrox ½ mg Tablets (10.2%) 984
Myochrysine Injection 1516
Naldecon CX Adult Liquid ⊡ 521
Naldecon DX Adult Liquid ⊡ 521
Naldecon DX Children's Syrup ⊡ 522
Naldecon DX Pediatric Drops ⊡ 522
Naldecon EX Children's Syrup ⊡ 522
Naldecon EX Pediatric Drops ⊡ 523
Naldecon Syrup, Tablets, Pediatric Drops and Pediatric Syrup 709
▲Nalfon Pulvules & Tablets (6.5%) 919
Naphcon Forte ⊙ 226
▲Naprosyn (3 to 9%) 2297
Nardil (Common) 1742
Naturetin Tablets (Occasional) 1789
Nebcin Vials, Hyporets & ADD-Vantage 1286
▲NebuPent for Inhalation Solution (31 to 47%) 1017
NegGram 2062
Nembutal Sodium Capsules (Less than 1%) 534
Nembutal Sodium Solution (Less than 1%) 536
Nembutal Sodium Suppositories (Less than 1%) 538
Nescaine/Nescaine MPF 629
Netromycin Injection 100 mg/ml 2104
Niclocide Chewable Tablets (1.4%) 1607
Nicorette (2.1%) 1335
Nimotop Capsules (Less than 1%) 1607
Nipride I.V. Infusion 1909
Nitro-Bid IV (Less than 1%) 1338
Nitro-Bid Ointment 1339
Nitro-Bid Capsules 1338
Nitrolingual Spray (Occasional) 1846
Nitrostat IV (Less than 1%) 1744
Nizoral Tablets (Less than 1%) 1145
Nolamine Tablets (Occasional) 838
Nolvadex Tablets (Infrequent) 1102
Nordette-21 Tablets 2481
Nordette-28 Tablets 2483
Norethin 2133
Norflex 1314
Norgesic 1314
Norinyl 2304
Norlestrin 1746
Norlutate 1754
Norlutin 1755
▲Normodyne Injection (2 to 16%) 2108
▲Normodyne Tablets (2% to 16%) 2110
▲Normozide Tablets (6 to 11%) 2112
Noroxin Tablets (1.8%) 1519
▲Norpace (3 to 9%) 2177
Norplant System 2484
Norpramin Tablets 1340
Nor-Q D Tablets 2304
Norzine (Occasional) 1818
Novafed A Capsules 1342
Novafed Capsules 1342
Novahistine DH 1342
Novahistine DMX ⊡ 595
Novahistine Elixir ⊡ 596
Novahistine Expectorant 1343
Novocain Hydrochloride for Spinal Anesthesia 2065
▲Nubain Injection (5%) 934
Nucofed Capsules 2219
Nucofed Expectorant 2219
Nucofed Pediatric Expectorant 2220
Nucofed Syrup 2219
Ogen 540
Omnipaque (2%) 2552
▲Optimine Tablets (Among most frequent) 2115
OptiPranolol Sterile Ophthalmic Solution (A small number of patients) ⊙ 261
▲Oramorph SR (Morphine Sulfate Sustained Release Tablets) (Among most frequent) 1988
Orap Tablets 1020
Oretic Tablets 544
Oreticyl 545
Ornade Spansule Capsules 2221
Ornex Caplets ⊡ 618
Ortho Diaphragm Kit 1664
Ortho Dienestrol Cream 1664
Ortho-Cyclen Tablets 1658
Ortho-Novum 1667
Ortho-White Diaphragm Kit-Flat Spring 1664
Orudis Capsules (Greater than 1%) 2488
Ovcon 1391
Ovral Tablets 2490
Ovral-28 Tablets 2491
Ovrette Tablets 2492
Oxsoralen-Ultra Capsule 1117
PBZ Tablets & Elixir (Among most frequent) 1037
PBZ-SR Tablets (Among most frequent) 1037
PCE Dispertab Tablets (Isolated reports) 549
PMB 200 and PMB 400 2504
Pamelor 2019
Pantopon Injectable 1911
Paraflex Caplets 1378
Parafon Forte DSC Caplets 1379
▲Parlodel (Less than 2-17%) 2020
Parnate Tablets 2222
▲PediaProfen Suspension (3-9%) 1363
Peganone Tablets 551
Pentam 300 Injection (0.5%) 1018
Pentaspan Injection 949
Pepcid (1.3%) 1524
Peptavlon 2563
▲Percocet Tablets (Among most frequent) 950
▲Percodan (Among most frequent) 951
Pergonal (menotropins for injection, USP) 2184
Periactin 1525
Peritrate 1756
▲Permax Tablets (19.1%) 1291
▲Persantine Tablets (13.6%) 683
▲Phenaphen with Codeine Capsules (Among most frequent) 1865
▲Phenaphen-650 with Codeine Tablets (Among most frequent) 1866
Phenergan with Codeine 2497
Phenergan with Dextromethorphan 2499
Phenergan Injection 2493
Phenergan Suppositories 2496
Phenergan Syrup 2495
Phenergan Tablets 2496
Phenergan VC 2500
Phenergan VC with Codeine 2501
Phenobarbital Elixir and Tablets (Less than 1 in 100 patients) 1293
Phenurone Tablets (Less than 1%) 552
Phrenilin 838
Pipracil 1230
Placidyl Capsules 553
Plaquenil Sulfate Tablets 2067
Plegine Tablets 2504
Plendil Extended-Release Tablets (0.8%) 1526
Polaramine 2116
Polymyxin B Sulfate, Aerosporin Brand Sterile Powder 798
Pondimin Tablets 1867
Ponstel 1758
Pontocaine Hydrochloride for Spinal Anesthesia 2069
Prelu-2 Capsules 683
Premarin Intravenous 2508
Premarin with Methyltestosterone 2515
Premarin Tablets 2510
Premarin Vaginal Cream 2512
Prilosec Delayed-Release Capsules (1.5%) 1530
Primaxin I.M. 1532
Primaxin I.V. (0.3%) 1535
▲Prinivil Tablets (6.3% to 9.0%) 1538
▲Prinzide Tablets (7.5%) 1540
Pro-Banthīne Tablets 2141
Procan SR Tablets (Occasional) 1760
▲Procardia Capsules (Approximately 10%) 1781
▲Procardia XL Tablets (4.1% to 27%) 1783
▲Procrit for Injection (7% to 9%) 1647
Proglycem 649
Prolastin Alpha$_1$-Proteinase Inhibitor (Human) (0.19%) 1585
Pronestyl Capsules and Tablets (Occasional) 1800
Pronestyl Injection (Occasional) 1798
Pronestyl-SR Tablets (Occasional) 1801
Propagest 839
▲ProSom Tablets (7%) 554
Prostigmin Injectable 1120
Prostigmin Tablets 1121
Protopam Chloride for Injection 2518
Protostat Tablets 1674
Proventil Inhalation Aerosol (Less than 5%) 2117
Proventil Repetabs Tablets (2%) 2120
▲Proventil Solutions for Inhalation 0.5% and 0.083% (7%) 2118
▲Proventil Syrup (3 of 100) 2119
Proventil Tablets (2%) 2120
Provera Tablets 2356
▲Prozac Pulvules (5.7%) 920
▲Pyridium Plus (One-third to one-half of patients) 1764
Pyrroxate Capsules ⊡ 669
Quadrinal Tablets 1183
Quarzan Capsules 1937
Questran Light 711
Questran Powder 710
Quinidex Extentabs 1868
Raudixin Tablets 1803
Rauzide Tablets 1804
Regitine 878
Reglan (Less frequent) 1869
Renese Tablets 1785
Renese-R Tablets 1786
▲Restoril Capsules (7%) 2023
▲Retrovir Capsules (6%) 802
▲Retrovir I.V. Infusion (6%) 805
▲Retrovir Syrup (6%) 802
Rheumatrex Methotrexate Dose Pack (Frequent; 1% to 3%) 1234
Rifadin 1345
Rifamate Capsules 1347
Rimactane Capsules 879
Ritalin 880
Robaxin Injectable 1871
Robaxin Tablets 1872
▲Robaxisal Tablets (One in 20-25) 1872
Robinul Forte Tablets 1873
Robinul Injectable 1873
Robinul Tablets 1873
Robitussin ⊡ 676
Robitussin-CF ⊡ 676
Robitussin-DAC Syrup 1875
Rocephin Injectable Vials, ADD-Vantage (Occasional) 1914
▲Roferon-A Injection (21% to 40%) 1916
Rogaine Topical Solution (3.42%) 2357
Rondec 1975
Rondec-DM 1976
Rondec-TR Tablet 1975
Rowasa (1.84 to 3.0%) 2248
▲Roxanol (Among most frequent) 1991
▲Roxicodone Tablets, Oral Solution & Intensol (Oxycodone) (Among most frequent) 1992
▲Rufen Tablets (3-9%) 691
Ru-Tuss DE Tablets 694

Ru-Tuss II Capsules 693
Ru-Tuss with Hydrocodone 694
Ru-Tuss Tablets 693
Ryna ▣ 741
▲ Rythmol Tablets (3.6 to 15.1%) 1184
Saluron 718
Salutensin/Salutensin-Demi 719
Sandoglobulin I.V. (Less than 1%) 2027
Sandostatin Injection (1.6%) 2029
Sanorex Tablets 2030
Sansert Tablets 2031
Scleromate (Rare) 1685
Seconal Sodium Pulvules (Less than 1 in 100) 1296
▲ Sectral Capsules (6%) 2520
▲ Sedapap Tablets 50 mg/650 mg (Among most frequent) 1360
Seldane Tablets (1.5%) 1349
Seldane-D Extended-Release Tablets 1350
Sensorcaine (Rare) 631
Sensorcaine-MPF Spinal (Rare) 634
Ser-Ap-Es Tablets 881
Serax Capsules (In few instances) 2522
Serax Tablets (In few instances) 2522
Serentil 686
Serophene (clomiphene citrate tablets, USP) (Less than 1 in 100 patients) 2186
Serpasil Tablets 883
Serpasil-Apresoline Tablets 884
Serpasil-Esidrix Tablets 886
Sinarest ▣ 562
Sine-Aid Maximum Strength Sinus Headache Caplets 1365
Sine-Aid Maximum Strength Sinus Headache Tablets 1365
Sinemet Tablets (Less frequent) 952
Sinemet CR Tablets (2.9%) 953
Sine-Off Maximum Strength Allergy/Sinus Formula Caplets ▣ 721
Sine-Off Maximum Strength No Drowsiness Formula Caplets ▣ 722
Sine-Off Sinus Medicine Tablets-Aspirin Formula ▣ 722
Sinequan (Occasional) 1960
Singlet Tablets ▣ 598
Sinulin 840
Sinutab Allergy Formula Sustained Action Tablets ▣ 640
Skelaxin 840
Solganal Suspension 2122
Soma Compound w/Codeine Tablets 2390
Soma Compound Tablets 2389
Soma Tablets 2388
Sorbitrate 1103
Stadol (2%) 721
Stelazine 2226
Stilphostrol Tablets and Ampuls 1609
Sublimaze Injection 1146
Sudafed Children's Liquid ▣ 543
Sudafed Cough Syrup ▣ 543
Sudafed Plus Liquid ▣ 544
Sudafed Plus Tablets ▣ 545
Sudafed Sinus Caplets ▣ 545
Sudafed Sinus Tablets ▣ 545
Sudafed Tablets, 30 mg ▣ 544
Sudafed Tablets, Adult Strength, 60 mg ▣ 544
Sudafed 12 Hour Capsules ▣ 545
Suprax (Less than 2%) 1235
Surmontil Capsules 2524
Sus-Phrine Injection 1006
▲ Symmetrel Capsules & Syrup (5-10%) 936
Synalgos-DC Capsules 2525
TACE 12 and 25 mg 1353
Tacaryl 2409
Tagamet (Approximately 1 in 100) 2228
Talacen 2070
▲ Talwin Injection (Most common) 2071
Talwin Compound 2072
▲ Talwin Injection (Most common) 2071
Talwin Nx 2073
▲ Tambocor Tablets (18.9%) 1315
Taractan 1920
▲ Tavist Syrup (Among most frequent) 2033
▲ Tavist Tablets (Among most frequent) 2035
▲ Tavist-D Tablets (Among most frequent) 2035
Tazicef for Injection (Less than 1%) 2231
Tazidime Vials, Faspak & ADD-Vantage 1299
▲ Tegison Capsules (1-10%) 1881
▲ Tegretol Chewable Tablets (Among most frequent) 654
▲ Tegretol Suspension (Among most frequent) 656
▲ Tegretol Tablets (Among most frequent) 654
Temaril Tablets, Syrup and Spansule Sustained Release Capsules 1085
▲ Tenex Tablets (2% to 4%) 1875
▲ Tenoretic Tablets (4 to 13%) 1105
▲ Tenormin Tablets and I.V. Injection (4 to 13%) 1107
Tenuate 1354
Tessalon Perles 1006
Thalitone Tablets 687
TheraCys BCG Live (Intravesical) (Up to 0.9%) 898
Thiotepa Parenteral 1240
Thorazine 2234
Tigan 2239
Timentin for Injection 2239
Timolide Tablets (1.2%) 1547
Timoptic in Ocudose 1552
Timoptic Sterile Ophthalmic Solution 1550
Tofranil Ampuls 1038
Tofranil Tablets 1039
Tofranil-PM Capsules 1041
▲ Tolectin (200, 400 and 600 mg) (3 to 9%) 1379
Tolinase Tablets (Infrequently) 2365
▲ Tonocard Tablets (8.0-25.3%) 1554
Toradol IM Injection (1% to 3%) 2302
Torecan (Occasional) 1993
▲ Tornalate (3%) 2074
Trancopal Caplets 2075
▲ Trandate HCT Tablets (6% in 208 patients) 579
▲ Trandate Injection (9 of 100 patients) 577
▲ Trandate Tablets (20%) 579
Transderm Scōp Transdermal Therapeutic System (Infrequent) 887
Tranxene (Less common) 556
▲ Trental (1.9% to 11.9%) 1099
▲ Trexan Tablets (Less than 10%) 937
Triaminic Allergy Tablets ▣ 688
Triaminic Chewables ▣ 688
Triaminic Cold Tablets ▣ 688
▲ Triaminic Expectorant DH (Among most frequent) 1995
▲ Triaminic Oral Infant Drops (Among most frequent) 1996
Triaminic Syrup (Occasional) ▣ 689
Triaminic-12 Tablets ▣ 690
Triaminic-DM Syrup ▣ 689
Triaminicin Tablets ▣ 690
Triaminicol Multi-Symptom Cold Tablets ▣ 691
Triaminicol Multi-Symptom Relief ▣ 691
Triavil Tablets 1556
Trilafon (Rare) 2123
Levlen/Tri-Levlen 665
Trilisate (Less than 2%) 1822
▲ Trinalin Repetabs Tablets (Among most frequent) 1170
Tri-Norinyl 2304
Triphasil-21 Tablets 2527
Triphasil-28 Tablets 2532
Trobicin Sterile Powder 2366
Tussionex Extended-Release Suspension 988
Tuss-Ornade Liquid 2242
Tuss-Ornade Spansule Capsules 2242
Tylenol with Codeine 1381
Children's Tylenol Cold Liquid Formula and Chewable Tablets 1368
Tylenol Cold & Flu Hot Medication, Packets 1369
Tylenol Cold & Flu No Drowsiness Hot Medication, Packets 1371
Tylenol Cold Medication Caplets and Tablets 1370
Tylenol Cold Medication No Drowsiness Formula Caplets 1370
Tylenol Cold Night Time Medication Liquid 1371
Tylenol Cough Medication Liquid with Decongestant, Maximum Strength 1372
Tylenol, Maximum Strength, Sinus Medication Gelcaps, Caplets and Tablets 1373
▲ Tylox Capsules (Among most frequent) 1382
Urecholine 1558
Urised Tablets 2396
Uroqid-Acid (Less frequent) 661
Ursinus Inlay-Tabs ▣ 691
Valpin 50 Tablets 941
Vancocin HCl, Oral Solution & Pulvules (Rare) 1304
Vancocin HCl, Vials & ADD-Vantage (Rare) 1302
▲ Vascor (200, 300 and 400 mg) Tablets (11.63 to 27.27%) 1383
▲ Vaseretic Tablets (8.6%) 1559
Vasocon-A ⊙ 278
Vasotec I.V. (0.5 to 1%) 1562
▲ Vasotec Tablets (4.3% to 7.9%) 1564
Velban Vials 1305
Velosef Capsules and for Oral Suspension 606
▲ Ventolin (Less than 5 in 100 patients) 583
▲ Verelan Capsules (3.3% to 4.2%) 1243
Versed Injection (Less than 1%) 1924
Vicks Daycare ▣ 660
Vicks Formula 44D Decongestant Cough Medicine ▣ 662
Vicks Formula 44M Multi-Symptom Cough Medicine ▣ 662
Vicks NyQuil Nighttime Colds Medicine-Original & Cherry Flavor ▣ 664
▲ Vicodin ES Tablets (Among most frequent) 1189
Vira-A for Injection 1766
▲ Visken Tablets (9%) 2036
Vivactil Tablets 1567
▲ Voltaren Tablets (About 3%) 1042
Vontrol Tablets (Rare) 2243
▲ Wellbutrin Tablets (22.3%) 821
▲ Wygesic Tablets (Most frequent) 2540
▲ Wytensin Tablets (12% to 17%) 2542
▲ Xanax Tablets (29.8%) 2367
▲ Xylocaine Injections (Among most common) 637
Xylocaine Injections for Ventricular Arrhythmias 639
Xylocaine 2% Jelly 643
Xylocaine 5% Ointment 644
Xylocaine 10% Oral Spray 645
4% Xylocaine-MPF Sterile Solution 641
Xylocaine 2% Viscous Solution 646
Yocon 1686
Yohimex Tablets 1190
Zantac Injection and Zantac Injection Premixed (Rare) 1063
Zantac (Rare) 1065
Zarontin Capsules 1768
Zarontin Syrup 1769
Zaroxolyn Tablets 989
▲ Zestoretic (7.5%) 2274
▲ Zestril Tablets (6.3%) 2277
▲ Zoladex (5%) 1110
Zovirax (0.3%) 824
▲ Zydone Capsules (Most frequent) 941
Zyloprim Tablets (Less than 1%) 830

Down's syndrome

Pergonal (menotropins for injection, USP) 2184
Serophene (clomiphene citrate tablets, USP) (Six cases) 2186

Dreaming

▲ Eldepryl (2 of 49 patients) 2250
Endep Tablets 1927
Limbitrol (Less common) 1933
MS Contin Tablets (Infrequent) 1814
MSIR (Infrequent) 1817
Milontin Kapseals 1741
▲ Orudis Capsules (Greater than 3%) 2488
Temaril Tablets, Syrup and Spansule Sustained Release Capsules 1085
Tenoretic Tablets (Up to 3%) 1105
Tenormin Tablets and I.V. Injection (Up to 3%) 1107
Versed Injection (Less than 1%) 1924

Dreaming, abnormalities

Aldomet Ester HCl Injection 1417
Anafranil Capsules (Up to 3%) 650
Anaprox and Anaprox DS Tablets (Less than 1%) 2288
Blocadren Tablets (Less than 1%) 1429
BuSpar (Frequent) 1401
Cardene Capsules (0.4%) 2290
Cardizem Tablets-30 mg, 60 mg, 90 mg and 120 mg (Less than 1%) 1329
Cardizem SR Capsules-60 mg, 90 mg and 120 mg (Less than 1%) 1327
Cartrol Tablets (Rare) 507
Catapres Tablets 676
Catapres-TTS 677
Centrax (Less frequent) 1693
Children's Advil Suspension (Less than 1%) 2426
Combipres Tablets 678
Cytovene Sterile Powder (1% or less) 2292
Desyrel and Desyrel Dividose (Less than 1%) 1404
Dilaudid-HP Injection 1175
Diprivan Injection (Less than 1%) 2267
Duragesic Transdermal System (1% or greater) 1133
Etrafon 2087
Feldene Capsules (Less than 1%) 1777
Flexeril Tablets (Less than 1%) 1471
Floxin Tablets (Less than 1%) 1652
Halcion Tablets (Rare) 2340
Inderal 2459
Inderal LA Long Acting Capsules 2461
Inderide Tablets 2463
IOPIDINE ⊙ 232
Kerlone Tablets (1.0%) 2172
Mellaril 2011
Motrin Tablets (Less than 1%) 2351
Naprosyn (Less than 1%) 2297
Norzine 1818
Nubain Injection (Less than 1%) 934
Oramorph SR (Morphine Sulfate Sustained Release Tablets) (Less frequent) 1988
PediaProfen Suspension (Less than 1%) 1363
Permax Tablets (2.7%) 1291
Prilosec Delayed-Release Capsules (Less than 1%) 1530
Prolixin Decanoate 1795
Prolixin Elixir 1793
Prolixin Enanthate 1796
Prolixin Injection 1791
Prolixin Oral Concentrate 1792
Prolixin Tablets 1793
ProSom Tablets (2%) 554
Prozac Pulvules (Frequent) 920
Rufen Tablets (Less than 1%) 691
Rythmol Tablets (Less than 1%) 1184
Sectral Capsules (2%) 2520
Serentil 686
Sinemet CR Tablets (1.8%) 953
Stadol (Less than 1%) 721
Talacen (Infrequent) 2070
Talwin Injection (Infrequent) 2071
Talwin Compound (Infrequent) 2072
Talwin Injection 2071
Talwin Nx 2073
Tambocor Tablets (Less than 1%) 1315
Tonocard Tablets (Less than 1%) 1554
Torecan 1993
Trexan Tablets (Less than 1%) 937
Triavil Tablets 1556
Trilafon 2123
▲ Visken Tablets (5%) 2036
Wellbutrin Tablets 821
Xanax Tablets (1.8%) 2367

Drowsiness

A.R.M. Allergy Relief Medicine Caplets ▣ 615
Accutane Capsules 1878
Actidil Tablets ▣ 538
Actifed Capsules ▣ 539
Actifed Plus Caplets ▣ 539
Actifed Plus Tablets ▣ 540
Actifed Syrup ▣ 540
Actifed Tablets ▣ 540
Actifed 12-Hour Capsules ▣ 539
Akineton 1171
Albalon Solution with Liquifilm ⊙ 238
Albalon-A Liquifilm (Some patients) ⊙ 238
Aldactazide 2150
Aldactone 2152
Alfenta Injection (2%) 1131
▲ Alferon N Injection (3% to 10%) 1809
Alka-Seltzer Plus Cold Medicine ▣ 623
Alka-Seltzer Plus Night-Time Cold Medicine ▣ 623
Allerest ▣ 559
Altace Capsules (Less than 1%) 1086
Alurate Elixir (1 to 3 per 100) 1883
Amen 833
▲ Anafranil Capsules (46% to 54%) 650
Ana-Kit Anaphylaxis Emergency Treatment Kit 1100
▲ Anaprox and Anaprox DS Tablets (3-9%) 2288
▲ Anestacon Solution (Among most common) 2394
Anexsia 5/500 Tablets 2196
Anexsia 7.5/650 Tablets 2197
Ansaid Tablets (1-3%) 2319
Antabuse Tablets (Small number of patients) 2429

Antivert, Antivert/25 Tablets, Antivert/25 Chewable Tablets & Antivert/50 Tablets 1940
Artane 1195
▲Asendin Tablets (14%) 1196
Atarax Tablets & Syrup 1941
▲Ativan Injection (6%) 2432
Atrohist Sprinkle Capsules 558
Atromid-S Capsules 2435
Atrovent Inhalation Aerosol (Less than 1 in 100) 675
Axid Pulvules (2.4%) 1246
Azdōne Tablets 844
Azo Gantrisin Tablets 1888
Azulfidine Tablets, EN-tabs, Oral Suspension (Rare) 1157
BC Cold Powder Multi-Symptom Formula ...... ▣ 517
B & O No. 15A & No. 16A Supprettes 2395
Bellergal-S Tablets (Rare) 1998
▲Benadryl Capsules (Among most frequent) 1691
Benadryl Decongestant Elixir ...... ▣ 635
Benadryl Decongestant ...... ▣ 635
Benadryl Elixir ...... ▣ 636
▲Benadryl Kapseals (Among most frequent) 1691
Benadryl 25 Kapseals ...... ▣ 636
▲Benadryl Parenteral (Among most frequent) 1692
Benadryl Plus ...... ▣ 636
Benadryl Plus Nighttime ...... ▣ 637
▲Benadryl Steri-Vials, Ampoules, and Steri-Dose Syringe (Among most frequent) 1692
Benadryl 25 Tablets ...... ▣ 636
▲Bentyl (9%) 1322
Benylin Cough Syrup ...... ▣ 637
Benylin Decongestant ...... ▣ 638
Blocadren Tablets (Less than 1%) 1429
Bonine Tablets 1773
Brethaire Inhaler 1024
▲Brethine Ampuls (9.8 to 11.7%) 1026
Brethine Tablets 1026
▲Brevibloc Injection (3%) 942
Brexin L.A. Capsules 2078
Bricanyl Injection 1324
Bricanyl Tablets 1325
Bromfed Capsules (Timed Release) 1615
Bromfed Syrup ...... ▣ 628
Bromfed 1615
Bronkolixir ...... ▣ 761
Bronkotabs Tablets ...... ▣ 762
Bucladin-S Softab Chewable Tablets (Occasional) 2264
▲BuSpar (10%) 1401
Butazolidin Capsules & Tablets (Less than 1%) 1027
Butisol Sodium Elixir & Tablets (1 to 3 patients per 100) 2377
Calan SR Caplets (1% or less) 2157
Calan Tablets (1% or less) 2155
Calcijex Calcitriol Injection 506
Calderol Capsules 1635
Cantil Tablets 1326
Capoten 2255
Capozide 2258
Carafate Tablets (Less than 0.5%) 1326
Carbocaine Hydrochloride 3% Injection 956
Carbocaine Hydrochloride Injection 2043
Carbocaine Hydrochloride 2% with Neo-Cobefrin 956
Cardene Capsules (1.1-1.4%) 2290
Cardizem Tablets-30 mg, 60 mg, 90 mg and 120 mg (Less than 1%) 1329
Cardizem SR Capsules-60 mg, 90 mg and 120 mg (1.3%) 1327
▲Cardura Tablets (5%) 1941
Cartrol Tablets (1%-7.4%) 507
▲Catapres Tablets (About 33 in 100 patients) 676
▲Catapres-TTS (About 35%) 677
Ceclor Pulvules & Suspension (Rare) 1251
Celontin (Frequent) 1692
▲Centrax (6.8%) 1693
Cerose-DM 2443
▲CHEMET (succimer) Capsules (1.0 to 12.7%) 1361
Children's Advil Suspension (Less than 1%) 2426
Chlor-Trimeton Allergy Syrup, Tablets & Long-Acting Repetabs Tablets ...... ▣ 693
Chlor-Trimeton Decongestant ...... ▣ 694
Cholybar 1705
Cibalith-S 870
Cipro I.V. (1% or less) 1592
Cipro Tablets (Less than 1%) 1589
Clinoril Tablets (Less than 1%) 1433
▲Clozaril Tablets (More than 5 to 39%) 2000
Codiclear DH Syrup 845
Codimal 846
Colestid Granules (Fewer than 1 in 1,000) 2328
▲Combipres Tablets (About 33%) 678
Compazine 2201
Allergy-Sinus Comtrex Multi-Symptom Allergy Sinus Formula Tablets & Caplets 746
Comtrex Multi-Symptom Cold Reliever Tablets/Caplets/Liqui-Gels/Liquid- 745
Day-Night Comtrex 747
Contac Continuous Action Decongestant/Antihistamine Capsules ...... ▣ 710
Contac Maximum Strength Continuous Action Decongestant/Antihistamine Caplets ...... ▣ 709
Contac Nighttime Cold Medicine ...... ▣ 713
Contac Severe Cold and Flu Formula Caplets ...... ▣ 711
Coricidin 'D' Decongestant Tablets ...... ▣ 695
Coricidin Demilets Tablets for Children ...... ▣ 696
Coricidin Tablets ...... ▣ 695
Corzide Tablets 702
Cyclogyl ...... ⊙ 215
Cycrin Tablets 2449
Cylert Tablets 510
Cystospaz 2395
▲Cytadren Tablets (1 in 3) 861
Cytosar-U Sterile Powder 2329
Cytotec (Infrequent) 2159
Cytovene Sterile Powder (1% or less) 2292
Dalmane Capsules 1927
Damason-P 1356
▲Dantrium Capsules (Among most frequent) 1619
Daranide Tablets (Among the most common effects) 1445
Darbid Tablets 2205
Decadron Phosphate with Xylocaine Injection, Sterile 1451
Deconamine 663
Demazin Nasal Decongestant/ Antihistamine Repetabs Tablets & Syrup ...... ▣ 697
Depo-Provera Sterile Aqueous Suspension (Occasional) 2336
Deprol Tablets 2382
Desyrel and Desyrel Dividose (Greater than 1%) 1404
Diamox Parenteral (Occasional) 1200
Diamox Sequels (Sustained Release) (Occasional) 1201
Diamox Tablets (Occasional) 1200
Dibenzyline Capsules 2207
▲Dilantin with Phenobarbital Kapseals (Among most common) 1715
Dilaudid Cough Syrup 1174
Dilaudid 1173
Dimetane Decongestant ...... ▣ 673
Dimetane ...... ▣ 672
Dimetapp Elixir ...... ▣ 673
Dimetapp Extentabs ...... ▣ 674
Dimetapp Plus Caplets ...... ▣ 675
Dimetapp Tablets ...... ▣ 675
Dipentum Capsules (1.8%) 1160
Diphtheria and Tetanus Toxoids and Pertussis Vaccine Adsorbed USP (For Pediatric Use) (Frequent) 892
Diprivan Injection (Less than 1%) 2267
Disophrol Chronotab Sustained-Action Tablets ...... ▣ 698
Ditropan 1332
Diulo 2129
Diuril Sodium Intravenous 1463
Dolobid Tablets (Greater than 1 in 100) 1465
Donnatal (In elderly patients) 1858
Donnatal Extentabs (In elderly patients) 1859
Donnatal Tablets (In elderly patients) 1858
Donnazyme Tablets (In elderly patients) 1860
▲Doral Tablets (12%) 2383
Dorcol Children's Cough Syrup ...... ▣ 685
Dorcol Children's Decongestant Liquid ...... ▣ 685
Dorcol Children's Liquid Cold Formula (Occasional) ...... ▣ 686
Dristan Cold Nasal Decongestant/ Antihistamine/ Analgesic Coated Tablets 2419
Drixoral Antihistamine/Nasal Decongestant Syrup ...... ▣ 698
Drixoral Plus Extended-Release Tablets ...... ▣ 699
Drixoral Sinus ...... ▣ 700
Drixoral Sustained-Action Tablets ...... ▣ 698
▲Duragesic Transdermal System (10% or more) 1133
Duranest Injections 624
Dyclone 0.5% and 1% Topical Solutions, USP 626
DynaCirc Capsules (0.5% to 1%) 2004
Easprin 1719
Elavil 2269
Eldepryl 2250
Elspar 1470
▲Emete-con Intramuscular/Intravenous (Most common) 1950
▲Empirin with Codeine Phosphate Nos. 2, 3 & 4 (Among most frequent) 764
Endep Tablets 1927
Enduronyl 518
Engerix-B Unit-Dose Vials (Less than 1%) 2213
Equagesic Tablets 2451
Ergamisol Tablets (2 to 3%) 1136
▲Esgic-Plus Tablets (Among most frequent) 1002
▲Esgic Tablets & Capsules (Among most frequent) 1001
Eskalith 2214
Ethmozine Tablets (Less than 2%) 946
Etrafon 2087
Eulexin Capsules (1%) 2089
Extendryl 994
4-Way Cold Tablets 750
Fedahist Gyrocaps 2145
Fedahist Timecaps 2145
Feldene Capsules (1 to 3%) 1777
▲Fioricet Tablets (Among most frequent) 2006
▲Fiorinal Capsules (Among most frequent) 2007
Fiorinal with Codeine Capsules (2.4%) 2008
▲Fiorinal Tablets (Among most frequent) 2007
▲Flexeril Tablets (16% to 39%) 1471
Floxin Tablets (1% to 3%) 1652
Glucotrol (1 in 50) 1952
Guaifed 1615
▲Halcion Tablets (14%) 2340
Haldol Decanoate 1375
Haldol Injection, Tablets and Concentrate 1373
Harmonyl Tablets 528
HibTITER (91 of 1,118 vaccinations) 1206
▲Hismanal Tablets (7.1%) 1138
Hycodan Syrup, Tablets 927
Hycomine Compound Tablets 929
Hycomine Syrup 927
Hycotuss Expectorant Syrup 930
Hydrea Capsules 728
Hydrocet Capsules 835
Hydromox R Tablets 1209
▲Hylorel Tablets (15.3%) 975
Hyperstat I.V. Injection 2095
▲Hytrin Tablets (0.6% to 5.4%) 529
▲IFEX (Among most common) 729
Imodium Capsules 1139
Inapsine Injection (Frequent) 1140
Indocin (Less than 1%) 1487
Innovar Injection (Frequent) 1141
Intal Inhaler (Rare) 979
Intal Nebulizer Solution 980
▲Intron A (Up to 5%) 2097
IPOL Poliovirus Vaccine Inactivated 894
Isoclor Timesule Capsules ...... ▣ 561
Isoptin Injectable (Few) 1177
Isoptin Oral Tablets (Less than 1%) 1179
Isoptin SR Sustained Release Tablets (Less than 1%) 1181
Isopto Hyoscine ...... ⊙ 222
Kerlone Tablets (Less than 1%) 2172
Kinesed Tablets 2272
▲Klonopin Tablets (50%) 1902
Kutrase Capsules 2146
Lamprene Capsules (Less than 1%) 1030
Levsin/Levsinex 2147
Librax Capsules 1929
Libritabs Tablets 1930
Librium Capsules (Some patients) 1931
Librium Injectable 1932
▲Limbitrol (Among most frequent) 1933
▲Lioresal Tablets (10-63%) 1031
Lithane Tablets 1596
Lithium Carbonate Capsules & Tablets 1984
Lithobid Tablets 870
Lodine Capsules (Less than 1%) 2468
Lomotil 2174
Lopid Capsules and Tablets 1736
▲Lopressor HCT Tablets (10 in 100 patients) 1034
Lortab ASA Tablets 2414
Lortab 2412
Loxitane 1213
Lozol Tablets (Less than 5%) 1843
▲Ludiomil Tablets (16%) 874
▲Lysodren (25%) 731
Macrodantin Capsules (Less frequent) 1624
Marax Tablets & DF Syrup (Occasional) 1954
Marcaine Hydrochloride 0.5% with Epinephrine 1:200,000 (as bitartrate) 958
Marcaine Hydrochloride with Epinephrine 1:200,000 2055
Marcaine Hydrochloride Injection 2055
Marcaine Spinal 2058
Marezine Tablets ...... ▣ 541
Marinol (Dronabinol) Capsules 1985
Matulane Capsules 1907
Maxzide 1215
Mebaral Tablets (1 to 3 in 100) 2061
Medi-Flu Caplet, Liquid ...... ▣ 640
Mellaril (Occasional) 2011
Menrium Tablets (Particularly in elderly or debilitated) 1934
Mesantoin Tablets 2013
Methotrexate Tablets, Parenteral, LPF Parenteral 1217
Midamor Tablets (Less than or equal to 1%) 1508
Maximum Strength Midol Multi-Symptom Menstrual Formula ...... ▣ 571
Maximum Strength Midol PMS Premenstrual Syndrome Formula ...... ▣ 570
Regular Strength Midol Multi-Symptom Menstrual Formula ...... ▣ 570
Milontin Kapseals 1741
Miltown Tablets 2386
▲Minipress Capsules (7.6%) 1778
▲Minizide Capsules (7.6%) 1779
Mintezol 1510
Mithracin 1602
▲Moban Tablets & Concentrate (Among most frequent) 932
Mobigesic Analgesic Tablets ...... ▣ 507
Moduretic Tablets (Less than or equal to 1%) 1510
Momentum Muscular Backache Formula ...... ▣ 751
Monistat I.V. 1143
Mono-Gesic Tablets 846
Monopril Tablets (0.2 to 1.0%) 1406
Motofen Tablets (1 in 25) 836
Motrin Tablets (Less than 1%) 2351
Mutamycin 733
Mykrox ½ mg Tablets 984
Mysoline (Occasional) 2480
Naldecon Syrup, Tablets, Pediatric Drops and Pediatric Syrup 709
▲Nalfon Pulvules & Tablets (8.5%) 919
Naphcon Forte ...... ⊙ 226
Naprosyn 2297
Nardil (Common) 1742
Navane Capsules and Concentrate 1954
Navane Intramuscular 1956
NebuPent for Inhalation Solution (1% or less) 1017
NegGram 2062
Nembutal Sodium Capsules (1% to 3%) 534
Nembutal Sodium Solution (1%-3%) 536
Nembutal Sodium Suppositories (1%-3%) 538
Neptazane Tablets ...... ⊙ 311
Nescaine/Nescaine MPF 629
Niclocide Chewable Tablets (1.4%) 1607
Nizoral Tablets (Less than 1%) 1145
Nolahist 837
Nolamine Tablets (Occasional) 838
Norflex 1314

Norgesic 1314
▲ Normodyne Injection (3%) 2108
Normodyne Tablets (Less than 1%) 2110
Normozide Tablets (Less than 1%) 2112
Noroxin Tablets (0.3% to 1%) 1519
Norpramin Tablets 1340
Norzine (Occasional) 1818
Novafed A Capsules 1342
Novocain Hydrochloride for Spinal Anesthesia 2065
Nucofed Capsules 2219
Nucofed Expectorant 2219
Nucofed Pediatric Expectorant 2220
Nucofed Syrup 2219
Numorphan Hydrochloride Injection 935
Numorphan Suppositories 935
Omnipaque (Less than 0.1%) 2552
Opcon-A Ophthalmic Solution .... ⊙ 262
▲ Optimine Tablets (Among most frequent) 2115
OptiPranolol Sterile Ophthalmic Solution (A small number of patients) .... ⊙ 261
Oreticyl 545
Ornade Spansule Capsules 2221
Orudis Capsules (Greater than 1%) 2488
▲ PBZ Tablets & Elixir (Among most frequent) 1037
▲ PBZ-SR Tablets (Among most frequent) 1037
PMB 200 and PMB 400 2504
Pamelor 2019
Paradione Capsules 548
Paraflex Caplets 1378
Parafon Forte DSC Caplets 1379
▲ Parlodel (3%) 2020
Parnate Tablets 2222
Pavabid Capsules (Rare) 1344
Pavabid HP Capsulets (Rare) 1344
PediaCare 1362
PediaCare Night Rest Cough-Cold Formula Liquid 1362
PediaProfen Suspension (Less than 1%) 1363
▲ PedvaxHIB (Among most frequent) 1521
Pepcid (Infrequent) 1524
Peptavlon 2563
Periactin 1525
▲ Permax Tablets (10.1%) 1291
Phenergan with Codeine 2497
Phenergan with Dextromethorphan 2499
Phenergan Injection 2493
Phenergan Suppositories 2496
Phenergan Syrup 2495
Phenergan Tablets 2496
Phenergan VC 2500
Phenergan VC with Codeine 2501
Phenobarbital Elixir and Tablets (1 to 3 patients per 100) 1293
▲ Phenurone Tablets (4%) 552
Phrenilin 838
Plendil Extended-Release Tablets (0.5% to 1.5%) 1526
▲ Polaramine (Among most frequent) 2116
Polymyxin B Sulfate, Aerosporin Brand Sterile Powder 798
▲ Pondimin Tablets (Among most common) 1867
Ponstel 1758
Pontocaine Hydrochloride for Spinal Anesthesia 2069
Prēmsyn PMS Capsules & Caplets .... ■ 547
Prilosec Delayed-Release Capsules (Less than 1%) 1530
Primaxin I.M. 1532
Primaxin I.V. (0.2%) 1535
Prinivil Tablets (1% or less) 1538
Prinzide Tablets (0.3% to 1%) 1540
Pro-Banthīne Tablets 2141
Procardia XL Tablets (Less than 3%) 1783
▲ ProHIBiT Haemophilus b Conjugate Vaccine (Diphtheria Toxoid Conjugate) (16.1%) 896
Prolixin Decanoate 1795
Prolixin Elixir 1793
Prolixin Enanthate 1796
Prolixin Injection 1791
Prolixin Oral Concentrate 1792
Prolixin Tablets 1793
▲ ProSom Tablets (42%) 554
Prostigmin Injectable 1120
Prostigmin Tablets 1121
Protopam Chloride for Injection 2518
Proventil (Less than 1%) 2120
Provera Tablets 2356
▲ Prozac Pulvules (11.6%) 920
▲ Pyridium Plus (One-third to one-half of patients) 1764
Pyrroxate Capsules .... ■ 669
Quarzan Capsules 1937
Quelidrine Syrup 556
Questran Light 711
Questran Powder 710
Raudixin Tablets 1803
Rauzide Tablets 1804
▲ Reglan (10%) 1869
Renese-R Tablets 1786
▲ Restoril Capsules (17%) 2023
▲ Retrovir Capsules (8%) 802
▲ Retrovir I.V. Infusion (8%) 805
▲ Retrovir Syrup (8%) 802
Rheumatrex Methotrexate Dose Pack 1234
Rifadin 1345
Rifamate Capsules 1347
Rimactane Capsules 879
Ritalin 880
Robaxin Injectable 1871
Robaxin Tablets 1872
Robaxisal Tablets 1872
Robinul Forte Tablets 1873
Robinul Injectable 1873
Robinul Tablets 1873
Robitussin Night Relief .... ■ 677
Robitussin-DM .... ■ 676
Rocaltrol Capsules 1913
Rondec-DM 1976
Rufen Tablets (Less than 1%) 691
Ru-Tuss with Hydrocodone 694
Ru-Tuss Tablets 693
Ryna .... ■ 741
▲ Rynatan (Among most common) 2387
▲ Rynatuss (Among most common) .. 2388
Rythmol Tablets (0.6 to 1.4%) 1184
Sandostatin Injection (Less than 1%) 2029
Sanorex Tablets 2030
Sansert Tablets 2031
Scleromate (Rare) 1685
▲ Seconal Sodium Pulvules (Most common) 1296
▲ Sedapap Tablets 50 mg/650 mg (Among most frequent) 1360
▲ Seldane Tablets (8.5%) 1349
▲ Seldane-D Extended-Release Tablets (7.2%) 1350
Sensorcaine 631
Sensorcaine-MPF Spinal 634
Ser-Ap-Es Tablets 881
Serax Capsules 2522
Serax Tablets 2522
Serentil 686
Seromycin Pulvules 1298
Serpasil Tablets 883
Serpasil-Apresoline Tablets 884
Serpasil-Esidrix Tablets 886
Sinarest .... ■ 562
Sinemet Tablets 952
Sinemet CR Tablets 953
Sine-Off Maximum Strength Allergy/Sinus Formula Caplets .... ■ 721
▲ Sinequan (Most common) 1960
Singlet Tablets .... ■ 598
Sinulin 840
Sinutab Allergy Formula Sustained Action Tablets .... ■ 640
Sinutab Maximum Strength .... ■ 641
Skelaxin 840
Sleep-eze 3 Tablets .... ■ 755
▲ Soma Compound w/Codeine Tablets (Most frequent) 2390
▲ Soma Compound Tablets (Most frequent) 2389
▲ Soma Tablets 2388
St. Joseph Nighttime Cold Medicine .... ■ 705
Stelazine 2226
▲ Sublimaze Injection (Frequent) 1146
Sudafed Plus Liquid .... ■ 544
Sudafed Plus Tablets .... ■ 545
Surmontil Capsules 2524
Synalgos-DC Capsules 2525
▲ Tacaryl (Most prominent) 2409
Tagamet (Approximately 1 in 100) 2228
Tambocor Tablets (1-3%) 1315
Tapazole Tablets 1298
Taractan (Most frequent CNS reaction) 1920
▲ Tavist Syrup (Among most frequent) 2033
▲ Tavist Tablets (Among most frequent) 2035
▲ Tavist-D Tablets (Among most frequent) 2035
Tedral SA 1765
▲ Tegretol Chewable Tablets (Among most frequent) 654
▲ Tegretol Suspension (Among most frequent) 656
▲ Tegretol Tablets (Among most frequent) 654
Teldrin Timed-Release Allergy Capsules, 12 mg. 2192
▲ Temaril Tablets, Syrup and Spansule Sustained Release Capsules (Most common) 1085
▲ Tenex Tablets (33%) 1875
Tenoretic Tablets (0.6 to 2%) 1105
Tenormin Tablets and I.V. Injection (0.6 to 2%) 1107
Tenuate 1354
Thalitone Tablets 687
TheraFlu Flu and Cold Medicine .. ■ 687
Thorazine 2234
Tigan 2239
Timolide Tablets (Less than 1%) 1547
Timoptic in Ocudose 1552
Timoptic Sterile Ophthalmic Solution 1550
Tofranil Ampuls 1038
Tofranil Tablets 1039
Tofranil-PM Capsules 1041
Tolectin (200, 400 and 600 mg) (1 to 3%) 1379
Tonocard Tablets (0.8-1.6%) 1554
▲ Toradol IM Injection (3% to 9%) 2302
Torecan 1993
Trancopal Caplets 2075
Trandate HCT Tablets (Less than 1% in 208 patients) 579
▲ Trandate Injection (3 of 100 patients) 577
Trandate Tablets (Less than 1% of 227 patients) 579
▲ Transderm Scōp Transdermal Therapeutic System (Less than one-sixth) 887
▲ Tranxene (Most frequent) 556
Trental (1.1%) 1099
Trexan Tablets (Less than 1%) 937
Triaminic Allergy Tablets .... ■ 688
Triaminic Chewables .... ■ 688
Triaminic Cold Tablets .... ■ 688
Triaminic Expectorant .... ■ 688
Triaminic Expectorant DH 1995
Triaminic Nite Light .... ■ 689
Triaminic Oral Infant Drops 1996
Triaminic Syrup (Occasional) .... ■ 689
Triaminic-12 Tablets .... ■ 690
Triaminicin Tablets .... ■ 690
Triaminicol Multi-Symptom Cold Tablets .... ■ 691
Triaminicol Multi-Symptom Relief .... ■ 691
Triavil Tablets 1556
Tridione 557
Tri-Immunol Diphtheria & Tetanus Toxoids & Pertussis Vaccine, Adsorbed (Rare) 1241
Trilafon 2123
Trilisate (Less than 2%) 1822
▲ Trinalin Repetabs Tablets (Among most frequent) 1170
Tussionex Extended-Release Suspension 988
Tussi-Organidin DM Liquid (Rare) .. 2392
Tussi-Organidin Liquid 2391
Tuss-Ornade Liquid 2242
Tuss-Ornade Spansule Capsules 2242
Tylenol Allergy Sinus Medication Caplets and Gelcaps, Maximum Strength 1372
Children's Tylenol Cold Liquid Formula and Chewable Tablets 1368
Tylenol Cold & Flu Hot Medication, Packets 1369
Tylenol Cold & Flu No Drowsiness Hot Medication, Packets 1371
Tylenol Cold Medication Caplets and Tablets 1370
Tylenol Cold Night Time Medication Liquid 1371
Tylenol PM, Extra Strength Caplets and Tablets 1368
Urispas Tablets 2242
▲ Valium Injectable (Among most common) 1937
▲ Valium Tablets (Among most common) 1939
Valpin 50 Tablets 941
▲ Valrelease Capsules (Among most common) 1923
Vascor (200, 300 and 400 mg) Tablets (0.5 to 6.98%) 1383
Vaseretic Tablets (0.5% to 2.0%) 1559
Vasocon-A .... ⊙ 278
Vasotec I.V. 1562
Vasotec Tablets (0.5% to 1%) 1564
Ventolin (Less than 1%) 583
Verelan Capsules (Less than 1%) .. 1243
Versed Injection (1.2%) 1924
Vicks Formula 44 Cough Medicine .... ■ 661
Vicks NyQuil Nighttime Colds Medicine-Original & Cherry Flavor .... ■ 664
Vicodin Tablets 1187
Vicodin ES Tablets 1189
Vistaril Capsules 1789
Vistaril Intramuscular Solution 1970
Vistaril Oral Suspension 1789
Vivactil Tablets 1567
Voltaren Tablets (Less than 1%) 1042
Vontrol Tablets 2243
▲ Wytensin Tablets (12%) 2542
▲ Xanax Tablets (76.8%) 2367
▲ Xylocaine Injections (Among most common) 637
Xylocaine Injections for Ventricular Arrhythmias 639
Xylocaine 2% Jelly 643
Xylocaine 5% Ointment 644
Xylocaine 10% Oral Spray 645
4% Xylocaine-MPF Sterile Solution 641
Xylocaine 2% Viscous Solution 646
Yutopar (1 to 3% (with IV administration)) 647
Zantac Injection and Zantac Injection Premixed 1063
Zantac (Rare) 1065
Zarontin Capsules 1768
Zarontin Syrup 1769
Zaroxolyn Tablets 989
Zestoretic (0.3 to 1%) 2274
Zestril Tablets (Less than 1%) 2277
Zovirax 824
Zydone Capsules 941
Zyloprim Tablets (Less than 1%) 830

Drug administration site reactions, unspecified

Alferon N Injection 1809
Duragesic Transdermal System (1% or greater) 1133
Engerix-B Unit-Dose Vials 2213
▲ Intron A (3%) 2097
Nuromax Injection 794
Staphage Lysate (SPL) 905

Drug effect, unspecified, prolonged

Nuromax Injection 794

Drug fever

Aldactazide 2150
Aldactone 2152
Aldoclor Tablets 1413
Aldomet Oral 1415
Aldoril Tablets 1418
Amikin Injectable (Rare) 602
Ancef Injection 2194
Asendin Tablets (Less than 1%) 1196
Azo Gantanol Tablets 1887
Bactrim DS Tablets 1891
Bactrim I.V. Infusion 1889
Bactrim 1891
Cefobid Intravenous/Intramuscular (1 in 260) 1943
Cefobid Pharmacy Bulk Package - Not for Direct Infusion (1 in 260) 1945
Ceftin Tablets 575
Coly-Mycin M Parenteral 1706
Compazine 2201
Depen Titratable Tablets 2379
Ethmozine Tablets (0.3-less than 2%) 946
Fansidar Tablets 1896
Gantrisin Ophthalmic Ointment/Solution 1900
Kefzol Vials, Faspak & ADD-Vantage 1279
Leukeran Tablets 788
Ludiomil Tablets (Rare) 874
Macrodantin Capsules 1624
Mandol Vials, Faspak & ADD-Vantage 1281
Mezlin 1597
Mezlin Pharmacy Bulk Package 1599
Norpramin Tablets 1340
Orap Tablets 1020
Pamelor 2019
Pediazole 1973
Polymyxin B Sulfate, Aerosporin Brand Sterile Powder (Occasional) 798
Prolixin Decanoate 1795
Prolixin Elixir 1793

Prolixin Enanthate 1796
Prolixin Injection 1791
Prolixin Tablets 1793
Septra 813
Septra I.V. Infusion 808
Septra I.V. Infusion ADD-Vantage Vials 810
Septra 813
Stelazine 2226
Suprax (Less than 2%) 1235
Tapazole Tablets 1298
Thiosulfil Forte Tablets 2526
Ticar for Injection 2236
Timentin for Injection 2239
Tofranil Ampuls 1038
Tofranil Tablets 1039
Tofranil-PM Capsules 1041
Unipen 2533
Urobiotic-250 Capsules 1968
Vancocin HCl, Oral Solution & Pulvules (Infrequent) 1304
Vancocin HCl, Vials & ADD-Vantage (Infrequent) 1302
Vivactil Tablets 1567
Zinacef (Rare) 1066

Drug idiosyncrasies (see under Allergic reactions)

Dry mouth (see under Xerostomia)

Dryness

A/T/S Topical Gel and Topical Solution 1089
Aclovate (1 in 100 patients) 1053
AK-Taine ⊙ 207
Alcaine ⊙ 210
Analpram-HC Rectal Cream 1% and 2.5% 970
Anusol-HC Cream (Infrequent) 1690
Anusol-HC Suppositories 1691
Benzac 5 & 10 Gel 1682
Benzac AC Wash 2½%, 5%, 10% Water-Base Cleanser 1681
Benzac 1682
Carmol HC Cream 1% (Infrequent) 2296
Catapres Tablets 676
Clear by Design Medicated Acne Gel ■ 709
Condylox (Less than 5%) 1630
Cortisporin Cream 757
Cortisporin Ointment 758
Cortisporin Otic Solution Sterile 760
Cortisporin Otic Suspension Sterile 760
Cutivate Cream 0.05% (1.2%) 1054
Cutivate Ointment 0.005% 1054
Decadron Phosphate Topical Cream 1455
Decaspray Topical Aerosol 1459
DesOwen Cream, Ointment and Lotion (Infrequent) 1682
▲ Desquam-E Gel (2 in 50 patients) 2397
▲ Desquam-X Gel (2 in 50 patients) 2397
▲ Desquam-X 5 Wash (2 in 50 patients) 2397
▲ Desquam-X 10 Bar (2 in 50 patients) 2397
▲ Desquam-X 10 Wash (2 in 50 patients) 2397
ETS-2% 1685
Elocon Lotion 0.1% 2084
Erycette (erythromycin 2%) Topical Solution 1678
Florone/Florone E 908
Fluoracaine ⊙ 208
Kenalog Cream, Lotion & Ointment (Infrequent) 2401
Lidex (Infrequent) 2296
Locoid Cream, Ointment and Topical Solution (Infrequent) 970
Maxivate Cream, Lotion & Ointment 0.05% 2406
Mycolog II Cream and Ointment (Infrequent) 2407
▲ Naftin Cream 1% (3%) 1084
NeoDecadron Topical Cream 1518
Neo-Synalar Cream (Infrequent) 2296
Neutrogena Melanex Topical Solution 1618
Nutracort Cream & Lotion (Infrequent) 1684
Ophthetic ⊙ 249
Otic Tridesilon Solution 0.05% (Infrequent) 1612
PediOtic Suspension Sterile 797
Pramosone Cream, Lotion & Ointment 971
ProctoCream-HC (Infrequent) 1834
Stri-Dex Maximum ■ 573
Stri-Dex Dual Textured Regular Strength Pads ■ 573
Stri-Dex Dual Textured Regular Strength Big Pads ■ 573
Synacort Creams 1%, 2.5% (Infrequent) 2296
Synalar (Infrequent) 2296
T-Stat 2.0% Topical Solution and Pads 2409
Temovate 1056
Theramycin Z Topical Solution 2% 1410
Theroxide 1411
Topicort (Infrequent) 1098
Tridesilon Creme 0.05% (Infrequent) 1611
Tridesilon Ointment 0.05% (Infrequent) 1611
Westcort 2411

Dryness, mucous membrane

Dolobid Tablets (Less than 1 in 100) 1465
Lomotil 2174
Mintezol Chewable Tablets 1510
Myleran Tablets (Rare) 790
Nasacort Nasal Inhaler (Less than 5%) 1844
Ru-Tuss with Hydrocodone 694
Ru-Tuss Tablets 693
▲ Rynatan (Among most common) 2387
▲ Rynatuss (Among most common) 2388
Timolide Tablets (Less than 1%) 1547
Trinalin Repetabs Tablets 1170
Voltaren Tablets (Less than 1%) 1042

Dryness, nose (see under Xeromycteria)

Dry sockets

Demulen 2161
Enovid 2161
Norethin 2133

Duodenal infarction

Gelfoam Sterile Sponge 2338

Duodenitis

Anafranil Capsules (Infrequent) 650
Sterile FUDR 1898
Permax Tablets (Rare) 1291

Dysarthria

CeeNU 725
Clozaril Tablets (Less than 1%) 2000
Depakene Capsules & Syrup 511
Depakote 512
Doral Tablets 2383
Elavil 2269
Enlon Injection 598
Flexeril Tablets (Less than 1%) 1471
Halcion Tablets 2340
Indocin Capsules (Less than 1%) 1487
Indocin I.V. (Less than 1%) 1490
Indocin (Less than 1%) 1487
Klonopin Tablets 1902
Lioresal Tablets 1031
Ludiomil Tablets (Rare) 874
Mesantoin Tablets 2013
Pondimin Tablets 1867
Prostigmin Injectable 1120
Prostigmin Tablets 1121
Prozac Pulvules (Rare) 920
Roferon-A Injection (Less than 0.5%) 1916
Seromycin Pulvules 1298
Soma Compound w/Codeine Tablets (Very rare) 2390
Soma Compound Tablets (Very rare) 2389
Soma Tablets 2388
Tensilon Injectable 1123
Tonocard Tablets (Less than 1%) 1554
Triavil Tablets 1556
Valium Injectable 1937
Valium Tablets (Infrequent) 1939
Valrelease Capsules (Occasional) 1923
Wellbutrin Tablets (Infrequent) 821
▲ Xanax Tablets (23.3%) 2367

Dyscrasias, blood (see under Blood dyscrasias)

Dysdiadochokinesia

Klonopin Tablets 1902

Dysesthesia

Halcion Tablets (Rare) 2340

Dysesthesia, hemifacial

Prilosec Delayed-Release Capsules (Less than 1%) 1530

Dysgeusia

Capoten (Approximately 2 to 4 of 100 patients) 2255
Capozide (Approximately 2 to 4 of 100 patients) 2258
Cardizem Tablets-30 mg, 60 mg, 90 mg and 120 mg (Less than 1%) 1329
Cardizem SR Capsules-60 mg, 90 mg and 120 mg (Less than 1%) 1327
Eskalith 2214
Floxin Tablets (1% to 3%) 1652
Mevacor Tablets (0.8%) 1505
Ridaura Capsules (1-3%) 2224
Rocephin Injectable Vials, ADD-Vantage (Less than 1%) 1914
Trilisate (Less than 1%) 1822

Dyskinesia

Anafranil Capsules (Infrequent) 650
Bentyl 1322
Compazine 2201
Cylert Tablets 510
Dexedrine 2206
Dilantin Infatabs (Rare) 1710
Dilantin Kapseals (Rare) 1708
Dilantin Parenteral (Rare) 1712
Dilantin-30 Pediatric/Dilantin-125 Suspension (Rare) 1713
Dilantin with Phenobarbital Kapseals (Rare) 1715
▲ Eldepryl (2 of 49 patients) 2250
Ethmozine Tablets (Less than 2%) 946
Etrafon 2087
Haldol Decanoate 1375
Haldol Injection, Tablets and Concentrate 1373
Loxitane (Less frequent) 1213
MS Contin Tablets (Infrequent) 1814
MSIR (Infrequent) 1817
Orap Tablets 1020
▲ Permax Tablets (62.4%) 1291
Prolixin Decanoate 1795
Prolixin Elixir 1793
Prolixin Enanthate 1796
Prolixin Injection 1791
▲ Prolixin Oral Concentrate (Among most frequent) 1792
Prolixin Tablets 1793
Prozac Pulvules 920
Ritalin 880
▲ Sinemet CR Tablets (16.5%) 953
Stelazine 2226
Tenuate 1354
Triavil Tablets 1556
Trilafon 2123
Vistaril Capsules 1789
Vistaril Oral Suspension 1789
Wellbutrin Tablets (Frequent) 821

Dyskinesia, tardive (see under Tardive dyskinesia)

Dyskinesia, transient

Orap Tablets 1020

Dysmenorrhea

▲ Anafranil Capsules (10% to 12%) 650
Clozaril Tablets (Less than 1%) 2000
Cytotec (0.1%) 2159
Demulen 2161
Diethylstilbestrol Tablets 1258
Enovid 2161
Estinyl Tablets 2085
Estrace 1385
Estrace Vaginal Cream 1388
Estratest 2245
Estrovis 1721
Floxin Tablets (Less than 1%) 1652
Levlen/Tri-Levlen 665
Lippes Loop Intrauterine Double-S 1654
Lo/Ovral Tablets 2471
Lo/Ovral-28 Tablets 2476
Mediatric Capsules 2476
Menrium Tablets 1934
Nordette-21 Tablets 2481
Nordette-28 Tablets 2483
Norethin 2133
Ogen 540
Ortho Dienestrol Cream 1664
Ovcon 1391
Ovral Tablets 2490
Ovral-28 Tablets 2491
Ovrette Tablets 2492
PMB 200 and PMB 400 2504
ParaGard T380A Intrauterine Copper Contraceptive 411
Permax Tablets (Frequent) 1291
Premarin Intravenous 2508
Premarin with Methyltestosterone 2515
Premarin Vaginal Cream 2512
Seldane Tablets 1349
Seldane-D Extended-Release Tablets 1350
TACE 12 and 25 mg 1353
▲ Terazol 3 Vaginal Cream (6%) 1676
Levlen/Tri-Levlen 665
Triphasil-21 Tablets 2527
Triphasil-28 Tablets 2532

Dyspareunia

Flagyl I.V. 2131
Flagyl Tablets 2170
Lippes Loop Intrauterine Double-S 1654
Mycelex-G 500 mg Vaginal Tablets (1 in 149 patients) 1606
ParaGard T380A Intrauterine Copper Contraceptive 411
Protostat Tablets 1674
Prozac Pulvules (Rare) 920
Vagistat (Less than 1%) 1397
Wellbutrin Tablets (Rare) 821

Dyspepsia

Actigall Capsules 2280
AeroBid Inhaler System (1-3%) 995
Alferon N Injection (1% to 3%) 1809
Altace Capsules (Less than 1%) 1086
▲ Anafranil Capsules (13% to 22%) 650
Anaprox and Anaprox DS Tablets (Less than 3%) 2288
▲ Ansaid Tablets (3-9%) 2319
Atromid-S Capsules 2435
Azdōne Tablets (Occasional) 844
Blocadren Tablets (0.6%) 1429
Brevibloc Injection (Less than 1%) 942
Butazolidin Capsules & Tablets (Greater than 1%) 1027
Capoten 2255
Capozide 2258
Cardene Capsules (0.8-1.5%) 2290
Cardizem Tablets-30 mg, 60 mg, 90 mg and 120 mg (Less than 1%) 1329
Cardizem SR Capsules-60 mg, 90 mg and 120 mg (1.3%) 1327
Cardura Tablets (1%) 1941
Cartrol Tablets (Rare) 507
Cipro I.V. 1592
Cipro Tablets 1589
▲ Clinoril Tablets (3-9%) 1433
Cytotec (2.0%) 2159
Damason-P (Occasional) 1356
▲ Dipentum Capsules (4.0%) 1160
▲ Dolobid Tablets (3% to 9%) 1465
Doral Tablets (1.1%) 2383
▲ Duragesic Transdermal System (3% to 10%) 1133
Easprin 1719
Empirin with Codeine Phosphate Nos. 2, 3 & 4 (Occasional) 764
Ergamisol Tablets (Less than 1 to 2%) 1136
▲ Ethmozine Tablets (2%-5%) 946
Feldene Capsules (Common) 1777
Flexeril Tablets (1 to 3%) 1471
Floxin Tablets (Less than 1%) 1652
▲ Fungizone Intravenous (Among most common) 2262
Haldol Decanoate 1375
Haldol Injection, Tablets and Concentrate 1373
Hytrin Tablets (At least 1%) 529
▲ Indocin (3% to 9%) 1487
Intron A (2% to 3%) 2097
Keflex Pulvules, Oral Suspension & Pediatric Drops 916
Keftab Tablets 917
▲ Kerlone Tablets (3.9% to 4.7%) 2172
Levatol (2.7%) 1832
▲ Lodine Capsules (10%) 2468
▲ Lopid Capsules and Tablets (19.6%) 1736
Lortab ASA Tablets (Occasional) 2414
Meclomen Capsules (Common) 1739
▲ Mevacor Tablets (3.9%) 1505
Midamor Tablets (Less than or equal to 1%) 1508
Moduretic Tablets 1510
▲ Nalfon Pulvules & Tablets (10.3%) 919
Naprosyn (Less than 3%) 2297
NebuPent for Inhalation Solution (1% or less) 1017
▲ Normodyne Injection (1 to 4%) 2108
▲ Normodyne Tablets (1% to 4%) 2110
Normozide Tablets (Less than 1 to 3%) 2112
Noroxin Tablets (0.3% to 1%) 1519
Nubain Injection (Less than 1%) 934
Omnipaque (Less than 0.3%) 2552
▲ Orudis Capsules (11.5%) 2488

▲ Parlodel (4%) 2020
▲ Permax Tablets (6.4%) 1291
Plendil Extended-Release Tablets 1526
Ponstel (Common) 1758
Prinivil Tablets (1.0%) 1538
Prinzide Tablets (1.3%) 1540
Procardia XL Tablets (Less than 3%) 1783
ProSom Tablets (2%) 554
Proventil Repetabs Tablets (2%) 2120
Proventil Solutions for Inhalation 0.5% and 0.083% (1%) 2118
Proventil Tablets (2%) 2120
▲ Prozac Pulvules (6.4%) 920
Recombivax HB (Less than 1%) 1544
▲ Retrovir Capsules (5%) 802
▲ Retrovir I.V. Infusion (5%) 805
▲ Retrovir Syrup (5%) 802
▲ Ridaura Capsules (3 to 9%) 2224
Rocephin Injectable Vials, ADD-Vantage (Rare) 1914
Rufen Tablets (Common) 691
▲ Rythmol Tablets (1.3 to 3.4%) 1184
▲ Sectral Capsules (4%) 2520
Sinemet CR Tablets (0.6%) 953
▲ Suprax (3%) 1235
Tambocor Tablets (1-3%) 1315
Tenex Tablets (Less than 3%) 1875
Timolide Tablets (Less than 1%) 1547
Timoptic in Ocudose 1552
Timoptic Sterile Ophthalmic Solution 1550
▲ Tolectin (200, 400 and 600 mg) (3 to 9%) 1379
Tonocard Tablets (Less than 1%) 1554
▲ Toradol IM Injection (3% to 9%) 2302
Tornalate (0.5%) 2074
Trandate HCT Tablets (Less than 1% in 208 patients) 579
Trandate Injection (1 of 100 patients) 577
▲ Trandate Tablets (3% of 227 patients) 579
▲ Trental (2.8% to 9.6%) 1099
▲ Vascor (200, 300 and 400 mg) Tablets (6.81 to 22%) 1383
Vaseretic Tablets (0.5% to 2.0%) 1559
Vasotec I.V. 1562
Vasotec Tablets (0.5% to 1%) 1564
Ventolin Inhalation Solution (1.5%) 583
Verelan Capsules (2.5%) 1243
Voltaren Tablets (Common) 1042
▲ Wellbutrin Tablets (3.1%) 821
Zestoretic (1.3%) 2274
Zestril Tablets (1%) 2277
Zyloprim Tablets (Less than 1%) 830

Dysphagia

Achromycin V Capsules 1193
Altace Capsules (Less than 1%) 1086
Anafranil Capsules (Up to 2%) 650
Cholybar 1705
Cipro I.V. (1% or less) 1592
Cipro Tablets (Less than 1%) 1589
Cosmegen Injection 1440
Cytotec (Infrequent) 2159
Darbid Tablets 2205
Declomycin Capsules, Tablets 1199
Doryx Capsules 1717
Edecrin 1468
Eldepryl 2250
Enlon Injection 598
Ethmozine Tablets (Less than 2%) 946
Etrafon 2087
Gastrocrom Capsules (Infrequent) 974
Intron A (2 patients) 2097
Kerlone Tablets (Less than 2%) 2172
Larodopa Tablets (Relatively frequent) 1905
Ludiomil Tablets (Rare) 874
▲ Lupron Depot 3.75 mg (Among most frequent) 2312
Lupron Depot 7.5 mg 2311
Lupron Injection (Less than 5%) 2310
Mexitil Capsules (About 2 in 1,000) 680
Minocin Intravenous 1221
Minocin Oral Suspension 1224
Minocin Pellet-Filled Capsules 1222
Monodox Capsules 1630
Monopril Tablets (0.2 to 1.0%) 1406
Parlodel 2020
Prozac Pulvules (Infrequent) 920
Questran Light 711
Questran Powder 710
Retrovir Capsules (Less than 5%) 802
Retrovir I.V. Infusion (Less than 5%) 805
Retrovir Syrup (Less than 5%) 802
Ridaura Capsules (Less than 0.1%) 2224
Sinemet Tablets 952
Sinemet CR Tablets 953
Tenex Tablets (Less than 3%) 1875
Tensilon Injectable 1123
Terramycin Capsules 1786
Terramycin Intramuscular Solution 1964
Tonocard Tablets (Less than 1%) 1554
Triavil Tablets 1556
Trilafon 2123
VePesid Capsules and Injection (Infrequent) 741
Vibramycin Hyclate Capsules 1787
Vibramycin Hyclate Intravenous 1968
Vibramycin 1787
Wellbutrin Tablets (Infrequent) 821

Dysphasia

Cipro I.V. (1% or less) 1592
Cipro Tablets 1589
Floxin Tablets 1652
Omnipaque 2552
Roferon-A Injection (Less than 1%) 1916

Dysphonia

Anafranil Capsules (Infrequent) 650
Empirin with Codeine Phosphate Nos. 2, 3 & 4 764
Enlon Injection 598
Tegison Capsules (Less than 1%) 1881
Tensilon Injectable 1123
Versed Injection (Less than 1%) 1924

Dysphoria

A.P.L. 2431
Actifed with Codeine Cough Syrup 752
Adipex-P Tablets and Capsules 1019
AK-Pentolate ⊙ 204
Aldactazide 2150
Aldoclor Tablets 1413
Aldoril Tablets 1418
Aminophyllin Tablets 2153
Ana-Kit Anaphylaxis Emergency Treatment Kit 1100
Anatuss LA Tablets 1359
Anexsia 5/500 Tablets 2196
Anexsia 7.5/650 Tablets 2197
Apresazide Capsules 854
Apresoline-Esidrix Tablets 857
Arfonad Ampuls 1887
Arm-a-Med Isoetharine Inhalation Solution, USP 616
Asbron G 1997
Asendin Tablets (Greater than 1%) 1196
Astramorph/PF Injection, USP (Preservative-Free) 618
Ativan Injection (1.3%) 2432
Atrohist Sprinkle Capsules 558
Azdone Tablets 844
Benadryl Capsules 1691
Benadryl Injection 1692
Biphetamine Capsules 973
Bontril Slow-Release 834
Brevital Sodium Vials 1248
Bronkaid Tablets ▣ 757
Bronkolixir ▣ 761
Bronkometer Aerosol 2042
Bronkosol Solution 2042
Bronkotabs Tablets ▣ 762
BuSpar (Infrequent) 1401
Capozide 2258
Carbocaine Hydrochloride Injection 2043
Cardilate Oral/Sublingual Tablets (Occasional) 757
Catapres Tablets 676
Catapres-TTS 677
Choledyl Pediatric Elixir 1702
Choledyl Tablets 1700
Choledyl SA Tablets 1704
Cibalith-S 870
▲ Cipro I.V. (Among most frequent) 1592
Cipro Tablets (1.1%) 1589
▲ Clozaril Tablets (4%) 2000
Cocaine Hydrochloride Topical Solution 620
Combipres Tablets 678
Allergy-Sinus Comtrex Multi-Symptom Allergy Sinus Formula Tablets & Caplets 746
Constant-T Tablets 1029
Corzide Tablets (Not uncommon) 702
Cyclogyl (Common) ⊙ 215
Cyclomydril ⊙ 216
Dalmane Capsules (Rare) 1927
Damason-P 1356
Darvon-N/Darvocet-N 1254
Darvon 1256
Darvon-N Suspension & Tablets 1254
Deconamine 663
Deconsal 559
Demerol 2047
Desoxyn Gradumet Tablets (Rare) 514
Dexedrine 2206
Didrex Tablets 2338
Dilatrate-SR 1827
Dilaudid Cough Syrup 1174
Dilaudid 1173
Dilaudid-HP Injection 1175
Dilor 2079
Dimetane-DC Cough Syrup 1857
Dimetane-DX Cough Syrup 1858
Ditropan 1332
Diucardin Tablets 2450
Diulo 2129
Diupres Tablets 1461
Diuril Oral Suspension 1464
Diuril Sodium Intravenous 1463
Diuril Tablets 1464
Dolophine Hydrochloride Ampoules & Vials 1260
Dolophine Hydrochloride Tablets 1261
Duramorph 960
Duranest Injections 624
Elavil 2269
Eldepryl 2250
Emete-con Intramuscular/Intravenous 1950
Endep Tablets 1927
Enduron Tablets 517
Enduronyl 518
Entex Capsules 1623
Entex LA Tablets 1623
Entex Liquid 1623
EpiPen—Epinephrine Auto-Injector 843
Esidrix Tablets 863
Esimil Tablets 864
Eskalith 2214
Etrafon 2087
Exna Tablets 1862
Fastin Capsules 2216
Fedahist Gyrocaps 2145
Fedahist Timecaps 2145
Guaifed Syrup ▣ 629
Halcion Tablets 2340
Haldol Decanoate 1375
Haldol Injection, Tablets and Concentrate 1373
Hycodan Syrup, Tablets 927
Hycomine Compound Tablets 929
Hycomine Syrup 927
Hycotuss Expectorant Syrup 930
Hydrocet Capsules 835
HydroDIURIL Tablets 1484
Hydromox R Tablets 1209
Hydromox Tablets 1208
Hydropres Tablets 1485
Inapsine Injection 1140
Inderide LA Long Acting Capsules 2465
Infumorph 200 and Infumorph 500 Sterile Solutions 962
Innovar Injection 1141
Ionamin Capsules 981
IPOL Poliovirus Vaccine Inactivated 894
Isordil (Occasional) 2467
Lariam Tablets 1904
Lasix 1093
Limbitrol 1933
Lithane Tablets 1596
Lithium Carbonate Capsules & Tablets 1984
Lithobid Tablets 870
Lomotil 2174
Lortab ASA Tablets 2414
Lortab 2412
Ludiomil Tablets (Rare) 874
Lufyllin & Lufyllin-400 Tablets 2384
Lufyllin-GG Elixir & Tablets 2385
▲ MS Contin Tablets (Among most frequent) 1814
▲ MSIR (Among most frequent) 1817
Marcaine Hydrochloride with Epinephrine 1:200,000 2055
Marcaine Hydrochloride Injection 2055
Marcaine Spinal 2058
Maxzide 1215
Mellaril (Extremely rare) 2011
Mepergan Injection 2479
Methadone Hydrochloride Diskets 1284
Methadone Hydrochloride Oral Solution & Tablets 1987
Minizide Capsules 1779
Moduretic Tablets 1510
Mykrox ½ mg Tablets 984
Naldecon Syrup, Tablets, Pediatric Drops and Pediatric Syrup 709
Naturetin Tablets (Common) 1789
Navane Capsules and Concentrate 1954
Navane Intramuscular 1956
Neo-Synephrine Hydrochloride 1% Carpuject 2063
Neo-Synephrine Hydrochloride 1% Injection 2063
Nescaine/Nescaine MPF 629
Nipride I.V. Infusion 1909
Nitro-Bid IV (Less than 1%) 1338
Nitro-Bid Ointment 1339
Nitrolingual Spray 1846
Nitrostat IV (Less than 1%) 1744
Nolex LA Tablets 838
Normodyne Tablets 2110
Normozide Tablets 2112
Noroxin Tablets 1519
Norpramin Tablets 1340
Norzine (Occasional) 1818
Novafed A Capsules 1342
Novafed Capsules 1342
Novahistine DH 1342
Novahistine DMX ▣ 595
Novahistine Elixir ▣ 596
Novahistine Expectorant 1343
Nubain Injection (Less than 1%) 934
Nucofed Capsules 2219
Nucofed Expectorant 2219
Nucofed Pediatric Expectorant 2220
Nucofed Syrup 2219
Numorphan Hydrochloride Injection 935
Numorphan Suppositories 935
Omnipaque 2552
Optimine Tablets 2115
▲ Oramorph SR (Morphine Sulfate Sustained Release Tablets) (Among most frequent) 1988
Oretic Tablets 544
Oreticyl 545
Ornade Spansule Capsules 2221
Orudis Capsules (Less than 1%) 2488
Oxsoralen-Ultra Capsule 1117
PBZ Tablets & Elixir 1037
PBZ-SR Tablets 1037
Pamelor 2019
Pantopon Injectable 1911
Parnate Tablets 2222
Percocet Tablets 950
Percodan 951
Periactin 1525
Peritrate (Occasional) 1756
Phenaphen with Codeine Capsules 1865
Phenaphen-650 with Codeine Tablets 1866
Phenergan with Codeine 2497
Phenergan VC 2500
Phenergan VC with Codeine 2501
Phenobarbital Elixir and Tablets 1293
Plegine Tablets 2504
Polaramine 2116
Pregnyl 1644
Prelu-2 Capsules 683
Prinzide Tablets 1540
Profasi (human chorionic gonadotropin, USP) 2186
Prolixin Decanoate 1795
Prolixin Elixir 1793
Prolixin Enanthate 1796
Prolixin Injection 1791
Prolixin Oral Concentrate 1792
Prolixin Tablets 1793
Proventil (Less than 1%) 2120
Quadrinal Tablets 1183
Quibron Capsules 713
Quibron-T 714
Quibron-T/SR 716
Quinamm Tablets 1344
Rauzide Tablets 1804
▲ Reglan (10%) 1869
Renese Tablets 1785
Respbid Tablets 684
Robitussin Night Relief ▣ 677
Robitussin-CF ▣ 676
Robitussin-PE ▣ 677
Roxanol 1991
Roxicodone Tablets, Oral Solution & Intensol (Oxycodone) 1992
Ru-Tuss II Capsules 693
Saluron 718
Salutensin/Salutensin-Demi 719
Sanorex Tablets 2030
Seldane-D Extended-Release Tablets (2.1%) 1350
Sensorcaine 631
Sensorcaine-MPF Spinal 634
Ser-Ap-Es Tablets 881
Serentil 686
Serpasil-Esidrix Tablets 886
Slo-bid Gyrocaps 1847
Sorbitrate (Occasional) 1103
Sublimaze Injection 1146
Surmontil Capsules 2524
Sus-Phrine Injection 1006

T-PHYL (Uniphyl) 200 mg Tablets 1820
Tavist Syrup 2033
Tavist Tablets 2035
Tavist-D Tablets 2035
Tenoretic Tablets 1105
Tenuate 1354
Thalitone Tablets 687
Theo-24 2179
Theo-Dur Sprinkle 1168
Theo-Dur Extended-Release Tablets 1166
Theolair 1317
Theolair-SR Tablets 1319
Theo-Organidin Elixir 2391
▲ TheoX Extended-Release Tablets (Among most consistent) 841
Timolide Tablets 1547
Tofranil Ampuls 1038
Tofranil Tablets 1039
Tofranil-PM Capsules 1041
Torecan 1993
Trandate HCT Tablets 579
Transderm Scōp Transdermal Therapeutic System (Infrequent) 887
Trexan Tablets (Less than 1%) 937
Triaminic Expectorant DH 1995
Triaminic Oral Infant Drops 1996
Triavil Tablets 1556
Trilafon 2123
Tussionex Extended-Release Suspension 988
Tylenol with Codeine 1381
Tylox Capsules 1382
Uniphyl 400 mg Tablets 1823
Vaseretic Tablets 1559
Ventolin Tablets (1 of 100 patients) 583
Versed Injection (Less than 1%) 1924
Vicodin Tablets 1187
Vicodin ES Tablets 1189
Vivactil Tablets 1567
Wellbutrin Tablets (Infrequent) 821
Wygesic Tablets 2540
Xylocaine Injections 637
Yutopar (Infrequent) 647
Zaroxolyn Tablets 989
Zestoretic 2274
Zydone Capsules 941

Dysplasia, bone marrow (see under Bone marrow dysplasia)

Dysplasia, cervical

Anafranil Capsules (Rare) 650
TACE 12 and 25 mg 1353

Dyspnea

▲ Adalat Capsules (10 mg and 20 mg) (6%) 1587
▲ Adenocard Injection (12%) 1007
AeroBid Inhaler System (1-3%) 995
Altace Capsules (Less than 1%) 1086
Anafranil Capsules (Up to 2%) 650
▲ Anaprox and Anaprox DS Tablets (3-9%) 2288
Ancobon Capsules 1886
Ansaid Tablets (Less than 1%) 2319
Antivenin (Crotalidae) Polyvalent 2430
Apresazide Capsules (Less frequent) 854
Apresoline Hydrochloride Parenteral (Ampuls) 856
Apresoline Hydrochloride Tablets (Less frequent) 855
Apresoline-Esidrix Tablets 857
AquaMEPHYTON Injection 1422
▲ Atgam Sterile Solution (More than 1% to 10%) 2320
Azactam for Injection (1 patient) 2252
Bentyl 1322
Betoptic Sterile Ophthalmic Solution (Rare) 569
Betoptic S Sterile Ophthalmic Suspension (Rare) 570
Blenoxane 724
Blocadren Tablets (1.7%) 1429
Brethaire Inhaler 1024
Brethine Ampuls (0.0 to 2.0%) 1026
Brevibloc Injection (Less than 1%) 942
Brevital Sodium Vials 1248
Calan SR Caplets (1.4%) 2157
Calan Tablets (1.4%) 2155
Capoten (0.5 to 2%) 2255
Capozide (0.5 to 2%) 2258
Cardene Capsules (0.6%) 2290
Cardizem Tablets-30 mg, 60 mg, 90 mg and 120 mg (Less than 1%) 1329
Cardizem SR Capsules-60 mg, 90 mg and 120 mg (Less than 1%) 1327
Cardura Tablets (1%) 1941
Cartrol Tablets (Less common) 507
Cipro I.V. (1% or less) 1592
Cipro Tablets (Less than 1%) 1589
Clinoril Tablets (Less than 1%) 1433
Clozaril Tablets (1%) 2000
Contac Nighttime Cold Medicine.. ▣ 713
▲ Cordarone Tablets (2% to 7%) 2446
Coumadin Injection & Tablets 944
Cytotec (Infrequent) 2159
Cytovene Sterile Powder (1% or less) 2292
Dantrium Capsules 1619
Depen Titratable Tablets 2379
Diapid Nasal Spray 2003
Diphtheria and Tetanus Toxoids and Pertussis Vaccine Adsorbed USP (For Pediatric Use) (Rare) 892
Diprivan Injection (Less than 1%) 2267
Diupres Tablets 1461
Dolobid Tablets (Rare) 1465
Dopram Injectable 1860
▲ Duragesic Transdermal System (3% to 10%) 1133
Duvoid Tablets 1853
DynaCirc Capsules (1.8%) 2004
▲ Emcyt Capsules (11%) 1161
▲ Eminase (Less than 10%) 2211
Enduronyl 518
Esimil Tablets 864
▲ Ethmozine Tablets (5.7%) 946
Feldene Capsules (Less than 1%) 1777
Flexeril Tablets (Rare) 1471
Floropryl Sterile Ophthalmic Ointment (Rare) 1473
Fungizone Intravenous 2262
Furoxone (Rare) 1855
Gamimune N Immune Globulin Intravenous (Human) 1572
Ganite Injection 1016
Gastrocrom Capsules (Infrequent) 974
Guaifed 1615
Harmonyl Tablets 528
Humorsol Sterile Ophthalmic Solution 1475
Hydropres Tablets 1485
Hyperstat I.V. Injection 2095
Hyskon Hysteroscopy Fluid (Rare) 1162
▲ Hytrin Tablets (0.9% to 3.1%) 529
Beef Regular, 100 Units 1275
Imferon 976
Indocin Capsules (Less than 1%) 1487
Indocin I.V. (Less than 1%) 1490
Indocin (Less than 1%) 1487
▲ Intron A (Up to 34%) 2097
▲ Intropin Injection (Among most frequent) 930
Ismelin Tablets 869
Isoptin Oral Tablets (1.4%) 1179
Isoptin SR Sustained Release Tablets (1.4%) 1181
K-Phos Neutral Tablets 660
K-Phos Original Formula 'Sodium Free' Tablets (Less frequent) 660
Kerlone Tablets (2.4%) 2172
Leukine for IV Infusion (Occasional) 1127
Levatol (2.1%) 1832
Lioresal Tablets (Rare) 1031
Lodine Capsules (Less than 1%) 2468
Lopressor Ampuls (1%) 1032
Lopressor HCT Tablets (1 in 100 patients) 1034
Lopressor Tablets (1%) 1032
Lotensin Tablets 872
Loxitane 1213
▲ Lupron Depot 3.75 mg (Among most frequent) 2312
▲ Lupron Depot 7.5 mg (5.4%) 2311
Lupron Injection (5% or more) 2310
Macrodantin Capsules (Common) 1624
Megace Tablets 732
Mephyton Tablets (Rare) 1503
Methadone Hydrochloride Diskets 1284
Methergine (Rare) 2016
Methotrexate Tablets, Parenteral, LPF Parenteral 1217
Metrodin (urofollitropin for injection) 2182
Mevacor Tablets (Rare) 1505
▲ Mexitil Capsules (3.3% to 5.7%) 680
Midamor Tablets (Between 1% and 3%) 1508
Minipress Capsules (1-4%) 1778
Minizide Capsules 1779
Miochol with Iocare Steri-Tags, Miochol System Pak and Miochol System Pak Plus (Rare) ⊙ 274
Moduretic Tablets (Greater than 1%, less than 3%) 1510
Mutamycin 733
Myochrysine Injection 1516
Nalfon Pulvules & Tablets (2.8%) 919
▲ Naprosyn (3 to 9%) 2297
▲ Neupogen for Injection (9%) 595
Nicorette 1335
Nimotop Capsules (Up to 1.2%) 1607
Nolvadex Tablets 1102
Normodyne Tablets (2%) 2110
Normozide Tablets (2%) 2112
Noroxin Tablets 1519
▲ Novantrone for Injection Concentrate (6 to 18%) 1226
Nubain Injection (Less than 1%) 934
Nucofed Capsules 2219
Nucofed Expectorant 2219
Nucofed Pediatric Expectorant 2220
Nucofed Syrup 2219
Omnipaque (0.1 to 0.2%) 2552
Oncovin Solution Vials & Hyporets 1288
OptiPranolol Sterile Ophthalmic Solution (A small number of patients) ⊙ 261
Oreticyl 545
▲ Orthoclone OKT3 Sterile Solution (21%) 1645
Orudis Capsules (Less than 1%) 2488
Pergonal (menotropins for injection, USP) 2184
▲ Permax Tablets (4.8%) 1291
Plendil Extended-Release Tablets (0.5% to 1.5%) 1526
Ponstel (Rare) 1758
Pre-Pen 2148
Primaxin I.M. 1532
Primaxin I.V. (Less than 0.2%) 1535
Prinivil Tablets (1.1%) 1538
Prinzide Tablets (0.3% to 1%) 1540
▲ Procardia XL Tablets (Less than 3% to 6%) 1783
Prokine for I.V. Infusion 1096
ProSom Tablets (Infrequent) 554
Prostigmin Injectable 1120
Prostigmin Tablets 1121
Protamine Sulfate Ampoules & Vials 1295
Prozac Pulvules (1.4%) 920
Quinamm Tablets 1344
Raudixin Tablets 1803
Rauzide Tablets 1804
Recombivax HB (Less than 1%) 1544
Reglan (Rare) 1869
▲ Retrovir Capsules (5%) 802
▲ Retrovir I.V. Infusion (5%) 805
▲ Retrovir Syrup (5%) 802
Rheumatrex Methotrexate Dose Pack 1234
▲ Roferon-A Injection (11%) 1916
▲ Rythmol Tablets (2.0 to 5.3%) 1184
Salutensin/Salutensin-Demi 719
Sandimmune 2024
Sansert Tablets 2031
▲ Sectral Capsules (4%) 2520
Ser-Ap-Es Tablets 881
Serophene (clomiphene citrate tablets, USP) 2186
Serpasil Tablets 883
Serpasil-Apresoline Tablets 884
Serpasil-Esidrix Tablets 886
Sinemet Tablets 952
Sinemet CR Tablets (1.6%) 953
Streptase for Infusion 635
Symmetrel Capsules & Syrup (0.1-1%) 936
Talwin Injection (Infrequent) 2071
▲ Tambocor Tablets (10.3%) 1315
▲ Tegison Capsules (1 to 10%) 1881
Tegretol Chewable Tablets 654
Tegretol Suspension 656
Tegretol Tablets 654
Tenex Tablets (Less than 3%) 1875
▲ Tenoretic Tablets (0.6 to 6%) 1105
▲ Tenormin Tablets and I.V. Injection (0.6 to 6%) 1107
Tenuate 1354
Timolide Tablets (1.2%) 1547
Timoptic in Ocudose 1552
Timoptic Sterile Ophthalmic Solution 1550
Tonocard Tablets (Less than 1%) 1554
Toradol IM Injection (1% or less) 2302
Tornalate (Less than 1%) 2074
Tracrium Injection 817
Trandate HCT Tablets (Rare) 579
Trandate Injection (Rare) 577
Trandate Tablets (Rare) 579
Trental (Less than 1%) 1099
Trexan Tablets (Less than 1%) 937
Tri-Immunol Diphtheria & Tetanus Toxoids & Pertussis Vaccine, Adsorbed 1241
Uroqid-Acid (Less frequent) 661
Valium Injectable 1937
Vancocin HCl, Vials & ADD-Vantage 1302
▲ Vascor (200, 300 and 400 mg) Tablets (3.5 to 8.70%) 1383
Vaseretic Tablets (0.5% to 2.0%) 1559
Vasotec I.V. 1562
Vasotec Tablets (0.5% to 1%) 1564
Velban Vials 1305
Ventolin Inhalation Solution (1.5%) 583
VePesid Capsules and Injection (0.7 to 2%) 741
Verelan Capsules (1.4%) 1243
Versed Injection (Less than 1%) 1924
Virazole 1126
▲ Visken Tablets (5%) 2036
Voltaren Tablets (Less than 1%) 1042
Wellbutrin Tablets (Infrequent) 821
Wytensin Tablets (3% or less) 2542
Yutopar (1 to 3% (with IV administration)) 647
Zefazone Sterile Powder 2372
Zestoretic (0.3 to 1%) 2274
Zestril Tablets (1.1%) 2277
Zydone Capsules 941

Dysrhythmia

Abbokinase 503
Asendin Tablets 1196
▲ Brethaire Inhaler (About 4%) 1024
Loxitane 1213
Mellaril 2011
Monistat I.V. 1143
Procardia XL Tablets (About 1 patient in 150) 1783

Dystonia

Anafranil Capsules (Rare) 650
BuSpar (Rare) 1401
Cibalith-S 870
Clozaril Tablets 2000
Compazine 2201
Dilantin Infatabs (Rare) 1710
Dilantin Kapseals (Rare) 1708
Dilantin Parenteral (Rare) 1712
Dilantin-30 Pediatric/Dilantin-125 Suspension (Rare) 1713
Dilantin with Phenobarbital Kapseals (Rare) 1715
Diprivan Injection (Less than 1%) 2267
Doral Tablets 2383
Eldepryl 2250
Eskalith (One report in a child) 2214
Etrafon 2087
Halcion Tablets 2340
Haldol Decanoate (Less frequent) 1375
Haldol Injection, Tablets and Concentrate 1373
Inapsine Injection 1140
Innovar Injection 1141
Larodopa Tablets (Frequent) 1905
Lioresal Tablets 1031
Lithane Tablets 1596
Lithium Carbonate Capsules & Tablets 1984
Lithobid Tablets 870
Loxitane 1213
Mellaril 2011
Moban Tablets & Concentrate (Infrequent) 932
Navane Capsules and Concentrate 1954
Navane Intramuscular 1956
Norzine 1818
Orap Tablets (Less frequent) 1020
▲ Permax Tablets (11.6%) 1291
Prolixin Decanoate 1795
Prolixin Elixir 1793
Prolixin Enanthate 1796
Prolixin Injection 1791
▲ Prolixin Oral Concentrate (Among most frequent) 1792
Prolixin Tablets 1793
Prozac Pulvules (Rare) 920
Reglan (0.2%) 1869
Serentil 686
▲ Sinemet Tablets (Among most common) 952
Sinemet CR Tablets (1.8%) 953
Stelazine 2226
Sublimaze Injection 1146
Taractan (Common) 1920
Thorazine 2234
Torecan 1993
Triavil Tablets 1556
Trilafon 2123
Wellbutrin Tablets (Frequent) 821
Xanax Tablets 2367
Zofran Injection 1069

Dystonia, tardive
Compazine ... 2201
Haldol Decanoate ... 1375
Haldol Injection, Tablets and Concentrate ... 1373
Thorazine ... 2234

Dystonic reactions (see under Dystonia)

Dysuria
Alferon N Injection (1%) ... 1809
Anafranil Capsules (Up to 2%) ... 650
Atrohist Sprinkle Capsules ... 558
Atromid-S Capsules ... 2435
Bontril Slow-Release ... 834
BuSpar (Infrequent) ... 1401
Cholybar ... 1705
Clinoril Tablets ... 1433
Cogentin ... 1435
Combipres Tablets (Rare) ... 678
Cytotec (Infrequent) ... 2159
Deconamine ... 663
Deconsal ... 559
Demser Capsules (A few patients) .. 1460
Desferal Vials ... 862
Dipentum Capsules (Rare) ... 1160
Diupres Tablets ... 1461
Dolobid Tablets (Less than 1 in 100) ... 1465
Ethmozine Tablets (Less than 2%) 946
Fedahist Gyrocaps ... 2145
Fedahist Timecaps ... 2145
Feldene Capsules (Less than 1%) .. 1777
Flagyl Tablets ... 2170
Floxin Tablets (Less than 1%) ... 1652
Gastrocrom Capsules (Infrequent).. 974
Harmonyl Tablets ... 528
Hiprex Tablets (Less than 3.5%) ... 1333
Hydrea Capsules (Very rare) ... 728
Hydropres Tablets ... 1485
IFEX ... 729
Intal Capsules (Less than 1 in 10,000 patients) ... 978
Intal Inhaler (Infrequent) ... 979
Intal Nebulizer Solution ... 980
Kerlone Tablets (Less than 2%) ... 2172
Klonopin Tablets ... 1902
Lioresal Tablets (Rare) ... 1031
Lodine Capsules (More than 1% but less than 3%) ... 2468
▲Lupron Depot 3.75 mg (Among most frequent) ... 2312
Lupron Depot 7.5 mg (Less than 5%) ... 2311
Lupron Injection (Less than 5%) ... 2310
Marplan Tablets (Rare) ... 1906
Methotrexate Tablets, Parenteral, LPF Parenteral (Less common) ... 1217
Midamor Tablets (Less than or equal to 1%) ... 1508
Moduretic Tablets (Less than or equal to 1%) ... 1510
Naldecon Syrup, Tablets, Pediatric Drops and Pediatric Syrup ... 709
Nalfon Pulvules & Tablets (Less than 1%) ... 919
Norpace (Less than 1%) ... 2177
Novafed A Capsules ... 1342
Novafed Capsules ... 1342
Novahistine DH ... 1342
Novahistine DMX ... ▣ 595
Novahistine Elixir ... ▣ 596
Novahistine Expectorant ... 1343
Oncovin Solution Vials & Hyporets 1288
Oreticyl ... 545
Ornade Spansule Capsules ... 2221
Permax Tablets (Infrequent) ... 1291
Plegine Tablets ... 2504
Plendil Extended-Release Tablets (0.5% to 1.5%) ... 1526
Pondimin Tablets ... 1867
Ponstel ... 1758
Procardia XL Tablets (1% or less).. 1783
Protostat Tablets ... 1674
Prozac Pulvules (Infrequent) ... 920
Questran Light ... 711
Questran Powder ... 710
Raudixin Tablets ... 1803
Rauzide Tablets ... 1804
Recombivax HB (Less than 1%) ... 1544
Retrovir Capsules (Less than 5%).. 802
Retrovir I.V. Infusion (Less than 5%) ... 805
Retrovir Syrup (Less than 5%) ... 802
Rheumatrex Methotrexate Dose Pack (Less common) ... 1234
Rondec ... 1975
Rondec-DM ... 1976
Rondec-TR Tablet ... 1975
Ru-Tuss with Hydrocodone ... 694
Ru-Tuss Tablets ... 693
Salutensin/Salutensin-Demi ... 719
Sansert Tablets ... 2031
Sectral Capsules (Up to 2%) ... 2520
Seldane-D Extended-Release Tablets ... 1350
Ser-Ap-Es Tablets ... 881
Serpasil Tablets ... 883
Serpasil-Apresoline Tablets ... 884
Serpasil-Esidrix Tablets ... 886
Tacaryl ... 2409
Tegison Capsules (Less than 1%) .. 1881
Temaril Tablets, Syrup and Spansule Sustained Release Capsules ... 1085
Tenuate ... 1354
▲TheraCys BCG Live (Intravesical) (3.6% to 51.8%) ... 898
Tolectin (200, 400 and 600 mg) (Less than 1%) ... 1379
Trinalin Repetabs Tablets ... 1170
Tuss-Ornade Liquid ... 2242
Tuss-Ornade Spansule Capsules ... 2242
Ultracef Capsules, Tablets & Oral Suspension ... 722
Unasyn (Less than 1%) ... 1965
Urispas Tablets ... 2242
Uroqid-Acid ... 661
Vagistat (Less than 1%) ... 1397
Wellbutrin Tablets (Rare) ... 821

E

Ear, discomfort
AeroBid Inhaler System (1-3%) ... 995
Ansaid Tablets (Less than 1%) ... 2319
Bumex (0.1%) ... 1895
Cytotec (Infrequent) ... 2159
Kerlone Tablets (Less than 2%) ... 2172
Ponstel ... 1758
▲Tegison Capsules (1-10%) ... 1881
Versed Injection (Less than 1%) ... 1924

Ear, drainage
Tegison Capsules (Less than 1%) .. 1881

Ear, external abnormalities, fetal
Accutane Capsules ... 1878
Depen Titratable Tablets ... 2379

Ear disease, unspecified
Ansaid Tablets (Less than 1%) ... 2319
Clozaril Tablets (Less than 1%) ... 2000

Ears, blocked
▲CHEMET (succimer) Capsules (1.0 to 3.7%) ... 1361
Dalgan Injection ... 620
Doxorubicin Hydrochloride for Injection, USP (Less than 1%) ... 622
Trexan Tablets (Less than 1%) ... 937
Versed Injection (Less than 1%) ... 1924

Ears, ringing (see under Tinnitus)

Ebstein's anomaly
Cibalith-S ... 870
Eskalith ... 2214
Lithane Tablets ... 1596
Lithium Carbonate Capsules & Tablets ... 1984
Lithobid Tablets ... 870

Ebriety, feeling of
Intron A (1% or less) ... 2097

Ecchymoses
Activase (Less than 1%) ... 1047
▲Anaprox and Anaprox DS Tablets (3-9%) ... 2288
Ansaid Tablets (Less than 1%) ... 2319
BuSpar (Rare) ... 1401
Calan SR Caplets (1% or less) ... 2157
Calan Tablets (1% or less) ... 2155
Celestone Soluspan Suspension ... 2081
Cholybar ... 1705
Clinoril Tablets (Less than 1%) ... 1433
Cordarone Tablets (Less than 1%) 2446
Cortenema ... 2244
Cortifoam ... 1827
Cortone Acetate Sterile Suspension ... 1437
Cortone Acetate Tablets ... 1439
Corzide Tablets (Occasional) ... 702
Dalalone D.P. Injectable ... 999
Decadron Elixir ... 1445
Decadron Phosphate Injection ... 1449
Decadron Phosphate Respihaler ... 1454
Decadron Phosphate Turbinaire ... 1456
Decadron Phosphate with Xylocaine Injection, Sterile ... 1451
Decadron-LA Sterile Suspension ... 1457
Depo-Medrol Sterile Aqueous Suspension ... 2334
Deprol Tablets ... 2382
Engerix-B Unit-Dose Vials (Less than 1%) ... 2213
Equagesic Tablets ... 2451
Feldene Capsules (Less than 1%) .. 1777
Hydeltrasol Injection, Sterile ... 1476
Hydeltra-T.B.A. Sterile Suspension 1478
Hydrocortone Acetate Sterile Suspension ... 1479
Hydrocortone Phosphate Injection, Sterile ... 1481
Hydrocortone Tablets ... 1482
Indocin Capsules (Less than 1%) ... 1487
Indocin I.V. (Less than 1%) ... 1490
Indocin (Less than 1%) ... 1487
Isoptin Oral Tablets (Less than 1%) ... 1179
Isoptin SR Sustained Release Tablets (Less than 1%) ... 1181
Kenalog-10 Injection ... 2402
Kenalog-40 Injection ... 2403
Lodine Capsules (Less than 1%) ... 2468
Lorelco Tablets ... 1333
▲Lupron Depot 3.75 mg (Among most frequent) ... 2312
Lupron Depot 7.5 mg ... 2311
Lupron Injection (Less than 5%) ... 2310
Medrol ... 2348
Methotrexate Tablets, Parenteral, LPF Parenteral ... 1217
Miltown Tablets ... 2386
▲Naprosyn (3 to 9%) ... 2297
Naturetin Tablets (Occasional) ... 1789
▲Novantrone for Injection Concentrate (7 to 11%) ... 1226
Omnipaque ... 2552
PMB 200 and PMB 400 ... 2504
Paraflex Caplets (Rare) ... 1378
Parafon Forte DSC Caplets (Rare) .. 1379
Pediapred Oral Liquid ... 987
Pipracil (Less frequent) ... 1230
Prozac Pulvules ... 920
Questran Light ... 711
Questran Powder ... 710
Rauzide Tablets ... 1804
Rheumatrex Methotrexate Dose Pack ... 1234
Roferon-A Injection (Rare) ... 1916
Solatene Capsules (Rare) ... 1881
Solu-Medrol Sterile Powder ... 2363
Tenuate ... 1354
Trilisate (Rare) ... 1822
Verelan Capsules (Less than 1%) .. 1243
Wellbutrin Tablets ... 821
Zyloprim Tablets (Less than 1%) ... 830

Echoacousia
Omnipaque ... 2552

Echolalia
Omnipaque ... 2552

Ectodactylia
Neosar for Injection (Two cases) ... 566

Ectropion
Oculinum for Injecton (Less than 1%) ... 587

Eczema
Accutane Capsules (Less than 1 in 10) ... 1878
▲AeroBid Inhaler System (3-9%) ... 995
Anafranil Capsules (Infrequent) ... 650
Ansaid Tablets (Less than 1%) ... 2319
Cardura Tablets (Less than 0.5% of 3960 patients) ... 1941
Cerumenex Drops (1% of 2,700 patients) ... 1813
Clozaril Tablets (Less than 1%) ... 2000
Compazine ... 2201
Dantrium Capsules (Less frequent) 1619
Engerix-B Unit-Dose Vials ... 2213
ERYC ... 1720
Etrafon ... 2087
Glucotrol (1 in 70) ... 1952
Kwell Cream (Rare) ... 1830
Kwell Lotion (Rare) ... 1831
Kwell Shampoo (Rare) ... 1832
Lopid Capsules and Tablets (1.9%) ... 1736
Macrodantin Capsules ... 1624
Micro-Guard Cream, Antiseptic, Antifungal Skin Cream (Occasional) ... 2286
Mulvidren-F Softab Tablets ... 2273
Orudis Capsules (Less than 1%) ... 2488
Permax Tablets (Infrequent) ... 1291
Prolixin Decanoate ... 1795
Prolixin Elixir ... 1793
Prolixin Enanthate ... 1796
Prolixin Injection ... 1791
Prolixin Oral Concentrate ... 1792
Prolixin Tablets ... 1793
Prozac Pulvules (Rare) ... 920
Quinidex Extentabs ... 1868
Rogaine Topical Solution ... 2357
Stelazine ... 2226
Taractan ... 1920
Triavil Tablets ... 1556
Trilafon ... 2123
Voltaren Tablets (Less than 1%) ... 1042

Eczematous reactions (see under Eczema)

Edema
A.P.L. ... 2431
Accutane Capsules (Less than 1%) ... 1878
▲AeroBid Inhaler System (3-9%) ... 995
Aldoclor Tablets ... 1413
Aldomet Ester HCl Injection ... 1417
Aldomet Oral ... 1415
Aldoril Tablets ... 1418
Alferon N Injection (One patient) ... 1809
Altace Capsules (Less than 1%) ... 1086
Amen ... 833
Americaine Anesthetic Lubricant ... 972
Americaine Otic Topical Anesthetic Ear Drops ... 973
Anadrol-50 Tablets ... 2287
Anafranil Capsules (Infrequent) ... 650
▲Anaprox and Anaprox DS Tablets (3-9%) ... 2288
Android ... 1111
▲Anestacon Solution (Among most common) ... 2394
▲Ansaid Tablets (3-9%) ... 2319
Antivenin (Crotalidae) Polyvalent ... 2430
Apresazide Capsules (Less frequent) ... 854
Apresoline Hydrochloride Parenteral (Ampuls) ... 856
Apresoline Hydrochloride Tablets (Less frequent) ... 855
Apresoline-Esidrix Tablets ... 857
Aristocort Suspension ... 1008
Aristospan Suspension ... 1011
Asendin Tablets (Greater than 1%) ... 1196
Atgam Sterile Solution (Less than 1% to less than 5%) ... 2320
Atropine Sulfate Sterile Ophthalmic Solution and S.O.P. Sterile Ophthalmic Ointment ... ⊙ 239
Aygestin Tablets ... 2437
Azo Gantrisin Tablets ... 1888
BSS (15 mL & 30 mL) Sterile Irrigation Solution ... ⊙ 230
BSS (250 mL) Sterile Irrigation Solution ... ⊙ 231
BSS (500 mL) Sterile Irrigation Solution ... ⊙ 231
BSS PLUS (500 mL) Sterile Irrigation Solution ... ⊙ 231
Bicillin C-R Injection ... 2438
Bicillin C-R 900/300 Injection ... 2440
Bicillin L-A Injection ... 2442
Blocadren Tablets (0.6%) ... 1429
Brevibloc Injection (Less than 1%) 942
Brevicon ... 2304
BuSpar (Infrequent) ... 1401
▲Butazolidin Capsules & Tablets (3-9%) ... 1027
Calan SR Caplets (1.9%) ... 2157
Calan Tablets (1.9%) ... 2155
Capozide ... 2258
Carbocaine ... 956
Cardene Capsules (0.6-1.0%) ... 2290
Cardizem Tablets-30 mg, 60 mg, 90 mg and 120 mg (2.4%) ... 1329
▲Cardizem SR Capsules-60 mg, 90 mg and 120 mg (5.4-9%) ... 1327
▲Cardura Tablets (4%) ... 1941
▲Catapres-TTS (3 of 101 patients) .. 677
Celestone Soluspan Suspension ... 2081
Children's Advil Suspension (Less than 3%) ... 2426
Cholybar ... 1705
Clinoril Tablets (Greater than 1%) 1433
Clozaril Tablets (Less than 1%) ... 2000
Cordarone Tablets (1 to 3%) ... 2446
Cortenema ... 2244
Cortifoam ... 1827

Cortone Acetate Sterile Suspension 1437
Cortone Acetate Tablets 1439
Creon Capsules 2245
Cycrin Tablets (Occasional) 2449
Cytotec (Infrequent) 2159
Cytovene Sterile Powder (1% or less) 2292
Dalalone D.P. Injectable 999
Dalgan Injection (Less than 1%) 620
Danocrine Capsules 2046
Decadron Elixir 1445
Decadron Phosphate Injection 1449
Decadron Phosphate Respihaler 1454
Decadron Phosphate Turbinaire 1456
Decadron Phosphate with Xylocaine Injection, Sterile 1451
Decadron Tablets 1447
Decadron-LA Sterile Suspension 1457
Deltasone Tablets 2332
Demulen 2161
Depakote Sprinkle Capsules 512
Depo-Medrol Sterile Aqueous Suspension 2334
Depo-Provera Sterile Aqueous Suspension 2336
Deprol Tablets 2382
Desquam-E Gel 2397
Desquam-X Gel 2397
Desquam-X 5 Wash 2397
Desquam-X 10 Bar 2397
Desquam-X 10 Wash 2397
Desyrel and Desyrel Dividose (Greater than 1%) 1404
Diethylstilbestrol Tablets 1258
Diphtheria & Tetanus Toxoids, Adsorbed Purogenated (Mild) 1202
Diphtheria and Tetanus Toxoids and Pertussis Vaccine Adsorbed USP (For Pediatric Use) 892
Diprivan Injection (Less than 1%) 2267
Dolobid Tablets (Less than 1 in 100) 1465
Dolophine Hydrochloride Ampoules & Vials 1260
Dolophine Hydrochloride Tablets 1261
Duragesic Transdermal System (1% or greater) 1133
Duranest Injections 624
Duricef 1405
Dyclone 0.5% and 1% Topical Solutions, USP 626
▲DynaCirc Capsules (1.2% to 7.2%) 2004
Elavil 2269
▲Emcyt Capsules (19%) 1161
Endep Tablets 1927
Enovid 2161
▲Epogen for Injection (9.0%) 591
Ergamisol Tablets (1%) 1136
Esimil Tablets 864
Estinyl Tablets 2085
Estrace 1385
Estrace Vaginal Cream 1388
Estraderm Transdermal System 866
Estradurin 2452
Estratest 2245
Estrovis 1721
▲Eulexin Capsules (4%) 2089
Feldene Capsules (Approximately 2%) 1777
Fiorinal with Codeine Capsules 2008
Flexeril Tablets (Rare) 1471
Floxin Tablets (Less than 1%) 1652
Gantanol 1899
Gantrisin 1901
Gastrocrom Capsules (Infrequent) 974
Halotestin Tablets 2341
Harmonyl Tablets (Rare) 528
Hemopad Absorbable Collagen Hemostat 627
Hismanal Tablets (Less frequent) 1138
Humatrope Vials (2.5%) 1266
Hydeltrasol Injection, Sterile 1476
Hydeltra-T.B.A. Sterile Suspension 1478
Hydrocortone Acetate Sterile Suspension 1479
Hydrocortone Phosphate Injection, Sterile 1481
Hydrocortone Tablets 1482
Hytrin Tablets (0.9%) 529
Indocin Capsules (Less than 1%) 1487
Indocin I.V. (Less than 1%) 1490
Indocin (Less than 1%) 1487
INSTAT Collagen Absorbable Hemostat 1151
Intron A (Less than 1%) 2097
Ismelin Tablets 869
Isoptin Oral Tablets (1.9%) 1179
Isoptin SR Sustained Release Tablets (1.9%) 1181
Isopto Atropine ◉ 218
Isopto Homatropine ◉ 221
Isopto Hyoscine ◉ 222
Jenest-28 Tablets 1636
Kenalog-10 Injection 2402
Kenalog-40 Injection 2403
Kerlone Tablets (1.3% to 1.8%) 2172
Klonopin Tablets 1902
Lamprene Capsules (Less than 1%) 1030
Larodopa Tablets (Rare) 1905
Leukine for IV Infusion 1127
Levlen/Tri-Levlen 665
Librax Capsules (Rare) 1929
Libritabs Tablets (Isolated cases) 1930
Librium Capsules (Isolated cases) 1931
Librium Injectable (Isolated cases) 1932
Lincocin 2344
Lioresal Tablets 1031
Lodine Capsules (Less than 1%) 2468
Lo/Ovral Tablets 2471
Lo/Ovral-28 Tablets 2476
Loestrin 1728
▲Loniten Tablets (7%) 2346
Lopressor HCT Tablets (1 in 100 patients) 1034
Lotrimin 2102
Lotrisone Cream (1 of 270 patients) 2103
Ludiomil Tablets (Rare) 874
▲Lupron Depot 7.5 mg (12.5%) 2311
MS Contin Tablets (Infrequent) 1814
MSIR (Infrequent) 1817
Marcaine Hydrochloride 0.5% with Epinephrine 1:200,000 (as bitartrate) 958
Matulane Capsules 1907
Maxair Inhaler (Less than 1%) 1311
Meclomen Capsules (Greater than 1%) 1739
Mediatric Capsules 2476
Medrol 2348
Megace Tablets 732
Mellaril 2011
Menrium Tablets 1934
Mesantoin Tablets 2013
Metandren Linguets and Tablets 875
Methadone Hydrochloride Diskets 1284
Methadone Hydrochloride Oral Solution & Tablets 1987
Metubine Iodide Vials 1285
Mevacor Tablets 1505
▲Mexitil Capsules (About 2 in 1,000 to 3.8%) 680
Micronor Tablets 1667
Minipress Capsules (1-4%) 1778
Minizide Capsules 1779
Modicon 1667
Monopril Tablets (0.2 to 1.0%) 1406
Motrin Tablets (Less than 3%) 2351
Mutamycin 733
Mycelex 1% Cream and Topical Solution 1% 1604
Mykrox ½ mg Tablets (Less than 2%) 984
▲Naprosyn (3 to 9%) 2297
Nardil (Common) 1742
NebuPent for Inhalation Solution (Greater than 1%, up to 5%) 1017
Nicorette 1335
Nimotop Capsules (Up to 1.2%) 1607
▲Nolvadex Tablets (3.8%) 1102
Nordette-21 Tablets 2481
Nordette-28 Tablets 2483
Norethin 2133
Norinyl 2304
Norlestrin 1746
Norlutate 1754
Norlutin 1755
Normodyne Injection (1 to 2%) 2108
Normodyne Tablets (1% to 2%) 2110
Normozide Tablets (1%) 2112
Norpace (1 to 3%) 2177
Norpramin Tablets 1340
Nor-Q D Tablets 2304
Novocain Hydrochloride for Spinal Anesthesia 2065
Ogen 540
Oncovin Solution Vials & Hyporets (Rare) 1288
OptiPranolol Sterile Ophthalmic Solution (A small number of patients) ◉ 261
Oramorph SR (Morphine Sulfate Sustained Release Tablets) (Less frequent) 1988
Ortho Diaphragm Kit 1664
Ortho Dienestrol Cream 1664
Ortho-Cyclen Tablets 1658
Ortho-Novum 1667
▲Orudis Capsules (Greater than 3%) 2488
Ovcon 1391
Ovral Tablets 2490
Ovral-28 Tablets 2491
Ovrette Tablets 2492
Oxsoralen-Ultra Capsule 1117
PMB 200 and PMB 400 2504
Pamelor 2019
Parnate Tablets 2222
Pediapred Oral Liquid 987
PediaProfen Suspension (Less than 3%) 1363
Pentaspan Injection 949
Permax Tablets (1.6%) 1291
Pfizerpen for Injection 1957
Pfizerpen-AS Aqueous Suspension 1959
Plague Vaccine 1584
Pontocaine Hydrochloride for Spinal Anesthesia 2069
Pregnyl 1644
Premarin Intravenous 2508
Premarin with Methyltestosterone 2515
Premarin Tablets 2510
Premarin Vaginal Cream 2512
Priscoline Hydrochloride Ampuls 877
▲Procardia XL Tablets (10% to about 30%) 1783
▲Procrit for Injection (9%) 1647
Profasi (human chorionic gonadotropin, USP) 2186
Proglycem (Frequent) 649
Prokine for I.V. Infusion 1096
ProSom Tablets (Rare) 554
Prostin VR Pediatric Sterile Solution (1%) 2355
Provera Tablets 2356
Prozac Pulvules (Infrequent) 920
Quadrinal Tablets 1183
Questran Light 711
Questran Powder 710
Raudixin Tablets (Rare) 1803
Rauzide Tablets (Rare) 1804
Recombivax HB (Less than 1%) 1544
Reglan 1869
Retrovir (0.8%) 802
▲Roferon-A Injection (9%) 1916
Rogaine Topical Solution (1.24 to 1.53%) 2357
Rowasa 2248
Roxanol 1991
Rufen Tablets (1 to 3%) 691
Rythmol Tablets (0.6 to 1.4%) 1184
Salutensin/Salutensin-Demi 719
Sandimmune (2% or less) 2024
Sandostatin Injection (1.0%) 2029
Sansert Tablets 2031
Sectral Capsules (2%) 2520
Ser-Ap-Es Tablets 881
Serax Capsules 2522
Serax Tablets 2522
Serentil 686
Serpasil Tablets 883
Serpasil-Apresoline Tablets 884
Serpasil-Esidrix Tablets 886
Sinemet Tablets 952
Sinemet CR Tablets 953
Sinequan (Occasional) 1960
Solu-Cortef Sterile Powder 2361
Solu-Medrol Sterile Powder 2363
Soma Compound w/Codeine Tablets 2390
Soma Compound Tablets 2389
Stilphostrol Tablets and Ampuls 1609
▲Synarel Nasal Solution (8% of patients) 2300
TACE 12 and 25 mg 1353
▲Tambocor Tablets (3.5%) 1315
Tapazole Tablets 1298
▲Tegison Capsules (1 to 10%) 1881
Tegretol Chewable Tablets 654
Tegretol Suspension 656
Tegretol Tablets 654
Tenex Tablets 1875
Tetanus Toxoid, Adsorbed Purogenated 1238
Theroxide 1411
Timolide Tablets 1547
Timoptic in Ocudose 1552
Timoptic Sterile Ophthalmic Solution 1550
Tofranil Ampuls 1038
Tofranil Tablets 1039
Tofranil-PM Capsules 1041
▲Tolectin (200, 400 and 600 mg) (3 to 9%) 1379
Tonocard Tablets (Less than 1%) 1554
Toradol IM Injection (1% to 3%) 2302
Trancopal Caplets 2075
Trandate Injection 577
Trandate Tablets (1% of 227 patients) 579
Trental (Less than 1%) 1099
Trexan Tablets (Less than 1%) 937
Triavil Tablets 1556
Levlen/Tri-Levlen 665
Trilisate (Less than 1%) 1822
Tri-Norinyl 2304
Triphasil-21 Tablets 2527
Triphasil-28 Tablets 2532
Unasyn (Less than 1%) 1965
Vascor (200, 300 and 400 mg) Tablets (0.5 to 2.0%) 1383
Verelan Capsules (1.9%) 1243
▲Visken Tablets (6%) 2036
Vivactil Tablets 1567
Voltaren Tablets (B 3% to 9%) 1042
Wellbutrin Tablets (Frequent) 821
Winstrol Tablets 2075
Wycillin Injection 2537
Wytensin Tablets (3% or less) 2542
▲Xanax Tablets (4.9%) 2367
Xylocaine Injections (Extremely rare) 637
Xylocaine 2% Jelly (Extremely rare) 643
Xylocaine 5% Ointment 644
Xylocaine 10% Oral Spray (Extremely rare) 645
4% Xylocaine-MPF Sterile Solution (Extremely rare) 641
▲Zoladex (7%) 1110
Zovirax Capsules (0.3%) 824
Zovirax Sterile Powder (Less than 1%) 828
Zovirax (0.3%) 824

Edema, allergic

Cytosar-U Sterile Powder (Less frequent) 2329
Periactin 1525
Retin-A (tretinoin) Cream/Gel/Liquid 1680

Edema, angioneurotic

Achromycin V Capsules 1193
Altace Capsules (0.3%) 1086
Anaprox and Anaprox DS Tablets (Rare) 2288
Ansaid Tablets (Less than 1%) 2319
Augmentin Tablets, Powder for Oral Suspension, and Chewable Tablets 2198
Azactam for Injection (Less than 1%) 2252
Azdōne Tablets 844
Azo Gantrisin Tablets 1888
Carafate Tablets 1326
Carbocaine Hydrochloride Injection 2043
Catapres Tablets (About 5 in 1,000 patients) 676
Catapres-TTS (5 per 1,000) 677
Ceptaz for Injection (Rare) 1057
Chloromycetin Cream, 1% 1694
Chloromycetin Otic 1697
Chloroptic S.O.P. ◉ 243
Chloroptic Sterile Ophthalmic Solution ◉ 243
Clinoril Tablets (Less than 1 in 100) 1433
Combipres Tablets (5 in 1,000) 678
Compazine 2201
Cortone Acetate Sterile Suspension 1437
Cortone Acetate Tablets 1439
CytoGam 891
Damason-P 1356
Decadron Elixir 1445
Decadron Phosphate Injection 1449
Decadron Phosphate Respihaler 1454
Decadron Phosphate Turbinaire 1456
Decadron Phosphate with Xylocaine Injection, Sterile 1451
Decadron Tablets 1447
Decadron-LA Sterile Suspension 1457
Declomycin Capsules, Tablets 1199
Depo-Provera Sterile Aqueous Suspension (Occasional) 2336
Dolobid Tablets (Less than 1 in 100) 1465
Doryx Capsules 1717
Elase-Chloromycetin Ointment 1015
Eminase 2211
Engerix-B Unit-Dose Vials 2213
Equagesic Tablets 2451
Etrafon 2087
Flexeril Tablets 1471
Flu-Imune Influenza Virus Vaccine (Rare) 1204
Fulvicin P/G Tablets (Rare) 2090

Fulvicin P/G 165 & 330 Tablets (Rare) 2091
Fulvicin-U/F Tablets (Rare) 2092
Gastrocrom Capsules (Infrequent).. 974
Grifulvin V (griseofulvin microsize) Tablets/Suspension (Rare) 1678
Grisactin (Rare) 2454
Grisactin Ultra Tablets (Rare) 2455
Gris-PEG Tablets, 125 mg & 250 mg (Rare) 1083
Hismanal Tablets (Less frequent) 1138
Hydeltrasol Injection, Sterile 1476
Hydeltra-T.B.A. Sterile Suspension 1478
Hydrocortone Acetate Sterile Suspension 1479
Hydrocortone Phosphate Injection, Sterile 1481
Hydrocortone Tablets 1482
Hyperab Rabies Immune Globulin (Human) (Rare) 1574
HyperHep Hepatitis B Immune Globulin (Human) 1575
Hyper-Tet Tetanus Immune Globulin (Human) (Few cases) 1576
Intal Nebulizer Solution 980
Lodine Capsules (Less than 1%) 2468
Lomotil 2174
Lopid Capsules and Tablets 1736
Lorelco Tablets 1333
Lortab ASA Tablets 2414
Lotensin Tablets 872
Marcaine Hydrochloride with Epinephrine 1:200,000 (Rare) 2055
Marcaine Hydrochloride Injection (Rare) 2055
Marcaine Spinal (Rare) 2058
Mellaril 2011
Mevacor Tablets (Rare) 1505
Micronase Tablets 2350
Miltown Tablets (Rare) 2386
Minocin Intravenous 1221
Minocin Oral Suspension 1224
Minocin Pellet-Filled Capsules 1222
Monodox Capsules 1630
Monopril Tablets (0.2 to 1.0%) 1406
Motofen Tablets 836
Myochrysine Injection 1516
Nalfon Pulvules & Tablets (Less than 1%) 919
Naprosyn (Rare) 2297
Nescaine/Nescaine MPF 629
Noroxin Tablets 1519
Norzine 1818
PMB 200 and PMB 400 (Rare) 2504
Paraflex Caplets (Extremely rare) 1378
Parafon Forte DSC Caplets (Extremely rare) 1379
Pepcid (Infrequent) 1524
Phenergan with Codeine (Infrequent) 2497
Phenergan Injection 2493
Phenergan Tablets 2496
Phenergan VC with Codeine 2501
Pre-Pen 2148
Prinzide Tablets 1540
Procan SR Tablets (Occasional) 1760
Prolixin Decanoate 1795
Prolixin Elixir 1793
Prolixin Enanthate 1796
Prolixin Injection 1791
Prolixin Oral Concentrate 1792
Prolixin Tablets 1793
Pronestyl Capsules and Tablets (Occasional) 1800
Pronestyl Injection (Occasional) 1798
Pronestyl-SR Tablets 1801
Quadrinal Tablets 1183
Robaxisal Tablets 1872
Salflex 839
Seldane-D Extended-Release Tablets 1350
Sensorcaine (Rare) 631
Sensorcaine-MPF Spinal (Rare) 634
Serentil 686
Solganal Suspension 2122
Soma Compound w/Codeine Tablets 2390
Soma Compound Tablets 2389
Soma Tablets 2388
Stelazine 2226
Streptase for Infusion 635
Tacaryl 2409
Talwin Compound 2072
Taractan 1920
Temaril Tablets, Syrup and Spansule Sustained Release Capsules 1085
Terramycin Capsules 1786
Terramycin Intramuscular Solution 1964
Thorazine 2234
Torecan 1993
Trandate HCT Tablets (Rare) 579
Trandate Injection (Rare) 577
Trandate Tablets (Rare) 579
Triavil Tablets 1556
Trilafon 2123
Vibramycin Hyclate Capsules 1787
Vibramycin Hyclate Intravenous 1968
Vibramycin 1787
Wellbutrin Tablets 821
Zantac Injection and Zantac Injection Premixed (Rare) 1063
Zantac (Rare) 1065
Zestoretic 2274
Zyloprim Tablets 830

Edema, ankle

Android 1111
Verelan Capsules (1.4%) 1243

Edema, aphakic cystoid macular

Timoptic in Ocudose 1552
Timoptic Sterile Ophthalmic Solution 1550

Edema, arm

Niclocide Chewable Tablets 1607
Torecan 1993

Edema, cerebral

Betoptic Sterile Ophthalmic Solution (Small numbers of patients) 569
Betoptic S Sterile Ophthalmic Suspension (Small numbers of patients) 570
Compazine 2201
Etrafon (Extremely rare) 2087
Navane Capsules and Concentrate 1954
Navane Intramuscular 1956
Permax Tablets (Rare) 1291
Prolixin Decanoate 1795
Prolixin Elixir 1793
Prolixin Enanthate 1796
Prolixin Injection 1791
Prolixin Oral Concentrate 1792
Prolixin Tablets 1793
Stelazine 2226
Taractan 1920
Thorazine 2234
Triavil Tablets 1556
Trilafon (Extremely rare) 2123

Edema, corneal

AMVISC Plus ◉ 323
Atabrine Hydrochloride Tablets 2041
BSS (15 mL & 30 mL) Sterile Irrigation Solution ◉ 230
BSS (250 mL) Sterile Irrigation Solution ◉ 231
BSS (500 mL) Sterile Irrigation Solution ◉ 231
BSS PLUS (500 mL) Sterile Irrigation Solution ◉ 231
Healon (Rare) ◉ 279
Miochol with Iocare Steri-Tags, Miochol System Pak and Miochol System Pak Plus (Infrequent) ◉ 274
▲ Rēv-Eyes Ophthalmic Eyedrops 0.5% (10% to 40%) ◉ 312
Zolyse ◉ 236

Edema, crusting

Condylox (Less than 5%) 1630

Edema, dependent

Anafranil Capsules (Rare) 650

Edema, extremities

Cipro I.V. (1% or less) 1592
Cipro Tablets (Less than 1%) 1589
Depakene Capsules & Syrup 511
Depakote Tablets 512
Norzine 1818
Parlodel 2020
Rifadin 1345
Teslac Tablets 741

Edema, facial

Antivenin (Crotalidae) Polyvalent 2430
Azmacort Inhaler (Infrequent) 1837
BuSpar (Infrequent) 1401
Cardura Tablets (1%) 1941
Cipro I.V. (1% or less) 1592
Cipro Tablets (Less than 1%) 1589
Elavil 2269
Endep Tablets 1927
Etrafon 2087
Flexeril Tablets (Less than 1%) 1471
Hytrin Tablets (At least 1%) 529
▲ Intron A (Up to 10%) 2097
Klonopin Tablets 1902
Limbitrol 1933
Loxitane 1213
Noroxin Tablets 1519
Norpramin Tablets 1340
Orudis Capsules (Less than 1%) 2488
Pamelor 2019
Pepcid (Infrequent) 1524
Permax Tablets (1.1%) 1291
Platinol 737
Platinol-AQ Injection (Occasional) 738
Plendil Extended-Release Tablets (0.5% to 1.5%) 1526
Ponstel 1758
Primaxin I.M. 1532
Primaxin I.V. (Less than 0.2%) 1535
Procardia XL Tablets (1% or Less) 1783
Prozac Pulvules (Infrequent) 920
Quinamm Tablets (Occasional) 1344
Rifadin 1345
Rogaine Topical Solution (1.27%).. 2357
Surmontil Capsules 2524
Talacen (Rare) 2070
Talwin Injection (Rare) 2071
Talwin Compound (Rare) 2072
Talwin Injection (Rare) 2071
Talwin Nx 2073
Tofranil Ampuls 1038
Tofranil Tablets 1039
Tofranil-PM Capsules 1041
Torecan 1993
Triavil Tablets 1556
Zyloprim Tablets 830

Edema, fibrinous

▲ Blenoxane (10%) 724

Edema, heart failure (see under Congestive heart failure)

Edema, laryngeal

Antivenin (Crotalidae) Polyvalent 2430
Axid Pulvules (Rare) 1246
Bicillin C-R Injection 2438
Bicillin C-R 900/300 Injection 2440
Bicillin L-A Injection 2442
Capoten (Approximately 1 in 1,000 patients) 2255
Capozide (1 case) 2258
Carbocaine Hydrochloride Injection 2043
Cipro I.V. (1% or less) 1592
Cipro Tablets (Less than 1%) 1589
Compazine 2201
Etrafon 2087
Garamycin Injectable 2093
Intal Capsules (Less than 1 in 10,000 patients) 978
Intal Inhaler (Rare) 979
Intal Nebulizer Solution (Rare) 980
Lopid Capsules and Tablets 1736
Marcaine Hydrochloride with Epinephrine 1:200,000 (Rare) 2055
Marcaine Hydrochloride Injection (Rare) 2055
Marcaine Spinal (Rare) 2058
Mellaril 2011
Nardil 1742
Nescaine/Nescaine MPF 629
Norzine 1818
Omnipaque 2552
Orudis Capsules (Less than 1%) 2488
Permax Tablets (Rare) 1291
Phenergan with Codeine (Infrequent) 2497
Phenergan VC with Codeine 2501
Prinivil Tablets 1538
Prinzide Tablets 1540
Prolixin Decanoate 1795
Prolixin Elixir 1793
Prolixin Enanthate 1796
Prolixin Injection 1791
Prolixin Oral Concentrate 1792
Prolixin Tablets 1793
Prozac Pulvules (Rare) 920
Reglan (Few) 1869
Sensorcaine 631
Sensorcaine-MPF Spinal 634
Serentil 686
Stelazine 2226
Tacaryl 2409
Taractan 1920
Temaril Tablets, Syrup and Spansule Sustained Release Capsules 1085
Thorazine 2234
Torecan 1993
Triavil Tablets 1556
Trilafon 2123
Vaseretic Tablets 1559
Vasotec Tablets 1564
Voltaren Tablets (Less than 1%) 1042
Zestoretic 2274
Zestril Tablets 2277

Edema, lips

Cipro I.V. (1% or less) 1592
Cipro Tablets (Less than 1%) 1589
Retrovir Capsules (Less than 5%).. 802
Retrovir I.V. Infusion (Less than 5%) 805
Retrovir Syrup (Less than 5%) 802

Edema, local

Anafranil Capsules (Up to 2%) 650
Cafergot/Cafergot P-B 1999
D.H.E. 45 Injection 2003
Ergostat 1719
Furacin Soluble Dressing (Approximately 1%) 1854
Furacin Topical Cream (Approximately 1%) 1854
Furacin Topical Solution 0.2% 1855
Medihaler Ergotamine Aerosol 1312
Omnipaque 2552
Retin-A (tretinoin) Cream/Gel/Liquid 1680
Rogaine Topical Solution 2357
Wigraine Tablets & Suppositories .. 1645
Zovirax Ointment 5% 827

Edema, lower extremities

▲ Cardene Capsules (7.1-8.0%) 2290
Eldepryl 2250
Eminase 2211
Ganite Injection 1016
Miacalcin Injection 2017
Sansert Tablets 2031

Edema, macular

Meclomen Capsules (Rare) 1739

Edema, non-specific (see under Edema)

Edema, oropharyngeal

Anafranil Capsules (Rare) 650
Cipro I.V. (1% or less) 1592
Cipro Tablets (Less than 1%) 1589
Proventil Inhalation Aerosol (Rare) 2117
Ventolin (Rare) 583
Voltaren Tablets (Less than 1%) 1042

Edema, palpebral

▲ AK-Poly-Bac Ointment (Among most frequent) ◉ 205
Aralen Phosphate Tablets 2039
Cipro I.V. (1% or less) 1592
Cipro Tablets (Less than 1%) 1589
DDAVP (Up to 2%) 1841
Feldene Capsules (Less than 1%) .. 1777
Herplex Liquifilm ◉ 248
Opticrom 4% (Infrequent) 986
ProSom Tablets (Infrequent) 554
Quadrinal Tablets 1183
Tobrex Ophthalmic Ointment and Solution (Less than 3 in 100 patients) 572
Viroptic Ophthalmic Solution, 1% Sterile (2.8%) 820
Zestoretic 2274
Zestril Tablets 2277

Edema, periorbital (see under Edema, peripheral)

Edema, perimacular

Meclomen Capsules (Rare) 1739

Edema, peripheral

▲ Adalat Capsules (10 mg and 20 mg) (7% to about 10%) 1587
AeroBid Inhaler System (1-3%) 995
Atgam Sterile Solution (At least 1 patient and less than 5% of total patients) 2320
Azo Gantanol Tablets 1887
Azo Gantrisin Tablets 1888
Azulfidine Tablets, EN-tabs, Oral Suspension (Rare) 1157
Cartrol Tablets (1.7%) 507
Celontin 1692
Compazine 2201
Demser Capsules (Rare) 1460
Deprol Tablets 2382
Diapid Nasal Spray 2003
Dipentum Capsules (Rare) 1160
Eldepryl 2250
Equagesic Tablets 2451
Ergamisol Tablets (Less frequent) .. 1136
Ethmozine Tablets (Less than 2%) 946
Etrafon 2087

Fansidar Tablets 1896
Feldene Capsules (Approximately 2%) 1777
Gantanol 1899
Gantrisin Ophthalmic Ointment/Solution 1900
Hespan Injection 948
▲Hylorel Tablets (28.6%) 975
Hyskon Hysteroscopy Fluid (Rare) 1162
▲Hytrin Tablets (0.6% to 5.5%) 529
Infumorph 200 and Infumorph 500 Sterile Solutions (Several reports) 962
Intron A (Less than 1%) 2097
▲Leukine for IV Infusion (11%) 1127
Lopressor (1%) 1032
Lotensin Tablets 872
▲Lupron Injection (5% or more) 2310
▲Marplan Tablets (Among most frequent) 1906
Mellaril 2011
Miltown Tablets 2386
▲Nalfon Pulvules & Tablets (5%) 919
Navane Capsules and Concentrate 1954
Navane Intramuscular 1956
Nolvadex Tablets (Infrequent) 1102
Orap Tablets 1020
Orudis Capsules 2488
PMB 200 and PMB 400 2504
Pediazole 1973
Pepcid (Infrequent) 1524
▲Permax Tablets (7.4%) 1291
▲Plendil Extended-Release Tablets (1.4% to 36.0%) 1526
Prilosec Delayed-Release Capsules (Less than 1%) 1530
Prinivil Tablets (1% or less) 1538
Prinzide Tablets 1540
▲Procardia Capsules (Approximately 10%) 1781
▲Procardia XL Tablets (1% or less to about 30%) 1783
▲Prokine for I.V. Infusion (11%) 1096
Prolixin Decanoate 1795
Prolixin Elixir 1793
Prolixin Enanthate 1796
Prolixin Injection 1791
Prolixin Oral Concentrate 1792
Prolixin Tablets 1793
Prozac Pulvules (Infrequent) 920
Rowasa (0.61%) 2248
Sansert Tablets 2031
Stelazine 2226
Symmetrel Capsules & Syrup (1-5%) 936
Taractan 1920
Temaril Tablets, Syrup and Spansule Sustained Release Capsules 1085
Thiosulfil Forte Tablets 2526
Thorazine 2234
Tolectin (200, 400 and 600 mg) (Some patients) 1379
Torecan 1993
Triavil Tablets 1556
Trilafon 2123
Zestoretic 2274
Zestril Tablets (Less than 1%) 2277
Zovirax 824

Edema, pharyngeal

Noroxin Tablets 1519

Edema, pulmonary

Adalat Capsules (10 mg and 20 mg) (About 2%) 1587
Aldoclor Tablets 1413
Aldoril Tablets 1418
Atgam Sterile Solution (Less than 1% to less than 5%) 2320
Blocadren Tablets 1429
Brevibloc Injection (Less than 1%) 942
Calan SR Caplets (1.8%) 2157
Calan Tablets (1.8%) 2155
Cipro I.V. (1% or less) 1592
Cipro Tablets (Less than 1%) 1589
Dantrium Intravenous (Rare) 1620
Diupres Tablets 1461
Diuril Oral Suspension 1464
Diuril Sodium Intravenous 1463
Diuril Tablets 1464
Dyazide Capsules 2208
▲Eminase (Less than 10%) 2211
Enduron Tablets 517
Esidrix Tablets 863
Fungizone Intravenous 2262
Hespan Injection 948
HydroDIURIL Tablets 1484
Hydropres Tablets 1485
Hyskon Hysteroscopy Fluid (Rare) 1162
Indocin Capsules (Less than 1%) 1487
Indocin I.V. (Less than 1%) 1490
Indocin (Less than 1%) 1487
Inversine Tablets 1492
Isoptin Oral Tablets (1.8%) 1179
Isoptin SR Sustained Release Tablets (1.8%) 1181
Isuprel Hydrochloride Injection 1:5000 2050
Moduretic Tablets 1510
Mutamycin 733
Nalfon Pulvules & Tablets (Less than 1%) 919
Narcan Injection 933
Normodyne Tablets 2110
Normozide Tablets 2112
Nubain Injection 934
Omnipaque 2552
▲Orthoclone OKT3 Sterile Solution (Up to 4.7%) 1645
Permax Tablets (Infrequent) 1291
Pilocar (Extremely rare) ⊙ 275
Pilostat Sterile Ophthalmic Solution 0.5%, 1%, 2%, 3%, 4%, 5%, 6% (Extremely rare) ⊙ 263
Prinzide Tablets 1540
Procardia Capsules (Approximately 2%) 1781
Procardia XL Tablets (About 2%) 1783
Protamine Sulfate Ampoules & Vials 1295
Prozac Pulvules (Rare) 920
Roferon-A Injection (Rare) 1916
Salutensin/Salutensin-Demi 719
Timolide Tablets 1547
Timoptic in Ocudose 1552
Timoptic Sterile Ophthalmic Solution 1550
Tonocard Tablets (Less than 1%) 1554
Trandate HCT Tablets 579
Vaseretic Tablets 1559
Vasotec I.V. 1562
Vasotec Tablets 1564
Verelan Capsules (1.8%) 1243
Yutopar 647
Zestoretic 2274
Zovirax Sterile Powder (Less than 1%) 828

Edema, pulmonary, non-cardiogenic

Streptase for Infusion (Rare) 635

Edema, retinal

Aralen Phosphate Tablets 2039
Lariam Tablets 1904
Lopid Capsules and Tablets 1736
Plaquenil Sulfate Tablets 2067

Edema, skin (see under Edema, angioneurotic)

Edema, tongue

Antivenin (Crotalidae) Polyvalent 2430
Elavil 2269
Endep Tablets 1927
Etrafon 2087
Flexeril Tablets (Less than 1%) 1471
Limbitrol 1933
Norpramin Tablets 1340
Pamelor 2019
Prozac Pulvules (Rare) 920
Retrovir Capsules (Less than 5%) 802
Retrovir I.V. Infusion (Less than 5%) 805
Retrovir Syrup (Less than 5%) 802
Surmontil Capsules 2524
Tofranil Ampuls 1038
Tofranil Tablets 1039
Tofranil-PM Capsules 1041
Triavil Tablets 1556
Voltaren Tablets (Less than 1%) 1042
Zyloprim Tablets (Less than 1%) 830

Edema effusive, corneal stroma

AK-Taine ⊙ 207

Efficacy, lack of

▲Syntocinon Nasal Spray (Most frequent) 2033

Ejaculation, inhibition

Demser Capsules (Infrequent) 1460
Dibenzyline Capsules 2207
Esimil Tablets 864
Etrafon 2087
Ismelin Tablets 869
Lioresal Tablets (Rare) 1031
Mellaril 2011
Normodyne Injection (Up to 5%) 2108
▲Normodyne Tablets (Up to 5%) 2110
Normozide Tablets (Less than 1% to 2%) 2112
Parnate Tablets 2222
Serentil 686
Tacaryl 2409
Taractan 1920
Temaril Tablets, Syrup and Spansule Sustained Release Capsules 1085
Trandate HCT/Trandate (Less than 1% in 108 patients) 579
Triavil Tablets 1556
Trilafon 2123
Wellbutrin Tablets (Infrequent) 821

Ejaculation, premature

Anafranil Capsules (Rare) 650
Bumex (0.1%) 1895

Ejaculation disturbances

Amicar Syrup, Tablets, and Injection (Rare) 1194
▲Anafranil Capsules (6% to 42%) 650
Asendin Tablets (Less than 1%) 1196
BuSpar (Rare) 1401
Clozaril Tablets (1%) 2000
Compazine 2201
Desyrel and Desyrel Dividose (Less than 1%) 1404
▲Hylorel Tablets (7.0%) 975
Nardil 1742
Norpramin Tablets 1340
Prozac Pulvules (Infrequent) 920
Stelazine 2226
Surmontil Capsules 2524
Thorazine 2234
Trandate Injection 577
▲Trexan Tablets (Less than 10%) 937
Wellbutrin Tablets (Rare) 821

Ejection fraction reduction

Adriamycin PFS 561
Adriamycin RDF 562
Doxorubicin Hydrochloride Injection, USP 848
Novantrone for Injection Concentrate 1226
Rubex 739

Elastosis perforans, serpiginosa

Cuprimine Capsules (Rare) 1442
Depen Titratable Tablets (Rare) 2379

Elation

▲Marinol (Dronabinol) Capsules (24%) 1985

Electrocardiographic changes (see under EKG changes)

Electroencephalographic changes (see under EEG changes)

Electrolyte disturbances (see under Electrolyte imbalance)

Electrolyte imbalance

Aldactone 2152
Aldoclor Tablets 1413
Aldoril Tablets 1418
Anadrol-50 Tablets 2287
Atromid-S Capsules 2435
Capastat Sulfate Vials (1 patient) 1250
Corzide Tablets 702
Cytosar-U Sterile Powder (Less than 7 patients) 2329
Daranide Tablets 1445
Decadron Elixir 1445
Decadron Phosphate Injection 1449
Decadron Phosphate Respihaler 1454
Decadron Phosphate Turbinaire 1456
Decadron Phosphate with Xylocaine Injection, Sterile 1451
Depo-Medrol Sterile Aqueous Suspension 2334
Diamox Parenteral 1200
Diamox Sequels (Sustained Release) 1201
Diamox Tablets 1200
Diupres Tablets 1461
Diuril Oral Suspension 1464
Diuril Sodium Intravenous 1463
Diuril Tablets 1464
Dyazide Capsules (Uncommon) 2208
Enduron Tablets 517
HydroDIURIL Tablets 1484
Hydropres Tablets 1485
Medrol 2348
Metandren Linguets and Tablets 875
Modane Plus Tablets ▣ 504
Modane Tablets ▣ 503
Moduretic Tablets 1510
Normozide Tablets (Rare) 2112
Permax Tablets (Rare) 1291
Platinol 737
Platinol-AQ Injection 738
Premarin with Methyltestosterone 2515
Prinzide Tablets 1540
Rauzide Tablets 1804
Serophene (clomiphene citrate tablets, USP) 2186
Sodium Polystyrene Sulfonate Suspension 1993
Tenoretic Tablets 1105
Thalitone Tablets 687
Timolide Tablets 1547
Trandate HCT Tablets 579
Vaseretic Tablets 1559
Winstrol Tablets 2075
Zestoretic 2274

Elevated bilirubin levels (see under Hyperbilirubinemia)

Embolism

Amen 833
Cycrin Tablets 2449
▲Eminase (Less than 10%) 2211
Sterile FUDR 1898
Metrodin (urofollitropin for injection) 2182
Norlutate 1754
Norlutin 1755
Ortho-Cyclen Tablets 1658
Paraplatin for Injection 735
Pronestyl Capsules and Tablets 1800
Pronestyl Injection 1798
Provera Tablets 2356

Embolism, arterial

Cardioquin Tablets 1812
Metrodin (urofollitropin for injection) 2182
Quinaglute Dura-Tabs Tablets 663
Quinidex Extentabs 1868

Embolism, lower extremities

Gelfoam Sterile Sponge 2338

Embolism, pulmonary

Actimmune (Rare) 1046
Amen 833
Ansaid Tablets (Less than 1%) 2319
Brevicon 2304
Calciparine Injection 925
Cipro I.V. (1% or less) 1592
Cipro Tablets (Less than 1%) 1589
Cycrin Tablets (Occasional) 2449
Demulen 2161
Depo-Provera Sterile Aqueous Suspension 2336
Emcyt Capsules (2%) 1161
Enovid 2161
Estrace 1385
Estrace Vaginal Cream 1388
Estradurin 2452
Estratest 2245
Ethmozine Tablets (Less than 2%) 946
Gelfoam Sterile Sponge 2338
Heparin Lock Flush Solution 2456
Heparin Sodium Vials 1264
Heparin Sodium Injection 2457
Heparin Sodium Injection, USP, Sterile Solution 2342
Jenest-28 Tablets 1636
Levlen/Tri-Levlen 665
Lo/Ovral Tablets 2471
Lo/Ovral-28 Tablets 2476
Loestrin 1728
▲Lupron Depot 3.75 mg (Among most frequent) 2312
Lupron Depot 7.5 mg 2311
Lupron Injection (Less than 5%) 2310
Megace Tablets (Rare) 732
Metrodin (urofollitropin for injection) 2182
Micronor Tablets 1667
Modicon 1667
Nordette-21 Tablets 2481
Nordette-28 Tablets 2483
Norethin 2133
Norinyl 2304
Norlestrin 1746
Norlutate 1754
Norlutin 1755
Nor-Q D Tablets 2304
Ortho Dienestrol Cream 1664
Ortho-Cyclen Tablets 1658
Ortho-Novum 1667

Ovcon 1391
Ovral Tablets 2490
Ovral-28 Tablets 2491
Ovrette Tablets 2492
PMB 200 and PMB 400 2504
Permax Tablets (Infrequent) 1291
Premarin Intravenous 2508
Premarin with Methyltestosterone 2515
Premarin Tablets 2510
Premarin Vaginal Cream 2512
Provera Tablets 2356
Scleromate 1685
Serophene (clomiphene citrate tablets, USP) 2186
Sotradecol (Sodium Tetradecyl Sulfate Injection) (One patient) 964
Stilphostrol Tablets and Ampuls 1609
TACE 12 and 25 mg 1353
Tenormin Tablets and I.V. Injection (1.2%) 1107
Tonocard Tablets (Less than 1%) 1554
Levlen/Tri-Levlen 665
Tri-Norinyl 2304
Triphasil-21 Tablets 2527
Triphasil-28 Tablets 2532
Vaseretic Tablets 1559
Vasotec I.V. 1562
Vasotec Tablets (0.5% to 1.0%) 1564
Wellbutrin Tablets (Rare) 821

Embryotoxicity

Adriamycin RDF 562
Cytovene Sterile Powder 2292
Methotrexate Tablets, Parenteral, LPF Parenteral 1217
Rheumatrex Methotrexate Dose Pack 1234
Terramycin Intramuscular Solution 1964

Emergence delirium

Versed Injection (Less than 1%) 1924

Emesis (see under Vomiting)

Emotional disturbances

Accutane Capsules 1878
Atabrine Hydrochloride Tablets (Infrequent) 2041
Depakene Capsules & Syrup 511
Depakote 512
Lariam Tablets (Less than 1%) 1904
Mysoline (Occasional) 2480
Norplant System 2484
Phenobarbital Elixir and Tablets 1293
Plaquenil Sulfate Tablets 2067
Tofranil Ampuls 1038
Tofranil Tablets 1039
▲ Yutopar (5 to 6% with IV administration) 647

Emotional lability

Anafranil Capsules (Up to 2%) 650
Ansaid Tablets (Less than 1%) 2319
Blocadren Tablets 1429
Bretylol Injection (1 in 1000) 923
BuSpar (Rare) 1401
Cardura Tablets (Less than 0.5% of 3960 patients) 1941
Cartrol Tablets 507
Children's Advil Suspension (Less than 1%) 2426
Corgard Tablets 701
Corzide Tablets 702
Danocrine Capsules 2046
Diprivan Injection (Less than 1%) 2267
Emcyt Capsules (2%) 1161
Inderal 2459
Inderal LA Long Acting Capsules 2461
Inderide Tablets 2463
Inderide LA Long Acting Capsules 2465
Intron A (1% or less) 2097
Kerlone Tablets (Less than 2%) 2172
Levatol 1832
Lopressor HCT Tablets 1034
Motrin Tablets (Less than 1%) 2351
NebuPent for Inhalation Solution (1% or less) 1017
Normodyne Tablets 2110
Normozide Tablets 2112
PediaProfen Suspension (Less than 1%) 1363
Permax Tablets (Infrequent) 1291
ProSom Tablets (Infrequent) 554
Proventil Syrup (Children 2-6: 1%) 2119
Prozac Pulvules (Infrequent) 920
Retrovir Capsules (Less than 5%) 802
Retrovir I.V. Infusion (Less than 5%) 805
Retrovir Syrup (Less than 5%) 802
Roferon-A Injection (Less than 3%) 1916
Rufen Tablets (Less than 1%) 691
Sectral Capsules 2520
▲ Synarel Nasal Solution (15% of patients) 2300
Tegison Capsules (Less than 1%) 1881
Tenoretic Tablets 1105
Tenormin Tablets and I.V. Injection 1107
Timolide Tablets 1547
Timoptic in Ocudose 1552
Timoptic Sterile Ophthalmic Solution 1550
Trandate HCT/Trandate 579
Ventolin Syrup (1% of children) 583
Visken Tablets 2036

Emphysema

▲ Exosurf Neonatal for Intratracheal Suspension (7% to 43%) 765
Permax Tablets (Infrequent) 1291

Endocardial fibrosis

Myleran Tablets (One case) 790

Encephalitis

Atgam Sterile Solution (At least 1 patient and less than 5% of total patients) 2320
Attenuvax 1424
Biavax II 1427
M-M-R II (Very rare) 1494
M-R-VAX II (Rare) 1496
Mumpsvax (Very rare) 1513
Solganal Suspension 2122
Vira-A for Injection 1766

Encephalopathy

Anafranil Capsules (Infrequent) 650
Bumex (0.6%) 1895
Ceptaz for Injection (Fewer than 1%) 1057
Diphtheria and Tetanus Toxoids and Pertussis Vaccine Adsorbed USP (For Pediatric Use) 892
Ergamisol Tablets (Less frequent) 1136
Garamycin Injectable 2093
Lariam Tablets 1904
M-M-R II (Very rare) 1494
M-R-VAX II (Once for every million doses) 1496
Methotrexate Tablets, Parenteral, LPF Parenteral 1217
Midamor Tablets (Between 1% and 3%) 1508
Moduretic Tablets 1510
Netromycin Injection 100 mg/ml 2104
Orthoclone OKT3 Sterile Solution 1645
Primaxin I.M. 1532
Primaxin I.V. (Less than 0.2%) 1535
Rheumatrex Methotrexate Dose Pack 1234
Roferon-A Injection (Less than 1%) 1916
Tapazole Tablets (Rare) 1298
Tri-Immunol Diphtheria & Tetanus Toxoids & Pertussis Vaccine, Adsorbed (Rare) 1241
Zovirax Sterile Powder (Approximately 1%) 828

Encephalopathy, hepatic

Eulexin Capsules 2089

Encephalopathy, hypertensive

Combipres Tablets 678
Epogen for Injection 591
Procrit for Injection 1647

Encephalopathy, post-viral

Atgam Sterile Solution (At least 1 patient and less than 5% of total patients) 2320

Encephalopathy, toxic

INH Tablets (Uncommon) 868
Rifamate Capsules (Uncommon) 1347

Endocrine disturbances

Compazine 2201
Permax Tablets (Rare) 1291
Rogaine Topical Solution (0.47%) 2357
Stelazine 2226

Endometrial carcinoma (see under Carcinoma, endometrial)

Endometrial hyperplasia

Anafranil Capsules (Rare) 650
Nolvadex Tablets (Isolated cases) 1102

Endometriosis

Anafranil Capsules (Infrequent) 650

Endometritis

Lippes Loop Intrauterine Double-S 1654
ParaGard T380A Intrauterine Copper Contraceptive 411

Endotracheal tube, reflux into

Exosurf Neonatal for Intratracheal Suspension 765
Survanta Beractant Intratracheal Suspension 1978

Energy, loss of

▲ Lozol Tablets (Greater than or equal to 5%) 1843
Micronor Tablets 1667
▲ Minipress Capsules (6.9%) 1778
▲ Minizide Capsules (6.9%) 1779
Modicon 1667
Ortho-Novum 1667
▲ Trexan Tablets (Greater than 10%) 937

Enteritis

Anafranil Capsules (Rare) 650
▲ Sterile FUDR (Among more common) 1898
Lamprene Capsules (Less than 1%) 1030
Lincocin 2344
Methotrexate Tablets, Parenteral, LPF Parenteral 1217
Prozac Pulvules (Rare) 920
Rheumatrex Methotrexate Dose Pack 1234

Enteritis, hemorrhagic

Methotrexate Tablets, Parenteral, LPF Parenteral 1217
Rheumatrex Methotrexate Dose Pack 1234

Enteritis, staphylococci

Furoxone 1855

Enterocolitis

Achromycin V Capsules 1193
Augmentin Tablets, Powder for Oral Suspension, and Chewable Tablets 2198
Chloromycetin Kapseals 1695
Chloromycetin Palmitate, Oral Suspension 1697
Chloromycetin Sodium Succinate 1698
Declomycin Capsules, Tablets 1199
Doryx Capsules 1717
Indocin I.V. (Less than 3%) 1490
Minocin Intravenous 1221
Minocin Oral Suspension 1224
Minocin Pellet-Filled Capsules 1222
Monodox Capsules 1630
Myochrysine Injection (Rare) 1516
ProSom Tablets (Rare) 554
Spectrobid Tablets & Powder for Oral Suspension 1961
Terramycin Capsules 1786
Terramycin Intramuscular Solution 1964
Unasyn 1965
Vibramycin Hyclate Capsules 1787
Vibramycin Hyclate Intravenous 1968
Vibramycin 1787

Enterocolitis, hemorrhagic

Velban Vials 1305

Enterocolitis, necrotizing

▲ Exosurf Neonatal for Intratracheal Suspension (Up to 6%) 765
▲ Survanta Beractant Intratracheal Suspension (6.1%) 1978

Enterocolitis, ulcerative

Ridaura Capsules (Less than 1%) 2224
Solganal Suspension (Rare) 2122

Entropion

Idamycin for Injection (Rare) 564
Oculinum for Injecton (Less than 1%) 587

Enuresis

BuSpar (Rare) 1401
Klonopin Tablets 1902
Lioresal Tablets (Rare) 1031
Mintezol 1510
Serentil 686
Wellbutrin Tablets (Rare) 821

Eosinophilia

Achromycin V Capsules 1193
Altace Capsules (Scattered incidents) 1086
Amikin Injectable (Rare) 602
Amoxil 2193
Anaprox and Anaprox DS Tablets (Less than 1%) 2288
Ancef Injection 2194
Ancobon Capsules 1886
Ansaid Tablets (Less than 1%) 2319
Apresazide Capsules (Less frequent) 854
Apresoline Hydrochloride Tablets (Less frequent) 855
Apresoline-Esidrix Tablets 857
Asendin Tablets (Very rare) 1196
Atgam Sterile Solution (Less than 5%) 2320
Atromid-S Capsules 2435
Augmentin Tablets, Powder for Oral Suspension, and Chewable Tablets 2198
Axid Pulvules (Rare) 1246
Azactam for Injection 2252
Azo Gantanol Tablets 1887
Azo Gantrisin Tablets 1888
Azulfidine Tablets, EN-tabs, Oral Suspension (Rare) 1157
Bactrim DS Tablets 1891
Bactrim I.V. Infusion 1889
Bactrim 1891
Beclovent Inhalation Aerosol and Refill 572
Bicillin C-R Injection 2438
Bicillin C-R 900/300 Injection 2440
Bicillin L-A Injection 2442
BuSpar (Rare) 1401
Butazolidin Capsules & Tablets 1027
Capastat Sulfate Vials 1250
▲ Capoten (About 4 to 7 of 100 patients) 2255
▲ Capozide (4 to 7 of 100 patients) 2258
Ceclor Pulvules & Suspension (1 in 50) 1251
▲ Cefizox Injection (1 to 5%) 1012
▲ Cefobid Intravenous/Intramuscular (1 in 10) 1943
▲ Cefobid Pharmacy Bulk Package - Not for Direct Infusion (1 in 10) 1945
Cefotan (1 in 200) 2265
Ceftin Tablets (1.1%) 575
Celontin 1692
Ceptaz for Injection (One in 13) 1057
CHEMET (succimer) Capsules (0.5 to 1.5%) 1361
Children's Advil Suspension (Less than 1%) 2426
▲ Cipro I.V. (Among most frequent) 1592
Cipro Tablets (0.6%) 1589
Claforan Sterile Injection (2.4%) 1089
Cleocin Pediatric Flavored Granules 2324
Cleocin Phosphate Injection 2325
Clinoril Tablets (Less than 1 in 100) 1433
Clozaril Tablets (1%) 2000
Compazine 2201
Cuprimine Capsules 1442
Cytosar-U Sterile Powder (Less than 7 patients) 2329
Cytovene Sterile Powder (1% or less) 2292
Danocrine Capsules 2046
Declomycin Capsules, Tablets 1199
Demser Capsules (Rare) 1460
Depakene Capsules & Syrup 511
Depakote 512
Depen Titratable Tablets 2379
Deprol Tablets 2382
Diabinese Tablets 1775
Dilantin Infatabs 1710
Dilantin Kapseals 1708
Dilantin-30 Pediatric/Dilantin-125 Suspension 1713
Dilantin with Phenobarbital Kapseals 1715
Dipentum Capsules (Rare) 1160
Dobutrex Solution Vials (Occasionally) 1259
Dolobid Tablets (Less than 1 in 100) 1465
Doryx Capsules 1717
Efudex 1880
Elavil 2269
Eminase (Occasional) 2211
Endep Tablets 1927
Equagesic Tablets 2451
Etrafon 2087
Fansidar Tablets 1896
Feldene Capsules (1 to 3%) 1777

Flexeril Tablets (Rare) ... 1471
Floxin Tablets (More than or equal to 1.0%) ... 1652
▲Fortaz (1 in 13) ... 1060
Fungizone Intravenous ... 2262
Gantanol ... 1899
Gantrisin ... 1901
Garamycin Injectable ... 2093
Geocillin Tablets ... 1951
INH Tablets ... 868
Intal Capsules (Less than 1 in 100,000 patients) ... 978
Intal Inhaler (Infrequent) ... 979
Intal Nebulizer Solution (Rare) ... 980
Keflex Pulvules, Oral Suspension & Pediatric Drops ... 916
Keftab Tablets ... 917
▲Kefurox Vials, Faspak & ADD-Vantage (1 in 14) ... 1277
Kefzol Vials, Faspak & ADD-Vantage ... 1279
Klonopin Tablets ... 1902
Lamprene Capsules (Less than 1%) ... 1030
Limbitrol ... 1933
Lopid Capsules and Tablets ... 1736
Lorelco Tablets ... 1333
Lotensin Tablets (Scattered incidents) ... 872
Ludiomil Tablets ... 874
Macrodantin Capsules (Less often) 1624
Mandol Vials, Faspak & ADD-Vantage ... 1281
Matulane Capsules ... 1907
Meclomen Capsules (Less than 1%) ... 1739
Mefoxin ... 1498
Mefoxin Premixed Intravenous Solution ... 1500
Mellaril ... 2011
Mesantoin Tablets ... 2013
Mezlin ... 1597
Mezlin Pharmacy Bulk Package ... 1599
Miltown Tablets ... 2386
Minocin Intravenous ... 1221
Minocin Oral Suspension ... 1224
Minocin Pellet-Filled Capsules ... 1222
Monocid Injection (2.9%) ... 2217
Monodox Capsules ... 1630
Monopril Tablets (2 patients) ... 1406
Motrin Tablets (Less than 1%) ... 2351
Myochrysine Injection ... 1516
Naprosyn (Less than 1%) ... 2297
Navane Capsules and Concentrate 1954
Navane Intramuscular ... 1956
Nebcin Vials, Hyporets & ADD-Vantage ... 1286
NebuPent for Inhalation Solution (1% or less) ... 1017
NegGram ... 2062
Netromycin Injection 100 mg/ml (4 of 1000 patients) ... 2104
Noroxin Tablets (1.8%) ... 1519
Norpramin Tablets ... 1340
Norzine ... 1818
PMB 200 and PMB 400 ... 2504
Pamelor ... 2019
Paradione Capsules ... 548
PediaProfen Suspension (Less than 1%) ... 1363
Permax Tablets (Rare) ... 1291
Pipracil ... 1230
Ponstel (Occasional) ... 1758
Primaxin I.M. ... 1532
Primaxin I.V. (Less than 0.2%) ... 1535
Procan SR Tablets ... 1760
Proglycem ... 649
Prolixin Elixir ... 1793
Prolixin Enanthate ... 1796
Prolixin Injection ... 1791
Prolixin Oral Concentrate ... 1792
Prolixin Tablets ... 1793
Quadrinal Tablets ... 1183
Rifadin (Occasional) ... 1345
Rifamate Capsules ... 1347
Rimactane Capsules ... 879
▲Rocephin Injectable Vials, ADD-Vantage (6%) ... 1914
Rufen Tablets (Less than 1%) ... 691
Sansert Tablets ... 2031
Septra ... 813
Septra I.V. Infusion ... 808
Septra I.V. Infusion ADD-Vantage Vials ... 810
Septra ... 813
Ser-Ap-Es Tablets ... 881
Serentil ... 686
Serpasil-Apresoline Tablets ... 884
Sinequan (A few patients) ... 1960
Solganal Suspension (Rare) ... 2122
Soma Compound w/Codeine Tablets ... 2390
Soma Compound Tablets ... 2389
Soma Tablets ... 2388
Spectrobid Tablets & Powder for Oral Suspension ... 1961
Stelazine ... 2226
Suprax (Less than 2%) ... 1235
Surmontil Capsules ... 2524
▲Synarel Nasal Solution (10% to 15%) ... 2300
Talacen (Rare) ... 2070
Talwin Injection (Rare) ... 2071
Talwin Compound ... 2072
Talwin Injection (Rare) ... 2071
Talwin Nx (Rare) ... 2073
Tao Capsules ... 1963
Taractan (Very rare) ... 1920
▲Tazicef for Injection (1 in 13 patients) ... 2231
▲Tazidime Vials, Faspak & ADD-Vantage (1 in 13) ... 1299
Tegretol Chewable Tablets ... 654
Tegretol Suspension ... 656
Tegretol Tablets ... 654
Terramycin Capsules ... 1786
Terramycin Intramuscular Solution 1964
Thorazine ... 2234
Ticar for Injection ... 2236
Timentin for Injection ... 2239
Tofranil Ampuls ... 1038
Tofranil Tablets ... 1039
Tofranil-PM Capsules ... 1041
Tonocard Tablets (Less than 1%) .. 1554
Torecan ... 1993
Triavil Tablets ... 1556
Tridione ... 557
Trilafon ... 2123
Unasyn ... 1965
Urispas Tablets ... 2242
Vancocin HCl, Oral Solution & Pulvules ... 1304
Vancocin HCl, Vials & ADD-Vantage ... 1302
Vaseretic Tablets ... 1559
Vasotec I.V. ... 1562
Vasotec Tablets ... 1564
Velosef Capsules and for Oral Suspension ... 606
Vibramycin Hyclate Capsules ... 1787
Vibramycin Hyclate Intravenous ... 1968
Vibramycin ... 1787
Vivactil Tablets ... 1567
Voltaren Tablets ... 1042
Wellbutrin Tablets ... 821
▲Xanax Tablets (3.2% to 9.5%) ... 2367
Zantac Injection and Zantac Injection Premixed ... 1063
Zantac (Rare) ... 1065
Zarontin Capsules ... 1768
Zarontin Syrup ... 1769
Zefazone Sterile Powder ... 2372
▲Zinacef (1 in 14 patients) ... 1066
Zyloprim Tablets (Less than 1%) ... 830

Eosinophilia, myoclonus

Tegretol Chewable Tablets ... 654
Tegretol Suspension ... 656
Tegretol Tablets ... 654

Eosinophilia, peripheral

Tegretol Chewable Tablets ... 654
Tegretol Suspension ... 656
Tegretol Tablets ... 654

Eosinophilia, pulmonary

Daraprim Tablets (Rare) ... 761

Eosinophilic pneumonitis

Anaprox and Anaprox DS Tablets (Less than 1%) ... 2288
Capoten ... 2255
Capozide ... 2258
Naprosyn (Less than 1%) ... 2297
NebuPent for Inhalation Solution (1% or less) ... 1017

Epidermal necrolysis (see also under Necrolysis, epidermal)

Aldoclor Tablets ... 1413
Aldomet Ester HCl Injection ... 1417
Aldomet Oral ... 1415
Aldoril Tablets ... 1418
Bactrim DS Tablets (Rare) ... 1891
Bactrim I.V. Infusion (Rare) ... 1889
Bactrim (Rare) ... 1891
Clinoril Tablets (Less than 1%) ... 1433
Cuprimine Capsules ... 1442
Diamox ... 1200
Dilantin Parenteral ... 1712
Fansidar Tablets ... 1896
Gantanol ... 1899
Gantrisin ... 1901
Keflex Pulvules, Oral Suspension & Pediatric Drops (Rare) ... 916
Keftab Tablets (Rare) ... 917
Naprosyn (Rare) ... 2297
Neptazane Tablets ... ⊙ 311
Septra DS Tablets ... 813
Tagamet (Very rare) ... 2228
Talacen (Rare) ... 2070
Talwin Injection (Rare) ... 2071
Talwin Compound ... 2072
Talwin Injection ... 2071
Tenoretic Tablets ... 1105
Thalitone Tablets ... 687
Thiosulfil Forte Tablets ... 2526
Trancopal Caplets (Rare) ... 2075
Vasotec I.V. ... 1562

Epidermolysis bullosa

Anaprox and Anaprox DS Tablets ... 2288
Naprosyn ... 2297

Epididymitis

Anadrol-50 Tablets ... 2287
Anafranil Capsules (Infrequent) ... 650
Cordarone Tablets (Rare) ... 2446
Permax Tablets (Rare) ... 1291
Prozac Pulvules (Rare) ... 920
Rogaine Topical Solution (0.91%) .. 2357
Winstrol Tablets ... 2075

Epigastric pain (see under Distress, epigastric)

Epilation

Colchicine Ampoules ... 1252
Velban Vials ... 1305

Epilepsy, aggravation

Indocin Capsules (Less than 1%) ... 1487
Indocin I.V. (Less than 1%) ... 1490
Indocin (Less than 1%) ... 1487

Epileptiform movements, unspecified

Clozaril Tablets (Less than 1%) ... 2000

Epinephrine effect, reversal

Compazine ... 2201
Etrafon ... 2087
Stelazine ... 2226
Taractan Concentrate ... 1920
Triavil Tablets ... 1556

Epiphyseal closure

Anadrol-50 Tablets ... 2287
Estratest ... 2245
Winstrol Tablets ... 2075

Epistaxis

▲Accutane Capsules (80%) ... 1878
Activase (Less than 1%) ... 1047
AeroBid Inhaler System (1-3%) ... 995
Alferon N Injection (1%) ... 1809
Altace Capsules (Less than 1%) ... 1086
Anafranil Capsules (Up to 2%) ... 650
Ansaid Tablets (Less than 1%) ... 2319
Atgam Sterile Solution (Less than 5%) ... 2320
Beconase AQ Nasal Spray (Fewer than 3 per 100 patients) ... 574
Beconase Inhalation Aerosol & Refill (Less than 2 in 100 patients) ... 574
BuSpar (Rare) ... 1401
Cardizem Tablets-30 mg, 60 mg, 90 mg and 120 mg (Less than 1%) ... 1329
Cardizem SR Capsules-60 mg, 90 mg and 120 mg (Less than 1%) 1327
Cardura Tablets (1%) ... 1941
Children's Advil Suspension (Less than 1%) ... 2426
Cipro I.V. (1% or less) ... 1592
Cipro Tablets (Less than 1%) ... 1589
Clinoril Tablets (Less than 1%) ... 1433
Clozaril Tablets (Less than 1%) ... 2000
Coumadin Injection & Tablets ... 944
Cytotec (Infrequent) ... 2159
DDAVP (Up to 3%) ... 1841
Decadron Phosphate Turbinaire ... 1456
Diupres Tablets ... 1461
Eminase (Less than 1%) ... 2211
Ergamisol Tablets (Up to 1%) ... 1136
Sterile FUDR (Remote possibility) .. 1898
Feldene Capsules (Less than 1%) .. 1777
Fiorinal with Codeine Capsules ... 2008
Fluorouracil Injection ... 1897
Hismanal Tablets (Less frequent) ... 1138
Hydropres Tablets ... 1485
Hytrin Tablets (At least 1%) ... 529
Indocin Capsules (Less than 1%) ... 1487
Indocin I.V. (Less than 1%) ... 1490
Indocin (Less than 1%) ... 1487
Intal Inhaler (Rare) ... 979
Intal Nebulizer Solution ... 980
Intron A (Up to 3%) ... 2097
Kerlone Tablets (Less than 2%) ... 2172
Matulane Capsules ... 1907
Methotrexate Tablets, Parenteral, LPF Parenteral (Less common) ... 1217
Minipress Capsules (1-4%) ... 1778
Minizide Capsules ... 1779
Mithracin ... 1602
Monopril Tablets (0.2 to 1.0%) ... 1406
Motrin Tablets (Less than 1%) ... 2351
Mykrox ½ mg Tablets (Less than 2%) ... 984
Nasacort Nasal Inhaler (Less than 5%) ... 1844
Nasalcrom Nasal Solution (Less than 1%) ... 986
Nasalide Nasal Solution 0.025% (5% or less) ... 2299
OptiPranolol Sterile Ophthalmic Solution (A small number of patients) ... ⊙ 261
Orudis Capsules (Less than 1%) ... 2488
Paradione Capsules ... 548
PediaProfen Suspension (Less than 1%) ... 1363
Permax Tablets (1.6%) ... 1291
Plendil Extended-Release Tablets (0.5% to 1.5%) ... 1526
Prilosec Delayed-Release Capsules (Less than 1%) ... 1530
Procardia XL Tablets (1% or less) .. 1783
ProSom Tablets (Rare) ... 554
Proventil Syrup (1 of 100) ... 2119
Prozac Pulvules (Infrequent) ... 920
Raudixin Tablets ... 1803
Rauzide Tablets ... 1804
Retrovir Capsules (Less than 5%) .. 802
Retrovir I.V. Infusion (Less than 5%) ... 805
Retrovir Syrup (Less than 5%) ... 802
Rheumatrex Methotrexate Dose Pack (Less common) ... 1234
Rocephin Injectable Vials, ADD-Vantage (Rare) ... 1914
Roferon-A Injection (Rare) ... 1916
Rufen Tablets (Less than 1%) ... 691
Salutensin/Salutensin-Demi ... 719
Seldane Tablets (0.7%) ... 1349
Seldane-D Extended-Release Tablets ... 1350
Ser-Ap-Es Tablets ... 881
Serpasil Tablets ... 883
Serpasil-Apresoline Tablets ... 884
Serpasil-Esidrix Tablets ... 886
▲Tegison Capsules (25-50%) ... 1881
Tolectin (200, 400 and 600 mg) (Less than 1%) ... 1379
Trental (Less than 1%) ... 1099
Trexan Tablets (Less than 1%) ... 937
Tridione ... 557
Trilisate (Less than 1%) ... 1822
Unasyn (Less than 1%) ... 1965
Vancenase AQ Nasal Spray 0.042% (Fewer than 3 per 100 patients) ... 2127
Vancenase Nasal Inhaler (2 per 100 patients) ... 2126
Ventolin (2% to 3%) ... 583
Voltaren Tablets (Less than 1%) ... 1042
Wellbutrin Tablets (Rare) ... 821
Zefazone Sterile Powder ... 2372
Zyloprim Tablets (Less than 1%) ... 830

Epithelial cells, atypical

▲Blenoxane (10%) ... 724
Cytoxan for Injection ... 726
Neosar for Injection ... 566

Epithelial punctate, staining

Profenal Sterile Ophthalmic Solution (Less than 0.5%) ... ⊙ 234

Equilibrium, dysfunction

Calan SR Caplets (1% or less) ... 2157
Calan Tablets (1% or less) ... 2155
Isoptin Oral Tablets (Less than 1%) ... 1179
Isoptin SR Sustained Release Tablets (Less than 1%) ... 1181
Lariam Tablets ... 1904
Restoril Capsules (Less than 1%) .. 2023
Tegison Capsules (Less than 1%) .. 1881

Transderm Scōp Transdermal Therapeutic System (Few patients) 887
Verelan Capsules (Less than 1%) 1243

Erection disturbances
Aldactazide 2150
Aldactone 2152
Bumex (0.1%) 1895
Dantrium Capsules (Less frequent) 1619
Desyrel and Desyrel Dividose 1404
Wellbutrin Tablets (Infrequent) 821
Winstrol Tablets 2075
▲Zoladex (18%) 1110

Ergotism
Cafergot/Cafergot P-B (Rare) 1999
Ergotrate Maleate Ampoules 1263
Parlodel (Rare) 2020

Erosion, genital
▲Condylox (67%) 1630

Eructation
Anafranil Capsules (Up to 2%) 650
Arfonad Ampuls 1887
Clozaril Tablets (Less than 1%) 2000
Colestid Granules (1 in 30 to 1 in 100 patients) 2328
Dolobid Tablets (Less than 1 in 100) 1465
Duvoid Tablets 1853
Intron A (Less than 5%) 2097
Lodine Capsules (Less than 1%) 2468
▲Nicorette (6%) 1335
Orap Tablets 1020
Orudis Capsules (Less than 1%) 2488
Permax Tablets (Infrequent) 1291
Prozac Pulvules (Infrequent) 920
Retrovir Capsules (Less than 5%) 802
Retrovir I.V. Infusion (Less than 5%) 805
Retrovir Syrup (Less than 5%) 802
▲Trental (0.6 to 9%) 1099

Eruptions
Cuprimine Capsules 1442
Diabinese Tablets (Approximately 1% or less) 1775
Monodox Capsules 1630
Norpace (1 to 3%) 2177
Renese-R Tablets 1786
Vibramycin 1787

Eruptions, acneiform (see under Acneiform eruptions)

Eruptions, bullous
ERYC 1720
Eulexin Capsules 2089
Loniten Tablets (Rare) 2346
Lozol Tablets 1843
▲Tegison Capsules (1-10%) 1881
Voltaren Tablets (Rare) 1042
Yodoxin 1072

Eruptions, cutaneous
Aldactazide 2150
Aldactone 2152
Dilantin with Phenobarbital Kapseals 1715
Seldane-D Extended-Release Tablets 1350

Eruptions, eczematoid (see under Eczema)

Eruptions, erythema annulare centrifugum
Plaquenil Sulfate Tablets 2067

Eruptions, erythematous
Aldactazide 2150
Aldactone 2152
Macrodantin Capsules 1624

Eruptions, exfoliative
INH Tablets 868
Quinidex Extentabs 1868

Eruptions, fixed drug
Depen Titratable Tablets 2379
Deprol Tablets 2382
Equagesic Tablets 2451
Miltown Tablets 2386
PMB 200 and PMB 400 2504
Soma Compound w/Codeine Tablets 2390
Soma Compound Tablets 2389
Soma Tablets 2388

Eruptions, hemorrhagic
Amen 833
Brevicon 2304
Cycrin Tablets 2449
Demulen 2161
Depo-Provera Sterile Aqueous Suspension 2336
Diethylstilbestrol Tablets 1258
Enovid 2161
Estinyl Tablets 2085
Estradurin 2452
Estratest 2245
Estrovis 1721
Jenest-28 Tablets 1636
Levlen/Tri-Levlen 665
Lo/Ovral Tablets 2471
Lo/Ovral-28 Tablets 2476
Loestrin 1728
Mediatric Capsules 2476
Menrium Tablets 1934
Micronor Tablets 1667
Modicon 1667
Nordette-21 Tablets 2481
Nordette-28 Tablets 2483
Norethin 2133
Norinyl 2304
Norlestrin 1746
Norlutate 1754
Norlutin 1755
Nor-Q D Tablets 2304
Ogen 540
Ortho Diaphragm Kit 1664
Ortho Dienestrol Cream 1664
Ortho-Cyclen Tablets 1658
Ortho-Novum 1667
Ovral Tablets 2490
Ovral-28 Tablets 2491
Ovrette Tablets 2492
PMB 200 and PMB 400 2504
Premarin Intravenous 2508
Premarin with Methyltestosterone 2515
Premarin Tablets 2510
Premarin Vaginal Cream 2512
Provera Tablets 2356
Stilphostrol Tablets and Ampuls 1609
TACE 12 and 25 mg 1353
Levlen/Tri-Levlen 665
Tri-Norinyl 2304
Triphasil-21 Tablets 2527
Triphasil-28 Tablets 2532

Eruptions, herpetic
▲CHEMET (succimer) Capsules (2.6 to 11.2%) 1361

Eruptions, lichenoid
Plaquenil Sulfate Tablets 2067

Eruptions, maculopapular
Aldactazide 2150
Aldactone 2152
Bicillin C-R Injection 2438
Bicillin C-R 900/300 Injection 2440
Bicillin L-A Injection 2442
DiaBeta (1.5%) 1091
Glucotrol (1 in 70) 1952
Haldol Decanoate 1375
Haldol Injection, Tablets and Concentrate 1373
INH Tablets 868
Macrodantin Capsules 1624
Micronase Tablets 2350
Mustargen (Occasional) 1514
Orinase Tablets 2354
Pfizerpen for Injection 1957
Pfizerpen-AS Aqueous Suspension 1959
Plaquenil Sulfate Tablets 2067
Tolinase Tablets (0.4%) 2365
Wycillin Injection 2537

Eruptions, morbilliform
Ceclor Pulvules & Suspension (1 in 100) 1251
DiaBeta (1.5%) 1091
Glucotrol (1 in 70) 1952
INH Tablets 868
Micronase Tablets 2350
Mysoline 2480
Paradione Capsules 548
Plaquenil Sulfate Tablets 2067
Tolinase Tablets (0.4%) 2365

Eruptions, mucocutaneous
▲CHEMET (succimer) Capsules (2.6 to 11.2%) 1361

Eruptions, purpuric
INH Tablets 868
Plaquenil Sulfate Tablets 2067

Eruptions, vascular
Pipracil (Less frequent) 1230

Erythema
A/T/S Topical Gel and Topical Solution 1089
Accutane Capsules (Less than 1 in 10) 1878
Aclovate (1 in 100 patients) 1053
Adriamycin RDF 562
Americaine Anesthetic Lubricant 972
Americaine Otic Topical Anesthetic Ear Drops 973
Anaprox and Anaprox DS Tablets 2288
Ativan Injection 2432
Bactroban Ointment (Less than 1%) 2200
Benzamycin Topical Gel 907
Betoptic Sterile Ophthalmic Solution (Small numbers of patients) 569
Betoptic S Sterile Ophthalmic Suspension (Small numbers of patients) 570
Biavax ‖ 1427
▲Blenoxane (50%) 724
Brevibloc Injection (Less than 1%) 942
Brevital Sodium Vials 1248
Brevoxyl Gel 2264
Calcimar Injection, Synthetic 1839
Calciparine Injection 925
Carbocaine Hydrochloride Injection 2043
▲Catapres-TTS (26 of 101 patients) 677
Ceftin Tablets 575
Cerumenex Drops (1% of 2,700 patients) 1813
Cholera Vaccine 2445
Cipro I.V. (1% or less) 1592
Cleocin T Topical 2327
Clozaril Tablets (Less than 1%) 2000
Collagenase Santyl Ointment 1172
Compazine 2201
Cortone Acetate Sterile Suspension 1437
Cortone Acetate Tablets 1439
Cosmegen Injection 1440
Cutivate Ointment 0.005% (Less than 1%) 1054
Dalalone D.P. Injectable 999
Dalgan Injection (Less than 1%) 620
Dantrium Intravenous (Rare) 1620
Debrisan 1150
Decadron Elixir 1445
Decadron Phosphate Injection 1449
Decadron Phosphate Respihaler 1454
Decadron Phosphate Turbinaire 1456
Decadron Phosphate with Xylocaine Injection, Sterile 1451
Decadron Tablets 1447
Decadron-LA Sterile Suspension 1457
Depo-Provera Sterile Aqueous Suspension 2336
Desferal Vials 862
Desquam-E Gel 2397
Desquam-X Gel 2397
Desquam-X 5 Wash 2397
Desquam-X 10 Bar 2397
Desquam-X 10 Wash 2397
DiaBeta (1.5%) 1091
Digibind (One patient) 762
Dipentum Capsules (Rare) 1160
Diphtheria & Tetanus Toxoids, Adsorbed Purogenated (Mild) 1202
Diphtheria and Tetanus Toxoids and Pertussis Vaccine Adsorbed USP (For Pediatric Use) 892
Diprivan Injection (Rare) 2267
Diprolene (Less than 1%) 2083
Duragesic Transdermal System (1% or greater) 1133
ETS-2% 1685
Elimite (permethrin) 5% Cream (1 to 2% or less) 1082
Engerix-B Unit-Dose Vials (Less than 1%) 2213
Erycette (erythromycin 2%) Topical Solution 1678
Etrafon 2087
Eulexin Capsules 2089
Exelderm Cream 1.0% (1%) 2398
▲Sterile FUDR (Among more common) 1898
Feldene Capsules (Less than 1%) 1777
Fiorinal with Codeine Capsules 2008
Fluorouracil Injection 1897
Formalyde-10 Spray 1769
Fungizone Cream, Lotion and Ointment 2261
Gamimune N Immune Globulin Intravenous (Human) (Some cases) 1572
Glucotrol (1 in 70) 1952
G-myticin Creme and Ointment 0.1% 1770
Halotex Cream & Solution (1 in 977 patients) 2400
Heparin Lock Flush Solution 2456
Heparin Sodium Vials 1264
Heparin Sodium Injection 2457
Heparin Sodium Injection, USP, Sterile Solution 2342
▲HibTITER (2.0% to 3.3%) 1206
Hydeltrasol Injection, Sterile 1476
Hydeltra-T.B.A. Sterile Suspension 1478
Hydrocortone Acetate Sterile Suspension 1479
Hydrocortone Phosphate Injection, Sterile 1481
Hydrocortone Tablets 1482
Beef Regular, 100 Units 1275
Intron A (Up to 2%) 2097
▲IPOL Poliovirus Vaccine Inactivated (3.2%) 894
Keralyt Gel 2405
Ketalar 1726
Kutapressin Injection 2146
Lamprene Capsules (Less than 1%) 1030
Lincocin (Rare) 2344
Lotrimin 2102
Lotrisone Cream 2103
Lupron Injection 2310
M-M-R ‖ 1494
M-R-VAX ‖ 1496
Marcaine Hydrochloride with Epinephrine 1:200,000 (Rare) 2055
Marcaine Hydrochloride Injection (Rare) 2055
Marcaine Spinal (Rare) 2058
Medrol 2348
Mellaril 2011
Meruvax ‖ 1503
MetroGel (Less than 2%) 903
Metubine Iodide Vials 1285
Micro-Guard Cream, Antiseptic, Antifungal Skin Cream (Occasional) 2286
Micronase Tablets (1.5%) 2350
Mini-Gamulin Rh, Rh_o(D) Immune Globulin (Human) (Occasional) 612
Minocin Oral Suspension 1224
Monocid Injection (Less than 1%) 2217
Mutamycin 733
Mycelex 1% Cream and Topical Solution 1% 1604
Mycelex-G 1% Vaginal Cream (0.5%) 1605
Naftin Cream 1% (2%) 1084
Naftin Gel 1% (0.5%) 1084
NebuPent for Inhalation Solution (1% or less) 1017
NegGram 2062
Nescaine/Nescaine MPF 629
Neutrogena Melanex Topical Solution 1618
Nicorette 1335
Nolvadex Tablets 1102
Noroxin Tablets (Less frequent) 1519
Norzine 1818
Orinase Tablets (1.1%) 2354
Oxistat Cream (0.2%) 1055
Oxsoralen-Ultra Capsule 1117
Paraplatin for Injection 735
PedvaxHIB 1521
Pipracil (2%) 1230
▲Plague Vaccine (10%) 1584
Plendil Extended-Release Tablets (0.5% to 1.5%) 1526
▲Pneumovax 23 (Common) 1528
Pre-Pen 2148
Primaxin I.V. (0.4%) 1535
ProHIBiT Haemophilus b Conjugate Vaccine (Diphtheria Toxoid Conjugate) (2.9%) 896
Prolixin Decanoate 1795
Prolixin Elixir 1793
Prolixin Enanthate 1796
Prolixin Injection 1791
Prolixin Oral Concentrate 1792
Prolixin Tablets 1793
Provera Tablets 2356
Recombivax HB (Equal to or greater than 1%) 1544
Retin-A (tretinoin) Cream/Gel/Liquid 1680
Rogaine Topical Solution 2357
Sandostatin Injection (1.0%) 2029
Sensorcaine (Rare) 631
Sensorcaine-MPF Spinal (Rare) 634

Serentil ... 686
Solganal Suspension ... 2122
▲Spectazole (econazole nitrate) Cream (3%) ... 1681
Stelazine ... 2226
Sufenta Injection (Less than 1%) ... 1147
T-Stat 2.0% Topical Solution and Pads ... 2409
Taractan ... 1920
Tegretol ... 654
Temaril Tablets, Syrup and Spansule Sustained Release Capsules ... 1085
Temovate (1 of 366 patients) ... 1056
Tenuate ... 1354
Tetanus Toxoid, Adsorbed Purogenated ... 1238
Theramycin Z Topical Solution 2% ... 1410
Theroxide ... 1411
Tolinase Tablets (0.4%) ... 2365
Torecan ... 1993
Tracrium Injection (0.6%) ... 817
Trandate HCT/Trandate ... 579
Transderm Scōp Transdermal Therapeutic System (Infrequent) ... 887
Triavil Tablets ... 1556
Trilafon ... 2123
Ultravate Cream 0.05% (Less frequent) ... 2410
Ultravate Ointment 0.05% (Less frequent) ... 2411
Unasyn (Less than 1%) ... 1965
▲Yutopar (10 to 15% with IV administration) ... 647
Zefazone Sterile Powder ... 2372

Erythema at injection site

▲Actimmune (14%) ... 1046
Attenuvax ... 1424
DDAVP Injection (Occasional) ... 1840

Erythema, conjunctival

▲AK-Poly-Bac Ointment (Among most frequent) ... ◉ 205
▲AK-Spore H.C. (Among most often) ... ◉ 206
▲AK-Spore (Among most frequent) ... ◉ 205
FML Forte Liquifilm ... ◉ 245
▲Rēv-Eyes Ophthalmic Eyedrops 0.5% (10% to 40%) ... ◉ 312
TobraDex Ophthalmic Suspension and Ointment (Less than 4%) ... ◉ 228
Tobrex Ophthalmic Ointment and Solution (Less than 3 in 100 patients) ... 572

Erythema, facial

Aristospan Suspension (Intra-articular) ... 1011
Celestone Soluspan Suspension ... 2081
Cortenema ... 2244
Deltasone Tablets ... 2332
Depo-Medrol Sterile Aqueous Suspension ... 2334
Hydrea Capsules ... 728
Kenalog-10 Injection ... 2402
Kenalog-40 Injection ... 2403
Normodyne Tablets ... 2110
Normozide Tablets ... 2112
Pediapred Oral Liquid ... 987
Solu-Cortef Sterile Powder ... 2361
Solu-Medrol Sterile Powder ... 2363
Trandate HCT/Trandate ... 579

Erythema, hemorrhagic exudative (see under Henoch-Schonlein purpura)

Erythema, maculopapular

Deprol Tablets ... 2382
Teslac Tablets ... 741

Erythema multiforme

Aldactazide ... 2150
Amen ... 833
Anaprox and Anaprox DS Tablets (Rare) ... 2288
Attenuvax (Rare) ... 1424
Augmentin Tablets, Powder for Oral Suspension, and Chewable Tablets ... 2198
Azactam for Injection (Less than 1%) ... 2252
Azo Gantanol Tablets ... 1887
Azo Gantrisin Tablets ... 1888
Azulfidine Tablets, EN-tabs, Oral Suspension (Rare) ... 1157
Bactrim DS Tablets ... 1891
Bactrim I.V. Infusion ... 1889
Bactrim ... 1891
Biavax II (Rare) ... 1427
Brevicon ... 2304
Butazolidin Capsules & Tablets (Less than 1%) ... 1027
Calan SR Caplets (1% or less) ... 2157
Calan Tablets (1% or less) ... 2155
Capoten ... 2255
Capozide ... 2258
Cardizem Tablets-30 mg, 60 mg, 90 mg and 120 mg (Infrequent) 1329
Cardizem SR Capsules-60 mg, 90 mg and 120 mg (Infrequent) ... 1327
Ceclor Pulvules & Suspension ... 1251
Ceftin Tablets ... 575
Ceptaz for Injection ... 1057
Children's Advil Suspension (Less than 1%) ... 2426
Cipro I.V. (1% or less) ... 1592
Cipro Tablets ... 1589
Cleocin HCl Capsules (Rare) ... 2322
Cleocin Pediatric Flavored Granules (Rare) ... 2324
Cleocin Phosphate Injection (Rare) 2325
Clinoril Tablets (Less than 1%) ... 1433
Cycrin Tablets ... 2449
Decadron Phosphate with Xylocaine Injection, Sterile ... 1451
Demulen ... 2161
Depakene Capsules & Syrup ... 511
Depakote ... 512
Deprol Tablets (Rare) ... 2382
Diabinese Tablets ... 1775
Diamox ... 1200
Diethylstilbestrol Tablets ... 1258
Dolobid Tablets (Less than 1 in 100) ... 1465
Engerix-B Unit-Dose Vials ... 2213
Enovid ... 2161
Estinyl Tablets ... 2085
Estrace ... 1385
Estrace Vaginal Cream ... 1388
Estradurin ... 2452
Estratest ... 2245
Estrovis ... 1721
Fansidar Tablets ... 1896
Feldene Capsules (Less than 1%) .. 1777
Fiorinal Capsules (Several cases) ... 2007
Fiorinal with Codeine Capsules ... 2008
Fiorinal Tablets (Several cases) ... 2007
Fortaz ... 1060
Gantanol ... 1899
Gantrisin Ophthalmic Ointment/Solution ... 1900
Gantrisin ... 1901
Indocin Capsules (Less than 1%) ... 1487
Indocin I.V. (Less than 1%) ... 1490
Indocin (Less than 1%) ... 1487
Isoptin Oral Tablets (Less than 1%) ... 1179
Isoptin SR Sustained Release Tablets (Less than 1%) ... 1181
Jenest-28 Tablets ... 1636
Keflex Pulvules, Oral Suspension & Pediatric Drops (Rare) ... 916
Keftab Tablets (Rare) ... 917
Kefurox Vials, Faspak & ADD-Vantage ... 1277
Lasix ... 1093
Levlen/Tri-Levlen ... 665
Lo/Ovral Tablets ... 2471
Lo/Ovral-28 Tablets ... 2476
Loestrin ... 1728
M-M-R II (Rare) ... 1494
M-R-VAX II (Rare) ... 1496
Macrodantin Capsules (Rare) ... 1624
Meclomen Capsules (Less than 1%) ... 1739
Mediatric Capsules ... 2476
Menrium Tablets ... 1934
Meruvax II (Rare) ... 1503
Mesantoin Tablets (Rare) ... 2013
Mevacor Tablets ... 1505
Micronor Tablets ... 1667
Milontin Kapseals ... 1741
Miltown Tablets (Rare) ... 2386
Minocin Intravenous ... 1221
Minocin Oral Suspension ... 1224
Minocin Pellet-Filled Capsules ... 1222
Mintezol ... 1510
Modicon ... 1667
Motrin Tablets (Less than 1%) ... 2351
Mumpsvax (Rare) ... 1513
Mustargen ... 1514
Myleran Tablets (Rare) ... 790
Naprosyn (Rare) ... 2297
Neptazane Tablets ... ◉ 311
Nordette-21 Tablets ... 2481
Nordette-28 Tablets ... 2483
Norethin ... 2133
Norinyl ... 2304
Norlestrin ... 1746
Norlutate ... 1754
Norlutin ... 1755
Noroxin Tablets ... 1519
Nor-Q D Tablets ... 2304
Ogen ... 540
Ortho Diaphragm Kit ... 1664
Ortho Dienestrol Cream ... 1664
Ortho-Cyclen Tablets ... 1658
Ortho-Novum ... 1667
Ovcon ... 1391
Ovral Tablets ... 2490
Ovral-28 Tablets ... 2491
Ovrette Tablets ... 2492
PMB 200 and PMB 400 ... 2504
Paradione Capsules ... 548
PediaProfen Suspension (Less than 1%) ... 1363
Pediazole ... 1973
Pipracil (Rare) ... 1230
Premarin Intravenous ... 2508
Premarin with Methyltestosterone .. 2515
Premarin Tablets ... 2510
Premarin Vaginal Cream ... 2512
Primaxin I.M. ... 1532
Primaxin I.V. (Less than 0.2%) ... 1535
Proloprim Tablets (Rare) ... 799
Provera Tablets ... 2356
Prozac Pulvules (Rare) ... 920
Ritalin ... 880
Rocaltrol Capsules (One case) ... 1913
Rufen Tablets (Less than 1%) ... 691
SSD RP Cream (Infrequent) ... 690
Septra ... 813
Septra I.V. Infusion ... 808
Septra I.V. Infusion ADD-Vantage Vials ... 810
Septra ... 813
Silvadene Cream 1% (Infrequent) .. 1352
Soma Compound w/Codeine Tablets ... 2390
Soma Compound Tablets ... 2389
Soma Tablets ... 2388
Spectrobid Tablets & Powder for Oral Suspension ... 1961
Stilphostrol Tablets and Ampuls ... 1609
Suprax (Rare) ... 1235
TACE 12 and 25 mg ... 1353
Tagamet (Very rare) ... 2228
Tegretol Chewable Tablets ... 654
Tegretol Suspension ... 656
Tegretol Tablets ... 654
Thiosulfil Forte Tablets ... 2526
Tolectin (200, 400 and 600 mg) (Less than 1%) ... 1379
Tonocard Tablets (Less than 1%) .. 1554
Trancopal Caplets (Rare) ... 2075
Tridione ... 557
Tri-Immunol Diphtheria & Tetanus Toxoids & Pertussis Vaccine, Adsorbed ... 1241
Levlen/Tri-Levlen ... 665
Trilisate (Rare) ... 1822
Trimpex Tablets (Rare) ... 1922
Tri-Norinyl ... 2304
Triphasil-21 Tablets ... 2527
Triphasil-28 Tablets ... 2532
Unasyn ... 1965
Vaseretic Tablets ... 1559
Vasotec I.V. ... 1562
Vasotec Tablets ... 1564
Verelan Capsules (Less than 1%) .. 1243
Voltaren Tablets (Rare) ... 1042
Zantac Injection and Zantac Injection Premixed (Rare) ... 1063
Zantac ... 1065
Zefazone Sterile Powder ... 2372
Zinacef (Rare) ... 1066
Zyloprim Tablets (Less than 1%) ... 830

Erythema nodosum

Accutane Capsules (Less than 1%) ... 1878
Amen ... 833
Brevicon ... 2304
Butazolidin Capsules & Tablets (Less than 1%) ... 1027
Cipro I.V. (1% or less) ... 1592
Cipro Tablets (Less than 1%) ... 1589
Cycrin Tablets ... 2449
Demulen ... 2161
Diethylstilbestrol Tablets ... 1258
Dipentum Capsules (Rare) ... 1160
Enovid ... 2161
Estradurin ... 2452
Estratest ... 2245
Estrovis ... 1721
Indocin Capsules (Less than 1%) ... 1487
Indocin I.V. (Less than 1%) ... 1490
Indocin (Less than 1%) ... 1487
Jenest-28 Tablets ... 1636
Levlen/Tri-Levlen ... 665
Lo/Ovral Tablets ... 2471
Lo/Ovral-28 Tablets ... 2476
Loestrin ... 1728
Meclomen Capsules (Rare) ... 1739
Mediatric Capsules ... 2476
Menrium Tablets ... 1934
Micronor Tablets ... 1667
Modicon ... 1667
Myleran Tablets (Rare) ... 790
Nordette-21 Tablets ... 2481
Nordette-28 Tablets ... 2483
Norethin ... 2133
Norinyl ... 2304
Norlestrin ... 1746
Norlutate ... 1754
Norlutin ... 1755
Nor-Q D Tablets ... 2304
Ogen ... 540
Ortho Diaphragm Kit ... 1664
Ortho Dienestrol Cream ... 1664
Ortho-Cyclen Tablets ... 1658
Ortho-Novum ... 1667
Ovral Tablets ... 2490
Ovral-28 Tablets ... 2491
Ovrette Tablets ... 2492
PMB 200 and PMB 400 ... 2504
Premarin Intravenous ... 2508
Premarin with Methyltestosterone .. 2515
Premarin Tablets ... 2510
Premarin Vaginal Cream ... 2512
Provera Tablets ... 2356
Recombivax HB (Less than 1%) ... 1544
Stilphostrol Tablets and Ampuls ... 1609
TACE 12 and 25 mg ... 1353
Tegretol Chewable Tablets ... 654
Tegretol Suspension ... 656
Tegretol Tablets ... 654
Levlen/Tri-Levlen ... 665
Tri-Norinyl ... 2304
Triphasil-21 Tablets ... 2527
Triphasil-28 Tablets ... 2532

Erythematous streaking

Doxorubicin Hydrochloride for Injection, USP ... 622
Doxorubicin Hydrochloride Injection, USP ... 848
Rubex ... 739

Erythrocyte survival time, shortened

Easprin ... 1719

Erythrocytes, aggregation on blood smears

Monistat I.V. ... 1143

Erythrocytosis

Danocrine Capsules ... 2046
Pergonal (menotropins for injection, USP) (One patient) ... 2184
Ponstel ... 1758

Erythrocyturia

Asbron G ... 1997
Choledyl SA Tablets ... 1704
Primaxin I.V. ... 1535
Quadrinal Tablets ... 1183
Quibron-T/SR ... 716
Respbid Tablets ... 684
Theo-Dur Sprinkle ... 1168

Erythroderma, exfoliative

Tagamet (Very rare) ... 2228

Erythromelalgia

Adalat Capsules (10 mg and 20 mg) (Less than 0.5%) ... 1587
Parlodel ... 2020
Procardia Capsules (Less than 0.5%) ... 1781

Erythropenia

Accutane Capsules (1 in 5 to 1 in 10) ... 1878
Apresazide Capsules (Less frequent) ... 854
Apresoline-Esidrix Tablets ... 857
Dopram Injectable ... 1860
Loniten Tablets ... 2346
Mustargen ... 1514
Ponstel ... 1758
Primaxin I.M. ... 1532
Ser-Ap-Es Tablets ... 881
Serpasil-Apresoline Tablets ... 884
Unasyn ... 1965
Zefazone Sterile Powder ... 2372

Esophageal disease, unspecified

Ansaid Tablets (Less than 1%) ... 2319

Myleran Tablets 790

Esophageal stricture

Ethamolin (0.1% to 1.3%) 1829
Lodine Capsules (Less than 1%) 2468

Esophageal tearing

Ethamolin (0.1% to 0.4%) 1829

Esophageal ulceration

Cytosar-U Sterile Powder (Less frequent) 2329
Doryx Capsules (Rare) 1717
Ethamolin (2.1%) 1829
Mexitil Capsules (About 1 in 10,000) 680
Micro-K 1863
Micro-K LS Packets 1864
Minocin Pellet-Filled Capsules (Rare) 1222
Pediapred Oral Liquid 987
Slow-K Tablets 2281

Esophagitis

Adriamycin RDF 562
Anafranil Capsules (Up to 1%) 650
Butazolidin Capsules & Tablets (Less than 1%) 1027
Cleocin HCl Capsules 2322
Cosmegen Injection 1440
Cytosar-U Sterile Powder (Less frequent) 2329
Doryx Capsules (Rare) 1717
Doxorubicin Hydrochloride for Injection, USP 622
Doxorubicin Hydrochloride Injection, USP 848
Ethamolin (0.1% to 0.4%) 1829
Fiorinal with Codeine Capsules 2008
Intron A (Less than 1%) 2097
Lodine Capsules (Less than 1%) 2468
Minocin Pellet-Filled Capsules (Rare) 1222
Monodox Capsules (Rare) 1630
NebuPent for Inhalation Solution (1% or less) 1017
Permax Tablets (Infrequent) 1291
Prozac Pulvules (Infrequent) 920
Quinaglute Dura-Tabs Tablets (Rare) 663
▲ Quinidex Extentabs (Among most frequent) 1868
Rubex 739
Rythmol Tablets (1.9%) 1184
Solu-Cortef Sterile Powder 2361
Solu-Medrol Sterile Powder 2363
Terramycin Capsules (Rare) 1786
Trilisate (Rare) 1822
Urobiotic-250 Capsules (Rare) 1968
Vibramycin (Rare) 1787

Esophagitis, ulcerative

Adriamycin PFS 561
Aristocort Suspension 1008
Aristospan Suspension 1011
Celestone Soluspan Suspension 2081
Cortenema 2244
Cortone Acetate Sterile Suspension 1437
Cortone Acetate Tablets 1439
Dalalone D.P. Injectable 999
Decadron Elixir 1445
Decadron Phosphate Injection 1449
Decadron Phosphate Respihaler 1454
Decadron Phosphate Turbinaire 1456
Decadron Phosphate with Xylocaine Injection, Sterile 1451
Depo-Medrol Sterile Aqueous Suspension 2334
Hydeltrasol Injection, Sterile 1476
Medrol 2348

Esophagopharyngitis

Ergamisol Tablets 1136
Sterile FUDR 1898
Fluorouracil Injection (Common) 1897

Esophagospasm

Gastrocrom Capsules (Infrequent) 974

Estrogen, decrease

Neosar for Injection 566

Euphoria

Actifed with Codeine Cough Syrup 752
Adipex-P Tablets and Capsules 1019
Akineton 1171
Alfenta Injection (Less than 1%) 1131
Anafranil Capsules (Infrequent) 650
▲ Anestacon Solution (Among most common) 2394
Aristospan Suspension (Intra-articular) 1011
Benadryl Capsules 1691
Benadryl Injection 1692
Biphetamine Capsules 973
BuSpar (Infrequent) 1401
Dalmane Capsules (Rare) 1927
Darvon-N/Darvocet-N 1254
Darvon 1256
Darvon-N Suspension & Tablets 1254
Deconamine 663
Demerol 2047
Depo-Medrol Sterile Aqueous Suspension 2334
Deprol Tablets 2382
Desoxyn Gradumet Tablets 514
Dexedrine 2206
Dilaudid-HP Injection 1175
Dimetane-DC Cough Syrup 1857
Dimetane-DX Cough Syrup 1858
Diprivan Injection (Less than 1%) 2267
Dolophine Hydrochloride Ampoules & Vials 1260
Dolophine Hydrochloride Tablets 1261
Doral Tablets 2383
▲ Duragesic Transdermal System (3% to 10%) 1133
Duranest Injections 624
Dyclone 0.5% and 1% Topical Solutions, USP 626
Empirin with Codeine Phosphate Nos. 2, 3 & 4 764
Equagesic Tablets 2451
Ergamisol Tablets 1136
Ethmozine Tablets (Less than 2%) 946
Sterile FUDR (Remote possibility) 1898
Fastin Capsules 2216
Floxin Tablets (Less than 1%) 1652
Fluorouracil Injection 1897
Halcion Tablets (Less frequent) 2340
Haldol Decanoate 1375
Haldol Injection, Tablets and Concentrate 1373
Hydrocortone Acetate Sterile Suspension 1479
Hyperstat I.V. Injection 2095
Infumorph 200 and Infumorph 500 Sterile Solutions 962
Ionamin Capsules 981
Larodopa Tablets (Relatively frequent) 1905
Limbitrol 1933
Lioresal Tablets 1031
Lomotil 2174
▲ MS Contin Tablets (Among most frequent) 1814
▲ MSIR (Among most frequent) 1817
Marplan Tablets (Rare) 1906
Mepergan Injection 2479
Methadone Hydrochloride Diskets 1284
Methadone Hydrochloride Oral Solution & Tablets 1987
Miltown Tablets 2386
Moban Tablets & Concentrate (Less frequent) 932
Motofen Tablets 836
Nardil (Less common) 1742
Nicorette 1335
Nubain Injection (Less than 1%) 934
Optimine Tablets 2115
▲ Oramorph SR (Morphine Sulfate Sustained Release Tablets) (Among most frequent) 1988
Ornade Spansule Capsules 2221
PBZ Tablets & Elixir 1037
PBZ-SR Tablets 1037
PMB 200 and PMB 400 2504
Pantopon Injectable 1911
Percocet Tablets 950
Percodan 951
Periactin 1525
Permax Tablets (Infrequent) 1291
Phenaphen with Codeine Capsules 1865
Phenaphen-650 with Codeine Tablets 1866
Phenergan with Codeine 2497
Phenergan Injection 2493
Phenergan Tablets 2496
Phenergan VC with Codeine 2501
Polaramine 2116
Prelu-2 Capsules 683
ProSom Tablets (Infrequent) 554
Prozac Pulvules (Infrequent) 920
Restoril Capsules (2-3%) 2023
Roxanol 1991
Roxicodone Tablets, Oral Solution & Intensol (Oxycodone) 1992
Ru-Tuss II Capsules 693
Sansert Tablets 2031
Serax Capsules 2522
Serax Tablets 2522
Sinemet Tablets 952
Sinemet CR Tablets 953
Soma Compound w/Codeine Tablets 2390
Soma Compound Tablets 2389
Soma Tablets 2388
Stadol (Less than 1%) 721
Tacaryl 2409
Talacen 2070
▲ Talwin Injection (Most common) 2071
Talwin Compound 2072
▲ Talwin Injection (Most common) 2071
Talwin Nx 2073
Tambocor Tablets (Less than 1%) 1315
Tavist Syrup 2033
Tavist Tablets 2035
Tavist-D Tablets 2035
Temaril Tablets, Syrup and Spansule Sustained Release Capsules 1085
Tenuate 1354
Toradol IM Injection (1% or less) 2302
Triaminic Expectorant DH 1995
Triaminic Oral Infant Drops 1996
Trinalin Repetabs Tablets 1170
Tussionex Extended-Release Suspension 988
Tylenol with Codeine 1381
Tylox Capsules 1382
Versed Injection (Less than 1%) 1924
Wellbutrin Tablets (1.2%) 821
Wygesic Tablets 2540
▲ Xylocaine Injections (Among most common) 637
Xylocaine Injections for Ventricular Arrhythmias 639
Xylocaine 2% Jelly 643
Xylocaine 5% Ointment 644
Xylocaine 10% Oral Spray 645
4% Xylocaine-MPF Sterile Solution 641
Xylocaine 2% Viscous Solution 646
Zarontin Capsules 1768
Zarontin Syrup 1769

Exanthema

Calan SR Caplets (1% or less) 2157
Calan Tablets (1% or less) 2155
Isoptin Oral Tablets (Less than 1%) 1179
Isoptin SR Sustained Release Tablets (Less than 1%) 1181
Ketalar 1726
Verelan Capsules (Less than 1%) 1243

Excitability

A.R.M. Allergy Relief Medicine Caplets .... ▣ 615
Actidil Tablets .... ▣ 538
Actifed Capsules .... ▣ 539
Actifed Plus Caplets .... ▣ 539
Actifed Plus Tablets .... ▣ 540
Actifed with Codeine Cough Syrup 752
Actifed Syrup .... ▣ 540
Actifed Tablets .... ▣ 540
Actifed 12-Hour Capsules .... ▣ 539
Alka-Seltzer Plus Cold Medicine .... ▣ 623
Alka-Seltzer Plus Night-Time Cold Medicine .... ▣ 623
Allerest .... ▣ 559
▲ Anestacon Solution (Among most common) 2394
Arm-a-Med Isoetharine Inhalation Solution, USP 616
Asendin Tablets (Greater than 1%) 1196
Astramorph/PF Injection, USP (Preservative-Free) 618
Benadryl Capsules 1691
Benadryl Decongestant Elixir .... ▣ 635
Benadryl Decongestant .... ▣ 635
Benadryl Elixir .... ▣ 636
Benadryl Kapseals 1691
Benadryl 25 Kapseals .... ▣ 636
Benadryl Parenteral 1692
Benadryl Plus .... ▣ 636
Benadryl Steri-Vials, Ampoules, and Steri-Dose Syringe 1692
Benadryl 25 Tablets .... ▣ 636
Bentyl 1322
Benylin Cough Syrup .... ▣ 637
Benylin Decongestant .... ▣ 638
Brexin L.A. Capsules 2078
Bromfed Capsules (Timed Release) 1615
Bromfed Syrup .... ▣ 628
Bromfed 1615
Bronkometer Aerosol 2042
Bronkosol Solution 2042
BuSpar (2%) 1401
Carbocaine 956
Cardioquin Tablets 1812
Cerose-DM 2443
Cheracol Plus Head Cold/Cough Formula .... ▣ 667
Chlor-Trimeton Allergy Syrup, Tablets & Long-Acting Repetabs Tablets .... ▣ 693
Chlor-Trimeton Decongestant .... ▣ 694
Cocaine Hydrochloride Topical Solution 620
Codimal 846
Cogentin 1435
Comhist LA Capsules 1618
Allergy-Sinus Comtrex Multi-Symptom Allergy Sinus Formula Tablets & Caplets 746
Comtrex Multi-Symptom Cold Reliever Tablets/Caplets/Liqui-Gels/Liquid- 745
Day-Night Comtrex 747
Contac Continuous Action Decongestant/Antihistamine Capsules .... ▣ 710
Contac Maximum Strength Continuous Action Decongestant/Antihistamine Caplets .... ▣ 709
Contac Nighttime Cold Medicine .... ▣ 713
Contac Severe Cold and Flu Formula Caplets .... ▣ 711
Coricidin 'D' Decongestant Tablets .... ▣ 695
Coricidin Demilets Tablets for Children .... ▣ 696
Coricidin Tablets .... ▣ 695
Dalmane Capsules (Rare) 1927
Darbid Tablets 2205
Deconamine 663
Demazin Nasal Decongestant/ Antihistamine Repetabs Tablets & Syrup .... ▣ 697
Deprol Tablets 2382
Desyrel and Desyrel Dividose (Greater than 1%) 1404
Dimetane Decongestant .... ▣ 673
Dimetane .... ▣ 672
Dimetapp Elixir .... ▣ 673
Dimetapp Extentabs .... ▣ 674
Dimetapp Plus Caplets .... ▣ 675
Dimetapp Tablets .... ▣ 675
Disophrol Chronotab Sustained-Action Tablets .... ▣ 698
Donnatal (In elderly patients) 1858
Donnatal Extentabs (In elderly patients) 1859
Donnatal Tablets (In elderly patients) 1858
Donnazyme Tablets (In elderly patients) 1860
Dristan Cold Nasal Decongestant/ Antihistamine/ Analgesic Coated Tablets 2419
Drixoral Antihistamine/Nasal Decongestant Syrup .... ▣ 698
Drixoral Plus Extended-Release Tablets .... ▣ 699
Drixoral Sinus .... ▣ 700
Drixoral Sustained-Action Tablets .... ▣ 698
Duramorph 960
Elavil 2269
Emete-con Intramuscular/Intravenous 1950
Endep Tablets 1927
Etrafon 2087
4-Way Cold Tablets 750
Flexeril Tablets (Less than 1%) 1471
Guaifed 1615
Hydromox R Tablets 1209
Infumorph 200 and Infumorph 500 Sterile Solutions 962
Isoclor Timesule Capsules .... ▣ 561
Kinesed Tablets 2272
Levsin/Levsinex 2147
Lioresal Tablets 1031
Lufyllin & Lufyllin-400 Tablets 2384
Lufyllin-GG Elixir & Tablets 2385
Marax Tablets & DF Syrup 1954
Marcaine Hydrochloride 0.5% with Epinephrine 1:200,000 (as bitartrate) 958
Marcaine Hydrochloride with Epinephrine 1:200,000 2055
Marcaine Hydrochloride Injection 2055
Marcaine Spinal 2058
Mebaral Tablets 2061
Medi-Flu Caplet, Liquid .... ▣ 640
Mellaril 2011
Narcan Injection 933
Neo-Synephrine Hydrochloride 1% Carpuject 2063

Neo-Synephrine Hydrochloride 1% Injection 2063
Nescaine/Nescaine MPF 629
Nolahist (More frequent in children) 837
Optimine Tablets 2115
Ornade Spansule Capsules 2221
Orthoxicol Cough Syrup ▣ 668
Orudis Capsules (Greater than 1%) 2488
PBZ Tablets & Elixir 1037
PBZ-SR Tablets 1037
PediaCare 1362
PediaCare Night Rest Cough-Cold Formula Liquid 1362
Periactin 1525
Phenergan Injection 2493
Phenergan Tablets 2496
Phenobarbital Elixir and Tablets 1293
Polaramine 2116
Pontocaine Hydrochloride for Spinal Anesthesia 2069
Prolixin Decanoate 1795
Prolixin Elixir 1793
Prolixin Enanthate 1796
Prolixin Injection 1791
Prolixin Oral Concentrate 1792
Prolixin Tablets 1793
Protopam Chloride for Injection (Several cases) 2518
▲ Proventil Syrup (2 of 100; children 2-6: 20%) 2119
Pyrroxate Capsules ▣ 669
Quadrinal Tablets 1183
Quinaglute Dura-Tabs Tablets 663
Quinidex Extentabs 1868
Robinul Injectable 1873
Rondec (Rare) 1975
Rondec-DM (Rare) 1976
Rondec-TR Tablet (Rare) 1975
Ru-Tuss DE Tablets 694
Ru-Tuss II Capsules 693
Ryna ▣ 741
Rynatuss 2388
Sensorcaine 631
Sensorcaine-MPF Spinal 634
Serentil 686
Sinarest ▣ 562
Sine-Off Maximum Strength Allergy/Sinus Formula Caplets ▣ 721
Sine-Off Sinus Medicine Tablets-Aspirin Formula ▣ 722
Singlet Tablets ▣ 598
Sinutab Allergy Formula Sustained Action Tablets ▣ 640
St. Joseph Nighttime Cold Medicine ▣ 705
Sudafed Plus Liquid ▣ 544
Sudafed Plus Tablets ▣ 545
Tacaryl 2409
Talacen (Rare) 2070
Talwin Injection (Rare) 2071
Talwin Compound (Rare) 2072
Talwin Injection (Rare) 2071
Talwin Nx 2073
Tavist Syrup 2033
Tavist Tablets 2035
Tavist-D Tablets 2035
Temaril Tablets, Syrup and Spansule Sustained Release Capsules 1085
TheraFlu Flu and Cold Medicine (In children) ▣ 687
Torecan 1993
Trancopal Caplets 2075
Triaminic Allergy Tablets ▣ 688
Triaminic Chewables ▣ 688
Triaminic Expectorant DH 1995
Triaminic Nite Light ▣ 689
Triaminic Oral Infant Drops 1996
Triaminic-12 Tablets ▣ 690
Triaminicin Tablets ▣ 690
Triaminicol Multi-Symptom Relief ▣ 691
Triavil Tablets 1556
Trinalin Repetabs Tablets 1170
Tylenol Allergy Sinus Medication Caplets and Gelcaps, Maximum Strength 1372
Children's Tylenol Cold Liquid Formula and Chewable Tablets 1368
Tylenol Cold & Flu Hot Medication, Packets 1369
Tylenol Cold & Flu No Drowsiness Hot Medication, Packets 1371
Tylenol Cold Medication Caplets and Tablets 1370
Tylenol Cold Night Time Medication Liquid 1371
Ventolin Syrup (2%) 583
Vicks Formula 44 Cough Medicine ▣ 661
Vicks NyQuil Nighttime Colds Medicine-Original & Cherry Flavor ▣ 664
Winstrol Tablets 2075
Xylocaine Injections for Ventricular Arrhythmias 639
Xylocaine 2% Jelly 643
Xylocaine 10% Oral Spray 645
4% Xylocaine-MPF Sterile Solution 641
Xylocaine 2% Viscous Solution 646
Yohimex Tablets 1190

Excitement, paradoxical

Equagesic Tablets 2451
Etrafon 2087
Halcion Tablets 2340
Libritabs Tablets 1930
Librium Capsules 1931
Miltown Tablets 2386
Norzine 1818
PMB 200 and PMB 400 2504
Placidyl Capsules 553
ProSom Tablets 554
Restoril Capsules (Less than 0.5%) 2023
Serax Capsules 2522
Serax Tablets 2522
Triavil Tablets 1556
Valium Injectable 1937
Valium Tablets 1939
Valrelease Capsules (Infrequent) 1923

Excoriation

▲ Catapres-TTS (3 of 101 patients) 677

Exercise tolerance, decreased

Blocadren Tablets 1429

Exophthalmos

Anafranil Capsules (Rare) 650
Aristocort Suspension 1008
Aristospan Suspension 1011
Celestone Soluspan Suspension 2081
Cortenema 2244
Cortone Acetate Sterile Suspension 1437
Cortone Acetate Tablets 1439
Dalalone D.P. Injectable 999
Decadron Elixir 1445
Decadron Phosphate Injection 1449
Decadron Phosphate Respihaler 1454
Decadron Phosphate Turbinaire 1456
Decadron Phosphate with Xylocaine Injection, Sterile 1451
Decadron Tablets 1447
Decadron-LA Sterile Suspension 1457
Deltasone Tablets 2332
Depo-Medrol Sterile Aqueous Suspension 2334
Hydeltrasol Injection, Sterile 1476
Hydeltra-T.B.A. Sterile Suspension 1478
Hydrocortone Acetate Sterile Suspension 1479
Hydrocortone Phosphate Injection, Sterile 1481
Hydrocortone Tablets 1482
Kenalog-10 Injection 2402
Kenalog-40 Injection 2403
Medrol 2348
Pediapred Oral Liquid 987
Solu-Cortef Sterile Powder 2361
Solu-Medrol Sterile Powder 2363

Extrapyramidal symptoms

Anafranil Capsules (Infrequent) 650
Asendin Tablets (Less than 1%) 1196
Cardizem Tablets-30 mg, 60 mg, 90 mg and 120 mg 1329
Cardizem SR Capsules-60 mg, 90 mg and 120 mg (Less than 1%) 1327
Clozaril Tablets 2000
Compazine 2201
▲ Demser Capsules (10%) 1460
Desyrel and Desyrel Dividose 1404
Elavil 2269
Endep Tablets 1927
Enduronyl 518
Eskalith 2214
Etrafon 2087
Flexeril Tablets (Rare) 1471
Haldol Decanoate (Frequent) 1375
Haldol Injection, Tablets and Concentrate (Frequent) 1373
Harmonyl Tablets 528
Inapsine Injection 1140
Innovar Injection 1141
Intron A (Less than 1%) 2097
Librax Capsules (Rare) 1929
Libritabs Tablets (Isolated cases) 1930
Librium Capsules (Isolated cases) 1931
Librium Injectable (Isolated cases) 1932
Limbitrol 1933
▲ Loxitane (Frequent) 1213
Ludiomil Tablets (Rare) 874
Mellaril (Infrequent) 2011
Menrium Tablets (Rare) 1934
Mepergan Injection (Rare) 2479
Moban Tablets & Concentrate 932
Navane Capsules and Concentrate 1954
Navane Intramuscular 1956
Norpramin Tablets 1340
Norzine 1818
Orap Tablets (Less frequent) 1020
Oreticyl 545
Pamelor 2019
Permax Tablets (1.6%) 1291
Phenergan with Codeine 2497
Phenergan Injection 2493
Phenergan Suppositories 2496
Phenergan Syrup 2495
Phenergan Tablets 2496
Proglycem 649
Prolixin Decanoate 1795
Prolixin Elixir 1793
Prolixin Enanthate 1796
Prolixin Injection 1791
▲ Prolixin Oral Concentrate (Among most frequent) 1792
Prolixin Tablets 1793
Prozac Pulvules (Rare) 920
Raudixin Tablets 1803
Rauzide Tablets 1804
Reglan (0.2%) 1869
Ser-Ap-Es Tablets (Rare) 881
Serpasil Tablets 883
Serpasil-Apresoline Tablets 884
Serpasil-Esidrix Tablets 886
Sinemet CR Tablets 953
Sinequan (Infrequent) 1960
Stelazine 2226
Sublimaze Injection 1146
Surmontil Capsules 2524
Tacaryl 2409
Taractan 1920
Temaril Tablets, Syrup and Spansule Sustained Release Capsules 1085
Thorazine 2234
Tigan 2239
Tofranil Ampuls 1038
Tofranil Tablets 1039
Tofranil-PM Capsules 1041
Torecan 1993
Triavil Tablets 1556
Trilafon 2123
Vivactil Tablets 1567
Zofran Injection (Two reports) 1069

Extrasystoles

Actifed with Codeine Cough Syrup 752
Aminophyllin Tablets 2153
Anafranil Capsules (Infrequent) 650
Asbron G 1997
Benadryl Capsules 1691
Benadryl Injection 1692
Cardene Capsules (Rare) 2290
Choledyl Pediatric Elixir 1702
Choledyl Tablets 1700
Choledyl SA Tablets 1704
Constant-T Tablets 1029
Deconamine 663
Dilor 2079
Glaucon ⊙ 218
Intron A (1% or less) 2097
Lariam Tablets (Less than 1%) 1904
Lopid Capsules and Tablets 1736
Lufyllin & Lufyllin-400 Tablets 2384
Lufyllin-GG Elixir & Tablets 2385
Murocoll-2 Sterile Ophthalmic Solution ⊙ 261
Optimine Tablets 2115
Ornade Spansule Capsules 2221
PBZ Tablets & Elixir 1037
PBZ-SR Tablets 1037
Periactin 1525
Polaramine 2116
Quadrinal Tablets 1183
Quibron Capsules 713
Quibron-T 714
Quibron-T/SR 716
Quinidex Extentabs 1868
Respbid Tablets 684
Ru-Tuss II Capsules 693
Slo-bid Gyrocaps 1847
T-PHYL (Uniphyl) 200 mg Tablets 1820
Tavist Syrup 2033
Tavist Tablets 2035
Tavist-D Tablets 2035
Theo-24 2179
Theo-Dur Sprinkle 1168
Theo-Dur Extended-Release Tablets 1166
Theolair 1317
Theolair-SR Tablets 1319
▲ TheoX Extended-Release Tablets (Among most consistent) 841
Triaminic Expectorant DH 1995
Triaminic Oral Infant Drops 1996
Trinalin Repetabs Tablets 1170
Uniphyl 400 mg Tablets 1823

Extravasation

Adriamycin PFS 561
Adriamycin RDF 562
Brevibloc Injection (Less than 1%) 942
Cerubidine 2443
Cosmegen Injection 1440
Doxorubicin Hydrochloride for Injection, USP 622
Doxorubicin Hydrochloride Injection, USP 848
Fluorescite ⊙ 217
Fungizone Intravenous 2262
Hyperstat I.V. Injection 2095
Idamycin for Injection 564
Intropin Injection 930
Levophed Bitartrate Injection 2054
Mutamycin 733
Oncovin Solution Vials & Hyporets 1288
Rubex 739
Velban Vials 1305

Exudate, increased

Bactroban Ointment (Less than 1%) 2200

Eye abnormalities, fetal

Accutane Capsules 1878

Eye globe, perforation (see under Bulbus oculi, perforation)

Eye movements, abnormal

Klonopin Tablets 1902

Eyeball, perforation (see under Bulbus oculi, perforation)

Eyelashes, matting of

Betoptic Sterile Ophthalmic Solution (Small numbers of patients) 569
Betoptic S Sterile Ophthalmic Suspension (Small numbers of patients) 570
Lacrisert Sterile Ophthalmic Insert 1493

Eyelids, edema of

Ciloxan Sterile Ophthalmic Solution (Less than 1%) ⊙ 214
Lacrisert Sterile Ophthalmic Insert 1493
Oculinum for Injecton (2 cases) 587
Phenobarbital Elixir and Tablets 1293
Polytrim Ophthalmic Solution Sterile (Less than 2 of 100) 588
▲ Rēv-Eyes Ophthalmic Eyedrops 0.5% (10% to 40%) ⊙ 312

Eyes, burning

AK-NaCl 5% Ointment & Solution ⊙ 204
AK-Taine (Occasional) ⊙ 207
▲ Betagan (1 in 3 patients) ⊙ 239
Bleph-10 Liquifilm Sterile Ophthalmic Solution 586
Bleph-10 Ophthalmic Ointment 10% 586
Blephamide 586
Catapres Tablets 676
Catapres-TTS 677
▲ Ciloxan Sterile Ophthalmic Solution (Among most frequent) ⊙ 214
Combipres Tablets 678
Cyclogyl ⊙ 215
Dalmane Capsules (Rare) 1927
Dexacidin ⊙ 272
Fluoracaine (Occasional) ⊙ 208
Genoptic S.O.P. Sterile Ophthalmic Ointment (Occasional) ⊙ 247
Gentacidin Ointment (Occasional) ⊙ 273
Gentacidin Solution (Occasional) ⊙ 273
HMS Liquifilm ⊙ 247
Inflamase ⊙ 274
IOPIDINE ⊙ 232
Isopto Carbachol ⊙ 219
Isopto Carpine ⊙ 219
Isopto Homatropine ⊙ 221

Lamprene Capsules (Greater than 1%) ... 1030
Motofen Tablets (Less frequent) ... 836
Muro 128 Sodium Chloride Ophthalmic Ointment ... ⊙ 260
Muro 128 Solution 2% and 5% ... ⊙ 260
▲ Ocufen (Among most frequent) ... ⊙ 237
Ophthetic ... ⊙ 249
Opticrom 4% (Frequent) ... 986
Phospholine Iodide ... ⊙ 315
Pilopine HS Gel ... ⊙ 227
Polytrim Ophthalmic Solution Sterile (Less than 4 of 100) ... 588
▲ Profenal Sterile Ophthalmic Solution (Among most frequent) ... ⊙ 234
▲ Propine with C Cap Compliance Cap (6%) ... ⊙ 255
Sandostatin Injection (Less than 1%) ... 2029
Sodium Sulamyd ... 2122
Soma Compound w/Codeine Tablets ... 2390
Soma Compound Tablets ... 2389
Tessalon Perles ... 1006
TobraDex Ophthalmic Suspension and Ointment ... ⊙ 228
Trexan Tablets (Less than 1%) ... 937
Vasocidin Ointment ... ⊙ 275
Vasocon-A ... ⊙ 278
Vasosulf ... ⊙ 279
Visken Tablets (2% or fewer patients) ... 2036
▲ Voltaren Ophthalmic Sterile Ophthalmic Solution (15%) ... ⊙ 268

Eyes, dilatation of pupil (see under Mydriasis)

Eyes, disorders

Ativan Tablets (Less frequent) ... 2434
Aureomycin Ophthalmic Ointment 1.0% ... ⊙ 308
Cartrol Tablets (Less common) ... 507
Clinoril Tablets (Less than 1%) ... 1433
Cordarone Tablets ... 2446
Depakene Capsules & Syrup (Rare) ... 511
Depakote Tablets ... 512
Desferal Vials ... 862
Desyrel and Desyrel Dividose (Greater than 1%) ... 1404
Fiorinal with Codeine Capsules (Infrequent) ... 2008
Loxitane ... 1213
Lupron Depot 3.75 mg ... 2312
Lupron Depot 7.5 mg ... 2311
Lupron Injection (Less than 5%) ... 2310
Mintezol ... 1510
Nasalide Nasal Solution 0.025% (5% or less) ... 2299
▲ Novantrone for Injection Concentrate (2 to 7%) ... 1226
Permax Tablets (1.1%) ... 1291
Tacaryl ... 2409
Tambocor Tablets ... 1315
▲ Tegison Capsules (50-75%) ... 1881
Tegretol Chewable Tablets ... 654
Tegretol Suspension ... 656
Tegretol Tablets ... 654
Urispas Tablets ... 2242
Versed Injection (Less than 1%) ... 1924

Eyes, dry (see also under Xerophthalmia)

Accutane Capsules (Rare) ... 1878
Blocadren Tablets ... 1429
Cordarone Tablets ... 2446
Corgard Tablets ... 701
Corzide Tablets (1 to 5 of 1000 patients) ... 702
Inderal ... 2459
Inderal LA Long Acting Capsules (Rare) ... 2461
Inderide LA Long Acting Capsules (Rare) ... 2465
Kerlone Tablets (Less than 2%) ... 2172
Lamprene Capsules (Greater than 1%) ... 1030
Lopressor (Rare) ... 1032
Motrin Tablets (Less than 1%) ... 2351
Normodyne Tablets ... 2110
Normozide Tablets ... 2112
▲ Norpace (3 to 9%) ... 2177
Opticrom 4% (Infrequent) ... 986
Rufen Tablets (Less than 1%) ... 691
Sectral Capsules (Up to 2%) ... 2520
Tenoretic Tablets ... 1105
Tenormin Tablets and I.V. Injection ... 1107
Trandate HCT/Trandate ... 579
Transderm Scōp Transdermal Therapeutic System (Infrequent) ... 887

Eyes, irritation

Adsorbonac 2% and 5% ... ⊙ 210
Adsorbotear ... ⊙ 210
AK-NaCl 5% Ointment & Solution ... ⊙ 204
AK-Poly-Bac Ointment ... ⊙ 205
AK-Spore H.C. ... ⊙ 206
AK-Spore ... ⊙ 205
Allergan Eyewash ... ⊙ 238
Allergy Drops ... ▣ 511
Atropine Sulfate Sterile Ophthalmic Solution and S.O.P. Sterile Ophthalmic Ointment ... ⊙ 239
Bleph-10 Liquifilm Sterile Ophthalmic Solution ... 586
Bleph-10 Ophthalmic Ointment 10% ... 586
Blocadren Tablets (1.1%) ... 1429
Cardizem Tablets-30 mg, 60 mg, 90 mg and 120 mg (Less than 1%) ... 1329
Cardizem SR Capsules-60 mg, 90 mg and 120 mg (Less than 1%) ... 1327
Celluvisc Lubricant Ophthalmic Solution ... ⊙ 243
Clear Eyes ACR ... ⊙ 305
Clearasil Double Textured Pads - Regular and Maximum Strength ... ▣ 658
Cleocin T Topical ... 2327
Cyclogyl ... ⊙ 215
Duratears Naturale ... ⊙ 216
Eye Wash ... ▣ 511
Eye-Stream ... 571
Feldene Capsules (Less than 1%) ... 1777
Genoptic Liquifilm Sterile Ophthalmic Solution ... ⊙ 247
Genoptic S.O.P. Sterile Ophthalmic Ointment ... ⊙ 247
Gentacidin Ointment ... ⊙ 273
Gentacidin Solution ... ⊙ 273
Glaucon ... ⊙ 218
Herplex Liquifilm (Occasional) ... ⊙ 248
Ilotycin Ophthalmic Ointment (Infrequent) ... 915
Isopto Atropine ... ⊙ 218
Isopto Cetamide Solution ... ⊙ 220
Isopto Homatropine ... ⊙ 221
Isopto Hyoscine ... ⊙ 222
Lacril Lubricant Ophthalmic Solution ... ⊙ 248
Lamprene Capsules (Greater than 1%) ... 1030
Methotrexate Tablets, Parenteral, LPF Parenteral ... 1217
Moisture Drops ... ▣ 512
Muro 128 Sodium Chloride Ophthalmic Ointment ... ⊙ 260
Muro 128 Solution 2% and 5% ... ⊙ 260
Naphcon ... ⊙ 226
NebuPent for Inhalation Solution (1% or less) ... 1017
Ocufen ... ⊙ 237
▲ Oculinum for Injecton (10.0%) ... 587
Ocusert Pilo-20 and Pilo-40 Ocular Therapeutic Systems (Infrequent) ... ⊙ 256
Ophthalgan ... ⊙ 315
Opticrom 4% (Infrequent) ... 986
▲ Polytrim Ophthalmic Solution Sterile (Most frequent) ... 588
Pondimin Tablets ... 1867
Ponstel ... 1758
Profenal Sterile Ophthalmic Solution (Less than 0.5%) ... ⊙ 234
Quadrinal Tablets ... 1183
Rheumatrex Methotrexate Dose Pack ... 1234
Roferon-A Injection (Less than 1%) ... 1916
Sween Prep, Protective Skin Barrier ... 2287
T-Stat 2.0% Topical Solution and Pads ... 2409
Tambocor Tablets (Less than 1%) ... 1315
▲ Tegison Capsules (50-75%) ... 1881
Theramycin Z Topical Solution 2% ... 1410
Timolide Tablets ... 1547
Vasosulf ... ⊙ 279
Visine L.R. Eye Drope ... ⊙ 303
Visken Tablets (2% or fewer patients) ... 2036

Eyes, redness

Adsorbonac 2% and 5% ... ⊙ 210
Adsorbotear ... ⊙ 210
AK-NaCl 5% Ointment & Solution ... ⊙ 204
AK-Poly-Bac Ointment ... ⊙ 205
AK-Spore H.C. ... ⊙ 206
AK-Spore ... ⊙ 205
AK-Taine (Occasional) ... ⊙ 207
Albalon Solution with Liquifilm ... ⊙ 238
Allergan Eyewash ... ⊙ 238
BuSpar (Infrequent) ... 1401
Celluvisc Lubricant Ophthalmic Solution ... ⊙ 243
Clozaril Tablets (Less than 1%) ... 2000
Duratears Naturale ... ⊙ 216
Eye Wash ... ▣ 511
Eye-Stream ... 571
Floropryl Sterile Ophthalmic Ointment ... 1473
Fluoracaine (Occasional) ... ⊙ 208
Humorsol Sterile Ophthalmic Solution ... 1475
Lacril Lubricant Ophthalmic Solution ... ⊙ 248
Moisture Drops ... ▣ 512
Ortho Diaphragm Kit ... 1664
Polytrim Ophthalmic Solution Sterile (Less than 4 of 100) ... 588
Transderm Scōp Transdermal Therapeutic System (Infrequent) ... 887
Visine L.R. Eye Drope ... ⊙ 303

Eyes, "spots" before the

Depakene Capsules & Syrup ... 511
Depakote Sprinkle Capsules ... 512

Eyes, swollen (see under Edema, palpebral)

Eyes, tearing

Beconase AQ Nasal Spray (Fewer than 3 per 100 patients) ... 574
Betoptic Sterile Ophthalmic Solution (Small numbers of patients) ... 569
Betoptic S Sterile Ophthalmic Suspension (Small numbers of patients) ... 570
▲ CHEMET (succimer) Capsules (1.0 to 3.7%) ... 1361
Ciloxan Sterile Ophthalmic Solution (Less than 1%) ... ⊙ 214
Dantrium Capsules (Less frequent) 1619
Dipentum Capsules (Rare) ... 1160
Emcyt Capsules (1%) ... 1161
Lorelco Tablets ... 1333
MetroGel (Less than 2%) ... 903
Nasalide Nasal Solution 0.025% ... 2299
Polytrim Ophthalmic Solution Sterile ... 588
Rēv-Eyes Ophthalmic Eyedrops 0.5% (Less frequently) ... ⊙ 312
Vancenase AQ Nasal Spray 0.042% (Fewer than 3 per 100 patients) ... 2127
Vasocon-A ... ⊙ 278

Eyes, winking increased

Alcaine ... ⊙ 210

ECG changes (see under EKG changes)

EEG changes

Anafranil Capsules (Infrequent) ... 650
Asendin Tablets (Greater than 1%) ... 1196
Cibalith-S ... 870
Compazine ... 2201
Deprol Tablets ... 2382
Diphtheria and Tetanus Toxoids and Pertussis Vaccine Adsorbed USP (For Pediatric Use) ... 892
Elavil ... 2269
Endep Tablets ... 1927
Equagesic Tablets ... 2451
Eskalith ... 2214
Etrafon ... 2087
Flexeril Tablets (Rare) ... 1471
Librax Capsules ... 1929
Libritabs Tablets (Isolated cases) ... 1930
Librium Capsules (Isolated cases) ... 1931
Librium Injectable ... 1932
Limbitrol ... 1933
Lithane Tablets ... 1596
Lithium Carbonate Capsules & Tablets ... 1984
Lithobid Tablets ... 870
Ludiomil Tablets (Rare) ... 874
Menrium Tablets (Rare) ... 1934
Miltown Tablets ... 2386
Norpramin Tablets ... 1340
Omnipaque ... 2552
PMB 200 and PMB 400 ... 2504
Pamelor ... 2019
Prolixin Decanoate ... 1795
Prolixin Elixir ... 1793
Prolixin Enanthate ... 1796
Prolixin Injection ... 1791
Prolixin Oral Concentrate ... 1792
Prolixin Tablets ... 1793
ProSom Tablets ... 554
Prozac Pulvules (Rare) ... 920
Serax Capsules ... 2522
Serax Tablets ... 2522
Solganal Suspension ... 2122
Surmontil Capsules ... 2524
Tofranil Ampuls ... 1038
Tofranil Tablets ... 1039
Tofranil-PM Capsules ... 1041
Triavil Tablets ... 1556
Valium Injectable ... 1937
Valium Tablets (Infrequent) ... 1939
Valrelease Capsules (Rare) ... 1923
Vivactil Tablets ... 1567
Wellbutrin Tablets (Rare) ... 821

EKG changes

Adriamycin PFS ... 561
Adriamycin RDF ... 562
Anafranil Capsules (Infrequent) ... 650
Aralen Hydrochloride Injection (Rare) ... 2038
Aralen Phosphate with Primaquine Phosphate Tablets (Rare) ... 2040
Aralen Phosphate Tablets (Rare) ... 2039
Azactam for Injection (Less than 1%) ... 2252
Bumex (0.4%) ... 1895
Cardene Capsules (0.6%) ... 2290
Cardizem Tablets-30 mg, 60 mg, 90 mg and 120 mg (Less than 1%) ... 1329
▲ Cardizem SR Capsules-60 mg, 90 mg and 120 mg (4.1%) ... 1327
Catapres Tablets (Rare) ... 676
Catapres-TTS (Rare) ... 677
Cibalith-S ... 870
Clozaril Tablets (1%) ... 2000
Combipres Tablets (Rare) ... 678
Compazine ... 2201
Demulen ... 2161
Deprol Tablets ... 2382
Diprivan Injection (Less than 1%) ... 2267
Elavil ... 2269
Enovid ... 2161
Equagesic Tablets ... 2451
Eskalith ... 2214
Ethmozine Tablets (1.6%) ... 946
Etrafon ... 2087
Haldol Decanoate ... 1375
Haldol Injection, Tablets and Concentrate ... 1373
Hyperstat I.V. Injection ... 2095
Kenalog-10 Injection ... 2402
Kenalog-40 Injection ... 2403
Lanoxicaps ... 772
Lanoxin Elixir Pediatric ... 775
Lanoxin Injection ... 778
Lanoxin Injection Pediatric ... 781
Lanoxin Tablets ... 783
Lithane Tablets ... 1596
Lithium Carbonate Capsules & Tablets ... 1984
Lithobid Tablets ... 870
Lotensin Tablets (Scattered incidents) ... 872
Loxitane (A few cases) ... 1213
▲ Lupron Depot 3.75 mg (Among most frequent) ... 2312
Lupron Depot 7.5 mg ... 2311
▲ Lupron Injection (5% or more) ... 2310
Mellaril ... 2011
Metaprel Inhalation Aerosol Bronchodilator ... 2014
Midamor Tablets ... 1508
Miltown Tablets ... 2386
Moban Tablets & Concentrate (Rare) ... 932
Nalfon Pulvules & Tablets (Less than 1%) ... 919
Navane Capsules and Concentrate ... 1954
Navane Intramuscular ... 1956
Nimotop Capsules (Up to 1.4%) ... 1607
Nipride I.V. Infusion ... 1909
Norethin ... 2133
Norzine ... 1818
Novantrone for Injection Concentrate ... 1226
Omnipaque ... 2552
Orap Tablets ... 1020
PMB 200 and PMB 400 ... 2504
Permax Tablets (Infrequent) ... 1291
Polycitra-K ... 2424
Prolixin Decanoate ... 1795
Prolixin Elixir ... 1793
Prolixin Enanthate ... 1796
Prolixin Injection ... 1791

Prolixin Oral Concentrate 1792
Prolixin Tablets 1793
Prostigmin Injectable 1120
Prostigmin Tablets 1121
Quinidex Extentabs 1868
Retrovir (2.4%) 802
Stelazine 2226
Tacaryl 2409
Taractan 1920
Tenuate 1354
Thorazine 2234
Tofranil Ampuls 1038
Tofranil Tablets 1039
Tofranil-PM Capsules 1041
Torecan 1993
Trexan Tablets (Less than 1%) 937
Triavil Tablets 1556
Trilafon (Occasional) 2123
Wellbutrin Tablets (Infrequent) 821
Zofran Injection (Rare) 1069

EKG changes, Q wave disturbances

Compazine 2201
Stelazine 2226
Thorazine 2234

EKG changes, QRS interval prolonged

Aralen Hydrochloride Injection (Rare) 2038
Aralen Phosphate with Primaquine Phosphate Tablets 2040
Aralen Phosphate Tablets (Rare) 2039
Cardioquin Tablets 1812
Doxorubicin Hydrochloride for Injection, USP 622
Doxorubicin Hydrochloride Injection, USP 848
Intropin Injection (Frequent) 930
Norpace (1 to 3%) 2177
Pronestyl Capsules and Tablets 1800
Pronestyl Injection 1798
Quinaglute Dura-Tabs Tablets 663
Quinidex Extentabs 1868
Rubex 739
Rum-K Syrup 995
Rythmol Tablets (0.5 to 1.9%) 1184
Tonocard Tablets (Less than 1%) 1554

EKG changes, QT interval prolonged

Lorelco Tablets 1333
Mellaril 2011
Norpace (1 to 3%) 2177
Orap Tablets 1020
Quinidex Extentabs 1868
Seldane Tablets 1349
Seldane-D Extended-Release Tablets 1350
Serentil 686
Tacaryl 2409
Temaril Tablets, Syrup and Spansule Sustained Release Capsules 1085
Tonocard Tablets (Less than 1%) 1554
Vascor (200, 300 and 400 mg) Tablets (0.5 to 2.0%) 1383

EKG changes, reversible flattening

Eskalith 2214
Lithane Tablets 1596
Lithium Carbonate Capsules & Tablets 1984

EKG changes, sinus pause

Brethaire Inhaler 1024
Ethmozine Tablets (1.6%) 946
Tambocor Tablets (1-3%) 1315

EKG changes, ST section

Adriamycin PFS 561
Adriamycin RDF 562
Brethaire Inhaler 1024
Clozaril Tablets 2000
Diprivan Injection (Less than 1%) 2267
Doxorubicin Hydrochloride for Injection, USP 622
Doxorubicin Hydrochloride Injection, USP 848
Lanoxicaps 772
Lanoxin Elixir Pediatric 775
Lanoxin Injection 778
Lanoxin Injection Pediatric 781
Lanoxin Tablets 783
Pentam 300 Injection (1 patient) 1018
Rubex 739
Rum-K Syrup 995

EKG changes, T-wave

Adriamycin PFS 561
Adriamycin RDF 562
Aralen Hydrochloride Injection (Rare) 2038
Aralen Phosphate with Primaquine Phosphate Tablets 2040
Aralen Phosphate Tablets (Rare) 2039
Brethaire Inhaler 1024
Cibalith-S 870
Clozaril Tablets 2000
Compazine 2201
Dopram Injectable 1860
Doxorubicin Hydrochloride for Injection, USP 622
Doxorubicin Hydrochloride Injection, USP 848
Eskalith 2214
Flagyl I.V. 2131
Flagyl Tablets 2170
Lithane Tablets 1596
Lithium Carbonate Capsules & Tablets 1984
Lithobid Tablets 870
▲Loniten Tablets (Approximately 60%) 2346
Mellaril 2011
Moban Tablets & Concentrate (Rare) 932
Orap Tablets 1020
Protostat Tablets 1674
Rubex 739
Rum-K Syrup 995
Serentil 686
Stelazine 2226
Tacaryl 2409
Temaril Tablets, Syrup and Spansule Sustained Release Capsules 1085
Thorazine 2234

ESR, elevation

Capoten 2255
Capozide 2258
Cipro I.V. (Rare) 1592
Cytotec (Infrequent) 2159
Floxin Tablets (More than or equal to 1.0%) 1652
Lamprene Capsules (Greater than 1%) 1030
Mevacor Tablets (Rare) 1505
Monopril Tablets (0.2 to 1.0%) 1406
Prinivil Tablets (1% or less) 1538
Prinzide Tablets 1540
Prozac Pulvules (Rare) 920
Recombivax HB 1544
Sansert Tablets 2031
▲Tegison Capsules (25-50%) 1881
Vaseretic Tablets 1559
Vasotec I.V. (0.5 to 1%) 1562
Vasotec Tablets (0.5% to 1%) 1564
Zestoretic 2274
Zestril Tablets 2277

F

Face, red scaly

▲Tegison Capsules (50-75%) 1881

Face, rhythmical involuntary movements

Compazine 2201
Etrafon 2087
Mellaril 2011
Orap Tablets 1020
Prolixin Oral Concentrate 1792
Reglan 1869
Stelazine 2226
Taractan 1920
Thorazine 2234

Facial angioedema

Catapres-TTS (2 of 3,539 patients) 677

Facial cramps

Omnipaque 2552

Facial dysmorphia, fetal

Accutane Capsules 1878

Facial features, coarsening

Dilantin Infatabs 1710
Dilantin Kapseals 1708
Dilantin Parenteral 1712
Dilantin-30 Pediatric/Dilantin-125 Suspension 1713
Dilantin with Phenobarbital Kapseals 1715

Facial swelling

Carbocaine 956
Corgard Tablets (1 to 5 of 1000 patients) 701
Cortifoam 1827
Corzide Tablets (1 to 5 of 1000 patients) 702
Lupron Injection (Less than 3%) 2310
Marcaine Hydrochloride 0.5% with Epinephrine 1:200,000 (as bitartrate) 958
Prinzide Tablets 1540
Stelazine 2226
Tambocor Tablets (Less than 1%) 1315
Unasyn (Less than 1%) 1965
Zestoretic 2274
Zestril Tablets 2277

Facies, mask-like

Compazine 2201
Loxitane 1213
Reglan 1869
Stelazine 2226
Taractan 1920
Thorazine 2234

Factors II, V, VII, X, decrease

Android 1111
Estratest 2245
Halotestin Tablets 2341
Metandren Linguets and Tablets 875
Premarin with Methyltestosterone 2515
Testred Capsules 1124

Factors VII, VIII, IX, X, increase

Amen 833
Aygestin Tablets 2437
Brevicon 2304
Estrace 1385
Estrace Vaginal Cream 1388
Estratest 2245
Micronor Tablets 1667
Modicon 1667
Norinyl 2304
Ortho-Novum 1667
Tri-Norinyl 28-Day Tablets 2304

Fainting (see under Syncope)

Fanconi syndrome

IFEX 729

Fasciculations

Anectine 755
Cibalith-S 870
Enlon Injection 598
Eskalith 2214
Lithane Tablets 1596
Lithium Carbonate Capsules & Tablets 1984
Lithobid Tablets 870
Mestinon Injectable 1115
Mestinon 1116
Myochrysine Injection (Rare) 1516
Omnipaque (Unusual) 2552
▲Prostigmin Injectable (Among most common) 1120
▲Prostigmin Tablets (Among most common) 1121
Tensilon Injectable 1123

Fatality, hepatic related

Cylert Tablets (Rare) 510

Fatigue

A.P.L. 2431
▲Accutane Capsules (Approximately 1 in 20) 1878
Actifed with Codeine Cough Syrup 752
Actigall Capsules 2280
▲Actimmune (14%) 1046
AeroBid Inhaler System (1-3%) 995
▲Alferon N Injection (6% to 14%) 1809
Altace Capsules (2.0%) 1086
Amen 833
Amicar Syrup, Tablets, and Injection 1194
▲Anafranil Capsules (35% to 39%) 650
Ancobon Capsules 1886
Antabuse Tablets (Small number of patients) 2429
Aquasol A Vitamin A Capsules, USP 615
Aquasol A Parenteral, USP 615
Asendin Tablets (Greater than 1%) 1196
Atromid-S Capsules (Less often) 2435
Atrovent Inhalation Aerosol (Less than 1%) 675
Azdōne Tablets 844
Azo Gantrisin Tablets 1888
Bactrim DS Tablets 1891
Bactrim I.V. Infusion 1889
Bactrim 1891
Benadryl Capsules 1691
Benadryl Injection 1692
▲Blocadren Tablets (3.4% to 5%) 1429
Brevibloc Injection (1%) 942
Bumex (0.1%) 1895
▲BuSpar (4%) 1401
Calan SR Caplets (1.7%) 2157
Calan Tablets (1.7%) 2155
Capoten (0.5 to 2%) 2255
Capozide (0.5 to 2%) 2258
▲Cardura Tablets (12%) 1941
▲Cartrol Tablets (0.5-7.1%) 507
Catapres Tablets (About 4 in 100 patients) 676
▲Catapres-TTS (4% to 6%) 677
▲Centrax (11.6%) 1693
▲CHEMET (succimer) Capsules (5.2 to 15.7%) 1361
Children's Advil Suspension 2426
Cholybar 1705
Cibalith-S 870
Clinoril Tablets (Less than 1 in 100) 1433
Clozaril Tablets (2%) 2000
Colestid Granules (1-3 patients in 1,000) 2328
▲Combipres Tablets (About 4%) 678
Compazine Ampuls 2201
▲Cordarone Tablets (4 to 9%) 2446
Corgard Tablets (2 in 100 patients) 701
Cortifoam 1827
Corzide Tablets (2%) 702
Cosmegen Injection 1440
Cycrin Tablets 2449
Cytotec (Infrequent) 2159
Damason-P (Occasional) 1356
Danocrine Capsules 2046
▲Dantrium Capsules (Among most frequent) 1619
Deconamine 663
Demulen 2161
Depo-Provera Sterile Aqueous Suspension (Occasional) 2336
Desyrel and Desyrel Dividose (Greater than 1%) 1404
Dibenzyline Capsules 2207
Dipentum Capsules (1.8%) 1160
Diprivan Injection (Less than 1%) 2267
Diulo 2129
Dolobid Tablets (Greater than 1 in 100) 1465
Doral Tablets (1.9%) 2383
Dyazide Capsules 2208
▲DynaCirc Capsules (0.4% to 3.9%) 2004
Dyrenium Capsules (Rare) 2210
Edecrin 1468
Elavil 2269
Eldepryl 2250
Elspar 1470
Emete-con Intramuscular/Intravenous 1950
Empirin with Codeine Phosphate Nos. 2, 3 & 4 (Occasional) 764
Endep Tablets 1927
▲Engerix-B Unit-Dose Vials (14%) 2213
Enovid 2161
▲Epogen for Injection (9.0% to 25%) 591
▲Ergamisol Tablets (6 to 11%) 1136
Esimil Tablets 864
Eskalith 2214
▲Ethmozine Tablets (5.9%) 946
Etrafon 2087
Fansidar Tablets 1896
Feldene Capsules (Occasional) 1777
Fiorinal with Codeine Capsules (Infrequent) 2008
Flexeril Tablets (1% to 3%) 1471
Floxin Tablets (1% to 3%) 1652
Fulvicin P/G Tablets 2090
Fulvicin P/G 165 & 330 Tablets 2091
Fulvicin-U/F Tablets 2092
Gammagard Immune Globulin, Intravenous (Human) (Occasional) 658
Gantanol 1899
Gantrisin 1901
Gastrocrom Capsules (Infrequent) 974
Grifulvin V (griseofulvin microsize) Tablets/Suspension (Occasional) 1678
Grisactin (Occasional) 2454
Grisactin Ultra Tablets (Occasional) 2455
Gris-PEG Tablets, 125 mg & 250 mg (Occasional) 1083
Halcion Tablets (Less frequent) 2340
Hexalen Capsules (1%) 2316
▲Hismanal Tablets (4.2%) 1138
Humulin 70/30, 100 Units 1267

(▣ Described in PDR For Nonprescription Drugs) Incidence data in parenthesis; ▲ 3% or more (◉ Described in PDR For Ophthalmology)

Humulin BR, 100 Units 1268
Humulin L, 100 Units 1268
Humulin U, 100 Units 1272
Hydromox R Tablets 1209
▲ Hylorel Tablets (25.7% to 63.6%) 975
▲ Hytrin Tablets (11.3%) 529
INH Tablets 868
IFEX (Less than 1%) 729
Imodium Capsules 1139
Inderal 2459
Inderal LA Long Acting Capsules 2461
Inderide Tablets 2463
Inderide LA Long Acting Capsules .. 2465
Indocin (Greater than 1%) 1487
▲ Intron A (18% to 84%) 2097
Inversine Tablets 1492
IOPIDINE ..... ⊙ 232
Ismelin Tablets 869
Isoptin Injectable (Few) 1177
Isoptin Oral Tablets (1.7%) 1179
Isoptin SR Sustained Release Tablets (1.7%) 1181
K-Lyte 707
K-Phos M.F. Tablets 659
K-Phos Neutral Tablets 660
K-Phos Original Formula 'Sodium Free' Tablets (Less frequent) 660
K-Phos No. 2 Tablets 659
Keflex Pulvules, Oral Suspension & Pediatric Drops 916
Keftab Tablets 917
Kenalog-10 Injection 2402
Kenalog-40 Injection 2403
▲ Kerlone Tablets (2.9% to 9.7%) 2172
Lamprene Capsules (Less than 1%) 1030
▲ Lariam Tablets (Among most frequent) 1904
Larodopa Tablets (Relatively frequent) 1905
▲ Levatol (4.4%) 1832
Limbitrol 1933
Lioresal Tablets (2-4%) 1031
Lithane Tablets 1596
Lithium Carbonate Capsules & Tablets 1984
Lithobid Tablets 870
▲ Lopid Capsules and Tablets (3.8%) 1736
▲ Lopressor Ampuls (10%) 1032
▲ Lopressor HCT Tablets (10 in 100 patients) 1034
▲ Lopressor Tablets (10%) 1032
Lortab ASA Tablets (Occasional) ... 2414
Lotensin Tablets (2.6%) 872
▲ Lozol Tablets (Greater than or equal to 5%) 1843
▲ Ludiomil Tablets (4%) 874
Lupron Injection (Less than 5%) 2310
▲ Marplan Tablets (Among most frequent) 1906
Matulane Capsules 1907
Maxair Inhaler (Less than 1%) 1311
Maxzide 1215
Meclomen Capsules (Rare) 1739
Mesantoin Tablets 2013
▲ Mesnex Injection (33%) 733
Methotrexate Tablets, Parenteral, LPF Parenteral (Frequent) 1217
Metrodin (urofollitropin for injection) 2182
▲ Mexitil Capsules (1.9% to 3.8%) .. 680
Micronor Tablets 1667
Midamor Tablets (Between 1% and 3%) 1508
Mintezol 1510
Modicon 1667
Moduretic Tablets (Greater than 1%, less than 3%) 1510
Monopril Tablets 1406
Motofen Tablets (1 in 200 to 1 in 600) 836
Motrin Tablets 2351
Mutamycin 733
▲ Mykrox ½ mg Tablets (4.4%) 984
Myleran Tablets 790
Mysoline (Occasional) 2480
Nalfon Pulvules & Tablets (1.7%) .. 919
Nardil (Common) 1742
Navane Capsules and Concentrate 1954
Navane Intramuscular 1956
▲ NebuPent for Inhalation Solution (53 to 72%) 1017
Neptazane Tablets ..... ⊙ 311
▲ Neupogen for Injection (11%) 595
▲ Nolvadex Tablets (3.8%) 1102
Norethin 2133
Norlutate 1754
Norlutin 1755
▲ Normodyne Injection (2 to 10%) 2108
▲ Normodyne Tablets (2% to 10%) .. 2110
Normozide Tablets (1 to 5%) 2112
Noroxin Tablets (0.3% to 1%) 1519
▲ Norpace (3 to 9%) 2177
Norpramin Tablets 1340
Optimine Tablets 2115
Ornade Spansule Capsules 2221
Ortho-Novum 1667
PBZ Tablets & Elixir 1037
PBZ-SR Tablets 1037
Pamelor 2019
Paradione Capsules 548
▲ Parlodel (1-7%) 2020
PediaProfen Suspension 1363
Peganone Tablets 551
Pentaspan Injection 949
Pepcid (Infrequent) 1524
Peptavlon 2563
Periactin 1525
Phenergan Injection 2493
Phenurone Tablets (Less than 1%) 552
Pipracil 1230
Plendil Extended-Release Tablets (0.5% or greater) 1526
Polaramine 2116
Pondimin Tablets 1867
Pregnyl 1644
Prilosec Delayed-Release Capsules (Less than 1%) 1530
▲ Prinivil Tablets (3.3% to 3.9%) 1538
▲ Prinzide Tablets (3.7%) 1540
▲ Procardia XL Tablets (5.9%) 1783
▲ Procrit for Injection (9% to 25%) .. 1647
Profasi (human chorionic gonadotropin, USP) 2186
Proventil Syrup (Children 2-6: 1%) 2119
Provera Tablets 2356
▲ Prozac Pulvules (4.2%) 920
Quadrinal Tablets 1183
Questran Light 711
Questran Powder 710
Recombivax HB (Equal to or greater than 1%) 1544
▲ Reglan (10%) 1869
Renese-R Tablets 1786
Rheumatrex Methotrexate Dose Pack (Frequent) 1234
RhoGAM $Rh_0(D)$ Immune Globulin (Human) 1651
Rifadin 1345
Rifamate Capsules 1347
Rimactane Capsules 879
▲ Roferon-A Injection (89% to 95%) 1916
Rogaine Topical Solution (0.36%) .. 2357
▲ Rowasa (3.44%) 2248
Ru-Tuss II Capsules 693
▲ Rythmol Tablets (1.8 to 6.0%) 1184
Sandostatin Injection (1.4%) 2029
Sansert Tablets 2031
▲ Sectral Capsules (11%) 2520
▲ Seldane Tablets (4.5%) 1349
Seldane-D Extended-Release Tablets (2.1%) 1350
Septra 813
Septra I.V. Infusion 808
Septra I.V. Infusion ADD-Vantage Vials 810
Septra 813
Serophene (clomiphene citrate tablets, USP) (Less than 1 in 100 patients) 2186
Sinemet Tablets 952
Sinemet CR Tablets 953
Sinequan (Occasional) 1960
Stelazine 2226
Stilphostrol Tablets and Ampuls 1609
Surmontil Capsules 2524
Symmetrel Capsules & Syrup (0.1-1%) 936
Tacaryl 2409
▲ Tambocor Tablets (7.7%) 1315
Tavist Syrup 2033
Tavist Tablets 2035
Tavist-D Tablets 2035
▲ Tegison Capsules (50-75%) 1881
Tegretol Chewable Tablets 654
Tegretol Suspension 656
Tegretol Tablets 654
Temaril Tablets, Syrup and Spansule Sustained Release Capsules 1085
▲ Tenex Tablets (3% to 4%) 1875
▲ Tenoretic Tablets (0.6 to 26%) 1105
▲ Tenormin Tablets and I.V. Injection (0.6 to 26%) 1107
Thalitone Tablets 687
TheraCys BCG Live (Intravesical) (Up to 0.9%) 898
Timolide Tablets (1.9%) 1547
Timoptic in Ocudose 1552
Timoptic Sterile Ophthalmic Solution 1550
Tofranil Ampuls 1038
Tofranil Tablets 1039
Tofranil-PM Capsules 1041
Tolinase Tablets (Infrequent) 2365
Tonocard Tablets (0.8-1.6%) 1554
Trandate HCT Tablets (1% in 208 patients) 579
Trandate Injection 577
▲ Trandate Tablets (11%) 579
Tranxene 556
Trexan Tablets (Less than 1%) 937
Triaminic Expectorant DH 1995
Triaminic Oral Infant Drops 1996
Triavil Tablets 1556
Tridione 557
Trinalin Repetabs Tablets 1170
Unasyn (Less than 1%) 1965
Uroqid-Acid (Less frequent) 661
Valium Injectable (Among most common) 1937
Valium Tablets (Among most common) 1939
▲ Valrelease Capsules (Among most common) 1923
▲ Vaseretic Tablets (3.9%) 1559
Vasotec I.V. (0.5 to 1%) 1562
Vasotec Tablets (1.8% to 3.0%) 1564
Ventolin Syrup (1% of children) 583
Verelan Capsules (1.7%) 1243
▲ Visken Tablets (8%) 2036
Vivactil Tablets 1567
Voltaren Tablets 1042
▲ Wellbutrin Tablets (5.0%) 821
▲ Xanax Tablets (48.6%) 2367
Zarontin Capsules 1768
Zarontin Syrup 1769
Zaroxolyn Tablets 989
▲ Zestoretic (3.7%) 2274
▲ Zestril Tablets (3.3%) 2277
Zovirax (0.3%) 824

Fatigue, muscular

Capozide 2258
Corzide Tablets 702
Fiorinal with Codeine Capsules (Infrequent) 2008
Prinzide Tablets 1540
Rauzide Tablets 1804
▲ Tenoretic Tablets (3 to 6%) 1105
▲ Tenormin Tablets and I.V. Injection (3 to 6%) 1107
Zestoretic 2274

Fat intolerance

Anafranil Capsules (Rare) 650

Fear

▲ Adrenalin Chloride Solution 1:100 & 1:1,000 (Often) 1689
Anexsia 5/500 Tablets 2196
Anexsia 7.5/650 Tablets 2197
Atrohist Sprinkle Capsules 558
Azdōne Tablets 844
BuSpar (Infrequent) 1401
Cipro Tablets (Less than 1%) 1589
Damason-P 1356
Deconamine 663
Deconsal 559
Dilaudid Cough Syrup 1174
Dilaudid 1173
EpiPen—Epinephrine Auto-Injector 843
Fedahist Gyrocaps 2145
Fedahist Timecaps 2145
Hycodan Syrup, Tablets 927
Hycomine Compound Tablets 929
Hycomine Syrup 927
Hycotuss Expectorant Syrup 930
Hydrocet Capsules 835
Lortab ASA Tablets 2414
Lortab 2412
Murocoll-2 Sterile Ophthalmic Solution ..... ⊙ 261
Novafed A Capsules 1342
Novafed Capsules 1342
Novahistine DH 1342
Novahistine DMX ..... ▣ 595
Novahistine Elixir ..... ▣ 596
Novahistine Expectorant 1343
Pfizerpen-AS Aqueous Suspension (Approximately 1 in 500) 1959
Phenobarbital Elixir and Tablets 1293
Ru-Tuss DE Tablets 694
Seldane-D Extended-Release Tablets 1350
Trinalin Repetabs Tablets 1170
Tussionex Extended-Release Suspension 988
Vicodin Tablets 1187
Vicodin ES Tablets 1189
Xanax Tablets (1.4%) 2367
Zydone Capsules 941

Febrile reactions

Albuminar-5, Albumin (Human) U.S.P. 5% 608
Albuminar-25, Albumin (Human) U.S.P. 25% 608
Capastat Sulfate Vials 1250
Digibind 762
Diphtheria and Tetanus Toxoids and Pertussis Vaccine Adsorbed USP (For Pediatric Use) 892
Fungizone Intravenous 2262
Imferon 976
Metrodin (urofollitropin for injection) (Less than 1 in 50) 2182
Monistat I.V. 1143
Mumpsvax (Very rare) 1513
Pergonal (menotropins for injection, USP) 2184
Thrombostat 1765
Tri-Immunol Diphtheria & Tetanus Toxoids & Pertussis Vaccine, Adsorbed 1241

Fecal fat, increase (see under Steatorrhea)

Fecal impaction

Etrafon 2087
Kayexalate (At large doses in elderly individuals) 2053
Prolixin Decanoate 1795
Prolixin Elixir 1793
Prolixin Enanthate 1796
Prolixin Injection 1791
Prolixin Oral Concentrate 1792
Prolixin Tablets 1793
Sodium Polystyrene Sulfonate Suspension 1993
Trilafon (Occasional) 2123

Feces, color change

Modane Plus Tablets ..... ▣ 504
Modane Tablets ..... ▣ 503
Prilosec Delayed-Release Capsules (Less than 1%) 1530

Feces, discoloration

Brevicon 2304
Derifil Tablets 1994
Evac-U-Gen Mild Laxative ..... ▣ 739
Lamprene Capsules (Greater than 1%) 1030
Norinyl 2304
Tri-Norinyl 28-Day Tablets 2304
Urised Tablets 2396

Feeling, intoxicated

Fiorinal with Codeine Capsules (1%) 2008

Feelings, unworldly (see under Alice in Wonderland syndrome)

Fertility, impairment of

Halotestin Tablets 2341

Festination

Eldepryl 2250

Fetal circulation, persistent

Exosurf Neonatal for Intratracheal Suspension (1%) 765

Fetal death

Capoten 2255
Capozide 2258
Methotrexate Tablets, Parenteral, LPF Parenteral 1217
Pitocin Injection, Ampoules, Steri-Dose Syringes 1757
Rheumatrex Methotrexate Dose Pack 1234

Fetal defects

▲ Accutane Capsules (Potentially all exposed fetuses) 1878
Butisol Sodium Elixir & Tablets 2377
Cytovene Sterile Powder 2292
Cytoxan for Injection 726
Demulen 2161
Enovid 2161
Estinyl Tablets 2085
Halcion Tablets 2340
Lupron Depot 7.5 mg 2311
Megace Tablets 732
Methotrexate Tablets, Parenteral, LPF Parenteral 1217

Nembutal Sodium Capsules 534
Nembutal Sodium Solution 536
Nembutal Sodium Suppositories........ 538
Neosar for Injection (One case)....... 566
Premarin with Methyltestosterone .. 2515
Rheumatrex Methotrexate Dose Pack............................. 1234
TACE 12 and 25 mg 1353
Tegison Capsules.............................. 1881

Fetal harm

A.P.L.. 2431
▲ Accutane Capsules (Potentially all exposed fetuses) 1878
Advil Cold & Sinus Caplets (formerly CoAdvil)............................. 2416
Advil Ibuprofen Tablets and Caplets.. 2416
Alkeran Tablets................................ 754
Alurate Elixir 1883
Amen.. 833
Amikin Injectable 602
Anadrol-50 Tablets.......................... 2287
Android-10 Tablets 1111
Aquasol A Vitamin A Capsules, USP 615
Aquasol A Parenteral, USP 615
Arfonad Ampuls 1887
Ativan Injection................................ 2432
Aygestin Tablets.............................. 2437
BiCNU 723
Butisol Sodium Elixir & Tablets 2377
Calcidrine Syrup................................ 506
CeeNU 725
Cerubidine 2443
Cibalith-S... 870
Colchicine Ampoules 1252
Cycrin Tablets.................................. 2449
Cytadren Tablets 861
Cytosar-U Sterile Powder 2329
Cytotec... 2159
Cytoxan for Injection 726
Danocrine Capsules 2046
Depen Titratable Tablets 2379
Depo-Provera Sterile Aqueous Suspension 2336
Didrex Tablets.................................. 2338
Diethylstilbestrol Tablets 1258
Diucardin Tablets............................. 2450
Doral Tablets 2383
Enduron Tablets................................ 517
Enduronyl 518
Ergostat.. 1719
Eskalith 2214
Estinyl Tablets.................................. 2085
Estrace 1385
Estrace Vaginal Cream 1388
Estraderm Transdermal System 866
Estratest 2245
Estrovis 1721
Eulexin Capsules 2089
Exna Tablets 1862
Sterile FUDR 1898
Fluoroplex Topical Solution & Cream 1% 1082
Fluorouracil Injection 1897
Garamycin Injectable 2093
Hydrocet Capsules 835
IFEX 729
Imuran Tablets 768
Leukeran Tablets 788
Lithane Tablets................................ 1596
Lithium Carbonate Capsules & Tablets 1984
Lithobid Tablets 870
Lupron Depot 3.75 mg.................... 2312
Lysodren 731
Marplan Tablets 1906
Matulane Capsules 1907
Maxzide 1215
Mebaral Tablets 2061
Megace Tablets 732
Metandren Linguets and Tablets...... 875
Metrodin (urofollitropin for injection) 2182
Mevacor Tablets.............................. 1505
Minocin Oral Suspension 1224
Minocin Pellet-Filled Capsules 1222
Mithracin.. 1602
Mustargen.. 1514
Myleran Tablets 790
Nebcin Vials, Hyporets & ADD-Vantage 1286
Nembutal Sodium Capsules 534
Nembutal Sodium Solution 536
Nembutal Sodium Suppositories...... 538
Neosar for Injection 566
Neosporin G.U. Irrigant Sterile......... 793
Netromycin Injection 100 mg/ml... 2104
Nicorette 1335
Nipride I.V. Infusion 1909
Nolvadex Tablets 1102
Norethin... 2133
Norlestrin 1746
Norlutate 1754
Norlutin 1755
Novantrone for Injection Concentrate 1226
Oncovin Solution Vials & Hyporets 1288
Oretic Tablets 544
Oreticyl... 545
Organidin Elixir, Solution & Tablets 2387
Ortho Dienestrol Cream 1664
Ovcon 1391
PMB 200 and PMB 400 2504
ParaGard T380A Intrauterine Copper Contraceptive 411
Paraplatin for Injection 735
Peganone Tablets 551
Pergonal (menotropins for injection, USP) 2184
Phenobarbital Elixir and Tablets 1293
Phenurone Tablets 552
Premarin Intravenous 2508
Premarin with Methyltestosterone .. 2515
Premarin Tablets 2510
ProSom Tablets 554
Purinethol Tablets 800
Quadrinal Tablets 1183
Quinamm Tablets 1344
Restoril Capsules 2023
Seconal Sodium Pulvules 1296
Serax Capsules 2522
Serax Tablets................................... 2522
Soma Compound w/Codeine Tablets 2390
Soma Compound Tablets................ 2389
Tapazole Tablets 1298
Terramycin Capsules 1786
Testred Capsules 1124
Thioguanine Tablets, Tabloid Brand 815
Velban Vials 1305
VePesid Capsules and Injection....... 741
Virazole 1126
Wigraine Tablets & Suppositories .. 1645
Winstrol Tablets 2075
Xanax Tablets 2367
Zorprin Tablets 698

Fetal hemorrhage

Coumadin Injection & Tablets 944
Dicumarol Tablets 516
Lortab ASA Tablets 2414
Panwarfin Tablets 547
Soma Compound w/Codeine Tablets 2390
Soma Compound Tablets................ 2389

Fetal hydantoin syndrome

Dilantin Infatabs.............................. 1710
Dilantin Kapseals 1708
Dilantin Parenteral 1712
Dilantin-30 Pediatric/Dilantin-125 Suspension 1713
Dilantin with Phenobarbital Kapseals 1715

Fetal problems, unspecified

Alka-Seltzer Plus Cold Medicine .. ▣ 623
Alka-Seltzer Plus Night-Time Cold Medicine .... ▣ 623
BC Powder .... ▣ 517
Genuine Bayer Aspirin Tablets & Caplets .... ▣ 564
Maximum Bayer Aspirin Tablets & Caplets..................................... ▣ 566
Bayer Plus Aspirin Tablets.............. ▣ 567
Therapy Bayer Aspirin Caplets .... ▣ 568
8 Hour Bayer Timed-Release Aspirin .... ▣ 566
Capoten 2255
Cipro I.V. 1592
Cipro Tablets 1589
Cytovene Sterile Powder................. 2292
Dalmane Capsules.......................... 1927
Empirin Aspirin............................. ▣ 541
Floropryl Sterile Ophthalmic Ointment 1473
Haltran Tablets............................. ▣ 668
Humorsol Sterile Ophthalmic Solution 1475
Medipren ibuprofen Caplets and Tablets 1362
Midol 200 Cramp Relief Formula ▣ 570
Motrin IB Caplets and Tablets ...... ▣ 736
Norwich Extra-Strength Aspirin.... ▣ 546
Norwich Regular Strength Aspirin .... ▣ 547
Nuprin Ibuprofen/Analgesic Tablets & Caplets 752
PediaProfen Suspension................. 1363
Polytrim Ophthalmic Solution Sterile 588
Rufen Tablets 691
Sine-Off Sinus Medicine Tablets-Aspirin Formula .... ▣ 722
Synarel Nasal Solution.................... 2300
Trendar Ibuprofen Tablets............ ▣ 756
Ursinus Inlay-Tabs......................... ▣ 691
Vaseretic Tablets 1559
Vasotec I.V. 1562
Vasotec Tablets 1564

Fever

Abbokinase (2%-3%) 503
Abbokinase Open-Cath (2%-3%) .. 505
▲ Actimmune (52%) 1046
Activase 1047
Adalat Capsules (10 mg and 20 mg) (2% or less) 1587
Adriamycin PFS (Occasional).......... 561
Adriamycin RDF (Occasional).......... 562
▲ AeroBid Inhaler System (3-9%) 995
Aldomet Ester HCl Injection 1417
Aldomet Oral 1415
Aldoril Tablets.................................. 1418
▲ Alferon N Injection (19% to 81%) 1809
Alurate Elixir 1883
Amen (Rare) 833
▲ Anafranil Capsules (2% to 4%) 650
Anaprox and Anaprox DS Tablets (Less than 1%)............................ 2288
Ancobon Capsules.......................... 1886
Ansaid Tablets (Less than 1%)....... 2319
Antivenin (Crotalidae) Polyvalent 2430
Apresazide Capsules (Less frequent) 854
Apresoline Hydrochloride Parenteral (Ampuls) 856
Apresoline Hydrochloride Tablets (Less frequent) 855
Apresoline-Esidrix Tablets 857
Asendin Tablets 1196
▲ Atgam Sterile Solution (1 in 3 patients; 51%) 2320
Attenuvax (Occasional) 1424
Augmentin Tablets, Powder for Oral Suspension, and Chewable Tablets (Frequent)........................ 2198
Axid Pulvules................................... 1246
Azactam for Injection (Less than 1%) 2252
Azo Gantrisin Tablets...................... 1888
▲ Azulfidine Tablets, EN-tabs, Oral Suspension (3 to 4%) 1157
▲ BAL in Oil Ampules (30% of children) 661
Benemid Tablets 1426
Biavax II (Occasional) 1427
Bicillin C-R Injection 2438
Bicillin C-R 900/300 Injection 2440
Bicillin L-A Injection 2442
▲ Blenoxane (Frequent)...................... 724
Blocadren Tablets 1429
Brevibloc Injection (Less than 1%) 942
BuSpar (Rare) 1401
Butazolidin Capsules & Tablets (Less than 1%)............................ 1027
Butisol Sodium Elixir & Tablets (1 to 3 patients per 100) 2377
Calan SR Caplets 2157
Calan Tablets................................... 2155
Calciparine Injection.......................... 925
▲ Capoten (About 4 to 7 of 100)....... 2255
▲ Capozide (4 to 7 of 100 patients).. 2258
Carbocaine Hydrochloride Injection 2043
Cardioquin Tablets 1812
Cardura Tablets (Less than 0.5% of 3960 patients) 1941
Cartrol Tablets (Less common)........ 507
Catapres Tablets 676
Catapres-TTS..................................... 677
Ceclor Pulvules & Suspension (Frequently) 1251
▲ Cefizox Injection (1 to 5%)............ 1012
Cefotan... 2265
Ceftin Tablets 575
Ceptaz for Injection (2% of patients) 1057
Ceredase Injection.......................... 1052
Cerose-DM 2443
Cerubidine (Rare) 2443
Cetamide Ointment........................ ⊙ 220
▲ CHEMET (succimer) Capsules (5.2 to 15.7%)..................................... 1361
Children's Advil Suspension (Less than 1%)...................................... 2426
Chloromycetin Kapseals 1695
Chloromycetin Palmitate, Oral Suspension 1697
Cipro I.V. (1% or less)..................... 1592
Cipro Tablets (Less than 1%) 1589
Claforan Sterile Injection (2.4%) 1089
Clinoril Tablets (Less than 1%)....... 1433
▲ Clozaril Tablets (More than 5%) 2000
Cogentin 1435
ColBENEMID Tablets 1436
Combipres Tablets 678
Compazine 2201
Corgard Tablets 701
Corzide Tablets 702
Cosmegen Injection 1440
Coumadin Injection & Tablets (Infrequent) 944
Cuprimine Capsules (Rare)............. 1442
Cyclogyl .... ⊙ 215
Cyclomydril .... ⊙ 216
Cycrin Tablets.................................. 2449
Cytadren Tablets (Several) 861
▲ CytoGam (Less than 5.0%) 891
Cytosar-U Sterile Powder (One case) 2329
Cytotec (Infrequent)........................ 2159
Cytovene Sterile Powder (2%) 2292
DTIC-Dome (Infrequent) 1595
Danocrine Capsules (Rare) 2046
Dantrium Capsules (Less frequent) 1619
Dapsone USP................................... 1130
Daranide Tablets 1445
Daraprim Tablets (Rare)................... 761
Darbid Tablets 2205
Depen Titratable Tablets (Rare) 2379
Depo-Provera Sterile Aqueous Suspension 2336
Deprol Tablets................................. 2382
Desferal Vials..................................... 862
Diamox 1200
Dicumarol Tablets (Infrequent) 516
Dilantin Infatabs.............................. 1710
Dilantin Kapseals 1708
Dilantin Parenteral 1712
Dilantin-30 Pediatric/Dilantin-125 Suspension 1713
Dilantin with Phenobarbital Kapseals 1715
Dilor... 2079
Dipentum Capsules (Rare).............. 1160
Diphtheria & Tetanus Toxoids, Adsorbed Purogenated (Mild) 1202
Diphtheria and Tetanus Toxoids and Pertussis Vaccine Adsorbed USP (For Pediatric Use) (Frequent).. 892
Diprivan Injection (Greater than 1%) 2267
Diucardin Tablets............................. 2450
Diupres Tablets 1461
Diuril Oral Suspension.................... 1464
Diuril Sodium Intravenous 1463
Diuril Tablets 1464
Dobutrex Solution Vials (Occasionally) 1259
Dolobid Tablets (Less than 1 in 100) 1465
Dopram Injectable 1860
Doxorubicin Hydrochloride for Injection, USP (Occasional)........... 622
Doxorubicin Hydrochloride Injection, USP (Occasional)........... 848
Easprin 1719
Edecrin 1468
Elavil 2269
Elspar 1470
Emete-con Intramuscular/Intravenous (Rare) 1950
▲ Eminase (Less than 10%).............. 2211
Enduron Tablets................................ 517
▲ Engerix-B Unit-Dose Vials (1% to 10%) 2213
▲ Epogen for Injection (38%) 591
Equagesic Tablets 2451
▲ Ergamisol Tablets (3 to 5%) 1136
Eskalith 2214
Ethamolin (2.1%) 1829
Etrafon 2087
Sterile FUDR 1898
Feldene Capsules (Less than 1%) .. 1777
Fiorinal with Codeine Capsules (Infrequent) 2008
Flagyl I.V. 2131
Flagyl Tablets 2170
Floxin Tablets (1% to 3%) 1652
Flu-Imune Influenza Virus Vaccine (Infrequent) 1204
Fluothane 2453
Fortaz (2%) 1060
▲ Fungizone Intravenous (Among most common) 2262
Furoxone 1855
Gamimune N Immune Globulin Intravenous (Human)................... 1572

Gammagard Immune Globulin, Intravenous (Human) (Occasional) ... 658
Gammar-IV, Immune Globulin Intravenous (Human) ... 610
Gamulin Rh, Rh$_0$(D) Immune Globulin (Human) (Infrequent) ... 610
Ganite Injection ... 1016
Gantanol ... 1899
Gantrisin ... 1901
Garamycin Injectable ... 2093
Gelfoam Sterile Sponge ... 2338
Haldol Decanoate ... 1375
Haldol Injection, Tablets and Concentrate ... 1373
Heparin Lock Flush Solution ... 2456
▲Heparin Sodium Vials (Among most common) ... 1264
Heparin Sodium Injection ... 2457
Heparin Sodium Injection, USP, Sterile Solution ... 2342
HibTITER (Up to 1.4%) ... 1206
Hydrea Capsules ... 728
HydroDIURIL Tablets ... 1484
Hydropres Tablets ... 1485
Hyperstat I.V. Injection ... 2095
Hyskon Hysteroscopy Fluid (Rare) ... 1162
Hytrin Tablets (At least 1%) ... 529
INH Tablets ... 868
▲Idamycin for Injection (26%) ... 564
IFEX (1%) ... 729
Imuran (Less than 1%) ... 768
Inderal ... 2459
Inderal LA Long Acting Capsules ... 2461
Inderide Tablets ... 2463
Inderide LA Long Acting Capsules ... 2465
Inocor Lactate Injection (0.9%) ... 2048
▲Intron A (37% to 68%) ... 2097
▲IPOL Poliovirus Vaccine Inactivated (38%) ... 894
Isoptin SR Sustained Release Tablets ... 1181
Keftab Tablets ... 917
Kefurox Vials, Faspak & ADD-Vantage ... 1277
Kerlone Tablets (Less than 2%) ... 2172
Klonopin Tablets ... 1902
Konÿne 80 Factor IX Complex ... 1571
Konÿne-HT Factor IX Complex ... 1583
Koro-Flex Arcing Spring Diaphragm ... 2142
Koromex Coil Spring Diaphragm ... 2142
Lamprene Capsules (Less than 1%) ... 1030
▲Lariam Tablets (Among most frequent) ... 1904
Lasix Tablets and Injection ... 1093
▲Leukine for IV Infusion (Among most frequent) ... 1127
Levatol ... 1832
Lodine Capsules ... 2468
Lopressor HCT Tablets ... 1034
Loxitane ... 1213
Lozol Tablets ... 1843
▲Lupron Depot 3.75 mg (Among most frequent) ... 2312
Lupron Depot 7.5 mg (Less than 5%) ... 2311
Lupron Injection (Less than 5%) ... 2310
M-M-R$_{II}$ ... 1494
M-R-VAX$_{II}$ ... 1496
Macrodantin Capsules (Rare) ... 1624
Matulane Capsules ... 1907
Maxzide ... 1215
Mebaral Tablets (Less than 1 in 100) ... 2061
Mefoxin ... 1498
Mefoxin Premixed Intravenous Solution ... 1500
Mellaril ... 2011
Meruvax$_{II}$ ... 1503
Methadone Hydrochloride Diskets ... 1284
Methotrexate Tablets, Parenteral, LPF Parenteral (Less common to frequent) ... 1217
Mevacor Tablets ... 1505
Mexitil Capsules (1.2%) ... 680
Miltown Tablets (Rare) ... 2386
Mini-Gamulin Rh, Rh$_0$(D) Immune Globulin (Human) (Occasional) ... 612
Minipress Capsules ... 1778
Minizide Capsules ... 1779
Mintezol ... 1510
Mithracin ... 1602
Moban Tablets & Concentrate ... 932
Moduretic Tablets ... 1510
▲Monistat I.V. (10%) ... 1143
Monocid Injection (Less than 1%) ... 2217
Monopril Tablets (0.2 to 1.0%) ... 1406
Motrin Tablets (Less than 1%) ... 2351
Mumpsvax (Uncommon) ... 1513
▲Mutamycin (14%) ... 733
Myambutol Tablets ... 1225
Myochrysine Injection ... 1516
Nalfon Pulvules & Tablets (Less than 1%) ... 919
Naprosyn (Less than 1%) ... 2297
Nardil (Less frequent) ... 1742
Naturetin Tablets (Occasional) ... 1789
Navane Capsules and Concentrate ... 1954
Navane Intramuscular ... 1956
Nebcin Vials, Hyporets & ADD-Vantage ... 1286
Nembutal Sodium Capsules ... 534
Nembutal Sodium Solution (Less than 1%) ... 536
Nembutal Sodium Suppositories (Less than 1%) ... 538
Neptazane Tablets ... ◉ 311
Netromycin Injection 100 mg/ml (1 of 1000 patients) ... 2104
▲Neupogen for Injection (12%) ... 595
Niclocide Chewable Tablets ... 1607
Nizoral Tablets (Less than 1%) ... 1145
Normodyne Tablets ... 2110
Normozide Tablets ... 2112
Noroxin Tablets (Less frequent) ... 1519
Norpace (Infrequent) ... 2177
Norzine (Occasional) ... 1818
▲Novantrone for Injection Concentrate (24 to 78%) ... 1226
Nuromax Injection ... 794
Omnipaque (Less than 0.7 to 3%) ... 2552
Oncovin Solution Vials & Hyporets ... 1288
Orap Tablets ... 1020
Ortho Diaphragm Kit ... 1664
▲Orthoclone OKT3 Sterile Solution (89% to 90%) ... 1645
Ortho-White Diaphragm Kit-Flat Spring ... 1664
PMB 200 and PMB 400 (Rare) ... 2504
Panhematin ... 546
Panwarfin Tablets (Infrequent) ... 547
ParaGard T380A Intrauterine Copper Contraceptive ... 411
PediaProfen Suspension (Less than 1%) ... 1363
PedvaxHIB ... 1521
Peganone Tablets ... 551
▲Pentam 300 Injection (3.5%) ... 1018
Pentaspan Injection ... 949
Pepcid (Infrequent) ... 1524
Pergonal (menotropins for injection, USP) ... 2184
Pfizerpen for Injection ... 1957
Pfizerpen-AS Aqueous Suspension ... 1959
Phenobarbital Elixir and Tablets (Less than 1 in 100 patients) ... 1293
Phenurone Tablets (Less than 1%) ... 552
▲Plague Vaccine (10%) ... 1584
Pneumovax 23 (Rare) ... 1528
Pnu-Imune 23 Pneumococcal Vaccine Polyvalent (Occasional) ... 1233
Polymyxin B Sulfate, Aerosporin Brand Sterile Powder ... 798
Pondimin Tablets ... 1867
Potaba (Infrequent) ... 1071
Prilosec Delayed-Release Capsules (Less than 1%) ... 1530
Primaxin I.M. ... 1532
Primaxin I.V. (0.5%) ... 1535
Prinivil Tablets (1% or less) ... 1538
Prinzide Tablets (0.3 to 1%) ... 1540
Procan SR Tablets (Common) ... 1760
Procardia Capsules (2% or less) ... 1781
Procardia XL Tablets (1% or less) ... 1783
▲Procrit for Injection (38%) ... 1647
Proglycem ... 649
▲ProHIBiT Haemophilus b Conjugate Vaccine (Diphtheria Toxoid Conjugate) (3.9%) ... 896
Prokine for I.V. Infusion ... 1096
Prolastin Alpha$_1$-Proteinase Inhibitor (Human) ... 1585
Prolixin Decanoate ... 1795
Prolixin Elixir ... 1793
Prolixin Enanthate ... 1796
Prolixin Injection ... 1791
Prolixin Tablets ... 1793
Proloprim Tablets ... 799
Pronestyl Capsules and Tablets ... 1800
Pronestyl Injection ... 1798
Pronestyl-SR Tablets ... 1801
ProSom Tablets (Infrequent) ... 554
▲Prostin VR Pediatric Sterile Solution (14%) ... 2355
Protostat Tablets ... 1674
Provera Tablets ... 2356
Prozac Pulvules (1.4%) ... 920
Quadrinal Tablets ... 1183
Quinaglute Dura-Tabs Tablets ... 663
Quinamm Tablets ... 1344
Quinidex Extentabs ... 1868
Rauzide Tablets ... 1804
▲Retrovir Capsules (3.2% to 16%) ... 802
▲Retrovir I.V. Infusion (16%) ... 805
▲Retrovir Syrup (3.2% to 16%) ... 802
Rheumatrex Methotrexate Dose Pack (Less common to frequent) ... 1234
▲RhoGAM Rh$_0$(D) Immune Globulin (Human) (25% in one study) ... 1651
Ridaura Capsules (Rare) ... 2224
Rifadin ... 1345
Rifamate Capsules ... 1347
Rimactane Capsules ... 879
Ritalin ... 880
Robaxin Injectable ... 1871
Robaxin Tablets ... 1872
Robaxisal Tablets ... 1872
Rocephin Injectable Vials, ADD-Vantage (Less than 1%) ... 1914
▲Roferon-A Injection (74% to 98%) ... 1916
▲Rowasa (1.2 to 3.19%) ... 2248
Rubex (Ocacsional) ... 739
Rufen Tablets (Less than 1%) ... 691
Ru-Tuss Tablets ... 693
Rythmol Tablets (1.9%) ... 1184
Salutensin/Salutensin-Demi ... 719
Sandimmune (2% or less) ... 2024
Sandoglobulin I.V. (Less than 1%) ... 2027
Sandostatin Injection (Less than 1%) ... 2029
Sansert Tablets ... 2031
Seconal Sodium Pulvules (Less than 1 in 100) ... 1296
Sectral Capsules ... 2520
Ser-Ap-Es Tablets ... 881
Serax Capsules ... 2522
Serax Tablets ... 2522
Serentil ... 686
Serpasil-Apresoline Tablets ... 884
Solganal Suspension ... 2122
Soma Compound w/Codeine Tablets ... 2390
Soma Compound Tablets ... 2389
Soma Tablets ... 2388
Staphage Lysate (SPL) ... 905
Stelazine ... 2226
▲Streptase for Infusion (0 to 21%) ... 635
Tagamet (Rare) ... 2228
Tambocor Tablets (1-3%) ... 1315
Tao Capsules ... 1963
Taractan ... 1920
Tazicef for Injection (2%) ... 2231
Tazidime Vials, Faspak & ADD-Vantage ... 1299
▲Tegison Capsules (10-25%) ... 1881
Tegretol Chewable Tablets ... 654
Tegretol Suspension ... 656
Tegretol Tablets ... 654
Tenoretic Tablets ... 1105
Tenormin Tablets and I.V. Injection ... 1107
Terazol 3 Vaginal Cream (1%) ... 1676
Terazol 3 Vaginal Suppositories (2.8% of 284 patients) ... 1677
Terazol 7 Vaginal Cream (1.7% of 521 patients) ... 1677
Tetanus & Diphtheria Toxoids, Adsorbed Purogenated (Rare) ... 1237
Tetanus Toxoid, Adsorbed Purogenated ... 1238
▲TheraCys BCG Live (Intravesical) (2.6% to 38.4%) ... 898
Thiotepa Parenteral ... 1240
Thorazine (Occasional) ... 2234
Timolide Tablets ... 1547
Timoptic in Ocudose ... 1552
Timoptic Sterile Ophthalmic Solution ... 1550
Tolectin (200, 400 and 600 mg) (Less than 1%) ... 1379
Tonocard Tablets (Less than 1%) ... 1554
Torecan (Occasional) ... 1993
Trandate HCT/Trandate (Less common) ... 579
Trexan Tablets (Less than 1%) ... 937
Triavil Tablets ... 1556
Tridione ... 557
▲Tri-Immunol Diphtheria & Tetanus Toxoids & Pertussis Vaccine, Adsorbed (50%) ... 1241
Trilafon ... 2123
Trimpex Tablets ... 1922
Trobicin Sterile Powder ... 2366
Urispas Tablets ... 2242
Vascor (200, 300 and 400 mg) Tablets (0.5 to 2.0%) ... 1383
Vaseretic Tablets ... 1559
Vasotec I.V. (0.5 to 1%) ... 1562
Vasotec Tablets (0.5% to 1%) ... 1564
VePesid Capsules and Injection (0.7 to 2%) ... 741
Verelan Capsules (1% or less) ... 1243
Visken Tablets ... 2036
Vivactil Tablets ... 1567
Wellbutrin Tablets (1.2%) ... 821
Wycillin Injection ... 2537
Yodoxin ... 1072
Zantac Injection and Zantac Injection Premixed ... 1063
Zantac (Rare) ... 1065
Zefazone Sterile Powder ... 2372
Zestoretic (0.3 to 1%) ... 2274
Zestril Tablets (Less than 1%) ... 2277
Zoladex (1% to 5%) ... 1110
Zovirax Capsules ... 824
Zovirax Sterile Powder ... 828
Zovirax ... 824
Zyloprim Tablets (Less than 1%) ... 830

Fever, neutropenic

▲Neupogen for Injection (13%) ... 595

Fibrillations

Cardioquin Tablets ... 1812
Narcan Injection ... 933
Nicolar Tablets ... 1846
Nicorette ... 1335
Pronestyl-SR Tablets ... 1801
Tambocor Tablets ... 1315
Tenex Tablets ... 1875

Fibrillations, atrial

Cardene Capsules (Less than 0.4%) ... 2290
Desyrel and Desyrel Dividose ... 1404
DynaCirc Capsules (0.5% to 1%) ... 2004
Emete-con Intramuscular/Intravenous ... 1950
Ethmozine Tablets (Less than 2%) ... 946
Idamycin for Injection ... 564
Intron A (Less than 1%) ... 2097
Lopid Capsules and Tablets (0.7%) ... 1736
Nalfon Pulvules & Tablets (Less than 1%) ... 919
Niacor Tablets ... 2376
Nicolar Tablets ... 1846
OptiPranolol Sterile Ophthalmic Solution (A small number of patients) ... ◉ 261
Permax Tablets (Infrequent) ... 1291
Rythmol Tablets (0.7 to 1.2%) ... 1184
Tegison Capsules (Less than 1%) ... 1881
▲Tenormin Tablets and I.V. Injection (5%) ... 1107
Vaseretic Tablets ... 1559
Vasotec I.V. ... 1562
Vasotec Tablets (0.5% to 1.0%) ... 1564

Fibrillations, ventricular

Dilantin Parenteral ... 1712
Diprivan Injection (Less than 1%) ... 2267
DynaCirc Capsules (0.5% to 1%) ... 2004
Fungizone Intravenous ... 2262
Isoptin SR Sustained Release Tablets ... 1181
Lanoxicaps ... 772
Lorelco Tablets ... 1333
Marcaine Hydrochloride with Epinephrine 1:200,000 ... 2055
Marcaine Hydrochloride Injection ... 2055
Norpace ... 2177
Norpramin Tablets ... 1340
Nuromax Injection ... 794
Procan SR Tablets (Common) ... 1760
Pronestyl Capsules and Tablets ... 1800
▲Pronestyl Injection (More common) ... 1798
Pronestyl-SR Tablets ... 1801
Prostin VR Pediatric Sterile Solution (Less than 1%) ... 2355
Quinaglute Dura-Tabs Tablets ... 663
Quinidex Extentabs ... 1868
Seldane Tablets (Rare) ... 1349
Seldane-D Extended-Release Tablets (Rare) ... 1350
Sensorcaine ... 631
Sensorcaine-MPF Spinal ... 634
Tonocard Tablets (Less than 1%) ... 1554

Fibrosis

Gelfoam Sterile Sponge ... 2338
Imferon ... 976
INSTAT Collagen Absorbable Hemostat ... 1151
Inversine Tablets ... 1492
Methotrexate Tablets, Parenteral, LPF Parenteral ... 1217
Myochrysine Injection ... 1516
Rheumatrex Methotrexate Dose Pack ... 1234
Ridaura Capsules (Rare) ... 2224
Solganal Suspension ... 2122

Fibrosis, bladder
Cytoxan for Injection ... 726
Neosar for Injection ... 566

Fibrosis, interstitial pulmonary (see under Pulmonary fibrosis)

Fibrosis, macular
Meclomen Capsules ... 1739

Fibrosis, ovary
Cytoxan for Injection ... 726
Neosar for Injection ... 566

Fibrosis, pelvic
Lupron Depot 7.5 mg ... 2311
Lupron Injection ... 2310

Fibrosis, periportal
Tagamet (Rare) ... 2228

Fibrosis, pleural
D.H.E. 45 Injection ... 2003

Fingernails, brittle
Sandimmune (2% or less) ... 2024
Trental (Less than 1%) ... 1099

Fingernails, darkening
Drithocreme ... 590
Dritho-Scalp ... 591

Fingers, discoloration
Cibalith-S ... 870
Eskalith ... 2214
Lithane Tablets (Single case) ... 1596
Lithium Carbonate Capsules & Tablets (A single report) ... 1984
Lithobid Tablets ... 870

Fissuring
AK-Taine ... ⊚ 207
Alcaine ... ⊚ 210
Ergamisol Tablets ... 1136
Sterile FUDR (Remote possibility) ... 1898
Fluoracaine ... ⊚ 208
Fluorouracil Injection ... 1897
Ophthetic ... ⊚ 249
Oxistat Cream (0.1%) ... 1055

Fistula, regional lymph node
BCG Vaccine, USP (Tice) (Rare) ... 1632
Tice BCG Vaccine, USP (Rare) ... 1632

Flaccidity
Omnipaque ... 2552

Flare
▲ Atgam Sterile Solution (1 in 8 patients; 27%) ... 2320
Dipentum Capsules ... 1160

Flare, postinjection
Aristospan Suspension (Intra-articular) ... 1011
Attenuvax (Rare) ... 1424
Biavax II ... 1427
Celestone Soluspan Suspension ... 2081
Decadron Phosphate Injection ... 1449
Decadron-LA Sterile Suspension ... 1457
Demerol ... 2047
Depo-Medrol Sterile Aqueous Suspension ... 2334
Hydeltrasol Injection, Sterile ... 1476
Hydeltra-T.B.A. Sterile Suspension ... 1478
Hydrocortone Acetate Sterile Suspension ... 1479
Kenalog-10 Injection ... 2402
Kenalog-40 Injection ... 2403
M-M-R II ... 1494
M-R-VAX II ... 1496
Mepergan Injection ... 2479
Meruvax II ... 1503
Mumpsvax (Rare) ... 1513
Stilphostrol Tablets and Ampuls ... 1609

Flatulence
Actigall Capsules ... 2280
Adalat Capsules (10 mg and 20 mg) (2% or less) ... 1587
AeroBid Inhaler System (1-3%) ... 995
Aldoclor Tablets ... 1413
Aldomet Ester HCl Injection ... 1417
Aldomet Oral ... 1415
Aldoril Tablets ... 1418
▲ Anafranil Capsules (Up to 6%) ... 650
Ansaid Tablets (1-3%) ... 2319
Asendin Tablets (Less than 1%) ... 1196
Atromid-S Capsules (Less frequent) ... 2435
Augmentin Tablets, Powder for Oral Suspension, and Chewable Tablets (Less frequent) ... 2198
Azo Gantrisin Tablets ... 1888
BuSpar (Infrequent) ... 1401
Butazolidin Capsules & Tablets (Less than 1%) ... 1027
Carafate Tablets (Less than 0.5%) ... 1326
Cardura Tablets (1%) ... 1941
Cartrol Tablets (Rare) ... 507
▲ Cephulac Syrup (20%) ... 1331
Children's Advil Suspension (Less than 3%) ... 2426
Cholybar (Less frequent) ... 1705
Chronulac Syrup ... 1332
Cipro I.V. (1% or less) ... 1592
Cipro Tablets ... 1589
Clinoril Tablets (1-3%) ... 1433
Colestid Granules (1 in 30 to 1 in 100 patients) ... 2328
Corgard Tablets (1 to 5 of 1000 patients) ... 701
Corzide Tablets (1 to 5 of 1000 patients) ... 702
Cytotec (2.9%) ... 2159
Desyrel and Desyrel Dividose (Less than 1%) ... 1404
Dipentum Capsules (Rare) ... 1160
Dolobid Tablets (Greater than 1 in 100) ... 1465
Duragesic Transdermal System (1% or greater) ... 1133
Emcyt Capsules (2%) ... 1161
Ergamisol Tablets (Less than 1 to 2%) ... 1136
Esgic-Plus Tablets (Less frequent) ... 1002
Esgic Tablets & Capsules (Less frequent) ... 1001
Eskalith ... 2214
Ethmozine Tablets (Less than 2%) ... 946
Feldene Capsules (1 to 3%) ... 1777
Fioricet Tablets (Less frequent) ... 2006
Fiorinal (Less frequent) ... 2007
Flexeril Tablets (Less than 1%) ... 1471
Floxin Tablets (1% to 3%) ... 1652
Gastrocrom Capsules (Infrequent) ... 974
Geocillin Tablets ... 1951
Hytrin Tablets (At least 1%) ... 529
Indocin Capsules (Less than 1%) ... 1487
Indocin I.V. (Less than 1%) ... 1490
Indocin (Less than 1%) ... 1487
Intron A (Less than 1%) ... 2097
K-Dur Microburst Release System (potassium chloride, USP) E.R. Tablets ... 1163
▲ K-Lor Powder Packets (Most common) ... 531
▲ K-Tab Filmtab (Most common) ... 532
▲ Klor-Con 8/Klor-Con 10 Extended-release Tablets (Among most common) ... 2374
Larodopa Tablets (Infrequent) ... 1905
▲ Lodine Capsules (3-9%) ... 2468
Lopressor Ampuls (1%) ... 1032
Lopressor HCT Tablets (1 in 100) ... 1034
Lopressor Tablets (1%) ... 1032
Lorelco Tablets ... 1333
▲ Meclomen Capsules (3-9%) ... 1739
▲ Mevacor Tablets (6.4%) ... 1505
▲ Micro-K LS Packets (Most common) ... 1864
Midamor Tablets (Less than or equal to 1%) ... 1508
Moduretic Tablets (Less than or equal to 1%) ... 1510
Monopril Tablets (0.2 to 1.0%) ... 1406
Motrin Tablets (Less than 3%) ... 2351
Nalfon Pulvules & Tablets (Less than 1%) ... 919
Normozide Tablets (Less than 1%) ... 2112
Noroxin Tablets (0.3% to 1%) ... 1519
▲ Norpace (3 to 9%) ... 2177
▲ Omnipaque (1 to 10%) ... 2552
▲ Orudis Capsules (Greater than 3%) ... 2488
PediaProfen Suspension (Less than 3%) ... 1363
Permax Tablets (Infrequent) ... 1291
Phrenilin ... 838
Plendil Extended-Release Tablets (0.5% to 1.5%) ... 1526
Ponstel (Less frequent) ... 1758
Prilosec Delayed-Release Capsules (Less than 1 to 2.7%) ... 1530
Prinivil Tablets (1% or less) ... 1538
Prinzide Tablets ... 1540
Procardia Capsules (2% or less) ... 1781
Procardia XL Tablets (Less than 3%) ... 1783
ProSom Tablets (Infrequent) ... 554
Prostigmin Injectable ... 1120
Prostigmin Tablets ... 1121
Prozac Pulvules (1.6%) ... 920
Questran Light (Less frequent) ... 711
Questran Powder ... 710
Retrovir Capsules (Less than 5%) ... 802
Retrovir I.V. Infusion (Less than 5%) ... 805
Retrovir Syrup (Less than 5%) ... 802
▲ Ridaura Capsules (3 to 9%) ... 2224
Rifadin (Some patients) ... 1345
Rifamate Capsules (Some patients) ... 1347
Rimactane Capsules ... 879
Rocephin Injectable Vials, ADD-Vantage (Rare) ... 1914
Roferon-A Injection (Less than 3%) ... 1916
▲ Rowasa (3.6 to 6.13%) ... 2248
Rufen Tablets (1 to 3%) ... 691
Rythmol Tablets (0.3 to 1.9%) ... 1184
Sandostatin Injection (Less than 1%) ... 2029
▲ Sectral Capsules (3%) ... 2520
Sedapap Tablets 50 mg/650 mg (Less frequent) ... 1360
Sinemet Tablets ... 952
Sinemet CR Tablets ... 953
▲ Suprax (4%) ... 1235
Tambocor Tablets (Less than 1%) ... 1315
Tegison Capsules (Less than 1%) ... 1881
Timentin for Injection ... 2239
▲ Tolectin (200, 400 and 600 mg) (3 to 9%) ... 1379
Toradol IM Injection (1% or less) ... 2302
Trandate HCT Tablets (Less than 1% in 208 patients) ... 579
Trexan Tablets (Less than 1%) ... 937
Unasyn (Less than 1%) ... 1965
Urecholine ... 1558
Vascor (200, 300 and 400 mg) Tablets (0.5 to 2.0%) ... 1383
Vaseretic Tablets (0.5% to 2.0%) ... 1559
Voltaren Tablets (1-3%) ... 1042
Zestoretic ... 2274
Zestril Tablets (Less than 1%) ... 2277

Flatus
Pitressin Synthetic, Ampoules ... 1758
▲ Trental (0.6 to 9%) ... 1099

Floating feeling
Dilaudid-HP Injection ... 1175
MS Contin Tablets (Infrequent) ... 1814
MSIR (Infrequent) ... 1817
Nubain Injection (Less than 1%) ... 934
▲ Stadol (3%) ... 721

Fluid, encapsulation
Gelfoam Sterile Sponge ... 2338

Fluid depletion
Capoten ... 2255
Capozide ... 2258
Cephulac Syrup ... 1331
Chronulac Syrup ... 1332

Fluid imbalance
Corzide Tablets ... 702
Modane Plus Tablets ... ▣ 504
Modane Tablets ... ▣ 503
Normozide Tablets (Rare) ... 2112
Premarin with Methyltestosterone ... 2515
Prinzide Tablets ... 1540
Tenoretic Tablets ... 1105
Trandate HCT Tablets ... 579
Vaseretic Tablets ... 1559
Zestoretic ... 2274

Fluid overload
Orthoclone OKT3 Sterile Solution ... 1645

Fluid retention (see under Edema)

Flu-like symptoms
▲ Actimmune (Most common) ... 1046
▲ AeroBid Inhaler System (10%) ... 995
▲ Alferon N Injection (30%) ... 1809
Altace Capsules ... 1086
Atromid-S Capsules ... 2435
Cartrol Tablets (Less common) ... 507
▲ CHEMET (succimer) Capsules (5.2 to 15.7%) ... 1361
DTIC-Dome ... 1595
Engerix-B Unit-Dose Vials (Less than 1%) ... 2213
Epogen for Injection (Rare) ... 591
Ergamisol Tablets (5 patients) ... 1136
Eulexin Capsules ... 2089
Feldene Capsules (Less than 1%) ... 1777
Hytrin Tablets (At least 1%) ... 529
▲ Intron A (37% to 79%) ... 2097
Kerlone Tablets (Less than 2%) ... 2172
▲ Lopressor HCT Tablets (10 in 100 patients) ... 1034
Normodyne Injection ... 2108
Normodyne Tablets ... 2110
ParaGard T380A Intrauterine Copper Contraceptive ... 411
Pergonal (menotropins for injection, USP) ... 2184
▲ Permax Tablets (3.2%) ... 1291
Procrit for Injection (Rare) ... 1647
▲ ProSom Tablets (3%) ... 554
Prozac Pulvules (2.8%) ... 920
Retrovir Capsules (Less than 5%) ... 802
Retrovir I.V. Infusion (Less than 5%) ... 805
Retrovir Syrup (Less than 5%) ... 802
Rifadin ... 1345
Roferon-A Injection ... 1916
▲ Rowasa (5.28%) ... 2248
Tegison Capsules (Less than 1%) ... 1881
Trandate HCT Tablets ... 579
Trandate Injection ... 577
Trandate Tablets ... 579
Trental (Less than 1%) ... 1099
Vascor (200, 300 and 400 mg) Tablets (0.5 to 2.08%) ... 1383
Voltaren Tablets ... 1042
Wellbutrin Tablets (Frequent) ... 821

Fluorosis, dental
Mulvidren-F Softab Tablets ... 2273
Poly-Vi-Flor ... 1397
Poly-Vi-Flor Drops ... 1398
Poly-Vi-Flor with Iron ... 1399
Poly-Vi-Flor with Iron Drops ... 1399
Tri-Vi-Flor 1.0 mg Vitamins with Fluoride Chewable Tablets ... 1400
Tri-Vi-Flor Drops ... 1400
Tri-Vi-Flor 0.25 mg Vitamins with Iron and Fluoride Drops ... 1401

Flushing
Accutane Capsules (Less than 1%) ... 1878
▲ Adalat Capsules (10 mg and 20 mg) (About 10% to 25%) ... 1587
Americaine Hemorrhoidal Ointment ... ▣ 558
Aminohippurate Sodium Injection ... 1421
Aminophyllin Tablets ... 2153
▲ Anafranil Capsules (7% to 8%) ... 650
Antivenin (Crotalidae) Polyvalent ... 2430
Apresazide Capsules (Less frequent) ... 854
Apresoline Hydrochloride Parenteral (Ampuls) ... 856
Apresoline Hydrochloride Tablets (Less frequent) ... 855
Apresoline-Esidrix Tablets ... 857
AquaMEPHYTON Injection ... 1422
Asbron G ... 1997
Atrovent Inhalation Aerosol (Less than 1 in 100) ... 675
Azactam for Injection (1 patient) ... 2252
Azo Gantrisin Tablets ... 1888
Bellergal-S Tablets (Rare) ... 1998
Benemid Tablets ... 1426
BiCNU ... 723
Bontril Slow-Release ... 834
Brethine Ampuls (0.0 to 2.4%) ... 1026
Bretylol Injection (1 in 1000) ... 923
Brevibloc Injection (Less than 1%) ... 942
Brexin L.A. Capsules ... 2078
Bromfed ... 1615
BuSpar (Infrequent) ... 1401
Calan SR Caplets (0.6%) ... 2157
Calan Tablets (0.6%) ... 2155
▲ Calcimar Injection, Synthetic (2 to 5%) ... 1839
Capoten (2 to 5 of 1000 patients) ... 2255
Capozide (2 to 5 of 1000 patients) ... 2258
▲ Cardene Capsules (5.6-9.7%) ... 2290
Cardilate Oral/Sublingual Tablets ... 757
Cardizem Tablets-30 mg, 60 mg, 90 mg and 120 mg (Less than 1%) ... 1329
Cardizem SR Capsules-60 mg, 90 mg and 120 mg (1.7-3%) ... 1327
Cardura Tablets (Less than 0.5% of 3960 patients) ... 1941
Choledyl Pediatric Elixir ... 1702
Choledyl Tablets ... 1700
Choledyl SA Tablets ... 1704
Chromagen Capsules ... 2078
▲ Cibacalcin Double-chambered Syringes (16-21%) ... 859
Cipro I.V. (1% or less) ... 1592
Cipro Tablets (Less than 1%) ... 1589

Clear By Design Medicated Cleansing Pads ▣ 709
Clinoril Tablets (Less than 1 in 100) 1433
Codimal 846
ColBENEMID Tablets 1436
Constant-T Tablets 1029
Cordarone Tablets (1 to 3%) 2446
▲CytoGam (Less than 5.0%) 891
DDAVP (Occasional) 1841
Dalgan Injection (Less than 1%) 620
Dalmane Capsules (Rare) 1927
Danocrine Capsules 2046
Dayto Himbin Tablets and Liquid 905
Dilatrate-SR 1827
Dilaudid-HP Injection 1175
Dilor 2079
Diprivan Injection (Greater than 1%) 2267
Donnagel (Rare) ▣ 675
Donnagel-PG (Rare) 1858
Dopram Injectable 1860
Duvoid Tablets 1853
▲DynaCirc Capsules (Up to 3.3%) 2004
Emcyt Capsules (1%) 1161
Emete-con Intramuscular/Intravenous 1950
Eminase (Occasional) 2211
Engerix-B Unit-Dose Vials (Less than 1%) 2213
Factrel (Rare) 2561
Fiorinal with Codeine Capsules 2008
Flagyl I.V. 2131
Flagyl Tablets 2170
Flex-all 454 Pain Relieving Gel ▣ 546
Fungizone Intravenous 2262
Furoxone (Rare) 1855
Gamimune N Immune Globulin Intravenous (Human) 1572
Gammagard Immune Globulin, Intravenous (Human) (Occasional) 658
Gammar-IV, Immune Globulin Intravenous (Human) 610
Gastrocrom Capsules (Infrequent) 974
Hyperstat I.V. Injection 2095
Hyskon Hysteroscopy Fluid (Rare) 1162
Imferon 976
Indocin Capsules (Less than 1%) 1487
Indocin I.V. (Less than 1%) 1490
Indocin (Less than 1%) 1487
Intron A (Up to 5%) 2097
Isoptin Oral Tablets (0.6%) 1179
Isoptin SR Sustained Release Tablets (0.6%) 1181
Isordil 2467
Kerlone Tablets (Less than 2%) 2172
Konӯne 80 Factor IX Complex 1571
Konӯne-HT Factor IX Complex 1583
Larodopa Tablets (Infrequent) 1905
Lodine Capsules (Less than 1%) 2468
Lomotil 2174
Lotensin Tablets 872
Lozol Tablets (Less than 5%) 1843
Ludiomil Tablets 874
Lufyllin & Lufyllin-400 Tablets 2384
Lufyllin-GG Elixir & Tablets 2385
Lutrepulse for Injection 1655
Lysodren 731
Matulane Capsules 1907
Maxair Inhaler (Less than 1%) 1311
Mephyton Tablets 1503
Metubine Iodide Vials 1285
Mevacor Tablets (Rare) 1505
Miochol with Iocare Steri-Tags, Miochol System Pak and Miochol System Pak Plus (Rare) ⊙ 274
MIOSTAT ⊙ 233
Moduretic Tablets (Less than or equal to 1%) 1510
Monistat I.V. 1143
Monopril Tablets (0.2 to 1.0%) 1406
Motofen Tablets 836
Myochrysine Injection 1516
Nicobid 1846
Nicorette 1335
Nimotop Capsules (Less than 1% to 2.1%) 1607
Nipride I.V. Infusion 1909
Nitro-Bid IV 1338
Nitro-Bid Ointment 1339
Nitrolingual Spray 1846
▲Nolvadex Tablets (32.7%) 1102
Norcuron (Rare) 1642
Normodyne Injection (1%) 2108
Norpramin Tablets 1340
Nubain Injection (Less than 1%) 934
Nuromax Injection 794
Omnipaque 2552
Pamelor 2019
Pantopon Injectable 1911
Pepcid (Infrequent) 1524
Peptavlon 2563
Persantine Tablets 683
Plegine Tablets 2504
▲Plendil Extended-Release Tablets (1.0% to 20.0%) 1526
Polymyxin B Sulfate, Aerosporin Brand Sterile Powder 798
Primaxin I.M. 1532
Primaxin I.V. (Less than 0.2%) 1535
Prinivil Tablets (1% or less) 1538
Prinzide Tablets (0.3 to 1%) 1540
Priscoline Hydrochloride Ampuls 877
Procan SR Tablets (Occasional) 1760
Procardia Capsules (1%) 1781
▲Procardia XL Tablets (Less than 3% to 25%) 1783
ProHIBiT Haemophilus b Conjugate Vaccine (Diphtheria Toxoid Conjugate) 896
Pronestyl Capsules and Tablets (Occasional) 1800
Pronestyl Injection (Occasional) 1798
Pronestyl-SR Tablets 1801
ProSom Tablets (Infrequent) 554
Prostigmin Injectable 1120
Prostigmin Tablets 1121
▲Prostin VR Pediatric Sterile Solution (10%) 2355
Protamine Sulfate Ampoules & Vials 1295
Protostat Tablets 1674
Proventil (Less than 1%) 2120
Quadrinal Tablets 1183
Quibron Capsules 713
Quibron-T 714
Quibron-T/SR 716
Recombivax HB (Less than 1%) 1544
Regitine 878
Reglan 1869
Renese-R Tablets 1786
Respbid Tablets 684
Rifadin 1345
Robaxin Injectable 1871
Rocephin Injectable Vials, ADD-Vantage (Occasional) 1914
Roferon-A Injection (Less than 0.5%) 1916
Rythmol Tablets (Less than 1%) 1184
Salutensin/Salutensin-Demi 719
Sandimmune (Less than 1 to 4%) 2024
Sandostatin Injection (1.4%) 2029
Ser-Ap-Es Tablets 881
Serpasil-Apresoline Tablets 884
Sinemet Tablets 952
Sinemet CR Tablets 953
Sinequan (Occasional) 1960
Slo-bid Gyrocaps 1847
Slo-Niacin Tablets 2376
Solganal Suspension 2122
Sorbitrate 1103
Stadol (Less than 1%) 721
Streptase for Infusion 635
Surmontil Capsules 2524
T-PHYL (Uniphyl) 200 mg Tablets 1820
Talacen (Infrequent) 2070
Talwin Compound (Infrequent) 2072
Talwin Nx (Infrequent) 2073
Tambocor Tablets (1-3%) 1315
Theo-24 2179
Theo-Dur Sprinkle 1168
Theo-Dur Extended-Release Tablets 1166
Theolair 1317
Theolair-SR Tablets 1319
▲TheoX Extended-Release Tablets (Among most consistent) 841
Tofranil Ampuls 1038
Tofranil Tablets 1039
Tofranil-PM Capsules 1041
Tornalate (Rare) 2074
Trancopal Caplets 2075
Trandate Injection (1 of 100 patients) 577
Trental (2.3%) 1099
Uniphyl 400 mg Tablets 1823
Urised Tablets 2396
Vancocin HCl, Vials & ADD-Vantage 1302
Vaseretic Tablets 1559
Vasotec I.V. 1562
Vasotec Tablets (0.5% to 1%) 1564
Ventolin Tablets (1 of 100 patients) 583
VePesid Capsules and Injection 741
Verelan Capsules (0.6%) 1243
Vivactil Tablets 1567
Voltaren Tablets (Rare) 1042
Wellbutrin Tablets (Rare) 821
Yocon 1686
Yohimex Tablets 1190
Zestoretic (0.3 to 1%) 2274
Zestril Tablets (Less than 1%) 2277

Flushing, cutaneous

Actibine 900
Baron-X Tablets 650
Cardioquin Tablets 1812
Diupres Tablets 1461
Duvoid Tablets 1853
Hydropres Tablets 1485
Isuprel Hydrochloride Injection 1:5000 2050
Isuprel Hydrochloride Mistometer 2051
Isuprel Hydrochloride Solution 1:200 & 1:100 2052
Nicotinex Elixir ▣ 563
Nitro-Bid IV 1338
Nitro-Bid Capsules 1338
Nitrolingual Spray 1846
Nitrostat IV 1744
Peritrate 1756
Quinaglute Dura-Tabs Tablets 663
Quinamm Tablets 1344
Quinidex Extentabs 1868
Roferon-A Injection (Less than 0.5%) 1916
Talwin Nx 2073
▲Tracrium Injection (5%) 817
Urecholine 1558

Flushing, ears

▲Cibacalcin Double-chambered Syringes (16-21%) 859

Flushing, facial

▲Adenocard Injection (18%) 1007
Adriamycin PFS 561
Adriamycin RDF 562
Alferon N Injection (One patient) 1809
▲Calcimar Injection, Synthetic (2 to 5%) 1839
Chromagen Capsules 2078
▲Cibacalcin Double-chambered Syringes (16-21%) 859
DDAVP Injection (Occasional) 1840
DTIC-Dome 1595
Demerol 2047
Dolophine Hydrochloride Ampoules & Vials 1260
Dolophine Hydrochloride Tablets 1261
Doxorubicin Hydrochloride for Injection, USP 622
Doxorubicin Hydrochloride Injection, USP 848
Duvoid Tablets 1853
Geref (sermorelin acetate for injection) 2560
Loxitane 1213
MS Contin Tablets (Infrequent) 1814
MSIR (Infrequent) 1817
Mepergan Injection 2479
Methadone Hydrochloride Diskets 1284
Methadone Hydrochloride Oral Solution & Tablets 1987
Miacalcin Injection (About 2-5%) 2017
Mintezol 1510
Mithracin 1602
Oramorph SR (Morphine Sulfate Sustained Release Tablets) (Less frequent) 1988
Papaverine Hydrochloride Vials and Ampoules 1290
Phenergan with Codeine 2497
Phenergan VC with Codeine 2501
Roxanol 1991
Rubex 739
Sandimmune 2024
Sandoglobulin I.V. (Less than 1%) 2027
Sansert Tablets (Rare) 2031
Soma Compound w/Codeine Tablets 2390
Soma Compound Tablets 2389
Tonocard Tablets (Less than 1%) 1554
Urecholine 1558

Flushing, generalized

Calcimar Injection, Synthetic 1839
Niacor Tablets 2376
Nicolar Tablets 1846

Flushing, hands

▲Calcimar Injection, Synthetic (2 to 5%) 1839
▲Cibacalcin Double-chambered Syringes (16-21%) 859
Miacalcin Injection (About 2-5%) 2017

Flushing, upper thorax

Sandimmune 2024

Focal sensorimotor signs, unspecified

Methotrexate Tablets, Parenteral, LPF Parenteral 1217
Rheumatrex Methotrexate Dose Pack 1234

Folic acid absorption, impaired

Azulfidine Tablets, EN-tabs, Oral Suspension 1157

Follicle development, multiple

Lutrepulse for Injection 1655

Follicular atresia, delayed

Norplant System 2484

Follicular staining

Meclan (meclocycline sulfosalicylate) Cream 1679

Folliculitis

Aclovate 1053
Alphatrex Cream, Ointment & Lotion (Infrequent) 2076
Anafranil Capsules (Rare) 650
Analpram-HC Rectal Cream 1% and 2.5% 970
Anusol-HC Cream (Infrequent) 1690
Anusol-HC Suppositories 1691
Aristocort A (Infrequent) 1010
Betatrex Cream, Ointment & Lotion 2077
Carmol HC Cream 1% (Infrequent) 2296
Cibalith-S 870
Cleocin T Topical 2327
Cortisporin Cream 757
Cortisporin Ointment 758
Cortisporin Otic Solution Sterile 760
Cortisporin Otic Suspension Sterile 760
Cutivate Cream 0.05% 1054
Cutivate Ointment 0.005% (Infrequent to more frequent) 1054
Cyclocort Lotion (Infrequent) 1198
Decadron Phosphate Topical Cream 1455
Decaspray Topical Aerosol 1459
DesOwen Cream, Ointment and Lotion (Infrequent) 1682
Diprolene (Less than 1%) 2083
Eldecort Cream 1.0% (Infrequent) 1113
Eldecort Cream 1.0% and 2.5% (Infrequent) 1113
Elocon (Infrequent) 2084
Epifoam 1828
Eskalith 2214
Florone/Florone E 908
Halog (Infrequent) 2399
Halotex Cream & Solution (1 in 977 patients) 2400
Hytone 909
Kenalog Cream, Lotion & Ointment (Infrequent) 2401
Lidex (Infrequent) 2296
Lithane Tablets 1596
Lithium Carbonate Capsules & Tablets 1984
Lithobid Tablets 870
Locoid Cream, Ointment and Topical Solution (Infrequent) 970
Lotrisone Cream (Infrequent) 2103
Mantadil Cream 789
Maxivate Cream, Lotion & Ointment 0.05% 2406
Mycolog II Cream and Ointment (Infrequent) 2407
Mytrex Cream & Ointment (Infrequent) 2080
NeoDecadron Topical Cream 1518
Neo-Synalar Cream (Infrequent) 2296
Nutracort Cream & Lotion (infrequent) 1684
Otic Tridesilon Solution 0.05% (infrequent) 1612
Oxsoralen-Ultra Capsule 1117
PediOtic Suspension Sterile 797
Pramosone Cream, Lotion & Ointment 971
ProctoCream-HC (Infrequent) 1834
Proctofoam-HC 1835
Psorcon Ointment 0.05% 909
Psorion Cream 0.05% (Infrequent) 1121
Synacort Creams 1%, 2.5% (Infrequent) 2296
Synalar (Infrequent) 2296
Temovate (1 of 366 patients) 1056
Topicort (Infrequent) 1098
Tridesilon Creme 0.05% (infrequent) 1611

Tridesilon Ointment 0.05% (infrequent) 1611
Ultravate Cream 0.05% (Infrequent) 2410
Ultravate Ointment 0.05% (Less frequent) 2411
Vanoxide-HC Acne Lotion 911
Vioform-Hydrocortisone Cream and Mild Cream 889
Vioform-Hydrocortisone Ointment 889
Vytone Cream 1% 911
Westcort 2411
Zetar Emulsion 911

Fontanels, bulging

Achromycin V Capsules 1193
Declomycin Capsules, Tablets 1199
Doryx Capsules 1717
Minocin Intravenous 1221
Minocin Oral Suspension 1224
Minocin Pellet-Filled Capsules 1222
Monodox Capsules 1630
NegGram (Occasional) 2062
Nizoral Tablets (Less than 1%) 1145
Terramycin Capsules 1786
Terramycin Intramuscular Solution 1964
Tri-Immunol Diphtheria & Tetanus Toxoids & Pertussis Vaccine, Adsorbed 1241
Urobiotic-250 Capsules 1968
Vibramycin Hyclate Capsules 1787
Vibramycin Hyclate Intravenous 1968
Vibramycin 1787

Foot drop

Matulane Capsules 1907
Oncovin Solution Vials & Hyporets 1288

Forceps delivery, increased incidence

Carbocaine Hydrochloride Injection 2043
Marcaine Hydrochloride with Epinephrine 1:200,000 2055
Marcaine Hydrochloride Injection 2055
Sensorcaine 631

Foreign body reaction

Anafranil Capsules (Infrequent) 650
▲Ciloxan Sterile Ophthalmic Solution (Less than 10%) ◉ 214
Gelfoam Sterile Sponge 2338
Hemopad Absorbable Collagen Hemostat 627
INSTAT Collagen Absorbable Hemostat 1151
Surgicel 1151

Foreskin irretraction (see under Preputium, irretraction of)

Foveal reflex, loss of

Aralen Phosphate Tablets 2039
Plaquenil Sulfate Tablets 2067

Fracture, pathological

Prozac Pulvules (Rare) 920

Fractures, long bones

Aristocort Suspension 1008
Aristospan Suspension 1011
Celestone Soluspan Suspension 2081
Cortenema 2244
Cortifoam 1827
Cortone Acetate Sterile Suspension 1437
Cortone Acetate Tablets 1439
Dalalone D.P. Injectable 999
Decadron Phosphate Injection 1449
Decadron Phosphate Respihaler 1454
Decadron Phosphate Turbinaire 1456
Decadron Tablets 1447
Decadron-LA Sterile Suspension 1457
Deltasone Tablets 2332
Depo-Medrol Sterile Aqueous Suspension 2334
Hydeltrasol Injection, Sterile 1476
Hydeltra-T.B.A. Sterile Suspension 1478
Hydrocortone Acetate Sterile Suspension 1479
Hydrocortone Phosphate Injection, Sterile 1481
Hydrocortone Tablets 1482
Kenalog-40 Injection 2403
Medrol 2348
Pediapred Oral Liquid 987
Solu-Cortef Sterile Powder 2361
Solu-Medrol Sterile Powder 2363

Fractures, unspecified

Rogaine Topical Solution (2.59%) 2357

Fractures, vertebral compression

Aristocort Suspension 1008
Aristospan Suspension 1011
Celestone Soluspan Suspension 2081
Cortenema 2244
Dalalone D.P. Injectable 999
Decadron Tablets 1447
Decadron-LA Sterile Suspension 1457
Hydeltrasol Injection, Sterile 1476
Hydeltra-T.B.A. Sterile Suspension 1478
Hydrocortone Acetate Sterile Suspension 1479
Hydrocortone Phosphate Injection, Sterile 1481
Hydrocortone Tablets 1482
Kenalog-10 Injection 2402
Kenalog-40 Injection 2403

Freckling

Cytosar-U Sterile Powder (Less frequent) 2329

Free fatty acids, elevation

▲Yutopar (80 to 100% with IV administration) 647

Free T3 resin uptake, decrease (see under T3, decrease)

Frigidity, unspecified

Sandostatin Injection (Less than 1%) 2029

Fullness, abdominal (see under Abdominal bloating)

Fungal invasion

Cetapred Ointment ◉ 220
FML-S Sterile Ophthalmic Suspension ◉ 246
Isopto Cetapred Suspension ◉ 220
Pred-G Liquifilm Sterile Ophthalmic Suspension ◉ 252
Pred-G S.O.P. Sterile Ophthalmic Ointment ◉ 253
TobraDex Ophthalmic Suspension and Ointment ◉ 228
Vasocidin Ophthalmic Solution ◉ 276

Furunculosis

Elocon Ointment 0.1% (3 of 812 patients) 2084
Intron A (Less than 1%) 2097
Methotrexate Tablets, Parenteral, LPF Parenteral 1217
Rheumatrex Methotrexate Dose Pack 1234
Zyloprim Tablets (Less than 1%) 830

G

Gait, abnormal

Actimmune (Rare) 1046
Anafranil Capsules (Infrequent) 650
Ativan Injection 2432
Cardizem Tablets-30 mg, 60 mg, 90 mg and 120 mg (Less than 1%) 1329
Cardizem SR Capsules-60 mg, 90 mg and 120 mg (Less than 1%) 1327
Compazine 2201
▲Cordarone Tablets (4 to 9%) 2446
Duragesic Transdermal System (1% or greater) 1133
Eldepryl 2250
Ethmozine Tablets (Less than 2%) 946
Flexeril Tablets (Rare) 1471
Intron A (1% or less) 2097
Loxitane 1213
NebuPent for Inhalation Solution (1% or less) 1017
Norzine 1818
Oncovin Solution Vials & Hyporets 1288
Permax Tablets (1.6%) 1291
Prozac Pulvules (Infrequent) 920
Roferon-A Injection (Less than 1%) 1916
Sinemet CR Tablets 953
Stelazine 2226
Thorazine 2234
Torecan 1993

Galactorrhea

Amen (Rare) 833
Asendin Tablets (Less than 1%) 1196
BuSpar (Rare) 1401
Calan SR Caplets (1% or less) 2157
Calan Tablets (1% or less) 2155
Compazine 2201
Cycrin Tablets (Rare) 2449
Demser Capsules (Infrequent) 1460
Demulen 2161
Depakene Capsules & Syrup 511
Depakote Sprinkle Capsules 512
Depo-Provera Sterile Aqueous Suspension (Few instances) 2336
Elavil 2269
Endep Tablets 1927
Enovid 2161
Etrafon 2087
Flexeril Tablets (Rare) 1471
Limbitrol 1933
Loxitane (Rare) 1213
Ludiomil Tablets 874
Mellaril 2011
Moban Tablets & Concentrate (Infrequent) 932
Norethin 2133
Norpramin Tablets 1340
Pamelor 2019
Proglycem 649
Prolixin Oral Concentrate 1792
Provera Tablets 2356
Reglan 1869
Sandostatin Injection (Less than 1%) 2029
Seldane Tablets 1349
Seldane-D Extended-Release Tablets 1350
Sinequan 1960
Stelazine 2226
Surmontil Capsules 2524
Taractan (Few) 1920
Tofranil Ampuls 1038
Tofranil Tablets 1039
Tofranil-PM Capsules 1041
Triavil Tablets 1556
Trilafon 2123
Vivactil Tablets 1567
Xanax Tablets 2367

Gallbladder, calcification

Cholybar (Occasional) 1705
Questran Light 711

Gallbladder, sonographic abnormalities

Rocephin Injectable Vials, ADD-Vantage (Rare) 1914

Gallbladder disease

Brevicon 2304
Demulen 2161
Diethylstilbestrol Tablets 1258
Enovid 2161
Estinyl Tablets 2085
▲Estrace (2 to 3 fold increase) 1385
Estrace Vaginal Cream 1388
Estraderm Transdermal System 866
Estradurin 2452
Estratest 2245
Estrovis 1721
Jenest-28 Tablets 1636
Levlen/Tri-Levlen 665
Lo/Ovral Tablets 2471
Lo/Ovral-28 Tablets 2476
Loestrin 1728
Lopid Capsules and Tablets (0.9%) 1736
Mediatric Capsules 2476
Menrium Tablets 1934
Micronor Tablets 1667
Modicon 1667
Nordette-21 Tablets 2481
Nordette-28 Tablets 2483
Norethin 2133
Norinyl 2304
Norlestrin 1746
Nor-Q D Tablets 2304
Ortho Diaphragm Kit 1664
Ortho Dienestrol Cream 1664
Ortho-Cyclen Tablets 1658
Ortho-Novum 1667
Ovcon 1391
Ovral Tablets 2490
Ovral-28 Tablets 2491
Ovrette Tablets 2492
PMB 200 and PMB 400 2504
Premarin Intravenous 2508
Premarin with Methyltestosterone 2515
Premarin Tablets 2510
Premarin Vaginal Cream 2512
Rocephin Injectable Vials, ADD-Vantage (Rare) 1914
Sandostatin Injection 2029
Stilphostrol Tablets and Ampuls 1609
TACE 12 and 25 mg 1353
Levlen/Tri-Levlen 665
Tri-Norinyl 2304
Triphasil-21 Tablets 2527
Triphasil-28 Tablets 2532

Gallstones

Atromid-S Capsules 2435
▲Sandostatin Injection (15 to 20%) 2029

Gamma-glutamyl transpeptidase, elevation

Fungizone Intravenous 2262
Prilosec Delayed-Release Capsules (Less than 1%) 1530

Gangrene

Calciparine Injection 925
Dicumarol Tablets 516
Heparin Lock Flush Solution 2456
Heparin Sodium Vials 1264
Heparin Sodium Injection 2457
Heparin Sodium Injection, USP, Sterile Solution 2342
Mepergan Injection 2479
Phenergan Injection 2493
Pitressin Synthetic, Ampoules 1758

Gangrene, cutaneous

Pitressin Synthetic, Ampoules 1758

Gastric acid, regurgitation

Prilosec Delayed-Release Capsules (1.9%) 1530

Gastric dilation

Anafranil Capsules (Infrequent) 650

Gastric discomfort (see under Distress, gastrointestinal)

Gastric disorder (see under Distress, gastrointestinal)

Gastric erosion

Azdōne Tablets 844
Empirin with Codeine Phosphate Nos. 2, 3 & 4 764
Lortab ASA Tablets 2414
Robaxisal Tablets 1872
Soma Compound w/Codeine Tablets (Rare) 2390
Soma Compound Tablets (Rare) 2389

Gastric regurgitation

Prostin VR Pediatric Sterile Solution (Less than 1%) 2355

Gastric secretions, increase

Enlon Injection 598
Renese-R Tablets 1786
Sansert Tablets 2031
Tensilon Injectable 1123

Gastritis

Aldactazide 2150
Aldactone 2152
Anafranil Capsules (Infrequent) 650
Ansaid Tablets (Less than 1%) 2319
Atromid-S Capsules 2435
Augmentin Tablets, Powder for Oral Suspension, and Chewable Tablets 2198
Butazolidin Capsules & Tablets (Less than 1%) 1027
Children's Advil Suspension (Less than 1%) 2426
Clinoril Tablets (Less than 1%) 1433
Dolobid Tablets (Less than 1 in 100) 1465
Eskalith 2214
Sterile FUDR 1898
Flexeril Tablets (Less than 1%) 1471
Keftab Tablets 917
Klonopin Tablets 1902
Lodine Capsules (More than 1% but less than 3%) 2468
Lotensin Tablets 872
Motrin Tablets (Less than 1%) 2351
Nalfon Pulvules & Tablets (Less than 1%) 919
NebuPent for Inhalation Solution (1% or less) 1017
Normozide Tablets (1%) 2112
Orudis Capsules (Less than 1%) 2488
PediaProfen Suspension (Less than 1%) 1363
Permax Tablets (Infrequent) 1291
ProSom Tablets (Infrequent) 554
Prozac Pulvules (Infrequent) 920
Robaxisal Tablets 1872
Rufen Tablets (Less than 1%) 691
Sandimmune (2% or less) 2024
Solganal Suspension 2122

Soma Compound w/Codeine Tablets ... 2390
Soma Compound Tablets ... 2389
Tolectin (200, 400 and 600 mg) (1 to 3%) ... 1379
Trandate HCT Tablets (1% in 208 patients) ... 579
Unasyn ... 1965
Vascor (200, 300 and 400 mg) Tablets (0.5 to 2.0%) ... 1383
Zyloprim Tablets (Less than 1%) ... 830

Gastroenteritis

Altace Capsules (Less than 1%) ... 1086
Cardura Tablets (Less than 0.5% of 3960 patients) ... 1941
Clinoril Tablets (Less than 1%) ... 1433
Clozaril Tablets (Less than 1%) ... 2000
Cytosar-U Sterile Powder (One case) ... 2329
Danocrine Capsules ... 2046
Sterile FUDR ... 1898
Fiorinal with Codeine Capsules ... 2008
Indocin Capsules (Less than 1%) ... 1487
Indocin I.V. (Less than 1%) ... 1490
Indocin (Less than 1%) ... 1487
Permax Tablets (Infrequent) ... 1291
Primaxin I.M. ... 1532
Primaxin I.V. (Less than 0.2%) ... 1535
Prozac Pulvules (1.0%) ... 920
Rythmol Tablets (1.9%) ... 1184

Gastroenteritis, hemorrhagic

Ansaid Tablets (1-3%) ... 2319
Fungizone Intravenous ... 2262

Gastroesophageal reflux

Anafranil Capsules (Infrequent) ... 650
Procardia XL Tablets (1% or less) .. 1783

Gastrointestinal bleeding (see under Bleeding, gastrointestinal)

Gastrointestinal disorders

▲ Accutane Capsules (Approximately 1 in 20) ... 1878
Adipex-P Tablets and Capsules ... 1019
Aldactone ... 2152
Aldoclor Tablets ... 1413
▲ Alka-Seltzer Effervescent Antacid and Pain Reliever (4.9% at doses of 1000 mg/day) ... 1568
▲ Alka-Seltzer (Flavored) Effervescent Antacid and Pain Reliever (4.9% at doses of 1000 mg/day) ... 1569
Alkeran Tablets (Infrequent) ... 754
Anafranil Capsules (Up to 2%) ... 650
Ana-Kit Anaphylaxis Emergency Treatment Kit ... 1100
Anaprox and Anaprox DS Tablets (Less than 3%) ... 2288
▲ Anturane (Most frequent) ... 853
Aralen Hydrochloride Injection ... 2038
Aralen Phosphate Tablets ... 2039
Atabrine Hydrochloride Tablets ... 2041
Ativan Tablets ... 2434
Atromid-S Capsules (Less frequent) ... 2435
▲ Genuine Bayer Aspirin Tablets & Caplets (4.9% at doses of 1000 mg/day) ... ▣ 564
▲ Bayer Plus Aspirin Tablets (4.9% of 4500 people treated) .. ▣ 567
▲ Therapy Bayer Aspirin Caplets (4.9% of 4500 people tested) ... ▣ 568
Benemid Tablets ... 1426
Berocca Plus Tablets ... 1894
Biphetamine Capsules ... 973
Brethaire Inhaler ... 1024
Brevicon ... 2304
▲ Bufferin Analgesic Tablets and Caplets (4.8%) ... 743
BuSpar ... 1401
Capoten ... 2255
Capozide (0.5-2%) ... 2258
Carnitor ... 2188
Cartrol Tablets (Rare) ... 507
Ceclor Pulvules & Suspension (2.5%) ... 1251
Cefotan (1.5%) ... 2265
Ceftin Tablets ... 575
▲ Ceptaz for Injection (Most common) ... 1057
Cetamide Ointment ... ◉ 220
Cleocin T Topical ... 2327
▲ Clinoril Tablets (3-9%) ... 1433
Colchicine Ampoules ... 1252
Corzide Tablets ... 702
▲ Cuprimine Capsules (17%) ... 1442
Cyklokapron Tablets and Injection .. 1159
DDAVP (Up to 2%) ... 1841
Dalmane Capsules ... 1927
Daranide Tablets (Among the most common effects) ... 1445
Decadron Elixir ... 1445
Decadron Phosphate Injection ... 1449
Decadron Phosphate Respihaler ... 1454
Decadron Phosphate Turbinaire ... 1456
Decadron Phosphate with Xylocaine Injection, Sterile ... 1451
Demulen ... 2161
Deprol Tablets ... 2382
Desyrel and Desyrel Dividose (Greater than 1%) ... 1404
Dexedrine ... 2206
Diamox Parenteral ... 1200
Diamox Sequels (Sustained Release) ... 1201
Diamox Tablets ... 1200
Didrex Tablets ... 2338
Didronel Tablets ... 1621
Dorcol Children's Cough Syrup ... ▣ 685
Dorcol Children's Decongestant Liquid ... ▣ 685
Dorcol Children's Liquid Cold Formula (Occasional) ... ▣ 686
Duricef ... 1405
▲ Ecotrin (4.9% at 1000 mg/day) ... 2189
Eminase ... 2211
Enovid ... 2161
Esgic-Plus Tablets (Less frequent) .. 1002
Esgic Tablets & Capsules (Less frequent) ... 1001
Ethmozine Tablets (0.3%-0.4%) ... 946
▲ Eulexin Capsules (6%) ... 2089
▲ Feldene Capsules (20%) ... 1777
Fioricet Tablets (Less frequent) ... 2006
Fiorinal (Less frequent) ... 2007
▲ Fortaz (Most common) ... 1060
Haltran Tablets (Occasional) ... ▣ 668
Hydrea Capsules ... 728
▲ Ilosone (Most frequent) ... 913
Ionamin Capsules ... 981
Isoptin Oral Tablets (Less than 1%) ... 1179
Jenest-28 Tablets ... 1636
K-Dur Microburst Release System (potassium chloride, USP) E.R. Tablets ... 1163
K-Phos M.F. Tablets ... 659
K-Phos Neutral Tablets ... 660
K-Phos No. 2 Tablets ... 659
Kefurox Vials, Faspak & ADD-Vantage (1 in 150) ... 1277
Kemadrin Tablets ... 771
Klor-Con 8/Klor-Con 10 Extended-release Tablets ... 2374
Klotrix ... 708
▲ Lactaid (Most frequent) ... 1191
▲ Lamprene Capsules (40-50%) ... 1030
Lanoxicaps ... 772
Lanoxin Elixir Pediatric ... 775
Lanoxin Injection ... 778
Lanoxin Injection Pediatric ... 781
Lanoxin Tablets ... 783
Leukeran Tablets ... 788
Leukine for IV Infusion ... 1127
▲ Lopid Capsules and Tablets (34.2%) ... 1736
Lupron Injection (Less than 5%) ... 2310
▲ Marplan Tablets (Among most frequent) ... 1906
▲ Meclomen Capsules (10%) ... 1739
Metrodin (urofollitropin for injection) ... 2182
Micronor Tablets ... 1667
Midamor Tablets (Less than or equal to 1%) ... 1508
Modicon ... 1667
Moduretic Tablets (Less than or equal to 1%) ... 1510
Mulvidren-F Softab Tablets ... 2273
Myambutol Tablets ... 1225
Mycostatin Oral Suspension (Occasional) ... 605
Mycostatin Oral Tablets (Occasional) ... 605
Mycostatin Pastilles (Occasional) ... 734
Nalfon Pulvules & Tablets ... 919
Neo-Calglucon Syrup (Extremely rare) ... 2018
Niacor Tablets ... 2376
Nicolar Tablets ... 1846
Nicorette ... 1335
Nimotop Capsules (Up to 2.4%) ... 1607
Norinyl ... 2304
Novahistine DMX ... ▣ 595
▲ Novantrone for Injection Concentrate (58 to 88%) ... 1226
Orap Tablets ... 1020
Orinase Tablets (1.4%) ... 2354
Ortho-Cyclen Tablets ... 1658
Ortho-Novum ... 1667
Oxsoralen-Ultra Capsule ... 1117
Pancrease Capsules ... 1377
▲ Pancrease MT Capsules (Most frequent) ... 1378
Paraflex Caplets (Occasional) ... 1378
Parafon Forte DSC Caplets ... 1379
▲ Paraplatin for Injection (17% to 21%) ... 735
Phenergan with Dextromethorphan 2499
Pima Syrup ... 994
Plaquenil Sulfate Tablets ... 2067
Prinzide Tablets (0.3 to 1%) ... 1540
Proglycem (Frequent) ... 649
Prokine for I.V. Infusion ... 1096
Proventil Syrup (Children 2-6: 2%) ... 2119
Pyridium Plus (Occasional) ... 1764
Quadrinal Tablets ... 1183
Renese-R Tablets ... 1786
▲ Retrovir Capsules (20%) ... 802
▲ Retrovir I.V. Infusion (20%) ... 805
▲ Retrovir Syrup (20%) ... 802
Rifadin ... 1345
Rimactane Capsules ... 879
Robaxin Injectable ... 1871
Rondec-DM ... 1976
▲ Rynatan (Among most common) ... 2387
▲ Rynatuss (Among most common) .. 2388
SSD RP Cream ... 690
Serophene (clomiphene citrate tablets, USP) ... 2186
Silvadene Cream 1% ... 1352
Skelaxin ... 840
Slo-Niacin Tablets ... 2376
Solu-Cortef Sterile Powder ... 2361
Solu-Medrol Sterile Powder ... 2363
St. Joseph Adult Chewable Aspirin (81 mg.) ... ▣ 703
▲ Suprax (30%) ... 1235
▲ Tazicef for Injection (Most common) ... 2231
Tenoretic Tablets ... 1105
Tenuate ... 1354
Tessalon Perles ... 1006
Thalitone Tablets ... 687
Theo-Dur Sprinkle ... 1168
Theragran Hematinic Tablets ... 605
Tofranil Ampuls ... 1038
Tofranil Tablets ... 1039
Tofranil-PM Capsules ... 1041
▲ Tolectin (200, 400 and 600 mg) (10%) ... 1379
Tolinase Tablets (1%) ... 2365
Tonocard Tablets (Less than 1%) .. 1554
▲ Toradol IM Injection (Less than 1% to 9%) ... 2302
Tranxene (Less common) ... 556
▲ Trecator-SC Tablets (Among most common) ... 2527
Triaminic Cold Tablets ... ▣ 688
Triaminic Expectorant ... ▣ 688
Triaminic Syrup (Occasional) ... ▣ 689
Triaminic-DM Syrup ... ▣ 689
Triaminicol Multi-Symptom Relief ... ▣ 691
▲ Trilisate (Less than 20%) ... 1822
Tri-Norinyl ... 2304
Trinsicon Capsules (Rare) ... 2415
Trisoralen Tablets ... 1125
Troph-Iron Liquid (Occasional) ... ▣ 619
Tussi-Organidin DM Liquid (Rare) .. 2392
Tuss-Ornade Liquid ... 2242
Tuss-Ornade Spansule Capsules ... 2242
Uroqid-Acid ... 661
▲ Vascor (200, 300 and 400 mg) Tablets (4.35 to 6.98%) ... 1383
Vaseretic Tablets ... 1559
Ventolin Syrup (2% of children) ... 583
Viokase ... 1877
▲ Voltaren Tablets (About 20%) ... 1042
Zestoretic (0.3 to 1.0%) ... 2274
Zinacef (1 in 150 patients) ... 1066
Zyloprim Tablets (Less than 1%) ... 830

Gastrointestinal motility, decreased

Cyclogyl ... ◉ 215
Cyclomydril ... ◉ 216
Ditropan ... 1332

Gastrointestinal obstruction

K-Dur Microburst Release System (potassium chloride, USP) E.R. Tablets ... 1163
K-Norm Capsules ... 982
K-Tab Filmtab ... 532
Klor-Con 8/Klor-Con 10 Extended-release Tablets ... 2374
Klotrix ... 708
Micro-K ... 1863
Micro-K LS Packets ... 1864
Slow-K Tablets ... 2281

Gastrointestinal perforation

Anaprox and Anaprox DS Tablets (Less than 1%) ... 2288
Atgam Sterile Solution (Less than 5%) ... 2320
Butazolidin Capsules & Tablets (Aproximately 1%) ... 1027
Children's Advil Suspension (Less than 1%) ... 2426
Clinoril Tablets (Rare) ... 1433
Cortone Acetate Sterile Suspension ... 1437
Cortone Acetate Tablets ... 1439
Decadron Phosphate Respihaler ... 1454
Decadron Phosphate Turbinaire ... 1456
Dolobid Tablets (Less than 1 in 100) ... 1465
Feldene Capsules (Less than 1%) .. 1777
Indocin (Approximately 1%) ... 1487
K-Dur Microburst Release System (potassium chloride, USP) E.R. Tablets ... 1163
K-Norm Capsules ... 982
K-Tab Filmtab ... 532
Klor-Con 8/Klor-Con 10 Extended-release Tablets ... 2374
Klotrix ... 708
Lodine Capsules ... 2468
Meclomen Capsules (Less than 1%) ... 1739
Micro-K ... 1863
Micro-K LS Packets ... 1864
Motrin Tablets (Less than 1%) ... 2351
Naprosyn (Less than 1%) ... 2297
Oncovin Solution Vials & Hyporets 1288
Orudis Capsules (Less than 1%) ... 2488
PediaProfen Suspension (Less than 1%) ... 1363
Ponstel ... 1758
Slow-K Tablets ... 2281
Solu-Cortef Sterile Powder ... 2361
Solu-Medrol Sterile Powder ... 2363
Tolectin (200, 400 and 600 mg) (Less than 1%) ... 1379
Toradol IM Injection (Approximately 1% to 4%) ... 2302
Voltaren Tablets (Approximately 1%) ... 1042

Gastrointestinal reactions (see under Gastrointestinal disorders)

Gastrointestinal reflux

Cytotec (Infrequent) ... 2159

Gastrointestinal symptoms (see under Gastrointestinal disorders)

Gastrointestinal toxicity

BiCNU ... 723
Butazolidin Capsules & Tablets ... 1027
CeeNU ... 725
Children's Advil Suspension ... 2426
Cytosar-U Sterile Powder (With experimental doses) ... 2329
Motrin Tablets ... 2351
PediaProfen Suspension ... 1363
Toradol IM Injection ... 2302

Gastrointestinal upset (see under Gastrointestinal disorders)

Genital abnormalities

Megace Tablets ... 732

Genital moniliasis

Duricef ... 1405

Genitalia, external, labial fusion of

Danocrine Capsules ... 2046

Genitourinary disturbances

Centrax ... 1693
Dalmane Capsules ... 1927
Eulexin Capsules (2%) ... 2089
Paraplatin for Injection (2%) ... 735
Tranxene ... 556

Germinal aplasia

Mustargen ... 1514

Gestation, increased length

Lortab ASA Tablets ... 2414

Giddiness (see under Dizziness)

Gingival hyperplasia
- Adalat Capsules (10 mg and 20 mg) (Less than 0.5%) 1587
- Calan SR Caplets (1% or less) 2157
- Calan Tablets (1% or less) 2155
- Cardizem Tablets-30 mg, 60 mg, 90 mg and 120 mg (Infrequent) 1329
- Cardizem SR Capsules-60 mg, 90 mg and 120 mg (Infrequent) 1327
- Dilantin Infatabs 1710
- Dilantin Kapseals 1708
- Dilantin Parenteral 1712
- Dilantin-30 Pediatric/Dilantin-125 Suspension 1713
- Dilantin with Phenobarbital Kapseals 1715
- Intron A (1 patient) 2097
- Isoptin Oral Tablets (Less than 1%) 1179
- Isoptin SR Sustained Release Tablets (Less than 1%) 1181
- Mesantoin Tablets 2013
- Plendil Extended-Release Tablets (Less than 0.5%) 1526
- Procardia Capsules (Less than 0.5%) 1781
- Procardia XL Tablets (1% or less) 1783
- ▲ Sandimmune (Up to 16%) 2024
- Verelan Capsules (Less than 1%) 1243

Gingival swelling
- Lomotil 2174
- Motofen Tablets 836

Gingival ulcer
- Children's Advil Suspension (Less than 1%) 2426
- Depen Titratable Tablets (Rare) 2379
- Motrin Tablets (Less than 1%) 2351
- PediaProfen Suspension (Less than 1%) 1363
- Rufen Tablets (Less than 1%) 691

Gingivitis
- Accutane Capsules (Less than 1%) 1878
- Anafranil Capsules (Infrequent) 650
- Benemid Tablets 1426
- ColBENEMID Tablets 1436
- Cytotec (Infrequent) 2159
- Demulen 2161
- Enovid 2161
- ▲ Intron A (Up to 14%) 2097
- Klonopin Tablets 1902
- Methotrexate Tablets, Parenteral, LPF Parenteral 1217
- Myochrysine Injection 1516
- NebuPent for Inhalation Solution (1% or less) 1017
- Nicorette 1335
- Norethin 2133
- Permax Tablets (Infrequent) 1291
- Prozac Pulvules (Infrequent) 920
- Rheumatrex Methotrexate Dose Pack 1234
- Ridaura Capsules (0.1 to 1%) 2224
- Solganal Suspension 2122
- Tegison Capsules (1-10%) 1881

Gingivostomatitis
- Cuprimine Capsules (Rare) 1442
- Depen Titratable Tablets (Rare) 2379

Glandular enlargement
- Cholybar 1705
- Etrafon (Rare) 2087
- Hespan Injection 948
- Intal Inhaler (Frequent) 979
- Questran Light 711
- Trexan Tablets (Less than 1%) 937

Glassy-eyed appearance
- Klonopin Tablets 1902

Glaucoma (see also under IOP, elevation)
- AK-Cide Sterile Ophthalmic Ointment & Suspension ◉ 202
- AK-Con ◉ 202
- AK-Dex ◉ 203
- AK-Pred ◉ 205
- AK-Spore H.C. ◉ 206
- AK-Trol Ointment & Suspension ◉ 207
- Anafranil Capsules (Rare) 650
- Anectine 755
- Aristocort Suspension 1008
- Aristospan Suspension 1011
- Artane 1195
- Beconase AQ Nasal Spray (Extremely rare) 574
- Beconase Inhalation Aerosol & Refill (Extremely rare) 574
- Blephamide 586
- Celestone Soluspan Suspension 2081
- ▲ Cetapred Ointment (Most often) ◉ 220
- Chloromycetin Hydrocortisone Ophthalmic 1694
- Cortenema 2244
- Cortifoam 1827
- Cortisporin Ophthalmic Ointment Sterile 758
- Cortisporin Ophthalmic Suspension Sterile 759
- Cortone Acetate Sterile Suspension 1437
- Cortone Acetate Tablets 1439
- Dalalone D.P. Injectable 999
- Decadron Elixir 1445
- Decadron Phosphate Injection 1449
- Decadron Phosphate Respihaler 1454
- Decadron Phosphate Sterile Ophthalmic Ointment 1453
- Decadron Phosphate Sterile Ophthalmic Solution 1453
- Decadron Phosphate Turbinaire 1456
- Decadron Phosphate with Xylocaine Injection, Sterile 1451
- Decadron Tablets 1447
- Decadron-LA Sterile Suspension 1457
- Deltasone Tablets 2332
- Depo-Medrol Sterile Aqueous Suspension 2334
- Dexacidin ◉ 272
- Diupres Tablets 1461
- ⅛% Econopred & 1% Econopred Plus ◉ 217
- Elavil 2269
- Endep Tablets 1927
- Enduronyl 518
- Etrafon 2087
- FML Forte Liquifilm ◉ 245
- FML S.O.P. ◉ 245
- ▲ FML-S Sterile Ophthalmic Suspension (Among most often) ◉ 246
- Fluor-Op Ophthalmic Suspension ◉ 272
- HMS Liquifilm (Rare) ◉ 247
- Harmonyl Tablets 528
- Healon ◉ 279
- Humorsol Sterile Ophthalmic Solution 1475
- Hydeltrasol Injection, Sterile 1476
- Hydeltra-T.B.A. Sterile Suspension 1478
- Hydrocortone Acetate Sterile Suspension 1479
- Hydrocortone Phosphate Injection, Sterile 1481
- Hydrocortone Tablets 1482
- Hydropres Tablets 1485
- Inflamase ◉ 274
- ▲ Isopto Cetapred Suspension (Most often) ◉ 220
- Kenalog-10 Injection 2402
- Kenalog-40 Injection 2403
- Kinesed Tablets 2272
- Maxidex Sterile Ophthalmic Ointment ◉ 222
- Maxidex Sterile Ophthalmic Suspension ◉ 223
- ▲ Maxitrol Ophthalmic Ointment/Suspension (Most often) ◉ 223
- Medrol 2348
- Metimyd ◉ 306
- Midamor Tablets (Less than or equal to 1%) 1508
- Moduretic Tablets 1510
- Naphcon-A Ophthalmic Solution 571
- Nardil (Less common) 1742
- NeoDecadron Sterile Ophthalmic Ointment 1517
- NeoDecadron Sterile Ophthalmic Solution 1518
- Norpramin Tablets 1340
- Ophthocort ◉ 301
- Oreticyl 545
- Ornade Spansule Capsules 2221
- Pediapred Oral Liquid 987
- Poly-Pred Liquifilm ◉ 250
- Pred-G Liquifilm Sterile Ophthalmic Suspension ◉ 252
- Pred-G S.O.P. Sterile Ophthalmic Ointment ◉ 253
- Prolixin Decanoate 1795
- Prolixin Elixir 1793
- Prolixin Enanthate 1796
- Prolixin Injection 1791
- Prolixin Oral Concentrate 1792
- Prolixin Tablets 1793
- Prozac Pulvules (Rare) 920
- Raudixin Tablets 1803
- Rauzide Tablets 1804
- Renese-R Tablets 1786
- Salutensin/Salutensin-Demi 719
- Ser-Ap-Es Tablets 881
- Serpasil Tablets 883
- Serpasil-Apresoline Tablets 884
- Serpasil-Esidrix Tablets 886
- Solu-Cortef Sterile Powder 2361
- Solu-Medrol Sterile Powder 2363
- Terra-Cortril Ophthalmic Suspension 1963
- TobraDex Ophthalmic Suspension and Ointment ◉ 228
- Transderm Scōp Transdermal Therapeutic System (Infrequent) 887
- Triavil Tablets 1556
- Trilafon (Occasional) 2123
- Vancenase AQ Nasal Spray 0.042% (Extremely rare) 2127
- Vancenase Nasal Inhaler (Extremely rare) 2126
- Vasocidin Ointment ◉ 275
- Vasocidin Ophthalmic Solution ◉ 276
- Viroptic Ophthalmic Solution, 1% Sterile 820
- Vivactil Tablets 1567

Glaucoma, angle closure precipitation
- Mydriacyl ◉ 225
- Ocusert Pilo-20 and Pilo-40 Ocular Therapeutic Systems ◉ 256

Glaucoma, corticosteroid-induced
- AK-Cide Sterile Ophthalmic Ointment & Suspension ◉ 202
- AK-Spore H.C. ◉ 206
- AK-Trol Ointment & Suspension ◉ 207
- Blephamide 586
- Cetapred Ointment ◉ 220
- Dexacidin ◉ 272
- ⅛% Econopred & 1% Econopred Plus ◉ 217
- FML Forte Liquifilm ◉ 245
- FML Liquifilm ◉ 244
- FML-S Sterile Ophthalmic Suspension ◉ 246
- Fluor-Op Ophthalmic Suspension ◉ 272
- HMS Liquifilm ◉ 247
- Inflamase ◉ 274
- Isopto Cetapred Suspension ◉ 220
- Maxidex Sterile Ophthalmic Ointment ◉ 222
- Maxidex Sterile Ophthalmic Suspension ◉ 223
- Maxitrol Ophthalmic Ointment/Suspension ◉ 223
- Ophthocort ◉ 301
- Poly-Pred Liquifilm ◉ 250
- Pred Forte ◉ 252
- Pred-G Liquifilm Sterile Ophthalmic Suspension ◉ 252
- TobraDex Ophthalmic Suspension and Ointment ◉ 228
- Vasocidin Ointment ◉ 275
- Vasocidin Ophthalmic Solution ◉ 276

Glaucoma, secondary
- AMO Vitrax Solution ◉ 236

Glaucoma, worsening of narrow angle
- Atrovent Inhalation Aerosol 675

Globus hystericus
- Daranide Tablets 1445

Glomerular filtration rate, decrease
- Capoten 2255
- Capozide 2258
- Monopril Tablets 1406

Glomerulitis
- Feldene Capsules (Less than 1%) 1777
- Ridaura Capsules 2224
- Solganal Suspension 2122

Glomerulonephritis
- Anaprox and Anaprox DS Tablets (Less than 3%) 2288
- Butazolidin Capsules & Tablets (Less than 1%) 1027
- Corzide Tablets (Occasional) 702
- Cuprimine Capsules 1442
- Depen Titratable Tablets (Rare) 2379
- Myochrysine Injection 1516
- Naprosyn (Less than 1%) 2297
- Naturetin Tablets (Occasional) 1789
- Rauzide Tablets 1804

Glossitis
- Achromycin V Capsules 1193
- AeroBid Inhaler System (1-3%) 995
- Anafranil Capsules (Infrequent) 650
- Augmentin Tablets, Powder for Oral Suspension, and Chewable Tablets 2198
- Azo Gantrisin Tablets 1888
- Bactrim DS Tablets 1891
- Bactrim I.V. Infusion 1889
- Bactrim 1891
- Betoptic Sterile Ophthalmic Solution (Rare) 569
- Betoptic S Sterile Ophthalmic Suspension (Rare) 570
- Capoten 2255
- Capozide 2258
- Chloromycetin Kapseals 1695
- Chloromycetin Palmitate, Oral Suspension 1697
- Chloromycetin Sodium Succinate 1698
- Clinoril Tablets (Less than 1%) 1433
- Cuprimine Capsules 1442
- Daraprim Tablets 761
- Declomycin Capsules, Tablets 1199
- Depen Titratable Tablets (Rare) 2379
- Doryx Capsules 1717
- Sterile FUDR 1898
- Fansidar Tablets 1896
- Flagyl I.V. 2131
- Flagyl Tablets 2170
- Gantanol 1899
- Gantrisin 1901
- Geocillin Tablets 1951
- Halcion Tablets 2340
- ▲ Hylorel Tablets (8.4%) 975
- Inversine Tablets 1492
- Lincocin 2344
- Maxair Inhaler (Less than 1%) 1311
- Minocin Intravenous 1221
- Minocin Oral Suspension 1224
- Minocin Pellet-Filled Capsules 1222
- Monodox Capsules 1630
- Myochrysine Injection 1516
- Nicorette 1335
- Permax Tablets (Rare) 1291
- Primaxin I.M. 1532
- Primaxin I.V. (Less than 0.2%) 1535
- Proloprim Tablets 799
- Protostat Tablets 1674
- Prozac Pulvules (Infrequent) 920
- Ridaura Capsules (1 to 3%) 2224
- Septra 813
- Septra I.V. Infusion 808
- Septra I.V. Infusion ADD-Vantage Vials 810
- Septra 813
- Solganal Suspension 2122
- Spectrobid Tablets & Powder for Oral Suspension 1961
- Tegretol Chewable Tablets 654
- Tegretol Suspension 656
- Tegretol Tablets 654
- Terramycin Capsules 1786
- Terramycin Intramuscular Solution 1964
- Teslac Tablets 741
- Tolectin (200, 400 and 600 mg) (Less than 1%) 1379
- Trimpex Tablets 1922
- Unasyn (Less than 1%) 1965
- Urobiotic-250 Capsules (Rare) 1968
- Vaseretic Tablets 1559
- Vasotec I.V. 1562
- Vasotec Tablets (0.5% to 1%) 1564
- Vibramycin Hyclate Capsules 1787
- Vibramycin Hyclate Intravenous 1968
- Vibramycin 1787
- Wellbutrin Tablets (Rare) 821

Glossodynia
- Aldoclor Tablets 1413
- Aldomet Ester HCl Injection 1417
- Aldomet Oral 1415
- Aldoril Tablets 1418
- Clozaril Tablets (1%) 2000
- Etrafon 2087
- Questran Light (Less frequent) 711
- Rifadin (Occasional) 1345
- Rifamate Capsules (Occasional) 1347
- Rimactane Capsules 879
- ▲ Tegison Capsules (10-25%) 1881
- Trilafon 2123

Glossoncus
- Calcimar Injection, Synthetic (A few cases) 1839
- Capozide 2258
- Miacalcin Injection (A few cases) 2017
- Myochrysine Injection 1516
- Prinzide Tablets 1540
- Solganal Suspension 2122

Tambocor Tablets (Less than 1%) 1315
Voltaren Tablets (Less than 1%) 1042
Zarontin Capsules 1768
Zarontin Syrup 1769
Zestoretic 2274
Zestril Tablets 2277

Glossotrichia

Aldomet Ester HCl Injection 1417
Augmentin Tablets, Powder for Oral Suspension, and Chewable Tablets 2198
Endep Tablets 1927
Etrafon 2087
Klonopin Tablets 1902
Limbitrol 1933
Ludiomil Tablets 874
Marplan Tablets (Rare) 1906
Norpramin Tablets 1340
Pamelor 2019
Spectrobid Tablets & Powder for Oral Suspension 1961
Surmontil Capsules 2524
Tofranil Ampuls 1038
Tofranil Tablets 1039
Tofranil-PM Capsules 1041
Unasyn 1965
Vivactil Tablets 1567

Glucose tolerance, changes

Anadrol-50 Tablets 2287
Brevicon 2304
Cortifoam 1827
Danocrine Capsules 2046
Demulen (Significant percentage of patients) 2161
Enovid (Significant percentage of patients) 2161
Estinyl Tablets 2085
Estrace 1385
Estrace Vaginal Cream 1388
Estradurin 2452
Estratest 2245
Kenalog in Orabase 604
Loestrin 1728
Mediatric Capsules 2476
Micronor Tablets 1667
Modicon 1667
Nicolar Tablets 1846
Norinyl 2304
Norlestrin 1746
Nor-Q D Tablets 2304
Ortho Dienestrol Cream 1664
Ortho-Novum 1667
Ovcon 1391
PMB 200 and PMB 400 2504
Phenergan Injection 2493
Premarin Intravenous 2508
▲ Premarin with Methyltestosterone (Significant percentage of patients) 2515
Stilphostrol Tablets and Ampuls 1609
TACE 12 and 25 mg 1353
Temaril Tablets, Syrup and Spansule Sustained Release Capsules 1085
Tri-Norinyl 28-Day Tablets 2304
Winstrol Tablets 2075
Zanosar Sterile Powder (Some patients) 2371

Glucose tolerance, decreased

Emcyt Capsules 1161
Jenest-28 Tablets 1636
Lo/Ovral Tablets 2471
Lo/Ovral-28 Tablets 2476
Niacor Tablets 2376
Nordette-21 Tablets 2481
Nordette-28 Tablets 2483
Ovral Tablets 2490
Ovral-28 Tablets 2491
Ovrette Tablets 2492
PMB 200 and PMB 400 2504
Premarin Intravenous 2508
Premarin with Methyltestosterone 2515
Premarin Vaginal Cream 2512
Triphasil-21 Tablets 2527
Triphasil-28 Tablets 2532

Glucosuria

Aclovate 1053
Alphatrex Cream, Ointment & Lotion 2076
Combipres Tablets (Rare) 678
Diprolene 2083
Elspar (Low) 1470
Floxin Tablets (More than or equal to 1.0%) 1652
Humatrope Vials (Infrequent) 1266
Maxivate Cream, Lotion & Ointment 0.05% 2406
Rythmol Tablets (Less than 1%) 1184
Sinemet CR Tablets 953
Temovate 1056
Ultravate Cream 0.05% 2410
Ultravate Ointment 0.05% 2411

Glycosuria

Aldoclor Tablets 1413
Aldoril Tablets 1418
Anafranil Capsules (Rare) 650
Apresazide Capsules 854
Apresoline-Esidrix Tablets 857
Capozide 2258
Cibalith-S 870
Combipres Tablets 678
Compazine 2201
Corzide Tablets 702
Cytotec (Infrequent) 2159
Diamox Parenteral (Occasional) 1200
Diamox Sequels (Sustained Release) 1201
Diamox Tablets (Occasional) 1200
Diucardin Tablets 2450
Diulo 2129
Diupres Tablets 1461
Diuril Oral Suspension 1464
Diuril Sodium Intravenous 1463
Diuril Tablets 1464
Dyazide Capsules 2208
Enduron Tablets 517
Enduronyl 518
Esidrix Tablets 863
Esimil Tablets 864
Eskalith 2214
Etrafon 2087
Exna Tablets 1862
HydroDIURIL Tablets 1484
Hydromox R Tablets 1209
Hydromox Tablets 1208
Hydropres Tablets 1485
Inderide Tablets 2463
Inderide LA Long Acting Capsules 2465
Indocin Capsules (Less than 1%) 1487
Indocin I.V. (Less than 1%) 1490
Indocin (Less than 1%) 1487
Kenalog-10 Injection 2402
Kenalog-40 Injection 2403
Lasix 1093
Lithane Tablets 1596
Lithium Carbonate Capsules & Tablets 1984
Lithobid Tablets 870
Lopressor HCT Tablets 1034
Lozol Tablets (Less than 5%) 1843
Maxzide 1215
Minizide Capsules 1779
Moduretic Tablets 1510
Mykrox ½ mg Tablets 984
Naturetin Tablets (Occasional) 1789
Navane Capsules and Concentrate 1954
Navane Intramuscular 1956
Normodyne Tablets 2110
Normozide Tablets 2112
Oretic Tablets 544
Oreticyl 545
Prilosec Delayed-Release Capsules (Less than 1%) 1530
Proglycem (Frequent) 649
Rauzide Tablets 1804
Renese Tablets 1785
Rocephin Injectable Vials, ADD-Vantage (Rare) 1914
Saluron 718
Salutensin/Salutensin-Demi 719
Ser-Ap-Es Tablets 881
Serpasil-Esidrix Tablets 886
Stelazine 2226
Taractan 1920
▲ Tegison Capsules (1-10%) 1881
Tegretol Chewable Tablets 654
Tegretol Suspension 656
Tegretol Tablets 654
Temaril Tablets, Syrup and Spansule Sustained Release Capsules 1085
Tenoretic Tablets 1105
Thalitone Tablets 687
Thorazine 2234
Timolide Tablets 1547
Trandate HCT Tablets 579
Trilafon 2123
Wellbutrin Tablets (Rare) 821
Yutopar (Infrequent) 647
Zanosar Sterile Powder 2371
Zaroxolyn Tablets 989

Goiter

Anafranil Capsules (Rare) 650
Azo Gantanol Tablets (Rare) 1887
Azo Gantrisin Tablets (Rare) 1888
Azulfidine Tablets, EN-tabs, Oral Suspension (Rare) 1157
Butazolidin Capsules & Tablets (Less than 1%) 1027
Gantrisin Ophthalmic Ointment/Solution 1900
Pediazole (Rare) 1973
Pima Syrup (Rare) 994
Prozac Pulvules (Rare) 920
Quadrinal Tablets 1183
Thiosulfil Forte Tablets (Rare) 2526

Goiter, diffuse

Cibalith-S 870
Lithane Tablets 1596
Lithium Carbonate Capsules & Tablets 1984
Lithobid Tablets 870

Goiter, euthyroid

Cibalith-S 870
Eskalith 2214
Lithane Tablets 1596
Lithium Carbonate Capsules & Tablets 1984
Lithobid Tablets 870

Goiter, fetal

Calcidrine Syrup 506
Organidin Elixir, Solution & Tablets (Rare) 2387
Quadrinal Tablets 1183
Tapazole Tablets 1298
Theo-Organidin Elixir 2391
Tussi-Organidin DM Liquid (Rare) 2392
Tussi-Organidin Liquid 2391

Goiter production (see under Goiter)

Gold deposits, ocular

Ridaura Capsules 2224

Gold toxicity

Myochrysine Injection (Common) 1516
Ridaura Capsules 2224

Gonadal suppression

Cytoxan for Injection (Reported in a number of patients) 726

Gonadotropin secretion, increase

Neosar for Injection 566

Gonadotropin secretion, inhibition

Android 1111
▲ Estratest (Among most common) 2245
Halotestin Tablets 2341
Metandren Linguets and Tablets 875
Premarin with Methyltestosterone (Among most common) 2515
Testred Capsules 1124

Goodpasture's syndrome

Cuprimine Capsules 1442
Depen Titratable Tablets (Rare) 2379

Gout

Anafranil Capsules (Infrequent) 650
Azdöne Tablets 844
Capozide 2258
Cardura Tablets (Less than 0.5% of 3960 patients) 1941
Cartrol Tablets (Rare) 507
Cipro I.V. (1% or less) 1592
Cipro Tablets (Less than 1%) 1589
Combipres Tablets 678
Cytotec (Infrequent) 2159
Diulo 2129
Edecrin 1468
Hytrin Tablets (At least 1%) 529
Lopressor HCT Tablets (1 in 100 patients) 1034
Lortab ASA Tablets 2414
Maxzide 1215
Moduretic Tablets (Less than or equal to 1%) 1510
Monopril Tablets (0.2 to 1.0%) 1406
Myambutol Tablets 1225
Mykrox ½ mg Tablets 984
Normozide Tablets (Less than 1%) 2112
Permax Tablets (Infrequent) 1291
Prinivil Tablets (1% or less) 1538
Prinzide Tablets 1540
Procardia XL Tablets (1% or less) 1783
Proglycem 649
Prozac Pulvules (Rare) 920
Rauzide Tablets 1804
Tegison Capsules (Less than 1%) 1881
Thalitone Tablets 687
Timolide Tablets 1547
Trandate HCT Tablets (Less than 1% in 208 patients) 579
Vaseretic Tablets (0.5% to 2.0%) 1559
Zaroxolyn Tablets 989
Zestoretic 2274
Zestril Tablets (Less than 1%) 2277
Zoladex (1% to 5%) 1110
Zyloprim Tablets (Less than 1%) 830

Granulocytopenia

Aldoclor Tablets 1413
Aldomet Ester HCl Injection (Rare) 1417
Aldomet Oral 1415
Aldoril Tablets 1418
Anaprox and Anaprox DS Tablets (Less than 1%) 2288
Atgam Sterile Solution (Less than 5%) 2320
Butazolidin Capsules & Tablets 1027
Chloromycetin Kapseals 1695
Chloromycetin Palmitate, Oral Suspension 1697
Chloromycetin Sodium Succinate 1698
Claforan Sterile Injection (Less than 1%) 1089
Cytosar-U Sterile Powder 2329
▲ Cytovene Sterile Powder (Approximately 40%) 2292
Dalmane Capsules (Rare) 1927
Dilantin Infatabs (Occasional) 1710
Dilantin Kapseals (Occasional) 1708
Dilantin Parenteral (Occasional) 1712
Dilantin-30 Pediatric/Dilantin-125 Suspension 1713
Dilantin with Phenobarbital Kapseals (Occasional) 1715
Ergamisol Tablets (Less than 1 to 2%) 1136
Fulvicin P/G Tablets 2090
Fulvicin P/G 165 & 330 Tablets 2091
Fulvicin-U/F Tablets 2092
Garamycin Injectable 2093
Grifulvin V (griseofulvin microsize) Tablets/Suspension 1678
Grisactin 2454
Grisactin Ultra Tablets 2455
Gris-PEG Tablets, 125 mg & 250 mg 1083
Intron A (2 patients) 2097
Limbitrol (Rare) 1933
Macrodantin Capsules 1624
Meclomen Capsules (Rare) 1739
Mefoxin 1498
Mefoxin Premixed Intravenous Solution 1500
Methotrexate Tablets, Parenteral, LPF Parenteral 1217
Milontin Kapseals 1741
Mustargen 1514
Myochrysine Injection 1516
Mysoline (Rare) 2480
Naprosyn (Less than 1%) 2297
Nebcin Vials, Hyporets & ADD-Vantage 1286
Procan SR Tablets (Infrequent) 1760
▲ Retrovir Capsules (10% to 47%) 802
▲ Retrovir I.V. Infusion (10% to 55%) 805
▲ Retrovir Syrup (10% to 47%) 802
Rheumatrex Methotrexate Dose Pack 1234
Ridaura Capsules 2224
Rythmol Tablets (Less than 1%) 1184
Solganal Suspension (Rare) 2122
Talacen 2070
Talwin Injection 2071
Talwin Compound (Rare) 2072
Talwin Injection 2071
Talwin Nx 2073
Tapazole Tablets 1298
Tolectin (200, 400 and 600 mg) (Less than 1%) 1379
Unipen (Infrequent) 2533
▲ Velban Vials (Among most common) 1305
Zantac Injection and Zantac Injection Premixed (Few patients) 1063
Zantac (A few patients) 1065

Granulocytosis

▲ Intron A (26% to 39%) 2097
Zefazone Sterile Powder 2372

Granulomatosis, Wegener's

Accutane Capsules (Few) 1878

Gray syndrome

Chloromycetin Kapseals (Two cases) 1695

Chloromycetin Palmitate, Oral Suspension (2 cases) 1697
Chloromycetin Sodium Succinate (2 cases) 1698

Grogginess
Versed Injection (Less than 1%) 1924

Groin, itch
Equagesic Tablets 2451
Miltown Tablets 2386
PMB 200 and PMB 400 2504

Groin, rash
Equagesic Tablets 2451
Miltown Tablets 2386
PMB 200 and PMB 400 2504

Growth, retardation
Aristocort Suspension 1008
Aristospan Suspension (Intralesional) 1011
Depen Titratable Tablets (One infant) 2379
Medrol 2348
Metubine Iodide Vials 1285
Prinivil Tablets 1538
Prinzide Tablets 1540
Solu-Cortef Sterile Powder 2361
Solu-Medrol Sterile Powder 2363
Vasotec I.V. 1562
Vasotec Tablets 1564
Yutopar 647
Zestoretic 2274
Zestril Tablets 2277

Growth, retardation, intrauterine
Vaseretic Tablets 1559

Growth, suppression in children
Android 1111
Aristospan Suspension (Intra-articular) 1011
Azmacort Inhaler 1837
Celestone Soluspan Suspension 2081
Cortenema 2244
Cortifoam 1827
Cortone Acetate Sterile Suspension 1437
Cortone Acetate Tablets 1439
Cylert Tablets 510
Dalalone D.P. Injectable 999
Decadron Elixir 1445
Decadron Phosphate Injection 1449
Decadron Phosphate Respihaler 1454
Decadron Phosphate Turbinaire 1456
Decadron Phosphate with Xylocaine Injection, Sterile 1451
Decadron Tablets 1447
Decadron-LA Sterile Suspension 1457
Deltasone Tablets 2332
Depo-Medrol Sterile Aqueous Suspension 2334
Desoxyn Gradumet Tablets 514
Hydeltrasol Injection, Sterile 1476
Hydeltra-T.B.A. Sterile Suspension 1478
Hydrocortone Acetate Sterile Suspension 1479
Hydrocortone Phosphate Injection, Sterile 1481
Hydrocortone Tablets 1482
Kenalog-10 Injection 2402
Kenalog-40 Injection 2403
Pediapred Oral Liquid 987

Guillain-Barré syndrome
Attenuvax (Rare) 1424
Biavax II (Isolated reports) 1427
Cuprimine Capsules 1442
Danocrine Capsules (Rare) 2046
Depen Titratable Tablets 2379
Engerix-B Unit-Dose Vials (Less than 1%) 2213
Flu-Imune Influenza Virus Vaccine 1204
HibTITER 1206
IPOL Poliovirus Vaccine Inactivated 894
M-M-R II (Rare) 1494
M-R-VAX II (Rare) 1496
Meruvax II (Isolated reports) 1503
Myochrysine Injection (Rare) 1516
Omnipaque (One case) 2552
Orimune Poliovirus Vaccine Live Oral Trivalent 1228
PedvaxHIB 1521
Pneumovax 23 (Rare) 1528
Pnu-Imune 23 Pneumococcal Vaccine Polyvalent 1233
ProHIBiT Haemophilus b Conjugate Vaccine (Diphtheria Toxoid Conjugate) (Rare) 896
Recombivax HB 1544
Tri-Immunol Diphtheria & Tetanus Toxoids & Pertussis Vaccine, Adsorbed 1241

Gums, sore
Prolixin Oral Concentrate 1792

Gustatory sensation
Norzine (Occasional) 1818
Torecan 1993
▲ Wellbutrin Tablets (3.1%) 821

Gynecomastia
A.P.L. 2431
Adalat Capsules (10 mg and 20 mg) (Less than 0.5%) 1587
Aldactazide (Not infrequent) 2150
Aldactone (Not infrequent) 2152
Aldoclor Tablets 1413
Aldomet Ester HCl Injection 1417
Aldomet Oral 1415
Aldoril Tablets 1418
Anadrol-50 Tablets 2287
Anafranil Capsules (Rare) 650
Android 1111
Asendin Tablets 1196
Atromid-S Capsules 2435
Axid Pulvules (Rare) 1246
Calan SR Caplets (1% or less) 2157
Calan Tablets (1% or less) 2155
Capoten 2255
Capozide 2258
Catapres Tablets (About 1 in 1,000 patients) 676
Catapres-TTS (1 per 1,000) 677
Children's Advil Suspension (Less than 1%) 2426
Cipro I.V. (1% or less) 1592
Clinoril Tablets (Rare) 1433
Combipres Tablets (About 1 in 1,000) 678
Compazine 2201
Elavil 2269
Endep Tablets 1927
Etrafon 2087
▲ Eulexin Capsules (9% with LHRH-agonist) 2089
Flexeril Tablets (Rare) 1471
Haldol Decanoate 1375
Haldol Injection, Tablets and Concentrate 1373
Halotestin Tablets 2341
INH Tablets 868
Indocin Capsules (Less than 1%) 1487
Indocin I.V. (Less than 1%) 1490
Indocin (Less than 1%) 1487
Intron A (Less than 5%) 2097
Isoptin Oral Tablets (Less than 1%) 1179
Isoptin SR Sustained Release Tablets (Less than 1%) 1181
Lanoxicaps (Occasional) 772
Lanoxin Elixir Pediatric (Occasional) 775
Lanoxin Injection (Occasional) 778
Lanoxin Injection Pediatric (Occasional) 781
Lanoxin Tablets (Occasional) 783
Limbitrol 1933
Loxitane (Rare) 1213
Ludiomil Tablets 874
▲ Lupron Depot 3.75 mg (Among most frequent) 2312
Lupron Depot 7.5 mg (Less than 5%) 2311
▲ Lupron Injection (5% or more) 2310
Matulane Capsules (In prepubertal and early pubertal boys) 1907
Mediatric Capsules (Rare) 2476
Mellaril 2011
Metandren Linguets and Tablets 875
Moban Tablets & Concentrate (Infrequent) 932
Motrin Tablets (Less than 1%) 2351
Myleran Tablets (Rare) 790
Navane Capsules and Concentrate 1954
Navane Intramuscular 1956
Nizoral Tablets (Less than 1%) 1145
Norpace (Rare) 2177
Norpramin Tablets 1340
Norzine 1818
Orudis Capsules (Less than 1%) 2488
Pamelor 2019
PediaProfen Suspension (Less than 1%) 1363
Pergonal (menotropins for injection, USP) (Occasionally) 2184
Pregnyl 1644
Prilosec Delayed-Release Capsules (Less than 1%) 1530
Profasi (human chorionic gonadotropin, USP) 2186
Prolixin Decanoate 1795
Prolixin Elixir 1793
Prolixin Enanthate 1796
Prolixin Injection 1791
Prolixin Oral Concentrate 1792
Prolixin Tablets 1793
Raudixin Tablets 1803
Rauzide Tablets 1804
Reglan 1869
Rifamate Capsules 1347
Rufen Tablets (Less than 1%) 691
▲ Sandimmune (Up to 4%) 2024
Ser-Ap-Es Tablets 881
Serentil 686
Serpasil Tablets 883
Serpasil-Apresoline Tablets 884
Serpasil-Esidrix Tablets 886
Sinequan 1960
Stelazine 2226
Surmontil Capsules 2524
Tacaryl 2409
Tagamet 2228
Taractan 1920
Temaril Tablets, Syrup and Spansule Sustained Release Capsules 1085
Tenuate 1354
Testred Capsules 1124
Thorazine 2234
Tofranil Ampuls 1038
Tofranil Tablets 1039
Tofranil-PM Capsules 1041
Torecan 1993
Trecator-SC Tablets 2527
Triavil Tablets 1556
Trilafon 2123
Verelan Capsules (Less than 1%) 1243
Vivactil Tablets 1567
Wellbutrin Tablets (Infrequent) 821
Winstrol Tablets 2075
Wytensin Tablets (3% or less) 2542
Xanax Tablets 2367
Zantac Injection and Zantac Injection Premixed 1063
Zantac (Occasional) 1065
Zyloprim Tablets (Less than 1%) 830

GGTP, elevation
▲ Accutane Capsules (1 in 5 to 1 in 10) 1878
Ceptaz for Injection (One in 19) 1057
Cipro I.V. (Infrequent) 1592
Cipro Tablets (Less than 0.1%) 1589
Fortaz (B 1 in 19) 1060
Monocid Injection (1.6%) 2217
▲ Tegison Capsules (10-25%) 1881

H

Haemophilus B disease
PedvaxHIB 1521

Hair, abnormal growth (see under Hirsutism)

Hair, dry brittle
Atromid-S Capsules (Less often) 2435
Cibalith-S 870
Eskalith 2214
Lithane Tablets 1596
Lithium Carbonate Capsules & Tablets 1984
Lithobid Tablets 870
Nizoral 2% Shampoo 1144
Sandimmune (Rare) 2024
Selsun Rx 2.5% Selenium Sulfide Lotion, USP 1977

Hair, oily
Nizoral 2% Shampoo 1144
Selsun Rx 2.5% Selenium Sulfide Lotion, USP 1977

Hair discoloration
Clear by Design Medicated Acne Gel ◘ 709
Clearasil 10% Benzoyl Peroxide Acne Medication Vanishing Lotion ◘ 658
Clearasil Maximum Strength ◘ 658
Drithocreme 590
Dritho-Scalp 591
MG 217 Psoriasis Shampoo and Conditioner ◘ 734
Oxy 10 Daily Face Wash Antibacterial Skin Wash ◘ 721
Oxy-5 and Oxy-10 Tinted and Vanishing Formulas with Sorboxyl ◘ 719
Plaquenil Sulfate Tablets 2067
Sebutone and Sebutone Cream Antiseborrheic Tar Shampoos 2408
Selsun Rx 2.5% Selenium Sulfide Lotion, USP 1977
Theraplex T Shampoo (Rare) 1411
Wellbutrin Tablets (Rare) 821

Hair loss (see under Alopecia)

Hair problems, unspecified
Accutane Capsules 1878
Emcyt Capsules (1%) 1161
▲ Lupron Depot 3.75 mg (Among most frequent) 2312

Hair texture, abnormal
Intron A (1 patient) 2097
Nizoral 2% Shampoo (One occurrence in 41 patients) 1144

Hair thinning
▲ Accutane Capsules (Less than 1 in 10) 1878
Actigall Capsules 2280
Cibalith-S 870
Combipres Tablets 678
Cortifoam 1827
Eskalith 2214
Lithane Tablets 1596
Lithium Carbonate Capsules & Tablets 1984
Lithobid Tablets 870
Monocid Injection (Less than 1%) 2217
Seldane Tablets 1349
Seldane-D Extended-Release Tablets 1350
Trilafon Tablets 2123

Halitosis
Anafranil Capsules (Up to 2%) 650
Azactam for Injection (Less than 1%) 2252

Hallucinations
Actifed with Codeine Cough Syrup 752
Actimmune (Rare) 1046
AK-Pentolate ⊙ 204
Alurate Elixir (Less than 1 in 100) 1883
Anafranil Capsules (Infrequent) 650
Ancobon Capsules 1886
Artane (Rare) 1195
Asendin Tablets (Very rare) 1196
Ativan Injection (1%) 2432
Atrohist Sprinkle Capsules 558
Azo Gantanol Tablets 1887
Azo Gantrisin Tablets 1888
Azulfidine Tablets, EN-tabs, Oral Suspension (Rare) 1157
Bactrim DS Tablets 1891
Bactrim I.V. Infusion 1889
Bactrim 1891
Blocadren Tablets (Less than 1%) 1429
BuSpar (Infrequent) 1401
Butisol Sodium Elixir & Tablets (Less than 1 in 100) 2377
Cardizem Tablets-30 mg, 60 mg, 90 mg and 120 mg (Less than 1%) 1329
Cardizem SR Capsules-60 mg, 90 mg and 120 mg (Less than 1%) 1327
Catapres Tablets 676
Celontin (Rare) 1692
Children's Advil Suspension (Less than 1%) 2426
Cipro I.V. (1% or less) 1592
Cipro Tablets (Less than 1%) 1589
Clozaril Tablets (Less than 1%) 2000
Cogentin 1435
Corgard Tablets 701
Corzide Tablets 702
Cyclogyl (Common) ⊙ 215
Cyclomydril ⊙ 216
Dalmane Capsules (Rare) 1927
Darvon-N/Darvocet-N 1254
Darvon 1256
Darvon-N Suspension & Tablets 1254
Deconamine 663
Deconsal 559
Demerol 2047
Demser Capsules 1460
Desyrel and Desyrel Dividose (Less than 1%) 1404
Dilaudid-HP Injection 1175
Dimetane-DC Cough Syrup 1857
Dimetane-DX Cough Syrup 1858
Ditropan 1332
Dolobid Tablets (Less than 1 in 100) 1465
Doral Tablets (Rare) 2383

▲ Duragesic Transdermal System (3% to 10%) 1133
E.E.S. (Isolated reports) 522
Elavil 2269
▲ Eldepryl (3 of 49 patients) 2250
Elspar 1470
Endep Tablets 1927
Ergamisol Tablets (Less frequent) .. 1136
EryPed (Isolated reports) 519
Ery-Tab Tablets (Isolated reports) .. 521
Erythrocin Stearate Filmtab (Isolated reports) 523
Erythromycin Base Filmtab (Isolated reports) 525
Erythromycin Delayed-Release Capsules, USP (Isolated reports) 526
Eskalith 2214
Ethmozine Tablets (Less than 2%) 946
Etrafon 2087
Fansidar Tablets 1896
Fedahist Gyrocaps 2145
Fedahist Timecaps 2145
Feldene Capsules (Less than 1%) .. 1777
Fiorinal with Codeine Capsules 2008
Flexeril Tablets (Less than 1%) 1471
Floxin Tablets (Less than 1%) 1652
Gantanol 1899
Gantrisin Ophthalmic Ointment/Solution 1900
Gantrisin 1901
Gastrocrom Capsules (Infrequent) .. 974
Halcion Tablets 2340
Haldol Decanoate 1375
Haldol Injection, Tablets and Concentrate 1373
Hydrea Capsules (Extremely rare) .. 728
▲ IFEX (Among most common) 729
Inapsine Injection 1140
Inderal 2459
Inderal LA Long Acting Capsules 2461
Inderide Tablets 2463
Inderide LA Long Acting Capsules .. 2465
Innovar Injection 1141
Keflex Pulvules, Oral Suspension & Pediatric Drops 916
Keftab Tablets 917
Kerlone Tablets (Less than 2%) 2172
Klonopin Tablets 1902
Lariam Tablets 1904
Larodopa Tablets (Relatively frequent) 1905
Leukeran Tablets (Rare) 788
Limbitrol 1933
Lioresal Tablets 1031
Lopressor Ampuls 1032
Lopressor HCT Tablets 1034
Lopressor Tablets 1032
Ludiomil Tablets (Rare) 874
MS Contin Tablets (Infrequent) 1814
MSIR (Infrequent) 1817
▲ Marinol (Dronabinol) Capsules (5%) 1985
Marplan Tablets (Rare) 1906
Matulane Capsules 1907
Mebaral Tablets (Less than 1 in 100) 2061
Mepergan Injection 2479
Methergine (Rare) 2016
Mexitil Capsules (About 3 in 1,000) 680
Minipress Capsules (Less than 1%) 1778
Minizide Capsules (Rare) 1779
Motrin Tablets (Less than 1%) 2351
Myambutol Tablets 1225
Myochrysine Injection (Rare) 1516
Naldecon Syrup, Tablets, Pediatric Drops and Pediatric Syrup 709
NebuPent for Inhalation Solution (1% or less) 1017
Nembutal Sodium Capsules (Less than 1%) 534
Nembutal Sodium Solution (Less than 1%) 536
Nembutal Sodium Suppositories (Less than 1%) 538
Norflex 1314
Norgesic (Occasional) 1314
Noroxin Tablets 1519
Norpramin Tablets 1340
Novafed A Capsules 1342
Novafed Capsules 1342
Novahistine DH 1342
Novahistine DMX .... ▣ 595
Novahistine Elixir .... ▣ 596
Novahistine Expectorant 1343
Nubain Injection (Less than 1%) 934
Omnipaque (Less than 0.7%) 2552
Oramorph SR (Morphine Sulfate Sustained Release Tablets) (Less frequent) 1988
Orthoclone OKT3 Sterile Solution .. 1645
Orudis Capsules (Less than 1%) 2488
PCE Dispertab Tablets (Isolated reports) 549
Pamelor 2019
Pantopon Injectable 1911
Parlodel 2020
PediaProfen Suspension (Less than 1%) 1363
Pediazole 1973
Pentam 300 Injection (1.7%) 1018
Pepcid (Infrequent) 1524
Periactin 1525
▲ Permax Tablets (13.8%) 1291
Pfizerpen-AS Aqueous Suspension (Approximately 1 in 500) 1959
Phenergan with Codeine 2497
Phenergan VC with Codeine 2501
Phenobarbital Elixir and Tablets (Less than 1 in 100 patients) 1293
Prilosec Delayed-Release Capsules (Less than 1%) 1530
Procan SR Tablets (Occasional) 1760
Pronestyl Capsules and Tablets (Occasional) 1800
Pronestyl Injection (Occasional) 1798
Pronestyl-SR Tablets (Occasional) .. 1801
ProSom Tablets 554
Prozac Pulvules (Infrequent) 920
Reglan (Rare) 1869
Restoril Capsules (Less than 0.5%) 2023
Roferon-A Injection (Less than 1%) 1916
Rondec 1975
Rondec-DM 1976
Rondec-TR Tablet 1975
Rufen Tablets (Less than 1%) 691
Ru-Tuss DE Tablets 694
Sansert Tablets 2031
Seconal Sodium Pulvules (Less than 1 in 100) 1296
Seldane-D Extended-Release Tablets 1350
Septra 813
Septra I.V. Infusion 808
Septra I.V. Infusion ADD-Vantage Vials 810
Septra 813
Serax Capsules 2522
Serax Tablets 2522
Sinemet Tablets 952
▲ Sinemet CR Tablets (3.9%) 953
Sinequan (Infrequent) 1960
Stadol (Less than 1%) 721
Sublimaze Injection 1146
Surmontil Capsules 2524
Symmetrel Capsules & Syrup (1-5%) 936
Tagamet 2228
Talacen 2070
Talwin Injection 2071
Talwin Compound 2072
Talwin Injection 2071
Talwin Nx 2073
Tenoretic Tablets 1105
Tenormin Tablets and I.V. Injection 1107
Thiosulfil Forte Tablets 2526
Timolide Tablets 1547
Timoptic in Ocudose 1552
Timoptic Sterile Ophthalmic Solution 1550
Tofranil Ampuls 1038
Tofranil Tablets 1039
Tofranil-PM Capsules 1041
▲ Tonocard Tablets (2.1-11.2%) 1554
Transderm Scōp Transdermal Therapeutic System (Infrequent) 887
Tranxene 556
Trexan Tablets (Less than 1%) 937
Triaminic Expectorant DH 1995
Triaminic Oral Infant Drops 1996
Triavil Tablets 1556
Trilisate (Rare) 1822
Trinalin Repetabs Tablets 1170
Valium Injectable 1937
Valium Tablets 1939
Valrelease Capsules (Infrequent) 1923
Vira-A for Injection 1766
Visken Tablets (Less than 1%) 2036
Vivactil Tablets 1567
Vontrol Tablets (Approximately 1 in 350) 2243
Wellbutrin Tablets (Frequent) 821
Xanax Tablets (Rare) 2367
Zantac Injection and Zantac Injection Premixed 1063
Zantac (Rare) 1065
Zovirax Capsules 824
Zovirax Sterile Powder 828
Zovirax 824

Hallucinations, auditory

Catapres-TTS 677
Combipres Tablets 678
Vontrol Tablets (Less than 1/2%) .. 2243

Hallucinations, hypnagogic

Anafranil Capsules (Infrequent) 650

Hallucinations, visual

Catapres-TTS 677
Combipres Tablets 678
Isopto Hyoscine .... ⊙ 222
Parlodel (Less than 1%) 2020
Talwin Compound 2072
Talwin Nx 2073
Tegretol Chewable Tablets 654
Tegretol Suspension 656
Tegretol Tablets 654
Vontrol Tablets (Less than 1/2%) .. 2243

Halos

Atabrine Hydrochloride Tablets 2041
Cordarone Tablets 2446

Hand-foot syndrome (see under Palmar-plantar erythrodysesthesia syndrome)

Hangover

Phenobarbital Elixir and Tablets 1293
Placidyl Capsules 553
▲ ProSom Tablets (3%) 554
Prozac Pulvules (Infrequent) 920

Headache

A.P.L. 2431
▲ Accutane Capsules (Approximately 1 in 20) 1878
Achromycin V Capsules 1193
Actibine 900
Actifed with Codeine Cough Syrup .. 752
Actigall Capsules 2280
▲ Actimmune (33%) 1046
Adagen Injection (One patient) 967
▲ Adalat Capsules (10 mg and 20 mg) (About 10% to 23%) 1587
Adenocard Injection (2%) 1007
Adipex-P Tablets and Capsules 1019
▲ Adrenalin Chloride Solution 1:100 & 1:1,000 (Often) 1689
▲ AeroBid Inhaler System (25%) 995
Aerolate 994
AK-Fluor Injection 10% and 25% .... ⊙ 204
AK-NaCl 5% Ointment & Solution .... ⊙ 204
Albalon Solution with Liquifilm .... ⊙ 238
Aldactazide 2150
Aldactone 2152
Aldoclor Tablets 1413
Aldomet Ester HCl Injection 1417
Aldomet Oral 1415
Aldoril Tablets 1418
Alfenta Injection (Less than 1%) .. 1131
▲ Alferon N Injection (15% to 31%) 1809
▲ Altace Capsules (5.4%) 1086
Alupent (1 to 4%) 674
Alurate Elixir (Less than 1 in 100) 1883
Amen (Rare) 833
Amicar Syrup, Tablets, and Injection (Occasional) 1194
Amikin Injectable (Rare) 602
Aminophyllin Tablets 2153
▲ Anafranil Capsules (28% to 52%) 650
Ana-Kit Anaphylaxis Emergency Treatment Kit 1100
▲ Anaprox and Anaprox DS Tablets (3-9%) 2288
Anatuss LA Tablets 1359
Ancobon Capsules 1886
Android 1111
▲ Ansaid Tablets (3-9%) 2319
Antabuse Tablets (Small number of patients) 2429
Apresazide Capsules (Common) 854
Apresoline Hydrochloride Parenteral (Ampuls) 856
Apresoline Hydrochloride Tablets (Common) 855
Apresoline-Esidrix Tablets 857
Aquasol A Vitamin A Capsules, USP 615
Aquasol A Parenteral, USP 615
Aralen Hydrochloride Injection 2038
Aralen Phosphate Tablets 2039
Aristocort Suspension 1008
Aristospan Suspension 1011
Arm-a-Med Isoetharine Inhalation Solution, USP 616
Artane 1195
Asbron G 1997
Asendin Tablets (Greater than 1%) 1196
Astramorph/PF Injection, USP (Preservative-Free) 618
Atabrine Hydrochloride Tablets 2041
▲ Atgam Sterile Solution (More than 1% to 10%; 1 patient in 6) 2320
Ativan Tablets (Less frequent) 2434
Atrohist Sprinkle Capsules 558
Atromid-S Capsules (Less often) .. 2435
Atrovent Inhalation Aerosol (2.4%) 675
Augmentin Tablets, Powder for Oral Suspension, and Chewable Tablets (Less frequent) 2198
Azactam for Injection (Less than 1%) 2252
Azdōne Tablets 844
Azo Gantanol Tablets 1887
Azo Gantrisin Tablets 1888
▲ Azulfidine Tablets, EN-tabs, Oral Suspension (Approximately one-third of patients) 1157
BAL in Oil Ampules 661
Bactrim DS Tablets 1891
Bactrim I.V. Infusion 1889
Bactrim 1891
Baron-X Tablets 650
▲ Beconase AQ Nasal Spray (Fewer than 5 per 100 patients) 574
Benadryl Capsules 1691
Benadryl Injection 1692
Benemid Tablets 1426
Bentyl 1322
Betagan (Rare) .... ⊙ 239
Betoptic Sterile Ophthalmic Solution (Rare) 569
Betoptic S Sterile Ophthalmic Suspension (Rare) 570
Biavax II 1427
Biltricide 1589
Biphetamine Capsules 973
Blocadren Tablets (Greater than 1%) 1429
Bontril Slow-Release 834
Brethaire Inhaler 1024
Brethine Ampuls 1026
Brethine Tablets 1026
Brevibloc Injection (2%) 942
Brevicon 2304
Brevital Sodium Vials 1248
Bricanyl Injection 1324
Bricanyl Tablets 1325
Bronkephrine Injection 2042
Bronkometer Aerosol 2042
Bronkosol Solution 2042
Bucladin-S Softab Chewable Tablets (Occasional) 2264
Bumex (0.6%) 1895
▲ BuSpar (6%) 1401
Butazolidin Capsules & Tablets (Less than 1%) 1027
Butisol Sodium Elixir & Tablets (Less than 1 in 100) 2377
Calan SR Caplets (2.2%) 2157
Calan Tablets (2.2%) 2155
Calcijex Calcitriol Injection 506
Calciparine Injection (Rare) 925
Calderol Capsules 1635
Cantil Tablets 1326
Capoten (0.5 to 2%) 2255
Capozide (0.5 to 2%) 2258
Carafate Tablets (Less than 0.5%) 1326
Carbocaine Hydrochloride Injection 2043
Cardene Capsules (B 6.4-8.2%) 2290
Cardilate Oral/Sublingual Tablets .. 757
Cardioquin Tablets 1812
Cardizem Tablets-30 mg, 60 mg, 90 mg and 120 mg (2.1%) 1329
▲ Cardizem SR Capsules-60 mg, 90 mg and 120 mg (4.5-12%) 1327
▲ Cardura Tablets (14%) 1941
Cartrol Tablets (0.7%) 507
Catapres Tablets (About 1 in 100 patients) 676
Catapres-TTS (1% to 5%) 677
Ceftin Tablets (Less than 0.7%) 575
Celestone Soluspan Suspension 2081
Celontin 1692
Centrax (Less frequent) 1693
Ceptaz for Injection (Fewer than 1%) 1057
Cerose-DM 2443
▲ CHEMET (succimer) Capsules (5.2 to 15.7%) 1361
Children's Advil Suspension (Less than 3%) 2426
Chloromycetin Kapseals 1695
Chloromycetin Palmitate, Oral Suspension 1697
Chloromycetin Sodium Succinate 1698

Choledyl Pediatric Elixir ... 1702
Choledyl Tablets ... 1700
Choledyl SA Tablets ... 1704
Cholera Vaccine ... 2445
Cholybar ... 1705
Cibacalcin Double-chambered Syringes (Rare) ... 859
Cibalith-S ... 870
▲ Cipro I.V. (Among most frequent) ... 1592
Cipro Tablets (1.2%) ... 1589
Claforan Sterile Injection (Less than 1%) ... 1089
▲ Clinoril Tablets (3-9%) ... 1433
▲ Clozaril Tablets (More than 5 to 7%) ... 2000
ColBENEMID Tablets ... 1436
Colestid Granules (1 in 300) ... 2328
Combipres Tablets (About 1 in 100) ... 678
Comhist LA Capsules ... 1618
Compazine ... 2201
Constant-T Tablets ... 1029
Cordarone Tablets (1 to 3%) ... 2446
Corgard Tablets (1 to 5 of 1000 patients) ... 701
Cortenema ... 2244
Cortifoam ... 1827
Cortone Acetate Sterile Suspension ... 1437
Cortone Acetate Tablets ... 1439
Corzide Tablets (1 to 5 of 1000 patients) ... 702
Coumadin Injection & Tablets ... 944
Cylert Tablets ... 510
▲ Cytadren Tablets (1 in 20) ... 861
Cytosar-U Sterile Powder (Less frequent) ... 2329
Cytotec (2.4%) ... 2159
Cytovene Sterile Powder (1% or less) ... 2292
DDAVP Injection (Infrequent) ... 1840
▲ DDAVP (2 to 5%) ... 1841
Dalalone D.P. Injectable ... 999
Dalgan Injection (Less than 1%) ... 620
Dalmane Capsules ... 1927
Danocrine Capsules ... 2046
Dantrium Capsules (Less frequent) ... 1619
Dapsone USP ... 1130
Daranide Tablets ... 1445
Daraprim Tablets (Rare) ... 761
Darbid Tablets ... 2205
Darvon-N/Darvocet-N ... 1254
Darvon ... 1256
Darvon-N Suspension & Tablets ... 1254
Dayto Himbin Tablets and Liquid ... 905
Decadron Elixir ... 1445
Decadron Phosphate Injection ... 1449
Decadron Phosphate Respihaler ... 1454
Decadron Phosphate Turbinaire ... 1456
Decadron Phosphate with Xylocaine Injection, Sterile ... 1451
Decadron Tablets ... 1447
Decadron-LA Sterile Suspension ... 1457
Declomycin Capsules, Tablets ... 1199
Deconamine ... 663
Deconsal ... 559
Deltasone Tablets ... 2332
Demerol ... 2047
Demser Capsules (Infrequent) ... 1460
Demulen ... 2161
Depakene Capsules & Syrup ... 511
Depakote ... 512
Depo-Medrol Sterile Aqueous Suspension ... 2334
▲ Deponit NTG Transdermal Delivery System (Most common) ... 2143
Depo-Provera Sterile Aqueous Suspension (Rare) ... 2336
Deprol Tablets ... 2382
Desoxyn Gradumet Tablets ... 514
Desyrel and Desyrel Dividose (Greater than 1%) ... 1404
Dexatrim ... ▣ 733
Dexedrine ... 2206
Diapid Nasal Spray (Infrequent) ... 2003
Didrex Tablets ... 2338
Diethylstilbestrol Tablets ... 1258
Diflucan Injection and Tablets (1.9% in 4048 patients) ... 1948
Dilantin Infatabs ... 1710
Dilantin Kapseals ... 1708
Dilantin Parenteral ... 1712
▲ Dilantin-30 Pediatric/Dilantin-125 Suspension (Among most common) ... 1713
▲ Dilantin with Phenobarbital Kapseals (Among most common) ... 1715
▲ Dilatrate-SR (Approximately 25%) ... 1827
Dilaudid-HP Injection ... 1175
Dilor ... 2079
Dilor-G Tablets & Liquid ... 2079
Dimetane-DC Cough Syrup ... 1857
Dimetane-DX Cough Syrup ... 1858
▲ Dipentum Capsules (Up to 5%) ... 1160
Diprivan Injection (Greater than 1%) ... 2267
Diucardin Tablets ... 2450
Diulo ... 2129
Diupres Tablets ... 1461
Diuril Oral Suspension ... 1464
Diuril Sodium Intravenous ... 1463
Diuril Tablets ... 1464
Dobutrex Solution Vials (1 to 3%) ... 1259
▲ Dolobid Tablets (3% to 9%) ... 1465
Dolophine Hydrochloride Ampoules & Vials ... 1260
Dolophine Hydrochloride Tablets ... 1261
Donnatal ... 1858
Donnatal Extentabs ... 1859
Donnatal Tablets ... 1858
Donnazyme Tablets ... 1860
Dopram Injectable ... 1860
▲ Doral Tablets (4.5%) ... 2383
Dorcol Children's Cough Syrup ... ▣ 685
Dorcol Children's Decongestant Liquid ... ▣ 685
▲ Duragesic Transdermal System (3% to 10%) ... 1133
Duramorph ... 960
Duranest Injections ... 624
Duvoid Tablets ... 1853
Dyazide Capsules ... 2208
▲ DynaCirc Capsules (1.9% to 13.7%) ... 2004
Dyrenium Capsules (Rare) ... 2210
Easprin ... 1719
Edecrin ... 1468
Elavil ... 2269
▲ Eldepryl (2 of 49 patients) ... 2250
Elspar ... 1470
Emcyt Capsules (1%) ... 1161
Emete-con Intramuscular/Intravenous ... 1950
▲ Eminase (Less than 10%) ... 2211
Empirin with Codeine Phosphate Nos. 2, 3 & 4 ... 764
Endep Tablets ... 1927
Enduron Tablets ... 517
Enduronyl ... 518
▲ Engerix-B Unit-Dose Vials (1% to 10%) ... 2213
Enovid ... 2161
Entex Capsules ... 1623
Entex LA Tablets ... 1623
Entex Liquid ... 1623
Epifrin ... ⊙ 244
EpiPen ... 843
▲ Epogen for Injection (0.4% to 19%) ... 591
Equagesic Tablets ... 2451
▲ Ergamisol Tablets (3 to 4%) ... 1136
Ergotrate Maleate Ampoules (Uncommon) ... 1263
Esidrix Tablets ... 863
Esimil Tablets ... 864
Eskalith ... 2214
Estinyl Tablets ... 2085
Estrace ... 1385
Estrace Vaginal Cream ... 1388
Estraderm Transdermal System ... 866
Estradurin ... 2452
Estratest ... 2245
Estrovis ... 1721
▲ Ethmozine Tablets (8.0%) ... 946
Etrafon ... 2087
Exna Tablets ... 1862
Sterile FUDR (Remote possibility) ... 1898
Factrel (Rare) ... 2561
Fansidar Tablets ... 1896
Fastin Capsules ... 2216
Fedahist Gyrocaps ... 2145
Fedahist Timecaps ... 2145
Feldene Capsules (1 to 3%) ... 1777
Fiorinal with Codeine Capsules (Infrequent) ... 2008
Flagyl I.V. ... 2131
Flagyl Tablets ... 2170
Flexeril Tablets (1% to 3%) ... 1471
Floropryl Sterile Ophthalmic Ointment ... 1473
▲ Floxin Tablets (1% to 9%) ... 1652
Fluorescite ... ⊙ 217
Fluorouracil Injection ... 1897
Fortaz (Less than 1%) ... 1060
Fulvicin P/G Tablets ... 2090
Fulvicin P/G 165 & 330 Tablets ... 2091
Fulvicin-U/F Tablets ... 2092
▲ Fungizone Intravenous (Among most common) ... 2262
Furoxone (Occasional) ... 1855
Gamimune N Immune Globulin Intravenous (Human) ... 1572
Gammagard Immune Globulin, Intravenous (Human) (Occasional) ... 658
Gammar-IV, Immune Globulin Intravenous (Human) ... 610
Gantanol ... 1899
Gantrisin Ophthalmic Ointment/Solution ... 1900
Gantrisin ... 1901
Garamycin Injectable ... 2093
▲ Gastrocrom Capsules (4 of 87 patients) ... 974
Gelfoam Sterile Sponge ... 2338
Geocillin Tablets ... 1951
Geref (sermorelin acetate for injection) ... 2560
Glaucon ... ⊙ 218
Glucotrol (1 in 50) ... 1952
Grifulvin V (griseofulvin microsize) Tablets/Suspension (Occasional) ... 1678
Grisactin (Occasional) ... 2454
Grisactin Ultra Tablets (Occasional) ... 2455
Gris-PEG Tablets, 125 mg & 250 mg (Occasional) ... 1083
Guaifed ... 1615
Guaifed Syrup ... ▣ 629
▲ Halcion Tablets (9.7%) ... 2340
Haldol Decanoate 50 (50 mg/mL) Injection ... 1375
Haldol Injection, Tablets and Concentrate ... 1373
Halotestin Tablets ... 2341
Harmonyl Tablets ... 528
Heparin Lock Flush Solution ... 2456
Heparin Sodium Vials (Rare) ... 1264
Heparin Sodium Injection ... 2457
Heparin Sodium Injection, USP, Sterile Solution ... 2342
Hespan Injection ... 948
▲ Hismanal Tablets (6.7%) ... 1138
Humatrope Vials (Infrequent) ... 1266
Humorsol Sterile Ophthalmic Solution ... 1475
Humulin 70/30, 100 Units ... 1267
Humulin BR, 100 Units ... 1268
Humulin L, 100 Units ... 1268
Humulin U, 100 Units ... 1272
Hydeltrasol Injection, Sterile ... 1476
Hydeltra-T.B.A. Sterile Suspension ... 1478
Hydrea Capsules (Extremely rare) ... 728
Hydrocortone Acetate Sterile Suspension ... 1479
Hydrocortone Phosphate Injection, Sterile ... 1481
Hydrocortone Tablets ... 1482
HydroDIURIL Tablets ... 1484
Hydromox R Tablets ... 1209
Hydromox Tablets ... 1208
Hydropres Tablets ... 1485
▲ Hylorel Tablets (58.1%) ... 975
Hyperstat I.V. Injection ... 2095
▲ Hytrin Tablets (1.3% to 16.2%) ... 529
▲ Idamycin for Injection (20%) ... 564
Imferon ... 976
Inderide Tablets ... 2463
Inderide LA Long Acting Capsules ... 2465
▲ Indocin (11.7%) ... 1487
Infumorph 200 and Infumorph 500 Sterile Solutions (A significant minority of cases) ... 962
Intal Capsules (Less than 1 in 10,000 patients) ... 978
Intal Inhaler (Infrequent) ... 979
Intal Nebulizer Solution ... 980
▲ Intron A (21% to 43%) ... 2097
▲ Intropin Injection (Among most frequent) ... 930
Ionamin Capsules ... 981
IOPIDINE ... ⊙ 232
ISMOTIC ... ⊙ 233
Isoptin Injectable (1.2%) ... 1177
Isoptin Oral Tablets (2.2%) ... 1179
Isoptin SR Sustained Release Tablets (2.2%) ... 1181
Isopto Carbachol ... ⊙ 219
▲ Isordil (25%) ... 2467
Isuprel Hydrochloride Injection 1:5000 ... 2050
Isuprel Hydrochloride Mistometer ... 2051
Isuprel Hydrochloride Solution 1:200 & 1:100 ... 2052
Jenest-28 Tablets ... 1636
K-Phos M.F. Tablets ... 659
K-Phos Neutral Tablets ... 660
K-Phos No. 2 Tablets ... 659
Keflex Pulvules, Oral Suspension & Pediatric Drops ... 916
Keftab Tablets ... 917
Kenalog-10 Injection ... 2402
Kenalog-40 Injection ... 2403
▲ Kerlone Tablets (6.5% to 14.8%) ... 2172
Kinesed Tablets ... 2272
Klonopin Tablets ... 1902
Konȳne 80 Factor IX Complex ... 1571
Konȳne-HT Factor IX Complex ... 1583
Kutrase Capsules ... 2146
Lamprene Capsules (Less than 1%) ... 1030
Lanoxicaps ... 772
Lanoxin Elixir Pediatric ... 775
Lanoxin Injection ... 778
Lanoxin Injection Pediatric ... 781
Lanoxin Tablets ... 783
▲ Lariam Tablets (Among most frequent) ... 1904
Larodopa Tablets (Relatively frequent) ... 1905
Lasix ... 1093
▲ Leukine for IV Infusion (Among most frequent) ... 1127
▲ Levatol (7.8%) ... 1832
Levlen/Tri-Levlen ... 665
Levophed Bitartrate Injection ... 2054
Levsin/Levsinex ... 2147
Limbitrol ... 1933
▲ Lioresal Tablets (4-8%) ... 1031
Lithane Tablets ... 1596
Lithium Carbonate Capsules & Tablets ... 1984
Lithobid Tablets ... 870
Lo/Ovral Tablets ... 2471
Lo/Ovral-28 Tablets ... 2476
Loestrin ... 1728
Lomotil ... 2174
Lopid Capsules and Tablets (1.2%) ... 1736
Lopressor Ampuls ... 1032
▲ Lopressor HCT Tablets (10 in 100 patients) ... 1034
Lopressor Tablets ... 1032
Lorelco Tablets ... 1333
Lortab ASA Tablets ... 2414
▲ Lotensin Tablets (5%) ... 872
Loxitane ... 1213
▲ Lozol Tablets (Greater than or equal to 5%) ... 1843
▲ Ludiomil Tablets (4%) ... 874
Lufyllin & Lufyllin-400 Tablets ... 2384
Lufyllin-GG Elixir & Tablets ... 2385
Lupron Depot 7.5 mg ... 2311
▲ Lupron Injection (5% or more) ... 2310
M-M-R II ... 1494
M-R-VAX II ... 1496
MS Contin Tablets (Infrequent) ... 1814
MSIR (Infrequent) ... 1817
Macrodantin Capsules (Less frequent) ... 1624
Marax Tablets & DF Syrup ... 1954
Marcaine Hydrochloride with Epinephrine 1:200,000 ... 2055
Marcaine Hydrochloride Injection ... 2055
Marcaine Spinal ... 2058
▲ Marinol (Dronabinol) Capsules (6%) ... 1985
▲ Marplan Tablets (Among most frequent) ... 1906
Matulane Capsules ... 1907
Maxair Inhaler (2.0%) ... 1311
Maxzide ... 1215
Mebaral Tablets (Less than 1 in 100) ... 2061
▲ Meclomen Capsules (3-9%) ... 1739
Mediatric Capsules ... 2476
Medrol ... 2348
Mellaril (Extremely rare) ... 2011
Menrium Tablets ... 1934
Mepergan Injection ... 2479
Meruvax II ... 1503
▲ Mesnex Injection (50%) ... 733
Metaprel Inhalation Aerosol Bronchodilator (1 to 4%) ... 2014
Methadone Hydrochloride Diskets ... 1284
Methadone Hydrochloride Oral Solution & Tablets ... 1987
Methergine ... 2016
Methotrexate Tablets, Parenteral, LPF Parenteral (Less common) ... 1217
Metopirone Tablets ... 876
Metrodin (urofollitropin for injection) ... 2182
▲ Mevacor Tablets (9.3%) ... 1505
▲ Mexitil Capsules (5.7% to 7.5%) ... 680
Micronor Tablets ... 1667
▲ Midamor Tablets (3% to 8%) ... 1508
Milontin Kapseals ... 1741
Miltown Tablets ... 2386
▲ Minipress Capsules (7.8%) ... 1778
▲ Minitran Transdermal Delivery System (63%) ... 1312
▲ Minizide Capsules (7.8%) ... 1779
Minocin Intravenous (Rare) ... 1221

Minocin Oral Suspension (Rare) 1224
Minocin Pellet-Filled Capsules 1222
Mintezol 1510
MIOSTAT .... ⊙ 233
Mithracin 1602
Modicon 1667
▲ Moduretic Tablets (3% to 8%) 1510
Monistat Dual-Pak (1.3%) 1657
Monistat 3 Vaginal Suppositories (1.3%) 1657
Mono-Gesic Tablets 846
Monopril Tablets 1406
Motofen Tablets (1 in 40) 836
Motrin Tablets (Less than 3%) 2351
Mulvidren-F Softab Tablets 2273
Murocoll-2 Sterile Ophthalmic Solution (Frequent) .... ⊙ 261
Mutamycin 733
Myambutol Tablets 1225
Mydriacyl .... ⊙ 225
▲ Mykrox ½ mg Tablets (9.3%) 984
Myochrysine Injection 1516
Naldecon Syrup, Tablets, Pediatric Drops and Pediatric Syrup 709
▲ Nalfon Pulvules & Tablets (8.7%) .. 919
Naphcon Forte .... ⊙ 226
▲ Naprosyn (3 to 9%) 2297
Nardil (Common) 1742
▲ Nasacort Nasal Inhaler (Approximately 18%) 1844
Nasalcrom Nasal Solution (1 in 50) 986
Nasalide Nasal Solution 0.025% (5% or less) 2299
Naturetin Tablets (Occasional) 1789
Nebcin Vials, Hyporets & ADD-Vantage 1286
NebuPent for Inhalation Solution (Greater than 1%, up to 5%) 1017
NegGram 2062
Nembutal Sodium Capsules (Less than 1%) 534
Nembutal Sodium Solution (Less than 1%) 536
Nembutal Sodium Suppositories (Less than 1%) 538
Neo-Synephrine Hydrochloride 1% Carpuject 2063
Neo-Synephrine Hydrochloride 1% Injection 2063
Neptazane Tablets .... ⊙ 311
Nescaine/Nescaine MPF 629
Netromycin Injection 100 mg/ml (Fewer than 1 of 1000 patients) 2104
▲ Neupogen for Injection (7%) 595
Niacor Tablets 2376
Niclocide Chewable Tablets (1.4%) 1607
Nicorette (1.1%) 1335
▲ Nimotop Capsules (Up to 4.1%) 1607
Nipride I.V. Infusion 1909
Nitro-Bid IV (2%) 1338
▲ Nitro-Bid Ointment (50%) 1339
Nitro-Bid Capsules 1338
▲ Nitrodisc (63%) 2176
▲ Nitro-Dur (nitroglycerin) Transdermal Infusion System (Most common) 1164
▲ Nitrogard Tablets (Among most common) 1004
▲ Nitrolingual Spray (50%) 1846
Nitrostat IV (2%) 1744
Nizoral Tablets (Less than 1%) 1145
Nolex LA Tablets 838
Nolvadex Tablets (Infrequent) 1102
Nordette-21 Tablets 2481
Nordette-28 Tablets 2483
Norethin 2133
Norflex 1314
Norgesic 1314
Norinyl 2304
Norisodrine Aerotrol 540
Norlestrin 1746
Norlutate 1754
Norlutin 1755
Normodyne Tablets (2%) 2110
Normozide Tablets (Less than 1 to 2%) 2112
Noroxin Tablets (2.7%) 1519
▲ Norpace (3 to 9%) 2177
Norplant System 2484
Norpramin Tablets 1340
Nor-Q D Tablets 2304
Norzine (Occasional) 1818
Novafed A Capsules 1342
Novafed Capsules 1342
Novahistine DH 1342
Novahistine DMX .... ▣ 595
Novahistine Elixir .... ▣ 596
▲ Novantrone for Injection Concentrate (10 to 13%) 1226
Novocain Hydrochloride for Spinal Anesthesia 2065
▲ Nubain Injection (3%) 934
Nucofed Capsules 2219
Nucofed Expectorant 2219
Nucofed Pediatric Expectorant 2220
Nucofed Syrup 2219
Numorphan Hydrochloride Injection 935
Numorphan Suppositories 935
Ogen 540
▲ Omnipaque (Less than 0.01 to approximately 18%) 2552
Oncovin Solution Vials & Hyporets 1288
OptiPranolol Sterile Ophthalmic Solution (A small number of patients) .... ⊙ 261
Oramorph SR (Morphine Sulfate Sustained Release Tablets) 1988
Orap Tablets 1020
Oretic Tablets 544
Oreticyl 545
Orinase Tablets (Occasional) 2354
Ornade Spansule Capsules 2221
Ortho Dienestrol Cream 1664
▲ Orthoclone OKT3 Sterile Solution (11% to 44%) 1645
Ortho-Cyclen Tablets 1658
Ortho-Novum 1667
▲ Orudis Capsules (Greater than 3%) 2488
OSM_GLYN .... ⊙ 234
Ovcon 1391
Ovral Tablets 2490
Ovral-28 Tablets 2491
Ovrette Tablets 2492
Oxsoralen-Ultra Capsule 1117
PBZ Tablets & Elixir 1037
PBZ-SR Tablets 1037
PMB 200 and PMB 400 2504
Pamelor 2019
Pantopon Injectable 1911
Papaverine Hydrochloride Vials and Ampoules 1290
Paradione Capsules 548
▲ Parlodel (Less than 2-19%) 2020
Parnate Tablets 2222
Pavabid Capsules (Rare) 1344
Pavabid HP Capsulets (Rare) 1344
Pediapred Oral Liquid 987
PediaProfen Suspension (Less than 3%) 1363
Pediazole 1973
Peganone Tablets 551
Pentaspan Injection 949
▲ Pepcid (4.7%) 1524
Peptavlon 2563
Pergonal (menotropins for injection, USP) 2184
Periactin 1525
Peritrate 1756
▲ Permax Tablets (5.3%) 1291
Persantine Tablets (2.3%) 683
Phenergan with Codeine 2497
Phenergan VC with Codeine 2501
Phenobarbital Elixir and Tablets (Less than 1 in 100 patients) 1293
Phenurone Tablets (2%) 552
Pipracil 1230
▲ Plague Vaccine (10%) 1584
Plaquenil Sulfate Tablets 2067
Plegine Tablets 2504
▲ Plendil Extended-Release Tablets (2.1% to 28.0%) 1526
Polaramine 2116
Polymyxin B Sulfate, Aerosporin Brand Sterile Powder 798
Pondimin Tablets 1867
Ponstel 1758
Pontocaine Hydrochloride for Spinal Anesthesia 2069
Pregnyl 1644
Prelu-2 Capsules 683
Premarin Intravenous 2508
Premarin with Methyltestosterone .. 2515
Premarin Tablets 2510
Premarin Vaginal Cream 2512
Prilosec Delayed-Release Capsules (2.4 to 2.9%) 1530
Primaxin I.M. 1532
Primaxin I.V. (Less than 0.2%) 1535
▲ Prinivil Tablets (4.3% to 5.3%) 1538
▲ Prinzide Tablets (5.2%) 1540
Pro-Banthīne Tablets 2141
Procardia Capsules (1%) 1781
▲ Procardia XL Tablets (15.8% to 23%) 1783
▲ Procrit for Injection (0.40% to 19%) 1647
Profasi (human chorionic gonadotropin, USP) 2186
Proglycem 649
Prolixin Decanoate 1795
Prolixin Elixir 1793
Prolixin Enanthate 1796
Prolixin Injection 1791
Prolixin Oral Concentrate 1792
Prolixin Tablets 1793
▲ ProSom Tablets (16%) 554
Prostigmin Injectable 1120
Prostigmin Tablets 1121
Protopam Chloride for Injection 2518
Protostat Tablets 1674
Proventil Inhalation Aerosol 2117
▲ Proventil Repetabs Tablets (7%) 2120
▲ Proventil Solutions for Inhalation 0.5% and 0.083% (3%) 2118
▲ Proventil Syrup (4 of 100) 2119
▲ Proventil Tablets (7%) 2120
Provera Tablets 2356
Provocholine for Inhalation (1 occurrence) 1911
▲ Prozac Pulvules (20.3%) 920
Pyridium 1763
Pyridium Plus 1764
Quadrinal Tablets 1183
Quarzan Capsules 1937
Questran Light 711
Questran Powder 710
Quibron Capsules 713
Quibron-T 714
Quibron-T/SR 716
Quinaglute Dura-Tabs Tablets 663
Quinamm Tablets 1344
Quinidex Extentabs 1868
Raudixin Tablets 1803
Rauzide Tablets 1804
Recombivax HB (Equal to or greater than 1%) 1544
Reglan 1869
Renese Tablets 1785
Renese-R Tablets 1786
Respbid Tablets 684
▲ Retrovir Capsules (1.6% to 42%) 802
▲ Retrovir I.V. Infusion (42%) 805
▲ Retrovir Syrup (1.6% to 42%) 802
▲ Rēv-Eyes Ophthalmic Eyedrops 0.5% (10% to 40%) .... ⊙ 312
Rheumatrex Methotrexate Dose Pack (Less common) 1234
Rifadin 1345
Rifamate Capsules 1347
Rimactane Capsules 879
Ritalin 880
Robaxin Injectable 1871
Robaxin Tablets 1872
Robaxisal Tablets 1872
Robinul Forte Tablets 1873
Robinul Injectable 1873
Robinul Tablets 1873
Robitussin .... ▣ 676
Robitussin-CF .... ▣ 676
Robitussin-PE .... ▣ 677
Rocaltrol Capsules 1913
Rocephin Injectable Vials, ADD-Vantage (Occasional) 1914
▲ Roferon-A Injection (66% to 71%) 1916
▲ Rogaine Topical Solution (3.42%) .. 2357
Rondec 1975
Rondec-DM 1976
Rondec-TR Tablet 1975
▲ Rowasa (6.50%) 2248
Roxanol 1991
Rufen Tablets (1 to 3%) 691
Ru-Tuss DE Tablets 694
Ru-Tuss II Capsules 693
Ru-Tuss with Hydrocodone 694
Ru-Tuss Tablets 693
▲ Rythmol Tablets (1.5 to 4.5%) 1184
Saluron 718
Salutensin/Salutensin-Demi 719
▲ Sandimmune (Less than 1 to 15%) 2024
Sandostatin Injection (2.0%) 2029
Sanorex Tablets 2030
Scleromate (Rare) 1685
Seconal Sodium Pulvules (Less than 1 in 100) 1296
▲ Sectral Capsules (6%) 2520
▲ Seldane Tablets (15.8%) 1349
▲ Seldane-D Extended-Release Tablets (17.4%) 1350
Sensorcaine 631
Sensorcaine-MPF Spinal 634
Septra 813
Septra I.V. Infusion 808
Septra I.V. Infusion ADD-Vantage Vials 810
Septra 813
Ser-Ap-Es Tablets 881
Serax Capsules (In few instances) .. 2522
Serax Tablets (In few instances) 2522
Seromycin Pulvules 1298
Serophene (clomiphene citrate tablets, USP) (Less than 1 in 100 patients) 2186
Serpasil Tablets 883
Serpasil-Apresoline Tablets 884
Serpasil-Esidrix Tablets 886
Sinemet Tablets 952
Sinemet CR Tablets (2.0%) 953
Sinequan (Occasional) 1960
Skelaxin 840
Slo-bid Gyrocaps 1847
Slo-Niacin Tablets 2376
Solganal Suspension (Rare) 2122
Solu-Cortef Sterile Powder 2361
Solu-Medrol Sterile Powder 2363
Soma Compound w/Codeine Tablets (Infrequent or rare) 2390
Soma Compound Tablets (Infrequent or rare) 2389
Soma Tablets 2388
▲ Sorbitrate (25%) 1103
Sotradecol (Sodium Tetradecyl Sulfate Injection) 964
▲ Stadol (3%) 721
Stelazine 2226
Stilphostrol Tablets and Ampuls 1609
Streptase for Infusion 635
▲ Suprax (3%) 1235
Surgicel 1151
Surital Ampoules, Steri-Vials 1764
Surmontil Capsules 2524
Sus-Phrine Injection 1006
Symmetrel Capsules & Syrup (1-5%) 936
▲ Synarel Nasal Solution (19% of patients) 2300
TACE 12 and 25 mg 1353
T-PHYL (Uniphyl) 200 mg Tablets 1820
Tagamet (2.1% to 3.5%) 2228
Talacen 2070
Talwin Injection 2071
Talwin Compound 2072
Talwin Injection 2071
Talwin Nx 2073
▲ Tambocor Tablets (9.6%) 1315
Tapazole Tablets 1298
Taractan 1920
Tavist Syrup 2033
Tavist Tablets 2035
Tavist-D Tablets 2035
Tazicef for Injection (Less than 1%) 2231
Tazidime Vials, Faspak & ADD-Vantage (Less than 1%) 1299
▲ Tegison Capsules (25-50%) 1881
Tegretol Chewable Tablets 654
Tegretol Suspension 656
Tegretol Tablets 654
Temaril Tablets, Syrup and Spansule Sustained Release Capsules 1085
Temovate Scalp Application (1 of 294 patients) 1056
▲ Tenex Tablets (2% to 4%) 1875
Tenuate 1354
▲ Terazol 3 Vaginal Cream (21%) 1676
▲ Terazol 3 Vaginal Suppositories (30.3% of 284 patients) 1677
▲ Terazol 7 Vaginal Cream (26% of 521 patients) 1677
Tessalon Perles 1006
Testred Capsules 1124
Thalitone Tablets 687
Theo-24 2179
Theo-Dur Sprinkle 1168
Theo-Dur Extended-Release Tablets 1166
Theolair 1317
Theolair-SR Tablets 1319
▲ TheoX Extended-Release Tablets (Among most consistent) 841
TheraCys BCG Live (Intravesical) (Up to 1.8%) 898
Thiosulfil Forte Tablets 2526
Thiotepa Parenteral 1240
Tigan 2239
Timentin for Injection 2239
Timolide Tablets (Less than 1%) 1547
Timoptic in Ocudose 1552
Timoptic Sterile Ophthalmic Solution 1550
Tofranil Ampuls 1038
Tofranil Tablets 1039
Tofranil-PM Capsules 1041
▲ Tolectin (200, 400 and 600 mg) (3 to 9%) 1379
Tolinase Tablets (Infrequent) 2365
Tonocard Tablets (2.1-4.6%) 1554
Toradol IM Injection (1% to 3%) 2302
Torecan (Occasional) 1993

▲Tornalate (4%) 2074
Trancopal Caplets 2075
Trandate HCT/Trandate (Less than 1% in 208 patients) 579
Transderm Scōp Transdermal Therapeutic System (Few patients) 887
▲Transderm-Nitro Transdermal Therapeutic System (63%) 2283
Tranxene 556
▲Trental (1.2% to 6.2%) 1099
▲Trexan Tablets (Greater than 10%) 937
Triaminic Expectorant ▣ 688
Triaminic Expectorant DH 1995
Triaminic Oral Infant Drops 1996
Triaminic-DM Syrup ▣ 689
Triavil Tablets 1556
▲Tridil Ampuls & Vials (Among most common) 939
Tridione 557
Trilafon 2123
Levlen/Tri-Levlen 665
Trilisate (Less than 2%) 1822
Trinalin Repetabs Tablets 1170
Tri-Norinyl 2304
Triphasil-21 Tablets 2527
Triphasil-28 Tablets 2532
Tropicacyl ◉ 209
Tuss-Ornade Liquid 2242
Tuss-Ornade Spansule Capsules 2242
Typhoid Vaccine 2533
Unasyn (Less than 1%) 1965
Uniphyl 400 mg Tablets 1823
Urecholine 1558
Urispas Tablets 2242
Uroqid-Acid (Less frequent) 661
Valium Injectable 1937
Valium Tablets (Infrequent) 1939
Valpin 50 Tablets 941
Valrelease Capsules (Infrequent) 1923
Vancenase AQ Nasal Spray 0.042% (Fewer than 5 per 100 patients) 2127
▲Vascor (200, 300 and 400 mg) Tablets (11.34 to 13.64%) 1383
▲Vaseretic Tablets (5.5%) 1559
Vasocon-A ◉ 278
Vasosulf ◉ 279
Vasotec I.V. (2.9%) 1562
▲Vasotec Tablets (1.8% to 5.2%) 1564
Vasoxyl Injection 819
Velban Vials 1305
▲Ventolin (2% to 5%) 583
▲Verelan Capsules (2.5% to 5.3%) 1243
Versed Injection (1.3% to 1.5%) 1924
Vira-A for Injection 1766
Vivactil Tablets 1567
▲Voltaren Tablets (About 7%) 1042
Vontrol Tablets (Rare) 2243
Wygesic Tablets 2540
▲Wytensin Tablets (5%) 2542
▲Xanax Tablets (12.9% to 29.2%) 2367
▲Xylocaine Injections (3%) 637
Yocon 1686
Yohimex Tablets 1190
▲Yutopar (10 to 15% (with IV administration)) 647
Zantac Injection and Zantac Injection Premixed 1063
Zantac 1065
Zarontin Capsules 1768
Zarontin Syrup 1769
Zaroxolyn Tablets 989
Zefazone Sterile Powder 2372
▲Zestoretic (5.2%) 2274
▲Zestril Tablets (5.3%) 2277
▲Zofran Injection (16%) 1069
Zoladex (1% to 5%) 1110
▲Zovirax Capsules (0.6 to 5.9%) 824
Zovirax Sterile Powder (Less than 1%) 828
▲Zovirax (0.6% to 5.9%) 824
Zyloprim Tablets (Less than 1%) 830

Headache, migraine

Prozac Pulvules (Rare) 920
Stilphostrol Tablets and Ampuls 1609
▲Wellbutrin Tablets (25.7%) 821

Headache, periorbital

Pilopine HS Gel ◉ 227

Headache, positional

▲Xylocaine Injections (3%) 637

Headache, sinus

▲CHEMET (succimer) Capsules (5.2 to 15.7%) 1361
Prozac Pulvules (2.3%) 920

Headache, supraorbital

Isopto Carpine ◉ 219
Pilocar ◉ 275
Pilostat Sterile Ophthalmic Solution 0.5%, 1%, 2%, 3%, 4%, 5%, 6% ◉ 263

Headache, temporal

Isopto Carpine ◉ 219
Pilocar ◉ 275
Pilopine HS Gel ◉ 227
Pilostat Sterile Ophthalmic Solution 0.5%, 1%, 2%, 3%, 4%, 5%, 6% ◉ 263

Headache, throbbing

Hyperstat I.V. Injection 2095
Pitressin Synthetic, Ampoules 1758
Sandostatin Injection (Less than 1%) 2029

Headache, transient

Aralen Hydrochloride Injection 2038
Aralen Phosphate Tablets 2039
Atabrine Hydrochloride Tablets 2041
DDAVP Injection (Infrequent) 1840
DDAVP (Infrequent) 1841
Levophed Bitartrate Injection 2054
▲Minitran Transdermal Delivery System (Most common) 1312
Niacor Tablets 2376
Nicobid 1846
Nicolar Tablets 1846
Nitrodisc 2176
Nitrostat Tablets 1743
Plaquenil Sulfate Tablets 2067
▲Transderm-Nitro Transdermal Therapeutic System (Most common) 2283

Headedness, heavy

Parlodel 2020

Hearing, decrease

Anaprox and Anaprox DS Tablets (Less than 3%) 2288
Aralen Hydrochloride Injection 2038
Aralen Phosphate with Primaquine Phosphate Tablets 2040
Aralen Phosphate Tablets 2039
Ativan Injection (Infrequent) 2432
Cardioquin Tablets 1812
Clinoril Tablets (Less than 1%) 1433
Nalfon Pulvules & Tablets (1.6%) 919
Naprosyn Tablets (Less than 3%) 2297
ProSom Tablets (Rare) 554

Hearing, disturbances

Diamox 1200
Indocin Capsules (Less than 1%) 1487
Indocin I.V. (Less than 1%) 1490
Indocin (Less than 1%) 1487
Intron A (Less than 5%) 2097
▲Lupron Depot 3.75 mg (Among most frequent) 2312
Lupron Depot 7.5 mg 2311
Lupron Injection 2310
Omnipaque (A few cases) 2552

Hearing, impaired

Arthritis Strength Bufferin Analgesic Caplets 744
Bumex (0.5%) 1895
Desferal Vials 862
Diamox Sequels (Sustained Release) 1201
Disalcid 1310
Ecotrin 2189
Kefurox Vials, Faspak & ADD-Vantage 1277
Lasix Oral Solution 1093
Mustargen 1514
Naprosyn Suspension (Less than 3%) 2297
Orudis Capsules (Less than 1%) 2488
Quinaglute Dura-Tabs Tablets 663
Salflex 839
Trilisate (Less than 2%) 1822

Hearing, loss of

Altace Capsules 1086
Amikin Injectable 602
Ancobon Capsules 1886
Aralen Hydrochloride Injection (1 patient) 2038
Ascriptin A/D Caplets 1850
Regular Strength Ascriptin Tablets 1850
Azo Gantrisin Tablets 1888
Azulfidine Tablets, EN-tabs, Oral Suspension (Rare) 1157
Children's Bayer Chewable Aspirin ▣ 564
Genuine Bayer Aspirin Tablets & Caplets ▣ 564
Maximum Bayer Aspirin Tablets & Caplets ▣ 566
Bayer Plus Aspirin Tablets ▣ 567
Therapy Bayer Aspirin Caplets ▣ 568
8 Hour Bayer Timed-Release Aspirin ▣ 566
Bumex Tablets (0.5%) 1895
Butazolidin Capsules & Tablets (Less than 1%) 1027
Cama Arthritis Pain Reliever ▣ 685
▲Capastat Sulfate Vials (3%) 1250
Children's Advil Suspension (Less than 1%) 2426
Cipro I.V. (1% or less) 1592
Cipro Tablets 1589
Desferal Vials 862
Empirin with Codeine Phosphate Nos. 2, 3 & 4 764
Floxin Tablets (Less than 1%) 1652
Fungizone Intravenous 2262
Garamycin Injectable 2093
Gelfoam Sterile Sponge 2338
Lasix 1093
Matulane Capsules 1907
Mono-Gesic Tablets 846
Motrin Tablets (Less than 1%) 2351
Nebcin Vials, Hyporets & ADD-Vantage 1286
Netromycin Injection 100 mg/ml (1 of 250 patients) 2104
PediaProfen Suspension (Less than 1%) 1363
Platinol (Occasional) 737
Quinidex Extentabs 1868
Retrovir Capsules (Less than 5%) 802
Retrovir I.V. Infusion (Less than 5%) 805
Retrovir Syrup (Less than 5%) 802
Rufen Tablets (Less than 1%) 691
Salflex 839
Sandimmune (2% or less) 2024
Tegison Capsules (Less than 1%) 1881
Tonocard Tablets (0.4-1.5%) 1554
Trilisate (Rare) 1822
Vancocin HCl, Oral Solution & Pulvules (A few dozen cases) 1304
Vancocin HCl, Vials & ADD-Vantage (Few dozen cases) 1302
Zinacef (A few pediatric patients) 1066

Hearing loss, reversible

Ansaid Tablets (Less than 1%) 2319
E.E.S. 522
E-Mycin Tablets (Isolated reports) 688
Easprin 1719
EryPed (Isolated reports) 519
Ery-Tab Tablets (Isolated reports) 521
Erythrocin Stearate Filmtab (Isolated reports) 523
Erythromycin Base Filmtab (Isolated reports) 525
Erythromycin Delayed-Release Capsules, USP (Isolated reports) 526
Feldene Capsules (Less than 1%) 1777
Hyperstat I.V. Injection 2095
Ilosone (Isolated reports) 913
Ilotycin Gluceptate, IV, Vials (Rare) 915
Noroxin Tablets 1519
Omnipaque (A few cases) 2552
PCE Dispertab Tablets (Isolated reports) 549
Pediazole (Isolated reports) 1973
Primaxin I.M. 1532
Primaxin I.V. (Less than 0.2%) 1535
Salflex 839
Voltaren Tablets (Less than 1%) 1042

Heart beat, irregular

Brethaire Inhaler 1024
▲Intropin Injection (Among most frequent) 930
K-Phos M.F. Tablets 659
K-Phos Neutral Tablets 660
K-Phos Original Formula 'Sodium Free' Tablets (Less frequent) 660
K-Phos No. 2 Tablets 659
Lozol Tablets (Less than 5%) 1843
Maxair Inhaler (Less than 1%) 1311
Quadrinal Tablets 1183
Uroqid-Acid (Less frequent) 661

Heart block

Actimmune (Rare) 1046
Adenocard Injection 1007
Anafranil Capsules (Rare) 650
Asendin Tablets (Very rare) 1196
Betagan ◉ 239
Betoptic Sterile Ophthalmic Solution (Rare) 569
Betoptic S Sterile Ophthalmic Suspension (Rare) 570
Brevibloc Injection (Less than 1%) 942
Carbocaine Hydrochloride Injection 2043
Cardene Capsules (Less than 0.4%) 2290
Cartrol Tablets (Rare) 507
Cordarone Tablets (2 to 5%) 2446
Corgard Tablets (Single instance) 701
Corzide Tablets (Single instance) 702
Diprivan Injection (Less than 1%) 2267
Elavil 2269
Endep Tablets 1927
Etrafon 2087
Flexeril Tablets (Rare) 1471
Klorvess Effervescent Granules 2010
Klorvess Effervescent Tablets 2011
Klorvess 10% Liquid 2010
Limbitrol 1933
Ludiomil Tablets (Rare) 874
Marcaine Hydrochloride with Epinephrine 1:200,000 2055
Marcaine Hydrochloride Injection 2055
Marcaine Spinal 2058
Normodyne Injection 2108
Normodyne Tablets 2110
Normozide Tablets (Rare) 2112
Norpace 2177
Norpramin Tablets 1340
Omnipaque (0.5 to 0.6%) 2552
Pamelor 2019
Permax Tablets (Rare) 1291
Procan SR Tablets (2 of almost 500) 1760
Pronestyl Capsules and Tablets (2 of almost 500 patients) 1800
Pronestyl-SR Tablets (2 of almost 500 patients) 1801
Provocholine for Inhalation 1911
Rum-K Syrup 995
Sensorcaine 631
Sensorcaine-MPF Spinal 634
Surmontil Capsules 2524
Tenex Tablets 1875
▲Tenormin Tablets and I.V. Injection (4.5%) 1107
Timoptic in Ocudose 1552
Timoptic Sterile Ophthalmic Solution 1550
Tofranil Ampuls 1038
Tofranil Tablets 1039
Tofranil-PM Capsules 1041
Trandate HCT Tablets (Rare) 579
Trandate Injection (Rare) 577
Trandate Tablets (Rare) 579
Triavil Tablets 1556
Vascor (200, 300 and 400 mg) Tablets 1383
Visken Tablets (2% or fewer patients) 2036
Vivactil Tablets 1567

Heart block, second degree

Dipentum Capsules (Rare) 1160
Prostin VR Pediatric Sterile Solution (Less than 1%) 2355

Heartburn

▲Adalat Capsules (10 mg and 20 mg) (11%) 1587
▲AeroBid Inhaler System (3-9%) 995
Alferon N Injection (1% to 3%) 1809
▲Alka-Seltzer Effervescent Antacid and Pain Reliever (11.9% at doses of 1000 mg/day) 1568
▲Alka-Seltzer (Flavored) Effervescent Antacid and Pain Reliever (11.9% at doses of 1000 mg/day) 1569
▲Anaprox and Anaprox DS Tablets (3-9%) 2288
Arfonad Ampuls 1887
Azdōne Tablets (Occasional) 844
▲Genuine Bayer Aspirin Tablets & Caplets (11.9% at doses of 1000 mg/day) ▣ 564
▲Bayer Plus Aspirin Tablets (11.9% of 4500 people treated) ▣ 567
▲Therapy Bayer Aspirin Caplets (11.9% of 4500 people tested) ▣ 568
▲Bufferin Analgesic Tablets and Caplets (11.9%) 743
Butazolidin Capsules & Tablets (Greater than 1%) 1027
▲Children's Advil Suspension (3-9%) 2426
Cholybar (Less frequent) 1705
▲Clozaril Tablets (4%) 2000
Dalmane Capsules 1927

Damason-P (Occasional) 1356
DiaBeta (1.8%) 1091
Diapid Nasal Spray (Infrequent) 2003
Dipentum Capsules (1 out of 441 patients) 1160
▲Ecotrin (11.9% at 1000 mg/day) 2189
Eldepryl 2250
Empirin with Codeine Phosphate Nos. 2, 3 & 4 (Occasional) 764
Etrafon 2087
Fedahist Gyrocaps 2145
Fedahist Timecaps 2145
Fiorinal with Codeine Capsules (Infrequent) 2008
Haltran Tablets (Occasional) ⊞ 668
▲Indocin (3% to 9%) 1487
Lopressor Ampuls (1%) 1032
Lopressor HCT Tablets (1 in 100) 1034
Lopressor Tablets (1%) 1032
Lortab ASA Tablets (Occasional) 2414
▲Meclomen Capsules (3-9%) 1739
Mevacor Tablets (1.6%) 1505
▲Mexitil Capsules (39.3% to 39.6%) 680
Micronase Tablets (1.8%) 2350
Midamor Tablets (Less than or equal to 1%) 1508
Moduretic Tablets 1510
Monopril Tablets (0.2 to 1.0%) 1406
▲Motrin Tablets (3-9%) 2351
Naldecon Syrup, Tablets, Pediatric Drops and Pediatric Syrup 709
▲Naprosyn (3 to 9%) 2297
Noroxin Tablets (0.3% to 1%) 1519
Novafed A Capsules 1342
Novahistine DH 1342
Novahistine Elixir ⊞ 596
Orinase Tablets (1.4%) 2354
▲PediaProfen Suspension (3-9%) 1363
Ponstel (Less frequent) 1758
Primaxin I.M. 1532
Primaxin I.V. (Less than 0.2%) 1535
Prinzide Tablets (0.3% to 1%) 1540
Procardia Capsules 1781
▲Procardia XL Tablets (11%) 1783
Proventil Inhalation Aerosol (Less than 5%) 2117
Questran Light (Less frequent) 711
Questran Powder 710
Rifadin (Some patients) 1345
Rifamate Capsules (Some patients) 1347
Rimactane Capsules 879
Rondec 1975
Rondec-DM 1976
Rondec-TR Tablet 1975
▲Rufen Tablets (3-9%) 691
Sandostatin Injection (Less than 1%) 2029
Sansert Tablets 2031
Sinemet CR Tablets 953
▲St. Joseph Adult Chewable Aspirin (81 mg.) (11.9% of 4500 patients) ⊞ 703
Syprine Capsules 1546
Tolinase Tablets (1%) 2365
▲Trilisate (Less than 20%) 1822
▲Ventolin (Less than 5 in 100 patients) 583
Vontrol Tablets (Rare) 2243
Zestoretic (0.3 to 1%) 2274
Zorprin Tablets 698

Heart defects, congenital
Amen 833
Depo-Provera Sterile Aqueous Suspension 2336
Menrium Tablets 1934
Ogen 540
Premarin with Methyltestosterone 2515
Provera Tablets 2356

Heart failure
Actimmune (Rare) 1046
Adriamycin PFS 561
Ansaid Tablets (Less than 1%) 2319
Calan SR Caplets 2157
Calan Tablets 2155
Cartrol Tablets (Rare) 507
DynaCirc Capsules (0.5% to 1%) 2004
Intron A (Less than 1%) 2097
Isoptin Oral Tablets (1.8%) 1179
Isoptin SR Sustained Release Tablets 1181
Kerlone Tablets (Less than 2%) 2172
Nicorette 1335
Procardia XL Tablets (Rare) 1783
Sectral Capsules (Up to 2%) 2520
▲Tenormin Tablets and I.V. Injection (19%) 1107
Vascor (200, 300 and 400 mg) Tablets (1.9%) 1383
Verelan Capsules 1243
Visken Tablets (Less than 1%) 2036

Heart failure, congestive (see under Congestive heart failure)

Heart murmur
Cipro I.V. (1% or less) 1592
Sansert Tablets 2031
Yutopar (Infrequent) 647

Heart rate, changes
▲Blocadren Tablets (5%) 1429
Dopram Injectable 1860
Ergostat 1719
Nucofed Capsules 2219
Nucofed Expectorant 2219
Nucofed Pediatric Expectorant 2220
Nucofed Syrup 2219
▲Yutopar (80 to 100% with IV administration) 647

Heart rate, changes fetal
Brethine Ampuls 1026
Brethine Tablets 1026
Sectral Capsules 2520
▲Yutopar (80 to 100% with IV administration) 647

Heart rate, decrease
Betagan ⊙ 239
Cocaine Hydrochloride Topical Solution 620
Guaifed 1615
Levatol (1 in 25%) 1832
Tracrium Injection (0.6%) 817

Heart rate, increase
Actibine 900
Baron-X Tablets 650
Brethine Tablets 1026
Bricanyl Injection (Common) 1324
Bricanyl Tablets (Common) 1325
Bronkaid Mist ⊞ 757
Bronkaid Mist Suspension ⊞ 757
Cocaine Hydrochloride Topical Solution 620
DDAVP Injection 1840
Darbid Tablets 2205
Dayto Himbin Tablets and Liquid 905
▲Dobutrex Solution Vials (7.5 to approximately 10%) 1259
Papaverine Hydrochloride Vials and Ampoules 1290
Pentaspan Injection 949
Pro-Banthīne Tablets 2141
Rondec 1975
Rondec-DM 1976
Rondec-TR Tablet 1975
Thalitone Tablets 687
Tracrium Injection (2.1%) 817
Transderm-Nitro Transdermal Therapeutic System 2283
Vivarin Stimulant Tablets (Occasional) ⊞ 726
Yohimex Tablets 1190
Yutopar ((With oral administration)) 647

Heart spasms (see under Cardiospasm)

Heat intolerance
Alferon N Injection (1%) 1809

Heat stroke
Asendin Tablets 1196
Cogentin 1435
Compazine 2201
Haldol Decanoate 1375
Haldol Injection, Tablets and Concentrate 1373
Loxitane 1213
Orap Tablets 1020
Prolixin Decanoate 1795
Prolixin Elixir 1793
Prolixin Enanthate 1796
Prolixin Injection 1791
Prolixin Tablets 1793
Stelazine 2226

Heavy sensation, arms
Adenocard Injection (Less than 1%) 1007
Nubain Injection (Less than 1%) 934
Peptavlon 2563

Heavy sensation, legs
Eldepryl 2250
K-Phos M.F. Tablets 659
K-Phos Neutral Tablets 660
K-Phos Original Formula 'Sodium Free' Tablets (Less frequent) 660
K-Phos No. 2 Tablets 659
Nubain Injection (Less than 1%) 934
Peptavlon 2563
Uroqid-Acid (Less frequent) 661

Hebetude
▲Dilantin with Phenobarbital Kapseals (Among most common) 1715

Hematemesis
Aminophyllin Tablets 2153
Anaprox and Anaprox DS Tablets (Less than 1%) 2288
Ansaid Tablets (Less than 1%) 2319
Asbron G 1997
Choledyl Pediatric Elixir 1702
Choledyl Tablets 1700
Choledyl SA Tablets 1704
Clozaril Tablets (Less than 1%) 2000
Constant-T Tablets 1029
Dilor 2079
Feldene Capsules (Less than 1%) 1777
Lufyllin & Lufyllin-400 Tablets 2384
Lufyllin-GG Elixir & Tablets 2385
Matulane Capsules 1907
Methotrexate Tablets, Parenteral, LPF Parenteral 1217
Mithracin 1602
Mutamycin 733
Naprosyn (Less than 1%) 2297
Orudis Capsules (Less than 1%) 2488
Permax Tablets (Infrequent) 1291
Prozac Pulvules (Rare) 920
Quadrinal Tablets 1183
Quibron Capsules 713
Quibron-T 714
Quibron-T/SR 716
Respbid Tablets 684
Rheumatrex Methotrexate Dose Pack 1234
Slo-bid Gyrocaps 1847
T-PHYL (Uniphyl) 200 mg Tablets 1820
Theo-24 2179
Theo-Dur Sprinkle 1168
Theo-Dur Extended-Release Tablets 1166
Theolair 1317
Theolair-SR Tablets 1319
▲TheoX Extended-Release Tablets (Among most consistent) 841
Uniphyl 400 mg Tablets 1823
Vira-A for Injection 1766

Hematochezia
Anafranil Capsules (Infrequent) 650
Coumadin Injection & Tablets 944
Dipentum Capsules (Rare) 1160
Doxorubicin Hydrochloride for Injection, USP 622
Doxorubicin Hydrochloride Injection, USP 848
Nalfon Pulvules & Tablets (Less than 1%) 919
NebuPent for Inhalation Solution (1% or less) 1017
Orudis Capsules (Less than 1%) 2488
Ridaura Capsules (0.1 to 1%) 2224
Rowasa 2248
Rubex 739
Voltaren Tablets (Less than 1%) 1042

Hematocrit, decrease
Altace Capsules (0.4% to 1.5%) 1086
Ansaid Tablets (Less than 1%) 2319
Blocadren Tablets 1429
Butazolidin Capsules & Tablets 1027
Cefobid Pharmacy Bulk Package - Not for Direct Infusion (1 in 20) 1945
Children's Advil Suspension (Less than 1%) 2426
▲Cipro I.V. (Among most frequent) 1592
Dopram Injectable 1860
▲Feldene Capsules (3 to 9%) 1777
▲Kefurox Vials, Faspak & ADD-Vantage (1 in 10) 1277
▲Lariam Tablets (Most frequent) 1904
Larodopa Tablets 1905
Loniten Tablets 2346
Lopid Capsules and Tablets 1736
Lorelco Tablets 1333
Meclomen Capsules (1 of 6) 1739
Methotrexate Tablets, Parenteral, LPF Parenteral (Less common) 1217
Mezlin 1597
Mezlin Pharmacy Bulk Package 1599
Monistat I.V. 1143
Monopril Tablets 1406
Motrin Tablets (Less than 1%) 2351
Noroxin Tablets (Less frequent) 1519
Norpace (Less than 1%) 2177
PediaProfen Suspension (Less than 1%) 1363
▲Ponstel (2-5%) 1758
Primaxin I.M. 1532
Primaxin I.V. 1535
Prinivil Tablets (Frequent) 1538
Prinzide Tablets (Frequent) 1540
Proglycem 649
Rheumatrex Methotrexate Dose Pack (Less common) 1234
Rufen Tablets (Less than 1%) 691
Sinemet CR Tablets (1% or greater) 953
Timentin for Injection 2239
Tolectin (200, 400 and 600 mg) (1 to 3%) 1379
Tranxene 556
Trobicin Sterile Powder 2366
Unasyn 1965
Vaseretic Tablets (0.5% to 2.0%) 1559
Vasotec I.V. (0.5 to 1%) 1562
Vasotec Tablets (0.5% to 1%) 1564
Vira-A for Injection 1766
Xanax Tablets (Less than 1%) 2367
Zanosar Sterile Powder 2371
Zefazone Sterile Powder 2372
Zestoretic (Approximately 1.5%) 2274
Zestril Tablets (Frequent) 2277
▲Zinacef (1 in 10 patients) 1066

Hematocrit, increase
Epogen for Injection 591
Procrit for Injection 1647

Hematocrit, transient decrease
Cytosar-U Sterile Powder (Less than 7 patients) 2329

Hematocrit content, deviation
Bumex (0.6%) 1895
Doral Tablets (1.5%) 2383

Hematologic reactions
Ana-Kit Anaphylaxis Emergency Treatment Kit 1100
Aralen Phosphate with Primaquine Phosphate Tablets 2040
Dapsone USP 1130
Daraprim Tablets 761
Feldene Capsules 1777
Lopid Capsules and Tablets 1736
Marplan Tablets (Rare) 1906
Procan SR Tablets (Common) 1760
Pronestyl Capsules and Tablets 1800
Pronestyl Injection 1798
Pronestyl-SR Tablets 1801
Tegretol Suspension 656

Hematologic toxicity
Adriamycin PFS 561
Adriamycin RDF 562
Ana-Kit Anaphylaxis Emergency Treatment Kit (Rare) 1100
Butazolidin Capsules & Tablets 1027
Depen Titratable Tablets 2379
Doxorubicin Hydrochloride for Injection, USP 622
Doxorubicin Hydrochloride Injection, USP 848
Sterile FUDR 1898
Imuran Tablets 768
Rubex 739
Solganal Suspension 2122
Zanosar Sterile Powder (Rare) 2371

Hematoma
Anadrol-50 Tablets 2287
Calciparine Injection 925
Depakene Capsules & Syrup 511
Depakote Tablets 512
Eldepryl 2250
Eminase (2.8%) 2211
Gelfoam Sterile Sponge 2338
Hemopad Absorbable Collagen Hemostat 627
Heparin Lock Flush Solution 2456
Heparin Sodium Vials 1264
Heparin Sodium Injection 2457
Heparin Sodium Injection, USP, Sterile Solution 2342
INSTAT Collagen Absorbable Hemostat 1151
Lutrepulse for Injection 1655
Netromycin Injection 100 mg/ml (4 of 1000 patients) 2104
Nimotop Capsules (Less than 1%) 1607

Omnipaque (0.7%) 2552
Pipracil 1230
Versed Injection (Less than 1%) 1924

Hematoma, pelvic

Oxytocin Injection 2492
Pitocin Injection, Ampoules, Steri-Dose Syringes 1757
Syntocinon Injection 2032

Hematopoietic depression

Cosmegen Injection 1440
▲ DTIC-Dome (Among most common) 1595
Methotrexate Tablets, Parenteral, LPF Parenteral 1217
Mustargen (Occasional) 1514
Rheumatrex Methotrexate Dose Pack 1234

Hematuria

▲ Accutane Capsules (Less than 1 in 10) 1878
Anafranil Capsules (Infrequent) 650
Anaprox and Anaprox DS Tablets (Less than 1%) 2288
Ansaid Tablets (Less than 1%) 2319
Atromid-S Capsules 2435
Azo Gantrisin Tablets 1888
Azulfidine Tablets, EN-tabs, Oral Suspension (Rare) 1157
Benemid Tablets 1426
Butazolidin Capsules & Tablets (Less than 1%) 1027
Children's Advil Suspension (Less than 1%) 2426
Cholybar 1705
Cipro I.V. (1% or less) 1592
Cipro Tablets 1589
Clinoril Tablets (Less than 1%) 1433
ColBENEMID Tablets 1436
Condylox (Less than 5%) 1630
Constant-T Tablets 1029
Coumadin Injection & Tablets 944
Cuprimine Capsules 1442
Cytotec (Infrequent) 2159
Cytovene Sterile Powder (1% or less) 2292
Cytoxan for Injection 726
Danocrine Capsules 2046
Dantrium Capsules (Less frequent) 1619
Daraprim Tablets 761
Demser Capsules (A few patients) .. 1460
Depen Titratable Tablets 2379
Desyrel and Desyrel Dividose (Less than 1%) 1404
Diamox Parenteral (Occasional) 1200
Diamox Sequels (Sustained Release) 1201
Diamox Tablets (Occasional) 1200
Dipentum Capsules (Rare) 1160
Diuril Sodium Intravenous (1 case following intravenous use) 1463
Dolobid Tablets (Less than 1 in 100) 1465
Edecrin 1468
Eminase 2211
Feldene Capsules (Less than 1%) .. 1777
Floxin Tablets (More than or equal to 1.0%) 1652
Hylorel Tablets (2.3%) 975
▲ IFEX (6% to 92%) 729
Imferon 976
Indocin Capsules (Less than 1%) 1487
Indocin I.V. (Less than 1%) 1490
Indocin (Less than 1%) 1487
Intron A (Less than 1%) 2097
Lioresal Tablets (Rare) 1031
Lodine Capsules (Less than 1%) 2468
Lufyllin & Lufyllin-400 Tablets 2384
Lufyllin-GG Elixir & Tablets 2385
▲ Lupron Depot 3.75 mg (Among most frequent) 2312
Lupron Depot 7.5 mg (Less than 5%) 2311
▲ Lupron Injection (5% or more) 2310
Lysodren (Infrequent) 731
Mandelamine (Rare) 1738
Matulane Capsules 1907
Meclomen Capsules 1739
Methergine (Rare) 2016
Methotrexate Tablets, Parenteral, LPF Parenteral 1217
Milontin Kapseals 1741
Mintezol 1510
Motrin Tablets (Less than 1%) 2351
Myochrysine Injection 1516
Nalfon Pulvules & Tablets (Less than 1%) 919
Naprosyn (Less than 1%) 2297
Neosar for Injection 566
Neupogen for Injection (Less frequent) 595
Orudis Capsules (Less than 1%) 2488
PediaProfen Suspension (Less than 1%) 1363
Permax Tablets (1.1%) 1291
Ponstel 1758
Prilosec Delayed-Release Capsules (Less than 1%) 1530
Primaxin I.M. 1532
Primaxin I.V. 1535
Priscoline Hydrochloride Ampuls 877
Procardia XL Tablets (1% or less) .. 1783
Proglycem 649
ProSom Tablets (Rare) 554
Prostin VR Pediatric Sterile Solution (Less than 1%) 2355
Prozac Pulvules (Rare) 920
Questran Light 711
Questran Powder 710
Retrovir (0.8%) 802
Rheumatrex Methotrexate Dose Pack 1234
Ridaura Capsules (1 to 3%) 2224
Rifadin (Rare) 1345
Rifamate Capsules (Rare) 1347
Rimactane Capsules 879
Rocephin Injectable Vials, ADD-Vantage (Rare) 1914
Rufen Tablets (Less than 1%) 691
Sandimmune (Rare) 2024
Sinemet CR Tablets (1% or greater) 953
Solganal Suspension 2122
T-PHYL (Uniphyl) 200 mg Tablets 1820
Tazicef for Injection 2231
▲ Tegison Capsules (1-10%) 1881
▲ TheraCys BCG Live (Intravesical) (17.0% to 39.3%) 898
Tolectin (200, 400 and 600 mg) (Less than 1%) 1379
Toradol IM Injection 2302
Unasyn 1965
Uniphyl 400 mg Tablets 1823
Urobiotic-250 Capsules 1968
Uroqid-Acid (Rare) 661
Voltaren Tablets (Less than 1%) 1042
Zarontin Capsules 1768
Zarontin Syrup 1769
Zovirax Sterile Powder (Less than 1%) 828
Zyloprim Tablets (Less than 1%) 830

Hematuria, genitourinary

Eminase (2.4%) 2211

Hematuria, microscopic

Celontin 1692

Hemeralopia

Paradione Capsules 548
Tridione 557

Hemiparesis

Anafranil Capsules (Rare) 650
Klonopin Tablets 1902
Methotrexate Tablets, Parenteral, LPF Parenteral 1217
Omnipaque (Less than 0.3%) 2552
Rheumatrex Methotrexate Dose Pack 1234

Hemiplegia

Omnipaque 2552
Permax Tablets (Rare) 1291

Hemoconcentration

Diulo 2129
Mykrox ½ mg Tablets 984
Serophene (clomiphene citrate tablets, USP) 2186
Zaroxolyn Tablets 989

Hemodilution

Hespan Injection 948

Hemoglobin, decrease

Altace Capsules (0.4% to 1.5%) 1086
Ansaid Tablets (Less than 1%) 2319
Apresazide Capsules (Less frequent) 854
Apresoline Hydrochloride Parenteral (Ampuls) 856
Apresoline Hydrochloride Tablets (Less frequent) 855
Apresoline-Esidrix Tablets 857
Blocadren Tablets 1429
▲ Cefobid Intravenous/Intramuscular (1 in 20) 1943
▲ Cefobid Pharmacy Bulk Package - Not for Direct Infusion (1 in 20) 1945
▲ Children's Advil Suspension (Less than 1% to 22.8%) 2426
▲ Cipro I.V. (Among most frequent) .. 1592
Cipro Tablets (Less than 0.1%) 1589
Cytadren Tablets (1 patient) 861
▲ Dapsone USP (Almost all patients) 1130
Dopram Injectable 1860
Easprin 1719
▲ Feldene Capsules (3 to 9%) 1777
▲ Kefurox Vials, Faspak & ADD-Vantage (1 in 10) 1277
Larodopa Tablets (Occasional) 1905
Loniten Tablets 2346
Lopid Capsules and Tablets 1736
Lorelco Tablets 1333
Lotensin Tablets (Rare; 1 of 2014 patients) 872
Meclomen Capsules (1 of 6) 1739
Mezlin 1597
Mezlin Pharmacy Bulk Package 1599
Mithracin 1602
Monopril Tablets 1406
Motrin Tablets (Less than 1%) 2351
Mustargen 1514
Norpace (1 to 3%) 2177
▲ PediaProfen Suspension (Less than 1 to 22.8%) 1363
Primaxin I.M. 1532
Primaxin I.V. 1535
Prinivil Tablets (Frequent) 1538
Prinzide Tablets (Frequent) 1540
Proglycem 649
Ridaura Capsules 2224
Rifadin 1345
Rifamate Capsules 1347
Rimactane Capsules (Rare) 879
▲ Roferon-A Injection (27%) 1916
Rufen Tablets 691
Serpasil-Apresoline Tablets 884
Sinemet CR Tablets (1% or greater) 953
▲ Tegison Capsules (10-25%) 1881
Timentin for Injection 2239
Tolectin (200, 400 and 600 mg) (1 to 3%) 1379
Unasyn 1965
Vaseretic Tablets (0.5% to 2.0%) 1559
Vasotec I.V. (0.5 to 1%) 1562
Vasotec Tablets (0.5% to 1%) 1564
Vira-A for Injection 1766
Voltaren Tablets (Less than 1%) 1042
Zefazone Sterile Powder 2372
Zestoretic (Approximately 0.5%) 2274
Zestril Tablets (Frequent) 2277
▲ Zinacef (1 in 10 patients) 1066

Hemoglobin content, deviation

Bumex (0.8%) 1895
Doral Tablets (1.4%) 2383
▲ Intron A (1% to 15%) 2097
Xanax Tablets (Less than 1%) 2367
Zovirax Sterile Powder 828

Hemoglobinemia

Zovirax Sterile Powder (Less than 1%) 828

Hemoglobinuria

Quinamm Tablets 1344
Rifadin (Rare) 1345
Rifamate Capsules 1347
Rimactane Capsules (Rare) 879
▲ Tegison Capsules (1-10%) 1881

Hemolysis

Atgam Sterile Solution (Less than 5%) 2320
▲ Dapsone USP (Most common) 1130
Furoxone 1855
Kefurox Vials, Faspak & ADD-Vantage 1277
Orudis Capsules (Less than 1%) 2488
Plaquenil Sulfate Tablets 2067
Platinol 737
Quinamm Tablets 1344
Rifadin (Rare) 1345
Rifamate Capsules (Rare) 1347
Rimactane Capsules 879
Synkayvite Injection 1919
Synkayvite Tablets 1920
Vaseretic Tablets (A few cases) 1559
Vasotec I.V. 1562
Vasotec Tablets (A few cases) 1564

Hemolysis, neonatal

AquaMEPHYTON Injection 1422
Dapsone USP 1130
Konakion Injection 1903
Mephyton Tablets 1503

Hemolytic anemia

Achromycin V Capsules 1193
Actifed with Codeine Cough Syrup .. 752
Aldoclor Tablets 1413
Aldomet Ester HCl Injection 1417
Aldomet Oral 1415
Aldoril Tablets 1418
Alkeran Tablets 754
Anaprox and Anaprox DS Tablets (Rare) 2288
Ansaid Tablets (Rare) 2319
Aralen Phosphate with Primaquine Phosphate Tablets 2040
Atgam Sterile Solution (Less than 5%) 2320
Azdōne Tablets 844
Azo Gantanol Tablets 1887
Azo Gantrisin Tablets 1888
▲ Azulfidine Tablets, EN-tabs, Oral Suspension (3 to 4%) 1157
Bactrim DS Tablets 1891
Bactrim I.V. Infusion 1889
Bactrim 1891
Benadryl Capsules 1691
Benadryl Injection 1692
Benemid Tablets 1426
Bicillin C-R Injection 2438
Bicillin C-R 900/300 Injection 2440
Bicillin L-A Injection (Infrequent) 2442
Butazolidin Capsules & Tablets (Less than 1%) 1027
Capoten 2255
Capozide 2258
Cardioquin Tablets 1812
Cardizem Tablets-30 mg, 60 mg, 90 mg and 120 mg 1329
Cardizem SR Capsules-60 mg, 90 mg and 120 mg (Less than 1%) 1327
Ceclor Pulvules & Suspension (Rare) 1251
Cefotan 2265
Ceftin Tablets 575
Ceptaz for Injection 1057
Children's Advil Suspension (Less than 1%) 2426
Cipro I.V. (Rare) 1592
Cipro Tablets 1589
Claforan Sterile Injection (Rare) 1089
Clinoril Tablets (Less than 1 in 100) 1433
ColBENEMID Tablets 1436
Compazine 2201
Corzide Tablets 702
Cuprimine Capsules 1442
Damason-P 1356
Declomycin Capsules, Tablets 1199
Deconamine 663
Depen Titratable Tablets 2379
Desyrel and Desyrel Dividose 1404
DiaBeta 1091
Diabinese Tablets 1775
Diamox 1200
Dimetane-DC Cough Syrup 1857
Dimetane-DX Cough Syrup 1858
Diucardin Tablets 2450
Diupres Tablets 1461
Diuril Oral Suspension 1464
Diuril Sodium Intravenous 1463
Diuril Tablets 1464
Dolobid Tablets (Less than 1 in 100) 1465
Doryx Capsules 1717
Dyazide Capsules 2208
Empirin with Codeine Phosphate Nos. 2, 3 & 4 764
Enduron Tablets 517
Etrafon 2087
Eulexin Capsules 2089
Fansidar Tablets 1896
Feldene Capsules (Less than 1%) .. 1777
Fiorinal with Codeine Capsules 2008
Fortaz 1060
Gantanol 1899
Gantrisin Ophthalmic Ointment/Solution 1900
Gantrisin 1901
Glucotrol 1952
HydroDIURIL Tablets 1484
Hydropres Tablets 1485
INH Tablets 868
Indocin Capsules (Less than 1%) 1487
Indocin I.V. (Less than 1%) 1490
Indocin (Less than 1%) 1487
Larodopa Tablets (Rare) 1905
Lasix 1093
Lortab ASA Tablets 2414
Macrodantin Capsules 1624
Matulane Capsules 1907
Maxzide 1215
Meclomen Capsules (Less than 1%) 1739

Mefoxin 1498
Mefoxin Premixed Intravenous Solution 1500
Mesantoin Tablets (Uncommon) 2013
Mevacor Tablets (Rare) 1505
Micronase Tablets 2350
Minocin Intravenous 1221
Minocin Oral Suspension 1224
Minocin Pellet-Filled Capsules 1222
Moduretic Tablets 1510
Monodox Capsules 1630
Monopril Tablets (0.2 to 1.0%) 1406
Motrin Tablets (Less than 1%) 2351
Mustargen (Rare) 1514
Mutamycin 733
Nalfon Pulvules & Tablets (Less than 1%) 919
Naturetin Tablets 1789
Navane Capsules and Concentrate 1954
Navane Intramuscular 1956
NegGram (Rare) 2062
Neptazane Tablets ◉ 311
Nizoral Tablets (Less than 1%) 1145
Normozide Tablets 2112
Optimine Tablets 2115
Orap Tablets 1020
Ornade Spansule Capsules 2221
PBZ Tablets & Elixir 1037
PBZ-SR Tablets 1037
PediaProfen Suspension (Less than 1%) 1363
Pediazole 1973
Periactin 1525
Pfizerpen for Injection (Rare) 1957
Platinol 737
Platinol-AQ Injection 738
Polaramine 2116
Ponstel 1758
Prilosec Delayed-Release Capsules 1530
Prinzide Tablets 1540
Procan SR Tablets (Rare) 1760
Procardia XL Tablets 1783
Pronestyl Capsules and Tablets (Rare) 1800
Pronestyl Injection (Rare) 1798
Pronestyl-SR Tablets (Rare) 1801
Pyridium 1763
Pyridium Plus 1764
Quinaglute Dura-Tabs Tablets 663
Quinidex Extentabs 1868
Rauzide Tablets 1804
Rifadin 1345
Rifamate Capsules 1347
Rimactane Capsules (Rare) 879
Rufen Tablets (Less than 1%) 691
Ru-Tuss II Capsules 693
SSD RP Cream 690
Septra 813
Septra I.V. Infusion 808
Septra I.V. Infusion ADD-Vantage Vials 810
Septra 813
Silvadene Cream 1% 1352
Sinemet Tablets (Rare) 952
Sinemet CR Tablets 953
Skelaxin 840
Stelazine 2226
Suprax 1235
Synkayvite Injection 1919
Synkayvite Tablets 1920
Talacen (Rare) 2070
Taractan (Very rare) 1920
Tavist Syrup 2033
Tavist Tablets 2035
Tavist-D Tablets 2035
Terramycin Capsules 1786
Terramycin Intramuscular Solution 1964
Thiosulfil Forte Tablets 2526
Thorazine 2234
Timolide Tablets 1547
Tolectin (200, 400 and 600 mg) (Less than 1%) 1379
Tolinase Tablets 2365
Tonocard Tablets (Less than 1%) 1554
Trandate HCT Tablets 579
Triaminic Expectorant DH 1995
Triaminic Oral Infant Drops 1996
Trilafon 2123
Trinalin Repetabs Tablets 1170
Vaseretic Tablets 1559
Vibramycin Hyclate Capsules 1787
Vibramycin Hyclate Intravenous 1968
Vibramycin 1787
Voltaren Tablets (Less than 1%) 1042
Zefazone Sterile Powder 2372
Zestoretic 2274
Zinacef 1066
Zyloprim Tablets (Less than 1%) 830

Hemolytic icterus (see under Jaundice)

Hemolytic sideroblastic anemia
Rifamate Capsules 1347

Hemolytic-uremic syndrome
Brevicon 2304
Demulen 2161
Enovid 2161
Jenest-28 Tablets 1636
Levlen/Tri-Levlen 665
Lo/Ovral Tablets 2471
Lo/Ovral-28 Tablets 2476
Loestrin 1728
Micronor Tablets 1667
Modicon 1667
Mutamycin 733
Nordette-21 Tablets 2481
Nordette-28 Tablets 2483
Norethin 2133
Norinyl 2304
Norlestrin 1746
Nor-Q D Tablets 2304
Ortho Diaphragm Kit 1664
Ortho-Cyclen Tablets 1658
Ortho-Novum 1667
Ovral Tablets 2490
Ovral-28 Tablets 2491
Ovrette Tablets 2492
Paraplatin for Injection (Rare) 735
Levlen/Tri-Levlen 665
Tri-Norinyl 2304

Hemopericardium
Cytoxan for Injection 726

Hemoperitoneum
Metrodin (urofollitropin for injection) 2182
Pergonal (menotropins for injection, USP) 2184
Serophene (clomiphene citrate tablets, USP) 2186

Hemoptysis
Anafranil Capsules (Rare) 650
Cipro I.V. (1% or less) 1592
Cipro Tablets (Less than 1%) 1589
Duragesic Transdermal System (1% or greater) 1133
Eminase (2.2%) 2211
Intal Capsules (Less than 1 in 100,000 patients) 978
Intal Inhaler (Rare) 979
Intal Nebulizer Solution (Rare) 980
▲Lupron Depot 3.75 mg (Among most frequent) 2312
Lupron Depot 7.5 mg (Less than 5%) 2311
Lupron Injection 2310
Matulane Capsules 1907
NebuPent for Inhalation Solution (1% or less) 1017
Orudis Capsules (Less than 1%) 2488
Permax Tablets (Infrequent) 1291
Prozac Pulvules (Rare) 920

Hemorrhage (see under Bleeding)

Hemorrhage, adrenal
Calciparine Injection 925
Heparin Lock Flush Solution 2456
Heparin Sodium Injection 2457
Heparin Sodium Injection, USP, Sterile Solution 2342

Hemorrhage, cerebral (see under Cerebral hemorrhage)

Hemorrhage, eyes
Eminase (Less than 1%) 2211
Ocufen ◉ 237
Permax Tablets (Infrequent) 1291
Proglycem 649
Prozac Pulvules (Rare) 920

Hemorrhage, gastrointestinal (see under Bleeding, gastrointestinal)

Hemorrhage, intra-alveolar
Depen Titratable Tablets 2379

Hemorrhage, intramuscular
Abbokinase 503
Abbokinase Open-Cath 505

Hemorrhage, intraventricular
▲Exosurf Neonatal for Intratracheal Suspension (Up to 57%) 765

Hemorrhage, muscle
Prozac Pulvules (Rare) 920

Hemorrhage, neonatal
Lortab ASA Tablets 2414
Mebaral Tablets 2061
Mysoline 2480
Quadrinal Tablets 1183
Rifadin 1345

Hemorrhage, ovarian
Calciparine Injection 925
Dicumarol Tablets 516
Heparin Lock Flush Solution 2456
Heparin Sodium Vials 1264
Heparin Sodium Injection 2457
Heparin Sodium Injection, USP, Sterile Solution 2342
Panwarfin Tablets 547

Hemorrhage, postpartum
Oxytocin Injection 2492
Pitocin Injection, Ampoules, Steri-Dose Syringes 1757
Rifadin 1345
Syntocinon Injection 2032

Hemorrhage, pulmonary
▲Exosurf Neonatal for Intratracheal Suspension (Up to 10%) 765
▲Survanta Beractant Intratracheal Suspension (7.2%) 1978

Hemorrhage, purpuric
Tegretol Chewable Tablets 654
Tegretol Suspension 656
Tegretol Tablets 654

Hemorrhage, renal pelvic
Cytoxan for Injection 726

Hemorrhage, retinal
Ansaid Tablets (Rare) 2319
Butazolidin Capsules & Tablets (Less than 1%) 1027
Matulane Capsules 1907
Orudis Capsules (Less than 1%) 2488
Oxytocin Injection 2492
Paradione Capsules 548
Tridione 557

Hemorrhage, retroperitoneal
Abbokinase 503
Abbokinase Open-Cath 505
Activase (Less than 1%) 1047
Calciparine Injection 925
Eminase 2211
Heparin Lock Flush Solution 2456
Heparin Sodium Injection 2457
Heparin Sodium Injection, USP, Sterile Solution 2342

Hemorrhage, subarachnoid
Ansaid Tablets (Less than 1%) 2319
Brevicon 2304
Demulen 2161
Enovid 2161
Mydfrin 2.5% ◉ 224
Norinyl 2304
Tri-Norinyl 28-Day Tablets 2304

Hemorrhage, subcutaneous
Mustargen 1514

Hemorrhagic colitis
Cytoxan for Injection (Isolated reports) 726
Neosar for Injection (Isolated reports) 566
Primaxin I.M. 1532
Primaxin I.V. (Less than 0.2%) 1535

Hemorrhagic complications
Calciparine Injection 925
Coumadin Injection & Tablets 944
Heparin Sodium Vials 1264

Hemorrhagic diathesis
Butazolidin Capsules & Tablets 1027
▲Mithracin (5.4 to 11.9%) 1602
Solganal Suspension (Rare) 2122

Hemorrhagic eruptions (see under Eruptions, hemorrhagic)

Hemorrhagic syndrome (see under Bleeding syndrome)

Hemorrhagic tendency
Mithracin 1602
Mustargen 1514

Hemorrhoids
Anafranil Capsules (Infrequent) 650
▲CHEMET (succimer) Capsules (12 to 20.9%) 1361
Rowasa (1.35%) 2248
Trexan Tablets (Less than 1%) 937

Hemorrhoids, aggravation
Colestid Granules 2328
Questran Light 711

Hemostasis, interference
Depakote Sprinkle Capsules 512
Zorprin Tablets 698

Hemothorax
Permax Tablets (Rare) 1291

Henoch-Schonlein purpura
Bactrim DS Tablets 1891
Bactrim I.V. Infusion 1889
Bactrim 1891
Children's Advil Suspension (Less than 1%) 2426
Septra 813

Henoch-Schonlein vasculitis
PediaProfen Suspension (Less than 1%) 1363
Rufen Tablets (Less than 1%) 691

Hepatic adenoma
Brevicon 2304
Danocrine Capsules 2046
Estinyl Tablets 2085
Estrace 1385
Estrace Vaginal Cream 1388
Estradurin 2452
Estratest (Rare) 2245
Jenest-28 Tablets 1636
Lo/Ovral Tablets 2471
Lo/Ovral-28 Tablets 2476
Loestrin 1728
Mediatric Capsules 2476
Nordette-21 Tablets 2481
Nordette-28 Tablets 2483
Norinyl 2304
Norlestrin 1746
Nor-Q D Tablets 2304
Ortho-Cyclen Tablets 1658
Ovral Tablets 2490
Ovral-28 Tablets 2491
Ovrette Tablets 2492
PMB 200 and PMB 400 2504
Premarin Intravenous 2508
Premarin with Methyltestosterone 2515
Premarin Vaginal Cream 2512
Stilphostrol Tablets and Ampuls 1609
TACE 12 and 25 mg 1353
Tri-Norinyl 2304
Triphasil-21 Tablets 2527
Triphasil-28 Tablets 2532

Hepatic coma
Anadrol-50 Tablets 2287
Prinzide Tablets 1540
Rauzide Tablets 1804
Vaseretic Tablets 1559
Zestoretic 2274

Hepatic dysfunction
Anadrol-50 Tablets 2287
Anafranil Capsules (Infrequent) 650
Ancobon Capsules 1886
Augmentin Tablets, Powder for Oral Suspension, and Chewable Tablets (Rare) 2198
Azo Gantrisin Tablets 1888
Butazolidin Capsules & Tablets 1027
Butisol Sodium Elixir & Tablets (Less than 1 in 100) 2377
Cardioquin Tablets 1812
Ceftin Tablets 575
Ceptaz for Injection 1057
Children's Advil Suspension (Less than 1%) 2426
▲Cipro I.V. (Among most frequent) 1592
Cuprimine Capsules 1442
Cylert Tablets 510

▲ Cytosar-U Sterile Powder (Among most frequent) 2329
Cytotec (Infrequent) 2159
Cytovene Sterile Powder (2%) 2292
Danocrine Capsules 2046
Dantrium Capsules 1619
Daranide Tablets 1445
Darvon-N/Darvocet-N 1254
Darvon 1256
Darvon-N Suspension & Tablets 1254
Depakote Sprinkle Capsules 512
Depen Titratable Tablets (Isolated cases) 2379
Diamox Parenteral (Occasional) 1200
Diamox Sequels (Sustained Release) 1201
Diamox Tablets (Occasional) 1200
Dilantin Infatabs 1710
Dilantin Kapseals 1708
Dilantin-30 Pediatric/Dilantin-125 Suspension 1713
Dilantin with Phenobarbital Kapseals 1715
Disalcid 1310
Dolobid Tablets (Less than 1 in 100) 1465
Dyazide Capsules 2208
E.E.S. 522
ERYC 1720
EryPed 519
Ery-Tab Tablets 521
Erythrocin Stearate Filmtab 523
Erythromycin Base Filmtab 525
Erythromycin Delayed-Release Capsules, USP 526
Feldene Capsules (Less than 1%) 1777
Fluothane 2453
Fortaz 1060
Halcion Tablets (Rare) 2340
▲ IFEX (3%) 729
Intron A (2 patients) 2097
Keftab Tablets 917
Librax Capsules (Occasional) 1929
Libritabs Tablets (Occasional) 1930
Librium Capsules (Occasional) 1931
Librium Injectable (Occasional) 1932
Limbitrol (Rare) 1933
▲ Lupron Depot 3.75 mg (Among most frequent) 2312
Lupron Depot 7.5 mg 2311
Lupron Injection 2310
Matulane Capsules 1907
Meclomen Capsules (Less than 1%) 1739
Menrium Tablets (Occasional) 1934
Moban Tablets & Concentrate (Rare) 932
Naprosyn Tablets (Less than 1%) 2297
NebuPent for Inhalation Solution (1% or less) 1017
Nizoral Tablets (Rare) 1145
Normodyne Injection 2108
Normodyne Tablets 2110
Normozide Tablets 2112
▲ Novantrone for Injection Concentrate (10 to 14%) 1226
Orudis Capsules (Less than 1%) 2488
PCE Dispertab Tablets 549
PediaProfen Suspension (Less than 1%) 1363
Persantine Tablets (Rare) 683
Salflex 839
Serax Capsules 2522
Serax Tablets 2522
Suprax 1235
Tagamet (Rare) 2228
Tambocor Tablets (Rare) 1315
Tapazole Tablets 1298
Tegretol Chewable Tablets 654
Tegretol Suspension 656
Tegretol Tablets 654
Tenex Tablets 1875
TheraCys BCG Live (Intravesical) (Up to 2.7%) 898
Tolectin (200, 400 and 600 mg) (Less than 1%) 1379
Toradol IM Injection 2302
Trandate HCT Tablets 579
Trandate Injection 577
Wygesic Tablets 2540
Zanosar Sterile Powder 2371
Zefazone Sterile Powder 2372
Zinacef 1066
Zorprin Tablets 698

Hepatic enzymes, elevation (see also under SGOT elevation; SGPT elevation; Serum transaminase, elevation)

Accutane Capsules (1 in 5 to 5 in 10) 1878
Altace Capsules (Rare) 1086
Biltricide 1589
Brethine Ampuls 1026
Brethine Tablets 1026
Butazolidin Capsules & Tablets 1027
Calan SR Caplets 2157
Calan Tablets 2155
Cefobid Pharmacy Bulk Package - Not for Direct Infusion (1 patient in 1285) 1945
Cefotan (1.2%) 2265
Corgard Tablets 701
Corzide Tablets 702
Danocrine Capsules 2046
Dyrenium Capsules (Rare) 2210
Hydrea Capsules 728
▲ IFEX (3%) 729
Inocor Lactate Injection 2048
Isoptin Oral Tablets 1179
Isoptin SR Sustained Release Tablets 1181
Lodine Capsules (Less than 1%) 2468
Lotensin Tablets (Scattered incidents) 872
Ludiomil Tablets 874
Maxzide 1215
Methotrexate Tablets, Parenteral, LPF Parenteral 1217
Minocin Intravenous 1221
Minocin Oral Suspension 1224
Minocin Pellet-Filled Capsules 1222
Normodyne Injection 2108
Norpace (Less than 1%) 2177
Norpramin Tablets 1340
Pipracil (Less frequent) 1230
Prinzide Tablets (Rare) 1540
Rheumatrex Methotrexate Dose Pack 1234
Ridaura Capsules (Less than 1%) 2224
Roferon-A Injection (Frequent) 1916
Rowasa 2248
Sandostatin Injection (Less than 1%) 2029
Sinemet Tablets 952
Symmetrel Capsules & Syrup (Occasional) 936
Tenoretic Tablets 1105
Tenormin Tablets and I.V. Injection 1107
Thioguanine Tablets, Tabloid Brand (Occasional) 815
▲ Toradol IM Injection (Up to 15%) 2302
Trandate HCT Tablets 579
Trandate Injection 577
Trandate Tablets 579
Vascor (200, 300 and 400 mg) Tablets (Approximately 1%) 1383
Vaseretic Tablets (Rare) 1559
Verelan Capsules 1243
Voltaren Tablets (Rare) 1042
Xanax Tablets 2367
▲ Zanosar Sterile Powder (A number of patients) 2371
Zestoretic (Rare) 2274
Zestril Tablets (Rare) 2277

Hepatic failure

Depakene Capsules & Syrup 511
Depakote 512
Elavil 2269
Monopril Tablets (0.2 to 1.0%) 1406
Prilosec Delayed-Release Capsules (Rare) 1530
Zofran Injection (One report) 1069

Hepatic function tests, impaired (see under Liver function, impaired)

Hepatic veno-occlusive disease, life threatening

Imuran (Rare) 768
Myleran Tablets 790
Thioguanine Tablets, Tabloid Brand 815

Hepatitis

Accutane Capsules (Several cases) 1878
Aldoclor Tablets 1413
Aldomet Ester HCl Injection 1417
Aldomet Oral 1415
Aldoril Tablets 1418
Anafranil Capsules (Infrequent) 650
Ansaid Tablets (Less than 1%) 2319
Apresazide Capsules (Rare) 854
Apresoline Hydrochloride Parenteral (Ampuls) (Rare) 856
Apresoline Hydrochloride Tablets (Rare) 855
Apresoline-Esidrix Tablets (Rare) 857
Asendin Tablets (Less than 1%) 1196
Atabrine Hydrochloride Tablets 2041
Augmentin Tablets, Powder for Oral Suspension, and Chewable Tablets (Rare) 2198
Axid Pulvules (Rare) 1246
Azactam for Injection (Less than 1%) 2252
Azo Gantanol Tablets 1887
Azo Gantrisin Tablets 1888
Azulfidine Tablets, EN-tabs, Oral Suspension (Rare) 1157
Bactrim DS Tablets 1891
Bactrim I.V. Infusion 1889
Bactrim 1891
Butazolidin Capsules & Tablets (Less than 1%) 1027
Capoten 2255
Capozide 2258
Cartrol Tablets (Rare) 507
Catapres Tablets (Rare) 676
Catapres-TTS (Rare) 677
Ceclor Pulvules & Suspension (Rare) 1251
Children's Advil Suspension (Less than 1%) 2426
Clinoril Tablets (Less than 1%) 1433
Combipres Tablets (Rare) 678
Corzide Tablets (Occasional) 702
Cosmegen Injection 1440
Cylert Tablets 510
Demulen 2161
DiaBeta (Rare) 1091
Dilantin Parenteral 1712
Dipentum Capsules (Rare) 1160
Disalcid 1310
Diulo 2129
Dolobid Tablets (Less than 1 in 100) 1465
Elavil (Rare) 2269
Endep Tablets (Rare) 1927
Enovid 2161
Etrafon (Rare) 2087
Eulexin Capsules (Less than 1%) 2089
Fansidar Tablets 1896
Feldene Capsules (Less than 1%) 1777
Fiorinal with Codeine Capsules 2008
Flexeril Tablets (Rare) 1471
Fungizone Intravenous 2262
Gantanol 1899
Gantrisin Ophthalmic Ointment/Solution 1900
Gantrisin 1901
Halotestin Tablets 2341
INH Tablets (Occasional) 868
Keflex Pulvules, Oral Suspension & Pediatric Drops (Rare) 916
Keftab Tablets (Rare) 917
Kefzol Vials, Faspak & ADD-Vantage (Rare) 1279
Konÿne 80 Factor IX Complex 1571
Lamprene Capsules (Less than 1%) 1030
Lodine Capsules (Less than 1%) 2468
Loxitane (Rare) 1213
Macrodantin Capsules (Rare) 1624
Mandol Vials, Faspak & ADD-Vantage (Rare) 1281
Meclomen Capsules (Rare) 1739
Mesantoin Tablets 2013
Mevacor Tablets 1505
Mexitil Capsules (Rare) 680
Micronase Tablets (Rare) 2350
Minocin Intravenous (Rare) 1221
Minocin Oral Suspension (Rare) 1224
Minocin Pellet-Filled Capsules (Rare) 1222
Monopril Tablets (0.2 to 1.0%) 1406
Motrin Tablets (Less than 1%) 2351
Myochrysine Injection 1516
Naturetin Tablets (Occasional) 1789
NebuPent for Inhalation Solution (1% or less) 1017
Nimotop Capsules (Less than 1%) 1607
Norethin 2133
Normodyne Injection 2108
Normodyne Tablets 2110
Normozide Tablets 2112
Noroxin Tablets 1519
Norpramin Tablets 1340
Papaverine Hydrochloride Vials and Ampoules (Infrequent) 1290
Paradione Capsules (Rare) 548
Paraflex Caplets 1378
Parafon Forte DSC Caplets 1379
Parnate Tablets (Rare) 2222
PediaProfen Suspension (Less than 1%) 1363
Pediazole 1973
Permax Tablets (Infrequent) 1291
Phenurone Tablets (2%) 552
Prilosec Delayed-Release Capsules (Less than 1%) 1530
Primaxin I.M. 1532
Primaxin I.V. (Rare) 1535
Prinivil Tablets 1538
Prinzide Tablets 1540
Priscoline Hydrochloride Ampuls 877
Prozac Pulvules (Rare) 920
Quinamm Tablets 1344
Rauzide Tablets 1804
Rifadin (Rare) 1345
Rifamate Capsules (Rare) 1347
Rimactane Capsules (Rare) 879
Roferon-A Injection (Less than 1%) 1916
Rufen Tablets (Less than 1%) 691
Rythmol Tablets (0.3%) 1184
SSD RP Cream 690
Salflex 839
Sandostatin Injection (Less than 1%) 2029
Seldane Tablets (Isolated reports) 1349
Seldane-D Extended-Release Tablets 1350
Septra 813
Septra I.V. Infusion 808
Septra I.V. Infusion ADD-Vantage Vials 810
Septra 813
Ser-Ap-Es Tablets 881
Serpasil-Apresoline Tablets 884
Silvadene Cream 1% 1352
Solganal Suspension 2122
Stelazine 2226
Tapazole Tablets 1298
▲ Tegison Capsules (1-10%) 1881
Tegretol Chewable Tablets 654
Tegretol Suspension 656
Tegretol Tablets 654
Thiosulfil Forte Tablets 2526
Timentin for Injection (Rare) 2239
Tolectin (200, 400 and 600 mg) (Less than 1%) 1379
Tonocard Tablets (Less than 1%) 1554
Trandate HCT Tablets (Less common) 579
Trandate Injection (Less common) 577
Trandate Tablets (Less common) 579
Trecator-SC Tablets 2527
Trental (Rare) 1099
Triavil Tablets (Rare) 1556
Tridione (Rare) 557
Trilisate (Rare) 1822
Urobiotic-250 Capsules 1968
Vaseretic Tablets 1559
Vasotec I.V. 1562
Vasotec Tablets (0.5% to 1%) 1564
Voltaren Tablets (Less than 1%) 1042
Wellbutrin Tablets 821
Yutopar (Less than 1% (with IV administration)) 647
Zantac Injection and Zantac Injection Premixed 1063
Zantac (Occasional) 1065
Zaroxolyn Tablets 989

Hepatitis, allergic

Adalat Capsules (10 mg and 20 mg) (Less than 0.5%) 1587
Procardia Capsules (Less than 0.5%) 1781
Procardia XL Tablets (Rare instances) 1783

Hepatitis, cholestatic

Antabuse Tablets 2429
Ceptaz for Injection 1057
Cordarone Tablets (Rare) 2446
Dipentum Capsules (One case) 1160
Estratest 2245
Mediatric Capsules 2476
Metandren Linguets and Tablets 875
Nalfon Pulvules & Tablets (Less than 1%) 919
Pipracil (Less frequent) 1230
Premarin with Methyltestosterone 2515
Seldane Tablets (Isolated reports) 1349
Seldane-D Extended-Release Tablets 1350
Tao Capsules 1963

Hepatitis, fulminant

Antabuse Tablets 2429
Tapazole Tablets (Rare) 1298

Hepatitis, granulomatous

Dipentum Capsules (Rare) 1160
Quinaglute Dura-Tabs Tablets 663
Quinidex Extentabs 1868
Zyloprim Tablets (Less than 1%) 830

Hepatitis, overt

Dantrium Capsules 1619

Hepatitis, reactive
Dipentum Capsules (Rare) 1160

Hepatitis, symptomatic
Dantrium Capsules 1619

Hepatitis, toxic
Cuprimine Capsules (Rare) 1442
Dapsone USP 1130
Depen Titratable Tablets (Rare) 2379
Dilantin Infatabs 1710
Dilantin Kapseals 1708
Dilantin-30 Pediatric/Dilantin-125 Suspension 1713
Dilantin with Phenobarbital Kapseals 1715
Indocin Capsules (Less than 1%) 1487
Indocin I.V. (Less than 1%) 1490
Indocin (Less than 1%) 1487
Rifamate Capsules 1347
Solganal Suspension 2122

Hepatitis, viral
Atgam Sterile Solution (Less than 5%) 2320
Koāte-HP Antihemophilic Factor (Human) 1581
Konyne-HT Factor IX Complex 1583
Prolastin Alpha$_1$-Proteinase Inhibitor (Human) 1585

Hepatobiliary dysfunction
Azactam for Injection (Less than 1%) 2252

Hepatomas
Anadrol-50 Tablets 2287
Brevicon 2304
Demulen (Very rare) 2161
Enovid (Very rare) 2161
Loestrin 1728
Lopid Capsules and Tablets 1736
Micronor Tablets (Rare) 1667
Modicon (Rare) 1667
Norinyl 2304
Ortho-Novum (Rare) 1667
PMB 200 and PMB 400 2504
Premarin Intravenous 2508
Premarin with Methyltestosterone 2515
Premarin Vaginal Cream 2512
Tri-Norinyl 2304

Hepatomas, benign
Jenest-28 Tablets 1636
Levlen/Tri-Levlen 665
Lo/Ovral Tablets 2471
Lo/Ovral-28 Tablets 2476
Loestrin 1728
Micronor Tablets 1667
Modicon 1667
Nordette-21 Tablets 2481
Nordette-28 Tablets 2483
Norlestrin 1746
Ortho-Novum 1667
Ovral Tablets 2490
Ovral-28 Tablets 2491
Ovrette Tablets 2492
Levlen/Tri-Levlen 665
Triphasil-21 Tablets 2527
Triphasil-28 Tablets 2532

Hepatomas, malignant
Demulen 2161
Enovid 2161
Norethin 2133

Hepatomegaly
Atromid-S Capsules 2435
Blocadren Tablets 1429
Cosmegen Injection 1440
Garamycin Injectable 2093
Klonopin Tablets 1902
NebuPent for Inhalation Solution (1% or less) 1017
Permax Tablets (Infrequent) 1291
Procan SR Tablets 1760
Pronestyl Capsules and Tablets 1800
Pronestyl-SR Tablets 1801
Prozac Pulvules (Rare) 920
Thioguanine Tablets, Tabloid Brand 815
Timolide Tablets 1547
Timoptic in Ocudose 1552
Timoptic Sterile Ophthalmic Solution 1550
Zyloprim Tablets (Less than 1%) 830

Hepatosplenomegaly
Atgam Sterile Solution (At least 1 patient and less than 5% of total patients) 2320
Paradione Capsules 548
Tridione Capsules 557

Hepatotoxicity
▲Accutane Capsules (1 in 5 to 1 in 10) 1878
Anadrol-50 Tablets 2287
Android 1111
Azdone Tablets 844
BiCNU 723
CeeNU 725
Cosmegen Injection 1440
Cytadren Tablets (Less than 1 in 1000) 861
Damason-P 1356
Dantrium Capsules 1619
Depakene Capsules & Syrup 511
Depakote 512
Easprin 1719
Empirin with Codeine Phosphate Nos. 2, 3 & 4 764
Estratest 2245
Ethrane (Rare) 599
Fulvicin P/G Tablets 2090
Fulvicin P/G 165 & 330 Tablets 2091
Fulvicin-U/F Tablets 2092
Furoxone 1855
Imuran (Less than 1%) 768
Inocor Lactate Injection (0.2%) 2048
Leukeran Tablets 788
Lortab ASA Tablets 2414
Loxitane 1213
Methotrexate Tablets, Parenteral, LPF Parenteral 1217
Minocin Oral Suspension 1224
Nizoral Tablets 1145
▲Purinethol Tablets (Frequent) 800
Quinaglute Dura-Tabs Tablets 663
Quinidex Extentabs 1868
Reglan (Rare) 1869
Rheumatrex Methotrexate Dose Pack 1234
Roferon-A Injection (Rare) 1916
▲Sandimmune (Less than 1 to 7%) 2024
Tagamet (Rare) 2228
Terramycin Capsules 1786
Tigan 2239
Torecan 1993
Trexan Tablets 937
VePesid Capsules and Injection (0 to 3%) 741
▲Zanosar Sterile Powder (A number of patients) 2371
Zyloprim Tablets 830

Hernia, unspecified
Permax Tablets (Infrequent) 1291

Heroin withdrawal syndrome
Methadone Hydrochloride Diskets 1284

Herpes labialis
Alferon N Injection (1%) 1809

Herpes, precipitation
Demulen 2161
⅛% Econopred & 1% Econopred Plus ◉ 217
Enovid 2161
Matulane Capsules 1907
Norethin 2133
Oxsoralen-Ultra Capsule 1117
▲Roferon-A Injection (8%) 1916

Herpes gestationis
Demulen 2161
Enovid 2161

Herpes simplex
Ansaid Tablets (Less than 1%) 2319
Atgam Sterile Solution 2320
Permax Tablets (Infrequent) 1291
Proglycem 649
Prozac Pulvules (Infrequent) 920
Tegison Capsules (Less than 1%) 1881

Herpes simplex, disseminated
Accutane Capsules (Less than 1%) 1878

Herpes zoster
Ansaid Tablets (Less than 1%) 2319
Engerix-B Unit-Dose Vials 2213
Mustargen 1514
Permax Tablets (Infrequent) 1291
Prozac Pulvules (Rare) 920
Recombivax HB 1544
Vaseretic Tablets 1559
Vasotec I.V. 1562

Herxheimer's reaction
Bicillin L-A Injection 2442
Chloromycetin Kapseals 1695
Chloromycetin Palmitate, Oral Suspension 1697
Chloromycetin Sodium Succinate 1698
Pfizerpen for Injection 1957
Pfizerpen-AS Aqueous Suspension 1959
Wycillin Injection 2537

Hiccups
Anafranil Capsules (Rare) 650
Atgam Sterile Solution (Less than 1%) 2320
Bretylol Injection (1 in 1000) 923
Brevital Sodium Vials 1248
BuSpar (Rare) 1401
Celontin 1692
Cholybar 1705
Cipro I.V. (1% or less) 1592
Cipro Tablets (Less than 1%) 1589
Dalalone D.P. Injectable 999
Dalgan Injection (Less than 1%) 620
Decadron Elixir 1445
Decadron Phosphate Injection 1449
Decadron Phosphate Respihaler 1454
Decadron Phosphate Turbinaire 1456
Decadron Phosphate with Xylocaine Injection, Sterile 1451
Decadron Tablets 1447
Decadron-LA Sterile Suspension (Low) 1457
Diprivan Injection (Greater than 1%) 2267
Dopram Injectable 1860
Duragesic Transdermal System (1% or greater) 1133
Emete-con Intramuscular/Intravenous 1950
Fiorinal with Codeine Capsules 2008
ISMOTIC (Very rare) ◉ 233
Larodopa Tablets (Rare) 1905
Mexitil Capsules (About 1 in 1,000) 680
Moduretic Tablets (Less than or equal to 1%) 1510
▲Nicorette (14.9%) 1335
Paradione Capsules 548
Permax Tablets (1.1%) 1291
Prozac Pulvules (Infrequent) 920
Questran Light 711
Questran Powder 710
Sandimmune (2% or less) 2024
Sinemet Tablets 952
Sinemet CR Tablets 953
Soma Compound w/Codeine Tablets 2390
Soma Compound Tablets 2389
Soma Tablets 2388
Surital Ampoules, Steri-Vials 1764
Tonocard Tablets (Less than 1%) 1554
Tridione 557
Valium Injectable 1937
▲Versed Injection (3.9%) 1924
Zarontin Capsules 1768
Zarontin Syrup 1769

Hidradenitis suppurativa
Demulen 2161
Enovid 2161

Hidrocephalies
Prozac Pulvules (Rare) 920

Hirsutism
Accutane Capsules (Less than 1%) 1878
Aldactazide 2150
Aldactone 2152
Amen (Few cases) 833
Anadrol-50 Tablets 2287
Android 1111
Brevicon 2304
Cortone Acetate Sterile Suspension 1437
Cortone Acetate Tablets 1439
Cycrin Tablets 2449
Cytadren Tablets (Rare) 861
Danocrine Capsules 2046
Dantrium Capsules (Less frequent) 1619
Decadron Elixir 1445
Decadron Phosphate Injection 1449
Decadron Tablets 1447
Decadron-LA Sterile Suspension 1457
Demulen 2161
Depo-Provera Sterile Aqueous Suspension (Few cases) 2336
Diethylstilbestrol Tablets 1258
Dilantin Kapseals 1708
Eldepryl 2250
Enovid 2161
Estinyl Tablets 2085
Estrace 1385
Estrace Vaginal Cream 1388
Estradurin 2452
Estratest 2245
Estrovis 1721
Halotestin Tablets 2341
Hydeltrasol Injection, Sterile 1476
Hydeltra-T.B.A. Sterile Suspension 1478
Hydrocortone Acetate Sterile Suspension 1479
Hydrocortone Phosphate Injection, Sterile 1481
Hydrocortone Tablets 1482
Hyperstat I.V. Injection 2095
Intron A (1% or less) 2097
Jenest-28 Tablets 1636
Kenalog-10 Injection 2402
Kenalog-40 Injection 2403
Klonopin Tablets 1902
Levlen/Tri-Levlen 665
Lo/Ovral Tablets 2471
Lo/Ovral-28 Tablets 2476
Loestrin 1728
Lupron Depot 7.5 mg (Less than 5%) 2311
Lupron Injection 2310
Mediatric Capsules 2476
Menrium Tablets 1934
Metandren Linguets and Tablets 875
Micronor Tablets 1667
Modicon 1667
Nordette-21 Tablets 2481
Nordette-28 Tablets 2483
Norethin 2133
Norinyl 2304
Norlestrin 1746
Norlutate 1754
Norlutin 1755
Norplant System 2484
Nor-Q D Tablets 2304
Ogen 540
Ortho Dienestrol Cream 1664
Ortho-Cyclen Tablets 1658
Ortho-Novum 1667
Ovcon 1391
Ovral Tablets 2490
Ovral-28 Tablets 2491
Ovrette Tablets 2492
PMB 200 and PMB 400 2504
Permax Tablets (Infrequent) 1291
Premarin Intravenous 2508
Premarin with Methyltestosterone 2515
Premarin Tablets 2510
Premarin Vaginal Cream 2512
Proglycem (Frequent) 649
Provera Tablets 2356
Prozac Pulvules (Rare) 920
▲Sandimmune (Less than 1 to 45%) 2024
Stilphostrol Tablets and Ampuls 1609
Synarel Nasal Solution (2.5% of patients) 2300
TACE 12 and 25 mg 1353
▲Tegison Capsules (1-10%) 1881
Testred Capsules 1124
Levlen/Tri-Levlen 665
Tri-Norinyl 2304
Triphasil-21 Tablets 2527
Triphasil-28 Tablets 2532
Wellbutrin Tablets (Rare) 821
Winstrol Tablets 2075
Zarontin Capsules 1768
Zarontin Syrup 1769

Hives
(see also under Urticaria)
AeroBid Inhaler System (1-3%) 995
Atrovent Inhalation Aerosol (Less than 1 in 100) 675
Betoptic Sterile Ophthalmic Solution (Rare) 569
Betoptic S Sterile Ophthalmic Suspension (Rare) 570
Bumex (0.2%) 1895
Carafate Tablets 1326
Catapres Tablets (About 5 in 1,000 patients) 676
Catapres-TTS (5 per 1,000 patients) 677
Combipres Tablets (About 5 in 1,000) 678
Cutivate Ointment 0.005% (Less than 1%) 1054
Diphtheria and Tetanus Toxoids and Pertussis Vaccine Adsorbed USP (For Pediatric Use) (Rare) 892
Diprivan Injection (Less than 1%) 2267
Emete-con Intramuscular/Intravenous 1950
Fiorinal with Codeine Capsules 2008

Flu-Imune Influenza Virus Vaccine (Rare) 1204
Fluorescite (Very rare) ◉ 217
HibTITER 1206
Lozol Tablets (Less than 5%) 1843
Metrodin (urofollitropin for injection) 2182
Monistat Dual-Pak (Less than 0.5%) 1657
Monistat 3 Vaginal Suppositories (Less than 0.5%) 1657
Omnipaque (Less than 0.7%) 2552
Quadrinal Tablets 1183
Rogaine Topical Solution (1.27%) 2357
Soma Compound w/Codeine Tablets 2390
Soma Compound Tablets 2389
Sotradecol (Sodium Tetradecyl Sulfate Injection) 964
Stadol (Less than 1%) 721
Thiotepa Parenteral (Rare) 1240
Tracrium Injection (0.1%) 817
Versed Injection (Less than 1%) 1924
Zorprin Tablets 698
Zovirax Sterile Powder (Approximately 2%) 828

Hives at injection site

Idamycin for Injection 564

Hoarseness

▲ AeroBid Inhaler System (3-9%) 995
Android 1111
Atrovent Inhalation Aerosol (Less than 1%) 675
Azmacort Inhaler 1837
Beclovent Inhalation Aerosol and Refill (A few patients) 572
Capoten 2255
Capozide 2258
Decadron Phosphate Respihaler 1454
Emcyt Capsules (1%) 1161
Intal Capsules (Less than 1 in 100,000 patients) 978
Intal Inhaler (Rare) 979
Intal Nebulizer Solution (Rare) 980
Larodopa Tablets (Rare) 1905
Matulane Capsules 1907
Monopril Tablets (0.2 to 1.0%) 1406
Nicorette 1335
Retrovir Capsules (Less than 5%) 802
Retrovir I.V. Infusion (Less than 5%) 805
Retrovir Syrup (Less than 5%) 802
Sinemet Tablets 952
Sinemet CR Tablets 953
Trexan Tablets (Less than 1%) 937
Vanceril Inhaler (Few patients) 2128
Vaseretic Tablets 1559
Vasotec I.V. 1562
Vasotec Tablets 1564
Ventolin Rotacaps for Inhalation (2%) 583

Hodgkin's disease

Dilantin Infatabs 1710
Dilantin Kapseals 1708
Dilantin Parenteral 1712
Dilantin-30 Pediatric/Dilantin-125 Suspension 1713
Dilantin with Phenobarbital Kapseals 1715

Hormonal imbalance

ParaGard T380A Intrauterine Copper Contraceptive 411
Wellbutrin Tablets (Rare) 821

Horner's syndrome

Larodopa Tablets (Rare) 1905
Sinemet Tablets 952
Sinemet CR Tablets 953

Hostility

Anafranil Capsules (Infrequent) 650
BuSpar (2%) 1401
Desyrel and Desyrel Dividose (Greater than 1%) 1404
Duragesic Transdermal System (Less than 1%) 1133
Nubain Injection (Less than 1%) 934
Omnipaque 2552
Permax Tablets (Infrequent) 1291
ProSom Tablets (Infrequent) 554
Prozac Pulvules (Infrequent) 920
▲ Wellbutrin Tablets (5.6%) 821

Hot flashes

Alferon N Injection (1%) 1809
▲ Anafranil Capsules (2% to 5%) 650
Cardene Capsules (Rare) 2290
Clozaril Tablets (Less than 1%) 2000
Dipentum Capsules (Rare) 1160
▲ Eulexin Capsules (61% with LHRH-agonist) 2089
Fiorinal with Codeine Capsules (Infrequent) 2008
Intron A (Less than 1%) 2097
Larodopa Tablets (Infrequent) 1905
▲ Lupron Depot 7.5 mg (58.9%) 2311
▲ Lupron Injection (5% or more) 2310
Mexitil Capsules (Less than 1% or about 2 in 1,000) 680
▲ Nolvadex Tablets (Up to 25%) 1102
Procardia XL Tablets (1% or less) 1783
Prozac Pulvules (1.8%) 920
Roferon-A Injection (Less than 1%) 1916
Rythmol Tablets (Less than 1%) 1184
Sinemet Tablets 952
Sinemet CR Tablets 953
▲ Synarel Nasal Solution (90% of patients) 2300
Zefazone Sterile Powder 2372
▲ Zoladex (62%) 1110

Hydrocephalus

Pergonal (menotropins for injection, USP) (One report) 2184
Prozac Pulvules (Rare) 920

Hydrocephalus, fetal

Accutane Capsules 1878

Hydrothorax

Serophene (clomiphene citrate tablets, USP) 2186

Hyperactive deep tendon reflexes

Cibalith-S 870
Eskalith 2214
Lithium Carbonate Capsules & Tablets 1984
Lithobid Tablets 870

Hyperactivity

AeroBid Inhaler System (1-3%) 995
Amoxil (Rare) 2193
Augmentin Tablets, Powder for Oral Suspension, and Chewable Tablets (Rare) 2198
Ceclor Pulvules & Suspension (Rare) 1251
Cyclogyl (Common) ◉ 215
Cyclomydril ◉ 216
Dalmane Capsules (Rare) 1927
Depakene Capsules & Syrup 511
Depakote 512
Dopram Injectable 1860
Etrafon 2087
Fiorinal with Codeine Capsules 2008
Inapsine Injection 1140
Infumorph 200 and Infumorph 500 Sterile Solutions 962
Innovar Injection 1141
Ludiomil Tablets (Rare) 874
▲ Marplan Tablets (Among most frequent) 1906
Mellaril (Extremely rare) 2011
Moban Tablets & Concentrate (Less frequent) 932
Phenobarbital Elixir and Tablets 1293
Proventil Syrup (2 of 100) 2119
Roferon-A Injection (Less than 1%) 1916
Taractan 1920
Trilafon 2123
Ventolin (Less than or equal to 1%) 583
Versed Injection 1924
Yocon 1686
Zarontin Capsules 1768
Zarontin Syrup 1769

Hyperactivity, paradoxical

Restoril Capsules (Less than 0.5%) 2023

Hyperacusis

Anafranil Capsules (Infrequent) 650
Tegretol Chewable Tablets 654
Tegretol Suspension 656
Tegretol Tablets 654

Hyperalgesia

Retrovir Capsules (Less than 5%) 802
Retrovir I.V. Infusion (Less than 5%) 805
Retrovir Syrup (Less than 5%) 802

Hyperammonemia

Depakene Capsules & Syrup 511
Depakote 512

Hyperbilirubinemia

Altace Capsules (Rare) 1086
Anadrol-50 Tablets 2287
Ancobon Capsules 1886
AquaMEPHYTON Injection 1422
Bactrim DS Tablets 1891
Bactrim I.V. Infusion 1889
Bactrim 1891
BiCNU 723
Calan SR Caplets (1% or less) 2157
Calan Tablets (1% or less) 2155
Capoten 2255
Capozide 2258
CeeNU (Small percentage) 725
Cefizox Injection (Less than 1%) 1012
Ceftin Tablets 575
Ceptaz for Injection 1057
▲ Cipro I.V. (Among most frequent) 1592
Cipro Tablets (0.3%) 1589
Cytosar-U Sterile Powder (With experimental doses) 2329
Dalmane Capsules (Rare) 1927
Dapsone USP 1130
Depakene Capsules & Syrup (Occasional) 511
Depakote (Occasional) 512
Desyrel and Desyrel Dividose 1404
Elspar 1470
Ergamisol Tablets (Up to 1%) 1136
Eulexin Capsules 2089
▲ Exosurf Neonatal for Intratracheal Suspension (20% to 21%) 765
▲ Sterile FUDR (Among more common) 1898
Fortaz 1060
Fungizone Intravenous 2262
Garamycin Injectable 2093
Hyperstat I.V. Injection 2095
INH Tablets 868
▲ IFEX (31%) 729
Inocor Lactate Injection (Rare) 2048
Isoptin Oral Tablets 1179
Isoptin SR Sustained Release Tablets 1181
Konakion Injection 1903
Lamprene Capsules (Less than 1%) 1030
Larodopa Tablets (Rare) 1905
Leukine for IV Infusion 1127
Lopid Capsules and Tablets (Occasional) 1736
Lotensin Tablets 872
Mephyton Tablets (Rare) 1503
Mevacor Tablets 1505
Mezlin 1597
Mezlin Pharmacy Bulk Package 1599
Mithracin 1602
Monopril Tablets 1406
Netromycin Injection 100 mg/ml (15 of 1000 patients) 2104
▲ Paraplatin for Injection (5%) 735
Pipracil (Less frequent) 1230
Prilosec Delayed-Release Capsules (Less than 1%) 1530
Primaxin I.M. 1532
Primaxin I.V. 1535
Prinivil Tablets (Rare) 1538
Prinzide Tablets (Rare) 1540
Proglycem 649
Proloprim Tablets 799
Prostin VR Pediatric Sterile Solution (Less than 1%) 2355
RhoGAM $Rh_0(D)$ Immune Globulin (Human) 1651
Rifadin 1345
Rifamate Capsules 1347
Rimactane Capsules (Rare) 879
Rocephin Injectable Vials, ADD-Vantage (Less than 1%) 1914
Sectral Capsules 2520
Septra 813
Septra I.V. Infusion 808
Septra I.V. Infusion ADD-Vantage Vials 810
Septra 813
Sinemet Tablets 952
Synkayvite Injection 1919
Synkayvite Tablets 1920
Tenoretic Tablets 1105
Tenormin Tablets and I.V. Injection 1107
Timentin for Injection 2239
Trimpex Tablets 1922
Vaseretic Tablets (Rare) 1559
Vasotec I.V. (0.5 to 1%) 1562
Vasotec Tablets (Rare) 1564
Velosef Capsules and for Oral Suspension 606
Verelan Capsules 1243
Winstrol Tablets 2075
Xanax Tablets 2367
Zefazone Sterile Powder 2372
Zestoretic (Rare) 2274
Zestril Tablets (Rare) 2277
Zinacef (1 in 500 patients) 1066
Zyloprim Tablets (Less than 1%) 830

Hypercalcemia

Calderol Capsules 1635
Capozide (A few patients) 2258
Cibacalcin Double-chambered Syringes (Rare) 859
Cipro I.V. (Infrequent) 1592
Corzide Tablets 702
Enduron Tablets 517
Enduronyl 518
Eskalith 2214
Estinyl Tablets 2085
Estrace 1385
Estrace Vaginal Cream 1388
Estradurin 2452
Estratest 2245
Intron A (Less than 1%) 2097
Lupron Depot 7.5 mg (Less than 5%) 2311
Maxzide 1215
Mediatric Capsules 2476
Megace Tablets 732
Metandren Linguets and Tablets 875
Neo-Calglucon Syrup 2018
Nolvadex Tablets (Infrequent) 1102
Oretic Tablets 544
Oreticyl 545
Ortho Dienestrol Cream 1664
PMB 200 and PMB 400 2504
PhosLo Tablets 700
Premarin Intravenous 2508
Premarin with Methyltestosterone 2515
Premarin Tablets 2510
Premarin Vaginal Cream 2512
Prinzide Tablets 1540
Rauzide Tablets (Few patients) 1804
▲ Rocaltrol Capsules (1 in 3) 1913
Stilphostrol Tablets and Ampuls 1609
Vaseretic Tablets 1559
Winstrol Tablets 2075
Zestoretic 2274
Zyloprim Tablets (Less than 1%) 830

Hypercalciuria

Aristospan Suspension (Intra-articular) 1011
Calderol Capsules 1635
▲ Rocaltrol Capsules (1 in 7) 1913

Hypercapnia

Prostin VR Pediatric Sterile Solution (Less than 1%) 2355

Hypercarbia

Alfenta Injection (Less than 1%) 1131
Survanta Beractant Intratracheal Suspension (Less than 1%) 1978

Hyperchloremia

Android 1111
Colestid Granules 2328
Daranide Tablets 1445
Metandren Linguets and Tablets 875
Primaxin I.M. 1532
Primaxin I.V. 1535
Winstrol Tablets 2075

Hyperchloremic acidosis

Cholybar (Less frequent) 1705
Colestid Granules 2328
Questran Light 711
Questran Powder 710

Hyperchlorhydria

Prozac Pulvules (Rare) 920

Hypercholesterolemia

▲ Accutane Capsules (About 7%) 1878
Anafranil Capsules (Infrequent) 650
Android 1111
Calcijex Calcitriol Injection 506
Calderol Capsules 1635
▲ CHEMET (succimer) Capsules (4.2 to 10.4%) 1361
Cipro I.V. (Infrequent) 1592
Cipro Tablets 1589
Estratest 2245
Floxin Tablets 1652
Kerlone Tablets (Less than 2%) 2172
Metandren Linguets and Tablets 875
Micronor Tablets 1667
Modicon 1667
Norpace (1 to 3%) 2177
Ortho-Novum 1667
Permax Tablets (Infrequent) 1291

Premarin with Methyltestosterone .. 2515
Prinzide Tablets 1540
Prozac Pulvules (Rare) 920
Rocaltrol Capsules 1913
Synarel Nasal Solution 2300
▲Tegison Capsules (19%) 1881
Tegretol Chewable Tablets (Occasional) 654
Tegretol Suspension (Occasional) .. 656
Tegretol Tablets (Occasional) 654
Temaril Tablets, Syrup and Spansule Sustained Release Capsules 1085
Testred Capsules 1124
Vaseretic Tablets 1559

Hypercorticism

Beconase AQ Nasal Spray 574
Beconase Inhalation Aerosol & Refill 574
Nasacort Nasal Inhaler 1844
Nasalide Nasal Solution 0.025% 2299
Vasocidin Ophthalmic Solution (Rare) .... ⊙ 276

Hyperemia

Atropine Sulfate Sterile Ophthalmic Solution and S.O.P. Sterile Ophthalmic Ointment .... ⊙ 239
Celontin 1692
Cyclogyl .... ⊙ 215
Lacrisert Sterile Ophthalmic Insert 1493
Prostin VR Pediatric Sterile Solution (Less than 1%) 2355
TACE 12 and 25 mg 1353
Vaseretic Tablets (0.5% to 2.0%) 1559
Vasosulf .... ⊙ 279
Viroptic Ophthalmic Solution, 1% Sterile 820

Hyperemia, conjunctival

Chibroxin Sterile Ophthalmic Solution 1431
Diprivan Injection (Less than 1%) .. 2267
Enlon Injection 598
Tensilon Injectable 1123

Hyperesthesia

Anafranil Capsules (Rare) 650
Omnipaque 2552
Sandostatin Injection (Less than 1%) 2029
Sansert Tablets 2031
Sectral Capsules (Up to 2%) 2520

Hyperesthesia, tongue

Alferon N Injection (1%) 1809

Hyperestrogenism

Lupron Depot 3.75 mg 2312

Hyperexcitability, reflex

Aminophyllin Tablets 2153
Asbron G 1997
Choledyl Pediatric Elixir 1702
Choledyl Tablets 1700
Choledyl SA Tablets 1704
Constant-T Tablets 1029
Dilor 2079
Quadrinal Tablets 1183
Quibron Capsules 713
Quibron-T 714
Quibron-T/SR 716
Respbid Tablets 684
Slo-bid Gyrocaps 1847
T-PHYL (Uniphyl) 200 mg Tablets 1820
Theo-24 2179
Theo-Dur Sprinkle 1168
Theo-Dur Extended-Release Tablets 1166
Theolair 1317
Theolair-SR Tablets 1319
▲TheoX Extended-Release Tablets (Among most consistent) 841
Uniphyl 400 mg Tablets 1823

Hypergammaglobulinemia

Procan SR Tablets 1760

Hyperglycemia

▲Accutane Capsules (Less than 1 in 10) 1878
Aclovate 1053
Actimmune (Rare) 1046
AK-Con .... ⊙ 202
AK-Con-A .... ⊙ 203
Albalon Solution with Liquifilm .... ⊙ 238
Albalon-A Liquifilm (Rare) .... ⊙ 238
Aldoclor Tablets 1413
Aldoril Tablets 1418
Altace Capsules (Rare) 1086
Aminophyllin Tablets 2153
Anafranil Capsules (Infrequent) 650
Anaprox and Anaprox DS Tablets (Rare) 2288
Apresazide Capsules 854
Apresoline-Esidrix Tablets 857
Asbron G 1997
Atgam Sterile Solution (Less than 1% to less than 5%) 2320
Blocadren Tablets 1429
▲Bumex (6.6%) 1895
Butazolidin Capsules & Tablets (Less than 1%) 1027
Capozide 2258
Cardizem Tablets-30 mg, 60 mg, 90 mg and 120 mg (Less than 1%) 1329
Cardizem SR Capsules-60 mg, 90 mg and 120 mg (Less than 1%) 1327
Catapres Tablets (Rare) 676
Catapres-TTS (Rare) 677
Celestone Soluspan Suspension 2081
Choledyl Pediatric Elixir 1702
Choledyl Tablets 1700
Choledyl SA Tablets 1704
Cibalith-S 870
▲Cipro I.V. (Among most frequent) .. 1592
Cipro Tablets 1589
Clinoril Tablets (Rare) 1433
Combipres Tablets 678
Compazine 2201
Constant-T Tablets 1029
Corzide Tablets 702
Diprolene 2083
Diucardin Tablets 2450
Diulo 2129
Diupres Tablets 1461
Diuril Oral Suspension 1464
Diuril Sodium Intravenous 1463
Diuril Tablets 1464
Dyazide Capsules 2208
Edecrin 1468
Elavil 2269
Elspar (Low) 1470
Endep Tablets 1927
Enduron Tablets 517
Enduronyl 518
Esidrix Tablets 863
Esimil Tablets 864
Etrafon 2087
Exna Tablets 1862
Feldene Capsules (Less than 1%) .. 1777
Flexeril Tablets (Rare) 1471
Floxin Tablets (More than or equal to 1.0%) 1652
Haldol Decanoate 1375
Haldol Injection, Tablets and Concentrate 1373
Humatrope Vials (Infrequent) 1266
HydroDIURIL Tablets 1484
Hydromox R Tablets 1209
Hydromox Tablets 1208
Hydropres Tablets 1485
Hyperstat I.V. Injection 2095
INH Tablets 868
Inderide LA Long Acting Capsules .. 2465
Indocin Capsules (Less than 1%) 1487
Indocin I.V. (1% to 3%) 1490
Indocin (Less than 1%) 1487
Kenalog-10 Injection 2402
Kenalog-40 Injection 2403
Kerlone Tablets (Less than 2%) 2172
Lamprene Capsules (Greater than 1%) 1030
Lasix 1093
Limbitrol 1933
Lioresal Tablets 1031
Lithane Tablets 1596
Lithobid Tablets 870
Lo/Ovral Tablets 2471
Lo/Ovral-28 Tablets 2476
Lopressor HCT Tablets 1034
Lorelco Tablets 1333
Lozol Tablets (Less than 5%) 1843
Ludiomil Tablets (Rare) 874
Lufyllin & Lufyllin-400 Tablets 2384
Lufyllin-GG Elixir & Tablets 2385
Maxivate Cream, Lotion & Ointment 0.05% 2406
Maxzide 1215
Megace Tablets 732
Minizide Capsules 1779
Mintezol 1510
Moduretic Tablets 1510
Mykrox ½ mg Tablets 984
Naphcon Forte .... ⊙ 226
Naphcon-A Ophthalmic Solution 571
Naprosyn (Rare) 2297
Naturetin Tablets (Occasional) 1789
Navane Capsules and Concentrate 1954
Navane Intramuscular 1956
NebuPent for Inhalation Solution (1% or less) 1017
Nimotop Capsules (0.8%) 1607
Normodyne Tablets 2110
Normozide Tablets 2112
Norpramin Tablets 1340
Opcon-A Ophthalmic Solution .... ⊙ 262
Oretic Tablets 544
Oreticyl 545
Ovral Tablets 2490
Ovral-28 Tablets 2491
Ovrette Tablets 2492
Pamelor 2019
Pentam 300 Injection (1 patient) 1018
Permax Tablets (Infrequent) 1291
Prinzide Tablets 1540
Proglycem (Frequent) 649
Prozac Pulvules (Rare) 920
Quadrinal Tablets 1183
Quibron Capsules 713
Quibron-T 714
Quibron-T/SR 716
Rauzide Tablets 1804
Renese Tablets 1785
Respbid Tablets 684
Rifamate Capsules 1347
Saluron 718
Salutensin/Salutensin-Demi 719
Sandimmune (2% or less) 2024
Sandostatin Injection (1.6%) 2029
Ser-Ap-Es Tablets 881
Serpasil-Esidrix Tablets 886
Sinemet CR Tablets (1% or greater) 953
Sinequan 1960
Slo-bid Gyrocaps 1847
Stelazine 2226
Surmontil Capsules 2524
T-PHYL (Uniphyl) 200 mg Tablets 1820
Taractan 1920
Temovate 1056
Tenoretic Tablets 1105
Thalitone Tablets 687
Theo-24 2179
Theo-Dur Sprinkle 1168
Theo-Dur Extended-Release Tablets 1166
Theolair 1317
Theolair-SR Tablets 1319
▲TheoX Extended-Release Tablets (Among most consistent) 841
Thorazine 2234
Timolide Tablets 1547
Timoptic in Ocudose 1552
Timoptic Sterile Ophthalmic Solution 1550
Tofranil Ampuls 1038
Tofranil Tablets 1039
Tofranil-PM Capsules 1041
Trandate HCT Tablets 579
Triavil Tablets 1556
Trilafon 2123
Triphasil-21 Tablets 2527
Triphasil-28 Tablets 2532
Ultravate Cream 0.05% 2410
Ultravate Ointment 0.05% 2411
Uniphyl 400 mg Tablets 1823
Vaseretic Tablets (0.5% to 2.0%) 1559
Vasocon-A .... ⊙ 278
Vivactil Tablets 1567
Zaroxolyn Tablets 989
Zestoretic 2274
Zoladex (1% to 5%) 1110

Hyperglycemia, transient

Eskalith 2214
Lithium Carbonate Capsules & Tablets 1984

Hyperglycinemia

Asendin Tablets (Very rare) 1196
Depakene Capsules & Syrup 511
Depakote 512
Lotensin Tablets 872

Hyperheparinemia

Mustargen (Rare) 1514

Hyperhidrosis

Accutane Capsules (Less than 1%) 1878
Actibine 900
Decadron Phosphate with Xylocaine Injection, Sterile 1451
DynaCirc Capsules (0.5% to 1%) .. 2004
Fiorinal with Codeine Capsules (Infrequent) 2008
Lorelco Tablets 1333
▲Marplan Tablets (Among most frequent) 1906
Plendil Extended-Release Tablets (0.5% or greater) 1526
Prilosec Delayed-Release Capsules (Less than 1%) 1530
Primaxin I.M. 1532
Primaxin I.V. (Less than 0.2%) 1535
Prinzide Tablets (0.3 to 1%) 1540
Quadrinal Tablets 1183
Sandostatin Injection (Less than 1%) 2029
Vaseretic Tablets (0.5% to 2.0%) 1559
Visken Tablets (2% or fewer patients) 2036
Zestoretic (0.3 to 1%) 2274

Hyperirritability

Mintezol 1510
Mysoline (Occasional) 2480
Prostin VR Pediatric Sterile Solution (Less than 1%) 2355
Ru-Tuss with Hydrocodone 694
Ru-Tuss Tablets 693
Seromycin Pulvules 1298

Hyperirritability, muscle

Cibalith-S 870
Eskalith 2214
Lithane Tablets 1596
Lithium Carbonate Capsules & Tablets 1984
Lithobid Tablets 870

Hyperirritability, neuromuscular

Mezlin 1597
Mezlin Pharmacy Bulk Package 1599
Timentin for Injection 2239

Hyperkalemia

Altace Capsules 1086
Anaprox and Anaprox DS Tablets (Less than 1%) 2288
Android 1111
Anectine 755
Ansaid Tablets (Less than 1%) 2319
Atromid-S Capsules 2435
Blocadren Tablets 1429
Capoten 2255
Capozide 2258
Cipro I.V. (Infrequent) 1592
Cipro Tablets 1589
Clinoril Tablets (Less than 1 in 100) 1433
Dyazide Capsules 2208
Dyrenium Capsules (Rare) 2210
Epogen for Injection (0.11%) 591
Estratest 2245
Feldene Capsules (Less than 1%) .. 1777
Floxin Tablets (More than or equal to 1.0%) 1652
Fungizone Intravenous 2262
Halotestin Tablets 2341
Indocin Capsules (Less than 1%) 1487
Indocin I.V. (Less than 1%) 1490
Indocin (Less than 1%) 1487
K-Dur Microburst Release System (potassium chloride, USP) E.R. Tablets 1163
▲K-Lor Powder Packets (Most severe) 531
K-Lyte (Rare) 707
K-Norm Capsules 982
▲K-Tab Filmtab (Most common) 532
Kerlone Tablets (Less than 2%) 2172
▲Klor-Con 8/Klor-Con 10 Extended-release Tablets (Most severe) 2374
Klorvess Effervescent Granules 2010
Klorvess Effervescent Tablets 2011
Klorvess 10% Liquid 2010
Klotrix 708
Kolyum Liquid 983
Lotensin Tablets 872
Maxzide 1215
Metandren Linguets and Tablets 875
Micro-K 1863
▲Micro-K LS Packets (Most severe) .. 1864
Midamor Tablets (Between 1% and 3%) 1508
Moduretic Tablets (Greater than 1%, less than 3%) 1510
Monopril Tablets 1406
Naprosyn (Less than 1%) 2297
Netromycin Injection 100 mg/ml (Fewer than 1 of 1000 patients) 2104
Pentam 300 Injection (0.7%) 1018
Polycitra Syrup 2424
Polycitra-K 2424
Polycitra-LC—Sugar-Free 2424
Primaxin I.M. 1532
Primaxin I.V. 1535
Prinivil Tablets (2.2%) 1538

Prinzide Tablets 1540
Procrit for Injection (0.11%) 1647
Prostin VR Pediatric Sterile Solution (Less than 1%) 2355
Rum-K Syrup 995
Sandimmune (Occasional) 2024
Slow-K Tablets 2281
▲ Tegison Capsules (25-50%) 1881
Ten-K Controlled-Release Tablets 2282
Testred Capsules 1124
Vaseretic Tablets (0.5% to 2.0%) 1559
Vasotec I.V. (0.5 to 1%) 1562
Vasotec Tablets (0.5% to 1%) 1564
Winstrol Tablets 2075
Zestoretic (1.4%) 2274
Zestril Tablets (Less than 1%) 2277

Hyperkeratosis
Blenoxane 724
Calan SR Caplets (1% or less) 2157
Calan Tablets (1% or less) 2155
Isoptin Oral Tablets (Less than 1%) 1179
Isoptin SR Sustained Release Tablets (Less than 1%) 1181
Verelan Capsules (Less than 1%) 1243

Hyperkinesia
Alurate Elixir (Less than 1 in 100) 1883
Anafranil Capsules (Infrequent) 650
Butisol Sodium Elixir & Tablets (Less than 1 in 100) 2377
Cardene Capsules (Rare) 2290
Clozaril Tablets (1%) 2000
Doral Tablets 2383
Intron A (1% or less) 2097
Maxair Inhaler (Less than 1%) 1311
Mebaral Tablets (Less than 1 in 100) 2061
Nembutal Sodium Capsules (Less than 1%) 534
Nembutal Sodium Solution (Less than 1%) 536
Nembutal Sodium Suppositories (Less than 1%) 538
Permax Tablets (Infrequent) 1291
Phenobarbital Elixir and Tablets (Less than 1 in 100 patients) 1293
▲ Proventil Syrup (Children 2-6: 4%) 2119
Prozac Pulvules (Infrequent) 920
Seconal Sodium Pulvules (Less than 1 in 100) 1296
Seldane-D Extended-Release Tablets (1.1%) 1350
Tegison Capsules (Less than 1%) 1881
Tornalate (Less than 1%) 2074
▲ Ventolin Syrup (4% in children) 583

Hyperlipidemia
Calciparine Injection 925
Heparin Lock Flush Solution 2456
Heparin Sodium Vials 1264
Heparin Sodium Injection 2457
Heparin Sodium Injection, USP, Sterile Solution 2342
Kerlone Tablets (Less than 2%) 2172
Monistat I.V. 1143
Prozac Pulvules (Rare) 920
Sandimmune 2024

Hypermenorrhea
Cytotec (0.5%) 2159
Intron A (Less than 1%) 2097

Hypermetabolic syndrome
Nardil (Less frequent) 1742

Hypermotility, gastrointestinal
Roferon-A Injection (Less than 1%) 1916

Hypernatremia
Cephulac Syrup 1331
Chronulac Syrup 1332
Fleet Enema 991
ISMOTIC (Very rare) ⊙ 233
Nardil (Less common) 1742
Timentin for Injection 2239

Hyperosmolarity
ISMOTIC (Very rare) ⊙ 233
Sandostatin Injection (Less than 1%) 2029

Hyperostosis, skeletal
Accutane Capsules 1878
Anafranil Capsules (Rare) 650
▲ Tegison Capsules (Greater than 75%) 1881

Hyperoxemia, venous
Nipride I.V. Infusion 1909

Hyperoxia
Exosurf Neonatal for Intratracheal Suspension 765

Hyperparathyroidism
Eskalith 2214
Prinzide Tablets 1540
Vaseretic Tablets 1559

Hyperphenylalaninemia
Daraprim Tablets (Rare) 761

Hyperphosphatemia
Android 1111
Estratest 2245
▲ Lupron Depot 3.75 mg (5% to 8%) 2312
Metandren Linguets and Tablets 875
Minocin Oral Suspension 1224
Premarin with Methyltestosterone 2515
Roferon-A Injection (Less than 5%) 1916
▲ Synarel Nasal Solution (10% to 15%) 2300
Terramycin Capsules 1786
Testred Capsules 1124
Winstrol Tablets 2075

Hyperpigmentation
Accutane Capsules (Less than 1%) 1878
Adriamycin RDF (A few cases) 562
Aristospan Suspension (Intra-articular) 1011
BiCNU 723
▲ Blenoxane (50%) 724
Blocadren Tablets 1429
▲ Catapres-TTS (5 of 101 patients) 677
Celestone Soluspan Suspension 2081
Cipro I.V. (1% or less) 1592
Cipro Tablets (Less than 1%) 1589
Cortone Acetate Sterile Suspension 1437
Dalalone D.P. Injectable 999
Decadron Phosphate Injection 1449
Decadron Phosphate with Xylocaine Injection, Sterile 1451
Decadron-LA Sterile Suspension 1457
Deltasone Tablets 2332
Depo-Medrol Sterile Aqueous Suspension 2334
▲ Efudex (Among most frequent) 1880
Fluoroplex Topical Solution & Cream 1% (Occasional) 1082
Hydeltrasol Injection, Sterile 1476
Hydeltra-T.B.A. Sterile Suspension 1478
Hydrocortone Acetate Sterile Suspension 1479
Hydrocortone Phosphate Injection, Sterile 1481
Kenalog-10 Injection 2402
Kenalog-40 Injection 2403
▲ Lamprene Capsules (75-100%) 1030
Lodine Capsules (Less than 1%) 2468
Matulane Capsules 1907
▲ Myleran Tablets (5-10%) 790
Purinethol Tablets 800
Retin-A (tretinoin) Cream/Gel/Liquid 1680

Hyperpigmentation, dermal creases
Adriamycin PFS (A few cases primarily in children) 561
Adriamycin RDF (A few cases) 562

Hyperpigmentation, nail beds
Adriamycin PFS (A few cases primarily in children) 561
Adriamycin RDF (A few cases) 562
Doxorubicin Hydrochloride for Injection, USP (A few cases) 622
Doxorubicin Hydrochloride Injection, USP (A few cases) 848
Rubex (A few cases) 739

Hyperplasia, endocervical
Demulen 2161
Enovid 2161
Nolvadex Tablets (Isolated cases) 1102
Norethin 2133

Hyperplasia, gingival (see under Gingival hyperplasia)

Hyperplasia, mammary
Cuprimine Capsules (Rare) 1442
Depen Titratable Tablets (Rare) 2379

Hyperpnea
Azdōne Tablets 844
Damason-P 1356
Lortab ASA Tablets 2414

Hyperprolactinemia
Aldoclor Tablets 1413
Aldomet Ester HCl Injection 1417
Aldomet Oral 1415
Aldoril Tablets 1418
Asendin Tablets (Greater than 1%) 1196
Calan SR Caplets (1% or less) 2157
Calan Tablets (1% or less) 2155
Compazine 2201
Haldol Injection, Tablets and Concentrate 1373
Moban Tablets & Concentrate 932
Prolixin Oral Concentrate 1792
Prozac Pulvules 920
Rauzide Tablets 1804
Reglan 1869
Stelazine 2226
Thorazine 2234
Trilafon 2123

Hyperprothrombinemia
Eminase 2211
Estrace 1385
Estrace Vaginal Cream 1388
Estratest 2245
Jenest-28 Tablets 1636
Micronor Tablets 1667
Modicon 1667
Ortho-Novum 1667
Zyloprim Tablets (Less than 1%) 830

Hyperpyrexia (see under Fever)

Hyperreflexia
Anafranil Capsules (Rare) 650
Ansaid Tablets 2319
Compazine 2201
Etrafon 2087
Haldol Decanoate (Less frequent) 1375
Haldol Injection, Tablets and Concentrate 1373
Lithane Tablets 1596
▲ Marplan Tablets (Among most frequent) 1906
Nardil (Common) 1742
Navane Capsules and Concentrate 1954
Navane Intramuscular 1956
Nipride I.V. Infusion 1909
Omnipaque 2552
Orap Tablets (Less frequent) 1020
Pfizerpen for Injection 1957
Prolixin Decanoate 1795
Prolixin Elixir 1793
Prolixin Enanthate 1796
Prolixin Injection 1791
▲ Prolixin Oral Concentrate (Among most frequent) 1792
Prolixin Tablets 1793
Seromycin Pulvules 1298
Stelazine 2226
Temaril Tablets, Syrup and Spansule Sustained Release Capsules 1085
Triavil Tablets 1556
Trilafon 2123

Hyperreflexia, neonatal
Compazine 2201
Etrafon 2087
Stelazine 2226
Tacaryl Chewable Tablets 2409
Thorazine 2234

Hypersecretion
Diupres Tablets 1461
Enduronyl 518
Harmonyl Tablets 528
Hydropres Tablets 1485
Oreticyl 545
Raudixin Tablets 1803
Rauzide Tablets 1804
Renese-R Tablets 1786
Ser-Ap-Es Tablets 881
Serpasil Tablets 883
Serpasil-Apresoline Tablets 884
Serpasil-Esidrix Tablets 886

Hypersensitivity
Activase (Occasional) 1047
AK-Cide Sterile Ophthalmic Ointment & Suspension ⊙ 202
AK-Con ⊙ 202
AK-Dex ⊙ 203
AK-Fluor Injection 10% and 25% (Rare) ⊙ 204
AK-Mycin Ointment ⊙ 204
AK-NaCl 5% Ointment & Solution ⊙ 204
AK-Poly-Bac Ointment ⊙ 205
AK-Pred ⊙ 205
AK-Spore H.C. ⊙ 206
AK-Spore ⊙ 205
Albalon-A Liquifilm ⊙ 238
Alcaine ⊙ 210
Americaine Otic Topical Anesthetic Ear Drops 973
Amoxil 2193
Anectine (Rare) 755
Augmentin Tablets, Powder for Oral Suspension, and Chewable Tablets 2198
Axid Pulvules (Rare) 1246
Azulfidine Tablets, EN-tabs, Oral Suspension 1157
Beclovent Inhalation Aerosol and Refill 572
Beconase AQ Nasal Spray (Rare) 574
Beconase Inhalation Aerosol & Refill (Rare) 574
Betagan ⊙ 239
Bicillin C-R Injection 2438
Bicillin C-R 900/300 Injection 2440
Bicillin L-A Injection 2442
Bleph-10 Liquifilm Sterile Ophthalmic Solution 586
Bleph-10 Ophthalmic Ointment 10% 586
Blephamide Liquifilm Sterile Ophthalmic Suspension 586
Butisol Sodium Elixir & Tablets (Less than 1 in 100) 2377
Calciparine Injection 925
Carafate Tablets 1326
Ceclor Pulvules & Suspension 1251
Cefobid Intravenous/Intramuscular 1943
Cefobid Pharmacy Bulk Package - Not for Direct Infusion 1945
Cefotan (1.2%) 2265
Ceftin Tablets (2.9%) 575
Ceptaz for Injection (Immediate in 1 in 285 patients) 1057
Cetamide Ointment ⊙ 220
Cetapred Ointment ⊙ 220
Chloromycetin Ophthalmic Ointment, 1% 1696
Cleocin HCl Capsules 2322
Cleocin Pediatric Flavored Granules 2324
Cleocin Phosphate Injection 2325
Clinoril Tablets (Less than 1%) 1433
Cocaine Hydrochloride Topical Solution 620
Collagenase Santyl Ointment (One case) 1172
Cortisporin Ophthalmic Suspension Sterile 759
Cortone Acetate Sterile Suspension 1437
Cortone Acetate Tablets 1439
Coumadin Injection & Tablets (Infrequent) 944
Dalalone D.P. Injectable 999
Daranide Tablets 1445
Daraprim Tablets 761
Decadron Elixir 1445
Decadron Phosphate Injection 1449
Decadron Phosphate Respihaler 1454
Decadron Phosphate Turbinaire 1456
Decadron Phosphate with Xylocaine Injection, Sterile 1451
Decadron Tablets 1447
Decadron-LA Sterile Suspension 1457
Demser Capsules (Rare) 1460
Depo-Medrol Sterile Aqueous Suspension (Rare) 2334
Diapid Nasal Spray 2003
Dicumarol Tablets (Infrequent) 516
Digibind 762
Dilantin with Phenobarbital Kapseals (Rare) 1715
Dolobid Tablets (Less than 1 in 100) 1465
Elspar 1470
Estratest (Rare) 2245
FML-S Sterile Ophthalmic Suspension ⊙ 246
Factrel (Rare) 2561
Flexeril Tablets 1471
Fluorescite ⊙ 217
Fortaz (Immediate in 1 in 285 patients) 1060
Gammagard Immune Globulin, Intravenous (Human) (Possible) 658
Gentak Ointment & Solution ⊙ 208

Geocillin Tablets 1951
Glaucon ◉ 218
Gordochom Solution 1072
Grisactin 2454
Grisactin Ultra Tablets 2455
Gris-PEG Tablets, 125 mg & 250 mg 1083
Halotestin Tablets 2341
Heparin Sodium Vials 1264
Heparin Sodium Injection, USP, Sterile Solution 2342
Hep-B-Gammagee (Rare) 1474
Hibistat Germicidal Hand Rinse (Very rare) 2272
Hydeltrasol Injection, Sterile 1476
Hydeltra-T.B.A. Sterile Suspension 1478
Hydrocortone Acetate Sterile Suspension 1479
Hydrocortone Phosphate Injection, Sterile 1481
Hydrocortone Tablets 1482
Hyperstat I.V. Injection 2095
Imodium Capsules 1139
Inderide Tablets 2463
Indocin (Less than 1%) 1487
Inocor Lactate Injection 2048
ISMOTIC ◉ 233
Isopto Atropine ◉ 218
Isopto Cetamide Solution ◉ 220
Isopto Cetapred Suspension ◉ 220
Kefurox Vials, Faspak & ADD-Vantage (Less than 1%) 1277
Lacrisert Sterile Ophthalmic Insert 1493
Leukeran Tablets 788
Lincocin 2344
Lopressor HCT Tablets 1034
Lupron Injection 2310
Maxitrol Ophthalmic Ointment/Suspension ◉ 223
Mediatric Capsules (Rare) 2476
Medrol 2348
Metandren Linguets and Tablets 875
Metrodin (urofollitropin for injection) 2182
Metubine Iodide Vials 1285
Miacalcin Injection 2017
Miltown Tablets 2386
Mustargen 1514
Nembutal Sodium Capsules 534
Nembutal Sodium Solution (Less than 1%) 536
Nembutal Sodium Suppositories (Less than 1%) 538
NeoDecadron Topical Cream 1518
Nizoral Tablets (Several cases) 1145
Norflex 1314
Noroxin Tablets 1519
Novocain Hydrochloride for Spinal Anesthesia (Rare) 2065
Ogen 540
Organidin Elixir, Solution & Tablets (Rare) 2387
PBZ Tablets & Elixir 1037
PBZ-SR Tablets 1037
Panwarfin Tablets (Infrequent) 547
Paraplatin for Injection (2%) 735
Pentaspan Injection 949
Peptavlon 2563
Peridex (Rare) 1808
Pfizerpen-AS Aqueous Suspension 1959
Phenobarbital Elixir and Tablets 1293
Pontocaine Hydrochloride for Spinal Anesthesia 2069
Premarin with Methyltestosterone 2515
Prinzide Tablets 1540
Procardia XL Tablets 1783
Proloprim Tablets 799
Pronestyl Capsules and Tablets 1800
Pronestyl Injection 1798
Quinamm Tablets 1344
Recombivax HB 1544
Rifadin 1345
Rimactane Capsules 879
Rimso-50 (Occasional) 1836
Ritalin 880
Sandoglobulin I.V. (Less than 1%) 2027
Seromycin Pulvules 1298
Sodium Sulamyd (Single instance) 2122
Solu-Cortef Sterile Powder 2361
Synarel Nasal Solution (0.2%) 2300
Talacen (A few cases) 2070
Tazicef for Injection (1 in 285 patients) 2231
Tenoretic Tablets 1105
Tessalon Perles 1006
Tetanus Toxoid, Adsorbed Purogenated 1238
Theo-Organidin Elixir (Rare) 2391
TheraCys BCG Live (Intravesical) (Up to 1.8%) 898
Tigan 2239
Timoptic in Ocudose 1552
Timoptic Sterile Ophthalmic Solution 1550
TobraDex Ophthalmic Suspension and Ointment (Less than 4%) ◉ 228
Tobrex Ophthalmic Ointment and Solution (Less than 3 in 100 patients) 572
Tonocard Tablets (Less than 1%) 1554
Trandate HCT Tablets (Rare) 579
Trandate Injection (Rare) 577
Trandate Tablets (Rare) 579
Trimpex Tablets (Rare) 1922
Tussi-Organidin DM Liquid (Rare) 2392
Tussi-Organidin Liquid (Rare) 2391
Unasyn 1965
Urobiotic-250 Capsules 1968
Vancenase AQ Nasal Spray 0.042% (Rare) 2127
Vancenase Nasal Inhaler (Rare) 2126
Vanceril Inhaler (Rare) 2128
Vaseretic Tablets 1559
Vasocidin Ophthalmic Solution (Single instance) ◉ 276
Vasosulf (Rare) ◉ 279
Vioform-Hydrocortisone Cream and Mild Cream (Few) 889
Vioform-Hydrocortisone Ointment (Few) 889
Viroptic Ophthalmic Solution, 1% Sterile 820
Xylocaine Injections 637
Xylocaine Injections for Ventricular Arrhythmias 639
Xylocaine 2% Jelly 643
Xylocaine 10% Oral Spray 645
4% Xylocaine-MPF Sterile Solution 641
Xylocaine 2% Viscous Solution 646
Zantac Injection and Zantac Injection Premixed (Rare) 1063
Zantac (Rare) 1065
Zefazone Sterile Powder 2372
Zephiran (Rare) ▣ 762
Zestoretic 2274
Zinacef (Less than 1%) 1066
Zyloprim Tablets (Less than 1%) 830

Hypersensitivity pancreatitis

Imuran 768

Hypersensitivity pneumonitis

Fungizone Intravenous 2262

Hypersensitivity reactions, Arthus-type

Diphtheria and Tetanus Toxoids and Pertussis Vaccine Adsorbed USP (For Pediatric Use) 892

Hypersensitivity reactions, general

Alkeran Tablets 754
Altace Capsules (Less than 1%) 1086
Arm-a-Med Metaproterenol Sulfate Inhalation Solution, USP (Rare) 617
Brethine Ampuls 1026
Brethine Tablets 1026
Ceptaz for Injection (2% of patients) 1057
Didronel Tablets (Rare) 1621
Dobutrex Solution Vials (Occasionally) 1259
Flu-Imune Influenza Virus Vaccine 1204
Grifulvin V (griseofulvin microsize) Tablets/Suspension 1678
Heparin Lock Flush Solution 2456
Heparin Sodium Injection 2457
Keflex Pulvules, Oral Suspension & Pediatric Drops 916
Lotensin Tablets 872
Maxzide 1215
Mebaral Tablets (Less than 1 in 100) 2061
Mevacor Tablets 1505
Minocin Pellet-Filled Capsules 1222
Monocid Injection (Less than 1%) 2217
Phenobarbital Elixir and Tablets (Less than 1 in 100 patients) 1293
Polytrim Ophthalmic Solution Sterile (Less than 2 of 100) 588
Seconal Sodium Pulvules (Less than 1 in 100) 1296
Skelaxin 840
Streptase for Infusion 635
Terramycin Capsules 1786
Thiosulfil Forte Tablets 2526

Hypersensitivity vasculitis

Aldoclor Tablets 1413
Aldomet Ester HCl Injection 1417
Aldomet Oral Suspension 1415
Aldoril Tablets 1418
Brethine Ampuls (Rare) 1026
Brethine Tablets (Rare) 1026
Clinoril Tablets (Less than 1 in 100) 1433
Dolobid Tablets (Less than 1 in 100) 1465
Tagamet (Rare) 2228

Hypersomnia

Nardil (Common) 1742

Hypertension

Actibine 900
Adipex-P Tablets and Capsules 1019
AeroBid Inhaler System (1-3%) 995
AK-Con ◉ 202
AK-Con-A ◉ 203
AK-Dilate Solution 2.5% and 10% ◉ 203
Albalon Solution with Liquifilm ◉ 238
Albalon-A Liquifilm (Rare) ◉ 238
▲ Alfenta Injection (18%) 1131
Alupent 674
Amen 833
Ana-Kit Anaphylaxis Emergency Treatment Kit 1100
Anectine 755
Ansaid Tablets (Less than 1%) 2319
Aristocort Suspension 1008
Aristospan Suspension 1011
Arm-a-Med Metaproterenol Sulfate Inhalation Solution, USP (Less frequent) 617
Asendin Tablets (Less than 1%) 1196
Atgam Sterile Solution (Less than 1% to less than 5%) 2320
Ativan Injection (0.1%) 2432
BAL in Oil Ampules 661
Baron-X Tablets 650
Biphetamine Capsules 973
Bontril Slow-Release 834
Brethaire Inhaler (Fewer than 1 per 100) 1024
Bretylol Injection (1-2 in 1000) 923
Brevicon 2304
Bronkephrine Injection 2042
BuSpar (Infrequent) 1401
Butazolidin Capsules & Tablets (Less than 1%) 1027
Calcijex Calcitriol Injection 506
Calderol Capsules 1635
Capoten 2255
Capozide 2258
Carbocaine Hydrochloride Injection 2043
Celestone Soluspan Suspension 2081
Ceptaz for Injection (Very rare) 1057
Children's Advil Suspension (Less than 1%) 2426
Cipro I.V. (1% or less) 1592
Cipro Tablets 1589
Clinoril Tablets (Less than 1%) 1433
▲ Clozaril Tablets (4%) 2000
Coricidin 'D' Decongestant Tablets ▣ 695
Coricidin Demilets Tablets for Children ▣ 696
Cortenema 2244
Cortifoam 1827
Cortone Acetate Sterile Suspension 1437
Cortone Acetate Tablets 1439
Cycrin Tablets 2449
Cytotec (Infrequent) 2159
Cytovene Sterile Powder (1% or less) 2292
DDAVP Injection (Infrequent) 1840
Dalalone D.P. Injectable 999
Dalgan Injection (Less than 1%) 620
Danocrine Capsules 2046
Dayto Himbin Tablets and Liquid 905
Decadron Elixir 1445
Decadron Phosphate Injection 1449
Decadron Phosphate Respihaler 1454
Decadron Phosphate Turbinaire 1456
Decadron Phosphate with Xylocaine Injection, Sterile 1451
Decadron Tablets 1447
Decadron-LA Sterile Suspension 1457
Deltasone Tablets 2332
Demulen 2161
Depo-Medrol Sterile Aqueous Suspension 2334
Desoxyn Gradumet Tablets 514
Desyrel and Desyrel Dividose (Greater than 1%) 1404
Dexedrine 2206
Diapid Nasal Spray 2003
Didrex Tablets 2338
Dilaudid-HP Injection 1175
Dimetane-DC Cough Syrup 1857
Dimetane-DX Cough Syrup 1858
Dipentum Capsules (Rare) 1160
Diprivan Injection (Greater than 1%) 2267
▲ Dobutrex Solution Vials (Most patients) 1259
Dopram Injectable 1860
Duragesic Transdermal System (1% to 3%) 1133
Ecotrin 2189
Elavil 2269
Eldepryl 2250
Emete-con Intramuscular/Intravenous 1950
Endep Tablets 1927
Enovid 2161
▲ Epogen for Injection (0.75% to approximately 25%) 591
Ergotrate Maleate Ampoules (Small percentage of patients) 1263
Estinyl Tablets 2085
Estrace 1385
Estrace Vaginal Cream 1388
Estradurin 2452
Estratest (Common) 2245
Ethmozine Tablets (Less than 2%) 946
Etrafon 2087
Eulexin Capsules (1%) 2089
Fastin Capsules 2216
Feldene Capsules (Less than 1%) 1777
Flexeril Tablets (Rare) 1471
Floxin Tablets (Less than 1%) 1652
Fortaz (Very rare) 1060
Fungizone Intravenous 2262
Gammagard Immune Globulin, Intravenous (Human) (Occasional) 658
Garamycin Injectable 2093
Glaucon ◉ 218
Haldol Decanoate 1375
Haldol Injection, Tablets and Concentrate 1373
Hycomine Compound Tablets 929
Hycomine Syrup 927
Hycotuss Expectorant Syrup 930
Hydeltrasol Injection, Sterile 1476
Hydeltra-T.B.A. Sterile Suspension 1478
Hydrocortone Acetate Sterile Suspension 1479
Hydrocortone Phosphate Injection, Sterile 1481
Hydrocortone Tablets 1482
IFEX (Less than 1%) 729
Inapsine Injection 1140
Indocin Capsules (Less than 1%) 1487
Indocin I.V. (Less than 1%) 1490
Indocin (Less than 1%) 1487
Innovar Injection 1141
Intron A (2%) 2097
Intropin Injection (Infrequent) 930
Ionamin Capsules 981
Isuprel Hydrochloride Injection 1:5000 2050
Jenest-28 Tablets 1636
Kenalog-10 Injection 2402
Kenalog-40 Injection 2403
Kerlone Tablets (Less than 2%) 2172
Ketalar 1726
Larodopa Tablets (Rare) 1905
Levlen/Tri-Levlen 665
Levophed Bitartrate Injection 2054
Limbitrol 1933
Lodine Capsules (Less than 1%) 2468
Lo/Ovral Tablets 2471
Lo/Ovral-28 Tablets 2476
Loestrin 1728
Loxitane 1213
Ludiomil Tablets (Rare) 874
▲ Lupron Depot 3.75 mg (Among most frequent) 2312
Lupron Depot 7.5 mg 2311
▲ Lupron Injection (5% or more) 2310
Lysodren (Infrequent) 731
MS Contin Tablets (Infrequent) 1814
MSIR (Infrequent) 1817
Mediatric Capsules 2476
Medrol 2348
Megace Tablets 732
Mepergan Injection (Rare) 2479
Metaprel Inhalation Aerosol Bronchodilator 2014
Metaprel Inhalation Solution (Less frequent) 2015
Metaprel 2015
▲ Methergine (Most common) 2016
Mexitil Capsules (Less than 1% or about 1 in 1,000) 680
Micronor Tablets 1667
Modicon 1667
Motrin Tablets (Less than 1%) 2351

Murocoll-2 Sterile Ophthalmic Solution ⊙ 261
Mutamycin 733
Mydfrin 2.5% ⊙ 224
Naphcon Forte ⊙ 226
Naphcon-A Ophthalmic Solution 571
Narcan Injection 933
NebuPent for Inhalation Solution (1% or less) 1017
Neo-Synephrine Hydrochloride (Ophthalmic) (Rare) 2064
Nicorette 1335
Nimotop Capsules (Less than 1%) 1607
Nordette-21 Tablets 2481
Nordette-28 Tablets 2483
Norethin 2133
Norinyl 2304
Norlestrin 1746
Norlutate 1754
Norlutin 1755
Norplant System 2484
Norpramin Tablets 1340
Nor-Q D Tablets 2304
Novocain Hydrochloride for Spinal Anesthesia 2065
Nubain Injection (Less than 1%) 934
Omnipaque (Less than 0.1%) 2552
Oncovin Solution Vials & Hyporets 1288
Opcon-A Ophthalmic Solution ⊙ 262
Oramorph SR (Morphine Sulfate Sustained Release Tablets) (Less frequent) 1988
Orap Tablets 1020
Ornade Spansule Capsules 2221
Ortho Dienestrol Cream 1664
▲ Orthoclone OKT3 Sterile Solution (8%) 1645
Ortho-Cyclen Tablets 1658
Ortho-Novum 1667
Orudis Capsules (Less than 1%) 2488
Ovcon 1391
Ovral Tablets 2490
Ovral-28 Tablets 2491
Ovrette Tablets 2492
PMB 200 and PMB 400 2504
Pamelor 2019
Papaverine Hydrochloride Vials and Ampoules 1290
Parlodel 2020
Pediapred Oral Liquid 987
PediaProfen Suspension (Less than 1%) 1363
Permax Tablets (1.6%) 1291
Phenergan with Codeine 2497
Phenergan with Dextromethorphan 2499
Phenergan Injection 2493
Phenergan Suppositories 2496
Phenergan Syrup 2495
Phenergan Tablets 2496
Phenergan VC 2500
Phenergan VC with Codeine 2501
Pilocar (Extremely rare) ⊙ 275
Pilostat Sterile Ophthalmic Solution 0.5%, 1%, 2%, 3%, 4%, 5%, 6% (Extremely rare) ⊙ 263
Plegine Tablets 2504
Pondimin Tablets 1867
Prelu-2 Capsules 683
Premarin Intravenous 2508
Premarin with Methyltestosterone 2515
Premarin Tablets 2510
Premarin Vaginal Cream 2512
Priscoline Hydrochloride Ampuls 877
▲ Procrit for Injection (0.75% to approximately 25%) 1647
Proglycem (Rare) 649
Prolixin Decanoate 1795
Prolixin Elixir 1793
Prolixin Enanthate 1796
Prolixin Injection 1791
Prolixin Oral Concentrate 1792
Prolixin Tablets 1793
Propagest 839
Propine with C Cap Compliance Cap ⊙ 255
Protopam Chloride for Injection 2518
Proventil Inhalation Aerosol (Less than 5%) 2117
Proventil Repetabs Tablets 2120
Proventil Solutions for Inhalation 0.5% and 0.083% (1%) 2118
Proventil Syrup 2119
Proventil Tablets 2120
Provera Tablets 2356
Prozac Pulvules (Infrequent) 920
Reglan 1869
Rocaltrol Capsules 1913
Roferon-A Injection (Less than 3%) 1916
Rogaine Topical Solution (1.53%) 2357
Rondec 1975
Rondec-DM 1976
Rondec-TR Tablet 1975
Rufen Tablets (Less than 1%) 691
Ru-Tuss II Capsules 693
Ru-Tuss with Hydrocodone 694
Ru-Tuss Tablets 693
▲ Sandimmune (13 to 53%) 2024
Sandostatin Injection (Less than 1%) 2029
Sinemet Tablets (Rare) 952
Sinemet CR Tablets 953
Sinequan 1960
Sinulin 840
Solu-Cortef Sterile Powder 2361
Solu-Medrol Sterile Powder 2363
Stadol (Rare to less than 1%) 721
Stilphostrol Tablets and Ampuls 1609
Sublimaze Injection 1146
▲ Sufenta Injection (3%) 1147
Surmontil Capsules 2524
Survanta Beractant Intratracheal Suspension (Less than 1%) 1978
TACE 12 and 25 mg 1353
Talwin Injection (Infrequent) 2071
Tambocor Tablets (Less than 1%) 1315
Tegretol Chewable Tablets 654
Tegretol Suspension 656
Tegretol Tablets 654
Tenuate 1354
Teslac Tablets 741
Timoptic in Ocudose 1552
Timoptic Sterile Ophthalmic Solution 1550
Tofranil Ampuls 1038
Tofranil Tablets 1039
Tofranil-PM Capsules 1041
▲ Tolectin (200, 400 and 600 mg) (3 to 9%) 1379
Tonocard Tablets (Less than 1%) 1554
Trexan Tablets (Less than 1%) 937
Triavil Tablets 1556
Trilafon (Occasional) 2123
Levlen/Tri-Levlen 665
Trinalin Repetabs Tablets 1170
Tri-Norinyl 2304
Triphasil-21 Tablets 2527
Triphasil-28 Tablets 2532
Tuss-Ornade Liquid 2242
Tuss-Ornade Spansule Capsules 2242
Vascor (200, 300 and 400 mg) Tablets (0.5 to 2.0%) 1383
Vasocon-A ⊙ 278
Vasotec I.V. 1562
Vasoxyl Injection 819
Velban Vials (Among most common) 1305
▲ Ventolin (Less than 5 in 100 patients) 583
VePesid Capsules and Injection 741
Versed Injection 1924
Vivactil Tablets 1567
Voltaren Tablets (Less than 1%) 1042
▲ Wellbutrin Tablets (4.3%) 821
Yocon 1686
Yohimex Tablets 1190
Zoladex (1% to 5%) 1110

Hypertension, aggravation

Tegretol Chewable Tablets 654
Tegretol Suspension 656
Tegretol Tablets 654

Hypertension, intracranial

Azo Gantrisin Tablets 1888
Cutivate Cream 0.05% 1054
Cutivate Ointment 0.005% 1054
Danocrine Capsules (Rare) 2046
Doryx Capsules 1717
Minocin Oral Suspension 1224
Minocin Pellet-Filled Capsules 1222
Monodox Capsules 1630
Permax Tablets (Rare) 1291
Terramycin Capsules 1786
Terramycin Intramuscular Solution 1964
Urobiotic-250 Capsules 1968
Vibramycin Hyclate Capsules 1787
Vibramycin Hyclate Intravenous 1968
Vibramycin 1787

Hypertension, malignant

Demulen 2161
Enovid 2161

Hypertension, neonatal

Mydfrin 2.5% ⊙ 224

Hypertension, rebound

Deponit NTG Transdermal Delivery System 2143
Minitran Transdermal Delivery System (Uncommon) 1312
Nitrodisc (Uncommon) 2176
Nitro-Dur (nitroglycerin) Transdermal Infusion System 1164
Nitrogard Tablets (Uncommon) 1004
Transderm-Nitro Transdermal Therapeutic System (Uncommon) 2283
Tridil Ampuls & Vials (Uncommon) 939

Hypertensive crises

Corzide Tablets 702
Emete-con Intramuscular/Intravenous 1950
Monopril Tablets (0.2 to 1.0%) 1406

Hyperthermia

Anectine Flo-Pack 755
Asendin Tablets (Less than 1%) 1196
Biltricide 1589
Bretylol Injection (1 in 1000) 923
Calcijex Calcitriol Injection 506
Calderol Capsules 1635
Cholera Vaccine 2445
Cogentin 1435
Elspar 1470
Emete-con Intramuscular/Intravenous 1950
Furoxone (Rare) 1855
Geocillin Tablets 1951
Hespan Injection 948
Hyperab Rabies Immune Globulin (Human) 1574
Hyper-Tet Tetanus Immune Globulin (Human) 1576
HypRho-D Mini-Dose Rh_0-D Immune Globulin (Human) 1578
Lomotil 2174
MICRhoGAM Rh_0(D) Immune Globulin (Human) (Reported in a small number of women) 1650
Marcaine Hydrochloride with Epinephrine 1:200,000 (Rare) 2055
Marcaine Hydrochloride Injection (Rare) 2055
Marcaine Spinal (Rare) 2058
Motofen Tablets 836
Nescaine/Nescaine MPF 629
Prolixin Decanoate 1795
Prolixin Elixir 1793
Prolixin Enanthate 1796
Prolixin Injection 1791
Prolixin Tablets 1793
Reglan 1869
Rocaltrol Capsules 1913
Sensorcaine (Rare) 631
Sensorcaine-MPF Spinal (Rare) 634
Stelazine 2226
Typhoid Vaccine 2533

Hyperthyroidism

Anafranil Capsules (Rare) 650
Butazolidin Capsules & Tablets 1027
Cibalith-S (Rare) 870
Cordarone Tablets (1 to 3%) 2446
Cytomel Tablets 2203
Eskalith (Rare) 2214
Euthroid 1724
Intron A (1% or less) 2097
Levothroid Tablets (Rare) 1003
Levoxine Tablets 904
Lithane Tablets (Rare) 1596
Lithium Carbonate Capsules & Tablets (Rare cases) 1984
Lithobid Tablets (Rare) 870
Prozac Pulvules (Rare) 920
Synthroid 695

Hypertonia

▲ Anafranil Capsules (2% to 4%) 650
Ansaid Tablets (Less than 1%) 2319
Cardura Tablets (1%) 1941
Ceclor Pulvules & Suspension (Rare) 1251
Diprivan Injection (Less than 1%) 2267
Duragesic Transdermal System (Less than 1%) 1133
Eskalith 2214
Flexeril Tablets (Less than 1%) 1471
Intron A (Up to 5%) 2097
Lotensin Tablets 872
Omnipaque (Less than 0.1%) 2552
Permax Tablets (1.1%) 1291
Procardia XL Tablets (1% or less) 1783
Prozac Pulvules (Rare) 920
Tegison Capsules (Less than 1%) 1881

Hypertrichosis

Aclovate Cream 1053
Alphatrex Cream, Ointment & Lotion (Infrequent) 2076
Anafranil Capsules (Rare) 650
Analpram-HC Rectal Cream 1% and 2.5% 970
Anusol-HC Cream (Infrequent) 1690
Aristocort A (Infrequent) 1010
Betatrex Cream, Ointment & Lotion 2077
Carmol HC Cream 1% (Infrequent) 2296
Cortifoam 1827
Cortisporin Cream 757
Cortisporin Ointment 758
Cortisporin Otic Solution Sterile 760
Cortisporin Otic Suspension Sterile 760
Cutivate Ointment 0.005% (Less than 1%) 1054
Cyclocort Lotion (Infrequent) 1198
Decadron Phosphate Topical Cream 1455
Decaspray Topical Aerosol 1459
DesOwen Cream, Ointment and Lotion (Infrequent) 1682
Dilantin Infatabs 1710
Dilantin Kapseals 1708
Dilantin Parenteral 1712
Dilantin-30 Pediatric/Dilantin-125 Suspension 1713
Dilantin with Phenobarbital Kapseals 1715
Diprolene (Infrequent) 2083
Eldecort Cream 1.0% (Infrequent) 1113
Eldecort Cream 1.0% and 2.5% (Infrequent) 1113
Elocon (Infrequent) 2084
Florone/Florone E 908
Halog (Infrequent) 2399
Hytone 909
Kenalog Cream, Lotion & Ointment (Infrequent) 2401
Lidex (Infrequent) 2296
Locoid Cream, Ointment and Topical Solution (Infrequent) 970
▲ Loniten Tablets (80%) 2346
Lotrisone Cream (Infrequent) 2103
Mantadil Cream 789
Maxivate Cream, Lotion & Ointment 0.05% 2406
Mycolog II Cream and Ointment (Infrequent) 2407
Mytrex Cream & Ointment (Infrequent) 2080
NeoDecadron Topical Cream 1518
Neo-Synalar Cream (Infrequent) 2296
Norplant System 2484
Nutracort Cream & Lotion (Infrequent) 1684
Otic Tridesilon Solution 0.05% (Infrequent) 1612
PediOtic Suspension Sterile 797
Pramosone Cream, Lotion & Ointment 971
ProctoCream-HC (Infrequent) 1834
Proctofoam-HC 1835
Proglycem 649
Psorcon Ointment 0.05% 909
Psorion Cream 0.05% (Infrequent) 1121
Rogaine Topical Solution 2357
Synacort Creams 1%, 2.5% (Infrequent) 2296
Synalar (Infrequent) 2296
Temovate 1056
Topicort (Infrequent) 1098
Tridesilon Creme 0.05% (Infrequent) 1611
Tridesilon Ointment 0.05% (Infrequent) 1611
Ultravate Cream 0.05% (Infrequent) 2410
Ultravate Ointment 0.05% 2411
Vanoxide-HC Acne Lotion 911
Vioform-Hydrocortisone Cream and Mild Cream 889
Vioform-Hydrocortisone Ointment 889
Vytone Cream 1% 911
Westcort 2411

Hypertriglyceridemia

▲ Accutane Capsules (1 in 4) 1878
Blocadren Tablets 1429
Brevicon 2304
▲ Cipro I.V. (Among most frequent) 1592
Cipro Tablets 1589
Demulen 2161
Enovid 2161
Estrace 1385
Estrace Vaginal Cream 1388
Estratest 2245
Floxin Tablets 1652
Jenest-28 Tablets (A small proportion of women) 1636

Levlen/Tri-Levlen (A small portion of women) 665
Lo/Ovral Tablets 2471
Lo/Ovral-28 Tablets 2476
▲Lupron Depot 3.75 mg (12%) 2312
Micronor Tablets 1667
Modicon 1667
Nordette-21 Tablets 2481
Nordette-28 Tablets 2483
Norinyl 2304
Norpace (1 to 3%) 2177
Nor-Q D Tablets 2304
Ortho-Novum 1667
Ovcon 1391
Ovral Tablets 2490
Ovral-28 Tablets 2491
Ovrette Tablets 2492
Prinzide Tablets 1540
▲Synarel Nasal Solution (12%) 2300
▲Tegison Capsules (46%) 1881
Tegretol Chewable Tablets (Occasional) 654
Tegretol Suspension (Occasional) 656
Tegretol Tablets (Occasional) 654
Levlen/Tri-Levlen (A small portion of women) 665
Tri-Norinyl 28-Day Tablets 2304
Triphasil-21 Tablets 2527
Triphasil-28 Tablets 2532
Vaseretic Tablets 1559
Zestoretic 2274

Hypertrophic papillae of the tongue

Primaxin I.M. 1532
Primaxin I.V. (Less than 0.2%) 1535
Serentil 686

Hypertrophy, gum

Peganone Tablets 551
Zarontin Capsules 1768
Zarontin Syrup 1769

Hyperuricemia

▲Accutane Capsules (1 in 10 patients) 1878
Adriamycin PFS 561
Adriamycin RDF 562
Aldoclor Tablets 1413
Aldoril Tablets 1418
Altace Capsules (Rare) 1086
Anafranil Capsules (Infrequent) 650
Ansaid Tablets (Less than 1%) 2319
Apresazide Capsules 854
Apresoline-Esidrix Tablets 857
Axid Pulvules 1246
Benemid Tablets 1426
Blocadren Tablets 1429
Bufferin Analgesic Tablets and Caplets 743
▲Bumex (18.4%) 1895
Capozide 2258
Cardizem Tablets-30 mg, 60 mg, 90 mg and 120 mg 1329
Cardizem SR Capsules-60 mg, 90 mg and 120 mg (Less than 1%) 1327
Cerubidine 2443
▲Cipro I.V. (Among most frequent) 1592
Cipro Tablets (Less than 0.1%) 1589
Combipres Tablets 678
Corzide Tablets 702
Cotazym 1636
Creon Capsules 2245
Cytosar-U Sterile Powder 2329
Daranide Tablets 1445
Diucardin Tablets 2450
Diulo 2129
Diupres Tablets 1461
Diuril Oral Suspension 1464
Diuril Sodium Intravenous 1463
Diuril Tablets 1464
Doxorubicin Hydrochloride for Injection, USP 622
Doxorubicin Hydrochloride Injection, USP 848
Dyazide Capsules 2208
Ecotrin 2189
Edecrin 1468
Enduron Tablets 517
Enduronyl 518
Esidrix Tablets 863
Esimil Tablets 864
Exna Tablets 1862
Hydrea Capsules (Occasional) 728
HydroDIURIL Tablets 1484
Hydropres Tablets 1485
Inderide Tablets 2463
Inderide LA Long Acting Capsules 2465
Kerlone Tablets (Less than 2%) 2172
Larodopa Tablets 1905
Lasix 1093
Lopressor HCT Tablets 1034
Lorelco Tablets 1333
Lotensin Tablets 872
Lozol Tablets (Less than 5%) 1843
Lupron Depot 7.5 mg (Less than 5%) 2311
Lupron Injection 2310
Maxzide 1215
Minizide Capsules 1779
Moduretic Tablets 1510
Myambutol Tablets 1225
Mykrox ½ mg Tablets 984
Myleran Tablets 790
Naturetin Tablets (Occasional) 1789
▲Neupogen for Injection (27 to 58%) 595
Niacor Tablets 2376
Nicolar Tablets 1846
Normodyne Tablets 2110
Normozide Tablets 2112
Novantrone for Injection Concentrate 1226
Oretic Tablets 544
Oreticyl 545
Pancrease Capsules 1377
Pancrease MT Capsules (With extremely high dose) 1378
Parlodel 2020
Permax Tablets (Rare) 1291
Platinol 737
Platinol-AQ Injection 738
Prinzide Tablets 1540
Proglycem (Common) 649
Purinethol Tablets 800
Rauzide Tablets 1804
Renese Tablets 1785
Rifadin 1345
Rifamate Capsules 1347
Rimactane Capsules 879
Roferon-A Injection (Less than 5%) 1916
Rubex 739
Saluron 718
Sandimmune (Occasional) 2024
Ser-Ap-Es Tablets 881
Serpasil-Esidrix Tablets 886
Tenoretic Tablets 1105
Thalitone Tablets 687
Thioguanine Tablets, Tabloid Brand (Frequent) 815
Timolide Tablets 1547
Trandate HCT Tablets 579
Vaseretic Tablets (0.5% to 2.0%) 1559
Viokase 1877
Zaroxolyn Tablets 989
Zestoretic 2274
Zymase Capsules (With extremely high doses) 1645

Hyperuricosuria

Creon Capsules 2245

Hyperuricuria

Cotazym 1636
Myleran Tablets 790
Pancrease Capsules 1377
Pancrease MT Capsules (With extremely high dose) 1378
Viokase 1877
Zymase Capsules (With extremely high doses) 1645

Hyperventilation

Adenocard Injection (Less than 1%) 1007
Anafranil Capsules (Infrequent) 650
Ansaid Tablets (Less than 1%) 2319
Azdōne Tablets 844
Bumex (0.1%) 1895
BuSpar (Infrequent) 1401
Clozaril Tablets (Less than 1%) 2000
Damason-P 1356
Diprivan Injection (Less than 1%) 2267
Empirin with Codeine Phosphate Nos. 2, 3 & 4 764
Ethmozine Tablets (Less than 2%) 946
Lortab ASA Tablets 2414
Mono-Gesic Tablets 846
NebuPent for Inhalation Solution (1% or less) 1017
Orthoclone OKT3 Sterile Solution 1645
Permax Tablets (Infrequent) 1291
Primaxin I.M. 1532
Primaxin I.V. (Less than 0.2%) 1535
ProSom Tablets (Rare) 554
Protopam Chloride for Injection 2518
Prozac Pulvules (Infrequent) 920
Valium Injectable 1937
Versed Injection (Less than 1%) 1924
Voltaren Tablets (Less than 1%) 1042
▲Xanax Tablets (9.7%) 2367
Yutopar (Infrequent) 647

Hypervitaminosis A syndrome

Aquasol A Vitamin A Capsules, USP 615
Aquasol A Parenteral, USP 615

Hypesthesia

▲Ethmozine Tablets (2%-5%) 946
Lopid Capsules and Tablets 1736
NebuPent for Inhalation Solution (1% or less) 1017
Prozac Pulvules (Infrequent) 920

Hypnotic effects

Placidyl Capsules 553
Trilafon 2123

Hypoactivity

AeroBid Inhaler System (1-3%) 995
Valium Injectable 1937

Hypoadrenalism, neonatal

Aristocort Suspension 1008
Aristospan Suspension 1011
Azmacort Inhaler 1837
Celestone Soluspan Suspension 2081
Cortone Acetate Tablets 1439
Decadron Elixir 1445
Decadron Phosphate Injection 1449
Decadron Phosphate Respihaler 1454
Decadron Phosphate Turbinaire 1456
Decadron Phosphate with Xylocaine Injection, Sterile 1451
Decadron Tablets 1447
Decadron-LA Sterile Suspension 1457
Depo-Medrol Sterile Aqueous Suspension 2334
Hydeltrasol Injection, Sterile 1476
Hydeltra-T.B.A. Sterile Suspension 1478
Hydrocortone Acetate Sterile Suspension 1479
Hydrocortone Phosphate Injection, Sterile 1481
Hydrocortone Tablets 1482
Kenalog-40 Injection 2403
Maxidex Sterile Ophthalmic Ointment ◉ 222
Medrol 2348
Solu-Cortef Sterile Powder 2361
Solu-Medrol Sterile Powder 2363
Vancenase AQ Nasal Spray 0.042% 2127
Vancenase Nasal Inhaler 2126
Vanceril Inhaler 2128

Hypoalbuminemia

Dapsone USP 1130
▲Zanosar Sterile Powder (A number of patients) 2371

Hypoalbuminuria

Elspar 1470
Unasyn 1965

Hypocalcemia

Cortifoam 1827
Cosmegen Injection 1440
Fungizone Intravenous 2262
Ganite Injection 1016
Garamycin Injectable 2093
Kayexalate 2053
Mithracin 1602
Nebcin Vials, Hyporets & ADD-Vantage 1286
NebuPent for Inhalation Solution (1% or less) 1017
▲Paraplatin for Injection (22% to 31%) 735
Pentam 300 Injection (0.2%) 1018
Platinol 737
Platinol-AQ Injection 738
Roferon-A Injection (Less than 5%) 1916
Sodium Polystyrene Sulfonate Suspension 1993
Synarel Nasal Solution 2300
Yutopar 647

Hypocarbia

Exosurf Neonatal for Intratracheal Suspension 765
Survanta Beractant Intratracheal Suspension (Less than 1%) 1978

Hypochloremia

▲Bumex (14.9%) 1895
Diulo 2129
Dyazide Capsules 2208
Enduron Tablets 517
Enduronyl 518
Lozol Tablets (Less than 5%) 1843
Maxzide 1215
Mykrox ½ mg Tablets 984
Oretic Tablets 544
Oreticyl 545
Zaroxolyn Tablets 989

Hypochloremic alkalosis

Corzide Tablets 702
Diulo 2129
Diuril Sodium Intravenous 1463
Mykrox ½ mg Tablets 984
Prinzide Tablets 1540
Rauzide Tablets 1804
Tenoretic Tablets 1105
Thalitone Tablets 687
Vaseretic Tablets (0.5% to 2.0%) 1559
Zaroxolyn Tablets 989
Zestoretic 2274

Hypocoagulability

Orudis Capsules (Less than 1%) 2488

Hypoesthesia

Anafranil Capsules (Rare) 650
Cardura Tablets (0.5% to 1%) 1941
Engerix-B Unit-Dose Vials 2213
▲Intron A (1% to 10%) 2097
Normodyne Injection (1%) 2108
Procardia XL Tablets (1% or less) 1783
Sectral Capsules (Up to 2%) 2520
Tambocor Tablets (1-3%) 1315
Trandate Injection (1 of 100 patients) 577

Hypoestrogeneism

Danocrine Capsules 2046
▲Lupron Depot 3.75 mg (Among most frequent) 2312
▲Synarel Nasal Solution (Most frequent) 2300

Hypofibrinogenemia

Azo Gantrisin Tablets 1888
Depakene Capsules & Syrup 511
Depakote 512
Elspar 1470
Panhematin 546
Pitocin Injection, Ampoules, Steri-Dose Syringes 1757
Trental (Less than 1%) 1099

Hypogammaglobulinemia

Methotrexate Tablets, Parenteral, LPF Parenteral (Rare) 1217
Rheumatrex Methotrexate Dose Pack (Rare) 1234

Hypogeusia

Cuprimine Capsules (Some patients) 1442
Depen Titratable Tablets (Some patients) 2379

Hypoglycemia

Anaprox and Anaprox DS Tablets (Rare) 2288
Ancobon Capsules 1886
Azo Gantanol Tablets (Rare) 1887
Azo Gantrisin Tablets (Rare) 1888
Azulfidine Tablets, EN-tabs, Oral Suspension (Rare) 1157
Bactrim DS Tablets (Rare) 1891
Bactrim I.V. Infusion (Rare) 1889
Bactrim (Rare) 1891
Blocadren Tablets 1429
Children's Advil Suspension (Less than 1%) 2426
Cipro I.V. (Rare) 1592
Cipro Tablets (Less than 0.1%) 1589
Compazine 2201
Cuprimine Capsules 1442
Cytovene Sterile Powder (1% or less) 2292
Depen Titratable Tablets (Extremely rare) 2379
DiaBeta 1091
Diabinese Tablets 1775
Edecrin (In 2 uremic patients) 1468
Elavil 2269
Endep Tablets 1927
Etrafon 2087
Fansidar Tablets (Rare) 1896
Feldene Capsules (Less than 1%) 1777
Flexeril Tablets (Rare) 1471
Floxin Tablets (More than or equal to 1.0%) 1652
Furoxone 1855
Gantanol (Rare) 1899
Gantrisin Ophthalmic Ointment/Solution 1900
Gantrisin (Rare) 1901
Haldol Decanoate 1375

Haldol Injection, Tablets and Concentrate 1373
Humulin 70/30, 100 Units 1267
Humulin BR, 100 Units 1268
Humulin L, 100 Units 1268
Humulin U, 100 Units 1272
Beef Regular, 100 Units 1275
Indocin I.V. (1% to 3%) 1490
Limbitrol 1933
Ludiomil Tablets (Rare) 874
▲Lupron Depot 3.75 mg (Among most frequent) 2312
Lupron Depot 7.5 mg 2311
Lupron Injection (Less than 5%) 2310
Micronase Tablets 2350
Mithracin 1602
Motrin Tablets (Less than 1%) 2351
Naprosyn (Rare) 2297
Navane Capsules and Concentrate 1954
Navane Intramuscular 1956
NebuPent for Inhalation Solution (1% or less) 1017
Normodyne Injection 2108
Norpace 2177
Norpramin Tablets 1340
Omnipaque (0.3%) 2552
Orinase Tablets 2354
Pamelor 2019
PediaProfen Suspension (Less than 1%) 1363
Pediazole (Rare) 1973
Pentam 300 Injection (2.4 to 3.5%) 1018
Permax Tablets (Infrequent) 1291
Prilosec Delayed-Release Capsules (Less than 1%) 1530
Prostin VR Pediatric Sterile Solution (Less than 1%) 2355
Prozac Pulvules (Infrequent) 920
Rufen Tablets (Less than 1%) 691
Sandostatin Injection (1.2%) 2029
Septra (Rare) 813
Septra I.V. Infusion (Rare) 808
Septra I.V. Infusion ADD-Vantage Vials (Rare) 810
Septra (Rare) 813
Sinequan 1960
Stelazine 2226
Surmontil Capsules 2524
Taractan 1920
Thiosulfil Forte Tablets (Rare) 2526
Thorazine 2234
Timolide Tablets 1547
Timoptic in Ocudose 1552
Timoptic Sterile Ophthalmic Solution 1550
Tofranil Ampuls 1038
Tofranil Tablets 1039
Tofranil-PM Capsules 1041
Triavil Tablets 1556
Trilafon 2123
Vivactil Tablets 1567
Voltaren Tablets (Less than 1%) 1042
Yutopar 647
Zanosar Sterile Powder 2371

Hypoglycemia, neonatal

Brethine Ampuls 1026
Brethine Tablets 1026
Bricanyl Injection 1324
DiaBeta 1091
Normodyne Tablets (Rare) 2110

Hypohidrosis

Bellergal-S Tablets (Rare) 1998
Bentyl 1322
Cantil Tablets 1326
Cyclogyl ◉ 215
Cyclomydril ◉ 216
Darbid Tablets 2205
Ditropan 1332
Donnatal 1858
Donnatal Extentabs 1859
Donnatal Tablets 1858
Donnazyme Tablets 1860
Kinesed Tablets 2272
Kutrase Capsules 2146
Levsin/Levsinex 2147
Pro-Banthīne Tablets 2141
Quarzan Capsules 1937
Robinul Forte Tablets 1873
Robinul Injectable 1873
Robinul Tablets 1873
Valpin 50 Tablets 941

Hypokalemia

Aldactazide 2150
Aldoril Tablets 1418
Anafranil Capsules (Infrequent) 650
Ancobon Capsules 1886
Arfonad Ampuls 1887
Aristocort Suspension 1008
Aristospan Suspension 1011
▲Bumex (14.7%) 1895
Cardura Tablets (Less than 0.5% of 3960 patients) 1941
Celestone Soluspan Suspension 2081
Cephulac Syrup 1331
Chronulac Syrup 1332
Cipro I.V. (Infrequent) 1592
Colestid Granules 2328
Combipres Tablets 678
Cortenema 2244
Cortifoam 1827
Cortone Acetate Sterile Suspension 1437
Cortone Acetate Tablets 1439
Corzide Tablets 702
Dalalone D.P. Injectable 999
Daranide Tablets 1445
Decadron Elixir 1445
Decadron Phosphate Injection 1449
Decadron Phosphate Respihaler 1454
Decadron Phosphate Turbinaire 1456
Decadron Phosphate with Xylocaine Injection, Sterile 1451
Decadron Tablets 1447
Decadron-LA Sterile Suspension 1457
Deltasone Tablets 2332
Depo-Medrol Sterile Aqueous Suspension 2334
Digibind 762
Diulo 2129
Diuril Sodium Intravenous 1463
Dobutrex Solution Vials (Rare) 1259
Dyazide Capsules 2208
Dyrenium Capsules (Rare) 2210
Enduron Tablets 517
Enduronyl 518
Fungizone Intravenous (Common) 2262
Garamycin Injectable 2093
Hydeltrasol Injection, Sterile 1476
Hydeltra-T.B.A. Sterile Suspension 1478
Hydrocortone Acetate Sterile Suspension 1479
Hydrocortone Phosphate Injection, Sterile 1481
Hydrocortone Tablets 1482
HydroDIURIL Tablets 1484
Kayexalate 2053
Kenalog-10 Injection 2402
Kenalog-40 Injection 2403
Kerlone Tablets (Less than 2%) 2172
Lamprene Capsules (Less than 1%) 1030
Lanoxicaps 772
Lopressor HCT Tablets (Less than 10 in 100 patients) 1034
▲Lozol Tablets (3 to 7%) 1843
Maxzide 1215
Medrol 2348
Mezlin (Rare) 1597
Mezlin Pharmacy Bulk Package 1599
Mithracin 1602
Mykrox ½ mg Tablets 984
Nebcin Vials, Hyporets & ADD-Vantage 1286
Normozide Tablets (1%) 2112
Norpace (1 to 3%) 2177
Oretic Tablets 544
Oreticyl 545
▲Paraplatin for Injection (20% to 28%) 735
Pediapred Oral Liquid 987
Permax Tablets (Infrequent) 1291
Pipracil (Rare with high doses) 1230
Platinol 737
Platinol-AQ Injection 738
Prinzide Tablets 1540
Prostin VR Pediatric Sterile Solution (1%) 2355
Prozac Pulvules (Rare) 920
Rauzide Tablets 1804
Renese Tablets 1785
Sinemet CR Tablets 953
Sodium Polystyrene Sulfonate Suspension 1993
Solu-Cortef Sterile Powder 2361
Solu-Medrol Sterile Powder 2363
▲Tegison Capsules (25-50%) 1881
Tenoretic Tablets 1105
Thalitone Tablets 687
Timentin for Injection 2239
Trandate HCT Tablets (1% in 208 patients) 579
Vaseretic Tablets (0.5% to 2.0%) 1559
Zaroxolyn Tablets 989
Zestoretic 2274
Zofran Injection (Rare) 1069
Zovirax Sterile Powder (Less than 1%) 828

Hypokalemic alkalosis

Aristocort Suspension 1008
Aristospan Suspension 1011
Celestone Soluspan Suspension 2081
Cortenema 2244
Cortone Acetate Sterile Suspension 1437
Cortone Acetate Tablets 1439
Dalalone D.P. Injectable 999
Decadron Elixir 1445
Decadron Phosphate Injection 1449
Decadron Phosphate Respihaler 1454
Decadron Phosphate Turbinaire 1456
Decadron Phosphate with Xylocaine Injection, Sterile 1451
Decadron Tablets 1447
Decadron-LA Sterile Suspension 1457
Deltasone Tablets 2332
Depo-Medrol Sterile Aqueous Suspension 2334
Hydeltrasol Injection, Sterile 1476
Hydeltra-T.B.A. Sterile Suspension 1478
Hydrocortone Acetate Sterile Suspension 1479
Hydrocortone Phosphate Injection, Sterile 1481
Hydrocortone Tablets 1482
Kenalog-10 Injection 2402
Kenalog-40 Injection 2403
Medrol 2348
Pediapred Oral Liquid 987
Solu-Cortef Sterile Powder 2361
Solu-Medrol Sterile Powder 2363

Hypokinesia

Anafranil Capsules (Infrequent) 650
▲Clozaril Tablets (4%) 2000
Doral Tablets 2383
Permax Tablets (Infrequent) 1291
▲ProSom Tablets (8%) 554
Tenex Tablets (Less than 3%) 1875

Hypomagnesemia

Capozide 2258
Corzide Tablets 702
Diuril Sodium Intravenous 1463
Fungizone Intravenous 2262
Garamycin Injectable 2093
HydroDIURIL Tablets 1484
Lanoxicaps 772
Maxzide 1215
Nebcin Vials, Hyporets & ADD-Vantage 1286
▲Paraplatin for Injection (29% to 43%) 735
Platinol 737
Platinol-AQ Injection 738
Prinzide Tablets 1540
Rauzide Tablets 1804
Sandimmune (In some patients) 2024
Vaseretic Tablets (0.5% to 2.0%) 1559
Zestoretic 2274

Hypomania

Asendin Tablets (Less than 1%) 1196
Desyrel and Desyrel Dividose (Less than 1%) 1404
Endep Tablets (Rare) 1927
Limbitrol 1933
Ludiomil Tablets (Rare) 874
▲Marplan Tablets (Among most frequent) 1906
Norpramin Tablets 1340
Pamelor 2019
Surmontil Capsules 2524
Tofranil Ampuls 1038
Tofranil Tablets 1039
Tofranil-PM Capsules 1041
Triavil Tablets (Rare) 1556
Vivactil Tablets 1567
Wellbutrin Tablets (Frequent) 821
Xanax Tablets 2367

Hypomenorrhea

Prozac Pulvules (Rare) 920

Hyponatremia

Actimmune (Rare) 1046
Aldactone 2152
▲Bumex (9.2%) 1895
Capoten 2255
Capozide 2258
Colestid Granules 2328
Corzide Tablets 702
DDAVP Injection 1840
DDAVP 1841
DiaBeta 1091
Diulo 2129
Diuril Sodium Intravenous 1463
Dyazide Capsules 2208
Enduron Tablets 517
Enduronyl 518
Garamycin Injectable 2093
Glucotrol 1952
Haldol Decanoate 1375
Haldol Injection, Tablets and Concentrate 1373
▲Indocin I.V. (3% to 9%) 1490
Lotensin Tablets (Scattered incidents) 872
Lozol Tablets (Less than 5%) 1843
Maxzide 1215
Micronase Tablets 2350
Moduretic Tablets 1510
Monopril Tablets (0.2 to 1.0%) 1406
Mykrox ½ mg Tablets 984
Nebcin Vials, Hyporets & ADD-Vantage 1286
Nimotop Capsules (Less than 1%) 1607
Oncovin Solution Vials & Hyporets 1288
Oretic Tablets 544
Oreticyl 545
Orinase Tablets 2354
Orudis Capsules (Less than 1%) 2488
▲Paraplatin for Injection (29% to 47%) 735
Platinol 737
Platinol-AQ Injection 738
Primaxin I.M. 1532
Primaxin I.V. 1535
Prinzide Tablets 1540
Prozac Pulvules (Rare) 920
Rauzide Tablets 1804
Rythmol Tablets (Less than 1%) 1184
Tegretol Chewable Tablets 654
Tegretol Suspension 656
Tegretol Tablets 654
Tenoretic Tablets 1105
Thalitone Tablets 687
Tolinase Tablets 2365
Vaseretic Tablets (0.5% to 2.0%) 1559
Vasotec I.V. (0.5 to 1%) 1562
Vasotec Tablets (0.5% to 1%) 1564
Zaroxolyn Tablets 989
Zestoretic 2274

Hyponatremia, dilutional

Capozide 2258
Corzide Tablets 702
Diuril Sodium Intravenous 1463
Prinzide Tablets 1540
Rauzide Tablets 1804
Renese Tablets 1785
Vaseretic Tablets 1559
Zestoretic 2274

Hypophosphatemia

ALternaGEL Liquid 1154
Basaljel 2438
Capozide (A few patients) 2258
Corzide Tablets 702
Diulo 2129
▲Ganite Injection (Up to 79%) 1016
Gelusil Liquid & Tablets ■ 639
Maalox Plus Extra Strength 1850
Maxzide 1215
Mithracin 1602
Mykrox ½ mg Tablets 984
Mylanta 1155
Mylanta • Double Strength 1155
Platinol 737
Platinol-AQ Injection 738
Rauzide Tablets (Few patients) 1804
Rolaids ■ 743
Zanosar Sterile Powder 2371
Zaroxolyn Tablets 989

Hypopigmentation

Accutane Capsules (Less than 1%) 1878
Aclovate Cream 1053
Alphatrex Cream, Ointment & Lotion (Infrequent) 2076
Analpram-HC Rectal Cream 1% and 2.5% 970
Anusol-HC Cream (Infrequent) 1690
Anusol-HC Suppositories 1691
Aristospan Suspension (Intra-articular) 1011
Betatrex Cream, Ointment & Lotion 2077
Carmol HC Cream 1% (Infrequent) 2296
Celestone Soluspan Suspension 2081
Cortisporin Cream 757
Cortisporin Ointment 758
Cortisporin Otic Solution Sterile 760
Cortisporin Otic Suspension Sterile 760
Cortone Acetate Sterile Suspension 1437
Cutivate Cream 0.05% 1054

Cutivate Ointment 0.005% (Infrequent to more frequent) 1054
Cyclocort Lotion (Infrequent) 1198
Dalalone D.P. Injectable 999
Decadron Phosphate Injection 1449
Decadron Phosphate Topical Cream 1455
Decadron Phosphate with Xylocaine Injection, Sterile 1451
Decadron-LA Sterile Suspension 1457
Decaspray Topical Aerosol 1459
Depo-Medrol Sterile Aqueous Suspension 2334
DesOwen Cream, Ointment and Lotion (Infrequent) 1682
Diprolene (Infrequent) 2083
Eldecort Cream 1.0% (Infrequent) 1113
Eldecort Cream 1.0% and 2.5% (Infrequent) 1113
Elocon (Infrequent) 2084
Epifoam 1828
Florone/Florone E 908
Halog (Infrequent) 2399
Hydeltrasol Injection, Sterile 1476
Hydeltra-T.B.A. Sterile Suspension 1478
Hydrocortone Acetate Sterile Suspension 1479
Hydrocortone Phosphate Injection, Sterile 1481
Hytone 909
Kenalog Cream, Lotion & Ointment (Infrequent) 2401
Kenalog-10 Injection 2402
Kenalog-40 Injection 2403
Lidex (Infrequent) 2296
Locoid Cream, Ointment and Topical Solution (Infrequent) 970
Lotrisone Cream (Infrequent) 2103
Mantadil Cream 789
Maxivate Cream, Lotion & Ointment 0.05% 2406
Mycolog II Cream and Ointment (Infrequent) 2407
Mytrex Cream & Ointment (Infrequent) 2080
NeoDecadron Topical Cream 1518
Neo-Synalar Cream (Infrequent) 2296
Nutracort Cream & Lotion (Infrequent) 1684
Orabase HCA Oral Paste (Infrequent) 890
Otic Tridesilon Solution 0.05% (Infrequent) 1612
Oxsoralen-Ultra Capsule 1117
PediOtic Suspension Sterile 797
Pramosone Cream, Lotion & Ointment 971
ProctoCream-HC (Infrequent) 1834
Proctofoam-HC 1835
Psorcon Ointment 0.05% 909
Psorion Cream 0.05% (Infrequent) 1121
Retin-A (tretinoin) Cream/Gel/Liquid 1680
Solu-Cortef Sterile Powder 2361
Solu-Medrol Sterile Powder 2363
Synacort Creams 1%, 2.5% (Infrequent) 2296
Synalar (Infrequent) 2296
Temovate 1056
Topicort (Infrequent) 1098
Tridesilon Creme 0.05% (Infrequent) 1611
Tridesilon Ointment 0.05% (Infrequent) 1611
Ultravate Cream 0.05% (Infrequent) 2410
Ultravate Ointment 0.05% 2411
Vanoxide-HC Acne Lotion 911
Vioform-Hydrocortisone Cream and Mild Cream 889
Vioform-Hydrocortisone Ointment 889
Vytone Cream 1% 911
Westcort 2411

Hypoplasia, enamel

Achromycin V Capsules 1193
Declomycin Capsules, Tablets 1199
Doryx Capsules 1717
Minocin Intravenous 1221
Minocin Oral Suspension 1224
Monodox Capsules 1630
Terramycin Capsules 1786
Terramycin Intramuscular Solution 1964
Vibramycin Hyclate Capsules 1787
Vibramycin Hyclate Intravenous 1968
Vibramycin 1787

Hypoplasia, myeloid

Capoten 2255
Capozide 2258

Hypoplastic anemia

Chloromycetin Kapseals 1695
Cytovene Sterile Powder (2%) 2292
Depakote Sprinkle Capsules 512
Diulo 2129
Eminase (Less than 1%) 2211
Mykrox ½ mg Tablets 984
Myochrysine Injection 1516
Optimine Tablets 2115
Paradione Capsules 548
Polaramine 2116
Prilosec Delayed-Release Capsules (Less than 1%) 1530
Procan SR Tablets 1760
Pronestyl Capsules and Tablets (Approximately 0.5%) 1800
Pronestyl Injection (Approximately 0.5%) 1798
Pronestyl-SR Tablets (0.5%) 1801
▲ Retrovir Capsules (3% to 29%) 802
▲ Retrovir I.V. Infusion (1% to 45%) 805
▲ Retrovir Syrup (3% to 29%) 802
Rythmol Tablets (Less than 1%) 1184
Solganal Suspension (Rare) 2122
Tonocard Tablets (Less than 1%) 1554
Tridione 557
Trinalin Repetabs Tablets 1170
Zaroxolyn Tablets 989
Zovirax Sterile Powder (Less than 1%) 828

Hypopnea

Humulin 70/30, 100 Units 1267
Humulin BR, 100 Units 1268
Humulin L, 100 Units 1268
Humulin U, 100 Units 1272
Stadol (Less than 1%) 721

Hypoproteinemia

Cipro I.V. 1592
Lupron Depot 7.5 mg 2311
Lupron Injection 2310
Unasyn 1965
Zefazone Sterile Powder 2372

Hypoprothrombinemia

Azo Gantanol Tablets 1887
Azo Gantrisin Tablets 1888
Azulfidine Tablets, EN-tabs, Oral Suspension (Rare) 1157
Bactrim DS Tablets 1891
Bactrim I.V. Infusion 1889
Bactrim 1891
Cardioquin Tablets 1812
Cipro I.V. (Rare) 1592
Fansidar Tablets 1896
Gantanol 1899
Gantrisin Ophthalmic Ointment/Solution 1900
Gantrisin 1901
Limbitrol DS Tablets (Rare) 1933
Mithracin 1602
Pediazole 1973
Questran Light 711
Quinaglute Dura-Tabs Tablets 663
Quinamm Tablets 1344
Quinidex Extentabs 1868
Rocephin Injectable Vials, ADD-Vantage (Rare) 1914
Septra 813
Septra I.V. Infusion 808
Septra I.V. Infusion ADD-Vantage Vials 810
Septra 813
Tapazole Tablets 1298
Thiosulfil Forte Tablets 2526
Zefazone Sterile Powder 2372

Hypoprothrombinemia, paradoxical

Konakion Injection 1903

Hypopyon

Healon (Rare) ◉ 279

Hyporeflexia

Compazine 2201
Matulane Capsules 1907
ProSom Tablets (Rare) 554
Prozac Pulvules (Rare) 920
▲ Retrovir (5.6%) 802
Stelazine 2226
Tegretol 654
Thorazine 2234

Hyporeflexia, neonatal

Compazine 2201
Stelazine Concentrate 2226
Thorazine 2234

Hyporesponsive episode, unspecified

HibTITER (One case) 1206

Hypospadias

Megace Tablets 732

Hyposthenuria

Fungizone Intravenous (Common) 2262

Hypotension

Abbokinase 503
Abbokinase Open-Cath 505
Actifed with Codeine Cough Syrup 752
Actimmune (Rare) 1046
Activase 1047
▲ Adalat Capsules (10 mg and 20 mg) (Approximately 5%) 1587
Adenocard Injection (Less than 1%) 1007
AK-Fluor Injection 10% and 25% ◉ 204
Aldoclor Tablets 1413
Aldomet Oral 1415
Aldoril Tablets 1418
▲ Alfenta Injection (10%) 1131
▲ Alferon N Injection (6%) 1809
Altace Capsules (Rare to more frequent) 1086
Alurate Elixir (Less than 1 in 100) 1883
Amicar Syrup, Tablets, and Injection (Occasional) 1194
Amikin Injectable (Rare) 602
Aminophyllin Tablets 2153
Anectine 755
▲ Anestacon Solution (Among most common) 2394
Apresazide Capsules (Less frequent) 854
Apresoline Hydrochloride Parenteral (Ampuls) 856
Apresoline Hydrochloride Tablets (Less frequent) 855
Apresoline-Esidrix Tablets 857
AquaMEPHYTON Injection 1422
Aralen Hydrochloride Injection (Rare) 2038
Aralen Phosphate with Primaquine Phosphate Tablets (Rare) 2040
Aralen Phosphate Tablets (Rare) 2039
Asbron G 1997
Asendin Tablets (Less than 1%) 1196
Atgam Sterile Solution (At least 1 patient and less than 5% of total patients) 2320
Ativan Injection (0.1%) 2432
Ativan Tablets (Rare) 2434
Atrohist Sprinkle Capsules 558
Atrovent Inhalation Aerosol 675
Azactam for Injection (Less than 1%) 2252
Benadryl Capsules 1691
Benadryl Injection 1692
Betagan ◉ 239
Blenoxane (1%) 724
▲ Blocadren Tablets (3%) 1429
▲ Bretylol Injection (3%) 923
▲ Brevibloc Injection (20% to 50%) 942
Brevital Sodium Vials 1248
Bronkephrine Injection 2042
Bumex (0.8%) 1895
BuSpar (Infrequent) 1401
Butisol Sodium Elixir & Tablets (Less than 1 in 100) 2377
Calan SR Caplets (2.5%) 2157
Calan Tablets (2.5%) 2155
Capoten 2255
Capozide 2258
Carbocaine Hydrochloride Injection 2043
Cardene Capsules (Rare) 2290
Cardilate Oral/Sublingual Tablets 757
Cardioquin Tablets 1812
Cardizem Tablets-30 mg, 60 mg, 90 mg and 120 mg (Less than 1%) 1329
Cardizem SR Capsules-60 mg, 90 mg and 120 mg (1%) 1327
Cardura Tablets (1%) 1941
Centrax 1693
Ceptaz for Injection (Rare) 1057
Choledyl Pediatric Elixir 1702
Choledyl Tablets 1700
Choledyl SA Tablets 1704
Cibalith-S 870
Cipro I.V. (1% or less) 1592
Cleocin Phosphate Injection (Rare) 2325
Clinoril Tablets (Less than 1 in 100) 1433
▲ Clozaril Tablets (More than 5 to 9%) 2000
Comhist LA Capsules 1618
Compazine 2201
Constant-T Tablets 1029
Cordarone Tablets (Less than 1%) 2446
Corgard Tablets (1 in 100 patients) 701
Corzide Tablets (1%) 702
Cyklokapron Tablets and Injection 1159
▲ Cytadren Tablets (1 in 30) 861
CytoGam 891
Cytotec (Infrequent) 2159
Cytovene Sterile Powder (1% or less) 2292
DDAVP Injection 1840
Dalgan Injection (Less than 1%) 620
Dalmane Capsules (Rare) 1927
Decadron Phosphate with Xylocaine Injection, Sterile 1451
Deconamine 663
Deconsal 559
Demerol 2047
Deponit NTG Transdermal Delivery System (Less frequent) 2143
Deprol Tablets 2382
Desferal Vials 862
Desyrel and Desyrel Dividose (Greater than 1%) 1404
Dilantin Parenteral 1712
Dilatrate-SR 1827
Dilaudid 1173
Dilaudid-HP Injection 1175
Dilor 2079
Dimetane-DC Cough Syrup 1857
Dimetane-DX Cough Syrup 1858
Diphtheria and Tetanus Toxoids and Pertussis Vaccine Adsorbed USP (For Pediatric Use) (Rare) 892
▲ Diprivan Injection (3% to 10%) 2267
Disalcid 1310
Diupres Tablets 1461
Diuril Oral Suspension 1464
Diuril Sodium Intravenous 1463
Diuril Tablets 1464
Dobutrex Solution Vials (Occasionally) 1259
Duragesic Transdermal System (1% to 3%) 1133
Duranest Injections 624
Duvoid Tablets 1853
Dyazide Capsules 2208
Dyclone 0.5% and 1% Topical Solutions, USP 626
DynaCirc Capsules (0.5% to 1%) 2004
Elavil 2269
Eldepryl 2250
Emete-con Intramuscular/Intravenous 1950
▲ Eminase (10.4%) 2211
Endep Tablets 1927
Engerix-B Unit-Dose Vials (Less than 1%) 2213
Enlon Injection 598
Esidrix Tablets 863
Esimil Tablets 864
Eskalith 2214
Ethmozine Tablets (Less than 2%) 946
Ethrane 599
Etrafon 2087
▲ Exosurf Neonatal for Intratracheal Suspension (54% to 77%) 765
Fedahist Gyrocaps 2145
Fedahist Timecaps 2145
Flexeril Tablets (Less than 1%) 1471
Fluorescite ◉ 217
Fluothane 2453
Forane 600
Fortaz (Rare) 1060
▲ Fungizone Intravenous (Among most common) 2262
Furoxone 1855
Gamimune N Immune Globulin Intravenous (Human) (Rare) 1572
Gammar-IV, Immune Globulin Intravenous (Human) 610
Ganite Injection 1016
Garamycin Injectable 2093
Haldol Decanoate 1375
Haldol Injection, Tablets and Concentrate 1373
Humulin 70/30, 100 Units (Less common) 1267
Humulin BR, 100 Units (Less common) 1268
Humulin L, 100 Units (Less common) 1268
Humulin U, 100 Units (Less common) 1272
HydroDIURIL Tablets 1484
Hydromox R Tablets 1209
Hydromox Tablets 1208
Hydropres Tablets 1485
▲ Hyperstat I.V. Injection (7%) 2095

Hyskon Hysteroscopy Fluid (Rare).. 1162
Hytrin Tablets 529
IFEX (Less than 1%) 729
Imferon 976
Inapsine Injection 1140
Inderal 2459
Inderal LA Long Acting Capsules 2461
Inderide Tablets 2463
Inderide LA Long Acting Capsules .. 2465
Indocin Capsules (Less than 1%) 1487
Indocin I.V. (Less than 1%) 1490
Indocin (Less than 1%) 1487
▲ Innovar Injection (Most common) 1141
Inocor Lactate Injection (1.3%) 2048
Insulatard NPH 1626
Insulatard NPH Human 1627
▲ Intron A (Up to 8%) 2097
▲ Intropin Injection (Among most frequent) 930
Ismelin Tablets 869
Isoptin Injectable (1.5%) 1177
Isoptin Oral Tablets (2.5%) 1179
Isoptin SR Sustained Release Tablets (2.5%) 1181
Isopto Atropine ◉ 218
▲ Isordil (2 to 36%) 2467
Isuprel Hydrochloride Injection 1:5000 2050
Kerlone Tablets (Less than 2%) 2172
Ketalar 1726
Klorvess Effervescent Granules 2010
Klorvess Effervescent Tablets 2011
Klorvess 10% Liquid 2010
Levo-Dromoran (Infrequent) 1906
Librium Injectable (Isolated cases) 1932
Limbitrol 1933
Lincocin (Rare) 2344
▲ Lioresal Tablets (0-9%) 1031
Lithane Tablets 1596
Lithium Carbonate Capsules & Tablets 1984
Lithobid Tablets 870
Lopressor Ampuls (1%) 1032
Lopressor HCT Tablets 1034
Lopressor Tablets (1%) 1032
Loxitane 1213
Ludiomil Tablets (Rare) 874
Lufyllin & Lufyllin-400 Tablets 2384
Lufyllin-GG Elixir & Tablets 2385
▲ Lupron Depot 3.75 mg (Among most frequent) 2312
Lupron Depot 7.5 mg 2311
Lupron Injection 2310
MS Contin Tablets (Infrequent) 1814
MSIR (Infrequent) 1817
Marcaine Hydrochloride 0.5% with Epinephrine 1:200,000 (as bitartrate) 958
Marcaine Hydrochloride with Epinephrine 1:200,000 2055
Marcaine Hydrochloride Injection 2055
Marcaine Spinal 2058
Matulane Capsules 1907
Maxair Inhaler (Less than 1%) 1311
Mebaral Tablets (Less than 1 in 100) 2061
Mefoxin 1498
Mefoxin Premixed Intravenous Solution 1500
Mellaril 2011
Mepergan Injection (Rare) 2479
Mephyton Tablets (Rare) 1503
▲ Mesnex Injection (17%) 733
Methergine 2016
Metubine Iodide Vials 1285
Mexitil Capsules (Less than 1% or about 6 in 1,000) 680
▲ Minitran Transdermal Delivery System (4%) 1312
Mintezol 1510
Miochol with Iocare Steri-Tags, Miochol System Pak and Miochol System Pak Plus (Rare) ◉ 274
Mixtard 70/30 1627
Mixtard Human 70/30 1628
Moban Tablets & Concentrate (Rare) 932
Monopril Tablets (0.2 to 1.0%) 1406
Naldecon Syrup, Tablets, Pediatric Drops and Pediatric Syrup 709
Narcan Injection 933
Navane Capsules and Concentrate 1954
Navane Intramuscular 1956
NebuPent for Inhalation Solution (1% or less) 1017
Nembutal Sodium Capsules (Less than 1%) 534
Nembutal Sodium Solution (Less than 1%) 536
Nembutal Sodium Suppositories (Less than 1%) 538
Nescaine/Nescaine MPF 629
Netromycin Injection 100 mg/ml (Fewer than 1 of 1000 patients) 2104
Niacor Tablets 2376
Nicolar Tablets 1846
▲ Nimotop Capsules (1.2%-50.0%) 1607
Nitro-Bid IV 1338
Nitro-Bid Ointment 1339
Nitrodisc (Infrequent) 2176
Nitro-Dur (nitroglycerin) Transdermal Infusion System (Infrequent) 1164
Nitrogard Tablets (Infrequent) 1004
Nitrolingual Spray 1846
Norcuron (Rare) 1642
Normodyne Injection 2108
Normozide Tablets (Less common) 2112
Norpace (1 to 3%) 2177
Norpramin Tablets 1340
Norzine 1818
Novafed A Capsules 1342
Novafed Capsules 1342
Novahistine DH 1342
Novahistine DMX ▣ 595
Novahistine Elixir ▣ 596
Novahistine Expectorant 1343
Novantrone for Injection Concentrate (Occasional) 1226
Novocain Hydrochloride for Spinal Anesthesia 2065
Nubain Injection (Less than 1%) 934
Nuromax Injection 794
Omnipaque (Less than 0.1%) 2552
Oncovin Solution Vials & Hyporets 1288
Optimine Tablets 2115
OptiPranolol Sterile Ophthalmic Solution (A small number of patients) ◉ 261
Oramorph SR (Morphine Sulfate Sustained Release Tablets) (Less frequent) 1988
Orap Tablets 1020
Ornade Spansule Capsules 2221
Orthoclone OKT3 Sterile Solution .. 1645
Oxsoralen-Ultra Capsule 1117
PBZ Tablets & Elixir 1037
PBZ-SR Tablets 1037
Pamelor 2019
Pantopon Injectable 1911
Paraplatin for Injection (Rare) 735
Parlodel 2020
Pentam 300 Injection (0.9%, 4.0%) 1018
Periactin 1525
Permax Tablets (2.1%) 1291
Phenergan with Codeine 2497
Phenergan with Dextromethorphan 2499
Phenergan Injection 2493
Phenergan Suppositories 2496
Phenergan Syrup 2495
Phenergan Tablets 2496
Phenergan VC 2500
Phenergan VC with Codeine 2501
Phenobarbital Elixir and Tablets (Less than 1 in 100 patients) 1293
Placidyl Capsules 553
Plague Vaccine (Rare) 1584
Plasma-Plex Plasma Protein Fraction (Human) 613
Platinol (Occasional) 737
Platinol-AQ Injection (Occasional) .. 738
Plendil Extended-Release Tablets (0.5% to 1.5%) 1526
Polaramine 2116
Pondimin Tablets 1867
Pontocaine Hydrochloride for Spinal Anesthesia 2069
Pre-Pen 2148
Primaxin I.M. 1532
Primaxin I.V. (0.4%) 1535
Prinivil Tablets (1.2%) 1538
Prinzide Tablets (1.4%) 1540
Priscoline Hydrochloride Ampuls 877
Procan SR Tablets (Rare) 1760
▲ Procardia Capsules (5%) 1781
Procardia XL Tablets (1% or less).. 1783
Proglycem (Rare) 649
Prolixin Decanoate (Rare) 1795
Prolixin Elixir (Rare) 1793
Prolixin Enanthate (Rare) 1796
Prolixin Injection (Rare) 1791
Prolixin Oral Concentrate (Rare) 1792
Prolixin Tablets (Rare) 1793
Pronestyl Capsules and Tablets (Rare) 1800
▲ Pronestyl Injection (More common) 1798
Pronestyl-SR Tablets (Rare) 1801
Prostigmin Injectable 1120
Prostigmin Tablets 1121
▲ Prostin VR Pediatric Sterile Solution (4%) 2355
Protamine Sulfate Ampoules & Vials 1295
Provocholine for Inhalation 1911
Prozac Pulvules (Infrequent) 920
Quadrinal Tablets 1183
Quibron Capsules 713
Quibron-T 714
Quibron-T/SR 716
Quinaglute Dura-Tabs Tablets 663
Quinidex Extentabs 1868
Rauzide Tablets 1804
Recombivax HB (Less than 1%) 1544
Regitine 878
Reglan 1869
Respbid Tablets 684
Rifadin 1345
Robaxin Injectable 1871
▲ Roferon-A Injection (4%) 1916
Rogaine Topical Solution (1.53%).. 2357
Roxanol 1991
Rum-K Syrup 995
Ru-Tuss II Capsules 693
Ru-Tuss with Hydrocodone 694
Ru-Tuss Tablets 693
Rythmol Tablets (0.1 to 1.1%) 1184
Salflex 839
Sandoglobulin I.V. (Less than 1%).. 2027
Seconal Sodium Pulvules (Less than 1 in 100) 1296
Sectral Capsules (Up to 2%) 2520
Seldane Tablets (Rare) 1349
Seldane-D Extended-Release Tablets (Rare) 1350
Sensorcaine (Rare) 631
Sensorcaine-MPF Spinal (Rare) 634
Ser-Ap-Es Tablets 881
Serentil 686
Serpasil-Apresoline Tablets 884
Sinemet CR Tablets 953
Sinequan (Occasional) 1960
Slo-bid Gyrocaps 1847
Solu-Medrol Sterile Powder 2363
Soma Compound w/Codeine Tablets 2390
Soma Compound Tablets 2389
Soma Tablets 2388
Sorbitrate 1103
Stadol (Less than 1%) 721
Stelazine 2226
▲ Streptase for Infusion (1 to 10%).. 635
Sublimaze Injection 1146
▲ Sufenta Injection (7%) 1147
Surital Ampoules, Steri-Vials 1764
Surmontil Capsules 2524
Survanta Beractant Intratracheal Suspension (Less than 1%) 1978
T-PHYL (Uniphyl) 200 mg Tablets 1820
Talacen (Infrequent) 2070
Talwin Compound (Infrequent) 2072
Talwin Nx 2073
Tambocor Tablets (Less than 1%) 1315
Taractan (Common) 1920
Tavist Syrup 2033
Tavist Tablets 2035
Tavist-D Tablets 2035
Tegretol Chewable Tablets 654
Tegretol Suspension 656
Tegretol Tablets 654
▲ Tenormin Tablets and I.V. Injection (25%) 1107
Tensilon Injectable 1123
Thalitone Tablets 687
Theo-24 2179
Theo-Dur Sprinkle 1168
Theo-Dur Extended-Release Tablets 1166
Theolair 1317
Theolair-SR Tablets 1319
▲ TheoX Extended-Release Tablets (Among most consistent) 841
Timolide Tablets (1.6%) 1547
Timoptic in Ocudose 1552
Timoptic Sterile Ophthalmic Solution 1550
Tonocard Tablets (1.8-3.4%) 1554
Torecan 1993
Tracrium Injection (5 out of 875) .. 817
Trandate HCT Tablets 579
Trandate Injection (Less common) 577
Trandate Tablets 579
▲ Transderm-Nitro Transdermal Therapeutic System (4%) 2283
Tranxene 556
Trental (Less than 1%) 1099
Triaminic Expectorant DH 1995
Triaminic Oral Infant Drops 1996
Triavil Tablets 1556
Tridil Ampuls & Vials 939
Tri-Immunol Diphtheria & Tetanus Toxoids & Pertussis Vaccine, Adsorbed (Rare) 1241
Trilafon (Rare) 2123
Trinalin Repetabs Tablets 1170
Tuss-Ornade Liquid 2242
Tuss-Ornade Spansule Capsules 2242
Uniphyl 400 mg Tablets 1823
Urecholine 1558
Valium Injectable 1937
Valium Tablets (Infrequent) 1939
Valrelease Capsules (Infrequent) 1923
Vancocin HCl, Vials & ADD-Vantage 1302
Vaseretic Tablets (0.9%) 1559
▲ Vasotec I.V. (1.8 to 5.2%) 1562
Vasotec Tablets (0.9% to 6.7%) 1564
Velosulin 1627
Velosulin Human 1628
VePesid Capsules and Injection (0.7 to 2%) 741
Verelan Capsules (2.5%) 1243
Versed Injection 1924
Virazole 1126
Visken Tablets (2% or fewer patients) 2036
Vivactil Tablets 1567
Voltaren Tablets 1042
Vontrol Tablets (Few) 2243
Wellbutrin Tablets (2.5%) 821
▲ Xanax Tablets (4.7%) 2367
▲ Xylocaine Injections (3%) 637
Xylocaine Injections for Ventricular Arrhythmias 639
Xylocaine 2% Jelly 643
Xylocaine 5% Ointment 644
Xylocaine 10% Oral Spray 645
4% Xylocaine-MPF Sterile Solution 641
Xylocaine 2% Viscous Solution 646
▲ Yutopar (80 to 100% (with IV administration)) 647
Zefazone Sterile Powder 2372
Zestoretic (1.4%) 2274
Zestril Tablets (1.8%) 2277
Zovirax Sterile Powder (Less than 1%) 828

Hypotension, asymptomatic

▲ Neupogen for Injection (7 of 176 patients) 595
▲ Verelan Capsules (5%) 1243

Hypotension, exertional

Cardene Capsules (Rare) 2290

Hypotension, neonatal

Altace Capsules 1086
Capoten 2255
Capozide 2258
Normodyne Tablets (Rare) 2110
Prinivil Tablets 1538
Prinzide Tablets 1540
Sectral Capsules 2520
Vaseretic Tablets 1559
Vasotec I.V. 1562
Vasotec Tablets 1564
Yutopar 647
Zestoretic 2274
Zestril Tablets 2277

Hypotension, orthostatic

▲ Adalat Capsules (10 mg and 20 mg) (Approximately 5%) 1587
Aldactazide 2150
Aldoclor Tablets 1413
Aldomet Ester HCl Injection 1417
Aldomet Oral 1415
Aldoril Tablets 1418
Apresazide Capsules 854
Apresoline-Esidrix Tablets 857
Capoten (Infrequent) 2255
Capozide 2258
▲ Cardura Tablets (Up to 23%) 1941
Catapres-TTS 677
Clozaril Tablets 2000
Combipres Tablets (About 3 in 100) 678
Corzide Tablets 702
Desyrel and Desyrel Dividose 1404
▲ Dilatrate-SR (2-36%) 1827
Dipentum Capsules (Rare) 1160
Diucardin Tablets 2450
Diulo 2129
Diupres Tablets 1461
Diuril Oral Suspension 1464
Diuril Sodium Intravenous 1463
Diuril Tablets 1464
Dolophine Hydrochloride Tablets 1261
Elavil 2269
Eldepryl 2250
Endep Tablets 1927

Enduron Tablets 517
Enduronyl 518
Esidrix Tablets 863
Esimil Tablets 864
Exna Tablets 1862
Furoxone 1855
HydroDIURIL Tablets 1484
Hydromox R Tablets 1209
Hydromox Tablets 1208
Hydropres Tablets 1485
▲ Hylorel Tablets (6.6%) 975
Hyperstat I.V. Injection 2095
Hytrin Tablets 529
Inderide Tablets 2463
Inderide LA Long Acting Capsules 2465
IOPIDINE ◉ 232
Larodopa Tablets 1905
Lasix 1093
Loniten Tablets 2346
Lopressor HCT Tablets 1034
Loxitane 1213
Lozol Tablets (Less than 5%) 1843
Lysodren (Infrequent) 731
▲ Marplan Tablets (Among most frequent) 1906
Maxzide 1215
Methadone Hydrochloride Diskets 1284
Midamor Tablets (Less than or equal to 1%) 1508
Minipress Capsules (1-4%) 1778
Minizide Capsules 1779
Moduretic Tablets (Less than or equal to 1%) 1510
Monopril Tablets (1.4%) 1406
Mykrox ½ mg Tablets (Less than 2%) 984
Naturetin Tablets 1789
Normozide Tablets 2112
Oretic Tablets 544
Oreticyl 545
▲ Parlodel (6%) 2020
Phenergan with Codeine 2497
Phenergan VC with Codeine 2501
Prinivil Tablets (1% or less) 1538
Prinzide Tablets (0.5%) 1540
Rauzide Tablets 1804
Regitine 878
Renese Tablets 1785
Renese-R Tablets 1786
Saluron 718
Salutensin/Salutensin-Demi 719
Sandostatin Injection (Less than 1%) 2029
Ser-Ap-Es Tablets 881
Serpasil-Esidrix Tablets 886
Sinemet Tablets (Less frequent) 952
Sinemet CR Tablets (1.0%) 953
Symmetrel Capsules & Syrup (1-5%) 936
Tenex Tablets 1875
Tenoretic Tablets 1105
Thalitone Tablets 687
Timolide Tablets 1547
Tofranil Ampuls 1038
Tofranil Tablets 1039
Tofranil-PM Capsules 1041
Tonocard Tablets (Less than 1%) 1554
Trandate HCT Tablets 579
Triavil Tablets 1556
Vaseretic Tablets (0.5% to 2.0%) 1559
Vasotec I.V. 1562
Vasotec Tablets (0.5% to 1%) 1564
Vivactil Tablets 1567
Wellbutrin Tablets 821
Zaroxolyn Tablets 989
Zestoretic (0.5%) 2274
Zestril Tablets (Less than 1%) 2277

Hypotension, postural
Akineton 1171
▲ Anafranil Capsules (4% to 6%) 650
Bretylol Injection (7 in 1000) 923
Cardene Capsules (Rare) 2290
Cardura Tablets (0.3%) 1941
Cipro Tablets 1589
Dibenzyline Capsules 2207
Dyazide Capsules 2208
Esimil Tablets 864
Etrafon 2087
Floxin Tablets 1652
Hycomine Compound Tablets 929
Hycomine Syrup 927
Hycotuss Expectorant Syrup 930
Hytrin Tablets (0.5% to 1.3%) 529
Intron A (Less than 1%) 2097
Inversine Tablets 1492
Ismelin Tablets 869
▲ Isordil (2% to 36%) 2467
Lotensin Tablets (0.4%) 872
Marinol (Dronabinol) Capsules (1%) 1985
Nardil (Common) 1742
Nitro-Bid Ointment 1339
Nitrolingual Spray (Occasional) 1846
Nitrostat Tablets (Occasional) 1743
▲ Normodyne Injection (58%) 2108
Normodyne Tablets (1%) 2110
Normozide Tablets (1%) 2112
Orap Tablets 1020
▲ Parlodel (6%) 2020
Peritrate (Occasional) 1756
▲ Permax Tablets (9.0%) 1291
Prozac Pulvules (Infrequent) 920
Sansert Tablets 2031
Soma Compound w/Codeine Tablets 2390
Soma Compound Tablets 2389
Soma Tablets 2388
Sorbitrate 1103
▲ Tacaryl (Most common) 2409
Taractan 1920
Tegison Capsules (Less than 1%) 1881
▲ Temaril Tablets, Syrup and Spansule Sustained Release Capsules (Most common) 1085
▲ Tenoretic Tablets (2 to 4%) 1105
▲ Tenormin Tablets and I.V. Injection (2 to 4%) 1107
Thorazine 2234
▲ Trandate Injection (58%) 577
Trecator-SC Tablets 2527
Trilafon 2123
Vasotec I.V. (2.3%) 1562

Hypotension, secondary to spinal block
Duranest Injections 624
Marcaine Hydrochloride with Epinephrine 1:200,000 2055
Marcaine Hydrochloride Injection 2055
Sensorcaine 631
Sensorcaine-MPF Spinal 634
Xylocaine Injections 637

Hypotension, symptomatic
Altace Capsules 1086
Calan SR Caplets 2157
Cardizem Tablets-30 mg, 60 mg, 90 mg and 120 mg (Occasional) 1329
Cardizem SR Capsules-60 mg, 90 mg and 120 mg (Less than 1%) 1327
Lotensin Tablets (Rare to 0.3%) 872

Hypotensive crisis
Dalalone D.P. Injectable 999
Equagesic Tablets 2451
Fiorinal with Codeine Capsules 2008
Miltown Tablets 2386
PMB 200 and PMB 400 (One instance) 2504

Hypothalamic-pituitary dysfunction
Sandostatin Injection 2029

Hypothermia
Clozaril Tablets (Less than 1%) 2000
Ethmozine Tablets (Less than 2%) 946
Ganite Injection 1016
Permax Tablets (Infrequent) 1291
Prostin VR Pediatric Sterile Solution (Less than 1%) 2355
Prozac Pulvules (Rare) 920

Hypothyroidism
Anafranil Capsules (Infrequent) 650
Butazolidin Capsules & Tablets 1027
Cibalith-S 870
Cordarone Tablets (1 to 3%) 2446
Eskalith 2214
Intron A (1% or less) 2097
Lithane Tablets 1596
Lithium Carbonate Capsules & Tablets 1984
Lithobid Tablets 870
Nipride I.V. Infusion 1909
Permax Tablets (Infrequent) 1291
Protropin 1049
Prozac Pulvules (Infrequent) 920
Sandostatin Injection (Less than 1%) 2029

Hypotonia
Duragesic Transdermal System (Less than 1%) 1133
Klonopin Tablets 1902
Permax Tablets (Infrequent) 1291

Hypouresis
Atromid-S Capsules 2435
▲ CHEMET (succimer) Capsules (Up to 3.7%) 1361
Dilaudid-HP Injection 1175
▲ Indocin I.V. (41% of infants) 1490
K-Phos M.F. Tablets 659
K-Phos Neutral Tablets 660
K-Phos No. 2 Tablets 659
Proglycem 649
Uroqid-Acid (Less frequent) 661
Yocon 1686

Hypouricemia
Cipro I.V. (Infrequent) 1592
Timentin for Injection 2239

Hypoventilation
Alurate Elixir (Less than 1 in 100) 1883
Anafranil Capsules (Rare) 650
Butisol Sodium Elixir & Tablets (Less than 1 in 100) 2377
Carbocaine Hydrochloride Injection 2043
Dopram Injectable 1860
▲ Duragesic Transdermal System (2% to 10%) 1133
Marcaine Hydrochloride with Epinephrine 1:200,000 2055
Marcaine Hydrochloride Injection 2055
Marcaine Spinal 2058
Mebaral Tablets (Less than 1 in 100) 2061
Nembutal Sodium Capsules (Less than 1%) 534
Nembutal Sodium Solution (Less than 1%) 536
Nembutal Sodium Suppositories (Less than 1%) 538
Nesacaine Injections 629
Permax Tablets (Rare) 1291
Phenobarbital Elixir and Tablets (Less than 1 in 100 patients) 1293
Seconal Sodium Pulvules (Less than 1 in 100) 1296
Versed Injection 1924

Hypovolemia
Diulo 2129
Estratest 2245
Inapsine Injection 1140
Mykrox ½ mg Tablets 984
Serophene (clomiphene citrate tablets, USP) 2186
Zaroxolyn Tablets 989

Hypoxemia
Inocor Lactate Injection (1 case) 2048
Methotrexate Tablets, Parenteral, LPF Parenteral 1217
Rheumatrex Methotrexate Dose Pack 1234

Hypoxia
Depakote Sprinkle Capsules 512
Diprivan Injection (Less than 1%) 2267
Levophed Bitartrate Injection 2054
Nardil (Less frequent) 1742
Permax Tablets (Rare) 1291
Prozac Pulvules (Rare) 920
Tegretol Chewable Tablets 654
Tegretol Suspension 656
Tegretol Tablets 654

Hysteria
Actifed with Codeine Cough Syrup 752
Deconamine 663
Diprivan Injection (Less than 1%) 2267
Klonopin Tablets 1902
Optimine Tablets 2115
Ornade Spansule Capsules 2221
PBZ Tablets & Elixir 1037
PBZ-SR Tablets 1037
Periactin 1525
Phenergan Injection 2493
Phenergan Tablets 2496
Placidyl Capsules 553
Polaramine 2116
Prozac Pulvules (Rare) 920
Ru-Tuss II Capsules 693
Tacaryl 2409
Tavist Syrup 2033
Tavist Tablets 2035
Tavist-D Tablets 2035
Temaril Tablets, Syrup and Spansule Sustained Release Capsules 1085
Triaminic Expectorant DH 1995
Triaminic Oral Infant Drops 1996
Trinalin Repetabs Tablets 1170

HPA axis suppression
Aclovate 1053
Alphatrex Cream, Ointment & Lotion 2076
Cutivate Cream 0.05% 1054
Cutivate Ointment 0.005% 1054
Diprolene 2083
Maxivate Cream, Lotion & Ointment 0.05% 2406
Temovate 1056
Ultravate Cream 0.05% 2410
Ultravate Ointment 0.05% 2411

HPA function suppression
Azmacort Inhaler 1837
Beclovent Inhalation Aerosol and Refill 572
Vanceril Inhaler 2128

I

Ichthyosis
▲ Lamprene Capsules (8-28%) 1030

Idiosyncrasy
Anestacon Solution 2394
Berocca Plus Tablets (Possible) 1894
Berocca Tablets (Possible) 1893
Blenoxane (1%) 724
Cocaine Hydrochloride Topical Solution 620
Deprol Tablets 2382
Donnatal 1858
Donnatal Extentabs 1859
Donnatal Tablets 1858
Donnazyme Tablets 1860
Duricef 1405
Larobec Tablets 1905
Luride Drops (Rare) 889
Luride Lozi-Tabs Tablets (Rare) 890
Miltown Tablets 2386
Novocain Hydrochloride for Spinal Anesthesia (Rare) 2065
Omnipaque 2552
PMB 200 and PMB 400 2504
Poly-Vi-Flor 1397
Poly-Vi-Flor Drops 1398
Poly-Vi-Flor with Iron 1399
Poly-Vi-Flor with Iron Drops 1399
Pontocaine Hydrochloride for Spinal Anesthesia 2069
Pro-Banthīne Tablets 2141
Quinamm Tablets 1344
Robinul Forte Tablets 1873
Robinul Injectable 1873
Robinul Tablets 1873
Soma Compound w/Codeine Tablets (Very rare) 2390
Soma Compound Tablets (Very rare) 2389
Soma Tablets (Very rare) 2388
Tri-Vi-Flor 1.0 mg Vitamins with Fluoride Chewable Tablets 1400
Tri-Vi-Flor Drops 1400
Tri-Vi-Flor 0.25 mg Vitamins with Iron and Fluoride Drops 1401
Xylocaine Injections 637
Xylocaine Injections for Ventricular Arrhythmias 639
Xylocaine 2% Jelly 643
Xylocaine 10% Oral Spray 645
4% Xylocaine-MPF Sterile Solution 641
Xylocaine 2% Viscous Solution 646

Idiosyncratic reactions (see under Idiosyncrasy)

Idioventricular rhythms
Cardioquin Tablets 1812
Eminase 2211

Ileitis, regional
Accutane Capsules 1878
Indocin (Less than 1%) 1487

Ileus
Atgam Sterile Solution (Less than 1%) 2320
Cipro I.V. (1% or less) 1592
Cogentin 1435
Ethmozine Tablets (Less than 2%) 946
Forane 600
Hyperstat I.V. Injection 2095
Indocin I.V. (1% to 3%) 1490
Inversine Tablets 1492
Nipride I.V. Infusion 1909
Proglycem (Frequent) 649
Vaseretic Tablets 1559
Vasotec I.V. 1562
Vasotec Tablets (0.5% to 1%) 1564
Velban Vials 1305
Yutopar (Infrequent) 647

Ileus, adynamic
Compazine 2201
Etrafon 2087
Navane Capsules and Concentrate 1954

Navane Intramuscular 1956
Stelazine 2226
Taractan 1920
Thorazine 2234
Trilafon (Occasional) 2123

Ileus, neonatal

Yutopar 647

Ileus, paralytic

Anafranil Capsules (Rare) 650
Apresazide Capsules (Less frequent) 854
Apresoline Hydrochloride Parenteral (Ampuls) 856
Apresoline Hydrochloride Tablets (Less frequent) 855
Apresoline-Esidrix Tablets 857
Arfonad Ampuls 1887
Artane (Rare) 1195
Asendin Tablets (Very rare) 1196
Calan SR Caplets (Infrequent) 2157
Calan Tablets (Infrequent) 2155
Cogentin 1435
Dicumarol Tablets 516
Elavil 2269
Endep Tablets 1927
Flexeril Tablets (Rare) 1471
Limbitrol 1933
Lomotil 2174
Loxitane 1213
Ludiomil Tablets 874
Meclomen Capsules (Rare) 1739
Mellaril 2011
Motofen Tablets 836
Norpramin Tablets 1340
Norzine 1818
Oncovin Solution Vials & Hyporets 1288
Pamelor 2019
Panwarfin Tablets 547
Prolixin Decanoate 1795
Prolixin Elixir 1793
Prolixin Enanthate 1796
Prolixin Injection 1791
Prolixin Oral Concentrate 1792
Prolixin Tablets 1793
Ser-Ap-Es Tablets 881
Serentil 686
Serpasil-Apresoline Tablets 884
Surmontil Capsules 2524
Tofranil Ampuls 1038
Tofranil Tablets 1039
Tofranil-PM Capsules 1041
Torecan 1993
Triavil Tablets 1556
Verelan Capsules (Infrequent) 1243
Vivactil Tablets 1567

Illusion, unspecified

Anafranil Capsules (Rare) 650

Immobility

Moban Tablets & Concentrate 932

Immunoglobulin, abnormalities

Dilantin Infatabs 1710
Dilantin Kapseals 1708
Dilantin Parenteral 1712
Dilantin-30 Pediatric/Dilantin-125 Suspension 1713
Dilantin with Phenobarbital Kapseals 1715

Immunosuppression

Cytoxan for Injection 726
Neosar for Injection 566
Purinethol Tablets 800
Rifamate Capsules 1347
Rimactane Capsules 879

Impotence

Adipex-P Tablets and Capsules 1019
Aldoclor Tablets 1413
Aldomet Ester HCl Injection 1417
Aldomet Oral 1415
Aldoril Tablets 1418
Altace Capsules (Less than 1%) 1086
Anadrol-50 Tablets 2287
▲ Anafranil Capsules (Up to 20%) 650
Antabuse Tablets (Small number of patients) 2429
Asendin Tablets (Less than 1%) 1196
Atromid-S Capsules 2435
Axid Pulvules 1246
Bentyl 1322
Biphetamine Capsules 973
Blocadren Tablets (Less than 1%) 1429
BuSpar (Rare) 1401
Calan SR Caplets (1% or less) 2157
Calan Tablets (1% or less) 2155
Cantil Tablets 1326
Capoten 2255
Capozide 2258
Cardene Capsules (Rare) 2290
Cardizem Tablets-30 mg, 60 mg, 90 mg and 120 mg 1329
Cardizem SR Capsules-60 mg, 90 mg and 120 mg (Less than 1%) 1327
Cartrol Tablets (Less common) 507
Catapres Tablets (About 3 in 100 patients) 676
Catapres-TTS (Up to 3%) 677
Clozaril Tablets (Less than 1%) 2000
Combipres Tablets (About 3%) 678
Compazine 2201
Corgard Tablets (1 to 5 of 1000 patients) 701
Corzide Tablets (1 to 5 of 1000 patients) 702
Cytotec (Infrequent) 2159
Darbid Tablets 2205
Demser Capsules (Infrequent) 1460
Desoxyn Gradumet Tablets 514
Desyrel and Desyrel Dividose (Greater than 1%) 1404
Dexedrine 2206
Dipentum Capsules (Rare) 1160
Ditropan 1332
Diupres Tablets 1461
Dolophine Hydrochloride Ampoules & Vials 1260
Donnatal 1858
Donnatal Extentabs 1859
Donnatal Tablets 1858
Donnazyme Tablets 1860
Doral Tablets 2383
Dyazide Capsules (A few patients) 2208
DynaCirc Capsules (0.5% to 1%) 2004
Enduronyl 518
Esimil Tablets 864
Eskalith 2214
Ethmozine Tablets (Less than 2%) 946
▲ Eulexin Capsules (33% with LHRH-agonist) 2089
Fastin Capsules 2216
Flexeril Tablets (Rare) 1471
Gelfoam Sterile Sponge 2338
Haldol Decanoate 1375
Haldol Injection, Tablets and Concentrate 1373
Harmonyl Tablets 528
Hydropres Tablets 1485
Hytrin Tablets (1.2%) 529
Inderal (Rare) 2459
Inderal LA Long Acting Capsules (Rare) 2461
Inderide Tablets (Rare) 2463
Inderide LA Long Acting Capsules (Rare) 2465
Intron A (Less than 1%) 2097
Inversine Tablets 1492
Ionamin Capsules 981
Ismelin Tablets 869
Isoptin Oral Tablets (Less than 1%) 1179
Isoptin SR Sustained Release Tablets (Less than 1%) 1181
Kerlone Tablets (1.2%) 2172
Kinesed Tablets 2272
Levatol (0.5%) 1832
Levsin/Levsinex 2147
Limbitrol (Less common) 1933
Lioresal Tablets (Rare) 1031
Lopid Capsules and Tablets 1736
Lopressor HCT Tablets (1 in 100 patients) 1034
Lorelco Tablets 1333
Lotensin Tablets 872
Lozol Tablets (Less than 5%) 1843
Ludiomil Tablets (Rare) 874
▲ Lupron Depot 3.75 mg (Among most frequent) 2312
▲ Lupron Depot 7.5 mg (5.4%) 2311
▲ Lupron Injection (5% or more) 2310
MS Contin Tablets (Infrequent) 1814
MSIR (Infrequent) 1817
Methadone Hydrochloride Diskets 1284
Methotrexate Tablets, Parenteral, LPF Parenteral 1217
Mexitil Capsules (Less than 1% or about 4 in 1,000) 680
Midamor Tablets (Between 1% and 3%) 1508
Minipress Capsules (Less than 1%) 1778
Minizide Capsules (Rare) 1779
Moduretic Tablets (Less than or equal to 1%) 1510
Mykrox ½ mg Tablets (Less than 2%) 984
Mysoline (Occasional) 2480
Navane Capsules and Concentrate 1954
Navane Intramuscular 1956
Neosar for Injection 566
Nizoral Tablets (Less than 1%) 1145
▲ Normodyne Injection (1 to 4%) 2108
▲ Normodyne Tablets (1% to 4%) 2110
Normozide Tablets (1%) 2112
Norpace (1 to 3%) 2177
Norpramin Tablets 1340
Orap Tablets 1020
Oreticyl 545
Orudis Capsules (Less than 1%) 2488
Pamelor 2019
Parnate Tablets 2222
Pepcid (Rare) 1524
Permax Tablets (Infrequent) 1291
Plendil Extended-Release Tablets (0.5% to 1.5%) 1526
Prelu-2 Capsules 683
Prinivil Tablets (0.7%) 1538
Prinzide Tablets (1.2%) 1540
Pro-Banthīne Tablets 2141
Procardia XL Tablets (Less than 3%) 1783
Prolixin Decanoate 1795
Prolixin Elixir 1793
Prolixin Enanthate 1796
Prolixin Injection 1791
Prolixin Oral Concentrate 1792
Prolixin Tablets 1793
Prozac Pulvules (Infrequent) 920
Quarzan Capsules 1937
Raudixin Tablets 1803
Rauzide Tablets 1804
Reglan 1869
Renese-R Tablets 1786
Rheumatrex Methotrexate Dose Pack 1234
Robinul Forte Tablets 1873
Robinul Injectable 1873
Robinul Tablets 1873
▲ Roferon-A Injection (6%) 1916
Rythmol Tablets (Less than 1%) 1184
Salutensin/Salutensin-Demi 719
Sanorex Tablets (Rare) 2030
Sectral Capsules (Up to 2%) 2520
Ser-Ap-Es Tablets 881
Serentil 686
Serpasil Tablets 883
Serpasil-Apresoline Tablets 884
Serpasil-Esidrix Tablets 886
Stelazine 2226
Surmontil Capsules 2524
Tagamet 2228
Tambocor Tablets (Less than 1%) 1315
Tegretol Chewable Tablets 654
Tegretol Suspension 656
Tegretol Tablets 654
Tenex Tablets (1% to 4%) 1875
Tenoretic Tablets 1105
Tenormin Tablets and I.V. Injection 1107
Tenuate 1354
Thalitone Tablets 687
Thorazine 2234
Timolide Tablets 1547
Timoptic in Ocudose 1552
Timoptic Sterile Ophthalmic Solution 1550
Tofranil Ampuls 1038
Tofranil Tablets 1039
Tofranil-PM Capsules 1041
Trandate HCT Tablets (1% in 108 patients) 579
Trandate Injection 577
Trandate Tablets (1% of 227 patients) 579
Trecator-SC Tablets 2527
▲ Trexan Tablets (Less than 10%) 937
Trilafon 2123
Valpin 50 Tablets 941
Vascor (200, 300 and 400 mg) Tablets (0.5 to 2.0%) 1383
Vaseretic Tablets (2.2%) 1559
Vasotec I.V. 1562
Vasotec Tablets (0.5% to 1%) 1564
Verelan Capsules (Less than 1%) 1243
Visken Tablets (2% or fewer patients) 2036
Vivactil Tablets 1567
Voltaren Tablets (Less than 1%) 1042
▲ Wellbutrin Tablets (3.4%) 821
Winstrol Tablets 2075
Wytensin Tablets (3% or less) 2542
Zantac Injection and Zantac Injection Premixed 1063
Zantac (Occasional) 1065
Zaroxolyn Tablets 989
Zestoretic (1.2%) 2274
Zestril Tablets (0.7%) 2277
Zyloprim Tablets (Less than 1%) 830

Impulse control, impaired

Anafranil Capsules (Rare) 650

Incontinence

Doral Tablets 2383
Etrafon 2087
Halcion Tablets 2340
▲ Lupron Depot 3.75 mg (Among most frequent) 2312
Lupron Depot 7.5 mg 2311
Lupron Injection (Less than 5%) 2310
Marplan Tablets (Rare) 1906
Minipress Capsules (Less than 1%) 1778
Minizide Capsules (Rare) 1779
Moduretic Tablets (Less than or equal to 1%) 1510
Norzine 1818
Protostat Tablets 1674
Serax Capsules 2522
Serax Tablets 2522
Serentil 686
Tensilon Injectable 1123
Valium Injectable 1937
Valium Tablets (Infrequent) 1939
Valrelease Capsules (Infrequent) 1923
Xanax Tablets (1.5%) 2367

Incontinence, fecal

Carbocaine Hydrochloride Injection 2043
Cardura Tablets (Less than 0.5% of 3960 patients) 1941
Cibalith-S 870
Eskalith 2214
Klonopin Tablets 1902
Lithane Tablets 1596
Lithium Carbonate Capsules & Tablets 1984
Lithobid Tablets 870
Marcaine Hydrochloride with Epinephrine 1:200,000 2055
Marcaine Hydrochloride Injection 2055
Marcaine Spinal 2058
Permax Tablets (Rare) 1291
Prozac Pulvules (Rare) 920

Incontinence, urinary

Anafranil Capsules (Infrequent) 650
Carbocaine Hydrochloride Injection 2043
Cardura Tablets (1%) 1941
Cibalith-S 870
Clozaril Tablets (1%) 2000
Dantrium Capsules (Less frequent) 1619
Desyrel and Desyrel Dividose 1404
Doral Tablets 2383
Esimil Tablets 864
Eskalith 2214
Ethmozine Tablets (Less than 2%) 946
Flagyl I.V. 2131
Flagyl Tablets 2170
Floropryl Sterile Ophthalmic Ointment (Rare) 1473
Humorsol Sterile Ophthalmic Solution (Rare) 1475
Hytrin Tablets (At least 1%) 529
Ismelin Tablets 869
Larodopa Tablets (Infrequent) 1905
Lithane Tablets 1596
Lithium Carbonate Capsules & Tablets 1984
Lithobid Tablets 870
Marcaine Hydrochloride with Epinephrine 1:200,000 2055
Marcaine Hydrochloride Injection 2055
Marcaine Spinal 2058
Mellaril 2011
Parlodel 2020
ProSom Tablets (Rare) 554
Prozac Pulvules (Infrequent) 920
Reglan 1869
Serentil 686
Sinemet Tablets 952
Sinemet CR Tablets 953
Tenex Tablets 1875
Tensilon Injectable 1123
▲ TheraCys BCG Live (Intravesical) (Up to 6.3%) 898
Torecan 1993
Wellbutrin Tablets (Rare) 821

Incoordination (see under Ataxia)

Indecisiveness

Anafranil Capsules (Rare) 650

Indigestion

Augmentin Tablets, Powder for Oral Suspension, and Chewable Tablets 2198

Butazolidin Capsules & Tablets (Greater than 1%) ... 1027
Carafate Tablets (Less than 0.5%) 1326
Children's Advil Suspension (Less than 3%) ... 2426
Cholybar (Less frequent) ... 1705
Corgard Tablets (1 to 5 of 1000 patients) ... 701
Corzide Tablets (1 to 5 of 1000 patients) ... 702
▲ Depakene Capsules & Syrup (Among most common) ... 511
▲ Depakote (Among most common) .. 512
Eskalith ... 2214
Feldene Capsules (1 to 3%) ... 1777
▲ Hylorel Tablets (23.7%) ... 975
▲ Indocin (3% to 9%) ... 1487
Lopressor HCT Tablets (1 in 100 patients) ... 1034
Lorelco Tablets ... 1333
Motrin Tablets (Less than 3%) ... 2351
Nicorette ... 1335
Parlodel ... 2020
PediaProfen Suspension (Less than 3%) ... 1363
Questran Light (Less frequent) ... 711
Questran Powder ... 710
Rufen Tablets (1 to 3%) ... 691
Sinequan ... 1960
▲ Trilisate (Less than 20%) ... 1822
Ventolin Rotacaps for Inhalation (Less than 1%) ... 583
▲ Voltaren Tablets (3% to 9%) ... 1042
Vontrol Tablets ... 2243

Induration at injection site

Ancef Injection ... 2194
Biavax II ... 1427
▲ Brevibloc Injection (8%) ... 942
Capastat Sulfate Vials ... 1250
▲ Cefizox Injection (1 to 5%) ... 1012
Cholera Vaccine ... 2445
▲ Claforan Sterile Injection (4.7%) ... 1089
Cleocin Phosphate Injection ... 2325
Dalalone D.P. Injectable ... 999
Decadron-LA Sterile Suspension ... 1457
Demerol ... 2047
Desferal Vials ... 862
Diphtheria and Tetanus Toxoids and Pertussis Vaccine Adsorbed USP (For Pediatric Use) ... 892
Dolophine Hydrochloride Ampoules & Vials ... 1260
▲ Engerix-B Unit-Dose Vials (1% to 10 %) ... 2213
Factrel (Rare) ... 2561
▲ Flu-Imune Influenza Virus Vaccine (Less than one-third of recipients) .. 1204
IPOL Poliovirus Vaccine Inactivated (1%) ... 894
Kefzol Vials, Faspak & ADD-Vantage (Infrequent) ... 1279
Lupron Injection ... 2310
Lutrepulse for Injection ... 1655
M-M-R II ... 1494
M-R-VAX II ... 1496
Mefoxin ... 1498
Mepergan Injection ... 2479
Meruvax II ... 1503
Netromycin Injection 100 mg/ml (4 of 1000 patients) ... 2104
PedvaxHIB ... 1521
Pentam 300 Injection ... 1018
Pipracil (2%) ... 1230
▲ Plague Vaccine (10%) ... 1584
Pneumovax 23 ... 1528
Primaxin I.V. (0.2%) ... 1535
ProHIBiT Haemophilus b Conjugate Vaccine (Diphtheria Toxoid Conjugate) (1.4%) ... 896
Rocephin Injectable Vials, ADD-Vantage (1%) ... 1914
Talwin Injection ... 2071
Tetanus & Diphtheria Toxoids, Adsorbed Purogenated ... 1237
Ticar for Injection ... 2236
Timentin for Injection ... 2239
Tri-Immunol Diphtheria & Tetanus Toxoids & Pertussis Vaccine, Adsorbed (Common) ... 1241
Trobicin Sterile Powder ... 2366
Typhoid Vaccine ... 2533
Versed Injection (1.7%) ... 1924

Infantile spasms

Diphtheria and Tetanus Toxoids and Pertussis Vaccine Adsorbed USP (For Pediatric Use) ... 892

Infection, bacterial

Cytosar-U Sterile Powder ... 2329
Cytovene Sterile Powder ... 2292
Lopid Capsules and Tablets ... 1736
Maxidex Sterile Ophthalmic Ointment ... ⊙ 222
Neosar for Injection ... 566
Orthoclone OKT3 Sterile Solution .. 1645
▲ Paraplatin for Injection (5%) ... 735

Infection, body as a whole

▲ Atgam Sterile Solution (Less than 1% to 13%) ... 2320
Capoten ... 2255
Cardene Capsules (Rare) ... 2290
Cardura Tablets (Less than 0.5% of 3960 patients) ... 1941
Cartrol Tablets (Less common) ... 507
Compazine ... 2201
Coumadin Injection & Tablets ... 944
Cytovene Sterile Powder (1% or less) ... 2292
▲ Ergamisol Tablets (5 to 12%) ... 1136
Etrafon ... 2087
Gelfoam Sterile Sponge ... 2338
▲ Idamycin for Injection (95%) ... 564
▲ IFEX (8%) ... 729
Lodine Capsules (Less than 1%) 2468
Lotensin Tablets ... 872
Lupron Depot 7.5 mg ... 2311
Lupron Injection (Less than 5%) ... 2310
Orudis Capsules (Less than 1%) 2488
Permax Tablets (1.1%) ... 1291
Pronestyl Capsules and Tablets ... 1800
Pronestyl Injection ... 1798
Stelazine ... 2226
TheraCys BCG Live (Intravesical) (2.0% to 2.7%) ... 898
Xanax Tablets (1.3%) ... 2367

Infection, cecum

Adriamycin RDF ... 562

Infection, colon

Adriamycin RDF ... 562

Infection, conjunctiva

Urobiotic-250 Capsules ... 1968

Infection, cryptococcus

Orthoclone OKT3 Sterile Solution (1.6%) ... 1645

Infection, cytomegalovirus

▲ Orthoclone OKT3 Sterile Solution (19%) ... 1645
▲ Sandimmune (4.8 to 12.3%) ... 2024

Infection, decreased resistance

Anafranil Capsules (Infrequent) ... 650
Cytoxan for Injection ... 726
▲ Methotrexate Tablets, Parenteral, LPF Parenteral (Among most frequent) ... 1217
Orthoclone OKT3 Sterile Solution .. 1645
▲ Rheumatrex Methotrexate Dose Pack (Among most frequent) ... 1234

Infection, ears

▲ AeroBid Inhaler System (3-9%) ... 995
▲ PedvaxHIB (Among most frequent) 1521
Rogaine Topical Solution (1.17%).. 2357
Tegison Capsules (Less than 1%) .. 1881

Infection, eyes

AeroBid Inhaler System (1-3%) ... 995
Depo-Medrol Sterile Aqueous Suspension ... 2334

Infection, eyes, fungal

AK-Cide Sterile Ophthalmic Ointment & Suspension ... ⊙ 202
AK-Spore H.C. ... ⊙ 206
Blephamide ... 586
Cetapred Ointment ... ⊙ 220
Cortisporin Ophthalmic Ointment Sterile ... 758
Cortisporin Ophthalmic Suspension Sterile ... 759
Dexacidin ... ⊙ 272
Isopto Cetapred Suspension ... ⊙ 220
Maxidex Sterile Ophthalmic Ointment ... ⊙ 222
Maxidex Sterile Ophthalmic Suspension ... ⊙ 223
Pred-G S.O.P. Sterile Ophthalmic Ointment ... ⊙ 253
Vasocidin Ointment ... ⊙ 275
Vasocidin Ophthalmic Solution ... ⊙ 276

Infection, fungal

AK-Trol Ointment & Suspension .. ⊙ 207
Blephamide ... 586
Cytosar-U Sterile Powder ... 2329
Cytovene Sterile Powder ... 2292
⅛% Econopred & 1% Econopred Plus ... ⊙ 217
FML Forte Liquifilm ... ⊙ 245
FML Liquifilm ... ⊙ 244
FML S.O.P. ... ⊙ 245
FML-S Sterile Ophthalmic Suspension ... ⊙ 246
Humatin Capsules ... 1726
Intron A (Less than 1%) ... 2097
Maxidex Sterile Ophthalmic Ointment ... ⊙ 222
Maxitrol Ophthalmic Ointment/Suspension ... ⊙ 223
Neosar for Injection ... 566
▲ Novantrone for Injection Concentrate (9 to 15%) ... 1226
Ophthocort ... ⊙ 301
Orthoclone OKT3 Sterile Solution .. 1645
Poly-Pred Liquifilm ... ⊙ 250

Infection, fungal, local

▲ Sandimmune (7.5 to 9.6%) ... 2024

Infection, fungal, systemic

Sandimmune (2.2 to 3.9%) ... 2024

Infection, gastrointestinal

Adriamycin PFS ... 561
Cytotec (Infrequent) ... 2159
Doxorubicin Hydrochloride for Injection, USP ... 622
Doxorubicin Hydrochloride Injection, USP ... 848
Rubex ... 739

Infection, gram-negative bacteria

Orthoclone OKT3 Sterile Solution (1.6%) ... 1645

Infection, helminthic

Neosar for Injection ... 566

Infection, herpes simplex

Inflamase ... ⊙ 274
Intron A (Up to 3%) ... 2097
▲ Orthoclone OKT3 Sterile Solution (27%) ... 1645

Infection, Legionella

Orthoclone OKT3 Sterile Solution (1.6%) ... 1645

Infection, localized

Atgam Sterile Solution (Less than 1%) ... 2320
Depo-Medrol Sterile Aqueous Suspension ... 2334

Infection, masking signs of

AK-Cide Sterile Ophthalmic Ointment & Suspension ... ⊙ 202
AK-Dex ... ⊙ 203
AK-Pred ... ⊙ 205
AK-Spore H.C. ... ⊙ 206
AK-Trol Ointment & Suspension .. ⊙ 207
Blephamide ... 586
FML Liquifilm ... ⊙ 244
FML S.O.P. ... ⊙ 245
FML-S Sterile Ophthalmic Suspension ... ⊙ 246
Kenalog-10 Injection ... 2402
Kenalog-40 Injection ... 2403
Maxidex Sterile Ophthalmic Ointment ... ⊙ 222
Maxitrol Ophthalmic Ointment/Suspension ... ⊙ 223
NeoDecadron Topical Cream ... 1518
TobraDex Ophthalmic Suspension and Ointment ... ⊙ 228
Vasocidin Ophthalmic Solution .... ⊙ 276

Infection, nasal

Beconase Inhalation Aerosol & Refill (Rare) ... 574

Infection, non-pulmonary

▲ Exosurf Neonatal for Intratracheal Suspension (Up to 35%) ... 765

Infection, parasitic

Cytosar-U Sterile Powder ... 2329

Infection, pelvis

Lippes Loop Intrauterine Double-S.. 1654
ParaGard T380A Intrauterine Copper Contraceptive ... 411
Wellbutrin Tablets (Rare) ... 821

Infection, pharyngeal

Beconase Inhalation Aerosol & Refill (Rare) ... 574
Decadron Phosphate Respihaler ... 1454

Infection, Pneumocystis carinii (see under Pneumocystis carinii, susceptibility)

Infection, post-treatment, unspecified

▲ Survanta Beractant Intratracheal Suspension (10.2 to 20.7%) ... 1978

Infection, potentiation

Hemopad Absorbable Collagen Hemostat ... 627
INSTAT Collagen Absorbable Hemostat ... 1151
Kenalog-10 Injection ... 2402
Kenalog-40 Injection ... 2403

Infection, protozoan

Neosar for Injection ... 566

Infection, respiratory

Accutane Capsules ... 1878
DDAVP ... 1841
Nalfon Pulvules & Tablets (1.5%) .. 919
Plendil Extended-Release Tablets (0.5% to 1.5%) ... 1526
TheraCys BCG Live (Intravesical) (Up to 2.7%) ... 898
Vascor (200, 300 and 400 mg) Tablets (2.84%) ... 1383

Infection, sapraphytic

Cytosar-U Sterile Powder ... 2329

Infection, secondary

Aclovate Cream ... 1053
AK-Cide Sterile Ophthalmic Ointment & Suspension ... ⊙ 202
AK-Dex ... ⊙ 203
AK-Pred ... ⊙ 205
AK-Spore H.C. ... ⊙ 206
AK-Trol Ointment & Suspension ... ⊙ 207
Alphatrex Cream, Ointment & Lotion (Infrequent) ... 2076
Analpram-HC Rectal Cream 1% and 2.5% ... 970
Anusol-HC Cream (Infrequent) ... 1690
Anusol-HC Suppositories ... 1691
Aristocort A (Infrequent) ... 1010
Betatrex Cream, Ointment & Lotion ... 2077
Blephamide ... 586
Carmol HC Cream 1% (Infrequent) ... 2296
Cetamide Ointment ... ⊙ 220
Cetapred Ointment ... ⊙ 220
Cortisporin Cream ... 757
Cortisporin Ointment ... 758
Cortisporin Ophthalmic Ointment Sterile ... 758
Cortisporin Ophthalmic Suspension Sterile ... 759
Cortisporin Otic Solution Sterile ... 760
Cortisporin Otic Suspension Sterile 760
Cutivate Cream 0.05% ... 1054
Cutivate Ointment 0.005% (Infrequent to more frequent) ... 1054
Cyclocort Lotion (Infrequent) ... 1198
Decadron Phosphate Sterile Ophthalmic Ointment ... 1453
Decadron Phosphate Sterile Ophthalmic Solution ... 1453
Decadron Phosphate Topical Cream ... 1455
Decaspray Topical Aerosol ... 1459
DesOwen Cream, Ointment and Lotion (Infrequent) ... 1682
Dexacidin ... ⊙ 272
Diprolene (Infrequent) ... 2083
E.E.S. ... 522
Eldecort Cream 1.0% (Infrequent) 1113
Eldecort Cream 1.0% and 2.5% (Infrequent) ... 1113
Elocon (Infrequent) ... 2084
Epifoam ... 1828
EryPed 200 & EryPed 400 Granules ... 519
Ery-Tab Tablets ... 521
Erythrocin Stearate Filmtab ... 523
FML Forte Liquifilm ... ⊙ 245
FML Liquifilm ... ⊙ 244
FML S.O.P. ... ⊙ 245
FML-S Sterile Ophthalmic Suspension ... ⊙ 246
Florone/Florone E ... 908

Fluor-Op Ophthalmic Suspension ⊙ 272
Halog (Infrequent) 2399
Hytone 909
Ilosone 913
Ilotycin Gluceptate, IV, Vials 915
Imuran 768
Inflamase ⊙ 274
Isopto Cetamide Solution ⊙ 220
Isopto Cetapred Suspension ⊙ 220
Kenalog Cream, Lotion & Ointment (Infrequent) 2401
Lidex (Infrequent) 2296
Locoid Cream, Ointment and Topical Solution (Infrequent) 970
Lotrisone Cream (1 of 270 patients) 2103
Mantadil Cream 789
Maxidex Sterile Ophthalmic Ointment ⊙ 222
Maxitrol Ophthalmic Ointment/Suspension ⊙ 223
Metimyd ⊙ 306
Mycolog II Cream and Ointment (Infrequent) 2407
Mytrex Cream & Ointment (Infrequent) 2080
NeoDecadron Topical Cream 1518
Neo-Synalar Cream (Infrequent) 2296
Nutracort Cream & Lotion (Infrequent) 1684
Orabase HCA Oral Paste (Infrequent) 890
Otic Tridesilon Solution 0.05% (Infrequent) 1612
PediOtic Suspension Sterile 797
Pipracil 1230
Poly-Pred Liquifilm ⊙ 250
Pramosone Cream, Lotion & Ointment 971
Pred Forte ⊙ 252
Pred Mild ⊙ 254
Pred-G Liquifilm Sterile Ophthalmic Suspension ⊙ 252
Pred-G S.O.P. Sterile Ophthalmic Ointment ⊙ 253
ProctoCream-HC (Infrequent) 1834
Proctofoam-HC 1835
Psorcon Ointment 0.05% 909
Psorion Cream 0.05% (Infrequent) 1121
Synacort Creams 1%, 2.5% (Infrequent) 2296
Synalar (Infrequent) 2296
Temovate 1056
TobraDex Ophthalmic Suspension and Ointment ⊙ 228
Topicort (Infrequent) 1098
Tridesilon Creme 0.05% (Infrequent) 1611
Tridesilon Ointment 0.05% (Infrequent) 1611
Ultravate Cream 0.05% (Infrequent) 2410
Ultravate Ointment 0.05% 2411
Vanoxide-HC Acne Lotion 911
Vasocidin Ointment ⊙ 275
Vasocidin Ophthalmic Solution ⊙ 276
Vioform-Hydrocortisone Cream and Mild Cream 889
Vioform-Hydrocortisone Ointment 889
Vytone Cream 1% 911
Westcort 2411

Infection, Serratia
Orthoclone OKT3 Sterile Solution (1.6%) 1645

Infection, Staphylococcus epidermidis
▲ Orthoclone OKT3 Sterile Solution (4.8%) 1645

Infection, unspecified
Humatin Capsules 1726
▲ Imuran (1% to 10%) 768
Methotrexate Tablets, Parenteral, LPF Parenteral 1217
Rheumatrex Methotrexate Dose Pack 1234

Infection, upper respiratory
▲ AeroBid Inhaler System (25%) 995
Altace Capsules 1086
Cytotec (Infrequent) 2159
Decadron Phosphate Respihaler 1454
Dipentum Capsules (1.5%) 1160
Kerlone Tablets (2.6%) 2172
Levatol (2.5%) 1832
Methotrexate Tablets, Parenteral, LPF Parenteral (Less common) 1217
▲ PedvaxHIB (Among most frequent) 1521
Plendil Extended-Release Tablets (0.1%) 1526
Prilosec Delayed-Release Capsules 1530
Prinzide Tablets (2.2%) 1540
Procardia XL Tablets (1% or less) 1783
Prolixin Oral Concentrate 1792
▲ Prozac Pulvules (7.6%) 920
Recombivax HB (Equal to or greater than 1%) 1544
Rheumatrex Methotrexate Dose Pack (Less common) 1234
▲ Rogaine Topical Solution (7.16%) 2357
Rowasa 2248
Seldane-D Extended-Release Tablets (1.3%) 1350
Sinemet CR Tablets (1.8%) 953
Vaseretic Tablets 1559
Vasotec I.V. 1562
▲ Xanax Tablets (4.3%) 2367
Zestoretic (2.2%) 2274
▲ Zoladex (7%) 1110

Infection, urinary tract
Ergamisol Tablets (2 patients) 1136
Hytrin Tablets (At least 1%) 529
Lopid Capsules and Tablets 1736
Lotensin Tablets 872
▲ Lupron Injection (5% or more) 2310
▲ Novantrone for Injection Concentrate (7%) 1226
Prilosec Delayed-Release Capsules (Less than 1%) 1530
Prinivil Tablets (1% or less) 1538
Prinzide Tablets (0.3 to 1%) 1540
Prozac Pulvules (1.2%) 920
Rogaine Topical Solution (0.93%) 2357
▲ Sandimmune (20.2 to 21.1%) 2024
Sinemet CR Tablets (2.2%) 953
Tolectin (200, 400 and 600 mg) (1 to 3%) 1379
Vaseretic Tablets (0.5% to 2.0%) 1559
Vasotec I.V. 1562
Wellbutrin Tablets (Infrequent) 821
Zestoretic (0.3 to 1%) 2274
Zestril Tablets (Less than 1%) 2277

Infection, vagina
Micronor Tablets 1667
Modicon 1667
Ortho-Novum 1667

Infection, viral
Cytosar-U Sterile Powder 2329
⅛% Econopred & 1% Econopred Plus ⊙ 217
Intron A (Less than 1%) 2097
Koāte-HP Antihemophilic Factor (Human) 1581
Konȳne 80 Factor IX Complex 1571
Konȳne-HT Factor IX Complex 1583
Maxidex Sterile Ophthalmic Ointment ⊙ 222
Neosar for Injection 566
Prinzide Tablets (0.3% to 1%) 1540
Prolastin Alpha$_1$-Proteinase Inhibitor (Human) 1585
▲ Prozac Pulvules (3.4%) 920
▲ Sandimmune (15.9 to 18.4%) 2024
Vasocidin Ophthalmic Solution ⊙ 276
Zestoretic (0.3 to 1%) 2274

Infectious-mononucleosis-like syndrome
Dapsone USP 1130

Infertility
Cytovene Sterile Powder 2292
Demulen 2161
Enovid 2161
Leukeran Tablets 788
Lippes Loop Intrauterine Double-S 1654
Lo/Ovral Tablets 2471
Lo/Ovral-28 Tablets 2476
Lopid Capsules and Tablets 1736
Methotrexate Tablets, Parenteral, LPF Parenteral 1217
Nordette-21 Tablets (discontinued) 2481
Nordette-28 Tablets 2483
Norethin 2133
Ovral Tablets 2490
Ovral-28 Tablets 2491
Ovrette Tablets 2492
ParaGard T380A Intrauterine Copper Contraceptive 411
Rheumatrex Methotrexate Dose Pack 1234
Zyloprim Tablets (Less than 1%) 830

Infertility, male
Dapsone USP 1130

Infertility, temporary
Brevicon 2304
Jenest-28 Tablets 1636
Levlen/Tri-Levlen 665
Loestrin 1728
Micronor Tablets 1667
Modicon 1667
Norinyl 2304
Norlestrin 1746
Nor-Q D Tablets 2304
Ortho-Cyclen Tablets 1658
Ortho-Novum 1667
Ovcon 1391
Levlen/Tri-Levlen 665
Tri-Norinyl 2304
Triphasil-21 Tablets 2527
Triphasil-28 Tablets 2532

Infertility, tubal
Lippes Loop Intrauterine Double-S 1654

Inflammation
AMVISC Plus (Rare) ⊙ 323
Adalat Capsules (10 mg and 20 mg) (2% or less) 1587
▲ Calcimar Injection, Synthetic (10%) 1839
Ceptaz for Injection (1 in 69 patients) 1057
Chloromycetin Ophthalmic Ointment, 1% 1696
Dalalone D.P. Injectable 999
Decadron-LA Sterile Suspension 1457
Diphtheria and Tetanus Toxoids and Pertussis Vaccine Adsorbed USP (For Pediatric Use) 892
Fluoroplex Topical Solution & Cream 1% 1082
Fortaz (1 in 69 patients) 1060
Hemopad Absorbable Collagen Hemostat 627
Herplex Liquifilm ⊙ 248
Humulin 70/30, 100 Units (Occasional) 1267
Humulin BR, 100 Units (Occasional) 1268
Humulin L, 100 Units (Occasional) 1268
Humulin U, 100 Units (Occasional) 1272
INSTAT Collagen Absorbable Hemostat 1151
▲ Lupron Depot 3.75 mg (Among most frequent) 2312
Lupron Depot 7.5 mg 2311
Lupron Injection (Less than 5%) 2310
ParaGard T380A Intrauterine Copper Contraceptive 411
Pre-Pen 2148
Prilosec Delayed-Release Capsules (Less than 1%) 1530
Procardia Capsules (2% or less) 1781
Terramycin with Polymyxin B Sulfate Ophthalmic Ointment (Rare) 1965
Zestoretic (0.3 to 1%) 2274

Inflammation, genital
▲ Condylox (63% to 71%) 1630

Inflammation, ocular
AMO Vitrax Solution ⊙ 236
Betoptic Sterile Ophthalmic Solution (Small numbers of patients) 569
Betoptic S Sterile Ophthalmic Suspension (Small numbers of patients) 570
Depo-Medrol Sterile Aqueous Suspension 2334

Inflammation, oral (see under Stomatitis)

Inflammation, perianal
Creon Capsules (Rare) 2245
▲ Cytosar-U Sterile Powder (Among most frequent) 2329
Doryx Capsules 1717

Inflammation, periocular
Depo-Medrol Sterile Aqueous Suspension 2334

Inflammation, upper respiratory tract
Solganal Suspension 2122

Inflammation, uterine
Anafranil Capsules (Rare) 650

Inflammation at injection site
Atgam Sterile Solution (Less than 5%) 2320
▲ Brevibloc Injection (8%) 942
▲ Calcimar Injection, Synthetic (10%) 1839
Ceptaz for Injection (One in 69 patients) 1057
▲ Claforan Sterile Injection (4.3%) 1089
Cytovene Sterile Powder (1% or less) 2292
▲ Dalgan Injection (3 to 9%) 620
Dilantin Parenteral 1712
Diprivan Injection (Less than 1%) 2267
Dobutrex Solution Vials 1259
Estratest 2245
▲ Flu-Imune Influenza Virus Vaccine (Less than one-third of recipients) 1204
▲ Fortaz (Most common) 1060
Geref (sermorelin acetate for injection) 2560
Imferon 976
▲ Intron A (6% to 7%) 2097
Lutrepulse for Injection 1655
▲ Miacalcin Injection (About 10%) 2017
Mini-Gamulin Rh, Rho(D) Immune Globulin (Human) (Infrequent) 612
Premarin with Methyltestosterone 2515
Roferon-A Injection (Less than 3%) 1916
Staphage Lysate (SPL) 905
Tazicef for Injection (Less than 2%) 2231
Testred Capsules 1124
Tetanus & Diphtheria Toxoids, Adsorbed Purogenated (Mild to moderate) 1237
Vancocin HCl, Vials & ADD-Vantage 1302
Versed Injection (0.5%-2.6%) 1924
▲ Zovirax Sterile Powder (Approximately 9%) 828

Influenza-like symptoms
Cardura Tablets (Less than 0.5% of 3960 patients) 1941
Engerix-B Unit-Dose Vials (Less than 1%) 2213
Hespan Injection 948
Plendil Extended-Release Tablets (0.5% to 1.5%) 1526
Prinzide Tablets (0.3% to 1%) 1540
Prozac Pulvules (1.2%) 920
Recombivax HB (Less than 1%) 1544
Zestoretic (0.3 to 1%) 2274

Insomnia
A.R.M. Allergy Relief Medicine Caplets ▣ 615
Accutane Capsules 1878
Actifed Capsules ▣ 539
Actifed Plus Caplets ▣ 539
Actifed Plus Tablets (At higher doses) ▣ 540
▲ Actifed with Codeine Cough Syrup (Among most frequent) 752
Actifed Syrup ▣ 540
Actifed Tablets ▣ 540
Actifed 12-Hour Capsules ▣ 539
Acutrim ▣ 548
Adipex-P Tablets and Capsules 1019
Advil Cold & Sinus Caplets (formerly CoAdvil) 2416
AeroBid Inhaler System (1-3%) 995
Afrin Tablets ▣ 693
Alferon N Injection (1% to 2%) 1809
Alka-Seltzer Plus Cold Medicine ▣ 623
Alka-Seltzer Plus Night-Time Cold Medicine ▣ 623
Allerest ▣ 559
Altace Capsules (Less than 1%) 1086
Alurate Elixir (Less than 1 in 100) 1883
Amen 833
Aminophyllin Tablets 2153
Amoxil (Rare) 2193
Anadrol-50 Tablets 2287
▲ Anafranil Capsules (11% to 25%) 650
Anaprox and Anaprox DS Tablets (Less than 1%) 2288
Anatuss LA Tablets 1359
Ansaid Tablets (1-3%) 2319
Aristospan Suspension (Intra-articular) 1011
Arm-a-Med Isoetharine Inhalation Solution, USP 616
Asbron G 1997
Asendin Tablets (Greater than 1%) 1196
Atrohist Sprinkle Capsules 558
Atrovent Inhalation Aerosol (Less than 1%) 675

Augmentin Tablets, Powder for Oral Suspension, and Chewable Tablets (Rare) 2198
Azactam for Injection (Less than 1%) 2252
Azo Gantanol Tablets 1887
Azo Gantrisin Tablets 1888
Azulfidine Tablets, EN-tabs, Oral Suspension (Rare) 1157
Bactrim DS Tablets 1891
Bactrim I.V. Infusion 1889
Bactrim 1891
▲Benadryl Capsules (Among most frequent) 1691
Benadryl Decongestant Elixir ▣ 635
Benadryl Decongestant ▣ 635
▲Benadryl Kapseals (Among most frequent) 1691
Benadryl Parenteral 1692
Benadryl Plus ▣ 636
Benadryl Plus Nighttime ▣ 637
Benadryl Steri-Vials, Ampoules, and Steri-Dose Syringe 1692
Bentyl 1322
Benylin Decongestant ▣ 638
Betoptic Sterile Ophthalmic Solution (Rare) 569
Betoptic S Sterile Ophthalmic Suspension (Rare) 570
Biphetamine Capsules 973
Blocadren Tablets (Less than 1%) 1429
Bontril Slow-Release 834
Brethaire Inhaler 1024
Bromfed 1615
Bronkaid Mist ▣ 757
Bronkaid Mist Suspension ▣ 757
Bronkaid Tablets ▣ 757
Bronkolixir ▣ 761
Bronkometer Aerosol 2042
Bronkosol Solution 2042
Bronkotabs Tablets ▣ 762
▲BuSpar (3%) 1401
Butisol Sodium Elixir & Tablets (Less than 1 in 100) 2377
Calan SR Caplets (1% or less) 2157
Calan Tablets (1% or less) 2155
Cantil Tablets 1326
Capoten (0.5 to 2%) 2255
Capozide (0.5 to 2%) 2258
Cardene Capsules (0.6%) 2290
Cardizem Tablets-30 mg, 60 mg, 90 mg and 120 mg (Less than 1%) 1329
Cardizem SR Capsules-60 mg, 90 mg and 120 mg (1%) 1327
Cardura Tablets (1%) 1941
Cartrol Tablets (1.7%) 507
Catapres Tablets (About 5 in 1,000 patients) 676
Catapres-TTS (5 per 1,000) 677
Ceclor Pulvules & Suspension (Rare) 1251
Celontin 1692
Cerose-DM 2443
Children's Advil Suspension (Less than 1%) 2426
Chlor-Trimeton Decongestant ▣ 694
Choledyl Pediatric Elixir 1702
Choledyl Tablets 1700
Choledyl SA Tablets 1704
Cipro I.V. (1% or less) 1592
Cipro Tablets (Less than 1%) 1589
Clinoril Tablets (Less than 1%) 1433
Clozaril Tablets (2%) 2000
Codimal 846
Combipres Tablets (About 5 in 1,000) 678
Comhist LA Capsules 1618
Compazine (Sometimes) 2201
Allergy-Sinus Comtrex Multi-Symptom Allergy Sinus Formula Tablets & Caplets 746
Cough Formula Comtrex (At higher doses) 746
Comtrex Multi-Symptom Cold Reliever Tablets/Caplets/Liqui-Gels/Liquid- 745
Day-Night Comtrex 747
Non-Drowsy Comtrex 747
Condylox (Less than 5%) 1630
Constant-T Tablets 1029
Contac Continuous Action Decongestant/Antihistamine Capsules ▣ 710
Contac Jr. Children's Cold Medicine ▣ 712
Contac Maximum Strength Continuous Action Decongestant/Antihistamine Caplets ▣ 709
Contac Nighttime Cold Medicine ▣ 713
Contac Severe Cold and Flu Formula Caplets ▣ 711
Contac Sinus Caplets Maximum Strength Non-Drowsy Formula ▣ 710
Contac Sinus Tablets Maximum Strength Non-Drowsy Formula ▣ 710
Cordarone Tablets (1 to 3%) 2446
Coricidin 'D' Decongestant Tablets ▣ 695
Coricidin Demilets Tablets for Children ▣ 696
Cortifoam 1827
Cycrin Tablets 2449
▲Cylert Tablets (Most frequent) 510
Dantrium Capsules (Less frequent) 1619
Dapsone USP 1130
Daraprim Tablets (Rare) 761
Darbid Tablets 2205
Deconamine 663
Deconsal 559
Demazin Nasal Decongestant/ Antihistamine Repetabs Tablets & Syrup ▣ 697
Demser Capsules 1460
Depo-Medrol Sterile Aqueous Suspension 2334
Depo-Provera Sterile Aqueous Suspension (Occasional) 2336
Desoxyn Gradumet Tablets 514
Desyrel and Desyrel Dividose (Greater than 1%) 1404
Dexatrim ▣ 733
Dexedrine 2206
Didrex Tablets 2338
Dilantin Infatabs 1710
Dilantin Kapseals 1708
Dilantin Parenteral 1712
Dilantin-30 Pediatric/Dilantin-125 Suspension 1713
Dilantin with Phenobarbital Kapseals 1715
Dilaudid-HP Injection 1175
Dimacol Caplets ▣ 672
Dimetane Decongestant ▣ 673
Dimetane-DC Cough Syrup 1857
Dimetane-DX Cough Syrup 1858
Dimetapp Elixir ▣ 673
Dimetapp Extentabs ▣ 674
Dimetapp Plus Caplets ▣ 675
Dimetapp Tablets ▣ 675
Dipentum Capsules (Rare) 1160
Disophrol Chronotab Sustained-Action Tablets ▣ 698
Ditropan 1332
Diulo 2129
Dolobid Tablets (Greater than 1 in 100) 1465
Dolophine Hydrochloride Ampoules & Vials 1260
Dolophine Hydrochloride Tablets 1261
Donnatal 1858
Donnatal Extentabs 1859
Donnatal Tablets 1858
Donnazyme Tablets 1860
Dristan Cold Nasal Decongestant/ Antihistamine/ Analgesic Coated Tablets 2419
Dristan Sinus Caplets 2419
Drixoral Antihistamine/Nasal Decongestant Syrup ▣ 698
Drixoral Plus Extended-Release Tablets ▣ 699
Drixoral Sustained-Action Tablets ▣ 698
DynaCirc Capsules (0.5% to 1%) 2004
Efudex 1880
Elavil 2269
Eldepryl (1 of 49 patients) 2250
▲Emcyt Capsules (3%) 1161
Emete-con Intramuscular/Intravenous 1950
Endep Tablets 1927
Engerix-B Unit-Dose Vials (Less than 1%) 2213
Entex Capsules 1623
Entex LA Tablets 1623
Entex Liquid 1623
Ergamisol Tablets (1%) 1136
Etrafon 2087
Sinus Excedrin Analgesic, Decongestant Tablets & Caplets 750
4-Way Cold Tablets 750
Fansidar Tablets 1896
Fastin Capsules 2216
Fedahist Gyrocaps 2145
Fedahist Timecaps 2145
Feldene Capsules (Less than 1%) 1777
Fiorinal with Codeine Capsules 2008
Flagyl I.V. 2131
Flagyl Tablets 2170
Flexeril Tablets (Less than 1%) 1471
▲Floxin Tablets (3% to 7%) 1652
Fulvicin P/G Tablets 2090
Fulvicin P/G 165 & 330 Tablets 2091
Fulvicin-U/F Tablets 2092
Gantanol 1899
Gantrisin Ophthalmic Ointment/Solution 1900
Gantrisin 1901
Gastrocrom Capsules (Infrequent) 974
Grifulvin V (griseofulvin microsize) Tablets/Suspension (Occasional) 1678
Grisactin (Occasional) 2454
Grisactin Ultra Tablets (Occasional) 2455
Gris-PEG Tablets, 125 mg & 250 mg (Occasional) 1083
Halcion Tablets (Rare) 2340
Haldol Decanoate 1375
Haldol Injection, Tablets and Concentrate 1373
Hydromox R Tablets 1209
Hytrin Tablets (At least 1%) 529
Inderal 2459
Inderal LA Long Acting Capsules 2461
Inderide Tablets 2463
Inderide LA Long Acting Capsules 2465
Indocin (Less than 1%) 1487
▲Intron A (Up to 5%) 2097
Ionamin Capsules 981
IOPIDINE ⊙ 232
Isoclor Timesule Capsules ▣ 561
Isoptin Oral Tablets (Less than 1%) 1179
Isoptin SR Sustained Release Tablets (Less than 1%) 1181
Kenalog-10 Injection 2402
Kenalog-40 Injection 2403
▲Kerlone Tablets (1.2% to 5%) 2172
Kinesed Tablets 2272
Klonopin Tablets 1902
Larodopa Tablets (Relatively frequent) 1905
Levatol (1.9%) 1832
Levsin/Levsinex 2147
▲Lioresal Tablets (2-7%) 1031
Lodine Capsules (Less than 1%) 2468
Lopressor Ampuls 1032
Lopressor HCT Tablets 1034
Lopressor Tablets 1032
Lorelco Tablets 1333
Lotensin Tablets 872
Loxitane 1213
Lozol Tablets (Less than 5%) 1843
Ludiomil Tablets (2%) 874
Lufyllin & Lufyllin-400 Tablets 2384
Lufyllin-GG Elixir & Tablets 2385
Lupron Depot 7.5 mg (Less than 5%) 2311
▲Lupron Injection (5% or more) 2310
MS Contin Tablets (Infrequent) 1814
MSIR (Infrequent) 1817
Marax Tablets & DF Syrup 1954
▲Marplan Tablets (Among most frequent) 1906
Matulane Capsules 1907
Maxair Inhaler (Less than 1%) 1311
Maxzide 1215
Mebaral Tablets (Less than 1 in 100) 2061
Meclomen Capsules (Rare) 1739
Medi-Flu Caplet, Liquid ▣ 640
Mesantoin Tablets 2013
Methadone Hydrochloride Diskets 1284
Methadone Hydrochloride Oral Solution & Tablets 1987
Mevacor Tablets 1505
Micronor Tablets 1667
Midamor Tablets (Less than or equal to 1%) 1508
Modicon 1667
Moduretic Tablets (Less than or equal to 1%) 1510
Motofen Tablets (1 in 200 to 1 in 600) 836
Motrin Tablets (Less than 1%) 2351
Mykrox ½ mg Tablets 984
Naldecon CX Adult Liquid ▣ 521
Naldecon DX Adult Liquid ▣ 521
Naldecon DX Children's Syrup ▣ 522
Naldecon DX Pediatric Drops ▣ 522
Naldecon EX Children's Syrup ▣ 522
Naldecon EX Pediatric Drops ▣ 523
Naldecon Syrup, Tablets, Pediatric Drops and Pediatric Syrup 709
Nalfon Pulvules & Tablets (Less than 1%) 919
Naprosyn (Less than 1%) 2297
Nardil (Common) 1742
Navane Capsules and Concentrate 1954
Navane Intramuscular 1956
NebuPent for Inhalation Solution (1% or less) 1017
Nembutal Sodium Capsules (Less than 1%) 534
Nembutal Sodium Solution (Less than 1%) 536
Nembutal Sodium Suppositories (Less than 1%) 538
Neo-Synephrine (Rare) ▣ 759
Nicorette (1.1%) 1335
Nolamine Tablets (Occasional) 838
Nolex LA Tablets 838
Norisodrine Aerotrol 540
Normozide Tablets 2112
Noroxin Tablets (0.3% to 1%) 1519
Norpace (Less than 1%) 2177
Norpramin Tablets 1340
Novafed A Capsules 1342
Novafed Capsules 1342
Novahistine DH 1342
Novahistine DMX ▣ 595
Novahistine Elixir ▣ 596
Novahistine Expectorant 1343
Nucofed Capsules 2219
Nucofed Expectorant 2219
Nucofed Pediatric Expectorant 2220
Nucofed Syrup 2219
Omnipaque 2552
Optimine Tablets 2115
Oramorph SR (Morphine Sulfate Sustained Release Tablets) (Less frequent) 1988
Orap Tablets 1020
Ornade Spansule Capsules 2221
Ornex Caplets ▣ 618
Ortho-Novum 1667
▲Orudis Capsules (Greater than 3%) 2488
Oxsoralen-Ultra Capsule 1117
PBZ Tablets & Elixir 1037
PBZ-SR Tablets 1037
Pamelor 2019
Paradione Capsules 548
Parlodel (Less than 1%) 2020
Parnate Tablets 2222
PediaProfen Suspension (Less than 1%) 1363
Pediazole 1973
Peganone Tablets 551
Pentaspan Injection 949
Pepcid (Infrequent) 1524
Periactin 1525
▲Permax Tablets (7.9%) 1291
Phenergan with Dextromethorphan 2499
Phenergan Injection 2493
Phenergan VC 2500
Phenobarbital Elixir and Tablets (Less than 1 in 100 patients) 1293
Phenurone Tablets (1%) 552
Plegine Tablets 2504
Plendil Extended-Release Tablets (0.5% to 1.5%) 1526
Polaramine 2116
Pondimin Tablets 1867
Ponstel 1758
Prelu-2 Capsules 683
Prilosec Delayed-Release Capsules (Less than 1%) 1530
Primatene Tablets 2421
Prinivil Tablets (1% or less) 1538
Prinzide Tablets 1540
Pro-Banthine Tablets 2141
Procardia XL Tablets (Less than 3%) 1783
Proglycem 649
Propagest 839
Protostat Tablets 1674
Proventil Inhalation Aerosol 2117
Proventil Repetabs Tablets (2%) 2120
Proventil Solutions for Inhalation 0.5% and 0.083% (1%) 2118
Proventil Syrup (Children 2-6: 2%) 2119
Proventil Tablets (2%) 2120
Provera Tablets 2356
▲Prozac Pulvules (13.8%) 920
Pyrroxate Capsules ▣ 669
Quadrinal Tablets 1183
Quarzan Capsules 1937
Quelidrine Syrup 556
Quibron Capsules 713
Quibron-T 714
Quibron-T/SR 716
Recombivax HB (Less than 1%) 1544
Reglan 1869
Respbid Tablets 684
▲Retrovir Capsules (2.4% to 5%) 802
▲Retrovir I.V. Infusion (5%) 805
▲Retrovir Syrup (2.4% to 5%) 802
▲Ritalin (Among most common) 880
Robinul Forte Tablets 1873

(▣ Described in PDR For Nonprescription Drugs) Incidence data in parenthesis; ▲ 3% or more (⊙ Described in PDR For Ophthalmology)

Robinul Injectable 1873
Robinul Tablets 1873
Robitussin Night Relief ■ 677
Robitussin-CF ■ 676
Robitussin-DAC Syrup 1875
Rondec 1975
Rondec-DM 1976
Rondec-TR Tablet 1975
Rowasa (0.12%) 2248
Roxanol 1991
Rufen Tablets (Less than 1%) 691
Ru-Tuss DE Tablets 694
Ru-Tuss II Capsules 693
Ru-Tuss with Hydrocodone 694
Ru-Tuss Tablets 693
Ryna ■ 741
Rythmol Tablets (0.3 to 1.5%) 1184
Sandostatin Injection (Less than 1%) 2029
▲Sanorex Tablets (Among most common) 2030
Sansert Tablets 2031
Seconal Sodium Pulvules (Less than 1 in 100) 1296
▲Sectral Capsules (3%) 2520
Seldane Tablets 1349
▲Seldane-D Extended-Release Tablets (25.9%) 1350
Septra 813
Septra I.V. Infusion 808
Septra I.V. Infusion ADD-Vantage Vials 810
Septra 813
Serophene (clomiphene citrate tablets, USP) (Approximately 1 in 50 patients) 2186
Sinarest ■ 562
Sine-Aid Maximum Strength Sinus Headache Caplets 1365
Sine-Aid Maximum Strength Sinus Headache Tablets 1365
Sinemet Tablets 952
Sinemet CR Tablets (1.2%) 953
Sine-Off Maximum Strength Allergy/Sinus Formula Caplets ■ 721
Sine-Off Maximum Strength No Drowsiness Formula Caplets ■ 722
Sine-Off Sinus Medicine Tablets-Aspirin Formula ■ 722
Singlet Tablets ■ 598
Sinulin 840
Sinutab Allergy Formula Sustained Action Tablets ■ 640
Slo-bid Gyrocaps 1847
Soma Compound w/Codeine Tablets (Infrequent or rare) 2390
Soma Compound Tablets (Infrequent or rare) 2389
Soma Tablets 2388
Stelazine (Sometimes) 2226
Sudafed Children's Liquid ■ 543
Sudafed Cough Syrup ■ 543
Sudafed Plus Liquid ■ 544
Sudafed Plus Tablets ■ 545
Sudafed Sinus Caplets ■ 545
Sudafed Sinus Tablets ■ 545
Sudafed Tablets, 30 mg ■ 544
Sudafed Tablets, Adult Strength, 60 mg ■ 544
Sudafed 12 Hour Capsules ■ 545
Surmontil Capsules 2524
Symmetrel Capsules & Syrup (5-10%) 936
▲Synarel Nasal Solution (8% of patients) 2300
T-PHYL (Uniphyl) 200 mg Tablets 1820
Tacaryl 2409
Talacen (Infrequent) 2070
Talwin Injection 2071
Talwin Compound (Infrequent) 2072
Talwin Injection 2071
Talwin Nx 2073
Tambocor Tablets (1-3%) 1315
Taractan 1920
Tavist Syrup 2033
Tavist Tablets 2035
Tavist-D Tablets 2035
Tedral SA 1765
Temaril Tablets, Syrup and Spansule Sustained Release Capsules 1085
▲Tenex Tablets (4%) 1875
Tenuate 1354
Theo-24 2179
Theo-Dur Sprinkle 1168
Theo-Dur Extended-Release Tablets 1166
Theolair 1317
Theolair-SR Tablets 1319
Theo-Organidin Elixir 2391
▲TheoX Extended-Release Tablets (Among most consistent) 841
Thiosulfil Forte Tablets 2526
Thorazine 2234
Timolide Tablets (Less than 1%) 1547
Timoptic in Ocudose 1552
Timoptic Sterile Ophthalmic Solution 1550
Tofranil Ampuls 1038
Tofranil Tablets 1039
Tofranil-PM Capsules 1041
Tonocard Tablets (Less than 1%) 1554
Toradol IM Injection (1% or less) 2302
Tornalate (Less than 1%) 2074
Trandate HCT Tablets (Less than 1%) 579
Tranxene 556
Trental (2.3%) 1099
Triaminic Allergy Tablets ■ 688
Triaminic Chewables ■ 688
Triaminic Expectorant DH 1995
Triaminic Oral Infant Drops 1996
Triaminic-12 Tablets ■ 690
Triaminicin Tablets ■ 690
Triaminicol Multi-Symptom Cold Tablets ■ 691
Triavil Tablets 1556
Tridione 557
Trilafon 2123
Trinalin Repetabs Tablets 1170
Trobicin Sterile Powder 2366
Tuss-Ornade Liquid 2242
Tuss-Ornade Spansule Capsules 2242
Children's Tylenol Cold Liquid Formula and Chewable Tablets 1368
Tylenol Cold & Flu Hot Medication, Packets 1369
Tylenol Cold & Flu No Drowsiness Hot Medication, Packets 1371
Tylenol Cold Medication Caplets and Tablets 1370
Tylenol Cold Medication No Drowsiness Formula Caplets 1370
Tylenol Cold Night Time Medication Liquid 1371
Tylenol Cough Medication Liquid with Decongestant, Maximum Strength 1372
Tylenol, Maximum Strength, Sinus Medication Gelcaps, Caplets and Tablets 1373
Uniphyl 400 mg Tablets 1823
Ursinus Inlay-Tabs ■ 691
Valium Injectable 1937
Valium Tablets 1939
Valpin 50 Tablets 941
Valrelease Capsules (Infrequent) 1923
Vascor (200, 300 and 400 mg) Tablets (0.5 to 2.65%) 1383
Vaseretic Tablets (0.5% to 2.0%) 1559
Vasotec I.V. 1562
Vasotec Tablets (0.5% to 1%) 1564
Ventolin (Less than 1%) 583
Verelan Capsules (Less than 1%) 1243
Versed Injection (Less than 1%) 1924
Vicks Daycare ■ 660
Vicks Formula 44D Decongestant Cough Medicine ■ 662
Vicks Formula 44M Multi-Symptom Cough Medicine ■ 662
Vicks NyQuil Nighttime Colds Medicine-Original & Cherry Flavor ■ 664
▲Visken Tablets (10%) 2036
Vivactil Tablets 1567
Vivarin Stimulant Tablets ■ 726
Voltaren Tablets (Less than 1%) 1042
▲Wellbutrin Tablets (18.6%) 821
Winstrol Tablets 2075
▲Xanax Tablets (29.4%) 2367
Zantac Injection and Zantac Injection Premixed 1063
Zantac (Rare) 1065
Zaroxolyn Tablets 989
Zestoretic 2274
Zestril Tablets (Less than 1%) 2277
▲Zoladex (5%) 1110
Zyloprim Tablets (Less than 1%) 830

Insulin allergy
Insulatard NPH (Rare) 1626
Insulatard NPH Human (Very rare) 1627
Mixtard 70/30 (Very rare) 1627
Mixtard Human 70/30 (Rare) 1628
Velosulin (Very rare) 1627
Velosulin Human (Very rare) 1628

Insulin autoimmune syndrome
Tapazole Tablets 1298

Insulin reaction
Dalalone D.P. Injectable 999
Insulatard NPH 1626
Insulatard NPH Human 1627
Mixtard 70/30 1627
Mixtard Human 70/30 1628
Velosulin 1627
Velosulin Human 1628

Insulin requirement, changes
Aristocort Suspension 1008
Aristospan Suspension 1011
Celestone Soluspan Suspension 2081
Cortenema 2244
Cortone Acetate Sterile Suspension 1437
Cortone Acetate Tablets 1439
Danocrine Capsules 2046
Decadron Elixir 1445
Decadron Phosphate Injection 1449
Decadron Phosphate Respihaler 1454
Decadron Phosphate Turbinaire 1456
Decadron Phosphate with Xylocaine Injection, Sterile 1451
Decadron Tablets 1447
Decadron-LA Sterile Suspension 1457
Deltasone Tablets 2332
Hydrocortone Phosphate Injection, Sterile 1481
Hydrocortone Tablets 1482
Kenalog-10 Injection 2402
Kenalog-40 Injection 2403
Pediapred Oral Liquid 987
Solu-Cortef Sterile Powder 2361
Solu-Medrol Sterile Powder 2363
Tenoretic Tablets 1105

Insulin shock
Zanosar Sterile Powder 2371

Intercourse, sexual, painful (see under Pain with coitus)

Intestinal motility, decrease
Bellergal-S Tablets (Rare) 1998

Intestinal motility, increase
Raudixin Tablets 1803
Rauzide Tablets 1804
Salutensin/Salutensin-Demi 719

Intestinal obstruction
Anafranil Capsules (Rare) 650
Dicumarol Tablets 516
Kayexalate 2053
Lamprene Capsules (Less than 1%) 1030
Lippes Loop Intrauterine Double-S 1654
Panwarfin Tablets 547
ParaGard T380A Intrauterine Copper Contraceptive 411
Permax Tablets (Infrequent) 1291
Sodium Polystyrene Sulfonate Suspension (Rare) 1993
Ten-K Controlled-Release Tablets 2282

Intestinal perforation
Butazolidin Capsules & Tablets 1027
Cipro I.V. (Less than 1%) 1592
Cipro Tablets (Less than 1%) 1589
Hydrocortone Tablets 1482
Methotrexate Tablets, Parenteral, LPF Parenteral 1217
ParaGard T380A Intrauterine Copper Contraceptive 411
Rheumatrex Methotrexate Dose Pack 1234
Ten-K Controlled-Release Tablets 2282
Thioguanine Tablets, Tabloid Brand 815
Wellbutrin Tablets (Rare) 821

Intoxication, chronic
Miltown Tablets 2386

Intracranial pressure, increase
Aristocort Suspension 1008
Aristospan Suspension (Intralesional) 1011
Celestone Soluspan Suspension 2081
Cibalith-S 870
Cipro I.V. 1592
Cortenema 2244
Cortifoam 1827
Cortone Acetate Sterile Suspension 1437
Cortone Acetate Tablets 1439
Dalalone D.P. Injectable 999
Decadron Elixir 1445
Decadron Phosphate Injection 1449
Decadron Phosphate Respihaler 1454
Decadron Phosphate Turbinaire 1456
Decadron Phosphate with Xylocaine Injection, Sterile 1451
Decadron Tablets 1447
Decadron-LA Sterile Suspension 1457
Depo-Medrol Sterile Aqueous Suspension 2334
Dilaudid Cough Syrup 1174
Dilaudid 1173
Dilaudid-HP Injection 1175
Eskalith 2214
Floxin Tablets 1652
Hydeltrasol Injection, Sterile 1476
Hydeltra-T.B.A. Sterile Suspension 1478
Hydrocortone Acetate Sterile Suspension 1479
Hydrocortone Phosphate Injection, Sterile 1481
Hydrocortone Tablets 1482
Ketalar 1726
Lithane Tablets 1596
Lithium Carbonate Capsules & Tablets 1984
Lithobid Tablets 870
MS Contin Tablets (Infrequent) 1814
MSIR (Infrequent) 1817
NegGram (Occasional) 2062
Nipride I.V. Infusion 1909

Intracranial pressure with papilledema
Aristospan Suspension (Intra-articular) 1011
Deltasone Tablets 2332

Intraocular pressure, increase (see under Glaucoma)

Intraocular pressure, paradoxical increase
Floropryl Sterile Ophthalmic Ointment 1473
Humorsol Sterile Ophthalmic Solution 1475
Phospholine Iodide ◎ 315

Intravascular coagulation, disseminated
Clinoril Tablets (Less than 1 in 100) 1433
Dolobid Tablets (Less than 1 in 100) 1465
Indocin Capsules (Less than 1%) 1487
Indocin I.V. 1490
Indocin (Less than 1%) 1487
Parlodel 2020
Prostin VR Pediatric Sterile Solution (1%) 2355
TheraCys BCG Live (Intravesical) (Up to 2.7%) 898

Involuntary movements, abnormal
Atgam Sterile Solution (Less than 5%) 2320
Clozaril Tablets (Less than 1%) 2000
Cordarone Tablets 2446
Dopram Injectable 1860
Elavil 2269
Eldepryl 2250
Moban Tablets & Concentrate 932
Orap Tablets 1020
Parlodel 2020
Prolixin Oral Concentrate 1792
Roferon-A Injection (Less than 0.5%) 1916
Tegretol Chewable Tablets 654
Tegretol Suspension 656
Tegretol Tablets 654

Involuntary movements, extremities
Compazine 2201
Haldol Decanoate 1375
Haldol Injection, Tablets and Concentrate 1373
Moban Tablets & Concentrate 932
Navane Capsules and Concentrate 1954
Navane Intramuscular 1956
Orap Tablets 1020
Prolixin Decanoate 1795
Prolixin Enanthate 1796
Prolixin Oral Concentrate 1792
Reglan 1869
Serentil 686
Stelazine 2226
Thorazine 2234

Involuntary movements, trunk
Haldol Decanoate 1375
Mellaril 2011
Orap Tablets 1020
Prolixin Decanoate 1795

Prolixin Enanthate ... 1796
Reglan ... 1869
Serentil ... 686

Iodine uptake, elevated

Lithobid/Cibalith ... 870

Iodism

Calcidrine Syrup ... 506
Omnipaque (Infrequent) ... 2552
Quadrinal Tablets ... 1183
Theo-Organidin Elixir ... 2391
Tussi-Organidin DM Liquid ... 2392
Tussi-Organidin Liquid ... 2391

Iridocyclitis (see also under Iritis)

Betagan (Rare) ... ◉ 239

Iris cysts

Floropryl Sterile Ophthalmic Ointment ... 1473
Humorsol Sterile Ophthalmic Solution ... 1475
Phospholine Iodide (Rare) ... ◉ 315

Iritis (see also under Uveitis)

AK-Cide Sterile Ophthalmic Ointment & Suspension ... ◉ 202
AK-Taine (Sometimes) ... ◉ 207
Alcaine (Occasional) ... ◉ 210
Fluoracaine ... ◉ 208
Healon (Rare) ... ◉ 279
Kerlone Tablets (Less than 2%) ... 2172
Meclomen Capsules (Rare) ... 1739
MIOSTAT (Occasional) ... ◉ 233
Myochrysine Injection (Rare) ... 1516
Ophthetic (Sometimes) ... ◉ 249
Profenal Sterile Ophthalmic Solution (Less than 0.5%) ... ◉ 234
Prozac Pulvules (Rare) ... 920
Solganal Suspension (Rare) ... 2122
Tenex Tablets (Less than 3%) ... 1875
Zyloprim Tablets (Less than 1%) ... 830

Iritis, activation of latent

Floropryl Sterile Ophthalmic Ointment ... 1473
Humorsol Sterile Ophthalmic Solution ... 1475
Phospholine Iodide ... ◉ 315

Iron deficiency

Cuprimine Capsules ... 1442
Syprine Capsules ... 1546

Iron deficiency anemia

Lortab ASA Tablets (Infrequent) ... 2414
Permax Tablets (Infrequent) ... 1291

Irritability

A.P.L. ... 2431
Actibine ... 900
Actifed with Codeine Cough Syrup ... 752
▲ AeroBid Inhaler System (3-9%) ... 995
Aminophyllin Tablets ... 2153
Anafranil Capsules (2%) ... 650
Aquasol A Vitamin A Capsules, USP ... 615
Aquasol A Parenteral, USP ... 615
Asbron G ... 1997
Atabrine Hydrochloride Tablets (Infrequent) ... 2041
Baron-X Tablets ... 650
Benadryl Capsules ... 1691
Benadryl Injection ... 1692
Brexin L.A. Capsules ... 2078
Bromfed ... 1615
Calderol Capsules ... 1635
Celontin ... 1692
Choledyl Pediatric Elixir ... 1702
Choledyl Tablets ... 1700
Choledyl SA Tablets ... 1704
Cipro I.V. (1% or less) ... 1592
Cipro Tablets (Less than 1%) ... 1589
Clozaril Tablets (Less than 1%) ... 2000
Codimal ... 846
Constant-T Tablets ... 1029
Cylert Tablets ... 510
Dalmane Capsules ... 1927
Dayto Himbin Tablets and Liquid ... 905
Deconamine ... 663
Dilor ... 2079
Dimetane-DC Cough Syrup ... 1857
Dimetane-DX Cough Syrup ... 1858
Dipentum Capsules (Rare) ... 1160
Diphtheria and Tetanus Toxoids and Pertussis Vaccine Adsorbed USP (For Pediatric Use) (1 in 2 doses) ... 892
Doral Tablets ... 2383
Efudex ... 1880
Eldepryl ... 2250
Elspar ... 1470
Endep Tablets ... 1927
Engerix-B Unit-Dose Vials (Less than 1%) ... 2213
Fiorinal with Codeine Capsules ... 2008
Flagyl I.V. ... 2131
Flagyl Tablets ... 2170
Gastrocrom Capsules (2 of 87 patients) ... 974
Guaifed ... 1615
Halcion Tablets ... 2340
HibTITER (133 of 1,118 vaccinations) ... 1206
▲ Intron A (4% to 10%) ... 2097
IOPIDINE ... ◉ 232
ISMOTIC (Very rare) ... ◉ 233
▲ Lozol Tablets (Greater than or equal to 5%) ... 1843
Lufyllin & Lufyllin-400 Tablets ... 2384
Lufyllin-GG Elixir & Tablets ... 2385
▲ Marinol (Dronabinol) Capsules (7%) ... 1985
Mebaral Tablets ... 2061
Mesantoin Tablets ... 2013
Methadone Hydrochloride Diskets ... 1284
Methotrexate Tablets, Parenteral, LPF Parenteral ... 1217
Niclocide Chewable Tablets ... 1607
Nicorette (1.1%) ... 1335
Optimine Tablets ... 2115
Ornade Spansule Capsules ... 2221
PBZ Tablets & Elixir ... 1037
PBZ-SR Tablets ... 1037
Paradione Capsules ... 548
Periactin ... 1525
Phenobarbital Elixir and Tablets ... 1293
Plaquenil Sulfate Tablets ... 2067
Plendil Extended-Release Tablets (0.5% to 1.5%) ... 1526
Polaramine ... 2116
Pregnyl ... 1644
Profasi (human chorionic gonadotropin, USP) ... 2186
▲ ProHIBiT Haemophilus b Conjugate Vaccine (Diphtheria Toxoid Conjugate) (16.1%) ... 896
Protostat Tablets ... 1674
Proventil Repetabs Tablets (Less than 1%) ... 2120
Proventil Syrup (1 of 100) ... 2119
Proventil Tablets (Less than 1%) ... 2120
Quadrinal Tablets ... 1183
Quibron Capsules ... 713
Quibron-T ... 714
Quibron-T/SR ... 716
Respbid Tablets ... 684
Retrovir (1.5%) ... 802
Rheumatrex Methotrexate Dose Pack ... 1234
Roferon-A Injection (Less than 1%) ... 1916
Ru-Tuss DE Tablets ... 694
Ru-Tuss II Capsules ... 693
Sandostatin Injection (Less than 1%) ... 2029
Seldane-D Extended-Release Tablets (1.1%) ... 1350
Skelaxin ... 840
Slo-bid Gyrocaps ... 1847
Soma Compound w/Codeine Tablets (Infrequent or rare) ... 2390
Soma Compound Tablets (Infrequent or rare) ... 2389
Soma Tablets ... 2388
Symmetrel Capsules & Syrup (1-5%) ... 936
T-PHYL (Uniphyl) 200 mg Tablets ... 1820
Talacen (Rare) ... 2070
Talwin Injection ... 2071
Talwin Compound (Rare) ... 2072
Talwin Injection ... 2071
Talwin Nx ... 2073
Tavist Syrup ... 2033
Tavist Tablets ... 2035
Tavist-D Tablets ... 2035
Theo-24 ... 2179
Theo-Dur Sprinkle ... 1168
Theo-Dur Extended-Release Tablets ... 1166
Theolair ... 1317
Theolair-SR Tablets ... 1319
▲ TheoX Extended-Release Tablets (Among most consistent) ... 841
Tranxene ... 556
▲ Trexan Tablets (Less than 10%) ... 937
Triaminic Expectorant DH ... 1995
Triaminic Oral Infant Drops ... 1996
Triavil Tablets ... 1556
Tridione ... 557
Trinalin Repetabs Tablets ... 1170
Tuss-Ornade Liquid ... 2242
Tuss-Ornade Spansule Capsules ... 2242
Uniphyl 400 mg Tablets ... 1823
Ventolin (Less than 1 of 100 patients) ... 583
Vivarin Stimulant Tablets ... ▣ 726
Voltaren Tablets (Less than 1%) ... 1042
▲ Xanax Tablets (33.1%) ... 2367
Yocon ... 1686
Yohimex Tablets ... 1190
Zarontin Capsules ... 1768
Zarontin Syrup ... 1769

Irritation

Aclovate (1 in 100 patients) ... 1053
Adsorbonac 2% and 5% ... ◉ 210
Alcaine ... ◉ 210
Americaine Hemorrhoidal Ointment ... ▣ 558
Analpram-HC Rectal Cream 1% and 2.5% ... 970
Anusol Ointment ... ▣ 634
Anusol-HC Cream (Infrequent) ... 1690
Anusol-HC Suppositories ... 1691
Aqua Care Cream ... ▣ 616
Aqua Care Lotion ... ▣ 616
Atrovent Inhalation Aerosol (1.6%) ... 675
Benoquin Cream 20% (Occasional) ... 1112
5 Benzagel (5% benzoyl peroxide) & 10 Benzagel (10% benzoyl peroxide), Acne Gels, Microgel Formula ... 907
BiCozene Creme ... ▣ 684
Bleph-10 Ophthalmic Ointment 10% ... 586
Calciparine Injection ... 925
Carmol HC Cream 1% (Infrequent) ... 2296
Chloresium (A few instances) ... 1994
Clear by Design Medicated Acne Gel ... ▣ 709
Cleocin T Topical ... 2327
Cortisporin Otic Solution Sterile ... 760
Cortisporin Otic Suspension Sterile ... 760
Cutivate Cream 0.05% ... 1054
Cutivate Ointment 0.005% ... 1054
Decadron Phosphate Topical Cream ... 1455
Decaspray Topical Aerosol ... 1459
Denorex ... 2418
Denorex Medicated Shampoo, Extra Strength ... ▣ 748
Denorex ... 2418
Desenex ... ▣ 561
DesOwen Cream, Ointment and Lotion (Infrequent) ... 1682
Dyclone 0.5% and 1% Topical Solutions, USP ... 626
Elocon Lotion 0.1% ... 2084
Eurax Cream & Lotion ... 2398
Florone/Florone E ... 908
Floxin Tablets (Less than 1%) ... 1652
Fluoroplex Topical Solution & Cream 1% ... 1082
Formalyde-10 Spray ... 1769
Fungizone Cream, Lotion and Ointment (Occasional) ... 2261
Garamycin Ophthalmic Solution—Sterile ... ◉ 305
Gentak Ointment & Solution ... ◉ 208
Hibiclens Antimicrobial Skin Cleanser ... 2271
Hibistat Towelette ... 2272
Hytone ... 909
Kenalog Cream, Lotion & Ointment (Infrequent) ... 2401
Lidex (Infrequent) ... 2296
Locoid Cream, Ointment and Topical Solution (Infrequent) ... 970
Lotrisone Cream (Infrequent) ... 2103
Luroscrub Antimicrobial Skin Cleanser ... 912
Maxivate Cream, Lotion & Ointment 0.05% ... 2406
Monistat 3 Vaginal Suppositories ... 1657
Monistat-Derm (miconazole nitrate) Cream (Isolated reports) ... 1679
Mycelex 1% Cream and Topical Solution 1% ... 1604
Mycelex OTC Antifungal Cream and Solution ... 1571
Mycelex-G 1% Vaginal Cream (0.5%) ... 1605
Mycolog II Cream and Ointment (Rare) ... 2407
Mycostatin Pastilles (Rare) ... 734
NeoDecadron Topical Cream ... 1518
Neo-Synalar Cream (Infrequent) ... 2296
▲ Nizoral 2% Cream (5%) ... 1143
Nizoral 2% Shampoo (Less than 1%) ... 1144
Nutracort Cream & Lotion (Infrequent) ... 1684
Oncovin Solution Vials & Hyporets ... 1288
Orabase HCA Oral Paste (Infrequent) ... 890
Otic Tridesilon Solution 0.05% (Infrequent) ... 1612
Oxistat Cream (0.4%) ... 1055
PediOtic Suspension Sterile ... 797
Persa-Gel (benzoyl peroxide) ... 1680
Pramosone Cream, Lotion & Ointment ... 971
Pred-G Liquifilm Sterile Ophthalmic Suspension ... ◉ 252
PreSun 15 Facial Sunscreen ... ▣ 537
PreSun 8, 15 and 39 Creamy Sunscreens ... ▣ 537
PreSun 15 and 29 Sensitive Skin Sunscreen ... ▣ 537
ProctoCream-HC (Infrequent) ... 1834
Psorcon Ointment 0.05% ... 909
Selsun Blue Dandruff Shampoo ... 1978
Shade Oil-Free ... ▣ 705
Super Shade ... ▣ 705
Synacort Creams 1%, 2.5% (Infrequent) ... 2296
Synalar (Infrequent) ... 2296
Temovate (2 of 366 patients) ... 1056
Thera-Gesic ... 1614
Theraplex T Shampoo ... 1411
Theraplex Z Shampoo ... 1411
Tinactin ... ▣ 706
Tridesilon Creme 0.05% (Infrequent) ... 1611
Tridesilon Ointment 0.05% (Infrequent) ... 1611
Vagistat (Less than 1%) ... 1397
Vanoxide-HC Acne Lotion (Among most frequent) ... 911
Vytone Cream 1% ... 911
Westcort ... 2411

Irritation, anal

Anusol Ointment ... ▣ 634
Cholybar (Less frequent) ... 1705
Colyte ... 1826
Creon Capsules ... 2245
GoLYTELY (Infrequent) ... 699
Questran Light (Less frequent) ... 711
Questran Powder ... 710

Irritation, gastric

Akineton ... 1171
Aldoclor Tablets ... 1413
Aldoril Tablets ... 1418
Apresazide Capsules ... 854
Apresoline-Esidrix Tablets ... 857
Capoten (0.5 to 2%) ... 2255
Capozide (0.5 to 2%) ... 2258
Combipres Tablets ... 678
Corzide Tablets ... 702
Dantrium Capsules (Less frequent) ... 1619
Diucardin Tablets ... 2450
Diupres Tablets ... 1461
Diuril Oral Suspension ... 1464
Diuril Sodium Intravenous ... 1463
Diuril Tablets ... 1464
Enduron Tablets ... 517
Enduronyl ... 518
Entex Capsules ... 1623
Entex LA Tablets ... 1623
Entex Liquid ... 1623
Esidrix Tablets ... 863
Esimil Tablets ... 864
Exna Tablets ... 1862
HydroDIURIL Tablets ... 1484
Hydromox R Tablets ... 1209
Hydromox Tablets ... 1208
Hydropres Tablets ... 1485
Inderide Tablets ... 2463
Inderide LA Long Acting Capsules ... 2465
Kayexalate ... 2053
Lasix ... 1093
Lopressor HCT Tablets ... 1034
Lozol Tablets (Less than 5%) ... 1843
Marax Tablets & DF Syrup ... 1954
Maxzide ... 1215
Minizide Capsules ... 1779
Moduretic Tablets ... 1510
Nalfon Pulvules & Tablets (Less than 1%) ... 919
Naturetin Tablets (Occasional) ... 1789
Nolex LA Tablets ... 838
Norflex ... 1314
Oretic Tablets ... 544
Oreticyl ... 545
Prinzide Tablets ... 1540

Quadrinal Tablets ... 1183
Rauzide Tablets ... 1804
Renese Tablets ... 1785
Saluron ... 718
Salutensin/Salutensin-Demi ... 719
Ser-Ap-Es Tablets ... 881
Serpasil-Esidrix Tablets ... 886
Synkayvite Tablets (Rare) ... 1920
Thalitone Tablets ... 687
Theo-Organidin Elixir ... 2391
Timolide Tablets ... 1547
Trandate HCT Tablets ... 579
Vaseretic Tablets ... 1559
Zestoretic ... 2274

Irritation, gastrointestinal

Colestid Granules (Fewer than 1 in 500) ... 2328
Dibenzyline Capsules ... 2207
▲K-Lor Powder Packets (Most common) ... 531
▲K-Norm Capsules (Among most common) ... 982
Organidin Elixir, Solution & Tablets (Rare) ... 2387
Procardia XL Tablets (Less than 1%) ... 1783
Ten-K Controlled-Release Tablets ... 2282
Tenoretic Tablets ... 1105
Theo-Organidin Elixir (Rare) ... 2391
Tussi-Organidin DM Liquid (Rare) ... 2392
Tussi-Organidin Liquid (Rare) ... 2391

Irritation, glossal (see under Irritation, oral)

Irritation, local

AK-Spore H.C. ... ◉ 206
AK-Spore ... ◉ 205
▲Anthra-Derm Ointment 1%, ½%, ¼%, 1/10% (Most frequent) ... 907
Aristocort A (Infrequent) ... 1010
Aspercreme Creme & Lotion Analgesic Rub ... ▣ 732
Astramorph/PF Injection, USP (Preservative-Free) ... 618
Atrac-Tain, Moisturizing Cream ... 2285
Attrac-Tain, Moisturizing Lotion ... 2285
Auralgan Otic Solution ... 2437
BAZA Cream, Occlusive Skin Protectant ... 2285
Bentyl Injection ... 1322
BenzaShave Medicated Shave Cream 5% and 10% ... 1409
Bleph-10 Liquifilm Sterile Ophthalmic Solution ... 586
Bleph-10 Ophthalmic Ointment 10% ... 586
Calciparine Injection ... 925
Carmol 20 Cream ... ▣ 732
Carmol 10 Lotion ... ▣ 732
Cetamide Ointment ... ◉ 220
Chloromycetin Cream, 1% ... 1694
Chloromycetin Otic ... 1697
Cholybar (Less frequent) ... 1705
Clearasil Adult Care Medicated Blemish Cream ... ▣ 657
Cortisporin Ophthalmic Ointment Sterile ... 758
Critic-Aid, Antimicrobial Skin Paste ... 2286
Cyclocort Lotion (Infrequent) ... 1198
Demerol ... 2047
Deponit NTG Transdermal Delivery System ... 2143
Desferal Vials ... 862
Dilantin Parenteral ... 1712
Drithocreme ... 590
Dritho-Scalp ... 591
Duramorph ... 960
Edecrin (Occasionally) ... 1468
Elase-Chloromycetin Ointment ... 1015
Eldecort Cream 1.0% (Infrequenty) ... 1113
Eldecort Cream 1.0% and 2.5% (Infrequent) ... 1113
▲Estraderm Transdermal System (17%) ... 866
Eurax Cream & Lotion ... 2398
Halotex Cream & Solution (0.8 to 1.7%) ... 2400
Heparin Lock Flush Solution ... 2456
Heparin Sodium Vials ... 1264
Heparin Sodium Injection ... 2457
Heparin Sodium Injection, USP, Sterile Solution ... 2342
HibTITER ... 1206
Infumorph 200 and Infumorph 500 Sterile Solutions ... 962
Isopto Atropine ... ◉ 218
Isopto Cetamide Solution ... ◉ 220
Kenalog-10 Injection (Occasional) ... 2402
Luroscrub Antimicrobial Skin Cleanser ... 912
Meclan (meclocycline sulfosalicylate) Cream (Isolated Reports) ... 1679
Mepergan Injection ... 2479
Minitran Transdermal Delivery System ... 1312
Monistat Dual-Pak ... 1657
Mycelex 1% Cream and Topical Solution 1% ... 1604
NP-27 Cream, Solution, Spray Powder & Powder Antifungal ... ▣ 734
Naftin Cream 1% (2%) ... 1084
Nitrodisc (Rare) ... 2176
Nitro-Dur (nitroglycerin) Transdermal Infusion System ... 1164
▲Nizoral 2% Cream (5%) ... 1143
Occlusal-HP ... 1045
Ogen ... 540
Otic Domeboro Solution ... 1609
Oxy Clean ... ▣ 720
Oxy Clean Medicated Pads - Regular, Sensitive Skin, and Maximum Strength ... ▣ 720
Oxy Clean Medicated Soap ... ▣ 720
Oxy 10 Daily Face Wash Antibacterial Skin Wash ... ▣ 721
Oxy-5 and Oxy-10 Tinted and Vanishing Formulas with Sorboxyl ... ▣ 719
Paplex/Paplex Ultra ... 1410
▲Polytrim Ophthalmic Solution Sterile (Most frequent) ... 588
Psorion Cream 0.05% (Infrequent) ... 1121
Questran Powder ... 710
Retin-A (tretinoin) Cream/Gel/Liquid ... 1680
Sebulex Antiseborrheic Treatment Shampoo ... 2408
Sebulex Shampoo with Conditioners ... 2408
Sebutone and Sebutone Cream Antiseborrheic Tar Shampoos ... 2408
Selsun Rx 2.5% Selenium Sulfide Lotion, USP ... 1977
Sodium Sulamyd ... 2122
Stri-Dex Maximum ... ▣ 573
Stri-Dex Dual Textured Regular Strength Pads ... ▣ 573
Stri-Dex Dual Textured Regular Strength Big Pads ... ▣ 573
Sulfacet-R Acne Lotion (Rare) ... 910
Sultrin (Frequent) ... 1675
Terramycin Intramuscular Solution ... 1964
Theroxide ... 1411
Topicort (Infrequent) ... 1098
Transderm-Nitro Transdermal Therapeutic System ... 2283
Trans-Plantar ... 2315
Trans-Ver-Sal Wart Remover Dermal Patch Delivery System ... 2315
Tronothane Hydrochloride Cream ... 558
Vascor (200, 300 and 400 mg) Tablets (0.5 to 2.0%) ... 1383
Vasocidin Ointment ... ◉ 275
Vasocidin Ophthalmic Solution ... ◉ 276
Vioform-Hydrocortisone Cream and Mild Cream ... 889
Vioform-Hydrocortisone Ointment ... 889
Viranol Gel ... 591
Viroptic Ophthalmic Solution, 1% Sterile ... 820
VōSol (Rare) ... 2392

Irritation, nasal

AeroBid Inhaler System (1-3%) ... 995
Beconase AQ Nasal Spray ... 574
▲Beconase Inhalation Aerosol & Refill (11 in 100 patients) ... 574
▲Decadron Phosphate Turbinaire (Most common) ... 1456
Diapid Nasal Spray (Infrequent) ... 2003
Nasacort Nasal Inhaler (2.8%) ... 1844
Nasalcrom Nasal Solution (1 in 40) ... 986
Nasalide Nasal Solution 0.025% (5% or less) ... 2299
▲Synarel Nasal Solution (3% of patients) ... 2300
Syntocinon Nasal Spray ... 2033
Vancenase AQ Nasal Spray 0.042% ... 2127
▲Vancenase Nasal Inhaler (11 per 100 patients) ... 2126

Irritation, nasopharyngeal

▲Beconase AQ Nasal Spray (24% of patients) ... 574
Intal Inhaler (Rare) ... 979
Intal Nebulizer Solution ... 980
▲Vancenase AQ Nasal Spray 0.042% (Up to 24%) ... 2127

Irritation, ocular

▲A/T/S Topical Gel and Topical Solution (17 out of 90) ... 1089
Albalon Solution with Liquifilm ... ◉ 238
ETS-2% ... 1685
Erycette (erythromycin 2%) Topical Solution ... 1678
Gantrisin Ophthalmic Ointment/Solution ... 1900
Lacrisert Sterile Ophthalmic Insert ... 1493
Monopril Tablets (0.2 to 1.0%) ... 1406
Naphcon Forte ... ◉ 226
Oncovin Solution Vials & Hyporets ... 1288
ProSom Tablets (Infrequent) ... 554
Rythmol Tablets (Less than 1%) ... 1184
Temovate Scalp Application (1 of 294 patients) ... 1056
Timoptic in Ocudose ... 1552
Timoptic Sterile Ophthalmic Solution ... 1550
Vasocon-A ... ◉ 278
Vira-A Ophthalmic Ointment, 3% ... 1767

Irritation, oral

AeroBid Inhaler System (1-3%) ... 995
Anbesol ... 2417
Cholybar (Less frequent) ... 1705
Hydergine Sublingual Tablets ... 2010
Lasix ... 1093
Niclocide Chewable Tablets ... 1607
Peridex ... 1808
Questran Powder ... 710
Sandimmune (Rare) ... 2024

Irritation, oropharyngeal

Proventil Inhalation Aerosol ... 2117
Ventolin ... 583

Irritation, oropharynx

Brethaire Inhaler ... 1024
Proventil ... 2120
Ventolin ... 583

Irritation, penile

Conceptrol ... ▣ 631
Emko Because Contraceptor Vaginal Contraceptive Foam ... ▣ 700
Emko Vaginal Contraceptive Foam ... ▣ 701
Gynol II Extra Strength Contraceptive Jelly (Occasional) ... ▣ 632

Irritation, perianal (see under Irritation, anal)

Irritation, skin (see under Irritation, local)

Irritation, vaginal

Conceptrol (Occasional) ... ▣ 631
Emko Because Contraceptor Vaginal Contraceptive Foam ... ▣ 700
Emko Vaginal Contraceptive Foam ... ▣ 701
Encare Vaginal Contraceptive Suppositories ... ▣ 733
Gynol II Extra Strength Contraceptive Jelly (Occasional) ... ▣ 632
Monistat Dual-Pak (2%) ... 1657
Monistat 3 Vaginal Suppositories (2%) ... 1657
Mycelex-G 100 mg Vaginal Tablets (Rare) ... 1606
Mycelex-G 500 mg Vaginal Tablets (1 in 149 patients) ... 1606
Semicid Vaginal Contraceptive Inserts ... 2422
Sultrin (Frequent) ... 1675
▲Terazol 3 Vaginal Cream (5%) ... 1676
▲Terazol 7 Vaginal Cream (3.1% of 521 patients) ... 1677

Irritation, vulvovaginal (see under Irritation, vaginal)

Irritation at injection site

Bactrim I.V. Infusion (Infrequent) ... 1889
Bentyl Injection ... 1322
▲Eulexin Capsules (3%) ... 2089
Kenalog-40 Injection ... 2403
Metrodin (urofollitropin for injection) ... 2182
Nembutal Sodium Capsules ... 534
Nembutal Sodium Solution (Less than 1%) ... 536
Nembutal Sodium Suppositories (Less than 1%) ... 538
Nipride I.V. Infusion ... 1909
Oreticyl ... 545
Pepcid I.V. (Infrequent) ... 1524
Pergonal (menotropins for injection, USP) ... 2184
Septra I.V. Infusion (Infrequent) ... 808
Septra I.V. Infusion ADD-Vantage Vials (Infrequent) ... 810

Ischemia

Brevibloc Injection (1%) ... 942
Calciparine Injection ... 925
Heparin Sodium Vials ... 1264
Heparin Sodium Injection, USP, Sterile Solution ... 2342
▲Lupron Depot 3.75 mg (Among most frequent) ... 2312
Lupron Depot 7.5 mg ... 2311
▲Lupron Injection (5% or more) ... 2310
Roferon-A Injection (Less than 1%) ... 1916
Sandostatin Injection (Less than 1%) ... 2029
Sensorcaine ... 631
Sensorcaine-MPF Spinal ... 634

Ischemia, arteria basilaris

AK-Fluor Injection 10% and 25% ... ◉ 204
Fluorescite ... ◉ 217

Ischemia, cerebral

Ansaid Tablets (Less than 1%) ... 2319
Betagan ... ◉ 239
Cardene Capsules (Less than 0.4%) ... 2290
Cardilate Oral/Sublingual Tablets ... 757
▲Dilatrate-SR (2-36%) ... 1827
Nitrolingual Spray (Occasional) ... 1846
Peritrate (Occasional) ... 1756
Sorbitrate (Ocasional) ... 1103

Ischemia, myocardial

Anafranil Capsules (Rare) ... 650
Diprivan Injection (Less than 1%) ... 2267
Ergamisol Tablets ... 1136
Sterile FUDR (Remote possibility) ... 1898
Fluorouracil Injection ... 1897
Hyperstat I.V. Injection ... 2095
Omnipaque ... 2552
Pitressin Synthetic, Ampoules ... 1758

Ischemia, peripheral

Anafranil Capsules (Rare) ... 650
Cardura Tablets (0.3%) ... 1941
Intron A (Less than 1%) ... 2097
Kerlone Tablets (Less than 2%) ... 2172

Ischemia of digits

Zovirax Sterile Powder (Less than 1%) ... 828

Ischemic attacks, transient

Actimmune (Rare) ... 1046
Clozaril Tablets ... 2000
Demulen ... 2161
DynaCirc Capsules (0.5% to 1%) ... 2004
Enovid ... 2161
Epogen for Injection (0.4%) ... 591
▲Lupron Depot 3.75 mg (Among most frequent) ... 2312
Lupron Depot 7.5 mg ... 2311
Lupron Injection ... 2310
Omnipaque (Less than 0.3 to 1.6%) ... 2552
Procrit for Injection (0.4%) ... 1647
Tonocard Tablets ... 1554

Ischemic colitis

Corgard Tablets ... 701
Corzide Tablets ... 702
Inderal ... 2459
Inderal LA Long Acting Capsules ... 2461
Inderide Tablets ... 2463
Inderide LA Long Acting Capsules ... 2465
Kerlone Tablets ... 2172
Levatol ... 1832
Normodyne Tablets ... 2110
Sectral Capsules ... 2520
Timolide Tablets ... 1547
Timoptic in Ocudose ... 1552
Timoptic Sterile Ophthalmic Solution ... 1550

Ischemic injury

Levophed Bitartrate Injection ... 2054

Itching (see under Pruritus)

Itching, eyes

▲ AK-Poly-Bac Ointment (Amomg most frequent) ⊙ 205
▲ AK-Spore H.C. (Among most often) ⊙ 206
▲ AK-Spore (Among most frequent) ⊙ 205
Betoptic Sterile Ophthalmic Solution (Small numbers of patients) 569
Betoptic S Sterile Ophthalmic Suspension (Small numbers of patients) 570
BuSpar (Infrequent) 1401
Chloroptic Sterile Ophthalmic Solution ⊙ 243
▲ Ciloxan Sterile Ophthalmic Solution (Less than 10%) ⊙ 214
Combipres Tablets 678
Geocillin Tablets 1951
Lamprene Capsules (Greater than 1%) 1030
Mykrox ½ mg Tablets (Less than 2%) 984
TobraDex Ophthalmic Suspension and Ointment (Less than 4%) ⊙ 228
Tobrex Ophthalmic Ointment and Solution (Less than 3 in 100 patients) 572

Itching, vulvovaginal

Clozaril Tablets (Less than 1%) 2000
Femstat Prefill Vaginal Cream 2% (0.9%) 2295
Femstat Vaginal Cream 2% (0.9%) 2295
Kefzol Vials, Faspak & ADD-Vantage 1279
Monistat Dual-Pak (2%) 1657
Monistat 3 Vaginal Suppositories (2%) 1657
Rogaine Topical Solution (0.91%) 2357
Terazol 3 Vaginal Cream 1676
Terazol 7 Vaginal Cream (2.3% of 521 patients) 1677

IOP, elevation

AMO Vitrax Solution ⊙ 236
AMVISC Plus ⊙ 323
AK-Cide Sterile Ophthalmic Ointment & Suspension ⊙ 202
AK-Con ⊙ 202
AK-Con-A ⊙ 203
AK-Pentolate ⊙ 204
AK-Spore H.C. ⊙ 206
AK-Trol Ointment & Suspension ⊙ 207
Albalon Solution with Liquifilm ⊙ 238
Albalon-A Liquifilm ⊙ 238
Ansaid Tablets (Less than 1%) 2319
Aristospan Suspension (Intra-articular) 1011
Blephamide 586
Cetapred Ointment ⊙ 220
Cyclogyl ⊙ 215
Cyclomydril ⊙ 216
Darbid Tablets 2205
Deltasone Tablets 2332
Depo-Medrol Sterile Aqueous Suspension 2334
Dexacidin ⊙ 272
FML Forte Liquifilm ⊙ 245
FML Liquifilm ⊙ 244
FML S.O.P. ⊙ 245
FML-S Sterile Ophthalmic Suspension ⊙ 246
HMS Liquifilm ⊙ 247
Healon (Some cases) ⊙ 279
Isopto Cetapred Suspension ⊙ 220
Maxidex Sterile Ophthalmic Ointment ⊙ 222
▲ Maxitrol Ophthalmic Ointment/Suspension (Most often) ⊙ 223
Mydriacyl ⊙ 225
Naphcon Forte ⊙ 226
Occucoat (Some cases) ⊙ 312
Opcon-A Ophthalmic Solution ⊙ 262
Ophthocort ⊙ 301
Oramorph SR (Morphine Sulfate Sustained Release Tablets) (Less frequent) 1988
Orcolon (Some cases) ⊙ 325
Permax Tablets (Infrequent) 1291
Poly-Pred Liquifilm ⊙ 250
Pred Forte ⊙ 252
Pred Mild ⊙ 254
Pred-G Liquifilm Sterile Ophthalmic Suspension ⊙ 252
TobraDex Ophthalmic Suspension and Ointment ⊙ 228
Tropicacyl ⊙ 209
Vasocidin Ointment ⊙ 275
Vasocidin Ophthalmic Solution ⊙ 276
Vasocon-A ⊙ 278
Viroptic Ophthalmic Solution, 1% Sterile 820
Viscoat Sterile Viscoelastic Ophthalmic ⊙ 235
▲ Voltaren Ophthalmic Sterile Ophthalmic Solution (15%) ⊙ 268
Zolyse ⊙ 236

IUD, difficult removal

Lippes Loop Intrauterine Double-S 1654
ParaGard T380A Intrauterine Copper Contraceptive 411

IUD, embedment

ParaGard T380A Intrauterine Copper Contraceptive 411

IUD, expulsion (complete)

Lippes Loop Intrauterine Double-S 1654
ParaGard T380A Intrauterine Copper Contraceptive 411

IUD, expulsion (partial)

Lippes Loop Intrauterine Double-S 1654
ParaGard T380A Intrauterine Copper Contraceptive 411

IUD, fragmentation

Lippes Loop Intrauterine Double-S 1654
ParaGard T380A Intrauterine Copper Contraceptive 411

J

Jaundice

Aldactazide 2150
Aldoclor Tablets 1413
Aldomet Ester HCl Injection 1417
Aldomet Oral 1415
Aldoril Tablets 1418
Amen (A few instances) 833
Anaprox and Anaprox DS Tablets (Less than 1%) 2288
Ancobon Capsules 1886
Ansaid Tablets (Rare) 2319
Apresazide Capsules 854
AquaMEPHYTON Injection 1422
Asendin Tablets (Very rare) 1196
Axid Pulvules (Rare) 1246
Azactam for Injection (Less than 1%) 2252
Azo Gantrisin Tablets 1888
Brevicon 2304
Butazolidin Capsules & Tablets (Rare) 1027
Capoten 2255
Capozide 2258
Cartrol Tablets (Less common) 507
Children's Advil Suspension (Less than 1%) 2426
Cipro I.V. (1% or less) 1592
Cipro Tablets 1589
Cleocin HCl Capsules 2322
Cleocin Pediatric Flavored Granules 2324
Cleocin Phosphate Injection 2325
Clinoril Tablets (Less than 1%) 1433
Combipres Tablets 678
Corzide Tablets 702
Cylert Tablets 510
Cytosar-U Sterile Powder (Less frequent) 2329
Cytoxan for Injection (Isolated reports) 726
Danocrine Capsules 2046
Dantrium Capsules 1619
Dapsone USP 1130
Darvon-N/Darvocet-N (Rare) 1254
Darvon 1256
Darvon-N Suspension & Tablets 1254
Depo-Provera Sterile Aqueous Suspension (Few cases) 2336
Desyrel and Desyrel Dividose 1404
Dilantin with Phenobarbital Kapseals 1715
Diucardin Tablets 2450
Diuril Sodium Intravenous 1463
Dolobid Tablets (Less than 1 in 100) 1465
Doral Tablets 2383
Dyazide Capsules 2208
Dyrenium Capsules (Rare) 2210
E.E.S. 522
Edecrin (Rare) 1468
Enduron Tablets 517
ERYC (A few reports) 1720
EryPed 200 & EryPed 400 Granules 519
Ery-Tab Tablets 521
Erythrocin Stearate Filmtab 523
Esidrix Tablets 863
Esimil Tablets 864
Estrace 1385
Estrace Vaginal Cream 1388
Etrafon 2087
Eulexin Capsules (Less than 1%) 2089
Exna Tablets 1862
Feldene Capsules (Less than 1%) 1777
Flexeril Tablets (Rare) 1471
Fungizone Intravenous 2262
Glucotrol (Rare) 1952
Halcion Tablets 2340
Haldol Decanoate 1375
Haldol Injection, Tablets and Concentrate 1373
Halotestin Tablets 2341
HydroDIURIL Tablets 1484
Hydromox R Tablets 1209
Hydromox Tablets 1208
Hydropres Tablets 1485
INH Tablets 868
Inderide Tablets 2463
Inderide LA Long Acting Capsules 2465
Indocin Capsules (Less than 1%) 1487
Indocin I.V. (Less than 1%) 1490
Indocin (Less than 1%) 1487
Inocor Lactate Injection (Rare) 2048
Intron A (1% or less) 2097
Jenest-28 Tablets 1636
Lamprene Capsules (Less than 1%) 1030
Lasix 1093
Leukeran Tablets 788
Levlen/Tri-Levlen 665
Librax Capsules (Occasional) 1929
Libritabs Tablets (Occasional) 1930
Librium Capsules (Occasional) 1931
Librium Injectable (Occasional) 1932
Limbitrol (Rare) 1933
Lincocin 2344
Lodine Capsules (Rare) 2468
Lopressor HCT Tablets 1034
Loxitane (Rare) 1213
Lozol Tablets 1843
Ludiomil Tablets 874
Matulane Capsules 1907
Maxzide 1215
Meclomen Capsules (Rare) 1739
Mefoxin 1498
Mefoxin Premixed Intravenous Solution 1500
Mellaril 2011
Menrium Tablets 1934
Mesantoin Tablets 2013
Micronase Tablets (Rare) 2350
Micronor Tablets 1667
Midamor Tablets (Less than or equal to 1%) 1508
Mintezol 1510
Modicon 1667
Moduretic Tablets 1510
Monopril Tablets (0.2 to 1.0%) 1406
Motrin Tablets (Less than 1%) 2351
Mustargen (Infrequent) 1514
Myochrysine Injection 1516
Nalfon Pulvules & Tablets (Less than 1%) 919
Naprosyn (Less than 1%) 2297
Nardil (Less frequent) 1742
Naturetin Tablets (Occasional) 1789
Neosar for Injection (Isolated reports) 566
Niacor Tablets 2376
Nicolar Tablets 1846
Nimotop Capsules (Less than 1%) 1607
Norinyl 2304
Normodyne Injection 2108
Normodyne Tablets 2110
Normozide Tablets 2112
Norpramin Tablets 1340
Nor-Q D Tablets 2304
Norzine 1818
▲ Novantrone for Injection Concentrate (3 to 7%) 1226
Orinase Tablets 2354
Ortho-Novum 1667
Orudis Capsules (Less than 1%) 2488
Ovcon 1391
Pamelor 2019
Paraflex Caplets (Rare) 1378
Parafon Forte DSC Caplets (Rare) 1379
PediaProfen Suspension (Less than 1%) 1363
Periactin 1525
Permax Tablets (Rare) 1291
Phenergan Injection 2493
Phenergan Tablets 2496
Prilosec Delayed-Release Capsules (Less than 1%) 1530
Primaxin I.M. 1532
Primaxin I.V. 1535
Prinzide Tablets 1540
Pronestyl Capsules and Tablets 1800
Pronestyl Injection 1798
Prozac Pulvules (Rare) 920
Rauzide Tablets 1804
Reglan (Rare) 1869
Renese Tablets 1785
Ridaura Capsules (Less than 1%) 2224
Rifadin (Some patients) 1345
Rifamate Capsules 1347
Rocephin Injectable Vials, ADD-Vantage (Rare) 1914
Rufen Tablets (Less than 1%) 691
Saluron 718
Salutensin/Salutensin-Demi 719
Sandostatin Injection (Less than 1%) 2029
Seldane Tablets (Isolated reports) 1349
Seldane-D Extended-Release Tablets 1350
Ser-Ap-Es Tablets 881
Serax Capsules 2522
Serax Tablets 2522
Serentil 686
Serpasil-Esidrix Tablets 886
Sinequan (Occasional) 1960
Skelaxin 840
Solganal Suspension 2122
Stelazine 2226
Surmontil Capsules 2524
Tacaryl 2409
Tambocor Tablets 1315
Tao Capsules 1963
Tapazole Tablets 1298
Taractan (Occasional) 1920
Temaril Tablets, Syrup and Spansule Sustained Release Capsules 1085
Tenoretic Tablets 1105
Thalitone Tablets 687
Thioguanine Tablets, Tabloid Brand 815
Thorazine 2234
Tigan 2239
Tofranil Ampuls 1038
Tofranil Tablets 1039
Tofranil-PM Capsules 1041
Tolinase Tablets (Rare) 2365
Tonocard Tablets (Less than 1%) 1554
Torecan 1993
Trancopal Caplets (Rare) 2075
Trandate HCT Tablets 579
Trandate Injection (Rare) 577
Trandate Tablets 579
Trecator-SC Tablets 2527
Trental (Rare) 1099
Triavil Tablets 1556
Trilafon (Low incidence) 2123
Levlen/Tri-Levlen 665
Tri-Norinyl 28-Day Tablets 2304
Valium Injectable (Isolated reports) 1937
Valium Tablets (Isolated reports) 1939
Valrelease Capsules (Occasional) 1923
Vaseretic Tablets 1559
Vivactil Tablets 1567
Voltaren Tablets (Less than 1%) 1042
Vontrol Tablets 2243
Wellbutrin Tablets (Infrequent) 821
Wygesic Tablets (Rare) 2540
Xanax Tablets 2367
Yutopar (Infrequent) 647
Zantac Injection and Zantac Injection Premixed 1063
Zantac (Occasional) 1065
Zestoretic 2274

Jaundice, cholestatic

Amen 833
Anadrol-50 Tablets 2287
Android 1111
Ansaid Tablets (Rare) 2319
Augmentin Tablets, Powder for Oral Suspension, and Chewable Tablets (Rare) 2198
Axid Pulvules (Rare) 1246
Aygestin Tablets 2437
Bactrim DS Tablets 1891
Bactrim I.V. Infusion 1889
Bactrim 1891
Brevicon 2304
Capozide (Rare) 2258
Ceclor Pulvules & Suspension (Rare) 1251
Cipro Tablets 1589

Compazine 2201
Cycrin Tablets 2449
Danocrine Capsules 2046
Dapsone USP 1130
Darvon-N/Darvocet-N (Rare) 1254
Darvon 1256
Darvon-N Suspension & Tablets (Rare) 1254
Demulen 2161
DiaBeta (Rare) 1091
Diabinese Tablets (Rare) 1775
Diethylstilbestrol Tablets 1258
Enovid 2161
Estinyl Tablets 2085
Estraderm Transdermal System 866
Estradurin 2452
Estratest 2245
Estrovis 1721
Eulexin Capsules (Less than 1%) 2089
Glucotrol (Rare) 1952
Jenest-28 Tablets 1636
Keflex Pulvules, Oral Suspension & Pediatric Drops (Rare) 916
Keftab Tablets (Rare) 917
Kefzol Vials, Faspak & ADD-Vantage (Rare) 1279
Leukeran Tablets 788
Levlen/Tri-Levlen 665
Lo/Ovral Tablets 2471
Lo/Ovral-28 Tablets 2476
Loestrin 1728
Lopid Capsules and Tablets 1736
Macrodantin Capsules (Rare) 1624
Mandol Vials, Faspak & ADD-Vantage (Rare) 1281
Meclomen Capsules (Less than 1%) 1739
Mediatric Capsules 2476
Menrium Tablets 1934
Metandren Linguets and Tablets 875
Mevacor Tablets 1505
Micronor Tablets 1667
Modicon 1667
Monopril Tablets (0.2 to 1.0%) 1406
Myleran Tablets (Rare) 790
Myochrysine Injection 1516
Nordette-21 Tablets 2481
Nordette-28 Tablets 2483
Norethin 2133
Norinyl 2304
Norlestrin 1746
Norlutate 1754
Norlutin 1755
Normodyne Injection 2108
Normodyne Tablets 2110
Norpace (Infrequent) 2177
Nor-Q D Tablets 2304
Norzine (Occasional) 1818
Ogen 540
Ortho Dienestrol Cream 1664
Ortho-Cyclen Tablets 1658
Ortho-Novum 1667
Ovral Tablets 2490
Ovral-28 Tablets 2491
Ovrette Tablets 2492
PMB 200 and PMB 400 2504
Pepcid (Infrequent) 1524
Placidyl Capsules 553
Premarin Intravenous 2508
Premarin with Methyltestosterone 2515
Premarin Tablets 2510
Premarin Vaginal Cream 2512
Prinivil Tablets 1538
Prinzide Tablets 1540
Procardia XL Tablets 1783
Prolixin Decanoate 1795
Prolixin Elixir 1793
Prolixin Enanthate 1796
Prolixin Injection 1791
Prolixin Oral Concentrate 1792
Prolixin Tablets 1793
Proloprim Tablets (Rare) 799
Provera Tablets 2356
Renese-R Tablets 1786
Ridaura Capsules (Rare) 2224
Septra 813
Septra I.V. Infusion 808
Septra I.V. Infusion ADD-Vantage Vials 810
Septra 813
Stelazine 2226
Stilphostrol Tablets and Ampuls 1609
TACE 12 and 25 mg 1353
Tegretol Chewable Tablets 654
Tegretol Suspension 656
Tegretol Tablets 654
Testred Capsules 1124
Timentin for Injection (Rare) 2239
Torecan 1993
Trancopal Caplets 2075
Trandate HCT Tablets 579
Trandate Injection (Less common) 577
Trandate Tablets 579
Levlen/Tri-Levlen 665
Tri-Norinyl 2304
Triphasil-21 Tablets 2527
Triphasil-28 Tablets 2532
Vaseretic Tablets 1559
Vasotec I.V. 1562
Vasotec Tablets (0.5% to 1%) 1564
Winstrol Tablets (Rare) 2075
Zyloprim Tablets (Less than 1%) 830

Jaundice, hepatocellular

Augmentin Tablets, Powder for Oral Suspension, and Chewable Tablets (Rare) 2198
Axid Pulvules (Rare) 1246
Monopril Tablets (0.2 to 1.0%) 1406
Prinivil Tablets 1538
Prinzide Tablets 1540
Tegretol Chewable Tablets 654
Tegretol Suspension 656
Tegretol Tablets 654
Vaseretic Tablets 1559
Vasotec I.V. 1562
Vasotec Tablets 1564

Jaundice, intrahepatic

Minizide Capsules 1779
Renese Tablets 1785
Solganal Suspension 2122
Tegretol Chewable Tablets 654

Jaundice, intrahepatic cholestatic

Aldoclor Tablets 1413
Apresazide Capsules 854
Apresoline-Esidrix Tablets (Less frequent) 857
Augmentin Tablets, Powder for Oral Suspension, and Chewable Tablets (Rare) 2198
Capozide 2258
Combipres Tablets 678
Corzide Tablets 702
Diucardin Tablets 2450
Diulo 2129
Diupres Tablets 1461
Diuril Oral Suspension 1464
Diuril Sodium Intravenous 1463
Diuril Tablets 1464
Enduron Tablets 517
Enduronyl 518
Esidrix Tablets 863
Esimil Tablets 864
Exna Tablets 1862
HydroDIURIL Tablets 1484
Hydromox R Tablets 1209
Hydromox Tablets 1208
Hydropres Tablets 1485
Inderide Tablets 2463
Inderide LA Long Acting Capsules 2465
Lasix 1093
Lopressor HCT Tablets 1034
Lozol Tablets 1843
Maxzide 1215
Moduretic Tablets 1510
Mykrox ½ mg Tablets 984
Naturetin Tablets (Occasional) 1789
Normozide Tablets 2112
Oretic Tablets 544
Oreticyl 545
Prinzide Tablets 1540
Rauzide Tablets 1804
Saluron 718
Salutensin/Salutensin-Demi 719
Ser-Ap-Es Tablets 881
Serpasil-Esidrix Tablets 886
Solganal Suspension 2122
Tenoretic Tablets 1105
Thalitone Tablets 687
Timolide Tablets 1547
Trandate HCT Tablets 579
Vaseretic Tablets 1559
Zaroxolyn Tablets 989
Zestoretic 2274

Jaundice, neonatal

Aldactazide 2150
Aldoclor Tablets 1413
Aldoril Tablets 1418
Amen (A few cases) 833
Apresazide Capsules 854
Apresoline-Esidrix Tablets 857
AquaMEPHYTON Injection 1422
Capozide 2258
Compazine 2201
Corzide Tablets 702
Diucardin Tablets 2450
Diulo 2129
Diupres Tablets 1461
Diuril Oral Suspension 1464
Diuril Sodium Intravenous 1463
Diuril Tablets 1464
Dyazide Capsules 2208
Enduron Tablets 517
Enduronyl 518
Esidrix Tablets 863
Esimil Tablets 864
Exna Tablets 1862
HydroDIURIL Tablets 1484
Hydromox R Tablets 1209
Hydromox Tablets 1208
Hydropres Tablets 1485
Inderide Tablets 2463
Inderide LA Long Acting Capsules 2465
Konakion Injection 1903
Lopressor HCT Tablets 1034
Lozol Tablets 1843
Maxzide 1215
Mephyton Tablets 1503
Micronor Tablets 1667
Modicon 1667
Moduretic Tablets 1510
Mykrox ½ mg Tablets 984
Naturetin Tablets 1789
Normozide Tablets 2112
Oretic Tablets 544
Oreticyl 545
Ortho-Novum 1667
Oxytocin Injection 2492
Pitocin Injection, Ampoules, Steri-Dose Syringes 1757
Prinzide Tablets 1540
Rauzide Tablets 1804
Renese Tablets 1785
Renese-R Tablets 1786
Saluron 718
Salutensin/Salutensin-Demi 719
Ser-Ap-Es Tablets 881
Serpasil-Esidrix Tablets 886
Stelazine 2226
Syntocinon Injection 2032
Tacaryl Chewable Tablets 2409
Temaril Tablets, Syrup and Spansule Sustained Release Capsules 1085
Tenoretic Tablets 1105
Thalitone Tablets 687
Thorazine 2234
Timolide Tablets 1547
Trandate HCT/Trandate 579
Vaseretic Tablets 1559
Zestoretic 2274

Jaundice, obstructive

Tacaryl 2409
Thorazine 2234
Tofranil Ampuls 1038
Tofranil Tablets 1039
Tofranil-PM Capsules 1041

Jerks (see under Twitching)

Jitteriness

Adalat Capsules (10 mg and 20 mg) (2% or less) 1587
Bucladin-S Softab Chewable Tablets (Occasional) 2264
Compazine 2201
Etrafon 2087
▲ Marplan Tablets (Among most frequent) 1906
Nardil (Less common) 1742
Procardia Capsules (2% or less) 1781
Prostin VR Pediatric Sterile Solution (Less than 1%) 2355
Reglan 1869
Stelazine 2226
Tenuate 1354
Thorazine 2234
▲ Yutopar (5 to 8% (with oral administration) 5 to 6% (with IV administration)) 647

Joint pain (see under Arthralgia)

Joint stiffness

Adalat Capsules (10 mg and 20 mg) (2% or less) 1587
Atgam Sterile Solution (At least 1 patient and less than 5% of total patients) 2320
Cipro I.V. (1% or less) 1592
Cipro Tablets 1589

K

Keratitis

Anafranil Capsules (Rare) 650
Betagan ⊙ 239
Betoptic Sterile Ophthalmic Solution (Rare) 569
Betoptic S Sterile Ophthalmic Suspension (Rare) 570
Ciloxan Sterile Ophthalmic Solution (Less than 1%) ⊙ 214
Engerix-B Unit-Dose Vials 2213
Oculinum for Injecton (Less than 1%) 587
Pilopine HS Gel ⊙ 227
Timoptic Sterile Ophthalmic Solution 1550
▲ Voltaren Ophthalmic Sterile Ophthalmic Solution (28%) ⊙ 268

Keratitis, epithelial

AK-Taine ⊙ 207
Alcaine (Rare) ⊙ 210
Fluoracaine (Rare) ⊙ 208
Ophthetic ⊙ 249
Vasosulf ⊙ 279

Keratitis, punctate

Albalon Solution with Liquifilm ⊙ 238
Cyclogyl ⊙ 215
Naphcon Forte ⊙ 226
Pred-G Liquifilm Sterile Ophthalmic Suspension (Occasional) ⊙ 252
Pred-G S.O.P. Sterile Ophthalmic Ointment ⊙ 253
▲ Rēv-Eyes Ophthalmic Eyedrops 0.5% (10% to 40%) ⊙ 312
Vasocon-A ⊙ 278

Keratitis, superficial punctate

Vira-A Ophthalmic Ointment, 3% 1767
Viroptic Ophthalmic Solution, 1% Sterile 820

Keratitis nigricans

Niacor Tablets 2376
Timoptic in Ocudose 1552

Keratoconjunctivitis

Viroptic Ophthalmic Solution, 1% Sterile 820

Keratocystic response

Zetar Emulsion 911

Keratopathy

Ciloxan Sterile Ophthalmic Solution (Less than 1%) ⊙ 214
Trilafon 2123

Keratopathy, bullous

BSS (15 mL & 30 mL) Sterile Irrigation Solution ⊙ 230
BSS (250 mL) Sterile Irrigation Solution ⊙ 231
BSS (500 mL) Sterile Irrigation Solution ⊙ 231
Balanced Salt Solution ⊙ 239
MIOSTAT ⊙ 233

Keratopathy, epithelial

Compazine 2201
Etrafon 2087
Stelazine 2226
Tacaryl 2409
Thorazine 2234
Viroptic Ophthalmic Solution, 1% Sterile 820

Keratosis, nigricans

Nicolar Tablets 1846

Kernicterus

Konakion Injection 1903
Synkayvite Injection 1919
Synkayvite Tablets 1920

Kernicterus, neonatal

Azo Gantanol Tablets 1887
Azo Gantrisin Tablets 1888
Azulfidine Tablets, EN-tabs, Oral Suspension 1157
Bactrim DS Tablets 1891
Bactrim I.V. Infusion 1889
Bactrim 1891
Fansidar Tablets 1896
Gantanol 1899
Gantrisin Ophthalmic Ointment/Solution 1900
Gantrisin 1901
Pediazole 1973
Septra 813
Silvadene Cream 1% 1352
Thiosulfil Forte Tablets 2526

Kidney, decrease in size
BiCNU 723
CeeNU 725

Kidney, enlarged
Atgam Sterile Solution 2320

Kidney, ruptured
Atgam Sterile Solution 2320

Kidney damage
BiCNU (Occasional) 723
CeeNU (Occasional) 725
Coly-Mycin M Parenteral 1706
Milontin Kapseals 1741

Kidney stones
Tegison Capsules (Less than 1%) .. 1881

L

Labor, preterm, delayed
Ventolin 583

Labor, slowing
Astramorph/PF Injection, USP (Preservative-Free) 618
Carbocaine Hydrochloride Injection 2043
Marcaine Hydrochloride with Epinephrine 1:200,000 2055
Marcaine Hydrochloride Injection 2055
Marcaine Spinal 2058
Proventil Repetabs Tablets (Some reports) 2120
Proventil Solutions for Inhalation 0.5% and 0.083% (Some reports) 2118
Proventil Syrup (Some patients) 2119
Proventil Tablets (Some patients) .. 2120
Sensorcaine 631
Sensorcaine-MPF Spinal 634

Laboratory abnormalities, unspecified
Ethmozine Tablets (0.3%-0.4%) 946

Labyrinth disorder
Anafranil Capsules (Rare) 650

Labyrinthitis
Actifed with Codeine Cough Syrup.. 752
Kerlone Tablets (Less than 2%) 2172
Optimine Tablets 2115
Ornade Spansule Capsules 2221
Periactin 1525
Polaramine 2116
Ru-Tuss II Capsules 693
Tavist Syrup 2033
Tavist Tablets 2035
Tavist-D Tablets 2035
Triaminic Expectorant DH 1995
Triaminic Oral Infant Drops 1996
Trinalin Repetabs Tablets 1170

Labyrinthitis hysteria, acute
Benadryl Capsules 1691
Benadryl Injection 1692

Lacrimal duct, stenosis
Ergamisol Tablets 1136
Sterile FUDR (Remote possibility) .. 1898
Fluorouracil Injection 1897

Lacrimal gland, disorders
DDAVP (Up to 2%) 1841
Intron A (Less than 1%) 2097

Lacrimation
Adriamycin PFS (Rare) 561
Adriamycin RDF (Rare) 562
Albalon Solution with Liquifilm ◉ 238
Alcaine ◉ 210
Apresazide Capsules (Less frequent) 854
Apresoline Hydrochloride Parenteral (Ampuls) 856
Apresoline Hydrochloride Tablets (Less frequent) 855
Apresoline-Esidrix Tablets 857
Asendin Tablets (Less than 1%) 1196
BAL in Oil Ampules 661
Calciparine Injection (Rare) 925
Doxorubicin Hydrochloride for Injection, USP (Rare) 622
Doxorubicin Hydrochloride Injection, USP (Rare) 848
Duvoid Tablets 1853
Efudex 1880
Emcyt Capsules (Approximately 1%) 1161
Enlon Injection 598
Sterile FUDR (Remote possibility) .. 1898
Floropryl Sterile Ophthalmic Ointment 1473
Fluorouracil Injection 1897
Heparin Lock Flush Solution 2456
Heparin Sodium Vials (Rare) 1264
Heparin Sodium Injection 2457
Heparin Sodium Injection, USP, Sterile Solution 2342
Humorsol Sterile Ophthalmic Solution 1475
Hyperstat I.V. Injection 2095
Intal Capsules (Less than 1 in 10,000 patients) 978
Intal Inhaler (Infrequent) 979
Intal Nebulizer Solution 980
Lorelco Tablets 1333
Methadone Hydrochloride Diskets .. 1284
Naphcon Forte ◉ 226
▲ Oculinum for Injecton (10.0%) 587
Omnipaque 2552
OptiPranolol Sterile Ophthalmic Solution (A small number of patients) ◉ 261
Phospholine Iodide ◉ 315
Pilocar ◉ 275
Pilopine HS Gel ◉ 227
Pilostat Sterile Ophthalmic Solution 0.5%, 1%, 2%, 3%, 4%, 5%, 6% ◉ 263
Procardia XL Tablets (1% or less).. 1783
Proglycem 649
Rubex (Rare) 739
Ser-Ap-Es Tablets 881
Serpasil-Apresoline Tablets 884
Syntocinon Nasal Spray 2033
▲ Tegison Capsules (1-10%) 1881
Tensilon Injectable 1123
Urecholine 1558
Vaseretic Tablets 1559
Vasocon-A ◉ 278
Vasotec I.V. 1562
Vasotec Tablets 1564
Vira-A Ophthalmic Ointment, 3% 1767

Lacrimation, abnormal
Anafranil Capsules (Up to 3%) 650
Cardura Tablets (Less than 0.5% of 3960 patients) 1941
▲ Ergamisol Tablets (Up to 4%) 1136
Kerlone Tablets (Less than 2%) 2172

Lacrimation, decrease
Ditropan 1332

Lactation
Aldoclor Tablets 1413
Aldomet Ester HCl Injection 1417
Aldomet Oral 1415
Aldoril Tablets 1418
Compazine 2201
Desyrel and Desyrel Dividose 1404
Etrafon 2087
Haldol Decanoate 1375
Haldol Injection, Tablets and Concentrate 1373
▲ Lupron Depot 3.75 mg (Among most frequent) 2312
Mellaril 2011
Navane Capsules and Concentrate 1954
Navane Intramuscular 1956
Permax Tablets (Infrequent) 1291
Prozac Pulvules (Rare) 920
Serentil 686
Stelazine 2226
Synarel Nasal Solution (Less than 1%) 2300
Tacaryl 2409
Taractan 1920
Temaril Tablets, Syrup and Spansule Sustained Release Capsules 1085
Thorazine 2234
Triavil Tablets 1556
Trilafon 2123

Lactation, non-puerperal
▲ Anafranil Capsules (Up to 4%) 650
Diupres Tablets 1461
Hydropres Tablets 1485
Salutensin/Salutensin-Demi 719

Lactation, possible diminution
Brevicon 2304
Demulen 2161
Enovid 2161
Jenest-28 Tablets 1636
Levlen/Tri-Levlen 665
Lo/Ovral Tablets 2471
Lo/Ovral-28 Tablets 2476
Loestrin 1728
Micronor Tablets 1667
Modicon 1667
Nordette-21 Tablets 2481
Nordette-28 Tablets 2483
Norinyl 2304
Norlestrin 1746
Nor-Q D Tablets 2304
Ortho Diaphragm Kit/All-Flex Arcing Spring 1664
Ortho-Cyclen Tablets 1658
Ortho-Novum 1667
Ovral Tablets 2490
Ovral-28 Tablets 2491
Ovrette Tablets 2492
Levlen/Tri-Levlen 665
Tri-Norinyl 2304
Triphasil-21 Tablets 2527
Triphasil-28 Tablets 2532

Lactation, pseudo
Serpasil Tablets 883
Serpasil-Apresoline Tablets 884

Lactation, suppression
Bentyl 1322
Cantil Tablets 1326
Darbid Tablets 2205
Ditropan 1332
Donnatal 1858
Donnatal Extentabs 1859
Donnatal Tablets 1858
Donnazyme Tablets 1860
Kinesed Tablets 2272
Kutrase Capsules 2146
Levsin/Levsinex 2147
Norethin 2133
Ovcon 1391
Pro-Banthīne Tablets 2141
Quarzan Capsules 1937
Robinul Forte Tablets 1873
Robinul Injectable 1873
Robinul Tablets 1873
Valpin 50 Tablets 941

Lactation abnormalities
Demulen 2161
Enovid 2161
Norethin 2133
Prolixin Decanoate 1795
Prolixin Elixir 1793
Prolixin Enanthate 1796
Prolixin Injection 1791
Prolixin Oral Concentrate 1792
Prolixin Tablets 1793
Serpasil Tablets 883
Serpasil-Apresoline Tablets 884

Lactic acidosis
Yutopar (Infrequent) 647

Lactose, intolerance to
Levothroid Tablets 1003

Lagophthalmos
Oculinum for Injecton 587

Laryngeal changes
Mexitil Capsules (About 1 in 1,000) 680

Laryngitis
AeroBid Inhaler System (1-3%) 995
Anafranil Capsules (Up to 2%) 650
Ansaid Tablets (Less than 1%) 2319
Clozaril Tablets (Less than 1%) 2000
Monopril Tablets (0.2 to 1.0%) 1406
NebuPent for Inhalation Solution (1% or less) 1017
Omnipaque (0.1 to 0.2%) 2552
Permax Tablets (Infrequent) 1291
ProSom Tablets (Rare) 554
Trental (Less than 1%) 1099

Laryngospasm
Alfenta Injection (Less than 1%) 1131
Anafranil Capsules (Rare) 650
Atgam Sterile Solution (Less than 1% to less than 5%) 2320
Blocadren Tablets 1429
Brevital Sodium Vials 1248
Cartrol Tablets 507
Corgard Tablets 701
Corzide Tablets 702
Dilaudid-HP Injection 1175
Diprivan Injection (Less than 1%) .. 2267
Dopram Injectable 1860
Enlon Injection 598
Haldol Decanoate 1375
Haldol Injection, Tablets and Concentrate 1373
Inapsine Injection 1140
Inderal 2459
Inderal LA Long Acting Capsules 2461
Inderide Tablets 2463
Inderide LA Long Acting Capsules .. 2465
Innovar Injection 1141
Isoptin Injectable (Rare) 1177
Kerlone Tablets 2172
Ketalar 1726
Levatol 1832
Lopressor HCT Tablets 1034
MS Contin Tablets (Infrequent) 1814
MSIR (Infrequent) 1817
NebuPent for Inhalation Solution (1% or less) 1017
Normodyne Tablets 2110
Normozide Tablets 2112
Oramorph SR (Morphine Sulfate Sustained Release Tablets) (Less frequent) 1988
Reglan 1869
Sectral Capsules 2520
Sublimaze Injection 1146
Surital Ampoules, Steri-Vials 1764
Tenoretic Tablets 1105
Tenormin Tablets and I.V. Injection 1107
Tensilon Injectable 1123
Timolide Tablets 1547
Timoptic in Ocudose 1552
Timoptic Sterile Ophthalmic Solution 1550
Tracrium Injection 817
Trandate HCT/Trandate 579
Valium Injectable 1937
Versed Injection (Less than 1.0%) 1924
Visken Tablets 2036

Lassitude
Azo Gantrisin Tablets 1888
Brexin L.A. Capsules 2078
Bromfed 1615
▲ Cartrol Tablets (0.5-7.1%) 507
Codiclear DH Syrup 845
Codimal 846
Daranide Tablets 1445
Dexedrine 2206
Esimil Tablets 864
▲ Hytrin Tablets (11.3%) 529
Inderal 2459
Inderal LA Long Acting Capsules 2461
Inderide Tablets 2463
Inderide LA Long Acting Capsules .. 2465
Ismelin Tablets 869
▲ Mykrox ½ mg Tablets (4.4%) 984
Parlodel (Less than 1%) 2020
Phenergan Injection 2493
Phenergan Tablets 2496
Plaquenil Sulfate Tablets 2067
Protamine Sulfate Ampoules & Vials 1295
▲ Reglan (10%) 1869
Ru-Tuss with Hydrocodone 694
Ru-Tuss Tablets 693
Tacaryl 2409
Temaril Tablets, Syrup and Spansule Sustained Release Capsules 1085
Tonocard Tablets (0.8-1.6%) 1554
Triavil Tablets 1556

Laughing, easy
▲ Marinol (Dronabinol) Capsules (24%) 1985

Laxative effect
Beelith Tablets 659
Charcoaid ▣ 653
Derifil Tablets 1994
Entozyme Tablets 1862
Mag-Ox 400 673
Neutra-Phos (Occasional) 2423
Concentrated Phillips' Milk of Magnesia ▣ 573
Phillips' Milk of Magnesia Liquid.. ▣ 572
Phillips' Milk of Magnesia Tablets ▣ 573
Uro-Mag 673

Left ventricular ejection fraction, asymptomatic declines in
Idamycin for Injection 564

Left ventricular ejection fraction, change
Novantrone for Injection Concentrate 1226

Legs, heaviness
K-Lyte 707
Rum-K Syrup 995

Legs, stiffness
Gastrocrom Capsules (Infrequent).. 974

Legs, weakness
▲ Ergostat (Frequent) 1719
Gastrocrom Capsules (Infrequent).. 974
K-Lyte 707

Lens, pigmentation
Triavil Tablets 1556

Lens opacities, changes
Etrafon 2087
Floropryl Sterile Ophthalmic Ointment 1473
Humorsol Sterile Ophthalmic Solution 1475
Isopto Carpine ⊙ 219
Mevacor Tablets 1505
Norzine 1818
Pilocar ⊙ 275
Pilostat Sterile Ophthalmic Solution 0.5%, 1%, 2%, 3%, 4%, 5%, 6% ⊙ 263
Tacaryl 2409

Lens opacities, irregular
Lysodren (Infrequent) 731
Mellaril 2011
Moban Tablets & Concentrate 932
Prolixin Decanoate 1795
Prolixin Elixir 1793
Prolixin Enanthate 1796
Prolixin Injection 1791
Prolixin Tablets 1793
Serentil 686
Thorazine 2234
Torecan 1993

Lenticular deposits
Compazine 2201
Lariam Tablets 1904
Prolixin Oral Concentrate 1792
Ridaura Capsules (Less than 1%) .. 2224
Stelazine 2226
Thorazine 2234
Trilafon 2123

Leriche's syndrome
Sansert Tablets 2031

Lesions, anogenital
Achromycin V Capsules 1193
Declomycin Capsules, Tablets 1199
Minocin Intravenous 1221
Minocin Oral Suspension 1224
Minocin Pellet-Filled Capsules 1222
Monodox Capsules 1630
Terramycin Capsules 1786
Vibramycin 1787

Lesions, cardiac
Amicar Syrup, Tablets, and Injection (One case) 1194

Lesions, cutaneous
▲ Anestacon Solution (Among most common) 2394
Duranest Injections 624
Dyclone 0.5% and 1% Topical Solutions, USP 626
Lupron Depot 7.5 mg 2311
Novocain Hydrochloride for Spinal Anesthesia 2065
Pontocaine Hydrochloride for Spinal Anesthesia 2069
Pronestyl Capsules and Tablets 1800
Pronestyl Injection 1798
Pronestyl-SR Tablets 1801
Quadrinal Tablets 1183
▲ Tonocard Tablets (0.4-12.2%) 1554
Xylocaine Injections (Extremely rare) 637
Xylocaine 2% Jelly (Extremely rare) 643
Xylocaine 5% Ointment 644
Xylocaine 10% Oral Spray (Extremely rare) 645
4% Xylocaine-MPF Sterile Solution (Extremely rare) 641

Lesions, erythema perstans-like
AquaMEPHYTON Injection 1422

Lesions, esophageal
Voltaren Tablets (Less than 1%) 1042

Lesions, gastrointestinal
K-Dur Microburst Release System (potassium chloride, USP) E.R. Tablets 1163
K-Norm Capsules 982
K-Tab Filmtab 532
Klotrix 708
Micro-K 1863
Micro-K LS Packets 1864
Slow-K Tablets 2281

Lesions, hepatic
Amicar Syrup, Tablets, and Injection (One case) 1194

Lesions, macular
Aralen Phosphate with Primaquine Phosphate Tablets 2040

Lesions, neuro-ocular
Cycrin Tablets 2449
Micronor Tablets 1667
Modicon 1667
Ortho-Novum 1667
Provera Tablets 2356

Lesions, retinal vascular
Brevicon 2304
Cycrin Tablets 2449
Demulen 2161
Enovid 2161
Levlen/Tri-Levlen 665
Micronor Tablets 1667
Modicon 1667
Norinyl 2304
Ortho-Novum 1667
Levlen/Tri-Levlen 665
Tri-Norinyl 28-Day Tablets 2304

Lesions, sceloderma-like
AquaMEPHYTON Injection 1422

Lesions, stenotic
K-Norm Capsules 982

Lethargy
Accutane Capsules 1878
Aldactazide 2150
Aldactone 2152
Anexsia 5/500 Tablets 2196
Anexsia 7.5/650 Tablets 2197
Aquasol A Vitamin A Capsules, USP 615
Aquasol A Parenteral, USP 615
Atgam Sterile Solution (At least 1 patient and less than 5% of total patients) 2320
Azdōne Tablets 844
Bentyl 1322
Betagan (Rare) ⊙ 239
Betoptic Sterile Ophthalmic Solution (Rare) 569
Betoptic S Sterile Ophthalmic Suspension (Rare) 570
Bretylol Injection (1 in 1000) 923
Butazolidin Capsules & Tablets (Less than 1%) 1027
▲ Catapres-TTS (3 of 101 patients) .. 677
CeeNU 725
Cibalith-S 870
Cipro I.V. (1% or less) 1592
Cipro Tablets (Less than 1%) 1589
Clozaril Tablets (1%) 2000
Corzide Tablets 702
Cosmegen Injection 1440
Dalmane Capsules 1927
Damason-P 1356
Depakote Sprinkle Capsules 512
Dilaudid Cough Syrup 1174
Dilaudid 1173
Dipentum Capsules (1.8%) 1160
Diupres Tablets 1461
Diuril Sodium Intravenous 1463
DynaCirc Capsules (0.5% to 1%) .. 2004
Eldepryl (1 of 49 patients) 2250
▲ Emcyt Capsules (4%) 1161
Eskalith 2214
Etrafon 2087
Sterile FUDR 1898
Fiorinal with Codeine Capsules 2008
Ganite Injection 1016
Garamycin Injectable 2093
Gastrocrom Capsules (Infrequent).. 974
Haldol Decanoate 1375
Haldol Injection, Tablets and Concentrate 1373
Hycodan Syrup, Tablets 927
Hycomine Compound Tablets 929
Hycomine Syrup 927
Hycotuss Expectorant Syrup 930
Hydrocet Capsules 835
Hydropres Tablets 1485
Hyperstat I.V. Injection 2095
Inderal 2459
Inderal LA Long Acting Capsules 2461
Inderide Tablets 2463
ISMOTIC (Very rare) ⊙ 233
Kerlone Tablets (2.8%) 2172
Limbitrol 1933
Lithane Tablets 1596
Lithium Carbonate Capsules & Tablets 1984
Lithobid Tablets 870
Lomotil 2174
▲ Lopressor HCT Tablets (10 in 100 patients) 1034
Lortab ASA Tablets 2414
Lortab 2412
▲ Lozol Tablets (Greater than or equal to 5%) 1843
Lupron Depot 7.5 mg 2311
Lupron Injection (Less than 5%) 2310
▲ Lysodren (25%) 731
Matulane Capsules 1907
Mellaril (Extremely rare) 2011
Milontin Kapseals 1741
Mithracin 1602
▲ Mykrox ½ mg Tablets (4.4%) 984
Nebcin Vials, Hyporets & ADD-Vantage 1286
Orthoclone OKT3 Sterile Solution .. 1645
Parlodel 2020
Phenobarbital Elixir and Tablets 1293
Prinzide Tablets 1540
Prolixin Decanoate 1795
Prolixin Elixir 1793
Prolixin Enanthate 1796
Prolixin Injection 1791
Prolixin Oral Concentrate 1792
Prolixin Tablets 1793
Prostin VR Pediatric Sterile Solution (Less than 1%) 2355
Rauzide Tablets 1804
▲ Restoril Capsules (5%) 2023
▲ RhoGAM Rh_0(D) Immune Globulin (Human) (25% in one study) 1651
Roferon-A Injection (Less than 0.5%) 1916
Salutensin/Salutensin-Demi 719
Sandimmune (Rare) 2024
Serax Capsules 2522
Serax Tablets 2522
Solganal Suspension (Rare) 2122
Stadol (2%) 721
▲ Tegison Capsules (1-10%) 1881
Tenoretic Tablets (1 to 3%) 1105
Tenormin Tablets and I.V. Injection (1 to 3%) 1107
Thalitone Tablets 687
Tonocard Tablets (0.8-1.6%) 1554
Trexan Tablets (Less than 1%) 937
Trilafon 2123
Trilisate (Less than 2%) 1822
Tussionex Extended-Release Suspension 988
Vaseretic Tablets 1559
▲ Verelan Capsules (3.2%) 1243
Versed Injection (Less than 1.0%) 1924
Vicodin Tablets 1187
Vicodin ES Tablets 1189
Visken Tablets (2% or fewer patients) 2036
Voltaren Tablets 1042
Zarontin Capsules 1768
Zarontin Syrup 1769
Zestoretic 2274
▲ Zoladex (8%) 1110
Zovirax Sterile Powder (1%) 828
Zydone Capsules 941

Leucoencephalopathy
Methotrexate Tablets, Parenteral, LPF Parenteral 1217
Rheumatrex Methotrexate Dose Pack 1234

Leukemia, acute
Anadrol-50 Tablets 2287
BiCNU 723
Butazolidin Capsules & Tablets (Less than 1%) 1027
CeeNU 725
Leukeran Tablets 788
VePesid Capsules and Injection (Rare) 741

Leukemia, lymphoblastic
Permax Tablets (Rare) 1291

Leukemia, lymphocytic
Mustargen 1514

Leukemia, unspecified
Humatrope Vials (Small number) 1266
Indocin (Rare) 1487
Protropin 1049

Leukemoid reaction
Anafranil Capsules (Rare) 650
Netromycin Injection 100 mg/ml (Fewer than 1 in 1000 patients) 2104

Leukocytosis
▲ Adriamycin RDF (High incidence).... 562
Azactam for Injection (Less than 1%) 2252
Capastat Sulfate Vials 1250
Cibalith-S 870
Cipro I.V. (Rare) 1592
Cipro Tablets (Less than 0.1%) 1589
Clozaril Tablets (Less than 1%) 2000
Cuprimine Capsules 1442
Danocrine Capsules (Rare) 2046
Depen Titratable Tablets 2379
Efudex 1880
Eskalith 2214
Ethrane 599
Floxin Tablets (More than or equal to 1.0%) 1652
Forane 600
Fungizone Intravenous 2262
Haldol Decanoate 1375
Haldol Injection, Tablets and Concentrate 1373
Imferon 976
Kerlone Tablets (Less than 2%) 2172
Lariam Tablets (Occasional) 1904
Lithane Tablets 1596
Lithium Carbonate Capsules & Tablets 1984
Lithobid Tablets 870
Mesantoin Tablets 2013
Moban Tablets & Concentrate (Rare) 932
Monopril Tablets (0.2 to 1.0%) 1406
Navane Capsules and Concentrate (Occasional) 1954
Navane Intramuscular 1956
Nebcin Vials, Hyporets & ADD-Vantage 1286
Norzine 1818
Omnipaque 2552
Panhematin 546
Permax Tablets (Infrequent) 1291
Plague Vaccine 1584
Prilosec Delayed-Release Capsules (Less than 1%) 1530
Primaxin I.V. 1535
Prolastin Alpha$_1$-Proteinase Inhibitor (Human) 1585
Prolixin Decanoate 1795
Prolixin Elixir 1793
Prolixin Enanthate 1796
Prolixin Injection 1791
Prolixin Oral Concentrate 1792
Prolixin Tablets 1793
Quinidex Extentabs 1868
Rocephin Injectable Vials, ADD-Vantage (Rare) 1914
Tao Capsules 1963
▲ Tegison Capsules (10-25%) 1881
Tegretol Chewable Tablets 654
Tegretol Suspension 656
Tegretol Tablets 654
Torecan 1993
Vaseretic Tablets 1559
Vasotec I.V. 1562
Vasotec Tablets 1564
Wellbutrin Tablets 821
Zefazone Sterile Powder 2372
Zovirax Sterile Powder (Less than 1%) 828
Zyloprim Tablets (Less than 1%) 830

Leukocyturia
Amikin Injectable 602
Primaxin I.M. 1532
Primaxin I.V. 1535
Sinemet CR Tablets (1% or greater) 953

Leukoderma
Ultravate Cream 0.05% (Less frequent) 2410
Ultravate Ointment 0.05% 2411

Leukonychia
Desyrel and Desyrel Dividose 1404

Leukopenia
▲ Accutane Capsules (1 in 5 to 1 in 10) 1878
Adalat Capsules (10 mg and 20 mg) (Less than 0.5%) 1587
Adriamycin PFS (High incidence) 561
Adriamycin RDF 562
Aldactazide 2150
Aldoclor Tablets 1413

Aldomet Ester HCl Injection 1417
Aldomet Oral 1415
Aldoril Tablets 1418
▲ Alferon N Injection (11%) 1809
Altace Capsules (Scattered incidents) 1086
Amoxil 2193
Anaprox and Anaprox DS Tablets (Less than 1%) 2288
Ancef Injection 2194
Ancobon Capsules 1886
Ansaid Tablets (Less than 1%) 2319
Anturane (Rare) 853
Apresazide Capsules (Less frequent) 854
Apresoline Hydrochloride Parenteral (Ampuls) 856
Apresoline Hydrochloride Tablets (Less frequent) 855
Apresoline-Esidrix Tablets 857
Aralen Phosphate with Primaquine Phosphate Tablets 2040
Asendin Tablets (Less than 1%) 1196
▲ Atgam Sterile Solution (1 in 7 patients; 14%) 2320
Atromid-S Capsules 2435
Augmentin Tablets, Powder for Oral Suspension, and Chewable Tablets 2198
Azo Gantanol Tablets 1887
Azo Gantrisin Tablets 1888
Azulfidine Tablets, EN-tabs, Oral Suspension (Rare) 1157
Bactrim DS Tablets 1891
Bactrim I.V. Infusion 1889
Bactrim 1891
Benemid Tablets 1426
Bicillin C-R Injection 2438
Bicillin C-R 900/300 Injection 2440
Bicillin L-A Injection (Infrequent) 2442
BiCNU 723
BuSpar (Rare) 1401
Butazolidin Capsules & Tablets (Less than 1%) 1027
Capastat Sulfate Vials 1250
Capozide 2258
Cardizem Tablets-30 mg, 60 mg, 90 mg and 120 mg (Infrequent) 1329
Cardizem SR Capsules-60 mg, 90 mg and 120 mg (Infrequent) 1327
Cardura Tablets 1941
Ceclor Pulvules & Suspension 1251
CeeNU 725
Cefizox Injection (Rare) 1012
Cefotan 2265
Ceftin Tablets 575
Celontin 1692
Ceptaz for Injection (Very rare) 1057
Chloromycetin Kapseals 1695
Chloromycetin Palmitate, Oral Suspension 1697
Chloromycetin Sodium Succinate 1698
Cipro I.V. (Infrequent) 1592
Cipro Tablets (0.4%) 1589
Claforan Sterile Injection (Less than 1%) 1089
Cleocin HCl Capsules 2322
Cleocin Pediatric Flavored Granules 2324
Cleocin Phosphate Injection 2325
Clinoril Tablets (Less than 1%) 1433
▲ Clozaril Tablets (3%) 2000
ColBENEMID Tablets 1436
Combipres Tablets 678
Comhist LA Capsules 1618
Compazine 2201
Corzide Tablets 702
Cosmegen Injection 1440
Cuprimine Capsules (2%) 1442
Cytadren Tablets (Rare) 861
▲ Cytosar-U Sterile Powder (Among most frequent) 2329
Cytovene Sterile Powder 2292
Cytoxan for Injection 726
Dalmane Capsules (Rare) 1927
Danocrine Capsules 2046
Daranide Tablets 1445
Daraprim Tablets 761
Depakene Capsules & Syrup 511
Depakote 512
Depen Titratable Tablets (2%) 2379
Deprol Tablets 2382
DiaBeta 1091
Diabinese Tablets 1775
Diamox 1200
Dicumarol Tablets (Infrequent) 516
Diflucan Injection and Tablets 1948
Dilantin Infatabs (Occasional) 1710
Dilantin Kapseals (Occasional) 1708
Dilantin Parenteral (Occasional) 1712
Dilantin-30 Pediatric/Dilantin-125 Suspension (Occasional) 1713
Dilantin with Phenobarbital Kapseals (Occasional) 1715
Dipentum Capsules (Rare) 1160
Diucardin Tablets 2450
Diulo 2129
Diupres Tablets 1461
Diuril Oral Suspension 1464
Diuril Sodium Intravenous 1463
Diuril Tablets 1464
Dolobid Tablets (Less than 1 in 100) 1465
Doxorubicin Hydrochloride Injection, USP 848
Dyazide Capsules 2208
DynaCirc Capsules (0.5% to 1%) .. 2004
Easprin 1719
Elavil 2269
Elspar 1470
▲ Emcyt Capsules (4%) 1161
Endep Tablets 1927
Enduron Tablets 517
Enduronyl 518
Equagesic Tablets 2451
▲ Ergamisol Tablets (Up to 33%) 1136
Esidrix Tablets 863
Esimil Tablets 864
Etrafon 2087
▲ Eulexin Capsules (3%) 2089
Exna Tablets 1862
▲ Sterile FUDR (Among more common) 1898
Fansidar Tablets 1896
Feldene Capsules (1 to 3%) 1777
Flagyl I.V. 2131
Flagyl Tablets 2170
Flexeril Tablets (Rare) 1471
Fluorouracil Injection 1897
Fortaz (Rare) 1060
Fulvicin P/G Tablets 2090
Fulvicin P/G 165 & 330 Tablets 2091
Fulvicin-U/F Tablets 2092
Fungizone Intravenous 2262
Ganite Injection 1016
Gantanol 1899
Gantrisin Ophthalmic Ointment/Solution 1900
Gantrisin 1901
Garamycin Injectable 2093
Geocillin Tablets 1951
Glucotrol 1952
Grifulvin V (griseofulvin microsize) Tablets/Suspension (Rare) 1678
Grisactin (Rare) 2454
Grisactin Ultra Tablets (Rare) 2455
Gris-PEG Tablets, 125 mg & 250 mg (Rare) 1083
Haldol Decanoate 1375
Haldol Injection, Tablets and Concentrate 1373
▲ Hexalen Capsules (1% to 15%) 2316
Hydrea Capsules 728
HydroDIURIL Tablets 1484
Hydromox R Tablets 1209
Hydromox Tablets 1208
Hydropres Tablets 1485
Hyperstat I.V. Injection 2095
IFEX 729
▲ Imuran (28% to more than 50%) .. 768
Inderide Tablets 2463
Inderide LA Long Acting Capsules .. 2465
Indocin Capsules (Less than 1%) 1487
Indocin I.V. (Less than 1%) 1490
Indocin (Less than 1%) 1487
Intron A (2 patients) 2097
Ismelin Tablets 869
Keftab Tablets 917
Kefurox Vials, Faspak & ADD-Vantage (1 in 750) 1277
Kefzol Vials, Faspak & ADD-Vantage 1279
Klonopin Tablets 1902
Lariam Tablets 1904
Larodopa Tablets 1905
Lasix 1093
Lincocin 2344
Lodine Capsules (Less than 1%) 2468
Loniten Tablets (Rare) 2346
Lopid Capsules and Tablets (Rare) 1736
Lopressor HCT Tablets 1034
Lotensin Tablets (Scattered incidents) 872
Loxitane (Rare) 1213
Lozol Tablets 1843
Lupron Depot 7.5 mg 2311
Lupron Injection 2310
Macrodantin Capsules 1624
▲ Matulane Capsules (Frequent) 1907
Maxzide 1215
Meclomen Capsules (Less than 1%) 1739
Mefoxin 1498
Mefoxin Premixed Intravenous Solution 1500
Mellaril (Increased risk in aged) 2011
Mepergan Injection (Very rare) 2479
Mesantoin Tablets 2013
▲ Methotrexate Tablets, Parenteral, LPF Parenteral (Among most frequent; 1 to 3%) 1217
Mevacor Tablets (Rare) 1505
Mexitil Capsules (About 1 in 1,000) 680
Mezlin 1597
Mezlin Pharmacy Bulk Package 1599
Micronase Tablets 2350
Milontin Kapseals 1741
Minizide Capsules 1779
Mintezol 1510
▲ Mithracin (6%) 1602
Moban Tablets & Concentrate (Rare) 932
Moduretic Tablets 1510
Monocid Injection (Less than 1%) .. 2217
Monopril Tablets 1406
Mutamycin 733
Mykrox ½ mg Tablets 984
Myleran Tablets 790
Naprosyn (Less than 1%) 2297
Nardil (Less frequent) 1742
Naturetin Tablets 1789
Navane Capsules and Concentrate (Occasional) 1954
Navane Intramuscular (Occasional) 1956
Nebcin Vials, Hyporets & ADD-Vantage 1286
NegGram (Rare) 2062
Neosar for Injection (Frequent) 566
Neptazane Tablets .... ◉ 311
Netromycin Injection 100 mg/ml (Fewer than 1 in 1000 patients) 2104
Nizoral Tablets (Less than 1%) 1145
Normodyne Tablets 2110
Normozide Tablets 2112
Noroxin Tablets (1.2%) 1519
Norzine 1818
Oncovin Solution Vials & Hyporets 1288
Oretic Tablets 544
Oreticyl 545
Orinase Tablets 2354
Ornade Spansule Capsules 2221
PBZ Tablets & Elixir 1037
PBZ-SR Tablets 1037
PMB 200 and PMB 400 2504
Panwarfin Tablets (Infrequent) 547
Paradione Capsules 548
▲ Paraplatin for Injection (26% to 85%) 735
Parnate Tablets 2222
Pediazole 1973
▲ Pentam 300 Injection (2.8 to 7.5%) 1018
Pepcid (Rare) 1524
Periactin 1525
Permax Tablets (Infrequent) 1291
Pfizerpen for Injection (Rare) 1957
Phenergan with Codeine (Rare) 2497
Phenergan with Dextromethorphan (Rare) 2499
Phenergan Injection 2493
Phenergan Suppositories (Rare) 2496
Phenergan Syrup (Rare) 2495
Phenergan Tablets (Rare) 2496
Phenergan VC (Rare) 2500
Phenergan VC with Codeine (Rare) 2501
Phenurone Tablets (2%) 552
Pipracil 1230
Plaquenil Sulfate Tablets 2067
Platinol 737
Platinol-AQ Injection 738
Ponstel (Occasional) 1758
Primaxin I.M. 1532
Primaxin I.V. (Less than 0.2%) 1535
Prinzide Tablets 1540
Priscoline Hydrochloride Ampuls 877
Procardia Capsules (Less than 0.5%) 1781
Prolixin Decanoate 1795
Prolixin Elixir 1793
Prolixin Enanthate 1796
Prolixin Injection 1791
Prolixin Oral Concentrate 1792
Prolixin Tablets 1793
Proloprim Tablets 799
ProSom Tablets (Rare) 554
Protostat Tablets 1674
Prozac Pulvules (Rare) 920
Purinethol Tablets (Frequent) 800
Rauzide Tablets 1804
Reglan (A few cases) 1869
Renese Tablets 1785
Renese-R Tablets (Rare) 1786
▲ Rheumatrex Methotrexate Dose Pack (Among most frequent) 1234
Ridaura Capsules 2224
Rifadin 1345
Rifamate Capsules 1347
Rimactane Capsules (Rare) 879
Ritalin 880
Rocephin Injectable Vials, ADD-Vantage (2.1%) 1914
▲ Roferon-A Injection (49%) 1916
Rubex 739
Ru-Tuss Tablets 693
Rythmol Tablets (Less than 1%) 1184
▲ SSD (20%) 694
SSD RP Cream 690
Saluron 718
Salutensin/Salutensin-Demi 719
▲ Sandimmune (Up to 19%) 2024
Septra 813
Septra I.V. Infusion 808
Septra I.V. Infusion ADD-Vantage Vials 810
Septra 813
Ser-Ap-Es Tablets 881
Serax Capsules (Rare) 2522
Serax Tablets (Rare) 2522
Serentil 686
Serpasil-Apresoline Tablets 884
Serpasil-Esidrix Tablets 886
Silvadene Cream 1% (Infrequent) .. 1352
Sinemet Tablets (Rare) 952
Sinemet CR Tablets 953
Sinequan (Occasional) 1960
Skelaxin 840
Solganal Suspension (Rare) 2122
Soma Compound w/Codeine Tablets (Very rare) 2390
Soma Compound Tablets (Very rare) 2389
Soma Tablets 2388
Spectrobid Tablets & Powder for Oral Suspension 1961
Stelazine 2226
Suprax (Less than 2%) 1235
Symmetrel Capsules & Syrup (Less than 0.1%) 936
Tacaryl 2409
Tagamet (Approximately 1 per 100,000) 2228
Tambocor Tablets (Less than 1%) 1315
Taractan (Very rare) 1920
Tazicef for Injection (Very rare) 2231
▲ Tegison Capsules (10-25%) 1881
Tegretol Chewable Tablets 654
Tegretol Suspension 656
Tegretol Tablets 654
Temaril Tablets, Syrup and Spansule Sustained Release Capsules 1085
Tenoretic Tablets 1105
Tenuate 1354
Thalitone Tablets 687
▲ TheraCys BCG Live (Intravesical) (Up to 5.4%) 898
Thiosulfil Forte Tablets 2526
Thiotepa Parenteral 1240
Thorazine 2234
Ticar for Injection 2236
Timentin for Injection 2239
Timolide Tablets 1547
Tolinase Tablets 2365
Tonocard Tablets (Less than 1%) .. 1554
Torecan 1993
Trandate HCT Tablets 579
Trental (Less than 1%) 1099
Triavil Tablets 1556
Tridione 557
Trilafon 2123
Trimpex Tablets 1922
Unasyn 1965
Unipen 2533
Urispas Tablets (1 case) 2242
Vascor (200, 300 and 400 mg) Tablets (2 cases) 1383
Vaseretic Tablets 1559
▲ Velban Vials (Among most common) 1305
Velosef Capsules and for Oral Suspension 606
▲ VePesid Capsules and Injection (3 to 17%) 741
Vivactil Tablets 1567
Voltaren Tablets (Less than 1%) 1042
Wellbutrin Tablets 821
Zanosar Sterile Powder 2371
Zantac Injection and Zantac Injection Premixed (Few patients) 1063
Zantac (A few patients) 1065

Zarontin Capsules 1768
Zarontin Syrup 1769
Zaroxolyn Tablets 989
Zefazone Sterile Powder 2372
Zestoretic 2274
Zinacef (1 in 750 patients) 1066
Zovirax Capsules 824
Zovirax Sterile Powder 828
Zovirax 824
Zyloprim Tablets (Less than 1%) 830

Leukopenia, transient

▲SSD RP Cream (20%) 690

Leukoplakia, oral

Intron A (1 patient) 2097

Leukorrhea

Anafranil Capsules (Up to 2%) 650
Intron A (Less than 1%) 2097
Lippes Loop Intrauterine Double-S 1654
Lodine Capsules (Less than 1%) 2468
Norplant System 2484
Permax Tablets (Rare) 1291
Prozac Pulvules (Infrequent) 920

Lhermitte's sign

Platinol 737
Platinol-AQ Injection 738

Libido, changes

Adipex-P Tablets and Capsules 1019
Amen 833
▲Anafranil Capsules (Up to 21%) 650
Asendin Tablets (Less than 1%) 1196
Biphetamine Capsules 973
Brevicon 2304
Cycrin Tablets 2449
Danocrine Capsules 2046
Demulen 2161
Depo-Provera Sterile Aqueous Suspension 2336
Desoxyn Gradumet Tablets 514
Desyrel and Desyrel Dividose (Greater than 1%) 1404
Dexedrine 2206
Didrex Tablets 2338
Diethylstilbestrol Tablets 1258
Doral Tablets 2383
Elavil 2269
Endep Tablets 1927
Enovid 2161
Estinyl Tablets 2085
Estrace 1385
Estrace Vaginal Cream 1388
Estraderm Transdermal System 866
Estradurin 2452
Estratest 2245
Estrovis 1721
Etrafon 2087
Fastin Capsules 2216
Flexeril Tablets (Rare) 1471
Halcion Tablets 2340
Halotestin Tablets 2341
Ionamin Capsules 981
Jenest-28 Tablets 1636
Levlen/Tri-Levlen 665
Librax Capsules (Rare) 1929
Libritabs Tablets (Isolated cases) 1930
Librium Capsules (Isolated cases) 1931
Librium Injectable (Isolated cases) 1932
Limbitrol 1933
Lo/Ovral Tablets 2471
Lo/Ovral-28 Tablets 2476
Loestrin 1728
Mediatric Capsules 2476
Mellaril 2011
Menrium Tablets 1934
Metandren Linguets and Tablets 875
Micronor Tablets 1667
Modicon 1667
Nordette-21 Tablets 2481
Nordette-28 Tablets 2483
Norethin 2133
Norinyl 2304
Norlestrin 1746
Norlutate 1754
Norlutin 1755
Norpramin Tablets 1340
Nor-Q D Tablets 2304
Norzine 1818
Ogen 540
Ortho Dienestrol Cream 1664
Ortho-Cyclen Tablets 1658
Ortho-Novum 1667
Orudis Capsules (Less than 1%) 2488
Ovral Tablets 2490
Ovral-28 Tablets 2491
Ovrette Tablets 2492
PMB 200 and PMB 400 2504
Plegine Tablets 2504
Pondimin Tablets 1867
Prelu-2 Capsules 683
Premarin Intravenous 2508
Premarin with Methyltestosterone 2515
Premarin Tablets 2510
Premarin Vaginal Cream 2512
Provera Tablets 2356
Sanorex Tablets (Rare) 2030
Serax Capsules 2522
Serax Tablets 2522
Serentil 686
Sinequan 1960
Stilphostrol Tablets and Ampuls 1609
TACE 12 and 25 mg 1353
Tenuate 1354
Tofranil Ampuls 1038
Tofranil Tablets 1039
Tofranil-PM Capsules 1041
Torecan 1993
Trexan Tablets (Less than 1%) 937
Triavil Tablets 1556
Trilafon 2123
Levlen/Tri-Levlen 665
Tri-Norinyl 2304
Triphasil-21 Tablets 2527
Triphasil-28 Tablets 2532
Valium Injectable 1937
Valium Tablets (Infrequent) 1939
Valrelease Capsules (Occasional) 1923
Vivactil Tablets 1567
▲Xanax Tablets (7.1%) 2367

Libido, decrease

Aldoclor Tablets 1413
Aldomet Ester HCl Injection 1417
Aldomet Oral 1415
Aldoril Tablets 1418
Anadrol-50 Tablets 2287
Android 1111
Atromid-S Capsules 2435
Axid Pulvules 1246
Blocadren Tablets (0.6%) 1429
Bontril Slow-Release 834
BuSpar (Infrequent) 1401
Calcijex Calcitriol Injection 506
Calderol Capsules 1635
Clozaril Tablets (Less than 1%) 2000
Cordarone Tablets (1 to 3%) 2446
Corgard Tablets (1 to 5 of 1000 patients) 701
Corzide Tablets (1 to 5 of 1000 patients) 702
Cytotec (Infrequent) 2159
Diupres Tablets 1461
Dolophine Hydrochloride Ampoules & Vials 1260
Dolophine Hydrochloride Tablets 1261
DynaCirc Capsules (0.5% to 1%) 2004
Enduronyl 518
Ethmozine Tablets (Less than 2%) 946
Fiorinal with Codeine Capsules 2008
Flagyl Tablets 2170
Harmonyl Tablets 528
Hydropres Tablets 1485
Hyperstat I.V. Injection 2095
Hytrin Tablets (0.6%) 529
Intron A (Less than 5%) 2097
Inversine Tablets 1492
IOPIDINE ◉ 232
Kerlone Tablets (Less than 2%) 2172
Lopid Capsules and Tablets 1736
Lopressor 1032
Lotensin Tablets 872
Lozol Tablets (Less than 5%) 1843
Ludiomil Tablets (Rare) 874
Lupron Depot 7.5 mg (Less than 5%) 2311
Lupron Injection (Less than 5%) 2310
MS Contin Tablets 1814
MSIR 1817
Metandren Linguets and Tablets 875
Methadone Hydrochloride Diskets 1284
Methadone Hydrochloride Oral Solution & Tablets 1987
Mexitil Capsules (Less than 1% or about 4 in 1,000) 680
Midamor Tablets (Less than or equal to 1%) 1508
Moduretic Tablets 1510
Monopril Tablets (0.2 to 1.0%) 1406
Normozide Tablets (Less than 1%) 2112
Norpramin Tablets 1340
Oramorph SR (Morphine Sulfate Sustained Release Tablets) (Less frequent) 1988
Oreticyl 545
Pamelor 2019
Pepcid (Infrequent) 1524
Permax Tablets (Infrequent) 1291
Plendil Extended-Release Tablets (0.5% to 1.5%) 1526
Pondimin Tablets 1867
Prinivil Tablets (0.2%) 1538
Prinzide Tablets (0.3% to 1%) 1540
Procardia XL Tablets (1% or less) 1783
ProSom Tablets (Rare) 554
Protostat Tablets 1674
Prozac Pulvules (1.6%) 920
Raudixin Tablets 1803
Rauzide Tablets 1804
Renese-R Tablets 1786
Rocaltrol Capsules 1913
Roxanol 1991
Salutensin/Salutensin-Demi 719
Sandostatin Injection (Less than 1%) 2029
Ser-Ap-Es Tablets 881
Serpasil Tablets 883
Serpasil-Apresoline Tablets 884
Serpasil-Esidrix Tablets 886
Surmontil Capsules 2524
▲Synarel Nasal Solution (22% of patients) 2300
Tacaryl 2409
Tambocor Tablets (Less than 1%) 1315
Temaril Tablets, Syrup and Spansule Sustained Release Capsules 1085
Tenex Tablets (Less than 3%) 1875
Testred Capsules 1124
Timolide Tablets (Less than 1%) 1547
Timoptic in Ocudose 1552
Timoptic Sterile Ophthalmic Solution 1550
Tofranil Ampuls 1038
Tofranil Tablets 1039
Tofranil-PM Capsules 1041
Trandate HCT Tablets (Less than 1% in 208 patients) 579
Vaseretic Tablets (0.5% to 2.0%) 1559
▲Wellbutrin Tablets (3.1%) 821
Winstrol Tablets 2075
Wytensin Tablets (3% or less) 2542
▲Xanax Tablets (14.4%) 2367
Zantac Injection and Zantac Injection Premixed 1063
Zantac (Occasional) 1065
Zestoretic (0.3 to 1%) 2274
Zestril Tablets (0.2%) 2277
Zyloprim Tablets (Less than 1%) 830

Libido, increase

Anadrol-50 Tablets 2287
Android 1111
Bontril Slow-Release 834
BuSpar (Infrequent) 1401
Cholybar 1705
Clozaril Tablets (Less than 1%) 2000
Etrafon 2087
Haldol Decanoate 1375
Haldol Injection, Tablets and Concentrate 1373
Klonopin Tablets 1902
Ludiomil Tablets (Rare) 874
▲Lupron Depot 3.75 mg (Among most frequent) 2312
Lupron Depot 7.5 mg 2311
Lupron Injection 2310
Metandren Linguets and Tablets 875
Moban Tablets & Concentrate 932
Norpramin Tablets 1340
Pamelor 2019
Permax Tablets (Infrequent) 1291
Pondimin Tablets 1867
Prolixin Decanoate 1795
Prolixin Elixir 1793
Prolixin Enanthate 1796
Prolixin Injection 1791
Prolixin Oral Concentrate 1792
Prolixin Tablets 1793
Prozac Pulvules (1.6%) 920
Questran Light 711
Questran Powder 710
Surmontil Capsules 2524
Synarel Nasal Solution (1% of patients) 2300
Taractan 1920
Testred Capsules 1124
Tofranil Ampuls 1038
Tofranil Tablets 1039
Tofranil-PM Capsules 1041
Wellbutrin Tablets (Frequent) 821
Winstrol Tablets 2075
▲Xanax Tablets (7.7%) 2367
Zarontin Capsules (Rare) 1768
Zarontin Syrup (Rare) 1769

Libido, loss

Catapres Tablets (About 3 in 100 patients) 676
▲Catapres-TTS (3%) 677
Combipres Tablets (About 3%) 678
▲Eulexin Capsules (36% with LHRH-agonist) 2089
Methotrexate Tablets, Parenteral, LPF Parenteral 1217
Orap Tablets 1020
Rheumatrex Methotrexate Dose Pack 1234
Roferon-A Injection (Less than 1%) 1916
Vascor (200, 300 and 400 mg) Tablets (0.5 to 2.0%) 1383

Lichen planus

Aralen Hydrochloride Injection 2038
Aralen Phosphate Tablets 2039
Atabrine Hydrochloride Tablets 2041
Cuprimine Capsules 1442
Depen Titratable Tablets (Rare) 2379
Minipress Capsules (Less than 1%) 1778
Minizide Capsules (Rare) 1779
Trandate HCT/Trandate 579

Lichen planus, bullous

Normodyne Tablets 2110
Normozide Tablets 2112
Trandate Tablets 579

Light-headedness

▲Adalat Capsules (10 mg and 20 mg) (About 10% to 27%) 1587
Adenocard Injection (2%) 1007
Aldoclor Tablets 1413
Aldomet Ester HCl Injection 1417
Aldomet Oral 1415
▲Alferon N Injection (3%) 1809
Anaprox and Anaprox DS Tablets (Less than 3%) 2288
▲Anestacon Solution (Among most common) 2394
▲Anexsia 5/500 Tablets (Among most frequent) 2196
▲Anexsia 7.5/650 Tablets (Among most frequent) 2197
Atgam Sterile Solution (At least 1 patient and less than 5% of total patients) 2320
▲Azdōne Tablets (Among most frequent) 844
▲Beconase AQ Nasal Spray (Fewer than 5 per 100 patients) 574
▲Bentyl (11%) 1322
Bretylol Injection (7 in 1000) 923
Brevibloc Injection (Less than 1%) 942
BuSpar (3%) 1401
Capoten 2255
▲Cardura Tablets (Up to 23%) 1941
▲Centrax (6.8%) 1693
Cipro I.V. (1% or less) 1592
Cipro Tablets (Less than 1%) 1589
Cutivate Ointment 0.005% (Less than 1%) 1054
Dalmane Capsules 1927
▲Damason-P (Among most frequent) 1356
Dantrium Capsules (Less frequent) 1619
Daraprim Tablets (Rare) 761
Darvon-N/Darvocet-N 1254
Darvon 1256
Darvon-N Suspension & Tablets 1254
Decadron Phosphate Turbinaire 1456
Deconamine 663
Demerol 2047
Deponit NTG Transdermal Delivery System (Occasional) 2143
Desyrel and Desyrel Dividose 1404
Dilaudid-HP Injection 1175
Dipentum Capsules (1 out of 441 patients) 1160
Diulo 2129
Dolobid Tablets (Less than 1 in 100) 1465
▲Dolophine Hydrochloride Ampoules & Vials (Among most frequent) 1260
▲Dolophine Hydrochloride Tablets (Among most frequent) 1261
Dorcol Children's Decongestant Liquid ▣ 685
Duranest Injections 624
Duvoid Tablets 1853
Dyclone 0.5% and 1% Topical Solutions, USP 626
▲Eldepryl (7 of 49 patients) 2250
▲Empirin with Codeine Phosphate Nos. 2, 3 & 4 (Among most frequent) 764
Esgic-Plus Tablets (Less frequent) 1002
Esgic Tablets & Capsules (Less frequent) 1001
Factrel (Rare) 2561

Fioricet Tablets (Less frequent) 2006
Fiorinal Capsules (Less frequent).... 2007
Fiorinal with Codeine Capsules (2.6%) 2008
Fiorinal Tablets (Less frequent)....... 2007
Gammagard Immune Globulin, Intravenous (Human) (Occasional).... 658
Gastrocrom Capsules (Infrequent).. 974
▲ Halcion Tablets (4.9%) 2340
Hydrocet Capsules 835
Hyperstat I.V. Injection 2095
▲ Hytrin Tablets (28%) 529
Inderal 2459
Inderal LA Long Acting Capsules 2461
Inderide Tablets 2463
Inderide LA Long Acting Capsules .. 2465
Indocin (Less than 1%) 1487
Inversine Tablets 1492
ISMOTIC (Very rare).... ◉ 233
Kemadrin Tablets 771
▲ Lortab ASA Tablets (Among most frequent) 2414
▲ Lortab (Among most frequent) 2412
Loxitane 1213
Lozol Tablets (Less than 5%) 1843
Lupron Depot 7.5 mg 2311
▲ Lupron Injection (5% or more) 2310
▲ MS Contin Tablets (Among most frequent) 1814
▲ MSIR (Among most frequent) 1817
Marcaine Spinal 2058
▲ Mepergan Injection (Among most frequent) 2479
▲ Methadone Hydrochloride Diskets (Among most frequent) 1284
Methadone Hydrochloride Oral Solution & Tablets.... 1987
▲ Mexitil Capsules (10.5 to 26.4%).. 680
▲ Minitran Transdermal Delivery System (6%) 1312
Minocin Intravenous 1221
Minocin Oral Suspension 1224
Motofen Tablets (1 in 20) 836
▲ Mykrox ½ mg Tablets (10.2%) 984
Naprosyn (Less than 3%) 2297
Navane Capsules and Concentrate 1954
Navane Intramuscular 1956
Nicorette (2.1%) 1335
Nimotop Capsules (Less than 1%) 1607
▲ Nitrodisc (6%) 2176
Nitro-Dur (nitroglycerin) Transdermal Infusion System (Occasional) 1164
Nitrogard Tablets.... 1004
Nolvadex Tablets (Infrequent) 1102
Norflex 1314
Norgesic.... 1314
Noroxin Tablets 1519
Nucofed Capsules 2219
Nucofed Expectorant 2219
Nucofed Pediatric Expectorant 2220
Nucofed Syrup 2219
Numorphan Hydrochloride Injection 935
Numorphan Suppositories 935
Omnipaque (Less than or equal to 1%) 2552
▲ Oramorph SR (Morphine Sulfate Sustained Release Tablets) (Among most frequent) 1988
Paraflex Caplets (Rare) 1378
Parafon Forte DSC Caplets (Rare) .. 1379
Parlodel (Less than 1-5%) 2020
Peptavlon 2563
▲ Percocet Tablets (Among most frequent) 950
▲ Percodan (Among most frequent) .. 951
▲ Phenaphen with Codeine Capsules (Among most frequent) 1865
▲ Phenaphen-650 with Codeine Tablets (Among most frequent) 1866
Phenergan with Codeine.... 2497
Phenergan VC with Codeine 2501
Phrenilin 838
Prinzide Tablets 1540
Procan SR Tablets (Infrequent).... 1760
▲ Procardia Capsules (Approximately 10%) 1781
▲ Procardia XL Tablets (27%) 1783
Prolastin Alpha$_1$-Proteinase Inhibitor (Human) (0.19%) 1585
Provocholine for Inhalation (1 occurrence) 1911
Prozac Pulvules (1.6%) 920
Quadrinal Tablets 1183
Quinidex Extentabs 1868
Rauzide Tablets 1804
Recombivax HB (Less than 1%).... 1544
Robaxin Injectable 1871
Robaxin Tablets 1872
▲ Robaxisal Tablets (One in 20-25) .. 1872
▲ Rogaine Topical Solution (3.42%).. 2357
▲ Roxanol (Among most frequent).... 1991
▲ Roxicodone Tablets, Oral Solution & Intensol (Oxycodone) (Among most frequent) 1992
Ru-Tuss DE Tablets 694
Sandostatin Injection (1.6%) 2029
Sansert Tablets.... 2031
Sedapap Tablets 50 mg/650 mg (Less frequent) 1360
Sensorcaine 631
Sensorcaine-MPF Spinal 634
Serophene (clomiphene citrate tablets, USP) (Less than 1 in 100 patients) 2186
Stadol (1%) 721
▲ Symmetrel Capsules & Syrup (5-10%) 936
Synalgos-DC Capsules.... 2525
Talacen.... 2070
▲ Talwin Injection (Most common).... 2071
Talwin Compound 2072
▲ Talwin Injection (Most common).... 2071
Talwin Nx.... 2073
▲ Tambocor Tablets (18.9%) 1315
Tenoretic Tablets (1 to 3%).... 1105
Tenormin Tablets and I.V. Injection (1 to 3%) 1107
▲ Tornalate (3%).... 2074
▲ Transderm-Nitro Transdermal Therapeutic System (6%) 2283
Tridil Ampuls & Vials 939
Trilisate (Less than 2%).... 1822
Tylenol with Codeine 1381
▲ Tylox Capsules (Among most frequent) 1382
Urecholine.... 1558
Vancenase AQ Nasal Spray 0.042% (Fewer than 5 per 100 patients) 2127
Vaseretic Tablets 1559
Ventolin Rotacaps for Inhalation (1%) 583
Versed Injection (Less than 1%) 1924
▲ Vicodin Tablets (Most frequent) 1187
▲ Vicodin ES Tablets (Among most frequent) 1189
Wygesic Tablets 2540
▲ Xanax Tablets (20.8% to 29.8%).. 2367
▲ Xylocaine Injections (Among most common).... 637
Xylocaine Injections for Ventricular Arrhythmias 639
Xylocaine 2% Jelly 643
Xylocaine 5% Ointment 644
Xylocaine 10% Oral Spray 645
4% Xylocaine-MPF Sterile Solution 641
Xylocaine 2% Viscous Solution 646
Zaroxolyn Tablets 989
Zestoretic 2274
Zestril Tablets 2277
Zovirax Sterile Powder (Less than 1%).... 828
▲ Zydone Capsules (Most frequent) .. 941

Limb reduction defects

Amen.... 833
Depo-Provera Sterile Aqueous Suspension (Less than 1 per 1,000) 2336
Diethylstilbestrol Tablets 1258
Estinyl Tablets.... 2085
Estrovis 1721
Lo/Ovral Tablets 2471
Lo/Ovral-28 Tablets.... 2476
Mediatric Capsules (Less than 1 per 1,000).... 2476
Menrium Tablets (Somewhat less than 1 per 1,000).... 1934
Metubine Iodide Vials.... 1285
Nordette-21 Tablets.... 2481
Nordette-28 Tablets.... 2483
Norinyl 2304
Ogen 540
Ovral Tablets 2490
Ovral-28 Tablets 2491
Ovrette Tablets.... 2492
Parlodel (3 infants).... 2020
Provera Tablets (Less than 1 in 1,000).... 2356
Tri-Norinyl.... 2304
Vaseretic Tablets 1559

Lipoprotein levels, changes

▲ Accutane Capsules (Approximately 15%) 1878
Anadrol-50 Tablets.... 2287
Danocrine Capsules 2046
Demulen 2161
Enovid.... 2161
Jenest-28 Tablets 1636
Levlen/Tri-Levlen.... 665
Loestrin 1728
Lupron Depot 3.75 mg (2%).... 2312
Norlestrin 1746
Synarel Nasal Solution.... 2300
Tegretol Chewable Tablets (Occasional).... 654
Tegretol Suspension (Occasional) .. 656
Tegretol Tablets (Occasional) 654
Timolide Tablets.... 1547
Levlen/Tri-Levlen.... 665
Triphasil-21 Tablets.... 2527
Winstrol Tablets 2075

Lipoproteins, electrophoretic abnormalities

Sandimmune 2024

Lips, enlargement

Dilantin Infatabs.... 1710
Dilantin Kapseals 1708
Dilantin Parenteral 1712
Dilantin-30 Pediatric/Dilantin-125 Suspension.... 1713
Dilantin with Phenobarbital Kapseals 1715
Eskalith 2214

Lips, swelling

▲ Intron A (Less than 14%) 2097
Phenobarbital Elixir and Tablets 1293
Prinzide Tablets 1540
Quadrinal Tablets 1183
Tambocor Tablets (Less than 1%) 1315
Voltaren Tablets (less than 1%).... 1042
Zestoretic 2274
Zestril Tablets 2277

Listlessness

Atgam Sterile Solution (At least 1 patient and less than 5% of total patients) 2320
Indocin (Greater than 1%) 1487
Klorvess Effervescent Granules.... 2010
Klorvess Effervescent Tablets 2011
Klorvess 10% Liquid 2010
Polycitra Syrup 2424
Polycitra-K 2424
Polycitra-LC—Sugar-Free.... 2424
Rum-K Syrup 995

Livedo reticularis

Symmetrel Capsules & Syrup (1-5%).... 936

Liver abnormalities

Anaprox and Anaprox DS Tablets.... 2288
Cardene Capsules (Rare) 2290
Catapres Tablets (About 1 in 100 patients) 676
Clozaril Tablets (1%).... 2000
Combipres Tablets 678
Compazine (A few observations) 2201
Cytadren Tablets (Rare) 861
Lamprene Capsules (Less than 1%).... 1030
Methotrexate Tablets, Parenteral, LPF Parenteral 1217
Pepcid (Infrequent).... 1524
Rheumatrex Methotrexate Dose Pack.... 1234
Ridaura Capsules (1 to 3%).... 2224
Rythmol Tablets (Less than 1%) 1184
Sectral Capsules 2520

Liver abscess

Cytosar-U Sterile Powder (With experimental doses).... 2329

Liver damage

Alurate Elixir 1883
Butisol Sodium Elixir & Tablets (Less than 1 in 100).... 2377
Compazine 2201
Cytosar-U Sterile Powder 2329
Dilantin Infatabs.... 1710
Dilantin Kapseals 1708
Dilantin Parenteral 1712
Dilantin-30 Pediatric/Dilantin-125 Suspension.... 1713
Dilantin with Phenobarbital Kapseals 1715
Dimetapp Plus Caplets .... ▣ 675
Etrafon.... 2087
INH Tablets (Occasional).... 868
Leukine for IV Infusion.... 1127
Mebaral Tablets (Less than 1 in 100).... 2061
Mintezol.... 1510
Nardil (Very few patients) 1742
Nembutal Sodium Capsules 534
Nembutal Sodium Solution (Less than 1%).... 536
Nembutal Sodium Suppositories (Less than 1%).... 538
Parafon Forte DSC Caplets (One case).... 1379
Phenobarbital Elixir and Tablets (Less than 1 in 100 patients) 1293
Prokine for I.V. Infusion 1096
Prolixin Decanoate 1795
Prolixin Enanthate 1796
Prolixin Oral Concentrate.... 1792
Seconal Sodium Pulvules (Less than 1 in 100) 1296
Stelazine 2226
Synkayvite Injection 1919
Synkayvite Tablets 1920
Tegretol Chewable Tablets 654
Tegretol Suspension.... 656
Tegretol Tablets 654
Triavil Tablets 1556
Trilafon.... 2123
Wellbutrin Tablets (Infrequent) 821

Liver disorders

Aldoclor Tablets.... 1413
Aldomet Oral 1415
Aldoril Tablets.... 1418
Butazolidin Capsules & Tablets.... 1027
Cosmegen Injection 1440
Intal Inhaler (Rare) 979
Lo/Ovral Tablets 2471
Lo/Ovral-28 Tablets.... 2476
Ludiomil Tablets (Rare) 874
Ovral Tablets.... 2490
Ovral-28 Tablets 2491
Ovrette Tablets.... 2492
Prozac Pulvules (Rare) 920
Triphasil-21 Tablets.... 2527
Triphasil-28 Tablets.... 2532

Liver dysfunction (see under Hepatic dysfunction)

Liver function, changes

Aldoclor Tablets.... 1413
Aldomet Ester HCl Injection 1417
Aldomet Oral 1415
Aldoril Tablets.... 1418
Asendin Tablets (Less than 1%).... 1196
Aygestin Tablets.... 2437
Blocadren Tablets 1429
Capoten 2255
Capozide 2258
Cefobid Intravenous/Intramuscular (1 patient in 1285) 1943
Centrax.... 1693
Clinoril Tablets (Less than 1 in 100) 1433
Cosmegen Injection 1440
Cytovene Sterile Powder (2%) 2292
Dantrium Capsules 1619
Depakene Capsules & Syrup (Occasional).... 511
Depakote Sprinkle Capsules (Occasional).... 512
DiaBeta (Isolated cases) 1091
Dolobid Tablets (Less than 1 in 100) 1465
Emcyt Capsules 1161
Engerix-B Unit-Dose Vials.... 2213
EryPed Drops and Chewable Tablets 519
Erythromycin Base Filmtab 525
Erythromycin Delayed-Release Capsules, USP.... 526
Estratest 2245
Feldene Capsules (Less than 1%) .. 1777
Ilotycin Gluceptate, IV, Vials 915
▲ Methotrexate Tablets, Parenteral, LPF Parenteral (15%).... 1217
Mevacor Tablets.... 1505
Micronor Tablets 1667
Minipress Capsules (Less than 1%) 1778
Minizide Capsules (Rare) 1779
Mithracin 1602
Modicon 1667
Niacor Tablets.... 2376
Nicolar Tablets 1846
Nicorette 1335
Normodyne Injection 2108
Ortho-Novum.... 1667
▲ Pentam 300 Injection (8.7%) 1018
Pipracil (Less than 2%) 1230
Prinivil Tablets (Rare) 1538
Prolixin Decanoate 1795
Prolixin Elixir 1793
Prolixin Enanthate 1796
Prolixin Injection.... 1791

Prolixin Oral Concentrate 1792
Prolixin Tablets 1793
Provera Tablets 2356
Reglan (Rare) 1869
Retrovir Capsules 802
Retrovir I.V. Infusion 805
Retrovir Syrup 802
▲ Rheumatrex Methotrexate Dose Pack (15%) 1234
Rufen Tablets (Less than 1%) 691
Surmontil Capsules 2524
Tegretol Chewable Tablets 654
Tegretol Suspension 656
Tegretol Tablets 654
Timolide Tablets 1547
Tonocard Tablets (Less than 1%) 1554
Toradol IM Injection (1% or less) 2302
Trental (Rare) 1099
Vasotec I.V. 1562
Vasotec Tablets (Rare) 1564
Voltaren Tablets (1-3%) 1042
Winstrol Tablets 2075
Zestril Tablets (Rare) 2277
Zovirax Capsules 824
Zovirax Sterile Powder 828
Zovirax 824

Liver function, impaired

Actimmune (Rare) 1046
Aldoclor Tablets 1413
Aldomet Ester HCl Injection 1417
Aldomet Oral 1415
Aldoril Tablets 1418
Anaprox and Anaprox DS Tablets (Less than 1%) 2288
Android 1111
Atgam Sterile Solution (Less than 5%) 2320
Atromid-S Capsules 2435
Catapres Tablets 676
Catapres-TTS (1%) 677
Children's Advil Suspension (Less than 1%) 2426
Cleocin HCl Capsules 2322
Cleocin Pediatric Flavored Granules 2324
Cleocin Phosphate Injection 2325
▲ Cordarone Tablets (4 to 9%) 2446
Cycrin Tablets 2449
DTIC-Dome (Few reports) 1595
Desyrel and Desyrel Dividose 1404
DynaCirc Capsules (0.5% to 1%) 2004
E.E.S. 522
Edecrin (Rare) 1468
ERYC 1720
EryPed 200 & EryPed 400 Granules 519
Ery-Tab Tablets 521
Erythrocin Stearate Filmtab 523
Estrace 1385
Estrace Vaginal Cream 1388
Etrafon 2087
Eulexin Capsules 2089
Flexeril Tablets (Less than 1%) 1471
Gastrocrom Capsules (Infrequent) 974
Haldol Decanoate 1375
Haldol Injection, Tablets and Concentrate 1373
Halotestin Tablets 2341
Idamycin for Injection (No more than 1%) 564
Konakion Injection 1903
Lincocin (Few instances) 2344
Lopid Capsules and Tablets 1736
Meclomen Capsules (Less than 1%) 1739
Mediatric Capsules 2476
Metandren Linguets and Tablets 875
Mevacor Tablets 1505
Mexitil Capsules (About 5 in 1,000) 680
Micronase Tablets 2350
Midamor Tablets (Rare) 1508
Moduretic Tablets 1510
Motrin Tablets (Less than 1%) 2351
Myambutol Tablets 1225
Mycelex Troches 1605
Nimotop Capsules (Up to 1.2%) 1607
Normodyne Tablets 2110
Norpramin Tablets 1340
▲ Orudis Capsules (Greater than 3%) 2488
PCE Dispertab Tablets 549
Pamelor 2019
Paraflex Caplets (Rare) 1378
PediaProfen Suspension (Less than 1%) 1363
Permax Tablets (Infrequent) 1291
Premarin with Methyltestosterone 2515
Premarin Vaginal Cream 2512
Prozac Pulvules (Infrequent) 920
Rifadin (Rare) 1345
Rifamate Capsules 1347
Rimactane Capsules (Rare) 879
Tegretol Chewable Tablets 654
Tegretol Suspension 656
Tegretol Tablets 654
Thioguanine Tablets, Tabloid Brand (Occasional) 815
Tofranil Ampuls 1038
Tofranil Tablets 1039
Tofranil-PM Capsules 1041
Trandate HCT Tablets (Less common) 579
Trandate Injection (Less common) 577
Trandate Tablets (Less common) 579
Triavil Tablets (Rare) 1556
Vascor (200, 300 and 400 mg) Tablets (0.5 to 2.0%) 1383
Vivactil Tablets 1567
Wygesic Tablets 2540
Yutopar (Less than 1% (with IV administration)) 647

Liver injury

Cordarone Tablets (Common) 2446
Ethrane (Rare) 599
Eulexin Capsules 2089

Liver tumors (see under Hepatomas)

Liver, degenerative changes in

Phenobarbital Elixir and Tablets 1293

Loss of balance

Adalat Capsules (10 mg and 20 mg) (2% or less) 1587
Amikin Injectable 602
Eldepryl 2250
Rythmol Tablets (1.2%) 1184
Versed Injection (Less than 1%) 1924

Lower spinal segments deficit

Duranest Injections 624

Lung, carcinoma

Permax Tablets (Rare) 1291

Lung consolidation

Survanta Beractant Intratracheal Suspension 1978

Lung development, hypoplastic

Prinivil Tablets 1538
Prinzide Tablets 1540
Vaseretic Tablets 1559
Vasotec I.V. 1562
Vasotec Tablets 1564
Zestoretic 2274
Zestril Tablets 2277

Lupus erythematosus

Aldoclor Tablets 1413
Aldomet Ester HCl Injection 1417
Aldomet Oral 1415
Aldoril Tablets 1418
Anafranil Capsules (Rare) 650
Azo Gantanol Tablets 1887
Dapsone USP 1130
Demulen 2161
Dilantin Infatabs 1710
Dilantin Kapseals 1708
Dilantin Parenteral 1712
Dilantin-30 Pediatric/Dilantin-125 Suspension 1713
Dilantin with Phenobarbital Kapseals 1715
Enovid 2161
Fansidar Tablets 1896
Grisactin 2454
Grisactin Ultra Tablets 2455
Gris-PEG Tablets, 125 mg & 250 mg 1083
Inderal (Rare) 2459
Inderal LA Long Acting Capsules (Rare) 2461
Inderide LA Long Acting Capsules (Rare) 2465
Kenalog-10 Injection 2402
Norethin 2133
Paradione Capsules 548
Pediazole 1973
Peganone Tablets 551
Quinaglute Dura-Tabs Tablets (Rare) 663
Rufen Tablets (Less than 1%) 691
Rythmol Tablets (Less than 1%) 1184
Tegretol Chewable Tablets 654
Tegretol Suspension 656
Tegretol Tablets 654
Thiosulfil Forte Tablets 2526
Tonocard Tablets (1.6%) 1554
Tridione 557

Lupus erythematosus, systemic

Achromycin V Capsules 1193
AK-Cide Sterile Ophthalmic Ointment & Suspension .... ◉ 202
Atromid-S Capsules 2435
Azo Gantrisin Tablets 1888
Bactrim DS Tablets 1891
Bactrim I.V. Infusion 1889
Bactrim 1891
Butazolidin Capsules & Tablets (Less than 1%) 1027
Capozide 2258
Celontin 1692
Compazine 2201
Declomycin Capsules, Tablets 1199
Dilantin Infatabs 1710
Dilantin Kapseals 1708
Dilantin Parenteral 1712
Dilantin-30 Pediatric/Dilantin-125 Suspension 1713
Dilantin with Phenobarbital Kapseals 1715
Doryx Capsules 1717
Dyazide Capsules 2208
Etrafon 2087
Gantanol 1899
Gantrisin 1901
Inderal (Extremely rare) 2459
Inderal LA Long Acting Capsules (Extremely rare) 2461
Inderide Tablets (Extremely rare) 2463
Inderide LA Long Acting Capsules (Extremely rare) 2465
Mellaril 2011
Metimyd .... ◉ 306
Mexitil Capsules (About 4 in 10,000) 680
Milontin Kapseals 1741
Minocin Intravenous 1221
Minocin Oral Suspension 1224
Minocin Pellet-Filled Capsules 1222
Monodox Capsules 1630
Normodyne Tablets 2110
Normozide Tablets 2112
Prinzide Tablets 1540
Procan SR Tablets 1760
Prolixin Decanoate 1795
Prolixin Elixir 1793
Prolixin Enanthate 1796
Prolixin Injection 1791
Prolixin Oral Concentrate 1792
Prolixin Tablets 1793
Quinidex Extentabs 1868
Sectral Capsules 2520
Septra 813
Septra I.V. Infusion 808
Septra I.V. Infusion ADD-Vantage Vials 810
Septra 813
Serentil 686
Stelazine 2226
Syprine Capsules 1546
Taractan 1920
Terramycin Capsules 1786
Terramycin Intramuscular Solution 1964
Thalitone Tablets 687
Thorazine 2234
Trandate HCT/Trandate 579
Trilafon 2123
Vaseretic Tablets 1559
Vasocidin Ophthalmic Solution .... ◉ 276
Vasosulf (One case) .... ◉ 279
Vibramycin Hyclate Capsules 1787
Vibramycin Hyclate Intravenous 1968
Vibramycin 1787
Zarontin Capsules 1768
Zarontin Syrup 1769
Zestoretic 2274

Lupus erythematosus, systemic, exacerbation or activation of

Rauzide Tablets 1804

Lupus erythematosus syndrome

Azulfidine Tablets, EN-tabs, Oral Suspension (Rare) 1157
Children's Advil Suspension (Less than 1%) 2426
Cuprimine Capsules 1442
Depen Titratable Tablets 2379
Fulvicin P/G 165 & 330 Tablets 2091
Fulvicin-U/F Tablets 2092
Gantrisin Ophthalmic Ointment/Solution 1900
INH Tablets 868
Kenalog-40 Injection 2403
Mesantoin Tablets 2013
Mexitil Capsules (About 4 in 10,000) 680
Motrin Tablets (Less than 1%) 2351
Navane Capsules and Concentrate 1954
Navane Intramuscular 1956
Norpace (Some cases) 2177
PediaProfen Suspension (Less than 1%) 1363
Permax Tablets (Rare) 1291
▲ Pronestyl Capsules and Tablets (1 in 500 to 30%) 1800
Pronestyl Injection (1 in 500 to 30%) 1798
Pronestyl-SR Tablets (1 in 500 to 30%) 1801
Prozac Pulvules (Rare) 920
Rifamate Capsules 1347
Tegretol Chewable Tablets (Isolated cases) 654
Tegretol Suspension (Isolated cases) 656
Tegretol Tablets (Isolated cases) 654
Temaril Tablets, Syrup and Spansule Sustained Release Capsules 1085
Thorazine 2234

Lupus-like syndrome

Aldoclor Tablets 1413
Aldomet Ester HCl Injection 1417
Aldomet Oral 1415
Aldoril Tablets 1418
BCG Vaccine, USP (Tice) (Rare) 1632
Cetamide Ointment .... ◉ 220
Cuprimine Capsules 1442
Depen Titratable Tablets 2379
Elavil 2269
Fulvicin P/G 165 & 330 Tablets 2091
Fulvicin-U/F Tablets 2092
Grisactin 2454
Grisactin Ultra Tablets 2455
Gris-PEG Tablets, 125 mg & 250 mg 1083
Levlen/Tri-Levlen 665
Lopid Capsules and Tablets 1736
Macrodantin Capsules 1624
Meclomen Capsules (Less than 1%) 1739
Mevacor Tablets (Rare) 1505
Sodium Sulamyd 2122
Tacaryl 2409
Tapazole Tablets 1298
Tice BCG Vaccine, USP (Rare) 1632
Tonocard Tablets (1.6%) 1554
Levlen/Tri-Levlen 665
Vasocidin Ophthalmic Solution (Single instance) .... ◉ 276

Lyell's syndrome

Azulfidine Tablets, EN-tabs, Oral Suspension (Rare) 1157
Butazolidin Capsules & Tablets (Less than 1%) 1027
Combipres Tablets 678
Proloprim Tablets (Rare) 799
Tegretol Chewable Tablets (Extremely rare) 654
Tegretol Suspension (Extremely rare) 656
Tegretol Tablets (Extremely rare) 654
Tenoretic Tablets 1105
Thalitone Tablets 687
Trimpex Tablets (Rare) 1922
Zyloprim Tablets (Less than 1%) 830

Lymph nodes, tender

Atgam Sterile Solution (At least 1 patient and less than 5% of total patients) 2320
ProSom Tablets (Rare) 554

Lymphadenopathy

Accutane Capsules (Less than 1%) 1878
AeroBid Inhaler System (1-3%) 995
Alferon N Injection (1%) 1809
Anafranil Capsules (Infrequent) 650
Ansaid Tablets (Less than 1%) 2319
Antivenin (Crotalidae) Polyvalent 2430
Apresazide Capsules (Less frequent) 854
Apresoline Hydrochloride Parenteral (Ampuls) 856
Apresoline Hydrochloride Tablets (Less frequent) 855
Apresoline-Esidrix Tablets 857
Atgam Sterile Solution (Less than 1% to less than 5%) 2320
Attenuvax (Less common) 1424
BCG Vaccine, USP (Tice) (Occasional) 1632

Biavax II ... 1427
Cardura Tablets (Less than 0.5% of 3960 patients) ... 1941
Ceclor Pulvules & Suspension (Infrequent) ... 1251
Cuprimine Capsules ... 1442
Depen Titratable Tablets ... 2379
Dilantin Infatabs ... 1710
Dilantin Kapseals ... 1708
Dilantin Parenteral ... 1712
Dilantin-30 Pediatric/Dilantin-125 Suspension ... 1713
Dilantin with Phenobarbital Kapseals ... 1715
Engerix-B Unit-Dose Vials (Less than 1%) ... 2213
INH Tablets ... 868
Imferon ... 976
Intron A (1% or less) ... 2097
Kerlone Tablets (Less than 2%) ... 2172
Klonopin Tablets ... 1902
Lamprene Capsules (Less than 1%) ... 1030
▲ Lupron Depot 3.75 mg (Among most frequent) ... 2312
M-M-R II ... 1494
M-R-VAX II ... 1496
Meruvax II ... 1503
Mesantoin Tablets ... 2013
Mintezol ... 1510
Monopril Tablets (0.2 to 1.0%) ... 1406
Mumpsvax ... 1513
Nalfon Pulvules & Tablets (Less than 1%) ... 919
Paradione Capsules ... 548
Peganone Tablets ... 551
Permax Tablets (Infrequent) ... 1291
▲ Plague Vaccine (10%) ... 1584
Proglycem ... 649
Prozac Pulvules (Infrequent) ... 920
Quadrinal Tablets ... 1183
Recombivax HB (Less than 1%) ... 1544
Retrovir Capsules (Less than 5%) ... 802
Retrovir I.V. Infusion (Less than 5%) ... 805
Retrovir Syrup (Less than 5%) ... 802
Rifamate Capsules ... 1347
Rogaine Topical Solution (0.31%) ... 2357
Ser-Ap-Es Tablets ... 881
Serpasil-Apresoline Tablets ... 884
Tapazole Tablets ... 1298
Tegretol Chewable Tablets ... 654
Tegretol Suspension ... 656
Tegretol Tablets ... 654
Tice BCG Vaccine, USP (Occasional) ... 1632
Tolectin (200, 400 and 600 mg) (Less than 1%) ... 1379
Tridione ... 557
Wellbutrin Tablets (Rare) ... 821
Zovirax ... 824
Zyloprim Tablets (Less than 1%) ... 830

Lymphadenopathy, post-cervical
Atgam Sterile Solution (At least 1 patient and less than 5% of total patients) ... 2320

Lymphocytes, decrease (see under Lymphocytopenia)

Lymphocytes, increase (see under Lymphocytosis)

Lymphocytopenia
Dipentum Capsules (Rare) ... 1160
Floxin Tablets (More than or equal to 1.0%) ... 1652
▲ Intron A (17%) ... 2097
Lopid Capsules and Tablets ... 1736
Metopirone Tablets (Rare) ... 876
Mustargen ... 1514
Stelazine Tablets ... 2226
Tagamet Injection (Approximately 1 per 100,000) ... 2228
Talwin Injection (Rare) ... 2071
Unasyn ... 1965
▲ Xanax Tablets (5.5% to 7.4%) ... 2367
Zefazone Sterile Powder ... 2372

Lymphocytosis
Ceclor Pulvules & Suspension ... 1251
Ceptaz for Injection (Very rare) ... 1057
Cipro I.V. (Infrequent) ... 1592
Depakene Capsules & Syrup ... 511
Depakote ... 512
Fortaz (Rare) ... 1060
Permax Tablets (Rare) ... 1291
Primaxin I.M. ... 1532
Primaxin I.V. ... 1535
Prozac Pulvules (Rare) ... 920
Rocephin Injectable Vials, ADD-Vantage (Rare) ... 1914
Tazicef for Injection (Very rare) ... 2231
Unasyn ... 1965
Zefazone Sterile Powder ... 2372
Zyloprim Tablets (Less than 1%) ... 830

Lymphoma
Dilantin Infatabs ... 1710
Dilantin Kapseals ... 1708
Dilantin Parenteral ... 1712
Dilantin-30 Pediatric/Dilantin-125 Suspension ... 1713
Dilantin with Phenobarbital Kapseals ... 1715
Imuran (0.5%) ... 768
Orthoclone OKT3 Sterile Solution (2 patients) ... 1645
▲ Sandimmune (Up to 6%) ... 2024

Lymphoma-like disorder
Anafranil Capsules (Rare) ... 650

Lymphomonocytosis
Haldol Decanoate ... 1375
Haldol Injection, Tablets and Concentrate ... 1373

LDH abnormalities
Bumex (1.0%) ... 1895
Ceftin Tablets (1.0%) ... 575
▲ Emcyt Capsules (33 to 34%) ... 1161
Intron A (Up to 3%) ... 2097
Nimotop Capsules (0.4%) ... 1607
Sinemet CR Tablets ... 953

LDH increase
Accutane Capsules ... 1878
Cardizem Tablets-30 mg, 60 mg, 90 mg and 120 mg (Less than 1%) ... 1329
Cardizem SR Capsules-60 mg, 90 mg and 120 mg (Less than 1%) ... 1327
Cefotan (1 in 700) ... 2265
Ceptaz for Injection (One in 18) ... 1057
▲ Cipro I.V. (Among most frequent) ... 1592
Cipro Tablets (0.4%) ... 1589
Claforan Sterile Injection (Less than 1%) ... 1089
Cuprimine Capsules (Few cases) ... 1442
Depakene Capsules & Syrup (Frequent) ... 511
Depakote (Frequent) ... 512
Depen Titratable Tablets (Few reports) ... 2379
▲ Sterile FUDR (Among more common) ... 1898
▲ Fortaz (1 in 18) ... 1060
Garamycin Injectable ... 2093
Inderide Tablets ... 2463
Kefurox Vials, Faspak & ADD-Vantage (1 in 75) ... 1277
Kerlone Tablets (Less than 2%) ... 2172
Larodopa Tablets ... 1905
Lopid Capsules and Tablets (Occasional) ... 1736
▲ Lupron Depot 3.75 mg (5% to 8%) ... 2312
▲ Lupron Depot 7.5 mg (19.6%) ... 2311
Mefoxin ... 1498
Monocid Injection (1.6%) ... 2217
Monopril Tablets ... 1406
Nalfon Pulvules & Tablets (Less than 1%) ... 919
Nebcin Vials, Hyporets & ADD-Vantage ... 1286
▲ Neupogen for Injection (27 to 58%) ... 595
Noroxin Tablets (Less frequent) ... 1519
Pipracil (Less frequent) ... 1230
Primaxin I.M. ... 1532
Primaxin I.V. ... 1535
Procardia XL Tablets (Rare) ... 1783
▲ Roferon-A Injection (10% to 13%) ... 1916
Sectral Capsules ... 2520
Sinemet Tablets ... 952
Sinemet CR Tablets ... 953
▲ Tazicef for Injection (1 in 18 patients) ... 2231
▲ Tegison Capsules (15%) ... 1881
Timentin for Injection ... 2239
Unasyn ... 1965
▲ Zanosar Sterile Powder (A number of patients) ... 2371
Zefazone Sterile Powder ... 2372
Zinacef (1 in 75 patients) ... 1066

LE cells test positive (see under Lupus erythematosus)

LE-like reactions (see under Lupus erythematosus)

M

Maceration
Monistat-Derm (miconazole nitrate) Cream (Isolated reports) ... 1679
Oxistat Cream (0.1%) ... 1055

Maceration, skin
Anusol-HC Cream (Infrequent) ... 1690
Cortisporin Otic Solution Sterile ... 760
Cortisporin Otic Suspension Sterile ... 760
DesOwen Cream, Ointment and Lotion (Infrequent) ... 1682
Locoid Cream, Ointment and Topical Solution (Infrequent) ... 970
Nutracort Cream & Lotion (Infrequent) ... 1684
PediOtic Suspension Sterile ... 797
ProctoCream-HC (Infrequent) ... 1834

Macrocytic anemia
Dilantin Infatabs ... 1710
Dilantin Kapseals ... 1708
Dilantin Parenteral ... 1712
Dilantin-30 Pediatric/Dilantin-125 Suspension ... 1713
Dilantin with Phenobarbital Kapseals ... 1715
Eulexin Capsules ... 2089
Imuran (2 cases) ... 768

Macrophages, reactive
▲ Blenoxane (10%) ... 724

Maculae
Calan SR Caplets (1% or less) ... 2157
Calan Tablets (1% or less) ... 2155
Isoptin Oral Tablets (Less than 1%) ... 1179
Isoptin SR Sustained Release Tablets (Less than 1%) ... 1181
Verelan Capsules (Less than 1%) ... 1243

Maculopathy
Tolectin (200, 400 and 600 mg) (Less than 1%) ... 1379

Malabsorption syndrome
Elspar ... 1470
Gelfoam Sterile Sponge ... 2338
Sandostatin Injection (1.6%) ... 2029

Malaise
Accutane Capsules ... 1878
AeroBid Inhaler System (1-3%) ... 995
▲ Alferon N Injection (9% to 65%) ... 1809
Altace Capsules (Less than 1%) ... 1086
Amicar Syrup, Tablets, and Injection (Occasional) ... 1194
Anafranil Capsules (Infrequent) ... 650
Anaprox and Anaprox DS Tablets (Less than 1%) ... 2288
Ansaid Tablets (1-3%) ... 2319
Antivenin (Crotalidae) Polyvalent ... 2430
Aquasol A Vitamin A Capsules, USP ... 615
Aquasol A Parenteral, USP ... 615
Atgam Sterile Solution (Less than 1% to less than 5%) ... 2320
Azactam for Injection (Less than 1%) ... 2252
Biavax II ... 1427
Biltricide ... 1589
BuSpar (Rare) ... 1401
Calan SR Caplets ... 2157
Calan Tablets ... 2155
Capoten (0.5 to 2%) ... 2255
Capozide (0.5 to 2%) ... 2258
Cardene Capsules (0.6%) ... 2290
▲ Cardura Tablets (12%) ... 1941
Cartrol Tablets (Less common) ... 507
Catapres Tablets (About 1 in 100 patients) ... 676
Catapres-TTS (1%) ... 677
Children's Advil Suspension ... 2426
Cholera Vaccine ... 2445
Cipro I.V. (1% or less) ... 1592
Cipro Tablets (Less than 1%) ... 1589
Clinoril Tablets (Less than 1 in 100) ... 1433
Clozaril Tablets (Less than 1%) ... 2000
Combipres Tablets (About 1%) ... 678
▲ Cordarone Tablets (4 to 9%) ... 2446
Cortone Acetate Sterile Suspension ... 1437
Cortone Acetate Tablets ... 1439
Cosmegen Injection ... 1440
Cytosar-U Sterile Powder (Occasional) ... 2329
Cytovene Sterile Powder (1% or less) ... 2292
DTIC-Dome (Infrequent) ... 1595
Dalalone D.P. Injectable ... 999
▲ Dantrium Capsules (Among most frequent) ... 1619
Daraprim Tablets (Rare) ... 761
Decadron Elixir ... 1445
Decadron Phosphate Injection ... 1449
Decadron Phosphate Respihaler ... 1454
Decadron Phosphate Turbinaire ... 1456
Decadron Phosphate with Xylocaine Injection, Sterile ... 1451
Decadron Tablets ... 1447
Decadron-LA Sterile Suspension ... 1457
Depakote Sprinkle Capsules ... 512
Desyrel and Desyrel Dividose (Greater than 1%) ... 1404
Diphtheria & Tetanus Toxoids, Adsorbed Purogenated (Mild) ... 1202
Dolobid Tablets (Less than 1 in 100) ... 1465
Doral Tablets ... 2383
Duvoid Tablets ... 1853
Edecrin ... 1468
Eldepryl ... 2250
Endep Tablets ... 1927
Engerix-B Unit-Dose Vials (Less than 1%) ... 2213
Sterile FUDR ... 1898
Feldene Capsules (1 to 3%) ... 1777
Flexeril Tablets (Less than 1%) ... 1471
Floxin Tablets (Less than 1%) ... 1652
Flu-Imune Influenza Virus Vaccine (Infrequent) ... 1204
▲ Fungizone Intravenous (Among most common) ... 2262
Furoxone (Occasional) ... 1855
Gamimune N Immune Globulin Intravenous (Human) ... 1572
Gastrocrom Capsules (1 report) ... 974
Hydeltrasol Injection, Sterile ... 1476
Hydeltra-T.B.A. Sterile Suspension ... 1478
Hydrea Capsules ... 728
Hydrocortone Acetate Sterile Suspension ... 1479
Hydrocortone Phosphate Injection, Sterile ... 1481
Hydrocortone Tablets ... 1482
Hyperstat I.V. Injection ... 2095
INH Tablets ... 868
IFEX (Less than 1%) ... 729
Imuran ... 768
Indocin (Greater than 1%) ... 1487
▲ Intron A (2% to 14%) ... 2097
Isoptin SR Sustained Release Tablets ... 1181
Kerlone Tablets (Less than 2%) ... 2172
Larodopa Tablets (Relatively frequent) ... 1905
Leukine for IV Infusion ... 1127
▲ Lodine Capsules (3-9%) ... 2468
Lomotil ... 2174
Lopid Capsules and Tablets ... 1736
▲ Lozol Tablets (Greater than or equal to 5%) ... 1843
M-M-R II ... 1494
M-R-VAX II ... 1496
Macrodantin Capsules (Common) ... 1624
Meclomen Capsules (Rare) ... 1739
Meruvax II ... 1503
Methotrexate Tablets, Parenteral, LPF Parenteral (Frequent) ... 1217
Metrodin (urofollitropin for injection) (Less than 1 in 50) ... 2182
Mevacor Tablets (Rare) ... 1505
Mexitil Capsules (Less than 1% or about 3 in 1,000) ... 680
Mithracin ... 1602
Moduretic Tablets (Less than or equal to 1%) ... 1510
Motrin Tablets ... 2351
Myambutol Tablets ... 1225
▲ Mykrox ½ mg Tablets (4.4%) ... 984
Myochrysine Injection ... 1516
Nalfon Pulvules & Tablets (Less than 1%) ... 919
Naprosyn (Less than 1%) ... 2297
Nardil ... 1742
Neptazane Tablets ... ⊙ 311
Normozide Tablets (Less than 1%) ... 2112
▲ Norpace (3 to 9%) ... 2177
Norpramin Tablets ... 1340
Omnipaque ... 2552
Orudis Capsules (Greater than 1%) ... 2488
Oxsoralen-Ultra Capsule ... 1117

Pamelor 2019
Papaverine Hydrochloride Vials and Ampoules 1290
Paradione Capsules 548
Paraflex Caplets (Rare) 1378
Parafon Forte DSC Caplets (Rare) 1379
Pavabid Capsules (Rare) 1344
Pavabid HP Capsulets (Rare) 1344
PediaProfen Suspension 1363
Pentaspan Injection 949
Pergonal (menotropins for injection, USP) 2184
Permax Tablets (Infrequent) 1291
▲ Plague Vaccine (10%) 1584
Pneumovax 23 1528
Prilosec Delayed-Release Capsules (Less than 1%) 1530
Prinivil Tablets (1% or less) 1538
Prinzide Tablets 1540
Procardia XL Tablets (1% or less) 1783
Proglycem 649
Prokine for I.V. Infusion 1096
▲ ProSom Tablets (5%) 554
Prozac Pulvules (Infrequent) 920
Recombivax HB (Equal to or greater than 1%) 1544
▲ Retrovir Capsules (8%) 802
▲ Retrovir I.V. Infusion (8%) 805
▲ Retrovir Syrup (8%) 802
Rheumatrex Methotrexate Dose Pack (Frequent) 1234
Rifamate Capsules 1347
Sandostatin Injection (Less than 1%) 2029
Sansert Tablets 2031
Sectral Capsules 2520
Sinemet Tablets 952
Sinemet CR Tablets 953
Solganal Suspension 2122
Staphage Lysate (SPL) 905
Surmontil Capsules 2524
Tambocor Tablets (1-3%) 1315
Tenex Tablets (Less than 3%) 1875
Tenuate 1354
Tetanus & Diphtheria Toxoids, Adsorbed Purogenated (Rare) 1237
Tetanus Toxoid, Adsorbed Purogenated 1238
▲ TheraCys BCG Live (Intravesical) (2.0% to 40.2%) 898
Tofranil Ampuls 1038
Tofranil Tablets 1039
Tofranil-PM Capsules 1041
Tolinase Tablets 2365
Tonocard Tablets (Less than 1%) 1554
Trandate HCT Tablets (Less than 1% in 208 patients) 579
Trental (Less than 1%) 1099
Triavil Tablets 1556
Tridione 557
Typhoid Vaccine 2533
Unasyn (Less than 1%) 1965
Urecholine 1558
▲ Velban Vials (Most common) 1305
Ventolin Inhalation Solution (1.5%) 583
Verelan Capsules 1243
Vira-A for Injection 1766
Voltaren Tablets (Less than 1%) 1042
Vontrol Tablets (Rare) 2243
▲ Yutopar (5 to 6% (with IV administration)) 647
Zantac Injection and Zantac Injection Premixed (Rare) 1063
Zantac (Rare) 1065
Zestril Tablets (0.3% to 1.0%) 2277
▲ Zovirax (11.5%) 824
Zyloprim Tablets (Less than 1%) 830

Malaria relapse
Aramine Injection 1424

Male pattern baldness (see under Alopecia, hereditaria)

Malignancies, secondary
Leukeran Tablets 788
Neosar for Injection 566

Malignant hyperthermia
Anectine 755
Ethrane 599
Forane 600

Malignant hyperthermia, familial
Sensorcaine 631
Sensorcaine-MPF Spinal 634

Malignant melanoma
Demulen 2161
Enovid 2161
Norethin 2133
Sinemet Tablets 952
Sinemet CR Tablets 953

Malignant neoplasms
Estinyl Tablets 2085
Estrace 1385
Estrace Vaginal Cream 1388
Estraderm Transdermal System 866
▲ Tegison Capsules (1 to 10%) 1881

Malodor, unspecified
Condylox (Less than 5%) 1630

Manic behavior
Anafranil Capsules (Infrequent) 650
Cipro I.V. (1% or less) 1592
Cipro Tablets (Less than 1%) 1589
Endep Tablets 1927
Halcion Tablets 2340
Ludiomil Tablets (Rare) 874
▲ Marplan Tablets (Among most frequent) 1906
Nardil (Less frequent) 1742
Parnate Tablets 2222
Permax Tablets (Infrequent) 1291
Protopam Chloride for Injection (Several cases) 2518
Prozac Pulvules (Infrequent) 920
Rythmol Tablets (Less than 1%) 1184
Triavil Tablets (Rare) 1556
Wellbutrin Tablets (Frequent) 821
Xanax Tablets 2367

Mass, abdominal (see under Abdominal mass)

Mastalgia (see under Mastodynia)

Mastodynia
Estrace 1385
Estrace Vaginal Cream 1388
Estratest 2245
Haldol Decanoate 1375
Nalfon Pulvules & Tablets (Less than 1%) 919
Norplant System 2484
Premarin Intravenous 2508
Premarin with Methyltestosterone 2515
Premarin Tablets 2510
Premarin Vaginal Cream 2512
TACE 12 and 25 mg 1353

Medullary hypoplasia
Novantrone for Injection Concentrate 1226

Medullary paralysis
Cyclogyl ◉ 215
Cyclomydril ◉ 216

Megacolon, toxic
Lomotil 2174
Motofen Tablets 836

Megaloblastic anemia
Alurate Elixir 1883
Azulfidine Tablets, EN-tabs, Oral Suspension (Rare) 1157
Bactrim DS Tablets 1891
Bactrim I.V. Infusion 1889
Bactrim 1891
Cytovene Sterile Powder (2%) 2292
Depakote 512
Dilantin Infatabs 1710
Dilantin Kapseals 1708
Dilantin Parenteral 1712
Dilantin-30 Pediatric/Dilantin-125 Suspension 1713
Dilantin with Phenobarbital Kapseals 1715
Dyazide Capsules 2208
Dyrenium Capsules (Rare) 2210
Eminase (Less than 1%) 2211
Fansidar Tablets 1896
Macrodantin Capsules 1624
Mebaral Tablets (Less than 1 in 100) 2061
Mesantoin Tablets (Uncommon) 2013
Mysoline (Rare idiosyncrasy) 2480
Nembutal Sodium Capsules 534
Nembutal Sodium Solution (Less than 1%) 536
Nembutal Sodium Suppositories (Less than 1%) 538
Permax Tablets (Infrequent) 1291
Phenobarbital Elixir and Tablets (A few cases) 1293
Prilosec Delayed-Release Capsules (Less than 1%) 1530
Proloprim Tablets 799
▲ Retrovir Capsules (3% to 29%) 802
▲ Retrovir I.V. Infusion (1% to 45%) 805
▲ Retrovir Syrup (3% to 29%) 802
Rythmol Tablets (Less than 1%) 1184
Seconal Sodium Pulvules 1296
Septra 813
Septra I.V. Infusion 808
Septra I.V. Infusion ADD-Vantage Vials 810
Septra 813
Trimpex Tablets 1922
Zovirax Sterile Powder (Less than 1%) 828

Megaloblastosis
Cytosar-U Sterile Powder 2329
Maxzide 1215

Melanoma, malignant, activation of
Larodopa Tablets 1905

Melanosis
Intron A (1% or less) 2097

Melasma
Amen 833
Aygestin Tablets 2437
Depo-Provera Sterile Aqueous Suspension 2336
Diethylstilbestrol Tablets 1258
Estinyl Tablets 2085
Estrace 1385
Estrace Vaginal Cream 1388
Estratest 2245
Estrovis 1721
Menrium Tablets 1934
Micronor Tablets 1667
Modicon 1667
Norethin 2133
Norlutate 1754
Norlutin 1755
Ortho Dienestrol Cream 1664
Ortho-Novum 1667
Ovcon 1391
Stilphostrol Tablets and Ampuls 1609
TACE 12 and 25 mg 1353

Melasma, possibly persistent
Brevicon 2304
Demulen 2161
Enovid 2161
Estradurin 2452
Jenest-28 Tablets 1636
Levlen/Tri-Levlen 665
Loestrin 1728
Mediatric Capsules 2476
Micronor Tablets 1667
Modicon 1667
Norinyl 2304
Norlestrin 1746
Nor-Q D Tablets 2304
Ogen 540
Ortho-Cyclen Tablets 1658
Ortho-Novum 1667
PMB 200 and PMB 400 2504
Premarin Intravenous 2508
Premarin with Methyltestosterone 2515
Premarin Tablets 2510
Premarin Vaginal Cream 2512
Levlen/Tri-Levlen 665
Tri-Norinyl 2304

Melena
Anaprox and Anaprox DS Tablets (Less than 1%) 2288
Azo Gantrisin Tablets 1888
Children's Advil Suspension (Less than 1%) 2426
Diamox Parenteral (Occasional) 1200
Diamox Sequels (Sustained Release) 1201
Diamox Tablets (Occasional) 1200
Feldene Capsules (Less than 1%) 1777
Fungizone Intravenous 2262
Intron A (Less than 1%) 2097
Lodine Capsules (More than 1% but less than 3%) 2468
Lotensin Tablets 872
Methotrexate Tablets, Parenteral, LPF Parenteral 1217
Motrin Tablets (Less than 1%) 2351
Naprosyn (Less than 1%) 2297
NebuPent for Inhalation Solution (1% or less) 1017
Orudis Capsules (Less than 1%) 2488
PediaProfen Suspension (Less than 1%) 1363
Permax Tablets (Infrequent) 1291
Procardia XL Tablets (1% or less) 1783
ProSom Tablets 554
Prozac Pulvules (Infrequent) 920
Rheumatrex Methotrexate Dose Pack 1234
Ridaura Capsules (0.1 to 1%) 2224
Rufen Tablets (Less than 1%) 691
Tegison Capsules (Less than 1%) 1881
Toradol IM Injection (1% or less) 2302
Vaseretic Tablets 1559
Vasotec I.V. 1562
Vasotec Tablets (0.5% to 1.0%) 1564
Voltaren Tablets (Less than 1%) 1042

Memory impairment
▲ Anafranil Capsules (7% to 9%) 650
Cogentin 1435
Desyrel and Desyrel Dividose (Greater than 1%) 1404
Eldepryl 2250
Eskalith 2214
Halcion Tablets (Less frequent) 2340
INH Tablets 868
Klonopin Tablets 1902
Lopressor Ampuls 1032
Lopressor HCT Tablets 1034
Lopressor Tablets 1032
Ludiomil Tablets (Rare) 874
▲ Lupron Depot 3.75 mg (Among most frequent) 2312
Lupron Depot 7.5 mg 2311
Lupron Injection (Less than 5%) 2310
▲ Marplan Tablets (Among most frequent) 1906
Monopril Tablets (0.2 to 1.0%) 1406
Rifamate Capsules (Uncommon) 1347
Roferon-A Injection (Less than 3%) 1916
Sandostatin Injection (Less than 1%) 2029
Serax Capsules 2522
Serax Tablets 2522
Seromycin Pulvules 1298
Sinemet CR Tablets 953
Timolide Tablets 1547
Tonocard Tablets (Less than 1%) 1554
Trandate Tablets 579
Transderm Scōp Transdermal Therapeutic System (Infrequent) 887
Voltaren Tablets (Less than 1%) 1042
Wellbutrin Tablets (Infrequent) 821
▲ Xanax Tablets (33.1%) 2367

Memory loss, short-term
Blocadren Tablets 1429
Cartrol Tablets 507
Clozaril Tablets (Less than 1%) 2000
Corgard Tablets 701
Corzide Tablets 702
Ergamisol Tablets (10 patients) 1136
Ethmozine Tablets (Less than 2%) 946
Inderal 2459
Inderal LA Long Acting Capsules 2461
Inderide Tablets 2463
Inderide LA Long Acting Capsules 2465
Kerlone Tablets 2172
Levatol 1832
Lopressor HCT Tablets 1034
Mexitil Capsules (About 9 in 1,000) 680
NebuPent for Inhalation Solution (1% or less) 1017
Normodyne Tablets 2110
Normozide Tablets 2112
Rythmol Tablets (Less than 1%) 1184
Sectral Capsules 2520
Tenoretic Tablets 1105
Tenormin Tablets and I.V. Injection 1107
Timoptic in Ocudose 1552
Timoptic Sterile Ophthalmic Solution 1550
Trandate HCT Tablets 579
Visken Tablets 2036

Meniere's syndrome
Netromycin Injection 100 mg/ml 2104

Meningism
Antivenin (Crotalidae) Polyvalent (Occasional) 2430
Marcaine Hydrochloride with Epinephrine 1:200,000 2055
Marcaine Hydrochloride Injection 2055
Marcaine Spinal 2058
Novocain Hydrochloride for Spinal Anesthesia 2065
Omnipaque (Less than 0.01%) 2552
Pontocaine Hydrochloride for Spinal Anesthesia 2069
Sensorcaine 631
Sensorcaine-MPF Spinal 634

Meningitis

Ansaid Tablets (Less than 1%) 2319
Carbocaine Hydrochloride Injection 2043
Depo-Medrol Sterile Aqueous Suspension 2334
▲ Exosurf Neonatal for Intratracheal Suspension (3% to 4%) 765
Gelfoam Sterile Sponge 2338
Marcaine Hydrochloride with Epinephrine 1:200,000 2055
Marcaine Spinal 2058
Motrin Tablets (Less than 1%) 2351
Permax Tablets (Infrequent) 1291
Sensorcaine 631
Sensorcaine-MPF Spinal 634

Meningitis, aseptic

Anaprox and Anaprox DS Tablets 2288
Bactrim 1891
Naprosyn 2297
Omnipaque (Rare) 2552
Proloprim Tablets 799
Septra 813
Septra I.V. Infusion 808
Septra I.V. Infusion ADD-Vantage Vials 810
Septra 813
Tegretol Chewable Tablets 654
Tegretol Suspension 656
Tegretol Tablets 654

Meningitis, septic

Carbocaine Hydrochloride Injection 2043
Marcaine Hydrochloride with Epinephrine 1:200,000 2055
Marcaine Hydrochloride Injection 2055
Omnipaque (Rare) 2552

Menometrorrhagia

Orudis Capsules (Less than 1%) 2488

Menopause

Permax Tablets (Infrequent) 1291
Prozac Pulvules (Infrequent) 920
Wellbutrin Tablets (Rare) 821

Menorrhagia

Children's Advil Suspension (Less than 1%) 2426
Dipentum Capsules (Rare) 1160
Floxin Tablets (Less than 1%) 1652
▲ Intron A (Less than 14%) 2097
Motrin Tablets (Less than 1%) 2351
PediaProfen Suspension (Less than 1%) 1363
Permax Tablets (Infrequent) 1291
Prozac Pulvules (Infrequent) 920
Rufen Tablets (Less than 1%) 691

Menstrual disorders

▲ Anafranil Capsules (Up to 4%) 650
Anaprox and Anaprox DS Tablets (Less than 1%) 2288
Ansaid Tablets (Less than 1%) 2319
Cytotec (0.3%) 2159
Danocrine Capsules 2046
Depo-Medrol Sterile Aqueous Suspension 2334
Depo-Provera Sterile Aqueous Suspension 2336
Etrafon 2087
Halcion Tablets 2340
Halotestin Tablets 2341
Kerlone Tablets (Less than 2%) 2172
Medrol 2348
Mustargen 1514
Naprosyn (Less than 1%) 2297
▲ Nolvadex Tablets (5.7%) 1102
ParaGard T380A Intrauterine Copper Contraceptive 411
Rimactane Capsules 879
Seldane-D Extended-Release Tablets 1350
Solu-Cortef Sterile Powder 2361
Solu-Medrol Sterile Powder 2363
Tegison Capsules (Less than 1%) 1881
Tenuate 1354
Trilafon 2123
▲ Wellbutrin Tablets (4.7%) 821
▲ Xanax Tablets (10.4%) 2367

Menstrual dysfunction

Methotrexate Tablets, Parenteral, LPF Parenteral 1217
Rheumatrex Methotrexate Dose Pack 1234

Menstrual flow, changes

Amen 833
Aygestin Tablets 2437
Coumadin Injection & Tablets 944
Cycrin Tablets 2449
Danocrine Capsules 2046
Demulen 2161
Enovid 2161
Estinyl Tablets 2085
Estraderm Transdermal System 866
Estratest 2245
Estrovis 1721
Jenest-28 Tablets 1636
Levlen/Tri-Levlen 665
Lippes Loop Intrauterine Double-S 1654
Lo/Ovral Tablets 2471
Lo/Ovral-28 Tablets 2476
Loestrin 1728
Meclomen Capsules 1739
Mediatric Capsules 2476
Menrium Tablets 1934
Micronor Tablets 1667
Moban Tablets & Concentrate 932
Modicon 1667
Nordette-21 Tablets 2481
Nordette-28 Tablets 2483
Norethin 2133
Norlestrin 1746
Norlutate 1754
Norlutin 1755
Ogen 540
Ortho Dienestrol Cream 1664
Ortho-Cyclen Tablets 1658
Ortho-Novum 1667
Ovral Tablets 2490
Ovral-28 Tablets 2491
Ovrette Tablets 2492
PMB 200 and PMB 400 2504
ParaGard T380A Intrauterine Copper Contraceptive 411
Premarin Intravenous 2508
Premarin with Methyltestosterone 2515
Premarin Vaginal Cream 2512
Provera Tablets 2356
Rogaine Topical Solution (0.47%) 2357
TACE 12 and 25 mg 1353
Levlen/Tri-Levlen 665
Triphasil-21 Tablets 2527
Triphasil-28 Tablets 2532

Menstrual irregularities

Accutane Capsules (Less than 1%) 1878
▲ AeroBid Inhaler System (3-9%) 995
Aldactazide 2150
Aldactone 2152
Anadrol-50 Tablets 2287
Android 1111
Aristocort Suspension 1008
Aristospan Suspension 1011
Asendin Tablets (Less than 1%) 1196
Brevicon 2304
BuSpar (Infrequent) 1401
Calan SR Caplets (1% or less) 2157
Calan Tablets (1% or less) 2155
Celestone Soluspan Suspension 2081
Compazine 2201
Cortenema 2244
Cortifoam 1827
Cortone Acetate Sterile Suspension 1437
Cortone Acetate Tablets 1439
Dalalone D.P. Injectable 999
Decadron Elixir 1445
Decadron Phosphate Injection 1449
Decadron Phosphate Respihaler 1454
Decadron Phosphate Turbinaire 1456
Decadron Phosphate with Xylocaine Injection, Sterile 1451
Decadron Tablets 1447
Decadron-LA Sterile Suspension 1457
Deltasone Tablets 2332
Demulen 2161
Depakene Capsules & Syrup 511
Depakote 512
Desyrel and Desyrel Dividose (Less than 1%) 1404
Doral Tablets 2383
Enovid 2161
Estrace 1385
Estrace Vaginal Cream 1388
▲ Estratest (Among most common) 2245
Fulvicin P/G Tablets (Rare) 2090
Fulvicin P/G 165 & 330 Tablets (Rare) 2091
Fulvicin-U/F Tablets (Rare) 2092
Haldol Decanoate 1375
Haldol Injection, Tablets and Concentrate 1373
Hydeltrasol Injection, Sterile 1476
Hydeltra-T.B.A. Sterile Suspension 1478
Hydrocortone Acetate Sterile Suspension 1479
Hydrocortone Phosphate Injection, Sterile 1481
Hydrocortone Tablets 1482
Isoptin Oral Tablets (Less than 1%) 1179
Isoptin SR Sustained Release Tablets (Less than 1%) 1181
Kenalog-10 Injection 2402
Kenalog-40 Injection 2403
Librax Capsules (Rare) 1929
Libritabs Tablets (Isolated cases) 1930
Librium Capsules (Isolated cases) 1931
Librium Injectable (Isolated cases) 1932
Limbitrol (Rare) 1933
Loxitane (Rare) 1213
Mellaril 2011
Menrium Tablets (Rare) 1934
▲ Metandren Linguets and Tablets (Most common) 875
▲ Nolvadex Tablets (12.5%) 1102
Norethin 2133
Norinyl 2304
Norzine 1818
Ovcon 1391
ParaGard T380A Intrauterine Copper Contraceptive 411
Pediapred Oral Liquid 987
Premarin with Methyltestosterone 2515
Prolixin Decanoate 1795
Prolixin Elixir 1793
Prolixin Enanthate 1796
Prolixin Injection 1791
Prolixin Oral Concentrate 1792
Prolixin Tablets 1793
Rifadin 1345
Rifamate Capsules 1347
Rimactane Capsules 879
Seldane Tablets 1349
Serax Capsules 2522
Serax Tablets 2522
Serentil 686
Stelazine 2226
Tacaryl 2409
Taractan 1920
Testred Capsules 1124
Torecan 1993
Triavil Tablets 1556
Tri-Norinyl 2304
Winstrol Tablets 2075

Menstruation, early

Actifed with Codeine Cough Syrup 752
Benadryl Capsules 1691
Benadryl Injection 1692
Deconamine 663
Optimine Tablets 2115
Ornade Spansule Capsules 2221
Periactin 1525
Polaramine 2116
Ru-Tuss II Capsules 693
Tacaryl 2409
Tavist Syrup 2033
Tavist Tablets 2035
Tavist-D Tablets 2035
Temaril Tablets, Syrup and Spansule Sustained Release Capsules 1085
Triaminic Expectorant DH 1995
Trinalin Repetabs Tablets 1170

Menstruation, painful

Prozac Pulvules (1.9%) 920

Mental acuity, loss of

Retrovir Capsules (Less than 5%) 802
Retrovir I.V. Infusion (Less than 5%) 805
Retrovir Syrup (Less than 5%) 802
Sinemet CR Tablets 953

Mental clouding

Anexsia 5/500 Tablets 2196
Anexsia 7.5/650 Tablets 2197
Azdone Tablets 844
Compazine 2201
Damason-P 1356
Halcion Tablets 2340
Hycodan Syrup, Tablets 927
Hycomine Compound Tablets 929
Hycomine Syrup 927
Hycotuss Expectorant Syrup 930
Hydrocet Capsules 835
Lortab ASA Tablets 2414
Lortab 2412
Tussionex Extended-Release Suspension 988
Vicodin Tablets 1187
Vicodin ES Tablets 1189
Zydone Capsules 941

Mental confusion (see under Confusion)

Mental depression (see under Depression, mental)

Mental perception, altered

Mykrox ½ mg Tablets 984

Mental performance, impairment

Aldoclor Tablets 1413
Aldomet Ester HCl Injection 1417
Aldomet Oral 1415
Aldoril Tablets 1418
Alferon N Injection (1%) 1809
Anafranil Capsules (Up to 5%) 650
Anaprox and Anaprox DS Tablets (Less than 1%) 2288
Anexsia 5/500 Tablets 2196
Anexsia 7.5/650 Tablets 2197
Asendin Tablets (Less than 1%) 1196
Ativan Injection 2432
Azdone Tablets 844
Bentyl 1322
Cardura Tablets (Less than 0.5% of 3960 patients) 1941
Cibalith-S 870
Clozaril Tablets 2000
Compazine 2201
Damason-P 1356
Demerol 2047
Desyrel and Desyrel Dividose 1404
Dilaudid Cough Syrup 1174
Dilaudid 1173
Elavil 2269
Endep Tablets 1927
Equagesic Tablets 2451
Eskalith 2214
Etrafon 2087
Fulvicin P/G Tablets 2090
Fulvicin P/G 165 & 330 Tablets 2091
Fulvicin-U/F Tablets 2092
Grifulvin V (griseofulvin microsize) Tablets/Suspension 1678
Grisactin 2454
Grisactin Ultra Tablets 2455
Hycodan Syrup, Tablets 927
Hycomine Compound Tablets 929
Hycomine Syrup 927
Hycotuss Expectorant Syrup 930
Hydrocet Capsules 835
▲ Intron A (Less than 14%) 2097
Inversine Tablets 1492
Libritabs Tablets 1930
Limbitrol 1933
Lithobid Tablets 870
Lortab ASA Tablets 2414
Lortab 2412
Loxitane 1213
Marinol (Dronabinol) Capsules 1985
Mebaral Tablets 2061
Naprosyn Suspension (Less than 1%) 2297
Norpramin Tablets 1340
Omnipaque (Rare) 2552
Orap Tablets 1020
PBZ-SR Tablets 1037
PMB 200 and PMB 400 2504
Phenergan with Codeine 2497
Phenergan with Dextromethorphan 2499
Phenergan Injection 2493
Phenergan Suppositories 2496
Phenergan Syrup 2495
Phenergan Tablets 2496
Phenergan VC 2500
Phenergan VC with Codeine 2501
Prozac Pulvules (1.5%) 920
Rauzide Tablets 1804
Restoril Capsules (Less than 1%) 2023
Rifadin 1345
Rifamate Capsules 1347
Rimactane Capsules 879
Ryna ▣ 741
Surmontil Capsules 2524
Synalgos-DC Capsules 2525
Timolide Tablets 1547
Timoptic in Ocudose 1552
Timoptic Sterile Ophthalmic Solution 1550
Tussionex Extended-Release Suspension 988
Tylox Capsules 1382
Vicodin Tablets 1187
Vistaril Intramuscular Solution (Seldom) 1970
Wygesic Tablets 2540
Xanax Tablets 2367
Zarontin Capsules 1768
Zarontin Syrup 1769
Zydone Capsules 941

Mental slowness
Celontin 1692
Tonocard Tablets (Less than 1%) 1554

Mental status, altered
Clozaril Tablets 2000
Eldepryl 2250
▲Idamycin for Injection (41%) 564
Mellaril 2011
Moban Tablets & Concentrate 932
Navane Capsules and Concentrate 1954
Navane Intramuscular 1956
Orap Tablets 1020
Orthoclone OKT3 Sterile Solution 1645
▲Roferon-A Injection (17%) 1916
Sinemet CR Tablets 953
Stelazine 2226
Triavil Tablets 1556

Mesenteric arterial thrombosis
Blocadren Tablets 1429
Corgard Tablets 701
Corzide Tablets 702
Inderal 2459
Inderal LA Long Acting Capsules 2461
Inderide Tablets 2463
Inderide LA Long Acting Capsules 2465
Kerlone Tablets 2172
Levatol 1832
Lo/Ovral Tablets 2471
Lo/Ovral-28 Tablets 2476
Loestrin 1728
Nordette-21 Tablets 2481
Nordette-28 Tablets 2483
Norlestrin 1746
Normodyne Tablets 2110
Ovral Tablets 2490
Ovral-28 Tablets 2491
Ovrette Tablets 2492
Sectral Capsules 2520
Tenoretic Tablets 1105
Tenormin Tablets and I.V. Injection 1107
Timolide Tablets 1547
Timoptic in Ocudose 1552
Timoptic Sterile Ophthalmic Solution 1550
Triphasil-21 Tablets 2527
Triphasil-28 Tablets 2532

Metabolic acidosis (see under Acidosis, metabolic)

Metabolic changes
Methotrexate Tablets, Parenteral, LPF Parenteral 1217
Rheumatrex Methotrexate Dose Pack 1234

Metaplasia, bronchiolar squamous
▲Blenoxane (10%) 724

Methemoglobinemia
Americaine Anesthetic Lubricant (Rare) 972
Americaine Otic Topical Anesthetic Ear Drops (Rare) 973
Aralen Phosphate with Primaquine Phosphate Tablets 2040
Azo Gantanol Tablets 1887
Azo Gantrisin Tablets 1888
Azulfidine Tablets, EN-tabs, Oral Suspension (Rare) 1157
Bactrim DS Tablets 1891
Bactrim I.V. Infusion 1889
Bactrim 1891
Deponit NTG Transdermal Delivery System (Extremely rare) 2143
Desyrel and Desyrel Dividose 1404
Eulexin Capsules 2089
Fansidar Tablets 1896
Gantanol 1899
Gantrisin Ophthalmic Ointment/Solution 1900
Gantrisin 1901
Isordil (Rare) 2467
Minitran Transdermal Delivery System (Infrequent) 1312
Nipride I.V. Infusion (Rare) 1909
Nitrodisc (Extremely rare) 2176
Nitrogard Tablets (Extremely rare) 1004
Pediazole 1973
Proloprim Tablets 799
Pyridium 1763
Pyridium Plus 1764
Reglan 1869
Septra 813
Septra I.V. Infusion 808
Septra I.V. Infusion ADD-Vantage Vials 810
Septra 813
Thiosulfil Forte Tablets 2526
Transderm-Nitro Transdermal Therapeutic System (Extremely rare) 2283
Tridil Ampuls & Vials (Extremely rare) 939
Trimpex Tablets 1922

Metrorrhagia
Floxin Tablets (Less than 1%) 1652
Permax Tablets (Infrequent) 1291
Prozac Pulvules (Rare) 920

Metyrapone test, altered results
Aygestin Tablets 2437
Cycrin Tablets 2449
Estratest 2245
Provera Tablets 2356

Microcephaly, fetal
Accutane Capsules 1878
Dilantin Infatabs 1710
Dilantin Parenteral 1712
Dilantin-30 Pediatric/Dilantin-125 Suspension 1713
Dilantin with Phenobarbital Kapseals 1715

Microembolizatiion of systemic cholesterol
Coumadin Injection & Tablets 944

Microphthalmia, fetal
Accutane Capsules 1878

Micropinna, fetal
Accutane Capsules 1878

Micturition, difficulty
Actifed with Codeine Cough Syrup 752
Apresazide Capsules (Less frequent) 854
Apresoline Hydrochloride Parenteral (Ampuls) 856
Apresoline Hydrochloride Tablets (Less frequent) 855
Apresoline-Esidrix Tablets 857
Astramorph/PF Injection, USP (Preservative-Free) 618
Atrovent Inhalation Aerosol (Less than 1%) 675
Benadryl Capsules 1691
Benadryl Injection 1692
Blocadren Tablets 1429
Catapres Tablets (About 2 in 1,000 patients) 676
Catapres-TTS (2 per 1,000) 677
▲CHEMET (succimer) Capsules (Up to 3.7%) 1361
Combipres Tablets (About 2 in 1,000) 678
Dantrium Capsules (Less frequent) 1619
Deconamine 663
Dimetane-DC Cough Syrup 1857
Dimetane-DX Cough Syrup 1858
Donnagel (Rare) ▣ 675
Donnagel-PG (Rare) 1858
Fiorinal with Codeine Capsules 2008
Flexeril Tablets (Rare) 1471
▲Hylorel Tablets (33.6%) 975
Kutrase Capsules 2146
Normodyne Tablets 2110
Normozide Tablets 2112
Norpramin Tablets 1340
Nucofed Capsules 2219
Nucofed Expectorant 2219
Nucofed Pediatric Expectorant 2220
Nucofed Syrup 2219
Omnipaque (Less than 0.1%) 2552
Optimine Tablets 2115
PBZ Tablets & Elixir 1037
PBZ-SR Tablets 1037
Periactin 1525
Polaramine 2116
Proventil (Less than 1%) 2120
Quadrinal Tablets 1183
Ru-Tuss II Capsules 693
Ser-Ap-Es Tablets 881
Serpasil-Apresoline Tablets 884
Surgicel 1151
Tavist Syrup 2033
Tavist Tablets 2035
Tavist-D Tablets 2035
Tedral SA 1765
Timolide Tablets 1547
Timoptic in Ocudose 1552
Timoptic Sterile Ophthalmic Solution 1550
Tofranil Ampuls 1038
Tofranil Tablets 1039
Tofranil-PM Capsules 1041
Trancopal Caplets 2075
Trandate HCT/Trandate (Less than 1% in 208 patients) 579
Transderm Scōp Transdermal Therapeutic System (Infrequent) 887
Trexan Tablets (Less than 1%) 937
Triaminic Expectorant DH 1995
Triaminic Oral Infant Drops 1996
Tuss-Ornade Liquid 2242
Tuss-Ornade Spansule Capsules 2242
Urised Tablets 2396
Uroqid-Acid (Occasional) 661
Valpin 50 Tablets 941
Ventolin Tablets (1 of 100 patients) 583
Vivactil Tablets 1567
▲Xanax Tablets (12.2%) 2367
Zovirax Sterile Powder (Less than 1%) 828

Micturition, obstructed
Lasix 1093

Micturition, painful
Nucofed Capsules 2219
Nucofed Expectorant 2219
Nucofed Pediatric Expectorant 2220
Nucofed Syrup 2219
Uroqid-Acid (Occasional) 661
Zovirax Sterile Powder (Less than 1%) 828

Micturition disturbances
Actifed with Codeine Cough Syrup 752
▲Anafranil Capsules (4% to 14%) 650
Asendin Tablets (Very rare) 1196
Benadryl Capsules 1691
Benadryl Injection 1692
Benemid Tablets 1426
Bontril Slow-Release 834
BuSpar (Infrequent) 1401
Calan SR Caplets (1% or less) 2157
Calan Tablets (1% or less) 2155
Capoten (Approximately 1 to 2 of 1000 patients) 2255
Capozide (Approximately 1 to 2 of 1000 patients) 2258
Cardene Capsules (Rare) 2290
Cardura Tablets (0%) 1941
Cartrol Tablets (Less common) 507
▲Cibacalcin Double-chambered Syringes (5-10%) 859
Cipro I.V. (1% or less) 1592
Clozaril Tablets (1%) 2000
ColBENEMID Tablets 1436
Comhist LA Capsules 1618
Dalgan Injection (Less than 1%) 620
Dantrium Capsules (Less frequent) 1619
Daranide Tablets 1445
Deconamine 663
Desyrel and Desyrel Dividose (Less than 1%) 1404
Diapid Nasal Spray 2003
Dimetane-DC Cough Syrup 1857
Dimetane-DX Cough Syrup 1858
Dipentum Capsules (Rare) 1160
Dolophine Hydrochloride Ampoules & Vials 1260
Dolophine Hydrochloride Tablets 1261
Dopram Injectable 1860
Duragesic Transdermal System (Less than 1%) 1133
Elavil 2269
Eldepryl 2250
Endep Tablets 1927
Enlon Injection 598
Eskalith 2214
Ethmozine Tablets (Less than 2%) 946
Etrafon 2087
Flexeril Tablets (Less than 1%) 1471
Floxin Tablets (Less than 1%) 1652
Hydrocet Capsules 835
Hytrin Tablets (At least 1%) 529
IFEX 729
Indocin (Rare) 1487
Intal Capsules (Less than 1 in 10,000 patients) 978
Intal Inhaler (Infrequent) 979
Intal Nebulizer Solution 980
Intron A (Less than 1%) 2097
Isoptin Oral Tablets (Less than 1%) 1179
Isoptin SR Sustained Release Tablets (Less than 1%) 1181
Limbitrol 1933
▲Lioresal Tablets (2-6%) 1031
Lodine Capsules (More than 1% but less than 3%) 2468
Lozol Tablets (Less than 5%) 1843
Ludiomil Tablets 874
▲Lupron Depot 3.75 mg (Among most frequent) 2312
▲Lupron Injection (5% or more) 2310
Matulane Capsules 1907
Methadone Hydrochloride Diskets 1284
Midamor Tablets (Less than or equal to 1%) 1508
Milontin Kapseals 1741
Minipress Capsules (1-4%) 1778
Minizide Capsules (Rare) 1779
Moduretic Tablets 1510
Monopril Tablets (0.2 to 1.0%) 1406
Mycelex-G 100 mg Vaginal Tablets (Rare) 1606
Mycelex-G 500 mg Vaginal Tablets (Rare) 1606
Normozide Tablets 2112
▲Norpace (3 to 9%) 2177
Norpramin Tablets 1340
Nubain Injection (Less than 1%) 934
Optimine Tablets 2115
Orap Tablets 1020
Ornade Spansule Capsules 2221
PBZ Tablets & Elixir 1037
PBZ-SR Tablets 1037
Pamelor 2019
Parlodel 2020
Permax Tablets (2.7%) 1291
Plegine Tablets 2504
Plendil Extended-Release Tablets (0.5% to 1.5%) 1526
Polaramine 2116
Pondimin Tablets 1867
Prilosec Delayed-Release Capsules (Less than 1%) 1530
ProSom Tablets (Infrequent) 554
Prostigmin Injectable 1120
Prostigmin Tablets 1121
Prozac Pulvules (1.6%) 920
Reglan 1869
Retrovir Capsules (Less than 5%) 802
Retrovir I.V. Infusion (Less than 5%) 805
Retrovir Syrup (Less than 5%) 802
Ru-Tuss II Capsules 693
Ru-Tuss with Hydrocodone 694
Ru-Tuss Tablets 693
▲Sectral Capsules (3%) 2520
Seldane Tablets 1349
Seldane-D Extended-Release Tablets 1350
Serophene (clomiphene citrate tablets, USP) (Less than 1 in 100 patients) 2186
Sinemet CR Tablets (0.8%) 953
Stilphostrol Tablets and Ampuls 1609
Surmontil Capsules 2524
Tacaryl 2409
Tavist Syrup 2033
Tavist Tablets 2035
Tavist-D Tablets 2035
Tegretol Chewable Tablets 654
Tegretol Suspension 656
Tegretol Tablets 654
Temaril Tablets, Syrup and Spansule Sustained Release Capsules 1085
Tenex Tablets 1875
Tensilon Injectable 1123
▲TheraCys BCG Live (Intravesical) (1.8% to 40.2%) 898
Tofranil Ampuls 1038
Tofranil Tablets 1039
Tofranil-PM Capsules 1041
Toradol IM Injection (1% or less) 2302
Trexan Tablets (Less than 1%) 937
Triaminic Expectorant DH 1995
Triaminic Oral Infant Drops 1996
Triavil Tablets 1556
Trinalin Repetabs Tablets 1170
Urecholine 1558
Vasoxyl Injection 819
Verelan Capsules (Less than 1%) 1243
Vivactil Tablets 1567
Voltaren Tablets (Less than 1%) 1042
Wellbutrin Tablets (2.5%) 821
Wytensin Tablets (3% or less) 2542

Migraine
Anafranil Capsules (Up to 3%) 650
Brevicon 2304
Cardura Tablets (Less than 0.5% of 3960 patients) 1941
Cycrin Tablets 2449
Demulen 2161
Diethylstilbestrol Tablets 1258
Eldepryl 2250
Engerix-B Unit-Dose Vials 2213
Enovid 2161
Estinyl Tablets 2085
Estraderm Transdermal System 866
Estradurin 2452
Estratest 2245

Estrovis 1721
Gastrocrom Capsules (Infrequent) 974
Intron A (Less than 5%) 2097
Jenest-28 Tablets 1636
Levlen/Tri-Levlen 665
Lo/Ovral Tablets 2471
Lo/Ovral-28 Tablets 2476
Loestrin 1728
Maxair Inhaler (Less than 1%) 1311
Mediatric Capsules 2476
Menrium Tablets 1934
Micronor Tablets 1667
Modicon 1667
Nordette-21 Tablets 2481
Nordette-28 Tablets 2483
Norethin 2133
Norinyl 2304
Norlestrin 1746
Nor-Q D Tablets 2304
Ogen 540
Ortho Dienestrol Cream 1664
Ortho-Cyclen Tablets 1658
Ortho-Novum 1667
Orudis Capsules (Less than 1%) 2488
Ovral Tablets 2490
Ovral-28 Tablets 2491
Ovrette Tablets 2492
PMB 200 and PMB 400 2504
Permax Tablets (Rare) 1291
Premarin Intravenous 2508
Premarin with Methyltestosterone 2515
Premarin Tablets 2510
Premarin Vaginal Cream 2512
Procardia XL Tablets (1% or less) 1783
Prozac Pulvules (Infrequent) 920
Stilphostrol Tablets and Ampuls 1609
TACE 12 and 25 mg 1353
Levlen/Tri-Levlen 665
Tri-Norinyl 2304
Triphasil-21 Tablets 2527
Triphasil-28 Tablets 2532

Miliaria
Aclovate Cream 1053
Alphatrex Cream, Ointment & Lotion (Infrequent) 2076
Analpram-HC Rectal Cream 1% and 2.5% 970
Anusol-HC Cream (Infrequent) 1690
Aristocort A (Infrequent) 1010
Betatrex Cream, Ointment & Lotion 2077
Carmol HC Cream 1% (Infrequent) 2296
Cortisporin Cream 757
Cortisporin Ointment 758
Cortisporin Otic Solution Sterile 760
Cortisporin Otic Suspension Sterile 760
Cutivate Cream 0.05% 1054
Cutivate Ointment 0.005% (Infrequent to more frequent) 1054
Cyclocort Lotion (Infrequent) 1198
Decadron Phosphate Topical Cream 1455
Decaspray Topical Aerosol 1459
DesOwen Cream, Ointment and Lotion (Infrequent) 1682
Diprolene (Infrequent) 2083
Eldecort Cream 1.0% (Infrequent) 1113
Eldecort Cream 1.0% and 2.5% (Infrequent) 1113
Elocon 2084
Epifoam 1828
Florone/Florone E 908
Halog (Infrequent) 2399
Hytone 909
Kenalog Cream, Lotion & Ointment (Infrequent) 2401
Lidex (Infrequent) 2296
Locoid Cream, Ointment and Topical Solution (Infrequent) 970
Lotrisone Cream (Infrequent) 2103
Mantadil Cream 789
Maxivate Cream, Lotion & Ointment 0.05% 2406
Mycolog II Cream and Ointment (Infrequent) 2407
Mytrex Cream & Ointment (Infrequent) 2080
NeoDecadron Topical Cream 1518
Neo-Synalar Cream (Infrequent) 2296
Nutracort Cream & Lotion (Infrequent) 1684
Orabase HCA Oral Paste (Infrequent) 890
Oxsoralen-Ultra Capsule 1117
PediOtic Suspension Sterile 797
Pramosone Cream, Lotion & Ointment 971
ProctoCream-HC (Infrequent) 1834
Proctofoam-HC 1835
Psorcon Ointment 0.05% 909
Psorion Cream 0.05% (Infrequent) 1121
Synacort Creams 1%, 2.5% (Infrequent) 2296
Synalar (Infrequent) 2296
Temovate 1056
Topicort (Infrequent) 1098
Tridesilon Creme 0.05% (Infrequent) 1611
Tridesilon Ointment 0.05% (Infrequent) 1611
Ultravate Cream 0.05% (Infrequent) 2410
Ultravate Ointment 0.05% 2411
Vanoxide-HC Acne Lotion 911
Vioform-Hydrocortisone Cream and Mild Cream 889
Vioform-Hydrocortisone Ointment 889
Vytone Cream 1% 911
Westcort 2411

Miosis
Carbocaine Hydrochloride Injection 2043
Compazine 2201
Dibenzyline Capsules 2207
Dilaudid-HP Injection 1175
Duvoid Tablets 1853
Enlon Injection 598
Fiorinal with Codeine Capsules 2008
Lioresal Tablets 1031
MS Contin Tablets (Infrequent) 1814
MSIR (Infrequent) 1817
Marcaine Hydrochloride 0.5% with Epinephrine 1:200,000 (as bitartrate) 958
Marcaine Hydrochloride with Epinephrine 1:200,000 2055
Marcaine Hydrochloride Injection 2055
Mellaril 2011
Mestinon Injectable 1115
Mestinon 1116
Navane Capsules and Concentrate 1954
Navane Intramuscular 1956
Nipride I.V. Infusion 1909
Norzine 1818
Numorphan Hydrochloride Injection 935
Numorphan Suppositories 935
Oramorph SR (Morphine Sulfate Sustained Release Tablets) (Less frequent) 1988
Pantopon Injectable 1911
Pilagan ◉ 250
Pontocaine Hydrochloride for Spinal Anesthesia 2069
Prostigmin Injectable 1120
Prostigmin Tablets 1121
Renese-R Tablets 1786
Sensorcaine 631
Sensorcaine-MPF Spinal 634
Serentil 686
Soma Compound w/Codeine Tablets 2390
Stelazine 2226
Talwin Injection (Rare) 2071
Tensilon Injectable 1123
Thorazine 2234
Torecan 1993
Tussi-Organidin Liquid 2391
Urecholine 1558
Versed Injection (Less than 1%) 1924

Miosis, rebound
Mydfrin 2.5% ◉ 224

Miscarriage
Cytotec 2159
Levlen/Tri-Levlen 665
NebuPent for Inhalation Solution (1% or less) 1017
Nicorette (Rare) 1335
Levlen/Tri-Levlen 665

Mitral valve prolapse
Loestrin 1728
Norlestrin 1746

Moaning
Diprivan Injection (Less than 1%) 2267

Moniliasis
▲CHEMET (succimer) Capsules (5.2 to 15.7%) 1361
▲Intron A (Less than 14%) 2097
Monodox Capsules 1630
Permax Tablets (Infrequent) 1291
Prozac Pulvules (Rare) 920
Vibramycin 1787

Moniliasis, genital
Ancef Injection 2194
Claforan Sterile Injection (Less than 1%) 1089
Keflex Pulvules, Oral Suspension & Pediatric Drops 916
Keftab Tablets 917
Kefzol Vials, Faspak & ADD-Vantage 1279
Minocin Oral Suspension 1224
Minocin Pellet-Filled Capsules 1222
Rocephin Injectable Vials, ADD-Vantage (Occasional) 1914
Ultracef Capsules, Tablets & Oral Suspension 722

Monoclonal B-lymphoproliferative disorder
Orthoclone OKT3 Sterile Solution (1 of 22 Bone marrow transplants) 1645

Monocytosis
Celontin 1692
Cipro Tablets (Less than 0.1%) 1589
Cuprimine Capsules 1442
Depen Titratable Tablets 2379
Mesantoin Tablets 2013
Primaxin I.M. 1532
Primaxin I.V. 1535
Rocephin Injectable Vials, ADD-Vantage (Rare) 1914
Unasyn 1965
Zefazone Sterile Powder 2372

Mononeuropathy
Tri-Immunol Diphtheria & Tetanus Toxoids & Pertussis Vaccine, Adsorbed 1241

Mood changes
▲Adalat Capsules (10 mg and 20 mg) (7%) 1587
AeroBid Inhaler System (1-3%) 995
Anexsia 5/500 Tablets 2196
Anexsia 7.5/650 Tablets 2197
Aristospan Suspension (Intra-articular) 1011
Azdōne Tablets 844
Damason-P 1356
Dilaudid Cough Syrup 1174
Dilaudid 1173
Dilaudid-HP Injection 1175
Dipentum Capsules (Rare) 1160
Eldepryl 2250
Feldene Capsules (Less than 1%) 1777
Hexalen Capsules 2316
Hycodan Syrup, Tablets 927
Hycomine Compound Tablets 929
Hycomine Syrup 927
Hycotuss Expectorant Syrup 930
Hydrocet Capsules 835
Lortab ASA Tablets 2414
Lortab 2412
Lupron Depot 7.5 mg 2311
Lupron Injection (Less than 5%) 2310
MS Contin Tablets (Infrequent) 1814
MSIR (Infrequent) 1817
Methotrexate Tablets, Parenteral, LPF Parenteral 1217
Micronor Tablets 1667
Modicon 1667
Monopril Tablets (0.2 to 1.0%) 1406
Oramorph SR (Morphine Sulfate Sustained Release Tablets) (Less frequent) 1988
Ortho-Novum 1667
Pondimin Tablets 1867
▲Procardia XL Tablets (7%) 1783
Rheumatrex Methotrexate Dose Pack 1234
Stilphostrol Tablets and Ampuls 1609
▲Tonocard Tablets (1.5-11.0%) 1554
Tussionex Extended-Release Suspension 988
Vicodin Tablets 1187
Vicodin ES Tablets 1189
Wellbutrin Tablets (Infrequent) 821
Zydone Capsules 941

Moro reflex, depressed
Diupres Tablets 1461
Hydropres Tablets 1485
Salutensin/Salutensin-Demi 719

Motor and phonic tics, exacerbations
Dexedrine 2206

Motor restlessness
Compazine 2201
Haldol Decanoate (Less frequent) 1375
Haldol Injection, Tablets and Concentrate 1373
Mellaril 2011
Navane Capsules and Concentrate 1954
Navane Intramuscular 1956
Norzine 1818
Orap Tablets 1020
Prolixin Decanoate 1795
Prolixin Enanthate 1796
Reglan 1869
Serentil 686
Stelazine 2226
Taractan 1920
Thorazine 2234

Motor skills, impairment
Cogentin 1435
Compazine 2201
Dapsone USP 1130
Desyrel and Desyrel Dividose (Greater than 1%) 1404
Dilaudid Cough Syrup 1174
Doral Tablets 2383
Halcion Tablets 2340
Kinesed Tablets 2272
Moban Tablets & Concentrate 932
Novafed A Capsules 1342
Novahistine DH 1342
Omnipaque (Rare) 2552
Oncovin Solution Vials & Hyporets 1288
Orap Tablets 1020
Platinol 737
Platinol-AQ Injection 738
Robaxin Injectable 1871
Soma Compound w/Codeine Tablets 2390
Soma Compound Tablets 2389
Tonocard Tablets (0.0-1.2%) 1554

Mouth, burning
Fiorinal with Codeine Capsules 2008
Gastrocrom Capsules (Infrequent) 974

Mouth, cauterization
Eldepryl 2250

Mouth, dry (see under Xerostomia)

Mouth, puckering
Compazine 2201
Etrafon 2087
Haldol Decanoate 1375
Haldol Injection, Tablets and Concentrate 1373
Mellaril 2011
Moban Tablets & Concentrate 932
Navane Capsules and Concentrate 1954
Navane Intramuscular 1956
Orap Tablets 1020
Prolixin Decanoate 1795
Prolixin Enanthate 1796
Prolixin Oral Concentrate 1792
Serentil 686
Stelazine 2226
Taractan 1920
Thorazine 2234
Triavil Tablets 1556
Trilafon 2123

Mouth, sore
Atgam Sterile Solution (Less than 5%) 2320
Prolixin Decanoate 1795
Prolixin Enanthate 1796
Prolixin Oral Concentrate 1792
Pronestyl Capsules and Tablets 1800
Pronestyl Injection 1798
Rifadin (Occasional) 1345
Rifamate Capsules 1347
Rimactane Capsules 879
Tegison Capsules 1881

Movement, abnormal
▲Diprivan Injection (3% to 10%) 2267
Oramorph SR (Morphine Sulfate Sustained Release Tablets) (Less frequent) 1988
▲Xanax Tablets (14.8%) 2367

Mucha-Habermann syndrome
Azulfidine Tablets, EN-tabs, Oral Suspension (Rare) 1157

Mucosal pigmentation, changes
Aralen Hydrochloride Injection 2038
Aralen Phosphate with Primaquine Phosphate Tablets 2040

Aralen Phosphate Tablets ... 2039
Intron A ... 2097
Minocin Oral Suspension ... 1224
Minocin Pellet-Filled Capsules ... 1222
Plaquenil Sulfate Tablets ... 2067

Mucositis

▲ Neupogen for Injection (12%) ... 595

Mucous plugs

Exosurf Neonatal for Intratracheal Suspension ... 765

Mucous membrane, abnormalities

Adriamycin PFS ... 561
Adriamycin RDF ... 562
Alferon N Injection (One patient) ... 1809
Cerubidine ... 2443
Clinoril Tablets ... 1433
Doxorubicin Hydrochloride for Injection, USP ... 622
Doxorubicin Hydrochloride Injection, USP ... 848
Hydrea Capsules ... 728
▲ Idamycin for Injection (50%) ... 564
Leukine for IV Infusion ... 1127
Mexitil Capsules (About 1 in 1,000) ... 680
Minocin Intravenous ... 1221
Minocin Oral Suspension ... 1224
Minocin Pellet-Filled Capsules ... 1222
▲ Novantrone for Injection Concentrate (18 to 29%) ... 1226
Paraplatin for Injection (1%) ... 735
Prokine for I.V. Infusion ... 1096
Rubex ... 739
▲ Tegison Capsules (1-10%) ... 1881

Mucus, blood-tinted

Peptavlon ... 2563

Mucus, excess

▲ Trexan Tablets (Less than 10%) ... 937

Mucus secretion, decreased

Tegison Capsules (Less than 1%) ... 1881

Multinodular goiter, enlargement

Lorelco Tablets ... 1333

Murmur

▲ Lupron Depot 3.75 mg (Among most frequent) ... 2312
Lupron Depot 7.5 mg ... 2311
▲ Lupron Injection (5% or more) ... 2310

Muscle cramp (see under Cramping, muscular)

Muscle hypotonia

Anectine Flo-Pack ... 755
Pipracil (Rare) ... 1230
▲ Xanax Tablets (6.3%) ... 2367

Muscle mass, loss

Aristocort Suspension ... 1008
Aristospan Suspension ... 1011
Celestone Soluspan Suspension ... 2081
Cortenema ... 2244
Cortone Acetate Sterile Suspension ... 1437
Cortone Acetate Tablets ... 1439
Dalalone D.P. Injectable ... 999
Decadron Elixir ... 1445
Decadron Phosphate Injection ... 1449
Decadron Phosphate Respihaler ... 1454
Decadron Phosphate Turbinaire ... 1456
Decadron Phosphate with Xylocaine Injection, Sterile ... 1451
Decadron Tablets ... 1447
Decadron-LA Sterile Suspension ... 1457
Deltasone Tablets ... 2332
Depo-Medrol Sterile Aqueous Suspension ... 2334
Hydeltrasol Injection, Sterile ... 1476
Hydeltra-T.B.A. Sterile Suspension ... 1478
Hydrocortone Phosphate Injection, Sterile ... 1481
Hydrocortone Tablets ... 1482
Kenalog-10 Injection ... 2402
Kenalog-40 Injection ... 2403
Medrol ... 2348
Oncovin Solution Vials & Hyporets ... 1288
Pediapred Oral Liquid ... 987
Solu-Cortef Sterile Powder ... 2361
Solu-Medrol Sterile Powder ... 2363

Muscle movement, intraoperative

Sufenta Injection (Less than 1%) ... 1147

Muscle rigidity

▲ Alfenta Injection (Most common) ... 1131
Asendin Tablets ... 1196
Brevibloc Injection (Less than 1%) ... 942
BuSpar (Infrequent) ... 1401
Compazine ... 2201
Cytotec (Infrequent) ... 2159
Dilaudid-HP Injection ... 1175
Ethrane ... 599
▲ Innovar Injection (Most common) ... 1141
Loxitane ... 1213
MS Contin Tablets (Infrequent) ... 1814
MSIR (Infrequent) ... 1817
Mellaril ... 2011
Moban Tablets & Concentrate ... 932
Navane Capsules and Concentrate ... 1954
Navane Intramuscular ... 1956
Norzine ... 1818
Oramorph SR (Morphine Sulfate Sustained Release Tablets) (Less frequent) ... 1988
Orap Tablets ... 1020
Prolixin Decanoate ... 1795
Prolixin Elixir ... 1793
Prolixin Enanthate ... 1796
Prolixin Injection ... 1791
Prolixin Tablets ... 1793
ProSom Tablets (1%) ... 554
Prostin VR Pediatric Sterile Solution (Less than 1%) ... 2355
Reglan ... 1869
Serentil ... 686
Stelazine ... 2226
Sublimaze Injection (Infrequent) ... 1146
Sufenta Injection (Infrequent) ... 1147
Thorazine ... 2234
Torecan ... 1993
Trilafon ... 2123
Valrelease Capsules (Infrequent) ... 1923
Versed Injection (0.3%) ... 1924
Wellbutrin Tablets ... 821
Xanax Tablets (2.2%) ... 2367

Muscle spasms

Aldactazide ... 2150
Aldoclor Tablets ... 1413
Aldoril Tablets ... 1418
Apresazide Capsules ... 854
Apresoline-Esidrix Tablets ... 857
BuSpar (Infrequent) ... 1401
Capozide ... 2258
Clozaril Tablets (1%) ... 2000
Combipres Tablets ... 678
Corzide Tablets (Not uncommon) ... 702
Danocrine Capsules ... 2046
Diucardin Tablets ... 2450
Diulo ... 2129
Diupres Tablets ... 1461
Diuril Oral Suspension ... 1464
Diuril Sodium Intravenous ... 1463
Diuril Tablets ... 1464
Dopram Injectable ... 1860
Doral Tablets (Rare) ... 2383
Enduron Tablets ... 517
Enduronyl ... 518
Esidrix Tablets ... 863
Esimil Tablets ... 864
Etrafon ... 2087
Exna Tablets ... 1862
Halcion Tablets ... 2340
HydroDIURIL Tablets ... 1484
Hydromox R Tablets ... 1209
Hydromox Tablets ... 1208
Hydropres Tablets ... 1485
Inderide Tablets ... 2463
Inderide LA Long Acting Capsules ... 2465
Indocin I.V. (Less than 1%) ... 1490
Lasix ... 1093
Lopressor HCT Tablets ... 1034
Loxitane ... 1213
▲ Lozol Tablets (Greater than or equal to 5%) ... 1843
▲ Lupron Injection (Greater than 3%) ... 2310
Mestinon Injectable ... 1115
Mestinon ... 1116
Minizide Capsules ... 1779
Moban Tablets & Concentrate (Infrequent) ... 932
Moduretic Tablets (Less than or equal to 1%) ... 1510
Naturetin Tablets (Common) ... 1789
Normozide Tablets ... 2112
Oretic Tablets ... 544
Oreticyl ... 545
Parnate Tablets ... 2222
Prinzide Tablets ... 1540
ProSom Tablets (Infrequent) ... 554
Prostigmin Injectable ... 1120
Prostigmin Tablets ... 1121
Proventil Syrup (Less than 1 of 100) ... 2119
Rauzide Tablets ... 1804
Renese Tablets ... 1785
Retrovir Capsules (Less than 5%) ... 802
Retrovir I.V. Infusion (Less than 5%) ... 805
Retrovir Syrup (Less than 5%) ... 802
Saluron ... 718
Salutensin/Salutensin-Demi ... 719
Ser-Ap-Es Tablets ... 881
Serpasil-Esidrix Tablets ... 886
Tenoretic Tablets ... 1105
Thalitone Tablets ... 687
Timolide Tablets ... 1547
Tonocard Tablets (Less than 1%) ... 1554
Trandate HCT Tablets ... 579
Valium Injectable ... 1937
Valium Tablets ... 1939
Vancocin HCl, Vials & ADD-Vantage (Infrequent) ... 1302
Vaseretic Tablets ... 1559
Ventolin Syrup (Less than 1 of 100 patients) ... 583
Wellbutrin Tablets (1.9%) ... 821
Xanax Tablets (Rare) ... 2367
Zestoretic ... 2274

Muscle twitching

Aminophyllin Tablets ... 2153
Asbron G ... 1997
Choledyl Pediatric Elixir ... 1702
Choledyl Tablets ... 1700
Choledyl SA Tablets ... 1704
Clozaril Tablets (Less than 1%) ... 2000
Constant-T Tablets ... 1029
Dalalone D.P. Injectable ... 999
Decadron-LA Sterile Suspension (Low) ... 1457
Desyrel and Desyrel Dividose (Less than 1%) ... 1404
Dilaudid-HP Injection ... 1175
Dilor ... 2079
Dopram Injectable ... 1860
Flexeril Tablets (Less than 1%) ... 1471
Floropryl Sterile Ophthalmic Ointment ... 1473
Garamycin Injectable ... 2093
Humorsol Sterile Ophthalmic Solution ... 1475
Larodopa Tablets (Infrequent) ... 1905
Loxitane ... 1213
Lufyllin & Lufyllin-400 Tablets ... 2384
Lufyllin-GG Elixir & Tablets ... 2385
▲ Marplan Tablets (Among most frequent) ... 1906
Netromycin Injection 100 mg/ml ... 2104
Nipride I.V. Infusion ... 1909
Nitro-Bid IV (Less than 1%) ... 1338
Nitrostat IV (Less than 1%) ... 1744
Quadrinal Tablets ... 1183
Quibron Capsules ... 713
Quibron-T ... 714
Quibron-T/SR ... 716
Respbid Tablets ... 684
Retrovir Capsules (Less than 5%) ... 802
Retrovir I.V. Infusion (Less than 5%) ... 805
Retrovir Syrup (Less than 5%) ... 802
Sinemet Tablets ... 952
Sinemet CR Tablets ... 953
T-PHYL (Uniphyl) 200 mg Tablets ... 1820
Theo-Dur Sprinkle ... 1168
Theo-Dur Extended-Release Tablets ... 1166
Theolair ... 1317
Theolair-SR Tablets ... 1319
▲ TheoX Extended-Release Tablets (Among most consistent) ... 841
Tonocard Tablets (Less than 1%) ... 1554
Uniphyl 400 mg Tablets ... 1823
▲ Xanax Tablets (7.9%) ... 2367

Muscle weakness (see also under Asthenia; Weakness, muscle)

Anaprox and Anaprox DS Tablets (Less than 1%) ... 2288
▲ Antivenin (Crotalidae) Polyvalent (Frequent) ... 2430
Aristocort Suspension ... 1008
Aristospan Suspension ... 1011
BuSpar (Rare) ... 1401
Celestone Soluspan Suspension ... 2081
Clozaril Tablets (1%) ... 2000
Cortenema ... 2244
Dalalone D.P. Injectable ... 999
Decadron Tablets ... 1447
Decadron-LA Sterile Suspension ... 1457
Deltasone Tablets ... 2332
Depakene Capsules & Syrup ... 511
Depakote Tablets ... 512
Depo-Medrol Sterile Aqueous Suspension ... 2334
Deprol Tablets ... 2382
Enduron Tablets ... 517
Etrafon ... 2087
Fansidar Tablets ... 1896
Garamycin Injectable ... 2093
Hydrocortone Acetate Sterile Suspension ... 1479
Intron A (Less than 1%) ... 2097
Kenalog-40 Injection ... 2403
Klonopin Tablets ... 1902
Klorvess Effervescent Granules ... 2010
Klorvess Effervescent Tablets ... 2011
Klorvess 10% Liquid ... 2010
Medrol ... 2348
Mestinon Injectable ... 1115
Mestinon ... 1116
Milontin Kapseals ... 1741
Naprosyn Tablets (Less than 1%) ... 2297
▲ Norpace (3 to 9%) ... 2177
Omnipaque (Rare) ... 2552
Pediapred Oral Liquid ... 987
Placidyl Capsules ... 553
Plaquenil Sulfate Tablets ... 2067
Prostigmin Injectable ... 1120
Prostigmin Tablets ... 1121
Proventil Repetabs Tablets (2%) ... 2120
Proventil Syrup (Less than 1%) ... 2119
Proventil Tablets (2%) ... 2120
Rifadin ... 1345
Rifamate Capsules ... 1347
Solu-Cortef Sterile Powder ... 2361
Solu-Medrol Sterile Powder ... 2363
Tensilon Injectable ... 1123
Triavil Tablets ... 1556
Trilafon ... 2123
Xanax Tablets ... 2367

Muscular disturbances

Roferon-A Injection (Less than 0.5%) ... 1916

Musculoskeletal symptoms, unspecified

Seldane Tablets ... 1349
Seldane-D Extended-Release Tablets ... 1350

Mutism

Anafranil Capsules (Rare) ... 650

Myalgia

Actigall Capsules ... 2280
▲ Actimmune (6%) ... 1046
Aldoclor Tablets ... 1413
Aldomet Ester HCl Injection ... 1417
Aldomet Oral ... 1415
Aldoril Tablets ... 1418
Alferon N Injection (One patient to 3%) ... 1809
Altace Capsules (Less than 1%) ... 1086
Amicar Syrup, Tablets, and Injection ... 1194
▲ Anafranil Capsules (Up to 13%) ... 650
Anaprox and Anaprox DS Tablets (Less than 1%) ... 2288
Anectine ... 755
▲ Atgam Sterile Solution (At least 1 patient; less than 5% to 10% of total patients) ... 2320
Atromid-S Capsules (Less often) ... 2435
Augmentin Tablets, Powder for Oral Suspension, and Chewable Tablets ... 2198
Azactam for Injection (Less than 1%) ... 2252
Azo Gantrisin Tablets ... 1888
Bactrim DS Tablets ... 1891
Bactrim I.V. Infusion ... 1889
Bactrim ... 1891
Biavax II ... 1427
Bumex (0.2%) ... 1895
Cafergot/Cafergot P-B ... 1999
Calcijex Calcitriol Injection ... 506
Calderol Capsules ... 1635
Capoten ... 2255
Capozide ... 2258
Cardene Capsules (1.0%) ... 2290
Cardura Tablets (1%) ... 1941
Catapres Tablets (About 6 in 1,000 patients) ... 676
Catapres-TTS (6 per 1,000) ... 677
Cholybar ... 1705
Clinoril Tablets (Less than 1 in 100) ... 1433
Clozaril Tablets (1%) ... 2000
Colestid Granules (Less than 1 in 1,000) ... 2328

Combipres Tablets (About 6 in 1,000) ... 678
Corzide Tablets ... 702
Cosmegen Injection ... 1440
Cytosar-U Sterile Powder ... 2329
Cytotec (Infrequent) ... 2159
D.H.E. 45 Injection ... 2003
DTIC-Dome (Infrequent) ... 1595
Dalgan Injection (Less than 1%) ... 620
Dantrium Capsules (Less frequent) 1619
Diprivan Injection (Less than 1%) .. 2267
Diupres Tablets ... 1461
Dolobid Tablets (Less than 1 in 100) ... 1465
Donnatal ... 1858
Donnatal Extentabs ... 1859
Donnatal Tablets ... 1858
Donnazyme Tablets ... 1860
Dyazide Capsules ... 2208
Engerix-B Unit-Dose Vials (Less than 1%) ... 2213
Epogen for Injection (Rare) ... 591
Ergamisol Tablets (2 to 3%) ... 1136
Esimil Tablets ... 864
▲Ethmozine Tablets (2%-5%) ... 946
Flexeril Tablets (Rare) ... 1471
Floxin Tablets (Less than 1%) ... 1652
Flu-Imune Influenza Virus Vaccine (Infrequent) ... 1204
▲Fungizone Intravenous (Among most common) ... 2262
Gamimune N Immune Globulin Intravenous (Human) ... 1572
Gammar-IV, Immune Globulin Intravenous (Human) ... 610
Gantanol ... 1899
Gantrisin ... 1901
▲Gastrocrom Capsules (3 of 87 patients) ... 974
Harmonyl Tablets ... 528
Hespan Injection ... 948
Hismanal Tablets (Less frequent) ... 1138
Humatrope Vials (Infrequent) ... 1266
Hytrin Tablets (At least 1%) ... 529
Imferon ... 976
Imuran ... 768
Intal Capsules (Less than 1 in 100,000 patients) ... 978
Intal Inhaler (Rare) ... 979
Intal Nebulizer Solution (Rare) ... 980
▲Intron A (28% to 44%) ... 2097
Ismelin Tablets ... 869
▲Kerlone Tablets (3.2%) ... 2172
Koro-Flex Arcing Spring Diaphragm ... 2142
Koromex Coil Spring Diaphragm ... 2142
▲Lariam Tablets (Among most frequent) ... 1904
▲Leukine for IV Infusion (Among most frequent) ... 1127
Lioresal Tablets ... 1031
Lopid Capsules and Tablets ... 1736
Lopressor Ampuls ... 1032
Lopressor HCT Tablets (1 in 100 patients) ... 1034
Lopressor Tablets ... 1032
Lotensin Tablets ... 872
Lupron Depot 7.5 mg (Less than 5%) ... 2311
▲Lupron Injection (5% or more) ... 2310
M-M-R II ... 1494
M-R-VAX II ... 1496
Macrodantin Capsules ... 1624
Matulane Capsules ... 1907
Medihaler Ergotamine Aerosol ... 1312
Meruvax II ... 1503
Methotrexate Tablets, Parenteral, LPF Parenteral (Rare) ... 1217
Metrodin (urofollitropin for injection) (Less than 1 in 50) ... 2182
Mevacor Tablets (2.4%) ... 1505
Micronase Tablets ... 2350
Monocid Injection (Less than 1%) .. 2217
Monopril Tablets (0.2 to 1.0%) ... 1406
Naprosyn (Less than 1%) ... 2297
NebuPent for Inhalation Solution (Greater than 1%, up to 5%) ... 1017
Nimotop Capsules (Up to 1.4%) ... 1607
Nolvadex Tablets (2.8%) ... 1102
Noroxin Tablets ... 1519
Norplant System ... 2484
Oncovin Solution Vials & Hyporets 1288
OptiPranolol Sterile Ophthalmic Solution (A small number of patients) ... ⊙ 261
Oreticyl ... 545
Ortho Diaphragm Kit ... 1664
Orthoclone OKT3 Sterile Solution .. 1645
Ortho-White Diaphragm Kit-Flat Spring ... 1664
Orudis Capsules (Less than 1%) ... 2488
Pepcid (Infrequent) ... 1524
Permax Tablets (1.1%) ... 1291
Phenobarbital Elixir and Tablets (Rare) ... 1293
Phenurone Tablets (Less than 1%) 552
Plague Vaccine ... 1584
Plendil Extended-Release Tablets (0.5% to 1.5%) ... 1526
Pneumovax 23 ... 1528
Pnu-Imune 23 Pneumococcal Vaccine Polyvalent (Occasional) .. 1233
Pondimin Tablets ... 1867
Prilosec Delayed-Release Capsules (Less than 1%) ... 1530
Prinivil Tablets (1% or less) ... 1538
Prinzide Tablets (0.3% to 1%) ... 1540
Procan SR Tablets (Common) ... 1760
Procardia XL Tablets (1% or less) .. 1783
Procrit for Injection (Rare) ... 1647
Pronestyl Capsules and Tablets ... 1800
Pronestyl Injection ... 1798
Pronestyl-SR Tablets ... 1801
ProSom Tablets (Infrequent) ... 554
Prozac Pulvules (1.2%) ... 920
Questran Light ... 711
Questran Powder ... 710
Quinidex Extentabs ... 1868
Raudixin Tablets ... 1803
Rauzide Tablets ... 1804
Recombivax HB (Less than 1%) ... 1544
▲Retrovir Capsules (8%) ... 802
▲Retrovir I.V. Infusion (8%) ... 805
▲Retrovir Syrup (8%) ... 802
Rheumatrex Methotrexate Dose Pack (Rare) ... 1234
▲RhoGAM $Rh_0(D)$ Immune Globulin (Human) (25% in one study) ... 1651
Rocaltrol Capsules ... 1913
▲Roferon-A Injection (69% to 73%) 1916
Salutensin/Salutensin-Demi ... 719
Sandimmune (2% or less) ... 2024
Sandostatin Injection (Less than 1%) ... 2029
Sansert Tablets ... 2031
Sectral Capsules (2%) ... 2520
Septra ... 813
Septra I.V. Infusion ... 808
Septra I.V. Infusion ADD-Vantage Vials ... 810
Septra ... 813
Serpasil-Apresoline Tablets ... 884
Serpasil-Esidrix Tablets ... 886
Streptase for Infusion ... 635
▲Synarel Nasal Solution (10% of patients) ... 2300
Tagamet (Rare) ... 2228
Tambocor Tablets (Less than 1%) 1315
Tapazole Tablets ... 1298
▲Tegison Capsules (1-10%) ... 1881
Tegretol Chewable Tablets ... 654
Tegretol Suspension ... 656
Tegretol Tablets ... 654
Tenex Tablets ... 1875
Tenoretic Tablets ... 1105
Tenuate ... 1354
Thalitone Tablets ... 687
▲TheraCys BCG Live (Intravesical) (1.0% to 7.1%) ... 898
Timentin for Injection ... 2239
Timolide Tablets (Less than 1%) ... 1547
Tonocard Tablets (1.7%) ... 1554
Toradol IM Injection (1% or less) ... 2302
▲Trexan Tablets (Greater than 10%) ... 937
Typhoid Vaccine ... 2533
Vaseretic Tablets ... 1559
Vasotec I.V. (0.5 to 1%) ... 1562
Vasotec Tablets (0.5% to 1%) ... 1564
Verelan Capsules (1.1%) ... 1243
▲Visken Tablets (10%) ... 2036
Wellbutrin Tablets ... 821
Wigraine Tablets & Suppositories .. 1645
Wytensin Tablets (3% or less) ... 2542
Zestoretic (0.3 to 1%) ... 2274
Zestril Tablets ... 2277
Zovirax ... 824
Zyloprim Tablets (Less than 1%) ... 830

Myasthenia gravis

Ansaid Tablets (Less than 1%) ... 2319
Blocadren Tablets (Less than 1%) 1429
Capoten ... 2255
Capozide ... 2258
Cipro Tablets ... 1589
Cuprimine Capsules ... 1442
Depen Titratable Tablets ... 2379
Garamycin Injectable ... 2093
Myleran Tablets (Rare) ... 790
Netromycin Injection 100 mg/ml ... 2104
Paradione Capsules ... 548
Timolide Tablets ... 1547
Timoptic in Ocudose ... 1552
Timoptic Sterile Ophthalmic Solution ... 1550
Tonocard Tablets (Less than 1%) .. 1554
Tridione Capsules ... 557

Myasthenia gravis, exacerbation of

Cipro I.V. ... 1592
Floxin Tablets ... 1652
Norpace ... 2177

Mydriasis

AK-Cide Sterile Ophthalmic Ointment & Suspension (Occasional) ... ⊙ 202
AK-Con ... ⊙ 202
AK-Con-A ... ⊙ 203
Albalon Solution with Liquifilm ... ⊙ 238
Albalon-A Liquifilm ... ⊙ 238
Alcaine ... ⊙ 210
Anafranil Capsules (Up to 2%) ... 650
Arfonad Ampuls ... 1887
Artane ... 1195
Asendin Tablets (Less than 1%) ... 1196
Bentyl ... 1322
Cantil Tablets ... 1326
Cardioquin Tablets ... 1812
Clozaril Tablets (Less than 1%) ... 2000
Cocaine Hydrochloride Topical Solution ... 620
Cogentin ... 1435
Compazine ... 2201
Darbid Tablets ... 2205
Ditropan ... 1332
Donnatal ... 1858
Donnatal Extentabs ... 1859
Donnatal Tablets ... 1858
Donnazyme Tablets ... 1860
Dopram Injectable ... 1860
Elavil ... 2269
Endep Tablets ... 1927
Etrafon ... 2087
Inversine Tablets ... 1492
IOPIDINE (0.4%) ... ⊙ 232
Kemadrin Tablets ... 771
Kinesed Tablets ... 2272
Kutrase Capsules ... 2146
Larodopa Tablets (Infrequent) ... 1905
Levsin/Levsinex ... 2147
Limbitrol Tablets ... 1933
Lioresal Tablets ... 1031
Ludiomil Tablets (Rare) ... 874
Metimyd ... ⊙ 306
Naphcon Forte ... ⊙ 226
Naphcon-A Ophthalmic Solution ... 571
Navane Capsules and Concentrate 1954
Navane Intramuscular ... 1956
Norflex ... 1314
Norgesic ... 1314
Opcon-A Ophthalmic Solution ... ⊙ 262
Pamelor ... 2019
Pro-Banthīne Tablets ... 2141
Propine with C Cap Compliance Cap (Infrequent) ... ⊙ 255
Proventil Syrup (Less than 1%) ... 2119
Prozac Pulvules (Infrequent) ... 920
Quarzan Capsules ... 1937
Quinaglute Dura-Tabs Tablets ... 663
Quinidex Extentabs ... 1868
Robinul Forte Tablets ... 1873
Robinul Injectable ... 1873
Robinul Tablets ... 1873
Ru-Tuss with Hydrocodone ... 694
Ru-Tuss Tablets ... 693
Sinemet Tablets ... 952
Soma Compound w/Codeine Tablets (Very rare) ... 2390
Soma Compound Tablets (Very rare) ... 2389
Soma Tablets ... 2388
Stelazine ... 2226
Surmontil Capsules ... 2524
Tenuate ... 1354
Thorazine ... 2234
Tofranil Ampuls ... 1038
Tofranil Tablets ... 1039
Tofranil-PM Capsules ... 1041
Transderm Scōp Transdermal Therapeutic System ... 887
Triavil Tablets ... 1556
Trilafon (Occasional) ... 2123
Trinalin Repetabs Tablets ... 1170
Tropicacyl ... ⊙ 209
Valpin 50 Tablets ... 941
Vasocidin Ointment (Occasional) ⊙ 275
Vasocidin Ophthalmic Solution (Occasional) ... ⊙ 276
Vasocon-A ... ⊙ 278
Ventolin Syrup (Less than 1 of 100 patients) ... 583
Vivactil Tablets ... 1567
Wellbutrin Tablets (Infrequent) ... 821

Myelitis

Omnipaque (Rare) ... 2552
Permax Tablets (Rare) ... 1291
Recombivax HB ... 1544

Myelitis, transverse

Azulfidine Tablets, EN-tabs, Oral Suspension (Rare) ... 1157
Engerix-B Unit-Dose Vials ... 2213
Recombivax HB ... 1544

Myelofibrosis

Mexitil Capsules (About 2 in 10,000) ... 680

Myeloproliferative syndrome

Alkeran Tablets ... 754

Myelosuppression

Adriamycin PFS ... 561
Adriamycin RDF ... 562
▲BiCNU (Most frequent) ... 723
CeeNU ... 725
▲Cerubidine (All patients) ... 2443
Cytosar-U Sterile Powder ... 2329
Doxorubicin Hydrochloride for Injection, USP ... 622
Doxorubicin Hydrochloride Injection, USP ... 848
Hexalen Capsules ... 2316
Idamycin for Injection ... 564
IFEX ... 729
Mutamycin ... 733
Myleran Tablets ... 790
Novantrone for Injection Concentrate ... 1226
▲Platinol (25 to 30%) ... 737
▲Platinol-AQ Injection (25% to 30% of patients) ... 738
Purinethol Tablets ... 800
Roferon-A Injection (Rare) ... 1916
▲Thioguanine Tablets, Tabloid Brand (Most frequent) ... 815
Velban Vials ... 1305
VePesid Capsules and Injection ... 741

Myelosuppression, persistent severe

Adriamycin PFS ... 561
Doxorubicin Hydrochloride Injection, USP ... 848
Novantrone for Injection Concentrate ... 1226
Rubex ... 739

Myocardial failure

Protamine Sulfate Ampoules & Vials ... 1295

Myocardial infarction

Actimmune (Rare) ... 1046
▲Adalat Capsules (10 mg and 20 mg) (About 4%) ... 1587
Altace Capsules (Less than 1%) ... 1086
Anafranil Capsules (Rare) ... 650
Ansaid Tablets (Less than 1%) ... 2319
Apresoline Hydrochloride Parenteral (Ampuls) ... 856
Asendin Tablets (Very rare) ... 1196
Blenoxane (Rare) ... 724
Brevicon ... 2304
BuSpar (Rare) ... 1401
Calan SR Caplets (1% or less) ... 2157
Calan Tablets (1% or less) ... 2155
Calciparine Injection ... 925
Capoten (2 to 3 of 1000 patients) 2255
Capozide (2 to 3 of 1000 patients) ... 2258
Cardene Capsules (Less than 0.4%) ... 2290
Cardizem Tablets-30 mg, 60 mg, 90 mg and 120 mg ... 1329
Cardura Tablets (Less than 0.5% of 3960 patients) ... 1941
Cipro I.V. (1% or less) ... 1592
Cipro Tablets (Less than 1%) ... 1589
Clozaril Tablets ... 2000
DDAVP Injection (Rare) ... 1840
Demulen ... 2161
Desyrel and Desyrel Dividose ... 1404
Diapid Nasal Spray ... 2003
DynaCirc Capsules (0.5% to 1%) .. 2004
Elavil ... 2269
▲Emcyt Capsules (3%) ... 1161
Endep Tablets ... 1927
Enovid ... 2161
Epogen for Injection (0.4%) ... 591
Ergotrate Maleate Ampoules (Rare) ... 1263

Estrace 1385
Estrace Vaginal Cream 1388
Estradurin 2452
Estratest 2245
Ethmozine Tablets (Less than 2%) 946
Etrafon 2087
Flexeril Tablets (Rare) 1471
Heparin Lock Flush Solution 2456
Heparin Sodium Vials 1264
Heparin Sodium Injection 2457
Heparin Sodium Injection, USP, Sterile Solution 2342
Hyperstat I.V. Injection 2095
Idamycin for Injection 564
Isoptin Oral Tablets (Less than 1%) 1179
Isoptin SR Sustained Release Tablets (Less than 1%) 1181
Jenest-28 Tablets 1636
Kerlone Tablets (Less than 2%) 2172
Levlen/Tri-Levlen 665
Limbitrol 1933
Lodine Capsules (Less than 1%) 2468
Lo/Ovral Tablets 2471
Lo/Ovral-28 Tablets 2476
Loestrin 1728
Ludiomil Tablets 874
▲Lupron Depot 3.75 mg (Among most frequent) 2312
Lupron Depot 7.5 mg 2311
Lupron Injection (Less than 5%) 2310
Micronor Tablets 1667
Modicon 1667
Monopril Tablets (0.2 to 1.0%) 1406
Mydfrin 2.5% ⊛ 224
Nicorette 1335
Nordette-21 Tablets 2481
Nordette-28 Tablets 2483
Norethin 2133
Norinyl 2304
Norlestrin 1746
Normodyne Injection 2108
Norpramin Tablets 1340
Nor-Q D Tablets 2304
Nuromax Injection 794
Omnipaque 2552
Oncovin Solution Vials & Hyporets 1288
OptiPranolol Sterile Ophthalmic Solution (A small number of patients) ⊛ 261
Ortho Dienestrol Cream 1664
Ortho-Cyclen Tablets 1658
Ortho-Novum 1667
Orudis Capsules (Less than 1%) 2488
Ovcon 1391
Ovral Tablets 2490
Ovral-28 Tablets 2491
Ovrette Tablets 2492
PMB 200 and PMB 400 2504
Pamelor 2019
Parlodel (3 cases) 2020
Permax Tablets (1.1%) 1291
Platinol (Rare) 737
Platinol-AQ Injection (Rare) 738
Plendil Extended-Release Tablets (0.5% to 1.5%) 1526
Premarin Intravenous 2508
Premarin with Methyltestosterone 2515
Premarin Tablets 2510
Premarin Vaginal Cream 2512
Prinivil Tablets (1% or less) 1538
Prinzide Tablets 1540
▲Procardia Capsules (4%) 1781
Procardia XL Tablets (About 1 patient in 15) 1783
Procrit for Injection (0.4%) 1647
Prozac Pulvules (Rare) 920
Roferon-A Injection (Less than 1%) 1916
Sandimmune (Rare) 2024
Sinemet CR Tablets 953
Stilphostrol Tablets and Ampuls 1609
Surmontil Capsules 2524
TACE 12 and 25 mg 1353
Tegretol 654
Tenex Tablets 1875
Tofranil Ampuls 1038
Tofranil Tablets 1039
Tofranil-PM Capsules 1041
Tonocard Tablets (Less than 1%) 1554
Triavil Tablets 1556
Levlen/Tri-Levlen 665
Tri-Norinyl 2304
Triphasil-21 Tablets 2527
Triphasil-28 Tablets 2532
Vascor (200, 300 and 400 mg) Tablets (About 3% of patients) 1383
Vaseretic Tablets 1559
Vasotec I.V. (0.5 to 1%) 1562
Vasotec Tablets (0.5% to 1%) 1564
Velban Vials 1305
Verelan Capsules (Less than 1%) 1243
Vivactil Tablets 1567
Voltaren Tablets (Less than 1%) 1042
Wellbutrin Tablets (Rare) 821
Zestoretic 2274
Zestril Tablets 2277
Zoladex (1% to 5%) 1110

Myocardial insufficiency

Idamycin for Injection 564

Myocardial necrosis

Cytoxan for Injection 726

Myocardial rupture, following recent MI

Cortone Acetate Sterile Suspension 1437
Cortone Acetate Tablets 1439
Decadron Elixir 1445
Decadron Phosphate Injection 1449
Decadron Phosphate Respihaler 1454
Decadron Phosphate Turbinaire 1456
Decadron Phosphate with Xylocaine Injection, Sterile 1451
Decadron Tablets 1447
Decadron-LA Sterile Suspension 1457
Hydeltrasol Injection, Sterile 1476
Hydeltra-T.B.A. Sterile Suspension 1478
Hydrocortone Acetate Sterile Suspension 1479
Hydrocortone Phosphate Injection, Sterile 1481
Hydrocortone Tablets 1482

Myocarditis

Aldoclor Tablets 1413
Aldomet Ester HCl Injection 1417
Aldomet Oral 1415
Aldoril Tablets 1418
Atgam Sterile Solution (At least 1 patient and less than 5% of total patients) 2320
Cerubidine (Rare) 2443
Gantrisin 1901

Myocarditis, allergic

Azo Gantanol Tablets 1887
Azo Gantrisin Tablets 1888
Azulfidine Tablets, EN-tabs, Oral Suspension 1157
Bactrim DS Tablets 1891
Bactrim I.V. Infusion 1889
Bactrim 1891
Fansidar Tablets 1896
Gantanol 1899
Gantrisin Ophthalmic Ointment/Solution 1900
Pediazole 1973
Septra 813
Septra I.V. Infusion 808
Septra I.V. Infusion ADD-Vantage Vials 810
Septra 813
Thiosulfil Forte Tablets 2526

Myocarditis, hemorrhagic

Cytoxan for Injection 726
Neosar for Injection 566

Myocarditis, interstitial

Butazolidin Capsules & Tablets (Less than 1%) 1027

Myocardium, depression

Carbocaine Hydrochloride 3% Injection 956
Carbocaine Hydrochloride Injection 2043
Carbocaine Hydrochloride 2% with Neo-Cobefrin 956
Decadron Phosphate with Xylocaine Injection, Sterile 1451
Marcaine Hydrochloride 0.5% with Epinephrine 1:200,000 (as bitartrate) 958
Marcaine Hydrochloride with Epinephrine 1:200,000 2055
Marcaine Hydrochloride Injection 2055
Marcaine Spinal 2058
Nesacaine Injections 629
Normodyne Tablets 2110
Novocain Hydrochloride for Spinal Anesthesia 2065
Pontocaine Hydrochloride for Spinal Anesthesia 2069
Sensorcaine 631
Sensorcaine-MPF Spinal 634

Myoclonia

▲Anafranil Capsules (2% to 13%) 650
Clozaril Tablets (1%) 2000
Diprivan Injection (Greater than 1%) 2267
Eldepryl 2250
Infumorph 200 and Infumorph 500 Sterile Solutions 962
Nardil (Common) 1742
Noroxin Tablets 1519
Omnipaque (Unusual) 2552
Permax Tablets (Infrequent) 1291
Primaxin I.M. 1532
Primaxin I.V. (Less than 0.2%) 1535
Prozac Pulvules (Rare) 920
Wellbutrin Tablets (Frequent) 821

Myoglobinemia

Anectine Injection 755

Myoglobinuria

Amicar Syrup, Tablets, and Injection (Rare) 1194
Anectine 755
Orap Tablets 1020

Myopathy

Amicar Syrup, Tablets, and Injection (Occasional) 1194
Anafranil Capsules (Rare) 650
Atromid-S Capsules 2435
Celestone Soluspan Suspension 2081
Colchicine Ampoules 1252
Cortenema 2244
Cortone Acetate Tablets 1439
Dalalone D.P. Injectable 999
Darvon-N/Darvocet-N 1254
Darvon 1256
Darvon-N Suspension & Tablets 1254
Decadron Phosphate Respihaler 1454
Decadron Phosphate Turbinaire 1456
Depo-Medrol Sterile Aqueous Suspension 2334
Hydeltrasol Injection, Sterile 1476
Intal Inhaler (Infrequent) 979
Lopid Capsules and Tablets 1736
Medrol 2348
Mevacor Tablets (0.5%) 1505
Normodyne Tablets 2110
Normozide Tablets 2112
Pediapred Oral Liquid 987
Retrovir Capsules 802
Retrovir I.V. Infusion 805
Retrovir Syrup 802
Rifadin (Rare) 1345
Solu-Cortef Sterile Powder 2361
Solu-Medrol Sterile Powder 2363
Trandate HCT/Trandate 579
Zyloprim Tablets (Less than 1%) 830

Myopathy, steroid

Aristocort Suspension 1008
Aristospan Suspension 1011
Cortone Acetate Sterile Suspension 1437
Decadron Elixir 1445
Decadron Phosphate Injection 1449
Decadron Phosphate with Xylocaine Injection, Sterile 1451
Decadron Tablets 1447
Decadron-LA Sterile Suspension 1457
Deltasone Tablets 2332
Hydeltra-T.B.A. Sterile Suspension 1478
Hydrocortone Acetate Sterile Suspension 1479
Hydrocortone Phosphate Injection, Sterile 1481
Hydrocortone Tablets 1482
Kenalog-10 Injection 2402
Kenalog-40 Injection 2403

Myopia

Floropryl Sterile Ophthalmic Ointment 1473
Humorsol Sterile Ophthalmic Solution 1475
Isopto Carpine ⊛ 219
Phospholine Iodide ⊛ 315
Pilocar ⊛ 275
Pilopine HS Gel ⊛ 227
Pilostat Sterile Ophthalmic Solution 0.5%, 1%, 2%, 3%, 4%, 5%, 6% ⊛ 263
Zarontin Capsules 1768
Zarontin Syrup 1769

Myopia, transient

Combipres Tablets (Occasional) 678
Diamox Parenteral 1200
Diamox Sequels (Sustained Release) 1201
Diamox Tablets 1200

Myosis

Etrafon 2087
Trilafon 2123

Myositis

Anafranil Capsules (Rare) 650
Atromid-S Capsules 2435
Inocor Lactate Injection (1 case) 2048
Lopid Capsules and Tablets 1736
Permax Tablets (Infrequent) 1291
Prozac Pulvules (Rare) 920

Myxedema

Cibalith-S 870
Eskalith 2214
Lithane Tablets 1596
Lithium Carbonate Capsules & Tablets 1984
Lithobid Tablets 870
Quadrinal Tablets 1183

N

Nails, changes

Accutane Capsules (Less than 1%) 1878
Ansaid Tablets (Less than 1%) 2319
Blenoxane 724
BuSpar (Rare) 1401
Cytoxan for Injection 726
Ergamisol Tablets 1136
Sterile FUDR (Remote possibility) 1898
Fluorouracil Injection 1897
Intron A (Less than 1%) 2097
Neosar for Injection 566
▲Tegison Capsules (10-25%) 1881
Teslac Tablets 741

Nails, discoloration

Retrovir Capsules 802
Retrovir I.V. Infusion 805
Retrovir Syrup 802

Nails, loss of

Sterile FUDR (Remote possibility) 1898
Fluorouracil Injection 1897

Nasal burning

▲Beconase Inhalation Aerosol & Refill (11 in 100 patients) 574
Intal Inhaler (Rare) 979
Intal Nebulizer Solution 980
IOPIDINE ⊛ 232
Nasacort Nasal Inhaler (Rare) 1844
▲Nasalcrom Nasal Solution (1 in 25) 986
▲Nasalide Nasal Solution 0.025% (Approximately 45%) 2299
▲Vancenase Nasal Inhaler (11 per 100 patients) 2126

Nasal congestion

▲Adalat Capsules (10 mg and 20 mg) (2% or less to 6%) 1587
▲AeroBid Inhaler System (15%) 995
Aldoclor Tablets 1413
Aldomet Ester HCl Injection 1417
Aldomet Oral 1415
Aldoril Tablets 1418
Apresazide Capsules (Less frequent) 854
Apresoline Hydrochloride Parenteral (Ampuls) 856
Apresoline Hydrochloride Tablets (Less frequent) 855
Apresoline-Esidrix Tablets 857
Azactam for Injection (Less than 1%) 2252
Bentyl 1322
Brevibloc Injection (Less than 1%) 942
BuSpar (Frequent) 1401
Cardizem Tablets-30 mg, 60 mg, 90 mg and 120 mg (Less than 1%) 1329
Cardizem SR Capsules-60 mg, 90 mg and 120 mg (Less than 1%) 1327
Cartrol Tablets (1.1%) 507
▲CHEMET (succimer) Capsules (0.7 to 3.7%) 1361
Cibacalcin Double-chambered Syringes (Rare) 859
Clozaril Tablets (1%) 2000
Comhist LA Capsules 1618
Compazine 2201
Corgard Tablets (1 to 5 of 1000 patients) 701
DDAVP (Occasional) 1841
Danocrine Capsules (Rare) 2046
Darbid Tablets 2205
Deconamine 663
Demser Capsules (Infrequent) 1460

Desyrel and Desyrel Dividose ... 1404
Diapid Nasal Spray (Infrequent) ... 2003
Dibenzyline Capsules ... 2207
Diupres Tablets ... 1461
Enduronyl ... 518
Esimil Tablets ... 864
Etrafon ... 2087
Fiorinal with Codeine Capsules (Infrequent) ... 2008
Flagyl I.V. ... 2131
Flagyl Tablets ... 2170
Harmonyl Tablets ... 528
Hydromox R Tablets ... 1209
Hydropres Tablets ... 1485
Hyskon Hysteroscopy Fluid (Rare) .. 1162
▲ Hytrin Tablets (0.6% to 5.9%) ... 529
Intal Capsules (Less than 1 in 10,000 patients) ... 978
Intal Inhaler (Infrequent) ... 979
Intal Nebulizer Solution ... 980
▲ Intron A (Up to 10%) ... 2097
Ismelin Tablets ... 869
Limbitrol (Less common) ... 1933
Lioresal Tablets ... 1031
Loxitane ... 1213
Ludiomil Tablets ... 874
Mellaril ... 2011
Methergine (Rare) ... 2016
Midamor Tablets (Less than or equal to 1%) ... 1508
Minipress Capsules (1-4%) ... 1778
Minizide Capsules ... 1779
Moduretic Tablets (Less than or equal to 1%) ... 1510
Nasalcrom Nasal Solution (Less than 1%) ... 986
Nasalide Nasal Solution 0.025% (5% or less) ... 2299
Navane Capsules and Concentrate 1954
Navane Intramuscular ... 1956
Omnipaque ... 2552
Optimine Tablets ... 2115
Oreticyl ... 545
Ornade Spansule Capsules ... 2221
▲ Parlodel (3-4%) ... 2020
Pentaspan Injection ... 949
Periactin ... 1525
Polaramine ... 2116
Prinivil Tablets (0.3%) ... 1538
Prinzide Tablets (0.3% to 1%) ... 1540
Procardia Capsules (2%) ... 1781
▲ Procardia XL Tablets (6%) ... 1783
Prolixin Decanoate ... 1795
Prolixin Elixir ... 1793
Prolixin Enanthate ... 1796
Prolixin Injection ... 1791
Prolixin Oral Concentrate ... 1792
Prolixin Tablets ... 1793
Protostat Tablets ... 1674
Proventil Solutions for Inhalation 0.5% and 0.083% (1%) ... 2118
Prozac Pulvules (2.6%) ... 920
Raudixin Tablets ... 1803
Rauzide Tablets ... 1804
Regitine ... 878
▲ Renese-R Tablets (Frequent) ... 1786
Robaxin Injectable ... 1871
Robaxin Tablets ... 1872
Salutensin/Salutensin-Demi ... 719
Ser-Ap-Es Tablets ... 881
Serentil ... 686
Serpasil Tablets ... 883
Serpasil-Apresoline Tablets ... 884
Serpasil-Esidrix Tablets ... 886
Stelazine ... 2226
Tacaryl ... 2409
Tavist Syrup ... 2033
Tavist Tablets ... 2035
Tavist-D Tablets ... 2035
Tessalon Perles ... 1006
Thorazine ... 2234
Timoptic in Ocudose ... 1552
Timoptic Sterile Ophthalmic Solution ... 1550
Trental (Less than 1%) ... 1099
Trexan Tablets (Less than 1%) ... 937
Triaminic Expectorant DH ... 1995
Triaminic Oral Infant Drops ... 1996
Trilafon (Occasional) ... 2123
Ventolin (2%) ... 583
Wytensin Tablets (3% or less) ... 2542
▲ Xanax Tablets (7.3% to 17.4%) ... 2367
Zestoretic (0.3 to 1%) ... 2274
Zestril Tablets (0.3%) ... 2277

Nasal drainage

Alferon N Injection (2%) ... 1809

Nasal itching (see under Pruritus, rhinal)

Nasal mucosa, dryness (see under Xeromycteria)

Nasal septum, perforation

Beconase AQ Nasal Spray (Extremely rare) ... 574
Beconase Inhalation Aerosol & Refill (Extremely rare) ... 574
Decadron Phosphate Turbinaire ... 1456
Nasalide Nasal Solution 0.025% (Rare) ... 2299
Vancenase AQ Nasal Spray 0.042% (Extremely rare) ... 2127
Vancenase Nasal Inhaler (Extremely rare) ... 2126

Nasal stinging

Nasacort Nasal Inhaler (Rare) ... 1844
▲ Nasalcrom Nasal Solution (1 in 20) ... 986

Nasal stuffiness

Actifed with Codeine Cough Syrup.. 752
Amicar Syrup, Tablets, and Injection (Occasional) ... 1194
Asendin Tablets (Less than 1%) ... 1196
Beconase AQ Nasal Spray (Fewer than 3 per 100 patients) ... 574
Benadryl Capsules ... 1691
Benadryl Injection ... 1692
Bentyl ... 1322
Bretylol Injection (1 in 1000) ... 923
Corzide Tablets (1 to 5 of 1000 patients) ... 702
Loxitane ... 1213
▲ Normodyne Injection (1 to 6%) ... 2108
▲ Normodyne Tablets (1% to 6%) ... 2110
▲ Normozide Tablets (3%) ... 2112
PBZ Tablets & Elixir ... 1037
PBZ-SR Tablets ... 1037
Phenergan Injection ... 2493
Phenergan Tablets ... 2496
Ru-Tuss II Capsules ... 693
Taractan (Occasional) ... 1920
Temaril Tablets, Syrup and Spansule Sustained Release Capsules ... 1085
▲ Trandate HCT Tablets (3%) ... 579
Trandate Injection ... 577
▲ Trandate Tablets (3% of 227 patients) ... 579
Trinalin Repetabs Tablets ... 1170
Vancenase AQ Nasal Spray 0.042% (Fewer than 3 per 100 patients) ... 2127

Nasal ulceration

Beconase AQ Nasal Spray (Rare) ... 574
Beconase Inhalation Aerosol & Refill (Rare) ... 574
Diapid Nasal Spray (Infrequent) ... 2003
Vancenase Nasal Inhaler (Rare) ... 2126

Nasolacrimal canals, obstruction

Floropryl Sterile Ophthalmic Ointment ... 1473
Humorsol Sterile Ophthalmic Solution ... 1475
Phospholine Iodide ... ⊙ 315

Nasopharyngitis

Nalfon Pulvules & Tablets (1.2%).. 919

Nausea

Abbokinase ... 503
Abbokinase Open-Cath ... 505
Accutane Capsules ... 1878
Achromycin V Capsules ... 1193
Actibine ... 900
Actifed with Codeine Cough Syrup.. 752
Actigall Capsules ... 2280
▲ Actimmune (10%) ... 1046
Activase ... 1047
▲ Adalat Capsules (10 mg and 20 mg) (About 10% to 11%) ... 1587
▲ Adenocard Injection (3%) ... 1007
▲ Adriamycin RDF (Frequent) ... 562
▲ AeroBid Inhaler System (25%) ... 995
Aerolate ... 994
AK-Fluor Injection 10% and 25% ... ⊙ 204
Albalon Solution with Liquifilm ... ⊙ 238
Albuminar-5, Albumin (Human) U.S.P. 5% ... 608
Albuminar-25, Albumin (Human) U.S.P. 25% ... 608
Aldactazide ... 2150
Aldoclor Tablets ... 1413
Aldomet Ester HCl Injection ... 1417
Aldomet Oral ... 1415
Aldoril Tablets ... 1418
▲ Alfenta Injection (28%) ... 1131
▲ Alferon N Injection (4% to 48%) ... 1809
▲ Alka-Seltzer Effervescent Antacid and Pain Reliever (7.6% at doses of 1000 mg/day) ... 1568
▲ Alka-Seltzer (Flavored) Effervescent Antacid and Pain Reliever (7.6% at doses of 1000 mg/day) ... 1569
Alkeran Tablets (Infrequent) ... 754
Allbee C-800 Plus Iron Tablets ... ▣ 670
Altace Capsules (1.1%) ... 1086
Alupent (1 to 4%) ... 674
Alurate Elixir (Less than 1 in 100) 1883
Amen (Rare) ... 833
Amicar Syrup, Tablets, and Injection (Occasional) ... 1194
Amikin Injectable (Rare) ... 602
Aminohippurate Sodium Injection .. 1421
Aminophyllin Tablets ... 2153
Amoxil ... 2193
Anadrol-50 Tablets ... 2287
▲ Anafranil Capsules (9% to 33%) ... 650
Ana-Kit Anaphylaxis Emergency Treatment Kit ... 1100
▲ Anaprox and Anaprox DS Tablets (3-9%) ... 2288
Anatuss LA Tablets ... 1359
Ancef Injection (Rare) ... 2194
Ancobon Capsules ... 1886
Android ... 1111
▲ Anexsia 5/500 Tablets (Among most frequent) ... 2196
▲ Anexsia 7.5/650 Tablets (Among most frequent) ... 2197
▲ Ansaid Tablets (3-9%) ... 2319
Antabuse Tablets ... 2429
Antilirium Injectable ... 998
Antivenin (Crotalidae) Polyvalent ... 2430
Apresazide Capsules (Common) ... 854
Apresoline Hydrochloride Parenteral (Ampuls) ... 856
Apresoline Hydrochloride Tablets (Common) ... 855
Apresoline-Esidrix Tablets ... 857
Aralen Hydrochloride Injection ... 2038
Aralen Phosphate with Primaquine Phosphate Tablets ... 2040
Aralen Phosphate Tablets ... 2039
Arfonad Ampuls ... 1887
Arm-a-Med Isoetharine Inhalation Solution, USP ... 616
Arm-a-Med Metaproterenol Sulfate Inhalation Solution, USP (1 in 50 patients) ... 617
▲ Artane (30% to 50%) ... 1195
Asbron G ... 1997
Asendin Tablets (Greater than 1%) ... 1196
Astramorph/PF Injection, USP (Preservative-Free) (Frequent) ... 618
Atabrine Hydrochloride Tablets ... 2041
▲ Atgam Sterile Solution (1 patient in 15; more than 1% to 10%) ... 2320
Ativan Injection (Occasional) ... 2432
Ativan Tablets (Less frequent) ... 2434
Atrohist Sprinkle Capsules ... 558
▲ Atromid-S Capsules (Most common) ... 2435
Atrovent Inhalation Aerosol (2.8%) ... 675
▲ Augmentin Tablets, Powder for Oral Suspension, and Chewable Tablets (3%) ... 2198
Axid Pulvules ... 1246
Azactam for Injection (1-1.3%) ... 2252
▲ Azdōne Tablets (Among most frequent) ... 844
Azo Gantanol Tablets ... 1887
Azo Gantrisin Tablets ... 1888
▲ Azulfidine Tablets, EN-tabs, Oral Suspension (Approximately one-third of patients) ... 1157
BAL in Oil Ampules ... 661
B & O No. 15A & No. 16A Supprettes ... 2395
▲ Bactrim DS Tablets (Among most common) ... 1891
▲ Bactrim I.V. Infusion (Among most common) ... 1889
▲ Bactrim (Among most common) ... 1891
Bactroban Ointment (Less than 1%) ... 2200
Baron-X Tablets ... 650
▲ Genuine Bayer Aspirin Tablets & Caplets (7.3% at doses of 1000 mg/day) ... ▣ 564
▲ Bayer Plus Aspirin Tablets (7.6% of 4500 people treated) .. ▣ 567
▲ Therapy Bayer Aspirin Caplets (7.6% of 4500 people tested) ... ▣ 568
▲ Beconase AQ Nasal Spray (5 in 100 patients) ... 574
Benadryl Capsules ... 1691
Benadryl Injection ... 1692
Benemid Tablets ... 1426
▲ Bentyl (14%) ... 1322
Betagan ... ⊙ 239
Biavax II ... 1427
BiCNU (Frequent) ... 723
Biltricide ... 1589
Blocadren Tablets (0.6%) ... 1429
Bontril Slow-Release ... 834
Brethaire Inhaler ... 1024
Brethine Ampuls (1.3 to 3.9%) ... 1026
Brethine Tablets ... 1026
▲ Bretylol Injection (3%) ... 923
▲ Brevibloc Injection (7%) ... 942
Brevicon ... 2304
Brevital Sodium Vials ... 1248
Brexin L.A. Capsules ... 2078
Bricanyl Injection ... 1324
Bricanyl Tablets ... 1325
Bromfed ... 1615
Bronkephrine Injection ... 2042
Bronkometer Aerosol ... 2042
Bronkosol Solution ... 2042
▲ Bufferin Analgesic Tablets and Caplets (7.6%) ... 743
Bumex (0.6%) ... 1895
▲ BuSpar (8%) ... 1401
Butazolidin Capsules & Tablets (Greater than 1%) ... 1027
Butisol Sodium Elixir & Tablets (Less than 1 in 100) ... 2377
Cafergot/Cafergot P-B ... 1999
Calan SR Caplets (2.7%) ... 2157
Calan Tablets (2.7%) ... 2155
Calcidrine Syrup ... 506
Calcijex Calcitriol Injection ... 506
▲ Calcimar Injection, Synthetic (10%) ... 1839
Calciparine Injection (Rare) ... 925
Calderol Capsules ... 1635
Cantil Tablets ... 1326
Capoten (0.5 to 2%) ... 2255
Capozide (0.5 to 2%) ... 2258
Carafate Tablets (Less than 0.5%) 1326
Carbocaine Hydrochloride Injection 2043
Cardene Capsules (1.9-2.2%) ... 2290
Cardilate Oral/Sublingual Tablets .. 757
Cardioquin Tablets ... 1812
Cardizem Tablets-30 mg, 60 mg, 90 mg and 120 mg (1.9%) ... 1329
Cardizem SR Capsules-60 mg, 90 mg and 120 mg (1.3-1.6%) ... 1327
▲ Cardura Tablets (3%) ... 1941
Carnitor ... 2188
Cartrol Tablets (0.4-2.1%) ... 507
Catapres Tablets (About 5 in 100 patients) ... 676
▲ Catapres-TTS (5%) ... 677
Ceclor Pulvules & Suspension (Rare) ... 1251
CeeNU ... 725
Cefizox Injection (Occasional) ... 1012
Cefobid Intravenous/Intramuscular (Rare) ... 1943
Cefobid Pharmacy Bulk Package - Not for Direct Infusion (Rare) ... 1945
Cefotan (1 in 700) ... 2265
Ceftin Tablets (2.4%) ... 575
Celontin (Frequent) ... 1692
Cephulac Syrup ... 1331
Ceptaz for Injection (One in 156 patients) ... 1057
Ceredase Injection ... 1052
Cerubidine ... 2443
▲ CHEMET (succimer) Capsules (12-20.9%) ... 1361
▲ Children's Advil Suspension (Up to 9%) ... 2426
Chloromycetin Kapseals ... 1695
Chloromycetin Palmitate, Oral Suspension ... 1697
Chloromycetin Sodium Succinate ... 1698
Choledyl Pediatric Elixir ... 1702
Choledyl Tablets ... 1700
Choledyl SA Tablets ... 1704
Cholybar (Less frequent) ... 1705
Chromagen Capsules ... 2078
Chronulac Syrup ... 1332
▲ Cibacalcin Double-chambered Syringes (14-21%) ... 859
Cibalith-S ... 870
Ciloxan Sterile Ophthalmic Solution (Less than 1%) ... ⊙ 214
▲ Cipro I.V. (Among most frequent) .. 1592

(▣ Described in PDR For Nonprescription Drugs) Incidence data in parenthesis; ▲ 3% or more (⊙ Described in PDR For Ophthalmology)

▲ Cipro Tablets (5.2%) 1589
Claforan Sterile Injection (1.4%) 1089
Cleocin HCl Capsules 2322
Cleocin Pediatric Flavored Granules 2324
Cleocin Phosphate Injection 2325
▲ Clinoril Tablets (3-9%) 1433
▲ Clozaril Tablets (More than 5%) 2000
Codiclear DH Syrup 845
Codimal 846
Cogentin 1435
Colace (Exceedingly small) 1403
ColBENEMID Tablets 1436
Colchicine Ampoules 1252
Colestid Granules (1 in 30 to 1 in 100 patients) 2328
Colyte 1826
▲ Combipres Tablets (About 5%) 678
Comhist LA Capsules 1618
Compazine 2201
Constant-T Tablets 1029
▲ Cordarone Tablets (10 to 33%) 2446
Corgard Tablets (1 to 5 of 1000 patients) 701
Cortone Acetate Sterile Suspension 1437
Cortone Acetate Tablets 1439
Corzide Tablets (1 to 5 of 1000 patients) 702
Cosmegen Injection (Common) 1440
Coumadin Injection & Tablets (Infrequent) 944
▲ Creon Capsules (Among most frequent) 2245
Crystodigin Tablets 1253
Cuprimine Capsules (Greater than 1%) 1442
Cycrin Tablets 2449
Cyklokapron Tablets and Injection 1159
Cylert Tablets 510
▲ Cytadren Tablets (1 in 8) 861
▲ CytoGam (Less than 5.0%) 891
▲ Cytosar-U Sterile Powder (Among most frequent) 2329
Cytotec (3.2%) 2159
Cytovene Sterile Powder (1% or less) 2292
Cytoxan for Injection 726
DDAVP Injection (Infrequent) 1840
DDAVP (Up to 2%) 1841
D.H.E. 45 Injection 2003
▲ DTIC-Dome (90% with the initial few doses) 1595
Dalalone D.P. Injectable 999
▲ Dalgan Injection (3 to 9%) 620
Dalmane Capsules 1927
▲ Damason-P (Among most frequent) 1356
Danocrine Capsules 2046
Dapsone USP 1130
Daranide Tablets (Among the most common effects) 1445
Darbid Tablets 2205
▲ Darvon-N/Darvocet-N (Among most frequent) 1254
▲ Darvon (Among most frequent) 1256
▲ Darvon-N Suspension & Tablets (Among most frequent) 1254
Decadron Elixir 1445
Decadron Phosphate Injection 1449
Decadron Phosphate Respihaler 1454
Decadron Phosphate Turbinaire 1456
Decadron Phosphate with Xylocaine Injection, Sterile 1451
Decadron Tablets 1447
Decadron-LA Sterile Suspension 1457
Declomycin Capsules, Tablets 1199
Deconamine 663
Deconsal 559
Demerol 2047
Demser Capsules (Infrequent) 1460
▲ Demulen (Among most common) 2161
▲ Depakene Capsules & Syrup (Among most common) 511
▲ Depakote (Among most common) 512
▲ Depen Titratable Tablets (17%) 2379
Depo-Provera Sterile Aqueous Suspension (Rare) 2336
Deprol Tablets 2382
Desyrel and Desyrel Dividose (Greater than 1%) 1404
DiaBeta (1.8%) 1091
▲ Diabinese Tablets (Less than 5%) 1775
Diamox Parenteral 1200
Diamox Sequels (Sustained Release) 1201
Diamox Tablets 1200
Dicumarol Tablets (Infrequent) 516
Didrex Tablets 2338
Didronel Tablets 1621
Diethylstilbestrol Tablets 1258
▲ Diflucan Injection and Tablets (3.7% in 4048 patients) 1948
Dilantin Infatabs 1710
Dilantin Kapseals 1708
Dilantin Parenteral 1712
Dilantin-30 Pediatric/Dilantin-125 Suspension 1713
Dilantin with Phenobarbital Kapseals 1715
Dilatrate-SR (Uncommon) 1827
Dilaudid Cough Syrup 1174
Dilaudid 1173
Dilaudid-HP Injection 1175
Dilor 2079
Dilor-G Tablets & Liquid 2079
Dimacol Caplets ⊡ 672
Dimetane-DC Cough Syrup 1857
Dimetane-DX Cough Syrup 1858
▲ Dipentum Capsules (Up to 5%) 1160
▲ Diprivan Injection (10% or greater) 2267
Disalcid (Occasional) 1310
Ditropan 1332
Diucardin Tablets 2450
Diulo 2129
Diupres Tablets 1461
Diuril Oral Suspension 1464
Diuril Sodium Intravenous 1463
Diuril Tablets 1464
Dobutrex Solution Vials (1 to 3%) 1259
▲ Dolobid Tablets (3% to 9%) 1465
▲ Dolophine Hydrochloride Ampoules & Vials (Among most frequent) 1260
▲ Dolophine Hydrochloride Tablets (Among most frequent) 1261
Donnatal 1858
Donnatal Extentabs 1859
Donnatal Tablets 1858
Donnazyme Tablets 1860
Dopram Injectable 1860
Doral Tablets 2383
Dorcol Children's Decongestant Liquid ⊡ 685
Doryx Capsules 1717
Doxorubicin Hydrochloride for Injection, USP 622
▲ Duragesic Transdermal System (10% or more) 1133
Duramorph 960
Duricef 1405
Duvoid Tablets 1853
Dyazide Capsules 2208
DynaCirc Capsules (1.8%) 2004
Dyrenium Capsules (Rare) 2210
E.E.S. 522
E-Mycin Tablets (Infrequent) 688
Easprin 1719
▲ Ecotrin (7.6% at 1000 mg/day) 2189
Edecrin 1468
Elavil 2269
▲ Eldepryl (10 of 49 patients) 2250
Elspar 1470
▲ Emcyt Capsules (15%) 1161
Emete-con Intramuscular/Intravenous 1950
▲ Eminase (Less than 10%) 2211
▲ Empirin with Codeine Phosphate Nos. 2, 3 & 4 (Among most frequent) 764
Endep Tablets 1927
Enduron Tablets 517
Enduronyl 518
Engerix-B Unit-Dose Vials (Less than 1%) 2213
Enlon Injection 598
▲ Enovid (Among most common) 2161
Enrich Liquid Nutrition with Fiber 1971
Ensure Liquid Nutrition 1971
Ensure Plus High Calorie Liquid Nutrition 1971
Entex Capsules 1623
Entex LA Tablets 1623
Entex Liquid 1623
EpiPen Jr. 843
▲ Epogen for Injection (0.26% to 15%) 591
Equagesic Tablets 2451
▲ Ergamisol Tablets (9 to 65%) 1136
▲ Ergostat (10% of patients) 1719
▲ ERYC (Among most frequent) 1720
▲ EryPed (Among most frequent) 519
▲ Ery-Tab Tablets (Among most frequent) 521
▲ Erythrocin Stearate Filmtab (Among most frequent) 523
▲ Erythromycin Base Filmtab (Among most frequent) 525
▲ Erythromycin Delayed-Release Capsules, USP (Among most frequent) 526
Esgic-Plus Tablets (Less frequent) 1002
Esgic Tablets & Capsules 1001
Esidrix Tablets 863
Esimil Tablets 864
Eskalith 2214
Estinyl Tablets 2085
Estrace 1385
Estrace Vaginal Cream 1388
Estraderm Transdermal System 866
Estradurin 2452
Estratest 2245
Estrovis 1721
▲ Ethmozine Tablets (3.2%-9.6%) 946
Ethrane 599
Etrafon 2087
▲ Eulexin Capsules (11% with LHRH-agonist) 2089
Exna Tablets 1862
▲ Sterile FUDR (Among more common) 1898
Factrel (Rare) 2561
Fansidar Tablets 1896
Fedahist Gyrocaps 2145
Fedahist Timecaps 2145
▲ Feldene Capsules (3 to 9%) 1777
Feosol Elixir (Occasional) 2191
Feosol Tablets (Occasional) 2191
Fioricet Tablets (Less frequent) 2006
Fiorinal Capsules (Less frequent) 2007
▲ Fiorinal with Codeine Capsules (3.7%) 2008
Fiorinal Tablets (Less frequent) 2007
Flagyl I.V. 2131
▲ Flagyl Tablets (12.0%) 2170
Flexeril Tablets (1% to 3%) 1471
Floropryl Sterile Ophthalmic Ointment (Rare) 1473
▲ Floxin Tablets (3% to 10%) 1652
Fluorescite ⊙ 217
Fluorouracil Injection (Common) 1897
Fluothane 2453
Forane 600
Fortaz (1 in 156 patients) 1060
Fulvicin P/G Tablets 2090
Fulvicin P/G 165 & 330 Tablets 2091
Fulvicin-U/F Tablets 2092
▲ Fungizone Intravenous (Among most common) 2262
Furoxone (Occasional) 1855
Gamimune N Immune Globulin Intravenous (Human) 1572
Gammagard Immune Globulin, Intravenous (Human) (Occasional) 658
Gammar-IV, Immune Globulin Intravenous (Human) 610
Ganite Injection 1016
Gantanol 1899
Gantrisin Ophthalmic Ointment/Solution 1900
Gantrisin 1901
Garamycin Injectable 2093
▲ Gastrocrom Capsules (3 of 87 patients) 974
Geocillin Tablets 1951
Geref (sermorelin acetate for injection) 2560
Glucagon for Injection Vials and Emergency Kit (Occasional) 1263
Glucotrol (1 in 70) 1952
▲ GoLYTELY (Up to 50%) 699
Grifulvin V (griseofulvin microsize) Tablets/Suspension (Occasional) 1678
Grisactin (Occasional) 2454
Grisactin Ultra Tablets 2455
Gris-PEG Tablets, 125 mg & 250 mg (Occasional) 1083
Guaifed 1615
Guaifed Syrup ⊡ 629
▲ Halcion Tablets (4.6%) 2340
Haldol Decanoate 1375
Haldol Injection, Tablets and Concentrate 1373
Halotestin Tablets 2341
Harmonyl Tablets 528
Heparin Lock Flush Solution 2456
Heparin Sodium Vials (Rare) 1264
Heparin Sodium Injection 2457
Heparin Sodium Injection, USP, Sterile Solution 2342
▲ Hexalen Capsules (1% to 33%) 2316
Hiprex Tablets (Less than 3.5%) 1333
Hismanal Tablets (2.5%) 1138
Humatin Capsules 1726
Humorsol Sterile Ophthalmic Solution (Rare) 1475
Humulin 70/30, 100 Units 1267
Humulin BR, 100 Units 1268
Humulin L, 100 Units 1268
Humulin U, 100 Units 1272
Hycodan Syrup, Tablets 927
Hycomine Compound Tablets 929
Hycomine Syrup 927
Hycotuss Expectorant Syrup 930
Hydeltrasol Injection, Sterile 1476
Hydeltra-T.B.A. Sterile Suspension 1478
Hydergine 2010
Hydrea Capsules 728
Hydrocet Capsules 835
Hydrocortone Acetate Sterile Suspension 1479
Hydrocortone Phosphate Injection, Sterile 1481
Hydrocortone Tablets 1482
HydroDIURIL Tablets 1484
Hydromox R Tablets 1209
Hydromox Tablets 1208
Hydropres Tablets 1485
▲ Hylorel Tablets (3.9%) 975
▲ Hyperstat I.V. Injection (4%) 2095
Hyskon Hysteroscopy Fluid (Rare) 1162
▲ Hytrin Tablets (0.8% to 4.4%) 529
INH Tablets 868
▲ Idamycin for Injection (82%) 564
▲ IFEX (58%) 729
Ilosone (Infrequent) 913
Imferon 976
Imodium Capsules 1139
▲ Imuran (Approximately 12%) 768
Inderal 2459
Inderal LA Long Acting Capsules 2461
Inderide Tablets 2463
Inderide LA Long Acting Capsules 2465
▲ Indocin (3% to 9%) 1487
Infumorph 200 and Infumorph 500 Sterile Solutions 962
Innovar Injection 1141
Inocor Lactate Injection (1.7%) 2048
Intal Capsules (Less than 1 in 10,000 patients) 978
▲ Intal Inhaler (Among most frequent) 979
Intal Nebulizer Solution 980
▲ Intron A (17% to 28%) 2097
▲ Intropin Injection (Among most frequent) 930
Inversine Tablets 1492
Ismelin Tablets 869
ISMOTIC ⊙ 233
Isoptin Injectable (0.9%) 1177
Isoptin Oral Tablets (2.7%) 1179
Isoptin SR Sustained Release Tablets (2.7%) 1181
Isordil (Uncommon) 2467
Isuprel Hydrochloride Mistometer 2051
Isuprel Hydrochloride Solution 1:200 & 1:100 2052
Jenest-28 Tablets 1636
K-Dur Microburst Release System (potassium chloride, USP) E.R. Tablets 1163
▲ K-Lor Powder Packets (Most common) 531
▲ K-Lyte (Among most common) 707
▲ K-Norm Capsules (Among most common) 982
K-Phos M.F. Tablets 659
K-Phos Neutral Tablets 660
K-Phos Original Formula 'Sodium Free' Tablets 660
K-Phos No. 2 Tablets 659
▲ K-Tab Filmtab (Most common) 532
Kato Potassium Supplement 1114
Kayexalate 2053
Keflex Pulvules, Oral Suspension & Pediatric Drops (Rare) 916
Keftab Tablets (Rare) 917
Kefurox Vials, Faspak & ADD-Vantage (1 in 440) 1277
Kefzol Vials, Faspak & ADD-Vantage (Rare) 1279
Kemadrin Tablets 771
▲ Kerlone Tablets (1.6% to 5.8%) 2172
Ketalar 1726
Kinesed Tablets 2272
Klonopin Tablets 1902
▲ Klor-Con 8/Klor-Con 10 Extended-release Tablets (Among most common) 2374
Klorvess Effervescent Granules 2010
Klorvess Effervescent Tablets 2011
Klorvess 10% Liquid 2010
▲ Klotrix (Most common) 708
▲ Kolyum Liquid (Among most common) 983
Ku-Zyme HP Capsules 2147
▲ Lamprene Capsules (40-50%) 1030
Lanoxicaps (Common) 772
Lanoxin Elixir Pediatric (Common) 775
Lanoxin Injection (Common) 778
Lanoxin Injection Pediatric (Common) 781

Lanoxin Tablets (Common) 783
▲ Lariam Tablets (Among most frequent) 1904
Larodopa Tablets (Relatively frequent) 1905
Lasix 1093
Legatrin .... ▣ 556
Leukeran Tablets 788
Leukine for IV Infusion 1127
▲ Levatol (4.3%) 1832
Levlen/Tri-Levlen 665
Levo-Dromoran (Common) 1906
Levsin/Levsinex 2147
Librax Capsules (Infrequent) 1929
Libritabs Tablets (Isolated cases) 1930
Librium Capsules (Isolated cases) 1931
Librium Injectable (Isolated cases) 1932
Limbitrol 1933
Lincocin 2344
▲ Lioresal Tablets (4-12%) 1031
Lithane Tablets 1596
Lithium Carbonate Capsules & Tablets 1984
Lithobid Tablets 870
▲ Lodine Capsules (3-9%) 2468
▲ Lo/Ovral Tablets (10% or less) 2471
▲ Lo/Ovral-28 Tablets (10% or less) 2476
Loestrin 1728
Lomotil 2174
Loniten Tablets 2346
Lopid Capsules and Tablets (2.5%) 1736
Lopressor Ampuls (1%) 1032
Lopressor HCT Tablets (1 in 100 patients) 1034
Lopressor Tablets (1%) 1032
Lorelco Tablets 1333
▲ Lortab ASA Tablets (Among most frequent) 2414
▲ Lortab (Among most frequent) 2412
Lotensin Tablets (1.4%) 872
Loxitane 1213
Lozol Tablets (Less than 5%) 1843
Ludiomil Tablets (2%) 874
Lufyllin & Lufyllin-400 Tablets 2384
Lufyllin-GG Elixir & Tablets 2385
▲ Lupron Depot 7.5 mg (5.4%) 2311
▲ Lupron Injection (5% or more) 2310
Lysodren 731
M-M-R II 1494
M-R-VAX II 1496
▲ MS Contin Tablets (Among most frequent) 1814
▲ MSIR (Among most frequent) 1817
▲ Macrodantin Capsules (Most often) 1624
Mandol Vials, Faspak & ADD-Vantage (Rare) 1281
Marax Tablets & DF Syrup (Frequent, on empty stomach) 1954
Marcaine Hydrochloride 0.5% with Epinephrine 1:200,000 (as bitartrate) 958
Marcaine Hydrochloride with Epinephrine 1:200,000 2055
Marcaine Hydrochloride Injection (Rare) 2055
Marcaine Spinal (Rare) 2058
▲ Matulane Capsules (Frequent) 1907
Maxair Inhaler (1.7%) 1311
Maxzide 1215
Mebaral Tablets (Less than 1 in 100) 2061
▲ Meclomen Capsules (11%) 1739
Mediatric Capsules 2476
Medihaler Ergotamine Aerosol 1312
Mefoxin (Rare) 1498
Mefoxin Premixed Intravenous Solution (Rare) 1500
Megace Tablets 732
Mellaril 2011
Menrium Tablets 1934
▲ Mepergan Injection (Among most frequent) 2479
Meruvax II 1503
Mesantoin Tablets 2013
▲ Mesnex Injection (33%) 733
Mestinon Injectable 1115
Mestinon 1116
Metandren Linguets and Tablets 875
Metaprel Inhalation Aerosol Bronchodilator (1 to 4%) 2014
Metaprel Inhalation Solution (1 in 50 patients) 2015
Metaprel 2015
▲ Methadone Hydrochloride Diskets (Among most frequent) 1284
Methadone Hydrochloride Oral Solution & Tablets 1987
Methergine (Occasional) 2016
▲ Methotrexate Tablets, Parenteral, LPF Parenteral (Among most frequent; 10%) 1217
Metopirone Tablets 876
Metrodin (urofollitropin for injection) (Less than 1 in 50) 2182
▲ Mevacor Tablets (4.7%) 1505
▲ Mexitil Capsules (39.3% to 39.6%) 680
Mezlin 1597
Mezlin Pharmacy Bulk Package 1599
▲ Miacalcin Injection (About 10%) 2017
Micro-K 1863
▲ Micro-K LS Packets (Most common) 1864
▲ Micronase Tablets (Most common) 2350
Micronor Tablets 1667
▲ Midamor Tablets (3% to 8%) 1508
Milontin Kapseals (Frequent) 1741
Miltown Tablets 2386
▲ Minipress Capsules (4.9%) 1778
▲ Minizide Capsules (4.9%) 1779
Minocin Intravenous 1221
Minocin Oral Suspension 1224
Minocin Pellet-Filled Capsules 1222
Mintezol 1510
Mithracin 1602
Moban Tablets & Concentrate (Occasional) 932
Modane Plus Tablets .... ▣ 504
Modane Tablets .... ▣ 503
Modicon 1667
▲ Moduretic Tablets (3% to 8%) 1510
▲ Monistat I.V. (18%) 1143
Monoclate-P Factor VIII:C, Pasteurized, Antihemophilic Factor (Human) 612
Monodox Capsules 1630
Monopril Tablets 1406
Motofen Tablets (1 in 15) 836
Motrin Tablets (Less than 3%) 2351
Mustargen 1514
▲ Mutamycin (14%) 733
Myambutol Tablets 1225
▲ Mycelex Troches (1 in 20 patients) 1605
Mycostatin Oral Suspension (Occasional) 605
Mycostatin Oral Tablets (Occasional) 605
Mycostatin Pastilles (Occasional) 734
Mykrox ½ mg Tablets (Less than 2%) 984
Myleran Tablets 790
Myochrysine Injection 1516
Mysoline (Occasional) 2480
Naldecon Syrup, Tablets, Pediatric Drops and Pediatric Syrup 709
▲ Nalfon Pulvules & Tablets (7.7%) 919
Naphcon Forte .... ◉ 226
▲ Naprosyn (3 to 9%) 2297
Narcan Injection 933
Nardil 1742
Nasalide Nasal Solution 0.025% (5% or less) 2299
Naturetin Tablets (Common) 1789
Navane Capsules and Concentrate 1954
Navane Intramuscular 1956
Nebcin Vials, Hyporets & ADD-Vantage 1286
▲ NebuPent for Inhalation Solution (10 to 23%) 1017
NegGram 2062
Nembutal Sodium Capsules (Less than 1%) 534
Nembutal Sodium Solution (Less than 1%) 536
Nembutal Sodium Suppositories (Less than 1%) 538
Neo-Calglucon Syrup 2018
Neosar for Injection (Common) 566
Neptazane Tablets .... ◉ 311
Nescaine/Nescaine MPF 629
Netromycin Injection 100 mg/ml 2104
▲ Neupogen for Injection (57%) 595
▲ Niclocide Chewable Tablets (4.1%) 1607
▲ Nicorette (18.1%) 1335
Nimotop Capsules (0-1.4%) 1607
Nipride I.V. Infusion 1909
Nitro-Bid IV (Less than 1%) 1338
Nitro-Bid Ointment (Uncommon) 1339
Nitro-Bid Capsules 1338
Nitrolingual Spray (Uncommon) 1846
Nitrostat IV (Less than 1%) 1744
▲ Nizoral Tablets (3%) 1145
Nolex LA Tablets 838
▲ Nolvadex Tablets (4.8% to 25%) 1102
▲ Nordette-21 Tablets (10% or less) 2481
▲ Nordette-28 Tablets (10% or less) 2483
▲ Norethin (10% or fewer patients during first cycle) 2133
Norflex 1314
Norgesic 1314
Norinyl 2304
Norisodrine Aerotrol 540
Norlestrin 1746
▲ Normodyne Injection (Less than 1 to 19%) 2108
▲ Normodyne Tablets (Less than 1% to 19%) 2110
▲ Normozide Tablets (2 to 6%) 2112
Noroxin Tablets (2.8%) 1519
▲ Norpace (3 to 9%) 2177
Norplant System 2484
Norpramin Tablets 1340
Nor-Q D Tablets 2304
Novafed A Capsules 1342
Novafed Capsules 1342
Novahistine DH 1342
Novahistine DMX .... ▣ 595
Novahistine Elixir .... ▣ 596
Novahistine Expectorant 1343
Novocain Hydrochloride for Spinal Anesthesia 2065
▲ Nubain Injection (6%) 934
Nucofed Capsules 2219
Nucofed Expectorant 2219
Nucofed Pediatric Expectorant 2220
Nucofed Syrup 2219
▲ NuLYTELY (Up to 50% of patients) 699
Numorphan Hydrochloride Injection 935
Numorphan Suppositories 935
Nystatin, USP for Extemporaneous Preparation of Oral Suspension (Occasional) 1685
Ogen 540
▲ Omnipaque (About 6%) 2552
Oncovin Solution Vials & Hyporets 1288
OptiPranolol Sterile Ophthalmic Solution (A small number of patients) .... ◉ 261
▲ Oramorph SR (Morphine Sulfate Sustained Release Tablets) (Among most frequent) 1988
Orap Tablets 1020
Oretic Tablets 544
Oreticyl 545
▲ Orinase Tablets (Most common) 2354
Ornade Spansule Capsules 2221
Ortho Dienestrol Cream 1664
▲ Orthoclone OKT3 Sterile Solution (19%) 1645
Ortho-Cyclen Tablets 1658
Ortho-Novum 1667
▲ Orudis Capsules (Greater than 3%) 2488
OSM_GLYN .... ◉ 234
Osmolite Isotonic Liquid Nutrition 1972
Osmolite HN High Nitrogen Isotonic Liquid Nutrition 1972
▲ Ovcon (10% or less) 1391
▲ Ovral Tablets (10% or less) 2490
▲ Ovral-28 Tablets (10% or less) 2491
▲ Ovrette Tablets (10% or less) 2492
▲ Oxsoralen-Ultra Capsule (10%) 1117
Oxytocin Injection 2492
PBZ Tablets & Elixir 1037
PBZ-SR Tablets 1037
▲ PCE Dispertab Tablets (Among most frequent) 549
PMB 200 and PMB 400 2504
Pamelor 2019
Pantopon Injectable 1911
Panwarfin Tablets (Infrequent) 547
Papaverine Hydrochloride Vials and Ampoules 1290
Paradione Capsules 548
▲ Paraplatin for Injection (92%) 735
▲ Parlodel (7-49%) 2020
Parnate Tablets 2222
Pavabid Capsules (Rare) 1344
Pavabid HP Capsules (Rare) 1344
▲ PediaProfen Suspension (Up to 9%) 1363
Pediazole 1973
Peganone Tablets 551
▲ Pentam 300 Injection (5.9%) 1018
Pentaspan Injection 949
Pepcid (Infrequent) 1524
Peptavlon 2563
▲ Percocet Tablets (Among most frequent) 950
▲ Percodan (Among most frequent) 951
Pergonal (menotropins for injection, USP) 2184
Periactin 1525
Peri-Colace (Exceedingly small) 1409
Peritrate (Occasional) 1756
▲ Permax Tablets (24.3%) 1291
▲ Phenaphen with Codeine Capsules (Among most frequent) 1865
▲ Phenaphen-650 with Codeine Tablets (Among most frequent) 1866
Phenergan with Codeine 2497
Phenergan with Dextromethorphan 2499
Phenergan Injection 2493
Phenergan Suppositories 2496
Phenergan Syrup 2495
Phenergan Tablets 2496
Phenergan VC 2500
Phenergan VC with Codeine 2501
Phenobarbital Elixir and Tablets (Less than 1 in 100 patients) 1293
PhosChol 568
PhosLo Tablets (Occasional) 700
Phrenilin 838
Pilocar (Extremely rare) .... ◉ 275
Pilostat Sterile Ophthalmic Solution 0.5%, 1%, 2%, 3%, 4%, 5%, 6% (Extremely rare) ◉ 263
Pima Syrup 994
Pipracil (Less frequent) 1230
Pitocin Injection, Ampoules, Steri-Dose Syringes 1757
Pitressin Synthetic, Ampoules 1758
Placidyl Capsules 553
Plague Vaccine 1584
Plaquenil Sulfate Tablets 2067
Plasma-Plex Plasma Protein Fraction (Human) 613
▲ Platinol (Almost all patients) 737
▲ Platinol-AQ Injection (Almost all patients) 738
Plegine Tablets 2504
Plendil Extended-Release Tablets (0.8%) 1526
Polaramine 2116
Pondimin Tablets 1867
Ponstel 1758
Pontocaine Hydrochloride for Spinal Anesthesia 2069
Potaba (Infrequent) 1071
Premarin Intravenous 2508
Premarin with Methyltestosterone 2515
Premarin Tablets 2510
Premarin Vaginal Cream 2512
Prilosec Delayed-Release Capsules (0.9 to 4.0%) 1530
Primaxin I.M. (0.6%) 1532
Primaxin I.V. (2.0%) 1535
Prinivil Tablets (2.3% to 2.5%) 1538
Prinzide Tablets (2.2%) 1540
Priscoline Hydrochloride Ampuls 877
Pro-Banthine Tablets 2141
▲ Procan SR Tablets (3-4%) 1760
▲ Procardia Capsules (Approximately 10%) 1781
▲ Procardia XL Tablets (3.3% to 11%) 1783
▲ Procrit for Injection (0.26% to 15%) 1647
Proglycem (Frequent) 649
Prokine for I.V. Infusion 1096
Prolixin Decanoate 1795
Prolixin Elixir 1793
Prolixin Enanthate 1796
Prolixin Injection 1791
Prolixin Oral Concentrate 1792
Prolixin Tablets 1793
Proloprim Tablets 799
▲ Pronestyl Capsules and Tablets (3-4%) 1800
Pronestyl Injection 1798
▲ Pronestyl-SR Tablets (3 to 4%) 1801
▲ ProSom Tablets (4%) 554
Prostigmin Injectable 1120
Prostigmin Tablets 1121
Protamine Sulfate Ampoules & Vials 1295
Protopam Chloride for Injection 2518
▲ Protostat Tablets (About 12% of patients) 1674
▲ Proventil Inhalation Aerosol (Less than 15%) 2117
Proventil Repetabs Tablets (2%) 2120
▲ Proventil Solutions for Inhalation 0.5% and 0.083% (4%) 2118
Proventil Tablets (2%) 2120
Provera Tablets 2356
Provocholine for Inhalation 1911
▲ Prozac Pulvules (21.1%) 920
Pulmocare Specialized Nutrition for Pulmonary Patients 1975
Purinethol Tablets (Uncommon) 800
Quadrinal Tablets 1183
Quarzan Capsules 1937
Quelidrine Syrup 556
Questran Light (Less frequent) 711
Questran Powder 710
Quibron Capsules 713

Quibron-T ... 714
Quibron-T/SR ... 716
Quinaglute Dura-Tabs Tablets ... 663
Quinamm Tablets ... 1344
▲ Quinidex Extentabs (Among most frequent) ... 1868
Q-vel Muscle Relaxant Pain Reliever ... ▣ 552
Raudixin Tablets ... 1803
Rauzide Tablets ... 1804
Recombivax HB (Equal to or greater than 1%) ... 1544
Regitine ... 878
Reglan ... 1869
Renese Tablets ... 1785
Renese-R Tablets ... 1786
Respbid Tablets ... 684
▲ Retrovir Capsules (0.8% to 46%) ... 802
▲ Retrovir I.V. Infusion (46%) ... 805
▲ Retrovir Syrup (0.8% to 46%) ... 802
▲ Rheumatrex Methotrexate Dose Pack (Among most frequent) ... 1234
▲ Ridaura Capsules (10%) ... 2224
Rifadin (Some patients) ... 1345
Rifamate Capsules (Some patients) ... 1347
Rimactane Capsules ... 879
Ritalin ... 880
Robaxin Tablets ... 1872
▲ Robaxisal Tablets (One in 20-25) .. 1872
Robinul Forte Tablets ... 1873
Robinul Injectable ... 1873
Robinul Tablets ... 1873
Robitussin ... ▣ 676
Robitussin Cough Calmers ... ▣ 677
Robitussin Pediatric ... ▣ 678
Robitussin-CF ... ▣ 676
Robitussin-DM ... ▣ 676
Robitussin-PE ... ▣ 677
Rocaltrol Capsules ... 1913
Rocephin Injectable Vials, ADD-Vantage (Less than 1%) ... 1914
▲ Roferon-A Injection (32% to 51%) 1916
▲ Rogaine Topical Solution (4.33%).. 2357
Rondec ... 1975
Rondec-DM ... 1976
Rondec-TR Tablet ... 1975
▲ Rowasa (1.2 to 5.77%) ... 2248
▲ Roxanol (Among most frequent) ... 1991
▲ Roxicodone Tablets, Oral Solution & Intensol (Oxycodone) (Among most frequent) ... 1992
▲ Rufen Tablets (3-9%) ... 691
Rum-K Syrup ... 995
Ru-Tuss DE Tablets ... 694
Ru-Tuss II Capsules ... 693
Ru-Tuss with Hydrocodone ... 694
Ru-Tuss Tablets ... 693
▲ Rythmol Tablets (2.4 to 10.7%) ... 1184
Salflex ... 839
Saluron ... 718
Salutensin/Salutensin-Demi ... 719
▲ Sandimmune (Less than 1 to 10%) ... 2024
Sandoglobulin I.V. (Less than 1%).. 2027
▲ Sandostatin Injection (9.6%) ... 2029
Sanorex Tablets ... 2030
Sansert Tablets ... 2031
Seconal Sodium Pulvules (Less than 1 in 100) ... 1296
▲ Sectral Capsules (4%) ... 2520
Sedapap Tablets 50 mg/650 mg (Less frequent) ... 1360
▲ Seldane Tablets (7.6%) ... 1349
▲ Seldane-D Extended-Release Tablets (4.5%) ... 1350
Senna X-Prep Bowel Evacuant Liquid ... 1073
Sensorcaine (Rare) ... 631
Sensorcaine-MPF Spinal (Rare) ... 634
▲ Septra (Most common) ... 813
▲ Septra I.V. Infusion (Most common) ... 808
▲ Septra I.V. Infusion ADD-Vantage Vials (Most common) ... 810
▲ Septra (Most common) ... 813
Ser-Ap-Es Tablets ... 881
Serax Capsules ... 2522
Serax Tablets ... 2522
Serentil ... 686
Serophene (clomiphene citrate tablets, USP) (Approximately 1 in 50 patients) ... 2186
Serpasil Tablets ... 883
Serpasil-Apresoline Tablets ... 884
Serpasil-Esidrix Tablets ... 886
Sinemet Tablets (Common) ... 952
▲ Sinemet CR Tablets (5.5%) ... 953
Sinequan ... 1960
Skelaxin ... 840
Slo-bid Gyrocaps ... 1847
▲ Slow-K Tablets (Among most common) ... 2281
Sodium Polystyrene Sulfonate Suspension ... 1993
Solganal Suspension (Rare) ... 2122
Solu-Medrol Sterile Powder ... 2363
Soma Compound w/Codeine Tablets ... 2390
Soma Compound Tablets ... 2389
Soma Tablets ... 2388
Sorbitrate (Uncommon) ... 1103
Sotradecol (Sodium Tetradecyl Sulfate Injection) ... 964
Spectrobid Tablets & Powder for Oral Suspension (2%) ... 1961
▲ St. Joseph Adult Chewable Aspirin (81 mg.) (7.3% of 4500 patients) ... ▣ 703
▲ Stadol (6%) ... 721
Stelazine ... 2226
Stilphostrol Tablets and Ampuls ... 1609
Streptase for Infusion ... 635
Sublimaze Injection ... 1146
Sufenta Injection (Less than 1%) ... 1147
▲ Suprax (7%) ... 1235
Surital Ampoules, Steri-Vials ... 1764
Surmontil Capsules ... 2524
Sus-Phrine Injection ... 1006
▲ Symmetrel Capsules & Syrup (5-10%) ... 936
Synalgos-DC Capsules ... 2525
Syntocinon Injection ... 2032
TACE 12 and 25 mg ... 1353
T-PHYL (Uniphyl) 200 mg Tablets 1820
Tacaryl ... 2409
Talacen (Rare) ... 2070
▲ Talwin Injection (Most common) ... 2071
Talwin Compound ... 2072
▲ Talwin Injection (Most common) ... 2071
Talwin Nx ... 2073
▲ Tambocor Tablets (8.9%) ... 1315
Tao Capsules (Infrequent) ... 1963
Tapazole Tablets ... 1298
Tavist Syrup ... 2033
Tavist Tablets ... 2035
Tavist-D Tablets ... 2035
Tazicef for Injection (Less than 2%; 1 in 156 patients) ... 2231
Tazidime Vials, Faspak & ADD-Vantage (1 in 156) ... 1299
▲ Tegison Capsules (10-25%) ... 1881
▲ Tegretol Chewable Tablets (Among most frequent) ... 654
▲ Tegretol Suspension (Among most frequent) ... 656
▲ Tegretol Tablets (Among most frequent) ... 654
Temaril Tablets, Syrup and Spansule Sustained Release Capsules ... 1085
Tenex Tablets (Less than 3%) ... 1875
▲ Ten-K Controlled-Release Tablets (Among most common) ... 2282
▲ Tenoretic Tablets (3 to 4%) ... 1105
▲ Tenormin Tablets and I.V. Injection (3 to 4%) ... 1107
Tensilon Injectable ... 1123
Tenuate ... 1354
Terramycin Capsules ... 1786
Terramycin Intramuscular Solution 1964
Teslac Tablets ... 741
Tessalon Perles ... 1006
Testred Capsules ... 1124
Thalitone Tablets ... 687
Theo-24 ... 2179
Theo-Dur Sprinkle ... 1168
Theo-Dur Extended-Release Tablets ... 1166
Theolair ... 1317
Theolair-SR Tablets ... 1319
Theo-Organidin Elixir ... 2391
▲ TheoX Extended-Release Tablets (Among most consistent) ... 841
▲ TheraCys BCG Live (Intravesical) (Up to 16.1%) ... 898
Thera-Gesic ... 1614
Theragran Hematinic Tablets ... 605
Thioguanine Tablets, Tabloid Brand (Infrequent) ... 815
Thiosulfil Forte Tablets ... 2526
Thiotepa Parenteral ... 1240
Thorazine ... 2234
Ticar for Injection ... 2236
Timentin for Injection ... 2239
Timolide Tablets (Less than 1%) ... 1547
Timoptic in Ocudose ... 1552
Timoptic Sterile Ophthalmic Solution ... 1550
Tofranil Ampuls ... 1038
Tofranil Tablets ... 1039
Tofranil-PM Capsules ... 1041
▲ Tolectin (200, 400 and 600 mg) (11%) ... 1379
Tolinase Tablets (1%) ... 2365
▲ Tonocard Tablets (14.5-24.6%) ... 1554
▲ Toradol IM Injection (3% to 9%) ... 2302
▲ Tornalate (3%) ... 2074
Trancopal Caplets ... 2075
Trandate HCT Tablets (2% in 208 patients) ... 579
▲ Trandate Injection (13 of 100 patients) ... 577
▲ Trandate Tablets (14%) ... 579
Transderm Scōp Transdermal Therapeutic System (Few patients) ... 887
▲ Trental (2.2% to 28.8%) ... 1099
▲ Trexan Tablets (Greater than 10%) ... 937
Triaminic Expectorant DH ... 1995
Triaminic Oral Infant Drops ... 1996
Triavil Tablets ... 1556
Tridione ... 557
Trilafon (Occasional) ... 2123
Levlen/Tri-Levlen ... 665
▲ Trilisate (Less than 20%) ... 1822
Trimpex Tablets ... 1922
Trinalin Repetabs Tablets ... 1170
Tri-Norinyl ... 2304
▲ Triphasil-21 Tablets (10% or less) 2527
▲ Triphasil-28 Tablets (10% or less) 2532
Trobicin Sterile Powder ... 2366
Troph-Iron Liquid (Occasional) ... ▣ 619
Tussionex Extended-Release Suspension ... 988
Tussi-Organidin Liquid ... 2391
Tuss-Ornade Liquid ... 2242
Tuss-Ornade Spansule Capsules ... 2242
Tylenol with Codeine ... 1381
▲ Tylox Capsules (Among most frequent) ... 1382
Ultracef Capsules, Tablets & Oral Suspension (Rare) ... 722
Unasyn (Less than 1%) ... 1965
Unipen ... 2533
Uniphyl 400 mg Tablets ... 1823
Urecholine ... 1558
Urispas Tablets ... 2242
Urobiotic-250 Capsules (Rare) ... 1968
Uroqid-Acid ... 661
Valium Injectable ... 1937
Valium Tablets (Infrequent) ... 1939
Valpin 50 Tablets ... 941
Valrelease Capsules (Occasional) ... 1923
Vancenase AQ Nasal Spray 0.042% (Fewer than 5 per 100 patients) ... 2127
Vancocin HCl, Oral Solution & Pulvules (Infrequent) ... 1304
▲ Vascor (200, 300 and 400 mg) Tablets (12.29 to 26.09%) ... 1383
Vaseretic Tablets (2.5%) ... 1559
Vasocon-A ... ◉ 278
Vasotec I.V. (1.1%) ... 1562
Vasotec Tablets (1.3% to 1.4%) ... 1564
Vasoxyl Injection ... 819
Velban Vials (Not common) ... 1305
Velosef Capsules and for Oral Suspension (Rare) ... 606
▲ Ventolin (Less than 15 in 100 patients) ... 583
▲ VePesid Capsules and Injection (31 to 43%) ... 741
Verelan Capsules (2.7%) ... 1243
Versed Injection (2.8%) ... 1924
Vibramycin Hyclate Capsules ... 1787
Vibramycin Hyclate Intravenous ... 1968
Vibramycin ... 1787
▲ Vicodin Tablets (Most frequent) ... 1187
▲ Vicodin ES Tablets (Among most frequent) ... 1189
Vira-A for Injection ... 1766
▲ Visken Tablets (5%) ... 2036
Vivactil Tablets ... 1567
Voltaren Ophthalmic Sterile Ophthalmic Solution (1%) ... ◉ 268
▲ Voltaren Tablets (3% to 9%) ... 1042
Vontrol Tablets ... 2243
▲ Wellbutrin Tablets (22.9%) ... 821
Wigraine Tablets & Suppositories .. 1645
Winstrol Tablets ... 2075
▲ Wygesic Tablets (Most frequent) ... 2540
Wytensin Tablets (3% or less) ... 2542
▲ Xanax Tablets (9.6% to 22%) ... 2367
Xylocaine Injections (Less than 1%) ... 637
▲ Yocon (Common) ... 1686
Yodoxin ... 1072
▲ Yutopar (5 to 8% (with oral administration); 10 to 15% (with IV administration)) ... 647
▲ Zanosar Sterile Powder (Most patients) ... 2371
Zantac Injection and Zantac Injection Premixed ... 1063
Zantac ... 1065
Zarontin Capsules (Frequent) ... 1768
Zarontin Syrup (Frequent) ... 1769
Zaroxolyn Tablets ... 989
Zefazone Sterile Powder (1%) ... 2372
Zestoretic (2.2%) ... 2274
Zestril Tablets (2.3%) ... 2277
Zinacef (1 in 440 patients) ... 1066
▲ Zoladex (5%) ... 1110
▲ Zovirax Capsules (2.7% to 8%) ... 824
Zovirax Sterile Powder ... 828
▲ Zovirax (2.7% to 8%) ... 824
▲ Zydone Capsules (Most frequent) .. 941
Zyloprim Tablets (Less than 1%) ... 830

Nausea, acute/severe

▲ Adriamycin PFS (Frequent) ... 561
Doxorubicin Hydrochloride for Injection, USP (Frequent) ... 622
Doxorubicin Hydrochloride Injection, USP (Frequent) ... 848
▲ Novantrone for Injection Concentrate (31 to 72%) ... 1226
Rubex (Frequent) ... 739

Neck, hyperextension of

Prostin VR Pediatric Sterile Solution (Less than 1%) ... 2355

Neck, rigidity of

Prozac Pulvules (Infrequent) ... 920

Necrolysis, digitus

▲ Tegison Capsules (Greater than 75%) ... 1881

Necrolysis, epidermal

▲ Accutane Capsules (Approximately 1 in 20) ... 1878
Anaprox and Anaprox DS Tablets (Rare) ... 2288
Ansaid Tablets (Rare) ... 2319
Atromid-S Capsules ... 2435
Azo Gantanol Tablets ... 1887
Azo Gantrisin Tablets ... 1888
Azulfidine Tablets, EN-tabs, Oral Suspension (Rare) ... 1157
Betoptic Sterile Ophthalmic Solution (Rare) ... 569
Betoptic S Sterile Ophthalmic Suspension (Rare) ... 570
Brevoxyl Gel ... 2264
Ceclor Pulvules & Suspension (Rare) ... 1251
Ceftin Tablets ... 575
Ceptaz for Injection ... 1057
Children's Advil Suspension (Less than 1%) ... 2426
Cipro I.V. (1% or less) ... 1592
Cipro Tablets ... 1589
Clearasil 10% Benzoyl Peroxide Acne Medication Vanishing Lotion ... ▣ 658
Clearasil Double Textured Pads - Regular and Maximum Strength ... ▣ 658
Clearasil Maximum Strength ... ▣ 658
Cleocin T Topical ... 2327
Combipres Tablets ... 678
Condylox (Less than 5%) ... 1630
Depakene Capsules & Syrup (One case) ... 511
Depen Titratable Tablets (Rare) ... 2379
Desquam-E Gel ... 2397
Desquam-X Gel ... 2397
Desquam-X 5 Wash ... 2397
Desquam-X 10 Bar ... 2397
Desquam-X 10 Wash ... 2397
Diamox Sequels (Sustained Release) ... 1201
Dilantin Infatabs ... 1710
Dilantin Kapseals ... 1708
Dilantin-30 Pediatric/Dilantin-125 Suspension ... 1713
Dilantin with Phenobarbital Kapseals ... 1715
Dolobid Tablets (Less than 1 in 100) ... 1465
Emcyt Capsules (1%) ... 1161
Eulexin Capsules ... 2089
FML-S Sterile Ophthalmic Suspension ... ◉ 246
Feldene Capsules (Less than 1%) .. 1777
Fiorinal Capsules (Several cases) ... 2007
Fiorinal with Codeine Capsules ... 2008
Fiorinal Tablets (Several cases) ... 2007
Floxin Tablets ... 1652

Fortaz 1060
Gantrisin Ophthalmic Ointment/Solution 1900
Indocin Capsules (Less than 1%) 1487
Indocin I.V. (Less than 1%) 1490
Indocin (Less than 1%) 1487
Intron A (Less than 1%) 2097
Lactinol-E Creme 1770
Lodine Capsules (Less than 1%) 2468
Lotrimin 2102
Lotrisone Cream 2103
Mesantoin Tablets (Rare) 2013
Mevacor Tablets 1505
Motrin Tablets (Less than 1%) 2351
Mycelex 1% Cream and Topical Solution 1% 1604
Nalfon Pulvules & Tablets (Less than 1%) 919
Noroxin Tablets 1519
Oxy-5 and Oxy-10 Tinted and Vanishing Formulas with Sorboxyl ■ 719
PediaProfen Suspension (Less than 1%) 1363
Pediazole 1973
Phenobarbital Elixir and Tablets (Rare) 1293
Primaxin I.M. 1532
Primaxin I.V. (Rare) 1535
Proloprim Tablets 799
Retin-A (tretinoin) Cream/Gel/Liquid 1680
Rufen Tablets (Less than 1%) 691
Septra 813
Septra I.V. Infusion 808
Septra I.V. Infusion ADD-Vantage Vials (Rare) 810
Septra 813
Suprax 1235
▲Tegison Capsules (Greater than 75%) 1881
Tegretol Chewable Tablets (Extremely rare) 654
Tegretol Suspension (Extremely rare) 656
Tegretol Tablets (Extremely rare) 654
Theroxide 1411
Tolectin (200, 400 and 600 mg) (Less than 1%) 1379
Vaseretic Tablets 1559
Vasosulf ⊙ 279
Vasotec I.V. 1562
Vasotec Tablets 1564
Zefazone Sterile Powder 2372
Zinacef (Rare) 1066

Necrosis
Adrenalin Chloride Solution 1:100 & 1:1,000 1689
Aplisol (tuberculin PPD, diluted) 2550
Aplitest (tuberculin PPD, multiple-puncture device) 2551
Benadryl Parenteral 1692
Brevibloc Injection (Less than 1%) 942
Capoten (Rare) 2255
Capozide (Rare) 2258
Coumadin Injection & Tablets 944
Dicumarol Tablets 516
Ethamolin (0.1% to 0.4%) 1829
Garamycin Injectable (Rare) 2093
Gelfoam Sterile Sponge 2338
Heparin Sodium Injection, USP, Sterile Solution 2342
Imferon 976
Levophed Bitartrate Injection 2054
Medrol 2348
PPD Tine Test 2548
Scleromate 1685
Solu-Cortef Sterile Powder 2361
Solu-Medrol Sterile Powder 2363
▲Tegison Capsules (Greater than 75%) 1881
Tuberculin, Old, Tine Test 2549

Necrosis, aseptic
Aristocort Suspension 1008
Aristospan Suspension (Intralesional) 1011
Cortone Acetate Tablets 1439
Dalalone D.P. Injectable 999
Kenalog-10 Injection 2402
Kenalog-40 Injection 2403
Pediapred Oral Liquid 987

Necrosis, bone
Prozac Pulvules (Rare) 920

Necrosis, bowel
Cytosar-U Sterile Powder (Less frequent) 2329

Necrosis, buccal
Orudis Capsules (Less than 1%) 2488

Necrosis, cecal
Adriamycin PFS 561
Adriamycin RDF 562
Doxorubicin Hydrochloride Injection, USP 848
Rubex 739

Necrosis, colon
Kayexalate 2053
Sodium Polystyrene Sulfonate Suspension (Rare) 1993

Necrosis, cortical
Butazolidin Capsules & Tablets (Less than 1%) 1027

Necrosis, cutaneous
Aramine Injection 1424
Atgam Sterile Solution (Less than 1%) 2320
Calciparine Injection 925
Dicumarol Tablets 516
Heparin Lock Flush Solution 2456
Heparin Sodium Vials 1264
Heparin Sodium Injection 2457
Heparin Sodium Injection, USP, Sterile Solution 2342
Mutamycin 733
Panwarfin Tablets 547
SSD RP Cream (Infrequent) 690

Necrosis, hepatic
Anadrol-50 Tablets (Rare) 2287
Azo Gantanol Tablets 1887
Azo Gantrisin Tablets 1888
Azulfidine Tablets, EN-tabs, Oral Suspension (Rare) 1157
Bactrim DS Tablets (Rare) 1891
Bactrim I.V. Infusion (Rare) 1889
Bactrim (Rare) 1891
Benemid Tablets 1426
Cipro I.V. (1% or less) 1592
Cipro Tablets 1589
ColBENEMID Tablets 1436
DTIC-Dome 1595
Darvon-N/Darvocet-N 1254
Darvon Compound-65 Pulvules 1256
Darvon-N Suspension & Tablets 1254
Diamox Parenteral (Occasional) 1200
Diamox Sequels (Sustained Release) 1201
Diamox Tablets (Occasional) 1200
Eulexin Capsules 2089
FML-S Sterile Ophthalmic Suspension ⊙ 246
Sterile FUDR 1898
Fansidar Tablets 1896
Floxin Tablets 1652
Fluothane 2453
Gantanol 1899
Gantrisin Ophthalmic Ointment/Solution 1900
Gantrisin 1901
Mexitil Capsules (Rare) 680
Nardil (Less frequent) 1742
Normodyne Injection 2108
Normodyne Tablets 2110
Normozide Tablets 2112
Paraflex Caplets 1378
Parafon Forte DSC Caplets 1379
Pediazole 1973
SSD RP Cream 690
Septra 813
Septra I.V. Infusion 808
Septra I.V. Infusion ADD-Vantage Vials (Rare) 810
Septra 813
Silvadene Cream 1% 1352
Tapazole Tablets (Rare) 1298
Trandate HCT Tablets 579
Trandate Injection (Less common) 577
Trandate Tablets 579
Winstrol Tablets (Rare) 2075
Wygesic Tablets 2540
Zyloprim Tablets (Less than 1%) 830

Necrosis, intestinal
Adriamycin PFS 561
Adriamycin RDF 562
Lanoxicaps (Very rare) 772
Lanoxin Elixir Pediatric (Very rare) 775
Lanoxin Injection (Very rare) 778
Lanoxin Injection Pediatric (Very rare) 781
Lanoxin Tablets (Very rare) 783
Oncovin Solution Vials & Hyporets 1288
Thioguanine Tablets, Tabloid Brand 815

Necrosis, papillary
Butazolidin Capsules & Tablets 1027
Dapsone USP (Rare) 1130
Feldene Capsules (Less than 1%) 1777
Nalfon Pulvules & Tablets (Less than 1%) 919
Ponstel 1758
Rufen Tablets (Less than 1%) 691
Voltaren Tablets (Rare) 1042

Necrosis, renal papillary
Anaprox and Anaprox DS Tablets (Less than 1%) 2288
Children's Advil Suspension (Less than 1%) 2426
Darvon-N/Darvocet-N 1254
Darvon 1256
Darvon-N Suspension & Tablets 1254
Meclomen Capsules 1739
Motrin Tablets (Less than 1%) 2351
Naprosyn (Less than 1%) 2297
PediaProfen Suspension (Less than 1%) 1363

Necrosis, renal tubular
Butazolidin Capsules & Tablets 1027
Calcium Disodium Versenate Injection 1309
Cytoxan for Injection 726
Neosar for Injection 566

Necrosis, tissue
Adriamycin PFS 561
Adriamycin RDF 562
Cerubidine 2443
Doxorubicin Hydrochloride for Injection, USP (Occasional) 622
Doxorubicin Hydrochloride Injection, USP 848
Idamycin for Injection 564
Intropin Injection 930
Mepergan Injection 2479
Novantrone for Injection Concentrate (Rare reports) 1226
Phenergan Injection 2493
Phenergan Tablets 2496
Rubex 739
Silvadene Cream 1% (Infrequent) 1352
Sotradecol (Sodium Tetradecyl Sulfate Injection) 964

Necrotizing angiitis
Aldactazide 2150
Aldoclor Tablets 1413
Aldoril Tablets 1418
Apresazide Capsules 854
Apresoline-Esidrix Tablets 857
Capozide 2258
Combipres Tablets 678
Cortifoam 1827
Corzide Tablets (Occasional) 702
Diucardin Tablets 2450
Diulo 2129
Diupres Tablets 1461
Diuril Sodium Intravenous 1463
Dyazide Capsules 2208
Enduron Tablets 517
Enduronyl 518
Esidrix Tablets 863
Esimil Tablets 864
Exna Tablets 1862
HydroDIURIL Tablets 1484
Hydromox R Tablets 1209
Hydromox Tablets 1208
Hydropres Tablets 1485
Inderide Tablets 2463
Inderide LA Long Acting Capsules 2465
Kenalog-10 Injection 2402
Kenalog-40 Injection 2403
Lasix 1093
Lopressor HCT Tablets 1034
Lozol Tablets 1843
Maxzide 1215
Minizide Capsules 1779
Moduretic Tablets 1510
Mykrox ½ mg Tablets 984
Naturetin Tablets (Occasional) 1789
Normozide Tablets 2112
Oretic Tablets 544
Oreticyl 545
Prinzide Tablets 1540
Rauzide Tablets 1804
Renese Tablets 1785
Renese-R Tablets 1786
Saluron 718
Salutensin/Salutensin-Demi 719
Ser-Ap-Es Tablets 881
Serpasil-Esidrix Tablets 886
Tenoretic Tablets 1105
Thalitone Tablets 687
Trandate HCT Tablets 579
Vaseretic Tablets 1559
Zaroxolyn Tablets 989
Zestoretic 2274

Neonatal prematurity
Prinivil Tablets 1538
Prinzide Tablets 1540
Vaseretic Tablets 1559
Vasotec I.V. 1562
Vasotec Tablets 1564
Zestoretic 2274
Zestril Tablets 2277

Neoplasm (see under Carcinoma)

Neoplasm, malignant
Estratest 2245
Ortho Dienestrol Cream 1664
Stilphostrol Tablets and Ampuls 1609

Neoplasms, hepatic
Anadrol-50 Tablets 2287
Android (Rare) 1111
Brevicon 2304
Estratest (Rare) 2245
Metandren Linguets and Tablets 875
Norinyl 2304
Norlestrin 1746
Nor-Q D Tablets 2304
Ortho-Cyclen Tablets 1658
Premarin with Methyltestosterone 2515
Testred Capsules (Rare) 1124
Tri-Norinyl 2304
Winstrol Tablets 2075

Nephritis
Azo Gantrisin Tablets 1888
Capastat Sulfate Vials (1 patient) 1250
Cipro Tablets (Less than 1%) 1589
Disalcid 1310
Naprosyn Tablets (Less than 1%) 2297
NebuPent for Inhalation Solution (1% or less) 1017
Phenurone Tablets (1%) 552
Quinidex Extentabs 1868
Salflex 839
Solganal Suspension 2122
Tapazole Tablets (Very rare) 1298
Zyloprim Tablets (Less than 1%) 830

Nephritis, interstitial
Aldoclor Tablets 1413
Aldoril Tablets 1418
Anaprox and Anaprox DS Tablets (Less than 3%) 2288
Ansaid Tablets (Rare) 2319
Bactrim DS Tablets 1891
Bactrim I.V. Infusion 1889
Bactrim 1891
Butazolidin Capsules & Tablets (Less than 1%) 1027
Capoten 2255
Capozide 2258
Ceclor Pulvules & Suspension (Rare) 1251
Children's Advil Suspension 2426
Cipro I.V. (1% or less) 1592
Cipro Tablets (Less than 1%) 1589
Clinoril Tablets (Less than 1 in 100) 1433
Diupres Tablets 1461
Diuril Oral Suspension 1464
Diuril Sodium Intravenous 1463
Diuril Tablets 1464
Dolobid Tablets (Less than 1 in 100) 1465
Dyazide Capsules 2208
Dyrenium Capsules (Rare) 2210
Feldene Capsules (Less than 1%) 1777
HydroDIURIL Tablets 1484
Hydropres Tablets 1485
Indocin (Less than 1%) 1487
Keflex Pulvules, Oral Suspension & Pediatric Drops (Rare) 916
Keftab Tablets (Rare) 917
Kefzol Vials, Faspak & ADD-Vantage 1279
Lodine Capsules (Less than 1%) 2468
Maxzide (Rare) 1215
Meclomen Capsules 1739
Mezlin (Rare) 1597
Mezlin Pharmacy Bulk Package (Rare) 1599
Moduretic Tablets 1510
Monocid Injection (Rare) 2217
Motrin Tablets 2351
Nalfon Pulvules & Tablets (Less than 1%) 919
Naprosyn Suspension (Less than 1%) 2297

Noroxin Tablets 1519
Orudis Capsules (Less than 1%) 2488
PediaProfen Suspension 1363
Pipracil (Rare) 1230
Prinzide Tablets 1540
Rifadin 1345
Rifamate Capsules (Rare) 1347
SSD (Rare) 694
SSD RP Cream (Infrequent) 690
Septra 813
Septra I.V. Infusion 808
Septra I.V. Infusion ADD-Vantage Vials 810
Septra 813
Silvadene Cream 1% (One case) 1352
Streptase for Infusion 635
Tagamet (Rare) 2228
Vancocin HCl, Oral Solution & Pulvules (Rare) 1304
Vancocin HCl, Vials & ADD-Vantage (Rare) 1302
Vaseretic Tablets 1559
Voltaren Tablets (Rare) 1042
Zestoretic 2274

Nephritis, lupus

Quinidex Extentabs 1868

Nephrocalcinosis

Fungizone Intravenous (Common) 2262
Rocaltrol Capsules 1913

Nephropathy

Bicillin C-R Injection 2438
Bicillin C-R 900/300 Injection 2440
Bicillin L-A Injection (Infrequent) 2442
Ceftin Tablets 575
Ceptaz for Injection 1057
Fortaz 1060
Intal Capsules (Less than 1 in 100,000 patients) 978
Keftab Tablets 917
Pfizerpen for Injection (Rare) 1957
Suprax 1235
Zefazone Sterile Powder 2372
Zinacef 1066

Nephropathy, acute uric acid

Oncovin Solution Vials & Hyporets 1288

Nephropathy, severe

Methotrexate Tablets, Parenteral, LPF Parenteral 1217
Rheumatrex Methotrexate Dose Pack 1234

Nephrosis, toxic

Azo Gantanol Tablets 1887
Azo Gantrisin Tablets 1888
Azulfidine Tablets, EN-tabs, Oral Suspension (Rare) 1157
Bactrim DS Tablets 1891
Bactrim I.V. Infusion 1889
Bactrim 1891
Cortisporin Cream 757
Cortisporin Ointment 758
Fansidar Tablets 1896
Fulvicin P/G Tablets 2090
Fulvicin P/G 165 & 330 Tablets 2091
Fulvicin-U/F Tablets 2092
Gantanol 1899
Gantrisin Ophthalmic Ointment/Solution 1900
Gantrisin 1901
Intal Inhaler (Rare) 979
Intal Nebulizer Solution (Rare) 980
Mesantoin Tablets 2013
Nalfon Pulvules & Tablets (Less than 1%) 919
Paradione Capsules 548
Pediazole 1973
Permax Tablets (Rare) 1291
SSD RP Cream 690
Septra 813
Septra I.V. Infusion 808
Septra I.V. Infusion ADD-Vantage Vials 810
Septra 813
Silvadene Cream 1% 1352
Thiosulfil Forte Tablets 2526
Tridione 557

Nephrotic syndrome

Anaprox and Anaprox DS Tablets (Less than 1%) 2288
Azulfidine Tablets, EN-tabs, Oral Suspension (Rare) 1157
Benemid Tablets 1426
Butazolidin Capsules & Tablets (Occasional) 1027
Capoten (1 to 2 of 1000 patients) 2255
Capozide (Approximately 1 to 2 of 1000 patients) 2258
Children's Advil Suspension (Occasional) 2426
Clinoril Tablets (Less than 1 in 100) 1433
ColBENEMID Tablets 1436
Cuprimine Capsules 1442
Dapsone USP 1130
Depen Titratable Tablets 2379
Dolobid Tablets (Rare) 1465
Feldene Capsules (Less than 1%) 1777
Hyperab Rabies Immune Globulin (Human) (Rare) 1574
Hyper-Tet Tetanus Immune Globulin (Human) (Few cases) 1576
Indocin (Less than 1%) 1487
Meclomen Capsules (Occasionally) 1739
Motrin Tablets (Occasional) 2351
Myochrysine Injection 1516
Naprosyn (Less than 1%) 2297
Orudis Capsules (Less than 1%) 2488
PediaProfen Suspension (Occasional) 1363
Proglycem 649
Ridaura Capsules 2224
Rythmol Tablets (Less than 1%) 1184
Solganal Suspension 2122
Voltaren Tablets (Rare) 1042

Nephrotoxicity

Amikin Injectable 602
BiCNU 723
Capastat Sulfate Vials 1250
CeeNU 725
Cortisporin Otic Solution Sterile 760
Cortisporin Otic Suspension Sterile 760
Furoxone 1855
Garamycin Injectable 2093
Methotrexate Tablets, Parenteral, LPF Parenteral 1217
Nebcin Vials, Hyporets & ADD-Vantage 1286
NeoDecadron Topical Cream 1518
Neosporin Cream 792
Neosporin G.U. Irrigant Sterile 793
Neosporin Ointment 793
Netromycin Injection 100 mg/ml 2104
PediOtic Suspension Sterile 797
Platinol 737
Platinol-AQ Injection 738
Polymyxin B Sulfate, Aerosporin Brand Sterile Powder 798
Rheumatrex Methotrexate Dose Pack 1234
Rowasa 2248
▲Sandimmune (25 to 38%) 2024
Vancocin HCl, Oral Solution & Pulvules (A few dozen cases) 1304
Vancocin HCl, Vials & ADD-Vantage (A few dozen cases) 1302
Zanosar Sterile Powder 2371

Nerve damage

Surgicel 1151

Nerve deafness

Biavax II 1427
M-M-R II 1494
Mumpsvax 1513
Plaquenil Sulfate Tablets 2067

Nerve injury at injection site

Brevital Sodium Vials 1248

Nervousness

A.R.M. Allergy Relief Medicine Caplets ▣ 615
Accutane Capsules 1878
Actifed Capsules ▣ 539
Actifed Plus Caplets ▣ 539
Actifed Plus Tablets ▣ 540
Actifed with Codeine Cough Syrup 752
Actifed Syrup ▣ 540
Actifed Tablets ▣ 540
Actifed 12-Hour Capsules ▣ 539
Acutrim ▣ 548
▲Adalat Capsules (10 mg and 20 mg) (2% or less to 7%) 1587
Advil Cold & Sinus Caplets (formerly CoAdvil) 2416
▲AeroBid Inhaler System (3-9%) 995
Afrin Tablets ▣ 693
Albalon Solution with Liquifilm ◉ 238
Alferon N Injection (1%) 1809
Alka-Seltzer Plus Cold Medicine ▣ 623
Alka-Seltzer Plus Night-Time Cold Medicine ▣ 623
Allerest ▣ 559
Altace Capsules (Less than 1%) 1086
▲Alupent (6.8%) 674
Alurate Elixir (Less than 1 in 100) 1883
Amen 833
▲Anafranil Capsules (4% to 18%) 650
Anatuss LA Tablets 1359
▲Anestacon Solution (Among most common) 2394
Ansaid Tablets (1-3%) 2319
▲Arm-a-Med Metaproterenol Sulfate Inhalation Solution, USP (1 in 7 patients) 617
▲Artane (30% to 50%) 1195
Asendin Tablets (Greater than 1%) 1196
Atabrine Hydrochloride Tablets (Infrequent) 2041
Atrohist Sprinkle Capsules 558
▲Atrovent Inhalation Aerosol (3.1%) 675
Bactrim DS Tablets 1891
Bactrim I.V. Infusion 1889
Bactrim 1891
Benadryl Capsules 1691
Benadryl Decongestant Elixir ▣ 635
Benadryl Decongestant ▣ 635
Benadryl Kapseals 1691
Benadryl Parenteral 1692
Benadryl Plus ▣ 636
Benadryl Plus Nighttime ▣ 637
Benadryl Steri-Vials, Ampoules, and Steri-Dose Syringe 1692
▲Bentyl (6%) 1322
Benylin Decongestant ▣ 638
Blocadren Tablets (Less than 1%) 1429
Brethaire Inhaler 1024
▲Brethine Ampuls (16.9 to 38.0%) 1026
Brethine Tablets (Common) 1026
Brevicon 2304
▲Bricanyl Injection (Among most common) 1324
▲Bricanyl Tablets (Among most common) 1325
Bromfed 1615
Bronkaid Mist ▣ 757
Bronkaid Mist Suspension ▣ 757
Bronkaid Tablets ▣ 757
Bronkolixir ▣ 761
Bronkotabs Tablets ▣ 762
▲BuSpar (5%) 1401
Butisol Sodium Elixir & Tablets (Less than 1 in 100) 2377
Cantil Tablets 1326
Capoten 2255
Capozide 2258
Carbocaine 956
Cardene Capsules (0.6%) 2290
Cardizem Tablets-30 mg, 60 mg, 90 mg and 120 mg (Less than 1%) 1329
Cardizem SR Capsules-60 mg, 90 mg and 120 mg (Less than %) 1327
Cardura Tablets (2%) 1941
Cartrol Tablets (Less common) 507
Catapres Tablets (About 3 in 100 patients) 676
Catapres-TTS (1% to 3%) 677
Ceclor Pulvules & Suspension (Rare) 1251
Celontin 1692
Cerose-DM 2443
Children's Advil Suspension (Less than 3%) 2426
Chlor-Trimeton Decongestant ▣ 694
Clinoril Tablets (Greater than 1%) 1433
Cocaine Hydrochloride Topical Solution 620
Codimal 846
Cogentin 1435
Combipres Tablets (About 3%) 678
Comhist LA Capsules 1618
Compazine 2201
Allergy-Sinus Comtrex Multi-Symptom Allergy Sinus Formula Tablets & Caplets 746
Cough Formula Comtrex (At higher doses) 746
Comtrex Multi-Symptom Cold Reliever Tablets/Caplets/Liqui-Gels/Liquid- 745
Day-Night Comtrex 747
Non-Drowsy Comtrex 747
Contac Continuous Action Decongestant/Antihistamine Capsules ▣ 710
Contac Jr. Children's Cold Medicine ▣ 712
Contac Maximum Strength Continuous Action Decongestant/Antihistamine Caplets ▣ 709
Contac Nighttime Cold Medicine ▣ 713
Contac Severe Cold and Flu Formula Caplets ▣ 711
Contac Sinus Caplets Maximum Strength Non-Drowsy Formula ▣ 710
Contac Sinus Tablets Maximum Strength Non-Drowsy Formula ▣ 710
Coricidin 'D' Decongestant Tablets ▣ 695
Coricidin Demilets Tablets for Children ▣ 696
Cycrin Tablets 2449
Cytovene Sterile Powder (1% or less) 2292
Dalmane Capsules 1927
Danocrine Capsules 2046
Dantrium Capsules (Less frequent) 1619
Daranide Tablets 1445
Darbid Tablets 2205
Dayto Himbin Tablets and Liquid 905
Decadron Phosphate with Xylocaine Injection, Sterile 1451
Deconamine 663
Deconsal 559
Demazin Nasal Decongestant/Antihistamine Repetabs Tablets & Syrup ▣ 697
Demulen 2161
Depo-Provera Sterile Aqueous Suspension (Occasional) 2336
Deprol Tablets (One case) 2382
Desyrel and Desyrel Dividose (Greater than 1%) 1404
Dexatrim ▣ 733
Dilantin Infatabs 1710
Dilantin Kapseals 1708
Dilantin Parenteral 1712
Dilantin-30 Pediatric/Dilantin-125 Suspension 1713
Dilantin with Phenobarbital Kapseals 1715
Dilaudid-HP Injection 1175
Dimacol Caplets ▣ 672
Dimetane Decongestant ▣ 673
Dimetane-DC Cough Syrup 1857
Dimetane-DX Cough Syrup 1858
Dimetapp Elixir ▣ 673
Dimetapp Extentabs ▣ 674
Dimetapp Plus Caplets ▣ 675
Dimetapp Tablets ▣ 675
Disophrol Chronotab Sustained-Action Tablets ▣ 698
Diupres Tablets 1461
Dolobid Tablets (Less than 1 in 100) 1465
Donnatal 1858
Donnatal Extentabs 1859
Donnatal Tablets 1858
Donnazyme Tablets 1860
Doral Tablets 2383
Dristan Cold Nasal Decongestant/Antihistamine/ Analgesic Coated Tablets 2419
Dristan Sinus Caplets 2419
Drixoral Antihistamine/Nasal Decongestant Syrup ▣ 698
Drixoral Plus Extended-Release Tablets ▣ 699
Drixoral Sinus ▣ 700
Drixoral Sustained-Action Tablets ▣ 698
▲Duragesic Transdermal System (3% to 10%) 1133
Duranest Injections 624
Dyclone 0.5% and 1% Topical Solutions, USP 626
DynaCirc Capsules (0.5% to 1%) 2004
Eldepryl 2250
Emete-con Intramuscular/Intravenous 1950
Enduronyl 518
Enovid 2161
Entex Capsules 1623
Entex LA Tablets 1623
Entex Liquid 1623
EpiPen Jr. 843
Ergamisol Tablets (1 to 2%) 1136
▲Ethmozine Tablets (2%-5%) 946
Eulexin Capsules (1%) 2089
Sinus Excedrin Analgesic, Decongestant Tablets & Caplets 750
4-Way Cold Tablets 750
Fansidar Tablets 1896
Fedahist Gyrocaps 2145
Fedahist Timecaps 2145
Feldene Capsules (Less than 1%) 1777
Fiorinal with Codeine Capsules 2008
Flexeril Tablets (1% to 3%) 1471
Floxin Tablets (1% to 3%) 1652
Guaifed Syrup ▣ 629
▲Halcion Tablets (5.2%) 2340

Harmonyl Tablets 528
Hismanal Tablets (2.1%) 1138
Humulin 70/30, 100 Units 1267
Humulin BR, 100 Units 1268
Humulin L, 100 Units 1268
Humulin U, 100 Units 1272
Hydropres Tablets 1485
Hytrin Tablets (2.3%) 529
Indocin (Less than 1%) 1487
Intron A (Up to 1%) 2097
Isoclor Timesule Capsules ▣ 561
Isuprel Hydrochloride Injection 1:5000 2050
Isuprel Hydrochloride Mistometer .. 2051
Isuprel Hydrochloride Solution 1:200 & 1:100 2052
Jenest-28 Tablets 1636
Kerlone Tablets (0.8%) 2172
Kinesed Tablets 2272
Kutrase Capsules 2146
Levlen/Tri-Levlen 665
Levsin/Levsinex 2147
Lodine Capsules (More than 1% but less than 3%) 2468
Lo/Ovral Tablets 2471
Lo/Ovral-28 Tablets 2476
Loestrin 1728
Lotensin Tablets 872
▲ Lozol Tablets (Greater than or equal to 5%) 1843
▲ Ludiomil Tablets (6%) 874
Lupron Depot 7.5 mg 2311
Lupron Injection (Less than 5%) 2310
MS Contin Tablets (Infrequent) 1814
MSIR (Infrequent) 1817
Marax Tablets & DF Syrup 1954
Marcaine Hydrochloride 0.5% with Epinephrine 1:200,000 (as bitartrate) 958
Matulane Capsules 1907
▲ Maxair Inhaler (6.9%) 1311
Mebaral Tablets (Less than 1 in 100) 2061
Medi-Flu Caplet, Liquid ▣ 640
Mesantoin Tablets 2013
▲ Metaprel Inhalation Aerosol Bronchodilator (6.8%) 2014
▲ Metaprel Inhalation Solution (1 in 7 patients) 2015
Metaprel 2015
▲ Mexitil Capsules (5% to 11.3%) 680
Micronor Tablets 1667
Midamor Tablets (Less than or equal to 1%) 1508
Minipress Capsules (1-4%) 1778
Minizide Capsules 1779
Modicon 1667
Moduretic Tablets (Less than or equal to 1%) 1510
Motofen Tablets (1 in 200 to 1 in 600) 836
Motrin Tablets (1-3%) 2351
Mykrox ½ mg Tablets (Less than 2%) 984
Naldecon CX Adult Liquid ▣ 521
Naldecon DX Adult Liquid ▣ 521
Naldecon DX Children's Syrup ▣ 522
Naldecon DX Pediatric Drops ▣ 522
Naldecon EX Children's Syrup ▣ 522
Naldecon EX Pediatric Drops ▣ 523
Naldecon Syrup, Tablets, Pediatric Drops and Pediatric Syrup 709
▲ Nalfon Pulvules & Tablets (5.7%) .. 919
Naphcon Forte ⊙ 226
Nembutal Sodium Capsules (Less than 1%) 534
Nembutal Sodium Solution (Less than 1%) 536
Nembutal Sodium Suppositories (Less than 1%) 538
Nolamine Tablets (Occasional) 838
Nolex LA Tablets 838
Nordette-21 Tablets 2481
Nordette-28 Tablets 2483
Norethin 2133
Norinyl 2304
Norlestrin 1746
Norlutate 1754
Norlutin 1755
Norpace (1 to 3%) 2177
Norplant System 2484
Nor-Q D Tablets 2304
Novafed A Capsules 1342
Novahistine DH 1342
Novahistine DMX ▣ 595
Novahistine Elixir ▣ 596
Novocain Hydrochloride for Spinal Anesthesia 2065
Nubain Injection (Less than 1%) 934
Nucofed Capsules 2219
Nucofed Expectorant 2219
Nucofed Pediatric Expectorant 2220
Nucofed Syrup 2219
Optimine Tablets 2115
OptiPranolol Sterile Ophthalmic Solution (A small number of patients) ⊙ 261
Oramorph SR (Morphine Sulfate Sustained Release Tablets) (Less frequent) 1988
Oreticyl 545
Ornade Spansule Capsules 2221
Ornex Caplets ▣ 618
Ortho-Cyclen Tablets 1658
Ortho-Novum 1667
▲ Orudis Capsules (Greater than 3%) 2488
Ovcon 1391
Ovral Tablets 2490
Ovral-28 Tablets 2491
Ovrette Tablets 2492
Oxsoralen-Ultra Capsule 1117
PBZ Tablets & Elixir 1037
PBZ-SR Tablets 1037
Parlodel 2020
PediaProfen Suspension (Less than 3%) 1363
Periactin 1525
Permax Tablets (Frequent) 1291
Phenergan Injection 2493
Phenergan Tablets 2496
Phenergan VC 2500
Phenergan VC with Codeine 2501
Phenobarbital Elixir and Tablets (Less than 1 in 100 patients) 1293
Plaquenil Sulfate Tablets 2067
Plendil Extended-Release Tablets (0.5% to 1.5%) 1526
Polaramine 2116
Pondimin Tablets 1867
Ponstel 1758
Pontocaine Hydrochloride for Spinal Anesthesia 2069
Prilosec Delayed-Release Capsules (Less than 1%) 1530
Primatene Tablets 2421
Prinivil Tablets (1% or less) 1538
Prinzide Tablets 1540
Pro-Banthīne Tablets 2141
Procardia Capsules (2% or less) 1781
▲ Procardia XL Tablets (Less than 3% to 7%) 1783
Propagest 839
▲ ProSom Tablets (8%) 554
▲ Proventil Inhalation Aerosol (Less than 10%) 2117
▲ Proventil Repetabs Tablets (20%) 2120
▲ Proventil Solutions for Inhalation 0.5% and 0.083% (4%) 2118
▲ Proventil Syrup (9 of 100; children 2-6: 15%) 2119
▲ Proventil Tablets (20%) 2120
Provera Tablets 2356
▲ Prozac Pulvules (14.9%) 920
Pyrroxate Capsules ▣ 669
Quadrinal Tablets 1183
Quarzan Capsules 1937
Quelidrine Syrup 556
Raudixin Tablets 1803
Rauzide Tablets 1804
Renese-R Tablets 1786
Retrovir Capsules (1.5% to 5%) 802
Retrovir I.V. Infusion (Less than 5%) 805
Retrovir Syrup (1.5% to 5%) 802
▲ Ritalin (Among most common) 880
Robinul Forte Tablets 1873
Robinul Injectable 1873
Robinul Tablets 1873
Robitussin Night Relief ▣ 677
Robitussin-CF ▣ 676
Robitussin-DAC Syrup 1875
Robitussin-PE ▣ 677
Roferon-A Injection (Less than 3%) 1916
Rondec 1975
Rondec-DM 1976
Rondec-TR Tablet 1975
Rufen Tablets (1 to 3%) 691
Ru-Tuss DE Tablets 694
Ru-Tuss II Capsules 693
Ru-Tuss with Hydrocodone 694
Ru-Tuss Tablets 693
Ryna ▣ 741
Salutensin/Salutensin-Demi 719
Sandostatin Injection (Less than 1%) 2029
▲ Sanorex Tablets (Among most common) 2030
Seconal Sodium Pulvules (Less than 1 in 100) 1296
Seldane Tablets (1.7%) 1349
▲ Seldane-D Extended-Release Tablets (6.7%) 1350
Septra 813
Septra I.V. Infusion 808
Septra I.V. Infusion ADD-Vantage Vials 810
Septra 813
Ser-Ap-Es Tablets 881
Serophene (clomiphene citrate tablets, USP) (Approximately 1 in 50 patients) 2186
Serpasil Tablets 883
Serpasil-Apresoline Tablets 884
Serpasil-Esidrix Tablets 886
Sinarest ▣ 562
Sine-Aid Maximum Strength Sinus Headache Caplets 1365
Sine-Aid Maximum Strength Sinus Headache Tablets 1365
Sinemet CR Tablets 953
Sine-Off Maximum Strength Allergy/Sinus Formula Caplets ▣ 721
Sine-Off Maximum Strength No Drowsiness Formula Caplets ▣ 722
Sine-Off Sinus Medicine Tablets-Aspirin Formula ▣ 722
Singlet Tablets ▣ 598
Sinulin 840
Sinutab Allergy Formula Sustained Action Tablets ▣ 640
Skelaxin 840
Stadol (Less than 1%) 721
Stilphostrol Tablets and Ampuls 1609
Sudafed Children's Liquid ▣ 543
Sudafed Cough Syrup ▣ 543
Sudafed Plus Liquid ▣ 544
Sudafed Plus Tablets ▣ 545
Sudafed Sinus Caplets ▣ 545
Sudafed Sinus Tablets ▣ 545
Sudafed Tablets, 30 mg ▣ 544
Sudafed Tablets, Adult Strength, 60 mg ▣ 544
Sudafed 12 Hour Capsules ▣ 545
Tacaryl 2409
Tavist Syrup 2033
Tavist Tablets 2035
Tavist-D Tablets 2035
Temaril Tablets, Syrup and Spansule Sustained Release Capsules 1085
Tenex Tablets 1875
Tenuate 1354
Timolide Tablets (Less than 1%) 1547
Timoptic in Ocudose 1552
Timoptic Sterile Ophthalmic Solution 1550
Tofranil Ampuls 1038
Tofranil Tablets 1039
▲ Tonocard Tablets (0.4-11.5%) 1554
Toradol IM Injection (1% or less) 2302
▲ Tornalate (5%) 2074
Tranxene (Less common) 556
Trental (1.7%) 1099
▲ Trexan Tablets (Greater than 10%) 937
Triaminic Allergy Tablets ▣ 688
Triaminic Chewables ▣ 688
Triaminic Expectorant DH 1995
Triaminic Oral Infant Drops 1996
Triaminic-12 Tablets ▣ 690
Triaminicin Tablets ▣ 690
Triaminicol Multi-Symptom Cold Tablets ▣ 691
Levlen/Tri-Levlen 665
Trinalin Repetabs Tablets 1170
Tri-Norinyl 2304
Triphasil-21 Tablets 2527
Triphasil-28 Tablets 2532
Tuss-Ornade Liquid 2242
Tuss-Ornade Spansule Capsules 2242
Children's Tylenol Cold Liquid Formula and Chewable Tablets 1368
Tylenol Cold & Flu Hot Medication, Packets 1369
Tylenol Cold & Flu No Drowsiness Hot Medication, Packets 1371
Tylenol Cold Medication Caplets and Tablets 1370
Tylenol Cold Medication No Drowsiness Formula Caplets 1370
Tylenol Cold Night Time Medication Liquid 1371
Tylenol Cough Medication Liquid with Decongestant, Maximum Strength 1372
Tylenol, Maximum Strength, Sinus Medication Gelcaps, Caplets and Tablets 1373
Urispas Tablets 2242
Ursinus Inlay-Tabs ▣ 691
Valpin 50 Tablets 941
▲ Vascor (200, 300 and 400 mg) Tablets (7.37 to 11.36%) 1383
Vaseretic Tablets (0.5% to 2.0%) 1559
Vasocon-A ⊙ 278
Vasotec I.V. 1562
Vasotec Tablets (0.5% to 1%) 1564
▲ Ventolin (Less than 10 in 100 patients) 583
Versed Injection (Less than 1%) 1924
Vicks Daycare ▣ 660
Vicks Formula 44D Decongestant Cough Medicine.. ▣ 662
Vicks Formula 44M Multi-Symptom Cough Medicine ▣ 662
Vicks NyQuil Nighttime Colds Medicine-Original & Cherry Flavor ▣ 664
▲ Visken Tablets (7%) 2036
Vivarin Stimulant Tablets ▣ 726
▲ Xanax Tablets (4.1%) 2367
▲ Xylocaine Injections (Among most common) 637
Xylocaine Injections for Ventricular Arrhythmias 639
Xylocaine 2% Jelly 643
Xylocaine 5% Ointment 644
Xylocaine 10% Oral Spray 645
4% Xylocaine-MPF Sterile Solution 641
Xylocaine 2% Viscous Solution 646
▲ Yutopar (5 to 6% (with IV administration)) 647
Zaroxolyn Tablets (Less than 2%).. 989
Zestoretic 2274
Zestril Tablets 2277

Neuralgia

Altace Capsules (Less than 1%) 1086
Anafranil Capsules (Infrequent) 650
Lamprene Capsules (Less than 1%) 1030
NebuPent for Inhalation Solution (1% or less) 1017
▲ Omnipaque (Less than 0.1 to about 8%) 2552
Pentam 300 Injection (0.9%) 1018
Permax Tablets (1.1%) 1291
Phenobarbital Elixir and Tablets (Rare) 1293
Prozac Pulvules (Infrequent) 920

Neuritis

Actifed with Codeine Cough Syrup.. 752
Benadryl Capsules 1691
Benadryl Injection 1692
Clinoril Tablets (Rare) 1433
Cytosar-U Sterile Powder (Less frequent) 2329
Deconamine 663
Kenalog-10 Injection 2402
Kenalog-40 Injection 2403
Marplan Tablets (Rare) 1906
Optimine Tablets 2115
Ornade Spansule Capsules 2221
Periactin 1525
Permax Tablets (Rare) 1291
Polaramine 2116
ProSom Tablets 554
Ru-Tuss II Capsules 693
Tacaryl 2409
Tapazole Tablets 1298
Tavist Syrup 2033
Tavist Tablets 2035
Tavist-D Tablets 2035
Temaril Tablets, Syrup and Spansule Sustained Release Capsules 1085
Triaminic Expectorant DH 1995
Triaminic Oral Infant Drops 1996
Trinalin Repetabs Tablets 1170
Zyloprim Tablets (Less than 1%) 830

Neuritis, optic

Accutane Capsules (Less than 1%) 1878
Amen 833
Attenuvax 1424
Biavax II 1427
Butazolidin Capsules & Tablets (Less than 1%) 1027
Cardioquin Tablets 1812
Children's Advil Suspension (Less than 1%) 2426
Chloromycetin Kapseals 1695
Chloromycetin Palmitate, Oral Suspension 1697
Chloromycetin Sodium Succinate 1698
Cordarone Tablets (Rare) 2446
Cuprimine Capsules 1442
Cycrin Tablets 2449

(▣ Described in PDR For Nonprescription Drugs) Incidence data in parenthesis; ▲ 3% or more (⊙ Described in PDR For Ophthalmology)

Decadron Phosphate Sterile Ophthalmic Ointment 1453
Decadron Phosphate Sterile Ophthalmic Solution 1453
Demulen 2161
Depen Titratable Tablets 2379
Engerix-B Unit-Dose Vials 2213
Enovid 2161
Estrace 1385
Estrace Vaginal Cream 1388
Estradurin 2452
Estratest 2245
Ganite Injection 1016
INH Tablets (Uncommon) 868
Levlen/Tri-Levlen 665
Lo/Ovral Tablets 2471
Lo/Ovral-28 Tablets 2476
M-M-R ‖ (Infrequent) 1494
M-R-VAX ‖ 1496
Motrin Tablets (Less than 1%) 2351
Mumpsvax 1513
Myambutol Tablets 1225
Nalfon Pulvules & Tablets (Less than 1%) 919
Nordette-21 Tablets 2481
Nordette-28 Tablets 2483
Norethin 2133
Norlutate 1754
Norlutin 1755
Ortho Dienestrol Cream 1664
Ovcon 1391
Ovral Tablets 2490
Ovral-28 Tablets 2491
Ovrette Tablets 2492
PMB 200 and PMB 400 2504
PediaProfen Suspension (Less than 1%) 1363
Platinol (Infrequent) 737
Platinol-AQ Injection (Infrequent) 738
Premarin Intravenous 2508
Premarin with Methyltestosterone 2515
Premarin Vaginal Cream 2512
Provera Tablets 2356
Quinaglute Dura-Tabs Tablets 663
Quinidex Extentabs 1868
Rifamate Capsules (Uncommon) 1347
Rufen Tablets (Less than 1%) 691
Stilphostrol Tablets and Ampuls 1609
TACE 12 and 25 mg 1353
Trecator-SC Tablets 2527
Levlen/Tri-Levlen 665
Yodoxin 1072

Neuritis, peripheral
Antabuse Tablets 2429
Antivenin (Crotalidae) Polyvalent (Occasional) 2430
Apresazide Capsules (Less frequent) 854
Apresoline Hydrochloride Parenteral (Ampuls) 856
Apresoline Hydrochloride Tablets (Less frequent) 855
Apresoline-Esidrix Tablets 857
Azo Gantanol Tablets 1887
Azo Gantrisin Tablets 1888
Bactrim DS Tablets 1891
Bactrim I.V. Infusion 1889
Bactrim 1891
Chloromycetin Kapseals 1695
Chloromycetin Palmitate, Oral Suspension 1697
Chloromycetin Sodium Succinate 1698
ColBENEMID Tablets 1436
Colchicine Ampoules 1252
Fansidar Tablets 1896
Gantanol 1899
Gantrisin Ophthalmic Ointment/Solution 1900
Gantrisin 1901
Intal Capsules (Less than 1 in 100,000 patients) 978
Intal Inhaler (Rare) 979
Intal Nebulizer Solution (Rare) 980
Lopid Capsules and Tablets 1736
Lorelco Tablets 1333
Myambutol Tablets 1225
Nasalcrom Nasal Solution (Rare) 986
Pediazole 1973
Septra 813
Septra I.V. Infusion 808
Septra I.V. Infusion ADD-Vantage Vials 810
Septra 813
Ser-Ap-Es Tablets 881
Serpasil-Apresoline Tablets 884
Solganal Suspension 2122
Tegretol Chewable Tablets 654
Tegretol Suspension 656
Tegretol Tablets 654
Thiosulfil Forte Tablets 2526

Trecator-SC Tablets 2527
Velban Vials 1305

Neuritis, retrobulbar
Ansaid Tablets (Less than 1%) 2319
Attenuvax 1424
Biavax ‖ 1427
M-M-R ‖ 1494
M-R-VAX ‖ 1496
Meruvax ‖ 1503
Mumpsvax (Infrequent) 1513

Neuroleptic malignant syndrome
Asendin Tablets (Less than 1%) 1196
Clozaril Tablets 2000
Compazine 2201
Etrafon 2087
Haldol Decanoate 1375
Haldol Injection, Tablets and Concentrate 1373
Loxitane 1213
Mellaril 2011
Moban Tablets & Concentrate 932
Navane Capsules and Concentrate (Rare) 1954
Navane Intramuscular (Rare) 1956
Orap Tablets 1020
Prolixin Decanoate 1795
Prolixin Elixir 1793
Prolixin Enanthate 1796
Prolixin Injection 1791
Prolixin Oral Concentrate 1792
Prolixin Tablets 1793
Reglan (Rare) 1869
Sinemet Tablets 952
Sinemet CR Tablets 953
Stelazine 2226
Taractan 1920
Temaril Tablets, Syrup and Spansule Sustained Release Capsules (Rare) 1085
Thorazine 2234
Triavil Tablets 1556
Trilafon 2123

Neuromuscular block reversal, difficult
Nuromax Injection 794

Neuromuscular blockade
Amikin Injectable 602
Coly-Mycin M Parenteral 1706
Netromycin Injection 100 mg/ml 2104

Neuromuscular excitability
Ceptaz for Injection 1057
Ticar for Injection (With very high doses) 2236

Neuromuscular symptoms
Eulexin Capsules (2%) 2089

Neuromyopathy
Aralen Hydrochloride Injection 2038
Aralen Phosphate Tablets 2039
Prozac Pulvules (Infrequent) 920

Neuro-ocular lesions
Amen 833
Demulen 2161
Enovid 2161
Levlen/Tri-Levlen 665
Loestrin 1728
Norethin 2133
Norlestrin 1746
Norlutate 1754
Norlutin 1755
Levlen/Tri-Levlen 665
Triphasil-21 Tablets 2527
Triphasil-28 Tablets 2532

Neuropathy
Altace Capsules (Less than 1%) 1086
Anafranil Capsules (Rare) 650
Bicillin C-R Injection 2438
Bicillin C-R 900/300 Injection 2440
Bicillin L-A Injection (Infrequent) 2442
▲CHEMET (succimer) Capsules (1.0 to 12.7%) 1361
Cortifoam 1827
Cuprimine Capsules 1442
Cytosar-U Sterile Powder 2329
Cytotec (Infrequent) 2159
Depen Titratable Tablets 2379
Diulo 2129
Engerix-B Unit-Dose Vials 2213
Fiorinal with Codeine Capsules 2008
Fungizone Intravenous 2262
Gelfoam Sterile Sponge 2338
Intron A (1 patient) 2097
Kerlone Tablets (Less than 2%) 2172

Matulane Capsules 1907
Mutamycin 733
Mykrox ½ mg Tablets (Less than 2%) 984
NebuPent for Inhalation Solution (1% or less) 1017
Nimotop Capsules (Less than 1%) 1607
Omnipaque (Less than 0.1 to 0.7%) 2552
Permax Tablets (Infrequent) 1291
Pfizerpen for Injection (Rare) 1957
Prozac Pulvules (Rare) 920
Roferon-A Injection (Less than 0.5%) 1916
Urobiotic-250 Capsules 1968
Zaroxolyn Tablets 989

Neuropathy, autonomic
Platinol 737
Platinol-AQ Injection 738

Neuropathy, optic
Decadron Phosphate Injection 1449
Decadron Phosphate Sterile Ophthalmic Ointment 1453
Decadron Phosphate Sterile Ophthalmic Solution 1453
Tolectin (200, 400 and 600 mg) (Less than 1%) 1379
Yodoxin 1072

Neuropathy, peripheral
Ancobon Capsules 1886
Azulfidine Tablets, EN-tabs, Oral Suspension (Rare) 1157
Cordarone Tablets (Common) 2446
Cuprimine Capsules 1442
Dapsone USP 1130
Depen Titratable Tablets 2379
Diphtheria and Tetanus Toxoids and Pertussis Vaccine Adsorbed USP (For Pediatric Use) (A few cases) 892
Elavil 2269
Endep Tablets 1927
Etrafon 2087
Flagyl I.V. 2131
Flagyl Tablets 2170
Flexeril Tablets (Rare) 1471
Fungizone Intravenous 2262
Garamycin Injectable 2093
▲Hexalen Capsules (9% to 31%) 2316
▲INH Tablets (Most common) 868
▲Idamycin for Injection (7%) 564
Indocin Capsules (Less than 1%) 1487
Indocin I.V. (Less than 1%) 1490
Indocin (Less than 1%) 1487
Leukeran Tablets 788
Ludiomil Tablets 874
▲Lupron Depot 3.75 mg (Among most frequent) 2312
Lupron Depot 7.5 mg 2311
Lupron Injection (Less than 5%) 2310
Macrodantin Capsules 1624
Mevacor Tablets 1505
Myochrysine Injection (Rare) 1516
Netromycin Injection 100 mg/ml 2104
Norpramin Tablets 1340
Omnipaque (Rare) 2552
Pamelor 2019
▲Paraplatin for Injection (6%) 735
Platinol 737
Platinol-AQ Injection 738
Protostat Tablets 1674
Recombivax HB 1544
Ridaura Capsules (Less than 1%) 2224
Rifamate Capsules 1347
Surmontil Capsules 2524
Tofranil Ampuls 1038
Tofranil Tablets 1039
Tofranil-PM Capsules 1041
Triavil Tablets 1556
Vivactil Tablets 1567
Zyloprim Tablets (Less than 1%) 830

Neuropsychometrics performance, decrease
Blocadren Tablets 1429
Cartrol Tablets 507
Corgard Tablets 701
Corzide Tablets 702
Inderal 2459
Inderal LA Long Acting Capsules 2461
Inderide Tablets 2463
Inderide LA Long Acting Capsules 2465
Kerlone Tablets 2172
Levatol 1832
Normodyne Tablets 2110
Normozide Tablets 2112
Sectral Capsules 2520
Tenoretic Tablets 1105

Tenormin Tablets and I.V. Injection 1107
Timoptic in Ocudose 1552
Timoptic Sterile Ophthalmic Solution 1550
Trandate HCT/Trandate 579
Visken Tablets 2036

Neuroretinitis
BiCNU 723

Neurosis, unspecified
Intron A (1 patient) 2097
Permax Tablets (Infrequent) 1291

Neurotoxicity
Cytosar-U Sterile Powder (Less frequent) 2329
Garamycin Injectable 2093
Hexalen Capsules 2316
INH Tablets 868
Nebcin Vials, Hyporets & ADD-Vantage 1286
Netromycin Injection 100 mg/ml 2104
Nipride I.V. Infusion 1909
Oncovin Solution Vials & Hyporets 1288
▲Paraplatin for Injection (5%) 735
Platinol 737
Platinol-AQ Injection 738
Polymyxin B Sulfate, Aerosporin Brand Sterile Powder 798
Velban Vials (Not common) 1305

Neurotoxicity, peripheral
VePesid Capsules and Injection (1 to 2%) 741

Neurovascular episodes
Lippes Loop Intrauterine Double-S 1654

Neutropenia
Achromycin V Capsules 1193
Altace Capsules (Rare to more frequent) 1086
Ancef Injection 2194
Atgam Sterile Solution (Less than 5%) 2320
Azactam for Injection (Less than 1%) 2252
Bactrim DS Tablets 1891
Bactrim I.V. Infusion 1889
Bactrim 1891
Capoten 2255
Capozide 2258
Cardura Tablets 1941
Ceclor Pulvules & Suspension 1251
Cefizox Injection (Rare) 1012
Cefobid Intravenous/Intramuscular (1 in 50) 1943
Cefobid Pharmacy Bulk Package - Not for Direct Infusion (1 in 50) 1945
Ceftin Tablets 575
Ceptaz for Injection (Very rare) 1057
Children's Advil Suspension (Less than 1%) 2426
Claforan Sterile Injection (Less than 1%) 1089
Cleocin Phosphate Injection 2325
Clinoril Tablets (Less than 1 in 100) 1433
▲Clozaril Tablets (3%) 2000
▲Cytovene Sterile Powder (Approximately 40%) 2292
Declomycin Capsules, Tablets 1199
Desyrel and Desyrel Dividose (Occasional) 1404
Dipentum Capsules (Rare) 1160
Doryx Capsules 1717
Duricef 1405
Edecrin 1468
Ergamisol Tablets (2 patients) 1136
Flagyl Tablets 2170
Fortaz (Rare) 1060
Gantanol 1899
Gastrocrom Capsules (Infrequent) 974
Geocillin Tablets 1951
Halcion Tablets (1.5%) 2340
Keflex Pulvules, Oral Suspension & Pediatric Drops 916
Keftab Tablets 917
Kefurox Vials, Faspak & ADD-Vantage (Less than 1 in 100) 1277
Kefzol Vials, Faspak & ADD-Vantage 1279
Lincocin 2344
Lotensin Tablets 872
Mandol Vials, Faspak & ADD-Vantage 1281
Meclomen Capsules (Less than 1%) 1739
Mefoxin 1498

Mefoxin Premixed Intravenous Solution ... 1500
Mesantoin Tablets ... 2013
Mexitil Capsules (About 1 in 1,000) ... 680
Mezlin ... 1597
Mezlin Pharmacy Bulk Package ... 1599
Midamor Tablets (Rare) ... 1508
Minocin Intravenous ... 1221
Minocin Oral Suspension ... 1224
Minocin Pellet-Filled Capsules ... 1222
Moduretic Tablets ... 1510
Monocid Injection (Less than 1%) .. 2217
Monodox Capsules ... 1630
Monopril Tablets (0.2 to 1.0%) ... 1406
Motrin Tablets (Less than 1%) ... 2351
NebuPent for Inhalation Solution (1% or less) ... 1017
Neosar for Injection ... 566
Noroxin Tablets (1.2%) ... 1519
Omnipaque ... 2552
Paradione Capsules ... 548
▲Paraplatin for Injection (21% to 67%) ... 735
PediaProfen Suspension (Less than 1%) ... 1363
Pipracil ... 1230
Prilosec Delayed-Release Capsules (Less than 1%) ... 1530
Primaxin I.M. ... 1532
Primaxin I.V. (Less than 0.2%) ... 1535
Prinivil Tablets (Rare) ... 1538
Prinzide Tablets (Rare) ... 1540
Procan SR Tablets (Rare) ... 1760
Proglycem ... 649
Proloprim Tablets ... 799
Pronestyl Capsules and Tablets (Approximately 0.5%) ... 1800
Pronestyl Injection (Approximately 0.5%) ... 1798
Pronestyl-SR Tablets (0.5%) ... 1801
Protostat Tablets ... 1674
Quinidex Extentabs ... 1868
Reglan (A few cases) ... 1869
Renese-R Tablets (Rare) ... 1786
Ridaura Capsules (0.1 to 1%) ... 2224
Rocephin Injectable Vials, ADD-Vantage (Less than 1%) ... 1914
▲Roferon-A Injection (52%) ... 1916
Rufen Tablets (Less than 1%) ... 691
SSD ... 694
Sansert Tablets ... 2031
Septra ... 813
Septra I.V. Infusion ... 808
Septra I.V. Infusion ADD-Vantage Vials ... 810
Septra ... 813
Symmetrel Capsules & Syrup (Less than 0.1%) ... 936
Tazicef for Injection (Very rare) ... 2231
Terramycin Capsules ... 1786
Terramycin Intramuscular Solution 1964
Ticar for Injection ... 2236
Timentin for Injection ... 2239
Tonocard Tablets (Less than 1%) .. 1554
Tridione ... 557
Trimpex Tablets ... 1922
Ultracef Capsules, Tablets & Oral Suspension ... 722
Unasyn ... 1965
Unipen (Infrequent) ... 2533
Valium Injectable (Isolated reports) 1937
Valium Tablets (Isolated reports) ... 1939
Valrelease Capsules (Rare) ... 1923
Vancocin HCl, Oral Solution & Pulvules (Several dozen cases) ... 1304
Vancocin HCl, Vials & ADD-Vantage (Several dozen cases) ... 1302
Vascor (200, 300 and 400 mg) Tablets (2 cases) ... 1383
Vaseretic Tablets (Rare) ... 1559
Vasotec I.V. (Rare) ... 1562
Vasotec Tablets (Rare) ... 1564
Velosef Capsules and for Oral Suspension ... 606
Vibramycin Hyclate Capsules ... 1787
Vibramycin Hyclate Intravenous ... 1968
Vibramycin ... 1787
Xanax Tablets (2.3% to 3.0%) ... 2367
Zefazone Sterile Powder ... 2372
Zestoretic ... 2274
Zestril Tablets ... 2277
Zinacef (Less than 1 in 100) ... 1066
Zovirax Sterile Powder (Less than 1%) ... 828

Neutropenia, irreversible
Cytovene Sterile Powder (Some patients) ... 2292

Neutrophilia
Zovirax Sterile Powder (Less than 1%) ... 828

Neutrophils, decrease (see under Neutropenia)

Nicotine intoxication
Nicorette ... 1335

Night blindness (see under Nyctalopia)

Nightmares
Aldoclor Tablets ... 1413
Aldomet Ester HCl Injection ... 1417
Aldomet Oral ... 1415
Aldoril Tablets ... 1418
Alurate Elixir (Less than 1 in 100) 1883
Asendin Tablets (Greater than 1%) ... 1196
Atabrine Hydrochloride Tablets (Infrequent) ... 2041
Blocadren Tablets ... 1429
Butisol Sodium Elixir & Tablets (Less than 1 in 100) ... 2377
Catapres Tablets ... 676
Catapres-TTS ... 677
Cipro I.V. (1% or less) ... 1592
Cipro Tablets (Less than 1%) ... 1589
▲Clozaril Tablets (4%) ... 2000
Combipres Tablets ... 678
Diupres Tablets ... 1461
Doral Tablets ... 2383
Elavil ... 2269
Eldepryl ... 2250
Endep Tablets ... 1927
Enduronyl ... 518
Etrafon ... 2087
Halcion Tablets (Rare) ... 2340
Harmonyl Tablets ... 528
Hydromox R Tablets ... 1209
Hydropres Tablets ... 1485
Larodopa Tablets (Relatively frequent) ... 1905
Lopressor Ampuls ... 1032
Lopressor HCT Tablets (1 in 100 patients) ... 1034
Lopressor Tablets ... 1032
Ludiomil Tablets (Rare) ... 874
Matulane Capsules ... 1907
Mebaral Tablets (Less than 1 in 100) ... 2061
Nardil (Infrequent) ... 1742
Nembutal Sodium Capsules (Less than 1%) ... 534
Nembutal Sodium Solution (Less than 1%) ... 536
Nembutal Sodium Suppositories (Less than 1%) ... 538
Norpramin Tablets ... 1340
Oreticyl ... 545
Orudis Capsules (Less than 1%) ... 2488
Pamelor ... 2019
Parlodel ... 2020
Phenobarbital Elixir and Tablets (Less than 1 in 100 patients) ... 1293
Plaquenil Sulfate Tablets ... 2067
Raudixin Tablets ... 1803
Rauzide Tablets ... 1804
Renese-R Tablets ... 1786
Salutensin/Salutensin-Demi ... 719
Seconal Sodium Pulvules (Less than 1 in 100) ... 1296
Seldane Tablets ... 1349
Seldane-D Extended-Release Tablets ... 1350
Ser-Ap-Es Tablets ... 881
Serpasil Tablets ... 883
Serpasil-Apresoline Tablets ... 884
Serpasil-Esidrix Tablets ... 886
Sinemet Tablets ... 952
Surmontil Capsules ... 2524
Temaril Tablets, Syrup and Spansule Sustained Release Capsules ... 1085
Tenex Tablets ... 1875
Timolide Tablets ... 1547
Timoptic in Ocudose ... 1552
Timoptic Sterile Ophthalmic Solution ... 1550
Tofranil Ampuls ... 1038
Tofranil Tablets ... 1039
Tofranil-PM Capsules ... 1041
Trexan Tablets (Less than 1%) ... 937
Triavil Tablets ... 1556
Ventolin (1%) ... 583
Versed Injection (Less than 1%) ... 1924
Vivactil Tablets ... 1567
Voltaren Tablets (Less than 1%) ... 1042

Night sweat
▲NebuPent for Inhalation Solution (10 to 23%) ... 1017

Night terrors (see under Pavor nocturnus)

Nitritoid reactions
Myochrysine Injection ... 1516

Nitrogen balance, changes (see under BUN levels, changes)

Nocturia
Anafranil Capsules (Infrequent) ... 650
BuSpar (Rare) ... 1401
Calcijex Calcitriol Injection ... 506
Calderol Capsules ... 1635
Cardene Capsules (0.4%) ... 2290
Cardizem Tablets-30 mg, 60 mg, 90 mg and 120 mg (Less than 1%) ... 1329
Cardizem SR Capsules-60 mg, 90 mg and 120 mg (Less than 1%) 1327
Catapres Tablets (About 1 in 100 patients) ... 676
Catapres-TTS (1%) ... 677
Combipres Tablets (About 1%) ... 678
Dantrium Capsules (Less frequent) 1619
DynaCirc Capsules (0.5% to 1%) .. 2004
Eldepryl ... 2250
Esimil Tablets ... 864
▲Hylorel Tablets (48.4%) ... 975
Hyperstat I.V. Injection ... 2095
Intron A (Less than 1%) ... 2097
Ismelin Tablets ... 869
Klonopin Tablets ... 1902
Lioresal Tablets (Rare) ... 1031
Lorelco Tablets ... 1333
Lozol Tablets (Less than 5%) ... 1843
Matulane Capsules ... 1907
Meclomen Capsules (Rare) ... 1739
Miacalcin Injection ... 2017
Moduretic Tablets (Less than or equal to 1%) ... 1510
Mykrox ½ mg Tablets (Less than 2%) ... 984
Normozide Tablets (Less than 1%) 2112
Norpramin Tablets ... 1340
Orap Tablets ... 1020
Pamelor ... 2019
Plendil Extended-Release Tablets (0.5% or greater) ... 1526
Procardia XL Tablets (1% or less).. 1783
ProSom Tablets (Rare) ... 554
Rocaltrol Capsules ... 1913
Sectral Capsules (Up to 2%) ... 2520
Tenex Tablets ... 1875
Trandate HCT Tablets (Less than 1% in 208 patients) ... 579
Trilafon ... 2123
Vagistat (Less than 1%) ... 1397
Vivactil Tablets ... 1567
Voltaren Tablets (Less than 1%) ... 1042
Wellbutrin Tablets (Frequent) ... 821

Nodal rhythm
Isoptin SR Sustained Release Tablets ... 1181
Lanoxicaps (Common) ... 772
Lanoxin Elixir Pediatric (Common).. 775
Lanoxin Injection (Common) ... 778
Lanoxin Injection Pediatric (Common) ... 781
Lanoxin Tablets (Common) ... 783
Prostigmin Injectable ... 1120
Prostigmin Tablets ... 1121
Sodium Polystyrene Sulfonate Suspension ... 1993
Versed Injection (Less than 1%) ... 1924

Nodule, subcutaneous
Prozac Pulvules (Rare) ... 920

Noise intolerance
BuSpar (Infrequent) ... 1401

Nuchal rigidity
Methotrexate Tablets, Parenteral, LPF Parenteral ... 1217
Rheumatrex Methotrexate Dose Pack ... 1234

Numbness
Adenocard Injection (1%) ... 1007
AeroBid Inhaler System (1-3%) ... 995
Alferon N Injection (One patient to 3%) ... 1809
▲Anestacon Solution (Among most common) ... 2394
Apresazide Capsules (Less frequent) ... 854
Apresoline Hydrochloride Parenteral (Ampuls) ... 856
Apresoline Hydrochloride Tablets (Less frequent) ... 855
Apresoline-Esidrix Tablets ... 857
Asendin Tablets (Less than 1%) ... 1196
Bentyl ... 1322
BuSpar (2%) ... 1401
Butazolidin Capsules & Tablets (Less than 1%) ... 1027
Cefizox Injection (Rare) ... 1012
Clozaril Tablets (Less than 1%) ... 2000
Desyrel and Desyrel Dividose (Less than 1%) ... 1404
Diprivan Injection (Greater than 1%) ... 2267
DynaCirc Capsules (0.5% to 1%) .. 2004
Elavil ... 2269
Elimite (permethrin) 5% Cream (1 to 2% or less) ... 1082
Endep Tablets ... 1927
Fiorinal with Codeine Capsules (Infrequent) ... 2008
Flagyl I.V. ... 2131
Garamycin Injectable ... 2093
K-Phos Neutral Tablets ... 660
K-Phos Original Formula 'Sodium Free' Tablets (Less frequent) ... 660
Kerlone Tablets (Less than 2%) ... 2172
Larodopa Tablets (Relatively frequent) ... 1905
Limbitrol ... 1933
Loxitane ... 1213
Ludiomil Tablets (Rare) ... 874
Lupron Depot 7.5 mg ... 2311
Lupron Injection (Less than 5%) ... 2310
▲Mexitil Capsules (2.4% to 3.8%) .. 680
Mintezol ... 1510
Moduretic Tablets (Less than or equal to 1%) ... 1510
Netromycin Injection 100 mg/ml... 2104
Nicorette ... 1335
Normodyne Injection (1%) ... 2108
Norpace (Less than 1%) ... 2177
Norpramin Tablets ... 1340
Nubain Injection (Less than 1%) ... 934
Pamelor ... 2019
Parlodel ... 2020
Parnate Tablets ... 2222
Peganone Tablets ... 551
Rifadin ... 1345
Rifamate Capsules ... 1347
Rimactane Capsules ... 879
▲Roferon-A Injection (3% to 6%) ... 1916
Rythmol Tablets (Less than 1%) ... 1184
Sandostatin Injection (Less than 1%) ... 2029
Ser-Ap-Es Tablets ... 881
Serpasil-Apresoline Tablets ... 884
Sinemet Tablets ... 952
Sinemet CR Tablets ... 953
Sinequan (Infrequent) ... 1960
Surmontil Capsules ... 2524
Tessalon Perles ... 1006
Tofranil Ampuls ... 1038
Tofranil Tablets ... 1039
Tofranil-PM Capsules ... 1041
Tonocard Tablets (Less than 1%) .. 1554
Trandate Injection (1 of 100 patients) ... 577
Triavil Tablets ... 1556
Uroqid-Acid (Less frequent) ... 661
Vivactil Tablets ... 1567
Xylocaine 5% Ointment ... 644

Numbness, buccal mucosa
Azactam for Injection (Less than 1%) ... 2252
Clozaril Tablets (1%) ... 2000
Marcaine Spinal ... 2058
Stilphostrol Tablets and Ampuls ... 1609

Numbness, extremities
Cogentin ... 1435
Coly-Mycin M Parenteral ... 1706
Etrafon ... 2087
Flagyl I.V. RTU ... 2131
Flagyl Tablets ... 2170
IOPIDINE ... ⊙ 232
Lomotil ... 2174
▲Lozol Tablets (Greater than or equal to 5%) ... 1843
Maxair Inhaler (Less than 1%) ... 1311
Micronor Tablets ... 1667
Modicon ... 1667
Myambutol Tablets ... 1225
Norpramin Tablets ... 1340
Ortho-Novum ... 1667
Protostat Tablets ... 1674

Sansert Tablets 2031
Trilafon 2123

Numbness, face

Placidyl Capsules 553

Numbness, feet

K-Lyte 707
K-Phos M.F. Tablets 659
K-Phos No. 2 Tablets 659

Numbness, fingers

Aclovate Ointment (1 of 366 patients) 1053
Alferon N Injection (One patient) 1809
Cutivate Cream 0.05% (1.0%) 1054
D.H.E. 45 Injection 2003
Temovate (1 of 366 patients) 1056
Wigraine Tablets & Suppositories 1645

Numbness, hands

Alferon N Injection (One patient) 1809
Hyperstat I.V. Injection 2095
K-Lyte 707
K-Phos M.F. Tablets 659
K-Phos No. 2 Tablets 659

Numbness, lips

K-Lyte 707
K-Phos M.F. Tablets 659
K-Phos Neutral Tablets 660
K-Phos Original Formula 'Sodium Free' Tablets (Less frequent) 660
K-Phos No. 2 Tablets 659
Marcaine Spinal 2058
Sensorcaine 631
Sensorcaine-MPF Spinal 634
Uroqid-Acid (Less frequent) 661

Numbness, mouth (see under Numbness, buccal mucosa)

Numbness, nose

Stilphostrol Tablets and Ampuls 1609

Numbness, skin

Cibalith-S 870
Eskalith 2214
Lithane Tablets 1596
Lithium Carbonate Capsules & Tablets 1984
Lithobid Tablets 870

Numbness, toes

D.H.E. 45 Injection 2003
Wigraine Tablets & Suppositories 1645

Numbness, tongue (see under Numbness, buccal mucosa)

Numbness/tingling, fingers and toes

Eldepryl 2250
Ergostat 1719

Nyctalopia

Accutane Capsules (Rare) 1878
Anafranil Capsules (Rare) 650
Aralen Hydrochloride Injection 2038
Aralen Phosphate Tablets 2039
Cardioquin Tablets 1812
Cholybar (One case) 1705
Questran Light (1 case) 711
Questran Powder (1 case) 710
Quinaglute Dura-Tabs Tablets 663
Quinidex Extentabs 1868
Tegison Capsules (Less than 1%) 1881
Voltaren Tablets (Less than 1%) 1042

Nystagmus

Anafranil Capsules (Rare) 650
Cibalith-S 870
Cipro I.V. (1% or less) 1592
Cipro Tablets 1589
Clozaril Tablets (Less than 1%) 2000
Cylert Tablets 510
Dalalone D.P. Injectable 999
Decadron-LA Sterile Suspension (Low) 1457
Depakene Capsules & Syrup 511
Depakote 512
▲ Dilantin Infatabs (Among most common) 1710
▲ Dilantin Kapseals (Among most common) 1708
▲ Dilantin Parenteral (Among most common) 1712
▲ Dilantin-30 Pediatric/Dilantin-125 Suspension (Among most common) 1713
▲ Dilantin with Phenobarbital Kapseals (Among most common) 1715
Dilaudid-HP Injection 1175
Diprivan Injection (Less than 1%) 2267
Ergamisol Tablets 1136
Eskalith 2214
Ethmozine Tablets (Less than 2%) 946
Sterile FUDR (Remote possibility) 1898
Floxin Tablets 1652
Fluorouracil Injection 1897
Isoptin Injectable (Few) 1177
Ketalar 1726
Klonopin Tablets 1902
Lioresal Tablets 1031
Lithane Tablets 1596
Lithium Carbonate Capsules & Tablets 1984
Lithobid Tablets 870
MS Contin Tablets (Infrequent) 1814
MSIR (Infrequent) 1817
Macrodantin Capsules (Less frequent) 1624
Matulane Capsules 1907
Mebaral Tablets 2061
Mesantoin Tablets 2013
Mysoline (Occasional) 2480
Nardil (Less common) 1742
Netromycin Injection 100 mg/ml 2104
Omnipaque (Less than 0.3%) 2552
Oramorph SR (Morphine Sulfate Sustained Release Tablets) (Less frequent) 1988
Peganone Tablets 551
Plaquenil Sulfate Tablets 2067
ProSom Tablets 554
Prozac Pulvules (Rare) 920
Robaxin Injectable 1871
Talwin Injection (Rare) 2071
Tambocor Tablets (Less than 1%) 1315
Tegretol Chewable Tablets 654
Tegretol Suspension 656
Tegretol Tablets 654
Tonocard Tablets (0.0-1.1%) 1554
Valium Injectable 1937
Versed Injection (Less than 1%) 1924

Nystagmus, horizontal (see also under Nystagmus)

Restoril Capsules (Less than 0.5%) 2023

NMS (see under Neuroleptic malignant syndrome)

NPN elevation

▲ Capastat Sulfate Vials (36%) 1250
Garamycin Injectable 2093
Nebcin Vials, Hyporets & ADD-Vantage 1286

O

Obstipation

Compazine 2201
Etrafon 2087
Mellaril 2011
Norzine 1818
Serentil 686
Stelazine 2226
Taractan 1920
Thorazine 2234
Torecan 1993
Triavil Tablets 1556
Trilafon (Occasional) 2123

Obtundation

Intron A (Some patients) 2097
Roferon-A Injection (Rare) 1916
Zovirax Sterile Powder 828

Occult bleeding

Azdone Tablets (Occasional) 844
Damason-P (Occasional) 1356
Fiorinal with Codeine Capsules 2008
Lortab ASA Tablets (Occasional) 2414
Soma Compound w/Codeine Tablets 2390
Soma Compound Tablets 2389
Zorprin Tablets 698

Occult blood in stool, positive test

Children's Advil Suspension 2426
Lioresal Tablets 1031
PediaProfen Suspension 1363

Ocular allergy

Anafranil Capsules (Up to 2%) 650
Aureomycin Ophthalmic Ointment 1.0% ◉ 308
Murocoll-2 Sterile Ophthalmic Solution (Rare) ◉ 261
Profenal Sterile Ophthalmic Solution (Less than 0.5%) ◉ 234

Ocular discomfort

Betoptic Sterile Ophthalmic Solution 569
Betoptic S Sterile Ophthalmic Suspension 570

Ocular, foreign body sensation

Betoptic Sterile Ophthalmic Solution (Small numbers of patients) 569
Betoptic S Sterile Ophthalmic Suspension (Small numbers of patients) 570
IOPIDINE ◉ 232

Ocular exudate

Betoptic Sterile Ophthalmic Solution (Small numbers of patients) 569
Betoptic S Sterile Ophthalmic Suspension (Small numbers of patients) 570
Isopto Atropine ◉ 218
Isopto Homatropine ◉ 221
Isopto Hyoscine ◉ 222

Ocular hypotony

IOPIDINE ◉ 232

Ocular infection

Metimyd ◉ 306
NeoDecadron Sterile Ophthalmic Ointment 1517
NeoDecadron Sterile Ophthalmic Solution 1518
Opticrom 4% (Infrequent) 986
Terra-Cortril Ophthalmic Suspension 1963
Trilafon 2123

Ocular lesions

Brevicon 2304
Decadron Phosphate Sterile Ophthalmic Ointment 1453
Decadron Phosphate Sterile Ophthalmic Solution 1453
Lariam Tablets 1904
Norinyl 2304
Ovcon 1391
Tri-Norinyl 28-Day Tablets 2304

Ocular palsies

Attenuvax (Rare) 1424
Butazolidin Capsules & Tablets (Less than 1%) 1027
M-M-R $_{II}$ (Rare) 1494
M-R-VAX $_{II}$ (Rare) 1496
Plaquenil Sulfate Tablets 2067

Ocular perforation

Decadron Phosphate Sterile Ophthalmic Ointment 1453
Decadron Phosphate Sterile Ophthalmic Solution 1453

Ocular tension, increase

Bentyl 1322
Cantil Tablets 1326
Darbid Tablets 2205
Decadron Phosphate Sterile Ophthalmic Ointment 1453
Decadron Phosphate Sterile Ophthalmic Solution 1453
Donnatal 1858
Donnatal Extentabs 1859
Donnatal Tablets 1858
Donnazyme Tablets 1860
Kinesed Tablets 2272
Kutrase Capsules 2146
Levsin/Levsinex 2147
Medrol 2348
Norflex 1314
Norgesic 1314
Pro-Banthīne Tablets 2141
Robinul Forte Tablets 1873
Robinul Injectable 1873
Robinul Tablets 1873
Solu-Cortef Sterile Powder 2361
Solu-Medrol Sterile Powder 2363
Urispas Tablets 2242
Valpin 50 Tablets 941

Ocular toxicity

Nolvadex Tablets 1102
Plaquenil Sulfate Tablets 2067
Platinol 737
Platinol-AQ Injection 738
Ridaura Capsules 2224
TobraDex Ophthalmic Suspension and Ointment ◉ 228
Tobrex Ophthalmic Ointment and Solution (Less than 3 in 100 patients) 572

Oculogyric crises

Anafranil Capsules (Rare) 650
Compazine 2201
Cylert Tablets 510
Etrafon 2087
Haldol Decanoate (Less frequent) 1375
Haldol Injection, Tablets and Concentrate 1373
Inapsine Injection 1140
Innovar Injection 1141
Larodopa Tablets (Rare) 1905
Mellaril 2011
Norzine 1818
Orap Tablets (Less frequent) 1020
Phenergan with Codeine 2497
Phenergan with Dextromethorphan 2499
Phenergan Injection 2493
Phenergan Suppositories 2496
Phenergan Syrup 2495
Phenergan Tablets 2496
Phenergan VC 2500
Phenergan VC with Codeine 2501
Prolixin Decanoate 1795
Prolixin Elixir 1793
Prolixin Enanthate 1796
Prolixin Injection 1791
▲ Prolixin Oral Concentrate (Among most frequent) 1792
Prolixin Tablets 1793
Reglan 1869
Serentil 686
Sinemet Tablets 952
Stelazine 2226
Sublimaze Injection 1146
Symmetrel Capsules & Syrup (Less than 0.1%) 936
Taractan 1920
Temaril Tablets, Syrup and Spansule Sustained Release Capsules 1085
Thorazine 2234
Timolide Tablets 1547
Torecan 1993
Triavil Tablets 1556
Trilafon 2123

Oculomotor disturbances

Omnipaque (Less than 0.01%) 2552
Tegretol Chewable Tablets 654
Tegretol Suspension 656
Tegretol Tablets 654

Oiliness

A/T/S Topical Gel and Topical Solution 1089
ETS-2% 1685
Erycette (erythromycin 2%) Topical Solution 1678
T-Stat 2.0% Topical Solution and Pads 2409
Theramycin Z Topical Solution 2% 1410

Oligohydramnios

Altace Capsules 1086
Clinoril Tablets 1433
Dolobid Tablets 1465
Prinivil Tablets 1538
Prinzide Tablets 1540
Vaseretic Tablets 1559
Vasotec I.V. 1562
Vasotec Tablets 1564
Zestoretic 2274
Zestril Tablets 2277

Oligomenorrhea

Brevicon 2304
Jenest-28 Tablets 1636
Levlen/Tri-Levlen 665
Micronor Tablets 1667
Modicon 1667
Mustargen 1514
▲ Nolvadex Tablets (8.7%) 1102
Norinyl 2304
Ortho-Novum 1667
Levlen/Tri-Levlen 665
Tri-Norinyl 28-Day Tablets 2304

Oligospermia

Anadrol-50 Tablets 2287
Android 1111
▲ Azulfidine Tablets, EN-tabs, Oral

Suspension (Approximately one-third of patients) ... 1157
Cytoxan for Injection ... 726
Halotestin Tablets ... 2341
Metandren Linguets and Tablets ... 875
Methotrexate Tablets, Parenteral, LPF Parenteral ... 1217
Neosar for Injection ... 566
Nizoral Tablets (Infrequent) ... 1145
Rheumatrex Methotrexate Dose Pack ... 1234
Testred Capsules ... 1124
Winstrol Tablets ... 2075

Oliguria

Amikin Injectable ... 602
Anafranil Capsules (Infrequent) ... 650
Astramorph/PF Injection, USP (Preservative-Free) ... 618
Azo Gantanol Tablets ... 1887
Azo Gantrisin Tablets ... 1888
Azulfidine Tablets, EN-tabs, Oral Suspension (Rare) ... 1157
Bactrim DS Tablets ... 1891
Bactrim I.V. Infusion ... 1889
Bactrim ... 1891
Capastat Sulfate Vials (1 patient) ... 1250
Capoten (Approximately 1 to 2 of 1000 patients) ... 2255
Capozide (Approximately 1 to 2 of 1000 patients) ... 2258
Cibalith-S ... 870
Cleocin Phosphate Injection (Rare) 2325
ColBENEMID Tablets ... 1436
Corzide Tablets ... 702
Deprol Tablets (Rare) ... 2382
Duragesic Transdermal System (Less than 1%) ... 1133
Duramorph ... 960
Equagesic Tablets (Rare) ... 2451
Eskalith ... 2214
Fansidar Tablets ... 1896
Fungizone Intravenous ... 2262
Gantanol ... 1899
Gantrisin Ophthalmic Ointment/Solution ... 1900
Gantrisin ... 1901
Garamycin Injectable ... 2093
Hyskon Hysteroscopy Fluid (Rare) .. 1162
Infumorph 200 and Infumorph 500 Sterile Solutions ... 962
Lithane Tablets ... 1596
Lithium Carbonate Capsules & Tablets ... 1984
Lithobid Tablets ... 870
Metrodin (urofollitropin for injection) ... 2182
Miltown Tablets (Rare) ... 2386
Nalfon Pulvules & Tablets (Less than 1%) ... 919
Nebcin Vials, Hyporets & ADD-Vantage ... 1286
Netromycin Injection 100 mg/ml ... 2104
Omnipaque (Rare) ... 2552
PMB 200 and PMB 400 (Rare) ... 2504
Pediazole ... 1973
Phenergan with Codeine ... 2497
Phenergan VC with Codeine ... 2501
Primaxin I.M. ... 1532
Primaxin I.V. (Less than 0.2%) ... 1535
Prinivil Tablets (1% or less) ... 1538
Prinzide Tablets ... 1540
Priscoline Hydrochloride Ampuls ... 877
ProSom Tablets (Rare) ... 554
Rauzide Tablets ... 1804
Sandostatin Injection (Less than 1%) ... 2029
Sansert Tablets ... 2031
Septra ... 813
Septra I.V. Infusion ... 808
Septra I.V. Infusion ADD-Vantage Vials ... 810
Septra ... 813
Serophene (clomiphene citrate tablets, USP) ... 2186
Tegretol Chewable Tablets ... 654
Tegretol Suspension ... 656
Tegretol Tablets ... 654
Tenoretic Tablets ... 1105
Thalitone Tablets ... 687
Thiosulfil Forte Tablets ... 2526
Toradol IM Injection (1% or less) ... 2302
Vaseretic Tablets ... 1559
Vasotec I.V. ... 1562
Vasotec Tablets (0.5% to 1%) ... 1564
Voltaren Tablets (Rare) ... 1042
Zestoretic ... 2274
Zestril Tablets (Less than 1%) ... 2277

"On-off" phenomenon

Larodopa Tablets ... 1905
Parlodel ... 2020
Sinemet Tablets ... 952
Sinemet CR Tablets (1.6%) ... 953

Onycholysis

Adriamycin PFS (Few cases) ... 561
Adriamycin RDF (A few cases) ... 562
Doxorubicin Hydrochloride for Injection, USP (A few cases) ... 622
Doxorubicin Hydrochloride Injection, USP (A few cases) ... 848
Feldene Capsules (Less than 1%) .. 1777
Orudis Capsules (Less than 1%) ... 2488
Rubex (A few cases) ... 739
▲ Tegison Capsules (1-10%) ... 1881
Zyloprim Tablets (Less than 1%) ... 830

Oogenesis, defective

Methotrexate Tablets, Parenteral, LPF Parenteral ... 1217
Rheumatrex Methotrexate Dose Pack ... 1234

Opisthotonos

Compazine ... 2201
Diprivan Injection (Less than 1%) .. 2267
Etrafon ... 2087
Haldol Decanoate ... 1375
Haldol Injection, Tablets and Concentrate ... 1373
Mellaril ... 2011
Norzine ... 1818
Orap Tablets (Less frequent) ... 1020
Prolixin Decanoate ... 1795
Prolixin Elixir ... 1793
Prolixin Enanthate ... 1796
Prolixin Injection ... 1791
▲ Prolixin Oral Concentrate (Among most frequent) ... 1792
Prolixin Tablets ... 1793
Reglan ... 1869
Serentil ... 686
Stelazine ... 2226
Thorazine ... 2234
Tigan ... 2239
Torecan ... 1993
Triavil Tablets ... 1556
Trilafon ... 2123

Optic atrophy

Aralen Phosphate with Primaquine Phosphate Tablets ... 2040
Aralen Phosphate Tablets ... 2039
Cibalith-S ... 870
Diupres Tablets ... 1461
Enduronyl ... 518
Eskalith ... 2214
Harmonyl Tablets ... 528
Hydropres Tablets ... 1485
INH Tablets (Uncommon) ... 868
Lithane Tablets ... 1596
Lithium Carbonate Capsules & Tablets ... 1984
Lithobid Tablets ... 870
Oncovin Solution Vials & Hyporets 1288
Oreticyl ... 545
Plaquenil Sulfate Tablets ... 2067
Raudixin Tablets ... 1803
Rauzide Tablets ... 1804
Renese-R Tablets ... 1786
Salutensin/Salutensin-Demi ... 719
Ser-Ap-Es Tablets ... 881
Serpasil Tablets ... 883
Serpasil-Apresoline Tablets ... 884
Serpasil-Esidrix Tablets ... 886
Yodoxin ... 1072

Optic disorders

Medrol ... 2348
Provera Tablets ... 2356
Solu-Cortef Sterile Powder ... 2361
Solu-Medrol Sterile Powder ... 2363

Optic nerve, damage

AK-Cide Sterile Ophthalmic Ointment & Suspension (Infrequent) ... ⊙ 202
AK-Dex ... ⊙ 203
AK-Pred ... ⊙ 205
AK-Spore H.C. (Infrequent) ... ⊙ 206
AK-Trol Ointment & Suspension (Infrequent) ... ⊙ 207
Aristospan Suspension (Intra-articular) ... 1011
Blephamide (Infrequent) ... 586
Cetapred Ointment (Infrequent) .. ⊙ 220
Chloromycetin Hydrocortisone Ophthalmic (Infrequent) ... 1694
Cortisporin Ophthalmic Ointment Sterile (Infrequent) ... 758
Cortisporin Ophthalmic Suspension Sterile ... 759
Dapsone USP ... 1130
Dexacidin (Infrequent) ... ⊙ 272
⅛% Econopred & 1% Econopred Plus ... ⊙ 217
FML Forte Liquifilm ... ⊙ 245
FML Liquifilm ... ⊙ 244
FML S.O.P. ... ⊙ 245
FML-S Sterile Ophthalmic Suspension (Infrequent) ... ⊙ 246
Fluor-Op Ophthalmic Suspension ⊙ 272
HMS Liquifilm (Rare) ... ⊙ 247
Inflamase ... ⊙ 274
Isopto Cetapred Suspension (Infrequent) ... ⊙ 220
Maxidex Sterile Ophthalmic Ointment ... ⊙ 222
Maxidex Sterile Ophthalmic Suspension ... ⊙ 223
Maxitrol Ophthalmic Ointment/Suspension (Infrequent) ... ⊙ 223
Metimyd ... ⊙ 306
NeoDecadron Sterile Ophthalmic Ointment ... 1517
NeoDecadron Sterile Ophthalmic Solution ... 1518
Ophthocort ... ⊙ 301
Poly-Pred Liquifilm (Infrequent) .. ⊙ 250
Pred Forte ... ⊙ 252
Pred Mild ... ⊙ 254
Pred-G Liquifilm Sterile Ophthalmic Suspension (Infrequent) ... ⊙ 252
Pred-G S.O.P. Sterile Ophthalmic Ointment ... ⊙ 253
Terra-Cortril Ophthalmic Suspension (Infrequent) ... 1963
TobraDex Ophthalmic Suspension and Ointment (Infrequent) ... ⊙ 228
Vasocidin Ointment (Infrequent) .. ⊙ 275
Vasocidin Ophthalmic Solution (Infrequent) ... ⊙ 276

Optic nerve, infarction

Hyperstat I.V. Injection ... 2095

Orchitis

Biavax ǁ ... 1427
M-M-R ǁ ... 1494
Mumpsvax (Rare) ... 1513
Prozac Pulvules (Rare) ... 920

Organic brain syndrome

Cibalith-S ... 870
Eskalith ... 2214
Garamycin Injectable ... 2093
Lithane Tablets ... 1596
Lithium Carbonate Capsules & Tablets ... 1984
Lithobid Tablets ... 870

Oropharyngitis

▲ Roferon-A Injection (14% to 16%) 1916

Oropharynx, dry

▲ Atrovent Inhalation Aerosol (About 5 in 100) ... 675
Brethaire Inhaler ... 1024
Proventil Repetabs Tablets ... 2120
Proventil Syrup ... 2119
Proventil Tablets ... 2120
▲ Roferon-A Injection (14% to 16%) 1916
Tussionex Extended-Release Suspension ... 988
Ventolin ... 583

Osteoarticular pain

Cardizem Tablets-30 mg, 60 mg, 90 mg and 120 mg (Less than 1%) ... 1329
Cardizem SR Capsules-60 mg, 90 mg and 120 mg (Less than 1%) 1327

Osteomalcia

Phenobarbital Elixir and Tablets ... 1293

Osteomalacia syndromes

Aludrox Oral Suspension ... 2428
Amphojel ... 2429
Basaljel ... 2438
Gelusil Liquid & Tablets ... ▣ 639
Maalox Plus Extra Strength ... 1850
Mylanta ... 1155
Mylanta • Double Strength ... 1155
Rolaids ... ▣ 743

Osteomalacia, phosphate-induced

K-Phos M.F. Tablets ... 659
K-Phos Neutral Tablets ... 660
K-Phos Original Formula 'Sodium Free' Tablets ... 660
K-Phos No. 2 Tablets ... 659
Uroqid-Acid ... 661

Osteomyelitis

BCG Vaccine, USP (Tice) (1 per 1,000,000 vaccinees) ... 1632
Permax Tablets (Rare) ... 1291
Tice BCG Vaccine, USP (1 per 1,000,000 vaccines) ... 1632

Osteoporosis

Aristocort Suspension ... 1008
Aristospan Suspension ... 1011
Calciparine Injection ... 925
Celestone Soluspan Suspension ... 2081
Cholybar (Less frequent) ... 1705
Cortenema ... 2244
Cortifoam ... 1827
Cortone Acetate Sterile Suspension ... 1437
Cortone Acetate Tablets ... 1439
Dalalone D.P. Injectable ... 999
Decadron Elixir ... 1445
Decadron Phosphate Injection ... 1449
Decadron Phosphate Respihaler ... 1454
Decadron Phosphate Turbinaire ... 1456
Decadron Phosphate with Xylocaine Injection, Sterile ... 1451
Decadron Tablets ... 1447
Decadron-LA Sterile Suspension ... 1457
Deltasone Tablets ... 2332
Depo-Medrol Sterile Aqueous Suspension ... 2334
Heparin Lock Flush Solution ... 2456
Heparin Sodium Vials ... 1264
Heparin Sodium Injection ... 2457
Heparin Sodium Injection, USP, Sterile Solution ... 2342
Hydeltrasol Injection, Sterile ... 1476
Hydeltra-T.B.A. Sterile Suspension 1478
Hydrocortone Acetate Sterile Suspension ... 1479
Hydrocortone Phosphate Injection, Sterile ... 1481
Hydrocortone Tablets ... 1482
Kenalog-10 Injection ... 2402
Kenalog-40 Injection ... 2403
Medrol ... 2348
Methotrexate Tablets, Parenteral, LPF Parenteral ... 1217
Neupogen for Injection (Less frequent) ... 595
Pediapred Oral Liquid ... 987
Permax Tablets (Rare) ... 1291
Prozac Pulvules (Rare) ... 920
Questran Light (Less frequent) ... 711
Questran Powder ... 710
Rheumatrex Methotrexate Dose Pack ... 1234
Solu-Cortef Sterile Powder ... 2361
Solu-Medrol Sterile Powder ... 2363

Otitis, externa

▲ Tegison Capsules (1-10%) ... 1881

Otitis, media

▲ Anafranil Capsules (Up to 4%) ... 650
Cardura Tablets (Less than 0.5% of 3960 patients) ... 1941
▲ CHEMET (succimer) Capsules (1.0 to 3.7%) ... 1361
M-M-R ǁ ... 1494
▲ PedvaxHIB (Among most frequent) 1521
Permax Tablets (Infrequent) ... 1291

Ototoxicity

Amikin Injectable ... 602
Bumex ... 1895
Cortisporin Cream ... 757
Cortisporin Ointment ... 758
Cortisporin Otic Solution Sterile (Occasional) ... 760
Cortisporin Otic Suspension Sterile 760
Garamycin Injectable ... 2093
Nebcin Vials, Hyporets & ADD-Vantage ... 1286
NeoDecadron Topical Cream ... 1518
Neosporin Cream ... 792
Neosporin G.U. Irrigant Sterile ... 793
Neosporin Ointment ... 793
Netromycin Injection 100 mg/ml ... 2104
Paraplatin for Injection (1%) ... 735
PediOtic Suspension Sterile ... 797
▲ Platinol (Up to 31%) ... 737
▲ Platinol-AQ Injection (Up to 31% of patients) ... 738
Vancocin HCl, Oral Solution & Pulvules ... 1304

Vancocin HCl, Vials & ADD-Vantage 1302

Ovarian cyst formation
Anafranil Capsules (Infrequent) 650
Metrodin (urofollitropin for injection) 2182
Nolvadex Tablets (2.8%) 1102
Pergonal (menotropins for injection, USP) 2184
Profasi (human chorionic gonadotropin, USP) 2186
Serophene (clomiphene citrate tablets, USP) (Less than 1 in 100 patients) 2186

Ovarian cysts, enlargement of existing
A.P.L. 2431
Synarel Nasal Solution 2300

Ovarian disorder
Prozac Pulvules (Infrequent) 920
Wellbutrin Tablets (Rare) 821

Ovarian enlargement
Lutrepulse for Injection (Rare) 1655
▲ Metrodin (urofollitropin for injection) (Approximately 20%) 2182
▲ Pergonal (menotropins for injection, USP) (Approximately 20%) 2184
▲ Serophene (clomiphene citrate tablets, USP) (Approximately 1 in 7 patients) 2186

Ovarian hyperstimulation syndrome
A.P.L. 2431
Lutrepulse for Injection (One case) 1655
▲ Metrodin (urofollitropin for injection) (6%) 2182
Pergonal (menotropins for injection, USP) 2184
Profasi (human chorionic gonadotropin, USP) 2186

Oversedation
Versed Injection (1.6%) 1924

Overstimulation
Adipex-P Tablets and Capsules 1019
Biphetamine Capsules 973
Bontril Slow-Release 834
Deprol Tablets 2382
Desoxyn Gradumet Tablets 514
Dexedrine 2206
Didrex Tablets 2338
Eldepryl 2250
Equagesic Tablets 2451
Fastin Capsules 2216
Halcion Tablets 2340
Ionamin Capsules 981
Miltown Tablets 2386
PMB 200 and PMB 400 2504
Paraflex Caplets (Occasional) 1378
Parafon Forte DSC Caplets 1379
Parnate Tablets 2222
Plegine Tablets 2504
Prelu-2 Capsules 683
Sanorex Tablets 2030
Tenuate 1354
Vontrol Tablets 2243

P

Pain
Americaine Hemorrhoidal Ointment ▣ 558
▲ Anafranil Capsules (3% to 4%) 650
▲ Antivenin (Crotalidae) Polyvalent (Frequent) 2430
Aplisol (tuberculin PPD, diluted) 2550
Aplitest (tuberculin PPD, multiple-puncture device) 2551
BAL in Oil Ampules 661
Bactroban Ointment (1.5%) 2200
Calan SR Caplets 2157
Calan Tablets 2155
Calciparine Injection 925
Cardura Tablets (2%) 1941
Cartrol Tablets (Less common) 507
▲ CHEMET (succimer) Capsules (5.2-15.7%) 1361
▲ Claforan Sterile Injection (4.3%) 1089
Cleocin Phosphate Injection 2325
▲ Condylox (50% to 72%) 1630
Coumadin Injection & Tablets 944
Cytotec (Infrequent) 2159
Dalalone D.P. Injectable 999
Dalmane Capsules 1927
Danocrine Capsules 2046
Debrisan 1150
Decadron-LA Sterile Suspension 1457
Desferal Vials 862
Diphtheria and Tetanus Toxoids and Pertussis Vaccine Adsorbed USP (For Pediatric Use) (Frequent) 892
▲ Diprivan Injection (10% or greater) 2267
▲ Efudex (Among most frequent) 1880
Feldene Capsules (Less than 1%) 1777
Floxin Tablets (Less than 1%) 1652
Fluorescite Injection ⊙ 217
Fluoroplex Topical Solution & Cream 1% 1082
Fluorouracil Injection 1897
▲ Fungizone Intravenous (Among most common) 2262
Gamimune N Immune Globulin Intravenous (Human) 1572
Gelfoam Sterile Sponge 2338
Halcion Tablets (Less frequent) 2340
Heparin Sodium Vials 1264
Heparin Sodium Injection, USP, Sterile Solution 2342
Herplex Liquifilm ⊙ 248
▲ Intron A (Up to 18%) 2097
K-Phos Neutral Tablets 660
K-Phos Original Formula 'Sodium Free' Tablets (Less frequent) 660
Kenalog-10 Injection 2402
Kenalog-40 Injection (Few) 2403
Kerlone Tablets (Less than 2%) 2172
Klonopin Tablets 1902
Konakion Injection (Rare) 1903
Kutapressin Injection 2146
Lamprene Capsules (Less than 1%) 1030
Librium Injectable 1932
Lippes Loop Intrauterine Double-S 1654
▲ Lupron Depot 7.5 mg (7.1%) 2311
▲ Lupron Injection (5% or more) 2310
Marax Tablets & DF Syrup 1954
Matulane Capsules 1907
Mutamycin 733
Neupogen for Injection (2%) 595
Nolvadex Tablets (2.8%) 1102
Normozide Tablets (Less than 1%) 2112
▲ Norpace (3 to 9%) 2177
▲ Norplant System (3.7%) 2484
▲ Omnipaque (0.6 to 49%) 2552
Orudis Capsules (Less than 1%) 2488
PPD Tine Test 2548
ParaGard T380A Intrauterine Copper Contraceptive 411
▲ Paraplatin for Injection (23%) 735
Pergonal (menotropins for injection, USP) 2184
▲ Permax Tablets (7.0%) 1291
Prilosec Delayed-Release Capsules (Less than 1%) 1530
Procardia XL Tablets (Less than 3%) 1783
Profenal Sterile Ophthalmic Solution (Less than 0.5%) ⊙ 234
ProSom Tablets (2%) 554
Rogaine Topical Solution (2.59%) 2357
Rowasa (1.35%) 2248
Rythmol Tablets (Less than 1%) 1184
▲ Tegison Capsules (1-10%) 1881
▲ Terazol 3 Vaginal Suppositories (3.9% of 284 patients) 1677
Terazol 7 Vaginal Cream (2.1% of 521 patients) 1677
Tetanus Toxoid, Adsorbed Purogenated 1238
Theo-24 2179
Trandate HCT Tablets (Less than 1% in 208 patients) 579
Travase Ointment 697
Trexan Tablets (Less than 1%) 937
Tuberculin, Old, Tine Test 2549
Vancocin HCl, Vials & ADD-Vantage 1302
Vascor (200, 300 and 400 mg) Tablets (0.5 to 2.0%) 1383
Versed Injection (0.5%-1.7%) 1924
Vira-A Ophthalmic Ointment, 3% 1767
Wellbutrin Tablets (Infrequent) 821
Zovirax Capsules 824
Zovirax Ointment 5% 827
Zovirax 824

Pain, abdominal (see under Abdominal pain/cramps)

Pain, back (see under Backache)

Pain, biliary
Actigall Capsules 2280

Pain, bone
Calcijex Calcitriol Injection 506
Calderol Capsules 1635
Cytosar-U Sterile Powder (Occasional) 2329
Didronel Tablets 1621
K-Phos M.F. Tablets 659
K-Phos Original Formula 'Sodium Free' Tablets (Less frequent) 660
K-Phos No. 2 Tablets 659
Lamprene Capsules (Less than 1%) 1030
▲ Leukine for IV Infusion (Among most frequent) 1127
Levatol (2.4%) 1832
▲ Lupron Depot 3.75 mg (Among most frequent) 2312
Lupron Depot 7.5 mg (Less than 5%) 2311
▲ Lupron Injection (5% or more) 2310
▲ Neupogen for Injection (22%) 595
▲ Nolvadex Tablets (5.7%) 1102
Oncovin Solution Vials & Hyporets 1288
Permax Tablets (Infrequent) 1291
Prozac Pulvules (Infrequent) 920
Rifadin 1345
Rocaltrol Capsules 1913
▲ Tegison Capsules (50-75%) 1881
Uroqid-Acid 661
▲ Velban Vials (Among most common) 1305
Zoladex (Small number of patients) 1110

Pain, breast
Cytotec (Infrequent) 2159
Kerlone Tablets (Less than 2%) 2172
▲ Lupron Injection (5% or more) 2310
Permax Tablets (Infrequent) 1291

Pain, cancer related
Zoladex (Small number of patients) 1110

Pain, ear
Anafranil Capsules (Infrequent) 650
Diprivan Injection (Less than 1%) 2267
Fiorinal with Codeine Capsules (Infrequent) 2008
Intron A (Less than 1%) 2097
Lopressor HCT Tablets (1 in 100 patients) 1034
Permax Tablets (Infrequent) 1291
Prinzide Tablets (0.3 to 1%) 1540
ProSom Tablets (Infrequent) 554
Prozac Pulvules (Infrequent) 920
Recombivax HB (Less than 1%) 1544
Roferon-A Injection (Less than 1%) 1916
Timolide Tablets 1547
Tonocard Tablets (Less than 1%) 1554
Trental (Less than 1%) 1099
Zestoretic (0.3 to 1%) 2274

Pain, epigastric (see under Distress, epigastric)

Pain, extremities
Blocadren Tablets 1429
Calciparine Injection 925
Cartrol Tablets (Rare) 507
Danocrine Capsules 2046
Diprivan Injection (Less than 1%) 2267
Floxin Tablets (Less than 1%) 1652
Fluorouracil Injection 1897
Heparin Sodium Vials 1264
▲ Hytrin Tablets (3.5%) 529
IOPIDINE ⊙ 232
▲ Mesnex Injection (50%) 733
Sansert Tablets 2031
Teslac Tablets 741
Trexan Tablets (Less than 1%) 937
Wytensin Tablets 2542

Pain, eye
Adsorbonac 2% and 5% ⊙ 210
Adsorbotear ⊙ 210
AK-NaCl 5% Ointment & Solution ⊙ 204
AK-Poly-Bac Ointment ⊙ 205
AK-Spore ⊙ 205
Allergan Eyewash ⊙ 238
Allergy Drops ▣ 511
Anafranil Capsules (Infrequent) 650
Atrovent Inhalation Aerosol 675
Betoptic Sterile Ophthalmic Solution (Small numbers of patients) 569
Betoptic S Sterile Ophthalmic Suspension (Small numbers of patients) 570
BuSpar (Rare) 1401
Cardura Tablets (1%) 1941
Celluvisc Lubricant Ophthalmic Solution ⊙ 243
Cipro I.V. (1% or less) 1592
Cipro Tablets (Less than 1%) 1589
Clear Eyes ACR ⊙ 305
Collyrium for Fresh Eyes 2445
Collyrium Fresh 2445
Diprivan Injection (Less than 1%) 2267
Duratears Naturale ⊙ 216
Eldepryl 2250
Epifrin ⊙ 244
Ethmozine Tablets (Less than 2%) 946
Eye Wash ▣ 511
Eye-Stream 571
Herplex Liquifilm ⊙ 248
Intron A (Up to 3%) 2097
Lacril Lubricant Ophthalmic Solution ⊙ 248
Miacalcin Injection 2017
Moisture Drops ▣ 512
Naphcon ⊙ 226
Ophthalgan ⊙ 315
Orudis Capsules (Less than 1%) 2488
Permax Tablets (Infrequent) 1291
ProSom Tablets (Infrequent) 554
Prozac Pulvules (Infrequent) 920
Sectral Capsules (Up to 2%) 2520
Soma Tablets 2388
Synarel Nasal Solution (Less than 1%) 2300
Tambocor Tablets (Less than 1%) 1315
Tegison Capsules (Frequent) 1881
Visine L.R. Eye Drope ⊙ 303
Zincfrin ⊙ 230

Pain, female genitalia
Floxin Tablets (Less than 1%) 1652

Pain, femoral nerve
Cholybar 1705
Questran Light 711
Questran Powder 710

Pain, flank
Sansert Tablets 2031

Pain, genital
▲ Condylox (50% to 72%) 1630
▲ TheraCys BCG Live (Intravesical) (Up to 9.8%) 898

Pain, hip
Plendil Extended-Release Tablets (0.5% to 1.5%) 1526

Pain, jaw
Cipro I.V. (1% or less) 1592
▲ Nicorette (37%) 1335
Oncovin Solution Vials & Hyporets 1288
Permax Tablets (Infrequent) 1291
ProSom Tablets (Rare) 554
Prozac Pulvules (Infrequent) 920
▲ Velban Vials (Among most common) 1305

Pain, lower extremities
Atgam Sterile Solution (Less than 5%) 2320
Cartrol Tablets (1.2%) 507
Catapres Tablets (About 3 in 1,000 patients) 676
CHEMET (succimer) Capsules (Up to 3%) 1361
Clozaril Tablets (1%) 2000
Eldepryl (1 of 49 patients) 2250
Fiorinal with Codeine Capsules (Infrequent) 2008
Lopid Capsules and Tablets 1736
Midamor Tablets (Less than or equal to 1%) 1508
Moduretic Tablets 1510
NebuPent for Inhalation Solution (1% or less) 1017
Omnipaque (Rare) 2552
Oncovin Solution Vials & Hyporets 1288
Plendil Extended-Release Tablets (0.5% to 1.5% or greater) 1526
Prilosec Delayed-Release Capsules (Less than 1%) 1530

Prinzide Tablets (0.3% to 1%)........ 1540
▲ProSom Tablets (3%)........ 554
Rifadin........ 1345
Rifamate Capsules........ 1347
Rimactane Capsules........ 879
Rowasa (2.09%)........ 2248
Sandostatin Injection (Less than 1%)........ 2029
Sinemet CR Tablets........ 953
Tegretol Chewable Tablets........ 654
Tegretol Suspension........ 656
Tegretol Tablets........ 654
Tenex Tablets........ 1875
Tenoretic Tablets (Up to 3%)........ 1105
▲Tenormin Tablets and I.V. Injection (Up to 3%)........ 1107
Timolide Tablets........ 1547
Timoptic in Ocudose........ 1552
Timoptic Sterile Ophthalmic Solution........ 1550
Zestoretic (0.3 to 1%)........ 2274
Zovirax (0.3%)........ 824

Pain, medullary bone

▲Neupogen for Injection (24%)........ 595

Pain, Mittelschmerz

Serophene (clomiphene citrate tablets, USP)........ 2186

Pain, muscle (see under Myalgia)

Pain, neck (see under Torticollis)

Pain, neuritic

Oncovin Solution Vials & Hyporets........ 1288

Pain, nostril

DDAVP (Up to 2%)........ 1841

Pain, oral mucosa

▲Alferon N Injection (1% to 6%)........ 1809
Cipro Tablets (Less than 1%)........ 1589

Pain, parotid gland

Oncovin Solution Vials & Hyporets........ 1288

Pain, pelvic

Danocrine Capsules........ 2046
Metrodin (urofollitropin for injection)........ 2182
Permax Tablets (Infrequent)........ 1291
Prozac Pulvules (Infrequent)........ 920

Pain, perineal

Anafranil Capsules (Infrequent)........ 650

Pain, pharynx

Oncovin Solution Vials & Hyporets........ 1288
Prilosec Delayed-Release Capsules (Less than 1%)........ 1530
Primaxin I.M.........1532
Primaxin I.V. (Less than 0.2%)........ 1535
Prinivil Tablets (1% or less)........ 1538
Prinzide Tablets (0.3% to 1%)........ 1540
Sinemet CR Tablets........ 953
Zestoretic (0.3 to 1%)........ 2274
Zestril Tablets (Less than 1%)........ 2277

Pain, precordium

Cafergot/Cafergot P-B........ 1999
Chromagen Capsules........ 2078
D.H.E. 45 Injection........ 2003
Mykrox ½ mg Tablets (2.7%)........ 984
Phenergan VC with Codeine........ 2501
Tenuate........ 1354
Wigraine Tablets & Suppositories........ 1645

Pain, prostate

▲Lupron Depot 3.75 mg (Among most frequent)........ 2312
Lupron Depot 7.5 mg........ 2311
Lupron Injection........ 2310

Pain, rectum

Cholybar........ 1705
Cortenema (Rare)........ 2244
Questran Light........ 711
Questran Powder........ 710
Rowasa (1.8 to 1.23%)........ 2248

Pain, renal

Anafranil Capsules (Infrequent)........ 650

Pain, right upper quadrant

Tapazole Tablets........ 1298

Pain, shoulder

Brevibloc Injection (Less than 1%)........ 942
Cartrol Tablets (Less common)........ 507
Engerix-B Unit-Dose Vials (Less than 1%)........ 2213
Hytrin Tablets (At least 1%)........ 529
Moduretic Tablets........ 1510
Plendil Extended-Release Tablets (0.5% or greater)........ 1526
Prinivil Tablets (1% or less)........ 1538
Prinzide Tablets (0.3% to 1%)........ 1540
Recombivax HB (Less than 1%)........ 1544
Sandostatin Injection (Less than 1%)........ 2029
Sinemet CR Tablets (1.0%)........ 953
Tonocard Tablets (Less than 1%)........ 1554
Trexan Tablets (Less than 1%)........ 937
Zestoretic (0.3 to 1%)........ 2274
Zestril Tablets (Less than 1%)........ 2277

Pain, stomach (see under Stomachache)

Pain, testicular

▲Lupron Depot 3.75 mg (Among most frequent)........ 2312
Lupron Depot 7.5 mg (Less than 5%)........ 2311
Lupron Injection (Less than 5%)........ 2310
Prilosec Delayed-Release Capsules (Less than 1%)........ 1530

Pain, thoracic spine

▲CHEMET (succimer) Capsules (5.2-15.7%)........ 1361
Primaxin I.M.........1532
Primaxin I.V. (Less than 0.2%)........ 1535

Pain, throat

DDAVP........ 1841

Pain, tingling

Uroqid-Acid (Less frequent)........ 661

Pain, trunk

Diprivan Injection (Less than 1%)........ 2267
Floxin Tablets (1% to 3%)........ 1652

Pain, tumor site

Blenoxane (Infrequent)........ 724
Nolvadex Tablets........ 1102
Velban Vials........ 1305

Pain, upper extremities

Cipro I.V. (1% or less)........ 1592
Engerix-B Unit-Dose Vials (Less than 1%)........ 2213
Lopid Capsules and Tablets........ 1736
Midamor Tablets (Less than or equal to 1%)........ 1508
Moduretic Tablets........ 1510
Plendil Extended-Release Tablets (0.5% to 1.5%)........ 1526
ProSom Tablets (Infrequent)........ 554
Rifadin........ 1345
Rifamate Capsules........ 1347
Rimactane Capsules........ 879
Sandostatin Injection (Less than 1%)........ 2029
Timolide Tablets........ 1547
Timoptic in Ocudose........ 1552
Timoptic Sterile Ophthalmic Solution........ 1550

Pain, urethral

Permax Tablets (Rare)........ 1291
Prozac Pulvules (Rare)........ 920

Pain, urinary bladder

Duragesic Transdermal System (Less than 1%)........ 1133

Pain, vaginal

Vagistat (Less than 1%)........ 1397

Pain, vascular

Lamprene Capsules (Less than 1%)........ 1030

Pain, vulva

DDAVP Injection (Occasional)........ 1840
▲Terazol 3 Vaginal Suppositories (4.2% of 284 patients)........ 1677

Pain at application site

Zovirax Ointment 5%........ 827

Pain at injection site

A.P.L.........2431
Actimmune........ 1046
Adagen Injection (Two patients)........ 967
Alfenta Injection (Less than 1%)........ 1131
▲Alferon N Injection (12%)........ 1809
Ancef Injection (Infrequent)........ 2194
AquaMEPHYTON Injection........ 1422
Atgam Sterile Solution (More than 1%; less than 5%)........ 2320
▲Ativan Injection (17%)........ 2432
Attenuvax........ 1424
BAL in Oil Ampules........ 661
Bactrim I.V. Infusion (Infrequent)........ 1889
Biavax II........ 1427
Brethine Ampuls (0.5 to 2.6%)........ 1026
Brevital Sodium Vials........ 1248
Calcijex Calcitriol Injection........ 506
Capastat Sulfate Vials........ 1250
▲Cefizox Injection (1 to 5%)........ 1012
Cefobid Intravenous/Intramuscular (Occasional)........ 1943
Cefobid Pharmacy Bulk Package - Not for Direct Infusion (Occasional)........ 1945
Ceftin Tablets........ 575
Cholera Vaccine........ 2445
Cipro I.V. (1% or less)........ 1592
Cytovene Sterile Powder (1% or less)........ 2292
Demerol........ 2047
Desferal Vials........ 862
Dilaudid-HP Injection........ 1175
Dolophine Hydrochloride Ampoules & Vials........ 1260
Edecrin (Occasional)........ 1468
Engerix-B Unit-Dose Vials (Less than 1%)........ 2213
Factrel (Occasional)........ 2561
Fluorescite........ ⊙ 217
▲Fungizone Intravenous (Among most common)........ 2262
Gammar, Immune Globulin (Human) U.S.P.........609
Garamycin Injectable (Occasional)........ 2093
Hep-B-Gammagee........ 1474
Humatrope Vials (Infrequent)........ 1266
HyperHep Hepatitis B Immune Globulin (Human)........ 1575
Hyperstat I.V. Injection........ 2095
HypRho-D Rh_0-D Immune Globulin (Human)........ 1578
HypRho-D Mini-Dose Rh_0-D Immune Globulin (Human)........ 1578
Imferon........ 976
▲Intron A (Up to 20%)........ 2097
▲IPOL Poliovirus Vaccine Inactivated (13%)........ 894
Kefzol Vials, Faspak & ADD-Vantage (Infrequent)........ 1279
Ketalar........ 1726
Konakion Injection (Rare)........ 1903
Lasix........ 1093
Lincocin (Infrequent)........ 2344
Mandol Vials, Faspak & ADD-Vantage (Infrequent)........ 1281
Mefoxin........ 1498
Mepergan Injection........ 2479
Meruvax II........ 1503
Metrodin (urofollitropin for injection)........ 2182
Mezlin........ 1597
Mezlin Pharmacy Bulk Package........ 1599
▲Monocid Injection (5.7%)........ 2217
Nebcin Vials, Hyporets & ADD-Vantage........ 1286
Netromycin Injection 100 mg/ml (4 of 1000 patients)........ 2104
Pantopon Injectable........ 1911
▲Pentam 300 Injection (11.1%)........ 1018
Peptavlon........ 2563
Pergonal (menotropins for injection, USP)........ 2184
Pipracil (2%)........ 1230
▲Pneumovax 23 (Common)........ 1528
▲Pnu-Imune 23 Pneumococcal Vaccine Polyvalent (72%)........ 1233
Polymyxin B Sulfate, Aerosporin Brand Sterile Powder (Occasional)........ 798
Pregnyl........ 1644
Premarin with Methyltestosterone........ 2515
Primaxin I.M. (1.2%)........ 1532
Primaxin I.V. (0.7%)........ 1535
Profasi (human chorionic gonadotropin, USP)........ 2186
Recombivax HB (Equal to or greater than 1%)........ 1544
Robaxin Injectable........ 1871
Rocephin Injectable Vials, ADD-Vantage (1%)........ 1914
Roferon-A Injection (Less than 1%)........ 1916
▲Sandostatin Injection (7.5%)........ 2029
Septra I.V. Infusion (Infrequent)........ 808
Septra I.V. Infusion ADD-Vantage Vials (Infrequent)........ 810
Sotradecol (Sodium Tetradecyl Sulfate Injection)........ 964
Surital Ampoules, Steri-Vials........ 1764
Tazidime Vials, Faspak & ADD-Vantage (Less than 2%)........ 1299
Testred Capsules........ 1124
Thiotepa Parenteral........ 1240
Ticar for Injection........ 2236
Timentin for Injection........ 2239
Toradol IM Injection (2%)........ 2302
▲Unasyn (16%)........ 1965
▲Versed Injection (3.7% to 5.0%)........ 1924
Vira-A for Injection........ 1766
Zantac Injection and Zantac Injection Premixed........ 1063
Zefazone Sterile Powder........ 2372

Pain with coitus

Condylox (Less than 5%)........ 1630

Paleness, unusual

Geref (sermorelin acetate for injection)........ 2560
Humulin 70/30, 100 Units........ 1267
Humulin BR, 100 Units........ 1268
Humulin L, 100 Units........ 1268
Humulin U, 100 Units........ 1272
Nucofed Capsules........ 2219
Nucofed Expectorant........ 2219
Nucofed Pediatric Expectorant........ 2220
Nucofed Syrup........ 2219

Palilalia

Nardil (Less common)........ 1742

Pallor

AK-Dilate Solution 2.5% and 10% (Rare)........ ⊙ 203
Anafranil Capsules (Infrequent)........ 650
Ana-Kit Anaphylaxis Emergency Treatment Kit........ 1100
Atrohist Sprinkle Capsules........ 558
Azo Gantrisin Tablets........ 1888
Brevibloc Injection (Less than 1%)........ 942
Capoten (2 to 5 of 1000 patients)........ 2255
Capozide (2 to 5 of 1000 patients)........ 2258
Cardilate Oral/Sublingual Tablets (Occasional)........ 757
Cardura Tablets (Less than 0.5% of 3960 patients)........ 1941
Catapres Tablets........ 676
Catapres-TTS........ 677
Clozaril Tablets (Less than 1%)........ 2000
Combipres Tablets........ 678
Cytotec (Infrequent)........ 2159
Dalgan Injection (Less than 1%)........ 620
Dapsone USP........ 1130
Deconamine........ 663
Deconsal........ 559
Dilatrate-SR........ 1827
EpiPen........ 843
Etrafon........ 2087
Fedahist Gyrocaps........ 2145
Fedahist Timecaps........ 2145
Isordil (Occasional)........ 2467
Levophed Bitartrate Injection........ 2054
Mellaril........ 2011
Murocoll-2 Sterile Ophthalmic Solution........ ⊙ 261
Naldecon Syrup, Tablets, Pediatric Drops and Pediatric Syrup........ 709
Nitro-Bid Ointment........ 1339
Nitrolingual Spray........ 1846
Novafed A Capsules........ 1342
Novafed Capsules........ 1342
Novahistine DH........ 1342
Novahistine DMX........ ▣ 595
Novahistine Elixir........ ▣ 596
Novahistine Expectorant........ 1343
Omnipaque........ 2552
Peritrate (Occasional)........ 1756
Proventil Syrup (Children 2-6: 1%)........ 2119
Rondec........ 1975
Rondec-DM........ 1976
Rondec-TR Tablet........ 1975
Seldane-D Extended-Release Tablets........ 1350
Sorbitrate (Occasional)........ 1103
Survanta Beractant Intratracheal Suspension (Less than 1%)........ 1978
Sus-Phrine Injection........ 1006
Tonocard Tablets (Less than 1%)........ 1554
Toradol IM Injection (1% or less)........ 2302
Trilafon (Occasional)........ 2123
Trinalin Repetabs Tablets........ 1170
Ventolin Syrup (1% of children)........ 583
Wellbutrin Tablets (Rare)........ 821

Pallor, facial

Parlodel (Less than 1%) 2020

Pallor, optic disc

Aralen Phosphate with Primaquine Phosphate Tablets 2040
Aralen Phosphate Tablets 2039
Plaquenil Sulfate Tablets 2067

Pallor, perioral

Pitressin Synthetic, Ampoules 1758

Palmar-plantar erythrodysesthesia syndrome

Fluorouracil Injection 1897

Palpebra superior, elevation

IOPIDINE (1.3%) ..... ◉ 232

Palpitations

Accutane Capsules (Less than 1%) 1878
Actifed with Codeine Cough Syrup.. 752
▲ Adalat Capsules (10 mg and 20 mg) (2% or less to 7%) 1587
Adenocard Injection (Less than 1%) 1007
Adipex-P Tablets and Capsules 1019
▲ Adrenalin Chloride Solution 1:100 & 1:1,000 (Often) 1689
▲ AeroBid Inhaler System (3-9%) 995
Aerolate 994
AK-Dilate Solution 2.5% and 10% (Rare) ..... ◉ 203
Altace Capsules (Less than 1%) 1086
Alupent (1 to 4%) 674
Aminophyllin Tablets 2153
▲ Anafranil Capsules (4%) 650
Ana-Kit Anaphylaxis Emergency Treatment Kit 1100
Anaprox and Anaprox DS Tablets (Less than 3%) 2288
Apresazide Capsules (Common) 854
Apresoline Hydrochloride Parenteral (Ampuls) 856
Apresoline Hydrochloride Tablets (Common) 855
Apresoline-Esidrix Tablets 857
Arm-a-Med Isoetharine Inhalation Solution, USP 616
Arm-a-Med Metaproterenol Sulfate Inhalation Solution, USP (Less frequent) 617
Asbron G 1997
Asendin Tablets (Greater than 1%) 1196
Atrohist Sprinkle Capsules 558
Atrovent Inhalation Aerosol (1.8%) 675
Azo Gantrisin Tablets 1888
Bellergal-S Tablets (Rare) 1998
Benadryl Capsules 1691
Benadryl Injection 1692
Bentyl 1322
Betagan ..... ◉ 239
Biphetamine Capsules 973
Blocadren Tablets 1429
Bontril Slow-Release 834
▲ Brethine Ampuls (7.8 to 22.9%) 1026
Brethine Tablets 1026
Brexin L.A. Capsules 2078
Bricanyl Injection (Common) 1324
Bricanyl Tablets (Common) 1325
Bromfed 1615
Bronkephrine Injection 2042
Bronkometer Aerosol 2042
Bronkosol Solution 2042
BuSpar (1%) 1401
Calan SR Caplets (1% or less) 2157
Calan Tablets (1% or less) 2155
Cantil Tablets 1326
Capoten (Approximately 1 of 100 patients) 2255
Capozide (Approximately 1 of 100 patients) 2258
▲ Cardene Capsules (3.3-4.1%) 2290
Cardizem Tablets-30 mg, 60 mg, 90 mg and 120 mg (Less than 1%) 1329
Cardizem SR Capsules-60 mg, 90 mg and 120 mg (1.3%) 1327
Cardura Tablets (2%) 1941
Cartrol Tablets (Less common) 507
Catapres Tablets (About 5 in 1,000 patients) 676
Catapres-TTS (5 per 1,000) 677
Centrax (Less frequent) 1693
Children's Advil Suspension (Less than 1%) 2426
Choledyl Pediatric Elixir 1702
Choledyl Tablets 1700
Choledyl SA Tablets 1704
Cipro I.V. (1% or less) 1592
Cipro Tablets (Less than 1%) 1589
Clinoril Tablets (Less than 1 in 100) 1433
Clozaril Tablets (Less than 1%) 2000
Codimal 846
Combipres Tablets (About 5 in 1,000) 678
Comhist LA Capsules 1618
Constant-T Tablets 1029
Dalmane Capsules 1927
Darbid Tablets 2205
Deconamine 663
Deconsal 559
Demerol 2047
Deprol Tablets 2382
Desoxyn Gradumet Tablets 514
Desyrel and Desyrel Dividose (Greater than 1%) 1404
Dexatrim ..... ▣ 733
Dexedrine 2206
Didrex Tablets 2338
Dilaudid-HP Injection 1175
Dilor 2079
Dimetane-DX Cough Syrup 1858
Dipentum Capsules (Rare) 1160
Ditropan 1332
Diulo 2129
Dobutrex Solution Vials (1 to 3%).. 1259
Dolobid Tablets (Rare) 1465
Dolophine Hydrochloride Ampoules & Vials 1260
Dolophine Hydrochloride Tablets 1261
Donnatal 1858
Donnatal Extentabs 1859
Donnatal Tablets 1858
Donnazyme Tablets 1860
Doral Tablets 2383
▲ DynaCirc Capsules (0.8% to 4.0%) 2004
E.E.S. (Isolated reports) 522
Elavil 2269
Eldepryl (1 of 49 patients) 2250
Endep Tablets 1927
Engerix-B Unit-Dose Vials 2213
EpiPen 843
Equagesic Tablets 2451
EryPed (Isolated reports) 519
Ery-Tab Tablets (Isolated reports) .. 521
Erythrocin Stearate Filmtab (Isolated reports) 523
Erythromycin Base Filmtab (Isolated reports) 525
Erythromycin Delayed-Release Capsules, USP (Isolated reports) 526
▲ Ethmozine Tablets (5.8%) 946
Etrafon 2087
Fastin Capsules 2216
Fedahist Gyrocaps 2145
Fedahist Timecaps 2145
Feldene Capsules (Less than 1%) .. 1777
Fiorinal with Codeine Capsules 2008
Flexeril Tablets (Less than 1%) 1471
Floxin Tablets (Less than 1%) 1652
Glaucon ..... ◉ 218
Guaifed 1615
Hismanal Tablets (Less frequent) 1138
Hycomine Compound Tablets 929
Hycomine Syrup 927
Hycotuss Expectorant Syrup 930
▲ Hylorel Tablets (29.5%) 975
Hyperstat I.V. Injection 2095
▲ Hytrin Tablets (1.4% to 4.3%) 529
Indocin (Less than 1%) 1487
Intron A (Less than 1%) 2097
▲ Intropin Injection (Among most frequent) 930
Ionamin Capsules 981
IOPIDINE ..... ◉ 232
Isoptin Oral Tablets (Less than 1%) 1179
Isoptin SR Sustained Release Tablets (Less than 1%) 1181
Isuprel Hydrochloride Injection 1:5000 2050
Isuprel Hydrochloride Mistometer .. 2051
Isuprel Hydrochloride Solution 1:200 & 1:100 2052
Kerlone Tablets (1.9%) 2172
Kinesed Tablets 2272
Klonopin Tablets 1902
Kutrase Capsules 2146
Larodopa Tablets (Infrequent) 1905
Levsin/Levsinex 2147
Limbitrol 1933
Lioresal Tablets (Rare) 1031
Lodine Capsules (Less than 1%) 2468
Lopressor Ampuls (1%) 1032
Lopressor HCT Tablets 1034
Lopressor Tablets (1%) 1032
Lorelco Tablets 1333
Lotensin Tablets 872
Lozol Tablets (Less than 5%) 1843
Ludiomil Tablets (Rare) 874
Lufyllin & Lufyllin-400 Tablets 2384
Lufyllin-GG Elixir & Tablets 2385
▲ Lupron Depot 3.75 mg (Among most frequent) 2312
MS Contin Tablets (Infrequent) 1814
MSIR (Infrequent) 1817
Marax Tablets & DF Syrup 1954
Maxair Inhaler (1.7%) 1311
Meclomen Capsules (Rare) 1739
Mepergan Injection 2479
Metaprel Inhalation Aerosol Bronchodilator (1 to 4%) 2014
Metaprel Inhalation Solution (Less frequent) 2015
Metaprel 2015
Methadone Hydrochloride Diskets .. 1284
Methadone Hydrochloride Oral Solution & Tablets 1987
Methergine (Rare) 2016
▲ Mexitil Capsules (4.3% to 7.5%) .. 680
Midamor Tablets (Less than or equal to 1%) 1508
Miltown Tablets 2386
▲ Minipress Capsules (5.3%) 1778
▲ Minizide Capsules (5.3%) 1779
Modane Plus Tablets ..... ▣ 504
Modane Tablets ..... ▣ 503
Moduretic Tablets 1510
Monopril Tablets (0.2 to 1.0%) 1406
Motrin Tablets (Less than 1%) 2351
Murocoll-2 Sterile Ophthalmic Solution ..... ◉ 261
Mykrox ½ mg Tablets (Less than 2%) 984
Naldecon Syrup, Tablets, Pediatric Drops and Pediatric Syrup 709
Nalfon Pulvules & Tablets (2.5%) .. 919
Naprosyn (Less than 3%) 2297
NebuPent for Inhalation Solution (1% or less) 1017
Neo-Synephrine (Rare) ..... ▣ 759
Netromycin Injection 100 mg/ml (Fewer than 1 of 1000 patients) 2104
Niclocide Chewable Tablets 1607
Nicorette 1335
Nimotop Capsules (Less than 1%) 1607
Nipride I.V. Infusion 1909
Nitro-Bid IV (Less than 1%) 1338
Nitrostat IV (Less than 1%) 1744
Nitrostat Tablets (Occasional) 1743
Norflex 1314
Norgesic 1314
Norisodrine Aerotrol 540
Normozide Tablets 2112
Norpramin Tablets 1340
Novafed A Capsules 1342
Novafed Capsules 1342
Novahistine DH 1342
Novahistine DMX ..... ▣ 595
Novahistine Elixir ..... ▣ 596
Novahistine Expectorant 1343
Optimine Tablets 2115
OptiPranolol Sterile Ophthalmic Solution (A small number of patients) ..... ◉ 261
Oramorph SR (Morphine Sulfate Sustained Release Tablets) (Less frequent) 1988
Orap Tablets 1020
Ornade Spansule Capsules 2221
Orudis Capsules (Less than 1%) 2488
PBZ Tablets & Elixir 1037
PBZ-SR Tablets 1037
PCE Dispertab Tablets (Isolated reports) 549
PMB 200 and PMB 400 2504
Pamelor 2019
Pantopon Injectable 1911
Parnate Tablets 2222
PediaProfen Suspension (Less than 1%) 1363
Pepcid (Infrequent) 1524
Periactin 1525
Permax Tablets (2.1%) 1291
Phenergan with Codeine 2497
Phenergan VC with Codeine 2501
Phenurone Tablets (Less than 1%) 552
Plegine Tablets 2504
▲ Plendil Extended-Release Tablets (0.5% to 12.0%) 1526
Polaramine 2116
Pondimin Tablets 1867
Ponstel (Rare) 1758
Prelu-2 Capsules 683
Prilosec Delayed-Release Capsules (Less than 1%) 1530
Primaxin I.M. 1532
Primaxin I.V. (Less than 0.2%) 1535
Prinivil Tablets (1% or less) 1538
Prinzide Tablets (0.3 to 1%) 1540
Pro-Banthīne Tablets 2141
Procardia Capsules (2% or less) 1781
▲ Procardia XL Tablets (Less than 3% to 7%) 1783
Proglycem (Common) 649
Pronestyl Capsules and Tablets 1800
Pronestyl Injection 1798
ProSom Tablets (Infrequent) 554
▲ Proventil Inhalation Aerosol (Less than 10%) 2117
▲ Proventil Repetabs Tablets (5%) 2120
Proventil Syrup (Less than 1 of 100) 2119
▲ Proventil Tablets (5%) 2120
Prozac Pulvules (1.3%) 920
Quadrinal Tablets 1183
Quarzan Capsules 1937
Quelidrine Syrup 556
Quibron Capsules 713
Quibron-T 714
Quibron-T/SR 716
Recombivax HB (Less than 1%) 1544
Respbid Tablets 684
Restoril Capsules (Less than 1%) .. 2023
Ritalin 880
Robinul Forte Tablets 1873
Robinul Injectable 1873
Robinul Tablets 1873
Rocephin Injectable Vials, ADD-Vantage (Rare) 1914
Roferon-A Injection (Less than 3%) 1916
Rogaine Topical Solution (1.53%).. 2357
Rondec 1975
Roxanol 1991
Rufen Tablets (Less than 3%) 691
Ru-Tuss DE Tablets 694
Ru-Tuss II Capsules 693
Ru-Tuss with Hydrocodone 694
Ru-Tuss Tablets 693
▲ Rythmol Tablets (0.6 to 3.4%) 1184
Sandostatin Injection (Less than 1%) 2029
Sanorex Tablets 2030
Seldane Tablets (Rare) 1349
Seldane-D Extended-Release Tablets (2.4%) 1350
Ser-Ap-Es Tablets 881
Serpasil-Apresoline Tablets 884
Sinemet Tablets (Less frequent) 952
Sinemet CR Tablets 953
Slo-bid Gyrocaps 1847
Stadol (Less than 1%) 721
Surmontil Capsules 2524
Sus-Phrine Injection 1006
Synarel Nasal Solution (Less than 1%) 2300
T-PHYL (Uniphyl) 200 mg Tablets 1820
▲ Tambocor Tablets (6.1%) 1315
Tavist Syrup 2033
Tavist Tablets 2035
Tavist-D Tablets 2035
Tedral SA 1765
Tenex Tablets (Less than 3%) 1875
Tenuate 1354
Theo-24 2179
Theo-Dur Sprinkle 1168
Theo-Dur Extended-Release Tablets 1166
Theolair 1317
Theolair-SR Tablets 1319
Theo-Organidin Elixir 2391
▲ TheoX Extended-Release Tablets (Among most consistent) 841
Timolide Tablets 1547
Timoptic in Ocudose 1552
Timoptic Sterile Ophthalmic Solution 1550
Tofranil Ampuls 1038
Tofranil Tablets 1039
Tofranil-PM Capsules 1041
Tonocard Tablets (0.4-1.8%) 1554
▲ Tornalate (Approximately 3%) 2074
Trandate HCT Tablets 579
Trental (1.7%) 1099
Trexan Tablets (Less than 1%) 937
Triaminic Expectorant DH 1995
Triaminic Oral Infant Drops 1996
Triavil Tablets 1556
Trinalin Repetabs Tablets 1170
Tuss-Ornade Liquid 2242
Tuss-Ornade Spansule Capsules 2242
Uniphyl 400 mg Tablets 1823
Urispas Tablets 2242
Valpin 50 Tablets 941
▲ Vascor (200, 300 and 400 mg) Tablets (2.27 to 6.52%) 1383
Vaseretic Tablets (0.5% to 2.0%) 1559

Vasotec I.V. 1562
Vasotec Tablets (0.5% to 1%) 1564
▲ Ventolin (Less than 10 in 100 patients) 583
Verelan Capsules (Less than 1%) .. 1243
Visken Tablets (Less than 1%) 2036
Vivactil Tablets 1567
Voltaren Tablets (Less than 1%) 1042
▲ Wellbutrin Tablets (3.7%) 821
Wytensin Tablets (3% or less) 2542
▲ Xanax Tablets (7.7%) 2367
▲ Yutopar Intravenous Injection (10 to 15%) 647
Zaroxolyn Tablets 989
Zestoretic (0.3 to 1%) 2274
Zestril Tablets (Less than 1%) 2277

Palsy, cranial nerve

Carbocaine Hydrochloride Injection 2043
Marcaine Spinal 2058
NegGram (A few cases) 2062
Omnipaque (Rare) 2552
Pontocaine Hydrochloride for Spinal Anesthesia 2069
Sensorcaine 631
Sensorcaine-MPF Spinal 634

Pancolitis

Rowasa 2248

Pancreatic enzymes, increased

Norpramin Tablets 1340

Pancreatic infarction

Gelfoam Sterile Sponge 2338

Pancreatitis

Actimmune (Rare) 1046
Aldactazide 2150
Aldoclor Tablets 1413
Aldomet Ester HCl Injection 1417
Aldomet Oral 1415
Aldoril Tablets 1418
Altace Capsules (Less than 1%) 1086
Apresazide Capsules 854
Apresoline-Esidrix Tablets 857
Aristocort Suspension 1008
Aristospan Suspension 1011
Asendin Tablets (Very rare) 1196
Azo Gantanol Tablets 1887
Azo Gantrisin Tablets 1888
Azulfidine Tablets, EN-tabs, Oral Suspension (Rare) 1157
Bactrim DS Tablets 1891
Bactrim I.V. Infusion 1889
Bactrim 1891
Butazolidin Capsules & Tablets (Less than 1%) 1027
Calcijex Calcitriol Injection 506
Calderol Capsules 1635
Capoten 2255
Capozide 2258
Celestone Soluspan Suspension 2081
Children's Advil Suspension (Less than 1%) 2426
Cholybar 1705
Cipro I.V. (1% or less) 1592
Cipro Tablets 1589
Clinoril Tablets (Less than 1 in 100) 1433
Combipres Tablets 678
Cortenema 2244
Cortifoam 1827
Cortone Acetate Sterile Suspension 1437
Cortone Acetate Tablets 1439
Corzide Tablets 702
Cuprimine Capsules 1442
Cytosar-U Sterile Powder 2329
Dalalone D.P. Injectable 999
Danocrine Capsules (Rare) 2046
Decadron Elixir 1445
Decadron Phosphate Injection 1449
Decadron Phosphate Respihaler 1454
Decadron Phosphate Turbinaire 1456
Decadron Phosphate with Xylocaine Injection, Sterile 1451
Decadron Tablets 1447
Decadron-LA Sterile Suspension 1457
Declomycin Capsules, Tablets 1199
Deltasone Tablets 2332
Demulen 2161
Depakene Capsules & Syrup (Rare) 511
Depakote (Rare) 512
Depen Titratable Tablets (Isolated cases) 2379
Depo-Medrol Sterile Aqueous Suspension 2334
Dipentum Capsules (Rare) 1160
Diucardin Tablets 2450
Diulo 2129
Diupres Tablets 1461
Diuril Oral Suspension 1464
Diuril Sodium Intravenous 1463
Diuril Tablets 1464
Dyazide Capsules 2208
Edecrin (Rare) 1468
Elspar 1470
Enduron Tablets 517
Enduronyl 518
Enovid 2161
Esidrix Tablets 863
Esimil Tablets 864
Exna Tablets 1862
Fansidar Tablets 1896
Feldene Capsules (Less than 1%) .. 1777
Flagyl I.V. (Rare) 2131
Flagyl Tablets (Rare) 2170
Gantanol 1899
Gantrisin Ophthalmic Ointment/Solution 1900
Gantrisin 1901
Hydeltrasol Injection, Sterile 1476
Hydeltra-T.B.A. Sterile Suspension 1478
Hydrocortone Acetate Sterile Suspension 1479
Hydrocortone Phosphate Injection, Sterile 1481
Hydrocortone Tablets 1482
HydroDIURIL Tablets 1484
Hydromox R Tablets 1209
Hydromox Tablets 1208
Hydropres Tablets 1485
Hyperstat I.V. Injection 2095
Inderide Tablets 2463
Inderide LA Long Acting Capsules .. 2465
Kenalog-10 Injection 2402
Kenalog-40 Injection 2403
Lasix 1093
Lomotil 2174
Lopid Capsules and Tablets 1736
Lopressor HCT Tablets 1034
Macrodantin Capsules 1624
Maxzide 1215
Medrol 2348
Mevacor Tablets 1505
Minipress Capsules (Less than 1%) 1778
Minizide Capsules (Rare) 1779
Minocin Oral Suspension 1224
Minocin Pellet-Filled Capsules 1222
Moduretic Tablets 1510
Monopril Tablets (0.2 to 1.0%) 1406
Motofen Tablets 836
Motrin Tablets (Less than 1%) 2351
Mykrox ½ mg Tablets 984
Nalfon Pulvules & Tablets (Less than 1%) 919
Naturetin Tablets 1789
NebuPent for Inhalation Solution (1% or less) 1017
Norethin 2133
Normozide Tablets 2112
Noroxin Tablets (Rare) 1519
Ogen 540
Oretic Tablets 544
Oreticyl 545
Pediapred Oral Liquid 987
PediaProfen Suspension (Less than 1%) 1363
Pediazole 1973
Permax Tablets (Rare) 1291
Prinivil Tablets (1% or less) 1538
Prinzide Tablets 1540
Proglycem 649
Prozac Pulvules 920
Questran Light 711
Questran Powder 710
Rauzide Tablets 1804
Renese Tablets 1785
Renese-R Tablets 1786
Rocaltrol Capsules 1913
Rowasa 2248
Rufen Tablets (Less than 1%) 691
Saluron 718
Salutensin/Salutensin-Demi 719
Sandimmune (Rare) 2024
Septra 813
Septra I.V. Infusion 808
Septra I.V. Infusion ADD-Vantage Vials 810
Septra 813
Ser-Ap-Es Tablets 881
Serpasil-Esidrix Tablets 886
Solu-Cortef Sterile Powder 2361
Solu-Medrol Sterile Powder 2363
Tagamet (Rare) 2228
Tenoretic Tablets 1105
Thalitone Tablets 687
Thiosulfil Forte Tablets 2526
Timolide Tablets 1547
Tonocard Tablets (Less than 1%) .. 1554
Trandate HCT Tablets 579
Tridione 557
Urobiotic-250 Capsules 1968
Vaseretic Tablets 1559
Vasotec I.V. 1562
Vasotec Tablets (0.5% to 1%) 1564
Voltaren Tablets (Less than 1%) 1042
Zantac Injection and Zantac Injection Premixed (Rare) 1063
Zantac (Rare) 1065
Zaroxolyn Tablets 989
Zestoretic 2274

Pancytopenia

Ancobon Capsules 1886
Atgam Sterile Solution (Less than 5%) 2320
Azactam for Injection (Less than 1%) 2252
Butazolidin Capsules & Tablets (Less than 1%) 1027
Capoten 2255
Capozide 2258
Ceftin Tablets 575
Celontin 1692
Ceptaz for Injection 1057
Chloromycetin Kapseals 1695
Chloromycetin Sodium Succinate 1698
Cipro I.V. (Rare) 1592
Cipro Tablets (0.1%) 1589
Compazine 2201
Cosmegen Injection 1440
Cytosar-U Sterile Powder (Less than 7 patients) 2329
Daraprim Tablets 761
DiaBeta 1091
Diabinese Tablets 1775
Diamox 1200
Dilantin Infatabs (Occasional) 1710
Dilantin Kapseals (Occasional) 1708
Dilantin Parenteral (Occasional) 1712
Dilantin-30 Pediatric/Dilantin-125 Suspension (Occasional) 1713
Dilantin with Phenobarbital Kapseals (Occasional) 1715
Ergamisol Tablets 1136
Etrafon 2087
Sterile FUDR (Remote possibility) .. 1898
Fluorouracil Injection 1897
Fortaz 1060
Glucotrol 1952
Kefurox Vials, Faspak & ADD-Vantage 1277
Lincocin 2344
Matulane Capsules 1907
Mellaril 2011
Mesantoin Tablets 2013
Methotrexate Tablets, Parenteral, LPF Parenteral (1 to 3%) 1217
Micronase Tablets 2350
Milontin Kapseals 1741
Monopril Tablets (0.2 to 1.0%) 1406
Mustargen 1514
Nalfon Pulvules & Tablets (Less than 1%) 919
Navane Capsules and Concentrate 1954
Navane Intramuscular 1956
NebuPent for Inhalation Solution (1% or less) 1017
Neptazane Tablets .... ⊙ 311
Norzine 1818
Orinase Tablets 2354
Paradione Capsules 548
Pepcid (Rare) 1524
Ponstel (Occasional) 1758
Prilosec Delayed-Release Capsules (Less than 1%) 1530
Prolixin Decanoate 1795
Prolixin Elixir 1793
Prolixin Enanthate 1796
Prolixin Injection 1791
Prolixin Oral Concentrate 1792
Prolixin Tablets 1793
Prozac Pulvules 920
Retrovir Capsules 802
Retrovir I.V. Infusion 805
Retrovir Syrup 802
Rheumatrex Methotrexate Dose Pack (1% to 3%) 1234
Ridaura Capsules (Less than 0.1%) 2224
Serentil 686
Soma Compound w/Codeine Tablets (Very rare) 2390
Soma Compound Tablets (Very rare) 2389
Soma Tablets 2388
Stelazine 2226
Taractan (Very rare) 1920
Tegretol Chewable Tablets 654
Tegretol Suspension 656
Tegretol Tablets 654
Temaril Tablets, Syrup and Spansule Sustained Release Capsules 1085
▲ Thioguanine Tablets, Tabloid Brand (Nearly all patients) 815
Thorazine 2234
Tolinase Tablets 2365
Torecan 1993
Trental (Rare) 1099
Triavil Tablets 1556
Tridione 557
Trilafon 2123
Wellbutrin Tablets (Rare) 821
Zantac Injection and Zantac Injection Premixed (Rare) 1063
Zantac (Rare) 1065
Zarontin Capsules 1768
Zarontin Syrup 1769
Zefazone Sterile Powder 2372
Zinacef 1066
Zyloprim Tablets (Less than 1%) 830

Panencephalitis, sclerosing, subacute

M-M-R II 1494

Panic

Anafranil Capsules (1% to 2%) 650
Pamelor 2019

Panmyelopathy

Solganal Suspension (Rare) 2122

Papilledema

Accutane Capsules 1878
Aquasol A Vitamin A Capsules, USP 615
Aquasol A Parenteral, USP 615
Brevicon 2304
Celestone Soluspan Suspension 2081
Cibalith-S 870
Cortenema 2244
Cortone Acetate Sterile Suspension 1437
Cortone Acetate Tablets 1439
Cycrin Tablets 2449
Decadron Elixir 1445
Decadron Phosphate Injection 1449
Decadron Phosphate Respihaler 1454
Decadron Phosphate Turbinaire 1456
Decadron Phosphate with Xylocaine Injection, Sterile 1451
Decadron Tablets 1447
Decadron-LA Sterile Suspension 1457
Demulen 2161
Depo-Medrol Sterile Aqueous Suspension 2334
Enovid 2161
Eskalith 2214
Hydeltrasol Injection, Sterile 1476
Hydeltra-T.B.A. Sterile Suspension 1478
Hydrocortone Acetate Sterile Suspension 1479
Hydrocortone Phosphate Injection, Sterile 1481
Hydrocortone Tablets 1482
Hyperstat I.V. Injection (1 patient) .. 2095
Levlen/Tri-Levlen 665
Lithane Tablets 1596
Lithium Carbonate Capsules & Tablets 1984
Lithobid Tablets 870
Matulane Capsules 1907
Micronor Tablets 1667
Modicon 1667
NegGram (Occasional) 2062
Norinyl 2304
Ortho-Novum 1667
Ovcon 1391
Platinol (Infrequent) 737
Platinol-AQ Injection (Infrequent) 738
Solu-Cortef Sterile Powder 2361
Solu-Medrol Sterile Powder 2363
Levlen/Tri-Levlen 665
Tri-Norinyl 28-Day Tablets 2304

Papillitis

Attenuvax 1424
Biavax II 1427
M-M-R II (Infrequent) 1494
M-R-VAX II 1496
Mumpsvax (Infrequent) 1513

Papules

Catapres-TTS (1 of 101 patients) .. 677
Duragesic Transdermal System (1% or greater) 1133
Yodoxin 1072

Paralysis
Calciparine Injection ... 925
Carbocaine Hydrochloride Injection 2043
Coumadin Injection & Tablets ... 944
Hyperstat I.V. Injection ... 2095
▲ Lupron Depot 3.75 mg (Among most frequent) ... 2312
Lupron Depot 7.5 mg ... 2311
Lupron Injection ... 2310
Novocain Hydrochloride for Spinal Anesthesia ... 2065
Omnipaque ... 2552
Oncovin Solution Vials & Hyporets 1288
Orimune Poliovirus Vaccine Live Oral Trivalent (Rare) ... 1228
Permax Tablets (Infrequent) ... 1291
Pontocaine Hydrochloride for Spinal Anesthesia ... 2069
Prozac Pulvules (Rare) ... 920
Sodium Polystyrene Sulfonate Suspension ... 1993
Surgicel ... 1151
Tegretol Chewable Tablets ... 654
Tegretol Suspension ... 656
Tegretol Tablets ... 654

Paralysis, acute muscular
Amikin Injectable ... 602
Netromycin Injection 100 mg/ml ... 2104

Paralysis, bladder
Etrafon ... 2087
Prolixin Decanoate ... 1795
Prolixin Enanthate ... 1796
Prolixin Oral Concentrate ... 1792

Paralysis, extraocular muscles
Plaquenil Sulfate Tablets ... 2067

Paralysis, flaccid
Diamox Parenteral (Occasional) ... 1200
Diamox Sequels (Sustained Release) ... 1201
Diamox Tablets (Occasional) ... 1200
Klorvess Effervescent Granules ... 2010
Klorvess Effervescent Tablets ... 2011
Klorvess 10% Liquid ... 2010
Rum-K Syrup ... 995

Paralysis, legs (see under Paralysis, lower extremities)

Paralysis, lower extremities
Carbocaine Hydrochloride Injection 2043
Marcaine Hydrochloride with Epinephrine 1:200,000 ... 2055
Marcaine Hydrochloride Injection ... 2055
Marcaine Spinal ... 2058
Sensorcaine ... 631
Sensorcaine-MPF Spinal ... 634

Paralysis, oculomotor nerve
Anafranil Capsules (Rare) ... 650

Paralysis, radial nerve
Diphtheria and Tetanus Toxoids and Pertussis Vaccine Adsorbed USP (For Pediatric Use) ... 892

Paralysis, respiratory
Amikin Injectable ... 602
Carbocaine Hydrochloride Injection 2043
Diphtheria and Tetanus Toxoids and Pertussis Vaccine Adsorbed USP (For Pediatric Use) ... 892
Enlon Injection ... 598
Marcaine Hydrochloride with Epinephrine 1:200,000 ... 2055
Marcaine Hydrochloride Injection ... 2055
Marcaine Spinal ... 2058
Novocain Hydrochloride for Spinal Anesthesia ... 2065
Pontocaine Hydrochloride for Spinal Anesthesia ... 2069
Sensorcaine ... 631
Sensorcaine-MPF Spinal ... 634
Tensilon Injectable ... 1123

Paralysis, sensory motor
Demerol ... 2047
Pantopon Injectable ... 1911

Paralysis, skeletal muscle
Norcuron ... 1642
Nuromax Injection ... 794

Paralysis, spinal cord
Ethamolin ... 1829

Paralysis, spinal nerve
Novocain Hydrochloride for Spinal Anesthesia ... 2065
Pontocaine Hydrochloride for Spinal Anesthesia ... 2069

Paralysis agitans (see under Parkinsonism)

Paranoia
Adalat Capsules (10 mg and 20 mg) (Less than 0.5%) ... 1587
Anafranil Capsules (Infrequent) ... 650
Artane (One) ... 1195
Cipro I.V. (1% or less) ... 1592
Clozaril Tablets (Less than 1%) ... 2000
Doral Tablets ... 2383
Duragesic Transdermal System (1% or greater) ... 1133
Etrafon ... 2087
Larodopa Tablets (Infrequent) ... 1905
Marinol (Dronabinol) Capsules (2%) ... 1985
NebuPent for Inhalation Solution (1% or less) ... 1017
Parlodel (Less than 1%) ... 2020
Permax Tablets (Frequent) ... 1291
Prozac Pulvules (Infrequent) ... 920
Sinemet Tablets ... 952
Sinemet CR Tablets ... 953
Trexan Tablets (Less than 1%) ... 937
Trilafon ... 2123
Wellbutrin Tablets (Infrequent) ... 821

Paraparesis
Depo-Medrol Sterile Aqueous Suspension ... 2334

Paraplegia
Depo-Medrol Sterile Aqueous Suspension ... 2334
Methotrexate Tablets, Parenteral, LPF Parenteral ... 1217
Rheumatrex Methotrexate Dose Pack ... 1234

Parapsoriasis varioliformis acuta
Azulfidine Tablets, EN-tabs, Oral Suspension (Rare) ... 1157

Parasympathetic stimulation
Mydriacyl ... ⊙ 225
Tropicacyl ... ⊙ 209

Parathyroid hormone deficiency, fetal
Accutane Capsules ... 1878

Parenchymatous organs, toxic damage
Dilantin with Phenobarbital Kapseals ... 1715
Phenobarbital Elixir and Tablets ... 1293

Paresis
Anafranil Capsules (Up to 2%) ... 650
Cardura Tablets (Less than 0.5% of 3960 patients) ... 1941
Engerix-B Unit-Dose Vials ... 2213
Gelfoam Sterile Sponge ... 2338
Intron A (Less than 1%) ... 2097
Leukeran Tablets (Rare) ... 788
Methotrexate Tablets, Parenteral, LPF Parenteral ... 1217
Omnipaque ... 2552
Oncovin Solution Vials & Hyporets 1288
Rheumatrex Methotrexate Dose Pack ... 1234
Seromycin Pulvules ... 1298
Tambocor Tablets (1-3%) ... 1315
Tenex Tablets ... 1875

Paresthesia
Accutane Capsules ... 1878
Actifed with Codeine Cough Syrup ... 752
Aldactazide ... 2150
Aldoclor Tablets ... 1413
Aldomet Ester HCl Injection ... 1417
Aldomet Oral ... 1415
Aldoril Tablets ... 1418
Altace Capsules (Less than 1%) ... 1086
Amikin Injectable (Rare) ... 602
▲ Anafranil Capsules (2% to 9%) ... 650
Ancobon Capsules ... 1886
Android ... 1111
Ansaid Tablets (Less than 1%) ... 2319
Apresazide Capsules (Less frequent) ... 854
Apresoline Hydrochloride Parenteral (Ampuls) ... 856
Apresoline Hydrochloride Tablets (Less frequent) ... 855
Apresoline-Esidrix Tablets ... 857
Atgam Sterile Solution (Less than 1% to less than 5%) ... 2320
Atrovent Inhalation Aerosol (Less than 1 in 100) ... 675
Azactam for Injection (Less than 1%) ... 2252
Azo Gantrisin Tablets ... 1888
Benadryl Capsules ... 1691
Benadryl Injection ... 1692
Biavax II ... 1427
Blocadren Tablets (0.6%) ... 1429
Brevibloc Injection (Less than 1%) 942
BuSpar (1%) ... 1401
Calan SR Caplets (1% or less) ... 2157
Calan Tablets (1% or less) ... 2155
Capoten (0.5 to 2%) ... 2255
Capozide (0.5 to 2%) ... 2258
Carbocaine Hydrochloride Injection 2043
Cardene Capsules (1.0%) ... 2290
Cardizem Tablets-30 mg, 60 mg, 90 mg and 120 mg (Less than 1%) ... 1329
Cardizem SR Capsules-60 mg, 90 mg and 120 mg (Less than 1%) 1327
Cardura Tablets (1%) ... 1941
Cartrol Tablets (2.0%) ... 507
▲ Cefizox Injection (1 to 5%) ... 1012
Ceptaz for Injection (Fewer than 1%) ... 1057
▲ CHEMET (succimer) Capsules (1.0 to 12.7%) ... 1361
Children's Advil Suspension (Less than 1%) ... 2426
Cholybar ... 1705
Cibacalcin Double-chambered Syringes (Rare) ... 859
Cipro I.V. (1% or less) ... 1592
Cipro Tablets (Less than 1%) ... 1589
Clinoril Tablets (Less than 1%) ... 1433
Combipres Tablets ... 678
▲ Cordarone Tablets (4 to 9%) ... 2446
Corgard Tablets (6 of 1000 patients) ... 701
Corzide Tablets (Approximately 6 of 1000 patients) ... 702
Cytovene Sterile Powder (1% or less) ... 2292
Dalalone D.P. Injectable ... 999
Danocrine Capsules ... 2046
Daranide Tablets (Among the most common effects) ... 1445
Decadron-LA Sterile Suspension ... 1457
Deconamine ... 663
Demulen ... 2161
Deprol Tablets ... 2382
Desyrel and Desyrel Dividose (Greater than 1%) ... 1404
Diamox Sequels (Sustained Release) ... 1201
Dilaudid-HP Injection ... 1175
Dipentum Capsules (Rare) ... 1160
Diprivan Injection (Less than 1%) ... 2267
Diucardin Tablets ... 2450
Diulo ... 2129
Diupres Tablets ... 1461
Diuril Oral Suspension ... 1464
Diuril Sodium Intravenous ... 1463
Diuril Tablets ... 1464
Dolobid Tablets (Less than 1 in 100) ... 1465
Duragesic Transdermal System (1% or greater) ... 1133
Dyazide Capsules ... 2208
DynaCirc Capsules (0.5% to 1%) ... 2004
▲ Eminase (Less than 10%) ... 2211
Enduron Tablets ... 517
Enduronyl ... 518
Engerix-B Unit-Dose Vials ... 2213
Enovid ... 2161
Equagesic Tablets ... 2451
Ergamisol Tablets (2 to 3%) ... 1136
Esidrix Tablets ... 863
Esimil Tablets ... 864
Estratest ... 2245
▲ Ethmozine Tablets (2%-5%) ... 946
Exna Tablets ... 1862
Feldene Capsules (Less than 1%) ... 1777
Flagyl I.V. ... 2131
Flexeril Tablets (Less than 1%) ... 1471
Floxin Tablets (Less than 1%) ... 1652
Fortaz (Less than 1%) ... 1060
Ganite Injection ... 1016
Gastrocrom Capsules (Infrequent) ... 974
Gelfoam Sterile Sponge ... 2338
Halcion Tablets (Rare) ... 2340
Halotestin Tablets ... 2341
HydroDIURIL Tablets ... 1484
Hydromox R Tablets ... 1209
Hydromox Tablets ... 1208
Hydropres Tablets ... 1485
▲ Hylorel Tablets (25.1%) ... 975
Hytrin Tablets (0.8% to 2.9%) ... 529
Imferon ... 976
Inderide Tablets ... 2463
Inderide LA Long Acting Capsules ... 2465
Indocin (Less than 1%) ... 1487
▲ Intron A (Up to 21%) ... 2097
Inversine Tablets ... 1492
IOPIDINE ... ⊙ 232
Ismelin Tablets ... 869
Isoptin Oral Tablets (Less than 1%) ... 1179
Isoptin SR Sustained Release Tablets (Less than 1%) ... 1181
Kenalog-10 Injection ... 2402
Kenalog-40 Injection ... 2403
Kerlone Tablets (1.9%) ... 2172
Klorvess Effervescent Granules ... 2010
Klorvess Effervescent Tablets ... 2011
Klorvess 10% Liquid ... 2010
Lasix ... 1093
Lioresal Tablets ... 1031
Lodine Capsules (Less than 1%) ... 2468
Lopid Capsules and Tablets ... 1736
Lopressor HCT Tablets ... 1034
Lorelco Tablets ... 1333
Lotensin Tablets ... 872
Lotrisone Cream (5 of 270 patients) ... 2103
Loxitane ... 1213
Lupron Depot 7.5 mg (Less than 5%) ... 2311
▲ Lupron Injection (Greater than 5%) ... 2310
M-M-R II ... 1494
M-R-VAX II ... 1496
MS Contin Tablets (Infrequent) ... 1814
MSIR (Infrequent) ... 1817
Marcaine Spinal ... 2058
▲ Marinol (Dronabinol) Capsules (3%) ... 1985
Matulane Capsules ... 1907
Maxzide ... 1215
Meclomen Capsules (Rare) ... 1739
Meruvax II ... 1503
Metandren Linguets and Tablets ... 875
Mevacor Tablets ... 1505
▲ Mexitil Capsules (2.4% to 3.8%) ... 680
Midamor Tablets (Less than or equal to 1%) ... 1508
Miltown Tablets ... 2386
Minipress Capsules (Less than 1%) ... 1778
Minizide Capsules (Rare) ... 1779
Moduretic Tablets (Less than or equal to 1%) ... 1510
Monopril Tablets (0.2 to 1.0%) ... 1406
Motrin Tablets (Less than 1%) ... 2351
Mykrox ½ mg Tablets ... 984
Nardil (Less common) ... 1742
NebuPent for Inhalation Solution (1% or less) ... 1017
NegGram (Rare) ... 2062
Neptazane Tablets ... ⊙ 311
Netromycin Injection 100 mg/ml (Fewer than 1 of 1000 patients) 2104
Nicorette ... 1335
Norethin ... 2133
▲ Normodyne Injection (2 to 5%) ... 2108
Normodyne Tablets (Less than 1% to 5%) ... 2110
Normozide Tablets (Less than 1%) 2112
Noroxin Tablets ... 1519
Omnipaque (Less than 0.1%) ... 2552
Oncovin Solution Vials & Hyporets 1288
Oramorph SR (Morphine Sulfate Sustained Release Tablets) (Less frequent) ... 1988
Oretic Tablets ... 544
Oreticyl ... 545
Ornade Spansule Capsules ... 2221
Orudis Capsules (Less than 1%) ... 2488
PMB 200 and PMB 400 ... 2504
Paradione Capsules ... 548
Paraplatin for Injection (1%) ... 735
Parlodel (Less than 1%) ... 2020
Parnate Tablets ... 2222
PediaProfen Suspension (Less than 1%) ... 1363
Pentaspan Injection ... 949
Pepcid (Infrequent) ... 1524
Periactin ... 1525
Permax Tablets (1.6%) ... 1291
Phenurone Tablets (Less than 1%) 552
Platinol ... 737
Platinol-AQ Injection ... 738
Plendil Extended-Release Tablets (0.1%) ... 1526
Pneumovax 23 (Rare) ... 1528

- Pnu-Imune 23 Pneumococcal Vaccine Polyvalent 1233
- Polaramine 2116
- Polymyxin B Sulfate, Aerosporin Brand Sterile Powder 798
- Premarin with Methyltestosterone 2515
- Prilosec Delayed-Release Capsules (Less than 1%) 1530
- Primaxin I.M. 1532
- Primaxin I.V. (Less than 0.2%) 1535
- Prinivil Tablets (0.8%) 1538
- Prinzide Tablets (1.5%) 1540
- Proglycem 649
- ProSom Tablets (Infrequent) 554
- Prozac Pulvules (1.7%) 920
- Questran Light 711
- Questran Powder 710
- Rauzide Tablets 1804
- Renese Tablets 1785
- Renese-R Tablets 1786
- ▲Retrovir Capsules (6%) 802
- ▲Retrovir I.V. Infusion (6%) 805
- ▲Retrovir Syrup (6%) 802
- ▲Roferon-A Injection (6% to 8%) 1916
- Rufen Tablets (Less than 1%) 691
- Ru-Tuss II Capsules 693
- Rythmol Tablets (Less than 1%) 1184
- Saluron 718
- Salutensin/Salutensin-Demi 719
- Sandimmune (Up to 3%) 2024
- Sansert Tablets 2031
- Seldane Tablets 1349
- Seldane-D Extended-Release Tablets 1350
- Ser-Ap-Es Tablets 881
- Seromycin Pulvules 1298
- Serpasil-Apresoline Tablets 884
- Serpasil-Esidrix Tablets 886
- Sinemet CR Tablets (0.8%) 953
- Sinequan (Infrequent) 1960
- Synarel Nasal Solution (Less than 1%) 2300
- Talacen (Rare) 2070
- Talwin Injection (Infrequent) 2071
- Talwin Compound 2072
- Talwin Injection 2071
- Talwin Nx 2073
- Tambocor Tablets (1-3%) 1315
- Tapazole Tablets 1298
- Tavist Syrup 2033
- Tavist Tablets 2035
- Tavist-D Tablets 2035
- Tazicef for Injection (Less than 1%) 2231
- Tazidime Vials, Faspak & ADD-Vantage (Less than 1%) 1299
- ▲Tegison Capsules (1-10%) 1881
- Tegretol Chewable Tablets 654
- Tegretol Suspension 656
- Tegretol Tablets 654
- Tenex Tablets (Less than 3%) 1875
- Tenoretic Tablets 1105
- Teslac Tablets 741
- Testred Capsules 1124
- Thalitone Tablets 687
- Timolide Tablets 1547
- Timoptic in Ocudose 1552
- Timoptic Sterile Ophthalmic Solution 1550
- ▲Tonocard Tablets (3.5-9.2%) 1554
- Toradol IM Injection (1% or less) 2302
- Trandate HCT Tablets (Less than 1% in 208 patients) 579
- Trandate Injection 577
- Trandate Tablets (Less than 1% of 227 patients) 579
- Travase Ointment 697
- Triaminic Expectorant DH 1995
- Triaminic Oral Infant Drops 1996
- Tridione 557
- Trinalin Repetabs Tablets 1170
- Ultravate Ointment 0.05% 2411
- Vascor (200, 300 and 400 mg) Tablets (2.46%) 1383
- Vaseretic Tablets (0.5% to 2.0%) 1559
- Vasotec I.V. 1562
- Vasotec Tablets (0.5% to 1%) 1564
- Velban Vials 1305
- Verelan Capsules (Less than 1%) 1243
- Versed Injection (Less than 1%) 1924
- ▲Visken Tablets (3%) 2036
- Voltaren Tablets (Less than 1%) 1042
- Wellbutrin Tablets 821
- Xanax Tablets (2.4%) 2367
- Zaroxolyn Tablets 989
- Zestoretic (1.5%) 2274
- Zestril Tablets (0.8%) 2277
- Zovirax (0.8% to 1.2%) 824
- Zyloprim Tablets (Less than 1%) 830

Paresthesia, chest
- Esimil Tablets 864
- Ismelin Tablets 869

Paresthesia, extremities
- Asendin Tablets (Less than 1%) 1196
- Bellergal-S Tablets (Rare) 1998
- Cafergot/Cafergot P-B 1999
- Diamox 1200
- Elavil 2269
- Endep Tablets 1927
- Etrafon 2087
- Flagyl I.V. 2131
- Flagyl Tablets 2170
- Fulvicin P/G Tablets (Rare) 2090
- Fulvicin P/G 165 & 330 Tablets (Rare) 2091
- Fulvicin-U/F Tablets (Rare) 2092
- Gelfoam Sterile Sponge 2338
- Limbitrol 1933
- Medihaler Ergotamine Aerosol 1312
- Motofen Tablets 836
- Norpramin Tablets 1340
- Pamelor 2019
- Protostat Tablets 1674
- Rum-K Syrup 995
- Surmontil Capsules 2524
- Tofranil Ampuls 1038
- Tofranil Tablets 1039
- Tofranil-PM Capsules 1041
- Triavil Tablets 1556
- Velban Vials 1305
- Vivactil Tablets 1567

Paresthesia, facial
- DTIC-Dome 1595

Paresthesia, feet
- Grifulvin V (griseofulvin microsize) Tablets/Suspension (Rare) 1678
- Grisactin (Rare) 2454
- Grisactin Ultra Tablets (Rare) 2455
- Gris-PEG Tablets, 125 mg & 250 mg (Rare) 1083
- INH Tablets 868
- Rifamate Capsules 1347

Paresthesia, hands
- Grifulvin V (griseofulvin microsize) Tablets/Suspension (Rare) 1678
- Grisactin (Rare) 2454
- Grisactin Ultra Tablets (Rare) 2455
- Gris-PEG Tablets, 125 mg & 250 mg (Rare) 1083
- INH Tablets 868
- Inderal 2459
- Inderal LA Long Acting Capsules 2461
- Inderide Tablets 2463
- Inderide LA Long Acting Capsules 2465
- Rifamate Capsules 1347

Paresthesia, circumoral
- Coly-Mycin M Parenteral 1706
- ProSom Tablets (Rare) 554
- Prozac Pulvules (Rare) 920

Parkinsonism
- Aldoclor Tablets 1413
- Aldomet Ester HCl Injection 1417
- Aldomet Oral 1415
- Aldoril Tablets 1418
- Ancobon Capsules 1886
- Clozaril Tablets (Less than 1%) 2000
- Compazine 2201
- Demser Capsules 1460
- Diupres Tablets 1461
- Etrafon 2087
- Hydromox R Tablets 1209
- Hydropres Tablets 1485
- Indocin (Less than 1%) 1487
- Moban Tablets & Concentrate 932
- Orap Tablets 1020
- Raudixin Tablets 1803
- Rauzide Tablets (Rare) 1804
- Salutensin/Salutensin-Demi 719
- Serentil 686
- Stelazine 2226
- Tigan 2239
- Trilafon 2123

Parkinson-like symptoms
- Actimmune (Rare) 1046
- Compazine 2201
- Elspar (Rare) 1470
- Haldol Decanoate (Less frequent) 1375
- Haldol Injection, Tablets and Concentrate 1373
- Mellaril (Infrequent) 2011
- Navane Capsules and Concentrate 1954
- Navane Intramuscular 1956
- Orap Tablets (Frequent) 1020
- Prolixin Decanoate 1795
- Prolixin Elixir 1793
- Prolixin Enanthate 1796
- Prolixin Injection 1791
- ▲Prolixin Oral Concentrate (Among most frequent) 1792
- Prolixin Tablets 1793
- Reglan 1869
- Renese-R Tablets (Rare) 1786
- Ser-Ap-Es Tablets (Rare) 881
- Serpasil Tablets (Rare) 883
- Serpasil-Apresoline Tablets (Rare) 884
- Serpasil-Esidrix Tablets (Rare) 886
- ▲Taractan (Common) 1920
- Triavil Tablets 1556

Paroniria
- Cardura Tablets (Less than 0.5% of 3960 patients) 1941
- Intron A (2 patients) 2097
- Normozide Tablets 2112
- Procardia XL Tablets (1% or less) 1783
- Trandate HCT Tablets 579

Paronychia
- Accutane Capsules (Less than 1%) 1878
- ▲Tegison Capsules (1-10%) 1881

Parosmia
- Anafranil Capsules (Infrequent) 650
- Ansaid Tablets (Less than 1%) 2319
- Cardura Tablets (Less than 0.5% of 3960 patients) 1941
- ▲Intron A (Less than 14%) 2097

Parotid gland, enlargement
- Depakene Capsules & Syrup 511
- Depakote Sprinkle Capsules 512
- Etrafon (Rare) 2087
- Hyperstat I.V. Injection 2095
- Intal Capsules (Less than 1 in 10,000 patients) 978
- Intal Nebulizer Solution 980
- Limbitrol 1933
- Mellaril (Rare) 2011
- Pamelor 2019
- Surmontil Capsules 2524
- Taractan 1920
- Tofranil Ampuls 1038
- Tofranil Tablets 1039
- Tofranil-PM Capsules 1041

Parotid tenderness
- Catapres Tablets 676
- Esimil Tablets 864
- Ismelin Tablets 869
- Trilafon (Rare) 2123

Parotitis
- Artane (Rare) 1195
- Biavax II 1427
- Catapres Tablets (Rare) 676
- Catapres-TTS (Rare) 677
- Combipres Tablets (Rare) 678
- Kemadrin Tablets 771
- M-M-R II 1494
- Mumpsvax (Very low) 1513
- Norpramin Tablets 1340
- Organidin Elixir, Solution & Tablets (Rare) 2387
- Peridex 1808
- Theo-Organidin Elixir (Rare) 2391
- Tussi-Organidin DM Liquid (Rare) 2392
- Tussi-Organidin Liquid (Rare) 2391
- Vivactil Tablets 1567

Patent ductus arteriosus
- ▲Exosurf Neonatal for Intratracheal Suspension (Up to 59%) 765
- Prinivil Tablets 1538
- Prinzide Tablets 1540
- ▲Survanta Beractant Intratracheal Suspension (46.9%) 1978
- Vaseretic Tablets 1559
- Vasotec I.V. 1562
- Vasotec Tablets 1564
- Zestoretic 2274
- Zestril Tablets 2277

Pavor nocturnus
- Zarontin Capsules 1768
- Zarontin Syrup 1769

Peeling (see under Necrolysis, epidermal)

Peliosis hepatis
- Anadrol-50 Tablets 2287
- Android (Rare) 1111
- Danocrine Capsules 2046
- Estratest 2245
- Metandren Linguets and Tablets (Rare) 875
- Premarin with Methyltestosterone 2515
- Testred Capsules (Rare) 1124
- Winstrol Tablets 2075

Pellagra
- INH Tablets 868
- Rifamate Capsules 1347
- Trecator-SC Tablets 2527

Pelvic inflammatory disease
- BuSpar (Rare) 1401
- Lippes Loop Intrauterine Double-S 1654
- ParaGard T380A Intrauterine Copper Contraceptive 411

Pelvic pressure
- Flagyl Tablets 2170
- Protostat Tablets 1674

Pemphigoid-like lesion
- Capoten 2255
- Capozide 2258
- Corzide Tablets 702
- Depen Titratable Tablets 2379

Pemphigus
- Capozide 2258
- Cuprimine Capsules 1442
- Depen Titratable Tablets 2379
- Rifadin (Occasional) 1345
- Rifamate Capsules (Occasional) 1347
- Rimactane Capsules 879

Pemphigus, bullous
- Monopril Tablets (0.2 to 1.0%) 1406

Penile discharge, unspecified
- ProSom Tablets (Rare) 554

Penile erection, decrease
- ▲Zoladex (18%) 1110

Penile erection, prolonged or inappropriate
- Android 1111
- Desyrel and Desyrel Dividose 1404

Penile erections, increase (see under Priapism)

Penis, burning
- BAL in Oil Ampules 661
- Conceptrol (Occasional) ▣ 631
- Delfen Contraceptive Foam (Occasional) ▣ 631
- Gynol II Extra Strength Contraceptive Jelly (Occasional) ▣ 632
- Ortho-Gynol/Gynol II (Occasional) ▣ 632

Penis, decreased sensation
- Eldepryl 2250

Penis, enlargement
- A.P.L. 2431
- Anadrol-50 Tablets 2287
- ▲Lupron Depot 3.75 mg (Among most frequent) 2312
- Lupron Depot 7.5 mg 2311
- Lupron Injection 2310
- Winstrol Tablets 2075

Penis, fibrotic plaques (see under Peyronie's disease)

Perforation, cervix (partial)
- Lippes Loop Intrauterine Double-S 1654

Perforation, cervix (total)
- Lippes Loop Intrauterine Double-S 1654

Perforation, uterine wall
- ParaGard T380A Intrauterine Copper Contraceptive 411

Perforation, uterine wall (partial)
- Lippes Loop Intrauterine Double-S 1654
- ParaGard T380A Intrauterine Copper Contraceptive 411

Perforation, uterine wall (total)
- Lippes Loop Intrauterine Double-S 1654
- ParaGard T380A Intrauterine Copper Contraceptive 411

Perianal sensation, loss of

Carbocaine Hydrochloride Injection 2043
Marcaine Hydrochloride with Epinephrine 1:200,000 2055
Marcaine Hydrochloride Injection 2055
Marcaine Spinal 2058
Sensorcaine 631
Sensorcaine-MPF Spinal 634
Xylocaine Injections 637

Periarteritis

Nasalcrom Nasal Solution (Rare) 986
Tapazole Tablets 1298

Periarteritis nodosum

Azo Gantrisin Tablets 1888
Bactrim DS Tablets 1891
Bactrim I.V. Infusion 1889
Bactrim 1891
Dilantin Infatabs 1710
Dilantin Kapseals 1708
Dilantin Parenteral 1712
Dilantin-30 Pediatric/Dilantin-125 Suspension 1713
Dilantin with Phenobarbital Kapseals 1715
Fansidar Tablets 1896
Gantanol 1899
Gantrisin Ophthalmic Ointment/Solution 1900
Gantrisin 1901
Pediazole 1973
Septra 813
Septra I.V. Infusion 808
Septra I.V. Infusion ADD-Vantage Vials 810
Septra 813
Thiosulfil Forte Tablets 2526

Pericardial effusion

▲ Leukine for IV Infusion (4%) 1127
▲ Loniten Tablets (3%) 2346
▲ Prokine for I.V. Infusion (4%) 1096
Rogaine Topical Solution 2357

Pericardial tamponade

Azulfidine Tablets, EN-tabs, Oral Suspension 1157
Loniten Tablets 2346

Pericarditis

Achromycin V Capsules 1193
Aldoclor Tablets 1413
Aldomet Ester HCl Injection 1417
Aldomet Oral 1415
Aldoril Tablets 1418
Azulfidine Tablets, EN-tabs, Oral Suspension 1157
Butazolidin Capsules & Tablets (Less than 1%) 1027
Cardene Capsules (Less than 0.4%) 2290
Cerubidine (Rare) 2443
Cytoxan for Injection 726
Declomycin Capsules, Tablets 1199
Dipentum Capsules (Rare) 1160
Doryx Capsules 1717
Inocor Lactate Injection (1 case) 2048
Intal Capsules (Less than 1 in 100,000 patients) 978
Intal Inhaler (Rare) 979
Intal Nebulizer Solution (Rare) 980
Loniten Tablets 2346
Minocin Intravenous 1221
Minocin Oral Suspension 1224
Minocin Pellet-Filled Capsules 1222
Monodox Capsules 1630
Permax Tablets (Rare) 1291
Procan SR Tablets (Common) 1760
Pronestyl Capsules and Tablets 1800
Pronestyl Injection 1798
Pronestyl-SR Tablets 1801
Rogaine Topical Solution 2357
Rowasa (Rare) 2248
Terramycin Capsules 1786
Terramycin Intramuscular Solution 1964
Tonocard Tablets (Less than 1%) 1554
Vibramycin Hyclate Capsules 1787
Vibramycin Hyclate Intravenous 1968
Vibramycin 1787
Zyloprim Tablets (Less than 1%) 830

Peripheral nerve symptoms

Xylocaine Injections (Less than 1%) 637

Peripheral vascular disorder, unspecified

Cardene Capsules (Rare) 2290
Lopid Capsules and Tablets 1736
Orudis Capsules (Less than 1%) 2488
Zoladex (1% to 5%) 1110

Peripheral vascular insufficiency

Corgard Tablets (2 in 100 patients) 701
Corzide Tablets (Approximately 2 of 100 patients) 702
Pitressin Synthetic, Ampoules 1758

Peristalsis, increase

Enlon Injection 598
Mestinon Injectable 1115
Mestinon 1116
Prostigmin Injectable 1120
Prostigmin Tablets 1121
Tensilon Injectable 1123

Peritonitis

Cytosar-U Sterile Powder 2329
ParaGard T380A Intrauterine Copper Contraceptive 411
Prostin VR Pediatric Sterile Solution (Less than 1%) 2355

Personality changes

Aristospan Suspension (Intra-articular) 1011
Cardizem Tablets-30 mg, 60 mg, 90 mg and 120 mg (Less than 1%) 1329
Cardizem SR Capsules-60 mg, 90 mg and 120 mg (Less than 1%) 1327
Cytosar-U Sterile Powder (With experimental doses) 2329
Depo-Medrol Sterile Aqueous Suspension 2334
Eldepryl 2250
▲ Lupron Depot 3.75 mg (Among most frequent) 2312
Nalfon Pulvules & Tablets (Less than 1%) 919
Orudis Capsules (Less than 1%) 2488
Paradione Capsules 548
Permax Tablets (2.1%) 1291
Tridione 557

Perspiration (see under Diaphoresis)

Petechiae

Asendin Tablets (Very rare) 1196
Azactam for Injection (Less than 1%) 2252
Cardizem Tablets-30 mg, 60 mg, 90 mg and 120 mg (Less than 1%) 1329
Cardizem SR Capsules-60 mg, 90 mg and 120 mg (Less than 1%) 1327
Celestone Soluspan Suspension (No incidence in labeling) 2081
Clozaril Tablets (Less than 1%) 2000
Cortenema 2244
Cortone Acetate Sterile Suspension 1437
Cortone Acetate Tablets 1439
Dalalone D.P. Injectable 999
Danocrine Capsules 2046
Decadron Elixir 1445
Decadron Phosphate Injection 1449
Decadron Phosphate Respihaler 1454
Decadron Phosphate Turbinaire 1456
Decadron Phosphate with Xylocaine Injection, Sterile 1451
Decadron-LA Sterile Suspension 1457
Depakene Capsules & Syrup 511
Depakote 512
Depo-Medrol Sterile Aqueous Suspension 2334
Deprol Tablets 2382
Engerix-B Unit-Dose Vials (Less than 1%) 2213
Equagesic Tablets 2451
Feldene Capsules (Less than 1%) 1777
Hydeltrasol Injection, Sterile 1476
Hydeltra-T.B.A. Sterile Suspension 1478
Hydrocortone Acetate Sterile Suspension 1479
Hydrocortone Phosphate Injection, Sterile 1481
Hydrocortone Tablets 1482
Indocin Capsules (Less than 1%) 1487
Indocin I.V. (Less than 1%) 1490
Indocin (Less than 1%) 1487
Kenalog-10 Injection 2402
Kenalog-40 Injection 2403
Lorelco Tablets 1333
Ludiomil Tablets (Rare) 874
Matulane Capsules 1907
Medrol 2348
Miltown Tablets 2386
Mustargen 1514
Norpramin Tablets 1340
▲ Novantrone for Injection Concentrate (7 to 11%) 1226
PMB 200 and PMB 400 2504
Pamelor (No incidence in labeling) 2019
Paraflex Caplets (Rare) 1378
Parafon Forte DSC Caplets 1379
Pediapred Oral Liquid 987
Permax Tablets (Infrequent) 1291
Prozac Pulvules (Rare) 920
Roferon-A Injection (Less than 3%) 1916
Solganal Suspension 2122
Solu-Cortef Sterile Powder 2361
Solu-Medrol Sterile Powder 2363
Surmontil Capsules 2524
Tofranil Ampuls 1038
Tofranil Tablets 1039
Tofranil-PM Capsules 1041
Urobiotic-250 Capsules 1968
Vivactil Tablets 1567

Petechiae and ecchymosis

Aristocort Suspension 1008
Aristospan Suspension 1011
Decadron Tablets 1447
Deltasone Tablets 2332

Petechial hemorrhage

Paradione Capsules 548
Tegretol Chewable Tablets 654
Tegretol Suspension 656
Tegretol Tablets 654
Tridione 557

Peyronie's disease

Blocadren Tablets 1429
Cartrol Tablets 507
Corgard Tablets 701
Corzide Tablets 702
Dilantin Infatabs 1710
Dilantin Kapseals 1708
Dilantin Parenteral 1712
Dilantin-30 Pediatric/Dilantin-125 Suspension 1713
Dilantin with Phenobarbital Kapseals 1715
Inderal (Rare) 2459
Inderal LA Long Acting Capsules (Rare) 2461
Inderide Tablets (Rare) 2463
Inderide LA Long Acting Capsules (Rare) 2465
Kerlone Tablets 2172
Levatol 1832
Lopressor Ampuls (1 of 100,000 patients) 1032
Lopressor HCT Tablets (1 in 100,000) 1034
Lopressor Tablets (1 of 100,000 patients) 1032
Normodyne Tablets 2110
Normozide Tablets 2112
Sansert Tablets 2031
Sectral Capsules 2520
Tenoretic Tablets 1105
Tenormin Tablets and I.V. Injection 1107
Timolide Tablets 1547
Timoptic in Ocudose 1552
Timoptic Sterile Ophthalmic Solution 1550
Trandate HCT/Trandate 579
Visken Tablets 2036

Pharyngeal changes

Diapid Nasal Spray 2003
Mexitil Capsules (About 1 in 1,000) 680
Prinzide Tablets (0.3% to 1%) 1540

Pharyngeal secretion, increase

IOPIDINE ◉ 232
Prostigmin Injectable 1120
Prostigmin Tablets 1121

Pharyngitis

AeroBid Inhaler System (1-3%) 995
▲ Anafranil Capsules (Up to 14%) 650
Cardura Tablets (Less than 0.5% of 3960 patients) 1941
Cartrol Tablets (1.1%) 507
Cosmegen Injection 1440
Duragesic Transdermal System (1% or greater) 1133
Ethmozine Tablets (Less than 2%) 946
Sterile FUDR 1898
Hismanal Tablets (1.7%) 1138
Hytrin Tablets (At least 1%) 529
Inderal 2459
Inderal LA Long Acting Capsules 2461
Inderide Tablets 2463
Inderide LA Long Acting Capsules 2465
Intal Inhaler (Infrequent) 979
▲ Intron A (Up to 31%) 2097
Kerlone Tablets (2.0%) 2172
Lodine Capsules (Less than 1%) 2468
Methotrexate Tablets, Parenteral, LPF Parenteral 1217
Mexitil Capsules (Less than 1%) 680
Monopril Tablets (0.2 to 1.0%) 1406
▲ NebuPent for Inhalation Solution (10 to 23%) 1017
Nicorette 1335
Orudis Capsules (Less than 1%) 2488
Permax Tablets (Frequent) 1291
Plendil Extended-Release Tablets 1526
ProSom Tablets (1%) 554
Proventil Solutions for Inhalation 0.5% and 0.083% (Less than 1%) 2118
Prozac Pulvules (2.7%) 920
Recombivax HB (Equal to or greater than 1%) 1544
Retrovir Capsules (Less than 5%) 802
Retrovir I.V. Infusion (Less than 5%) 805
Retrovir Syrup (Less than 5%) 802
Rheumatrex Methotrexate Dose Pack 1234
Sectral Capsules (Up to 2%) 2520
Solganal Suspension 2122
Tegison Capsules (Less than 1%) 1881
Vascor (200, 300 and 400 mg) Tablets (0.5 to 2.0%) 1383
Velban Vials 1305
Ventolin Inhalation Solution (Less than 1%) 583
Zyloprim Tablets (Less than 1%) 830

Pharyngoxerosis

Tegretol Chewable Tablets 654
Tegretol Suspension 656
Tegretol Tablets 654

Pharynx, secretion decreased

Cyclogyl ◉ 215
Cyclomydril ◉ 216

Pheochromocytoma

Demulen 2161
Enovid 2161

Phlebitis

Ancef Injection (Rare) 2194
▲ Atgam Sterile Solution (1 in 20 patients) 2320
Atromid-S Capsules 2435
Azactam for Injection (1.9%) 2252
Blenoxane (Infrequent) 724
▲ Cefizox Injection (1 to 5%) 1012
Cefobid Intravenous/Intramuscular (1 in 120) 1943
Cefobid Pharmacy Bulk Package - Not for Direct Infusion (1 in 120) 1945
Cefotan (1 in 300) 2265
Ceftin Tablets 575
Ceptaz for Injection (Fewer than 2%) 1057
Clozaril Tablets (Less than 1%) 2000
Cytotec (Infrequent) 2159
Cytovene Sterile Powder (1% or less) 2292
Dantrium Capsules (Less frequent) 1619
Demerol 2047
Diprivan Injection (Less than 1%) 2267
Dobutrex Solution Vials (Occasional) 1259
Dopram Injectable 1860
Estrace 1385
Estrace Vaginal Cream 1388
Fluorescite Syringe ◉ 217
Fortaz (1 in 69 patients) 1060
▲ Fungizone Intravenous (Among most common) 2262
IFEX (2%) 729
Imferon 976
Kefzol Vials, Faspak & ADD-Vantage 1279
Larodopa Tablets (Rare) 1905
▲ Lupron Depot 3.75 mg (Among most frequent) 2312
Lupron Depot 7.5 mg 2311
▲ Lupron Injection (5% or more) 2310
Lutrepulse for Injection 1655
Mithracin 1602
▲ Monistat I.V. (29%) 1143
Monocid Injection (Less than 1%) 2217
Novantrone for Injection Concentrate (Infrequent) 1226
Ovcon 1391
Panhematin 546

Pentam 300 Injection (0.7%) 1018
▲Primaxin I.V. (3.1%) 1535
Provera Tablets 2356
Retrovir (1.6%) 802
Rocephin Injectable Vials, ADD-Vantage (Less than 1%) 1914
Serophene (clomiphene citrate tablets, USP) 2186
Sinemet Tablets (Rare) 952
Sinemet CR Tablets 953
Tazicef for Injection (Less than 2%) 2231
Tazidime Vials, Faspak & ADD-Vantage (Less than 2%) 1299
Tegison Capsules (Less than 1%) .. 1881
Ticar for Injection 2236
Trexan Tablets (Less than 1%) 937
Valium Injectable (Among most common) 1937
Vancocin HCl, Vials & ADD-Vantage 1302
Velban Vials 1305
Versed Injection (0.4%) 1924
Wellbutrin Tablets (Rare) 821
Zefazone Sterile Powder 2372
▲Zovirax Sterile Powder (Approximately 9%) 828

Phlebosclerosis

Adriamycin PFS 561
Adriamycin RDF 562
Doxorubicin Hydrochloride for Injection, USP 622
Doxorubicin Hydrochloride Injection, USP 848
Rubex 739

Phobic disorder

Anafranil Capsules (Infrequent) 650
Cipro I.V. (1% or less) 1592

Phosphaturia

Daranide Tablets 1445

Phosphenes

Serophene (clomiphene citrate tablets, USP) 2186

Phospholipid concentration, increase

Demulen 2161
Enovid 2161
Estrace 1385
Estrace Vaginal Cream 1388
Estratest 2245
Ovcon 1391
Triphasil-21 Tablets 2527
Triphasil-28 Tablets 2532

Photodynamic reaction

Urobiotic-250 Capsules 1968

Photomas

▲Omnipaque (2 to 15%) 2552

Photophobia

Accutane Capsules (Less than 1%) 1878
Anafranil Capsules (Infrequent) 650
B & O No. 15A & No. 16A Supprettes 2395
Betoptic Sterile Ophthalmic Solution (Small numbers of patients) 569
Betoptic S Sterile Ophthalmic Suspension (Small numbers of patients) 570
BuSpar (Rare) 1401
Calcijex Calcitriol Injection 506
Calderol Capsules 1635
Cardioquin Tablets 1812
Cardura Tablets (Less than 0.5% of 3960 patients) 1941
Celontin 1692
Chibroxin Sterile Ophthalmic Solution 1431
Ciloxan Sterile Ophthalmic Solution (Less than 1%) .... ⊙ 214
▲Cordarone Tablets (4 to 9%) 2446
Cyclogyl .... ⊙ 215
Cystospaz 2395
Ergamisol Tablets 1136
Etrafon 2087
Sterile FUDR (Remote possibility) .. 1898
Floxin Tablets (Less than 1%) 1652
Fluorouracil Injection 1897
Herplex Liquifilm .... ⊙ 248
Intron A (Less than 1%) 2097
Lacrisert Sterile Ophthalmic Insert 1493
Levophed Bitartrate Injection 2054
Lodine Capsules (Less than 1%) 2468
Matulane Capsules 1907
Mesantoin Tablets 2013
Mydriacyl .... ⊙ 225
Nizoral Tablets (Less than 1%) 1145
Oculinum for Injecton 587
Omnipaque (Less than 0.1%) 2552
OptiPranolol Sterile Ophthalmic Solution (A small number of patients) .... ⊙ 261
▲Orthoclone OKT3 Sterile Solution (10%) 1645
Paradione Capsules 548
Permax Tablets (Infrequent) 1291
Plaquenil Sulfate Tablets 2067
Profenal Sterile Ophthalmic Solution .... ⊙ 234
ProSom Tablets (Infrequent) 554
Prozac Pulvules (Infrequent) 920
Quinaglute Dura-Tabs Tablets 663
Quinamm Tablets 1344
Quinidex Extentabs 1868
Retrovir Capsules (Less than 5%) .. 802
Retrovir I.V. Infusion (Less than 5%) 805
Retrovir Syrup (Less than 5%) 802
▲Rēv-Eyes Ophthalmic Eyedrops 0.5% (10% to 40%) .... ⊙ 312
Rocaltrol Capsules 1913
Serentil 686
Serophene (clomiphene citrate tablets, USP) 2186
Tambocor Tablets (Less than 1%) 1315
Tegison Capsules (Less than 1%) .. 1881
Triavil Tablets 1556
Tridione 557
Trilafon 2123
Tropicacyl .... ⊙ 209
Vira-A Ophthalmic Ointment, 3% 1767

Photosensitivity

Achromycin V Capsules 1193
Actifed with Codeine Cough Syrup.. 752
Aldactazide 2150
Aldoclor Tablets 1413
Aldoril Tablets 1418
Alferon N Injection (1%) 1809
Altace Capsules 1086
Anafranil Capsules (Infrequent) 650
Anaprox and Anaprox DS Tablets 2288
Ancobon Capsules 1886
Ansaid Tablets (Rare) 2319
Apresazide Capsules 854
Apresoline-Esidrix Tablets 857
Asendin Tablets (Less than 1%) 1196
Azo Gantanol Tablets 1887
Azo Gantrisin Tablets 1888
Azulfidine Tablets, EN-tabs, Oral Suspension (Rare) 1157
Bactrim DS Tablets 1891
Bactrim I.V. Infusion 1889
Bactrim 1891
Benadryl Capsules 1691
Benadryl Injection 1692
Capoten 2255
Capozide 2258
Cardizem Tablets-30 mg, 60 mg, 90 mg and 120 mg (Less than 1%) 1329
Cardizem SR Capsules-60 mg, 90 mg and 120 mg (Less than 1%) 1327
Children's Advil Suspension (Less than 1%) 2426
Cipro I.V. (1% or less) 1592
Cipro Tablets (Less than 1%) 1589
Clinoril Tablets (Less than 1 in 100) 1433
Combipres Tablets 678
Compazine 2201
▲Cordarone Tablets (4 to 9%) 2446
Corzide Tablets 702
Dantrium Capsules 1619
Declomycin Capsules, Tablets 1199
Deconamine 663
Depakene Capsules & Syrup 511
Depakote Sprinkle Capsules 512
DiaBeta 1091
Diabinese Tablets 1775
Diamox Parenteral (Occasional) 1200
Diamox Sequels (Sustained Release) 1201
Diamox Tablets (Occasional) 1200
Dimetane-DC Cough Syrup 1857
Dimetane-DX Cough Syrup 1858
Dipentum Capsules (Rare) 1160
Diucardin Tablets 2450
Diulo 2129
Diupres Tablets 1461
Diuril Oral Suspension 1464
Diuril Sodium Intravenous 1463
Diuril Tablets 1464
Dolobid Tablets (Less than 1 in 100) 1465
Doryx Capsules 1717
Dyazide Capsules 2208
Dyrenium Capsules (Rare) 2210
Efudex 1880
Elavil 2269
Eldepryl 2250
Endep Tablets 1927
Enduron Tablets 517
Enduronyl 518
Ergamisol Tablets 1136
Esidrix Tablets 863
Esimil Tablets 864
Etrafon 2087
Eulexin Capsules 2089
Exna Tablets 1862
Sterile FUDR (Remote possibility) .. 1898
Fansidar Tablets 1896
Flexeril Tablets (Rare) 1471
Fluorouracil Injection 1897
Fulvicin P/G 165 & 330 Tablets 2091
Fulvicin-U/F Tablets 2092
Gantanol 1899
Gantrisin Ophthalmic Ointment/Solution 1900
Gantrisin 1901
Glucotrol 1952
Grifulvin V (griseofulvin microsize) Tablets/Suspension 1678
Grisactin (Occasional) 2454
Grisactin Ultra Tablets 2455
Gris-PEG Tablets, 125 mg & 250 mg 1083
Haldol Decanoate 1375
Haldol Injection, Tablets and Concentrate 1373
Hibistat Germicidal Hand Rinse (Rare) 2272
Hismanal Tablets (Less frequent) 1138
HydroDIURIL Tablets 1484
Hydromox R Tablets 1209
Hydromox Tablets 1208
Hydropres Tablets 1485
Inderide Tablets 2463
Inderide LA Long Acting Capsules .. 2465
Intal Inhaler (Rare) 979
Intron A (Less than 1%) 2097
Lasix 1093
Limbitrol 1933
Lodine Capsules (Less than 1%) 2468
Lopressor HCT Tablets 1034
Lozol Tablets 1843
Ludiomil Tablets (Rare) 874
Marplan Tablets (Rare) 1906
Maxzide 1215
Mellaril 2011
Mepergan Injection (Extremely rare) 2479
Methotrexate Tablets, Parenteral, LPF Parenteral 1217
Mevacor Tablets (Rare) 1505
Micronase Tablets 2350
Minizide Capsules 1779
Minocin Intravenous (Rare) 1221
Minocin Oral Suspension (Rare) 1224
Minocin Pellet-Filled Capsules (Rare) 1222
Moduretic Tablets 1510
Monodox Capsules 1630
Monopril Tablets (0.2 to 1.0%) 1406
Motrin Tablets (Less than 1%) 2351
Mykrox ½ mg Tablets 984
Naprosyn (Less than 1%) 2297
Naturetin Tablets 1789
Navane Capsules and Concentrate 1954
Navane Intramuscular 1956
NegGram 2062
Neptazane Tablets (Rare) .... ⊙ 311
Normodyne Tablets 2110
Normozide Tablets 2112
Noroxin Tablets 1519
Norpramin Tablets 1340
Optimine Tablets 2115
Oretic Tablets 544
Oreticyl 545
Orinase Tablets 2354
Ornade Spansule Capsules 2221
Orudis Capsules (Less than 1%) 2488
PBZ Tablets & Elixir 1037
PBZ-SR Tablets 1037
pHisoHex 2066
P & S Plus Tar Gel .... ▣ 510
Pamelor (No incidence in labeling).. 2019
PediaProfen Suspension (Less than 1%) 1363
Pediazole 1973
Periactin 1525
Phenergan with Codeine (Rare) 2497
Phenergan with Dextromethorphan (Rare) 2499
Phenergan Injection 2493
Phenergan Suppositories (Rare) 2496
Phenergan Syrup (Rare) 2495
Phenergan Tablets (Rare) 2496
Phenergan VC (Rare) 2500
Phenergan VC with Codeine (Rare) 2501
Polaramine 2116
Polytrim Ophthalmic Solution Sterile 588
Prinzide Tablets 1540
Prolixin Decanoate 1795
Prolixin Elixir 1793
Prolixin Enanthate 1796
Prolixin Injection 1791
Prolixin Oral Concentrate 1792
Prolixin Tablets 1793
ProSom Tablets (Rare) 554
Quinaglute Dura-Tabs Tablets 663
Quinidex Extentabs 1868
Rauzide Tablets 1804
Renese Tablets 1785
Renese-R Tablets 1786
Rheumatrex Methotrexate Dose Pack 1234
Ru-Tuss II Capsules 693
Saluron 718
Salutensin/Salutensin-Demi 719
Seldane Tablets 1349
Seldane-D Extended-Release Tablets 1350
Septra 813
Septra I.V. Infusion 808
Septra I.V. Infusion ADD-Vantage Vials 810
Septra 813
Ser-Ap-Es Tablets 881
Serpasil-Esidrix Tablets 886
Sinequan (Occasional) 1960
Solganal Suspension 2122
Stelazine (Occasional) 2226
Surmontil Capsules 2524
Tacaryl 2409
Taractan (Rare) 1920
Tavist Syrup 2033
Tavist Tablets 2035
Tavist-D Tablets 2035
Tegretol Chewable Tablets 654
Tegretol Suspension 656
Tegretol Tablets 654
Temaril Tablets, Syrup and Spansule Sustained Release Capsules 1085
Tenoretic Tablets 1105
Terramycin Capsules 1786
Terramycin Intramuscular Solution 1964
Thalitone Tablets 687
Thiosulfil Forte Tablets 2526
Thorazine (Occasional) 2234
Timolide Tablets 1547
Tofranil Ampuls 1038
Tofranil Tablets 1039
Tofranil-PM Capsules 1041
Tolinase Tablets 2365
Trandate HCT Tablets 579
Triaminic Expectorant DH 1995
Triaminic Oral Infant Drops 1996
Triavil Tablets 1556
Trilafon 2123
Trinalin Repetabs Tablets 1170
Vaseretic Tablets 1559
Vasosulf .... ⊙ 279
Vasotec I.V. 1562
Vasotec Tablets (0.5% to 1%) 1564
Velban Vials (1 case) 1305
Vibramycin Hyclate Capsules 1787
Vibramycin Hyclate Intravenous 1968
Vibramycin 1787
Vivactil Tablets 1567
Voltaren Tablets (Less than 1%) 1042
X-Seb T Shampoo .... ▣ 510
Zaroxolyn Tablets 989
Zestoretic 2274

Phototoxicity

Dapsone USP 1130
Floxin Tablets 1652
Lamprene Capsules (Less than 1%) 1030
Noroxin Tablets 1519

Physical performance, impairment

Adipex-P Tablets and Capsules 1019
Anexsia 5/500 Tablets 2196
Anexsia 7.5/650 Tablets 2197
Azdōne Tablets 844
Clozaril Tablets 2000
Compazine 2201
Damason-P 1356
Demerol 2047
Desyrel and Desyrel Dividose 1404
Equagesic Tablets 2451

Grisactin Ultra Tablets 2455
Hycodan Syrup, Tablets 927
Hycomine Compound Tablets 929
Hycomine Syrup 927
Hycotuss Expectorant Syrup 930
Hydrocet Capsules 835
Libritabs Tablets 1930
Lortab ASA Tablets 2414
Lortab 2412
Loxitane 1213
Mebaral Tablets 2061
Miltown Tablets 2386
Norpramin Tablets 1340
PMB 200 and PMB 400 2504
Phenergan with Codeine 2497
Phenergan with Dextromethorphan 2499
Phenergan Injection 2493
Phenergan Suppositories 2496
Phenergan Syrup 2495
Phenergan Tablets 2496
Phenergan VC 2500
Phenergan VC with Codeine 2501
Rauzide Tablets 1804
Surmontil Capsules 2524
Synalgos-DC Capsules 2525
Trandate HCT/Trandate 579
Tussionex Extended-Release Suspension 988
Tylenol with Codeine 1381
Tylox Capsules 1382
Vicodin Tablets 1187
Wygesic Tablets 2540
Zydone Capsules 941

Pigmentary deposits, conjuctiva
Mellaril 2011
Murocoll-2 Sterile Ophthalmic Solution ⊙ 261
Norzine 1818

Pigmentary deposits, cornea
Lamprene Capsules (Greater than 1%) 1030
Murocoll-2 Sterile Ophthalmic Solution ⊙ 261
Triavil Tablets 1556

Pigmentation
Accutane Capsules (Less than 1%) 1878
Cortifoam 1827
Cosmegen Injection 1440
Etrafon 2087
Glaucon ⊙ 218
Lupron Depot 7.5 mg 2311
Lupron Injection (Less than 5%) 2310
Mesantoin Tablets 2013
Minipress Capsules (Single report) 1778
Minizide Capsules (Single report) 1779
Norzine 1818
Plaquenil Sulfate Tablets 2067
Prolixin Decanoate 1795
Prolixin Elixir 1793
Prolixin Enanthate 1796
Prolixin Injection 1791
Prolixin Oral Concentrate 1792
Prolixin Tablets 1793
Solu-Cortef Sterile Powder 2361
Tacaryl 2409
Taractan 1920
Timolide Tablets (Less than 1%) 1547
Timoptic in Ocudose 1552
Timoptic Sterile Ophthalmic Solution 1550
Triavil Tablets 1556
Trilafon 2123
VePesid Capsules and Injection (Infrequent) 741

Pigmentation disorders
Accutane Capsules (Less than 1%) 1878
Aralen Hydrochloride Injection 2038
Aralen Phosphate Tablets 2039
Cordarone Tablets (Occasional) 2446
Daraprim Tablets (Rare) 761
Ethyl Chloride, U.S.P. 1022
Sterile FUDR (Remote possibility) 1898
Fluori-Methane 1022
Fluorouracil Injection 1897
Fluro-Ethyl 1023
Mellaril 2011
Methotrexate Tablets, Parenteral, LPF Parenteral 1217
Minocin Intravenous 1221
Minocin Oral Suspension 1224
Minocin Pellet-Filled Capsules 1222
Neosar for Injection 566
Orudis Capsules (Less than 1%) 2488
Quinidex Extentabs 1868
Rheumatrex Methotrexate Dose Pack 1234
Tapazole Tablets 1298
Tegretol Chewable Tablets 654
Tegretol Suspension 656
Tegretol Tablets 654
Thorazine 2234

Pill rolling motion
Compazine 2201
Stelazine 2226
Thorazine 2234

Piloerection
Anafranil Capsules (Rare) 650
Intropin Injection (Infrequent) 930
Yohimex Tablets 1190

Pituitary tumors
Demulen 2161
Enovid 2161
Norethin 2133

Pituitary unresponsiveness, secondary
Aristospan Suspension (Intra-articular) 1011
Celestone Soluspan Suspension 2081
Cortenema 2244
Cortone Acetate Sterile Suspension 1437
Cortone Acetate Tablets 1439
Decadron Elixir 1445
Decadron Phosphate Injection 1449
Decadron Phosphate Respihaler 1454
Decadron Phosphate Turbinaire 1456
Decadron Phosphate with Xylocaine Injection, Sterile 1451
Decadron Tablets 1447
Decadron-LA Sterile Suspension 1457
Deltasone Tablets 2332
Depo-Medrol Sterile Aqueous Suspension 2334
Hydeltrasol Injection, Sterile 1476
Hydeltra-T.B.A. Sterile Suspension 1478
Hydrocortone Acetate Sterile Suspension 1479
Hydrocortone Phosphate Injection, Sterile 1481
Hydrocortone Tablets 1482
Kenalog-40 Injection 2403
Medrol 2348
Pediapred Oral Liquid 987
Solu-Cortef Sterile Powder 2361
Solu-Medrol Sterile Powder 2363

Plaques, erythematous
AquaMEPHYTON Injection 1422

Plaques, indurated
AquaMEPHYTON Injection 1422

Plaques, pruritic
AquaMEPHYTON Injection 1422

Plasma dilution
Butazolidin Capsules & Tablets 1027

Platelet, decrease (see under Thrombocytopenia)

Platelet, increase (see under Thrombocytosis)

Plethora
Talwin Injection 2071
Talwin Nx 2073

Pleural effusion
Atgam Sterile Solution (At least 1 patient and less than 5% of total patients) 2320
Cipro I.V. (1% or less) 1592
Clinoril Tablets (Less than 1 in 100) 1433
Ethamolin (2.1%) 1829
Ganite Injection 1016
Hyskon Hysteroscopy Fluid (Rare) 1162
Leukine for IV Infusion (1%) 1127
Macrodantin Capsules 1624
Matulane Capsules 1907
Permax Tablets (Infrequent) 1291
Procan SR Tablets (Common) 1760
Prokine for I.V. Infusion (1%) 1096
Pronestyl Capsules and Tablets 1800
Pronestyl Injection 1798
Pronestyl-SR Tablets 1801
Prozac Pulvules (Rare) 920
Sansert Tablets 2031
Serophene (clomiphene citrate tablets, USP) 2186
Zefazone Sterile Powder 2372

Pleural effusion with pericarditis
Dantrium Capsules (Less frequent) 1619

Pleural friction rubs
▲Lupron Depot 3.75 mg (Among most frequent) 2312
Lupron Depot 7.5 mg 2311
Lupron Injection (Less than 5%) 2310
Sansert Tablets 2031

Pleural infiltration
Ethamolin (2.1%) 1829

Pleuralgia
Intron A (2 patients) 2097
Procan SR Tablets (Common) 1760

Pleurisy
AeroBid Inhaler System (1-3%) 995
Tonocard Tablets (Less than 1%) 1554

Pleuritis
Azulfidine Tablets, EN-tabs, Oral Suspension 1157
Inocor Lactate Injection (1 case) 2048
NebuPent for Inhalation Solution (1% or less) 1017

Pneumocystis carinii, susceptibility
▲Orthoclone OKT3 Sterile Solution (3.1%) 1645

Pneumocystosis, extrapulmonary
NebuPent for Inhalation Solution (1% or less) 1017

Pneumomediastinum
Exosurf Neonatal for Intratracheal Suspension (1%) 765

Pneumonia
AeroBid Inhaler System (1-3%) 995
Anafranil Capsules (Infrequent) 650
Clozaril Tablets (Less than 1%) 2000
Compazine 2201
Cytosar-U Sterile Powder (Less frequent) 2329
Cytotec (Infrequent) 2159
Ethamolin (1.2%) 1829
Intron A (Less than 1%) 2097
Kerlone Tablets (Less than 2%) 2172
▲Lupron Depot 3.75 mg (Among most frequent) 2312
Lupron Depot 7.5 mg 2311
Lupron Injection (Less than 5%) 2310
▲Novantrone for Injection Concentrate (9%) 1226
Permax Tablets (Frequent) 1291
Prolixin Oral Concentrate 1792
Prozac Pulvules (Infrequent) 920
▲Sandimmune (6.2 to 9.2%) 2024
Stelazine 2226
Tegretol Chewable Tablets 654
Tegretol Suspension 656
Tegretol Tablets 654
Tonocard Tablets (Less than 1%) 1554
Vaseretic Tablets 1559
Vasotec I.V. 1562
Virazole 1126
Wellbutrin Tablets (Rare) 821

Pneumonia, congenital
Exosurf Neonatal for Intratracheal Suspension (Up to 4%) 765

Pneumonia, eosinophilic
Prozac Pulvules 920

Pneumonia, fatal aspiration
Ethamolin 1829

Pneumonia, nosocomial
▲Exosurf Neonatal for Intratracheal Suspension (Up to 14%) 765

Pneumonitis
Aldoclor Tablets 1413
Aldoril Tablets 1418
Azo Gantrisin Tablets 1888
Azulfidine Tablets, EN-tabs, Oral Suspension 1157
▲Blenoxane (Up to 10%) 724
Capozide 2258
Clinoril Tablets (Less than 1 in 100) 1433
Corzide Tablets (Occasional) 702
Diucardin Tablets 2450
Diulo 2129
Diupres Tablets 1461
Diuril Oral Suspension 1464
Diuril Sodium Intravenous 1463
Diuril Tablets 1464
Dyazide Capsules 2208
Enduron Tablets 517
Esidrix Tablets 863
HydroDIURIL Tablets 1484
Hydropres Tablets 1485
Inderide Tablets 2463
Inderide LA Long Acting Capsules 2465
Leukeran Tablets 788
Lozol Tablets 1843
Matulane Capsules 1907
Maxzide 1215
Methotrexate Tablets, Parenteral, LPF Parenteral 1217
Moduretic Tablets 1510
Mykrox ½ mg Tablets 984
Myochrysine Injection 1516
Naturetin Tablets (Occasional) 1789
Normozide Tablets 2112
Prinzide Tablets 1540
Prolixin Oral Concentrate 1792
Rauzide Tablets 1804
Rheumatrex Methotrexate Dose Pack 1234
Salutensin/Salutensin-Demi 719
Solganal Suspension 2122
Tegretol Chewable Tablets 654
Tegretol Suspension 656
Tegretol Tablets 654
Timolide Tablets 1547
Trandate HCT Tablets 579
Vaseretic Tablets 1559
Zaroxolyn Tablets 989
Zestoretic 2274

Pneumonitis, eosinophilic
Monopril Tablets (0.2 to 1.0%) 1406

Pneumonitis, interstitial
Actimmune (Rare) 1046
Alkeran Tablets 754
Cordarone Tablets 2446
Cuprimine Capsules (Rare) 1442
Cytosar-U Sterile Powder (Two patients) 2329
Depen Titratable Tablets 2379
Ludiomil Tablets 874
Macrodantin Capsules (Common) 1624
Methotrexate Tablets, Parenteral, LPF Parenteral 1217
NebuPent for Inhalation Solution (1% or less) 1017
Rheumatrex Methotrexate Dose Pack 1234
Ridaura Capsules (Less than 0.1%) 2224
Tonocard Tablets (Less than 1%) 1554

Pneumopericardium
Exosurf Neonatal for Intratracheal Suspension (1-4%) 765

Pneumothorax
▲Exosurf Neonatal for Intratracheal Suspension (10% to 11%) 765
NebuPent for Inhalation Solution (Greater than 1%, up to 5%) 1017
Permax Tablets (Rare) 1291
Virazole 1126

Pollakiuria
DynaCirc Capsules (1.5%) 2004
Sandostatin Injection (Less than 1%) 2029
Visken Tablets (2% or fewer patients) 2036

Polyarteritis nodosa
Anafranil Capsules (Rare) 650
Azo Gantanol Tablets 1887
Azulfidine Tablets, EN-tabs, Oral Suspension (Rare) 1157

Polyarthralgia
Depen Titratable Tablets 2379
Eskalith 2214
Minocin Intravenous 1221
Minocin Oral Suspension 1224
Minocin Pellet-Filled Capsules 1222
Primaxin I.M. 1532
Primaxin I.V. (Less than 0.2%) 1535

Polyarthralgia, migratory
Cuprimine Capsules (Some patients) 1442
Depen Titratable Tablets 2379

Polyarthritis
Cleocin HCl Capsules (Rare) 2322

Cleocin Pediatric Flavored Granules (Rare) 2324
Cleocin Phosphate Injection (Rare) 2325

Polyarthropathy
Mesantoin Tablets 2013

Polycythemia
Android 1111
Danocrine Capsules 2046
Estratest 2245
Gastrocrom Capsules (Infrequent) 974
Halotestin Tablets 2341
Metandren Linguets and Tablets 875
Permax Tablets (Rare) 1291
Premarin with Methyltestosterone 2515
Testred Capsules 1124

Polydipsia
Calcijex Calcitriol Injection 506
Calderol Capsules 1635
Clozaril Tablets (Less than 1%) 2000
Eskalith 2214
Lithane Tablets 1596
Lithium Carbonate Capsules & Tablets 1984
Loxitane 1213
Navane Capsules and Concentrate 1954
Navane Intramuscular 1956
Rocaltrol Capsules 1913

Polymyalgia rheumatica
Mevacor Tablets (Rare) 1505

Polymyositis
Cuprimine Capsules (Rare) 1442
Depen Titratable Tablets (Rare) 2379
Intal Capsules (Less than 1 in 100,000 patients) 978
Intal Inhaler (Rare) 979
Intal Nebulizer Solution (Rare) 980
Tagamet (Rare) 2228

Polyneuritis
Antabuse Tablets 2429
Biavax II 1427
M-M-R II 1494
M-R-VAX II 1496
Meruvax II 1503
Proglycem 649

Polyneuropathy
Biavax II (Isolated reports) 1427
Dilantin Infatabs 1710
Dilantin Kapseals 1708
Dilantin Parenteral 1712
Dilantin-30 Pediatric/Dilantin-125 Suspension 1713
Dilantin with Phenobarbital Kapseals 1715
IFEX (Less than 1%) 729
M-M-R II 1494
M-R-VAX II 1496
Meruvax II (Isolated reports) 1503
Streptase for Infusion (Rare) 635
Tri-Immunol Diphtheria & Tetanus Toxoids & Pertussis Vaccine, Adsorbed 1241

Polyphagia
Atromid-S Capsules 2435
Etrafon 2087
Triavil Tablets 1556
Trilafon 2123

Polyps, endometrial
Nolvadex Tablets (Isolated cases) 1102

Polyps, rectal
▲Lupron Depot 3.75 mg (Among most frequent) 2312
Lupron Depot 7.5 mg 2311
Lupron Injection (Less than 5%) 2310

Polyradiculoneuropathy
Depen Titratable Tablets 2379

Polyuria
Anafranil Capsules (Infrequent) 650
Atrohist Sprinkle Capsules 558
Calcijex Calcitriol Injection 506
Calderol Capsules 1635
Capoten (Approximately 1 to 2 of 1000 patients) 2255
Capozide (Approximately 1 to 2 of 1000 patients) 2258
Cardizem Tablets-30 mg, 60 mg, 90 mg and 120 mg (Less than 1%) 1329
Cardizem SR Capsules-60 mg, 90 mg and 120 mg (1.3%) 1327
Cardura Tablets (2%) 1941
Children's Advil Suspension (Less than 1%) 2426
Cibalith-S 870
Cipro I.V. (1% or less) 1592
Cipro Tablets (Less than 1%) 1589
Cytotec (Infrequent) 2159
Diamox Parenteral 1200
Diamox Sequels (Sustained Release) 1201
Diamox Tablets 1200
Elspar (Low) 1470
Eskalith 2214
Etrafon 2087
Flagyl I.V. 2131
Flagyl Tablets 2170
Intron A (Less than 1%) 2097
Lithane Tablets 1596
Lithium Carbonate Capsules & Tablets 1984
Lithobid Tablets 870
Lozol Tablets (Less than 5%) 1843
Midamor Tablets (Less than or equal to 1%) 1508
Moduretic Tablets 1510
Motrin Tablets (Less than 1%) 2351
Naldecon Syrup, Tablets, Pediatric Drops and Pediatric Syrup 709
Neo-Calglucon Syrup 2018
Normozide Tablets (Less than 1%) 2112
Novahistine DH 1342
Novahistine Elixir ▣ 596
Oncovin Solution Vials & Hyporets 1288
PediaProfen Suspension (Less than 1%) 1363
Primaxin I.M. 1532
Primaxin I.V. (Less than 0.2%) 1535
Procardia XL Tablets (Less than 3%) 1783
Prolixin Decanoate 1795
Prolixin Elixir 1793
Prolixin Enanthate 1796
Prolixin Injection 1791
Prolixin Oral Concentrate 1792
Prolixin Tablets 1793
Protostat Tablets 1674
Prozac Pulvules (Rare) 920
Retrovir Capsules (Less than 5%) 802
Retrovir I.V. Infusion (Less than 5%) 805
Retrovir Syrup (Less than 5%) 802
Rocaltrol Capsules 1913
Rondec 1975
Rondec-DM 1976
Rondec-TR Tablet 1975
Rufen Tablets (Less than 1%) 691
Sansert Tablets 2031
Tambocor Tablets (Less than 1%) 1315
Tegison Capsules (Less than 1%) 1881
Tenuate 1354
Tonocard Tablets (Less than 1%) 1554
Trandate HCT Tablets (Less than 1% in 208 patients) 579
Trilafon (Occasional) 2123

Porphyria
Brevicon 2304
Demulen 2161
Deprol Tablets 2382
Enovid 2161
Estrace 1385
Estrace Vaginal Cream 1388
Glucotrol 1952
Jenest-28 Tablets 1636
Levlen/Tri-Levlen 665
Lo/Ovral Tablets 2471
Lo/Ovral-28 Tablets 2476
Menrium Tablets 1934
Micronor Tablets 1667
Modicon 1667
Nordette-21 Tablets 2481
Nordette-28 Tablets 2483
Norethin 2133
Norinyl 2304
Norlestrin 1746
Nor-Q D Tablets 2304
Orinase Tablets 2354
Ortho-Cyclen Tablets 1658
Ortho-Novum 1667
Ovcon 1391
Ovral Tablets 2490
Ovral-28 Tablets 2491
Ovrette Tablets 2492
Plaquenil Sulfate Tablets 2067
Reglan 1869
Tolinase Tablets 2365
Levlen/Tri-Levlen 665
Tri-Norinyl 2304
Triphasil-21 Tablets 2527
Triphasil-28 Tablets 2532

Porphyria, aggravation
Atabrine Hydrochloride Tablets 2041
Dilantin Infatabs 1710
Dilantin Kapseals (Isolated reports) 1708
Dilantin-30 Pediatric/Dilantin-125 Suspension (Isolated reports) 1713
Dilantin with Phenobarbital Kapseals 1715
Epogen for Injection 591
Equagesic Tablets 2451
Estinyl Tablets 2085
Estradurin 2452
Estratest 2245
Estrovis 1721
Libritabs Tablets 1930
Loestrin 1728
Mediatric Capsules 2476
Menrium Tablets 1934
Miltown Tablets 2386
Ogen 540
Ortho Dienestrol Cream 1664
PMB 200 and PMB 400 2504
Plaquenil Sulfate Tablets 2067
Premarin Intravenous 2508
Premarin with Methyltestosterone 2515
Premarin Tablets 2510
Premarin Vaginal Cream 2512
Stilphostrol Tablets and Ampuls 1609
TACE 12 and 25 mg 1353

Porphyria, hepatic cutaneous
DiaBeta 1091
Diabinese Tablets 1775
Glucotrol 1952

Porphyria, intermittent, acute
Tegretol Chewable Tablets 654
Tegretol Suspension 656
Tegretol Tablets 654

Porphyria cutanea tarda
Anaprox and Anaprox DS Tablets 2288
DiaBeta 1091
Diabinese Tablets 1775
Micronase Tablets 2350
Myleran Tablets (Rare) 790
Naprosyn 2297

Potassium loss (see under Hypokalemia)

Potassium retention (see under Hyperkalemia)

Potentia, decrease
Arfonad Ampuls 1887

Precocious puberty
A.P.L. 2431
Pregnyl 1644
Profasi (human chorionic gonadotropin, USP) 2186

Pregnancy, ectopic
Demulen 2161
Enovid 2161
Lippes Loop Intrauterine Double-S 1654
Metrodin (urofollitropin for injection) 2182
Micronor Tablets 1667
Modicon 1667
Norplant System 2484
Ortho-Novum 1667
Ovcon 1391
Pergonal (menotropins for injection, USP) 2184

Pregnancy, multiple
Lutrepulse for Injection 1655

Pregnancy, spontaneous termination of
Lutrepulse for Injection 1655

Pregnancy tests, false positive
Compazine 2201
Mellaril 2011
Navane Capsules and Concentrate 1954
Navane Intramuscular 1956
Norzine 1818
Phenergan Injection 2493
Serentil 686
Stelazine 2226
Thorazine 2234
Triavil Tablets 1556

Pregnancy tests, false results
Etrafon 2087
Phenergan Injection 2493
Prolixin Decanoate 1795
Prolixin Elixir 1793
Prolixin Enanthate 1796
Prolixin Injection 1791
Prolixin Oral Concentrate 1792
Prolixin Tablets 1793
Temaril Tablets, Syrup and Spansule Sustained Release Capsules 1085
Torecan 1993
Trilafon 2123

Premature ventricular contractions
Demulen 2161
Diprivan Injection (Less than 1%) 2267
Enovid 2161
Mexitil Capsules (1.0% to 1.9%) 680
Norethin 2133
Norpramin Tablets 1340
▲Omnipaque (2 to 16%) 2552
Rythmol Tablets (0.6 to 1.5%) 1184
Versed Injection (Less than 1%) 1924

Premenstrual-like syndrome
Amen 833
Brevicon 2304
Cycrin Tablets 2449
Demulen 2161
Depo-Provera Sterile Aqueous Suspension 2336
Diethylstilbestrol Tablets 1258
Enovid 2161
Estinyl Tablets 2085
Estrace 1385
Estrace Vaginal Cream 1388
Estratest 2245
Estrovis 1721
Jenest-28 Tablets 1636
Levlen/Tri-Levlen 665
Lo/Ovral Tablets 2471
Lo/Ovral-28 Tablets 2476
Loestrin 1728
Mediatric Capsules 2476
Menrium Tablets 1934
Micronor Tablets 1667
Modicon 1667
Nordette-21 Tablets 2481
Nordette-28 Tablets 2483
Norethin 2133
Norinyl 2304
Norlestrin 1746
Norlutate 1754
Norlutin 1755
Nor-Q D Tablets 2304
Ogen 540
Ortho Dienestrol Cream 1664
Ortho-Cyclen Tablets 1658
Ortho-Novum 1667
Ovcon 1391
Ovral Tablets 2490
Ovral-28 Tablets 2491
Ovrette Tablets 2492
PMB 200 and PMB 400 2504
Premarin Intravenous 2508
Premarin with Methyltestosterone 2515
Premarin Vaginal Cream 2512
Provera Tablets 2356
TACE 12 and 25 mg 1353
Levlen/Tri-Levlen 665
Tri-Norinyl 2304
Triphasil-21 Tablets 2527
Triphasil-28 Tablets 2532

Preputium, irretraction of
Condylox (Less than 5%) 1630

Pressor response, paradoxical
Aldomet Ester HCl Injection 1417
Apresazide Capsules (Less frequent) 854
Apresoline Hydrochloride Tablets (Less frequent) 855
Apresoline-Esidrix Tablets 857
Ser-Ap-Es Tablets 881
Serpasil Tablets 883
Serpasil-Apresoline Tablets 884

Priapism
Anadrol-50 Tablets 2287
Android 1111
Calciparine Injection 925
Compazine 2201
Coumadin Injection & Tablets 944
Desyrel and Desyrel Dividose (Greater than 1%) 1404
Dicumarol Tablets 516
Esimil Tablets 864
Haldol Decanoate 1375
Haldol Injection, Tablets and Concentrate 1373
Halotestin Tablets 2341
Heparin Lock Flush Solution 2456
Heparin Sodium Vials 1264

Heparin Sodium Injection 2457
Heparin Sodium Injection, USP, Sterile Solution 2342
Ismelin Tablets 869
Larodopa Tablets (Rare) 1905
Mediatric Capsules 2476
Mellaril 2011
Metandren Linguets and Tablets 875
Minipress Capsules (Less than 1%) 1778
Minizide Capsules (Rare) 1779
Moban Tablets & Concentrate (1 patient) 932
Panwarfin Tablets 547
Papaverine Hydrochloride Vials and Ampoules 1290
Permax Tablets (Infrequent) 1291
Sinemet Tablets 952
Sinemet CR Tablets 953
Stelazine 2226
Testred Capsules 1124
Thorazine 2234
Winstrol Tablets 2075

Proarrhythmia
▲Ethmozine Tablets (3.7% of 1072 patients) 946
▲Rythmol Tablets (1.2 to 4.7%) 1184

Proctitis
Cosmegen Injection 1440
Deprol Tablets (Rare) 2382
Equagesic Tablets (Rare) 2451
Flagyl Tablets 2170
Furoxone 1855
Indocin Capsules (Less than 1%) 1487
Indocin I.V. (Less than 1%) 1490
Indocin (Less than 1%) 1487
Miltown Tablets (Rare) 2386
PMB 200 and PMB 400 (Rare) 2504
Protostat Tablets 1674
Urobiotic-250 Capsules (Rare) 1968

Proctocolitis
Diabinese Tablets (Less than 1%) 1775

Prolactin levels, elevated (see under Hyperprolactinemia)

Prolactin secretion, inhibition of
Bellergal-S Tablets 1998

Proptosis
Brevicon 2304
Cycrin Tablets 2449
Demulen 2161
Enovid 2161
Levlen/Tri-Levlen 665
Micronor Tablets 1667
Modicon 1667
Norinyl 2304
Ortho-Novum 1667
Ovcon 1391
Levlen/Tri-Levlen 665
Tri-Norinyl 28-Day Tablets 2304

Prostate disease, unspecified
Ansaid Tablets (Less than 1%) 2319

Prostatic cancer, transient worsening symptoms
Zoladex (Small number of patients) 1110

Prostatic disorder
Anafranil Capsules (Infrequent) 650

Prostatic hypertrophy
Android 1111
Cystospaz 2395
Eldepryl 2250

Prostatitis
Kerlone Tablets (Less than 2%) 2172
Rogaine Topical Solution (0.91%) 2357
Sandostatin Injection (Less than 1%) 2029

Prostration
Bicillin C-R Injection 2438
Bicillin C-R 900/300 Injection 2440
Bicillin L-A Injection 2442
Pfizerpen for Injection 1957
Pfizerpen-AS Aqueous Suspension 1959
Wycillin Injection 2537

Protein bound iodine, lowered (see under PBI decrease)

Protein catabolism
Aristospan Suspension (Intra-articular) 1011
Hydeltrasol Injection, Sterile 1476
Hydeltra-T.B.A. Sterile Suspension 1478
Hydrocortone Acetate Sterile Suspension 1479
Hydrocortone Phosphate Injection, Sterile 1481
Hydrocortone Tablets 1482
Kenalog in Orabase 604

Proteinuria
▲Accutane Capsules (Less than 1 in 10) 1878
Altace Capsules (Scattered incidents) 1086
Anaprox and Anaprox DS Tablets 2288
Atgam Sterile Solution (At least 1 patient and less than 5% of total patients) 2320
Atromid-S Capsules 2435
Azulfidine Tablets, EN-tabs, Oral Suspension (Rare) 1157
Butazolidin Capsules & Tablets (Less than 1%) 1027
Capoten (About 1 of 100 patients) 2255
Capozide (About 1 of 100 patients) 2258
Ceclor Pulvules & Suspension (Infrequent) 1251
Celontin 1692
Children's Advil Suspension 2426
Cleocin HCl Capsules 2322
Cleocin Pediatric Flavored Granules 2324
Cleocin Phosphate Injection (Rare) 2325
Clinoril Tablets (Less than 1 in 100) 1433
▲Cuprimine Capsules (6%) 1442
▲Depen Titratable Tablets (6%) 2379
Dipentum Capsules (Rare) 1160
Dolobid Tablets (Less than 1 in 100) 1465
Elspar (Infrequent) 1470
Eminase 2211
Feldene Capsules (Less than 1%) 1777
Floxin Tablets (More than or equal to 1.0%) 1652
Fulvicin P/G Tablets 2090
Fulvicin P/G 165 & 330 Tablets 2091
Fulvicin-U/F Tablets 2092
Garamycin Injectable 2093
Grifulvin V (griseofulvin microsize) Tablets/Suspension (Rare) 1678
Grisactin (Rare) 2454
Grisactin Ultra Tablets (Rare) 2455
Gris-PEG Tablets, 125 mg & 250 mg (Rare) 1083
IFEX (Rare) 729
Indocin (Less than 1%) 1487
Kerlone Tablets (Less than 2%) 2172
Lincocin (Rare) 2344
Lotensin Tablets (Scattered incidents) 872
Meclomen Capsules 1739
Mithracin 1602
Motrin Tablets 2351
Myochrysine Injection 1516
Nebcin Vials, Hyporets & ADD-Vantage 1286
Netromycin Injection 100 mg/ml 2104
Neupogen for Injection (Less frequent) 595
Omnipaque 2552
PediaProfen Suspension 1363
Prilosec Delayed-Release Capsules (Less than 1%) 1530
Primaxin I.M. 1532
Primaxin I.V. 1535
Ridaura Capsules (0.9%) 2224
Roferon-A Injection (Less than 1%) 1916
Sinemet CR Tablets 953
Solganal Suspension 2122
▲Tegison Capsules (1-10%) 1881
Tolectin (200, 400 and 600 mg) (Less than 1%) 1379
Toradol IM Injection 2302
Voltaren Tablets (Less than 1%) 1042

Proteinuria, increased
▲CHEMET (succimer) Capsules (Up to 3.7%) 1361

Prothrombin, decrease (see under Hypoprothrombinemia)

Prothrombin, increase (see under Hyperprothrombinemia)

Prothrombin time, deviation
Bumex (0.8%) 1895
Depakote Sprinkle Capsules 512
Rythmol Tablets (Less than 1%) 1184

Prothrombin time, increase (see under Prothrombin time prolongation)

Prothrombin time prolongation
Azactam for Injection 2252
Cefotan 2265
Ceftin Tablets 575
Ceptaz for Injection 1057
Cholybar 1705
Cipro I.V. 1592
Cipro Tablets 1589
Clinoril Tablets 1433
Sterile FUDR 1898
Floxin Tablets (More than or equal to 1.0%) 1652
Fortaz 1060
Hespan Injection 948
Keftab Tablets 917
Kefurox Vials, Faspak & ADD-Vantage 1277
Netromycin Injection 100 mg/ml (1 of 1000 patients) 2104
Panhematin 546
Pentaspan Injection 949
Primaxin I.M. 1532
Primaxin I.V. 1535
Provera Tablets 2356
Questran Light 711
Questran Powder 710
Rocephin Injectable Vials, ADD-Vantage (Less than 1%) 1914
Streptase for Infusion (Rare) 635
Suprax (Rare) 1235
Synkayvite Injection 1919
Synkayvite Tablets 1920
▲Tegison Capsules (10-25%) 1881
Timentin for Injection 2239
Zefazone Sterile Powder 2372
Zinacef 1066

Pruritus
▲A/T/S Topical Gel and Topical Solution (17 out of 90) 1089
▲Accutane Capsules (80%) 1878
Aclovate (2 in 100 patients) 1053
Actigall Capsules 2280
Adalat Capsules (10 mg and 20 mg) (2% or less) 1587
▲AeroBid Inhaler System (3-9%) 995
AK-Spore H.C. ⊙ 206
AK-Spore ⊙ 205
Aldactazide 2150
Alfenta Injection (Less than 1%) 1131
Alferon N Injection (2%) 1809
Alphatrex Cream, Ointment & Lotion (Infrequent) 2076
Altace Capsules 1086
Amen (Occasional) 833
Americaine Anesthetic Lubricant 972
Americaine Otic Topical Anesthetic Ear Drops 973
▲Anafranil Capsules (2% to 6%) 650
Analpram-HC Rectal Cream 1% and 2.5% 970
▲Anaprox and Anaprox DS Tablets (3-9%) 2288
Ancef Injection 2194
Ancobon Capsules 1886
Ansaid Tablets (Less than 1%) 2319
Antivenin (Crotalidae) Polyvalent 2430
Anusol-HC Cream (Infrequent) 1690
Anusol-HC Suppositories 1691
Aplisol (tuberculin PPD, diluted) 2550
Aplitest (tuberculin PPD, multiple-puncture device) 2551
Apresazide Capsules (Less frequent) 854
Apresoline Hydrochloride Parenteral (Ampuls) 856
Apresoline Hydrochloride Tablets (Less frequent) 855
Apresoline-Esidrix Tablets 857
Aralen Hydrochloride Injection 2038
Aralen Phosphate Tablets 2039
Artonad Ampuls 1887
Aristocort A (Infrequent) 1010
Asendin Tablets (Less than 1%) 1196
▲Astramorph/PF Injection, USP (Preservative-Free) (High incidence) 618
▲Atgam Sterile Solution (1 in 8 patients; 27%) 2320
Atromid-S Capsules (Less often) 2435
Atrovent Inhalation Aerosol (Less than 1 in 100) 675
Aygestin Tablets 2437
Azactam for Injection (Less than 1%) 2252
Azo Gantanol Tablets 1887
Azo Gantrisin Tablets 1888
▲Azulfidine Tablets, EN-tabs, Oral Suspension (3 to 4%) 1157
B & O No. 15A & No. 16A Supprettes (Occasional) 2395
Bactrim DS Tablets 1891
Bactrim I.V. Infusion 1889
Bactrim 1891
Bactroban Ointment (1%) 2200
Benemid Tablets 1426
Bentyl 1322
Benzamycin Topical Gel 907
Betagan (Rare) ⊙ 239
Betatrex Cream, Ointment & Lotion 2077
Blenoxane 724
Blocadren Tablets (1.1%) 1429
Brevital Sodium Vials 1248
Bumex (0.4%) 1895
BuSpar (Infrequent) 1401
Butazolidin Capsules & Tablets (Less than 1%) 1027
Cafergot/Cafergot P-B 1999
Calcijex Calcitriol Injection 506
Calciparine Injection 925
Calderol Capsules 1635
Capoten (About 2 of 100 patients) 2255
Capozide (About 2 of 100 patients) 2258
Carafate Tablets (Less than 0.5%) 1326
Carbocaine Hydrochloride Injection 2043
Cardioquin Tablets 1812
Cardizem Tablets-30 mg, 60 mg, 90 mg and 120 mg (Less than 1%) 1329
Cardizem SR Capsules-60 mg, 90 mg and 120 mg (Less than 1%) 1327
Cardura Tablets (1%) 1941
Carmol HC Cream 1% (Infrequent) 2296
Catapres Tablets (About 7 in 1,000 patients) 676
▲Catapres-TTS (51 of 101 patients) 677
Ceclor Pulvules & Suspension (Less than 1 in 200) 1251
▲Cefizox Injection (1 to 5%) 1012
Cefotan (1 in 700) 2265
Ceftin Tablets (0.3%) 575
Centrax 1693
Ceptaz for Injection (2% of patients) 1057
Cerumenex Drops (1% of 2,700 patients) 1813
▲CHEMET (succimer) Capsules (2.6 to 11.2%) 1361
Children's Advil Suspension (Less than 3%) 2426
Chloresium (A few instances) 1994
Chloromycetin Cream, 1% 1694
Chloromycetin Otic 1697
Chloroptic S.O.P. ⊙ 243
Cibalith-S 870
Cipro I.V. (1% or less) 1592
Cipro Tablets (Less than 1%) 1589
Claforan Sterile Injection (2.4%) 1089
Clear by Design Medicated Acne Gel ▣ 709
Clear By Design Medicated Cleansing Pads ▣ 709
Clearasil 10% Benzoyl Peroxide Acne Medication Vanishing Lotion ▣ 658
Clearasil Maximum Strength ▣ 658
Clinoril Tablets (Greater than 1%) 1433
Clozaril Tablets (Less than 1%) 2000
ColBENEMID Tablets 1436
Coly-Mycin M Parenteral 1706
Compazine 2201
Corgard Tablets (1 to 5 of 1000 patients) 701
Cortisporin Cream 757
Cortisporin Ointment 758
Cortisporin Ophthalmic Ointment Sterile 758
Cortisporin Ophthalmic Suspension Sterile 759
Cortisporin Otic Suspension Sterile 760

Corzide Tablets (1 to 5 of 1000 patients) ... 702
▲ Cuprimine Capsules (5%) ... 1442
Cutivate Cream 0.05% (2.9%) ... 1054
Cutivate Ointment 0.005% (2.9%) ... 1054
Cyclocort Lotion (Infrequent) ... 1198
Cycrin Tablets (Occasional) ... 2449
▲ Cytadren Tablets (1 in 20) ... 861
Cytosar-U Sterile Powder (Less frequent) ... 2329
Cytovene Sterile Powder (1% or less) ... 2292
D.H.E. 45 Injection ... 2003
Dalgan Injection (Less than 1%) ... 620
Dalmane Capsules (Rare) ... 1927
Danocrine Capsules ... 2046
Dantrium Capsules (Less frequent) 1619
Daranide Tablets ... 1445
Decadron Phosphate Topical Cream ... 1455
Decaspray Topical Aerosol ... 1459
Demerol ... 2047
Demulen ... 2161
Depakene Capsules & Syrup ... 511
Depakote ... 512
▲ Depen Titratable Tablets (5%) ... 2379
Depo-Provera Sterile Aqueous Suspension (Occasional) ... 2336
Deprol Tablets ... 2382
Desferal Vials ... 862
DesOwen Cream, Ointment and Lotion (Infrequent) ... 1682
Desyrel and Desyrel Dividose ... 1404
DiaBeta (1.5%) ... 1091
Diabinese Tablets (Less than 3%) .. 1775
Didronel Tablets (Rare) ... 1621
Dilaudid-HP Injection ... 1175
Dimetane-DC Cough Syrup ... 1857
Dimetane-DX Cough Syrup ... 1858
Dipentum Capsules (1.1% to 1.3%) ... 1160
Diprivan Injection (Less than 1%) .. 2267
Diprolene (Infrequent) ... 2083
Diupres Tablets ... 1461
Dolobid Tablets (Less than 1 in 100) ... 1465
Dolophine Hydrochloride Tablets ... 1261
Dopram Injectable ... 1860
Doral Tablets ... 2383
▲ Duragesic Transdermal System (1% to 10%) ... 1133
▲ Duramorph (High incidence) ... 960
Duricef ... 1405
DynaCirc Capsules (0.5% to 1%) .. 2004
ETS-2% ... 1685
Easprin ... 1719
▲ Efudex (Among most frequent) ... 1880
Elase-Chloromycetin Ointment ... 1015
Eldecort Cream 1.0% (Infrequent) 1113
Eldecort Cream 1.0% and 2.5% (Infrequent) ... 1113
▲ Elimite (permethrin) 5% Cream (7%) ... 1082
Elocon (1 of 319 patients) ... 2084
Emcyt Capsules (2%) ... 1161
Eminase (Occasional) ... 2211
Empirin with Codeine Phosphate Nos. 2, 3 & 4 ... 764
Enduronyl ... 518
Engerix-B Unit-Dose Vials (Less than 1%) ... 2213
Enovid ... 2161
Equagesic Tablets ... 2451
Ergamisol Tablets (1 to 2%) ... 1136
Ergostat ... 1719
ERYC ... 1720
Erycette (erythromycin 2%) Topical Solution ... 1678
Ethmozine Tablets (Less than 2%) 946
Etrafon ... 2087
Eulexin Capsules ... 2089
▲ Exelderm Cream 1.0% (3%) ... 2398
Exelderm Solution 1.0% (Approximately 1%) ... 2399
Factrel (Occasional) ... 2561
Fansidar Tablets ... 1896
Feldene Capsules (1 to 3%) ... 1777
Femstat Prefill Vaginal Cream 2% (0.2%) ... 2295
Femstat Vaginal Cream 2% (0.2%) ... 2295
Fiorinal with Codeine Capsules (Infrequent) ... 2008
Flagyl I.V. ... 2131
Flexeril Tablets (Rare) ... 1471
Florone/Florone E ... 908
Floxin Tablets (1% to 3%) ... 1652
Fluorescite (Very rare) ... ⊚ 217
Fluoroplex Topical Solution & Cream 1% ... 1082
Fluorouracil Injection ... 1897
Fortaz (2%) ... 1060
Fungizone Cream, Lotion and Ointment ... 2261
Fungizone Intravenous ... 2262
Furacin Soluble Dressing (Approximately 1%) ... 1854
Furacin Topical Cream (Approximately 1%) ... 1854
Furacin Topical Solution 0.2% ... 1855
Gantanol ... 1899
Gantrisin Ophthalmic Ointment/Solution ... 1900
Gantrisin ... 1901
Garamycin Injectable ... 2093
▲ Gastrocrom Capsules (3 of 87 patients) ... 974
Geocillin Tablets (Infrequent) ... 1951
Glucotrol (1 in 70) ... 1952
G-myticin Creme and Ointment 0.1% ... 1770
Halcion Tablets ... 2340
Halog (Infrequent) ... 2399
Halotex Cream & Solution (1 in 819 patients) ... 2400
Harmonyl Tablets ... 528
Heparin Lock Flush Solution ... 2456
Heparin Sodium Vials ... 1264
Heparin Sodium Injection ... 2457
Heparin Sodium Injection, USP, Sterile Solution ... 2342
Herplex Liquifilm ... ⊚ 248
Hespan Injection ... 948
Hexalen Capsules (Less than 1%) .. 2316
Hismanal Tablets (Less frequent) ... 1138
Hycodan Syrup, Tablets ... 927
Hycomine Syrup ... 927
Hydropres Tablets ... 1485
Hyskon Hysteroscopy Fluid (Rare) .. 1162
Hytone ... 909
Hytrin Tablets (At least 1%) ... 529
Beef Regular, 100 Units ... 1275
Imferon ... 976
Indocin (Less than 1%) ... 1487
Infumorph 200 and Infumorph 500 Sterile Solutions (Occasional) ... 962
Insulatard NPH ... 1626
Insulatard NPH Human ... 1627
▲ Intron A (4% to 20%) ... 2097
IOPIDINE ... ⊚ 232
Isoptin Injectable (Rare) ... 1177
Kefurox Vials, Faspak & ADD-Vantage (Less than 1 in 250) ... 1277
Kenalog Cream, Lotion & Ointment (Infrequent) ... 2401
Kerlone Tablets (Less than 2%) ... 2172
▲ Lamprene Capsules (1-5%) ... 1030
Lariam Tablets (Less than 1%) ... 1904
Lasix ... 1093
Levo-Dromoran (Rare) ... 1906
Lidex (Infrequent) ... 2296
Limbitrol ... 1933
Lioresal Tablets ... 1031
Lithane Tablets ... 1596
Lithium Carbonate Capsules & Tablets ... 1984
Lithobid Tablets ... 870
Lodine Capsules (More than 1% but less than 3%) ... 2468
Locoid Cream, Ointment and Topical Solution (Infrequent) ... 970
Lomotil ... 2174
Lopid Capsules and Tablets ... 1736
▲ Lopressor Ampuls (5%) ... 1032
Lopressor HCT Tablets (Fewer than 1 in 100) ... 1034
▲ Lopressor Tablets (5%) ... 1032
Loprox Cream 1% and Lotion 1% (1 out of 514) ... 1095
Lorelco Tablets ... 1333
Lotensin Tablets ... 872
Lotrimin ... 2102
Lotrisone Cream ... 2103
Loxitane ... 1213
Lozol Tablets (Less than 5%) ... 1843
Ludiomil Tablets (Rare) ... 874
Lupron Depot 7.5 mg ... 2311
Lupron Injection (Less than 5%) ... 2310
MS Contin Tablets (Infrequent) ... 1814
MSIR (Infrequent) ... 1817
Macrodantin Capsules ... 1624
Marcaine Hydrochloride with Epinephrine 1:200,000 (Rare) ... 2055
Marcaine Hydrochloride Injection (Rare) ... 2055
Marcaine Spinal (Rare) ... 2058
Matulane Capsules ... 1907
Maxair Inhaler (Less than 1%) ... 1311
Maxivate Cream, Lotion & Ointment 0.05% ... 2406
Meclomen Capsules (Greater than 1%) ... 1739
Mefoxin ... 1498
Mefoxin Premixed Intravenous Solution ... 1500
Methadone Hydrochloride Diskets .. 1284
Methadone Hydrochloride Oral Solution & Tablets ... 1987
Methotrexate Tablets, Parenteral, LPF Parenteral (1 to 3%) ... 1217
▲ Mevacor Tablets (5.2%) ... 1505
Mezlin ... 1597
Mezlin Pharmacy Bulk Package ... 1599
Micronase Tablets (1.5%) ... 2350
Midamor Tablets (Less than or equal to 1%) ... 1508
Milontin Kapseals ... 1741
Minipress Capsules (Less than 1%) ... 1778
Minizide Capsules (Rare) ... 1779
Mintezol ... 1510
Mixtard 70/30 ... 1627
Mixtard Human 70/30 ... 1628
Moduretic Tablets (Greater than 1%, less than 3%) ... 1510
▲ Monistat I.V. (21%) ... 1143
Monocid Injection (Less than 1%) .. 2217
Monopril Tablets (0.2 to 1.0%) ... 1406
Motofen Tablets ... 836
Motrin Tablets (Less than 3%) ... 2351
Myambutol Tablets ... 1225
Mycelex 1% Cream and Topical Solution 1% ... 1604
Mycelex-G 100 mg Vaginal Tablets (Rare) ... 1606
Mycolog II Cream and Ointment (Infrequent) ... 2407
Mykrox ½ mg Tablets (Less than 2%) ... 984
Myochrysine Injection ... 1516
Mytrex Cream & Ointment (Infrequent) ... 2080
Naftin Cream 1% (2%) ... 1084
Naftin Gel 1% (1.0%) ... 1084
▲ Nalfon Pulvules & Tablets (4.2%) .. 919
▲ Naprosyn (3 to 9%) ... 2297
Naturetin Tablets (Occasional) ... 1789
Navane Capsules and Concentrate 1954
Navane Intramuscular ... 1956
Nebcin Vials, Hyporets & ADD-Vantage ... 1286
NebuPent for Inhalation Solution (1% or less) ... 1017
NegGram ... 2062
NeoDecadron Topical Cream ... 1518
Neo-Synalar Cream (Infrequent) ... 2296
Nescaine/Nescaine MPF ... 629
Netromycin Injection 100 mg/ml (4 or 5 of 1000 patients) ... 2104
Niacor Tablets ... 2376
Nicobid ... 1846
Nicolar Tablets ... 1846
Nicorette ... 1335
Nimotop Capsules (Less than 1%) 1607
▲ Nizoral 2% Cream (5%) ... 1143
Nizoral 2% Shampoo (One occurrence in 41 patients) ... 1144
Nizoral Tablets (1.5%) ... 1145
Norethin ... 2133
Norflex ... 1314
Norlutate ... 1754
Norlutin ... 1755
Normodyne Injection (1%) ... 2108
Normodyne Tablets ... 2110
Noroxin Tablets ... 1519
Norpace (1 to 3%) ... 2177
Norpramin Tablets ... 1340
Novahistine DH ... 1342
Novahistine Expectorant ... 1343
Nubain Injection (Less than 1%) ... 934
Numorphan Hydrochloride Injection ... 935
Numorphan Suppositories ... 935
Nutracort Cream & Lotion (Infrequent) ... 1684
Omnipaque (0.1%) ... 2552
Orabase HCA Oral Paste (Infrequent) ... 890
Oramorph SR (Morphine Sulfate Sustained Release Tablets) (Less frequent) ... 1988
Oreticyl ... 545
Orinase Tablets (1.1%) ... 2354
Orthoclone OKT3 Sterile Solution .. 1645
Orudis Capsules (Less than 1%) ... 2488
Otic Tridesilon Solution 0.05% (Infrequent) ... 1612
Oxistat Cream (1.6%) ... 1055
▲ Oxsoralen-Ultra Capsule (10%) ... 1117
Oxy-5 and Oxy-10 Tinted and Vanishing Formulas with Sorboxyl ... ▣ 719
PMB 200 and PMB 400 ... 2504
PPD Tine Test ... 2548
Pamelor ... 2019
Pantopon Injectable ... 1911
Paradione Capsules ... 548
Paraplatin for Injection ... 735
PediaProfen Suspension (Less than 3%) ... 1363
Pediazole ... 1973
PediOtic Suspension Sterile ... 797
Pepcid (Infrequent) ... 1524
Percocet Tablets ... 950
Percodan ... 951
Permax Tablets (Infrequent) ... 1291
Persantine Tablets ... 683
Phenaphen with Codeine Capsules 1865
Phenaphen-650 with Codeine Tablets ... 1866
Phenergan with Codeine (Infrequent) ... 2497
Phenergan VC with Codeine ... 2501
Pipracil (Less frequent) ... 1230
Plaquenil Sulfate Tablets ... 2067
Plendil Extended-Release Tablets (0.5% or greater) ... 1526
Pramosone Cream, Lotion & Ointment ... 971
Pre-Pen ... 2148
Prilosec Delayed-Release Capsules (Less than 1%) ... 1530
Primaxin I.M. ... 1532
Primaxin I.V. (0.3%) ... 1535
Prinivil Tablets (1% or less) ... 1538
Prinzide Tablets (0.3 to 1%) ... 1540
Procan SR Tablets (Occasional) ... 1760
Procardia Capsules (2% or less) ... 1781
Procardia XL Tablets (Less than 3%) ... 1783
ProctoCream-HC (Infrequent) ... 1834
Proglycem ... 649
Prolixin Decanoate ... 1795
Prolixin Elixir ... 1793
Prolixin Enanthate ... 1796
Prolixin Injection ... 1791
Prolixin Oral Concentrate ... 1792
Prolixin Tablets ... 1793
▲ Proloprim Tablets (Most often) ... 799
Pronestyl Capsules and Tablets (Occasional) ... 1800
Pronestyl Injection (Occasional) ... 1798
Pronestyl-SR Tablets ... 1801
ProSom Tablets (1%) ... 554
Provera Tablets ... 2356
Provocholine for Inhalation (1 occurrence) ... 1911
Prozac Pulvules (2.4%) ... 920
Psorcon Ointment 0.05% ... 909
Psorion Cream 0.05% (Infrequent) ... 1121
Pyridium ... 1763
Pyridium Plus ... 1764
Quinaglute Dura-Tabs Tablets ... 663
Quinamm Tablets ... 1344
Quinidex Extentabs ... 1868
Raudixin Tablets ... 1803
Rauzide Tablets ... 1804
Recombivax HB (Less than 1%) ... 1544
Renese-R Tablets ... 1786
Retrovir Capsules (Less than 5%) .. 802
Retrovir I.V. Infusion (Less than 5%) ... 805
Retrovir Syrup (Less than 5%) ... 802
▲ Rēv-Eyes Ophthalmic Eyedrops 0.5% (10% to 40%) ... ⊚ 312
Rheumatrex Methotrexate Dose Pack (1% to 3%) ... 1234
▲ Ridaura Capsules (17%) ... 2224
Rifadin (Occasional) ... 1345
Rifamate Capsules (Occasional) ... 1347
Rimactane Capsules (Occasional) .. 879
Robaxin Injectable ... 1871
Robaxin Tablets ... 1872
Robaxisal Tablets ... 1872
Rocaltrol Capsules ... 1913
Rocephin Injectable Vials, ADD-Vantage (Less than 1%) ... 1914
▲ Roferon-A Injection (5% to 13%) .. 1916
Rogaine Topical Solution ... 2357
Rowasa (1.23%) ... 2248
Roxanol ... 1991
Roxicodone Tablets, Oral Solution & Intensol (Oxycodone) ... 1992
Rufen Tablets (Less than 3%) ... 691
Rythmol Tablets (Less than 1%) ... 1184
SSD (Low) ... 694
Salutensin/Salutensin-Demi ... 719
Sandimmune (Rare) ... 2024

Sandostatin Injection (Less than 1%) 2029
Sectral Capsules (Up to 2%) 2520
Seldane Tablets (1.6%) 1349
Seldane-D Extended-Release Tablets 1350
Sensorcaine (Rare) 631
Sensorcaine-MPF Spinal (Rare) 634
Septra 813
Septra I.V. Infusion 808
Septra I.V. Infusion ADD-Vantage Vials 810
Septra 813
Ser-Ap-Es Tablets 881
Serentil 686
Serpasil Tablets 883
Serpasil-Apresoline Tablets 884
Serpasil-Esidrix Tablets 886
Silvadene Cream 1% (0.1%) 1352
Sinequan (Occasional) 1960
Skelaxin 840
Slo-Niacin Tablets 2376
Solganal Suspension 2122
Soma Compound w/Codeine Tablets (Rare) 2390
Soma Compound Tablets (Rare) 2389
Soma Tablets 2388
▲ Spectazole (econazole nitrate) Cream (3%) 1681
Stelazine 2226
Streptase for Infusion 635
Stri-Dex Maximum ▣ 573
Stri-Dex Dual Textured Regular Strength Pads ▣ 573
Stri-Dex Dual Textured Regular Strength Big Pads ▣ 573
Sufenta Injection (Less than 1%) 1147
Suprax (Less than 2%) 1235
Surmontil Capsules 2524
Synacort Creams 1%, 2.5% (Infrequent) 2296
Synalar (Infrequent) 2296
Synalgos-DC Capsules 2525
Synemol Cream 0.025% (Infrequent) 2296
T-Stat 2.0% Topical Solution and Pads 2409
Talwin Injection 2071
Talwin Nx 2073
Tambocor Tablets (Less than 1%) 1315
Tapazole Tablets 1298
Taractan 1920
Tazicef for Injection (2%) 2231
Tazidime Vials, Faspak & ADD-Vantage (2%) 1299
▲ Tegison Capsules (50-75%) 1881
Tegretol 654
Temovate (2 of 266 patients) 1056
Tenex Tablets (Less than 3%) 1875
Terazol 3 Vaginal Suppositories (1.8% of 284 patients) 1677
Tessalon Perles 1006
Theramycin Z Topical Solution 2% 1410
Thiosulfil Forte Tablets 2526
Ticar for Injection 2236
Timentin for Injection 2239
Timolide Tablets 1547
Timoptic in Ocudose 1552
Timoptic Sterile Ophthalmic Solution 1550
Tofranil Ampuls 1038
Tofranil Tablets 1039
Tofranil-PM Capsules 1041
Tolinase Tablets (0.4%) 2365
Tonocard Tablets (Less than 1%) 1554
Topicort (Infrequent) 1098
Toradol IM Injection (1% or less) 2302
Tracrium Injection (0.2%) 817
Trandate HCT Tablets (Rare) 579
Trandate Injection (Rare) 577
Trandate Tablets (Rare) 579
Trental (Less than 1%) 1099
Trexan Tablets (Less than 1%) 937
Triavil Tablets 1556
Tridesilon Creme 0.05% (Infrequent) 1611
Tridesilon Ointment 0.05% (Infrequent) 1611
Tridione 557
Trilafon 2123
Trilisate (Less than 1%) 1822
Trimpex Tablets 1922
Tuberculin, Old, Tine Test 2549
Tussionex Extended-Release Suspension 988
Tylenol with Codeine 1381
Tylox Capsules 1382
▲ Ultravate Cream 0.05% (4%) 2410
Ultravate Ointment 0.05% 2411
Unasyn (Less than 1%) 1965
Unipen 2533
▲ Vagistat (Approximately 5%) 1397
Vancocin HCl, Vials & ADD-Vantage 1302
Vanoxide-HC Acne Lotion 911
Vaseretic Tablets (0.5% to 2.0%) 1559
Vasotec I.V. 1562
Vasotec Tablets (0.5% to 1%) 1564
Velosef Capsules and for Oral Suspension (Few) 606
Velosulin 1627
Velosulin Human 1628
VePesid Capsules and Injection (Infrequent) 741
Versed Injection (Less than 1%) 1924
Vioform-Hydrocortisone Cream and Mild Cream 889
Vioform-Hydrocortisone Ointment 889
Vira-A for Injection 1766
Visken Tablets (1%) 2036
Vivactil Tablets 1567
Voltaren Tablets (1-3%) 1042
Vytone Cream 1% 911
Wellbutrin Tablets (2.2%) 821
Westcort 2411
Wigraine Tablets & Suppositories 1645
Wytensin Tablets (3% or less) 2542
Xanax Tablets 2367
Xerac AC 1773
Yodoxin 1072
Zantac Injection and Zantac Injection Premixed 1063
Zefazone Sterile Powder 2372
Zestoretic (0.3 to 1%) 2274
Zestril Tablets (Less than 1%) 2277
Zinacef (Less than 1 in 250 patients) 1066
Zovirax Capsules 824
Zovirax Ointment 5% 827
Zovirax Sterile Powder (Approximately 2%) 828
Zovirax 824
Zyloprim Tablets (Less than 1%) 830

Pruritus, ear lobes
Miacalcin Injection 2017

Pruritus, exacerbation of
Actigall Capsules (One patient) 2280

Pruritus, genital
Anafranil Capsules (Infrequent) 650
Ancef Injection 2194
Ceclor Pulvules & Suspension (Less than 1 in 100) 1251
▲ Condylox (50% to 65%) 1630
Floxin Tablets (1% to 3%) 1652
Keflex Pulvules, Oral Suspension & Pediatric Drops 916
Keftab Tablets 917
Kefzol Vials, Faspak & ADD-Vantage 1279
Nolvadex Tablets (Infrequent) 1102
Primaxin I.M. 1532
Primaxin I.V. (Less than 0.2%) 1535
ProSom Tablets (Infrequent) 554
Suprax (Les than 2%) 1235
▲ Terazol 3 Vaginal Cream (5%) 1676
Terazol 3 Vaginal Suppositories (1.8% of 284 patients) 1677
Terazol 7 Vaginal Cream (2.3% of 521 patients) 1677
Today Vaginal Contraceptive Sponge 2422
Ultracef Capsules, Tablets & Oral Suspension 722
▲ Vagistat (Approximately 5%) 1397

Pruritus, injection site
▲ Alferon N Injection (12%) 1809
Cipro I.V. (1% or less) 1592
Diprivan Injection (Less than 1%) 2267
Engerix-B Unit-Dose Vials (Less than 1%) 2213
Staphage Lysate (SPL) 905

Pruritus, localized
Calciparine Injection 925
Diapid Nasal Spray (Infrequent) 2003
Diprivan Injection (Less than 1%) 2267
Epifoam 1828
Eskalith 2214
Humulin 70/30, 100 Units (Occasional) 1267
Humulin BR, 100 Units (Occasional) 1268
Humulin L, 100 Units (Occasional) 1268
Humulin U, 100 Units (Occasional) 1272
▲ Norplant System (3.7%) 2484
Polytrim Ophthalmic Solution Sterile 588
Proctofoam-HC 1835

Pruritus, not associated with rash
Combipres Tablets (About 7 in 1,000) 678

Pruritus, rhinal
Intal Nebulizer Solution 980

Pruritus ani
Ancef Injection 2194
Furoxone 1855
Keflex Pulvules, Oral Suspension & Pediatric Drops 916
Keftab Tablets 917
Kefzol Vials, Faspak & ADD-Vantage 1279
Lincocin 2344
Niclocide Chewable Tablets (0.3%) 1607
Yodoxin 1072

Pseudolactation
Raudixin Tablets 1803
Rauzide Tablets 1804
Ser-Ap-Es Tablets 881
Serpasil-Esidrix Tablets 886

Pseudolymphoma
Dilantin Infatabs 1710
Dilantin Kapseals 1708
Dilantin Parenteral 1712
Dilantin-30 Pediatric/Dilantin-125 Suspension 1713
Dilantin with Phenobarbital Kapseals 1715

Pseudomembranous colitis
Ancef Injection 2194
Augmentin Tablets, Powder for Oral Suspension, and Chewable Tablets 2198
Azactam for Injection (Less than 1%) 2252
Azo Gantrisin Tablets 1888
Ceclor Pulvules & Suspension 1251
Cefizox Injection 1012
Cefobid Intravenous/Intramuscular 1943
Cefobid Pharmacy Bulk Package - Not for Direct Infusion 1945
Cefotan 2265
Ceftin Tablets 575
Ceptaz for Injection 1057
Cipro I.V. (1% or less) 1592
Cipro Tablets 1589
Claforan Sterile Injection 1089
Cleocin HCl Capsules 2322
Cleocin Pediatric Flavored Granules 2324
Cleocin Phosphate Injection 2325
Duricef 1405
E.E.S. (Rare) 522
EryPed (Rare) 519
Ery-Tab Tablets (Rare) 521
Erythrocin Stearate Filmtab (Rare) 523
Erythromycin Base Filmtab (Rare) 525
Erythromycin Delayed-Release Capsules, USP (Rare) 526
Floxin Tablets 1652
Fortaz (Less frequent) 1060
Gantrisin 1901
Keflex Pulvules, Oral Suspension & Pediatric Drops 916
Keftab Tablets 917
Kefurox Vials, Faspak & ADD-Vantage (1 in 440) 1277
Kefzol Vials, Faspak & ADD-Vantage 1279
Mandol Vials, Faspak & ADD-Vantage 1281
Mefoxin 1498
Mefoxin Premixed Intravenous Solution 1500
Mezlin 1597
Mezlin Pharmacy Bulk Package 1599
Monocid Injection 2217
Noroxin Tablets 1519
PCE Dispertab Tablets (Rare) 549
Pipracil (Rare) 1230
Primaxin I.M. 1532
Primaxin I.V. (Less than 0.2%) 1535
Rifadin 1345
Rocephin Injectable Vials, ADD-Vantage 1914
Spectrobid Tablets & Powder for Oral Suspension 1961
Suprax (Several patients) 1235
Tazicef for Injection 2231
Unasyn 1965
Velosef Capsules and for Oral Suspension 606
Zefazone Sterile Powder (Rare) 2372
Zinacef 1066

Pseudomembranous enterocolitis
Bactrim DS Tablets 1891
Bactrim I.V. Infusion 1889
Bactrim 1891
Gantanol 1899
Rimactane Capsules (Rare) 879
Septra 813
Septra I.V. Infusion 808
Septra I.V. Infusion ADD-Vantage Vials 810
Septra 813

Pseudoparkinsonism
Compazine 2201
Mellaril (Infrequent) 2011
Navane Capsules and Concentrate 1954
Navane Intramuscular 1956
Stelazine 2226
Taractan 1920
Thorazine 2234
Triavil Tablets 1556
Wellbutrin Tablets (1.5%) 821

Pseudoschizophrenia
Temaril Tablets, Syrup and Spansule Sustained Release Capsules 1085

Pseudotumor cerebri
Accutane Capsules 1878
Achromycin V Capsules 1193
Aristospan Suspension (Intra-articular) 1011
Celestone Soluspan Suspension 2081
Children's Advil Suspension (Less than 1%) 2426
Cibalith-S 870
Cordarone Tablets (Rare) 2446
Cortenema 2244
Cortone Acetate Sterile Suspension 1437
Cortone Acetate Tablets 1439
Decadron Elixir 1445
Decadron Phosphate Injection 1449
Decadron Phosphate Respihaler 1454
Decadron Phosphate Turbinaire 1456
Decadron Phosphate with Xylocaine Injection, Sterile 1451
Decadron Tablets 1447
Declomycin Capsules, Tablets 1199
Depo-Medrol Sterile Aqueous Suspension 2334
Eskalith 2214
Garamycin Injectable 2093
Hydeltrasol Injection, Sterile 1476
Hydrocortone Tablets 1482
Lithane Tablets 1596
Lithium Carbonate Capsules & Tablets 1984
Lithobid Tablets 870
Medrol 2348
Minocin Intravenous 1221
Minocin Oral Suspension 1224
Minocin Pellet-Filled Capsules 1222
Motrin Tablets (Less than 1%) 2351
Pediapred Oral Liquid 987
PediaProfen Suspension (Less than 1%) 1363
Rufen Tablets 691
Solu-Cortef Sterile Powder 2361
Tegison Capsules 1881

Psoriasis
Anafranil Capsules (Infrequent) 650
Eskalith 2214
Prozac Pulvules (Rare) 920
Quinidex Extentabs 1868

Psoriasis, exacerbation
Atabrine Hydrochloride Tablets 2041
Cibalith-S 870
Eskalith 2214
Lithane Tablets 1596
Lithium Carbonate Capsules & Tablets 1984
Lithobid Tablets 870
Methotrexate Tablets, Parenteral, LPF Parenteral 1217
Oxsoralen-Ultra Capsule 1117
Plaquenil Sulfate Tablets 2067
Rheumatrex Methotrexate Dose Pack 1234

Psoriasis, pustular
Cutivate Cream 0.05% 1054
Cutivate Ointment 0.005% 1054

Psychiatric disturbances
Aldoclor Tablets 1413
Aldomet Ester HCl Injection 1417
Aldomet Oral 1415
Aldoril Tablets 1418
Alurate Elixir (Less than 1 in 100) 1883
Anafranil Capsules (Up to 3%) 650
Apresoline-Esidrix Tablets 857
Aralen Hydrochloride Injection 2038
Aralen Phosphate Tablets 2039
Artane 1195
Atabrine Hydrochloride Tablets (Infrequent) 2041
Clinoril Tablets (Less than 1 in 100) 1433
Cogentin 1435
Cortone Acetate Sterile Suspension 1437
Cortone Acetate Tablets 1439
Cuprimine Capsules 1442
Decadron Elixir 1445
Decadron Phosphate Injection 1449
Decadron Phosphate Respihaler 1454
Decadron Phosphate Turbinaire 1456
Decadron Phosphate with Xylocaine Injection, Sterile 1451
Decadron Tablets 1447
Decadron-LA Sterile Suspension 1457
Depo-Medrol Sterile Aqueous Suspension 2334
Hydeltrasol Injection, Sterile 1476
Hydeltra-T.B.A. Sterile Suspension 1478
Hydrocortone Acetate Sterile Suspension 1479
Hydrocortone Phosphate Injection, Sterile 1481
Hydrocortone Tablets 1482
▲ Hylorel Tablets (3.8%) 975
Indocin (Less than 1%) 1487
Kenalog-10 Injection 2402
Kenalog-40 Injection 2403
Mebaral Tablets (Less than 1 in 100) 2061
Mevacor Tablets 1505
Mintezol 1510
Nembutal Sodium Capsules (Less than 1%) 534
Nembutal Sodium Solution (1-3%) 536
Nembutal Sodium Suppositories (Less than 1%) 538
Nizoral Tablets (Rare) 1145
Noroxin Tablets 1519
Pepcid (Infrequent) 1524
Pfizerpen-AS Aqueous Suspension (Approximately 1 in 500) 1959
Phenobarbital Elixir and Tablets (Less than 1 in 100 patients) 1293
▲ Phenurone Tablets (17%) 552
Prilosec Delayed-Release Capsules (Less than 1%) 1530
Primaxin I.M. 1532
Primaxin I.V. (Less than 0.2%) 1535
Seconal Sodium Pulvules (Less than 1 in 100) 1296
Ser-Ap-Es Tablets 881
Timoptic in Ocudose 1552
Timoptic Sterile Ophthalmic Solution 1550
Tonocard Tablets (Less than 1%) 1554
Trecator-SC Tablets 2527
Zarontin Capsules 1768
Zarontin Syrup 1769

Psychic dependence (see under Dependence, psychological)

Psychomotor retardation
Lithobid/Cibalith 870

Psychoses
Adipex-P Tablets and Capsules 1019
AK-Pentolate ⊙ 204
Aldoclor Tablets 1413
Aldomet Ester HCl Injection 1417
Aldomet Oral 1415
Aldoril Tablets 1418
Anafranil Capsules (Infrequent) 650
Ancobon Capsules 1886
Antabuse Tablets 2429
Apresazide Capsules 854
Aralen Phosphate Tablets (Rare) 2039
Aristospan Suspension (Intra-articular) 1011
Atabrine Hydrochloride Tablets (Infrequent) 2041
Azo Gantrisin Tablets 1888
Biphetamine Capsules (Rare) 973
Bontril Slow-Release (Rare) 834
BuSpar (Rare) 1401
Butisol Sodium Elixir & Tablets (Less than 1 in 100) 2377
Calan SR Caplets (1% or less) 2157
Calan Tablets (1% or less) 2155
Calderol Capsules (Rare) 1635
Cantil Tablets 1326
Celontin (Rare) 1692
Clinoril Tablets (Less than 1 in 100) 1433
Cyclogyl ⊙ 215
Cyclomydril ⊙ 216
Cytovene Sterile Powder (1% or less) 2292
Dapsone USP 1130
Depakene Capsules & Syrup 511
Depakote 512
Desoxyn Gradumet Tablets (Rare) 514
Desyrel and Desyrel Dividose 1404
Dexedrine (Rare at recommended doses) 2206
Duramorph 960
Fastin Capsules (Rare) 2216
Fiorinal with Codeine Capsules 2008
Gastrocrom Capsules (Infrequent) 974
Hydropres Tablets 1485
IFEX 729
Indocin (Less than 1%) 1487
Ionamin Capsules (Rare) 981
Isoptin Oral Tablets (Less than 1%) 1179
Isoptin SR Sustained Release Tablets (Less than 1%) 1181
Klonopin Tablets 1902
Lanoxicaps 772
Lanoxin Elixir Pediatric 775
Lanoxin Injection 778
Lanoxin Injection Pediatric 781
Lanoxin Tablets 783
Lariam Tablets 1904
Larodopa Tablets (Infrequent) 1905
Ludiomil Tablets (Rare) 874
Mellaril (Extremely rare) 2011
Mexitil Capsules (Less than 1% or about 2 in 1,000) 680
Mydriacyl ⊙ 225
Nardil (Infrequent) 1742
Noroxin Tablets 1519
Norpace (Rare) 2177
Omnipaque 2552
Parlodel (Less than 1%) 2020
Permax Tablets (2.1%) 1291
Plaquenil Sulfate Tablets 2067
Plegine Tablets 2504
Prelu-2 Capsules (Rare) 683
Procan SR Tablets (Occasional) 1760
Pronestyl Capsules and Tablets (Occasional) 1800
Pronestyl Injection (Occasional) 1798
Pronestyl-SR Tablets (Occasional) 1801
Prozac Pulvules (Infrequent) 920
Rocaltrol Capsules (Rare) 1913
Rythmol Tablets (Less than 1%) 1184
Seromycin Pulvules 1298
Sinemet Tablets 952
Sinemet CR Tablets 953
Symmetrel Capsules & Syrup (0.1-1%) 936
Syntocinon Nasal Spray (1 case) 2033
Tagamet 2228
Taractan 1920
Tenuate (Rare) 1354
Tonocard Tablets (Less than 1%) 1554
Trilafon 2123
Tropicacyl ⊙ 209
Verelan Capsules (Less than 1%) 1243
Vira-A for Injection 1766
Voltaren Tablets (Rare) 1042
Wellbutrin Tablets (Infrequent) 821
Zarontin Capsules 1768
Zarontin Syrup 1769
Zovirax Sterile Powder 828

Psychoses, aggravation
Aristospan Suspension (Intra-articular) 1011
Etrafon 2087
Mellaril 2011
Norpramin Tablets 1340
Norzine 1818
Pamelor 2019
Prolixin Decanoate 1795
Prolixin Elixir 1793
Prolixin Enanthate 1796
Prolixin Injection 1791
Prolixin Oral Concentrate 1792
Prolixin Tablets 1793
Serentil 686
Surmontil Capsules 2524
Tofranil Ampuls 1038
Tofranil Tablets 1039
Tofranil-PM Capsules 1041
Torecan 1993
Vivactil Tablets 1567

Psychoses, toxic
Astramorph/PF Injection, USP (Preservative-Free) 618
Atabrine Hydrochloride Tablets (Rare) 2041
Cipro I.V. (1% or less) 1592
Cipro Tablets 1589
Floxin Tablets 1652
INH Tablets 868
Infumorph 200 and Infumorph 500 Sterile Solutions 962
NegGram (Rare) 2062
Rifamate Capsules (Uncommon) 1347
Ritalin 880

Psychosis, activation
Compazine 2201
Prolixin Decanoate 1795
Prolixin Elixir 1793
Prolixin Enanthate 1796
Prolixin Injection 1791
Prolixin Oral Concentrate 1792
Prolixin Tablets 1793
Stelazine 2226
Tegretol 654
Triavil Tablets 1556

Psychosis, overt
Calcijex Calcitriol Injection (Rare) 506

Psychosis, paranoid
Bretylol Injection 923
Zarontin Capsules (Rare) 1768
Zarontin Syrup (Rare) 1769

Psychotic episodes (see under Psychoses)

Psychotic symptoms, paradoxical exacerbation
Haldol Decanoate 1375
Navane Capsules and Concentrate (Infrequent) 1954
Navane Intramuscular (Infrequent) 1956

Ptosis, eyelids
AK-Cide Sterile Ophthalmic Ointment & Suspension (Occasional) ⊙ 202
Betagan ⊙ 239
Blocadren Tablets 1429
Clozaril Tablets (Less than 1%) 2000
Depen Titratable Tablets 2379
Esimil Tablets 864
Ismelin Tablets 869
Loxitane 1213
Metimyd ⊙ 306
▲ Oculinum for Injecton (11.0 to 15.7%) 587
Prozac Pulvules (Rare) 920
▲ Rēv-Eyes Ophthalmic Eyedrops 0.5% (10% to 40%) ⊙ 312
Timolide Tablets 1547
Timoptic in Ocudose 1552
Timoptic Sterile Ophthalmic Solution 1550
Vasocidin Ointment (Occasional) ⊙ 275
Vasocidin Ophthalmic Solution (Occasional) ⊙ 276

Pubic hair, growth
A.P.L. 2431

Pulmonary air leak
▲ Exosurf Neonatal for Intratracheal Suspension (Up to 48%) 765
▲ Survanta Beractant Intratracheal Suspension (10.9%) 1978

Pulmonary allergy, unspecified
Idamycin for Injection (2%) 564

Pulmonary disease, chronic interstitial obstructive
Methotrexate Tablets, Parenteral, LPF Parenteral (Occasional) 1217
Rheumatrex Methotrexate Dose Pack (Occasional) 1234

Pulmonary disease, chronic obstructive
Zoladex (Small number of patients) 1110

Pulmonary distress
Betoptic Sterile Ophthalmic Solution (Rare) 569
Betoptic S Sterile Ophthalmic Suspension (Rare) 570
Serophene (clomiphene citrate tablets, USP) 2186

Pulmonary edema (see under Edema, pulmonary)

Pulmonary embolism (see under Embolism, pulmonary)

Pulmonary emphysema, interstitial
▲ Survanta Beractant Intratracheal Suspension (20.2%) 1978

Pulmonary fibrosis
Alkeran Tablets 754
BiCNU 723
▲ Blenoxane (10%) 724
CeeNU 725
▲ Cordarone Tablets (4 to 9%) 2446
Cuprimine Capsules (Rare) 1442
Cytoxan for Injection 726
Depen Titratable Tablets 2379
Garamycin Injectable 2093
Leukeran Tablets (Infrequent) 788
▲ Lupron Depot 3.75 mg (Among most frequent) 2312
Lupron Depot 7.5 mg 2311
Lupron Injection (Less than 5%) 2310
Macrodantin Capsules 1624
Mesantoin Tablets 2013
Mexitil Capsules (Isolated reports) 680
Myleran Tablets (Rare) 790
Neosar for Injection 566
Permax Tablets (Rare) 1291
Prozac Pulvules (Rare) 920
Sansert Tablets 2031
Tonocard Tablets (Less than 1%) 1554

Pulmonary function, changes
Eulexin Capsules (Less than 1%) 2089
IFEX (Less than 1%) 729
Macrodantin Capsules (Common) 1624
Mexitil Capsules (Isolated reports) 680
▲ Novantrone for Injection Concentrate (24 to 43%) 1226
Virazole 1126

Pulmonary hemorrhage (see under Hemorrhage, pulmonary)

Pulmonary hypersensitivity
Septra 813
Septra I.V. Infusion 808
Septra I.V. Infusion ADD-Vantage Vials 810
Septra 813
Tegretol 654

Pulmonary hypersensitivity, acute
Macrodantin Capsules 1624
Tegretol Suspension 656

Pulmonary hypersensitivity, chronic
Macrodantin Capsules 1624
Timolide Tablets 1547

Pulmonary hypersensitivity, subacute
Macrodantin Capsules 1624

Pulmonary hypertension
Cleocin Phosphate Injection (Rare) 2325
Demulen 2161
Enovid 2161
Indocin I.V. (1% to 3%) 1490
Norethin 2133
Permax Tablets (Rare) 1291
Pondimin Tablets 1867
Protamine Sulfate Ampoules & Vials 1295

Pulmonary infarction
Ansaid Tablets (Less than 1%) 2319
Metrodin (urofollitropin for injection) 2182
Vaseretic Tablets 1559
Vasotec I.V. 1562
Vasotec Tablets (0.5% to 1.0%) 1564

Pulmonary infiltrates
Azo Gantanol Tablets 1887
Azo Gantrisin Tablets 1888
Bactrim DS Tablets 1891
Bactrim I.V. Infusion 1889
Bactrim 1891
Beclovent Inhalation Aerosol and Refill 572

BiCNU ... 723
CeeNU ... 725
Fansidar Tablets ... 1896
Ganite Injection ... 1016
Gantanol ... 1899
Gantrisin ... 1901
Intal Capsules (Less than 1 in 100,000 patients) ... 978
Intal Nebulizer Solution (Rare) ... 980
Lupron Depot 7.5 mg ... 2311
Lupron Injection ... 2310
Macrodantin Capsules ... 1624
Minocin Intravenous (Rare) ... 1221
Minocin Oral Suspension (Rare) ... 1224
Minocin Pellet-Filled Capsules (Rare) ... 1222
Mutamycin ... 733
Septra (Rare) ... 813
Septra I.V. Infusion (Rare) ... 808
Septra I.V. Infusion ADD-Vantage Vials ... 810
Septra (Rare) ... 813

Pulmonary inflammation

Catapres-TTS (1%) ... 677
Cordarone Tablets ... 2446

Pulmonary toxicity, unspecified

BiCNU ... 723
CeeNU ... 725
▲Cordarone Tablets (10% to 17%) 2446
Fungizone Intravenous ... 2262
▲Idamycin for Injection (39%) ... 564
Leukine for IV Infusion ... 1127
Mutamycin ... 733

Pulse, fast

Arco-Lase Plus Tablets ... 607
B & O No. 15A & No. 16A Supprettes ... 2395
Cystospaz ... 2395
Dexatrim ... ▣ 733
Humulin 70/30, 100 Units (Less common) ... 1267
Humulin BR, 100 Units (Less common) ... 1268
Humulin L, 100 Units (Less common) ... 1268
Humulin U, 100 Units (Less common) ... 1272
Insulatard NPH ... 1626
Insulatard NPH Human ... 1627
Ketalar ... 1726
Mixtard 70/30 ... 1627
Mixtard Human 70/30 ... 1628
Propagest ... 839
Rogaine Topical Solution (1.53%) .. 2357
Sinulin ... 840
Urised Tablets ... 2396
Velosulin ... 1627
Velosulin Human ... 1628

Pulse changes

AquaMEPHYTON Injection ... 1422
Asendin Tablets ... 1196
Bronkephrine Injection ... 2042
Carbocaine ... 956
Clozaril Tablets ... 2000
Compazine ... 2201
Dalgan Injection (Less than 1%) ... 620
Etrafon ... 2087
Loxitane ... 1213
Mellaril ... 2011
Mephyton Tablets (Rare) ... 1503
Metaprel Inhalation Aerosol Bronchodilator ... 2014
Moban Tablets & Concentrate ... 932
Navane Capsules and Concentrate ... 1954
Navane Intramuscular ... 1956
Orap Tablets ... 1020
Prolixin Decanoate ... 1795
Prolixin Elixir ... 1793
Prolixin Enanthate ... 1796
Prolixin Injection ... 1791
Prolixin Tablets ... 1793
Ritalin ... 880
Stelazine ... 2226
Triavil Tablets ... 1556
Trilafon (Occasional) ... 2123
Versed Injection (Among most frequent) ... 1924
Vira-A Ophthalmic Ointment, 3% ... 1767

Pulse rate, depression

Cafergot/Cafergot P-B ... 1999
Lanoxicaps ... 772
Lanoxin Elixir Pediatric ... 775
Lanoxin Injection ... 778
Lanoxin Injection Pediatric ... 781
Lanoxin Tablets ... 783
Rogaine Topical Solution (1.53%) .. 2357
Sansert Tablets ... 2031

Purple toes syndrome

Coumadin Injection & Tablets (Infrequent) ... 944
Dicumarol Tablets (Infrequent) ... 516
Panwarfin Tablets ... 547

Purpura

Adalat Capsules (10 mg and 20 mg) (Less than 0.5%) ... 1587
Aldactazide ... 2150
Aldoclor Tablets ... 1413
Aldoril Tablets ... 1418
Altace Capsules ... 1086
Alurate Elixir (Less than 1 in 100) 1883
Anafranil Capsules (Up to 3%) ... 650
Anaprox and Anaprox DS Tablets (Less than 3%) ... 2288
Apresazide Capsules (Less frequent) ... 854
Apresoline Hydrochloride Parenteral (Ampuls) ... 856
Apresoline Hydrochloride Tablets (Less frequent) ... 855
Apresoline-Esidrix Tablets ... 857
Asendin Tablets (Very rare) ... 1196
Attenuvax (Rare) ... 1424
Azactam for Injection (Less than 1%) ... 2252
Azo Gantanol Tablets ... 1887
Azo Gantrisin Tablets ... 1888
Azulfidine Tablets, EN-tabs, Oral Suspension (Rare) ... 1157
Bactrim DS Tablets ... 1891
Bactrim I.V. Infusion ... 1889
Bactrim ... 1891
Biavax II ... 1427
Calan SR Caplets (1% or less) ... 2157
Calan Tablets (1% or less) ... 2155
Capozide ... 2258
Cardizem Tablets-30 mg, 60 mg, 90 mg and 120 mg ... 1329
Cardizem SR Capsules-60 mg, 90 mg and 120 mg (Less than 1%) 1327
Cardura Tablets (Less than 0.5% of 3960 patients) ... 1941
Cipro I.V. (1% or less) ... 1592
Clinoril Tablets (Less than 1 in 100) ... 1433
ColBENEMID Tablets ... 1436
Combipres Tablets (Few) ... 678
Corzide Tablets ... 702
Cytotec (Infrequent) ... 2159
Dapsone USP ... 1130
Diucardin Tablets ... 2450
Diulo ... 2129
Diupres Tablets ... 1461
Diuril Oral Suspension ... 1464
Diuril Sodium Intravenous ... 1463
Diuril Tablets ... 1464
Dyazide Capsules ... 2208
Easprin ... 1719
Elavil ... 2269
▲Eminase (Less than 10%) ... 2211
Endep Tablets ... 1927
Enduron Tablets ... 517
Enduronyl ... 518
Engerix-B Unit-Dose Vials ... 2213
Equagesic Tablets ... 2451
Esidrix Tablets ... 863
Esimil Tablets ... 864
Etrafon ... 2087
Exna Tablets ... 1862
Fansidar Tablets ... 1896
Flexeril Tablets (Rare) ... 1471
Gantanol ... 1899
Gantrisin Ophthalmic Ointment/Solution ... 1900
Gantrisin ... 1901
Garamycin Injectable ... 2093
HydroDIURIL Tablets ... 1484
Hydromox R Tablets ... 1209
Hydromox Tablets ... 1208
Hydropres Tablets ... 1485
Imferon ... 976
Inderide Tablets ... 2463
Inderide LA Long Acting Capsules .. 2465
Indocin Capsules (Less than 1%) ... 1487
Indocin I.V. (Less than 1%) ... 1490
Indocin (Less than 1%) ... 1487
Intron A (Less than 1%) ... 2097
Isoptin Oral Tablets (Less than 1%) ... 1179
Isoptin SR Sustained Release Tablets (Less than 1%) ... 1181
Kenalog-10 Injection ... 2402
Kenalog-40 Injection ... 2403
Lasix ... 1093
Limbitrol ... 1933
Lodine Capsules (Rare) ... 2468
Lopressor HCT Tablets (1 in 100 patients) ... 1034
Lozol Tablets ... 1843
Ludiomil Tablets ... 874
M-M-R II ... 1494
M-R-VAX II ... 1496
Matulane Capsules ... 1907
Maxzide ... 1215
Minizide Capsules ... 1779
Moduretic Tablets ... 1510
Mumpsvax (Extremely rare) ... 1513
Mykrox ½ mg Tablets ... 984
Myochrysine Injection ... 1516
Nalfon Pulvules & Tablets (Less than 1%) ... 919
Naprosyn (Less than 3%) ... 2297
Naturetin Tablets (Occasional) ... 1789
Normodyne Tablets ... 2110
Normozide Tablets ... 2112
Norpramin Tablets ... 1340
Omnipaque (0.1%) ... 2552
Oretic Tablets ... 544
Oreticyl ... 545
Orudis Capsules (Less than 1%) ... 2488
Pamelor ... 2019
Panwarfin Tablets (Infrequent) ... 547
Pediazole ... 1973
Permax Tablets (Rare) ... 1291
Prinzide Tablets ... 1540
Procardia Capsules (Less than 0.5%) ... 1781
Procardia XL Tablets (1% or less) .. 1783
ProSom Tablets (Rare) ... 554
Prozac Pulvules (Rare) ... 920
Quinaglute Dura-Tabs Tablets ... 663
Quinidex Extentabs ... 1868
Raudixin Tablets ... 1803
Rauzide Tablets ... 1804
Renese Tablets ... 1785
Renese-R Tablets (Rare) ... 1786
Rifadin ... 1345
Rythmol Tablets (Less than 1%) ... 1184
Saluron ... 718
Salutensin/Salutensin-Demi ... 719
Septra ... 813
Ser-Ap-Es Tablets ... 881
Serpasil Tablets ... 883
Serpasil-Apresoline Tablets ... 884
Serpasil-Esidrix Tablets ... 886
Sinequan (Occasional) ... 1960
Solganal Suspension (Rare) ... 2122
Spectrobid Tablets & Powder for Oral Suspension ... 1961
Surmontil Capsules ... 2524
Tegretol Chewable Tablets ... 654
Tegretol Suspension ... 656
Tegretol Tablets ... 654
Tenex Tablets (Less than 3%) ... 1875
Tenoretic Tablets ... 1105
Tenormin Tablets and I.V. Injection 1107
Thalitone Tablets ... 687
Thiosulfil Forte Tablets ... 2526
Timolide Tablets ... 1547
Tofranil Ampuls ... 1038
Tofranil Tablets ... 1039
Tofranil-PM Capsules ... 1041
Tolectin (200, 400 and 600 mg) (Less than 1%) ... 1379
Toradol IM Injection (1% or less) ... 2302
Trandate HCT/Trandate ... 579
Trental (Rare) ... 1099
Triavil Tablets ... 1556
Urobiotic-250 Capsules ... 1968
Vaseretic Tablets ... 1559
Verelan Capsules (Less than 1%) .. 1243
Vivactil Tablets ... 1567
Voltaren Tablets (Less than 1%) ... 1042
Zaroxolyn Tablets ... 989
Zestoretic ... 2274
Zyloprim Tablets (Less than 1%) ... 830

Purpura, allergic

Voltaren Tablets (Rare) ... 1042

Purpura, anaphylactoid

Achromycin V Capsules ... 1193
Declomycin Capsules, Tablets ... 1199
Doryx Capsules ... 1717
Minocin Intravenous ... 1221
Minocin Oral Suspension ... 1224
Minocin Pellet-Filled Capsules ... 1222
Monodox Capsules ... 1630
Terramycin Capsules ... 1786
Terramycin Intramuscular Solution 1964
Vibramycin Hyclate Capsules ... 1787
Vibramycin Hyclate Intravenous ... 1968
Vibramycin ... 1787

Purpura, fulminous

Zovirax Sterile Powder (Less than 1%) ... 828

Purpura, nonthrombocytopenic

Blocadren Tablets ... 1429
Butazolidin Capsules & Tablets (Less than 1%) ... 1027
Cartrol Tablets ... 507
Corgard Tablets ... 701
Corzide Tablets ... 702
Deprol Tablets ... 2382
Edecrin (Rare) ... 1468
Equagesic Tablets ... 2451
Inderal ... 2459
Inderal LA Long Acting Capsules ... 2461
Inderide Tablets ... 2463
Inderide LA Long Acting Capsules .. 2465
Kerlone Tablets ... 2172
Levatol ... 1832
Lopressor HCT Tablets ... 1034
Normodyne Tablets ... 2110
Normozide Tablets ... 2112
PMB 200 and PMB 400 ... 2504
Prolixin Decanoate ... 1795
Prolixin Elixir ... 1793
Prolixin Enanthate ... 1796
Prolixin Injection ... 1791
Prolixin Oral Concentrate ... 1792
Prolixin Tablets ... 1793
Sectral Capsules ... 2520
Septra I.V. Infusion ... 808
Septra I.V. Infusion ADD-Vantage Vials ... 810
Timolide Tablets ... 1547
Timoptic in Ocudose ... 1552
Timoptic Sterile Ophthalmic Solution ... 1550
Trandate HCT/Trandate ... 579
Visken Tablets ... 2036

Purpura, thrombocytopenic

Amoxil ... 2193
Atromid-S Capsules ... 2435
Augmentin Tablets, Powder for Oral Suspension, and Chewable Tablets ... 2198
Axid Pulvules (Rare) ... 1246
Blocadren Tablets ... 1429
Cardioquin Tablets ... 1812
Cartrol Tablets ... 507
Children's Advil Suspension (Less than 1%) ... 2426
Compazine ... 2201
Corgard Tablets ... 701
Corzide Tablets ... 702
Cuprimine Capsules ... 1442
Demulen ... 2161
Diamox ... 1200
Diupres Tablets ... 1461
Enduronyl ... 518
Enovid ... 2161
Equagesic Tablets ... 2451
Etrafon ... 2087
Harmonyl Tablets ... 528
Hydropres Tablets ... 1485
Inderal ... 2459
Inderal LA Long Acting Capsules ... 2461
Inderide Tablets ... 2463
Inderide LA Long Acting Capsules .. 2465
Indocin Capsules (Less than 1%) ... 1487
Indocin I.V. (Less than 1%) ... 1490
Indocin (Less than 1%) ... 1487
Kerlone Tablets ... 2172
Levatol ... 1832
Lincocin ... 2344
Lopressor HCT Tablets ... 1034
Meclomen Capsules (Less than 1%) ... 1739
Meruvax II ... 1503
Miltown Tablets (Rare) ... 2386
Motrin Tablets (Less than 1%) ... 2351
Neptazane Tablets ... ◉ 311
Norethin ... 2133
Normodyne Tablets ... 2110
Normozide Tablets ... 2112
PMB 200 and PMB 400 (Rare) ... 2504
PediaProfen Suspension (Less than 1%) ... 1363
Phenergan Injection ... 2493
Phenergan Tablets ... 2496
Ponstel (Occasional) ... 1758
Proglycem ... 649
Prolixin Decanoate ... 1795
Prolixin Elixir ... 1793
Prolixin Enanthate ... 1796
Prolixin Injection ... 1791
Prolixin Oral Concentrate ... 1792
Prolixin Tablets ... 1793
Prozac Pulvules ... 920
Quinamm Tablets ... 1344
Quinidex Extentabs ... 1868
Ritalin ... 880
Rufen Tablets (Less than 1%) ... 691
Salutensin/Salutensin-Demi ... 719

Sectral Capsules 2520
Stelazine 2226
Tacaryl 2409
Talacen (A few cases) 2070
Taractan (Very rare) 1920
Temaril Tablets, Syrup and Spansule Sustained Release Capsules 1085
Thorazine 2234
Timolide Tablets 1547
Timoptic in Ocudose 1552
Timoptic Sterile Ophthalmic Solution 1550
Trandate HCT/Trandate 579
Triavil Tablets 1556
Trilafon 2123
Visken Tablets 2036

Purpura, thrombocytopenic thrombotic
Cuprimine Capsules 1442
Depen Titratable Tablets 2379

Pustules, scalp
Nizoral 2% Shampoo (One occurrence in 41 patients) 1144

Pustules, unspecified
Duragesic Transdermal System (Less than 1%) 1133
Ultravate Ointment 0.05% (Less frequent) 2411

Pustulosis, provocation
Aclovate (Rare) 1053
Temovate (Rare) 1056

Pyelonephritis
Anafranil Capsules (Rare) 650
Permax Tablets (Rare) 1291
Prozac Pulvules (Rare) 920

Pyrexia (see under Fever)

Pyridoxine deficiency
INH Tablets 868
Rifamate Capsules 1347

Pyrogenic granuloma
▲ Accutane Capsules (A number of cases) 1878
▲ Tegison Capsules (1-10%) 1881

Pyrosis (see under Heartburn)

Pyuria
Anafranil Capsules (Rare) 650
Floxin Tablets (More than or equal to 1.0%) 1652
Permax Tablets (Infrequent) 1291
Prilosec Delayed-Release Capsules (Less than 1%) 1530
Prozac Pulvules (Rare) 920

PBI decrease
Capozide 2258
Estratest 2245
Lysodren (Infrequent) 731
Maxzide 1215
Mediatric Capsules 2476
Premarin with Methyltestosterone 2515
Rauzide Tablets 1804
Thalitone Tablets 687

PBI increase
Aygestin Tablets 2437
Corzide Tablets 702
Cycrin Tablets 2449
Etrafon 2087
Larodopa Tablets (Rare) 1905
Summer's Eve Medicated Douche 993
Trilafon 2123

PSP excretion, depression
▲ Capastat Sulfate Vials (Many instances) 1250

Q

Quadriplegia
Omnipaque 2552
Soma Compound w/Codeine Tablets (Very rare) 2390
Soma Compound Tablets (Very rare) 2389
Soma Tablets 2388

R

Radiculoneuropathy
Pneumovax 23 (Rare) 1528
Pnu-Imune 23 Pneumococcal Vaccine Polyvalent 1233
Recombivax HB 1544

Rage
Libritabs Tablets 1930
Librium Capsules 1931
Serax Capsules 2522
Serax Tablets 2522
Valium Tablets 1939
Xanax Tablets 2367

Rales
Blenoxane 724
Blocadren Tablets (0.6%) 1429
Brevibloc Injection (Less than 1%) 942
Ganite Injection 1016
NebuPent for Inhalation Solution (1% or less) 1017
Survanta Beractant Intratracheal Suspension 1978
Timolide Tablets (Less than 1%) 1547
Timoptic in Ocudose 1552
Timoptic Sterile Ophthalmic Solution 1550

Rash
Abbokinase (Rare) 503
Abbokinase Open-Cath (Rare) 505
▲ Accutane Capsules (Less than 1 in 10) 1878
Actigall Capsules 2280
▲ Actimmune (17%) 1046
▲ AeroBid Inhaler System (3-9%) 995
Agoral ▣ 634
AK-Spore H.C. ◉ 206
AK-Spore ◉ 205
AK-Trol Ointment & Suspension ◉ 207
Aldoclor Tablets 1413
Aldomet Ester HCl Injection 1417
Aldomet Oral 1415
Aldoril Tablets 1418
Altace Capsules 1086
Amen (Occasional) 833
Americaine Anesthetic Lubricant 972
Americaine Hemorrhoidal Ointment ▣ 558
Americaine Otic Topical Anesthetic Ear Drops 973
Aminophyllin Tablets 2153
Amoxil 2193
▲ Anafranil Capsules (4% to 8%) 650
Anaprox and Anaprox DS Tablets (Less than 1%) 2288
Ancobon Capsules 1886
Anectine 755
Ansaid Tablets (1-3%) 2319
Apresazide Capsules (Less frequent) 854
Apresoline Hydrochloride Parenteral (Ampuls) 856
Apresoline Hydrochloride Tablets (Less frequent) 855
Apresoline-Esidrix Tablets 857
▲ Atgam Sterile Solution (1 in 8 patients; 27%) 2320
Atrovent Inhalation Aerosol (1.2%) 675
Attenuvax (Occasional) 1424
Axid Pulvules (Rare) 1246
Azactam for Injection (1-1.3%) 2252
Azdōne Tablets 844
Azo Gantrisin Tablets 1888
▲ Bactrim DS Tablets (Among most common) 1891
▲ Bactrim I.V. Infusion (Among most common) 1889
▲ Bactrim (Among most common) 1891
Bactroban Ointment (Less than 1%) 2200
Bentyl 1322
Betagan ◉ 239
Biavax II (Infrequent) 1427
BiCozene Creme ▣ 684
▲ Blenoxane (50%) 724
Blocadren Tablets (Less than 1%) 1429
Brevicon 2304
Bumex (0.2%) 1895
Butazolidin Capsules & Tablets (Greater than 1%) 1027
Butesin Picrate Ointment 506
Butisol Sodium Elixir & Tablets (Less than 1 in 100) 2377
Caladryl Cream, Lotion, Spray ▣ 638
Calan SR Caplets (1.2%) 2157
Calan Tablets (1.2%) 2155
▲ Capoten (About 4 to 7 of 100 patients) 2255
▲ Capozide (4 to 7 of 100 patients) 2258
Carafate Tablets (Less than 0.5%) 1326
Cardene Capsules (0.4-1.2%) 2290
Cardizem Tablets-30 mg, 60 mg, 90 mg and 120 mg (1.3%) 1329
Cardizem SR Capsules-60 mg, 90 mg and 120 mg (1-1.5%) 1327
Cardura Tablets (1%) 1941
Cartrol Tablets (0.4-1.3%) 507
Catapres Tablets (About 1 in 100 patients) 676
Catapres-TTS (1 in 100) 677
Ceclor Pulvules & Suspension 1251
▲ Cefizox Injection (1 to 5%) 1012
Cefotan (1 in 150) 2265
Ceftin Tablets (0.6%) 575
Ceptaz for Injection (2% of patients) 1057
Cerose-DM 2443
Certain Dri Antiperspirant ▣ 630
Cerumenex Drops 1813
Cetamide Ointment ◉ 220
Chap Stick Petroleum Jelly Plus with Sunblock 15 ▣ 671
▲ CHEMET (succimer) Capsules (2.6 to 11.2%) 1361
▲ Children's Advil Suspension (3-9%) 2426
Choledyl Pediatric Elixir 1702
Choledyl Tablets 1700
Cholybar (Less frequent) 1705
Cipro I.V. (Greater than 1%) 1592
Cipro Tablets (1.1%) 1589
Cleocin HCl Capsules (Most frequent) 2322
Cleocin Pediatric Flavored Granules (Most frequent) 2324
▲ Cleocin Phosphate Injection (Most frequent) 2325
▲ Clinoril Tablets (3% to 9%) 1433
Clozaril Tablets (2%) 2000
Cogentin 1435
Colace (Exceedingly small) 1403
Combipres Tablets 678
Compazine 2201
Cordarone Tablets (Less than 1%) 2446
Corgard Tablets 701
Correctol Laxative Tablets ▣ 696
Corzide Tablets (1 to 5 of 1000 patients) 702
▲ Cuprimine Capsules (5%) 1442
Cyclogyl ◉ 215
Cycrin Tablets (Occasional) 2449
▲ Cytadren Tablets (1 in 6) 861
▲ Cytosar-U Sterile Powder (Among most frequent) 2329
Cytotec (Infrequent) 2159
Cytovene Sterile Powder (2%) 2292
DDAVP 1841
Dalgan Injection (Less than 1%) 620
Damason-P 1356
Danocrine Capsules 2046
Dantrium Capsules 1619
Depakene Capsules & Syrup 511
Depakote 512
▲ Depen Titratable Tablets (5%) 2379
Depo-Provera Sterile Aqueous Suspension (Occasional) 2336
Desferal Vials 862
Desyrel and Desyrel Dividose 1404
Didronel Tablets (Rare) 1621
Diflucan Injection and Tablets (1.8% in 4048 patients) 1948
Dilantin Infatabs 1710
Dilantin Kapseals 1708
Dilantin-30 Pediatric/Dilantin-125 Suspension 1713
Dilantin with Phenobarbital Kapseals 1715
Dilaudid-HP Injection 1175
Dimacol Caplets ▣ 672
Dipentum Capsules (1.1% to 2.3%) 1160
Diphtheria and Tetanus Toxoids and Pertussis Vaccine Adsorbed USP (For Pediatric Use) 892
Diprivan Injection (Less than 1%) 2267
Disalcid 1310
Ditropan 1332
Diucardin Tablets 2450
Diupres Tablets 1461
Diuril Oral Suspension 1464
Diuril Sodium Intravenous 1463
Diuril Tablets 1464
▲ Dolobid Tablets (3% to 9%) 1465
Doral Tablets 2383
Duragesic Transdermal System (1% or greater) 1133
Duricef 1405
Dyazide Capsules 2208
DynaCirc Capsules (1.5%) 2004
Dyrenium Capsules (Rare) 2210
E-Mycin Tablets 688
Eldepryl 2250
Elimite (permethrin) 5% Cream (1 to 2% or less) 1082
Emete-con Intramuscular/Intravenous 1950
Eminase (Occasional) 2211
Enduron Tablets 517
Enduronyl 518
Engerix-B Unit-Dose Vials (Less than 1%) 2213
▲ Epogen for Injection (Up to 16%) 591
Ergamisol Tablets (2%) 1136
ERYC 1720
Esidrix Tablets 863
Esimil Tablets 864
Eskalith 2214
Estrace 1385
Estrace Vaginal Cream 1388
Estraderm Transdermal System (Rare) 866
Ethmozine Tablets (0.3%-less than 2%) 946
Etrafon 2087
▲ Eulexin Capsules (3%) 2089
Evac-U-Gen Mild Laxative ▣ 739
Ex-Lax Chocolated Laxative ▣ 686
Ex-Lax Pills, Unflavored ▣ 686
Extra Gentle Ex-Lax ▣ 687
Exna Tablets 1862
Sterile FUDR 1898
Feldene Capsules (1 to 3%) 1777
Fiorinal with Codeine Capsules 2008
Floxin Tablets (1% to 3%) 1652
Fulvicin P/G Tablets 2090
Fulvicin P/G 165 & 330 Tablets 2091
Fulvicin-U/F Tablets 2092
Furacin Soluble Dressing (Approximately 1%) 1854
Furacin Topical Cream (Approximately 1%) 1854
Furacin Topical Solution 0.2% 1855
Gamimune N Immune Globulin Intravenous (Human) (Rare) 1572
Ganite Injection 1016
Gantanol 1899
Gantrisin 1901
Garamycin Injectable 2093
Gastrocrom Capsules (2 of 87 patients) 974
Guaifed Syrup ▣ 629
Haldol Decanoate 1375
Haldol Injection, Tablets and Concentrate 1373
Harmonyl Tablets 528
Hexalen Capsules (Less than 1%) 2316
HibTITER (133 of 1,118 vaccinations) 1206
Hiprex Tablets (Less than 3.5%) 1333
Hismanal Tablets (Less frequent) 1138
Humulin 70/30, 100 Units (Less common) 1267
Humulin BR, 100 Units (Less common) 1268
Humulin L, 100 Units (Less common) 1268
Humulin U, 100 Units (Less common) 1272
Hycomine Syrup 927
HydroDIURIL Tablets 1484
Hydromox R Tablets 1209
Hydromox Tablets 1208
Hydropres Tablets 1485
Hyperab Rabies Immune Globulin (Human) (Rare) 1574
Hyperstat I.V. Injection 2095
Hytrin Tablets (At least 1%) 529
Idamycin for Injection 564
Imferon 976
Inderide Tablets 2463
Inderide LA Long Acting Capsules 2465
Indocin Capsules (Less than 1%) 1487
Indocin I.V. (Less than 1%) 1490
Indocin (Less than 1%) 1487
Intal Capsules (Less than 1 in 10,000 patients) 978
Intal Inhaler (Infrequent) 979
Intal Nebulizer Solution 980
ISMOTIC (Very rare) ◉ 233
Isoptin Oral Tablets (1.2%) 1179
Isoptin SR Sustained Release Tablets (1.2%) 1181
Isopto Cetamide Solution ◉ 220
K-Lor Powder Packets (Rare) 531
K-Tab Filmtab (Rare) 532
Keflex Pulvules, Oral Suspension & Pediatric Drops 916
Keftab Tablets 917

Kefurox Vials, Faspak & ADD-Vantage (1 in 125) ... 1277
Kerlone Tablets (1.2%) ... 2172
Klotrix ... 708
Koro-Flex Arcing Spring Diaphragm ... 2142
Koromex Coil Spring Diaphragm ... 2142
▲ Lariam Tablets (Among most frequent) ... 1904
Leukine for IV Infusion (Infrequent) ... 1127
Lincocin ... 2344
Lithane Tablets ... 1596
Lithium Carbonate Capsules & Tablets ... 1984
Lodine Capsules (More than 1% but less than 3%) ... 2468
Lo/Ovral Tablets ... 2471
Lo/Ovral-28 Tablets ... 2476
Loestrin ... 1728
Loniten Tablets ... 2346
Lopid Capsules and Tablets (1.7%) ... 1736
Lopressor HCT Tablets ... 1034
Lorelco Tablets ... 1333
Lortab ASA Tablets ... 2414
Lotensin Tablets ... 872
Lozol Tablets (Less than 5%) ... 1843
Lupron Injection (Less than 3%) ... 2310
M-M-R II (Infrequent) ... 1494
M-R-VAX II (Infrequent) ... 1496
Macrodantin Capsules ... 1624
Mandelamine (Occasional) ... 1738
Matulane Capsules ... 1907
Maxair Inhaler (Less than 1%) ... 1311
Maxzide ... 1215
▲ Meclomen Capsules (3-9%) ... 1739
Mefoxin ... 1498
Mefoxin Premixed Intravenous Solution ... 1500
Megace Tablets ... 732
Meruvax II ... 1503
Mesantoin Tablets ... 2013
Methotrexate Tablets, Parenteral, LPF Parenteral (1 to 3%) ... 1217
Metrodin (urofollitropin for injection) ... 2182
▲ Mevacor Tablets (5.2%) ... 1505
▲ Mexitil Capsules (3.8% to 4.2%) ... 680
Miacalcin Injection ... 2017
Micro-K LS Packets (Rare) ... 1864
Micronor Tablets ... 1667
Modicon ... 1667
▲ Moduretic Tablets (3% to 8%) ... 1510
▲ Monistat I.V. (9%) ... 1143
Monocid Injection (Less than 1%) ... 2217
Monopril Tablets (0.2 to 1.0%) ... 1406
▲ Motrin Tablets (3-9%) ... 2351
Mutamycin (Rare) ... 733
Mykrox ½ mg Tablets (Less than 2%) ... 984
Naftin Gel 1% (0.5%) ... 1084
▲ Nalfon Pulvules & Tablets (3.7%) ... 919
Naprosyn Tablets (Less than 1%) ... 2297
Nasalcrom Nasal Solution (Less than 1%) ... 986
Naturetin Tablets ... 1789
Navane Capsules and Concentrate ... 1954
Navane Intramuscular ... 1956
▲ NebuPent for Inhalation Solution (31 to 47%) ... 1017
NegGram ... 2062
Neosar for Injection ... 566
Neptazane Tablets ... ⊙ 311
Netromycin Injection 100 mg/ml (4 or 5 of 1000 patients) ... 2104
▲ Neupogen for Injection (6%) ... 595
Neutrogena Sunblock ... ▣ 630
Nicorette ... 1335
Nimotop Capsules (Up to 2.4%) ... 1607
Nipride I.V. Infusion ... 1909
Nitro-Bid IV ... 1338
Nitro-Bid Ointment ... 1339
Nordette-21 Tablets ... 2481
Nordette-28 Tablets ... 2483
Norinyl ... 2304
Norlestrin ... 1746
Norlutate ... 1754
Norlutin ... 1755
Normodyne Tablets (1%) ... 2110
Normozide Tablets (1%) ... 2112
▲ Noroxin Tablets (Among most common) ... 1519
Norpace (1 to 3%) ... 2177
Nor-Q D Tablets ... 2304
Novantrone for Injection Concentrate (Occasional) ... 1226
Oculinum for Injecton (2 cases) ... 587
Omnipaque (0.3%) ... 2552
Oncovin Solution Vials & Hyporets (Rare) ... 1288
OptiPranolol Sterile Ophthalmic Solution (A small number of patients) ... ⊙ 261
Orap Tablets ... 1020
Oretic Tablets ... 544
Oreticyl ... 545
Organidin Elixir, Solution & Tablets (Rare) ... 2387
Ortho Diaphragm Kit ... 1664
Orthoclone OKT3 Sterile Solution ... 1645
Ortho-Novum ... 1667
Ortho-White Diaphragm Kit-Flat Spring ... 1664
Orudis Capsules (Greater than 1%) ... 2488
Ovcon ... 1391
Ovral Tablets ... 2490
Ovrette Tablets ... 2492
Oxsoralen-Ultra Capsule ... 1117
Pamelor ... 2019
Pantopon Injectable ... 1911
Paradione Capsules ... 548
Paraflex Caplets (Rare) ... 1378
Parafon Forte DSC Caplets ... 1379
Paraplatin for Injection ... 735
Pavabid Capsules (Rare) ... 1344
Pavabid HP Capsulets (Rare) ... 1344
▲ PediaProfen Suspension (3-9%) ... 1363
Pediazole ... 1973
▲ Pentam 300 Injection (3.3%) ... 1018
Pepcid (Infrequent) ... 1524
Percocet Tablets ... 950
Pergonal (menotropins for injection, USP) ... 2184
Peri-Colace (Exceedingly small) ... 1409
Peritrate ... 1756
▲ Permax Tablets (3.2%) ... 1291
Persantine Tablets (2.3%) ... 683
Phenergan with Codeine ... 2497
Phenergan with Dextromethorphan ... 2499
Phenergan Suppositories ... 2496
Phenergan Syrup ... 2495
Phenergan VC ... 2500
Phenergan VC with Codeine ... 2501
Placidyl Capsules ... 553
Platinol (Infrequent) ... 737
Platinol-AQ Injection (Infrequent) ... 738
Plendil Extended-Release Tablets (0.1%) ... 1526
Pneumovax 23 (Rare) ... 1528
Pnu-Imune 23 Pneumococcal Vaccine Polyvalent (Rare to infrequent) ... 1233
Poly-Vi-Flor (Rare) ... 1397
Poly-Vi-Flor Drops (Rare) ... 1398
Poly-Vi-Flor with Iron (Rare) ... 1399
Poly-Vi-Flor with Iron Drops (Rare) ... 1399
Pondimin Tablets ... 1867
Ponstel ... 1758
Premarin Tablets ... 2510
PreSun 15 Facial Sunscreen ... ▣ 537
PreSun 8, 15 and 39 Creamy Sunscreens ... ▣ 537
PreSun 15 and 29 Sensitive Skin Sunscreen ... ▣ 537
Prilosec Delayed-Release Capsules (1 to 1.5%) ... 1530
Primaxin I.M. (0.4%) ... 1532
Primaxin I.V. (0.9%) ... 1535
Prinivil Tablets (1.5%) ... 1538
Prinzide Tablets (1.2%) ... 1540
Priscoline Hydrochloride Ampuls ... 877
Procardia XL Tablets (Less than 3%) ... 1783
▲ Procrit for Injection (Up to 16%) ... 1647
Prokine for I.V. Infusion ... 1096
▲ Proloprim Tablets (2.9% to 6.7%) ... 799
ProSom Tablets (Infrequent) ... 554
Prostigmin Injectable ... 1120
Prostigmin Tablets ... 1121
Proventil Inhalation Aerosol (Rare) ... 2117
Proventil (2%) ... 2120
Provera Tablets ... 2356
Prozac Pulvules (2.7%) ... 920
Pyridium ... 1763
Pyridium Plus ... 1764
Questran Light (Less frequent) ... 711
Questran Powder ... 710
Quibron-T ... 714
Quibron-T/SR ... 716
Quinaglute Dura-Tabs Tablets ... 663
Quinidex Extentabs ... 1868
Q-vel Muscle Relaxant Pain Reliever ... ▣ 552
Raudixin Tablets ... 1803
Rauzide Tablets ... 1804
Recombivax HB (Less than 1%) ... 1544
Respbid Tablets ... 684
▲ Retrovir Capsules (17%) ... 802
▲ Retrovir I.V. Infusion (17%) ... 805
▲ Retrovir Syrup (17%) ... 802
Rheumatrex Methotrexate Dose Pack (1% to 3%) ... 1234
▲ Ridaura Capsules (24%) ... 2224
Rifadin (Occasional) ... 1345
Rifamate Capsules (Occasional) ... 1347
Rimactane Capsules ... 879
Robaxin Injectable ... 1871
Robaxin Tablets ... 1872
Robaxisal Tablets ... 1872
Robitussin ... ▣ 676
Robitussin-CF ... ▣ 676
Robitussin-DM ... ▣ 676
Robitussin-PE ... ▣ 677
Rocephin Injectable Vials, ADD-Vantage (1.7%) ... 1914
▲ Roferon-A Injection (11% to 18%) ... 1916
Rowasa (1.2 to 2.82%) ... 2248
▲ Rufen Tablets (3-9%) ... 691
Ru-Tuss Tablets ... 693
Rythmol Tablets (0.6 to 2.6%) ... 1184
SSD RP Cream (Infrequent) ... 690
Salflex ... 839
Saluron ... 718
Salutensin/Salutensin-Demi ... 719
Sandostatin Injection (Less than 1%) ... 2029
Sanorex Tablets ... 2030
Sansert Tablets (Rare) ... 2031
Sectral Capsules (2%) ... 2520
Seldane Tablets (1.6%) ... 1349
Seldane-D Extended-Release Tablets (1.1%) ... 1350
▲ Septra (Most common) ... 813
▲ Septra I.V. Infusion (Most common) ... 808
▲ Septra I.V. Infusion ADD-Vantage Vials (Most common) ... 810
▲ Septra (Most common) ... 813
Ser-Ap-Es Tablets ... 881
Serentil ... 686
Serpasil Tablets ... 883
Serpasil-Apresoline Tablets ... 884
Serpasil-Esidrix Tablets ... 886
Shade Oil-Free ... ▣ 705
Super Shade ... ▣ 705
Silvadene Cream 1% (0.2%) ... 1352
Sinemet CR Tablets ... 953
Skelaxin ... 840
Slo-bid Gyrocaps ... 1847
Slo-Niacin Tablets ... 2376
Slow-K Tablets (Rare) ... 2281
Solganal Suspension ... 2122
Soma Compound w/Codeine Tablets ... 2390
Soma Compound Tablets ... 2389
Stadol (Less than 1%) ... 721
Stelazine ... 2226
Suprax (Less than 2%) ... 1235
Symmetrel Capsules & Syrup (0.1-1%) ... 936
Tagamet (Approximately 1 in 100) ... 2228
Talacen (Infrequent) ... 2070
Talwin Carpuject (Infrequent) ... 2071
Talwin Compound (Infrequent) ... 2072
Talwin Injection (Infrequent) ... 2071
Talwin Nx (Infrequent) ... 2073
Tazicef for Injection (2%) ... 2231
▲ Tegison Capsules (50-75%) ... 1881
Tenex Tablets ... 1875
Tenuate ... 1354
Thalitone Tablets ... 687
Theo-24 ... 2179
Theo-Dur Sprinkle ... 1168
Theo-Dur Extended-Release Tablets ... 1166
Theolair ... 1317
Theolair-SR Tablets ... 1319
Theo-Organidin Elixir ... 2391
TheoX Extended-Release Tablets ... 841
Theragran Hematinic Tablets ... 605
Timolide Tablets (Less than 1%) ... 1547
Timoptic in Ocudose ... 1552
Timoptic Sterile Ophthalmic Solution ... 1550
Tolectin (200, 400 and 600 mg) ... 1379
▲ Tonocard Tablets (0.4-12.2%) ... 1554
Tracrium Injection ... 817
Trandate HCT Tablets (Rare) ... 579
Trandate Injection (Rare) ... 577
Trandate Tablets (Rare) ... 579
Transderm Scōp Transdermal Therapeutic System (Infrequent) ... 887
Trental (Less than 1%) ... 1099
▲ Trexan Tablets (Less than 10%) ... 937
Tridione Capsules ... 557
Tri-Immunol Diphtheria & Tetanus Toxoids & Pertussis Vaccine, Adsorbed ... 1241
Trilisate (Less than 1%) ... 1822
▲ Trimpex Tablets (2.6% to 6.7%) ... 1922
Tri-Norinyl 28-Day Tablets ... 2304
Triphasil-21 Tablets ... 2527
Triphasil-28 Tablets ... 2532
Tri-Vi-Flor 1.0 mg Vitamins with Fluoride Chewable Tablets (Rare) ... 1400
Tri-Vi-Flor Drops (Rare) ... 1400
Tri-Vi-Flor 0.25 mg Vitamins with Iron and Fluoride Drops (Rare) ... 1401
Tussionex Extended-Release Suspension ... 988
Tussi-Organidin DM Liquid (Rare) ... 2392
Tussi-Organidin Liquid (Rare) ... 2391
Tylox Capsules ... 1382
Ultracef Capsules, Tablets & Oral Suspension ... 722
Ultravate Cream 0.05% (Less frequent) ... 2410
Ultravate Ointment 0.05% ... 2411
Unasyn (Less than 2%) ... 1965
Urised Tablets ... 2396
Vancenase Nasal Inhaler (Rare) ... 2126
Vanceril Inhaler (Rare) ... 2128
Vancocin HCl, Oral Solution & Pulvules (Infrequent) ... 1304
Vancocin HCl, Vials & ADD-Vantage (Infrequent) ... 1302
Vascor (200, 300 and 400 mg) Tablets (0.5 to 2.0%) ... 1383
Vaseretic Tablets (0.5% to 2.0%) ... 1559
Vasotec I.V. (0.5 to 1%) ... 1562
Vasotec Tablets (1.3% to 1.4%) ... 1564
Velosef Capsules and for Oral Suspension (Few) ... 606
VePesid Capsules and Injection (Infrequent) ... 741
Verelan Capsules (Less than 1% to 1.4%) ... 1243
Versed Injection (Less than 1%) ... 1924
Vioform-Hydrocortisone Cream and Mild Cream (Few) ... 889
Vioform-Hydrocortisone Ointment (Few) ... 889
Vira-A for Injection ... 1766
Virazole ... 1126
Visken Tablets (Less than 1%) ... 2036
Voltaren Tablets (1-3%) ... 1042
▲ Wellbutrin Tablets (8.0%) ... 821
Wytensin Tablets (3% or less) ... 2542
▲ Xanax Tablets (10.8%) ... 2367
Yutopar (Infrequent) ... 647
Zaroxolyn Tablets ... 989
Zefazone Sterile Powder (1.1%) ... 2372
Zestoretic (1.2%) ... 2274
Zestril Tablets (1.5%) ... 2277
Ziradryl Lotion ... ▣ 643
Zofran Injection (Approximately 1%) ... 1069
▲ Zoladex (6%) ... 1110
Zorprin Tablets ... 698
Zovirax Capsules (1.3% to 1.7%) ... 824
Zovirax Ointment 5% ... 827
Zovirax Sterile Powder ... 828
Zovirax (1.3% to 1.7%) ... 824

Rash, actinic

Solganal Suspension ... 2122

Rash, allergic

Amen ... 833
Aygestin Tablets ... 2437
Brevicon ... 2304
Cycrin Tablets ... 2449
Demulen ... 2161
Depo-Provera Sterile Aqueous Suspension ... 2336
Empirin with Codeine Phosphate Nos. 2, 3 & 4 ... 764
Enovid ... 2161
Jenest-28 Tablets ... 1636
Levlen/Tri-Levlen ... 665
Loestrin ... 1728
Luride Drops (Rare) ... 889
Luride Lozi-Tabs Tablets (Rare) ... 890
Metopirone Tablets ... 876
Micronor Tablets ... 1667
Modicon ... 1667
Norethin ... 2133
Norinyl ... 2304
Norlestrin ... 1746
Norlutate ... 1754
Norlutin ... 1755
Nor-Q D Tablets ... 2304
Ortho Diaphragm Kit-Coil Spring ... 1664
Ortho-Cyclen Tablets ... 1658
Ortho-Novum ... 1667
Periactin ... 1525
Levlen/Tri-Levlen ... 665
Tri-Norinyl ... 2304

Rash, bullous

Corgard Tablets ... 701
Orudis Capsules (Less than 1%) ... 2488

Trandate HCT/Trandate 579

Rash, bullous erythrodermatous of the palms and soles

Idamycin for Injection 564

Rash, circumocular

Polytrim Ophthalmic Solution Sterile (2 of 100 patients) 588

Rash, drug

Actifed with Codeine Cough Syrup.. 752
Benadryl Capsules 1691
Benadryl Injection 1692
Cardilate Oral/Sublingual Tablets (Occasional) 757
Comhist LA Capsules 1618
Deconamine 663
Dimetane-DC Cough Syrup 1857
Dimetane-DX Cough Syrup 1858
Isordil (Occasional) 2467
Nitro-Bid IV 1338
Nitro-Bid Ointment 1339
Nitro-Bid Capsules 1338
Nitrolingual Spray 1846
Nitrostat IV (Occasional) 1744
Optimine Tablets 2115
Ornade Spansule Capsules 2221
PBZ Tablets & Elixir 1037
PBZ-SR Tablets 1037
Polaramine 2116
Ru-Tuss II Capsules 693
Sorbitrate (Occasional) 1103
Tavist Syrup 2033
Tavist Tablets 2035
Tavist-D Tablets 2035
Trancopal Caplets 2075
Triaminic Expectorant DH 1995
Triaminic Oral Infant Drops 1996
Trinalin Repetabs Tablets 1170

Rash, erythematous

Achromycin V Capsules 1193
Anafranil Capsules (Infrequent) 650
Blocadren Tablets 1429
Cartrol Tablets 507
Celontin 1692
DTIC-Dome (Infrequent) 1595
Declomycin Capsules, Tablets 1199
Dilantin with Phenobarbital Kapseals 1715
Doryx Capsules 1717
Flagyl I.V. 2131
Flagyl Tablets 2170
Inderal 2459
Inderal LA Long Acting Capsules 2461
Inderide Tablets 2463
Inderide LA Long Acting Capsules .. 2465
Kerlone Tablets 2172
Levatol 1832
Methotrexate Tablets, Parenteral, LPF Parenteral 1217
Milontin Kapseals 1741
Minocin Intravenous 1221
Minocin Oral Suspension 1224
Minocin Pellet-Filled Capsules 1222
Monodox Capsules 1630
Protostat Tablets 1674
Rheumatrex Methotrexate Dose Pack 1234
Sectral Capsules 2520
Tegretol Chewable Tablets 654
Tegretol Suspension 656
Tegretol Tablets 654
Tenoretic Tablets 1105
Tenormin Tablets and I.V. Injection 1107
Terramycin Capsules 1786
Terramycin Intramuscular Solution 1964
Timolide Tablets 1547
Timoptic in Ocudose 1552
Timoptic Sterile Ophthalmic Solution 1550
Vibramycin Hyclate Capsules 1787
Vibramycin Hyclate Intravenous 1968
Vibramycin 1787
Visken Tablets 2036
Zarontin Capsules 1768
Zarontin Syrup 1769

Rash, erythematous maculopapular

Aldactazide 2150
Amoxil 2193
Bretylol Injection (1 in 1000) 923
Equagesic Tablets 2451
Hydrea Capsules 728
Miltown Tablets 2386
PMB 200 and PMB 400 2504

Rash, exfoliative

Tenex Tablets (Few cases) 1875

Rash, female genitalia

Floxin Tablets (Less than 1%) 1652

Rash, herpetic (see under Eruptions, herpetic)

Rash, leg

DDAVP 1841

Rash, lichenoid

Normodyne Tablets 2110
Permax Tablets (Rare) 1291
Trandate HCT/Trandate 579

Rash, maculopapular

Achromycin V Capsules 1193
Aclovate Cream (1 in 100 patients) 1053
Anafranil Capsules (Infrequent) 650
Capastat Sulfate Vials 1250
Capoten 2255
Capozide 2258
Catapres-TTS (1 of 101 patients) .. 677
Children's Advil Suspension (Less than 3%) 2426
Chloromycetin Kapseals 1695
Chloromycetin Palmitate, Oral Suspension 1697
Chloromycetin Sodium Succinate 1698
Cleocin Pediatric Flavored Granules 2324
Cleocin Phosphate Injection 2325
Cytosar-U Sterile Powder 2329
Danocrine Capsules 2046
Declomycin Capsules, Tablets 1199
Doryx Capsules 1717
Sterile FUDR (Remote possibility) .. 1898
Fluorouracil Injection 1897
Fungizone Intravenous 2262
▲ Intron A (4%) 2097
Lanoxicaps (Rare) 772
Lanoxin Elixir Pediatric (Rare) 775
Lanoxin Injection (Rare) 778
Lanoxin Injection Pediatric (Rare) .. 781
Lanoxin Tablets (Rare) 783
Lodine Capsules (Less than 1%) 2468
Lotrisone Cream (1 of 270 patients) 2103
Mandol Vials, Faspak & ADD-Vantage 1281
Mesantoin Tablets 2013
Minocin Intravenous 1221
Minocin Oral Suspension 1224
Minocin Pellet-Filled Capsules 1222
Monodox Capsules 1630
Motrin Tablets (Less than 3%) 2351
Normodyne Tablets 2110
Normozide Tablets 2112
PediaProfen Suspension (Less than 3%) 1363
Procan SR Tablets (Occasional) 1760
Proloprim Tablets (Mild to moderate) 799
Pronestyl Capsules and Tablets (Occasional) 1800
Pronestyl Injection (Occasional) 1798
Pronestyl-SR Tablets 1801
Prozac Pulvules (Infrequent) 920
Rifamate Capsules 1347
▲ Rufen Tablets (3-9%) 691
Serax Capsules 2522
Serax Tablets 2522
Synarel Nasal Solution (Less than 1%) 2300
Terramycin Capsules 1786
Terramycin Intramuscular Solution 1964
Trandate HCT/Trandate 579
Vibramycin Hyclate Capsules 1787
Vibramycin Hyclate Intravenous 1968
Vibramycin Monohydrate for Oral Suspension 1787
Zyloprim Tablets (Less than 1%) 830

Rash, morbilliform

▲ Cleocin Phosphate Injection (Most frequent) 2325
▲ Dilantin Infatabs (Among most common) 1710
▲ Dilantin Kapseals (Among most common) 1708
Dilantin Parenteral (Among most common) 1712
▲ Dilantin-30 Pediatric/Dilantin-125 Suspension (Among most common) 1713
▲ Dilantin with Phenobarbital Kapseals (Among most common) 1715
Furoxone 1855
Ketalar 1726
Mesantoin Tablets 2013
Paradione Capsules 548
Proloprim Tablets (Mild to moderate) 799
Rifamate Capsules 1347
Serax Capsules 2522
Serax Tablets 2522
Tridione 557

Rash, papular

▲ CHEMET (succimer) Capsules (2.6 to 11.2%) 1361
Quinamm Tablets 1344

Rash, papular, neck

Alferon N Injection (1%) 1809

Rash, perianal

Mintezol 1510

Rash, pleomorphic

Omnipaque 2552

Rash, pruritic

Capoten 2255
▲ Capozide (About 4-7 of 100 patients) 2258
Cibalith-S 870
Cycrin Tablets 2449
Equagesic Tablets 2451
ERYC 1720
Sterile FUDR (Remote possibility) .. 1898
Lithobid Tablets 870
Miltown Tablets 2386
Norlutate 1754
Norlutin 1755
PMB 200 and PMB 400 2504
Proloprim Tablets (Mild to moderate) 799
Skelaxin 840
Spectazole (econazole nitrate) Cream (One case) 1681
Tegretol Chewable Tablets 654
Tegretol Suspension 656
Tegretol Tablets 654

Rash, psoriaform

Inderal (Rare) 2459
Inderal LA Long Acting Capsules (Rare) 2461
Inderide Tablets (Rare) 2463
Inderide LA Long Acting Capsules (Rare) 2465
Normodyne Tablets 2110
Normozide Tablets 2112
Tenoretic Tablets 1105
Tenormin Tablets and I.V. Injection 1107
Trandate HCT/Trandate 579

Rash, purpuric

Danocrine Capsules 2046
Dilantin Infatabs 1710
Dilantin Kapseals 1708
Dilantin-30 Pediatric/Dilantin-125 Suspension 1713
Dilantin with Phenobarbital Kapseals 1715
Eminase (0.3%) 2211
Mesantoin Tablets 2013
Orudis Capsules (Less than 1%) 2488
Prozac Pulvules (Rare) 920
Rifamate Capsules 1347

Rash, pustular

Anafranil Capsules (Infrequent) 650
Prozac Pulvules (Rare) 920

Rash, scarlatiniform

Dilantin Infatabs 1710
Dilantin Kapseals 1708
Dilantin Parenteral 1712
Dilantin-30 Pediatric/Dilantin-125 Suspension 1713
Dilantin with Phenobarbital Kapseals 1715
Mesantoin Tablets 2013
Quinamm Tablets 1344

Rash, skin (see also under Rash)

Alurate Elixir (Less than 1 in 100) 1883
Amicar Syrup, Tablets, and Injection (Occasional) 1194
Amikin Injectable (Rare) 602
Ancef Injection 2194
Anturane 853
Aristocort Suspension 1008
Artane 1195
Asendin Tablets (Greater than 1%) 1196
Ativan Injection (Occasional) 2432
Atromid-S Capsules (Less often) 2435
▲ Augmentin Tablets, Powder for Oral Suspension, and Chewable Tablets (3%) 2198
▲ Azulfidine Tablets, EN-tabs, Oral Suspension (3 to 4%) 1157
Beclovent Inhalation Aerosol and Refill (Rare) 572
Beconase AQ Nasal Spray (Rare) 574
Beconase Inhalation Aerosol & Refill (Rare) 574
Bicillin C-R Injection 2438
Bicillin C-R 900/300 Injection 2440
Bicillin L-A Injection 2442
BuSpar (1%) 1401
Butazolidin Capsules & Tablets (Greater than 1%) 1027
Calcimar Injection, Synthetic (Occasional) 1839
Centrax 1693
Ceptaz for Injection (2%) 1057
Cerubidine (Rare) 2443
Chromagen Capsules 2078
Cibacalcin Double-chambered Syringes (Rare) 859
Claforan Sterile Injection (2.4%) 1089
Combipres Tablets (About 1%) 678
Corgard Tablets (1 to 5 of 1000 patients) 701
Corzide Tablets (1 to 5 of 1000 patients) 702
Cyclogyl ..... ⊙ 215
Cylert Tablets 510
Cytosar-U Sterile Powder (Rare) 2329
Cytoxan for Injection (Occurs occasionally) 726
Dalmane Capsules (Rare) 1927
Danocrine Capsules 2046
Darvon-N/Darvocet-N 1254
Darvon 1256
Darvon-N Suspension & Tablets (Less than 1%) 1254
Demerol 2047
Dilatrate-SR (Occasional) 1827
Diulo 2129
Dobutrex Solution Vials (Occasionally) 1259
Dolophine Hydrochloride Ampoules & Vials 1260
Dolophine Hydrochloride Tablets 1261
Edecrin 1468
Elavil 2269
Elspar 1470
Emcyt Capsules (1%) 1161
Empirin with Codeine Phosphate Nos. 2, 3 & 4 764
Endep Tablets 1927
▲ Entozyme Tablets (Most frequent).. 1862
Ery-Tab Tablets 521
Factrel 2561
Feldene Capsules (1 to 3%) 1777
Flexeril Tablets (Less than 1%) 1471
Fortaz (2%) 1060
Geocillin Tablets (Infrequent) 1951
Grifulvin V (griseofulvin microsize) Tablets/Suspension 1678
Grisactin 2454
Grisactin Ultra Tablets 2455
Gris-PEG Tablets, 125 mg & 250 mg 1083
Hycodan Syrup, Tablets 927
Hydromox R Tablets 1209
Hydromox Tablets 1208
Hyskon Hysteroscopy Fluid (Rare).. 1162
Ilosone 913
Imodium Capsules 1139
Imuran (2%) 768
Insulatard NPH 1626
Insulatard NPH Human 1627
▲ Intron A (25%) 2097
K-Norm Capsules (Rare) 982
Kefzol Vials, Faspak & ADD-Vantage 1279
Kemadrin Tablets (Occasional) 771
Klonopin Tablets 1902
Lamprene Capsules (1-5%) 1030
Larodopa Tablets (Infrequent) 1905
Lasix 1093
Levo-Dromoran (Occasional) 1906
Limbitrol 1933
Lioresal Tablets 1031
▲ Lopressor Ampuls (5%) 1032
Lopressor HCT Tablets 1034
▲ Lopressor Tablets (5%) 1032
Loxitane 1213
Ludiomil Tablets (Rare) 874
Lysodren 731
MS Contin Tablets (Infrequent) 1814
MSIR (Infrequent) 1817
▲ Marplan Tablets (Among most frequent) 1906
Mebaral Tablets (Less than 1 in 100) 2061

Mepergan Injection 2479
Mestinon Injectable (Occasional) 1115
Mestinon (Occasional) 1116
Methadone Hydrochloride Diskets 1284
Methadone Hydrochloride Oral Solution & Tablets 1987
Mezlin 1597
Mezlin Pharmacy Bulk Package 1599
Midamor Tablets (Less than or equal to 1%) 1508
Midrin Capsules 836
Minipress Capsules (1-4%) 1778
Minizide Capsules 1779
Mintezol 1510
Mixtard 70/30 1627
Mixtard Human 70/30 1628
Moban Tablets & Concentrate (Occasional) 932
Modane Plus Tablets ▣ 504
Modane Tablets ▣ 503
Monistat Dual-Pak (Less than 0.5%) 1657
▲Monistat I.V. (9%) 1143
Monistat 3 Vaginal Suppositories (Less than 0.5%) 1657
Mycelex-G 100 mg Vaginal Tablets (Rare) 1606
Mycelex-G 500 mg Vaginal Tablets (Rare) 1606
Naprosyn Suspension (Less than 1%) 2297
Nardil (Less common) 1742
Naturetin Tablets 1789
Nebcin Vials, Hyporets & ADD-Vantage 1286
Nembutal Sodium Capsules 534
Nembutal Sodium Solution (Less than 1%) 536
Nembutal Sodium Suppositories (Less than 1%) 538
Neosporin Ophthalmic Ointment Sterile 793
Neosporin Ophthalmic Solution Sterile 794
Nicobid 1846
Nolvadex Tablets (Less frequent) 1102
Normozide Tablets 2112
Norpramin Tablets 1340
Oramorph SR (Morphine Sulfate Sustained Release Tablets) (Less frequent) 1988
Papaverine Hydrochloride Vials and Ampoules 1290
Parlodel 2020
Parnate Tablets (Rare) 2222
Pediazole 1973
Peganone Tablets 551
Pfizerpen for Injection 1957
Pfizerpen-AS Aqueous Suspension 1959
Phenobarbital Elixir and Tablets (Less than 1 in 100 patients) 1293
▲Phenurone Tablets (5%) 552
Pipracil (1%) 1230
Pnu-Imune 23 Pneumococcal Vaccine Polyvalent (Rare to infrequent) 1233
Pondimin Tablets 1867
Potaba (Infrequent) 1071
Proglycem 649
Proloprim Tablets 799
Purinethol Tablets 800
Quadrinal Tablets 1183
Quinamm Tablets 1344
Quinidex Extentabs 1868
Raudixin Tablets 1803
Rauzide Tablets 1804
Reglan (A few cases) 1869
Renese Tablets 1785
Renese-R Tablets 1786
Ritalin 880
Roxanol 1991
Roxicodone Tablets, Oral Solution & Intensol (Oxycodone) 1992
SSD (Low) 694
Seconal Sodium Pulvules (Less than 1 in 100) 1296
Serax Capsules (Rare) 2522
Serax Tablets (Rare) 2522
Seromycin Pulvules 1298
Sinemet Tablets 952
Sinequan (Occasional) 1960
Soma Compound w/Codeine Tablets 2390
Soma Compound Tablets 2389
Soma Tablets 2388
Spectrobid Tablets & Powder for Oral Suspension 1961
Stilphostrol Tablets and Ampuls 1609
Surital Ampoules, Steri-Vials 1764
Surmontil Capsules 2524
Synkayvite Injection (Occasional) 1919
Synkayvite Tablets (Occasional) 1920
T-PHYL (Uniphyl) 200 mg Tablets 1820
Talacen (A few cases) 2070
Tambocor Tablets (1-3%) 1315
Tao Capsules 1963
Tapazole Tablets 1298
Tazidime Vials, Faspak & ADD-Vantage (2%) 1299
Tegretol 654
Tenex Tablets 1875
Ten-K Controlled-Release Tablets (Rare) 2282
Tenoretic Tablets 1105
Tenormin Tablets and I.V. Injection 1107
TheraCys BCG Live (Intravesical) (Up to 1.8%) 898
Thiotepa Parenteral (Occasional) 1240
Ticar for Injection 2236
Timentin for Injection 2239
Tofranil Ampuls 1038
Tofranil Tablets 1039
Tofranil-PM Capsules 1041
Trandate HCT/Trandate (Less than 1% in 208 patients) 579
Tranxene 556
Trecator-SC Tablets 2527
Trental (Less than 1%) 1099
Triavil Tablets 1556
Trinsicon Capsules (Extremely rare) 2415
Unasyn 1965
Unipen 2533
Uniphyl 400 mg Tablets 1823
Urised Tablets 2396
Urobiotic-250 Capsules 1968
Uroqid-Acid 661
Valium Injectable 1937
Valium Tablets (Infrequent) 1939
Valrelease Capsules (Occasional) 1923
Vancocin HCl, Oral Solution & Pulvules (Infrequent) 1304
Vancocin HCl, Vials & ADD-Vantage (Infrequent) 1302
Velosulin 1627
Velosulin Human 1628
Ventolin (Rare) 583
Vivactil Tablets 1567
Vontrol Tablets (Rare) 2243
Wycillin Injection 2537
Wygesic Tablets 2540
Zantac Injection and Zantac Injection Premixed 1063
Zantac (Rare) 1065
Zaroxolyn Tablets 989
Zinacef (1 in 125 patients) 1066
Zovirax Capsules (0.3%) 824
Zovirax Ointment 5% (0.3%) 827
Zovirax (0.3%) 824
Zyloprim Tablets (Less than 1%) 830

Rash, urticarial

Capoten (Rare) 2255
Capozide (Rare) 2258
DTIC-Dome (Infrequent) 1595
Equagesic Tablets 2451
Mesantoin Tablets 2013
Miltown Tablets 2386
Normodyne Tablets 2110
Normozide Tablets 2112
PMB 200 and PMB 400 2504
Quinamm Tablets 1344
Serax Capsules 2522
Serax Tablets 2522
Trandate HCT/Trandate 579

Rash, vesiculobullous

Lodine Capsules (Less than 1%) 2468
Permax Tablets (Rare) 1291
Prozac Pulvules (Rare) 920

Raynaud's phenomenon

Blenoxane (Isolated reports) 724
Blocadren Tablets 1429
Capoten (2 to 3 of 1000 patients) 2255
Capozide (2 to 3 of 1000 patients) 2258
Catapres Tablets (Rare) 676
Catapres-TTS (Rare) 677
Cibalith-S 870
Combipres Tablets (Rare) 678
Corgard Tablets (2 of 100 patients) 701
Corzide Tablets (Approximately 2 of 100 patients) 702
Demulen 2161
Enovid 2161
Inderal 2459
Inderal LA Long Acting Capsules 2461
Inderide Tablets 2463
Inderide LA Long Acting Capsules 2465
Kerlone Tablets 2172
Lithobid Tablets 870
Loestrin 1728
Lopressor HCT Tablets 1034
Maxzide-25 MG Tablets 1215
Norethin 2133
Norlestrin 1746
Parlodel (Less than 2%) 2020
Roferon-A Injection (Less than 1%) 1916
Tenormin Tablets and I.V. Injection 1107
Timolide Tablets 1547
Timoptic in Ocudose 1552
Timoptic Sterile Ophthalmic Solution 1550
Velban Vials 1305

Rectal bleeding

Accutane Capsules 1878
Anafranil Capsules (Infrequent) 650
BuSpar (Infrequent) 1401
Cholybar 1705
Clozaril Tablets (Less than 1%) 2000
Cortenema (Rare) 2244
Dipentum Capsules (Rare) 1160
Eldepryl 2250
Geocillin Tablets 1951
Indocin Capsules (Less than 1%) 1487
Indocin I.V. (Less than 1%) 1490
Indocin (Less than 1%) 1487
Intron A (Less than 1%) 2097
Niclocide Chewable Tablets 1607
Orudis Capsules (Less than 1%) 2488
Questran Light 711
Questran Powder 710
Retrovir Capsules (Less than 5%) 802
Retrovir I.V. Infusion (Less than 5%) 805
Retrovir Syrup (Less than 5%) 802
Toradol IM Injection (1% or less) 2302
Velban Vials 1305

Rectal disorders, unspecified

Cytotec (Infrequent) 2159
Dipentum Capsules 1160
Kerlone Tablets (Less than 2%) 2172
Wellbutrin Tablets (Rare) 821

Rectal spasms

Sandostatin Injection (Less than 1%) 2029

Red blood cell, aplasia

Mysoline (Rare) 2480

Red blood cell, hypoplasia of

Mysoline (Rare) 2480

"Red neck" syndrome

Vancocin HCl, Vials & ADD-Vantage 1302

Reflexes, abnormal

Methotrexate Tablets, Parenteral, LPF Parenteral 1217
Rheumatrex Methotrexate Dose Pack 1234

Reflexes, increased (see under Hyperreflexia)

Regurgitation

IPOL Poliovirus Vaccine Inactivated 894

Renal agenesis, unilateral, neonatal

Leukeran Tablets 788

Renal calculi

Anafranil Capsules (Infrequent) 650
Butazolidin Capsules & Tablets (Less than 1%) 1027
Cardura Tablets (Less than 0.5% of 3960 patients) 1941
Cipro I.V. (1% or less) 1592
Cipro Tablets 1589
Clinoril Tablets (Rare) 1433
Daranide Tablets 1445
Diamox 1200
Floxin Tablets (More than or equal to 1.0%) 1652
Lodine Capsules (Less than 1%) 2468
Neptazane Tablets ◉ 311
Permax Tablets (Infrequent) 1291
Prozac Pulvules (Rare) 920
Rogaine Topical Solution (0.93%) 2357

Renal colic

Benemid Tablets 1426
ColBENEMID Tablets 1436
Daranide Tablets 1445
Ethmozine Tablets (Less than 2%) 946
Kerlone Tablets (Less than 2%) 2172
Timolide Tablets (Less than 1%) 1547

Renal disease

Anaprox and Anaprox DS Tablets (Less than 1%) 2288
Naprosyn (Less than 1%) 2297

Renal failure

Aldoclor Tablets 1413
Aldoril Tablets 1418
Amicar Syrup, Tablets, and Injection (Rare) 1194
Anaprox and Anaprox DS Tablets (Less than 1%) 2288
Ancobon Capsules 1886
Ansaid Tablets (Less than 1%) 2319
Bactrim DS Tablets 1891
Bactrim I.V. Infusion 1889
Bactrim 1891
BiCNU 723
Bumex (0.1%) 1895
Butazolidin Capsules & Tablets (Less than 1%) 1027
Capoten (Approximately 1 to 2 of 1000 patients) 2255
Capozide (Approximately 1 to 2 of 1000 patients) 2258
CeeNU 725
Cipro I.V. (1% or less) 1592
Cipro Tablets (Less than 1%) 1589
Clinoril Tablets (Less than 1 in 100) 1433
Diupres Tablets 1461
Diuril Oral Suspension 1464
Diuril Sodium Intravenous 1463
Diuril Tablets 1464
Dolobid Tablets (Less than 1 in 100) 1465
Dyazide Capsules 2208
Ergamisol Tablets (Less frequent) 1136
Feldene Capsules (Less than 1%) 1777
HydroDIURIL Tablets 1484
Hydropres Tablets 1485
IFEX (1 episode) 729
Indocin (Less than 1%) 1487
Meclomen Capsules (Less than 1%) 1739
Methotrexate Tablets, Parenteral, LPF Parenteral 1217
Moduretic Tablets (Less than or equal to 1%) 1510
Mutamycin 733
Naprosyn (Less than 1%) 2297
NebuPent for Inhalation Solution (1% or less) 1017
Noroxin Tablets 1519
▲Novantrone for Injection Concentrate (0 to 8%) 1226
Permax Tablets (Infrequent) 1291
Ponstel 1758
Prinzide Tablets 1540
ProHIBiT Haemophilus b Conjugate Vaccine (Diphtheria Toxoid Conjugate) 896
Rheumatrex Methotrexate Dose Pack 1234
Rythmol Tablets (Less than 1%) 1184
Septra 813
Septra I.V. Infusion 808
Septra I.V. Infusion ADD-Vantage Vials 810
Septra 813
Tegretol Chewable Tablets 654
Tegretol Suspension 656
Tegretol Tablets 654
Tenormin Tablets and I.V. Injection (0.4%) 1107
Tolectin (200, 400 and 600 mg) (Less than 1%) 1379
Tonocard Tablets 1554
Toradol IM Injection 2302
Vancocin HCl, Oral Solution & Pulvules (Rare) 1304
Vancocin HCl, Vials & ADD-Vantage (Rare) 1302
Vaseretic Tablets 1559
Vasotec I.V. 1562
Voltaren Tablets (Rare) 1042
Zovirax Sterile Powder 828

Renal failure, acute

Anectine 755
Atgam Sterile Solution (Less than 5%) 2320
Azo Gantrisin Tablets 1888
Children's Advil Suspension (Less than 1%) 2426
Demulen 2161
Elspar 1470
Enovid 2161

Ethamolin 1829
Fungizone Intravenous 2262
Ganite Injection 1016
Indocin I.V. (Less than 1%) 1490
Maxzide 1215
Mefoxin (Rare) 1498
Mefoxin Premixed Intravenous Solution (Rare) 1500
Methotrexate Tablets, Parenteral, LPF Parenteral 1217
Mevacor Tablets 1505
Monocid Injection (Rare) 2217
Monopril Tablets (0.2 to 1.0%) 1406
Motrin Tablets (Less than 1%) 2351
Norethin 2133
Orap Tablets 1020
Orudis Capsules (Less than 1%) 2488
PediaProfen Suspension (Less than 1%) 1363
Pentam 300 Injection (0.5%) 1018
Primaxin I.M. 1532
Primaxin I.V. (Rare) 1535
Prinivil Tablets (1% or less) 1538
Prinzide Tablets (Rare) 1540
Prolixin Decanoate 1795
Prolixin Elixir 1793
Prolixin Enanthate 1796
Prolixin Injection 1791
Prolixin Oral Concentrate 1792
Prolixin Tablets 1793
Rheumatrex Methotrexate Dose Pack 1234
Rifadin (Rare) 1345
Rifamate Capsules (Rare) 1347
Rimactane Capsules (Rare) 879
Rufen Tablets 691
Tenex Tablets 1875
Vaseretic Tablets (Rare) 1559
Vasotec Tablets (0.5% to 1%) 1564
Zestoretic (Rare) 2274
Zestril Tablets (Less than 1%) 2277

Renal failure, neonatal
Capoten 2255

Renal function impairment
Aldoclor Tablets 1413
Aldoril Tablets 1418
Amikin Injectable 602
Bretylol Injection (1 in 1000) 923
Brevicon 2304
Butazolidin Capsules & Tablets (Less than 1%) 1027
Ceftin Tablets 575
Ceptaz for Injection 1057
Cleocin HCl Capsules (Rare) 2322
Cleocin Pediatric Flavored Granules (Rare) 2324
Cleocin Phosphate Injection (Rare) 2325
Cytosar-U Sterile Powder (Less frequent) 2329
DTIC-Dome (Few reports) 1595
Demulen 2161
▲Didronel I.V. Infusion (Approximately 10%) 1307
Diupres Tablets 1461
Diuril Oral Suspension 1464
Diuril Sodium Intravenous 1463
Diuril Tablets 1464
Enovid 2161
Fiorinal with Codeine Capsules 2008
Fortaz 1060
Fungizone Intravenous (Common) 2262
HydroDIURIL Tablets 1484
Hydropres Tablets 1485
Idamycin for Injection (Less than 5%) 564
Jenest-28 Tablets 1636
Keftab Tablets 917
Kerlone Tablets (Less than 2%) 2172
Leukine for IV Infusion 1127
Levlen/Tri-Levlen 665
Loestrin 1728
Micronor Tablets 1667
Modicon 1667
Moduretic Tablets (Less than or equal to 1%) 1510
Mutamycin 733
Nebcin Vials, Hyporets & ADD-Vantage 1286
Nolvadex Tablets 1102
Norethin 2133
Norinyl 2304
Norlestrin 1746
Nor-Q D Tablets 2304
Ortho-Cyclen Tablets 1658
Ortho-Novum 1667
Platinol 737
Platinol-AQ Injection 738
Prinivil Tablets 1538
Prinzide Tablets 1540
▲Sandimmune (6 to 38%) 2024
Suprax 1235
Tegretol Chewable Tablets 654
Tegretol Suspension 656
Tegretol Tablets 654
Tonocard Tablets 1554
Levlen/Tri-Levlen 665
Tri-Norinyl 2304
Vaseretic Tablets 1559
Vasotec I.V. 1562
Zefazone Sterile Powder 2372
Zestoretic 2274

Renal impairment
Capozide 2258
Clinoril Tablets (Less than 1 in 100) 1433
ColBENEMID Tablets 1436
Dolobid Tablets (Less than 1 in 100) 1465
Garamycin Injectable 2093
Hydrea Capsules (Occasional) 728
▲IFEX (6%) 729
▲Indocin I.V. (41% of infants) 1490
▲Netromycin Injection 100 mg/ml (7%) 2104
Panhematin 546
Rauzide Tablets 1804
Vasotec Tablets (0.5% to 1%) 1564
Zestoretic 2274

Renal insufficiency
Capastat Sulfate Vials (1 patient) 1250
Capoten (Approximately 1 to 2 of 1000 patients) 2255
Capozide (Approximately 1 to 2 of 1000 patients) 2258
E.E.S. (Isolated reports) 522
Elspar 1470
Erythrocin Stearate Filmtab (Isolated reports) 523
Ganite Injection 1016
Indocin Capsules (Less than 1%) 1487
Indocin I.V. (Less than 1%) 1490
Indocin (Less than 1%) 1487
Monopril Tablets (0.2 to 1.0%) 1406
PCE Dispertab Tablets (Isolated reports) 549
▲Platinol (28 to 36%) 737
Rifadin (Rare) 1345
Rifamate Capsules (Rare) 1347
Rimactane Capsules (Rare) 879
Zoladex (1% to 5%) 1110

Renal insufficiency, reversible
Actimmune (Rare) 1046

Renal rickets
IFEX 729

Renal stones
Butazolidin Capsules & Tablets (Less than 1%) 1027
Clinoril Tablets 1433
Dyazide Capsules 2208
Dyrenium Capsules (Rare) 2210
Maxzide 1215

Renal tubular cells excretion, increase
Asbron G 1997
Choledyl SA Tablets 1704
Constant-T Tablets 1029
Dilor 2079
Quadrinal Tablets 1183
Quibron-T/SR 716
Theo-Dur Sprinkle 1168

Respiration, Cheyne-Stokes
Anexsia 5/500 Tablets 2196
Anexsia 7.5/650 Tablets 2197

Respiratory alkalosis
Butazolidin Capsules & Tablets (Less than 1%) 1027
Ganite Injection 1016

Respiratory arrest
Alfenta Injection 1131
Ancobon Capsules 1886
▲Anestacon Solution (Among most common) 2394
AquaMEPHYTON Injection 1422
Arfonad Ampuls 1887
Carbocaine Hydrochloride 3% Injection 956
Carbocaine Hydrochloride Injection 2043
Carbocaine Hydrochloride 2% with Neo-Cobefrin 956
Cardioquin Tablets 1812
Cipro I.V. (1% or less) 1592
Coly-Mycin M Parenteral 1706
Decadron Phosphate with Xylocaine Injection, Sterile 1451
Demerol 2047
Dilaudid-HP Injection 1175
Dilor 2079
Dolophine Hydrochloride Ampoules & Vials 1260
Dolophine Hydrochloride Tablets 1261
Duranest Injections 624
Dyclone 0.5% and 1% Topical Solutions, USP 626
Enlon Injection (Isolated instances) 598
Fluothane 2453
Innovar Injection 1141
MS Contin Tablets 1814
MSIR 1817
Marcaine Hydrochloride 0.5% with Epinephrine 1:200,000 (as bitartrate) 958
Marcaine Hydrochloride with Epinephrine 1:200,000 2055
Marcaine Hydrochloride Injection 2055
Marcaine Spinal 2058
Mepergan Injection 2479
Methadone Hydrochloride Diskets 1284
Methadone Hydrochloride Oral Solution & Tablets 1987
Nescaine/Nescaine MPF 629
Novocain Hydrochloride for Spinal Anesthesia 2065
Oramorph SR (Morphine Sulfate Sustained Release Tablets) 1988
Pantopon Injectable 1911
Pontocaine Hydrochloride for Spinal Anesthesia 2069
Prostigmin Injectable 1120
Prostigmin Tablets 1121
Quinaglute Dura-Tabs Tablets 663
Quinidex Extentabs 1868
Roxanol 1991
Sensorcaine 631
Sensorcaine-MPF Spinal 634
Sublimaze Injection 1146
Tonocard Tablets (Less than 1%) 1554
▲Xylocaine Injections (Among most common) 637
Xylocaine Injections for Ventricular Arrhythmias 639
Xylocaine 2% Jelly 643
Xylocaine 5% Ointment 644
4% Xylocaine-MPF Sterile Solution 641

Respiratory congestion, unspecified
▲Epogen for Injection (15%) 591
▲Procrit for Injection (15%) 1647

Respiratory depression (see under Depression, respiratory)

Respiratory depression, postoperative
Alfenta Injection (2%) 1131
Sublimaze Injection (Occasional) 1146
Sufenta Injection (Less than 1%) 1147

Respiratory difficulty
Ana-Kit Anaphylaxis Emergency Treatment Kit 1100
Atrohist Sprinkle Capsules 558
Carafate Tablets 1326
Deconamine 663
Deconsal 559
Diphtheria and Tetanus Toxoids and Pertussis Vaccine Adsorbed USP (For Pediatric Use) 892
EpiPen 843
Fedahist Gyrocaps 2145
Fedahist Timecaps 2145
Floropryl Sterile Ophthalmic Ointment (Infrequent) 1473
Haldol Decanoate 1375
Haldol Injection, Tablets and Concentrate 1373
Humorsol Sterile Ophthalmic Solution (Infrequent) 1475
Imferon 976
Levophed Bitartrate Injection 2054
Metubine Iodide Vials 1285
Naldecon Syrup, Tablets, Pediatric Drops and Pediatric Syrup 709
Norpace (Infrequent) 2177
Novafed A Capsules 1342
Novafed Capsules 1342
Novahistine DH 1342
Novahistine DMX ▣ 595
Novahistine Elixir ▣ 596
Novahistine Expectorant 1343
Novocain Hydrochloride for Spinal Anesthesia 2065
Papaverine Hydrochloride Vials and Ampoules 1290
Pontocaine Hydrochloride for Spinal Anesthesia 2069
Rondec 1975
Rondec-DM 1976
Rondec-TR Tablet 1975
Ru-Tuss DE Tablets 694
Seldane-D Extended-Release Tablets 1350
Solganal Suspension 2122
Sus-Phrine Injection 1006
Triavil Tablets 1556
Tri-Immunol Diphtheria & Tetanus Toxoids & Pertussis Vaccine, Adsorbed 1241
Trinalin Repetabs Tablets 1170
Versed Injection (Less than 1%) 1924

Respiratory discharge, upper, unspecified
Emcyt Capsules (1%) 1161

Respiratory distress
Aldoclor Tablets 1413
Aldoril Tablets 1418
Americaine Otic Topical Anesthetic Ear Drops 973
Atgam Sterile Solution (At least 1 patient and less than 5% of total patients) 2320
Betagan ⊙ 239
Blocadren Tablets 1429
Capozide 2258
Cartrol Tablets 507
Cipro I.V. (1% or less) 1592
Corgard Tablets 701
Corzide Tablets 702
Cytosar-U Sterile Powder 2329
Dalgan Injection (Less than 1%) 620
Dantrium Capsules (Less frequent) 1619
Diucardin Tablets 2450
Diulo 2129
Diupres Tablets 1461
Diuril Oral Suspension 1464
Diuril Sodium Intravenous 1463
Diuril Tablets 1464
Duragesic Transdermal System (Less than 1%) 1133
Dyazide Capsules 2208
Elspar 1470
Enduron Tablets 517
Esidrix Tablets 863
HydroDIURIL Tablets 1484
Hydropres Tablets 1485
Inderal 2459
Inderal LA Long Acting Capsules 2461
Inderide Tablets 2463
Inderide LA Long Acting Capsules 2465
Indocin Capsules (Less than 1%) 1487
Indocin I.V. (Less than 1%) 1490
Indocin (Less than 1%) 1487
▲Intron A (Less than 14%) 2097
Kerlone Tablets 2172
Levatol 1832
Lopressor HCT Tablets 1034
Lozol Tablets 1843
▲Lupron Depot 3.75 mg (Among most frequent) 2312
Lupron Depot 7.5 mg 2311
Maxzide 1215
Metrodin (urofollitropin for injection) 2182
▲Mexitil Capsules (3.3% to 5.7%) 680
Moduretic Tablets 1510
Mutamycin (Few cases) 733
Mykrox ½ mg Tablets 984
Naturetin Tablets (Occasional) 1789
Normodyne Tablets 2110
Normozide Tablets 2112
Nuromax Injection 794
▲Paraplatin for Injection (6%) 735
Phenergan VC 2500
Phenergan VC with Codeine 2501
Prinzide Tablets 1540
Procardia XL Tablets (1% or less) 1783
Prostin VR Pediatric Sterile Solution (Less than 1%) 2355
Protamine Sulfate Ampoules & Vials 1295
Rauzide Tablets 1804
Salutensin/Salutensin-Demi 719
Sandimmune 2024
Sectral Capsules 2520
Tenoretic Tablets 1105
Tenormin Tablets and I.V. Injection 1107
Timolide Tablets 1547
Timoptic in Ocudose 1552
Trandate HCT/Trandate 579
Triaminic Expectorant DH 1995
Vaseretic Tablets 1559

Virazole 1126
Visken Tablets 2036
Zaroxolyn Tablets 989
Zefazone Sterile Powder 2372
Zestoretic 2274

Respiratory distress, neonatal
Stadol (Less than 1%) 721

Respiratory failure
Betoptic Sterile Ophthalmic Solution (Rare) 569
Betoptic S Sterile Ophthalmic Suspension (Rare) 570
Cocaine Hydrochloride Topical Solution 620
Isoptin Injectable 1177
Survanta Beractant Intratracheal Suspension 1978
Timoptic in Ocudose 1552
Timoptic Sterile Ophthalmic Solution 1550

Respiratory tract, hypersensitivity
Septra 813
Septra I.V. Infusion 808
Septra I.V. Infusion ADD-Vantage Vials (Rare) 810
Septra 813

Restlessness (see under Dysphoria)

Retardation, psychomotor
Eskalith 2214
Lithane Tablets 1596
Lithium Carbonate Capsules & Tablets 1984
Roferon-A Injection (Less than 1%) 1916

Retching
Nipride I.V. Infusion 1909
Versed Injection (Less than 1%) 1924

Reticulocytopenia
Chloromycetin Palmitate, Oral Suspension 1697
Chloromycetin Sodium Succinate 1698
Cosmegen Injection 1440
Cytosar-U Sterile Powder 2329
Vira-A for Injection 1766

Reticulocytosis
▲ Dapsone USP (Almost all patients) 1130
Dipentum Capsules (Rare) 1160
Garamycin Injectable 2093
▲ Tegison Capsules (25-50%) 1881
Virazole 1126
Zyloprim Tablets (Less than 1%) 830

Retinal atrophy
Aralen Phosphate Tablets 2039
Clinoril Tablets 1433
Plaquenil Sulfate Tablets 2067

Retinal damage
Aralen Hydrochloride Injection 2038
Aralen Phosphate with Primaquine Phosphate Tablets 2040
Aralen Phosphate Tablets 2039
Dapsone USP 1130
Plaquenil Sulfate Tablets 2067

Retinal detachment
Butazolidin Capsules & Tablets (Less than 1%) 1027
Cytovene Sterile Powder 2292
Humorsol Sterile Ophthalmic Solution (Occasional) 1475
Isopto Carpine (Rare) ◉ 219
MIOSTAT ◉ 233
Ocusert Pilo-20 and Pilo-40 Ocular Therapeutic Systems ◉ 256
Permax Tablets (Rare) 1291
Phospholine Iodide (A few cases) ◉ 315
Pilocar ◉ 275
Pilopine HS Gel (Rare) ◉ 227
Pilostat Sterile Ophthalmic Solution 0.5%, 1%, 2%, 3%, 4%, 5%, 6% ◉ 263

Retinal hemorrhage, neonatal
Pitocin Injection, Ampoules, Steri-Dose Syringes 1757
Syntocinon Injection 2032

Retinal pigmentation disorders
Aralen Phosphate with Primaquine Phosphate Tablets 2040
Aralen Phosphate Tablets 2039
Desferal Vials 862
Plaquenil Sulfate Tablets 2067
Platinol 737

Retinitis
Attenuvax (Infrequent) 1424
Indocin (Less than 1%) 1487
M-M-R II (Infrequent) 1494
M-R-VAX II 1496

Retinopathy
Anafranil Capsules (Rare) 650
Aralen Hydrochloride Injection 2038
Aralen Phosphate Tablets 2039
Atabrine Hydrochloride Tablets (Rare) 2041
Cardizem Tablets-30 mg, 60 mg, 90 mg and 120 mg 1329
Cardizem SR Capsules-60 mg, 90 mg and 120 mg (Less than 1%) 1327
Clinoril Tablets 1433
Haldol Decanoate 1375
Haldol Injection, Tablets and Concentrate 1373
Lysodren (Infrequent) 731
Meclomen Capsules (Rare) 1739
Minipress Capsules (Single report) 1778
Minizide Capsules (Single report) 1779
Nolvadex Tablets 1102
Plaquenil Sulfate Tablets 2067
Prolixin Decanoate 1795
Prolixin Elixir 1793
Prolixin Enanthate 1796
Prolixin Injection 1791
Prolixin Oral Concentrate 1792
Prolixin Tablets 1793
▲ Tegison Capsules (10-25%) 1881
Tolectin (200, 400 and 600 mg) (Less than 1%) 1379

Retinopathy, pigmentary
Aralen Phosphate Tablets 2039
Compazine 2201
Etrafon 2087
Stelazine 2226
Tacaryl 2409
Taractan 1920
Thorazine 2234
Triavil Tablets 1556
Trilafon 2123

Retrocollis
Etrafon 2087
Trilafon 2123

Retrolental fibroplasia
▲ Indocin I.V. (3% to 9%) 1490

Retroperitoneal fibrosis
Blocadren Tablets 1429
D.H.E. 45 Injection 2003
Parlodel (A few cases) 2020
Sansert Tablets (Very rare) 2031
Timolide Tablets 1547
Timoptic in Ocudose 1552
Timoptic Sterile Ophthalmic Solution 1550

Retrosternal discomfort
Ethamolin (1.6%) 1829
IOPIDINE ◉ 232
Levophed Bitartrate Injection 2054
Nipride I.V. Infusion 1909
Nitro-Bid IV (Less than 1%) 1338
Nitrostat IV (Less than 1%) 1744

Rhabdomyolysis
Amicar Syrup, Tablets, and Injection (Rare) 1194
Anectine 755
Atromid-S Capsules 2435
Lopid Capsules and Tablets 1736
Mevacor Tablets (Rare) 1505
Orap Tablets 1020
Wellbutrin Tablets 821

Rheumatic syndrome
INH Tablets 868
Rifamate Capsules 1347

Rheumatoid arthritis
Atromid-S Capsules 2435
Demulen 2161
Enovid 2161
Norethin 2133
Prozac Pulvules (Rare) 920

Rheumatoid factor, positive
Aldoclor Tablets 1413
Aldomet Ester HCl Injection 1417
Aldomet Oral 1415
Aldoril Tablets 1418
Elavil 2269

Rhinitis
Actigall Capsules 2280
▲ AeroBid Inhaler System (3-9%) 995
▲ Anafranil Capsules (7% to 12%) 650
Anaprox and Anaprox DS Tablets 2288
Ansaid Tablets (1-3%) 2319
Brevital Sodium Vials 1248
Calciparine Injection (Rare) 925
Capoten 2255
Capozide 2258
Carafate Tablets 1326
Cardene Capsules (Rare) 2290
▲ Cardura Tablets (3%) 1941
Cartrol Tablets (Less common) 507
Children's Advil Suspension (Less than 1%) 2426
▲ DDAVP (3 to 8%) 1841
Demulen 2161
Depo-Medrol Sterile Aqueous Suspension 2334
Enovid 2161
Heparin Lock Flush Solution 2456
Heparin Sodium Vials (Rare) 1264
Heparin Sodium Injection 2457
Heparin Sodium Injection, USP, Sterile Solution 2342
Hytrin Tablets (At least 1%) 529
▲ Intron A (Less than 5%) 2097
Kerlone Tablets (1.4%) 2172
Lodine Capsules (Less than 1%) 2468
Monopril Tablets (0.2 to 1.0%) 1406
Motrin Tablets (Less than 1%) 2351
Mumpsvax 1513
NebuPent for Inhalation Solution (1% or less) 1017
Norethin 2133
Normozide Tablets (Less than 1%) 2112
Omnipaque (0.2% or less) 2552
OptiPranolol Sterile Ophthalmic Solution (A small number of patients) ◉ 261
Orudis Capsules (Less than 1%) 2488
PediaProfen Suspension (Less than 1%) 1363
▲ Permax Tablets (12.2%) 1291
Plendil Extended-Release Tablets (0.5% or greater) 1526
Prinzide Tablets (0.3 to 1%) 1540
ProSom Tablets (Infrequent) 554
Prozac Pulvules (Frequent) 920
Recombivax HB (Less than 1%) 1544
Retrovir Capsules (Less than 5%) 802
Retrovir I.V. Infusion (Less than 5%) 805
Retrovir Syrup (Less than 5%) 802
Roferon-A Injection (Less than 1%) 1916
Rogaine Topical Solution (1.27%) 2357
Rufen Tablets (Less than 1%) 691
Sectral Capsules 2520
Tenex Tablets (Less than 3%) 1875
Trandate HCT Tablets (Less than 1% in 208 patients) 579
Vascor (200, 300 and 400 mg) Tablets (0.5 to 2.0%) 1383
Zestoretic (0.3 to 1%) 2274
Zorprin Tablets 698
Zyloprim Tablets (Less than 1%) 830

Rhinorrhea
▲ AeroBid Inhaler System (3-9%) 995
Azdone Tablets 844
BAL in Oil Ampules 661
Beconase AQ Nasal Spray (Fewer than 3 per 100 patients) 574
Beconase Inhalation Aerosol & Refill (1 per 100 patients) 574
Calcijex Calcitriol Injection 506
Calderol Capsules 1635
▲ CHEMET (succimer) Capsules (0.7 to 3.7%) 1361
Clozaril Tablets (Less than 1%) 2000
Colyte 1826
Damason-P 1356
Diapid Nasal Spray (Infrequent) 2003
Dristan Long Lasting Nasal Spray, Regular and Regular with Metered Dose Pump 2419
Dristan Nasal Spray, Regular and Regular with Metered Pump 2419
Empirin with Codeine Phosphate Nos. 2, 3 & 4 764
4-Way Fast Acting Nasal Spray - Original Formula (regular & mentholated) & Metered Spray Pump (regular) 751
4-Way Long Lasting Nasal Spray & Metered Spray Pump 751
Floxin Tablets (Less than 1%) 1652
GoLYTELY (Isolated cases) 699
Intron A (2%) 2097
Klonopin Tablets 1902
Lortab ASA Tablets 2414
Lozol Tablets (Less than 5%) 1843
Methadone Hydrochloride Diskets 1284
NuLYTELY 699
Plendil Extended-Release Tablets 1526
Rocaltrol Capsules 1913
▲ Roferon-A Injection (4%) 1916
Sandostatin Injection (Less than 1%) 2029
Soma Compound w/Codeine Tablets 2390
Soma Compound Tablets 2389
Syntocinon Nasal Spray 2033
Tegison Capsules (Less than 1%) 1881
Trexan Tablets (Less than 1%) 937
Vancenase AQ Nasal Spray 0.042% (Fewer than 3 per 100 patients) 2127
Vancenase Nasal Inhaler (1 per 100 patients) 2126
Vaseretic Tablets 1559
Vasotec I.V. 1562
Vasotec Tablets (0.5% to 1%) 1564
Yohimex Tablets 1190

Rhonchi
Brevibloc Injection (Less 1%) 942
Ganite Injection 1016

Rigidity
Alfenta Injection 1131
Azo Gantrisin Tablets 1888
Cardura Tablets (Less than 0.5% of 3960 patients) 1941
▲ Clozaril Tablets (3%) 2000
Cytotec (Infrequent) 2159
Diprivan Injection (Less than 1%) 2267
▲ Intron A (16% to 30%) 2097
Kerlone Tablets (Less than 2%) 2172
Lioresal Tablets 1031
Moban Tablets & Concentrate 932
Nardil (Less frequent) 1742
Normozide Tablets 2112
Omnipaque (Rare) 2552
▲ Orthoclone OKT3 Sterile Solution (8%) 1645
Procardia XL Tablets (1% or less) 1783
▲ Sublimaze Injection (Most common) 1146
▲ Tegison Capsules (1-10%) 1881
▲ Xanax Tablets (4.2%) 2367
Zovirax Sterile Powder (Less than 1%) 828

S

Salicylism
Easprin 1719
Empirin with Codeine Phosphate Nos. 2, 3 & 4 764

Salivary gland enlargement
Anafranil Capsules (Rare) 650
Azo Gantrisin Tablets 1888
Butazolidin Capsules & Tablets (Less than 1%) 1027
Omnipaque 2552
Permax Tablets (Infrequent) 1291
Prozac Pulvules (Rare) 920

Salivation
Alferon N Injection (1%) 1809
Altace Capsules (Less than 1%) 1086
Anafranil Capsules (Infrequent) 650
Anectine 755
Antilirium Injectable 998
BAL in Oil Ampules 661
Brevital Sodium Vials 1248
BuSpar (Infrequent) 1401
▲ Clozaril Tablets (More than 5 to 31%) 2000
Cordarone Tablets (1 to 3%) 2446
Dalmane Capsules (Rare) 1927
Desyrel and Desyrel Dividose (Less than 1%) 1404
Diupres Tablets 1461
Duvoid Tablets 1853
Emete-con Intramuscular/Intravenous 1950
Eskalith 2214
Etrafon 2087
Fiorinal with Codeine Capsules 2008
Floropryl Sterile Ophthalmic Ointment (Rare) 1473
Garamycin Injectable 2093
Haldol Injection, Tablets and Concentrate 1373

Humorsol Sterile Ophthalmic Solution (Rare) ... 1475
Hydropres Tablets ... 1485
Hyperstat I.V. Injection ... 2095
IFEX (Less than 1%) ... 729
Intron A (Less than 1%) ... 2097
Isopto Carbachol ... ⊙ 219
Kerlone Tablets (Less than 2%) ... 2172
Loxitane ... 1213
Ludiomil Tablets ... 874
Mestinon Injectable ... 1115
Mestinon ... 1116
Mexitil Capsules (About 4 in 1,000) ... 680
Moban Tablets & Concentrate ... 932
Navane Capsules and Concentrate 1954
Navane Intramuscular ... 1956
Nicorette (2.1%) ... 1335
Orap Tablets ... 1020
Orudis Capsules (Less than 1%) ... 2488
PhosChol ... 568
Pilocar (Extremely rare) ... ⊙ 275
Pilostat Sterile Ophthalmic Solution 0.5%, 1%, 2%, 3%, 4%, 5%, 6% (Extremely rare) ⊙ 263
Primaxin I.M. ... 1532
Primaxin I.V. (Less than 0.2%) ... 1535
Prolixin Decanoate ... 1795
Prolixin Elixir ... 1793
Prolixin Enanthate ... 1796
Prolixin Injection ... 1791
Prolixin Oral Concentrate ... 1792
Prolixin Tablets ... 1793
Prostigmin Injectable (Among most common) ... 1120
Prostigmin Tablets (Among most common) ... 1121
Prozac Pulvules (Rare) ... 920
Quadrinal Tablets ... 1183
Roferon-A Injection (Less than 1%) ... 1916
Salutensin/Salutensin-Demi ... 719
Surital Ampoules, Steri-Vials ... 1764
Tensilon Injectable ... 1123
Trental (Less than 1%) ... 1099
Triavil Tablets ... 1556
Trilafon ... 2123
Urecholine ... 1558
Valium Injectable (Rare) ... 1937
Valium Tablets (Infrequent) ... 1939
Valrelease Capsules (Occasional) ... 1923
Versed Injection (Less than 1%) ... 1924
▲Wellbutrin Tablets (3.4%) ... 821
▲Xanax Tablets (4.2% to 5.6%) ... 2367

Salivation, increase (see under Salivation)

Salpingitis
Permax Tablets (Infrequent) ... 1291
Prozac Pulvules (Rare) ... 920

Sarcoma, bone
Permax Tablets (Infrequent) ... 1291

Scalp, dry
Nizoral 2% Shampoo ... 1144
Selsun Rx 2.5% Selenium Sulfide Lotion, USP ... 1977

Scalp, oily
Nizoral 2% Shampoo ... 1144
Selsun Rx 2.5% Selenium Sulfide Lotion, USP ... 1977

Scalp, tightness
Temovate Scalp Application (Less frequent) ... 1056

Scalp defects, fetal
Tapazole Tablets (Rare) ... 1298

Scarring
Aplisol (tuberculin PPD, diluted) ... 2550
Aplitest (tuberculin PPD, multiple-puncture device) ... 2551
Condylox (Less than 5%) ... 1630
Decadron-LA Sterile Suspension ... 1457
Efudex ... 1880
Fluoroplex Topical Solution & Cream 1% (Occasional) ... 1082

Schizophrenia, precipitation
Anafranil Capsules (Rare) ... 650
Nardil (Less frequent) ... 1742

Sciatica
Wellbutrin Tablets (Rare) ... 821

Sclera, discoloration
Mellaril ... 2011
Minipress Capsules (1-4%) ... 1778
Minizide Capsules ... 1779
Norzine ... 1818
Novantrone for Injection Concentrate ... 1226
Serentil ... 686
Torecan ... 1993

Sclera, infection
Azulfidine Tablets, EN-tabs, Oral Suspension (Rare) ... 1157
Urobiotic-250 Capsules ... 1968

Scleral injection
Azo Gantanol Tablets ... 1887
Azo Gantrisin Tablets ... 1888
Bactrim DS Tablets ... 1891
Bactrim I.V. Infusion ... 1889
Bactrim ... 1891
Fansidar Tablets ... 1896
Gantanol ... 1899
Gantrisin Ophthalmic Ointment/Solution ... 1900
Pediazole ... 1973
Septra ... 813
Septra I.V. Infusion ... 808
Septra I.V. Infusion ADD-Vantage Vials ... 810
Septra ... 813
Thiosulfil Forte Tablets ... 2526

Scleritis
Anafranil Capsules (Infrequent) ... 650

Sclerosis, skin
Talwin Injection ... 2071

Sclerosis, subcutaneous tissues
Talwin Injection ... 2071

Scotomata
Aralen Hydrochloride Injection ... 2038
Aralen Phosphate Tablets ... 2039
Butazolidin Capsules & Tablets (Less than 1%) ... 1027
Cardioquin Tablets ... 1812
Children's Advil Suspension (Less than 1%) ... 2426
Cibalith-S ... 870
Eskalith ... 2214
Lithane Tablets ... 1596
Lithium Carbonate Capsules & Tablets ... 1984
Lithobid Tablets ... 870
Motrin Tablets ... 2351
PediaProfen Suspension (Less than 1%) ... 1363
Plaquenil Sulfate Tablets ... 2067
Proglycem ... 649
ProSom Tablets (Rare) ... 554
Quinaglute Dura-Tabs Tablets ... 663
Quinamm Tablets ... 1344
Quinidex Extentabs ... 1868
Rufen Tablets (Less than 1%) ... 691
Tegison Capsules (Less than 1%) .. 1881
Trental (Less than 1%) ... 1099
Voltaren Tablets (Less than 1%) ... 1042

Scotomata, scintillating
Serophene (clomiphene citrate tablets, USP) ... 2186

Screaming, excessive
Tri-Immunol Diphtheria & Tetanus Toxoids & Pertussis Vaccine, Adsorbed (Rare) ... 1241

Seborrhea
Accutane Capsules (Less than 1 in 10) ... 1878
Anafranil Capsules (Rare) ... 650
Danocrine Capsules ... 2046
Halotestin Tablets ... 2341
Loxitane ... 1213
Permax Tablets (Infrequent) ... 1291
Prolixin Decanoate ... 1795
Prolixin Elixir ... 1793
Prolixin Enanthate ... 1796
Prolixin Injection ... 1791
Prolixin Oral Concentrate ... 1792
Prolixin Tablets ... 1793
Prozac Pulvules (Rare) ... 920
▲Synarel Nasal Solution (8% of patients) ... 2300

Sedation
▲Actifed with Codeine Cough Syrup (Among most frequent) ... 752
AK-Con ... ⊙ 202
Aldoclor Tablets ... 1413
Aldomet Ester HCl Injection ... 1417
Aldomet Oral ... 1415
Aldoril Tablets ... 1418
Ancobon Capsules ... 1886
▲Anexsia 5/500 Tablets (Among most frequent) ... 2196
▲Anexsia 7.5/650 Tablets (Among most frequent) ... 2197
Ativan Injection ... 2432
▲Ativan Tablets (15.9%) ... 2434
▲Azdōne Tablets (Among most frequent) ... 844
▲Benadryl Capsules (Among most frequent) ... 1691
▲Benadryl Injection (Among most frequent) ... 1692
BuSpar ... 1401
▲Catapres Tablets (About 10 in 100 patients) ... 676
▲Catapres-TTS (About 8%) ... 677
▲Clozaril Tablets (More than 5 to 39%) ... 2000
▲Combipres Tablets (About 10%) ... 678
Comhist LA Capsules ... 1618
Corgard Tablets (6 of 1000 patients) ... 701
Corzide Tablets (Approximately 6 of 1000 patients) ... 702
▲Dalgan Injection (3 to 9%) ... 620
Dalmane Capsules ... 1927
▲Damason-P (Among most frequent) ... 1356
▲Darvon-N/Darvocet-N (Among most frequent) ... 1254
▲Darvon (Among most frequent) ... 1256
▲Darvon-N Suspension & Tablets (Among most frequent) ... 1254
Deconamine ... 663
Demerol ... 2047
▲Demser Capsules (Almost all patients) ... 1460
Depakene Capsules & Syrup ... 511
Depakote ... 512
Dilaudid Cough Syrup ... 1174
Dilaudid ... 1173
Dilaudid-HP Injection ... 1175
▲Dimetane-DC Cough Syrup (Most frequent) ... 1857
Dimetane-DX Cough Syrup (Among most frequent) ... 1858
Diupres Tablets ... 1461
▲Dolophine Hydrochloride Ampoules & Vials (Among most frequent) ... 1260
▲Dolophine Hydrochloride Tablets (Among most frequent) ... 1261
Fedahist Gyrocaps ... 2145
Fedahist Timecaps ... 2145
Fiorinal with Codeine Capsules ... 2008
Halcion Tablets ... 2340
Hycodan Syrup, Tablets ... 927
Hycomine Compound Tablets ... 929
Hycomine Syrup ... 927
Hycotuss Expectorant Syrup ... 930
Hydrocet Capsules ... 835
Hydropres Tablets ... 1485
Lioresal Tablets ... 1031
Lomotil ... 2174
▲Lortab ASA Tablets (Among most frequent) ... 2414
▲Lortab (Among most frequent) ... 2412
▲MS Contin Tablets (Among most frequent) ... 1814
▲MSIR (Among most frequent) ... 1817
▲Mepergan Injection (Among most frequent) ... 2479
▲Methadone Hydrochloride Diskets (Among most frequent) ... 1284
Methadone Hydrochloride Oral Solution & Tablets ... 1987
Metopirone Tablets ... 876
Motofen Tablets ... 836
Naldecon Syrup, Tablets, Pediatric Drops and Pediatric Syrup ... 709
Navane Capsules and Concentrate 1954
Navane Intramuscular ... 1956
Novafed A Capsules ... 1342
Novahistine DH ... 1342
Novahistine Expectorant ... 1343
▲Nubain Injection (36%) ... 934
▲Optimine Tablets (Among most frequent) ... 2115
▲Oramorph SR (Morphine Sulfate Sustained Release Tablets) (Among most frequent) ... 1988
Orap Tablets ... 1020
Ornade Spansule Capsules ... 2221
Pantopon Injectable ... 1911
Papaverine Hydrochloride Vials and Ampoules ... 1290
▲Percocet Tablets (Among most frequent) ... 950
▲Percodan (Among most frequent) .. 951
Periactin ... 1525
▲Phenaphen with Codeine Capsules (Among most frequent) ... 1865
▲Phenaphen-650 with Codeine Tablets (Among most frequent) ... 1866
Phenergan with Codeine ... 2497
Phenergan with Dextromethorphan 2499
Phenergan Suppositories ... 2496
Phenergan Syrup ... 2495
Phenergan VC ... 2500
Phenergan VC with Codeine ... 2501
Phenobarbital Elixir and Tablets ... 1293
Polaramine ... 2116
Prozac Pulvules (1.9%) ... 920
Roferon-A Injection (Less than 1%) ... 1916
Rondec ... 1975
Rondec-DM ... 1976
Rondec-TR Tablet ... 1975
▲Roxanol (Among most frequent) ... 1991
▲Roxicodone Tablets, Oral Solution & Intensol (Oxycodone) (Among most frequent) ... 1992
Ru-Tuss II Capsules ... 693
▲Rynatan (Among most common) ... 2387
▲Rynatuss (Among most common) .. 2388
Salutensin/Salutensin-Demi ... 719
▲Seldane-D Extended-Release Tablets (7.2%) ... 1350
Soma Compound w/Codeine Tablets ... 2390
▲Stadol (40%) ... 721
Synalgos-DC Capsules ... 2525
Talacen ... 2070
Talwin Injection ... 2071
Talwin Compound ... 2072
Talwin Injection ... 2071
Talwin Nx ... 2073
Taractan (Common) ... 1920
▲Tavist Syrup (Among most frequent) ... 2033
▲Tavist Tablets (Among most frequent) ... 2035
▲Tavist-D Tablets (Among most frequent) ... 2035
▲Tenex Tablets (1% to 14%) ... 1875
Tessalon Perles ... 1006
▲Triaminic Expectorant DH (Among most frequent) ... 1995
▲Triaminic Oral Infant Drops (Among most frequent) ... 1996
Triavil Tablets ... 1556
▲Trinalin Repetabs Tablets (Among most frequent) ... 1170
Tussionex Extended-Release Suspension ... 988
Tylenol with Codeine ... 1381
▲Tylox Capsules (Among most frequent) ... 1382
Versed Injection (1.6%) ... 1924
▲Vicodin Tablets (Most frequent) ... 1187
▲Vicodin ES Tablets (Among most frequent) ... 1189
▲Wellbutrin Tablets (19.8%) ... 821
▲Wygesic Tablets (Most frequent) ... 2540
▲Wytensin Tablets (20%) ... 2542
Xanax Tablets ... 2367
▲Zydone Capsules (Most frequent) .. 941

Seizures (see also under Convulsions)
Accutane Capsules ... 1878
Actimmune (Rare) ... 1046
Adalat Capsules (10 mg and 20 mg) (Less than 0.5%) ... 1587
Asendin Tablets (Less than 1%) ... 1196
Atgam Sterile Solution (Less than 1% to less than 5%) ... 2320
Attenuvax (Rare) ... 1424
Azactam for Injection (Less than 1%) ... 2252
Brethine Ampuls (Rare) ... 1026
Brethine Tablets (Rare) ... 1026
Brevital Sodium Vials ... 1248
BuSpar (Infrequent) ... 1401
Carbocaine ... 956
Ceftin Tablets ... 575
Ceptaz for Injection (Fewer than 1%) ... 1057
▲Clozaril Tablets (3.5 to more than 5%) ... 2000
Cyclogyl (Common) ... ⊙ 215
Cyclomydril ... ⊙ 216
DDAVP Injection (Rare) ... 1840
DDAVP (Rare) ... 1841
Dantrium Capsules (Less frequent) 1619
Daraprim Tablets (Rare) ... 761
Depo-Medrol Sterile Aqueous Suspension ... 2334
Desyrel and Desyrel Dividose ... 1404

Diphtheria and Tetanus Toxoids and Pertussis Vaccine Adsorbed USP (For Pediatric Use) 892
Diprivan Injection (Less than 1%) 2267
E.E.S. (Isolated reports) 522
Elavil 2269
Eldepryl 2250
Endep Tablets 1927
Epogen for Injection (1.1% to 10%) 591
EryPed (Isolated reports) 519
Ery-Tab Tablets (Isolated reports) 521
Erythrocin Stearate Filmtab (Isolated reports) 523
Erythromycin Base Filmtab (Isolated reports) 525
Erythromycin Delayed-Release Capsules, USP (Isolated reports) 526
Ethmozine Tablets (Less than 2%) 946
Ethrane 599
Etrafon 2087
▲Exosurf Neonatal for Intratracheal Suspension (6% to 8%) 765
Fortaz (Less frequent) 1060
Guaifed 1615
Hexalen Capsules (1%) 2316
HibTITER (One case) 1206
▲Idamycin for Injection (4%) 564
IFEX (Occasional) 729
Isoptin Injectable (Occasional) 1177
K-Phos M.F. Tablets 659
K-Phos Neutral Tablets 660
K-Phos No. 2 Tablets 659
Lariam Tablets 1904
Leukeran Tablets (Rare) 788
Loxitane 1213
Ludiomil Tablets (Rare) 874
M-M-R II (Rare) 1494
M-R-VAX II (Rare) 1496
MS Contin Tablets (Infrequent) 1814
MSIR (Infrequent) 1817
Methergine 2016
Mexitil Capsules (About 2 in 1,000) 680
Myleran Tablets 790
Nalfon Pulvules & Tablets (Less than 1%) 919
Narcan Injection 933
Navane Capsules and Concentrate (Infrequent) 1954
Navane Intramuscular (Infrequent) 1956
NebuPent for Inhalation Solution (1% or less) 1017
Noroxin Tablets 1519
Norpramin Tablets 1340
▲Novantrone for Injection Concentrate (2 to 4%) 1226
Omnipaque 2552
Oramorph SR (Morphine Sulfate Sustained Release Tablets) (Less frequent) 1988
Orap Tablets 1020
Orthoclone OKT3 Sterile Solution (2 patients) 1645
PCE Dispertab Tablets (Isolated reports) 549
Pamelor 2019
Parlodel (38 cases) 2020
PedvaxHIB (Infrequent) 1521
Platinol 737
Platinol-AQ Injection 738
Primaxin I.M. 1532
Primaxin I.V. (0.4%) 1535
▲Procrit for Injection (1.1% to 10%) 1647
ProHIBiT Haemophilus b Conjugate Vaccine (Diphtheria Toxoid Conjugate) 896
ProSom Tablets (Infrequent) 554
▲Prostin VR Pediatric Sterile Solution (4%) 2355
Prozac Pulvules (12 among 6,000 patients) 920
Retrovir Capsules (0.8%) 802
Retrovir I.V. Infusion 805
Retrovir Syrup (0.8%) 802
Roferon-A Injection (Less than 1%) 1916
Rythmol Tablets (0.3%) 1184
Seldane Tablets 1349
Seldane-D Extended-Release Tablets 1350
Seromycin Pulvules 1298
Sinequan (Infrequent) 1960
Stadol (Less than 1%) 721
Suprax 1235
Surmontil Capsules 2524
Syntocinon Nasal Spray (1 case) 2033
Talwin Injection 2071
Talwin Compound 2072
Talwin Injection 2071
Tegretol Chewable Tablets 654
Tegretol Suspension 656
Tegretol Tablets 654
Tofranil Ampuls 1038
Tofranil Tablets 1039
Tofranil-PM Capsules 1041
Tonocard Tablets (Less than 1%) 1554
Trandate Injection 577
Trandate Tablets 579
Triavil Tablets 1556
Uroqid-Acid (Less frequent) 661
Vivactil Tablets 1567
Wellbutrin Tablets (Frequent) 821
Xanax Tablets 2367
Zefazone Sterile Powder 2372
Zinacef 1066
Zovirax Sterile Powder (Approximately 1%) 828

Seizures, convulsive
Aralen Hydrochloride Injection 2038
Aralen Phosphate Tablets 2039
Cipro I.V. (1% or less) 1592
Cipro Tablets (Less than 1%) 1589
Cylert Tablets 510
Flagyl I.V. 2131
Flagyl Tablets 2170
Mezlin 1597
Mezlin Pharmacy Bulk Package 1599
Phenergan Injection 2493
Phenergan Tablets 2496
Protostat Tablets 1674
Reglan (Rare) 1869
Robaxin Injectable 1871
Thorazine 2234
Timentin for Injection 2239
Trilafon 2123

Seizures, epileptiform
Cibalith-S 870
Eskalith 2214
Etrafon 2087
Lioresal Tablets 1031
Lithane Tablets 1596
Lithium Carbonate Capsules & Tablets 1984
Lithobid Tablets 870
Parlodel (4 cases) 2020

Seizures, grand mal
Brevibloc Injection (Less than 1%) 942
Haldol Decanoate 1375
Haldol Injection, Tablets and Concentrate 1373
Orap Tablets 1020
Paradione Capsules 548
Pepcid (Infrequent) 1524
Sodium Polystyrene Sulfonate Suspension (One case) 1993
Tacaryl 2409
Temaril Tablets, Syrup and Spansule Sustained Release Capsules 1085
Thorazine 2234
Tridione 557
Zofran Injection (Rare) 1069

Seminal volume, decrease in
Anadrol-50 Tablets 2287

Sensation, abnormal (see under Paresthesia)

Sensation, disturbance of temperature
▲Anestacon Solution (Among most common) 2394
Dopram Injectable 1860
Duranest Injections 624
Dyclone 0.5% and 1% Topical Solutions, USP 626
Ethmozine Tablets (Less than 2%) 946
IOPIDINE ⊙ 232
Omnipaque (Less than 0.1%) 2552
Tonocard Tablets (0.5-1.5%) 1554
Trexan Tablets (Less than 1%) 937
Xylocaine Injections 637
Xylocaine Injections for Ventricular Arrhythmias 639
Xylocaine 2% Jelly 643
Xylocaine 10% Oral Spray 645
4% Xylocaine-MPF Sterile Solution 641
Xylocaine 2% Viscous Solution 646

Sensation, heavy
Omnipaque (Less than 0.1%) 2552

Sensations, numbness
Duranest Injections 624
Dyclone 0.5% and 1% Topical Solutions, USP 626
Xylocaine Injections 637
Xylocaine Injections for Ventricular Arrhythmias 639
Xylocaine 2% Jelly 643
Xylocaine 10% Oral Spray 645
4% Xylocaine-MPF Sterile Solution 641
Xylocaine 2% Viscous Solution 646

Sensitivity, light
Isopto Atropine ⊙ 218
Isopto Homatropine ⊙ 221
Isopto Hyoscine ⊙ 222
Trexan Tablets (Less than 1%) 937
Tropicacyl ⊙ 209

Sensitivity, sun
Danocrine Capsules (Rare) 2046
Minocin Oral Suspension 1224
Retin-A (tretinoin) Cream/Gel/Liquid 1680
Terramycin Capsules 1786
Thorazine 2234

Sensitivity reactions
AVC 1322
AK-Mycin Ointment ⊙ 204
Alcaine (Occasional) ⊙ 210
Anestacon Solution (Rare) 2394
Anusol Ointment (Rare) ▣ 634
Auralgan Otic Solution 2437
Bactroban Ointment 2200
Betadine Skin Cleanser (Rare) 1812
Bleph-10 Liquifilm Sterile Ophthalmic Solution (Rare) 586
Bleph-10 Ophthalmic Ointment 10% (Rare) 586
Brevoxyl Gel 2264
Cetamide Ointment (Rare) ⊙ 220
Cleocin T Topical 2327
Coly-Mycin S Otic w/Neomycin & Hydrocortisone 1708
Congess 994
Cortisporin Otic Solution Sterile (Occasional) 760
Critic-Aid, Antimicrobial Skin Paste 2286
Cycrin Tablets (Occasional) 2449
Dorcol Children's Fever & Pain Reducer ▣ 686
Drithocreme 590
Dritho-Scalp 591
Dyclone 0.5% and 1% Topical Solutions, USP 626
Ethyl Chloride, U.S.P. (Extremely rare) 1022
FML-S Sterile Ophthalmic Suspension ⊙ 246
Fero-Folic-500 Filmtab 527
Fluori-Methane (Extremely rare) 1022
Fluro-Ethyl (Extremely rare) 1023
Gantrisin Ophthalmic Ointment/Solution 1900
Hibiclens Antimicrobial Skin Cleanser 2271
Hibistat Towelette 2272
Hyperab Rabies Immune Globulin (Human) 1574
Hyper-Tet Tetanus Immune Globulin (Human) (Rare) 1576
HypRho-D Mini-Dose Rh_0-D Immune Globulin (Human) (Rare) 1578
Iberet-Folic-500 Filmtab 527
Ilotycin Ophthalmic Ointment 915
Isopto Cetamide Solution (Rare) ⊙ 220
Luroscrub Antimicrobial Skin Cleanser 912
Metrodin (urofollitropin for injection) 2182
Mini-Gamulin Rh, Rh_0(D) Immune Globulin (Human) (Rare) 612
Monistat Dual-Pak 1657
Monistat 3 Vaginal Suppositories 1657
Mycelex 1% Cream and Topical Solution 1% 1604
Mycostatin Pastilles (Rare) 734
Naphcon Forte ⊙ 226
Nescaine/Nescaine MPF 629
Oreticyl 545
pHisoHex 2066
Pergonal (menotropins for injection, USP) 2184
Plague Vaccine (Rare) 1584
Polytrim Ophthalmic Solution Sterile (Rare) 588
Prinzide Tablets 1540
Provera Tablets 2356
Rauzide Tablets 1804
Renese Tablets 1785
Retrovir I.V. Infusion 805
Rogaine Topical Solution (1.27%) 2357
Sensorcaine 631
Sensorcaine-MPF Spinal 634
Thalitone Tablets 687
THROMBOGEN Topical Thrombin, USP, Transfer Needle 1153
Tylenol acetaminophen Children's Chewable Tablets & Elixir (Rare) 1366
Tylenol Allergy Sinus Medication Caplets and Gelcaps, Maximum Strength 1372
Tylenol Cold & Flu No Drowsiness Hot Medication, Packets (Rare) 1371
Tylenol Cold Medication No Drowsiness Formula Caplets (Rare) 1370
Tylenol Cold Night Time Medication Liquid (Rare) 1371
Tylenol, Extra Strength, acetaminophen Adult Liquid Pain Reliever (Rare) 1367
Tylenol, Extra Strength, acetaminophen Gelcaps, Caplets, Tablets (Rare) 1367
Tylenol, Infants' Drops (Rare) 1366
Tylenol, Junior Strength, acetaminophen Coated Caplets, Grape and Fruit Chewable Tablets (Rare) 1366
Tylenol, Maximum Strength, Sinus Medication Gelcaps, Caplets and Tablets (Rare) 1373
Tylenol, Regular Strength, acetaminophen Tablets and Caplets (Rare) 1367
Vasocidin Ointment (Rare) ⊙ 275
Vira-A Ophthalmic Ointment, 3% 1767
Zestoretic 2274

Sensorium, clouded
Blocadren Tablets 1429
Cartrol Tablets 507
Corgard Tablets 701
Corzide Tablets 702
Inderal 2459
Inderal LA Long Acting Capsules 2461
Inderide Tablets 2463
Inderide LA Long Acting Capsules 2465
Kerlone Tablets 2172
Levatol (Slight) 1832
Lopressor HCT Tablets 1034
Mexitil Capsules (1.9% to 2.6%) 680
Normodyne Tablets 2110
Normozide Tablets 2112
Sectral Capsules 2520
Tenoretic Tablets 1105
Tenormin Tablets and I.V. Injection 1107
Timolide Tablets 1547
Timoptic in Ocudose 1552
Timoptic Sterile Ophthalmic Solution 1550
Trandate HCT/Trandate 579
Visken Tablets 2036

Sensorium, dull
Diupres Tablets 1461
Enduronyl 518
Harmonyl Tablets 528
Hydropres Tablets 1485
Oreticyl 545
Raudixin Tablets 1803
Rauzide Tablets 1804
Salutensin/Salutensin-Demi 719
Ser-Ap-Es Tablets 881
Serpasil Tablets 883
Serpasil-Apresoline Tablets 884
Serpasil-Esidrix Tablets 886

Sensory deficit
Oncovin Solution Vials & Hyporets 1288

Sensory deficit, persistent
Duranest Injections 624

Sensory disturbances
Anafranil Capsules (Infrequent) 650
Carbocaine 956
Depo-Medrol Sterile Aqueous Suspension 2334

Sepsis
Cytosar-U Sterile Powder (One case) 2329
Cytovene Sterile Powder 2292
Ergamisol Tablets (1-2 patients) 1136
Exosurf Neonatal for Intratracheal Suspension (B 24% to 34%) 765
Intron A (Less than 1%) 2097
Leukine for IV Infusion 1127
▲Novantrone for Injection Concentrate (31 to 34%) 1226
Permax Tablets (Infrequent) 1291
Prokine for I.V. Infusion 1096

Prostin VR Pediatric Sterile Solution (2%) 2355
Rythmol Tablets 1184
Survanta Beractant Intratracheal Suspension 1978

Sepsis, intestinal

Cholybar (One case) 1705

Septicemia

Lippes Loop Intrauterine Double-S.. 1654
Orudis Capsules (Less than 1%) 2488
ParaGard T380A Intrauterine Copper Contraceptive 411
▲Sandimmune (4.8 to 5.3%) 2024
Tonocard Tablets (Less than 1%) 1554

Septic shock

ParaGard T380A Intrauterine Copper Contraceptive 411
Tonocard Tablets (Less than 1%) 1554

Seroma, subgaleal

Hemopad Absorbable Collagen Hemostat 627
INSTAT Collagen Absorbable Hemostat (Less than 1%) 1151

Serositis

Monopril Tablets (0.2 to 1.0%) 1406
Pronestyl Capsules and Tablets 1800
Pronestyl Injection 1798
Vaseretic Tablets 1559
Vasotec I.V. 1562
Vasotec Tablets 1564

Serum alkaline phosphatase, elevation

Accutane Capsules (1 in 5 to 1 in 10) 1878
Atgam Sterile Solution 2320
Axid Pulvules 1246
Azactam for Injection (Less than 1%) 2252
BiCNU 723
Bumex (0.4%) 1895
Calan SR Caplets 2157
Calan Tablets 2155
Capoten 2255
Capozide 2258
Cardizem Tablets-30 mg, 60 mg, 90 mg and 120 mg (Less than 1%) 1329
Cardizem SR Capsules-60 mg, 90 mg and 120 mg (1%) 1327
Ceclor Pulvules & Suspension (1 in 40) 1251
▲Cefizox Injection (1 to 5%) 1012
Cefotan (1 in 700) 2265
Ceftin Tablets 575
Ceptaz for Injection (One in 23) 1057
▲CHEMET (succimer) Capsules (4.2 to 10.4%) 1361
▲Cipro I.V. (Among most frequent) 1592
Cipro Tablets (0.8%) 1589
Claforan Sterile Injection (Less than 1%) 1089
Colestid Granules (One or more occasions) 2328
Cytotec (Infrequent) 2159
Dalgan Injection 620
Dalmane Capsules (Rare) 1927
Depen Titratable Tablets (Few reports) 2379
Elspar 1470
Ergamisol Tablets (Less frequent) 1136
▲Sterile FUDR (Among more common) 1898
▲Fortaz (1 in 23) 1060
Fungizone Intravenous 2262
▲Hexalen Capsules (9%) 2316
Imuran (Less than 1%) 768
Inderide Tablets 2463
▲Intron A (3% to 6%) 2097
Isoptin Oral Tablets 1179
Isoptin SR Sustained Release Tablets 1181
Keftab Tablets 917
Kefzol Vials, Faspak & ADD-Vantage (Rare) 1279
Klonopin Tablets 1902
Larodopa Tablets 1905
Loniten Tablets 2346
Lopid Capsules and Tablets (Occasional) 1736
Lorelco Tablets 1333
▲Lupron Depot 7.5 mg (5.4%) 2311
Mandol Vials, Faspak & ADD-Vantage 1281
Meclomen Capsules 1739
Mefoxin 1498
Mefoxin Premixed Intravenous Solution 1500
Mevacor Tablets 1505
Mezlin 1597
Mezlin Pharmacy Bulk Package 1599
Mithracin 1602
Monocid Injection (1.6%) 2217
Monopril Tablets 1406
Nalfon Pulvules & Tablets (Less than 1%) 919
Navane Capsules and Concentrate 1954
Navane Intramuscular 1956
▲Neupogen for Injection (27 to 58%) 595
Nimotop Capsules (0.2%) 1607
Noroxin Tablets (1.4%) 1519
Norpramin Tablets 1340
Parafon Forte DSC Caplets 1379
▲Paraplatin for Injection (24% to 37%) 735
Parlodel 2020
Prilosec Delayed-Release Capsules (Less than 1%) 1530
Primaxin I.M. 1532
Primaxin I.V. 1535
Procardia XL Tablets (Rare) 1783
Proglycem 649
Rifadin 1345
Rifamate Capsules 1347
Rimactane Capsules (Rare) 879
Rocephin Injectable Vials, ADD-Vantage (Less than 1%) 1914
▲Roferon-A Injection (8% to 11%) 1916
Rythmol Tablets (0.2%) 1184
Sectral Capsules 2520
Sinemet Tablets 952
Suprax (Less than 2%) 1235
Tambocor Tablets (Rare) 1315
▲Tazicef for Injection (1 in 23 patients) 2231
▲Tegison Capsules (10-25%) 1881
Timentin for Injection 2239
Unasyn 1965
Verelan Capsules 1243
Winstrol Tablets 2075
Xanax Tablets (Less than 1% to 1.7%) 2367
Zefazone Sterile Powder 2372
Zinacef (1 in 50 patients) 1066

Serum amylase, elevation

Cipro I.V. (Rare) 1592
Cipro Tablets (Less than 0.1%) 1589
Cuprimine Capsules (Few cases) 1442
Cytotec (Infrequent) 2159

Serum bicarbonate content, variations

▲Bumex (3.1%) 1895
▲Ganite Injection (40 to 50%) 1016

Serum bilirubin, elevation (see under Hyperbilirubinemia)

Serum bilirubin levels, abnormalities

Bumex (0.8%) 1895
Doral Tablets (Less than 1%) 2383
Emcyt Capsules (2 to 3%) 1161
Imuran 768
Kefurox Vials, Faspak & ADD-Vantage (1 in 500) 1277
Kefzol Vials, Faspak & ADD-Vantage (Rare) 1279
Nebcin Vials, Hyporets & ADD-Vantage 1286
Roferon-A Injection (Less than 1% to 2%) 1916
Sinemet Tablets 952
Sinemet CR Tablets 953
Xanax Tablets (Less than 1% to 1.6%) 2367

Serum calcium, depression (see under Hypocalcemia)

Serum calcium content, variations

Bumex (2.4%) 1895

Serum calcium decrease (see under Hypocalcemia)

Serum cholesterol, increase (see under Hypercholesterolemia)

Serum creatine phosphokinase, elevation

Catapres Tablets (Rare) 676
▲Cipro I.V. (Among most frequent) 1592
Combipres Tablets (Rare) 678
Normozide Tablets (Less than 1%) 2112
Quinidex Extentabs 1868
Xylocaine Injections for Ventricular Arrhythmias 639

Serum creatinine, elevation

Altace Capsules (Less than 1% to 1.5%) 1086
Amikin Injectable 602
Anadrol-50 Tablets 2287
Ancobon Capsules 1886
Atgam Sterile Solution 2320
Azactam for Injection 2252
Azo Gantrisin Tablets 1888
Bactrim DS Tablets 1891
Bactrim I.V. Infusion 1889
Bactrim 1891
▲Bumex (7.4%) 1895
Capoten 2255
Capozide 2258
Ceclor Pulvules & Suspension (Less than 1 in 500) 1251
Cefizox Injection (Occasional) 1012
Cefobid Intravenous/Intramuscular (1 in 48) 1943
Cefobid Pharmacy Bulk Package - Not for Direct Infusion (1 in 48) 1945
Ceftin Tablets 575
Ceptaz for Injection (Occasional) 1057
Children's Advil Suspension (Occasional) 2426
▲Cipro I.V. (Among most frequent) 1592
Cipro Tablets (1.1%) 1589
Cytovene Sterile Powder (1% or less) 2292
Didronel I.V. Infusion 1307
Diulo 2129
Dyazide Capsules 2208
Dyrenium Capsules (Rare) 2210
Ergamisol Tablets (Less frequent) 1136
Eulexin Capsules 2089
Feldene Capsules (1 to 3%) 1777
Fortaz (Occasional) 1060
Fungizone Intravenous 2262
▲Ganite Injection (12.5%) 1016
Gantanol 1899
Gantrisin 1901
Glucotrol 1952
▲Hexalen Capsules (7%) 2316
Hydrea Capsules (Occasional) 728
IFEX 729
Indocin I.V. 1490
Intron A (2%) 2097
Keftab Tablets 917
Kefurox Vials, Faspak & ADD-Vantage 1277
Leukine for IV Infusion 1127
Lodine Capsules (Less than 1%) 2468
Loniten Tablets 2346
Lotensin Tablets (About 2%) 872
Lozol Tablets (Less than 5%) 1843
▲Lupron Depot 3.75 mg (Among most frequent) 2312
Lupron Depot 7.5 mg 2311
Lupron Injection (Less than 5%) 2310
Mandol Vials, Faspak & ADD-Vantage 1281
Maxzide 1215
Mefoxin 1498
Mefoxin Premixed Intravenous Solution 1500
Mezlin 1597
Mezlin Pharmacy Bulk Package 1599
Mithracin 1602
Monocid Injection (Occasional) 2217
Monopril Tablets 1406
Motrin Tablets (Occasional) 2351
Mutamycin (2%) 733
Mykrox ½ mg Tablets 984
Nebcin Vials, Hyporets & ADD-Vantage 1286
▲Normodyne Injection (8%) 2108
Noroxin Tablets (Less frequent) 1519
Norpace (Less than 1%) 2177
▲Paraplatin for Injection (10%) 735
PediaProfen Suspension (Occasional) 1363
▲Pentam 300 Injection (23.1%) 1018
Pipracil 1230
Platinol 737
Platinol-AQ Injection 738
Prilosec Delayed-Release Capsules (Less than 1%) 1530
Primaxin I.M. 1532
Primaxin I.V. 1535
Prinivil Tablets (2%) 1538
Prinzide Tablets 1540
Procardia XL Tablets (Rare) 1783
Proloprim Tablets 799
▲Rocaltrol Capsules (1 in 6) 1913
Rocephin Injectable Vials, ADD-Vantage (Less than 1%) 1914
Roferon-A Injection (Less than 1% to 2%) 1916
Rufen Tablets 691
Septra 813
Septra I.V. Infusion 808
Septra I.V. Infusion ADD-Vantage Vials 810
Septra 813
Sinemet CR Tablets 953
Suprax (Less than 2%) 1235
Tagamet 2228
Tazicef for Injection (Occasional) 2231
Tazidime Vials, Faspak & ADD-Vantage (Occasional) 1299
▲Tegison Capsules (1-10%) 1881
Timentin for Injection 2239
▲Trandate Injection (8 of 100 patients) 577
Trilisate (Less than 1%) 1822
Trimpex Tablets 1922
Unasyn 1965
Vancocin HCl, Oral Solution & Pulvules (Rare) 1304
Vancocin HCl, Vials & ADD-Vantage (A few dozen cases) 1302
Vaseretic Tablets (About 0.6%) 1559
Vasotec I.V. (0.5 to 1%) 1562
Vasotec Tablets (0.5% to 1%) 1564
Xanax Tablets (1.9% to 2.2%) 2367
Zantac Injection and Zantac Injection Premixed 1063
Zantac 1065
Zaroxolyn Tablets 989
Zefazone Sterile Powder 2372
Zestoretic 2274
Zestril Tablets (About 2%) 2277
Zinacef 1066
▲Zovirax Sterile Powder (5% to 10%) 828

Serum electrolyte changes (see under Electrolyte imbalance)

Serum fibrogen, decrease

Trental (Rare) 1099

Serum PBI levels, decrease (see under PBI decrease)

Serum phosphorus content, variations

▲Bumex (4.5%) 1895
Colestid Granules 2328

Serum potassium, reduction (see under Hypokalemia)

Serum proteins, changes

Bumex (0.7%) 1895
Doral Tablets (Less than 1%) 2383

Serum sickness

Amoxil 2193
Antivenin (Black Widow Spider) 1422
Antivenin (Crotalidae) Polyvalent 2430
▲Atgam Sterile Solution (Less than 1% to a majority of patients) 2320
Augmentin Tablets, Powder for Oral Suspension, and Chewable Tablets 2198
Azo Gantanol Tablets 1887
Azo Gantrisin Tablets 1888
Azulfidine Tablets, EN-tabs, Oral Suspension (Rare) 1157
Bactrim DS Tablets 1891
Bactrim I.V. Infusion 1889
Bactrim 1891
Bicillin C-R Injection 2438
Bicillin C-R 900/300 Injection 2440
Bicillin L-A Injection 2442
Butazolidin Capsules & Tablets (Less than 1%) 1027
Ceclor Pulvules & Suspension (0.05%-0.024%) 1251
Children's Advil Suspension (Less than 1%) 2426
Fansidar Tablets 1896
Feldene Capsules (Less than 1%) 1777
Flagyl I.V. 2131
Gantanol 1899
Gantrisin Ophthalmic Ointment/Solution 1900
Gantrisin 1901
Intal Inhaler (Rare) 979
Intal Nebulizer Solution 980
Lincocin 2344

Meclomen Capsules (Less than 1%) 1739
Motrin Tablets (Less than 1%) 2351
Nasalcrom Nasal Solution (Rare) 986
Orthoclone OKT3 Sterile Solution (2 Patients) 1645
PediaProfen Suspension (Less than 1%) 1363
Pediazole 1973
Pfizerpen for Injection 1957
Pfizerpen-AS Aqueous Suspension 1959
Pneumovax 23 (Rare) 1528
Protostat Tablets 1674
Prozac Pulvules (Rare) 920
Quadrinal Tablets 1183
Recombivax HB (Less than 1%) 1544
Rocephin Injectable Vials, ADD-Vantage (Rare) 1914
Rufen Tablets (Less than 1%) 691
Septra 813
Septra I.V. Infusion 808
Septra I.V. Infusion ADD-Vantage Vials 810
Septra 813
Suprax (Rare) 1235
Thiosulfil Forte Tablets 2526
Tolectin (200, 400 and 600 mg) (Less than 1%) 1379
Unipen 2533
Wycillin Injection 2537

Serum transaminase, elevation

Atromid-S Capsules 2435
Bactrim DS Tablets 1891
Bactrim I.V. Infusion 1889
Bactrim 1891
BiCNU 723
Calan SR Caplets 2157
Calan Tablets 2155
Capoten 2255
CeeNU (Small percentage) 725
Cordarone Tablets 2446
Depakote Sprinkle Capsules (Frequent) 512
DiaBeta (Isolated cases) 1091
Diflucan Injection and Tablets (1% of 4048 patients) 1948
▲Eminase (Less than 10%) 2211
Ethrane 599
Eulexin Capsules 2089
▲Sterile FUDR (Among more common) 1898
Garamycin Injectable 2093
▲INH Tablets (10 to 20%) 868
Imuran 768
Inderide Tablets 2463
Inderide LA Long Acting Capsules 2465
Isoptin Oral Tablets (Less than 1%) 1179
Isoptin SR Sustained Release Tablets 1181
Klonopin Tablets 1902
Lariam Tablets (Occasional) 1904
Leukine for IV Infusion 1127
Lopid Capsules and Tablets 1736
Lorelco Tablets 1333
Lotensin Tablets (Scattered incidents) 872
Meclomen Capsules 1739
Methotrexate Tablets, Parenteral, LPF Parenteral 1217
Mevacor Tablets (1.9%) 1505
Micronase Tablets 2350
Mithracin 1602
Monopril Tablets 1406
Nardil (Common) 1742
Navane Capsules and Concentrate (Infrequent) 1954
Navane Intramuscular (Infrequent) 1956
Nebcin Vials, Hyporets & ADD-Vantage 1286
Netromycin Injection 100 mg/ml (15 of 1000 patients) 2104
▲Normodyne Injection (4%) 2108
▲Normodyne Tablets (4%) 2110
▲Normozide Tablets (4%) 2112
Plendil Extended-Release Tablets (2 episodes) 1526
Proloprim Tablets 799
Rheumatrex Methotrexate Dose Pack 1234
Rifadin 1345
▲Rifamate Capsules (10% to 20%) 1347
Rimactane Capsules (Rare) 879
Rythmol Tablets (0.2%) 1184
Seldane Tablets (1 case) 1349
Seldane-D Extended-Release Tablets 1350
Septra 813
Septra I.V. Infusion 808
Septra I.V. Infusion ADD-Vantage Vials 810
Septra 813
Seromycin Pulvules 1298
Tagamet 2228
Tambocor Tablets (Rare) 1315
▲Trandate HCT Tablets (4% of patients) 579
▲Trandate Injection (4% of patients) 577
Trilisate (Rare) 1822
Trimpex Tablets 1922
Ultracef Capsules, Tablets & Oral Suspension 722
Vascor (200, 300 and 400 mg) Tablets (Approximately 1%) 1383
Verelan Capsules 1243
Yutopar (Less than 1% (with IV administration)) 647
Zovirax Sterile Powder (1% to 2%) 828

Serum triglyceride, elevation (see under Hypertriglyceridemia)

Sexual activity, decrease

▲Catapres Tablets (About 3 in 100 patients) 676
▲Catapres-TTS (3%) 677
Combipres Tablets (About 3%) 678
Stilphostrol Tablets and Ampuls 1609
TACE 12 and 25 mg 1353

Sexual activity, increase

Fiorinal with Codeine Capsules 2008

Sexual dysfunction

Adalat Capsules (10 mg and 20 mg) (2% or less) 1587
Arfonad Ampuls 1887
Carbocaine Hydrochloride Injection 2043
Cardizem Tablets-30 mg, 60 mg, 90 mg and 120 mg (Less than 1%) 1329
Cardizem SR Capsules-60 mg, 90 mg and 120 mg (Less than 1%) 1327
Cardura Tablets (2%) 1941
Catapres-TTS (2 of 101 patients) 677
Duranest Injections 624
Eldepryl 2250
Eskalith 2214
Levatol (0.5%) 1832
Marcaine Hydrochloride with Epinephrine 1:200,000 2055
Marcaine Hydrochloride Injection 2055
Marcaine Spinal 2058
Marplan Tablets (Rare) 1906
Maxzide 1215
Monopril Tablets 1406
Nardil (Common) 1742
Nescaine/Nescaine MPF 629
Procardia Capsules (2% or less) 1781
Prozac Pulvules (1.9%) 920
Rogaine Topical Solution 2357
Sensorcaine 631
Sensorcaine-MPF Spinal 634
Trexan Tablets (Less than 1%) 937
Wellbutrin Tablets (Frequent) 821
Wytensin Tablets (3% or less) 2542
▲Xanax Tablets (7.4%) 2367
Xylocaine Injections 637
▲Zoladex (21%) 1110

Shivering (see under Trembling)

Shock

AK-Fluor Injection 10% and 25% ◎ 204
Antivenin (Crotalidae) Polyvalent 2430
AquaMEPHYTON Injection 1422
Aralen Hydrochloride Injection 2038
Calciparine Injection (Rare) 925
Coumadin Injection & Tablets 944
Demerol 2047
Demulen 2161
Desferal Vials 862
Dilaudid-HP Injection 1175
Diphtheria and Tetanus Toxoids and Pertussis Vaccine Adsorbed USP (For Pediatric Use) (Rare) 892
Dolophine Hydrochloride Ampoules & Vials 1260
Dolophine Hydrochloride Tablets 1261
▲Eminase (Less than 10%) 2211
Enovid 2161
Etrafon 2087
Floropryl Sterile Ophthalmic Ointment (Infrequent) 1473
Fluorescite ◎ 217
Fungizone Intravenous 2262
Heparin Lock Flush Solution (Rare) 2456
Heparin Sodium Vials (Rare) 1264
Heparin Sodium Injection (Rare) 2457
Heparin Sodium Injection, USP, Sterile Solution (Rare) 2342
Humorsol Sterile Ophthalmic Solution (Infrequent) 1475
Hyperstat I.V. Injection 2095
Imferon 976
Indocin Capsules (Less than 1%) 1487
Indocin I.V. (Less than 1%) 1490
Indocin (Less than 1%) 1487
Klorvess Effervescent Granules 2010
Klorvess Effervescent Tablets 2011
Klorvess 10% Liquid 2010
Lippes Loop Intrauterine Double-S 1654
MS Contin Tablets 1814
MSIR 1817
Mepergan Injection 2479
Methadone Hydrochloride Diskets 1284
Methadone Hydrochloride Oral Solution & Tablets 1987
Midamor Tablets 1508
Omnipaque 2552
Orudis Capsules (Less than 1%) 2488
Permax Tablets (Infrequent) 1291
Pitressin Synthetic, Ampoules 1758
Prostin VR Pediatric Sterile Solution (Less than 1%) 2355
Rifadin (Rare) 1345
Rifamate Capsules (Rare) 1347
Roxanol 1991
Sandoglobulin I.V. (Rare) 2027
Sus-Phrine Injection 1006
Talwin Injection (Infrequent) 2071
Thorazine 2234
Tri-Immunol Diphtheria & Tetanus Toxoids & Pertussis Vaccine, Adsorbed (1 per 1,750) 1241
Trilafon 2123
Vancocin HCl, Vials & ADD-Vantage 1302
Zefazone Sterile Powder 2372

Shock, anaphylactic (see under Anaphylactic shock)

Sialadenitis

Aldoclor Tablets 1413
Aldomet Ester HCl Injection 1417
Aldomet Oral 1415
Aldoril Tablets 1418
Apresazide Capsules 854
Apresoline-Esidrix Tablets 857
Capozide 2258
Corzide Tablets (Occasional) 702
Diucardin Tablets 2450
Diulo 2129
Diupres Tablets 1461
Diuril Oral Suspension 1464
Diuril Sodium Intravenous 1463
Diuril Tablets 1464
Dyazide Capsules 2208
Enduron Tablets 517
Esidrix Tablets 863
Esimil Tablets 864
HydroDIURIL Tablets 1484
Hydropres Tablets 1485
Inderide Tablets 2463
Inderide LA Long Acting Capsules 2465
Lopressor HCT Tablets 1034
Lozol Tablets 1843
Macrodantin Capsules 1624
Maxzide 1215
Moduretic Tablets 1510
Mykrox ½ mg Tablets 984
Naturetin Tablets (Occasional) 1789
Normozide Tablets 2112
Permax Tablets (Rare) 1291
Prinzide Tablets 1540
Rauzide Tablets 1804
Ser-Ap-Es Tablets 881
Serpasil-Esidrix Tablets 886
Timolide Tablets 1547
Trandate HCT Tablets 579
Vaseretic Tablets 1559
Zaroxolyn Tablets 989
Zestoretic 2274

Sialadenopathy

Tapazole Tablets 1298

Sialism (see under Salivation)

Sialorrhea

Albuminar-5, Albumin (Human) U.S.P. 5% 608
Albuminar-25, Albumin (Human) U.S.P. 25% 608
Diprivan Injection (Less than 1%) 2267
Haldol Decanoate 1375
Intron A (Less than 1%) 2097
Larodopa Tablets (Relatively frequent) 1905
Mestinon Injectable 1115
Mestinon 1116
NebuPent for Inhalation Solution (1% or less) 1017
Norzine (Occasional) 1818
Prostigmin Injectable 1120
Prostigmin Tablets 1121
Roferon-A Injection (Less than 1%) 1916
Sinemet Tablets 952
Sinemet CR Tablets 953
Tensilon Injectable 1123
Torecan (Occasional) 1993

Sialosis (see under Salivation)

Sickle cell disease

Levlen/Tri-Levlen 665
Loestrin 1728
Norlestrin 1746
Levlen/Tri-Levlen 665

Sinoatrial block

Blocadren Tablets (Less than 1%) 1429

Sinoatrial node dysfunction

Cordarone Tablets 2446
Eskalith 2214

Sinus arrest

Cordarone Tablets 2446
Rythmol Tablets (Less than 1%) 1184
Tambocor Tablets (1-3%) 1315
Tonocard Tablets (Less than 1%) 1554

Sinus bradycardia

Brethaire Inhaler 1024
▲Cardizem SR Capsules-60 mg, 90 mg and 120 mg (3%) 1327
Catapres Tablets (Rare) 676
Catapres-TTS (Rare) 677
Children's Advil Suspension (Less than 1%) 2426
Combipres Tablets (Rare) 678
Cordarone Tablets (2 to 5%) 2446
Desyrel and Desyrel Dividose (Occasional) 1404
Eldepryl 2250
Eminase 2211
Lanoxicaps 772
Lanoxin Elixir Pediatric 775
Lanoxin Injection 778
Lanoxin Injection Pediatric 781
Lanoxin Tablets 783
PediaProfen Suspension (Less than 1%) 1363
Rufen Tablets (Less than 1%) 691
Tambocor Tablets (1-3%) 1315
Vascor (200, 300 and 400 mg) Tablets (0.5 to 2.0%) 1383

Sinus congestion

▲AeroBid Inhaler System (3-9%) 995
Desyrel and Desyrel Dividose 1404
▲Lupron Depot 3.75 mg (Among most frequent) 2312
Lupron Depot 7.5 mg 2311
▲Lupron Injection (5% or more) 2310
Mykrox ½ mg Tablets (Less than 2%) 984
Nasacort Nasal Inhaler (Less than 5%) 1844

Sinus discomfort

AeroBid Inhaler System (1-3%) 995

Sinus drainage

Alferon N Injection (2%) 1809

Sinusitis

▲AeroBid Inhaler System (3-9%) 995
▲Anafranil Capsules (2% to 6%) 650
Brevibloc Injection (2 patients) 942
Cardene Capsules (Rare) 2290
Cardura Tablets (Less than 0.5% of 3960 patients) 1941
Cartrol Tablets (Less common) 507
Ethmozine Tablets (Less than 2%) 946
Hytrin Tablets (2.6%) 529
▲Intron A (Up to 21%) 2097
Kerlone Tablets (Less than 2%) 2172
Lodine Capsules (Less than 1%) 2468
Lotensin Tablets 872
Monopril Tablets (0.2 to 1.0%) 1406
Permax Tablets (Infrequent) 1291

Plendil Extended-Release Tablets (0.5% to 1.5%) 1526
Prinivil Tablets (1% or less) 1538
Prinzide Tablets (0.3 to 1%) 1540
Procardia XL Tablets (1% or less) 1783
ProSom Tablets (Infrequent) 554
Prozac Pulvules (2.1%) 920
Retrovir Capsules (Less than 5%) 802
Retrovir I.V. Infusion (Less than 5%) 805
Retrovir Syrup (Less than 5%) 802
Roferon-A Injection (Less than 3%) 1916
▲ Rogaine Topical Solution (7.16%) 2357
▲ Sandimmune (Up to 7%) 2024
Trexan Tablets (Less than 1%) 937
Zestoretic (0.3 to 1%) 2274
Zestril Tablets (Less than 1%) 2277

Sinus syndrome, sick

Rythmol Tablets (Less than 1%) 1184

Sinus tachycardia

Aramine Injection 1424
Children's Advil Suspension (Less than 1%) 2426
PediaProfen Suspension (Less than 1%) 1363
Rufen Tablets (Less than 1%) 691
Seldane Tablets 1349
Seldane-D Extended-Release Tablets 1350
Vascor (200, 300 and 400 mg) Tablets (0.5 to 2.0%) 1383

Skin, anesthesia (see under Numbness, skin)

Skin, burning

A/T/S Topical Gel and Topical Solution 1089
Clear By Design Medicated Cleansing Pads ▣ 709
Cleocin T Topical 2327
Cortenema (Rare) 2244
▲ Diprolene (6%) 2083
Drysol 1772
Efudex 1880
Epifoam 1828
▲ Exelderm Cream 1.0% (3%) 2398
Exelderm Solution 1.0% (Approximately 1%) 2399
Gastrocrom Capsules (Infrequent) 974
Halog (Infrequent) 2399
Halotex Cream & Solution 2400
Loprox Cream 1% and Lotion 1% 1095
MetroGel (Less than 2%) 903
Monistat Dual-Pak 1657
Oxsoralen Lotion 1% 1116
Oxsoralen-Ultra Capsule 1117
Proctofoam-HC 1835
Trisoralen Tablets 1125
Tronothane Hydrochloride Cream 558
▲ Ultravate Cream 0.05% (4%) 2410
Ultravate Ointment 0.05% (1.6%) 2411

Skin, cracking

Aclovate Ointment (1 of 366 patients) 1053
Sandostatin Injection (Less than 1%) 2029
Temovate (1 of 366 patients) 1056

Skin, darkening

Cytoxan for Injection 726

Skin, discoloration

AK-Fluor Injection 10% and 25% ⊙ 204
Anafranil Capsules (Infrequent) 650
Android 1111
Atabrine Hydrochloride Tablets 2041
Azulfidine Tablets, EN-tabs, Oral Suspension (Rare) 1157
Brevibloc Injection (Less than 1%) 942
Compazine 2201
Cordarone Tablets (Less than 1%) 2446
Drithocreme 590
Dritho-Scalp 591
Ergamisol Tablets (Up to 2%) 1136
Estrace 1385
Estrace Vaginal Cream 1388
Estratest 2245
Fluorescite Syringe ⊙ 217
Imferon 976
Intron A (Less than 1%) 2097
Lamprene Capsules (More than 1%) 1030
Minocin Oral Suspension 1224
Orudis Capsules (Less than 1%) 2488
Parlodel 2020
Permax Tablets (Infrequent) 1291
Prozac Pulvules (Rare) 920
Quadrinal Tablets 1183
Retin-A (tretinoin) Cream/Gel/Liquid 1680
SSD RP Cream (Infrequent) 690
Silvadene Cream 1% 1352
Sotradecol (Sodium Tetradecyl Sulfate Injection) 964
Stelazine 2226
Tegretol Chewable Tablets 654
Tegretol Suspension 656
Tegretol Tablets 654
Temaril Tablets, Syrup and Spansule Sustained Release Capsules 1085

Skin, dryness

▲ A/T/S Topical Gel and Topical Solution (17 out of 90) 1089
▲ Accutane Capsules (80%) 1878
Actigall Capsules 2280
Alphatrex Cream, Ointment & Lotion (Infrequent) 2076
Anafranil Capsules (Up to 2%) 650
Ansaid Tablets (Less than 1%) 2319
Aristocort A (Infrequent) 1010
Atromid-S Capsules 2435
Bactroban Ointment (Less than 1%) 2200
Benzac 5 & 10 Gel 1682
Benzac AC 1681
Benzac 1682
Benzamycin Topical Gel (3 out of 153) 907
Betatrex Cream, Ointment & Lotion 2077
BuSpar (Infrequent) 1401
Cardura Tablets (Less than 0.5% of 3960 patients) 1941
Clear By Design Medicated Cleansing Pads ▣ 709
Clearasil 10% Benzoyl Peroxide Acne Medication Vanishing Lotion ▣ 658
Clearasil Double Textured Pads - Regular and Maximum Strength ▣ 658
Clearasil Maximum Strength ▣ 658
Cleocin T Topical (Most common) 2327
Corgard Tablets (1 to 5 of 1000 patients) 701
Cortifoam 1827
Corzide Tablets (1 to 5 of 1000 patients) 702
Cyclocort Lotion (Infrequent) 1198
▲ Desquam-E Gel (2 in 50 patients) 2397
▲ Desquam-X Gel (2 in 50 patients) 2397
▲ Desquam-X 5 Wash (2 in 50 patients) 2397
▲ Desquam-X 10 Bar (2 in 50 patients) 2397
▲ Desquam-X 10 Wash (2 in 50 patients) 2397
▲ Diprolene (4%) 2083
Donnagel (Rare) ▣ 675
Donnagel-PG (Rare) 1858
Eldecort Cream 1.0% (Infrequent) 1113
Eldecort Cream 1.0% and 2.5% (Infrequent) 1113
Elocon (Infrequent) 2084
Emcyt Capsules (2%) 1161
Epifoam 1828
Ergamisol Tablets 1136
Ethmozine Tablets (Less than 2%) 946
Sterile FUDR (Remote possibility) 1898
Florone/Florone E 908
Fluorouracil Injection 1897
Fungizone Cream, Lotion and Ointment 2261
Halog (Infrequent) 2399
Hytone 909
▲ Intron A (Up to 10%) 2097
▲ Lamprene Capsules (8-28%) 1030
Lomotil 2174
Lotrisone Cream (Infrequent) 2103
Lupron Depot 7.5 mg 2311
Lupron Injection (Less than 5%) 2310
Metrodin (urofollitropin for injection) 2182
MetroGel (Less than 2%) 903
Mexitil Capsules (About 1 in 1,000) 680
Motofen Tablets 836
Mykrox ½ mg Tablets (Less than 2%) 984
Myleran Tablets (Rare) 790
Mytrex Cream & Ointment (Infrequent) 2080
NebuPent for Inhalation Solution (1% or less) 1017
Neutrogena Melanex Topical Solution 1618
Niacor Tablets 2376
Nicolar Tablets 1846
Nizoral 2% Shampoo (One occurrence in 41 patients) 1144
Orabase HCA Oral Paste (Infrequent) 890
Oxy Clean ▣ 720
Oxy 10 Daily Face Wash Antibacterial Skin Wash ▣ 721
Oxy-5 and Oxy-10 Tinted and Vanishing Formulas with Sorboxyl ▣ 719
pHisoHex 2066
Pepcid (Infrequent) 1524
Permax Tablets (Infrequent) 1291
Prilosec Delayed-Release Capsules (Less than 1%) 1530
Proctofoam-HC 1835
ProSom Tablets (Rare) 554
Prozac Pulvules (Infrequent) 920
Psorcon Ointment 0.05% 909
Psorion Cream 0.05% (Infrequent) 1121
▲ Roferon-A Injection (5% to 13%) 1916
Rogaine Topical Solution 2357
▲ Tegison Capsules (50-75%) 1881
Ultravate Cream 0.05% (Less frequent) 2410
Ultravate Ointment 0.05% 2411
Vanoxide-HC Acne Lotion 911
Vioform-Hydrocortisone Cream and Mild Cream 889
Vioform-Hydrocortisone Ointment 889
Vytone Cream 1% 911
Wellbutrin Tablets (Infrequent) 821

Skin, eruptions

▲ Anaprox and Anaprox DS Tablets (3-9%) 2288
Antabuse Tablets (Occasional) 2429
Aralen Hydrochloride Injection 2038
Atabrine Hydrochloride Tablets (Infrequent) 2041
Azo Gantanol Tablets 1887
Bactrim DS Tablets 1891
Bactrim I.V. Infusion 1889
Bactrim 1891
Calcidrine Syrup 506
Cosmegen Injection 1440
Cytosar-U Sterile Powder (Less frequent) 2329
Daranide Tablets 1445
Depen Titratable Tablets (Rare) 2379
Dilantin with Phenobarbital Kapseals 1715
E.E.S. 522
Easprin 1719
EryPed 200 & EryPed 400 Granules 519
Ery-Tab Tablets 521
Erythrocin Stearate Filmtab 523
Fansidar Tablets 1896
Gantanol 1899
Gantrisin Ophthalmic Ointment/Solution 1900
Gantrisin 1901
Halotestin Tablets 2341
INH Tablets 868
Ilotycin Gluceptate, IV, Vials 915
Librax Capsules (Rare) 1929
Libritabs Tablets (Isolated cases) 1930
Librium Capsules (Isolated cases) 1931
Librium Injectable (Isolated instances) 1932
Mellaril (Infrequent) 2011
Menrium Tablets (Rare) 1934
Micronase Tablets (1.5%) 2350
Milontin Kapseals 1741
Mysoline (Occasional) 2480
▲ Naprosyn (3 to 9%) 2297
Orinase Tablets (1.1%) 2354
PCE Dispertab Tablets 549
Pediazole 1973
Phenobarbital Elixir and Tablets (Rare) 1293
Pima Syrup 994
Plaquenil Sulfate Tablets 2067
Provera Tablets 2356
Rifamate Capsules 1347
Seldane Tablets (1.6%) 1349
Septra 813
Septra I.V. Infusion 808
Septra I.V. Infusion ADD-Vantage Vials 810
Septra 813
Tessalon Perles 1006
Thiosulfil Forte Tablets 2526
Tolinase Tablets (0.4%) 2365
Yodoxin 1072
Zyloprim Tablets (Less than 1%) 830

Skin, erythema

Gastrocrom Capsules (Infrequent) 974
pHisoHex 2066
Plaquenil Sulfate Tablets 2067
Terramycin Intramuscular Solution 1964
Vibramycin Hyclate Intravenous 1968

Skin, fluorescence

AK-Fluor Injection 10% and 25% ⊙ 204

Skin, fragile

▲ Accutane Capsules (Up to 80%) 1878
Sandostatin Injection (Less than 1%) 2029

Skin, fragility

Aristocort Suspension 1008
Aristospan Suspension 1011
Celestone Soluspan Suspension 2081
Cortenema 2244
Cortone Acetate Sterile Suspension 1437
Cortone Acetate Tablets 1439
Cuprimine Capsules 1442
Decadron Elixir 1445
Decadron Phosphate Injection 1449
Decadron Phosphate Respihaler 1454
Decadron Phosphate Turbinaire 1456
Decadron Phosphate with Xylocaine Injection, Sterile 1451
Decadron Tablets 1447
Decadron-LA Sterile Suspension 1457
Deltasone Tablets 2332
Depen Titratable Tablets (Rare) 2379
Depo-Medrol Sterile Aqueous Suspension 2334
Hydeltrasol Injection, Sterile 1476
Hydeltra-T.B.A. Sterile Suspension 1478
Hydrocortone Acetate Sterile Suspension 1479
Hydrocortone Phosphate Injection, Sterile 1481
Hydrocortone Tablets 1482
Kenalog-10 Injection 2402
Kenalog-40 Injection 2403
Medrol 2348
Pediapred Oral Liquid 987
Solu-Cortef Sterile Powder 2361
Solu-Medrol Sterile Powder 2363
▲ Tegison Capsules (50-75%) 1881

Skin, hypertrophy

Anafranil Capsules (Rare) 650
Prozac Pulvules (Rare) 920

Skin, infection

▲ Accutane Capsules (1 in 20) 1878
▲ Sandimmune (7.0 to 10.1%) 2024

Skin, irritation

Acnomel Cream ▣ 615
Alphatrex Cream, Ointment & Lotion (Infrequent) 2076
Betadine Solution 1812
Betadine Surgical Scrub (Rare) 1812
Betatrex Cream, Ointment & Lotion 2077
Blocadren Tablets 1429
Chap Stick Petroleum Jelly Plus with Sunblock 15 ▣ 671
Clear By Design Medicated Cleansing Pads ▣ 709
Clearasil Double Textured Pads - Regular and Maximum Strength ▣ 658
Compazine 2201
Cortisporin Cream 757
Cortisporin Ointment 758
Diprolene (1%) 2083
Drithocreme 590
Dritho-Scalp 591
Elocon (Infrequent) 2084
Epifoam 1828
Flex-all 454 Pain Relieving Gel ▣ 546
Halog (Infrequent) 2399
Icy Hot ▣ 659
Intron A 2097
Lotrimin 2102
Lotrisone Cream 2103
MG 217 ▣ 734
Mantadil Cream 789
MetroGel (Less than 2%) 903
Mycelex 1% Cream and Topical Solution 1% 1604
Mytrex Cream & Ointment (Rare) 2080
Neutrogena Melanex Topical Solution 1618
Neutrogena Sunblock ▣ 630

Occlusal 1045
Occlusal-HP 1045
Orap Tablets 1020
Oxy Night Watch Nighttime Acne Medication-Maximum Strength and Sensitive Skin Formulas ▣ 721
P & S Liquid ▣ 509
P & S Plus Tar Gel ▣ 510
Panafil (Occasional) 1995
Proctofoam-HC 1835
Questran Light (Less frequent) 711
SalAc 1045
Sebulex Antiseborrheic Treatment Shampoo 2408
Selsun Rx 2.5% Selenium Sulfide Lotion, USP 1977
Stelazine 2226
▲ Tegison Capsules (50-75%) 1881
Timolide Tablets 1547
Timoptic in Ocudose 1552
Timoptic Sterile Ophthalmic Solution 1550
Tolectin (200, 400 and 600 mg) (1 to 3%) 1379
Ultra Mide 25 ▣ 510
X-Seb Plus Conditioning Shampoo ▣ 510
X-Seb T Shampoo ▣ 510
X-Seb T Plus Conditioning Shampoo ▣ 510
Xerac AC 1773

Skin, lesions
Lupron Injection (Less than 5%) 2310
Procan SR Tablets (Common) 1760

Skin, maceration
Aclovate Cream 1053
Alphatrex Cream, Ointment & Lotion (Infrequent) 2076
Analpram-HC Rectal Cream 1% and 2.5% 970
Betatrex Cream, Ointment & Lotion 2077
Carmol HC Cream 1% (Infrequent) 2296
Cortisporin Cream 757
Cyclocort Lotion (Infrequent) 1198
Dalalone D.P. Injectable 999
Decadron Phosphate Topical Cream 1455
Decaspray Topical Aerosol 1459
Diprolene (Less than 1%) 2083
Eldecort Cream 1.0% (Infrequent) 1113
Eldecort Cream 1.0% and 2.5% (Infrequent) 1113
Elocon (Infrequent) 2084
Epifoam 1828
Florone/Florone E 908
Halog (Infrequent) 2399
Hytone 909
Kenalog Cream, Lotion & Ointment (Infrequent) 2401
Lidex (Infrequent) 2296
Lotrisone Cream (Infrequent) 2103
Maxivate Cream, Lotion & Ointment 0.05% 2406
Monistat Dual-Pak 1657
Mycolog II Cream and Ointment (Infrequent) 2407
Mytrex Cream & Ointment (Infrequent) 2080
NeoDecadron Topical Cream 1518
Neo-Synalar Cream (Infrequent) 2296
Otic Tridesilon Solution 0.05% (Infrequent) 1612
Pramosone Cream, Lotion & Ointment 971
Proctofoam-HC 1835
Psorcon Ointment 0.05% 909
Psorion Cream 0.05% (Infrequent) 1121
Synacort Creams 1%, 2.5% (Infrequent) 2296
Synalar (Infrequent) 2296
Temovate 1056
Topicort (Infrequent) 1098
Tridesilon Creme 0.05% (Infrequent) 1611
Tridesilon Ointment 0.05% (Infrequent) 1611
Vanoxide-HC Acne Lotion 911
Vioform-Hydrocortisone Cream and Mild Cream 889
Vioform-Hydrocortisone Ointment 889
Vytone Cream 1% 911
Westcort 2411

Skin, nodule
Permax Tablets (Rare) 1291

Skin, oiliness
Cleocin T Topical 2327
Trexan Tablets (Less than 1%) 937

Skin, photoallergic reactions
Feldene Capsules (Less than 1%) 1777
Rufen Tablets (Less than 1%) 691

Skin, phototoxic eruptions
Proloprim Tablets 799
Trimpex Tablets 1922

Skin, tenderness
▲ Blenoxane (50%) 724
Efudex 1880
Konakion Injection (Rare) 1903
Naftin Gel 1% (0.5%) 1084

Skin atrophy
Aclovate 1053
Alphatrex Cream, Ointment & Lotion (Infrequent) 2076
Analpram-HC Rectal Cream 1% and 2.5% 970
Anusol-HC Cream (Infrequent) 1690
Aristocort A (Infrequent) 1010
Betatrex Cream, Ointment & Lotion 2077
Carmol HC Cream 1% (Infrequent) 2296
Cortisporin Cream 757
Cortisporin Ointment 758
Cortisporin Otic Solution Sterile 760
Cortisporin Otic Suspension Sterile 760
Cutivate Cream 0.05% 1054
Cutivate Ointment 0.005% (Infrequent to more frequent) 1054
Cyclocort 1198
Decadron Phosphate Topical Cream 1455
Decaspray Topical Aerosol 1459
DesOwen Cream, Ointment and Lotion (Infrequent) 1682
Diprolene (Less than 1%) 2083
Eldecort Cream 1.0% (Infrequent) 1113
Eldecort Cream 1.0% and 2.5% (Infrequent) 1113
Elocon (3 of 319 patients) 2084
Epifoam 1828
Etrafon 2087
Florone/Florone E 908
Halog (Infrequent) 2399
Hytone 909
Kenalog Cream, Lotion & Ointment (Infrequent) 2401
Lidex (Infrequent) 2296
Locoid Cream, Ointment and Topical Solution (Infrequent) 970
Lotrisone Cream (Infrequent) 2103
Mantadil Cream 789
Maxivate Cream, Lotion & Ointment 0.05% 2406
Mycolog II Cream and Ointment (Infrequent) 2407
Mytrex Cream & Ointment (Infrequent) 2080
NeoDecadron Sterile Ophthalmic Ointment 1517
NeoDecadron Sterile Ophthalmic Solution 1518
NeoDecadron Topical Cream 1518
Neo-Synalar Cream (Infrequent) 2296
Nutracort Cream & Lotion (Infrequent) 1684
Otic Tridesilon Solution 0.05% (Infrequent) 1612
PediOtic Suspension Sterile 797
Pramosone Cream, Lotion & Ointment 971
ProctoCream-HC (Infrequent) 1834
Proctofoam-HC 1835
Psorcon Ointment 0.05% 909
Psorion Cream 0.05% (Infrequent) 1121
Synacort Creams 1%, 2.5% (Infrequent) 2296
Synalar (Infrequent) 2296
Tegison Capsules (Less than 1%) 1881
Temovate (1 of 366 patients) 1056
Topicort (Infrequent) 1098
Tridesilon Creme 0.05% (Infrequent) 1611
Tridesilon Ointment 0.05% (Infrequent) 1611
Ultravate Cream 0.05% (Less frequent) 2410
Ultravate Ointment 0.05% 2411
Vanoxide-HC Acne Lotion 911
Vioform-Hydrocortisone Cream and Mild Cream 889
Vioform-Hydrocortisone Ointment 889
Vytone Cream 1% 911
Westcort 2411

Skin eruptions, pleomorphic
Aralen Phosphate Tablets 2039

Skin odor, abnormal
Anafranil Capsules (Up to 2%) 650

Skin reactions
Adriamycin RDF 562
▲ Catapres-TTS (51 of 101 patients) 677
Cefobid Intravenous/Intramuscular (1 in 45) 1943
Cefobid Pharmacy Bulk Package - Not for Direct Infusion (1 in 45) 1945
Compazine 2201
Cortisporin Otic Suspension Sterile 760
Doxorubicin Hydrochloride Injection, USP 848
▲ Epogen for Injection (7.0% to 10%) 591
▲ Exelderm Cream 1.0% 2398
Exelderm Solution 1.0% (Infrequent) 2399
Furacin Topical Solution 0.2% (1.1%) 1855
Insulatard NPH 1626
Insulatard NPH Human 1627
Kutapressin Injection 2146
Lanoxicaps (Rare) 772
Lanoxin Elixir Pediatric (Rare) 775
Lanoxin Injection (Rare) 778
Lanoxin Injection Pediatric (Rare) 781
Lanoxin Tablets (Rare) 783
Lupron Depot 7.5 mg (Less than 5%) 2311
Lupron Injection (Less than 5%) 2310
Mixtard 70/30 1627
Mixtard Human 70/30 1628
ParaGard T380A Intrauterine Copper Contraceptive 411
Primaxin I.M. 1532
Primaxin I.V. (Less than 0.2%) 1535
▲ Procrit for Injection (7% to 10%) 1647
Rifadin 1345
Rubex 739
Synalgos-DC Capsules 2525
Tegison Capsules (Less than 1%) 1881
Velosulin 1627
Velosulin Human 1628

Skin test reactions, suppression
Aristocort Suspension 1008
Aristospan Suspension 1011
Celestone Soluspan Suspension 2081
Cortenema 2244
Cortone Acetate Sterile Suspension 1437
Cortone Acetate Tablets 1439
Decadron Elixir 1445
Decadron Phosphate Injection 1449
Decadron Phosphate Respihaler 1454
Decadron Phosphate Turbinaire 1456
Decadron Phosphate with Xylocaine Injection, Sterile 1451
Decadron Tablets 1447
Decadron-LA Sterile Suspension 1457
Deltasone Tablets 2332
Depo-Medrol Sterile Aqueous Suspension 2334
Hydeltrasol Injection, Sterile 1476
Hydeltra-T.B.A. Sterile Suspension 1478
Hydrocortone Acetate Sterile Suspension 1479
Hydrocortone Phosphate Injection, Sterile 1481
Hydrocortone Tablets 1482
Kenalog-10 Injection 2402
Kenalog-40 Injection 2403
Medrol 2348
Pediapred Oral Liquid 987

Skull abnormalities, fetal
Accutane Capsules 1878
Capoten 2255
Capozide 2258

Sleep, disturbances
Actigall Capsules 2280
Adalat Capsules (10 mg and 20 mg) (2% or less) 1587
▲ Anafranil Capsules (4% to 9%) 650
Ativan Tablets (Less frequent) 2434
Cibalith-S 870
▲ Clozaril Tablets (4%) 2000
Cordarone Tablets (1 to 3%) 2446
Corgard Tablets 701
Corzide Tablets 702
Dalgan Injection (Less than 1%) 620
Danocrine Capsules 2046
Deprol Tablets 2382
Doral Tablets (Rare) 2383
Eldepryl 2250
▲ Ethmozine Tablets (2%-5%) 946
Floxin Tablets (1% to 3%) 1652
Halcion Tablets 2340
HibTITER 1206
Hylorel Tablets (2.1%) 975
Lithium Carbonate Capsules & Tablets 1984
Lithobid Tablets 870
Lopressor 1032
Lupron Depot 7.5 mg 2311
▲ Lupron Injection (5% or more) 2310
▲ Mexitil Capsules (7.1% to 7.5%) 680
Monopril Tablets (0.2 to 1.0%) 1406
Nardil (Common) 1742
Parlodel 2020
Procardia Capsules (2% or less) 1781
ProSom Tablets (Infrequent) 554
Proventil Syrup (Less than 1 of 100) 2119
Recombivax HB (Less than 1%) 1544
▲ Roferon-A Injection (5%) 1916
Sinemet CR Tablets 953
Tofranil Ampuls 1038
Tofranil Tablets 1039
Tonocard Tablets (Less than 1%) 1554
▲ Trexan Tablets (Greater than 10%) 937
Triavil Tablets 1556
Trinalin Repetabs Tablets 1170
Valium Tablets 1939
Ventolin Syrup (Less than 1 of 100 patients) 583
Verelan Capsules (1.4%) 1243
Versed Injection (Less than 1%) 1924
Vontrol Tablets 2243
▲ Wellbutrin Tablets (4.0%) 821
Wytensin Tablets (3% or less) 2542
Xanax Tablets (Rare) 2367
Zarontin Capsules 1768
Zarontin Syrup 1769

Sleepiness (see under Drowsiness)

Sleeplessness (see under Insomnia)

Sloughing
AK-Taine (Rare) ⊙ 207
Alcaine (Rare) ⊙ 210
Aramine Injection 1424
Depo-Medrol Sterile Aqueous Suspension 2334
Dilantin Parenteral 1712
Efudex 1880
Fluoracaine (Rare) ⊙ 208
Fluorescite Syringe ⊙ 217
Intropin Injection 930
Ophthetic ⊙ 249
Robaxin Injectable 1871
Scleromate 1685
Sotradecol (Sodium Tetradecyl Sulfate Injection) 964
Talwin Injection 2071
Velban Vials 1305

Smell, disturbances
▲ AeroBid Inhaler System (3-9%) 995
BuSpar (Infrequent) 1401
Cordarone Tablets (1 to 3%) 2446
Intron A (Less than 1%) 2097
Lorelco Tablets 1333
Maxair Inhaler (Less than 1%) 1311
Nasalide Nasal Solution 0.025% (5% or less) 2299
NebuPent for Inhalation Solution (1% or less) 1017
Rythmol Tablets (Less than 1%) 1184
Timentin for Injection 2239
Tonocard Tablets (Less than 1%) 1554

Smell, loss of the sense (see under Anosmia)

Smoker's tongue (see under Leukoplakia, oral)

Sneezing
▲ AeroBid Inhaler System (3-9%) 995
Afrin ▣ 692
Azactam for Injection (Less than 1%) 2252
▲ Beconase AQ Nasal Spray (4%) 574
▲ Beconase Inhalation Aerosol & Refill (10 in 100 patients) 574
Bentyl 1322
Carbocaine Hydrochloride Injection 2043

Clozaril Tablets (Less than 1%) 2000
Diprivan Injection (Less than 1%) .. 2267
Dristan Long Lasting Nasal Spray, Regular and Regular with Metered Dose Pump 2419
Dristan Nasal Spray, Regular and Regular with Metered Pump 2419
4-Way Fast Acting Nasal Spray - Original Formula (regular & mentholated) & Metered Spray Pump (regular) 751
4-Way Long Lasting Nasal Spray & Metered Spray Pump 751
Intal Inhaler (Rare) 979
Intal Nebulizer Solution 980
Intron A (1% or less) 2097
Marcaine Hydrochloride with Epinephrine 1:200,000 (Rare) 2055
Marcaine Hydrochloride Injection (Rare) 2055
Marcaine Spinal (Rare) 2058
Methadone Hydrochloride Diskets .. 1284
Nasacort Nasal Inhaler (Less than 5%) 1844
▲ Nasalcrom Nasal Solution (1 in 10) 986
Nasalide Nasal Solution 0.025% (5% or less) 2299
Nescaine/Nescaine MPF 629
Nicorette 1335
Omnipaque 2552
Plendil Extended-Release Tablets (0.5% to 1.5%) 1526
Quadrinal Tablets 1183
Sensorcaine (Rare) 631
Sensorcaine-MPF Spinal (Rare) 634
Surgicel (Occasional) 1151
Trexan Tablets (Less than 1%) 937
▲ Vancenase AQ Nasal Spray 0.042% (About 4%) 2127
▲ Vancenase Nasal Inhaler (10 per 100 patients) 2126

Social reaction, anti See Sociopathy (see under Sociopathy)

Sociopathy
Prozac Pulvules (Rare) 920

Sodium depletion (see under Hyponatremia)

Sodium loss (see under Hyponatremia)

Sodium retention
Anadrol-50 Tablets 2287
Android 1111
Aristocort Suspension 1008
Aristospan Suspension 1011
Butazolidin Capsules & Tablets (Less than 1%) 1027
Celestone Soluspan Suspension 2081
Cortenema 2244
Cortone Acetate Sterile Suspension 1437
Cortone Acetate Tablets 1439
Dalalone D.P. Injectable 999
Decadron Elixir 1445
Decadron Phosphate Injection 1449
Decadron Phosphate Respihaler 1454
Decadron Phosphate Turbinaire 1456
Decadron Phosphate with Xylocaine Injection, Sterile 1451
Decadron Tablets 1447
Decadron-LA Sterile Suspension 1457
Deltasone Tablets 2332
Depo-Medrol Sterile Aqueous Suspension 2334
▲ Estratest (Among most common) .. 2245
Halotestin Tablets 2341
Hydeltrasol Injection, Sterile 1476
Hydeltra-T.B.A. Sterile Suspension 1478
Hydrocortone Acetate Sterile Suspension 1479
Hydrocortone Phosphate Injection, Sterile 1481
Hydrocortone Tablets 1482
Hyperstat I.V. Injection 2095
Kayexalate 2053
Kenalog-10 Injection 2402
Kenalog-40 Injection 2403
Loniten Tablets 2346
Mediatric Capsules 2476
Medrol 2348
Metandren Linguets and Tablets 875
Pediapred Oral Liquid 987
Premarin with Methyltestosterone .. 2515
Proglycem (Frequent) 649
Sodium Polystyrene Sulfonate Suspension 1993
Solu-Cortef Sterile Powder 2361
Solu-Medrol Sterile Powder 2363
Testred Capsules 1124
Winstrol Tablets 2075

Somnambulism
Anafranil Capsules (Infrequent) 650
Halcion Tablets 2340

Somnolence (see under Drowsiness)

Soreness, injection site
▲ Alferon N Injection (10%) 1809
▲ Engerix-B Unit-Dose Vials (22%) 2213
Hyperab Rabies Immune Globulin (Human) 1574
Hyper-Tet Tetanus Immune Globulin (Human) 1576

Soreness, vaginal
Femstat Prefill Vaginal Cream 2% (0.2%) 2295
Femstat Vaginal Cream 2% (0.2%) 2295
Mycelex-G 500 mg Vaginal Tablets (1 in 149 patients) 1606

Sore throat (see under Throat, soreness)

Spasm, biliary tract
Demerol 2047
Dilaudid-HP Injection 1175
Dolophine Hydrochloride Ampoules & Vials 1260
Dolophine Hydrochloride Tablets 1261
MS Contin Tablets (Infrequent) 1814
MSIR (Infrequent) 1817
Methadone Hydrochloride Diskets .. 1284
Methadone Hydrochloride Oral Solution & Tablets 1987
Oramorph SR (Morphine Sulfate Sustained Release Tablets) (Less frequent) 1988
Pantopon Injectable 1911
Phenergan with Codeine 2497
Phenergan VC with Codeine 2501
Roxanol 1991
Trilafon 2123

Spasm, blepharal tract
BAL in Oil Ampules 661

Spasm, gastrointestinal
Fiorinal with Codeine Capsules 2008

Spasm, generalized
Anafranil Capsules (Rare) 650

Spasm, vesical sphincters
Anexsia 5/500 Tablets 2196
Anexsia 7.5/650 Tablets 2197
Azdōne Tablets 844
Damason-P 1356
Hycodan Syrup, Tablets 927
Lortab ASA Tablets 2414
Tussionex Extended-Release Suspension 988
Vicodin ES Tablets 1189

Speech, bulbar type
Reglan 1869

Speech, incoherent
AK-Pentolate ...... ◉ 204
Clozaril Tablets (Less than 1%) 2000
Cyclogyl (Common) ...... ◉ 215
Cyclomydril ...... ◉ 216
Marcaine Spinal 2058
Sensorcaine 631
Sensorcaine-MPF Spinal 634

Speech, slurring
BuSpar (Rare) 1401
Centrax (Less frequent) 1693
Cibalith-S 870
Clozaril Tablets (1%) 2000
Coly-Mycin M Parenteral 1706
Corgard Tablets (1 to 5 of 1000 patients) 701
Corzide Tablets (1 to 5 of 1000 patients) 702
Dalgan Injection (Less than 1%) 620
Dalmane Capsules (Rare) 1927
Deprol Tablets 2382
Desyrel and Desyrel Dividose (Less than 1%) 1404
▲ Dilantin Infatabs (Among most common) 1710
▲ Dilantin Kapseals (Among most common) 1708
Dilantin Parenteral (Among most common) 1712
▲ Dilantin-30 Pediatric/Dilantin-125 Suspension (Among most common) 1713
▲ Dilantin with Phenobarbital Kapseals (Among most common) 1715
Doral Tablets 2383
Equagesic Tablets 2451
Eskalith 2214
Etrafon 2087
Fiorinal with Codeine Capsules 2008
Halcion Tablets 2340
Klonopin Tablets 1902
Lioresal Tablets 1031
Lithane Tablets 1596
Lithium Carbonate Capsules & Tablets 1984
Lithobid Tablets 870
Loxitane 1213
Matulane Capsules 1907
Mebaral Tablets 2061
Miltown Tablets 2386
PMB 200 and PMB 400 2504
Serax Capsules 2522
Serax Tablets 2522
Serentil 686
Symmetrel Capsules & Syrup (0.1-1%) 936
Tonocard Tablets (Less than 1%) .. 1554
Tranxene 556
Trilafon 2123
Valium Injectable 1937
Valium Tablets (Infrequent) 1939
Valrelease Capsules (Occasional) 1923
Versed Injection (Less than 1%) 1924
Xanax Tablets 2367

Speech difficulties
Clozaril Tablets (Less than 1%) 2000
▲ Demser Capsules (10%) 1460
Ethmozine Tablets (Less than 2%) 946
Mexitil Capsules (2.6%) 680
Nubain Injection (Less than 1%) 934

Speech disturbances
Anafranil Capsules (Up to 3%) 650
Bentyl 1322
Brevibloc Injection (Less than 1%) 942
Dantrium Capsules (Less frequent) 1619
Doral Tablets 2383
Duragesic Transdermal System (1% or greater) 1133
Eldepryl 2250
Intron A (Less than 1%) 2097
Kerlone Tablets (Less than 2%) 2172
Levsin/Levsinex 2147
Omnipaque 2552
Permax Tablets (1.1%) 1291
Rythmol Tablets (Less than 1%) 1184
Tambocor Tablets (Less than 1%) 1315
Tegretol Chewable Tablets 654
Tegretol Suspension 656
Tegretol Tablets 654
Tonocard Tablets (Less than 1%) .. 1554

Spermatogenesis, changes
Thiotepa Parenteral 1240

Spermatogenesis, defective
Methotrexate Tablets, Parenteral, LPF Parenteral 1217
Mustargen 1514
Rheumatrex Methotrexate Dose Pack 1234

Spermatogenesis, inhibition
Cytoxan for Injection 726

Spinal block
Carbocaine Hydrochloride Injection 2043
Duranest Injections 624
Marcaine Hydrochloride with Epinephrine 1:200,000 2055
Marcaine Hydrochloride Injection 2055
Marcaine Spinal 2058
Nescaine/Nescaine MPF 629
Novocain Hydrochloride for Spinal Anesthesia 2065
Xylocaine Injections 637

Spinal cord, compression
Gelfoam Sterile Sponge 2338
Zoladex (Isolated cases) 1110

Spinal fluid proteins, elevation
Temaril Tablets, Syrup and Spansule Sustained Release Capsules 1085

Spinal fracture
▲ Lupron Depot 3.75 mg (Among most frequent) 2312
Lupron Depot 7.5 mg 2311
Lupron Injection 2310

Spinal stenosis
Gelfoam Sterile Sponge 2338

Splenic infarction
Lamprene Capsules (Less than 1%) 1030

Splenomegaly
Apresazide Capsules (Less frequent) 854
Apresoline Hydrochloride Parenteral (Ampuls) 856
Apresoline Hydrochloride Tablets (Less frequent) 855
Apresoline-Esidrix Tablets 857
Garamycin Injectable 2093
NebuPent for Inhalation Solution (1% or less) 1017
▲ Neupogen for Injection (3%) 595
Permax Tablets (Rare) 1291
RhoGAM Rh_0(D) Immune Globulin (Human) (One patient) 1651
Ser-Ap-Es Tablets 881
Serpasil-Apresoline Tablets 884

Spotting
Amen 833
Aygestin Tablets 2437
Brevicon 2304
BuSpar (Infrequent) 1401
Cycrin Tablets 2449
Cytotec (0.7%) 2159
Danocrine Capsules 2046
Demulen 2161
Depo-Provera Sterile Aqueous Suspension 2336
Enovid 2161
Estinyl Tablets 2085
Estrace 1385
Estrace Vaginal Cream 1388
Estraderm Transdermal System 866
Estratest 2245
Estrovis 1721
Jenest-28 Tablets 1636
Levlen/Tri-Levlen 665
Lippes Loop Intrauterine Double-S.. 1654
Lo/Ovral Tablets 2471
Lo/Ovral-28 Tablets 2476
Loestrin 1728
Meclomen Capsules 1739
Mediatric Capsules 2476
Menrium Tablets 1934
Micronor Tablets 1667
Modicon 1667
Nordette-21 Tablets 2481
Nordette-28 Tablets 2483
Norethin 2133
Norinyl 2304
Norlestrin 1746
Norlutate 1754
Norlutin 1755
▲ Norplant System (17.1%) 2484
Nor-Q D Tablets 2304
Ogen 540
Ortho-Cyclen Tablets 1658
Ortho-Novum 1667
Ovral Tablets 2490
Ovral-28 Tablets 2491
Ovrette Tablets 2492
PMB 200 and PMB 400 2504
ParaGard T380A Intrauterine Copper Contraceptive 411
Premarin Intravenous 2508
Premarin with Methyltestosterone .. 2515
Premarin Tablets 2510
Premarin Vaginal Cream 2512
Provera Tablets 2356
TACE 12 and 25 mg 1353
Levlen/Tri-Levlen 665
Tri-Norinyl 2304
Triphasil-21 Tablets 2527
Triphasil-28 Tablets 2532
Verelan Capsules (1% or less) 1243

Sputum, discoloration
Lamprene Capsules (Greater than 1%) 1030

Sputum, increase
▲ AeroBid Inhaler System (3-9%) 995
Anafranil Capsules (Infrequent) 650
Tegison Capsules (Less than 1%) .. 1881
Ventolin Inhalation Solution (1.5%) 583

Status epilepticus

Depakote Sprinkle Capsules (Strong possibility) 512
Tegretol Chewable Tablets 654
Tegretol Suspension 656
Tegretol Tablets 654

Steatorrhea

Cholybar (Less frequent) 1705
Imuran (Less than 1%) 768
Questran Light (Less frequent) 711
Questran Powder 710

Stenosis, subglottic

Survanta Beractant Intratracheal Suspension 1978

Stevens-Johnson syndrome

AK-Cide Sterile Ophthalmic Ointment & Suspension ⊙ 202
Anaprox and Anaprox DS Tablets (Rare) 2288
Ancef Injection 2194
Apresazide Capsules 854
Apresoline-Esidrix Tablets 857
Augmentin Tablets, Powder for Oral Suspension, and Chewable Tablets (Rare) 2198
Azo Gantanol Tablets 1887
Azo Gantrisin Tablets 1888
Azulfidine Tablets, EN-tabs, Oral Suspension (Rare) 1157
Bactrim DS Tablets (Rare) 1891
Bactrim I.V. Infusion 1889
Bactrim (Rare) 1891
Bleph-10 Liquifilm Sterile Ophthalmic Solution (Isolated incident) 586
Bleph-10 Ophthalmic Ointment 10% (Isolated incident) 586
Butazolidin Capsules & Tablets (Less than 1%) 1027
Calan SR Caplets (1% or less) 2157
Calan Tablets (1% or less) 2155
Capoten 2255
Capozide 2258
Ceclor Pulvules & Suspension (Rare) 1251
Ceftin Tablets 575
Celontin 1692
Ceptaz for Injection 1057
Cetamide Ointment (Isolated incident) ⊙ 220
Children's Advil Suspension (Less than 1%) 2426
Cipro I.V. (1% or less) 1592
Cipro Tablets 1589
Cleocin HCl Capsules 2322
Cleocin Pediatric Flavored Granules 2324
Cleocin Phosphate Injection 2325
Clinoril Tablets (Less than 1 in 100) 1433
Danocrine Capsules 2046
Deprol Tablets (Rare) 2382
Diamox Parenteral 1200
Diamox Sequels (Sustained Release) 1201
Diamox Tablets 1200
Diflucan Injection and Tablets 1948
Dilantin Infatabs 1710
Dilantin Kapseals 1708
Dilantin Parenteral 1712
Dilantin-30 Pediatric/Dilantin-125 Suspension 1713
Dilantin with Phenobarbital Kapseals 1715
Dolobid Tablets (Less than 1 in 100) 1465
Enduron Tablets 517
Engerix-B Unit-Dose Vials 2213
Equagesic Tablets (Rare) 2451
Esidrix Tablets 863
Esimil Tablets 864
FML-S Sterile Ophthalmic Suspension (Rare) ⊙ 246
Fansidar Tablets 1896
Feldene Capsules (Less than 1%) 1777
Floxin Tablets 1652
Fortaz 1060
Gantanol 1899
Gantrisin Ophthalmic Ointment/Solution 1900
Gantrisin 1901
Indocin Capsules (Less than 1%) 1487
Indocin I.V. (Less than 1%) 1490
Indocin (Less than 1%) 1487
Isoptin Oral Tablets (Less than 1%) 1179
Isoptin SR Sustained Release Tablets (Less than 1%) 1181
Isopto Cetamide Solution (Isolated incident) ⊙ 220
Keflex Pulvules, Oral Suspension & Pediatric Drops (Rare) 916
Keftab Tablets (Rare) 917
Kefurox Vials, Faspak & ADD-Vantage 1277
Lincocin (Rare) 2344
Lodine Capsules (Rare) 2468
Loniten Tablets (Rare) 2346
Lopressor HCT Tablets 1034
Lozol Tablets 1843
Macrodantin Capsules (Rare) 1624
Meclomen Capsules (Less than 1%) 1739
Mesantoin Tablets 2013
Metimyd ⊙ 306
Mevacor Tablets 1505
Mexitil Capsules (Rare) 680
Milontin Kapseals 1741
Miltown Tablets (Rare) 2386
Minocin Intravenous (Rare) 1221
Minocin Oral Suspension (Rare) 1224
Minocin Pellet-Filled Capsules (Rare) 1222
Mintezol 1510
Motrin Tablets (Less than 1%) 2351
Nalfon Pulvules & Tablets (Less than 1%) 919
Naprosyn (Rare) 2297
Neptazane Tablets ⊙ 311
Noroxin Tablets 1519
PMB 200 and PMB 400 (Rare) 2504
PediaProfen Suspension (Less than 1%) 1363
Pediazole 1973
Pentam 300 Injection (0.2%) 1018
Phenobarbital Elixir and Tablets (Rare) 1293
Pipracil (Rare) 1230
Proloprim Tablets (Rare) 799
Rufen Tablets (Less than 1%) 691
SSD RP Cream 690
Septra 813
Septra I.V. Infusion 808
Septra I.V. Infusion ADD-Vantage Vials (Rare) 810
Septra 813
Ser-Ap-Es Tablets 881
Serpasil-Esidrix Tablets 886
Silvadene Cream 1% 1352
Sodium Sulamyd (Isolated incident) 2122
Sultrin (Frequent) 1675
Suprax (Rare) 1235
Tagamet (Very rare) 2228
Tegretol Chewable Tablets (Extremely rare) 654
Tegretol Suspension (Extremely rare) 656
Tegretol Tablets (Extremely rare) 654
Thiosulfil Forte Tablets 2526
Tonocard Tablets (Less than 1%) 1554
Trancopal Caplets (Rare) 2075
Trimpex Tablets (Rare) 1922
Ultracef Capsules, Tablets & Oral Suspension 722
Uniphyl 400 mg Tablets 1823
Vancocin HCl, Oral Solution & Pulvules 1304
Vancocin HCl, Vials & ADD-Vantage 1302
Vaseretic Tablets 1559
Vasocidin Ointment (Isolated incident) ⊙ 275
Vasocidin Ophthalmic Solution (Isolated incident) ⊙ 276
Vasosulf ⊙ 279
Vasotec I.V. 1562
Vasotec Tablets 1564
Verelan Capsules (Less than 1%) 1243
Voltaren Tablets (Rare) 1042
Zarontin Capsules 1768
Zarontin Syrup 1769
Zefazone Sterile Powder 2372
Zinacef (Rare) 1066

Stimulation

Anafranil Capsules (Infrequent) 650
Centrax (Less frequent) 1693
Dalmane Capsules (Rare) 1927
Placidyl Capsules 553
Proventil Repetabs Tablets 2120
Proventil Syrup 2119
Proventil Tablets 2120
Serax Capsules 2522
Serax Tablets 2522
Sinemet Tablets 952
Sinemet CR Tablets 953
Toradol IM Injection (1% or less) 2302
Valium Injectable 1937
Valium Tablets 1939
Valrelease Capsules (Infrequent) 1923
Xanax Tablets (Rare) 2367

Stinging

Aci-Jel Therapeutic Vaginal Jelly (Occasional cases) 1652
Aclovate Ointment (1 of 366 patients) 1053
Adriamycin PFS 561
Adriamycin RDF 562
Afrin ▣ 692
AK-Taine (Occasional) ⊙ 207
Alcaine ⊙ 210
Americaine Anesthetic Lubricant 972
Americaine Otic Topical Anesthetic Ear Drops 973
Attenuvax 1424
Bactroban Ointment (1.5%) 2200
▲ Betagan (1 in 3 patients) ⊙ 239
Biavax II 1427
Bleph-10 Liquifilm Sterile Ophthalmic Solution 586
Bleph-10 Ophthalmic Ointment 10% 586
Carmol 20 Cream ▣ 732
Chloromycetin Ophthalmic Ointment, 1% (Occasional) 1696
Chloromycetin Ophthalmic Solution 1696
Chloroptic S.O.P. ⊙ 243
Chloroptic Sterile Ophthalmic Solution ⊙ 243
Cortisporin Otic Solution Sterile 760
Cyclocort Lotion (Infrequent) 1198
▲ Diprivan Injection (10% or greater) 2267
▲ Diprolene (6%) 2083
Doxorubicin Hydrochloride Injection, USP 848
Dristan Long Lasting Nasal Spray, Regular and Regular with Metered Dose Pump 2419
Dristan Nasal Spray, Regular and Regular with Metered Pump 2419
Dyclone 0.5% and 1% Topical Solutions, USP 626
▲ Elimite (permethrin) 5% Cream (10%) 1082
Elocon Ointment 0.1% (7 of 812 patients) 2084
▲ Exelderm Cream 1.0% (3%) 2398
Exelderm Solution 1.0% (Approximately 1%) 2399
4-Way Fast Acting Nasal Spray - Original Formula (regular & mentholated) & Metered Spray Pump (regular) 751
4-Way Long Lasting Nasal Spray & Metered Spray Pump 751
Floropryl Sterile Ophthalmic Ointment 1473
Fluoracaine (Occasional) ⊙ 208
Garamycin Ophthalmic Ointment—Sterile ⊙ 305
Genoptic S.O.P. Sterile Ophthalmic Ointment (Occasional) ⊙ 247
Gentacidin Ointment (Occasional) ⊙ 273
Gentacidin Solution (Occasional) ⊙ 273
Gentak Ointment & Solution (Occasional) ⊙ 208
Glaucon ⊙ 218
HMS Liquifilm (Occasional) ⊙ 247
Humorsol Sterile Ophthalmic Solution 1475
Idamycin for Injection 564
Inflamase (Rare) ⊙ 274
Intron A 2097
Isopto Carbachol ⊙ 219
Isopto Carpine ⊙ 219
Isopto Homatropine ⊙ 221
Lactinol-E Creme 1770
Lotrimin 2102
Lotrisone Cream 2103
Lubraseptic Jelly (In some individuals) 1073
M-M-R II 1494
M-R-VAX II 1496
Maxidex Sterile Ophthalmic Ointment (Rare) ⊙ 222
Meruvax II 1503
Micro-Guard Cream, Antiseptic, Antifungal Skin Cream (Occasional) 2286
Monoclate-P Factor VIII:C, Pasteurized, Antihemophilic Factor (Human) 612
Mumpsvax 1513
Murocoll-2 Sterile Ophthalmic Solution ⊙ 261
Mutamycin 733
Mycelex 1% Cream and Topical Solution 1% 1604
Mydriacyl ⊙ 225
▲ Naftin Cream 1% (6%) 1084
▲ Naftin Gel 1% (5.0%) 1084
▲ Nasalide Nasal Solution 0.025% (Approximately 45%) 2299
Neutrogena Melanex Topical Solution 1618
▲ Nizoral 2% Cream (5%) 1143
▲ Ocufen (Among most frequent) ⊙ 237
Ophthetic (Occasional) ⊙ 249
Ophthochlor Ophthalmic Solution ⊙ 300
PediOtic Suspension Sterile 797
Phospholine Iodide ⊙ 315
Polytrim Ophthalmic Solution Sterile 588
Pred-G Liquifilm Sterile Ophthalmic Suspension ⊙ 252
▲ Profenal Sterile Ophthalmic Solution (Among most frequent) ⊙ 234
Propine with C Cap Compliance Cap (6%) ⊙ 255
Retin-A (tretinoin) Cream/Gel/Liquid 1680
Rubex 739
Sodium Sulamyd 2122
▲ Spectazole (econazole nitrate) Cream (3%) 1681
Surgicel (Occasional) 1151
Talwin Injection 2071
Temovate (1 of 366 patients) 1056
▲ Topicycline for Topical Solution (About 33%) 1856
Tropicacyl ⊙ 209
▲ Ultravate Cream 0.05% (4%) 2410
Ultravate Ointment 0.05% (1.6%) 2411
Vasocon-A ⊙ 278
Vasosulf ⊙ 279
▲ Viroptic Ophthalmic Solution, 1% Sterile (4.6%) 820
▲ Voltaren Ophthalmic Sterile Ophthalmic Solution (15%) ⊙ 268
VōSol (Occasional) 2392
Xerac AC 1773
Ziradryl Lotion ▣ 643
▲ Zovirax Ointment 5% (28.3%) 827

Stomach, nervous

Clozaril Tablets (Less than 1%) 2000

Stomachache

▲ AeroBid Inhaler System (10%) 995
▲ Alka-Seltzer Effervescent Antacid and Pain Reliever (14.5% at doses of 1000 mg/day) 1568
▲ Alka-Seltzer (Flavored) Effervescent Antacid and Pain Reliever (14.5% at doses of 1000 mg/day) 1569
Atgam Sterile Solution (Less than 5%) 2320
▲ Genuine Bayer Aspirin Tablets & Caplets (14.3% at doses of 1000 mg/day) ▣ 564
▲ Bayer Plus Aspirin Tablets (14.5% of 4500 people tested) ▣ 567
▲ Therapy Bayer Aspirin Caplets (14.5% of 4500 people tested) ▣ 568
Bontril Slow-Release 834
▲ Bufferin Analgesic Tablets and Caplets (14.5%) 743
▲ CHEMET (succimer) Capsules (5.2-15.7%) 1361
Cylert Tablets 510
▲ Ecotrin (14.5% at 1000 mg/day) 2189
Glucotrol (1 in 100) 1952
Guaifed 1615
Haltran Tablets (Occasional) ▣ 668
Hiprex Tablets (Less than 3.5%) 1333
Intal Inhaler (Rare) 979
Intal Nebulizer Solution 980
K-Phos M.F. Tablets 659
K-Phos Neutral Tablets 660
K-Phos Original Formula 'Sodium Free' Tablets 660
K-Phos No. 2 Tablets 659
Omnipaque (Less than 0.7%) 2552
PhosChol 568
Plegine Tablets 2504
Proventil Syrup (Less than 1 of 100) 2119
Sinemet CR Tablets 953
▲ St. Joseph Adult Chewable Aspirin (81 mg.) (14.3% of 4500 patients) ▣ 703
Uroqid-Acid 661

Ventolin (2% to 3%) 583

Stomatitis

Actigall Capsules 2280
Adriamycin PFS 561
Adriamycin RDF 562
▲ Alferon N Injection (6%) 1809
Anaprox and Anaprox DS Tablets (Less than 3%) 2288
Ansaid Tablets (Less than 1%) 2319
Atgam Sterile Solution (More than 1%; less than 5%) 2320
Atromid-S Capsules 2435
Augmentin Tablets, Powder for Oral Suspension, and Chewable Tablets 2198
Azo Gantanol Tablets 1887
Azo Gantrisin Tablets 1888
Azulfidine Tablets, EN-tabs, Oral Suspension (Rare) 1157
Bactrim DS Tablets 1891
Bactrim I.V. Infusion 1889
Bactrim 1891
Blenoxane 724
Butazolidin Capsules & Tablets (Less than 1%) 1027
CeeNU (Infrequent) 725
Chloromycetin Kapseals 1695
Chloromycetin Palmitate, Oral Suspension 1697
Chloromycetin Sodium Succinate 1698
Clinoril Tablets (Less than 1 in 100) 1433
▲ Cytosar-U Sterile Powder (Among most frequent) 2329
Depen Titratable Tablets 2379
Deprol Tablets (Rare) 2382
Dipentum Capsules (1.0%) 1160
Dolobid Tablets (Less than 1 in 100) 1465
Doxorubicin Hydrochloride for Injection, USP 622
Doxorubicin Hydrochloride Injection, USP 848
Efudex 1880
Elavil 2269
Endep Tablets 1927
Equagesic Tablets (Rare) 2451
▲ Ergamisol Tablets (9 to 39%) 1136
Estratest 2245
Etrafon 2087
▲ Sterile FUDR (Among more common) 1898
Fansidar Tablets 1896
Feldene Capsules (1 to 3%) 1777
Flagyl I.V. 2131
Flagyl Tablets 2170
Flexeril Tablets (Rare) 1471
Fluorouracil Injection (Common) 1897
Gantanol 1899
Gantrisin Ophthalmic Ointment/Solution 1900
Gantrisin 1901
Garamycin Injectable 2093
Halcion Tablets 2340
Hydrea Capsules 728
IFEX (Less than 1%) 729
▲ Intron A (Less than 5%) 2097
Leukine for IV Infusion 1127
Limbitrol 1933
Lincocin 2344
Ludiomil Tablets 874
Matulane Capsules 1907
Maxair Inhaler (Less than 1%) 1311
Meclomen Capsules (Greater than 1%) 1739
Metandren Linguets and Tablets 875
▲ Methotrexate Tablets, Parenteral, LPF Parenteral (3 to 10%) 1217
Mevacor Tablets 1505
Miltown Tablets (Rare) 2386
Mithracin 1602
▲ Mutamycin (Frequent) 733
Myochrysine Injection 1516
Naprosyn (Less than 3%) 2297
▲ Neupogen for Injection (5%) 595
Nicorette 1335
Noroxin Tablets 1519
Norpramin Tablets 1340
▲ Novantrone for Injection Concentrate (18 to 29%) 1226
Orudis Capsules (Greater than 1%) 2488
PMB 200 and PMB 400 (Rare) 2504
Pamelor 2019
Pediazole 1973
Premarin with Methyltestosterone 2515
Prokine for I.V. Infusion 1096
Pronestyl Capsules and Tablets 1800
Pronestyl Injection 1798
Pronestyl-SR Tablets 1801
Protostat Tablets 1674
Prozac Pulvules (Infrequent) 920
Quadrinal Tablets 1183
▲ Rheumatrex Methotrexate Dose Pack (3% to 10%) 1234
▲ Ridaura Capsules (13%) 2224
Rubex 739
Septra 813
Septra I.V. Infusion 808
Septra I.V. Infusion ADD-Vantage Vials 810
Septra 813
Sinequan 1960
Solganal Suspension 2122
Spectrobid Tablets & Powder for Oral Suspension 1961
Surmontil Capsules 2524
Tegretol Chewable Tablets 654
Tegretol Suspension 656
Tegretol Tablets 654
Temaril Tablets, Syrup and Spansule Sustained Release Capsules 1085
Testred Capsules 1124
Thioguanine Tablets, Tabloid Brand 815
Thiosulfil Forte Tablets 2526
Timentin for Injection 2239
Tofranil Ampuls 1038
Tofranil Tablets 1039
Tofranil-PM Capsules 1041
Tolectin (200, 400 and 600 mg) (Less than 1%) 1379
Tonocard Tablets (Less than 1%) 1554
Toradol IM Injection (1% or less) 2302
Trecator-SC Tablets 2527
Triavil Tablets 1556
Unasyn 1965
Urobiotic-250 Capsules (Rare) 1968
Vaseretic Tablets 1559
Vasotec I.V. 1562
Vasotec Tablets 1564
▲ VePesid Capsules and Injection (1 to 6%) 741
Vivactil Tablets 1567
Wellbutrin Tablets (Frequent) 821

Stomatitis, ulcerative

Anafranil Capsules (Up to 2%) 650
Anaprox and Anaprox DS Tablets (Rare) 2288
Cosmegen Injection 1440
Indocin Capsules (Less than 1%) 1487
Indocin I.V. (Less than 1%) 1490
Indocin (Less than 1%) 1487
Intron A (Less than 1%) 2097
Lodine Capsules (Less than 1%) 2468
▲ Methotrexate Tablets, Parenteral, LPF Parenteral (Among most frequent) 1217
Naprosyn (Rare) 2297
Permax Tablets (Rare) 1291
Prozac Pulvules (Infrequent) 920
▲ Rheumatrex Methotrexate Dose Pack (Among most frequent) 1234
Voltaren Tablets (Less than 1%) 1042

Stool, bloody (see under Hematochezia)

Stool, color changes

Anafranil Capsules (Rare) 650
Cholybar 1705
Coumadin Injection & Tablets 944
FemIron Multi-Vitamins and Iron ▣ 617
Geritol Complete Tablets ▣ 717
Geritol Liquid - High Potency Iron & Vitamin Tonic ▣ 717
Micronor Tablets 1667
Modicon 1667
Nullo Deodorant Tablets (Few cases) ▣ 547
Ortho-Novum 1667
Pepto-Bismol Liquid & Tablets 1807
Maximum Strength Pepto-Bismol Liquid 1808
Questran Light 711

Stools, abnormal

Clozaril Tablets (Less than 1%) 2000

Stools, loose

Atromid-S Capsules (Less frequent) 2435
▲ Augmentin Tablets, Powder for Oral Suspension, and Chewable Tablets (9%) 2198
Cefobid Pharmacy Bulk Package - Not for Direct Infusion (1 in 30) 1945
Ceftin Tablets (1.3%) 575
▲ CHEMET (succimer) Capsules (12-20.9%) 1361
▲ Dipentum Capsules (5.9%) 1160
Geocillin Tablets 1951
▲ Intron A (3%) 2097
Kutrase Capsules 2146
Ku-Zyme Capsules 2146
Lorelco Tablets 1333
Magonate Tablets and Liquid ▣ 563
▲ Mesnex Injection (70%) 733
Micro-K LS Packets (Frequent) 1864
Pipracil (2%) 1230
▲ Ridaura Capsules (approx. 50%) 2224
▲ Sandostatin Injection (4.3%) 2029
Solatene Capsules (Occasional) 1881
▲ Suprax (6%) 1235
▲ Tonocard Tablets (0.0-6.8%) 1554

Strabismus

Anafranil Capsules (Rare) 650
Lioresal Tablets 1031
Prozac Pulvules (Rare) 920

Striae

Aclovate Cream 1053
Alphatrex Cream, Ointment & Lotion (Infrequent) 2076
Analpram-HC Rectal Cream 1% and 2.5% 970
Anusol-HC Cream (Infrequent) 1690
Aristocort A (Infrequent) 1010
Betatrex Cream, Ointment & Lotion 2077
▲ Blenoxane (50%) 724
Carmol HC Cream 1% (Infrequent) 2296
Cortisporin Cream 757
Cortisporin Ointment 758
Cortisporin Otic Solution Sterile 760
Cortisporin Otic Suspension Sterile 760
Cutivate Cream 0.05% 1054
Cutivate Ointment 0.005% (Infrequent to more frequent) 1054
Cyclocort Lotion (Infrequent) 1198
Decadron Phosphate Topical Cream 1455
Decaspray Topical Aerosol 1459
DesOwen Cream, Ointment and Lotion (Infrequent) 1682
Diprolene (Infrequent) 2083
Eldecort Cream 1.0% (Infrequent) 1113
Eldecort Cream 1.0% and 2.5% (Infrequent) 1113
Elocon (Infrequent) 2084
Epifoam 1828
Florone/Florone E 908
Halog (Infrequent) 2399
Hytone 909
Kenalog Cream, Lotion & Ointment (Infrequent) 2401
Kenalog-10 Injection 2402
Kenalog-40 Injection 2403
Lidex (Infrequent) 2296
Locoid Cream, Ointment and Topical Solution (Infrequent) 970
Lotrisone Cream (Infrequent) 2103
Mantadil Cream 789
Maxivate Cream, Lotion & Ointment 0.05% 2406
Mycolog II Cream and Ointment (Infrequent) 2407
Mytrex Cream & Ointment (Infrequent) 2080
NeoDecadron Topical Cream 1518
Neo-Synalar Cream (Infrequent) 2296
Nutracort Cream & Lotion (Infrequent) 1684
Orabase HCA Oral Paste (Infrequent) 890
PediOtic Suspension Sterile 797
Pramosone Cream, Lotion & Ointment 971
ProctoCream-HC (Infrequent) 1834
Proctofoam-HC 1835
Psorcon Ointment 0.05% 909
Psorion Cream 0.05% (Infrequent) 1121
Synacort Creams 1%, 2.5% (Infrequent) 2296
Synalar (Infrequent) 2296
Temovate 1056
Topicort (Infrequent) 1098
Tridesilon Creme 0.05% (Infrequent) 1611
Tridesilon Ointment 0.05% (Infrequent) 1611
Ultravate Cream 0.05% (Infrequently) 2410
Ultravate Ointment 0.05% 2411
Vanoxide-HC Acne Lotion 911
Vioform-Hydrocortisone Cream and Mild Cream 889
Vioform-Hydrocortisone Ointment 889
Vytone Cream 1% 911
Westcort 2411
Zolyse ⊙ 236

Stridor

Reglan (Rare) 1869

Stroke

Activase (0.9%) 1047
Asendin Tablets (Very rare) 1196
Brevicon 2304
Calciparine Injection 925
Demulen 2161
DynaCirc Capsules (0.5% to 1%) 2004
Elavil 2269
Endep Tablets 1927
Enovid 2161
Estrace 1385
Estrace Vaginal Cream 1388
Estradurin 2452
Estratest 2245
Etrafon 2087
Flexeril Tablets (Rare) 1471
Heparin Lock Flush Solution 2456
Heparin Sodium Vials 1264
Heparin Sodium Injection 2457
Heparin Sodium Injection, USP, Sterile Solution 2342
Limbitrol 1933
Loestrin 1728
Ludiomil Tablets 874
▲ Lupron Depot 3.75 mg (Among most frequent) 2312
Lupron Depot 7.5 mg 2311
Lupron Injection 2310
Metrodin (urofollitropin for injection) 2182
Micronor Tablets 1667
Modicon 1667
Norinyl 2304
Norlestrin 1746
Norpramin Tablets 1340
Nor-Q D Tablets 2304
Ortho Dienestrol Cream 1664
Ortho-Cyclen Tablets 1658
Ortho-Novum 1667
Ovcon 1391
Pamelor 2019
Parlodel (15 cases) 2020
Premarin Intravenous 2508
Premarin with Methyltestosterone 2515
Premarin Vaginal Cream 2512
Prinivil Tablets (1% or less) 1538
Prinzide Tablets 1540
Roferon-A Injection (Less than 1%) 1916
Stilphostrol Tablets and Ampuls 1609
Surmontil Capsules 2524
TACE 12 and 25 mg 1353
Tofranil Ampuls 1038
Tofranil Tablets 1039
Tofranil-PM Capsules 1041
Triavil Tablets 1556
Tri-Norinyl 28-Day Tablets 2304
Vivactil Tablets 1567
Zestoretic 2274
Zestril Tablets (Less than 1%) 2277

Stroke, hemorrhagic

Demulen 2161
Enovid 2161
Micronor Tablets 1667
Modicon 1667
Ortho-Novum 1667
Triphasil-21 Tablets 2527
Triphasil-28 Tablets 2532

Stroke, thrombotic

Triphasil-21 Tablets 2527
Triphasil-28 Tablets 2532

Stuffiness, nasal (see under Nasal congestion)

Stupor

Anafranil Capsules (Rare) 650
BuSpar (Rare) 1401
Cibalith-S 870
Desyrel and Desyrel Dividose 1404
Dilantin with Phenobarbital Kapseals (Common) 1715
Duragesic Transdermal System (Less than 1%) 1133
Eskalith 2214
Kerlone Tablets (Less than 2%) 2172
Lithane Tablets 1596
Lithium Carbonate Capsules & Tablets 1984

Lithobid Tablets 870
Moduretic Tablets (Less than or equal to 1%) 1510
Omnipaque (Several instances) 2552
Permax Tablets (Rare) 1291
PhosLo Tablets 700
ProSom Tablets (Infrequent) 554
Prozac Pulvules (Rare) 920
Ru-Tuss Tablets 693
Serax Capsules 2522
Serax Tablets 2522
Tambocor Tablets (Less than 1%) 1315

Stye

Intron A (Less than 5%) 2097

Sudden Infant Death Syndrome

Diphtheria and Tetanus Toxoids and Pertussis Vaccine Adsorbed USP (For Pediatric Use) 892

Suicidal ideation

Anafranil Capsules (Infrequent) 650
BuSpar (Infrequent) 1401
Celontin (Rare) 1692
Desyrel and Desyrel Dividose 1404
Hydropres Tablets 1485
Intron A (1 patient) 2097
Klonopin Tablets 1902
Lamprene Capsules (Less than 1%) 1030
Larodopa Tablets (Infrequent) 1905
Miltown Tablets 2386
Nizoral Tablets (Rare) 1145
Pronestyl Injection 1798
Prozac Pulvules 920
Reglan 1869
Seromycin Pulvules 1298
Sinemet Tablets 952
Sinemet CR Tablets 953
Trilafon 2123
Wellbutrin Tablets (Rare) 821
Zarontin Capsules (Rare) 1768
Zarontin Syrup (Rare) 1769

Sulfhemoglobinemia

Azo Gantrisin Tablets 1888

Sulfite, sensitivity to

Aldomet Oral Suspension 1415
Amikin Injectable 602
Ana-Kit Anaphylaxis Emergency Treatment Kit 1100
Antilirium Injectable 998
Aramine Injection 1424
Arm-a-Med Isoetharine Inhalation Solution, USP 616
Bronkephrine Injection 2042
Bronkometer Aerosol 2042
Bronkosol Solution 2042
Carbocaine 956
Compazine 2201
Dalgan Injection 620
Decadron Phosphate Injection 1449
Decadron Phosphate with Xylocaine Injection, Sterile 1451
Dobutrex Solution Vials 1259
Enlon Injection 598
EpiPen 843
Garamycin Injectable 2093
Hydrocortone Phosphate Injection, Sterile 1481
Intropin Injection 930
Isuprel Hydrochloride Injection 1:5000 2050
Isuprel Hydrochloride Solution 1:200 & 1:100 2052
Marcaine Hydrochloride 0.5% with Epinephrine 1:200,000 (as bitartrate) 958
Mepergan Injection 2479
Minocin Oral Suspension 1224
Moban Tablets & Concentrate 932
Mydfrin 2.5% ◉ 224
Neo-Synephrine Hydrochloride 1% Carpuject 2063
Neo-Synephrine Hydrochloride 1% Injection 2063
Norflex Injectable 1314
Novocain Hydrochloride for Spinal Anesthesia 2065
Nubain Injection 934
Numorphan Hydrochloride Injection 935
Phenergan Injection 2493
Pontocaine Hydrochloride for Spinal Anesthesia 2069
Rowasa 2248
Septra I.V. Infusion 808
Stelazine 2226
Synkayvite Injection 1919
Talwin Injection 2071
Tensilon Injectable 1123
Theragran Hematinic Tablets 605
Topicycline for Topical Solution 1856
Torecan Injection (Thiethylperazine Malate) 1993
Tylenol with Codeine Phosphate Tablets 1381
Tylox Capsules 1382
Xylocaine with Epinephrine Injections 637

Sunburn

▲ Accutane Capsules (Approximately 1 in 20) 1878
Methotrexate Tablets, Parenteral, LPF Parenteral 1217
Rheumatrex Methotrexate Dose Pack 1234
▲ Tegison Capsules (25-50%) 1881

Superinfection

Adriamycin PFS 561
Ancef Injection 2194
Ceftin Tablets 575
Cipro Tablets 1589
Doxorubicin Hydrochloride Injection, USP 848
Macrodantin Capsules 1624
Pipracil 1230
Primaxin I.M. 1532
Rubex 739
Suprax 1235
Terramycin Capsules 1786
Vascor (200, 300 and 400 mg) Tablets (0.5 to 2.0%) 1383
Zefazone Sterile Powder 2372

Suppuration

Efudex 1880

Swallowing

Diprivan Injection (Less than 1%) 2267

Swallowing, impairment

Calciparine Injection 925
Capoten 2255
Capozide 2258
Compazine 2201
Coumadin Injection & Tablets 944
Dantrium Capsules (Less frequent) 1619
Fiorinal with Codeine Capsules (Infrequent) 2008
Myochrysine Injection 1516
Perdiem Fiber Granules 1852
Perdiem Granules 1852
Prinzide Tablets 1540
Sandimmune (Rare) 2024
Solganal Suspension 2122
Stelazine 2226
Thorazine 2234
Vaseretic Tablets 1559
Zestoretic 2274
Zestril Tablets 2277

Sweat discoloration

Lamprene Capsules (Greater than 1%) 1030
Sinemet Tablets 952
Sinemet CR Tablets 953

Sweating (see under Diaphoresis)

Sweats, night

Atgam Sterile Solution (More than 1%; less than 5%) 2320

Swelling

▲ AK-Spore H.C. (Among most often) ◉ 206
▲ AK-Spore (Among most frequent) ◉ 205
Americaine Hemorrhoidal Ointment ▣ 558
Atromid-S Capsules 2435
Bactroban Ointment (Less than 1%) 2200
Calciparine Injection 925
Clear by Design Medicated Acne Gel ▣ 709
Clear By Design Medicated Cleansing Pads ▣ 709
Cortisporin Ophthalmic Ointment Sterile 758
Cortisporin Ophthalmic Suspension Sterile 759
Coumadin Injection & Tablets 944
Desferal Vials 862
Diphtheria and Tetanus Toxoids and Pertussis Vaccine Adsorbed USP (For Pediatric Use) (2 in 5 doses) 892
Efudex 1880
Factrel 2561
Femstat Prefill Vaginal Cream 2% (0.2%) 2295
Femstat Vaginal Cream 2% (0.2%) 2295
Fluorouracil Injection 1897
▲ HibTITER (1.7% to 3.3%) 1206
Imferon 976
Intal Inhaler (Infrequent) 979
Konakion Injection (Rare) 1903
Kutapressin Injection 2146
▲ Mykrox ½ mg Tablets (3.1%) 984
Nasalcrom Nasal Solution 986
▲ Omnipaque (22 to 42%) 2552
PedvaxHIB 1521
Phenobarbital Elixir and Tablets 1293
Prinivil Tablets 1538
ProHIBiT Haemophilus b Conjugate Vaccine (Diphtheria Toxoid Conjugate) 896
Quadrinal Tablets 1183
Recombivax HB (Equal to or greater than 1%) 1544
Stri-Dex Maximum ▣ 573
Stri-Dex Dual Textured Regular Strength Pads ▣ 573
Stri-Dex Dual Textured Regular Strength Big Pads ▣ 573
TobraDex Ophthalmic Suspension and Ointment (Less than 4%) ◉ 228
Versed Injection (Less than 1%) 1924
Zestril Tablets 2277

Swelling, edematous, ankles

Android 1111
Cibalith-S 870
Eskalith 2214
Estratest 2245
Lithane Tablets 1596
Lithium Carbonate Capsules & Tablets 1984
Lithobid Tablets 870
Lo/Ovral Tablets 2471
Lo/Ovral-28 Tablets 2476
Ovral Tablets 2490
Ovral-28 Tablets 2491
Ovrette Tablets 2492
Triphasil-21 Tablets 2527
Triphasil-28 Tablets 2532

Swelling, edematous, wrists

Cibalith-S 870
Eskalith 2214
Lithane Tablets 1596
Lithium Carbonate Capsules & Tablets 1984
Lithobid Tablets 870

Swelling, extremities

Prinzide Tablets 1540
Stilphostrol Tablets and Ampuls 1609
Zestoretic 2274
Zestril Tablets 2277

Swelling, feet

Centrax 1693
K-Phos M.F. Tablets 659
K-Phos Neutral Tablets 660
K-Phos No. 2 Tablets 659
Uroqid-Acid (Less frequent) 661

Swelling, joint

Danocrine Capsules 2046
Intal Capsules (Less than 1 in 10,000 patients) 978
Intal Nebulizer Solution 980

Swelling, legs

K-Phos M.F. Tablets 659
K-Phos Neutral Tablets 660
K-Phos No. 2 Tablets 659
Uroqid-Acid (Less frequent) 661

Swelling, lower legs (see under Swelling, legs)

Swelling, mouth

Diphtheria and Tetanus Toxoids and Pertussis Vaccine Adsorbed USP (For Pediatric Use) (Rare) 892
Ethmozine Tablets (Less than 2%) 946

Swelling, periorbital

Streptase for Infusion 635

Swelling, salivary gland

Elavil 2269
Eskalith 2214
Flexeril Tablets (Rare) 1471

Swelling at injection site

Atgam Sterile Solution (Less than 5%) 2320
Attenuvax 1424
Azactam for Injection (2.4%) 2252
Ceredase Injection 1052
Cipro I.V. (1% or less) 1592
DDAVP Injection (Occasional) 1840
▲ Engerix-B Unit-Dose Vials (1% to 10%) 2213
Geref (sermorelin acetate for injection) 2560
Humulin 70/30, 100 Units (Occasional) 1267
Humulin BR, 100 Units (Occasional) 1268
Humulin L, 100 Units (Occasional) 1268
Humulin U, 100 Units (Occasional) 1272
Beef Regular, 100 Units 1275
Konakion Injection (Rare) 1903
M-M-R II 1494
M-R-VAX II 1496
Metrodin (urofollitropin for injection) 2182
Pergonal (menotropins for injection, USP) 2184
Pnu-Imune 23 Pneumococcal Vaccine Polyvalent (Rare) 1233
Staphage Lysate (SPL) 905
Timentin for Injection 2239
Zefazone Sterile Powder 2372

Syncope

Actimmune (Rare) 1046
Adalat Capsules (10 mg and 20 mg) (Approximately 0.5%) 1587
AeroBid Inhaler System (1-3%) 995
AK-Fluor Injection 10% and 25% ◉ 204
Altace Capsules (Less than 1%) 1086
Alurate Elixir (Less than 1 in 100) 1883
Anafranil Capsules (Up to 2%) 650
Antabuse Tablets 2429
Arfonad Ampuls 1887
Asendin Tablets (Less than 1%) 1196
Atgam Sterile Solution (Less than 1% to less than 5%) 2320
Azo Gantrisin Tablets 1888
Bentyl 1322
Betagan ◉ 239
Blocadren Tablets (0.6%) 1429
Bretylol Injection (7 in 1000) 923
Brevibloc Injection (Less than 1%) 942
BuSpar (Infrequent) 1401
Butisol Sodium Elixir & Tablets (Less than 1 in 100) 2377
Calan SR Caplets (1% or less) 2157
Calan Tablets (1% or less) 2155
Capoten 2255
Capozide 2258
Carbocaine Hydrochloride 3% Injection 956
Carbocaine Hydrochloride Injection 2043
Carbocaine Hydrochloride 2% with Neo-Cobefrin 956
Cardene Capsules (0.8%) 2290
Cardioquin Tablets 1812
Cardizem Tablets-30 mg, 60 mg, 90 mg and 120 mg (Less than 1%) 1329
Cardizem SR Capsules-60 mg, 90 mg and 120 mg (Less than 1%) 1327
▲ Cardura Tablets (0.5% to 23%) 1941
Centrax 1693
Cholybar 1705
Cipro I.V. (1% or less) 1592
Cipro Tablets (Less than 1%) 1589
Clinoril Tablets (Less than 1%) 1433
▲ Clozaril Tablets (More than 5 to 6%) 2000
Cytotec (Infrequent) 2159
Dalmane Capsules (Rare) 1927
Danocrine Capsules 2046
Demerol 2047
Deponit NTG Transdermal Delivery System (Less frequent) 2143
Deprol Tablets 2382
Desyrel and Desyrel Dividose (Greater than 1%) 1404
Dilaudid-HP Injection 1175
Diprivan Injection (Less than 1%) 2267
Diulo 2129
Diupres Tablets 1461
Dolobid Tablets (Rare) 1465
Dolophine Hydrochloride Ampoules & Vials 1260
Dolophine Hydrochloride Tablets 1261

Duragesic Transdermal System (1% or greater) ... 1133
Duvoid Tablets ... 1853
DynaCirc Capsules (0.5% to 1%) .. 2004
Elavil ... 2269
▲Eldepryl (7 of 49 patients) ... 2250
Engerix-B Unit-Dose Vials ... 2213
Equagesic Tablets ... 2451
Esimil Tablets ... 864
Eskalith ... 2214
Ethmozine Tablets (Less than 2%) ... 946
Etrafon ... 2087
Fiorinal with Codeine Capsules (Infrequent) ... 2008
Flagyl I.V. ... 2131
Flexeril Tablets (Less than 1%) ... 1471
Floxin Tablets (Less than 1%) ... 1652
Fluorescite ... ⊙ 217
Gamimune N Immune Globulin Intravenous (Human) ... 1572
Glaucon ... ⊙ 218
Halcion Tablets ... 2340
Hydropres Tablets ... 1485
Hylorel Tablets (0.4%) ... 975
Hytrin Tablets (0.5%) ... 529
Imferon ... 976
Indocin (Less than 1%) ... 1487
Intron A (Less than 1%) ... 2097
Inversine Tablets ... 1492
Ismelin Tablets ... 869
ISMOTIC (Very rare) ... ⊙ 233
Isoptin Oral Tablets (Less than 1%) ... 1179
Isoptin SR Sustained Release Tablets (Less than 1%) ... 1181
Isopto Carbachol ... ⊙ 219
Kenalog-10 Injection ... 2402
Kenalog-40 Injection ... 2403
Kerlone Tablets (Less than 2%) ... 2172
Koro-Flex Arcing Spring Diaphragm ... 2142
Koromex Coil Spring Diaphragm ... 2142
Lariam Tablets (Less than 1%) ... 1904
Larodopa Tablets (Relatively frequent) ... 1905
Librax Capsules (Few) ... 1929
Libritabs Tablets (Few instances) ... 1930
Librium Capsules (Few instances) .. 1931
Librium Injectable (Isolated instances) ... 1932
Limbitrol ... 1933
Lioresal Tablets (Rare) ... 1031
Lippes Loop Intrauterine Double-S .. 1654
Lodine Capsules (Less than 1%) ... 2468
Lopid Capsules and Tablets ... 1736
Lorelco Tablets ... 1333
Lotensin Tablets (0.1%) ... 872
Loxitane ... 1213
Ludiomil Tablets (Rare) ... 874
▲Lupron Depot 3.75 mg (Among most frequent) ... 2312
Lupron Depot 7.5 mg ... 2311
Lupron Injection (Less than 5%) ... 2310
MS Contin Tablets (Infrequent) ... 1814
MSIR (Infrequent) ... 1817
Marcaine Hydrochloride with Epinephrine 1:200,000 (Rare) ... 2055
Marcaine Hydrochloride Injection (Rare) ... 2055
Marcaine Spinal (Rare) ... 2058
Matulane Capsules ... 1907
Maxair Inhaler (Less than 1%) ... 1311
Mebaral Tablets (Less than 1 in 100) ... 2061
Menrium Tablets (Occasional) ... 1934
Mepergan Injection ... 2479
Methadone Hydrochloride Diskets .. 1284
Methadone Hydrochloride Oral Solution & Tablets ... 1987
Mexitil Capsules (Less than 1% or about 6 in 1,000) ... 680
Miltown Tablets ... 2386
Minipress Capsules (1-4%) ... 1778
▲Minitran Transdermal Delivery System (4%) ... 1312
Minizide Capsules (Rare) ... 1779
Modane Plus Tablets ... ▣ 504
Modane Tablets ... ▣ 503
Moduretic Tablets (Less than or equal to 1%) ... 1510
Monopril Tablets (0.2 to 1.0%) ... 1406
Mumpsvax ... 1513
Mutamycin ... 733
Mydfrin 2.5% ... ⊙ 224
Mykrox ½ mg Tablets ... 984
Myochrysine Injection ... 1516
Navane Capsules and Concentrate ... 1954
Navane Intramuscular ... 1956
NebuPent for Inhalation Solution (1% or less) ... 1017
Nembutal Sodium Capsules (Less than 1%) ... 534
Nembutal Sodium Solution (Less than 1%) ... 536
Nembutal Sodium Suppositories (Less than 1%) ... 538
Nicorette ... 1335
Nitrodisc (Uncommon) ... 2176
Nitro-Dur (nitroglycerin) Transdermal Infusion System (Uncommon) ... 1164
Nitrogard Tablets (Uncommon) ... 1004
Nitrostat Tablets ... 1743
Norflex ... 1314
Norgesic ... 1314
Normodyne Injection ... 2108
Normodyne Tablets (Rare) ... 2110
Normozide Tablets (Rare) ... 2112
Norpace (1 to 3%) ... 2177
Nubain Injection (Less than 1%) ... 934
Omnipaque (Less than or equal to 1%) ... 2552
Oramorph SR (Morphine Sulfate Sustained Release Tablets) (Less frequent) ... 1988
Orap Tablets ... 1020
Ortho Diaphragm Kit ... 1664
PMB 200 and PMB 400 ... 2504
ParaGard T380A Intrauterine Copper Contraceptive ... 411
Parlodel (0.7%) ... 2020
Peptavlon ... 2563
Periactin ... 1525
Permax Tablets (2.1%) ... 1291
Phenergan with Codeine ... 2497
Phenergan Injection ... 2493
Phenergan Tablets ... 2496
Phenergan VC with Codeine ... 2501
Phenobarbital Elixir and Tablets (Less than 1 in 100 patients) ... 1293
Placidyl Capsules ... 553
Plendil Extended-Release Tablets (0.5% to 1.5%) ... 1526
Pondimin Tablets ... 1867
Prinivil Tablets (0.1%) ... 1538
Prinzide Tablets (0.8%) ... 1540
Procardia Capsules (Approximately 0.5%) ... 1781
Procardia XL Tablets (Approximately 1 patient in 250) ... 1783
ProSom Tablets (Rare) ... 554
Prostigmin Injectable ... 1120
Prostigmin Tablets ... 1121
Provocholine for Inhalation ... 1911
Prozac Pulvules (Infrequent) ... 920
Questran Light ... 711
Questran Powder ... 710
Quinaglute Dura-Tabs Tablets ... 663
Quinamm Tablets ... 1344
Quinidex Extentabs ... 1868
Retrovir Capsules (Less than 5%) .. 802
Retrovir I.V. Infusion (Less than 5%) ... 805
Retrovir Syrup (Less than 5%) ... 802
Robaxin Injectable ... 1871
Roferon-A Injection (Less than 0.5%) ... 1916
▲Rogaine Topical Solution (3.42%) .. 2357
Roxanol ... 1991
Ru-Tuss with Hydrocodone ... 694
Ru-Tuss Tablets ... 693
Rythmol Tablets (0.8 to 2.2%) ... 1184
Salutensin/Salutensin-Demi ... 719
Sandostatin Injection (Less than 1%) ... 2029
Seldane-D Extended-Release Tablets (Rare) ... 1350
Ser-Ap-Es Tablets ... 881
Serax Capsules (Rare) ... 2522
Serax Tablets (Rare) ... 2522
Serentil ... 686
Serpasil Tablets ... 883
Serpasil-Apresoline Tablets ... 884
Serpasil-Esidrix Tablets ... 886
Sinemet Tablets ... 952
Sinemet CR Tablets ... 953
Solganal Suspension ... 2122
Soma Compound w/Codeine Tablets (Infrequent or rare) ... 2390
Soma Compound Tablets (Infrequent or rare) ... 2389
Soma Tablets ... 2388
Tacaryl ... 2409
Talacen (Infrequent) ... 2070
Talwin Injection (Rare) ... 2071
Talwin Compound (Infrequent) ... 2072
Talwin Injection ... 2071
Talwin Nx ... 2073
Tambocor Tablets (1-3%) ... 1315
Taractan ... 1920
Tegison Capsules (Less than 1%) .. 1881
Tegretol Chewable Tablets ... 654
Tegretol Suspension ... 656
Tegretol Tablets ... 654
Temaril Tablets, Syrup and Spansule Sustained Release Capsules ... 1085
Tenex Tablets ... 1875
Thorazine ... 2234
Timolide Tablets (Less than 1%) ... 1547
Timoptic in Ocudose ... 1552
Timoptic Sterile Ophthalmic Solution ... 1550
Tofranil Ampuls ... 1038
Tofranil Tablets ... 1039
Tonocard Tablets (Less than 1%) .. 1554
Trandate HCT Tablets (Rare) ... 579
Trandate Injection (Rare) ... 577
Trandate Tablets (Rare) ... 579
▲Transderm-Nitro Transdermal Therapeutic System (4%) ... 2283
Tridil Ampuls & Vials (Uncommon) ... 939
Urecholine ... 1558
Valium Injectable ... 1937
Vascor (200, 300 and 400 mg) Tablets (0.5 to 2.0%) ... 1383
Vaseretic Tablets (0.5% to 2.0%) ... 1559
Vasotec I.V. ... 1562
Vasotec Tablets (0.5% to 1%) ... 1564
Verelan Capsules (Less than 1%) .. 1243
Versed Injection (Less than 1%) ... 1924
Visken Tablets (2% or fewer patients) ... 2036
Wellbutrin Tablets (1.2%) ... 821
▲Xanax Tablets (3.1% to 3.8%) ... 2367
Zaroxolyn Tablets ... 989
Zestoretic (0.8%) ... 2274
Zestril Tablets (0.1%) ... 2277

Synechiae

Cyclogyl ... ⊙ 215

Synovia, immunological destruction

Solganal Suspension ... 2122

Synovitis

Cuprimine Capsules (Some patients) ... 1442
Depen Titratable Tablets ... 2379
Lopid Capsules and Tablets ... 1736

Systemic lupus erythematosus (see under Lupus erythematosus, systemic)

SGOT changes

Alferon N Injection ... 1809
Atgam Sterile Solution ... 2320
Bumex (0.6%) ... 1895
Doral Tablets (1.3%) ... 2383
▲Emcyt Capsules (33 to 34%) ... 1161
▲Intron A (11% to 41%) ... 2097
▲Roferon-A Injection (42% to 46%) 1916
Sinemet Tablets ... 952
Sinemet CR Tablets ... 953

SGOT elevation

Accutane Capsules ... 1878
Amoxil ... 2193
Anadrol-50 Tablets ... 2287
Ancef Injection ... 2194
Ansaid Tablets (Less than 1%) ... 2319
Atromid-S Capsules ... 2435
Augmentin Tablets, Powder for Oral Suspension, and Chewable Tablets ... 2198
Axid Pulvules ... 1246
Azactam for Injection (Less than 1%) ... 2252
BuSpar (Infrequent) ... 1401
Butazolidin Capsules & Tablets (Less than 1%) ... 1027
Calan SR Caplets ... 2157
Calan Tablets ... 2155
Calcijex Calcitriol Injection ... 506
Calciparine Injection ... 925
Calderol Capsules ... 1635
Cardizem Tablets-30 mg, 60 mg, 90 mg and 120 mg (Less than 1%) ... 1329
Cardizem SR Capsules-60 mg, 90 mg and 120 mg (Less than 1%) 1327
Ceclor Pulvules & Suspension (1 in 40) ... 1251
▲Cefizox Injection (1 to 5%) ... 1012
Cefotan (1 in 300) ... 2265
Ceftin Tablets (2.0%) ... 575
Ceptaz for Injection (One in 16) ... 1057
▲CHEMET (succimer) Capsules (4.2 to 10.4%) ... 1361
Children's Advil Suspension (Less than 1%) ... 2426
▲Cipro I.V. (Among most frequent) .. 1592
Cipro Tablets (1.7%) ... 1589
Claforan Sterile Injection (Less than 1%) ... 1089
Colestid Granules (One or more occasions) ... 2328
Cordarone Tablets ... 2446
Dalgan Injection (Less than 1%) ... 620
Dalmane Capsules (Rare) ... 1927
Demser Capsules (Rare) ... 1460
Depakene Capsules & Syrup (Frequent) ... 511
Depakote (Frequent) ... 512
Diflucan Injection and Tablets ... 1948
Dipentum Capsules (Rare) ... 1160
Elspar ... 1470
Eulexin Capsules ... 2089
Feldene Capsules (Less than 1%) .. 1777
▲Fortaz (1 in 16) ... 1060
Fungizone Intravenous ... 2262
Geocillin Tablets ... 1951
Glucotrol ... 1952
Heparin Lock Flush Solution ... 2456
▲Heparin Sodium Vials (A high percentage of patients) ... 1264
Heparin Sodium Injection ... 2457
Heparin Sodium Injection, USP, Sterile Solution ... 2342
INH Tablets ... 868
Imuran ... 768
▲Intron A (4% to 12%) ... 2097
Isoptin Oral Tablets ... 1179
Isoptin SR Sustained Release Tablets ... 1181
Keflex Pulvules, Oral Suspension & Pediatric Drops ... 916
Keftab Tablets ... 917
▲Kefurox Vials, Faspak & ADD-Vantage (1 in 25) ... 1277
Kefzol Vials, Faspak & ADD-Vantage (Rare) ... 1279
Kerlone Tablets (Less than 2%) ... 2172
Lamprene Capsules (Less than 1%) ... 1030
Larodopa Tablets (Rare) ... 1905
Leukine for IV Infusion ... 1127
Lioresal Tablets ... 1031
Lopid Capsules and Tablets (Occasional) ... 1736
Lotensin Tablets (Scattered incidents) ... 872
Loxitane ... 1213
Lupron Depot 3.75 mg (Twice normal limit—one patient) ... 2312
▲Lupron Depot 7.5 mg (5.4%) ... 2311
Mandol Vials, Faspak & ADD-Vantage ... 1281
Meclomen Capsules (Less than 1%) ... 1739
Mefoxin ... 1498
Mefoxin Premixed Intravenous Solution ... 1500
Mezlin ... 1597
Mezlin Pharmacy Bulk Package ... 1599
Mithracin ... 1602
Monocid Injection (1.6%) ... 2217
Motrin Tablets (Less than 1%) ... 2351
▲Mycelex Troches (15%) ... 1605
Nalfon Pulvules & Tablets (Less than 1%) ... 919
Nebcin Vials, Hyporets & ADD-Vantage ... 1286
Niclocide Chewable Tablets (One case in a narcotic addict) ... 1607
Noroxin Tablets (1.8%) ... 1519
Orudis Capsules (Less than 1%) ... 2488
▲Paraplatin for Injection (15% to 19%) ... 735
Parlodel ... 2020
PediaProfen Suspension (Less than 1%) ... 1363
Pipracil (Less frequent) ... 1230
Platinol (Infrequent) ... 737
Platinol-AQ Injection (Infrequent) ... 738
Prilosec Delayed-Release Capsules (Less than 1%) ... 1530
Primaxin I.M. ... 1532
Primaxin I.V. ... 1535
Procan SR Tablets (One case) ... 1760
Procardia XL Tablets (Rare) ... 1783
Pronestyl Capsules and Tablets ... 1800
Pronestyl-SR Tablets ... 1801
ProSom Tablets (Rare) ... 554
Rifamate Capsules ... 1347
Rocaltrol Capsules ... 1913
▲Rocephin Injectable Vials, ADD-Vantage (3.1%) ... 1914
Rufen Tablets (Less than 1%) ... 691
Sectral Capsules ... 2520

Septra I.V. Infusion ADD-Vantage Vials.......... 810
Seromycin Pulvules.......... 1298
Sinemet Tablets.......... 952
Spectrobid Tablets & Powder for Oral Suspension.......... 1961
Suprax (Less than 2%).......... 1235
Synarel Nasal Solution.......... 2300
▲ Tazicef for Injection (1 in 16 patients).......... 2231
▲ Tazidime Vials, Faspak & ADD-Vantage (1 in 16).......... 1299
▲ Tegison Capsules (18%).......... 1881
Ticar for Injection.......... 2236
Timentin for Injection.......... 2239
Toradol IM Injection (Less than 1%).......... 2302
Tornalate (Rare).......... 2074
Unasyn.......... 1965
Velosef Capsules and for Oral Suspension.......... 606
Verelan Capsules.......... 1243
Vira-A for Injection.......... 1766
Voltaren Tablets (About 2%).......... 1042
Winstrol Tablets.......... 2075
Xanax Tablets (Less than 1% to 3.2%).......... 2367
▲ Zanosar Sterile Powder (A number of patients).......... 2371
Zefazone Sterile Powder.......... 2372
▲ Zinacef (1 in 25 patients).......... 1066
▲ Zofran Injection (Approximately 5%).......... 1069
Zyloprim Tablets (Less than 1%).......... 830

SGPT changes

Atgam Sterile Solution.......... 2320
Bumex (0.5%).......... 1895
▲ Intron A (10% to 15%).......... 2097
Septra I.V. Infusion ADD-Vantage Vials.......... 810
Sinemet Tablets.......... 952
Sinemet CR Tablets.......... 953
Voltaren Tablets (About 2%).......... 1042

SGPT elevation

Accutane Capsules.......... 1878
Ancef Injection.......... 2194
Atromid-S Capsules.......... 2435
Augmentin Tablets, Powder for Oral Suspension, and Chewable Tablets.......... 2198
Axid Pulvules.......... 1246
Azactam for Injection (Less than 1%).......... 2252
BuSpar (Infrequent).......... 1401
Butazolidin Capsules & Tablets (Less than 1%).......... 1027
Calan SR Caplets.......... 2157
Calan Tablets.......... 2155
Calcijex Calcitriol Injection.......... 506
Calciparine Injection.......... 925
Calderol Capsules.......... 1635
Cardizem Tablets-30 mg, 60 mg, 90 mg and 120 mg (Less than 1%).......... 1329
Cardizem SR Capsules-60 mg, 90 mg and 120 mg (Less than 1%) 1327
Ceclor Pulvules & Suspension (1 in 40).......... 1251
▲ Cefizox Injection (1 to 5%).......... 1012
Cefotan (1 in 150).......... 2265
Ceftin Tablets (1.6%).......... 575
Ceptaz for Injection (One in 15).......... 1057
▲ CHEMET (succimer) Capsules (4.2 to 10.4%).......... 1361
Children's Advil Suspension (Less than 1%).......... 2426
▲ Cipro I.V. (Among most frequent).. 1592
Cipro Tablets (1.9%).......... 1589
Claforan Sterile Injection (Less than 1%).......... 1089
Cordarone Tablets.......... 2446
Dalmane Capsules (Rare).......... 1927
Depakene Capsules & Syrup (Frequent).......... 511
Depakote (Frequent).......... 512
Dipentum Capsules (Rare).......... 1160
Doral Tablets (Less than 1%).......... 2383
Elspar.......... 1470
Eulexin Capsules.......... 2089
Feldene Capsules (Less than 1%).. 1777
Floxin Tablets (More than or equal to 1.0%).......... 1652
▲ Fortaz (1 in 15).......... 1060
Fungizone Intravenous.......... 2262
Heparin Lock Flush Solution.......... 2456
▲ Heparin Sodium Vials (A high percentage of patients).......... 1264
Heparin Sodium Injection.......... 2457
Heparin Sodium Injection, USP, Sterile Solution.......... 2342
INH Tablets.......... 868
Imuran.......... 768
▲ Intron A (10% to 13%).......... 2097
Isoptin Oral Tablets.......... 1179
Isoptin SR Sustained Release Tablets.......... 1181
Keflex Pulvules, Oral Suspension & Pediatric Drops.......... 916
Keftab Tablets.......... 917
▲ Kefurox Vials, Faspak & ADD-Vantage (1 in 25).......... 1277
Kefzol Vials, Faspak & ADD-Vantage (Rare).......... 1279
Kerlone Tablets (Less than 2%).......... 2172
Larodopa Tablets (Rare).......... 1905
Leukine for IV Infusion.......... 1127
Lopid Capsules and Tablets (Occasional).......... 1736
Lotensin Tablets (Scattered incidents).......... 872
Loxitane.......... 1213
Mandol Vials, Faspak & ADD-Vantage.......... 1281
Meclomen Capsules (Less than 1%).......... 1739
Mefoxin.......... 1498
Mefoxin Premixed Intravenous Solution.......... 1500
Mezlin.......... 1597
Mezlin Pharmacy Bulk Package.......... 1599
Mithracin.......... 1602
Monocid Injection (1.6%).......... 2217
Motrin Tablets (Less than 1%).......... 2351
Nebcin Vials, Hyporets & ADD-Vantage.......... 1286
Nimotop Capsules (0.2%).......... 1607
Noroxin Tablets (1.8%).......... 1519
Orudis Capsules (Less than 1%).... 2488
Parlodel.......... 2020
PediaProfen Suspension (Less than 1%).......... 1363
Pipracil (Less frequent).......... 1230
Prilosec Delayed-Release Capsules (Less than 1%).......... 1530
Primaxin I.M... 1532
Primaxin I.V... 1535
Procan SR Tablets (Rare).......... 1760
Procardia XL Tablets (Rare).......... 1783
Pronestyl Capsules and Tablets.......... 1800
Pronestyl-SR Tablets.......... 1801
Rifamate Capsules.......... 1347
Rocaltrol Capsules.......... 1913
▲ Rocephin Injectable Vials, ADD-Vantage (3.3%).......... 1914
Rufen Tablets (Less than 1%).......... 691
Sectral Capsules.......... 2520
Seromycin Pulvules.......... 1298
Sinemet Tablets.......... 952
Suprax (Less than 2%).......... 1235
Synarel Nasal Solution.......... 2300
▲ Tazicef for Injection (1 in 15 patients).......... 2231
▲ Tazidime Vials, Faspak & ADD-Vantage (1 in 15).......... 1299
▲ Tegison Capsules (23%).......... 1881
Ticar for Injection.......... 2236
Timentin for Injection.......... 2239
Toradol IM Injection (Less than 1%).......... 2302
Trobicin Sterile Powder.......... 2366
Unasyn.......... 1965
Velosef Capsules and for Oral Suspension.......... 606
Verelan Capsules.......... 1243
Zantac Injection and Zantac Injection Premixed.......... 1063
Zantac.......... 1065
Zefazone Sterile Powder.......... 2372
▲ Zinacef (1 in 25 patients).......... 1066
▲ Zofran Injection (Approximately 5%).......... 1069
Zyloprim Tablets (Less than 1%).... 830

SIADH secretion syndrome (see under ADH syndrome, inappropriate)

SLE-like syndrome (see under Lupus erythematosus, systemic)

ST section changes (see under EKG changes, ST section)

S_3 gallop (see under Ventricular gallop)

T

T-wave flattening (see under EKG changes, T-wave)

Tachyarrhythmia

Actimmune (Rare).......... 1046
Isuprel Hydrochloride Injection 1:5000.......... 2050
Nicorette (Occasional).......... 1335
Seldane Tablets.......... 1349

Tachyarrhythmia, ventricular

Seldane Tablets (Rare).......... 1349
Seldane-D Extended-Release Tablets (Rare).......... 1350

Tachycardia

Accutane Capsules (Less than 1%).......... 1878
Actifed with Codeine Cough Syrup.. 752
Adipex-P Tablets and Capsules.......... 1019
AeroBid Inhaler System (1-3%).......... 995
AK-Pentolate.......... ⊙ 204
▲ Alfenta Injection (12%).......... 1131
Alupent (Less than 1%).......... 674
Aminophyllin Tablets.......... 2153
▲ Anafranil Capsules (2% to 4%).......... 650
Anatuss LA Tablets.......... 1359
Anectine.......... 755
Apresazide Capsules (Common).......... 854
Apresoline Hydrochloride Parenteral (Ampuls).......... 856
Apresoline Hydrochloride Tablets (Common).......... 855
Apresoline-Esidrix Tablets.......... 857
Arfonad Ampuls.......... 1887
Arm-a-Med Isoetharine Inhalation Solution, USP.......... 616
▲ Arm-a-Med Metaproterenol Sulfate Inhalation Solution, USP (1 in 7 patients).......... 617
Artane.......... 1195
Asbron G.......... 1997
Asendin Tablets (Less than 1%).......... 1196
▲ Atgam Sterile Solution (More than 1% to 10%).......... 2320
Atrohist Sprinkle Capsules.......... 558
Atrovent Inhalation Aerosol (Less than 1 in 100).......... 675
Azdone Tablets.......... 844
Azo Gantrisin Tablets.......... 1888
BAL in Oil Ampules.......... 661
Bellergal-S Tablets (Rare).......... 1998
Benadryl Capsules.......... 1691
Benadryl Injection.......... 1692
Bentyl.......... 1322
Biphetamine Capsules.......... 973
Bontril Slow-Release.......... 834
▲ Brethaire Inhaler (About 5 per 100).......... 1024
Brethine Ampuls (1.3 to 1.5%).......... 1026
Bronkometer Aerosol.......... 2042
Bronkosol Solution.......... 2042
BuSpar (1%).......... 1401
Cafergot/Cafergot P-B.......... 1999
Cantil Tablets.......... 1326
Capoten (Approximately 1 of 100 patients).......... 2255
Capozide (Approximately 1 of 1000 patients).......... 2258
Carbocaine Hydrochloride Injection 2043
Cardene Capsules (0.8-3.4%).......... 2290
Cardizem Tablets-30 mg, 60 mg, 90 mg and 120 mg (Less than 1%).......... 1329
Cardizem SR Capsules-60 mg, 90 mg and 120 mg (Less than 1%) 1327
Cardura Tablets (0.3%).......... 1941
Catapres Tablets (About 5 in 1,000 patients).......... 676
Catapres-TTS (5 per 1,000 patients).......... 677
Choledyl Pediatric Elixir.......... 1702
Choledyl Tablets.......... 1700
Choledyl SA Tablets.......... 1704
Cipro I.V. (1% or less).......... 1592
Clinoril Tablets (Less than 1 in 100).......... 1433
▲ Clozaril Tablets (More than 5 to 25%).......... 2000
Cogentin.......... 1435
Combipres Tablets (About 5 in 1,000).......... 678
Compazine.......... 2201
Constant-T Tablets.......... 1029
Corzide Tablets.......... 702
Cyclogyl.......... ⊙ 215
Cyclomydril.......... ⊙ 216
Cytadren Tablets (1 in 40).......... 861
D.H.E. 45 Injection.......... 2003
Damason-P.......... 1356
Dantrium Capsules (Less frequent) 1619
Dapsone USP.......... 1130
Darbid Tablets.......... 2205
Deconamine.......... 663
Deconsal.......... 559
Demerol.......... 2047
Deprol Tablets.......... 2382
Desferal Vials.......... 862
Desoxyn Gradumet Tablets.......... 514
Desyrel and Desyrel Dividose (Greater than 1%).......... 1404
Dexedrine.......... 2206
Dibenzyline Capsules.......... 2207
Didrex Tablets.......... 2338
Dilaudid-HP Injection.......... 1175
Dilor.......... 2079
Dipentum Capsules (Rare).......... 1160
Diprivan Injection (Less than 1%).. 2267
Ditropan.......... 1332
Donnagel (Rare).......... ▣ 675
Donnatal.......... 1858
Donnatal Extentabs.......... 1859
Donnatal Tablets.......... 1858
Donnazyme Tablets.......... 1860
Dorcol Children's Liquid Cold Formula (Occasional).......... ▣ 686
Dyazide Capsules.......... 2208
DynaCirc Capsules (1.5%).......... 2004
Elavil.......... 2269
Eldepryl.......... 2250
Empirin with Codeine Phosphate Nos. 2, 3 & 4.......... 764
Endep Tablets.......... 1927
Engerix-B Unit-Dose Vials.......... 2213
EpiPen Jr... 843
Epogen for Injection (0.31%).......... 591
Equagesic Tablets.......... 2451
Ethrane.......... 599
Etrafon.......... 2087
Factrel (Rare).......... 2561
Fastin Capsules.......... 2216
Fedahist Gyrocaps.......... 2145
Fedahist Timecaps.......... 2145
Fiorinal with Codeine Capsules (Infrequent).......... 2008
Flexeril Tablets (Less than 1%).......... 1471
Gamimune N Immune Globulin Intravenous (Human).......... 1572
Ganite Injection.......... 1016
Glaucon.......... ⊙ 218
Guaifed.......... 1615
Halcion Tablets (Less frequent).......... 2340
Haldol Decanoate.......... 1375
Haldol Injection, Tablets and Concentrate.......... 1373
Humulin 70/30, 100 Units.......... 1267
Humulin BR, 100 Units.......... 1268
Humulin L, 100 Units.......... 1268
Humulin U, 100 Units.......... 1272
Hycomine Compound Tablets.......... 929
Hycomine Syrup.......... 927
Hytrin Tablets (0.6% to 1.9%).......... 529
Imferon.......... 976
Inapsine Injection.......... 1140
Indocin Capsules (Less than 1%).......... 1487
Indocin I.V. (Less than 1%).......... 1490
Indocin (Less than 1%).......... 1487
Innovar Injection.......... 1141
Intron A (Up to 3%).......... 2097
▲ Intropin Injection (Among most frequent).......... 930
Ionamin Capsules.......... 981
Isoptin Injectable (1.0%).......... 1177
Isuprel Hydrochloride Injection 1:5000.......... 2050
Isuprel Hydrochloride Mistometer.. 2051
Isuprel Hydrochloride Solution 1:200 & 1:100.......... 2052
K-Phos M.F. Tablets.......... 659
K-Phos Neutral Tablets.......... 660
K-Phos No. 2 Tablets.......... 659
Kinesed Tablets.......... 2272
Kutrase Capsules.......... 2146
Lanoxicaps.......... 772

Levsin/Levsinex 2147
Librium Injectable 1932
Limbitrol 1933
Lomotil 2174
Lortab ASA Tablets 2414
Loxitane 1213
Ludiomil Tablets (Rare) 874
Lufyllin & Lufyllin-400 Tablets 2384
Lufyllin-GG Elixir & Tablets 2385
▲Lupron Depot 3.75 mg (Among most frequent) 2312
Lutrepulse for Injection 1655
MS Contin Tablets (Infrequent) 1814
MSIR (Infrequent) 1817
Marax Tablets & DF Syrup 1954
Marcaine Hydrochloride with Epinephrine 1:200,000 (Rare) 2055
Marcaine Hydrochloride Injection (Rare) 2055
Marcaine Spinal (Rare) 2058
Marinol (Dronabinol) Capsules (1%) 1985
Matulane Capsules 1907
Maxair Inhaler (1.2%) 1311
Maxzide 1215
Medihaler Ergotamine Aerosol 1312
Mellaril 2011
Mepergan Injection 2479
Metaprel Inhalation Aerosol Bronchodilator (Less than 1%) 2014
▲Metaprel Inhalation Solution (1 in 7 patients) 2015
Metaprel 2015
Methadone Hydrochloride Diskets 1284
Metubine Iodide Vials 1285
Miltown Tablets 2386
Minipress Capsules (Less than 1%) 1778
Minizide Capsules (Rare) 1779
Moban Tablets & Concentrate (Occasional) 932
Moduretic Tablets (Less than or equal to 1%) 1510
Monistat I.V. 1143
Motofen Tablets 836
Motrin Tablets (Less than 1%) 2351
Murocoll-2 Sterile Ophthalmic Solution ⊙ 261
Mydfrin 2.5% ⊙ 224
Mydriacyl ⊙ 225
Naldecon Syrup, Tablets, Pediatric Drops and Pediatric Syrup 709
Nalfon Pulvules & Tablets (Less than 1%) 919
Narcan Injection 933
Nardil (Less frequent) 1742
Navane Capsules and Concentrate 1954
Navane Intramuscular 1956
NebuPent for Inhalation Solution (1% or less) 1017
Nescaine/Nescaine MPF 629
Nicorette 1335
Nimotop Capsules (Up to 1.4%) 1607
Nipride I.V. Infusion 1909
Nitro-Bid IV (Less than 1%) 1338
Nitrostat IV (Less than 1%) 1744
Norcuron (Rare) 1642
Norflex 1314
Norgesic 1314
Norisodrine Aerotrol 540
Normodyne Injection 2108
Norpramin Tablets 1340
Novafed A Capsules 1342
Novafed Capsules 1342
Novahistine DMX ⊡ 595
Novahistine Elixir ⊡ 596
Novantrone for Injection Concentrate 1226
Nubain Injection (Less than 1%) 934
Omnipaque (Less than 0.4 to 1.0%) 2552
Optimine Tablets 2115
Oramorph SR (Morphine Sulfate Sustained Release Tablets) (Less frequent) 1988
Orap Tablets 1020
Ornade Spansule Capsules 2221
▲Orthoclone OKT3 Sterile Solution (10%) 1645
Orudis Capsules (Less than 1%) 2488
PBZ Tablets & Elixir 1037
PBZ-SR Tablets 1037
PMB 200 and PMB 400 2504
Pamelor 2019
Pantopon Injectable 1911
Parnate Tablets 2222
Peptavlon 2563
Pergonal (menotropins for injection, USP) 2184
Periactin 1525
Permax Tablets (Infrequent) 1291
Phenergan with Codeine 2497
Phenergan Injection 2493
Phenergan Tablets 2496
Phenergan VC with Codeine 2501
Pilocar (Extremely rare) ⊙ 275
Pilostat Sterile Ophthalmic Solution 0.5%, 1%, 2%, 3%, 4%, 5%, 6% (Extremely rare) ⊙ 263
Plague Vaccine (Rare) 1584
Platinol (Occasional) 737
Platinol-AQ Injection (Occasional) 738
Plegine Tablets 2504
Plendil Extended-Release Tablets (0.5% to 1.5%) 1526
Polaramine 2116
Prelu-2 Capsules 683
Prilosec Delayed-Release Capsules (Less than 1%) 1530
Primaxin I.M. 1532
Primaxin I.V. (Less than 0.2%) 1535
Prinivil Tablets (1% or less) 1538
Prinzide Tablets 1540
Priscoline Hydrochloride Ampuls 877
Pro-Banthine Tablets 2141
Procardia XL Tablets (1% or less) 1783
Procrit for Injection (0.31%) 1647
Proglycem (Common) 649
Prolixin Decanoate 1795
Prolixin Elixir 1793
Prolixin Enanthate 1796
Prolixin Injection 1791
Prolixin Oral Concentrate 1792
Prolixin Tablets 1793
Propine with C Cap Compliance Cap ⊙ 255
Prostigmin Injectable 1120
Prostigmin Tablets 1121
▲Prostin VR Pediatric Sterile Solution (3%) 2355
Protopam Chloride for Injection 2518
▲Proventil Inhalation Aerosol (10%) 2117
▲Proventil Repetabs Tablets (5%) 2120
Proventil Solutions for Inhalation 0.5% and 0.083% (1%) 2118
Proventil Syrup (1 of 100; children 2-6: 2%) 2119
▲Proventil Tablets (5%) 2120
Prozac Pulvules (Infrequent) 920
Quadrinal Tablets 1183
Quarzan Capsules 1937
Quibron Capsules 713
Quibron-T 714
Quibron-T/SR 716
Rauzide Tablets 1804
Regitine 878
Respbid Tablets 684
Ritalin 880
Robinul Forte Tablets 1873
Robinul Injectable 1873
Robinul Tablets 1873
Rogaine Topical Solution 2357
Ru-Tuss DE Tablets 694
Ru-Tuss II Capsules 693
Ru-Tuss with Hydrocodone 694
Ru-Tuss Tablets 693
Sandimmune 2024
▲Sanorex Tablets (Among most common) 2030
Sansert Tablets 2031
Seldane Tablets 1349
Seldane-D Extended-Release Tablets 1350
Sensorcaine (Rare) 631
Sensorcaine-MPF Spinal (Rare) 634
Ser-Ap-Es Tablets 881
Serentil 686
Serpasil-Apresoline Tablets 884
Sinequan (Occasional) 1960
Slo-bid Gyrocaps 1847
Soma Compound w/Codeine Tablets 2390
Soma Compound Tablets 2389
Soma Tablets 2388
Stelazine 2226
Sufenta Injection (Less than 1%) 1147
Surmontil Capsules 2524
Survanta Beractant Intratracheal Suspension 1978
T-PHYL (Uniphyl) 200 mg Tablets 1820
Tacaryl 2409
Tagamet (Rare) 2228
Talacen (Infrequent) 2070
Talwin Injection (Rare) 2071
Talwin Compound (Infrequent) 2072
Talwin Injection 2071
Talwin Nx 2073
Tambocor Tablets (1-3%) 1315
Taractan 1920
Tavist Syrup 2033
Tavist Tablets 2035
Tavist-D Tablets 2035
Temaril Tablets, Syrup and Spansule Sustained Release Capsules 1085
Tenex Tablets 1875
Tenoretic Tablets 1105
Tenuate 1354
Thalitone Tablets 687
Theo-24 2179
Theo-Dur Sprinkle 1168
Theo-Dur Extended-Release Tablets 1166
Theolair 1317
Theolair-SR Tablets 1319
▲TheoX Extended-Release Tablets (Among most consistent) 841
Thorazine 2234
Tofranil Ampuls 1038
Tofranil Tablets 1039
Tofranil-PM Capsules 1041
▲Tonocard Tablets (3.2%) 1554
Tornalate (Less than 1%) 2074
Tracrium Injection 817
Trental (Rare) 1099
Trexan Tablets (Less than 1%) 937
Triaminic Cold Tablets ⊡ 688
Triaminic Expectorant DH 1995
Triaminic Oral Infant Drops 1996
Triaminic Syrup (Occasional) ⊡ 689
Triaminicol Multi-Symptom Relief ⊡ 691
Triavil Tablets 1556
Trilafon 2123
Trinalin Repetabs Tablets 1170
Tropicacyl ⊙ 209
Uniphyl 400 mg Tablets 1823
Urispas Tablets 2242
Uroqid-Acid 661
Valpin 50 Tablets 941
Vaseretic Tablets (0.5% to 2.0%) 1559
▲Ventolin (10 in 100 patients) 583
VePesid Capsules and Injection (0.7 to 2%) 741
Visken Tablets (Less than 2%) 2036
Vivactil Tablets 1567
Voltaren Tablets (Less than 1%) 1042
▲Wellbutrin Tablets (10.8%) 821
Wigraine Tablets & Suppositories 1645
▲Xanax Tablets (7.7% to 15.4%) 2367
Yocon 1686
Zantac Injection and Zantac Injection Premixed (Rare) 1063
Zantac (Rare) 1065
Zestoretic 2274
Zestril Tablets (Less than 1%) 2277
Zofran Injection (Rare) 1069

Tachycardia, paradoxical

Cardioquin Tablets 1812
Quinaglute Dura-Tabs Tablets 663

Tachycardia, persistent (maternal)

▲Yutopar (80 to 100% with IV administration) 647

Tachycardia, reflux

Duvoid Tablets 1853
Urecholine 1558

Tachycardia, supraventricular

Prostin VR Pediatric Sterile Solution (Less than 1%) 2355
Reglan 1869
Rythmol Tablets (Less than 1%) 1184
Sodium Polystyrene Sulfonate Suspension 1993
▲Tenormin Tablets and I.V. Injection (11.5%) 1107

Tachycardia, ventricular

Anafranil Capsules (Rare) 650
Aramine Injection 1424
Axid Pulvules (2 in 5,000 patients) 1246
Cardene Capsules (Less than 0.4%) 2290
Cardioquin Tablets 1812
Desyrel and Desyrel Dividose (Two patients) 1404
Dobutrex Solution Vials (Rare) 1259
E.E.S. (Occasional reports) 522
Eminase 2211
EryPed (Occasional reports) 519
Ery-Tab Tablets (Occasional reports) 521
Erythrocin Stearate Filmtab (Occasional reports) 523
Erythromycin Base Filmtab (Occasional reports) 525
Erythromycin Delayed-Release Capsules, USP (Occasional reports) 526
▲Ethmozine Tablets (2%-5%) 946
Hyperstat I.V. Injection 2095
Ilosone (Rare) 913
Ilotycin Gluceptate, IV, Vials (Rare) 915
Lanoxicaps 772
Lanoxin Elixir Pediatric 775
Lanoxin Injection 778
Lanoxin Injection Pediatric 781
Lanoxin Tablets 783
Lorelco Tablets 1333
Marcaine Hydrochloride with Epinephrine 1:200,000 2055
Marcaine Hydrochloride Injection 2055
Nalfon Pulvules & Tablets (Less than 1%) 919
Narcan Injection 933
Norpace 2177
Norpramin Tablets 1340
Omnipaque (0.5 to 0.6%) 2552
PCE Dispertab Tablets (Occasional reports) 549
Parlodel (Less than 1%) 2020
Pentam 300 Injection (0.2%) 1018
Permax Tablets (Infrequent) 1291
Quinaglute Dura-Tabs Tablets 663
Quinidex Extentabs 1868
▲Rythmol Tablets (1.4 to 3.4%) 1184
Sensorcaine 631
Sensorcaine-MPF Spinal 634
Sodium Polystyrene Sulfonate Suspension 1993
Survanta Beractant Intratracheal Suspension 1978
▲Tenormin Tablets and I.V. Injection (16%) 1107
Vascor (200, 300 and 400 mg) Tablets (0.5 to 2.0%) 1383
Versed Injection (Less than 1%) 1924

Tachyphylaxis

Diapid Nasal Spray 2003

Tachypnea

Actimmune (Rare) 1046
Aminophyllin Tablets 2153
Asbron G 1997
Choledyl Pediatric Elixir 1702
Choledyl Tablets 1700
Choledyl SA Tablets 1704
Constant-T Tablets 1029
Dilor 2079
Diprivan Injection (Less than 1%) 2267
Dopram Injectable 1860
Ethrane 599
▲Fungizone Intravenous (Among most common) 2262
Lufyllin & Lufyllin-400 Tablets 2384
Lufyllin-GG Elixir & Tablets 2385
Nardil (Less frequent) 1742
NebuPent for Inhalation Solution (1% or less) 1017
Pergonal (menotropins for injection, USP) 2184
Prostin VR Pediatric Sterile Solution (Less than 1%) 2355
Quadrinal Tablets 1183
Quibron Capsules 713
Quibron-T 714
Quibron-T/SR 716
Respbid Tablets 684
Roferon-A Injection (Less than 1%) 1916
Ru-Tuss Tablets 693
Sensorcaine 631
Sensorcaine-MPF Spinal 634
Slo-bid Gyrocaps 1847
T-PHYL (Uniphyl) 200 mg Tablets 1820
Theo-24 2179
Theo-Dur Sprinkle 1168
Theo-Dur Extended-Release Tablets 1166
Theolair 1317
Theolair-SR Tablets 1319
▲TheoX Extended-Release Tablets (Among most consistent) 841
Uniphyl 400 mg Tablets 1823
Versed Injection (Less than 1%) 1924

Talkativeness

Dalmane Capsules 1927
Tegretol Chewable Tablets 654
Tegretol Suspension 656
Tegretol Tablets 654
Xanax Tablets (2.2%) 2367

Tardive dyskinesia

Asendin Tablets (Rare) 1196
Clozaril Tablets 2000
Compazine 2201
Desyrel and Desyrel Dividose 1404
Elavil 2269

Eldepryl ... 2250
Etrafon ... 2087
Haldol Decanoate ... 1375
Haldol Injection, Tablets and Concentrate ... 1373
Loxitane ... 1213
Mellaril ... 2011
Moban Tablets & Concentrate ... 932
Navane Capsules and Concentrate ... 1954
Navane Intramuscular ... 1956
Orap Tablets ... 1020
Prolixin Decanoate ... 1795
Prolixin Elixir ... 1793
Prolixin Enanthate ... 1796
Prolixin Injection ... 1791
Prolixin Oral Concentrate ... 1792
Prolixin Tablets ... 1793
Reglan ... 1869
Serentil ... 686
Sinequan ... 1960
Stelazine ... 2226
Taractan ... 1920
Thorazine ... 2234
Triavil Tablets ... 1556
Trilafon ... 2123

Tardive dystonia (see under Dystonia, tardive)

Taste, altered

Alferon N Injection (1%) ... 1809
Altace Capsules (Less than 1%) ... 1086
Anadrol-50 Tablets ... 2287
▲Anafranil Capsules (4% to 8%) ... 650
Ansaid Tablets (Less than 1%) ... 2319
AquaMEPHYTON Injection ... 1422
Azactam for Injection (Less than 1%) ... 2252
Brevibloc Injection (Less than 1%) ... 942
BuSpar (Infrequent) ... 1401
Capoten (Approximately 2 to 4 of 100 patients) ... 2255
Capozide (Approximately 2 to 4 of 100 patients) ... 2258
Cardura Tablets (Less than 0.5% of 3960 patients) ... 1941
Catapres-TTS (1 of 101 patients) .. 677
Cordarone Tablets (1 to 3%) ... 2446
▲Cuprimine Capsules (12%) ... 1442
Cytotec (Infrequent) ... 2159
Dantrium Capsules (Less frequent) 1619
Diamox Parenteral ... 1200
Diamox Sequels (Sustained Release) ... 1201
Diamox Tablets ... 1200
▲Didronel I.V. Infusion (5%) ... 1307
Dilaudid-HP Injection ... 1175
Diprivan Injection (Less than 1%) .. 2267
Doral Tablets ... 2383
Eldepryl ... 2250
Endep Tablets ... 1927
▲Ergamisol Tablets (8%) ... 1136
Eskalith ... 2214
Gastrocrom Capsules (Infrequent).. 974
Geref (sermorelin acetate for injection) ... 2560
Halcion Tablets (Rare) ... 2340
Hyperstat I.V. Injection ... 2095
▲Intron A (Up to 13%) ... 2097
IOPIDINE ... ◎ 232
Kerlone Tablets (Less than 2%) ... 2172
Lamprene Capsules (Less than 1%) ... 1030
Limbitrol ... 1933
Lioresal Tablets (Rare) ... 1031
Lodine Capsules (Less than 1%) ... 2468
Lopid Capsules and Tablets ... 1736
Lupron Depot 7.5 mg ... 2311
Lupron Injection (Less than 5%) ... 2310
MS Contin Tablets (Infrequent) ... 1814
MSIR (Infrequent) ... 1817
Maxair Inhaler (Less than 1%) ... 1311
Maxzide ... 1215
Meclomen Capsules (Rare) ... 1739
Mexitil Capsules (About 5 in 1,000) ... 680
Mezlin ... 1597
Mezlin Pharmacy Bulk Package ... 1599
Monopril Tablets (0.2 to 1.0%) ... 1406
Nicorette ... 1335
Normodyne Injection (1%) ... 2108
Normodyne Tablets (1%) ... 2110
Normozide Tablets (1%) ... 2112
Omnipaque (0.5 to 1%) ... 2552
Oramorph SR (Morphine Sulfate Sustained Release Tablets) (Less frequent) ... 1988
Orinase Tablets (Occasional) ... 2354
Orudis Capsules (Less than 1%) ... 2488
Paraplatin for Injection (1%) ... 735
Pepcid (Infrequent) ... 1524
Permax Tablets (1.6%) ... 1291
Platinol ... 737
Prilosec Delayed-Release Capsules (Less than 1%) ... 1530
Primaxin I.M. ... 1532
Primaxin I.V. (Less than 0.2%) ... 1535
Procardia XL Tablets (1% or less).. 1783
ProSom Tablets (Infrequent) ... 554
Proventil Inhalation Aerosol ... 2117
Proventil Repetabs Tablets ... 2120
Proventil Syrup ... 2119
Proventil Tablets ... 2120
Prozac Pulvules (1.8%) ... 920
Quadrinal Tablets ... 1183
Quarzan Capsules ... 1937
▲Retrovir Capsules (5%) ... 802
▲Retrovir I.V. Infusion (5%) ... 805
▲Retrovir Syrup (5%) ... 802
▲Roferon-A Injection (13% to 25%) 1916
▲Rythmol Tablets (2.5 to 22.6%) 1184
Seldane-D Extended-Release Tablets (1.1%) ... 1350
Sinequan ... 1960
Surmontil Capsules ... 2524
Talwin Injection (Rare) ... 2071
Tambocor Tablets (Less than 1%) 1315
Tegison Capsules (Less than 1%) .. 1881
Tenex Tablets (Less than 3%) ... 1875
Timentin for Injection ... 2239
Tofranil Ampuls ... 1038
Tofranil Tablets ... 1039
Tofranil-PM Capsules ... 1041
Tonocard Tablets (Less than 1%) .. 1554
Toradol IM Injection (1% or less) ... 2302
Trandate HCT Tablets (1%) ... 579
Trandate Injection (1 of 100 patients) ... 577
Trandate Tablets (1% of 227 patients) ... 579
Triavil Tablets ... 1556
Vascor (200, 300 and 400 mg) Tablets (0.5 to 2.0%) ... 1383
Vaseretic Tablets ... 1559
Vasotec I.V. ... 1562
Vasotec Tablets (0.5% to 1%) ... 1564
Ventolin (2%) ... 583
Voltaren Tablets (Less than 1%) ... 1042
Wytensin Tablets (3% or less) ... 2542
Xanax Tablets ... 2367

Taste, bad

Arm-a-Med Metaproterenol Sulfate Inhalation Solution, USP (1 in 300 patients) ... 617
Cholybar ... 1705
▲Ciloxan Sterile Ophthalmic Solution (Less than 10%) ... ◎ 214
Cipro I.V. (1% or less) ... 1592
Cipro Tablets (Less than 1%) ... 1589
Cleocin Phosphate Injection ... 2325
Desyrel and Desyrel Dividose (Greater than 1%) ... 1404
Didrex Tablets ... 2338
Fluorescite ... ◎ 217
▲Intal Inhaler (Among most frequent) ... 979
Lupron Injection (Less than 3%) ... 2310
▲Mesnex Injection (100%) ... 733
Metaprel Inhalation Solution (Less frequent) ... 2015
Methergine (Rare) ... 2016
Moduretic Tablets (Less than or equal to 1%) ... 1510
Nasalcrom Nasal Solution (1 in 50) ... 986
Niclocide Chewable Tablets ... 1607
Pentam 300 Injection (1.7%) ... 1018
Pondimin Tablets ... 1867
Trental (Less than 1%) ... 1099
Zovirax (0.3%) ... 824

Taste, bitter

Ceftin Tablets ... 575
Chibroxin Sterile Ophthalmic Solution ... 1431
Clinoril Tablets (Less than 1 in 100) ... 1433
Clozaril Tablets (Less than 1%) ... 2000
Colace (Exceedingly small) ... 1403
Dalmane Capsules (Rare) ... 1927
Diulo ... 2129
Ethmozine Tablets (Less than 2%) 946
Larodopa Tablets (Infrequent) ... 1905
Ludiomil Tablets (Rare) ... 874
Mykrox ½ mg Tablets (Less than 2%) ... 984
Nubain Injection (Less than 1%) ... 934
▲Procan SR Tablets (3-4%) ... 1760
▲Pronestyl Capsules and Tablets (3-4%) ... 1800
▲Pronestyl-SR Tablets (3 to 4%) ... 1801
Sinemet Tablets ... 952
Sinemet CR Tablets ... 953
Versed Injection (Less than 1%) 1924
Zaroxolyn Tablets ... 989

Taste, changes (see under Taste, altered)

Taste, loss (see under Ageusia)

Taste, metallic

Actigall Capsules ... 2280
Adenocard Injection (Less than 1%) ... 1007
Antabuse Tablets (Small number of patients) ... 2429
Calcijex Calcitriol Injection ... 506
Calderol Capsules ... 1635
▲CHEMET (succimer) Capsules (12-20.9%) ... 1361
Cibacalcin Double-chambered Syringes (Rare) ... 859
Cibalith-S ... 870
Cleocin Phosphate Injection ... 2325
Clinoril Tablets (Less than 1 in 100) ... 1433
▲Didronel I.V. Infusion (5%) ... 1307
Eskalith ... 2214
Flagyl I.V. ... 2131
Flagyl Tablets (Not unusual) ... 2170
Lithane Tablets ... 1596
Lithium Carbonate Capsules & Tablets ... 1984
Lithobid Tablets ... 870
Marcaine Spinal ... 2058
Myochrysine Injection ... 1516
Nalfon Pulvules & Tablets (Less than 1%) ... 919
▲NebuPent for Inhalation Solution (53 to 72%) ... 1017
Omnipaque ... 2552
Pima Syrup ... 994
Protostat Tablets ... 1674
Ridaura Capsules ... 2224
Robaxin Injectable ... 1871
Rocaltrol Capsules ... 1913
Sensorcaine ... 631
Sensorcaine-MPF Spinal ... 634
Solganal Suspension ... 2122

Taste, salty

Miacalcin Injection ... 2017

Taste, unpleasant

Adipex-P Tablets and Capsules ... 1019
▲AeroBid Inhaler System (10%) ... 995
Asendin Tablets (Less than 1%) ... 1196
Biphetamine Capsules ... 973
Brethaire Inhaler ... 1024
Desoxyn Gradumet Tablets ... 514
Dexedrine ... 2206
Efudex ... 1880
Elavil ... 2269
Etrafon ... 2087
Fastin Capsules ... 2216
Flagyl I.V. ... 2131
Flagyl Tablets (Not unusual) ... 2170
Flexeril Tablets (1% to 3%) ... 1471
Ionamin Capsules ... 981
Mephyton Tablets ... 1503
Norpramin Tablets ... 1340
Pamelor ... 2019
Prelu-2 Capsules ... 683
Quadrinal Tablets ... 1183
Questran Light ... 711
Questran Powder ... 710
Rimso-50 ... 1836
Sanorex Tablets ... 2030
Tenuate ... 1354
Vivactil Tablets ... 1567

Teeth, discoloration

Achromycin V Capsules ... 1193
Declomycin Capsules, Tablets ... 1199
Doryx Capsules ... 1717
Feosol Elixir ... 2191
Minocin Intravenous (Rare) ... 1221
Minocin Oral Suspension (Rare) ... 1224
Minocin Pellet-Filled Capsules (Rare) ... 1222
Monodox Capsules ... 1630
Pediaflor Drops ... 1972
Peridex ... 1808
Terramycin Capsules ... 1786
Terramycin Intramuscular Solution 1964
Urobiotic-250 Capsules ... 1968
Ventolin (1%) ... 583
Vibramycin Hyclate Capsules ... 1787
Vibramycin Hyclate Intravenous ... 1968
Vibramycin ... 1787
Vi-Daylin/F ADC Vitamins Drops With Fluoride ... 1981
Vi-Daylin/F ADC Vitamins + Iron Drops With Fluoride ... 1981
Vi-Daylin/F Multivitamin Drops With Fluoride ... 1981
Vi-Daylin/F Multivitamin + Iron Drops With Fluoride ... 1981
Vi-Daylin/F Multivitamin Chewable Tablets With Fluoride ... 1982
Vi-Daylin/F Multivitamin + Iron Chewable Tablets With Fluoride .. 1982

Teeth, mottling of enamel (see under Teeth, discoloration)

Teeth, osseous changes

Pediaflor Drops ... 1972
Vi-Daylin/F ADC Vitamins Drops With Fluoride ... 1981
Vi-Daylin/F ADC Vitamins + Iron Drops With Fluoride ... 1981
Vi-Daylin/F Multivitamin Drops With Fluoride ... 1981
Vi-Daylin/F Multivitamin + Iron Drops With Fluoride ... 1981
Vi-Daylin/F Multivitamin Chewable Tablets With Fluoride ... 1982
Vi-Daylin/F Multivitamin + Iron Chewable Tablets With Fluoride .. 1982

Teeth grinding

Anafranil Capsules (Infrequent) ... 650

Telangiectasia

Aclovate Ointment (1 of 366 patients) ... 1053
Diprolene (Less than 1%) ... 2083
Efudex ... 1880
Fluoroplex Topical Solution & Cream 1% ... 1082
Marplan Tablets (Rare) ... 1906
Methotrexate Tablets, Parenteral, LPF Parenteral ... 1217
Rheumatrex Methotrexate Dose Pack ... 1234
Sansert Tablets (Rare) ... 2031
Temovate (1 of 366 patients) ... 1056
Ultravate Ointment 0.05% (Less frequent) ... 2411

Telogen effluvium

Lariam Tablets ... 1904

Temperature elevation (see under Hyperthermia)

Temporal arteritis, aggravation

Butazolidin Capsules & Tablets (Less than 1%) ... 1027

Temporal bone, swelling

Lupron Depot 7.5 mg ... 2311

Tenderness

A/T/S Topical Gel and Topical Solution ... 1089
Americaine Anesthetic Lubricant ... 972
Americaine Otic Topical Anesthetic Ear Drops ... 973
Bactroban Ointment (Less than 1%) ... 2200
Biavax II ... 1427
Bretylol Injection (1 in 1000) ... 923
▲Cefizox Injection (1 to 5%) ... 1012
Cibacalcin Double-chambered Syringes (Rare) ... 859
▲Claforan Sterile Injection (4.3%) 1089
Condylox (Less than 5%) ... 1630
Dilantin Parenteral ... 1712
Diphtheria and Tetanus Toxoids and Pertussis Vaccine Adsorbed USP (For Pediatric Use) ... 892
ETS-2% ... 1685
Gammar, Immune Globulin (Human) U.S.P. ... 609
Hep-B-Gammagee ... 1474
▲HibTITER (3.7%) ... 1206
HyperHep Hepatitis B Immune Globulin (Human) ... 1575
M-M-R II ... 1494
M-R-VAX II ... 1496
Mefoxin ... 1498
Mini-Gamulin Rh, $Rh_0(D)$ Immune Globulin (Human) (Occasional) 612
Plague Vaccine ... 1584
▲ProHIBiT Haemophilus b Conjugate Vaccine (Diphtheria Toxoid Conjugate) (5.3%) ... 896
Recombivax HB (Equal to or greater than 1%) ... 1544

T-Stat 2.0% Topical Solution and Pads 2409
Temovate Scalp Application (1 of 294 patients) 1056
Tetanus Toxoid, Adsorbed Purogenated 1238
Thioguanine Tablets, Tabloid Brand 815
▲ Versed Injection (5.6%) 1924

Tenderness at injection site
▲ Actimmune (14%) 1046
Cholera Vaccine 2445
▲ Flu-Imune Influenza Virus Vaccine (Less than one-third of recipients) 1204
Typhoid Vaccine 2533

Tendon fixation
Gelfoam Sterile Sponge 2338

Tendonitis
Kerlone Tablets (Less than 2%) 2172
Rogaine Topical Solution (2.59%) 2357

Tendon rupture
Celestone Soluspan Suspension 2081
Cortone Acetate Sterile Suspension 1437
Cortone Acetate Tablets 1439
Decadron Elixir 1445
Decadron Phosphate Injection 1449
Decadron Phosphate Respihaler 1454
Decadron Phosphate Turbinaire 1456
Decadron Phosphate with Xylocaine Injection, Sterile 1451
Decadron Tablets 1447
Decadron-LA Sterile Suspension 1457
Hydeltrasol Injection, Sterile 1476
Hydeltra-T.B.A. Sterile Suspension 1478
Hydrocortone Acetate Sterile Suspension 1479
Hydrocortone Phosphate Injection, Sterile 1481
Hydrocortone Tablets 1482

Tenosynovitis
Permax Tablets (Infrequent) 1291
Prozac Pulvules (Infrequent) 920

Tenseness
Bronkometer Aerosol 2042
Bronkosol Solution 2042
EpiPen—Epinephrine Auto-Injector 843
Fedahist Gyrocaps 2145
Fedahist Timecaps 2145
Loxitane 1213
▲ Lozol Tablets (Greater than or equal to 5%) 1843
Novafed A Capsules 1342
Novafed Capsules 1342
Novahistine DH 1342
Novahistine DMX ▣ 595
Novahistine Elixir ▣ 596
Novahistine Expectorant 1343
Seldane-D Extended-Release Tablets 1350
Trinalin Repetabs Tablets 1170

Testes, size decrease
▲ Lupron Depot 3.75 mg (Among most frequent) 2312
▲ Lupron Depot 7.5 mg (5.4%) 2311
▲ Lupron Injection (5% or more) 2310

Testicular atrophy
Anadrol-50 Tablets 2287
Neosar for Injection 566
Tegretol Chewable Tablets 654
Tenex Tablets 1875
Winstrol Tablets 2075

Testicular function, inhibited
Anadrol-50 Tablets 2287
Winstrol Tablets 2075

Testicular swelling
A.P.L. 2431
Asendin Tablets (Very rare) 1196
Elavil 2269
Endep Tablets 1927
Etrafon 2087
Flexeril Tablets (Rare) 1471
Limbitrol 1933
Ludiomil Tablets (Isolated cases) 874
Norpramin Tablets 1340
Pamelor 2019
Sinequan 1960
Surmontil Capsules 2524
Tofranil Ampuls 1038
Tofranil Tablets 1039
Tofranil-PM Capsules 1041
Triavil Tablets 1556
Vivactil Tablets 1567
Wellbutrin Tablets (Infrequent) 821

Testosterone, decreased physiologic effects
Lupron Injection 2310

Testosterone serum levels, transient increase
Zoladex 1110

Tetany
Cibacalcin Double-chambered Syringes (Rare) 859
Garamycin Injectable 2093
Platinol (Occasional) 737
Platinol-AQ Injection (Occasional) 738
Syntocinon Injection 2032

Thermoregulatory mechanisms, interference
Astramorph/PF Injection, USP (Preservative-Free) 618
Compazine 2201
Duramorph 960
Infumorph 200 and Infumorph 500 Sterile Solutions 962

Thinking, abnormality
Alurate Elixir (Less than 1 in 100) 1883
Anafranil Capsules (Frequent) 650
Brevibloc Injection (Less than 1%) 942
Butisol Sodium Elixir & Tablets (Less than 1 in 100) 2377
Cardura Tablets (Less than 0.5% of 3960 patients) 1941
Cytovene Sterile Powder (1% or less) 2292
Deprol Tablets 2382
Doral Tablets 2383
Duragesic Transdermal System (1% or greater) 1133
Flexeril Tablets (Less than 1%) 1471
Intron A (Less than 1%) 2097
Kerlone Tablets (Less than 2%) 2172
Marinol (Dronabinol) Capsules 1985
Mebaral Tablets (Less than 1 in 100) 2061
Nembutal Sodium Capsules (Less than 1%) 534
Nembutal Sodium Solution (Less than 1%) 536
Nembutal Sodium Suppositories (Less than 1%) 538
Permax Tablets (Frequent) 1291
Phenobarbital Elixir and Tablets (Less than 1 in 100 patients) 1293
ProSom Tablets (2%) 554
Seconal Sodium Pulvules (Less than 1 in 100) 1296
Tegison Capsules (Less than 1%) 1881
Toradol IM Injection (1% or less) 2302
Wellbutrin Tablets (Infrequent) 821

Thiocynate toxicity
Nipride I.V. Infusion 1909

Thirst (see under Dipsesis)

Thrashing
Diprivan Injection (Less than 1%) 2267

Throat, burning
Diprivan Injection (Less than 1%) 2267
Eldepryl 2250
Emcyt Capsules (1%) 1161
Gastrocrom Capsules (Infrequent) 974

Throat, congestion
Bentyl 1322

Throat, dryness
▲ Actifed with Codeine Cough Syrup (Among most frequent) 752
AeroBid Inhaler System (1-3%) 995
Azmacort Inhaler 1837
Benadryl Injection 1692
Catapres-TTS (2%) 677
Clozaril Tablets (Less than 1%) 2000
Comhist LA Capsules 1618
Daraprim Tablets (Rare) 761
▲ Dimetane-DC Cough Syrup (Most frequent) 1857
Dimetane-DX Cough Syrup (Among most frequent) 1858
Hylorel Tablets (1.7%) 975
Lopressor HCT Tablets 1034
Marax Tablets & DF Syrup 1954
▲ Norpace (3 to 9%) 2177
Optimine Tablets 2115
Ornade Spansule Capsules 2221
PBZ Tablets & Elixir 1037
PBZ-SR Tablets 1037
Periactin 1525
Polaramine 2116
Robinul Injectable 1873
Ru-Tuss II Capsules 693
▲ Seldane Tablets (4.8%) 1349
▲ Seldane-D Extended-Release Tablets (21.7%) 1350
Tavist Syrup 2033
Tavist Tablets 2035
Tavist-D Tablets 2035
Triaminic Expectorant DH 1995
Triaminic Oral Infant Drops 1996
Trinalin Repetabs Tablets 1170
Ventolin 583

Throat, irritation
AeroBid Inhaler System (1-3%) 995
Alupent (1 to 4%) 674
Azmacort Inhaler 1837
Clozaril Tablets (1%) 2000
Decadron Phosphate Respihaler 1454
▲ Intal Inhaler (Among most frequent) 979
Isuprel Hydrochloride Mistometer 2051
Metaprel Inhalation Aerosol Bronchodilator (1 to 4%) 2014
Nasacort Nasal Inhaler (Less than 5%) 1844
Provocholine for Inhalation (1 occurrence) 1911
▲ Tornalate (5%) 2074
▲ Ventolin Rotacaps for Inhalation (2% to 6%) 583

Throat, presence of hard nodule
Lupron Depot 7.5 mg (Less than 5%) 2311
Lupron Injection 2310

Throat, soreness
▲ Adalat Capsules (10 mg and 20 mg) (6%) 1587
▲ AeroBid Inhaler System (20%) 995
Atgam Sterile Solution (Less than 5%) 2320
Biavax II 1427
Blocadren Tablets 1429
BuSpar (Frequent) 1401
Butazolidin Capsules & Tablets 1027
Capoten 2255
Capozide 2258
Cardene Capsules (Rare) 2290
Cartrol Tablets 507
▲ CHEMET (succimer) Capsules (0.7 to 3.7%) 1361
Colace (Exceedingly small) 1403
Compazine 2201
Corgard Tablets 701
Corzide Tablets 702
Cytosar-U Sterile Powder (Less frequent) 2329
Danocrine Capsules 2046
Dapsone USP 1130
DynaCirc Capsules (0.5% to 1%) 2004
Inderal 2459
Inderal LA Long Acting Capsules 2461
Inderide Tablets 2463
Inderide LA Long Acting Capsules 2465
Kerlone Tablets 2172
Koro-Flex Arcing Spring Diaphragm 2142
Koromex Coil Spring Diaphragm 2142
Levatol 1832
M-M-R II 1494
M-R-VAX II 1496
Maxair Inhaler (Less than 1%) 1311
Meruvax II 1503
Mykrox ½ mg Tablets (Less than 2%) 984
Nasalide Nasal Solution 0.025% (5% or less) 2299
▲ Neupogen for Injection (4%) 595
▲ Nicorette (37.2%) 1335
Normodyne Tablets 2110
Normozide Tablets 2112
Ortho Diaphragm Kit 1664
Prinzide Tablets 1540
▲ Procardia XL Tablets (6%) 1783
Prolixin Decanoate 1795
Prolixin Enanthate 1796
Prolixin Oral Concentrate 1792
Pronestyl Capsules and Tablets 1800
Pronestyl Injection 1798
Pronestyl-SR Tablets 1801
Quadrinal Tablets 1183
Rowasa (2.33%) 2248
Sandostatin Injection (Less than 1%) 2029
Sectral Capsules 2520
▲ Seldane Tablets (3.2%) 1349
Seldane-D Extended-Release Tablets (1.9%) 1350
Stelazine 2226
Tegretol Chewable Tablets 654
Tenoretic Tablets 1105
Tenormin Tablets and I.V. Injection 1107
Timoptic in Ocudose 1552
Timoptic Sterile Ophthalmic Solution 1550
Tonocard Tablets 1554
Trandate HCT/Trandate 579
Trental (Less than 1%) 1099
Trexan Tablets (Less than 1%) 937
Valium Injectable 1937
Vaseretic Tablets 1559
Vasotec I.V. 1562
Vasotec Tablets 1564
Visken Tablets 2036
Zestoretic 2274
Zestril Tablets 2277
Zovirax (0.3%) 824

Throat, swelling of
Miacalcin Injection (A few cases) 2017

Throat, tightness
Adenocard Injection (Less than 1%) 1007
Alferon N Injection (1%) 1809
Etrafon 2087
Trilafon 2123
Unasyn (Less than 1%) 1965

Throbbing, head
EpiPen—Epinephrine Auto-Injector 843

Thrombocythemia (see under Thrombocytosis)

Thrombocytopenia
Accutane Capsules (Less than 1 in 10) 1878
Achromycin V Capsules 1193
Actifed with Codeine Cough Syrup 752
Adalat Capsules (10 mg and 20 mg) (Less than 0.5%) 1587
Adriamycin PFS 561
Adriamycin RDF 562
Aldactazide 2150
Aldoclor Tablets 1413
Aldomet Ester HCl Injection 1417
Aldomet Oral 1415
Aldoril Tablets 1418
Amoxil 2193
Anaprox and Anaprox DS Tablets (Less than 1%) 2288
Ancef Injection 2194
Ancobon Capsules 1886
Ansaid Tablets (Rare) 2319
Anturane (Rare) 853
Apresazide Capsules 854
Apresoline-Esidrix Tablets 857
Asendin Tablets (Very rare) 1196
▲ Atgam Sterile Solution (1 in 9 patients; 30%) 2320
Attenuvax (Rare) 1424
Augmentin Tablets, Powder for Oral Suspension, and Chewable Tablets 2198
Axid Pulvules 1246
Azactam for Injection (Less than 1%) 2252
Azo Gantanol Tablets 1887
Azo Gantrisin Tablets 1888
Azulfidine Tablets, EN-tabs, Oral Suspension (Rare) 1157
Bactrim DS Tablets 1891
Bactrim I.V. Infusion 1889
Bactrim 1891
Benadryl Capsules 1691
Benadryl Injection 1692
Biavax II 1427
Bicillin C-R Injection 2438
Bicillin C-R 900/300 Injection 2440
Bicillin L-A Injection (Infrequent) 2442
BiCNU 723
Bumex (0.2%) 1895
BuSpar (Rare) 1401
Butazolidin Capsules & Tablets (Less than 1%) 1027
▲ Calciparine Injection (0 to 30%) 925
Capastat Sulfate Vials (Rare) 1250
Capoten 2255
Capozide 2258
Cardizem Tablets-30 mg, 60 mg, 90 mg and 120 mg 1329

Cardizem SR Capsules-60 mg, 90 mg and 120 mg (Less than 1%) 1327
Ceclor Pulvules & Suspension (Rare) 1251
CeeNU 725
Cefizox Injection (Rare) 1012
Cefotan 2265
Ceftin Tablets 575
Ceptaz for Injection (Very rare) 1057
Children's Advil Suspension (Less than 1%) 2426
Chloromycetin Kapseals 1695
Chloromycetin Palmitate, Oral Suspension 1697
Chloromycetin Sodium Succinate 1698
▲Cipro I.V. (Among most frequent) 1592
Cipro Tablets (0.1%) 1589
Claforan Sterile Injection (Less than 1%) 1089
Cleocin HCl Capsules 2322
Cleocin Pediatric Flavored Granules 2324
Cleocin Phosphate Injection 2325
Clinoril Tablets (Less than 1 in 100) 1433
Colchicine Ampoules 1252
Combipres Tablets 678
Comhist LA Capsules 1618
Cordarone Tablets (Rare) 2446
Corzide Tablets 702
Cosmegen Injection 1440
▲Cuprimine Capsules (4%) 1442
Cytosar-U Sterile Powder (Less than 7 patients) 2329
Cytotec (Infrequent) 2159
▲Cytovene Sterile Powder (Approximately 20%) 2292
Cytoxan for Injection (A few patients) 726
Danocrine Capsules 2046
Daranide Tablets 1445
Daraprim Tablets 761
Declomycin Capsules, Tablets 1199
Deconamine 663
Demser Capsules (Rare) 1460
▲Depakene Capsules & Syrup (Among most common) 511
Depakote 512
▲Depen Titratable Tablets (4%) 2379
DiaBeta 1091
Diabinese Tablets 1775
Diflucan Injection and Tablets 1948
Dilantin Infatabs (Occasional) 1710
Dilantin Kapseals (Occasional) 1708
Dilantin Parenteral (Occasional) 1712
Dilantin-30 Pediatric/Dilantin-125 Suspension (Occasional) 1713
Dilantin with Phenobarbital Kapseals (Occasional) 1715
Dimetane-DC Cough Syrup 1857
Dimetane-DX Cough Syrup 1858
Dipentum Capsules (Rare) 1160
Diucardin Tablets 2450
Diulo 2129
Diupres Tablets 1461
Diuril Oral Suspension 1464
Diuril Sodium Intravenous 1463
Diuril Tablets 1464
Dolobid Tablets (Less than 1 in 100) 1465
Dolophine Hydrochloride Ampoules & Vials 1260
Dolophine Hydrochloride Tablets 1261
Doryx Capsules 1717
Dyazide Capsules 2208
Dyrenium Capsules (Rare) 2210
Easprin 1719
Edecrin (Rare) 1468
Efudex 1880
Elavil 2269
Emcyt Capsules (1%) 1161
▲Eminase (Less than 10%) 2211
Endep Tablets 1927
Enduron Tablets 517
Enduronyl 518
Engerix-B Unit-Dose Vials 2213
▲Ergamisol Tablets (Up to 10%) 1136
Esidrix Tablets 863
Esimil Tablets 864
Etrafon 2087
Eulexin Capsules (1%) 2089
▲Exosurf Neonatal for Intratracheal Suspension (12% to 25%) 765
Exna Tablets 1862
▲Sterile FUDR (Among more common) 1898
Fansidar Tablets 1896
Feldene Capsules (Less than 1%) 1777
Flagyl I.V. (Rare) 2131
Flagyl Tablets (Rare) 2170
Flexeril Tablets (Rare) 1471
Fluorouracil Injection 1897
Fortaz (Rare) 1060
Fungizone Intravenous 2262
Gantanol 1899
Gantrisin Ophthalmic Ointment/Solution 1900
Gantrisin 1901
Garamycin Injectable 2093
Geocillin Tablets 1951
Glucotrol 1952
▲Heparin Lock Flush Solution (0 to 30%) 2456
▲Heparin Sodium Vials (0 to 30%) 1264
▲Heparin Sodium Injection (0 to 30%) 2457
▲Heparin Sodium Injection, USP, Sterile Solution (0-30%) 2342
▲Hexalen Capsules (3% to 10%) 2316
Hydrea Capsules (Occasional) 728
HydroDIURIL Tablets 1484
Hydromox R Tablets 1209
Hydromox Tablets 1208
Hydropres Tablets 1485
Hyperstat I.V. Injection 2095
INH Tablets 868
▲IFEX (About 20%) 729
Imuran 768
Inderide Tablets 2463
Inderide LA Long Acting Capsules 2465
Indocin I.V. (1% to 3%) 1490
Inocor Lactate Injection (2.4%) 2048
▲Intron A (18%) 2097
Ismelin Tablets 869
Keflex Pulvules, Oral Suspension & Pediatric Drops 916
Keftab Tablets 917
Kefurox Vials, Faspak & ADD-Vantage 1277
Kerlone Tablets (Less than 2%) 2172
Klonopin Tablets 1902
Lariam Tablets 1904
Lasix 1093
Limbitrol 1933
Lodine Capsules (Less than 1%) 2468
Loniten Tablets (Rare) 2346
Lopid Capsules and Tablets (Rare) 1736
Lopressor HCT Tablets 1034
Lorelco Tablets 1333
Loxitane (Rare) 1213
Lozol Tablets 1843
Ludiomil Tablets 874
M-M-R II 1494
M-R-VAX II 1496
Macrodantin Capsules 1624
Mandol Vials, Faspak & ADD-Vantage (Rare) 1281
▲Matulane Capsules (Frequent) 1907
Maxzide 1215
Meclomen Capsules (Rare) 1739
Mefoxin 1498
Mefoxin Premixed Intravenous Solution 1500
Mellaril 2011
Mesantoin Tablets 2013
Methadone Hydrochloride Diskets (1 person) 1284
▲Methotrexate Tablets, Parenteral, LPF Parenteral (3 to 10%) 1217
Mevacor Tablets (Rare) 1505
Mexitil Capsules (About 2 in 1,000) 680
Mezlin 1597
Mezlin Pharmacy Bulk Package 1599
Micronase Tablets 2350
Minizide Capsules 1779
Minocin Intravenous 1221
Minocin Oral Suspension 1224
Minocin Pellet-Filled Capsules 1222
Mithracin 1602
Moduretic Tablets 1510
Monistat I.V. 1143
Monocid Injection (Less than 1%) 2217
Monodox Capsules 1630
Monopril Tablets (0.2 to 1.0%) 1406
Motrin Tablets (Less than 1%) 2351
Mustargen 1514
Mutamycin 733
Mykrox ½ mg Tablets 984
Myleran Tablets 790
Myochrysine Injection 1516
Nalfon Pulvules & Tablets (Less than 1%) 919
Naprosyn (Less than 1%) 2297
Naturetin Tablets 1789
Navane Capsules and Concentrate 1954
Navane Intramuscular 1956
Nebcin Vials, Hyporets & ADD-Vantage 1286
NebuPent for Inhalation Solution (1% or less) 1017
NegGram (Rare) 2062
Neosar for Injection (Occasional) 566
Netromycin Injection 100 mg/ml (1 per 1000 patients) 2104
Neupogen for Injection (Less frequent) 595
Nimotop Capsules (Less than 1%) 1607
Nipride I.V. Infusion 1909
Nizoral Tablets (Less than 1%) 1145
Norethin 2133
Normodyne Tablets 2110
Normozide Tablets 2112
Noroxin Tablets 1519
Norpace (Rare) 2177
Norpramin Tablets 1340
Norzine 1818
Oncovin Solution Vials & Hyporets 1288
Optimine Tablets 2115
Oretic Tablets 544
Oreticyl 545
Orinase Tablets 2354
Ornade Spansule Capsules 2221
Orudis Capsules (Less than 1%) 2488
PBZ Tablets & Elixir 1037
PBZ-SR Tablets 1037
Pamelor 2019
Panhematin 546
Paradione Capsules 548
▲Paraplatin for Injection (35% to 62%) 735
Parnate Tablets 2222
PediaProfen Suspension (Less than 1%) 1363
Pediazole 1973
PedvaxHIB (One child) 1521
Pentam 300 Injection (0.9 to 1.7%) 1018
Pepcid (Rare) 1524
Periactin 1525
Permax Tablets (Infrequent) 1291
Pfizerpen for Injection (Rare) 1957
Phenergan with Codeine (Rare) 2497
Phenergan with Dextromethorphan (Rare) 2499
Phenergan Suppositories (Rare) 2496
Phenergan Syrup 2495
Phenergan VC 2500
Phenergan VC with Codeine 2501
Pipracil 1230
Placidyl Capsules (One case) 553
Plaquenil Sulfate Tablets 2067
Platinol 737
Platinol-AQ Injection 738
Pneumovax 23 1528
Pnu-Imune 23 Pneumococcal Vaccine Polyvalent (Rare) 1233
Polaramine 2116
Prilosec Delayed-Release Capsules (Less than 1%) 1530
Primaxin I.M. 1532
Primaxin I.V. (Less than 0.2%) 1535
Prinzide Tablets 1540
Priscoline Hydrochloride Ampuls 877
Procan SR Tablets (Rare) 1760
Procardia Capsules (Less than .5%) 1781
Proglycem 649
ProHIBiT Haemophilus b Conjugate Vaccine (Diphtheria Toxoid Conjugate) (One adult) 896
Proloprim Tablets 799
Pronestyl Capsules and Tablets (Approximately 0.5%) 1800
Pronestyl Injection (Approximately 0.5%) 1798
Pronestyl-SR Tablets (0.5%) 1801
Prostin VR Pediatric Sterile Solution (Less than 1%) 2355
Protostat Tablets (Rare) 1674
Prozac Pulvules 920
Purinethol Tablets 800
Quinaglute Dura-Tabs Tablets 663
Quinidex Extentabs 1868
Rauzide Tablets 1804
Recombivax HB 1544
Renese Tablets 1785
Renese-R Tablets (Rare) 1786
▲Rheumatrex Methotrexate Dose Pack (3% to 10%) 1234
Ridaura Capsules (1 to 3%) 2224
Rifadin (Rare) 1345
Rifamate Capsules 1347
Rimactane Capsules (Rare) 879
Rocephin Injectable Vials, ADD-Vantage (Less than 1%) 1914
▲Roferon-A Injection (35%) 1916
Rogaine Topical Solution (0.31%) 2357
Rufen Tablets (Less than 1%) 691
Ru-Tuss II Capsules 693
Ru-Tuss Tablets 693
Rythmol Tablets (Less than 1%) 1184
SSD RP Cream 690
Saluron 718
Salutensin/Salutensin-Demi 719
Sandimmune (2% or less) 2024
Septra 813
Septra I.V. Infusion 808
Septra I.V. Infusion ADD-Vantage Vials 810
Septra 813
Ser-Ap-Es Tablets 881
Serentil 686
Serpasil-Esidrix Tablets 886
Silvadene Cream 1% 1352
Sinemet Tablets (Rare) 952
Sinemet CR Tablets 953
Sinequan (Occasional) 1960
Solganal Suspension (Rare) 2122
Spectrobid Tablets & Powder for Oral Suspension 1961
Stelazine 2226
Suprax (Less than 2%) 1235
Surmontil Capsules 2524
Tagamet (Approximately 3 per 1,000,000) 2228
Tambocor Tablets (Less than 1%) 1315
Tapazole Tablets 1298
Tavist Syrup 2033
Tavist Tablets 2035
Tavist-D Tablets 2035
Tazicef for Injection (Very rare) 2231
▲Tegison Capsules (1-10%) 1881
Tegretol Chewable Tablets (Not common) 654
Tegretol Suspension 656
Tegretol Tablets 654
Tenoretic Tablets 1105
Tenormin Tablets and I.V. Injection 1107
Terramycin Capsules 1786
Terramycin Intramuscular Solution 1964
Thalitone Tablets 687
TheraCys BCG Live (Intravesical) (Up to 0.9%) 898
Thiosulfil Forte Tablets 2526
Thiotepa Parenteral 1240
Ticar for Injection 2236
Timentin for Injection 2239
Timolide Tablets 1547
Tofranil Ampuls 1038
Tofranil Tablets 1039
Tofranil-PM Capsules 1041
Tolectin (200, 400 and 600 mg) (Less than 1%) 1379
Tolinase Tablets 2365
Tonocard Tablets (Less than 1%) 1554
Torecan 1993
Trandate HCT Tablets 579
Trecator-SC Tablets 2527
Trental (Rare) 1099
Triaminic Expectorant DH 1995
Triaminic Oral Infant Drops 1996
Triavil Tablets 1556
Tridione 557
Trimpex Tablets 1922
Trinalin Repetabs Tablets 1170
Unasyn 1965
Unipen (Infrequent) 2533
Vancocin HCl, Oral Solution & Pulvules (Rare) 1304
Vancocin HCl, Vials & ADD-Vantage (Rare) 1302
Vaseretic Tablets (Rare) 1559
Vasotec I.V. (Rare) 1562
Vasotec Tablets (Rare) 1564
Velban Vials 1305
▲VePesid Capsules and Injection (1 to 41%) 741
Vibramycin Hyclate Capsules 1787
Vibramycin Hyclate Intravenous 1968
Vibramycin 1787
Vira-A for Injection 1766
Vivactil Tablets 1567
Voltaren Tablets (Less than 1%) 1042
Zanosar Sterile Powder 2371
Zantac Injection and Zantac Injection Premixed (Few patients) 1063
Zantac (A few patients) 1065
Zaroxolyn Tablets 989
Zefazone Sterile Powder 2372
Zestoretic 2274
Zinacef 1066
Zovirax Sterile Powder (Less than 1%) 828
Zyloprim Tablets (Less than 1%) 830

Thrombocytopenic purpura (see under Purpura, thrombocytopenic)

Thrombocytosis

Accutane Capsules (1 in 5 to 1 in 10) 1878

Ancef Injection 2194
Augmentin Tablets, Powder for Oral Suspension, and Chewable Tablets (Less than 1%) 2198
Azactam for Injection (Less than 1%) 2252
▲Cefizox Injection (1 to 5%) 1012
Cefotan (1 in 300) 2265
Ceptaz for Injection (One in 45) 1057
CHEMET (succimer) Capsules (0.5 to 1.5%) 1361
▲Cipro I.V. (Among most frequent) 1592
Cipro Tablets (0.1%) 1589
Cuprimine Capsules 1442
Demser Capsules (Rare) 1460
Depen Titratable Tablets 2379
Estratest 2245
Fortaz (1 in 45) 1060
▲Intron A (Up to 9%) 2097
Kefzol Vials, Faspak & ADD-Vantage 1279
Monocid Injection (1.7%) 2217
Netromycin Injection 100 mg/ml (2 of 1000 patients) 2104
Permax Tablets (Rare) 1291
Primaxin I.M. 1532
Prozac Pulvules (Rare) 920
▲Rocephin Injectable Vials, ADD-Vantage (5.1%) 1914
Tazicef for Injection (1 in 45 patients) 2231
Unasyn 1965
Zefazone Sterile Powder 2372
Zovirax Sterile Powder (Less than 1%) 828

Thromboembolic complications

Atromid-S Capsules 2435
Brevicon 2304
Calciparine Injection 925
Cycrin Tablets 2449
Demulen 2161
Enovid 2161
Estinyl Tablets 2085
Estrace 1385
Estrace Vaginal Cream 1388
Estradurin 2452
Estratest 2245
Estrovis 1721
Heparin Lock Flush Solution 2456
Heparin Sodium Vials 1264
Heparin Sodium Injection 2457
Heparin Sodium Injection, USP, Sterile Solution 2342
Levlen/Tri-Levlen 665
Loestrin 1728
Mediatric Capsules 2476
Metrodin (urofollitropin for injection) 2182
Micronor Tablets 1667
Modicon 1667
Nolvadex Tablets (Infrequent) 1102
Nordette-21 Tablets 2481
Nordette-28 Tablets 2483
Norinyl 2304
Norlestrin 1746
Nor-Q D Tablets 2304
Ortho Dienestrol Cream 1664
Ortho-Cyclen Tablets 1658
Ortho-Novum 1667
Ovcon 1391
PMB 200 and PMB 400 2504
Premarin Intravenous 2508
Premarin with Methyltestosterone 2515
Premarin Vaginal Cream 2512
Provera Tablets 2356
Serophene (clomiphene citrate tablets, USP) 2186
Stilphostrol Tablets and Ampuls 1609
TACE 12 and 25 mg 1353
Levlen/Tri-Levlen 665
Tri-Norinyl 2304
Triphasil-21 Tablets 2527
Triphasil-28 Tablets 2532

Thromboembolic disease (see under Thromboembolic complications)

Thromboembolism

Amen 833
Brevicon 2304
Cortone Acetate Sterile Suspension 1437
Cortone Acetate Tablets 1439
Cycrin Tablets 2449
Dalalone D.P. Injectable 999
Danocrine Capsules 2046
Decadron Elixir 1445
Decadron Phosphate Injection 1449
Decadron Phosphate Respihaler 1454
Decadron Phosphate Turbinaire 1456
Decadron Phosphate with Xylocaine Injection, Sterile 1451
Decadron Tablets 1447
Decadron-LA Sterile Suspension 1457
Demulen 2161
Diethylstilbestrol Tablets 1258
Enovid 2161
Estrace 1385
Estrace Vaginal Cream 1388
Estraderm Transdermal System 866
Estratest 2245
Hydeltrasol Injection, Sterile 1476
Hydeltra-T.B.A. Sterile Suspension 1478
Hydrocortone Acetate Sterile Suspension 1479
Hydrocortone Phosphate Injection, Sterile 1481
Hydrocortone Tablets 1482
Kenalog-10 Injection 2402
Kenalog-40 Injection 2403
Lamprene Capsules (Less than 1%) 1030
Lo/Ovral Tablets 2471
Lo/Ovral-28 Tablets 2476
Loestrin 1728
Menrium Tablets 1934
Micronor Tablets 1667
Modicon 1667
Nordette-21 Tablets 2481
Nordette-28 Tablets 2483
Norinyl 2304
Norlestrin 1746
Nor-Q D Tablets 2304
Ortho Dienestrol Cream 1664
Ortho-Novum 1667
Ovcon 1391
Ovral Tablets 2490
Ovral-28 Tablets 2491
Ovrette Tablets 2492
Premarin Tablets 2510
Premarin Vaginal Cream 2512
Tri-Norinyl 28-Day Tablets 2304
Triphasil-21 Tablets 2527
Triphasil-28 Tablets 2532

Thromboembolism, arterial

A.P.L. 2431
Brevicon 2304
Demulen 2161
Enovid 2161
Jenest-28 Tablets 1636
Levlen/Tri-Levlen 665
Loestrin 1728
Metrodin (urofollitropin for injection) (Less than 1 in 50) 2182
Micronor Tablets 1667
Modicon 1667
Norethin 2133
Norinyl 2304
Norlestrin 1746
Nor-Q D Tablets 2304
Ortho-Cyclen Tablets 1658
Ortho-Novum 1667
Pergonal (menotropins for injection, USP) 2184
Levlen/Tri-Levlen 665
Tri-Norinyl 2304

Thrombopenia (see under Thrombocytopenia)

Thrombophlebitis

AK-Fluor Injection 10% and 25% ⊙ 204
Amen 833
Amicar Syrup, Tablets, and Injection 1194
Anafranil Capsules (Rare) 650
Atgam Sterile Solution (Less than 5%) 2320
Azactam for Injection (2.4%) 2252
Bactrim I.V. Infusion (Rare) 1889
Brevibloc Injection (Less than 1%) 942
Brevicon 2304
Brevital Sodium Vials 1248
Cipro I.V. (1% or less) 1592
Cleocin Phosphate Injection 2325
Clozaril Tablets (Less than 1%) 2000
Cortifoam 1827
Cuprimine Capsules (Rare) 1442
Cycrin Tablets (Occasional) 2449
▲Cytosar-U Sterile Powder (Among most frequent) 2329
Dalgan Injection (Less than 1%) 620
Dantrium Intravenous 1620
Demulen 2161
Depen Titratable Tablets (Rare) 2379
Depo-Provera Sterile Aqueous Suspension 2336
▲Emcyt Capsules (3%) 1161
Enovid 2161
Ergamisol Tablets 1136
Estradurin 2452
Estratest 2245
Ethmozine Tablets (Less than 2%) 946
Sterile FUDR 1898
Flagyl I.V. 2131
Fluorescite ⊙ 217
Fluorouracil Injection 1897
Fungizone Intravenous 2262
Indocin Capsules (Rare) 1487
Indocin I.V. 1490
Indocin (Rare) 1487
Jenest-28 Tablets 1636
Kefurox Vials, Faspak & ADD-Vantage (1 in 60) 1277
Kenalog-10 Injection 2402
Kenalog-40 Injection 2403
Kerlone Tablets (Less than 2%) 2172
Lasix 1093
Levlen/Tri-Levlen 665
Lo/Ovral Tablets 2471
Lo/Ovral-28 Tablets 2476
Loestrin 1728
Mandol Vials, Faspak & ADD-Vantage (Rare) 1281
Mefoxin 1498
Mefoxin Premixed Intravenous Solution 1500
Megace Tablets (Rare) 732
Mestinon Injectable 1115
Methergine (Rare) 2016
Mezlin 1597
Mezlin Pharmacy Bulk Package 1599
Micronor Tablets 1667
Modicon 1667
Mustargen 1514
Mutamycin 733
Nordette-21 Tablets 2481
Nordette-28 Tablets 2483
Norethin 2133
Norinyl 2304
Norlestrin 1746
Norlutate 1754
Norlutin 1755
Nor-Q D Tablets 2304
Omnipaque 2552
Ortho Dienestrol Cream 1664
Ortho-Cyclen Tablets 1658
Ortho-Novum 1667
Ovcon 1391
Ovral Tablets 2490
Ovral-28 Tablets 2491
Ovrette Tablets 2492
PMB 200 and PMB 400 2504
Permax Tablets (Infrequent) 1291
▲Pipracil (4%) 1230
Polymyxin B Sulfate, Aerosporin Brand Sterile Powder (Occasional) 798
Premarin Intravenous 2508
Premarin with Methyltestosterone 2515
Premarin Tablets 2510
Premarin Vaginal Cream 2512
▲Primaxin I.V. (3.1%) 1535
Provera Tablets 2356
Prozac Pulvules (Rare) 920
Robaxin Injectable 1871
Sandostatin Injection (Less than 1%) 2029
Sansert Tablets 2031
Septra I.V. Infusion (Rare) 808
Septra I.V. Infusion ADD-Vantage Vials (Rare) 810
Stilphostrol Tablets and Ampuls 1609
Surital Ampoules, Steri-Vials 1764
TACE 12 and 25 mg 1353
Tegretol Chewable Tablets 654
Tegretol Suspension 656
Tegretol Tablets 654
Timentin for Injection 2239
Levlen/Tri-Levlen 665
Tri-Norinyl 2304
Triphasil-21 Tablets 2527
Triphasil-28 Tablets 2532
▲Unasyn (3%) 1965
Zefazone Sterile Powder 2372
Zinacef (1 in 60 patients) 1066
Zyloprim Tablets (Less than 1%) 830

Thrombophlebitis, peripheral

Atgam Sterile Solution (More than 1%; less than 5%) 2320

Thromboplastin time, increase

Azactam for Injection 2252
Eminase 2211
Streptase for Infusion (Rare) 635
Zefazone Sterile Powder 2372

Thrombosis

BiCNU (Rare) 723
Demulen 2161
Dicumarol Tablets 516
Diprivan Injection (Less than 1%) 2267
Emcyt Capsules 1161
Enovid 2161
Estrace 1385
Estrace Vaginal Cream 1388
Estradurin 2452
Estratest 2245
Kerlone Tablets (Less than 2%) 2172
Konÿne 80 Factor IX Complex 1571
Konÿne-HT Factor IX Complex 1583
▲Lupron Depot 3.75 mg (Among most frequent) 2312
Lupron Depot 7.5 mg 2311
Lupron Injection (2%) 2310
Metrodin (urofollitropin for injection) 2182
Mustargen 1514
Norethin 2133
Ovcon 1391
PMB 200 and PMB 400 2504
Pipracil 1230
Premarin Intravenous 2508
Premarin with Methyltestosterone 2515
Premarin Vaginal Cream 2512
TACE 12 and 25 mg 1353
▲Valium Injectable (Among most common) 1937

Thrombosis of vascular access

Epogen for Injection 591
Procrit for Injection 1647

Thrombosis, cerebral (see under Cerebral thrombosis)

Thrombosis, coronary (see under Coronary thrombosis)

Thrombosis, glomerular capillary

Amicar Syrup, Tablets, and Injection 1194
Sandimmune 2024

Thrombosis, mesenteric

Brevicon 2304
Cartrol Tablets 507
Demulen 2161
Enovid 2161
Estradurin 2452
Estratest 2245
Levatol 1832
Levlen/Tri-Levlen 665
Norethin 2133
Norinyl 2304
Normozide Tablets 2112
Nor-Q D Tablets 2304
Ortho Dienestrol Cream 1664
PMB 200 and PMB 400 2504
Premarin Intravenous 2508
Premarin with Methyltestosterone 2515
Premarin Vaginal Cream 2512
Stilphostrol Tablets and Ampuls 1609
TACE 12 and 25 mg 1353
Trandate HCT/Trandate 579
Levlen/Tri-Levlen 665
Tri-Norinyl 2304
Visken Tablets 2036

Thrombosis, renal artery

Atgam Sterile Solution (Less than 1% to less than 5%) 2320

Thrombosis, retinal

Amen 833
Brevicon 2304
Cycrin Tablets (Occasional) 2449
Demulen 2161
Enovid 2161
Estradurin 2452
Estratest 2245
Jenest-28 Tablets 1636
Levlen/Tri-Levlen 665
Lo/Ovral Tablets 2471
Lo/Ovral-28 Tablets 2476
Loestrin 1728
Micronor Tablets 1667
Modicon 1667
Nordette-21 Tablets 2481
Nordette-28 Tablets 2483
Norethin 2133
Norinyl 2304
Norlestrin 1746
Norlutate 1754
Norlutin 1755
Nor-Q D Tablets 2304
Ortho Dienestrol Cream 1664
Ortho-Novum 1667

Ovral Tablets 2490
Ovral-28 Tablets 2491
Ovrette Tablets 2492
PMB 200 and PMB 400 2504
Premarin Intravenous 2508
Premarin with Methyltestosterone 2515
Premarin Vaginal Cream 2512
Provera Tablets 2356
Stilphostrol Tablets and Ampuls 1609
TACE 12 and 25 mg 1353
Levlen/Tri-Levlen 665
Tri-Norinyl 2304
Triphasil-21 Tablets 2527
Triphasil-28 Tablets 2532

Thrombosis, sagittal sinus
Danocrine Capsules 2046

Thrombosis, venous
Actimmune (Rare) 1046
Atgam Sterile Solution (Less than 5%) 2320
Demulen 2161
Diulo 2129
Enovid 2161
Jenest-28 Tablets 1636
Loestrin 1728
Mepergan Injection 2479
Micronor Tablets 1667
Modicon 1667
Mykrox ½ mg Tablets 984
Nimotop Capsules (Less than 1%) 1607
Norlestrin 1746
Ortho-Cyclen Tablets 1658
Ortho-Novum 1667
Phenergan Injection 2493
Pipracil (Less frequent) 1230
Zaroxolyn Tablets 989

Thrombotic events, unspecified
DDAVP Injection 1840
Danocrine Capsules 2046
Epogen for Injection 591
Procrit for Injection 1647

Thrombotic microangiopathy
Blenoxane (Rare) 724
Platinol (Rare) 737
Platinol-AQ Injection (Rare) 738

Thrombotic vascular disease
Ortho Dienestrol Cream 1664
TACE 12 and 25 mg 1353
▲ Tegison Capsules (1 to 10%) 1881

Thrush, oral (see under Candidiasis, oral)

Thymol turbidity test, positive
Atromid-S Capsules 2435
Cuprimine Capsules 1442
Depen Titratable Tablets (Few reports) 2379

Thymus gland abnormalities, fetal
Accutane Capsules 1878

Thyroid adenoma
Permax Tablets (Rare) 1291
Quadrinal Tablets 1183

Thyroid binding globulin, increase (see under T4, increase)

Thyroid disorders (see under T3 or T4)

Thyroid function test, abnormal
Mevacor Tablets (Rare) 1505
Provera Tablets 2356

Thyroid gland discoloration
Declomycin Capsules, Tablets 1199
Minocin Oral Suspension 1224
Minocin Pellet-Filled Capsules 1222
Monodox Capsules 1630
Terramycin Capsules 1786
Terramycin Intramuscular Solution 1964
Vibramycin Hyclate Capsules 1787
Vibramycin Hyclate Intravenous 1968
Vibramycin Monohydrate for Oral Suspension 1787

Thyroid gland enlargement
Lupron Depot 7.5 mg 2311
Lupron Injection (Less than 5%) 2310
Organidin Elixir, Solution & Tablets (Rare) 2387
Theo-Organidin Elixir (Rare) 2391
Tussi-Organidin DM Liquid (Rare) 2392
Tussi-Organidin Liquid (Rare) 2391

Thyroid hormone, changes (see under T3 or T4)

Thyroid hyperplasia
Butazolidin Capsules & Tablets (Less than 1%) 1027

Thyroid nodule
ProSom Tablets (Rare) 554

Thyroiditis
Cuprimine Capsules 1442
Depen Titratable Tablets (Extremely rare) 2379

Tingling
Apresazide Capsules (Less frequent) 854
Apresoline Hydrochloride Tablets (Less frequent) 855
Apresoline-Esidrix Tablets 857
Asendin Tablets (Less than 1%) 1196
Bentyl 1322
Cipro I.V. 1592
Cipro Tablets 1589
Condylox (Less than 5%) 1630
D.H.E. 45 Injection 2003
Decadron Phosphate Injection 1449
Diprivan Injection (Greater than 1%) 2267
DynaCirc Capsules (0.5% to 1%) 2004
Elimite (permethrin) 5% Cream (1 to 2% or less) 1082
Endep Tablets 1927
Engerix-B Unit-Dose Vials (Less than 1%) 2213
Fiorinal with Codeine Capsules (Infrequent) 2008
K-Phos Neutral Tablets 660
K-Phos Original Formula 'Sodium Free' Tablets (Less frequent) 660
Konÿne 80 Factor IX Complex 1571
Konÿne-HT Factor IX Complex 1583
Ludiomil Tablets (Rare) 874
Nicobid 1846
Noroxin Tablets 1519
Norpace (Less than 1%) 2177
Norpramin Tablets 1340
Nubain Injection (Less than 1%) 934
Pamelor 2019
Priscoline Hydrochloride Ampuls 877
Sandimmune (Rare) 2024
Ser-Ap-Es Tablets 881
Serpasil-Apresoline Tablets 884
Slo-Niacin Tablets 2376
Tofranil Ampuls 1038
Tofranil Tablets 1039
Tofranil-PM Capsules 1041

Tingling, ears
Parlodel (Less than 1%) 2020

Tingling, extremities
Bellergal-S Tablets (Rare) 1998
Coly-Mycin M Parenteral 1706
Diamox Sequels (Sustained Release) 1201
Elavil 2269
Etrafon 2087
Hydrocortone Phosphate Injection, Sterile 1481
Limbitrol 1933
Lozol Tablets (Less than 5%) 1843
Myambutol Tablets 1225
Norpramin Tablets 1340
Polycitra Syrup 2424
Polycitra-K 2424
Polycitra-LC—Sugar-Free 2424
Surmontil Capsules 2524
Tofranil Ampuls 1038
Tofranil Tablets 1039
Tofranil-PM Capsules 1041
Triavil Tablets 1556
Vivactil Tablets 1567

Tingling, feet
Alferon N Injection (1%) 1809
Fluorouracil Injection 1897
K-Lyte 707
K-Phos M.F. Tablets 659
K-Phos No. 2 Tablets 659

Tingling, fingers
D.H.E. 45 Injection 2003
Parlodel 2020
Peptavlon 2563
Wigraine Tablets & Suppositories 1645

Tingling, hands
Adenocard Injection (1%) 1007
BAL in Oil Ampules 661
Fluorouracil Injection 1897
K-Lyte 707
K-Phos M.F. Tablets 659
K-Phos No. 2 Tablets 659

Tingling, legs
Alferon N Injection (1%) 1809

Tingling, lips
K-Lyte 707
K-Phos M.F. Tablets 659
K-Phos Neutral Tablets 660
K-Phos Original Formula 'Sodium Free' Tablets (Less frequent) 660
K-Phos No. 2 Tablets 659
Marcaine Spinal 2058
Sensorcaine 631
Sensorcaine-MPF Spinal 634
Uroqid-Acid (Less frequent) 661

Tingling, mouth
Marcaine Spinal 2058
Sensorcaine 631
Sensorcaine-MPF Spinal 634
Stilphostrol Tablets and Ampuls 1609

Tingling, nose
Stilphostrol Tablets and Ampuls 1609

Tingling, perineal area
Hydeltrasol Injection, Sterile 1476

Tingling, scalp
▲ Normodyne Injection (7%) 2108
▲ Normodyne Tablets (Most frequent) 2110
Normozide Tablets (Less than 1%) 2112
Temovate Scalp Application (2 of 294 patients) 1056
Trandate HCT Tablets 579
▲ Trandate Injection (7 of 100 patients) 577
Trandate Tablets 579

Tingling, skin
Garamycin Injectable 2093
Netromycin Injection 100 mg/ml 2104
▲ Normodyne Injection (7%) 2108

Tingling, toes
D.H.E. 45 Injection 2003
Wigraine Tablets & Suppositories 1645

Tinnitus
Accutane Capsules (Less than 1%) 1878
Actifed with Codeine Cough Syrup 752
Alferon N Injection (One patient) 1809
Altace Capsules (Less than 1%) 1086
Amicar Syrup, Tablets, and Injection (Occasional) 1194
▲ Anafranil Capsules (4% to 6%) 650
▲ Anaprox and Anaprox DS Tablets (3-9%) 2288
▲ Anestacon Solution (Among most common) 2394
Ansaid Tablets (1-3%) 2319
Aralen Hydrochloride Injection (1 patient) 2038
Aralen Phosphate with Primaquine Phosphate Tablets (1 patient) 2040
Aralen Phosphate Tablets (1 patient) 2039
Arthritis Strength BC Powder ▣ 516
Ascriptin A/D Caplets 1850
Regular Strength Ascriptin Tablets 1850
Asendin Tablets (Less than 1%) 1196
Azactam for Injection (Less than 1%) 2252
Azo Gantanol Tablets 1887
Azo Gantrisin Tablets 1888
Azulfidine Tablets, EN-tabs, Oral Suspension (Rare) 1157
BC Powder ▣ 517
Bactrim DS Tablets 1891
Bactrim I.V. Infusion 1889
Bactrim 1891
Children's Bayer Chewable Aspirin ▣ 564
Genuine Bayer Aspirin Tablets & Caplets ▣ 564
Maximum Bayer Aspirin Tablets & Caplets ▣ 566
Bayer Plus Aspirin Tablets ▣ 567
Therapy Bayer Aspirin Caplets ▣ 568
▲ 8 Hour Bayer Timed-Release Aspirin (Among most frequent) ▣ 566
Benadryl Capsules 1691
Benadryl Injection 1692
Blocadren Tablets (Less than 1%) 1429
Arthritis Strength Bufferin Analgesic Caplets 744
BuSpar (Frequent) 1401
Butazolidin Capsules & Tablets (Less than 1%) 1027
Cama Arthritis Pain Reliever ▣ 685
Capastat Sulfate Vials 1250
Carbocaine Hydrochloride Injection 2043
Cardene Capsules (Rare) 2290
Cardioquin Tablets 1812
Cardizem Tablets-30 mg, 60 mg, 90 mg and 120 mg (Less than 1%) 1329
Cardizem SR Capsules-60 mg, 90 mg and 120 mg (Less than 1%) 1327
Cardura Tablets (1%) 1941
Cartrol Tablets (Less common) 507
Children's Advil Suspension (Less than 3%) 2426
Cholybar 1705
Cibalith-S 870
Cipro I.V. (1% or less) 1592
Cipro Tablets (Less than 1%) 1589
Clinoril Tablets (Greater than 1%) 1433
Corgard Tablets (1 to 5 of 1000 patients) 701
Corzide Tablets (1 to 5 of 1000 patients) 702
Cuprimine Capsules (Greater than 1%) 1442
Cytotec (Infrequent) 2159
Dalgan Injection (Less than 1%) 620
Dapsone USP 1130
Daranide Tablets 1445
Deconamine 663
Depen Titratable Tablets 2379
Desferal Vials 862
Desyrel and Desyrel Dividose (Greater than 1%) 1404
Diamox Parenteral 1200
Diamox Sequels (Sustained Release) 1201
Diamox Tablets 1200
Diprivan Injection (Less than 1%) 2267
Disalcid 1310
Dolobid Tablets (Greater than 1 in 100) 1465
Duranest Injections 624
Dyclone 0.5% and 1% Topical Solutions, USP 626
Easprin 1719
Ecotrin 2189
Edecrin 1468
Elavil 2269
Eldepryl 2250
Emcyt Capsules 1161
Empirin with Codeine Phosphate Nos. 2, 3 & 4 764
Endep Tablets 1927
Equagesic Tablets 2451
Eskalith 2214
Ethmozine Tablets (Less than 2%) 946
Etrafon 2087
Fansidar Tablets 1896
Feldene Capsules (1 to 3%) 1777
Fiorinal with Codeine Capsules (Infrequent) 2008
Flexeril Tablets (Less than 1%) 1471
Fungizone Intravenous 2262
Ganite Injection 1016
Gantanol 1899
Gantrisin Ophthalmic Ointment/Solution 1900
Gantrisin 1901
Garamycin Injectable 2093
Halcion Tablets (Rare) 2340
Hyperstat I.V. Injection 2095
Hytrin Tablets (At least 1%) 529
Ilosone 913
Indocin (Greater than 1%) 1487
▲ Intron A (Up to 4%) 2097
Kerlone Tablets (Less than 2%) 2172
▲ Lariam Tablets (Among most frequent) 1904
Lasix 1093
Legatrin ▣ 556
Lincocin (Occasional) 2344
Lioresal Tablets 1031
Lithane Tablets 1596
Lithium Carbonate Capsules & Tablets 1984
Lithobid Tablets 870
Lodine Capsules (More than 1% but less than 3%) 2468
Lopressor Ampuls 1032
Lopressor HCT Tablets 1034
Lopressor Tablets 1032
Lorelco Tablets 1333
Ludiomil Tablets (Rare) 874

Marcaine Hydrochloride 0.5% with Epinephrine 1:200,000 (as bitartrate) 958
Marcaine Hydrochloride with Epinephrine 1:200,000 2055
Marcaine Hydrochloride Injection 2055
Marcaine Spinal 2058
Meclomen Capsules (Greater than 1%) 1739
Methergine (Rare) 2016
Methotrexate Tablets, Parenteral, LPF Parenteral (Less common) 1217
Mexitil Capsules (1.9% to 2.4%) .. 680
Midamor Tablets (Less than or equal to 1%) 1508
Minipress Capsules (Less than 1%) 1778
Minizide Capsules (Rare) 1779
Mintezol 1510
Moduretic Tablets 1510
Mono-Gesic Tablets 846
Monopril Tablets (0.2 to 1.0%) 1406
Motrin Tablets (Less than 3%) 2351
Mustargen (Infrequent) 1514
Mykrox ½ mg Tablets (Less than 2%) 984
▲ Nalfon Pulvules & Tablets (4.5%) .. 919
▲ Naprosyn (3 to 9%) 2297
Nebcin Vials, Hyporets & ADD-Vantage 1286
Nescaine/Nescaine MPF 629
Netromycin Injection 100 mg/ml 2104
Nicorette 1335
Nipride I.V. Infusion 1909
Norpramin Tablets 1340
Norwich Extra-Strength Aspirin .... ▣ 546
Norwich Regular Strength Aspirin .... ▣ 547
Norzine 1818
Omnipaque (Less than 0.1%) 2552
Optimine Tablets 2115
Ornade Spansule Capsules 2221
Orudis Capsules (Greater than 1%) 2488
P-A-C Analgesic Tablets .... ▣ 669
PBZ Tablets & Elixir 1037
PBZ-SR Tablets 1037
Pamelor 2019
Parnate Tablets 2222
PediaProfen Suspension (Less than 3%) 1363
Pediazole 1973
Pepcid (Infrequent) 1524
Pepto-Bismol Liquid & Tablets 1807
Maximum Strength Pepto-Bismol Liquid 1808
Periactin 1525
Permax Tablets (Infrequent) 1291
Phenergan Injection 2493
Phenergan Tablets 2496
Plaquenil Sulfate Tablets 2067
Platinol 737
Platinol-AQ Injection 738
Plendil Extended-Release Tablets (0.5% or greater) 1526
Polaramine 2116
Pontocaine Hydrochloride for Spinal Anesthesia 2069
Prilosec Delayed-Release Capsules (Less than 1%) 1530
Primaxin I.M. 1532
Primaxin I.V. (Less than 0.2%) 1535
Prinzide Tablets (0.3 to 1%) 1540
Procardia XL Tablets (1% or less) .. 1783
ProSom Tablets (Infrequent) 554
Proventil (2%) 2120
Prozac Pulvules (Infrequent) 920
Questran Light 711
Questran Powder 710
Quinaglute Dura-Tabs Tablets 663
Quinamm Tablets 1344
Quinidex Extentabs 1868
Q-vel Muscle Relaxant Pain Reliever .... ▣ 552
Recombivax HB (Less than 1%) 1544
Rheumatrex Methotrexate Dose Pack (Less common) 1234
Rufen Tablets (1 to 3%) 691
Ru-Tuss II Capsules 693
Ru-Tuss with Hydrocodone 694
Ru-Tuss Tablets 693
Rythmol Tablets (1.9%) 1184
Salflex (Common) 839
Sandimmune (2% or less) 2024
Sensorcaine 631
Sensorcaine-MPF Spinal 634
Septra 813
Septra I.V. Infusion 808
Septra I.V. Infusion ADD-Vantage Vials 810
Septra 813
Sinequan (Occasional) 1960
Soma Compound w/Codeine Tablets 2390
Soma Compound Tablets 2389
Surmontil Capsules 2524
Tacaryl 2409
Talacen (Rare) 2070
Talwin Injection (Rare) 2071
Talwin Compound 2072
Talwin Injection 2071
Talwin Nx 2073
Tambocor Tablets (1-3%) 1315
Tavist Syrup 2033
Tavist Tablets 2035
Tavist-D Tablets 2035
Tegretol Chewable Tablets 654
Tegretol Suspension 656
Tegretol Tablets 654
Temaril Tablets, Syrup and Spansule Sustained Release Capsules 1085
Tenex Tablets (Less than 3%) 1875
Thera-Gesic 1614
Thiosulfil Forte Tablets 2526
Timolide Tablets 1547
Timoptic in Ocudose 1552
Timoptic Sterile Ophthalmic Solution 1550
Tofranil Ampuls 1038
Tofranil Tablets 1039
Tofranil-PM Capsules 1041
Tolectin (200, 400 and 600 mg) (1 to 3%) 1379
Tonocard Tablets (0.4-1.5%) 1554
Torecan 1993
Trexan Tablets (Less than 1%) 937
Triaminic Expectorant DH 1995
Triaminic Oral Infant Drops 1996
Triavil Tablets 1556
▲ Trilisate (Less than 20%) 1822
Trinalin Repetabs Tablets 1170
Ursinus Inlay-Tabs .... ▣ 691
Vancocin HCl, Oral Solution & Pulvules (Rare) 1304
Vancocin HCl, Vials & ADD-Vantage (Rare) 1302
▲ Vascor (200, 300 and 400 mg) Tablets (Up to 6.52%) 1383
Vaseretic Tablets (0.5% to 2.0%) 1559
Vasotec I.V. 1562
Vasotec Tablets (0.5% to 1%) 1564
Vivactil Tablets 1567
Voltaren Tablets (1-3%) 1042
Wellbutrin Tablets 821
▲ Xanax Tablets (6.6%) 2367
▲ Xylocaine Injections (Among most common) 637
Xylocaine Injections for Ventricular Arrhythmias 639
Xylocaine 2% Jelly 643
Xylocaine 5% Ointment 644
Xylocaine 10% Oral Spray 645
4% Xylocaine-MPF Sterile Solution 641
Zestoretic (0.3 to 1%) 2274
Zorprin Tablets 698
Zyloprim Tablets (Less than 1%) 830

Tiredness (see under Fatigue)

Tissue damage, ischemic
Sansert Tablets (Rare) 2031

Toes, discoloration
Cibalith-S 870
Eskalith (A few reports) 2214
Lithane Tablets (Single case) 1596
Lithium Carbonate Capsules & Tablets (A single report) 1984
Lithobid Tablets 870

Tolerance
Adipex-P Tablets and Capsules 1019
Alurate Elixir 1883
Astramorph/PF Injection, USP (Preservative-Free) 618
Biphetamine Capsules 973
Diapid Nasal Spray 2003
Dilatrate-SR 1827
Duramorph 960
Dyclone 0.5% and 1% Topical Solutions, USP 626
Infumorph 200 and Infumorph 500 Sterile Solutions 962
Isordil 2467
Mebaral Tablets 2061
Methadone Hydrochloride Oral Solution & Tablets 1987
Numorphan Hydrochloride Injection 935
Oramorph SR (Morphine Sulfate Sustained Release Tablets) 1988
Roxanol 1991
Seconal Sodium Pulvules 1296
Sorbitrate 1103
Tylenol with Codeine 1381

Tolerance, diminished
Anestacon Solution 2394
Cocaine Hydrochloride Topical Solution 620
Timolide Tablets 1547
Timoptic in Ocudose 1552
Timoptic Sterile Ophthalmic Solution 1550
Xylocaine Injections 637
Xylocaine Injections for Ventricular Arrhythmias 639
Xylocaine 2% Jelly 643
Xylocaine 10% Oral Spray 645
4% Xylocaine-MPF Sterile Solution 641
Xylocaine 2% Viscous Solution 646

Tongue, black "hairy" (see under Glossotrichia)

Tongue, burning
BuSpar (Rare) 1401
Halcion Tablets 2340
Larodopa Tablets (Infrequent) 1905
Nalfon Pulvules & Tablets (Less than 1%) 919
Sinemet Tablets 952
Sinemet CR Tablets 953

Tongue, discoloration
Aldomet Ester HCl Injection 1417
Aldomet Oral 1415
Pepto-Bismol Liquid & Tablets 1807
Maximum Strength Pepto-Bismol Liquid 1808
Prozac Pulvules (Rare) 920
Trilafon 2123

Tongue, fine vermicular movements
Compazine 2201
Eskalith 2214
Etrafon 2087
Haldol Decanoate 1375
Haldol Injection, Tablets and Concentrate 1373
Mellaril 2011
Navane Capsules and Concentrate 1954
Navane Intramuscular 1956
Orap Tablets 1020
Reglan 1869
Stelazine 2226
Taractan 1920
Thorazine 2234

Tongue, furry
Flagyl Tablets 2170
Geocillin Tablets 1951
Protostat Tablets 1674

Tongue, mucosal atrophy
Prilosec Delayed-Release Capsules (Less than 1%) 1530

Tongue, protrusion
Compazine 2201
Etrafon 2087
Haldol Decanoate 1375
Haldol Injection, Tablets and Concentrate 1373
Loxitane 1213
Mellaril 2011
Moban Tablets & Concentrate 932
Navane Capsules and Concentrate 1954
Navane Intramuscular 1956
Orap Tablets 1020
Phenergan with Codeine 2497
Phenergan with Dextromethorphan 2499
Phenergan Suppositories 2496
Phenergan Syrup 2495
Phenergan VC 2500
Phenergan VC with Codeine 2501
Prolixin Decanoate 1795
Prolixin Enanthate 1796
Prolixin Oral Concentrate 1792
Prozac Pulvules 920
Reglan 1869
Serentil 686
Stelazine 2226
Taractan 1920
Thorazine 2234
Triavil Tablets 1556
Trilafon 2123

Tongue, rounding
Trilafon 2123

Tongue, sore (see under Glossodynia)

Tongue, swelling (see under Glossoncus)

Tooth development, impaired
Mulvidren-F Softab Tablets 2273
Permax Tablets (Infrequent) 1291
Terramycin Capsules 1786
Terramycin Intramuscular Solution 1964
Urobiotic-250 Capsules 1968
Vibramycin Hyclate Intravenous 1968

Tooth discoloration
Urobiotic-250 Capsules (Contraindicated in pregnancy) 1968

Tooth disorder
▲ Anafranil Capsules (Up to 5%) 650

Torsade de pointes
Ilosone (Rare) 913
Ilotycin Gluceptate, IV, Vials (Rare) 915
Lorelco Tablets 1333
Norpace 2177
Quinidex Extentabs 1868
Seldane Tablets (Rare) 1349
Seldane-D Extended-Release Tablets (Rare) 1350
Vascor (200, 300 and 400 mg) Tablets 1383

Torticollis
Adenocard Injection (Less than 1%) 1007
Anafranil Capsules (Rare) 650
Cartrol Tablets (Less common) 507
Cipro I.V. (1% or less) 1592
Cipro Tablets (Less than 1%) 1589
Clozaril Tablets (1%) 2000
Compazine 2201
Danocrine Capsules 2046
Diprivan Injection (Less than 1%) .. 2267
Eldepryl 2250
Engerix-B Unit-Dose Vials (Less than 1%) 2213
Etrafon 2087
Gelfoam Sterile Sponge 2338
Hylorel Tablets (1.5%) 975
Hytrin Tablets (At least 1%) 529
Kerlone Tablets (Less than 2%) 2172
Mellaril 2011
Moduretic Tablets 1510
Norzine 1818
▲ Omnipaque (About 8%) 2552
Permax Tablets (2.7%) 1291
Phenergan with Codeine 2497
Phenergan with Dextromethorphan 2499
Phenergan Suppositories 2496
Phenergan Syrup 2495
Phenergan VC 2500
Phenergan VC with Codeine 2501
Plendil Extended-Release Tablets (0.5% or greater) 1526
Polymyxin B Sulfate, Aerosporin Brand Sterile Powder 798
ProSom Tablets (Infrequent) 554
Prozac Pulvules (Rare to infrequent) 920
Recombivax HB (Less than 1%) 1544
Reglan 1869
Serentil 686
Stelazine 2226
Thorazine 2234
Tonocard Tablets (Less than 1%) .. 1554
Torecan 1993
Triavil Tablets 1556
Trilafon 2123

Total proteins, decrease (see under Hypoproteinemia)

Tourette's syndrome
Cylert Tablets 510
Desoxyn Gradumet Tablets 514
Dexedrine 2206
Ritalin (Rare) 880

Toxic granulation
Efudex 1880

Toxicity, bone marrow
▲ Mutamycin (64.4%) 733

Toxicity, cutaneous
▲ Lysodren (15%) 731

Toxicity, hepatic
Achromycin V Capsules (Rare) 1193
BiCNU 723

CeeNU ... 725
Cordarone Tablets ... 2446
Danocrine Capsules ... 2046
Declomycin Capsules, Tablets (Rare) ... 1199
Hexalen Capsules (Less than 1%) .. 2316
Methotrexate Tablets, Parenteral, LPF Parenteral ... 1217
Ponstel ... 1758
Pyridium ... 1763
Pyridium Plus ... 1764
Rheumatrex Methotrexate Dose Pack ... 1234
Terramycin Intramuscular Solution 1964
Urobiotic-250 Capsules ... 1968
VePesid Capsules and Injection (0 to 3%) ... 741

Toxicity, renal

Achromycin V Capsules ... 1193
Butazolidin Capsules & Tablets ... 1027
Declomycin Capsules, Tablets (No incidence, dose related) ... 1199
Depen Titratable Tablets ... 2379
Fiorinal with Codeine Capsules ... 2008
Humatin Capsules ... 1726
▲IFEX (6%) ... 729
Minocin Intravenous ... 1221
Minocin Oral Suspension ... 1224
Minocin Pellet-Filled Capsules ... 1222
Mutamycin (2%) ... 733
▲Platinol (28 to 36%) ... 737
▲Platinol-AQ Injection (28% to 36% of patients) ... 738
Pyridium ... 1763
Pyridium Plus ... 1764
Roferon-A Injection (Rare) ... 1916
▲TheraCys BCG Live (Intravesical) (2.0% to 9.8%) ... 898
Toradol IM Injection ... 2302

Toxicity, vascular

Blenoxane (Rare) ... 724
Platinol ... 737
Platinol-AQ Injection (Rare) ... 738

Toxic shock syndrome

Gelfoam Sterile Sponge ... 2338
Koro-Flex Arcing Spring Diaphragm ... 2142
Koromex Coil Spring Diaphragm ... 2142
Ortho Diaphragm Kit ... 1664
Today Vaginal Contraceptive Sponge ... 2422

Tracheitis

PedvaxHIB (One case) ... 1521
Solganal Suspension ... 2122

Transaminase, elevation (see under Serum transaminase, elevation)

Trembling

Adalat Capsules (10 mg and 20 mg) (2% or less) ... 1587
▲AeroBid Inhaler System (3-9%) ... 995
Alfenta Injection (Less than 1%) ... 1131
Alferon N Injection (One patient) ... 1809
Clozaril Tablets (Less than 1%) ... 2000
Diprivan Injection (Less than 1%) .. 2267
Emete-con Intramuscular/Intravenous ... 1950
Ethrane ... 599
Fluothane ... 2453
Forane ... 600
Inapsine Injection ... 1140
Innovar Injection ... 1141
Marax Tablets & DF Syrup ... 1954
Marcaine Spinal ... 2058
Murocoll-2 Sterile Ophthalmic Solution ... ⊙ 261
Nucofed Capsules ... 2219
Nucofed Expectorant ... 2219
Nucofed Pediatric Expectorant ... 2220
Nucofed Syrup ... 2219
Omnipaque (Less than 0.3%) ... 2552
Procardia Capsules (2% or less) ... 1781
Quadrinal Tablets ... 1183
Sandostatin Injection (Less than 1%) ... 2029
Sublimaze Injection ... 1146
▲Ventolin Syrup (9 of 100 patients) 583
Xylocaine Injections (2%) ... 637

Tremor, fine hand

Cibalith-S ... 870
Eskalith ... 2214
Lithane Tablets ... 1596
Lithium Carbonate Capsules & Tablets ... 1984
Lithobid Tablets ... 870
Sinemet Tablets ... 952
Sinemet CR Tablets ... 953
▲Vascor (200, 300 and 400 mg) Tablets (3.02 to 9.30%) ... 1383

Tremors

Actibine ... 900
Actifed with Codeine Cough Syrup .. 752
▲Adalat Capsules (10 mg and 20 mg) (8%) ... 1587
Adipex-P Tablets and Capsules ... 1019
AK-Dilate Solution 2.5% and 10% (Rare) ... ⊙ 203
Altace Capsules (Less than 1%) ... 1086
Alupent (1 to 4%) ... 674
Amikin Injectable (Rare) ... 602
▲Anafranil Capsules (33% to 54%) 650
Ana-Kit Anaphylaxis Emergency Treatment Kit ... 1100
▲Anestacon Solution (Among most common) ... 2394
Ansaid Tablets (1-3%) ... 2319
Apresazide Capsules (Less frequent) ... 854
Apresoline Hydrochloride Parenteral (Ampuls) ... 856
Apresoline Hydrochloride Tablets (Less frequent) ... 855
Apresoline-Esidrix Tablets ... 857
Arm-a-Med Isoetharine Inhalation Solution, USP ... 616
▲Arm-a-Med Metaproterenol Sulfate Inhalation Solution, USP (1 in 20 patients) ... 617
Asendin Tablets (Greater than 1%) ... 1196
Atarax Tablets & Syrup ... 1941
Atgam Sterile Solution (Less than 5%) ... 2320
Atrohist Sprinkle Capsules ... 558
Atromid-S Capsules ... 2435
Atrovent Inhalation Aerosol (Less than 1 in 100) ... 675
Baron-X Tablets ... 650
Benadryl Capsules ... 1691
Benadryl Injection ... 1692
Biphetamine Capsules ... 973
Bontril Slow-Release ... 834
Brethaire Inhaler ... 1024
▲Brethine Ampuls (7.8 to 38.0%) ... 1026
Brethine Tablets (Common) ... 1026
▲Bricanyl Injection (Among most common) ... 1324
▲Bricanyl Tablets (Among most common) ... 1325
Bronkometer Aerosol ... 2042
Bronkosol Solution ... 2042
BuSpar (1%) ... 1401
Butazolidin Capsules & Tablets (Less than 1%) ... 1027
Calan SR Caplets (1% or less) ... 2157
Calan Tablets (1% or less) ... 2155
Carbocaine Hydrochloride 3% Injection ... 956
Carbocaine Hydrochloride Injection 2043
Carbocaine Hydrochloride 2% with Neo-Cobefrin ... 956
Cardene Capsules (0.6%) ... 2290
Cardizem Tablets-30 mg, 60 mg, 90 mg and 120 mg (Less than 1%) ... 1329
Cardizem SR Capsules-60 mg, 90 mg and 120 mg (Less than 1%) 1327
Cardura Tablets (Less than 0.5% of 3960 patients) ... 1941
Centrax (Less frequent) ... 1693
Cibalith-S ... 870
Cipro I.V. (1% or less) ... 1592
Cipro Tablets (Less than 1%) ... 1589
▲Clozaril Tablets (More than 5 to 6%) ... 2000
Cocaine Hydrochloride Topical Solution ... 620
Compazine ... 2201
▲Cordarone Tablets (4 to 9%) ... 2446
Cytovene Sterile Powder (1% or less) ... 2292
Danocrine Capsules ... 2046
Daranide Tablets ... 1445
Dayto Himbin Tablets and Liquid ... 905
Decadron Phosphate with Xylocaine Injection, Sterile ... 1451
Deconamine ... 663
Deconsal ... 559
Demerol ... 2047
▲Demser Capsules (10%) ... 1460
Depakene Capsules & Syrup ... 511
Depakote ... 512
Desoxyn Gradumet Tablets ... 514
Desyrel and Desyrel Dividose (Greater than 1%) ... 1404
Dexedrine ... 2206
Didrex Tablets ... 2338
Dilantin Infatabs (Rare) ... 1710
Dilantin Kapseals (Rare) ... 1708
Dilantin Parenteral (Rare) ... 1712
Dilantin-30 Pediatric/Dilantin-125 Suspension (Rare) ... 1713
Dilantin with Phenobarbital Kapseals (Rare) ... 1715
Dilaudid-HP Injection ... 1175
Dimetane-DC Cough Syrup ... 1857
Dimetane-DX Cough Syrup ... 1858
Dipentum Capsules (Rare) ... 1160
Diprivan Injection (Less than 1%) .. 2267
Doral Tablets ... 2383
Duragesic Transdermal System (1% or greater) ... 1133
Duranest Injections ... 624
Dyclone 0.5% and 1% Topical Solutions, USP ... 626
Elavil ... 2269
Eldepryl ... 2250
Elspar ... 1470
Emete-con Intramuscular/Intravenous ... 1950
▲Eminase (Less than 10%) ... 2211
Endep Tablets ... 1927
EpiPen ... 843
▲Ergamisol Tablets (3 to 5%) ... 1136
Esimil Tablets ... 864
Eskalith ... 2214
Ethmozine Tablets (Less than 2%) 946
Etrafon ... 2087
Fastin Capsules ... 2216
Fedahist Gyrocaps ... 2145
Fedahist Timecaps ... 2145
Fiorinal with Codeine Capsules ... 2008
Flexeril Tablets (Less than 1%) ... 1471
Intron A (2 patients) ... 2097
Inversine Tablets ... 1492
Ionamin Capsules ... 981
Ismelin Tablets ... 869
Isoptin Oral Tablets (Less than 1%) ... 1179
Isoptin SR Sustained Release Tablets (Less than 1%) ... 1181
Isuprel Hydrochloride Injection 1:5000 ... 2050
Isuprel Hydrochloride Mistometer .. 2051
Isuprel Hydrochloride Solution 1:200 & 1:100 ... 2052
Kerlone Tablets (Less than 2%) ... 2172
Klonopin Tablets ... 1902
Larodopa Tablets (Relatively frequent) ... 1905
Leukeran Tablets (Rare) ... 788
Limbitrol (Less common) ... 1933
Lioresal Tablets ... 1031
Lithane Tablets ... 1596
Lithium Carbonate Capsules & Tablets ... 1984
Lithobid Tablets ... 870
Loxitane ... 1213
▲Ludiomil Tablets (3%) ... 874
MS Contin Tablets (Infrequent) ... 1814
MSIR (Infrequent) ... 1817
Marcaine Hydrochloride 0.5% with Epinephrine 1:200,000 (as bitartrate) ... 958
Marcaine Hydrochloride with Epinephrine 1:200,000 ... 2055
Marcaine Hydrochloride Injection ... 2055
Marcaine Spinal ... 2058
▲Marplan Tablets (Among most frequent) ... 1906
Matulane Capsules ... 1907
▲Maxair Inhaler (6.0%) ... 1311
Mellaril ... 2011
Mepergan Injection ... 2479
Mesantoin Tablets ... 2013
Metaprel Inhalation Aerosol Bronchodilator (1 to 4%) ... 2014
▲Metaprel Inhalation Solution (1 in 20 patients) ... 2015
Metaprel ... 2015
Methadone Hydrochloride Diskets .. 1284
▲Mexitil Capsules (12.6%) ... 680
Midamor Tablets (Less than or equal to 1%) ... 1508
Moban Tablets & Concentrate ... 932
Moduretic Tablets ... 1510
Monopril Tablets (0.2 to 1.0%) ... 1406
Naldecon Syrup, Tablets, Pediatric Drops and Pediatric Syrup ... 709
Nalfon Pulvules & Tablets (2.2%) .. 919
Nardil (Common) ... 1742
NebuPent for Inhalation Solution (1% or less) ... 1017
Neo-Synephrine (Rare) ... ▣ 759
Nescaine/Nescaine MPF ... 629
Nolamine Tablets (Occasional) ... 838
Norflex ... 1314
Norisodrine Aerotrol ... 540
Noroxin Tablets ... 1519
Norpramin Tablets ... 1340
Norzine ... 1818
Novafed A Capsules ... 1342
Novafed Capsules ... 1342
Novahistine DH ... 1342
Novahistine DMX ... ▣ 595
Novahistine Elixir ... ▣ 596
Novahistine Expectorant ... 1343
Novocain Hydrochloride for Spinal Anesthesia ... 2065
Omnipaque (Less than or equal to 1%) ... 2552
Optimine Tablets ... 2115
Oramorph SR (Morphine Sulfate Sustained Release Tablets) (Less frequent) ... 1988
Orap Tablets ... 1020
Ornade Spansule Capsules ... 2221
▲Orthoclone OKT3 Sterile Solution (13%) ... 1645
Pamelor ... 2019
Pantopon Injectable ... 1911
Parnate Tablets ... 2222
Pentaspan Injection ... 949
Periactin ... 1525
▲Permax Tablets (4.2%) ... 1291
Phenergan Injection ... 2493
Phenergan Tablets ... 2496
Phenergan VC ... 2500
Phenergan VC with Codeine ... 2501
Pitressin Synthetic, Ampoules ... 1758
Plegine Tablets ... 2504
Plendil Extended-Release Tablets (0.5% or greater) ... 1526
Polaramine ... 2116
Pontocaine Hydrochloride for Spinal Anesthesia ... 2069
Prelu-2 Capsules ... 683
Primaxin I.M. ... 1532
Primaxin I.V. (Less than 0.2%) ... 1535
▲Procardia XL Tablets (1% or less to 8%) ... 1783
ProSom Tablets (Rare) ... 554
▲Proventil Inhalation Aerosol (Less than 15%) ... 2117
▲Proventil Repetabs Tablets (20%) 2120
▲Proventil Solutions for Inhalation 0.5% and 0.083% (20%) ... 2118
▲Proventil Syrup (10 of 100) ... 2119
▲Proventil Tablets (20%) ... 2120
▲Prozac Pulvules (7.9%) ... 920
Reglan ... 1869
Restoril Capsules (Less than 1%) .. 2023
Retrovir Capsules (Less than 5%) .. 802
Retrovir I.V. Infusion (Less than 5%) ... 805
Retrovir Syrup (Less than 5%) ... 802
Roferon-A Injection (Less than 0.5%) ... 1916
Rondec ... 1975
Rondec-DM ... 1976
Rondec-TR Tablet ... 1975
Ru-Tuss DE Tablets ... 694
Ru-Tuss II Capsules ... 693
Rythmol Tablets (0.3 to 1.4%) ... 1184
▲Sandimmune (Up to 55%) ... 2024
Sandostatin Injection (Less than 1%) ... 2029
Sanorex Tablets ... 2030
Seldane Tablets ... 1349
Seldane-D Extended-Release Tablets ... 1350
Sensorcaine ... 631
Sensorcaine-MPF Spinal ... 634
Ser-Ap-Es Tablets ... 881
Serax Capsules ... 2522
Serax Tablets ... 2522
Serentil ... 686
Seromycin Pulvules ... 1298
Serpasil-Apresoline Tablets ... 884
Sinequan ... 1960
Soma Compound w/Codeine Tablets (Infrequent or rare) ... 2390
Soma Compound Tablets (Infrequent or rare) ... 2389
Soma Tablets ... 2388
Stelazine ... 2226
Surmontil Capsules ... 2524
Sus-Phrine Injection ... 1006
Tacaryl ... 2409
Talacen (Rare) ... 2070
Talwin Injection (Rarely) ... 2071
Talwin Compound (Rare) ... 2072
Talwin Injection (Rare) ... 2071
Talwin Nx (Rare) ... 2073
▲Tambocor Tablets (4.7%) ... 1315

Tavist Syrup 2033
Tavist Tablets 2035
Tavist-D Tablets 2035
Tedral SA 1765
Temaril Tablets, Syrup and Spansule Sustained Release Capsules 1085
Tenex Tablets 1875
Tenuate 1354
Thorazine 2234
Tofranil Ampuls 1038
Tofranil Tablets 1039
Tofranil-PM Capsules 1041
▲ Tonocard Tablets (2.9-21.6%) 1554
Torecan 1993
▲ Tornalate (14%) 2074
Trancopal Caplets 2075
Tranxene 556
Trental (0.3%) 1099
Trexan Tablets (Less than 1%) 937
Triaminic Expectorant DH 1995
Triaminic Oral Infant Drops 1996
Triavil Tablets 1556
Trinalin Repetabs Tablets 1170
Tuss-Ornade Liquid 2242
Tuss-Ornade Spansule Capsules 2242
Valium Injectable 1937
Valium Tablets (Infrequent) 1939
Valrelease Capsules (Occasional) 1923
▲ Vascor (200, 300 and 400 mg) Tablets (0.5 to 6.98%) 1383
▲ Ventolin (Less than 15 in 100 patients) 583
Verelan Capsules (Less than 1%) 1243
Vira-A for Injection 1766
Vistaril Capsules (Rare) 1789
Vistaril Intramuscular Solution (Rare) 1970
Vistaril Oral Suspension (Rare) 1789
Vivactil Tablets 1567
Voltaren Tablets (Less than 1%) 1042
▲ Wellbutrin Tablets (21.1%) 821
▲ Xanax Tablets (4%) 2367
▲ Xylocaine Injections (Among most common) 637
Xylocaine Injections for Ventricular Arrhythmias 639
Xylocaine 2% Jelly 643
Xylocaine 5% Ointment 644
Xylocaine 10% Oral Spray 645
4% Xylocaine-MPF Sterile Solution 641
Xylocaine 2% Viscous Solution 646
Yocon 1686
Yohimex Tablets 1190
▲ Yutopar (10 to 15% (IV or oral)) 647
Zovirax Sterile Powder (Approximately 1%) 828

Tremulousness
Narcan Injection 933
Sandostatin Injection (Less than 1%) 2029

Trigeminal neuralgia
Nalfon Pulvules & Tablets (Less than 1%) 919
Norzine (Occasional) 1818
Torecan (Occasional) 1993

Triglycerides, increase (see under Hypertriglyceridemia)

Trismus
Compazine 2201
Demser Capsules 1460
Etrafon 2087
Larodopa Tablets (Infrequent) 1905
Mellaril 2011
Norzine 1818
Reglan 1869
Serentil 686
Sinemet Tablets 952
Sinemet CR Tablets 953
Stelazine 2226
Thorazine 2234
Torecan 1993
Triavil Tablets 1556
Trilafon 2123

Tubal damage
ParaGard T380A Intrauterine Copper Contraceptive 411

Tubulopathy
Orudis Capsules (Rare) 2488

Tumor flare
Megace Tablets 732

Twins, conjoined
Fulvicin P/G Tablets (Rare) 2090
Fulvicin P/G 165 & 330 Tablets (Rare) 2091
Fulvicin-U/F Tablets 2092
Gris-PEG Tablets, 125 mg & 250 mg 1083

Twitching
▲ Anafranil Capsules (4% to 7%) 650
▲ Anestacon Solution (Among most common) 2394
Ansaid Tablets (Less than 1%) 2319
Brevital Sodium Vials 1248
Cardura Tablets (Less than 0.5% of 3960 patients) 1941
Cibalith-S 870
Compazine 2201
Desoxyn Gradumet Tablets 514
Dilantin Infatabs 1710
Dilantin Kapseals 1708
Dilantin Parenteral 1712
Dilantin-30 Pediatric/Dilantin-125 Suspension 1713
Dilantin with Phenobarbital Kapseals 1715
Diprivan Injection (Greater than 1%) 2267
Duranest Injections 624
Dyclone 0.5% and 1% Topical Solutions, USP 626
Eskalith 2214
Ethrane 599
Fiorinal with Codeine Capsules 2008
Innovar Injection 1141
Kerlone Tablets (Less than 2%) 2172
Lithane Tablets 1596
Lithium Carbonate Capsules & Tablets 1984
Lithobid Tablets 870
Nardil (Common) 1742
Permax Tablets (1.1%) 1291
ProSom Tablets (Infrequent) 554
Prozac Pulvules (Infrequent) 920
Retrovir Capsules (Less than 5%) 802
Retrovir I.V. Infusion (Less than 5%) 805
Retrovir Syrup (Less than 5%) 802
Sensorcaine 631
Sensorcaine-MPF Spinal 634
Stelazine 2226
Tambocor Tablets (Less than 1%) 1315
Trexan Tablets (Less than 1%) 937
Trilafon 2123
▲ Xylocaine Injections (Among most common) 637
Xylocaine Injections for Ventricular Arrhythmias 639
Xylocaine 2% Jelly 643
Xylocaine 5% Ointment 644
Xylocaine 10% Oral Spray 645
4% Xylocaine-MPF Sterile Solution 641
Xylocaine 2% Viscous Solution 646

Twitching, lid muscle
Floropryl Sterile Ophthalmic Ointment 1473
Humorsol Sterile Ophthalmic Solution 1475
Phospholine Iodide ⊙ 315

Twitching, muscle
Eldepryl 2250
Leukeran Tablets (Rare) 788
Parnate Tablets 2222
Slo-bid Gyrocaps 1847
Theo-24 2179

Typhlitis
Doxorubicin Hydrochloride Injection, USP 848

T4, decrease
Android 1111
Cibalith-S 870
Depakene Capsules & Syrup 511
Eskalith 2214
Lithium Carbonate Capsules & Tablets 1984
Lithobid Tablets 870
Sandostatin Injection 2029

T4, increase
Brevicon 2304
Danocrine Capsules 2046
Depakene Capsules & Syrup 511
Estratest 2245
Micronor Tablets 1667
Modicon 1667
Norinyl 2304
Ortho-Novum 1667
Tri-Norinyl 28-Day Tablets 2304

T3, decrease
Aygestin Tablets 2437
Brevicon 2304
Cibalith-S 870
Depakene Capsules & Syrup 511
Eskalith 2214
Estratest 2245
Lithium Carbonate Capsules & Tablets 1984
Lithobid Tablets 870
Micronor Tablets 1667
Modicon 1667
Norinyl 2304
Ortho-Novum 1667
Tri-Norinyl 28-Day Tablets 2304

U

Ulceration
Adriamycin PFS 561
Adriamycin RDF 562
Aldactazide 2150
Aldactone 2152
Aplisol (tuberculin PPD, diluted) 2550
Aplitest (tuberculin PPD, multiple-puncture device) 2551
Calciparine Injection 925
Cerumenex Drops 1813
Condylox (Less than 5%) 1630
Cytosar-U Sterile Powder (Less frequent) 2329
Doxorubicin Hydrochloride Injection, USP 848
Easprin 1719
Ethamolin (0.1% to 0.4%) 1829
Eulexin Capsules 2089
Fluorouracil Injection (Common) 1897
Heparin Lock Flush Solution 2456
Heparin Sodium Vials 1264
Heparin Sodium Injection 2457
Heparin Sodium Injection, USP, Sterile Solution 2342
K-Norm Capsules 982
K-Tab Filmtab 532
Micro-K 1863
Mutamycin 733
PPD Tine Test 2548
Questran Powder 710
Rubex 739
Sotradecol (Sodium Tetradecyl Sulfate Injection) 964
Talwin Injection 2071
Ten-K Controlled-Release Tablets 2282
Tuberculin, Old, Tine Test 2549

Ulcerative esophagitis
Decadron Tablets 1447
Decadron-LA Sterile Suspension 1457
Deltasone Tablets 2332
Hydeltra-T.B.A. Sterile Suspension 1478
Hydrocortone Acetate Sterile Suspension 1479
Hydrocortone Phosphate Injection, Sterile 1481
Hydrocortone Tablets 1482
Indocin I.V. (Less than 1%) 1490
Kenalog-10 Injection 2402
Kenalog-40 Injection 2403
Monodox Capsules (Rare) 1630
Terramycin Capsules (Rare) 1786
Vibramycin (Rare) 1787

Ulcer attack
Questran Light 711
Questran Powder 710

Ulcers
Nicorette 1335
Trexan Tablets (Less than 1%) 937
Zoladex (1% to 5%) 1110

Ulcers, anal
▲ Cytosar-U Sterile Powder (Among most frequent) 2329

Ulcers, aphthous
Capoten (0.5 to 2%) 2255
Capozide (0.5 to 2%) 2258

Ulcers, corneal
AK-Cide Sterile Ophthalmic Ointment & Suspension ⊙ 202
AK-Dex ⊙ 203
AK-Pred ⊙ 205
AK-Spore H.C. ⊙ 206
Cetapred Ointment ⊙ 220
Dexacidin ⊙ 272
Isopto Cetapred Suspension ⊙ 220
Myochrysine Injection (Rare) 1516
Oncovin Solution Vials & Hyporets 1288
Ophthocort ⊙ 301
Poly-Pred Liquifilm ⊙ 250
Solganal Suspension (Rare) 2122
Vasocidin Ointment ⊙ 275
Vasocidin Ophthalmic Solution ⊙ 276

Ulcers, cutaneous
Anafranil Capsules (Rare) 650
Cytosar-U Sterile Powder (Less frequent) 2329
Eskalith 2214
Lithane Tablets 1596
Lithium Carbonate Capsules & Tablets 1984

Ulcers, duodenal
Ancobon Capsules 1886
Children's Advil Suspension (Less than 1%) 2426
Sterile FUDR 1898
Indocin Capsules (Less than 1%) 1487
Indocin I.V. (Less than 1%) 1490
Indocin (Less than 1%) 1487
Klor-Con 8/Klor-Con 10 Extended-release Tablets 2374
Larodopa Tablets (Rare) 1905
Motrin Tablets (Less than 1%) 2351
PediaProfen Suspension (Less than 1%) 1363
Prozac Pulvules (Rare) 920
Questran Light 711
Questran Powder 710
Rufen Tablets (Less than 1%) 691
Sinemet Tablets (Rare) 952
Sinemet CR Tablets 953
Trilisate (Rare) 1822

Ulcers, esophageal
Permax Tablets (Rare) 1291
Urobiotic-250 Capsules (Rare) 1968

Ulcers, gastrointestinal
Adriamycin PFS 561
Anafranil Capsules (Infrequent) 650
Anaprox and Anaprox DS Tablets 2288
Butazolidin Capsules & Tablets (Less than 1%) 1027
Children's Advil Suspension (Less than 1%) 2426
Clinoril Tablets 1433
Clozaril Tablets (Less than 1%) 2000
Cosmegen Injection 1440
Dolobid Tablets 1465
Ergamisol Tablets 1136
Sterile FUDR 1898
Feldene Capsules (Less than 1%) 1777
Fiorinal with Codeine Capsules 2008
Fluorouracil Injection 1897
Indocin Capsules (Less than 1%) 1487
Indocin I.V. (Less than 1%) 1490
Indocin (Less than 1%) 1487
Intron A (1 patient) 2097
K-Dur Microburst Release System (potassium chloride, USP) E.R. Tablets 1163
K-Tab Filmtab 532
▲ Klor-Con 8/Klor-Con 10 Extended-release Tablets (Among most common) 2374
Larodopa Tablets (Rare) 1905
Lodine Capsules 2468
Meclomen Capsules 1739
Methotrexate Tablets, Parenteral, LPF Parenteral 1217
Micro-K 1863
Micro-K LS Packets 1864
Motrin Tablets (Less than 1%) 2351
Nalfon Pulvules & Tablets 919
Naprosyn 2297
NebuPent for Inhalation Solution (1% or less) 1017
Orudis Capsules (Less than 1%) 2488
PediaProfen Suspension (Less than 1%) 1363
Ponstel 1758
Purinethol Tablets 800
Rheumatrex Methotrexate Dose Pack 1234
Rufen Tablets 691
Slow-K Tablets (1 per 100,000 patient-years) 2281
Tolectin (200, 400 and 600 mg) (Less than 1%) 1379
▲ Toradol IM Injection (1.2% to 5.4%) 2302
Trilisate (Less than 1%) 1822
Voltaren Tablets 1042
Wellbutrin Tablets (Rare) 821

Ulcers, intestinal
Dyazide Capsules 2208
Ten-K Controlled-Release Tablets 2282

Ulcers, oral mucosal
Alkeran Tablets (Infrequent) 754
Anafranil Capsules (Infrequent) 650
Atrovent Inhalation Aerosol (Less than 1 in 100) 675
Azactam for Injection (Less than 1%) 2252
Cipro I.V. (1% or less) 1592
Cuprimine Capsules (Some patients) 1442
▲ Cytosar-U Sterile Powder (Among most frequent) 2329
Cytoxan for Injection (Isolated reports) 726
Depen Titratable Tablets (Some patients) 2379
Kerlone Tablets (Less than 2%) 2172
Leukeran Tablets (Infrequent) 788
Myochrysine Injection 1516
Nalfon Pulvules & Tablets (Less than 1%) 919
NebuPent for Inhalation Solution (1% or less) 1017
Neosar for Injection (Isolated reports) 566
Oncovin Solution Vials & Hyporets 1288
ProSom Tablets 554
Prozac Pulvules (Rare) 920
Retrovir Capsules (Less than 5%) 802
Retrovir I.V. Infusion (Less than 5%) 805
Retrovir Syrup (Less than 5%) 802
Solganal Suspension 2122
Tegison Capsules (Less than 1%) 1881
Tegretol Chewable Tablets 654

Ulcers, peptic
Anafranil Capsules (Infrequent) 650
Anaprox and Anaprox DS Tablets (Less than 1%) 2288
Aristocort Suspension 1008
Aristospan Suspension (Intralesional) 1011
Atromid-S Capsules 2435
Butazolidin Capsules & Tablets (Less than 1%) 1027
Capoten (0.5 to 2%) 2255
Capozide (0.5 to 2%) 2258
Clinoril Tablets (Less than 1 in 100) 1433
Colestid Granules (Fewer than 1 in 500 patients) 2328
Cortenema 2244
Cortifoam 1827
Cuprimine Capsules (Less than 1%) 1442
Dalalone D.P. Injectable 999
Damason-P 1356
Depen Titratable Tablets (Isolated cases) 2379
Dolobid Tablets (Less than 1 in 100) 1465
Fiorinal with Codeine Capsules 2008
Hydeltra-T.B.A. Sterile Suspension 1478
Hydrocortone Acetate Sterile Suspension 1479
Hydrocortone Phosphate Injection, Sterile 1481
Hydrocortone Tablets 1482
Hydromox R Tablets 1209
Indocin Capsules (Less than 1%) 1487
Indocin I.V. (Less than 1%) 1490
Indocin (Less than 1%) 1487
Kenalog in Orabase 604
Klor-Con 8/Klor-Con 10 Extended-release Tablets 2374
Klotrix 708
▲ Lupron Depot 3.75 mg (Among most frequent) 2312
Lupron Depot 7.5 mg 2311
Lupron Injection (Less than 5%) 2310
Meclomen Capsules (Greater than 1%) 1739
Mexitil Capsules (About 8 in 10,000) 680
Midamor Tablets (Rare) 1508
Moduretic Tablets 1510
Niacor Tablets 2376
Nicolar Tablets 1846
Orudis Capsules (Less than 1%) 2488
Permax Tablets (Infrequent) 1291
Prozac Pulvules (Rare) 920
Sandimmune (2% or less) 2024
Solu-Cortef Sterile Powder 2361
Solu-Medrol Sterile Powder 2363
Tolectin (200, 400 and 600 mg) (1 to 3%) 1379
Toradol IM Injection (1% or less) 2302
Voltaren Tablets (1-2%) 1042
Zorprin Tablets 698

Ulcers, peptic, aggravation of
Anturane 853
Eldepryl 2250

Ulcers, peptic, reactivation of
Anturane 853
Rauzide Tablets 1804

Ulcers, peptic with or without perforation
Lodine Capsules (Less than 1%) 2468
Nalfon Pulvules & Tablets (Less than 1%) 919
Voltaren Tablets (1-3%) 1042

Ulcers, peptic with perforation and hemorrhage
Anaprox and Anaprox DS Tablets (Less than 3%) 2288
Ansaid Tablets (Less than 1%) 2319
Aristospan Suspension (Intra-articular) 1011
Celestone Soluspan Suspension 2081
Children's Advil Suspension 2426
Cortone Acetate Sterile Suspension 1437
Cortone Acetate Tablets 1439
Decadron Elixir 1445
Decadron Phosphate Injection 1449
Decadron Phosphate Respihaler 1454
Decadron Phosphate Turbinaire 1456
Decadron Phosphate with Xylocaine Injection, Sterile 1451
Decadron Tablets 1447
Decadron-LA Sterile Suspension 1457
Deltasone Tablets 2332
Depo-Medrol Sterile Aqueous Suspension 2334
Hydeltrasol Injection, Sterile 1476
Hydrocortone Tablets 1482
Kenalog-10 Injection 2402
Kenalog-40 Injection 2403
Lodine Capsules (Less than 1%) 2468
Meclomen Capsules (Less than 1%) 1739
Medrol 2348
Motrin Tablets 2351
Naprosyn (Less than 1%) 2297
Pediapred Oral Liquid 987
PediaProfen Suspension 1363
Rufen Tablets (Less than 1%) 691
Voltaren Tablets (1-3%) 1042

Ulcers, pharyngeal
Myochrysine Injection 1516

Unconsciousness (see under Consciousness, loss of)

Underventilation (see under Hypoventilation)

Unsteadiness
Ativan Injection 2432
▲ Ativan Tablets (3.4%) 2434
Restoril Capsules (Less than 1%) 2023
Tambocor Tablets 1315
▲ Tegretol Chewable Tablets (Among most frequent) 654
▲ Tegretol Suspension (Among most frequent) 656
▲ Tegretol Tablets (Among most frequent) 654
Tofranil Ampuls 1038
Tofranil Tablets 1039
Tofranil-PM Capsules 1041
Tonocard Tablets (0.0-1.2%) 1554

Upper respiratory symptoms
Engerix-B Unit-Dose Vials (Less than 1%) 2213
▲ Prinivil Tablets (3.0% to 4.5%) 1538
▲ Wellbutrin Tablets (5.0%) 821
▲ Zestril Tablets (3.0%) 2277

Urate excretion, impaired
Fiorinal with Codeine Capsules 2008

Uremia (see under Azotemia)

Ureteral obstruction
Butazolidin Capsules & Tablets (Less than 1%) 1027
Surgicel (One report) 1151
Zoladex (Isolated cases) 1110

Ureteral spasm
Anexsia 5/500 Tablets 2196
Anexsia 7.5/650 Tablets 2197
Azdōne Tablets 844
Damason-P 1356
Dilaudid Cough Syrup 1174
Dilaudid 1173
Hycodan Syrup, Tablets 927
Hycomine Compound Tablets 929
Hycomine Syrup 927
Hycotuss Expectorant Syrup 930
Hydrocet Capsules 835
Lortab ASA Tablets 2414
Tussionex Extended-Release Suspension 988
Vicodin Tablets 1187
Vicodin ES Tablets 1189
Zydone Capsules 941

Ureteritis, hemorrhagic
Cytoxan for Injection 726
Neosar for Injection 566

Urethral disorder
Anafranil Capsules (Infrequent) 650

Urethritis
Dyclone 0.5% and 1% Topical Solutions, USP 626
Prozac Pulvules (Rare) 920
Rogaine Topical Solution (0.93%) 2357

Uric acid level, increase (see under Hyperuricemia)

Uric acid stones
Benemid Tablets 1426
ColBENEMID Tablets 1436

Uricaciduria
Permax Tablets (Rare) 1291

Urinary bladder, irritability
MIOSTAT ⊙ 233
Winstrol Tablets 2075

Urinary bladder malignancies
Neosar for Injection 566
Permax Tablets (Rare) 1291

Urinary calculi
Neptazane Tablets (Rare) ⊙ 311

Urinary difficulty (see under Micturition, difficulty)

Urinary disturbances
Cibalith-S 870
Esimil Tablets 864
Ismelin Tablets 869
Lithobid Tablets 870
MIOSTAT ⊙ 233
Prozac Pulvules (Infrequent) 920
Sansert Tablets 2031
▲ TheraCys BCG Live (Intravesical) (Up to 17.9%) 898
Trilafon (Occasional) 2123

Urinary findings, abnormal
Capastat Sulfate Vials (Many cases) 1250
Ceclor Pulvules & Suspension (Less than 1 in 200) 1251
Clozaril Tablets (2%) 2000
Phenurone Tablets (1 in 100 patients or less) 552

Urinary frequency (see under Micturition disturbances)

Urinary glucose, false-positive
Ceftin Tablets 575
Ceptaz for Injection 1057
Fortaz 1060

Urinary hesitancy
Arfonad Ampuls 1887
Artane 1195
Bentyl 1322
BuSpar (Infrequent) 1401
Cantil Tablets 1326
Dalgan Injection (Less than 1%) 620
Darbid Tablets 2205
Ditropan 1332
Dolophine Hydrochloride Ampoules & Vials 1260
Dolophine Hydrochloride Tablets 1261
Donnatal 1858
Donnatal Extentabs 1859
Donnatal Tablets 1858
Donnazyme Tablets 1860
Eldepryl (1 of 49 patients) 2250
Kinesed Tablets 2272
Kutrase Capsules 2146
Levsin/Levsinex 2147
Librax Capsules 1929
Ludiomil Tablets (Rare) 874
MS Contin Tablets (Infrequent) 1814
MSIR (Infrequent) 1817
Marax Tablets & DF Syrup 1954
Methadone Hydrochloride Diskets 1284
Methadone Hydrochloride Oral Solution & Tablets 1987
Mexitil Capsules (Less than 1% or about 2 in 1,000) 680
Norflex 1314
Norgesic 1314
▲ Norpace (14%) 2177
Oramorph SR (Morphine Sulfate Sustained Release Tablets) (Less frequent) 1988
Pamelor 2019
Pro-Banthīne Tablets 2141
ProSom Tablets (Infrequent) 554
Quarzan Capsules (Among most frequent) 1937
Retrovir Capsules (Less than 5%) 802
Retrovir I.V. Infusion (Less than 5%) 805
Retrovir Syrup (Less than 5%) 802
Robinul Forte Tablets 1873
Robinul Injectable 1873
Robinul Tablets 1873
Roxanol 1991
Valium Injectable 1937
Valium Tablets (Infrequent) 1939
Valpin 50 Tablets 941

Urinary obstruction
▲ Lupron Depot 3.75 mg (Among most frequent) 2312

Urinary retention
Actifed with Codeine Cough Syrup 752
Akineton 1171
▲ Anafranil Capsules (2% to 7%) 650
Anatuss LA Tablets 1359
Anexsia 5/500 Tablets 2196
Anexsia 7.5/650 Tablets 2197
Asendin Tablets (Less than 1%) 1196
▲ Astramorph/PF Injection, USP (Preservative-Free) (90% of males; somewhat less in females) 618
Azdōne Tablets 844
Azo Gantrisin Tablets 1888
B & O No. 15A & No. 16A Supprettes 2395
Bellergal-S Tablets (Rare) 1998
Benadryl Capsules 1691
Benadryl Injection 1692
Bentyl 1322
Brevibloc Injection (Less than 1%) 942
Bronkolixir ▣ 761
Bronkotabs Tablets ▣ 762
BuSpar (Rare) 1401
Cantil Tablets 1326
Carbocaine Hydrochloride Injection 2043
Catapres Tablets (About 1 in 1,000 patients) 676
Catapres-TTS (1 per 1,000 patients) 677
Cipro I.V. (1% or less) 1592
Cipro Tablets (Less than 1%) 1589
Clozaril Tablets (1%) 2000
Cogentin 1435
Combipres Tablets (About 1 in 1,000) 678
Comhist LA Capsules 1618
Compazine 2201
Cyclogyl ⊙ 215
Cyclomydril ⊙ 216
Cystospaz 2395
Cytosar-U Sterile Powder (Less frequent) 2329
Dalgan Injection (Less than 1%) 620
Damason-P 1356
Dantrium Capsules (Less frequent) 1619
Darbid Tablets 2205
Deconamine 663
Demerol 2047
Desyrel and Desyrel Dividose (Less than 1%) 1404
Dilaudid Cough Syrup 1174
Dilaudid 1173
Dilaudid-HP Injection 1175
Diprivan Injection (Less than 1%) 2267
Ditropan 1332
Dolophine Hydrochloride Ampoules & Vials 1260
Dolophine Hydrochloride Tablets 1261
Donnatal 1858
Donnatal Extentabs 1859
Donnatal Tablets 1858

(▣ Described in PDR For Nonprescription Drugs) Incidence data in parenthesis; ▲ 3% or more (⊙ Described in PDR For Ophthalmology)

Donnazyme Tablets 1860
Dopram Injectable 1860
Doral Tablets 2383
▲ Duragesic Transdermal System (3% to 10%) 1133
▲ Duramorph (90% of males) 960
Elavil 2269
Eldepryl 2250
Endep Tablets 1927
Entex Capsules 1623
Entex LA Tablets 1623
Entex Liquid 1623
Ethmozine Tablets (0.3%-0.4%) 946
Etrafon 2087
Flexeril Tablets (Less than 1%) 1471
Halcion Tablets 2340
Haldol Decanoate 1375
Haldol Injection, Tablets and Concentrate 1373
Hycodan Syrup, Tablets 927
Hycomine Compound Tablets 929
Hycomine Syrup 927
Hycotuss Expectorant Syrup 930
Hydrocet Capsules 835
Infumorph 200 and Infumorph 500 Sterile Solutions (Frequent) 962
Inversine Tablets 1492
Kinesed Tablets 2272
Klonopin Tablets 1902
Kutrase Capsules 2146
Larodopa Tablets (Infrequent) 1905
Levo-Dromoran (Infrequent) 1906
Levsin/Levsinex 2147
Limbitrol 1933
Lioresal Tablets (Rare) 1031
Lomotil 2174
Lortab ASA Tablets 2414
Loxitane 1213
Ludiomil Tablets (Rare) 874
MS Contin Tablets (Infrequent) 1814
MSIR (Infrequent) 1817
Marax Tablets & DF Syrup (Occasional) 1954
Marcaine Hydrochloride with Epinephrine 1:200,000 2055
Marcaine Hydrochloride Injection 2055
Marcaine Spinal 2058
Marplan Tablets (Rare) 1906
Mellaril 2011
Mepergan Injection 2479
Methadone Hydrochloride Diskets 1284
Methadone Hydrochloride Oral Solution & Tablets 1987
Mexitil Capsules (Less than 1% or about 2 in 1,000) 680
Moban Tablets & Concentrate 932
Motofen Tablets 836
Nardil (Less common) 1742
Nolex LA Tablets 838
Norflex 1314
Norgesic 1314
Normodyne Tablets 2110
Normozide Tablets (Less than 1%) 2112
▲ Norpace (3 to 9%) 2177
Norpramin Tablets 1340
Norzine 1818
Oncovin Solution Vials & Hyporets 1288
Optimine Tablets 2115
Oramorph SR (Morphine Sulfate Sustained Release Tablets) (Less frequent) 1988
Ornade Spansule Capsules 2221
PBZ Tablets & Elixir 1037
PBZ-SR Tablets 1037
Pamelor 2019
Pantopon Injectable 1911
Parlodel 2020
Parnate Tablets 2222
Periactin 1525
Permax Tablets (Infrequent) 1291
Phenergan with Codeine 2497
Phenergan VC with Codeine 2501
Polaramine 2116
Pro-Banthine Tablets 2141
Prozac Pulvules (Infrequent) 920
Quarzan Capsules 1937
Robinul Forte Tablets 1873
Robinul Injectable 1873
Robinul Tablets 1873
Roxanol 1991
Ru-Tuss II Capsules 693
Sensorcaine 631
Sensorcaine-MPF Spinal 634
Serentil 686
Sinemet Tablets 952
Sinemet CR Tablets 953
Sinequan 1960
Stelazine 2226
Surmontil Capsules 2524
Symmetrel Capsules & Syrup (0.1-1%) 936
Tacaryl 2409
Tagamet (Rare) 2228
Talacen (Rare) 2070
Talwin Injection (Infrequent) 2071
Talwin Compound 2072
Talwin Injection 2071
Talwin Nx 2073
Tambocor Tablets (Less than 1%) 1315
Tavist Syrup 2033
Tavist Tablets 2035
Tavist-D Tablets 2035
Tegison Capsules (Less than 1%) 1881
Tegretol Chewable Tablets 654
Tegretol Suspension 656
Tegretol Tablets 654
Temaril Tablets, Syrup and Spansule Sustained Release Capsules 1085
Thorazine 2234
Tofranil Ampuls 1038
Tofranil Tablets 1039
Tofranil-PM Capsules 1041
Tonocard Tablets (Less than 1%) 1554
Torecan 1993
Trandate HCT/Trandate (Less than 1% in 208 patients) 579
Triaminic Expectorant DH 1995
Triaminic Oral Infant Drops 1996
Triavil Tablets 1556
Trinalin Repetabs Tablets 1170
Trobicin Sterile Powder 2366
Tussionex Extended-Release Suspension 988
Unasyn (Less than 1%) 1965
Urised Tablets 2396
Valpin 50 Tablets 941
Valrelease Capsules (Occasional) 1923
Vicodin Tablets 1187
Vicodin ES Tablets 1189
Vivactil Tablets 1567
Wellbutrin Tablets (1.9%) 821
Xanax Tablets 2367
Zydone Capsules 941

Urinary sediment, abnormalities
Dyazide Capsules 2208
Roferon-A Injection (Infrequent) 1916

Urinary tract, burning
Rowasa (0.61%) 2248

Urinary tract, infection
▲ Anafranil Capsules (Up to 6%) 650
▲ Ansaid Tablets (3-9%) 2319
Cartrol Tablets (Less common) 507
Cytotec (Infrequent) 2159
Koro-Flex Arcing Spring Diaphragm 2142
Koromex Coil Spring Diaphragm 2142
▲ Lupron Depot 3.75 mg (Among most frequent) 2312
Lupron Depot 7.5 mg 2311
Permax Tablets (2.7%) 1291
Rowasa (0.61%) 2248
▲ TheraCys BCG Live (Intravesical) (1.0% to 17.9%) 898
Zoladex (1% to 5%) 1110

Urinary tract, obstruction
Lupron Depot 7.5 mg 2311
Lupron Injection (A few cases) 2310
Zoladex (1% to 5%) 1110

Urinary tract dilatation
Endep Tablets 1927
Etrafon 2087
Limbitrol 1933
Norpramin Tablets 1340
Pamelor 2019
Surmontil Capsules 2524
Tofranil Ampuls 1038
Tofranil Tablets 1039
Tofranil-PM Capsules 1041
Triavil Tablets 1556

Urinary tract disorder, unspecified
Leukine for IV Infusion 1127
Prozac Pulvules (Infrequent) 920

Urinary tract irritation
Orudis Capsules (Greater than 1%) 2488

Urinary urgency
Duvoid Tablets 1853
▲ Lupron Depot 3.75 mg (Among most frequent) 2312
Plendil Extended-Release Tablets (0.5% to 1.5%) 1526
ProSom Tablets (Infrequent) 554
Prozac Pulvules (Infrequent) 920
▲ TheraCys BCG Live (Intravesical) (Up to 17.9%) 898

Urination, difficult (see under Micturition, difficulty)

Urination, painful (see under Micturition, painful)

Urine, abnormal
Diprivan Injection (Less than 1%) 2267

Urine, burnt odor
Questran Light 711
Questran Powder 710

Urine, cells in
TheraCys BCG Live (Intravesical) (Up to 0.9%) 898
Zovirax Sterile Powder (Less than 1%) 828

Urine, color change
Adriamycin PFS 561
Adriamycin RDF (Expected reaction) 562
AK-Fluor Injection 10% and 25% ..... ◉ 204
Atabrine Hydrochloride Tablets 2041
Azulfidine Tablets, EN-tabs, Oral Suspension (Rare) 1157
Cerubidine 2443
Clinoril Tablets (Less than 1%) 1433
Coumadin Injection & Tablets 944
Desferal Vials 862
Diprivan Injection (Less than 1%) 2267
Doxorubicin Hydrochloride for Injection, USP 622
Doxorubicin Hydrochloride Injection, USP 848
Eulexin Capsules 2089
Evac-U-Gen Mild Laxative ..... ▣ 739
Flagyl I.V. 2131
Flagyl Tablets (Approximately 1 in 100,000 patients) 2170
Fluorescite ..... ◉ 217
Lamprene Capsules (Greater than 1%) 1030
Larodopa Tablets (Infrequent) 1905
Maxzide 1215
Modane Plus Tablets ..... ▣ 504
Modane Tablets ..... ▣ 503
Normodyne Injection 2108
Normodyne Tablets 2110
Novantrone for Injection Concentrate 1226
Paraflex Caplets (Rare) 1378
Parafon Forte DSC Caplets (Rare) 1379
Pronestyl Capsules and Tablets 1800
Pronestyl Injection 1798
Protostat Tablets (Approximately one patient in 100,000) 1674
Pyridium 1763
Pyridium Plus 1764
Rubex 739
Sectral Capsules 2520
Sinemet Tablets 952
Sinemet CR Tablets 953
Trandate HCT Tablets 579
Trandate Injection 577
Urised Tablets 2396
Yellolax ..... ▣ 590

Urine, fluorescence
AK-Fluor Injection 10% and 25% ..... ◉ 204

Urine, microscopic deposits
Tegretol Chewable Tablets 654
Tegretol Suspension 656
Tegretol Tablets 654

Urine, output low (see under Hypouresis)

Urine, presence of granular casts
Amikin Injectable 602
Primaxin I.M. 1532
Primaxin I.V. 1535
Rocephin Injectable Vials, ADD-Vantage (Less than 1%) 1914
Unasyn 1965

Urine, presence of RBCs (see under Hematuria)

Urine, presence of urobilinogen
Primaxin I.M. 1532
Primaxin I.V. 1535

Urolithiasis
Permax Tablets (Infrequent) 1291
Prozac Pulvules (Rare) 920

Urticaria
A/T/S Topical Gel and Topical Solution 1089
Accutane Capsules (Less than 1%) 1878
Achromycin V Capsules 1193
Actifed with Codeine Cough Syrup 752
Actigall Capsules 2280
Activase (Occasional) 1047
Adalat Capsules (10 mg and 20 mg) (2% or less) 1587
Adipex-P Tablets and Capsules 1019
Adriamycin PFS (Occasional) 561
Adriamycin RDF (Occasional) 562
AeroBid Inhaler System (1-3%) 995
Albuminar-5, Albumin (Human) U.S.P. 5% 608
Albuminar-25, Albumin (Human) U.S.P. 25% 608
Aldactazide 2150
Aldactone 2152
Aldoclor Tablets 1413
Aldoril Tablets 1418
Alfenta Injection (Less than 1%) 1131
Amen (Occasional) 833
Americaine Anesthetic Lubricant 972
Americaine Otic Topical Anesthetic Ear Drops 973
Amoxil 2193
Anafranil Capsules (Up to 1%) 650
Anaprox and Anaprox DS Tablets (Rare) 2288
Ancobon Capsules 1886
▲ Anestacon Solution (Among most common) 2394
Ansaid Tablets (Less than 1%) 2319
Antivenin (Crotalidae) Polyvalent 2430
Apresazide Capsules (Less frequent) 854
Apresoline Hydrochloride Parenteral (Ampuls) 856
Apresoline Hydrochloride Tablets (Less frequent) 855
Apresoline-Esidrix Tablets 857
Arfonad Ampuls 1887
Asendin Tablets (Less than 1%) 1196
Astramorph/PF Injection, USP (Preservative-Free) 618
▲ Atgam Sterile Solution (1 in 8 patients; 27%) 2320
Atromid-S Capsules (Less often) 2435
Attenuvax (Rare) 1424
▲ Augmentin Tablets, Powder for Oral Suspension, and Chewable Tablets (3%) 2198
Axid Pulvules (0.5%) 1246
Azactam for Injection (Less than 1%) 2252
Azdone Tablets 844
Azo Gantanol Tablets 1887
Azo Gantrisin Tablets 1888
▲ Azulfidine Tablets, EN-tabs, Oral Suspension (3 to 4%) 1157
B & O No. 15A & No. 16A Supprettes (Occasional) 2395
▲ Bactrim DS Tablets (Among most common) 1891
▲ Bactrim I.V. Infusion (Among most common) 1889
▲ Bactrim (Among most common) 1891
Beclovent Inhalation Aerosol and Refill (Rare) 572
Beconase AQ Nasal Spray (Rare) 574
Beconase Inhalation Aerosol & Refill (Rare) 574
Benadryl Injection 1692
Benemid Tablets 1426
Bentyl 1322
Benzamycin Topical Gel (1 out of 153) 907
Betagan (Rare) ..... ◉ 239
Biavax II 1427
Bicillin C-R Injection 2438
Bicillin C-R 900/300 Injection 2440
Bicillin L-A Injection 2442
Biltricide (Rare) 1589
Brevital Sodium Vials 1248
Butazolidin Capsules & Tablets (Less than 1%) 1027
Calan SR Caplets (1% or less) 2157
Calan Tablets (1% or less) 2155
Calciparine Injection 925
Cantil Tablets 1326
Capastat Sulfate Vials 1250
Capozide 2258
Carafate Tablets 1326

Carbocaine Hydrochloride 3% Injection 956
Carbocaine Hydrochloride Injection 2043
Carbocaine Hydrochloride 2% with Neo-Cobefrin 956
Cardizem Tablets-30 mg, 60 mg, 90 mg and 120 mg (Less than 1%) 1329
Cardizem SR Capsules-60 mg, 90 mg and 120 mg (Less than 1%) 1327
Catapres Tablets (About 5 in 1,000 patients) 676
Catapres-TTS (5 per 1,000 patients) 677
Ceclor Pulvules & Suspension (Less than 1 in 200) 1251
Ceftin Tablets (0.2%) 575
Ceptaz for Injection 1057
Children's Advil Suspension (Less than 1%) 2426
Chloromycetin Otic 1697
Chloroptic S.O.P. ⊚ 243
Chloroptic Sterile Ophthalmic Solution ⊚ 243
Cholybar 1705
Cipro I.V. (1% or less) 1592
Cipro Tablets (Less than 1%) 1589
Cleocin HCl Capsules 2322
Cleocin Pediatric Flavored Granules 2324
Cleocin Phosphate Injection 2325
Clozaril Tablets (Less than 1%) 2000
ColBENEMID Tablets 1436
Colestid Granules (Fewer than 1 in 1,000) 2328
Coly-Mycin M Parenteral 1706
Colyte 1826
Combipres Tablets (About 5 in 1,000) 678
Comhist LA Capsules 1618
Compazine 2201
Cortone Acetate Sterile Suspension 1437
Cortone Acetate Tablets 1439
Corzide Tablets (Occasional) 702
Coumadin Injection & Tablets (Infrequent) 944
Cuprimine Capsules 1442
Cycrin Tablets (Occasional) 2449
Cytadren Tablets (Rare) 861
Cytosar-U Sterile Powder (Less frequent) 2329
Cytovene Sterile Powder (1% or less) 2292
Damason-P 1356
Danocrine Capsules 2046
Dantrium Capsules (Less frequent) 1619
Dantrium Intravenous (Rare) 1620
Darbid Tablets 2205
Decadron Elixir 1445
Decadron Phosphate Injection 1449
Decadron Phosphate Respihaler 1454
Decadron Phosphate Turbinaire 1456
Decadron Phosphate with Xylocaine Injection, Sterile 1451
Decadron Tablets 1447
Decadron-LA Sterile Suspension 1457
Declomycin Capsules, Tablets 1199
Deconamine 663
Demerol 2047
Demser Capsules (Rare) 1460
Depen Titratable Tablets 2379
Depo-Medrol Sterile Aqueous Suspension 2334
Depo-Provera Sterile Aqueous Suspension (Occasional) 2336
Deprol Tablets 2382
Desferal Vials 862
Desoxyn Gradumet Tablets 514
Desyrel and Desyrel Dividose 1404
Dexedrine 2206
DiaBeta (1.5%) 1091
Diabinese Tablets (Approximately 1% or less) 1775
Diamox Parenteral (Occasional) 1200
Diamox Sequels (Sustained Release) 1201
Diamox Tablets (Occasional) 1200
Dicumarol Tablets (Infrequent) 516
Didrex Tablets 2338
Didronel Tablets (Rare) 1621
Dilaudid-HP Injection 1175
Dimacol Caplets ▣ 672
Dimetane-DC Cough Syrup 1857
Dimetane-DX Cough Syrup 1858
Diprivan Injection (Less than 1%) 2267
Disalcid 1310
Diucardin Tablets 2450
Diulo 2129
Diupres Tablets 1461
Diuril Oral Suspension 1464
Diuril Sodium Intravenous 1463
Diuril Tablets 1464
Dolobid Tablets (Less than 1 in 100) 1465
Dolophine Hydrochloride Ampoules & Vials 1260
Dolophine Hydrochloride Tablets 1261
Donnatal 1858
Donnatal Extentabs 1859
Donnatal Tablets 1858
Donnazyme Tablets 1860
Doryx Capsules 1717
Doxorubicin Hydrochloride for Injection, USP (Occasional) 622
Doxorubicin Hydrochloride Injection, USP (Occasional) 848
Duramorph 960
Duranest Injections 624
Duricef 1405
Dyazide Capsules 2208
Dyclone 0.5% and 1% Topical Solutions, USP 626
DynaCirc Capsules (0.5% to 1%) 2004
E.E.S. 522
E-Mycin Tablets 688
Easprin 1719
Efudex 1880
Elase-Chloromycetin Ointment 1015
Elavil 2269
Elspar 1470
Emete-con Intramuscular/Intravenous (Rare) 1950
Eminase (Occasional) 2211
Empirin with Codeine Phosphate Nos. 2, 3 & 4 764
Endep Tablets 1927
Enduron Tablets 517
Enduronyl 518
Engerix-B Unit-Dose Vials (Less than 1%) 2213
Epogen for Injection (Rare) 591
Equagesic Tablets 2451
Ergamisol Tablets (Less than 1%) 1136
ERYC 1720
Erycette (erythromycin 2%) Topical Solution 1678
EryPed 519
Ery-Tab Tablets 521
Erythrocin Stearate Filmtab 523
Erythromycin Base Filmtab 525
Erythromycin Delayed-Release Capsules, USP 526
Esidrix Tablets 863
Esimil Tablets 864
Ethmozine Tablets (Less than 2%) 946
Etrafon 2087
Exna Tablets 1862
Factrel (Rare) 2561
Fansidar Tablets 1896
Fastin Capsules 2216
Feldene Capsules (Less than 1%) 1777
Flagyl I.V. 2131
Flagyl Tablets 2170
Flexeril Tablets (Less than 1%) 1471
Fortaz 1060
Fulvicin P/G Tablets 2090
Fulvicin P/G 165 & 330 Tablets 2091
Fulvicin-U/F Tablets 2092
Furoxone 1855
Gammagard Immune Globulin, Intravenous (Human) (Occasional) 658
Gammar, Immune Globulin (Human) U.S.P. 609
Gantanol 1899
Gantrisin Ophthalmic Ointment/Solution 1900
Gantrisin 1901
Garamycin Injectable 2093
Gastrocrom Capsules (Infrequent) 974
Geocillin Tablets (Infrequent) 1951
Geref (sermorelin acetate for injection) (One patient) 2560
Glucotrol (1 in 70) 1952
GoLYTELY (Isolated cases) 699
Grifulvin V (griseofulvin microsize) Tablets/Suspension (Occasional) 1678
Grisactin 2454
Grisactin Ultra Tablets 2455
Gris-PEG Tablets, 125 mg & 250 mg 1083
Guaifed Syrup ▣ 629
Heparin Lock Flush Solution 2456
▲ Heparin Sodium Vials (Among most common) 1264
Heparin Sodium Injection 2457
Heparin Sodium Injection, USP, Sterile Solution 2342
Hep-B-Gammagee 1474
Hespan Injection 948
Hydeltrasol Injection, Sterile 1476
Hydeltra-T.B.A. Sterile Suspension 1478
Hydrocortone Acetate Sterile Suspension 1479
Hydrocortone Phosphate Injection, Sterile 1481
Hydrocortone Tablets 1482
HydroDIURIL Tablets 1484
Hydromox R Tablets 1209
Hydromox Tablets 1208
Hydropres Tablets 1485
HyperHep Hepatitis B Immune Globulin (Human) 1575
Hyskon Hysteroscopy Fluid (Rare) 1162
Idamycin for Injection 564
Beef Regular, 100 Units 1275
Ilosone 913
Ilotycin Gluceptate, IV, Vials 915
Imferon 976
Inderide Tablets 2463
Inderide LA Long Acting Capsules 2465
Indocin Capsules (Less than 1%) 1487
Indocin I.V. (Less than 1%) 1490
Indocin (Less than 1%) 1487
Infumorph 200 and Infumorph 500 Sterile Solutions 962
Insulatard NPH 1626
Insulatard NPH Human 1627
Intal Capsules (Less than 1 in 10,000 patients) 978
Intal Inhaler (Infrequent) 979
Intal Nebulizer Solution 980
Intron A (Up to 5%) 2097
Ionamin Capsules 981
Isoptin Injectable (Rare) 1177
Isoptin Oral Tablets (Less than 1%) 1179
Isoptin SR Sustained Release Tablets (Less than 1%) 1181
Keflex Pulvules, Oral Suspension & Pediatric Drops 916
Keftab Tablets 917
Kefurox Vials, Faspak & ADD-Vantage (Less than 1 in 250) 1277
Kinesed Tablets 2272
Kutrase Capsules 2146
Lasix 1093
Leucovorin Calcium Injection 1210
Leucovorin Calcium Tablets 1212
Levo-Dromoran (Occasional) 1906
Levsin/Levsinex 2147
Limbitrol 1933
Lincocin 2344
Lodine Capsules (Less than 1%) 2468
Lomotil 2174
Lopid Capsules and Tablets 1736
Lopressor HCT Tablets 1034
Lortab ASA Tablets 2414
Lotrimin 2102
Lotrisone Cream 2103
Lutrepulse for Injection 1655
M-M-R II 1494
M-R-VAX II 1496
MS Contin Tablets (Infrequent) 1814
MSIR (Infrequent) 1817
Macrodantin Capsules 1624
Mandol Vials, Faspak & ADD-Vantage 1281
Marcaine Hydrochloride 0.5% with Epinephrine 1:200,000 (as bitartrate) 958
Marcaine Hydrochloride with Epinephrine 1:200,000 (Rare) 2055
Marcaine Hydrochloride Injection (Rare) 2055
Marcaine Spinal (Rare) 2058
Matulane Capsules 1907
Maxzide 1215
Meclomen Capsules (Greater than 1%) 1739
Medrol 2348
Mellaril (Infrequent) 2011
Mepergan Injection 2479
Meruvax II 1503
Methadone Hydrochloride Diskets 1284
Methadone Hydrochloride Oral Solution & Tablets 1987
Methotrexate Tablets, Parenteral, LPF Parenteral 1217
Mevacor Tablets (Rare) 1505
Mezlin 1597
Mezlin Pharmacy Bulk Package 1599
Micronase Tablets (1.5%) 2350
Minizide Capsules 1779
Minocin Intravenous 1221
Minocin Oral Suspension 1224
Minocin Pellet-Filled Capsules 1222
Mixtard 70/30 1627
Mixtard Human 70/30 1628
Moduretic Tablets 1510
Monodox Capsules 1630
Monopril Tablets (0.2 to 1.0%) 1406
Motofen Tablets 836
Motrin Tablets (Less than 1%) 2351
Mulvidren-F Softab Tablets 2273
Mumpsvax (Extremely rare) 1513
Mycelex 1% Cream and Topical Solution 1% 1604
Mykrox ½ mg Tablets 984
Myleran Tablets 790
Nalfon Pulvules & Tablets (Less than 1%) 919
Naprosyn (Rare) 2297
Nasalcrom Nasal Solution 986
Naturetin Tablets (Occasional) 1789
Navane Capsules and Concentrate 1954
Navane Intramuscular 1956
Nebcin Vials, Hyporets & ADD-Vantage 1286
NebuPent for Inhalation Solution (1% or less) 1017
NegGram 2062
Nescaine/Nescaine MPF 629
Niclocide Chewable Tablets (Two cases in patients with tape worm) 1607
Nicorette 1335
Nizoral Tablets (Several cases) 1145
Norflex (Rare) 1314
Norgesic (Rare) 1314
Normozide Tablets 2112
Noroxin Tablets 1519
Norpramin Tablets 1340
Novantrone for Injection Concentrate (Occasional) 1226
Novocain Hydrochloride for Spinal Anesthesia 2065
Nubain Injection (Less than 1%) 934
NuLYTELY (Isolated cases) 699
Nuromax Injection 794
Omnipaque (0.3%) 2552
Optimine Tablets 2115
Oramorph SR (Morphine Sulfate Sustained Release Tablets) (Less frequent) 1988
Oretic Tablets 544
Oreticyl 545
Orinase Tablets (1.1%) 2354
Ornade Spansule Capsules 2221
Orudis Capsules (Less than 1%) 2488
Oxsoralen-Ultra Capsule 1117
PBZ Tablets & Elixir 1037
PBZ-SR Tablets 1037
PCE Dispertab Tablets 549
Pamelor 2019
Pantopon Injectable 1911
Panwarfin Tablets (Infrequent) 547
Paraflex Caplets 1378
ParaGard T380A Intrauterine Copper Contraceptive 411
Paraplatin for Injection 735
PediaProfen Suspension (Less than 1%) 1363
Pediazole 1973
PedvaxHIB (Two children) 1521
Pentaspan Injection 949
Pepcid (Infrequent) 1524
Periactin 1525
Pfizerpen for Injection 1957
Pfizerpen-AS Aqueous Suspension 1959
Phenergan with Codeine 2497
Phenergan Injection 2493
Phenergan Tablets 2496
Phenergan VC with Codeine 2501
Pitressin Synthetic, Ampoules 1758
Placidyl Capsules 553
Plague Vaccine (Rare) 1584
Plaquenil Sulfate Tablets 2067
Plendil Extended-Release Tablets (0.5% to 1.5%) 1526
Pneumovax 23 (Rare) 1528
Pnu-Imune 23 Pneumococcal Vaccine Polyvalent (Rare) 1233
Polaramine 2116
Polymyxin B Sulfate, Aerosporin Brand Sterile Powder (Occasional) 798
Pondimin Tablets 1867
Ponstel 1758
Pontocaine Hydrochloride for Spinal Anesthesia 2069
Prelu-2 Capsules 683
Pre-Pen 2148
Prilosec Delayed-Release Capsules (Less than 1%) 1530
Primaxin I.M. 1532
Primaxin I.V. (0.2%) 1535
Prinivil Tablets (1% or less) 1538
Prinzide Tablets 1540
Pro-Banthine Tablets 2141
Procan SR Tablets (Occasional) 1760

Procardia Capsules (2% or less) 1781
Procardia XL Tablets (1% or less).. 1783
Procrit for Injection (Rare)................ 1647
ProHIBiT Haemophilus b Conjugate Vaccine (Diphtheria Toxoid Conjugate) (Infrequent) 896
Prolixin Decanoate 1795
Prolixin Elixir 1793
Prolixin Enanthate 1796
Prolixin Injection............................. 1791
Prolixin Oral Concentrate.................. 1792
Prolixin Tablets................................. 1793
Pronestyl Capsules and Tablets (Occasional)................................ 1800
Pronestyl Injection (Occasional) 1798
Pronestyl-SR Tablets 1801
ProSom Tablets (Infrequent) 554
Prostigmin Injectable 1120
Prostigmin Tablets 1121
Protostat Tablets 1674
Proventil Inhalation Aerosol (Rare) 2117
Provera Tablets 2356
Prozac Pulvules (Infrequent) 920
Quarzan Capsules 1937
Questran Light 711
Questran Powder 710
Quinaglute Dura-Tabs Tablets 663
Quinidex Extentabs 1868
Rauzide Tablets 1804
Recombivax HB (Less than 1%)....... 1544
Reglan (A few cases) 1869
Renese Tablets 1785
Retrovir Capsules (Less than 5%).. 802
Retrovir I.V. Infusion (Less than 5%)... 805
Retrovir Syrup (Less than 5%) 802
Rheumatrex Methotrexate Dose Pack.. 1234
Ridaura Capsules (1 to 3%)............ 2224
Rifadin (Occasional) 1345
Rifamate Capsules (Occasional) 1347
Rimactane Capsules 879
Ritalin 880
Robaxin Injectable............................ 1871
Robaxin Tablets 1872
Robaxisal Tablets.............................. 1872
Robinul Forte Tablets........................ 1873
Robinul Injectable 1873
Robinul Tablets................................. 1873
Robitussin.. ▣ 676
Robitussin-CF .... ▣ 676
Robitussin-DM.................................. ▣ 676
Robitussin-PE .... ▣ 677
Roferon-A Injection (Less than 3%)... 1916
Roxanol 1991
Rubex (Occasional)............................ 739
Rufen Tablets (Less than 1%)......... 691
Ru-Tuss II Capsules 693
Ru-Tuss Tablets 693
Salflex... 839
Saluron.. 718
Salutensin/Salutensin-Demi 719
Seldane Tablets (1.6%) 1349
Seldane-D Extended-Release Tablets 1350
Sensorcaine (Rare) 631
Sensorcaine-MPF Spinal (Rare) 634
▲Septra (Most common) 813
▲Septra I.V. Infusion (Most common) 808
▲Septra I.V. Infusion ADD-Vantage Vials (Most common) 810
▲Septra (Most common) 813
Ser-Ap-Es Tablets 881
Serax Capsules 2522
Serax Tablets.................................... 2522
Serophene (clomiphene citrate tablets, USP) (Less than 1 in 100 patients) 2186
Serpasil-Apresoline Tablets.............. 884
Serpasil-Esidrix Tablets.................... 886
Solu-Medrol Sterile Powder.............. 2363
Soma Compound w/Codeine Tablets 2390
Soma Compound Tablets (Rare)...... 2389
Sotradecol (Sodium Tetradecyl Sulfate Injection) 964
Spectrobid Tablets & Powder for Oral Suspension............................ 1961
Stelazine 2226
Streptase for Infusion 635
Suprax (Less than 2%)..................... 1235
Surital Ampoules, Steri-Vials............ 1764
Surmontil Capsules........................... 2524
Sus-Phrine Injection 1006
Synarel Nasal Solution (Less than 1%)... 2300
Synkayvite Injection (Occasional).... 1919
Synkayvite Tablets (Occasional) 1920
TACE 12 and 25 mg 1353
T-Stat 2.0% Topical Solution and Pads 2409
Tacaryl 2409
Talacen (Rare) 2070
Talwin Carpuject 2071
Talwin Compound (Rare) 2072
Talwin Injection................................. 2071
Talwin Nx (Rare) 2073
Tambocor Tablets (Less than 1%) 1315
Tao Capsules (Infrequent) 1963
Tapazole Tablets 1298
Taractan (Infrequent) 1920
Tavist Syrup...................................... 2033
Tavist Tablets 2035
Tavist-D Tablets 2035
Tegison Capsules (Less than 1%) .. 1881
Tegretol Chewable Tablets 654
Tegretol Suspension......................... 656
Tegretol Tablets 654
Temaril Tablets, Syrup and Spansule Sustained Release Capsules 1085
Tenoretic Tablets.............................. 1105
Tenuate 1354
Terramycin Capsules 1786
Terramycin Intramuscular Solution 1964
Thalitone Tablets 687
Thiosulfil Forte Tablets 2526
Thorazine (Occasional) 2234
Ticar for Injection 2236
Timentin for Injection........................ 2239
Timolide Tablets................................ 1547
Timoptic in Ocudose 1552
Timoptic Sterile Ophthalmic Solution 1550
Tofranil Ampuls 1038
Tofranil Tablets 1039
Tofranil-PM Capsules........................ 1041
Tolectin (200, 400 and 600 mg) (Less than 1%).............................. 1379
Tolinase Tablets (0.4%).................... 2365
Tonocard Tablets (Less than 1%) .. 1554
Toradol IM Injection (1% or less).... 2302
Tracrium Injection 817
Trandate HCT Tablets (Rare)........... 579
Trandate Injection (Rare).................. 577
Trandate Tablets (Rare) 579
Trental (Less than 1%).................... 1099
Triaminic Expectorant DH 1995
Triaminic Oral Infant Drops.............. 1996
Triavil Tablets 1556
Tri-Immunol Diphtheria & Tetanus Toxoids & Pertussis Vaccine, Adsorbed.. 1241
Trilafon... 2123
Trilisate (Rare) 1822
Trinalin Repetabs Tablets 1170
Trobicin Sterile Powder.................... 2366
Ultracef Capsules, Tablets & Oral Suspension..................................... 722
Ultravate Ointment 0.05% (Less frequent) 2411
Unasyn 1965
Unipen 2533
Urispas Tablets................................. 2242
Valium Injectable 1937
Valpin 50 Tablets 941
Vancenase Nasal Inhaler (Rare) 2126
Vanceril Inhaler (Rare)..................... 2128
Vancocin HCl, Vials & ADD-Vantage (Infrequent) 1302
Vaseretic Tablets 1559
Vasotec I.V.. 1562
Vasotec Tablets 1564
Velosef Capsules and for Oral Suspension (Few)............................ 606
Velosulin 1627
Velosulin Human 1628
Ventolin (Rare) 583
Verelan Capsules (Less than 1%) .. 1243
Vibramycin Hyclate Capsules 1787
Vibramycin Hyclate Intravenous 1968
Vibramycin 1787
Vivactil Tablets 1567
Voltaren Tablets (Less than 1%) 1042
Wellbutrin Tablets 821
Wycillin Injection 2537
Xylocaine Injections (Extremely rare) 637
Xylocaine 2% Jelly (Extremely rare) 643
Xylocaine 5% Ointment 644
Xylocaine 10% Oral Spray (Extremely rare).............................. 645
4% Xylocaine-MPF Sterile Solution (Extremely rare).............................. 641
Yodoxin 1072
Zarontin Capsules 1768
Zarontin Syrup 1769
Zaroxolyn Tablets 989
Zefazone Sterile Powder.................. 2372
Zestoretic 2274
Zestril Tablets 2277
Zinacef (Less than 1 in 250 patients) 1066
Zovirax 824
Zyloprim Tablets (Less than 1%).... 830

Urticaria, hemorrhagic

Dolophine Hydrochloride Ampoules & Vials (Rare) 1260
Dolophine Hydrochloride Tablets (Rare) 1261
Methadone Hydrochloride Diskets (Rare) 1284
Methadone Hydrochloride Oral Solution & Tablets (Rare)............. 1987
Roxanol (Rare) 1991

Urticarial reaction, generalized

Benadryl Capsules............................ 1691
Celontin 1692
Chloromycetin Cream, 1% 1694
Chloromycetin Kapseals 1695
Chloromycetin Palmitate, Oral Suspension..................................... 1697
Chloromycetin Sodium Succinate..... 1698
ETS-2% 1685
Scleromate 1685
T-Stat 2.0% Topical Solution and Pads (One case)............................ 2409
Theramycin Z Topical Solution 2% (One case) 1410

Uterine contractions, altered

Astramorph/PF Injection, USP (Preservative-Free) 618
Proventil Repetabs Tablets 2120
Proventil Solutions for Inhalation 0.5% and 0.083%........................ 2118
Proventil Syrup................................. 2119
Proventil Tablets 2120
Talwin Injection................................. 2071

Uterine contractions, cessation of

Proglycem... 649

Uterine contractions, production of

Cytotec... 2159

Uterine contractions, prolonged

Syntocinon Nasal Spray 2033
Wigraine Tablets & Suppositories .. 1645

Uterine fibromyomata, increase in size

Demulen 2161
Diethylstilbestrol Tablets 1258
Enovid.. 2161
Estinyl Tablets.................................. 2085
Estrace... 1385
Estrace Vaginal Cream 1388
Estraderm Transdermal System 866
Estratest 2245
Estrovis 1721
Loestrin 1728
Mediatric Capsules 2476
Menrium Tablets 1934
Norethin.. 2133
Norlestrin 1746
Ogen 540
Ortho Dienestrol Cream 1664
Ortho-Novum 7/7/7 □28 Tablets 1667
Ovcon 1391
PMB 200 and PMB 400 2504
Premarin Intravenous 2508
Premarin with Methyltestosterone .. 2515
Premarin Tablets 2510
Premarin Vaginal Cream.................. 2512
TACE 12 and 25 mg 1353

Uterine hypertonus

Oxytocin Injection 2492
Pitocin Injection, Ampoules, Steri-Dose Syringes.................... 1757
Syntocinon Injection 2032
Vasoxyl Injection 819

Uterine rupture

Oxytocin Injection 2492
Pitocin Injection, Ampoules, Steri-Dose Syringes.................... 1757
Syntocinon Injection 2032

Uterine spasm

Oxytocin Injection 2492
Prozac Pulvules (Rare) 920
Syntocinon Injection 2032

Uterotonic effect

Bellergal-S Tablets 1998
Cafergot/Cafergot P-B 1999
D.H.E. 45 Injection 2003
Syntocinon Nasal Spray 2033

Uveitis

AK-Cide Sterile Ophthalmic Ointment & Suspension .... ◉ 202
Cholybar 1705
Diupres Tablets 1461
Enduronyl 518
Floropryl Sterile Ophthalmic Ointment 1473
Harmonyl Tablets 528
Humorsol Sterile Ophthalmic Solution 1475
Hydropres Tablets............................. 1485
Metimyd.. ◉ 306
Oreticyl... 545
Phospholine Iodide .... ◉ 315
Questran Light 711
Questran Powder 710
Raudixin Tablets............................... 1803
Rauzide Tablets 1804
Renese-R Tablets 1786
Salutensin/Salutensin-Demi 719
Ser-Ap-Es Tablets 881
Serpasil Tablets 883
Serpasil-Apresoline Tablets.............. 884
Serpasil-Esidrix Tablets.................... 886
Vasocidin Ointment .... ◉ 275
Vasocidin Ophthalmic Solution .... ◉ 276
Zolyse .... ◉ 236

V

Vagina, dryness

Danocrine Capsules 2046
Flagyl I.V.. 2131
Flagyl Tablets 2170
Protostat Tablets 1674
▲Synarel Nasal Solution (19% of patients) 2300
Vagistat (Less than 1%).................. 1397

Vaginal adenosis

Estrace... 1385
Estrace Vaginal Cream 1388
Estrovis 1721
Premarin with Methyltestosterone .. 2515
Premarin Tablets 2510
TACE 12 and 25 mg 1353

Vaginal burning

Conceptrol (Occasional).................... ▣ 631
Delfen Contraceptive Foam (Occasional).................................. ▣ 631
Femstat Prefill Vaginal Cream 2% (2.3%).. 2295
Femstat Vaginal Cream 2% (2.3%).. 2295
Gynol II Extra Strength Contraceptive Jelly (Occasional).................................. ▣ 632
Gynol II Original Formula Contraceptive Jelly (Occasional).................................. ▣ 632
Monistat Dual-Pak (2%)................... 1657
Monistat 3 Vaginal Suppositories (2%) 1657
Mycelex-G 1% Vaginal Cream (0.5%) 1605
Mycelex-G 500 mg Vaginal Tablets (1 in 149 patients)........................ 1606
Ortho-Gynol Contraceptive Jelly (Occasional).................................. ▣ 632
▲Terazol 3 Vaginal Cream (5%) 1676
▲Terazol 3 Vaginal Suppositories (15.2% of 284 patients)............... 1677
▲Terazol 7 Vaginal Cream (5.2% of 521 patients) 1677
Today Vaginal Contraceptive Sponge 2422
▲Vagistat (Approximately 6%)........... 1397

Vaginal candidiasis

Azactam for Injection (Less than 1%)... 2252
Brevicon.. 2304
Cipro Tablets.................................... 1589
Clozaril Tablets (Less than 1%) 2000
Demulen 2161
Diethylstilbestrol Tablets 1258
Enovid... 2161
Estinyl Tablets.................................. 2085
Estrace 1385
Estrace Vaginal Cream 1388
Estratest 2245
Estrovis 1721
Floxin Tablets (More than or equal to 1.0%) 1652
Jenest-28 Tablets 1636
Levlen/Tri-Levlen............................. 665

Lo/Ovral Tablets 2471
Lo/Ovral-28 Tablets 2476
Loestrin 1728
Mediatric Capsules 2476
Menrium Tablets 1934
Micronor Tablets 1667
Modicon 1667
Nordette-21 Tablets 2481
Nordette-28 Tablets 2483
Norethin 2133
Norinyl 2304
Norlestrin 1746
Nor-Q D Tablets 2304
Ogen 540
Ortho Dienestrol Cream 1664
Ortho-Cyclen Tablets 1658
Ortho-Novum 1667
Ovral Tablets 2490
Ovral-28 Tablets 2491
Ovrette Tablets 2492
PMB 200 and PMB 400 2504
Premarin with Methyltestosterone 2515
Premarin Tablets 2510
Premarin Vaginal Cream 2512
Protostat Tablets 1674
TACE 12 and 25 mg 1353
Tazidime Vials, Faspak & ADD-Vantage (Less than 1%) 1299
Levlen/Tri-Levlen 665
Tri-Norinyl 2304
Triphasil-21 Tablets 2527
Triphasil-28 Tablets 2532
Velosef Capsules and for Oral Suspension 606
Zinacef 1066

Vaginal discharge
Floxin Tablets (1% to 3%) 1652
Keflex Pulvules, Oral Suspension & Pediatric Drops 916
Keftab Tablets 917
Methotrexate Tablets, Parenteral, LPF Parenteral (Less common) 1217
Nolvadex Tablets (Less frequent) 1102
ProSom Tablets (Infrequent) 554
Rheumatrex Methotrexate Dose Pack (Less common) 1234
Rogaine Topical Solution (0.91%) 2357
Vagistat (Less than 1%) 1397

Vaginitis
Anafranil Capsules (Up to 2%) 650
Ancef Injection 2194
Ansaid Tablets (Less than 1%) 2319
Augmentin Tablets, Powder for Oral Suspension, and Chewable Tablets (1%) 2198
Azactam for Injection (Less than 1%) 2252
Brevicon 2304
Ceclor Pulvules & Suspension (Less than 1 in 100) 1251
Cefizox Injection (Rare) 1012
Ceftin Tablets (1.9%) 575
Ceptaz for Injection (Fewer than 1%) 1057
Cipro I.V. (1% or less) 1592
Cipro Tablets (Less than 1%) 1589
Claforan Sterile Injection (Less than 1%) 1089
Danocrine Capsules 2046
Demulen 2161
Duricef 1405
Enovid 2161
Floxin Tablets (1% to 3%) 1652
Fortaz (Less than 1%) 1060
Geocillin Tablets 1951
Jenest-28 Tablets 1636
Keflex Pulvules, Oral Suspension & Pediatric Drops 916
Keftab Tablets 917
Kefzol Vials, Faspak & ADD-Vantage 1279
Levlen/Tri-Levlen 665
Lincocin 2344
Lippes Loop Intrauterine Double-S 1654
Lo/Ovral Tablets 2471
Lo/Ovral-28 Tablets 2476
Loestrin 1728
Micronor Tablets 1667
Modicon 1667
Nordette-21 Tablets 2481
Nordette-28 Tablets 2483
Norethin 2133
Norinyl 2304
Norlestrin 1746
Norplant System 2484
Nor-Q D Tablets 2304
Ortho-Cyclen Tablets 1658
Ortho-Novum 1667
Ovcon 1391
Ovral Tablets 2490
Ovral-28 Tablets 2491
Ovrette Tablets 2492
ParaGard T380A Intrauterine Copper Contraceptive 411
Permax Tablets (Infrequent) 1291
Prozac Pulvules (Infrequent) 920
Rocephin Injectable Vials, ADD-Vantage (Occasional) 1914
Rogaine Topical Solution (0.91%) 2357
Solganal Suspension 2122
Suprax (Less than 2%) 1235
Tazicef for Injection (Less than 1%) 2231
Tazidime Vials, Faspak & ADD-Vantage (Less than 1%) 1299
Tegison Capsules (Less than 1%) 1881
Levlen/Tri-Levlen 665
Tri-Norinyl 2304
Triphasil-21 Tablets 2527
Triphasil-28 Tablets 2532
Ultracef Capsules, Tablets & Oral Suspension 722
Urobiotic-250 Capsules (Rare) 1968
Wellbutrin Tablets (Infrequent) 821
Zefazone Sterile Powder 2372
Zinacef 1066

Varices, esophageal
Myleran Tablets 790
Thioguanine Tablets, Tabloid Brand 815

Vascular access, clotting
▲Epogen for Injection (0.25 to 7%) 591
▲Procrit for Injection (0.25 to 7%) 1647

Vascular collapse
Brevital Sodium Vials 1248
Cardioquin Tablets 1812
Quinaglute Dura-Tabs Tablets 663
Quinidex Extentabs 1868

Vascular insufficiency, lower extremities
Sansert Tablets 2031

Vascular stenosis
Surgicel 1151

Vasculitis
Accutane Capsules (A few isolated reports) 1878
Aldoclor Tablets 1413
Aldomet Ester HCl Injection 1417
Aldomet Oral 1415
Aldoril Tablets 1418
Alkeran Tablets 754
Anaprox and Anaprox DS Tablets (Rare) 2288
Asendin Tablets (Rare) 1196
Atgam Sterile Solution (Less than 5%) 2320
Azo Gantrisin Tablets 1888
Azulfidine Tablets, EN-tabs, Oral Suspension 1157
Butazolidin Capsules & Tablets (Less than 1%) 1027
Calan SR Caplets (1% or less) 2157
Calan Tablets (1% or less) 2155
Capoten 2255
Capozide 2258
Cipro I.V. (1% or less) 1592
Cipro Tablets 1589
ColBENEMID Tablets 1436
Combipres Tablets 678
Cordarone Tablets (Rare) 2446
Corzide Tablets 702
Depen Titratable Tablets (Rare) 2379
Diucardin Tablets 2450
Diupres Tablets 1461
Diuril Oral Suspension 1464
Diuril Sodium Intravenous 1463
Diuril Tablets 1464
Dyazide Capsules 2208
Enduron Tablets 517
Exna Tablets 1862
Feldene Capsules (Less than 1%) 1777
Floxin Tablets (Less than 1%) 1652
HydroDIURIL Tablets 1484
Hydromox R Tablets 1209
Hydromox Tablets 1208
Hydropres Tablets 1485
INH Tablets 868
Inderide Tablets 2463
Inderide LA Long Acting Capsules 2465
Inocor Lactate Injection (1 case) 2048
Intal Inhaler (Rare) 979
Isoptin Oral Tablets (Less than 1%) 1179
Isoptin SR Sustained Release Tablets (Less than 1%) 1181
Lasix 1093
Lopid Capsules and Tablets 1736
Lozol Tablets (Less than 5%) 1843
Maxzide 1215
Mevacor Tablets 1505
Micronase Tablets 2350
Minizide Capsules 1779
Moduretic Tablets 1510
Monopril Tablets (0.2 to 1.0%) 1406
Motrin Tablets (Less than 1%) 2351
Mumpsvax (Rare) 1513
Naprosyn (Rare) 2297
Naturetin Tablets (Occasional) 1789
NebuPent for Inhalation Solution (1% or less) 1017
Normodyne Tablets 2110
Normozide Tablets 2112
Permax Tablets (Rare) 1291
Prinivil Tablets (1% or less) 1538
Prinzide Tablets 1540
Quinidex Extentabs 1868
Rauzide Tablets 1804
Renese Tablets 1785
Rifamate Capsules 1347
Ritalin 880
Saluron 718
Salutensin/Salutensin-Demi 719
Streptase for Infusion 635
Tenoretic Tablets 1105
Thalitone Tablets 687
Timolide Tablets 1547
Tonocard Tablets (Less than 1%) 1554
Trandate HCT Tablets 579
Vancocin HCl, Oral Solution & Pulvules (Rare) 1304
Vancocin HCl, Vials & ADD-Vantage (Rare) 1302
Vaseretic Tablets 1559
Vasotec I.V. 1562
Vasotec Tablets (0.5% to 1.0%) 1564
Verelan Capsules (Less than 1%) 1243
Zestoretic 2274
Zestril Tablets (Less than 1%) 2277
Zyloprim Tablets (Less than 1%) 830

Vasculitis, cutaneous
Capozide 2258
Cardilate Oral/Sublingual Tablets 757
Combipres Tablets 678
Corzide Tablets 702
Diucardin Tablets 2450
Diulo 2129
Diupres Tablets 1461
Diuril Oral Suspension 1464
Diuril Sodium Intravenous 1463
Diuril Tablets 1464
Enduron Tablets 517
Exna Tablets 1862
HydroDIURIL Tablets 1484
Hydromox R Tablets 1209
Hydromox Tablets 1208
Hydropres Tablets 1485
Inderide Tablets 2463
Inderide LA Long Acting Capsules 2465
Isordil 2467
Lasix 1093
Lodine Capsules (Rare) 2468
Maxzide 1215
Minizide Capsules 1779
Moduretic Tablets 1510
Mykrox ½ mg Tablets 984
Naturetin Tablets (Occasional) 1789
Normodyne Tablets 2110
Normozide Tablets 2112
Prinzide Tablets 1540
Rauzide Tablets 1804
Renese Tablets 1785
Saluron 718
Salutensin/Salutensin-Demi 719
Tenoretic Tablets 1105
Thalitone Tablets 687
Timolide Tablets 1547
Trandate HCT Tablets 579
Vaseretic Tablets 1559
Zaroxolyn Tablets 989
Zestoretic 2274

Vasculitis, leukocytoclastic
Cardizem Tablets-30 mg, 60 mg, 90 mg and 120 mg 1329

Vasculitis, periarteritic
Intal Capsules (Less than 1 in 100,000 patients) 978
Intal Nebulizer Solution (Rare) 980

Vasculitis, renal
Cuprimine Capsules (Rare) 1442
Depen Titratable Tablets 2379

Vasoconstriction
Cocaine Hydrochloride Topical Solution 620

Vasodilation
Ansaid Tablets (Less than 1%) 2319
Cartrol Tablets (Less common) 507
Cyclogyl ⊙ 215
Cyclomydril ⊙ 216
DDAVP 1841
Desyrel and Desyrel Dividose 1404
Dilatrate-SR 1827
Ditropan 1332
Ethmozine Tablets (Less than 2%) 946
Flexeril Tablets (Less than 1%) 1471
Floxin Tablets (Less than 1%) 1652
Hyperstat I.V. Injection 2095
Hytrin Tablets (At least 1%) 529
Marcaine Spinal 2058
NebuPent for Inhalation Solution (1% or less) 1017
Nitro-Bid Ointment 1339
Novocain Hydrochloride for Spinal Anesthesia 2065
Omnipaque 2552
Orudis Capsules (Less than 1%) 2488
▲Permax Tablets (3.2%) 1291
Retrovir Capsules (Less than 5%) 802
Retrovir I.V. Infusion (Less than 5%) 805
Retrovir Syrup (Less than 5%) 802
Sorbitrate 1103
Timolide Tablets 1547
Timoptic in Ocudose 1552
Timoptic Sterile Ophthalmic Solution 1550
Toradol IM Injection (1% or less) 2302
Tracrium Injection (Rare) 817
Vascor (200, 300 and 400 mg) Tablets (0.5 to 2.0%) 1383
Zyloprim Tablets (Less than 1%) 830

Vasodilation, peripheral
Persantine Tablets 683

Vasomotor disturbances
Aminohippurate Sodium Injection 1421
Duvoid Tablets 1853
▲Intropin Injection (Among most frequent) 930
Xanax Tablets (2.0%) 2367

Vasomotor flushes
▲Serophene (clomiphene citrate tablets, USP) (Approximately 1 in 10 patients) 2186

Vasospasm, digital
▲Parlodel (3%) 2020

Vasospasm, rebound
Nimotop Capsules (Less than 1%) 1607

Vasospasm, unspecified
Anafranil Capsules (Rare) 650

Vasovagal episode
Alferon N Injection (Up to 2%) 1809
IOPIDINE ⊙ 232
Omnipaque (Less than 0.4%) 2552
Parlodel (Less than 1%) 2020
Tonocard Tablets (Less than 1%) 1554
Versed Injection (Less than 1%) 1924

Vein cramp
Omnipaque 2552

Vein, pigmentation of
Fluorouracil Injection 1897

Veins, varicosis
Permax Tablets (Infrequent) 1291

Venous infection at injection site
Primaxin I.V. (0.1%) 1535

Venous streaking
Nipride I.V. Infusion 1909

Venous thrombophlebitis
Metrodin (urofollitropin for injection) 2182

Ventilator dependence
Virazole 1126

Ventricular arrhythmias
Adalat Capsules (10 mg and 20 mg) (Fewer than 0.5%) 1587
Aminophyllin Tablets 2153
Asbron G 1997

Carbocaine Hydrochloride Injection 2043
Choledyl Pediatric Elixir 1702
Choledyl Tablets 1700
Choledyl SA Tablets 1704
Constant-T Tablets 1029
Diethylstilbestrol Tablets 1258
EpiPen—Epinephrine Auto-Injector 843
Hyperstat I.V. Injection 2095
Ilosone (Rare) 913
Ilotycin Gluceptate, IV, Vials (Rare) 915
▲ Intron A (5% or less) 2097
Isuprel Hydrochloride Injection 1:5000 2050
Lanoxicaps 772
Lanoxin Elixir Pediatric 775
Lanoxin Injection 778
Lanoxin Injection Pediatric (Less common) 781
Lanoxin Tablets (Less common) 783
Lufyllin-GG Elixir & Tablets 2385
Marcaine Hydrochloride with Epinephrine 1:200,000 2055
Marcaine Hydrochloride Injection 2055
Marcaine Spinal 2058
Mexitil Capsules (1.0% to 1.9%) 680
Nescaine/Nescaine MPF 629
Normodyne Injection (1%) 2108
Procardia Capsules (Less than 0.5%) 1781
Prozac Pulvules (Rare) 920
Quadrinal Tablets 1183
Quibron Capsules 713
Quibron-T 714
Quibron-T/SR 716
Respbid Tablets 684
Sensorcaine 631
Sensorcaine-MPF Spinal 634
Slo-bid Gyrocaps 1847
Streptase for Infusion 635
T-PHYL (Uniphyl) 200 mg Tablets 1820
▲ Tambocor Tablets (7%) 1315
Theo-24 2179
Theo-Dur Sprinkle 1168
Theo-Dur Extended-Release Tablets 1166
Theolair 1317
Theolair-SR Tablets 1319
▲ TheoX Extended-Release Tablets (Among most consistent) 841
▲ Tonocard Tablets (10.9%) 1554
Trandate Injection (1 of 100 patients) 577
Uniphyl 400 mg Tablets 1823

Ventricular block

Omnipaque 2552

Ventricular contractions

Sodium Polystyrene Sulfonate Suspension 1993
Versed Injection (Less than 1%) 1924

Ventricular contractions, premature

Brethaire Inhaler 1024
Clozaril Tablets (Less than 1%) 2000
Diupres Tablets 1461
▲ Dobutrex Solution Vials (5%) 1259
Emete-con Intramuscular/Intravenous 1950
Hydropres Tablets 1485
Lanoxicaps (Common) 772
Lanoxin Elixir Pediatric (Common) 775
▲ Lanoxin Injection (Most common) 778
Lanoxin Injection Pediatric (Common) 781
Lanoxin Tablets (Common) 783
Lozol Tablets (Less than 5%) 1843
Norpramin Tablets 1340
Oxytocin Injection 2492
Pitocin Injection, Ampoules, Steri-Dose Syringes 1757
Salutensin/Salutensin-Demi 719
Syntocinon Injection 2032
▲ Tonocard Tablets (10.9%) 1554
Tornalate (Rare) 2074
Vascor (200, 300 and 400 mg) Tablets (0.5 to 2.0%) 1383
Voltaren Tablets (Less than 1%) 1042
Zantac Injection and Zantac Injection Premixed (Rare) 1063
Zantac (Rare) 1065

Ventricular contractions, premature, multifocal

Lanoxicaps 772
Lanoxin Elixir Pediatric 775
Lanoxin Injection 778
Lanoxin Injection Pediatric 781
Lanoxin Tablets 783

Ventricular contractions, premature, unifocal

Lanoxicaps 772
Lanoxin Elixir Pediatric 775
Lanoxin Injection 778
Lanoxin Injection Pediatric 781
Lanoxin Tablets 783

Ventricular dilation, left-side

Retrovir (0.8%) 802

Ventricular ectopic beats

Cardioquin Tablets 1812
Cipro Tablets 1589
Desyrel and Desyrel Dividose 1404
Digibind 762
Dobutrex Solution Vials 1259
Quinaglute Dura-Tabs Tablets 663
Vasoxyl Injection 819

Ventricular extrasystoles

Cardene Capsules (Rare) 2290
Cardizem Tablets-30 mg, 60 mg, 90 mg and 120 mg (Less than 1%) 1329
Cardizem SR Capsules-60 mg, 90 mg and 120 mg (Less than 1%) 1327
Permax Tablets (Infrequent) 1291

Ventricular failure

Doxorubicin Hydrochloride for Injection, USP 622
Doxorubicin Hydrochloride Injection, USP (Uncommon) 848
Rubex (Uncommon) 739
Tonocard Tablets (0.0-1.4%) 1554

Ventricular fibrillation (see under Fibrillations, ventricular)

Ventricular flutter

Quinidex Extentabs 1868

Ventricular gallop

Retrovir (0.8%) 802

Ventricular irregularities

Adriamycin RDF (Uncommon) 562
▲ Calan SR Caplets (15%) 2157
▲ Calan Tablets (15%) 2155
Eminase 2211
Isoptin Injectable 1177
Isoptin Oral Tablets (Greater than 1%) 1179
Isoptin SR Sustained Release Tablets (Greater than 1%) 1181
Verelan Capsules (Less than 1%) 1243

Ventricular irritation

Vaseretic Tablets 1559

Ventricular response, rapid

Calan SR Caplets 2157
Calan Tablets 2155
Verelan Capsules 1243

Venus sequelae

Diprivan Injection (Less than 1%) 2267

Vertebral compression fractures

Cortone Acetate Sterile Suspension 1437
Cortone Acetate Tablets 1439
Decadron Elixir 1445
Decadron Phosphate Injection 1449
Decadron Phosphate Respihaler 1454
Decadron Phosphate Turbinaire 1456
Decadron Phosphate with Xylocaine Injection, Sterile 1451
Deltasone Tablets 2332
Depo-Medrol Sterile Aqueous Suspension 2334
Kenalog-40 Injection 2403
Medrol 2348
Pediapred Oral Liquid 987
Solu-Cortef Sterile Powder 2361
Solu-Medrol Sterile Powder 2363

Vertical deviation

▲ Oculinum for Injecton (16.9%) 587

Vertigo

Actifed with Codeine Cough Syrup 752
AeroBid Inhaler System (1-3%) 995
Aldactazide 2150
Aldoclor Tablets 1413
Aldoril Tablets 1418
Altace Capsules (Less than 1%) 1086
Anafranil Capsules (Frequent) 650
Anaprox and Anaprox DS Tablets (Less than 3%) 2288
Ancobon Capsules 1886
Apresazide Capsules 854
Apresoline-Esidrix Tablets 857
Aristocort Suspension 1008
Aristospan Suspension 1011
Atabrine Hydrochloride Tablets (Infrequent) 2041
Azactam for Injection (Less than 1%) 2252
Azo Gantanol Tablets 1887
Azo Gantrisin Tablets 1888
Azulfidine Tablets, EN-tabs, Oral Suspension (Rare) 1157
Bactrim DS Tablets 1891
Bactrim I.V. Infusion 1889
Bactrim 1891
Benadryl Capsules 1691
Benadryl Injection 1692
Betoptic Sterile Ophthalmic Solution (Rare) 569
Betoptic S Sterile Ophthalmic Suspension (Rare) 570
Blocadren Tablets (0.6%) 1429
Brethaire Inhaler 1024
Bretylol Injection (7 in 1000) 923
Bumex (0.1%) 1895
Capastat Sulfate Vials 1250
Capozide 2258
Carafate Tablets (Less than 0.5%) 1326
Cardene Capsules (Rare) 2290
Cardioquin Tablets 1812
▲ Cardura Tablets (2% to 23%) 1941
Celestone Soluspan Suspension 2081
Cholybar 1705
Cibalith-S 870
Clinoril Tablets (Less than 1 in 100) 1433
▲ Clozaril Tablets (More than 5 to 19%) 2000
Colestid Granules (Fewer than 1 in 1,000) 2328
Coly-Mycin M Parenteral 1706
Combipres Tablets 678
Cortenema 2244
Cortone Acetate Sterile Suspension 1437
Cortone Acetate Tablets 1439
Corzide Tablets 702
Dalalone D.P. Injectable 999
Dalgan Injection (1 to less than 3%) 620
Dapsone USP 1130
Decadron Elixir 1445
Decadron Phosphate Injection 1449
Decadron Phosphate Respihaler 1454
Decadron Phosphate Turbinaire 1456
Decadron Phosphate with Xylocaine Injection, Sterile 1451
Decadron Tablets 1447
Decadron-LA Sterile Suspension 1457
Deconamine 663
Deltasone Tablets 2332
Depo-Medrol Sterile Aqueous Suspension 2334
Deprol Tablets 2382
Desyrel and Desyrel Dividose 1404
Dilantin with Phenobarbital Kapseals 1715
Dipentum Capsules (1.0%) 1160
Disalcid 1310
Diucardin Tablets 2450
Diulo 2129
Diupres Tablets 1461
Diuril Oral Suspension 1464
Diuril Sodium Intravenous 1463
Diuril Tablets 1464
Dolobid Tablets (Less than 1 in 100) 1465
Duragesic Transdermal System (Less than 1%) 1133
Dyazide Capsules 2208
E.E.S. (Isolated reports) 522
Easprin 1719
Edecrin 1468
Eldepryl 2250
▲ Eminase (Less than 10%) 2211
Enduron Tablets 517
Enduronyl 518
Engerix-B Unit-Dose Vials 2213
Equagesic Tablets 2451
EryPed (Isolated reports) 519
Ery-Tab Tablets (Isolated reports) 521
Erythrocin Stearate Filmtab (Isolated reports) 523
Erythromycin Base Filmtab (Isolated reports) 525
Erythromycin Delayed-Release Capsules, USP (Isolated reports) 526
Esidrix Tablets 863
Esimil Tablets 864
Eskalith 2214
Ethmozine Tablets (Less than 2%) 946
Fansidar Tablets 1896
Feldene Capsules (1 to 3%) 1777
Fiorinal with Codeine Capsules 2008
Flagyl I.V. 2131
Flagyl Tablets 2170
Flexeril Tablets (Less than 1%) 1471
Floxin Tablets (Less than 1%) 1652
Fungizone Intravenous 2262
Gantanol 1899
Gantrisin Ophthalmic Ointment/Solution 1900
Gantrisin 1901
Garamycin Injectable 2093
Haldol Injection, Tablets and Concentrate 1373
Hexalen Capsules 2316
Hydeltrasol Injection, Sterile 1476
Hydeltra-T.B.A. Sterile Suspension 1478
Hydrocortone Acetate Sterile Suspension 1479
Hydrocortone Phosphate Injection, Sterile 1481
Hydrocortone Tablets 1482
HydroDIURIL Tablets 1484
Hydromox R Tablets 1209
Hydromox Tablets 1208
Hydropres Tablets 1485
Inderide Tablets 2463
Inderide LA Long Acting Capsules 2465
Indocin (Greater than 1%) 1487
Intal Capsules (Less than 1 in 100,000 patients) 978
Intal Inhaler (Rare) 979
Intal Nebulizer Solution (Rare) 980
Intron A (Up to 1%) 2097
ISMOTIC (Very rare) ⊙ 233
Isoptin Injectable (Few) 1177
Kenalog-10 Injection 2402
Kenalog-40 Injection 2403
Klonopin Tablets 1902
Lariam Tablets 1904
Lasix 1093
Lincocin (Occasional) 2344
Lithane Tablets 1596
Lithium Carbonate Capsules & Tablets 1984
Lithobid Tablets 870
Lopid Capsules and Tablets (1.5%) 1736
Lopressor Ampuls 1032
▲ Lopressor HCT Tablets (10 in 100 patients) 1034
Lopressor Tablets 1032
Lozol Tablets (Less than 5%) 1843
▲ Lysodren (15%) 731
Macrodantin Capsules (Less frequent) 1624
Marax Tablets & DF Syrup 1954
▲ Marplan Tablets (Among most frequent) 1906
Maxzide 1215
Medrol 2348
Midamor Tablets (Less than or equal to 1%) 1508
Miltown Tablets 2386
Minipress Capsules (1-4%) 1778
Minizide Capsules 1779
Minocin Intravenous 1221
Minocin Oral Suspension 1224
Minocin Pellet-Filled Capsules 1222
Moduretic Tablets (Less than or equal to 1%) 1510
Mono-Gesic Tablets 846
Mustargen (Infrequent) 1514
▲ Mysoline (Among most frequent) 2480
Naprosyn (Less than 3%) 2297
Naturetin Tablets (Occasional) 1789
Nebcin Vials, Hyporets & ADD-Vantage 1286
NebuPent for Inhalation Solution (1% or less) 1017
NegGram 2062
Neptazane Tablets ⊙ 311
Netromycin Injection 100 mg/ml 2104
Nitrostat Tablets (Occasional) 1743
Norisodrine Aerotrol 540
Normodyne Injection (1%) 2108
Normodyne Tablets (2%) 2110
Normozide Tablets (2%) 2112
▲ Nubain Injection (5%) 934
Omnipaque (Less than 0.1%) 2552
Optimine Tablets 2115
Oretic Tablets 544
Oreticyl 545
Ornade Spansule Capsules 2221
Orudis Capsules (Less than 1%) 2488
PBZ Tablets & Elixir 1037
PBZ-SR Tablets 1037

PCE Dispertab Tablets (Isolated reports) ... 549
PMB 200 and PMB 400 ... 2504
Papaverine Hydrochloride Vials and Ampoules ... 1290
Paradione Capsules ... 548
Parlodel (Less than 1%) ... 2020
Pavabid Capsules (Rare) ... 1344
Pavabid HP Capsulets (Rare) ... 1344
Pediapred Oral Liquid ... 987
Pediazole ... 1973
Periactin ... 1525
Permax Tablets (Infrequent) ... 1291
Phenobarbital Elixir and Tablets ... 1293
Pitressin Synthetic, Ampoules ... 1758
Plaquenil Sulfate Tablets ... 2067
Polaramine ... 2116
Prilosec Delayed-Release Capsules (Less than 1%) ... 1530
Primaxin I.M. ... 1532
Primaxin I.V. (Less than 0.2%) ... 1535
Prinivil Tablets (0.1%) ... 1538
Prinzide Tablets (0.3% to 1%) ... 1540
Procardia XL Tablets (1% or less) ... 1783
Protostat Tablets ... 1674
Proventil Inhalation Aerosol ... 2117
Proventil Repetabs Tablets ... 2120
Proventil Syrup ... 2119
Proventil Tablets ... 2120
Prozac Pulvules (Infrequent) ... 920
Questran Light ... 711
Questran Powder ... 710
Quinaglute Dura-Tabs Tablets ... 663
Quinamm Tablets ... 1344
Quinidex Extentabs ... 1868
Rauzide Tablets ... 1804
Renese Tablets ... 1785
Renese-R Tablets ... 1786
Retrovir Capsules (Less than 5%) ... 802
Retrovir I.V. Infusion (Less than 5%) ... 805
Retrovir Syrup (Less than 5%) ... 802
Robaxin Injectable ... 1871
Roferon-A Injection (Less than 3%) ... 1916
Rogaine Topical Solution (1.17%) ... 2357
Ru-Tuss II Capsules ... 693
Rythmol Tablets (Less than 1%) ... 1184
Salflex ... 839
Saluron ... 718
Salutensin/Salutensin-Demi ... 719
Sandostatin Injection (Less than 1%) ... 2029
Septra ... 813
Septra I.V. Infusion ... 808
Septra I.V. Infusion ADD-Vantage Vials ... 810
Septra ... 813
Ser-Ap-Es Tablets ... 881
Serax Capsules (In few instances) ... 2522
Serax Tablets (In few instances) ... 2522
Seromycin Pulvules ... 1298
Serpasil-Esidrix Tablets ... 886
Solu-Cortef Sterile Powder ... 2361
Solu-Medrol Sterile Powder ... 2363
Soma Compound w/Codeine Tablets ... 2390
Soma Compound Tablets ... 2389
Soma Tablets ... 2388
▲Stadol (3%) ... 721
Tambocor Tablets (1-3%) ... 1315
Tapazole Tablets ... 1298
Tavist Syrup ... 2033
Tavist Tablets ... 2035
Tavist-D Tablets ... 2035
Tenex Tablets ... 1875
Tenoretic Tablets (2%) ... 1105
Tenormin Tablets and I.V. Injection (2%) ... 1107
Thalitone Tablets ... 687
Thiosulfil Forte Tablets ... 2526
Timolide Tablets ... 1547
Timoptic in Ocudose ... 1552
Timoptic Sterile Ophthalmic Solution ... 1550
Tolinase Tablets (Infrequent) ... 2365
▲Tonocard Tablets (8.0-25.3%) ... 1554
Toradol IM Injection (1% or less) ... 2302
Trandate HCT Tablets ... 579
Trandate Injection (1 of 100 patients) ... 577
Trandate Tablets (2% of 227 patients) ... 579
Triaminic Expectorant DH ... 1995
Triaminic Oral Infant Drops ... 1996
Tridione ... 557
Trinalin Repetabs Tablets ... 1170
Urispas Tablets ... 2242
Valium Injectable ... 1937
Valium Tablets (Infrequent) ... 1939
Valrelease Capsules (Occasional) ... 1923
Vancocin HCl, Oral Solution & Pulvules (Rare) ... 1304
Vancocin HCl, Vials & ADD-Vantage (Rare) ... 1302
Vascor (200, 300 and 400 mg) Tablets (0.5 to 2.0%) ... 1383
Vaseretic Tablets (0.5% to 2.0%) ... 1559
Vasotec I.V. ... 1562
Ventolin ... 583
Wellbutrin Tablets (Infrequent) ... 821
Yodoxin ... 1072
Zantac Injection and Zantac Injection Premixed ... 1063
Zantac (Rare) ... 1065
Zaroxolyn Tablets ... 989
Zestoretic (0.3 to 1%) ... 2274
Zestril Tablets (0.1%) ... 2277
Zyloprim Tablets (Less than 1%) ... 830

Vesical spasm

Dilaudid Cough Syrup ... 1174
Dilaudid ... 1173
Hycomine Compound Tablets ... 929
Hycomine Syrup ... 927
Hycotuss Expectorant Syrup ... 930
Hydrocet Capsules ... 835
Vicodin Tablets ... 1187
Zydone Capsules ... 941

Vesiculation

Aplisol (tuberculin PPD, diluted) ... 2550
Aplitest (tuberculin PPD, multiple-puncture device) ... 2551
Attenuvax ... 1424
▲Blenoxane (50%) ... 724
▲Catapres-TTS (7 of 101 patients) ... 677
Cipro I.V. (1% or less) ... 1592
Condylox (Less than 5%) ... 1630
Doxorubicin Hydrochloride for Injection, USP ... 622
Halotex Cream & Solution (1 in 819 patients) ... 2400
M-M-R II ... 1494
M-R-VAX II ... 1496
Oxsoralen-Ultra Capsule ... 1117
PPD Tine Test ... 2548
Tuberculin, Old, Tine Test ... 2549
Ultravate Cream 0.05% (Less frequent) ... 2410
Velban Vials ... 1305

Vesiculo bullous reaction

Children's Advil Suspension (Less than 1%) ... 2426
Feldene Capsules (Less than 1%) ... 1777
Motrin Tablets (Less than 1%) ... 2351
PediaProfen Suspension (Less than 1%) ... 1363
Rufen Tablets (Less than 1%) ... 691

Vestibular dysfunction

Anafranil Capsules (Up to 2%) ... 650

Virilization

Android ... 1111
▲Estratest (Among most common) ... 2245
Halotestin Tablets ... 2341
Intron A (Less than 1%) ... 2097
Mediatric Capsules ... 2476
Metandren Linguets and Tablets ... 875
Premarin with Methyltestosterone (Among most common) ... 2515
Testred Capsules ... 1124
Winstrol Tablets ... 2075

Virilization, female fetus

Android ... 1111
Megace Tablets ... 732
Metandren Linguets and Tablets ... 875
Testred Capsules ... 1124

Vision, blurred (see under Blurred vision)

Vision, changes (see under Visual disturbances)

Vision, complete loss

Alcaine ... ⊚ 210
Demulen ... 2161
Depo-Medrol Sterile Aqueous Suspension ... 2334
Enovid ... 2161
Levlen/Tri-Levlen ... 665
Micronor Tablets ... 1667
Modicon ... 1667
Ortho-Novum ... 1667
Plaquenil Sulfate Tablets (One case) ... 2067
Levlen/Tri-Levlen ... 665

Vision, double (see under Diplopia)

Vision, loss of color

Cipro I.V. (1% or less) ... 1592
Cipro Tablets (Less than 1%) ... 1589
Meclomen Capsules (Rare) ... 1739
Ponstel (Rare) ... 1758

Vision, obscured by enlarged iris cysts

Floropryl Sterile Ophthalmic Ointment ... 1473
Humorsol Sterile Ophthalmic Solution ... 1475

Vision, partial loss

Brevicon ... 2304
Demulen ... 2161
Enovid ... 2161
Levlen/Tri-Levlen ... 665
Micronor Tablets ... 1667
Modicon ... 1667
Norinyl ... 2304
Ortho-Novum ... 1667
Levlen/Tri-Levlen ... 665
Tri-Norinyl 28-Day Tablets ... 2304

Vision, temporary loss

Depo-Medrol Sterile Aqueous Suspension ... 2334
Meclomen Capsules (Rare) ... 1739
Omnipaque (A few cases) ... 2552
Soma Compound w/Codeine Tablets ... 2390
Soma Compound Tablets (Very rare) ... 2389
Soma Tablets ... 2388

Vision, tunnel

BuSpar (Rare) ... 1401

Visual acuity, defects

AK-Cide Sterile Ophthalmic Ointment & Suspension ... ⊚ 202
AK-Dex ... ⊚ 203
AK-Pred ... ⊚ 205
AK-Spore H.C. ... ⊚ 206
AK-Trol Ointment & Suspension ... ⊚ 207
Atabrine Hydrochloride Tablets ... 2041
Betoptic Sterile Ophthalmic Solution (Small numbers of patients) ... 569
Betoptic S Sterile Ophthalmic Suspension (Small numbers of patients) ... 570
Blephamide ... 586
Cipro I.V. (1% or less) ... 1592
Cipro Tablets ... 1589
Dexacidin ... ⊚ 272
⅛% Econopred & 1% Econopred Plus ... ⊚ 217
FML Forte Liquifilm ... ⊚ 245
FML Liquifilm ... ⊚ 244
FML S.O.P. ... ⊚ 245
FML-S Sterile Ophthalmic Suspension ... ⊚ 246
Fluor-Op Ophthalmic Suspension ... ⊚ 272
HMS Liquifilm ... ⊚ 247
Inflamase ... ⊚ 274
Isopto Carbachol ... ⊚ 219
Maxidex Sterile Ophthalmic Ointment ... ⊚ 222
Maxidex Sterile Ophthalmic Suspension ... ⊚ 223
Maxitrol Ophthalmic Ointment/Suspension ... ⊚ 223
Meclomen Capsules (Rare) ... 1739
Myambutol Tablets ... 1225
Nolvadex Tablets ... 1102
Pilocar ... ⊚ 275
Pilopine HS Gel ... ⊚ 227
Pilostat Sterile Ophthalmic Solution 0.5%, 1%, 2%, 3%, 4%, 5%, 6% ... ⊚ 263
Plaquenil Sulfate Tablets ... 2067
Pred-G Liquifilm Sterile Ophthalmic Suspension ... ⊚ 252
Pred-G S.O.P. Sterile Ophthalmic Ointment ... ⊚ 253
Rogaine Topical Solution ... 2357
Serophene (clomiphene citrate tablets, USP) ... 2186
TobraDex Ophthalmic Suspension and Ointment ... ⊚ 228
Vasocidin Ointment ... ⊚ 275
Vasocidin Ophthalmic Solution ... ⊚ 276

Vision abnormalities (see under Visual disturbances)

Visual disturbances

Accutane Capsules ... 1878
Adsorbonac 2% and 5% ... ⊚ 210
Adsorbotear ... ⊚ 210
AK-Cide Sterile Ophthalmic Ointment & Suspension ... ⊚ 202
AK-Dex ... ⊚ 203
AK-NaCl 5% Ointment & Solution ... ⊚ 204
AK-Pred ... ⊚ 205
AK-Spore H.C. ... ⊚ 206
AK-Trol Ointment & Suspension ... ⊚ 207
Alferon N Injection (1%) ... 1809
Allergan Eyewash ... ⊚ 238
Allergy Drops ... ▣ 511
Altace Capsules (Less than 1%) ... 1086
▲Anafranil Capsules (7% to 18%) ... 650
Anaprox and Anaprox DS Tablets (Less than 3%) ... 2288
Ansaid Tablets (1-3%) ... 2319
Aralen Hydrochloride Injection ... 2038
Aralen Phosphate with Primaquine Phosphate Tablets (Occasional) ... 2040
Aralen Phosphate Tablets ... 2039
Betagan ... ⊚ 239
Blephamide ... 586
Blocadren Tablets ... 1429
Brevibloc Injection (Less than 1%) ... 942
Brevicon (Rare) ... 2304
Butazolidin Capsules & Tablets ... 1027
Cardene Capsules (Rare) ... 2290
Cardioquin Tablets ... 1812
Cardura Tablets (2%) ... 1941
Celluvisc Lubricant Ophthalmic Solution ... ⊚ 243
Children's Advil Suspension (Less than 1%) ... 2426
Cibalith-S ... 870
Cipro I.V. (1% or less) ... 1592
Cipro Tablets (Less than 1%) ... 1589
Clear Eyes ACR ... ⊚ 305
Clinoril Tablets (Less than 1 in 100) ... 1433
▲Clozaril Tablets (5% or more) ... 2000
Collyrium for Fresh Eyes ... 2445
Collyrium Fresh ... 2445
▲Cordarone Tablets (4 to 9%) ... 2446
Corgard Tablets ... 701
Corzide Tablets ... 702
Cuprimine Capsules ... 1442
Cyklokapron Tablets and Injection ... 1159
Cytotec (Infrequent) ... 2159
Danocrine Capsules ... 2046
Dantrium Capsules (Less frequent) ... 1619
Darvon-N/Darvocet-N ... 1254
Darvon ... 1256
Darvon-N Suspension & Tablets ... 1254
Demerol ... 2047
Demulen (Uncommon) ... 2161
Deprol Tablets ... 2382
Desferal Vials ... 862
Dilaudid-HP Injection ... 1175
Dimetane-DC Cough Syrup ... 1857
Dimetane-DX Cough Syrup ... 1858
Dolobid Tablets (Less than 1 in 100) ... 1465
Dolophine Hydrochloride Ampoules & Vials ... 1260
Dolophine Hydrochloride Tablets ... 1261
Doral Tablets ... 2383
Duolube Eye Ointment ... ▣ 511
Duratears Naturale ... ⊚ 216
DynaCirc Capsules (0.5% to 1%) ... 2004
Easprin ... 1719
⅛% Econopred & 1% Econopred Plus ... ⊚ 217
Empirin with Codeine Phosphate Nos. 2, 3 & 4 ... 764
Engerix-B Unit-Dose Vials ... 2213
Enovid (Uncommon) ... 2161
Equagesic Tablets ... 2451
Eye Wash ... ▣ 511
Eye-Stream ... 571
FML-S Sterile Ophthalmic Suspension ... ⊚ 246
Sterile FUDR (Remote possibility) ... 1898
Feldene Capsules ... 1777
Floxin Tablets (1% to 3%) ... 1652
Fluorouracil Injection ... 1897
Garamycin Injectable ... 2093
Halcion Tablets (Less frequent) ... 2340
Haldol Decanoate ... 1375
Haldol Injection, Tablets and Concentrate ... 1373
▲Hylorel Tablets (29.2%) ... 975
Hytrin Tablets (At least 1%) ... 529
Inderal ... 2459
Inderal LA Long Acting Capsules ... 2461

(▣ Described in PDR For Nonprescription Drugs) Incidence data in parenthesis; ▲ 3% or more (⊚ Described in PDR For Ophthalmology)

Inderide Tablets 2463
Inderide LA Long Acting Capsules 2465
▲Intron A (Up to 7%) 2097
Isopto Carbachol ⊙ 219
Isopto Cetapred Suspension ⊙ 220
Kerlone Tablets (Less than 2%) 2172
Lacril Lubricant Ophthalmic Solution ⊙ 248
Lamprene Capsules (Less than 1%) 1030
Lanoxicaps 772
Lanoxin Elixir Pediatric 775
Lanoxin Injection 778
Lanoxin Injection Pediatric 781
Lanoxin Tablets 783
Lariam Tablets 1904
Legatrin ▣ 556
Lodine Capsules (Less than 1%) 2468
Lopressor Ampuls 1032
Lopressor HCT Tablets 1034
Lopressor Tablets 1032
MS Contin Tablets (Infrequent) 1814
MSIR (Infrequent) 1817
Matulane Capsules 1907
Mepergan Injection 2479
Methadone Hydrochloride Diskets 1284
Methadone Hydrochloride Oral Solution & Tablets 1987
▲Mexitil Capsules (5.7% to 7.5%) 680
Micronor Tablets (Rare) 1667
Midamor Tablets (Less than or equal to 1%) 1508
Miltown Tablets 2386
Modicon (Rare) 1667
Moduretic Tablets (Less than or equal to 1%) 1510
Moisture Drops ▣ 512
Monopril Tablets (0.2 to 1.0%) 1406
Motrin Tablets (Less than 1%) 2351
Myambutol Tablets 1225
Naphcon ⊙ 226
▲Naprosyn (Less than 7%) 2297
NegGram (Infrequent) 2062
Nolvadex Tablets 1102
Norinyl (Rare) 2304
Normodyne Tablets (1%) 2110
Normozide Tablets (1%) 2112
Noroxin Tablets 1519
Nor-Q D Tablets 2304
Omnipaque 2552
Ophthocort ⊙ 301
Oramorph SR (Morphine Sulfate Sustained Release Tablets) (Less frequent) 1988
Ortho-Novum (Rare) 1667
Orudis Capsules (Greater than 1%) 2488
PMB 200 and PMB 400 2504
Pantopon Injectable 1911
Paraplatin for Injection (1%) 735
Parlodel 2020
PediaProfen Suspension (Less than 1%) 1363
▲Permax Tablets (5.8%) 1291
Phenergan with Codeine 2497
Phenergan VC with Codeine 2501
Phospholine Iodide (More frequent in children) ⊙ 315
Plaquenil Sulfate Tablets 2067
Prefrin Liquifilm Vasoconstrictor and Lubricant Eye Drops ⊙ 254
Procardia XL Tablets (1% or less) 1783
ProSom Tablets (Infrequent) 554
Prostigmin Injectable 1120
Prostigmin Tablets 1121
Prozac Pulvules (2.8%) 920
Quinaglute Dura-Tabs Tablets 663
Quinamm Tablets 1344
Quinidex Extentabs 1868
Q-vel Muscle Relaxant Pain Reliever ▣ 552
Recombivax HB (Less than 1%) 1544
Reglan 1869
Ridaura Capsules 2224
Rifadin 1345
Rifamate Capsules 1347
Rimactane Capsules 879
▲Roferon-A Injection (Less than 3% to 5%) 1916
Rogaine Topical Solution 2357
Roxanol 1991
Rufen Tablets (Less than 1%) 691
Ru-Tuss with Hydrocodone 694
Ru-Tuss Tablets 693
Rythmol Tablets (1.9%) 1184
Sandimmune (Rare) 2024
Sandostatin Injection (Less than 1%) 2029
Sectral Capsules (2%) 2520
Seldane Tablets 1349
Seldane-D Extended-Release Tablets 1350
Serophene (clomiphene citrate tablets, USP) (Approximately 1 in 50 patients) 2186
Stilphostrol Tablets and Ampuls 1609
Symmetrel Capsules & Syrup (0.1-1%) 936
Tacaryl 2409
Talacen (Infrequent) 2070
Talwin Injection 2071
Talwin Compound (Infrequent) 2072
Talwin Injection 2071
Talwin Nx 2073
▲Tambocor Tablets (15.9%) 1315
Taractan (Occasional) 1920
▲Tegison Capsules (10-25%) 1881
Temaril Tablets, Syrup and Spansule Sustained Release Capsules 1085
Tenex Tablets (Less than 3%) 1875
Tenormin Tablets and I.V. Injection 1107
Terra-Cortril Ophthalmic Suspension 1963
Thorazine 2234
Timolide Tablets 1547
Timoptic in Ocudose 1552
Timoptic Sterile Ophthalmic Solution 1550
Tolectin (200, 400 and 600 mg) (1 to 3%) 1379
▲Tonocard Tablets (1.3-10.0%) 1554
Toradol IM Injection (1% or less) 2302
Trandate HCT/Trandate (Less than 1% in 208 patients) 579
Tri-Norinyl 28-Day Tablets 2304
Tuss-Ornade Liquid 2242
Tuss-Ornade Spansule Capsules 2242
Urispas Tablets 2242
Versed Injection (Less than 1%) 1924
Visine L.R. Eye Drope ⊙ 303
Visken Tablets (2% or fewer patients) 2036
Wellbutrin Tablets (Infrequent) 821
Wygesic Tablets 2540
Zincfrin ⊙ 230
Zovirax 824

Visual fields, defects
AK-Dex ⊙ 203
AK-Pred ⊙ 205
AK-Spore H.C. ⊙ 206
AK-Trol Ointment & Suspension ⊙ 207
Anafranil Capsules (Rare) 650
Blephamide 586
Dexacidin ⊙ 272
⅛% Econopred & 1% Econopred Plus ⊙ 217
Eskalith 2214
FML Forte Liquifilm ⊙ 245
FML Liquifilm ⊙ 244
FML S.O.P. ⊙ 245
FML-S Sterile Ophthalmic Suspension ⊙ 246
Fluor-Op Ophthalmic Suspension ⊙ 272
HMS Liquifilm ⊙ 247
Inflamase ⊙ 274
Lithane Tablets 1596
Maxidex Sterile Ophthalmic Ointment ⊙ 222
Maxidex Sterile Ophthalmic Suspension ⊙ 223
Maxitrol Ophthalmic Ointment/Suspension ⊙ 223
Permax Tablets (Infrequent) 1291
Pred Forte ⊙ 252
Pred Mild ⊙ 254
Pred-G Liquifilm Sterile Ophthalmic Suspension ⊙ 252
Quinamm Tablets 1344
TobraDex Ophthalmic Suspension and Ointment ⊙ 228
Vasocidin Ointment ⊙ 275
Vasocidin Ophthalmic Solution ⊙ 276

Visual impairment
Ciloxan Sterile Ophthalmic Solution (Less than 1%) ⊙ 214
Ganite Injection (At least one case) 1016
Ocusert Pilo-20 and Pilo-40 Ocular Therapeutic Systems ⊙ 256
Ridaura Capsules 2224

Vitamin D, increased requirement
Mebaral Tablets 2061

Vitamins, fat-soluble, absorption impaired
Colestid Granules 2328
Questran Light 711
Questran Powder 710

Vitiligio
Intron A (1% or less) 2097

Vitreous floaters
Voltaren Tablets (Less than 1%) 1042

Voice, alteration
Accutane Capsules (Less than 1%) 1878
Danocrine Capsules 2046
Permax Tablets (Infrequent) 1291
Ventolin (Less than 1%) 583

Voice, deepening
Aldactazide 2150
Aldactone 2152
Anadrol-50 Tablets 2287
Android 1111
Danocrine Capsules 2046
Estratest 2245
Halotestin Tablets 2341
Metandren Linguets and Tablets 875
Premarin with Methyltestosterone (Among most common) 2515
Testred Capsules 1124
Winstrol Tablets 2075

Voice, hoarseness
Danocrine Capsules 2046
Estratest 2245

Voice, loss of (see under Aphonia)

Vola, burning of
Atgam Sterile Solution (At least 1 patient and less than 5% of total patients) 2320

Volar pain
Atgam Sterile Solution (At least 1 patient and less than 5% of total patients) 2320

Vomiting
Abbokinase 503
Abbokinase Open-Cath 505
Accutane Capsules 1878
Achromycin V Capsules 1193
Actifed with Codeine Cough Syrup 752
Actigall Capsules 2280
▲Actimmune (13%) 1046
Activase 1047
Adriamycin PFS 561
Adriamycin RDF (Frequent) 562
▲AeroBid Inhaler System (25%) 995
Aerolate 994
AK-Fluor Injection 10% and 25% ⊙ 204
Albuminar-5, Albumin (Human) U.S.P. 5% 608
Albuminar-25, Albumin (Human) U.S.P. 25% 608
Aldactazide 2150
Aldactone 2152
Aldoclor Tablets 1413
Aldomet Ester HCl Injection 1417
Aldomet Oral 1415
Aldoril Tablets 1418
▲Alfenta Injection (18%) 1131
▲Alferon N Injection (Up to 29%) 1809
▲Alka-Seltzer Effervescent Antacid and Pain Reliever (7.6% at doses of 1000 mg/day) 1568
▲Alka-Seltzer (Flavored) Effervescent Antacid and Pain Reliever (7.6% at doses of 1000 mg/day) 1569
Alkeran Tablets (Infrequent) 754
Altace Capsules (1.1%) 1086
Alupent (1 to 4%) 674
Alurate Elixir (Less than 1 in 100) 1883
Amikin Injectable (Rare) 602
Aminohippurate Sodium Injection 1421
Aminophyllin Tablets 2153
Amoxil 2193
Anadrol-50 Tablets 2287
▲Anafranil Capsules (7%) 650
Ana-Kit Anaphylaxis Emergency Treatment Kit 1100
Anaprox and Anaprox DS Tablets (Less than 1%) 2288
Ancef Injection (Rare) 2194
Ancobon Capsules 1886
▲Anestacon Solution (Among most common) 2394
▲Anexsia 5/500 Tablets (Among most frequent) 2196
▲Anexsia 7.5/650 Tablets (Among most frequent) 2197
Ansaid Tablets (1-3%) 2319
Antilirium Injectable 998
Antivenin (Crotalidae) Polyvalent 2430
Apresazide Capsules (Common) 854
Apresoline Hydrochloride Parenteral (Ampuls) 856
Apresoline Hydrochloride Tablets (Common) 855
Apresoline-Esidrix Tablets 857
Aquasol A Vitamin A Capsules, USP 615
Aquasol A Parenteral, USP 615
Aralen Hydrochloride Injection 2038
Aralen Phosphate with Primaquine Phosphate Tablets 2040
Aralen Phosphate Tablets 2039
Arfonad Ampuls 1887
Arm-a-Med Metaproterenol Sulfate Inhalation Solution, USP (1 in 300 patients) 617
Artane 1195
Asbron G 1997
Asendin Tablets (Less than 1%) 1196
Astramorph/PF Injection, USP (Preservative-Free) (Frequent) 618
Atabrine Hydrochloride Tablets (Rare) 2041
▲Atgam Sterile Solution (More than 1% to 10%) 2320
Ativan Injection (Occasional) 2432
Atrohist Sprinkle Capsules 558
Atromid-S Capsules (Less frequent) 2435
Atrovent Inhalation Aerosol 675
Augmentin Tablets, Powder for Oral Suspension, and Chewable Tablets (1%) 2198
Azactam for Injection (1-1.3%) 2252
▲Azdōne Tablets (Among most frequent) 844
Azo Gantanol Tablets 1887
Azo Gantrisin Tablets 1888
▲Azulfidine Tablets, EN-tabs, Oral Suspension (Approximately one-third of patients) 1157
BAL in Oil Ampules 661
B & O No. 15A & No. 16A Supprettes 2395
▲Bactrim DS Tablets (Among most common) 1891
▲Bactrim I.V. Infusion (Among most common) 1889
▲Bactrim (Among most common) 1891
Baron-X Tablets 650
▲Genuine Bayer Aspirin Tablets & Caplets (7.3% at doses of 1000 mg/day) ▣ 564
▲Bayer Plus Aspirin Tablets (7.6% of 4500 people tested) ▣ 567
▲Therapy Bayer Aspirin Caplets (7.6% of 4500 people tested) ▣ 568
Benadryl Capsules 1691
Benadryl Injection 1692
Benemid Tablets 1426
Bentyl 1322
Biavax II 1427
BiCNU (Frequent) 723
▲Blenoxane (Frequent) 724
Blocadren Tablets (Less than 1%) 1429
Brethaire Inhaler 1024
Brethine Ampuls (1.3 to 3.9%) 1026
Brethine Tablets 1026
▲Bretylol Injection (3%) 923
Brevibloc Injection (About 1%) 942
Brevicon 2304
Brevital Sodium Vials 1248
Bricanyl Injection 1324
Bricanyl Tablets 1325
▲Bufferin Analgesic Tablets and Caplets (7.6%) 743
Bumex (0.2%) 1895
BuSpar (1%) 1401
Butazolidin Capsules & Tablets (Less than 1%) 1027
Butisol Sodium Elixir & Tablets (Less than 1 in 100) 2377
Cafergot/Cafergot P-B 1999
Calcidrine Syrup 506
Calcijex Calcitriol Injection 506
▲Calcimar Injection, Synthetic (10%) 1839
Calciparine Injection (Rare) 925
Calderol Capsules 1635
Cantil Tablets 1326
Capoten (0.5 to 2%) 2255
Capozide (0.5 to 2%) 2258
Carafate Tablets (Less than 0.5%) 1326
Carbocaine Hydrochloride Injection 2043
Cardene Capsules (0.4%) 2290
Cardilate Oral/Sublingual Tablets (Occasional) 757
Cardioquin Tablets 1812

Cardizem Tablets-30 mg, 60 mg, 90 mg and 120 mg (Less than 1%) 1329
Cardizem SR Capsules-60 mg, 90 mg and 120 mg (Less than 1%) 1327
Cardura Tablets (0%) 1941
Carnitor 2188
Catapres Tablets (About 5 in 100 patients) 676
▲ Catapres-TTS (5%) 677
Ceclor Pulvules & Suspension (Rare) 1251
CeeNU 725
Cefizox Injection (Occasional) 1012
Cefobid Intravenous/Intramuscular (Rare) 1943
Cefobid Pharmacy Bulk Package - Not for Direct Infusion (Rare) 1945
Ceftin Tablets (2.0%) 575
Celontin (Frequent) 1692
Centrax 1693
Cephulac Syrup 1331
Ceptaz for Injection (One in 500 patients) 1057
Ceredase Injection 1052
Cerubidine 2443
▲ CHEMET (succimer) Capsules (12-20.9%) 1361
Children's Advil Suspension (Less than 3%) 2426
Chloromycetin Kapseals 1695
Chloromycetin Palmitate, Oral Suspension 1697
Chloromycetin Sodium Succinate 1698
Choledyl Pediatric Elixir 1702
Choledyl Tablets 1700
Choledyl SA Tablets 1704
Cholybar (Less frequent) 1705
Chromagen Capsules 2078
Chronulac Syrup 1332
▲ Cibacalcin Double-chambered Syringes (14-21%) 859
Cibalith-S 870
Cipro I.V. (1% or less) 1592
Cipro Tablets (2.0%) 1589
Claforan Sterile Injection (1.4%) 1089
Cleocin HCl Capsules 2322
Cleocin Pediatric Flavored Granules 2324
Cleocin Phosphate Injection 2325
Clinoril Tablets (Greater than 1%) 1433
▲ Clozaril Tablets (3%) 2000
Cocaine Hydrochloride Topical Solution 620
Cogentin 1435
ColBENEMID Tablets 1436
Colchicine Ampoules 1252
Colestid Granules (1 in 30 to 1 in 100 patients) 2328
Colyte 1826
▲ Combipres Tablets (About 5%) 678
Comhist LA Capsules 1618
Compazine 2201
Condylox (Less than 5%) 1630
Constant-T Tablets 1029
▲ Cordarone Tablets (10 to 33%) 2446
Corgard Tablets (1 to 5 of 1000 patients) 701
Corzide Tablets (1 to 5 of 1000 patients) 702
Cosmegen Injection (Common) 1440
Crystodigin Tablets 1253
Cuprimine Capsules (Greater than 1%) 1442
Cyklokapron Tablets and Injection 1159
▲ Cytadren Tablets (1 in 30) 861
▲ CytoGam (Less than 5.0%) 891
▲ Cytosar-U Sterile Powder (Among most frequent) 2329
Cytotec (1.3%) 2159
Cytovene Sterile Powder (1% or less) 2292
Cytoxan for Injection 726
D.H.E. 45 Injection 2003
▲ DTIC-Dome (90% with the initial few doses) 1595
▲ Dalgan Injection (3 to 9%) 620
Dalmane Capsules 1927
▲ Damason-P (Among most frequent) 1356
Danocrine Capsules 2046
Dapsone USP 1130
Daranide Tablets (Among the most common effects) 1445
Daraprim Tablets 761
Darbid Tablets 2205
▲ Darvon-N/Darvocet-N (Among most frequent) 1254
▲ Darvon (Among most frequent) 1256
▲ Darvon-N Suspension & Tablets (Among most frequent) 1254
Declomycin Capsules, Tablets 1199
Deconamine 663
Demerol 2047
Demser Capsules (Infrequent) 1460
▲ Demulen (Among most common) 2161
▲ Depakene Capsules & Syrup (Among most common) 511
▲ Depakote (Among most common) 512
▲ Depen Titratable Tablets (17%) 2379
Deprol Tablets 2382
Desyrel and Desyrel Dividose (Greater than 1%) 1404
Diabinese Tablets (Less than 2%) 1775
Diamox Parenteral 1200
Diamox Sequels (Sustained Release) 1201
Diamox Tablets 1200
Dicumarol Tablets (Infrequent) 516
Diethylstilbestrol Tablets 1258
Diflucan Injection and Tablets (1.7% in 4048 patients) 1948
Dilantin Infatabs 1710
Dilantin Kapseals 1708
Dilantin Parenteral 1712
Dilantin-30 Pediatric/Dilantin-125 Suspension 1713
Dilantin with Phenobarbital Kapseals 1715
Dilatrate-SR (Uncommon) 1827
Dilaudid Cough Syrup 1174
Dilaudid 1173
Dilaudid-HP Injection 1175
Dilor 2079
Dilor-G Tablets & Liquid 2079
Dimacol Caplets ▣ 672
Dimetane-DC Cough Syrup 1857
Dimetane-DX Cough Syrup 1858
Dipentum Capsules (1.0%) 1160
Diphtheria and Tetanus Toxoids and Pertussis Vaccine Adsorbed USP (For Pediatric Use) (1 in 15 doses) 892
▲ Diprivan Injection (3% to 10%) 2267
Diucardin Tablets 2450
Diulo 2129
Diupres Tablets 1461
Diuril Oral Suspension 1464
Diuril Sodium Intravenous 1463
Diuril Tablets 1464
Dolobid Tablets (Greater than 1 in 100) 1465
▲ Dolophine Hydrochloride Ampoules & Vials (Among most frequent) 1260
▲ Dolophine Hydrochloride Tablets (Among most frequent) 1261
Donnatal 1858
Donnatal Extentabs 1859
Donnatal Tablets 1858
Donnazyme Tablets 1860
Dopram Injectable 1860
Dorcol Children's Decongestant Liquid ▣ 685
Doryx Capsules 1717
Doxorubicin Hydrochloride for Injection, USP (Frequent) 622
Doxorubicin Hydrochloride Injection, USP (Frequent) 848
▲ Duragesic Transdermal System (10% or more) 1133
Duramorph 960
Duranest Injections 624
Duricef 1405
Dyazide Capsules 2208
Dyclone 0.5% and 1% Topical Solutions, USP 626
DynaCirc Capsules (1.1%) 2004
Dyrenium Capsules (Rare) 2210
E.E.S. 522
E-Mycin Tablets (Infrequent) 688
Easprin 1719
▲ Ecotrin (7.6% at 1000 mg/day) 2189
Edecrin 1468
Elavil 2269
Eldepryl 2250
Elspar 1470
Emcyt Capsules (1%) 1161
▲ Eminase (Less than 10%) 2211
▲ Empirin with Codeine Phosphate Nos. 2, 3 & 4 (Among most frequent) 764
Endep Tablets 1927
Enduron Tablets 517
Enduronyl 518
Engerix-B Unit-Dose Vials (Less than 1%) 2213
Enlon Injection 598
▲ Enovid (Among most common) 2161
▲ Epogen for Injection (0.26% to 8.0%) 591
Equagesic Tablets 2451
▲ Ergamisol Tablets (9 to 20%) 1136
▲ Ergostat (10% of patients) 1719
Ergotrate Maleate Ampoules (Uncommon) 1263
▲ ERYC (Among most frequent) 1720
▲ EryPed (Among most frequent) 519
▲ Ery-Tab Tablets (Among most frequent) 521
▲ Erythrocin Stearate Filmtab (Among most frequent) 523
▲ Erythromycin Base Filmtab (Among most frequent) 525
▲ Erythromycin Delayed-Release Capsules, USP (Among most frequent) 526
Esgic-Plus Tablets (Less frequent) 1002
Esgic Tablets & Capsules (Less frequent) 1001
Esidrix Tablets 863
Esimil Tablets 864
Eskalith 2214
Estinyl Tablets 2085
Estrace 1385
Estrace Vaginal Cream 1388
Estraderm Transdermal System 866
Estradurin 2452
Estratest 2245
Estrovis 1721
▲ Ethmozine Tablets (2%-5%) 946
Ethrane 599
Etrafon 2087
▲ Eulexin Capsules (11% with LHRH-agonist) 2089
Exna Tablets 1862
▲ Sterile FUDR (Among more common) 1898
Fansidar Tablets 1896
Feldene Capsules (Less than 1%) 1777
Fioricet Tablets (Less frequent) 2006
Fiorinal Capsules (Less frequent) 2007
Fiorinal with Codeine Capsules (Infrequent) 2008
Fiorinal Tablets (Less frequent) 2007
Flagyl I.V. 2131
Flagyl Tablets (Occasional) 2170
Flexeril Tablets (Less than 1%) 1471
Floropryl Sterile Ophthalmic Ointment (Rare) 1473
Floxin Tablets (1% to 3%) 1652
Fluorescite ⊙ 217
Fluorouracil Injection (Common) 1897
Fluothane 2453
Forane 600
Fortaz (1 in 500 patients) 1060
Fulvicin P/G Tablets 2090
Fulvicin P/G 165 & 330 Tablets 2091
Fulvicin-U/F Tablets 2092
▲ Fungizone Intravenous (Among most common) 2262
Furoxone (Occasional) 1855
Gamimune N Immune Globulin Intravenous (Human) 1572
Gammagard Immune Globulin, Intravenous (Human) (Occasional) 658
Ganite Injection 1016
Gantanol 1899
Gantrisin Ophthalmic Ointment/Solution 1900
Gantrisin 1901
Garamycin Injectable 2093
Geocillin Tablets 1951
Geref (sermorelin acetate for injection) 2560
Glucagon for Injection Vials and Emergency Kit (Occasional) 1263
GoLYTELY (Infrequent) 699
Grifulvin V (griseofulvin microsize) Tablets/Suspension (Occasional) 1678
Grisactin (Occasional) 2454
Grisactin Ultra Tablets (Occasional) 2455
Gris-PEG Tablets, 125 mg & 250 mg (Occasional) 1083
Guaifed Syrup ▣ 629
▲ Halcion Tablets (4.6%) 2340
Haldol Decanoate 1375
Haldol Injection, Tablets and Concentrate 1373
Harmonyl Tablets 528
Heparin Lock Flush Solution 2456
Heparin Sodium Vials (Rare) 1264
Heparin Sodium Injection 2457
Heparin Sodium Injection, USP, Sterile Solution 2342
Hespan Injection 948
▲ Hexalen Capsules (1% to 33%) 2316
HibTITER (9 of 1,118 vaccinations) 1206
Humorsol Sterile Ophthalmic Solution (Rare) 1475
Hycodan Syrup, Tablets 927
Hycomine Compound Tablets 929
Hycomine Syrup 927
Hycotuss Expectorant Syrup 930
Hydrea Capsules 728
Hydrocet Capsules 835
HydroDIURIL Tablets 1484
Hydromox R Tablets 1209
Hydromox Tablets 1208
Hydropres Tablets 1485
▲ Hylorel Tablets (3.9%) 975
▲ Hyperstat I.V. Injection (4%) 2095
Hyskon Hysteroscopy Fluid (Rare) 1162
Hytrin Tablets (At least 1%) 529
INH Tablets 868
▲ Idamycin for Injection (82%) 564
▲ IFEX (58%) 729
Ilosone (Infrequent) 913
Imferon 976
Imodium Capsules 1139
▲ Imuran (Approximately 12%) 768
Inderal 2459
Inderal LA Long Acting Capsules 2461
Inderide Tablets 2463
Inderide LA Long Acting Capsules 2465
Indocin I.V. (1% to 3%) 1490
Infumorph 200 and Infumorph 500 Sterile Solutions 962
Innovar Injection 1141
Inocor Lactate Injection (0.9%) 2048
▲ Intron A (2% to 14%) 2097
▲ Intropin Injection (Among most frequent) 930
Inversine Tablets 1492
IOPIDINE ⊙ 232
Ismelin Tablets 869
ISMOTIC ⊙ 233
Isopto Carbachol ⊙ 219
Isordil (Uncommon) 2467
Isuprel Hydrochloride Mistometer 2051
Isuprel Hydrochloride Solution 1:200 & 1:100 2052
Jenest-28 Tablets 1636
K-Dur Microburst Release System (potassium chloride, USP) E.R. Tablets 1163
▲ K-Lor Powder Packets (Most common) 531
▲ K-Lyte (Among most common) 707
▲ K-Norm Capsules (Among most common) 982
K-Phos M.F. Tablets 659
K-Phos Neutral Tablets 660
K-Phos Original Formula 'Sodium Free' Tablets 660
K-Phos No. 2 Tablets 659
▲ K-Tab Filmtab (Most common) 532
Kato Potassium Supplement 1114
Kayexalate 2053
Keflex Pulvules, Oral Suspension & Pediatric Drops (Rare) 916
Keftab Tablets (Rare) 917
Kefurox Vials, Faspak & ADD-Vantage 1277
Kefzol Vials, Faspak & ADD-Vantage (Rare) 1279
Kemadrin Tablets 771
Kerlone Tablets (Less than 2%) 2172
Ketalar 1726
Kinesed Tablets 2272
▲ Klor-Con 8/Klor-Con 10 Extended-release Tablets (Among most common) 2374
Klorvess Effervescent Granules 2010
Klorvess Effervescent Tablets 2011
Klorvess 10% Liquid 2010
▲ Klotrix (Most common) 708
▲ Kolyum Liquid (Among most common) 983
Koro-Flex Arcing Spring Diaphragm 2142
Koromex Coil Spring Diaphragm 2142
▲ Lamprene Capsules (40-50%) 1030
Lanoxicaps (Common) 772
Lanoxin Elixir Pediatric (Common) 775
Lanoxin Injection (Common) 778
Lanoxin Injection Pediatric (Common) 781
Lanoxin Tablets (Common) 783
▲ Lariam Tablets (Among most frequent) 1904
Larodopa Tablets (Relatively frequent) 1905
Lasix 1093
Leukeran Tablets (Infrequent) 788
Leukine for IV Infusion 1127
Levlen/Tri-Levlen 665
Levo-Dromoran (Common) 1906
Levophed Bitartrate Injection 2054
Levsin/Levsinex 2147
Limbitrol 1933

(▣ Described in PDR For Nonprescription Drugs) Incidence data in parenthesis; ▲ 3% or more (⊙ Described in PDR For Ophthalmology)

Lincocin 2344
Lioresal Tablets (Rare) 1031
Lithane Tablets 1596
Lithium Carbonate Capsules & Tablets 1984
Lithobid Tablets 870
Lodine Capsules (More than 1% but less than 3%) 2468
▲ Lo/Ovral Tablets (10% or less) 2471
▲ Lo/Ovral-28 Tablets (10% or less) 2476
Loestrin 1728
Lomotil 2174
Loniten Tablets 2346
Lopid Capsules and Tablets (2.5%) 1736
Lopressor HCT Tablets (1 in 100 patients) 1034
Lorelco Tablets 1333
▲ Lortab ASA Tablets (Among most frequent) 2414
▲ Lortab (Among most frequent) 2412
Lotensin Tablets 872
Loxitane 1213
Lozol Tablets (Less than 5%) 1843
Ludiomil Tablets (Rare) 874
Lufyllin & Lufyllin-400 Tablets 2384
Lufyllin-GG Elixir & Tablets 2385
▲ Lupron Depot 7.5 mg (5.4%) 2311
▲ Lupron Injection (5% or more) 2310
Lysodren 731
M-M-R II 1494
M-R-VAX II 1496
▲ MS Contin Tablets (Among most frequent) 1814
▲ MSIR (Among most frequent) 1817
Maalox TC Suspension (Occasional) 1851
▲ Macrodantin Capsules (Most often) 1624
Mandol Vials, Faspak & ADD-Vantage (Rare) 1281
Marax Tablets & DF Syrup (Frequent, on empty stomach) 1954
Marcaine Hydrochloride 0.5% with Epinephrine 1:200,000 (as bitartrate) 958
Marcaine Hydrochloride with Epinephrine 1:200,000 (Rare) 2055
Marcaine Hydrochloride Injection (Rare) 2055
Marcaine Spinal (Rare) 2058
▲ Matulane Capsules (Frequent) 1907
Maxair Inhaler (Less than 1%) 1311
Maxzide 1215
Mebaral Tablets (Less than 1 in 100) 2061
▲ Meclomen Capsules (11%) 1739
Mediatric Capsules 2476
Medihaler Ergotamine Aerosol 1312
Mefoxin (Rarely) 1498
Mefoxin Premixed Intravenous Solution (Rarely) 1500
Megace Tablets 732
Mellaril 2011
Menrium Tablets 1934
▲ Mepergan Injection (Among most frequent) 2479
Meruvax II 1503
Mesantoin Tablets 2013
Mesnex Injection 733
Mestinon Injectable 1115
Mestinon 1116
Metaprel Inhalation Aerosol Bronchodilator (1 to 4%) 2014
Metaprel Inhalation Solution (Less frequent) 2015
Metaprel 2015
▲ Methadone Hydrochloride Diskets (Among most frequent) 1284
Methadone Hydrochloride Oral Solution & Tablets 1987
Methergine (Occasional) 2016
▲ Methotrexate Tablets, Parenteral, LPF Parenteral (10%) 1217
Metrodin (urofollitropin for injection) (Less than 1 in 50) 2182
Mevacor Tablets 1505
▲ Mexitil Capsules (39.3% to 39.6%) 680
Mezlin 1597
Mezlin Pharmacy Bulk Package 1599
▲ Miacalcin Injection (About 10%) 2017
Micro-K 1863
▲ Micro-K LS Packets (Most common) 1864
Micronor Tablets 1667
▲ Midamor Tablets (3% to 8%) 1508
Milontin Kapseals (Frequent) 1741
Miltown Tablets 2386
Minipress Capsules (1-4%) 1778
Minizide Capsules (Rare) 1779
Minocin Intravenous 1221
Minocin Oral Suspension 1224
Minocin Pellet-Filled Capsules 1222
Mintezol 1510
Mithracin 1602
Modane Plus Tablets ⊞ 504
Modane Tablets ⊞ 503
Modicon 1667
Moduretic Tablets (Less than or equal to 1%) 1510
▲ Monistat I.V. (7%) 1143
Monodox Capsules 1630
Mono-Gesic Tablets 846
Monopril Tablets 1406
Motofen Tablets (1 in 30) 836
Motrin Tablets (Less than 3%) 2351
Mustargen 1514
▲ Mutamycin (14%) 733
Myambutol Tablets 1225
▲ Mycelex Troches (1 in 20 patients) 1605
Mycelex-G 500 mg Vaginal Tablets (1 in 149 patients) 1606
Mycostatin Oral Suspension (Occasional) 605
Mycostatin Oral Tablets (Occasional) 605
Mycostatin Pastilles (Occasional) 734
Mykrox ½ mg Tablets (Less than 2%) 984
Myleran Tablets 790
Myochrysine Injection 1516
Mysoline (Occasional) 2480
Naldecon Syrup, Tablets, Pediatric Drops and Pediatric Syrup 709
Nalfon Pulvules & Tablets (2.6%) 919
Naprosyn (Less than 1%) 2297
Narcan Injection 933
Nardil 1742
Nasalide Nasal Solution 0.025% (5% or less) 2299
Naturetin Tablets (Common) 1789
Navane Capsules and Concentrate 1954
Navane Intramuscular 1956
Nebcin Vials, Hyporets & ADD-Vantage 1286
▲ NebuPent for Inhalation Solution (10 to 23%) 1017
NegGram 2062
Nembutal Sodium Capsules (Less than 1%) 534
Nembutal Sodium Solution (Less than 1%) 536
Nembutal Sodium Suppositories (Less than 1%) 538
Neo-Calglucon Syrup 2018
Neosar for Injection (Common) 566
Neptazane Tablets ◉ 311
Nesacaine Injections 629
Netromycin Injection 100 mg/ml (1 in 1000 patients) 2104
▲ Neupogen for Injection (57%) 595
▲ Niclocide Chewable Tablets (4.1%) 1607
▲ Nicorette (18.1%) 1335
Nimotop Capsules (Less than 1%) 1607
Nitro-Bid IV (Less than 1%) 1338
Nitro-Bid Ointment (Uncommon) 1339
Nitro-Bid Capsules 1338
Nitrolingual Spray (Uncommon) 1846
Nitrostat IV (Less than 1%) 1744
▲ Nizoral Tablets (3%) 1145
▲ Nolvadex Tablets (Up to 25%) 1102
▲ Nordette-21 Tablets (10% or less) 2481
▲ Nordette-28 Tablets (10% or less) 2483
▲ Norethin (10% or fewer patients during first cycle) 2133
Norflex 1314
Norgesic 1314
Norinyl 2304
Norlestrin 1746
▲ Normodyne Injection (Up to 4%) 2108
Normodyne Tablets (Less than 1% to 3%) 2110
Normozide Tablets (Less than 1%) 2112
Noroxin Tablets (Less frequent) 1519
Norpace (1 to 3%) 2177
Norpramin Tablets 1340
Nor-Q D Tablets 2304
Novahistine DH 1342
Novahistine Elixir ⊞ 596
Novahistine Expectorant 1343
▲ Novantrone for Injection Concentrate (31 to 72%) 1226
Novocain Hydrochloride for Spinal Anesthesia 2065
▲ Nubain Injection (6%) 934
Nucofed Capsules 2219
Nucofed Expectorant 2219
Nucofed Pediatric Expectorant 2220
Nucofed Syrup 2219
NuLYTELY 699
Numorphan Hydrochloride Injection 935
Numorphan Suppositories 935
Nystatin, USP for Extemporaneous Preparation of Oral Suspension (Occasional) 1685
Ogen 540
▲ Omnipaque (3 to 6%) 2552
Oncovin Solution Vials & Hyporets 1288
Optimine Tablets 2115
▲ Oramorph SR (Morphine Sulfate Sustained Release Tablets) (Among most frequent) 1988
Orap Tablets 1020
Oretic Tablets 544
Oreticyl 545
Ornade Spansule Capsules 2221
Ortho Diaphragm Kit 1664
Ortho Dienestrol Cream 1664
▲ Orthoclone OKT3 Sterile Solution (19%) 1645
Ortho-Cyclen Tablets 1658
Ortho-Novum 1667
Ortho-White Diaphragm Kit-Flat Spring 1664
Orudis Capsules (Greater than 1%) 2488
OSM_GLYN ◉ 234
Ovcon (10% or less) 1391
▲ Ovral Tablets (10% or less) 2490
▲ Ovral-28 Tablets (10% or less) 2491
▲ Ovrette Tablets (10% or less) 2492
Oxytocin Injection 2492
PBZ Tablets & Elixir 1037
PBZ-SR Tablets 1037
▲ PCE Dispertab Tablets (Among most frequent) 549
PMB 200 and PMB 400 (Rare) 2504
Pamelor 2019
Pantopon Injectable 1911
Panwarfin Tablets (Infrequent) 547
Paradione Capsules 548
▲ Paraplatin for Injection (81% to 92%) 735
▲ Parlodel (2-5%) 2020
PediaProfen Suspension (Less than 3%) 1363
Pediazole 1973
Peganone Tablets 551
Pepcid (Infrequent) 1524
Peptavlon 2563
▲ Percocet Tablets (Among most frequent) 950
▲ Percodan (Among most frequent) 951
Perdiem Fiber Granules 1852
Perdiem Granules 1852
Pergonal (menotropins for injection, USP) 2184
Periactin 1525
Peritrate (Occasional) 1756
Permax Tablets (2.7%) 1291
Persantine Tablets 683
▲ Phenaphen with Codeine Capsules (Among most frequent) 1865
▲ Phenaphen-650 with Codeine Tablets (Among most frequent) 1866
Phenergan with Codeine 2497
Phenergan with Dextromethorphan 2499
Phenergan Injection 2493
Phenergan Suppositories 2496
Phenergan Syrup 2495
Phenergan Tablets 2496
Phenergan VC 2500
Phenergan VC with Codeine 2501
Phenobarbital Elixir and Tablets (Less than in 100 patients) 1293
PhosLo Tablets 700
Phrenilin 838
Pilocar (Extremely rare) ◉ 275
Pilostat Sterile Ophthalmic Solution 0.5%, 1%, 2%, 3%, 4%, 5%, 6% (Extremely rare) ◉ 263
Pima Syrup 994
Pipracil (Less than 2%) 1230
Pitocin Injection, Ampoules, Steri-Dose Syringes 1757
Pitressin Synthetic, Ampoules 1758
Placidyl Capsules 553
Plague Vaccine 1584
Plaquenil Sulfate Tablets (Rare) 2067
▲ Platinol (Almost all patients) 737
▲ Platinol-AQ Injection (Almost all patients) 738
Plendil Extended-Release Tablets (0.5% to 1.5%) 1526
Polaramine 2116
Ponstel 1758
Pontocaine Hydrochloride for Spinal Anesthesia 2069
Premarin Intravenous 2508
Premarin with Methyltestosterone 2515
Premarin Tablets 2510
Premarin Vaginal Cream 2512
Prilosec Delayed-Release Capsules (0.4 to 3.2%) 1530
Primaxin I.M. (0.3%) 1532
Primaxin I.V. (1.5%) 1535
Prinivil Tablets (1.3%) 1538
Prinzide Tablets (1.4%) 1540
Priscoline Hydrochloride Ampuls 877
Pro-Banthīne Tablets 2141
▲ Procan SR Tablets (3-4%) 1760
Procardia XL Tablets (1% or less) 1783
▲ Procrit for Injection (0.26% to 8%) 1647
Proglycem (Frequent) 649
ProHIBiT Haemophilus b Conjugate Vaccine (Diphtheria Toxoid Conjugate) (1.2% or less) 896
Prokine for I.V. Infusion 1096
Proloprim Tablets 799
▲ Pronestyl Capsules and Tablets (3-4%) 1800
Pronestyl Injection 1798
▲ Pronestyl-SR Tablets (3 to 4%) 1801
ProSom Tablets (Infrequent) 554
Prostigmin Injectable 1120
Prostigmin Tablets 1121
Prostin VR Pediatric Sterile Solution (Less than 1%) 2355
Protamine Sulfate Ampoules & Vials 1295
Protostat Tablets (Occasional) 1674
Proventil Inhalation Aerosol 2117
Proventil Repetabs Tablets (2%) 2120
Proventil Syrup 2119
Proventil Tablets (2%) 2120
Provocholine for Inhalation 1911
Prozac Pulvules (2.4%) 920
Purinethol Tablets (Uncommon) 800
Quadrinal Tablets 1183
Quarzan Capsules 1937
Quelidrine Syrup 556
Questran Light (Less frequent) 711
Questran Powder 710
Quibron Capsules 713
Quibron-T 714
Quibron-T/SR 716
Quinaglute Dura-Tabs Tablets 663
Quinamm Tablets 1344
Quinidex Extentabs (Frequent) 1868
Raudixin Tablets 1803
Rauzide Tablets 1804
Recombivax HB (Less than 1%) 1544
Regitine 878
Renese Tablets 1785
Renese-R Tablets 1786
Respbid Tablets 684
▲ Retrovir Capsules (4.8% to 6%) 802
▲ Retrovir I.V. Infusion (6%) 805
▲ Retrovir Syrup (4.8% to 6%) 802
▲ Rheumatrex Methotrexate Dose Pack (10%) 1234
▲ Ridaura Capsules (10%) 2224
Rifadin (Some patients) 1345
Rifamate Capsules (Some patients) 1347
Rimactane Capsules 879
Robaxisal Tablets 1872
Robinul Forte Tablets 1873
Robinul Injectable 1873
Robinul Tablets 1873
Robitussin ⊞ 676
Robitussin Night Relief ⊞ 677
Robitussin-CF ⊞ 676
Robitussin-DM ⊞ 676
Robitussin-PE ⊞ 677
Rocaltrol Capsules 1913
Rocephin Injectable Vials, ADD-Vantage (Less than 1%) 1914
▲ Roferon-A Injection (10% to 17%) 1916
▲ Rogaine Topical Solution (4.33%) 2357
Rondec 1975
Rondec-DM 1976
Rondec-TR Tablet 1975
▲ Roxanol (Among most frequent) 1991
▲ Roxicodone Tablets, Oral Solution & Intensol (Oxycodone) (Among most frequent) 1992
Rubex (Frequent) 739
Rufen Tablets (1 to 3%) 691
Rum-K Syrup 995
Ru-Tuss DE Tablets 694
Ru-Tuss II Capsules 693
Ru-Tuss with Hydrocodone 694
Ru-Tuss Tablets 693
▲ Rythmol Tablets (2.4 to 10.7%) 1184
Saluron 718
Salutensin/Salutensin-Demi 719

▲ Sandimmune (Less than 1 to 10%) 2024
Sandoglobulin I.V. 2027
▲ Sandostatin Injection (3.9%) 2029
Sansert Tablets 2031
Seconal Sodium Pulvules (Less than 1 in 100) 1296
Sectral Capsules (Up to 2%) 2520
Sedapap Tablets 50 mg/650 mg (Less frequent) 1360
▲ Seldane Tablets (7.6%) 1349
Seldane-D Extended-Release Tablets 1350
Senna X-Prep Bowel Evacuant Liquid (Rare) 1073
Sensorcaine (Rare) 631
▲ Septra (Most common) 813
▲ Septra I.V. Infusion (Most common) 808
▲ Septra I.V. Infusion ADD-Vantage Vials (Most common) 810
▲ Septra (Most common) 813
Ser-Ap-Es Tablets 881
Serentil 686
Serophene (clomiphene citrate tablets, USP) (Approximately 1 in 50 patients) 2186
Serpasil Tablets 883
Serpasil-Apresoline Tablets 884
Serpasil-Esidrix Tablets 886
Sinemet Tablets (Less frequent) 952
Sinemet CR Tablets (1.8%) 953
Sinequan 1960
Skelaxin 840
Slo-bid Gyrocaps 1847
▲ Slow-K Tablets (Among most common) 2281
Sodium Polystyrene Sulfonate Suspension 1993
Solganal Suspension (Rare) 2122
Solu-Medrol Sterile Powder 2363
Soma Compound w/Codeine Tablets 2390
Soma Compound Tablets 2389
Soma Tablets 2388
Sorbitrate (Uncommon) 1103
Sotradecol (Sodium Tetradecyl Sulfate Injection) 964
Spectrobid Tablets & Powder for Oral Suspension 1961
▲ St. Joseph Adult Chewable Aspirin (81 mg.) (7.3% of 4500 patients) ▣ 703
Stadol (Less than 1%) 721
Stelazine 2226
Stilphostrol Tablets and Ampuls 1609
Sublimaze Injection 1146
Sufenta Injection (Less than 1%) 1147
Suprax (Less than 2%) 1235
Surital Ampoules, Steri-Vials 1764
Surmontil Capsules 2524
Sus-Phrine Injection 1006
Symmetrel Capsules & Syrup (0.1-1%) 936
Synalgos-DC Capsules 2525
Syntocinon Injection 2032
TACE 12 and 25 mg 1353
T-PHYL (Uniphyl) 200 mg Tablets 1820
Tacaryl 2409
Talacen (Occasional) 2070
▲ Talwin Injection (Most common) 2071
Talwin Compound 2072
▲ Talwin Injection (Most common) 2071
Talwin Nx 2073
Tambocor Tablets (1-3%) 1315
Tao Capsules (Infrequent) 1963
Tapazole Tablets 1298
Tavist Syrup 2033
Tavist Tablets 2035
Tavist-D Tablets 2035
Tazicef for Injection (Less than 2%; 1 in 500 patients) 2231
Tazidime Vials, Faspak & ADD-Vantage (1 in 500) 1299
▲ Tegretol Chewable Tablets (Among most frequent) 654
▲ Tegretol Suspension (Among most frequent) 656
▲ Tegretol Tablets (Among most frequent) 654
Temaril Tablets, Syrup and Spansule Sustained Release Capsules 1085
▲ Ten-K Controlled-Release Tablets (Among most common) 2282
Tenoretic Tablets 1105
Tensilon Injectable 1123
Tenuate 1354
Terramycin Capsules 1786
Terramycin Intramuscular Solution 1964
Teslac Tablets 741
Thalitone Tablets 687
Theo-24 2179
Theo-Dur Sprinkle 1168
Theo-Dur Extended-Release Tablets 1166
Theolair 1317
Theolair-SR Tablets 1319
Theo-Organidin Elixir 2391
▲ TheoX Extended-Release Tablets (Among most consistent) 841
▲ TheraCys BCG Live (Intravesical) (Up to 16.1%) 898
Thera-Gesic 1614
Theragran Hematinic Tablets 605
Thioguanine Tablets, Tabloid Brand (Infrequent) 815
Thiosulfil Forte Tablets 2526
Thiotepa Parenteral 1240
Ticar for Injection 2236
Timentin for Injection 2239
Timolide Tablets 1547
Timoptic in Ocudose 1552
Timoptic Sterile Ophthalmic Solution 1550
Tofranil Ampuls 1038
Tofranil Tablets 1039
Tofranil-PM Capsules 1041
▲ Tolectin (200, 400 and 600 mg) (3 to 9%) 1379
▲ Tonocard Tablets (4.6-9.0%) 1554
Toradol IM Injection (1% or less) 2302
Trandate HCT Tablets 579
▲ Trandate Injection (4 of 100 patients) 577
Trandate Tablets (Less than 1% of 227 patients) 579
Transderm Scōp Transdermal Therapeutic System (Few patients) 887
▲ Trental (1.2% to 4.5%) 1099
▲ Trexan Tablets (Greater than 10%) 937
Triaminic Expectorant DH 1995
Triaminic Oral Infant Drops 1996
Triavil Tablets 1556
Tridione 557
Tri-Immunol Diphtheria & Tetanus Toxoids & Pertussis Vaccine, Adsorbed 1241
Trilafon (Occasional) 2123
Levlen/Tri-Levlen 665
▲ Trilisate (Less than 20%) 1822
Trimpex Tablets 1922
Trinalin Repetabs Tablets 1170
Tri-Norinyl 2304
▲ Triphasil-21 Tablets (10% or less) 2527
▲ Triphasil-28 Tablets (10% or less) 2532
Tussionex Extended-Release Suspension 988
Tussi-Organidin Liquid (Rare) 2391
Tylenol with Codeine 1381
▲ Tylox Capsules (Among most frequent) 1382
Ultracef Capsules, Tablets & Oral Suspension (Rarely) 722
Unasyn (Less than 1%) 1965
Unipen 2533
Uniphyl 400 mg Tablets 1823
Urecholine 1558
Urispas Tablets 2242
Urobiotic-250 Capsules 1968
Uroqid-Acid 661
Valpin 50 Tablets 941
Vaseretic Tablets (0.5% to 2.0%) 1559
Vasotec I.V. 1562
Vasotec Tablets (0.5% to 1%) 1564
Vasoxyl Injection 819
Velban Vials (Not common) 1305
Velosef Capsules and for Oral Suspension (Rare) 606
▲ Ventolin (6 of 104 patients) 583
▲ VePesid Capsules and Injection (31 to 43%) 741
Versed Injection (2.6%) 1924
Vibramycin Hyclate Capsules 1787
Vibramycin Hyclate Intravenous 1968
Vibramycin 1787
▲ Vicodin Tablets (Most frequent) 1187
▲ Vicodin ES Tablets (Among most frequent) 1189
Vira-A for Injection 1766
Visken Tablets (2% or fewer patients) 2036
Vivactil Tablets 1567
Voltaren Ophthalmic Sterile Ophthalmic Solution (1%) ◉ 268
Voltaren Tablets (Less than 1%) 1042
▲ Wellbutrin Tablets (22.9%) 821
Wigraine Tablets & Suppositories 1645
Winstrol Tablets 2075
▲ Wygesic Tablets (Most frequent) 2540
Wytensin Tablets (3% or less) 2542
▲ Xanax Tablets (9.6% to 22%) 2367
▲ Xylocaine Injections (Among most common) 637
Xylocaine Injections for Ventricular Arrhythmias 639
Xylocaine 2% Jelly 643
Xylocaine 5% Ointment 644
Xylocaine 10% Oral Spray 645
4% Xylocaine-MPF Sterile Solution 641
Xylocaine 2% Viscous Solution 646
▲ Yocon (Common) 1686
Yodoxin 1072
▲ Yutopar (10 to 15% (with IV administration)) 647
Zanosar Sterile Powder 2371
Zantac Injection and Zantac Injection Premixed 1063
Zantac 1065
Zarontin Capsules (Frequent) 1768
Zarontin Syrup (Frequent) 1769
Zaroxolyn Tablets 989
Zefazone Sterile Powder 2372
Zestoretic (1.4%) 2274
Zestril Tablets (1.3%) 2277
Zoladex (1% to 5%) 1110
Zovirax Capsules (2.5% to 2.7%) 824
▲ Zovirax Sterile Powder (Approximately 7%) 828
Zovirax (2.5% to 2.7%) 824
▲ Zydone Capsules (Most frequent) 941
Zyloprim Tablets (Less than 1%) 830

Vulva, dryness (see under Vagina, dryness)

Vulva, edema

Vagistat (Less than 1%) 1397

Vulva, swelling

Vagistat (Less than 1%) 1397

Vulvar disorder

Anafranil Capsules (Rare) 650

Vulvitis

Rogaine Topical Solution (0.91%) 2357
Zovirax Ointment 5% (0.3%) 827

Vulvovaginitis

Ansaid Tablets (Less than 1%) 2319

W

Walking disorders

Oncovin Solution Vials & Hyporets 1288
Tonocard Tablets (0.0-1.2%) 1554

Warmth

▲ Adalat Capsules (10 mg and 20 mg) (25%) 1587
Dopram Injectable 1860
Geref (sermorelin acetate for injection) 2560
Hyperstat I.V. Injection 2095
Marax Tablets & DF Syrup 1954
Miacalcin Injection 2017
Nicobid 1846
Nubain Injection (Less than 1%) 934
▲ Omnipaque (7 to 23%) 2552
Peptavlon 2563
Plendil Extended-Release Tablets (0.5% to 1.5%) 1526
▲ Procardia XL Tablets (25%) 1783
Protamine Sulfate Ampoules & Vials 1295
Quadrinal Tablets 1183
Recombivax HB (Less than 1%) 1544
Sandostatin Injection (Less than 1%) 2029
Slo-Niacin Tablets 2376
Stadol (Less than 1%) 721
Versed Injection (Less than 1%) 1924
Xanax Tablets (1.3%) 2367

Water intoxication

DDAVP Injection 1840
Methergine (Rare) 2016
Oxytocin Injection 2492
Pitocin Injection, Ampoules, Steri-Dose Syringes 1757
Syntocinon Injection 2032
Tegretol Chewable Tablets 654
Tegretol Suspension 656
Tegretol Tablets 654

Water retention (see also under Edema)

Android 1111
▲ Butazolidin Capsules & Tablets (3-9%) 1027
Hyperstat I.V. Injection 2095
Loniten Tablets 2346
Mediatric Capsules 2476
Premarin with Methyltestosterone 2515
Raudixin Tablets (Rare) 1803
Rogaine Topical Solution 2357
Solu-Medrol Sterile Powder 2363
Testred Capsules 1124

Weakness (see under Asthenia)

Weakness, feet

K-Phos Neutral Tablets 660
K-Phos Original Formula 'Sodium Free' Tablets (Less frequent) 660
Uroqid-Acid (Less frequent) 661

Weakness, hands

K-Phos Neutral Tablets 660
K-Phos Original Formula 'Sodium Free' Tablets (Less frequent) 660
Uroqid-Acid (Less frequent) 661

Weakness, legs

D.H.E. 45 Injection 2003
K-Phos M.F. Tablets 659
K-Phos Neutral Tablets 660
K-Phos Original Formula 'Sodium Free' Tablets (Less frequent) 660
K-Phos No. 2 Tablets 659
Lupron Injection (A few cases) 2310
Omnipaque (Rare) 2552
Uroqid-Acid (Less frequent) 661
Wigraine Tablets & Suppositories 1645

Weakness, local

Plendil Extended-Release Tablets (0.5% or greater) 1526
Timoptic Sterile Ophthalmic Solution 1550

Weakness, muscle

Amicar Syrup, Tablets, and Injection 1194
Atromid-S Capsules (Less often) 2435
Cardilate Oral/Sublingual Tablets 757
Cardura Tablets (1%) 1941
Cibalith-S 870
Compazine 2201
Decadron Phosphate Injection 1449
Depen Titratable Tablets 2379
Eskalith 2214
Floropryl Sterile Ophthalmic Ointment (Infrequent) 1473
Humorsol Sterile Ophthalmic Solution (Infrequent) 1475
Hydeltra-T.B.A. Sterile Suspension 1478
Hydrocortone Phosphate Injection, Sterile 1481
Hydrocortone Tablets 1482
Kemadrin Tablets 771
Lithane Tablets 1596
Lithium Carbonate Capsules & Tablets 1984
Lithobid Tablets 870
Metubine Iodide Vials 1285
Mevacor Tablets 1505
Naprosyn Suspension (Less than 1%) 2297
Norcuron 1642
Nuromax Injection 794
Omnipaque (Rare) 2552
Protopam Chloride for Injection 2518
Rimactane Capsules 879
Sodium Polystyrene Sulfonate Suspension 1993
Stelazine 2226

Weight change, increase or decrease

Asendin Tablets (Less than 1%) 1196
Cycrin Tablets 2449
Demulen 2161
Enovid 2161
Estratest 2245
Jenest-28 Tablets 1636
Norlutate 1754
Norlutin 1755
Ortho-Cyclen Tablets 1658
TACE 12 and 25 mg 1353
Trexan Tablets (Less than 1%) 937

Weight changes, unspecified

Amen 833
Ansaid Tablets (1-3%) 2319
Aygestin Tablets 2437
Cytotec (Infrequent) 2159
Depo-Provera Sterile Aqueous Suspension 2336
Diethylstilbestrol Tablets 1258

Elavil ... 2269
Estraderm Transdermal System ... 866
Estrovis ... 1721
Flexeril Tablets (Rare) ... 1471
Klonopin Tablets ... 1902
Larodopa Tablets (Infrequent) ... 1905
Levlen/Tri-Levlen ... 665
Lodine Capsules (Less than 1%) ... 2468
Lo/Ovral Tablets ... 2471
Lo/Ovral-28 Tablets ... 2476
Loestrin ... 1728
Loxitane ... 1213
Ludiomil Tablets ... 874
Marax Tablets & DF Syrup (Possible, with large doses) ... 1954
▲Marplan Tablets (Among most frequent) ... 1906
Menrium Tablets ... 1934
Moban Tablets & Concentrate ... 932
Monopril Tablets (0.2 to 1.0%) ... 1406
Nordette-21 Tablets ... 2481
Nordette-28 Tablets ... 2483
Norethin ... 2133
Norlestrin ... 1746
Norpramin Tablets ... 1340
Ovral Tablets ... 2490
Ovral-28 Tablets ... 2491
Ovrette Tablets ... 2492
Prolixin Decanoate ... 1795
Prolixin Elixir ... 1793
Prolixin Enanthate ... 1796
Prolixin Injection ... 1791
Prolixin Oral Concentrate ... 1792
Prolixin Tablets ... 1793
Provera Tablets ... 2356
Stilphostrol Tablets and Ampuls ... 1609
Trental (Less than 1%) ... 1099
Triavil Tablets ... 1556
Levlen/Tri-Levlen ... 665
Triphasil-21 Tablets ... 2527
Triphasil-28 Tablets ... 2532
Vivactil Tablets ... 1567

Weight decrease (see under Weight loss)

Weight gain

AeroBid Inhaler System (1-3%) ... 995
Aldoclor Tablets ... 1413
Aldomet Ester HCl Injection ... 1417
Aldomet Oral ... 1415
Aldoril Tablets ... 1418
Altace Capsules (Less than 1%) ... 1086
▲Anafranil Capsules (2% to 18%) ... 650
Atromid-S Capsules ... 2435
Brevicon ... 2304
BuSpar (Rare) ... 1401
Butazolidin Capsules & Tablets ... 1027
Cardizem Tablets-30 mg, 60 mg, 90 mg and 120 mg (Less than 1%) ... 1329
Cardizem SR Capsules-60 mg, 90 mg and 120 mg (Less than 1%) ... 1327
Cardura Tablets (0.5% to 1%) ... 1941
Catapres Tablets (About 1 in 100 patients) ... 676
Catapres-TTS (1%) ... 677
Centrax ... 1693
Children's Advil Suspension ... 2426
Cholybar ... 1705
Cibalith-S ... 870
▲Clozaril Tablets (4%) ... 2000
Combipres Tablets (About 1%) ... 678
Compazine ... 2201
Corgard Tablets (1 to 5 1000 patients) ... 701
Cortifoam ... 1827
Cortone Acetate Sterile Suspension ... 1437
Cortone Acetate Tablets ... 1439
Corzide Tablets (1 to 5 of 1000 patients) ... 702
Dalalone D.P. Injectable ... 999
Danocrine Capsules ... 2046
Decadron Elixir ... 1445
Decadron Phosphate Injection ... 1449
Decadron Phosphate Respihaler ... 1454
Decadron Phosphate Turbinaire ... 1456
Decadron Phosphate with Xylocaine Injection, Sterile ... 1451
Decadron Tablets ... 1447
Decadron-LA Sterile Suspension ... 1457
Depakene Capsules & Syrup ... 511
Depakote ... 512
Desyrel and Desyrel Dividose (Greatar than 1%) ... 1404
Diupres Tablets ... 1461
Endep Tablets ... 1927
Enduronyl ... 518
Esimil Tablets ... 864
Eskalith ... 2214
Estinyl Tablets ... 2085
Estrace ... 1385
Estrace Vaginal Cream ... 1388
Estradurin ... 2452
Etrafon ... 2087
Feldene Capsules (Less than 1%) ... 1777
Harmonyl Tablets ... 528
▲Hismanal Tablets (3.6%) ... 1138
Hydeltrasol Injection, Sterile ... 1476
Hydeltra-T.B.A. Sterile Suspension ... 1478
Hydrocortone Acetate Sterile Suspension ... 1479
Hydrocortone Phosphate Injection, Sterile ... 1481
Hydrocortone Tablets ... 1482
Hydromox R Tablets ... 1209
Hydropres Tablets ... 1485
▲Hylorel Tablets (44.3%) ... 975
Hytrin Tablets (0.5%) ... 529
Indocin Capsules (Less than 1%) ... 1487
Indocin I.V. (Less than 1%) ... 1490
Indocin (Less than 1%) ... 1487
Ismelin Tablets ... 869
K-Phos M.F. Tablets ... 659
K-Phos Neutral Tablets ... 660
K-Phos No. 2 Tablets ... 659
Kerlone Tablets (Less than 2%) ... 2172
Limbitrol ... 1933
Lioresal Tablets ... 1031
Lithane Tablets ... 1596
Lithium Carbonate Capsules & Tablets ... 1984
Lithobid Tablets ... 870
Lupron Depot 7.5 mg (Less than 5%) ... 2311
Lupron Injection ... 2310
Maxair Inhaler (Less than 1%) ... 1311
Mediatric Capsules ... 2476
Megace Tablets (Frequent) ... 732
Mellaril ... 2011
Mesantoin Tablets ... 2013
Metrodin (urofollitropin for injection) ... 2182
Micronor Tablets ... 1667
Modicon ... 1667
Motrin Tablets ... 2351
Nardil (Common) ... 1742
Navane Capsules and Concentrate ... 1954
Navane Intramuscular ... 1956
Norinyl ... 2304
Norpace (1 to 3%) ... 2177
Norplant System ... 2484
Nor-Q D Tablets ... 2304
Norzine ... 1818
Ogen ... 540
Orap Tablets ... 1020
Oreticyl ... 545
Ortho Dienestrol Cream ... 1664
Ortho-Novum ... 1667
Orudis Capsules (Less than 1%) ... 2488
Ovcon ... 1391
PMB 200 and PMB 400 ... 2504
Pamelor ... 2019
PediaProfen Suspension ... 1363
Pentaspan Injection ... 949
Permax Tablets (1.6%) ... 1291
Premarin Intravenous ... 2508
Premarin with Methyltestosterone ... 2515
Premarin Tablets ... 2510
Premarin Vaginal Cream ... 2512
Prilosec Delayed-Release Capsules (Less than 1%) ... 1530
Procardia XL Tablets (1% or less) ... 1783
ProSom Tablets (Rare) ... 554
Prozac Pulvules (Infrequent) ... 920
Questran Light ... 711
Questran Powder ... 710
Raudixin Tablets ... 1803
Rauzide Tablets ... 1804
Rogaine Topical Solution (1.24%) ... 2357
Salutensin/Salutensin-Demi ... 719
Sansert Tablets ... 2031
Ser-Ap-Es Tablets ... 881
Serentil ... 686
Serophene (clomiphene citrate tablets, USP) (Less than 1 in 100 patients) ... 2186
Serpasil Tablets ... 883
Serpasil-Apresoline Tablets ... 884
Serpasil-Esidrix Tablets ... 886
Sinemet Tablets ... 952
Sinemet CR Tablets ... 953
Sinequan (Occasional) ... 1960
Stelazine (Occasional) ... 2226
Stilphostrol Tablets and Ampuls ... 1609
Surmontil Capsules ... 2524
▲Synarel Nasal Solution (8% of patients) ... 2300
Tacaryl ... 2409
Taractan ... 1920
Temaril Tablets, Syrup and Spansule Sustained Release Capsules ... 1085
Tofranil Ampuls ... 1038
Tofranil Tablets ... 1039
Tofranil-PM Capsules ... 1041
▲Tolectin (200, 400 and 600 mg) (3 to 9%) ... 1379
Torecan ... 1993
Trilafon ... 2123
Trilisate (Less than 1%) ... 1822
Tri-Norinyl ... 2304
Uroqid-Acid (Less frequent) ... 661
Visken Tablets (2% or fewer patients) ... 2036
▲Wellbutrin Tablets (9.4% to 13.6%) ... 821
Xanax Tablets (2.7% to 27.2%) ... 2367
Zoladex (1% to 5%) ... 1110

Weight loss

Accutane Capsules (Less than 1%) ... 1878
▲Actimmune (6%) ... 1046
▲Anafranil Capsules (Up to 7%) ... 650
Blenoxane ... 724
Blocadren Tablets ... 1429
Brevicon ... 2304
BuSpar ... 1401
Calcijex Calcitriol Injection ... 506
Calderol Capsules ... 1635
Capoten ... 2255
Capozide ... 2258
Cardura Tablets (Less than 0.5% of 3960 patients) ... 1941
Celontin ... 1692
Cholybar ... 1705
Cibalith-S ... 870
Cogentin ... 1435
Cylert Tablets ... 510
Daranide Tablets ... 1445
Depakene Capsules & Syrup ... 511
Depakote ... 512
Desyrel and Desyrel Dividose ... 1404
Dexedrine ... 2206
Eldepryl (1 of 49 patients) ... 2250
Elspar ... 1470
Endep Tablets ... 1927
Eskalith ... 2214
Estinyl Tablets ... 2085
Estrace ... 1385
Estrace Vaginal Cream ... 1388
Estradurin ... 2452
Etrafon ... 2087
Feldene Capsules (Less than 1%) ... 1777
Floxin Tablets (Less than 1%) ... 1652
▲Fungizone Intravenous (Among most common) ... 2262
Garamycin Injectable ... 2093
▲Hylorel Tablets (42.2%) ... 975
▲Intron A (Up to 5%) ... 2097
Lamprene Capsules ... 1030
Limbitrol ... 1933
Lithane Tablets ... 1596
Lithium Carbonate Capsules & Tablets ... 1984
Lithobid Tablets ... 870
Lopid Capsules and Tablets ... 1736
Lozol Tablets ... 1843
Mediatric Capsules ... 2476
Methadone Hydrochloride Diskets ... 1284
Micronor Tablets ... 1667
Modicon ... 1667
Myleran Tablets ... 790
Norinyl ... 2304
Ogen ... 540
Oncovin Solution Vials & Hyporets ... 1288
Orap Tablets ... 1020
Ortho Dienestrol Cream ... 1664
Ortho-Novum ... 1667
Orudis Capsules (Less than 1%) ... 2488
Ovcon ... 1391
PMB 200 and PMB 400 ... 2504
Pamelor ... 2019
Paradione Capsules ... 548
Permax Tablets (Frequent) ... 1291
Phenurone Tablets ... 552
Plaquenil Sulfate Tablets ... 2067
Premarin Intravenous ... 2508
Premarin with Methyltestosterone ... 2515
Premarin Tablets ... 2510
Premarin Vaginal Cream ... 2512
ProSom Tablets (Rare) ... 554
Prozac Pulvules (Frequent) ... 920
Questran Light ... 711
Questran Powder ... 710
Retrovir (0.8%) ... 802
Ritalin ... 880
Rocaltrol Capsules ... 1913
▲Roferon-A Injection (14% to 25%) ... 1916
Sandimmune (Rare) ... 2024
Sansert Tablets ... 2031
Sinemet Tablets ... 952
Sinemet CR Tablets ... 953
Stilphostrol Tablets and Ampuls ... 1609
Surmontil Capsules ... 2524
Synarel Nasal Solution (1% of patients) ... 2300
Tegison Capsules ... 1881
Timolide Tablets ... 1547
Timoptic in Ocudose ... 1552
Timoptic Sterile Ophthalmic Solution ... 1550
Tofranil Ampuls ... 1038
Tofranil Tablets ... 1039
Tofranil-PM Capsules ... 1041
▲Tolectin (200, 400 and 600 mg) (3 to 9%) ... 1379
Tridione ... 557
Tri-Norinyl ... 2304
Vira-A for Injection ... 1766
Voltaren Tablets (Rare) ... 1042
▲Wellbutrin Tablets (23.2% to 28%) ... 821
▲Xanax Tablets (2.3% to 22.6%) ... 2367
Zarontin Capsules (Frequent) ... 1768
Zarontin Syrup (Frequent) ... 1769

Wenckebach block

Lanoxin Elixir Pediatric ... 775
Lanoxin Injection ... 778
Lanoxin Injection Pediatric ... 781
Lanoxin Tablets ... 783

Wenckebach's period (see under A-V conduction, prolongation)

Wheals

Astramorph/PF Injection, USP (Preservative-Free) ... 618
▲Atgam Sterile Solution (1 in 8 patients; 27%) ... 2320
Attenuvax (Rare) ... 1424
Biavax II ... 1427
Demerol ... 2047
Desferal Vials ... 862
Duramorph ... 960
Infumorph 200 and Infumorph 500 Sterile Solutions ... 962
M-M-R II ... 1494
M-R-VAX II ... 1496
Mepergan Injection ... 2479
Meruvax II ... 1503
Mumpsvax (Extremely rare) ... 1513
Sandostatin Injection (1.0%) ... 2029

Wheezing

Actifed with Codeine Cough Syrup ... 752
▲Adalat Capsules (10 mg and 20 mg) (6%) ... 1587
▲AeroBid Inhaler System (3-9%) ... 995
Azmacort Inhaler (Infrequent) ... 1837
Beconase AQ Nasal Spray (Extremely rare) ... 574
Beconase Inhalation Aerosol & Refill (Extremely rare) ... 574
Blenoxane (1%) ... 724
Brethaire Inhaler ... 1024
Brevibloc Injection (Less than 1%) ... 942
Cartrol Tablets (Rare) ... 507
Cholybar ... 1705
Clozaril Tablets (Less than 1%) ... 2000
Comhist LA Capsules ... 1618
▲CytoGam (Less than 5.0%) ... 891
Deconamine ... 663
Depen Titratable Tablets ... 2379
Dimetane-DC Cough Syrup ... 1857
Dimetane-DX Cough Syrup ... 1858
Diprivan Injection (Less than 1%) ... 2267
Fungizone Intravenous ... 2262
Gamimune N Immune Globulin Intravenous (Human) ... 1572
Hespan Injection ... 948
Humulin 70/30, 100 Units (Less common) ... 1267
Humulin BR, 100 Units (Less common) ... 1268
Humulin L, 100 Units (Less common) ... 1268
Humulin U, 100 Units (Less common) ... 1272
Hyskon Hysteroscopy Fluid (Rare) ... 1162
Beef Regular, 100 Units ... 1275
Intal Capsules (Less than 1 in 10,000 patients to 1 in 25 patients) ... 978
▲Intal Inhaler (Among most frequent) ... 979
Intal Nebulizer Solution ... 980
Intron A (Less than 1%) ... 2097
Lopressor Ampuls (1%) ... 1032

Lopressor HCT Tablets (1 in 100) 1034
Lopressor Tablets (1%) 1032
Maxair Inhaler (Less than 1%) 1311
Nasalcrom Nasal Solution 986
Nicorette 1335
Nimotop Capsules (Less than 1%) 1607
Normodyne Injection (1%) 2108
Nuromax Injection 794
Optimine Tablets 2115
Ornade Spansule Capsules 2221
▲ Orthoclone OKT3 Sterile Solution (13%) 1645
PBZ Tablets & Elixir 1037
PBZ-SR Tablets 1037
Pentaspan Injection 949
Periactin 1525
Platinol (Occasional) 737
Platinol-AQ Injection (Occasional) 738
Polaramine 2116
▲ Procardia XL Tablets (6%) 1783
Pronestyl Capsules and Tablets 1800
Pronestyl Injection 1798
Prostin VR Pediatric Sterile Solution (Less than 1%) 2355
Proventil Solutions for Inhalation 0.5% and 0.083% (1%) 2118
Quadrinal Tablets 1183
Questran Light 711
Questran Powder 710
Rifadin 1345
Ru-Tuss II Capsules 693
Sandimmune 2024
Sectral Capsules (Up to 2%) 2520
Tacaryl 2409
Tavist Syrup 2033
Tavist Tablets 2035
Tavist-D Tablets 2035
Temaril Tablets, Syrup and Spansule Sustained Release Capsules 1085
Tenoretic Tablets (Up to 3%) 1105
Tenormin Tablets and I.V. Injection (Up to 3%) 1107
Tonocard Tablets 1554
Tracrium Injection (1 out of 875) 817
Trandate Injection (1 of 100 patients) 577
Triaminic Expectorant DH 1995
Triaminic Oral Infant Drops 1996
Trinalin Repetabs Tablets 1170
Vancenase AQ Nasal Spray 0.042% (Extremely rare) 2127
Vancocin HCl, Vials & ADD-Vantage 1302
Ventolin Inhalation Solution (1%) 583
Versed Injection (Less than 1%) 1924
Visken Tablets (2% or fewer patients) 2036

White-clot syndrome

Calciparine Injection (Rare) 925
Heparin Lock Flush Solution 2456
Heparin Sodium Injection 2457
Heparin Sodium Injection, USP, Sterile Solution (Rare) 2342

Withdrawal reactions

Anafranil Capsules (Rare) 650
Astramorph/PF Injection, USP (Preservative-Free) 618
B & O No. 15A & No. 16A Supprettes 2395
Butisol Sodium Elixir & Tablets 2377
Calciparine Injection (Rare) 925
Catapres Tablets 676
Dalmane Capsules 1927
Darvon-N/Darvocet-N 1254
Darvon Compound-65 Pulvules 1256
Darvon-N Suspension & Tablets 1254
Dexedrine 2206
Dilaudid Cough Syrup 1174
Dilaudid 1173
[illegible]
Halcion Tablets 2340
Heparin Sodium Vials (Rare) 1264
Infumorph 200 and Infumorph 500 Sterile Solutions 962
Klonopin Tablets 1902
Libritabs Tablets 1930
Librium Capsules 1931
Librium Injectable 1932
Lortab ASA Tablets 2414
Lortab 2412
MS Contin Tablets 1814
MSIR 1817
Mebaral Tablets 2061
Nembutal Sodium Capsules 534
Nembutal Sodium Solution 536
Nembutal Sodium Suppositories 538
Pamelor 2019
Phenobarbital Elixir and Tablets 1293
Placidyl Capsules (One report in an infant) 553
Procardia XL Tablets 1783
ProSom Tablets 554
Tranxene 556
Valium Injectable 1937
Valium Tablets 1939
Valrelease Capsules 1923
Xanax Tablets 2367

Wound dehiscence

Atgam Sterile Solution (More than 1%, less than 5%) 2320
Hemopad Absorbable Collagen Hemostat 627
INSTAT Collagen Absorbable Hemostat 1151

Wound healing, impaired

AK-Cide Sterile Ophthalmic Ointment & Suspension ◎ 202
AK-Spore H.C. ◎ 206
AK-Taine ◎ 207
AK-Trol Ointment & Suspension ◎ 207
Aristocort Suspension 1008
Aristospan Suspension 1011
Blephamide 586
Celestone Soluspan Suspension 2081
Cetapred Ointment ◎ 220
Chloromycetin Hydrocortisone Ophthalmic 1694
Cortenema 2244
Cortifoam 1827
Cortisporin Ophthalmic Ointment Sterile 758
Cortisporin Ophthalmic Suspension Sterile 759
Cortone Acetate Sterile Suspension 1437
Cortone Acetate Tablets 1439
Dalalone D.P. Injectable 999
Decadron Elixir 1445
Decadron Phosphate Injection 1449
Decadron Phosphate Respihaler 1454
Decadron Phosphate Turbinaire 1456
Decadron Phosphate with Xylocaine Injection, Sterile 1451
Decadron Tablets 1447
Decadron-LA Sterile Suspension 1457
Deltasone Tablets 2332
Depo-Medrol Sterile Aqueous Suspension 2334
Dexacidin ◎ 272
FML Forte Liquifilm ◎ 245
FML Liquifilm ◎ 244
FML-S Sterile Ophthalmic Suspension ◎ 246
Fluoracaine ◎ 208
Hydeltrasol Injection, Sterile 1476
Hydeltra-T.B.A. Sterile Suspension 1478
Hydrocortone Acetate Sterile Suspension 1479
Hydrocortone Phosphate Injection, Sterile 1481
Hydrocortone Tablets 1482
Isopto Cetapred Suspension ◎ 220
Kenalog-10 Injection 2402
Kenalog-40 Injection 2403
Maxitrol Ophthalmic Ointment/Suspension ◎ 223
Medrol 2348
Metimyd ◎ 306
NeoDecadron Sterile Ophthalmic Ointment 1517
NeoDecadron Sterile Ophthalmic Solution 1518
Ophthocort ◎ 301
Pediapred Oral Liquid 987
Poly-Pred Liquifilm ◎ 250
Pred-G Liquifilm Sterile Ophthalmic Suspension ◎ 252
Pred-G S.O.P. Sterile Ophthalmic [illegible]
Solu-Cortef Sterile Powder 2361
Solu-Medrol Sterile Powder 2363
Terra-Cortril Ophthalmic Suspension 1963
TobraDex Ophthalmic Suspension and Ointment ◎ 228
Vasocidin Ointment ◎ 275
Vasocidin Ophthalmic Solution ◎ 276

Wound infection

▲ Sandimmune (7.0 to 10.1%) 2024

WBC, immature

Cipro I.V. (Infrequent) 1592
Clozaril Tablets (1%) 2000

WBC counts, fluctuation

Bumex (0.3%) 1895
Butazolidin Capsules & Tablets 1027
Cytotec (Infrequent) 2159
Dopram Injectable 1860
Doral Tablets (2.6%) 2383
Sterile FUDR 1898
Halcion Tablets (1.7 to 2.1%) 2340
▲ Intron A (10% to 22%) 2097
Lopid Capsules and Tablets 1736
Polymyxin B Sulfate, Aerosporin Brand Sterile Powder 798
Primaxin I.M. 1532
Quinidex Extentabs 1868
▲ Synarel Nasal Solution (10% to 15%) 2300
Talwin Compound (Rare) 2072
▲ Tegison Capsules (10-25%) 1881
Tornalate 2074
Xanax Tablets (1.4% to 2.3%) 2367

X

Xanthopsia

Aldactazide 2150
Aldoclor Tablets 1413
Aldoril Tablets 1418
Apresazide Capsules 854
Apresoline-Esidrix Tablets 857
Capozide 2258
Combipres Tablets 678
Corzide Tablets (Occasional) 702
Diucardin Tablets 2450
Diulo 2129
Diupres Tablets 1461
Diuril Oral Suspension 1464
Diuril Sodium Intravenous 1463
Diuril Tablets 1464
Dyazide Capsules 2208
Enduron Tablets 517
Enduronyl 518
Esidrix Tablets 863
Esimil Tablets 864
Exna Tablets 1862
HydroDIURIL Tablets 1484
Hydromox R Tablets 1209
Hydromox Tablets 1208
Hydropres Tablets 1485
Inderide Tablets 2463
Inderide LA Long Acting Capsules 2465
Lanoxicaps 772
Lanoxin Elixir Pediatric 775
Lanoxin Injection 778
Lanoxin Injection Pediatric 781
Lanoxin Tablets 783
Lasix 1093
Lopressor HCT Tablets 1034
Lozol Tablets 1843
Maxzide 1215
Minizide Capsules 1779
Mintezol 1510
Moduretic Tablets 1510
Mykrox ½ mg Tablets 984
Naturetin Tablets (Occasional) 1789
Normodyne Tablets 2110
Normozide Tablets 2112
Oretic Tablets 544
Oreticyl 545
Prinzide Tablets 1540
Quadrinal Tablets 1183
Rauzide Tablets 1804
Renese Tablets 1785
Renese-R Tablets 1786
Saluron 718
Salutensin/Salutensin-Demi 719
Ser-Ap-Es Tablets 881
Serpasil-Esidrix Tablets 886
Tenoretic Tablets 1105
Thalitone Tablets 687
Timolide Tablets 1547
Trandate HCT Tablets 579
Vaseretic Tablets 1559
Zaroxolyn Tablets 989
Zestoretic 2274

Xeromycteria

▲ Accutane Capsules (80%) 1878
▲ Actifed with Codeine Cough Syrup (Among most frequent) 752
Benadryl Capsules 1691
Benadryl Injection 1692
Catapres Tablets 676
Catapres-TTS 677
Combipres Tablets 678
Comhist LA Capsules 1618
Cyclomydril ◎ 216
▲ Decadron Phosphate Turbinaire (Most common) 1456
Deconamine 663
▲ Dimetane-DC Cough Syrup (Most frequent) 1857
Dimetane-DX Cough Syrup (Among most frequent) 1858
IOPIDINE ◎ 232
Marax Tablets & DF Syrup 1954
▲ Norpace (3 to 9%) 2177
Norzine 1818
Optimine Tablets 2115
Ornade Spansule Capsules 2221
PBZ Tablets & Elixir 1037
PBZ-SR Tablets 1037
Periactin 1525
Polaramine 2116
Ru-Tuss II Capsules 693
▲ Seldane Tablets (4.8%) 1349
▲ Seldane-D Extended-Release Tablets (21.7%) 1350
Tavist Syrup 2033
Tavist Tablets 2035
Tavist-D Tablets 2035
▲ Tegison Capsules (Greater than 75%) 1881
Torecan 1993
Triaminic Expectorant DH 1995
Triaminic Oral Infant Drops 1996
Trinalin Repetabs Tablets 1170

Xerophthalmia

Accutane Capsules (Rare) 1878
Betoptic Sterile Ophthalmic Solution (Small numbers of patients) 569
Betoptic S Sterile Ophthalmic Suspension (Small numbers of patients) 570
Blocadren Tablets 1429
Catapres Tablets 676
Catapres-TTS 677
Children's Advil Suspension (Less than 1%) 2426
Combipres Tablets 678
Corgard Tablets (1 to 5 1000 patients) 701
Corzide Tablets (1 to 5 of 1000 patients) 702
Dipentum Capsules (Rare) 1160
Inderal (Rare) 2459
Inderal LA Long Acting Capsules (Rare) 2461
Inderide Tablets (Rare) 2463
Inderide LA Long Acting Capsules 2465
Intron A (1% or less) 2097
IOPIDINE ◎ 232
Kerlone Tablets (Less than 2%) 2172
Mintezol 1510
Motrin Tablets 2351
Normozide Tablets 2112
Oculinum for Injecton 587
PediaProfen Suspension (Less than 1%) 1363
Rēv-Eyes Ophthalmic Eyedrops 0.5% (Less frequently) ◎ 312
Sectral Capsules (Up to 2%) 2520
▲ Tegison Capsules (1-10%) 1881
Tenormin Tablets and I.V. Injection 1107
Timolide Tablets 1547
Timoptic in Ocudose 1552
Timoptic Sterile Ophthalmic Solution 1550
Trandate HCT Tablets 579
Vaseretic Tablets 1559
Vasotec I.V. 1562
Vasotec Tablets 1564

Xerosis cutis

Cibalith-S 870
Eskalith 2214
Lithane Tablets 1596
Lithium Carbonate Capsules & Tablets 1984
Lithobid Tablets 870

Xerostomia

▲ Accutane Capsules (80%) 1878
▲ Actifed with Codeine Cough Syrup [illegible]
Adipex-P Tablets and Capsules 1019
Akineton 1171
Aldactone 2152
Aldoclor Tablets 1413
Aldomet Ester HCl Injection 1417
Aldomet Oral 1415
Aldoril Tablets 1418
Alferon N Injection (One patient) 1809
Altace Capsules (Less than 1%) 1086
▲ Anafranil Capsules (63% to 84%) 650
Ana-Kit Anaphylaxis Emergency Treatment Kit 1100
Anatuss LA Tablets 1359
Ancobon Capsules 1886
Ansaid Tablets (Less than 1%) 2319
Antivert, Antivert/25 Tablets, Antivert/25 Chewable Tablets & Antivert/50 Tablets 1940

Arco-Lase Plus Tablets 607
Arfonad Ampuls 1887
▲ Artane (30% to 50%) 1195
▲ Asendin Tablets (14%) 1196
Atarax Tablets & Syrup 1941
Atrohist Sprinkle Capsules 558
Atrovent Inhalation Aerosol (2.4%) 675
Azmacort Inhaler 1837
B & O No. 15A & No. 16A Supprettes 2395
Beclovent Inhalation Aerosol and Refill (A few patients) 572
Bellergal-S Tablets (Rare) 1998
Benadryl Capsules 1691
Benadryl Injection 1692
▲ Bentyl (33%) 1322
Biphetamine Capsules 973
Bonine Tablets 1773
Bontril Slow-Release 834
Brethine Ampuls (Less than 0.5%) 1026
Brevibloc Injection (Less than 1%) 942
Brexin L.A. Capsules 2078
Bromfed 1615
Bucladin-S Softab Chewable Tablets (Occasional) 2264
Bumex (0.1%) 1895
▲ BuSpar (3%) 1401
Calan SR Caplets (1% or less) 2157
Calan Tablets (1% or less) 2155
Calcijex Calcitriol Injection 506
Calderol Capsules 1635
Cantil Tablets 1326
Capoten (0.5 to 2%) 2255
Capozide (0.5 to 2%) 2258
Carafate Tablets (Less than 0.5%) 1326
Cardene Capsules (0.4-1.4%) 2290
Cardizem Tablets-30 mg, 60 mg, 90 mg and 120 mg 1329
Cardizem SR Capsules-60 mg, 90 mg and 120 mg (Less than 1%) 1327
Cardura Tablets (2%) 1941
▲ Catapres Tablets (40 of 100 patients) 676
▲ Catapres-TTS (About 40%) 677
Centrax (Less frequent) 1693
Children's Advil Suspension (Less than 1%) 2426
Cibalith-S 870
Cipro I.V. (1% or less) 1592
Clinoril Tablets (Less than 1%) 1433
▲ Clozaril Tablets (More than 5 to 6%) 2000
Codimal 846
Cogentin 1435
▲ Combipres Tablets (40%) 678
Comhist LA Capsules 1618
Compazine 2201
Corgard Tablets (1 to 5 1000 patients) 701
Corzide Tablets (1 to 5 of 1000 patients) 702
Cyclogyl ⊙ 215
Cyclomydril ⊙ 216
Cystospaz 2395
Dalgan Injection (Less than 1%) 620
Dalmane Capsules (Rare) 1927
Daraprim Tablets (Rare) 761
Darbid Tablets 2205
Deconamine 663
Demerol 2047
Demser Capsules (Infrequent) 1460
Deprol Tablets 2382
Desoxyn Gradumet Tablets 514
Desyrel and Desyrel Dividose (Greater than 1%) 1404
Dexedrine 2206
Didrex Tablets 2338
Dilaudid-HP Injection 1175
Dimacol Caplets ▣ 672
▲ Dimetane-DC Cough Syrup (Most frequent) 1857
Dimetane-DX Cough Syrup (Among most frequent) 1858
Dipentum Capsules (Rare) 1160
Diprivan Injection (Less than 1%) 2267
Ditropan 1332
Diulo 2129
Diupres Tablets 1461
Diuril Sodium Intravenous 1463
Dolophine Hydrochloride Ampoules & Vials 1260
Dolophine Hydrochloride Tablets 1261
Donnagel (Rare) ▣ 675
Donnagel-PG (Rare) 1858
Donnatal 1858
Donnatal Extentabs 1859
Donnatal Tablets 1858
Donnazyme Tablets 1860
Doral Tablets (1.5%) 2383
Dorcol Children's Liquid Cold Formula (Occasional) ▣ 686
▲ Duragesic Transdermal System (10% or more) 1133
Dyazide Capsules 2208
DynaCirc Capsules (0.5% to 1%) 2004
Dyrenium Capsules (Rare) 2210
Elavil 2269
▲ Eldepryl (3 of 49 patients) 2250
Emete-con Intramuscular/Intravenous 1950
Endep Tablets 1927
Enduronyl 518
Esimil Tablets 864
Eskalith 2214
▲ Ethmozine Tablets (2%-5%) 946
Etrafon 2087
Fastin Capsules 2216
Fedahist Gyrocaps 2145
Fedahist Timecaps 2145
Feldene Capsules (Less than 1%) 1777
Fiorinal with Codeine Capsules (Infrequent) 2008
Flagyl Tablets 2170
▲ Flexeril Tablets (7% to 27%) 1471
Floxin Tablets (1% to 3%) 1652
Geocillin Tablets 1951
Guaifed Syrup ▣ 629
Halcion Tablets (Rare) 2340
Haldol Decanoate 1375
Haldol Injection, Tablets and Concentrate 1373
Harmonyl Tablets 528
▲ Hismanal Tablets (5.2%) 1138
HydroDIURIL Tablets 1484
Hydropres Tablets 1485
Hylorel Tablets (1.7%) 975
Hyperstat I.V. Injection 2095
Hytrin Tablets (At least 1%) 529
Imodium Capsules 1139
▲ Intron A (2% to 28%) 2097
Inversine Tablets 1492
Ionamin Capsules 981
IOPIDINE ⊙ 2:2
Ismelin Tablets 869
Isoptin Oral Tablets (Less than 1%) 1179
Isoptin SR Sustained Release Tablets (Less than 1%) 1181
Isopto Hyoscine ⊙ 222
Kemadrin Tablets 771
Kerlone Tablets (Less than 2%) 2172
Kinesed Tablets 2272
Klonopin Tablets 1902
Kutrase Capsules 2146
Larodopa Tablets (Relatively frequent) 1905
Levsin/Levsinex 2147
Librax Capsules 1929
▲ Limbitrol (Among most frequent) 1933
Lioresal Tablets (Rare) 1031
Lithane Tablets 1596
Lithium Carbonate Capsules & Tablets 1984
Lithobid Tablets 870
Lodine Capsules (Less than 1%) 2468
Lopressor Ampuls (1%) 1032
Lopressor HCT Tablets (1 in 100 patients) 1034
Lopressor Tablets (1%) 1032
Loxitane 1213
Lozol Tablets (Less than 5%) 1843
▲ Ludiomil Tablets (22%) 874
▲ Lupron Depot 3.75 mg (Among most frequent) 2312
MS Contin Tablets (Infrequent) 1814
MSIR (Infrequent) 1817
Marax Tablets & DF Syrup (Occasional) 1954
▲ Marinol (Dronabinol) Capsules (3%) 1985
▲ Marplan Tablets (Among most frequent) 1906
Matulane Capsules 1907
Maxair Inhaler (Less than 1%) 1311
Maxzide 1215
Mellaril 2011
Mepergan Injection 2479
Methadone Hydrochloride Diskets 1284
Methadone Hydrochloride Oral Solution & Tablets 1987
Mexitil Capsules (2.8%) 680
Midamor Tablets (Less than or equal to 1%) 1508
Minipress Capsules (1-4%) 1778
Minizide Capsules (Rare) 1779
Mintezol 1510
Moban Tablets & Concentrate 932
Moduretic Tablets 1510
Monopril Tablets (0.2 to 1.0%) 1406
Motofen Tablets (1 in 30) 836
Motrin Tablets (Less than 1%) 2351
Mydriacyl ⊙ 225
Mykrox ½ mg Tablets (Less than 2%) 984
Naldecon Syrup, Tablets, Pediatric Drops and Pediatric Syrup 709
Nalfon Pulvules & Tablets (Less than 1%) 919
Nardil (Common) 1742
Navane Capsules and Concentrate 1954
Navane Intramuscular 1956
NebuPent for Inhalation Solution (1% or less) 1017
Neo-Calglucon Syrup 2018
Nicorette 1335
Norflex 1314
Norgesic 1314
Noroxin Tablets (Less frequent) 1519
▲ Norpace (32%) 2177
Norpramin Tablets 1340
Norzine 1818
Novafed A Capsules 1342
Novahistine DH 1342
Novahistine Elixir ▣ 596
▲ Nubain Injection (4%) 934
Omnipaque (Less than 0.1 to 0.2%) 2552
Optimine Tablets 2115
Oramorph SR (Morphine Sulfate Sustained Release Tablets) (Less frequent) 1988
Orap Tablets 1020
Oreticyl 545
Ornade Spansule Capsules 2221
Orudis Capsules (Less than 1%) 2488
PBZ Tablets & Elixir (Among most frequent) 1037
PBZ-SR Tablets (Among most frequent) 1037
Pamelor 2019
Pantopon Injectable 1911
▲ Parlodel (4%) 2020
Parnate Tablets 2222
PediaProfen Suspension (Less than 1%) 1363
Pepcid (Infrequent) 1524
Periactin 1525
▲ Permax Tablets (3.7%) 1291
Phenergan with Codeine 2497
Phenergan with Dextromethorphan 2499
Phenergan Injection 2493
Phenergan Suppositories 2496
Phenergan Syrup 2495
Phenergan Tablets 2496
Phenergan VC 2500
Phenergan VC with Codeine 2501
Plegine Tablets 2504
Plendil Extended-Release Tablets (0.5% to 1.5%) 1526
Polaramine 2116
Pondimin Tablets (Among most common) 1867
Prelu-2 Capsules 683
Prilosec Delayed-Release Capsules (Less than 1%) 1530
Prinivil Tablets (1% or less) 1538
Prinzide Tablets (0.3% to 1%) 1540
Pro-Banthīne Tablets 2141
Procardia XL Tablets (Less than 3%) 1783
Prolixin Decanoate 1795
Prolixin Elixir 1793
Prolixin Enanthate 1796
Prolixin Injection 1791
Prolixin Oral Concentrate 1792
Prolixin Tablets 1793
ProSom Tablets (Frequent) 554
Protostat Tablets 1674
▲ Prozac Pulvules (9.5%) 920
▲ Pyridium Plus (One-third to one-half of patients) 1764
Quarzan Capsules (Among most frequent) 1937
Raudixin Tablets 1803
Rauzide Tablets 1804
Renese-R Tablets 1786
Robinul Forte Tablets 1873
Robinul Injectable 1873
Robinul Tablets 1873
Robitussin-CF ▣ 676
Robitussin-PE ▣ 677
Rocaltrol Capsules 1913
Rondec 1975
Rondec-DM 1976
Rondec-TR Tablet 1975
Roxanol 1991
Rufen Tablets (Less than 1%) 691
Ru-Tuss II Capsules 693
Ru-Tuss with Hydrocodone 694
Ru-Tuss Tablets 693
▲ Rythmol Tablets (0.9 to 5.7%) 1184
Salutensin/Salutensin-Demi 719
Sandostatin Injection (Less than 1%) 2029
▲ Sanorex Tablets (Among most common) 2030
▲ Seldane Tablets (4.8%) 1349
▲ Seldane-D Extended-Release Tablets (21.7%) 1350
Ser-Ap-Es Tablets 881
Serentil 686
Serpasil Tablets 883
Serpasil-Apresoline Tablets 884
Serpasil-Esidrix Tablets 886
Sinemet Tablets 952
Sinemet CR Tablets (1.4%) 953
Sinequan 1960
Stadol (Less than 1%) 721
Stelazine 2226
Surmontil Capsules (Rare) 2524
Symmetrel Capsules & Syrup (1-5%) 936
Tacaryl 2409
Talwin Injection 2071
Tambocor Tablets (Less than 1%) 1315
Taractan (Occasional) 1920
Tavist Syrup 2033
Tavist Tablets 2035
Tavist-D Tablets 2035
▲ Tegison Capsules (1-10%) 1881
Tegretol Chewable Tablets 654
Tegretol Suspension 656
Tegretol Tablets 654
Temaril Tablets, Syrup and Spansule Sustained Release Capsules 1085
▲ Tenex Tablets (7% to 28%) 1875
Tenoretic Tablets 1105
Tenuate 1354
Thalitone Tablets 687
Thorazine (Occasional) 2234
Timoptic in Ocudose 1552
Timoptic Sterile Ophthalmic Solution 1550
Tofranil Ampuls 1038
Tofranil Tablets 1039
Tofranil-PM Capsules 1041
Tonocard Tablets (Less than 1%) 1554
Toradol IM Injection (1% or less) 2302
Torecan 1993
▲ Transderm Scōp Transdermal Therapeutic System (Two-thirds) 887
Tranxene (Less common) 556
Trental (Less than 1%) 1099
Trexan Tablets (Less than 1%) 937
Triaminic Cold Tablets ▣ 688
Triaminic Expectorant DH 1995
Triaminic Oral Infant Drops 1996
Triaminic Syrup (Occasional) ▣ 689
Triaminicol Multi-Symptom Relief ▣ 691
Triavil Tablets 1556
Trilafon 2123
Trinalin Repetabs Tablets 1170
Tropicacyl ⊙ 209
Urised Tablets 2396
Urispas Tablets 2242
Valpin 50 Tablets 941
Vanceril Inhaler (Few patients) 2128
Vascor (200, 300 and 400 mg) Tablets (0.5 to 3.40%) 1383
Vaseretic Tablets (0.5% to 2.0%) 1559
Vasotec I.V. 1562
Vasotec Tablets 1564
Ventolin (Less than 1%) 583
Verelan Capsules (Less than 1%) 1243
Vistaril Capsules 1789
Vistaril Intramuscular Solution 1970
Vistaril Oral Suspension 1789
Vivactil Tablets 1567
Voltaren Tablets (Less than 1%) 1042
Vontrol Tablets 2243
▲ Wellbutrin Tablets (27.6%) 821
▲ Wytensin Tablets (28% to 38%) 2542
▲ Xanax Tablets (32.8%) 2367
Zaroxolyn Tablets 989
Zestoretic (0.3 to 1%) 2274

Y

Yawning

Anafranil Capsules (Up to 3%) 650
Methadone Hydrochloride Diskets 1284
▲ Normodyne Injection (3%) 2108
Tonocard Tablets (Less than 1%) 1554
▲ Trandate Injection (3 of 100 patients) 577
Trexan Tablets (Less than 1%) 937
Versed Injection (Less than 1%) 1924

NOTES

NOTES

NOTES

Key to Controlled Substances Categories

Products listed with the symbols shown below are subject to the Controlled Substances Act of 1970. These drugs are categorized according to their potential for abuse. The greater the potential, the more severe the limitations on their prescription.

CATEGORY	INTERPRETATION
CII	**High potential for abuse.** Use may lead to severe physical or psychological dependence. Prescriptions must be written in ink, or typewritten and signed by the practitioner. Verbal prescriptions must be confirmed in writing within 72 hours, and may be given only in a genuine emergency. No renewals are permitted.
CIII	**Some potential for abuse.** Use may lead to low-to-moderate physical dependence or high psychological dependence. Prescriptions may be oral or written. Up to 5 renewals are permitted within 6 months.
CIV	**Low potential for abuse.** Use may lead to limited physical or psychological dependence. Prescriptions may be oral or written. Up to 5 renewals are permitted within 6 months.
CV	**Subject to state and local regulation.** Abuse potential is low; a prescription may not be required.

Key to FDA Use-in-pregnancy Ratings

The Food and Drug Administration's Pregnancy Categories are based on the degree to which available information has ruled out risk to the fetus, balanced against the drug's potential benefits to the patient. Ratings range from "A," for drugs that have been tested for teratogenicity under controlled conditions without showing evidence of damage to the fetus, to "D" and "X" for drugs that are definitely teratogenic. The "D" rating is generally reserved for drugs with no safer alternatives. The "X" rating means there is absolutely no reason to risk using the drug in pregnancy.

CATEGORY	INTERPRETATION
A	**Controlled studies show no risk.** Adequate, well-controlled studies in pregnant women have failed to demonstrate risk to the fetus.
B	**No evidence of risk in humans.** Either animal findings show risk, but human findings do not; or, if no adequate human studies have been done, animal findings are negative.
C	**Risk cannot be ruled out.** Human studies are lacking, and animal studies are either positive for fetal risk, or lacking as well. However, potential benefits may justify the potential risk.
D	**Positive evidence of risk.** Investigational or post-marketing data show risk to the fetus. Nevertheless, potential benefits may outweigh the potential risk.
X	**Contraindicated in pregnancy.** Studies in animals or human, or investigational or post-marketing reports have shown fetal risk which clearly outweighs any possible benefit to the patient.

Conversion Tables

Metric Doses With Approximate Apothecary Equivalents

The approximate dose equivalents represent the quantities usually prescribed by physicians using, respectively, the metric and apothecary system of weights and measures. When prepared dosage forms such as tablets, capsules, etc. are prescribed in the metric system, the pharmacist may dispense the corresponding approximate equivalent in the apothecary system and vice versa. (Note: A milliliter [mL] is the approximate equivalent of a cubic centimeter [cc]). Exact equivalents, which appear in the United States Pharmacopeia and the National Formulary, must be used to calculate quantities in pharmaceutical formulas and prescription compounding:

LIQUID MEASURE		LIQUID MEASURE		LIQUID MEASURE		LIQUID MEASURE	
Metric	Approximate Apothecary Equivalents	Metric	Approximate Apothecary Equivalents	Metric	Approximate Apothecary Equivalents	Metric	Approximate Apothecary Equivalents
1000 mL	1 quart	3 mL	45 minims	30 mL	1 fluid ounce	0.25 mL	4 minims
750 mL	1½ pints	2 mL	30 minims	15 mL	4 fluid drams	0.2 mL	3 minims
500 mL	1 pint	1 mL	15 minims	10 mL	2½ fluid drams	0.1 mL	1½ minims
250 mL	8 fluid ounces	0.75 mL	12 minims	8 mL	2 fluid drams	0.06 mL	1 minim
200 mL	7 fluid ounces	0.6 mL	10 minims	5 mL	1¼ fluid drams	0.05 mL	¾ minim
100 mL	3½ fluid ounces	0.5 mL	8 minims	4 mL	1 fluid dram	0.03 mL	½ minim
50 mL	1¾ fluid ounces	0.3 mL	5 minims				

WEIGHT		WEIGHT		WEIGHT		WEIGHT	
Metric	Approximate Apothecary Equivalents	Metric	Approximate Apothecary Equivalents	Metric	Approximate Apothecary Equivalents	Metric	Approximate Apothecary Equivalents
30g	1 ounce	30mg	1/2 grain	500mg	7½ grains	1.2 mg	1/50 grain
15g	4 drams	25mg	3/8 grain	400mg	6 grains	1 mg	1/60 grain
10g	2½ drams	20mg	1/3 grain	300mg	5 grains	800 μg	1/80 grain
7.5g	2 drams	15mg	1/4 grain	250mg	4 grains	600 μg	1/100 grain
6g	90 grains	12mg	1/5 grain	200mg	3 grains	500 μg	1/120 grain
5g	75 grains	10mg	1/6 grain	150mg	2½ grains	400 μg	1/150 grain
4g	60 grains (1 dram)	8mg	1/8 grain	125mg	2 grains	300 μg	1/200 grain
3g	45 grains	6mg	1/10 grain	100mg	1½ grains	250 μg	1/250 grain
2g	30 grains (½ dram)	5mg	1/12 grain	75mg	1¼ grains	200 μg	1/300 grain
1.5g	22 grains	4mg	1/15 grain	60mg	1 grain	150 μg	1/400 grain
1g	15 grains	3mg	1/20 grain	50mg	¾ grain	120 μg	1/500 grain
750mg	12 grains	2mg	1/30 grain	40mg	⅔ grain	100 μg	1/600 grain
600mg	10 grains	1.5mg	1/40 grain				

Approximate Household Equivalents

For household purposes, an American Standard Teaspoon is defined by the American National Standards Institute as containing 4.93 ± 0.24 mL. The USP states that in view of the almost universal practice of employing teaspoons ordinarily available in the household for administration of medicine, the teaspoon may be regarded as representing 5 mL. Household units of measure often are used to inform patients of the size of a liquid dose. Because of difficulties involved in measuring liquids under normal conditions of use, household spoons are not appropriate when accurate measurement of a liquid dose is required. When accurate measurement of a liquid dose is required, the USP recommends that a calibrated oral syringe or dropper be used.

1 fluid dram = 1 teaspoonful = 5 mL
2 fluid drams = 1 dessertspoonful = 10 mL
4 fluid drams = 1 tablespoonful = 15 mL
2 fluid ounces = 1 wineglassful = 60 mL
4 fluid ounces = 1 teacupful = 120 mL
8 fluid ounces = 1 tumblerful = 240 mL

Pounds—Kilograms (kg) Conversion

1 pound = 0.453592 kg
1 kg = 2.2 pounds

Temperature Conversion Table:

$$9 \times °C = (5 \times °F) - 160$$

Centigrade to Fahrenheit = $(°C \times 9/5) + 32 = °F$

Fahrenheit to Centigrade = $(°F - 32) \times 5/9 = °C$

Milliequivalents per Liter (mEq/L)

$$\text{mEq/L} = \frac{\text{weight of salt (g)} \times \text{valence of ion} \times 1000}{\text{molecular weight of salt}}$$

$$\text{weight of salt (g)} = \frac{\text{mEq/L} \times \text{molecular weight of salt}}{\text{valence of ion} \times 1000}$$

Put the power of PDR® in the palm of your hand with . . .

POCKET PDR™

Instant access to indications, contraindications, warnings, adverse reactions, dosage and how-supplied information on every Rx Drug in PDR. This convenient, easy-to-use pocket-sized electronic data bank folds down to 6" long x 3" wide, less than 1" thick — and weighs just 10 ounces. Use it for fast, on-the-spot look ups — for accurate, up-to-date information. As simple to use as a pocket calculator, the POCKET PDR gives you the information you need, when and where you need it!

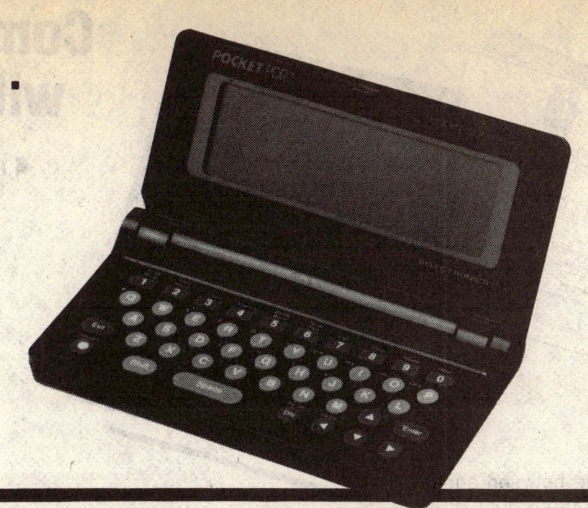

Also available with The Merck Manual!

Put the power of PDR on your personal computer!

◀ PDR® on CD-ROM

Fast, fail-safe access to the complete text of all 5 PDR volumes in one integrated program! Complete prescribing information on nearly 3,000 pharmaceuticals. Put the power of today's technology —and the vital information of a complete drug reference library — to work for you as never before!

Now with built-in Indications Index!

PDR® Drug Interactions and Side Effects Diskettes™ ▶

Search 5,000 brand and generic listings found in the PDR Library. Check 2,500 side effects as quickly as you can name the reaction. Find approved alternatives for more than 2,000 indications whenever you pinpoint a problem prescription.

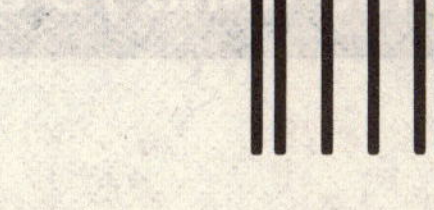

Use the order form on the reverse side.

NO POSTAGE NECESSARY IF MAILED IN THE UNITED STATES

BUSINESS REPLY MAIL

FIRST CLASS MAIL PERMIT NO. 28 MONTVALE NJ

POSTAGE WILL BE PAID BY ADDRESSEE

Physicians' Desk Reference
Medical Economics Data
P.O. Box 430
MONTVALE NJ 07645-9880